Fourth Edition

PHARMACOTHERAPY

A Pathophysiologic Approach

Fourth Edition

PHARMACOTHERAPY

A Pathophysiologic Approach

Editors

Joseph T. DiPiro, PharmD, FCCP
Panoz Professor, College of Pharmacy, Head, Department of Clinical and Administrative Sciences, University of Georgia College of Pharmacy;
Clinical Professor of Surgery, Medical College of Georgia, Augusta, Georgia

Robert L. Talbert, PharmD, FCCP, BCPS
Professor and Division Head, College of Pharmacy, University of Texas at Austin, Austin;
Professor, Departments of Medicine and Pharmacology, University of Texas Health Science Center at San Antonio, San Antonio, Texas

Gary C. Yee, PharmD, FCCP
Professor and Chair, Department of Pharmacy Practice, College of Pharmacy, University of Nebraska Medical Center, Omaha, Nebraska

Gary R. Matzke, PharmD, FCP, FCCP
Professor of Pharmaceutical Sciences and Medicine, Schools of Pharmacy and Medicine, Center of Clinical Pharmacology, University of Pittsburgh, Pittsburgh, Pennsylvania

Barbara G. Wells, PharmD, FASHP, FCCP, BCPP
Professor and Dean, Idaho State University College of Pharmacy, Pocatello, Idaho

L. Michael Posey, RPh
President, Pharmacy Editorial & News Services, Athens, Georgia

APPLETON & LANGE
Stamford, Connecticut

Notice: The authors and the publisher of this volume have taken care to make certain that the doses of drugs and schedules of treatment are correct and compatible with the standards generally accepted at the time of publication. Nevertheless, as new information becomes available, changes in treatment and in the use of drugs become necessary. The reader is advised to carefully consult the instruction and information material included in the package insert of each drug or therapeutic agent before administration. This advice is especially important when using, administering, or recommending new or infrequently used drugs. The authors and publisher disclaim all responsibility for any liability, loss, injury, or damage incurred as a consequence, directly or indirectly, of the use and application of any of the contents of this volume.

www.appletonlange.com

99 00 01 02 03 / 10 9 8 7 6 5 4 3 2 1

Prentice Hall International (UK) Limited, *London*
Prentice Hall of Australia Pty. Limited, *Sydney*
Prentice Hall Canada, Inc., *Toronto*
Prentice Hall Hispanoamericana, S.A., *Mexico*
Prentice Hall of India Private Limited, *New Delhi*
Prentice Hall of Japan, Inc., *Tokyo*
Simon & Schuster Asia Pte. Ltd., *Singapore*
Editora Prentice Hall do Brasil Ltda., *Rio de Janeiro*
Prentice Hall, *Upper Saddle River, New Jersey*

Library of Congress Catalog Card Number: 99-72672

Editor-in-Chief: Cheryl L. Mehalik
Development Editor: Kathleen McCullough
Production Editor: Lisa M. Guidone
Art Manager: Eve Siegel
Designer: Mary Skudlarek

ISBN 0-8385-7691-5

90000

9 780838 576915

PRINTED IN THE UNITED STATES OF AMERICA

Dedication

To those pharmacists who had the courage and perseverance to take the early steps that were needed to develop personally and professionally in the clinical practice of pharmacy.

To our mentors, whose wisdom provided educational and training programs that encouraged the professional growth of their students.

To the contemporary clinical pharmacy specialists and pharmacy care innovators who continue to advance the vision while clinging tenaciously to the highest standards of practice.

And to our families and faculty colleagues for their efforts and support for our endeavors.

CONTENTS

FOREWORD

We are in the midst of rapid changes as the 20th century comes to a close. Although these rapid changes are occurring in all aspects of our lives, the dynamic changes in health care have startled all health professionals. Not too long ago we had a clear and unquestioned goal of the highest possible quality of care for our patients. But as the cost of patient care increased significantly in excess of the costs of other goods and services, the concept of managed health care was developed. Some critics state that managed health care is, in reality, managed health costs, whereas supporters state that quality care can be achieved while being cost conscious. However, both critics and supporters of managed health care agree that the practices of clinicians will continue to be influenced by increased cost consciousness in health care reimbursed through both private and public programs. This is particularly the case in the area of pharmacotherapy.

We are also in a time when great advances in biomedical research are catalyzing the development of important new drugs that, in some cases, treat diseases that previously had no treatment, and in other cases, greatly improve upon previous therapies. But in some cases new drugs may not have benefits over older therapies that justify the often higher costs of the new therapy. The challenge is to welcome new drug therapies that are necessary for quality patient care and to reject those drug therapies that merely add cost without improving quality of care. Moreover, managed health care executives must realize that drug therapy, even when appearing expensive, is almost always the least costly alternative for patient care.

Just as rapid changes are occurring in health care and in drug therapies, rapid changes are also occurring in the profession of pharmacy. One hundred years ago pharmacists were compounders of prescriptions—a role now dominated by pharmaceutical manufacturers. Forty years ago pharmacists were primarily distributors of prescription drugs—a role of limited professional responsibility today. In 1966 Dean Linwood F. Tice of the Philadelphia College of Pharmacy stated,

> "I predict that the counting and pouring now often alleged to be the pharmacist's chief occupation will in time be done by technicians and eventually by automation. The pharmacist of tomorrow will function by reason of what he knows—increasing the efficiency and safety of drug therapy and working as a drug specialist in his own right. It is in this direction that pharmaceutical education must move without delay."

I was a faculty member at the Philadelphia College of Pharmacy in 1966 and I participated in Dean Tice's efforts to move pharmacy in a clinical direction toward what we now call pharmaceutical care.

Later, at the University of Kentucky, and for 20 years at the University of Texas, I had the good fortune to be a colleague and friend of Charles Walton. Charlie Walton wrote the Foreword to the first edition of this textbook. His Foreword eloquently addressed the importance of pharmacotherapy in the maturing of the profession of pharmacy. Charlie stated,

> "Within this book one will find the scientific foundation for the essential knowledge required of one who may aspire to specialty practice as a pharmacotherapist."

Note that Charlie stated, ". . . scientific foundation for the essential knowledge . . ." One thing Charlie Walton taught me was that the clinical pharmacy specialists he wanted to educate and train could not take any short cuts—the pharmacotherapist had to be a clinician who had a strong scientific foundation.

When we conceived our Texas clinical program in 1973, we committed to a three year post-baccalaureate PharmD program with an integrated residency program. These students took pathophysiology, along with medical students. No short cuts. The Texas PharmD program has evolved along with the adoption of the PharmD as the only professional degree in pharmacy. The principles that existed in the 1970s in a few schools have now generally been adopted by all colleges of pharmacy. However, specialty practice as a pharmacotherapist continues to require graduate pharmacy education beyond the PharmD, just as specialty practice in medicine requires graduate medical education beyond the MD. This text continues to be intended as "the scientific foundation for the essential knowledge required of one who may aspire to specialty practice as a pharmacotherapist."

It is interesting that Charlie Walton often stated that he was not a clinical pharmacist. I questioned his self-assessment because, in my view, he was a uniquely talented leader and motivator for patient-oriented concepts in pharmacy education and practice. However, Charlie Walton had very high standards for a pharmacist to be termed a clinical pharmacist or a pharmacotherapist. These standards should remain high as opportunities continue to expand for pharmacotherapists to enter one-on-one, collaborative practice with physicians and other health professionals. High standards will ensure the level of clinical competence needed in the pharmacotherapist to earn the respect of patients and medical colleagues.

William Miller wrote the Foreword in the second edition of *Pharmacotherapy*. Bill is a pioneer—a first generation clinical pharmacist and pharmacotherapist. He earned his PharmD at the University of Kentucky when Charlie Walton and I were on faculty. There were no pharmacy precedents for the education and training Bill received and there was no roadmap for him to follow in his career. Therefore, it was with a teacher's pride that I read his Foreword to the second edition. Bill's Foreword had the orientation of a practitioner that knew our recent successes in the evolution of pharmacotherapists are only a beginning. We have successfully demonstrated potential; the continuing challenge will be to broadly improve patient care through the specialty practice of more, and better trained, pharmacotherapists. Bill stated,

> "All pharmacotherapists additionally must document the effects of their actions on patient drug therapy outcomes. The relative value of Pharmacotheraphy Specialists in terms of costs and benefits must be compared with those of other professionals and technology, all these costs are driving up the price of health care. We must be avid supporters of continuous quality improvement which will encourage decisions about health care delivery systems based on fact and not simply opinion or perceptions."

In the Foreword to the third edition, Milo Gibaldi stated,

> "The idea of pharmaceutical ćare continues to enjoy near universal support in the profession, yet we have had critical lapses in organizational and academic leadership."

Practice as a clinical pharmacy specialist is no longer an experiment or pilot project. It has become a valued practice enhancing patient care. The time has come for a full commitment of organizational and academic leadership to the advancement of high quality clinical pharmacy specialty practice as well as the advancement of general practice oriented to pharmaceutical care. Strong leadership and a careful strategy will be required to advance the general and specialty practices of pharmacy in ways that do not advance one type of practice at the expense of the other.

The fourth edition of this textbook is strong evidence that the profession of pharmacy is continuing its exciting progress as a clinical profession. This text could not have been written in 1966. There were not pharmacists who could have authored the material, nor were there reasonable opportunities for pharmacists to utilize the material in practice even if, somehow, the book were authored. Today we have both the authors and the opportunity to improve patient care.

I hope that someday in the future, a leading pharmacotherapist will look back at this text and judge it to be "the text" that made the difference in pharmacists truly becoming pharmacotherapists. That is how I view the text. As dean of pharmacy at the University of Texas from 1973 to 1998, I participated, along with Charlie Walton, Bob Talbert, and others, in the development of faculty and programs that were based on pharmacy being a clinical profession. Other colleges and institutions made similar commitments. I look at this text as evidence that through these efforts the profession of pharmacy has joined medicine, nursing, and dentistry as a clinical profession.

We are in the midst of a wonderful journey.

James T. Doluisio, PhD
Hoechst Roussel Professor of Pharmacy
University of Texas
College of Pharmacy
Austin, Texas
February 1999

Preface

The publication of the fourth edition of *Pharmacotherapy: A Pathophysiologic Approach* continues the standards and philosophies set forth by the previous editions. *Pharmacotherapy* seeks to advance the level of pharmaceutical care through understanding of pharmacotherapeutic principles. We believe that this textbook will stimulate the pharmacy student to achieve a higher level of learning; motivate the young practitioner to perform more advanced patient care; challenge established pharmacists to learn concepts missed during years of practice; and inform the profession at large about the standards of pharmaceutical care toward which all should strive.

The authors and editors have attempted to impart a process of thinking about pharmacotherapy for the student and developing practitioner. The key to this process is the pathophysiology sections, which identify mechanisms of disease as a foundation for applying pharmacotherapeutic principles and strategies. By understanding pathophysiology and principles of therapy, the student and practitioner can assess more rigorously the place of new drugs or new therapeutic approaches.

In this edition, we have reached the limits of text that can be included in one volume and therefore made carefully considered decisions on chapters to be added and deleted. The present edition includes 132 chapters, an overall reduction of four chapters from the third edition. *New chapters* have been added on "Disorders of the Pituitary Gland" and "Substance-Related Disorders."

The *structure* of chapters and *design* of pages has continued to evolve to better meet user needs. In this edition, the following new features have been included: **more structured treatment sections**, containing a different type face which sets off the material in a visual way (**see example below**), a new section on **desired outcomes** of treatment, **redrawn flow diagrams**, disease states end-of-chapter reminders titled **principles of pharmacotherapy** which put the major points in perspective.

The overall organization of the book is retained from previous editions. The first seven chapters again provide *primers* on important fundamental information such as: **pharmacoeconomics, pharmacoepidemiology, pharmacokinetics, drug interactions,** and **clinical toxicology.**

Most of the remaining chapters specifically focus on disease states and maintain a *standard format* which includes the following headings: **epidemiology, pathophysiology, clinical presentation, desired outcomes, treatment,** and **evaluation of therapeutic outcomes.**

The textbook together with its companion works, *Pharmacotherapy Casebook: A Patient-focused Approach, Pharmacotheraphy Handbook,* and the *Pharmacotherapy.complete* CD-ROM provide a comprehensive package of tools useful for practice and instruction. New editions of each of the companion products should be available about the time that the fourth edition is published.

The editors recognize that many areas of this text will rapidly become outdated as our understanding of disease processes increases or as new therapies are adopted. The challenge for the student and the practitioner is to integrate information from a variety of sources, form a basis for application in pharmacotherapy, and be receptive to new information as it appears in the literature or as it is gained by personal experience.

The editors are deeply indebted to the contributors for the hours spent preparing accurate, thorough, and relevant discussions of each topic. A heartfelt thank you is well earned by the personnel at Appleton & Lange, especially Cheryl Mehalik, who provided critical support, insight, and motivation at every stage.

The Editors
April 1999

Example:

▶ TREATMENT: Syndrome X

Syndrome X refers to the occurrence of effort angina and exercise-induced ECG changes with a normal coronary arteriogram with no evidence of structural (stenosis) or functional (spasm) abnormalities. Although the basis for this syndrome is not yet established, it is thought that syndrome X may be a result of inducible myocardial ischemia caused by impaired functional coronary reserve at the microvascular level of intramural prearteriolar vessels. It has been proposed that this defect is caused by defective prearteriolar regulation of blood flow into the arteriolar bed with subsequent focal, sustained, compensatory release of adenosine; excessive local concentrations of adenosine are then responsible for the pain seen in this syndrome. Prearteriolar constriction may be the result of insufficient vasodilation or inappropriate vasoconstriction, or resetting of myogenic control on a segmental or generalized distribution basis.

Contributors

Betty J. Abate, PharmD, BCPS
Clinical Pharmacist Specialist, Infectious Diseases and Clinical Assistant Professor of Pharmacy, Grace Hospital and Wayne State University, Detroit, MI

Paul A. Abraham, MD
Associate Professor of Medicine, University of Minnesota, School of Medicine, Chief, Division of Nephrology, Department of Medicine Regions Hospital, St. Paul, MN

Val R. Adams, PharmD
Assistant Professor, College of Pharmacy, Department of Pharmacy Practice and Science, University of Kentucky, Lexington, KY

Jeffrey R. Aeschlimann, PharmD
Assistant Professor of Pharmacy Practice, School of Pharmacy University of Connecticut, Harwinton, CT

J. V. Anandan, PharmD, BCPS
Assistant Director and Adjunct Associate Professor, Department of Pharmacy, Henry Ford Hospital/Wayne State University College of Pharmacy and Allied Health Professions, Detroit, MI

Jan Dalke Anderson, PharmD, BCNSP
Medical Affairs Manager, Searle Pharmaceuticals, Denver, CO

Edward P. Armstrong, PharmD, BCPS, FASHP
Associate Professor, College of Pharmacy, Department of Pharmacy Practice and Science, University of Arizona, Tucson, AZ

George R. Bailie, MS, PharmD, PhD, FCCP
Professor of Pharmacy Practice, Adjunct Professor of Medicine, Albany College of Pharmacy and Albany Medical College, Albany, NY

Carol McManus Balmer, PharmD
Associate Professor, School of Pharmacy, University of Colorado, Denver, CO

Steven L. Barriere, PharmD, FCCP
Director, Clinical Affairs, Gilead Sciences, Foster City, CA

Larry A. Bauer, PharmD, FCP, FCCP
Associate Professor, Pharmacy & Lab Medicine, University of Washington, Seattle, WA

Jerry L. Bauman, PharmD, BCPS, FCCP, FACC
Professor and Head, Division of Clinical Pharmaceutical Sciences, College of Pharmacy, Professor Pediatrics, University of Illinois at Chicago, Chicago, IL

Terry J. Baumann, PharmD, BCPS
Clinical Manager, Pharmacy Munson Medical Center, Traverse City, MI

Eula D. Beasley, PharmD
Clinical Coordinator, Department of Pharmacy, Washington Hospital Center, Washington, DC

Brian E. Beckett, PharmD
Associate Professor of Pharmacy Practice, Department of Pharmacy Practice, McWhorter School of Pharmacy, Samford University, and Clinical Pharmacy Specialist, Lloyd Noland Hospital, Fairfield, AL

Susan E. Beltz, PharmD
Clinical Assistant Professor, Department of Pharmacy Practice, College of Pharmacy, University of Florida, and Pediatric Oncology Clinical Specialist, Department of Pharmacy Services, Shands Hospital at the University of Florida, Gainesville, FL

William H. Benefield, Jr., PharmD, FASCP, BCPP
Clinical Assistant Professor Pharmacology, Clinical Psychopharmacology Programs, The University of Texas Health Sciences Center at San Antonio, Clinical Assistant Professor of Pharmacy, College of Pharmacy, The University of Texas at Austin and Clinical Pharmacologist, San Antonio State School, San Antonio, TX

Rosemary R. Berardi, PharmD, FASHP
Professor of Pharmacy and Clinical Pharmacists in Gastroenterology, The University of Michigan, College of Pharmacy and Department of Pharmacy, University of Michigan Health System, Ann Arbor, MI

Richard C. Berchou, PharmD
Clinical Neuroscience Program, Sinai Hospital, Detroit, MI

Joseph S. Bertino, Jr., PharmD, FCCP
Co-Director, Clinical Pharmacology Research Center, Assistant Director, Clinical Pharmacy Service, and Associate Professor of Clinical Pharmacology, Bassett Healthcare/Columbia University College of Physicians and Surgeons, Cooperstown, NY

Larry E. Boh, MS
Professor and Chair, Pharmacy Practice Division, School of Pharmacy, University of Wisconsin, Madison, WI

John A. Bosso, PharmD, FCCP, BCPS
Professor and Head, Division of Clinical Pharmacy Sciences, College of Pharmacy, Professor of Pediatrics, College of Medicine, Medical University of South Carolina, Charleston, SC

Bradley A. Boucher, PharmD, BCPS, FCCP
Professor of Clinical Pharmacy and Neurosurgery, Department of Clinical Pharmacy, University of Tennessee, Memphis, TN

J. Chris Bradberry, PharmD
Department of Pharmacy Practice and Pharmacoeconomics, College of Pharmacy, The University of Tennessee-Memphis, Memphis, TN

Rex O. Brown, PharmD
Professor, Department of Clinical Pharmacy, College of Pharmacy, University of Tennessee, and Nutrition Support Pharmacist, Department of Pharmacy, Regional Medical Center at Memphis and UT Bowld Hospital, Memphis, TN

Kathryn K. Bucci, PharmD, BCPS
Associate Professor Family Medicine, Clinical Associate Professor of Pharmacy Practice, Medical University of South Carolina, Family Practice Residency Program, Self Memorial Hospital, Charleston, SC

Gilbert J. Burckart, PharmD, FCCP
Professor of Pharmaceutical Science, School of Pharmacy, University of Pittsburgh, Pittsburgh, PA

Mark B. Burlingame, PharmD, BCPS
Clinical Coordinator, Pharmacy Services, Department of Veterans Affairs Medical Center, and Clinical Associate Professor, Department of Pharmacy Practice, College

of Pharmacy, University of Florida, Gainesville, FL

Henry I. Bussey, PharmD
University of Texas Health Science Center-San Antonio, Clinical Pharmacy, Austin, TX

Karim A. Calis, PharmD, MPH, BCPS, BCNSP, FASHP
Clinical Specialist, Endocrinology and Women's Health, Coordinator, Drug Information Service, Warren G. Magnuson Clinical Center, National Institutes of Health, Bethesda, Maryland, Clinical Associate Professor, University of Maryland, Baltimore, MD, Associate Clinical Professor, Medical College of Virginia, Virginia Commonwealth University, Richmond, VA

Deborah Stier Carson, PharmD, BCPS
Associate Professor of Pharmacy Practice, Assistant Professor of Family Medicine, Medical University of South Carolina, Charleston, SC

Peggy L. Carver, PharmD
Associate Professor of Pharmacy, College of Pharmacy, University of Michigan, Ann Arbor, MI

Daniel T. Casto, PharmD, FCCP
Associate Professor of Pharmacy and Pedicatrics, College of Pharmacy, University of Texas Health Science Center, San Antonio, TX

Katherine Hammond Chessman, PharmD, BCNSP, BCPS
Associate Professor, Department of Pharmacy Practice, Medical University of South Carolina and Clinical Pharmacy Specialist, Pediatrics/Pediatric Surgery, Medical University of South Carolina, Children's Hospital, Charleston, SC

Marie A. Chisholm, PharmD
Assistant Professor Pharmacy Practice, The University of Georgia College of Pharmacy, Assistant Clinical Professor of Medicine, Medical College of Georgia, Augusta, GA

Susan K. Chuck, PharmD
Colleges of Pharmacy and Medicine, University of Illinois at Chicago, Chicago, IL

Peter A. Chyka, PharmD, ABAT, FAACT
Professor, Departments of Pharmacy Practice and Pharmacoeconomics and Clinical Pharmacy, College of Pharmacy, University of Tennessee, Memphis, and Executive Director, Southern Poison Center, Memphis, TN

Ann C. Collier, MD
Professor of Medicine, School of Medicine, University of Washington Health Science Center, Seattle, WA

Thomas J. Comstock, PharmD
Associate Professor, Department of Pharmacy & Pharmaceutics, School of Pharmacy, Medical College of Virginia, VA Commonwealth University, Richmond, VA

Stephen Joel Coons, PhD
Associate Professor, Division of Social and Administrative Sciences, College of Pharmacy, The University of Arizona, Tucson, AZ

Margaret K. Cramer, MD, FACOG
Division Chief, Obstetrics and Gynecology, Athens Regional Medical Center, Athens, GA

M. Lynn Crismon, PharmD, FCCP, BCPP
Professor and Southwestern Drug Corporation Centennial Fellow in Pharmacy, Co-Director, Texas Medication Algorithm Project, College of Pharmacy, The University of Texas at Austin, Austin, TX

Michael A. Crouch, PharmD, BCPS
Assistant Professor, School of Pharmacy, Virginia Commonwealth University, Richmond, VA

Clarence E. Curry, Jr., PharmD
Associate Professor, College of Pharmacy, Nursing and Allied Health Sciences, Howard University, Washington, DC

Christina Dalmady-Israel, PharmD, BCPS
Clinical Liaison, Medical Affairs, Roche Labs, Inc.

Larry H. Danziger, PharmD
Professor and Co-Director, Section of Infectious Diseases, College of Pharmacy, University of Illinois, Chicago, IL

Joseph F. Dasta, MS, FCCM
Professor, College of Pharmacy, Experimental and Clinical Pharmacology, The Ohio State University, Columbus, OH

Lisa E. Davis, PharmD, FCCP, BCPS
Associate Professor, Department of Pharmacy Practice, Philadelphia College of Pharmacy, Philadelphia, PA

Renee M. DeHart, PharmD
Assistant Professor, Department of Pharmacy Practice, Samford University, McWhorter School of Pharmacy, and Clinical Pharmacy Specialist, Department of Pharmacy, Birmingham Baptist Medical Center, Princeton, Birmingham, AL

Jeffrey C. Delafuente, MS, FCCP
Professor and Director of Geriatrics, School of Pharmacy, Virginia Commonwealth University, Richmond, VA

Michel Deschênes, MD
Chargé d'énseignement, Médecine D'Urgence, Chuq, Pavillon Chul, Quebec, Canada

Mariela Diaz-Linares, PharmD
Clinical Assistant Professor of Pharmacy, College of Pharmacy, University of Illinois at Chicago, Chicago, IL

Joseph T. DiPiro, PharmD, FCCP
Panoz Professor, College of Pharmacy, Head, Department of Clinical and Administrative Sciences, University of Georgia College of Pharmacy; Clinical Professor of Surgery, Medical College of Georgia, Augusta, Georgia

Paul L. Doering, MS
Distinguished Service Professor of Pharmacy Practice, University of Florida, Gainesville, FL

Julie A. Dopheide, PharmD, BCPP
Assistant Professor, Clinical Pharmacy, USC School of Pharmacy, Los Angeles, CA

Peter G. Dorson, PharmD, BCPP
Director of Psychiatric Pharmacy Services, Austin State Hospital, Austin, TX

Steve C. Ebert, PharmD
Clinical Specialist, Infectious Diseases and Clinical Associate Professor, Department of Pharmacy, Meriter Hospital and School of Pharmacy, University of Wisconsin, Madison, WI

Andrea E. Eggert, PharmD, BCPP
Research Scientist and Clinical Assistant Professor, College of Pharmacy, The University of Texas at Austin, Austin, TX

Victor A. Elsberry, PharmD, BCNSP
Assistant Professor, College of Pharmacy,

Department of Pharmacy Practice and Science, University of Arizona, Tucson, AZ

Sharon M. Erdman, PharmD
Department of Pharmacy Practice and Pharmacoeconomics, College of Pharmacy, Loyola Medical Center, Maywood, IL

Brian L. Erstad, PharmD
Associate Professor, College of Pharmacy, The University of Arizona, Tuscon, AZ

Susan C. Fagan, PharmD, BCPS, FCCP
Associate Professor of Pharmacy Practice, College of Pharmacy and Allied Health Professions, Wayne State University, Detroit, MI

Martha P. Fankhauser, MS Pharm, FASHP
Clinical Associate Professor, Department of Pharmacy Practice and Science, College of Pharmacy, The University of Arizona, Tuscon, AZ

Sally A. Felton, PharmD
Clinical Oncology Specialist, Director, Investigational Drug Section, Institute of Drug Development, San Antonio, TX

Rebecca S. Finley, PharmD, MS
Chairman, Department of Pharmacy Practice and Pharmacy Administration, Philadelphia College of Pharmacy, University of the Sciences in Philadelphia, Philadelphia, PA

Douglas N. Fish, PharmD, BCPS
Assistant Professor of Pharmacy, Department of Pharmacy Practice, School of Pharmacy, University of Colorado Health Sciences Center, Denver, CO

John O. Fleming, MD
Professor, Neurology, University of Wisconsin, Madison, WI

Courtney V. Fletcher, PharmD
Professor, College of Pharmacy, Experimental and Clinical Pharmacology, University of Minnesota, Minneapolis, MN

Reginald F. Frye, PharmD, PhD
Assistant Professor, Department of Pharmaceutical Sciences, School of Pharmacy, Center for Clinical Pharmacology, University of Pittsburgh, Pittsburgh, PA

Peter Gal, PharmD, BCPS, FCCP, FASHP
Director, Pharmacy Research, Pharmacotherapy and Education Greensboro Area Health Education Center, Moses Cone Health System, Greensboro, NC; Clinical Professor, School of Pharmacy, University of North Carolina, Chapel Hill, NC

William R. Garnett, PharmD, FCCP
Professor of Pharmacy and Pharmaceutics, Professor of Neurology, Medical College of Virginia, Richmond, VA

Stephen A. Geraci, MD
Assistant Professor, Departments of Medicine, Pharmacology, and Clinical Pharmacy, Colleges of Medicine and Pharmacy, University of Tennessee at Memphis, Memphis, TN

Barry E. Gidal, PharmD
Associate Professor, School of Pharmacy, Department of Neurology, University of Wisconsin, Madison, WI

Mark A. Gill, PharmD
Professor of Clinical Pharmacy, School of Pharmacy, University of Southern California, Los Angeles, CA

Mark L. Glover, PharmD
Assistant Professor, College of Pharmacy, Department of Pharmacy Practice and Science, Nova Southeastern University, Ft. Lauderdale, FL

Barry R. Goldspiel, PharmD, BCPS, FASHP
Oncology Clinical Pharmacy Specialist, Pharmacy Department, N. I. H. Clinical Center, Bethesda, MD

Nina M. Graves, PharmD, FCCP
Senior Clinical Evaluation Manager, Medtronic Neurological, Minneapolis, MN

John G. Gums, PharmD
Professor of Pharmacy and Medicine, Departments of Pharmacy Practice and Community Health Family Medicine, University of Florida Colleges of Pharmacy and Medicine, Gainesville, FL

Philip D. Hall, PharmD, BCPS
Associate Professor, College of Pharmacy, Medical University of South Carolina, Charleston, SC

Nina H. Han, PharmD
Clinical Assistant Professor, Department of Pharmacy Practice, University of Illinois College of Pharmacy, Chicago, IL

Joseph T. Hanlon, PharmD, MS, BCPS, FASCP, FASHP
Clinical Associate Professor, School of Pharmacy, University of North Carolina, Chapel Hill, NC; Coordinator of Pharmacogeriatrics, Center for the Study of Aging and Human Development, and Associate Research Professor, Department of Medicine, Duke University Medical Center; and Clinical Pharmacist Specialist in Geriatrics at the Geriatric Research, Education and Clinical Center and Senior Research Fellow, Center for Health Services Research in Primary Care, Durham Veterans Affairs Medical Center, Durham, NC

J. William Harbilas, PharmD, BCPS
Clinical Specialist, Ambulatory Services, Clinical Assistant Professor, Department of Pharmacy, Shands at the University of Florida, Gainesville, FL

Thomas C. Hardin, PharmD, FCCP
Clinical Coordinator, Pharmacy Services, South Texas Veterans Health Care System, San Antonio, TX

David W. Hawkins, PharmD
Professor of Pharmacy, University of Georgia, Athens Georgia; Clinical Professor of Medicine, Medical College of Georgia, Augusta, GA

Peggy E. Hayes, PharmD
Senior Strategic Consultant, Quintiles CNS Therapeutics, San Diego, CA

Thomas K. Hazlet, PharmD, DrPH
Assistant Professor of Pharmacy, Department of Pharmacy, School of Pharmacy, University of Washington, Seattle, WA

Amy M. Heck, PharmD
Specialized Resident in Drug Information Practice and Pharmacotherapy, Warren G. Magnuson Clinical Center, National Institutes of Health, Bethesda, MD

Karen L. Heim-Duthoy, PharmD, FCCP
Associate Professor, Department of Experiential and Clinical Pharmacology, College of Pharmacy, University of Minnesota, and Clinical Scientist, Hennepin County Medical Center, Division of Nephrology, Minneapolis, MN

Katherine C. Herndon, PharmD, BCPS
Assistant Professor of Pharmacy Practice, Department of Pharmacy Practice, McWhorter School of Pharmacy, Samford University and Clinical Pharmacy

Specialist, Department of Veterans Affairs Medical Center, Birmingham, AL

AnhThu D. Hoang, PharmD
Infectious Disease Fellow, University of Minnesota, St. Paul-Ramsey Medical Center, St. Paul, MN

Motria M. Horodysky, PharmD, BCPS
Assistant Professor of Clinical Pharmacy, Philadelphia College of Pharmacy, University of the Sciences in Philadelphia, Philadelphia, PA

Mark W. Jackson, MD
Staff Physician at Baptist Hospital of East Tennessee and Fort Sanders Regional Medical Center, Knoxville, TN

Stephen W. Janning, PharmD
Clinical Coordinator, Department of Pharmacy, Duke University Medical Center, Durham, NC

Douglas D. Janson, PharmD, BCNSP
Associate Professor, Department of Pharmacy and Therapeutics, University of Pittsburgh, School of Pharmacy and Nutrition Support Specialist, University of Pittsburgh Medical Center Health System, Pittsburgh, PA

Donna M. Jermain, PharmD, BCPP
Coordinator of Pharmacy Research and Education, Scott White Memorial Hospital, Assistant Professor, Department of Medicine and Psychiatry, College of Medicine, Texas A&M Health Science Center, and Clinical Associate Professor, College of Pharmacy, University of Texas at Austin, Austin, TX

Thomas E. Johns, PharmD, BCPS
Clinical Specialist, Infectious Diseases, Department of Pharmacy, Shands at the University of Florida, Gainesville, FL

Heather J. Johnson, PharmD
Associate Professor, Department of Pharmacy and Therapeutics, University of Pittsburgh and Clinical Pharmacist, Ambulatory Care Pharmacy, University of Pittsburgh Medical Center Health System, Pittsburgh, PA

Julie A. Johnson, PharmD, BCPS, FCCP
Associate Professor, Department of Pharmacy Practice, College of Pharmacy, University of Florida, Gainesville, FL

Lori A. Jones, PharmD
Director of Experience Programs, Clinical Assistant Professor, College of Pharmacy, University of Georgia, Augusta, GA

Thomas N. Kakuda, PharmD
Infectious Diseases Fellow, College of Pharmacy, Experimental and Clinical Pharmacology, University of Minnesota, Minneapolis, MN

Alan K. Kamada, PharmD
National Jewish Center of Immunology and Respiratory Disease, Department of Pediatrics, Denver, CO

Judith C. Kando, PharmD, BCPP
Executive Director, Massachusetts Project, Medical Management TM, Clinical Instructor, Harvard Medical School, Boston, MA

Janet L. Karlix, PharmD
Associate Professor, College of Pharmacy, University of Florida and Director, Transplant Clinical Pharmacology Research Center, Gainseville, FL

Peter W. Kazakoff, PharmD
Assistant Professor, School of Pharmacy, University of Colorado, Denver, CO

H. William Kelly, PharmD, FCCP, BCPS
Professor of Pharmacy and Pediatrics, College of Pharmacy, University of New Mexico Health Science, Albuquerque, MN

Mehmood A. Khan, MD, FACE
Assistant Professor, School of Medicine, University of Minnesota and Director, Division of Endocrinology, Department of Medicine, Hennepin County Medical Center, Minneapolis, MN

Robert A. Kilroy, PharmD, BCPS
Clinical Associate Professor, Department of Pharmacy Practice, University of Florida College of Pharmacy and Clinical Specialist, Department of Pharmacy Services, Shands Hospital at the University of Florida, Gainesville, FL

William R. Kirchain, PharmD, CDE
Associate Professor of Pharmacy Practice, University of the Sciences in Philadelphia, Philadelphia College of Pharmacy, Philadelphia, PA

Cynthia K. Kirkwood, PharmD
Assistant Professor, Pharmacy and Pharmaceutics, Virginia Commonwealth University, Richmond, VA

Leroy C. Knodel, PharmD
Clinical Associate Professor, University of Texas Health Science Center at San Antonio and College of Pharmacy, Austin, TX

Jill M. Kolesar, PharmD, BCPS
Assistant Professor, School of Pharmacy, University of Wisconsin, Madison, WI

Sherri L. Konzem, PharmD
Clinical Assistant Professor, Department of Clinical Sciences and Administration, University of Houston, College of Pharmacy and Department of Family Practice, Memorial Hospital Southwest, Houston, TX

Kathleen D. Lake, PharmD, FCCP, BCPS
Director, Clinical Research and Transplant Therapeutics, Division of Nephrology and Surgery, University of Michigan Medical Center, Ann Arbor, MI

Tom A. Larson PharmD, FCCP
Associate Professor of Pharmacy Practice, Department of Pharmacy Practice, University of Minnesota, Minneapolis, MN

Alan H. Lau, PharmD, FCCP
Associate Professor, Department of Pharmacy Practice, College of Pharmacy, University of Illinois, Chicago, IL

Timothy S. Lesar, PharmD
Director of Pharmacy, Department of Pharmacy, Albany Medical Center, Albany, NY

Matthew J. Lewis, PharmD, BCPS
Clinical Assistant Professor, Department of Pharmaceutical Care and Health Systems, College of Pharmacy, University of Minnesota and Clinical Scientist, Hennepin County Medical Center, Division of Nephrology, Minneapolis, MN

Peter A. LeWitt, MD
Associate Professor of Neurology, Clinical Neuroscience Program, Sinai Hospital, Wayne State University, Detroit, MI

Celeste M. Lindley, PharmD, MS, FCCP, BCPS
Associate Professor, School of Pharmacy, University of North Carolina, Chapel Hill, NC

Gwynn D. Long, MD
Associate Professor of Medicine, Bone Marrow Transplantation Program, Duke University Medical Center, Durham, NC

R. Leon Longe, PharmD
Professor, University of Georigia College of Pharmacy and Medical College of Georgia, Augusta, GA

Larry M. Lopez, PharmD, FCCP
Professor and Chairman, College of Pharmacy, University of Florida, Gainesville, FL

William L. Macias, MD, PhD
Associate Professor of Medicine, Department of Medicine, Indiana University School of Medicine, and Clinical Research Physician, Eli Lilly & Company, Indianapolis, IN

Patricia A. Marken, BS Pharm, PharmD, BCPP
University of Missouri-Kansas City, Associate Professor of Pharmacy Practice and Psychiatry and Psychopharmacy Specialist, Western Missouri Mental Health Center, Kansas City, MO

Patricia L. Marshik, PharmD
Assistant Professor of Pharmacy Practice, College of Pharmacy, Health Sciences Center, Albuquerque, NM

Todd W. Mattox, BCNSP
Nutritional Support Pharmacist, Department of Pharmacy, H. Lee Moffitt Cancer Center and Research Institute, Tampa, FL

Gary R. Matzke, PharmD, FCP, FCCP
Professor of Pharmaceutical Sciences and Medicine, Schools of Pharmacy and Medicine, Center of Clinical Pharmacology, University of Pittsburgh, Pittsburgh, PA

William N. May, MD
Assistant Professor, Pediatrics and Neurology, University of Tennessee, Memphis, Memphis, TN

J. Russel May, PharmD
Associate Director of Pharmacy, Department of Pharmacy, Medical College of Georgia Hospital and Clinics, Augusta, Georgia; Adjunct Associate Professor, Department of Clinical and Administrative Sciences, College of Pharmacy, University of Georgia, Athens, GA

Janet McCombs, PharmD
Clinical Assistant Professor, Department of Clinical and Administrative Sciences, University of Georgia, Athens, GA

Margaret E. McGuinness, PharmD
Assistant Professor, College of Pharmacy, Oregon State University, Portland, OR

Timothy R. McGuire, PharmD
Associate Professor, Department of Pharmacy Practice, College of Pharmacy, University of Nebraska Medical Center, Omaha, NE

Patricia A. Montgomery, PharmD
Clinical Assistant Professor of Pharmacy, College of Pharmacy and Clinical Pharmacist, Department of Pharmacy, University of Michigan Health System, The University of Michigan, Ann Arbor, MI

Ashley K. Morris, PharmD, BCPS, BCOP
Clinical Associate, Bone Marrow Transplant Program, Department of Medicine, Duke University Medical Center, Durham, NC

Bruce A. Mueller, PharmD, FCCP, BCPS
Associate Professor of Clinical Pharmacy, Department of Pharmacy Practice, School of Pharmacy and Pharmacal Science, Purdue University, Indianapolis, IN

Timothy A. Mullenix, PharmD, MS
Chairman and Associate Professor, College of Pharmacy, University of South Carolina, Columbia, SC

Patricia Moynahan Mullins, PharmD
Accountant Manager, Heritage Information Systems, Richmond, VA

Milap C. Nahata, PharmD, FCCP
Kimberly Professor of Pharmacy and Pediatrics, Colleges of Pharmacy and Medicine, Ohio State University, Columbus, OH

Jean Nappi, PharmD, FCCP, BCPS
Professor and Vice Chair, Department of Pharmacy Practice, College of Pharmacy, Medical University of South Carolina, Charleston, SC

Merlin V. Nelson, PharmD, MD
Affiliated Community Medical Center, Willmar, MN

Phillip A. Nowakowski, PharmD
Clinical Assistant Professor, Department of Pharmacy Practice, North Dakota State University, College of Pharmacy, and Director of Clinical Pharmacy Services University of Illinois College of Pharmacy, Chicago, IL

Mary Beth O'Connell, PharmD, BCPS, FASHP, FCCP
Associate Professor, Experimental and Clinical Pharmacology, College of Pharmacy, University of Minnesota, Minneapolis, MN

Laura J. Odell, PharmD
Clinical Pharmacist, Pharmacy/Family Practice, Paynesville Area Health Care System, Minneapolis, MN

Maria-Theresa Olivari, MD, FACC
Associate Cardiologist and Director, Heart Failure/Cardiac Transplant Program, Minneapolis Heart Institute, Minneapolis, MN

Shirley M. Palmer, PharmD
Assistant Professor, School of Pharmacy, Virginia Commonwealth University, Richmond, VA

Robert B. Parker, PharmD, FCCP
Associate Professor, Department of Clinical Pharmacy, College of Pharmacy, University of Tennessee at Memphis, Memphis, TN

Charles A. Peloquin, PharmD
Director, Infectious Disease Pharmacokinetics Laboratory, and Adjoint Associate Professor, National Jewish Medical/Research Center, Schools of Pharmacy and Medicine, University of Colorado, Denver, CO

Janelle B. Perkins, PharmD, BCPS
Manager, BMT Clinical Research, Blood and Marrow Transplant Program, H. Lee Moffitt Cancer Center, Tampa, FL

Jay I. Peters, MD
Professor, Division of Pulmonary Medicine, Department of Medicine, University of Texas Health Science Center, San Antonio, San Antonio, TX

Marnie L. Peterson, PharmD
Infectious Disease Fellow, University of Minnesota/St. Paul-Ramsey Medical Center, St. Paul, MN

William P. Petros, PharmD, FCCP
Assistant Clinical Professor, Department of Medicine, Duke University Medical Center, Durham, NC

Stephanie J. Phelps, PharmD, FCCP
Professor of Clinical Pharmacy, Associate Professor of Pediatrics, University of Tennessee, Memphis, Memphis, TN

Denise Walbrandt Pigarelli, PharmD
Clinical Professor, School of Pharmacy, University of Wisconsin, Madison, WI

Ron E. Polk, PharmD
Professor of Pharmacy and Medicine, School of Pharmacy, Virginia Commonwealth University, Richmond, VA

L. Michael Posey, RPh
President, Pharmacy Editorial & News Services, Athens, Georgia

Randall A. Prince, PharmD
Professor, College of Pharmacy, University of Houston, Houston, TX

L. Michael Prisant, MD
Associate Professor Medicine, Medical College of Georgia, Augusta, GA

Richard J. Ptachcinski, PharmD, FCCP
Associate Professor, Department of Pharmacy and Therapeutics, University of Pittsburgh and Director, Ambulatory and Managed Care Pharmacy, University of Pittsburgh Medical Center Health System, Pittsburgh, PA

Mark C. Pugh, PharmD
Pharmacists Manager, First Health Services, Corporation

Charles C. Pulliam, MS Pharm, FASHP
Associate Professor and Director, Program on Aging, School of Pharmacy, University of North Carolina, Chapel Hill, NC

Marsha A. Raebel, PharmD, FCCP, BCPS
Research and Education Administrator, Clinical Adjoint Associate Professor, Pharmacy Specialty Services, Kaiser Permanente Rocky Mountain Division and University of Colorado School of Pharmacy, Aurora, CO

Daniel W. Rahn, MD
Professor of Medicine, Vice Dean for Clinical Affairs, Medical College of Georgia, Augusta, GA

Charles A. Reasner, II, MD, FACE
Associate Professor and Head, Division of Clinical Endocrinology, Department of Medicine, University of Texas Health Science Center-San Antonio, San Antonio, TX

Michael D. Reed, PharmD, FCCP, FCP
Professor of Pediatrics, RB&C Hospital, Department of Pediatrics, Case Western Reserve University, Cleveland, OH

Pamela D. Reiter, PharmD, BCPS
Neonatal Clinical Specialist, Pediatrics, Department of Pharmacy, University Hospital, Denver, CO

Monique Richer, PharmD, MA (ed), BCPS
Assistant Professor, Faculté De Pharmacie, Université Laval, Quebec, Canada

Keith A. Rodvold, PharmD, FCCP, BCPS
Professor, Department of Pharmacy Practice, University of Illinois at Chicago, Chicago, IL

David A. Rogers, MD, FACS, FAAP
Associate Professor, Department of Surgery, Medical College of Georgia, Augusta, GA

Douglas F. Rose, MD
Associate Professor, Pediatrics and Neurology, University of Tennessee, Memphis, Memphis, TN

John C. Rotschafer, PharmD, FCCP
Professor, University of Minnesota/St. Paul-Ramsey Medical Center, St. Paul, MN

Christine M. Ruby, PharmD, BCPS
Adjunct Assistant Professor, School of Pharmacy, University of North Carolina, Chapel Hill, NC; Senior Fellow, Center for the Study of Aging and Human Development; and Clinical Pharmacists Specialist in Geriatrics, Department of Pharmacy, Durham Veterans Affaris Medical Center, Durham, NC

Maria I. Rudis, PharmD, ABAT, BCPS
Assistant Professor, Department of Clinical Pharmacy and Emergency Medicine, USC Schools of Pharmacy and Medicine, Los Angeles, CA

Michael J. Rybak, PharmD, FCCP, BCPS
Professor of Pharmacy and Medicine, Department of Pharmacy Practice, Wayne State University, Detroit, MI

Lisa A. Sanchez, PharmD, BCPS
President, PE Applications, Inc., Boston, MA

Robert R. Schade, MD
Professor and Chief, Department of Medicine, Section of Gastroenterology and Hepatology, Medical College of Georgia, Augusta, GA

Lauren S. Schlesselman, PharmD
Adult Internal Medicine Pharmacy Practice Resident, Veteran's Administration Medical Center, Gainesville, FL

Michael J. Schmidt, PharmD
Clinical Pharmacist, Pharmacy/Family Practice, Clement Zablocki VA Medical Center, Milwaukee, WI

Mark E. Schneiderhan, BS Pharm, PharmD, BCPP
Clinical Assistant Professor, Pharmacy Practice, University of Illinois, Chicago, IL

Marieke Dekker Schoen, PharmD, BCPS
Clinical Associate Professor, Department of Pharmacy Practice and Science, College of Pharmacy, University of Illinois at Chicago, Chicago, IL

Nathan J. Schultz, PharmD, BCPS
Clinical Assistant Professor, University of Minnesota, College of Pharmacy, and Vice President, Pharmaceutical Management Operation, Diversified Pharmaceutical Services, Inc, SmithKline Beecham, Edina, MN

Arthur A. Schuna, MS, FASHP
Clinical Professor, Clinical Pharmacy Coordinator, William S. Middleton VA Medical Center, University of Wisconsin, Madison, WI

Rowena N. Schwartz, PharmD
Associate Professor of Pharmacy and Therapeutics, Department of Pharmacy and Therapeutics, University of Pittsburgh, School of Pharmacy, Pittsburgh, PA

Christopher L. Shaffer, PharmD
Clinical Specialist, Intensive Care, Department of Pharmaceutical Services, Children's Hospital, Adjunct Assistant Professor, Department of Pharmacy Practice, Creighton University, Omaha, NE

David C. Shelledy, PhD
Associate Professor and Chairman, Department of Respiratory Care, Univer-

sity of Texas Health Science Center, San Antonio, TX

Penny S. Shelton, PharmD, FASCP
Assistant Professor, School of Pharmacy, Campbell University; and Clinical Specialist in Geriatrics, Dorothea Dix Hospital, Raleigh, NC

Ralph A. Slaker, PharmD
Clinical Assistnat Professor, Department of Pharmacy Practice, North Dakota State University, College of Pharmacy, and Director of Clincial Pharmacy Services, Chronimed Inc., Minnetonka, MN

Jerry D. Smith, PharmD
Clinical Fellow, Departments of Pharmacy Practice and Family Medicine, University of Florida, Gainesville, FL

Steven P. Smith, PharmD, BCPS
Adult Oncology Clinical Specialist, Department of Pharmacy, Shands at the University of Florida, Gainesville, FL

Alka Z. Somani, PharmD
Assistant Professor of Pharmacy and Therapeutics and Clincial Pharmacist, University of Pittsburgh and University of Pittsburgh Medical Center, Pittsburgh, PA

Roger W. Sommi, BS Pharm, PharmD, BCPP
Associate Professor of Pharmacy Practice and Psychiatry, Division of Pharmacy Practice, University of Missouri-Kansas City Schools of Pharmacy and Medicine, Kansas City, MO

Thomas T. Sproat, PharmD, BCPS, PA-C
Vice-President, Health Care Education, Cortex Communications, Inc., Tampa, FL

John V. St. Peter, PharmD, BCPS
Associate Professor, College of Pharmacy, University of Minnesota and Pharmacotherapy Specialist, Division of Endocrinology, Department of Medicine, Hennepin County Medical Center, Minneapolis, MN

Wendy L. St. Peter, PharmD, BCPS
Associate Dean for Professional Education, Department of Pharmaceutical Care and Health Systems, College of Pharmacy, University of Minnesota, and Clinical Scientist, Hennepin County Medical Center, Division of Nephrology, Minneapolis, MN

Chester T. Stafford, MD
Professor of Medicine and Pediatrics, Section of Allergy/Immunology, Medical College of Georgia, Augusta, GA

Condit F. Steil, PharmD, CDE
McWhorter School of Pharmacy, Samford University, Birmingham, AL

Andy Stergachis, PhD
Professor of Pharmacy and Epidemiology, Chairman, Department of Pharmacy, School of Pharmacy, University of Washington, Seattle, WA

Mark A. Stratton, PharmD, BCPS, FASHP
Professor and Chair, Department of Clinical Sciences and Amdinistration, College of Pharmacy, University of Houston, Houston, TX

Kathleen A. Stringer, PharmD, FCCP
Associate Professor, School of Pharmacy, University of Colorado, Denver, CO

Robert L. Talbert, PharmD, FCCP, BCPS
Professor and Division Head, College of Pharmacy, University of Texas at Austin, Austin; Professor, Departments of Medicine and Pharmacology, University of Texas Health Science Center at San Antonio, San Antonio, Texas

A. Thomas Tayler, PharmD
Associate Professor, University of Georgia College of Pharmacy and Clinical Professor, Medical College of Georgia, Augusta, GA

Kathleen M. Teasley-Strausburg, MS, RPh, BCNSP
Nutrition Support/Pharmacy Consultant, Lakewood, CO

Karen A. Theesen, PharmD, BCPP
Associate Professor of Pharmacy Practice and Psychiatry, Department of Pharmacy Practice, Creighton University, Omaha, NE

Philip Toltzis, MD
Assistant Professor of Pediatrics, RB&C Hospital, Department of Pediatrics, Case Western Reserve University, Cleveland, OH

Amy Wells Valley, PharmD, BCPS
Oncology Pharmacy Specialist, South Texas Veterans HealthCare System, Audie L. Murphy Division, San Antonio, TX

Bertil Wagner, PharmD, FCCM
College of Pharmacy, The State University of New Jersey, Piscataway, NJ

Sharon M. Watling, PharmD, BCPS
Clinical Specialist, Critical Care; Assistant Professor, Departments of Pharmacy and Medicine, University of Missouri, Columbia, MO

K. M. A. Welch, MD
Director, NMR and Headache Research Centers, Neurology, Henry Ford Hospital, Detroit, MI

Barbara G. Wells, PharmD, FASHP, FCCP, BCPP
Professor and Dean, Idaho State University College of Pharmacy, Pocatello, ID

Dennis P. West, PhD, FCCP
Professor of Dermatology, Northwestern University Medical School, Professor of Pharmacy Practice, University of Illinois College of Pharmacy, Chicago, IL

K. M. A. Welch, MD
Senior Associate Dean of Research and Graduate Studies, University of Kansas School of Medicine, KU Medical Center, Kansas City, KS

Dianne B. Williams, PharmD
Drug Information Specialist, Department of Pharmacy, Medical College of Georgia, Augusta, GA

David H. Wright, PharmD
Infectious Disease Resident, University of Minnesota/St. Paul-Ramsey Medical Center, St. Paul, MN

Jack A. Yanovski, MD, PhD
Chief, Unit of Growth and Obesity, Section on Women's Health, Developmental Endocrinology Branch, National Institute of Child Health and Human Development, National Institutes of Health, Bethesda, MD

Gary C. Yee, PharmD, FCCP
Professor and Chair, Department of Pharmacy Practice, College of Pharmacy, University of Nebraska Medical Center, Omaha, NE

William Zamboni, PharmD, BCPS, FASHP
Assistant Professor, Program of Molecular Therapeutics and Drug Delivery, University of Pittsburgh Cancer Institute, Pittsburgh, PA

Guiding Principles of Pharmacotherapy

1. There should be a justifiable indication for every medication that a patient receives.
2. A medication should be used at the lowest dosage and for the shortest duration that is likely to achieve the desired outcome.
3. Do not use more than one medication when one alone will be adequate.
4. Newly approved medications should be used only if there are clear advantages over older medications.
5. Whenever possible, the selection of a medication regimen should be based on evidence obtained from controlled clinical trials.
6. The timing of drug administration should be considered as a possible influence on drug efficacy, adverse effects, and interactions with other drugs and food.
7. A medication regimen should be simplified as much as possible to enhance patient compliance.
8. A patient's perception of illness or the risks and benefits of therapy should be recognized as possibly affecting compliance and treatment outcomes.
9. Careful observation of a patient's response to treatment is necessary to confirm efficacy, prevent, detect, or manage adverse effects, assess compliance, and determine the need for dosage adjustment or discontinuation of drug therapy.
10. To enhance compliance, choose a medication regimen that the patient can afford.
11. A medication should not be given by injection when giving it by mouth would be just as effective and safe.
12. Before medications are used, lifestyle modifications should be made, when indicated, to obviate the need for drug therapy or enahance pharmacotherapy outcomes.
13. Initiation of a drug regimen should be done with full recognition that a medication may cause a disease, sign, symptom, syndrome, or abnormal laboratory test.
14. When a variety of drugs are equally efficacious and equally safe, the drug which results in the lowest health care cost or is most convenient for the patient should be chosen.
15. When making a decision about drug therapy for individual patients, societal effects should be considered.
16. It is important to recognize the possible reasons for failure of medication regimens, which include poor compliance, improper drug dose or interval, misdiagnosis, concurrent illness, interactions with foods and drugs, environmental factors, or genetic factors.

Joseph T. DiPiro, PharmD, FCCP
Barbara G. Wells, PharmD, FASHP, FCCP, BCPP
David W. Hawkins, PharmD
August 17, 1998

1 PHARMACOECONOMICS: PRINCIPLES

Lisa A. Sanchez, PharmD, BCPS

Today's cost-sensitive health care environment has created a competitive and challenging workplace for clinicians. Competition for diminishing resources has necessitated that the appraisal of health care goods and services extend beyond evaluations of safety and efficacy and consider the economic impact of these goods and services on the cost of health care. A challenge for health care professionals is to provide quality patient care with minimal resources.

An interest in defining the "value" of medicine is a common thread joining today's health care professionals, especially pharmacists. With serious concerns about rising medication costs and consistent pressure to decrease pharmacy expenditures and budgets, pharmacists must answer the question, "What is the value of the pharmaceutical goods and services I provide?" *Pharmacoeconomics,* or the discipline of placing a value on drug therapy,[1] has evolved to provide an answer to this question.

Challenged to provide high-quality patient care in the least expensive way, pharmacists have developed strategies aimed at containing costs. However, most of these strategies focus solely on determining the least expensive alternative rather than the alternative that possesses the best value for the money. The "cheapest" alternative—with respect to drug acquisition cost—is not always the best value for patients, departments, institutions, and health care systems.

Quality patient care must not be compromised while attempting to contain costs. The products and services delivered by today's pharmacists should demonstrate "pharmacoeconomic value," that is, a balance of economic, humanistic, *and* clinical outcomes. Pharmacoeconomics can provide the systematic means for this quantification. This chapter discusses the principles and methods of pharmacoeconomics and how they can be applied to clinical pharmacy practice, and thereby how they can assist in evaluating the value of pharmacotherapy and other modalities of treatment in clinical practice.

PRINCIPLES OF PHARMACOECONOMICS

Pharmacoeconomics has been defined as the description and the analysis of the cost of drug therapy to health care systems and society.[2] More specifically, pharmacoeconomic research is the process of identifying, measuring, and comparing the costs, risks, and benefits of programs, services, or therapies and determining which alternative produces the best health outcome for the resource invested.[3] For most pharmacists this translates into weighing the cost of providing a pharmacy product or service against the consequences (outcomes) realized by using the product or service, to determine which alternative yields the optimal outcome per dollar spent. This information can assist clinical decision makers in choosing the most cost-effective treatment options.[4]

There is a distinct relationship between pharmacoeconomics, outcomes research, and pharmaceutical care. Pharmacoeconomics is not synonymous with outcomes research. Outcomes research is defined more broadly as studies that attempt to identify, measure, and evaluate the results of health care services in general.[5] Outcomes research is discussed further in Chapter 2. Pharmacoeconomics is a division of outcomes research that can be used to quantify the value of pharmaceutical care products and services. Pharmaceutical care has been defined as the responsible provision of drug therapy for the purposes of achieving definite outcomes.[6] By accepting this as the paradigm or vision for our profession, pharmacy is accepting responsibility for managing drug therapy so that positive outcomes are produced.

Cost is defined as the value of the resources consumed by a program or drug therapy of interest. *Consequence* is defined as the effects, outputs, or outcomes of the program of drug therapy of interest. Consideration of both costs and consequences differentiates most pharmacoeconomic evaluation methods from traditional cost-containment strategies and drug-use evaluations.

Assessing costs and consequences—the value of a pharmaceutical product or service—depends heavily on the perspective of the evaluation. Common perspectives include those of the patient; provider (hospital, managed care organization); payer (government, insurer, employer); and society. A pharmacoeconomic evaluation can assess the value of a product or service from single or multiple perspectives. However, clarification of the perspective is critical, because the results of a pharmacoeconomic evaluation depend heavily on the perspective taken. For example, if comparing the value of alteplase (tPA) to streptokinase from a patient or societal perspective, tPA may be the best-value alternative because a 1% reduction in mortality rates is observed in this large population. Yet from a small community hospital's perspective, streptokinase may represent a better value, because it provides similar outcomes for less money.

Once the perspective is clear, a full evaluation of the relevant costs and consequences can begin. Health care costs or economic outcomes can be grouped into several categories: direct medical, direct nonmedical, indirect nonmedical, and intangible costs.[7] *Direct medical costs* are those incurred for medical products and services used to prevent, detect, and/or treat a disease (e.g., drugs, laboratory tests, and hospitalizations).[7] *Direct nonmedical costs* are any costs for nonmedical services that are results of illness but do not involve purchasing medical services (e.g., costs of transportation and hotel rooms near a treatment center).[7] *Indirect nonmedical costs* are the costs of reduced productivity (e.g., morbidity and mortality costs).[7–9] *Intangible costs* are those costs incurred that represent other nonfinancial outcomes of disease and medical care, which are not appropriately expressed in a dollar value (e.g., pain, suffering, and grief).[7]

Costs can also be measured as opportunity costs. *Opportunity costs* represent the economic benefit forgone when using one therapy instead of the next best alternative therapy.[10] Therefore, if a resource has been used to purchase a program or treatment alternative, then the opportunity to use it for another purpose is lost. Table 1–1 contains examples of these costs. Again, the costs that are identified, measured, and ultimately compared will vary depending on the perspective. For example, from the patient perspective, costs are essentially what the patient pays for a product or service that is not covered by insurance. Whereas from the provider perspective, costs are essentially the true expense of providing a product or service, regardless of the charge.

The consequences (or outcomes) of medical care can also be categorized. One way is to separate outcomes into three categories: economic, clinical, and humanistic. Economic outcomes are the direct, indirect, and intangible costs compared to the consequences of medical treatment alternatives.[11] Clinical outcomes are the medical events that occur as a result of disease or treatment (e.g., safety and efficacy endpoints).[11] Humanistic outcomes are the consequences of disease or treatment on patient functional status or quality of life along several dimensions (e.g., physical function, social function, general health and well-being, and life satisfaction).[11] These consequences (outcomes) can also be categorized as positive or negative. An example of a positive outcome is a desired effect of a drug, possibly manifested as an efficacy or effectiveness measure of a drug. A negative outcome is an undesired or adverse effect of a drug, possibly manifested as a treatment failure or an adverse drug reaction (ADR). Pharmacoeconomic evaluations should include assessments of both positive and negative outcomes. Evaluating only positive outcomes may be misleading because of the detriment and expense associated with negative outcomes.

TABLE 1–1. Examples of Health Care Cost Categories

Cost Category	Costs
Direct medical costs	Drugs Supplies Laboratory tests Health care professionals' time Hospitalization
Direct nonmedical costs	Transportation Food Family care Home aides
Indirect costs	Lost wages (morbidity) Income forgone due to premature death (mortality)
Intangible costs	Pain Suffering Grief
Opportunity costs	Lost opportunity Revenue forgone

METHODS OF PHARMACOECONOMICS

The pharmacoeconomic methods of evaluation are listed in Figure 1–1. These methods or tools can be separated into two distinct categories: economic and humanistic evaluation techniques. These methods have been used in a variety of fields and are being applied increasingly to health care.[12] Those most commonly used by pharmacists are discussed in the next sections and briefly summarized in Table 1–2.

ECONOMIC EVALUATION METHODS

The basic task of economic evaluation is to identify, measure, value, and compare the costs and consequences of the alternatives being considered. The two distinguishing characteristics of economic evaluation are as follows: (1) Is there a comparison of two or more alternatives? and (2) Are both costs and consequences of the alternatives examined?[13] A full economic evaluation encompasses both characteristics, while a partial economic evaluation addresses only one.

Application of economic evaluation methods to health care products and services, especially pharmaceuticals, may increase their acceptance by health care professionals and society.[14] Popular economic evaluation methods include cost-of-illness evaluation, and cost-minimization, cost-benefit, cost-effectiveness, and cost-utility analyses. Each

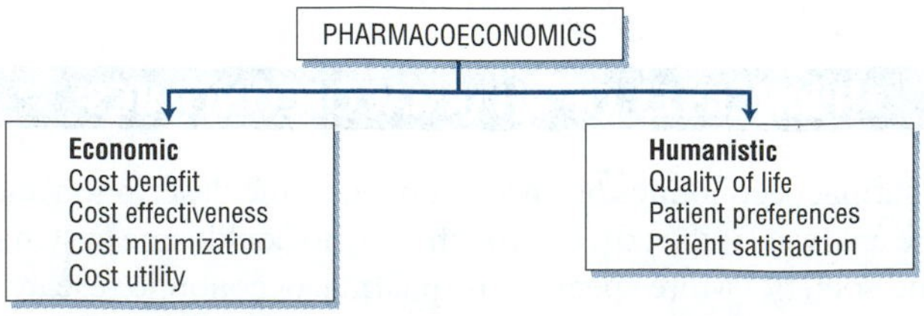

FIGURE 1–1. Components of pharmacoeconomics.

TABLE 1–2. Summary of Pharmacoeconomic Methodologies

Method	Description	Application	Cost Unit	Outcome Unit
COI	Estimates the cost of a disease on a defined population	Use to provide baseline to compare prevention/treatment options against	$$$	NA
CMA	Finds the least expensive cost alternative	Use when outcomes are the same	$$$	Assume to be equivalent
CBA	Measures benefit in monetary units and computes a net gain	Can compare programs with different objectives	$$$	$$$
CEA	Compares alternatives with therapeutic effects measured in physical units; computes a C/E ratio	Can compare drugs/programs that differ in clinical outcomes and use same unit of benefit	$$$	Natural units
CUA	Measures therapeutic consequences in utility units rather than physical units; computes a C/U ratio	Use to compare drugs/programs that are life extending with serious side effects or those producing reductions in morbidity	$$$	QALYs
QOL	Physical, social, and emotional aspects of patient's well-being that are relevant and important to the patient	Examines drug effects in areas not covered by laboratory or physiologic measurements	NA	QOL score

CBA = cost-benefit analysis; CEA = cost-effectiveness analysis; CMA = cost-minimization analysis; COI = cost-of-illness evaluation; CUA = cost-utility analysis; QOL = quality-of-life assessment; QALY = quality-adjusted life year gained.

method, except cost-of-illness evaluation, is used to compare competing programs or treatment alternatives. The methods are all similar in the way they measure cost (in dollars) and different in their measurement of outcomes. A brief discussion of each method is provided.

COST-OF-ILLNESS EVALUATION

A cost-of-illness (COI) evaluation identifies and estimates the overall cost of a particular disease for a defined population.[8] This evaluation method is often referred to as "burden-of-illness," and involves measuring the direct and indirect costs attributable to a specific disease. The costs of various diseases, including peptic ulcer disease, mental disorders, and cancer, in the United States have been estimated.

By successfully identifying the direct and indirect costs of an illness, one can determine the relative value of a treatment or prevention strategy. For example, by determining the cost of a particular disease to society, the cost of a prevention strategy could be subtracted from this to yield the benefit of implementing this strategy nationwide. COI is not used to compare competing treatment alternatives, but to provide an estimation of the financial burden of a disease. Thus, the value of prevention and treatment strategies can be measured against this illness cost.

COST-MINIMIZATION ANALYSIS

Cost-minimization analysis (CMA) involves the determination of the least costly alternative when comparing two or more treatment alternatives. With CMA, the alternatives must have an assumed or demonstrated equivalency in safety and efficacy (i.e., the two alternatives must be therapeutically equivalent). Once this equivalency in outcome is confirmed, the costs can be identified, measured, and compared in monetary units (dollars).

CMA is a relatively straightforward and simple method for comparing competing programs or treatment alternatives, as long as the therapeutic equivalence of the alternatives being compared has been established. If no evidence exists to support this, then a more comprehensive method such as cost-effectiveness analysis should be employed. Remember, CMA shows only a "cost savings" of one program or treatment over another.[15]

Employing CMA is appropriate when comparing two or more therapeutically equivalent agents or alternate dosing regimens of the same agent.[15] For example, if drugs A and B are antiulcer agents, documented to be equal in efficacy and incidence of ADRs, then the costs of using these drugs could be compared using CMA. These costs should extend beyond a comparison of drug acquisition costs and include costs of preparation, administration, and storage. The least expensive agent, considering all of these costs, should be preferred.

COST-BENEFIT ANALYSIS

Cost-benefit analysis (CBA) is a method that allows for the identification, measurement, and comparison of the benefits and costs of a program or treatment alternative. The benefits realized from a program or treatment alternative are compared with the costs of providing it. Both the costs and the benefits are measured and converted into equivalent dollars in the year in which they will occur.[8,12] Future cost and benefits are discounted or reduced to their current value.

These costs and benefits are expressed as a ratio (a benefit-to-cost ratio, B/C), a net benefit, or a net cost. A clinical decision maker would choose the program or treatment alternative with the highest net benefit or the greatest B/C ratio.[9] Guidelines for the interpretation of this ratio are indicated.[12,15,16]

- If B/C > 1, the program or treatment is of value. The benefits realized by the program or treatment alternative outweigh the cost of providing it.
- If B/C = 1, the benefits equal the cost. The benefits realized by the program or treatment alternative are equivalent to the cost of providing it.
- If B/C < 1, the program or treatment is not economically beneficial. The cost of providing the program or treatment alternative outweighs the benefits realized by it.

CBA should be employed when comparing treatment alternatives in which the costs and benefits do not occur simultaneously. CBA may also be used when comparing programs with different objectives, because all benefits are converted into dollars. CBA can also be used to evaluate a single program or compare multiple programs. However, valuing health benefits in monetary terms can be difficult and controversial. The expression of some health benefits as monetary units is neither appropriate nor widely accepted. Therefore, unless the benefits of a program or treatment alternative are appropriately expressed in dollars, CBA should not be employed.[15]

CBA may be an appropriate method to use in justifying and documenting the value of an existing health care service or the potential worth of a new one. For example, when competing for institutional resources, CBA can provide data to document that a clinical pharmacy service yields a high return on investment compared with other institutional services competing for the same resources. However, the relative magnitude of the costs and benefits for the service must be considered when making this resource allocation decision. If a service costs \$100 to implement and results in a benefit to the hospital of \$1000, and a service that costs \$100,000 to implement results in a benefit of \$1,000,000, both have a B/C ratio of 10.[15] Thus, caution should be exercised when using B/C ratios and CBA as a comparison tool.

COST-EFFECTIVENESS ANALYSIS

Cost-effectiveness analysis (CEA) is a way of summarizing the health benefits and resources used by competing health care programs so that policymakers can choose among them.[13] CEA involves comparing programs or treatment alternatives with different safety and efficacy profiles. Cost is measured in dollars, and outcomes in terms of obtaining a specific therapeutic outcome. These outcomes are often expressed in physical units, natural units, or nondollar units (lives saved, cases cured, life expectancy, or mm Hg drop in blood pressure).[8,17,18]

The results of CEA are also expressed as a ratio—either as an average cost-effectiveness ratio (ACER) or as an incremental cost-effectiveness (C/E) ratio. An ACER represents the total cost of a program or treatment alternative divided by its clinical outcome to yield a ratio representing the dollar cost per specific clinical outcome gained, independent of comparators. The AC/E ratio can be summarized as follows[7,15,18]:

$$\text{AC/E} = \frac{\text{Health care costs (\$)}}{\text{Clinical outcome (not in \$)}}$$

This allows the costs and outcomes to be reduced to a single value to allow for comparison. Using this ratio, the clinician would choose the alternative with the least cost per outcome gained.[9] The most cost-effective alternative is not always the least costly alternative for obtaining a specific therapeutic objective. In this regard, cost effectiveness need not be cost reduction, but rather cost optimization.[19]

Often clinical effectiveness is gained at an increased cost. Is the increased benefit worth the increased cost? Incremental cost-effectiveness analysis may be used to determine the additional cost and effectiveness gained when one treatment alternative is compared with the next best treatment alternative.[7] Thus, instead of comparing the average C/E ratios of each treatment alternative, the additional cost that a treatment alternative imposes over another treatment is compared with the additional effect, benefit, or outcome it provides. The incremental C/E ratio (ICER) can be summarized as follows:

$$\text{ICER} = \frac{\text{Cost (\$)}_a - \text{Cost (\$)}_b}{\text{Effect (\%)}_a - \text{Effect (\%)}_b}$$

This formula yields the additional cost required to obtain the additional effect gained by switching from drug A to drug B.

CEA is particularly useful in balancing cost with patient outcome, determining which treatment alternatives represent the best health outcome per dollar spent, and when it is appropriate to measure outcome in terms of obtaining a specific therapeutic objective. In addition, CEA may provide data to support drug policy, formulary management, and individual patient treatment decisions. Globally, CEA is being used to set public policies regarding the use of pharmaceutical products (national formularies) in countries such as Australia,[20] New Zealand, and Canada.[21]

When comparing antiemetic agents for development of a policy for the prevention of chemotherapy-induced emesis, CEA can be employed. Many of these agents differ with respect to effectiveness, safety, and cost. By performing a thorough CEA, these variables can be reduced to a single number (C/E ratio), which will allow for a meaningful comparison. The treatment alternative with a better C/E ratio than the others (i.e., lower cost per unit of outcome) would be selected and promoted for use.

COST-UTILITY ANALYSIS

Cost-utility analysis (CUA) is another method for comparing treatment alternatives. CUA integrates patient preferences and health-related quality of life (QOL). Cost is measured in dollars and therapeutic outcome in patient-weighted utilities, rather than in physical units. Often the utility measure used is a "quality-adjusted life year" (QALY) gained. QALY is a common measure of health status used in CUA, combining morbidity and mortality data.

Results of CUA are also expressed in a ratio, a cost-utility (C/U) ratio. Most often, this ratio is translated as the cost per quality-adjusted life year (QALY) gained."[8,12] The preferred treatment alternative is that with the lowest cost per QALY (or other health status utility).

CUA is the most appropriate method to use when comparing programs and treatment alternatives that are life extending with serious side effects (e.g., cancer chemotherapy), those that produce reductions in morbidity rather than mortality (e.g., medical treatment of arthritis),[19] and when QOL is the most important health outcome being examined. CUA is employed less frequently than other economic evaluation methods because of lack of agreement in measuring utilities, difficulty comparing QALYs across patients and populations, and difficulty quantifying patient preferences. Thus, CUA should be reserved for comparing treatment alternatives whose primary goal is improving QOL, and caution should be exercised when using this method.

HUMANISTIC EVALUATION METHODS

Pharmacoeconomic evaluations may also focus on humanistic concerns. Methods for evaluating the impact of disease and treatment of disease on patient's health-related QOL, patient preferences, and patient satisfaction are all growing in popularity and application to pharmacotherapy decisions. These methods can also assist clinicians in quantifying the value of pharmaceuticals.

QOL has been defined as the assessment of the functional effects of illness and its consequent therapy as perceived by the patient.[22] These effects are often displayed as physical, emotional, and social effects on the patient.[14] Measurement of health-related QOL is usually achieved through the use of patient-completed questionnaires. Many questionnaires are available, and most are either disease-specific or generic measures of health status.[23,24] Various overviews on QOL and its application to pharmacy have been published.[24–27] For further discussion, refer to Chapter 2.

APPLICATIONS OF PHARMACOECONOMICS

Pharmacists, regardless of practice setting, can benefit applying the principles and methods of pharmacoeconomics to their daily practice settings. Applied pharmacoeconomics is defined as putting pharmacoeconomic principles, methods, and theories into practice, to quantify the "value" of pharmacy products and pharmaceutical care services used in "real-world" environments. Today's pharmacy practitioners are increasingly required to justify the value of the products and services they provide. Applied pharmacoeconomics can provide the means or tools for this valuation.

One of the primary applications of pharmacoeconomics in clinical practice today is to aid clinical and policy decision making. Complete pharmacotherapy decisions should contain assessments of three basic outcome areas whenever appropriate: clinical, economic, and humanistic outcomes. Traditionally, most drug therapy decisions were based solely on the clinical outcomes (e.g., safety and efficacy) associated with a treatment alternative. Over the past 10 to 15 years, it has become quite popular to also include an assessment of the economic outcomes associated with a treatment alternative. The current trend is to also incorporate the humanistic outcomes associated with a treatment alternative, that is, to bring the patient back into this decision-making equation. In today's health care environment, it is no longer appropriate to make drug selection decisions based solely on acquisition costs. Thus, through the appropriate application of pharmacoeconomic principles and methods, incorporating these three critical components into clinical decisions can be accomplished.

Pharmacoeconomic data can be a powerful tool to support various clinical decisions, ranging from the level of the patient to the level of an entire health care system. Figure 1–2 shows various decisions that may be supported using pharmacoeconomics including effective formulary management, individual patient treatment, medication policy, and resource allocation.[15,18] For discussion purposes, the application of pharmacoeconomics to decision making is divided into two basic areas: drug therapy evaluation and clinical pharmacy service evaluation.

DRUG THERAPY EVALUATION

Historically, pharmacoeconomic principles and methods have been commonly applied to assist clinicians and practitioners in making more informed and complete decisions regarding drug therapy. For example, pharmacoeconomics can provide critical cost-effectiveness data to support the addition or deletion of a drug to or from the hospital formulary, with or without restriction. In fact, the pharmacoeconomic assessment of formulary actions is becoming a standardized part of many pharmacy and therapeutic (P&T) committees.

Selecting the most cost-effective drugs for an organizational formulary is important. However, it is equally important to determine the most appropriate way to use and prescribe these agents. Hence, developing and implementing appropriate use guidelines or policies, based on sound pharmacoeconomic data, can have a great impact on influencing prescribing patterns. Further, implementing sound drug use guidelines/policies will ensure the most appropriate and cost-effective use of pharmaceutical agents throughout the health care system.

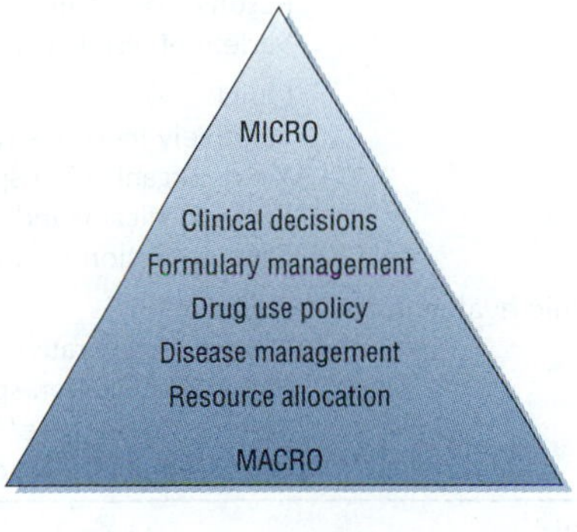

FIGURE 1–2. Decisions for pharmacoeconomic applications.

The application of pharmacoeconomics can also be useful for making a decision about an individual patient's therapy. Evaluating the impact a drug has on a patient's health-related quality of life can be useful when deciding between two agents for customizing a patient's pharmacotherapy. Although this can be one of the most difficult applications of pharmacoeconomics, it is also one of the most important.

CLINICAL PHARMACY SERVICE EVALUATION

The most recent application of pharmacoeconomic principles and methods has been for justifying the value of various health care services, particularly pharmacy services. When competing for hospital resources, pharmacoeconomics can provide the data necessary to justify that a specific service maximizes the resources allocated by health care system administrators. Pharmacoeconomics can be useful in determining the value of an existing service, estimating the potential worth of implementing a new service, or capturing the value of a "cognitive" clinical intervention. Practitioners and administrators can then use this data to make more informed resource allocation decisions.

For example, suppose you want to implement a pharmacy-based, therapeutic drug monitoring program. It is hypothesized that this service will improve quality of patient care and save money for the health care system. After negotiating with hospital administrators, the funding for this service is approved for a 1 year trial basis, after which you must document and justify the value of this practice. Theoretically, all of the relevant costs and benefits of the program should be measured, and if appropriate converted into dollars, using cost-benefit analysis. Potential benefits may include decreased total drug costs and decreased incidence of adverse drug reactions. Potential program costs are primarily the salary and benefits for a pharmacist and additional lab tests to monitor patients. Data documenting that the benefit of this pharmacy service yields a high return on investment (ROI) should increase the probability of your program being continually funded by the health care system.

Unfortunately, previous reviews of the literature have revealed a disappointing number of rigorous economic evaluations of clinical pharmacy services published to date.[28–30] McGhan and colleagues evaluated 35 potential cost-benefit or cost-effectiveness studies of pharmacy services, published before 1978, and concluded that only 5 of these studies were considered legitimate cost-benefit or cost-effectiveness analyses.[28] MacKeigan and Bootman, reviewed 22 cost-benefit or cost-effectiveness studies published between 1978 and 1987, and concluded that cost-benefit and cost-effectiveness analyses have not been extensively adopted for the evaluation of clinical pharmacy services.[29] Most recently, Schumock and associates[30] reviewed economic evaluations of pharmacy services published between 1988 and 1995. Of the studies reviewed, only 19 were considered "full" or legitimate economic analyses, and the authors concluded that although the number of articles published has increased over the years, there is still a need for improvement in the quality or rigor of study design.

STRATEGIES TO INCORPORATE PHARMACOECONOMICS INTO PHARMACOTHERAPY

Various strategies are available to incorporate pharmacoeconomics into pharmacotherapy. Popular strategies for using pharmacoeconomics to assess the value of pharmaceutical products and services include using the results of published pharmacoeconomic studies, using economic models, or conducting pharmacoeconomic research.[31] Advantages and disadvantages of these strategies are summarized in Table 1–3.

USE THE PHARMACOECONOMIC LITERATURE

Quantifying the value of pharmaceuticals through pharmacoeconomics has increased in popularity. Many pharmacoeconomic analyses are published in primary medical and pharmacy literature sources. However, the eagerness to

TABLE 1–3. Advantages and Disadvantages of Pharmacoeconomic Application Strategies

Strategy	Advantages	Disadvantages
Use published literature	Quick Inexpensive Subject to peer review Results may be from RCT Variety of results can be examined	Results from RCT (i.e., protocol-driven resource use) Difficult to generalize results May not be comparative Misuse of pharmacoeconomic terms Variations in rigor/quality
Build an economic model	Quick Relatively inexpensive Yields organization-specific results Bridges efficacy and effectiveness Data collection is unobtrusive	Results dependent on assumptions Potential for researcher bias Controversial Reluctance of decision makers to accept results
Conduct a pharmacoeconomic evaluation	Flexible Usually comparative Yields organization-specific data Reflects "usual care" or effectiveness Data from multiple sources can be used	Expensive Time consuming Difficult to control and randomize Potential for patient selection bias Potential for small sample size

RCT = randomized controlled trial.

conduct pharmacoeconomic evaluations of drugs often exceeds the quality of these evaluations. Variations in quality and indiscriminate use of pharmacoeconomic terminology are documented in medical and pharmacy literature sources.[4,28–30,32–34] To use this literature as an aid in clinical decision making, it must be (1) critically evaluated for quality and rigor and (2) interpreted correctly. Therefore, prior to using pharmacoeconomic data to make clinical and policy decisions, decision makers should recognize its potential limitations.

A primary consideration when evaluating and interpreting a study is the ability to generalize or transfer the results to other health care settings and countries. It can be difficult to generalize and transfer the results of a published study primarily due to wide variations in practice patterns, patient populations, and costs among health care systems and countries. Further, differences in study perspectives, data sources, and analytical styles may present a challenge for practitioners attempting to extrapolate or relate exact cost savings or cost ratios to their own practice setting. To enhance the ability to use pharmacoeconomic results published in the literature, consider the following points:

1. What is the technical merit of the study?
2. Are the results applicable to local decision making?
3. Do the results apply generally in different jurisdictions with different perspectives?[35]

Various guidelines, criteria, and consensus-based recommendations for evaluating, conducting, and reporting pharmacoeconomic literature have been published.[7,13,21,36–44] These guidelines and criteria have been combined and summarized into 11 categories most pertinent to pharmacotherapy.[39] A summary of these 11 criteria and pertinent questions for each category is given in Table 1–4. Each evaluation criterion is briefly discussed next.

STUDY OBJECTIVE

A clear statement of the purpose of the study should be given. This objective should be clear, concise, well defined, and measurable.

STUDY PERSPECTIVE

The researcher must select one or more perspectives (e.g., patient, provider, payer, or society) from which the analysis will be conducted.[9] This perspective should be appropriate given the scope of the pharmacoeconomic problem identified. An evaluation may be conducted from single or multiple perspectives, as long as the costs and consequences identified are relevant to the perspective(s) chosen.

PHARMACOECONOMIC METHOD

It should be clear which pharmacoeconomic method was employed (CEA, CMA, CBA, or CUA), and this method should be appropriate given the problem (e.g., CMA is appropriate if comparing two alternatives equivalent in therapeutic outcome, but not if the alternatives differ in therapeutic outcome). Also, a researcher may claim a specific method was employed (e.g., CEA) but actually employ another method (e.g., CMA).

STUDY DESIGN

Pharmacoeconomic evaluations can be prospective or retrospective. Although prospective designs are usually preferred, retrospective evaluations can be rich with information and reflective of usual care. Many pharmacoeconomic

TABLE 1–4. Basic Criteria for Evaluation of Pharmacoeconomic Literature

Objective
What is the question(s) being considered?
Is the question clear, defined, and measurable?
Perspective
What is the perspective(s) of the analysis?
Is it appropriate given the scope of the problem?
Pharmacoeconomic Method
What pharmacoeconomic tool was used?
Is it appropriate given the problem?
Is it actually what was conducted?
Study Design
What was the study design?
What were the data sources?
Is the evaluation suitable if carried out in a clinical trial?
Choice of Interventions
Were all appropriate alternatives considered and described?
Were any appropriate alternatives omitted?
Are the alternatives relevant to the perspective and clinical nature of the study?
Is there evidence that the alternatives' effectiveness has been established?
Costs and Consequences
What are the costs and consequences (outcomes) included?
Are the costs and outcomes relevant to the perspective chosen?
Do they include negative outcomes (failures, ADRs)?
How were they valued?
Were costs and consequences measured in the appropriate physical units?
Discounting
Was the study performed over time?
Were costs and consequences that occur in the future discounted to their present value?
Was any justification given for the discount rate used?
Results
Are the results accurate and practical for medical decision makers?
Were the appropriate statistical analyses performed?
Was an incremental analysis performed?
Are all the assumptions and limitations of the study discussed?
Sensitivity Analysis
Are cost ranges for significant variables tested for sensitivity?
Are the appropriate and relevant variables varied?
Do the findings follow the anticipated trend?
Conclusions
Are the conclusions of the study justified?
Is it possible to extrapolate the conclusions to daily clinical practice?
Sponsorship
Was there any bias due to the sponsorship of the study?

evaluations today are conducted as a part of randomized controlled clinical trials (RCTs). Two cautions for interpreting pharmacoeconomic data collected in this manner include (1) costs can be protocol driven, not necessarily reflective of using a drug in common practice[45]; and (2) control of subjects and decreased complications may yield greater costs and benefits than those observed in common practice.[36]

CHOICE OF INTERVENTIONS

All relevant available treatment options should be completely described or mentioned. The treatment alternatives and dosages being compared should be those used in common practice, and evidence of their effectiveness should be established. Because pharmacoeconomic methods are tools to aid in choosing between treatment alternatives, assessing the cost of a single alternative is considered a partial economic evaluation.

COSTS AND CONSEQUENCES

All of the important and relevant costs and consequences for each program or treatment alternative should be identified. The cost and consequences identified must be relevant to the study perspective(s), and measured in suitable terms, using the appropriate physical units. Costs should include direct, indirect, and intangible costs. Consequences should include the positive and negative clinical and humanistic outcomes associated with the program or treatment alternative. All of these costs and consequences must be valued credibly, with the data sources clearly identified.

DISCOUNTING

The comparison of programs or treatment alternatives should be made at one point in time; thus any costs and consequences not occurring in the present must be addressed. "Discounting," or adjusting for differential timing, is the process of reducing any costs and consequences that may occur in the future back to their present value. If a study is performed over time (more than 1 year), or if future cost savings are projected, discounting should be done using an appropriate discount rate. The rate typically used is 4% to 8%, representing annual inflation or bank interest rates. However, many researchers use a discount rate of 5%.

STUDY RESULTS

A full discussion of the study assumptions, limitations, and how to interpret the results in the context of different practice settings[13] should be provided. This discussion should include all relevant issues of concern to potential users of the study. The results should reflect that the appropriate statistical analyses were performed. Also, it may be appropriate to express the study results in terms of increases, that is, to use incremental cost analysis (additional cost of gaining an additional benefit by using one drug over another).

SENSITIVITY ANALYSIS

It is imperative that researchers test the sensitivity of study results using sensitivity analysis. Sensitivity analysis (SA) is the process of testing the robustness of an economic evaluation by examining changes in results. Specific variables such as percent effectiveness, incidence of ADRs, and dominant resources can be varied over a range of plausible values and the results recalculated. SA is of paramount importance because of the very common need for investigators to use assumptions and estimates for unknown variables.[34]

STUDY CONCLUSIONS

Researchers should assist the reader in extrapolating study conclusions to clinical practice. The conclusions drawn from the study results should be justified (internal validity) and able to be generalized (external validity).[39] Also, conclusions drawn from results that were "statistically" significant may or may not be "clinically" relevant, and vice versa.

SPONSORSHIP

Similar to evaluating the quality of a clinical trial, sponsorship of a study should be considered when evaluating the quality and usefulness of a pharmacoeconomic study.[37] Quality of studies conducted or sponsored by pharmaceutical companies will vary by company, product, or evaluation and the potential for bias should be neither ignored nor assumed. Many of the studies sponsored or conducted by the pharmaceutical industry to date have been academically rigorous as well as informative. A clear understanding of how to evaluate, critique, and use the pharmacoeconomic literature appropriately will minimize any potential effects of this criteria on clinical decision making.

BUILD AN ECONOMIC MODEL

Studies that "model" the economic impact of a pharmaceutical product or service on a defined population are increasing in popularity. Modeling studies use existing clinical and/or epidemiologic data to project future outcomes.[46] Use of economic models can provide support for various clinical decisions, especially those that are time contingent.[31] Identifying assumptions regarding the treatment alternatives being compared, the patient outcomes under study, and the probability of those outcomes occurring can provide the basis for an economic simulation to assist in the medication decision-making process.

Economic modeling often employs decision analysis, which has been defined as an explicit, quantitative, and prescriptive approach to choosing among alternative outcomes.[47,48] The tool used in decision analysis is a decision tree. A decision tree provides a framework to display graphically primary variables including treatment options, outcomes associated with those treatment options, and probabilities of the outcomes. The researcher can then algebraically reduce all of these factors into a single value, allowing for comparison.

Building an economic model can help the clinician to forecast the impact of medication-use decisions on a patient, institution, or health care system. Also, as new drugs are marketed that can displace older agents, an economic model can expedite the reappraisal process for formulary management and drug-use policy decisions.[49] For building an economic model to assist in clinical decision making, various published examples can be considered.[50,51]

CONDUCT A PHARMACOECONOMIC EVALUATION

Clinicians may need to conduct a pharmacoeconomic evaluation if there is insufficient literature, if published results cannot be extrapolated to clinical practice, or if building a model is not appropriate. Before conducting a pharmacoeconomic evaluation, clinicians should be familiar with the similarities, differences, and appropriate application of pharmacoeconomic methods, discussed earlier in the chapter.

The decision to conduct a local pharmacoeconomic study is not without its own costs. Because both time and monetary resources are consumed by these evaluations, specific pharmacy products and services for pharmacoeconomic evaluation should be targeted. Thus, this strategy should be reserved for pharmacy decisions that may have a significant impact on cost or quality of care.

Conducting pharmacoeconomic research in a hospital or managed care environment can be challenging. Lack of institutional resources, small sample sizes, difficulty randomizing, inability to compare with placebo, and difficulty generalizing results may all be limitations. For example, when asked to determine and recommend the most cost-effective antihypertensive agent for a formulary management decision, clinicians may lack monetary and time resources to conduct a scientifically rigorous study.

Conducting a pharmacoeconomic evaluation should be guided by the criteria for quality economic evaluations.[8,13,21,36–44] A 10-step process identified by Jolicoeur and associates,[52] and 4 additional steps identified by the author, can provide readers with guidance for conducting a local pharmacoeconomic study.[53] This process contains 14 fundamental steps for conducting a pharmacoeconomic evaluation in a health care system and can be applied to virtually any therapeutic area or health care service. Although some of these steps are similar to those evaluation criterion detailed earlier in this chapter, they will now be discussed briefly in the context of conducting an evaluation.

STEP 1: DEFINE THE PHARMACOECONOMIC PROBLEM

A broad problem might be "Which antiemetic regimen represents the best value for the prevention of chemotherapy-induced emesis (CIE)?" However, a more succinct and measurable problem would be "Which regimen is the best value for preventing acute CIE in patients receiving highly emetogenic chemotherapy?"

STEP 2: ASSEMBLE A CROSS-FUNCTIONAL STUDY TEAM

The study team can provide early "buy-in" and additional resources for a pharmacoeconomic evaluation. Team members vary depending on the analysis, but may include representatives from medicine, nursing, pharmacy, hospital administration, and information systems.

STEP 3: DEFINE THE APPROPRIATE STUDY PERSPECTIVE

Choose a study perspective(s) most relevant to the problem. For example, if the problem is as listed in step 1, then the perspective of the institution or health care system may be most appropriate.

STEP 4: IDENTIFY TREATMENT ALTERNATIVES AND OUTCOMES

Treatment alternatives can include pharmacologic and nonpharmacologic options, but should include all clinically relevant alternatives. The outcomes identified should include both positive and negative clinical outcomes.

STEP 5: IDENTIFY THE APPROPRIATE PHARMACOECONOMIC METHOD TO EMPLOY

Pharmacoeconomic methods to choose from include cost-minimization, cost-benefit, cost-effectiveness, and cost-utility analyses. Employing the incorrect method can adversely affect medication decisions influencing both cost and quality of care.

STEP 6: PLACE A MONETARY VALUE ON TREATMENT ALTERNATIVES AND OUTCOMES

Placing a monetary value on treatment alternatives and outcomes includes not only drug administration and acquisition costs but also the cost of positive and negative clinical outcomes (for example, determining the cost of ADRs and treatment failures). This can be measured prospectively or retrospectively, or estimated using comprehensive databases or expert panels.

STEP 7: IDENTIFY RESOURCES TO CONDUCT STUDY IN AN EFFICIENT MANNER

Resources necessary will vary by study, but may include access to medical or computerized records, average medical personnel wages, and specialty medical staff.

STEP 8: IDENTIFY PROBABILITIES THAT OUTCOMES MAY OCCUR IN STUDY POPULATION

What are the probabilities of the outcomes identified in step 4 actually occurring in clinical practice? Using primary literature and expert opinion, these probabilities can be obtained and may be manifested as efficacy rates and incidence of ADRs.

STEP 9: EMPLOY DECISION ANALYSIS

The use of decision analysis can assist in conducting various economic evaluations, including CEA. Although not necessary for all pharmacoeconomic evaluations, decision analysis and decision trees may provide a solid backbone or platform for the decision at hand. Using a decision tree, treatment alternatives, outcomes, and probabilities may be graphically presented and algebraically reduced to a single value for comparison (i.e., C/E ratio).

STEP 10: DISCOUNT COSTS OR PERFORM A SENSITIVITY OR INCREMENTAL COST ANALYSIS

Costs and consequences that occur in the future must be discounted back to their present value. Sensitive variables must be tested over a clinically relevant range and results recalculated. If appropriate, an incremental analysis of the costs and consequences should be performed.

STEP 11: PRESENT STUDY RESULTS

Results should be presented to the cross-functional team and the appropriate committees. Presentation style and content may vary depending on the audience.

STEP 12: DEVELOP A POLICY OR AN INTERVENTION

Take the study results and develop a policy or an intervention that can improve or maintain quality of care, possibly at a cost savings.

STEP 13: IMPLEMENT POLICY AND EDUCATE PROFESSIONALS

Spend adequate time and resources strategically implementing the policy or intervention. Educate those health care professionals most likely to be affected by this policy, using various strategies including verbal, written, and online communication.

STEP 14: FOLLOW-UP DOCUMENTATION

Once the intervention or policy has been implemented for a reasonable period of time, collect follow-up data. These data will provide feedback on the success and quality of the policy or intervention.

CONCLUSIONS

The principles and methods of pharmacoeconomics provide the means to quantify the value of pharmacotherapy through balancing costs and outcomes. Providing quality care with minimal resources is the future, and the future is here. By understanding the principles, methods, and application of pharmacoeconomics, pharmacists will be prepared to determine and quantify the value of pharmacotherapy to the health care system and society.

REFERENCES

1. Sanchez LA. Expanding the pharmacist's role in pharmacoeconomics: How and why? Pharmacoeconomics 1994;5:367–375.
2. Townsend RJ. Post-marketing drug research and development. Ann Pharmacother 1987;21:134–136.
3. Drummond M, Smith GT, Wells N. Economic Evaluation in the Development of Medicines. London, Office of Health Economics, 1988:33.
4. Lee JT, Sanchez LA. Interpretation of cost-effective and soundness of economic evaluations in the pharmacy literature. Am J Hosp Pharm 1991;48:2622–2627.
5. Bootman JL. Pharmacoeconomics and outcomes research. Am J Health System Pharm 1995;52(suppl 3):S16–S19.
6. Hepler CD, Strand LM. Opportunities and responsibilities in pharmaceutical care. Am J Hosp Pharm 1990;47:533–543.
7. Eisenberg JM. Clinical economics. A guide to economic analysis of clinical practices. JAMA 1989;262:2879–2886.
8. Bootman JL, Townsend RJ, McGhan WF. Principles of Pharmacoeconomics. Cincinnati, Harvey Whitney Books, 1991.
9. Freund DA, Dittus RS. Principles of pharmacoeconomic analysis of drug therapy. Pharmacoeconomics 1992;1:20–32.
10. Glossary of terms used in pharmacoeconomic and quality of life analysis. Pharmacoeconomics 1992;1:151.
11. Kozma CM, Reeder CE, Schulz RM. Economic, clinical, and humanistic outcomes: A planning model for pharmacoeconomic research. Clin Ther 1993;15:1121–1132.
12. Draugalis JR, Bootman LJ, Larson LN, McGhan WF. Current Concepts: Pharmacoeconomics. Kalamazoo, MI, Upjohn, 1989.
13. Drummond MF, Stoddart GL, Torrance GW. Methods for the Economic Evaluation of Health Care Programmes. Oxford, Oxford University Press, 1986:5–38, 74–111.
14. McGhan WF. Pharmacoeconomics and the evaluation of drugs and services. Hosp Formulary 1993;28:365–378.
15. Sanchez LA, Lee JT. Use and misuse of pharmacoeconomic terms. Top Hosp Pharm Manage 1994;13:11–22.
16. Sanchez LA. Pharmacoeconomic principles and methods: An introduction for hospital pharmacists. Hosp Pharm 1994;29:1035–1040.
17. Bootman JL, Larson LN, McGhan WF, Townsend RJ. Pharmacoeconomic research and clinical trials: Concepts and issues. Ann Pharmacother 1989;23:693–697.
18. Detsky AS, Nagiie IG. A clinician's guide to cost-effectiveness analysis. Ann Intern Med 1990;113:147–154.
19. Bootman JL. The basics of pharmacoeconomic analysis. Pharm Rep 1993;23:14–15.
20. Langley PC. The role of pharmacoeconomic guidelines for formulary approval: The Australian experience. Clin Ther 1993;15:1154–1176.
21. Detsky AS. Guidelines for economic analysis of pharmaceutical products: A draft document for Ontario and Canada. Pharmacoeconomics 1993;3:354–361.
22. Schipper H, Clinch J, Powell V. Definitions and conceptual issues. In: Spilker B, ed. Quality of Life Assessments in Clinical Trials. New York, Raven, 1990.
23. Spilker B. Quality of Life Assessments in Clinical Trials. New York, Raven, 1990.
24. Spilker B, et al. Quality of Life Bibliography and Indexes—1990 update. Clin Pharmacoepidemiology 1992;6:57–158.
25. Coons SJ. Quality of life assessment: Understanding its use as an outcome measure. Hosp Formulary 1993;28:486–498.
26. Jaeschke R, Guyatt GH, Cook D. Quality of life instruments in the evaluation of new drugs. Pharmacoeconomics 1992;1:84–94.
27. Mackeigan LD, Pathak DS. Overview of health-related quality-of-life measures. Am J Hosp Pharm 1992;49:2236–2245.
28. McGhan WF, Rowland CR, Bootman JL. Cost-benefit and cost-effectiveness: Methodologies for evaluating innovative pharmaceutical services. Am J Hosp Pharm 1978;35:133–140.

29. MacKeigan LD, Bootman JL. A review of cost-benefit and cost-effectiveness analyses of clinical pharmacy services. J Pharm Marketing and Manage 1988;2:63–84.
30. Schumock GT, Meek PD, Ploetz PA, Vermeulen LC. Economic evaluations of clinical pharmacy services—1988–1995. Pharmacotherapy 1996;16:1188–1208.
31. Sanchez LA. Pharmacoeconomic principles and methods: Including pharmacoeconomics into hospital pharmacy practice. Hosp Pharm 1994;29:1035–1040.
32. Doubilet P, et al. The use and misuse of the term "cost effective" in medicine. N Engl J Med 1986;314:253–256.
33. Bradley CA, Iskedjian M, Lanctot KL, et al. Quality assessment of economic evaluation in selected pharmacy, medical, and health economic journals. Ann Pharmacother 1995;29:681–689.
34. Udvarhelyi S, Colditz GA, Rai A, et al. Cost effectiveness and cost benefit analyses in the medical literature. Ann Intern Med 1992; 116:238–244.
35. Mason J. The generalisability of pharmacoeconomic studies. Pharmacoeconomics 1997;11:503–514.
36. Sacristan JA, Soto J, Galende I. Evaluation of pharmacoeconomic studies: Utilization of a checklist. Ann Pharmacother 1993;27: 1126–1133.
37. Hillman AL, Eisenberg JM, Pauly MV, et al. Avoiding bias in the conduct and reporting of cost-effectiveness research sponsored by pharmaceutical companies. N Engl J Med 1991;324:1362–1365.
38. McGhan WF, Lewis JV. Guidelines for pharmacoeconomic studies. Clin Ther 1992;14:486–494.
39. Sanchez LA. Pharmacoeconomic principles and methods: Evaluating the quality of published pharmacoeconomic evaluations. Hosp Pharm 1995;30:146–152.
40. Clemans K, Townsend R, Luscombe F, et al. Methodological and conduct principles for pharmacoeconomic research. Pharmacoeconomics 1995;8:169–174.
41. Task Force on Principles for Economic Analysis of Health Care Technology. Economic analysis of health care technology: A report on principles. Ann Intern Med 1995;122:61–70.
42. Russell LB, Gold MR, Siegel JE, et al. The role of cost-effectiveness analysis in health and medicine. JAMA 1996;276:1172–1177.
43. Weinstein MC, Siegel JE, Gold MR, et al. Recommendations of the Panel on Cost-Effectiveness in Health and Medicine. JAMA 1996; 276:1253–1258.
44. Siegel JE, Weinstein MC, Russell LB, et al. Recommendations for reporting cost-effectiveness analyses. JAMA 1996;276:1339–1341.
45. Eisenberg JM, Glick H, Koffer H. Pharmacoeconomics: Economic evaluation of pharmaceuticals. In: Strom BL, ed. Pharmacoepidemiology. New York, Churchill Livingstone, 1989:325–350.
46. Milne RJ. Evaluation of the pharmacoeconomic literature. Pharmacoeconomics 1994;6:337–345.
47. Sackett DL, Haynes RB, Tugwell P. Clinical Epidemiology: A Basic Science for Clinical Medicine. Boston, Little, Brown, 1985:126.
48. Barr JT, Schumacher GE. Applying decision analysis to pharmacy management and practice decisions. Top Hosp Pharm Manage 1994;13:60–71.
49. Schecter CB. Decision analysis in formulary decision making. Pharmacoeconomics 1993;3:454–461.
50. Crane VS. Economic aspects of clinical decision making: Applications of clinical decision analysis. Am J Hosp Pharm 1988;45:548–553.
51. Mutnick AH, Szymusiak-Mutnick B, Schumacher GE, Barr JT. Using decision analysis in the evaluation of drug therapy. Pharm Times 1990;59–66.
52. Jolicoeur LM, Jones-Grizzle AJ, Boyer JG. Guidelines for performing a pharmacoeconomic analysis. Am J Hosp Pharm 1992;49: 1741–1747.
53. Sanchez LA. Pharmacoeconomic principles and methods: Conducting pharmacoeconomic evaluations in a hospital setting. Hosp Pharm 1995;30:412–428.

2

Health Outcomes and Quality of Life

Stephen Joel Coons, PhD

Over the past decade, the medical care marketplace in the United States has undergone unprecedented change.[1] This change is evidenced by a variety of developments, including an increase in investor-owned organizations, numerous mergers and acquisitions, increasingly sophisticated clinical and administrative information systems, and new financing and organizational structures. In this dynamic and increasingly competitive environment, there is a concern that health care quality is being compromised in the rush to lower costs. As a consequence, there has been a growing movement to focus the evaluation of health care on the assessment of the end results, or *outcomes,* associated with medical care delivery systems as well as specific medical interventions. The primary objective of this effort is to maximize the net health benefit derived from the use of finite health care resources.[2] However, there is a serious lack of critical information as to what value is received for the tremendous amount of resources expended on medical care.[3] This lack of critical information as to the outcomes produced is an obstacle to optimal health care decision making at all levels.

HEALTH OUTCOMES

Although the implicit objective of medical care is to improve health outcomes, up until recently little attention was paid to the explicit measurement of them. An outcome is one of the three components of the conceptual framework articulated by Donabedian for assessing and assuring the quality of health care: *structure, process,* and *outcome.*[4] Traditionally, the approach to evaluating health care has emphasized the structure and processes involved in medical care delivery rather than the outcomes. However, health care regulators, payers, providers, manufacturers, and patients are placing increasing emphasis on the outcomes that medical care products and services produce.[5] As stated by Ellwood, outcomes research is "designed to help patients, payers, and providers make rational medical care–related choices based on better insight into the effect of these choices on the patient's life."[6]

TYPES OF OUTCOMES

The types of outcomes that result from medical care interventions can be described in a number of ways. One classic list, called "the five Ds," although quite negatively worded, captures a wide range of outcomes used in assessing the quality of medical care.[7] The five D's are death, disease, disability, discomfort, and dissatisfaction.

A more comprehensive conceptual framework, the ECHO model, places outcomes into three categories: economic, clinical, and humanistic outcomes.[8] The model covers the five D's within the clinical and humanistic outcomes, and provides an added economic outcomes dimension. As described by Kozma and associates, clinical outcomes are the medical events that occur as a result of the condition or its treatment. Economic outcomes are the direct, indirect, and intangible costs compared with the consequences of a medical intervention. Along with patient satisfaction, an essential humanistic outcome is patient function and well-being, or health-related quality of life. This chapter focuses on health-related quality of life as an outcome of pharmacotherapeutic interventions.

QUALITY OF LIFE

DEFINITION

As mentioned, one of the essential elements of outcomes research is the assessment of patient *health-related quality of life.* However, there is no consensus on the definition of quality of life or its overall conceptual framework.[9] In the literature, the term *quality of life* has been used in a variety of ways. It has been proposed that studies of health outcomes use the term *health-related quality of life* to distinguish health effects from the effects of job satisfaction, environment, and other factors on overall quality of life.[10] Only health outcomes are discussed in this chapter, so "quality of life" and "health-related quality of life" are used interchangeably, along with "health status."

Quality of life, like other aspects of the human experience, is hard to define. In much of the empiric literature, explicit definitions of quality of life are rare; readers must deduce the implicit definition of quality of life from the manner in which it is measured. However, some authors have provided definitions. For example, Schron and Shumaker define quality of life as "a multidimensional concept referring to a person's total well-being including his or her psychological, social, and physical health status."[11] Patrick and Erickson propose that quality of life is "the value assigned to duration of life as modified by the impairments, functional states, perceptions, and social opportunities that are influenced by disease, injury, treatment, or policy."[12] Although the two definitions differ in certain respects, a conceptual characteristic they share is the multidimensionality of quality of life. Although the terminology may vary with the author, commonly measured dimensions of health-related quality of life include the following:

- Physical health and functioning
- Psychological health and functioning
- Social and role functioning
- Perceptions of general well-being
- Disease or treatment-related symptomatology

RELEVANCE OF QUALITY OF LIFE AS AN OUTCOME

For medical care providers, quality of life is increasingly viewed as a therapeutic end point. An overriding factor leading to this has been the gradual shift in the focus of primary medical care from limiting mortality to limiting morbidity and the patient-reported impact of that morbidity. The pattern of illness in the United States has shifted from mostly acute disease to one in which chronic conditions predominate. In the early part of this century, many individuals died from infectious diseases for which cures (e.g., antibiotics) or effective preventive measures (e.g., increased sanitation, vaccines) were unavailable or underused. Although there are many diseases that may shorten life expectancy, it is more likely that a disease will have adverse health consequences leading to dysfunction and decreased well-being. For those conditions that shorten life expectancy and for which there are no cures, managing symptoms and maintaining function and well-being should be the primary objectives of medical care.

Because therapeutic interventions such as medications have the potential to increase or decrease quality of life, medical care providers must strive to achieve enhanced quality of life as an outcome of therapy. Although it must be assumed that quality of life has always played an implicit role in the provision of health care, it has not always been viewed as equal in importance to the more clinical or physiologic outcome parameters (e.g., blood pressure). The subjective nature of quality of life assessment has made many people uneasy with it as a measure of the patient outcomes produced by medical treatment.[13] However, there is growing awareness that in certain diseases, quality of life may be the most important health outcome to consider in assessing treatment.[14] Physiologic measures may change without improving functioning and well-being. Likewise, patients may feel better without measurable change in physiologic values.

QUALITY OF LIFE AND PHARMACOTHERAPY

As described by Smith, there are four possible quality of life outcomes associated with pharmacotherapy: (1) quality of life is improved; (2) quality of life is actively maintained; (3) quality of life decreases; or (4) quality of life remains unaffected.[15] To effectively assess these possible outcomes, moving beyond consideration of only the biologic or physical manifestations of a disease or its treatment is essential. The use of standardized measurement tools (e.g., self-reported quality of life instruments) to collect information regarding the impact of pharmacotherapy on the quality of patients' lives is increasing.[16,17] However, the vast majority of quality of life claims in prescription drug advertisements continue to be based on physiological parameters and/or clinician-assessed physical function rather than patient-reported functioning and well-being.[18]

A study by Croog and colleagues[19] was one of the first in a growing body of literature reporting the quality of life impact of pharmacotherapy, specifically the use of antihypertensive agents. Along with hypertension, examples of other therapeutic areas that are receiving increasing attention are arthritis, asthma, cancer, diabetes, end-stage renal disease, and migraine headache.[20–26]

Information about the impact of pharmacotherapy on quality of life can provide additional data for making medication-use policy decisions.[27] Pharmacy and therapeutics committees should incorporate quality of life data into the formulary and practice guideline decision-making process. Quality of life as an input to clinical decision making at the patient level is also very important. For example, alternative treatments may have equal efficacy based on traditional clinical parameters (e.g., blood pressure reduction) but produce very different effects on the patient's quality of life. Thus, a provider's selection among competing alternatives may hinge on documented differential impact on quality of life. A perceived decrease in quality of life attributed by the patient to an adverse effect of the drug may lead to a decrease in adherence to the medication regimen.[15]

MEASURING QUALITY OF LIFE

TYPES OF INSTRUMENTS

Hundreds of health-related quality of life instruments are available.[28–30] Table 2–1 gives a taxonomy of the different types of instruments.[31] A primary distinction among quality of life instruments is whether they are generic or specific.

GENERIC INSTRUMENTS

Generic, or general, quality of life instruments are designed to be applicable across all diseases or conditions, across different medical interventions, and across a wide variety of

TABLE 2–1. Taxonomy of Quality of Life Instruments

Generic Instruments
Health profiles
Utility–based measures
Specific Instruments
Disease specific (e.g., diabetes)
Population specific (e.g., frail elderly)
Function specific (e.g., sexual functioning)
Condition or problem specific (e.g., pain)

From Ref. 32.

populations.[32] Table 2–2 lists the dimensions or domains of five generic instruments. In choosing or evaluating the use of an instrument, the specific dimensions of functioning and well-being covered must be considered. The instruments in Table 2–2 share common dimensions, but they also reflect the diversity and range of dimensions covered. The two main types of generic instruments are health profiles and utility- or preference-based measures.

Health Profiles

Health profiles provide an array of scores representing individual dimensions or domains of quality of life or health status. An advantage of a health profile is that it provides multiple outcome scores that may be useful to clinicians and/or researchers attempting to measure differential effects of a condition or its treatment on various quality of life domains.

A commonly used profile instrument is the Medical Outcomes Study 36-Item Short-Form Health Survey (SF-36).[38] The instrument includes nine health concepts or scales (Table 2–3). The SF-36 can be self-administered or administered by a trained interviewer (face to face or via telephone). This instrument has several advantages. For example, it is brief (it takes about 5 to 10 minutes to complete) and its reliability and validity have been documented in many clinical situations and disease states.[39,40] A means of aggregating the items into physical (PCS) and mental (MCS) component summary scales is now available.[41] In addition, an abbreviated version of the SF-36, containing only 12 items (SF-12), has been introduced.[42] However, the scale scores and the mental and physical component summary scores derived from the SF-12 are based on fewer items and fewer defined levels of health and, as a result, are estimated with less precision and less reliable. The loss of precision and reliability in measurement can be a problem in small samples and/or with small expected effect sizes for an intervention.

TABLE 2–2. Domains Included in Selected Generic Instruments

EuroQol Group's EQ-5D[33]	
Mobility	Self-care
Usual activity	Pain/discomfort
Anxiety/depression	
Nottingham Health Profile (NHP)[34]	
Part I: Distress within the following domains	
Emotions	Energy
Sleep	Pain
Social isolation	Mobility
Part II: Health-related problems within the following domains	
Occupation	Sex life
Housework	Hobbies
Social life	Holidays
Home life	
Quality of Well-being Scale (QWB)[35]	
Symptoms/problems	Physical activity
Mobility	Social activity
Sickness Impact Profile (SIP)[36]	
Sleep and rest	Home management
Eating	Recreation and pastimes
Work	Body care and movement
Ambulation	Alertness behavior
Mobility	Emotional behavior
Communication	Social interaction
Health Utilities Index (HUI)—Mark III[37]	
Vision	Dexterity
Hearing	Cognition
Speech	Pain and discomfort
Ambulation	Emotion

TABLE 2–3. SF-36 Scales and Number of Items per Scale (SF-36/SF-12)

Physical functioning (10/2)
Role limitations attributed to physical problems (4/2)
Bodily pain (2/1)
General health (5/1)
Vitality (4/1)
Social functioning (2/1)
Role limitations attributed to emotional problems (3/2)
Mental health (5/2)
Health transition (1/0)

Compiled from Refs. 38 and 39.

Utility-based Measures

Quality of life as measured by utility-based (or preference-based) instruments is on a continuum from death (0.0) to perfect health (1.0). This approach incorporates the measurement of an individual's health status with an adjustment for the preference value, or utility, associated with that health state. The values or utilities are empirically measured or assigned through a variety of procedures.

Utility-based measures are useful in pharmacoeconomic research, specifically cost-utility analysis (CUA).[43] CUA, an economic technique discussed in Chapter 1, involves comparing the costs of an intervention (e.g., a medication) with its outcomes expressed in units such as quality-adjusted life years (QALYs) gained. QALYs gained is an outcome measure that incorporates both quantity and quality of life. This can be a key outcome measure, especially in diseases such as cancer, where the treatment itself can have a major impact on patient functioning and well-being.

QALYs can be produced by increases in quality of life and/or length of life. Figure 2–1 represents a case in which QALYs were gained through an increase in quality of life alone. The top curve represents the hypothetical life course of a cohort of individuals receiving a specific health care intervention compared with the life course of a cohort (i.e., lower curve) that did not receive the intervention. Average age at death did not differ between the two cohorts, but the intervention led to improvements in quality of life in the treatment cohort. The area between the curves represents the QALYs gained through the intervention. This hypothetical case reflects a chronic disease, such as osteoarthritis, in which functioning and well-being are increased but survival remains unchanged. Other hypothetical combinations of

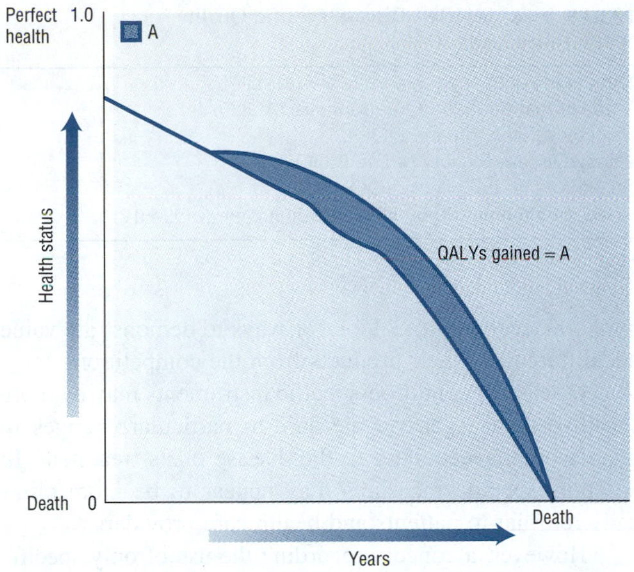

FIGURE 2–1. QALYs gained secondary to a hypothetical health care intervention, such as a drug.

quality and quantity of life can be graphed in this manner. For example, an alternative scenario could reflect a decrease in quality of life but an increase in survival that may result from a chemotherapeutic regimen for cancer.

Direct Measures of Health State Values/Utilities. The most commonly used direct measurement techniques include visual analog scales, standard gamble, and time trade-off.[44]

VISUAL ANALOG SCALES. The visual analog scale is a line, typically 100 cm in length, with the end points well defined (e.g., 0 = worst imaginable health state and 100 = best imaginable health state). The respondent is asked to mark the line where he or she would place one or more health states in relation to the two end points. If a subject rated his or her own health state, or a health state described in a hypothetical scenario, at the midpoint between 0 and 100 on the scale, the value for that health state would be 0.5.

STANDARD GAMBLE. The standard gamble offers a choice between two alternatives: choice A—living in health state *i* with certainty, or choice B—taking a gamble on a new treatment for which the outcome is uncertain. Figure 2–2 shows this gamble.[45] The subject is told that a hypothetical treatment will lead to perfect health, for a defined remaining lifetime, with a probability of p, or immediate death with a probability of $1 - p$. The subject can choose between remaining, for the same defined lifetime, in state *i*, which is intermediate between healthy and dead, or taking the gamble and trying the new treatment. The probability p is varied until the subject is indifferent between choices A and B. For example, if a subject is indifferent between the choices A and B when $p = 0.75$, the utility of state *i* is 0.75.

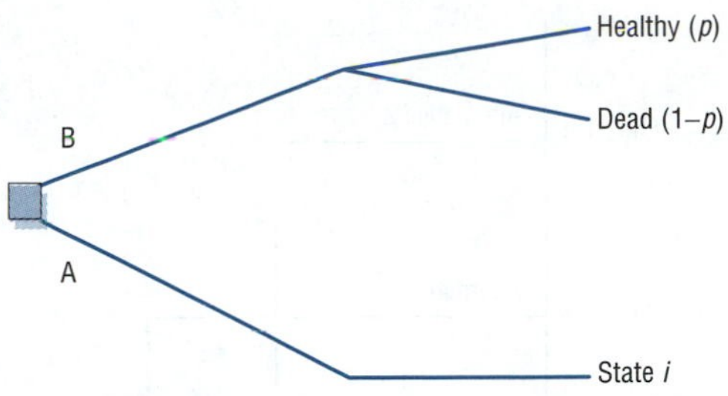

FIGURE 2–2. Standard gamble for a chronic health state. The subject is offered the choice between *A* and *B*. *A* involves the certainty of living in health state *i* (a suboptimal health state) for a specified period of time. *B* involves an intervention that could lead to full health for the same period of time or immediate death. The probabilities associated with the outcomes of healthy and dead are p and $1 - p$, respectively. As p is varied, the indifference point between choices *A* and *B* represents the utility of state *i*.

TIME TRADE-OFF. Figure 2–3 represents the time trade-off technique for a chronic disease state.[46] Here, the subject is offered a choice of living for a variable amount of time (x) in perfect health or a defined amount of time (t) in a health state (i) that is less desirable. By reducing the time x of being healthy (at 1.0) and leaving the time t in the suboptimal health state fixed, an indifference point can be determined ($h_i = x/t$). For example, a subject may indicate that undergoing chronic hemodialysis for 2 years is equivalent to perfect health for 1 year. Therefore, the value of that health state would be 0.5 ($h_i = 1/2$).

Multiattribute Utility Systems. In addition to direct measures, instruments are available for which the health state utilities/values have been empirically derived through population studies. The instruments are administered to measure respondents' health status, which is then mapped onto a multiattribute health status classification system. Examples of such instruments include the Quality of Well-being Scale (QWB),[35] the Health Utilities Index (HUI),[37] and the EuroQol Group's EQ-5D.[33]

The QWB is a generic quality of life instrument that includes symptoms or problems plus three dimensions of functional health status (Table 2–2). Standardized preference values for the health states represented by the QWB have been measured (via the category rating scale method, a technique related to visual analog scales) and validated on a general population sample.[35] Other investigators have reweighted the symptoms/problems and function levels of the QWB in specific populations such as arthritis patients[47] and human immunodeficiency virus (HIV)-infected subjects[48] and have found the generalizability of the original values to be very high. The QWB was originally available only as an interviewer-administered version, but a self-administered version is now available.[49]

The HUI is another generic instrument that describes the health status of a person at a point in time in terms of his or her ability to function on a set of attributes or dimensions of health status. The HUI Mark III is a 15-item self-administered form. The measurements for the development

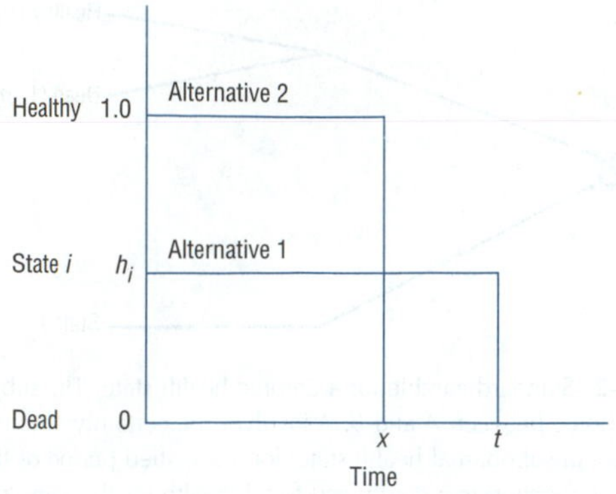

FIGURE 2–3. Time trade-off for a chronic health state. The subject chooses between living a varying amount of time in full health (x) and living a specified amount of time (t) in state i. The length of time in full health is shortened until the subject is indifferent between the two choices. The value of health state i (h_i) is then calculated by dividing x/t.

of the health state value system were made with visual analog scales and the standard gamble technique. The dimensions covered in the most recent version of the HUI (Mark III) are listed in Table 2–2.[37]

The EQ-5D was developed concurrently in five languages (Dutch, English, Finnish, Norwegian, and Swedish) by a multidisciplinary team of European researchers.[33] It was designed to be self-administered and short enough to be used in conjunction with other measures. The first of two parts classifies subjects into one of 243 health states within five dimensions. The health state values were derived using the time trade-off technique in a random sample of adults in the United Kingdom. The second part of the EQ-5D is a 20-cm visual analog scale (VAS) that has end points labeled "best imaginable health state" and "worst imaginable health state" anchored at 100 and 0, respectively. Respondents are asked to indicate how they rate their own health state by drawing a line from an anchor box to that point on the VAS that best represents their own health on that day.

SPECIFIC INSTRUMENTS

Specific instruments are intended to provide greater detail concerning particular outcomes, in terms of functioning and well-being, uniquely associated with a condition and/or its treatment. Several selected examples of disease-specific instruments are listed in Table 2–4. One of the instruments listed is the Asthma Quality of Life Questionnaire (AQLQ), a 32-item instrument developed to assess the impact of asthma on patients' everyday functioning and well-being.[51] Results from research in which the AQLQ was used have appeared in promotional materials for Glaxo Wellcome's salmeterol inhaler. As opposed to prior prescription drug advertisements that involved predominantly physiologic-based quality of life claims,[18] this is one of the first times a pharmaceutical firm has promoted a product based on data from trials involving quality of life as a primary outcome measure. (The study is referenced as "data on file" in a Serevent promotional brochure.) This is likely to occur with increasing frequency as pharmaceutical firms look for ways to demonstrate value and differentiate their products from the competition.

TABLE 2–4. Selected Disease-specific Quality of Life Instruments

Arthritis Impact Measurement Scale (AIMS)[50]
Asthma Quality of Life Questionnaire (AQLQ)[51]
Diabetes Quality of Life (DQOL)[52]
Kidney Disease Quality of Life (KDQOL)[53]
Quality of Life in Epilepsy (QOLIE)[54]
Medical Outcomes Study HIV Health Survey (MOS-HIV)[55]

Disease or condition-specific instruments may be more sensitive than a generic measure to particular changes in quality of life secondary to the disease or its treatment. In addition, specific measures may appear to be more clinically relevant to patients and health care providers.[31]

However, a concern regarding the use of only specific instruments is that, by focusing on the specific impact, the general or overall impact on functioning and well-being may be overlooked. In studies involving pharmacotherapy, the use of both a generic and a specific instrument may be the best approach. The generic instrument provides a more general outcome assessment and allows comparability across other disease states or conditions in which it has been used. An appropriately selected specific instrument should provide more detailed outcome information regarding expected changes in the particular patient population.

MEASUREMENT ISSUES

A number of issues must be considered when evaluating existing quality of life research and/or choosing the appropriate instrument to use when designing a study involving quality of life assessment. A thorough review of these issues is not within the scope of this chapter; more in-depth reviews of methodologic considerations are available in the literature.[12,56–58]

Of particular concern are the psychometric properties of a chosen instrument. Psychometrics refers to the measurement of psychological constructs, such as quality of life. Instruments should be developed and tested such that one can place confidence in the measurement made. Psychometric properties of measures (e.g., reliability and validity) are considered in the review criteria developed by the Scientific Advisory Committee of the Medical Outcomes Trust (MOT).[59] The MOT is a depository and distributor of standardized, health outcomes measurement instruments. Every instrument that is proposed for addition to the MOT list of approved instruments is reviewed against a rigorous set of eight attributes. These attributes provide a useful evaluative framework. The eight attributes of an instrument addressed by the review criteria are as follows: (1) conceptual and measurement model, (2) reliability, (3) validity, (4) responsiveness, (5) interpretability, (6) respondent and administrative burden, (7) alternative forms, and (8) cultural and language adaptations.

CONCEPTUAL AND MEASUREMENT MODELS

A conceptual model is the rationale for and description of the concepts that a measurement instrument is intended to assess and the interrelationships of those concepts. A measurement model is an instrument's scale and subscale structure, and the procedures followed to create scale and subscale scores. An example is the well-defined conceptual and measurement models for the scales and scale structure of the SF-36.[38] The SF-36 contains 36 items that cover nine theory-based health concepts. Eight of these health concepts are measured by multi-item scales. There is a clearly defined means of creating the individual scale scores and the physical and mental component summary scales.[41]

RELIABILITY

Reliability refers to the extent to which measures give consistent or accurate results.[60] The purpose of evaluating the reliability of a quality of life instrument is to estimate how much of the variation in a score is real as opposed to random. The two reliability assessment methods most often discussed in the quality of life literature are internal consistency and test–retest reliability. *Internal consistency* is an assessment of the performance of items within a scale. It is a function of the number of items and their covariation.[61] Internal consistency is commonly measured using Cronbach's alpha coefficient. Alpha coefficients above 0.90 are recommended for making comparisons between individuals and above 0.70 for comparisons between groups.[62]

Test–retest reliability refers to the relationship between scores obtained from the same instrument on two or more separate occasions when all pertinent conditions remain relatively unchanged.[61] It is usually evaluated using a Pearson product-moment correlation coefficient. However, quality of life is not assumed to be constant over the course of time. In fact, most clinical studies attempt to assess how quality of life changes. Test–retest reliability estimates may have limited value in evaluating measures that are designed to assess a dynamic process.

Interrater reliability and *equivalent-forms reliability* are two other approaches to reliability assessment that are not as commonly used in quality of life research. More in-depth discussions of these and the other reliability assessment methods are found elsewhere.[61,63]

VALIDITY

Reliability is necessary, but not sufficient for valid measurement.[61] Validity is an estimation of the extent to which the instrument is measuring what it is supposed to be measuring. Validity is not an absolute. Hence, a measurement instrument is not "valid," but empirical data can provide evidence to support its validity. Three types of validity commonly considered are criterion, content, and construct.

Criterion validity is demonstrated when a new measure corresponds to an established measure or observation that accurately reflects the phenomenon of interest. By definition, the criterion must be a superior measure of the phenomenon if it is to serve as a comparative norm. However, in quality of life assessment, gold standards or criterion measures rarely exist against which a new measure can be compared.

Content validity, which is infrequently tested statistically, refers to how adequately the questions/items capture the relevant aspects of the domain or concept being measured.

Construct validity refers to the relationship between measures purporting to measure the same underlying theoretical construct (convergent evidence) or purporting to measure different constructs (discriminant evidence). For example, convergent evidence for the validity of a new measure of emotional well-being could be established by showing a strong association between the new scale and the mental health scale from the SF-36. Ware and colleagues[60] have provided a substantial amount of data supporting the validity of the SF-36. Evidence for the construct validity of other aspects of the measure might be established through comparisons with physiologic measures, organ pathology, or clinical signs.

RESPONSIVENESS

Responsiveness, or sensitivity to change, is the ability or power of the measure to detect clinically important change when it occurs.[64] Although some authors have suggested that responsiveness is a psychometric property of a measure distinct from validity,[65] others argue that responsiveness is an aspect of validity rather than a separate property.[61,66]

INTERPRETABILITY

Interpretability is the degree to which one can assign qualitative meaning to an instrument's quantitative scores. Interpretability is facilitated by comparison of a score or change in scores to a qualitative category that has clinical or commonly understood meaning. For example, it would be helpful to know how scale scores obtained in a specific patient sample compare to the scale scores of the general population. Again, Ware and colleagues have provided a substantial amount of normative data for the SF-36.[60]

RESPONDENT AND ADMINISTRATIVE BURDEN

Respondent burden refers to the time, energy, and other demands placed on those to whom the instrument is administered. Administrative burden refers to the demands placed on those who administer the instrument. A practical aspect of the measurement of quality of life is length of the instrument or the administration time involved. Instruments should be as brief as possible without severely compromising the validity and reliability of the measurement. The longer an instrument, the greater the respondent burden. This can lead to an individual's unwillingness or refusal to complete the instrument or to incomplete responses.

ALTERNATIVE FORMS

Alternative forms of an instrument includes all modes of administration other than the original source instrument.

Evidence should be provided that supports the comparability of the alternative mode of administration with that of the original instrument.[67] Many quality of life measures can be administered in different ways. The primary modes of administration are (1) interviewer administered, either in person or over the telephone, or (2) self-administered.[31] Also used, but not recommended, are surrogate responders (i.e., using a health care provider, family member, or friend to respond for the subject when the subject is unable to complete the instrument. Because quality of life is such a subjective concept, patients must have the opportunity to provide their perspective on the impact of medical care on their functioning and well-being. The patient's perspective has been shown to be quite different from that of outside observers, including physicians and other health care professionals providing direct care to the patient.[68]

CULTURAL AND LANGUAGE ADAPTATIONS

Methods used to achieve conceptual and linguistic equivalence of cross-culturally adapted instruments should be explicitly stated.[69] Evidence should be provided that the measurement properties of the adaptation are comparable to the original instrument. It is obvious that this is an extremely important issue when planning cross-national quality of life assessment projects. However, it is also very important within countries that are multicultural, such as the United States. Many of the English-language instruments have been developed for the dominant U.S. culture and may not be appropriate for all patients.

OTHER MEASUREMENT ISSUES

Selection of an Appropriate Instrument

It is essential that the purpose of the measurement be well-defined before the selection of a quality of life instrument. Is the purpose of the measurement to describe the health status or quality of life of a patient population at a particular time or over time? Is it to document change in health outcomes associated with a particular intervention? These and other questions should be answered before quality of life instruments are selected. Too many practitioner-researchers attempting to demonstrate improvements in outcomes resulting from a pharmaceutical product or service select a commonly used generic instrument, such as the SF-36, with the expectation that it will be sufficiently responsive to changes that may occur. The best approach may be to use the SF-36 or other generic instrument in conjunction with a more targeted, disease-specific instrument.

Availability of Instruments

Many quality of life instruments are in the public domain. However, although they can be used for no or little cost, there may be a fee associated with the purchase of a user's guide or scoring manual. The Medical Outcomes Trust is a source of a wide array of instruments, including the SF-36, SF-12, QWB, MOS-HIV, AQLQ, and SIP. For further information, the MOT home page is http://www.outcomes-trust.org. Developers of particular instruments can often be contacted through addresses provided in other books referenced at the end of this chapter.[30,58]

CONCLUSIONS

The concept of quality of life has gained increasing attention in the evaluation of the outcomes associated with medical care, including pharmacotherapy. In fact, in certain diseases, quality of life may be the most important outcome to consider in assessing the effectiveness of health care interventions. Health care practitioners and policymakers must remember that efforts to increase quantity of life must not outstrip the ability to maintain or improve quality of life.

Health-related quality of life assessment is a relatively new field of endeavor and a number of theoretical and methodologic issues remain unresolved. However, some general concepts in the measurement of quality of life outcomes should be carefully considered when designing a study, evaluating existing research, or evaluating new programs or services. This chapter has provided only a brief overview of the concepts in an effort to sensitize students and health care practitioners to the importance of the area as well as to provide insight as to how these concepts can and should be incorporated into their practices.

REFERENCES

1. Corrigan JM, Ginsburg PB. Association leaders speak out on health system change. Health Affairs 1997;16:150–157.
2. Gold MR, Siegel JE, Russell LB, Weinstein MC, eds. Cost-Effectiveness in Health and Medicine. New York, Oxford University Press, 1996.
3. Sloan FA, ed. Valuing Health Care: Costs, Benefits, and Effectiveness of Pharmaceuticals and Other Medical Technologies. New York, Cambridge University Press, 1996.
4. Donabedian A. Explorations in Quality Assessment and Monitoring, vol I: The Definition of Quality and Approaches to Its Assessment. Ann Arbor, Health Administration Press, 1980.
5. Zitter M. Outcomes assessment: True customer focus comes to health care. Med Interface 1992;5:32–37.
6. Ellwood PM. Outcomes management: A technology of patient experience. N Engl J Med 1988;318:1551.
7. Lohr KN. Outcome measurement: Concepts and questions. Inquiry 1988;25:37–50.
8. Kozma CM, Reeder CE, Schulz RM. Economic, clinical, and humanistic outcomes: A planning model for pharmacoeconomic research. Clin Ther 1993;15:1121–1132.
9. Stewart AL. Conceptual and methodologic issues in defining quality of life: State of the art. Prog Cardiovasc Nurs 1992;7:3–11.
10. Kaplan RM, Bush JW. Health-related quality of life measurement for evaluation research and policy analysis. Health Psychol 1982;1:61–80.
11. Schron EB, Shumaker SA. The integration of health quality of life in clinical research: Experience from cardiovascular clinical trials. Prog Cardiovasc Nurs 1992;7(2):21.

12. Patrick DL, Erickson P. Health Status and Health Policy: Allocating Resources to Health Care. New York, Oxford University Press, 1993:22.
13. Schipper H, Clinch JJ, Olweny CLM. Quality of life studies: Definitions and conceptual issues. In: Spilker B, ed. Quality of Life and Pharmacoeconomics in Clinical Trials, 2nd ed. Philadelphia, Lippincott-Raven, 1996:11–23.
14. Staquet M, Aaronson NK, Ahmedzai S, et al. Health-related quality of life research. Qual Life Res 1992;1:3. Editorial.
15. Smith M. Medication, quality of life and compliance: The role of the pharmacist. PharmacoEconomics 1992;1:225–230.
16. Bungay KM, Boyer JG, Steinwald AB, Ware JE Jr. Health-related quality of life: An overview. In: Bootman JL, Townsend RJ, McGhan WF, eds. Principles of Pharmacoeconomics, 2nd ed. Cincinnati, Harvey Whitney Books, 1996:126–148.
17. Revicki DA, Rothman M, Luce B. Health-related quality of life assessment and the pharmaceutical industry. Pharmacoeconomics 1992; 1:394–408.
18. Rothermich EA, Pathak DS, Smeenk DA. Health-related quality of life claims in prescription drug advertisements. Am J Health Syst Pharm 1996;53:1565–1569.
19. Croog SH, Levine S, Testa MA, et al. The effects of antihypertensive therapy on quality of life. N Engl J Med 1986;319:1220–1221.
20. Gandhi SK, Kong SX. Quality of life measures in the evaluation of antihypertensive drug therapy: Reliability, validity, and quality of life domains. Clin Ther 1996;18:1276-1295.
21. Juniper EF. Quality of life considerations in the treatment of asthma. Pharmacoeconomics 1995;8:123–138.
22. Goodyear MDE, Fraumeni MA. Incorporating quality of life assessment into cancer clinical trials. In: Spilker B, ed. Quality of Life and Pharmacoeconomics in Clinical Trials, 2nd ed. Philadelphia, Lippincott-Raven, 1996:1003–1013.
23. Boyer JG, Earp JL. The development of an instrument for assessing the quality of life of people with diabetes. Med Care 1997;35: 440–453.
24. Gabriel SE, Matteson EL. Economic and quality of life impact of NSAIDs in rheumatoid arthritis: A conceptual framework and selected literature review. Pharmacoeconomics 1995;8:479–490.
25. Edgell ET, Coons SJ, Carter WB, et al. A review of health related quality of life measures used in end-stage renal disease. Clin Ther 1996;18:887–938.
26. Solomon GD, Litaker DG. The impact of drug therapy on quality of life in headache and migraine. Pharmacoeconomics 1997;11:334–342.
27. Bukstein DA. Incorporating quality of life data into managed care formulary decisions: A case study with salmeterol. Am J Man Care 1997;3:1701–1706.
28. Bowling A. Measuring Health: A Review of Quality of Life Measurement Scales, 2nd ed. Buckingham, Open University Press, 1997.
29. Bowling A. Measuring Disease: A Review of Disease–Specific Quality of Life Measurement Scales, 2nd ed. Buckingham, Open University Press, 1995.
30. McDowell I, Newell C. Measuring Health: A Guide to Rating Scales and Questionnaires, 2nd ed. New York, Oxford University Press, 1996.
31. Guyatt GH, Feeny DH, Patrick DL. Measuring health–related quality of life. Ann Intern Med 1993;118:622–629.
32. Patrick DL, Deyo RA. Generic and disease–specific measures in assessing health status and quality of life. Med Care 1989;27: S217–S232.
33. Kind P. The EuroQol instrument: An index of health–related quality of life. In: Spilker B, ed. Quality of Life and Pharmacoeconomics in Clinical Trials, 2nd ed. Philadelphia, Lippincott-Raven, 1996:191–201.
34. Hunt SM, McKewan J, McKenna SP. Measuring health status: A new tool for clinicians and epidemiologists. J R Coll Gen Prac 1985; 35:185–188.
35. Kaplan RM, Anderson JP. The general health policy model: An integrated approach. In: Spilker B, ed. Quality of Life and Pharmacoeconomics in Clinical Trials, 2nd ed. Philadelphia, Lippincott-Raven, 1996:309–322.
36. Bergner M, Bobbitt RA, Carter WB, Gilson BS. The sickness impact profile: Development and final revisions of a health status measure. Med Care 1976;14:57–67.
37. Feeny D, Furlong W, Boyle M, Torrance GW. Muliti–attribute health status classification systems: Health utilities index. Pharmacoeconomics 1995;7:490–502.
38. Ware JE Jr, Sherbourne CD. The MOS 36-item short-form health survey (SF-36): I. Conceptual framework and item selection. Med Care 1992;30:473–483.
39. McHorney CA, Ware JE Jr, Raczek AE. The MOS 36-item short-form health survey (SF-36): II. Psychometric and clinical tests of validity in measuring physical and mental health constructs. Med Care 1993; 31:247–263.
40. McHorney CA, Ware JE Jr, Raczek AE. The MOS 36-item short-form health survey (SF-36): III. Tests of data quality, scaling assumptions, and reliability across diverse patient groups. Med Care 1994; 32:40–66.
41. Ware JE Jr, Kosinski M, Keller SD. SF-36 Physical and Mental Health Summary Scales: A User's Manual. Boston, The Health Institute, 1994.
42. Ware JE Jr, Kosinski M, Keller SD. A 12-item short-form health survey: Construction of scales and preliminary test of reliability and validity. Med Care 1996;34:220.
43. Coons SJ, Kaplan RM. Cost–utility analysis. In: Bootman JL, Townsend RJ, McGhan WF, eds. Principles of Pharmacoeconomics, 2nd ed. Cincinnati, Harvey Whitney Books, 1996:102–126.
44. Feeny DH, Torrance GW, Labelle R. Integrating economic evaluations and quality of life assessments. In: Spilker B, ed. Quality of Life and Pharmacoeconomics in Clinical Trials, 2nd ed. Philadelphia, Lippincott-Raven, 1996:85–95.
45. Drummond MF, O'Brien B, Stoddart GL, Torrance GW. Methods for the Economic Evaluation of Health Care Programmes, 2nd ed. Oxford, Oxford University Press, 1997.
46. Torrance GW, Thomas WH, Sackett DL. Utility maximization model for evaluation of health care programmes. Health Serv Res 1972; 7:118–133.
47. Balaban DJ, Fagi PC, Goldfarb NI, Nettler S. Weights for scoring the quality of well-being instrument among rheumatoid arthritics. Med Care 1986;24:973–980.
48. Hughes TE, Coons SJ, Kaplan RM, Draugalis JR. Reweighting the quality of well-being scale in HIV-infected subjects. Qual Life Res 1994;3:79–80. Abstract.
49. Kaplan RM, Sieber WJ, Ganiats TG. The quality of well-being scale: Comparison of an interviewer-administered version with a self-administered questionnaire. Psychol Health 1997;12:783–791.
50. Meenan RF, Gertman PM, Mason JH. Measuring health status in arthritis: The arthritis impact measurement scales. Arthritis Rheum 1980;23:146–152.
51. Juniper EF, Guyatt GH, Epstein RS, et al. Evaluation of impairment of health-related quality of life in asthma: Development of a questionnaire for use in clinical trials. Thorax 1992;47:76–83.
52. Parkerson GR, Connis RT, Broadhead WE, et al. Disease-specific versus generic measurement of health-related quality of life in insulin-dependent diabetic patients. Med Care 1993;7:629–639.
53. Hays RD, Kallich JD, Mapes DL, et al. Development of the kidney disease quality of life (KDQOL) instrument. Qual Life Res 1994; 3:329–338.
54. Perrine KR. A new quality of life inventory for epilepsy patients: Interim results. Epilepsia 1993;34(suppl 4):S28–S33.
55. Wu AW, Revicki DA, Jacobson D, Malitz FE. Evidence for reliability, validity and usefulness of the medical outcomes study HIV health survey (MOS-HIV). Qual Life Res 1997;6:481–493.
56. Ware JE Jr. Standards for validating health measures: Definition and content. J Chron Dis 1987;40:473–480.
57. Pathak DS, MacKeigan LD. Assessment of quality of life and health status: Selected observations. J Res Pharm Econ 1992;4:31–52.

58. Spilker B, ed. Quality of Life and Pharmacoeconomics in Clinical Trials, 2nd ed. Philadelphia, Lippincott-Raven, 1996.
59. Lohr KN, Aaronson NK, Alonso J, et al. Evaluating quality of life and health status instruments: Development of scientific review criteria. Clin Ther 1996;18:979–992.
60. Ware JE Jr, Snow KK, Kosinski M, Gandek B. SF–36 Health Survey: Manual and Interpretation Guide. Boston, The Health Institute, 1993.
61. Hays RD, Anderson R, Revicki D. Psychometric considerations in evaluating health–related quality of life measures. Qual Life Res 1993;2:441–449.
62. Nunnally J. Psychometric Theory, 2nd ed. New York, McGraw-Hill, 1978.
63. Kaplan RM, Saccuzzo DP. Psychological Testing: Principles, Applications, and Issues, 3rd ed. Pacific Grove, CA, Brooks/Cole, 1993.
64. Juniper EF, Guyatt GH, Jaeschke R. How to develop and validate a new health–related quality of life instrument. In: Spilker B, ed. Quality of Life and Pharmacoeconomics in Clinical Trials, 2nd ed. Philadelphia, Lippincott-Raven, 1996:49–56.
65. Guyatt G, Walter S, Norman G. Measuring change over time: Assessing the usefulness of evaluative instruments. J Chron Dis 1987;40: 171–178.
66. Hays RD, Hadorn D. Responsiveness to change: An aspect of validity, not a separate dimension. Qual Life Res 1992;1:73–75.
67. Cook DJ, Guyatt GH, Juniper E, et al. Interviewer versus self–administered questionnaires in developing a disease–specific, health–related quality of life instrument for asthma. J Clin Epidemiol 1993;46:529–534.
68. Jachuck SJ, Brierly H, Jachuck S, Wilcox PM. The effect of hypotensive drugs on the quality of life. J R Coll Gen Prac 1982;32:103–105.
69. Bullinger M, Power MJ, Aaronson NK, et al. Creating and evaluating cross–cultural instruments. In: Spilker B, ed. Quality of Life and Pharmacoeconomics in Clinical Trials, 2nd ed. Philadelphia, Lippincott-Raven, 1996:659–668.

3

Clinical Pharmacokinetics and Pharmacodynamics

Larry A. Bauer, PharmD, FCP, FCCP

Pharmacokinetic concepts have been used successfully by pharmacists to individualize patient drug therapy for over 20 years. Pharmacokinetic consultant services and individual clinicians routinely provide patient-specific drug dosing recommendations that increase the efficacy and decrease the toxicity of many medications. Laboratories routinely measure patient serum or plasma samples for many drugs including antibiotics (aminoglycosides, vancomycin), theophylline, antiepileptics (phenytoin, carbamazepine, valproic acid, phenobarbital, ethosuximide), methotrexate, lithium, antiarrhythmics (lidocaine, procainamide, quinidine, digoxin), and immunosuppressants (cyclosporine, tacrolimus). Combined with a knowledge of the disease states and conditions that influence the disposition of a particular drug, kinetic concepts can be used to modify doses to produce serum drug concentrations that produce desirable pharmacologic effects without unwanted side effects. This narrow range of concentrations within which the pharmacologic response is produced and the adverse effects prevented in most patients is defined as the *therapeutic range* of the drug. Table 3–1 lists the therapeutic ranges for commonly used medications.

Although most individuals experience favorable effects with serum drug concentrations in the therapeutic range, the effects of a given serum concentration can vary widely among individuals. Clinicians should never assume that a serum concentration within the therapeutic range will be safe and effective for every patient. The response to the drug, such as number of seizures a patient experiences while taking an antiepileptic agent, should always be assessed when serum concentrations are measured.

Throughout this chapter, abbreviations for various pharmacokinetic parameters are used frequently. Commonly used abbreviations are listed in Table 3–2.

CLINICAL PHARMACOKINETIC CONCEPTS

Clinical pharmacokinetics is the discipline that describes the absorption, distribution, metabolism, and elimination of drugs in patients requiring drug therapy. When a drug is administered extravascularly to patients, it must be absorbed across biologic membranes to reach the systemic circulation. If the drug is given orally, the drug molecules must pass through the gastrointestinal tract wall into capillaries. For transdermal patches, the drug must penetrate the skin to enter the vascular system. In general, the pharmacologic effect of the drug is delayed when it is given extravascularly because time is required for the drug to be absorbed into the vascular system.

The vascular system generally provides the "transportation" for the drug molecule to its site of activity. After the drug reaches the systemic circulation, it can leave the vasculature and penetrate the various tissues or remain in the blood. If the drug remains in the blood it may bind to endogenous proteins such as albumin or α_1-acid glycoprotein. This binding is usually reversible, and an equilibrium is created between protein-bound drug and unbound drug. Unbound drug in the blood provides the driving force for distribution of the agent to body tissues. If unbound drug leaves the bloodstream and distributes to tissue it may become tissue bound, it may remain unbound in the tissue, or, if the tissue can metabolize or eliminate the drug, it may be rendered inactive and/or eliminated from the body. If the drug becomes tissue bound, it may bind to the receptor that causes its pharmacologic or toxic effect or to a nonspecific binding site that causes no effect. Again, tissue binding is usually reversible so that the tissue-bound drug is in equilibrium with unbound drug in the tissue.

Certain organs—such as the liver, gastrointestinal tract wall, and lung—possess enzymes that metabolize drugs. The resulting metabolite may be inactive or have a pharmacologic effect of its own. The blood also contains esterases, which cleave ester bonds in drug molecules and generally render them inactive.

Drug metabolism usually occurs in the liver through one or both of two types of reactions. Phase I reactions generally make the drug molecule more polar and water soluble so that it is prone to elimination by the kidney. Phase I modifications include oxidation, hydrolysis, and reduction. Phase II reactions involve conjugation to form glucuronides, acetates, or sulfates. These reactions generally inactivate the pharmacologic activity of the drug and may make it more prone to elimination by the kidney.

Other organs have the ability to eliminate drugs or metabolites from the body. The kidney can excrete drugs by glomerular filtration or by such active processes as proximal tubular secretion. Drugs can also be eliminated via bile produced by the liver or air expired by the lungs.

LINEAR PHARMACOKINETICS

Most drugs follow linear pharmacokinetics: Serum drug concentrations change proportionally with long-term daily dosing. As an example, if the drug dose were doubled from

TABLE 3–1. Selected Therapeutic Ranges

Drug	Therapeutic Range
Digoxin	0.9–2 ng/mL
Lidocaine	1.5–5 μg/mL
Procainamide/*N*-acetylprocainamide	10–30 μg/mL (total)
Quinidine	2–5 μg/mL
Amikacin[a]	20–30 μg/mL (peak)
	<5 μg/mL (trough)
Gentamicin, tobramycin, netilmicin[a]	5–10 μg/mL (peak)
	<2 μg/mL (trough)
Vancomycin	25–35 μg/mL (peak)
	5–10 μg/mL (trough)
Chloramphenicol	10–20 μg/mL
Lithium	0.6–1.4 mEq/L
Carbamazepine	4–12 μg/mL
Ethosuximide	40–100 μg/mL
Phenobarbital	15–40 μg/mL
Phenytoin	10–20 μg/mL
Primidone	5–12 μg/mL
Valproic acid	50–100 μg/mL
Theophylline	10–20 μg/mL
Cyclosporine	150-400 ng/mL (blood)

[a]Using a multiple dose per day dosage schedule, single daily dose therapeutic concentrations not yet established.

TABLE 3–2. Pharmacokinetic Abbreviations

Abbreviation	Definition
Cl	Clearance
k_0	Intravenous infusion rate
C_{ss}	Steady-state concentration
D	Dose
τ	Dosage interval
F	Fraction of drug absorbed into the systemic circulation
Q	Blood flow
E	Extraction ratio
f_b	Fraction of drug in the blood that is unbound
Cl_{int}	Intrinsic clearance
$C_{ss,u}$	Steady-state concentration of unbound drug
V_D	Volume of distribution
LD	Loading dose
MD	Maintenance dose
$t_{1/2}$	Half-life
k	Elimination rate constant
k_a	Absorption rate constant
α	Distribution rate constant
β	Terminal rate constant
t'	Postinfusion time
T	Duration of infusion
AUC	Area under serum or blood concentration-versus-time curve
V_{max}	Maximum rate of drug metabolism
K_m	Serum concentration at which the rate of metabolism equals $V_{max}/2$
C_{max}	Maximum serum or blood concentration
C_{min}	Minimum serum or blood concentration
DR	Dosage rate

300 to 600 mg/d, the patient's serum drug concentration would double.

When a drug is given by continuous intravenous infusion, serum concentrations increase until an equilibrium is established between the drug dosage rate and the rate of drug elimination. At that point, the rate of drug administration equals the rate of drug elimination and the serum concentrations therefore remain constant (Fig. 3–1). For example, if a patient were receiving a continuous intravenous infusion of theophylline at 40 mg/h, the theophylline serum concentration would increase until the patient's body was eliminating theophylline at 40 mg/h. When serum drug concentrations reach a constant value, steady state is achieved.

If the drug is given at intermittent dosage intervals, such as 250 mg every 6 hours, steady state is achieved when the serum concentration-versus-time curves for each dosage interval are superimposable. The amount of drug eliminated during the dosage interval equals the dose.

BIOAVAILABILITY AND BIOEQUIVALENCE

When drugs are administered extravascularly, drug molecules must be released from the dosage form (dissolution) and pass through several biologic barriers before reaching the vascular system (absorption). The fraction of drug absorbed into the systemic circulation (F) after extravascular administration is defined as its bioavailability and can be calculated after single intravenous and extravascular doses as[1]

$$F = D_{iv}(AUC_{0-\infty})/D(AUC_{iv0-\infty})$$

where D and D_{iv} are the extravascular and intravenous doses, respectively, and $AUC_{iv0-\infty}$ and $AUC_{0-\infty}$ are the intravenous and extravascular areas under the serum or blood concentration-versus-time curves, respectively, from time zero to infinity. The AUC represents the body's total exposure to the drug and is a function of the fraction of the drug dose that enters the systemic circulation via the administered route and clearance (Fig. 3–2). When F is less than one for a drug administered extravascularly, either the dosage form did not release all of the drug contained in it or some of the drug was eliminated or destroyed (by stomach acid or other means) before it reached the systemic circulation.

When the extravascular dose is administered orally, part of the dose may be metabolized by enzymes contained in the liver or gastrointestinal tract wall before it reaches the systemic circulation.[2,3] This commonly occurs when drugs have a high liver extraction ratio or are subject to gastrointestinal tract wall metabolism because, after oral administration, the drug must pass through the gastrointestinal tract wall and into the portal circulation of the liver. For example, if an orally administered drug is 100% absorbed from the gastrointestinal tract but has a hepatic extraction ratio of 0.75, only 25% of the original dose enters the systemic circulation. This "first-pass" effect through the liver and/or gastrointestinal tract wall is avoided when the drug is given by other routes of administration. The computation of F does not separate loss of oral drug metabolized by the first-pass effect and drug not absorbed by the gastrointestinal tract.

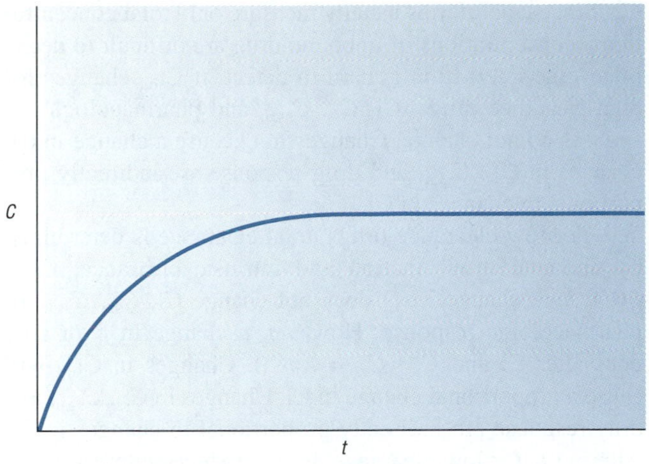

FIGURE 3–1. Normal serum concentration–time curve following a continuous intravenous infusion.

Special techniques are needed to determine the fraction of drug absorbed orally for drugs with high liver extraction ratios or substantial gut wall metabolism.

Two different dosage forms of the same drug are considered to be bioequivalent when the $AUC_{0-\infty}$, maximum serum or blood concentrations (C_{max}), and the times that C_{max} occurs (t_{max}) are neither clinically nor statistically different. When this occurs, the serum concentration-versus-time curves for the two dosage forms should be superimposable and, therefore, identical. Bioequivalence studies have become very important as many expensive drugs have recently become available in generic form. Most bioequivalence studies involve 18 to 25 healthy adults who are given the brand-name product and the generic product in a randomized, crossover study design.

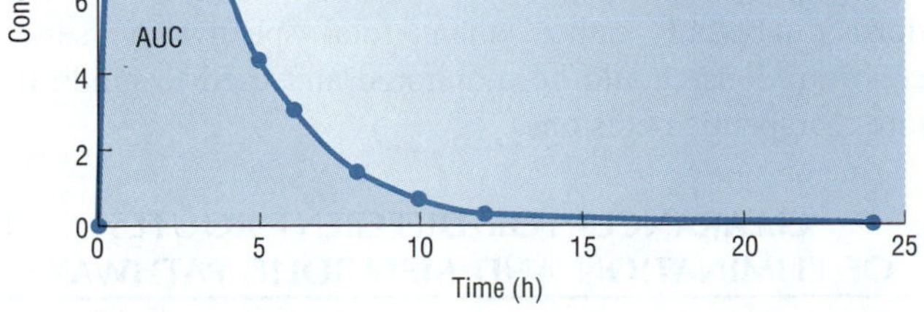

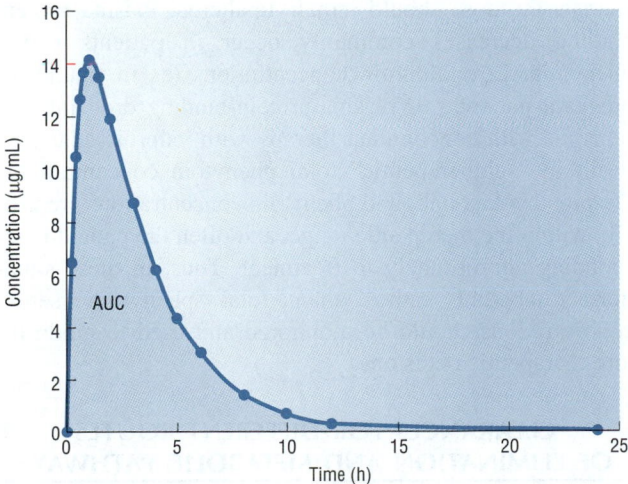

FIGURE 3–2. Area under the concentration–time curve (AUC) after the administration of an extravascular dose. The AUC is the function of the fraction of drug dose that enters the systemic circulation and clearance. AUCs measured after intravenous and extravascular doses can be used to determine bioavailability for the extravascular dose.

CLEARANCE

Clearance (Cl) is the most important pharmacokinetic parameter because it determines the steady-state concentration for a given dosage rate. When a drug is given at a continuous intravenous infusion rate equal to k_0 the steady-state concentration (C_{ss}) is determined by the quotient of k_0 and Cl ($C_{ss} = k_0/\text{Cl}$). If the drug is administered as individual doses (D) at a given dosage interval (τ), the average steady-state concentration (C_{ss}) over the dosage interval is given by the equation[4]:

$$C_{ss} = [F(D/\tau)]/\text{Cl}$$

where F is the fraction of dose absorbed into the systemic vascular system. The average steady-state concentration over the dosage interval is the steady-state concentration that would have occurred had the same dose been given as a continuous intravenous infusion (e.g., 300 mg every 6 hours would produce an average C_{ss} equivalent to the actual C_{ss} produced by a continuous infusion administered at a rate of 50 mg/h).

Physiologically, clearance is determined by (1) blood flow (Q) to the organ that metabolizes (liver) or eliminates (kidney) the drug and (2) the efficiency of the organ in extracting the drug from the bloodstream.[5] Efficiency is measured using an extraction ratio (E), calculated by subtracting the concentration in the blood leaving the extracting organ (C_{out}) from the concentration in the blood entering the organ (C_{in}) and then dividing the result by C_{in}:

$$E = (C_{in} - C_{out})/(C_{in})$$

Clearance for that organ is calculated by taking the product of Q and E: ($\text{Cl} = QE$). For example, if liver blood flow equals 1.5 L/min and the drug's extraction ratio is 0.33, hepatic clearance equals 0.5 L/min. Total clearance is computed by summing all of the individual organ clearance values. Clearance changes occur in patients when the blood flow to extracting organs changes or when the extraction ratio changes. Vasodilators like hydralazine or nifedipine increase liver blood flow, whereas congestive heart failure and hypotension can decrease hepatic blood flow. Extraction ratios can increase when enzyme inducers increase the amount of drug-metabolizing enzyme. Extraction ratios may decrease if enzyme inhibitors inhibit drug metabolizing enzymes or necrosis causes loss of parenchyma.

INTRINSIC CLEARANCE

The extraction ratio can also be thought of in terms of the unbound fraction of drug in the blood (f_b), the intrinsic ability of the extracting organ to clear unbound drug from the blood (Cl_{int}), and blood flow to the organ (Q)[6,7]:

$$E = [f_b(\text{Cl}_{int})]/\{Q + [f_b(\text{Cl}_{int})]\}$$

By substituting this equation for E, the clearance equation becomes:

$$\text{Cl} = Q[f_b(\text{Cl}_{int})]/\{Q + [f_b(\text{Cl}_{int})]\}$$

Clearance changes will occur when blood flow to the clearing organ changes (in conditions where blood flow is reduced [shock, congestive heart failure] or when medications such as vasodilators increase blood flow), binding in the blood changes (if highly protein-bound drugs are displaced), or intrinsic clearance of unbound drug changes (when metabolizing enzymes are induced or inhibited).

If Cl_{int} is large (enzymes have a high capacity to metabolize the drug), the product of f_b and Cl_{int} is much larger than Q. When $f_b(Cl_{int})$ is much greater than Q, the sum of Q and $f_b(Cl_{int})$ in the denominator of the clearance equation almost equals $f_b(Cl_{int})$:

$$f_b(Cl_{int}) \approx Q + f_b(Cl_{int})$$

Substituting this expression in the denominator of the clearance equation and canceling common terms leads to the following expression for drugs with a large Cl_{int}: $Cl \approx Q$. In this case the clearance of the drug is equal to blood flow to the organ; such drugs are called *high-clearance drugs* and have large extraction ratios. Propranolol, verapamil, morphine, and lidocaine are examples of high-clearance drugs. High-clearance drugs such as these typically exhibit high first-pass effects when adminstered orally.

If Cl_{int} is small (enzymes have a limited capacity to metabolize the drug), Q is much larger than the product of f_b and Cl_{int}. When Q is much greater than $f_b(Cl_{int})$, the sum of Q and $f_b(Cl_{int})$ in the denominator of the clearance equation becomes almost equal to Q: $Q \approx Q + f_b(Cl_{int})$. Substituting this expression in the denominator of the clearance equation and canceling common terms leads to the following expression for drugs with a small Cl_{int}: $Cl \approx f_b(Cl_{int})$. In this case, clearance of the drug is equal to the product of the fraction unbound in the blood and the intrinsic ability of the organ to clear unbound drug from the blood; such drugs are known as *low-clearance drugs* and have small extraction ratios. Warfarin, theophylline, diazepam, and phenobarbital are examples of low-clearance drugs.

As previously mentioned, the concentration of unbound drug in the blood is probably more important pharmacologically than the total (bound plus unbound) concentration. The unbound drug in the blood is in equilibrium with the unbound drug in the tissues and reflects the concentration of drug at its site of action. Therefore, the pharmacologic effect of a drug is thought to be a function of the concentration of unbound drug in the blood. The unbound steady-state concentration ($C_{ss,u}$) can be calculated by multiplying C_{ss} and f_b: $C_{ss,u} = C_{ss}f_b$. The effect that changes in Q, f_b, and Cl_{int} have on $C_{ss,u}$ and therefore on the pharmacologic response of a drug depends on whether a high- or low-clearance drug is involved. Because $Cl = Q$ for high-clearance drugs, a change in f_b or Cl_{int} does not change Cl or C_{ss} ($C_{ss} = k_0/Cl$). However, a change in unbound drug fraction does alter $C_{ss,u}$ ($C_{ss,u} = f_bC_{ss}$), thereby affecting the pharmacologic response. Plasma-protein-binding displacement drug interactions are thus very important clinically, but they are also dangerous because the changes in $C_{ss,u}$ are not reflected in changes in C_{ss}. Since laboratories usually measure only total concentrations (concentrations of unbound drug are difficult to determine), the interaction is hard to detect. If Cl_{int} changes for high-clearance drugs, Cl, C_{ss}, $C_{ss,u}$, and pharmacologic responses do not change. Changes in Q cause a change in Cl; changes in C_{ss}, $C_{ss,u}$, and drug response are indirectly proportional to changes in Cl.

For low-clearance drugs, total clearance is determined by unbound drug fraction and intrinsic clearance: $Cl = f_b(Cl_{int})$. A change in Q does not change Cl, C_{ss}, $C_{ss,u}$, or pharmacologic response. However, a change in f_b or Cl_{int} does alter Cl and C_{ss} ($C_{ss} = k_0/Cl$). Changes in Cl_{int} will cause a proportional change in Cl. Changes in C_{ss}, $C_{ss,u}$, and drug response are indirectly proportional to changes in Cl. Altering f_b for low-clearance drugs produces interesting results. A change in f_b alters Cl and C_{ss} ($C_{ss} = k_0/Cl$). As Cl and C_{ss} change in opposite directions with changes in f_b, $C_{ss,u}$ ($C_{ss,u} = f_bC_{ss}$) and pharmacologic responses do not change with alterations in the fraction of unbound drug in the blood. For example, a low-clearance drug is administered to a patient until steady-state is achieved:

$$Cl = f_b(Cl_{int})$$

$$C_{ss} = k_0/CL$$

Suppose another drug is administered to the patient that displaces the first drug from plasma protein binding sites and doubles f_b (f_b now equals $2f_b$). Cl doubles because of the protein binding displacement [$2Cl = 2f_b(Cl_{int})$], and C_{ss} decreases by one-half because of the change in clearance [$1/2(C_{ss}) = k_0/(2Cl)$]. $C_{ss,u}$ does not change because even though f_b is doubled, C_{ss} decreased by one-half ($C_{ss,u} = f_bC_{ss}$). The potential for error in this situation is that clinicians may increase the dose of a low-clearance drug after a protein-binding displacement interaction because C_{ss} decreased. Since $C_{ss,u}$ and the pharmacologic effect do not change, the dose should remain unaltered. Plasma protein binding decreases commonly occur in patients taking phenytoin. Low albumin concentrations (as in trauma or pregnant patients) or plasma-protein-binding drug interactions (as with concomitant therapy with valproic acid) can result in "subtherapeutic" total phenytoin concentrations. Despite this fact unbound phenytoin concentrations are usually within the therapeutic range, and often the patient is responding appropriately to treatment. Thus, in these situations, unbound rather than total phenytoin serum concentrations should be monitored and used to guide future therapeutic decisions.

CLEARANCES FOR DIFFERENT ROUTES OF ELIMINATION AND METABOLIC PATHWAYS

Clearances for individual organs can be computed if the excretion the organ produces can be obtained. For example, renal clearance can be calculated if urine is collected during a pharmacokinetic experiment. The patient empties his or her bladder immediately before the dose is given. Subsequent urine production is collected until the last serum concentration (C_{last}) is obtained. Renal clearance (Cl_R) is computed by dividing the amount of drug excreted in the urine by $AUC_{0-tlast}$. Biliary and other clearance values are computed in a similar fashion.

Clearances can also be calculated for each metabolite that is formed from the parent drug. This computation is particularly useful in drug interaction studies to determine which metabolic pathway is stimulated or inhibited. In the following metabolic scheme, the parent drug (D) is metabolized into two different metabolites (M_1, M_2), which are subsequently eliminated by the kidney (M_{1R}, M_{2R}):

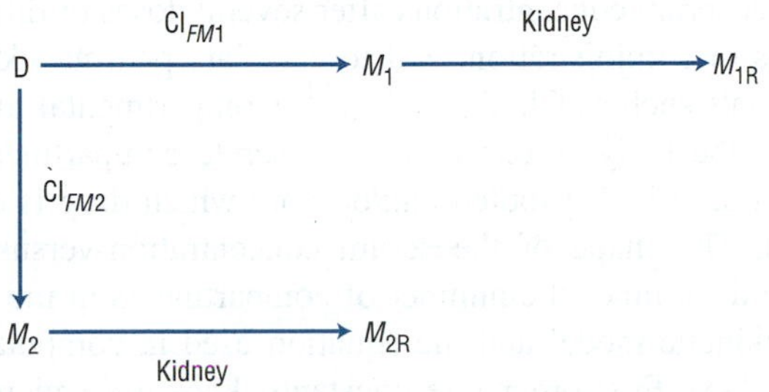

To compute the formation clearance of M_1 and M_2 (Cl_{FM1}, Cl_{FM2}), urine would be collected for five or more half-lives after a single dose or during a dosage interval at steady state. The amount of metabolite eliminated in the urine is then determined. The fraction of the dose (in moles, since the molecular weight of the parent drug and metabolites are not equal) eliminated by each metabolic pathway ($f_{M1} = M_{1R}/D$ and $f_{M2} = M_{2R}/D$) can then be computed. Formation clearance for each pathway can be calculated using the following equations: $Cl_{FM1} = f_{M1}Cl_M$ and $Cl_{FM2} = f_{M2}Cl_M$, where Cl_M is the metabolic clearance for the parent drug.

VOLUME OF DISTRIBUTION

The volume of distribution (V_D) is a proportionality constant that relates the amount of drug in the body to the serum concentration (amount in body = CV_D). V_D is used to calculate the loading dose (LD) of a drug that will immediately achieve a desired C_{ss} (LD = $C_{ss}V_D$). However, in practice the patient's own V_D is not known at the time the loading dose is administered. In this case an average V_D is assumed and used to calculate a loading dose. Because the patient's V_D is almost always different from the average V_D for the drug, a loading dose does not attain the calculated C_{ss}, but it hopefully achieves a therapeutic concentration.

The numeric value for the volume of distribution is determined by the physiologic volume of blood and tissues and how the drug binds in blood and tissues[8]:

$$V_D = V_b + (f_b/f_t)V_t$$

where V_b and V_t are the volumes of blood and tissues, respectively, and f_b and f_t are the fractions of unbound drug in blood and tissues, respectively.

HALF-LIFE

Half-life ($t_{1/2}$) is the time required for serum concentrations to decrease by one-half after absorption and distribution are complete. It takes the same amount of time for serum concentrations to drop from 200 to 100 mg/L as it does for concentrations to decline from 2 to 1 mg/L (Fig. 3–3).

Half-life is important because it determines the time required to reach steady state and the dosage interval. It takes approximately three to five $t_{1/2}$ to reach steady-state concentrations during continuous dosing. In three $t_{1/2}$, serum concentrations are at about 90% of their ultimate steady-state values. Because most serum drug assays have about a 10% error, it is difficult to differentiate concentrations that are within 10% of each other. For this reason, many clinicians consider concentrations obtained after three $t_{1/2}$ to be C_{ss}.

Half-life is also used to determine the dosage interval for a drug. For instance, it may be desirable to maintain maximum steady-state concentrations at 20 mg/L and minimum steady-state concentrations at 10 mg/L. In this case it would be necessary to administer the drug every $t_{1/2}$ because the minimum desirable concentration is one-half the maximum desirable concentration.

Half-life is a *dependent* kinetic variable because its value depends on the values of Cl and V_D.[8] The equation that describes the relationship among the three variables is $t_{1/2} = 0.693V_D/Cl$. Changes in $t_{1/2}$ can result from a change in either V_D or Cl; a change in $t_{1/2}$ does not necessarily indicate that Cl has changed. Half-life can change solely because of changes in V_D. The elimination rate constant (k) is related to the half-life by the following equation: $k = 0.693/t_{1/2}$. Both the half-life and elimination rate constant describe how quickly serum concentrations decrease in the serum or blood.

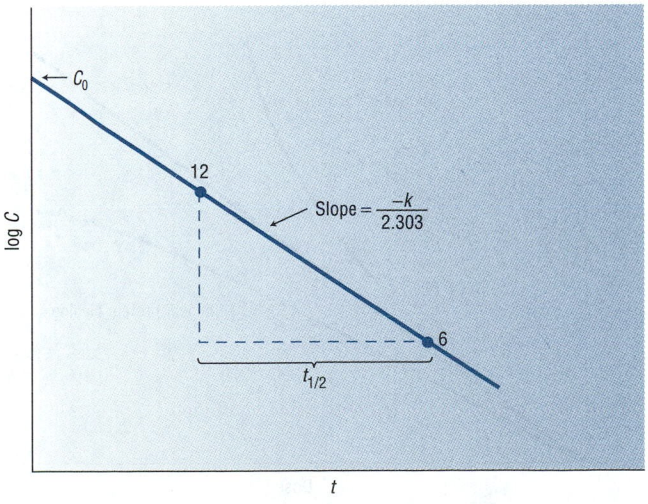

FIGURE 3–3. Calculation of the half-life of a drug following intravenous bolus dosing.

NONLINEAR PHARMACOKINETICS

MICHAELIS–MENTEN KINETICS

Some drugs do not follow the rules of linear pharmacokinetics. Instead of C_{ss} and AUC increasing proportionally with dose, serum concentrations change more or less than expected (Fig. 3–4). One explanation for the greater-than-expected increase in C_{ss} and AUC after an increase in dose is that the enzymes responsible for the metabolism or elimination of the drug may start to become saturated. When this occurs the maximum rate of metabolism (V_{max}) for the drug is approached. This is called Michaelis-Menten kinetics. The serum concentration at which the rate of metabolism equals $V_{max}/2$ is K_m. Practically speaking, K_m is the serum concentration at which nonproportional changes in C_{ss} and AUC start to occur when dose is increased. The Michaelis-Menten constants (V_{max} and K_m) determine the dosage rate (DR) needed to maintain a given C_{ss}: $DR = V_{max}C_{ss}/(K_m + C_{ss})$. Most drugs eliminated by the liver are metabolized by enzymes but still appear to follow linear kinetics. The reason for this disparity is that the therapeutic range for most drugs is well below the K_m of the enzyme system that metabolizes the agent. The therapeutic range is higher than K_m for some commonly used drugs. The average K_m for phenytoin is about 4 mg/L. The therapeutic range for phenytoin is usually 10–20 mg/L. Most patients experience Michaelis-Menten kinetics while taking phenytoin.

NONLINEAR PROTEIN BINDING

Another type of nonlinear kinetics can occur if C_{ss} and AUC increase less than expected after an increase in dose of a low-clearance drug. This usually indicates that plasma protein binding sites are starting to become saturated so that f_b increases with increases in dose (Fig. 3–4). For a low-clearance drug, Cl is dependent on the values of f_b and Cl_{int}($Cl = f_bCl_{int}$). When a dosage increase takes place, f_b increases because nearly all plasma protein binding sites are occupied and no binding sites are available. If f_b increases, Cl increases and C_{ss} increases less than expected with the dosage change ($C_{ss} = k_0/Cl$). However, $C_{ss,u}$ increases proportionally with dose since $C_{ss,u}$ depends on Cl_{int} for low-clearance drugs ($C_{ss,u} = k_0/Cl_{int}$). Valproic acid[9] and disopyramide[10] both follow saturable protein binding pharmacokinetics.

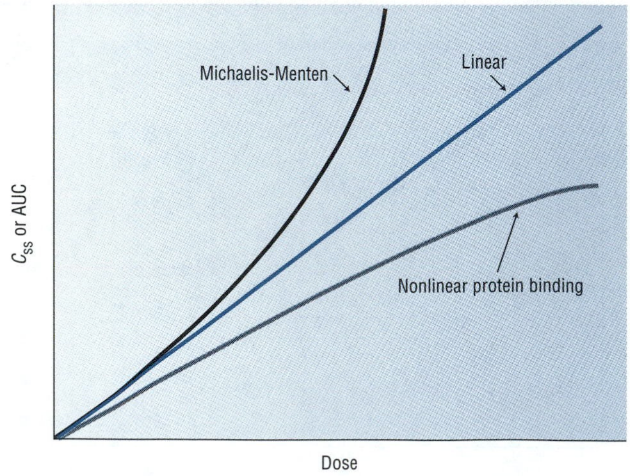

FIGURE 3–4. Relationship of dose and C_{ss} or AUC under linear and nonlinear conditions.

PHARMACOKINETIC MODELS AND EQUATIONS

Pharmacokinetic models are useful to describe data sets, to predict serum concentrations after several doses or different routes of administration, and to calculate pharmacokinetic constants such as Cl, V_D, and $t_{1/2}$.[11] Compartmental models depict the body as one or more discrete compartments to which drug is distributed and/or from which drug is eliminated. The shape of the serum concentration-versus-time curve determines the number of compartments in the pharmacokinetic model and the equation used in computations (Fig. 3–5). First-order rate constants, known as microconstants, describe the rate of transfer from one compartment to another. Each compartment also has its own V_D.

ONE-COMPARTMENT MODEL

The simplest case uses a single compartment to represent the entire body (Fig. 3–5). Drug enters the compartment by continuous intravenous infusion (k_0), absorption from an extravascular site with an absorption rate constant of k_a, or intravenous bolus (D). After an intravenous bolus, serum concentrations decline in a straight line when plotted on semilogarithmic coordinates (Fig. 3–3). The slope of the line is $-k/2.303$; $t_{1/2}$ can be computed by determining the time required for concentrations to decrease by one-half ($t_{1/2} = 0.693/k$). The equation that describes the data is $C = (D/V_D)e^{-kt}$. V_D is calculated by dividing the intravenous dose by the y intercept (the concentration at time zero, C_0) of the graph. CL is computed by taking the product of k and V_D.

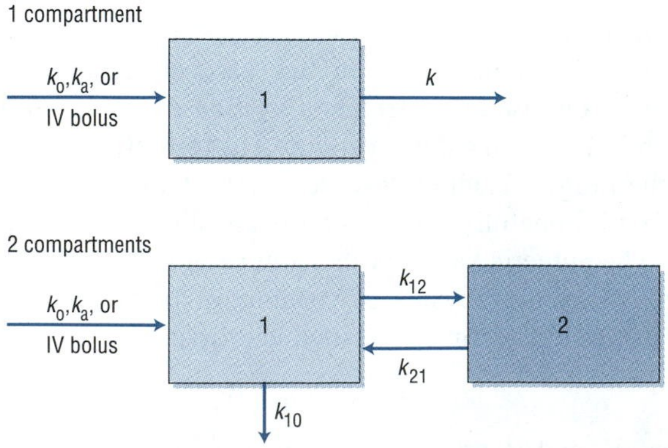

FIGURE 3–5. Visual representations of one- and two-compartment drug-distribution models.

Once V_D and k are known, concentrations at any time after the dose can be computed [$C = (D/V_D)e^{-kt}$].

When an extravascular dose is given, one-compartment model serum concentrations rise during absorption, reach C_{max}, and then decrease in a straight line with a slope equal to $-k/2.303$. The equation that describes the data is $C = [(FDk_a)/V_D(k_a - k)]\ (e^{-kt} - e^{-k_a t})$, where F is the fraction of the dose absorbed into the systemic circulation. The absorption rate constant (k_a) is obtained using the method of residuals.

The method of residuals is used to obtain the individual rate constants (Fig. 3–6). A is determined by extrapolating the terminal slope to the y axis; k can be obtained by calculating the slope or $t_{1/2}$ and using the formulas given for the intravenous bolus case. At each time point in the absorption portion of the curve, the concentration value from the extrapolated line is noted and called the extrapolated concentration. For each point the actual concentration is subtracted from the extrapolated concentration to compute the residual concentration. When the residual concentrations are plotted on semilogarithmic coordinates, a line with y intercept equal to A and slope equal to $-k_a/2.303$ is obtained. When these values are calculated, they can be placed into the equation ($C = Ae^{-kt} - Ae^{-k_a t}$, where $A = FDk_a/[V_D(k_a - k)]$) and used to compute the serum concentration at any time after the extravascular dose. The intercepts and rate constants can also be used to compute Cl and V_D: $Cl = FD/(A/k - A/k_a)$ and $V_D = Cl/k$, where F is the fraction of the dose absorbed into the systemic circulation.

During a continuous intravenous infusion, the serum concentrations in a one-compartment model change according to the following function: $C = (k_0/Cl)(1 - e^{-kt})$. If the infusion has been running for more than three to five half-lives, the patient will be at steady state and Cl can be calculated ($Cl = k_0/C_{ss}$). When the infusion is discontinued, serum concentrations appear to decline in a straight line when plotted on semilogarithmic paper with a slope of $-k/2.303$. V_D is computed by dividing Cl by k (Fig. 3–7).

MULTICOMPARTMENT MODEL

After an intravenous bolus dose, serum concentrations often decline in two or more phases. During the early phases, drug leaves the bloodstream by two mechanisms: (1) distribution into tissues and (2) metabolism and/or elimination. Because the drug is leaving the bloodstream through these two mechanisms, serum concentrations decline rapidly. After tissues and blood are in equilibrium, only metabolism and/or elimination remove drug from the blood. During this terminal phase serum concentrations decline more slowly. The half-life is measured during the terminal phase by determining the time required for concentrations to decline by one half.

After an intravenous bolus dose, serum concentrations decrease as if the drug were being injected into a central compartment that not only metabolizes and eliminates drug, but also distributes drug to one or more other compartments. Of these multicompartment models, the two-compartment model is most commonly encountered (Fig. 3–5). After an intravenous bolus injection, serum concentrations decrease in two distinct phases described by the equation:

$$C = D(\alpha - k_{21})/[V_{D1}(\alpha - \beta)]e^{-\alpha t} + D(k_{21} - \beta)/[V_{D1}(\alpha - \beta)]e^{-\beta t}$$

or $C = Ae^{-\alpha t} + Be^{-\beta t}$ where k_{21} is the first-order rate constant that reflects the transfer of drug from compartment 2 to compartment 1, V_{D1} is the V_D of compartment 1, $A = D(\alpha - k_{21})/[V_{D1}(\alpha - \beta)]$, and $B = D(k_{21} - \beta)/[V_{D1}(\alpha - \beta)]$. The rate constants α and β found in the exponents of the equations

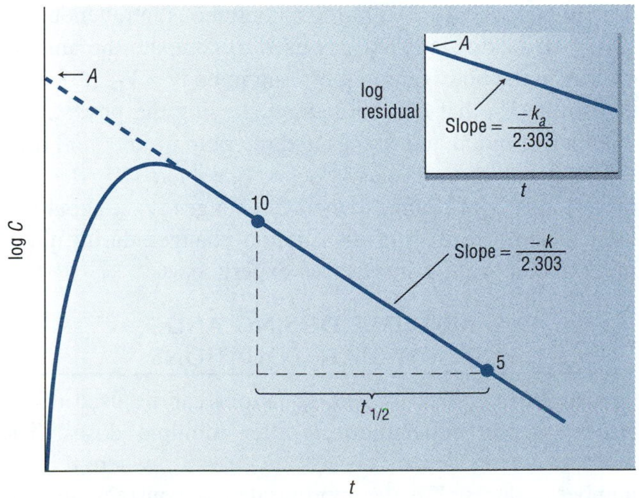

FIGURE 3–6. Calculation of the half-life of a drug following oral, intramuscular, or other extravascular dosing route.

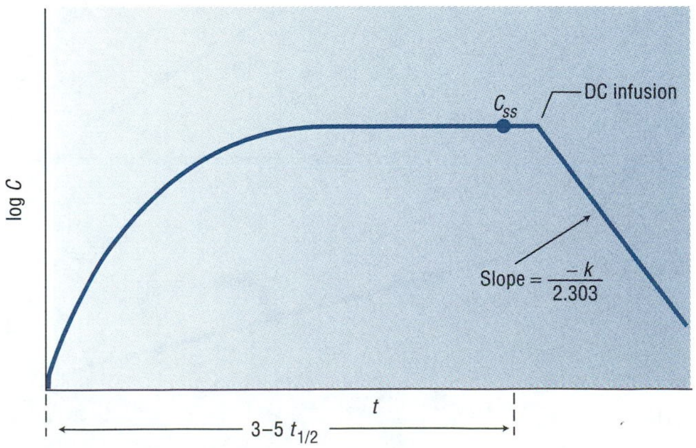

FIGURE 3–7. Achievement of steady-state serum concentrations after three to five half-lives of a drug. Note the elimination phase after discontinuance of the infusion.

describe the distribution and elimination of the drug, respectively (Fig. 3–8). A and B are the y intercepts of the lines that describe drug distribution and elimination, respectively, on the log concentration-versus-time plot.

The residual line is calculated as before using the method of residuals. The terminal line is extrapolated to the y axis, and extrapolated concentrations are determined for each time point. Because actual concentrations are greater in this case, residual concentrations are calculated by subtracting the extrapolated concentrations from the actual concentrations. When plotted on semilogarithmic paper the residual line has a y intercept equal to A. The slope of the residual line is used to compute α (slope = $-\alpha/2.303$). With the rate constants (α and β) and the intercepts (A and B), concentrations can be calculated for any time after the intravenous bolus dose ($C = Ae^{-\alpha t} + Be^{-\beta t}$) or pharmacokinetic constants can be computed: $Cl = D/[(A/\alpha) + (B/\beta)]$, $V_{D,\beta} = Cl/\beta$, $V_{D,ss} = D[(A/\alpha^2) + (B/\beta^2)]/[(A/\alpha) + (B/\beta)]^2$.

If serum concentrations of a drug given as a continuous intravenous infusion decline in a biphasic manner after the infusion is discontinued, a two-compartment model describes the data set[12,13] (Fig. 3–9). In this instance the postinfusion concentrations decrease according to the equation: $C = Re^{-\alpha t'} + Se^{-\beta t'}$, where t' is the postinfusion time ($t' = 0$ when infusion is discontinued) and R, S, α, and β are determined from the postinfusion concentrations using the method of residuals with the y axis set at $t' = 0$. R and S are used to compute A and B. A and B are the y intercepts that would have occurred had the total dose given during the infusion ($D = k_0T$) been administered as an intravenous bolus dose:

$$A = RD\alpha/[k_0(1 - e^{-\alpha T})]$$

$$B = SD\beta/[k_0(1 - e^{-\beta T})]$$

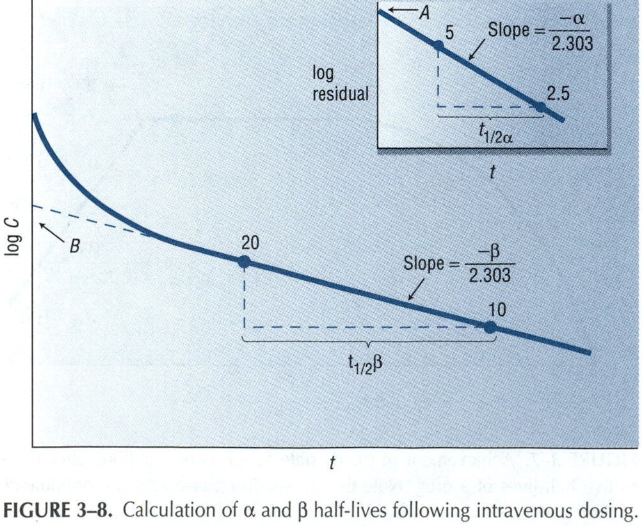

FIGURE 3–8. Calculation of α and β half-lives following intravenous dosing.

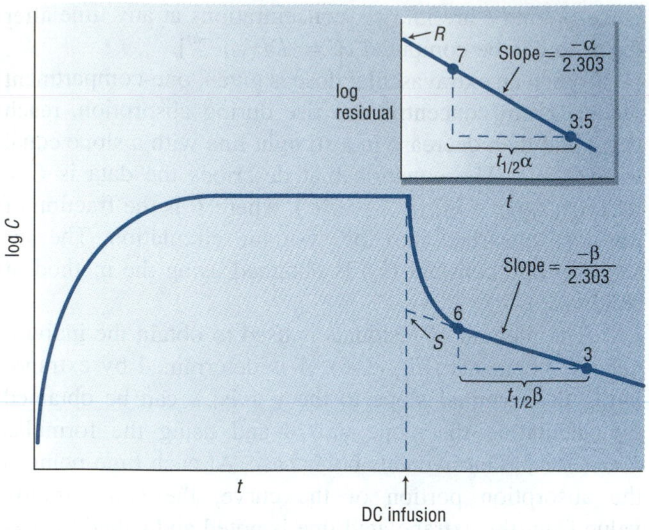

FIGURE 3–9. Calculation of α and β half-lives following a steady-state infusion.

where T is the duration of infusion. Once A, B, α, and β are known, the equations for an intravenous bolus are used to compute the pharmacokinetic constants. Often, when a drug is given as an intravenous bolus or continuous intravenous infusion, a two-compartment model is used to describe the data, but when the same agent is given extravascularly, a one-compartment model applies.[14] In this case, distribution occurs during the absorption phase so a distribution phase is not observed.

VOLUMES OF DISTRIBUTION IN MULTICOMPARTMENT MODELS

Two different V_D values are needed as proportionality constants for drugs that require multicompartment models to describe the serum concentration–time curve. The V_D that is used to compute the amount of drug in the body during the terminal (β) portion of the curve is called $V_{D,\beta}$ (amount of drug in body = $V_{D,\beta}C$). During a continuous intravenous infusion at steady state, $V_{D,ss}$ is used to compute the amount of drug in the body (amount of drug in body = $V_{D,ss}C$). $V_{D,ss}$ is also the V_D that can be computed using the physiologic volumes of blood and tissues and the ratio of unbound drug in blood to that in tissues [$V_{D,ss} = V_b + (f_b/f_t)V_t$]. Because the value of $V_{D,\beta}$ changes when Cl changes, $V_{D,ss}$ should be used to indicate if drug distribution changes during pharmacokinetic or drug-interaction experiments.

MULTIPLE DOSING AND STEADY-STATE EQUATIONS

Any of these compartmental equations can be used to determine serum concentrations after multiple doses. The multiple dosing factor, $(1 - e^{-nK\tau})/(1 - e^{-K\tau})$, where n is the number of doses, K is the appropriate rate constant, and τ is the dosage interval, is simply multiplied by each exponential term in the equation, substituting the rate constant of each exponent for K. Time (t) is set at 0 at the beginning of each dosage interval. For example, a single-dose two-compartment intravenous bolus is calculated as follows: $C = Ae^{-\alpha t} + Be^{-\beta t}$. The equation for a multiple dose two-compartment intravenous bolus is therefore

$$C = Ae^{-\alpha t}[(1 - e^{-n\alpha\tau})/(1 - e^{-\alpha\tau})] + Be^{-\beta t}[(1 - e^{-n\beta\tau})/(1 - e^{-\beta\tau})]$$

A single-dose one-compartment intravenous bolus is calculated as $C = (D/V_D)e^{-kt}$. For a multiple-dose one-compartment intravenous bolus the concentration is $C = (D/V_D)e^{-kt}[(1 - e^{-nk\tau})/(1 - e^{-k\tau})]$.

At steady state, the number of doses becomes large, $e^{-nk\tau}$ approaches zero, and the multiple dosing factor equals $1/(1 - e^{-K\tau})$. Therefore, the steady-state versions of the equations are simpler than their multiple dose counterparts:

$$C = [Ae^{-\alpha t}/(1 - e^{-\alpha\tau})] + [Be^{-\beta t}/(1 - e^{-\beta\tau})]$$

and

$$C = [(D/V_D)e^{-kt}]/(1 - e^{-k\tau})$$

for a steady-state two-compartment intravenous bolus and a steady-state one-compartment intravenous bolus, respectively.

USE OF PHARMACOKINETIC CONCEPTS FOR INDIVIDUALIZATION OF DRUG THERAPY

Many factors must be taken into consideration when deciding on the best drug dose for a patient. For example, the age of the patient is important because the dose (in mg per kg) for pediatric patients may be higher, and for geriatric patients may be lower, than the typically prescribed dose for young adults. Gender can also be a factor because males and females metabolize and eliminate some drugs differently. Patients who are significantly obese or cachectic may also require different drug doses because of clearance and volume of distribution changes. Other drug therapy that could cause drug interactions needs to be considered. Disease states and conditions may alter the drug-dosage regimen for a patient. Three disease states that deserve special mention are congestive heart failure, renal disease, and hepatic disease. Renal and hepatic disease cause loss of organ function and decreased drug elimination and metabolism. Congestive heart failure causes decreased blood flow to organs that clear the drug from the body.

Many drug compounds are racemic mixtures of stereoisomers. In most cases, one of the isomers is more pharmacologically active than the other isomer, and each isomer may exhibit different pharmacokinetic properties. Warfarin, propranolol, verapamil, and ibuprofen are all racemic mixtures of stereoisomers. Some drug interactions inhibit or increase the elimination of only one stereoisomer. The importance of the drug interaction depends on which isomer is affected. Other drugs, such as dextromethorphan, levofloxacin, and diltiazem, are composed of just one stereoisomer.

Genetics also plays a role in drug metabolism. Cytochrome P450 is a generic term for the group of enzymes that are responsible for most drug metabolism oxidation reactions. Several P450 isozymes have been identified that are responsible for the metabolism of many important drugs (Table 3–3). CYP2C19 ($P450IIC19$, $P450_{mp}$; formerly included in CYP2C9) is responsible for aromatic hydroxylation of mephenytoin and CYP2D6 (P450IID6, $P450_{db}$) oxidizes debrisoquine.[15] These subsets of the P450 enzyme family are also responsible for the metabolism of several other drugs (CYP2D6: most tricyclic antidepressants, encainide, metoprolol). Both of these isozymes appear to be under genetic control. As a consequence, there are "poor metabolizers" who lack the gene for the isozyme, cannot manufacture the isozyme and, therefore, cannot metabolize the drug substrate very well. "Extensive metabolizers" have the gene for the isozyme and metabolize the drugs normally. Poor metabolizers usually are a minority of the general population. They may achieve toxic concentrations of drug when usual doses are prescribed for them, or if the active drug moiety is a metabolite, may fail to have any pharmacologic effect from the drug. The ethnic background of the patient can affect the likelihood that they will be a poor metabolizer.[15] For

TABLE 3–3. Cytochrome P450 Enzyme Family and Selected Substrates

CYP1A2	Propafenone
Acetaminophen	Risperidone
Antipyrine	Thioridazine
Caffeine	Venlafaxine
Tacrine	CYP2E1
Theophylline	Ethanol
R-Warfarin	Isoniazid
CYP2C9	CYP3A4
Diclofenac	Alfentanil
Hexobarbital	Alprazolam
Ibuprofen	Astemizole
Naproxen	Carbamazepine
Phenytoin	Cisapride
Tolbutamide	Cyclosporine
S-Warfarin	Diltiazem
CYP2C19	Erythromycin
Diazepam	Felodipine
Mephenytoin	Fluconazole
Omeprazole	Itraconazole
CYP2D6	Ketoconazole
Codeine	Lidocaine
Debrisoquine	Lovastatin
Dextromethorphan	Midazolam
Encainide	Nifedipine
Fluoxetine	Quinidine
Haloperidol	Simvastatin
Loratadine	Tacrolimus
Metoprolol	Terfenadine
Paroxetine	Verapamil

example, the incidence of poor metabolizers for CYP2D6 is about 5% to 10% for Caucasians and about 0 to 1% for Asians, while for CYP2C19 poor metabolizers make up about 3% to 6% of the Caucasian population and about 20% of the Asian population.

Other P450 isozymes have been isolated.[15] CYP1A2 (P450IA2) is the enzyme that is responsible for the demethylation of caffeine and theophylline, CYP2C9 (P450IIC9) metabolizes phenytoin and tolbutamide, cyclosporine and nifedipine are metabolized by CYP3A4 (P450IIIA4), and ethanol is a substrate for CYP2E1 (P450IIE1). It is important to recognize that a drug may be metabolized by more than one P450 isozyme. While most tricyclic antidepressants are hydroxylated by CYP2D6, *N*-demethylation is probably mediated by a combination of CYP2C19, CYP1A2, and CYP3A4. Acetaminophen appears to be metabolized by both CYP1A2 and CYP2E1. The 4-hydroxy metabolite of propranolol is produced by CYP2D6, but side chain oxidation of propranolol is probably a product of CYP2C19.

Understanding which P450 isozyme is responsible for the metabolism of a drug is extraordinarily useful when predicting and understanding drug interactions. Some drug metabolism inhibitors and inducers are highly selective for certain P450 isozymes.[15] Quinidine is an extremely potent inhibitor of the CYP2D6 enzyme system[15]; a single 50-mg dose of quinidine can change a rapid metabolizer of debrisoquine into a poor metabolizer. Verapamil and diltiazem inhibit, while tobacco or marijuana smoke induce CYP1A2. Some drugs that are enzyme inhibitors are also substrates for that same enzyme system and appear to cause drug interactions by being a competitive inhibitor. For example, erythromycin is both a substrate for, and inhibitor of, CYP3A4. Obviously, if one knows that a new drug is metabolized by a given P450 enzyme system, it is logical to assume that the new drug will exhibit drug interactions with the known inducers and inhibitors of that P450 isozyme.

SELECTION OF INITIAL DRUG DOSES

When deciding on initial doses for drugs that are renally eliminated, the patient's renal function should be assessed. A common, useful way to do this is to measure the patient's serum creatinine concentration and convert this value into an estimated creatinine clearance ($CrCl_{est}$). Serum creatinine values alone should not be used to assess renal function because they do not include the effects of age, body weight, or gender. The Cockcroft–Gault equation[16] is probably the most widely used method to estimate creatinine clearance (in mL/min) in adults (18 years or older) who are within about 30% of their ideal body weight and have stable renal function:

$$\text{Male, } CrCl_{est} = [(140 - \text{age})BW]/(S_{cr} \cdot 72)$$

$$\text{Female, } CrCl_{est} = [0.85(140 - \text{age})BW]/(S_{cr} \cdot 72)$$

where BW is body weight (in kg), age is the patient's age (in yr), 0.85 is a correction factor to account for lower muscle mass in females, and S_{cr} is serum creatinine (in mg/dL). For children, the following estimation equations are available according to the age of the child[17]: age 0 to 1 years: $CrCl_{est}$ (in mL/min/1.73 m^2) = $(0.45 \cdot Lt)/S_{cr}$, age 1 to 20 years: $CrCl_{est}$ (in mL/min/1.73 m^2) = $(0.55 \cdot Lt)/S_{cr}$, where Lt is patient length in cm. Other methods to determine $CrCl_{est}$ for obese adults[18] and patients with rapidly changing renal function[19] are available. Creatinine is a byproduct of muscle breakdown in the body, so none of these estimation methods work well in patients with muscle disease, such as multiple sclerosis, or diseases that alter muscle mass, such as cachexia, malnutrition, cancer, or spinal cord injury. Nomograms that adjust initial doses according to a patient's renal function are available for several drugs including digoxin,[20] vancomycin,[21] and the aminoglycoside antibiotics.[22] For many other drugs, Dr. William M. Bennett[23,24] occasionally updates his monograph of drug dosing in renal disease, which includes suggested dosage adjustments.

A similar assessment of liver function should be made for drugs that are hepatically metabolized. Unfortunately, there is no single test that can accurately estimate liver drug metabolism capacity and those that are used don't always prove accurate. High aminotransferase (AST or SGOT and ALT or SGPT) and alkaline phosphatase concentrations usually indicate acute hepatic cellular damage and do not reliably establish poor liver drug metabolism. Abnormal values for three tests that *usually* indicate drugs will be poorly metabolized by the liver are high serum bilirubin, low serum albumin, and a prolonged prothrombin time. Bilirubin is metabolized by the liver, and albumin and clotting factors are manufactured by the liver, so aberrant values for all three of these tests are a more reliable indicator of abnormal liver drug metabolism. The Child–Pugh score,[25] a widely used clinical classification for liver disease that incorporates clinical signs and symptoms (ascites and hepatic encephalopathy) in addition to these three laboratory tests, can be used as an indicator of a patient's ability to metabolize drugs that are eliminated by the liver. A score in excess of 10 suggests very poor liver function. As a general rule, patients with cirrhosis have the most severe decreases in liver drug metabolism. Patients with acute or chronic hepatitis often retain relatively normal or slightly decreased hepatic drug metabolism capacity.

Since there are no good markers of liver function, clinicians have come to rely upon pharmacokinetic parameters derived in various patient populations to compute initial doses of drugs that are hepatically eliminated. Table 3–4 contains average pharmacokinetic parameters for theophylline in several disease states. Initial doses of many liver metabolized drugs are computed by determining which disease states and/or conditions the patient has that are known to alter the kinetics of the drug and by using these average pharmacokinetic constants to calculate doses. The patient is

TABLE 3–4. Theophylline Pharmacokinetic Parameters for Selected Disease States/Conditions

Disease State/Condition	Mean Clearance (mL/min/kg)	Mean Dose (mg/kg/h)
Children 1–9 yr	1.4	0.8
Children 9–12 yr or adult smokers	1.25	0.7
Adolescents 12–16 yr or elderly smokers (> 65 yr)	0.9	0.5
Adult nonsmokers	0.7	0.4
Elderly nonsmokers (> 65 yr)	0.5	0.3
Decompensated CHF, cor pulmonale, cirrhosis	0.35	0.2

Mean volume of distribution = 0.5 L/kg
Adapted from Reference 44.

then monitored for therapeutic and adverse effects, and drug serum concentrations are obtained to ensure that concentrations are appropriate and to adjust doses if necessary. The following computations illustrate the estimated intravenous loading and intravenous continuous infusion necessary to achieve a theophylline concentration of 10 mg/L for a 55-year-old, 70-kg male with liver cirrhosis (mean kinetic parameters obtained from Table 3–4):

$$V_D = (0.5 \text{ L/kg})(70 \text{ kg}) = 35 \text{ L}$$

$$\text{LD} = C_{ss}V_D = (10 \text{ mg/L})(35 \text{ L}) = 350 \text{ mg of theophylline infused over 20–30 min}$$

$$\text{Cl (in L/h)} = [(0.35 \text{ mL/min/kg})(70 \text{ kg})(60 \text{ min/h})]/1000 \text{ mL/L} = 1.5 \text{ L/h}$$

$$k_0 = C_{ss}\text{Cl} = (10 \text{ mg/L})(1.5 \text{ L/h}) = 15 \text{ mg/h of theophylline to begin after loading dose given}$$

If theophylline is to be given as the aminophylline salt form, each dose would need to be changed to reflect the fact that aminophylline contains only 85% theophylline (LD = 350 mg of theophylline/0.85 = 410 mg of aminophylline infused over 20–30 min, k_0 = 15 mg/h of theophylline/0.85 = 18 mg/h of aminophylline to begin after loading dose given).

Heart failure is often overlooked as a disease state that can alter drug disposition. Severe heart failure decreases cardiac output and, therefore, reduces liver blood flow. Theophylline,[26] lidocaine,[27] and drugs with high extraction ratios are compounds whose clearance declines with decreased liver blood flow. Initial dosages of these drugs should be reduced in patients with moderate to severe heart failure by 25% to 50% until steady-state concentrations and response can be determined.

USE OF STEADY-STATE DRUG CONCENTRATIONS

Serum drug concentrations are readily available to clinicians to use as guides for the individualization of drug therapy. The therapeutic ranges for several drugs have been identified, and it is likely that new drugs will also be monitored using serum concentrations. Although several individualization methods have been advocated for specific drugs, one simple, reliable method is commonly used. For drugs that exhibit linear pharmacokinetics, C_{ss} changes proportionally with dose. To adjust a patient's drug therapy, a reasonable starting dose is administered for an estimated three to five half-lives. A serum concentration is obtained assuming that it will reflect C_{ss}. Independent of the route of administration, the new dose (D_{new}) needed to attain the desired $C_{ss}(C_{ss,new})$ is calculated: $D_{new} = D_{old}\,(C_{ss,new}/C_{ss,old})$, where D_{old} and $C_{ss,old}$ are the old dose and old C_{ss}, respectively. To use this method $C_{ss,old}$ must reflect steady-state conditions. Often, patients are noncompliant with regard to their drug dosage and, therefore, are not at steady state. This occurs not only in outpatients, but in hospital inpatients as well. Inpatients can spit out oral doses or alter the infusion rates on intravenous pumps after the nurse leaves the hospital room. If $C_{ss,old}$ is much larger or smaller than expected for the D_{old} the patient is taking, one should suspect noncompliance and repeat the serum concentration after another three to five $t_{1/2}$ or change the patient's dose cautiously and monitor for signs of toxicity or lack of effect.

MEASUREMENT OF PHARMACOKINETIC PARAMETERS IN PATIENTS

If it is necessary to determine the kinetic constants for a patient to individualize his or her dose, a small kinetic evaluation is conducted in the individual. In these cases, the number of serum concentrations obtained from the patient is held to the minimum needed to calculate accurate pharmacokinetic parameters and doses. The reason for using fewer serum drug concentrations is to be as cost-effective as possible because these lab tests generally cost $20 to $50 each.

Although many drugs follow two-compartment model pharmacokinetics (especially after intravenous administration), a one-compartment model is used to compute kinetic parameters in patients since too many serum concentrations would be needed to accurately determine both the distribution and elimination phases found in the two-compartment model. Because of this, serum concentrations are not usually measured in patients during the distribution phase. Another important reason serum concentrations are not measured during the distribution phase for therapeutic drug monitoring purposes in patients is that drug in the blood and drug in the tissues are not in equilibrium during this time so that serum concentrations do not reflect tissue concentrations. When drug serum concentrations are obtained in patients for the purpose of assessing efficacy or toxicity, it is important that they be measured in the postdistribution phase when drug in the blood is in equilibrium with drug at the site of action.

In the case where the patient has received enough doses to be at steady state, pharmacokinetic parameters can be computed using a predose minimum concentration and a postdose maximum concentration. Under steady-state conditions, serum concentrations after each dose are identical so the predose minimum concentration is the same before each dose (Fig. 3–10). This situation allows the predose concentration to be used to compute both the patient's $t_{1/2}$ and V. If the drug was given extravascularly or has a significant distribution phase, the postdose concentration should be collected after absorption or distribution is finished. To assure that steady-state conditions have been achieved, the patient needs to receive the drug on schedule for at least three to five estimated half-lives. To make sure this is the case, inpatients should have their medication administration records checked, and the patient's nurse should be consulted regarding missed or late doses. Outpatients should be interviewed about compliance with the prescribed dosage regimen. When compliance with the dosage regimen has been verified, steady-state conditions can be reasonably assumed.

If the patient is not at steady state, an additional postdose serum concentration should be obtained to compute the patient's pharmacokinetic parameters. Ideally, the third concentration (C_3) should be acquired approximately one estimated $t_{1/2}$ after the postdose maximum concentration. Getting serum concentrations too close together will hamper the drug assay's ability to measure differences between them, and getting the third sample too late could result in

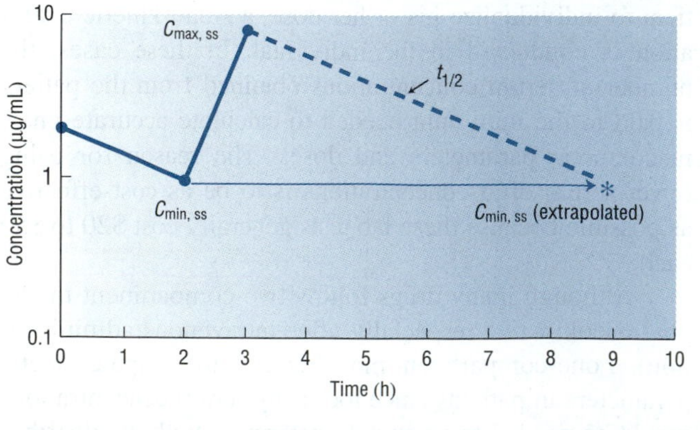

FIGURE 3–10. When a patient has received enough doses to be at steady state, steady-state maximum ($C_{max,ss}$) and minimum ($C_{min,ss}$) concentrations can be used to compute clearance, volume of distribution, and half-life. At steady state, consecutive $C_{min,ss}$ are equal, so the predose value can be extrapolated to the time before the next dose and be used to calculate half-life (dashed line).

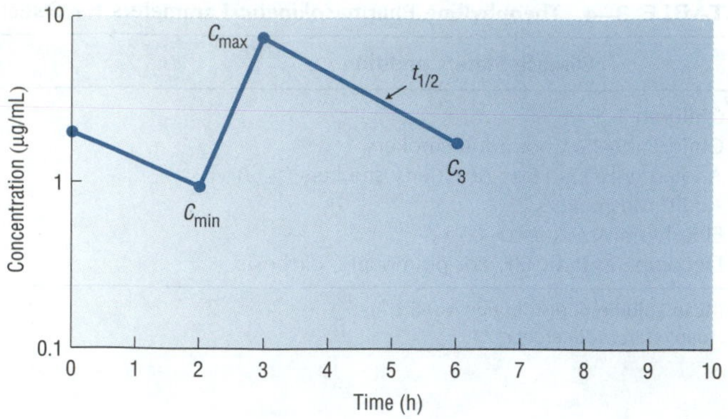

FIGURE 3–11. If a patient has not received enough doses to be at steady state, or doses have been given on an irregular schedule, the minimum concentration (C_{min}), maximum concentration (C_{max}), and an additional postdose concentration (C_3) can be used to compute clearance, volume of distribution, and half-life.

a concentration too low for the assay to detect. In this situation, the predose minimum and postdose maximum concentrations are used to compute V and both postdose concentrations are used to calculate $t_{1/2}$ (Fig. 3–11).

After Cl, V, and $t_{1/2}$ have been computed for a patient, the dose and dosage interval necessary to achieve desired steady-state serum concentrations can be calculated using one-compartment model equations. Specific examples of these methods to calculate initial doses and individualized doses using serum concentrations are discussed later in this chapter for the aminoglycoside antibiotics, vancomycin, digoxin, theophylline, and phenytoin.

COMPUTER PROGRAMS

Computer programs that aid in the individualization of therapy are available for many different drugs. The most sophisticated programs use nonlinear regression to fit Cl and V_D to actual serum concentrations obtained in a patient.[28] After drug doses and serum concentrations are entered into the computer, nonlinear least-squares regression programs adjust Cl and V_D until the sum of the squared error between actual (C_{act}) and computer-estimated concentrations (C_{est}) is at a minimum $[\Sigma(C_{est} - C_{act})^2]$. Once estimates of Cl and V_D are available, doses are easily calculated.

Many programs also take into account what the Cl and V_D should be on the basis of disease states and conditions present in the patient.[29] Incorporation of expected population-based parameters allows the computer to use a limited number of serum concentrations (one or two) to provide estimates of Cl and V_D. This type of computer program is called "Bayesian" because it incorporates portions of Bayes' theorem during the fitting routine.[30] Bayesian pharmacokinetic dosing programs are widely used to adjust the dose of a variety of drugs. In the case of renally eliminated drugs (aminoglycosides, vancomycin, digoxin), population estimates for kinetic parameters are generated by entering the patient's age, weight, height, gender, and serum creatinine concentration into the computer program. For hepatically eliminated drugs (theophylline, phenytoin) population estimates for kinetic parameters are computed using the patient's age, weight, and gender as well as other factors that might change hepatic clearance, such as the presence or absence of disease states (cirrhosis, congestive heart failure) or other drug therapy that might cause a drug interaction. The Bayesian estimates of the pharmacokinetic parameters are then modified using nonlinear least-squares regression fits of serum concentrations to result in individualized parameters for the patient. The individualized parameters are used to compute doses for the patient that will result in desired steady-state concentrations of the drug.

AMINOGLYCOSIDES

Although aminoglycoside pharmacokinetics follow multicompartment models,[31] a one-compartment model appears sufficient to individualize doses in patients.[32] Aminoglycosides are usually given as short-term intermittent intravenous infusions and administered as a single daily dose or multiple doses per day. Initial doses for aminoglycosides can be computed using estimated kinetic parameters derived from population pharmacokinetic data. The elimination rate constant is estimated using the patient's creatinine clearance in the following formula: k (in h^{-1}) = 0.00293 (CrCl) + 0.014, where CrCl is the measured or estimated creatinine clearance in mL/min. The volume of distribution is estimated using the average population value for normal-weight (within 30% of ideal weight) individuals equal to 0.26 L/kg [$V = 0.26$ (Wt), where Wt is patient weight] or for obese individuals (over 30% ideal weight)[33] by taking into account the patient's excess adipose tissue: $V = 0.26$ [IBW + 0.4(TBW − IBW)], where IBW is ideal body weight [IBW_{males} (in kg) = 50 + 2.3 (Ht − 60) or $IBW_{females}$ (in kg) = 45 + 2.3 (Ht − 60), where Ht is patient height in inches]. Additional volume of distribution population estimates are available for other disease states and conditions such as cystic fibrosis,[34] ascites,[35] or neonates.[36]

Appropriate $C_{max,ss}$ and $C_{min,ss}$ values are selected for the patient based on the site and severity of the infection and the sensitivity of the known or suspected pathogen as well as avoidance of adverse effects. For example, $C_{max,ss}$ values of 8–10 mg/L are generally selected for gram-negative pneumonia patients, whereas $C_{min,ss}$ less than 2 mg/L are usually chosen to avoid aminoglycoside-induced nephrotoxicity when tobramycin and gentamicin are prescribed using conventional multiple daily dosing regimens. Once appropriate steady-state serum concentrations are selected, the dosage interval required to achieve those concentrations is calculated and τ is rounded to a clinically acceptable value (e.g., 8, 12, 18, 24, 36, 48 hours): $\tau = [(\ln C_{max,ss} - \ln C_{min,ss})/k] + T$. Finally, a dose is computed for the patient using the one-compartment model intermittent intravenous infusion equation at steady state, and the dose is rounded off to the nearest 5–10 mg:

$$D = TkV_D C_{max,ss}[(1 - e^{-k\tau})/(1 - e^{-kT})]$$

The Hull and Sarrubi aminoglycoside dosage nomogram (Table 3–5) is based on this dosage calculation method and includes precalculated doses and dosage intervals for a variety of creatinine clearance values.[22] The nomogram assumes $V_D = 0.26$ L/kg and should not be used to compute doses for disease states with altered V_D.

An example of this initial dosage scheme for a typical case is provided to illustrate the use of the various equations. Mr. JJ is a 65-year-old, 80-kg, 6-ft tall male with the diagnosis of gram-negative pneumonia. His serum creatinine equals 2.1 mg/dL and is stable. Compute a gentamicin

TABLE 3–5. Aminoglycoside Dosage Chart

1. Compute patient's creatinine clearance (CrCl) using Cockcroft–Gault method: CrCl = [(140 − age)BW]/(Scr × 72). Multiply by 0.85 for females.
2. Use patient's weight if within 30% of IBW; otherwise use adjusted dosing weight = IBW + [0.40(TBW − IBW)].
3. Select loading dose in mg/kg to provide peak serum concentrations in range listed below for the desired aminoglycoside antibiotic:

Aminoglycoside	Usual Loading Doses	Expected Peak Serum Concentrations
Tobramycin Gentamicin Netilmicin	1.5 to 2.0 mg/kg	4 to 10 μg/mL
Amikacin Kanamycin	5.0 to 7.5 mg/kg	15 to 30 μg/mL

4. Select maintenance dose (as percentage of loading dose) to continue peak serum concentrations indicated above according to desired dosage interval and the patient's creatinine clearance. To maintain usual peak/trough ratio, use dosage intervals in clear areas.

Percentage of Loading Dose Required for Dosage Interval Selected

CrCl (mL/min)	Est. half-life (h)	8 h (%)	12 h (%)	24 h (%)
>90	2–3	90	—	—
90	3.1	84	—	—
80	3.4	80	91	—
70	3.9	76	88	—
60	4.5	71	84	—
50	5.3	65	79	—
40	6.5	57	72	92
30	8.4	48	63	86
25	9.9	43	57	81
20	11.9	37	50	75
17	13.6	33	46	70
15	15.1	31	42	67
12	17.9	27	37	61
10[a]	20.4	24	34	56
7[a]	25.9	19	28	47
5[a]	31.5	16	23	41
2[a]	46.8	11	16	30
0[a]	69.3	8	11	21

[a]Note: Dosing for patients with CrCl ≤ 10 mL/min should be assisted by measuring serum concentrations.

Adapted from Sarubbi, Hull.[22]

dosage regimen (infused over 1 hour) that would provide approximate peak and trough concentrations of $C_{max,ss}$ = 8 mg/L and $C_{min,ss}$ = 1.5 mg/L, respectively. The patient is within 30% of his ideal body weight (IBW_{male} = 50 + 2.3 (72 in. – 60) = 78 kg) and has stable renal function, so the Cockcroft–Gault creatinine clearance estimation equation can be used: $CrCl_{est}$ = [(140 – 65 y)80 kg]/[72(2.1 mg/dL)] = 40 mL/min. The patient's weight and estimated creatinine clearance are used to compute his V and k, respectively: V = 0.26 L/kg (80 kg) = 20.8 L, k = 0.00293 (40 mL/min) + 0.014 = 0.131 h^{-1} or $t_{1/2}$ = 0.693/0.131 h^{-1} = 5.3 h. The dosage interval and dose for the desired serum concentrations would then be calculated: τ = [(ln 8 mg/L – ln 1.5 mg/L)/0.131 h^{-1}] + 1 h = 13.7 h rounded to 12 h, D = (1 h)(0.131 h^{-1})(20.8 L)(8 mg/L)[(1 – $e^{-(0.131\ h^{-1})(12\ h)}$)/(1 – $e^{-(0.131\ h^{-1})(1\ h)}$)] = 140 mg. Thus, the prescribed dose would be gentamicin 140 mg every 12 hours administered as a 1-hour infusion. If a loading dose were deemed necessary, it would be given as the first dose [LD = (20.8 L)(8 mg/L) = 166 mg rounded to 170 mg infused over 1 hour], and the first maintenance dose administered 12 hours (e.g., one dosage interval) later.

If appropriate aminoglycoside serum concentrations are available, kinetic parameters can be calculated at any point in therapy. When the patient is not at steady-state, serum aminoglycoside concentrations are obtained before a dose (C_{min}), after a dose administered as an intravenous infusion of about 1 hour, or as a ½-hour infusion followed by a ½-hour waiting period to allow for drug distribution (C_{max}), and at one additional postdose time (C_3) approximately one estimated $t_{1/2}$ after C_{max}. The $t_{1/2}$ and k are computed using C_{max} and C_3: $k = (\ln C_{max} - \ln C_3)/\Delta t$ and $t_{1/2} = 0.693/k$, where Δt is the time that expired between the times C_{max} and C_3 were obtained. If the patient is at steady state, serum aminoglycoside concentrations are obtained before a dose ($C_{min,ss}$) and after a dose adminstered as an intravenous infusion of about 1 hour or as a ½-hour infusion followed by a ½-hour waiting period to allow for drug distribution ($C_{max,ss}$). The $t_{1/2}$ and k are computed using $C_{max,ss}$ and $C_{min,ss}$: $k = (\ln C_{max,ss} - \ln C_{min,ss})/(\tau - T)$ and $t_{1/2} = 0.693/k$, where τ is the dosage interval and T is the dose infusion time or dose infusion time plus waiting time.

Assuming a one-compartment model, the following equation is used to compute V_D[32]:

$$V_D = [(D/T)(1 - e^{-kT})]/\{k[C_{max} - (C_{min}e^{-kT})]\}$$

where D is dose and T is duration of infusion. Once these are known, the dose and dosage interval (τ) can be calculated for any desired maximum $C_{ss}(C_{max,ss})$ and minimum $C_{ss}(C_{min,ss})$:

$$\tau = [(\ln C_{max,ss} - \ln C_{min,ss})/k] + T$$

$$D = TkV_DC_{max,ss}[(1 - e^{-k\tau})/(1 - e^{-kT})]$$

The dose and dosage interval should be rounded to provide clinically accepted values (every 8, 12, 18, 24, 36, 48 hours for dosage interval, nearest 5–10 mg for dose). This method has also been used to individualize intravenous theophylline dosage regimens.[37]

To provide an example for this technique, the problem given previously will be extended to include steady-state concentrations. Mr. JJ was prescribed gentamicin 140 mg every 12 hours (infused over 1 hour) for the treatment of gram-negative pneumonia. Steady-state trough ($C_{min,ss}$) and peak ($C_{max,ss}$) were obtained before and after the fourth dose was given (> three to five estimated $t_{1/2}$), respectively, and equaled $C_{min,ss}$ = 2.8 mg/L and $C_{max,ss}$ = 8.5 mg/L. Clinically, the patient was improving with decreased white blood cell counts and body temperatures and a resolving chest x-ray. However, the serum creatinine value had increased to 2.5 mg/dL. Because of this, a new dosage regimen with a similar peak (to maintain high intrapulmonary levels) but lower trough (to decrease the risk of drug-induced nephrotoxicity) concentration was suggested. The patient's elimination rate constant and half-life can be computed using the following formulas: k = (ln 8.5 mg/L – ln 2.8 mg/L)/(12 h – 1 h) = 0.101 h^{-1}, $t_{1/2}$ = 0.693/0.101 h^{-1} = 6.9 h. The patient's volume of distribution can be calculated using the following equation:

$$V = [(140\ mg/1\ h)(1 - e^{-(0.101\ h^{-1})(1\ h)})]/\{0.101\ h^{-1}[8.5\ mg/L - ((2.8\ mg/L)e^{-(0.101\ h^{-1})(1\ h)})]\} = 22.3\ L$$

Thus, the patient's volume of distribution was larger and half-life was longer than originally estimated, and this led to higher serum concentrations than anticipated. To achieve the desired serum concentrations ($C_{min,ss}$ = 1.5 mg/L and $C_{max,ss}$ = 8 mg/L), the patient's actual kinetic parameters are used to compute a new dose and dosage interval: τ = [(ln 8 mg/L – ln 1.5 mg/L)/0.101 h^{-1}] + 1 h = 17.6 h, rounded to 18 h and

$$D = (1\ h)(0.101\ h^{-1})(22.3\ L)(8\ mg/L)[(1 - e^{-(0.101\ h^{-1})(18\ h)})/(1 - e^{-(0.101\ h^{-1})(1\ h)})] = 157\ mg, \text{ rounded to } 160\ mg$$

Thus, the new dose would be gentamicin 160 mg every 18 hours and infused over 1 hour; the first dose of the new dosage regimen would be given 18 hours (e.g., the new dosage interval) after the last dose of the old dosage regimen.

VANCOMYCIN

Vancomycin requires multicompartment models to completely describe its serum concentration-versus-time curves. However, if peak serum concentrations are obtained after the distribution phase is completed (usually ½ to 1 hour after a 1-hour intravenous infusion), a one-compartment model can be used for patient dosage calculation. Also, since vancomycin has a relatively long $t_{1/2}$ compared to the infusion time, only a small amount of drug is eliminated during infusion, and it is usually not necessary to use more complex intravenous infusion equations. Thus, simple IV bolus equations can be used to calculate vancomycin doses for most patients. Although a recent review paper[38] questioned the clinical usefulness of measuring vancomycin concentrations on a routine basis, research articles[39,40] have shown potential benefits in obtaining vancomycin concentrations in selected patient populations. The decision to conduct vancomycin concentration monitoring should be made on a patient-to-patient basis.

Initial doses of vancomycin can be computed for adult patients using estimated kinetic parameters derived from population pharmacokinetic data. Clearance is estimated using the patient's creatinine clearance in the following equation[41]: Cl (in mL/min/kg) = 0.695 (CrCl in mL/min/kg) + 0.05. The volume of distribution is computed assuming the standard value of 0.7 L/kg: $V_D = 0.7$ (Wt), where Wt is patient weight. In the case of obese patients, actual or total body weight is used in the calculations.[42] The elimination rate constant is calculated using clearance and volume of distribution estimates, correcting for possible differences in units for these parameters: $k = Cl/V_D$. A nomogram that uses this type of approach for vancomycin therapy is available to rapidly determine initial doses for patients (Table 3–6).[43]

Steady-state peak and trough concentrations are chosen for the patient based on the site and severity of the infection as well as the known or suspected pathogen and avoidance of potential side effects. $C_{max,ss}$ values between 25 and 35 mg/L and $C_{min,ss}$ values between 5 and 10 mg/L are typically used for patients with moderate-to-severe methicillin-resistant *Staphylococcus aureus* infections. After appropriate steady-state concentrations are chosen, the dosage interval required to attain those concentrations is computed, and τ is rounded to a clinically acceptable value (12, 18, 24, 36, 48, 72 hours): $\tau = [(\ln C_{max,ss} - \ln C_{min,ss})/k] + T_{max}$, where T_{max} is the combined infusion time (usually 1 hour) and waiting time after the end of the infusion (usually ½ to 1 hour) before $C_{max,ss}$ is obtained. Finally, the maintenance dose is computed for the patient using a one-compartment model intravenous bolus equation at steady state, and the dose is rounded off to the nearest 50 to 100 mg:

$$D = [C_{max,ss} V_D (1 - e^{-k\tau})]/e^{-kT_{max}}$$

If desired, a loading dose can be computed using the following equation: $LD = V_D C_{max,ss}$.

The following case will illustrate the use of this dosage methodology. Ms. HJ is a 65-year-old, 68-kg, 5-ft 4-in. tall S/P CABG surgery patient who has developed a surgical wound infection with *S. aureus* the suspected pathogen. Her serum creatinine is 1.8 mg/dL and stable. Compute a vancomycin dosage regimen that would provide approximate peak (obtained 1 hour after a 1-hour infusion) and trough concentrations of 30 mg/L and 7 mg/L, respectively. The patient is within 30% of her ideal body weight [IBW_{female} = 45 + 2.3 (64 in. – 60) = 54 kg] and has stable renal function, so the Cockcroft–Gault creatinine clearance estimation formula can be used: $CrCl_{est}$ = 0.85[(140 – 65 y) 68 kg]/ [72(1.8 mg/dL)] = 33 mL/min. The patient's weight and estimated creatinine clearance are used to calculate her estimated Cl, V_D, and k, respectively: Cl = 0.695 (33 mL/min/68 kg) + 0.05 = 0.387 mL/min/kg, V_D = 0.7 L/kg (68 kg) = 48 L, k = [(0.387 mL/min/kg)(68 kg)(60 min/h)]/[(48 L)(1000 mL/L)] = 0.033 h^{-1} or $t_{1/2}$ = 0.693/ 0.033 h^{-1} = 21 h. The dosage interval, maintenance dose, and loading dose for the desired serum concentrations can then be computed: τ = [(ln 30 mg/L – ln 7 mg/L)/0.033 h^{-1}] + 2 h = 46 h rounded to 48 h, $D = [(30\ mg/L)\ (48\ L)(1 - e^{-(0.033\ h-1)(48\ h)})]/e^{-(0.033\ h^{-1})(2\ h)}$ = 1222 mg rounded to 1200 mg, LD = (48 L)(30 mg/L) = 1440 mg rounded to 1450 mg. Therefore, the prescribed dosed would be vancomycin 1200 mg every 48 hours administered as a 1-hour infusion. If a loading dose was used, it would be given as the first dose, and the first maintenance dose administered 48 hours (one dosage interval) later.

If appropriate vancomycin serum concentrations are available, kinetic parameters can be computed at any point in therapy. When the patient is not at steady state, serum vancomycin concentrations are obtained before a dose (C_{min}), after a dose administered as an intravenous infusion of an hour followed by a ½- to 1-hour waiting period to allow for drug distribution (C_{max}), and at one additional postdose time (C_3) approximately one estimated $t_{1/2}$ after C_{max}. The $t_{1/2}$ and k are computed using C_{max} and C_3: $k = (\ln C_{max} - \ln C_3)/\Delta t$ and $t_{1/2} = 0.693/k$, where Δt is the time that expired between the times C_{max} and C_3 were obtained. If the patient is at steady state, serum vancomycin concentrations are obtained before a dose ($C_{min,ss}$) and after a dose adminstered as an intravenous infusion of about 1 hour followed by a ½- to 1-hour waiting period to allow for drug distribution ($C_{max,ss}$). The $t_{1/2}$ and k are computed using $C_{max,ss}$ and

TABLE 3–6. Vancomycin Dosage Chart

1. Compute patient's creatinine clearance (CrCl) using Cockcroft–Gault method: CrCl = [(140 – age)BW]/(S_{cr} × 72). Multiply by 0.85 for females.
2. Use patient's total body weight to compute doses.
3. Dosage chart designed to achieve peak serum concentrations of 30 µg/mL and trough concentrations of 7.5 µg/mL.
4. Compute loading dose of 25 mg/kg.
5. Compute maintenance dose of 19 mg/kg given at the dosage interval listed in the following chart for the patient's CrCl:

Cr Cl (mL/min)	Dosage interval (days)
≥120	0.5
100	0.6
80	0.75
60	1.0
40	1.5
30	2.0
20	2.5
10	4.0
5	6.0
0	12.0

Adapted from Ref. 43.

$C_{min,ss}$: $k = (\ln C_{max,ss} - \ln C_{min,ss})/(\tau - T_{max})$ and $t_{1/2} = 0.693/k$, where τ is the dosage interval and T_{max} is the dose infusion time plus waiting time.

Assuming a one-compartment model, the following equation is used to compute V_D:

$$V_D = D/[(C_{max}/e^{-kT_{max}}) - C_{min}]$$

where D is dose and T_{max} is the dose infusion time plus waiting time. Once these are known, the dose and dosage interval (τ) can be calculated for any desired maximum $C_{ss}(C_{max,ss})$ and minimum $C_{ss}(C_{min,ss})$:

$$\tau = [(\ln C_{max,ss} - \ln C_{min,ss})/k] + T_{max}$$

$$D = [C_{max,ss}V_D(1 - e^{-k\tau})]/e^{-kT_{max}}$$

The dose and dosage interval should be rounded to provide clinically accepted values (every 12, 18, 24, 36, 48, 72 hours for dosage interval, nearest 50 to 100 mg for dose).

To provide an example for this dosage-calculation method, the previous problem will be extended to include steady-state concentrations. Ms. HJ was prescribed vancomycin 1200 mg every 48 hours (infused over 1 hour) for the treatment of a surgical wound infection. Steady-state trough ($C_{min,ss}$) and peak ($C_{max,ss}$), obtained 1 hour after end of infusion, were obtained before and after the third dose was given (> three to five estimated $t_{1/2}$), respectively, and equaled $C_{min,ss}$ = 2.5 mg/L and $C_{max,ss}$ = 22.4 mg/L. Clinically, the patient had improved somewhat, but the WBC was still elevated and the patient was still febrile. Because of this, a modified dosage regimen with a $C_{max,ss}$ = 30 mg/L and $C_{min,ss}$ = 7 mg/L was suggested to maintain trough concentrations three to five times above the minimal inhibitory concentration (MIC) for the suspected pathogen. The patient's actual elimination rate constant and half-life can be calculated using the following formulas: $k = (\ln 22.4 \text{ mg/L} - \ln 2.5 \text{ mg/L})/(48 \text{ h} - 2 \text{ h}) = 0.048 \text{ h}^{-1}$, $t_{1/2} = 0.693/0.048 \text{ h}^{-1} = 14.4$ h. The patient's volume of distribution can be calculated using the following equation:

$$V_D = 1200 \text{ mg}/\{[(22.4 \text{ mg/L})/e^{-(0.048 \text{ h}^{-1})(2 \text{ h})}] - (2.5 \text{ mg/L})\} = 54 \text{ L}$$

Thus, the patient's volume of distribution was larger and half-life shorter than originally estimated, and this led to lower serum concentrations than anticipated. To achieve the desired serum concentrations ($C_{max,ss}$ = 30 mg/L and $C_{min,ss}$ = 7 mg/L), the patient's actual kinetic parameters are used to calculate a new dose and dosage interval:

$$\tau = [(\ln 30 \text{ mg/L} - \ln 7 \text{ mg/L})/0.048 \text{ h}^{-1}] + 2 \text{ h} = 32 \text{ h rounded to } 36 \text{ h}$$

$$D = [(30 \text{ mg/L})(54 \text{ L})(1 - e^{-(0.048 \text{ h}^{-1})(36 \text{ h})})]/e^{-(0.048 \text{ h}^{-1})(2 \text{ h})} = 1466 \text{ mg rounded to } 1500 \text{ mg}$$

The new dose would be vancomycin 1500 mg every 36 hours (infused over 1 hour); the first dose of the new dosage regimen would be given 36 hours (the new dosage interval) after the last dose of the old dosage regimen.

DIGOXIN

Digoxin pharmacokinetics are best described by a two-compartment model. However, because digoxin has a long half-life compared to its dosage interval and a very long distribution phase, simple pharmacokinetic equations can be used to individualize dosing when postdistribution serum concentrations are used. Digoxin can be given as an intravenous injection and orally as elixir (F = 0.8), tablets (F = 0.7), or capsules (F = 0.9). When given orally, the appropriate bioavailability fraction must be used to compute the correct dose. Initial doses of digoxin can be computed using population pharmacokinetic data obtained from published studies. Digoxin clearance is estimated using the patient's creatinine clearance in the following formula[20]: Cl (in mL/min) = 1.101 (CrCl in mL/min) + Cl_m, where Cl_m is metabolic clearance and equals 40 mL/min for patients with no or mild heart failure or 20 mL/min for patients with moderate-severe heart failure. The volume of distribution decreases with declining renal function and is estimated using the following equation[20]: V_D (in L) = 225 + {[298 (CrCl in mL/min)]/[29.1 + (CrCl in mL/min)]}. The elimination rate constant can be computed by taking the product of Cl and V_D: $k = Cl/V_D$. For obese individuals, digoxin dosing should be based on ideal body weight.[44]

Appropriate C_{ss} values are chosen for the patient based on the disease state being treated, the goal of therapy, and the avoidance of adverse effects. The inotropic effects of digoxin occur at lower concentrations than do the chronotropic effects. Therefore, initial serum concentrations of digoxin for the treatment of heart failure are generally ≤ 1 ng/mL and for the treatment of atrial fibrillation 1–1.5 ng/mL. Once the appropriate C_{ss} is selected, a dose is computed for the patient: $D/\tau = (C_{ss}Cl)/F$.

An example of this initial dosage scheme is provided in the following case. Mr. PO is a 72-year-old, 83-kg, 5-ft 11-in. male admitted to the hospital for the treatment of community-acquired pneumonia. While in the hospital, Mr. PO develops atrial fibrillation and the decision is made to treat him with digoxin to provide ventricular rate control. His serum creatinine is 2.5 mg/dL and stable. Calculate an intravenous loading dose and oral maintenance dose that will achieve a C_{ss} = 1.5 ng/mL. The Cockcroft–Gault equation can be used to estimate the patient's creatinine clearance since his serum creatinine is stable and he is within 30% of his ideal weight [IBW_{male} = 50 + 2.3 (71 in. – 60) = 75 kg]: CrCl = [(140 – 72 y)83 kg]/[72(2.5 mg/dL)] = 31 mL/min. Using the estimated CrCl, both Cl and V_D can be computed:

$$Cl = 1.101(31 \text{ mL/min}) + 40 = 74 \text{ mL/min}$$

$$V_D = 225 + \{[298\ (31 \text{ mL/min})]/[29.1 + (31 \text{ mL/min})]\} = 379 \text{ L}$$

The maintenance dose will be given as digoxin tablets, so F = 0.7 in the dosing equation: D/τ = [(1.5 μg/L)(74 mL/min)(60 min/h)(24 h/d)]/[0.7(1000 mL/L)] =

228 μg/d rounded to 250 μg/d. The loading dose will be given intravenously as digoxin injection: LD = (1.5 μg/L) (379 L) = 568 μg rounded to 500 μg. The loading dose would be given 50% now (250 μg), 25% (125 μg) in 4 to 6 hours after monitoring the patient's heart rate and blood pressure and assessing the patient for digoxin adverse effects, and the final 25% (125 μg) 4 to 6 hours later after monitoring the same clinical parameters. The first maintenance dose would be given one dosage interval (in this case 24 hours) after the first part of the loading dose was given.

Adjustment of digoxin doses using steady-state concentrations is accomplished using linear pharmacokinetics and dosage ratios: $D_{new} = D_{old}(C_{ss,new}/C_{ss,old})$. For example, Mr. PO's atrial fibrillation responded to digoxin therapy, and he was discharged after resolution of his pneumonia. A month later, he was followed up in the clinic with moderate nausea possibly due to digoxin toxicity. His heart rate was 55 beats/min. A steady-state digoxin concentration was obtained and reported by the clinic lab as 2.2 μg/L. Compute a new dose for the patient to achieve a C_{ss} = 1.5 μg/L. The digoxin C_{ss} and old dose would be used to calculate a new dose using the linear pharmacokinetic equation: D_{new} = 250 μg/d [(1.5 μg/L)/(2.2 μg/L)] = 170 μg/d. This approximate average daily dose could be achieved by having the patient alternate taking one 250-μg tablet and one-half 250-μg tablet (125 μg) daily giving an average dose equal to 187.5 μg/d ([250 μg + 125 μg]/ 2 = 187.5 μg/d).

THEOPHYLLINE

Theophylline disposition is most accurately described by nonlinear kinetics.[45,46] However, at the usual doses, theophylline acts as if it obeys linear kinetics in most patients. Initial theophylline doses are computed by taking a detailed medical history of the patient and noting disease states and conditions that are known to change theophylline disposition. Age, smoking of tobacco-containing products, heart failure, and liver disease are among the important factors that alter theophylline kinetic parameters and dosage requirements. Once the patient has been assessed, average theophylline kinetic parameters obtained from the literature for patients similar to the one being currently treated are used to compute either oral or intravenous doses. Dosage guidelines that take into account most common disease states and conditions that change theophylline kinetic parameters are available (Table 3–4).[47] Once theophylline is administered, the patient is monitored for the therapeutic effect and potential adverse effects. Theophylline concentrations are then used to individualize the theophylline dose that the patient receives. An example of this approach was given previously for a patient case in the section on drug dosing in patients with liver disease.

Continuous intravenous infusions of theophylline (or its salt, aminophylline) can be rapidly individualized by determining the patient's Cl before steady state occurs.[48] Assuming the patient receives theophylline only by continuous intravenous infusion (previous doses of sustained-release oral theophylline are completely absorbed), two serum theophylline concentrations are obtained 4 or more hours apart. The infusion rate (k_0) cannot be changed between the times the concentrations are drawn. With one-compartment model equations, the first (C_1) and second (C_2) theophylline concentrations are used to calculate theophylline Cl:

$$\mathrm{Cl} = 2k_0/(C_1 + C_2) + [2V_D(C_1 - C_2)/(C_1 + C_2)(t_2 - t_1)]$$

V_D is assumed to be 0.5 L/kg and t_1 and t_2 are the times at which C_1 and C_2, respectively, are obtained. Once Cl is known, k_0 can be easily computed for any desired C_{ss}(C_{ss} = k_0/Cl). This method can probably be applied to other drugs that are administered as continuous intravenous infusions, such as intravenous antiarrhythmics, when rapid individualization of drug dosage is desirable.

An example of this approach can be obtained by continuing the theophylline patient case from the section on drug dosing in liver disease. In this example, a 55-year-old, 70-kg male with liver cirrhosis was prescribed a loading dose of theophylline 350 mg IV over 20 to 30 minutes followed by a maintenance dose of 15 mg/h of theophylline as a continuous infusion. The infusion began at 0900H, blood samples were obtained at 1000H and 1600H, and the clinical lab reported the theophylline serum concentrations as 9.6 mg/L and 12.3 mg/L, respectively. The patient's theophylline clearance and revised continuous infusion to maintain a C_{ss} = 15 mg/L can be computed as follows (patient's V_D estimated at 0.5 L/kg):

$$\begin{aligned}\mathrm{Cl} = {} & 2(15\ \mathrm{mg/h})/(10.9\ \mathrm{mg/L} + 12.3\ \mathrm{mg/L}) \\ & + [2(0.5\ \mathrm{L/kg} \times 70\ \mathrm{kg})(10.9\ \mathrm{mg/L} - 12.3\ \mathrm{mg/L})/ \\ & (10.9\ \mathrm{mg/L} + 12.3\ \mathrm{mg/L})(16 - 10\ \mathrm{h})]\end{aligned}$$

$$\mathrm{Cl} = 0.59\ \mathrm{L/h}$$

$$k_0 = C_{ss}\mathrm{Cl} = (15\ \mathrm{mg/L})(0.59\ \mathrm{L/h}) = 9\ \mathrm{mg/h\ theophylline}$$

If theophylline is to be given as the aminophylline salt form, the doses would need to be changed to reflect the fact that aminophylline contains only 85% theophylline (k_0 = 9 mg/h theophylline/0.85 = 11 mg/h aminophylline).

If continuous intravenous infusions or oral dosage regimens are given long enough for steady state to occur (three to five estimated $t_{1/2}$ based on previous studies conducted in similar patients), linear pharmacokinetics can be used to adjust doses for either route of administration: $D_{new} = D_{old}(C_{ss,new}/C_{ss,old})$. For example, a patient receiving 200 mg of sustained-release oral theophylline every 12 hours with a theophylline steady-state serum concentration of 9.5 μg/mL can have the dose required to achieve a new steady-state concentration equal to 15 μg/mL computed by applying linear pharmacokinetics: D_{new} = 200 mg [(15 μg/mL)/(9.5 μg/mL)] = 316 mg, rounded to 300 mg. Thus, the new theophylline dose would be 300 mg every 12 hours.

PHENYTOIN

Phenytoin doses are very difficult to individualize because the drug follows Michaelis-Menten kinetics, and there is a large amount of interpatient variability in V_{max} and K_m. Initial maintenance doses of phenytoin in adults usually range between 4 and 7 mg/kg/d yielding starting doses of 300–400 mg/d in most individuals. If needed, loading doses of phenytoin or fosphenytoin (a prodrug of phenytoin used intravenously) can be administered in adults at a dose of 15 mg/kg, which is approximately 1000 mg in many individuals. Loading doses of phenytoin can be given orally, but need to be administered in divided doses separated by several hours in order to avoid decreased bioavailability (400 mg, 300 mg, then 300 mg with each dose separated by 4 to 6 hours). Since phenytoin is hepatically metabolized, decreased doses may be needed in patients with liver disease. Because phenytoin follows dose-dependent pharmacokinetics, the half-life of phenytoin increases for a patient as the maintenance dose increases. Therefore, the time to steady-state phenytoin concentrations increases with dose. On average, at a phenytoin dose of 300 mg/d it takes approximately 5 to 7 days to achieve steady state, at a dose of 400 mg/d it takes approximately 10 to 14 days to achieve steady state, and at a dose of 500 mg/d it takes approximately 21 to 28 days to achieve steady state. It should be noted that the injectable and capsule dosage forms of phenytoin are phenytoin sodium, and the labeled dosage amounts contain 92% of active phenytoin (300 mg of phenytoin sodium capsules contains 276 mg [300 mg × 0.92 = 276 mg] of active phenytoin). Unbound phenytoin concentrations are useful in patients with hypoalbuminemia (pregnancy, trauma, liver disease) or in patients receiving other drugs that may displace phenytoin from plasma-protein-binding sights (valproic acid, salicylates, warfarin).

After steady state has occurred, phenytoin serum concentrations can be obtained as an aid to dosage adjustment. A simple, easy way to approximate new serum concentrations after a dosage adjustment with phenytoin is to temporarily assume linear pharmacokinetics, then add 15% to 20% for a dosage increase or subtract 15% to 20% for a dosage decrease to account for Michaelis-Menten kinetics. For example, Ms. PP is a 35-year-old, 65-kg patient with grand mal seizures who is receiving phenytoin capsules 300 mg orally at bedtime. A steady-state concentration of 9.2 μg/mL is measured. It is observed that her seizure frequency decreased by only about 15% and that she has no adverse effects due to phenytoin treatment. Because of this, her phenytoin dose is increased to 400 mg orally at bedtime. The expected phenytoin steady-state concentration would be estimated using linear pharmacokinetics ($C_{new} = [D_{new}/D_{old}]C_{old}$ = [400 mg/300 mg]/(9.2 μg/mL) = 12.3 μg/mL) then increased by 15% to 20% to account for nonlinear kinetics (C_{new} = 1.15 (12.3 μg/mL) = 14.1 μg/mL. (Note: A 15% increase was chosen for an estimated concentration < 15 μg/mL; a 20% increase would be used if the estimated concentration was ≥ 15 μg/mL.) Thus, the patient

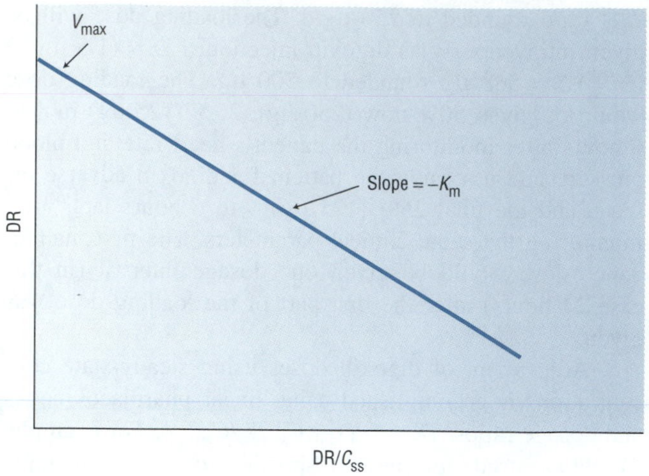

FIGURE 3–12. Relationship between dosage rate (DR) and steady-state serum concentrations (C_{ss}).

would be expected to have a steady-state phenytoin concentration of approximately 14 μg/mL due to the dosage increase. An alternative approach would be to use a graphical Bayesian method that allows an estimate of V_{max} and K_m from one steady-state phenytoin concentration and the prediction of new steady-state concentrations when doses are changed.[49]

Other methods used to individualize phenytoin doses involve rearrangements of the Michaelis-Menten equation [$DR = V_{max}C_{ss}/(K_m + C_{ss})$, in which DR is the dosage rate at steady state] so that two or more doses and C_{ss} values can be used to obtain graphic solutions for V_{max} and K_m. One rearrangement[50] is $DR = -K_m(DR/C_{ss}) + V_{max}$. When DR is plotted on the y axis and DR/C_{ss} is plotted on the x axis of Cartesian graph paper, a straight line with a y intercept of V_{max} and slope equal to $-K_m$ is found (Fig. 3–12). To use this method, patients are prescribed an initial phenytoin dose and C_{ss} is obtained. The phenytoin dose is then changed and a second C_{ss} from the new dose is obtained. Each dose is divided by its respective C_{ss} to derive DR/C_{ss} values. The DR/C_{ss} and C_{ss} values are plotted on the graph to calculate V_{max} (y intercept) and K_m (−slope). The steady-state Michaelis-Menten equation can be used to compute C_{ss} for a given DR or a DR for any C_{ss}.

CLINICAL PHARMACODYNAMICS

Pharmacodynamics is the study of the relationship between the concentration of a drug and the response obtained in a patient. Originally, investigators examined the dose–response relationship of drugs in humans, but found that the same dose of a drug usually resulted in different concentrations in individuals because of pharmacokinetic differences in clearance and volume of distribution. Examples of quantifiable pharmacodynamic measurements include changes in blood pressure during antihypertensive drug therapy, decreases in heart rate during β-blocker treatment, and alterations in prothrombin time or INR during warfarin therapy.

For drugs that exhibit a direct and reversible effect, the following diagram describes what occurs at the level of the drug receptor:

Drug + Receptor ↔ Drug–receptor complex ↔ Response

According to this scheme, there is a drug receptor located within the target organ or tissue. When a drug molecule "finds" the receptor, it forms a complex that causes the pharmacologic response to occur. The drug and receptor are in dynamic equilibrium with the drug–receptor complex.

THE E_{max} AND SIGMOID E_{max} MODELS

The mathematical model that comes from the classic drug receptor theory shown previously is known as the E_{max} model:

$$E = \frac{E_{max} \times C}{EC_{50} + C}$$

where E is the pharmacologic effect elicited by the drug, E_{max} is the maximum effect the drug can cause, EC_{50} is the concentration causing one-half of the maximum drug effect ($E_{max}/2$), and C is the concentration of drug at the receptor site. EC_{50} can be used as a measure of drug potency (a lower EC_{50} indicating a more potent drug), whereas E_{max} reflects the intrinsic efficacy of the drug (a higher E_{max} indicating greater efficacy). If pharmacologic effect is plotted versus concentration in the E_{max} equation, a hyperbola results with an asymptote equal to E_{max} (Fig. 3–13). At a concentration of zero, no measurable effect is present.

When dealing with human studies where a drug is administered to a patient and pharmacologic effect is measured, it is very difficult to determine the concentration of drug at the receptor site. Because of this, serum concentrations (total or unbound) are usually used as the concentration parameter in the E_{max} equation. Therefore, the values of E_{max} and EC_{50} are much different than if the drug were added to an isolated tissue contained in a laboratory beaker.

The result is that a much more empiric approach is used to describe the relationship between concentration and effect in clinical pharmacology studies. After a pharmacodynamic experiment has been conducted, concentration–effect plots are generated. The shape of the concentration–effect curve is used to determine which pharmacodynamic model will be used to describe the data. Because of this, the pharmacodynamic models used in a clinical pharmacology study are *deterministic* in the same way that the shape of the serum concentration-versus-time curve determines which pharmacokinetic model is used in clinical pharmacokinetic studies.

Sometimes a hyperbolic function does not adequately describe the concentration–effect relationship at lower concentrations. When this is the case, the sigmoid E_{max} equation may be superior to the E_{max} model:

$$E = \frac{E_{max} \times C^n}{EC_{50}{}^n + C^n}$$

where n is an exponent that changes the shape of the concentration–effect curve. When $n > 1$, the concentration–effect curve is S or sigmoid shaped at lower serum concentrations. When $n < 1$, the concentration–effect curve has a steeper slope at lower concentrations (Fig. 3–14).

With both the E_{max} and sigmoid E_{max} models, the largest changes in drug effect occur at the lower end of the concentration scale. Small changes in low serum concentrations cause large changes in effect. As serum concentrations become larger, further increases in serum concentration result in smaller changes in effect. Using the E_{max} model as

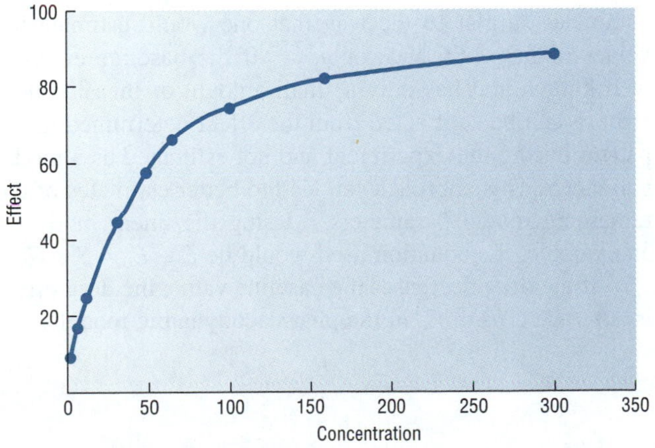

FIGURE 3–13. The E_{max} model [$E = (E_{max} \times C)/(EC_{50} + C)$] has the shape of a hyperbola with an asymptote equal to E_{max}. EC_{50} is the concentration where effect = $E_{max}/2$.

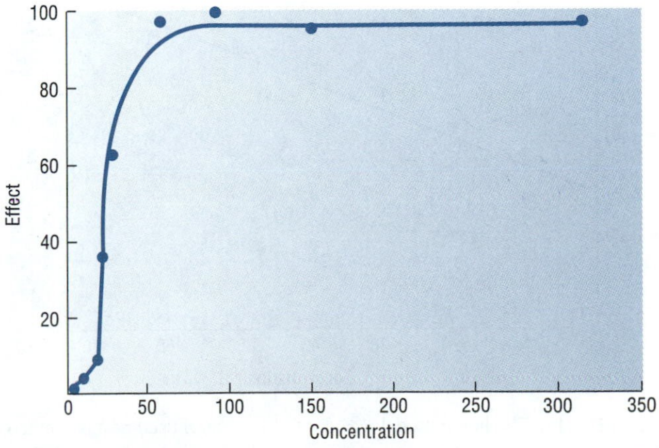

FIGURE 3–14. The sigmoid E_{max} model [$E = (E_{max} \times C_n)/(EC_{50}{}^n + C_n)$] has an S-shaped curve at lower concentrations. In this example, E_{max} and EC_{50} have the same values as in Fig. 3–13.

an example and setting E_{max} = 100 units and EC_{50} = 20 mg/L, doubling the serum concentration from 5 to 10 mg/L increases the effect from 20 to 33 units (a 67% increase), whereas doubling the serum concentration from 40 to 80 mg/L only increases the effect from 67 to 80 units (a 19% increase). This is an important concept for clinicians to remember when doses are being titrated in patients.

LINEAR MODELS

When serum concentrations obtained during a pharmacodynamic experiment are between 20% and 80% E_{max}, the concentration–effect curve may appear to be linear (Fig. 3–15). This occurs often because lower drug concentrations may not be detectable with the analytic technique used to assay serum samples and higher drug concentrations may be avoided to prevent toxic side effects. The equation used is that of a simple line: $E = S \times C + I$, where E is the drug effect, C is the drug concentration, S is the slope of the line, and I is the y intercept. In this situation, the value of S can be used as a measure of drug potency (the larger the value of S, the more potent the drug). The linear model can be derived from the E_{max} model. When EC_{50} is much greater than C, $E = (E_{max}/EC_{50})C = S \times C$, where $S = E_{max}/EC_{50}$.

The linear model allows a nonzero value for effect when the concentration equals zero. This may be a baseline value for the effect that is present without the drug, the result of measurement error when determining effect, or model misspecification. Also, this model does not allow the prediction of a maximum response.

Some investigators have used a log–linear model in pharmacodynamic experiments: $E = S \times (\log C) + I$, where the symbols have the same meaning as in the linear model. The advantages of this model are that the concentration scale is compressed on concentration–effect plots for experiments where wide concentration ranges were used, and the concentration values are transformed so that linear regression can be used to compute model parameters. The disadvantages are that the model cannot predict a maximum effect or an effect when the concentration equals zero. With the increased availability of nonlinear regression programs that can easily compute the parameters of nonlinear functions such as the E_{max} model, the use of the log–linear model has been discouraged.[51]

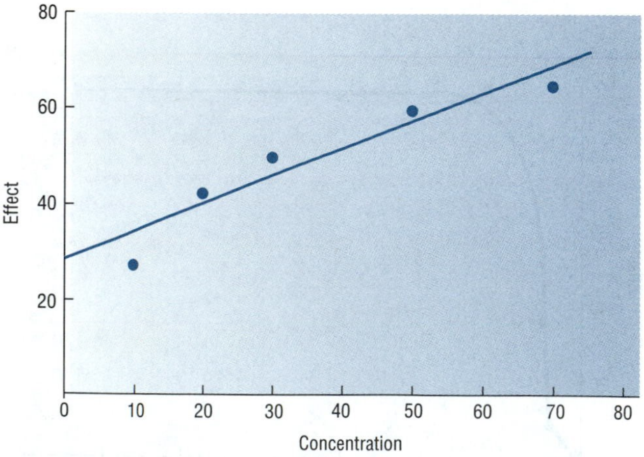

FIGURE 3–15. The linear model ($E = S \times C + I$) is often used as a pharmacodynamic model when the measured pharmacologic effect is 20% to 80% of E_{max}. In this situation, the determination of E_{max} and EC_{50} is not possible. To illustrate this, effect measurements from Fig. 3–2 between 20% and 80% of E_{max} are graphed using the linear pharmacodynamic model.

BASELINE EFFECTS

At times, the effect measured during a pharmacodynamic study has a value before the drug is administered to the patient. In these cases, the drug changes the patient's baseline value. Examples of these types of measurements are heart rate or blood pressure. In addition, a given drug may increase or decrease the baseline value. Two basic techniques are used to incorporate baseline values into pharmacodynamic data. One way incorporates the baseline value into the pharmacodynamic model; the other way transforms the effect data to take baseline values into account.

Incorporation of the baseline value into the pharmacodynamic model involves the addition of a new term to the previous equations. E_0 is the symbol used to denote the baseline value of the effect that will be measured. The form that these equations takes depends on whether the drug increases or decreases the pharmacodynamic effect. When the drug increases the baseline value, E_0 is added to the equations:

$$E = E_0 + \frac{E_{max} \times C}{EC_{50} + C}$$

$$E = E_0 + \frac{E_{max} \times C^n}{EC_{50}{}^n + C^n}$$

$$E = S \times C + E_0$$

When E_0 is not known with any better certainty than any other effect measurement, it should be estimated as a model parameter similar to the way that one would estimate the values of E_{max}, EC_{50}, S, or n.[52,53] If the baseline effect is well known and has only a small amount of measurement error, it can be subtracted from the effect determined in the patient during the experiment and not estimated as a model parameter. This approach can lead to better estimates of the remaining model parameters.[53] Using the linear model as an example, the equation used would be $E - E_0 = S \times C$.

If the drug decreases the baseline value, the drug effect is subtracted from E_0 in the pharmacodynamic models:

$$E = E_0 - \frac{E_{max} \times C}{IC_{50} + C}$$

$$E = E_0 - \frac{E_{max} \times C^n}{IC_{50}{}^n + C^n}$$

$$E = E_0 - S \times C$$

where E_{max} represents the maximum reduction in effect caused by the drug and IC_{50} is the concentration that produces a 50% inhibition of E_{max}. These forms of the equations have been called the inhibitory E_{max} and inhibitory sigmoidal E_{max} equations, respectively. In this arrangement of the pharmacodynamic model, E_0 is a model parameter and can be estimated. If the baseline effect is well known and has little measurement error, the effect in the presence of the drug can be subtracted from the baseline effect and not estimated as a model parameter. Using the inhibitory E_{max} model as an example, the formula would be $E_0 - E = (E_{max} \times C)/(IC_{50} + C)$.

When using the inhibitory E_{max} model, a special situation occurs if the baseline effect can be completely obliterated by the drug (decreased premature ventricular contractions during antiarrhythmic therapy). In this situation, $E_{max} = E_0$ and the equation simplifies to a rearrangement known as the fractional E_{max} equation:

$$E = E_0\left(1 - \frac{C}{IC_{50} + C}\right)$$

This form of the model relates drug concentration to the fraction of the maximum effect.

An alternative approach to the pharmacodynamic modeling of drugs that alter baseline effects is to transform the effect data so that it represents a percentage increase or decrease from the baseline value.[53] For drugs that increase the effect, the following transformation equation would be used: percent effect_t = [(treatment_t – baseline)/baseline] × 100. For drugs that decrease the effect, the following formula would be applied to the data: percent inhibition_t = [(baseline – treatment_t)/baseline] × 100. The subscript indicates the treatment, effect, or inhibition that occurred at time *t* during the experiment. If the study included a placebo control phase, baseline measurements made at the same time as treatment measurements (i.e., heart rate determined 2 hours after placebo and 2 hours after drug treatment) could be used in the appropriate transformation equation.[53] The appropriate model (excluding E_0) would then be used.

HYSTERESIS

Concentration–effect curves do not always follow the same pattern when serum concentrations increase as they do when serum concentrations decrease. In this situation the concentration–effect curves form a loop that is known as *hysteresis*. With some drugs, the effect is greater when serum concentrations are increasing, whereas with other drugs the effect is greater while serum concentrations are decreasing (Fig. 3–16). When individual concentration–effect pairs are joined in time sequence, this results in clockwise and counterclockwise hysteresis loops.

Clockwise hysteresis loops are usually caused by the development of tolerance to the drug. In this situation, the longer the patient is exposed to the drug, the smaller the pharmacologic effect for a given concentration. Therefore, after an extravascular or short-term infusion dose of the drug, the effect is smaller when serum concentrations are decreasing compared with the time when serum concentrations are increasing during the infusion or absorption phase. Accumulation of a drug metabolite that acts as an antagonist can also cause clockwise hysteresis.

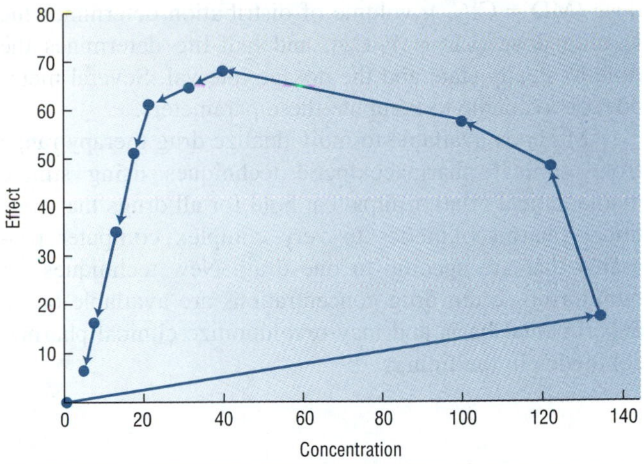

FIGURE 3–16. Hysteresis occurs when effect measurements are different at the same concentration. This is commonly seen after short-term intravenous infusions or extravascular doses where concentrations increase and subsequently decrease. Counterclockwise hysteresis loops are found when concentration–effect points are joined as time increases (shown by arrows) and effect is larger at the same concentration but at a later time. Clockwise hysteresis loops are similar, but the concentration–effect points are joined in clockwise order and the effect is smaller at a later time.

Counterclockwise hysteresis loops can be caused by the accumulation of an active metabolite, sensitization to the drug, or delay in time in equilibration between serum concentration and concentration of drug at the site of action. Combined pharmacokinetic–pharmacodynamic models have been devised that allow equilibration lag times to be taken into account.

CONCLUSIONS

The availability of inexpensive, rapidly available serum drug concentrations has changed the way clinicians monitor drug therapy in patients. The therapeutic range for many drugs is known, and it is likely that more drugs will be monitored using serum concentrations in the future. Clinicians need to remember that the therapeutic range is merely an average guideline and to take into account interindividual pharmacodynamic variability when treating patients. Individual patients may respond to smaller concentrations or require concentrations that are much greater to obtain a therapeutic effect. Conversely, patients may show toxic effects at concentrations within or below the therapeutic range. Serum concentrations should never replace clinical judgment.

Three kinetic constants determine the dosage requirements of patients. Clearance determines the maintenance dose (MD = ClC_{ss}), volume of distribution determines the loading dose (LD = V_DC_{ss}), and half-life determines the time to steady state and the dosage interval. Several methods are available to compute these parameters.

Methods available to individualize drug therapy range from clinical pharmacokinetic techniques using simple mathematical relationships that hold for all drugs that obey linear pharmacokinetics to very complex computer programs that are specific to one drug. New techniques for monitoring serum drug concentrations are available on an experimental basis and may revolutionize clinical pharmacokinetics in the future.

REFERENCES

1. Koup JR, Gibaldi M. Some comments on the evaluation of bioavailability data. Drug Intell Clin Pharm 1980;14:327–330.
2. Gibaldi M, Boyes RN, Feldman S. Influence of first pass effect on availability of drugs on oral administration. J Pharm Sci 1971; 60:1338–1340.
3. Wu C-Y, Benet LZ, Hebert MF, et al. Differentiation of absorption and first-pass gut and hepatic metabolism in humans—Studies with cyclosporine. Clin Pharmacol Ther 1995;58:492–497.
4. Wagner JG, Northam JI, Alway CD, et al. Blood levels of drug at the equilibrium state after multiple dosing. Nature 1965;207:1301–1302.
5. Rowland M, Benet LZ, Graham GG. Clearance concepts in pharmacokinetics. J Pharmacokinet Biopharm 1973;1:123–136.
6. Wilkinson GR, Shand DG. A physiological approach to hepatic drug clearance. Clin Pharmacol Ther 1975;18:377–390.
7. Nies AS, Shand DG, Wilkinson GR. Altered hepatic blood flow and drug disposition. Clin Pharmacokinet 1976;1:135–155.
8. Gibaldi M, Koup JR. Pharmacokinetic concepts—Drug binding, apparent volume of distribution and clearance. Eur J Clin Pharmacol 1981;20:299–305.
9. Bowdle TA, Patel IH, Levy RH, et al. Valproic acid dosage and plasma protein binding and clearance. Clin Pharmacol Ther 1980; 28:486–492.
10. Lima JJ, Boudonlas H, Blanford M. Concentration-dependence of disopyramide binding to plasma protein and its influence on kinetics and dynamics. J Pharmacol Exp Ther 1981;219:741–747.
11. Gibaldi M, Perrier D. Pharmacokinetics, 2nd ed. New York, Marcel Dekker, 1980.
12. Gibaldi M. Estimation of the pharmacokinetic parameters of the two-compartment open model from post-infusion plasma concentration data. J Pharm Sci 1969;58:1133–1135.
13. Loo JCK, Riegelman S. Assessment of pharmacokinetic constants from postinfusion blood curves obtained after IV infusion. J Pharm Sci 1970;59:53–55.
14. Wagner JG. Model-independent linear pharmacokinetics. Drug Intell Clin Pharm 1976;10:179–180.
15. Brosen K. Recent developments in hepatic drug oxidation—Implications for clinical pharmacokinetics. Clin Pharmacokinet 1990; 18:220–239.
16. Cockcroft DW, Gault MH. Prediction of creatinine clearance from serum creatinine. Nephron 1976;16:31–41.
17. Traub SL, Johnson CE. Comparison of methods of estimating creatinine clearance in children. Am J Hosp Pharm 1980;37:195–201.
18. Salazar DE, Corcoran GB. Predicting creatinine clearance and renal drug clearance in obese patients from estimated fat-free body mass. Am J Med 1988;84:1053–1060.
19. Jelliffe RW, Jelliffe SM. A computer program for estimation of creatinine clearance from unstable serum creatinine levels, age, sex, and weight. Math Biosci 1972;14:17–24.
20. Koup JR, Jusko WJ, Elwood CM, Kohli RK. Digoxin pharmacokinetics—Role of renal failure in dosage regimen design. Clin Pharmacol Ther 1975;18:9–21.
21. Matzke GR, McGory RW, Halstenson CE, Keane WF. Pharmacokinetics of vancomycin in patients with various degrees of renal function. Antimicrob Agents Chemother 1984;25:433–437.
22. Sarubbi FA, Hull JH. Amikacin serum concentrations—Predictions of levels and dosage guidelines. Ann Intern Med 1978;89:612–618.
23. Sivan SK, Bennett WM. Drug dosing guidelines in patients with renal failure. West J Med 1992;156:633–638.
24. Bennett WM, Aronoff GR, Golper TA, et al. Drug Prescribing in Renal Failure—Dosing Guidelines for Adults, 3rd ed. Philadelphia, American College of Physicians, 1994.
25. Pugh RNH, Murray-Lyon IM, Dawson JL, Pietroni MC, Williams R. Transection of the oesophagus for bleeding oesophageal varices. Br J Surg 1973;60:646–649.
26. Jusko WJ, Gardner MJ, Mangione A, et al. Factors affecting theophylline clearances—Age, tobacco, marijuana, cirrhosis, congestive heart failure, obesity, oral contraceptives, benzodiazepines, barbiturates, and ethanol. J Pharm Sci 1979;68:1358–1366.
27. Thomson PD, Melmon KL, Richardson JA, et al. Lidocaine pharmacokinetics in advanced heart failure, liver disease, and renal failure in humans. Ann Intern Med 1973;78:499–508.
28. Koup JR, Killen T, Bauer LA. Multiple-dose nonlinear regression analysis program—Aminoglycoside dose prediction. Clin Pharmacokinet 1983;8:456–462.
29. Sheiner LB, Beal S, Rosenberg B, et al. Forecasting individual pharmacokinetics. Clin Pharmacol Ther 1979;26:294–305.
30. Sheiner LB, Beal SL. Bayesian individualization of pharmacokinetics—Simple implementation and comparison with non-Bayesian methods. J Pharm Sci 1982;71:1344–1348.
31. Schentag JJ, Jusko WJ. Renal clearance and tissue accumulation of gentamicin. Clin Pharmacol Ther 1977;22:364–370.
32. Sawchuk RJ, Zaske DE, Cipolle RJ, et al. Kinetic model for gentamicin dosing with the use of individual patient parameters. Clin Pharmacol Ther 1977;21:362–369.
33. Bauer LA, Edwards WAD, Dellinger EP, Simonowitz DA. Influence of weight on aminoglycoside pharmacokinetics in normal weight and morbidly obese patients. Eur J Clin Pharmacol 1983;24: 643–647.
34. Bauer LA, Piecoro JJ, Wilson HD, Blouin RA. Gentamicin and tobramycin pharmacokinetics in patients with cystic fibrosis. Clin Pharm 1983;2:262–4.
35. Sampliner R, Perrier D, Powell R, Finley P. Influence of acities on tobramycin pharmacokinetics. J Clin Pharmacol 1984;24:43–46.
36. Zank KE, Miwa L, Cohen JL, Waffarin F, Huxtable RF. Effect of body weight on gentamicin pharmacokinetics in neonates. Clin Pharm 1984;3:170–173.
37. Pancorbo S, Sawchuk RJ, Dashe C, et al. Use of a pharmacokinetic model for individual intravenous doses of aminophylline. Eur J Clin Pharmacol 1979;16:251–254.
38. Cantu TG, Yamanaka-Yuen NA, Lietman PS. Serum vancomycin concentrations—Reappraisal of their clinical value. Clin Infect Dis 1994;18:533–543.
39. Welty TE, Copa AK. Impact of vancomycin therapeutic drug monitoring on patient care. Ann Pharmacother 1994;28:1335–1339.
40. Zimmermann AE, Katona BG, Plaisance KI. Association of vancomycin serum concentrations with outcomes in patients with gram-positive bacteremia. Pharmacotherapy 1995;85–91.
41. Moellering RC Jr, Krogstad DJ, Greenblatt DJ. Vancomycin therapy in patients with impaired renal function—A nomogram for dosage. Ann Intern Med 1981;94:343–346.
42. Blouin RA, Bauer LA, Miller DD, Record KE, Griffen WO. Vancomycin pharmacokinetics in normal and morbidly obese subjects. Antimicrob Agents Chemother 1982;21:575–580.
43. Matzke GR, McGory RW, Halstenson CE, Keane WF. Pharmacokinetics of vancomycin in patients with various degrees of renal function. Antimicrob Agents Chemother 1984;25:433–437.

44. Abernethy DR, Greenblatt DJ, Smith TW. Digoxin disposition in obesity—Clinical pharmacokinetic investigations. Am Heart J 1981;102: 740–744.
45. Sarrazin E, Hendeles L, Weinberger M, et al. Dose-dependent kinetics for theophylline—Observations among ambulatory asthmatic children. J Pediatr 1980;97:825–828.
46. Tang-Liu DDS, Williams RL, Riegelman S. Nonlinear theophylline elimination. Clin Pharmacol Ther 1982;31:358–369.
47. Edwards DJ, Zarowitz BJ, Slaughter RL. Theophylline. In: Evans WE, Schentag JJ, Jusko WJ, eds. Applied Pharmacokinetics—Principles of Therapeutic Drug Monitoring. Vancouver, WA, Applied Therapeutics, 1992.
48. Vozeh S, Kewitz G, Wenk M, et al. Rapid prediction of steady-state serum theophylline concentrations in patients treated with intravenous aminophylline. Eur J Clin Pharmacol 1980;18:473–477.
49. Vozeh S, Muir KT, Sheiner LB, Follath F. Predicting individual phenytoin dosage. J Pharmacokinet Biopharm 1991;9:131–146.
50. Ludden TM, Allen JP, Valutsky WA, et al. Individualization of phenytoin dosage regimens. Clin Pharmacol Ther 1977;21:287–293.
51. Holford NHG, Sheiner LB. Understanding the dose–effect relationship—Clinical application of pharmacokinetic–pharmacodynamic models. Clin Pharmacokinet 1981;6:429–453.
52. Schwinghammer TL, Kroboth PD. Basic concepts in pharmacodynamic modeling. J Clin Pharmacol 1988;28:388–394.

4
PEDIATRICS

Milap C. Nahata, PharmD, FCCP

Remarkable progress has been made in the management of pediatric patients. This chapter highlights important principles of pediatric drug therapy that must be considered when the diseases discussed in other chapters of this book occur in pediatric patients, defined as those less than 18 years of age. Newborn infants born before 37 weeks of gestational age are termed premature; those between 1 day and 1 month of age are neonates; 1 month to 1 year old, infants; 1 year to 12 years of age, children; and 12 to 18 years, adolescents. Covered are notable examples of problems in pediatrics, pharmacokinetic differences in pediatric patients, drug efficacy and toxicity in this patient group, and various factors affecting pediatric pharmacotherapy. Specific examples of problems and special considerations in pediatric patients are cited to enhance understanding.

Infant mortality has declined from 200 per 1000 births in the 19th century, to 75 per 1000 births in 1925, to 7.1 per 1000 births in 1997.[1] This success has resulted largely from improvements in identification, prevention, and treatment of diseases once common during delivery and the period of infancy. Although most marketed drugs are used in pediatric patients, only one-fourth of the drugs approved by the Food and Drug Administration have indications specific for use in the pediatric population. Data on the pharmacokinetics, pharmacodynamics, efficacy, and safety of drugs in infants and children are scarce. Lack of this type of information led to such disasters as gray baby syndrome from chloramphenicol, phocomelia from thalidomide, and kernicterus from sulfonamide therapy.

Gray syndrome was first reported in two neonates who died after excessive chloramphenicol doses (100 to 300 mg/kg/d); the serum concentrations of chloramphenicol immediately before death were 75 and 100 μg/mL. Patients with gray syndrome usually have abdominal distension, vomiting, diarrhea, a characteristic gray color, respiratory distress, hypotension, and progressive shock.

Thalidomide is well known for its teratogenic effects. Clearly implicated as the cause of multiple congenital fetal abnormalities (particularly limb deformities), it can also cause polyneuritis, nerve damage, and mental retardation. Isotretinoin (Accutane) is another teratogen. Because it is used to treat acne vulgaris, common in teenage patients who may be sexually active, isotretinoin has presented a difficult problem in patient education during the 1980s and 1990s.

Kernicterus was reported in infants receiving sulfonamides, which displaced bilirubin from protein-binding sites in the blood to cause a hyperbilirubinemia. This results in deposition of bilirubin in the brain and induces encephalopathy in infants.

Another area of concern in pediatrics is identifying an optimal dosage. Dosage regimens cannot be based simply on body weight or surface area of a pediatric patient extrapolated from adult data. Bioavailability, pharmacokinetics, pharmacodynamics, efficacy, and adverse effect information can markedly differ between pediatric and adult patients as well as among pediatric patients because of differences in age, organ function, and disease state. Significant progress has been made in the area of pediatric pharmacokinetics during the last two decades, but few such studies have correlated pharmacokinetics with pharmacodynamics.

Several additional factors should be considered in optimizing pediatric drug therapy. Many drugs widely prescribed for infants and children are not available in suitable dosage forms. For example, extemporaneous liquid dosage forms of acetazolamide, captopril, rifampin, and spironolactone are prepared for infants and children who cannot swallow tablets or capsules; and parenteral dosage forms of aminophylline, methylprednisolone, morphine, and phenobarbital are diluted to measure accurately small doses for infants. Alteration (dilution or reformulation) of dosage forms intended for adult patients raises questions about the stability and compatibility of these drugs. Because of low fluid volume requirements and limited access to intravenous sites, special methods must be used for the delivery of intravenous drugs to infants and children. As simple as it may seem, administration of oral drugs to young patients continues to be a difficult task for nurses and parents. Similarly, assuring compliance with drug therapy in pediatric patients poses a special challenge.

Finally, the need for additional pharmacologic or therapeutic research brings up the issue of ethical justification for conducting research. The investigators proposing studies and institutional review committees approving human studies must assess the risk–benefit ratio of each study to be fair to children who are not in a position to accept or reject the opportunity to participate in the research project.

Enormous progress has been made in characterization of drug pharmacokinetics in pediatric patients. Two factors have contributed to this progress: (1) the availability of sensitive and specific analytic methods to measure drugs and their metabolites in small volumes of biologic fluids and (2) awareness of the importance of clinical pharmacokinetics in optimization of drug therapy. Absorption, distribution, metabolism, and elimination of many drugs are different in premature infants, full-term infants, and older children.

ABSORPTION

GASTROINTESTINAL TRACT

Two factors affecting the absorption of drugs from the gastrointestinal tract are pH-dependent passive diffusion and gastric-emptying time. Both processes are strikingly different in premature infants compared with older children and adults. In a full-term infant, gastric pH ranges from 6 to 8 at birth, but declines to 1 to 3 within 24 hours.[2] In contrast, the gastric pH is elevated in premature infants because of immature acid secretion.[3]

Higher serum concentrations of acid-labile drugs such as penicillin,[4] ampicillin,[5] and nafcillin,[6] and lower serum concentrations of a weak acid such as phenobarbital,[7] in premature infants can be explained by the higher gastric pH. Because of a lack of extensive data comparing serum concentration–time profiles after oral versus intravenous drug administration, differences in the bioavailability of drugs in premature infants are poorly understood. Studies have also shown that gastric emptying is slow in a premature infant.[8] Thus, drugs with limited absorption in adults may be efficiently absorbed in a premature infant because of prolonged contact time with gastrointestinal mucosa.

INTRAMUSCULAR SITES

Drug absorption from an intramuscular site may also be altered in premature infants. Differences in relative muscle mass, blood flow to various muscles, peripheral vasomotor instability, and insufficient muscular contractions in premature infants compared with older children and adults can influence drug absorption from the intramuscular site. The net effect of these factors on drug absorption is impossible to predict; phenobarbital has been reported to be rapidly absorbed,[9] whereas diazepam absorption may be delayed.[10] Thus, this site is rarely used in neonates.

SKIN

Percutaneous absorption may be substantially increased in newborn infants because of an underdeveloped epidermal barrier (stratum corneum) and increased skin hydration. The increased permeability can produce toxic effects after the topical use of hexachlorophene soaps and powders,[11] salicylic acid ointment, and rubbing alcohol.[12] Interestingly, a study has shown that a therapeutic serum concentration of theophylline can be achieved to control apnea in premature infants of less than 30 weeks' gestation after a topical application of gel containing a standard dose of theophylline.[13] The use of this route of administration may minimize the unpredictability of oral and intramuscular absorption and complications of intravenous drug administration for certain drugs.

DISTRIBUTION

Drug distribution is determined by the physicochemical properties of the drug itself (pK_a, molecular weight, partition coefficient), and the physiologic factors specific to the patient. Although the physicochemical properties of the drug are constant, the physiologic functions often vary in different patient populations. Some important patient-specific factors include extracellular and total body water, protein binding by the drug in plasma, and presence of pathologic conditions modifying physiologic function. Total body water, as a percentage of total body weight, has been estimated to be 94% in the fetus, 85% in premature infants, 78% in full-term infants, and 60% in adults.[14] Extracellular fluid volume is also markedly different in premature infants compared with older children and adults; the extracellular fluid volume may account for 50% of body weight in premature infants, 35% in 4- to 6-month-old infants, 25% in children 1 year of age, and 19% in adults.[14] This conforms to the observed gentamicin distribution volumes of 0.48 L/kg in neonates and 0.20 L/kg in adults.[15] The studies have shown that the distribution volume of tobramycin is largest in the most premature infants and decreases with increases in the gestational age and birthweight of the infant.[16]

Binding of drugs to plasma proteins is also decreased in newborn infants, because of the decreased plasma protein concentration, lower binding capacity of protein, decreased affinity of proteins for drug binding, and competition for certain binding sites by endogenous compounds such as bilirubin. The plasma protein binding of many drugs—including phenobarbital, salicylates, and phenytoin—is significantly less in the neonate than in the adult.[17] The decrease in plasma protein binding of drugs can increase their apparent volumes of distribution. Therefore, premature infants require a larger loading dose than older children and adults to achieve a therapeutic serum concentration of such drugs as phenobarbital[18] and phenytoin.[19]

The consequences of increased concentrations of free or unbound drug in the serum and tissues must be considered. Pharmacologic and toxic effects are directly related to the concentration of free drug in the body. Increases in free drug concentrations may result directly from decreases in plasma protein binding or indirectly from, for example, drug displacement from binding sites. The increased mortality from the development of kernicterus secondary to displacement of bilirubin by sulfisoxazole in neonates has been well documented.[20] However, because drug bound to plasma proteins cannot be eliminated by the kidney, an increase in free drug concentration may also increase its clearance.[21]

The amount of body fat is substantially lower in neonates compared to adults, which may affect drug therapy. Certain highly lipid-soluble drugs are distributed less widely in infants than in adults. The apparent volume of distribution of diazepam has ranged from 1.4 to 1.8 L/kg in neonates and from 2.2 to 2.6 L/kg in adults.[22] In recent years, the numbers of mothers breast feeding their infants has climbed. Thus, certain drugs distributed in breast milk may pose problems for the infants. The American Academy of Pediatrics recommends that bromocriptine, cyclophosphamide, cyclosporine, doxorubicin, ergotamine, lithium, methotrexate, phenindione, and drugs of abuse (e.g., amphetamine, cocaine, heroin, marijuana, and phencyclidine or PCP) be contraindicated during breast feeding. Further, radiopharmaceuticals should be temporarily stopped during breast feeding.[23] Note that these recommendations are based on limited data; other drugs taken over a prolonged period by the mother may also be toxic to the infant. For example, acebutolol, aspirin, atenolol, clemastine, phenobarbital, primidone, sulfasalazine, and 5-aminosalicyclic acid have been associated with adverse effects in some nursing infants.[23,24] Ideally, the use of any drug should be avoided by the mother during pregnancy and while breast feeding.

METABOLISM

Drug metabolism is substantially slower in infants compared with older children and adults. There are important differences in the maturation of various pathways of metabolism within a premature infant. For example, the sulfation pathway is well developed, but the glucuronidation pathway has not developed in infants.[25] Although acetaminophen metabolism by glucuronidation is impaired in an infant compared with adults, it is partly compensated for by the sulfation pathway. The tragedy of the chloramphenicol-induced gray baby syndrome in newborn infants is directly related to a decreased metabolism of chloramphenicol by glucuronyl transferases to the inactive glucuronide metabolite.[26] This metabolic pathway appears to be age related[27] and may take several months to a year to develop fully. Evidence for this is the increase in clearance with age up to 1 year.[28]

Interestingly, higher serum concentrations of morphine are required to achieve efficacy in a premature infant than in an adult, because the infant is not able to metabolize morphine adequately to its 6-glucuronide (20 times more active than morphine).[29]

Metabolism of drugs such as theophylline, phenobarbital, and phenytoin by oxidation is also impaired in newborn infants. The rate of metabolism, however, is more rapid with phenobarbital and phenytoin than with theophylline, perhaps due to the involvement of different cytochrome P450 isozymes. Total clearance of phenytoin surpasses adult values by 2 weeks of age, whereas theophylline clearance is not fully developed for several months.[17] Two additional observations should be noted about theophylline metabolism in pediatric patients. First, in premature infants receiving theophylline for the treatment of apnea, a significant amount of its active metabolite caffeine may be present, unlike in older children and adults.[17] Second, theophylline clearance in children 1 to 9 years of age exceeds the values in young infants as well as adults. Thus, a child with asthma often requires markedly higher doses on a weight basis of theophylline compared with an adult.[30] Because of decreased metabolism, doses of such drugs as theophylline, phenobarbital, phenytoin, and diazepam should be decreased in premature infants.

ELIMINATION

Drugs and their metabolites are often eliminated by the kidney. The processes of glomerular filtration, tubular secretion, and tubular reabsorption determine the efficiency of renal excretion. These processes may take several weeks to 1 year after birth to develop fully.

Studies in infants have shown that tobramycin clearance during the first postnatal week may increase with an increase in gestational age.[16] Netilmicin studies in infants up to 1 month after birth have suggested that postnatal age is also directly correlated with netilmicin clearance.[28] Thus, premature infants require a lower daily dose of drugs eliminated by the kidney during the first week of life; the dosage requirement then increases with age.

Because of immature renal elimination, chloramphenicol succinate can accumulate in premature infants. Although chloramphenicol succinate is inactive, this accumulation may be the reason for an increased bioavailability of chloramphenicol in premature infants compared with older children.[27] These data indicate that dose-related toxicity may result from an underdeveloped glucuronidation pathway as well as increased bioavailability of chloramphenicol in premature infants.

DRUG EFFICACY AND TOXICITY

Besides the pharmacokinetic differences previously identified between pediatric and older patients, factors related to drug efficacy and toxicity should also be considered in planning pediatric pharmacotherapy. Unique pathophysiologic changes occur in pediatric patients with some disease states.

Examples of these pathophysiologic and pharmacodynamic differences are numerous. Clinical presentation of chronic asthma differs in children and adults.[31] Children present almost exclusively with a reversible extrinsic type of asthma, whereas adults have nonspecific, nonatopic bronchial irritability.[31] This explains the value of adjunctive-hyposensitization therapy in the management of pediatric patients with extrinsic asthma.[32,33]

The maintenance dose of digoxin is substantially higher in an infant than in an adult. This is explained by a lower binding affinity of receptors in the myocardium for digoxin and increased digoxin-binding sites on neonatal erythrocytes, compared with adult erythrocytes.[34] Insulin requirement is highest during adolescence, because of the individual's rapid growth. Growth hormone therapy has allowed children with growth hormone deficiency to attain greater adult height. However, a recent study has shown that in "normal" short children (without growth hormone deficiency), early and rapid pubertal progression by growth hormone therapy may lead to a shorter final adult height than might have been attained naturally.[35] This emphasizes the need for identifying specific indications for the effective and safe use of drugs in pediatric patients.

Certain adverse effects of drugs are most common in the newborn period, whereas other toxic effects may continue to be important for many years of childhood. Chloramphenicol toxicity is increased in a newborn infant because of immature metabolism and enhanced bioavailability. Similarly, propylene glycol—added to many injectable drugs, including phenytoin, phenobarbital, digoxin, diazepam, vitamin D, and hydralazine, to increase their stability—can cause hyperosmolality in infants.[36] Benzyl alcohol was a popular preservative in intravascular flush solutions until a syndrome of metabolic acidosis, seizures, neurologic deterioration, gasping respirations, hepatic and renal abnormalities, cardiovascular collapse, and death was described in premature infants. A decline in both mortality and the incidence of major intraventricular hemorrhage has been documented after the use of solutions containing benzyl alcohol was stopped in low-birthweight infants.[37]

Tetracyclines are also contraindicated in pregnant women, nursing mothers, and children less than 8 years of age because they can cause dental staining and defects in enamelization of deciduous and permanent teeth as well as a decrease in bone growth.[38]

The antibiotics of the fluoroquinolone class (e.g., ciprofloxacin) are not recommended for children or pregnant women, because of an association between these drugs and development of permanent lesions of the cartilage of weight-bearing joints and other signs of arthropathy in immature animals of various species.[39] Reversible arthralgia, sometimes accompanied by synovial effusion, was associated with ciprofloxacin in 1.8% of pediatric patients with cystic fibrosis.[40] Although these drugs are used to treat certain infections in pediatric populations, further safety data are needed before they can be routinely prescribed in infants and children.

Certain drugs may be less toxic in pediatric patients than in adults. Aminoglycosides appear to be less toxic in infants than in adults. In adults, aminoglycoside toxicity is related to both peripheral compartment accumulation and the individual patient's inherent sensitivity to these tissue concentrations.[41] Although neonatal peripheral tissue compartments for gentamicin have been reported to closely resemble those of adults with similar renal function,[15] gentamicin is rarely nephrotoxic in infants. This dissimilarity in the incidence of nephrotoxicity implies that newborn infants may have less inherent tissue sensitivity for toxicity than adults.

The differences in efficacy, toxicity, and protein binding of drugs in pediatric versus adult patients raise an important question about the acceptable therapeutic range in children. Therapeutic ranges for drugs are first established in adults and are often directly applied to pediatric patients, but specific studies should be conducted in pediatric patients to define optimal therapeutic ranges of drugs.

FACTORS AFFECTING PEDIATRIC THERAPY

DISEASE STATES

Because most drugs are either metabolized by the liver or eliminated by the kidney, hepatic and renal disease are expected to decrease the dosage requirements in patients. Nevertheless, not all diseases require lower doses of drugs; for instance, patients with cystic fibrosis require larger doses of certain drugs to achieve therapeutic concentrations.[42]

LIVER DISEASE

Because the liver is the main organ for drug metabolism, drug clearance is usually decreased in patients with hepatic disease; however, most studies on the influence of liver disease on dosage requirements have been carried out in adults, and these data may not be extrapolated uniformly to pediatric patients.

Drug metabolism by the liver depends on complex interactions among hepatic blood flow, ability of the liver to extract the drug from the blood, drug binding in the blood, and both type and severity of liver disease. Routine liver function tests—such as determination of serum aspartate transaminase, serum alanine transaminase, alkaline phosphatase, and bilirubin levels—have not consistently correlated with drug pharmacokinetics. Further, because of different pathologic changes in various types of liver diseases, patients with acute viral hepatitis may have different abilities to metabolize drugs compared with patients with alcoholic cirrhosis.[43]

On the basis of hepatic extraction characteristics, drugs can be divided into two categories. The first category consists of drugs with a high hepatic extraction ratio (> 0.7; such drugs include morphine, meperidine, lidocaine, and propranolol). Clearance of these drugs is affected by hepatic blood flow. A decreased hepatic blood flow in the presence of such disease states as cirrhosis and congestive heart failure is expected to decrease the clearance of drugs with high extraction ratios. The second category comprises drugs with a low extraction ratio (< 0.2) and a low affinity for plasma proteins. Metabolism of these drugs (e.g., theophylline, chloramphenicol, and acetaminophen) is influenced mainly by hepatocellular function and not as much by changes in hepatic blood flow or plasma protein binding. One report suggested that theophylline clearance may decrease by 45% in a child with acute viral hepatitis.[44] Because of a lack of specific data on dosage adjustment in liver disease, drug therapy should be closely monitored in pediatric patients to avoid potential toxicity from excessive doses, particularly for drugs with narrow therapeutic indices.

RENAL DISEASE

Renal failure decreases the dosage requirement of drugs eliminated by the kidney. Once again, because of limited studies, dosage adjustments in pediatric patients are based largely on data obtained in adults. For many important drugs—such as aminoglycoside antibiotics—renal clearance or rate of elimination is directly proportional to the glomerular filtration rate as measured by endogenous renal creatinine clearance. Serum drug concentrations should be monitored for drugs with narrow therapeutic indices and eliminated largely by the kidney (e.g., aminoglycosides and vancomycin) to optimize therapy in pediatric patients with renal dysfunction. For drugs with wide therapeutic ranges (e.g., penicillins, cephalosporins), dosage adjustment may be necessary only in moderate to severe renal failure.

CYSTIC FIBROSIS

Drug therapy in pediatric patients with cystic fibrosis has been reviewed.[45] For unknown reasons, these patients require increased doses of certain drugs. Studies have reported higher clearance of drugs including gentamicin, tobramycin, netilmicin, amikacin, dicloxacillin, cloxacillin, azlocillin, piperacillin, and theophylline in patients with cystic fibrosis compared to those without this disease; the apparent distribution volume of certain drugs may also be altered in cystic fibrosis.[45] Severity of the illness may influence the change in dosage requirements, but this is not certain. Chapter 28 reviews these changes in detail.

OTHER DISEASES

Although specific dosage guidelines are not available, pediatric patients with gastrointestinal disease (e.g., celiac disease, gastroenteritis, and severe malabsorption) may require dosage adjustments.[42] Hypoxemia has also been shown to decrease the elimination of amikacin in low-birthweight infants.[46] Critically ill adult and pediatric patients with severe head trauma require higher than normal doses of phenytoin, in part due to increased intrinsic clearance.[47]

DRUG ADMINISTRATION

Drugs are often given by the intravenous route to seriously ill patients. Flow rates and injection sites vary widely with pediatric intravenous drug-delivery sets. Effective serum concentrations are expected to be achieved rapidly after drug infusion. In 1979, a therapeutic drug monitoring service was made available at my institution. Soon thereafter, lower-than-predicted peak and higher-than-predicted trough serum concentrations of aminoglycosides and chloramphenicol were noted. Subsequently, several studies demonstrated that the method of drug infusion has a profound influence on peak serum concentration and time to attain peak concentrations of chloramphenicol and tobramycin.[48,49] This has practical implications for routine therapeutic drug monitoring in that anticipated serum concentrations may be inaccurate, leading to unjustified, costly, and potentially harmful alterations in doses. Proper recommendations for obtaining patient specimens can be made only with the knowledge of drug characteristics and infusion method.

Intravenous drugs are commonly infused in an antegrade fashion. By this method, the doses injected at various sites of the intravenous set (e.g., a Y-site and a volumetric chamber such as Metriset Buretrol) are expected to move directly toward the patient (Fig. 4–1).

In vitro studies with gentamicin and aminophylline have shown that the delivery of these drugs may be delayed substantially depending on the flow rate and injection site.[50] These observations were confirmed with infusion of

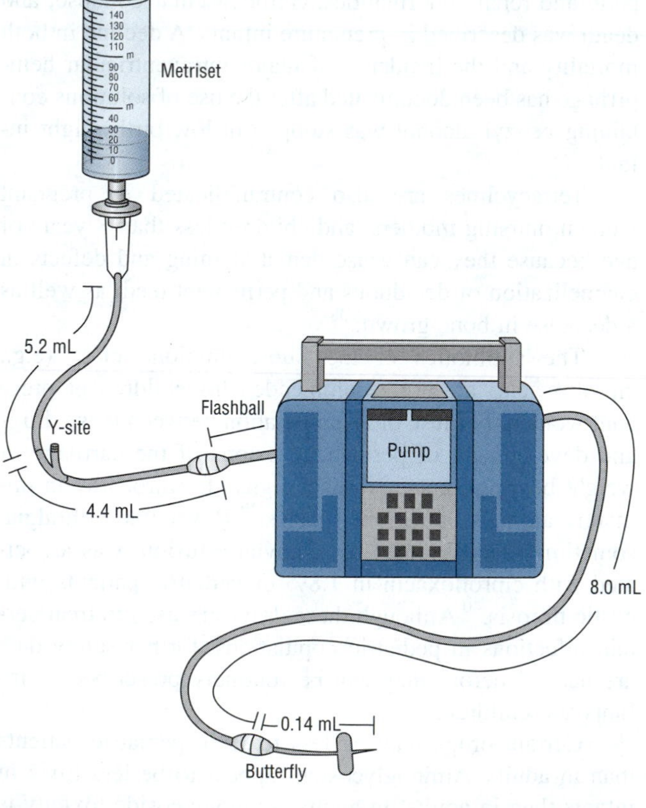

FIGURE 4–1. Schematic diagram of an intravenous set with a volumetric chamber (Metriset or Buretrol), Y-site, flashball, and butterfly. Values shown for the various components of the system are volume capacities. *(From Ref. 50, with permission.)*

chloramphenicol succinate[48] and tobramycin.[49] These studies have clearly demonstrated that the variables of intravenous drug infusion systems (e.g., flow rate, injection site, volume of drug, and fluid volume of the tubing) can markedly affect the serum concentrations of drugs after infusions into pediatric patients. For example, mean peak serum concentrations of chloramphenicol can be 5 μg/mL higher and occur 1 hour earlier after flashball injection compared with Buretrol injection in infants and children.[48] Similarly, the mean serum concentrations of tobramycin can be 2.3 to 2.5 μg/mL higher and occur 1 to 1.5 hours earlier after an infusion from a syringe pump compared with infusions from the Y-site of a system similar to that of Figure 4–1.[49] These differences can be important because of the narrow therapeutic indices of chloramphenicol and tobramycin. Furthermore, a lack of knowledge of these variables may result in inappropriate timing and interpretation of blood level data, leading to unnecessary dosage adjustments.

Specific gravity can also influence drug delivery at slow infusion rates.[51] For example, *in vitro* studies have indicated that drugs with a specific gravity lower than that of the maintenance fluid may layer at the top of the tubing where delivery would be prolonged by laminar-flow characteristics.[51] Similarly, injections into a filter chamber, Y-site, or T-site with dead space can also prolong drug delivery.

No single infusion system is ideal for drug delivery in all institutions for all patients. For example, a syringe pump with a microbore tubing may be preferred for the infusion of vancomycin to neonates. Each facility must be cognizant of problems of drug delivery and develop specific guidelines for intravenous infusions. At my institution, specific guidelines are provided for administration of each drug. These guidelines take into account various infusion rates and provide consistency of delivery with each dose. As long as the time for actual delivery can be anticipated, times to obtain blood samples can be adjusted accordingly to generate meaningful data.

ALTERNATION OF DOSAGE FORMS

Many drugs used in pediatric patients are not available in suitable dosage forms. This necessitates dilution of high concentrations of drugs intended for adult patients. Examples of these drugs include atropine, carbamazepine, diazepam, digoxin, epinephrine, hydralazine, insulin, morphine, phenobarbital, and phenytoin. Volumes ranging from 0.001 to 0.1 mL must be measured to dispense these drugs for use in infants. This can obviously be associated with large errors in measurements, and such errors have caused intoxication with digoxin[52] and morphine[53] in infants. One solution to this problem is to dilute these concentrated products, but such alterations can influence the stability or compatibility of these drugs. Because of limited data, pharmacists may justifiably be reluctant to alter dosage forms of certain drugs.

Selection of the appropriate vehicle to dilute the adult dosage forms for use in pediatric patients can also be difficult. Phenobarbital sodium contains propylene glycol in the original product to improve drug stability. Because propylene glycol can cause hyperosmolality in infants,[36] further addition of this vehicle may not be wise. Because of limited access to intravenous sites in pediatric patients, drugs must be administered through the same site; however, data on their compatibility are often missing. Newborn infants often require aminoglycosides for presumed or proven sepsis and calcium gluconate to correct hypocalcemia. Tobramycin and calcium gluconate have been found to be compatible at least during a 1-hour period of administration at the same site.[54]

Administration of oral drugs continues to challenge parents and nurses. Alteration of these drugs by crushing or mixing, refusal of patients to accept the medication, and loss of drug during administration are some factors that can affect pediatric therapy. A common practice is to mix medications in applesauce, syrup, ice cream, or other vehicles to make the drugs palatable.

A variety of extemporaneous formulations for oral, intravenous, and rectal administration are included in a recent publication for use in pediatric patients.[55] A specific reference on the stability of many drugs in these formulations, however, is still lacking. This emphasizes the need for continued research in this area. Drug administration into the middle ear, nose, and eye of a child requires special attention. Certain drugs (e.g., sodium valproate and morphine) can be administered rectally to infants who have limited access for intravenous drug administration or if oral drug administration cannot be accomplished.

Transdermal drug delivery can be used in pediatric patients (1) to avoid problems of drug absorption from the oral route and complications from the intravenous route and (2) to maximize duration of effect and minimize adverse effects of drugs. Unfortunately, the commercially available transdermal dosage forms (e.g., clonidine, scopolamine) are not intended for pediatric patients; these would deliver doses much higher than those needed for infants and children. Favorable results with percutaneous theophylline in infants with apnea[13] and with subcutaneous morphine in pediatric patients with cancer[56] form the basis for studies with additional drugs.

MEDICATION COMPLIANCE

The issue of medication compliance is more complex in pediatric patients than in adults. The parents must appreciate the importance of following the prescribing information. Among the factors that can negatively affect compliance are poor communication between the physician and patient or parent, insufficient prescribing information, lack of understanding about the severity of illness by the patient or parent, fear of side effects, failure of the patient or parent to remember to administer the drugs, inconvenient dosage forms or dosing schedules, and unpalatability of drug products.[57] Studies in pediatric volunteers have been done to compare the palatability of antibiotics.[58] These data may have important implications for compliance in children.

CONCLUSIONS

Although tremendous progress has been made in the area of pediatric pharmacotherapy, many questions remain unanswered. The pharmacokinetics of many important drugs have been elucidated, but correlation between pharmacokinetics and pharmacodynamics has not been explored fully. Similarly, effect of disease states, patient characteristics such as genetic status, and protein-binding alterations have not been studied for most drugs. Although pharmacokinetics studies are generally conducted once during therapy, data for certain drugs suggest that serum concentrations may change during a typical course of therapy in a patient receiving the same dose. Implications of such changes on patient outcome are unknown.

There will be a continued need to develop new methods and refine present techniques for measuring drug concentrations in small volumes of various body fluids of pediatric patients. These analytic methods should be easy to use, accurate, precise, sensitive, and specific for measuring drugs in biologic specimens.

The development of new drugs has contributed to improved patient care. However, greater emphasis should be placed on disease prevention. Millions of children die because of preventable diseases, particularly in developing countries of the world. Administration of vaccines and control of diarrhea alone could save millions of these lives annually. However, the developed countries face different problems. The infant mortality rate in the United States is nearly twice as high among blacks as with whites. In some cities, more than 30% of the infants admitted to neonatal intensive care units were born to cocaine-abusing mothers.[59] Improved prenatal care and educational programs, and avoidance of alcohol, smoking, and drugs of abuse during pregnancy, may decrease mortality as well as morbidity from illnesses, including acquired immunodeficiency syndrome.

Another exciting development is an identification of the genetic cause of common serious diseases such as cystic fibrosis. Nearly 70% of the gene mutations in cystic fibrosis are caused by the loss of a single trinucleotide codon, and the protein therefore lacks only one amino acid, phenylalanine. One day soon it may be possible to offer gene therapy to correct the gene defects that cause a multitude of diseases.[60] Finally, new procedures (extracorporeal membrane oxygenation, organ transplantation) and new drugs (colony stimulating factors, dornase alpha, epoetin alpha, immunoglobulins, surfactants, growth hormones) may improve quality of life or survival in patients in certain situations.

Although much needs to be learned about the optimization of pediatric therapy, it is encouraging to witness the continued growth in knowledge of this area.

▶ PRINCIPLES OF PHARMACOTHERAPY

- Assess patients, medication history, and clinical/laboratory data.
- Document the need for drug therapy.
- Confirm the accuracy of patient's age, body weight, and dosage regimens of drugs.
- Select the most appropriate dosage form and regimen.
- Prepare a stable extemporaneous dosage form if not commercially available.
- Use the most effective, safe, palatable, and economical medicines based on comparative data.
- Establish therapeutic end points and measure health outcomes.
- Monitor for adverse effects and drug interactions.
- Implement changes in drug(s), dose(s), or dosage interval(s) as needed.
- Simplify regimens to improve compliance.
- Counsel patients and caregivers.
- Periodically contact the patient and caregivers for continuity of care.

REFERENCES

1. Ventura SJ, Anderson RN, Martin JA, et al. Births and deaths: Preliminary data for 1997. National Vital Statistics Report. U.S. Department of Health and Human Services. Center for Disease Control. National Center for Health Statistics. 1998;47:27–28.
2. Avery GB, Randolph JG, Weaver T. Gastric acidity in the first day of life. Pediatrics 1966;37:1005–1007.
3. Agunod M, Yamaguchi N, Lopex R, et al. Correlative study of hydrochloric acid, pepsin, and intrinsic factor secretion in newborns and infants. Am J Dig Dis 1969;14:400–414.
4. Huang NN, High RN. Comparison of serum levels following the administration of oral and parenteral preparations of penicillin to infants and children of various age groups. J Pediatr 1953;42:657–668.
5. Silverio J, Poole JW. Serum concentrations of ampicillin in newborn infants after oral administration. Pediatrics 1973;51:578–580.
6. O'Connor WJ, Warren GH, Edrada LS, et al. Serum concentrations of sodium nafcillin in infants during the perinatal period. Antimicrob Agents Chemother 1965:220–222.
7. Jalling B. Plasma concentrations of phenobarbital in the treatment of seizures in newborns. Acta Paediatr Scand 1975;64:514–524.
8. Signer E, Fridrich R. Gastric emptying in newborns and young infants. Acta Paediatr Scand 1975;64:525–530.
9. Boreus IO. Plasma concentrations of phenobarbital in mother and child after combined prenatal and postnatal administration for prophylaxis of hyperbilirubinemia. J Pediatr 1978;93:695.
10. Morselli PL. Serum levels and pharmacokinetics of anticonvulsants in the management of seizure disorders. In: Merkin B, ed. Clinical Pharmacology. Chicago, Year Book, 1978:89.
11. Tyrala FF, Hillman LS, Hillman RE, et al. Clinical pharmacology of hexachlorophene in newborn infants. J Pediatr 1977;91:481–486.

12. McFadden S, Haddow JE. Coma produced by topical application of isopropanol. Pediatrics 1969;43:622–623.
13. Evans NJ, Rutter N, Hadgraft J, et al. Percutaneous administration of theophylline in preterm infant. J Pediatr 1985;107:307–311.
14. Friis-Hansen B. Body water compartments in children: Changes during growth and related changes in body composition. Pediatrics 1961;28:169–181.
15. Haughey DB, Hilligoss DM, Grassi A, et al. Two-compartment gentamicin pharmacokinetics in premature neonates: A comparison to adults with decreased glomerular filtration rates. J Pediatr 1980; 96:325–330.
16. Nahata MC, Powell DA, Durrell DE, et al. Effect of gestational age and birth weight on tobramycin kinetics in newborn infants. J Antimicrob Chemother 1984;14:59–65.
17. Roberts RJ. Pharmacologic principles in therapeutics in infants. In: Drug Therapy in Infants. Philadelphia, Saunders, 1984:3–12.
18. Pitlick W, Painter M, Pippenger C. Phenobarbital pharmacokinetics in neonates. Clin Pharmacol Ther 1978;23:346–350.
19. Painter MJ, Pippenger C, MacDonald H, et al. Phenobarbital and diphenylhydantoin levels in neonates with seizures. J Pediatr 1978; 92:315–319.
20. Silverman WA, Anderson DH, Blanc WA, et al. A difference in mortality rate and incidence of kernicterus among premature infants allotted to two prophylactic antibacterial regimens. Pediatrics 1956;18: 614–624.
21. Odell GB. The dissociation of bilirubin from albumin and its clinical implications. J Pediatr 1959;55:268–279.
22. Morselli PL. Clinical pharmacokinetics in neonates. Clin Pharmacokinet 1976;1:81–98.
23. Committee on Drugs, American Academy of Pediatrics. The transfer of drugs and other chemicals into human milk. Pediatrics 1994; 93:137–150.
24. Anderson PO. Drugs and breast milk. J Pediatr 1995;95:957.
25. Rane A. Basic principles of drug disposition and action in infants and children. In: Yaffe JF, ed. Pediatric Pharmacology: Therapeutic Principles in Practice. New York, Grune & Stratton, 1980:7–28.
26. Weiss CF, Glazko AJ, Weston JK. Chloramphenicol in the newborn infant. A physiologic explanation of its toxicity when given in excessive doses. N Engl J Med 1960;262:787–794.
27. Nahata MC, Powell DA. Comparative bioavailability and pharmacokinetics of chloramphenicol after intravenous chloramphenicol succinate in premature infants and older patients. Dev Pharmacol Ther 1983;6:23–32.
28. Kuhn R, Nahata MC, Powell DA, et al. Netilmicin pharmacokinetics in newborn infants. Eur J Clin Pharmacol 1986;29:635–637.
29. Chay PCW, Duffy BJ, Walker JS. Pharmacokinetic-pharmacodynamic relationships of morphine in neonates. Clin Pharmacol Ther 1992; 51:334–342.
30. Edwards DJ, Zarowitz BJ, Slaughter RL. Theophylline. In: Evans WE, Schentag JJ, Jusko WJ, eds. Applied Pharmacokinetics, 3rd ed. Vancouver, WA, Applied Therapeutics, 1992:1–47.
31. Leffert FL. The management of chronic asthma. J Pediatr 1980; 97:875–885.
32. Johnston DE. Immunotherapy in children: Past, present, and future. Part I. Ann Allergy 1981;46:1–7.
33. Johnston DE. Immunotherapy in children: Past, present, and future. Part II. Ann Allergy 1981;46:59–66.
34. Kearin M, Kelly JG, O'Malley K. Digoxin "receptors" in neonates: An explanation of less sensitivity to digoxin than in adults. Clin Pharmacol Ther 1980;28:346–349.
35. Kawai M, Momoi T, Yorifuji T, et al. Unfavorable effects of growth hormone therapy on the final height of boys with short stature not caused by growth hormone deficiency. J Pediatr 1997;130:205–209.
36. Glasgow AM, Boeckx RL, Miller MK, et al. Hyperosmolality in small infants due to propylene glycol. Pediatrics 1983;72:353–355.
37. Hiller JL, Benda GI, Rahatzad M, et al. Benzyl alcohol toxicity: Impact of mortality and intraventricular hemorrhage among very low birth weight infants. Pediatrics 1986;77:500–506.
38. Grossman ER, Walchek A, Freedman H. Tetracyclines and permanent teeth: The relation between dose and tooth color. Pediatrics 1971; 47:567–570.
39. Walker RC, Wright AJ. The quinolones. Mayo Clin Proc 1987; 62:1007–1012.
40. Chysky V, Kapla M, Hullman R, et al. Safety of ciprofloxacin in children: Worldwide clinical experience based on compassionate usage. Infection 1991;19:289–296.
41. Schentag JJ, Plaut ME, Cerra FB, et al. Aminoglycoside nephrotoxicity in critically ill surgical patients. J Surg Res 1979;26:270–279.
42. Kauffman RE, Habersange R. Modification of dosage regimens in disease states of childhood. In: Mirkin BL, ed. Clinical Pharmacology and Therapeutics: A Pediatric Perspective. Chicago, Year Book, 1978: 73–88.
43. Roberts RJ. Special considerations in drug therapy in infants. In: Drug Therapy in Infants. Philadelphia, Saunders, 1984:25–35.
44. Feinstein RA, Miles MV. The effect of acute viral hepatitis on theophylline clearance. Clin Pediatr 1985;24:357–358.
45. Wallace CS, Hall M, Kuhn RJ. Pharmacologic management of cystic fibrosis. Clin Pharm 1993;12:657–674.
46. Myers MG, Roberts JF, Mirhig NJ. Effect of gestational age, birth weight, and hypoxemia on the pharmacokinetics of amikacin in serum of infants. Antimicrob Agents Chemother 1977;11:1027.
47. Bahal-O'Mara N, Jones R, Nahata MC, et al. Pharmacokinetics of phenytoin in children with acute neurotrauma. Crit Care Med 1995; 23:1418–1424.
48. Nahata MC, Powell DA, Glazer JP, et al. Effect of intravenous flow rate and infection site on *in vitro* delivery of chloramphenicol succinate and *in vivo* kinetics. J Pediatr 1981;99:463–466.
49. Nahata MC, Powell DA, Durrell DE, et al. Effect of infusion methods on tobramycin serum concentrations in newborn infants. J Pediatr 1984;104:136–138.
50. Gould T, Roberts RJ. Therapeutic problems arising from the use of intravenous route for drug administration. J Pediatr 1979;95: 465–471.
51. Rajchgot P, Radde IC, MacLeod SM. Influence of specific gravity on intravenous drug delivery. J Pediatr 1981;99:658–661.
52. Berman W, Whitman V, Marks KH, et al. Inadvertent overadministration of digoxin to low birthweight infants. J Pediatr 1978;92:1024.
53. Zenk KE, Anderson S. Improving the accuracy of mini-volume injections. Infusion 1982;Jan/Feb:7–11.
54. Nahata MC, Durrell DE. Stability of tobramycin sulfate in admixtures containing calcium gluconate. Am J Hosp Pharm 1985;42:1987–1988.
55. Nahata MC, Hipple TF. Pediatric Drug Formulations, 3rd ed. Cincinnati, Harvey Whitney, 1997:1–118.
56. Nahata MC, Miser A, Miser J, et al. Analgesic plasma concentrations of morphine in children with terminal malignancy receiving a continuous subcutaneous infusion of morphine sulfate to control severe pain. Pain 1984;18:109–114.
57. Boreus LO. Drug compliance. In: Yaffe SJ, ed. Principles of Pediatric Pharmacology. New York, Churchill Livingstone, 1982:176–192.
58. Matsui D, Barron A, Rieder MJ. Assessment of the palatability of antistaphylococcal antibiotics in pediatric volunteers. Ann Pharmacother 1996;30:586–588.
59. Cherukuri R, Minkoff H, Feldman J, et al. A cohort study of alkaloidal cocaine (crack) in pregnancy. Obstet Gynecol 1988;72:147–151.
60. Nahata MC. Discovery of the gene defect in cystic fibrosis: Implications for diagnosis and treatment. Clin Pharm 1990;9:716–717.

5

GERIATRICS

Joseph T. Hanlon, PharmD, MS, BCPS, FASCP, FASHP, Christine M. Ruby, PharmD, BCPS, Penny S. Shelton, PharmD, FASCP, and Charles C. Pulliam, MS Pharm, FASHP

Pharmacotherapy for the elderly can cure or palliate disease as well as enhance health-related quality of life (HRQOL). Health-related quality of life considerations for the elderly include focusing on improvement in physical functioning (e.g., activities of daily living), psychological functioning (e.g., cognition, depression), social functioning (e.g., social activities, support systems), and overall health (e.g., general health perception).[1–4] Despite the benefits of pharmacotherapy, HRQOL can be compromised by drug-related problems. The avoidance of drug-related adverse consequences in the elderly requires health care practitioners to become knowledgeable about a number of age-specific issues. To address these knowledge needs, this chapter will discuss the epidemiology of aging, physiologic changes associated with aging with emphasis on those that could affect the pharmacokinetics and pharmacodynamics of drugs, common clinical conditions seen in geriatric patients, epidemiology of drug-related problems in the elderly, and an approach to reduce drug-related problems through the provision of comprehensive geriatric assessment.

EPIDEMIOLOGY OF AGING

In an era of limited resources, the importance of community assessment and population-based planning for clinical practice cannot be overstated. Not only does awareness of a population's social and health characteristics provide a rational basis for allocating present resources and skills, but it also makes possible prudent attention to future training, research, and resource needs. In considering the entire older American population, the terms "diversity" and "heterogeneity" are frequently and appropriately applied. It is teasing apart the various threads of wellness and illness, independence and dependence, wealth and poverty, and function and dysfunction that makes the available sociodemographic data valuable for clinical practice today and planning for the future.

A clamor of attention has been given to the aging of the "baby boomer" generation. However, during the 5 to 7 years following the publication of this fourth edition of *Pharmacotherapy,* the rate of increase in older Americans will slow. This has occurred because today's new elders were born during the Great Depression years, a time of low birth rate in the United States.[5] More relevant to today's practitioners will be the declining mortality rate among elders, which has lead to increasing numbers of older Americans living into advanced old age.[6] In the 20 years from 1990 to 2010, the population aged 65 years or older will grow 1.3% annually, its slowest 20-year rate of this century. In contrast, the age group 85 years or older is the fastest-growing segment of the population during the 1990s. According to the Census Bureau, the 85 and older population will grow from approximately 3 million in 1990 to 4.3 million in the year 2000, a 43% increase during the decade.[5]

When today's elders were young adults, America was less racially and ethnically diverse than it is today. Consequently there is less racial and ethnic diversity among elders than we see in society as a whole. By the middle of the 21st century the elderly black population will increase threefold and the elderly Hispanic population will increase fourfold, with a resulting decline in the proportion of elderly white citizens from 86% to 67%.[7]

Although life expectancy rose from 47 to 75 years through the first three-quarters of the 20th century, the rate of increase diminished during the 1980s.[8] At the start of this century 41% of newborns would live to see their 65th birthday; in 1991 the proportion who could expect the same had risen to 80%.[5] More relevant to providers of care for older Americans is life expectancy at age 65. In 1991, white women 65 years of age could expect an average additional 19.2 years of life; black women, 17.2 years; white men, 15.4 years; and black men, 13.4 years. Life expectancy at age 85 ranges from 6.5 to 5.1 years in the same race and gender order.[5]

The largest proportion of elders, both men and women, in every age strata live at home independently. Of course, a far larger proportion (89% for women, 90% for men) of 65- to 74-year-olds live independently than do elders 85 years of age or older (38% for women, 54% for men).[9] In 1991, 77% of elderly householders were homeowners, most living in single-family homes.[5] Only a small proportion (4%) of those 65 years of age and older reside in nursing homes.[10]

Maintenance of independence and prevention of disability are primary goals in the clinical care of persons 65 years of age or older. This is an important principle in geriatric care, one that ought to influence therapeutic decisions (e.g., prescribing). Recent data among older people suggest that disability rates, measured by ability to perform activities of daily living, are declining (21.3% in 1994 compared to 24.0% in 1982).[11] Moreover, disability among elders with functional problems may be less severe than that reported in previous research.[11] For elders between the ages of 65 and 80, the most common causes of disability are from chronic diseases.[6]

Persons suffering from chronic diseases account for 80% of hospital days, 69% of hospital admissions, and 83% of prescription drug use.[12] Rates of chronic disease are highest among those 65 or older compared to younger age groups. At least one chronic disease burdens almost 9 of 10 elders (88%); and two or more chronic diseases are suffered by 7 out of 10 (69%) in the senior age group.[12] These high figures are consistent with 1993 data indicating that 88.2% of elders had visited a physician in the previous year.[13] Moreover, because of these multiple comorbidities, the elderly take multiple prescription medications. Elderly prescription medications account for approximately 35% ($12.7 to 14.3 billion in 1991) of all drug expenditures in the United States.[14]

The most common chronic conditions of older Americans have changed little in the past decade.[15] Arthritic conditions remain the most prevalent (50%) of the chronic diseases in this age group. When taken together, the prevalence of hypertension and other heart diseases (36% and 32%, respectively) exceed the arthritic conditions. Other prevalent conditions among older Americans in rank order include hearing impairments (29%), cataracts (17%), orthopedic impairments (17%), sinusitis (15%), diabetes (10%), tinnitus (9%), and visual impairments (8%).[15] Common primary diagnoses for elderly patients admitted to a nursing home are cardiovascular or cerebrovascular disease, mental disorders, nervous system or sensory impairment, or complications secondary to injuries.[10] A recent study of patients in eight nursing homes found the five most frequent active chronic conditions to be cardiovascular and cerebrovascular disorders, arthritis, dementia, and depression.[16] Hospital admission diagnoses in the elderly have been studied as well. In a recent population-based study of hospital admissions in the elderly, investigators found that from one-half to approximately two-thirds of progressive disability or catastrophic patients were admitted with one of seven medical diagnoses: stroke, cancer, hip fracture, coronary artery disease, congestive heart failure, diabetes mellitus, or dehydration.[17] A common problem noted in elderly hospitalized patients is delirium, present in approximately 25% of this population.[18]

As mentioned previously, the mortality rate among elders is declining. Figure 5–1 shows the top ten causes of death in elders, which have changed little during the past decade. In 1980, heart diseases, cancers, or stroke accounted for 75% of death in those 65 or older; in 1995, these diagnoses accounted for 79% of deaths.[19] Among young elders (age 65 to 74), heart diseases and cancers each accounted for approximately one-third of all deaths in 1995, but among the old-old (85 years and older) heart diseases alone accounted for 42% of deaths.[19]

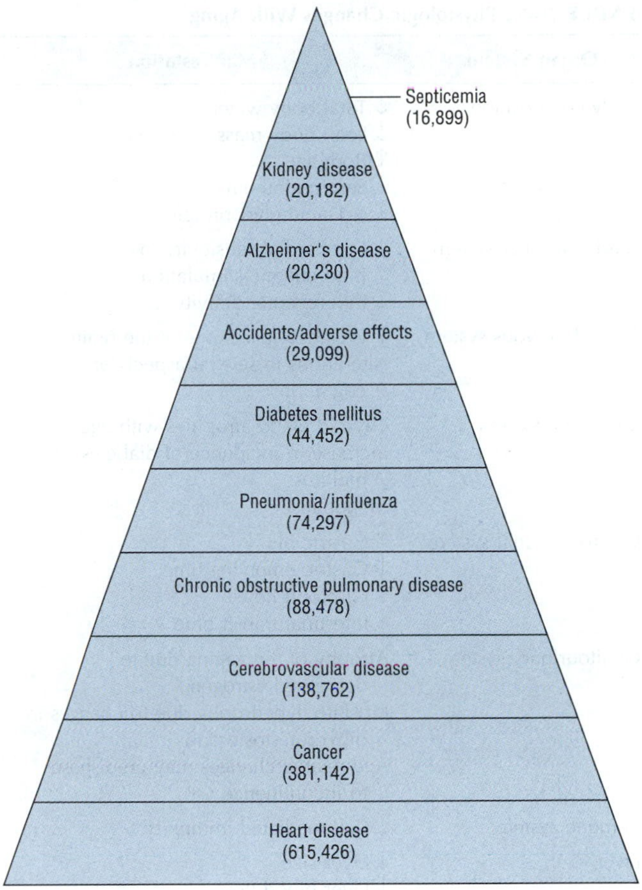

FIGURE 5–1. Leading causes of death in persons 65 years and older, 1995. (Rates per 100,000 population in parentheses.) *(Adapted from Ref. 19.)*

HUMAN AGING AND CHANGES IN DRUG PHARMACOKINETICS AND PHARMACODYNAMICS

There is a progressive functional decline in organ systems with advancing age. Table 5–1 reviews some common physiologic changes with emphasis on those that can affect pharmacotherapy. For more detailed information, readers are referred to discussions in several recent reviews.[20–22]

Age-associated physiologic changes may cause reductions in functional reserve capacity (or the ability to respond to physiologic challenges or stresses) and the homeostasis of the body.[23,24] In order to deal with physiologic challenges or stresses, an older individual may need 95% of their remaining reserve capacity.[21] However, physiologic aging slowly reduces functional reserve capacity and homeostatic control mechanisms, thus making an elder more susceptible to decompensation in a stressful situation. The cardiovascular, musculoskeletal, and central nervous system may be most affected.[21] An event resulting in functional impairment may involve an insult for which the body cannot compensate, and relatively small stresses may result in major morbidity and mortality.[23]

TABLE 5–1. Physiologic Changes With Aging

Organ System	Manifestation
Body composition	↓ Total body water ↓ Lean body mass ↑ Body fat ↓ Serum albumin ↑ α-1-acid glycoprotein
Cardiovascular system	↓ Myocardial sensitivity to β-adrenergic stimulation ↓ Baroreceptor activity
Central nervous system	↓ Weight and volume of the brain Alterations in several aspects of cognition
Endocrine system	Thyroid gland atrophies with age Increase in incidence of diabetes mellitus Menopause
Gastrointestinal system	↑ Gastric pH ↓ Gastric emptying time ↓ GI blood flow ↓ Intestinal transit time
Genitourinary system	Atrophy of the vagina due to decreased estrogen Prostate hypertrophy due to changes in dihydrotestosterone Age-related changes may predispose to incontinence
Immune system	↓ Cell-mediated immunity
Liver	↓ Liver size ↓ Liver blood flow
Oral changes	Altered dentition ↓ Ability to taste sweetness, sourness, and bitterness
Pulmonary system	↓ Respiratory muscle strength ↓ Chest wall compliance ↓ Total alveolar surface
Renal system	↓ Glomerular filtration rate ↓ Renal blood flow ↓ Tubular function
Sensory changes	↓ Accommodation of the lens of the eye, causing far-sightedness Presbycusis—a loss of auditory acuity
Skeletal system	Loss of skeletal bone mass (osteopenia)
Skin and hair	Skin dryness, wrinkling, and changes in pigmentation, epithelial thinning, loss of dermal thickness ↓ Number of hair follicles ↓ Number of melanocytes in the hair bulbs

There are a number of physiologic changes that occur with aging that could potentially affect pharmacokinetics and pharmacodynamics (Table 5–1). Unfortunately, limited data are available about the pharmacokinetics and pharmacodynamics of individual drugs that are commonly used in the elderly. This information gap may improve with the passage of new Food and Drug Administration (FDA) regulations establishing a "geriatric use" subsection in product labeling as well as voluntary adaption of the "Guidelines for the Study of Drugs Likely to Be Used in the Elderly" by pharmaceutical companies.[25,26]

ALTERED PHARMACOKINETICS

Table 5–2 and the following discussion summarizes what is known about each of the four major phases of pharmacokinetics.[27–29]

ABSORPTION

Most drugs are given orally, and thus a number of age-related changes in gastrointestinal physiology (Table 5–1) could potentially affect the absorption of medications. Fortunately, most drugs are absorbed via passive diffusion and age-related physiologic changes appear to have little influence on bioavailability.[30] There are a few drugs that require active transport and thus their bioavailability may be reduced (e.g., calcium in the setting of reduction in gastric acidity). However, there is evidence showing a decreased first-pass effect that results in increased bioavailability and higher plasma concentrations of drugs such as propranolol and morphine.[30]

The effect of age-related changes in skin physiology on the bioavailability of drugs delivered transdermally is poorly understood. One study found that the bioavailability of transdermal fentanyl was enhanced.[31] Whether this finding holds true for the currently marketed transdermal fentanyl dosage form or other drugs delivered transdermally remains to be determined.

DISTRIBUTION

The distribution of medications in the body depends on factors such as blood flow, plasma protein binding, and body composition, each of which may be altered with age (Table 5–1). For example, the volume of distribution of water-soluble drugs is decreased, whereas lipophilic drugs will exhibit an increased volume of distribution.[27–29] Changes in the volume of distribution of medications can have a direct impact on the amount of medication that needs to be given as a loading dose.

The two major plasma proteins to which medications can bind are albumin and α-1-acid glycoprotein, and these may change with age (see Table 5–1).[32] For acidic drugs such as naproxen, phenytoin, tolbutamide, and warfarin, decreased serum albumin may lead to an increased free fraction. The increase in α-1-acid glycoprotein levels may lead to a decreased free fraction of basic medications such as lidocaine, propranolol, quinidine, and imipramine. Although clinical effects of these potential changes are unlikely, they are important to consider when interpreting serum drug levels for these drugs, as usually only total concentrations (free and bound drug) are reported.

METABOLISM

The liver is the major organ responsible for drug metabolism, including phase I (preparative) or phase II (conjugative) reactions.[33] Recent data suggest that age-related declines in phase I metabolism are more likely due to reduced

TABLE 5–2. Age-related Changes in Drug Pharmacokinetics

Pharmacokinetic Phase	Pharmacokinetic Parameters
Gastrointestinal absorption	Unchanged passive diffusion and no change in bioavailability for most drugs ↓ Active transport and ↓ bioavailability for some drugs ↓ Decreased first-pass effect and ↑ bioavailability
Distribution	↓ Volume of distribution and ↑ concentration of water-soluble drugs ↑ Volume of distribution and ↑ half-life for fat-soluble drugs ↑ Or ↓ decreased free fraction of highly plasma protein bound drugs
Hepatic metabolism	↓ Clearance and ↑ half-life for some phase I oxidation drugs ↓ Clearance and ↑ half-life of drugs with high extraction ratio
Renal excretion	↓ Clearance and ↑ half-life of renally eliminated drugs

liver volume rather than reduced hepatic enzymatic activity.[34] Decreased phase I metabolism, producing decreased clearance and increased half-life, has been reported for medications such as diazepam, piroxicam, theophylline, and quinidine. Phase II metabolism of medications such as oxazepam appears to be relatively unaffected by age.

Age-related decreases in liver blood flow (Table 5–1) can also significantly decrease the metabolism of high hepatic extraction ratio drugs such as imipramine, lidocaine, morphine, and propranolol.[33] The effect that age has on drugs that undergo polymorphic drug metabolism is less clear, although a recent study suggests that age had no biologically important effect on acetylator phenotype.[35] Moreover, a number of potential confounding factors including race, gender, frailty, smoking, diet, and drug interactions may significantly affect hepatic metabolism in the elderly.[36]

ELIMINATION

Renal excretion is the primary route of elimination for many drugs. Although age-related reductions in glomerular filtration are well documented, as many as one-third of "normal" elderly subjects may have no decrease as measured by creatinine clearance.[27–29] Moreover, emerging information suggests that tubular secretion may not decline in proportion to other renal processes.[37] The estimation of creatinine clearance by using equations, although not entirely accurate in all patients, can serve as a useful screening approximation.[38] One of the most commonly used equations was created by Cockcroft and Gault.[39] It can be calculated by the following equation:

$$\text{Creatinine clearance (males)} = \frac{(140 - \text{age})(\text{actual body weight in kg})}{(72)(\text{serum creatinine})}$$

For females, multiply the above result times 0.85.

Medications that are primarily renally excreted for which there is evidence of age-related reduction in clearance include acetazolamide, amantadine, aminoglycosides, atenolol, captopril, cimetidine, digoxin, lithium, and vancomycin. Some hepatically metabolized medications can yield active, primarily renally excreted metabolites such as *N*-acetylprocainamide, normeperidine, and morphine-6-glucuronide, whose clearance is also reduced with advanced age.

ALTERED PHARMACODYNAMICS

There is some evidence in the elderly of enhanced drug response or "sensitivity." Four possible mechanisms have been suggested: changes in receptor numbers, changes in receptor affinity, postreceptor alterations, and age-related impairment of homeostatic mechanisms.[24,40] Evidence from epidemiologic and experimental studies suggests that, independent of pharmacokinetic alterations, the elderly are more sensitive to benzodiazepine's central nervous system effects. The elderly also have greater analgesic response to narcotics when compared with their younger counterparts. In addition, the elderly may have enhanced response to anticoagulants such as warfarin and heparin and thrombolytic therapy. Certain drugs (e.g., beta agonists and antagonists) exhibit decreased pharmacodynamic sensitivity. In addition, reflex tachycardia, commonly seen with vasodilator therapy, is often blunted in the elderly, perhaps due to dampened baroreceptor function. Moreover, for some drugs (calcium channel blockers), both enhanced pharmacodynamic sensitivity (as demonstrated by greater reduction in blood pressure) and decreased sensitivity (as demonstrated by reduced atrioventricular node blockade) occur simultaneously.[29]

CLINICAL GERIATRICS

As mentioned previously, maintenance of independence and prevention of disability are primary goals in the clinical care of persons 65 years of age or older. Because the elderly are not a homogeneous group, to achieve these goals it is necessary that clinicians understand the concept of functional status. Typically, functional status can be determined by inquiring about an elderly patient's ability to perform basic activities of daily living (feeding, dressing, ambulation, toileting, bathing, grooming) and instrumental activities of daily living (cooking, cleaning, shopping, using the telephone, managing money, and managing medications).[41,42] However, functional status depends not only on physical ailments but also on psychological and social circumstances.[2]

TABLE 5–3. The I's of Geriatrics: Common Problems in the Elderly

Immobility	Instability
Isolation	Intellectual impairment
Incontinence	Impotence
Infection	Immunodeficiency
Inanition (malnutrition)	Insomnia
Impaction	Iatrogenesis
Impaired senses	

One of the challenges of maintaining and improving functional status in geriatric patients is diagnosing and managing conditions primarily seen in the elderly. Common problems found in older patients are sometimes referred to as the "I's" of Geriatrics (Table 5–3).[20] Examples of diseases and syndromes that can present as these common problems include Parkinson's disease, falls, hip fractures, benign prostatic hypertrophy, dementia, glaucoma, postherpetic neuralgia, and tuberculosis.

Another factor that contributes to the challenge of clinical geriatrics is that approximately 50% of older patients present with atypical symptoms or complaints, making it difficult to use the classic medical model for diagnosis.[43–45] Such unusual presentations may be due to factors associated with age-related physiologic changes, the presence of multiple comorbid illnesses, compromised functioning, and the presence of psychological stressors.[43] Table 5–4 presents some examples of medical illnesses that often present atypically.[43–45] Other atypical symptoms are also often indicative of frailty, and commonly include delirium, falls, and nonspecific functional decline.[43–45]

TABLE 5–4. Atypical Disease Presentation in the Elderly

Disease	Presentation
Acute myocardial infarction	Only ~50% present with chest pain, and diaphoresis and vomiting are uncommon in the absence of chest pain. In general, the elderly present with weakness, confusion, syncope, and abdominal pain; however, ECG findings are similar to younger patients.
Gastrointestinal bleeding	Although the mortality rate is ~10%, the presenting symptoms are nonspecific, ranging from mental status change to syncope with hemodynamic collapse. Abdominal pain is often absent.
Congestive heart failure	Instead of dyspnea the patient may present with hypoxic symptoms, lethargy, restlessness, and confusion.
Urinary tract infection	Dysuria, fever, and flank pain may be absent. More commonly the elderly present with incontinence, confusion, abdominal pain, nausea/vomiting, and azotemia.
Upper respiratory infection	Older patients typically present with lethargy, confusion, anorexia, and decompensation of a preexisting medical condition. Fever, chills, and a productive cough may or may not be present.

Another common threat to independence that distinguishes elderly from younger patients is multiple coexisting chronic illnesses. It is not unusual for elderly patients to have multiple comorbidities such as osteoarthritis, heart disease, and diabetes. Although multiple comorbidities can have a substantial impact on a patient's functional status, the mere existence of multiple diseases alone does not determine functional impairment.

DRUG-RELATED PROBLEMS IN THE ELDERLY

Although medications used by the elderly can lead to improvement in HRQOL, negative outcomes due to drug-related problems are considerable.[46,47] Two important and potentially preventable negative outcomes due to drug-related problems that can occur in the elderly are therapeutic failure (inadequate drug therapy), and adverse drug reactions (ADRs).[48,49] There are limited data regarding the prevalence of therapeutic failure in the elderly. Grymonpre and coworkers reported that 19% of drug-associated hospital admissions in a group of older Canadians were related to therapeutic failure.[48] Adverse drug reactions are thought to occur more commonly among elders, compared with other age groups.[47] However, it is controversial whether age alone is a risk factor.[50] The reported rates of ADRs in the elderly range from 2.5% to 50.6%, depending on the study population and methodology employed.[47] In the nursing home setting, a recent cost of illness study estimated that drug-related problems cost $4 billion per year.[51]

RISK FACTORS

A number of factors increase the risk of drug-related problems in the elderly, including suboptimal prescribing (overuse of medications or polypharmacy, inappropriate use, and underuse); medication errors (both dispensing and administration problems); and patient medication noncompliance (both intentional and unintentional). The following sections address suboptimal prescribing and medication noncompliance, the most common problems.

OVERUSE

Overuse of medications refers to a type of polypharmacy in which several different agents are unnecessarily used concomitantly.[52,53] Polypharmacy is common in elderly persons; community-based surveys reveal that elders take an average of 2.7 to 3.9 prescription and nonprescription medications.[54,55] This figure is almost doubled for those elders who are hospitalized.[54] A recent nursing facility survey found that institutionalized elderly persons take an average of 8.9 routine and prn medications.[56] Drug-use studies have not routinely defined polypharmacy as a specific number of unnecessary medications. However, a recent critical evaluation concluded that up to 51% of medications for the elderly were "overused."[57] Moreover, population-based studies have shown that whites, women, and those with advanced age are more likely to use greater numbers of prescription and nonprescription drugs.[58,59]

Multiple medication use has been strongly associated with adverse drug reactions.[47] The increase in ADR risk rises with increasing drug use. The sequelae of multiple drug use may also increase use of health care resources and the associated costs.[52,53]

INAPPROPRIATE PRESCRIBING

Inappropriate prescribing is defined as prescribing of medications outside the bounds of accepted medical standards.[60–62] This phenomenon occurs commonly for elderly outpatients, as exemplified by a study in which explicit criteria were applied to make implicit judgments of prescribing appropriateness in 208 ambulatory elderly veterans with polypharmacy. The investigators found that 74% of drugs taken by these older patients had at least one inappropriate rating.[60]

Alternatively, inappropriate prescribing can be defined as those drugs whose use should be avoided, because the risk outweighs the benefit.[57,63] A critical evaluation of the literature concluded that as much as three fourths of medications for the elderly are inappropriately prescribed.[56] Applying explicit criteria developed by Beers and associates[63] for 20 medications or medication classes whose use should be avoided in the elderly, Wilcox and coworkers found that 23.5% of persons 65 years of age and older from the 1987 National Medical Expenditure Survey were taking one or more such drugs.[64] These explicit criteria were recently revised and have been expanded to consider drug–disease interactions.[65]

Inappropriate prescribing may pose important health risks. Limited retrospective data suggest that inappropriate prescribing is associated with drug-related hospital admissions and readmissions. A recent GAO report estimated that hospitalization due to inappropriate prescribing in the elderly costs $20 billion annually.[66] One study documented that 50% of adverse drug reactions causing hospital admissions in elderly patients were due to inappropriate prescribing of drugs with contraindications or interactions.[67] Doucet and colleagues,[68] in a prospective study of 1000 elderly people admitted to hospital, found that 12.9% were related to one type of inappropriate prescribing: drug–drug interactions. Finally, Bero and associates[69] found that 29% of drug-related hospital readmissions were due to medication inappropriateness.

UNDERUSE

Underuse of medications has not been well studied in the elderly. One study found that 55% of 236 ambulatory elderly patients had one or more necessary drugs omitted by lack of physician prescribing.[70] Other investigators have focused on the omission of treatment of certain conditions such as hypertension, cancer chemotherapy, depression, and myocardial infarction.[70,71] In particular, depression in the elderly is an illness that is underdiagnosed and undertreated by drugs.[72] For instance, 8% of community elders in one study were determined to be depressed, but only 11.2% of those with depression had received antidepressants in the previous year.[73] Recognition and treatment of depression may be improving in long-term care facilities, as evidenced by an increase in antidepressant usage from 16.3% to 26.3% over a 3-year period.[56]

Underuse may have an important relationship with negative health outcomes in the elderly. For example, untreated depression has been associated with functional disability, health services use, and death.[72] The risk from underuse of medication in general due to limiting Medicaid patients' access to medications resulted in a more than doubling of the risk of admission to a nursing home.[74]

MEDICATION COMPLIANCE

Medication noncompliance is a common problem in the elderly. The prevalence rate is reported to range from 40% to 70% of patients, with the average being approximately 50% of patients.[75,76] However, these patients may be compliant with up to 75% of their medications, overall.[77] It is commonly thought that the elderly have worse compliance than younger patients. However, this does not appear to be the case when the number of drugs taken by both groups is similar.[78] What does seem to be different is that intentional noncompliance may be more common in the elderly.[79] Some have speculated that this may be related to the occurrence of adverse drug reactions and may represent intelligent noncompliance.[76]

Limited retrospective data suggest that noncompliance is associated with drug-related hospital admissions. A meta-analysis of studies published before 1989 by Sullivan and associates that included patients of all ages determined that the rate of hospital admissions due to noncompliance was 5.5%.[80] A more recent study by Col and coworkers evaluated 315 consecutive elderly patients admitted to a hospital and determined that 11.4% of admissions were due to noncompliance.[81]

PROVISION OF COMPREHENSIVE GERIATRIC ASSESSMENT

Given that drug-related problems are common, costly, and clinically important, how can they be improved? A solution may lie in comprehensive geriatric assessment. The term "comprehensive geriatric assessment" has been applied to geriatric evaluation and management (GEM), where GEM clinicians manage the patient; and to consultative geriatric assessment, where the geriatric multidisciplinary team makes recommendations to other clinicians for the management of the patient.[82–84] Comprehensive geriatric assessment has become a cornerstone in the care of the elderly; its effectiveness was recently summarized in a meta-analysis of 28 controlled trials.[85–87]

A number of published papers describe the role of pharmacists in optimizing pharmacotherapy for the elderly.[88–92] One has specifically documented the contribution of a clinical pharmacist to the effectiveness of interdisciplinary specialized geriatric care on drug-related problems.[92] The following sections provide an approach to how pharmacists in any practice setting can optimize medication use through the provision of comprehensive geriatric assessment.

HISTORY TAKING

Several potential difficulties may occur while taking medication histories from the elderly. They include (1) communication problems (impaired hearing and vision); (2) underreporting (health beliefs, cognitive impairment); (3) vague or nonspecific symptoms (altered presentation); (4) multiple diseases and medications; (5) reliance on a caregiver for the history; and (6) lack of medical records to confirm findings. However, despite these potential difficulties, practitioners should find value in pursuing the collection of this vital medication history information. The importance of inquiry regarding nonprescription medication use in the elderly cannot be stressed enough, as one third of all medications used by the ambulatory elderly are sold without a prescription, including analgesics, nutritional supplements, and laxatives.[55] Asking elders and their caregivers about methods they use to keep track of medicines is also important. This will allow one to design solutions to problems that are detected, and prevent repeating ineffective and previously used methods. It is also prudent to question about risk factors for prescribing problems (e.g., multiple physicians and pharmacies) and for compliance problems (e.g., impaired hearing, vision, and cognition; ability to open safety caps, pay for medicines, and swallow medications).[93]

ASSESSING AND MONITORING DRUG THERAPY

It is important to assess the prescribing appropriateness of each medication, which can be accomplished using a variety of methods.[62,65,94,95] One standardized measure, with demonstrated reliability and validity, is the Medication Appropriateness Index (MAI).[94–98] The MAI consists of 10 questions that should be asked for each medication (Table 5–5). Other factors to consider when assessing prescribing appropriateness that are not included in the MAI include (1) suboptimal choice, (2) allergy (especially for new prescriptions), (3) undertreatment, and (4) drug–food/lab interactions.[94] Some additional factors to consider during drug regimen review include compliance, medication storage problems, therapeutic endpoints, and adverse drug reactions.

TABLE 5–5. Medication Appropriateness Index

1. Is there an indication for the drug?
2. Is the medication effective for the condition?
3. Is the dosage correct?
4. Are the directions correct?
5. Are the directions practical?
6. Are there clinically significant drug–drug interactions?
7. Are there clinically significant drug–disease/condition interactions?
8. Is there unnecessary duplication with other drug(s)?
9. Is the duration of therapy acceptable?
10. Is this drug the least expensive alternative compared to others of equal utility?

Complied from Refs. 94–97.

DOCUMENTING PROBLEMS AND FORMULATING A THERAPEUTIC PLAN

It is important to document the problems that have been detected, develop a therapeutic plan to resolve them, and establish reasonable therapeutic endpoints if these have not already been set. An important point to highlight is that what may be a reasonable endpoint for a 40-year-old patient may not be as reasonable for an 80-year-old person when comorbidities, functional status, and life expectancy are taken into consideration.

CONSULTING THE PHYSICIAN REGARDING PROBLEMS/CONCERNS

In some cases, it will be necessary to consult with the patients' physician regarding problems and concerns that have been detected and documented. The importance of optimizing the prescribing for elderly patients before implementing strategies to enhance their compliance cannot be over stressed. Otherwise, the compliance intervention, if effective, may result in patient harm. Similarly in institutional settings, strategies to reduce medication administration errors may not improve patient outcomes if prescribing is not improved beforehand.

COUNSELING AND COMPLIANCE AIDS

Some general factors to consider, before medication dispensing, to enhance compliance in the elderly include modifying medication schedules to fit patient life-style, considering generic agents to reduce costs, using easy-to-open bottles and easy-to-swallow dosage forms, and using larger type direction labels and auxiliary labels.[99,100] When dispensing medications (in particular, new medications or changes in old ones), both written and verbal drug information should be provided to the patient and family. To improve the likelihood of compliance, one should also recruit active patient and family involvement, stress the importance of compliance, and consider the use of compliance-enhancing aids (special packaging, medication record, drug calendar, medication boxes, magnification for insulin syringes, dose-measuring devices, and spacers for metered-dose inhalers).[101–103] In institutional settings, discussion of special considerations (medications that can be crushed and given via feeding tube) with health care professionals responsible for medication administration is also prudent.

DOCUMENTING INTERVENTIONS AND MONITORING PATIENT PROGRESS

All interventions must be documented, and the steps just outlined must be repeated over time with elderly patients. During follow-up contacts, minimum inquiry should include questions as to whether the patient has any questions or concerns regarding medicines and determining whether the therapeutic end points previously established have been achieved. Moreover, ask patients whether they are or have recently experienced any side effects, unwanted reactions, or other problems with their medications to assess potential adverse drug events.[104]

TARGETING HIGH-RISK ELDERLY

In busy practices, the approach outlined here may not be feasible for every patient. Therefore, practitioners may consider targeting these activities for patients at high risk for developing drug-related problems. A recent Delphi survey of geriatric experts identified 18 risk factors for drug-related problems in elderly nursing home patients.[105] These include (1) polypharmacy (9 or more medications or 12 or more doses per day); (2) taking specific high-risk drugs (intermediate and long half-life benzodiazepines, sedative/ hypnotics, antipsychotics, anticholinergics, narcotic analgesics, chlorpropamide); (3) certain patient characteristics (low body weight, age ≥ 85 years, decreased renal function); (4) use of narrow therapeutic range drugs (lithium, digoxin, warfarin, anticonvulsants); (5) a history of prior adverse drug reaction; and (6) presence of six or more illnesses. The applicability of these criteria to elderly persons in other care settings, and the relationship between identification of elderly patients with these potential risk factors and actual health outcomes, remain to be determined.

CONCLUSIONS

The number of people above age 65 years is growing in the United States and around the world. A number of physiologic changes with age can affect pharmacokinetics and pharmacodynamics of drugs, especially particular hepatic metabolism and renal excretion. Improving and maintaining functional status and managing comorbidities are hallmarks of clinical geriatrics. Certain medical conditions are restricted to the elderly, and drug-related problems represent a major concern for this group. Innovative approaches, such as the provision of comprehensive geriatric assessment by pharmacists, are needed to decrease the occurrence of these drug-related problems. Adherence to the principles outlined below may also result in more optimal pharmacotherapy for the elderly.

▶ PRINCIPLES OF PHARMACOTHERAPY

- Consider whether drug therapy is absolutely necessary.
- Streamline the number of medicines needed to treat common problems.
- Adjust doses and/or dosage intervals for medications.
- Establish reasonable therapeutic end points and monitor for these desired outcomes.
- Monitor for adverse drug reactions.
- Encourage compliance.
- Regularly review for long-term medications.

REFERENCES

1. Applegate WB, Blass JP, Williams TF. Instruments for the functional assessment of older patients. N Engl J Med 1990;322:1207–1214.
2. Kane RA. Instruments to assess functional status. In: Cassel CK, Cohen HJ, Larson EB, et al, eds. Geriatric Medicine, 3rd ed. New York, Springer-Verlag, 1997:169–179.
3. Ware JE, Sherbourne CD. The MOS 36-item short-form health survey (SF-36). Med Care 1992;30:473–483.
4. Weinberger M, Samsa GP, Hanlon JT, et al. Evaluation of a brief health status measure in elderly veterans. J Am Geriatr Soc 1991; 39:691–694.
5. U.S. Bureau of the Census. Current Population Reports, Special Studies, P23-190, 65+ in the United States. Washington DC, U.S. Government Printing Office, 1996.
6. Applegate WB, Burns R. Geriatric medicine. JAMA 1996;275: 1812–1813.
7. Institute of Medicine. Feasley JC, ed. Health outcomes for older people: Questions for the coming decade. Washington, DC, National Academy Press, 1996.
8. Fries JF, Green LW, Levine S. Health promotion and the compression of morbidity. Lancet 1989;1:481–483.
9. Guralnik JM, Simonsick EM. Physical disability in older Americans. J Gerontol 1993;48:3–10.
10. Dey AN. Characteristics of elderly nursing home residents: Data from the 1995 national nursing home survey. U.S. Department of Health and Human Services, Centers for Disease Control and Prevention, National Center for Health Statistics, Advance Data. 1997; 289:1–9.
11. Manton KG, Corder L, Stallard E. Chronic disability trends in elderly United States populations—1982–1994. Proc Natl Acad Sci USA 1997;94:2593–2598.
12. Hoffman C, Rice D, Sung HY. Persons with chronic conditions: Their prevalence and costs. JAMA 1996;276:1473–1479.
13. Rubenstein LZ . Contexts of care. In: Cassel CK, Cohen HJ, Larson EB, et al, eds. Geriatric Medicine, 3rd ed. New York, Springer-Verlag, 1997:73–80.
14. Long SH. Prescription drugs and the elderly: Issues and options. Health Affairs 1994;2:157–174.
15. National Center for Health Statistics. Current estimates from the National Health Interview Survey, 1994. Vital Health Stat 1995;10: 81–82.

16. Mulrow CD, Gerety MB, Cornell JE, et al. The relationship between disease and function and perceived health in very frail elders. J Am Geriatr Soc 1994;42:374–380.
17. Ferrucci L, Guralnik JM, Pahor M, et al. Hospital diagnoses, Medicare charges, and nursing home admissions in the year when older persons become severely disabled. JAMA 1997;277:728–734.
18. Francis J. Delirium in older patients. J Am Geriatr Soc 1992; 40:829–838.
19. Anderson RN, Kochanek KD, Murphy SL. Report of final mortality statistics, 1995. Monthly Vital Stat Rep 1997;25(S2):20–24.
20. Kane RL, Ouslander JG, Abrass IB. Clinical implications of the aging process. In: Essentials of Clinical Geriatrics, 3rd ed. New York, McGraw-Hill, 1994:3–18.
21. Lamy PP. Introduction to the aging process. In: Delafuente JC, Stewart RB, eds. Therapeutics in the Elderly, 2nd ed. Cincinnati, Harvey Whitney Books, 1995:1–30.
22. Taffet GE. Age-related physiologic changes. In: Reuben DB, Yoshikawa TT, Besdine RW, eds. Geriatrics Review Syllabus: A Core Curriculum in Geriatric Medicine, 3rd ed. Dubuque, IA, Kendall/Hunt for the American Geriatrics Society, 1996:11–24.
23. Becker PM, Cohen HJ. The functional approach to the care of the elderly: A conceptual framework. J Am Geriatr Soc 1984;32:923–929.
24. Swift CG. Pharmacodynamics: Changes in homeostatic mechanisms, receptor and target organ sensitivity in the elderly. Br Med Bull 1990;46:36–52.
25. U.S. Food and Drug Administration. Guidelines of the study for drugs likely to be used in the elderly. J Geriatr Drug Ther 1990; 5:5–17.
26. U.S. Food and Drug Administration. Specific requirements on content and format of labeling for human prescription drugs: Addition of "geriatric use" subsection in the labeling. Fed Reg 1997;62: 45313–45326.
27. Chapron DJ. Drug disposition and response in the elderly. In: Delafuente JC, Stewart RB, eds. Therapeutics in the Elderly, 2nd ed. Cincinnati; Harvey Whitney Books, 1995:190–211.
28. Parker BM, Cusack BJ, Vestal RE. Pharmacokinetic optimisation of drug therapy in elderly patients. Drugs Aging 1995;7:10–18.
29. Institute of Medicine. Pharmacokinetics and drug interactions in the elderly and special issues in elderly African-American populations. Washington, DC, National Academy Press, 1997:1–42.
30. Iber FL, Murphy PA, Connor ES. Age-related changes in the gastrointestinal system: Effects on drug therapy. Drugs Aging 1994;5: 34–48.
31. Holdsworth MT, Forman WB, Killilea TA, et al. Transdermal fentanyl disposition in elderly subjects. Gerontology 1994;40: 32–37.
32. Wallace SW, Verbeeck RK. Plasma protein binding in the elderly. Clin Pharmacokinet 1987;12:41–72.
33. Woodhouse K, Wynne HA. Age-related changes in hepatic function. Drugs Aging 1992;2:243–255.
34. Sotaniemi EA, Arranto AJ, Pelkonen O, Pasanen M. Age and cytochrome P450-linked drug metabolism in humans. Clin Pharmacol Ther 1997;61:331–339.
35. Korrapati MR, Sorkin JD, Andres R, et al. Acetylator phenotype in relation to age and gender in the Baltimore Longitudinal Study of Aging. J Clin Pharmacol 1997;37:83–91.
36. O'Mahony MS, Woodhouse KW. Age, environmental factors and drug metabolism. Pharmacol Ther 1994;61:279–284.
37. Ujhelyi MR, Bottorff MB, Schur M, et al. Aging effects on the organic base transporter and stereoselective renal clearance. Clin Pharmacol Ther 1997;62:117–128.
38. Malmrose LC, Gray SL, Pieper CF, et al. Measured versus estimated creatinine clearance in a high-functioning elderly sample: MacArthur Foundation Study of Successful Aging. J Am Geriatr Soc 1993;41: 715–721.
39. Cockcroft DW, Gault MH. Prediction of creatinine clearance from serum creatinine. Nephron 1976;16:31–41.
40. Feely J, Coakley D. Altered pharmacodynamics in the elderly. Clin Geriatr Med 1990;6:269–283.
41. Katz S, Akpom CA. A measure of primary sociobiologic functions. Int J Health Serv 1976;6:493–507.
42. Fillenbaum GG. Screening the elderly: A brief instrumental ADL measure. J Am Geriatr Soc 1985;33:698–706.
43. Fried LP, Storer DJ, King DE, et al. Diagnosis of illness presentation in the elderly. J Am Geriatr Soc 1991;39:117–23.
44. Jarrett PG, Rockwood K, Carver D, et al. Illness presentation in elderly patients. Arch Intern Med 1995;155:1060–1064.
45. Starer PJ. History and physical examination. In: Abrams WB, Beers MH, Berkow R, eds. Merck Manual of Geriatrics. Whitehouse Station, NJ, Merck, 1995:205–224.
46. Pulliam CC, Hanlon JT, Moore SR. Contemporary issues in geriatric drug therapy. J Geriatr Drug Ther 1989;4:43–86.
47. Hanlon JT, Schmader K, Gray SL. Adverse drug reactions. In: Delafuente JC, Stewart RB, eds. Therapeutics in the Elderly, 3rd ed. Cincinnati, Harvey Whitney Books. In press.
48. Grymonpre RE, Mitenko PA, Sitar DS, et al. Drug-associated hospital admissions in older medical patients. J Am Geriatr Soc 1988;36: 1092–1098.
49. Karch FE, Lasagna L. Adverse drug reactions: A critical review. JAMA 1975;234:1236–1241.
50. Gurwitz JH, Avorn J. The ambiguous relation between aging and adverse drug reactions. Ann Intern Med 1991;114:956–966.
51. Bootman JL, Harrison DL, Cox E. The health care cost of drug-related morbidity and mortality in nursing facilities. Arch Intern Med 1997;157:2089–2096.
52. Montamat SC, Cusack B. Overcoming problems with polypharmacy and drug misuse in the elderly. Clin Geriatr Med 1992;8: 143–158.
53. Stewart RB, Cooper JW. Polypharmacy in the aged: Practical solutions. Drugs Aging 1994;4:449–461.
54. Nolan L, O'Malley K. Prescribing for the elderly, part II. J Am Geriatr Soc 1988;36:245–254.
55. Hanlon JT, Fillenbaum GG, Burchett B, et al. Drug-use patterns among black and nonblack community dwelling elderly. Ann Pharmacother 1992;26:679–685.
56. Tobias DE, Pulliam CC. General and psychotherapeutic medication use in 878 nursing facilities: A 1997 national survey. Consult Pharm 1997;12:1401–1408.
57. Brook RH, Kamberg CJ, Mayer-Oakes A, et al. Appropriateness of acute medical care for the elderly: An analysis of the literature. Health Policy 1990;14:225–242.
58. Fillenbaum GG, Hanlon JT, Corder EH, et al. Prescription and nonprescription drug use among black and white community-residing elderly. Am J Public Health 1993;83:1577–1582.
59. Stewart RB, Marks RG, May FE, Hale WE. Factors which predict multiple drug use in the elderly. J Geriatr Drug Ther 1994;9:53–67.
60. Schmader K, Hanlon JT, Weinberger M, et al. Appropriateness of medication prescribing in ambulatory elderly patients. J Am Geriatr Soc 1994;42:1241–1247.
61. Murray MD. Medication Appropriateness Index: Putting a number on an old problem in older patients. Ann Pharmacother 1997;31: 643–644.
62. Buetow SA, Sibbald B, Cantrill JA, Halliwell S. Appropriateness in health care: Application to prescribing. Soc Sci Med 1997;45: 261–271.
63. Beers MH, Ouslander JG, Rollingher I, et al. Explicit criteria for determining inappropriate medication use in nursing home residents. Arch Intern Med 1991;151:1825–1832.
64. Wilcox SM, Himmelstein DU, Woolhandler S. Inappropriate drug prescribing for community dwelling elderly. JAMA 1994;272: 292–296.
65. Beers MH. Explicit criteria for determining potentially inappropriate medication use by the elderly: An update. Arch Intern Med 1997; 157:1531–1536.

66. Prescription drugs and the elderly: Many still receive potentially harmful drugs despite recent improvements. GAO Report, July 1995: 1–30 (GAO/HEHS-95-152).
67. Lindley CM, Tulley MP, Paramsothy V, Tallis RC. Inappropriate medication is a major cause of adverse drug reactions in elderly patients. Age Ageing 1992;21:294–300.
68. Doucet J, Chassagne P, Trivalle C, et al. Drug–drug interactions related to hospital admissions in older adults: A prospective study of 1000 patients. J Am Geriatr Soc 1996;44:944–948.
69. Bero LA, Lipton HL, Bird JA. Characterization of geriatric drug-related hospital readmissions. Med Care 1991;29:989–1003.
70. Lipton HL, Bero LA, Bird JA, McPhee SJ. Undermedication among geriatric outpatients: Results of a randomized controlled trial. Ann Rev Gerontol Geriatr 1992;12:95–108.
71. Gurwitz JH. Suboptimal medication use in the elderly. The tip of the iceberg. JAMA 1994;272:316–317.
72. National Institute of Health (NIH) consensus statement. Diagnosis and treatment of depression in late life: Consensus statement update. JAMA 1997;278:1186–1190.
73. Blazer D, Hughes DC, George LK. The epidemiology of depression in an elderly community population. Gerontologist 1987;27:281–287.
74. Soumerai SB, Ross-Degnan D, Avorn J, et al. Effects of Medicaid drug-payment limits on admission to hospitals and nursing homes. N Engl J Med 1991;325:1072–1077.
75. Stewart RB, Caranasos G. Medication compliance in the elderly. Med Clin North Am 1989;73:1551–1560.
76. Weintraub M. Compliance in the elderly. Clin Geriatr Med 1990; 6:445–452.
77. Lipton HL, Bird JA. The impact of clinical pharmacists' consultations on geriatric patients' compliance and medical care use: A randomized controlled trial. Gerontologist 1994;34:307–315.
78. German PS, Klein LE, McPhee SJ, et al. Knowledge of and compliance with drug regimens in the elderly. J Am Geriatr Soc 1982; 30:568–571.
79. Cooper JK, Love DW, Raffoul PR. International prescription nonadherence (noncompliance) by the elderly. J Am Geriatr Soc 1982; 30:329–333.
80. Sullivan SD, Kreling DH, Hazlet TK. Noncompliance with medication regimens and subsequent hospitalizations: Literature analysis and cost of hospitalization estimate. J Res Pharm Econ 1990;2: 19–33.
81. Col N, Fanale JE, Kronholm P. The role of medication noncompliance and adverse drug reactions in hospitalizations in the elderly. Arch Intern Med 1990;150:841–845.
82. Rubenstein LZ. Geriatric assessment: An overview of its impact. Clin Geriatr Med 1987;3:1–16.
83. Becker PM, McVey LJ, Saltz CC, et al. Hospital acquired complications in a randomized controlled clinical trial of a geriatric consultation team. JAMA 1987;257:2313–2317.
84. Epstein AM, Hall JA, Besdine R, et al. The emergence of geriatric assessment units. Ann Intern Med 1987;106:299–303.
85. American College of Physicians (ACP). Comprehensive functional assessment of the elderly. Ann Intern Med 1988;109:70–72
86. National Institute of Health (NIH) consensus development conference statement. Geriatric assessment methods for clinical decision-making. J Am Geriatr Soc 1988;36:342–347.
87. Stuck AE, Siu AL, Wieland GD, et al. Comprehensive geriatric assessment: A meta-analysis of controlled trials. Lancet 1993;342: 1032–1036.
88. Adamcik BA, Rhodes RS. The pharmacist's role in rational drug therapy of the aged. Drugs Aging 1993;3:481–486.
89. Dyer CC, Oles KS, Davis SW. The role of the pharmacist in a geriatric nursing home: A literature review. Drug Intell Clin Pharm 1984;18:428–433.
90. Hanlon JT, Weinberger M, Samsa GP, et al. A randomized controlled trial of a clinical pharmacist intervention with elderly outpatients with polypharmacy. Am J Med 1996;100:428–437.
91. Owens NJ, Silliman RA, Fretwell MD. The relationship between comprehensive functional assessment and optimal pharmacotherapy in the older patient. Drug Intell Clin Pharm 1989;23:847–854.
92. Owens NJ, Sherburne NJ, Silliman RA, Fretwell MD. The senior care study: The optimal use of medications in acutely ill older patients. J Am Geriatr Soc 1990;38:1082–1087.
93. Ruscin JM, Semla TP. Assessment of medication management skills in older outpatients. Ann Pharmacother 1996;30:1083–1087.
94. Lipton HL, Bird JA, Bero LA, McPhee SJ. Assessing the appropriateness of physician prescribing for geriatric outpatients: Development and testing of an instrument. J Pharm Technol 1993; 9:107–113.
95. Hanlon JT, Schmader KE, Samsa GP, et al. A method for assessing drug therapy appropriateness. J Clin Epidemiol 1992;45:1045–1051.
96. Samsa G, Hanlon JT, Schmader KE, et al. A summated score for the Medication Appropriateness Index: Development and assessment of clinimetric properties including content validity. J Clin Epidemiol 1994;47:891–896.
97. Fitzgerald LS, Hanlon JT, Shelton PS, et al. Reliability of a modified Medication Appropriateness Index in ambulatory older persons. Ann Pharmacother 1997;31:543–548.
98. Schmader K, Hanlon JT, Landsman PM, et al. Inappropriate prescribing and health outcomes in the elderly in a pharmacist intervention trial. Ann Pharmacother 1997;31:529–533.
99. Mallet L. Counseling in special populations: The elderly patient. Am Pharm 1992;NS32:71–81.
100. Opdycke RA, Ascione FJ, Shimp LA, Rosen RI. A systematic approach to educating elderly patients about their medications. Patient Educ Counsel 1992;19:43–60.
101. Murray MD, Birt JA, Manatunga AK, Darnell JC. Medication compliance in elderly outpatients using twice-daily dosing and unit-of-use packaging. Ann Pharmacother 1993;27:616–620.
102. Ascione FJ, Shrimp LA. The effectiveness of four education strategies in the elderly. Drug Intell Clin Pharm 1984;18:126–131.
103. Rivers PH. Compliance aids—Do they work? Drugs Aging 1992;2: 103–111.
104. Hanlon JT, Schmader KE, Koronkowski MJ, et al. Adverse drug events in high risk elderly outpatients. J Am Geriatr Soc 1997; 45:945–948.
105. Fouts MM, Hanlon JT, Pieper CF, et al. Identification of elderly nursing facility residents at high risk for drug-related problems. Consult Pharm 1997;12:1103–1111.

6

PHARMACOEPIDEMIOLOGY

Andy Stergachis, PhD, and Thomas K. Hazlet, PharmD, DrPH

The practice of pharmacotherapy requires knowledge of the benefits and risks of pharmaceuticals as applied to human populations. Much of our understanding about the efficacy and safety of drugs arises from well-controlled studies conducted during the drug development and approval process. However, many additional risks and, to a lesser degree, additional benefits are only identified after the drug is widely used by the general population. Benefits and risks learned following a drug's approval may range from relatively minor to clinically important effects that seriously alter an individual drug's benefit-to-risk ratio. The association between certain appetite-suppressant drugs and primary pulmonary hypertension and valvular heart disease is a recent example where serious adverse effects were discovered only after these drugs had come into widespread use.[1,2] This example highlights both the inherent limitations of the drug development process and the need to study populations receiving medications obtained through usual clinical practice. The purpose of this chapter is to describe the role of pharmacoepidemiology in drug development and therapeutics and to characterize the primary methods and issues in this field.

Pharmacoepidemiology is a discipline that provides valuable information about the health and cost outcomes of drugs, devices, and biologics, particularly after their approval for clinical use. Pharmacoepidemiology is defined as the study of the use of and the effects of drugs in large numbers of people.[3] The field as applied to the period after a drug enters the market is referred to as postmarketing drug surveillance (PMS) or pharmacovigilance. There is an ever-increasing number of health research reports that use epidemiologic study methodologies, such as case control and cohort study designs, to assess the association between drug exposures and health outcomes. One of the noteworthy developments in the field has been the use of automated, linked databases that permit efficient and rapid studies of drug effects.

Epidemiologic study designs are essential for evaluating drug safety and effectiveness in situations where it is either unfeasible or unethical to randomly assign patients to active treatment or placebo. While the randomized, controlled, blinded trial (RCT) is the standard against which other designs are measured, it is often not suitable for questions within the domain of pharmacoepidemiology. Randomized trials, for example, cannot contribute much to our understanding of the long-term or rare adverse effects associated with therapies. Clinical trials conducted prior to drug approval cannot uncover every important health effect of a pharmaceutical. For example, the adverse health effects of drugs on the human fetus can be estimated only through observational but not experimental methods. Epidemiologic studies of the patterns of drug prescribing and use are also essential to assess a drug's usefulness.[4] As a discipline, pharmacoepidemiology has traditionally concerned itself with the study of adverse drug effects. Epidemiologic study designs, such as case control and cohort studies, are also used to identify beneficial effects of drugs in populations. For example, to determine the relationship between patterns of use of inhaled corticosteroids and the risk of fatal or near fatal asthma, Ernst and colleagues conducted an epidemiologic study of 12,301 residents of Saskatchewan who were dispensed 10 or more asthma drugs over a 10-year period.[5] They found a 90% lower risk of fatal and near-fatal asthma among regular users of inhaled corticosteroids. These findings support practice guidelines that recommend the use of inhaled anti-inflammatories in moderate to severe asthmatics.

Whether or not a drug in fact achieves its desired effect in the real world is referred to as its effectiveness, not efficacy. Studies of drug effectiveness are generally conducted using observational study designs.[6] It is widely recognized that results from an RCT offer the best evidence that a drug will perform under ideal conditions and it is likely that the RCT, "well-controlled" design will continue to be required for New Drug Applications (NDAs) to the Food and Drug Administration (FDA). As described in regulations governing NDAs, reports of adequate and well-controlled investigations provide the primary basis for determining whether there is "substantial evidence" to support the claims of effectiveness for new drugs.[7] However, the rigorous circumstances surrounding design and implementation of the RCT do not necessarily extrapolate to the individual patient. Fletcher and associates draw a distinction between "efficacy"—does the treatment work? —and "effectiveness"—does the treatment's benefits outweigh its liabilities for those to whom it is offered in clinical practice?[8] The tension between the conflicting goals of validity in efficacy trials and generalizability in effectiveness trials is shown in Figure 6–1. For example, in an efficacy trial, subjects are selected using narrowly defined eligibility criteria, are monitored closely to assure that they use or are exposed to the intervention in the manner defined in the trial's protocol, and are cooperative with medical advice. In clinical practice, patients are not selected and the manner in which the patient uses the intervention may vary widely from the intended use for which it was approved. For instance, in an

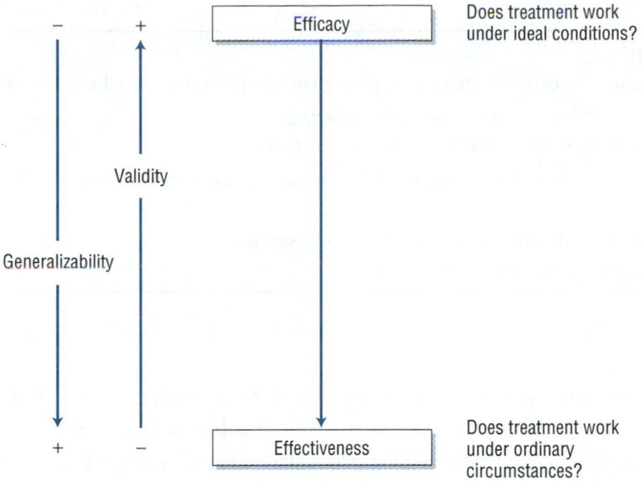

FIGURE 6–1. Schematic drawing showing the tension between conflicting goals of validity in efficacy trials and generalizalility in effectiveness trials. *(Adapted from Ref. 8.)*

effectiveness trial to compare stepped care beginning with niacin to the use of lovastatin in the treatment of elevated LDL-C, Oster and coworkers found that insurance status and out-of-pocket expenses for drugs, issues that would not often surface in a clinical trial, had a major impact on compliance and therapeutic response.[9] Clinical outcomes among RCT subjects are often better than in nontrial patients.[10] Finally, trials to evaluate effectiveness in clinical practice are difficult or expensive for researchers because, with diminished control over patient behavior, there is a risk that study results will be inconclusive.

LIMITS OF KNOWLEDGE AT THE TIME OF NEW DRUG APPROVAL

The new drug approval process and the role of pharmacoepidemiology in the United States have evolved since the Federal Food, Drug, and Cosmetic (FD&C) Act of 1938 was enacted into law. The FD&C Act was adopted following the deaths of more than 100 patients of renal failure from sulfanilamide prepared in a diethylene glycol vehicle.[11] For the first time in U.S. history, the act required a drug to be proven safe under conditions of use intended by the manufacturer prior to marketing. The act also required manufacturers to conduct preclinical toxicity testing and gather and submit clinical data about drug safety to the FDA prior to drug marketing under a New Drug Application. It also required new drugs to be labeled with adequate instructions and appropriate warnings for safe use. However, the FD&C act required no proof of drug efficacy.

The FD&C act was amended in 1962 following the epidemic of thalidomide-associated birth defects in Europe.[12] The Kefauver–Harris Amendments of 1962 strengthened the requirements for proof of drug safety and added a new requirement for demonstration of drug efficacy prior to marketing. Requiring "substantial evidence that the drug will have the effect it purports or is represented to have" resulted in the establishment of the randomized controlled clinical trial as the "gold standard" for proof of efficacy. The 1962 amendments also required manufacturers to report adverse drug events detected in the postmarketing setting to the FDA. Investigational New Drug Applications (INDs) were required to be submitted to the FDA before clinical testing could begin. In 1985, requirements for manufacturers' adverse drug event (ADE) reporting were clarified and specific regulations and guidelines were published to define the manufacturers' obligations in reviewing and reporting adverse drug reactions.

The Kefauver–Harris Amendments also identified explicit phases of preclinical animal testing followed by three phases of clinical testing (Fig. 6–2). In addition, there is a postapproval surveillance and phase 4 of drug development. Today, we are witnessing even more regulatory changes to our drug approval process as it pertains to pharmacoepidemiology. The Food and Drug Administration

	Early research preclinical testing		Clinical Trials: Phase I	Clinical Trials: Phase II	Clinical Trials: Phase III		FDA		Phase IV
Years	6.5		1.5	2	3.5		1.5	15 Total	Additional post-marketing testing required by FDA
Test population	Laboratory and animal studies	File IND at FDA	20–80 healthy volunteers	100–300 patient volunteers	1000–3000 patient volunteers	File NDA at FDA	Review process/ approval		
Purpose	Assess safety and biologic activity		Determine safety and dosage	Evaluate effectiveness, look for side effects	Confirm effectiveness, monitor adverse reactions from long-term use				
Success rate	5000 compounds evaluated		5 enter trials				1 approved		

FIGURE 6–2. The drug development and approval process in the United States.

TABLE 6–1. Limitations of Premarketing Clinical Trials

Short duration	Premarketing studies are limited in time Effects that develop following chronic use or those that have a long latency period cannot be detected
Small sample size	Few drugs are studied in more than 4000 subjects before FDA approval Effects that occur with a frequency of less than 1/1000 are difficult to detect
Narrowly defined population	Premarketing studies generally do not include special populations, such as children, women of child-bearing age, or the elderly
Narrow set of indications	Manufacturers pursue specific indications for use during premarketing studies
Limited comparison groups	The comparison group is often limited to placebo

Modernization Act of 1997 resulted in new provisions stating that substantial evidence of drug effectiveness may consist of data from one adequate and well-controlled clinical investigation plus confirmatory evidence. This indicates that two or more well-controlled trials (the previous standard) are not always necessary and the FDA should relate the number and type of trials to the specific product under development. The act of 1997 also calls on the FDA to establish a system for tracking manufacturer compliance with promises to conduct postapproval (phase 4) studies on new drugs.

Phase 3 controlled clinical trials required by the FDA as part of the process of drug approval and labeling are the primary source of information about new drugs. Although these studies help ensure that a drug is efficacious and does not cause unacceptable harm, premarketing studies fail to provide much of the information needed to make therapeutic decisions.[13] Table 6–1 describes the major limitations of premarketing controlled clinical trials, which lend support to the need for further evaluation of drugs after their approval for marketing by the FDA. Briefly, clinical trials performed during drug development cannot be depended on to detect rare adverse drug events. In addition, they cannot directly be used to address the performance of drugs in the populations that will use the drug in ways not studied in clinical trials, because clinical trials restrict the complexity of the patients tested. Thus, often not included in drug testing are many persons who are likely to eventually receive new medicines—the chronically ill, women of child-bearing age, and pregnant women. To improve the representativeness of populations included in clinical trials, the FDA has issued guidelines in support of inclusion of geriatric patients in phase 2 and phase 3 studies. Also, the FDA has issued guidelines to encourage manufacturers to provide efficacy, safety, pharmacokinetic, and pharmacodynamic information in support of the use of drugs and biologic products in pediatric populations.

Despite the rigorous process for drug approval and regulation, there have been numerous major adverse drug reactions over the past 30 years. Recent examples of serious but uncommon effects include arrhythmias linked to the use of antihistamines terfenadine and astemizole,[14] acute flank syndrome associated with suprofen,[15] and the gastrointestinal and other adverse effects associated with the use of non-steroidal anti-inflammatory drugs in the elderly.[16,17] Partially in response to concerns about adverse drug effects, a number of epidemiology programs were developed, beginning in the 1970s. An initial emphasis of early programs such as the Boston Collaborative Drug Surveillance Program was the estimation of drug use and adverse events among hospitalized patients.[18] The Drug Epidemiology Unit, now the Slone Epidemiology Unit, was also formed in the early 1970s to perform hospital-based case control studies.[19] In the United Kingdom, the Drug Surveillance Research Unit established the Prescription Event Monitoring program in 1980, now called the Drug Safety Research Trust.[20] Subsequent resources for pharmacoepidemiology evolved from the use of Medicaid data, followed by the use of databases from health maintenance organizations (HMOs) and other population-based data sources. Since the time of the 1980 report of the Joint Commission on Prescription Drug Use, there has been considerable interest in the use of HMO records for postmarketing drug surveillance.[21] Advantages to conducting PMS in an HMO setting include the availability of an identifiable population base for the estimation of rates, presence of a relatively stable population base, and access to medical records and computerized databases.[22]

ROLE OF FDA AND PHARMACOEPIDEMIOLOGY

Drug development should be viewed as a process that continues even after a drug is approved for marketing. As noted in the previous section, it is not possible to detect all potential risks and benefits during premarketing studies. The FDA's postmarketing surveillance program provides important information on the clinical experience of medical products. The FDA's involvement in postmarketing drug surveillance includes monitoring approved drug use, monitoring the occurrence of serious adverse drug events associated with the use of approved drugs, and the initiation of selected epidemiologic studies to estimate the risk or test specific hypotheses.[23] One of the primary uses of findings from PMS of drugs is modification of a drug's labeling or package insert. Other methods used to communicate the results of PMS efforts involve requiring the manufacturer to mail out a "Dear Doctor" letter, publishing in the *FDA Med-*

ical Bulletin, presentation of findings at professional meetings, and publication of findings in peer-reviewed journals.

As a condition of approval for marketing, drug manufacturers are required to notify the FDA of all adverse events of which they are aware. It is important for clinicians to report ADEs either to the manufacturer or to the MEDWATCH program at the FDA. This program depends on health care professionals and the lay public to report serious adverse events observed in the course of their practice as part of their professional responsibility. The MEDWATCH form can be used to report adverse events or product problems related to any medical product, with the exception of those occurring with vaccines. Reports concerning vaccines should be sent to the Vaccine Adverse Event Reporting System (VAERS), a joint program of the FDA and the Centers for Disease Control and Prevention. Table 6–2 describes the characteristics of the FDA's MEDWATCH program.

The FDA provides limited funding for investigators to use large, automated databases to conduct large-scale epidemiologic studies. Through its cooperative agreements program, the FDA has encouraged the development of databases for use in pharmacoepidemiology. These agreements provide the FDA with access to data on the safety of pharmaceuticals. The objectives of these programs include the rapid and efficient conduct of pharmacoepidemiologic research designed to test hypotheses, particularly those arising from the MEDWATCH program. Current programs receiving funding for postmarketing drug surveillance from the FDA include Brigham and Women's Hospital and United HealthCare/ University of Washington. Even though the FDA supports cooperative agreements for PMS, it lacks regulatory authority to require phase 4 studies for previously approved drugs. The FDA Modernization Act of 1997 does require any sponsor of a drug that agreed to conduct a postmarketing study to report annually to the FDA on the progress of the study.

TABLE 6–2. Characteristics of the FDA's MEDWATCH Program

Report experiences with:
- Medications (drugs or biologics)
- Medical devices (including *in vitro* diagnostics)
- Special nutritional products (dietary supplements, medical foods, infant formulas)
- Other products regulated by the FDA

Report SERIOUS adverse events. An event is serious when the patient outcome is:
- Death
- Life threatening (real risk of dying)
- Hospitalization (initial or prolonged)
- Disability (significant, persistent, or permanent)
- Congenital anomaly
- Required intervention to prevent permanent impairment or damage

Report even if:
- You're not certain that the product caused the event
- You don't have all the details

Report product problems—quality, performance, or safety concerns—such as:
- Suspected contamination
- Questionable stability
- Defective components
- Poor packaging or labeling
- Therapeutic failures

Important numbers:
- 1-899-FDA-0178 to Fax report
- 1-800-FDA-7737 to report by modem
- 1-800-FDA-1088 to report by phone, for more information, or to obtain software for reporting by modem
- 1-800-822-7967 for a VAERS form for vaccines
- FDA MedWatch Web site: http://www.fda.gov/medwatch/
  Download reporting forms (PDF format)
  MedWatch information

ADVERSE DRUG EVENTS

The field of pharmacoepidemiology primarily concerns itself with the study of adverse drug reactions. According to the World Health Organization, an adverse drug reaction (ADR) is any noxious, unintended, and undesired effect of a drug, which occurs at doses used in humans for prophylaxis, diagnosis, or therapy.[24] The term adverse drug event (ADE) is used to describe an injury resulting from administration of a drug. Virtually any drug can have adverse effects. Between 3% and 11% of hospital admissions have been attributed to adverse effects.[25] The likelihood that a patient will experience an adverse drug event during hospitalization ranges from 1% to 44%, depending on the type of hospital, definition of an adverse event, and study methodology.[26] The economic impact of adverse drug events is substantial and potentially avoidable.[27] Recently, the incidence of serious and fatal adverse drug reactions in hospital patients was reported to be as high as 6.7% and 0.32%, respectively.[28]

Although most adverse drug effects can be anticipated, others are unpredictable, especially rare idiosyncratic reactions. Adverse reactions have been separated into Type A and B reactions.[29] Type A reactions are expected exaggerations of a drug's known pharmacologic effects of the drug. Therefore, they are usually dose dependent and predictable. Type A reactions are responsible for the majority of adverse drug events encountered. Examples include hypotension with antihypertensive agents and anticholinergic effects with the tricyclic antidepressants. Type A reactions tend to occur in individuals who have one of three characteristics.[30] First, the individuals may have received more of a drug than is customarily required. Second, they may have received a conventional dose of the drug, but they may metabolize or excrete the drug unusually slowly, leading to drug levels that are too high, possibly due to concomitant disease or drug interactions. Third, they may have normal drug levels, but for some reason are overly sensitive to them. Most type A reactions are identified prior to drug marketing and listed in a product's labeling.

Type B reactions are idiosyncratic and tend to be unrelated to the known pharmacologic action of the drug. They are usually not related to dose, unpredictable, uncommon, and potentially more serious than type A reactions. They may be due to what are known as hypersensitivity reactions or immunologic reactions. Type B reactions may be the consequence of some other idiosyncratic reaction to the drug, such as an inherited susceptibility. These reactions may concentrate in certain body systems, including the liver, blood, skin, kidney, and nervous system.[31] Type B reactions represent a major focus of pharmacoepidemiologic studies of adverse drug reactions. Carcinogenic and teratogenic adverse drug events are considered type B reactions.

Because adverse drug reactions represent an important public health concern, institutions complying with the Joint Commission on Accreditation of Healthcare Organizations (JCAHO) are required to perform numerous steps pertaining to the surveillance and management of adverse drug reactions. They must define significant adverse drug reactions, initiate intensive assessments for adverse drug reactions meeting the institution's definition, and be able to provide evidence during accreditation surveys of sufficiently detailed follow-up on the causes of adverse drug reactions.[32] JCAHO has recently instituted an additional requirement for reporting of sentinel events, which are those involving the occurrence of risk of death or serious physical or psychological injury. In situations where the sentinel event indicates an ongoing possibility of threat to life or safety, the JCAHO may conduct an unscheduled survey and require that the institution undertake extensive systems and process reviews, and implement improvements to prevent recurrence of the sentinel event.

METHODOLOGIES FOR PHARMACOEPIDEMIOLOGIC STUDIES

A wide variety of study designs and methods are used to generate pharmacoepidemiologic data. Epidemiologic methods, such as case control, cohort, and cross-sectional studies, are used extensively. Large automated databases, meta-analysis, randomized controlled trials, and hybrid designs, such as nested case control studies, also play an important role in pharmacoepidemiology. Epidemiologic studies typically do not use randomization to determine who will receive a particular drug exposure. Rather, associations between exposure(s) and disease(s) under study are determined through the use of observational study designs and statistical analyses. Observational methods are used in most situations. Ethics and cost limit use of experimentation. A variety of methods are used to study health events associated with drug exposures. The usual approach to studying adverse drug reactions has been the collection of spontaneous reports of drug-related morbidity or mortality. There has been a growing interest in using computerized databases containing medical care information for pharmacoepidemiologic studies.[33] These databases usually consist of patient-level data from two or more separate files, which were originally developed for clinical or administrative applications.[34] Through record linkage, it is possible to create person-based longitudinal files on an ad hoc basis. Multipurpose databases used for pharmacoepidemiologic studies include data from health maintenance organizations, the Medicaid program, the Medicare program, and geographically defined populations. In general, these databases include information on patient demographics, outpatient drugs, hospital discharge diagnoses, and ambulatory care encounters. The advantages and disadvantages of linked databases for pharmacoepidemiologic studies have been the subject of numerous publications.[35,36]

CASE REPORTS AND CASE SERIES

Case reports describe a single patient who was exposed to a drug and experienced a particular, usually adverse, outcome. For example, within the first 3 months of marketing, hemolytic anemia and acute renal failure following use of the antibiotic temafloxacin were reported to the Spontaneous Report System, the predecessor of the MEDWATCH System. Case reports are useful for raising hypotheses about drug effects to be tested with more rigorous study designs. It is uncommon for a case report or a series of case reports to be used to make a statement about causation. Case series are collections of patients, all of who have a single exposure, whose clinical outcomes are then evaluated and described. They are useful for quantifying the incidence of an adverse reaction, particularly for a newly approved drug. Further, case series can be useful for being certain that the incidence rate of any particular adverse effect of concern does not occur in a population, which is larger than that studied prior to drug's marketing.

If the event is rare and the exposure combination is very specific, the cause of the adverse health event may be inferred from a case series study. In most situations, however, it is necessary to compare cases with a group of controls to identify risk factors. Thus, the major disadvantage of a case series study is the lack of a comparison group. However, recent methodologic advances in the analysis of case series data allow the estimation of relative incidence without the use of controls.[37]

CASE CONTROL STUDIES

A case control study assembles a group of cases (people who have the disease of interest) and controls (people who do not). The exposure histories of the cases and the controls are determined to establish the extent of association between exposure(s) of interest and disease. Case control studies compare patients with a specific disease to a control group composed of similar people but without the disease. Case control studies attempt to identify risk factors for a disease by examining differences in antecedent exposure variables between cases and controls. For example, one can select cases of women of child-bearing age with ovarian cysts and compare them to controls, looking for differences in prior use of oral contraceptives. Such a study was performed to determine if the then newly introduced triphasic oral contraceptives were associated with functional ovarian cysts.[38]

Case control studies have been extensively used to assess the safety of pharmaceuticals. There are many examples of case control studies that have identified important associations between drugs and adverse health events: vaginal cancer and diethylstilbestrol (DES), Reye's syndrome and aspirin, peptic ulcer disease and nonsteroidal anti-inflammatory drugs, and venous thromboembolism and oral contraceptives. Data from case control studies are used to calculate an odds ratio, which is the ratio of the odds of developing the disease for exposed patients to the odds of developing the disease for the unexposed patients.

A classic example is a study of DES given during pregnancy and the risk of vaginal adenocarcinoma among female offspring nearly a generation later.[39] A study of hip fracture risk in relation to the prescription of benzodiazepines exemplifies a nested case control design.[40] Hip fracture cases and controls were chosen from a large existing database on health care use among Saskatchewan residents. The use of a nested case control design to efficiently assess the role of potential confounding factors is further illustrated in the previously cited study of inhaled corticosteroids and the risk of fatal and near-fatal asthma.[5] A nested case control study is an efficient variation of a case control and a cohort study. In a nested case control study, all cases (or a sample of all cases) and only a random sample of all controls are chosen for study from the same defined population.

An advantage of the case control design for the study of drug–outcome relationships is its efficiency for the study of rare or delayed outcomes. Compared with other strategies, the case control study is relatively inexpensive. One potential problem with case control studies is their susceptibility to certain types of bias, including selection bias and information bias.

COHORT STUDIES

A cohort study assembles a group of persons without the disease(s) of interest at the onset of the study, ascertains the exposure status of each person, and then follows the cohort over time to determine the development of disease in exposed and nonexposed persons. Cohort studies involve the comparison of the incidence of one or more outcome events among those who received a drug or some other exposure of interest compared with the incidence of the event(s) for a comparison group. For example, much information about the risk of fatal cardiovascular diseases among oral contraceptive users has come from the Royal College of General Practitioners Oral Contraception Study, in which 23,000 oral contraceptive users were compared with 23,000 nonusers chosen from the same British general practices.[41] Death certificate records were used to ascertain instances of fatal events during the follow-up period.

Cohort studies can be prospective, as the RCGP study illustrates, or retrospective. Prospective cohort studies are one of the most valid types of observational study designs, because exposure is measured and recorded prior to the development of the health outcome(s) of interest. Using a prospective cohort study design, Hooton and colleagues determined the association between contraceptive methods and symptomatic urinary tract infections in young women.[42] The investigators recruited sexually active young women who were starting a new method of contraception and followed them for 6 months to determine the incidence of symptomatic urinary tract infections by contraceptive method.

An alternative to the prospective cohort design is the retrospective cohort study. Retrospective cohort studies are useful when comparison cohorts of persons exposed and not exposed to drugs of interest can be identified at some time in the past from large preexisting databases and followed from that time to the present with regard to the incidence of a given outcome. Recently, Soumerai and associates used a retrospective cohort design to study the determinants and adverse health outcomes of beta-blocker underuse in elderly patients with myocardial infarction.[43] Controlling for other predictors of survival, the mortality rate among beta-blocker recipients was 43% less than that for the comparison group (relative risk, 0.57; 95% confidence interval, 0.47 to 0.69), suggesting that use of beta blockers reduces the risk of death among elderly patients with myocardial infarction.

Prospective cohort studies can provide strong evidence of associations between drugs and diseases because the exposure is assessed before the outcome occurs. However, because many cohort studies require large numbers of people followed for long periods of time, they can be expensive and, in some instances, infeasible. Retrospective or historical cohort studies can overcome these limitations if high quality data have already been collected and recorded.

USE OF QUASI-EXPERIMENTAL DESIGNS IN PHARMACOEPIDEMIOLOGY

One of the opportunities that has emerged with increased computerization in health care is the use of large, linked databases for exploring pharmaceutical outcomes. The ability to use transaction or claims data from an insurance company or state Medicaid agency and link these data to files containing diagnosis and other patient-specific information has allowed researchers to explore outcomes questions at relative low expense. Because these studies do not rely upon random assignment of subjects, they have been described as "quasi-experimental." The typical design includes a treatment (exposed) group, a control (unexposed) group, and some type of posttest assessment for both. Although efforts may be made to match treatment and control groups for important patient characteristics, the groups are not "equivalent" in the sense of an RCT. A refinement to this design is one where an analysis of "secular trends"—factors that could influence study outcomes and are

TABLE 6–3. Criteria for the Causal Nature of an Association

1. **The association makes biologic sense.** In other words, the proposed association is consistent with our knowledge of the mechanism of disease. You can use data from other human or animal studies, or data from *in vitro* studies.
2. **The suspected cause precedes the disease.** Even though this is self-evident, it can be overlooked when interpreting findings from certain observational studies.
3. **The association is strong.** Associations with a relative risk of less than 2.0 are considered to be weak. Risks of 2.0 to 4.0 are considered moderate, while those greater than 4.0 are strong. You also need to consider the 95% confidence interval.
4. **The association is found consistently when studied using different methods or populations.** An important characteristic of science is that a finding is reproducible.
5. **There is a dose–response relationship.** For example, there is a higher risk among persons with greater exposure to a risk factor.

progress independent of the study—is made using interrupted time series methods. These studies are often used to evaluate the consequences of a change in policy, such as a prescription limit, or addition or removal of a drug from the marketplace. For instance, Soumerai and associates studied the effect of a prescription cap on the use of psychotropic drugs and emergency mental health services using claims data. They used claims data collected over a 42-month period, including the 11 months that the prescription cap was in effect, and found that drug usage decreased while costs to the state Medicaid program increased during the period of the cap.[44]

INTERPRETATION OF PHARMACOEPIDEMIOLOGIC STUDIES

Not all associations represent a cause–effect relationship. Because most epidemiologic studies of drug effects do not employ random allocation, it is important to determine if a reported association is causal. A central methodologic concern in observational studies is confounding—that is, the possibility that the apparent effect of an exposure or intervention is due wholly or partly to other factors associated with it that have their own impact on the outcome of interest. Criteria have been proposed to help determine if an association is causal. The fewer criteria that are met, the less likely it is that an association is causal. Table 6–3 is adapted from the work of Hill and Stolly.[45,46] Practitioners should ask the series of questions listed in the table to interpret findings from studies to determine if an association is likely to be causal.

FUTURE DIRECTIONS

Pharmacoepidemiologic studies conducted during the postapproval period provide important information to assist in optimizing therapeutic responses to drugs. These studies can provide valuable information about the relationship between therapeutic agents and adverse and beneficial health outcomes. Information from pharmacoepidemiologic studies also contributes to population-based care and drug regulatory and reimbursement decisions. At the level of individual patient care, a combination of medical and epidemiologic knowledge leads to the choice to use a particular medication. Moreover, patient monitoring to optimize the therapeutic response to drugs also involves epidemiologic data and logic to balance likely benefits against potential risks. Epidemiologic information can provide vital information regarding safety, patterns of drug use, and effectiveness to assist in the provision of evidence-based health care. There is an inherent trade-off between the need for more information about a drug's risks and the need to make a drug available for use. Because of limitations in the drug development process, more information emerges about a drug after its approval through postmarketing surveillance.

REFERENCES

1. Abenhaim L, Moride Y, Brenot F, et al. Appetite-suppressant drugs and the risk of primary pulmonary hypertension. N Engl J Med 1996; 335:609–616.
2. Connolly HM, Crary JL, McGoon MD, et al. Valvular heart disease associated with fenfluramine-phentermine. N Engl J Med 1997;337: 581–588.
3. Strom BL, ed. Pharmacoepidemiology. New York, Wiley, 1994.
4. Collett JP, Boissel JP. Pharmacoepidemiology: Epidemiologic approach to the study of drugs. Post Marketing Surveillance 1991;5: 3–14.
5. Ernst P, Spitzer WO, Suissa S, et al. Risk of fatal and near-fatal asthma in relation to inhaled corticosteroid use. JAMA 1992;268: 3462–3464.
6. Strom BL, Melmon KL. The use of pharmacoepidemiology to study beneficial drug effects. In: Strom BL, ed. Pharmacoepidemiology. New York, Wiley, 1994.
7. 21 CFR Part 314.126 Adequate and well-controlled studies.
8. Fletcher RH, Fletcher SW, Wagner EH. Clinical Epidemiology, The Essentials, 3rd ed. Baltimore, Williams & Wilkins, 1996.
9. Oster G, Borok GM, Menzin J, et al. Cholesterol-reduction intervention study (CRIS). A randomized trial to assess effectiveness and costs in clinical practice. Arch Intern Med 1996;156:731–739.
10. Fayers PM. Generalisation from phase III clinical trials: Survival, quality of life, and health economics. Lancet 1997;350:1025–1027.
11. Geiling EMK, Cannon PR. Pathogenic effects of elixir of sulfanilimide (diethylene glycol) poisoning. JAMA 1938;111:919–926.
12. Lenz W. Malformations caused by drugs in pregnancy. Am J Dis Child 1966;112:99–106.
13. Ray WA, Griffin MR, Avorn J. Evaluating drugs after their approval for clinical use. N Engl J Med 1993;329:2029–2032.
14. Honig PK, Wortham DC, Zamani K, et al. Terfenadine-ketoconazole interaction: Pharmacokinetic and electrocardiographic consequences. JAMA 1993;269:1535–1539.
15. Rossi AC, Bosco L, Faich GA, et al. The importance of adverse reaction reporting by physicians: Suprofen and the flank pain syndrome. JAMA 1988;259:1203–1204.
16. Griffin Mr, Piper JM, Daugherty JR, et al. Nonsteroidal anti-inflammatory drug use and increased risk for peptic ulcer disease in elderly persons. Ann Intern Med 1991;114:257–263.
17. Henry D, Page J, Whyte I, et al. Consumption of non-steroidal antiinflammatory drugs on glomerular filtration rate in elderly patients. Br J Clin Pharmacol 1997;44:85–90.
18. Jick H, Miettinen OS, Shapiro S, et al. Comprehensive drug surveillance. JAMA 1970;213:1455–1460.

19. Shapiro S. Case-control surveillance. In: Strom BL, ed. Pharmacoepidemiology. New York, Wiley, 1994.
20. Inman WHW. Prescription Event Monitoring. Acta Med Scand Suppl 1984;683:119–126.
21. Joint Commission on Prescription Drug Use, 96th Congress. Washington, DC, United States Government Printing Office, 1980.
22. Saunders KW, Stergachis A, Von Korff M. Group Health Cooperative. In: Strom BL, ed. Pharmacoepidemiology, 2nd ed. New York, Wiley, 1994:171–185.
23. Arrowsmith-Lowe JB, Anello C. A view from a regulatory agency. In: Strom BL, ed. Pharmacoepidemiology, 2nd ed. New York, Wiley, 1994:87–97.
24. World Health Organization. International Drug Monitoring: The Role of the Hospital. Geneva, World Health Organization, 1966. Technical report series no. 425.
25. Beard K. Adverse reactions as a cause of hospital admission in the aged. Drugs Aging 1992;2:356–367.
26. Koch KE. Adverse drug reactions. In: Brown T, ed. Handbook of institutional pharmacy practice, 3rd ed. Bethesda, American Society of Hospital Pharmacists, 1992:279–291.
27. Johnson JA, Bootman JL. Drug-related morbidity and mortality: A cost-of-illness model. Arch Intern Med 1995;155:1949–1956.
28. Lazarou J, Pomeranz BH, Corey PN. Incidence of adverse drug reactions in hospitalized patients. A meta-analysis of prospective studies. JAMA, 1998;279:1200–1205.
29. May JR. Adverse drug reactions and interactions. In: DiPiro JT, Talbert RL, Hayes PE, et al, eds. Pharmacotherapy: A Pathophysiologic Approach, 3rd ed. Norwalk, CT, Appleton & Lange, 1995:101–116.
30. Strom BL. In: Strom BL, ed. Pharmacoepidemiology. 2nd ed. New York: John Wiley & Sons, 1994:3–14.
31. Park BK, Pirmohamed M, Kitteringham NNR. Idiosyncratic drug reactions: a mechanistic evaluation of risk factors. Br J Clin Pharmacol 1992;34:377–95.
32. Joint Commission on Accreditation of Healthcare Organizations. Comprehensive accreditation manual for hospitals: The official handbook. Oakbrook Terrace, IL, JCAHO, 1996.
33. Strom BL, Carson JL. Use of automated databases for pharmacoepidemiology research. Epidemiologic Rev 1990;12:87–107.
34. Stergachis A. Evaluating the quality of linked automated data sets for use in pharmacoepidemiology. In: Hartzema AG, Porta MS, Tilson HH, eds. Pharmacoepidemiology: An Introduction, 2nd ed, Cincinnati, Harvey Whitney Books, 1991.
35. Shapiro S. The role of automated records linkage in the postmarketing surveillance of drug safety. A critique. Clin Pharmacol Ther 1989;46: 371–386.
36. Faich GA, Stadel BV. The future of automated record linkage for postmarketing surveillance: A response to Shapiro. Clin Pharmacol Ther 1989;46:387–389.
37. Farrington CP, Nash J, Miller E. Case series analysis of adverse reactions to vaccines: A comparative evaluation. Am J Epidemiol 1996; 143:1165–1173.
38. Holt VL, Daling JR, Weiss NS, et al. Functional ovarian cyst risk associated with use of monophasic and triphasic oral contraceptives. Obstet Gynecol 1992;79:529–533.
39. Herbst AL, Ulfelder H, Poskanzer DC. Adenocarcinoma of the vagina: association of maternal stilbestrol therapy with tumor appearance in young women. N Engl J Med 1971;284:878–881.
40. Ray WA, Griffin MR, Downey W. Benzodiazepines of long and short elimination half-life and the risk of hip fracture. JAMA 1989;262: 3303–3307.
41. Royal College of General Practitioners. Oral Contraceptives and Health. London, Pitman, 1974.
42. Hooten TM, Scholes D, Hughs JP, et al. A prospective study of risk factors for symptomatic urinary tract infection in young women. N Engl J Med 1996;335:468–474.
43. Soumerai SB, McLaughlin TJ, Spiegelman D, et al. Adverse outcomes of underuse of beta-blockers in elderly survivors of acute myocardial infarction. JAMA 1997;277:115–121.
44. Soumerai SB, McLaughlin TJ, Ross-Degnan D, et al. Effects of limiting Medicaid drug-reimbursement benefits on the use of psychotropic agents and acute mental health services by patients with schizophrenia. N Engl J Med 1994;441:650–655.
45. Hill, AB. The environment and disease: Association or causation? Proc R Soc Med 1965;58:295–300.
46. Stolly PD. How to interpret studies of adverse drug reactions. Clin Pharmacol Ther 1990;48:337–339.

7

Clinical Toxicology

Peter A. Chyka, PharmD, ABAT, FAACT

Poisoning is an adverse effect from a chemical that has been taken in excessive amounts. The body is able to tolerate, and in some cases detoxify, a certain dose of a chemical, but once a critical threshold is exceeded, toxicity results. Poisoning can produce minor local effects that are readily treated in the outpatient setting, or systemic life-threatening situations that require intensive medical intervention. This spectrum of toxicity is typical for chemicals with which people come in contact. Virtually any chemical can become a poison when taken in sufficient quantity, but the potency of some compounds leads to serious toxicity with small quantities (Table 7–1).[1] Poisoning by chemicals includes exposures to drugs, industrial chemicals, household products, plants, venomous animals, and agrichemicals. This chapter describes some examples of this spectrum of toxicity, outlines means to recognize poisoning risk, and presents principles of treatment.

EPIDEMIOLOGY

Each year poisonings account for approximately 15,000 deaths and 225,000 hospitalizations in the United States. Young adults aged 25 to 44 years are at greatest risk of a poisoning death, and males have a twofold higher risk of death than females. Nearly one-half of all poisoning deaths of adults are due to suicide. Poisoning deaths in adults most commonly involve motor vehicle exhaust (carbon monoxide), other gases or vapors, antidepressants, tranquilizers, barbiturates, alcohol, opioids, and local anesthetics including cocaine.[2,3] Approximately 1% of poisoning deaths involve children under the age of 6 years. The elderly, those 75 years old and older, children under 5 years of age, and adolescents and young adults 15 to 24 years of age have the highest risk for nonfatal poisonings requiring hospitalization. The circumstances surrounding nearly one-half of hospitalized injuries are unrecorded; however, nearly two-thirds of those in which the intent is recorded are deemed to be intentional. If deaths from the abuse of drugs by nondependent individuals are considered as poisonings, another 3000 deaths could be added to the yearly total.[3] The number of deaths from medication errors increased 2.6-fold from 3000 in 1983 to 7391 in 1993 (Fig. 7–1).[4] This categorization also includes unintentional poisonings by medicines that were taken in overdose and inadvertently.

There are several databases in the United States that provide different levels of insight and documentation of the poisoning problem (Table 7–2). Poisonings documented by U.S. poison centers are compiled in the annual report of the American Association of Poison Control Centers Toxic Exposure Surveillance System (AAPCC-TESS).[5,6] Although it represents the largest database on poisoning, it is not complete because it relies upon individuals contacting a poison control center and the center voluntarily reporting the incident. Despite this shortcoming, AAPCC-TESS provides valuable insight into the characteristics and frequency of poisonings. In the 1996 AAPCC-TESS summary 2,155,952 poisoning exposures were reported by 67 participating poison centers that served a population of 232 million people.[6] Children younger than 6 years of age accounted for 53% of the cases. The site of the exposure was the home in 91% of the cases, and a single substance was involved in 93% of the cases. An acute exposure accounted for 94% of the cases, 86% of which were unintentional or accidental exposures. Only 11% were intentional. Fatalities accounted for 726 (0.03%) cases, of which 4% were children younger than 6 years of age. The majority of fatalities (61%) occurred in 20- to 49-year-old individuals. The distribution of substances most frequently involved in pediatric and adult exposures differed; however, medicines were the most frequently involved substance (Table 7–3). In summary, children account for the majority of reported poisonings with morbidity, but adults account for a greater proportion of mortality from poisoning.

ECONOMIC IMPACT OF POISONING

The economic impact of poisoning can be inferred from the role of poison control centers in cost avoidance. Poison control centers can optimize the use of health care resources by triaging patients to receive the appropriate level of medical care and thereby reduce overall health care costs. In one example, the cost for managing a case ranged from $23 for those managed at home by a poison control center to $635 when a call was placed to the 911 emergency service that resulted in ambulance transport to an emergency department.[7,8] Another economic analysis estimated that for every dollar spent on poison control center services, at least $7.75 in medical spending was saved, a value comparable to that obtained from immunizations.[9]

Poisoning, which ranks fourth in cost of injury, accounted for 3% of the total injuries in this country, and a total lifetime cost of $8.5 billion. The average lifetime cost per person for a fatal poisoning is $372,691, ranking second to the cost of a firearm fatality per person.[2] Estimates of the lifetime cost of injury include related health care costs and lost lifetime earnings of the victim; however, they do not

TABLE 7–1. Serious Toxicity Associated With Ingestion of One Mouthful or One Dosage Unit

Methanol	Hydrocarbons
Caustics or alkalis[a]	Acids[a]
Cationic detergents[a]	Selenous acid
Cyanide[a]	Anticholinesterase insecticides[a]
Phencyclidine or LSD	Clonidine
Colchicine	Chloroquine

[a]Concentrated or undiluted form.

include the costs of suffering, reduced productivity of caregivers, or legal costs. The average cost per person hospitalized for poisoning is $17,631 versus $171 for those not hospitalized.[2]

POISON PREVENTION STRATEGIES

The number of poisoning deaths in children has dramatically declined over the past three decades in part due to several poison prevention approaches.[10] These included the Poison Prevention Packaging Act of 1970, the evolution of regional poison control centers, the application of prompt first-aid measures, improvements in overall critical care, development of less toxic product formulations, better clarity in the packaging and labeling of products, and public education on the risks and prevention of poisoning. Although all of these factors play a role in minimizing poisoning dangers, particularly in children, the Poison Prevention Packaging Act has perhaps had the most significant influence.[10] The intent of the Act was to develop packaging that is difficult for children under 5 years of age to open or to obtain harmful amounts within a reasonable period of time. However, the packaging was not to be difficult for normal adults to use properly. There are a number of products and product categories for which safety packaging is required (Table 7–4). Child-resistant containers are not totally childproof and may be opened by children, which can result in poisoning. Despite the success of child-resistant containers, many adults disable the hardware or simply use no safety cap and thus place children

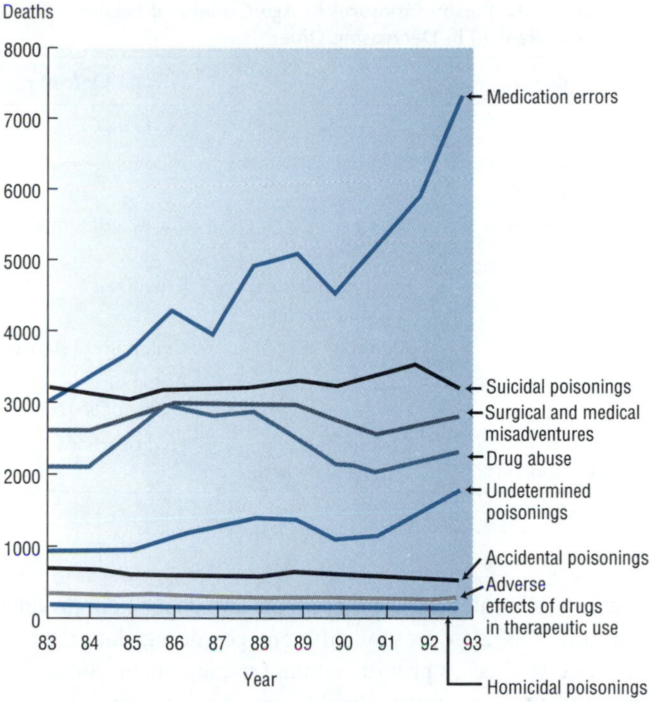

FIGURE 7–1. Trends in U.S. deaths from poisonings, medication errors, and other related causes. *(From Ref. 4, with permission.)*

at risk.[11] Fatigue of the packaging materials can also occur, which underscores the need for new prescription ware for refills, as required in the Act.[12] The compliance of pharmacists with the Act has not been complete. A compliance rate of 96.8% was estimated by a 1990 national survey of 193 pharmacies by the U.S. Consumer Product Safety Commission. Other studies with ferrous sulfate tablets[13] or amitriptyline tablets[14] found compliance rates of 77% and 89%, respectively. A printed reminder on the prescription order to dispense the drug in a child-resistant container did not improve compliance.[13]

Poison prevention requires constant vigilance, because there are new generations of families where parents and grandparents need to be educated on poisoning risks and

TABLE 7–2. Strengths of Various Poisoning Databases

Database (abbreviation)	Strength
Death certificates from state health departments compiled by the National Center for Health Statistics (NCHS)	Compiles all U.S. death certificates where the cause of death was by disease or external forces, such as poisoning. Data typically verified by laboratory and clinical observations.
National Electronic Injury Surveillance System of U.S. Consumer Product Safety Commission (NEISS)	Surveys electronically all injuries, including poisonings, treated daily at a sample of U.S. emergency departments. Used to identify first-time and recurring product-related injuries.
Drug Abuse Warning Network (DAWN) of the Federal Substance Abuse and Mental Health Services Administration	Identifies drug-of-abuse-related episodes and deaths that are reported to 685 hospitals and 145 medical examiners in the United States.
Toxic Exposure Surveillance System of American Association of Poison Control Centers (AAPCC-TESS)	Represents largest database of poisonings with high representation of children based on voluntary reporting by poison control centers.

TABLE 7–3. Poison Exposures by Age Group and Fatal Outcome, Ranked in Decreasing Order

Pediatric	Adult	Fatal Outcome
Medicines	Medicines	Medicines
Cosmetics and personal care items	Cleaning substances	Alcohols
Cleaning substances	Bites or envenomations	Gases and fumes
Plants	Food products or food poisoning	Chemicals
Foreign bodies	Alcohols	Cleaning substances
Pesticides	Gases and fumes	Automotive products
Arts and crafts or office supplies	Cosmetics and personal care items	Hydrocarbons

From Ref. 6.

TABLE 7–5. Psychosocial Characteristics of Poisoning Patients

Children	Young Adults	Elderly
Act purposefully or are poisoned by caretaker or sibling	Intentional abuse or suicidal intent is possible	Suicidal intent or unintentional misuse
Act with developmentally appropriate curiosity	Disregard or cannot read directions	Confuse product identity and directions for use
Attracted by product appearance	Do not recognize poisoning risk	Do not recognize poisoning risk
Ingest substances which adults find unpleasant	Reluctant to seek assistance until ill	Comorbid conditions complicate toxicity
React to stressful and disrupted household	Exaggerate or misrepresent situation	Unable or unwilling to describe situation
Imitate adult behaviors (e.g., taking medicine)	Peer pressure to experiment with drugs	Multiple drugs may lead to adverse reactions

prevention strategies. New products and changes in product formulations also present different poisoning dangers and must be studied to provide optimal management. Strategies to prevent poisonings should consider the various psychosocial circumstances of poisoning (Table 7–5), prioritize risk groups and behaviors, and customize an intervention for specific situations.[15–18]

RECOGNITION AND ASSESSMENT

The clinician's initial responsibility is to determine whether a poisoning has occurred or if there is a potential for one to develop. Some patients describe a clear account of an exposure that has occurred with a known quantity of a specific agent. In other cases, the patient may appear with only an unexplained illness characterized by nonspecific signs and symptoms and no immediate history of ingestion. Exposure to folk remedies, herbal medicines, nutritional supplements, and environmental toxins should also be considered. Patients with suicide gestures can deliberately give an unclear history and poisoning should be routinely suspected. Poisoning and drug overdoses should be suspected in any patient with a sudden, unexplained illness or with a puzzling combination of signs and symptoms, particularly in high-risk age groups. Nearly any symptom can be seen with poisoning; however, some signs and symptoms are suggestive of a particular toxin exposure.[19,20] Compounds that produce characteristic clinical pictures (toxidromes), such as organophosphate poisoning with pinpoint pupils, rales, bradycardia, central nervous system depression, sweating, excessive salivation, and diarrhea, are most readily recognizable.[21]

Assessment of the patient may be aided by consultation with a poison control center. These centers can provide information on product composition, typical symptoms, the range of toxicity, laboratory analysis, treatment options, and bibliographic references. Furthermore, the center will have specially trained physicians, pharmacists, and toxicologists on staff or on file to assist with difficult cases. Contact with a poison control center may also identify changes in currently recommended therapy. A list of active poison control centers may be found in references such as the *USP Drug Information*[22] or on the Internet (http://www.aapcc.org).

When the circumstances of a poison exposure indicate that it is minimally toxic, many poisonings can be successfully managed at the scene of the poisoning, usually the home.[6] Poison control centers typically monitor the victim by telephone during the first 2 to 6 hours of the exposure to assess the patient's status and outcome of first aid.

Once a poisoning is suspected and there is a need to confirm the diagnosis for medical or legal purposes, appropriate biologic material should be sent to the laboratory for analysis. Gastric contents may contain the greatest concentration of drug, but it is difficult to analyze. Blood or urine may be tested by qualitative screening in order to detect a drug's presence.[23,24] The results of a qualitative drug screen can be misleading due to interfering or low-level substances; it rarely guides therapy and thus has questionable value for nonspecific, general screening purposes.[21–23] Quantitative determination of serum concentrations may be important for the assessment of some poisonings such as acetaminophen, ethanol, methanol, iron, theophylline, and digoxin.

TABLE 7–4. Examples of Products Requiring Child-Resistant Closures

Aspirin	Acetaminophen
Ibuprofen	Diphenhydramine
Oral prescription drugs[a]	Iron pharmaceuticals
Turpentine	Kerosene
Ethylene glycol	Methanol
Sulfuric acid	Sodium hydroxide
Glue removers containing acetonitrile	Permanent hair wave neutralizers containing sodium bromate

[a]With certain exceptions such as nitrogylcerin and oral contraceptives.

PHARMACOKINETICS OF OVERDOSE

The pharmacokinetic characteristics of drugs taken in overdose may differ from those observed following therapeutic doses (Table 7–6).[25,26] These differences are due to dose-dependent changes in absorption, distribution, metabolism, or elimination; pharmacologic effects of the drug; or pathophysiologic consequences of the overdose. Dose-dependent changes may decrease the rate and extent of absorption, whereas the bioavailability of the agent may be increased due to saturation of first-pass metabolism. The distribution of a compound may be altered due to saturation of protein-binding sites. Metabolism and elimination of a compound may be retarded due to saturated biotransformation pathways leading to nonlinear elimination kinetics. Delayed gastric emptying by anticholinergic drugs or as the result of general central nervous system (CNS) depression caused by many drugs may alter the rate and extent of absorption. Drug-induced hypoperfusion may affect drug distribution and result in reduced hepatic or renal clearance. Changes in blood pH may alter the distribution of weak acids and bases. Drug-induced renal or hepatic injury can also significantly decrease clearance. Implications of these changes for poisoning management include the delayed achievement of peak concentrations with a corresponding longer period of time to remove drug from the gastrointestinal tract. The expected duration of effects may be much greater than those observed with therapeutic doses due to continued absorption and impaired clearance. The application of pharmacokinetic variables, such as percent protein binding and volume of distribution, from therapeutic doses may not be appropriate in poisoning cases.[25] Data on toxicokinetics are often difficult to interpret and compare because the doses and times of ingestion are uncertain, the duration of sampling is often inadequate, active metabolites may not be measured, protein binding is typically not assessed, and the severity of toxicity may vary dramatically.

TABLE 7–6. Examples of the Influence of Drug Overdosage on Pharmacokinetic and Pharmacodynamic Characteristics

Effect of Overdosage[a]	Examples
Slowed absorption due to formation of poorly soluble concretions in the gastrointestinal tract	Aspirin, lithium, phenytoin, sustained-release theophylline
Slowed absorption due to slowed gastrointestinal motility	Benztropine, nortriptyline
Slowed absorption due to toxin-induced hypoperfusion	Procainamide
Decreased serum protein binding	Lidocaine, salicylates, valproic acid
Increased volume of distribution associated with toxin-induced acidemia	Salicylates
Slowed elimination due to saturation of biotransformation pathways	Ethanol, phenytoin, salicylates, theophylline
Slowed elimination due to toxin-induced hypothermia (< 35°C)	Ethanol, propranolol
Prolonged toxicity due to formation of longer-acting metabolites	Carbamazepine, dapsone, glutethimide, meperidine

[a]Compared to characteristics following therapeutic doses or resolution of toxicity.

Adapted from Refs. 25 and 26.

MECHANISMS OF TOXICITY

Characterization of the mechanism of toxicity of poisons is often limited by our understanding of the pharmacology and cellular mechanism of action of an agent. Although many toxic effects are an exaggeration of typical actions and effects, some chemicals produce toxic effects that are not observed with lower or therapeutic doses. Tricyclic antidepressants produce a characteristically widened QRS-complex on ECG due to an exaggeration of their pharmacologic actions on the sodium channel of myocardium. Overdoses of acetaminophen lead to accumulation of a hepatotoxic metabolite, which is typically detoxified when taken in therapeutic doses. These and other examples will be more fully described later in the chapter. Poisons may exhibit local effects on skin, eye, lung, gastrointestinal mucosa, or other tissue as the result of their pharmacologic, irritant, or corrosive action. Once absorbed, systemic effects may be immediate or delayed in onset. Local and systemic effects may set the stage for secondary effects that are a consequence of the initial injury, such as infection, metabolic acidosis, or reflex tachycardia. Finally, a single poisoning incident may result in permanent or disabling effects, such as blindness from methanol poisoning.

▶ TREATMENT: Clinical Toxicology

GENERAL APPROACHES TO TREATMENT OF THE POISONED PATIENT

PREHOSPITAL CARE

First Aid

The presence of adequate airway, breathing, and circulation should be assessed and cardiopulmonary resuscitation should be started if needed. The most important step in preventing a minor exposure from progressing to a serious intoxication is early decontamination of the poison. Basic poisoning first-aid and decontamination measures (Table 7–7) should be instituted immediately at the scene of the poisoning.[27] If there is any question about the potential severity of the poison exposure, a poison control center should be consulted immediately. While awaiting transport, placing the patient on the left side may afford easier clearing of the airway if emesis occurs and may slow absorption of drug from the gastrointestinal tract.[28]

Ipecac Syrup

Ipecac syrup induces emesis typically within 15 to 30 minutes by direct irritation of the stomach and stimulation of the CNS chemoreceptor trigger zone. Emesis typically occurs in one to six episodes lasting up to 1 hour.[29] The dose of ipecac syrup is

TABLE 7–7. First Aid and Immediate Decontamination for Poison Exposures

Inhaled Poison
Immediately get the person to fresh air. Avoid breathing fumes. Open doors and windows. If victim is not breathing, start artificial respiration.
Poison on the Skin
Remove contaminated clothing and flood skin with water for 10 minutes. Wash gently with soap and water and rinse. Avoid further contamination of victim or first aid providers.
Poison in the Eye
Flood the eye with lukewarm or cool water poured from a glass 2 or 3 inches from the eye. Repeat for 10 to 15 continuous minutes. Keep eye open, but do not force the eyelid open.
Swallowed Poison
Unless the patient is unconscious, having convulsions, or cannot swallow, give 2 to 4 ounces of water immediately and then seek further help. Ipecac syrup should only be used on advice of a poison control center, emergency department, or physician.

5 to 10 mL for a child 6 months to 1 year of age, 15 mL for children 1 to 12 years old, and 15 to 30 mL for patients over 12 years of age.[30] To aid gastric evacuation, 6 to 8 ounces of water, fruit juice, or carbonated drinks should be administered with ipecac syrup. The same dose is repeated in 30 minutes if no emesis occurs. Ipecac syrup produces emesis in 98% of individuals within 60 minutes.[29,31] The adverse effects of ipecac syrup when given in therapeutic doses include drowsiness (10% to 21%), diarrhea (5% to 26%), and protracted vomiting beyond 1 hour (13% to 17%). Rare complications include Mallory–Weiss tears, pneumomediastinum, and aspiration pneumonia.[31] Ipecac syrup should be considered for poisonings of mild to moderate severity, when contraindications are not present, and it should be administered within 1 hour of the ingestion.

There are several contraindications to its use.[31] If the patient is without a gag reflex; is lethargic, comatose, or convulsing; or is expected to become unresponsive within the next 30 minutes, emesis should not be induced. If a fruitful emesis has spontaneously occurred shortly after ingestion, ipecac syrup may not be necessary. Ingestions of caustics, corrosives, ammonia, or bleach are definite contraindications to ipecac-induced emesis. The ingestion of aliphatic hydrocarbons (e.g., gasoline, kerosene, and charcoal lighter fluid) typically does not require emesis. When the agent is definitely known to be nontoxic, induction of emesis is purposeless and potentially dangerous. The rapid onset of coma or seizures or the potential to exaggerate the toxic effects of the poison may preclude the use of ipecac syrup. Some examples include diphenoxylate, propoxyphene, clonidine, tricyclic antidepressants, hypoglycemic agents, camphor, nicotine, lindane, strychnine, beta-blocking agents, calcium channel blockers, and pseudoephedrine. Debilitated, pregnant, and elderly patients may be further compromised by the induction of emesis. Ipecac syrup is not routinely used in the emergency department except for certain poisonings such as iron where alternatives to ipecac syrup, such as activated charcoal, are not useful. If treatment at an emergency department is imminent, within an hour of ingestion, use of ipecac syrup should be reconsidered.

HOSPITAL TREATMENT

General Care

Supportive and symptomatic care is the mainstay of treatment of the poisoned patient. In the search for specific antidotes and methods to increase excretion of the drug, attention to vital signs and organ functions should not be neglected. Establishment of adequate oxygenation and maintenance of adequate circulation are the highest priority. Other components of the acute supportive care plan include the management of seizures, arrhythmias, hypotension, acid–base balance, fluid status, electrolyte balance, and hypoglycemia. Placement of an intravenous and urinary catheter is typical to assure delivery of fluids and drugs when necessary and to monitor urine production, respectively.

Gastric Lavage

Gastric lavage involves the placement of an orogastric tube and washing out of the gastric contents through repetitive instillation and withdrawal of fluid. Gastric lavage should be considered only if a potentially toxic agent has been ingested within the past hour for most cases. If the patient is comatose or lacks a gag reflex, gastric lavage should be performed only after intubation with a cuffed or well-fitting endotracheal tube. The largest orogastric tube that can be passed (at least an external diameter of 12 mm in adults and 8 mm in children) should be used to ensure adequate evacuation, especially of undissolved tablets. Lavage should be performed with warm (37 to 38°C) normal saline or tap water until the gastric return is clear; this usually requires 2 to 4 L or more of fluid. Relative contraindications for gastric lavage include ingestion of a corrosive or hydrocarbon agent. Complications of gastric lavage include aspiration pneumonitis, laryngospasm, mechanical injury to the esophagus and stomach, hypothermia, and fluid and electrolyte imbalance.[32]

Single-dose Activated Charcoal

Reduction of toxin absorption can be achieved by the administration of activated charcoal. It is a highly purified, adsorbent form of carbon that prevents the absorption of a drug from the gastrointestinal tract by chemically binding (adsorbing) it to the charcoal surface. There are no contraindications to its use, but it is generally ineffective for iron, lead, lithium, simple alcohols, and corrosives. It is not indicated for aliphatic hydrocarbons due to increased risk of emesis and pulmonary aspiration. Activated charcoal is most effective when given within the first few hours after ingestion, ideally within the first hour.[33] The recommended dose of activated charcoal for a child (1 to 12 years old) is 25 to 50 g; for an adolescent or adult it is 25 to 100 g. Children under 1 year of age may receive 1 g/kg.[30] Activated charcoal is mixed with water to make a slurry, shaken vigorously, and administered orally or by means of a nasogastric tube. Activated charcoal is contraindicated when the gastrointestinal tract is not intact. Activated charcoal is relatively nontoxic, but there are two identified risks: (1) emesis following administration and (2) pulmonary aspiration of charcoal and gastric contents leading to pneumonitis in patients with an unprotected airway or absent gag reflex.[33] Some activated charcoal products contain sorbitol, a cathartic, which may be associated with an increased incidence of emesis following its use.[34]

Cathartics

Cathartics may decrease the rate of absorption by increasing gastrointestinal excretion of the poison and the poison-activated charcoal complex, but their value is unproven. Poisoned patients do not routinely require the administration of a cathartic, and it is rarely if ever given without concurrent activated charcoal administration.[35] If used, a cathartic should only be administered once and only if bowel sounds are present. The cathartics typically used are magnesium citrate, 4 mL/kg up to 300 mL/dose; 70% sorbitol 1 to 2 mL/kg for adults, and 35% sorbitol 4 mL/kg for children. Infants, the elderly, and patients with renal failure should be given saline cathartics cautiously, if at all.[35]

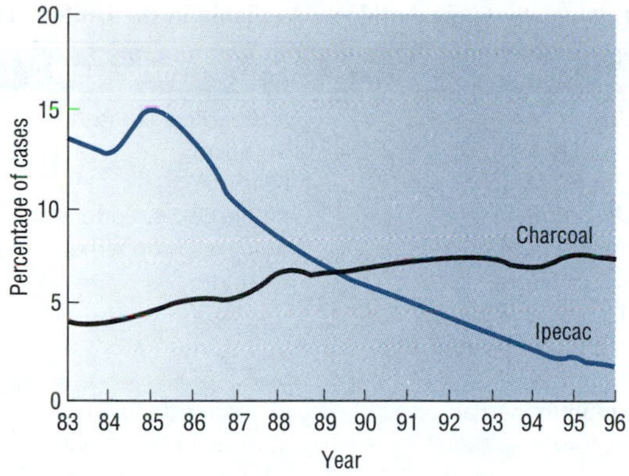

FIGURE 7–2. Trends in the use of ipecac syrup and activated charcoal based on cases reported by U.S. poison centers. *(From Ref. 6.)*

Whole-bowel Irrigation

Polyethylene glycol electrolyte solutions, such as GoLytely and Colyte, are routinely used as whole-bowel irrigants prior to colonoscopy and bowel surgery. [36] These solutions can also be used as a means to decontaminate the gastrointestinal tract of ingested toxins.[37] Large volumes of these osmotically balanced solutions are continuously administered through a nasogastric or duodenal tube for 4 to 12 hours or more. They quickly cause gastrointestinal evacuation and are continued until the rectal discharge is relatively clear. This procedure may be indicated for certain patients in whom the ingestion occurred several hours prior to hospitalization and the drug still is suspected to be in the gastrointestinal tract, such as cocaine smugglers who swallow condoms filled with cocaine.[38] In addition, patients who have ingested delayed-release or enteric-coated drug formulations, or have ingested substances such as iron that are not well-adsorbed by activated charcoal, may benefit from whole-bowel irrigation.[37] It should not be used in patients with a bowel perforation or obstruction, gastrointestinal hemorrhage, ileus, or intractable emesis. Emesis, abdominal cramps, and intestinal bloating have been reported with whole-bowel irrigation.[37] The safety and effectiveness of whole-bowel irrigation as a routine poisoning treatment are debatable and further studies are warranted before it is generally indicated.

Perspectives on Gastric Decontamination

Although there are a variety of options for gastric decontamination, two clinical toxicology groups (American Academy of Clinical Toxicology and the European Association of Poison Centres and Clinical Toxicologists) have concluded that no means of gastric decontamination should be routinely used for a poisoned patient without careful consideration.[31–33,35,37] They indicate that therapy is most effective within the first hour and effectiveness beyond this time cannot be supported or refuted with the available data. A clinical policy statement by the American College of Emergency Physicians concludes that, although no definitive recommendation can be made on the use of ipecac syrup, gastric lavage, cathartics, or whole-bowel irrigation, activated charcoal is advocated for most patients when appropriate.[39] In recent years the use of ipecac syrup has declined (Fig. 7–2) in part due to its apparent lower efficacy compared to activated charcoal in minimizing drug absorption.[31,33] Poison control centers may be a source of guidance on the contemporary application of gastric decontamination techniques for a specific patient.

Enhanced Elimination

Numerous methods have been used to increase the rate of excretion of poisons from the body. Of these, only diuresis, multiple-dose activated charcoal, and hemodialysis are occasionally useful. These approaches should only be considered if the risks of the procedure are significantly outweighed by the expected benefits or if the recovery of the patient is seriously in doubt and the method has been shown to be helpful.

Diuresis. Diuresis may be used for poisons excreted predominately by the renal route; however, most drugs and poisons are metabolized and only a good urine flow, such as 2 to 3 mL/kg/h, needs to be maintained for most patients. Fluid and electrolyte balance should be closely monitored. Ionized diuresis may increase excretion of certain chemicals that are weak acids or bases by trapping ionized drug in the renal tubule and minimizing reabsorption. Alkalinization of the urine to achieve a urine pH of 7.5 or greater for poisoning by weak acids such as salicylates or phenobarbital can be achieved by the intravenous administration of sodium bicarbonate 1 to 2 mEq/kg over a 1- to 2-hour period. Complications of urinary alkalinization include alkalosis, fluid and electrolyte disturbances, and inability to achieve target urinary pH values.[40] Acid diuresis may enhance the excretion of weak bases, such as amphetamines, but it is rarely if ever used because it risks worsening rhadomyolysis commonly associated with amphetamine overdose.[41] Generally, ionized diuresis is rarely indicated for poisoned patients, because it is inefficient relative to other methods of enhancing elimination, there is a risk of unacceptable adverse effects, and the renal elimination of most drugs is not dramatically enhanced.

Multiple-dose Activated Charcoal. Multiple doses of activated charcoal can augment the body's clearance of certain drugs by enhanced passage from the bloodstream into the gastrointestinal tract and subsequent adsorption. This process, termed "charcoal intestinal dialysis" or "charcoal-enhanced intestinal exorption," describes the attraction of drug molecules across the capillary bed of the intestine by activated charcoal in the intestinal lumen and subsequent adsorption of the drug to the charcoal.[42] Furthermore, it may interrupt the enterohepatic recirculation of certain drugs, such as tricylic antidepressants.[42,43] Once the drug is adsorbed to the charcoal, it is eliminated with the charcoal in the stool. The systemic clearance of several drugs has been shown to be enhanced by up to several-fold (Table 7–8). Although a prospective randomized study of the effects of multiple-dose activated charcoal on phenobarbital-overdosed patients demonstrated increased drug elimination, no demonstrable effect on patient outcome was observed.[44]

TABLE 7–8. Drugs Whose Elimination Half-Life is Reduced by Multiple-Dose Activated Charcoal

Drug	Percent Reduction in Half-life[a]
Phenobarbital	62
Digitoxin	54
Dapsone	53
Piroxicam	51
Phenytoin	50
Theophylline	47
Carbamazepine	45
Quinine	45
Nortriptyline	35
Digoxin	33
Propoxyphene	32
Phenylbutazone	29
Amitriptyline	23

[a]Increased elimination in normal volunteers compared to a control group not receiving activated charcoal.
Adapted from Ref. 42, with permission.

This approach provides a rapid onset of action that is limited by blood flow and a maximal "ceiling effect" related to the dose of charcoal present in the intestine. The response to multiple-dose activated charcoal is greatest for drugs with the following characteristics: good affinity for adsorption by activated charcoal, low intrinsic clearance, sufficient residence time in the body (long serum half-life), long distributive phase, and nonrestrictive protein binding. A small volume of distribution is also desirable, but it has a marginal influence as an isolated characteristic[45] particularly if multiple-dose activated charcoal is instituted during the toxin's distributive phase. Development of nonlinear kinetics due to overdose or disease may favor a response for drugs otherwise shown to be unaffected with subtoxic doses in human volunteer studies.[46]

A typical dosage schedule is 15 to 25 g of activated charcoal every 2 to 6 hours until serious symptoms abate or the serum concentration of the toxin is below the toxic range. This procedure has been used in premature and full-term infants in doses of 1 g/kg every 1 to 4 hours. Complications are the same as those for single-dose charcoal. The risks of aspiration pneumonitis in obtunded or uncooperative patients, and of intestinal obstruction in patients prone to ileus following a period of bowel ischemia, for example, after cardiopulmonary arrest in the elderly may be higher.[43] Contraindications are the same as those for single-dose charcoal.

Hemodialysis. Hemodialysis may be necessary for certain severe cases of poisoning. Dialysis should be considered when the duration of symptoms is expected to be prolonged, other pathways of excretion are unavailable, clinical deterioration is present, the drug is dialyzable, and appropriate personnel and equipment are available. Drugs that are effectively dialyzed possess a low molecular weight, are not highly or tightly protein bound, and are not highly distributed to tissues. The principles of therapeutic hemodialysis are described in Chapter 44. Hemodialysis and charcoal hemoperfusion are the most efficient methods of dialysis, but both pose serious risks related to anticoagulation, blood transfusions, loss of blood elements, fluid and electrolyte disturbances, and infection.[47] Hemodialysis may be life saving for methanol and ethylene glycol poisoning and quite effective for other poisons, such as lithium, salicylates, ethanol, and theophylline.[27] Charcoal hemoperfusion was popular in the 1970s and 1980s as a means to quickly remove toxins from the circulation, but this approach has fallen out of favor due to poor results, inappropriate use for drugs with large volumes of distribution, and limited commercial availability of charcoal hemoperfusion columns.

Antidotes

The search for and use of an antidote should never replace good supportive care. Specific systemic antidotes are available for many common poisonings (Table 7–9).[48,49] Inadequate availability of antidotes at acute care hospitals has been noted throughout the United States and can complicate the care of a poisoned patient. Studies performed in three regions of the United States have shown that less than 10% of hospitals stocked sufficient quantities of the antidotes required for 1 or 2 adult doses.[50–52] Some antidotes (e.g., alcohol for injection, crotalidae snake antivenin, and pralidoxime) were insufficiently stocked by two-thirds or more of the institutions. The use of drug-specific antibodies (e.g., digoxin-specific Fab antibody fragments)[53] has offered a new approach to the treatment of poisoning victims. With the development of other immunologic antidotes such as those directed against snake venom or antidepressants, this approach may prove useful in the treatment of other intoxications.

TABLE 7–9. Systemic Antidotes Available in the United States

Antidote	Toxic Agent
Atropine	Anticholinesterase insecticides
Botulism antitoxin	Botulism
Calcium EDTA	Lead
Crotalidae polyvalent antivenin	Rattlesnakes, cottonmouth snakes, copperhead snakes
Cyanide antidote kit (Amyl nitrite, sodium nitrate, and sodium thiosulfate)	Cyanide
Deferoxamine	Iron
Digoxin immune Fab	Digoxin, digitoxin
Dimercaprol	Various heavy metals
Ethanol	Ethylene glycol, methanol
Flumazenil	Benzodiazepines
Fomepizole	Ethylene glycol; possibly methanol
Lactrodectus mactans antivenin	Black widow spider
Methylene blue	Methemoglobinemia
Micrurus fulvius antivenin	Coral snake
N-acetylcysteine	Acetaminophen
Naloxone	Opioids
Oxygen	Carbon monoxide
Penicillamine	Various heavy metals
Phytonadione	Anticoagulants
Pralidoxime	Organophosphate insecticides
Succimer	Lead

Assessing the Effectiveness of Therapies

Our knowledge of poisoning treatment is derived from case reports, clinical studies, human volunteer studies, animal investigations, and *in vitro* tests. Each of these approaches has limited applicability to the care of humans who have been poisoned. Case reports are often difficult to assess, because they are uncontrolled, the histories are uncertain, and multiple therapies are often used. They can, however, be useful to describe unique or new toxicities or characterize adverse effects associated with a therapy. Although clinical studies may describe tens to hundreds of patients, they can exhibit serious shortcomings such as weak randomization procedures, no laboratory confirmation or correlation with history, insufficient number of severe cases, no control group, and no quantitative measure of outcome. Extrapolation of data from human volunteer studies to patients who overdose is difficult because of potential or unknown variations in pharmacokinetics (e.g., differing dissolution, gastric emptying, and absorption rates) seen with toxic as opposed to therapeutic doses[25,26]; differences in time to institute therapy in the emergency setting; and differences in absorption in fasted human volunteers compared with the full stomach of some patients who overdose. These studies, however, provide the most controlled and objective measures of the efficacy of a treatment. Experiences from animal studies cannot be directly applied to humans due to interspecies differences in toxicity and metabolism. *In vitro* tests serve to screen the efficacy of some approaches, such as activated charcoal adsorption, but they do not sufficiently mimic physiologic conditions to allow direct clinical application of the findings. Despite their limitations, these data comprise the basis for the therapy of poisoned patients and are tempered with the consideration of nonpoisoning-related factors, such as a particular patient's underlying medical condition, age, and need for concurrent supportive measures.

CLINICAL SPECTRUM OF POISONING

Poisoning and/or drug overdose with acetaminophen, anticholinesterase insecticides, iron, theophylline, and tricyclic antidepressants are the focus of the remainder of this chapter, because they represent commonly encountered poisonings for which pharmacotherapy is indicated. These agents were also chosen because they represent common examples with different mechanisms of toxicity, and they illustrate the application of general treatment approaches as well as some agent-specific interventions.

ACETAMINOPHEN

Signs and Symptoms. Acute acetaminophen poisoning characteristically results in hepatotoxicity.[54–57] Clinical presentation is determined by the time required for hepatic necrosis to occur, presence of risk factors, and the ingestion of other drugs. During the first 12 to 24 hours after ingestion, nausea, vomiting, anorexia, and diaphoresis may be observed; however, many patients are asymptomatic. During the next 1 to 3 days, a latent phase of lessened symptoms, patients often have an asymptomatic rise in liver enzymes and bilirubin. Signs and symptoms of hepatic injury become manifest 3 to 5 days after ingestion and include right upper quadrant abdominal tenderness, jaundice, hypoglycemia, and encephalopathy. Prolongation of the prothrombin time worsens as hepatic necrosis progresses and may lead to disseminated intravascular coagulapathy. By 7 to 8 days after ingestion, patients with hepatic damage may develop hepatic coma and hepatorenal syndrome. Death can occur, [55–57] but recovery is usually complete, even in patients with severe hepatotoxicity with no residual functional or histologic abnormalities of the liver noted within 1 to 6 months of the incident due to tissue regeneration and repair.[54,56]

In many cases of severe hepatotoxicity, renal injury is also present and may range from oliguria to acute renal failure. The etiology of the renal injury may be a direct effect of a toxic metabolite of acetaminophen, NAPQI (discussed in the next section), generated by renal cytochrome oxidase, or a consequence of hepatic injury resulting in hepatorenal syndrome.[58] Isolated cases of myocardial injury have rarely been reported.[59]

Mechanism of Toxicity. Acetaminophen is metabolized in the liver primarily to glucuronide or sulfate conjugates, which are excreted into the urine with small amounts (<5%) of unchanged drug. Approximately 5% of a therapeutic dose is metabolized by the cytochrome P450 mixed-function oxygenase system, primarily CYP2E1, to a reactive metabolite, *N*-acetyl-*p*-benzoquinone-imine (NAPQI). This metabolite normally is conjugated with glutathione, a sulfhydryl-containing compound, in the hepatocyte and excreted in the urine as a mercapturate conjugate (Fig. 7–3).

In an acute overdose situation, sulfate stores are depleted, shifting more drug through the cytochrome system, thereby depleting the available glutathione used to detoxify the reactive metabolite. The reactive metabolite, NAPQI, then reacts with other hepatocellular sulfhydryl compounds such as those in the cytosol, cell wall, and endoplasmic reticulum. This results in centrilobular hepatic necrosis.[54]

Causative Agents. Acetaminophen, also known as paracetamol in other countries, is widely available without prescription as an analgesic and antipyretic. It is available in various oral dosage forms including an extended release preparation. Acetaminophen may be combined with other drugs and marketed in cough and cold preparations, menstrual remedies, and allergy products.

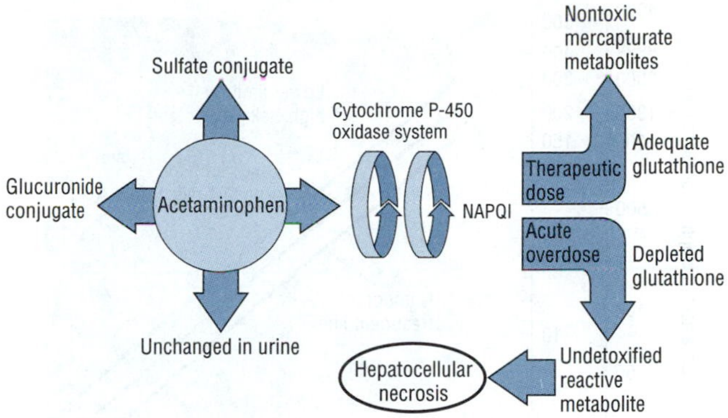

FIGURE 7–3. Pathway of acetaminophen metabolism and basis for hepatotoxicity. (NAPQI = *N*-acetyl-*p*-benzoquinone-imine, a reactive acetaminophen metabolite.)

Incidence. Acetaminophen is one of the most commonly ingested drugs by small children and is commonly used in suicide attempts by adolescents and adults. The 1996 AAPCC-TESS report documented 72,886 nonfatal exposures and 61 deaths from acetaminophen with 57% of the exposures under 6 years of age.[6]

Age-based differences in the metabolism of acetaminophen appear to be responsible for major differences in the incidence of serious toxicity. Despite the common ingestion of acetaminophen by young children, few develop hepatotoxicity.[60] In children under 9 to 12 years of age, acetaminophen undergoes more sulfation and less glucuronidation. The reduced fraction available for metabolism by the cytochrome system may explain the rare development of serious toxicity in young children who take large overdoses.[61] Earlier treatment intervention and spontaneous emesis may also reduce the risk of toxicity in children.

Risk Assessment. There is a risk of developing hepatotoxicity when adolescents or adults acutely ingest more than 5 to 7.5 g of acetaminophen or when children acutely ingest greater than 150 mg/kg.[55] The least amount reported to produce death is 10 g in an adult; but others have survived much larger doses, particularly with early treatment. Initial symptoms, if present, do not predict how serious the toxicity may eventually become.

Chronic exposure to drugs that induce the cytochrome oxidase system—specifically isoenzyme CYP2E1, which is responsible for most of formation of NAPQI—may increase the risk of acetaminophen hepatotoxicity. Poorer outcomes have been noted in patients who chronically ingest alcohol and those receiving anticonvulsants, both known to induce CYP2E1.[56,57,62,63]

Chronic, excessive acetaminophen consumption, defined as doses exceeding the recommended daily doses of 4 g for an adult and 90 mg/kg for a child for several days, has been associated with hepatotoxicity.[56,57] The incidence is unknown and the basis of this association is not well understood. Patients who are fasting or have ingested alcohol in the preceding 5 days appear to be at greater risk.[64] Young children who receive acetaminophen in excess of the recommended total daily dose of 50 to 75 mg/kg have a risk of developing hepatotoxicity particularly when they have been acutely fasting due to febrile illness or gastroenteritis.[65]

The risk of developing hepatotoxicity may be predicted from a nomogram (Fig. 7–4) comprised of a plot of the acetaminophen serum concentration and time after ingestion.[55] The treatment line of the nomogram (150 μg/mL at 4 hr), which allows a margin of error in laboratory analysis and time of ingestion, should

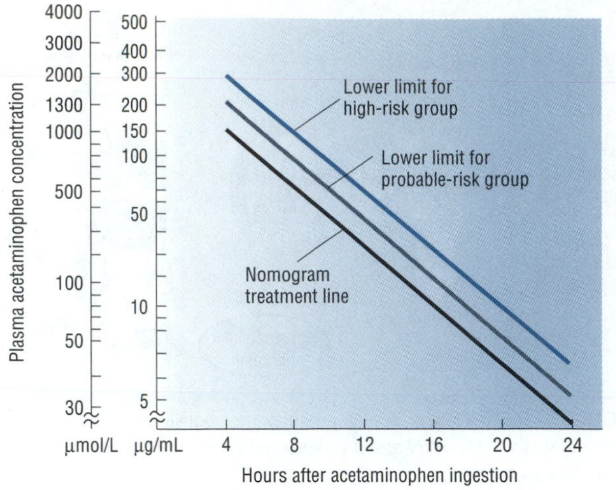

FIGURE 7–4. Nomogram for assessing hepatotoxic risk following acute ingestion of acetaminophen. *(Adapted from Ref. 55, with permission.)*

be used to make treatment decisions. The other lines on the nomogram indicate differing levels of risk for hepatotoxicity based on a multicenter study of 11,195 patients.[55]

If the plasma concentration plotted on the nomogram falls above the nomogram treatment line, indicating that hepatic damage is possible, a full course of treatment with *N*-acetylcysteine is indicated. When the results of the acetaminophen determination will be available later than 8 hours after the ingestion, *N*-acetylcysteine therapy should be initiated based on the history and later discontinued if the results indicate nontoxic concentrations. The nomogram has not been evaluated, and thus is not useful, for assessing chronic exposure to acetaminophen.

Management of Toxicity. Therapy of an acute acetaminophen overdose is dependent on the amount ingested, time after ingestion, and the serum concentration of acetaminophen. When adolescents or adults ingest excessive amounts, when the history is unclear or suggests an intentional ingestion, the patient must be evaluated at an emergency department and acetaminophen serum concentrations obtained. No prehospital care is generally indicated and ipecac syrup is typically avoided because emesis may complicate later therapy.

If the patient presents to the emergency department within 4 hours of the ingestion or other drugs are suspected, one dose of activated charcoal should be administered. There has been concern that charcoal may minimize the effectiveness of orally administered protective therapy (i.e., *N*-acetylcysteine) by adsorbing it in the gastrointestinal tract. Recent evidence suggests that activated charcoal may not interfere with *N*-acetylcysteine to the extent previously thought and it may be considered to be appropriate therapy.[33]

N-acetylcysteine, a sulfhydryl-containing compound, functionally replenishes the hepatic stores of glutathione, by serving as a glutathione surrogate that combines directly with reactive metabolites or by serving as a source of sulfate, thus preventing hepatic damage.[54,55] Hepatic injury is not reversed by *N*-acetylcysteine; it is ostensibly protective in nature. It should be started within 10 hours of the ingestion to be most effective.[55] Initiation of therapy 24 to 36 hours after the ingestion may be of value in some cases particularly those with measurable serum acetaminophen concentrations. Patients with fulminant hepatic failure may benefit through other mechanisms by the administration or initiation of *N*-acetylcysteine several days after ingestion.[66] Therapy is initiated with a loading dose of 140 g/kg orally followed in 4 hours by 70 mg/kg every 4 hours over a period of 68 hours (i.e., 17 maintenance doses). If the patient vomits a dose within an hour of administration, the dose should be repeated. *N*-acetylcysteine can be diluted with carbonated drinks, cola, juice, or water to a 5% solution and administered orally or through a nasogastric tube. Adverse effects of *N*-acetylcysteine therapy include nausea, vomiting, and rarely hypersensitivity reactions.[54,55,67]

The unpleasant odor and associated emesis of *N*-acetylcysteine can limit the delivery of the full course of therapy. Aggressive antiemetic therapy with metoclopramide, ondansetron, or droperidol may enhance patient tolerability of *N*-acetylcysteine.[68] Other approaches include administration by a nasogastric or duodenal tube over 30 to 60 minutes or use of an investigational intravenous form of *N*-acetylcysteine.[67] A 52-hour course of intravenous *N*-acetylcysteine may be as effective as the 72-hour oral regimen.[69] Intravenous administration of the oral *N*-acetylcysteine product is not generally recommended, because the product is not pyrogen-free. However, extemporaneous filtration with a 0.2-micron filter unit yields an intravenous product that has been associated with a limited number of adverse effects and may be potentially life saving when oral administration is not possible.[70] The local poison control center should be consulted for availability of the intravenous product.

When plasma concentrations are below the nomogram treatment line, there is little risk of toxicity, protective therapy with *N*-acetylcysteine is not necessary, and further medical therapy is unnecessary for the acetaminophen overdose.[55] The acetaminophen blood sample should be drawn no sooner than 4 hours after the ingestion, to assure that peak acetaminophen concentrations have been reached. If a concentration is obtained less than 4 hours after ingestion, it is uninterpretable and a second determination should be done at least 4 hours after ingestion. Serial determinations of a serum concentration are typically unnecessary unless there is some evidence of slowed gastrointestinal motility from other ingested drugs (e.g., opioids or anticholinergic drugs), or unless an extended-release product is involved.

An extended-release formulation of acetaminophen was introduced in 1995 and raised significant issues in the management of overdose. One formulation (Tylenol-ER) delivers 325 mg in immediate release and another 325 mg in extended release. The pharmacokinetics of the extended-release preparation on overdose are unknown, but one case exhibited a peak concentration at 16 hours after ingestion compared to the peak time of the standard-release preparation within 1 to 2 hours.[71] The validity of the toxic dose thresholds and the nomogram for extended-release formulation overdoses is untested to date. In 1994 a manufacturer, McNeil, suggested obtaining two serum acetaminophen concentrations 4 to 6 hours apart and continuing therapy with *N*-acetylcysteine if any concentration was above the treatment line of the nomogram and discontinuing therapy when both concentrations were below the treatment line. These provisional recommendations have yet to be validated.

Although young children have an inherently lower risk of acetaminophen-induced hepatotoxicity, these patients should be managed in the same manner as adults. When acetaminophen plasma concentrations predict that toxicity is probable, young children should receive *N*-acetylcysteine in the dosing regimen previously described.[60]

If fulminant hepatic failure develops, the approaches described in Chapter 35 should be considered. In unresponsive cases, liver transplantation is a life-saving option.[56]

Monitoring and Prevention. Baseline liver function tests (AST, ALT, bilirubin, prothrombin time), serum creatinine, and urinalysis should be obtained on admission and repeated at 24-hour intervals until at least 96 hours have elapsed for those at risk. Most patients with liver injury develop elevated transaminase concentrations within 24 hours of ingestion. Transaminase concentrations greater than 1000 IU/L are commonly associated with other signs of liver dysfunction and have been used as the threshold concentration in outcome studies to define severe liver toxicity.[55] The extent of transaminase elevation is not directly correlated with severity of the hepatic injury, with nonfatal cases demonstrating peak concentrations as high as 30,000 IU/L between 48 and 72 hours after ingestion.[56,57]

Prevention of acetaminophen poisoning is based on the recognition of the maximum daily therapeutic doses, observance of general poison prevention practices, and early intervention in cases of suspected overdose.

ANTICHOLINESTERASE INSECTICIDES

Signs and Symptoms. The clinical manifestations of anticholinesterase insecticide poisoning include any or all of the following: pinpoint pupils, excessive lacrimation, excessive salivation, bronchorrhea, bronchospasm and expiratory wheezes, hyperperistalsis producing abdominal cramps and diarrhea, bradycardia, excessive sweating, fasciculations and weakness of skeletal muscles, paralysis of skeletal muscles (particularly those involved with respiration), convulsions, and coma.[72,73] Symptoms of anticholinesterase poisoning and their response to antidotal therapy are dependent on the action of excessive acetylcholinesterase at different receptor types (Table 7–10).

The time of onset and severity of symptoms depend on the route of exposure, potency of the agent, and total dose received. Toxic signs and symptoms develop most rapidly after inhalation or intravenous injection and slowest after skin contact. Anticholinesterase insecticides are absorbed through the skin, lungs, conjunctivae, and gastrointestinal tract. Severe symptoms can occur from absorption by any route. Within 6 hours most patients are symptomatic, and without treatment death may occur within 24 hours.[72,73] Death is typically caused by respiratory failure due to the combination of pulmonary and cardiovascular effects (Fig. 7–5).[72,74]

Mechanism of Toxicity. Anticholinesterase insecticides phosphorylate the active site of cholinesterase in all parts of the body. Inhibition of this enzyme leads to accumulation of acetylcholine at affected receptors and results in widespread toxicity. Acetylcholine is the neurohormone responsible for physiologic transmission of nerve impulses from preganglionic and postganglionic neurons of the cholinergic (parasympathetic) nervous system, preganglionic adrenergic (sympathetic) neurons, the neuromuscular junction in skeletal muscles, and multiple nerve endings in the central nervous system (Fig. 7–6).

Causative Agents. Anticholinesterase insecticides include organophosphate and carbamate insecticides. These insecticides are currently in widespread use throughout the world for eradication of insects in dwellings and crops. Carbamates typically are less potent and inactivate cholinesterase in a more reversible fashion through carbamylation compared to organophosphates.[72–74] The prototype anticholinesterase agent is the organophosphate, which will be the focus of this discussion. A large number of organophosphates are used as pesticides (Table 7–11), and several have also been used as potent chemical warfare agents (e.g., sarin, tabun, and VX, which are known as nerve gases). The chemical warfare agents act like organophosphate insecticides, but as a group they are highly potent, quickly absorbed, and deadly to humans.[75] An anticholinesterase insecticide is typically stored in garage, chemical storage, or living areas. Anticholinesterase agents can also be found in occupational (e.g., pest exterminators) or agricultural (e.g., crop dusters or farm workers) settings. These agents have also been used as a means for suicide or homicide.

TABLE 7–10. Effects of Acetylcholinesterase Inhibition at Muscarinic, Nicotinic, and CNS Receptors

Muscarinic Receptors	**Nicotinic–Sympathetic Neurons**
Diarrhea	Increased blood pressure
Urination	Sweating and piloerection
Miosis[a]	Mydriasis[a]
Bronchorrhea	Hyperglycemia
Bradycardia[a]	Tachycardia[a]
Emesis	Priapism
Lacrimation	**Nicotinic–Neuromuscular Neurons**
Salivation	Muscular weakness
CNS Receptors (Mixed Type)	Cramps
	Fasciculations
Coma	Muscular paralysis
Seizures	

[a]Generally muscarinic effects predominate, but nicotinic effects can be observed.

Incidence. Anticholinesterase insecticides are among the most poisonous substances commonly used for pest control and are a frequent source of serious poisoning in children and adults in rural and urban settings. The 1996 AAPCC-TESS report documented 25,407 nonfatal exposures and 11 deaths from anticholinesterase insecticides alone or in combination with other pesticides with 36% of the exposures in children under 6 years of age.[6] The World Health Organization estimates more than 220,000 deaths each year are related to pesticide poisoning worldwide particularly, in developing countries.[76]

Risk Assessment. The triad of miosis, bronchial secretions, and muscle fasciculations should suggest the possibility of anticholinesterase insecticide poisoning and warrants a therapeutic trial of the antidote atropine. In cases of low-level exposure, failure to develop signs within 6 hours indicates a low likelihood of subsequent toxicity.[73]

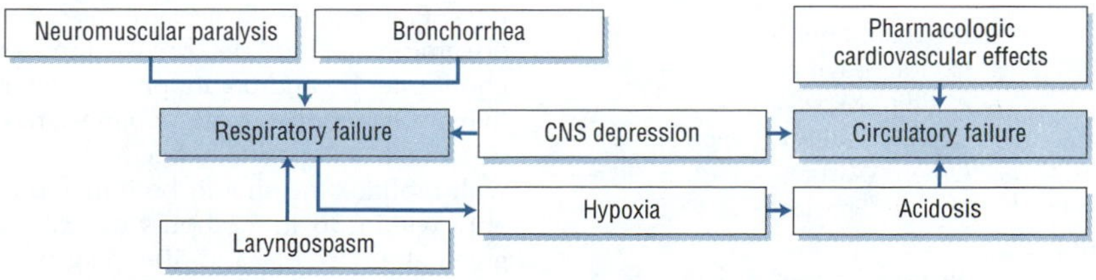

FIGURE 7–5. Pathogenesis of life-threatening effects of organophosphate poisoning.

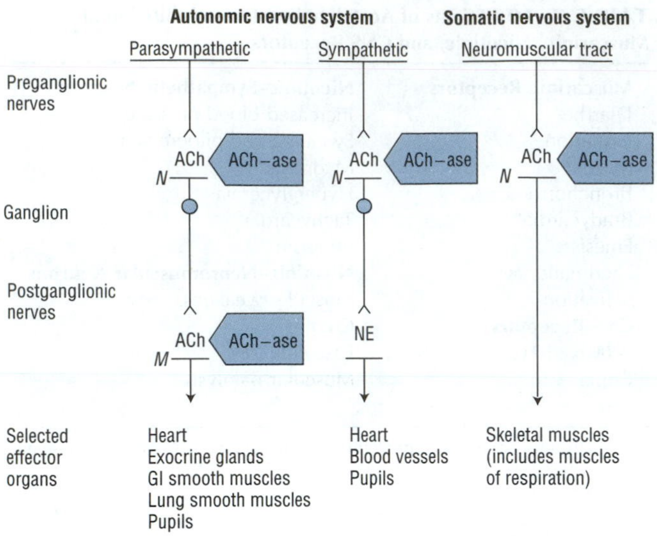

FIGURE 7–6. Organization and neurotransmitters of the peripheral nervous system and site of acetylcholinesterase action. (ACh = acetylcholine; ACh-ase = acetylcholinesterase; NE = norepinephrine; M = muscarinic receptor; N = nicotinic receptor.)

Although the lethal dose for parathion is approximately 4 mg/kg, as little as 10 to 20 mg can be lethal to an adult and 2 mg (0.1 mg/kg) to a child. Small children may be more susceptible to toxicity because less pesticide is required per body weight to produce toxicity.[73] Estimation of an exact dose is impossible in most cases of acute poisoning and tabulated "toxic" doses are thus generally not helpful in assessing risk of toxicity. Generally, ingestion of a small mouthful (5 mL or less) of the concentrated forms of an organophosphate intended to be diluted and for commercial or agricultural use will produce serious toxicity, whereas a mouthful of an already diluted household product such as Raid or Black Flag does not typically produce serious toxic effects.[75]

Measurement of acetylcholinesterase activity at the neuronal synapse is not clinically feasible. Cholinesterase activity can be measured in the blood as the pseudocholinesterase (butylcholinesterase) activity of the plasma and acetylcholinesterase activity in the erythrocyte. Both cholinesterases will be depressed with anticholinesterase insecticide poisoning.[72,74] Severity can be roughly estimated by the extent of depressed activity in relation to the low end of normal values. Because there are several methods to measure and report cholinesterase activity, each particular laboratory's normal range must be considered. Clinical toxicity is usually seen only after a 50% reduction in enzyme activity and severe toxicity typically is observed with levels at 20% or less of the normal range.[73] A clinical severity scoring system has been proposed as an alternative to cholinesterase activity determination.[72] The intrinsic activity of acetylcholinesterase may be depressed in some individuals, but the absence of any manifestations in most people does not permit the recognition of the relative deficiency in the general population. Therapy should not be delayed pending laboratory confirmation when the clinical suspicion of poisoning is present.

TABLE 7–11. Commonly Used Organophosphate Insecticides

Chemical Name	Product Name Examples
Agricultural Use: High Potency	
Disulfoton	Di-syston
Mevinphos	Phosdrin
Parathion	Niagara Phos Kil Dust
Animal Use: Intermediate Potency	
Chlorpyrifos	Dursban, Lorsban
Coumaphos	Co-Ral, Baymix
Dichlorphos	Agridip, Muscatox
Famphur	Brevinyl, DDVP, Vapona
Phosmet	Dovip, Warbex
Trichlorfon	Prolate, Smidan
Household Use: Low Potency	
Diazinon	Security Fire Ant Killer
Malathion	Ortho Malathion Insect Spray

Management of Toxicity. Those handling the patient should wear gloves and aprons to protect themselves against contaminated clothing, skin, or gastric fluid of the patient. Because many insecticides are dissolved in a hydrocarbon vehicle, there is an additional risk of pulmonary aspiration of the hydrocarbon leading to pneumonitis. The risks and benefits of prehospital ipecac-induced emesis should be carefully considered and should involve consultation with a poison control center or clinical toxicologist. Symptomatic cases of anticholinesterase insecticide exposure are typically referred to an emergency department for evaluation and treatment.

If the poison has been ingested, gastric lavage should be performed followed by the administration of activated charcoal. The patient with skin contamination should be washed with copious amounts of soap and water. An alcohol wash may be useful to remove residual insecticide due to its liphophillic nature. A surgical scrub kit for the hands, feet, and nails may be useful for exposure to those areas.

Supportive therapy should include maintenance of an airway, including bronchotracheal suctioning, provision of adequate ventilation, and establishment of an intravenous line. Based on a history of an exposure and presence of typical symptoms, the anticholinesterase syndrome should be recognized without difficulty.

The pharmacologic management of organophosphate intoxication relies on the administration of atropine and pralidoxime.[72,73,75] Atropine has no effect on inhibited cholinesterase, but it competitively blocks the actions of acetylcholine on cholinergic and some central nervous system receptors. It thereby alleviates bronchospasm and reduces bronchial secretions. Although atropine has little effect on the flaccid muscle paralysis or the central respiratory failure of severe poisoning, it is indicated in all symptomatic patients and can be used as a diagnostic aid. It should be given intravenously and, in larger than conventional, doses of 0.05 to 0.1 mg/kg in children under 12 years of age and 2 to 5 mg for adolescents and young adults.[73] It should be repeated at 5- to 10-minute intervals until bronchial secretions and pulmonary rales resolve. Therapy may require large doses over a period of several days until all absorbed organophosphate is metabolized and acetylcholinesterase activity is restored.

Restoration of enzyme activity is necessary for severe poisoning characterized by reduction of cholinesterase activity to less than 20% of normal, profound weakness, and respiratory distress. Pralidoxime (Protopam), also called 2-PAM or pyridine aldoxamine methiodide, breaks the covalent bond between the cholinesterase and organophosphate and regenerates enzyme activity. Organophosphate-cholinesterase binding is initially reversible, but it gradually becomes irreversible. Therefore, therapy with pralidoxime should be initiated as soon as possible, preferably within 36 to 72 hours of exposure.[73] The drug should be given at a dose of 25 to 50 mg/kg up to 1 g intravenously over 5 to 20 minutes. If muscle weakness persists or recurs, the dose may be repeated after an hour and again if needed. A continuous

TABLE 7–12. Comparative Characteristics of Atropine and Pralidoxime for Anticholinesterase Poisoning

Characteristic	Atropine	Pralidoxime
Interaction	Synergy with pralidoxime	Reduces atropine dose requirement
Indication	Any anticholinesterase agent	Typically needed for organophosphates
Primary sites of action	Muscarinic, CNS	Nicotinic > muscarinic > CNS
Adverse effects	Coma, hallucinations, tachycardia	Dizziness, diplopia, tachycardia, headache
Daily dose[a]	2–1600 mg	1–12 g
Total dose[a]	2–11,422 mg	1–92 g

[a]Range of some reported cases; higher doses may be required in rare cases.

infusion of pralidoxime has been shown to be effective in adults when administered at 3.2 mg/kg/h preceded by a loading dose of 4 mg/kg,[77] and in children at 10 to 20 mg/kg/h with a loading dose of 15 to 50 mg/kg.[78] Both atropine and pralidoxime should be given together due to their complementary roles (Table 7–12). Carbamate insecticide poisonings typically do not require the administration of pralidoxime.

One of the pitfalls of therapy is the delay in administering sufficient doses of atropine or pralidoxime.[73,75] The adverse effects of atropine and pralidoxime, predictable extensions of anticholinergic actions, are minimally important compared to the life-threatening effects of severe anticholinesterase poisoning, and can be easily minimized by decreasing the dose.

Monitoring and Prevention. Poisoned patients may require monitoring of vital signs, measurements of ventilatory adequacy such as blood gases and pulse oximetry, leukocyte count with differential to assess development of pneumonia, and chest radiographs to assess the degree of pulmonary edema or development of hydrocarbon pneumonitis. Workers involved in the formulation and application of pesticides should be monitored by periodic measurement of cholinesterase activity in their bloodstream. Untreated, anticholinesterase-depressed acetylcholinesterase activity returns to normal values in approximately 120 days.[73]

Many anticholinesterase insecticide poisonings are unintentional due to misuse, improper storage, failure to follow instructions for mixing or application or inability to read directions for use. Training and vigilant adherence to directions may minimize some poisonings. Storing pesticides in original or labeled containers can minimize the risk of unintentional ingestion. Keeping pesticides out of children's reach may decrease the risk of childhood poisoning.

IRON

Signs and Symptoms. In the first few hours of ingestion of toxic amounts of iron, symptoms of gastrointestinal irritation (e.g., nausea, vomiting, and diarrhea) are common. In certain severe cases, acidosis and shock can become manifest within 6 hours of ingestion. Some have observed a quiescent phase between 6 and 48 hours after ingestion where symptoms improve or abate, but this phenomenon is poorly characterized.[79] Continued gastrointestinal symptoms, poor perfusion, and oliguria should suggest the development of severe toxicity with other effects still to become manifest. Generally, within 24 to 36 hours after the ingestion, CNS involvement with coma and seizures; hepatic injury characterized by jaundice, increased prothrombin time, increased bilirubin, and hypoglycemia; cardiovascular shock; and acidosis also develop.[79] Adult respiratory distress syndrome (ARDS) may develop in patients with severe cardiovascular shock and further compromise recovery.[80] Coagulopathy with decreased thrombin formation is one of the early direct effects of excessive iron concentrations and later disturbances of coagulation (after 24 to 48 hours of ingestion) are a consequence of hepatotoxicity.[81] Mucosal injury, an iron-rich circulation, or deferoxamine therapy may promote septicemia with Yersinia enterocolitica during iron overdose[82]; other bacteria or viruses may also cause septicemia. The pathophysiologic relationships of acute iron toxicity are shown in Figure 7– 7. Two to four weeks after the exposure some patients experience persistent vomiting from gastric outlet obstruction due to pyloric and duodenal stenosis from the earlier gastric mucosal necrosis.

Mechanism of Toxicity. The toxicity of acute iron poisoning includes local effects on the gastrointestinal mucosa and systemic effects induced by excessive iron in the body.[79,80] Iron is irritating to the gastric and duodenal mucosa, which may result in hemorrhage and occasional perforations. Once absorbed, iron is taken up by tissues, particularly the liver, and acts as a mitochondrial poison. It occasionally causes hepatic injury. Iron may significantly inhibit aerobic glycolysis and perturb the electron transport system. Further, iron may shunt electrons away from the electron transport system, thereby reducing the efficiency of oxidative phosphorylation. These biochemical factors, along with the cardiovascular effects of iron, lead to metabolic acidosis. The pathogenesis of shock is not well understood, but may include development of hypovolemia and lactic acidosis, release of endogenous vasodilators, and direct vasodepressant effects of iron and ferritin on the circulation (Fig. 7– 7).

Causative Agents. Iron poisoning results from the ingestion and absorption of excessive amounts of iron from iron tablets, multiple vitamins with iron and prenatal vitamins. Different iron salts and formulations contain varying amounts of elemental iron (see Chap. 91). Generally, children's chewable vitamins are less likely to produce systemic iron poisoning due in part to lower iron content.

Incidence. Acute iron poisoning can produce death in children and adults.[83] In a hazard analysis of 3,810,405 pediatric poisonings reported to poison centers from 1985 to 1989, iron was found to be the most frequent cause of unintentional childhood poisoning death, accounting for 11,234 total cases and 16 deaths.[84] The 1996 AAPCC-TESS documented 29,091 nonfatal and 2 fatal cases, respectively, of iron poisoning with 80% of the exposures in children under 6 years of age. In the majority of cases (84%), multiple vitamins with iron were the source of iron.[6]

Risk Assessment. The minimum lethal and toxic doses for acute iron poisoning are not well established. The ingestion of 10 to 20 mg/kg of elemental iron usually elicits mild gastrointestinal

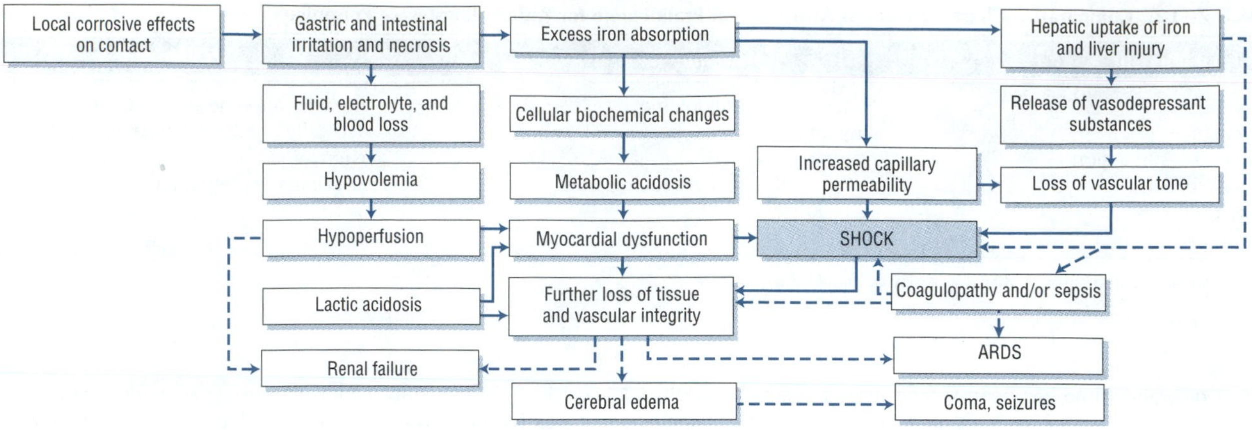

FIGURE 7–7. Pathophysiology of acute iron poisoning. Events indicated by dashed lines are not observed consistently in all serious poisonings. (ARDS = adult respiratory distress syndrome.)

symptoms. The ingestion of 20 to 60 mg/kg is not likely to produce systemic toxicity, and typically these cases can be managed at home with observation and ipecac syrup, if indicated. Ingestions of greater than 60 mg/kg are usually associated with serious systemic toxicity and require medical attention. Immediate psychiatric and medical intervention is indicated for adults and adolescents who acutely ingest greater than 20 mg/kg of elemental iron, because this suggests the overdose was intentional.[79,80]

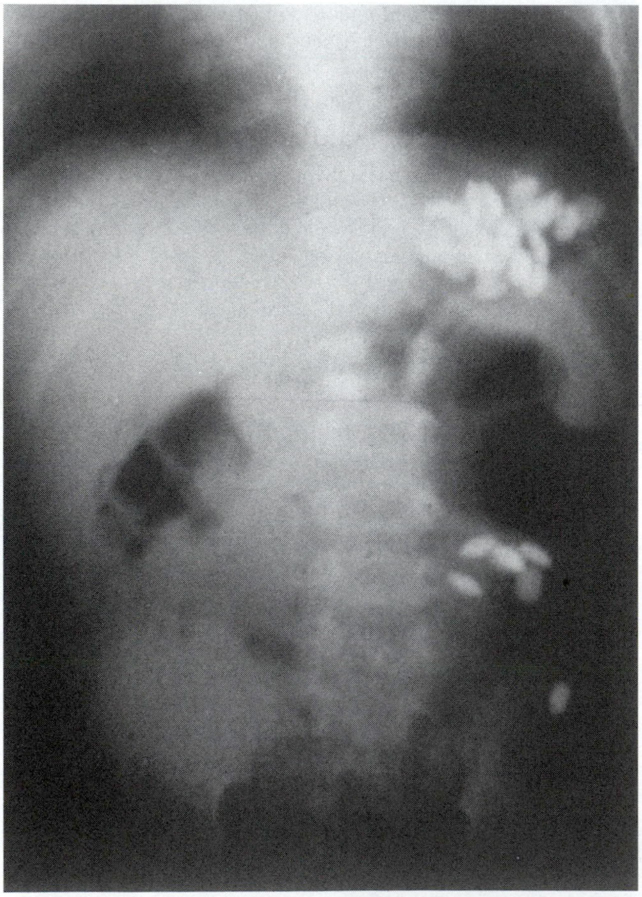

FIGURE 7–8. Abdominal radiograph of a 3-year-old boy who had ingested ferrous sulfate tablets.

An abdominal radiograph (Fig. 7–8) may help confirm the ingestion of iron tablets and indicate the need for aggressive gastrointestinal evacuation. An abdominal radiograph is most useful within 2 hours of ingestion. The visualization of radioopaque iron tablets is confounded by the presence of other hard-coated tablets and some extended-release tablets that are also radioopaque. Furthermore, the radioopacity of iron tablets diminishes as the tablets disintegrate, and chewable and liquid formulations not are typically radioopaque.[85]

Most iron poisoning results in vomiting and diarrhea; however, these symptoms are poor indicators of later serious toxicity. The presence of a combination of findings such as coma, radioopacities, leukocytosis, and increased anion gap, however, is associated with dangerously high serum concentrations greater than 500 μg/dL. The presence of single signs and symptoms, such as vomiting, leukocytosis, or hyperglycemia, is not a reliable indicator of the severity of iron poisoning in adults or children.[86,87]

Once iron is absorbed, it is only eliminated by bleeding or sloughing of the intestinal and epidermal cells. Thus, iron kinetics essentially represent a closed system with multiple compartments. The serum iron concentration represents a small fraction of the total body content of iron, and is at its greatest concentration in the postabsorptive and distributive phases, typically 2 to 10 hours after ingestion.[88] Serum iron concentrations in excess of 500 μg/dL have been associated with severe toxicity, while concentrations below 350 μg/dL are not typically associated with severe toxicity; however, there are exceptions reported for both thresholds. Serious toxicity is best determined by assessing the development of gross gastrointestinal bleeding, metabolic acidosis, shock, and coma regardless of the serum iron concentration. The serum iron concentration serves as a guide for further assessment and treatment options.

The ratio of the serum iron concentration to the total-iron-binding capacity has previously been advocated to assess acute iron poisoning, but it is no longer used. This procedure is unreliable, insensitive, and has little relationship to toxicity.[87]

A deferoxamine challenge test has been proposed, on the basis that the presence of ferrioxamine as orange-red-colored urine would indicate that excess iron is present and able to be chelated. This approach is attractive in its simplicity and potential utility, but there has been no evaluation of its relationship to toxicity, there is no standardized protocol, and the color change may not be perceptible.

Management of Toxicity. Unless the patient has vomited spontaneously, ipecac syrup should be considered for a recent ingestion of 10 to 60 mg/kg of elemental iron, unless contraindications for ipecac use are present. The patient can be managed on the scene with follow-up contact to ascertain that emesis was induced. If symptoms such as persistent vomiting, bloody emesis, diarrhea, or unresponsiveness develop, if the patient ingested greater than 60 mg/kg, or if intentional overdosage is suspected, immediate referral to an emergency department is indicated.[79]

At the emergency department, ipecac syrup may be used if no more than 2 hours have elapsed since ingestion and spontaneous emesis is not evident. Gastric lavage with normal saline may be used to remove iron in unresponsive patients. Activated charcoal administration is not routinely warranted because it poorly adsorbs iron. Lavage with normal saline may remove iron tablet fragments and dissolved iron, but because the lumen of the tube is often smaller than some whole tablets, effective removal is unlikely.[79] If abdominal radiographs reveal a large number of iron tablets, whole-bowel irrigation with polyethylene glycol electrolyte solution is typically necessary[37]; moreover, removal by gastrostomy has been used in a few cases.[89] Early and aggressive decontamination and evacuation of the gastrointestinal tract will minimize iron absorption and thereby reduce the risk of systemic toxicity.

Patients with systemic symptoms (shock, coma, or gross gastrointestinal bleeding or metabolic acidosis) should receive deferoxamine as soon as possible. If the serum iron concentration exceeds 500 µg/dL, deferoxamine is also indicated because serious systemic toxicity is likely.[79,80] Its use is less clear in patients with serum iron concentrations in the range of 350 to 500 µg/dL because many of these patients do not develop systemic symptoms.

Deferoxamine is a highly selective chelator of iron that theoretically binds ferric (Fe^{3+}) iron in a 1:1 molar ratio (100 mg of deferoxamine to 8.5 mg ferric iron) that is more stable than the binding of iron to transferrin. Deferoxamine removes excess iron from the circulation and some iron from transferrin by chelating ferric complexes in equilibrium with transferrin. The resultant iron–deferoxamine complex, ferrioxamine, is then excreted in the urine. Its action on intracellular iron is unclear, but it may have a protective intracellular effect or may chelate extramitochondrial iron.[90]

The parenteral administration of deferoxamine produces an orange-red colored urine within 3 to 6 hours due to the presence of ferrioxamine in the urine.[79] For mild to moderate cases of iron poisoning, where its use is unclear, the presence of discolored urine indicates the persistent presence of chelatable iron and the need to continue deferoxamine. The reliance of discolored urine has been challenged because it is not sensitive and is difficult to detect.[91]

An intravenous infusion of 15 mg/kg/h is indicated, and some have used up to 30 mg/kg/h for life-threatening cases by titrating the dose to minimize deferoxamine-induced hypotension.[79,80,92] Although the manufacturer states that the total dose in 24 hours should not exceed 6 g, the basis for this recommendation is unclear and daily doses as high as 16 to 37.1 g have been administered without incident.[92,93] Because ferrioxamine is more stable at a pH above 6, a slightly alkaline urine may be desirable.[79] Good hydration and urine output may moderate some of the secondary physiologic effects of iron toxicity and assure urinary elimination of ferrioxamine. In the patient who develops renal failure, hemodialysis or hemofiltration does not remove excess iron, but it will remove ferrioxamine.[79]

The rapid intravenous infusion of deferoxamine (> 15 mg/kg/h) has been associated with tachycardia, hypotension, shock, generalized erythema, and urticaria.[79,94] Anaphylaxis has been rarely reported. The use of deferoxamine for greater than 24 hours at doses used for the treatment of acute poisoning has been associated with the exacerbation or development of ARDS.[93–95]

The end point of deferoxamine therapy is not clear. Some have suggested that deferoxamine therapy should cease when the serum iron concentration falls below 150 µg/dL.[80] The decline of serum iron concentrations, however, may not account for the potential cellular action of deferoxamine irrespective of its effect on iron elimination. The cessation of orange-red urine production that is indicative of ferrioxamine excretion is also not reliable, because many individuals cannot distinguish its presence in the urine.[91] Considering these shortcomings, deferoxamine therapy should be continued for 12 hours after the patient is asymptomatic and the urine returns to normal color, or until the serum iron concentration falls below 350 µg/dL and approaches 150 µg/dL.

Other Therapies. Various fluids have been proposed to minimize the absorption of iron from the gastrointestinal tract. The oral administration of deferoxamine has been advocated by some to reduce iron absorption,[90] but the ferrioxamine complex is absorbable, increases the total iron body burden, is toxic in high concentrations, and may outstrip the hospital's supply that should be used for intravenous administration.[96] Lavage solutions of phosphate were proposed as a means to render iron insoluble, but they were found ineffective and could lead to dangerous hyperphosphatemia.[80,97] Lavage with 1% to 2% sodium bicarbonate or administration of milk of magnesia may increase intragastric pH and precipitate iron, but the precipitate is reversibly soluble in the acidic pH of the stomach.[97] Administering deferoxamine orally with activated charcoal has been shown in volunteers to decrease iron absorption, but its application to the poisoned patient requires further evaluation.[98] Oral iron chelating agents, such as deferiprone,[99] are under development for the treatment of chronic iron overload states and may have some application for the treatment of acute iron poisoning.

Monitoring and Prevention. Once a poisoning has occurred, acid–base balance (anion gap and arterial blood gases), fluid and electrolyte balance, and perfusion should be monitored. Other indicators of organ toxicity such as ALT, AST, bilirubin, prothrombin time, serum glucose, and creatinine, and markers of physiologic stress or infection such as leukocytosis, should also be monitored.

Iron poisoning is often not recognized as a potentially serious problem by parents or victims until symptoms develop, and thus valuable time to institute treatment is lost. Parents should be made aware of the potential risks and asked to observe basic poison-prevention measures. Many chewable vitamins with iron are shaped like animal or cartoon characters that can be attractive to children and can lead to poisoning. Some hard-coated iron tablets resemble candy-coated chocolates and are easily confused by children. Based on these considerations and the frequency of this poisoning, iron tablets are packaged in child-resistant containers. In 1998, iron products were required to be sold in special packages, such as blister packs, which limit the total dose and present additional physical barriers for children.[100] Although child-resistant containers are required for iron-containing drugs, failures in pharmacist compliance with their dispensing and patient adherence limit their proper use.[11,13]

THEOPHYLLINE

Signs and Symptoms. Gastrointestinal, cardiovascular, neurologic, and metabolic effects have been observed following acute and chronic poisoning with theophylline.[101] Gastrointestinal symptoms include nausea and vomiting in 60% to 100% of cases, abdominal pain, diarrhea, and acute gastritis with gastrointestinal bleeding. Vomiting may be difficult to control despite antiemetic therapy. Supraventricular tachycardia is present in most cases. Peripheral vasodilation typically leads to hypotension in severe cases. Premature ventricular beats are also commonly observed. Ventricular tachycardia and fibrillation are associated with more severe intoxications and may be life threatening. Atrial fibrillation is more frequently seen with chronic exposure.[102–104] Theophylline may produce tachypnea due to stimulation of CNS respiratory centers. Headache, hallucinations, disorientation, coma, ataxia, and tremor may be observed. Seizures are a common consequence of serious theophylline poisoning and are associated with increased mortality. The seizures are typically generalized, may occur without warning, and may be resistant to conventional anticonvulsant therapy. Irritability, vomiting, and headache may precede seizure activity. Neurologic complications of theophylline-induced seizure activity are more common with chronic toxicity and include amnesia, quadraplegia, persistent seizures, and intracerebral hemorrhage.[104,105] Theophylline poisoning typically produces marked hypokalemia, but its consequences are unclear. Blood glucose concentrations are elevated and in some cases may exceed 400 mg/dL. Hypercalcemia, hypophosphatemia, hypomagnesemia, and respiratory alkalosis have also been reported.[101–105] Metabolic acidosis is a common finding in cases of moderate to severe severity. Theophylline may also have a mild diuretic effect.

There are differences in onset and duration of toxic symptoms compared to effects at therapeutic doses. Peak effects from therapeutic doses may be observed in 1 to 2 hours, but with overdosage peak concentrations and effects may occur from 2 to 8 hours after ingestion. Sustained-release preparations may peak between 6 and 24 hours. Tablet concretions have been reported with sustained-release tablets.[106]

Mechanism of Toxicity. Theophylline relaxes smooth muscles, stimulates the CNS, reduces peripheral vascular resistance, increases the rate and force of myocardial contractions, and increases urine production. The exact mechanism for these actions is not known for theophylline at therapeutic or toxic levels, but several hypotheses exist. Inhibition of phosphodiesterase leading to increased cyclic AMP has been proposed. General sympathetic stimulation may occur as evidenced by increases in circulating catecholamines. The translocation of intracellular calcium as the result of increased permeability of the sarcoplasmic reticulum in striated muscles has also been observed. Another potential mechanism involves the competitive blockade of adenosine receptors thereby minimizing the effects of endogenous adenosine, a recognized bronchconstrictor, anticonvulsant, and regulator of cardiac rhythm.[101] Hypokalemia, one of the metabolic effects of theophylline toxicity, may result from cyclic-AMP mediated stimulation of the sodium-potassium-ATPase pump, resulting in decreased extracellular potassium.

Causative Agents. There are numerous theophylline-containing products on the market for the treatment of asthma and other pulmonary conditions (see Chaps. 24 and 25). Despite several different forms of theophylline, there is no apparent difference in toxicity with equivalent doses of theophylline. Theophylline is available as a liquid, and several solid dosage forms including sustained-release formulations.

Incidence. The 1996 AAPCC-TESS report documented 3100 patients with an exposure to theophylline of which 55% were greater than 19 years of age and 31% were intentional poisonings.[6] Of the 76 people who experienced a major effect and the 11 people who died, all were over 40 years of age. As the therapy of asthma shifts from the routine use of theophylline products (see Chap. 24), the availability of theophylline and incidence of poisoning are likely to decline.

Risk Assessment. The circumstances, symptoms, and toxic serum concentrations are different based on whether theophylline exposure is acute or chronic (Table 7–13). Theophylline toxicity is likely with the acute, single ingestion of 10 mg/kg or more of theophylline. Chronic theophylline toxicity typically results from overmedication, changes in metabolism of theophylline, or drug interactions (see Chap 24).[103–107]

Interpretation of serum theophylline concentrations should consider whether the exposure was acute or chronic. Ventricular tachycardia is associated with concentrations greater that 100 μg/mL with acute exposures and concentrations of 40 μg/mL or greater following chronic exposures. Convulsions are seen in 50% of patients following acute exposures with serum concentrations over 120 μg/mL or chronic exposures with concentrations exceeding 40 μg/mL.[101–104] Patients with acute theophylline poisoning typically exhibit signs of minor toxicity at serum theophylline concentrations of 20 to 40 μg/mL, moderate toxicity in the range of 40 to 80 μg/mL, and severe toxicity with concentrations greater than 70 to 80 μg/mL. The serum theophylline concentration is less predictive for chronic exposures[108,109]; patients have experienced seizures, arrhythmias, and death at serum concentrations as low as 20 to 30 μg/mL.[101,109]

With acute theophylline poisoning, few patient risk factors have been associated with the development of toxicity. The risk of toxicity from chronic exposure is increased by several factors including drug interactions and saturable biotransformation. Because theophylline is metabolized by the cytochrome oxidase system, inhibitors of this enzyme system, such as erythromycin, oral contraceptives, allopurinol, cimetidine, and ciprofloxin (see Chaps. 24 and 25), may lead to theophylline toxicity within several days of their concomitant use. Chronic toxicity is seen at lower serum concentrations than acute toxicity.[104,105,108] Possible explanations for chronic toxicity include CNS saturation or accu-

TABLE 7–13. Comparison of Acute and Chronic Theophylline Toxicity

Characteristic	Acute	Chronic
Circumstance	Intentional overdose Unintentional ingestion	Patient increased dose Drug interaction Altered elimination Dosing/dispensing error
Symptoms	Vomiting, tremor, tachycardia, hypotension, hypokalemia, acidosis, seizures	Occasional vomiting Tachycardia, seizures
Life-threatening serum theophylline concentration (μg/mL)	> 100	> 40–60
Predictor of life-threatening events	Serum concentration (> 100 μg/mL)	Extremes of age

mulation of 3-methylxanthine, an active metabolite of theophylline. Although seizures and serious dysrhythmias have been reported at concentrations of 15 to 20 μg/mL, they are more frequently seen with chronic serum theophylline concentrations of 35 to 70 μg/mL. Age rather than peak serum concentration is more predictive of major toxicity after chronic theophylline exposure, with the very young and the elderly at greatest risk.[103,104] Older patients with preexisting cardiopulmonary disease are more susceptible to the life-threatening complications of theophylline toxicity. Risk factors for life-threatening effects include the presence of seizures, hypotension, preexisting cardiac or hepatic disease, chronic exposure, and age over 50 years.[103,104,108,109]

Management of Toxicity. Routine supportive care and gastric decontamination procedures are typically indicated for theophylline poisoning. Due to the risk of theophylline-induced seizure activity, ipecac syrup is avoided. Activated charcoal adsorbs theophylline and may be useful for acute theophylline ingestions when the drug is still suspected to be present in the gastrointestinal tract. Vomiting is commonly associated with theophylline poisoning and may limit the ability to administer activated charcoal. Vomiting may be controlled by parenteral ranitidine, high-dose metoclopromide (0.5 to 1 mg/kg), ondansetron, and droperidol.[101,107] Whole-bowel irrigation has been used the evacuate the intestines following ingestion of sustained-release theophylline products.[37]

Because of the associated increase in mortality and resistance to anticonvulsant therapy, the anticipation and treatment of seizures are essential in the management of theophylline poisoning. Although phenobarbital prophylaxis for anticipated theophylline-induced seizures has been proposed,[102] it is based on animals pretreated with the anticonvulsant[110] and is not considered to be effective clinically for other drug-induced seizures.[111] Once seizures occur, they should be treated aggressively. Initially a benzodiazepine, such as diazepam or lorazepam, should be used, and may require large doses. Phenobarbital may be considered a second-line therapy; however, phenytoin is avoided due to its ineffectiveness for theophylline-induced seizures.[102,110] If anticonvulsants are ineffective in terminating seizures, skeletal muscle paralysis and general anesthesia may be necessary.

Cardiac dysrhythmias, such as supraventricular tachycardia, may require no treatment. Hemodynamically significant supraventricular tachycardia may be treated with esmolol, adenosine, or verapamil[101]; however, verapamil may exacerbate hypotension. Ventricular dysrhythmias may respond to lidocaine, beta-blockers, or other antiarrhythmics, depending upon the cardiac disturbance. Hypotension, with an increased pulse pressure and diastolic hypotension, is often due to decreased vascular resistance and may respond to a modest intravenous fluid bolus followed by conventional vasopressors, such as dopamine, dobutamine, and norepinephrine, if needed.[107]

Hypokalemia, hyperglycemia, hypophosphatemia, hypercalcemia and metabolic acidosis have been corrected by intravenous propranolol[107] and by specific replacement if indicated. Most metabolic disturbances do not require aggressive therapy. Propranolol or adensosine should be used cautiously in individuals susceptible to the risk of bronchoconstriction.

Multiple-dose activated charcoal has proven to be effective at enhancing elimination of theophylline from the bloodstream even after intravenous overdose.[101,111] It has been shown to reduce theophylline half-life by 50%. Repeat-dose activated charcoal should be considered if serum concentrations in acute overdose are over 40 μg/mL, when patients are symptomatic (acute or chronic exposures), or in chronic intoxication with serum concentrations over 20 μg/mL.[100]

Charcoal hemoperfusion and hemodialysis are very effective in removal of theophylline from the bloodstream,[100,106] but they are frequently unnecessary when repeat-dose charcoal can be successfully employed.[112] Although hemoperfusion and hemodialysis are nearly similar in effectiveness, hemoperfusion is associated with more complications whereas hemodialysis is more readily available.[113] Extracorporeal removal should be considered in acute overdose with serum concentrations over 100 μg/mL, for patients with seizure activity or hemodynamically significant dysrhythmias not responding to conventional therapy, or in chronic intoxication with serum concentrations over 40 μg/mL.[101,103]

Monitoring and Prevention. Theophylline may be reliably detected by enzyme-mediated immunoassays (EMIT) or high-performance liquid chromatography. Laboratory monitoring should include electrolytes, calcium, magnesium, phosphorus, arterial blood gases, and urine pH. Seizure activity should prompt the monitoring of serum creatine phosphokinase and myoglobinuria. When elevations occur, prophylactic treatment for rhabdomyolysis should be instituted, including alkaline diuresis to maintain a urine pH of 7.5 to 8 to minimize the risk of tubular deposition of myoglobin and resultant acute renal failure.

Theophylline poisoning may be prevented by recognition of its poisonous potential and institution of general poison prevention measures when young children are present. Monitoring of patients receiving theophylline for changes in health status (e.g., viral illness or cardiac disease, drug therapy leading to drug interactions, drug dosage by the patient or caregiver, and metabolism due to age-related changes in drug disposition) may identify patients at risk of developing chronic theophylline poisoning.[103,108]

TRICYCLIC ANTIDEPRESSANTS

Signs and Symptoms. Symptoms of tricyclic antidepressant poisoning typically occur within the first hour of ingestion and can rapidly progress to death in several hours. Patients may deteriorate rapidly and progress from no symptoms to life-threatening cardiotoxicity or seizures within 1 hour.[114,115] The principal effects of tricyclic antidepressant poisoning involve the cardiovascular and central nervous systems and can result in arrhythmias, hypotension, coma, and seizures.

Prolongation of the QRS complex on ECG indicating nonspecific intraventricular conduction delay or bundle-branch block is the most distinctive feature of tricyclic antidepressant overdose.[115] Sinus tachycardia with rates typically under 160 beats per minute is common and does not cause serious hemodynamic changes in most patients. Ventricular tachycardia is a common ventricular arrhythmia, but it may be difficult to distinguish from sinus tachycardia in the presence of QRS prolongation and the apparent absence of P waves. It often occurs in patients with marked QRS prolongation or hypotension and may be precipitated by seizures.[115–117] High rates of mortality are associated with ventricular tachycardia; ventricular fibrillation is the terminal rhythm. Torsades de pointes is infrequently observed with tricyclic antidepressant poisoning. With massive tricyclic antidepressant overdose, slow ventricular rhythms may be observed. A few cases of sudden death from presumed fatal arrhythmias have been reported 2 to 5 days after ingestion, but these cases are isolated events that have an unclear causal relationship to tricyclic antidepressant overdose.[114] Hypotension is a significant factor in most cases of tricyclic antidepressant poisoning. Refractory hypotension leading to death is due to vasodilation and impaired cardiac contractility.[115] Other factors—such as extreme heart rates, intravascular volume depletion, hypoxia, hyperthermia, seizures, and acidosis—may contribute to refractory hypotension.

Coma is usually present in patients with tricyclic antidepressant poisoning and may or may not be associated with QRS prolongation. In severe cases, coma is sufficient to depress respirations. Delirium, manifest as agitation or disorientation, may occur early in the course of severe poisoning or with poisoning of moderate severity. Seizures often occur within 2 hours of ingestion and are usually generalized, single, and brief. Seizures may result in acidosis, hyperthermia, or rhabdomyolysis, and 10% to 20% of patients may abruptly develop cardiovascular deterioration.[115] Myoclonus may also be observed with tricyclic antidepressant overdose.

Hyperthermia often results from seizure and myoclonic activity in the presence of decreased sweating and is associated with a high incidence of neurologic sequelae and mortality. Anticholinergic symptoms, such as urinary retention, ileus, and dry mucous membranes, are often observed with tricyclic antidepressant overdose.[114–116] Pupil size is variable.

Functional stages for tricyclic antidepressant overdose can be established based on the patient's symptoms and recovery time. In stage one, patients are responsive to pain, have sinus tachycardia, and recover within 24 hours. In the second stage, seizures, coma, and cardiac conduction problems are evident; respiratory support is typically needed. Patients recover within 24 to 48 hours of ingestion. Stage three is characterized by the features of stage two with the addition of respiratory arrest, hypotension, ventricular dysrhythmias, and asystole, which may occur within 1 to 24 hours of ingestion.

Amoxipine, buproprion, and maprotiline are atypical antidepressants associated with a higher incidence of seizures upon overdose; amoxipine produces minimal cardiotoxicity.[115,118]

The selective serotonin reuptake inhibitors (SSRIs) generally produce a common toxicity profile on overdose despite their structural and pharmacologic distinctions. The SSRIs inhibit the presynaptic neuronal uptake of serotonin, resulting in increased synaptic serotonin levels. When ingested in excess, SSRIs rarely cause death and typically produce nausea, vomiting, diarrhea, tremor, and decreased level of consciousness. Tachycardia and seizures are infrequent.[115,118,119] Serotonin syndrome is associated with the coingestion of drugs increasing serotonin levels, and develops within minutes to hours of the inciting action. It is characterized by a collection of neurobehavioral (confusion, agitation, coma, seizures), autonomic (hyperthermia, diaphoresis, tachycardia, hypertension), and neuromuscular (myoclonus, rigidity, tremor, ataxia, shivering, nystagmus) signs and symptoms.[120,121] Most cases are mild and resolve spontaneously within 24 to 72 hours. Cardiac arrest, coma, and multiple organ failure have been reported as consequences of serotonin syndrome.[120] Recognition of the syndrome is based on a high index of suspicion and identification of risk factors.

Mechanism of Toxicity. Many of the toxic effects of tricyclic antidepressants are associated with an exaggeration of their pharmacologic action. The tricyclic antidepressants inhibit the fast sodium channel so that phase 0 depolarization of the myocardium is slowed similar to type Ia antiarrhythmic drugs.[115] This action leads to QRS prolongation, atrioventricular block, ventricular tachycardia, and decreased myocardial contractility. Tricyclic antidepressants also block vascular alpha-adrenergic receptors, resulting in vasodilation, which contributes to hypotension. Sinus tachycardia is related to the inhibition of norepinephrine reuptake and anticholinergic effects. Other anticholinergic effects include urinary retention, ileus, dry mucous membranes, and impaired sweating. Inhibition of norepinephrine reuptake may also account for the early, transient, and self-limiting elevation of blood pressure observed in some patients. The CNS toxicity of tricyclic antidepressants is not well understood.

Causative Agents. Tricylic antidepressants and SSRIs are used to treat a variety of behavioral conditions (see Chaps. 65 and 66). The tricyclic antidepressants include drugs such as amitriptyline, desipramine, doxepin, imipramine, and nortriptyline. Atypical agents include amoxapine, buproprion, and maprotilene. The SSRIs include fluoxetine, nefazadone, paroxetine, sertraline, trazadone, and venlafaxine.

The tricyclic antidepressants are generally highly protein bound, exhibit a large volume of distribution, and possess elimination half-lives of 8 to 24 hours or more. Virtually none of the drug is eliminated unchanged in the urine. Metabolism of the parent drug produces active metabolites in most cases (e.g., amitriptyline to nortriptyline, which may contribute to toxicity after the first 12 to 24 hours).[115] Genetic polymorphism at CYP2D6 may lead to slower recovery in patients who are slow hydroxylators.[122]

Incidence. Tricyclic antidepressant poisoning is a common cause of death from drug overdose.[115,117] The 1996 AAPCC-TESS report documented 17,812 patients with exposures to tricyclic antidepressants of which 65% were intentional overdoses. A total of 1535 people experienced a major effect and 106 people died. Two of the deaths were children aged 6 years or less.[6]

Risk Assessment. Ingestion of greater that 1 g of a tricyclic antidepressant (> 10 mg/kg in children) typically results in life-threatening toxicity.[115] Because serious toxicity may occur within 1 to 2 hours of ingestion, prompt transport to an emergency department is crucial for overdoses. A QRS complex greater than 100 msec or progressive prolongation of the QRS are indicators of toxicity and often precede more serious symptoms.[115,117,123] Serum concentrations of tricyclic antidepressants in excess of 1000 ng/mL have been associated with a QRS complex of 100 msec or greater, but an ECG reading is more readily obtainable and serves as a more direct indicator of toxicity.[123] Although urine drug analyses routinely screen for tricyclic antidepressant, the qualitative result can only suggest or confirm a potential risk for the development of toxicity.

Patients with coexisting cardiovascular and pulmonary conditions (e.g., ARDS, pulmonary infection, pulmonary aspiration) may be more susceptible to the toxic effects or complications of tricyclic antidepressant poisoning. The influence of chronic exposure to tricyclic antidepressants on the risks of an acute overdose is unclear. Tricyclic antidepressants interact with other CNS depressant drugs, which together may lead to increased CNS and respiratory depression.

The risk of serotonin syndrome may be increased shortly after dosage increases of SSRIs or when drug interactions increase serotonin activity.[124] Concomitant or proximal use of SSRIs, tricyclic antidepressants, or monoamine oxidase inhibitors may cause serotonin syndrome. Further, the addition of certain drugs, such as tryptophan, dextromethorphan, cocaine, or sympathomimetics, to SSRI therapy may increase the risk of developing serotonin syndrome.[120,124]

Management of Toxicity. Once the ingestion of an overdose of tricyclic antidepressant is suspected, or for any intentional ingestion, medical evaluation and treatment should be promptly sought. If the patient is symptomatic, it may be prudent to call for an ambulance owing to the rapid progression of some cases. At the emergency department, the patient should be carefully monitored, have vital signs assessed regularly, and have an intravenous line started. Supportive and symptomatic care includes oxygen, intravenous fluids, and other treatments as indicated. Prompt administration of activated charcoal may decrease the absorption of any remaining tricyclic antidepressant. It may be useful beyond the first hour of ingestion due to decreased gastrointestinal motility from the anticholinergic action of tricyclic antidepressants. Gastric lavage may be considered if the time of the ingestion is unknown or if it occurred within the past 1 to 2 hours. Some avoid gastric lavage altogether.[115] Ipecac syrup should be avoided in patients who ingest tricyclic antidepressants due to the rapid onset of toxicity. Multiple-dose activated charcoal has been shown to increase the elimination of some tricyclic antidepressants in human volunteers[42] and has been used in poisoned patients.[114,115] It may be most useful during the first 12 hours after ingestion, while the drug is distributing to tissue compartments. Because the tricyclic antidepressants possess such a large volume of distribution and so little of the drug is present in the bloodstream, hemodialysis is not useful for the extracorporeal removal of tricyclic antidepressants.

Intravenous sodium bicarbonate is part of the first-line treatment of QRS prolongation, ventricular arrhythmias, and hypotension caused by tricyclic antidepressant overdose (Fig. 7–9).[115,125] Typically 1 to 2 mEq/kg of sodium bicarbonate (1 mEq/mL) is administered as a bolus infusion (usually a 50-mEq ampule in an adult) and repeated as necessary to achieve an arterial blood pH of 7.50 to 7.55 or abatement of toxicity.[114,115] A therapeutic effect is usually observed within minutes. Excessive use of sodium bicarbonate may produce dangerous alkalemia, which is by itself associated with ventricular arrhythmias.[115] The mechanism of action of sodium bicarbonate is unclear. Although some proposed that sodium bicarbonate increased protein binding of tricyclic antidepressants, this has been discounted. Sodium may play an important role by stabilizing tricyclic antidepressant-induced changes to the sodium gradient of the myocardium.[115] Regardless of its action, it is effective and generally safe. Hyperventilation to produce a mild state of respiratory alkalosis has been used to treat some dysrhythmias, but it is less widely used than sodium bicarbonate.[114,115]

Treatment of the complications of tricyclic antidepressant poisoning is outlined in Table 7–14 and includes pharmacologic and nonpharmacologic approaches.[115] Several agents should generally be avoided in the treatment of tricyclic antidepressant poisoning. Other drugs that inhibit the fast sodium channel, such as procainamide and quinidine, are contraindicated. Phenytoin has limited usefulness in treating tricyclic antidepressant seizures and has questionable efficacy in managing cardiotoxicity.[114] Physostigmine was used in the past as a treatment of tricyclic antidepressant cardiotoxicity and seizures, because it antagonizes anticholinergic actions. However, physostigmine is otherwise ineffective, is associated bradycardia and asystole,[115,126] and has no role in the contemporary treatment of tricyclic antidepressant

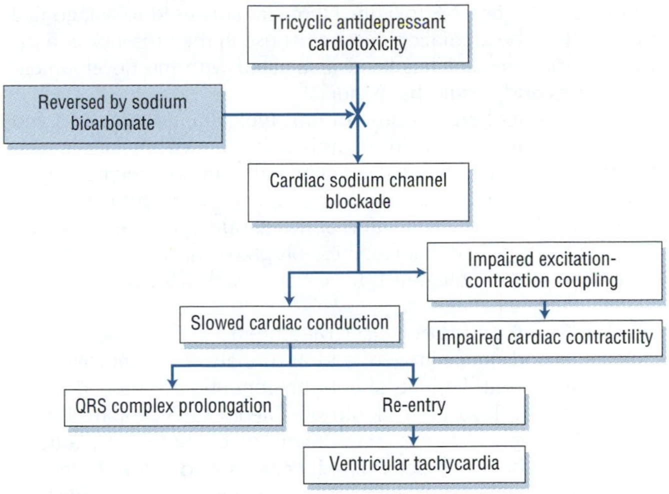

FIGURE 7–9. Role of sodium bicarbonate in limiting cardiotoxicity from tricyclic antidepressant poisoning. *(Adapted from Ref. 115, with permission.)*

TABLE 7–14. Treatment Options for Tricyclic Antidepressant Toxicity

Toxic Effect	Treatment
Cardiovascular Effects	
QRS prolongation	Intravenous sodium bicarbonate if QRS prolongation is marked or progressive (not clear if treatment is needed in the absence of hypotension or arrhythmias)
Hypotension	Intravascular volume expansion, intravenous sodium bicarbonate Vasopressors (norepinephrine) or inotropes (dopamine) Treat hyperthermia, acidosis, seizures Consider mechanical circulatory support
Ventricular tachycardia	Intravenous sodium bicarbonate, lidocaine, overdrive pacing Treat hypotension, hyperthermia, acidosis, seizures
Torsades de pointes	Overdrive cardiac pacing
Ventricular bradycardia	Chronotropes (epinephrine), cardiac pacemaker
Sinus tachycardia	Treatment rarely needed
Atrioventricular block—type II second or third degree	Cardiac pacemaker
Hypertension	If needed, rapidly titratable antihypertensive agent (nitroprusside)
CNS Effects	
Delirium and agitation	Physical restraints, benzodiazepines Neuromuscular blockade if hyperthermia or acidosis present
Seizures	Benzodiazepine Neuromuscular blockade if hyperthermia or acidosis present
Coma	Endotracheal intubation, mechanical ventilation if needed
Other Effects	
Hyperthermia	Treat seizures, agitation Cooling measures (cooling blanket, ice water lavage, cool water mist of body)
Acidosis	Intravenous sodium bicarbonate Treat hypotension, hypoventilation

Adapted from Ref. 115.

cardiovascular or CNS toxicity. Flumazemil is used to antagonize the effects of benzodiazepines, but its use in the presence of a tricyclic antidepressant has been associated with the development of seizures and should be avoided.[127]

Treatment of an overdose of the atypical antidepressants and SSRIs is primarily directed towards decontamination of the gastrointestinal tract with activated charcoal, symptomatic treatment, and general supportive care. Management of the serotonin syndrome involves discontinuation of the serotinergic agent and supportive therapy. Benzodiazepines, propranolol, and cyproheptadine, a serotonin antagonist, have been used successfully.[120]

Monitoring and Prevention. Measurement of vital signs, electrolytes, blood urea nitrogen, and an urinalysis are indicated for initial assessment. Patients should be continuously monitored by ECG, and a 12-lead ECG should obtained if QRS prolongation is noted. If patients start to show signs of cardiotoxicity, arterial blood gases should be determined. Patients who show no signs of toxicity during 6 hours of observation and have promptly received activated charcoal require no further medical monitoring. Psychiatric evaluation is indicated for adolescents and adults. When signs of tricyclic antidepressant are present in a patient, cardiac monitoring is generally recommended for at least 24 hours after the patient is without findings.[115]

Prevention of tricyclic antidepressant poisoning poses unique challenges. Many of the dosage forms are small in size, and large numbers can be easily consumed by adults and children. In the course of treating depression, several antidepressant agents may be tried to achieve results. Instead of discarding unused medicines, a storehouse of potentially deadly drugs may be kept for children to discover or for the despondent patient to use to attempt suicide. Although patients take tricyclic antidepressants for therapeutic relief of depression, they are also a group likely to contemplate suicide with tricyclic antidepressants. Strategies that would limit the amount of tricyclic antidepressant prescribed at one time would also potentially impair adherence to a dosage regimen and thereby compromise the therapeutic potential of these agents.[115,125] Patients with a history of suicidal gestures may be candidates for the atypical antidepressants or SSRIs, which possess less cardiotoxicity. General poison prevention measures may limit childhood poisonings, and monitoring depressed patients for suicidal ideation may identify patients at risk.

REFERENCES

1. Koren G. Medications which can kill a toddler with one tablet or teaspoonful. Clin Toxicol 1993;31:407–413.
2. Rice DJ, MacKenzie EJ. Cost of Injury in the United States: A Report to Congress. San Francisco, Institute for Health & Aging, University of California, and Injury Prevention Center, Johns Hopkins University, 1989:23–25, 37–85.
3. Fingerhut LA, Cox CS. Poisoning mortality. Public Health Rep 1998;113:218–233.
4. Phillips DP, Christenfeld N, Glynn LM. Increase in US medication-error deaths between 1983 and 1993. Lancet 1998;351:643–644
5. Litovitz T. The TESS database: Use in product safety assessment. Drug Saf 1998;18:9–19.
6. Litovitz TL, Smilkstein M, Felberg L, et al. 1996 annual report of the American Association of Poison Control Centers Toxic Exposure Surveillance System. Am J Emerg Med 1997;15:447–500.
7. Kearney TE, Olson KR, Heard SE, Blanc PD. Health care cost effects of public use of a regional poison control center. West J Med 1995;162:499–504.
8. Phillips KA, Homan RK, Hiatt PH, et al. The costs and outcomes of restricting public access to poison control centers. Results from a natural experiment. Med Care 1998;36:271–280.
9. Litovitz T. Listen, ye legislators, our children need you! West J Med 1995;162:552–553. Editorial.
10. Rodgers GB. The safety effects of child-resistant packaging for oral prescription drugs: Two decades of experience. JAMA 1996; 275:1661–1665.
11. King WD, Palmisano PA. Ingestion of prescription drugs by children: An epidemiologic study. South Med J 1989;82:1468–1478.
12. Poison Prevention Packaging: A textbook for pharmacists and physicians. Washington, DC, U.S. Consumer Product Safety Commission, 1993.
13. Dole EJ, Czajka PA, Rivara FP. Evaluation of pharmacists' compliance with the Poison Prevention Packaging Act. Am J Public Health 1986;76:1335–1336.
14. Slagle MA, Chyka PA, Holley JE. Pharmacists' use of safety caps on refilled prescriptions. Am Pharmacy 1994;34:37–40.
15. Beatrais AL, Fergusson DM, Shannon FT. Life events and childhood morbidity: A prospective study. Pediatrics 1982;70:935–940.
16. Rodgers GC, Tenenbien M. The role of aversive bittering agents in the prevention of pediatric poisonings. Pediatrics 1994;93:68–69.
17. Buckley NA, Whyte IM, Dawson AH, et al. Correlations between prescriptions and drugs taken in self-poisoning. Med J Aust 1995; 162:194–197.
18. Haselberger MB, Kroner BA. Drug poisoning in older patients: Preventative and management strategies. Drugs Aging 1995;7:292–297.
19. Olson K, Pentel P, Kelley M. Physical assessment and differential diagnosis of the poisoned patient. Med Toxicol 1987;2:52–81.
20. Nice A, Leikin JB, Maturen A, et al. Toxidrome recognition to improve efficiency of emergency uring drug screens. Ann Emerg Med 1988;17:676–680.
21. Liang HK. Clinical evaluation of the poisoned patient and toxic syndromes. Clin Chem 1996;42:1350–1355.
22. USP Drug Information. Volume II, Advice for the Patient, 18th ed. Rockville, MD, United States Pharmacopeial Convention, 1997.
23. Liu RH. Important considerations in the interpretation of forensic urine drug test results. Forensic Sci Rev 1992;4:51–64.
24. Woolf AD, Shannon MW. Clinical toxicology for the pediatrician. Pediatr Clin North Am 1995;42:317–333.
25. Rosenberg J, Benowitz NL, Pond S. Pharmacokinetics of drug overdose. Clin Pharmacokinet 1981;6:161–192.
26. Young-Jin S, Shannon M. Pharmacokinetics of drugs in overdose. Clin Pharmacokinet 1992;23:93–105.
27. Vernon DD, Gleich MC. Poisoning and drug overdose. Crit Care Clin North Am 1997;13:647–667.
28. Vance MV, Selden BS, Clark RF. Optimal patient position for transport and initial management of toxic ingestions. Ann Emerg Med 1992;21:243–246.
29. Mowry JB, Sketris IS, Czajka PA. Ipecac syrup for poisoning at home: availability, compliance, and response monitored by telephone. Am J Hosp Pharm 1981;38:1028–1030.
30. USP Drug Information. Volume I, Drug Information for the Health Care Professional, 18th ed. Rockville, MD, United States Pharmacopeial Convention, 1997.
31. American Academy of Clinical Toxicology, European Association of Poison Centres and Clinical Toxicologists. Position statement: Ipecac syrup. Clin Toxicol 1997;35:699–709.

32. American Academy of Clinical Toxicology, European Association of Poison Centres and Clinical Toxicologists. Position statement: Gastric lavage. Clin Toxicol 1997;35:711–719.
33. American Academy of Clinical Toxicology, European Association of Poison Centres and Clinical Toxicologists. Position statement: Single-dose activated charcoal. Clin Toxicol 1997;35:721–741.
34. McFarland AK, III, Chyka PA. Selection of activated charcoal products for the treatment of poisonings. Ann Pharmacother 1993;27:358–361.
35. American Academy of Clinical Toxicology, European Association of Poisons Centres and Clinical Toxicologists. Position statement: Cathartics. Clin Toxicol 1997;35:743–752.
36. Oral electrolyte solutions for colonic lavage before colonoscopy or barium enema. Med Lett Drugs Ther 1985;27:39–40.
37. American Academy of Clinical Toxicology, European Association of Poison Centres and Clinical Toxicologists. Position statement: Whole bowel irrigation. Clin Toxicol 1997;35:753–762.
38. Hoffman RS, Smilkstein MJ, Goldfrank LR. Whole bowel irrigation and the cocaine body-packer: A new approach to a common problem. Am J Emerg Med 1990;8:523–527.
39. American College of Emergency Physicians. Clinical policy for the initial approach to patients presenting with acute toxic ingestion or dermal or inhalation exposure. Ann Emerg Med 1995;25:570–585.
40. Elenbaas RM. Critical review of forced alkaline diuresis in acute salicylism. Crit Care Q 1982;4:89–95.
41. Scandling J, Spital A. Amphetamine-associated myoglobinuric renal failure. South Med J 1982;75:237–240.
42. Chyka PA. Multiple-dose activated charcoal and enhancement of systemic drug clearance: Summary of studies in animals and humans. J Toxicol Clin Toxicol 1995;33:399–405.
43. Neuvonen PJ, Olkkola KT. Oral activated charcoal in the treatment of intoxication. Role of single and repeated doses. Med Toxicol 1988;3:33–58.
44. Pond SM, Olson KR, Osterloh JD, et al. Randomized study of the treatment of phenobarbital overdose with repeated doses of activated charcoal. JAMA 1984;251:3104–3108.
45. Chyka PA, Holley JE, Mandrell TM, Sugathan P. Correlation of drug pharmacokinetics and effectiveness of multiple-dose activated charcoal therapy. Ann Emerg Med 1995;25:356–362.
46. Farrar HC, Herold DA, Reed MD. Acute valproic acid intoxication: Enhanced drug clearance with oral-activated charcoal. Crit Care Med 1993;21:299–301.
47. Pond SM. Extracorporeal techniques in the treatment of poisoned patients. Med J Aust 1991;154:617–622.
48. Bowden CA, Krenzelok EP. Clinical applications of commonly used contemporary antidotes. Drug Saf 1997;16:9–47.
49. Trujillo MH, Guerrero J, Fragachan C, Fernandez MA. Pharmacologic antidotes in critical care medicine: A practical guide for drug administration. Crit Care Med 1998;26:377–391.
50. Chyka P, Conner HG. Availability of antidotes in rural and urban hospitals in Tennessee. Am J Hosp Pharm 1994;51:1346–1348.
51. Woolf AD, Chrisanthus K. On-site availability of selected antidotes: Results of a survey of Massachusetts hospitals. Am J Emerg Med 1997;15:62–66.
52. Dart RC, Stark Y, Fulton B, et al. Insufficient stocking of poisoning antidotes in hospital pharmacies. JAMA 1996;276:1508–1510.
53. Antman EM, Wenger TL, Butler VP, et al. Treatment of 150 cases of life-threatening digitalis intoxication with digoxin-specific Fab antibody fragments. Circulation 1990;81:1744–1752.
54. Prescott LF. Paracetamol overdosage: Pharmacological considerations and clinical management. Drugs 1983;25:290–314.
55. Smilkstein MJ, Knapp GL, Kulig KW, Rumack BH. Efficacy of oral *N*-acetylcysteine in the treatment of acetaminophen overdose: Analysis of the national multicenter study (1976 to 1985). N Engl J Med 1988;319:1557–1562.
56. Makin AJ, Wendon J, Williams R. A 7-year experience of severe acetaminophen-induced hepatotoxicity (1987–1993). Gastroenterology 1995;109:1907–1916.
57. Schiodt FV, Rochling FA, Casey DL, Lee WM. Acetaminophen toxicity in an urban county hospital. N Engl J Med 1997;337:1112–1117.
58. Blantz RC. Acetaminophen: Acute and chronic effects on renal function. Am J Kid Dis 1996;28(suppl 1):S3–S6.
59. Smilkstein MJ. APAP-induced heart injury? Maybe yes, maybe no. Next question. Clin Toxicol 1996;34:145–147.
60. Peterson RG, Rumack BH. Age as a variable in acetaminophen overdose. Arch Intern Med 1981;141:390–393.
61. Miller RP, Roberts RJ, Fischer LJ. Acetaminophen elimination kinetics in neonates, children, and adults. Clin Pharmacol Ther 1976; 19:284–294.
62. Bray GP, Harrison PM, O'Grady JG, et al. Long-term anticonvulsant therapy worsens outcome in paracetamol-induced fulminant hepatic failure. Hum Exp Toxicol 1992;11:26–36.
63. Johnston SC, Pelletier LL Jr. Enhanced hepatotoxicity of acetaminophen in the alcoholic patient. Two case reports and a review of the literature. Medicine 1997;76:185–191.
64. Whitcomb DC, Block GD. Association of acetaminophen hepatotoxicity with fasting and ethanol use. JAMA 1994;272:1845–1850.
65. Heubi JE, Barbacci MB, Zimmerman HJ. Therapeutic misadventures with acetaminophen: Hepatotoxicity after multiple doses in children. J Pediatr 1998;132:22–27.
66. Harrison PM, Keays R, Bray GP, et al. Improved outcome of paracetamol-induced fulminant hepatic failure by late administration of acetylcysteine. Lancet 1990;335:1572–1573.
67. Dhawan A, Sorrell MF. Acetaminophen overdose: Need to consider intravenous preparation of *N*-acetylcysteine in the United States. Am J Gastroenterol 1996;91:1476.
68. Clark RF, Chen R, Williams SR, et al. The use of ondansetron in the treatment of nausea and vomiting associated with acetaminophen poisoning. Clin Toxicol 1996;34:163–167.
69. Perry HE, Shannon MW. Efficacy of oral versus intravenous *N*-acetylcysteine in acetaminophen overdose: Results of an open-label clinical trial. J Pediatr 1998;132:149–152.
70. Yip L, Dart RC, Hurlbut KM. Intravenous administration of oral *N*-acetylcysteine. Crit Care Med 1998;26:40–43.
71. Bizovi KE, Aks SE, Paloucek F, et al. Late increase in acetaminophen concentration after overdose of Tylenol Extended Relief. Ann Emerg Med 1996;28:549–551.
72. Bardin PG, van Eeden SF, Moolman JA, et al. Organophosphate and carbamate poisoning. Arch Intern Med 1994;154:1433–1441.
73. Namba T, Nolte CT, Jackrel J, Grob D. Poisoning due to organophosphate insecticides. Am J Med 1971;50:475–490.
74. Goswamy R, Chaudhuri A, Hahashur AA. Study of respiratory failure in organophosphate and carbamate poisoning. Heart Lung 1994;23:466–472.
75. Poisindex editorial staff. Organophosphates (management/treatment protocol). In: Rumack BH, Rider PK, Gelman CR, eds. Poisindex System. Englewood, CO, Micromedex vol. 96 (edition expired May 31, 1998).
76. World Health Organization. Public health impact of pesticides used in agriculture. Geneva, World Health Organization, 1990.
77. Medicic JJ, Stork CM, Howland MA, et al. Pharmacokinetics following a loading dose plus a continuous infusion of pralidoxime compared with the traditional short infusion regimen in human volunteers. Clin Toxicol 1996;34:289–295.
78. Farrar HC, Wells TG, Kearns GL. Use of continuous infusion of pralidoxime for treatment of organophosphate poisoning in children. J Pediatr 1989;116:658–661.
79. Banner W, Tong TG. Iron poisoning. Pediatr Clin North Am 1986;33:393–409.
80. Mills KC, Curry SC. Acute iron poisoning. Emerg Med Clin North Am 1994;12:397–413.
81. Tenenbein M, Israels SJ. Early coagulopathy in severe iron poisoning. J Pediatr 1988;113:695–697.

82. Melby K, Slordahl S, Gutteberg TJ, Nordbo SA. Septicaemia due to Yersinia enterocolitica after oral overdose of iron. Br Med J 1982;285:467–468.
83. Toddler deaths resulting from ingestion of iron supplements—Los Angeles, 1992–1993. MMWR 1993;42:111–113.
84. Litovitz T, Manoguerra A. Comparison of pediatric poisoning hazards: an analysis of 3.8 million exposure incidents. A report from the American Association of Poison Control Centers. Pediatrics 1992; 89:999–1006.
85. Everson GW, Oukjhane K, Young LW, et al. Effectiveness of abdominal radiographs in visualizing chewable iron supplements following overdose. Am J Emerg Med 1989;7:459–463.
86. Palatnick W, Tenenbein M. Leukocytosis, hyperglycemia, vomiting, and positive x-rays are not indicators of severity of iron overdose in adults. Am J Emerg Med 1996;4:454–455.
87. Chyka PA, Butler AY. Assessment of acute iron poisoning by laboratory and clinical observations. Am J Emerg Med 1993;11:99–103.
88. Chyka PA, Butler AY, Holley JE. Serum iron concentrations and symptoms of acute iron poisoning in children. Pharmacotherapy 1996;16:1053–1058.
89. Venturelli J, Kwee Y, Cameron G. Gastrotomy in the management of acute iron poisoning. J Pediatr 1982;100:787–789.
90. Robotham JL, Lietnams PS. Acute iron poisoning in children. Am J Dis Child 1980;134:875–879.
91. Eisen TF, Lacouture PG, Woolf A. Visual detection of ferrioxamine color changes in urine. Vet Hum Toxicol 1988;30:369–370.
92. Peck M, Rogers J, Riverbach J. Use of high doses of deferoxamine (Desferal) in an adult patient with acute iron overdosage. Clin Toxicol 1982;19:865–869.
93. Shannon M. Desferrioxamine in acute iron poisoning. Lancet 1992;339:1601. Letter.
94. Howland MA. Risks of parenteral deferoxamine for acute iron poisoning. Clin Toxicol 1996;34:491–497.
95. Tenenbein M, Kowalski S, Sienko A, et al. Pulmonary toxic effects of continuous desferrioxamine administration in acute iron poisoning. Lancet 1992;339:699–701.
96. Banner W, Czajka PA. Iron poisoning. Am J Dis Child 1981; 135:484–485. Letter.
97. Czajka PA, Konrad JD, Duffy JP. Iron poisoning: An *in vitro* comparison of bicarbonate and phosphate lavage solutions. J Pediatr 1981;98:491–494.
98. Gomez HF, McClafferty HH, Flory D, et al. Prevention of gastrointestinal iron absorption by chelation from an orally administered premixed deferoxamine/charcoal slurry. Ann Emerg Med 1997; 30:598–592.
99. Diav-Citrin O, Koren G. Oral iron chelation with deferiprone. Pediatr Clin North Am 1997;44:235–247.
100. Iron-containing supplements and drugs: Label warning statements and unit-dose packaging requirements; final rule. Federal Register. January 15, 1997;62:2217–2250.
101. Stork CM, Howland MA, Goldfrank LR. Concepts and controversies of bronchodilator overdose. Emerg Med Clin North Am 1994; 12:415–436.
102. Hendeles L, Jenkins J, Temple R. Revised FDA labeling guidelines for theophylline oral dosage forms. Pharmacotherapy 1995; 15:409–427.
103. Sessler CN. Theophylline toxicity: Clinical features of 116 consecutive cases. Am J Med 1990;88:567–576.
104. Olson KR, Benowitz NL, Woo OF, Pond SM. Theophylline overdose: Acute single ingestion versus chronic repeated over medication. Am J Emerg Med 1985;3:386–394.
105. Shannon M, Lovejoy FH Jr. Effect of acute versus chronic intoxication on clinical features of theophylline poisoning in children. J Pediatr 1992;121:125–130.
106. American Academy of Pediatrics Committee on Drugs. Precautions concerning the use of theophylline. Pediatrics 1992;89:781–783.
107. Minton NA, Henry JA. Treatment of theophylline overdose. Am J Emerg Med 1996;14:606–612.
108. Shannon M, Lovejoy FH Jr. The influence of age vs. peak serum concentration on life-threatening events after chronic theophylline intoxication. Arch Intern Med 1990;150:2045–2048.
109. Aitken ML, Martin TR. Life-threatening theophylline toxicity is not predictable by serum levels. Chest 1987;91:10–14.
110. Chyka PA, Hornfeldt CS, Howland MA, et al. Prophylaxis of seizures after theophylline overdose. Pharmacotherapy 1997; 17: 1044–1045.
111. Alldredge BK. Drug-induced seizures: Controversies in their identification and management. Pharmacotherapy 1997;17:857–860.
112. Gal P, Miller A. Oral activated charcoal to enhance theophylline elimination in an acute overdose. JAMA 1984;251:3130–3131.
113. Shannon MW. Comparative efficacy of hemodialysis and hemoperfusion in severe theophylline intoxication. Acad Emerg Med 1997; 4:674–678.
114. Pimentel L, Trommer L. Cyclic antidepressant overdose: A review. Emerg Clin North Am 1994;12:533–547.
115. Pentel PR, Keyler DE, Haddad LM. Tricyclic antidepressants and selective serotonin reuptake inhibitors. In: Haddad LM, Shannon MW, Winchester JI, eds. Clinical Management of Poisoning and Drug Overdose, 3rd ed. Philadelphia, Saunders, 1998:437–451.
116. Callaham M. Tricyclic antidepressant overdose. J Am Coll Emerg Physicians 1979;8:413–425.
117. James LP, Kearns GL. Cyclic antidepressant toxicity in children and adolescents. J Clin Pharmacol 1995;35:343–350.
118. Henry JA. Epidemiology and relative toxicity of antidepressant drugs in overdose. Drug Saf 1997;16:374–390.
119. Borys DJ, Setzer SC, Ling LJ, et al. Acute fluoxetine overdose: A report of 234 cases. Am J Emerg Med 1992;10:115–120.
120. Mills KC. Serotonin syndrome. Crit Care Clin 1997;13:763–783.
121. Corkeron MA. Serotonin syndrome—A potentially fatal complication of antidepressant therapy. Med J Aust 1995;163:481–482.
122. Spina E, Henthorn TK, Eleborg L, et al. Desmethylimipramine overdose: Nonlinear kinetics in a slow hydroxylator. Ther Drug Monit 1985;7:239–241.
123. Boehnert MT, Lovejoy FH. Value of QRS duration versus the serum drug level in predicting seizures and ventricular arrhthmias after an acute overdose of tricyclic antidepressants. N Engl J Med 1985; 313:474–479.
124. Mitchell PB. Drug interactions of clinical significance with selective serotonin reuptake inhibitors. Drug Saf 1997;17:390–406.
125. Smilkstein MJ. Reviewing cyclic antidepressant cardiotoxicity: Wheat and chaff. J Emerg Med 1990;8:645–648.
126. Newton RW. Physostigmine salicylate in the treatment of tricyclic antidepressant overdosage. JAMA 1975;231:941–943.
127. Weinbroum AA, Flaishon R, Sorkine P. A risk-benefit assessment of flumazenil in the management of benzodiazepine overdose. Drug Saf 1997;17:181–196.

8

CARDIOVASCULAR TESTING

Margaret E. McGuinness, PharmD, and Robert L. Talbert, PharmD, FCCP, BCPS

Cardiovascular disease (CVS disease) remains the leading cause of death in the United States. More than 50% of patients with ischemic heart disease (IHD) initially present with an acute myocardial infarction (AMI), and 50% of patients who suffer an AMI do not survive.[1] Although it may seem prudent to screen the population for CVS disease to prevent its development and reduce mortality, no tests available have adequate sensitivity or specificity to warrant their use in this fashion. An awareness of symptoms of cardiovascular disease and aggressive prevention and management of risk factors are more cost effective than expensive diagnostic tests.[1]

There is a plethora of tests available to evaluate CVS disease, many of which are very expensive and without comparative evaluation with "gold standard" tests. There are four principle properties of the CVS system that can be evaluated to provide diagnostic, prognostic, and therapeutic management information. These include (1) electrical conduction, (2) pump function, (3) myocardial perfusion and vasculature competence, and (4) anatomy.[2] Multiple test modalities are available to evaluate each of these functions, with many of the tests providing overlapping information, albeit with different parameters. For example, myocardial perfusion can be evaluated using the gold standard angiography, but can also be measured using echocardiography (ECHO), positron emission tomography (PET), computed axial tomography (CAT), magnetic resonance (MRI), and nuclear imaging, and it can be inferred from the exercise stress test (ET) and electrocardiogram (ECG). Although gold standards tests are recognized, in many cases it is unclear which test provides the best information.[2,3] One reason for this is lack of comparative data and the rapid development of new drugs and tests in CVS medicine. Results from ET done in the prethrombolytic era cannot be extrapolated to patients who have received thrombolytics. There is considerable debate as to how best to evaluate new tests; but for cost-effective use of tests, comparative head-to-head trials are essential. This chapter aims to outline each of the main groups of CVS testing modalities, highlight their advantages, and disadvantages and give basic interpretation of results, and where possible provide some comparative information. Tables 8–1 and 8–2 outline the use of different tests in CVS disease.[2,4]

PATIENT HISTORY AND INTERVIEW

In cardiovascular disease, the history taking, interview, and physical examination remain the most important elements of patient assessment.[4–6] Technologically advanced tests can only be used effectively in conjunction with a complete physical examination and history.

The history and patient interview provide valuable insight into the patient's condition and help in the planning and interpretation of tests performed at a later date. History taking enables the examiner to establish a relationship with the patient, develop an awareness of the patient's perception of problems and quality of life, and an assessment of the problem's acuity and severity. History taking covers elements such as chief complaint, present problems, past medical history, review of systems, and social and family history.

SIGNS AND SYMPTOMS

The primary signs and symptoms of cardiovascular disease include chest pain, dyspnea with or without orthopnea, paroxysmal nocturnal dyspnea, cyanosis, fatigue, palpitations, cough, edema, and syncope.[4–6] During the interview and physical exam, identification, elucidation of characteristics, and modulating factors for these cardiac-related signs and symptoms are obtained.

PHYSICAL EXAMINATION

The cardiovascular physical examination is divided into four categories:

1. Global examination of the patient for signs of cardiovascular disease and review of all body systems.
2. Observation and assessment of physical findings (e.g., jugular venous pressure).
3. Measurement of parameters of cardiovascular function (pulse, blood pressure).
4. Auscultation and palpation of the chest.[4–6]

Each physical finding allows the clinician to direct more specific questioning in order to define the differential diag-

TABLE 8–1. Types of Tests Used to Evaluate the Cardiovascular System

	Cardiac Function[a]			
	Myocardial Perfusion	*Pump*	*Electrical Rhythm*	*Anatomy*
Type of test	Stress tests Nuclear imaging Angiography Echocardiography	Angiography MUGA Echocardiography	ECG Electrophysiologic studies Holter monitoring	Echocardiography Angiography Intravascular ultrasound Angioscopy
Parameters evaluated	Coronary anatomy and blood flow Myocardial perfusion	Cardiac output Ejection fraction Valvular function Shunts	Rhythm Rate Conduction pathways	Chamber size Wall motion Valve function Valve structure Pericardium Coronary anatomy

[a]Not all tests for any one cardiac function are used to evaluate all parameters listed.
MUGA = multigated acquisition; ECG = electrocardiogram.

nosis more clearly (e.g., dyspnea may be a symptom of either pulmonary or cardiovascular disease). Accompanying symptoms and relief measures can help elucidate its etiology and relevance to cardiovascular disease. Chest pain, for example, may be a nonspecific indicator of cardiovascular disease and requires careful localization and characterization. Physical examination of the cardiovascular system includes observation, palpation, percussion, and auscultation of the heart and related structures.

Prior to auscultation of the heart, the precordium should be inspected and palpated for normal pulses, thrills (humming vibrations like the throat of a purring cat), and heaves (lifting of the chest wall). The apical pulse (also known as the point of maximum impulse or PMI) is helpful to estimate heart size and rotation. This is usually located in the fifth intercostal space, 7 to 9 cm from the midsternal line, and radiates in an arc of 1 to 2 cm. Heightened intensity and/or displacement laterally suggests left or right ventricle enlargement, and reduced intensity may be a sign of fluid overload or pericardial effusion. Factors such as obesity, large breasts, muscularity, and pulmonary disease can interfere with determination of the apical pulse. The carotid pulse can be examined for its intensity and, concurrently with the apical pulse, for concordance within the cardiac cycle. Decreased carotid pulsations may be due to reduced stroke volume or atherosclerotic narrowing of the carotid artery. Other characteristics observed are thrills, which may accompany murmurs (e.g., aortic stenosis); and heaves, which may indicate enlargement of one of the heart chambers or an abnormal vessel such as an aneurysm.

HEART SOUNDS

Auscultation with a stethoscope is used to characterize the location, timing, duration, pitch, and intensity of the normal heart sounds, S_1 (first heart sound) and S_2 (second heart sound), and to determine the presence or absence of other sounds, such as S_3 (third heart sound) and S_4 (fourth heart

TABLE 8–2. Types of Tests for Various Cardiac Disorders or Features

Feature/Disorder	CXR	Echo	Angiography	Nuclear Scan	CT	MRI	ET	ECG	PET
Ischemic	—	+++	++++	+++	++/+++[a]	++	++	++	+++
Valvular	+	++++	+++	+	+++	+++	++	+	+
Congential	++	++++	+++	+	+++	++++	+	+	+
Anatomy	+	+++	++	+	+++	++++	—	+	+
Cardiomyopathy	+	++++	+++	++	+++	+++	—	—	++
Pericardial	+	++++	++	—	++++	++++	—	±	—
Endocarditis	—	++++[b]	+	—	++	+++	—	±	—
Masses	—	++++	+	—	+++	+++	—	—	+
Metabolism	—	—	—	+	—	—	—	—	++++
Graft patency	—	±	+++	++	+	++	++	+	+++
CA anatomy	—	—	++++	++	+	++	++	+	+
Ventricular function	—	++++	+++	++	+++	+++	+	—	++

CXR = chest x-ray; Echo = echocardiography; CT = computed tomography; MRI = magnetic resonance imaging; ET = exercise testing; ECG = electrocardiogram; PET = positron emission tomography; CA = coronary artery.
[a]Ultrafast or cine-CT may be very useful in detecting ischemia based on calcium deposition.
[b]Transesophageal echocardiography is superior to transthoracic echocardiography.

sound) and murmurs.[4–6] The diaphragm of the stethoscope is better to identify and characterize high-pitched sounds such as S_1 and S_2, murmurs of aortic and mitral regurgitation, and pericardial friction rubs. The bell is preferred for low-pitched sounds such as S_3 and S_4. Auscultation is conducted in a systematic manner to ensure that all sites where normal and abnormal sounds are typically heard are reviewed (Fig. 8–1). Initially the patient is examined lying partially on the left side to accentuate left-sided S_3 and S_4 and mitral murmurs, with the bell on the PMI. To identify S_1 and S_2, the patient can be examined lying or sitting. The other areas that are auscultated are the apex or base of the heart (mitral sounds), lower left sternal border (tricuspid sounds), second left interspace (pulmonic sounds), and second right interspace (aortic sounds). At each of these locations, S_1 and S_2 should be heard.

Heart sounds are characterized by pitch, intensity, duration, and timing within the cardiac cycle. S_1 and S_2 are created by the closing of the mitral and tricuspid valves and the pulmonic and aortic valves, respectively. The sound of S_1 is thought to be generated by closure of the valvular leaflet. The sounds may be "spilt" if the two valves do not close synchronously. S_1 is heard as a click at the end of diastole and is usually synchronous with the apical pulse. The intensity of S_1 can be increased if systole begins prior to the mitral valve closing, which may occur in high output states (exercise, tachycardia, anemia, or hyperthyroidism) and mitral valve stenosis. S_1 intensity is decreased in first-degree heart block, mitral regurgitation, states of reduced myocardial contractility (such as congestive heart failure or coronary artery disease), obesity (difficult to hear), and systemic or pulmonary hypertension. S_2 is heard at the end of systole and is best heard at the tricuspid and mitral areas. Most of the sound arises from aortic valve closure. Splitting of S_2 creates a pulmonic (P_2) and aortic (A_2) sound. Physiologic splitting of S_1 or S_2 is accentuated by inspiration and may

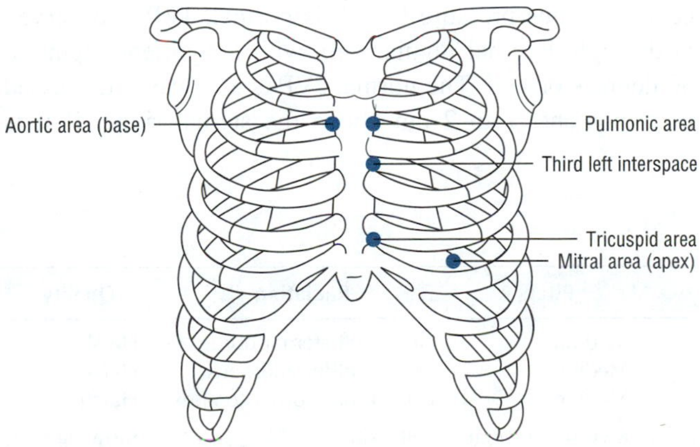

FIGURE 8–1. Schematic illustration of topographic areas on the precordium for cardiac auscultation. Auscultatory areas do not correspond to anatomic locations of the valves but to the sites at which particular valves are heard best. *(Redrawn from Kinney MR, Packa DR, eds. Andreoli's Comprehensive Cardiac Care, 8th ed. St. Louis: Mosby-Year Book, 1996, with permission.)*

disappear with expiration. S_2 is frequently heard as a split sound and is most predominant at the height of inspiration. Although S_1 may also be split, this is often difficult to hear.

Pathologic splitting of S_2 during expiration is described as wide splitting, fixed splitting, and paradoxical splitting and may be indicative of both stenosis and regurgitation, indicating that the valves did not close completely or synchronously with each cardiac cycle. Increased intensity of P_2 is seen in pulmonary hypertension, dilated pulmonary arteries, and atrial septal defect. Decreased or absent P_2 may be seen in aging and pulmonic stenosis. In the presence of right heart overload (pulmonary edema), right bundle branch block, pulmonic stenosis, and atrial septal defects, the S_2 sound may be split as closure of the pulmonic valve is delayed. Fixed splitting of S_2 may not be affected by respiration, and this is associated with large atrial–septal defects and right ventricular failure. The characteristics of the heart sounds are important because they have diagnostic implications; for example, an S_1 heard as a opening snap is characteristic of mitral stenosis. The loud snap heard in mitral stenosis indicates the valve is pliable but does not close as rapidly as a normal valve. A soft or absent S_1 may also be heard in mitral valve stenosis if the valve is so calcified that it is unable to snap shut, or in mitral regurgitation due to the backflow of blood through the valve.

Extra heart sounds in systole include early systolic ejection sounds and clicks and midsystolic clicks. Early ejection sounds such as aortic or pulmonic ejection sounds are often associated with valvular disease. Midsystolic to late systolic clicks are usually due to mitral valve prolapse (MVP). MVP is best heard at or medial to the apex, but may also be heard at the left lower sternal border.

The S_3 heart sound, or ventricular gallop, is an abnormal, low-pitched sound, usually heard at the apex of the heart. It is thought to be due to rapid filling and stretching of the left ventricle when the left ventricle is somewhat noncompliant. This heart sound is characteristic of volume overloading such as in congestive heart failure (especially left-sided heart failure), tricuspid or mitral valve insufficiency, and atrial and/or ventricular septal defects. A physiologic S_3 is commonly heard in children and may persist into young adulthood. Localization of the S_3 is helpful for determining heart rotation within the chest cavity.

The S_4 diastolic sound is a dull, low-pitched postsystolic atrial gallop (rapid blood flow), usually due to reduced ventricular compliance. It is best heard at the apex in the left lateral position. Like the S_3, it occurs with reduced ventricular compliance, and is present in conditions such as aortic stenosis, hypertension, hypertrophic cardiomyopathies, and coronary artery disease. It is less specific for congestive heart failure than S_3. Respiratory pattern, various maneuvers such as handgrip or the valsalva maneuver, sitting versus standing, and pharmacologic agents (e.g., amyl nitrate) may also be used in the evaluation of heart sounds to accentuate or diminish the intensity of these sounds.

Auscultation is an acquired art and requires considerable practice to become competent.

HEART MURMURS

Murmurs are auditory vibrations heard on auscultation, and occur because of turbulent blood flow within the heart chambers or through the valves.[5,6] They are classified by timing and duration within the cardiac cycle (systolic, diastolic, and continuous), location, intensity, shape (configuration or pattern), pitch (frequency), quality, and radiation (Table 8–3). Some murmurs are considered innocent or physiologic and result from rapid, turbulent flow of blood into the left ventricle during atrial systole and through the aorta during ventricular systole. Fever, anxiety, anemia, hyperthyroidism, and pregnancy exacerbate physiologic murmurs, and these murmurs need to be distinguished from those suggestive of valvular abnormalities. As with heart sounds, accurate determination of murmurs requires practice. The intensity or loudness or a murmur is graded using a scale of grade I to VI. Grade I is so faint that it is heard only with special effort. Grade VI may be heard with the stethoscope just off the chest wall. Determinants of the grade include the amount of blood ejected across a valve, severity of the lesion, and chest anatomy.

Systolic murmurs begin with or after S_1 and end at or before S_2 depending on the origin of the murmur. They are classified based on time of onset and termination within systole: midsystolic, holosystolic (pansystolic), early, or late. Pathologic midsystolic murmurs are associated with pulmonic stenosis, aortic stenosis, and hypertrophic cardiomyopathy. Midsystolic murmurs include obstruction to ventricular outflow, dilatation of the aortic root or pulmonary trunk, an increased flow in the great arteries, anatomic changes in the semilunar valves, and some forms of regurgitation. Holosystolic murmurs occur when blood flows from a chamber of higher pressure to one of lower pressure, such as with mitral or tricuspid regurgitation, and ventricular septal defects. Early systolic murmurs are decrescendo and may be associated with ventricular septal defects, mitral regurgitation, or tricuspid regurgitation. A late systolic murmur preceded by one or more midsystolic to late systolic clicks is the hallmark of MVP. Atherosclerotic obstruction of the carotid, subclavicular, or iliofemoral arteries can give rise to a crescendo–decrescendo extracardiac systolic arterial murmur.

Early diastolic murmurs are commonly heard with aortic regurgitation. This murmur begins with A_2, and is generally decrescendo, reflecting the progressive decline in volume and rate of regurgitant flow during diastole. Aortic regurgitation is best heard by having the patient lean forward while holding his or her breath and listening with the diaphragm at the midleft sternal border. Handgrip intensifies the murmur. Pulmonary hypertension (Graham Steell's murmur) may also cause an early diastolic murmur. Middiastolic murmurs occur across the atrioventricular valves during rapid filling and are consistent with pure mitral stenosis or mitral stenosis along with a ventricular septal defect or tricuspid regurgitation with an atrial septal defect. The Austin Flint murmur may be middiastolic or presystolic, and results from antegrade flow across the mitral valve that is closing rapidly because of simultaneous left ventricular filling from aortic regurgitation. Continuous murmurs begin in systole and continue without interruption into all or part of diastole. Such murmurs are mainly due to aortopulmonary connections (e.g., patent ductus arteriosus), arteriovenous connections (e.g., arteriovenous fistula, coronary artery fistula), and disturbances of flow patterns in arteries or veins.

Anatomic correlation of murmurs may require cardiac catheterization or echocardiography, where direct visualization of the blood flow abnormality and calculation of flow and chamber pressures can be obtained. PET and MRI scanning are also possible options to evaluate flow patterns and gradients of murmurs across heart valves.

JUGULAR VENOUS PRESSURE

The jugular venous pressure (JVP) is used as a measure of right atrial pressure.[5,6] The JVP is measured in centimeters from the sternal angle and is best visualized with the patient's head rotated to the left. For persons in whom the central venous pressure (CVP) is normal, JVP is observed in the right internal jugular vein with the patient supine at 30 degrees or less. The normal JVP is a V wave (discussed in a moment) 1 to 2 cm above the sternal ridge. If it is

TABLE 8–3. Characteristics of Heart Sounds

Type of Murmur	Examples	Location	Pitch	Radiation	Quality
Midsystolic	Aortic stenosis	2nd RICS	Medium	Neck, left sternal border	Harsh
	Pulmonic stenosis	2nd and 3rd LICS	Medium	Left shoulder and neck	Harsh
	Hypertrophic cardiomyopathy	3rd and 4th LICS	Medium	Left sternal border to apex	Harsh
Pansystolic	Mitral regurgitation	Apex	Medium to high	Left axilla	Blowing
	Tricuspid regurgitation	Lower left sternal border	Medium	Right sterum, xiphoid	Blowing
	Ventricular septal defect	3rd, 4th, and 5th LICS	High		Often harsh
Diastolic	Aortic regurgitation	2nd to 4th LICS	High	Apex	Blowing
	Mitral stensis	Apex	Low	Little or none	

RICS = right intercostal space; LICS = left intercostal space.

greater than halfway to the jaw angle, there is elevated CVP. When reporting a JVP, both the measure and the patient position must be reported. The JVP can be reported as actual centimeters above the manubrium or this value plus 5 to 7 cm to indicate the rise of the JVP above the right ventricle. In the presence of an elevated CVP, the JVP is measured at 60 to 90 degrees. In patients with poor myocardial function, the accuracy of the JVP as a measure of CVP is reduced, and is best measured directly by means of a Swan–Ganz catheter. The JVP is described for its quality and character, effects of respiration, and patient position-induced changes. Both the degree of elevation of the JVP and its wave flow in conjunction with the heart beat are noted. The first wave, or *A wave,* represents atrial contraction and occurs just prior to S_1, giving rise to an increased pressure. It is seen as an undulating pulsation in the internal jugular vein. The second and much larger wave, the *V wave,* represents the increased venous pressure that occurs during venous filling. To interpret the JVP accurately, the carotid pulse is concurrently palpated. The A wave occurs just before the pulse and the V wave just after.

PERIPHERAL CIRCULATION AND ARTERIAL PULSES

All arterial pulses are evaluated and characterized bilaterally by observation, palpation, and auscultation for presence, character, pattern, and rhythm.[4–6] Bruits and thrills are detected using the heel of the hand to sense the vibrations. Various arterial pulse patterns are described such as pulsus alterans (variation in amplitude beat to beat), bisferans pulse (increased arterial pulse with a double systolic peak), bigeminal pulse (reduced amplitude associated with premature ventricular beats), and paradoxical pulse (decrease in amplitude with inspiration). Although each may be associated with certain disorders (e.g., bigeminal pulse in premature ventricular contractions), none is sensitive or specific enough to be diagnostic. The status of the patient's overall peripheral circulation is recorded, especially the presence and degree of edema, or skin changes suggestive of venous or arterial insufficiency. Color, condition, and integrity of the skin are also recorded, including signs of thrombophlebitis, tenderness, or swelling. Capillary refill (normal < 2 seconds) is assessed by depressing the nail bed until it blanches, then releasing pressure and watching for the return of color indicating blood flow.

HEART RATE

The rate and rhythm of heart rate are both reported.[5,6] In healthy individuals, the heart rate is usually assessed by counting the radial pulse for 15 seconds and multiplying by four. In patients with irregular rhythms, the pulse should be taken over an extended period, approximately 1 to 2 minutes, to try to determine the patient's average pulse and rhythm because a 10- to 15-second measure may result in inaccurate estimates of the pulse rate.

Arterial pulses may be used to determine heart rate. The arterial pulse is usually taken at the radius, but carotid or other arterial pulses may be used. These are an accurate measure of the ventricular rate in the healthy person with good ventricular function. In patients with a rapid ventricular rate—because of supraventricular tachyarrhythmias such as atrial flutter or fibrillation or rapid ventricular rates (e.g., ventricular tachycardia or premature ventricular beats)—extremity pulses (e.g., radial pulse) may be considerably slower than the true ventricular rate. A more accurate ventricular rate is determined by listening to the ventricles with the stethoscope (usually at the apex) or counting from an electrocardiogram. In patients with atrial fibrillation and a fast ventricular rate, a pulse deficit (measure of the difference in true ventricular rate and peripheral pulse rate) may exist. This may be as much as 10 to 20 beats/min. So the location of the recorded pulse (radial or apical) should be recorded. The pulse deficit will be reduced as the ventricular rate is controlled with drug therapy or normal sinus rhythm is restored.

TESTING MODALITIES

CHEST X-RAY

The chest x-ray (CXR) provides supplemental information to the physical examination and is usually the first diagnostic test in a cardiac workup.[4–6] It does not provide details of internal cardiac structures but gives global information about position and size of the heart and chambers and surrounding anatomy. The standard CXRs for evaluation of lungs and heart are a standing posterior–anterior (PA) and lateral view taken at maximal inspiration. Portable CXRs are usually less satisfactory due to penetration difficulties, patient rotation, and poor inspiratory effort.

Initial assessment of the CXR evaluates the quality of film for patient rotation, inspiratory effort, and penetration. Rotation is assessed by evaluating symmetry of the clavicles and central placement of the carina. Inspiratory effect is considered adequate if the diaphragms are pulled below the ninth rib. Lack of inspiratory effort and obesity lead to a poor-quality CXR. These make it more difficult to assess presence of pleural effusions and fluid in the costophrenic angles. Comparison with previous or baseline films should be made to determine both quality of film and comparison of structures.

The PA CXR outlines the superior vena cava, right atrium on the right side and on the left, aortic knob, main pulmonary artery, left atrial appendage (especially if enlarged), and left ventricle. In the lateral view, the CXR visualizes the right ventricle, inferior vena cava, and left ventricle. These structures are visualized as shadows of differing density rather than discrete structures (Fig. 8–2).

The CXR is approached from two perspectives: (1) observation and (2) clinical correlation. Observation notes gross anatomic features such as size and placement of the cardiac silhouette, definition of cardiac border, chamber enlargement, pulmonary vasculature, air–fluid levels, and

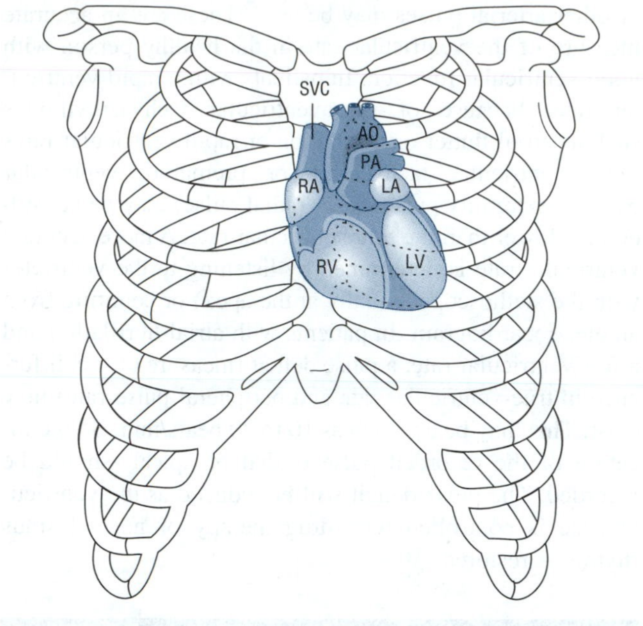

FIGURE 8–2. Schematic illustration of the parts of the heart. (AO = aorta; SVC = superior vena cava; RA = right atrium; PA = pulmonary artery; LA = left atrium; RV = right ventricle; LV = left ventricle.) *(Redrawn from Kinney MR, Packa DR, eds. Andreoli's Comprehensive Cardiac Care, 8th ed. St. Louis: Mosby-Year Book, 1996, with permission.)*

diaphragm. Cardiac enlargement is determined by the cardiothoracic (CT) ratio, which is the maximal transverse diameter of the heart divided by the maximal transverse diameter of the thorax of a PA view. Normal averages 0.45, but it may be up to 0.55 in subjects with large stroke volumes (e.g., highly trained athletes). Heart conditions such as ischemic heart disease do not alter cardiac size unless accompanied by other disorders such as congestive heart failure or hypertension. Individual chamber enlargement can be seen on the CXR. Right ventricle enlargement is best seen on the lateral film, where the heart appears to occupy the retrosternal space. Left atrial enlargement is suspected if there is elevation of the left bronchus or an increase in the atrial appendage bulge. Left ventricular enlargement is the most common feature identified on CXR, and is seen as an elongation and downward displacement of the apex of the heart. Sometimes a characteristic boot or water bottle outline is seen.

The pulmonary vessels are examined for plumpness and definition of vessel walls. Decreased pulmonary flow (e.g., tetralogy of Fallot) causes central and peripheral vessels to be decreased in size. Increased pulmonary flow is associated with high output states such as hyperthyroidism and atrial septal defects. This may lead to enlargement and tortuosity of the central and peripheral vessels. Pulmonary arterial hypertension (increased pulmonary resistance) is identified by enlargement of the central vessels and diminished peripheral vessels. Pulmonary venous hypertension is usually due to mitral stenosis or left ventricular failure. This is characterized by larger than normal vessels in the upper lung zones due to recruitment of upper vessels from blood diverted from the lower constricted vessels (cephalization of flow).

Heart failure causes Kerley's B lines (edema of interlobular septa), which appear as thin horizontal reticular lines in the costophrenic angles. At higher pressures, alveolar edema and pleural effusions appear in the pleural space or as blunting of the costophrenic angles. Pericardial effusions may also appear as a large heart, but because it usually occurs rapidly there is no evidence of pulmonary venous congestion.

ELECTROCARDIOGRAM

Measurement of electrical activity in the heart was introduced about 75 years ago by Willem Einthoven. The electrocardiogram reflects the electrical activity of the heart and is the most frequently used cardiovascular test.[7–10] The ECG also provides information about the anatomy, blood flow, and hemodynamics of the cardiovascular system. It is used as a diagnostic and prognostic tool and to characterize rhythms and conduction abnormalities.[3,8]

Few ECG recordings are highly specific or sensitive to a disease state. Sensitivity and specificity of ECG changes primarily depend on the clinical setting, recording technique, and skill of interpreters. Sensitivity and specificity of findings are increased by interpretation in conjunction with patient information such as age, gender, medical history, and medications. This is particularly important in patients with significant cardiac disease, or on medications that alter the ECG. The ECG is sensitive to detect rhythm abnormalities, but it does not record the actual activity of the conduction tissue.

Prior and/or serial ECGs significantly increase the sensitivity and specificity of findings. These should be obtained for comparison prior to identifying new findings on a current ECG as diagnostic.[7–9] As an example, initial ECGs are normal in about 10%, and abnormal but nondiagnostic in 40%, of patients having an acute myocardial infarction. Over time, more than 80% of patients will develop changes highly suggestive or diagnostic of myocardial ischemia.[10] Computer interpretation of the ECG provides a standardized reading, and records and calculates basic rhythm patterns, heart rate, and intervals but does not interpret arrhythmias. Independent review of the ECG is highly recommended for accurate translation of findings.[8]

In epidemiologic studies, the ECG is used to assess physical fitness, document the prevalence of ischemic heart disease, and identify subclinical heart disease. The sensitivity and specificity of ECG changes are highly dependent on the pretest probability of heart disease. As the pretest probability of heart disease increases, the sensitivity and specificity of ECG findings increases. As an example, in the elderly where there is a high incidence of heart disease, ECG abnormalities frequently correlate with the presence of disease. The use and value of the ECG as a screening tool is controversial. It is only used where the diagnosis of heart disease would preclude active employment, such as in airline pilots. The ECG is frequently used in conjunction with other diagnostic tests, to provide additional data, to monitor the patient, and to identify if abnormalities detected during tests correlate with ECG changes.[7,8,10] "Gating," or linkage of and simultaneous recording of an ECG and other diagnostic tests, such as echocardiography and computed tomography (CT), allow for correlation of images with the cardiac cycle. Gating is either prospective, where a certain portion of the cardiac cycle is predetermined as the time during which the images are obtained, or retrospective, where the ECG and image are recorded simultaneously but independently and later matched for concurrent events. This allows multiple cardiac cycles to be overlayed, thus increasing the sensitivity to detect abnormalities.

Electrocardiography is based on the measurement of change in summated, three-dimensional electrical vectors or forces, which result from depolarization and repolarization of cells in the conduction system and heart muscle. The standard external 12-lead ECG uses two sets of leads: limb and chest (Fig. 8–3) The 6 limb leads look at the heart in a single frontal plane. Limb lead nomenclature is as follows: lead I, right arm/left arm; lead II, right arm/left leg; lead III, left arm/left leg. Altering resistances create the augmented limb leads, which are called aVR, aVL, and aVF. Unipolar chest leads are positioned across the chest, and labeled V_1 to V_6. V_1 is positioned slightly to the right of the midline and V_6 is positioned in the left midaxillary line (Fig. 8–4) Leads aVR and V_1 are considered right-sided leads, so appear inverted; and leads aVL, I, II, and $V_{5,6}$ are left-sided leads, so appear upright on the ECG. Leads II, III, and aVF are inferior leads. Leads V_1 to V_4 are anterior wall leads. Single-lead ECGs or ECG monitors frequently use lead II.

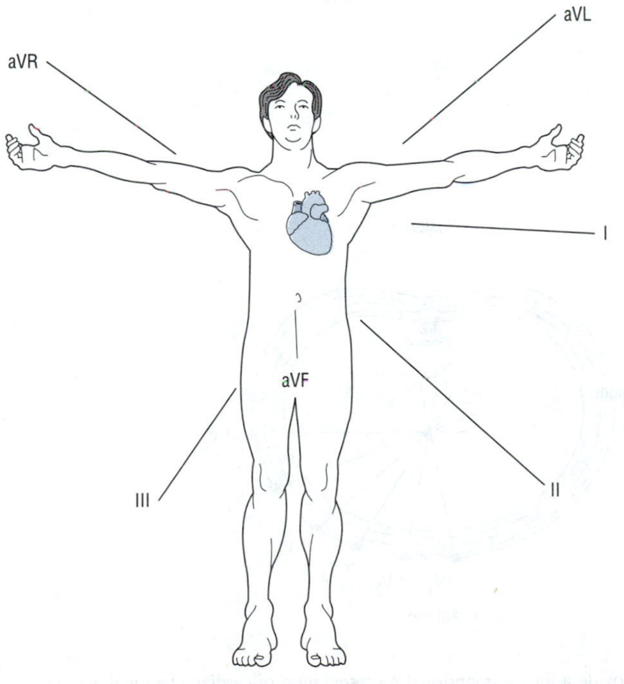

FIGURE 8–3. The torso with the 6 limb leads in a single frontal plane.

Recording of the ECG has several standard features. The paper is divided into squares of 1 mm; each 10 mm (10 small boxes) is equivalent to 1 mV. Paper speed is 25 mm/s. Each small box on the tracing paper equals 0.04 seconds (40 ms), and each big box is 0.2 seconds. If there is one QRS complex per 6 big boxes (6×0.20 seconds), the patient has a heart rate of 50 beats/min, while one QRS per big box indicates a heart rate of 300 beats/min.

The ECG pattern is named alphabetically and is read from left to right, beginning with the P wave. Electrical activation (depolarization) of the right and then left atria due to discharge from the sinoatrial (SA) nodes causes an upward or positive deflection in lead II called the P wave. The normal duration of the P wave is up to 0.12 seconds, and has an amplitude of 0.25 mV (i.e., 2.5 small boxes). The PR segment is created by passage of the impulse through the atrioventricular (AV) node and the bundle of His and its branches, and has a duration of 0.12 to 0.21 seconds. The QRS complex primarily traces the electrical depolarization of the ventricles. Initially there is a negative deflection, the Q wave; followed by a positive deflection, the R wave; and finally a negative deflection, the S wave. Q-wave duration is normally 0.4 seconds or less, and the amplitude is 25% or less of the overall height of the QRS complex. Normal duration of the QRS complex is 0.12 seconds. The QRS complex is positive in left-sided leads and negative in right-sided leads, because the left ventricle is much thicker than the right, and the forces going left during depolarization dominate.

Following the QRS is a plateau phase called the ST segment, which extends from the end of the QRS complex (called the J point) to the beginning of the T wave. The ST segment is evaluated for its position relevant to the baseline, configuration, and leads where changes occur. The ST segment is normally on or slightly above the baseline. Configuration changes, convexity upward or downward, identify the presence of myocardial ischemia. Lead localization of ST changes indicates the area of ischemia. The QT interval is measured from the start of the QRS complex to the end of the T wave. This varies with heart rate and is corrected (QTc) for heart rates greater than 60 beats/min. The corrected QT is less than 0.42 seconds in men and 0.43 seconds in women. Repolarization of the ventricle leads to the T wave. The T wave usually goes in the same direction as the QRS complex. The normal axis of the ECG is –30 degrees (above the horizontal) to +110 degrees (away from the horizontal) (Fig. 8–5).

The ECG is evaluated in a systematic manner, to avoid omission of important characteristics. All ECGs are interpreted for the following elements: rate, general rhythm, intervals, voltage, axis, waveforms, abnormal features (e.g., Q waves), and technical aspects such as adequacy of lead placement and calibration.[8] The number of

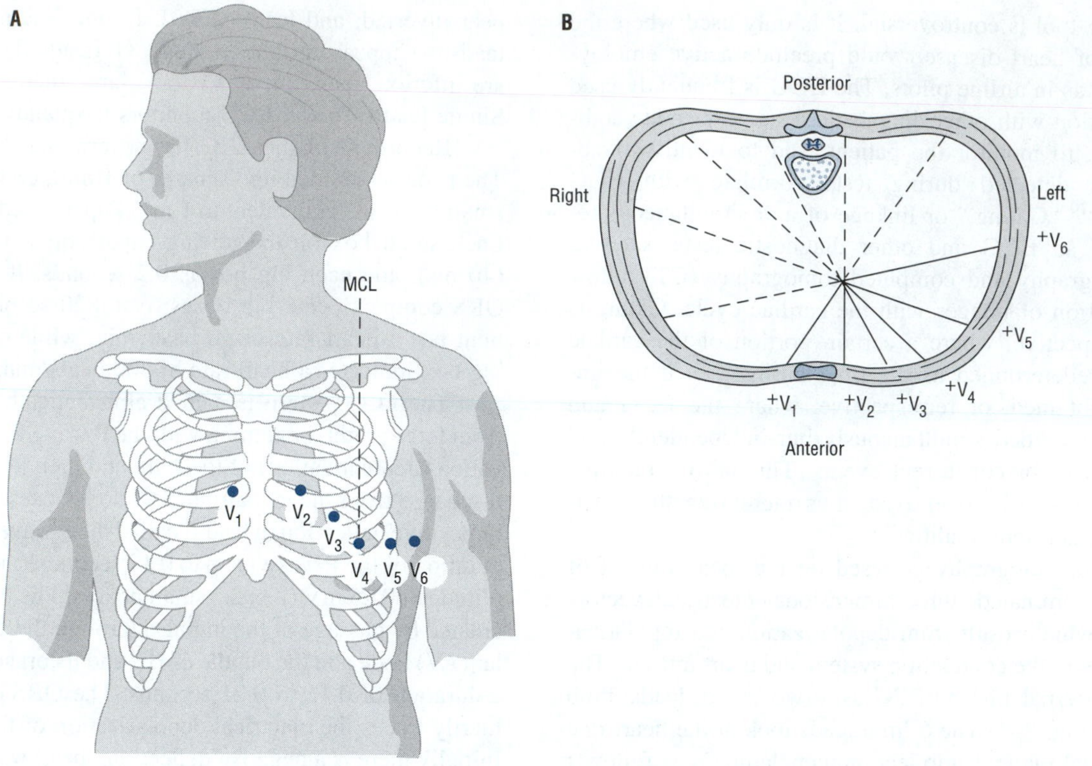

FIGURE 8–4. A. Electrode positions of the precordial leads (V_1 = fourth intercostal space at the right sternal border; V_2 = fourth intercostal space at the left sternal border; V_3 = halfway between V_2 and V_4; V_4 = fifth intercostal space at the midclavicular line; V_5 = anterior axillary line directly lateral to V_4; V_6 = anterior axillary space directly lateral to V_5.) **B.** The precordial reference figure. Leads V_1 and V_2 are called right-sided precordial leads; leads V_3 and V_4, midprecordial leads; and leads V_5 and V_6, left-sided precordial leads. *(Redrawn from Kinney MR, Packa DR, eds. Andreoli's Comprehensive Cardiac Care, 8th ed. St. Louis: Mosby-Year Book, 1996, with permission.)*

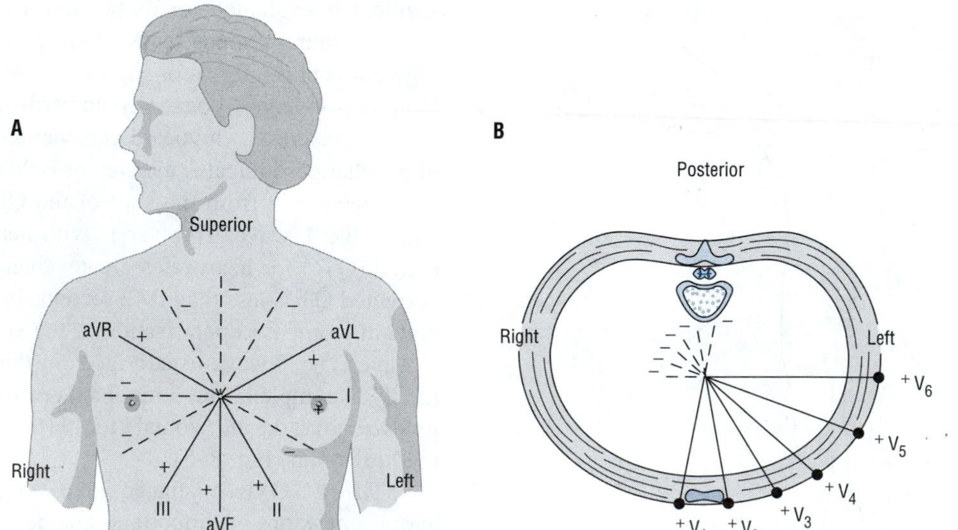

FIGURE 8–5. The 6 frontal plane **(A)** and the 6 horizontal plane **(B)** leads provide a three-dimensional representation of cardiac electrical activity. *(Redrawn from Ref. 7, with permission.)*

P waves and QRS complexes (RR interval) are also used to determine rate. QRS complexes may be more useful if heart block exists. The rhythm from the ECG is identified by the following features:

1. The rate of the QRS (> 100/min is tachycardia, and < 60/min is bradycardia).
2. The regularity of the QRS; the presence or absence of the QRS complex with each P wave helps identify if the rhythm is atrial or ventricular in origin, and if each atrial beat (P wave) is being conducted to the ventricles. The regularity of the QRS identifies conditions such as atrial fibrillation and extra beats.
3. Configuration of the QRS—wide or narrow, indicating if it is generated from electrical activity that arose in the atria or ventricles.

Always reported are the RR, PR, QRS, and QT intervals; and the duration, magnitude, and configuration of the P waves, QRS complexes, ST segments, T waves, and U waves. Abnormalities of the ECG include abnormal intervals, configuration of the wave forms, various forms of heart block, changes due to ischemia and infarction, atrial and ventricular enlargement and hypertrophy, atrial and ventricular rhythm disorders, pericarditis, metabolic abnormalities, drug-induced changes, and pacemaker-related changes. ECG patterns found on consecutive leads can help identify where a particular conduction defect or impulse generation is occurring, or anatomic problem is located. For example, ST elevation in V_2 to V_6 is indicative of anterior wall myocardial infarction from occlusion of the left anterior descending coronary artery. Single lead abnormalities most frequently are attributed to poor lead placement, position of the patient, or recording artifacts.

Examples of some common findings will be briefly discussed.[7,8] Short PR intervals are associated with the Wolff–Parkinson–White and the Lown–Ganong–Levine syndromes, and reflect the presence of accessory pathways. Long PR intervals are measures of heart block. The presence of a Q wave is a marker for loss of electrically functioning myocardium, and suggests a prior myocardial infarction. It may also be present in congenital heart disorders, hypertrophic cardiomyopathy, left ventricular hypertrophy, conduction defects such as Wolff–Parkinson–White syndrome, and intraventricular conduction defects. U waves are relatively nonspecific, the most common cause being hypertension. Bundle branch blocks are frequent findings and indicate conduction defects in one of the bundles of His. Their presence confounds the interpretation of important ECG findings such as ischemia. Right bundle branch block is associated with an R wave and the following abnormalities: QRS complex greater than or equal to 12 milliseconds; delayed right ventricular forces resulting in terminal R waves in the right-sided leads and S wave in the left-sided lead; and right-sided ST segment depression and T-wave inversion. Left bundle branch block is characterized by the following: QRS complex greater than or equal to 12 milliseconds; delayed left ventricular activation; loss of the normal "septal Q wave" in the left-sided leads; and left-sided ST depression and T-wave inversion. Intraventricular conduction delay usually causes a wide QRS complex and generally there are ST–T wave abnormalities.

Myocardial ischemia, ranging from injury to necrosis, results in T-wave changes, ST abnormalities, and changes in the QRS complex. Myocardial infarction results in a typical pattern of ECG changes, which begins with tall peaked T waves persisting up to several hours, followed by ST segment elevation with a coved (convexity upward) configuration, and inverted T waves. Development of a new Q wave has a high specificity but low sensitivity for acute myocardial ischemia. Q waves, which are 4 milliseconds or longer in duration and 25% or greater of the overall QRS height, are considered diagnostic, and occur within minutes to hours of occlusion. Although Q waves usually evolve within hours of infarction, they may not become evident for several days. The finding of new and significant Q waves on an ECG is indicative of a previous infarction. Q waves persist indefinitely in 80% to 90% of myocardial infarctions. The location of Q waves identifies the region of myocardium affected and the coronary artery blocked (e.g., inferior infarction will result in Q waves in II, III, and aVF, associated with blockage in the right coronary artery). Non-Q-wave (subendocardial) myocardial infarction implies the Q wave does not meet the diagnostic criteria for Q-wave infarction. ST segment depression may be present.

ST segment changes are very common, and should always be compared to a previous ECG. ST elevation may be seen in persons with no known coronary disease but is usually indicative of hyperacute ischemia. ST depression is never considered a normal finding. ST segment scooping (convexity downward) may be normal but coving (convexity upward) is abnormal. Depression of the ST segment that does not quickly return to normal and changes in multiple leads suggest clinically significant heart disease. Diffuse ST segment elevation in all leads except V_1 and aVR suggests the diagnosis of pericarditis. Exertion in normal individuals may cause J-point depression with rapid rise of the ST segment, and this may be confused with ST depression due to the configuration. Poor R-wave progression (usually increase in size moving from V_1 to V_6) suggests anterior myocardial infarction, but smaller R waves can also occur in diseases such as chronic obstructive pulmonary disease. T-wave changes are the most frequent and most sensitive abnormality on the ECG but are also the least specific and are frequently found in persons with no heart disease.

Left atrial enlargement is characterized by a P wave that is 12 mV in lead II or the negative component of the biphasic P is 4 mV in duration and 0.1 mV in depth in lead V_1. In right atrial enlargement, the P wave in lead II can exceed 0.25 mV and usually has a vertical axis. Ventricular hypertrophy results in increased deflection of the

QRS because of the increased muscle mass. Left ventricular hypertrophy (LVH) is diagnosed from the ECG using several different sets of criteria; none is considered highly sensitive or specific. LVH is often indicative of hypertension and resultant ventricular enlargement and strain. Voltage criteria indicating LVH commonly used are summation of the S wave in V_1 and the R wave in V_5, or the S wave in V_2 and the R wave in V_6, which exceeds 3.5 mV (35 small boxes); or the R wave in lead aVL exceeds 1.1 mV (11 small boxes). Right ventricular hypertrophy is characterized by an R wave in V_1 that is equal to or greater than the S wave in that lead. In persons who are obese, increased voltage may not be apparent, making voltage criteria a less useful tool to identify hypertrophy. LVH may also be assessed using echocardiography.

Electrolyte abnormalities have characteristic signs on the ECG and can be used as monitoring parameters. Hypokalemia may increase ventricular ectopy and causes ST segment depression, T-wave flattening, and appearance of a U wave (usually when serum potassium is less than 3.0 mEq/L). Hyperkalemia results in very characteristic changes in the ECG. Potassium concentrations above 6.0 mEq/L produce tall, peaked T waves. As the concentration rises further, intraventricular conduction becomes blocked, with widening of the QRS complex, and ultimately a sine wave develops. Hypercalcemia causes a short QT interval and, occasionally, ST segment depression, sinus arrest, and AV conduction blocks. Hypocalcemia causes a long QT interval and some broadening of the T wave.

A number of drugs cause characteristic changes in the ECG that may mask interpretation of other findings. A list of commonly used drugs that may alter the ECG is given in Table 8–4.[8] Pericardial effusion, obesity, and large breasts limit the amount of voltage, which is measured on the skin surface, and reduce the QRS voltage. In the presence of large pericardial effusions, rapid changes in the positive to negative deflection of the QRS or electrical alterans may occur because the heart is swinging on a beat-to-beat basis.

Signal-averaged ECG (SAEKG) may be used to help elucidate the presence of low-amplitude bioelectric potentials. Derangements of ventricular activation and late potentials can be detected in the ECG after the QRS and ST segments, and are thought to be associated with increased risk of ventricular arrhythmias. Traditional ECGs are unable to detect these potentials as they are "lost" in the noise of the ECG recording. SAECG improves the signal to noise ratio, enabling the low-amplitude potentials to be interpreted. SAEKG can be used to identify patients at risk for developing sustained ventricular tachycardia postmyocardial infarction. Patients with IHD and unexplained syncope who are at risk for SVT may also be candidates for SAEKG. Other potential uses of SAEKG include patients with nonischemic cardiomyopathy with sustained ventricular tachycardia, detection of acute rejection of heart transplant, and assessing proarrhythmia potential of antiarrhythmic drug therapy.[11]

TABLE 8–4. Drugs That May Affect the Electrocardiogram

Digoxin	Doxorubicin
Antiarrhythmics—Classes I–IV	Pentamidine
Tricyclic antidepressants	Lithium
H_1 antagonists (e.g., astemizole)	Catecholamines (e.g., dopamine, albuterol)
Methylxanthines	Diuretics (electrolyte abnormalities)

AMBULATORY ELECTROCARDIOGRAPHIC (HOLTER) MONITORING

Ambulatory electrocardiographic monitoring (AEM), commonly referred to as Holter monitoring after its inventor, is an aid to detect, document, characterize, and evaluate arrhythmias and other ECG abnormalities.[12–18] The main goals of AEM are to document and characterize occurrences of random and spontaneous ECG abnormalities that may have prognostic implications. Where possible, temporal relationship of abnormalities with symptoms and daily activities is sought. As a diagnostic or screening tool there is considerable controversy as to value of AEM because of low sensitivity and specificity. A patient's history and the results of other diagnostic tests increase the probability that observed ECG changes are correlated with disease.[6,12,13] As a prognostic tool it is primarily used to evaluate patients with known cardiovascular disease who have symptoms that may be associated with an arrhythmia. It is also frequently used in clinical trials to evaluate the efficacy of drug therapy, and as a monitoring tool for the presence of silent ischemia.[14,15]

Clinical examples of conditions where AEM is of benefit include detection of silent myocardial ischemia in patients with chest pain or a history suggestive of cardiac disease, assessment of symptoms possibly related to arrhythmias, evaluation of antiarrhythmic devices or drugs, and assessing risk of future cardiac events in patients with conditions known to be associated with sudden cardiac death.[13–15] AEM is considerably less expensive than electrophysiologic studies (EPS), but some studies suggest poor concordance of results for efficacy of antiarrhythmic drug therapy between EPS and AEM.[16] Patients in whom cardiovascular disease is suspected or needs to be ruled out as the etiology for symptoms (e.g., syncope due to neurologic disease) are also potential candidates for AEM.[17] Although somewhat controversial, AEM may be used in patients with ischemic heart disease to identify the frequency and pattern of ischemic changes and response to therapy. Repeat AEM may demonstrate as much as a 90% difference in the number of PVCs recorded.[13] When AEM is used for evaluating an intervention, there should be a 75% to 85% reduction in PVCs, and a 70% reduction in the frequency of complex ventricular ectopy, before the intervention is considered to be successful. The presence of silent ischemia, complex ventricular arrhythmias, and other abnormalities such as sinoatrial pauses, on AEM appear to be an independent marker of future cardiac events. The asymptomatic cardiac ischemia pilot (ACIP) study found that 75% of patients with asymptomatic evidence of ischemia on AEM had multivessel coronary disease on angiography.[18] Other uses of AEM include clinical trials to identify the effect of drug therapy (e.g., nicotine patches) on incidence of PVCs, to compare effects of different dosage forms on ECG abnormalities, and to identify factors that may precipitate ischemia. AEM, in conjunction with signal-averaged ECG and left ventricular function, is also part of the workup to identify patients at high risk for sudden cardiac death following myocardial infarction.[14,15,18]

In 1993, the American Heart Association (AHA) and American College of Cardiology (ACC) published guidelines as to the recommended uses of Holter monitoring.[12] Class I indications are defined as general agreement that ambulatory ECG monitoring is useful and reliable, such as evaluation of patients with sleep apnea, arrhythmias with characteristics suggestive of risk for sudden death, paroxysmal symptoms and pacemakers, left ventricular dysfunction postmyocardial infarction, and to evaluate pacing devices. Class II indications are defined as situations where there is divergence of opinion as to the usefulness of AEM. Examples in this category include patients with long QT intervals or Wolf–Parkinson–White syndrome, and to assess or evaluate pacemakers, proarrhythmias, and drug-induced arrhythmias.

AEM requires the patient to wear a portable electrocardiographic recorder with 2 to 4 thoracic leads for up to 24 hours. Usually at least 2 leads are used to reduce aberrant and artifact recordings being interpreted as ECG abnormalities. This also increases the sensitivity to identify ST abnormalities. Three types of monitors are available: (1) continuous monitors, which record an ECG strip over the duration of the test; (2) event or intermittent recorders, which continuously monitor the ECG but only record preprogrammed abnormal ECG events or are patient activated based on occurrence of symptoms; and (3) real-time analytical recorders, which record throughout the monitoring period and analyze each beat as it occurs. Monitors digitize, encode, and store the information in a solid-state memory. Event monitors are preprogrammed to record parameters such as the number of PVCs and heart rate During monitoring, the patient maintains a diary in which the occurrence, duration, and severity of symptoms (e.g., light-headedness, chest pain) are recorded, plus any specific activities undertaken, development of symptoms with the activity, and any interventions such as taking of medication. A clocking device in the recorder allows later correlation of the patient's diary and the recorded ECG.

Computer-assisted interpretation is used to scan the ECG and identify irregular rhythms, rates, and ST–T-wave changes. Sections identified by the computer as abnormal or those correlating with patient symptoms are then evaluated and characterized further (e.g., potentially pathologic rhythms) by technical personnel and physicians. The main advantages of computer analysis are to reduce interpretation of artifact recordings and identify areas of the ECG that require further analysis. Confounding factors when using AEM can arise from the patient and the device (Table 8–5).

EXERCISE "STRESS" TESTING

Exercise "stress" testing (ET) is a noninvasive test used to evaluate clinical and cardiovascular responses to exercise.[19–24] It is used as a diagnostic and prognostic assessment tool in patients with known or suspected IHD, and as a prognostic indicator in patients postmyocardial infarction and postrevascularization.[20–22] Theoretically, ET is a test of myocardial perfusion under stress, but it is primarily used to determine adequacy of cardiovascular function, and assess patients' functional capacity.

The principle behind ET is to increase myocardial oxygen demand above myocardial oxygen supply and coronary reserve, thereby provoking ischemia (inadequate myocardial perfusion), using exercise as a stressor.[19] ET is a controlled method to assess the balance between myocardial oxygen demand and coronary blood flow under stress. Ischemia can be detected by patient symptoms, ECG changes, or hemodynamic changes. ET can be used as a means to quantitate maximum oxygen uptake (Vo_2max) or amount of oxygen used before symptoms suggestive of ischemia. The type of ECG changes, leads affected, and patient performance can be used as an index of severity and location of disease.[19–22]

ET is widely available, can be conducted in a physician's office, and is about 20 times less expensive than an angiogram and almost three times less expensive than stress

TABLE 8–5. Confounding Factors in Ambulatory ECG Monitoring

Patient Factors	Equipment Factors
Electrolyte abnormalities	Battery failure
Hyperventilation	Loose lead
Lead interference by patient	Mechanical failure of recorder
Medications	Motor failure
Patient activities (e.g., bursts of exercise)	Overrecording
Lead interference by patient	Computer inability to detect arrhythmia
Physiologic variations in waveforms	
Medications	
Patient activities (e.g., sudden exercise)	
Physiologic variations in ECG waveforms	
Presence of atrial fibrillation	

echocardiography. Almost two-thirds of ETs billed to Medicare in 1996 were conducted in physician offices, and one-third were conducted by noncardiologists.[20] Specialized and calibrated equipment is necessary for the test result to be meaningful and reproducible.[23,24] Guidelines for conducting and interpreting the tests, and details of testing equipment and environment, are outlined in the ACC/AHA guidelines on exercise testing and exercise testing standards.[20,23,24]

Indications for ET, as defined by the ACC/AHA, can be classified into three groups according to the relative usefulness of the test based on clinical experience. Class I indications are those for which ET has been shown to provide useful information about the patient's condition. Examples of such subjects are males older than the age of 40 who have atypical symptoms suggestive of IHD, or where functional capacity needs to be assessed to determine prognosis in a patient with confirmed IHD. Class II indications are those where there is some disagreement as to the usefulness of ET. It includes patients with variant angina, or women with a history of typical or atypical chest pain. Class III conditions are those where ET has not been shown to be of any value or the patient's condition precludes successful or safe testing. Examples of class III indications are patients with simple PVCs on a resting ECG, with no other signs or symptoms of IHD.[20,24] Additional indications for stress testing include assessment of patients' functional capacity, and assessment of symptoms such as chest pain or breathlessness. There are no data to substantiate the ET as a screening tool for IHD or to detect early coronary artery disease in asymptomatic subjects.[19] ET is frequently used as an initial test, in conjunction with physical exam and patient symptoms, to aid in selection of additional testing modalities.[19,20] The ET should only be used if the results are able to alter patient management or to assess patient function.

Exercise testing is conducted on a treadmill or bicycle ergometer or by means of a handgrip. Dynamic forms of exercise, such as the treadmill or bicycle ergometer, are preferred to assess exercise tolerance, because they induce a volume and pressure load and not just a pressure load on the heart. Also the degree of "stress" can be delivered in a graded and calibrated manner. Treadmill walking is preferred over the ergometer because it involves more muscle mass.[20] Many patients cannot exercise to full capacity on the cycle ergometer because of leg fatigue, and the Vo_2max achieved with cycle ergometer is 10% to 15% lower than with the treadmill.

The ET is conducted according to an established protocol to decrease inter- and intrapatient variability and allow for standardization in the interpretation of the tests.[20] Numerous protocols have been developed, but the two most commonly used are the Bruce and Naughton protocols.[22] Protocols may be customized to individual patients, to ensure an exercise time of 6 to 12 minutes and a heart rate of 85% to 90% of maximum predicted (adjusted for age, sex, and gender). Protocols detail gradient, speed, and rates of change of these parameters during the test. In preparation for ET, patients fast for a minimum of 3 hours prior to the test, may not exercise 12 hours prior to the test, and must dress suitably for exercise. Baseline evaluation consists of history and physical, blood pressure, heart rate, and ECG. The test begins with a 1-minute warm-up period to orient the patient to the equipment. Each stage of the test is maintained for at least 3 minutes. Continuous blood pressure, heart rate, and ECG recordings are obtained with definitive readings 2 minutes into each stage. Patients are questioned 2 to 3 minutes into each stage of the test about symptoms such as headache, dizziness, and chest pain. Clinical symptoms assessed include color of skin, level of perspiration, and evidence of peripheral cyanosis and light-headedness. Patients are encouraged to exercise as vigorously as they can to ensure an optimal test result. Onset, nature, and duration of all changes in symptoms, hemodynamics, and ECG are noted. Following the test there is a cool-down period during which the patient is seated or lying and is observed for changes as described above.

Interpretation of the ET requires correlation of clinical, ECG, and other parameters measured during the test, with the patient's history (e.g., age, gender, concurrent risk factors, medical history) and concomitant therapy. Results of exercise testing can be used as a guide to future patient management, including suitability for interventional cardiology and selection of pharmacotherapy.[19,21,22] A positive ET is defined as 1 mm horizontal or downsloping depression or elevation of the ST segment for 60 to 80 milliseconds after the QRS complex. For patients with baseline ST depression, combinations of abnormal responses, (e.g., 2-mm ST depression with abnormal hemodynamic abnormalities) would be necessary to call a test positive. ST segment depression of 2 mm or more, especially in conjunction with heart rates of less than 120 beats/min, low levels of stress, or depression persisting for up to 6 minutes after the cessation of the ET, is associated with a poor prognosis.[21,22] Depression of the ST segment in multiple leads is also significant. Other electrocardiographic changes include development of U waves and increased complexity and/or frequency of PVCs or beats, especially if associated with bigeminy or periods of ventricular tachycardia.

Although ECG changes and heart rate responses are used as objective end points, and for interpretation of an ET; patient and clinical end points are actually preferred. Symptom-limited or patient-directed tests are continued to the predetermined end point(s) unless the patient tires or certain characteristics are noted. Clinical symptoms, exhaustion, chest pain, changes in blood pressure, heart rate, and the ECG (rhythm, configuration, and rate) are used as end points for such "open-ended" tests. Close-ended testing is the use of fixed end points such as time on the treadmill or maximal heart rate. The use of the 85% to 90% maximally predicted heart rate is highly variable between patients, and is often not achieved because of concomitant drug therapy and different levels of fitness. Patient performance—measured as exercise duration, time until symptoms, stress at which symptoms occur, and hemodynamic parameters—is a better indicator of an adequate test than heart rate response. Patients who are unable to progress beyond stage II of the Bruce protocol have a poor prognosis and more severe IHD. Other rating scales (e.g., Borg, which measures perceived exertion) may be used in conjunction with the objective results from the ET, to classify patients into high- and low-risk groups.[20]

The product of blood pressure and heart rate (double product) is a measure of myocardial oxygen demand (see Chap. 12). In patients with stable angina, the double product is reproducible on repeat ETs; thus it is used as an objective parameter to follow a patient's disease. Inappropriate or inadequate responses in blood pressure and/or heart rate to exercise suggest heart disease. A reduction in heart rate or a flat response (failure to increase heart rate above 120) with increasing levels of stress has a poor prognosis. Likewise, failure to increase the systolic blood pressure or the finding of a sustained decrease of more than 10 mm Hg are also associated with a worse prognosis. Such responses indicate the heart has an inadequate reserve to respond to stress.

To provide standardized comparability between tests and patients, metabolic equivalents (METs) are used as a measure of Vo_2max. A MET is a measure of resting oxygen uptake. Activity energy demands can then be calculated in terms of METs. For example, 4 METs is equivalent to walking at 4 mph. The number of METs a patient can undertake without symptoms of ischemia correlates with prognosis and helps guide appropriate management strategies.[20,23,24] Refer to Table 8–6 for examples of METs and activity correlations. Exercise capacities of less than 5 METs are associated with a poor prognosis; those greater than 13 METs have a good prognosis, despite presence of disease.[20,21]

Meta-analysis of more than 24,000 patients in 147 studies showed a mean sensitivity of 68% and specificity of 77% for ET as a diagnostic test. The specificity of ET to detect the presence of IHD, compared to angiography, is 84%. Sensitivity ranges from 40% to 90% depending on the number of vessels affected, with a mean of 66%.[20]

TABLE 8–6. MET Relationship to Activity and Function

METs	Level of Activity	ET Result
1	Resting	< 6 METs
2	Level walking at 2 mph	Symptom-limited life-style
4	Level walking at 4 mph	Sedentary life-style tolerated
13	Cycling 9–10 mph	Little or no activity-limited life-style
20	Shoveling heavy snow	No limitations on life-style

Five specific clinical groups have been identified as appropriate to be evaluated using ET[20]:

1. For patients with diagnosed IHD or with symptoms or signs suggestive of IHD,[18] the ET is used to confirm the diagnosis, assess the patient's functional capacity, and provide prognostic information.
2. In patients considered to be at risk for IHD, an ET can be used as a screening tool in certain situations. Males older than the age of 40 with symptoms suggestive of IHD and risk factors for coronary artery disease are the most suitable patients. Screening ETs may also be used in sedentary males older than 40 who are considering embarking on a vigorous exercise or activity program, or those who have high-risk occupations, such as pilots and firemen. False-positive tests are common in most other subjects and especially in women. The reason for the high rate of false positives in women is unclear, but may relate to a "digoxin"-like effect on the ECG from estrogen.
3. Postmyocardial infarction, the ET is of benefit to evaluate ventricular function, assess cardiovascular functional status, determine the degree of rehabilitation the patient has achieved, and assess adequacy of pharmacotherapy. This provides guidance for reentry into the workforce and resumption of normal activities. The ET is also of value in post-MI patients prognostically as an indicator for future cardiac events.[22]
4. The ET is essentially a functional assessment of cardiovascular performance, and can be employed before and after revascularization to assess patient status. It is recommended that stress-induced ischemia be documented prior to revascularization.
5. The ET is also used to assess exercise capability in patients with mitral or aortic valvular disease.[20]

In post-MI patients, the ET is often used to expedite hospital discharge. It can be used as a screening test to determine functional capacity, assess the degree of rehabilitation, and identify those patients at risk of further cardiovascular events. A modified protocol is used; termination of the test occurs when a heart rate of 70% to 75% of age- and gender-predicted maximum is reached (e.g., 140 beats/min for those under age 40, and 130 for those older than 40), or a MET level of 5 for patients older than 40 or 7 for those below 40.[1,20] Tests are usually done prior to discharge or within 6 weeks of infarction. Mortality and reinfarction rates are 0.02% and 0.09%, respectively.[1,20] Patients may be stratified into low-, intermediate-, and high-risk categories, depending on the evidence for ischemia and the level of

TABLE 8–7. Contraindications for Exercise Testing

Absolute	Relative
Unstable angina	Left main coronary artery disease
Syncope	Tachy or brady arrhythmias
< 72 hours post AMI	Electrolyte abnormalities
Uncontrolled CHF	Hypertension (SBP > 220 mm Hg)
Uncontrolled arrhythmias	High-degree AV block
Acute systemic illness	
Acute pulmonary embolism	
Acute myocarditis	
Thrombosis of lower extremity	

exercise tolerance. Post-MI, the ET is safe and may be performed as early as 3 days postevent in stable patients.[1]

Patients in whom ET is contraindicated are those who are unable or who should not exercise because of physiologic or psychological limitations (Table 8–7).[20] Patients with comorbid diseases such as chronic obstructive pulmonary disease (COPD) or peripheral vascular disease (PVD) may be limited in their exercise capacity, while lower limb amputees are unable to perform the standard treadmill test. For patients with disabilities, or other medical conditions that limit their exercise capacity independent of heart disease, ET is not possible. In these instances, pharmacologic stress testing with dipyridamole or other agents may be useful (see the section on pharmacologic stress testing later in the chapter). Unstable angina is usually a contraindication to ET, because of the instability of the patient's disease state and patients cannot exercise to a satisfactory level for the test to be considered adequate. However, once stable, ET is excellent for prognostic evaluation. In patients with untreated life-threatening arrhythmias or congestive heart failure, the ET is also contraindicated. ET is relatively safe with an estimated risk of MI or death of 10 per 10,000 tests overall. Most adverse effects are cardiac in nature including arrhythmias, (primarily bradyarrhythmias), sudden death, hypotension, and myocardial infarction.[1,20]

The ET requires considerable effort, with many patients requiring encouragement to perform to the best of their ability. Some patients use the test as a personal challenge, and perform better on repeated attempts. This is referred to as a training effect and may be a confounding factor in using ET to assess the effect of drug therapy or after interventions for IHD in clinical trials. Silent ischemia may also confound the interpretation of ET because blood pressure and ECG changes may occur in the absence of symptoms.

Drug therapy is rarely discontinued for the test primarily because few data exist to support better test results off drug therapy.[20] Some interference is known to occur, the most common being a decreased maximum heart rate and systolic blood pressure product for patients on β-blockers or calcium channel blockers. Although these patients may not achieve maximal heart rates, the ET helps demonstrate patients' exercise capacity on drug therapy. Nitrates do not alter exercise capacity directly and so need not be discontinued, but may theoretically improve patient response because they relieve or prevent symptoms of ischemia. Digoxin interferes with interpretation of ST segment changes, and patients rarely achieve ST segment changes greater than 1 mm even in the face of significant ischemia. Due its long half-life, digoxin need not be discontinued prior to the test.

CARDIAC CATHETERIZATION AND ANGIOGRAPHY

The development of the cardiac catheterization technique was a major milestone in the diagnosis and management of cardiovascular disease, because it provided a physiologic and anatomic approach to assess patency of coronary vessels and hemodynamic parameters of cardiac function.[25–37] Although cardiac catheterization is commonly referred to as the "test" a patient is to undergo, this term only describes the method of approach, that is, catheterization of the coronary arteries or heart chambers. Once the catheters are placed, other procedures are undertaken, be it angiography (ventriculography or arteriography) or determination of cardiac performance parameters.[25–27]

Cardiac catheterization is primarily undertaken as an aid to diagnose or confirm the presence of IHD, define the anatomy of the coronary arteries, evaluate cardiac performance using angiographic evidence by measuring cardiac chamber pressures, blood flow, and/or to visualize valvular abnormalities. Cardiac catheterization with arteriography is the "gold standard" in the diagnosis and assessment of IHD. New noninvasive methods are currently measured against cardiac catheterization.[25–28] Unlike most other procedures, catheterization determines the morphology of a stenotic lesion. Cardiac catheterization is also used for therapeutic maneuvers such as balloon angioplasty (PTCA) and for evaluation of success of thrombolytic therapy in MI.[25,29,30] Other therapeutic uses include nonsurgical closure of patent ductus arteriosus and transverse pulmonary embolectomy. Catheterization can be used for intracoronary administration of pharmacologic agents. This route of administration is primarily used in clinical trials (e.g., thrombolytics), where objective measures of coronary artery patency are being used as an end point in the trial; or for management of events (e.g., chest pain) during catheterization; or for diagnostic purposes (e.g., ergonovine).[25,28] Placement of cardiac pacemakers, selective internal mammary artery angiography, and aortic root angiography may also be completed during catheterization procedures.[28–30]

Ventricular function, chamber pressures during both systole and diastole, flow rates across the heart valves, and direct measurement or calculation of cardiac performance parameters (such as cardiac output, stroke volume, and systemic vascular resistance) can also be determined during catheterization. Measured and observed parameters obtained during catheterization are used to determine cardiac performance. Contractility, as judged by wall motion and ejection fraction, can be used to assess global cardiac performance and to plan and evaluate or assess therapy. Further applications of cardiac catheterization include aortic root angiography, pharmacologic studies, pulmonary angiography, retrieval of foreign bodies, PTCA, and atherectomy.[28]

The ACC and AHA have developed guidelines for the appropriate use of and criteria for cardiac catheterization, coronary angiography, and percutaneous transluminal coronary angioplasty (PTCA).[28,29] They classify appropriateness of catheterization into three groups. Class I includes patients in whom the procedure is justified based on findings from previous tests, risk factors, and the clinical presentation. Class II includes patients for whom the test may be justified but where there is divergence of opinion among physicians concerning the need for the procedure (e.g., post-MI patient with normal LV function, evidence of ischemia, and a positive ET but no history of heart disease). Class III includes patients in whom the test would not be considered justified but in certain circumstances may become the procedure of choice. Examples in this category include those who have had a coronary bypass graft and currently have no evidence of ischemia.[28,29]

Prior to the procedure the patient is given nothing by mouth (after midnight) except for oral medications. It is not necessary to stop any medications except warfarin prior to catheterization. Patients receiving warfarin are switched to a heparin product about 1 to 2 days prior to the procedure. It is stopped about 6 hours before the procedure to allow normalization of coagulation. Heparin is also used during the procedure to prevent thrombosis. Depending on the procedure undertaken, heparin is either discontinued almost immediately following the procedure, or continued for 12 to 24 hours. Patients frequently develop chest pain and/or vasospasm during introduction and manipulation of catheters and injection of angiography dyes. Nitroglycerin and/or morphine may be given for chest pain. Nitroglycerin can be used sublingually or by intravenous infusion. Most units routinely give this prior to the procedure to prevent vasospasm as the catheter is introduced. For patients undergoing PTCA, aspirin, ticlopidine, and calcium channel blockers may also be used prior to and following the procedure. Sedatives, such as midazolam or other short-acting benzodiazepines, are frequently given to ensure patient comfort and safety, but the patient is awake and aware of the procedure because patient cooperation is necessary to obtain the angiographic views and assess symptoms. The patient may even be able to view the procedure on a television screen. To reduce bleeding complications, the sheath is removed several hours after the procedure; and the patient remains still in bed for about 8 hours.[27–29,31] Despite the invasive nature of the procedure, there is some controversy as to the need for prophylactic antibiotics in patients at risk for bacterial endocarditis because of valvular prostheses or prior history of rheumatic fever.[27,28]

Right heart (venous) catheterization enables the right heart, coronary sinus pulmonary arteries, and pulmonary wedge position to be reached. Right-sided catheterization is primarily used for determination of cardiac performance parameters. Hemodynamic measurements are useful in patients with congestive heart failure, and in this setting they may be obtained with a Swan–Ganz flow-directed catheter.[27,32] Left-sided catheterization is performed using the brachial or femoral artery and passing the catheter, in a retrograde fashion, to the aorta, left ventricle, and left atrium. Less commonly, a transeptal approach may be used. High pressures in the left heart and the necessity of a retrograde catheter approach make left-sided heart catheterization more difficult than an arterial approach. This is especially so in patients with aortic stenosis or prosthetic aortic valves.

Measurements taken during catheterization are done after hemodynamic stabilization whether at baseline, after movement of the catheter, or during pharmacologic intervention.[27,32,33] During the procedure, hemodynamic parameters are continuously monitored, as well as blood pressure and heart rate. Continuous electrocardiographic monitoring with 12-lead ECGs is repeated at intervals throughout the procedure. Information obtained during catheterization is real time, but it is only that. It is assumed that these data reflect the ongoing status of the coronary circulation; however, the presence of vasospasm may be misleading, as the catheter itself is a powerful stimulus for spasm.[27,28,35]

The ACC and the AHA guidelines for catheterization, angiography, and PTCA also include such items as technique, procedures, facilities, personnel, and training.[27–29,31] Many catheterization procedures can be undertaken in the outpatient setting. However when interventional procedures are contemplated, these should be done on an inpatient basis. It is imperative that all facilities be in close liaison with a cardiothoracic surgery unit.

The incidence of complications is related to the expertise and experience of the operator, with case load being a good indicator of the latter. The AHA/ACC guidelines on catheterization and angioplasty include a description of the number of procedures necessary to maintain a minimum competence. The incidence of significant complications is reported to be 1.8%, with mortality ranging from 0.05% to 2.37%, based on the experience among operators. The AHA guidelines state that the risk to life should be less than 0.2% and the risk of adverse effects less than 0.5%. Various risk factors have been identified as being associated with an increased incidence of complications, some of which are considered direct contraindications to the procedure.[28,29,31] A list of contraindications is given in Table 8–8.[28,29] Complication rates increase with the duration of catheterization, in particular, thrombotic complications. The major complications during and after cardiac catheterization are development of an arterial thrombosis and bleeding complications

TABLE 8–8. Contraindications of Cardiac Catherization and Other Procedures[a]

Recent stroke	Patient noncompliance[b]
Advanced physiologic age	Digoxin intoxication
Severe anemia	Anaphylaxis to radiographic dyes
Severe hypertension	Active infection
Active gastrointestinal bleed	Severe electrolyte imbalances
Fever	Unstable condition
Other comorbid illnesses, e.g., COPD[c,d]	

[a]Primarily contraindications to procedures such as arteriography and PTCA.
[b]Patient not willing to undergo further treatment (e.g., surgery based on results of catherization).
[c]COPD = chronic obstructive pulmonary disease.
[d]Disease states that may prohibit or increase risk of other interventions (e.g., surgery).
[e]Patients in whom emergency cardiac surgery would pose a high risk (e.g., during acute asthma or acute exacerbation of COPD).

postprocedure. The use of heparin during the procedure and immediately after has not been shown to definitively reduce thrombotic complications, but it is commonly given, especially with arteriography, left-sided heart catheterization, and angioplasty. Bleeding complications can be reduced by ensuring that patients have normal coagulation studies prior to procedure, bed rest for several hours after the procedure, and frequent and careful observation of the entry site. In the event of a bleeding complication, direct pressure is required with sandbags, and if there is no resolution, emergency surgery may be necessary to prevent further complications. Heart perforation is an uncommon but potentially lethal complication. Emergency surgical intervention would be necessary. Dwell time of catheters is the major feature in thrombotic complications. The thrombogenicity of a catheter is determined primarily by the material, with factors such as hardness, friction coefficient, and moisture retention being important. During the procedure patients may experience a vagal reflex with development of hypotension, bradycardia, and nausea. This most frequently occurs in conjunction with patient anxiety and can be prevented or treated with atropine. An increased predisposition to MI during and after the procedure is seen in patients with unstable angina, recent subendocardial infarction, and in patients with insulin-dependent diabetes mellitus. Postcatheterization, patients may have elevated creatine phosphokinase due to tissue damage during the procedure, but usually this does not interfere with serial enzymes for detection of a myocardial infarction.[28,29,34]

Arteriography (injection of radiopaque dye into an artery) assesses the size of the artery, presence of collateral circulation, and the presence of dynamic abnormalities such as vasospasm. Arteriography is unique in that it determines the morphology but not the physiologic significance, or functional impact of the lesion. This is well demonstrated in diabetic patients, who may have significant microvascular coronary artery disease with apparently unaffected larger arteries at arteriography.[29,33,35]

The severity of the lesion may be assessed in several ways. Considerable controversy exists as to the best methodology. During angiography, there is an attempt to assess the severity of the lesion by visual comparison with surrounding vessels. There are inherent difficulties with such a method, because it assumes that surrounding vessels are in fact normal, which may not be so, especially if the patient has diffuse disease. Calipers can be used to actually document physical size, but generally the degree of stenosis is reported as a percent narrowing. Various grading scales are used to record the percent narrowing (25% to 100%) and a severity score assigned from 1 to 32 (see Chap. 12).[25,28,29] Anatomic problems compound these methods, as vessels may travel down into the myocardium for a time, leaving the epicardial surface appearing as narrowed; or two vessels may overlie one another, distorting the image obtained. Multiple views are required to obtain a good image of the vessel; the right anterior oblique planes are most commonly used (two views at 90 degrees to each other). Lesions may be described as concentric and smooth (simple lesions) or eccentric and broad with a rough surface (complicated lesions).[27,29,36]

Angiography is able to detect lesions that occlude the vessel by as little as 20%. Occlusions of 75% or more are almost always seen on angiography. Significant narrowing is usually assumed to be 50% or more, although some studies use 75% narrowing as the cutoff point.[29,36] As described in Chapter 13, coronary artery lesions most prone to rupture and thrombosis are those with 40% to 60% narrowing. The number of lesions is also considered of importance to the severity and prognosis of IHD, although there is considerable variation in the accuracy of such predictions, because angiographic and pathologic correlation of lesions is imperfect. The occurrence of spasm, variants in anatomy, and collateral filling also complicate interpretation of the angiogram.[37] The angiographic films are used to plan interventions. Arteriography is considered standard care prior to a procedure to ensure the best procedure is undertaken with a good outcome. The angiographic films may be used during both surgery and PTCA to guide the procedure.[29,33]

Ventriculography studies may be performed during cardiac catheterization to obtain information about the contours of the heart and to assess the global and segmental function. Regional wall motion, filling defects, and presence of mural thrombi may also be visualized. During this procedure, radiopaque dye is injected into the heart chambers and serial films are taken to follow the dye passage.[29,33,34] Left ventricular ventriculography is a routine part of left-sided catheterization unless ventricular function information is already available from other noninvasive studies or there are specific contraindications to the procedure.

Invasive cardiology is growing rapidly not only in terms of the numbers of patients undergoing such procedures, but the diversity of procedures. The development of electrophysiologic studies for the assessment and treatment of arrhythmias was made possible because of catheterization.

The diversity of techniques is "limited only by the imagination of the physician and inventiveness of the microtechnologist."[35]

COMPUTED TOMOGRAPHY

Computed tomography (CT) is not a primary diagnostic procedure in the evaluation of cardiovascular disease and function, because it identifies structural abnormalities that are well defined and visualized by other diagnostic procedures (e.g., echocardiography), and it is significantly more expensive.[38–41] The primary advantages of CT imaging are enhanced definition and spatial resolution of structures, and acquisition of three-dimensional images.[38] CT also overcomes the problems of background interference found with planar imaging techniques. CT imaging has found a special niche in evaluating aortic disease, pericardial disease, and assessing paracardiac and cardiac masses. More accurate determination of chamber volume and size, and mass calculations of myocardial wall thickness, can be obtained from tomographic imaging than with other methods such as echocardiography or angiography.[39]

New techniques, such as ultrafast CT (cine-CT), have largely overcome the problems of cardiac motion that distorts more conventional CT images. In this technique, complete tomograms can be completed in 50 milliseconds, which is within one cardiac cycle; the tomograms are thus real-time images.[38,40] Without cine-CT, images must be correlated with the cardiac cycle. This is achieved by gating the CT to the ECG, as described previously. Gating is not required for ultrafast CT scanners, but a set event within the cardiac cycle (determined by ECG) is usually used as initiator for imaging to ensure standardization. Cine-CT scans the heart at 10 to 14 tomographic levels in 10-mm slices. Although still in its infancy, cine-CT has been proposed as a screening tool for evaluating the risk of developing obstructive coronary artery disease. Cine-CT is more sensitive and specific than fluoroscopy to identify the extent and density of coronary artery calcification. The calcium score (calcium density and volume of calcium) in patients older than 30 to 70 years with known coronary artery disease is significantly higher than in subjects with no coronary artery disease, and appears to correlate well with the degree of coronary artery occlusion.[38,40]

CT is clearly more definitive and accurate in the diagnosis of aortic dissection, and evaluation of the pericardium, than echocardiography. Diagnostic accuracy of aortic dissections with CT scanning is at least 90%. Clear definition of the edges of the intimal flap of the dissection and true and false channels can be seen. CT scanning provides clear definition of the components of the myocardial wall from the inner endocardial wall through to the epicardial surface and pericardium. This allows precise visualization of abnormalities within and on either side of the wall, such as aneurysms, and thrombin. Detection of the presence of a thrombus on CT is comparable in accuracy to two-dimensional echocardiography.[39,40] CT scanning has also been used postcardiac transplant to view the coronary calcifications, which have been shown to be a predictor of cardiac events.

On a CT image, the pericardium appears as a distinct entity and can be evaluated for thickening (defined as a thickness greater than 4 mm) and calcification. It is the most sensitive technique to differentiate types of pericarditis and to estimate pericardial fluid volume. CT scanning compares well with echocardiographic imaging for defining loculated and hemorrhagic effusions.[39,40]

In the evaluation of cardiac masses, the main advantage that CT provides is that the mass is visualized as a distinct space-occupying entity. The shape, density, and tissue type may also be delineated, aiding in the determination of the nature of masses. Masses as small as 0.5 to 1 cm can be identified on CT. The three-dimensional image of CT also allows determination of the extent and distribution of left ventricular hypertrophy in patients with hypertrophic or congestive cardiomyopathy.[39]

Like radionuclide assessment, contrast angiography, and echocardiography, CT scanning can be used to calculate ejection fraction, left ventricular volume, and stroke volume. The blood pool is defined with IV iodinated contrast material. Ventricular volumes, ejection fraction, and stroke volume are determined directly from the blood pool on each image. Values obtained with CT are more accurate and reproducible than those obtained on angiography and echocardiography.[39]

Although not yet in common practice, CT scans have been used as a diagnostic tool in IHD, to localize areas of infarction and abnormal perfusion, and to quantify the extent and density of coronary artery calcification. Spatial separation of cardiac anatomic regions allows precise delineation and distribution of areas of wall thinning or thickening and/or the dynamics of wall-motion abnormalities during both diastole and systole. It has been shown that both gated and cine-CT scanning have a 94% sensitivity and 87% specificity when compared to left ventricular cineangiography from catheterization to detect regional wall abnormalities.[38]

CT perfusion scanning can also be used to assess coronary and myocardial perfusion following revascularization and myocardial infarction, but is not as popular as nuclear imaging or coronary angiography primarily because of lack of comparative data and availability of equipment. CT scans do not provide information regarding degree of stenosis or adequacy of blood flow.

CT scanning has proven to be an effective noninvasive method to visualize congenital heart disease, but its role is challenged by the higher-resolution capacity of magnetic resonance imaging. For measuring parameters in some congenital disorders, such as evaluation of ventricular function and estimation of the volume of cardiac shunts, CT scanning still remains the evaluation method of choice.[39]

In summary, CT scanning, especially cine-CT, is a rapidly evolving technique for evaluation of cardiovascular disease. It remains an expensive alternative to other methodologies, in many instances, but the high resolution and spatial capabilities means CT offers unique properties.

MAGNETIC RESONANCE IMAGING

In cardiovascular disease, magnetic resonance imaging (MRI) is primarily used to assess anatomy and blood flow velocities.[42–47] It is a noninvasive technique, where no ionizing radiation is used, and contrast is not required. MRI produces three-dimensional images with excellent anatomic resolution and differentiation between tissues (including different soft tissues and blood). There are few specific indications for MRI, as other less expensive techniques such as echocardiography provide comparable information to MRI. The main factors that limit the use of MRI are cost, time, the requirement for specialized equipment and environment, and the lack of comparative data with other techniques.[42]

MRI uses an external magnetic field that picks up the magnetic properties of nuclei or protons. Unpaired protons in nuclei, when placed in an electromagnetic field, are elevated to a higher energy state and emit energy, causing magnetic resonance. The magnetic field used in MRI is very strong, being on the order of 0.15 to 2 T, as compared to the earth's magnetic field of 0.0003 to 0.0007 T. These strengths are obtained by using a very small magnetic coil with a small internal diameter (as little as 60 cm).[42,43] Lack of motion is essential to prevent artifact and distortion of the MRI images. The patient must be able to cooperate by being completely motionless throughout the scanning procedure. To allow coordination with the cardiac cycle, images are gated to the ECG. Magnetic field imaging is contraindicated in patients with pacemakers or ferromagnetic intracerebral clips, in patients who cannot remain motionless, and in those who suffer from claustrophobia or have unstable conditions.[43]

MRI has found most use in evaluation of anatomic abnormalities, such as thoracic aortic aneurysms and aortic dissection, and coarctation of the aorta where it may be the procedure of choice.[44] In abdominal aortic aneurysms, MRI has been shown to be superior to ultrasound, but remains a second-line imaging technique due to the portability of ultrasound.[45] MRI offers similar benefits to CT in such conditions, in that thombi, the wall, and flap(s) of the aneurysm may be visualized.[45]

MRI is easily able to differentiate between viable and nonviable myocardium if the latter has been replaced by fibrous tissue. It cannot distinguish between ischemic and normal myocardium. It has been used postmyocardial infarction to assess complications such as aneurysm and intraventricular thrombi, and postrevascularization to assess graft patency.[46] In hypertrophic cardiomyopathy and left ventricular hypertrophy, MRI is a useful tool to assess extent of involvement, distribution of muscle mass, and wall thickness. MRI competes well with CT for assessment of paracardiac and cardiac masses, especially where there is mediastinal involvement and extension into the heart. It may be used following echocardiography for better definition of the mass. It has also been shown to be equal to CT for pericardial assessment, but is superior in identifying the type of pericardial fluid.

An interesting application of MRI is its utility to assess blood flow velocities and pathologic blood flows such as shunts. With MRI images, it is possible to calculate accurate measurements of gradients in shunts and across stenotic valves.[47] More recently, MRI has been used to assess cardiac function where ejection fraction, stroke volume, and chamber volumes can be accurately and reproducibly calculated.

An investigational use of MRI is to assess the presence and extent of rejection of cardiac transplantation by detecting abnormal relaxation properties and evidence of reduced high-energy phosphate levels. The obvious advantage of this technique is its noninvasive nature compared to transvenous endomyocardial biopsy. MRI remains an investigational and research tool in this area; only two studies in humans thus far have been published.[44]

POSITRON EMISSION TOMOGRAPHY

Positron emission tomography (PET) is a relatively new modality for diagnostic imaging in cardiovascular medicine.[48–54] It is primarily a research tool because of expense, availability, and lack of comparative data with other technologies.[48,49] Positron-emitting agents are linked with compounds known to have selective (e.g., biochemical property of substrate) or perfusion-dependent uptake into the tissue or cell in question. It is primarily used to assess myocardial tissue perfusion and to characterize physiologic and metabolic activity within the myocardium. PET scanning has been used to measure regional myocardial uptake of exogenous glucose and fatty acids, quantitate free fatty acid metabolism, define perfused myocardium energy source(s), and evaluate myocardial chemoreceptor sites.[50] The radiopharmaceutical's radioactivity (concentration) is detected by a rotating camera that obtains multiple simultaneous images and, with the aid of a computer, a planar image is produced. The primary advantages of PET over other imaging techniques are its noninvasive nature; the ability to do repeat scans within a short period of time, such as pre- and postpercutaneous transluminal coronary angioplasty; and the reproducibility of images over time.

In coronary artery disease, PET is used to assess and follow the physiologic significance of stenotic lesions. Postinfarction, PET myocardial substrate metabolism studies are used to evaluate the amount and activity of viable tissue around the infarcted area. PET scanning has also been linked with physiologic (exercise) or pharmacologic (dipyridamole) stress to allow assessment of the myocardium under stress conditions. It can also be used to detect ischemic versus nonischemic cardiomyopathy, and the site and extent of myocardial infarction. Limited studies in patients with more than 50% stenosis on angiography suggest that dipyridamole–stress single-photon emission computed tomography (SPECT) and ^{13}N ammonia PET are comparable tests to assess coronary artery perfusion, with respective sensitivities of 98% and 96% and specificity of 88% and 81%.[51]

Myocardial perfusion studies with PET are able to identify more accurately the viable and nonviable myocardium than other imaging agents such as technetium and thallium; this is probably due to the higher contrast resolution available with PET. PET also quantifies regional myocardial perfusion more accurately than other modalities. It has shown at least 70% accuracy in predicting functional recovery of myocardium postrevascularization.[52] PET scanning appears to provide increased sensitivity to detect hibernating myocardium, especially when compared to thallium scanning. Comparative studies with SPECT–thallium in conjunction with bicycle ergometer or dipyridamole versus PET perfusion scanning showed comparative sensitivities (76% to 79%) but improved specificity (90% versus 82%, $P < .005$).[53,54]

Substrates used in PET scanning are those that can be used as the markers for perfusion or metabolic activity. For myocardial perfusion studies, ^{82}Rubidium (^{82}Rh), ^{13}N ammonia ($^{13}NH_3$), and $^{15}O_2$-labeled water are used. For myocardial substrate metabolism studies, ^{11}C palmitate, ^{11}C acetate, and ^{18}F 2-deoxyglucose (FDG) are used.

Uptake of ^{82}Rb occurs preferentially in viable tissue, although uptake tends to decrease at high myocardial blood flows. Net uptake into tissue resolving from an ischemic insult and irreversibly injured tissue (infarcted) is reduced. Hence, viable tissue demonstrates an overall accumulation of ^{82}Rb. Although ^{82}Rb is primarily used to evaluate myocardial blood flow, it is also a marker of tissue viability, with viable tissue continuing to accumulate the compound. Comparative studies with ET, SPECT, and stress ECHO show PET scanning to be more accurate in the detection of IHD.

The substrate $^{13}NH_3$ is extracted into myocardium by glutamine synthetase. This product produces high-contrast images with a sensitivity of 88% to 97% and specificity of 90% to 100% to detect IHD. The overall uptake is still dependent on blood flow and, like rubidium, uptake decreases at high flow rates. Oxygen-15-labeled water has a high extraction ratio into myocardial tissue, which appears to be independent of blood flow or the metabolic state of the myocardium. Oxygen-15-labeled water studies are done in conjunction with ^{15}O carbon monoxide (labels red blood cells in the vascular space) studies to help eliminate some of the background activity that occurs as a result of the high extraction ratio.[54]

Tracers used for assessment of myocardial metabolism are selected based on the type of metabolism of interest; FDG traces glucose metabolism; ^{11}C palmitate, mitochondrial fatty acid metabolism; and ^{11}C acetate is an indirect marker for myocardial oxygen consumption, allowing assessment of ventricular performance. Carbon-11 palmitate is a useful marker for normal myocardial oxygen consumption, because baseline energy needs of the myocardium are met through fatty acid oxidation. Clearance of ^{11}C palmitate is biexponential, and studies in animals and in healthy men have shown clearance to be proportional to cardiac workload and myocardial oxygen consumption. Increased cardiac workload increases the first phase of clearance, reflecting an increased rate of fatty acid oxidation and decreases in the endogenous lipid pool. The second clearance phase is unrelated to cardiac workload, and is believed to merely represent uptake of ^{11}C palmitate into the endogenous lipid pool. The use of ^{11}C palmitate to assess myocardial metabolism in ischemic tissue is limited because there is altered transport and storage of the compound, and significant back diffusion of the agent into the vascular space. Carbon-11 hydroxyephedrine has recently been used as an investigational tool in assessment of the autonomic innervation (sympathetic) of the myocardium, as it accumulates in the presynaptic cleft. Global decreases in uptake are found in cardiomyopathy and in congestive heart failure suggesting decreased neuronal function.

FDG accumulates in the heart proportional to glucose use by the myocardial cell, and so is a marker of cell viability. FDG studies help identify the affected vascular bed and allow evaluation as to whether angioplasty or surgery might be used.[50] Detection of hibernating myocardium is decreased, but viable metabolic activity can be readily seen on PET scans. This gives a more definitive evaluation of overall myocardial function, as it identifies the degree of hibernating myocardium. Patients with a significant degree of jeopardized or hibernating myocardium identified on PET scanning could then undergo vascularization procedures with restoration to functional myocardium. In contrast, perfusion studies do not show good differentiation of infarcted or hibernating tissue, and based on perfusion scans, revascularization would not have been considered. FDG has an 85% positive predictive accuracy to determine improvement of wall abnormalities postrevascularization. It has also been shown of value to detect hibernating myocardium. PET scanning with FDG has been used in assessment of perfusion and/or metabolic states in cardiomyopathies. In ischemic cardiomyopathy, discrete regional ischemia is seen as a patchy nonhomogeneous uptake of the tracers; dilated cardiomyopathies tend to show global decreased uptake of tracers.

The future of PET appears promising. Improved tomographic scanners, development of new radiopharmaceuticals, and improved understanding of substrate metabolism and its relationship to myocardial tissue viability, will provide new dimensions to assess and evaluate myocardial function. Research enterprises are developing agents to label receptors as a tool to determine cardiovascular physiology and how altered receptor function, biochemical abnormalities, substrate metabolism, or other as-yet unrecognized abnormalities impair cardiac function.

ECHOCARDIOGRAPHY

Echocardiography is the use of ultrasound to visualize anatomic structures such as the valves within the heart, and to describe wall motion.[6,55–61] Images obtained from echocardiography can be used to estimate wall thickness and ejection fraction, assess ventricular function, and detect abnormalities of the pericardium such as effusions or thickening.[55–57] It is a simple, noninvasive test, and is the procedure of choice in the diagnosis and evaluation of a number of conditions such as valvular dysfunction (aortic and mitral stenosis and regurgitation, endocarditis), wall motion abnormalities associated with ischemia, and congenital abnormalities, such as ventricular or atrial septal defects. Echocardiography can be linked with the various stress tests (ET, dipyridamole) to assess stress-induced structural or functional abnormalities (e.g., changes in wall motion). However, for best resolution, static images obtained with the patient at rest allow for best visualization of heart structures.

Echocardiography is based on the principle of differential acoustic impedance (or tissue density) and the laws of reflection and refraction.[57] Sound waves directed across tissues from a transducer will reflect back sound waves of different frequencies. The ability of the ultrasonic beam to penetrate chest wall structures is inversely proportional to the frequency of the signal. When using transthoracic echocardiography, frequencies of 2.0 to 5.0 MHz are commonly used in adults, and 3.5 to 10.0 MHz are used in children.[55] Corrections are made for impedance of the ultrasound wave through structures that are not part of the test, and for depth of structures that are part of the test to improve the image viewed on the oscilloscope. Successful echocardiography is highly dependent on operator technique and the quality of equipment. Serial determinations in a given patient using the same conditions and echocardiographic images (windows) provide the best form of internal control to allow comparison of test results. In clinical trials, echocardiograms are read and interpreted independently by two or three clinicians to provide a means of control.

Several types of echocardiography are used in clinical practice. The transducer can be placed on the chest wall (transthoracic) or in the esophagus (transesophageal, TEE). In the transthoracic approach, the most common modes are M-mode (motion) and two-dimensional (2-D) imaging. Both M-mode and 2-D echocardiography provide visualization of heart structures and can indicate numerous structural abnormalities such as aneurysms, wall thickness abnormalities, chamber collapse (e.g., tamponade), and valvular stenosis.[55,56] Transesophageal echocardiography is primarily used for assessment of valvular anatomy and function or to image abnormal masses such as tumors or thrombi.[58,59] Doppler and color flow Doppler technology can be added to improve resolution of structures, identify patterns of blood flow, and calculate flow gradients. The Doppler principle involves reflecting sound off a moving object; in the case of echocardiography, the red blood cell.[55–57] As the red cell moves in relation to the transducer, a frequency shift occurs in the reflected wave. Color enhancement allows flow direction to be visualized, as different colors are used for antegrade and retrograde flow. Newer, but less commonly used, forms are contrast and epicardial echocardiography.

In M-mode, the transducer is placed at a single site on the chest (usually along the sternal border) with the ultrasound being directed posteriorly. M-mode echocardiography records only static objects in one plane, producing a single picture of a small region of the heart or an "icepick" view. Results depend on the exact placement of the transducer with respect to the underlying structures. Conventional M-mode echocardiography provides visualization of the right ventricle, left ventricle, and posterior left ventricular wall and pericardium. If the transducer is swept in an arc from the apex to the base of the heart, virtually the whole heart can be visualized; including the valves and left atrium.

Two-dimensional echocardiography employs multiple windows of the heart; each view provides a wedge-shaped image. Windows most commonly used include parasternal long and short axis, and apical two- and four-chamber views (Fig. 8–6). These views are processed onto a videotape to produce a motion picture of the heart. Two-dimensional echocardiography renders increased accuracy in calculating ventricular volumes, wall thickness, and degree of valvular stenosis compared to M-mode echocardiography.[57]

Using 2-D echocardiography, patient-specific derived and calculated parameters such as ejection fraction and wall

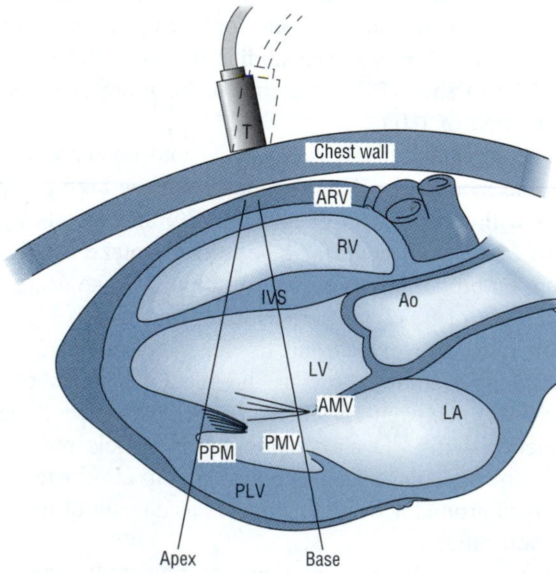

FIGURE 8–6. Schematic drawing of two-dimensional echocardiography to illustrate location of cardiac structures as "seen" by the transducer. The transducer is swept in an arc so several pictures of the heart are obtained to generate the final electrocardiogram. *(Redrawn from Corya BC et al. Applications of echocardiography in acute myocardial infarction. Cardiovasc Clin 1995; 2:113,1975, with permission.)*

thickness can be compared to standardized values (population based) or to previously obtained values from the patient. The latter are of more use clinically, as population values are not derived for specific populations or disease states. Serial determinations in a given patient, especially following a change in clinical condition or a procedure, allow evaluation of progression of disease over time. Baseline characterization of a newly diagnosed abnormality is an essential part of the cardiovascular evaluation (e.g., mitral stenosis, congestive heart failure).

In TEE, the transducer is advanced into the esophagus and allowed to rest just behind the heart. Images are obtained in either horizontal or vertical planes.[58] There is also some experience with passing the transducer into the fundus of the stomach to obtain better images of the ventricles. The procedure is considered to be a low-risk invasive procedure by the AHA, and does not require routine antibiotic prophylaxis for patients at risk of developing endocarditis.[57] Patients require sedation with a short-acting benzodiazepine and pharyngeal anesthesia prior to the procedure. Complications such as esophageal tears or perforation, esophageal burns, transient ventricular tachycardia, minor throat irritation, and transient vocal cord paralysis have rarely been reported.[59] In one series of 10,218 studies, only 1 death (0.0098%) was reported, comparable to that with esophageal gastroduodenoscopy (0.004%).[58] TEE is contraindicated in patients with esophageal abnormalities where passage of the transducer might be limited (e.g., esophageal strictures or varices).

TEE has become popular because higher resolution and improved visualization of structures within the heart is possible compared to transthoracic echocardiography.[58,59] These structures include the pulmonary veins, thoracic aorta heart chambers, and valves. Interference of ribs, lungs, and subcutaneous tissues is minimized, enabling TEE to be more useful in patients where the conventional transthoracic approach has been limited because of pulmonary disease, mechanical ventilation, or obesity. Better resolution is also obtained by using a higher frequency transducer (5 MHz for adults). TEE essentially has the same indications as transthoracic echocardiography, but improved image resolution gives it wider clinical application. Visualization of the heart valves—in particular, the mitral valve—is superior, allowing more accurate evaluation of both native and prosthetic valves.[55] Visualization of valvular vegetations as small as 5 mm is possible with TEE.[58,60,61] In a study of 80 patients with infective endocarditis, TEE detected vegetations in 90% of patients compared to 58% with transthoracic echocardiography.[60] It can also help define complications of endocarditis such as thrombosis or valve leakage.[61] In aortic dissection, TEE is able to identify the initial flap and origin of dissection, and has an overall sensitivity and specificity of 97% and 100%, respectively.[58] Computed tomography remains the diagnostic method of choice for aortic dissection but TEE offers a sensitive and fast test that can be conducted in the emergency room.

Other uses of TEE include identification of cardiac thrombus, especially those in the left atrium, and assessment of atrial dilation. After transient ischemic attacks or cerebrovascular accident, TEE may enable identification of the site of cardiac emboli by providing excellent images of likely sources of such, namely, ventricular or atrial thrombus, valvular vegetation, cardiac shunts, cardiac tumors, or atrial and ventricular septal defects. In particular, TEE provides good visualization of the left atrial appendage. In a study of almost 1500 patients with cerebral ischemia or nonvalvular atrial fibrillation, atrial thrombi were seen in 183 patients when evaluated by TEE versus only 2 patients using transthoracic echocardiography.[58] Intraoperative TEE with Doppler flow during valvular surgery is useful in planning and monitoring surgical corrections. TEE is also the procedure of choice if intraoperative cardiac imaging is required to ascertain development of ischemia.

Doppler echocardiography is primarily used in conjunction with traditional echocardiography when valvular function or blood flow patterns need to be determined. It allows measurement of transvalvular pressure gradients, valve area, and pressure changes on either side of the valve.[55,57] Doppler echocardiography is either continuous or pulsed; the former is used to assess pressure changes, while the latter is used to localize points of origin and creation of turbulent and high blood flow. Assessment with Doppler echocardiography combines structural images and hemodynamic monitoring. Thus, it is possible to evaluate the impact of structural disease on cardiac function and quantify the associated hemodynamics. Color Doppler is used to visualize blood flow (e.g., regurgitation). Turbulence associated with valvular abnormalities and wall motion abnormalities can be clearly visualized and quantified.[55,57]

In aortic regurgitation, Doppler echocardiography is the best noninvasive technique to assess the pressure and severity of regurgitation.[57] Color flow mapping allows tracing of the jet direction and an indication of its volume, point of wall contact, and width.[57] Because Doppler echocardiography distinguishes different types of turbulence, it can simultaneously identify more than one type of valvular abnormality (e.g., aortic regurgitation and mitral stenosis) and the source of concomitant heart murmur.

Ischemia is seen on echocardiography as alterations and abnormalities of wall motion.[55] It is used in ischemic heart disease to localize regions of ischemia at both rest and under stress. Wall motion abnormalities are seen as altered thickness of various segments of the heart and decreased anterior and septal wall movement between diastolic and systolic contraction. Wall motion abnormalities are graded using descriptive terms such as akinetic, hypokinetic, dyskinetic, and hyperkinetic.[57] Loss of myocardial thickness is also indirect evidence of scar formation. Post-MI, echocardiography is a useful noninvasive diagnostic tool for detection of ventricular aneurysms, and can be used serially for diagnostic and prognostic information.[57] Because it is possible to visualize the complete ventricle (in segments), both global left ventricular function and regional function can be assessed as well as ejection fraction. Response of the myocardium to stress (induction of ischemia) can also be evaluated using echocardiography. Echocardiography can be linked to either the exercise or pharmacologic stress tests to determine myocardial response to stress. Further discussion is included in the section on pharmacologic stress testing later in the chapter.

NUCLEAR CARDIOLOGY

Nuclear cardiology has been a major breakthrough in terms of noninvasive testing methods.[62–68] Development of new radionuclides with short half-lives—which can be either used alone, such as technetium 99m (^{99m}Tc), or combined with other substances to form agents with particular properties, such as ^{99m}Tc-pyrophosphate—has expanded the role for nuclear imaging in cardiology. Factors important in extending the utility of nuclear medicine in cardiovascular medicine include cost and availability of equipment, personnel, and the sensitivity and specificity of such tests in comparison to the current gold standard testing methods. The main limitation of nuclear cardiology is the availability of suitable radionuclides and correlation of nuclear images with cardiovascular function.

Despite the availability of many new radionuclides, ^{99m}Tc remains one of the two most commonly used radionuclides. Its characteristics are ideal for clinical imaging, as it has a short half-life of about 6 hours; a single 140-keV photon peak, which is suitable for available imaging systems; emits primarily γ-rays; and is able to be combined with multiple pharmaceuticals. It is generated "in-house" by a bench-top generator, which helps to reduce transportation costs and provides immediate availability.[63,64] Thallium-201 (^{201}Tl), is also commonly used, as its perfusion properties allow assessment of coronary and myocardial perfusion. Its uptake into cells is dependent on blood flow. It has a relatively long half-life of 73 hours, which prevents the use of multiple doses close together, but this property allows for delayed imaging. The energy from thallium-201 is x-ray, with an energy level of 69 to 83 keV. Production of thallium requires a cyclotron. Images are obtained with a conventional gamma camera. Thallium scanning may also be done using alternate scanning techniques, such as SPECT, which yield better images in terms of spatial orientation. The gamma camera is still the most widely used in nuclear imaging techniques and provides good images for most studies.[63,64]

TECHNETIUM SCANNING

Technetium scanning is used for evaluation of blood pool (angiography) and myocardial perfusion, and as an infarct-avid agent to identify damaged myocardium.[64,67,68] Analysis of the blood pool, as in a multigated angiography (MUGA), uses technetium either alone or as a red blood cell complex. The former obtains images following a bolus of technetium, and traces its passage from the venous system through the heart to the aorta and is known as first-pass angiography. Equilibrium tests where technetium is bound to red blood cells provide an imaging time of several hours and are gated to the ECG. The main advantage of equilibrium tests is the ability to obtain serial images. These tests are used to determine right and left ventricular ejection fractions, assess ventricular volumes and wall motion, and detect cardiac shunts.[64]

Infarct-avid radionuclides such as technetium-pyrophosphate (^{99m}Tc-PYP) are used to evaluate the presence and extent of damaged myocardium[67] such as post-MI, in suspected myocardial contusion, and following chest wall injuries. Imaging with ^{99m}Tc-PYP is applicable when patient history, ECGs changes, and laboratory evidence of MI are not definitive but MI is clinically suspected.[64] Uptake of ^{99m}Tc-PYP into infarcted tissue depends on regional blood flow, myocardial calcium concentration, the degree of irreversible myocardial injury, and time after infarction.[64,67] Technetium-pyrophosphate attaches to calcium deposited in the infarcted area, so is known as "hot spot" scanning.[64,66] False "hot spots" may occur where there is necrotic myocardial tissue as may be found in myocarditis, myocardial abscesses, old myocardial infarctions, and myocardial trauma. Calcium concentration appears to play the major role in the localizing of ^{99m}Tc-PYP in infarcted tissue (and bone).[67,68] In infarcted tissue, ^{99m}Tc-PYP levels can be as high as 18 to 20 times that of normal myocardium, which gives rise to very distinct borders between the infarcted and normal myocardium.[67] The central core of infarcted myocardium may have a lower density of radiopharmaceutical due to absence of blood flow.[67,68] Although sensitivity and specificity of ^{99m}Tc-PYP for necrotic tissue is high, there are reports of myocardial uptake in unstable angina at sites of ventricular aneurysms and during ventricular dyskinesia, presumably because of marked ischemia occurring in such conditions.[68] Uptake of ^{99m}Tc-PYP into necrotic myocardium is delayed and not measurable until after about 4 hours of coronary occlusion. Scans during the first hours postinfarction may be negative. Scans become positive about 12 hours after occlusion, and peak intensity of ^{99m}Tc-PYP is reached at 48 hours. Washout occurs over 5 to 7 days so ^{99m}Tc-PYP is a useful late marker of infarction, especially in patients who present late or with a silent infarction.[67] Images are viewed by comparing sternum and rib uptake to that seen in the myocardium. After coronary artery bypass surgery, ^{99m}Tc-PYP imaging can be used to assess graft patency. Certain characteristics of the images obtained have been linked with various prognostic values, but as yet these remain observations and have not stood the test of comparative and long-term prognostic trials.

Other agents using technetium include technetium *t*-butyl isonitrile (^{99m}Tc-TIBI); technetium carboxy isopropyl isonitrile (^{99m}Tc-CPI); technetium sestamibi, also known as methoxy-isobutyl isonitrile (^{99m}Tc-MIBI), and technetium-teboroxime. Technetium-sestamibi has a similar myocardial uptake pattern to thallium, and has been shown to provide similar results. It generates a much higher photon yield, which improves image quality. Technetium-teboroxime is being evaluated in clinical trials to assess its safety and efficacy. The main advantages of the newer technetium compounds are their lack of redistribution perfusion and delayed imaging.[67] This is particularly useful in acute clinical settings; the radiopharmaceutical can be injected during the acute event, with imaging undertaken when the patient is more stable. The short half-life and favorable pharmacokinetic profile allow for individual high doses with repeat injections to evaluate efficacy of interventional therapy.[64,67,68]

THALLIUM SCANNING

Thallium is a potassium analog taken up into normal myocardium by passive diffusion and possibly by active transport via the Na^+/K^+-ATPase pump.[64,65,67,69] Uptake is dependent on regional blood flow and occurs in a linear fashion up to very high blood flow rates. Thallium uptake primarily occurs in perfused myocardium. Thallium uptake into ischemic myocardium occurs at a reduced rate. Scans taken during ischemia (e.g., stress testing with thallium) or infarction will show areas of poor or nil distribution of thallium. Scans taken 4 to 6 hours after the initial scan may show a redistribution of the thallium into areas that previously had little to no thallium uptake. These defects are referred to as partial defects, and demonstrate areas of hypoperfused but viable myocardium. Redistribution occurs because there is delayed (compared to normal tissue) washout of thallium from poorly perfused myocardium, resulting in less contrast between the density of thallium in different areas of the heart. This gives the appearance of "redistribution" of the radionuclide into the previously ischemic area when viewed on the scan. To enhance evaluation of potential partial defects, a second injection of thallium can be used. Late redistribution areas have improved perfusion after revascularization.[64,65] Areas of nil distribution are called "cold spots," or fixed defects and reflect infarcted myocardium.

Thallium scanning with the aid of computer analysis segregates the images into anatomic regions and specifically localizes areas of dead or necrotic myocardial tissue. In conjunction with echocardiography, thallium scans can correlate areas of abnormal wall motion with areas of poor perfusion. Sensitivity and specificity of thallium scanning to detect IHD disease is comparable to exercise stress testing (75% and 80%, respectively).[64,69] When used in conjunction with exercise ECG, sensitivity increases to about 80%. Thallium scanning can be used in conjunction with exercise testing, where thallium is injected at the peak of the exercise test, and exercise continues for another 30 to 60 seconds, when the initial images are taken. Repeat images are taken at 3 to 4 hours. Such testing allows detection of lower levels of ischemia than may be determined from ECG abnormalities or patient symptoms.[64,65,69]

Thallium scanning is useful in patients with atypical chest pain and ambiguous or false-positive ET to determine if IHD is the cause of symptoms and the ET abnormalities. Thallium scanning is also used for postoperative evaluation of revascularization or angioplasty procedures and for preoperative evaluation for prognostic stratification for persons with IHD. A normal thallium scan heralds a benign outcome, even in patients who have angiographically evident coronary disease.[64] The finding of redistribution is a marker of jeopardized but viable myocardium and has been shown to have important prognostic value. Major cardiac events such as myocardial infarction in patients with normal thallium-201 studies average less than 1% per year.[64] The best predictor of coronary events, which correlate thallium scans with clinical significance, are the number of myocardial segments with transient (redistribution) defects.

A number of other radiopharmaceuticals have found some use in cardiovascular testing, such as labeled antimyosin antibodies.[67] Theoretically, these antibodies should be more specific markers of myocyte necrosis. The currently used antibodies are a murine Fab fragment. Phase I, II, and III trials suggest that these are highly specific for irreversibly injured myocytes, but they have limitations in terms of pharmacokinetic properties. Uptake into myocardial tissues is very slow, with a prolonged blood pool activity seen for at least 24 hours. In clinical use, the antibody is given within 24 hours of the infarction, and planar or SPECT imaging undertaken 24 to 48 hours later. Despite the supposed specificity of the antibody to myosin, localization is more dependent on blood flow than myosin concentration, so accurate measurement of infarction size is not as accurate as expected. Another investigational agent, ^{123}-I-phenylpentadecanoic acid, is able to assess both myocardial perfusion and metabolism by virtue of its affinity for fatty acid metabolism.[67]

PHARMACOLOGIC STRESS TESTING

Pharmacologic stress testing is an alternative to ET in patients who are unable or unwilling to undergo ET.[64,69–75] The pharmacologic agent produces stress by a hyperemic (vasodilator) response or by increasing myocardial oxygen demand (heart rate and myocardial contractility). Agents currently used include dipyridamole and adenosine (hyperemic stress), and dobutamine (myocardial stress). Initially, pharmacologic stress tests were linked to thallium planar scanning as a means to detect ischemic response. Thallium scanning remains the most common modality for evaluating hyperemic response, but dobutamine is most frequently linked to echocardiography. Pharmacologic stress testing evaluates wall motion abnormalities and is comparable to exercise stress testing followed by ECG and echocardiography.[64]

The principle of dipyridamole and adenosine thallium imaging is related to their coronary arteriolar vasodilator properties. Dipyridamole inhibits adenosine cellular reuptake, resulting in increased concentrations of adenosine in the blood and tissues. Adenosine is a potent coronary artery vasodilator and can increase perfusion 4 to 5 times over baseline. Areas distal to a coronary artery obstruction will show a relative hypoperfusion compared to normal coronary arteries, as there is reduced perfusion pressure due to preferential perfusion of normal segments over stenotic segments. Acutely, such areas will appear as cold spots, but on the redistribution scans, such defects will fill if the area is viable but jeopardized myocardium.[69]

Both dipyridamole and adenosine can be used in conjunction with thallium scanning to detect areas of ischemia and jeopardized myocardium under stress. Thallium is given at the end of drug infusion in a dose of 2.5 to 4 mCi.[64] The maximum effect of dipyridamole occurs in about 5 minutes and adenosine at about 30 seconds after intravenous infusion. The heart is scanned about 5 minutes after thallium administration, with repeat scans done 4 hours later. Delayed images after 24 hours, as in thallium scanning, can be used to heighten the redistribution defects from fixed or partial defects.[64,70]

Like exercise thallium scanning, dipyridamole and adenosine scanning are used to detect IHD, evaluate prognosis of patients with known disease, and assess patients post-MI, and as a risk stratification method prior to vascular, cardiac, and noncardiac surgery.[71] Using planar scanning and dipyridamole, sensitivity to detect IHD is 90% with a 70% specificity, which is comparable to exercise thallium scanning.[64] Sensitivity to detect IHD with adenosine thallium planar scanning is 85% with a specificity of 90%. Adenosine may identify more ischemic segments, have fewer late adverse reactions, and cost less than dipyridamole.[63] Both agents may be used in conjunction with exercise testing, echocardiography, or the newer tomographic imaging techniques like SPECT.[69,70] SPECT scanning has at least comparable sensitivity and specificity to planar imaging, but produces higher-quality imaging which may enhance quantitative interpretation.

Dipyridamole testing has been shown to be safe and effective in the elderly and in those with unstable angina immediately post-MI (within days). It may also be used to assess the status of revascularization procedures.[70] Adverse effects with dipyridamole thallium testing are minimal, the main adverse effects being chest pain (with or without ischemic changes on the ECG), headache, dizziness, and nausea. Chest pain may not only be due to ischemia because not all patients demonstrate ECG changes.[70] Although systolic blood pressure decreases and heart rate increases during the test, these hemodynamic changes are not felt to interfere significantly with interpretation of the test to assess coronary blood flow. Adverse effects are related to the increased adenosine activity and can be ameliorated by xanthine compounds such as theophylline and caffeine. Xanthines are direct competitive antagonists of adenosine at the receptor level. Their use in dipyridamole testing to offset adverse effects is of questionable value, because adverse effects rapidly dissipate on completion of dipyridamole infusion. Pentoxifylline, also a methylxanthine, has been shown not to interfere with the test. Adenosine is associated with a higher incidence of adverse effects (80% versus 50%), but these are very transient.[64,73] Both agents are relatively contraindicated in patients with a history of bronchospasm.

The current dosage recommendation for dipyridamole is derived from investigational work in dogs, which demonstrated the maximum hyperemic response occurred with doses of 0.56 mg/kg given as a 4-minute intravenous infusion.[64,70,71] This dose has been shown to increase baseline coronary blood flow in the normal tissues up to four to five times over control. Some studies have used doses up to 0.84 mg/kg, to try and enhance further vasodilator response.[64] At the higher dose, adverse effects such as chest pain are more common, but cease within a few minutes of the end of the infusion.[64,69]

Use of adenosine for stress testing remains an unlabeled use of this drug. Studies are promising and correlate well with the experience of dipyridamole and coronary angiography.[69,73] The main advantage of adenosine is its short duration of action (approximately 10 seconds).

Dobutamine, a synthetic catecholamine increases heart rate and cardiac output, resulting in an increase in myocardial oxygen demand. Ischemia will develop in areas where stenosis prevents the increase in oxygen demand being met with increased blood flow. Ischemia can be detected by echocardiography as regional wall motion abnormalities.[64,74]

Dobutamine, when used as a stress test, is given in doses of 20 to 40 μg/kg/min. The dose is titrated up in 10 μg/kg/min increments, at 3-minute intervals. To increase heart rate to 85% of the patient's calculated maximum, atropine 0.6 to 2 mg may be used.[64] ECG and blood pressure are recorded continuously throughout the test, and echocardiographic recordings are made during the last minute of each dose level and during recovery.

Beta blocker and calcium channel blocker therapy may interfere with the heart rate response to dobutamine stress tests, and are recommended to be discontinued prior to the test. Dobutamine stress testing (DST) is relatively well tolerated. Reasons to discontinue the test include development of severe chest pain, extensive new wall motion abnormalities, ST elevation and depression suggestive of significant ischemia, tachyarrhythmias, and symptomatic reductions in blood pressure.[64,74] Beta blockers can be used to reverse most adverse effects if adverse effects persist. Dobutamine stress tests are contraindicated in patients with aortic stenosis, uncontrolled hypertension, and severe ventricular arrhythmias. Ventricular fibrillation and myocardial infarction occur at a rate of about 0.05%.[64,74]

Dobutamine stress testing has been studied as a diagnostic, prognostic, and therapy assessment tool postmyocardial infarction and for unstable and chronic angina.[75–78] One of the few comparative studies with dipyridamole and exercise stress testing compared to coronary angiography for diagnostic accuracy in patients with IHD showed an overall accuracy of 87% for exercise, 82% for dobutamine, and 77% for dipyridamole.[79] A recent review of 28 studies for the detection of IHD with DST calculated the sensitivity to be about 80% with an 84% specificity. Sensitivities were highest for detection of three-vessel disease (92%).[74] Comparative studies with ET and dipyridamole echocardiography show dobutamine to be more sensitive. Postmyocardial infarction, DST prognostically identifies patients at high risk of subsequent cardiac events. In patients with suspected or known IHD, a positive DST is an independent predictor of cardiac events, and a negative test affords protection from cardiac death.[75–78]

INTRAVASCULAR ULTRASOUND

Intravascular ultrasound (IVUS) combines braided polyethylene catheter technology with miniaturized ultrasound transducers that can be inserted into a variety of vascular beds within the body, including the coronary artery vasculature.[80,81] Catheter configuration varies and may include over-the-wire, monorail, and fixed guidewire tip configurations, resulting in different torqueability, steerability, and pushability characteristics for each type of catheter. There are two basic types of transducers, the solid-state, phased array or a rotating mechanical transducer. In general, the phased array transducers are smaller and may be mounted on more flexible catheters so that smaller vessels (such as coronary arteries) can be visualized, but require a more complex system for image reconstruction and show more artifact in imaging.

In contrast to angiography, IVUS provides quantitative information from within the vessel on diameter, circumference, luminal diameter, and percent stenosis. Qualitative information regarding the amount of plaque elevation, plaque composition (calcific, fibrous, or fatty plaque), and the presence of plaque versus thrombus, thrombus versus tumor, and aneurysm and hematoma can be provided with IVUS. IVUS is also used as a therapeutic adjunct with PTCA, atherectomy, stent or graft placement, and fibrinolysis. These combination procedures may be monitored in real time as the procedure (e.g., atherectomy) is being performed.

CORONARY ANGIOSCOPY

Percutaneous coronary angioscopy permits direct visualization of the luminal surface of coronary blood vessels.[82] The coronary angioscope is composed of a flexible catheter with a fiber-optic imaging bundle coupled with a video monitor and video recorder for live and archival viewing. Because a blood-free field is necessary for viewing, an occlusion catheter on the end of the catheter can be inflated for 45 to 90 seconds in a disease-free portion of the artery of interest and flushed with saline or lactated Ringer's solution to view diseased segments.

Although the role of angioscopy is still being developed, the recognized uses include guiding saphenous vein bypass graft interventions, postinterventional evaluation of lesions, identification of culprit and borderline lesions, stent deployment, and directing of procedures to achieve better outcomes with fewer complications. The limitations of angioscopy include lack of cross-sectional information, large fluid boluses to clear the field, large introducer size, and length of the procedure. Currently, this technology is not widely available but it holds promise for future applications.

REFERENCES

1. Ryan TJ, Anderson JL, Rapaport E, et al. ACC/AHA guidelines for the management of patients with acute myocardial infarction: A report of the American College of Cardiology/American Heart Association task force on practice guidelines (committee on management of acute myocardial infarction.) J Am Coll Cardiol 1996;28:1328–1428.
2. American Heart Association. AHA medical/scientific statement. Classification of functional capacity and objective assessment of patients with diseases of the heart. Circulation 1994;90:644–645.
3. Bernstein SJ, Hilborne LH, Leape LL, et al. The appropriateness of use of cardiovascular procedures in women and men. Arch Intern Med 1994;1554:2759–2765.
4. Braunwald E. Physical examination. In: Braunwald E, ed. Heart Disease: A Textbook of Cardiovascular Medicine, 4th ed. Philadelphia, Saunders, 1992:13–42.
5. O'Rourke RA, Braunwald E. Physical examination of the cardiovascular system. In Fauci AS, Braunwald E, Isselbacher KJ, et al, eds. Harrison's Principles of Internal Medicine, 14th ed. New York, McGraw-Hill, 1998:1231–1237.
6. Come PC, Lee RT, Braunwald E. Noninvasive methods of cardiac examination. In Isselbacher KJ, Braunwald E, Wilson JD, et al, eds. Harrison's Principles of Internal Medicine, 13th ed. New York, McGraw-Hill, 1994:966–972.
7. Goldberger AL. Electrocardiography. In: Fauci AS, Braunwald E, Isselbacher KJ, et al, eds. Harrison's Principles of Internal Medicine, 14th ed. New York, McGraw-Hill, 1998:1237–1247.
8. Davis D. How to Quickly and accurately master ECG Interpretation, 2nd ed. Philadelphia, Lippincott, 1992:89–95, 235–273.
9. Fisch C. Evolution of the clinical electrocardiogram. J Am Coll Cardiol 1989;14:1127–1138.
10. Garland JL, Wolfson AB. Routine admission electrocardiography in emergency department patients. Ann Emerg Med 1994;23:275–280.
11. ACC expert consensus document: Signal averaged electrocardiography. J Am Coll Cardiol 1996;27:238–249.
12. Clinical competence in ambulatory electrocardiography. A statement for physicians from the ACP/ACC/AHA task force on clinical privileges in cardiology. J Am Coll Cardiol 1993;22:331–335.
13 Fisch C, DeSanctis RW, Dodge HT, et al. Guidelines for ambulatory electrocardiography. J Am Coll Cardiol 1989;13:249–258.
14. DiMarco JP, Philbrick JT. Ambulatory electrocardiographic (Holter) monitoring. Ann Intern Med 1990;113:77–79.
15. Resch DD. Diagnostic and prognostic value of ambulatory electrocardiographic monitoring in older patients. J Am Geriatr Soc 1996; 43:66–70.
16. Reiter MJ, Karagounis LA, Mann De, et al. Reproducibility of drug efficacy predictions by Holter monitoring in the electrophysiologic study versus electrocardiographic monitoring (ESVEM) trial. Am J Cardiol 1997;79:315–322.
17. Linzer M, Yang EH, Estes M, et al. Diagnosing syncope. Part 1: Value of history, physical examination and electrocardiography. Ann Intern Med 1997;126:989–996.
18. Sharaf BL, Williams DO, Miele RP, et al. A detailed angiographic analysis of patients with ambulatory electrocardiographic ischemia: Results from the Asymptomatic Cardiac Ischemia Pilot (ACIP) study of angiographic core laboratory. J Am Coll Cardiol 1997;29:78–84.

19. Chaitman B. Exercise stress testing. In: Braunwald E, ed. Heart Disease: A Textbook of Cardiovascular Medicine, 4th ed. Philadelphia, Saunders, 1992:161–179.
20. Gibbins RJ, Balady GJ, Beasley JW, et al. ACC/AHA guidelines for exercise testing: A report of the American College of Cardiology/American Heart Association task force on practice guidelines on exercise testing. J Am Coll Cardiol 1997;30:260–315.
21. Mark D. Prognostic value of a treadmill exercise score in outpatients with suspected coronary artery disease. N Engl J Med 1991;325: 849–853.
22. Seceri S, Michelassi C. Prognostic impact of stress testing in coronary artery disease. Circulation 1991;83(suppl 3):82–89.
23. Pina IL, Balady GJ, Hanson P, et al. Guidelines for clinical exercise testing laboratories: A statement for healthcare professionals from the committee on exercise and cardiac rehabilitation, American Heart Association. Circulation 1995;91:912–921.
24. Fletcher GF, Balady G, Froelicher VF, et al. Exercise standards: A statement for healthcare professionals from the American Heart Association. Circulation 1995;91:580–615.
25. Grossman W, Barry WH. Cardiac catheterization. In: Braunwald E, ed. Heart Disease: A Textbook of Cardiovascular Medicine, 4th ed. Philadelphia, Saunders, 1992:180–205.
26. Baim DS, Grossman W. Diagnostic cardiac catheterization and angiography. In: Fauci AS, Braunwald E, Isselbacher KJ, et al, eds. Harrison's Principles of Internal Medicine, 14th ed. New York, McGraw-Hill, 1998:1247–1253.
27. Levin DC, Gardiner GA. Cardiac arteriography. In Braunwald E, ed. Heart Disease: A Textbook of Cardiovascular Medicine, 4th ed. Philadelphia, Saunders, 1992:235–275.
28. Report of the American College of Cardiology/American Heart Association task force on assessment of diagnostic and therapeutic cardiovascular procedures (subcommittee on cardiac catheterization). Guidelines for cardiac catheterization and cardiac catheterization laboratories. J Am Coll Cardiol 1991;18:1149–1182.
29. Report of the American College of Cardiology/American Heart Association task force on assessment of diagnostic and therapeutic cardiovascular procedures (subcommittee on coronary angiography). Guidelines for coronary angiography. J Am Coll Cardiol 1987;10:935–950.
30. Walder LA, Schaller FA. Diagnostic cardiac catheterization. When is it appropriate? Postgrad Med 1995;97:37–42.
31. Ryan TJ, Bauman WB, Kennedy JW, et al. Guidelines for percutaneous transluminal coronary 81 angioplasty: A report of the ACC/AHA task force on assessment of diagnostic and therapeutic cardiovascular procedures (committee on percutaneous transluminal coronary angioplasty). J Am Coll Cardiol 1993;22:2033–2054.
32. Foley DP, Escaned J, Strauss BH, et al. Quantitative coronary angiography (QCA) in interventional cardiology: clinical application of QCA measurements. Prog Cardiovasc Dis 1994;36:363–384.
33. Reagan K, Boxt LM, Katz J. Introduction to coronary arteriography. Radiol Clin North Am 1994;32:419–433.
35. Gorlin R. Perspectives on invasive cardiology: The 24th Louis F. Bishop lecture. J Am Coll Cardiol 1994;23:525–532.
36. Topol EJ, Nissen SE. Our preoccupation with coronary luminology. The dissociation between clincial and angiographic findings on ischemic heart disease. Circulation 1995; 92:2333–2342.
36. Landau C, Lange RA, Hillis LD. Percutaneous transluminal coronary angioplasty. N Engl J Med 1994;330:981–993.
37. Strauss BH, Escaned J, Foley DP, et al. Technological considerations and practical limitations in the use of quantitative angiography during percutaneous coronary recanalization. Prog Cardiovasc Dis 1994; 36:343–362
38. Higgins CB. Newer cardiac imaging techniques: CT, MRI. In Braunwald E, ed. Heart Disease: A Textbook of Cardiovascular Medicine, 4th ed. Philadelphia, Saunders, 1992,312–341.
39. Higgins CB. New cardiac imaging techniques. In Isselbacher KJ, Braunwald E, Wilson JD, et al, eds. Harrison's Principles of Internal Medicine, 13th ed. New York, McGraw-Hill, 1994:972–979.
40. Thompson BH, Stanford W. Evaluation of cardiac function with ultrafast computed tomography. Radiol Clin North Am 1995;32:537–554.
41. Lazem F, Barbir M, Banner N, et al. Coronary calcification detected by ultrafast computed tomography is a predictor of cardiac events in heart transplant recipients. Transplant Proc 1997;29:572–575.
42. Ganz W, Serafini A, Lerner D. et al. Cardiovascular magnetic resonance imaging goes beyond anatomy. Crit Rev Diagn Imaging 1995; 36:479–503.
43. Hartiala J, Knuuti J. Imaging of the heart by MRI and PET. Ann Med 1995;27:35–45.
44. Hartiala J, Sakuma H, Higgins CB. Magnetic resonance imaging and spectroscopy of the human heart. Scand J Clin Lab Invest 1993; 53:425–437.
45. McMillan RM. Cardiac magnetic resonance imaging. Cardiovasc Clin 1003;23:125–135.
46. De Roos A, van der Wall EE. Evaluation of ischemic heart disease by magnetic resonance imaging and spectroscopy. Radiol Clin North Am 1994;32:581–592.
47. Globits S, Higgins CB. Assessment of valvular heart disease by magnetic resonance imaging. Am Heart J 1995;129:369–381.
48. McGhie AI. Positron emission tomography. In: Raizner AE, ed. Topics in Cardiology: Indications for Diagnostic Procedures. New York, Igaku-Shoin, 1997:81–98.
49. Go RT, MacIntyre WJ, Chen EQ, et al. Current status of the clinical applications of cardiac positron emission tomography. Radiol Clin North Am 1995;32:501–520.
50. Schelbert HR. Metabolic imaging to assess myocardial viability. J Nucl Med 1994;35(suppl):8s–14s.
51. Schwaiger M, Beanlands R, vom Dahl J. Metabolic tissue characterization in the failing heart by positron emission tomography. Eur Hear J 1994;15 (suppl D):14.
52. Canmici PG, Gropler RJ, Jones T, et al. The impact of myocardial blood flow quantification with PET on the understanding of heart diseases. Eur Heart J 1996;17:25–34.
53. Schwaiger M, Hutchins G. Quantification of regional myocardial perfusion by PET: Rationale and first clinical results. Eur Heart J 1995;16 (suppl J):84–91.
54. Schwaiger M, Muzik O. Assessment of myocardial perfusion by perfusion emission tomography. Am J Cardiol 1991;67:35D–43D.
55. Feigenbaum H. Echocardiography. In Braunwald E, ed. Heart Disease: A Textbook of Cardiovascular Medicine, 4th ed. Philadelphia, Saunders, 1992:64–115.
56. Popp RL. Echocardiography. In: Bennett JC, Plum F, Gill GN, et al, eds. Cecil Textbook of Medicine, 20th ed. Philadelphia, Saunders 1996:194–199.
57. Cheitlin MD, Alpert JS, Armstrong WF, et al. ACC/AHA guidelines for the clincial application of echocardiography: A report of the American College of Cardiology/American Heart Association task force on practice guidelines (committee on clinical application of echocardiography). Circulation 1997;95:1686–1744.
58. Fisher EA, Stahl JA, Budd JH, et al. Transesophageal echocardiography: Procedures and clinical application. J Am Coll Cardiol 1991; 18:1333–1348.
59. Seward JB, Khandheria BK, Oh JK, et al. Critical appraisal of transesophageal echocardiography: Limitations, pitfalls, and complications. J Am Soc Echocardiogr 1992;5:288–305.
60. Shively BK, Gurule FT, Roldan CA, et al. Diagnostic value of transesophageal compared with transthoracic echocardiography in infective endocarditis. J Am Coll Cardiol 1991;18:391–397.
61. Birmingham GD, Rahko PS, Ballantyne F III. Improved detection of infective endocarditis with transesophageal echocardiography. Am Heart J 1992;123:774–781.
62. Zaret BL, Wachers FJ, Soufer R. Nuclear cardiology. In:Braunwald E, ed. Heart Disease: A Textbook of Cardiovascular Medicine, 4th ed. Philadelphia, Saunders, 1992:276–311.
63. Taillefer R, Amyot R, Turpin S, Lambert R. Comparison between dipyridamole and adenosine as pharmacologic coronary vasodilators

in detection of coronary artery disease with thallium 201 imaging. J Nucl Cardiol 1996;3:204–11.
64. Report of the American College of Cardiology/American Heart Association task force on assessment of diagnostic and therapeutic cardiovascular procedures (committee on radionuclide imaging, developed in collaboration with the American Society of Nuclear Cardiology). Guidelines for clinical use of cardiac radionuclide imaging. Circulation 1995;91:1278–1303.
65. Zaret BL, Wackers FJ. Nuclear imaging in cardiology. Part I. N Engl J Med 1993;329:775–783.
66. Zaret BL, Wackers FJ. Nuclear imaging in cardiology. Part II. N Engl J Med 1993;329:855–863.
67. Kahn JK, Pippin JJ, Corbett JR. New radionuclides for cardiac imaging: Descriptive applications. Cardiol Clin 1989;7:589–591.
68. Khan BA, Heber E. Imaging necrotic myocardium with 99m technetium-pyrophosphate and radiolabeled antibodies. Cardiol Clin 1989; 7:577–588.
69. Beller GA. Pharmacological stress testing. JAMA 1991;265:633–638.
70. Iskandrian AS, Heo J, Askenase A, et al. Dipyridamole cardiac imaging. Am Heart J 1988;115:432–443.
71. Stratmann HG, Kennedy HL. Evaluation of coronary artery disease in the patient unable to exercise: Alternatives to exercise stress testing. Am Heart J 1989;117:1344–1365.
72. Mahmarian JJ, Verani MS. Exercise thallium-201 perfusion scintigraphy in the assessment of coronary artery disease. Am J Cardiol 1991; 67:2D–11D.
73. Verani MS. Adenosine thallium-201 myocardial perfusion scintigraphy. Am Heart J 1991;122:269–277.
74. Geleijnse ML, Fioretti PM, Roelandt JRTC. Methodology, feasibility, safety and diagnostic accuracy of dobutamine stress echocardiography. J Am Coll Cardiol 1997;30:595–606.
75. Sicari R, Picano E, Landi P, et al. Prognostic value of dobutamine–atropine stress echocardiography early after acute myocardial infarction. J Am Coll Cardiol 1997;29:254–260.
76. Greco CA, Salustri A, Seccareccia F, et al. Prognostic value of dobutamine echocardiography early after uncomplicated acute myocardial infarction: A comparison with exercise electrocardiography. J Am Coll Cardiol 1997;29:261–267.
77. Rallidis L, Cokkinos P, Tousoulis D, Nihoyannopoulos P. Comparison of dobutamine and treadmill exercise echocardiogrpahy in inducing ischemia in patients with coronary artery disease. J Am Coll Cardiol 1997;30:1660–1668.
78. Steinberg EH, Madmon L, Patel CP, et al. Long term prognostic significance of dobutamine echocardiography in patients with suspected coronary artery disease: Results of a 5 year follow up study. J Am Coll Cardiol 1997;29:969–973.
79. Beleslin BD, Ostojic M, Stepanovic J, et al. Stress echocardiography in the detection of myocardial ischemia. Head to toe comparison of exercise, dobutamine, and dipyridamole test. Circulation 1994; 90:1168–1176.
80. Metz JA, Yock PG, Fitzgerald PJ. Intravascular ultrasound: Basic interpretation. Cardiol Clin 1997;15:1–16.
81. Benenati JF. Intravascular ultrasound. The role in diagnostic and therapeutic procedures. Cardiol Clin 1997;15:141–159.
82. Annex BH. Coronary angioscopy: Clinical applications. Cardiol Clin 1997;15:131–140.

9

CARDIOPULMONARY RESUSCITATION

Lori A. Jones, PharmD

Sudden death has been described as the leading medical emergency in the United States.[1] Of the 300,000 to 750,000 individuals in the United States who experience a cardiac arrest each year, approximately 200,000 receive cardiopulmonary resuscitation (CPR) attempts.[2,3] By definition, cardiopulmonary arrest occurs when spontaneous and effective ventilation and circulation abruptly terminate following a cardiac or respiratory event.[4]

Resuscitation attempts are thought to date back to Egyptian mythology and the biblical era.[5] These early efforts at restoring life centered on the sole provision of providing artificial resuscitation. The modern era of CPR began in the late 1950s and early 1960s.[4,6] In 1958, Safar and colleagues[7] demonstrated that adequate artificial ventilation could be provided using a mouth-to-mouth resuscitation technique. Later in 1960, Kouwenhoven and colleagues proved in animal models that administering closed-chest compressions enabled successful defibrillation following prolonged ventricular fibrillation.[8] Subsequently, resuscitation methods combining variations of mouth-to-mouth ventilation and closed-chest compressions led to the development of modern CPR techniques.

EPIDEMIOLOGY AND ETIOLOGY

The etiology of cardiopulmonary arrest varies depending on patient age and the presence of comorbidities. In adults, sudden death usually results from the development of cardiac arrhythmias. For those individuals possessing underlying coronary artery disease, sudden death most often occurs outside the hospital and within hours of developing related symptoms.[1] It has been estimated that approximately 80% to 90% of all nontraumatic adult cardiac arrests are initiated by either ventricular tachycardia (VT) or ventricular fibrillation (VF).[1] Several researchers have recently challenged the validity of this statement and suggest that the true incidence of VT or VF is lower than initially predicted.[1] They argue that early estimates were biased since studies dealt primarily with patients undergoing ambulatory electrocardiographic (ECG) monitoring. Regardless of the initiating rhythm, only 35% to 55% of all adults suffering out of hospital cardiac arrests are actually found in either VF or VT.[9] In addition, the percentage of patients presenting with VF or VT declines as patient age increases.[10] The importance of this issue is based on improved survival rates for these rhythms as compared with other presenting arrhythmias. Approximately 20% of patients found initially in VF or VT survive to hospital discharge versus 1% to 7% of those found in asystole or pulseless electrical activity (PEA).[11]

Pediatric arrests most commonly result from primary respiratory arrests that if not treated successfully then progress to full cardiopulmonary arrest. Most pediatric arrests occur subsequent to the following: sudden infant death syndrome, trauma, drowning, pulmonary infection, or aspiration.[12] Primary cardiac arrests are uncommon in pediatric patients except in the presence of underlying cardiac abnormalities.[13] As a result of their etiology, most pediatric patients with cardiopulmonary arrest present with initial rhythms of asystole or PEA.[12] Less than 15% of these patients present with either VF or VT. Subsequently, survival from pediatric cardiopulmonary arrest is quite dismal. Although most studies have demonstrated survival rates between 3% and 17%, many survivors have poor neurologic outcomes.[13]

PATHOPHYSIOLOGY AND OUTCOME MEASURES OF CPR

Two theories exist regarding the mechanism of blood flow in CPR.[4,14] The initial theory, known as the *cardiac pump theory,* explains forward blood flow based on active compression of the heart between the sternum and vertebrae. During compression, an "artificial systole" is produced in which intraventricular pressure increases, the atrioventricular valves close, the aortic valve opens, and blood is forced from the right and left ventricles. When ventricular compression ends, the atrioventricular valves reopen to allow blood to fill the ventricles passively during an analogous diastole. Alternatively, the *thoracic pump theory* gained prominence in the late 1970s after the discovery of cough CPR.[4,14] The thoracic pump theory is founded on the belief that blood flow during CPR results from intrathoracic pressure alterations induced by chest compressions. During compression, or systole, a pressure gradient develops between the intrathoracic arteries and extrathoracic veins, causing forward blood flow from the lungs into the systemic circulation. Retrograde blood flow is inhibited by the operation of venous valves. After compression ends, or in diastole, intrathoracic pressure declines. This subsequently reverses the pressure gradient and results in blood return to the lungs. Therefore, in the thoracic pump theory, the heart acts merely as a passive organ through which blood flows.

Both the cardiac pump and the thoracic pump theories have been challenged since their inception. In reality, components of both theories may operate during CPR.[4,14] Despite the controversy, experimental methods of performing CPR have been developed based on the assertions of these divergent theories. As discussed previously, cough CPR follows the thoracic pump theory.[15] This technique is primarily used in closely monitored situations, such as the cardiac catheterization laboratory, in which ventricular fibrillation occurs. During vigorous coughing, intrathoracic pressures increase secondary to contraction of the diaphragm, abdominal, and intracostal muscles while the glottis remains closed. During this "cough systole," forward blood flow is achieved, which maintains cerebral perfusion. "Cough diastole" is initiated upon inhalation. At this time, declining intrathoracic and intraabdominal pressures promote ventricular filling, coronary perfusion, and venous return. By increasing cerebral blood flow, consciousness can be maintained until definitive therapy can be given.[15]

Adequately performed standard CPR techniques provide cerebral and myocardial blood flow rates comparable to 30% and 10% of their prearrest values, respectively.[2] Consequently, superior methods of providing CPR have been sought. Three investigational methods that have been studied use either a pneumatic vest, interposed abdominal compression, or active compression–decompression (ACD).[14] Although preliminary studies suggested that each of these techniques achieves significantly higher initial resuscitation rates than standard CPR techniques,[16–18] these results have not been demonstrated in large-scale trials. In fact, Stiell and colleagues recently published a trial comparing standard CPR and ACD in 773 in-hospital and 1011 prehospital cardiac arrest patients.[19] These investigators found no improvement in either immediate or long-term survival. Additionally, neurologic outcome of survivors was not different between the two methods.[19] Therefore, further research is necessary to document the relative advantages and disadvantages of each investigational CPR technique before their use can be endorsed on a widespread basis.

That brings us to the issue of outcome measures. Until recently, a myriad of outcome measures had been selected as end points for published CPR research. Due to the variability in definitions assigned to these end points, great difficulty exists in comparing results obtained by different investigators. The most obvious end point of CPR is survival. Although seemingly unambiguous, survival has been defined in terms of initial resuscitation, 24-hour survival, hospital discharge, and 1-year survival. Neurologic outcome has been similarly determined at varying timepoints and by nonstandard methods. Two hemodynamic parameters often studied are coronary and cerebral perfusion pressure. Coronary perfusion pressure is defined as aortic diastolic pressure minus right atrial diastolic pressure. Physiologically, raising aortic diastolic pressure shunts blood toward the heart and brain. Paradis and colleagues demonstrated that obtaining coronary perfusion pressures above 15 mm Hg is a positive predictor of return of spontaneous circulation (ROSC) in humans.[20] ROSC has been one of the most frequently employed outcome measures but has also been defined in many ways. Arbitrary definitions for ROSC have included the attainment of either a predetermined heart rate and/or blood pressure measurement for varying lengths of time (e.g., 1 to 5 minutes). In an effort to standardize both resuscitation definitions and data collection forms, guidelines have been introduced for prehospital, in-hospital, and pediatric cardiopulmonary arrests.[21–23]

▶ Treatment: Cardiopulmonary Resuscitation

DESIRED OUTCOME

The goal of attempting cardiopulmonary resuscitation is to return effective ventilation and circulation as quickly as possible to minimize hypoxic damage to vital organs. It is not sufficient to merely return spontaneous circulation if the patient is left neurologically devastated or incurs severe morbidity in the process. Therefore, it is necessary to determine factors that predict successful resuscitation as well as those that predict futility. Factors proven to enhance prehospital survival include the following: occurrence of a witnessed arrest, presence of VF or VT, rapid implementation of bystander CPR, early administration of defibrillation therapy for VF, and early application of prehospital advanced cardiac life support (ACLS).[11,24] Considerable controversy, however, surrounds the identification of patient-specific factors affecting resuscitation survival. Much of the disagreement is probably related to the relatively small populations examined, many of which are not generalizable due to specific inclusion and exclusion criteria applied in these studies.

GENERAL APPROACH TO TREATMENT

Since the mid-1960s, organized committees have convened periodically to encourage widespread competency in CPR techniques. In 1966, the National Academy of Sciences–National Research Council (NAS–NRC) recommended that all health care professionals be proficient in current CPR procedures. Since that time, five additional conferences have been organized by the American Heart Association (AHA) to update philosophies for providing CPR and emergency cardiac care (ECC) to the general population. The most recent guidelines are the result of the 1997 National Conference on CPR and ECC.[1] In addition to developing guidelines for providing basic life support (BLS) and ACLS, the committee recognized the importance of increasing public education on the prevention of cardiovascular and cerebrovascular disease. Likewise, emphasis has been placed on educating patients to identify early warning signs and symptoms so that medical care can be accessed earlier. Committee recommendations for all therapeutic interventions are classified into three

TABLE 9–1. Responsibilities for Cardiac Resuscitation Team Members

Team Member	Responsibilities
Physician-in-charge	Team leader; determines appropriate therapy; directs and oversees order implementation including provision of CPR, electrical therapy, endotracheal intubation, intravenous access, EKG monitoring, and drug administration; arranges postresuscitation care
Surgeon	Identifies surgically correctable causes for arrest
Anesthesiologist	Performs endotracheal intubation; provides adequate oxygenation; may assist with obtaining vascular access
Respiratory therapist	Maintains adequate oxygenation and ventilation
Nurse	Records timing and outcome of therapeutic interventions; may assist with chest compressions, obtaining peripheral venous access, administering fluids and medications, and acquiring blood samples for laboratory determination
Pharmacist	Prepares medications for administration; provides drug information; documents medication administration including name, dose, route, and time; may assist with chest compressions

(Adapted from Ref. 28).

categories according to the significance of available scientific literature.[1] Class I recommendations are considered to be appropriate and efficacious. Class II recommendations are subdivided into the following: IIa, probably beneficial and efficacious; and IIb, possibly beneficial without causing harm. Recommendations in Class III are considered to be inappropriate and potentially harmful. These recommendations have additionally been organized into treatment algorithms based on the underlying cardiac arrhythmia.

As discussed above, the guidelines supplied by the National Conference on CPR and ECC primarily address the provision of BLS and ACLS for adults, children, and neonates. BLS is based on the assessment and application of the ABCs: airway, breathing, and circulation. Initially, an unconscious victim should be assessed for the presence of spontaneous breathing. If absent, the airway should be opened and rescue breathing attempted. After successfully securing the airway, the individual should be examined for the presence of a palpable carotid or femoral pulse. A series of closed-chest compressions combined with rescue breathing should be performed only if the victim is deemed pulseless. Once begun, BLS should be continued until ROSC is achieved, ACLS is obtained, or exhaustion prohibits continued efforts. There has been discussion of incorporating defibrillation into BLS training for two reasons: (1) early defibrillation is known to improve survival from cardiac arrest for patients in VF or VT, and (2) automatic electronic defibrillators (AEDs) are becoming more common within the community setting.[25] It should be stated, however, that application of AEDs is currently inappropriate in pediatric patients due to the weight-based energy requirements advocated for these victims.[13] In contrast to BLS, ACLS incorporates all the following: CPR, electrical defibrillation, airway management, ECG monitoring, and drug administration.

In an effort to highlight crucial components for successful resuscitation, the National Council on CPR and ECC has orchestrated the "chain of survival."[1] Based on the concept that "a chain is only as strong as its weakest link," each element incorporated into the chain is essential for improving resuscitation outcomes. The four components in the "chain of survival" are swift emergency system entry (enhanced 911), prompt bystander CPR, early defibrillation of VF or VT, and rapid ACLS.[1] One avenue for implementing the chain of survival concept is through the development of in-hospital cardiac resuscitation teams. The idea of a team approach toward cardiac resuscitation has existed since the early 1960s.[26] It was not until the late 1960s, however, that pharmacists began participating as cardiac resuscitation team members.[27] By defining roles for specific health care professionals, it is hoped that resuscitation attempts will become more efficient and consequently more effective. A representative code team may consist of the following persons: physician-in-charge, surgeon, anesthesiologist, respiratory therapist, nurse, and pharmacist.[28] Team composition varies though among institutions. Typical roles for each team member are listed in Table 9–1.[28] Overall, the physician-in-charge coordinates the cardiac resuscitation effort and decides which therapeutic interventions are appropriate for the given situation. In addition, the physician-in-charge directs and oversees the actions of all other team members. With regard to participation of pharmacists, their roles have greatly expanded from the primary drug-preparation focus prevalent in the late 1960s.[27] Unfortunately, in a 1992 survey conducted in 1597 United States hospital-based pharmacies, only 30% of all hospitals possessing cardiac resuscitation teams included pharmacists.[29] These results are similar to those reported by Shimp and colleagues.[30] Alarmingly, these investigators found that 59% of hospitals with pharmacists participating on resuscitation teams did not require BLS certification for pharmacists.[30] This is in direct opposition to the current national guidelines, which advocate that all health care members responding to cardiopulmonary emergencies be trained in providing BLS and defibrillation using AEDs.[31]

VENTRICULAR FIBRILLATION AND PULSELESS VENTRICULAR TACHYCARDIA

NONPHARMACOLOGIC THERAPY

Cardiac arrest victims found in either pulseless ventricular tachycardia (PVT) or VF should receive immediate electrical defibrillation using up to three countershocks. In adult victims, the initial defibrillation attempt should begin with 200 J. If PVT or VF persists, a second and third attempt is recommended using 200 to 300 J and 360 J, respectively. In pediatric patients, defibrillation energy is applied using a weight-based dose. For pediatric patients, the initial defibrillation attempt should begin with 2 J/kg, whereas all successive attempts should use 4 J/kg. Following unsuccessful defibrillation, the patient should receive CPR, endotracheal intubation, and intravenous (IV) access. Once an airway is achieved, patients should be ventilated with 100% oxygen. Pharmacologic agents, such as sympathomimetics and antiarrhythmics, are not recommended until an airway is obtained and IV access is attempted (see Fig. 9–1).

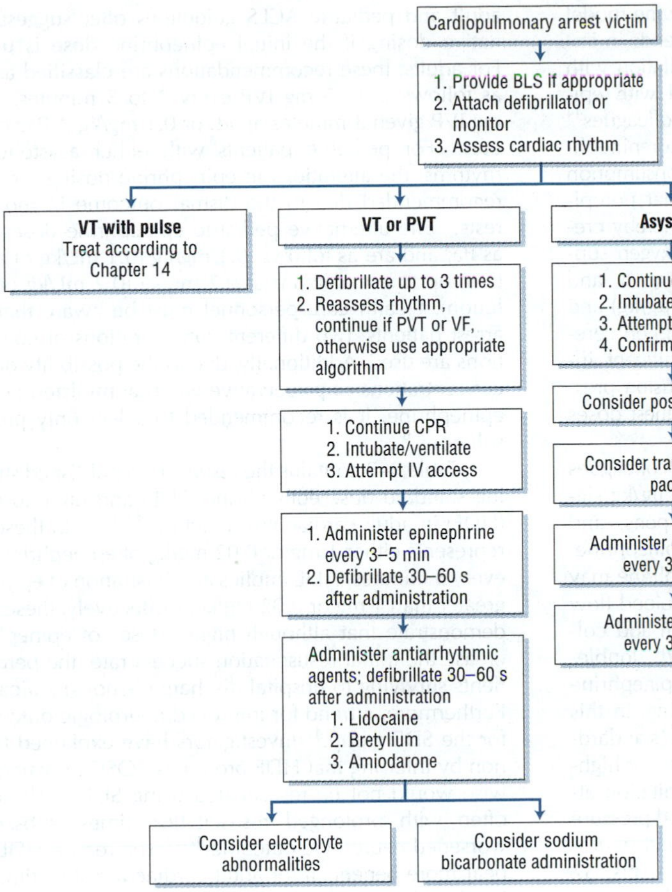

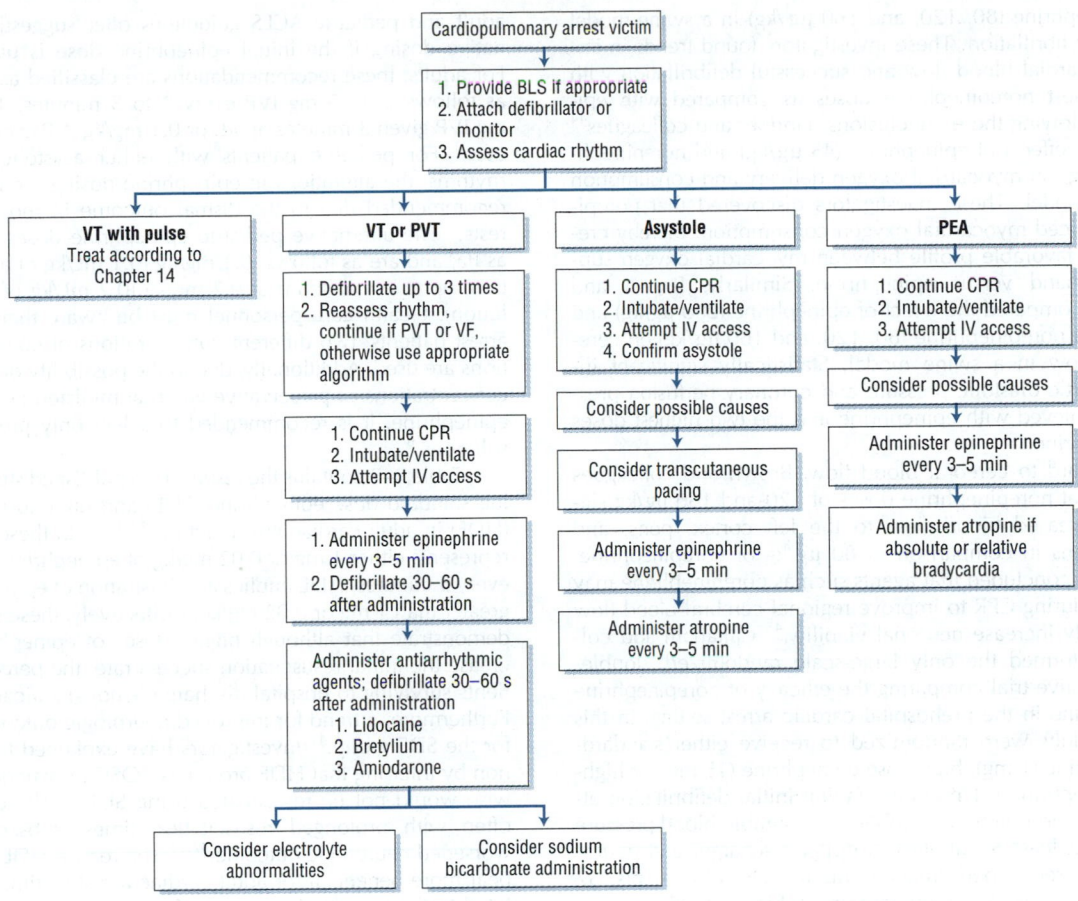

FIGURE 9–1. Treatment algorithm for adult cardiopulmonary arrest.

PHARMACOLOGIC THERAPY

SYMPATHOMIMETICS

The goal of using adrenergic agonist agents is to augment both coronary and cerebral blood flow present during the low-flow state associated with CPR.[2] Animal studies have demonstrated that coronary perfusion pressure averages between 10 and 15 mm Hg with CPR alone following 10 minutes of ventricular fibrillation.[32] This inability to raise coronary perfusion pressure results from the fact that standard CPR is unable to increase aortic diastolic pressure significantly. Following administration of epinephrine or norepinephrine, aortic diastolic pressure significantly increases without altering right atrial diastolic pressure.[32] Therefore, by definition, these agents successfully raise coronary perfusion pressure. In addition, agents possessing α-adrenergic activity prevent carotid artery collapse, thereby increasing cerebral blood flow.[33]

Although cardiac arrest is associated with high concentrations of endogenous catecholamines, aortic diastolic pressure, myocardial blood flow, and cerebral blood flow remain low.[34] Several theories addressing the need for exogenous catecholamine administration during CPR include reduced myocardial sensitivity with acidosis or hypoxemia, decreased number of available receptors, and reduced receptor affinity.[35–41] As yet, the optimal adrenergic agent has not been identified. Currently, epinephrine (an α_1, α_2, β_1, and β_2 agonist) is recommended as first-line pharmacologic therapy in the treatment of VF, PVT, asystole, and PEA. A multitude of studies, however, have compared sympathomimetic agents during CPR to distinguish desirable properties.[34] Pure α_1-agonist agents, such as phenylephrine and methoxamine, have been compared with epinephrine to determine whether β-agonist–related increases in myocardial oxygen demand impact negatively on cardiac arrest outcome. To date, superiority of these agents over epinephrine has not been demonstrated in human studies.[42] One reason for this finding may be related to the postsynaptic α_2 activity of epinephrine. Postsynaptic α_1-receptors, which reside in the adventitia–medial border of vascular smooth muscle, respond primarily to neuronally released norepinephrine.[43] Conversely, postsynaptic α_2-receptors are located extrajunctionally on the intimal region of the vessel lumen.[43] Since IV medications are in contact with the intimal blood vessel layer, it is thought that postsynaptic α_2-receptors may be responsible for mediating much of the vasopressor response from exogenous catecholamine administration.[43] Furthermore, during ischemia, the number of postsynaptic α_1-receptors decreases, which suggests a greater role for postsynaptic α_2-agonist activity during CPR.[34]

Another agent possessing postsynaptic α_2-agonist activity is norepinephrine (an α_1, α_2, and β_1 agonist). Since it has been hypothesized that β_2-agonist–induced vasodilation might counteract the efficacy of α-agonist–induced vasoconstriction, investigators have compared exogenous administration of epinephrine and norepinephrine to determine the impact of β_2-agonist activity during CPR.[32,44–47] In 1989, Robinson and colleagues[32] conducted a study comparing the effects of epinephrine (200 μg/kg) and norepinephrine (80, 120, and 160 μg/kg) in a swine model of ventricular fibrillation. These investigators found trends in improved myocardial blood flow and successful defibrillation with the two highest norepinephrine doses as compared with epinephrine. Following these conclusions, Lindner and colleagues[44] examined the effects of epinephrine (45 μg/kg) and norepinephrine (45 μg/kg) on myocardial oxygen delivery and consumption in a swine model. These investigators discovered that norepinephrine reduced myocardial oxygen consumption, thereby creating a more favorable profile between myocardial oxygen supply and demand versus epinephrine. Similarly, Brown and colleagues[45] compared the effect of epinephrine (200 μg/kg) and three doses of norepinephrine (80, 120, and 160 μg/kg) on cerebral blood flow in a swine model. Statistically significant increases in aortic diastolic pressure and coronary perfusion pressure were achieved with epinephrine and the two highest doses of norepinephrine.

With regard to cerebral blood flow, Brown and colleagues discovered that norepinephrine doses of 120 and 160 μg/kg significantly increased blood flow to the left cortex, pons, and medulla regions in comparison to 80 μg/kg of norepinephrine. These authors concluded that agents such as norepinephrine may be preferred during CPR to improve regional cerebral blood flow and potentially increase neuronal viability.[45] Callaham and colleagues[47] performed the only large-scale randomized, double-blind, prospective trial comparing the efficacy of norepinephrine and epinephrine in the prehospital cardiac arrest setting. In this study, 816 adults were randomized to receive either standard-dose epinephrine (1 mg), high-dose epinephrine (15 mg), or high-dose norepinephrine (11 mg) after failing initial defibrillation attempts. Study end points were ROSC (measurable blood pressure or pulse for at least 5 minutes), hospital discharge, and neurologic status (cerebral performance criteria). Of 286 patients, 37 (12.9%) receiving 15 mg of epinephrine achieved ROSC prior to reaching the hospital versus 21 of 260 patients (8.1%) randomized to 1 mg of epinephrine ($P < .01$). ROSC was not statistically different for either high-dose epinephrine or norepinephrine. Overall, only 1.8% of all patients enrolled survived to hospital discharge. Due to the small numbers involved, statistical analysis was not performed on hospital discharge or neurologic status on discharge. The percentage of patients discharged from the standard-dose epinephrine, high-dose epinephrine, and high-dose norepinephrine groups were 1.2%, 1.7%, and 2.6%, respectively. Neurologic survival was most favorable in the standard-dose epinephrine group.[47] Therefore, it appears that although norepinephrine demonstrates preferred effects over epinephrine on myocardial oxygen balance and regional cerebral blood flow in animals, human studies have not confirmed this beneficial effect. Consequently, epinephrine remains the first-line adrenergic agent for CPR until more definitive information becomes available.

Considerable controversy surrounds the idea of the optimal epinephrine dose in CPR. Currently, the standard epinephrine dose for adults is 1 mg (10 mL of 1:10,000 solution) administered by IVP every 3 to 5 minutes.[1] This epinephrine dose, derived from animal studies, equates to approximately 0.015 mg/kg for a 70-kg human. In pediatric patients, the standard epinephrine dose is 0.01 mg/kg (0.1 mL/kg of a 1:10,000 solution) administered by IVP or the intraosseous route every 3 to 5 minutes.[1] Gonzalez and coworkers[48] demonstrated a dose-dependent vasopressor effect for epinephrine (1 mg–3 mg–5 mg) administered late in adult prehospital cardiac arrest victims. Goetting and Paradis published a small study in pediatric cardiac arrest patients that found improved rates of ROSC, survival to discharge, and neurologic outcome in patients receiving 0.2 mg/kg epinephrine versus 0.01 mg/kg of epinephrine late in the arrest sequence.[49]

Along with other published case reports suggesting increased efficacy resulting from higher epinephrine doses, the current adult and pediatric ACLS guidelines offer suggestions for alternative dosing if the initial epinephrine dose is unsuccessful.[1,6] For adults, these recommendations are classified as IIb. They are as follows: 2 to 5 mg IVP every 3 to 5 minutes, 1 mg–3 mg–5 mg IVP given 3 minutes apart, or 0.1 mg/kg IVP every 3 to 5 minutes.[1] For pediatric patients with either asystolic or pulseless rhythms, the alterations in epinephrine dosing are more strongly recommended due to the dismal outcome in most of these arrests.[6] The alternative pediatric epinephrine doses are classified as IIa, and are as follows: 0.1 mg/kg (0.1 mL/kg of a 1:1000 solution) up to a maximum of 0.2 mg/kg (0.2 mL/kg of a 1:1000 solution). Health care personnel must be aware that for pediatric arrest patients, two different concentrations of epinephrine solutions are used. Additionally, due to the possibility of creating high concentrations of preservative when administering high doses of epinephrine, it is recommended to select only preservative-free solutions.[6]

Table 9–2 contains the results from published studies comparing standard dose epinephrine (SDE) and high-dose epinephrine (HDE) in adult cardiac arrest victims.[47,50–54] In these studies, SDE represents either 1 mg or 0.02 mg/kg of epinephrine administered every 5 minutes. HDE implies administration of epinephrine doses greater than 1 mg or 0.02 mg/kg. Collectively, these studies[47,50–54] demonstrate that although higher doses of epinephrine may increase the initial resuscitation success rate, the percentage of patients surviving to hospital discharge is not significantly different. Furthermore, a trend for improved neurologic outcome is present for the SDE group.[47] Investigators have explained this phenomenon by inferring that HDE promotes ROSC in patients who otherwise would not be resuscitated using SDE.[47] These individuals, often with prolonged resuscitation times, subsequently have worsened neurologic outcome.[47,53] The reason HDE does not appear more beneficial for adult cardiac arrest victims might be related to the increased presence of coronary artery disease in the population.[53] Consequently, the beneficial effects derived from raising aortic diastolic pressure and cerebral blood flow may be outweighed by increasing myocardial oxygen demand with higher epinephrine doses.[53]

VASOPRESSIN

Recently there has been interest in administering vasopressin in adult patients with refractory cardiac arrest. In a swine model of ventricular fibrillation, Lindner and coworkers compared the effects of epinephrine (0.2 mg/kg) with three doses of vasopressin (0.2, 0.4, and 0.8 U/kg) on blood flow to vital organs.[55] These investigators discovered that 0.8 U/kg of vasopressin resulted in improved myocardial blood flow as compared with epinephrine. Additionally, they found that the duration of vasoconstriction was significantly longer in those animals receiving both medium- and high-dose vasopressin. Of concern, they also noted marked skin pallor and reduced intestinal blood flow in vasopressin-treated animals. In a subsequent study, Lindner and colleagues discovered that high circulating concentrations of endogenous vasopressin were present in adults undergoing cardiac arrest.[56] Additionally, higher vasopressin concentrations appeared to correlate with improved rates of ROSC. Most recently, Lindner and coworkers published an article containing eight case reports of refractory cardiac arrest patients in whom 40-U boluses of vasopressin were administered intravenously. ROSC (undefined) was achieved in all cases.[57] The authors stated that three of the patients survived until discharge. All of these were said to have "good neurologic recovery," although this was not defined.

It is theorized that in cardiac arrest, vasopressin acts by raising systemic vascular resistance.[55] This action is thought to occur either through a direct effect on the "V_1" receptor or by potentiation of the vasoconstrictor effects of other endogenous cate-

TABLE 9–2. Summary of Adult High-Dose Epinephrine Studies

Author	Design[a]	Epinephrine Dosing[b] SDE vs HDE	*N*	Initial Resuscitation[c] SDE vs HDE (*P* value)	Hospital Discharge SDE vs HDE (*P* value)	Discharge Neurologic Status SDE vs HDE
Lindner et al.[50]	P, R, DB	1 mg vs 5 mg, then 1 mg doses	68	6/40 vs 16/28 ($P < .001$)	2/40 vs 4/28	Not addressed
Callaham et al.[51]	Ret (survived 6 h)	HDE: ≥ 50 μg/kg bolus or total dose greater than 2.8 μg/kg/min	68	N/A	11/35 vs 6/33 ($P = .32$)	Intact 8/11 vs 4/6[d] Impaired 2/11 vs 2/6 Vegetative 1/11 vs 0/6
Stiell et al.[52]	P, R, DB	1 mg vs 7 mg up to 5 doses	650	76/333 vs 56/317 ($P = .12$)	16/333 vs 10/317 ($P = .38$)	Best CPC[e] 94% vs 90%
Brown et al.[53]	P, R, DB, MC	0.02 mg/kg vs 0.2 mg/kg	1280	217/648 vs 190/632	31/648 vs 26/632	CPC[e] 1–3:29/31 vs 24/26 4–5:2/31 vs 2/26
Callaham et al.[47]	P, R, DB	1 mg vs 15 mg	546	22/270 vs 37/286 ($P < .01$)	3/270 vs 5/286	Mean CPC[e] 2.3 vs 3.2
Lipman et al.[54]	P, R, DB	1 mg vs 10 mg up to 3 doses	35	11/16 vs 15/19	1/16 vs 0/19	Not addressed

[a]P = prospective; R = randomized; DB = double-blind; MC = multicenter; Ret = retrospective.
[b]SDE = standard dose epinephrine; HDE = high-dose epinephrine.
[c]Defined by investigators: Lindner et al.: systolic blood pressure ≥ 80 mm Hg for 12 h with or without dopamine; Stiell et al.: regain pulse and blood pressure for ≥ 1 h; Brown et al.: palpable pulse and blood pressure for ≥ 1 min after first epinephrine dose; Callaham et al.: palpable pulse or blood pressure for ≥ 5 min; Lipman et al.: regain spontaneous rhythm.
[d]Unknown criteria
[e]Cerebral performance category: 1 = normal; 2 = moderate disability; 3 = severe disability, dependent; 4 = coma; 5 = brain death.

cholamines.[55] As a consequence of the vasoconstrictive effects of vasopressin, blood in shunted away from skeletal muscle, small intestine, and fatty tissue.[55] Consequently, there should be concern regarding ischemic damage resulting from vasopressin administration. Along these lines, there have been documented cases of acute myocardial infarction in patients receiving vasopressin for the treatment of GI bleeds. Therefore, it is reasonable to assume that vasopressin administration in patients with coronary artery disease could result in further myocardial damage. With these concerns in mind, widespread administration of vasopressin during cardiac arrest should not occur until further studies document the benefits and adverse effects associated with this therapy.

ANTIARRHYTHMICS

Antiarrhythmic agents are administered in the treatment of persistent PVT or VF following unsuccessful defibrillation with initial epinephrine administration. Due to the scarcity of randomized, placebo-controlled trials examining the efficacy of antiarrhythmic agents during CPR, these agents received a IIa classification in the 1997 ACLS guidelines.[1] The first-line antiarrhythmic agent in the treatment of PVT or VF is lidocaine, followed by bretylium. Within the past several years, intravenous amiodarone has become available and has been shown to be beneficial in the treatment of refractory VT and VF.[58,59] However, due to the limited information available with its use in patients with VF and PVT, amiodarone was not included in the current AHA treatment algorithm.[1] With regard to the treatment of pediatric cardiac arrests, practitioners should be aware that there are no data to support the use of bretylium or amiodarone.[1] Procainamide is no longer used in the treatment of PVT or VF due to the excessive time required for drug administration. Current recommendations suggest administering successive doses of antiarrhythmic agents at a more frequent interval during cardiac arrest in an effort to increase circulating blood concentrations and hopefully improve efficacy.[1]

Lidocaine

In adult patients, current AHA guidelines suggest that lidocaine therapy be initiated with a 1.5 mg/kg IVP bolus.[1] If defibrillation is unsuccessful, an additional 1.5 mg/kg bolus can be administered in 3 to 5 minutes (total dose of 3 mg/kg). A continuous lidocaine infusion of 2 to 4 mg/min should be started once the arrhythmia is suppressed. In pediatric patients, the recommended dose of lidocaine is 1 mg/kg.[6] Additionally, there are no recommendations for subsequent bolus doses if defibrillation is unsuccessful. If the arrhythmia is suppressed, however, a continuous lidocaine infusion should be started at a rate of 20 to 50 μg/kg/min. Although lidocaine is considered to be the first-line antiarrhythmic agent for the treatment of PVT or VF in adults, superiority over bretylium has not been demonstrated in human clinical trials.[60,61] The selection of lidocaine over bretylium is based on the increased familiarity and preferred adverse-effect profile of lidocaine.[1]

Evidence suggests that lidocaine may reduce arrhythmia recurrence following successful defibrillation.[1] Chow and colleagues found that plasma lidocaine concentrations > 6 μg/mL may be necessary for antifibrillatory effects in an animal model.[62] In this study, they demonstrated that lidocaine (2 mg/kg) raised the ventricular fibrillation threshold (VFT) within 5 minutes of drug administration compared to the 10 minutes required for bretylium (5 mg/kg). The duration of effect, however, was greater for bretylium. In a similar animal model, Hanyok and colleagues demonstrated that a combination of bretylium (5 mg/kg) and lidocaine (2 mg/kg) possessed both a rapid onset of action and prolonged duration of VFT elevation.[63] Therefore, combination therapy may be rational for persistent or recurrent VF. Controversy continues to exist, however, regarding the effect of lidocaine on defibrillation energy requirements for VF.[64]

The pharmacokinetic characteristics of lidocaine, a type Ib antiarrhythmic agent, have not been extensively studied during cardiac arrest.[65] It is known, however, that hepatic blood flow is the primary determinant for the rate of hepatic lidocaine metabolism. Therefore, as cardiac output and hepatic blood flow decline during cardiac arrest, lidocaine clearance is reduced.[65] Additionally, during myocardial ischemia, lidocaine protein binding increases as α_1-acid glycoprotein is released. Consequently, while total plasma lidocaine concentrations are elevated, the percentage of unbound lidocaine (free fraction) may be reduced.[65] With more aggressive lidocaine loading, as recommended by the AHA guidelines, increased toxicity may be encountered.[1] Dosage reductions are suggested for lidocaine maintenance infusions in patients with reduced cardiac output (e.g., myocardial infarction, congestive heart failure, cardiogenic shock), hepatic dysfunction, or age greater than 70 years.[1] With prolonged maintenance infusions, plasma concentrations should be monitored and patients should be assessed for adverse effects such as slurred speech, altered consciousness, muscle twitching, and seizures.[1]

Bretylium Tosylate

Bretylium is classified as a type III antiarrhythmic agent. As discussed previously, two randomized controlled trials comparing the efficacy of lidocaine and bretylium in adult prehospital cardiac arrests found no statistical difference.[60,61] In one study, composed of 146 cardiac arrests, 60% of patients treated with lidocaine were successfully resuscitated compared with 58% in the bretylium-treated group.[60] Hospital discharge rates were 26% and 34% for the lidocaine and bretylium groups, respectively. In a study of 91 prehospital cardiac arrest victims, Olson and colleagues[61] found that 56% of lidocaine-treated patients achieved ROSC in contrast to 35% in the bretylium group. In this study, 10% of patients receiving lidocaine survived to hospital discharge compared with 5% receiving bretylium. Therefore, in the absence of efficacy differences, the choice of bretylium as a second-line agent is based largely on the preferred adverse-effect profile of lidocaine. For those patients nonresponsive to lidocaine, early administration of bretylium is desirable to increase the chance of successful defibrillation given the time required to raise VFT.[62–64]

In the 1950s, bretylium was used as an antihypertensive agent due to its adrenergic blocking properties. With the discovery of its antifibrillatory properties in the 1960s, there was a renewed interest in bretylium.[66] The antiarrhythmic actions of bretylium result from a complex combination of direct myocardial and indirect adrenergic effects. Apart from its ability to raise the ventricular fibrillation threshold, bretylium reduces differences in action potential duration and refractory periods between infarcted and noninfarcted myocardium.[66] In addition, bretylium improves the conduction velocity within infarcted areas, which may reduce the development of VF.[66] As for effects on adrenergic nerve terminals, these vary with the time course following drug administration. Initially, bretylium administration potentiates norepinephrine release, which can be manifested clinically by increases in blood pressure, heart rate, and cardiac output. It is hypothesized that this sympathomimetic response may be important in achieving ROSC with bretylium since coronary blood flow may be augmented.[64] Approximately 15 to 20 minutes following administration, bretylium blocks further release of norepinephrine. Clinically, hypotension may occur, which requires the administration of fluids and vasopressors.[66] This profound hypotensive effect, however, may have a detrimental effect on coronary perfusion pressure.[64] In addition, bretylium blocks norepinephrine reuptake into adrenergic nerve endings, which blocking may intensify effects obtained from exogenous catecholamine administration.[66]

In both pediatric and adult patients with PVT or VT, AHA guidelines recommend initiating bretylium with a 5 mg/kg IVP bolus.[1,6] The drug should then be allowed to circulate 1 or 2 minutes prior to defibrillation. If the defibrillation attempt is unsuccessful in pediatric patients, an additional bolus dose of 10 mg/kg can be administered.[6] If the defibrillation attempt is unsuccessful in adults, subsequent bolus doses of 10 mg/kg may be administered at 5-minute intervals up to a total dose of 30 to 35 mg/kg. If arrhythmia suppression is achieved in adults, a continuous infusion may be initiated at 1 to 2 mg/min.[1] For the treatment of persistent VT, 5 to 10 mg/kg should be diluted in 50 mL of fluid and infused over 8 to 10 minutes. Because the occurrence of nausea and vomiting are related to peak serum concentrations, intravenous infusions should be used in conscious patients.[65] Serum concentration monitoring is not useful with bretylium therapy because antifibrillatory activity correlates better with myocardial drug concentrations.[65]

Amiodarone

Amiodarone is officially classified as a type III antiarrhythmic agent; however, it exerts characteristics of all four Vaughn Williams classifications. In the acute setting, intravenous amiodarone displays mainly antiadrenergic (Class II) and calcium channel blocking (Class IV) properties.[67] Consequently, the most frequently reported adverse effects associated with intravenous amiodarone use in VF and VT are hypotension (18% to 27%) and bradycardia (4% to 6%).[58,59] Other adverse effects noted acutely are fever, elevated liver function tests, confusion, nausea, and thrombocytopenia. It is hypothesized that hypotension may be directly proportional to the infusion rate. Similarly, the hypotension may result from polysorbate 80, the diluent for the amiodarone solution, since it is known to cause vasodilation.[58] Although amiodarone has a major active metabolite, the effects from *N*-desesthyl-amiodarone (DEA) are negligible in the acute setting.[67]

Few studies have examined the efficacy of intravenous amiodarone in the setting of cardiac arrest. Within the framework of two published clinical studies, patients undergoing cardiac arrest were enrolled.[58,59] Based on the information contained within these studies, it appears that approximately 10% of study patients from both trials could be classified as cardiac arrest victims. The primary end point for both studies was prevention of recurrent VF or VT episodes. As a result of the primary study focus and the small number of cardiac arrest patients included, very little information is available regarding the initial effectiveness of amiodarone in these patients. It is interesting to note that in a study comparing amiodarone and bretylium in patients with recurrent hemodynamically destabilizing VF and VT, amiodarone (1000 mg/24 h) had similar efficacy to bretylium (2500 mg/24 h) in terms of preventing recurrent VF or VT.[59] Additionally, the incidence of hypotension was 32% in the bretylium group as compared with 18% in the amiodarone-treated patients. As discussed previously, amiodarone is not currently included in the AHA treatment algorithm of VF/PVT. However, once more experience is obtained with this agent in VF and VT, amiodarone may well replace bretylium as the preferred second-line agent based upon the preferable side-effect profile of amiodarone. Until that time, however, bretylium will remain the second-line antiarrhythmic agent of choice in the treatment of VF and PVT (see Fig. 9–1).

For the treatment of VT or VF, adults should initially receive 150 mg of amiodarone administered over 10 minutes. This initial infusion should be followed by a maintenance infusion of amiodarone given at a rate of 1 mg/min. After completing 6 hours of the maintenance infusion, the rate should be decreased to 0.5 mg/min. Supplemental rapid infusions (150 mg amiodarone in 100 mL D_5W over 10 minutes) can be administered for recurrent VT or VF. Clinicians should be aware that D_5W is the only recommended diluent for amiodarone. Additionally, due to adsorption of amiodarone to polyvinylchloride, infusions greater than 2 hours should be prepared in either glass or polyolefin containers. Special IV tubing, however, is not required. Once prepared, infusions with concentrations exceeding 2 mg/mL should only be given centrally since peripheral administration could result in phlebitis. Last, aside from the drug interactions known to occur with oral amiodarone, clinicians should be aware of the potential for elevated serum concentrations of lidocaine and cyclosporine to occur when either drug is administered to patients receiving intravenous amiodarone.[67]

THERAPEUTIC ALTERNATIVES FOR REFRACTORY VF OR VT

Patients with persistent or recurrent VT or VF following antiarrhythmic administration should be assessed for underlying electrolyte abnormalities as a cause for their refractory arrhythmia. Ideally, therapeutic decisions should be based on the patient's measured electrolyte concentrations. The primary electrolyte abnormalities associated with refractory ventricular arrhythmias include hyperkalemia, hypokalemia, and hypomagnesemia.[1] Adults with known or suspected hyperkalemia ($[K^+] > 6.0$ mEq/L) should receive 4 mg/kg IV of a 10% calcium chloride solution.[1] Sodium bicarbonate (1 mEq/kg) may also be given to drive potassium intracellularly until more definitive therapy is available.[1]

In one study of prehospital cardiac arrests, 49% of resuscitated patients were found to be hypokalemic ($[K^+] < 3.6$ mEq/L) on hospital admission.[68] Although frequently debated, it is unknown whether the hypokalemia most often precedes cardiac arrest or is a consequence of cardiac resuscitation.[68-72] Preexisting hypokalemia is primarily associated with diuretic use.[69,71,72] Hypokalemia identified during cardiac arrest may also result from conditions present during resuscitation. For example, intracellular potassium shifts may occur secondarily to metabolic derangements or elevated circulating catecholamine concentrations.[68-70] With the association of hypokalemia and sudden death, it has been recommended to administer potassium (10 mEq IV over 30 minutes) to patients with refractory VF in whom hypokalemia is known or suspected.[1] Similarly, hypomagnesemia has been associated with ventricular arrhythmias.[73] Investigators have found that in hospitalized patients, approximately 40% of hypokalemic patients have coexisting hypomagnesemia.[74,75] This is important since uncorrected hypomagnesemia may prevent successful potassium repletion.[74] It is recommended (class IIa) that patients in refractory VF with either known ($[Mg^{2+}] < 1.4$ mEq/L) or suspected hypomagnesemia receive 1 to 2 g of magnesium sulfate diluted in 10 mL of fluid over 1 to 2 minutes.[1] Caution should be used since rapid magnesium supplementation may produce significant hypotension or asystole.[64]

ASYSTOLE AND PEA

NONPHARMACOLOGIC THERAPY

As discussed previously, hospital discharge rates are usually < 5% for patients presenting with either asystole or PEA.[2,4] Within the pediatric population, asystole is a much more common presenting arrhythmia than VF or VT. In adults, asystole usually signals degeneration of a ventricular arrhythmia. Asystole may, however, occur from increased parasympathetic tone. On the ECG monitor, asystole is defined by the presence of "flat line." Rarely, fine VF can resemble asystole if the patient is monitored with a single ECG lead. If this occurs, a second lead should be selected to confirm the cardiac rhythm.[1] Asystolic patients should receive the following: CPR, intubation, and IV access. Defibrillation should be avoided because it may increase parasympathetic tone, which, in turn, might worsen survival from asystole.[1] If available, attempts could be made to pace the heart using transcutaneous pacing.[1]

PEA encompasses all pulseless rhythms associated with electrical activity other than VT or VF.[1] Since these rhythms may result from underlying treatable conditions, it is first necessary to exclude all possible causes. Specifically, these include hypoxia, hypovolemia, cardiac tamponade, tension pneumothorax, hypothermia, pulmonary embolism, drug overdose, hyperkalemia, acidosis, and acute myocardial infarction.[1]

PHARMACOLOGIC THERAPY

The primary pharmacologic agents used in the treatment of asystole are epinephrine and atropine. Recommended epinephrine dosing is identical to that used in the treatment of VF and PVT.[1] The use of atropine in asystole will be discussed below.

For the treatment of PEA, epinephrine should be administered if attempts to correct potential underlying disorders are unsuccessful. Atropine may be used in the presence of absolute bradycardia (i.e., heart rate < 60 beats/min).[1]

ATROPINE

Atropine, an antimuscarinic agent, improves sinus node and atrioventricular node conduction by inhibiting vagal activity. Possible reasons for high vagal tone during cardiac arrest include: (1) oropharyngeal stimulation with endotracheal intubation, (2) the presence of hypoxia and acidosis, and (3) alterations in the contribution of parasympathetic and sympathetic control.[76] To date, there have not been any large randomized trials demonstrating benefit from atropine in the treatment of asystole. The majority of human data was compiled from either small case series or retrospective studies.[76-82]

Gupta and colleagues[77] published four case reports in which atropine was used for "cardiac standstill." The response time for treating asystole in these patients was ≤ 22.5 seconds. Although all patients survived, only one patient was in asystole at the time of atropine administration.[77] In 1978, Iseri and colleagues[78] published a retrospective case series of 33 patients with prehospital bradyasystole. Of the 15 asystolic patients, only two received atropine (0.5-mg dose). None of the patients with asystole survived.[78] Brown and coworkers[76] reported results from eight asystolic cases receiving atropine. The initial atropine dose ranged from 0.5 to 1 mg, with a maximum dose limit of 2 mg. In this case series, three of eight (37.5%) survived to hospital discharge. It should be noted, however, that asystole was related to cardiac catheterization in two of these surviving patients.[76] In 1981, Coon and associates[79] published a prospective study of 21 prehospital patients with either asystole or pulseless idioventricular rhythm. Of the 10 patients who received atropine, none survived to hospital discharge. In comparison, 1 of 11 patients in the control group was discharged.[79] Stueven and colleagues[80] compared the results of patients receiving atropine (n = 43) with control (n = 41) patients in the treatment of prehospital refractory asystole. The investigators did not specify the atropine dose used. Although 6 of 43 (14%) atropine-treated patients achieved ROSC, none survived to hospital discharge. In contrast, ROSC was not obtained for any patients in the control group.[80] In 1985, Ornato and associates[81] published a retrospective study containing 24 prehospital patients with asystole as the presenting rhythm. The purpose of this study was to identify the ability of defibrillation and medications to transform the cardiac rhythm. Of the 22 patients receiving atropine, asystole was abolished in 4 of them. Unfortunately, none of these patients was discharged from the hospital.[81] Last, Tortolani and colleagues[82] conducted a retrospective study of 123 in-hospital cardiac arrest patients with asystole as their initial cardiac rhythm. Atropine was administered in 101 of these patients. For those receiving atropine, 24 were alive

24 hours postresuscitation. It is unclear how many of these patients were eventually discharged.[82] Therefore, with little documentation of efficacy, atropine remains to be recommended (class IIa) for the treatment of asystole.[1]

Until recently, it was recommended that atropine be initiated with a 1-mg IV bolus in the treatment of asystole in adults. If unsuccessful, a second 1-mg bolus could be administered.[66] Although not well substantiated in the medical literature, 2 mg of atropine has been touted to be a maximally vagolytic dose for the majority of adults.[83] With the 1992 revision of the ACLS guidelines, atropine dosing was changed based on previous scientific evidence.[6] In 1967, Chamberlain and colleagues[83] published a prospective study of 10 healthy volunteers that examined the effects of heart rate and blood pressure to incremental dosage increases of atropine. Prior to receiving atropine, these individuals were given propranolol as a means to achieve chemical sympathetic denervation. For these 10 subjects, maximal heart rate increases were obtained with the following total atropine doses: 1.8 mg (3 patients), 2.4 mg (4 patients), and 3.0 mg (3 patients). On a weight basis, the maximum vagolytic dose for atropine in these healthy adults ranged from 0.025 to 0.04 mg/kg. The authors did note, however, that the maximum vagolytic dose was higher for those subjects with lower baseline heart rates.[83] Subsequently, the current 1997 ACLS guidelines reflect the information identified by the above clinical studies and recommend that atropine be initiated at a dose of 1 mg. This dose should be repeated, if necessary, at 3- to 5-minute intervals up to a total dose of 0.04 mg/kg (approximately 3 mg in a 70-kg adult).[1] In comparison, for the treatment of symptomatic bradycardia in adults, atropine dosing should begin with 0.5 to 1 mg (class I). The recommended total dose in this situation is 0.03 to 0.04 mg/kg (approximately 2 to 3 mg in a 70-kg adult).[1] Administration of atropine doses < 0.5 mg in adults should be avoided since a paradoxical vagotonic effect may result.[66]

In pediatric patients with asystole, atropine administration should be initiated with single doses of 0.02 mg/kg.[6] Within this guideline, it is suggested that the minimum dose be no less than 0.1 mg and the maximum single dose should not exceed 0.5 mg in a child and 1.0 mg in an adolescent. Doses may be repeated at 5-minute intervals. Maximum total doses of atropine in the treatment of pediatric asystole should not exceed 1 mg in children or 2 mg in adolescents.[6]

CALCIUM CHLORIDE

Although once encouraged, calcium administration during cardiac resuscitation has declined during the past decade. Calcium is a positive inotropic agent. Released in response to electrical stimulation of the muscle, calcium interacts with actin and myosin filaments to augment myocardial contractility.[66] Although initially advocated for the treatment of asystole and electromechanical dissociation, investigators have demonstrated no beneficial effects from using calcium in these disorders.[84,85] Furthermore, calcium administration has been associated with causing reperfusion injury and postischemic cerebral hypoperfusion.[86,89] As a result, the indications for calcium administration during cardiac arrest are limited. Calcium is recommended (class IIa) only for hyperkalemia, hypocalcemia, and calcium antagonist toxicity.[1]

ACID–BASE MANAGEMENT DURING CPR

During cardiac arrest, acid–base imbalances result from decreased perfusion and ineffective ventilation. As established previously, approximately 30% of the baseline cardiac output is achieved during standard CPR.[2] In the presence of reduced tissue perfusion and oxygen delivery, anaerobic metabolism predominates, thereby raising P_{CO_2} concentrations. Elimination of P_{CO_2} is hampered by this state of diminished blood flow. Subsequently, attempts to correct the acidosis should be directed at improving blood flow (i.e., optimizing cardiac compressions) and ventilation.

SODIUM BICARBONATE

At one time, sodium bicarbonate ($NaHCO_3$) administration was recommended during cardiac resuscitation to correct systemic acidosis. It was believed that alkali administration would reduce detrimental effects associated with acidosis such as reduced myocardial contractility and VF threshold.[90] The majority of available data, however, do not support sodium bicarbonate use in CPR.[1,90,91] Aside from the lack of efficacy on survival,[1,91] administration of sodium bicarbonate can have detrimental results.[66,91] For example, sodium bicarbonate can generate CO_2 production by the following equation:

$$[H^+] + [HCO_3^-] \leftrightarrow H_2CO_3 \leftrightarrow CO_2 + H_2O$$

thereby worsening acidosis. In the absence of effective CO_2 elimination, rapid intracellular diffusion of CO_2 can result in the development of intracellular acidosis. Likewise, cerebrospinal and central venous acidosis can occur with sodium bicarbonate administration. Other possible adverse effects include decreased oxygen release secondary to alterations in the oxyhemoglobin dissociation curve and production of hyperosmolality and hypernatremia.[66]

Currently, sodium bicarbonate has a limited role during cardiac resuscitation attempts.[1] A proportion of patients, however, may benefit from bicarbonate therapy (class IIa).[1] These individuals include those with (1) known bicarbonate-responsive acidosis, (2) hyperkalemia, or (3) tricyclic antidepressant or phenobarbital overdose. The remaining indication (class IIb) for sodium bicarbonate administration involves cases with prolonged arrest times (> 10 minutes).[1] In this situation, patients should first receive adequate CPR, intubation, ventilation, and multiple epinephrine doses prior to considering sodium bicarbonate administration. If the decision is made to institute bicarbonate therapy, the initial recommended dose for adults and children is 1 mEq/kg.[1] If necessary, subsequent doses of 0.5 mEq/kg can be administered at 10-minute intervals. To reduce the adverse effects associated with alkalosis, it is recommended that bicarbonate use be guided by results obtained from blood gas analysis.[1]

GUIDELINES FOR DRUG ADMINISTRATION DURING EMERGENCY SITUATIONS

During cardiac resuscitation, several routes for drug administration are available. Each route, however, is associated with various advantages and disadvantages. Ideally, the drug administration route should be easily accessible during CPR and provide rapid entry into the central circulation. Although central venous administration results in both earlier and higher peak drug concentrations compared with peripheral venous administration,[92,93] it may be unavailable early in the cardiac arrest event. Additionally, attempts to obtain central access may necessitate unwanted interruptions in performing CPR. Peripheral venous access, using the antecubital vein, is acceptable if central access is unavailable. It is recommended that all peripheral IV injections be followed immediately with a 20-mL fluid bolus and elevation of the extremity in an effort to speed drug entry into the central circulation.[1,94] If ROSC is not achieved following the first peripherally administered dose, central access should be attempted.[6]

In the event that neither central nor peripheral access is available, endotracheal administration of atropine, lidocaine, and epinephrine may be utilized. The AHA mnemonic for drugs that can be administered via the endotracheal route is A-L-E.[1] Practitioners should be aware that it is not recommended to administer either sodium bicarbonate or bretylium endotracheally.[95] The rationale for this recommendation is that sodium bicarbonate administration would require excessive volumes to be given endotracheally, whereas bretylium is poorly absorbed by the endotracheal route. Within the medical literature, great debate surrounds the optimal dose conversion from IV to endotracheal administration. Recommendations for the endotracheal dose have varied from equivalent doses to as much as 10 times the intravenous dose.[95] For adults, the 1997 ACLS guidelines suggest that endotracheal doses of 2 to 2.5 times the recommended IV dose be used.[1] Within the pediatric guidelines, dosage adjustments vary based on the drug. For epinephrine, it is suggested to use 10 times the IV dose except when administering high-dose epinephrine. In the latter case, the endotracheal dose should equal the IV dose. With other endotracheally administered drugs, the pediatric guidelines only state that higher doses should probably be used.[6] Because endotracheal administration is associated with delayed onset and prolonged duration of action, rescuers should be aware that increased drug effects may be seen if spontaneous circulation is achieved.[95]

The recommended method for endotracheal administration is as follows: (1) dilution of dose (for adults: 10 mL of distilled water or normal saline; for pediatrics: 1 to 2 mL of normal or half-normal saline), (2) interruption of CPR, (3) rapid drug administration beyond the tip of the endotracheal tube, (4) three to five quick insufflations using a bag-valve device to aerosolize the drug, and (5) resumption of CPR.[1] In pediatric patients, the intraosseous route may be used temporarily if no other routes of drug administration are available. Last, intracardiac drug administration is not recommended during closed-chest CPR.

Related to the issue of drug administration, the current 1997 AHA guidelines address the appropriateness of administering various IV fluids.[1] For years, dextrose-containing solutions have been used during cardiac resuscitation to keep IV lines patent as well as to provide a drug-delivery vehicle. Concern over the use of dextrose-containing fluids during ischemic events stems from information linking hyperglycemia with worsened neurologic survival.[96] Controversy exists, however, regarding whether hyperglycemia produces neurologic deficits or whether it is merely a marker of prolonged resuscitative efforts.[96–98] Until further clarification is available, use of normal saline or lactated Ringer's is recommended for all intravenous infusions.[1,96] Dextrose solutions should be reserved for patients with documented or suspected hypoglycemia.[1] It is worth noting, however, that fingerstick glucose determinations have been shown to be misleading in cardiac arrest victims.[99,100] Studies have shown that up to one-third of hypotensive patients are misclassified as hypoglycemic. Although the mechanism is unknown, researchers have hypothesized that the finding may result from the combination of increased glucose usage and decreased peripheral blood flow.[99] Therefore, venous blood samples should be obtained.

ETHICAL AND ECONOMIC CONSIDERATIONS IN CPR

Should CPR be instituted on demand? Are physicians required to initiate CPR in terminally ill patients? Can resuscitation efforts be terminated prior to reaching the hospital? These are among the many questions currently facing emergency care providers. Most agree that attaining "neurologic survival" is the primary objective of cardiac resuscitation. Since this often is not attainable, many health care professionals are attempting to identify patients unlikely to benefit from cardiac resuscitation. The initial obstacle to accomplishing this task is defining the term "medical futility." The current AHA guidelines suggest that medical futility occurs only when there are no reported survivors for a population subgroup.[1] Others object to the stringent nature of this definition, recommending instead that medical futility be defined by an acceptable threshold value (< 0.1%, 1%, or 2% survivors) determined from outcome data in the medical literature.[1,101,102] By withholding CPR attempts in futile cases, the following benefits may be achieved: (1) reduced number of suboptimal outcomes, (2) decreased injuries incurred while delivering rapid emergency care, and (3) provision of more cost-effective health care.[103] For example, investigators have shown that victims not regaining a pulse with ACLS prior to hospital arrival rarely survive, with the exception of those patients with refractory VT or VF.[103] Furthermore, it has been estimated that in the United States, yearly costs incurred for continued ER resuscitation efforts in these individuals approaches half a billion dollars.[103]

To decrease the number of futile resuscitation attempts, information must be gathered that documents the probabilities of successful resuscitation in given population subsets. As discussed previously, current attempts to accomplish this objective include standardizing resuscitation definitions[21–23] and developing prearrest morbidity indices.[104] Once survival probabilities are known, patients should be presented with information specific to their situation. In the meantime, efforts to establish resuscitation status prior to hospitalization should be continued, especially in the elderly and terminally ill.

EVALUATION OF THERAPEUTIC OUTCOMES

In the most basic sense, successful CPR is often described as the restoration of a stable heart rate, cardiac rhythm, and blood pressure (SBP > 70 mm Hg). However, to truly be successful, patients should remain neurologically intact with minimal morbidity following resuscitation. To gauge the success of resuscitation outcomes, therapeutic outcome monitoring should occur during the resuscitation attempt and in the postresuscitation phase. Use of standardized guidelines to document resuscitation events is essential. For all patients undergoing CPR, the following parameters should be assessed and documented throughout the resuscitation attempt and subsequent to each intervention: respiratory rate, heart rate, cardiac rhythm, and blood pressure. Determination of the presence or absence of respirations, heart rate, and the associated cardiac rhythm is paramount to deciding which interventions may be appropriate. In addition, nonresponse to an array of suitable interventions may signal a patient incapable of being resuscitated. Determination of coronary and cerebral perfusion pressures during the resuscitation attempt is desirable, although not realistic in most institutions.

Following successful resuscitation, the primary goals include optimizing tissue oxygenation, identifying the precipitating cause(s) of the arrest, and preventing subsequent episodes of cardiopulmonary arrest. In an effort to determine causation, a prearrest history should be obtained, which includes documentation of any medications. During the postresuscitation period, patients should receive a 12-lead ECG, chest x-ray, arterial blood gas, blood chemistry determinations, frequent vital sign monitoring, continuous ECG monitoring, and ventilatory support if necessary. Special attention should be given to altered cardiac, hepatic, and renal function resulting from ischemic damage during the cardiopulmonary arrest. The following assessments of neurologic function should also be completed: (1) Glasgow Coma Scale determined at 24 hours post-ROSC, hospital discharge, 6 months postevent, and 1 year postevent; and (2) Cerebral Performance Category recorded at hospital discharge, 6 months postevent, and 1 year postevent.

▶ PRINCIPLES OF PHARMACOTHERAPY

- Cardiopulmonary arrest can occur as a result of either a primary cardiac or respiratory event. The etiology of cardiopulmonary arrest varies depending on patient age and the presence of comorbidities.
- The goal of attempting cardiopulmonary resuscitation is to return effective ventilation and circulation as quickly as possible to minimize hypoxic damage to vital organs.
- Patients presenting with VF or PVT should receive rapid defibrillation, CPR, endotracheal intubation, and IV access. Pharmacologic agents are not recommended until an airway is obtained and IV access is attempted.
- Epinephrine is recommended as first-line pharmacologic therapy in the treatment of VF, PCT, asystole, and PEA.
- Documentation of cardiac resuscitation attempts should follow standardized guidelines.

REFERENCES

1. 1997–1999 Emergency Cardiovascular Care Programs, Advanced Cardiac Life Support. American Heart Association, 1997.
2. O'Nunain S, Ruskin J. Cardiac arrest. Lancet 1993;341:1641–1647.
3. Madl C, Grimm G, Kramer L, et al. Early prediction of individual outcome after cardiopulmonary resuscitation. Lancet 1993;341: 855–858.
4. Niemann DT. Cardiopulmonary resuscitation. N Engl J Med 1992; 327:1075–1080.
5. Varon J, Sternbach GL. Cardiopulmonary resuscitation: Lessons from the past. J Emerg Med 1991;9:503–507.
6. Emergency Cardiac Care Committee and Subcommittees, American Heart Association. Guidelines for cardiopulmonary resuscitation and emergency cardiac care. JAMA 1992:268:2171–2302.
7. Safar P, Escarraga L, Elam JO. A comparison of the mouth-to-mouth and mouth-to-airway methods of artificial respiration with chest pressure arm-life method. N Engl J Med 1958;258:671–677.
8. Kouwenhoven WB, Jude JR, Knickerbocker GG. Closed-chest cardiac massage. JAMA 1960;173:1064–1067.
9. Pepe PE, Levine RL, Fromm R. Cardiac arrest presenting with rhythms other than ventricular fibrillation: Contribution of resuscitative efforts toward total survivorship. Crit Care Med 1993;21: 1838–1843.
10. Bonnin MJ, Pepe PE, Clark PS. Survival in the elderly after out-of-hospital cardiac arrest. Crit Care Med 1993;21:1645–1651.
11. Joslyn SA, Pomrehn PR, Brown DD. Survival from out-of-hospital cardiac arrest: Effects of patient age and presence of 911 emergency medical services phone access. Am J Emerg Med 1993; 11:200–206.
12. Kuisma M, Suominen P, Korpela R. Paediatric out-of-hospital cardiac arrests—Epidemiology and outcome. Resuscitation 1995;30: 141–150.
13. Nadkarni V, Hazinski MF, Zideman D, et al. Pediatric resuscitation: An advisory statement from the Pediatric Working Group of the International Liaison Committee on Resuscitation. Circulation 1997; 95:2185–2195.
14. Tucker KJ, Savitt MA, Idris A, Redberg RF. Cardiopulmonary resuscitation: Historical perspectives, physiology, and future directions. Arch Intern Med 1994;154:2141–2150.
15. Eorgan PA, Greer JL, Cough CPR: A consideration for high-risk cardiac patient discharge teaching. Crit Care Nurse 1992;12:21–27.
16. Sack JB, Kesselbrenner MB, Anwar J. Interposed abdominal compression–cardiopulmonary resuscitation and outcome during asystole and electromechanical dissociation. Circulation 1992;86: 1692–1700.
17. Cohen TJ, Goldner BG, Maccaro PC, et al. A comparison of active compression–decompression cardiopulmonary resuscitation with standard cardiopulmonary resuscitation for cardiac arrests occurring in the hospital. N Engl J Med 1993;329:1918–1921.
18. Halperin HR, Tsitlik JE, Gelfand M, et al. A preliminary study of cardiopulmonary resuscitation by circumferential compression of the chest with use of a pneumatic vest. N Engl J Med 1993;329: 762–768.
19. Stiell IG, Hebert PC, Wells GA, et al. Compression–decompression cardiopulmonary resuscitation for in-hospital and prehospital cardiac arrest. JAMA 1996;275:1417–1423.
20. Paradis NA, Martin GB, Rivers EP, et al. Coronary perfusion pressure and the return of spontaneous circulation in human cardiopulmonary resuscitation. JAMA 1990;263:1106–1113.
21. Cummins RO, Chamberlain DA, Abramson NS, et al. Recommended guidelines for uniform reporting of data from out-of-hospital cardiac arrest: The Utstein style. A statement for health professionals from a task force of the American Heart Association, the European Resuscitation Council, the Heart and Stroke Foundation of Canada, and the Australian Resuscitation Council. Circulation 1991;84:960–975.
22. Cummins RO, Chamberlain D, Hazinski MF, et al. Recommended guidelines for reviewing, reporting, and conducting research on in-hospital resuscitation: The in-hospital "Utstein style." A statement for healthcare professionals from the American Heart Association, the European Resuscitation Council, the Heart and Stroke Foundation of Canada, the Australian Resuscitation Council, and the Resuscitation Councils of South Africa. Circulation 1997;95: 2213–2239.
23. Zaritsky A, et al. Recommended guidelines for uniform reporting of pediatric advanced life support: The pediatric Utstein style. Circulation 1995;92:2006–2020.
24. Kellermann AL, Hackman BB, Somes G. Predicting the outcome of unsuccessful prehospital advanced cardiac life support. JAMA 1993; 270:1433–1436.
25. Handley AJ, Becker LB, Allen M, et al. Single-rescuer adult basic life support: An advisory statement from the basic life support working group of the international liaison committee on resuscitation. Circulation 1997;95:2174–2179.
26. Ayers SM. Preventing cardiac arrest. Crit Care Med 1994;22: 189–191.
27. Edwards GA, Samuels TM. The role of the hospital pharmacist in emergency situations. Am J Hosp Pharm 1968;25:128–133.
28. Bardas SL. Demystifying the cardiopulmonary code team response. J Pharm Technol 1992;8:151–154.
29. Bond CA, Raehl CL, Pitterle ME. 1992 national clinical pharmacy services study. Pharmacotherapy 1994;14:282–304.

30. Shimp LA, Mason NA, Toedter NM, et al. Pharmacist participation in cardiopulmonary resuscitation. Am J Health Syst Pharm 1995; 52:980–984.
31. Cummins RO, Sanders A, Mancini E, Hazinski MF. In-hospital resuscitation: A statement for healthcare professionals from the American Heart Association Emergency Cardiac Care Committee and the Advanced Cardiac Life Support, Basic Life Support, Pediatric Resuscitation, and Program Administration Subcommittees. Circulation 1997;95:2211–2212.
32. Robinson LA, Brown CG, Jenkins J, et al. The effect of norepinephrine versus epinephrine on myocardial hemodynamics during CPR. Ann Emerg Med 1989;18:336–340.
33. Berkowitz ID, Rogers MC. The physiology of cerebral blood flow during cardiopulmonary resuscitation. Can J Anaesth 1988;35: S23–S29.
34. Brown CG, Weman HA. Collective review. Adrenergic agonists during cardiopulmonary resuscitation. Resuscitation 1990;1:1–16.
35. Darby TD, Aldinger EE, Gadsen RH, et al. Effects of metabolic acidosis on ventricular isometric systolic tension and the response to epinephrine and levarterenol. Circ Res 1980;8:1242–1253.
36. Houle OB, Weil MH, Brown EB, et al. Influence of respiratory acidosis on ECG and pressor response to epinephrine, norepinephrine, and metaraminol. Proc Soc Exp Biol Med 1957;94:561–564.
37. Camilton de Hurtado MC, Argel MI, Cingoliani HE. Influence of acid–base alterations on myocardial sensitivity to catecholamines. Arch Pharmacol 1981;317:219–224.
38. Burget DE, Visscher MB. Variations of the pH of the blood and the response of the vascular system to adrenalin. Am J Physiol 1927; 81:113–123.
39. Motulsky HJ, Insel PA. Adrenergic receptors in man. Direct identification, physiologic regulation, and clinical alterations. N Engl J Med 1982;307:18–28.
40. Lefkowitz RJ, Caron MC, Stiles GI. Mechanisms of membrane-receptor regulation. Biochemical, physiological, and clinical insights derived from studies of the adrenergic receptor. N Engl J Med 1984;310:1570–1579.
41. Leftowitz RJ. Beta-adrenergic receptors: Recognition and regulation. N Engl J Med 1979;295:323–328.
42. Ornato JP. Use of adrenergic agonists during CPR in adults. Ann Emerg Med 1993;22(part 2):411–416.
43. Langer SZ, Shepperson NB. Postjunctional α_1- and α_2-adrenoceptors: Preferential innervation of α_1-adrenoceptors and the role of neuronal uptake. J Cardiovasc Pharmacol 1982;4:S8–S13.
44. Lindner KH, Ahnefeld FW, Schuermann W, et al. Epinephrine and norepinephrine in cardiopulmonary resuscitation. Chest 1990;97: 1458–1462.
45. Brown CG, Robinson LA, Jenkins, J, et al. The effect of norepinephrine on regional cerebral blood flow during cardiopulmonary resuscitation. Am J Emerg Med 1989;7:278–282.
46. Lindner KH, Ahnefeld FW, Grünert A. Epinephrine versus norepinephrine in prehospital ventricular fibrillation. Am J Cardiol 1991; 678:427–428.
47. Callaham M, Madsen CD, Barton CW, et al. A randomized clinical trial of high-dose epinephrine and norepinephrine versus standard-dose epinephrine in prehospital cardiac arrest. JAMA 1992;268: 2667–2672.
48. Gonzalez ER, Ornato JP, Garnett AR, et al. Dose-dependent vasopressor response to epinephrine during CPR in human beings. Ann Emerg Med 1989;19:920–925.
49. Goetting MG, Paradis NA. High-dose epinephrine improves outcome from pediatric cardiac arrest. Ann Emerg Med 1991;20:22–26.
50. Lindner KH, Ahnefeld FW, Prengel AW. Comparison of standard and high-dose adrenaline in the resuscitation of asystole and electromechanical dissociation. Acta Anaesthesiol Scand 1991;35:253–256.
51. Callaham M, Barton CW, Kayser S. Potential complications of high-dose epinephrine therapy in patients resuscitated from cardiac arrest. JAMA 1991;265:1117–1122.
52. Stiell IG, Hebert PC, Weitzman BN, et al. High-dose epinephrine in adult cardiac arrest. N Engl J Med 1992;327:1045–1050.
53. Brown CG, Martin DR, Pepe PE, et al. A comparison of standard-dose and high-dose epinephrine in cardiac arrest outside the hospital. N Engl J Med 1992;327:1051–1055.
54. Lipman J, Wilson W, Kobilski S, et al. High-dose adrenaline in adult in-hospital asystolic cardiopulmonary resuscitation: A double-blind randomised trial. Anaesth Intensive Care 1993;21:192–196.
55. Lindner KH, Prengel AW, Pfenninger EG, et al. Vasopressin improves vital organ blood flow during closed-chest cardiopulmonary resuscitation in pigs. Circulation 1995;91:215–221.
56. Lindner KH, Haak T, Keller A, et al. Release of endogenous vasopressor during and after cardiopulmonary resuscitation. Heart 1996; 75:145–150.
57. Lindner KH, Prengel AW, Brinkmann, et al. Vasopressin administration in refractory cardiac arrest. Ann Intern Med 1996;124: 1061–1064.
58. Scheinman MM, Levine JH, Cannom DS, et al. Dose-ranging study of intravenous amiodarone in patients with life-threatening ventricular tachyarrhythmias. Circulation 1995;92:3264–3272.
59. Kowey PR, Levine JH, Herre JM, et al. Randomized, double-blind comparison of intravenous amiodarone and bretylium in the treatment of patients with recurrent, hemodynamically destabilizing ventricular tachycardia or fibrillation. Circulation 1995;92:3255–3262.
60. Haynes RE, Chinn TI, Copass MK, et al. Comparison of bretylium tosylate and lidocaine in the management of out-of-hospital ventricular fibrillation: A randomized clinical trial. Am J Cardiol 1981; 48:353–356.
61. Olson DW, Thompson BM, Daqrin JC, et al. A randomized comparison study of bretylium tosylate and lidocaine in the resuscitation of patients with out-of-hospital ventricular fibrillation in a paramedic system. Ann Emerg Med 1984;13:807–810.
62. Chow MSS, Kluger J, DiPersio DM, et al. Antifibrillatory effects of lidocaine and bretylium immediately post cardiopulmonary resuscitation. Am Heart J 1985;110:938–943.
63. Hanyok JJ, Chow MSS, Kluger J, et al. Antifibrillatory effects of high dose bretylium and a lidocaine–bretylium combination during cardiopulmonary resuscitation. Crit Care Med 1988;16:691–694.
64. Jaffe AS. The use of antiarrhythmics in advanced cardiac life support. Ann Emerg Med 1993;22(2 part 2):307–316.
65. Pentel P, Benowitz N. Pharmacokinetic and pharmacodynamic considerations in drug therapy of cardiac emergencies. Clin Pharmacokinet 1984;9:273–308.
66. Advanced Cardiac Life Support Working Group. Cardiovascular pharmacology I. In: Jaffe AS, ed: Textbook of Advanced Cardiac Life Support. Dallas, American Heart Association, 1987:97–113.
67. Chow MSS. Intravenous amiodarone: Pharmacology, pharmacokinetics, and clinical use. Ann Pharmacother 1996;30:637–643.
68. Thompson RG, Cobb LA. Hypokalemia after resuscitation from out-of-hospital ventricular fibrillation. JAMA 1982;248:2860–2863.
69. Ornato JP, Gonzalez ER, Starke H, et al. Incidence and causes of hypokalemia associated with cardiac resuscitation. Am J Emerg Med 1985;3:503–506.
70. Higham PD, Adams PC, Murray, et al. Plasma potassium, serum magnesium and ventricular fibrillation: A prospective study. Q J Med 1993;86:609–617.
71. Singh BN, Hollenberg NK, Poole-Wilson PA, et al. Diuretic induced potassium and magnesium deficiency: Relation to drug-induced QT prolongation, cardiac arrhythmias and sudden death. J Hypertens 1992;10:301–316.
72. McInnes, GT, Yeo WW, Ramsay LE, et al. Cardiotoxicity and diuretics: Much speculation—little substance. J Hypertens 1992;10: 317–335.
73. Eisenberg MJ. Magnesium deficiency and sudden death. Am Heart J 1992;124:544–549.

74. Whang R, Flink EB, Dyckner T, et al. Magnesium depletion as a cause of refractory potassium repletion. Arch Intern Med 1985;145:1686–1689.
75. Boyd JC, Bruns DE, Wills MR. Occurrence of hypomagnesemia in hypokalemic states. Clin Chem 1983;29:178–179.
76. Brown DC, Lewis AJ, Criley JM. Asystole and its treatment: The possible role of the parasympathetic nervous system in cardiac arrest. JACEP 1979;8:448–452.
77. Gupta PK, Lichstein E, Chadda KD. Transient atrioventricular standstill: Etiology and management. JAMA 1975:234:1038–1042.
78. Iseri LT, Humphrey SB, Siner EJ. Prehospital brady-asystolic cardiac arrest. Ann Intern Med 1978:88:741–745.
79. Coon GA, Clinton JE, Ruiz E. Use of atropine from bradyasystolic prehospital cardiac arrest. Ann Emerg Med 1981;10:462–467.
80. Stueven HA, Tonsfeldt DJ, Thompson BM, et al. Atropine in asystole: Human studies. Ann Emerg Med 1984;13(part 2):815–817.
81. Ornato JP, Gonzalez ER, Morkunas AR, et al. Treatment of presumed asystole during prehospital cardiac arrest: Superiority of electrical countershock. Am J Emerg Med 1985:3:395–399.
82. Tortolani AJ, Risucci DA, Powell SR, et al. In-hospital cardiopulmonary resuscitation during asystole: Therapeutic factors associated with 24-hour survival. Chest 1989;96:622–632.
83. Chamberlain DA, Turner P, Sneddon JM. Effects of atropine on heart-rate in healthy man. Lancet 1967;2:12–15.
84. Stueven HA, Thompson B, Aprahamian C, et al. Lack of effectiveness of calcium chloride in refractory asystole. Ann Emerg Med 1985;14:630–632.
85. Harrison EE, Arney BD. Use of calcium in electromechanical dissociation. Ann Emerg Med 1984;13(part 2):844–845.
86. Dembo DH. Calcium in advanced life support. Crit Care Med 1981; 9:358–359.
87. Schanne FAX, Kane AB, Young EE, et al. Calcium dependence of toxic cell death: A final common pathway. Science 1979;206:700–702.
88. Kirsch JR, Dean JM, Rogers MC. Current concepts in brain resuscitation. Arch Intern Med 1986;146:1413–1419.
89. Follette DM, Key K, Buckberg GD, et al. Reducing postischemic damage by temporary modification of reperfusate calcium, potassium, pH, and osmolarity. J Thorac Cardiovasc Surg 1981;82:221–238.
90. Bleske BE, Chow MSS, Zhao H, et al. Effects of different dosages and modes of sodium bicarbonate administration during cardiopulmonary resuscitation. Am J Emerg Med 1992;10:525–532.
91. Von Planta M, Bar-Joseph G, Wiklund L, et al. Pathophysiologic and therapeutic implications of acid–base changes during CPR. Ann Emerg Med 1993;22(part 2):404–410.
92. Kuhn GJ, White BC, Swetnam RE, et al. Peripheral vs central circulation time during CPR: A pilot study. Ann Emerg Med 1981;10:417–419.
93. Barsan WG, Levy RC, Weir H. Lidocaine levels during CPR: Differences after peripheral venous, central venous and intracardiac injection. Ann Emerg Med 1981;10:73–78.
94. Emerman CL, Pinchak AC, Hancock D, et al. The effect of bolus injection on circulation times during cardiac arrest. Am J Emerg Med 1990;8:190–193.
95. Raehl CL. Endotracheal drug therapy in cardiopulmonary resuscitation. Clin Pharm 1986;5:572–579.
96. Grillo JA, Gonzalez ER. Changes in the pharmacotherapy of CPR. Heart Lung 1993;22:548–553.
97. Longstreth WT, Diehr P, Cobb LA, et al. Neurologic outcome and blood glucose levels during out-of-hospital cardiopulmonary resuscitation. Neurology 1986;36:1186–1191.
98. Martin GB, O'Brien JF, Best R, et al. Insulin and glucose levels during CPR in the canine model. Ann Emerg Med 1985;14:293–297.
99. Thomas SH, Gough JE, Benson N, et al. Accuracy of fingerstick glucose determination in patients receiving CPR. South Med J 1994;87:1072–1075.
100. Harling DW, Wilson RM. Misleading result from a capillary blood sugar sample during acute resuscitation. Resuscitation 1995;29:139–141.
101. Murphy DF, Finucan TE. New do-not-resuscitate policies: A first step in cost control. Arch Intern Med 1993;153:1641–1648.
102. Jecker NS, Schneiderman LJ. Ceasing futile resuscitation in the field: Ethical considerations. Arch Intern Med 1992;152:2392–2397.
103. Bonnin MJ, Pepe PE, Kimball KT, et al. Distinct criteria for termination of resuscitation in the out-of-hospital setting. JAMA 1993;270:1457–1462.
104. George AL, Folk BP, Crecelius PK, et al. Pre-arrest morbidity and other correlates of survival after in-hospital cardiopulmonary arrest. Am J Med 1989;87:28–34.

10
HYPERTENSION

David W. Hawkins, PharmD, Henry I. Bussey, PharmD, and L. Michael Prisant, MD

Arterial blood pressure is generated by the interplay between blood flow and the resistance to blood flow. It reaches a peak during cardiac systole (systolic pressure) and a nadir at the end of diastole (diastolic pressure). Arterial blood pressure is conventionally measured in millimeters of mercury and recorded as systolic pressure over diastolic pressure (120/80 mm Hg). The difference between systolic and diastolic pressure, pulse pressure, is an indicator of the tone of arterial walls. The mean arterial pressure is the average pressure throughout the cardiac cycle. Mean arterial pressure (MAP) can be estimated by adding one-third of the pulse pressure (PP) to the diastolic blood pressure (DBP): $MAP = \frac{1}{3}PP + DBP$.

Under normal physiologic conditions, the arterial blood pressure stays within narrow limits. It may reach its height during physical or emotional stress and it usually falls to its lowest level during sleep. Blood pressure tends to be lower in women than men, it tends to be higher in blacks than whites, and it rises with age.

Arterial blood pressure (BP) can be defined hemodynamically as the product of cardiac output (CO) and total peripheral resistance (TPR): $BP = CO \times TPR$. Cardiac output is the major determinant of systolic pressure while total peripheral resistance largely determines the level of diastolic pressure. In turn, cardiac output is a function of stroke volume, heart rate, and venous capacitance. Factors that increase stroke volume or heart rate may increase cardiac output and, consequently, systolic blood pressure. Venous capacitance affects the volume of blood (or preload) that is returned to the heart through the central venous circulation. Venous dilatation increases venous capacitance and decreases preload and systolic pressure. Contraction of the peripheral veins, of course, would cause the opposite effect.

Total peripheral resistance is regulated chiefly by contraction and dilation of the arterioles. Arteriolar constriction increases peripheral resistance and thus diastolic blood pressure. Other factors that affect intravascular resistance include the elasticity of aortic and arterial walls and blood viscosity.

Because arterial blood pressure is a continuous variable, it is impossible to define a cut point below which the blood pressure is normal and above which the pressure is abnormally high. Nevertheless, evidence from epidemiologic studies clearly indicates a strong correlation between blood pressure and cardiovascular morbidity and mortality.[1] The higher the pressure, the more likely it is that an individual will experience stroke, myocardial infarction, angina, heart failure, renal failure, or early death from a cardiovascular cause. In addition, large-scale clinical studies have shown that the increased risk of stroke and heart failure and death associated with elevated blood pressure is substantially reduced by interventions that lower blood pressure.[2–8]

The Sixth Joint National Committee on the Detection, Evaluation, and Treatment of High Blood Pressure (JNC-VI)[9] classifies hypertension in adults as follows:

Category	Systolic (mm Hg)	Diastolic (mm Hg)
Optimal	<120	<80
Normal	<130	<85
High normal	130–139	85–89
Hypertension		
Stage 1	140–159	90–99
Stage 2	160–179	100–109
Stage 3	≥180	≥110

If the diastolic blood pressure is less than 90 mm Hg and the systolic blood pressure is 140 mm Hg or higher, then the term *isolated systolic hypertension* is applicable. Isolated systolic hypertension is believed to result from the pathophysiology of aging and portends an increased risk of cardiovascular morbidity and mortality.

A marked or sharp increase in diastolic blood pressure is considered a hypertensive crisis. Hypertensive crises represent either a hypertensive emergency or a hypertensive urgency. If the elevation of diastolic blood pressure is accompanied by acute target organ injury, then a hypertensive emergency exists. Examples of acute target organ injury include encephalopathy, intracranial hemorrhage, acute left ventricular failure with pulmonary edema, dissecting aortic aneurysm, unstable angina, and eclampsia or severe hypertension associated with pregnancy. Such hypertensive situations require an immediate but gradual reduction in blood pressure over a period of several minutes to several hours. A reasonable goal is to lower the diastolic blood pressure gradually down to 100 to 110 mm Hg. Hypertensive urgencies, on the other hand, usually signify severe hypertension without signs or symptoms of acute target organ complications. In these situations, reduction in blood pressure may proceed safely over several hours to several days.

EPIDEMIOLOGY

As many as 50 million Americans have high blood pressure (≥140/90 mm Hg).[9] Blood pressure increases with age, but the onset of hypertension most often occurs during the third, fourth, and fifth decades of life. The prevalence of hypertension is 17% among white women, 26% among white men, 37% among black women, and 44% among black men 35 to 45 years of age.[10] In the elderly population (age > 65 years), gender differences in blood pressure are less marked, and the prevalence of hypertension is approximately 63% in whites and 76% in blacks.

ETIOLOGY

Hypertension is a heterogeneous disorder that may result from either a specific cause (secondary hypertension) or some underlying pathophysiologic mechanism stemming from an unknown etiology (primary or essential hypertension). Fewer than 5% of people who suffer from high blood pressure have secondary hypertension. In most of these, chronic renal disease or renovascular disease is the cause of hypertension. Other conditions that are known to cause secondary hypertension include pheochromocytoma, Cushing's syndrome, hyperthyroidism, hypothyroidism, hyperparathyroidism, primary aldosteronism, and coarctation of the aorta. In some instances, exposure to various exogenous substances may produce hypertension. The most notable of these are estrogens, glucocorticoids, licorice, sympathomimetic amines, nonsteroidal anti-inflammatory agents, chronic alcohol use, and tyramine-containing foods in combination with monoamine oxidase (MAO) inhibitors.

In the vast majority of individuals with high blood pressure, a specific cause of sustained hypertension cannot be found. A vigorous search for a single underlying abnormality that eventuates into high blood pressure has led to the discovery of numerous mechanisms that may contribute to the pathogenesis of hypertension.

The fact that hypertension often runs in families suggests that genetic factors may play an important pathogenic role in the development of essential hypertension. There is even some evidence that single genes might be responsible for specific subtypes of hypertension. These include genetic traits for high sodium–lithium countertransport, a low urinary kallikrein excretion, increased aldosterone and other adrenal steroids, and high angiotensinogen levels.[11,12] Identifying individuals with these traits could lead to more direct approaches for preventing or treating hypertension.

PATHOPHYSIOLOGY[1,13–22]

Multiple factors may contribute to the development of primary hypertension including abnormal neural mechanisms; defects in peripheral autoregulation; malfunctions in either humoral or vasodepressor mechanisms; and disturbances in sodium, calcium, and natriuretic hormone.

NEURAL COMPONENTS

Both the central (CNS) and the autonomic nervous systems are intricately involved in the maintenance of arterial blood pressure.

Stimulation of certain areas within the CNS (nucleus tractus solitarius, vagal nuclei, vasomotor center, and the area postrema) can result in either an increase or a decrease in blood pressure. For example, α_2-adrenergic stimulation within the CNS decreases blood pressure through an inhibitory effect on the vasomotor center. Increased angiotensin II, however, increases sympathetic outflow from the vasomotor center, which eventuates in an increase in blood pressure.

Located on the presynaptic surface of sympathetic terminals are a variety of receptors that either enhance or inhibit norepinephrine release. The α and β presynaptic receptors play a role in negative and positive feedback to the norepinephrine-containing vesicles located near the neuronal ending. Stimulation of presynaptic α (α_2) receptors exerts a negative inhibition on norepinephrine release. Stimulation of presynaptic β-receptors facilitates further release of norepinephrine.

The α- and β-receptors are also located on the surface of effector cells innervated by sympathetic neuronal fibers. Stimulation of postsynaptic α- (α_1)-receptors on arterioles and venules results in vasoconstriction. There are two types of postsynaptic β-receptors, β_1 and β_2. Both types of β-adrenergic receptors are present in all tissue innervated by the sympathetic nervous system; however, the distribution of β_1- and β_2-receptors is such that in some tissue β_1-receptors predominate and in other tissue β_2-receptors predominate. Stimulation of β_1-receptors in the heart results in an increase in heart rate and contractility. When β_2-receptors in the arterioles and venules are stimulated, vasodilation occurs.

The major negative-feedback mechanism controlling sympathetic activity is the system of baroreceptor reflexes. Baroreceptors are nerve endings lying in the walls of large arteries, especially in the carotid arteries and aortic arch. The baroreceptors respond extremely rapidly to changes in arterial pressure. Baroreceptor impulses are transmitted to the brainstem primarily through the ninth cranial nerve and vagus nerves. In this reflex system, an acute elevation in arterial pressure increases the rate of baroreceptor discharge, which results in vasodilation throughout the peripheral circulatory system and a decrease in heart rate and myocardial contractility. Conversely, low pressure has the opposite effect, causing reflex vasoconstriction and an increase in heart rate and force of contraction. These baroreceptor reflex mechanisms may be blunted in elderly individuals.

A pathologic disturbance in any of these neural components that modulate arterial blood pressure could conceivably lead to a sustained elevation in blood pressure. It is reasonable to postulate that the primary defect can occur in any of the four major components: CNS, autonomic nerve fibers, adrenergic receptors, or baroreceptors. Also, because they are so physiologically interrelated, a defect in one component may disturb the normal function in another, and the combined abnormalities may then cause hypertension.

PERIPHERAL AUTOREGULATORY COMPONENTS

Abnormalities in either the renal or tissue autoregulatory processes could cause hypertension. In fact, it seems reasonable to postulate that individuals may first develop a renal defect for sodium excretion and then reset their tissue autoregulatory processes to a higher arterial blood pressure.

Normally, the volume–pressure adaptive mechanism of the kidney works well to maintain a normal blood pressure. When the blood pressure drops, the kidneys adapt by retaining more sodium and water. This leads to plasma volume expansion, which increases blood pressure. Conversely, when blood pressure rises above normal, sodium and water excretion are increased, plasma volume and cardiac output are reduced, and the blood pressure returns to normal.

Local autoregulatory processes operate to maintain adequate tissue oxygenation. When oxygen demand is low, the arteriolar bed is in a relatively constricted state. Peripheral vascular resistance is maintained at a sufficient level to regulate adequate blood flow (flow = pressure/resistance). An increase in metabolic demand triggers arteriolar vasodilation through autoregulation. This then lowers peripheral vascular resistance to increase blood flow and oxygen delivery.

An initial defect in the renal adaptive mechanism could lead to plasma volume expansion and increase blood flow to peripheral tissues even when blood pressure is normal. To offset the increase in blood flow, local tissue autoregulatory processes would induce arteriolar constriction to raise the peripheral vascular resistance. In time, a thickening of the arteriolar walls may occur, resulting in a sustained elevation in peripheral vascular resistance. An increase in total peripheral vascular resistance is a common underlying problem in patients with primary hypertension.

HUMORAL MECHANISMS

At least three possible humoral abnormalities may be responsible for causing primary hypertension in some individuals. One involves the renin–angiotensin–aldosterone system (RAS), which has been well described. Another entails the presence of a natriuretic hormone that modulates sodium transport. A third is associated with the possible link between hyperinsulinemia and hypertension.

The RAS is important to the regulation of sodium, potassium, and fluid balance, and it significantly influences vascular tone and sympathetic nervous system activity. Of course, all of these factors contribute to blood pressure homeostasis.

In the kidney, renin is synthesized and stored in the juxtaglomerular cells, which are located primarily in the media of the renal afferent arterioles. Several factors are known to control renin release. These can be grouped into intrarenal factors (such as perfusion pressure, catecholamines, angiotensin II) and extrarenal factors (such as sodium, chloride, and potassium).

The juxtaglomerular cells function as a baroreceptor sensing device in the afferent arteriole. Decreased perfusion pressure leads to an increase in renin secretion. The juxtaglomerular apparatus also contains a group of specialized distal tubule cells referred to collectively as the macula densa. The flux of sodium and chloride across the cells influences renin release. A decrease in the amount of sodium and chloride delivered in the distal tubule stimulates renin release.

Angiotensin II has been shown to directly inhibit the release of renin through negative feedback. Catecholamines increase renin release probably by directly stimulating the juxtaglomerular cells through an action involving the formation of cyclic AMP. Both potassium and calcium may also play a direct role in renin release. Decreased serum potassium or intracellular calcium stimulates renin release by the juxtaglomerular cells.

In blood, renin catalyzes the conversion of angiotensinogen to angiotensin I, which is then converted to angiotensin II by angiotensin-converting enzyme (ACE). Angiotensin II exerts its biologic effects in various tissues following binding to specific receptors classified as AT_1 or AT_2 subtypes. The AT_1 receptor is located in brain, renal, myocardial, vascular, and adrenal tissue. The AT_2 receptor is located in adrenal medullary tissue, uterus, and brain. AT_1 receptors mediate the majority of responses critical to cardiovascular and renal function. An increase in circulating angiotensin II can cause an elevation in blood pressure through both pressor and volume effects. The pressor effects of angiotensin II include direct vasoconstriction, stimulation of catecholamine release from the adrenal medulla, and a centrally mediated increase in sympathetic nervous system activity. Angiotensin II also stimulates the release of aldosterone from the adrenal gland, which leads to retention of both sodium and fluid, with a resultant increase in plasma volume and blood pressure. Clearly, any disturbance in the RAS that leads to an increase in any or all three components could produce hypertension.

The kidney is not the only organ involved in the activation of the RAS. Recent studies have shown that other organs and tissues have the capacity to produce and secrete biologically active forms of angiotensin peptides.

Both the heart and brain contain a local RAS. In the heart, angiotensin II is also generated by a second enzyme, angiotensin I convertase (human chymase), which is not blocked by ACE inhibition. Activation of the myocardial RAS leads to increased cardiac contractility and stimulation of cardiac hypertrophy. The brain RAS has at least two functions. Angiotensin II modulates the production and release of hypothalamic and pituitary hormones. Angiotensin II also enhances sympathetic outflow from the medulla oblongata.

Local generation of biologically active angiotensin peptides in peripheral tissues may play an important role in the increased vascular resistance often observed in hypertensive individuals. There is also some evidence that angiotensin produced by local tissue may interact with other humoral regulators and endothelium-derived growth factors to stimulate vascular smooth muscle growth and metabolism. This in situ generation of angiotensin peptides may, in fact, underlie the development of increased vascular resistance in forms of hypertension that are associated with low plasma renin activity. Components of tissue RAS may be responsible for long-term adaptation to hypertension (i.e., left ventricular hypertrophy, smooth muscle hypertrophy of blood vessels, and glomerular hypertrophy).

Another humoral factor that may be involved in the development of primary hypertension is the increased concentration of natriuretic hormone. The proposed role of natriuretic hormone is to inhibit Na^+/K^+-ATPase and, thus, to interfere with sodium transport across cell membranes. It has been suggested that an inherited defect in the kidney's ability to eliminate sodium would cause an increase in extracellular fluid and plasma volume, as discussed earlier. This may cause a compensatory increase in the concentration of circulating natriuretic hormone, which would increase urinary excretion of sodium and water. This same hormone, however, is also thought to block the active transport of sodium out of arteriolar smooth muscle cells. The increased intracellular concentration of sodium would ultimately lead to increased vascular tone and hypertension.

Evidence linking insulin resistance and hyperinsulinemia to the development of hypertension is mounting. Several possibilities by which hyperinsulinemia may lead to hypertension include renal sodium retention, enhanced sympathetic nervous system activity, and induction of vascular smooth muscle hypertrophy. Another possible way by which insulin could raise blood pressure is by increasing intracellular calcium concentration, which leads to increased vascular resistance. Hyperinsulinemia often accompanies upper body obesity, but even nonobese hypertensive individuals have been shown to be insulin resistant, glucose intolerant, and hyperinsulinemic. The mechanism by which insulin resistance and hyperinsulinemia occur in hypertension is unknown. Hyperinsulinemia is also associated with hypertriglyceridemia, which results in a decreased concentration of HDL cholesterol.

VASCULAR ENDOTHELIAL MECHANISMS

The vascular endothelium plays an important role in regulating blood vessel tone. These regulating functions are mediated through a variety of vasoactive substances synthesized by the endothelial cells including prostacyclin, bradykinin, endothelium-derived relaxing factor (nitric oxide), angiotensin II, and endothelin I.

It has been postulated that a deficiency in the local synthesis of vasodilating substances such as prostacyclin, bradykinin, and nitric oxide, or an increase in the production of vasoconstricting substances such as angiotensin II and endothelin I contribute to the pathogenesis of hypertension, atherosclerosis, and other diseases.

INFLUENCE OF DIETARY SODIUM, CALCIUM, AND POTASSIUM ON BLOOD PRESSURE

The evidence linking excess sodium to the development of hypertension is based on both epidemiologic studies and clinical experiments. In general, population studies indicate that high salt intake is associated with a high prevalence of stroke and hypertension and low salt intake is associated with a low prevalence of hypertension. Clinical studies have consistently shown that restriction of salt intake in the diet lowers blood pressure in many (but not all) subjects with hypertension. The exact mechanism by which excess sodium leads to hypertension is not known, but it is thought to be linked to the natriuretic hormone hypothesis discussed before. It has been proposed that an increased sodium intake together with an inherited defect in the kidney's ability to excrete sodium leads to a substantial increase in circulating natriuretic hormone. As previously mentioned, natriuretic hormone inhibits intracellular sodium transport, which causes increased vascular reactivity and, consequently, a rise in blood pressure.

Altered calcium homeostasis may also play an important role in the pathogenesis of hypertension. The calcium hypothesis states that a lack of calcium in the diet leads to a disturbance in the balance between intracellular and extracellular calcium. This imbalance is characterized by an increased intracellular concentration of calcium, which leads to altered vascular smooth muscle function and increased peripheral vascular resistance. Some studies have shown that supplementing the diet with calcium results in a modest decrease in the blood pressure of hypertensive subjects. More research is needed to clarify the role of altered calcium homeostasis in causing hypertension in humans.

The role of potassium fluctuations is also inadequately understood. Potassium depletion may cause an increase in peripheral vascular resistance, but the clinical impact of small changes in the serum potassium concentration is not clearly defined. Furthermore, very limited data have suggested that potassium supplementation is associated with a reduced incidence of stroke, but this issue needs further study before supplementation can be endorsed.

CLINICAL PRESENTATION[1,9,13]

Patients with uncomplicated, primary hypertension are usually asymptomatic initially. While a complete history and physical examination may help identify concerns that warrant further evaluation, a few basic tests should be performed in all hypertensive patients prior to initiating drug therapy. These include hemoglobin and hematocrit, urinalysis, serum potassium and creatinine, liver function tests, and electrocardiogram. Total and high-density-lipoprotein cholesterol, plasma glucose, and serum uric acid are indicated to assess other risk factors and to develop baseline data for monitoring drug-induced metabolic changes. As the hypertension progresses, however, symptoms characteristic of cardiovascular, cerebrovascular, or renal disease may occur as the patient develops target organ damage. Patients with secondary hypertension usually complain of symptoms suggestive of the underlying disorder. For example, many patients with pheochromocytoma have a history of paroxysmal headaches, sweating, tachycardia, and palpitations occurring singly or in combinations. More than half of the patients with this form of secondary hypertension suffer episodes of orthostatic dizziness or syncope. In primary aldosteronism, hypokalemic symptoms usually include muscle cramps and muscle weakness. Patients who present with hypertension secondary to Cushing's syndrome may complain of weight gain, polyuria, edema, menstrual irregularities, recurrent acne, or muscular weakness.

Frequently, the only sign of primary hypertension is an elevated blood pressure. The rest of the physical examination may be completely normal. Again, as the hypertension progresses, signs of end-organ damage begin to appear. These are chiefly related to pathologic changes in the eye, brain, heart, kidneys, and peripheral blood vessels.

The funduscopic exam may reveal arteriolar narrowing reflective of increased peripheral vascular resistance and/or arteriovenous nicking, which is a consequence of long-standing arteriosclerosis. Retinal hemorrhages and infarcts reflect serious vasculitis secondary to high arterial blood pressure indicative of accelerated hypertension. Papilledema in hypertensive patients suggests a malignant stage of high blood pressure requiring rapid treatment.

The neurologic examination will reveal gross neurologic deficits in patients with previous cerebral infarcts or encephalopathy. A slight hemiparesis with some incoordination and hyperreflexia may also be found upon careful neurologic examination.

Auscultation of the heart may identify an accentuated second heart sound (S_2) created by a high intra-aortic diastolic pressure, a systolic ejection murmur caused by a hyperdynamic state, an S_4 gallop rhythm indicative of decreased ventricular compliance, or an S_3 gallop sound associated with congestive heart failure.

The physical examination may provide clues for diagnosing secondary hypertension. For example, patients with coarctation of the aorta may have diminished or even absent femoral pulses and patients with renal artery stenosis may have an abdominal systolic–diastolic bruit. Of course, patients with Cushing's syndrome may have the classic physical features (i.e., moon face, buffalo hump, hirsutism, abdominal striae) that characterize individuals with this endocrine disorder.

Certain routine laboratory tests may help identify patients with secondary hypertension. A low serum potassium before antihypertensive therapy is begun may suggest mineralocorticoid-induced hypertension. The presence of protein, blood cells, and casts in the urine may indicate an underlying parenchymal kidney disease as the cause of hypertension.

More specific laboratory tests are used to diagnose secondary hypertension. These include plasma norepinephrine and urinary metanephrine for pheochromocytoma, plasma and urinary aldosterone levels for primary aldosteronism, and plasma renin activity, captopril stimulation test, renal vein renins, and renal artery angiography for renovascular disease.

BLOOD PRESSURE MEASUREMENT

The usual, indirect method of measuring blood pressure is with the sphygmomanometer cuff on the patient's arm at the level of the heart. It is important to use a proper size cuff to avoid overestimating the actual pressure when the cuff is too small. The inflatable rubber bag should encircle at least 80% of the arm and the width of the cuff should be at least two-thirds the length of the upper arm. It is also imperative to use equipment that meets certification criteria.[23]

Proper technique requires rapid inflation of the cuff to about 30 mm Hg above the point at which the radial pulse disappears, and then released at a rate of 2 to 3 mm Hg per second. As the pressure falls, the Korotkoff sounds become audible through the bell of the stethoscope applied over the brachial artery in the antecubital fossa. The first sounds consist of clear tapping sounds. Systolic blood pressure should be recorded at the level the first tapping sound is heard. Diastolic blood pressure should be read at the moment all sounds disappear (i.e., at the fifth Korotkoff phase).

It should be emphasized that a single reading of blood pressure elevation does not constitute a diagnosis of hypertension. If the blood pressure taken on two or more subsequent days is 140/90 mm Hg or higher, then a diagnosis of hypertension is confirmed.

Several factors, in addition to those mentioned previously, may give misleading blood pressure measurements. A falsely high blood pressure may be recorded in elderly patients with a rigid, calcified brachial artery. This is one cause of pseudohypertension, because the actual pressure as determined by direct intraarterial measurement is much lower than that obtained by the indirect cuff method. To test for this cause of pseudohypertension, the blood pressure cuff should be inflated above peak systolic blood pressure. If the radial artery remains palpable, the patient has rigid arteries. This is known as a positive Osler's maneuver.

The occurrence of an "auscultatory gap" in some patients may result in an erroneous underestimation of systolic or overestimation of diastolic measurement. As the cuff pressure falls from the true systolic value, the Korotkoff sound may sequentially disappear (a false diastolic measurement), "reappear" (a false systolic measurement), and then disappear again at the true diastolic value. A third factor that may produce misleading values is an irregular ventricular rate. Because systolic and diastolic pressures may vary from one heartbeat to the next, the correct recording of the patient's blood pressure requires that the highest and lowest systolic and diastolic values be carefully identified and then averaged to yield a "mean" systolic and a "mean" diastolic value. In all instances, it is recommended that the stethoscope bell, rather than the diaphragm, be used. Otherwise, the low-frequency Korotkoff sounds may not be heard clearly and accurately, especially if the patient has faint or "distant" sounds.

Blood pressure varies with environmental temperature, the time of day, the timing of meals, physical activity, posture, and emotions. An individual who exhibits a defense reflex in a medical setting may experience a rise in blood pressure that returns to normal outside the medical setting. This is known as "white coat" hypertension. White coat hypertension appears to occur in approximately 20% of newly diagnosed hypertensive patients. Interestingly, such a rise in blood pressure gradually dissipates over several hours after leaving the office and usually is not precipitated by other stresses in the patient's daily life. White coat hypertension is more likely to occur in young, female patients who do not have a long history of hypertension. Suspected white coat hypertension is one of a limited number of indications for which ambulatory blood pressure monitoring may be warranted. Recently the National High Blood Pressure Education Program Coordinating Committee published a report from their working group on ambulatory blood pressure monitoring.[24] This report reviewed the technical, logistic, and financial constraints of utilizing currently available 24-hour blood pressure monitoring systems. Although it appears that a patient's 24-hour blood pressure profile correlates better with end-organ damage than do casual office measurements, current limitations prohibit routine use of such technology. For a more thorough discussion of this area, the reader is referred to the committee's report and other reviews.[25,26]

NATURAL COURSE

Early in the course of primary hypertension, the blood pressure may fluctuate between abnormal and normal levels. This stage of the disease is usually referred to as labile hypertension. It may begin as early as the second decade of life. During this stage, many patients have a hyperdynamic circulation with increased cardiac output and normal or even low peripheral vascular resistance.

As the disease progresses, peripheral vascular resistance increases and patients develop a sustained increase in blood pressure. In most cases the diastolic blood pressure does not exceed 115 mm Hg. Individuals with secondary hypertension are more likely to experience severe elevations in blood pressure. Only a small proportion of patients suffering from primary hypertension develop accelerated or severe hypertension.

The main causes of death in hypertensive subjects are cerebrovascular accidents, cardiovascular events, and renal failure. The probability of premature death from any of these causes increases with increasing systolic or diastolic blood pressure.

Hypertension accelerates atherosclerosis and stimulates left ventricular and vascular hypertrophy. These pathologic changes are thought to be secondary to both a chronic pressure overload and a variety of nonhemodynamic stimuli. Some of the nonhemodynamic disturbances that have been implicated in the pathogenesis of cardiac and vascular hypertrophy include the adrenergic and renin–angiotensin systems, increased synthesis and secretion of endothelin I, and a decreased production of prostacyclin and endothelial-derived relaxing factor. The mechanisms of accelerated atherogenesis in hypertension include proliferation of smooth muscle cells, lipid infiltration into the vascular endothelium, and an enhancement of vascular calcium accumulation.

The target organ damage secondary to chronic hypertension principally involves the brain, the eye, the heart, and the kidney.

Hypertension is the major cause of stroke. The types of cerebrovascular lesions most commonly seen in hypertensive individuals include lacunar infarcts caused by thrombotic occlusion of small vessels, intracerebral hemorrhage resulting from ruptured microaneurysms, and transient ischemic attacks secondary to atherosclerotic disease in the carotid arteries.

The damage hypertension does to the eye is characterized by a variety of retinopathies. Nonspecific changes include an increased light reflex, increased tortuosity of vessels, and arteriovenous nicking. These are all associated with the accelerated arteriosclerosis that accompanies hypertension. Focal arteriolar narrowing, retinal infarcts, and flame-shaped hemorrhages are usually pathognomonic of an accelerated or malignant phase of hypertension and are associated with increased arteriolar resistance and fibrinoid necrosis. Papilledema is a swelling of the optic disc and is caused by a breakdown in autoregulation of capillary blood flow in the presence of high pressure. Its presence is indicative of severe hypertension.

The principal cardiac complications of hypertension are left ventricular hypertrophy, coronary heart disease, and congestive heart failure. These complications may lead to cardiac arrhythmias, angina, myocardial infarction, and sudden death. Coronary heart disease is the most common cause of death in hypertensive patients.

The renal damage caused by hypertension is pathologically characterized by hyaline arteriosclerosis, hyperplastic arteriosclerosis, arteriolar hypertrophy, fibrinoid necrosis, and atheroma of the major renal arteries. Glomerular hyperfiltration and intraglomerular hypertension may be the earliest stage of hypertensive nephropathy followed by microalbuminuria and a gradual decline in renal function. Frank renal failure is rare unless accelerated hypertension occurs in which fibrinoid necrosis of renal arterioles is the pathologic hallmark. The primary renal complication in hypertension is nephrosclerosis, which is secondary to accelerated arteriosclerosis. Atheromatous disease of a major renal artery may give rise to renal artery stenosis. Although renal failure is an uncommon complication of essential hypertension, it remains an important cause of end-stage renal disease, especially in blacks.

▶ TREATMENT: Hypertension

DESIRED OUTCOME AND GENERAL APPROACH TO TREATMENT

The treatment plan for hypertension should include measures to minimize contributing factors and to reduce or prevent other known risk factors. Obesity, hyperlipidemia, glucose intolerance, excessive salt intake, cigarette smoking, and alcohol consumption are important risk factors that should be addressed in formulating a rational antihypertensive treatment program. The JNC-VI treatment algorithm is presented in Figure 10–1.

It seems reasonable that the first step in the treatment of hypertension would consist of a carefully constructed, aggressively promoted modification in life-style. A sensible dietary program should be designed for gradual weight reduction, if appropriate, and for reducing the saturated fat and salt content of the diet. The rationale for dietary treatment of hypertension is based on the following observations and facts:

1. Hypertension is two to three times more prevalent in overweight as compared to lean persons.
2. Sixty percent of hypertensive persons are overweight.
3. Weight loss, even as little as 10 pounds, decreases blood pressure in 60% to 80% of hypertensive, overweight individuals.
4. Upper body obesity is associated with insulin resistance and hyperinsulinemia. Hyperinsulinemia may be involved in the pathogenesis of hypertension as well as hyperlipidemia.
5. Diets rich in fruits and vegetables and low in saturated fat have been shown to lower blood pressure in hypertensive individuals.[27]
6. Thirty percent to 60% of hypertensive patients are salt sensitive. In this group, blood pressure will fall by an average of 10 mm Hg if salt intake is reduced from 12 g daily to 6 g daily.

In addition to these dietary measures, it is also important to reduce the intake of alcohol, because excessive alcohol intake may either cause or worsen hypertension. Hypertensive patients who drink alcoholic beverages should restrict their intake to one ounce or less per day. One ounce of alcohol is contained in 2 ounces of 100 proof whiskey, 8 ounces of wine, or 24 ounces of beer. Because cigarette smoking is another major independent risk factor of coronary heart disease, patients who smoke should undergo counseling and take advantage of any available smoking-cessation programs.

Another useful life-style modification for hypertensive patients is a carefully designed program of regular physical exercise. Studies have shown that aerobic exercise, such as jogging, swimming, walking, and bicycling, can reduce blood pressure even in the absence of weight loss. Patients should consult their physicians before starting an exercise program.

The coexistence of hypertension and diabetes mellitus occurs more than chance alone would predict. This fact has led some to propose that these two chronic conditions may share a common etiologic factor. As stated earlier, insulin resistance may play a role in the pathogenesis of hypertension. Insulin resistance is, of course, an important pathogenic lesion in non-insulin-dependent diabetes mellitus. Just what causes insulin resistance to occur in the first place in either diabetes or

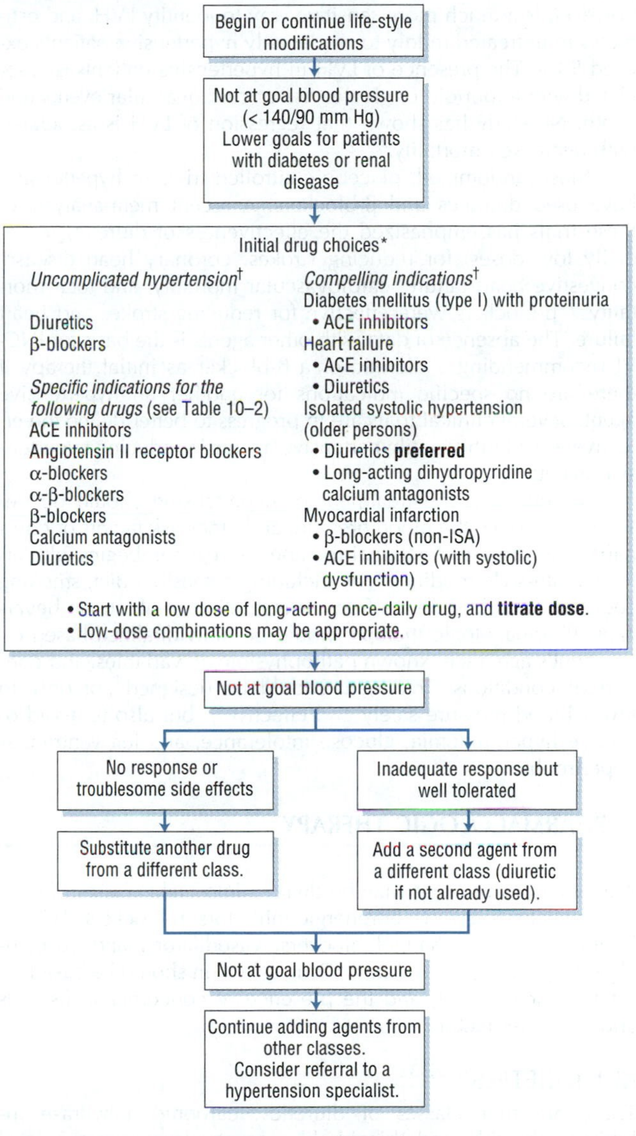

FIGURE 10–1. Algorithm for the treatment of hypertension *Unless contraindicated. ACE, angiotensin-converting enzyme; ISA, intrinsic sympathomimetic activity. †Based on randomized controlled trials. *(From the Sixth Report of the Joint National Committee on Prevention, Detection, Evaluation, and Treatment of High Blood Pressure. NIH Publication No. 98-4080, November 1997.)*

hypertension is not known. Any intervention that increases insulin resistance or glucose intolerance may adversely affect control of blood pressure. Conversely, measures that ameliorate insulin resistance or reduce glucose intolerance should help in the overall management of hypertension.[28]

One of the major independent risk factors associated with the development of coronary heart disease, congestive heart failure, and sudden death in hypertensive patients is left ventricular hypertrophy (LVH). In past years, the prevalence of LVH was considerably underestimated because its detection depended on electrocardiographic interpretation. The electrocardiogram is a very insensitive method for detecting LVH. The echocardiogram, however, is a much more sensitive way to identify LVH, and estimates in untreated mildly to moderately hypertensive patients exceed 50%. The presence of LVH in hypertensive patients is associated with a fourfold or greater risk of cardiovascular events and death. No study has shown that regression of LVH is associated with decreased mortality.[29,30]

Most randomized, placebo-controlled trials in hypertension have used diuretics and β-blockers. A recent meta-analysis of these trials has emphasized the effectiveness of diuretics (especially low doses) for reducing strokes, coronary heart disease, congestive heart failure, cardiovascular mortality, and total mortality.[31] β-blockers were effective for reducing strokes and heart failure. The absence of data with other agents is the basis for JNC-VI recommending a diuretic or a β-blocker as initial therapy if there are no specific indications for another antihypertensive agent. Several clinical trials are in progress to better define the effectiveness of other antihypertensive agents in reducing hypertensive events.

In summary, the treatment of hypertension should be designed to reduce the blood pressure and other risk factors of coronary heart disease. A rational therapeutic regimen begins with effective life-style modifications including a sensible diet, smoking cessation, and abstinence from or restriction of alcoholic beverages. Pharmacologic therapy should be individualized based on a patient's age, race, known pathophysiologic variables, and concurrent conditions. Treatment should be designed not only to lower blood pressure safely and effectively, but also to avoid or reverse hyperlipidemia, glucose intolerance, and left ventricular hypertrophy.

PHARMACOLOGIC THERAPY

Antihypertensive drugs may be divided into eight classes: diuretics, central α_2-agonists, adrenergic inhibitors, β-blockers, ACE inhibitors, calcium channel blockers, vasodilators, and postganglionic sympathetic inhibitors. Drug selection should be based on safety, efficacy, cost, and the presence of concomitant diseases and other risk factors.

DIURETICS[1,32,33]

There are four classes of diuretics: carbonic anhydrase inhibitors, thiazide and thiazide-like agents, loop diuretics, and potassium-sparing diuretics. In general, carbonic anhydrase inhibitors are weak antihypertensive agents and therefore are not used in the treatment of hypertension. The potassium-sparing diuretics are also weak antihypertensive agents when used alone, but provide an additive hypotensive effect when used in combination with thiazide or loop diuretics. Moreover, they counteract the potassium- and magnesium-losing properties of other diuretic agents.

In patients with adequate renal function (i.e., a glomerular filtration rate greater than 30 mL/min), thiazide diuretics appear to be more effective hypotensive agents than loop diuretics such as furosemide. As renal function declines, however, sodium and fluid accumulate and the use of a more potent diuretic is necessary to counter the effects that volume and sodium expansion have on arterial blood pressure.

All thiazide diuretics are equally effective in lowering blood pressure. The major differences between the various thiazides are the serum half-life and the duration of diuretic effect. These differences may not be clinically relevant, however, because the serum half-life of most antihypertensive agents does not correlate with the hypotensive duration of action. Moreover, diuretics may lower blood pressure primarily through extrarenal mechanisms.

Mechanism of Action

The exact hypotensive mode of action of diuretics is not known. Of course, acutely, diuretics lower blood pressure by causing a diuresis. The reduction in plasma volume and stroke volume associated with a diuresis decreases cardiac output and, consequently, blood pressure. The initial drop in cardiac output produced by the diuresis causes a compensatory increase in peripheral vascular resistance. With continuing diuretic therapy, the extracellular fluid volume and plasma volume return almost to pretreatment levels, and peripheral vascular resistance falls below its pretreatment baseline. It is the reduction in peripheral vascular resistance that accompanies chronic use of diuretics that is responsible for their long-term hypotensive effectiveness.

Evidently, diuretic-induced total body sodium depletion is necessary for blood pressure reduction, because a high dietary sodium intake can reverse the antihypertensive effect and a low salt intake will potentiate the effect of diuretics on blood pressure.

It has been postulated that thiazide diuretics lower blood pressure by mobilizing sodium and water from arteriolar walls. This action would lessen the amount of physical encroachment on the lumen of the vessel created by excessive accumulation of intracellular fluid. Of course, as the diameter of the lumen increases (opens up), there is less resistance to the flow of blood through the vessel (i.e., peripheral vascular resistance drops).

Another postulated hypotensive mechanism of action stems from the possible association between changes in the electrolyte composition of intraarteriolar walls and vascular responsiveness. The alterations in sodium, potassium, calcium, and magnesium intracellular concentrations may decrease vascular response to pressor substances and increase vascular response to depressor substances.

Still another possible antihypertensive mode of action of the thiazide diuretics is direct relaxation of vascular smooth muscle. This theory is based on the known mechanism of action of diazoxide, a chemical closely related to the thiazide diuretics. Diazoxide is a direct vasodilator, and it is possible that the thiazide diuretics exert a similar action.

When diuretics are used in combination with other antihypertensive agents, an additive hypotensive effect is usually observed. This occurs as a result of two independent pharmacodynamic properties. First, it is a well-known pharmacologic principle that when two drugs cause the same effect through different mechanisms of action, their combined use results in an additive or synergistic response. Second, many nondiuretic antihypertensive agents induce salt and water retention, which, of course, is counteracted by the concurrent use of a diuretic.

Side Effects

The side effects of thiazide diuretics include hypokalemia, hypomagnesemia, hypercalcemia, hyperuricemia, hyperglycemia, hyperlipidemia, and sexual dysfunction. Loop diuretics may cause the same side effects, although the effect on serum lipids and glucose is not as significant and hypocalcemia may occur. Short-term studies indicate that indapamide does not adversely effect lipids or glucose tolerance, or cause sexual dysfunction.

The hypokalemia and hypomagnesemia caused by diuretics may lead to cardiac arrhythmias in susceptible patients. Patients at greatest risk are those receiving digitalis therapy, those with left ventricular hypertrophy, and those with ischemic heart disease. Low-dose diuretic therapy (i.e., 25 mg of hydrochlorthiazide or chlorthalidone daily) seldom causes electrolyte disturbances in patients with uncomplicated hypertension.

Diuretic-induced hyperuricemia may produce gouty arthritis or uric acid stones, especially in individuals who are predisposed to gout. In patients with no previous history of gout, acute gouty arthritis and nephrolithiasis are extremely unlikely consequences of diuretic-induced hyperuricemia. If some manifestation of gout does occur in a patient who requires diuretic therapy for effective treatment of hypertension, allopurinol or a uricosuric agent can be given to prevent recurrent gouty attacks without compromising the antihypertensive effects of the diuretic.

At high doses, thiazide and loop diuretics may adversely affect glucose control and serum lipids. These effects, however, are usually transient and often inconsequential. Low-dose diuretic therapy has not been shown to produce metabolic abnormalities.

Potassium-sparing diuretics have the potential for causing hyperkalemia, especially in patients with renal insufficiency or diabetes, and in patients receiving concurrent treatment with an ACE inhibitor, NSAIDs, or potassium supplements. The potassium-sparing drug spironolactone may cause gynecomastia.

CENTRAL α_2-RECEPTOR AGONISTS[1,34]

Clonidine, guanabenz, guanfacine, and methyldopa all lower blood pressure primarily by stimulating α_2-adrenergic receptors in the brain. Such action leads to a reduction in sympathetic outflow from the vasomotor center in the brain and an associated increase in vagal tone. It is also possible that stimulation of presynaptic α_2-receptors peripherally may contribute to the reduction in sympathetic tone. As a consequence of reduced sympathetic activity together with some enhancement of parasympathetic activity, heart rate is decreased, cardiac output decreases slightly, total peripheral resistance is lowered, plasma renin activity is reduced, and baroreceptor reflexes are blunted.

Chronic use of the centrally acting α-agonists results in sodium and fluid retention, which appears to be most prominent with methyldopa. Low doses of either clonidine, guanfacine, or guanabenz can be used to treat mild hypertension without the addition of a diuretic; however, methyldopa, even at low doses, usually leads to enough sodium and fluid accumulation that tolerance to its hypotensive effect soon develops in the absence of concurrent diuretic therapy.

Sedation and dry mouth are common side effects of these antihypertensive agents. These symptoms may diminish or completely abate with chronic use of low doses. As with other centrally acting antihypertensive drugs, these agents may cause depression.

Abrupt cessation of any antihypertensive agent may lead to rebound hypertension or overshoot hypertension. Rebound hypertension is characterized by a sudden increase in blood pressure to the pretreatment level, whereas overshoot implies an increase in excess of the pretreatment level. In most cases, abrupt withdrawal of antihypertensive therapy leads to a gradual increase in blood pressure. Rebound hypertension may rarely occur when a central α-receptor agonist is stopped. This is thought to occur secondary to a compensatory increase in norepinephrine release that follows a discontinuation of presynaptic α-receptor stimulation. The propensity for this is increased in patients receiving concurrent β-blocker therapy due to unopposed β-receptor stimulation.

In addition to the side effects already mentioned, methyldopa rarely may cause hepatitis or hemolytic anemia. A transient elevation in liver function tests is occasionally associated with methyldopa therapy and is clinically unimportant. But a persistent increase in serum transaminases or alkaline phosphatase may herald the onset of a fulminant hepatitis, which can be fatal. A Coombs-positive hemolytic anemia occurs in less than 1% of patients receiving methyldopa, although 20% exhibit a positive direct Coombs test without anemia.

One pharmaceutical formulation that may be associated with fewer side effects and increased compliance is the transdermal delivery system for clonidine. This device, which is applied to the skin and left in place for 1 week before being replaced, appears to reduce blood pressure while avoiding the high peak serum drug concentrations that are seen with oral dosing and are thought to contribute to the adverse effects. The delivery system is ideal for patients who cannot take medication by mouth, such as the perioperative patient. The disadvantages of this system are cost, a 20% incidence of local skin rash or irritation, and a 2- or 3-day delay of onset of effect so that oral medications should be overlapped for this period of time when patch therapy is first started. A similar delay in "offset" of action also may be seen when the patch is removed and the blood pressure returns to pretreatment values over a 2- or 3-day period.

PERIPHERAL α_1-RECEPTOR BLOCKERS[1,34,35]

Prazosin, terazosin, and doxazosin are selective α_1-receptor blockers. These selective α_1-blockers differ from phentolamine and phenoxybenzamine in that the latter block both α_1- and α_2-receptors. The severe reflex tachycardia associated with the use of nonselective α-blockers renders them of no value in the treatment of essential hypertension. They are, however, useful for the initial management of pheochromocytoma. Since the selective α-blockers do not alter α_2-receptor activity, they do not usually cause reflex tachycardia.

At low doses, selective α-blockers may be used as monotherapy in the treatment of mild hypertension. At higher doses, and sometimes with chronic administration of even low doses, fluid and sodium accumulate and concurrent diuretic therapy is then required to maintain the hypotensive efficacy of the α-receptor blocker.

Even though the antihypertensive effect of these drugs is achieved through a peripheral mechanism of action, they do cross the blood–brain barrier and may cause CNS side effects such as lassitude, vivid dreams, and depression. The most interesting side effect of selective α_1-blockers is the so-called first-dose phenomenon. This is characterized by transient dizziness or faintness, palpitations, and even syncope occurring within 1 to 3 hours of the first dose, or subsequently after the first increased dose. These episodes are accompanied by orthostatic hypotension and can be obviated by having the patient take the first dose, and first increased dose, at bedtime. Occasionally, orthostatic dizziness persists with chronic administration. α_1-blockers may also cause priapism. α_1-Blockers provide symptomatic benefit to patients with benign prostatic hypertrophy.

β-ADRENOCEPTOR BLOCKERS[1,36,37]

The hypotensive mechanism of β-adrenoceptor blockers (β-blockers) is not exactly known. Several mechanisms of action have been proposed, but none of them has been shown to be consistently associated with a reduction in arterial blood pressure.

β-Blockers reduce cardiac output through their negative chronotropic and inotropic effects on the heart. It is reasonable to postulate that drugs that lower cardiac output lower blood pressure, because blood pressure is the product of cardiac output and peripheral vascular resistance; however, even though cardiac output is reduced after both intravenous and oral administration of propranolol therapy, blood pressure falls only when propranolol is given orally. Furthermore, cardiac output falls to the same degree in patients whose blood pressure is not lowered by these drugs as in patients who respond with a fall in blood pressure. Finally, β-blockers with intrinsic sympathomimetic activity do not reduce cardiac output in the resting state and yet they lower blood pressure and decrease peripheral resistance.

Another possible explanation of the hypotensive action of β-blockers is related to a central action. Within the brain there are both α- and β-receptors. Stimulation of α_2-adrenergic receptors causes a reduction in sympathetic outflow from the vasomotor center. It seems plausible that blocking β-adrenergic receptors in the brain might produce the same effect. All β-blockers traverse the blood–brain barrier, but the extent to which they enter the brain depends on their degree of lipophilicity. At one end of the spectrum is propranolol, a highly lipophilic drug; at the other end is atenolol, which is weakly lipophilic. One would therefore expect a much higher concentration of propranolol in the brain than atenolol after equivalent doses of the two drugs are given, and this indeed is the case. Despite this difference in CNS concentration, there is no difference in their hypotensive effectiveness. Of course, one cannot rule out the possibility that CNS β-blockade is optimally achieved with atenolol even though it penetrates the blood–brain barrier much more poorly than propranolol.

Blockade of β-adrenoceptors located on the surface membranes of juxtaglomerular cells leads to a reduction in the release of renin. This, in turn, may result in the attenuation of the RAS, which should reduce blood pressure. Some studies, in fact, have shown a correlation between pretreatment plasma renin activity and reduction in blood pressure by β-blocker therapy. The higher the plasma renin activity, the greater the reduction in blood pressure. Other studies, however, have not shown an association between pretreatment plasma renin activity and degree of blood pressure reduction achieved by β-blockers. Furthermore, some β-blockers (e.g., pindolol, acebutolol) lower blood pressure without reducing plasma renin levels. Therefore, alternative or additional mechanisms need to be invoked to account for the antihypertensive effect of β-adrenoceptor blocking agents.

It has been suggested that a peripheral mechanism common to all β-blockers may be responsible for the long-term reduction in blood pressure. The proposed peripheral mechanism involves the possible presence of β-adrenoceptors on the surface of sympathetic neuronal endings. Blocking these presynaptic β-receptors could lead to a reduction in the release of norepinephrine into the synaptic cleft. This intriguing hypothesis is based on the theory that norepinephrine release from neuronal endings is regulated to some extent by presynaptic adrenergic feedback loops. Stimulation of presynaptic α_2-receptors would provoke a negative inhibition on the release of norepinephrine, whereas stimulation of presynaptic β-receptors would engender a positive-feedback increase in norepinephrine release. If presynaptic β-receptors do indeed exist, blocking them would interrupt the positive-feedback loop and thus reduce the release of norepinephrine from the neuronal ending. A diminution in the release of norepinephrine from peripheral sympathetic nerve endings should lower blood pressure.

Pharmacodynamics/Pharmacokinetics

Even though there are important pharmacodynamic and pharmacokinetic differences among the various β-blockers (Table 10–1), there is no difference in their clinical antihypertensive efficacy. Three pharmacodynamic properties of the β-blockers differentiate them to some extent. The first of these is cardioselectivity. β-blockers that possess a much greater affinity for β_1-receptors than β_2-receptors are said to be *cardioselective*. The β_1- and β_2-adrenoceptors are distributed throughout the body, but in certain organs and tissues β_1-receptors predominate and in other organs and tissues β_2-receptors predominate. There is a preponderance of β_1-receptors in the heart and kidney and a preponderance of β_2-receptors in the lungs, liver, pancreas, and arteriolar smooth muscle. Stimulation of β_1-receptors produces an increase in heart rate, contractility, and renin release. β_2-receptor stimulation results in bronchodilation and vasodilation. β-Adrenergic blockers that bind more avidly to β_1-receptors than to β_2-receptors are therefore less likely to provoke bronchospasm and vasoconstriction. Also, because both insulin secretion and glycogenolysis are adrenergically mediated, blockade of β_2-receptors may reduce either process and cause hyperglycemia or blunt recovery from hypoglycemia, respectively.

TABLE 10–1. Pharmacodynamic and Pharmacokinetic Properties of the β-Adrenoceptor Blocking Agents

	α-Blockade	β_1-Selectivity	MSA	ISA	Lipid Solubility	Bioavailability (%)	Half-life (h)
Acebutolol	0	+	+	+	Low	20–60	3–4
Atenolol	0	+	0	0	Low	50	6–9
Betaxalol	0	+	±	0	Low	100	14–24
Bisoprolol	0	++	0	0	Low	80	9–12
Carteolol	0	0	0	+	Low	50	6
Carvedilol	+	0	0	0	High	25–35	7–10
Labetalol	+	0	+	0	Moderate	40	3–5
Metoprolol	0	+	0	0	Moderate	50	3–4
Nadolol	0	0	0	0	Low	30	14–24
Penbutolol	0	0	0	+	High	100	5
Pindolol	0	0	+	+++	Moderate	100	3–4
Propranolol	0	0	+	0	High	35	4–6
Timolol	0	0	0	0	Low	75	3–4

MSA = membrane stabilizing activity; ISA = intrinsic sympathomimetic activity.

At low doses, bisoprolol, metoprolol, atenolol, and acebutolol are cardioselective β-blockers. For this reason they may be safer than nonselective β-blockers to use in patients with asthma, chronic obstructive pulmonary disease (COPD), peripheral vascular disease, and diabetes; however, it should be pointed out that cardioselectivity is a dose-dependent phenomenon. At higher doses, metoprolol, bisoprolol, atenolol, and acebutolol lose their relative selectivity for β_1-receptors and block β_2-receptors as effectively as they block β_1-receptors. The dose at which cardioselectivity is lost varies from patient to patient.

Another pharmacodynamic difference among the β-blockers is the intrinsic sympathomimetic activity (ISA) that pindolol, penbutolol, carteolol, and acebutolol possess. These four β-blockers are partial β-receptor agonists and are capable therefore of maintaining normal basal sympathetic tone while blocking the effects of excessive adrenergic stimulation. Unlike cardioselectivity, this property is manifested at all dosage levels and varies in significance only with the intrinsic sympathetic tone. When sympathetic tone is low, as it is during resting states, β-receptors are partially stimulated. Therefore, resting heart rate, cardiac output, and peripheral blood flow are not reduced when receptors are blocked. Theoretically, pindolol, penbutolol, carteolol, and acebutolol would be less hazardous β-blockers to use in patients with borderline congestive heart failure, sinus bradycardia, or perhaps even peripheral vascular disease; however, clinical studies have not confirmed a clear-cut advantage in patients with the aforementioned disorders.

All β-blockers are capable of exerting a membrane-stabilizing action on cardiac cells if large enough doses are given. It was once thought that this membrane-stabilizing or quinidine-like effect was responsible for the antidysrhythmic effect of β-blockers (see Chap. 14). It is now known that the effectiveness of β-blockers in treating or preventing cardiac arrhythmias is due primarily to their β-blockade property. Only propranolol, sotolol, and acebutolol are indicated for arrhythmias. The dose of β-blockers required to achieve membrane-stabilizing activity usually greatly exceeds that used in treating hypertension or cardiac arrhythmias.

Pharmacokinetic differences among β-blockers can be found in first-pass metabolism, serum half-lives, degree of lipophilicity, and route of elimination. Propranolol and metoprolol undergo extensive first-pass metabolism. Therefore, the dose required to achieve β-blockade with either drug is quite variable from patient to patient. Atenolol and nadolol, which have relatively long half-lives, are renally excreted and the dosage of each may need to be adjusted in patients with renal insufficiency. Even though the half-lives of the other β-blockers are much shorter, once-daily administration may still be effective. As is the case with most other antihypertensive agents, the serum half-life does not correlate with the drug's hypotensive duration of action. β-Blockers also vary in terms of their lipophilic properties and thus CNS penetration.

Numerous trials have shown a reduction in mortality and nonfatal reinfarction using β-blockers following an acute myocardial infarction. β-Blockers with ISA (with the exception of acebutolol) do not afford this protection and, in fact, may lead to an increased risk of mortality. Thus, in hypertensive patients surviving an acute myocardial infarction, the use of β-blockers without ISA may be beneficial not only in reducing blood pressure but also in reducing the risk of myocardial reinfarction and mortality.

Studies in hypertensive patients with LVH show that β-blockers reduce blood pressure and produce LVH regression. All β-blockers, with the possible exception of pindolol, appear to reduce left ventricular mass, irrespective of their different pharmacodynamic properties. Recent evidence also indicates that β-blockers may exhibit antiatherosclerotic effects. Whether such effects are due to a reduction in stress forces at artery bifurcations, alteration in cholesterol binding in the arterial wall, an antiplatelet effect, or other mechanisms is not known at this time.

Since sympathetic nervous system activation plays an important role in the progression of heart failure, β-blockers may be helpful in the management of patients with chronic heart failure. Carvedilol has been shown to reduce the mortality in patients with heart failure who are receiving treatment with digoxin, diuretics, and an angiotensin-converting enzyme inhibitor (see Chap. 11).

Side Effects

Most of the side effects of β-blockers represent physiologic consequences of antagonizing β-adrenoceptors in various organs and tissues. For example, β-blockade in the myocardium can be associated with bradycardia, atrioventricular conduction abnormalities, and the development of congestive heart failure. Antagonism of β_2-receptors in the lung may lead to acute exacerbations of bronchospasm in patients with asthma or COPD. Blocking β_2-receptors in arteriolar smooth muscle may aggravate intermittent claudication or Raynaud's phenomenon and may cause cold extremities as a result of decreased peripheral blood flow. In addition, an increase of sympathetic tone during periods of acute stress (or hypoglycemia) may result in a significant increase in blood pressure because of unopposed α-receptor-mediated vasoconstriction.

Abrupt cessation of β-blocker therapy may produce unstable angina, myocardial infarction, or even death in patients predisposed to ischemic myocardial events. For this reason, it is always prudent to gradually taper the dose of β-blocker over 14 days before eventually discontinuing the drug. The acute withdrawal syndrome is believed to be secondary to a combination of factors, including progression of underlying coronary artery disease, hypersensitivity of β-adrenergic receptors, and failure to recognize the need to restrict physical activity upon withdrawal of a drug that decreases myocardial oxygen requirements. The hypersensitivity of β-receptors results partly from an increased synthesis of β-receptors that occurs in the presence of long-term β-receptor antagonism. In patients without coronary artery disease, abrupt discontinuation of β-blocker therapy may be associated with sinus tachycardia, increased sweating, and generalized malaise.

The adverse effects β-blockers have on serum lipids and glucose tolerance may unfortunately offset some of their beneficial effects on cardiovascular morbidity and mortality. β-blockers increase serum triglyceride levels and decrease HDL cholesterol levels. These adverse lipid effects are brought on by the inhibitory effect that unopposed α-stimulation has on the activity of lipoprotein lipase and lecithin cholesterol acyltransferase. Lipoprotein lipase enhances VLDL and triglyceride catabolism. HDL cholesterol is one of the by-products of VLDL catabolism. Lecithin cholesterol acyltransferase is also involved in the production of HDL cholesterol. β-Blockers with α-blocking properties produce no appreciable change in serum lipid concentration. Also, β-blockers with ISA do not adversely affect serum lipids and may even increase HDL cholesterol.

β-Blockers may induce glucose intolerance by inhibiting insulin secretion and by generating insulin resistance. As in the case with lipids, these adverse effects on glucose tolerance usually are not associated with the use of β-blockers that possess ISA or α-receptor blocking properties.

ANGIOTENSIN-CONVERTING ENZYME INHIBITORS[1,38,39]

Currently, there are nine ACE inhibitors on the U.S. market. Enalapril is metabolized to enalaprilat, which has a long half-life and duration of hypotensive action, and is therefore given once daily in the treatment of hypertension. Lisinopril has an even longer duration of action but does not require metabolic conversion to exert its effect. Captopril, which has a much shorter half-life than enalapril, is usually administered two to three times daily. Recent studies, however, indicate that once-daily administration of captopril may be adequate for the treatment of hypertension in salt-restricted patients. All three of these drugs are excreted in the urine and therefore an adjustment in dosage may be necessary in patients with renal dysfunction. The absorption of captopril, but not enalapril or lisinopril, is reduced by 30% to 40% by the presence of food in the stomach.

Benazepril, fosinopril, moexipril, quinapril, ramipril, and trandolapril can provide 24-hour blood pressure reduction with once- or twice-daily dosing. Benazepril, quinapril, and ramipril have the greatest effect on tissue ACE.

ACE is widely distributed in many tissues. It is present in several different cell types, but its principal location is in endothelial cells. Since the vascular endothelium covers a large surface area, the major site for angiotensin II production in the body is the blood vessels, not the kidney. ACE inhibitors block the conversion of angiotensin I to angiotensin II. This latter substance is a potent vasoconstrictor and stimulator of aldosterone secretion. ACE inhibitors also block the degradation of bradykinin and stimulate the synthesis of other vasodilating substances, including prostaglandin E_2 and prostacyclin. It is conceivable that different ACE inhibitors exert different effects on these various local vasoactive substances, but that remains to be proven. The observation that ACE inhibitors lower blood pressure in patients with normal plasma renin and ACE activity clearly indicates the importance of tissue production of ACE as a cause of increased vascular resistance.

Recent experiments and clinical studies have demonstrated that the blockade of angiotensin II production by ACE inhibitors increased the compliance of large arteries. The distensibility of these vessels determines the impedance of ventricular ejection, which is important in determining end-systolic ventricular wall stress. Increased wall stress gives rise to left ventricular hypertrophy and failure. Therefore, by increasing compliance of large arteries ACE inhibitors may effectively prevent or reverse left ventricular hypertrophy. They may also help prevent or slow down the rate of arteriosclerosis in these large vessels, which is the major cause of cardiovascular complications.

The most worrisome adverse effects of the ACE inhibitors are neutropenia and agranulocytosis, proteinuria, glomerulonephritis, and angioedema. Fortunately, these serious adverse effects are rare, occurring in fewer than 1% of patients exposed. Patients with preexisting renal or connective tissue diseases appear to be most vulnerable to the renal and hematologic side effects. Patients with bilateral renal artery stenosis or unilateral stenosis of a solitary functioning kidney and patients dependent on the vasoconstrictive effect of angiotensin II on the efferent arteriole are particularly susceptible to developing acute renal failure on ACE inhibitors.

Approximately 10% of patients who receive captopril develop a skin rash. In most cases the rash is transient and disappears despite continued treatment with the drug. Another fairly common side effect of captopril is a reversible loss of taste or taste disturbance (dysgeusia), which has been reported in about 6% of patients who receive the drug. The higher incidence of skin rash, dysgeusia, and proteinuria with captopril has been attributed to its sulfhydryl group, which is not present on enalapril or lisinopril. Approximately 10% to 20% of patients will develop a persistent cough while on ACE inhibitors. These patients may be switched to an angiotensin II receptor antagonist, which is less likely to produce cough.

Acute hypotension may occur at the onset on ACE inhibitor therapy, especially in patients who are severely sodium or volume depleted. It may be necessary to discontinue diuretics and reduce the dosage of other antihypertensive agents before initiating therapy with either captopril, enalapril, or lisinopril. One may also choose to begin ACE inhibitors at the lowest dose possible and administer the first dose at bedtime.

ACE inhibitors are absolutely contraindicated in pregnancy because serious neonatal problems, including renal failure and death, have been reported when mothers took these agents during the second and third trimesters of pregnancy.

Angioneurotic edema is a feared complication of ACE inhibitor therapy. It is more likely to occur in blacks than whites. Facial involvement is most common and only requires drug withdrawl. Laryngeal edema occasionally occurs and requires emergent medical care. Patients sensitive to one ACE inhibiotr may be sensitive to another.

Finally, hyperkalemia has been observed in patients treated with ACE inhibitors. This propensity for hyperkalemia is seen primarily in patients with renal disease or diabetes mellitus (especially with type IV renal tubular acidosis), or patients on concomitant NSAIDs, potassium supplements, or potassium-sparing diuretics. A uricosuric effect may warrant measures to decrease the risk of uric acid precipitation in patients with hyperuricemia or gout.

ANGIOTENSIN II RECEPTOR BLOCKERS[40–43]

This is a new class of antihypertensive drugs that are clearly distinct from ACE inhibitors. These drugs directly block the angiotensin AT_1 receptor that mediates the known effects of angiotensin II in humans: vasoconstriction, aldosterone release, sympathetic activation, ADH release, and constriction of the efferent arteriole of the glomerulus. Angiotensin II is generated by two enzymatic pathways: the renin–angiotensin pathway, which involves angiotensin converting enzyme, and an alternative pathway that utilizes other enzymes such as chymases. ACE inhibitors can block only the effects of angiotensin II produced by the renin–angiotensin system, whereas angiotensin II receptor blockers antagonize angiotensin II generated by either pathway. Unlike ACE inhibitors, with angiotensin II receptor blockers the breakdown of bradykinin is not blocked. Like ACE inhibitors, angiotensin II receptor blockers may cause renal insufficiency and hyperkalemia. Cough and angioneurotic edema are less likely to occur.

Currently four angiotensin II receptor blockers are marketed for the treatment of hypertension: irbesartan, losartan, candesartan, and valsartan. Several others are under development including eprosartan, tazosartan, telmisartan, and zolasartan.

VASODILATORS[1,44]

Hydralazine and minoxidil cause direct arteriolar smooth muscle relaxation through mechanisms that increase the intracellular concentration of cyclic GMP. They exert little effect, if any, on the venous side of the circulation. By decreasing the amount of systemic pressure in the arterial system, they reduce impedance to myocardial contractility.

The reduction in perfusion pressure brought on by direct arteriolar vasodilation activates the baroreceptor reflexes, which results in an increase in sympathetic outflow from the vasomotor center. This leads to an increase in heart rate, cardiac output, and renin release. Consequently, the hypotensive effectiveness of direct vasodilators diminishes in time unless the patient is also taking a sympathetic inhibitor and a diuretic to counteract the compensatory changes created by the baroreceptor reflexes. In older patients, however, baroreceptor mechanisms may be blunted enough that blood pressure may be lowered with vasodilatory therapy without causing sympathetic overactivity.

Direct vasodilator use can precipitate angina in patients with underlying coronary artery disease unless the baroreceptor reflex mechanism is completely blocked. To accomplish this, any sympathetic inhibitor may work, but the β-adrenergic blocking agents are most effective.

One side effect that is unique to hydralazine is a lupus-like syndrome. This adverse effect is associated with a chronic accumulation of hydralazine and is therefore dose related. The elimination of hydralazine involves hepatic *N*-acetyltransferase activity. As the activity of this enzyme system is predetermined genetically, the rate of acetylation may vary considerably. "Slow" acetylators are especially prone to develop a lupus-like reaction to hydralazine. The syndrome, which is more common in women, seldom progresses to the extent that systemic lupus erythematosus does, and it is reversible upon discontinuation of the drug. By keeping the total daily dose below 200 mg, lupus-like reactions can usually be avoided. Other side effects associated with hydralazine include dermatitis, drug fever, peripheral neuropathy, hepatitis, and vascular headaches.

Because minoxidil is a more potent vasodilator, the compensatory increases in heart rate, cardiac output, renin release, and sodium retention are even more dramatic than those observed with hydralazine. It therefore may be necessary to coadminister a β-adrenergic blocker and a loop diuretic with minoxidil. Other sympathetic inhibitors and thiazide diuretics may prove inadequate in counteracting the minoxidil-induced baroreceptor reflex and intrarenal compensatory mechanisms.

A very troublesome side effect of minoxidil is hypertrichosis. Increased hair growth occurs on the face, arms, back, and chest. This drug-induced hirsutism ceases with discontinuation of the drug. Other minoxidil side effects include pericardial effusion and a nonspecific T-wave change on the electrocardiogram.

CALCIUM CHANNEL ANTAGONISTS[45–52]

An increase in the level of free intracellular calcium from the extracellular fluid is required for the contraction of cardiac and smooth muscle cells, but not skeletal muscle cells. When cardiac or vascular smooth muscle is stimulated, voltage-sensitive channels in the cell membrane are opened, allowing calcium to enter the cells. The influx of extracellular calcium into the cell initiates a release of stored calcium from the sarcoplasmic reticulum. As the intracellular concentration of free calcium increases, it binds to a protein, calmodulin, which then activates myosin kinase. Activation of myosin kinase enables myosin to interact with actin to induce contraction. There are two types of voltage-gated calcium channels: a high-voltage channel (L-type) and a low-voltage channel (T-type). Blockade of the L-type channel leads to coronary and peripheral vasodilation. L-channel blockade may cause reflex sympathetic activation and a possible negative inotropic effect. T-channel blockade also leads to coronary and peripheral vasodilation but, in contrast to L-channel blockade, it does not cause a negative inotropic effect or reflex increase in sympathetic activity.

Currently there are seven L-type calcium channel antagonists in use for the treatment of hypertension: verapamil, diltiazem, and five dihydropyridines: amlodipine, felodipine, nifedipine, nicardipine, and isradipine. Mibefradil is a T-channel calcium antagonist. They are all similar in their antihypertensive effectiveness, but they differ somewhat in other pharmacodynamic effects. For example, verapamil decreases heart rate and slows atrioventricular nodal conduction. These properties make it an excellent drug for the treatment of supraventricular tachyarrhythmias. Verapamil also produces a negative inotropic effect that is responsible for its propensity to cause heart failure in subjects with borderline cardiac reserve. Diltiazem also decreases atrioventricular conduction and heart rate, but to a lesser extent than verapamil. Nifedipine, because of its potent peripheral vasodilating effects, causes a baroreceptor-mediated reflex increase in heart rate. It does not usually alter conduction through the atrioventricular node. The reason that pharmacodynamic differences exist among the three major classes of calcium channel antagonists—verapamil, diltiazem, and the dihydropyridines—is that they all act at specific receptors. The density and distribution of these receptors varies from tissue to tissue.

Nifedipine rarely may cause an increase in the frequency, intensity, and duration of angina in association with acute hypotension. This effect may be obviated by the administration of nifedipine with meals or by using sustained-release formulations of nifedipine. Other side effects of nifedipine include dizziness, flushing, headache, gingival hyperplasia peripheral edema, mood changes, and various gastrointestinal complaints. The short-acting nifedipine is not indicated for hypertension because it may be linked to increased mortality.

Diltiazem and verapamil rarely cause cardiac conduction abnormalities such as bradycardia, atrioventricular block, and congestive heart failure. Both can cause anorexia, nausea, peripheral edema, and hypotension. Verapamil causes constipation in about 7% of patients.

Verapamil, diltiazem, felodipine, nicardipine, and nifedipine are now marketed in sustained-release formulations. These new formulations allow for less frequent daily dosing and may result in fewer adverse drug reactions. Amlodipine is given once daily due to its long half-life.

There is some suggestive evidence from case control studies and a meta-analysis of several controlled trials that short-acting calcium channel anatgonists may be associated with an increase risk of acute myocardial infarction. Since evidence from such studies can only implicate an association, proper randomized trials are needed to determine if a cause-and-effect relationship actually exists. These studies are underway but the results will not be available for several years. In the meantime, it may be prudent to avoid short-acting calcium channel antagonists in the managment of hypertension.

POSTGANGLIONIC SYMPATHETIC INHIBITORS[1,34]

Guanethidine and guanadrel deplete norepinephrine from postganglionic sympathetic nerve terminals and they inhibit the release of norepinephrine in response to sympathetic nerve stimulation.

Hemodynamic studies indicate that the fall in blood pressure produced by postganglionic inhibitors is associated with a reduction in cardiac output and peripheral vascular resistance. Because reflex-mediated vasoconstriction is blocked by these drugs, a much greater hypotensive effect occurs in the upright posture, and postural hypotension is common. The use of postganglionic sympathetic inhibitors is associated with many other unwarranted side effects including impotence, diarrhea, and weight gain. The gastrointestinal side effects occur as a result of unopposed parasympathetic activity.

Long-term norepinephrine depletion leads to postsynaptic receptor supersensitivity. Therefore, the administration of drugs that compete with postganglionic inhibitors for uptake into the nerve terminals (such as tricyclic antidepressants and sympathomimetics) may occasionally provoke acute severe hypertensive episodes.

Because of their potential to cause explosive diarrhea, impotence, and orthostatic hypotension and syncope, the postganglionic sympathetic inhibitors are usually restricted to use in patients with refractory hypertension.

RESERPINE[1,34,53]

Reserpine lowers blood pressure through several different mechanisms. It depletes norepinephrine from sympathetic nerve endings and it blocks the transport of norepinephrine into its storage granules. When the nerve is stimulated, less than the usual amount of norepinephrine is released into the synapse. This causes diminution in sympathetic tone with a resulting decrease in peripheral vascular resistance and blood pressure.

Reserpine also depletes catecholamines from the brain and the myocardium. Consequently, the use of reserpine may lead to sedation and depression and decreased cardiac output.

Reserpine is a very long-acting drug and it may take 2 to 6 weeks before the maximal effect of the drug is realized. Its use is associated with significant sodium and fluid retention and therefore it should be administered in combination with a diuretic.

Reserpine's strong inhibition of sympathetic activity allows increased parasympathetic activity to occur, which is responsible for some of its side effects including nasal stuffiness, increased gastric acid secretion, diarrhea, and bradycardia.

The most important side effect of reserpine, however, is mental depression, which is a consequence of CNS depletion of catecholamines and serotonin. Patients may complain of sadness, loss of appetite, loss of self-confidence, gradual loss of energy, impotence, and early morning awakening. The incidence of reserpine-induced depression is dose related. The problem can be minimized by not exceeding a dose of 0.25 mg daily. At low doses the rate of depression with reserpine is equivalent to that of β-blockers, diuretics, or placebo.[53]

Reserpine is an inexpensive antihypertensive agent and has enjoyed the distinction of being chosen as the sympathetic inhibitor in many of the major clinical trials that have documented the benefit in treating hypertension.

DIFFERENTIAL APPROACH TO THE MANAGEMENT OF HYPERTENSION

Hypertension is a heterogeneous disorder that poses special therapeutic problems in several specific clinical situations. These situations are discussed briefly in this section, which attempts to integrate the pathophysiology of hypertension in certain subgroups of patients with the pharmacology of the various antihypertensive agents. Table 10–2 summarizes some of the key points.

HYPERTENSION IN CHILDHOOD[54–56]

In most cases, the factors associated with hypertension in children are identical to those in adults. Hypertensive children often have a family history of high blood pressure. There is, however, one important distinction between hypertension in children and in adults: Secondary hypertension is much more common in children.

Renal disease is the most common cause of secondary hypertension in children. Pyelonephritis, glomerulonephritis, renal artery stenosis, and renal cysts may all produce hypertension in children. Medical or surgical management of the underlying renal disorder usually restores normal blood pressure. Pheochromocytoma and coarctation of the aorta are more often discovered during childhood and are fortunately amenable to corrective surgery. Less common causes of secondary hypertension in children include congenital defects of adrenal steroid synthesis, Wilms' tumor, and neuroblastoma.

Primary hypertension is much more common in children than was once thought. In many young people, primary hypertension is associated with an increased cardiac output and a normal plasma volume and total peripheral vascular resistance. This is often referred to as a hyperdynamic or a hyperkinetic circulatory state. It would seem that this form of hypertension would best be treated with a β-adrenergic blocking agent. An alternative treatment might be clonidine, guanfacine, or guanabenz, which are known to lower serum norepinephrine levels and thus reduce hyperadrenergic activity.

HYPERTENSION IN PREGNANCY[57–62]

In 1990, the National High Blood Pressure Education Program Working Group Report on High Blood Pressure in Pregnancy was published. This report clearly emphasizes the importance of separating preeclampsia from chronic or transient hypertension of pregnancy since preeclampsia can lead rapidly to life-threatening complications for both mother and fetus. Preeclampsia usually presents after 20 weeks' gestation in primigravid women. The di-

TABLE 10–2. Differential Antihypertensive Therapy in Specific Clinical Situations

	Advantageous	Disadvantageous
Heart failure	ACE inhibitor,[a] diuretic	β-Blockers (except carvedilol), Ca channel antagonists (except amlodipine)
Angina	β-Blocker, Ca channel antagonist	Hydralazine, minoxidil
Elderly	Diuretic, α-agonist, Ca channel antagonist	
Black	Diuretic, Ca channel antagonist	β-Blocker as initial agent
Young	β-Blocker, α-agonist, ACE inhibitor	Diuretic
Diabetes	ACE inhibitor, α-agonist Ca channel antagonist	β-Blocker, diuretic
Broncospasm	Ca channel antagonist	β-Blocker, ACE inhibitor
Pregnancy	Methyldopa, hydralazine, labetolol	Diuretic, β-blocker
Renal insufficinecy	α-Agonist, Ca channel antagonist, minoxidil, hydralazine, loop diuretic	Thiazide diuretic, potassium-sparing agents
Tachycardia	β-Blocker, α-agonist, verapamil, diltiazem	Nifedipine, hydralazine, minoxidil
Hyperlipidemia	α-Blocker, ACE inhibitor, Ca channel antagonist	Diuretic, β-blocker
Gout/hyperuricemia	α-Agonist, α-blocker, Ca channel antagonist, ACE inhibitor	Diuretic, ACE inhibitor

ACE = angiotensin-converting enzyme; COPD = chronic obstructive pulmonary disease.

[a]ACE inhibitors may increase urinary clearance of uric acid thereby reducing hyperuricemia but increasing the risk of uric acid deposition in the urine or kidneys.

agnosis of preeclampsia is based on the appearance of hypertension, or a significant increase in blood pressure, with proteinuria, edema, or both. An increase of 30 mm Hg systolic or 15 mm Hg diastolic is also considered diagnostic even if the measured values do not exceed 140/90 mm Hg. Since the diastolic blood pressure usually decreases by 7 to 10 mm Hg during the early weeks of pregnancy, preeclampsia patients may demonstrate the required increase in blood pressure without achieving hypertensive readings. The hypertension and other signs of preeclampsia are thought to reflect pathophysiologic changes that induce vasospasm and may cause hematologic, renal, hepatic, brain, and uteroplacental damage. It is important to realize that it is the underlying pathology, not simply the blood pressure elevation, that is responsible for the terrible complications of this condition. It is uncertain whether blood pressure reduction is of any benefit in reducing the complications of preeclampsia.

Definitive treatment of preeclampsia is delivery or abortion, and this is clearly indicated if pending or frank eclampsia (preeclampsia plus convulsions) is present. Otherwise, such measures as restriction of activity, bed rest, and close monitoring are in order. Salt restriction, or any other measures that may contract blood volume, should not be employed. If drug treatment of hypertension is indicated (DBP > 100 mm Hg), methyldopa (or perhaps another α-agonist) is still the recommended drug of choice; and ACE inhibitors are specifically contraindicated because of reports of animal teratogenicity and acute renal failure in neonates. β-Blockers appear safe and effective in simple hypertension of pregnancy even though there is some concern about effects on fetal heart rate, glucose intolerance, and growth retardation. Since preeclampsia is thought to involve vasospasm, it would seem logical to avoid blockade of β-receptors in the vascular system since this could potentiate such vasospasm. Calcium channel blockers have been used extensively in Europe and would seem to be a good choice except, perhaps, for nifedipine. Nifedipine may induce proteinuria and has been shown to be teratogenic in rats. These agents also have been used successfully to treat preterm labor.

In 1989, two placebo-controlled studies reported beneficial results with either 60 or 100 mg of aspirin per day in pregnant women at risk of preeclampsia. The study using the lower dose started therapy at week 12 of gestation and continued until delivery. In the other study, therapy was started around week 30 of gestation and continued until 10 days before anticipated delivery. Pregnancy-induced hypertension, proteinuria, length of pregnancy, and fetal outcome were improved with aspirin therapy.[58] In a more recent study, low-dose aspirin was shown to decrease the incidence of preeclampsia among nulliparous women, primarily through its effect in those who have elevated systolic blood pressure initially.[61] However, in a multicenter study involving 9364 women, the use of aspirin was associated with a reduction of only 12% in the incidence of preeclampsia, which was not significant.[62] Thus, low-dose aspirin is not recommended in the general pregnant population.

HYPERTENSION IN THE ELDERLY[63–65]

The elderly may present with either isolated systolic hypertension or an elevation in both systolic and diastolic blood pressure. Epidemiologic data indicate that cardiovascular morbidity and mortality are more closely related to systolic blood pressure than to diastolic blood pressure. In a double-blind placebo-controlled trial, the Systolic Hypertension in the Elderly Program (SHEP), active treatment of isolated systolic hypertension resulted in a 36% reduction in the incidence of total stroke and a 27% reduction in the total number of cardiovascular events.[66]

In another placebo-controlled trial, the European Working Party Hypertension in the Elderly (EWPHE) study, a subgroup analysis of patients with isolated systolic hypertension revealed that treatment reduced overall mortality by 25% and cardiovascular mortality by 27%. However, these results were obtained from a small number of subjects in that trial and statistical analysis of the result was not reported.

The Joint National Committee on Detection, Evaluation, and Treatment of High Blood Pressure recommends a reduction in the systolic blood pressure (SBP) to less than 160 mm Hg for those with a SBP greater than 180 mm Hg and a reduction in blood pressure by 20 mm Hg for those with SBP between 160 and 179 mm Hg.

Elderly patients are usually more sensitive to volume depletion and sympathetic inhibition than their younger counterparts. Therefore, antihypertensive treatment should be initiated with smaller-than-usual dosages. Most authorities agree that the initial drug should be a diuretic. The starting dose should be low (e.g., 12.5 mg of hydrochlorothiazide) and gradually increased, but probably not to the maximum dosage. If diuretic therapy alone does not achieve the desired reduction in systolic blood pressure, a sympathetic inhibitor can be added. Again, it is best to start off with a low dose and slowly increase the dose, if necessary, but avoid excessive doses. Calcium channel blockers or β-blockers should be considered in elderly patients with hypertension and angina, and ACE inhibitors might be preferred for hypertensive patients with congestive heart failure. The pharmacologic management of diastolic hypertension in the elderly should be similar to that outlined for isolated systolic hypertension.

HYPERTENSION IN BLACKS[67]

Hypertension is common in all races, but it affects blacks at a disproportionately higher rate. It is also more severe in blacks than nonblacks. The reasons for the increased prevalence and severity of hypertension in blacks are not fully understood. Differences in electrolyte homeostasis, glomerular filtration rate, sodium excretion and transport mechanisms, plasma renin activity, and blood pressure response to plasma volume expansion have been noted. These differences may help explain the propensity for blacks to develop hypertension, but they do not account for the increased severity of hypertension in blacks as compared with whites. Further investigations in this area are needed.

Although dietary sodium intake is similar in blacks and whites, blacks ingest less potassium and calcium than whites. Supplemental potassium and calcium have both been shown to cause a modest reduction in blood pressure in some studies. It would therefore seem reasonable to assess the effect of increasing the amount of potassium and calcium in the diet as part of the nonpharmacologic management of hypertension in blacks.

The lower plasma renin activity and increased blood pressure response to sodium and fluid loading observed in blacks suggest a more sodium- and volume-dependent hypertension than exists in nonblacks. Several clinical studies have shown that blacks are hyperresponsive to diuretic therapy, a finding that is entirely consistent with the previously mentioned physiologic observations. These findings also point out the rationale of using diuretic therapy or calcium antagonist as the initial treatment of hypertension in blacks.

If diuretic therapy alone does not adequately control blood pressure in black hypertensives, then the addition of a sympathetic inhibitor is appropriate. Some clinicians have the misconception that β-blockers and ACE inhibitors are not effective in blacks. Although diuretics may be more effective as the initial treatment, diuretic therapy combined with β-blockers or ACE inhibitors is equally efficacious in hypertensive blacks and whites.

Controlled clinical trials have shown that calcium channel antagonists are as effective as diuretics in the initial pharmacologic treatment of hypertension in blacks. Thus, an alternative to diuretic therapy for this group is available and might, under certain conditions, be preferable.

HYPERTENSION AND CONCOMITANT DISORDERS

When hypertension is associated with other medical problems, the approach to its treatment should reflect proper consideration for the interactions that may occur between the antihypertensive drug regimen and the other disease states. These interactions consist of both positive and negative effects.

ASTHMA, COPD, AND PERIPHERAL VASCULAR DISEASE

β-Blockers, even those with β_1 selectivity, should be avoided in hypertensive patients with asthma, COPD, and peripheral vascular disease.

DIABETES[68–74]

The blood pressure treatment goal in diabetic patients with hypertension is 130/85 mm Hg or less, if tolerated. No antihypertensive agent is specifically contraindicated for use in the diabetic population, but caution is needed with most drugs.

Problems posed by β-blocker therapy in the diabetic hypertensive stem from the effects β-adrenergic blockade produces during hypoglycemic episodes. Since most of the symptoms of hypoglycemia (tremor, tachycardia, palpitations) are mediated through the sympathetic nervous system, these signs and symptoms are masked in the presence of β-adrenergic blockade. Sweating, another symptom of hypoglycemia, is cholinergically mediated, and therefore increases during a hypoglycemic episode. Since recovery of hypoglycemia depends on various compensatory mechanisms, including those produced by catecholamine input, then another consequence of β-adrenergic blockade is a delay in recovery time. Finally, hypertensive patients may experience marked elevations in blood pressure due to vasoconstrictor caused by unopposed α-receptor stimulation during the hypoglycemic recovery phase.

The α_1 antagonists may increase the risk of orthostatic hypotension and the α_2-agonists may cause a paradoxical increase in blood pressure. Both of these effects appear to be secondary to a more sensitive autonomic nervous system in patients with diabetic neuropathy.

Some evidence indicates that ACE inhibitors may increase insulin sensitivity, and there are a few case reports of hypoglycemia resulting from the combination of an ACE inhibitor and an oral hypoglycemic agent. While such interactions may occur and could be detrimental in some patients, the fact that ACE inhibitors improve insulin sensitivity could be taken advantage of in the diabetic patient inadequately controlled. Another potential benefit of ACE inhibitors in diabetic patients is their renal protective effects. In animal studies, ACE inhibitors and nondihydropyridine calcium channel antagonists have been shown to reduce intraglomerular hypertension. An increased glomerular pressure, hyperfiltration, and the accompanying microalbuminuria appear to be the earliest signs of diabetic nephropathy. Recent clinical studies support the renal protective effect of ACE inhibitors. Thus these agents may be considered the preferred pharmacologic treatment of hypertension in the diabetic subject. One possible adverse side effect that may attend the use of ACE inhibitors in diabetics is hyperkalemia. This is particularly likely to occur in diabetic patients with type 4 renal tubular acidosis, or in any diabetic on potassium supplements or potassium-sparing diuretics.

HYPERLIPIDEMIA[75,76]

As with glucose intolerance, hyperlipidemia compounds the risk of coronary artery disease attributed to hypertension. Therefore, every effort should be made to not only control high blood pressure but also to effectively manage or prevent hyperlipidemia. As discussed earlier, some antihypertensive agents may adversely affect serum lipids, namely, thiazide diuretics and β-blockers without ISA or α-blocking properties. These effects, however, may only be transient and of no clinical consequence. On the other hand, α-adrenergic antagonists have been shown to decrease LDL cholesterol levels and increase HDL cholesterol levels, giving them some advantage over other agents. ACE inhibitors and calcium channel antagonists have no effect on serum lipids.

LEFT VENTRICULAR HYPERTROPHY

LVH is another independent risk factor for coronary artery disease. LVH is present in about 50% of hypertensive patients. With the exception of vasodilators, most classes of antihypertensive agents have been shown to prevent or regress LVH. Prevention or regression of LVH should be considered an important objective in the overall management of hypertension. One study showed that the long-term use of diuretics led to the most regression.[77]

SMOKING

Smoking essentially doubles the cardiovascular risks associated with hypertension. Data from the MRC trial demonstrated that smoking eliminated any beneficial effect of propranolol in reducing cardiac events. Smoking induces catecholamine release, which, in the presence of β_2-receptor blockade, may lead to an increase in vascular resistance and therefore blood pressure and cardiac workload. The α-agonist clonidine has been shown to be useful in smoking cessation (particularly in women) and this may provide cause to consider this antihypertensive agent in smokers who are trying to kick the habit. Otherwise, there is little guidance in the literature as to how best to treat hypertension in patients who smoke.

CORONARY ARTERY DISEASE

For hypertensive patients with ischemic heart disease, β-blockers and calcium channel antagonists offer the advantage of lowering blood pressure and reducing myocardial oxygen demand. The cardiac stimulation that may occur with nifedipine or β-blockers with ISA, however, may make these agents less desirable in this clinical setting.

In patients with coronary artery disease, overtreating high blood pressure may bring about more harm than good. Since coronary blood flow occurs during diastole, the rate of flow is directly influenced by the diastolic blood pressure. Reducing the diastolic blood pressure excessively may therefore compromise coronary perfusion, especially in patients with fixed coronary artery stenosis, and lead to myocardial infarction. Thus in hypertensive patients with preexisting coronary artery disease, the risk of infarction increases at high diastolic blood pressures, decreases as diastolic blood pressure is lowered, then increases again at less than optimal diastolic blood pressures. This phenomenon is referred to as the "J curve." A meta-analysis of several published studies showed that the break point in this J-curve relationship between diastolic blood pressure and cardiac events occurs at a pressure of 85 mm Hg.[78]

For secondary prevention of infarction in hypertensive patients, calcium channel blockers do not afford the same degree of benefit as β-blockers. Diltiazem has been shown to reduce reinfarction in patients with non-Q-wave infarcts and may reduce cardiac events in post-MI patients who do not have CHF. However, diltiazem was shown to be harmful if pulmonary congestion was present. Similarly, verapamil offers some protection to post-MI patients with normal left ventricular ejection fractions. Studies evaluating the use of calcium channel antagonists post-MI were not carried out in hypertensive patients per se, although one would expect the same degree of protection for such patients.

HEART FAILURE

In patients with heart failure, captopril, enalapril, and ramipril have been shown to improve symptomatology and reduce mortality. Although heart failure, not hypertension, was the focus of these studies, it seems logical to use ACE inhibitors to treat hypertension in the setting of concomitant heart failure. Because of the high renin and angiotensin II status of patients with heart failure, therapy with an ACE inhibitor should be initiated at low doses to avoid a profound drop in blood pressure.

A β-blocker or nondihydropyridine calcium channel antagonist may improve left ventricular filling and cardiac output in patients with reduced cardiac output due to diastolic dysfunction. On the other hand, these agents may worsen heart failure in patients with systolic decompensation (see Chap. 11).

RENOVASCULAR DISEASE

In managing patients with hypertension due to renal artery stenosis or renal artery hyperplasia, ACE inhibitors and angiotensin II receptor blockers may be particularly advantageous. This is due to the fact that these conditions are associated with an increase in plasma renin and angiotensin activity. Two important cautions, however, are that patients may experience a rapid and profound drop in blood pressure or acute renal failure. The potential for ACE inhibitors to produce acute renal failure is particularly noted in patients with bilateral renal artery stenosis or a solitary functioning kidney with stenosis. Functional renal failure may occur in patients whose kidneys are dependent on angiotensin II for perfusion.

ACE inhibitors have also been shown to be effective for controlling the accelerated hypertension of sclerodermal renal crisis. If treatment is begun early, progressive deterioration in renal function can be prevented and occasional improvement in renal function results.

HYPERTENSIVE URGENCIES AND EMERGENCIES[79–81]

Oral antihypertensive loading with clonidine or captopril has been found to be effective in treating hypertensive urgencies. With oral clonidine loading, 0.2 mg of clonidine is given initially followed by 0.2 mg hourly until the diastolic pressure falls below 110 mm Hg or a total of 0.7 mg of clonidine has been administered. A single dose may be all that is necessary. Captopril is usually administered in doses of 25 to 50 mg orally at 1- to 2-hour intervals. The onset of action of oral captopril is 15 to 30 minutes, and a marked fall in blood pressure is unlikely to occur if no hypotensive response is observed within 30 to 60 minutes. Even though short-acting nifedipine has been used to treat hypertensive urgencies and emergencies, it may cause more harm than good and therefore is not recommended.[52]

There are no data confirming that the rapid reduction of blood pressure in patients with severe asymptomatic hypertension is more beneficial than the gradual reduction of blood pressure in these patients.[79] Since autoregulation of blood flow in chronically hypertensive patients occurs at a much higher range of pressure than in normotensive persons, there are some inherent risks in reducing blood pressure too precipitously, resulting in cerebrovascular accidents, myocardial infarction, and acute renal failure.

A hypertensive emergency is defined as a severe elevation in diastolic blood pressure, usually higher than 120 mm Hg, in the presence of target organ damage. Immediate treatment with an intravenous antihypertensive agent is needed to salvage viable tissue. These events are thought to be precipitated by an abrupt increase in vascular resistance as a result of an acute rise in circulating or local tissue levels of vasoconstricting substances. The marked elevation in blood pressure leads to arteriolar fibrinoid necrosis, endothelial damage, platelet and fibrin deposition in the media of smooth muscle, and loss of autoregulatory function. The end result is end-organ ischemia, which triggers a vicious cycle of further release of vasoactive substances, vasoconstriction, and endothelial proliferation. The goal in treatment is to interrupt this vicious cycle by lowering the diastolic blood pressure.

Just how rapidly to lower the pressure and to what level is somewhat controversial. Most authorities agree that the diastolic blood pressure should not be lowered below 100 to 110 mm Hg over several minutes to several hours depending on the clinical situation. Precipitous drops in blood pressure to the normotensive range or lower may lead to end-organ ischemia or infarction. After the goal diastolic blood pressure is reached, treatment should be designed to hold that level of pressure for several days to allow physiologic adjustments in autoregulatory function. Then, the blood pressure can be further reduced to normotensive levels.

The treatment of hypertensive emergencies can be accomplished with any one of several antihypertensive agents. The clinical situation may dictate which agent is preferred and which is contraindicated.

Nitroprusside is widely considered the agent of choice for the minute-to-minute control in most cases of severe hypertension. It is a direct-acting vasodilator that decreases peripheral vascular resistance, but does not increase cardiac output unless left ventricular failure is present. It is usually given as a continuous intravenous infusion at a rate of 0.5 to 8.0 mg/kg/min. Its onset of hypotensive action is immediate and its effect disappears within 2 to 5 minutes of discontinuation of the infusion. Nitroprusside can be given to treat any hypertensive emergency, but in aortic dissection propranolol should be given first to prevent reflex sympathetic activation. Nitroprusside is metabolized to cyanide and then to thiocyanate and eliminated by the kidneys. When the infusion must be continued longer than 72 hours, serum thiocyanate levels should be measured, and the infusion should be discontinued if the level exceeds 12 mg/dL. The risk of thiocyanate toxicity is increased in patients with impaired renal function. Other side effects of nitroprusside include fatigue, nausea, anorexia, disorientation, psychotic behavior, muscle spasms, and, rarely, hypothyroidism. Nitroprusside administration requires constant intraarterial pressure monitoring.

Intravenous nitroglycerin shares many of the advantages of sodium nitroprusside. In large doses, nitroglycerin dilates both arterioles and venous capacitance vessels, thereby producing both afterload- and preload-reducing effects. By reducing end-diastolic volume and pressure, the drug decreases myocardial oxygen demand. It also dilates collateral coronary blood vessels and improves perfusion to ischemic myocardium. These properties make intravenous nitroglycerin particularly beneficial in the management of severe hypertension in the presence of myocardial ischemia. The dose of intravenous nitroglycerin is 5 to 100 μg/min. As in the case with oral nitrates, intravenous nitroglycerin is associated with tolerance over 24 to 48 hours.

Diazoxide is also a direct-acting arteriolar vasodilator that decreases peripheral resistance, increases cardiac output, and maintains or increases renal plasma flow. Because diazoxide increases plasma volume, it is common practice to give a diuretic concurrently unless the patient is volume depleted. It has quick onset and a duration of action ranging from 4 to 12 hours. Diazoxide occasionally causes overshoot hypotension, which can be reversed by pressor agents. To avoid the precipitous fall in pressure that occurs when diazoxide is given as a 300-mg rapid bolus, smaller bolus doses (50 to 100 mg every 5 to 10 minutes) or slow infusion over 15 to 30 minutes should be used. Other side effects of diazoxide include nausea, vomiting, tachycardia, hyperglycemia, and hyperuricemia.

Trimethaphan camsylate is a ganglionic blocking agent. It dilates both arterioles and veins, with hypotension potential in the upright position. It reduces cardiac output and renal plasma flow and increases plasma volume. Trimethaphan is particularly useful for treating hypertension in patients with acute aortic dissection.

Like nitroprusside, trimethaphan is administered by continuous intravenous infusion, which requires constant or frequent intraarterial pressure monitoring. The initial infusion rate is 1 mg/min and the dose can be adjusted up to 10 mg/min. Its onset of action is immediate and its effects disappear within 10 minutes of discontinuation of the infusion. Besides profound orthostatic hypotension, trimethaphan may cause ileus, urinary retention, dry mouth, and visual impairment. Respiratory arrest has been reported at infusion rates greater than 5 mg/min.

Labetolol is a combination nonselective β-adrenergic and α-adrenergic blocker. It reduces blood pressure by decreasing peripheral vascular resistance. It does not significantly affect heart rate or cardiac output. The initial dose is 20 mg by slow intravenous injection over a 2-minute period, followed by repeated injections of 40 to 80 mg at 10-minute intervals, up to a total dose of 300 mg. Alternatively, the drug can be administered by continuous infusion at an initial rate of 2 mg/min and adjusted according to blood pressure response. Because of its α-blocking effects, labetolol can cause orthostatic hypotension. Other side effects include nausea, vomiting, paresthesias, sweating, dizziness, flushing, and headaches.

Hydralazine is an arteriolar vasodilator. It causes a marked reflex tachycardia and an increase in myocardial oxygen demand, which can cause ischemic chest pain in patients with coronary artery disease. Its onset of action ranges from 10 to 30 minutes and its effects last 2 to 4 hours. When given intravenously, 10 to 20 mg is diluted in 20 mL of 5% dextrose in water (D_5W) and administered at a rate of 0.5 to 1.0 mL/min. Because the hypotensive response is less predictable than with other parenteral agents, its major role is in the treatment of eclampsia or hypertensive encephalopathy associated with renal insufficiency. It has a good track record in the treatment of these two types of hypertensive emergencies.

An intravenous form of nicardipine has recently been approved for short-term treatment of hypertension. It is administered at 5 to 15 mg/h, which is adjusted by 1 to 2.5 mg/h after 15 minutes. Headaches, nausea, and vomiting are common side effects, and the use of the agent increases heart rate by 8 to 18 beats per minute.

PHARMACOECONOMIC CONSIDERATIONS

Hypertension affects approximately 50 million persons in the United States. Just over half of them are being treated for their high blood pressure. Less than 30% of patients are controlled at levels < 140/90 mm Hg.[82] The cost of antihypertensive therapy has been estimated at $8 to $10 billion per year. The economic impact of aggressively treating all Americans with hypertension to goal blood pressure (< 140/90 mm Hg) is mind-boggling. But this has to be offset from the cost savings that would be realized by reducing the frequency of morbid events in hypertensive individuals, which can drive health care costs up substantially.[83]

The cost per life-year saved from treating hypertension has been estimated to be $40,000 for younger adults and even less for older adults.[84] Treatments that cost less than $75,000 per life-year saved are generally considered favorable by health economists.

Drug costs can account for 70% to 80% of the total cost of hypertensive care. It is therefore crucial to identify ways to reduce the cost of care without increasing the morbidity and mortality associated with uncontrolled hypertension. The logical first step is to convince the patient of the need for life-style modification. A carefully designed program for smoking cessation, weight reduction, exercise, and moderation of dietary sodium and alcohol intake can be quite effective at preventing and treating hypertension at little cost.

If nonpharmacologic measures prove inadequate, either a diuretic or a β-blocker should be initiated. Both of these are available in generic forms and as such are far less expensive than alternative antihypertensive agents. One model for calculating the cost-effectiveness of various initial monotherapies for mild to moderate hypertension found that the cost of life-year saved was $10,900 for propranolol, $16,400 for hydrochlorothiazide, $31,600 for nifedipine, $61,900 for prazosin, and $72,100 for captopril.[85] In a cost minimization study that included the cost of drug acquisition, supplemental drugs, laboratory tests, clinic visits, and complications, the total costs of treating hypertension were $895 for β-blockers, $1043 for diuretics, $1165 for α-agonists, $1243 for ACE inhibitors, $1288 for α-blockers, and $1425 for calcium channel blockers.[86]

When a second-line antihypertensive agent that has been preferentially selected for initial treatment does not adequately control blood pressure, adding low-dose diuretic should be considered. Adding a diuretic will not only keep the cost down, but it will likely prove more effective than the addition of an alternative antihypertensive agent.

EVALUATION OF THERAPEUTIC OUTCOMES

The goals of antihypertensive therapy are to control blood pressure and to prevent cardiovascular morbidity and mortality. This can be achieved by maintaining arterial blood pressure below 140 mm Hg systolic and 90 mm Hg diastolic, while controlling other modifiable cardiovascular risk factors, such as smoking, hyperlipidemia, and diabetes mellitus. An attempt to lower blood pressure to the optimal range (< 120/80) may be pursued, with the caution that excessive lowering in patients with coronary heart disease may precipitate ischemic myocardial events. Another consideration is the impact aggressive treatment may have on various quality-of-life measures. Patients undergoing antihypertensive therapy should be questioned periodically about changes in their general health perception, energy level, physical functioning, and overall satisfaction with their treatment. A careful history for chest pain, palpitations, dizziness, dyspnea, orthopnea, slurred speech, and loss of balance should be taken to assess the likelihood of cardiovascular and cerebrovascular hypertensive complications.

Either self-recorded measurements of blood pressure or automatic ambulatory blood pressure monitoring should be performed to establish effective 24-hour control. This is especially important during the early morning hours when patients are particularly vulnerable to cardiac events. Blood pressure readings should be taken after 2 to 4 weeks of initiating or making changes in therapy. Once the goal of therapy is achieved and the patient is asymptomatic, blood pressure readings need be evaluated only every 3 to 6 months. More frequent evaluations are required in patients with poor control, advancing target-organ damage, or symptoms of adverse drug effects.

Other clinical monitoring parameters that may be used to assess therapeutic efficacy include changes in funduscopic findings, left ventricular hypertrophy regression on ECG or echocardiogram, resolution of proteinuria, and improvement in renal function.

Since hypertension is a relatively asymptomatic disease and the antihypertensive agents are not without adverse side effects, it is imperative to assess patient compliance with the therapeutic regimen on a regular basis. Detection of noncompliance should be followed up with appropriate patient education and counseling.

Patients should be monitored routinely for adverse drug effects. The most common side effects that attend each class of antihypertensive agents are discussed in the Treatment section of this chapter. The occurrence of an adverse drug event may require dosage reduction or substitution with an alternative antihypertensive agent.

CONCLUSION

Hypertension is a very common chronic medical disorder. It affects more than 50 million Americans. In more than 90% of cases the etiology of hypertension is unknown. Several pathophysiologic mechanisms have been proposed in the causation of hypertension. These include central and peripheral nervous system abnormalities, autoregulatory dysfunction, renal defects, humoral aberrancies, and deficiencies in various endogenous vasodepressor substances.

TABLE 10–3. The Antihypertensive Agents

Drug	Dose Range (mg/d)	
	Initial	*Maximum*
Diuretics		
Thiazides and related sulfonamide diuretics		
Bendroflumethiazide	2.5	5
Benzthiazide	25	50
Chlorothiazide sodium	250	500
Chlorthalidone	12.5	50
Cyclothiazide	1	2
Hydrochlorothiazide	12.5	50
Hydroflumethiazide	25	50
Indapamide	1.25	5
Methyclothiazide	2.5	5
Metolazone	2.5	5
Polythiazide	2	4
Quinethazone	50	100
Trichlormethiazide	2	4
Loop diuretics		
Bumetanide	0.5	10
Ethacrynic acid	25	200
Furosemide	40	240
Potassium-sparing agents		
Amiloride hydrochloride	5	10
Spironolactone	25	100
Triamterene	25	100
Adrenergic Inhibitors		
β-Adrenergic blockers		
Acebutolol	200	800
Atenolol	25	100
Betaxolol	5	40
Bisoprolol	2.5	20
Carteolol	2.5	10
Metoprolol tartrate	50	300
Nadolol	20	320
Oxprenolol hydrochloride	160	480
Penbutolol	10	80
Pindolol	10	60
Propranolol hydrochloride	40	480
Propranolol, long-acting (LA)	80	480
Timolol maleate	20	60
Central-acting adrenergic inhibitors		
Clonidine hydrochloride	0.2	1.2
Guanabenz acetate	8	32
Guanfacine	1	3.0
Methyldopa	500	2000
Peripheral-acting adrenergic antagonists		
Guanadrel sulfate	10	150
Guanethidine monosulfate	10	300
Rauwolfia alkaloids		
Rauwolfia (whole root)	50	100
Reserpine	0.05	0.25
α_1-Adrenergic blocker		
Doxazosin	1	16
Prazosin hydrochloride	2	20
Terazosin	1	5.0
Combined α- and β-adrenergic blockers		
Carvedilol	12.5	50
Labetolol	200	1200
Vasodilators		
Hydralazine hydrochloride	50	300
Minoxidil	5	100
Angiotensin-converting Enzyme Inhibitors		
Benazepril	5	40
Captopril	25	150
Enalapril maleate	5	40
Fosinopril	10	80
Lisinopril	5	80
Moexipril	7.5	30
Quinapril	5	80
Ramipril	1.25	20
Trandolapril	1	4
Calcium Channel Antagonists		
Amlodipine	2.5	10
Diltiazem hydrochloride	120	360
Felodipine	2.5	20
Isradipine	5	20
Mibefradil	50	100
Nicardipine	60	120
Nifedipine	30	180
Nislodipine	20	60
Verapamil hydrochloride	120	480

Untreated or inadequately controlled hypertension is a major risk factor in the morbidity and mortality of cardiovascular, cerebrovascular, and renovascular diseases. Antihypertensive drug therapy should be individualized according to various patient characteristics and underlying pathophysiologic circumstances. Table 10–3 provides a list of agents currently available for the treatment of hypertension in the United States.

▶ PRINCIPLES OF PHARMACOTHERAPY

- Carefully perform blood pressure measurements on three separate occasions to confirm the diagnosis of hypertension. A single elevated blood pressure does not necessarily mean that someone is hypertensive.
- Inquire as to self-medication as a cause of high blood pressure (e.g., NSAIDs, weight-reducing agents or sinus preparations containing phenylpropanolamine, greater than 2 ounces of ethanol per day).
- Investigate heavy sodium intake as a factor for hypertension.
- Implement life-style changes as the initial treatment for hypertension unless target-organ damage is present. This should include sodium restriction, weight reduction, ethanol abstinence or reduction, increased physical activity.
- Evaluate the patient carefully in terms of target-organ damage (angina, heart failure, renal insufficiency), comorbid diseases (e.g., asthma, gout, diabetes, lipid disorder, BPH), and life-style (jogger, restricted finances, intelligence).
- In the uncomplicated patient and the elderly patient, diuretics and β-blockers should be considered as initial therapy. Other drug choices are dictated by target-organ damage, comorbid diseases, contraindications, and life-style issues.
- Use small doses of a single drug initially. Consider low-dose combinations if it is unlikely that a single drug will suffice. Wait 4 to 6 weeks to assess the response of the drug.
- Failure to control blood pressure after an additional titration should result in the addition of a second antihypertensive drug. Wait 4 to 6 weeks to assess the response of the combination
- Failure to control blood pressure after an additional titration of the second drug should result in a reassessment of compliance, sodium intake, secondary causes of hypertension, alcohol abuse, drug–drug interactions, or the need to use a diuretic.
- If these issues are resolved, then add a diuretic. If the patient is already on a diuretic, add a rational third drug. Wait 4 to 6 weeks to assess the response of the new regimen.

REFERENCES

1. Kaplan MN. Clinical Hypertension, 6th ed. Baltimore, Williams & Wilkins, 1994.
2. Hypertension Detection and Follow-up Program Cooperative Group. Five year findings of the Hypertension Detection and Follow-up Program. 1: Reduction in mortality of persons with high blood pressure, including mild hypertension. JAMA 1979;242:2567–2571.
3. Veterans Administration Cooperative Study Group on Antihypertensive Agents. Effects of treatment on morbidity in hypertension. JAMA 1967;202:1028–1034.
4. Management Committee. The Australian therapeutic trial in mild hypertension. Lancet 1980;1:1261–1269.
5. SHEP Cooperative Research Group. Prevention of stroke by antihypertensive drug treatment in older persons with isolated systolic hypertension. JAMA 1991;265:3255–3264.
6. Dahöf B, Lindholm FH, Hansson L, et al. Morbidity and mortality in the Swedish trial in old patients with hypertension (STOP–Hypertension). Lancet 1991;338:1281–1285.
7. MRC Working Party. Medical Research Council trial of treatment of hypertension in older adults: Principal results. Br Med J 1992;304: 405–412.
8. Staessen JA, Fagard R, Lutgarde T, et al. Randomised double-blind comparison of placebo and active treatment for older patients with isolated systolic hypertension. Lancet 1997;350:757–764.
9. The Sixth Report of the National Committee on detection, evaluation, and treatment of high blood pressure (JNC-VI). Arch Intern Med 1997;157:2413–2446.
10. Burt VL, Whelton P, Roccella EJ, et al. Prevalence of hypertension in the US adult population: Results from the third National Health and Nutrition Examination Survey, 1988–1991. Hypertension 1995;25: 305–313.
11. Caulfield M, Lavender P, Farrall M, et al. Linkage of the angiotensinogen gene to essential hypertension. N Engl J Med 1994; 330:1629–1633.
12. Williams RR, Hunt SC, Hopkins PN, et al. Evidence for single gene contributions to hypertension and lipid disturbances: Definition, genetics, and clinical significance. Clin Genet 1994;46:80–87.
13. Laragh JH, Brenner BM eds. Hypertension: Pathophysiology, Diagnosis, and Management, 2nd ed. New York, Raven Press, 1995.
14. Sowers JR, Messerli FH. Pathophysiological mechanisms in hypertension and target organ damage. In: Izzlo JL, Black HR, eds. Hypertension Primer. Dallas, American Heart Association, 1993:61–142.
15. Haffner SM. Epidemiology of hypertension and insulin resistance syndrome. J Hypertens 1997;15(suppl):S25–30.
16. Sowers JR. Insulin and insulin-like growth factor in normal and pathological cardiovascular physiology. Hypertension 1997;29:691–699.
17. Bhanot S, McNeil JH. Insulin and hypertension: A causal relationship? Cardiovasc Res 1996;31:212–221.
18. Reaven GM, Lithell H, Landsberg L. Hypertension and associated metabolic abnormalities—the role of insulin resistance and the sympathoadrenal system. N Engl J Med 1996;334:374–381.
19. Ferrario CM. Importance of the renin–angiotensin–aldosterone system (RAS) in the physiology and pathology of hypertension. Drugs 1990;39(suppl 2):1–8.
20. Reaven GM. Role of insulin resistance in human disease. Diabetes 1988;37:1595–1607.
21. Marigliano A, Tedde R, Sechi LA, et al. Insulinemia and blood pressure. Am J Hypertens 1990;3:521–526.
22. Vane JR, Änggard EE, Botting RM. Regulatory functions of the vascular endothelium. N Engl J Med 1990;323:27–36.
23. Prisant LM, Albert BS, Robbins CB, et al. American National Standard for nonautomated sphygmomanometers: Summary report. Am J Hypertens 1995;8:210–213.
24. The National High Blood Pressure Education Program Coordinating Committee. National High Blood Pressure Education Program Work-

ing Group report on ambulatory blood pressure monitoring. Arch Intern Med 1990;150:2270–2280.
25. Smolensky MH, Portaluppi F. Ambulatory blood pressure monitoring. Application to clinical medicine and antihypertensive medication trials. Ann NY Acad Sci 1996;783:278–294.
26. Prisant LM, Bottini PB, Carr AA. Ambulatory blood pressure monitoring: Methodological issues. Am J Nephrol 1996;16:190–201.
27. Appel LJ, Moore TJ, Obarzanek E, et al. A clinical trial of the effects of dietary patterns on blood pressure. N Engl J Med 1997; 36: 1117–1124.
28. Epstein M, Sowers JR. Diabetes mellitus and hypertension. Hypertension 1992;19:403–418.
29. Eselin JA, Carter BC. Hypertension and left ventricular hypertrophy: Is drug therapy beneficial? Pharmacotherapy 1994;14:60–88.
30. Masserli FH, Aristizabal D, Soria F. Reduction of left ventricular hypertrophy: How beneficial? Am Heart J 1993;125:1520–1524.
31. Psaty BM, Smith NL, Siscovick DS, et al. Health outcomes associated with antihypertensive therapies used as first-line agents. A systematic review and meta-analysis. JAMA 1997;277:739–745.
32. Valvo E, D'Angelo G. Diuretics in hypertension. Kidney Int 1997; 59(suppl):S36–S38.
33. Puschett JB. Diuretics. In: Izzlo JL, Black HR, eds. Hypertension Primer. Dallas, American Heart Association, 1993:294–296.
34. Perry HM. Central and peripheral sympatholytics. In: Izzlo JL, Black HR, eds. Hypertension Primer. Dallas, American Heart Association, 1993:306–308.
35. Veelken R, Schmieder RE. Overview of alpha 1-adrenocepter antagonism and recent advances in hypertensive therapy. Am J Hypertens 1996;9:139S–149S.
36. Nadelmann J, Frishman WH. Clinical use of β-adrenoceptor blockade in systemic hypertension. Drugs 1990;39:862–876.
37. Goldstein S. Beta-blockers in hypertensive and coronary heart disease. Arch Intern Med 1996;156:1267–1276.
38. Dzau VJ. Mechanism of action of angiotensin-converting enzyme (ACE) inhibitors in hypertension and heart failure: Role of plasma versus tissue ACE. Drugs 1990;39(suppl 2):11–16.
39. Hanssens M, Keirse MJNC, Vankelecom F, et al. Fetal and neonatal effects of treatment with angiotensin-converting-enzyme inhibitors in pregnancy. Obstet Gynecol 1991;78:128–135.
40. Goa KL, Wagstaff AJ. Losartan potassium: A review of its pharmacology, clinical efficacy and tolerability in the management of hypertension. Drugs 1996;51:820–845.
41. Carr AA, Prisant LM. Losartan: First of a new class of angiotensin antagonists for the management of hypertension. J Clin Pharmacol 1996;36:3–12.
42. Messerli FH, Weber MA, Brunner HR. Angiotensin II receptor inhibition. A new therapeutic principle. Arch Intern Med 1996;156: 1957–1965.
43. Goodfriend TL, Elliott ME, Catt KJ. Angiotensin receptors and their antagonists. N Engl J Med 1996;334:1649–1654.
44. Venkata C, Ram S, Featherston WE. Vasodilators. In Izzlo JL, Black HR, eds Hypertension Primer. Dallas, American Heart Association, 1993:314–316.
45. Kaplan NM. Calcium entry blockers in the treatment of hypertension. JAMA 1989;262:817–823.
46. Ferrari R. Major differences among the three classes of calcium antagonists. Eur Heart J 1997;18(suppl A):A56–A70.
47. van Zwieten PA. Clinical pharmacology of calcium antagonists as antihypertensive and anti-anginal drugs. J Hypertens 1996;14 (suppl): S3–S9.
48. Palma-Gamiz JL. High blood pressure and calcium antagonism. Cardiology 1997;88(suppl 1):39–46.
49. Triggle DJ. Pharmacologic and therapeutic differences among calcium channel antagonists: Profile of mebefradil, a new calcium antagonist. Am J Cardiol 1996;78:7–12.
50. Opie LH. Calcium channel blockers for hypertension: Dissecting the evidence for adverse effects. Am J Hypertens 1997;10:565–577.
51. Michalewicz L, Messerli FH. Cardiac effects of calcium antagonists in systemic hypertension. Am J Cardiol 1997;79:39–46.
52. Grossman E, Messerli FH, Grodzicki T, Kowey P. Should a moratorium be placed on sublingual nifedipine capsules given for hypertensive emergencies and pseudoemergencies? JAMA 1996;276:1328–1331.
53. Prisant LM, Spruill WJ, Fincham J, et al. Depression associated with antihypertensive drugs. J Fam Pract 1991;33:481–485.
54. Hohn AR. Diagnosis and management of hypertension in childhood. Pediatr Ann 1997;26:105–110.
55. Feld LG. Hypertension in children. Boston, Butterworth-Heinemann, 1997.
56. Sinaiko AR. Hypertension in children. N Engl J Med 1996;335: 1968–1973.
57. Cunningham FG, Lindheimer MD. Hypertension in pregnancy. N Engl J Med 1992;326:927–932.
58. National High Blood Pressure Education Program Working Group report on high blood pressure in pregnancy. Am J Obstet Gynecol 1990;163:1689–1712.
59. Henriksen T. Hypertension in pregnancy: Use of antihypertensive drugs. Acta Obstet Gynecol Scand 1997;76:96–106.
60. Sibai BM. Treatment of hypertension in pregnant women. N Engl J Med 1996;335:257–265.
61. Sibai BM, Caritis SN, Thom E, et al. Prevention of preeclampsia with low-dose aspirin in healthy, nulliparous pregnant women. N Engl J Med 1993;329:1213–1218.
62. CLASP: A randomized trial of low-dose aspirin for the prevention and treatment of preeclampsia among 9364 pregnant women. Lancet 1994;343:619–629.
63. Amery A, Birkenhager W, Brixko P, et al. Mortality and morbidity results from the European Working Party on High Blood Pressure in the Elderly trial. Lancet 1985;1:1349–1354.
64. Insug JT, Sacks HS, Lau Tai-Shing, et al. Drug treatment of hypertension in the elderly: A meta-analysis. Ann Intern Med 1994;121:355–362.
65. Hansson L. Hypertension in the elderly. J Hypertens 1996;14 (suppl): S17–S21.
66. SHEP Cooperative Research Group. Prevention of stroke by antihypertensive drug treatment in older persons with isolated systolic hypertension: Final results of the Systolic in the Elderly Program (SHEP). JAMA 1991;265:3255–3264.
67. Rahman M, Douglas JG, Wright JT Jr. Pathophysiology and treatment implications of hypertension in the African-American population. Endocrinol Metab Clin North Am 1997;26:125–144.
68. Christlieb AR. Treatment section considerations for the hypertensive diabetic patient. Arch Intern Med 1990;150:1167–1174.
69. National High Blood Pressure Education Program Working Group report on hypertension in diabetes. Hypertension 1994;23:145–158.
70. Houston MC. New insights and approaches to reduce end-organ damage in the treatment of hypertension: Subsets of hypertension approach. Am Heart J 1992;123:1337–1367.
71. Lebovitz H, Wiegmann T, Canan A, et al. Renal protective effects of enalapril in hypertensive NIDDM: Role of baseline albuminuria. Kidney Int 1994;45:S150–S155.
72. Arauz-Pacheco C, Raskin P. Hypertension in diabetes mellitus. Endocrinol Metab Clin North Am 1996;25:401–423.
73. Leese GP, Savage MW, Chattington PD, Voar JP. The diabetic patient with hypertension. Postgrad Med J 1996;72:263–268.
74. Fatourechi V, Kennedy FP, Rizza RA, Hogan MJ. A practical guide for management of hypertension in patients with diabetes. Mayo Clin Proc 1996;71:53–58.
75. Working Group on Management of Patients with Hypertension and High Blood Cholesterol. National education programs working group report on the management of patients with hypertension and high blood cholesterol. Ann Intern Med 1991;114:224–237.
76. Chobanian AV, Alexander RW. Exacerbation of atherosclerosis by hypertension: Potential mechanisms and clinical implications. Arch Intern Med 1996;156:1952–1956.

77. Neaton JD, Grimm RH, Prineas RJ, et al. Treatment of mild hypertension study (TOHMS). Final results. JAMA 1993;270:713–721.
78. Farnett L, Mulrow CD, Linn WD, et al. The J-curve phenomenon and the treatment of hypertension. JAMA 1991;265:489–495.
79. Zeller KR, Kuhnert LLV, Matthews C. Rapid reduction of severe asymptomatic hypertension. Arch Intern Med 1989;149:2186–2189.
80. Calhoun DA, Oparil S. Treatment of hypertensive crisis. N Engl J Med 1990;323:1177–1183.
81. Prisant LM, Car AA, Hawkins DW. Treating hypertensive emergencies. Postgrad Med 1993;93:92–110.
82. Burt VL, Cutler JA, Higgins M, et al. Trends in the prevalence, awareness, treatment, and control of hypertension in the adult US population: Data from the health examination surveys, 1960–1991. Hypertension 1995;26:60–69.
83. Moser M. Hypertension can be treated effectively without increasing the cost of care. J Hum Hypertens 1996;10(suppl 2):533–538.
84. Barrie W. Cost-effective therapy for hypertension. West J Med 1996;164:303–309.
85. Edelson JT, Weinstein MC, Tosteson AN, et al. Long-term cost-effectiveness of various initial monotherapies for mild to moderate hypertension. JAMA 1990;263:407–413.
86. Hilleman DE, Mohjuddin SM, Lucas BD, et al. Cost-minimization analysis of initial antihypertensive therapy in patients with mild-to-moderate essential diastolic hypertension. Clin Ther 1994;16:88–102.

11
HEART FAILURE

Julie A. Johnson, PharmD, BCPS, FCCP, Robert B. Parker, PharmD, FCCP, and Stephen A. Geraci, MD

Heart failure is a pathophysiologic state in which the heart is unable to pump blood at a rate sufficient to meet the metabolic needs of the body.[1] In the past it was commonly referred to as congestive heart failure (CHF); the preferred nomenclature is now *heart failure* because a patient can have the clinical syndrome of heart failure without having symptoms of congestion. Heart failure is not a specific disease entity, but a clinical syndrome that may be caused by numerous different cardiac disorders. The normal cardiac cycle is comprised of two main components, ventricular diastole and ventricular systole. Diseases that adversely affect either component may lead to heart failure. Filling of the ventricle occurs during ventricular diastole while ventricular contraction and ejection of blood occur during ventricular systole. For many years it was believed that reduced myocardial contractility, or systolic dysfunction, was the sole disturbance in cardiac function responsible for heart failure. However, it is now recognized that disturbances in relaxation (lusitropic) properties of the heart, or diastolic dysfunction, account for symptoms of heart failure in approximately one-third of patients.[1] A diagnosis of isolated diastolic dysfunction is usually made in patients with symptoms of heart failure but normal systolic function. The remaining two-thirds of patients with heart failure symptoms have systolic dysfunction alone or systolic plus diastolic dysfunction.[1]

EPIDEMIOLOGY

It is estimated that 3 to 4 million Americans have been diagnosed with heart failure, and approximately 400,000 new cases are diagnosed each year.[2,3] The incidence doubles with each decade of life, and heart failure is the most common hospital discharge diagnosis in individuals over age 65. Heart failure is more common in men than in women, which is thought to be due to the greater incidence of ischemic heart disease in men. Unlike most other cardiovascular diseases, the incidence and morbidity/mortality from heart failure have not decreased over the last two decades and the prevalence is expected to double in the next 40 years. This is ascribed to the aging population, and the fact that more people are surviving early cardiovascular death (from myocardial infarction). Heart failure hospitalizations increased fourfold in two decades, with over 2 million hospitalizations for heart failure as the primary or secondary diagnosis in 1990.[2] NHLBI estimates that in 1989 $10.4 billion were spent in the United States on direct and indirect health care costs of heart failure and more recent estimates are that the economic impact of heart failure exceeds $34 billion.[4] Thus heart failure is a major medical problem which is expected to become even more significant with time.

The overall 5-year survival is 30% to 40% for all patients with a diagnosis of heart failure, and 1-year survival is only 50% for those with class IV heart failure.[2] Death is classified as sudden in 20% to 50% of patients,[5,6] implicating serious ventricular arrhythmias as the underlying cause in many patients with heart failure.

ETIOLOGY

Heart failure is a pathophysiologic state which can result from many cardiac diseases or disorders; common causes of heart failure are shown in Table 11–1.[1,7] The common cardiovascular diseases cause both systolic and diastolic dysfunction, thus many patients have heart failure as a result of abnormal ventricular filling and reduced myocardial contractility.

Systolic contractile dysfunction is a cardinal feature of dilated cardiomyopathies. Although the cause of reduced contractility is frequently unknown, abnormalities such as interstitial fibrosis, cellular infiltrates, cellular hypertrophy, and myocardial cell degeneration are commonly seen on histologic examination.[7] Dilated cardiomyopathies are discussed in detail in Chap. 15.

Pressure or volume overload causes ventricular hypertrophy, which helps return contractility to a near-normal state. However, if the pressure or volume overload persists, the hypertrophied myocardial cells eventually become fibrotic, and contractility decreases. Ventricular hypertrophy also increases ventricular stiffness and slows relaxation, therefore impairing diastolic function.[1] Examples of pressure overload include systemic or pulmonary hypertension and aortic or pulmonic valve stenosis. Volume overload may occur in the presence of valvular regurgitation, shunts, or high-output states such as anemia or pregnancy.

Another cause of systolic dysfunction is reduction in muscle mass due to acute myocardial infarction (AMI). AMI leads to death of affected myocardial cells, and the degree to which contractility is decreased will depend on the size of the infarction. Myocardial ischemia and infarction also affect the diastolic properties of the heart by slowing ventricular relaxation and increasing ventricular stiffness. Thus, AMI frequently results in systolic and diastolic dysfunction. Less common causes of diastolic dysfunction are listed in Table 11–1 and include infiltrative myocardial diseases, mitral or tricuspid valve stenosis, and pericardial disease.

TABLE 11–1. Causes of Heart Failure

Systolic dysfunction (decreased contractility)
1. Reduction in muscle mass (e.g., myocardial infarction)
2. Dilated cardiomyopathies
3. Ventricular hypertrophy
   a. Pressure overload (e.g., systemic or pulmonary hypertension, aortic or pulmonic valve stenosis)
   b. Volume overload (e.g., valvular regurgitation, shunts, high-output states)

Diastolic dysfunction (restriction in ventricular filling)
1. Increased ventricular stiffness
   a. Ventricular hypertrophy (e.g., hypertrophic cardiomyopathy, other examples above)
   b. Infiltrative myocardial diseases (e.g., amyloidosis, sarcoidosis, endomyocardial fibrosis)
   c. Myocardial ischemia and infarction
2. Mitral or tricuspid valve stenosis
3. Pericardial disease (e.g., pericarditis, pericardial tamponade)

Compiled from Refs. 1 and 6.

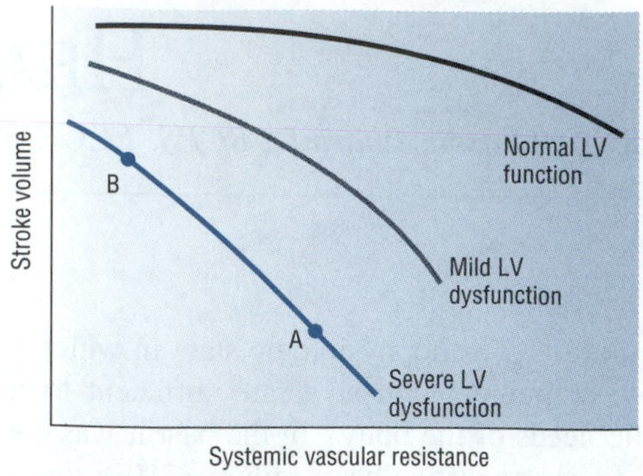

FIGURE 11–1. Relationship between stroke volume and systemic vascular resistance. In an individual with normal left ventricular (LV) function, increasing systemic vascular resistance has little effect on stroke volume. As the extent of LV dysfunction increases, the negative, inverse relationship between stroke volume and systemic vascular resistance becomes more important (B to A).

In the most recently published Framingham study of patients with heart failure, ischemic heart disease alone was present in 19% of men and 7% of women with heart failure.[3] Hypertension alone was present in 30% of men and 37% of women, and hypertension plus ischemic heart disease was present in 40% of both genders. Thus, ischemic heart disease and/or hypertension contribute to development of heart failure in the majority of patients. Hypertension and ischemic heart disease were absent in 11% to 15% of patients[3] suggesting their heart failure was due to less common etiologies including cardiomyopathies (idiopathic dilated, viral, alcoholic, hypertrophic) and valvular disease.[3,7] Many patients with pure diastolic dysfunction will have hypertension as their primary etiology, whereas in patients with any systolic dysfunction, ischemic heart disease is present in approximately 70% of patients. The role of hypertension should not, however, be underestimated based on this statistic because hypertension is an important risk factor for ischemic heart disease.

PATHOPHYSIOLOGY

NORMAL CARDIAC FUNCTION

To understand the pathophysiologic processes in heart failure, a basic understanding of normal cardiac function is necessary. Cardiac output (CO) is defined as the volume of blood ejected per unit time (L/min) and is the product of heart rate (HR) and stroke volume (SV):

$$CO = HR \times SV$$

The relationship between CO and mean arterial pressure (MAP) is:

$$MAP = CO \times SVR$$

where SVR is systemic vascular resistance. Heart rate is controlled by the autonomic nervous system. Stroke volume, or the volume of blood ejected during systole, is dependent on preload, afterload, and contractility.[1] As defined by the Frank-Starling mechanism, the ability of the heart to alter the force of contraction is dependent on changes in preload. As myocardial sarcomere length is stretched, the number of cross bridges between thick and thin myofilaments increases, resulting in an increase in the force of contraction. The length of the sarcomere is determined primarily by the volume of blood in the ventricle, therefore left ventricular end-diastolic volume (LVEDV) is the primary determinant of preload. In normal hearts, the preload response is the primary compensatory mechanism such that a small increase in end-diastolic volume results in a large increase in cardiac output. Because of the relationship between pressure and volume in the heart, left ventricular end diastolic pressure (LDEVP) is often used in the clinical setting to estimate preload. The hemodynamic measurement used to estimate LVEDP is the pulmonary artery occlusion pressure (PAOP). Afterload is a more complex physiologic concept which can be viewed pragmatically as the sum of forces preventing active forward ejection of blood by the ventricle. Major components of global ventricular afterload are ejection impedance, wall tension, and regional wall geometry. In patients with left ventricular systolic dysfunction, an inverse relationship exists between afterload (or SVR) and stroke volume such that increasing afterload causes a decrease in stroke volume (Fig. 11–1). Contractility is the intrinsic property of cardiac muscle describing fiber shortening and tension development.

COMPENSATORY MECHANISMS IN HEART FAILURE

As cardiac function decreases secondary to one or more of the disorders described above, the heart relies on compensatory responses to maintain an adequate cardiac output. They are (1) tachycardia and increased contractility through sympathetic nervous system (SNS) activation; (2) the

TABLE 11–2. Beneficial and Detrimental Effects of the Compensatory Responses in Heart Failure

Compensatory Response	Beneficial Effects of Compensation	Detrimental Effects of Compensation
Increased preload (through Na^+ and water retention)	Optimize stroke volume via Frank–Starling mechanism	Pulmonary and systemic congestion and edema formation Increased $M\dot{V}O_2$
Vasoconstriction	Maintain BP in face of reduced CO Shunt blood from nonessential organs to brain and heart	Increased $M\dot{V}O_2$ Increases afterload, decreases stroke volume, and further activates the compensatory responses
Tachycardia and increased contractility (due to SNS activation)	Helps maintain CO	Increased $M\dot{V}O_2$ Shortened diastolic filling time β_1-receptor down-regulation, decreased receptor sensitivity Precipitation of ventricular arrhythmias (?)
Ventricular hypertrophy	Helps maintain CO Reduces myocardial wall stress Decreases $M\dot{V}O_2$	Diastolic dysfunction Systolic dysfunction Increased risk of myocardial cell death Increased risk of myocardial ischemia Increased arrhythmia risk

Abbreviations: SNS = sympathetic nervous system, BP = blood pressure; $M\dot{V}O_2$ = myocardial oxygen demand, CO = cardiac output.

Frank-Starling mechanism, whereby an increase in preload results in an increase in stroke volume; (3) vasoconstriction; and (4) ventricular hypertrophy and remodeling. The benefits and detrimental consequences of these compensatory responses are described below and are summarized in Table 11–2.

TACHYCARDIA AND INCREASED CONTRACTILITY THROUGH SNS ACTIVATION

The change in heart rate and contractility which occurs in response to a drop in cardiac output is primarily due to release of norepinephrine from adrenergic nerve terminals. Because cardiac output equals the product of heart rate and stroke volume, one might expect cardiac output to change linearly with heart rate, but the relationship is much more complex. Because systolic time intervals change comparatively little with changing heart rate, almost all cardiac cycle shortening occurs during diastole. Cardiac output continues to increase with heart rate until diastolic filling becomes compromised, which in the normal heart is 170 to 200 beats per minute. When preexisting or acute diastolic dysfunction is present, however, the ventricle's need for more complete (longer) diastolic filling results in reduction of effective preload at significantly lower heart rates. Loss of atrial contribution to ventricular filling can also occur (atrial fibrillation, ventricular tachycardia), reducing ventricular performance even more. Because ionized calcium is sequestered into the sarcoplasmic reticulum and pumped out of the cell during diastole, shortened diastolic time also results in a higher average intracellular calcium concentration during diastole, increasing actin–myosin interaction, augmenting the active resistance to fibril stretch, and reducing lusitropy. Conversely, the higher average calcium concentration translates into greater filament interaction during systole, generating more tension.[8]

Increasing heart rate greatly increases myocardial oxygen demand. If ischemia is induced or worsened, both diastolic and systolic function may become impaired, and stroke volume can drop precipitously.

INCREASED PRELOAD

Augmentation of preload is another compensatory response which is rapidly activated in response to decreased cardiac output. Renal perfusion in heart failure is reduced due to both depressed cardiac output and redistribution of blood away from nonvital organs. The kidney interprets the reduced perfusion as an ineffective blood volume, thus stimulating sodium and water retention. Reduced renal perfusion and increased sympathetic tone also stimulate renin release from juxtaglomerular cells in the kidney. As shown in Figure 11–2, renin is responsible for conversion of angiotensinogen to angiotensin I. Angiotensin I is converted to angiotensin II by angiotensin-converting enzyme (ACE). Angiotensin II feeds back on the adrenal gland to stimulate aldosterone release, thereby providing an additional mechanism for sodium and water retention in the kidney. As intravascular volume increases secondary to sodium and water retention, left ventricular volume and pressure (preload) increase, sarcomeres are stretched, and the force of contraction is enhanced.[1] While the preload response is the primary compensatory mechanism in normal hearts, the chronically failing heart has usually exhausted its preload reserve.[1] As

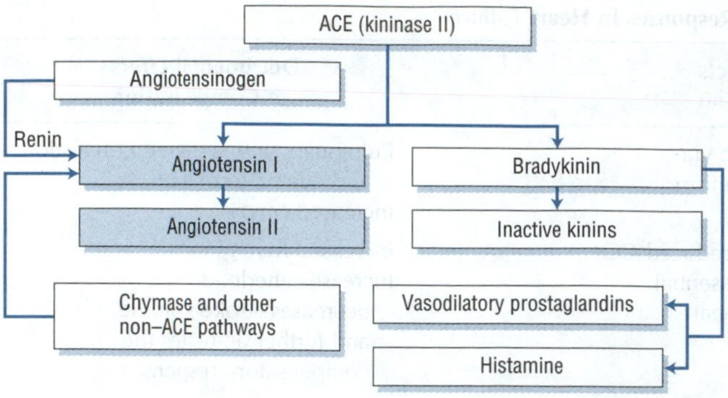

FIGURE 11–2. Activity of angiotensin-converting enzyme (ACE), which is identical to kininase II, on angiotensin and bradykinin.

can be seen in Figure 11–3, increases in preload will increase stroke volume only to a certain point. Once the flat portion of the curve is reached, further increases in preload will only lead to pulmonary or systemic congestion, a detrimental result.[1] Figure 11–3 also shows that the curve is flatter in patients with left ventricular dysfunction. Consequently, a given increase in preload in a patient with heart failure will produce a smaller increment in stroke volume than in an individual with normal ventricular function.

In addition to causing symptoms of congestion, augmentation of preload in the heart failure patient will increase afterload because increasing the radius of the ventricle elevates wall tension. Because the failing ventricle is highly afterload dependent, increases in performance by augmented preload may at times be offset by the attendant increase in afterload. Additionally, the effects of increased preload on force of contraction and afterload will increase myocardial oxygen consumption. Thus an increase in preload can induce ischemia in the coronary patient, with subsequent lusitropic and inotropic compromise.[8]

VASOCONSTRICTION

Vasoconstriction occurs in patients with heart failure to help redistribute blood flow away from nonessential organs to coronary and cerebral circulations to support blood pressure which may be reduced secondary to a decrease in cardiac output (MAP = CO × SVR).[1] A number of neurohormones likely contribute to the vasoconstriction including norepinephrine, angiotensin II, endothelin-1, and arginine vasopressin (AVP).[1,8] Vasoconstriction impedes forward ejection of blood from the ventricle, further depressing cardiac output and heightening the compensatory responses. Because the failing ventricle has usually exhausted its preload reserve (unless the patient is intravascularly depleted), its performance is exquisitely sensitive to changes in afterload. Thus, increases in afterload often potentiate a vicious cycle of continued worsening and downward spiraling of the heart failure state.

VENTRICULAR HYPERTROPHY AND REMODELING

Whereas sympathetic activation and increased preload are compensatory responses of rapid onset, ventricular hypertrophy occurs chronically. An increase in ventricular muscle mass (ventricular hypertrophy) is induced by increases in preload or afterload or by decreases in contractility or myocardial muscle mass. A number of neurohormones and/or autocrine/paracrine factors initiate the signal transduction cascade for ventricular hypertrophy. Ventricular hypertrophy provides an important mechanism for improving contractile function, and the type of hypertrophy is dependent upon the stressor. Pressure overload (and probably hormonal activation) associated with hypertension produces a concentric hypertrophy (increase in the ventricular wall thickness without chamber enlargement). Eccentric left ventricular hypertrophy (LVH, myocyte lengthening with increased chamber size, with minimal increase in wall thickness) characterizes the hypertrophy seen in patients with systolic dysfunction or previous myocardial infarction (MI). In post-MI patients, the risk of development of heart failure is largely dependent on the degree of chamber enlargement (dilatation) and remodeling. While myocyte hypertrophy is occurring, many patients, especially post-MI patients, also develop hyperplasia (increased cell number) of the cardiac interstitium.[9] This extracellular matrix remodeling contributes significantly to abnormal myocardial stiffness and systolic and diastolic dysfunction. Thus, while ventricular hypertrophy is designed to be an important compensatory response in heart failure it often leads to increased myocardial ischemia, impaired ventricular relaxation (causing diastolic dysfunction), systolic dysfunction through ineffective myocyte function and/or cell loss, and increased risk of ventricular arrhythmias and sudden cardiac death. Based on clinical trials (especially with the ACE inhibitors) continued LVH and remodeling probably determines the progressive nature of heart failure.

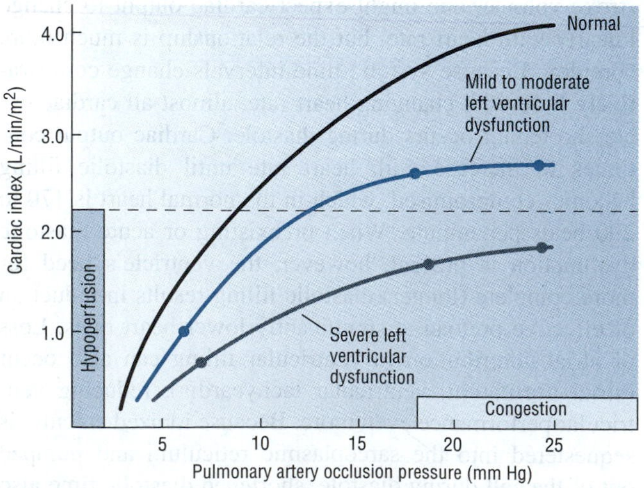

FIGURE 11–3. Relationship between cardiac output (shown as cardiac index which is CO/BSA) and preload (shown as pulmonary artery occlusion pressure).

ROLE OF NEUROHORMONES AND AUTOCRINE/PARACRINE FACTORS IN COMPENSATORY RESPONSES

ANGIOTENSIN II[1]

The effects of angiotensin II are highlighted in Figure 11–4 and most contribute to its detrimental effects in heart failure. Angiotensin II increases systemic vascular resistance in heart failure through direct, potent vasoconstriction. Its ability to cause release of AVP and endothelin-1 may also contribute to vasoconstriction. Angiotensin II also facilitates release of norepinephrine from adrenergic nerve terminals, heightening SNS activation. It promotes sodium retention through direct effects on the renal tubules and by stimulating aldosterone release. Its vasoconstriction of the efferent glomerular arteriole helps to maintain perfusion pressure in patients with severe heart failure or impaired renal function. Thus, in patients dependent on angiotensin II for maintenance of perfusion pressure, initiation of an ACE inhibitor and angiotensin II type 1 (AT_1) receptor blocker causes efferent arteriole vasodilation, decreased perfusion pressure, and decreased glomerular filtration. This explains the risk of impairment in renal function associated with initiation of ACE inhibitor or AT_1-receptor blocker therapy. Finally, angiotensin II in cardiac tissue plays an important role in stimulating ventricular hypertrophy and remodeling. Clinical data suggest blocking these effects contributes substantially to the prolonged survival of ACE inhibitor-treated heart failure patients. The favorable effects of ACE inhibitors on hemodynamics, symptoms, quality of life, and survival in heart failure suggest angiotensin II is an important peptide in the pathophysiology of heart failure.

NOREPINEPHRINE[1,10]

Many of the detrimental effects of norepinephrine (NE) in heart failure are described above. It plays a central role in

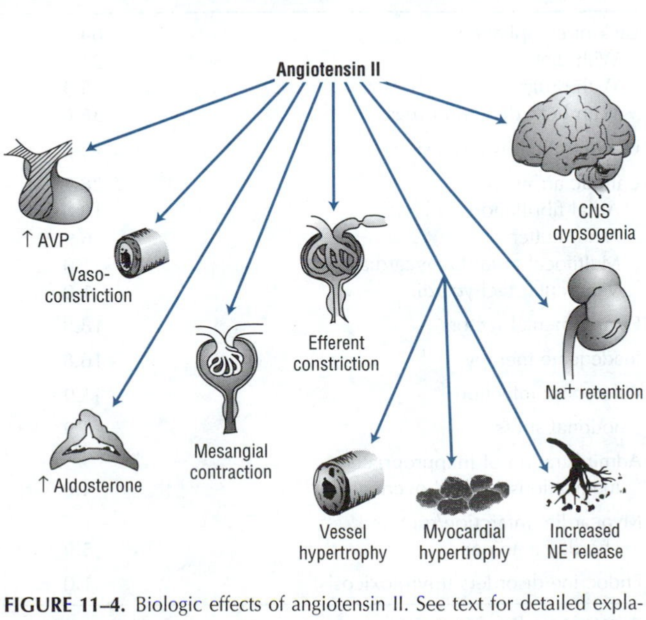

FIGURE 11–4. Biologic effects of angiotensin II. See text for detailed explanation. AVP = arginine vasopressin, NE = norepinephrine. *(From Ref. 104, with permission.)*

the tachycardia, vasoconstriction, and increased contractility observed in heart failure. Plasma NE concentrations are elevated in correlation with the degree of heart failure and patients with the highest plasma NE concentrations have the poorest prognosis. In addition to the detrimental effects described, excessive SNS activation causes down-regulation of β-receptors, with a subsequent loss of sensitivity to receptor stimulation. Excess catecholamines may also be cardiotoxic and produce additional myonecrosis and play a role in the increased risk of arrhythmias. Finally, NE may contribute to ventricular hypertrophy. The detrimental effects of SNS activation are further highlighted by the clinical trials with chronic β-agonists, phosphodiesterase inhibitors, or other drugs which cause SNS activation, as they have uniformly been shown to increase mortality in heart failure (discussed under "Chronic Heart Failure"). Additionally, β-blockers, ACE inhibitors, and digoxin all help to decrease SNS activation, through various mechanisms, and are beneficial in heart failure. Thus, NE plays a critical role in the pathophysiology of the heart failure state.

NATRIURETIC PEPTIDES[11] AND ARGININE VASOPRESSIN[1]

The natriuretic peptide family has three members, atrial natriuretic peptide (ANP), brain natriuretic peptide (BNP), and C-type natriuretic peptide (CNP). ANP is stored mainly in the right atrium whereas BNP is found mainly in the ventricles. Both are released in response to pressure or volume overload. CNP is found mainly in the brain and has very low plasma concentrations. ANP and BNP are thought to balance the effects of the renin–angiotensin–aldosterone (RAA) system by causing natriuresis and vasodilation. Additionally, ANP and CNP have antitrophic effects in cell culture, and may help to slow ventricular hypertrophy in heart failure.

Plasma levels of ANP and BNP are elevated in patients with heart failure in relation to the severity of the disease and can be followed to assess response to therapy. A recent study found ANP and BNP to be highly sensitive and specific in identifying patients with left ventricular systolic dysfunction, regardless of whether the patient was symptomatic or asymptomatic.[12] The authors suggested that measurement of ANP or BNP may be useful in screening the general population for LV systolic dysfunction.

The elevation of ANP or BNP in heart failure appears to have no detrimental effects, but resistance to ANP's actions occurs in heart failure, possibly due to down regulation of the natriuretic-peptide receptors. Additionally, the effects of the RAA and other counter-regulatory systems probably overwhelm the beneficial effects of the natriuretic peptide family. Although there is interest in the therapeutic potential of these peptides, there has been little success with orally active agents for chronic heart failure therapy.

Arginine vasopressin (AVP) is an antidiuretic hormone that regulates free water metabolism and plasma osmolality and is typically elevated in patients with heart failure. AVP has potent vasoconstrictor properties, although its clinical importance in heart failure is unclear.

ENDOTHELIN[13]

There are three distinct endothelin peptides, endothelin-1 (ET-1), endothelin-2 (ET-2), and endothelin-3 (ET-3), which bind to two distinct G-protein coupled receptors, endothelin-A (ET_A) and endothelin B (ET_B). ET-1 is the most potent known vasoconstrictor (5 to 10 times as potent as angiotensin II). ET-1 may be involved in heart failure pathophysiology through a number of mechanisms. Its arterial and venous constrictive effects would increase preload and afterload, and its vasoconstriction of both efferent and afferent renal arterioles may decrease renal plasma flow and induce sodium retention. ET-1 also appears to modulate many other neurohormones involved in heart failure pathophysiology, as it enhances production of angiotensin II, aldosterone, and epinephrine. Based on *in vitro* and animal studies, ET-1 also appears to be an important modulator of ventricular hypertrophy.

Like other peptides and hormones described above, ET-1 plasma concentrations are elevated in heart failure in relation to the severity of disease and it is estimated that ET-1 plasma concentrations are the most sensitive known predictors of prognosis in heart failure. ET-1 plasma concentrations are also directly correlated with New York Heart Association functional class, various hemodynamic parameters, extent of pulmonary hypertension, need for cardiac transplant, 1-year postinfarction mortality, and risk of death.

Both animal and clinical studies with ET-receptor antagonists also suggest ET-1 may play an important role in the pathophysiology of heart failure. Clinical studies of the acute and short-term (2 weeks) hemodynamic effects of ET-receptor blockers have shown favorable effects on most hemodynamic parameters. Beneficial effects have also been noted with ET-receptor blockers in animal models of heart failure, including beneficial modulation of left ventricular hypertrophy. The most promising animal data come from a 12-week study using a coronary artery ligation rat model of heart failure.[14] In this study an ET_A-receptor blocker decreased mortality by over 70%, had marked beneficial effects on hemodynamics, and decreased left ventricular dilatation and remodeling postinfarction.

The clinical and animal data suggest ET-1 is an important factor in heart failure pathophysiology. Limited studies suggest that ET_B blockade is not beneficial and may be detrimental in heart failure.[12] Further investigations will clarify the role of ET-1 in heart failure, the potential place in therapy for ET-receptor antagonists, and whether ET_A-blockers are preferred over nonselective ET-blockers.

CYTOKINES[15]

As described above, a number of hormones appear to play an important role in the pathophysiology and disease progression in heart failure. Recent animal and clinical evidence suggests that cytokines may also play an important role in heart failure. The inflammatory cytokine, tumor necrosis factor α is increased in heart failure and has negative inotropic effects. Natural killer cells and other cytokines may also contribute to heart failure pathophysiology and ongoing work in the field should help clarify whether cytokines play an important role in heart failure and thus may be a therapeutic target.

PRECIPITATING FACTORS

Patients may have a diagnosis of heart failure, yet appropriate therapy can maintain them in a "compensated" state, indicating that they are relatively symptom free. However, there are many aggravating or precipitating factors that may cause a previously compensated patient to decompensate. Factors involved in precipitating a decompensation were evaluated prospectively in patients admitted to the study hospital with heart failure.[16] The results are shown in Table 11–3. Multiple factors were identified in some patients. A number of the decompensating factors can be minimized through pharmacist intervention. Specifically, patient education and counseling by a pharmacist should help to decrease the most common reason for heart failure exacerbation: noncompliance with dietary sodium restrictions, drug therapy, or both. Pharmacists should also be able to identify and address poorly controlled hypertension, administration of inappropriate or inadequate heart failure therapy, and administration of drugs with negative inotropic, cardiotoxic, or sodium-retaining properties. Specific examples of drugs that can worsen heart failure are given in Table 11–4. The value of the pharmacist's role in careful and repeated education of patients, and monitoring of the drug regimen should not be underestimated.

TABLE 11–3. Precipitating Factors in Chronic Heart Failure

Factor	% of Patients
Lack of compliance	64.3
With diet	21.8
With drugs	5.9
With both diet and drugs	36.6
Uncontrolled hypertension	43.6
Cardiac arrhythmias	28.7
Atrial fibrillation	19.8
Atrial flutter	6.9
Multifocal atrial tachycardia	1.0
Ventricular tachycardia	1.0
Environmental factors	18.8
Inadequate therapy	16.8
Pulmonary infection	11.9
Emotional stress	6.9
Administration of inappropriate medications or fluid overload	4.0
Myocardial infarction/ruptured chordae tendinae	5.9
Endocrine disorders (thyrotoxicosis)	1.0

Adapted from Ref. 14.

TABLE 11–4. Drugs That May Precipitate or Exacerbate Heart Failure

Negative inotropic effect
Antiarrhythmics (e.g., disopyramide, flecainide, and others)
β-Blockers (e.g., propranolol, metoprolol, atenolol, and others)
Calcium channel blockers (e.g., verapamil and others)
Cardiotoxic
Doxorubicin
Daunomycin
Cyclophosphamide
Sodium and water retention
Glucocorticoids
Androgens
Estrogens
Nonsteroidal anti-inflammatory agents
Salicylates (high dose)
Sodium-containing drugs (e.g., carbenicillin disodium, ticarcillin disodium)

CLINICAL PRESENTATION[17]

An understanding of the pathophysiologic and compensatory processes in heart failure makes it easy to understand the clinical signs and symptoms. The underlying pathophysiology in heart failure typically causes a reduction in cardiac output. In an attempt to compensate for reduced cardiac output, the SNS activates as do mechanisms that increase preload. However, an overshoot of preload augmentation and an inability of the heart to efficiently accept or eject the increased blood volume results in systemic and/or pulmonary congestion, the most common signs and symptoms in heart failure. Peripheral hypoperfusion and increased SNS activity are responsible for the remaining clinical findings in heart failure patients. Table 11–5 contains a summary of the signs and symptoms of CHF.

Congestion develops behind the failing ventricle with left ventricular failure causing signs and symptoms of pulmonary congestion and right ventricular failure causing signs and symptoms of systemic congestion. Most patients initially have left ventricular failure. However, because the ventricles share a septal wall and left heart failure increases the workload of the right ventricle, both ventricles eventually fail. Many heart failure patients will therefore present with symptoms of both right and left ventricular failure.

SIGNS AND SYMPTOMS OF LEFT VENTRICULAR FAILURE

When the left ventricle fails, it is unable to accept and eject the increased blood volume that is delivered to it. Consequently, pulmonary venous and capillary pressures rise, leading to interstitial and bronchial edema, increased airway resistance, and dyspnea. The associated signs and symptoms may include (1) dyspnea on exertion (DOE), (2) orthopnea, (3) paroxysmal nocturnal dyspnea (PND), (4) dyspnea at rest, and (5) pulmonary edema. Exertional dyspnea is a symptom of heart failure when there is a reduction in the level of exertion that causes breathlessness. This is typically described as more breathlessness than was previously associated with a specific activity (vacuuming, stair climbing). As heart failure progresses, many patients eventually have dyspnea at rest.

Orthopnea is dyspnea that occurs with assumption of the supine position. It occurs within minutes of recumbency and is due to reduced pooling of blood in the lower extremities and abdomen. Orthopnea is relieved almost immediately by sitting upright and is typically prevented by elevating the head with pillows. A change in the number of pillows required to prevent orthopnea (e.g., a change from "two-pillow" to "three-pillow" orthopnea) suggests worsening heart failure. Pulmonary congestion may also cause a nonproductive cough, either with exertion or at night. Attacks of PND typically occur after 2 to 4 hours of sleep; the patient awakens from sleep with a sense of suffocation. The attacks are due to severe pulmonary and bronchial congestion, leading to shortness of breath and wheezing. Unlike orthopnea, the patient may have to sit upright for 30 minutes or more to obtain relief from an attack of PND. The reasons these attacks occur at night are unclear but may include (1) reduced pooling of blood in the lower extremities and abdomen (as in orthopnea), (2) slow resorption of interstitial fluid from sites of dependent edema, (3) normal reduction in sympathetic activity that occurs with sleep (e.g., less support for the failing ventricle), and (4) normal depression in respiratory drive that occurs with sleep.

Pulmonary edema is the most severe form of pulmonary congestion, and is caused by accumulation of fluid in the interstitial spaces and alveoli. In heart failure patients, it is the result of increased pulmonary venous pressure. The

TABLE 11–5. Signs and Symptoms of Congestive Heart Failure

Symptoms	Signs
Right ventricular dysfunction	
Abdominal pain	Peripheral edema
Anorexia	Jugular venous distension
Nausea	Hepatojugular reflux
Bloating	Hepatomegaly
Constipation	
Ascites	
Left ventricular dysfunction	
Dyspnea on exertion	Bibasilar rales
Paroxysmal nocturnal dyspnea	Pulmonary edema
Orthopnea	S_3 gallop
Tachypnea	Pleural effusion
Cough	Cheyne-Stokes respiration
Hemoptysis	
Nonspecific findings	
Exercise intolerance	Tachycardia
Fatigue	Pallor
Weakness	Cyanosis of digits
Nocturia	Cardiomegaly
CNS symptoms	

patient experiences extreme breathlessness, anxiety, and may cough pink, frothy sputum. Pulmonary edema can be terrifying for the patient, causing a feeling of suffocation or drowning.

Rales (crackling sounds heard on auscultation) are present in the lung bases in patients with left-sided heart failure due to transudation of fluid into alveoli. The rales are typically bibasilar, but if heard unilaterally, are usually right sided. A third heart sound, or S3 gallop, is frequently heard in patients with left ventricular failure and may be due to elevated atrial pressure and altered distensibility of the ventricle. Patients with very severe heart failure may have Cheyne-Stokes respiration, alternating between hyperventilation and apnea.

SIGNS AND SYMPTOMS OF RIGHT VENTRICULAR FAILURE

Signs and symptoms of right ventricular failure are the result of systemic venous congestion. Examination of the right internal jugular vein with the patient at a 45° angle is a simple method for assessing jugular venous pressure (JVP). Elevation of JVP more than 4 cm above the sternal angle suggests systemic venous congestion. In patients with mild right heart failure, JVP may be normal at rest but application of pressure to the abdomen will cause an elevation of JVP (hepatojugular reflux). Abdominal (especially hepatic) congestion and an inability of the right ventricle to accept or eject the increased blood volume causes this finding. Development of ascites uncommonly occurs in patients with longstanding systemic venous congestion.

Peripheral edema is a cardinal finding in right-sided heart failure. Edema usually occurs in dependent parts of the body, and thus is seen as ankle or pedal edema in ambulatory patients although it may be manifested as sacral edema in bedridden patients. Adults typically have a 10-lb fluid weight gain before trace peripheral edema is evident, therefore patients with acute heart failure may have no clinical evidence of systemic congestion except weight gain.

Symptoms associated with right-sided heart failure are less common than those of left-sided heart failure. These symptoms are related to hepatic and intestinal congestion and may include abdominal pain, anorexia, nausea, bloating, and constipation.

NONSPECIFIC FINDINGS IN HEART FAILURE

Physical examination and chest x-ray findings that suggest cardiomegaly are found in most patients with heart failure but are considered nonspecific. There are no specific electrocardiographic (ECG) findings associated with heart failure. Many patients will, however, have left ventricular hypertrophy by ECG. The remaining signs and symptoms of heart failure are primarily a result of reduced cardiac output or elevated SNS activity. Weakness, fatigue, and exercise intolerance are present in most patients with heart failure, related in part to inadequate oxygen delivery to skeletal muscles from reduced cardiac output. It must be kept in mind, however, that these symptoms may also be seen in many noncardiac disorders. Symptoms of central nervous system (CNS) hypoperfusion such as confusion, lethargy, hallucinations, nightmares, insomnia, and headache may occur in patients with severe heart failure, especially if they have underlying cerebral arteriosclerosis.

Increased SNS activity is responsible for the tachycardia often observed in heart failure. As previously described, numerous factors contribute to peripheral vasoconstriction which manifests as pallor, cool extremities, or cyanosis of the digits. Vasoconstriction also serves to shunt blood away from nonvital organs such as the kidney. Nocturia is frequently noted in heart failure patients because of the reductions in sympathetic activation and cardiac output demands at night. Consequently, renal vasoconstriction diminishes, increasing renal blood flow and urine formation.

CLASSIFICATION OF CONGESTIVE HEART FAILURE PATIENTS

Systems that classify patients according to their level of disability are useful from several perspectives. They can be used to follow the progress of the patient longitudinally, to assess the impact of therapeutic maneuvers, or to provide a reference point for comparison with other patients. The most widely used classification system is the New York Heart Association (NYHA) Functional Classification System.[16] It divides patients into four categories (Table 11–6). There are obvious limitations to assigning a numerical score to subjective findings; however, this system is fairly useful for monitoring patients and is widely used in heart failure studies.

TABLE 11–6. New York Heart Association Functional Classification

Functional Class	
I	Patients with cardiac disease but without limitations of physical activity. Ordinary physical activity does not cause undue fatigue, dyspnea, or palpitation.
II	Patients with cardiac disease that results in slight limitations of physical activity. Ordinary physical activity results in fatigue, palpitation, dyspnea, or angina.
III	Patients with cardiac disease that results in marked limitation of physical activity. Although patients are comfortable at rest, less than ordinary activity will lead to symptoms.
IV	Patients with cardiac disease that results in an inability to carry on physical activity without discomfort. Symptoms of congestive heart failure are present even at rest. With any physical activity, increased discomfort is experienced.

▶ TREATMENT: Acute/Severe Heart Failure

PATHOPHYSIOLOGY AND CLINICAL PRESENTATION

Patients requiring intensive care for severe heart failure may arrive at this stage via several pathways. Patients with chronic progressive heart failure can become refractory to available oral therapy and acutely decompensate following a relatively mild insult (e.g., dietary indiscretion), from medical noncompliance, or a noncardiac concurrent illness (e.g., infection). A new cardiac event, such as recurrent MI, myocarditis or acute valvular insufficiency can also cause a patient with previously compensated heart failure to develop shock, pulmonary edema, or both. A third group of patients are those with acute, massive MI whose initial presentation is severe heart failure.

Patients should be admitted to an intensive care unit (ICU) for severe heart failure when they show signs of significant systemic hypoperfusion (altered mental status, depressed renal function, hypotension), develop pulmonary vascular congestion requiring mechanical ventilation, manifest symptomatic sustained tachyarrhythmias, or require potent intravenous vasoactive or inotropic drugs or mechanical ventricular assistance. Reversible causes of the patient's decompensation should be sought early and aggressively; correction of problems such as hypothyroidism, hypocalcemia, drug-induced cardiotoxicity, hypoxia, or concurrent sepsis will be necessary for successful resuscitation and eventual unit discharge.[18]

The general pathophysiologic determinants of myocardial systolic (preload, afterload, inotropy) and diastolic (ventricular compliance or lusitropic) function in these patients are essentially the same as described earlier in this chapter. However, the severity of their symptoms, paucity of cardiopulmonary reserve, and potential for adverse responses to intervention makes a more detailed examination of these factors, their mutual interaction, and reflex responses essential to sophisticated support decisions. Many adult patients requiring ICU management of heart failure have significant coronary artery disease, whether as the primary cause of their heart failure or as stable but flow-limiting chronic stenoses present as a concurrent cardiac illness. When interventions for heart failure augment myocardial oxygen demand beyond supply, the induction of ischemic dysfunction may blunt or even negate the intended beneficial effects on ventricular performance.

HEMODYNAMIC MONITORING AND IMAGING

Patients with severe heart failure typically have critically reduced cardiac output, usually with low arterial blood pressure and systemic hypoperfusion resulting in organ system dysfunction. They may also show hydrostatic pulmonary edema with hypoxemia, respiratory acidosis, and markedly increased work of breathing. As cardiopulmonary support must be instituted and adjusted rapidly, immediate assessment of the results of an intervention permit risks to be limited and advances in therapy to be made more promptly. ECG monitoring, continuous pulse oximetry, urimetry, and automated sphygmomanometric blood pressure recording are now the minimal noninvasive standard of care for critically ill patients with cardiopulmonary embarrassment. Peripheral or femoral arterial catheters provide beat-to-beat assessment of arterial pressure which is more accurate than cuff pressures in patients with severely depressed cardiac output. Central venous catheters are helpful in assessing volume status in patients without primary pulmonary vascular or right heart disease, and right heart filling pressures in all circumstances.

Flow-directed pulmonary artery (PA) catheters are typically placed percutaneously through a central vein, right heart, and into the pulmonary artery. Inflation of a balloon proximal to the endport allows the catheter to "wedge," yielding the PAOP, which estimates the pulmonary venous (left atrial) pressure and, in the absence of intracardiac shunt or mitral valve disease, left ventricular diastolic pressure. Normal values for hemodynamic monitoring are listed in Table 11–7. Although the routine use of pulmonary artery catheters has recently come under scrutiny, it will provide essential information in the most critically ill patients during exacting dose titration of rapidly-acting medications. Hemodynamic monitoring is extensively reviewed in Chap. 8.

Imaging techniques including transthoracic and transesophageal echo-Doppler cardiography, thallium-201 perfusion imaging, and radionuclide ventriculography can all be performed at the bedside and provide valuable information about cardiac structure and function. A detailed description is beyond the scope of this chapter, but is summarized in Chap. 8 and elsewhere.[19]

GENERAL APPROACH TO TREATMENT

The wide spectra of etiologies, presentations, complications, and concurrent illnesses make the concepts of first choice and alternative therapies for severe heart failure inadequate for sophisticated therapeutic decision making. A joint task force of the American College of Cardiology and the American Heart Association has produced the most widely accepted consensus statement to date.[20] Like all such works, however, it must be viewed as a general guideline, and its suggestions modified based on individual patient needs. A thorough understanding of pathophysiology and pharmacology leads to the general approach to therapy given in Fig. 11–5.

Initial stabilization may require oxygen, mechanical ventilatory support, direct current cardioversion, or antiarrhythmic drugs if sustained tachyarrhythmias are present. Temporary transvenous pacing for significant bradyarrhythmias may also be necessary. Echocardiography is often necessary if physical examination fails to exclude structural abnormalities such as tamponade, valvular insufficiency, or intracardiac shunt.

To select the most appropriate therapy, the following issues should be addressed in the initial assessment.

TABLE 11–7. Hemodynamic Monitoring: Normal Values

Central venous (right atrial) pressure, mean	< 5 mm Hg
Right ventricular pressure	25/0 mm Hg
Pulmonary artery pressure	25/10 mm Hg
PAP, mean	< 18 mm Hg
Pulmonary artery occlusion pressure, mean	< 12 mm Hg
Systemic arterial pressure	120/80 mm Hg
Mean arterial pressure	90–110 mm Hg
Cardiac index	2.8–4.2 $L/min/m^2$
Stroke volume index	30–65 $mL/b/m^2$
Systemic vascular resistance	900–1400 $dyne\cdot sec\cdot cm^{-5}$
Pulmonary vascular resistance	150–250 $dyne\cdot sec\cdot cm^{-5}$
Arterial oxygen content	20 mL/dL
Mixed venous oxygen content	15 mL/dL
Arteriovenous oxygen content difference	3–5 mL/dL

PAP = pulmonary artery pressure.

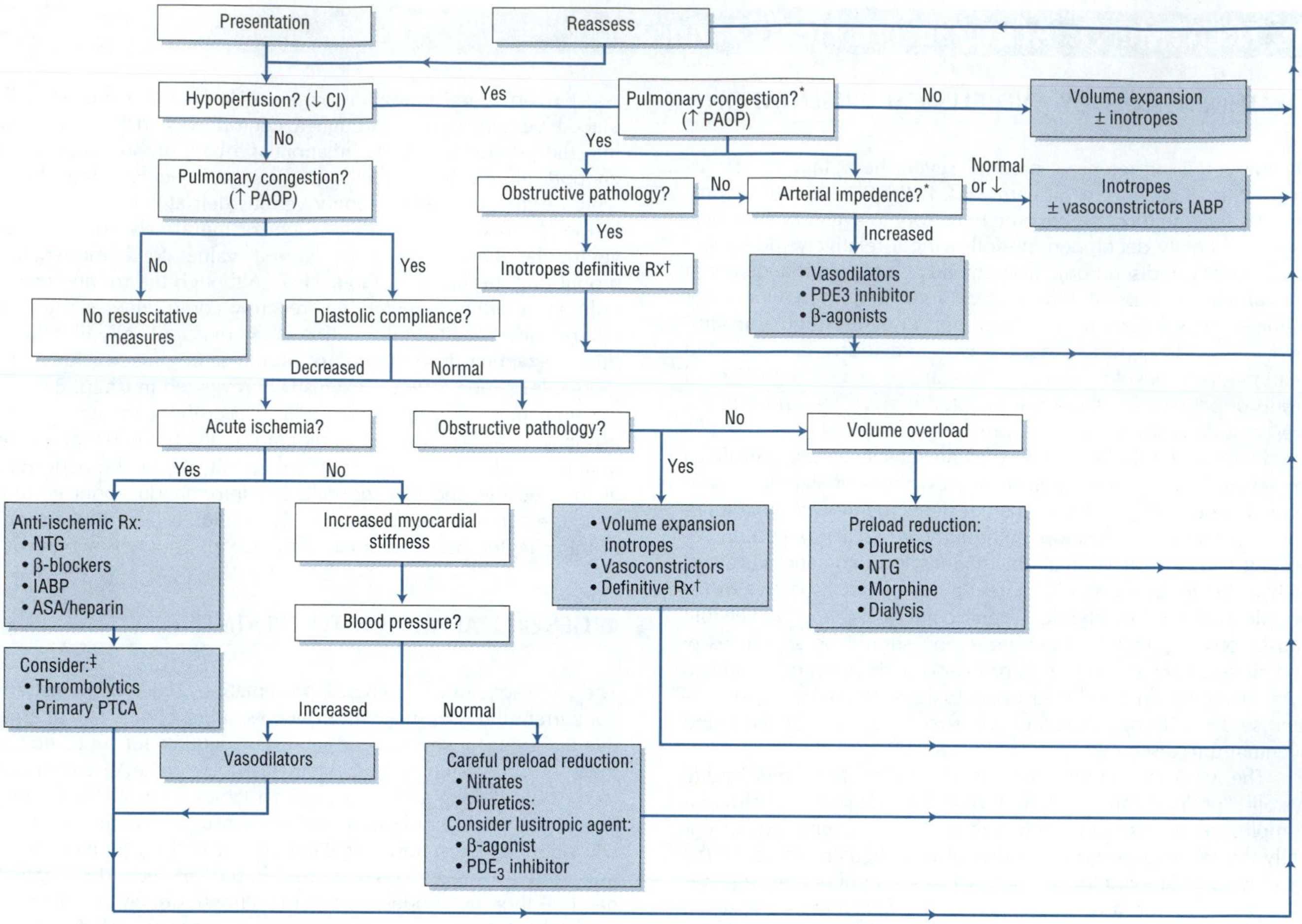

FIGURE 11–5. Treatment algorithm for patients with acute/severe heart failure. See text for details. CI = cardiac index, PAOP = pulmonary artery occlusion pressure, IABP = intra-aortic balloon pump, PDE = phosphodiesterase, NTG = nitroglycerin, ASA = aspirin, PTCA = percutaneous transluminal coronary angioplasty. *Evaluation for contributory ischemia is indicated. †See text for details or diagnostic methods/differential. ‡See chapter for indications.

IS THE PATIENT MANIFESTING INADEQUATE SYSTEMIC PERFUSION, VENOUS HYPERTENSION, OR BOTH?

Signs of insufficient systemic perfusion (insufficient cardiac output) are discussed above. In the most severely ill patients, findings in profound shock include depressed mental status, prerenal or ischemic renal failure, shock liver, ileus, and lactic acidosis. Hydrostatic pulmonary edema can compromise oxygenation, carbon dioxide excretion, or both, increasing the work of breathing and placing additional demands on the already overtaxed heart. On initial assessment, and in the absence of obstructive pathology (tamponade, mitral stenosis, pulmonary veno-occlusive disease), the presence of pulmonary venous (pulmonary or systemic) hypertension suggests that preload reserve is exhausted, and maneuvers to increase cardiac output via Starling mechanisms are unlikely to benefit and may even worsen the patient's overall condition. The absence of systemic venous hypertension (associated with elevated right ventricular end-diastolic pressure) implies that the patient is either volume contracted, suffering from a process affecting only the left heart, or is amidst a new catastrophic event affecting primarily the left ventricle (e.g., massive anterior MI).

In the absence of pulmonary edema, intravascular volume expansion to increase preload is usually the first maneuver attempted to raise cardiac output. When this is not possible or fails, inotropic agents or vasodilators will be needed to improve perfusion. If systemic perfusion appears adequate but the primary manifestation is pulmonary edema, careful reduction in end-diastolic pressure with venodilators should be performed. It is essential to remember that a precipitous drop in filling pressure can cause a catastrophic reduction in cardiac performance if significant diastolic dysfunction is present, and short-acting, titratable agents (e.g., IV nitroglycerin) are preferable in this setting.

IS OBSTRUCTIVE PATHOLOGY PRESENT?

Obstructive pathology includes such things as cardiac tamponade, mitral stenosis, and pulmonary veno-occlusive disease. The important points here are that ventricular systolic and diastolic function may be normal even though the patient is manifesting shock and/or pulmonary edema. Volume expansion as tolerated, and, if needed, positive inotropes with vasoconstricting actions are used to stabilize the patient until definitive therapy can be performed. Administration of drugs with vasodilatory effects must be avoided in these disorders; sudden, profound shock and cardiac arrest often result, with little hope of successful resuscitation.

IS ARTERIAL IMPEDENCE HIGH, NORMAL, OR LOW?

Any disorder that results in a significant reduction in cardiac output or systemic perfusion pressure will cause reflex vasoconstriction, and occasionally high peripheral resistance may be the primary disorder (hypertensive emergency). In patients with underlying left ventricular dysfunction, small doses of arterial vasodilators will often result in impressive improvement of cardiac output in this setting (Fig. 11–1). The response to vasodilator therapy in the absence of high peripheral resistance will be minimal, and its use in this setting may critically reduce systemic perfusion pressure.

Is Diastolic Compliance Reduced or Normal?

Absolute *intravascular* volume overload is relatively uncommon in the absence of significant renal failure or severe longstanding biventricular failure. As such, pulmonary venous hypertension is most often due to diastolic dysfunction. This may be acute in the presence of active myocardial ischemia (impaired active relaxation), or chronic in the setting of a host of disorders associated with myocardial hypertrophy, fibrosis, or infiltration (see above). Chronic severe diastolic dysfunction is associated with a steep compliance curve (Fig. 11–6) and is not generally amenable to acute modulation. Therefore, preload reduction with venodilating or diuretic agents should be performed with extreme caution using short-acting, titratable drugs; a small decrease in ventricular pressure can result in a much greater reduction in diastolic volume, critically compromising preload and cardiac output.

IS ACTIVE OR CHRONIC ISCHEMIC HEART DISEASE PRESENT?

As discussed above, acute ischemia may cause severe diastolic dysfunction, systolic dysfunction, or both. Anti-ischemic therapy to reduce myocardial oxygen demand and improve coronary blood flow is paramount, as most other pharmacologic interventions employed in treatment of nonischemic heart failure carry the risk of increasing $M\dot{V}O_2$ (inotropes), reducing coronary perfusion pressure (vasodilators), or critically lowering preload in the severely noncompliant ventricle (diuretics, narcotics). Treatment of acute myocardial ischemia is discussed in Chap. 13.

IS THERE A REVERSIBLE ETIOLOGY FOR THE ACUTE HEART FAILURE?

Investigation of reversible etiologies of cardiopulmonary decompensation should begin early in the treatment course; otherwise, chances for long-term recovery will be severely compromised. A detailed listing of reversible causes for acute heart failure is provided elsewhere.

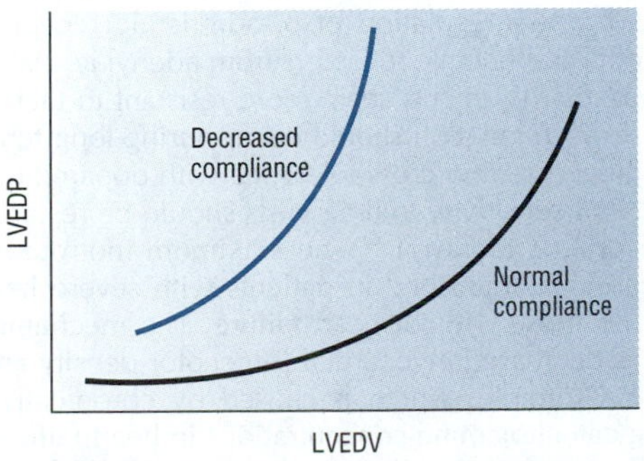

FIGURE 11–6. Relationship between left ventricular end diastolic volume (LVEDV) and pressure (LVEDP). A fixed increase in volume produces a larger increase in pressure when the LVEDV is elevated. Various disease states will decrease ventricular compliance and cause a shift in the curve and yield higher LVEDP for any given LVEDV.

PHARMACOLOGIC THERAPY OF SEVERE HEART FAILURE

The pharmacotherapeutic agents used to treat patients with severe heart failure rarely if ever produce a single cardiovascular action. Even when intended for a single purpose (e.g., a positive inotrope), other drug effects (tachycardia, vasodilation, or vasoconstriction) may either add to the therapeutic effect or cause adverse events that negate or even outweigh the intended therapeutic benefit. It can often be difficult to anticipate how an individual patient will respond to a given intervention. For this reason, cardiovascular monitoring is usually employed during resuscitation, and many drugs are considered first-line therapy due in part to their short half-lives and titratability. The description of expected drug actions outlined below should be viewed as a guide to the clinician, who must remain vigilant for outcomes other than those sought in these tenuous patients.

POSITIVE INOTROPIC AGENTS

Drugs that increase intracellular cyclic adenosine monophosphate (cAMP) are the only positive inotropic agents used for the treatment of acute/severe heart failure. β-agonists activate adenylate cyclase through stimulation of β-adrenergic receptors with the enzyme then catalyzing the conversion of ATP to cAMP. Phosphodiesterase inhibitors raise cAMP concentrations by reducing its degradation. Thus both drug classes increase intracellular cAMP which enhances phospholipase (and subsequently phosphorylase) activity, increasing the rate and extent of calcium influx during systole and enhancing contractility. Additionally, cAMP enhances reuptake of calcium by the sarcoplasmic reticulum during diastole, improving active relaxation.[18]

Digoxin has little if any place in the treatment of patients with acute heart failure who are hemodynamically unstable. The delay in peak inotropic effect, limited maximal efficacy, long duration of action, and significant toxicity (arrhythmic, vasoconstrictive, neurologic) are major disadvantages in the acute setting.

Adrenergic Agonists

Several adrenergic agents are used for the treatment of patients with severe heart failure. These compounds vary in their affinities for adrenergic receptors in the heart and peripheral tissues, and consequently lead to different pharmacologic effects (Table 11–8). Hemodynamic effects in patients will be the result of direct receptor-mediated effects plus reflex-mediated sequelae. These compounds have half-lives of a few minutes, and must be administered by continuous intravenous infusion.

Dopamine.[21] Dopamine, the endogenous precursor of NE, exerts its effects by directly stimulating adrenergic receptors as well as causing release of NE from adrenergic nerve terminals.

TABLE 11–8. Relative Effects of Adrenergic Drugs on Receptors

Drug	α_1	β_1	β_2	Dopamine$_1$
Norepinephrine	++++	++++	0	0
Epinephrine	++++	++++	++	0
Dopamine[a]	++++	++++	++	++
Isoproterenol	0	++++	++++	0
Dobutamine[b]	+	++++	++	0

[a]See text for a more detailed description of the dose-dependent hemodynamic effects.

[b]Combined effects of the commercially available recemic mixture (see text).

TABLE 11–9. Usual Hemodynamic Effects of Intravenous Agents Commonly Used for Treatment of Acute/Severe Heart Failure[a]

Drug	Dose	HR	MAP	PAOP	CO	SVR
Dopamine	0.5–3 μg/kg/min	0	0	0	0/+	–
Dopamine	3–10 μg/kg/min	+	+	0	+	0
Dopamine	>10 μg/kg/min	+	+	+	+	+
Dobutamine	2.5–20 μg/kg/min	0/+	0	–	+	–
Amrinone	5–10 μg/kg/min	0/+	0/–	–	+	–
Milrionone	0.375–0.75 μg/kg/min	0/+	0/–	–	+	–
Nitroprusside	0.25–3 mg/kg/min	0/+	0/–	–	+	–
Nitroglycerin	5–200 μg/min	0/+	0/–	–	0/+	0/–
Furosemide	20–80 mg, repeated as needed up to 4–6 times/d	0	0	–	0	0
Enalaprilat	1.25–2.5 mg q6–8h	0	0/–	–	+	+

[a]See text for a more detailed description of the interpatient variability in response.
Abbreviations: + = increase, – = decrease, 0 = no change, HR = heart rate, MAP = mean arterial pressure, PAOP = pulmonary artery occlusion pressure, CO = cardiac output, SVR = systemic vascular resistance.

Dopamine produces dose-dependent hemodynamic effects because of its relative affinity for α_1-, β_1-, β_2-, and D_1- (vascular dopaminergic) receptors (Table 11–9). At low doses (0.5 to 3—average 1—μg/kg/min), stimulation of D_1-receptors predominates and leads to selective dilation of renal, mesenteric, cerebral, and coronary vascular beds. The result is increased renal blood flow, glomerular filtration and urine output, natriuresis, and kaliuresis. The renal effects are accentuated by an increase in cardiac index which may be evident even with low doses.

Positive inotropic effects mediated primarily by β_1-receptors become more prominent with dopamine doses of 3 to 10 μg/kg/min. Cardiac index is increased because of an increase in stroke volume and a variable increase in heart rate, which is partially dose dependent. There is usually little change in systemic vascular resistance, presumably because neither vasodilation (D_1- and β_2-receptor-mediated) nor vasoconstriction (α_1-receptor-mediated) predominates. Renal effects of dopamine may still be evident at these higher doses and are caused by a combination of D_1-mediated renovascular effects, increased cardiac index, and altered sodium tubular reabsorption. At doses above 10 μg/kg/min, chronotropic and α_1-receptor-mediated vasoconstricting effects become more prominent. Mean arterial pressure usually elevates because of an increase in both cardiac index and (SVR) (Table 11–9). The vasoconstricting effects of higher doses could indirectly limit the increase in cardiac index by increasing afterload and PAOP, thus complicating the management of patients with preexisting high afterload. In such patients, alternative agents (dobutamine, amrinone, milrinone) or the addition of diuretics and/or vasodilators may be necessary.

Dopamine, particularly at higher doses, will alter several parameters that increase myocardial oxygen demand (increased heart rate, contractility, and systolic pressure) and potentially decrease myocardial blood flow (coronary vasoconstriction and increased wall tension), worsening ischemia in some patients with coronary disease. Arrhythmogenesis is more common at higher doses.

Dobutamine.[21] Dobutamine, a synthetic catecholamine, is a β_1- and β_2-receptor agonist with some α_1-agonist effects. Unlike dopamine, dobutamine does not cause release of NE from nerve terminals. The overall hemodynamic effects of dobutamine are the result of its effects on adrenergic receptors and reflex-mediated actions. Its β_2-receptor-mediated effects are greater than those from dopamine and β_2-receptor-mediated vasodilation will tend to offset some of the α_1-receptor-mediated vasoconstriction. Thus, the net vascular effect is usually vasodilation. The positive inotropy is a β_1-receptor mediated effect with some inotropy effects through stimulation of cardiac α_1- and β_2-receptors. Cardiac α_1-receptor stimulation by dobutamine causes an increase in contractility but no significant change in heart rate, and may provide an explanation for the apparently more modest chronotropic actions of dobutamine compared to dopamine.

The overall hemodynamic effects of dobutamine are those of a potent inotropic agent with vasodilating action. Initial doses of 2.5 to 5 μg/kg/min can be progressively increased to 20 μg/kg/min or higher based on clinical and hemodynamic responses and duration of therapy. Cardiac index is increased because of inotropic stimulation, arterial vasodilation, and a variable increase in heart rate. In patients with heart failure and high peripheral resistance, the decrease in SVR provides another mechanism to increase cardiac index. Because of the offsetting changes in arteriolar resistance and cardiac index, dobutamine will usually cause relatively little change in mean arterial pressure compared to the more consistent increase observed with dopamine. This smaller effect on blood pressure is beneficial in patients with heart failure and ischemic heart disease as it will minimize the increase in myocardial oxygen demand. However, the absence of a consistent hypertensive effect with dobutamine will be a disadvantage in patients with heart failure and hypotension. Dobutamine's vasodilating action will usually decrease PAOP, making it particularly useful in the presence of low cardiac index and an elevated filling pressure.

Attenuation of dobutamine's hemodynamic effects has been reported after 72 hours of continuous infusion and may be a consequence of down-regulation of β_1-adrenergic receptors or uncoupling of β2-adrenergic receptors from adenylate cyclase.[23] Peripheral vascular β_2 effects seem more resistant to tachyphylaxis. Receptor down-regulation should occur during long-term therapy with any β-agonist, and cross-tolerance with dopamine would be predicted. Full sensitivity to β-agonists should be restored 7 to 10 days after drug withdrawal.[23] The maximum inotropic effects of dobutamine are diminished in patients with severe heart failure compared to those without heart failure. The mechanism of this tolerance is decreased myocardial β-receptor density and uncoupling from G-protein, which is caused by chronically elevated circulating catecholamine concentrations in heart failure patients.

Despite the fact that dobutamine has a half-life of approximately 2.5 minutes, some patients may display sustained hemodynamic and symptomatic benefits for several days to months after a treatment course.[24,25] These beneficial effects have been associated with widely different dobutamine dosage regimens (4- to 72-hour infusions of 7.4 to 25.3 μg/kg/min every 3 to 7 days for 4 to 24 weeks). The mechanism is unclear, but the drug may promote cardiovascular conditioning analogous to exercise training.[24] However, a randomized placebo-controlled multicenter trial in outpatients with chronic heart failure showed increased mortality in dobutamine-treated patients.[26] Thus, despite symptomatic benefits, the potential for increased mortality should preclude the chronic scheduled administration of intermittent dobutamine infusions in most patients.

Norepinephrine.[21] As a pharmacologic agent, intravenous NE displays primarily β_1- and α_1-agonist effects, with little or no β_2 effect. This catecholamine is also taken up presynaptically into adrenergic nerve terminals, and enhances neurotransmitter release. With virtually no vasodilatory effect, the combination of profound arteriolar constriction and tachycardia can result in excessive increases in afterload and arrhythmias when the drug is used alone, making it a suboptimal agent in most patients with severe heart failure.

NE is administered at rates of 0.1 to 1.0 μg/kg/min, titrated to desired effect. Except in the special circumstances described above, this agent should probably be reserved for the profoundly hypotensive patient, and preferably used in combination with a vasodilating drug.

Epinephrine.[21] Epinephrine is a naturally occurring adrenal medullary hormone with both α- and β-agonist effects. At infusion rates of 0.03 μg/kg/min, this drug displays primarily nonspecific β-agonist properties. At doses in excess of 0.3 μg/kg/min, however, the α-receptor effects predominate while myocardial β_1-receptor stimulation increases. Although rarely used in the heart failure patient, it is more often employed in short-term support of profound but reversible inotropic suppression, as seen after cardiopulmonary bypass, β-blocker overdose, and drug intoxications.

Phosphodiesterase Inhibitors

Drugs from this class produce their hemodynamic effects by inhibiting phosphodiesterase fraction III (PDE3) and increasing cAMP concentrations. The consequences, as described above, are enhanced inotropic and lusitropic myocardial function. In vascular smooth muscle cells, the increase in cAMP produces relaxation, causing venous and arteriolar dilation. These drugs are therefore referred to as *inodilators.* The IV formulations of amrinone and milrinone are the only agents from this class currently approved in the United States for use in heart failure.

Amrinone and Milrinone.[27,28] These bipyridine derivatives have very similar pharmacologic and hemodynamic effects during IV administration. Both positive inotropic and vasodilating effects contribute to the therapeutic response in heart failure patients. Their relative importance in a particular patient may vary with dose and underlying cardiovascular pathology.

During IV administration, there is an increase in stroke volume with little change in heart rate (Table 11–9). Despite the increase in cardiac index, mean arterial pressure generally remains constant because of the concomitant decrease in arteriolar resistance. However, the vasodilating effects may predominate in certain patients and lead to a decrease in blood pressure and a reflex tachycardia. The drugs lower PAOP by venodilation and thus are particularly useful in patients with a low cardiac index and an elevated end-diastolic pressure. Such a reduction in preload, however, can be hazardous for patients without excessive filling pressure, leading to a decrease in cardiac index. Such an effect would blunt the improvement in cardiac output that would otherwise be produced by the positive inotropic and arterial dilating actions. These drugs should rarely be used as single agents in severely hypotensive heart failure patients because they will not increase, and may even decrease, arterial blood pressure.

The results of controlled studies comparing dobutamine to amrinone or milrinone indicate that they produce generally similar hemodynamic effects to dobutamine.[28,29] A clinically insignificant but greater increase in heart rate with dobutamine is the most consistent difference in these studies. The combination of dobutamine and a bipyridine produces additive effects on cardiac index and PAOP reduction,[30] suggesting this regimen as an option in patients who have dose-limiting adverse effects with either class of drugs. It is unclear, however, if this combination provides a therapeutic advantage over the combination of a positive inotrope and a traditional pure vasodilator such as nitroprusside.

It is often assumed that phosphodiesterase inhibitors will avoid the pharmacodynamic tolerance associated with continuous β-agonist infusions. In one study, hemodynamic tolerance to amrinone was documented after 72 hours of continuous infusion.[31] Tachyphylaxis to amrinone was associated with a downregulation and uncoupling of β-receptors from adenylate cyclase, similar to that seen with β-agonists.[31]

Amrinone and milrinone have much longer terminal elimination half-lives than adrenergic agonists. The average half-life for milrinone is 2.3 hours; for amrinone it is 2 to 4 hours in healthy subjects and up to 12 hours in patients with severe heart failure. The long elimination half-lives of these drugs are a distinct disadvantage in this patient population because a loading dose is necessary to obtain a prompt initial response, minute-to-minute titrations in dose cannot be made based on response, and adverse effects (arrhythmias or hypotension) will persist much longer after drug discontinuation. Peak hemodynamic effects are generally obtained within 15 minutes of the loading dose. The usual loading dose of amrinone is 0.75 mg/kg administered over 2 to 3 minutes, followed by a continuous infusion of 5 to 10 μg/kg/min. An additional loading dose of 0.75 mg/kg may be repeated after 30 minutes. Maintenance doses above 20 μg/kg/min do not produce additional hemodynamic benefits and clearly enhance toxicity.[31] The recommended loading dose of milrinone is 50 μg/kg administered over 10 minutes, followed by a continuous infusion of 0.5 μg/kg/min (range; 0.375 to 0.75 μg/kg/min). Over 80% of a dose of milrinone is excreted unchanged in urine and, unlike amrinone, its infusion rate should be decreased by 50% to 70% in patients with significant renal impairment.

In addition to undesirable hemodynamic effects, the most notable adverse events associated with amrinone and milrinone are arrhythmias and thrombocytopenia. Thrombocytopenia is reported to occur in 2.4% of patients who have received IV amrinone, with decreased platelet survival from nonimmunologic platelet damage as the postulated mechanism. This adverse effect is dose dependent and generally completely reversible within 5 to 7 days of drug discontinuation. The incidence of thrombocytopenia associated with milrinone therapy is very low (< 0.5%).[27] Milrinone is therefore preferable to amrinone because of its better side-effect profile. Patients who receive either drug should be monitored for signs of bleeding and have platelet counts determined before and during therapy.

Generally, milrinone or amrinone should be considered for patients who have not responded adequately to dobutamine, dopamine, IV vasodilators, or a combination of these agents, or when hypertension is part of the clinical picture. Their combination with dopamine or dobutamine may also be helpful in patients with dose-limiting adverse effects to single drug therapy.

Vasodilators

Activation of the SNS, the RAA system, AVP, and endothelial and platelet-derived mediators all cause vasoconstriction and increase SVR. In patients with heart failure, stroke volume varies inversely with SVR (Fig. 11–1) such that an increase in peripheral resistance leads to a severe decline in stroke volume and cardiac output.

Vasodilators are typically described by their prominent site of action (arterial or venous). Arterial vasodilators act as impedance-reducing agents and typically cause an increase in cardiac output. Venodilators act as preload reducers by increasing venous capacitance, reducing symptoms of pulmonary congestion in patients with high cardiac filling pressures. Mixed vasodilators act on both resistance and capacitance vessels, reducing congestive symptoms while increasing cardiac output. Nitroprusside and nitroglycerin are the most widely studied and commonly used IV vasodilating agents in acute/severe heart failure, with parenteral ACE inhibitors next most commonly used. Other vasodilators have shown either tachyphylaxis, excessive reflex tachycardia, or refractory hypotension compromising coronary blood flow; they are rarely if ever used in this setting.

Nitroprusside.[27] Sodium nitroprusside, a mixed arterial-venous vasodilator, acts on vascular smooth muscle, increasing synthesis of nitric oxide to produce its balanced vasodilating action. As such, it both increases cardiac index and decreases venous pressure. Nitroprusside's effects on these parameters are qualitatively similar to those produced by dobutamine and amrinone/milrinone, despite the fact that it has no direct inotropic activity (Table 11–9). However, nitroprusside generally causes a greater decrease in PAOP, SVR, and blood pressure than dobutamine. Mean arterial pressure may remain fairly constant but often decreases depending on the relative increase in cardiac output and reduction in arteriolar tone. Hypotension is an important dose-limiting adverse effect of nitroprusside and other vasodilators. Therefore, this drug is primarily used in patients who have a significantly elevated SVR.

Patients with normal left ventricular function will not have an increase in stroke volume when SVR falls, as the normal ventricle is fairly insensitive to small changes in afterload (Fig 11–1). Consequently, these patients experience a significant decrease in blood pressure after administration of arterial vasodilators. This explains why nitroprusside is a potent antihypertensive agent in patients without heart failure but causes less hypotension and reflex tachycardia in patients with left ventricular dysfunction. Nonetheless, even a modest increase in heart rate could have adverse consequences in patients with underlying ischemic heart disease and/or resting tachycardia, and close monitoring is necessary during therapy.

Nitroprusside has been extensively studied and shown to be effective in the short-term management of patients with severe heart failure in a variety of settings (i.e., AMI, valvular regurgitation, postcoronary bypass surgery, decompensated chronic heart failure).[22] The combination of nitroprusside and dopamine or dobutamine is particularly useful for patients with pulmonary edema and cardiogenic shock who fail to respond to either agent alone. Furthermore, if the initial blood pressure is relatively low (a relative contraindication to vasodilator therapy) or if significant hypotension develops during nitroprusside therapy, the addition of dopamine to raise mean arterial pressure may allow optimal use of both inotropic and vasodilator drugs. Generally, nitroprusside will not worsen, and may improve, the balance between myocardial oxygen demand and supply. This is mainly due to a decrease in oxygen demand caused by the lowering of left ventricular wall tension and a possible increase in subendocardial blood flow resulting from decreased left ventricular diastolic pressure. However, an excessive decrease in systemic arterial pressure can reduce coronary perfusion and worsen ischemia, leading to concern about coronary steal.[32]

Nitroprusside has a rapid onset of action and a duration of action of less than 10 minutes, necessitating its administration by continuous IV infusion. This allows for precise dose titration based on measured clinical and hemodynamic parameters. It, like other vasodilators used in heart failure, should be initiated at a low dose (0.1 to 0.25 μg/kg/min) to avoid excessive hypotension, and then increased by small increments (0.1 to 0.2 μg/kg/min) every 5 to 10 minutes as needed and tolerated. Usually effective doses range from 0.5 to 3.0 μg/kg/min. A rebound phenomenon has been reported after abrupt withdrawal of nitroprusside in patients with heart failure and is apparently due to reflex neurohumoral activation during therapy.[33] If renal perfusion pressure is compromised by the drug, salt and water retention can contribute to volume expansion and tachyphylaxis; this is typically seen only in patients with chronic hypertension, baseline azotemia or when therapeutic augmentation of cardiac output during therapy is minimal. It is usually advisable to taper doses slowly when stopping nitroprusside and switching to oral drugs, or to add diuretics during prolonged therapy. Nitroprusside can cause cyanide and thiocyanate toxicity but these are very unlikely when doses less than 3 μg/kg/min are administered for less than 3 days, except in patients with a serum creatinine greater than 3 mg/dL.[34]

Nitroglycerin.[27] Intravenous nitroglycerin is often considered the preferred agent for preload reduction in patients with severe heart failure. Because of its short half-life, IV nitroglycerin is administered by continuous infusion. Its major hemodynamic actions are reductions in preload and PAOP via functional venodilation, and mild arterial vasodilation which is particularly evident in patients with heart failure and elevated SVR, or when given in doses approaching 200 μg/min (Table 11–9). IV nitroglycerin is used primarily as a preload reducer for patients with pulmonary congestion and low-normal cardiac output, or in combination with inotropic agents for patients with severely depressed systolic function and pulmonary edema. Combination therapy with nitroglycerin and dobutamine or dopamine produces complementary effects to increase cardiac index and decrease PAOP. As indicated previously, excessive PAOP reduction should be avoided to prevent suboptimal ventricular filling pressure and maintain cardiac index while relieving symptoms of pulmonary congestion. In higher doses, nitroglycerin displays potent coronary vasodilating properties and overall beneficial effects on myocardial oxygen demand and supply, making it the vasodilator of choice for patients with severe heart failure and ischemic heart disease.

Nitroglycerin should be initiated at a dose of 5 to 10 μg/min (0.1 μg/kg/min) and increased every 5 to 10 minutes as necessary and tolerated. Hypotension and an excessive decrease in PAOP are important dose-limiting side effects. Maintenance doses usually vary from 35 to 200 μg/min (0.5 to 3.0 μg/kg/min), although doses over 1000 μg/min (15 μg /kg/min) have been used in rare cases. Tolerance to the hemodynamic effects of nitroglycerin develops in most patients over 12 to 72 hours of continuous administration,[35] but some patients have a sustained response.[36] The drug may inhibit the anticoagulant action of heparin, rarely results in methemoglobinemia, and can worsen shunt in patients with pulmonary vascular disease.[37] Neither nitroglycerin nor nitroprusside should be used in the presence of elevated intracranial pressure, as either may worsen cerebral edema in this setting.

Enalaprilat. Enalaprilat is the active diacid metabolite of enalapril. Like other ACE inhibitors, enalaprilat is a mixed arterial-venous vasodilator but generally has a quicker onset of action than oral drugs in this class. The hemodynamic response to bolus and continuous infusions of enalaprilat have been documented in several studies.[38] IV enalaprilat should be used mainly for the short-term management of relatively stable patients who cannot take oral medications or to initiate ACE inhibitor therapy later in a treatment course to facilitate weaning from nitroprusside or inodilator therapy. The usual dose is 1.25 to 2.5 mg every 6 to 8 hours.

Hydralazine. Although IV hydralazine is available, individual patient sensitivity to parenteral administration is highly variable. This results in a narrow and unpredictable toxic:therapeutic ratio. IV hydralazine should not be used in critically ill patients with heart failure.

DIURETICS

Intravenous loop diuretics, including furosemide, ethacrynic acid, bumetanide, and torsemide, are used in the management of acute/severe heart failure, with furosemide by far the most widely used and studied agent in this setting. Bolus administration of diuretics decreases preload by functional venodilation within 5 to 15 minutes, and later (> 20 min) via salt and water excretion,[39,40] thereby improving pulmonary congestion. However, the acute reduction in venous return may severely compromise effective preload in patients with significant diastolic dysfunction or intravascular depletion, resulting in a reflex increased sympathetic activation, renin release, NE and AVP elevations, and the expected consequences of arteriolar and coronary constriction, tachycardia, and increased PAOP and myocardial oxygen consumption.[40] Unlike arterial dilators and positive inotropic agents, diuretics do not cause an upward shift in the Starling curve or increase cardiac index significantly in most patients (Table 11–9). Excessive preload reduction with diuretics can lead to a decline in cardiac output (Fig. 11–3). Thus, diuretics must be used judiciously to obtain the desired improvement in symptoms of congestion while avoiding a reduction in cardiac output.

Diuretic Resistance

Occasionally, patients respond poorly to large doses of loop diuretics, and heart failure is the most common clinical setting in which diuretic resistance is observed.[41,42] The mechanisms responsible for diuretic resistance in heart failure patients appear to be both pharmacokinetic and pharmacodynamic in nature. Brater[42] showed that bioavailability of furosemide is normal in heart failure patients, but the rate of absorption is prolonged approximately twofold and peak concentrations are about half of normal. Because loop diuretics have a sigmoid-shaped urine concentration–response curve, prolonged absorption may result in concentrations that fail to reach the steep portion of this curve, resulting in diminished responsiveness. Thus, diuretic resistance with oral therapy might be overcome by IV administration or by giving larger oral doses.

In spite of normal pharmacokinetics following IV administration, diuretic resistance is also observed with this route, suggesting an important pharmacodynamic component to diuretic resistance. The decreased responsiveness in heart failure patients is explained in large part by the high concentrations of sodium reaching the distal tubule as a result of the blockade of sodium reabsorption in the loop of Henle. As a consequence, the distal tubule hypertrophies, increasing its ability to reabsorb sodium.[41,42]

Several maneuvers can be attempted to overcome diuretic resistance. Treatment of heart failure by other maneuvers (e.g., afterload reduction) may improve diuresis. Administration of low doses of dopamine with the hope of enhancing diuresis is also a common practice. However, recent data suggest addition of dopamine to furosemide provides no additional diuresis.[43] Larger IV bolus doses may achieve concentrations closer to the top of the concentration–response curve or a continuous IV infusion may be administered to maintain more constant concentrations in the steep portion of the concentration–response curve. Recent studies of continuous infusion furosemide suggest greater natriuretic effect and no difference in metabolic adverse effects when compared to the same total daily dose given by IV bolus.[44] Infusions may also limit adverse hemodynamic events.

Another approach to improving diuresis is addition of a second diuretic with a different mechanism of action. Combining a loop diuretic with distal tubule blocker (most commonly metolazone, a thiazide-type diuretic, or hydrochlorothiazide) produces a synergistic diuretic effect.[41,42] The synergism is not a pharmacokinetic interaction, but is related to the increased delivery of sodium to the distal convoluted tubule. Enhanced sodium delivery to (and reabsorption in) the distal tubule can then be blocked by the thiazide-type diuretic. Thus, when thiazide-type diuretics are added to a loop diuretic, they block more than their normal 5% to 8% of filtered sodium and the combination results in synergistic natriuresis.[41,42]

The loop diuretic–thiazide combination should generally be reserved for the inpatient setting where the patient can be closely monitored as it can induce a profound diuresis, with severe sodium, potassium, and volume depletion. When used in the outpatient setting, very low doses or only occasional doses of the thiazide-type diuretic should be used to avoid serious adverse events.

MECHANICAL CIRCULATORY SUPPORT

The intra-aortic balloon pump (IABP) is the most widely used form of mechanical circulatory assistance and is typically employed in patients with acute/severe heart failure who do not respond adequately to drug therapy, or who have intractable myocardial ischemia as part of their presentation. The IABP is placed percutaneously into the high descending thoracic aorta. During counterpulsation, the balloon inflates during diastole, displacing aortic blood and thereby increasing aortic diastolic pressure and coronary perfusion. It deflates just prior to aortic valve opening and causes a sudden decrease in aortic pressure, allowing the left ventricle to pump against a reduced arterial impedance. IABP support results in increased cardiac index and coronary perfusion wtih decreased myocardial oxygen demand,[45] and is particularly useful for patients with acute/severe heart failure in the setting of myocardial ischemia (evolving infarction, patients awaiting emergency coronary bypass surgery). It is also used as a bridge to cardiac transplantation.[45] IV vasodilators and inotropic agents are generally used in conjunction with the IABP to maximize hemodynamic and clinical benefits.

Several different ventricular assist devices and total artificial hearts are currently under investigation for the support of patients who cannot be sustained with pharmacologic therapy and IABP counterpulsation. These devices are approved for use as a temporary bridge to transplantation.[45] Investigators also continue to study the use of assist devices for long-term management in selected patients.

SURGICAL THERAPY

Orthotopic cardiac transplantation remains the best therapeutic option for patients with chronic irreversible NYHA Class IV heart failure, with a 5-year survival of approximately 75% in well-selected patients.[46] Unfortunately, the paucity of acceptable donor hearts has resulted in an average waiting time for transplant of more than 6 months, with only about one in five approved potential recipients receiving a heart before succumbing to their disease. Another large percentage of patients are rejected from consideration for transplant because of age, concurrent illnesses, psychosocial factors, and other reasons. The shortage of donor hearts has prompted development of new surgical techniques, including ventricular aneurysm resection, ventricular myoplasty, and latissimus dorsi wraps, which have shown variable degrees of symptomatic improvement.[47] Further development of these and other techniques may offer additional options in patients unable to receive transplantation. See Chap. 16 for additional details on cardiac transplantation.

EVALUATION OF THERAPEUTIC OUTCOMES

Assessment of adequacy of therapy in the critically ill heart failure patient can be separated into two general categories: initial improvement of physiologic parameters and safe discharge from the ICU following conversion to a chronic therapeutic regimen. Both goals must be achieved, because improvement of hemodynamics with IV medications and mechanical support is not per se correlated with prolonged symptom improvement or enhanced survival.

Initial stabilization requires achievement of adequate arterial oxygen saturation and content ($Sao_2 \geq 0.90$, $Cao_2 \geq 18$ mL/dL). Cardiac index and blood pressure must be sufficient to assure adequate organ perfusion, as assessed by alert mental status, creatinine clearance sufficient to prevent metabolic azotemic complications, hepatic function adequate to maintain synthetic and excretory functions, a stable heart rate (generally between 50 and 110 bpm) and rhythm (predominately sinus rhythm, rate-stabilized atrial fibrillation or flutter, or paced rhythm), absence of ongoing myocardial ischemia or infarction, skeletal muscle and skin blood flow sufficient to prevent ischemic injury, and normal arterial pH (7.34 to 7.47) with a normal serum lactate concentration. Although these goals are most often achieved with a cardiac index greater than 2.2 L/min/m^2, a mean arterial blood pressure greater than 60 mm Hg, and PAOP $\leq$ 25 mm Hg, the absolute values are highly variable and depend on chronicity of illness, efficacy of chronic compensatory mechanisms, previous chronic therapy, and concurrent illness.

Discharge from the intensive care unit requires maintenance of the above parameters in the absence of ongoing intravenous infusion therapy, mechanical circulatory support or positive pressure ventilation. Some patients may achieve this goal with markedly lower blood pressure or higher filling pressure than suggested above; hence, numerical goals cannot always be substituted for clinical status. Nonpharmacologic treatments aimed at the precipitants of a patient's heart failure exacerbation include permanent pacing, coronary angioplasty or valvuloplasty, pericardial drainage, cardiac surgery (coronary bypass, valve replacement or reconstruction, closure of intracardiac shunts), or even cardiac transplantation to achieve initial stabilization, definitive therapy, or both.

▶ TREATMENT: Chronic Heart Failure

DESIRED OUTCOME

The goals of therapy in management of chronic heart failure are to improve the patient's quality of life, reduce symptoms, reduce hospitalizations, slow progression of the disease process, and prolong survival. Drug therapies clearly proven to affect one or more of these goals of therapy include vasodilators (specifically ACE inhibitors and hydralazine/nitrate combination), diuretics, digoxin, and carvedilol. These therapies are described below under "Drug Treatments of First Choice." Alternative treatments which may positively impact the goals of therapy are also described and include antiarrhythmics, angiotensin II-receptor blockers, and the dihydropyridine calcium channel blockers amlodipine and felodipine. Somewhat unique to chronic heart failure therapy is the large number of drugs shown to be ineffective or detrimental. These will be described briefly as they provide insight into the pathophysiologic process in heart failure.

Clinical practice guidelines for management of heart failure have been published recently by three independent groups. Guidelines for management of left ventricular systolic dysfunction were published by the Agency for Health Care Policy and Research (AHCPR) through the U.S. Public Health Service in 1994.[48] Pharmacotherapy recommendations for systolic dysfunction represent only a small portion of the guidelines, which also provide extensive information on patient evaluation and assessment of left ventricular dysfunction, patient and family education and counseling, outcomes assessment, and the role of revascularization. In 1995 the American College of Cardiology and the American Heart Association published practice guidelines for the evaluation and management of heart failure.[19] These recommendations are more comprehensive than the AHCPR guidelines, covering both acute and chronic heart failure and systolic and diastolic dysfunction. The Canadian Cardiovascular Society's Consensus report is largely in agreement with the other publications, although less detailed.[49] In general the drug therapy recommendations from the different consensus statements are very similar. The discussions and recommendations in this chapter are based largely on these published guidelines, with incorporation of new, relevant clinical data published subsequent to the guidelines.

GENERAL APPROACH TO TREATMENT

The first step in management of chronic heart failure is to determine the etiology (Table 11–1) and/or precipitating factors (Table 11–3) of the syndrome. Treatment of underlying disorders such as anemia or hyperthyroidism may obviate the need for treatment of heart failure. Patients with valvular diseases may derive significant benefit from valve replacement or repair. Revascularization or anti-ischemic therapy in patients with coronary disease may reduce heart failure symptoms. Drugs that aggravate heart failure (Table 11–4) should be discontinued if possible.

Restriction of physical activity reduces cardiac workload and is recommended for virtually all patients with acute congestive symptoms. However, once the patient's symptoms have stabilized and excess fluid is removed, restrictions on physical activity are discouraged. In fact, recent data suggest low intensity exercise training programs in stable heart failure patients improve exercise tolerance and functional capacity.[50]

Because a major compensatory response in heart failure is sodium and water retention, restriction of dietary sodium is an important nonpharmacologic intervention. The typical American diet contains 3 to 6 g of sodium per day, which should be reduced by half (1.5 to 3 g of sodium per day). This can be accomplished by not adding salt to prepared foods and eliminating foods high in sodium (salt-cured meats, salted snack foods, pickles, soups, delicatessen meats). Further reductions in dietary sodium can be achieved by eliminating salt from cooking. However, this is not recommended for most heart failure patients because excessive sodium restriction produces an unpalatable diet which leads to poor dietary compliance and compromised nutritional status. Additionally, the availability of potent diuretics makes excessive sodium restriction unnecessary in most cases. Although dietary sodium restriction should be instituted in all heart failure patients, pharmacologic therapy is required for

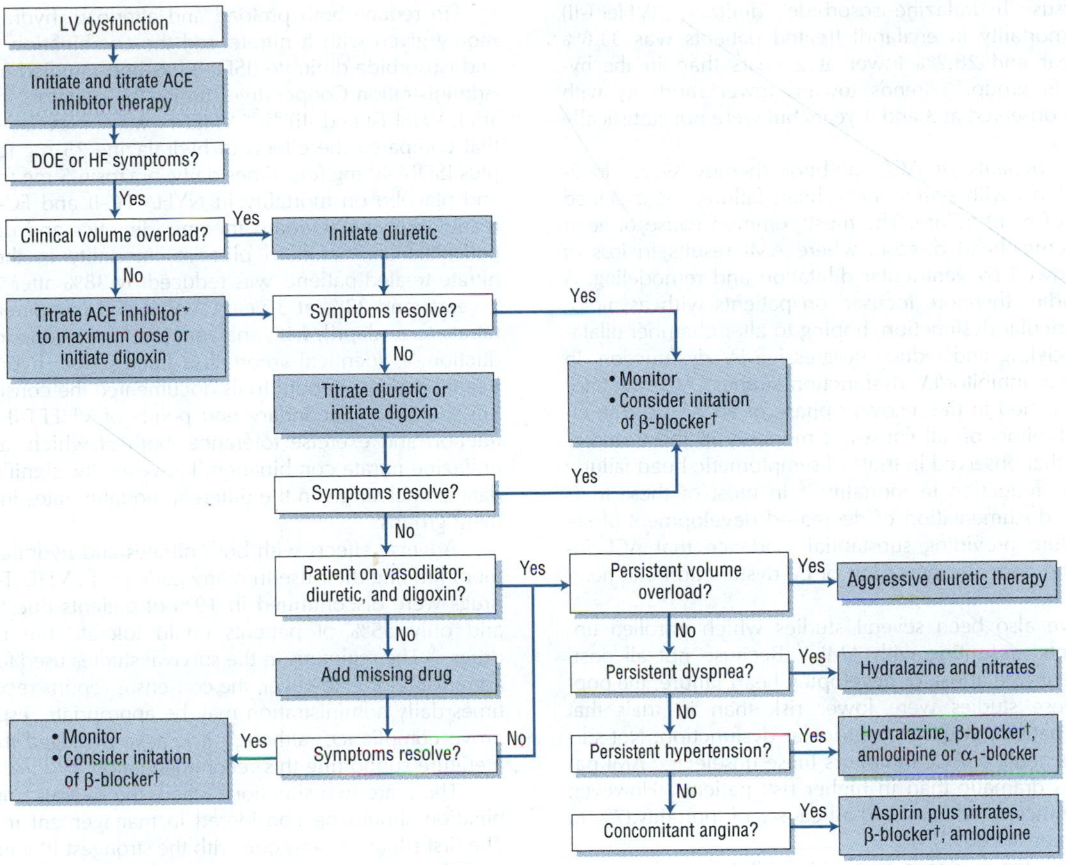

FIGURE 11–7. Treatment algorithm for patients with chronic heart failure. See text for details. Abbreviations: LV = left ventricular, ACE = angiotensin-converting enzyme, DOE = dyspnea on exertion, HF = heart failure. *If ACEI not started when LV dysfunction recognized, start now. If ACEI not started previously due to contraindication or patient intolerance, initiate hydralazine and nitrates now. †Initiation of β-blocker should be with appropriately low doses with slow, upward titration. *(Adapted from Ref. 43, with permission.)*

survival prolongation and is usually necessary for control of symptoms. A treatment algorithm for management of chronic heart failure is shown in Figure 11–7.

PHARMACOLOGIC THERAPY

DRUG TREATMENTS OF FIRST CHOICE

Vasodilators

The vasodilators represent a cornerstone of heart failure therapy, having been documented to positively impact all therapeutic goals in heart failure. All patients with symptomatic heart failure should be on either an ACE inhibitor or hydralazine/nitrate combination. The basis for this recommendation follows.

ACE Inhibitors. ACE inhibitors cause arterial and venous dilatation, reducing both preload and afterload. The vasodilation they produce appears to be due to both reduced activation of angiotensin II, a potent vasoconstrictor, and reduced breakdown of bradykinin, a vasodilator (see Fig. 11–2). Bradykinin, which is inactivated by ACE (identical to kininase II), also enhances release of vasodilatory prostaglandins and histamine. The contribution of antibradykinin effects to the efficacy of ACE inhibitors in heart failure is unknown, but will be clarified to some extent as angiotensin II receptor blockers (which lack bradykinin effects) are compared to ACE inhibitors in treatment of heart failure.

Numerous placebo-controlled trials have documented the favorable effects of ACE inhibitor therapy on hemodynamic variables, clinical status, and symptoms in heart failure.[51] Hemodynamic effects observed with long-term therapy include significant increases in cardiac index, stroke work index, and stroke volume index as well as significant reductions in left ventricular filling pressure, SVR, mean arterial pressure, and heart rate. Significant improvements in clinical status, functional class, exercise tolerance, and left ventricular size are also well documented. When compared with placebo, patients treated with ACE inhibitors have fewer treatment failures, fewer hospitalizations, fewer increases in diuretic dosages, and fewer ventricular premature beats on ambulatory ECG monitoring.[5,6,51] The acute response to ACE inhibitor therapy is greater in patients with high levels of plasma renin activity. However, long-term hemodynamic and clinical responses to ACE inhibition cannot be predicted from the plasma renin activity or from response to the initial dose of ACE inhibitor.

The beneficial effect of ACE inhibitors on mortality has been conclusively documented. Since the publication of the Cooperative North Scandinavian Enalapril Survival Study (CONSENSUS) in 1987,[5] over a dozen mortality trials have documented the survival benefit associated with ACE inhibitor therapy.[52] Early trials of patients with symptomatic heart failure showed enalapril therapy reduced mortality by 20% to 30%.[5,6] ACE inhibitors are clearly superior in mortality reduction to the other vasodilator regimen shown to reduce mortality in heart failure, specifically the hydralazine-nitrate combination.[53] A comparative trial of enalapril versus hydralazine-isosorbide dinitrate (VHeFT-II) showed that mortality in enalapril treated patients was 33.6% lower at 1 year and 28.2% lower at 2 years than in the hydralazine-nitrate group.[53] Trends toward lower mortality with enalapril were observed at 3 and 4 years but were not statistically significant.

Once the benefits of ACE inhibitor therapy were documented in patients with symptomatic heart failure, focus shifted to prevention of heart failure. The most common cause of heart failure is ischemic heart disease, where AMI results in loss of myocytes, followed by ventricular dilatation and remodeling. A number of studies therefore focused on patients with asymptomatic left ventricular dysfunction, hoping to alter chamber dilatation and remodeling and reduce progressive LV dysfunction. In most of the ACE inhibitor/LV dysfunction studies, ACE inhibitor therapy was initiated in the recovery phase of an AMI.[52] The effect of ACE inhibitors on all causes of mortality in these studies was similar to that observed in trials of symptomatic heart failure: a 20% to 30% reduction in mortality.[52] In most of these trials there was also documentation of decreased development of severe heart failure providing substantial evidence that ACE inhibitors alter the normal progression of LV dysfunction and heart failure.

There have also been several studies which enrolled unselected patients presenting with AMI.[52] Because not all post-infarction patients are at risk of developing heart failure, the populations in these studies were lower risk than in trials that included only patients with left ventricular dysfunction. Not surprisingly, the benefits of ACE inhibitors these unselected AMI patients were less dramatic than in higher risk patients. However, statistically significant reductions in all causes of mortality (7% to 11%) were demonstrated.

In summary, the evidence that ACE inhibitors slow disease progression and decrease mortality in heart failure is unequivocal. As such, all patients with documented left ventricular dysfunction, irrespective of symptomatology, should receive ACE inhibitors, unless there are contraindications or intolerance is present.[19]

The mechanisms by which ACE inhibitors slow disease progression and decrease mortality are not entirely clear. Substantial evidence suggests these effects are due in part to inhibition of angiotensin II's growth promoting effects on cardiac muscle and interstitium. Both clinical and animal studies provide compelling evidence that angiotensin II modulates LVH, dilatation, and remodeling.[9,52,54,55] Thus, ACE inhibitor therapy appears to play an important role in preventing angiotensin II-mediated progressive worsening of myocardial function. Whether the hemodynamic effects of ACE inhibitors also contribute to its effects on disease progression and mortality is unclear. Hydralazine/nitrates lack the effects of ACE inhibitors on LVH, yet have been shown to reduce mortality in heart failure. This would suggest that preload and afterload reduction contribute to some degree to the beneficial effects of ACE inhibitors on disease progression and mortality.

Nitrates and Hydralazine. Nitrates activate guanylate cyclase to increase cyclic guanosine monophosphate (cGMP) in vascular smooth muscle, with preferential vasodilatory effects in the venous bed.[26] The predominant hemodynamic effect of nitrates is preload reduction, although a mild reduction in SVR may be seen.

Hydralazine is a direct-acting vasodilator that acts predominantly on arterial smooth muscle.[26] It causes a significant reduction in SVR, increasing stroke volume and cardiac output (Fig. 11–1); its effects on preload are minimal. By reducing afterload, hydralazine theoretically interrupts the cycle of worsening heart failure.

To reduce both preload and afterload, hydralazine is commonly given with a nitrate and the combination of hydralazine and isosorbide dinitrate (ISDN) has been studied in two Veterans Administration Cooperative studies (Vasodilators in Heart Failure Trial, VHEFT-I and -II).[53,56] VHEFT-I was a placebo-controlled trial that compared the effects of hydralazine 75 mg four times daily plus ISDN 40 mg four times daily, prazosin 5 mg four times daily, and placebo on mortality in NYHA FC-II and FC-III patients already receiving standard therapy (diuretics and digoxin in most patients). Compared to placebo, mortality in the hydralazine/nitrate treated patients was reduced by 38% after 1 year, 25% at 2 years, and 23% at 3 years.[56] VHEFT-II compared hydralazine-nitrate to enalapril, with enalapril producing superior mortality reduction.[53] Identical mortality curves for hydralazine-nitrate treated patients in both trials documented the consistent effects of this therapy.[53] Secondary end points of VHEFT-II were ejection fraction and exercise tolerance, both of which favored the hydralazine-nitrate combination. However, the significance of these data is unclear given the different mortality rates in the two treatment groups.

Adverse effects with both nitrates and hydralazine are common, limiting their use in many patients. In VHEFT-I, one or both drugs were discontinued in 19% of patients due to side effects, and only 55% of patients could tolerate full doses of both drugs.[56] The regimens in the survival studies used four times daily administration. However, the consensus reports recommend three times daily administration may be appropriate, especially to improve compliance, although it is acknowledged that there is no literature supporting this recommendation.[19,48]

There are two situations where the hydralazine-nitrate combination should be considered in management in heart failure. The first situation, and one with the strongest literature support, is in patients with symptomatic heart failure who are unable to take ACE inhibitors. The other setting is in patients who remain symptomatic on optimal dose ACE inhibitor therapy.[19,48]

Summary. Vasodilators represent the cornerstone of therapy in patients with symptomatic heart failure, and all such patients should be treated with a vasodilator. ACE inhibitors are clearly the vasodilator of choice, with hydralazine-nitrates substituted when ACE inhibitors cannot be given. This therapy will provide significant symptomatic benefits, slow disease progression, and decrease mortality. Patients with asymptomatic left ventricular dysfunction should also be treated with ACE inhibitors to prevent symptomatic heart failure and reduce mortality.

Diuretics

The compensatory mechanisms in heart failure stimulate excessive sodium and water retention, often leading to signs and symptoms of systemic and pulmonary congestion. Consequently, diuretic therapy is recommended for all patients with clinical evidence of fluid retention.[19,48] Although a majority of heart failure patients require chronic diuretic therapy, some may be well controlled without them. Therefore, diuretic therapy is a common component of a heart failure pharmacologic regimen, but should not be viewed as mandatory. The primary goal of diuretic therapy is to decrease edema and pulmonary congestion by reduction of preload. Although preload is a determinant of cardiac output, the Frank-Starling curve (Fig. 11–3) shows that patients with congestive symptoms have reached the flat portion of the curve. A reduction in filling pressure improves symptoms but has little effect on the patient's stroke volume or cardiac output until the steep portion of the curve is reached. Once diuretic therapy is initiated, dosage adjustments are based on symptomatic improvement and daily body weight. Change in body weight is a sensitive marker of fluid retention or loss.

Thiazide Diuretics. Thiazide diuretics such as hydrochlorothiazide block sodium and chloride reabsorption in the distal convoluted tubule (approximately 5% to 8% of filtered sodium).[41] The thiazides are therefore relatively weak diuretics and are used infrequently in heart failure.

Loop Diuretics. Loop diuretics are the most widely used diuretics in heart failure. Loop diuretics such as furosemide and bumetanide act in the thick ascending limb of the loop of Henle, where 20% to 25% of filtered sodium is normally reabsorbed.[41] Because loop diuretics are highly bound to plasma proteins, they are not highly filtered at the glomerulus. They reach the tubular lumen by active transport via the organic acid transport pathway. Competitors for this pathway (probenecid or organic byproducts of uremia) can inhibit delivery of loop diuretics to their site of action and decrease effectiveness. Loop diuretics also induce a prostaglandin-mediated increase in renal blood flow, which contributes to their natriuretic effect. Coadministration of nonsteroidal anti-inflammatory drugs (NSAIDs) blocks this prostaglandin-mediated effect and can diminish diuretic efficacy.[42] Unlike thiazides, loop diuretics maintain their effectiveness in the presence of impaired renal function although higher doses are often necessary. The appropriate dose is that which maintains the patient at a stable weight. For furosemide this will typically range from 40 to 240 mg/d given once or twice daily.

Diuretic-induced Hypokalemia in Heart Failure. Diuretics cause a variety of metabolic abnormalities with the severity related to the potency of the diuretic. The reader is referred to Chap. 10 for a detailed discussion on the adverse effects of diuretic therapy.

The most common metabolic disturbance associated with both thiazide and loop diuretics is hypokalemia, which in heart failure patients may be exacerbated by hyperaldosteronism. Hypokalemia is especially worrisome in this setting as it can precipitate ventricular arrhythmias, a common mode of death in CHF. Digitalis-associated arrhythmias are also more common with concurrent hypokalemia. Concomitant ACE inhibitor therapy may help minimize diuretic-induced hypokalemia because these drugs tend to increase serum potassium through their effects on aldosterone. Nonetheless, serum potassium should be monitored closely in heart failure patients, and supplemented appropriately when needed, either with potassium replacement or use of a potassium sparing diuretic.

Digitalis Glycosides

In 1785, William Withering was the first to report extensively on the use of foxglove or *Digitalis purpurea* for the treatment of dropsy (i.e., edema). Although digitalis glycosides have been in clinical use for more than 200 years, not until the 1920s were they clearly demonstrated to have a positive inotropic effect on the heart.[22,51] Furthermore, it was not until the late 1980s that clinical trials were conducted to critically evaluate the role of digoxin in the therapy of chronic heart failure. The recently published results of the Digitalis Investigation Group (DIG) trial helped clarify the role of digoxin in this setting.[58] The following discussion focuses on digoxin because it is by far the most widely studied and frequently prescribed digitalis glycoside in the United States.

Clinical Efficacy and Role in Therapy. The efficacy of digoxin in patients with heart failure and supraventricular tachyarrhythmias such as atrial fibrillation is well established and widely accepted.[51] Its role in heart failure patients with normal sinus rhythm has been considerably more controversial. Until the 1980s, most data supporting efficacy of digoxin in these patients came from anecdotal evidence and seriously flawed or uncontrolled studies. Since then, a number of clinical trials have shown that digoxin improves left ventricular ejection fraction, quality of life, exercise tolerance, and heart failure symptoms.[59–61] However, these studies involved small numbers of patients followed for short time periods with many of the patients being withdrawn from preexisting digoxin treatment upon entering the trial.[60,61] In these withdrawal studies, the observed beneficial effects of digoxin could be due to the poor response to abrupt discontinuation of the drug in patients receiving placebo. Although these trials demonstrated hemodynamic and symptomatic improvement in heart failure patients receiving digoxin, a more important question was the unknown effect of digoxin on mortality. This was of particular concern given the increased mortality seen with other positive inotropic drugs and finally led to organization and performance of the DIG trial to determine the effects of digoxin on survival in patients with heart failure and sinus rhythm.[58]

The DIG trial was a double-blind, randomized, placebo-controlled trial with the primary end point of all-cause mortality. Patients (n = 6800) with heart failure symptoms and a left ventricular ejection fraction of ≤ 0.45 were eligible and were followed for a mean of 37 months. Approximately 85% of patients were in NYHA functional class II or III and ischemic cardiomyopathy was the primary cause of heart failure in 70% of patients. Most patients received background therapy with diuretics and ACE inhibitors. The mean serum digoxin concentration achieved was 0.80 ng/mL after 12 months of therapy. No significant difference in all cause mortality was found between patients receiving digoxin and placebo (34.8% and 35.1%, respectively). A trend toward lower mortality due to worsening heart failure was observed in the digoxin group, although this was offset by a trend toward an increased mortality from other cardiovascular causes (presumably arrhythmias) in patients receiving digoxin. Hospitalizations for worsening heart failure were reduced 28% by digoxin compared to placebo ($P < .001$) while hospitalizations for other cardiovascular causes was increased in the digoxin group. In all, 64.3% of digoxin treated patients were hospitalized compared to 67.1% of patients receiving placebo ($P = .006$). Therefore, DIG is the first trial to show that a positive inotropic agent does not increase mortality in patients with heart failure. Although these results also suggest that digoxin should be routinely used because it reduces hospitalizations for progressive heart failure, it is important to keep in mind that hospitalizations for presumed arrhythmia increased. Therefore, there was little difference in overall hospitalization rates between the groups (absolute difference of 2.8%). Given the subjectivity associated with classifying the reason for hospital admission, the important end point should be a reduction in the total number of hospital admissions, regardless of cause. A mere shifting of the admitting diagnosis, with little difference in the overall number of hospitalizations, is insufficient justification for routine use of the drug.

Digoxin's place in the pharmacotherapy of chronic heart failure can therefore be summarized for two patient groups. In patients with left ventricular systolic dysfunction and supraventricular tachyarrhythmias such as atrial fibrillation, it should be considered early in therapy to help control ventricular response rate. For patients in normal sinus rhythm, digoxin is not first line therapy because it does not improve survival. Its positive inotropic effects, symptom reduction, and quality of life improvement may be most evident in patients with moderate-to-severe left ventricular systolic function. Thus, digoxin is indicated for patients in sinus rhythm who remain symptomatic after optimization of therapies known to improve survival.

The appropriate dose or target plasma concentration for digoxin remains unclear. Little information is available on the relationship between digoxin plasma concentration and either the drug's neurohormonal or positive inotropic effects. Two recent studies evaluated the dose response to digoxin in heart failure patients receiving ACE inhibitors and diuretics.[62,63] One reported that an increase in the digoxin plasma concentration from a mean of 0.67 to 1.22 ng/mL resulted in a minor increase in left ventricular ejection fraction (23.7% to 27.1%), but no improvement in symptoms, exercise tolerance, or neurohormone levels.[62] The other study found that an increase in digoxin plasma concentration from 0.8 to 1.5 ng/mL produced no additional effect on ejection fraction and likewise did not improve other hemodynamic variables or indices of neurohormonal function.[63]

These results suggest most of the benefit from digoxin is achieved at low plasma concentrations and little additional effect is achieved with higher doses. Thus, for most patients, the target digoxin plasma concentration should be ~ 1.0 ng/mL. This more conservative target would also be expected to decrease the risk of adverse effects. An ongoing subgroup analysis of the DIG study, evaluating the relationship between digoxin plasma concentration and sudden death, should provide additional information on the proper target digoxin plasma concentration. Most patients can achieve 1.0 ng/mL with 0.125 to 0.25 mg/d digoxin, although lower doses may be necessary in patients with significant renal impairment. Several equations and nomograms have been proposed to estimate digoxin maintenance doses based on estimated renal function for a particular patient and population pharmacokinetic parameters. These methods are extensively reviewed elsewhere.[64] In the absence of tachyarrhythmias, a loading dose is not indicated because digoxin is a mild inotropic agent that will produce gradual effects over several hours, even after loading.

β-Blockers

It may seem paradoxical that, within this chapter, β-blockers are listed as drugs that may exacerbate or worsen heart failure (Table 11–4) and as first-line therapy for management of chronic heart failure, but both are true. Administration of normal doses of β-blockers to patients with heart failure can lead to symptomatic worsening or decompensation. However, there is mounting clinical evidence that if stable patients are initiated on low doses of a β-blocker with upward dose titration over several weeks, they may derive significant benefits.[65,66] As of 1997, over 3000 heart failure patients had been studied in 24 randomized, controlled clinical trials of β-blockers.[65] Although many different agents have been studied (including acebutolol, bucindolol, bisoprolol, carvedilol, labetalol, metoprolol, and nebivolol), over half the patients were enrolled in studies of carvedilol, the first β-blocker approved by the Food and Drug Administration to treat heart failure. Carvedilol is indicated in patients with NYHA-FC II or III heart failure, added to standard heart failure therapy, to reduce the progression of disease and thus affect cardiovascular death, hospitalizations, and need for upward titration of other heart failure medications.

The effects of β-blockers in heart failure have been assessed using several end points. Following several weeks of therapy, β-blockers have been consistently documented to increase ejection fraction (EF) by 5 to 10 units (e.g., from an EF of 20% to 25% or 30%).[65,67] These hemodynamic changes have not consistently translated into improved exercise tolerance as assessed by standardized protocols such as treadmill exercise, but β-blockers also did not impair exercise tolerance, as might be predicted.[65,67] Global assessments by patients or physicians have more consistently suggested symptomatic improvement with β-blocker therapy. Additionally, β-blockers have positive benefits on the markers of progression of heart failure, such as decreasing hospitalizations, need for increased heart failure medications, and heart transplantation.[65,67]

Of final consideration is the effect of β-blockers on mortality. The strongest mortality data come from four carvedilol treatment protocols that included mortality assessment as a safety measure, and from the Cardiac Insufficiency Bisoprolol Study II (CIBIS II). The carvedilol studies were halted prematurely by the Data Safety Monitoring Board due to a marked (67%) decrease in mortality in the carvedilol groups.[68] Although this mortality reduction is clearly impressive, these data were not considered definitive evidence that carvedilol, or β-blockers in general, reduce mortality in heart failure. The reasons are that the data come from several studies, none of which was designed to assess mortality; the duration of follow-up was only 6 months, and the actual number of deaths was relatively small. The CIBIS II study was the first β-blocker in heart failure study designed with mortality as a primary end point.[68a] In this study, the β_1-selective blocker bisoprolol was compared to placebo in 2647 patients with ejection fraction < 35% and NYHA-FC III or IV heart failure. The trial was halted prematurely due to decreased mortality associated with bisoprolol. Based on preliminary reports of the study, bisoprolol produced a 32% relative reduction of all-cause mortality compared to placebo (11.8% vs. 17.3% respectively).[68b] All-cause hospital admission rates were also significantly lower in the bisoprolol group (33.6% vs. 39.8%). These data provide the most convincing evidence of the mortality benefits of β-blocker therapy in heart failure. They are also very consistent with two different meta-analyses (performed prior to the CIBIS II study) which both estimated an overall 31% reduction in mortality associated with β-blocker therapy.[66,68]

The CIBIS II study also helps clarify questions about the role of ancillary properties of β-blockers and benefit in heart failure. Prior to announcement of the CIBIS II results, the β-blocker with the strongest data in heart failure was carvedilol, a nonselective β-blocker with α_1-receptor blockade and mild antioxidant effects. This raised questions about whether the ancillary properties of carvedilol contributed to its benefit in heart failure. Data from the meta-analyses also suggested that β-blockers wtih the ancillary property of vasodilation may provide greater benefits in heart failure.[66,69] However, CIBIS II data would suggest the ancillary properties of β-blockers are unimportant since bisoprolol is a β_1-selective blocker with no ancillary properties. Thus, it seems likely that all β-blockers (except those with intrinsic sympathomimetic activity) would likely be beneficial in heart failure.

One of the keys to successful use of β-blockers in heart failure is initiation of therapy at very low doses, with slow upward titration. In general, initial doses are 1/10 to 1/20 that of the target dose, with doubling of the dose every 1 to 2 weeks until the target dose is reached or further dose titrations cannot be tolerated.[70] For carvedilol, the recommended initial dose is 3.125 mg twice daily, with doubling of the dose every 2 weeks to the highest level tolerated or a target dose of 25 mg twice daily for those weighing up to 85 kg or 50 mg twice daily if over 85 kg.

A number of potential mechanisms have been suggested to explain the beneficial effects of β-blockers in heart failure patients. These include: blockade of the detrimental effects of sympathetic stimulation, decreased sympathetic stimulation due to decreased plasma NE, and antiarrhythmic actions.[65] β-blockers may also improve diastolic dysfunction by prolonging diastolic filling time. It is not clear if one or many of these mechanisms is responsible for the observed clinical improvements.

In summary, data suggest β-blockers slow the progression of heart failure, and reduce hospitalizations, the need for adjustments of other heart failure medications and heart transplantation, and mortality. Although they have not typically improved exercise performance or formal quality of life assessments, patients and their physicians often rate β-blockers as beneficial in global assessments. The available data on β-blockers appear stronger than those for digoxin or hydralazine-nitrate, thus qualifying β-blockers (specifically carvedilol) as first-line therapy for heart failure. However, it may require positive results from the ongoing mortality trials for β-blockers to be widely embraced as first-line therapy for heart failure. Nonetheless, the current data suggest that β-blockers should be strongly considered in patients with symptomatic heart failure with the primary goal of therapy being slowed disease progression.

ALTERNATIVE DRUG TREATMENTS

Angiotensin II Receptor Antagonists

ACE inhibitors decrease the synthesis of angiotensin II and reduce bradykinin breakdown. However, angiotensin II can be formed in a number of tissues, including the heart, through non-ACE–dependent pathways.[71,72] Therefore, blockade of the detrimental effects of angiotensin II by ACE inhibition is incomplete. The angiotension II receptor antagonists losartan and valsartan and irbesartan block the angiotensin II receptor subtype, AT_1, preventing the effects of angiotensin II, regardless of its origin. Thus, these agents offer a theoretical advantage for the treatment of heart failure over ACE inhibitors by more complete block of the effects of angiotensin II. Whether AT_1 receptor antagonists are superior to ACE inhibitors or if more complete blockade of angiotensin II actions with combination therapy could further decrease morbidity and mortality are presently unknown.

Although the AT_1 antagonists are only approved for the treatment of hypertension, there is much interest in their use in heart failure. A recent short-term study comparing losartan to enalapril in patients with heart failure indicates that these agents produce similar hemodynamic effects.[73] The effects of losartan and captopril in 722 patients with NYHA class II to IV heart failure were compared in the Evaluation of Losartan in the Elderly (ELITE) study.[74] The primary end point of this trial, frequency of elevations in serum creatinine, was not different between the two groups. The secondary end point, all-cause mortality, was significantly reduced (P = .035) in patients receiving losartan compared to captopril (8.7% versus 4.8%, respectively; risk reduction, 46%). However, these mortality results should be interpreted cautiously as they were based on only 49 total deaths (17 in losartan and 32 in captopril treated patients). Losartan was generally better tolerated than captopril with no losartan treated patients experiencing cough or angioedema. The results of the prospective mortality trial (ELITE-II) are needed before angiotension II blockers can be considered first-line therapy in heart failure. Until then, these agents may be most useful in patients intolerant to ACE inhibitors due to severe cough or those with persistent heart failure symptoms and/or hypertension despite maximal ACE inhibitor doses.

Antiarrhythmic Therapy

Sudden cardiac death, presumably due to ventricular arrhythmias, kills up to 50% of heart failure patients.[4–6] The value of antiarrhythmic therapy in reducing heart failure mortality is therefore of interest. Based on data from the Cardiac Arrhythmia Suppression Trials (CAST),[75,76] class I antiarrhythmics should be avoided in all patients with coronary disease and/or left ventricular dysfunction. Recent attention has therefore focused on alternative therapies, namely class III antiarrhythmic drugs and implantable cardioverter defibrillators (ICD).

Amiodarone is a class III antiarrhythmic drug with many pharmacologic effects that may contribute to its antiarrhythmic actions, including noncompetitive block of both α- and β-adrenergic receptors, inhibition of L-type calcium channels, and interference with thyroid metabolism. Several studies with amiodarone in patients with heart failure have yielded conflicting results. The GESICA study randomized 516 patients with moderate to severe heart failure to amiodarone 300 mg/d or placebo and found that amiodarone reduced total mortality by 28%.[77] In contrast, the CHF-STAT trial found that amiodarone had no effect on total mortality in 674 patients with ejection fractions of 40% or lower.[78] Subgroup analysis showed a trend (P = .07) toward improved survival in amiodarone treated patients with nonischemic cardiomyopathy, but not in those with ischemic cardiomyopathy.

Similar to the results of CHF-STAT, the EMIAT trial found that amiodarone had no effect on total mortality compared to placebo in patients within 5 to 21 days of an MI and an ejection fraction of 40% or lower.[79] The reason for the conflicting results is unclear but may be related to differences in heart failure etiologies (ischemic versus nonischemic) in the trials. If amiodarone is more effective in nonischemic than ischemic cardiomyopathy, as suggested by CHF-STAT, the greater percentage of patients with nonischemic cardiomyopathy in GESICA may account for this difference. Also, patients in GESICA had more severe heart failure (lower mean ejection fraction on trial entry) and were older, suggesting amiodarone may be of greatest benefit in the sickest patients. This concept is supported by a retrospective analysis of the GESICA results showing that amiodarone improved survival only in patients with baseline heart rates of at least 90 bpm.[80] Because heart rate correlates with disease severity, the mean baseline heart rate of 90 bpm in GESICA compared to 80 bpm in CHF-STAT may account for the disparate results. In contrast to other antiarrhythmic drugs, amiodarone does not appear to increase mortality, making it the first-line agent when antiarrhythmic therapy is needed (e.g., maintenance of sinus rhythm in heart failure patients with atrial fibrillation). However, the lack of proven benefit on survival and the potential for serious adverse effects argues against its routine use in this population.

The frequency and severity of adverse effects with amiodarone fostered interest in sotalol for heart failure patients. Sotalol has class III antiarrhythmic activity and blocks β-adrenergic receptors. The drug is marketed as a mixture of the *d* and *l* isomers with the *d* isomer lacking clinically significant β-blocking actions. Thus, *d*-sotalol would be expected to be well tolerated in heart failure patients and served as the basis for the Survival with Oral *d*-Sotalol (SWORD) trial that randomly assigned post-MI patients with an ejection fraction of 40% or less to receive either *d*-sotalol or placebo.[81] This trial was terminated early because of increased mortality in the active treatment group (relative risk, 1.65; P = .006). Thus, antiarrhythmic agents with pure class III effects do not appear to be effective in patients with heart failure.

Initial reports with ICD implantation in patients with left ventricular dysfunction suggested the device markedly reduced the rate of sudden cardiac death, but did not improve total mortality. The Multicenter Automatic Defibrillator Implantation Trial (MADIT) randomized post-MI patients with ejection fractions of 35% or lower, no history of spontaneous sustained ventricular tachycardia (VT) or ventricular fibrillation (VF), and inducible sustained VT on electrophysiologic study that was not suppressed by IV procainamide to ICD implantation or conventional medical therapy.[82] The trial was stopped early because of a 54% reduction in total mortality in the ICD group. These results led the FDA to approve the ICD for use in this high-risk population; however, these findings should be confirmed in other ongoing trials before the ICD is widely used in this setting. Clinically, prophylactic use of the ICD may be considered in post-MI heart failure patients who are unable to tolerate β-blockers or ACE inhibitors. In heart failure patients that have experienced an episode of sustained VT/VF, the ICD may be preferred over drug therapy. The Antiarrhythmics versus Implantable Defibrillator (AVID) trial randomized patients with an ejection fraction of 40% or less experiencing sustained VT/VF to ICD implantation or drug therapy with amiodarone or sotalol. Although the results have not been published yet, the study was stopped early because of a 38% reduction in 1 year mortality in patients receiving the ICD compared to the drug therapy group.[83] Publication and review of the results of this trial are needed, however, to establish the ICD as first-line therapy in heart failure patients with VT/VF.

Amlodipine/Felodipine

A number of previous studies demonstrate that calcium channel blockers worsen heart failure and increase mortality, most likely due to their negative inotropic effects and SNS activation.[84,85] However, the second-generation dihydropyridine agents, amlodipine and felodipine, offer theoretical advantages over other calcium antagonists for the treatment of heart failure including more vascular selectivity, weak negative inotropic effects, lack of SNS activation, and minimal reflex tachycardia. These potential advantages led to their investigation in patients with heart failure. The VHeFT-III trial compared felodipine to placebo in 450 male patients with NYHA class II to III heart failure receiving concurrent treatment with ACE inhibitors and diuretics.[86] Although felodipine improved ejection fraction in the short term, there was no improvement in exercise capacity, quality of life, or survival, although the study was not powered to detect mortality differences. No differences in outcome based on heart failure etiology (ischemic versus nonischemic) were noted. Disturbingly, a trend toward increased hospitalizations and worsening heart failure was observed during the first 3 months of felodipine therapy. The PRAISE trial randomized 1153 patients with NYHA class III to IV heart failure treated with ACE inhibitors, diuretics, and digoxin to amlodipine 10 mg/d or placebo.[87] The randomization was stratified by heart failure etiology (ischemic versus nonischemic). Amlodipine had no significant effect on the primary (combined risk of all-cause mortality plus cardiovascular morbidity) or secondary end points (all-cause mortality). Amlodipine had no significant effect on either end point in patients with ischemic cardiomyopathy. However, in patients with nonischemic cardiomyopathy, amlodipine reduced the primary end point by 31% ($P = .04$) and the secondary end point by 46% ($P < .001$). These results suggest that amlodipine can be safely administered to heart failure patients, making it the agent of choice in patients with another indication for calcium channel blocker therapy (hypertension or angina). However, current data fail to support its routine use specifically to treat heart failure. The effects of amlodipine in nonischemic cardiomyopathy are being further investigated in the PRAISE-2 trial.

Therapies Proven to Be Ineffective or Detrimental

Clinical trials of therapeutic modalities for the management of heart failure have revealed drugs that improve symptoms and decrease mortality. Clinical trials have also proven a number of drugs to be ineffective or to increase mortality in heart failure. Most of these drugs never received FDA approval and therefore are not available for clinical use. Nonetheless, an understanding of the types of drugs that increase mortality provides insight into pathophysiologic processes in heart failure.

Ineffective/Detrimental Vasodilators. Prazosin is an α_1-adrenergic receptor antagonist that causes both arterial and venous dilation. It is not indicated for heart failure because long-term prazosin therapy in VHeFT-I failed to produce sustained hemodynamic effects or impact mortality.[56]

Calcium channel blockers cause direct vasodilation in arterial resistance vessels, but are also associated with varying degrees of direct negative inotropic activity. Like many other vasodilators, their short-term hemodynamic effects did not translate into long-term symptomatic benefits. In fact, clinical trial data suggest chronic calcium channel blocker therapy (with nifedipine or diltiazem) may be harmful in heart failure patients, potentially increasing their risk of cardiac events (e.g., death or MI) and worsened heart failure.[81,85] As described, newer dihydropyridine calcium channel blockers (felodipine and amlodipine) may be safe to use in these patients when another indication for calcium channel blocker therapy exists, but none are currently recommended as a treatment modality for heart failure.

Drugs That Increase Mortality in Heart Failure. Reduced contractility is the underlying pathophysiology for many patients with heart failure. This fact, coupled with the dramatic hemodynamic improvements produced by β-agonists and phosphodiesterase inhibitors in acute heart failure, stimulated research with these agents for management of chronic heart failure. These drug classes are similar in that they act to increase intracellular levels of the second messenger cAMP, although by different mechanisms. Despite theoretical benefits of these agents in treatment of heart failure, studies have consistently shown that they increase mortality.

Phosphodiesterase inhibitors shown to increase mortality in heart failure when used chronically include amrinone, milrinone, enoximone, and vesnarinone.[88] Studies of chronic β-agonist therapy (or adrenergic agonist therapy) have resulted in similarly disappointing results. Xamoterol, dobutamine, and ibopamine have also been shown to increase mortality when used as chronic heart failure therapies.[88] The magnitude of detrimental effect of β-agonists and phosphodiesterase inhibitors was estimated in a meta-analysis of β-agonists and phosphodiesterase III inhibitors,[89] although this meta-analysis was performed prior to publication of the milrinone, vesnarinone, and ibopamine data. The authors reviewed 21 randomized, placebo-controlled trials involving a total of 1124 patients in phosphodiesterase inhibitor studies and 1234 patients in β-agonist studies. The analysis revealed an overall 58% increase in mortality with phosphodiesterase inhibitors and a greater than two-fold increase in mortality with β-agonists. Although increasing myocardial contractility in patients with heart failure seems theoretically sound, the clinical trials suggest that doing so by increasing intracellular AMP decreases patient survival.

Other therapies shown to increase mortality in chronic heart failure are flosequinan and prostacyclin.[86] Although both therapies produced vasodilation by mechanisms independent of the adrenergic system, both were associated with increases in heart rate, suggesting that the drugs caused SNS activation. Data from studies on the numerous drugs described above all suggest that long-term stimulation of the SNS in patients with chronic heart failure is detrimental.

DRUG CLASS INFORMATION

ACE Inhibitors

A number of ACE inhibitors are currently available in the United States; those approved for use in heart failure in the United States are summarized in Table 11–10. The major differences in the ACE inhibitors are not in their pharmacologic properties but their pharmacokinetic properties. Although it appears that mortality reduction with ACE inhibitors is probably a drug class effect, not all ACE inhibitors approved by the FDA for treatment of heart failure have been tested for their effects on mortality in heart failure. Thus it seems most prudent to use clinically those ACE inhibitors that have been documented to prolong survival, because the dose required for this effect has been documented. Table 11–10 also contains a summary of the target doses for survival benefit.

There is some evidence that coadministration of aspirin with an ACE inhibitor may negatively impact both the hemodynamic and survival benefits of ACE inhibitors.[90,91] However, the data in

TABLE 11–10. ACE Inhibitors Approved for Use in Heart Failure

Generic Name	Brand Name	Usual Daily Dose (mg)	Dosing Frequency	Target Dosing—Survival Benefit	Prodrug	Elimination[b]	$t_{1/2}$ (h)
Captopril	Capoten	18.75–150	tid	50 mg tid	No	Renal	2
Enalapril	Vasotec	2.5–400	bid	10 mg bid	Yes	Renal	10[c]
Lisinopril	Zestril Prinivil	5–400	qd	10 mg qd	No	Renal	12[c]
Quinapril	Accupril	5–800	bid	No data	Yes	Renal	25[c]
Ramipril	Altace	1.25–200	qd or bid	5 mg bid	Yes	Renal	9–18[c]

Abbreviations: tid = three times daily, bid = twice daily, qd = once daily.
[a]Target doses associated with survival benefits in clinical trials.
[b]Primary route of elimination.
[c]Half-life of active metabolite.

this area are sparse, thus the true impact of aspirin on efficacy of ACE inhibitors is unclear. At present it seems logical to avoid use of aspirin in heart failure patients when possible, but there is no compelling evidence to support withholding aspirin in patients with heart failure and a clear indication for aspirin, such as ischemic heart disease.

Adverse Effects of ACE Inhibitors. The primary adverse effects of ACE inhibitor therapy in heart failure are hypotension and functional renal insufficiency. Hypotension may be manifested as dizziness, lightheadedness, presyncope, or syncope. It occurs most commonly with the first dose, although it may occur at any time during therapy.[5] Patients at increased risk of developing hypotension are those with hyponatremia (serum sodium < 130 mEq/L), and recent increases in diuretic dose. The occurrence of hypotension may be minimized by initiating therapy with lower ACE inhibitor doses and/or temporarily withholding or reducing the dose of diuretic.

Functional renal insufficiency is manifested as increases in serum creatinine and blood urea nitrogen. As cardiac output and renal blood flow decline, renal perfusion is maintained by the vasoconstrictor effect of angiotensin II on the efferent arteriole. Patients most dependent on this system for maintenance of renal perfusion (and therefore most likely to develop functional renal insufficiency with ACE inhibitors) are those with severe heart failure, hyponatremia, and dehydration.[5] Sodium depletion (usually secondary to diuretic therapy) is the most important factor in the development of functional renal insufficiency with ACE inhibitor therapy. Renal insufficiency can therefore be minimized in many cases by reduction in diuretic dosage or liberalization of sodium intake.

Careful dose titration can minimize the risks of hypotension and transient worsening of renal function. Thus, usual initial doses should be about one-fourth the final target dose with slow upward dose titration over several days, based on blood pressure and serum creatinine. In certain patients, especially those hospitalized patients who seem at high risk for hypotension or worsening of renal function, it may also be advisable to initiate therapy with a short-acting agent like captopril. This will help minimize the duration of adverse effects should they occur. Once the patient is stabilized on ACE inhibitor therapy with captopril, they can then be switched to a longer half-life drug.

Retention of potassium with ACE inhibitor therapy is common and is due to the reduced feedback of angiotensin II to stimulate aldosterone release. Hyperkalemia rarely develops, although caution is necessary in patients with renal insufficiency and in patients taking concomitant potassium supplementation, potassium containing salt substitutes, or potassium-sparing diuretic therapy.[5,51]

Rash and dysgeusia are troublesome side effects of ACE inhibitor therapy which appear to be more common with high doses; the rash may resolve with continued therapy. A dry, hacking cough occurs with a similar frequency with all the agents and may be related to accumulation of tissue bradykinins. Cough occurs in up to 40% of patients with heart failure, independent of ACE inhibitor use, although ACE inhibitors significantly increase its incidence. However, in large clinical trials, only about 1% of participants discontinued ACE inhibitor therapy because of cough. Because cough is a bradykinin mediated effect, replacement of ACE inhibitor therapy with an AT_1-receptor blocker would be reasonable in those patients who discontinue ACE inhibitor therapy due to cough.

Nitrates

The nitrate product most extensively studied in the treatment of chronic CHF is ISDN, although all oral nitroglycerin products are probably equally effective. Recommended doses of ISDN range from 20 to 80 mg every 6 hours and the mortality trials administered 40 mg every 6 hours.[53,56]

Tolerance to the effects of nitrates is seen during both heart failure and antianginal therapy. Intravenous and transdermal nitroglycerin administration result in relatively constant plasma concentrations and tolerance can occur with these routes of administration.[35,36] However, the literature is not highly suggestive of tolerance to chronic ISDN in heart failure. Large clinical trials with ISDN in patients with heart failure have used every-6-hour administration and have shown symptomatic benefits after months to years of therapy.[53,56] Thus, nitrate tolerance does not appear to be as problematic in heart failure as in angina. The mechanism of nitrate tolerance is still poorly understood. When seen in a heart failure patient, the best treatment option appears to be daily 8- to 12-hour nitrate-free intervals (see Chap. 12).

Digoxin

Pharmacology. Digoxin exerts its positive inotropic effect by binding to sodium- and potassium-activated adenosine triphosphatase (NaK-ATPase or sodium pump).[57] Inhibition of NaK-ATPase decreases outward transport of sodium and leads to increased intracellular sodium concentrations. Higher intracellular sodium concentrations favor calcium entry and reduce calcium extrusion from the cell through effects on the sodium-calcium exchanger.[57] The result is increased storage of intracellular calcium in the sarcoplasmic reticulum and, with each action potential, a greater release of calcium to activate contractile elements.

Digoxin also has beneficial neurohumoral actions. These effects occur at low doses, where little inotropic effect is seen, and are independent of inotropic activity.[92] Unlike other positive

TABLE 11–11. Clinical Pharmacokinetics of Digoxin

Oral bioavailability	
Tablets	0.5–0.9 (0.65)[a]
Elixir	0.75–0.85 (0.80)
Capsules	0.9–1.0 (0.95)
Onset of action	
Oral	1.5–6 h
Intravenous	15–30 min
Peak effect	
Oral	4–6 h
Intravenous	1.5–4 h
Terminal half-life	
Normal renal function	36 h
Anuric patients	5 d
Volume of distribution at steady state	7.3 L/kg
Fraction unbound in plasma	0.75–0.80
Fraction excreted unchanged in urine	0.65–0.70

[a]Range and mean value in parenthesis.
Compiled from Ref. 63.

inotropes that increase intracellular cAMP, digoxin blunts the excessive SNS activation present in heart failure patients.[92] Although the precise mechanism is unknown, a digoxin-mediated reduction in central sympathetic outflow and improvement in impaired baroreceptor function appear to play an important role.[92] Because mortality and progression of heart failure are linked to the extent of SNS activation, these sympathoinhibitory effects may be an important component of the clinical response to the drug. Chronic heart failure is also marked by autonomic dysfunction, most notably suppression of the parasympathetic (vagal) system.[92] Digoxin increases parasympathetic activity in heart failure patients and may lead to a variable decrease in heart rate, enhancing diastolic filling.[57,94] The vagal effects also result in slowed conduction and prolongation of atrioventricular node refractoriness, thus slowing the ventricular response in patients with atrial fibrillation. Because atrial fibrillation is a common complication of heart failure, the combined positive inotropic, neurohormonal, and negative dromotropic effects of digoxin can be particularly beneficial for such patients. The overall response to digoxin is usually an increase in cardiac index, a decrease in SVR, PAOP, and plasma NE, but relatively little change in arterial blood pressure.[57] The diuretic effect is presumably mediated by the both an increase in cardiac index and a decrease in RAA activity.[57]

■ *Pharmacokinetics.* Numerous studies of digoxin pharmacokinetics have been published and are summarized in Table 11–11.[64] Digoxin has a large volume of distribution and is extensively bound to various tissues, most notably to NaK-ATPase in skeletal and cardiac muscles. Because it does not distribute appreciably to body fat, loading doses of digoxin should be calculated based on estimates of lean body weight. There is a long "distribution phase" after administration of oral or IV digoxin resulting in a lag time before maximum pharmacologic response is observed

TABLE 11–12. Potentially Significant Pharmacokinetic/Pharmacodynamic Drug Interactions with Digoxin

Drug	Mechanism/Effect	Suggested Clinical Management
Amiodarone	Decrease in renal and nonrenal clearance can increase SDC by 70–100%	Monitor SDC and adverse effects; anticipate the need to reduce the dose by 50%
Antacids	Concurrent administration may decrease digoxin bioavailability by 20–35%	Space doses at least 2 h apart to avoid concurrent use if possible
Neomycin, sulfasalazine	Decrease in bioavailability by 20%–25%	Space doses at least 2 h apart to avoid concurrent use if possible
Erythromycin, tetracycline	Alter gut bacterial flora; bioavailability and SDC increase 40–100% in about 10% of patients who extensively metabolize digoxin in the gut	Monitor SDC and anticipate the need to reduce the dose; avoid concurrent use if possible
Cholestrayramine, colestipol	Bind digoxin in gut and decrease bioavailability 20–35%; may also decrease enterohepatic recycling	Space doses at least 2 h apart to avoid concurrent use if possible
Diurectics	Thiazides or loop diuretics may cause hypokalemia and hypomagnesemia thereby increasing the risk of digitalis toxicity	Monitor and replace electrolytes if necessary
Kaolin-pectin	Large dose (30–60 mL) may decrease digoxin bioavailability by about 60%	Space drugs at least 2 h apart or avoid concurrent use if possible
Metoclopramide	Increase in gut mobility may decrease bioavailability of slow-dissolving tablets; unknown significance	Effect is minimized by administration of digoxin capsules
Quinidine	Decrease in renal and nonrenal clearance; also displacement of digoxin from tissue binding and decrease in the volume of distrubution; SDC generally increases about twofold	Monitor SDC and adverse effects; anticipate the need to reduce the dose by 50%
Spironolactone	Decrease in renal and nonrenal clearance; also interference with some digoxin assays thus increasing apparent SDC	Monitor SDC and anticipate the need to reduce dose; check assay for interference
Verapamil	Decrease in renal and nonrenal clearance; SDC may increase 70–100%	Monitor SDC and anticipate the need to reduce the dose by 50%; consider using another calcium channel blocker
Propafenone	Decrease in renal clearance; SDC may increase 30–40%	Monitor SDC and anticipate the need to reduce the dose

SDC = serum digoxin concentration.

(Table 11–11). Transiently elevated serum digoxin concentrations (SDCs) during the distribution phase are not associated with increased therapeutic or adverse effects, although they can mislead the clinician who is unaware of the timing of blood sampling relative to the previous digoxin dose. Consequently, blood samples for measurement of SDCs should be collected at least 6 hours and preferably 12 hours or more after the last dose.

In patients with normal renal function, 60% to 80% of a dose of digoxin is eliminated unchanged in urine via glomerular filtration and tubular secretion. The terminal half-life of digoxin is approximately 1.5 days in subjects with normal renal function but approximately 5 days in anuric patients (Table 11–11). It is important to emphasize that most studies of digoxin pharmacokinetics used immunoassays to measure digoxin concentrations in serum and urine. Lack of specificity with the immunoassays used in many studies of digoxin pharmacokinetics led to variable cross-reactivity with certain metabolites as well as endogenous digoxin-like immunoreactive substance(s) and probably affected the estimates of certain pharmacokinetic parameters.[64] Clinically important pharmacokinetic/pharmacodynamic drug interactions are summarized in Table 11–12. An extensive review of pharmacokinetics and pharmacodynamics of digoxin is available.[64]

Adverse Effects. Digoxin produces a variety of cardiac and noncardiac adverse effects (Table 11–13).[94] Noncardiac adverse effects frequently involve the CNS or gastrointestinal systems, but may also be nonspecific (e.g., fatigue or weakness). Cardiac manifestations include numerous different arrhythmias caused by enhanced automaticity, slowed or accelerated conduction, or delayed afterdepolarizations (Table 11–13). Cardiac arrhythmias may be the first evidence of toxicity in a patient (before any noncardiac symptoms occur). Rhythm disturbances are of particular concern because patients with chronic heart failure are already at increased risk for sudden cardiac death, presumably due to ventricular arrhythmias. Hypokalemia, hypercalcemia, and hypomagnesemia will predispose patients to cardiac manifestations of digoxin toxicity. Concomitant therapy with diuretics may lead to electrolyte abnormalities and increase the likelihood of cardiac arrhythmias. Similarly, hypothyroidism, myocardial ischemia, and acidosis will increase the risk of cardiac adverse effects. Usual treatment of digoxin toxicity includes drug withdrawal or dose reduction, and treatment of cardiac arrhythmias and electrolyte abnormalities. In patients with life-threatening digoxin toxicity, purified digoxin-specific Fab antibody fragments provide reversal of adverse effects within 1 hour in over 90% of cases.

Older case-control studies suggest that digoxin increases mortality after MI, although it could not be determined if digoxin was the cause of death or was just a marker for patients with more severe heart disease. A recent multivariate analysis that attempted to control for other confounding factors found a relative mortality risk of 1.8 for patients receiving digoxin after MI.[95] These findings are supported by those of the recently completed DIG trial that reported an increased risk of cardiac death (defined as death from a cardiac cause other than worsening heart failure) in patients receiving digoxin.[58] Although not conclusive, the expected benefit of digoxin should be carefully weighed against the potential risk in a patient with recent MI.

TABLE 11–13. Signs and Symptoms of Digitalis Toxicity

Noncardiac (mostly CNS) adverse effects[a]
Anorexia, nausea, vomiting, abdominal pain
Visual disturbances
Halos, photophobia, problems with color perception (red–green or yellow–green vision), scotomata
Fatigue, weakness, dizziness, headache, neuralgia, confusion, delirium, psychosis
Cardiac adverse effects[a,b]
Ventricular arrhythmias
Premature ventricular depolarizations, bigeminy, trigeminy, ventricular tachycardia, ventricular fibrillation
Atrioventricular (A-V) block
First degree, second degree (Mobitz type I), third degree block
A-V junctional escape rhythms, junctional tachycardia
Atrial arrhythmias with slowed A-V conduction or A-V block
Particularly paroxysmal atrial tachycardia with A-V block
Sinus bradycardia

[a]Some adverse effects may be difficult to distinguish from the signs/symptoms of heart failure.

[b]Digitalis toxicity has been associated with almost every known rhythm abnormality (only the more common manifestations are listed).

Compiled from Refs. 20, 56, and 63.

PHARMACOECONOMIC CONSIDERATIONS

Heart failure imposes a tremendous economic burden on the health care system. In patients over the age of 65, it is the most common reason for hospitalization with hospital admission rates for this disorder continuing to increase. Heart failure is also associated with 30% to 50% readmission rates during the 3 to 6 months after initial discharge. In 1989 the estimated costs of heart failure in the United States were greater than $10 billion,[2] with more recent estimates as high as $34 billion.[4] The prevalence of heart failure and the costs associated with patient care are expected to increase as the population ages and as survival from ischemic heart disease is improved. Thus, approaches to improve the quality and cost-effectiveness of care for these patients may have a significant impact on health care costs.

Several studies have attempted to assess the cost-effectiveness of drug therapy for heart failure. Carvedilol reduced the number of cardiovascular-related hospital admissions by 62% compared to placebo resulting in a significant savings in hospital costs.[96] In the DIG trial, patients treated with digoxin had fewer hospitalizations for heart failure, but digoxin produced an absolute decrease of only 2.8% in hospitalizations for any cause.[58] One study compared the cost-effectiveness of therapy with digoxin plus diuretics (standard therapy) to standard therapy plus hydralazine and isosorbide dinitrate, and standard therapy plus enalapril.[97] These investigators found that the additional cost per year of life saved with the hydralazine-isosorbide dinitrate combination was $5600 compared to $9700 for patients receiving enalapril. The authors concluded that the additional cost with enalapril was justified because enalapril saves more lives. Similarly, captopril therapy after MI in patients with an ejection fraction of 40% or lower was also shown to be cost effective, with cost-effectiveness of therapy increasing with increasing age.[98] It should be noted that cost-effectiveness analyses comparing regimens with different effects on mortality have limited clinical significance. Specifically, hydralazine-isosorbide dinitrate treatment may be slightly more cost effective than an ACE inhibitior; however, the use of this combination therapy over an ACE inhibitor could not be ethically justified because ACE inhibitors produce a greater improvement in survival.

Several studies have recently documented the benefits of multidisciplinary specialty care of heart failure patients over conventional care.[99] For example, in a comparison of heart failure patients receiving conventional care versus AHCPR guideline-guided care by a multidisciplinary team (consisting of nurses, dieticians, social services personnel, and cardiologists),[100] overall hospital readmissions for heart failure were reduced by 56% in the multidisciplinary versus conventional care groups. Quality of life also significantly improved in treatment group patients. Cost of care was reduced by $460 per patient because of the reduction in hospital admissions.

The impact of a pharmacist as a member of a multidisciplinary heart failure team was recently described.[101] These investigators randomly assigned 181 heart failure patients seen in an outpatient clinic to receive either conventional treatment (control group) or pharmacist intervention that included medication evaluation and therapeutic recommendations, patient education, and follow-up telephone monitoring. The primary end point, consisting of a composite of total mortality plus hospitalizations for heart failure, was significantly reduced in the pharmacist intervention group compared to the control group (4 versus 16 events, respectively; $P = .005$). This benefit was primarily due to a reduction in hospitalization for heart failure, mortality was not different between the groups. Target ACE inhibitor doses were more frequently achieved in patients in the intervention group and, in patients intolerant to ACE inhibitors, 75% of patients in the intervention group received alternative vasodilators compared to 26% of the control group. These results suggest that pharmacists can play an important role in improving therapeutic outcomes in heart failure patients.

It is estimated that of the more than $10 billion spent per year on heart failure, 73% is spent on hospitalizations while only 2% is spent on drugs;[48] thus efforts aimed at reducing costs of heart failure should be aimed at reducing hospitalizations. This is probably most easily accomplished through appropriate drug therapy. However, it is well documented that many heart failure patients are not treated according to consensus guidelines[102] or fail to receive adequate doses of medications with documented survival benefits.[103] The role and cost benefits of pharmacist involvement in the multidisciplinary care of heart failure patients is now apparent and should include optimizing doses of heart failure drug therapy, screening for drugs that exacerbate heart failure, and monitoring for adverse drug effects and drug interactions, educating patients, and patient follow up.

EVALUATION OF THERAPEUTIC OUTCOMES

Some of the more important therapeutic outcomes in heart failure management, such as prolonged survival or prevention or slowing of the progression of heart failure, cannot be measured in an individual patient. However, symptomatic improvement is readily measurable in the heart failure patient. The cardinal signs and symptoms of heart failure are caused by excess fluid retention and symptomatic improvement can be documented by the disappearance of these signs and symptoms (Table 11–5). Specifically, in a patient with pulmonary congestion, monitoring is indicated for resolution of rales and pulmonary edema, and improvement or resolution of DOE, orthopnea, and PND. For patients with systemic congestion, a decrease or disappearance in peripheral edema, jugular venous distension, and hepatojugular reflux is sought. Other therapeutic outcomes include an improvement in exercise tolerance and fatigue, decreased nocturia, and a decrease in heart rate. Clinicians will also want to monitor blood pressure and ensure that the patient does not develop symptomatic hypotension as a result of drug therapy. Body weight is a sensitive marker of fluid loss or retention, and patients should be counseled to weigh themselves daily, reporting changes to their health care provider.

▶ PRINCIPLES OF PHARMACOTHERAPY

- Heart failure is a clinical syndrome caused by the inability of the heart to pump sufficient blood to meet the metabolic needs of the body. Heart failure can result from reduced ventricular filling (diastolic dysfunction) and/or reduced myocardial contractility (systolic dysfunction).
- In patients with heart failure, a number of compensatory responses are activated in an attempt to maintain adequate cardiac output including the SNS, increased preload, vasoconstriction, and ventricular hypertrophy. These compensatory mechanisms are responsible for the symptoms of heart failure and contribute to disease progression.
- No therapy for acute/severe heart failure studied to date has been conclusively shown to influence mortality. Treatment goals are directed toward restoration of systemic oxygen transport and tissue perfusion, relief of pulmonary edema, and limitation of further cardiac damage. Combinations of short-acting IV medications with different cardiovascular actions are often needed to optimize cardiac output, relieve pulmonary edema, and limit myocardial ischemia. Invasive hemodynamic monitoring is usually required to provide immediate feedback on treatment efficacy and adverse effects.
- All patients with symptomatic heart failure should receive vasodilator therapy with the goals of improving survival, slowing disease progression, reducing hospitalizations, and improving quality of life. ACE inhibitors are the vasodilator of choice, but the combination of hydralazine and isosorbide dinitrate can be used if ACE inhibitors are contraindicated or not tolerated. Vasodilator doses should be targeted at the doses shown in clinical trials to improve survival.
- Patients with asymptomatic left ventricular dysfunction should be treated with ACE inhibitors with the goal of preventing symptomatic heart failure and reducing mortality.
- Although chronic diuretic therapy is frequently used in heart failure patients, it is not mandatory and required only in those patients with peripheral edema and/or pulmonary congestion.
- Digoxin does not improve survival in patients with heart failure. Therefore it should not automatically be considered first-line therapy in patients in normal sinus rhythm, but rather reserved for patients remaining

symptomatic after optimization of therapies known to improve survival. Digoxin doses should be adjusted to achieve plasma concentrations of approximately 1 ng/mL; higher plasma concentrations are not associated with additional benefits. Digoxin should be considered early in therapy in patients with heart failure and supraventricular tachyarrhythmias as it will help control the ventricular response rate.

- β-blockers slow the progression of heart failure, decrease hospitalizations, and improve survival. Carvedilol, a nonselective β-blocker with vasodilating properties, is the only β-blocker approved for use in patients with heart failure and should be considered first-line therapy in symptomatic patients in conjunction with ACE inhibitors, diuretics, and digoxin. The key to the successful use of any β-blocker in heart failure is initiation of therapy with low doses followed by slow upward dosage titration.
- Amiodarone and amlodipine appear to be safe for use in heart failure patients with another indication for use of these drugs. However, neither of these agents should be routinely used specifically for treatment of heart failure.
- Pharmacists should play an important role as part of a multidisciplinary team to optimize therapy in heart failure. The pharmacist should be responsible for such activities as optimizing doses of heart failure drug therapy, screening for drugs that exacerbate heart failure, and monitoring for adverse drug effects and drug interactions.

REFERENCES

1. Colucci WS, Braunwald E. Pathophysiology of congestive heart failure. In Braunwald E, ed. Heart Disease, A Textbook of Cardiovascular Medicine. Philadelphia, Saunders, 1997:394–420.
2. Kannel WB. Need and prospects for prevention of cardiac failure. Eur J Clin Pharmacol 1996;49:S3–S9.
3. Ho KKL, Pinsky JL, Kannel WB, Levy D. The epidemiology of heart failure: The Framingham Study. J Am Coll Cardiol 1993; 22(suppl A):6A–13A.
4. O'Connell JB, Bristow MR. Economic impact of heart failure in the United States: Time for a different approach. J Heart Lung Transplant 1994;13:S107–S111.
5. The CONSENSUS Trial Study Group. Effects of enalapril on mortality in severe congestive heart failure. Results of the Cooperative North Scandinavian Enalapril Survival Study (CONSENSUS). N Engl J Med 1987;316:1429–1435.
6. The SOLVD Investigators. Effect of enalapril on survival in patients with reduced left ventricular ejection fractions and congestive heart failure. N Engl J Med 1991;325:293–302.
7. Wynne J, Braunwald E. The cardiomyopathies and myocarditides. In Braunwald E, ed. Heart Disease, A Textbook of Cardiovascular Medicine. Philadelphia, Saunders, 1997:1404–1463.
8. Opie LH. Normal and abnormal contraction and relaxation. In Braunwald E, ed. Heart Disease, A Textbook of Cardiovascular Medicine. Philadelphia, Saunders, 1997:360–393.
9. Brilla CG, Miasch B. Regulation of the structural remodelling of the myocardium: From hypertrophy to heart failure. Eur Heart J 1994 (suppl D):45–52.
10. Francis GS, Cohn JN, Johnson G, et al. Plasma norepinephrine, plasma renin activity and congestive heart failure. Relations to survival and the effects of therapy in V-HeFT II. The V-HeFT VA Cooperative Studies Group. Circulation 1993;87(suppl 6): VI40–VI48.
11. Wilkins MR, Redondo J, Brown LA. The natriuretic-peptide family. Lancet 1997;349:1307–1310.
12. McDonagh TA, Robb SD, Murdoch DR, et al. Biochemical detection of left-ventricular systolic dysfunction. Lancet 1998;351:9-13.
13. Nguyen BNT, Johnson JA. Role of endothelin-1 in cardiovascular disease. Pharmacotherapy. 1998;18:706–719.
14. Sakai S, Moyauchi T, Kobayashi M, et al. Inhibition of myocardial endothelin pathway improves long-term survival in heart failure. Nature 1996;384:353–355.
15. Seta Y, Shan K, Bozkurt B, et al. Basic mechanisms in heart failure: The cytokine hypothesis. J Cardiac Failure 1996;2:243–249.
16. Ghali JK, Kadakia S, Cooper R, et al. Precipitating factors leading to decompensation of heart failure. Arch Intern Med 1988;148: 2013–2016.
17. Braunwald E, Colucci WS, Grossman W. Clinical aspects of heart failure: High output heart failure; pulmonary edema. In: Braunwald E ed. Heart Disease, A Textbook of Cardiovascular Medicine. Philadelphia, Saunders, 1997:445–470.
18. McCall D. Epidemiology, etiology and natural history. In McCall D, Rahimtoola SH, eds. Heart Failure: Current Topics in Cardiology. New York: Chapman & Hall, 1995:1–13.
19. Marcus ML, Schelbert HR, Skorton DJ, Wolf GL, eds. Cardiac imaging: A companion to Braunwald's Heart Disease. Philadelphia, Saunders, 1991.
20. American College of Cardiology/American Heart Association Task Force on Practice Guidelines. Guidelines for the evaluation and management of heart failure. Circulation 1995;92:2764–84.
21. Hoffman BB, Lefkowitz RJ. Catecholamines, sympathomimetic drugs and adrenergic receptor antagonists. In: Hardman JG, Limbird LE, Molinoff PB, et al, eds. Goodman and Gilman's Pharmacological Basis of Therapeutics, 9th ed. New York, McGraw Hill, 1996: 199–248.
22. Smith TW, Kelly RA, Stevenson LW, Braunwald E. The management of heart failure. In: Braunwald E, ed. Heart Disease A Textbook of Cardiovascular Medicine. Philadelphia, Saunders, 1997: 492–514.
23. Unverferth DV, Blanford M, Kates RE, et al. Tolerance to dobutamine after a 72 hour continuous infusion. Am J Med 1980;69: 262–266.
24. Leier CV, Huss P, Lewis RP, Unverferth DV. Drug-induced conditioning in congestive heart failure. Circulation 1982;65:1382–1387.
25. Erlemeier HH, Kupper W, Bleifeld W. Intermittent infusion of dobutamine in the therapy of severe congestive heart failure—Long-term effects and lack of tolerance. Cardiovasc Drugs Ther 1992;6:391–398.
26. Dies F, Krell MJ, Whitlow P, et al. Intermittent dobutamine in ambulatory outpatients with chronic cardiac failure. Circulation 1986;74(suppl II):II–38. Abstract.
27. Kelly RA, Smith TW. Pharmacologic treatment of heart failure. In: Hardman JG, Limbird LE, Molinoff PB, et al, eds. Goodman and Gilman's Pharmacological Basis of Therapeutics, 9th ed. New York, McGraw Hill, 1996:875–898.
28. Arnold JM. The role of phosphodiesterase inhibitors in heart failure. Pharmacol Ther 1993;57:161–170.
29. Anderson JL, and the United States Milrinone Multicenter Investigators. Hemodynamic and clinical benefits with intravenous milrinone in severe chronic heart failure: Results of a multicenter study in the United States. Am Heart J 1991;121:1956–1964.
30. Meissner A, Herrmann G, Gerdesmeyer L, Simon R. Additive effects of milrinone and dobutamine in patients with congestive heart failure. Z Kardiol 1992;81:266–271.
31. Amisel AS, Wright CM, Carter SM, et al. Tachyphylaxis with amrinone therapy: Association with sequestration and down-regulation of lymphocyte β-adrenergic receptors. Ann Intern Med 1989;110: 195–201.

32. Opie LH. Pharmacologic options for treatment of ischemic heart disease. In Smith TW, ed. Cardiovascular Therapeutics. Philadelphia, Saunders, 1996:22–57.
33. Packer M, Meller J, Medina N, et al. Rebound hemodynamic events after abrupt withdrawal of nitroprusside in patients with severe heart failure. New Engl J Med 1979;301:1193–1197.
34. Cohn JN, Burke LP. Nitroprusside. Ann Intern Med 1979;91:752–757.
35. Packer M, Lee WH, Kessler PD, et al. Prevention and reversal of nitrate tolerance in patients with congestive heart failure. N Engl J Med 1987;317:799–804.
36. Elkayam U, Kulick D, McIntosh N, et al. Incidence of early tolerance to hemodynamic effects of continuous infusion of nitroglycerin in patients with coronary heart disease and heart failure. Circulation 1987;76:577–588.
37. Jugdutt BI. Nitrates as anti-ischemic and cardioprotective agents. In: Singh BN, Dzau VJ, Vanhoutte PM, Woosley RL, eds. Cardiovascular Pharmacology and Therapeutics. New York, Churchill Livingstone, 1994:449–465.
38. MacFadyen RJ, Lees KR, Reid JL. Double blind controlled study of low dose intravenous perindoprilat or enalaprilat infusion in elderly patients with heart failure. Br Heart J 1993;69:293–297.
39. Francis GS, Siegel RM, Goldsmith SR, et al. Acute vasoconstrictor response to intravenous furosemide in patients with chronic congestive heart failure. Ann Intern Med 1985;103:1–6.
40. Kraus PA, Lipman J, Becker PJ. Acute preload effects of furosemide. Chest 1990;98:124–128.
41. Ellison DH. The physiologic basis of diuretic synergism: Its role in treating diuretic resistance. Ann Intern Med 1991;114:886–894.
42. Brater DC. Diuretic resistance: Mechanisms and therapeutic strategies. Cardiology 1994;84(suppl 2):57–67.
43. Vargo DL, Brater DC, Rudy DW, Swan SK. Dopamine does not enhance furosemide-induced natriuresis in patients with congestive heart failure. J Am Soc Nephrol 1996;7:1032–1037.
44. Dormans TP, van Meyel JJM, Gerlag PGG, et al. Diuretic efficacy of high dose furosemide in severe heart failure: Bolus injection versus continuous infusion. J Am Coll Cardiol 1996;28:376–382.
45. Richenbacher WE, Pierce WS. Assisted circulation and mechanical heart. In: Braunwald E, ed. Heart Disease, A Textbook of Cardiovascular Medicine. Philadelphia, Saunders, 1997:534–547.
46. Twenty-Fourth Bethesda Conference: Cardiac Transplantation. J Am Coll Cardiol 1993;22:1–64.
47. Elefteriades JA, Lee FA, Letsou GV. Advanced treatment options for the failing left ventricle. Cardiol Clinics 1995;13:1–147.
48. Konstam M, Dracup K, Baker D, et al. Heart failure: Evaluation and care of patients with left-ventricular systolic dysfunction. Clinical practice guideline #11. Rockville, MD: Agency for Health Care Policy and Research Publication #94-0612, Public Health Services. U.S. Department of Health and Human Services, 1994.
49. Vantrimpont P, Rouleau JL. Medical treatment of heart failure: The Canadian Cardiovascular Society's Consensus Conference revisited. Cardiovasc Drugs Ther 1997;10:711–716.
50. Belardinelli R, Deorgiou D, Scocco V, et al. Low intensity exercise training in patients with chronic heart failure. J Am Coll Cardiol 1995;26:975–982.
51. Deedwania PC. Angiotensin-converting enzyme inhibitors in congestive heart failure. Arch Intern Med 1990;150:1798–1805.
52. Latini R, Maggioni AP, Flather M, et al. ACE inhibitor use in patients with myocardial infarction. Summary of evidence from clinical trials. Circulation 1995;92:3132–3137
53. Cohn JN, Johnson G, Ziesche S, et al. A comparison of enalapril with hydralazine-isosorbide dinitrate in the treatment of chronic congestive heart failure. N Engl J Med 1991;325:303–310.
54. Wilke A, Funck R, Rupp H, Brilla CG. Effect of the renin–angiotensin–aldosterone system on the cardiac interstitium in heart failure. Basic Res Cardiol 1996;91(suppl 2):79–84.
55. Ertl G, Gaudron P, Hu K. Ventricular remodeling after myocardial infarction: Experimental and clinical studies. Basic Res Cardiol 1993; 88(suppl 1):125–137.
56. Cohn JN, Archibald DG, Ziesche S, et al. Effect of vasodilator therapy on mortality in chronic congestive heart failure. N Engl J Med 1986;314:1547–1552.
57. Smith TW. Digitalis. Mechanism of action and clinical use. N Engl J Med 1988;318:358–365.
58. The Digitalis Investigation Group. The effect of digoxin on mortality and morbidity in patients with heart failure. N Engl J Med 1997; 336:525–533.
59. The Captopril–Digoxin Multicenter Research Group. Comparative effects of therapy with captopril and digoxin in patients with mild to moderate heart failure. JAMA 1988;259:539–544.
60. Packer M, Gheorghiade M, Young JB, et al. Withdrawal of digoxin from patients with chronic heart failure treated with angiotensin-converting-enzyme inhibitors. N Engl J Med 1993;329:1–7.
61. Uretsky B, Young JB, Shahidi FE, et al. Randomized study assessing the effect of digoxin withrawal in patients with mild to moderate chronic congestive heart failure: Results of the PROVED trial. J Am Coll 1993;22:955–962.
62. Gheorghiade M, Hall VB, Jacobsen G, et al. Effects of increasing maintenance doses of digoxin on left ventricular function and neurohormones in patients with chronic heart failure treated with diuretics and angiotensin-converting enzyme inhibitors. Circulation 1995; 92:1801–1807.
63. Slatton ML, Irani WN, Hall SA, et al. Does digoxin provide additional hemodynamic and autonomic benefit at higher doses in patients with mild to moderate heart failure and normal sinus rhythm? J Am Coll Cardiol 1997;29:1206–1213.
64. Reuning RH, Geraets GR, Rocci ML, Vlasses PH. Digoxin. In: Evans WE, Schentag JJ, Jusko WJ, eds. Applied Pharmacokinetics: Principles of Therapeutic Drug Monitoring, 3rd ed. Spokane, WA, Applied Therapeutics, 1992:20-1–20-48.
65. Doughty RN, Sharpe N. β-adrenergic blocking agents in the treatment of congestive heart failure: Mechanisms and clinical results. Annu Rev Med 1997;48:103–114.
66. Doughty RN, Rodgers A, Shape N, MacMahon S. Effects of β-blocker therapy on mortality in patients with heart failure. A systematic overview of randomized controlled trials. Eur Heart J 1997; 18:560–565.
67. Chatterjee K. Heart failure therapy in evolution. Circulation 1996; 94:2689–2693. (Editorial.)
68. Packer M, Bristow MR, Cohn JN, et al. The effect of carvedilol on morbidity and mortality in patients with chronic heart failure. N Engl J Med 1996;334:1349–1355.
68a. The CIBIS Scientific Committee. Design of the cardiac insufficiency bisoprolol study II (CIBIS II). Fundam Clin Pharmacol 1997;11: 138–142.
68b. McMenemy MC. β-blockers given the go-ahead for treatment of heart failure (News). Lancet 1998;352:793.
69. Heidenreich PA, Lee TT, Massie BM. Effect of β-blockade on mortality in patients with heart failure: A meta-analysis of randomized clinical trials. J Am Coll Cardiol 1997;30:27–34.
70. Eichhorm EJ, Bristow MR. Practical guidelines for initiation of β-adrenergic blockade in patients with chronic heart failure. Am J Cardiol 1997;79:794–798.
71. Goodfriend TL, Elliot ME, Catt KJ. Angiotensin receptors and their antagonists. N Engl J Med 1996;334:1649–1654.
72. Messerli FH, Weber MA, Brunner HR. Angiotensin II receptor inhibition. A new therapeutic prinicple. Arch Intern Med 1996; 156:1957–1965.
73. Dickstein K, Chang P, Willenheimer R, et al. Comparison of the effects of losartan and enalapril on clinical status and exercise performance in patients with moderate or severe chronic heart failure. J Am Coll Cardiol 1995;26:438–445.
74. Pitt B, Segal R, Martinez FA, et al, on behalf of the ELITE Study investigators. Randomised trial of losartan versus captopril in patients over 65 with heart failure (Evaluation of Losartan in the Elderly Study, ELITE). Lancet 1997;349:747–752.

75. Echt DS, Liebson PR, Mitchell LB, et al. Mortality and morbidity in patients receiving encainide, flecainide or placebo. The Cardiac Arrhythmia Suppression Trial. N Engl J Med 1991;324:781–788.
76. The Cardiac Arrhythmia Suppression Trial II Investigators. Effect of the antiarrhythmic agent moricizine on survival after myocardial infarction. N Engl J Med 1992;327:227–233.
77. Doval HC, Nul DR, Grancelli HO, et al. Randomised trial of low-dose amiodarone in severe congestive heart failure. Lancet 1994; 344:493–498.
78. Singh SN, Fletcher RD, Fisher SG, et al, for the Survival Trial of Antiarrhythmic Therapy in Congestive Heart Failure. Amiodarone in patients with congestive heart failure and asymptomatic ventricular arrhythmia. N Engl J Med 1995;333:77–82.
79. Julian DG, Camm AJ, Frangin G, et al, for the European Myocardial Infarct Amiodarone Trial Investigators. Lancet 1997;349: 667–674.
80. Nul DR, Doval HC, Grancelli HO, et al, on behalf of the GESICA-GEMA investigators. Heart rate is a marker of amiodarone mortality reduction in severe heart failure. J Am Coll Cardiol 1997; 29:1199–1205.
81. Waldo AL, Camm AJ, deRuyter J, et al. for the SWORD Investigators. Effect of *d*-sotalol on mortality in patients with left ventricular dysfunction after recent and remote myocardial infarction. Lancet 1996;348:7–12.
82. Moss AJ, Hall WJ, Cannom DS, et al. Improved survival with an implanted defibrillator in patients with coronary artery disease at high risk for ventricular arrhythmia. N Engl J Med 1996;335: 1933–1940.
83. The Antiarrhythmic Versus Implantable Defibrillators (AVID) Investigators. A comparison of antiarrhythmic-drug therapy with implantable defibrillators in patients resuscitated from near-fatal ventricular arrhythmias. N Engl J Med 1997;337:1576–1583.
84. Goldstein RE, Boccuzzi SJ, Cruess D, et al. Diltiazem increases late-onset congestive heart failure in postinfarction patients with early reduction in ejection fraction. Circulation 1991;83:52–60.
85. Elkayam U, Amin J, Mehra A, et al. A prospective, randomized, double-blind, crossover study to compare the efficacy and safety of chronic nifedipine therapy with that of isosorbide dinitrate and their combination in the treatment of chronic congestive heart failure. Circulation 1990;82:1954–1961.
86. Cohn JN, Ziesche S, Smith R, for the V-HeFT Study Group. Effect of the calcium antagonist felodipine as supplementary vasodilator therapy in patients with chronic heart failure treated with enalapril, V-HeFT III. Circulation 1997;96:856–863.
87. Packer M, O'Connor CM, Ghali JK, et al, for the Prospective Randomized Amlodipine Survival Evaluation Study Group. Effect of amlodipine on morbidity and mortality in severe chronic heart failure. N Engl J Med 1996;335;1107–1114.
88. Niebauer J, Coats AJS. Treating chronic heart failure: Time to take stock. Lancet 1997;349:966–967.
89. Yusuf S, Teo K. Inotropic agents increase mortality in patients with congestive heart failure. Circulation 1990;82:III–673. Abstract.
90. Hall D, Zeitler H, Rudolph W. Counteraction of the vasodilator effects of enalapril by aspirin in severe heart failure. J Am Coll Cardiol 1992;20:1549–1555.
91. Nguyen KN, Aursnes I, Kjekshus J. Interaction between enalapril and aspirin on mortality after acute myocardial infarction: Subgroup analysis of the Cooperative New Scandinavian Enalapril Survival Study II (CONSENSUS II). Am J Cardiol 1997;79:115–119.
92. van Veldhuisen DJ, de Graeff PA, Remme WJ, Lie KI. Value of digoxin in heart failure and sinus rhythm: New features of an old drug? J Am Coll Cardiol 1996;28:813–819.
93. Krum H, Bigger JT, Goldsmith RL, Packer M. Effect of long-term digoxin therapy on autonomic function in patients with chronic heart failure. J Am Coll Cardiol 1995;25:289–294.
94. Smith TW, Antman EA, Friedman PL, et al. Digitalis glycosides: Mechanism and manifestations of toxicity. Prog Cardiovasc Dis 1984;26:413–441.
95. Kober L, Torp-Pedersen C, Gadsoll N, et al. Is digoxin an independent risk factor for long-term mortality after acute myocardial infarction? Eur Heart J 1994;15:382–388.
96. Oster G, Menzin J, Richner RE, et al. Impact of carvedilol therapy for heart failure on costs of cardiovascular-related hospitalization. J Am Coll Cardiol 1997;29(suppl A);326A. Abstract.
97. Paul SD, Kuntz KM, Eagle KA, Weinstein MC. Costs and effectiveness of angiotensin converting enzyme inhibition in patients with congestive heart failure. Arch Intern Med 1994;154: 1143–1149.
98. Tsevat J, Duke D, Goldman L, et al. Cost-effectiveness of captopril therapy after myocardial infarction. J Am Coll Cardiol 1995;26: 914–919.
99. Abraham WT, Bristow MR. Specialized centers for heart failure management. Circulation 1997;96:2755–2757.
100. Rich MW, Beckham V, Wittenberg C, et al. A multidisciplinary intervention to prevent the readmission of elderly patients with congestive heart failure. N Engl J Med 1995;333:1190–1195.
101. Gattis WA, Hasselblad V, Larsen RL, et al. Reduction in heart failure events by clinical pharmacist intervention: Pharmacist in Heart Failure Assessment Recommendation and Monitoring (PHARM Study). (Abstract.) J Am Coll Cardiol 1998;31:69A.
102. Edep ME, Shah NB, Tateo IM, Massie BM. Differences between primary care physicians and cardiologists in management of congestive heart failure: Relation to practice guidelines. J Am Coll Cardiol 1997;30:518–526.
103. Clark AL, Coats AJS. Severity of heart failure and dosage of angiotensin converting enzyme inhibitors. Br Med J 1995;310:973–974.
104. Francis GS. The relationship of the sympathetic nervous system and the renin-angiotensin system in congestive heart failure. Am Heart J 1989;118:642.

12

Ischemic Heart Disease

Robert L. Talbert, PharmD, FCCP, BCPS

There is a disorder of the breast, marked with strong and peculiar symptoms, considerable for the kind of danger belonging to it, and not extremely rare, of which I do not recollect any mention among medical authors. The seat of it and sense of strangling and anxiety with which it is attended may make it not improper to be called angina pectoris.

Some Account of a Disorder of the Breast

William Heberden, 1768

The history and evolution of our current understanding of ischemic heart disease (IHD) and all of its manifestations is long and quite colorful.[1] Although Heberden did not understand the pathogenesis of IHD, it is now appreciated that atherosclerosis is the main etiology of IHD and that this process begins early in life, often not being clinically manifest until the middle-aged years and beyond. IHD may present as acute myocardial infarction, angina pectoris occurring on exertion or at rest, or only as ischemia without clinical symptoms. Other manifestations of atherosclerosis include heart failure, arrhythmias, cerebrovascular disease, and peripheral vascular disease.

EPIDEMIOLOGY

The syndrome of angina pectoris is reported to occur with an average annual incidence rate (number of new cases per time period/total number of persons in the population for the same time period) of about 1.5% (range 0.1 to 5/1000) depending on the patient's age, gender, and risk factor profile.[2] The presenting manifestation in women is more commonly angina whereas men more frequently have myocardial infarction as the initial event. Estimates of the incidence and prevalence of angina are not entirely accurate owing to waxing and waning of symptoms; angina may disappear in up to 30% of patients with angina that is less severe and of recent onset.

Data from the Framingham study show that the prevalence was 5.9% for the 16-year period studied from earlier reports.[3] More recent data from the Framingham study show that the prevalence in a 1970 cohort followed for 10 years was about 1.5% for women and 4.3% for men aged 50 to 59 years at inception.[2] Other interesting trends noted included a 21% decline in the incidence of cardiovascular disease in women but only a 6% decline in men over two cohorts from 1950 and 1970. Cardiovascular mortality was reduced by 59% in women and 53% in men from the same cohorts. The risk of developing ischemic heart disease is not the same worldwide. Countries such as Japan and France are on the low end of the spectrum whereas Finland, Northern Ireland, Scotland, and South Africa have very high rates of IHD.[4,5]

Death resulting from IHD continues to be a major contributing source of mortality in this country (Table 12–1). IHD was responsible for 20.8% of total mortality whereas acute myocardial infarction (AMI) caused 9.4% of all deaths; other major cardiovascular disease was responsible for 41.1% of total mortality in 1995. Men die earlier from IHD and AMI than women, and aging of both sexes is associated with a higher incidence of these afflictions. The disparity in mortality from IHD between men and women decreases with aging, being about four to five times more common in men from the age of the mid-30s to a preponderance of female deaths in the very elderly.

Angina may be classified according to symptom severity, disability induced, or a specific activity scale (Tables 12–2 and 12–3). The specific activity scale developed by Goldman and coworkers[6] may be preferable because it has been shown to be equal to or better than the New York Heart Association or Canadian Cardiovascular Society functional classifications for reproducibility and provides better agreement with treadmill testing.

An important determinate of outcome for the angina patient is the number of vessels obstructed. Twelve-year survival from the Coronary Artery Surgery Study (CASS) for patients with zero-, one-, two-, and three-vessel disease was 88%, 74%, 59%, and 40%, respectively.[7] Other factors that increase the risk of death in medically managed patients include the presence of heart failure (or markers such as poor ventricular wall motion and low ejection fraction), smoking, left main or left main equivalent coronary artery disease, diabetes, or prior myocardial infarction. Twelve-year survival for patients with at least one diseased vessel and ejection fractions in the ranges of 50% to 100%, 35% to 49%, and 0% to 34% is 73%, 54%, and 21%, respectively. Of particular note, patients with left main coronary artery disease (or left main equivalent) are at extremely high risk and constitute a unique group for therapeutic consideration.[8,9] In the CASS, at 15 years of follow-up, 37% of the surgery group and 27% of the medical group are surviving; median survival is 13.3 years versus 6.7 years, respectively ($P < .0001$). If systolic function was normal, then median survival and percent surviving were not different between the surgery and medical groups (median survival of about 15 years). Patients screened but not randomized to CASS had similar survival rates, suggesting that results

TABLE 12–1. Causes of Death in the United States, 1995

	All Ages	35–44 y	45–54 y	55–64 y	65–74 y	75–84 y	85 y +
Death from all causes							
Number	2,312,123	102,270	143,000	235,512	480,890	652,177	561,259
Rate/100,000		240.8	460.1	1,114.5	2,563.5	5,851.8	15,469.5
Male	914.1						
Female	847.3						
Major cardiovascular disease							
Number	951,406	17,234	41,656	82,036	187,284	301,970	313,751
Rate/100,000		32.0	111.0	322.9	799.9	2,064.7	6,484.1
Male	351.1						
Female	372.6						
Ischemic heart disease							
Number	481,287	6,892	20,998	44,345	102,069	155,050	150,648
Rate/100,000		16.2	67.6	209.9	544.1	1,391.2	4,152.2
Male	190.8						
Female	175.9						
Acute myocardial infarction							
Number	218,229	3,773	11,962	24,472	51,575	70,711	55,062
Rate/100,000		8.9	38.5	115.8	274.9	634.5	1,517.6
Male	90.4						
Female	76.0						
Old myocardial infarction and other forms of chronic ischemic heart disease							
Number	259,478						
Rate/100,000		7.1	28.2	91.9	265.1	748.5	2,605.8
Male	99.0						
Female	98.6						

From Ref. 110.

TABLE 12–2. Criteria for Determination of the Specific Activity Scale Functional Class[a]

	Any yes	*No*
1. Can you walk down a flight of steps without stopping (4.5–5.2 mets)?	Go to #2	Go to #4
2. Can you carry anything up a flight of 8 steps without stopping (5–5.5 mets) Or can you: a. Have sexual intercourse without stopping (5–5.5 mets) b. Garden, rake, weed (5.6 mets) c. Roller skate, dance fox trot (5–6 mets) d. Walk at a 4-mph rate on level ground (5–6 mets)	Go to #3	Class III
3. Can you carry at least 24 pounds up 8 steps (10 mets)? Or can you: a. Carry objects that are at least 80 pounds (18 mets) b. Do outdoor work—shovel snow, spade soil (7 mets) c. Do recreational activities such as skiing, basketball, touch football, squash, handball (7–10 mets) d. Jog/walk 5 mph (9 mets)	Class I	Class II
4. Can you shower without stopping (3.6–4.2 mets)? Or can you: a. Strip and make bed (3.9–5 mets) b. Mop floors (4.2 mets) c. Hang washed clothes (4.4 mets) d. Clean windows (3.7 mets) e. Walk 2.5 mph (3–3.5 mets) f. Bowl (3–4.4 mets) g. Play golf—walk and carry clubs (4.5 mets) h. Push power lawn mower (4 mets)	Class III	Go to #5
5. Can you dress without stopping because of symptoms (2–2.3 mets)?	Class III	Class IV

[a]mets = metabolic equivalents of activity.
From Ref. 6, with permission.

TABLE 12–3. Grading of Angina Pectoris by the Canadian Cardiovascular Society Classification System

Class	Description of Stage
Class I	Ordinary physical activity does not cause angina, such as walking, climbing stairs. Angina occurs with stenous, rapid, or prolonged exertion at work or recreation.
Class II	Slight limitation or ordinary activity. Angina occurs on walking or climbing stairs rapidly, walking uphill, walking or stair climbing after meals, or in cold, or in wind, or under emotional stress, or only during the few hours after wakening. Walking more than two blocks on the level and climbing more than one flight of ordinary stairs at a normal pace and in normal condition.
Class III	Marked limitations of ordinary physical activity. Angina occurs on walking one to two blocks on the level and climbing one flight of stairs in normal conditions and at a normal pace.
Class IV	Inability to carry on any physical activity without discomfort—anginal symptoms may be present at rest.

From Ref. 111, with permission.

from randomized patients may be applicable to more generalized populations as a measure of external reliability.

PATHOPHYSIOLOGY

IHD has many clinical expressions including the following syndromes: stable exertional angina; unstable (rest, preinfarction, crescendo) angina; silent myocardial ischemia; acute coronary insufficiency; coronary vasomotion or vasospasm associated with atypical, variant, or Prinzmetal's angina; and myocardial infarction. The pathophysiology that underlies this disease process is dynamic, evolutionary, and complex. To better understand the rationale for the selection and use of pharmacotherapy for IHD, one must appreciate the importance of the determinants of myocardial oxygen demand (MVO_2), regulation of coronary blood flow, the effects of ischemia on the mechanical and metabolic function of the myocardium, and how ischemia may be recognized so that treatment may be instituted.

Ischemia may be defined as lack of oxygen and decreased or no blood flow in the myocardium. In contrast, anoxia, defined as the absence of oxygen to the myocardium, results in continued perfusion with washout of acid by-products of glycolysis, thereby preserving the mechanical and metabolic status of the heart to a greater extent than does ischemia for short periods of time.

DETERMINANTS OF OXYGEN DEMAND (MVO_2)

The major determinants of MVO_2 are (1) heart rate, (2) contractility, and (3) intramyocardial wall tension during systole. Overall, intramyocardial wall tension is thought to be the most important among these three factors. As the consequences of IHD are a result of increased demand in the face of a fixed supply of oxygen in most situations, alterations in MVO_2 are critically important in producing ischemia and for interventions intended to alleviate ischemia. MVO_2 cannot be directly measured in patients; however, an indirect assessment that correlates reasonably well with MVO_2 as determined in experimental animal models is the tension–time index (TTI). This is a measure of the area under the curve of the left ventricular (LV) pressure curve. Tension in the ventricle wall is a function of the radius of the LV and intraventricular pressure. These factors are related through Laplace's law, which states that wall stress is related directly to the product of intraventricular pressure and internal radius and inversely to wall thickness multiplied by a factor of two. Increasing systemic blood pressure or ventricular dilation would increase wall tension and oxygen demand whereas ventricular hypertrophy would tend to minimize increasing MVO_2. Clinical application of these principles has led to the use of the double product (DP), which is heart rate (HR) multiplied by systolic blood pressure (SBP) ($DP = HR \times SBP$). Although this is a clinically useful indirect estimate of MVO_2, it does not consider changes in contractility (an independent variable), and because only changes in pressure are considered with the double product, volume loading of the LV and increased MVO_2 related to ventricular dilation are underestimated.

REGULATION OF CORONARY BLOOD FLOW

Coronary blood flow is influenced by multiple factors; however, the caliber of the resistance vessels delivering blood to the myocardium and MVO_2 are the prime determinants in the occurrence of ischemia. The anatomy of the vascular bed will affect oxygen supply and, subsequently, myocardial metabolism and mechanical function.

ANATOMIC FACTORS

The normal coronary system (see Fig. 12–1 for normal anatomy) consists of large epicardial or surface vessels (R_1) that normally offer little intrinsic resistance to myocardial flow and intramyocardial arteries and arterioles (R_2), which branch into a dense capillary network (about 4000 capillaries per mm^2) to supply basal blood flow of 60 to 90 mL/min per 100 g of myocardium (Fig. 12–2). R_1 and R_2 are in series and total resistance is the algebraic sum; however, under normal circumstances, the resistance in R_2 is much greater. Myocardial blood flow is inversely related to arteriolar resistance and directly related to the coronary driving pressure. The arterioles dynamically alter their intrinsic tone in response to demands for oxygen and other factors, and as a result, myocardial oxygen delivery and myocardial oxygen demand are tightly coupled in a rapidly responsive system.

Atherosclerotic lesions encroaching on the luminal cross-sectional area of the larger epicardial vessels (R_1) transform the relationships among R_1, R_2, and blood flow.

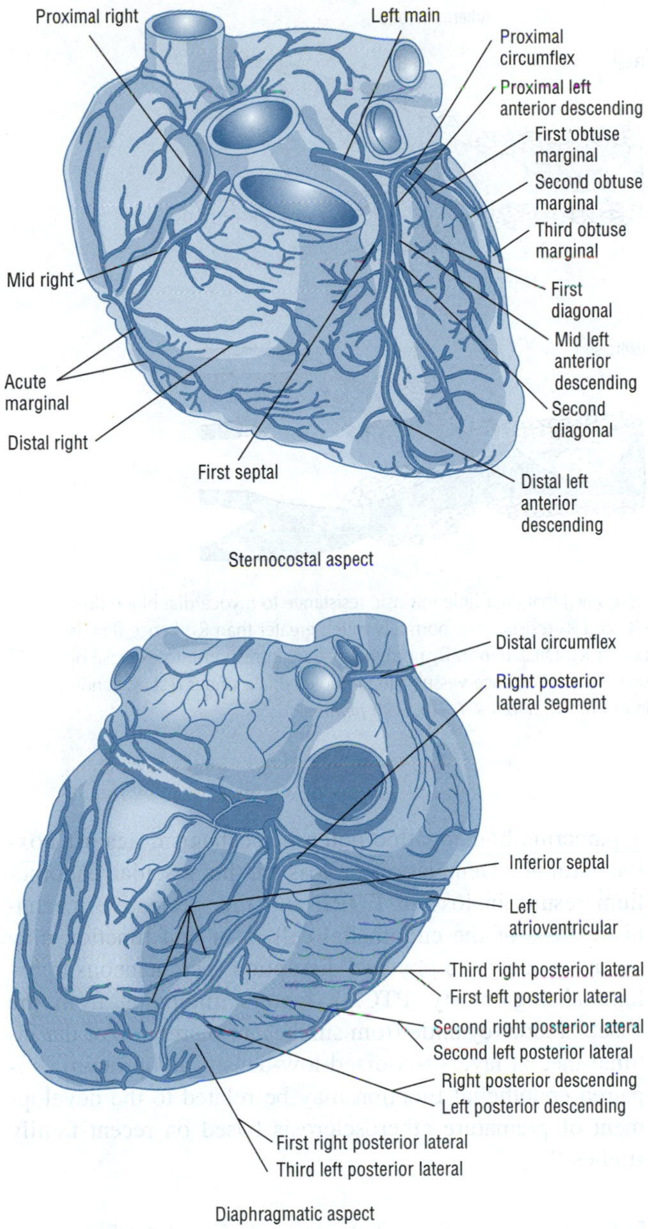

FIGURE 12–1. Coronary artery anatomy with sternocostal and diaphragmatic views.

As resistance increases in R_1 owing to occlusion, R_2 can vasodilate to maintain coronary blood flow (Fig. 12–2). This response is inadequate with greater degrees of obstruction, and the coronary flow reserve afforded by R_2 vasodilation is insufficient to meet oxygen demand (also referred to as autoregulation). The extent of functional obstruction is important in the limitation of coronary blood flow, and the presence of relatively severe stenosis (80% to 85%) may provoke ischemia and symptoms at rest, whereas less severe stenosis may allow a reserve of coronary blood flow for exertion[10]

The diameter of the lesion impeding blood flow through a vessel is important, but other factors such as length of the lesion and the influence of pressure drop across an area of stenosis also affect coronary blood flow and function of the collateral circulation. Resistance to flow in a vessel is directly related to length of the obstructing lesion, but resistance is inversely related to the diameter of the vessel to the fourth power. Diameter is, therefore, much more important. As blood flows across a stenotic lesion the pressure drops (energy losses) owing to friction between blood and the lesion and owing to the abrupt turbulent expansion as blood emerges from the stenosis. This pressure drop is dynamic and directly related to flow giving rise to a resistance that is not fixed, but rather fluctuates, as flow is changed. This relationship can dramatically affect collateral blood flow and its response to exercise, resulting in what has been called "coronary steal." A similar situation may also occur when the epicardial or subepicardial vessels "steal" blood flow from the endocardium in the presence of a stenotic lesion.

Large and small coronary arteries may undergo dynamic changes in coronary vascular resistance and coronary blood flow. Dynamic coronary obstruction can occur in normal vessels and vessels with stenosis in which vasomotion or spasm may be superimposed on a fixed stenosis. Although it is possible that these changes may be "active" in small coronary arteries, it is also possible that the observed changes may reflect collapse owing to poststenotic intraluminal pressure drop or increased intramyocardial compressive forces associated with inadequate ventricular relaxation.

Collateral blood flow exists to a certain extent from birth as native collaterals, but persisting ischemia may promote collateral growth as developed collaterals. These two types of collaterals differ in anatomy and in their ability to regulate coronary blood flow. Collateral development is dependent on the severity of obstruction, the presence of various growth factors (basic fibroblast growth factor, b-FGF, and vascular endothelial growth factor, VEGF), endogenous vasodilators (e.g., nitrous oxide, prostacyclin), hormones such as estrogen, and potentially exercise. Collateral development is highly species dependent and this should be considered when reading experimental literature.

METABOLIC REGULATION

Coronary blood flow is closely tied to oxygen needs of the heart. Changes in oxygen balance lead to very rapid changes in coronary blood flow. Although a number of mediators may contribute to these changes, the most important ones are likely to be adenosine, other nucleotides, nitric oxide, prostaglandins, CO_2, and H^+. Adenosine, which is formed from adenosine triphosphate (ATP) and adenosine monophosphate (AMP) under conditions of ischemia and stress, is a potent vasodilator that links decreased perfusion to metabolically induced vasodilation or "reactive hyperemia." The

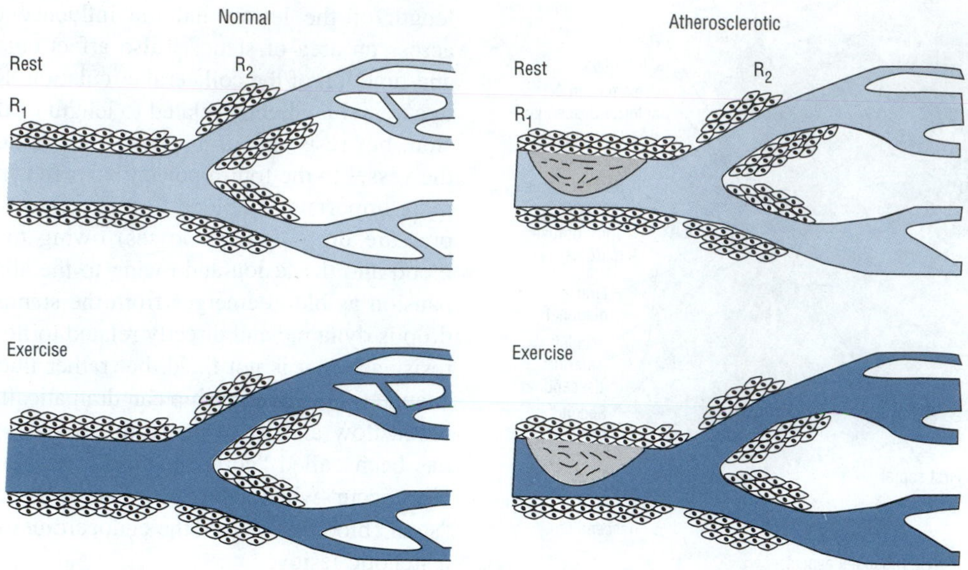

FIGURE 12–2. The coronary circulation with large epicardial conductance vessels (R_1) that offer little intrinsic resistance to myocardial blood flow and intramyocardial resistance arterioles (R_2). Resistance to flow equals $R_1 + R_2$ and R_2 resistance is normally much greater than R_1; hence flow is equal to the driving pressure across the coronary bed divided by the resistance in R_2. Dilatation in R_2 normally occurs in response to exercise or increased myocardial oxygen demand. When an atherosclerotic lesion narrows the conductance vessel, the arterioles dilate under resting conditions to prevent ischemia; however, with stress, the vasodilator reserve becomes limited. *(From Ref. 113, with permission.)*

synthesis and release of adenosine into coronary sinus venous effluent occurs within seconds after coronary artery occlusion, and about 30% of the hyperemic response can be blocked by metabolic blockers of adenosine.

ENDOTHELIAL CONTROL OF CORONARY VASCULAR TONE[11]

The vascular endothelium, a single-cell tissue with a enormous surface area separating the blood from vascular smooth muscle of the artery wall, is capable of a broad range of metabolic functions. In general, the endothelium should be considered as a protective surface for the artery wall, and as long as it remains intact and functional, it promotes vascular smooth muscle relaxation and inhibits thrombogenesis and atherosclerotic plaque formation; damaged endothelium reacts to numerous stimuli with vasoconstriction, thrombosis, and plaque formation. The vascular endothelium of the coronary arteries synthesizes large molecules such as fibronectin, interleukin-1, tissue plasminogen activator, and various growth factors. Small molecules that are also produced include prostacyclin, platelet-activating factor, endothelin-1, and endothelium-derived relaxing factor (EDRF) that is now characterized as nitric oxide. EDRF is synthesized from 1-arginine via nitric oxide synthase and released by shear force on the endothelium as well as through interaction with many biochemical stimuli such as acetylcholine, histamine, arginine, catecholamines, arachidonic acid, ADP, endothelin-1, bradykinin, serotonin, and thrombin. EDRF or nitric oxide then causes relaxation of the underlying smooth muscle and may be thought of as a paracrine homeopathic defense mechanism against noxious stimuli. Denudation or loss of the vascular endothelium results in loss of EDRF and this protective mechanism. Loss of the endothelial cell layer and function may occur secondary to physical disruption (percutaneous transluminal angioplasty, PTCA), factors impinging from the vascular side (cyanide from smoke), or disruption of the intimal-medial layers (oxidized low-density lipoprotein). Impaired endothelial function may be related to the development of premature atherosclerosis based on recent family studies.[11]

FACTORS EXTRINSIC TO THE VASCULAR BED

Blood flow to the coronary arteries arises from orifices located immediately distal to the aorta valve. Perfusion pressure is equal to the difference between the aortic pressure at an instantaneous point in time minus the intramyocardial pressure. Coronary vascular resistance is influenced by phasic systolic compression of the vascular bed. The driving force for perfusion is, therefore, not constant throughout the cardiac cycle. Opening of the aortic valve may also lead to a Venturi effect, which can slightly decrease perfusion pressure. If perfusion pressure is elevated for a period of time, coronary vascular resistance declines and blood flow increases; however, continued perfusion pressure increases lead, within limits, to a return of coronary blood flow back toward baseline levels through autoregulation.

Alterations in intramyocardial wall tension throughout the cardiac cycle will also impose significant changes in coronary blood flow. Diastole is the period during which coronary artery filling can occur due to these pressure differences and little or no coronary blood flow occurs to the left ventricle during systole. The extent of pressure development in the ventricle and heart rate have a major effect on the development of wall tension, time for diastolic coronary artery filling, and myocardial oxygen demand.

Under normal conditions, the average global distribution of blood flow between the epicardial and endocardial layer is about 1:1 at rest and remains approximately even during exercise secondary to autoregulatory changes. Regional disparity of blood flow distribution does exist normally, and these disparities are magnified in the presence of diseased coronary arteries and with increased cardiac work as the vasodilator reserve in the resistance vessels of the subendocardium layers is exhausted. Factors that favor a reduction in subendocardial blood flow include decreased perfusion pressure due to decreased diastolic blood pressure or coronary artery obstruction by atherosclerotic plaques with or without vasomotion, abbreviation of diastole (increased heart rate), and increased intraventricular diastolic pressure (e.g., valvular obstruction to flow).

Extravascular resistance may decrease coronary blood flow, primarily during systole. This effect is much more pronounced in the LV compared with the right ventricle (RV). When the effect of increased contractility is separated from the effect of ventricular pressure, about 75% of extravascular resistance is accounted for by passive stretch in equilibrium with ventricular pressure whereas only 25% results from active myocardial contraction.

FACTORS INTRINSIC TO THE VASCULAR BED

Metabolic factors, myogenic responses, neural reflexes, and humoral substances within the vascular bed of the coronary circulation function in an orchestrated fashion to maintain relative consistency in blood flow to the myocardium in the face of imposed changes in perfusion pressures. Autoregulation, mediated primarily through the effects of myogenic responses and metabolic factors, is thought to be responsible for maintaining regional blood flow in a narrow range while systemic pressure varies over a range of approximately 50 to 150 mm Hg.

Myogenic control (also known as the Bayliss effect) of coronary artery tone occurs when the vessel is stretched secondary to an increase in pressure and contracts to return blood flow to normal. It is thought that the myogenic response to stretching in coronary arteries is a modest one and that metabolic factors such as nitric oxide play a much larger role in autoregulation.

There are three well-studied metabolic factors that have the ability to modify coronary artery resistance and blood flow at the local level. Basal coronary blood flow meets oxygen demands of 8 to 10 mL/min per 100 g of myocardium with essentially complete extraction of oxygen from the blood. As cardiac output or mean arterial blood pressure increases, the increased demand for oxygen is met by increasing blood flow because little additional oxygen is available from hemoglobin. Decreased oxygen availability causes vasodilation of vascular smooth muscle and relaxation of precapillary sphincters, which increase tissue oxygen and help maintain blood flow on a regional basis.

At perfusion pressures below 60 mm Hg, as the coronary arteries are maximally dilated and the buffering effect of autoregulation has reached its capacity, further reduction in coronary blood flow will decrease perfusion pressure and tissue oxygenation. It is thought that autoregulation works more efficiently in the epicardial layers than in subendocardial layers, and this may contribute to coronary steal.

Neural components that participate in the regulation of coronary blood flow include the sympathetic nervous system, the parasympathetic nervous system, coronary reflexes, and possibly, central control of coronary blood flow. Within the sympathetic system, stimulation of the stellate ganglion elicits coronary vasodilation, which is associated with tachycardia and enhanced contractility. This indirect coronary vasodilation is secondary to increased $M\text{VO}_2$ related to increased heart rate, contractility, and aortic pressure and occurs following stellate stimulation. The direct effect of the sympathetic system is α_1-mediated vasoconstriction at rest and during exercise. Other receptor types, α_2 and β_1, have little influence on tone, whereas β_2 stimulation produces a modest vasodilatory effect. Although coronary atherosclerosis may decrease blood flow secondary to obstruction, severe coronary atherosclerosis and obstruction may also increase the sensitivity of coronary arteries to the effects of α_1 stimulation and vasoconstriction.

Vagal stimulation within the parasympathetic system produces a small to moderate increase in coronary blood flow, which involves the coronary efferent and afferent parasympathetic components (Bezold–Jarish reflex). Indirectly, vasoconstriction may result, with vagal stimulation as the result of bradycardia and decreased contractility reducing myocardial oxygen demand.

Coronary reflexes have an undetermined role in the regulation of coronary blood flow. Based on experimental data, coronary reflexes that may be important include the baroreceptor, the chemoreceptor, Bezold–Jarish reflex, and the pulmonary inhalation reflex.

FACTORS LIMITING CORONARY PERFUSION

During exercise and pacing, as $M\text{VO}_2$ increases, coronary vascular resistance can be reduced to about 25% of basal values, which results in a fourfold to fivefold increase in coronary blood flow. The cross-sectional area can be reduced by about 80% prior to any mechanical or biochemical changes in the myocardium, reflecting a margin of safety for coronary blood flow. The extent of cross-sectional obstruction, the length of the lesion, lesion composition, and the geometry of the obstructing lesion can each affect flow across coronary arteries with atherosclerosis. Bernoulli's theorem states that the pressure drop across a lesion is directly related to the length of the lesion and inversely related to the radius of the lesion to the fourth power; critical stenosis occurs when the obstructing lesion encroaches on the luminal diameter and exceeds 70% to 80%. Lesions creating obstruction of 50% to 70% may reduce blood flow; however, these obstructions are not consistent and vasospasm and thrombosis superimposed on a "noncritical" lesion may lead to clinical events such as myocardial infarction. If the lesion enlarges from 80% to 90%, resistance in that vessel is tripled. Coronary reserve is diminished at about 85% obstruction owing to vasoconstriction. Exaggerated responsiveness can be seen when coronary stenosis reaches this critical level and the role of vasoactive substances such as prostaglandins, thromboxanes, and serotonin may play more of a role in the regulation of coronary vascular tone and thrombosis.

Little reserve exists for coronary blood flow and a relatively small reduction of 10% to 20% results in decreased myocardial fiber shortening as the first evidence for abnormal function. The subendocardial layers are affected to a greater extent than the epicardium by ischemia, considering changes in fiber shortening, arteriovenous (AV) difference in oxygen saturation, and lactate production. A reduction of 80% gives rise to akinesis and a 95% reduction of coronary blood flow produces dyskinesis during contraction of the ventricles. Although these abnormalities of contraction are associated with transient impaired function, depletion of high-energy phosphate compounds and ultrastructural changes may last for days even after transient ischemia; this has been referred to as "stunned myocardium." Chronic hypoperfusion may lead to "hibernation," in which ventricular function is impaired over longer time intervals. Hibernating myocardium can be differentiated from necrosis with various techniques (see Chap. 10) and revascularization of hibernating myocardium is useful in improving ventricular function. Regional loss of contractility may impose a burden on the remaining myocardial tissue, resulting in heart failure, increased $M\dot{V}O_2$, and rapid depletion of oxygen stores. Consequently, zones of tissue with marginal blood flow may develop in a lateral or transmural fashion; such development puts this tissue at risk for more severe damage if the ischemic episode persists or becomes more severe. Nonischemic areas of myocardium may compensate for the severely ischemic and border zones of ischemia by developing more tension than usual in an attempt to maintain cardiac output. At the cellular level, ischemia and the attendant acidosis are thought to alter calcium release from storage sites such as the sarcolemma and the sarcoplasmic reticulum as well as inhibiting the binding of calcium to troponin, thereby impairing the association of actin and myosin. The clinical correlates of these cellular biochemical events leading to the development of LV or RV dysfunction include an S_3, dyspnea, orthopnea, tachycardia, fluctuating blood pressure, transient murmurs, and mitral or tricuspid regurgitation.

Calcium accumulation and overload secondary to ischemia impairs ventricular relaxation as well as contraction. This is apparently a result of impaired calcium uptake after systole from the myofilaments, leading to a less negative decline of the pressure in the ventricle over time. Impaired relaxation is associated with enhanced diastolic stiffness, decreased rate of wall thinning, and slowed pressure decay, producing an upward shift in the ventricular pressure–volume relationship; put more simply, $M\dot{V}O_2$ is likely to be increased secondary to increased wall tension. Impairment of both diastolic and systolic function leads to elevation of the filling pressure of the left ventricle.

CLINICAL PRESENTATION AND DIAGNOSIS

The classical symptoms associated with typical chest pain and angina caused by IHD appear in Table 12–4. Important aspects of the clinical history for chest pain in patients with angina include the nature or quality of the pain, precipitating factors, duration, pain radiation, and the response to nitroglycerin or rest. Because there can be considerable variation in the manifestations of angina, it is more accurate to refer to these symptoms as an anginal syndrome. For some patients with significant coronary disease, their presenting symptoms may differ from the classical symptoms, yet the symptoms

TABLE 12–4. Characteristics of Angina Pectoris

Quality
Sensation of pressure or heavy weight on the chest
Burning sensation
Feeling of tightness
Shortness of breath with feeling of constriction about the larynx or upper trachea
Visceral quality (deep, heavy, squeezing, aching)
Gradual increase in intensity followed by gradual fading away
Location
Over the sternum or very near to it
Anywhere between epigastrium and pharynx
Occasionally limited to left shoulder and left arm
Rarely limited to right arm
Limited to lower jaw
Lower cervical or upper thoracic spine
Left interscapular or suprascapular area
Duration
0.5–30 min
Precipitating factors
Relationship to exercise
Effort that involves use of arms above the head
Cold environment
Walking against the wind
Walking after a large meal
Emotional factors involved with physical exercise
Fright, anger
Coitus
Nitroglycerin relief
Relief of pain occurring within 45 s to 5 min of taking nitroglycerin
Radiation
Medial aspect of left arm
Left shoulder
Jaw
Occasionally right arm

From Ref. 114, with permission.

are due to ischemic pain, and these are often referred to as anginal equivalents. Obtaining an accurate and detailed family history is useful in placing symptoms in perspective. Significant positive information includes premature coronary heart disease (< 55 years in men and < 65 years in women) as manifested as fatal and nonfatal MI, stroke, peripheral vascular disease as well as other risk factors such as hypertension, smoking, familial lipid disorders, and diabetes mellitus. Typical pain radiation patterns include anterior chest pain (96%), left upper arm pain (83.7%), left lower arm pain (29.3%), and neck pain at some time (22%). Pain from other areas is less common. Ischemia detected by ECG monitoring is more likely to be detected in the morning hours (6 AM to 12 noon) than other periods throughout the day. Patients suffering from variant or Prinzmetal's angina secondary to coronary spasm are more likely to experience pain at rest and in the early morning hours, and the pain is not usually brought on by exertion or emotional stress nor relieved by rest; the ECG pattern is that of current injury with ST elevation rather than depression.

It is also important to differentiate the pattern of pain for stable angina from that of unstable angina. The definition of unstable angina is controversial, but includes the presence of one or more of the following: (1) new onset (< 2 months) exertional angina of at least Canadian Cardiovascular Society Classification (CCSC) class III (Table 12–3) in severity; (2) recent (< 2 months) acceleration of angina as reflected by an increase in severity of at least one CCSC class to at least CCSC class III; or (3) pain at rest which lasts for more than 20 minutes.[12,13] Ischemia may also be painless or "silent" in 60% to 100% of patients depending on the series cited and the patient population.[14,15] In patients with myocardial ischemia, approximately 70% of the episodes of documented ischemia are painless as determined by ambulatory ECG monitoring, and the ST segment changes associated with these episodes can be ST elevation or depression. The mechanism of silent ischemia is unclear, but studies have shown that patients not experiencing pain have altered pain perception, with the threshold and tolerance for pain being higher than that of patients who have pain more frequently. Although diabetics tend to have more extensive coronary disease than nondiabetics and may suffer from autonomic neuropathy, asymptomatic ischemia is not more prevalent based on the Asymptomatic Cardiac Ischemia Pilot (ACIP) study.[16] Reduced endorphin release is a plausible explanation but investigations with naloxone to block endorphins do not consistently show altered pain thresholds to various stimuli compared with patients with sympotmatic ischemia.[17] Alternatively, adenosine and substance P release during ischemia and mechanical stretch on coronary arteries may play a role in the perception of pain.

TABLE 12–5. Differential Diagnosis of Episodic Chest Pain Resembling Angina Pectoris

	Duration	Quality	Provocation	Relief	Location	Comment
Effort angina	5–15 min	Visceral (pressure)	During effort or emotion	Rest, NTG	Substernal, radiates	First episode vivid
Rest angina	5–15 min	Visceral (pressure)	Spontaneous (? with exercise)	NTG	Substernal, radiates	Often nocturnal
Mitral prolapse	Min–h	Superficial (rarely visceral)	Spontaneous (no pattern)	Time	Left anterior	No pattern, variable
Esophageal reflux	10 min–1 h	Visceral	Spontaneous, cold liquids, exercise, lying down	Foods, antacids, H_2-blockers and proton pump inhibitors, NTG	Substernal, radiates	Mimics angina
Peptic ulcer	H	Visceral, burning	Lack of food, "acid" foods	Foods, antacids, H_2-blockers and proton pump inhibitors	Epigastric, substernal	
Biliary disease	H	Visceral (wax and wane)	Spontaneous, food	Time, analgesia	Epigastric, radiates	Colic
Cervical disc	Variable (gradually subsides)	Superficial	Head and neck, movement and palpation	Time, analgesia	Arm, neck	Not relieved by rest
Hyperventilation	2–3 min	Visceral	Emotion, tachypnea	Stimulus removed	Substernal	Facial paraesthesia
Musculoskeletal	Variable	Superficial	Movement, palpation	Time, analgesia	Multiple	Tenderness
Pulmonary	30 min	Visceral (pressure)	Often spontaneous	Rest, time bronchodilator	Substernal	Dyspneic

Last, it should be recognized that the threshold for pain owing to exertion is fixed in some patients and variable in others and that the amount of exercise or stress necessary to provoke symptoms can change over time. A fixed threshold for the induction of pain or ECG evidence of ischemia means these indicators of ischemia occur at the same, or nearly so, double rate–pressure product. This is apparently owing to at least two factors. Over long periods of time atherosclerosis may progress, leading to more severe stenosis, reduced oxygen supply, and less of an increase in demand to precipitate ischemic symptoms. Once stenotic lesions reach a critical level of about 80% or greater, vasomotion, vasospasm, and thrombotic occlusion become significant factors impairing blood flow to the myocardium. Consequently, anatomic considerations and vasoactive substances may interact to provide an environment amenable to changing thresholds for the production of angina.

There appears to be little relationship between the historical features of angina and the severity or extent of coronary artery vessel involvement. Therefore, one may speculate that severe symptoms might be associated with multivessel disease, but no predictive markers exist on a routine basis.

Chest pain may resemble pain arising from a variety of noncardiac sources and the differential diagnosis of anginal pain from other etiologies may be quite difficult based on history alone. Table 12–5 outlines other common problems that may present with episodic chest pain. Although much less common, nonatherosclerotic etiologies of coronary artery disease do exist and should be excluded with appropriate tests.

There are few signs apparent on physical examination to indicate the presence of coronary artery disease and usually only the cardiovascular system reveals any useful information. Elevated heart rate or blood pressure can yield an increased double product and may be associated with angina, and it would be important to correct extreme tachycardia or hypertension if present. Other noncardiac physical findings that suggest that significant cardiovascular disease may be associated with angina include abdominal aortic aneurysms or peripheral vascular disease. A controversial finding is that of a diagonal ear lobe crease, which is said by some to be associated with significant coronary disease. Findings on the cardiac examination that may be seen in patients with coronary artery disease are noted in Table 12–6. During an angina attack these findings may appear or become more prominent, making them more valuable if present.

Other than risk-factor screening, there are no specific laboratory tests that are useful in diagnosing coronary artery disease. Lipid profiling with total cholesterol, high-density cholesterol, lipoprotein (a), and triglycerides will identify individuals susceptible to atherosclerosis. Of particular importance, total cholesterol concentrations of greater than 280 mg/dL are associated with multivessel disease and should be aggressively treated with diet and possibly drug therapy (see Chap. 19). Knowledge of other lipoprotein fractions is useful to select appropriate therapy but they have little predictive value for IHD. Fasting glucose determinations to exclude diabetes and glucose monitoring for concurrent diabetes should be performed routinely. Other risk factors that may be important for some patients include homocysteine level, evidence of chylamdia infection, low levels of endogenous antioxidants, and elevations in lipoprotein (a), fibrinogen, and plasminogen activator inhibitor.[18] Cardiac enzymes, creatine phosphokinase (CPK), lactate dehydrogenase (LDH), and serum glutamic-oxaloacetic transaminase (SGOT) should all be normal in the angina patient. Troponin T may be elevated in patients

TABLE 12–6. Cardiac Findings in Patients with Coronary Artery Disease

Sign	Clinical Significance	Frequency
Abnormal precordial systolic bulge	Left ventricular wall motion abnormality	Not usually present unless patient has sustained a prior MI (especially anterior wall) or is experiencing angina at time of examination
Decreased intensity of S_1	Decrease in left ventricular contractility	Difficult to evaluate in resting state, but can be commonly demonstrated during angina
Paradoxical splitting of S_2	Left ventricular wall motion abnormality	Very uncommon but occasionally noted during angina
S_3 (ventricular gallop)	Increased left ventricular diastolic pressure, with or without clinical CHF	Not usually present unless patient sustained extensive MI; may occasionally be present during angina
S_4 (atrial gallop)	Reduced ventricular compliance ("stiff heart")	Common; very common in patients who have sustained a prior MI as well as during angina
Apical systolic murmur (in absence of rheumatic mitral regurgitation or Barlow's syndome	Papillary muscle dysfunction	Not usually present unless patient has sustained prior MI
Diastolic murmur (in absence of aortic regurgitation)	Coronary artery stenosis	Rare

Abbreviations: S_1 = first heart sound; S_2 = second heart sound; S_3 = third heart sound; S_4 = fourth heart sound; MI = myocardial infarction.
From Ref. 115, with permission.

with unstable angina, and interventions such as anticoagulation have been shown to reduce cardiac end points when this marker for injury is elevated.[19] Chest x-ray findings of coronary artery calcification will be associated with critical stenosis in 90% of patients, but there is little correlation to clinical manifestations.

DIAGNOSTIC TESTS

See also Chap. 8, Cardiovascular Testing.

ELECTROCARDIOGRAM

The ECG is normal in about one-half of patients with angina who are not experiencing an acute attack. Typical ST-T-wave changes include depression, T-wave inversion, and ST-segment elevation. Forms of ischemia other than exertional angina may have ECG manifestations that are different; variant angina is associated with ST-segment elevation whereas silent ischemia may produce elevation or depression. Significant ischemia is associated with ST-segment depression of greater than 2 mm, exertional hypotension, and reduced exercise tolerance.

EXERCISE TOLERANCE TESTING

Exercise tolerance (stress) testing (ETT) is useful for a history of chest pain that is equivocal, for risk stratification, for implementation of medical versus surgical therapy, and to assess the efficacy of treatment. Although ETT is insensitive for predicting coronary artery anatomy, it does correlate well with outcome owing to IHD such as the likelihood of progressing to angina, the occurrence of acute MI, and cardiovascular death.[16] Ischemic ST depression that occurs during ETT is an independent risk factor for cardiac events and cardiovascular mortality. Thallium (^{201}Tl) myocardial perfusion scintigraphy may be used in conjunction with ETT to detect reversible and irreversible defects in blood flow to the myocardium because it is more sensitive than ETT.

CARDIAC IMAGING

Radionuclide angiocardiography (performed with technetium-99^{m}, a radioisotope) is used to measure ejection fraction, regional ventricular performance, cardiac output, ventricular volumes, valvular regurgitation, asynchrony or wall motion abnormalities, and intracardiac shunts. Technetium pyrophosphate scans are used routinely for detection and quantification of acute myocardial infarction (see Chap. 13). Positron emission tomography (PET) is useful for quantifying ischemia with metabolically important substrates such as oxygen, carbon, and nitrogen. Other metabolic probes use radiolabeled fatty acids and glucose to study metabolic processes that may be deranged during ischemia in animals and for investigative purposes in man.

A new method using ultra-rapid computerized tomography (cine-CT, ultrafast CT, electron beam CT) minimized artifact owing to motion of the heart during contraction and relaxation and provides a semiquantitative assessment of calcium content in coronary arteries.[20] If calcium is detected, then coronary disease is suspected; if no calcium is present, then coronary artery disease is unlikely.

ECHOCARDIOGRAPHY

Echocardiography has been shown to be useful for direct visualization of lesions in the left main coronary artery and in providing information concerning some of the complications of IHD, including the presence of ventricular aneurysms, and assessing ejection fraction as well as detecting regional or global LV function abnormalities or hypertrophy or associated valvular lesions. In patients unable to exercise, pharmacologic stress echocardiography (dobutamine, dipyridamole, or adenosine) or pacing may be done to identify abnormalities during stress.

AMBULATORY ELECTROCARDIOGRAPHIC (HOLTER MONITORING)

Ambulatory ECG monitoring is useful in detecting ischemia during symptomatic and asymptotic episodes and provides information for an extended period of time. This approach allows estimation of the total ischemic burden of the myocardium rather than only reported episodes of angina.

CARDIAC CATHETERIZATION AND CORONARY ARTERIOGRAPHY

Cardiac catheterization and angiography in patients with suspected coronary artery disease are used diagnostically to document the presence and severity of disease as well as for prognostic purposes. High-risk features during ETT suggesting the need for coronary arteriography include early and significant ($\geq$ 2 mm) changes on the ECG during ETT as well as multiple lead involvement, prolonged recovery from ischemia, low workload performance, abnormal blood pressure response (reduction in blood pressure), or ventricular arrhythmias. Multiple defects with thallium scans as well as lung uptake during exercise or postexercise ventricular cavity dilation are also high-risk indications for catheterization. Interventional catheterization is used for thrombolytic therapy in patients with acute myocardial infarction and for the management of patients with significant coronary artery disease to relieve obstruction through percutaneous transluminal anzioplasty (PTCA), atherectomy, or stent placement. Catheterization and arteriography may be done after coronary artery bypass grafting (CABG) to determine if the graft has closed or if coronary artery disease has progressed. Coronary artery intravascular ultrasound is useful for directly imaging anatomy, calcified and fatty plaques, and thrombosis superimposed on plaque as well as determining patency following revascularization procedures.[21]

▶ TREATMENT: Ischemic Heart Disease

MODIFICATION OF RISK FACTORS

Primary prevention of ischemic heart disease through the identification and modification of risk factors prior to the initial morbid event would be the optimal management approach and should result in a significant impact on the prevalence of IHD. However, early recognition of some risk factors may not be possible in all cases, and in others, the patient may not be willing to undertake intervention until overt evidence of coronary disease is apparent. Secondary intervention continues to be more commonly pursued by both health care professionals and patients, and it is important to recognize this type of intervention as effective in reducing subsequent morbidity and mortality. The presence of risk factors in individual patients plays a major role in determining the occurrence and severity of IHD.[22] Risk factors are additive in nature and can be classified as alterable or unalterable (see Table 12–7). Unalterable risk factors include gender; age; family history or genetic composition; environmental influences such as climate, air pollution, trace metal composition of drinking water; and to some extent, diabetes mellitus. Improved glycemic control reduces the microvascular complications of diabetes mellitus (see Chapter 70, Diabetes Mellitus) and reduces coronary end points; however, based on the Diabetes Control and Complications study, the reduction was impressive (40 vs 23 major events) but not significant because the trial was underpowered to detect these changes.[23] Risk factors that can be altered include smoking, hypertension, hyperlipidemia, obesity, sedentary life-style, hyperuricemia, psychosocial factors such as stress and type A behavior patterns, and the use of certain drugs that may be detrimental including progestins, corticosteroids, cyclosporine, thiazide diuretics, and β-adrenergic blocking agents.

Cigarette smoking is common; some 50 million people are regular smokers in this country, and the evidence for increased coronary mortality of smokers over nonsmokers of twofold to threefold is unequivocal.[7] Of the 325,000 premature deaths each year due to smoking, one-third are due to coronary heart disease. Risk due to smoking is related to the number of cigarettes smoked per day and the duration of smoking; however, even nonsmokers may be affected: passive smoking in angina pectoris patients has been shown to decrease exercise time.[4,24] Pipe and cigar smokers are at increased risk compared with nonsmokers, but their risk is somewhat less than that of cigarette smokers.[25] The direct effects of cigarette smoke that are detrimental to patients with angina include (1) elevated heart rate and blood pressure from nicotine, which increases MVO_2, and impaired myocardial oxygen delivery owing to carboxyhemoglobin generation from carbon monoxide inhalation in smoke; (2) the negative inotropic effect of carboxyhemoglobin; (3) increased platelet adhesiveness and promotion of aggregation resulting in thrombotic tendencies owing to nicotine and carboxyhemoglobin; (4) lowered threshold for ventricular fibrillation during ischemia owing to carboxyhemoglobin; and (5) impaired endothelial function owing to smoking.[26,27] Similar changes have been noted for marihuana smoking as well. Smoking also accelerates the risk for myocardial infarction, sudden death, cerebrovascular disease, peripheral vascular disease, and hypertension, and it reduces high-density lipoprotein concentrations. Clearly, primary prevention is needed for this risk factor and much of the education effort to discourage initiation of smoking should be targeted for teenagers. Techniques for cessation of smoking that may be useful include aversive conditioning, group programs, self-help programs, hypnosis, "cold turkey," and the use of nicotine substitutes (lobeline) or other sources of nicotine (Nicorette chewing gum and transdermal nicotine systems) for short-term substitution during withdrawal syndrome. Cessation of smoking reduces the incidence of coronary events to about one-half of that associated with continued smoking and these benefits are noted within 2 years of cessation.

Hypertension, whether labile or fixed, borderline or definite, casual or basal, systolic or diastolic, at any age regardless of gender, is the most common and a powerful contributor to atherosclerotic coronary vascular disease.[28] Morbidity and mortality increase progressively with the degree of blood pressure elevation of either systolic or diastolic pressure, and no discernible critical value exists (see Chapter 10, Hypertension). Numerous trials have documented the reduction in risk associated with blood pressure lowering; however, most of these studies show that mortality and morbidity reduction is a result of fewer strokes and less renal failure and heart failure. The reduction in coronary heart disease end points is significant but not as dramatic.[29] The reasons for this are unclear but perhaps relate to the multifactorial etiology of IHD.

Hypercholesterolemia is a significant cardiovascular risk factor, and risk is directly related to the degree of cholesterol elevation.[22] As with hypertension, there is no critical value that defines risk, but rather, risk is incrementally related to the degree of elevation and the presence of other risk factors (see Chapter 19, Hyperlipidemia for a detailed discussion). The role of triglycerides in coronary artery disease remains a controversial issue; however, most would agree that gross elevations, greater than 500 mg/dL, should be treated. A fasting lipoprotein panel should be obtained in all patients with known coronary artery disease (CAD). All patients should be on a Step I or II American Heart Association diet based on the presence or absence of CAD and the number of risk factors. The goals for lipid reduction in primary and secondary intervention are described in Chapter 19. Reductions in LDL cholesterol for primary prevention and secondary intervention have been shown to reduce total and CAD mortality as well as the need for interventions such as PTCA and CABG. Supplemental vitamin E or other antioxidants reduce the susceptibility of LDL cholesterol to oxidation and may retard or reduce the risk of atherosclerosis.[30,31]

TABLE 12–7. Risk Factors for Coronary Heart Disease

Positive risk factors
Age
Men: ≥ 45 years
Women: ≥ 55 years or premature menopause without estrogen replacement therapy
Family history of premature CHD (definite myocardial infarction or sudden death before 55 years of age in father or other male first-degree relative, or before 65 years of age in mother or other female first-degree relative)
Total and LDL cholesterol—ratio to HDL cholesterol may also be used
Current cigarette smoking
Hypertension (≥ 140/90 mm Hg or on antihypertensive medication)
Low HDL cholesterol (< 35 mg/dL)
Diabetes mellitus
Negative risk factor
High HDL cholesterol (≥ 60 mg/dL)

Based on recommendations provided by Ref. 22.

The prevalence of obesity, defined as greater than 20% over ideal body weight, ranges from 7.4% to 17% in men and from 9.6% to 34.7% in women in this country. Body mass index, weight (kg) divided by height (m) squared, greater than about 32 is associated with an increased mortality ratio compared with individuals of normal body weight, and the objective for patients with IHD is to maintain or reduce to a normal body weight. This may be accomplished through dietary modification, exercise, pharmacologic therapy, or surgical therapy. Frequently associated with obesity is a sedentary life-style, and inactivity may contribute to higher blood pressure, elevated blood lipid levels, and insulin resistance associated with glucose intolerance in diabetics (insulin resistance syndrome). Exercise to the level of about 300 kcal three times a week is useful in improving maximal oxygen uptake, improving cardiorespiratory efficiency, promoting collateral artery formation, and promoting potential alterations in the risk of ventricular fibrillation, coronary thrombosis, and improved tolerance to stress. Although a regular exercise program may not prevent the occurrence of IHD, participants feel better and their overall cardiovascular risk may be reduced.

Competitiveness, intense striving for achievement, easily provoked hostility, a sense of urgency about doing things quickly and being punctual, impatience, abrupt and rapid speech and gestures, and concentration on self-selected goals to the point of not perceiving and attending to other aspects of the environment are traits that characterize the behavioral pattern known as the type A or coronary prone personality. Although the issue is somewhat controversial, type A individuals may have increased cardiovascular risk with risk ratios ranging from insignificant to three times that of a matched population. The mechanism by which personality affects the cardiovascular system is not understood, but may reflect the activity of the sympathetic system and enhanced responsiveness of other stress hormones when compared with non-type A personalities. Gout or hyperuricemia appears to be indirectly atherogenic, an effect most likely mediated through associated hypertension, hyperlipidemia, and obesity. Attempts at normalizing uric acid levels are rational and may alter the risk of cardiovascular disease.

Alcohol ingestion in small to moderate amounts (< 40 g/d of pure ethanol) reduces the risk of coronary heart disease; however, consumption of large amounts (> 50 g/d) or binge drinking of alcohol is associated with increased mortality from stroke, malignant neoplasms, vehicular accidents, and cirrhosis. The mechanisms for the presumed protective effects of alcohol are not known but the effects may be related to increased high-density lipoprotein levels, impaired platelet function, or associations between the amount of alcohol ingested and personality type. Whatever the relationship, it is well to remember that alcohol drinking is implicated in over 40% of all fatal automobile accidents and consumption of alcohol predisposes to hepatic cirrhosis, the sixth to seventh most common cause of death in middle age in the United States. With this in mind, it seems illogical to suggest alcohol ingestion as a prophylactic measure for coronary disease but rather advise moderation of alcohol consumption, if it is the preference of the individual.

Thiazide diuretics have been shown to elevate serum cholesterol and triglyceride levels whereas β-blockers tend to lower HDL and raise LDL slightly; however, a direct association between these drugs and cardiovascular risk is tenuous and based on aggregating results rather than randomized clinical trials. Conjugated equine estrogen alone or in combination with a progestin lowers LDL and raises HDL based on the Postmenopausal Estrogen/Progestin Interventions (PEPI) study.[32] Unopposed estrogen is the optimal regimen for elevation of HDL, but the high rate of endometrial hyperplasia restricts use to women without a uterus. In women with a uterus, estrogen with cyclic medroxyprogesterone has the most favorable effect on HDL and no excess risk of endometrial hyperplasia. Other mechanisms for cardiovascular protection with estrogens include restoration of endothelial function and reduced oxidation of LDL cholesterol.[32] Use of oral contraceptives in women who smoke and are over the age of 35 years increases the risk of myocardial infarction, stroke, and venous thromboembolism by threefold or higher. Alternative forms of contraception and cessation of smoking should be promoted in these patients. The risk for nonsmoking oral contraceptive users under the age of 35 is very small. Estrogen replacement therapy (ERT) in the observational Nurses' Health Study reduced the risk of death in current or previous users of ERT compared with never users.[33] In women with a uterus, concurrent progestins (HRT) should be used to offset the risk of endometrial carcinoma. The relative risk of breast cancer is increased but in the absence of risk factors for breast cancer, the relative risk is approximately 1.3 (30% increase). Coffee consumption has also been linked to coronary heart disease and caffeine does transiently elevate blood pressure; however, the overall risk, if any, appears to be low. Although thiazide diuretics and β-blockers (nonselective without intrinsic sympathomimetic activity) may elevate both cholesterol and triglycerides by some 10% to 20%, and these effects may be detrimental, no objective evidence exists from prospective well-controlled studies to support avoiding these drugs at this time.[29] This controversy is most pertinent in the treatment of mild hypertension and it is discussed in greater detail in Chapter 10, Hypertension.

PHARMACOLOGIC THERAPY[34]

PLACEBO EFFECT

Historically, about 30% of anginal syndrome symptoms have responded regardless of which therapy was instituted. Examples of these placebo responses include drug therapies such as xanthines and khellin, as well as surgical procedures such as ligation of the internal mammary artery. These observations stem from two problems inherent in clinical trials undertaken to assess the efficacy of any therapy for angina: (1) adequate trial design incorporating appropriate controls and washout periods, and (2) assessment of treatment effects using objective measures of efficacy including improvement in exercise performance, resting and ambulatory ECG improvement in ischemic changes, or other objective tests to address other aspects of myocardial function or metabolism. The use of pain episode frequency and nitroglycerin consumption is subjective, and their use as sole measures of efficacy should be avoided. Objective assessment using ETT has shown that placebo does not provide improvement in patients with exertional angina, substantiating this as a valid means to assess efficacy.

β-ADRENERGIC BLOCKING AGENTS[35]

Decreased heart rate, decreased contractility, and a slight to moderate decrease in blood pressure with β-adrenergic receptor antagonism reduce $M\dot{V}O_2$. The predominant receptor type in the heart is the β_1-receptor, and competitive blockade minimizes the influence of endogenous catecholamines on the chronotropic and inotropic state of the myocardium. These beneficial effects may be countered to some degree with increased ventricular volume and ejection time seen with β-blockade; however, the overall effect of β-blockers in patients with effort-induced angina is a reduction in oxygen demand (Table 12–8). The β-blockers do not improve oxygen supply, and in certain instances, unopposed α-adrenergic stimulation following the use of β-blockers may lead to coronary vasoconstriction. For patients with chronic exertional stable angina, β-blockers improve symptoms about 80% of the time and objective measures of efficacy demonstrate improved exercise duration and delay in the time at which

TABLE 12–8. Effect of Drug Therapy on Myocardial Oxygen Demand[a]

			LV[b] Wall Tension	
	Heart Rate	Myocardial Contractility	*Systolic Pressure*	*LV Volume*
Nitrates	⇑	0	⇓	⇓⇓
β-Blockers	⇓⇓	⇓	⇓	⇑
Nifedipine	⇑	0 or ⇓	⇓⇓	0 or ⇓
Verapamil	⇓	⇓	⇓	0 or ⇓
Diltiazem	⇓⇓	0 or ⇓	⇓	0 or ⇓

[a]Calcium channel antagonists and nitrates may also increase myocardial oxygen supply through coronary vasodilation. Diastolic function may also be improved with verapamil, nifedipine, and, perhaps, diltiazem. These effects may vary from those indicated in the table depending on individual patient baseline hemodynamics.
[b]LV = left ventricular.

ST-segment changes and initial or limiting symptoms occur. β-Blockers do not alter the rate–pressure product (double product) for maximal exercise, therefore substantiating reduced demand rather than improved supply as the major consequence of their actions. Reflex tachycardia from nitrate therapy can be blunted with β-blocker therapy, making this a common and useful combination. Some patients with preexisting LV dysfunction who would be prone to heart failure may receive digitalis glycosides to maintain cardiac output if β-blockade is necessary for IHD. Although β-blockade may decrease exercise capacity in healthy individuals or in patients with hypertension, it may allow angina patients previously limited by symptoms to perform more exercise and ultimately improve overall cardiovascular performance through a training effect. Ideal candidates for β-blockers include patients in whom physical activity figures prominently in their anginal attacks, those who have coexistent hypertension, those with a history of supraventricular arrhythmias or post-MI angina, and those who have a component of anxiety associated with angina.[36]

Pertinent pharmacokinetics for the β-blockers include half-life and route elimination, which are reviewed in Chapter 10. Drugs with longer half-lives need to be dosed less frequently than ones with shorter half-lives; however, disparity exists between half-life and duration of action for several β-blockers (e.g., metoprolol) and this may reflect attenuation of the central nervous system–mediated effects on the sympathetic system as well as the direct effects of this category on heart rate and contractility. Renal and hepatic dysfunction can affect the disposition of β-blockers, but these agents are dosed to effect, either hemodynamic or symptomatic, and route of elimination is not a major consideration in drug selection.

Guidelines for the use of β-blockers in treating angina include the objective of lowering resting heart rate to 50 to 60 beats per minute and limiting maximal exercise heart rate to about 100 beats per minute or less. It has also been suggested that exercise heart rate should be no more than about 20 beats per minute or a 10% increment over resting heart rate with modest exercise. Because β-blockade is competitive and circulating catecholamine concentrations vary depending on the intensity of exercise and other factors, and cholinergic tone may be important in controlling heart rate in some patients, these guidelines are general in nature. These effects are generally dose and plasma concentration related, and for propranolol, plasma concentrations of 30 ng/mL are needed for a 25% reduction of anginal frequency. Initial doses of β-blockers should be at the lower end of the usual dosing range and titrated to response as indicated above.

There is little evidence to suggest superiority of any β-blocker; however, the duration of β-blockade is dependent partially on the half-life of the agent used, and those with longer half-lives may be dosed less frequently.[1] Of note, propranolol may be dosed twice a day in most patients with angina and the efficacy is similar to that seen with more frequent dosing. The ancillary property of membrane stabilizing activity is irrelevant in the treatment of angina, and intrinsic sympathomimetic activity appears to be detrimental in patients with rest or severe angina because the reduction in heart rate would be minimized, therefore limiting a reduction in MVO_2. Cardioselective β-blockers may be used in some patients to minimize adverse effects such as bronchospasm in asthmatic or chronic obstructive pulmonary disease patients, intermittent claudication, and sexual dysfunction. It should be remembered that cardioselectivity is a relative property and the use of larger doses (e.g., metoprolol 200 mg/d) is associated with the loss of selectivity and with adverse effects. Post-acute-MI patients with angina are particularly good candidates for β-blockade both because anginal symptoms may be treated as well as reducing the risk of post-MI reinfarction, and because mortality has been demonstrated with timolol, propranolol, and metoprolol (see Chap. 13). Combined β- (nonselective) and α-blockade with labetolol may be useful in some patients with marginal LV reserve, and fewer deleterious effects on coronary blood flow are seen when compared with other β-blockers.

Extension of pharmacologic effect is the underlying reason for many of the adverse effects seen with β-blockade. Hypotension, heart failure, bradycardia and heart block, bronchospasm, peripheral vasoconstriction and intermittent claudication, and altered glucose metabolism are directly related to β-adrenoreceptor antagonism. Patients with preexisting LV dysfunction and the use of other negative inotropic agents are most prone to developing overt heart failure, and in the absence of these, heart failure is uncommon (less than 5%). Other drugs that depress conduction are additive to β-blockade, and intrinsic conduction system disease predisposes the patient to conduction abnormalities. Altered glucose metabolism is most likely to be seen in insulin-dependent diabetics, and β-blockade obscures the symptoms of hypoglycemia except for sweating. β-Blockers may also aggravate the lipid abnormalities seen in patients with diabetes; however, these changes are dose related, are more common with normal baseline lipids than dyslipidemia, and may be of short-term significance only. One of the more common reasons for discontinuation of β-blocker therapy is related to central nervous system adverse effects of fatigue, malaise, and depression. Cognition changes seen with β-blockers are usually minimal and comparable to other categories of drugs based on studies done in hypertension.[37,38] Abrupt withdrawal of β-blocker therapy in patients with angina has been associated with increased severity and number of pain episodes and myocardial infarction. The mechanism of this effect is unknown but may be related to increased receptor sensitivity or disease progression during therapy, which becomes apparent following discontinuation of β-blockade. In any event, tapering of β-blocker therapy over about 2 days should minimize the risk of withdrawal reactions for those patients in whom therapy is being discontinued.

β-Adrenoreceptor blockade is effective in chronic exertional angina as monotherapy and in combination with nitrates and/or calcium channel antagonists. β-Blockers should be the first-line drug in chronic angina requiring daily maintenance therapy because β-blockers are more effective in reducing episodes of silent ischemia, reducing early morning peak of ischemic activity, and improving mortality after Q-wave MI than nitrates or calcium channel blockers. If β-blockers are ineffective or not tolerated, then monotherapy with a calcium channel blocker or combination therapy if monotherapy is ineffective for either alone may be instituted. Patients with severe angina, rest angina, or variant angina (i.e., a component of coronary artery spasm) may be better treated with calcium channel blockers.

NITRATES[39,40]

Nitroglycerin has a well-documented role in the alleviation of anginal attacks when used as rapidly absorbed and readily available preparations by the oral and intravenous routes (see Table 12–9). Sublingual, buccal, or spray products are the products of choice for this indication. Prevention of symptoms may be accomplished by the prophylactic use of oral or transdermal products; however, recent concern has been expressed over the long-term efficacy of many of these preparations and the development of tolerance.

Nitrates have multiple potential mechanisms of action, and for a given patient it is not always clear which of these is most important. In general, the major action appears to be indirectly mediated through a reduction of myocardial oxygen demand secondary to venodilation and arterial–arteriolar dilation, leading to a reduction in wall stress from reduced ventricular volume and pressure (see Table 12–8). Systemic venodilation also promotes increased flow to deep myocardial muscle by reducing the gradient between intraventricular pressure and coronary arteriolar (R_2) pressure. Direct actions on the coronary circulation include dilation of large and small intramural coronary arteries, collateral dilation, coronary artery stenosis dilation, abolition of normal tone in narrowed vessels, and relief of spasm; these actions occur even if the endothelium is denuded or dysfunctional. It is likely that depending on the underlying pathophysiology, different mechanisms become operative. For example, in the presence of a 60% to 70% stenosis, venodilation with $M\text{VO}_2$ reduction is most important; however, with higher grade lesions, direct effects on the coronary circulation and vessel tone are the predominant effects. Although the cellular mechanism of vasodilation by nitrates is not entirely understood, organic nitrates are converted intracellularly to nitric oxide (EDRF) and 5-nitrosothiol via interaction with sulfhydryl groups. Nitric oxide, and perhaps 5-nitrosothiol, activates soluble guanylate cyclase to increase intracellular concentrations of cyclic GMP. Increased cyclic GMP induces a sequence of protein phosphorylation associated with reduced intracellular calcium release from the sarcoplasmic reticulum or reduced permeability to extracellular calcium and, consequently, smooth muscle relaxation.

Pharmacokinetic characteristics common to the organic nitrates used for angina include a large first-pass effect of hepatic metabolism, short to very short half-lives (except for isosorbide mononitrate), large volumes of distribution, high clearance rates, and large interindividual variations in plasma or blood concentrations. Pharmacodynamic-pharmacokinetic relationships for the entire class remain poorly defined, presumably owing to methodologic difficulty in characterizing the parent drug and metabolite concentrations at or within vascular smooth muscle and secondary to counterregulatory or adaptive mechanisms from the drug's effects as well as the occurrence of tolerance. Nitroglycerin is extracted by a variety of tissues and metabolized locally; differential extraction and metabolite generation occur depending on the tissue site. There are also numerous technical problems limiting the generation of reliable pharmacokinetic parameter estimates including the following: assay sensitivity; arterial-venous extraction gradients and therefore extrahepatic metabolism; *in vitro* degradation; drug adsorption to polyvinyl chloride tubing and syringes; potentially saturable metabolism; accumulation of metabolites (some of which are active) with multiple doses; postural and exercise-induced changes in pharmacokinetics; a variety of variables associated with transdermal delivery including the delivery system (matrix, membrane-limited, ointment), vehicle used, the surface area and thickness of application, the site application, and other skin variables (temperature, moisture content).

Nitroglycerin concentrations are affected by the route of administration, with the highest concentrations usually obtained with intravenous administration, the lowest seen with lower oral doses. Peak concentrations with sublingual nitroglycerin appear within 2 to 4 minutes, with the oral route producing peaks at about 15 to 30 minutes and by the transdermal route at 1 to 2 hours. The half-life of nitroglycerin is 1 to 5 minutes regardless of route; hence the potential advantage of sustained-release and transdermal products. Transdermal nitroglycerin does produce sufficient concentrations for acute hemodynamic effects to occur and these concentrations are maintained for long intervals; however, the hemodynamic and antianginal effects are minimal after 1 week or less on chronic, continuous (24 h/d) therapy.

Isosorbide dinitrate (ISDN) is metabolized to isosorbide 2-mono- and 5-mononitrate (isosorbide mononitrate, ISMN). ISMN is well absorbed and has a half-life of about 5 hours and may be given once or twice daily depending on the product chosen. Multiple, larger doses of ISDN lead to disproportionate increases in the area under the plasma time profile, suggesting that metabolic pathways are being saturated or that metabolite accumulation may influence the disposition of ISDN. Little pharmacokinetic information is available for other nitrate compounds.

TABLE 12–9. Nitrate Products

Product	Onset (min)	Duration (min/h)	Initial Dose
Nitroglycerin			
IV	1–2	3–5	5 μg/min
SL/lingual	1–3	30–60	0.3 mg
PO	40	3–6	2.5–9 mg tid
Ointment	20–60	2–8	½–1 inch
Patch	40–60	> 8	1 patch
Erythritol tetranitrate	5–30	4–6	5–10 mg tid
Penterythritol tetranitrate	30	4–8	10–20 mg tid
Isosorbide dinitrate			
SL/chewable	2–5	1–2	2.5–5 mg tid
PO	20–40	4–6	5–20 mg tid
Isosorbide mononitrate	30–60	6–8	20 mg qd, bid[a]

[a]Product dependent.

Nitrate therapy may be used to terminate an acute anginal attack, to prevent effort or stress-induced attacks, or for long-term prophylaxis, usually in combination with β-blockers or calcium channel blockers. Sublingual nitroglycerin 0.3 to 0.4 mg will relieve pain in about 75% of patients within 3 minutes, with another 15% becoming pain free in 5 to 15 minutes. Pain persisting beyond about 20 to 30 minutes following the use of two or three nitroglycerin tablets is suggestive of evolving myocardial infarction or unstable angina and the patient should be instructed to seek emergency aid. Patients should be instructed to keep nitroglycerin in the original, tightly closed glass container and to avoid mixing with other medication, because mixing may reduce nitroglycerin adsorption and vaporization. Additional counseling should include the facts that nitroglycerin is not an analgesic but rather it partially corrects the underlying problem and that repeated use is not harmful or addicting. Patients should also be aware that enhanced venous pooling in the sitting or standing positions may improve the effect as well as the symptoms of postural hypotension, and that inadequate saliva may slow or prevent tablet disintegration and dissolution. An acceptable albeit expensive alternative is lingual spray, which may be more convenient and has a shelf-life of 3 years compared with 6 months or so for some forms of nitroglycerin tablets.

Chewable, oral, and transdermal products are acceptable for the long-term prophylaxis of angina; however, considerable controversy surrounds their use and it appears that the development of tolerance or adaptive mechanisms limits the efficacy of all chronic nitrate therapies regardless of route. Dosing of the longer acting preparations should be adjusted to provide a hemodynamic response, and as an example, this may require doses of oral ISDN ranging from 10 to 60 mg as often as every 3 to 4 hours owing to tolerance or first-pass metabolism, and similar large doses are required for other products. Nitroglycerin ointment seems to have a duration of up to 6 hours, but it is difficult to apply in a cosmetically acceptable fashion over a consistent surface area, and response varies depending on the epidermal thickness, vascularity, and amount of hair. Percutaneous adsorption of nitroglycerin ointment may occur unintentionally if someone other than the patient applies the ointment, and limiting exposure through the use of gloves or some other means is advisable. Peripheral edema may also impair the response to nitroglycerin because venodilation cannot increase capacitance to a maximum and pooling may be reduced. Transdermal patch delivery systems were approved on the basis of sustained and equivalent plasma concentrations to other forms of therapy. Trials required by the Food and Drug Administration using transdermal patches as a continuous 24-hour delivery system revealed a lack of efficacy for improved exercise tolerance. Subsequently, large, randomized, double-blind, placebo-controlled trials of intermittent (10 to 12 hours on; 12 to 14 hours off) transdermal nitroglycerin therapy in chronic stable angina demonstrated modest but significant improvement in exercise time after 4 weeks for the highest doses at 8 to 12 hours after patch placement.[30,41,42] Subjective assessment methods for nitrate effects include reduction in the number of painful episodes and the amount of nitroglycerin consumed. Objective assessment includes the resolution of ECG changes at rest, during exercise, or with ambulatory ECG monitoring. Because nitrates work primarily through a reduction in $M\dot{V}O_2$, the double product can be used to optimize the dose of sublingual and oral nitrate products. It is important to realize that reflex tachycardia may offset the beneficial reduction in systolic blood pressure and calculation of the observed changes is necessary. The double product is best assessed in the sitting position and at intervals of 5 to 10 minutes and 30 to 60 minutes following sublingual and oral therapy, respectively. Owing to the placebo effect, unpredictable and variable course of angina, numerous pharmacologic effects of nitroglycerin, diurnal variation in pain patterns, stringent investigative protocols, and interindividual sensitivity to nitroglycerin, assessment with transdermal and sustained-release products is difficult. ETT provides valuable information concerning efficacy and mechanism of action for nitrates but its use is usually reserved for clinical investigation rather than routine patient care. Most ETT studies have shown nitrates to delay the onset of ischemia (ST-segment changes or initial chest discomfort) at submaximal exercise but the threshold for maximal exercise is unaltered, suggesting a reduction in oxygen demand rather than an improved oxygen supply. More sophisticated studies of myocardial function such as wall motion abnormalities and myocardial metabolism could be used to document efficacy; however, these studies are generally only for investigative purposes.

Adverse effects of nitrates are related most commonly to an extension of their pharmacologic effects and include postural hypotension with associated central nervous system symptoms, headaches and flushing secondary to vasodilation, and occasional nausea from smooth muscle relaxation. If hypotension is excessive, coronary filling may be compromised and myocardial infarction can result as well as underfilling of the cerebral circulation and stroke. While reflex tachycardia is most common, bradycardia with nitroglycerin has been reported. Other noncardiovascular adverse effects include rash with all products but particularly with transdermal nitroglycerin, the production of methemoglobinemia with high doses given for extended periods, and measurable concentrations of ethanol (intoxication has been reported) and propylene glycol (found in the diluent) with intravenous nitroglycerin.

Tolerance with nitrate therapy was first described in 1867 with the initial experience using amyl nitrate for angina and later widely recognized in munition workers who underwent withdrawal reactions during periods of absence from exposure.[1] Tolerance to nitrates is associated with a reduction in tissue cyclic GMP, which results from decreased production (guanylate cyclase) and increased breakdown via cyclic GMP-phosphodiesterase and increased superoxide levels. One proposed mechanism for the lack of cyclic GMP is lack of conversion of organic nitrates to nitric oxide due to depletion of intracellular sulfhydryl cofactors (cysteine) in cells following chronic exposure to nitrates. This effect is more pronounced on the venous system than the arterial system. Activation of neurohormonal systems following vasodilation with nitrates may result in vasoconstriction and sodium retention. The major systems thought to be involved in this second mechanism are the sympathoadrenal axis and the renin–angiotensin system. Concomitant use of captopril (25 mg tid) may attenuate increased sensitivity to phenylephrine and angiotensin II noted in patients with stable CAD.[43,44] Nitroglycerin administration is accompanied by a fall in hematocrit (caused by hemodilution rather than renal water conservation) and intravascular volume expansion, minimizing the ability of nitrates to decrease ventricular filling pressures, as a third mechanism of tolerance. Logically, a diuretic would minimize this mechanism; however, Parker et al.[45] found no effect on the development of tolerance to continuous transdermal nitroglycerin. Diuretic therapy itself has important antianginal effects and improves exercise capacity in patients with stable angina.[45] Supplemental vitamin E has also been studied to restore cyclic GMP production and the vasodilatory response to nitroglycerin.[46] Most of the published information from controlled trials examining nitrate tolerance have been done with either ISDN or transdermal nitroglycerin, and these studies demonstrate the development of tolerance within as little as 24 hours of therapy. While the onset of tolerance is rapid, the offset may be just as rapid, and one alternative dosing strategy to circumvent or minimize tolerance is to provide a daily nitrate-free interval of 6 to 8 hours. Studies with a variety of nitrate preparations and dosing schedules demonstrate that this approach is useful and the nitrate-free interval should be a minimum of 8 hours and perhaps 12 hours for even better effects.[41] Another concern for intermittent transdermal nitrate therapy is the occurrence of rebound ischemia during the nitrate-free interval. Freedman et al.[47] found more silent ischemia during the patch-free interval during a randomized, double-blind, placebo-controlled trial than during the placebo patch phase, although others have not noted this effect[41,47] ISDN, for example, should not be used more often than three times per day if tolerance is to be avoided. Interestingly, hemodynamic tolerance does not always coincide with antianginal efficacy, but this is not well studied.[48]

Nitrates may be combined with other drugs for anginal therapy including β-adrenergic blocking agents and calcium channel antagonists.[36,49] These combinations are usually instituted for chronic prophylactic therapy based on complimentary or offsetting mechanisms of action (Table 12–9). Combination therapy is generally used in patients with more frequent or symptoms not responding to β-blockers alone (nitrates plus β-blockers or calcium blockers), in patients intolerant of β-blockers or calcium channel blockers, and in patients having an element of vasospasm leading to decreased supply (nitrates plus calcium blockers).[47,50]

CALCIUM CHANNEL ANTAGONISTS[51]

Modulation of calcium entry into vascular smooth muscle and myocardium as well as a variety of other tissues is the principle action of the calcium antagonists. The cellular mechanism of these drugs is not completely understood and it differs among the available classes of the phenylalkylamines (verapamil-like), dihydropyridines (nifedipine-like), benzothiazepines (diltiazem-like), bepridil, and a recent class referred to as T-channel blockers with mibefradil as the first drug in the category.[52] Receptor-operated channels stimulated by norepinephrine and other neurotransmittors, and potential-dependent channels activated by membrane depolarization, control the entry of calcium, and consequently the cytosolic concentration of calcium responsible for activation of actin–myosin complex leading to contraction of vascular smooth muscle and myocardium. In the myocardium, calcium entry triggers the release of intracellular stores of calcium to increase cytosolic calcium, whereas in smooth muscle calcium derived from the extracellular fluid may do this directly. Binding proteins within the cell, calmodulin and troponin, after binding with calcium, participate in phosphorylation reactions leading to contraction. Decreased calcium availability, through the actions of calcium antagonists, inhibits these reactions.

Direct actions of the calcium antagonists include vasodilation of systemic arterioles and coronary arteries, leading to a reduction of arterial pressure and coronary vascular resistance as well as depression of the myocardial contractility and conduction velocity of the sinoatrial and atrioventricular nodes (see Chapter 14, Arrhythmias). Reflex β-adrenergic stimulation overcomes much of the negative inotropic effect, and depression of contractility becomes clinically apparent only in the presence of LV dysfunction and when other negative inotropic drugs are used concurrently. Verapamil and diltiazem cause less peripheral vasodilation than nifedipine, and, consequently, the risk of myocardial depression is greater with these two agents. Conduction through the AV node is predictably depressed with verapamil and diltiazem, and they must be used with caution in patients with preexisting conduction abnormalities or in the presence of other drugs with negative chronotropic properties. Bepridil, in addition to having calcium channel-blocking properties, also has class I and III antiarrhythmic activity. $M\dot{V}O_2$ is reduced with all of the calcium channel antagonists because of reduced wall tension secondary to reduced arterial pressure and, to a minor extent, depressed contractility (Table 12–9). Heart rate changes are dependent on the drug used and the state of the conduction system. Nifedipine generally increases heart rate or causes no change whereas either no change or decreased heart rate is seen with verapamil and diltiazem because of the interaction of these direct and indirect effects. Mibefradil does not result in reflex tachycardia nor does it have significant myocardial depressant effects. In contrast to the β-blockers, calcium channel antagonists have the potential to improve coronary blood flow through areas of fixed coronary obstruction and by inhibiting coronary artery vasomotion and vasospasm. Beneficial redistribution of blood flow from well-perfused myocardium to ischemic areas and from epicardium to endocardium may also contribute to improvement in ischemic symptoms. Overall, the benefit provided by calcium channel antagonists is related to reduced $M\dot{V}O_2$ rather than improved oxygen supply based on lack of alteration in the rate pressure product at maximal exercise in most studies performed to date. However, as coronary artery disease progresses and vasospasm becomes superimposed on critical stenotic lesions, improved oxygen supply through coronary vasodilation may become more important.

Absorption of the calcium channel antagonists is characterized by excellent absorption and large, variable first-pass metabolism resulting in oral bioavailability ranging from about 20% to 50% or greater for diltiazem, nicardipine, nifedipine, verapamil, felodipine, and isradipine. Amlodipine and bepridil have a range of bioavailability of ~60% to 80%. Saturation of this effect may occur with verapamil and diltiazem, resulting in greater amounts of drug being absorbed with chronic dosing. Nifedipine may have slow or fast absorption patterns, and the ingestion of food delays and impairs its absorption as well as potential enhanced absorption in elderly patients. This variability in absorption produces fluctuation in the hemodynamic response with nifedipine. Sublingual nifedipine is frequently used to provide a more rapid response; however, the rationale for this application is suspect because little nifedipine is absorbed from the buccal mucosa and the swallowed drug is responsible for the observed plasma concentrations. Absorption of verapamil in sustained-release products may be influenced by food, and when used in the fasted state, dose dumping may occur, resulting in high peak concentrations with some products. The approved sustained-release products for nifedipine, verapamil, and diltiazem are approved primarily for the treatment of hypertension (see Chapter 10, Hypertension). The presence of severe liver disease (e.g., alcoholic liver disease with cirrhosis) has been shown to reduce the first-pass metabolism of verapamil, and this shunting of drug around the liver gives rise to higher plasma concentrations and lower dose requirements in these patients. Interestingly, this effect appears to be stereoselective for the more active isomer of verapamil. Verapamil may also reduce liver blood flow; however, evidence for this reduction is based primarily on animal experiments. Few data are available regarding the influence of liver disease on the kinetics of calcium blockers; however, these drugs undergo extensive hepatic metabolism with little unchanged drug being renally excreted, and liver disease can be expected to alter the pharmacokinetics. Nifedipine has no active metabolites whereas norverapamil possesses 20% or less activity of the parent compound. Desacetyldiltiazem has not been studied in man, but canine studies suggest its potency ranges from 100% to 40% of the parent compound for various cardiovascular effects; the clinical importance of these observations remains to be determined. With chronic dosing of verapamil and diltiazem, apparent saturation of metabolism occurs, producing higher plasma concentrations of each drug than those seen with single-dose administration. Consequently, the elimination half-life for verapamil is prolonged, and less frequent dosing intervals may be used in some patients. The elimination half-life for diltiazem is also somewhat prolonged and the half-life of desacetyldiltiazem is longer than that of the parent drug, but it is not clear if less frequent dosing may be used. Bepridil also undergoes hepatic elimination and an active metabolite, 4-hydroxyphenyl bepridil, is produced; the parent compound has a long half-life of 30 to 40 hours. Nifedipine does not accumulate with chronic dosing; however, it is eliminated via oxidative pathways that may be polymorphic, and slow and fast metabolizers have been described for nifedipine. Because oxidative pathways are important for the elimination of these drugs, inhibition or induction by drugs such as cimetidine or rifampin can alter the kinetics and pharmacodynamic response. Conversely, inhibition of hepatic microsomal drug metabolism by diltiazem and verapamil has been demonstrated, and interactions with drugs (e.g., theophylline) eliminated through oxidation may be expected. Renal insufficiency has little or no effect on the pharmacokinetics of these three drugs. Although disease alterations in kinetics have been described, the most important quantitative alteration is the influence of liver disease on bioavailability and elimination. Aging has been shown to reduce the clearance of verapamil and diltiazem, and dosing in this population should be done with caution. Altered protein binding owing to renal disease, decreased protein concentration, or increased α_1-acid glycoprotein has been noted, but the clinical import of these changes is unknown.

Good candidates for calcium channel blockers in angina include patients with contraindications or intolerance of β-blockers, coexisting conduction system disease (except for verapamil and possibly diltiazem), patients with Prinzmetal's angina (vasospastic or variable threshold angina), the presence of peripheral vascular disease, severe ventricular dysfunction (amlodipine is probably calcium channel blocker of choice and others need to be used with caution if the ejection fraction is < 40%), and concurrent hypertension.

▶ TREATMENT: Stable Exertional Angina Pectoris[34,53–55]

After assessing and manipulating the alterable risk factors as discussed previously, the next intervention that could be undertaken is the institution of a regular exercise program. Training is possible in many patients with angina and the observed benefits include decreased heart rate and systolic blood pressure as well as increased ejection fraction and duration of exercise. Although the mechanism of these effects has been debated, improved overall cardiovascular and muscular condition are probably most important. The intensity of exercise influences training and more vigorous programs provide better overall results.[56] Obviously, an exercise program should be undertaken with caution and in a graded fashion with adequate supervision. Although national guidelines for the pharmacotherapeutic management of stable angina do not currently exist, they are being formulated by the American Heart Association/American College of Cardiology; guidelines from other groups are referenced above.

Chronic prophylactic therapy for patients with more than one angina episode per day may also be instituted with β-adrenergic blocking agents, and in many instances β-blockers may be preferable because of less frequent dosing and other properties inherent in β-blockade (e.g., potential cardioprotective effects, antiarrhythmic effects, lack of tolerance, and antihypertensive effects), as well as their antianginal effects and documented protective effects in post-MI patients. Patients who continue to smoke have reduced antianginal efficacy of β-blockers. This may be due to enhanced hepatic metabolism of drugs that are eliminated through this route or related to the effects of smoking on $M\dot{V}O_2$ and oxygenation. As discussed previously, ancillary properties such as cardioselectivity are useful in patients with concurrent problems, but these properties do not contribute to the antianginal efficacy of β-blockers. The one characteristic that is relevant is the duration of effect on the double product. β-Blockers with longer half-lives (e.g., nadolol) are more likely to affect the double product for a longer period of time and require fewer doses per day. The choice of β-blocker for angina rests on choosing the appropriate dose to achieve the goals outlined for heart rate and double product, and choosing an agent that is well tolerated by individual patients and cost. Selective use may incorporate ancillary properties but these are secondary considerations in overall drug product selection. Patients most likely to respond well to β-blockade are those who have a high resting heart rate and those having a relatively fixed anginal threshold. In other words, their symptoms appear at the same level of exercise or work load on a consistent basis. Symptoms appearing with variable work loads suggest fluctuations in myocardial oxygen supply, perhaps due to coronary artery vasomotion, and these patients are more likely to respond to calcium channel antagonists.

Nitrate therapy should be the first step in managing acute attacks for patients with chronic stable angina if the attacks are infrequent (i.e., a few times per month) or for prophylaxis of symptoms when undertaking activities known to precipitate attacks. In general, if angina occurs no more often than once every few days, then sublingual (SL) nitroglycerin tablets or spray or buccal products may be sufficient to allow the patient to maintain an adequate life-style. For episodes of "first-effort" angina occurring in a predictable fashion, nitroglycerin may be used in a prophylactic manner with the patient taking 0.3 to 0.4 mg sublingually about 5 minutes prior to the anticipated time of activity. Nitroglycerin spray may be useful when inadequate saliva is produced to rapidly dissolve SL nitroglycerin or if a patient has difficulty opening the container. Most patients have a response that lasts about 30 minutes or so, but this is subject to interindividual variability. Obtaining the appropriate dose for a particular patient can be facilitated by the use of the double product to assess the hemodynamic effect of nitroglycerin. When angina occurs more frequently than once a day, a chronic prophylactic regimen using β-blockers as the first line of therapy should be considered (see Fig. 12–3 for the stable angina algorithm). Chronic prophylactic therapy with long-acting forms of nitroglycerin (oral or transdermal), isosorbide dinitrate, 5-mononitrate, and pentaerythritol trinitrate may be effective; however, the development of tolerance is a major limiting step in their continued effectiveness. Since long-acting nitrates are not as effective as β-blockers and do not have beneficial effects, monotherapy with nitrates should not be first-line therapy unless β-blockers and calcium channel blockers are contraindicated or not tolerated. As described previously, providing a nitrate-free interval of 8 hours per day or longer appears to be the most promising approach to maintaining the efficacy of chronic nitrate therapy. Oral administration of nitrates is susceptible to a saturable first-pass effect; therefore, larger doses can produce a measurable hemodynamic effect and dose titration should be based on these changes in the double product. There are few well-controlled studies comparing oral or sublingual nitrate efficacy, and the choice among these products should be based on familiarity with the preparation, cost, and patient acceptance.

Calcium channel antagonists have the potential advantage of improving coronary blood flow through coronary artery vasodilation as well as decreasing $M\dot{V}O_2$ and may be used instead of β-blockers for chronic prophylactic therapy; however, in

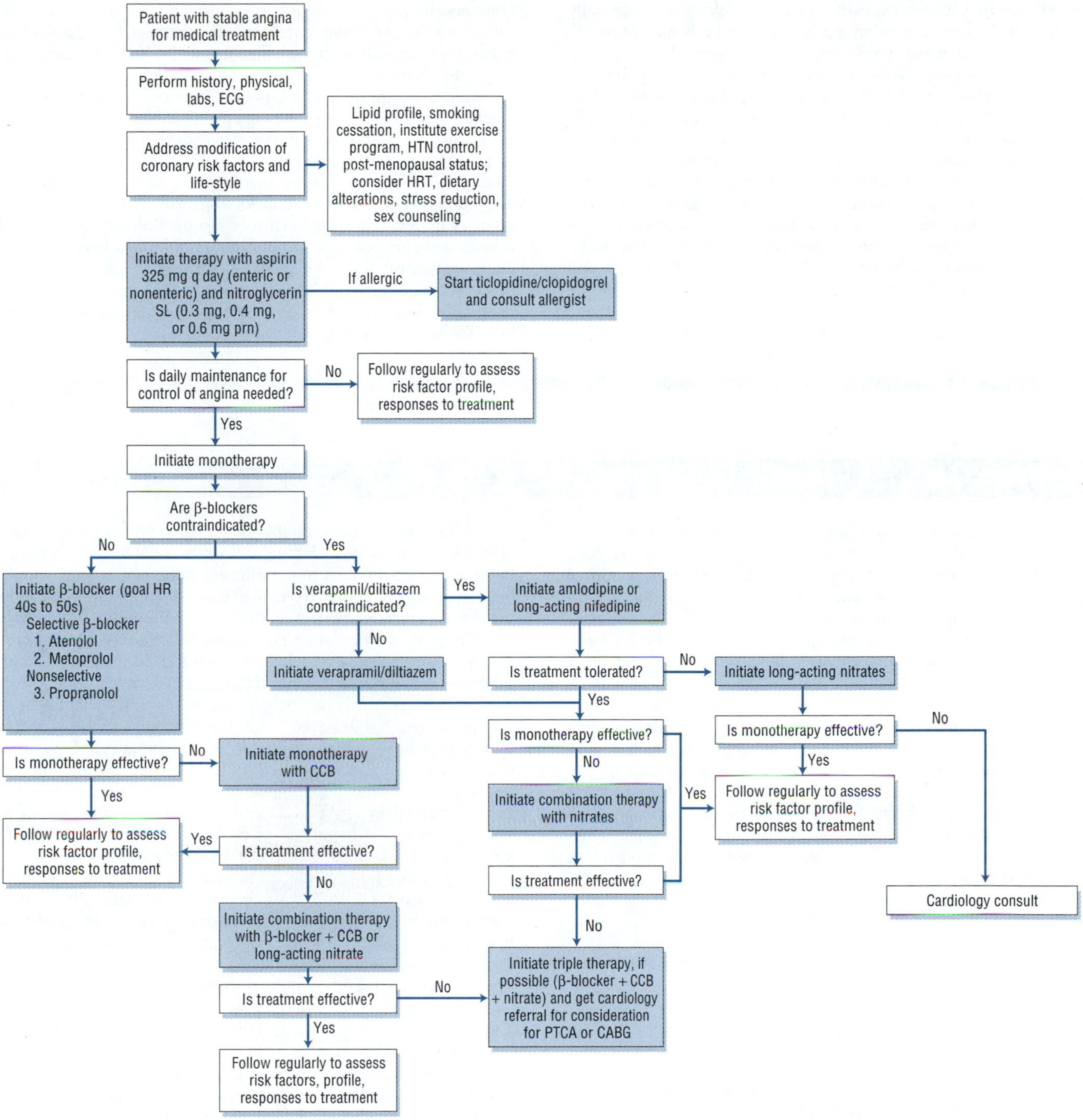

FIGURE 12–3. Algorithm for chronic stable angina. Abbreviations: HR = heart rate; HTN = hypertensive nephropathy; HRT = hormone replacement therapy; CCB = calcium channel blocker; PTCA = percutaneous transluminal angioplasty; CABG = coronary artery bypass grafting.

chronic stable angina comparative trials of long-acting calcium channel blockers with β-blockers do not show significant differences in response.[57,58] They are as effective as β-blockers and are most useful in patients who have a variable threshold for exertional angina. Calcium antagonists may provide better skeletal muscle oxygenation, resulting in decreased fatigue and better exercise tolerance. Additionally, if contraindications exist to β-blocker therapy, calcium antagonists can be safely used in many patients. The available calcium channel blockers appear to have similar efficacy in the management of chronic stable angina. Differences in their electrophysiology, peripheral and central hemodynamic effects, and adverse effect profiles are useful in selecting the appropriate agent. Patients with conduction abnormalities and moderate to severe LV dysfunction (ejection fraction < 35%) should be treated cautiously with verapamil whereas amlodipine and nifedipine may be safely used in many of these patients. Diltiazem has significant effects on the AV node and can produce heart block in patients with preexisting conduction disease or when other drugs, such as digoxin or β-blockers, with effects on conduction are used concurrently.

Nifedipine may cause excessive heart rate elevation, especially if the patient is not receiving a β-blocker, and this may offset the beneficial effect it has on MvO_2. Gingival hyperplasia has also been reported with nifedipine, and some dental authorities say this may be seen in as many as 20% of patients on nifedipine. Bepridil prolongs the QT interval in patients with certain conditions (hypokalemia, advanced age, preexisting QT interval prolongation) and because of this potential proarrhythmic effect, it is indicated only in patients who have been inadequately controlled with other antianginal therapy. Case control studies with calcium blockers suggest an increased risk for myocardial infarction and cancer.[59,60] The relationship to cancer appears to be weak to nonexistent whereas the risk for MI is probably real and related to the type of drug used and relationship to recent MI. Shorter acting calcium blockers can activate the sympathetic nervous system and in patients with recent MI or significant coronary disease, may induce ischemia. This effect has not been shown for longer acting products. The hemodynamic effect of calcium antagonists is complementary to β-blockade, and, consequently, combination therapy is rational.

Studies examining combination therapy have shown that calcium channel blockers when used with β-blockers provide objective evidence of improvement by increasing exercise duration and decreasing ECG evidence of ischemia. The addition of a calcium antagonist to β-blocker therapy may be more useful than the addition of nitrates, considering exercise duration and changes in global and regional ejection fraction in ischemic and nonischemic myocardium.[49] Because both β-blockers and calcium antagonists have the potential for depressing contractility, this combination should be used with care in patients with poor ventricular function; however, in well-preserved ventricular function, the combination is well tolerated.

▶ TREATMENT: Unstable Angina Pectoris[12,13,61,62]

Clinical and autopsy studies indicate that most patients who present with unstable angina or acute myocardial infarction have significant underlying coronary atherosclerosis. Precipitation of these acute ischemic syndromes are thought to be due to progression of atherosclerosis, acute coronary thrombosis, coronary artery vasoconstriction, and platelet aggregation.[36] The interrelationship of these mechanisms and potential therapeutic interventions are outlined in Fig. 12–4. Patients at high risk of death or nonfatal MI are those presenting with prolonged ongoing (> 20 minutes) rest pain, pulmonary edema related to ischemia, angina at rest with dynamic ST changes of ≥ 1 mm, angina with new or worsening mitral regurgitation, S_3 or rales, and angina with hypotension.[12,13] Unstable angina differs from stable angina in that the primary event is thought to be a reduction in coronary blood flow rather than an increase in MvO_2, with corresponding ischemic changes in the ECG occurring prior to changes in heart rate and blood pressure.

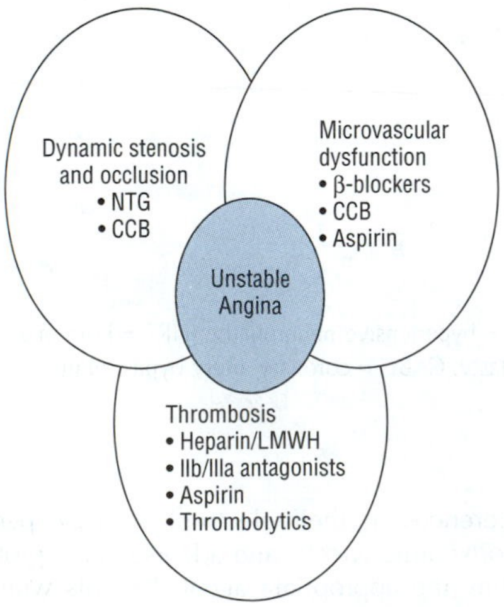

FIGURE 12–4. Pathophysiologic components of unstable angina and potentially useful therapeutic interventions. Dynamic stenosis or occlusion, microvascular dysfunction, and thrombosis interact equally to bring about unstable angina. NTG = nitroglycerin; CCB = calcium channel blocker; LMWH = low-molecular-weight heparin.

Initial management of the patient should include history, physical examination, electrocardiogram (within 20 minutes), bedrest with continuous monitoring for ischemia and arrhythmia detection, supplemental oxygen if cyanotic or hypoxemic, and immediate consideration of the use of IV nitroglycerin, aspirin, heparin, β-blockers (oral or IV depending on severity), and narcotics if pain is not relieved by nitrates and β-blockers (see Fig. 12–5 for the unstable angina algorithm). Morphine sulfate at a dose of 2 to 5 mg IV is recommended for any patient whose symptoms are not relieved after three serial sublingual NTG tablets or whose symptoms recur with adequate antiischemic therapy unless contraindicated by hypotension or intolerance. Because aspirin and heparin are used in AMI, their use is not contraindicated in unstable angina. Aspirin should be dosed at 160 to 325 mg and heparin is given as a bolus of 80 units/kg followed by a continuous infusion of 18 units/kg/h to maintain the activated partial thromboplastin time at 1.5 to 2.5 times control and continued for 2 to 5 days or until revascularization is performed. Based on anecdotal observations, this dosing regimen for heparin may overdose very obese patients, and these doses should be used with caution in the very obese patient. Acutely heparin may be useful to prevent further thrombosis formation, and aspirin acutely and chronically inhibits platelet aggregation. The combination of heparin and nitroglycerin has been shown in earlier studies to result in heparin resistance and more than typical heparin doses may be needed; however, more recent information suggest this interaction is not significant. Low-molecular-weight heparin (e.g., enoxaparin, nadroparin) may be useful along with aspirin instead of unfractionated heparin.[63–66] Thrombolysis is not indicated in patients who do not have evidence of acute ST-segment elevation or left bundle branch block on ECG. Long-term antiplatelet therapy with aspirin has been unequivocally shown to reduce the occurrence of mortality and nonfatal infarction in unstable angina by about 50% in doses ranging from 324 to 1300 mg/d in two well-controlled studies.[61] Earlier studies examined the effect of sulfinpyrazone alone and in combination with aspirin and found no benefit from sulfinpyrazone. Ticlopidine (250 mg bid) or clopidogrel (75 mg/d) may be considered in patients with aspirin hypersensitivity or recent major gastrointestinal bleeding.

If three doses of sublingual nitroglycerin do not relieve the patient's pain, then intravenous nitroglycerin provides a convenient method of titrating the dose and avoids uncertainty

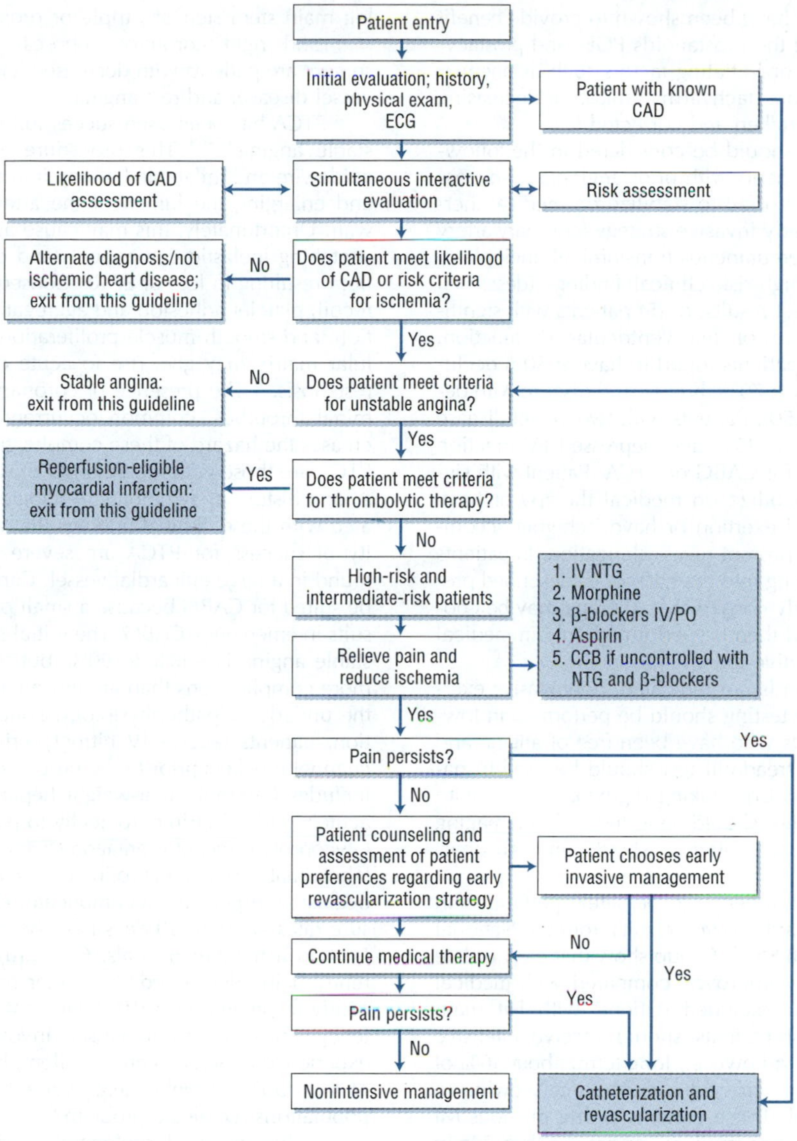

FIGURE 12–5. Algorithm for unstable angina. CAD = coronary artery disease; NTG = nitroglycerin.

concerning drug delivery. Dosing should be started low (5 to 10 μg/kg/min) and titrated upward by 10 μg/min every 5 to 10 minutes until symptoms are relieved or limiting adverse effects occur. A reduction in systolic blood pressure is expected and should be about 15 mm Hg or to a systolic pressure of 100 to 110 mm Hg. Caution is necessary in preload-dependent patients (with right ventricular infarct, hypovolemia, pericardial constriction or effusion) to avoid hypotension and decreased coronary perfusion pressure as well as excessive heart rate elevation if the patient is not receiving β-blockers. After 24 hours free of symptoms, patients may be switched over to oral or topical nitrates.

Intravenous β-blockers are recommended for high-risk patients (oral for intermediate- and low-risk patients) in the absence of contraindications. Regimens are similar to those used in AMI. Unstable patients with persisting or recurring pain while on nitrates and β-blockers should receive a calcium antagonist. β-blockers in unstable angina reduce the risk of progression to MI slightly but have not been shown to reduce mortality. β-Blockers do have strong evidence supporting their use in AMI and in post-MI patients, and this is sufficient evidence to recommend their routine use. β-Blocker therapy may prevent ischemia caused by tachycardia and reduce cardiac work. Patients should be screened for contraindications to therapy (see Table 13–3 in Chap. 13).

Several studies suggest efficacy of calcium channel blockers in unstable angina, and their effects are mediated via inhibition of increased coronary tone and through reduction in $M\dot{V}O_2$. Calcium antagonists may be added to nitrates and β-blockers, and some authors suggest that they are most useful in combination with pretreatment β-blockade. ST-segment elevation appears to respond better to calcium antagonism than does depression. Calcium channel blockers should be avoided in patients with pulmonary edema or evidence of left ventricular dysfunction. Nifedipine should not be used in the absence of concurrent β-blockade. The largest randomized trial with nifedipine and metoprolol found metoprolol to be more effective than placebo whereas nifedipine increased the risk of MI and recurrent angina compared to placebo; the combination was no better than metoprolol alone. Diltiazem may be more useful than other agents in the setting of unstable angina and non-Q-wave myocardial infarction because it has been shown to reduce reinfarction and refractory angina (see Chap. 13).

Other interventions that have been shown to provide benefit in short-term studies include the prostanoids PGE_1 and prostacyclin. A search for reversible or initiating factors such as anemia, thyroid dysfunction, infection, tachyarrhythmias, or increasing heart failure should be undertaken and corrected.

Cardiac catheterization should be considered in the following groups of patients: (1) patients with prior angioplasty, bypass surgery or MI; (2) patients who fail to stabilize on medical therapy; (3) patients opting for early invasive strategy (coronary artery bypass surgery [CABG] or percutaneous transluminal angioplasty [PTCA]); (4) patients with high-risk clinical findings (described previously) or noninvasive test results; or (5) patients with significant congestive heart failure or left ventricular dysfunction. CABG is recommended for patients found to have ≥ 50% occlusion of the left main artery or ≥ 70% three-vessel disease with depressed LV function (EF < 0.50). Patients with two-vessel disease with proximal LAD stenosis ≥ 95% and depressed LV function should be referred promptly for CABG or PTCA. Patient with significant CAD who fail to stabilize on medical therapy or have symptoms with low levels of exertion or have ischemia accompanied by CHF should have prompt revascularization. In patients with significant CAD not falling into the categories described previously, early invasive or early conservative therapy may be chosen. Revascularization would then be performed only in medical failures in the early conservative-therapy group.

If cardiac catheterization is not indicated, noninvasive exercise or pharmacologic stress testing should be performed in low- and intermediate-risk patients who have been free of angina and CHF for 48 hours. Exercise treadmill test should be used in patients with a normal ECG and not taking digoxin. Patients with significant resting ECG changes should be tested with an imaging modality. Those with physical limitations should undergo pharmacologic stress testing.

Coronary artery bypass surgery can be safely performed in patients with unstable angina; however, results from the National Cooperative Unstable Angina Study Group show that early or late infarction is not significantly improved compared with medical therapy.[1] This study, which excluded patients with left main stenosis, suggests that most patients should receive intensive medical management initially; however, long term, about 36% of the medically treated patients crossed over to surgery owing to inadequate symptom control. Those patients with a previous MI or hypertension, resting ST abnormalities, or greater than 3 mm ST-segment depression on exercise are likely to fail maximal medical therapy (about 3%) and become candidates for surgery as are those initially controlled with high-risk factors including left main stem stenosis, triple or proximal left anterior descending, and right coronary stenoses. Additional candidates for surgery are patients with decreased left ventricular function, three vessel disease, and rest angina.

PTCA has been used successfully in the management of unstable angina.[67–69] This procedure involves the insertion of a guidewire and inflatable balloon into the affected coronary artery and enlarging the lumen of the artery by stretching the vessel wall. Unfortunately, this may cause atheroma plaque fracture by stretching inelastic components and denudation of the endothelium resulting in loss of EDRF. Consequently, immediate vascular recoil, platelet adhesion and aggregation, mural thrombus formation, and smooth muscle proliferation, and synthesis of extracellular matrix may give rise to acute occlusion and early or late restenosis.[70] The presence of coronary artery spasm and intraluminal thrombus, common occurrences in unstable angina, increases the hazard of these complications. Patients best suited for PTCA are those with recent onset of worsening of angina without a long history of symptoms. Angiographic characteristics associated with these clinical findings that allow the greatest probability of success for PTCA are severe, discrete, proximal lesions found in a large epicardial vessel. Candidates for PTCA must also be suited for CABG because a small percentage of procedures results in emergency CABG. The initial success rate for PTCA in unstable angina is ~80% to 90%, but these patients are at risk for more complications than are those with stable angina because of the underlying pathophysiology. Following a period of stabilization, patients receive IV nitroglycerin with or without calcium channel blockers prior to the procedure, and follow-up treatment includes low-molecular-weight heparin or unfractioned heparin acutely and warfarin chronically to prevent coronary thrombosis. Glycoprotein receptor antagonists for the IIb/IIIa platelet receptor (abciximab, eptifatide, tirofiban) have been shown to prevent early occlusion, especially in complication PTCA procedures.[71–74] Closure rates at about 30 days have been reduced by about 30% to 50% in a number of trials. Oral drugs in this category are currently being developed.[75,76] Other methods have been tried recently to prevent post-PTCA late restenosis (see later). Initial patency rates for single-vessel involvement in the hands of experienced operators are excellent; however, a restenosis rate of 15% to 30% or higher (e.g., variant angina) in selected patient populations remains a problem.[75]

In the event of prolonged chest pain and ischemic ECG changes unrelieved by nitrate therapy or calcium channel antagonists, one may assume total occlusion of a coronary vessel and steps should be taken to restore blood flow.

▶ TREATMENT: Coronary Artery Spasm and Variant Angina Pectoris[54]

Prinzmetal, in his original description of variant angina pectoris, noted the waxing and waning course of this syndrome.[1] This has been observed by others, and it appears that the most severe symptoms and the greatest risk for mortality and morbidity occur within the first 6 months after the onset of symptoms. Following this initial rocky course, spontaneous remissions have been reported to occur. The cyclic nature of variant angina create difficulties in assessing the value of any therapeutic intervention. The exact cause of variant angina is not well understood, but there appears to be an imbalance of autonomic control characterized by parasympathetic dominance as well as endothelial dysfunction associated with increased secretion of vascular adhesion molecules, deficiencies of vitamin E and magnesium, supersensitivity to serotonin, and hyperinsulinemia.[77–79]

The merit of any intervention may be assessed by several methods, and a combination of these most likely will provide information for rational decisions concerning therapy. Reduction in symptoms and nitroglycerin consumption as documented by a patient diary can assist the interpretation of objective data obtained from ambulatory ECG recordings. This method may underestimate the number of ischemic episodes because of the variable nature of variant angina, and serial recordings may be of great value. Evidence of efficacy includes the reduction of ischemic events, both ST-segment depression and elevation, which may be symptomatic or asymptomatic with the latter being overall more common. Additional evidence would be reduced number of attacks of angina requiring hospitalization, absence of myocardial infarction, and sudden death. Ergonovine provocative testing has been suggested by some as a means for determining the effectiveness of therapy; however, not all investigators have found this method to be reliable because of the fluctuating course of variant angina, and provocation may be associated with drug-resistant vasospasm and ventricular arrhythmias.

Optimization of therapy includes dose titration using sufficiently high doses to obtain clinical efficacy without unacceptable adverse effects in individual patients. All patients should be treated for acute attacks and maintained on prophylactic treatment for 6 to 12 months following the initial episode. The occurrence of serious arrhythmias during attacks is associated with a greater risk of sudden death, and these patients should be treated more aggressively and for prolonged periods. In patients without arrhythmias who become asymptomatic and remain so for several months after treatment has been instituted, withdrawal of therapy may be safe after first ascertaining that disease activity is quiescent. Aggravating factors such as alcohol or cocaine use or cigarette smoking should be eliminated when instituting treatment.

Nitrates have been the mainstay of therapy for the acute attacks of variant angina and coronary artery spasm for many years. Most patients respond rapidly to SL nitroglycerin or isosorbide dinitrate; however, intravenous and intracoronary nitroglycerin may be very useful for patients not responding to SL preparations. In particular, vasospasm provoked by ergonovine may require intracoronary nitroglycerin. Other nitrate products including intravenous isosorbide dinitrate and nitroglycerin ointment have been shown to be effective for acute attacks of variant angina. Although studies with nitrates generally show them to be efficacious, high does are often required and it is unclear if they reduce mortality. Because calcium antagonists may be more effective, have few serious adverse effects in effective doses, and can be given less frequently than nitrates, some consider them the agents of choice for variant angina.

Nifedipine, verapamil, and diltiazem are all equally effective as single agents for the initial management of variant angina and coronary artery spasm. Dose titration is important to maximize the response with calcium antagonists. Comparative trials, which are few in number, do not reveal significant differences among these three drugs for variant angina. In patients unresponsive to calcium antagonists alone, nitrates may be added with a good response. Combination therapy with nifedipine–diltiazem or nifedipine–verapamil has been reported useful in patients unresponsive to single-drug regimens. This is probably rational because, at the cellular level, the drugs have different receptors, but the combination of verapamil–diltiazem should be used cautiously owing to their potential additive effects on contractility and conduction.

β-Adrenergic blockade has little or no role in the management of variant angina according to most authorities.[39,59] Although not all studies report increased painful episodes of variant angina with the addition of β-blockers, they may induce coronary vasoconstriction and prolong ischemia, as documented by continuous ECG monitoring.

Other approaches to therapy have attempted modification of α-adrenergic tone by α-antagonists such as phentolamine, phenoxybenzamine, or prazosin. The overall response to α-blockers is variable and long-term results are discouraging. Anticholinergic agents have also been administered to diminish enhanced parasympathetic activity leading to stimulation of sympathetic nerves and coronary vasospasm; however, only parenteral atropine has been studied and the role for chronic therapy is undetermined. Labetalol, because of its α-blocking properties, may be useful, but very little information is available. Adverse effects limit the utility of amiodarone and perhexilene, and only small numbers of patients with variant angina have been treated with these agents. Plexectomy, surgical interruption of the sympathetic innervation of the heart, with and without CABG, has been reported to benefit a few patients.

Agents to modify platelet aggregation and arachidonic acid metabolism have undergone preliminary clinical trials as sole interventions, but dramatic responses have not been seen. The effects of aspirin in variant angina have not been as successful as in unstable angina, perhaps reflecting differences in the underlying pathophysiology. The role of thromboxane synthesis inhibition, thromboxane receptor antagonism, prostacyclin, lipoxygenase inhibition, and ticlopidine is being clarified through ongoing studies, but these drugs do not occupy a major place in therapy at the present time. Dietary supplementation with fish oil can influence lipid levels, platelet aggregation, and possibly cardiovascular mortality, but because most of the available studies are either in animals or of an epidemiologic nature, routine use cannot be recommended for the prevention or treatment of variant angina. As mentioned previously, vitamin E or magnesism supplementation may also be useful.

▶ TREATMENT: Silent Myocardial Ischemia[36]

The objective in the treatment of silent myocardial ischemia is to reduce the total number of ischemic episodes, both symptomatic and asymptomatic, regardless of the direction of ST-segment shift. The incidence of silent ischemia in the general, asymptomatic population is not known. Significant day-to-day variability in the number of episodes, the duration of ischemia, and the amount of ST-segment deviation complicates both the understanding of this process and the utility of various therapeutic interventions. Silent ischemia in patients with known CAD is common (~80% of all ischemic episodes) and associated with the extent of disease as well as a high risk for myocardial infarction and sudden death when compared with symptomatic episodes of ischemia. Although the underlying mechanisms for silent ischemia are continuing to be defined, increased physical activity, activation of the sympathetic nervous system, increased cortisol secretion, increased coronary artery tone, and enhanced platelet aggregation due to the loss of EDRF leading to intermittent coronary obstruction may be additive in lowering the threshold for ischemia. Platelet aggregability is increased in the morning hours (7 AM to 11 AM), corresponding to circadian rhythms noted for the peak frequency of ischemia, acute myocardial infarction, and sudden death. Silent ischemia is associated with ST-segment elevation or depression and frequently occurs without antecedent changes in heart rate or blood pressure, suggesting that this form of ischemia is a result of primary reduction in oxygen supply in many instances whereas at other times in the same patient oxygen demand is increased prior to the onset ischemia. Silent ischemia is classified into Class I, patients who do not experience angina at any time, and Class II, patients who have both asymptomatic and symptomatic ischemia. Patients with silent ischemia have a defective warning system for angina pain that may encourage excessive myocardial demand. Regardless of the exact mechanism, there is increasing concern that painless ischemia carries considerable risk for myocardial perfusion defects, detrimental hemodynamic changes, arrhythmogenesis, and sudden death. Silent ischemia is associated with reduced survival and increased need for

PTCA and CABG as well as increased risk of AMI.[80] Because it is apparently very common in some settings, major emphasis should be placed on its management. A consensus has not been reached for the most appropriate method of detecting and quantifying the magnitude of silent ischemia; however, ambulatory electrocardiogram monitoring is felt by many to be the most useful tool at the present time.

The initial step in management is to modify the major risk factors for IHD, hypertension, hypercholesterolemia, and smoking, and data from the Multiple Risk Factor Intervention Trial (MRFIT) show these interventions to be useful in patients with silent ischemia. In a subset of the study population who had abnormal baseline exercise ECG responses, the special intervention group had a 57% reduction in coronary heart disease death (22.2/1000 vs 51.8/1000) and a reduction in sudden death resulting from cessation of smoking and lowering of blood pressure and cholesterol when compared with the usual-care group.[1]

Several studies with β-blockers have shown improvement in the number of ischemic episodes, primarily ST-segment depression and those associated with effort, compared with placebo; however, this benefit is not seen with all β-blockers. The Atenolol Silent Ischemia Study (ASIST) demonstrated that atenolol treatment reduced daily life ischemia and was associated with reduced risk for adverse outcome in asymptomatic and mildly symptomatic patients compared with placebo.[1] ACIP (Asymptomatic Cardiac Ischemia Pilot), a randomized trial of medical therapy versus revascularization (PTCA or CABG), at the 2-year follow-up demonstrates that total mortality was 6.6% in the angina-guided strategy, 4.4% in the ischemia-guided strategy, and 1.1% in the revascularization strategy ($P < .02$). The rate of death or myocardial infarction was 12.1% in the angina-guided strategy, 8.8% in the ischemia-guided strategy, and 4.7% in the revascularization strategy ($P < .04$).[81] The rate of death, myocardial infarction, or recurrent cardiac hospitalization was 41.8% in the angina-guided strategy, 38.5% in the ischemia-guided strategy, and 23.1% in the revascularization strategy ($P < .001$). Post-MI patients and those with a high level of sympathetic nervous system activity are perhaps the best candidates for β-blocker therapy.

Calcium channel antagonists alone and in combination have been shown to be effective in reducing symptomatic and asymptomatic ischemia; however, they do not interrupt the diurnal surge in ischemia observed on ambulatory monitoring and, in general, they are somewhat less effective than β-blockers for silent ischemia.[82] Nifedipine in particular seems to provide less protection and provides wide fluctuations in response with approximate reductions in the number of episodes ranging from 0% to 93% and in duration from 23% to 65% unless combined with β-blockers. Fewer studies are available with other calcium blockers and comparative trials are uncommon. Tzivoni et al. compared mibefradil 100 mg and 150 mg to amlodipine 10 mg/d and found that mibefradil was more effective in decreasing the number and duration of silent ischemic episodes; since amlodipine may dose up to 20 mg/d, this study may be flawed.[83] Earlier studies have shown that combination therapy with calcium and β-blockers provides a better response than calcium blockers and nitrates or monotherapy.[1,49]

Surgical intervention using CABG does not appear warranted in asymptomatic patients *without* significant coronary artery disease. Based on the CASS 12-year follow-up results, survival following CABG was enhanced in men with three vessel disease compared to medical therapy (61% vs 46%) but not for women (45% vs 50%) with silent ischemia.[14] The role for PTCA is promising in silent ischemia, and improvement in exercise tolerance and freedom from MI, CABG, and PTCA for new lesions or death may be seen in patients becoming asymptomatic after PTCA. However, exercise-induced silent myocardial ischemia is frequently seen early after successful PTCA and is more prevalent in patients undergoing multivessel angioplasty and incomplete revascularization. Both silent and symptomatic ischemia early after PTCA are predictors of an unfavorable prognosis.

▶ TREATMENT: Syndrome X

Syndrome X refers to the occurrence of effort angina and exercise-induced ECG changes with a normal coronary arteriogram with no evidence of structural (stenosis) or functional (spasm) abnormalities. Although the basis for this syndrome is not yet established, it is thought that syndrome X may be a result of inducible myocardial ischemia caused by impaired functional coronary reserve at the microvascular level of intramural prearteriolar vessels. It has been proposed that this defect is caused by defective prearteriolar regulation of blood flow into the arteriolar bed with subsequent focal, sustained, compensatory release of adenosine; excessive local concentrations of adenosine are then responsible for the pain seen in this syndrome. Prearteriolar constriction may be the result of insufficient vasodilation or inappropriate vasoconstriction, or resetting of myogenic control on a segmental or generalized distribution basis.[84] Cardiomyopathy and left bundle block may result from ischemia in some patients. Follow-up studies have shown that the occurrence of left bundle branch block in response to stress is associated with a greater likelihood of deterioration of left ventricular performance whereas stress-induced ST-segment depression does not predict a detrimental outcome in ventricular function. Esophageal abnormalities may be seen in these patients, and acid refluxing into the esophagus may reduce coronary blood flow.

β-Adrenergic blockers are much less effective in many studies in syndrome X than in exertional angina, and one characteristic, if present, that may predict a good response to β-blockers is increased sympathetic nervous system activity. Angiotensin-converting enzyme inhibitors (ACEI) have been shown to improve coronary reserve, exercise capacity, and exercise time in patients with microvascular angina.[85,86] Estrogen replacement therapy in postmenopausal women has been shown to restore endothelial responsiveness to acetylcholine and this has potential in the management of syndrome X patients but has not been tested.

▶ TREATMENT: Revascularization

CORONARY ARTERY BYPASS GRAFTING

Following the introduction of saphenous vein graft replacement for the severely occluded coronary arteries by Favorolo and Garrett in 1967, coronary artery bypass grafting (CABG) became an accepted and commonly used alternative approach for the management of IHD.[1] The objectives in performing CABG are twofold: (1) reduce the number of symptomatic anginal attacks not controlled with medical management or angioplasty and improve the life-style of the patient and (2) reduce the mortality associated with coronary artery disease. Surgery is effective in providing pain relief in large numbers of patients, with about 70% to 95% being pain-free at 1 year and 46% to 55% being pain-free at 5 years. This compares favorably with medical management, with which only about 30% are free of symptoms at 5 years. The second objective is met in certain patients and this has been addressed in three large, well-controlled trials of bypass surgery. These three studies, the Veterans Administration (VA), European Cooperative Surgery Study (ECSS), and the Coronary Artery Surgery Study (CASS), are not directly comparable because the inclusion and exclusion criteria for entry into each study were different and patients were followed for different periods of time.[1] They have also been criticized for not being representative of the population that may be candidates for surgery, lacking women or late-middle aged or elderly patients, and for crossover of medically managed patients to the surgical group. A major change in medical practice that influences the interpretation of these older studies is the common procedure of stent placement at the time of angioplasty.[87] There are about 20 different types of stents available and their use is associated with greater luminal diameter after angioplasty and fewer reocclusions and less restenosis after stent placement. Consequently, the validity of generalizing the results from these studies to routine practice has been questioned, but these studies are useful for providing a basis for decisions concerning surgery. In general, those patients who have left main stem stenosis of greater than 70%, proximal stenosis of the left anterior descending artery greater than 70% to 75%, poor left ventricular function, or severe three-vessel disease are most likely to have improved survival with surgical therapy. A notable exception to these observations is the lack of difference in any subgroup for CASS, and although trends suggesting improved survival were observed, no significant ($P < .05$) differences were found. This is probably related to patient selection, with patients in CASS having less severe disease compared with the other studies. As these studies have been followed out to 15 years or more, the difference in survival for any subgroup including left main or left main equivalent coronary artery disease becomes insignificant. In addition to survival, other aspects evaluated include exercise capacity, evidence of ischemia, need for drugs to treat angina, and quality of life, including employment status. Exercise capacity may be improved early after CABG; however, at 5 years no significant difference was noted between the medical and surgical groups in CASS and ECSS. The need for nitrates and β-blockers is clearly reduced by surgery, with only 30% of CABG patients requiring chronic medication whereas 70% of their medical counterparts received anginal drugs. Employment status after surgery has been shown in CASS to be more dependent on the pretreatment status than an effect induced by the treatment arm, and about 70% of patients are employed before and after surgery. Recent follow-up analyses of these studies suggest that patients who have diabetes or peripheral vascular disease, who are African-Americans, or who continued to smoke are at high risk for CAD events, and diabetics, in particular, are more likely to have a better outcome with CABG than PTCA.[24,88–90] The overall benefit noted after CABG is similar in men and women, and elderly patients appear to have outcomes similar to younger patients.[91,92]

Indications for bypass surgery should not be rigidly defined although general recommendations can be made based on the available data.[93] Indications may be based on symptoms, coronary anatomy, ventricular function, or evidence for myocardial ischemia with noninvasive stress testing. Based on symptoms, patients with unacceptable limitation of life-style because of symptoms despite optimum medical treatment or inability to tolerate drug therapy because of side effects are considered candidates. Regardless of symptoms, patients with significant stenosis (> 50% to 70%) of left main coronary artery or triple-vessel disease when the proximal left anterior descending coronary has > 70% stenosis or left ventricular function is impaired should be considered. High-risk clinical variables include early positive (> 1.5 mm depression) exercise test, fall in ejection fraction > 5% on exercise, large exercise-induced wall motion abnormality, or large or multiple thallium perfusion defects. In patients 65 years of age or older, surgical benefit is greatest in high-risk patients, 62% surviving compared with 33% in the medical group at 6 years' follow-up, whereas significant improvement was also seen overall (surgical 79% vs medical 64%). Corresponding differences were also noted in patients with chest pain. Left main stem disease or left main equivalent (combined proximal left anterior descending and proximal left circumflex) coronary disease patients are clearly benefited by surgical intervention if the patient has depressed ventricular function. Mortality is related to the severity of stenosis in this situation and perioperative mortality is also increased. Survival at 3 years in the surgical group averages about 85% to 90%, whereas in the medical group survival is significantly lower, about 60% to 70%. In left main equivalent disease, survival at 5 years in CASS was reported to be 85% in the surgical group versus 55% in the medical group, and those patients with ejection fraction less than 50% were the patients with the greatest improvement in survival (69% vs 26%). Similar trends have been noted in patients with three-vessel disease and abnormal ventricular function, with 4-year survival rates of 89% and 55% in the surgical and medical groups, respectively, and with longer follow-up intervals.[8,9]

Operative mortality is reported to range from 1% to 3% and is related to the number of vessels involved and preoperative ventricular function. Patients in CASS with one-, two-, or three-vessel disease had operative mortalities of 1.4%, 2.1%, and 2.8%, respectively. The relationship to left ventricular ejection fraction follows a similar trend with ejection fractions of greater than 50%, 20% to 40%, and less than 20% having operative mortality rates of 1.9%, 4.4%, and 6.7%, respectively. Perioperative infarction averages 5% depending on the sensitivity of the method for assessment, and the occurrence of an infarct reduces long-term survival. Neurologic dysfunction is relatively common postoperatively in CABG patients, but many of the deficits are clinically insignificant and resolve with time. Fatal brain damage occurs in 0.3% to 0.7%, stroke in about 5%, and ophthalmologic defects occur in 25%, but only 3% have clinically apparent field defects. Peripheral nerve lesions (12%) and brachial plexopathy (7%) are also reported to occur. Other complications include constrictive pericarditis (0.2%), cellulitis at the site of vein graft, and mediastinal infections.

Graft patency influences the success for symptom control, and survival and the mechanism for early graft occlusion is probably different from that associated with late closure. Early occlusion is related to platelet adhesion and aggregation whereas late occlusion may be related to endothelial proliferation and progression of atherosclerosis. Patency of grafts early on after the CABG are reported to range from 88% to 97% in at least one graft and 58% to 81% in all grafts at 1 year. Long-term patency based on the CASS Montreal Heart Institute experience suggests that 60% to 67% of all grafts remain patent at 5 to 11 years. Antiplatelet therapy has been demonstrated to improve early and late patency rates and should probably be used in all patients who do not have any contraindications. Aspirin with or without other antiplatelet agents (dipyridamole) reduces the late development of vein-graft occlusions. Late graft closure is related to elevated lipid levels and the progression of atherosclerosis in the grafted vessels as well as the native circulation. Elevation of very low-density lipoprotein (VLDL), low-density lipoprotein (LDL), and LDL apolipoprotein B is correlated to disease progression and graft closure. Aggressive lipid lowering can stablize the progression of CAD and may induce regression in selected coronary artery segments within a patient following CABG. Cessation of smoking is an important preoperative and postoperative objective as well as in the management of other coronary risk factors (e.g., hypertension) and institution of a supervised, daily exercise program is recommended. Internal mammary artery grafts should be used for revascularizing the left anterior descending artery system when possible owing to better graft survival and clinical outcomes.[36]

Valvular heart disease can coexist with coronary heart disease, although this is relatively uncommon with rheumatic valve disease, usually the mitral valve, and more common with aortic stenosis and regurgitation. Angina may occur in 35% to 65% of patients with aortic stenosis or regurgitation, and if severe, may be the cause of angina in the absence of coronary artery disease. Patients being evaluated for possible CABG should also be evaluated for valvular disease to determine if valve replacement needs to be performed along with bypass grafting.

PERCUTANEOUS TRANSLUMINAL CORONARY ANGIOPLASTY

Since the introduction into clinical cardiology of PTCA[94–96] by Gruentzig in 1977, this procedure has gained rapid acceptance as a safe and effective means of managing coronary artery disease. It is estimated that more than 300,000 PTCA procedures are done each year in this country. The proposed mechanisms of reduced stenosis with PTCA include (1) compression and redistribution of the atherosclerotic plaque; (2) embolization of plaque contents; (3) aneurysm formation; and (4) disruption of the plaque and arterial wall with distortion and tearing of the intima and media, which leads to denudation of the endothelium, platelet adhesion and aggregation, thrombus formation, and smooth muscle proliferation. Of these mechanisms, the last one is felt to be the most important, but the others may contribute to opening of the lesions in some situations.

The indications for PTCA have been provided by the ACC/AHA and now span single or multivessel disease as well as asymptomatic and symptomatic patients.[93] PTCA generally is *not* useful if only a small area of viable myocardium is at risk, when ischemia cannot be demonstrated in the laboratory, [a borderline (< 50%) stenosis, or patients are at high risk for] morbidity or mortality or both (e.g., left main or equivalent disease or three-vessel disease). PTCA alone or when used in conjunction or sequentially with thrombolysis for acute myocardial infarction is discussed in Chapter 13, Myocardial Infarction.

Assessment of outcome with PTCA can be based on several clinical and functional factors. It is important to remember that the success of PTCA is dependent on the experience of the operator, on complicating factors for the patient (including the number of vessels to be dilated), and on technical advances in the equipment used (e.g., steerable and low-profile catheters). The initial success rate for immediate opening of uncomplicated stenotic lesions averages ~90% in experienced hands, and angina is decreased or eliminated in about 75% and 85% of cases, respectively. The success rate for more complicated lesions (Type C, see below) is somewhat less (~65%). Mortality at 1 year is 1% and 3% for single-vessel disease and multiple-vessel involvement, respectively, reflecting the good prognosis associated with this degree of coronary artery disease. At 6 years, survival is 98% and 92% for single and multiple disease, respectively.[8,9] Most patients remain event-free (no death, MI, or CABG) for an extended period. Symptomatic status, as measured by the New York Heart Association (NYHA) classification, is improved in many patients. Restenosis is noted in about 30% of patients at 6 months, and two-thirds of these patients will have angina associated with restenosis. A few late restenotic events occur, but most restenosis occurs within the first 6 months. Factors that predict restenosis include little improvement (< 5%) in ejection fraction post-PTCA, continuing wall motion abnormalities, continued smoking, high cholesterol, diabetes, and positive exercise thallium scintigraphy. Increased likelihood for failure or complications with PTCA include female gender, age over 65 years, duration of angina more than 6 months, operator experience with fewer than 50 cases, eccentric stenosis, stenosis severity greater than 90%, calcified stenosis, intraluminal thrombus, involvement of branch vessels, and stenosis located on acute bend in vessel. Lesions are graded from A to C based on these characteristics, Type C being the worst type of lesion.

The overall complication rate ranges from 2% to 21% depending on the lesion type.[68] Coronary occlusion, dissection, or spasm occurs in 4% to 8% of patients, whereas myocardial infarction occurs in 5%. Prolonged angina and ventricular tachycardia or fibrillation occurs in 6.9% and 2.3%, respectively. Mortality was reported to be 0.9% overall and high-risk events for mortality included ventricular arrhythmias and myocardial infarction. The frequency of urgent CABG because of complications ranges from 1% to 4%.

During PTCA patients are usually heparinized to prevent immediate thrombus formation during the procedure, and systemic anticoagulation is continued for up to 24 hours. Some authors have advocated heparin alternatives such as hirudin or hirulog but there is no apparent long-term advantage with these agents.[97–99] In addition to anticoagulation with heparin, abciximab (RheoPro, a IIb/IIIa platelet glycoprotein inhibitor) given as a bolus and constant infusion has been shown in the EPIC trial (Evaluation of 7E3 for the Prevention of Ischemic Complications) to reduce the need for urgent repeat PTCA.[72,100] Abciximab works by preventing platelet binding to adhesive glycoproteins such as fibrinogen, von Willebrand factor, and others. Abciximab reduces the risk of death, MI, or need for revascularization by > 50% and the effect is most pronounced in patients with unstable angina. This improvement, however, came at the cost of a twofold increase in major bleeding complications (from 7% to 14%) and this drug costs more than $1400 per treatment course; however, an economic analysis has shown that during the 6-month follow-up, c7E3 Fab decreased repeat hospitalization rates by 23% (P = .004) and repeat revascularization by 22% (P = .04), producing a mean $1270 savings per patient (exclusive of drug cost) (P = .018).[101] Eptifibatide (Integrilin), another IIb/IIIa antagonist, also reduces the risk of death, myocardial infarction, unplanned surgical or repeat percutaneous revascularization, or coronary stent implantation for abrupt closure by about 20%.[71] Mechanisms that result in restenosis include acute lumen loss owing to "recoil," mural thrombosis formation, and smooth muscle cell proliferation with synthesis of extracellular matrix.[96] Approaches to prevent restenosis may be aimed at altering the underlying mechanisms. Recoil and loss of luminal diameter may be reduced by the use of stent placement; however, this beneficial effect is offset by an increased number of vascular complications. Cracking of the plaque leads to severe damage to the arterial wall, exposure of collagen, and endothelial dysfunction. These factors promote mural thrombi, and the propensity for thrombus formation is related, in part, to the composition of the plaque as well as the depth of injury. Heparin has been the traditional antithrombotic used to prevent thrombosis in this setting and recently abciximab has been approved as well; the results of the EPIC trial are described previously. Aspirin is typically used post-PTCA to minimize the platelet contribution to thrombosis formation with the usual dose 325 mg/d; however, antithrombotic therapy (warfarin, aspirin, dipyridamole, ticlopidine, prostacyclin, unfractioned heparin, LMWH, hirudin, or antiplatelet combinations) has little effect on long-term restenosis rates.[102] Most of the trials of lipid-lowering drugs or omega-3 fatty acids also show little benefit for prevention of restenosis. Small studies of antiproliferative agents (trapidil, angiopeptin, tranilast) show some promise in limiting restenosis.[103,104] Other investigational approaches continue to be explored.[102]

Smooth muscle activation leads to late restenosis (2 weeks to 3 months), which occurs in three waves. The first wave is medial smooth muscle activation, followed by medial smooth muscle cell migration secondary to the liberation of various chemoattractants, and finally, intimal proliferation and synthesis of extracellular matrix. Most of the pharmacologic interventions to prevent the third phase of restenosis have not been effective with the exception of trapidil, which is a platelet-derived growth factor antagonist as well as an inhibitor of platelet aggregation and smooth muscle cell proliferation. Other approaches include local drug delivery through double-balloon techniques or through barophoretic and inotophoretic methods.[105] Future approaches may include altering gene expression with specific growth factor inhibitors, intracoronary radiation therapy (ICRT), cyclin regulators or antisense nucleotides, enhancement of reendothelialization with gene transfer or natural endothelial-derived inhibitors, and, last, photodynamic therapy to produce locally active oxygen species to alter smooth muscle cell function.

Other agents such as thromboxanes A_2 synthetase inhibitor or receptor antagonists, ticlopidine, and others might be useful. Some studies with fish oil are positive whereas others are negative, and lovastatin does not alter restenosis. Corticosteroids and nonsteroidal agents may inhibit inflammation involved in restenosis but no large randomized trials exist supporting their use. Calcium antagonists may also be given to prevent coronary artery spasm during PTCA, and some centers also pretreat patients with antiplatelet therapy for PTCA. Following PTCA, calcium antagonists are given for 2 to 4 weeks to prevent coronary artery spasm and for their other antiischemic effects, and some believe they may also prevent restenosis. Individual studies with follow-up at 10 months have shown little difference between placebo and calcium antagonists on restenosis rates, but a meta-analysis of five trials shows about a 30% reduction in restenosis.[102,106] Antiplatelet therapy with aspirin or aspirin plus dipyridamole does not reduce or prevent restenosis, but the combination may reduce the incidence of acute complications during or immediately after angioplasty. Antiplatelet therapy with aspirin with or without dipyridamole is recommended by some for 1 year following PTCA to delay or prevent restenosis. Trials to test the effectiveness of ACEI in preventing intimal proliferation after angioplasty demonstrated no benefit on restenosis or clinical end points, which result may be related to lack of complete inhibition of ACE.

Alternatives to PTCA include directional coronary atherectomy (DCA), excimer laser, rotational atherectomy (rotablator), and intracoronary stents or some combination of these interventions.[94] Based on three randomized trials, DCA produces greater initial luminal diameter but results in a higher rate of post-procedural complications such as non-Q-wave MI and death and is more expensive. Consequently, PTCA is considered to be superior to DCA for most patients. The use of abciximab may improve these results. Excimer laser angioplasty followed by balloon angioplasty or rotational atherectomy provides no benefit additional to balloon angioplasty alone.[107–109] Intracoronary stents result in larger initial minimal lumen diameter, improved clinical outcome, and less restenosis than PTCA; however, these benefits are offset by loss of luminal diameter differences later and a two- to fourfold increase in bleeding and vascular complications owing to the need for anticoagulation.

When medical therapy, PTCA, and CABG have been compared, low-risk patients with single-vessel coronary artery disease and normal left ventricular function had greater alleviation of symptoms with PTCA than with medical treatment; mortality rates and rates of myocardial infarction were unchanged. In high-risk patients (risk was defined by severity of ischemia, number of diseased vessels, and presence of left ventricular dysfunction), improvement of survival was greater with CABG than with medical therapy. In moderate-risk patients with multivessel coronary artery disease (most had two-vessel disease and normal left ventricular function), PTCA and CABG produced equivalent mortality rates and rates of myocardial infarction.[95]

▶ PRINCIPLES OF PHARMACOTHERAPY

- IHD is primarily caused by atherosclerosis and is very common in the US population.
- Risk factor identification and modification are important for individual patients with known or suspected IHD and as a population-based policy to reduce the impact of this disease.
- Major risk factors that can be altered include dyslipidemia (high total and LDL cholesterol and low HDL cholesterol), smoking, glycemic control in diabetes mellitus, hypertension, and HRT in appropriate patients.
- Nitroglycerin and other nitrate products are useful for prophylaxis of angina when patients are undertaking activities know to provoke angina; however, when angina is occurring on a regular, routine basis, other therapies should be used for chronic prophylaxis.
- Chronic stable angina should be managed initially with β-blockers because they provide better symptomatic control at least as well as nitrates or calcium channel blockers and decrease the risk of recurrent MI and CAD mortality.
- Although calcium channel blockers are effective as monotherapy, they are generally used in combination with β-blockers or as monotherapy if patients are intolerant of β-blockers; most patients with moderate to severe angina will require two drugs to control their symptoms.
- Pharmacologic management is as effective as revascularization (PTCA, CABG, etc.) if one or two

vessels are involved and there are no differences in survival, recurrent MI, or other measures of effectiveness.

- Multivessel involvement, especially if the patient has left main coronary artery disease or left main equivalent disease, or two to three vessel involvement with significant left ventricular dysfunction is best managed with revascularization.
- PTCA and CABG produce similar results overall but certain patient subsets (e.g., diabetics) should have CABG done.

REFERENCES

1. Talbert R. Ischemic Heart Disease. In: DiPiro JT, Wells BG, Yee GC, Matzke GR, Posey LM eds. Pharmacotherapy: A Pathophysiologic Approach, 2nd ed. Samford, CT, Appleton & Lange, 1996:257–294.
2. Sytkowski PA, D'Agostino RB, Belanger A, Kannel WB. Sex and time trends in cardiovascular disease incidence and mortality: the Framingham Heart Study, 1950–1989. Am J Epidemiol 1996;143:338–350.
3. Kannel WB, Feinleib M. Natural history of angina pectoris in the Framingham study: Prognosis and survival. Am J Cardiol 1972;29:154–163.
4. Menotti A, Keys A, Blackburn H, et al. Comparison of multivariate predictive power of major risk factors for coronary heart diseases in different countries: Results from eight nations of the Seven Countries Study, 25-year follow-up. J Cardiovasc Risk 1996;3:69–75.
5. Keys A. Mediterranean diet and public health: Personal reflections. Am J Clin Nutr 1995;61:1321S–1323S.
6. Goldman L, Hashimoto B, Cook EF, et al. Comparative reproducibility and validity of systems for assessing cardiovascular functional class: Advantages of a new specific activity scale. Circulation 1981;64:1227–1234.
7. Emond M, Mock MB, Davis KB, et al. Long-term survival of medically treated patients in the Coronary Artery Surgery Study (CASS) Registry. Circulation 1994;90:2645–2657.
8. Caracciolo EA, Davis KB, Sopko G, et al. Comparison of surgical and medical group survival in patients with left main equivalent coronary artery disease. Long-term CASS experience. Circulation 1995;91:2335–2344.
9. Caracciolo EA, Davis KB, Sopko G, et al. Comparison of surgical and medical group survival in patients with left main coronary artery disease. Long-term CASS experience. Circulation 1995;91:2325–2334.
10. Epstein SE CRI, Talbot TL. Hemodynamic principles in the control of coronary blood flow. Am J Cardiol 1985;56:4E–10E.
11. Hasdai D, Gibbons RJ, Holmes DR Jr, Higano ST, Lerman A. Coronary endothelial dysfunction in humans is associated with myocardial perfusion defects. Circulation 1997;96:3390–3395.
12. Crawford M. Unstable Angina. Diagnosis and Management. Commentary on the AHCPR Clinical Practice Guidelines. New York, Chapman & Hall, 1997:1–143.
13. Braunwald E, Jones RH, Mark DB, et al. Diagnosing and managing unstable angina. Agency for Health Care Policy and Research. Circulation 1994; 90:613–622.
14. Weiner DA, Ryan TJ, Parsons L, et al. Significance of silent myocardial ischemia during exercise testing in women: Report from the Coronary Artery Surgery Study. Am Heart J 1995;129:465–470.
15. Stone PH, Chaitman BR, Forman S, et al. Prognostic significance of myocardial ischemia detected by ambulatory electrocardiography, exercise treadmill testing, and electrocardiogram at rest to predict cardiac events by one year (the Asymptomatic Cardiac Ischemia Pilot [ACIP] study). Am J Cardiol 1997;80:1395–1401.
16. Caracciolo EA, Chaitman BR, Forman SA, et al. Diabetics with coronary disease have a prevalence of asymptomatic ischemia during exercise treadmill testing and ambulatory ischemia monitoring similar to that of nondiabetic patients. An ACIP database study. ACIP Investigators. Asymptomatic Cardiac Ischemia Pilot Investigators. Circulation 1996;93:2097–2105.
17. Glusman M, Coromilas J, Clark WC, et al. Pain sensitivity in silent myocardial ischemia. Pain 1996;64:477–483.
18. Hoeg JM. Evaluating coronary heart disease risk. Tiles in the mosaic. JAMA 1997; 277:1387–1390. Clinical conference.
19. Lindahl B, Venge P, Wallentin L. Troponin T identifies patients with unstable coronary artery disease who benefit from long-term antithrombotic protection. Fragmin in Unstable Coronary Artery Disease (FRISC) Study Group. J Am Coll Cardiol 1997;29:43–48.
20. Thompson GR, Forbat S, Underwood R. Electron-beam CT scanning for detection of coronary calcification and prediction of coronary heart disease. Q J Med 1996;89:565–570.
21. Abizaid A, Mintz GS, Pichard AD, et al. Is intravascular ultrasound clinically useful or is it just a research tool? Heart 1997;78:27–30.
22. National Cholesterol Education Program. Second Report of the Expert Panel on Detection, Evaluation, and Treatment of High Blood Cholesterol in Adults (Adult Treatment Panel II). Circulation 1994; 89:1333–1445.
23. Effect of intensive diabetes management on macrovascular events and risk factors in the Diabetes Control and Complications Trial. Am J Cardiol 1995;75:894–903.
24. Cavender JB, Rogers WJ, Fisher LD, et al. Effects of smoking on survival and morbidity in patients randomized to medical or surgical therapy in the Coronary Artery Surgery Study (CASS): 10-year follow-up. CASS Investigators. J Am Coll Cardiol 1992;20: 287–294.
25. Wald NJ, Watt HC. Prospective study of effect of switching from cigarettes to pipes or cigars on mortality from three smoking related diseases. BMJ 1997;314:1860–1863.
26. Hung J, Lam JY, Lacoste L, Letchacovski G. Cigarette smoking acutely increases platelet thrombus formation in patients with coronary artery disease taking aspirin. Circulation 1995; 92:2432–2436.
27. Vogel RA. Coronary risk factors, endothelial function, and atherosclerosis: a review. Clin Cardiol 1997;20:426–432.
28. Kannel WB. Blood pressure as a cardiovascular risk factor: Prevention and treatment. JAMA 1996;275:1571–1576.
29. Mulrow CD, Cornell JA, Herrera CR, et al. Hypertension in the elderly. Implications and generalizability of randomized trials. JAMA 1994;272:1932–1938.
30. Mosca L, Rubenfire M, Mandel C, et al. Antioxidant nutrient supplementation reduces the susceptibility of low density lipoprotein to oxidation in patients with coronary artery disease. J Am Coll Cardiol 1997;30:392–399.
31. Paolisso G, Gambardella A, Giugliano D, et al. Chronic intake of pharmacological doses of vitamin E might be useful in the therapy of elderly patients with coronary heart disease. Am J Clin Nutr 1995; 61:848–852.
32. Subbiah MT. Mechanisms of cardioprotection by estrogens. Proc Soc Exp Biol Med 1998;217:23–29.
33. Grodstein F, Stampfer MJ, Colditz GA, et al. Postmenopausal hormone therapy and mortality. N Engl J Med 1997;336:1769–1775. See comments.
34. Gersh BJ, Braunwald E, Rutherford JD. Chronic coronary artery disease. In: Braunwald E, ed. Heart Disease. A Textbook of Cardiovascular Medicine. Philadelphia, Saunders, 1997:1289–1365.
35. Goldstein S. Beta-blocking drugs and coronary heart disease. Cardiovas Drugs Ther 1997;11:219–225.
36. Carbajal EV, Deedwania PC. Contemporary approaches in medical management of patients with stable coronary artery disease. Med Clin North Am 1995;79:1063–1084.
37. Prince MJ, Bird AS, Blizard RA, Mann AH. Is the cognitive function of older patients affected by antihypertensive treatment? Results

from 54 months of the Medical Research Council's trial of hypertension in older adults. BMJ 1996;312:801–805.
38. Rosenthal J, Bahrmann H, Benkert K, et al. Analysis of adverse effects among patients with essential hypertension receiving an ACE inhibitor or a beta-blocker. Cardiology 1996;87:409–414.
39. Abrams J. The role of nitrates in coronary heart disease. Arch Intern Med 1995;155:357–364.
40. Thadani U. Oral nitrates: More than symptomatic therapy in coronary artery disease? Cardiovasc Drugs Ther 1997;11:213–218.
41. Parker JO, Amies MH, Hawkinson RW, et al. Intermittent transdermal nitroglycerin therapy in angina pectoris. Clinically effective without tolerance or rebound. Minitran Efficacy Study Group. Circulation 1995;91:1368–1374.
42. DeMots H, Glasser SP on behalf of the Transderm-Nitro Study Group. Intermittent transdermal nitroglycerin therapy in the treatment of chronic stable angina. J Am Coll Cardiol 1989:786–793.
43. Heitzer T, Just H, Brockhoff C, et al. Long-term nitroglycerin treatment is associated with supersensitivity to vasoconstrictors in men with stable coronary artery disease: Prevention by concomitant treatment with captopril. J Am Coll Cardiol 1998;31:83–88.
44. Pizzulli L, Hagendorff A, Zirbes M, et al. Influence of captopril on nitroglycerin-mediated vasodilation and development of nitrate tolerance in arterial and venous circulation. Am Heart J 1996;131: 342–349.
45. Parker JD, Parker AB, Farrell B, Parker JO. Effects of diuretic therapy on the development of tolerance to nitroglycerin and exercise capacity in patients with chronic stable angina. Circulation 1996; 93:691–696.
46. Watanabe H, Kakihana M, Ohtsuka S, Sugishita Y. Randomized, double-blind, placebo-controlled study of supplemental vitamin E on attenuation of the development of nitrate tolerance. Circulation 1997;96:2545–2550.
47. Freedman SB, Daxini BV, Noyce D, Kelly DT. Intermittent transdermal nitrates do not improve ischemia in patients taking beta-blockers or calcium antagonists: Potential role of rebound ischemia during the nitrate-free period. J Am Coll Cardiol 1995;25:349–355.
48. Munzel T, Heitzer T, Kurz S, et al. Dissociation of coronary vascular tolerance and neurohormonal adjustments during long-term nitroglycerin therapy in patients with stable coronary artery disease. J Am Coll Cardiol 1996;27:297–303.
49. Pratt CM, McMahon RP, Goldstein S, et al. Comparison of subgroups assigned to medical regimens used to suppress cardiac ischemia (the Asymptomatic Cardiac Ischemia Pilot [ACIP] Study). Am J Cardiol 1996;77:1302–1309.
50. Parmley WW. Optimal treatment of stable angina. Cardiology 1997; 88:27–31.
51. Opie LH. Calcium channel antagonists in the treatment of coronary artery disease: Fundamental pharmacological properties relevant to clinical use. Prog Cardiovasc Dis 1996;38:273–290.
52. Brogden RN, Markham A. Mibefradil. A review of its pharmacodynamic and pharmacokinetic properties, and therapeutic efficacy in the management of hypertension and angina pectoris. Drugs 1997; 54:774–793.
53. North of England Stable Angina Guideline Development Group. North of England evidence based guidelines development project: Summary version of evidence based guideline for the primary care management angina. BMJ 1996;312:827–832.
54. The investigation and management of stable angina. Report of a working party of the Joint Audit Committee of the British Cardiac Society and the Royal College of Physicians of London. J R Coll Phys London 1993;27:267–273.
55. Management of stable angina pectoris. Recommendations of the Task Force of the European Society of Cardiology. Eur Heart J 1997;18:394–413.
56. Jensen BE, Fletcher BJ, Rupp JC, et al. Training level comparison study. Effect of high and low intensity exercise on ventilatory threshold in men with coronary artery disease. J Cardpulm Rehabil 1996; 16:227–232.
57. Fox KM, Mulcahy D, Findlay I, Ford I, Dargie HJ. The Total Ischaemic Burden European Trial (TIBET). Effects of atenolol, nifedipine SR and their combination on the exercise test and the total ischaemic burden in 608 patients with stable angina. The TIBET Study Group. Eur Heart J 1996;17:96–103.
58. Dargie HJ, Ford I, Fox KM. Total Ischaemic Burden European Trial (TIBET). Effects of ischaemia and treatment with atenolol, nifedipine SR and their combination on outcome in patients with chronic stable angina. The TIBET Study Group. Eur Heart J 1996;17:104–112.
59. Howes LG, Edwards CT. Calcium antagonists and cancer. Is there really a link? Drug Saf 1998;18:1–7.
60. Effects of calcium antagonists on the risks of coronary heart disease, cancer and bleeding. Ad Hoc Subcommittee of the Liaison Committee of the World Health Organisation and the International Society of Hypertension. Hyperten Res 1997;20:61–73.
61. Brunelli C, Spallarossa P, Rossettin P, Caponnetto S. Recognition and treatment of unstable angina. Drugs 1996;52:196–208.
62. Tonkin AM, Aroney CN. Guidelines for managing patients with unstable angina. Rating the evidence and rationale for treatment. Med J Aust 1997;166:644–647.
63. Gurfinkel EP, Manos EJ, Majail RI, et al. Low molecular weight heparin versus regular heparin or aspirin in the treatment of unstable angina and silent ischemia. J Am Coll Cardiol 1995;26:313–318.
64. Cohen M, Demers C, Gurfinkel EP, et al. A comparison of low-molecular-weight heparin with unfractionated heparin for unstable coronary artery disease. Efficacy and Safety of Subcutaneous Enoxaparin in Non-Q-Wave Coronary Events Study Group. N Engl J Med 1997;337:447–452.
65. Dose-ranging trial of enoxaparin for unstable angina: Results of TIMI 11A. The Thrombolysis in Myocardial Infarction (TIMI) 11A Trial Investigators. J Am Coll Cardiol 1997;29:1474–1482.
66. Breddin HK. Coronary heart disease, unstable angina, PTCA: New indications for low molecular weight heparins? Thromb Res 1996; 81:S47–51.
67. Williams DO, Braunwald E, Thompson B, et al. Results of percutaneous transluminal coronary angioplasty in unstable angina and non-Q-wave myocardial infarction. Observations from the TIMI IIIB Trial. Circulation 1996;94:2749–2755.
68. Keelan ET, Nunez BD, Grill DE, et al. Comparison of immediate and long-term outcome of coronary angioplasty performed for unstable angina and rest pain in men and women. Mayo Clin Proc 1997; 72:5–12.
69. Condado JA, Waksman R, Gurdiel O, et al. Long-term angiographic and clinical outcome after percutaneous transluminal coronary angioplasty and intracoronary radiation therapy in humans. Circulation 1997;96:727–732. See comments.
70. Libby P, Egan D, Skarlatos S. Roles of infectious agents in atherosclerosis and restenosis: An assessment of the evidence and need for future research. Circulation 1997;96:4095–5103.
71. Randomised placebo-controlled trial of effect of eptifibatide on complications of percutaneous coronary intervention: IMPACT-II. Integrilin to Minimise Platelet Aggregation and Coronary Thrombosis—II. Lancet 1997;349:1422–1428. See comments.
72. Platelet glycoprotein IIb/IIIa receptor blockade and low-dose heparin during percutaneous coronary revascularization. The EPILOG Investigators. N Engl J Med 1997;336:1689–1696. See comments.
73. Randomised placebo-controlled trial of abciximab before and during coronary intervention in refractory unstable angina: the CAPTURE Study. (published erratum appears in Lancet 1997;350:744). Lancet 1997;349:1429–1435.
74. Effects of platelet glycoprotein IIb/IIIa blockade with tirofiban on adverse cardiac events in patients with unstable angina or acute myocardial infarction undergoing coronary angioplasty. The RESTORE Investigators. Randomized Efficacy Study of Tirofiban for Outcomes and REstenosis. Circulation 1997;96:1445–1453.
75. Cannon CP, McCabe CH, Borzak S, et al. Randomized trial of an oral platelet glycoprotein IIb/IIIa antagonist, sibrafiban, in patients after

an acute coronary syndrome: Results of the TIMI 12 trial. Thrombolysis in Myocardial Infarction. Circulation 1998;97: 340–349.
76. Kereiakes DJ, Runyon JP, Kleiman NS, et al. Differential dose-response to oral xemilofiban after antecedent intravenous abciximab. Administration for complex coronary intervention. Circulation 1996; 94:906–910.
77. Tsuchiya T, Okumura K, Yasue H, Kugiyama K, Ogawa H. Heart period variability in patients with variant angina. Am J Cardiol 1996; 77:932–936.
78. Ishida T, Hirata K, Sakoda T, et al. 5-HT1D beta receptor mediates the supersensitivity of isolated coronary artery to serotonin in variant angina. Chest 1998;113:243–244.
79. Lanza GA, Pedrotti P, Pasceri V, et al. Autonomic changes associated with spontaneous coronary spasm in patients with variant angina. J Am Coll Cardiol 1996;28:1249–1256.
80. Conti CR, Geller NL, Knatterud GL, et al. Anginal status and prediction of cardiac events in patients enrolled in the Asymptomatic Cardiac Ischemia Pilot (ACIP) study. ACIP Investigators. Am J Cardiol 1997;79:889–892.
81. Davies RF, Goldberg AD, Forman S, et al. Asymptomatic Cardiac Ischemia Pilot (ACIP) study two-year follow-up: Outcomes of patients randomized to initial strategies of medical therapy versus revascularization. Circulation 1997;95:2037–2043. See comments.
82. Singh N, Mironov D, Goodman S, Morgan CD, Langer A. Treatment of silent ischemia in unstable angina: A randomized comparison of sustained-release verapamil versus metoprolol. Clin Cardiol 1995; 18:653–658.
83. Tzivoni D, Kadr H, Braat S, et al. Efficacy of mibefradil compared with amlodipine in suppressing exercise-induced and daily silent ischemia: Results of a multicenter, placebo-controlled trial. Circulation 1997;96:2557–2564.
84. Bund SJ, Tweddel A, Hutton I, Heagerty AM. Small artery structural alterations of patients with microvascular angina (syndrome X). Clin Sci 1996;91:739–743.
85. Motz W, Strauer BE. Improvement of coronary flow reserve after long-term therapy with enalapril. Hypertension 1996;27:1031–1038.
86. Iriarte M, Caso R, Murga N, et al. Enalapril-induced regression of hypertensive left ventricular hypertrophy, regional ischemia, and microvascular angina. Am J Cardiol 1995;75:850–852.
87. Serruys P. Handbook of Coronary Stents. St. Louis, Mosby, 1997: 1–163.
88. Comparison of coronary bypass surgery with angioplasty in patients with multivessel disease. The Bypass Angioplasty Revascularization Investigation (BARI) Investigators (published erratum appears in N Engl J Med 1997;336:147). N Engl J Med 1996;335:217–225. See comments.
89. Barzilay JI, Kronmal RA, Bittner V, et al. Coronary artery disease in diabetic patients with lower-extremity arterial disease: Disease characteristics and survival. A report from the Coronary Artery Surgery Study (CASS) registry. Diabetes Care 1997;20:1381–1387.
90. Taylor HA Jr, Mickel MC, Chaitman BR, et al. Long-term survival of African Americans in the Coronary Artery Surgery Study (CASS). J Am Coll Cardiol 1997;29:358–364.
91. Davis KB, Chaitman B, Ryan T, Bittner V, Kennedy JW. Comparison of 15-year survival for men and women after initial medical or surgical treatment for coronary artery disease: A CASS registry study. Coronary Artery Surgery Study. J Am Coll Cardiol 1995;25:1000–1009. See comments.
92. Morrison DA, Bies RD, Sacks J. Coronary angioplasty for elderly patients with "high risk" unstable angina: Short-term outcomes and long-term survival. J Am Coll Cardiol 1997;29:339–344.
93. Lee T. Practice guidelines in cardiovascular medicine. In: Braunwald E, ed. Heart Disease. A Textbook of Cardiovascular Medicine. Philadelphia, Saunders, 1997:1939–1996.
94. Moliterno DJ, Elliott JM. Randomized trials of myocardial revascularization. Curr Probl Cardiol 1995;20:125–190.
95. Solomon AJ, Gersh BJ. Management of chronic stable angina: Medical therapy, percutaneous transluminal coronary angioplasty, and coronary artery bypass graft surgery. Lessons from the randomized trials. Ann Intern Med 1998;128:216–223.
96. Landzberg BR, Frishman WH, Lerrick K. Pathophysiology and pharmacological approaches for prevention of coronary artery restenosis following coronary artery balloon angioplasty and related procedures. Prog Cardiovasc Dis 1997;39:361–398.
97. Shah PB, Ahmed WH, Ganz P, Bittl JA. Bivalirudin compared with heparin during coronary angioplasty for thrombus-containing lesions. J Am Coll Cardiol 1997;30:1264–1269.
98. A clinical trial comparing primary coronary angioplasty with tissue plasminogen activator for acute myocardial infarction. The Global Use of Strategies to Open Occluded Coronary Arteries in Acute Coronary Syndromes (GUSTO IIb) Angioplasty Substudy Investigators. N Engl J Med 1997;336:1621–1628.
99. Bittl JA, Strony J, Brinker JA, et al. Treatment with bivalirudin (Hirulog) as compared with heparin during coronary angioplasty for unstable or postinfarction angina. Hirulog Angioplasty Study Investigators. N Engl J Med 1995;333:764–769.
100. Lincoff AM, Califf RM, Anderson KM, et al. Evidence for prevention of death and myocardial infarction with platelet membrane glycoprotein IIb/IIIa receptor blockade by abciximab (c7E3 Fab) among patients with unstable angina undergoing percutaneous coronary revascularization. EPIC Investigators. Evaluation of 7E3 in Preventing Ischemic Complications. J Am Coll Cardiol 1997;30:149–156.
101. Mark DB, Talley JD, Topol EJ, et al. Economic assessment of platelet glycoprotein IIb/IIIa inhibition for prevention of ischemic complications of high-risk coronary angioplasty. EPIC Investigators. Circulation 1996;94:629–635.
102. Lefkovits J, Topol EJ. Pharmacological approaches for the prevention of restenosis after percutaneous coronary intervention. Prog Cardiovasc Dis 1997;40:141–158.
103. Kosuga K, Tamai H, Ueda K, et al. Effectiveness of tranilast on restenosis after directional coronary atherectomy. Am Heart J 1997;134:712–718.
104. Emanuelsson H, Beatt KJ, Bagger JP, et al. Long-term effects of angiopeptin treatment in coronary angioplasty. Reduction of clinical events but not angiographic restenosis. European Angiopeptin Study Group. Circulation 1995;91:1689–1696.
105. Bailey SR. Local drug delivery: Current applications. Prog Cardiovasc Dis 1997;40:183–204.
106. Hillegass WB, Ohman EM, Leimberger JD, Califf RM. A meta-analysis of randomized trials of calcium antagonists to reduce restenosis after coronary angioplasty. Am J Cardiol 1994;73: 835–839.
107. Appelman YE, Piek JJ, Strikwerda S, et al. Randomised trial of excimer laser angioplasty versus balloon angioplasty for treatment of obstructive coronary artery disease. Lancet 1996;347:79–84. See comments.
108. Reifart N, Vandormael M, Krajcar M, et al. Randomized comparison of angioplasty of complex coronary lesions at a single center. Excimer Laser, Rotational Atherectomy, and Balloon Angioplasty Comparison (ERBAC) Study. Circulation 1997;96:91–98.
109. Stone GW, de Marchena E, Dageforde D, et al. Prospective, randomized, multicenter comparison of laser-facilitated balloon angioplasty versus stand-alone balloon angioplasty in patients with obstructive coronary artery disease. The Laser Angioplasty Versus Angioplasty (LAVA) Trial Investigators. J Am Coll Cardiol 1997;30:1714–1721.
110. Monthly Vital Statistics Report 1997;45(suppl). Centers for Disease Control, National Centers for Health Statistics.
111. Campeau L. Grading of angina. Circulation 1976;54:522–523. Letter.
112. Principal Investigators of CASS and their associates. The National Heart, Lung, and Blood Institute coronary artery surgery study (CASS). Circulation 1981;62:I-1.
113. Epstein SE, Talbot, TL. Dynamic coronary tone in precipitation, exacerbation and relief of angina pectoris. Am J Cardiol 1981;48:798.
114. Helfant RH, Banka VS. A Clinical and Angiographic Approach to Coronary Heart Disease. Philadelphia, Davis, 1978:47.
115. Cohn PF, ed. Diagnosis and Therapy of Coronary Artery Disease, 2nd ed. Boston, Martin Nijhoff, 1985:101.

13

MYOCARDIAL INFARCTION

Kathleen A. Stringer, PharmD, FCCP, and Larry M. Lopez, PharmD, FCCP

Myocardial infarction is the number one killer of both men and women in the United States. Approximately 900,000 people experience acute myocardial infarction (MI) each year.[1] Of these, nearly 225,000 die, 125,000 of whom do so prior to receiving medical care.[1]

The cardiac mortality during hospitalization for first MI patients is 7% to 12% and approximately 6% per year thereafter.[2] Patients with larger MI such as anterior wall infarction, left ventricular dysfunction, and complex ventricular ectopy carry the highest 1-year mortality post-MI (22%).

The cost of coronary disease in the United States is steep.[1,3] In 1997, the estimated financial consequence of coronary artery disease to the U.S. health care system was severe, approximately $91 billion (direct and indirect costs).[1] Therefore, therapeutic interventions that reduce mortality and improve morbidity, as well as primary and secondary prevention strategies, will have a significant impact on the U.S. health care system.

Drug therapy and the approach to the management of MI patients has changed and improved dramatically since the mid-1980s. Technological and therapeutic advancements as well as a greater understanding of the pathophysiology of acute coronary syndromes have prompted the progress and development of pharmacotherapy for MI. One of the most important advancements has been the introduction of thrombolytic therapy. Though initially suggested as a potential therapeutic tool in the 1950s, thrombolytic therapy was not evaluated in clinical trials until the early 1980s. This delay was most likely due to the controversy that surrounded the etiology of MI.

Although it was suggested as early as 1912 that thrombus formation played a critical role in the pathophysiology of MI, it was not until 1980, when, using acute angiography, DeWood et al.[4] definitively demonstrated that thrombus formation was the principal etiology of MI. Once this pathology was established, a flurry of intracoronary thrombolytic trials followed. Subsequently, the feasibility and usefulness of peripherally administered intravenous (IV) thrombolytic therapy was demonstrated and is now widely accepted. Progress continues in the development of new thrombolytic agents, anticoagulants, and antiplatelet drugs to enhance patient care and outcome. Further, the role of primary angioplasty continues to evolve.

This chapter provides the clinician with an in-depth overview of the pathophysiology and current pharmacotherapeutic management of patients with uncomplicated MI. Also included is a brief discussion of the principles of secondary prevention and the management of the post-MI patient.

ETIOLOGY

Coronary artery disease (CAD) is the primary underlying process that leads to MI.[5–7] The process of CAD begins early in life, usually within the first decade. Fatty streaks deposit on coronary artery endothelium and may progress to form atherosclerotic plaques depending on the absence or presence of specific risk factors. These include hypertension, diabetes mellitus, smoking, and hyperlipidemia. Recent data also suggest that plasma homocysteine levels correlate to mortality associated with CAD.[8] However, there is yet insufficient data to confirm elevated homocysteine as an independent risk factor for CAD.

If progression occurs, atherosclerotic plaques develop, proliferate, and eventually disrupt the integrity and function of the endothelium.[9] Subsequently, myocardial ischemia may occur due to the narrowing of one or more coronary arteries. However, coronary artery narrowing is not the etiology of MI. Thrombus formation precipitated by atherosclerotic plaque rupture or fissure is the cause of more than 85% of acute MIs.[5–7] Upon plaque rupture, the thrombogenic, lipid-rich core is exposed, initiating platelet and thrombin activation, release of vasoactive substances such as thromboxane A_2 and endothelin, and subsequent thrombus formation.[9]

Myocardial ischemia most likely precedes MI, but there are two distinct characteristics that differentiate MI from myocardial ischemia. First, MI is precipitated by a sudden interruption of blood supply to an area of myocardium due to complete, or near complete, occlusion of a coronary artery. Second, the occlusion persists long enough that myocardial function is compromised and myocardium becomes necrotic (nonviable). Infarction is characterized by a "wavefront" of ischemia that progresses from the endocardium to the epicardium (Fig. 13–1).[10] Subsequently, if coronary blood flow is not restored, myocardium dies, the time course for which is approximately 3 hours in animal models. Therefore, the primary difference between ischemia and infarction is viable myocardium. However, despite this rapid time course, it has been demonstrated that a significant percentage of myocardium "hibernates" in response to ischemia and is salvageable after as long as 12 to 24 hours of ischemia. This phenomenon may also be due in part to the presence of collateral blood flow within the

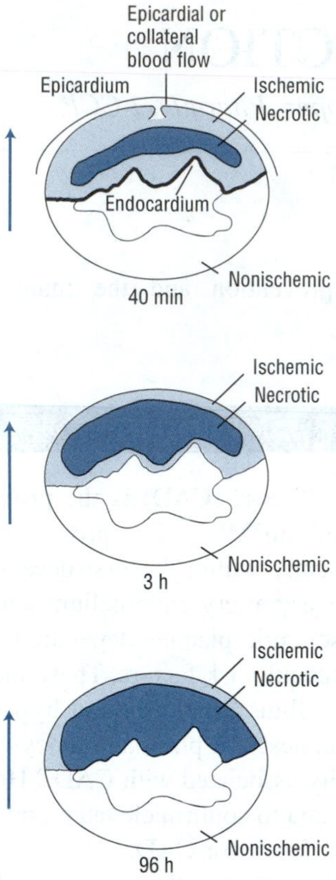

FIGURE 13–1. Wavefront of myocardial ischemia.

infarcted area.[11,12] Full recovery of systolic function after complete restoration of blood flow may nevertheless be delayed due to a process called myocardial "stunning." These features of MI have important implications for the therapeutic management, prognosis, and outcome of patients with MI.

INFARCT LOCATION AND TYPE

The type and location of MI play a very important role in determining the therapeutic management and predicting the prognosis of the patient. Anterior wall MI (AWMI) involves the anterior wall of the left ventricle and most often represents occlusion of the left anterior descending artery (LAD).[13] Location of the occlusion within the LAD determines whether or not other areas of the myocardium, such as the lateral wall or septum, are involved. Typically, AWMI involves a much larger area of myocardium than inferior wall MI (IWMI) and, consequently, there is a risk of a greater loss of myocardium and myocardial function. Patients with AWMI typically have the highest mortality of MI patients.

The clinical significance of a right ventricular (RV) MI was not considered important until recently. Although isolated RV infarction accounts for less than 3% of all MI, infarction of the right ventricle occurs in nearly 50% of the patients with IWMI.[14] The right ventricle is supplied by the right coronary artery (RCA). Although the oxygen demand of the RV is considerably less, the incidence of atherosclerotic disease is similar to that of the left circulation. Due to the lower oxygen demand of the RV, there tends to be a lower incidence of RV MI. However, this may not be the case in as many as 30% to 40% of the population in whom the RCA is a large, dominant vessel that not only supplies the right ventricle but also supplies a significant portion of inferior wall of the left ventricle. Therefore, in these individuals, occlusion of the RCA may result in an IWMI or the combination of an IWMI and RV infarction depending on where the occlusion in the RCA occurs. Because approximately 50% of IWMI patients may have RV involvement, a right-sided electrocardiogram (ECG) should be obtained and assessed in all patients who present with IWMI. The presence of ST-segment elevation in V_4R supports the diagnosis of RV infarction, as does the presence of right bundle branch block or complete heart block.[14]

In addition to the ECG, patients with RV infarction may be differentiated from patients with left ventricular (LV) infarction by their initial presentation and clinical course.[14] Hypotension, clear lung fields, and an elevated jugular venous pressure in a patient with an IWMI is an indication of RV involvement. Patients with RV infarct may present with or quickly develop hemodynamic compromise or cardiogenic shock. Due to RV dysfunction, there is inadequate filling of the left ventricle. Therefore, patients with RV infarct usually require IV volume loading with normal saline to maintain RV preload and cardiac output. If several liters of IV fluid are not effective in improving the hemodynamic status of the patient, use of inotropic and/or blood pressure support with dopamine may be necessary. Medications such as nitroglycerin, diuretics, and other drugs that reduce either preload or blood pressure should be avoided in patients with RV infarction. In patients with RV infarction that is accompanied by LV dysfunction, IV nitroprusside may be used cautiously to decrease the afterload of the left ventricle, and in severe cases where nitroprusside is not effective or tolerated, placement of an intra-aortic balloon pump (IABP) may be necessary.

Other than these exceptions, patients with RV infarction should be managed in the same manner as patients with LV infarction, particularly with regard to reperfusion therapy, which is discussed later in this chapter. In general, the prognosis of patients with RV infarction is favorable. Though patients with IWMI and RV involvement may have an in-hospital mortality as high as 31%, long-term survival is usually good.

In addition to location, the type of MI also has implications for therapeutic management. Q-wave MI, previously termed transmural, usually results in injury that transects the entire thickness of the myocardial wall.[5,6,13] Subsequently, most of these patients develop pathologic "Q waves" on the ECG. Non–Q-wave MI, previously termed nontransmural, only involves the subendocardial myocardium; these patients do not develop a pathologic Q-wave on the ECG. Patients with non–Q-wave MI present differently from patients with Q-wave MI in that the ECG may not show ST-segment elevation but may only have subtle findings such as T-wave inversion, nonspecific ST-T-wave changes, or ST-segment depression. To confirm the diagnosis, cardiac enzymes are needed. More important, the prognosis and therapeutic management of patients with non–Q-wave MI is different from patients with Q-wave MI. This chapter focuses primarily on the pharmacotherapy of Q-wave MI and briefly discusses the management of non–Q-wave MI when applicable.

POSTINFARCTION CHANGES IN THE LEFT VENTRICLE

One of the most serious complications of MI is heart failure. Enlargement of the left ventricle plays a critical role in the development of post-MI heart failure and subsequent mortality.[15–20] Heart failure following MI is directly related to the size of the MI and LV function (LV ejection fraction). However, the evolution of heart failure appears to involve additional processes other than loss of viable tissue. Following MI, a series of events occurs that relate to the response of the LV to injury. This process is called *ventricular remodeling*.[15–20] Activation of the neurohumoral and renin–angiotensin systems and the release of vasopressin ensue once a decrease in cardiac output occurs. Sinus tachycardia, mediated by activation of the adrenergic system, occurs first as a response to a drop in cardiac output and, within hours of infarction, expansion of the infarcted area occurs due to thinning and stretching of the infarcted segment, which is followed by acute dilatation and hypertrophy of the noninfarcted myocardium. This initial process precipitates chronic changes in ventricular volume leading to further ventricular dilatation and hypertrophy and eventually the development of LV failure. The entire process takes several months. Recently, clinical trials evaluating the impact of early drug therapy intervention on this remodeling process and the subsequent development of heart failure have been completed.[18–20] These trials are reviewed later in this chapter.

PROGNOSIS

The highest risk of death for an MI patient is early, within the first 48 hours.[21] This is true even in the era of reperfusion therapy, which has little impact on the risk of early death.[22] Rapid identification of MI patients and early risk stratification can reduce mortality and the likelihood of long-term complications.[21] For patients who have experienced their first MI, the prognosis for survival is generally good.[2] However, patients with a second or third MI have approximately a twofold higher incidence of early mortality compared to patients with first MI. Furthermore, long-term survival is substantially better in first-time MI patients than in those who have had more than one MI.

Several factors have been implicated in predicting outcome of patients with MI. The most significant predictors of death within 30 days are age, systolic blood pressure, heart rate at presentation, heart failure, infarct location, and previous MI.[21] Low-risk patients (a 2.5% 1-year cardiac mortality) are those patients less than 71 years of age with an LV ejection fraction of at least 40%. Subsequently, patients who develop heart failure post-MI have approximately a 50% 5-year mortality. In addition, 30-day and 5-year mortality correlate with the degree of patency of the infarct-related artery. Specifically, patients with Thrombolysis in Myocardial Infarction (TIMI) grade 3 flow (Table 13–1) have a substantially lower mortality rate than patients with TIMI grades 0–2 flow (Table 13–2).[23–25]

TABLE 13–1. Definitions of Thrombolysis in Myocardial Infarction (TIMI) Grade Flows

TIMI Grade	Definition
0	No perfusion; there is no antegrade flow beyond the obstruction
1	Penetration without flow (minimal perfusion); contrast passes beyond the occlusion but "hangs up" and fails to opacify the entire coronary bed distal to the occlusion
2	Partial perfusion; the contrast passes across the occlusion and opacifies the distal coronary bed but the rate of entry of contrast into distal vessels is slower than in normal vessels
3	Complete perfusion; antegrade flow to the distal coronary bed occurs as promptly as it does to the bed proximal to the occlusion; clearance of the contrast is rapid

Adapted from Ref 25.

TABLE 13–2. 90-Minute TIMI Grade Flow and the Corresponding Mortality Rate in Patients Enrolled in the GUSTO-I Study

TIMI Grade Flow	Mortality Rate (%)
0 or 1	8.9
2	7.4^a
3	4.4^b

Values are the mean ± SD. Difference between the mortality rate in patients with TIMI grade 3 flow versus TIMI grade 0 or 1 was significant ($P = .009$).
$^aP = .04$ vs TIMI grade 0 or 1.
$^bP = .08$ vs TIMI grade 2.
$^cP < .001$ vs TIMI grade 0 or 1.
$^dP < .001$ vs TIMI grade 2.
Adapted from Ref 23.

Controversy exists, however, about the importance of achieving TIMI grade 3 flow at 90 minutes versus another time point (i.e., 24 hours).[26]

The overall prognosis for patients with non–Q-wave MI is worse than for those with Q-wave MI; non–Q-wave MI is associated with a higher incidence of post-MI angina and reinfarction. Otherwise, similar outcome factors apply to non–Q-wave patients as do to Q-wave MI.[2] Location of the infarct correlates similarly to outcome in these patients as it does in patients with Q-wave MI.

Careful evaluation of MI patients, including an assessment of LV function, plays a key role in the therapeutic management and prognosis of these patients. To address these issues, aspects of secondary prevention and other post-MI management are discussed.

CLINICAL PRESENTATION

Chest pain is the predominant symptom that brings a patient with MI to the emergency department.[7,27] Patients will, however, frequently describe their symptom as chest pressure or a squeezing sensation rather than pain. Unfortunately, the presence of chest pain alone is not sufficient to make the diagnosis of MI, particularly since it is a subjective parameter and is often difficult to distinguish from a variety of other cardiac and noncardiac events. Furthermore, absence of pain has been reported in as many as 15% to 25% of patients with MI, particularly in patients with diabetes mellitus who may have autonomic dysfunction. Consequently, additional objective criteria are necessary to confirm the diagnosis of MI.

In addition to chest pain, patients may present with physical findings such as diaphoresis, nausea and vomiting, arm tingling/numbness, and shortness of breath. These symptoms too are not specific enough to confirm the diagnosis. Therefore, objective criteria must be used to confirm the diagnosis. These parameters include the 12-lead ECG, and characteristic changes in concentrations of the cardiac enzymes creatine kinase (CK), its MB isoenzyme fraction (CK-MB), and/or troponin T or I.[28,29]

The electrocardiographic diagnostic feature of MI is the Q wave associated with a pattern of ST-segment changes.[14,27] It is critical not to base the diagnosis on a single ECG but to obtain serial ECGs, to assess changes accurately. This strategy significantly enhances the sensitivity of the ECG in making the diagnosis. The earliest change in the ECG is associated with the T wave; it may be prolonged, peaked, or inverted. T-wave alterations are soon followed by ST-segment elevation (Fig. 13–2). A pathologic Q wave may or may not be present on the initial ECG or may appear hours or sometimes days after MI. Pathologic Q waves are those that are approximately one-third as deep the size of the QRS complex and are at least 1 mm (0.04 second) wide.

Serial blood samples for the determination of cardiac enzyme concentrations should be obtained from patients who present with suspected MI.[27–29] Peak concentrations of CK usually occur within 24 hours after MI followed by a decline and return to baseline by the third or fourth day. There must be an elevation of the total CK with at least a 4% CK-MB fraction to confirm the diagnosis of Q-wave MI. The higher the total CK and percent MB, the larger the infarct. Patients with non–Q-wave MI do not have as high a rise in total CK and may not have much more than a 4% MB fraction. Though the utility of LDH is limited and probably unnecessary in patients who present within 24 hours of the onset of symptoms, it may be useful in patients who present late (> 24 hours).[27] Peak concentrations should be at least two times above normal with an increase in the LDH-1 fraction that dominates in the heart. Troponin T or I is considered a more sensitive marker of myocardial injury than CK. In this respect, troponin has been shown to be a strong predictor of mortality in patients with acute myocardial ischemia.[28,29] Currently, the laboratory assay for troponin is not standardized so the reference range varies from institution to institution based on the assay that is being used.

Ultimately, the diagnosis of Q-wave MI is made if the following criteria are met: the presence of ischemic chest pain for at least 30 minutes and/or ST-segment elevation (or new left bundle branch block [LBBB]) on the ECG with the subsequent development of pathologic Q waves. New LBBB on the ECG can also be diagnostic of acute MI in the milieu of cardiac chest pain and other supportive symptomatology. The presence of LBBB makes it difficult to assess the ST segment but it is suggestive of injury to the left septum and therefore is considered indicative of acute MI. The diagnosis is then confirmed by a rise in cardiac enzymes as described above.

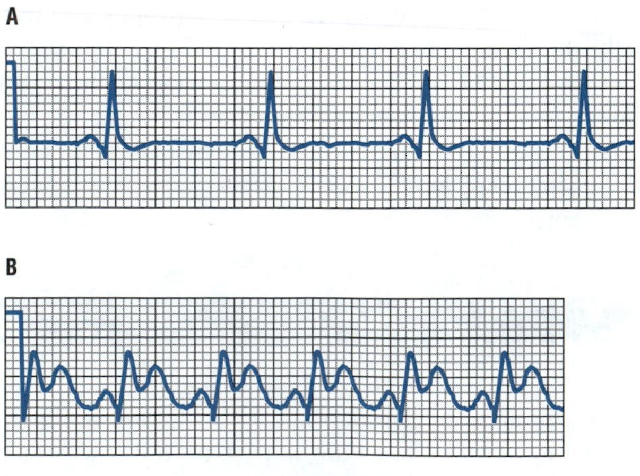

FIGURE 13–2. (A) Normal (isoelectric) ST segment with normal cardiac complexes and **(B)** ST-segment elevation with pathologic Q waves. Both rhythm strips are lead II.

▶ TREATMENT: Myocardial Infarction

DESIRED OUTCOME

The primary goals of therapy for patients with MI are to (1) minimize infarct size, (2) salvage ischemic myocardium, (3) prevent or minimize complications, and (4) improve outcome.

Admission to an intensive care or coronary care unit is mandatory for close observation and the acute care of MI patients. Close monitoring of vital signs, symptoms, and the ECG is recommended for the first 48 to 72 hours after MI in uncomplicated patients.[27] This includes patients who have received thrombolytic therapy or have undergone primary percutaneous revascularization. Continued intensive monitoring is recommended beyond 72 hours if the patient is hemodynamically unstable, has persistent ischemia, and/or has hemodynamically significant cardiac arrhythmias. The highest incidence of MI complications and death is during the first 48 hours after the onset of symptoms.[21,22]

In addition to intensive care, a number of other factors related to myocardial oxygen consumption should be aggressively controlled. Activity should be restricted for the first 2 to 3 days and gradually increased as tolerated by the patient. The hospital diet should include use of multiple small meals, sodium restriction, and reduced content of saturated fats and cholesterol. To avoid the stress associated with defecation, a stool softener, either docusate sodium 100 mg or docusate calcium 240 mg once or twice a day, is recommended.

In the following section, a treatment plan for the management of acute MI is discussed. Even though therapies are presented sequentially, most interventions for MI are "acute" in nature and frequently occur simultaneously or in close proximity to each other. Patients should be considered candidates for each therapy described based on a careful assessment of the risk and potential benefit of each intervention.

LEVELS OF EVIDENCE

Knowledge of pharmacotherapy stems primarily from information generated by clinical research trials. Though research is a vital mechanism by which knowledge is gained, the validity and usefulness of data in clinical practice requires further scrutiny. The development and publication of guidelines allows for this evaluation using a system by which data are ranked based on supportive evidence from clinical trials. The American College of Cardiology (ACC) and the American Heart Association (AHA) have published *Guidelines for the Management of Patients with Acute Myocardial Infarction*.[27] These guidelines serve as the basis for the recommendations made in the following treatment plan of acute MI. The committee that developed the guidelines based their recommendations on levels of evidence. The evidence was ranked as one of three levels:

- **A:** highest ranking; data that were acquired from multiple randomized clinical trials involving a large number of individuals;
- **B:** intermediate ranking; data derived from a limited number of trials with smaller numbers of patients or data from nonrandomized or observational trials;
- **C:** lowest ranking; consensus and/or opinion from experts in the field.

The evidence and its quality were analyzed and recommendations were subjected to the following scale.[27] The committee also noted when no evidence was available.

- **Class I:** Conditions for which there is evidence and/or general agreement that a given procedure or treatment is beneficial, useful, and effective.
- **Class II:** Conditions for which there is conflicting evidence and/or a divergence of opinion about the usefulness/efficacy of a procedure or treatment.
- **Class IIa:** Weight of evidence/opinion is in favor of usefulness/ efficacy.
- **Class IIb:** Usefulness/efficacy is less well established by evidence/opinion.
- **Class III:** Conditions for which there is evidence and/or general agreement that a procedure/treatment is not useful/effective and in some cases may be harmful.

The recommendations for treatment made in this chapter are based on the ACC/AHA guidelines; the classification of each recommendation is also noted based on those made in the guidelines where applicable.

NONPHARMACOLOGIC THERAPY

CLINICAL LABORATORIES

Patients with presumed acute MI should, if possible, have three large-bore (18-gauge) peripheral intravenous (IV) lines placed upon admission to the emergency department. Early establishment of IV access ensures prompt therapy with important drugs that have impact on the morbidity and mortality of the patient. In addition, IV access facilitates collection of blood for tests that are imperative to the diagnosis and assessment of a patient's suitability for thrombolytic therapy. One IV line should be reserved, if possible, for obtaining the frequent blood samples required. Pertinent laboratory tests on admission should include, but are not limited to, complete blood count (CBC) with platelet count, CK, CK-MB, activated partial thromboplastin time (aPTT), prothrombin time (PT), and International Normalized Ratio (INR). Serial CK and CK-MB and/or troponin T or I should be obtained every 6 to 8 hours for 24 hours. The utility of serial LDH determinations is limited unless that patient presents late (beyond 24 hours) from the onset of symptoms. If this is the case, determination of serial LDH concentrations every 6 to 8 hours may be useful in confirming the diagnosis. If the patient receives thrombolytic and/or heparin therapy, a regular assessment of hemoglobin, hematocrit, and platelets should also be obtained. Details regarding appropriate laboratory monitoring of drug therapy are given in the following discussions of each agent when applicable.

OXYGEN

Patients may be moderately hypoxic even during an uncomplicated MI. This may be due, in part, to a ventilation–perfusion mismatch.[27] Therefore, for the first 2 to 3 hours of MI, supplemental oxygen (2 to 4 L/min by nasal cannula) should be administered. Use of oxygen is even more important for patients with pulmonary edema or evidence of CHF because these patients will be more hypoxic. In severe cases of pulmonary edema or CHF, the patient may require mechanical ventilation. Administration of oxygen to MI patients with overt pulmonary edema is a Class I recommendation, whereas routine oxygen administration to all acute MI patients is a Class IIa recommendation.

PHARMACOLOGIC THERAPY

ANALGESIA

Pain control and relief of anxiety are the most immediate objectives in the management of acute MI. Notably, recent experience with thrombolytic agents strongly suggests that pain associated with MI is due mainly to continuing ischemia of viable myocardium rather than to necrosis. IV morphine sulfate is the drug of choice for acute management of pain associated with MI.[27,30] Morphine blocks sympathetic efferent discharge from the central nervous system, resulting in peripheral arterial dilation, making it particularly effective in the setting of acute MI. Overall, morphine reduces myocardial oxygen demand by decreasing systemic vascular resistance and afterload and decreasing circulating concentrations of catecholamines which may, in turn, reduce the likelihood of ventricular arrhythmias.

Dosing Guidelines

IV morphine should be administered slowly in small doses of 2 to 5 mg every 5 to 15 minutes as needed for pain. Dosage is often guided by blood pressure in that patients who are normotensive or hypertensive will tolerate higher morphine doses. A small number of patients whose pain persists may require maintenance doses of 4 to 8 mg every 4 to 6 hours.

Evaluation of Therapeutic Outcomes

Morphine therapy should be continued until pain relief is achieved or an unacceptable end point, such as hypotension (systolic blood pressure < 90 mm Hg), is reached. While receiving morphine, patients should be monitored closely for adverse effects such as hypotension, respiratory depression, and allergic reactions as well as the primary outcome, pain relief.

NITROGLYCERIN

The purpose of therapy with nitroglycerin (NTG) is to relieve myocardial ischemia via coronary vasodilation.[27] The benefit of NTG was established in several clinical trials during the prethrombolytic era.[31,32] Recent data from the Third Gruppo Italiano per lo Studio della Sopravvivenza nell'Infarto Miocardico (GISSI-3) suggest that IV NTG administered for 24 hours followed by transdermal NTG (10 mg) for 6 weeks has no impact on mortality.[20] Similarly, the Fourth International Study of Infarct Survival (ISIS-4) showed no effect of isosorbide dinitrate on 35-day mortality.[33] However, there was a lower incidence of death during day 0 to 1 in patients who received nitrate, suggesting that it might reduce the risk of early death in MI patients. Furthermore, there was substantial early use of NTG (≥ 50%) in the control groups of both studies. The incidence of adverse effects in nitrate-treated patients did not differ from the control group in either the GISSI-3 or the ISIS-4 studies. Thus, use of NTG to manage ischemia for the first 24 hours is justified and safe. Use beyond 48 hours should be reserved for patients with persistent chest pain, heart failure, or hypertension. Use of IV NTG for the first 24 to 48 hours in MI patients with heart failure, large or AWMI, persistent ischemia, or hypertension is a Class I recommendation. Routine use of IV NTG in all MI patients without hypotension (systolic BP < 90 mm Hg), bradycardia, or tachycardia is a Class IIb recommendation.

Dosing Guidelines and Evaluation of Therapeutic Outcomes

Sublingual (SL) NTG (0.4 mg) is frequently used to determine whether chest pain is due to either MI or ischemia. Typically, 0.4 mg SL NTG is administered and chest pain intensity and the ECG are assessed. For the purpose of diagnosis, this dose of NTG may be repeated three times, once every 5 minutes, as long as heart rate and blood pressure are stable.

Following SL administration, heart rate and blood pressure should be closely monitored and the ECG should be evaluated. It is possible that SL NTG will relieve some or all of the patient's initial chest pain, but ST-segment elevation on the ECG may remain. If the ECG changes persist despite relief of chest pain, the diagnosis is MI.

IV NTG, rather than oral or transdermal, is preferred in the management of MI because it is easily titrated.[27] Therapy may be initiated with an infusion of 5 to 10 μg/min via an infusion pump; a bolus dose is not necessary due to the very brief elimination half-life of NTG. The NTG infusion may be increased every 5 to 10 minutes by 5 to 10 μg/min based on the therapeutic end points described below. Duration of NTG therapy for an uncomplicated MI should not exceed 48 hours. Use beyond this time point should be reserved for patients with persistent post-MI angina, heart failure, or hypertension.[27]

During IV NTG administration, it is also critical that heart rate and blood pressure be monitored. The NTG infusion may be increased every 5 to 10 minutes by 5 to 10 μg/min increments for chest pain relief, resolution of ECG abnormalities, or until the systolic blood pressure is between 90 and 100 mm Hg. One or more of these therapeutic end points should be expected within 30 minutes of initiating therapy.

Reduction of the systolic blood pressure to less than 90 mm Hg is not recommended since a low systolic pressure will compromise coronary perfusion pressure, resulting in extension of the infarcted area. If a patient develops hypotension, the rate of the NTG infusion should be reduced or gradually discontinued. If upon discontinuation the patient remains hypotensive, IV fluids should be administered.

Patients with RV infarction or whose systolic blood pressure is less than 90 mm Hg should receive NTG cautiously or not at all. Tachycardic (heart rate > 100 beats/min) or bradycardic (heart rate < 60 beats/min) patients, particularly if in combination with hypotension (systolic blood pressure < 90 mm Hg), should not receive NTG. Furthermore, NTG should be used cautiously in patients who present with bradycardia associated with IWMI.

NTG administration may be associated with either tachycardia or bradycardia. If the patient becomes either symptomatically tachycardic or bradycardic, the NTG infusion rate should be decreased. The ECG should also be closely monitored for reemergence of ischemia even if the patient does not have recurrent chest pain.

Headache associated with NTG administration is common (> 50%), and a small percentage of patients (< 5%) may experience intolerable headache, which may require discontinuation of the drug. Decreasing the infusion rate and acetaminophen may be effective in relieving NTG headache and should be given consideration prior to discontinuation of the NTG infusion.

LIDOCAINE

Cardiac arrhythmias, specifically, ventricular tachycardia (VT) and ventricular fibrillation (VF), are the most common early consequences of MI.[21,22,27] However, the incidence of VT/VF declines linearly to nearly zero within the first 24 hours after MI. Since the incidence of VF is approximately 11% with a mortality rate of nearly 50%, it would seem reasonable to administer prophylactic antiarrhythmic therapy to these patients. However, there are no data to substantiate the prophylactic use of lidocaine in this setting.[27,34] Lidocaine has no role in the early management (within 48 hours) of MI unless the patient experiences VF and/or unsustained VT. The reader is referred to Chapter 14 for details regarding the use of lidocaine and other antiarrhythmic drugs in the management of VT/VF.

EARLY ADMINISTRATION OF β-ADRENERGIC BLOCKERS

Results of numerous clinical trials have established that early administration (within 12 hours of the onset of symptoms) of a β-blocker reduces the likelihood of ventricular arrhythmias, recurrent ischemia, and reinfarction, and, most importantly, mortality in patients with acute MI.[34] It is thought that these benefits occur primarily as a result of β-blocker–induced reduction in myocardial work load secondary to reductions in heart rate, systemic blood pressure, and myocardial contractility.[27] Also, perfusion to ischemic or injured areas of the myocardium may be improved as a consequence of a prolonged diastole in association with β-blocker–induced reduction in heart rate. Though many studies have been conducted evaluating the use of β-blockers in MI, most were conducted prior to the thrombolytic era. The usefulness of β-blockers in MI patients receiving thrombolytic therapy was not known until the completion of the Thrombolysis in Myocardial Infarction (TIMI) II-B, which showed that patients who received early therapy with IV metoprolol had a lower incidence of reinfarction and recurrent ischemia than patients who did not receive IV metoprolol.[35]

In the TIMI II-B study patients (n = 1434) treated with tPA and aspirin were randomized to receive either immediate metoprolol (three IV injections of 5 mg at 2-minute intervals followed by 50 to 100 mg orally twice daily) or delayed metoprolol (50 to 100 mg orally twice daily beginning 6 to 8 days after admission).[35] Use of immediate metoprolol was associated with a marked 90% and 30% reduction in the incidence of recurrent infarction and ischemia, respectively (both P = .02). Importantly, use of IV metoprolol resulted in a lower incidence of early death (within the first 6 days). Consequently, it appears that patients who are treated with a thrombolytic agent will also benefit from early administration of a β-blocker. The choice of β-blocker does not appear to be an issue since benefits of early administration have been observed with several different agents. Those agents with intrinsic sympathomimetic activity (ISA) should be avoided, however, since they have not been shown to be beneficial.[27,36] In patients without contraindications to β-blocker therapy, in whom a β-blocker can be administered within 12 hours of the onset of symptoms, regardless of the use of thrombolytic therapy, use of IV β-blocker therapy is a Class I recommendation.

Dosing Guidelines and Evaluation of Therapeutic Outcomes

Administration of a β-blocker is recommended for patients without evidence of moderate to severe LV dysfunction and other contraindications whether or not a thrombolytic agent has been administered (Tables 13–3 and 13–4). Such use may be especially beneficial for those patients with elevated blood pressure or a tachyarrhythmia. Notably, patients with signs of mild heart failure should still be considered candidates for β-blockade since they also benefit from this therapy with minimal accompanying risk.

Prior to starting a β-blocker, heart rate and blood pressure should be determined. Systolic blood pressure and heart rate should be greater than 100 mm Hg and 60 beats per minute, respectively.[27] After each IV dose, heart rate and blood pressure should be carefully reassessed and the ECG reviewed for AV block. Additionally, the patient should be carefully observed for signs of worsening heart failure. It may require up to 5 to 10 minutes between doses to fully assess these hemodynamic and ECG responses. If the heart rate falls below 55 beats per minute and/or systolic blood pressure falls below 90 mm Hg or if the PR interval becomes > 0.24 seconds, IV administration of β-blocker should be discontinued while hemodynamic and electrocardiographic monitoring continues. In some cases, bradycardia, hypotension, and AV block are transient and the IV regimen may be resumed once these problems resolve. If any of these problems persists, however, then IV β-blocker should be terminated. Approximately 10% to 15% of patients will not tolerate the full IV regimen.[35] This intolerance, however, does not preclude a patient from continuing with an oral regimen, which can be initiated 6 to 12 hours after the last IV dose. An algorithm outlining the decision-making process for acute β-blocker therapy is outlined in Figure 13–3.

TABLE 13–3. Recommendations and Doses for Early Use of IV β-Blockers in Acute Myocardial Infarction

Recommendations	
1. Patients, including those receiving thrombolytic agents, with tachycardia, systolic hypertension, or both without contraindications to β-blocker therapy	
2. Patients with continuing or recurrent ischemia without contraindications to β-blocker therapy	
3. Patients with postinfarction angina without contraindications to β-blocker therapy	
IV Doses	
Propranolol	0.1 mg/kg in two to three divided doses every 10 minutes
Metoprolol	15 mg in three divided doses every 5 minutes
Atenolol	5 to 10 mg in two divided doses every 5 to 10 minutes

LATE ADMINISTRATION OF A β-ADRENERGIC BLOCKER

The goal of late administration of a β-blocker (at least 24 hours after MI) is prevention of recurrent infarction and death. Patients who are not eligible for early IV β-blocker therapy should still be considered candidates for late administration. Such therapy, begun as early as 24 hours and as late as 28 days after myocardial infarction, is associated with 23% and 32% reductions in occurrences of death and recurrent infarction, respectively, for at least 2 to 3 years.[34,37] In spite of these impressive results, only 36% to 42% of patients eligible for β-blockade receive such therapy following MI.[38]

Notably, patients with mild CHF appear to benefit as much as and, in some cases, to a greater extent than patients with normal LV function.[39,40] Specifically, use of a β-blocker in such patients is associated with a 43% to 47% reduction in likelihood of sudden cardiac death compared with similar patients who did not receive a β-blocker, illustrating the importance of this class of drugs in these patients. These observations serve as the basis for the use of β-blockers in heart failure. For a more detailed

TABLE 13–4. Relative Contraindications to β-Blocker Therapy in Patients with Acute Myocardial Infarction

Relative Contraindications
Heart rate less than 60 beats/min
Systolic blood pressure less than 100 mm Hg
Moderate or severe left ventricular dysfunction
Signs of peripheral hypoperfusion
PR interval greater than 0.24 s
Second- or third-degree heart block
Severe chronic obstructive pulmonary disease
History of asthma
Type I diabetes mellitus

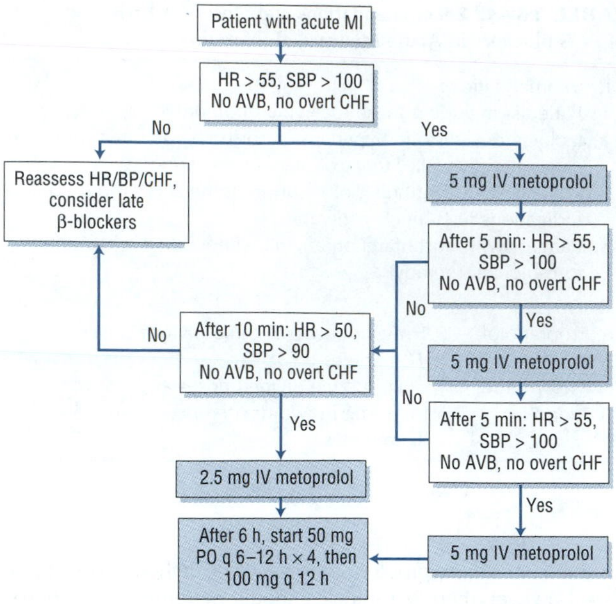

FIGURE 13–3. Algorithm for the administration of early IV metoprolol to patients with acute myocardial infarction. HR = heart rate; SBP = systolic blood pressure; AVB = atrioventricular block; CHF = congestive heart failure.

discussion of the use of β-blockers in heart failure the reader is referred to Chapter 11.

In patients with an uncomplicated MI, benefits of long-term β-blockade are less obvious. These are those patients *without* any of the following: previous MI, AWMI, age > 65, ventricular ectopy, or hemodynamic evidence of heart failure. Such patients have a very favorable prognosis for the first year after MI and adverse effects of β-blockade may be bothersome enough in this group to outweigh benefits.[27] Use of long-term (indefinite) β-blocker therapy is a Class I recommendation in all but low-risk patients and those with a contraindication to β-blocker therapy.

Dosing Guidelines

The FDA-approved β-blockers for use during and/or after MI are atenolol, metoprolol, propranolol, and timolol. Although other β-blockers may also be used in selected patients, use of agents with ISA should be avoided. Also, even though some patients may not tolerate maximum recommended doses, this problem should not preclude a patient from receiving a β-blocker at a lower tolerable dose. Whenever possible, however, the β-blocker dose should be maximized (Table 13–5) unless intolerable to the patient.

Contraindications (relative and absolute) to the late administration of β-blockers are the same as those described under early administration. For secondary prevention of recurrent ischemia and reinfarction, β-blocker therapy should be continued indefinitely.[27]

TABLE 13–5. β-Blockers for Late Administration in Acute Myocardial Infarction

Oral Doses	
Propranolol	180 to 240 mg/d in four divided doses
Metoprolol	200 mg/d in two divided doses
Atenolol	100 mg/d as a single dose
Timolol	22 mg/d in two divided doses

Evaluation of Therapeutic Outcomes

As mentioned under dosing guidelines, heart rate is an important tool in assessing a patient's response to a β-blocker. In addition, the patient should be followed closely for the development of CHF and/or hypotension. Although patients who leave the hospital with some degree of LV compromise (e.g., an ejection fraction < 40%) derive the greatest mortality benefit from use of a β-blocker, they also may be more prone to these adverse effects. If they occur, either β-blocker dose should be decreased or therapy discontinued. Patients should also be monitored for symptomatic bradycardia and for long-term adverse reactions such as impotence, depression, and claudication. In low-risk patients, those who had a small MI (IWMI and/or a CK enzyme peak < 1000 IU/L), the side effect profile of β-blockers may outweigh the small benefit they would receive.

CALCIUM ANTAGONISTS

Although enthusiasm for use of a calcium antagonist for management of acute MI was initially high, subsequent clinical experiences have revealed that their respective roles are actually quite limited.[27] In the acute phase of MI, only diltiazem or verapamil may be used and only then in circumstances where there is a clear indication such as persistent angina or hypertension that is unresponsive to a β-blocker, or when a β-blocker is contraindicated in either of these scenarios. Use of either diltiazem or verapamil may also be appropriate for patients with a rapid ventricular rate associated with atrial fibrillation. Even in these circumstances, there must be no evidence of CHF, LV dysfunction, or AV block. Importantly, there is no evidence that either diltiazem or verapamil confers a mortality benefit in the setting of acute MI.

Besides diltiazem and verapamil, there have been numerous attempts to justify usefulness of nifedipine in the acute phase of MI as well.[41] Results of these clinical trials have revealed that such use of nifedipine is associated with an increase in likelihood of early mortality and no change in occurrence of late mortality when used either as monotherapy or with a thrombolytic agent or a β-blocker. As a consequence of these observations, use of nifedipine is now contraindicated for management of acute MI.[27]

Notably, in spite of these observations, it has been estimated that approximately 47% of patients routinely receive a calcium antagonist as part of the acute care of their MI.[42] It appears that use of a calcium antagonist for management of an acute MI is much too frequent even though a β-blocker is usually the preferred choice in most patients. Use of verapamil or diltiazem in patients in whom a β-blocker is ineffective or contraindicated for relief of persistent ischemia or control of a rapid ventricular response in atrial fibrillation, in the absence of heart failure or AV block, is a Class IIa recommendation.

Calcium Channel Antagonists in the Management of Non–Q-Wave MI

An estimated 25% to 40% of patients with an MI have a non–Q-wave MI.[27,43] Typically, the in-hospital mortality rate of non–Q-wave MI is lower than that associated with a Q-wave MI. Long-term survival, however, is not as favorable for these patients as it is for patients with a Q-wave MI. This unfavorable long-term prognosis is believed to be due primarily to a higher incidence of recurrent ischemia in patients with non–Q-wave MI.

During the past 10 years, a number of clinical trials have been conducted evaluating the efficacy of calcium antagonists in MI.[36,41] However, only two clinical trials have addressed the use of a calcium antagonist following a non–Q-wave MI.[43,44] In the first one, the likelihood of recurrent MI was reduced by 51.2% in patients receiving diltiazem compared with those receiving placebo (5.2% vs 9.3%, respectively; $P < .03$).[44] This reduction in frequency of recurrent MI was found to be associated with a marked 49.7% ($P = .035$) reduction in occurrence of post-MI angina and an 80% ($P < .0007$) reduction in occurrence of angina associated with ECG changes in patients taking diltiazem compared with those taking placebo. Unfortunately, there was only a minimal effect on likelihood of mortality and the beneficial effect on recurrent MI was lost after 1 year of therapy.[44] Interpretation of these observations is confounded by the relatively infrequent use of aspirin in these patients as well as the relatively frequent concomitant use of a β-blocker. Nevertheless, diltiazem is currently recommended for prevention of post-MI angina and recurrent MI in patients with preserved LV function following a non–Q-wave MI.

Dosing Guidelines

The contraindications for use of a calcium antagonist are similar to those of β-blockers. Patients with evidence of compromised LV function should be treated cautiously or not at all with diltiazem, and diltiazem should be avoided in patients with heart block and/or hypotension. In patients with non–Q-wave MI who do not have any contraindications to a calcium antagonist, diltiazem 90 mg every 6 hours should be initiated between 24 and 72 hours after the onset of MI and continued for 1 year. There are at present no data to support or refute use of sustained-release diltiazem in such patients. It is expected that results of the INTERCEPT trial (Incomplete Infarction Trial of European Research Collaborators Evaluation Prognosis Post Thrombolysis) will provide this information soon.[45]

Evaluation of Therapeutic Outcomes

Heart rate and blood pressure should be monitored closely in patients receiving a calcium channel blocker. In particular, patients should be questioned about signs and symptoms of bradycardia, heart failure, and the frequency and severity of anginal episodes. The most common side effects of calcium channel blockade include constipation, nausea, and dizziness.

Secondary Prevention with Calcium Channel Antagonists

Routine use of a calcium antagonist for prevention of recurrent MI is currently not recommended. Overall, no mortality benefit has been observed following MI in patients receiving diltiazem, verapamil, or nifedipine.[41,46–48] A small mortality benefit has been observed, however, in these trials in patients with normal LV function who received either verapamil or diltiazem. Notably, all of these studies were conducted prior to the era of thrombolytic therapy and all were conducted using immediate-release formulations. Consequently, effects of either thrombolysis or use of a sustained-release formulation of any of these agents on occurrence of a second MI is unknown. Nevertheless, use of either diltiazem or verapamil may be appropriate for patients who are intolerant of a β-blocker or in whom β-blockade is contraindicated.

AMIODARONE

Post-MI patients who continue to manifest frequent premature ventricular contractions (PVCs) and/or ventricular arrhythmias represent a subgroup of patients at high risk for sudden cardiac death, the etiology of which is believed to be VT/VF.[21,22,27] The Cardiac Arrhythmia Suppression Trial (CAST) evaluated the efficacy of encainide, flecainide, and moricizine in this subgroup of post-MI patients.[49,50] This study clearly showed that antiarrhythmic therapy was associated with a significantly higher mortality than placebo. However, since CAST only evaluated the efficacy of Class Ic drugs, the possibility exists that other antiarrhythmic agents have different effects.

Amiodarone, a Class III antiarrhythmic drug, possesses unique characteristics such as mild calcium channel and β-blocking properties that suggest that it may be useful in post-MI patients at high risk for sudden cardiac death. During the last 5 years, several studies have been conducted to determine the effect of amiodarone on mortality in these patients. Most recently, the Canadian Amiodarone Myocardial Infarction Arrhythmia Trial (CAMIAT) and the European Myocardial Infarction Amiodarone Trial (EMIAT) studies were completed.[51,52] Both trials showed a significant reduction in the risk of arrhythmic death and resuscitated ventricular fibrillation but no reduction in overall mortality. Importantly, neither of these trials were powered sufficiently to detect less than a 33% reduction in total mortality. The recent Amiodarone Trials Meta-Analysis Investigators evaluated data from 13 randomized controlled trials of prophylactic amiodarone in patients post-MI or with heart failure.[53] In this analysis, amiodarone reduced total mortality by 13% and sudden death by 29% in both patient groups. However, how amiodarone might compare with β-blockers in preventing sudden death in high-risk post-MI patients is unknown. A trial large enough to confirm the results of this meta-analysis has not been conducted.

MAGNESIUM

The use of IV magnesium has been evaluated as part of the continuing search for new therapeutic modalities for the management of MI. Though magnesium was used as an antiarrhythmic in management of MI in the 1960s, only small studies were conducted. With the attention of most clinical trials focused on thrombolytic and antithrombotic therapy, the potential role of magnesium was not aggressively pursued until recently. Several small studies have been conducted and a meta-analysis of them shows that when compared with placebo, IV magnesium significantly reduces the mortality associated with MI.[54,55] As a note of caution, however, this meta-analysis included trials that were performed prior to the routine use of thrombolytic therapy and aspirin. Regardless, this triggered a renewed interest in the potential benefit of magnesium in MI and as a result a large prospective study was conducted.

The Fourth International Study of Infarct Survival (ISIS-4) is the largest trial to date evaluating the usefulness of magnesium in the management of MI.[33] In this study of 58,050 patients with suspected MI, 29,011 were allocated to IV magnesium and 29,039 to control. The mortality rate of patients who received magnesium did not differ significantly from that observed in patients who did not (7.28 vs 6.92%). So, despite a large difference in mortality in early studies, the results of ISIS-4 do not support routine use of magnesium in patients with MI. However, there are sources of heterogeneity between ISIS-4 and previous trials that may explain the lack of benefit observed in ISIS-4. First, magnesium was administered late in the ISIS-4 trial relative to the administration of thrombolytic therapy. This is relevant since one of the presumed benefits of magnesium is a reduction in myocardial reperfusion injury. Further, the mortality rate in the control group was lower than anticipated; a slightly higher mortality rate in the control group would have detected a significant benefit of magnesium. The ongoing Magnesium in Coronary Disease (MAGIC) study is designed to further evaluate the role of magnesium in high-risk acute MI patients, specifically early administration prior to thrombolytic therapy in higher risk patients.[56] Until results of this trial are known, however, routine administration of magnesium in MI is not recommended.[27]

THROMBOLYTIC THERAPY

Thrombolytic therapy probably represents the most important advancement in the treatment of MI in the last decade. Currently, streptokinase (SK [Streptase/Kabikinase]), recombinant tissue-type plasminogen activator (tPA, alteplase [Activase]), anisoylated plasminogen streptokinase activator complex (APSAC, anistreplase [Eminase]), urokinase, and most recently reteplase (rPA, [Retevase]), are approved for use by the FDA in patients with MI in the United States. These agents do not alter myocardial oxygen demand. Instead, they improve myocardial oxygen supply by dissolving the thrombus associated with acute MI, reestablishing blood flow to ischemic myocardium. Consequently, the extent of myocardial necrosis and infarct size is limited and the likelihood of survival is significantly improved if thrombolysis is achieved in a timely fashion.

All of these agents are plasminogen activators.[57] They act by converting, either directly or indirectly, plasminogen to the nonspecific proteolytic enzyme, plasmin (Fig. 13–4). Plasmin is the enzyme responsible for clot lysis, which results in the liberation of fibrin(ogen) degradation products. In addition, clotting factors I, II, V, and VIII break down and fibrinogen is depleted, resulting in a "lytic" state that inhibits further clotting (Fig. 13–4).

Many clinical trials have established the efficacy, safety, and mortality benefit of thrombolytic therapy in patients with MI. However, controversy still exists regarding the superiority of one agent over the others. Subsequently, the focus of more recent studies has been the direct comparison of the agents to one another.[58-61] The GUSTO-I (Global Utilization of Streptokinase and Tissue Plasminogen Activator for Occluded Coronary Arteries) trial, put forth the open-artery hypothesis: *Early and sustained infarct-related artery patency is associated with better survival in patients with MI* and evaluated the efficacy of accelerated tPA (bolus of 15 mg, 0.75 mg/kg over 30 minutes, not to exceed 50 mg followed by 0.5 mg/kg over 60 minutes, not to exceed 35 mg) in an open-label study, compared to three other strategies: SK, 1.5 mU over 1 hour with IV heparin; SK, 1.5 mU over 1 hour with SQ heparin; or the combination of SK, 1.5 mU over 1 hour, and tPA (1 mg/kg over 1 hour not to exceed 90 mg with 10% given as a bolus).[61] Intravenous heparin was administered as a 5000 U bolus followed by a 1000 U/h infusion, which was adjusted based on the activated partial thromboplastin time (aPTT). Subcutaneous heparin was given as 12,500 U twice a day starting 4 hours after the initiation of thrombolytic therapy. All patients received aspirin and patients without contraindications received 5 mg IV atenolol in two divided doses followed by oral therapy of 50 to 100 mg/d. The primary end point of the study was 30-day mortality. More than 41,000 patients were enrolled into GUSTO-I, approximately 10,000 in each treatment arm. The 30-day mortality significantly favored accelerated tPA and there was no significant difference between the two SK regimens (P = .731). The benefit observed with accelerated tPA translates to approximately 10 lives saved per 1000 patients, a risk reduction of 14%. However, there was a slightly higher incidence of stroke in patients who received accelerated tPA.

In addition to these findings, probably the most important observation made in the GUSTO-I was the relationship between TIMI grade flow and mortality (Table 13–2). Other studies have also demonstrated that TIMI grade 3 flow is a strong predictor of mortality.[24,26] This premise served as the basis for the GUSTO-III trial, which compared rPA to tPA.[62,63] Because previous data showed a higher incidence of TIMI grade 3 flow at 90 minutes with rPA, it was presumed that this would translate into a difference in mortality rates between the two agents.[62] This, however, was not the case and the validity of the open-artery hypothesis remains controversial.[26] Since the controversy is not likely to be settled in the near future, it is more important to rapidly identify eligible patients for thrombolysis and treat them expeditiously regardless of what agent is chosen. Thrombolysis (regardless of agent) is a Class I recommendation in patients with ST-segment elevation who present within 12 hours of the onset of symptoms and who are less than 75 years old. Thrombolytic therapy in patients older than 75 years is a Class IIa recommendation due to the overall higher rate of mortality in this patient group.

Hemorrhagic Complications

Stroke remains a concern though its overall incidence is low (≤ 1%). In GUSTO-I, strokes of all types occurred in 1.6% of accelerated tPA patients and 1.4% of SK/IV heparin patients and 1.2% of SK/SQ heparin patients.[23] However, hemorrhagic stroke occurred more often in patients who received accelerated tPA than either of the SK groups (0.72% vs 0.54% SK/IV vs 0.49% SK/SQ). Though there was no significant difference in severe or life-threatening bleeding between the treatment groups, moderate bleeding was slightly higher in the SK groups.

Additional important findings made in the GUSTO-I trial included age-related differences in the incidence of hemorrhagic stroke. In patients more than 75 years of age, there was a 71% higher incidence of hemorrhagic stroke in accelerated tPA-treated patients versus those treated with SK. Furthermore, the mortality rate of patients greater than age 75 was approximately fourfold

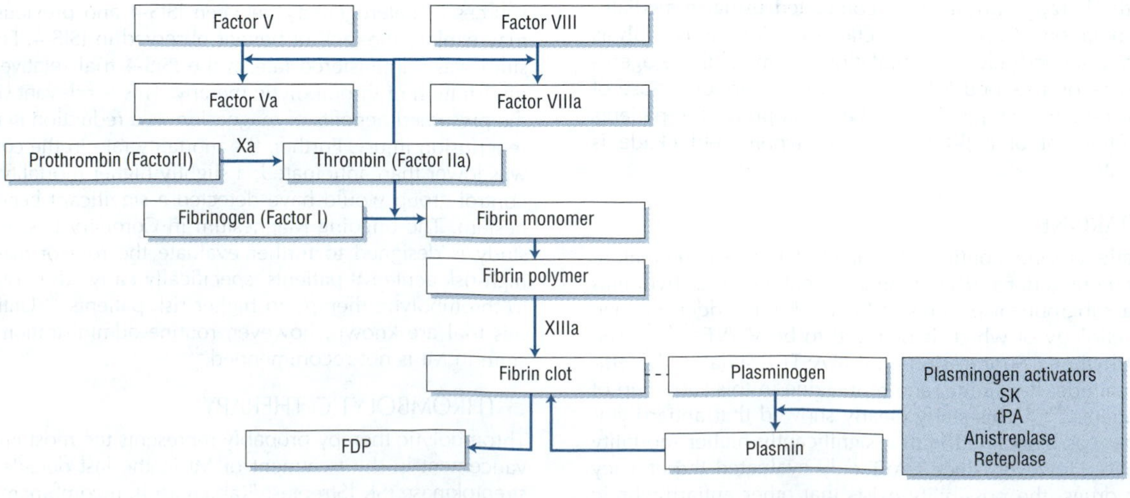

FIGURE 13–4. Clot formation and thrombolysis. SK = streptokinase; tPA = tissue plasminogen activator; FDP = fibrin degradation products.

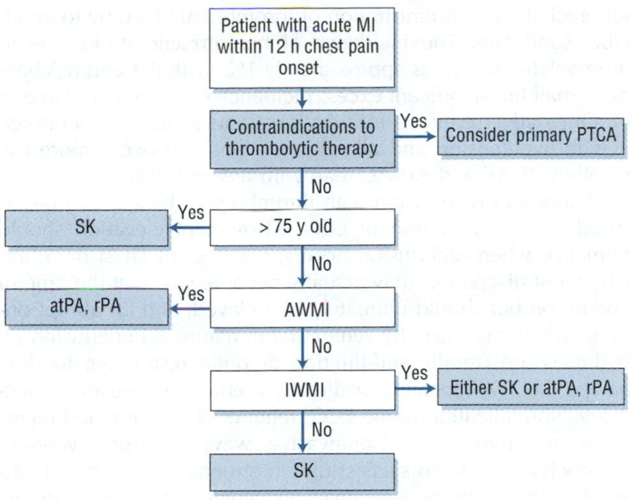

FIGURE 13–5. Algorithm for the administration of either streptokinase or accelerated tissue plasminogen to patients with acute myocardial infarction. AWMI = anterior wall myocardial infarction; IWMI = inferior wall myocardial infarction; SK = streptokinase, 1.5 million units over 60 minutes; rPA = retaplase.

higher than those age 75 or less, regardless of the thrombolytic agent they received (SK: 22.6% vs 5.5%, respectively, $P < .05$; tPA: 23.3% vs 4.4%, respectively, $P < .05$).

Patient Eligibility

Patients who present within the first 12 hours after the onset of chest pain should be evaluated as candidates for reperfusion therapy.[27] There are data, however, to support administration of thrombolytic therapy as far out as 24 hours after the onset of chest pain.[60] Patients who present after 24 hours should not be considered eligible for thrombolytic therapy. Patients who present between 12 and 24 hours are typically only considered for thrombolytic therapy if they have signs and symptoms of ongoing ischemia such as persistent ST-segment elevation and chest pain. Some of these patients may give a history of "stuttering" chest pain that has come and gone and come again in the last 6 to 12 hours. These patients represent a unique subgroup and need to be carefully evaluated. The risks and benefits of thrombolytic therapy need to be weighed before the decision to treat the patient with a lytic agent can be made. Currently, the recommendation for consideration of thrombolytic therapy is 12 hours from the onset of chest pain.[27]

Contraindications need to be carefully considered when determining whether an MI patient should receive thrombolytic therapy. So that therapy is not delayed, evaluation of potential contraindications needs to be made quickly. The sooner patients are treated with thrombolytic therapy, the better the outcome.[64] Good outcome is optimally achieved if eligible patients are treated with thrombolytic therapy within 70 minutes from the time of emergency department admission.[64]

Absolute and relative contraindications to thrombolytic therapy are outlined in Table 13–6. The decision to administer thrombolytic therapy should be made on a timely assessment of risks and benefits. The presence of more than one relative contraindication is considered an *absolute* contraindication to therapy. Of significant importance is the issue of the patient's age. Age is neither an absolute nor relative contraindication. Older individuals, particularly those over the age of 75, have a significantly higher mortality from MI and a higher risk of hemorrhagic stroke if treated with accelerated tPA, than younger individuals.[61] Importantly though, older patients still derive a mortality benefit from thrombolytic therapy. Therefore, in the absence of an absolute contraindication, older patients should not be excluded as candidates for thrombolytic therapy but they should probably not receive accelerated tPA due to a higher risk of hemorrhagic stroke.

The choice of thrombolytic agent is another consideration in the decision-making process. A 1% mortality benefit of accelerated tPA compared to SK is supported by data from the GUSTO-I study.[61] However, AWMI derived the greatest benefit from accelerated tPA. When deciding between agents, these factors should be taken into consideration (Fig. 13–5). In addition, a component of the decision process should also include cost. On average, tPA and rPA cost approximately $2400 compared to SK, which is about $220 for 1.5 million units. Is the 1% mortality benefit observed with accelerated tPA worth the difference in cost between the two agents? The economic analysis of GUSTO-I determined the cost-effectiveness ratio of tPA to be approximately $33,000 per year of life saved.[65] This ratio varied considerably depending on a number of different factors including patient age and infarct location. Patients with AWMI had the lowest cost-effectiveness ratio (greatest cost-effectiveness). Using these data, other cost-effectiveness data, and efficacy and adverse event data may guide clinicians in determining the most appropriate reperfusion strategy for their institution. Cost-effectiveness data are anticipated from the GUSTO-III study. As part of developing this strategy, clinicians should work together to facilitate the rapid identification of eligible MI patients and timely administration of therapy. Rapid administration of thrombolytic therapy can be facilitated, in part, by the availability of pharmacy services in the emergency room. Alternatively, pharmacists can assist in the development of thrombolytic therapy "kits" that contain the agent, diluent, and instructions for preparation and administration.

Dosing Guidelines

Though controversy still surrounds which thrombolytic agent is the drug of choice, it is not as important an issue as the

TABLE 13–6. Relative and Absolute Contraindications for Thrombolytic Therapy in Patients with Acute Myocardial Infarction

Contraindications
- History of hemorrhagic stroke at any time; other strokes or cerebrovascular events within 1 yr
- Possible aortic dissection
- Acute pericarditis
- Active internal bleeding (does not include menses)
- Known intracranial neoplasm

Relative Contraindications/Cautions
- Severe uncontrolled hypertension (BP >180/110 mm Hg) or history of chronic severe hypertension
- Recent trauma or surgery (i.e., within 2 to 4 wk)
- History of cerebrovascular accident
- Active peptic ulcer
- Current use of anticoagulation therapy (INR ≥ 2 to 3)
- Known bleeding diathesis
- Previous allergic reaction to streptokinase or anistreplase; use tPA
- Significant liver dysfunction
- Pregnancy
- Recent internal bleeding
- Prolonged CPR (>10 min)
- Noncompressible vascular punctures

underutilization of these drugs. Fewer than 30% of patients who are eligible for thrombolytic therapy actually receive it.[66] It has been suggested that increasing this number could save an additional 5000 lives annually. Therefore, the current recommendations call for the administration of thrombolytic therapy to patients with ECG evidence of Q-wave MI who present within 12 hours of the onset of chest pain without contraindications to therapy. In patients who present beyond 6 hours, SK may be the preferred thrombolytic agent.[27,61]

Eligible patients should be treated as soon as possible, but preferably within 70 minutes from the time they present to the emergency department, with one of the following regimens:

1. Tissue plasminogen activator (tPA, [Activase, Genentech]), 15-mg bolus followed by 0.75 mg/kg infusion (not to exceed 50 mg) over 30 minutes followed by 0.5 mg/kg infusion (not to exceed 35 mg) over 1 hour.
2. Streptokinase (SK), 1.5 million units in 50 mL of normal saline or D_5W over 60 minutes.
3. Anistreplase (APSAC, [Eminase, SmithKline Beecham]), 30 mg IVP over 2 minutes.
4. Reteplase (rPA, [Retevase, Centocor]), 10 U IVP over 2 minutes followed 30 minutes later with another 10 U IVP over 2 minutes.

Evaluation of Therapeutic Outcomes

Following thrombolytic therapy administration, the patient should be carefully monitored for adverse events as well as signs and symptoms of reperfusion. A lytic state develops rapidly after administration and may persist for up to 24 hours. It may be somewhat longer in patients who receive APSAC. During this time, the risk of bleeding is the greatest. The lytic state is characterized clinically by a fall in fibrinogen concentration, an increase in fibrin degradation products, and prolongation of the aPTT.[57] If the patient begins to bleed during this period, timely management is essential. Utilization of the algorithm outlined in Figure 13–6, for the management of bleeding that is not immediately life threatening provides guidelines for intervention and assists in the decision-making process. Hemorrhagic stroke causes the greatest concern and is the most serious adverse effect associated with thrombolytic therapy.[67] However, this concern should not preclude the administration of thrombolytic therapy to an eligible candidate. The incidence of hemorrhagic stroke due to thrombolytic therapy is approximately 1%, with tPA and rPA having a small but significant excess incidence of stroke compared to SK. Other adverse effects for which patients should be monitored include hypotension and allergic reactions that occur more frequently with SK and APSAC than with tPA and rPA.

Successful reperfusion with thrombolytic therapy can be assessed by (1) evaluation of ECG; ST-segment elevation should normalize when reperfusion occurs; (2) relief of chest pain; initially chest discomfort may actually become worse at the time of reperfusion but should ultimately be relieved; and (3) abrupt onset of arrhythmias, usually ventricular in nature.[68] Reperfusion arrhythmias are usually self-limiting or quite responsive to drug therapy (i.e., IV lidocaine) or direct current cardioversion, if necessary. Normalization of the ECG, relief of chest pain, and reperfusion arrhythmias are noninvasive ways to assess whether thrombolysis has been successful. Unfortunately, presence or absence of these observations may not always be an accurate assessment of thrombolytic success or failure since thrombolytic therapy is unsuccessful in approximately 22% to 30% of patients.[68] In addition, approximately 5% to 10% of patients will spontaneously reperfuse. This explains the difference in rates between patency and reperfusion in that patency rates tend to be approximately 5% to 10% higher than reperfusion rates.

PRIMARY PTCA

Ever since the first report describing use of primary PTCA as an alternative or adjunct to thrombolysis, its role has been debated.[69] Until recently, there were very few clinical trials comparatively evaluating the relative merits and problems of these two modalities of therapy. These early clinical trials comparing primary PTCA with thrombolysis were statistically underpowered to detect differences between these two treatment modalities, and results were inconsistent and inconclusive.[70–72] While the mortality rate was lower in patients randomized to PTCA in these studies, none of the observed differences achieved statistical significance. Also, a reduction in recurrent MI was observed in some of these trials but not in others. Even though a subsequent meta-analysis revealed that use of primary PTCA compared with thrombolysis was associated with a significant reduction in likeli-

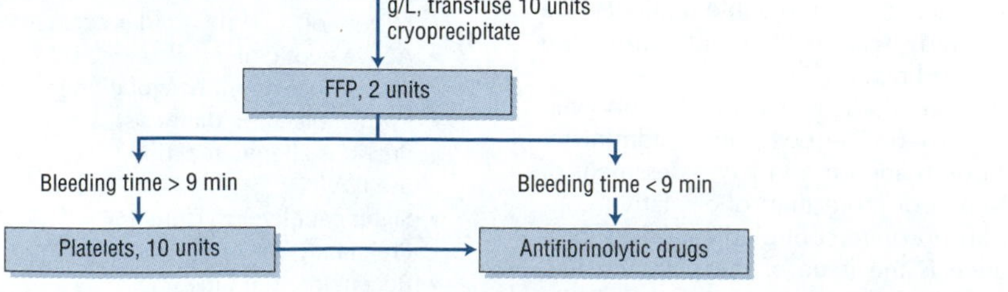

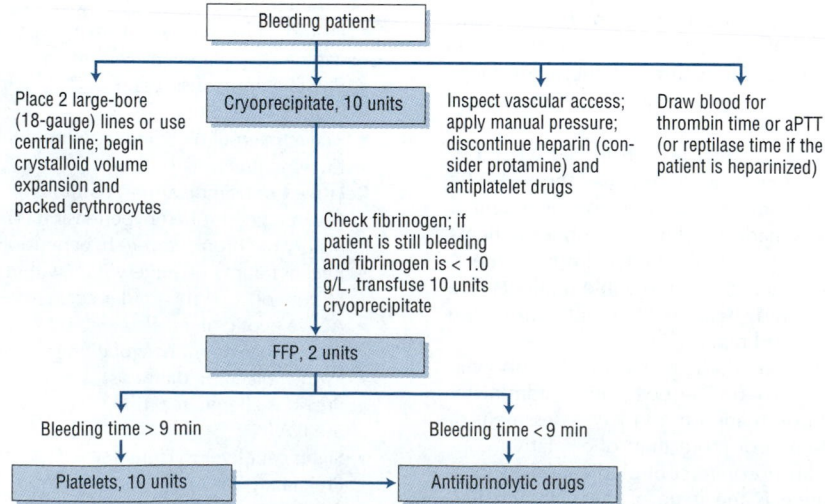

FIGURE 13–6. Algorithm for the management of bleeding associated with the administration of thrombolytic therapy. FFP = fresh frozen plasma. *(Adapted from Ref. 67.)*

hood of short-term (6-week) mortality and recurrent nonfatal MI, its role in management of acute MI was still debated.[73]

Recently, however, a number of randomized clinical trials have been completed that were large enough in size and scope to allow appropriate interpretation of results as well as extrapolation to a larger group of patients.[74–77] Overall, use of primary PTCA in these trials was found to be associated with a 55% reduction in mortality rate when compared with thrombolysis and a corresponding 64% reduction in recurrent MI. Notably, the extent of these beneficial effects of PTCA are similar to those previously observed only in patients with cardiogenic shock or severe LV dysfunction.[78,79] Additionally, another more recent meta-analysis revealed that use of primary PTCA compared with thrombolysis was associated with a 34% reduction (P = .02) in all-cause mortality at 30 days as well as a 42% reduction (P < .001) in death or nonfatal recurrent MI also at 30 days.[80] Notably, these beneficial effects of primary PTCA were observed regardless of the thrombolytic agent used. Based on these observations it would seem that primary PTCA should be considered the treatment-of-choice for acute management of MI for all patients, not just those with severe LV dysfunction.

Before embracing this conclusion it is important to keep in mind that fewer than 20% of hospitals in the United States have a cardiac catheterization laboratory and only a fraction of these are capable of providing an emergency PTCA service. Although a patient may be transferred to one of these facilities, the accompanying delay in initiation of therapy for these patients will likely offset any benefit associated with use of the procedure.

As a consequence of these practical limitations, primary PTCA as an alternative to thrombolysis is now thought to be most beneficial for patients with cardiogenic shock or severe left ventricular dysfunction.[27] Additionally, it is recommended as an alternative to thrombolysis only if it can be accomplished in a timely manner by skilled practitioners in a high-volume center that specializes in the procedure or in circumstances where thrombolysis is otherwise contraindicated. Obviously, the limitations of primary PTCA are that it is labor intensive and not feasible for use on a routine basis in many institutions. In addition, larger trials are still needed to determine the long-term mortality benefit of primary PTCA. Primary PTCA is a Class I recommendation as an alternative to thrombolytic therapy only if it is performed in a timely manner, by skilled individuals (those who perform more than 75 PTCA/year) at high-volume (> 200 PTCA/year) centers. Use of PTCA as an alternative to thrombolytic therapy in patients who are at high risk of bleeding or in patients with cardiogenic shock is a Class IIb recommendation.

ANGIOPLASTY FOLLOWING THROMBOLYTIC THERAPY

Though thrombolysis is effective in the majority of patients with acute MI, approximately 75% to 90% of patients will have a residual stenosis following clot lysis.[81,82] PTCA has been shown to be very effective in reducing this residual stenosis. However, several studies have shown that PTCA immediately following thrombolytic therapy is not beneficial and actually may contribute to morbidity and mortality.[81,82] Thus, PTCA following thrombolytic therapy should be reserved for patients who have symptomatic or objective evidence of ischemia.

ANTITHROMBOTIC THERAPY

Aspirin

Antithrombotic therapy with agents such as aspirin, heparin, and an oral anticoagulant such as warfarin, has played an important role in the management of patients with acute MI. Aspirin, in particular, has become a critical component of acute MI therapy due in no small part to observations from the Second International Study of Infarct Survival (ISIS-2) trial.[83] In this study 17,187 patients with suspected MI were assigned in a randomized, double-blind fashion to receive either SK (1.5 million units IV over 1 hour), aspirin (160 mg daily for 1 month), both aspirin and SK, or placebo. Compared with placebo, use of aspirin was associated with a highly significant 23% reduction (P < .00001) in mortality. Furthermore, in patients assigned to receive both aspirin and SK, mortality rate was 39% lower than that observed in the placebo group (P < .00001). This study clearly established the beneficial contribution of early aspirin administration with concomitant thrombolysis in patients with acute MI.

Inhibition of cyclooxygenase-dependent platelet activation is the most likely mechanism responsible for these beneficial effects. There is no evidence, however, that other platelet inhibitors, such as dipyridamole, ticlopidine, or clopidogrel have any advantage over aspirin with respect to effect on the likelihood of mortality.[84] Nevertheless, any of these agents may be used in place of aspirin in patients with a history of allergy to aspirin. Notably, there is also no evidence of differential effects of aspirin on any particular subgroup of patients and its beneficial effects on mortality are evident whether or not a patient receives a thrombolytic agent.[85] The use of aspirin (160 to 325 mg) for the acute management of MI and for continued use indefinitely is a Class I recommendation.

Aspirin for Secondary Prevention. Results of numerous studies have revealed that aspirin is useful for prevention of recurrent cardiovascular events following acute MI. Aspirin, when started within days to years of MI, significantly reduces frequency of recurrent events. The Antiplatelet Trialists' Collaboration has shown that the use of aspirin following MI reduces the risk of death from cardiovascular causes (including MI and stroke) by one-sixth, while the risk of a second nonfatal MI is reduced by one-third.[86]

Eight studies involving more than 16,000 MI patients have demonstrated that aspirin (300 to 1500 mg/d) alone or in combination with dipyridamole, decreases the risk of recurrent MI by 30% to 49%. Results of another trial revealed that use of a daily dose of 75 mg was associated with a 34% reduction in the combined end point of nonfatal MI and sudden death in patients with chronic stable angina. These observations suggest that a low dose of aspirin may also be effective and the likelihood of aspirin-related adverse effects would be diminished as well.

Dosing Guidelines. ASPIRIN AS ADJUNCTIVE THERAPY TO THROMBOLYTIC THERAPY. Current recommendations for aspirin therapy in patients with acute MI call for immediate initiation of non-enteric-coated aspirin 160 to 325 mg that should be chewed and swallowed to achieve a rapid antiplatelet effect.[27] Patients who present to the emergency department with suspected MI, whether or not they are considered candidates for thrombolysis, should also receive aspirin. The only exceptions to this recommendation are an aspirin allergy or aspirin intolerance due to gastrointestinal (GI) problems. When given, aspirin (160 to 325 mg) should be chewed and swallowed as soon as possible after the onset of symptoms.[27]

ASPIRIN FOR SECONDARY PREVENTION

To achieve an immediate antiplatelet effect, aspirin should be given as a single loading dose of 300 to 325 mg in patients not already receiving aspirin as part of their MI care. Subsequently, long-term aspirin therapy for prevention of a second MI should be dosed at 75 or 80 mg. There is no evidence that higher doses are more efficacious.[86] This recommendation is based on the studies that have been conducted to date evaluating the role of aspirin in secondary prevention. Enteric-coated aspirin may be used because it helps reduce the incidence of GI side effects.

Evaluation of Therapeutic Outcomes. Following acute MI, patients should be followed on a regular basis and evaluated for signs and symptoms of recurrent ischemia. Though aspirin is very effective in preventing recurrent ischemia, as many as 30% to 40% of patients will experience recurrent ischemia or reinfarction despite aspirin therapy.

Bleeding and GI side effects of aspirin are the most common, although the risk of these adverse events is dose dependent. Use of a daily dose < 325 mg is associated with an incidence of such adverse events that is indistinguishable from placebo. The incidence of GI complications such as stomach pain, heartburn, and nausea is as high as 40% to 60% in patients receiving 900 to 1300 mg/d of aspirin, while the incidence of these side effects is 4% to 13% in patients receiving 75 mg/d. The overall incidence of hemorrhagic stroke with low-dose aspirin is 0.3%, which increases as the dose of aspirin increases. The use of enteric-coated aspirin also reduces the incidence of GI side effects.

Heparin

Heparin in Combination with Thrombolytic Therapy. The primary justification for the use of heparin together with thrombolysis is the prevention of recurrent coronary thrombosis.[85] Unfortunately, when thrombolytic trials began in the early 1980s, it was assumed that concomitant administration of heparin was necessary to maintain infarct-related artery patency regardless of the thrombolytic agent used. As a consequence, the role and efficacy of heparin in this setting has not been rigorously evaluated. Current recommendations for use of heparin vary with thrombolytic agent chosen. For example, routine use of heparin with agents such as SK or APSAC does not appear necessary since these agents produce a prolonged state of systemic anticoagulation (a "lytic" state). This prolonged duration of action is probably related to depletion of clotting factors (especially factors V and VIII) as well as fibrinogen depletion and the production of fibrinogen degradation products, which are themselves anticoagulants. By comparison, the duration of action of agents such as tPA and rPA is shorter and their effects on systemic coagulation considerably more variable. Consequently, use of heparin in patients receiving either of these thrombolytic agents is conceptually more reasonable. The GISSI-2 and ISIS-3 trials have shown that heparin (high-dose SQ) confers a small added mortality benefit to thrombolysis; however, this benefit may be at the expense of an increased risk of bleeding.[58,60] To date there are no data to show that heparin has a favorable impact on mortality regardless of the thrombolytic agent used.[87]

Part of the difficulty in assessing the role of heparin has been the failure to use weight-adjusted dosing followed by appropriate monitoring. Results of several studies have clearly demonstrated the importance of using weight-adjusted heparin dosing and the benefit of a standardized nomogram for achieving maximum benefit and minimizing risk.[88]

Until more information is acquired, the current recommendation for concomitant heparin administration with thrombolytic therapy is as follows: Patients who receive tPA (accelerated or standard) or rPA should also receive a 70 U/kg bolus of heparin followed by a constant infusion of 15 U/kg/h at the time tPA or rPA therapy is initiated. For patients who receive SK or APSAC, use of IV heparin is recommended for those patients who are at high risk for systemic embolization. These patients include those with a large or AWMI, atrial fibrillation, history of previous thromboembolic event, or visualized LV thrombus. Additionally, a delay of 4 hours or until aPTT returns to less than two times control is recommended before initiation of heparin in these patients. At that time, use of a loading dose is probably unnecessary and a constant infusion of 15 U/kg/h can be initiated. For those patients who are not at such high risk, use of 7500 to 12,500 U SQ is preferred. Use of IV heparin with thrombolytic therapy is a Class IIa recommendation.

Heparin in the Prevention of Thromboembolism. There are data that support the use of heparin in the absence of a thrombolytic agent in MI patients. Such use of heparin is based on a 17% to 22% reduction in occurrence of recurrent MI in patients receiving heparin compared with those who did not.[89] Notably, the control groups in these trials did not reliably receive other therapies routinely used today such as aspirin, a β-blocker, nitrates, or an angiotensin-converting enzyme inhibitor (ACEI). Consequently, use of heparin for patients not receiving a thrombolytic agent as part of acute MI care is now reserved for two distinct clinical circumstances.

First, use of heparin has been shown to reduce risk of systemic thromboembolization in patients at high risk for deep vein thrombosis or pulmonary embolism. These patients include those with a visualized LV mural thrombus following MI, a large AWMI, previous history of an embolic event, or atrial fibrillation. The incidence of mural thrombus in patients with AWMI may be as high as 70% and appropriate use of heparin as well as warfarin in these patients has been shown to reduce the frequency of this complication to approximately 22%.[90] Recent observations suggest, however, that patients who are not treated early (within 10 days) with IV heparin have a higher incidence of LV thrombus even with concomitant warfarin.[91] Thus, the greatest benefit from IV heparin is gained if it is given early to patients with AWMI since formation of LV thrombus occurs within this time period after MI. Second, heparin, preferably via the subcutaneous route, is also useful for prevention of deep vein thrombosis and pulmonary embolus, complications that may occur as a consequence of MI or prolonged immobility and in association with a number of other risk factors as well. Most of these embolic complications occur within 3 days of MI, and the risk of occurrence is greatest in patients with heart failure or cardiogenic shock, massive or recurrent MI, patients > 70 years of age, or those immobilized for a prolonged period of time. Such early initiation of subcutaneous heparin (within 12 to 18 hours) has been shown to be associated with an 83% reduction in frequency of deep vein thrombosis.[92] Use of IV heparin in MI patients who are at high risk for thromboembolism (large or AWMI, atrial fibrillation, history of embolus, or known LV thrombus) is a Class IIa recommendation.

Dosing Guidelines. HEPARIN FOR ANTERIOR WALL MYOCARDIAL INFARCTION. Use of full-dose IV heparin as described previously is preferred for these patients because of their increased risk for LV thrombus formation. Heparin therapy should continue for approximately 48 hours and should be followed by warfarin for 1 to 3 months. Warfarin should be initiated during heparin therapy and titrated to an INR of 2.0 to 3.0.[27]

HEPARIN FOR PREVENTION OF THROMBOEMBOLISM

In these patients, use of subcutaneous heparin (7500 twice daily) is recommended to begin within 12 to 18 hours after onset of chest pain to prevent thromboembolic complications of MI. This regimen should be continued until the patient is ambulatory and follow-up therapy with warfarin is not necessary.[27]

Evaluation of Treatment Outcomes. During continuous IV or high-dose SQ heparin therapy, each patient should be monitored closely for signs and symptoms of bleeding, recurrent ischemia, and thromboembolism. Recurrent MI can still occur even in a patient receiving appropriate anticoagulation.

The aPTT is the coagulation test most commonly used to assess the level of heparin anticoagulation. Since therapeutic heparin concentrations correlate well to aPTT levels, the aPTT should not be measured until at least 6 hours after initiating a heparin infusion and, due to delayed distribution of SQ heparin, 12 hours after a SQ dose.[93] So-called therapeutic aPTTs vary substantially between institutions due to the number and variety of aPTT reagents and instruments available. The clinical laboratory should be contacted to determine the aPTT that corresponds to therapeutic levels of heparin (0.2 to 0.4 U/mL).[93] On average, this usually corresponds to an aPTT of 60 to 80 seconds but can range to as low as 50 seconds to as high as 110 seconds. Once an infusion rate is established, the aPTT should be checked once a day and at 6 hours following an infusion rate change.

Warfarin

Long-Term Anticoagulation. Whether or not anticoagulant therapy with warfarin should be continued following MI to prevent recurrent ischemia or reinfarction remains controversial. A number of studies have been conducted comparing warfarin with conventional therapy following MI.[94–96] Most of these trials were too small or poorly designed and controlled and aspirin was not included in any of them for comparison. Consequently, it is difficult to comparatively assess relative merits of aspirin and warfarin for secondary prevention of recurrent ischemia events following MI using these studies.

There has been only one clinical trial that prospectively evaluated effects of aspirin and warfarin on the secondary prevention of ischemic events following MI. The Antithrombotics in the Prevention of Reocclusion in Coronary Thrombolysis (APRICOT) study compared aspirin, warfarin, and placebo in MI patients successfully treated with thrombolytic therapy in regard to recurrent ischemic events, LV function, and infarct artery patency, 3 months after MI.[95] Patients were randomized to receive either aspirin 325 mg daily, placebo, or warfarin dosed to achieve an INR of 2.8 to 4.0. After 3 months of therapy, the rate of infarct-related artery reocclusion occurred with similar frequency in all three treatment groups (25%, 32%, and 30%, respectively; P = NS). Recurrent MI occurred in 30% of the patients regardless of antithrombotic therapy although the use of aspirin was associated with a significant reduction in the incidence of reinfarction when compared with placebo ($P < .025$). A 3-month event-free clinical course was observed in 93%, 82%, and 76% of the aspirin-treated patients, warfarin-treated patients, and placebo patients, respectively (aspirin vs placebo, $P < .001$; aspirin vs warfarin, $P < .05$). Based on these clinical observations and results of subsequent cost-effectiveness analyses, it appears that aspirin is preferred over warfarin for prevention of recurrent ischemic events following MI.

Although aspirin provides a benefit following MI, there is still an unacceptably high incidence of recurrent MI. Thus, a theoretical rationale would seem to exist to justify combination therapy with aspirin and warfarin. Unfortunately, observations from a large clinical trial designed to more clearly decipher this issue revealed that such combination therapy was not associated with a reduction in subsequent events following MI compared with aspirin alone.[97] Furthermore, the likelihood of spontaneous major hemorrhage was nearly twofold higher in patients receiving aspirin and warfarin as compared with those receiving aspirin alone (1.4% vs 0.74%, respectively; $P = .014$).

As a consequence of these observations, warfarin is currently recommended for secondary prevention in MI patients who are intolerant or allergic to aspirin. The combination of aspirin and warfarin is not recommended for secondary prevention. Additionally, patients with persistent or paroxysmal atrial fibrillation, extensive LV wall motion abnormalities, or severe LV dysfunction (LVEF < 35%) may also benefit from use of warfarin for prevention of subsequent thromboembolic phenomena, including stroke, following MI.[27,98] The recommendation for the use of warfarin for secondary prevention in aspirin-intolerant patients is Class I, as is the use of warfarin in post-MI patients with persistent atrial fibrillation and those with LV thrombus.

In patients unable to tolerate aspirin, the dose of warfarin should be titrated to an INR of 2.0 to 3.0 and continued for up to 2 years. Once stabilized, patients should be monitored closely for signs and symptoms of bleeding as well as recurrent ischemia. The reader is referred to Chapter 17 for detailed guidelines for appropriate follow-up of these patients.

ANGIOTENSIN-CONVERTING ENZYME INHIBITORS (ACEI)

Results of two large, randomized clinical trials reveal that early initiation (within 24 hours) of an ACEI is associated with a number of favorable outcomes.[20,33] Notably, in both of these trials, patients were administered a thrombolytic agent as part of their routine care for acute MI and, as a consequence, observations from these trials are directly applicable to current care of patients with acute MI.

In the first of these, the GISSI-3 evaluated 19,394 patients with acute MI who received, in addition to standard care, either placebo or lisinopril 5 to 10 mg daily, begun within 24 hours of admission.[20] After 42 days of therapy, a 12% reduction in mortality rate was observed in patients receiving lisinopril as compared with those randomized to receive placebo ($P = .03$). In the second study, the ISIS-4, patients ($n = 58{,}050$) with acute MI, also within 24 hours of onset of symptoms, were randomly assigned to receive either placebo or captopril 6.25 to 50 mg twice daily.[33] All patients received standard care as well and were followed for 35 days. Use of captopril in this study was associated with a modest but significant 7% reduction in mortality compared with placebo ($P = .02$).

Preliminary subgroup analyses of these trials suggests that maximum benefit from such early administration of an ACEI occurs in patients with an AWMI, evidence of a previous MI, LV dysfunction, or tachycardia. Experience from these trials also suggests that therapy should be initiated within 24 hours of onset of symptoms of MI, preferably after completion of thrombolytic therapy and subsequent stabilization of blood pressure. The importance of stable blood pressure in these patients became readily apparent with the completion of a third clinical trial. Notably, this trial evaluated early administration of enalapril and reported considerably different findings. Specifically, in CONSENSUS-II 6090 patients received either placebo or enalaprilat 1.0 mg IV over 2 hours followed by oral enalapril 2.5 to 10 mg twice daily for 6 months.[18] The trial was stopped prematurely due to a higher mortality rate in the enalapril group as compared with placebo at 1 and 6 months (6.3% and 10.2% in the placebo group vs 7.2% and 11.0% in the enalapril group, respectively; $P = .26$). Additionally, unacceptable adverse effects, primarily hypotension, occurred more frequently in the enalapril group compared with the placebo group (12% vs 3%; respectively; $P < .001$), even though patients treated with enalapril were found to be less likely to develop heart failure than patients in the placebo group (28% vs 25%; respectively; $P = .012$). It was hypothesized that enalaprilat-induced hypotension may have exacerbated ischemia, which increased the likelihood of mortality. As a consequence of these observations, current recommendations advise against use of an ACEI in patients whose systolic blood pressure is < 100 mm Hg.[27] Use of an ACEI within the first 24 hours of a suspected AWMI or MI associated with clinical heart failure, in patients without contraindications to an ACEI, is a Class I recommendation. In addition, use of ACEI in MI patients with asymptomatic heart failure (LVEF ≤ 40%) is a Class I recommendation.

Secondary Prevention with ACEI

During the past several years, results of a number of studies have shown that use of an ACEI following MI is associated with a reduced incidence of recurrent MI and CHF.[99] In the Survival and Ventricular Enlargement trial (SAVE), for example, use of captopril 6.25 to 50 mg three times daily initiated 3 to 16 days following MI and continued for 42 months was associated with a 25% reduction in risk of recurrent MI compared with placebo ($P = .015$) as well as a 19% reduction in all-cause mortality ($P = .019$) and a 21% reduction in risk of death from cardiovascular causes ($P = .014$) in post-MI patients with an LVEF of ≤ 40%.[19] These observations were similar to those from the Studies of Left Ventricular Dysfunction (SOLVD) trial. In this study use of enalapril was associated with a 23% reduction in risk of acute MI and 20% reduction in risk of hospitalization for unstable angina.[100] Additionally, when ramipril or placebo was administered to 1986 patients with Class II–III heart failure 2 to 10 days following MI, a 27% reduction in all-cause mortality compared with placebo ($P = .002$) was observed after 15 months of therapy.[101] Finally, in the Trandolapril Cardiac Evaluation (TRACE) trial, trandolapril 1 to 4 mg daily or placebo was given to 1749 patients with LV ejection fractions ≤ 35% 3 to 7 days following MI.[102] After 24 to 50 months of therapy, use of trandolapril was associated with 17% reduction in all-cause mortality and a 21% reduction in cardiovascular mortality (both $P < .001$) and a 30% reduction in occurrence of severe CHF ($P < .003$). Secondary analyses of some of these results revealed that benefit of therapy from an ACEI following MI occurs primarily in patients with AWMI or those with an ejection fraction ≤ 40%.[99] As a consequence of these observations, administration of an ACEI within the first 24 hours of MI is now recommended if there is no significant hypotension and there are no other contraindications to use of an ACEI. In patients with clinical evidence of heart failure or in asymptomatic patients with an ejection fraction ≤ 40%, therapy should be continued indefinitely. In those without evidence of LV dysfunction, however, ACEI can be discontinued after 4 to 6 weeks of therapy.[27] For a more detailed discussion of ACEI in heart failure, the reader is referred to Chapter 11.

Dosing Guidelines

To achieve maximal benefit and minimize adverse effects, dosing strategies and doses of individual agents should be restricted to those used in clinical trials described above. Specifically, ACEI therapy should be withheld until thrombolytic therapy has been completed and the patient's blood pressure has stabilized, preferably with a systolic blood pressure > 100 mm Hg. Additionally, initial doses of lisinopril, captopril, or trandolapril should not exceed 5 mg, 6.25 mg, and 1.0 mg, respectively. Goal of therapy with respect to dose should be the maximum dose used in these same trials, that is 10 mg daily, 50 mg twice or three times daily, and 4 mg once daily, respectively. Notably, although there will be an appreciable number of patients who will not be able to tolerate these maximal doses, therapy with the chosen ACEI should continue at maximally tolerated dose anyway. Future studies and further subgroup analyses will help clarify specific patient subgroups who may or may not benefit from ACEI therapy following MI.

Evaluation of Therapeutic Outcomes

When initiating ACEI therapy, blood pressure should be monitored closely. Usually if patients are going to have a hypotensive response to an ACEI, it will occur following the initial dose. Patients who are hyponatremic and/or hypertensive tend to be at greater risk for a hypotensive response to ACEI. Blood pressure should continue to be monitored regularly on an outpatient basis during therapy.

Other monitoring parameters for ACEI therapy include signs and symptoms of worsening heart failure, renal function, and serum potassium, particularly if the patient is concomitantly taking a diuretic and potassium supplementation. Common side effects of ACEI that patients should be questioned about and observed for are altered taste, dizziness, cough, and diarrhea.

ANTIHYPERLIPIDEMIC DRUGS

Secondary Prevention with Antihyperlipidemic Drugs

A history of CAD that includes previous MI is a major risk factor for recurrent MI. Recurrent MI is four to seven times more likely to occur in a patient with clinically apparent CAD than in an individual without such evidence. Given the intimate association between elevated concentrations of lipids and CAD, it would seem intuitive that, following MI, aggressive management of hyperlipidemia would be associated with beneficial outcomes. A summary of secondary prevention trials provided by the last report of the National Cholesterol Education Program (NCEP) revealed that use of both drugs and diet was associated with an overall 25% reduction in recurrent nonfatal MI and a 14% reduction in fatal MI.[103] Notably, none of the studies included in this overview evaluated effects of an HMG CoA reductase inhibitor on recurrent MI. Since publication of that report, two such studies have been completed.

In the first one, the Scandinavian Simvastatin Survival Study (4S), 4444 patients with stable angina and/or history of previous MI were randomly assigned to receive either placebo or simvastatin 10 to 40 mg every evening.[104] Additionally, each patient adhered to a step I/II diet and was followed for 5.4 years. Use of simvastatin in this trial was associated with a 42% reduction in cardiovascular mortality and a 30% reduction in all-cause mortality compared with placebo. Observations from the second study, the Cholesterol and Recurrent Events (CARE) trial, were quite similar. Specifically, patients (n = 4159) adhered to a step I/II diet and were given either placebo or pravastatin 40 mg every evening beginning 3 to 20 months after MI.[105] After 5 years of therapy, a 24% reduction in the primary end point of fatal CAD and nonfatal MI was observed in those taking pravastatin compared with those taking placebo. Notably, beneficial effects of cholesterol reduction observed in these two trials were in patients with only mild to moderate elevations in serum cholesterol. Average total- and LDL-cholesterol values in these two trials were 261 mg/dL and 188 mg/dL, respectively, in the 4S trial and 209 mg/dL and 139 mg/dL, respectively, in the CARE trial. These observations firmly established the benefits of cholesterol reduction following MI even in patients without profound elevations in total- and LDL-cholesterol concentrations.

Current recommendations for management of lipids following MI are consistent with those of NCEP.[27] Specifically, such patients should achieve and maintain an LDL-concentration of < 100 mg/dL through application of a step I/II diet and use of appropriate lipid-lowering agents(s). Considering the impressive findings of the 4S and CARE trials, use of either simvastatin or pravastatin to achieve this goal would seem to be more than a little prudent. Use of either niacin or gemfibrozil is currently recommended in patients whose triglyceride concentrations exceed 400 mg/dL. The reader is referred to Chapter 19 for details regarding dosing guidelines and evaluation of therapeutic outcomes for these agents. Use of the AHA step II diet and initiation of lipid-lowering drug therapy in patients with LDL-cholesterol > 125 mg/dL is a Class I recommendation. In patients with normal cholesterol levels but with high-density lipoprotein (HDL)-cholesterol levels < 35 mg/dL, the use of nonpharmacologic therapy (smoking cessation, exercise) to raise the HDL is a Class I recommendation.

RISK STRATIFICATION POST-MI

Patients with uncomplicated MI are usually discharged from the hospital within 1 week. In the era of cost containment, patients are now discharged after an uncomplicated MI within 3 to 4 days. Although in-hospital management plays a critical role in the outcome of MI patients, what happens after hospital discharge is also important. Risk stratification of MI patients should begin at the time of admission and continue through hospital discharge.[2,21] This strategy is important since approximately 25% of deaths during the first year post-MI occur within the first 48 hours of hospitalization.[21,22] Despite this statistic, patients after their first MI have a very good prognosis. Therefore, ensuring that all aspects of their post-MI care are discussed and understood is important. Prior to discharge, a discussion between health care practitioners, the patient, and the patient's family regarding medications, particularly secondary prevention; modification of risk factors such as smoking, cholesterol, and hypertension; an exercise program; and diet should be held. Guidelines for safe resumption of customary activities, such as returning to work or recreational activities, should be discussed in detail. All questions should be answered to the patient's satisfaction.

In addition to post-MI counseling, an objective assessment of a patient's prognosis and stratification for risk of recurrent cardiovascular events should be made. This should include an evaluation of the patient's exercise tolerance and determination of LV function. Assessment of LV function is critical since it is a primary determinant of long-term mortality post-MI (Fig. 13–7).[21] These parameters will assist in guiding further evaluation and treatment. A multitude of procedures and tests are available to assist in the stratification of post-MI patients.[21] However, many have limited utility and are extremely expensive. It is important to select a procedure/test that is cost effective and will provide useful and prognostic information about the patient.

Probably the most common noninvasive test that is performed post-MI is the exercise tolerance test.[2,21] This is typically done using a treadmill or bicycle and continuous ECG and blood pressure monitoring. This procedure will determine the patient's overall exercise capacity, blood pressure response to exercise, and if angina occurs, at what point during exercise it occurs, as well as if activity precipitates arrhythmias. Submaximal exercise testing can usually be performed just prior to hospital discharge and can then be followed by a full exercise test 1 month after infarction.

High-risk patients are easily identified by their low exercise capability, failure of the systolic blood pressure to rise above the resting value during exercise (frequently referred to as an inadequate blood pressure response to exercise), and chest pain associated with ischemic changes on the ECG.[2,21] In some cases, these patients may experience ventricular ectopy during or shortly after exercise. These patients require further evaluation by invasive means (coronary angiography) to assess coronary anatomy. In patients without these findings, no further diagnostic evaluation is necessary and the risk of a subsequent cardiac event is very low.

Many procedures exist to evaluate left ventricular function. Though no one test is considered the "gold standard," the type of test used depends on the expertise that exists at the given institution. Echocardiography, coronary angiography, and radionuclear ventriculograms are a few examples of methods to assess left ventricular function.

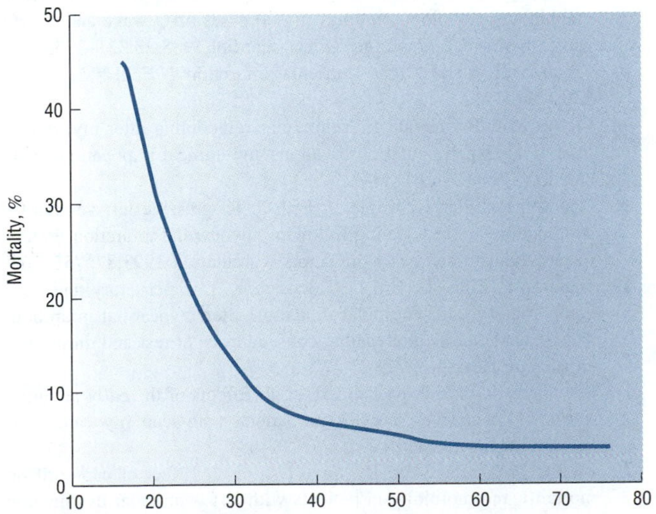

FIGURE 13–7. Relationship between left ventricular ejection fraction (%) at hospital discharge and mortality in patients following an acute myocardial infarction. *(Adapted from Ref. 21.)*

THERAPEUTIC PRINCIPLES

Despite the advancements in the pharmacotherapy of acute MI, approximately 5% to 9% of patients treated with thrombolytic therapy die.[58–61] Interestingly, the majority of these patients die during the first 24 hours following MI, suggesting that thrombolytic therapy may not prevent early death, and other factors may contribute to the demise of these patients.[22] The most important complications that signal for an increased risk for early death are recurrent ischemia, reinfarction, VT/VF, and clinical evidence of LV dysfunction.[21] In addition, patients who leave the hospital with TIMI grade 3 flow versus those who leave with TIMI grade 0 to 1 have a much lower long-term mortality rate. Thus, drug therapy during the early course of MI should be directed toward preventing and limiting early complications and maintaining infarct artery patency.

Though many pharmacotherapeutic advances have been made that have substantially lowered the mortality associated with MI, acute MI is still a leading cause of death in the United States today. A better understanding of the pathophysiology of MI has provided the basis for the advancement in therapeutic interventions such as thrombolytic therapy and new antithrombotic agents. Other therapies, such as β-blockers, ACEI, aspirin, and nitroglycerin also contribute to an improved outcome.

Probably the most significant advance made in the last decade has been thrombolytic therapy. These drugs have become the cornerstone of management for patients with MI. Unfortunately, only a small fraction of eligible patients are treated with thrombolytic drugs. Continuing to educate the general public as well as health care providers as to the importance of quickly recognizing and responding to MI will hopefully improve the use of these important drugs. Though the battle of the clot busters will most likely continue, enhanced use of any one of the thrombolytic drugs will save lives.

The role of primary PTCA in acute MI and how it compares to thrombolytic therapy will continue to evolve, as will research to evaluate a multitude of new agents such as the platelet glycoprotein IIb/IIIa inhibitors, low-molecular-weight heparins, and other modalities for the treatment of MI. Studies are ongoing to further assess the utilization of third and fourth generation thrombolytic agents and novel antithrombotic drugs. This continuum of information will surely provide new treatments and approaches to the therapeutic management of MI patients.

Though the management of MI has changed and improved dramatically over the past decade, progress continues. In the next 10 years, more therapies and strategies will be evaluated and become available. Insight as to the most appropriate management of patients with cardiogenic shock and postinfarction heart failure will be delineated. So, just as such advances have been made during the last several years, they will continue and the management of these patients will remain a dynamic process.

Evidence continues to mount supporting primary PTCA over thrombolysis as the reperfusion therapy of choice in acute MI. However, data are still lacking regarding the sustained morbidity and mortality benefit of this invasive procedure. Further, with the increasing use of coronary stents, this issue may become a mute point. Ongoing studies are evaluating the outcome of MI patients who receive a coronary stent. Recent data from the ISIS-2 study, however, show that the mortality benefit of SK, aspirin, or both is maintained over a 10-year period, whereas other data support a conservative, ischemia-guided approach to patients with non–Q-wave MI.[106,107] Long-term (> 1 year) mortality data for primary PTCA or coronary stenting are still lacking.

The platelet glycoprotein IIb/IIIa receptor (GP IIb/IIIa) antagonists represent the newest and most potent antiplatelet agents available.[108] The recent FDA approval of two additional GP IIb/IIIa antagonists along with recently published clinical trials expands the market of these agents. Presently three agents (c7Ec, abciximab [Reopro], tirofiban [Aggrastat], and eptifibatide [Integrilin]) are approved for use. Although the wording of the approved indications for each agent varies slightly, these drugs are indicated in the management of unstable angina and non–Q-wave MI. In combination with heparin and aspirin, a GP IIb/IIIa inhibitor reduces the incidence of the combined end point of death, MI, and recurrent ischemia in patients undergoing PTCA.[109] Tirofiban and eptifibatide also reduce the incidence of this combined end point in patients with unstable angina or non–Q-wave MI. None of these agents has been shown to reduce the single end point of mortality. Further, long-term data (30 days to 6 months) suggest that the benefit of a GP IIb/IIIa diminishes over time. Since the primary benefit of these agents is a reduction in recurrent ischemia or MI, and this effect diminishes with time, the specific role these agents will play in the management of unstable angina and non–Q-wave MI remains somewhat unclear. In addition, the superiority of one agent over the others has neither been evaluated in a clinical trial nor established from the clinical data presently available. Phase III trials of the platelet GP IIb/IIIa agents (abciximab and eptifibatide) in MI patients with ST segment elevation are ongoing.

Abciximab, tirofiban, and eptifibatide are intravenous agents. Oral platelet GP IIb/IIIa agents are currently undergoing clinical investigation. Most of these drugs are prodrugs, and they appear to have variable interpatient pharmacokinetic profiles. In addition, the safety and long-term tolerability of these agents is still unknown.[110,111]

In addition to the platelet GP IIb/IIIa antagonists, low-molecular-weight heparin, specifically enoxaparin (Lovenox), has been shown to improve the outcome of patients with unstable angina or non–Q-wave MI.[112] Similar to the GP IIb/IIIa trials, the Efficacy and Safety of Subcutaneous Enoxaparin in Non–Q wave Coronary Events (ESSENCE) trial utilized a composite end point of death, MI, or recurrent angina. Also similar to the GP IIb/IIIa data, the primary benefit of enoxaparin was a reduction in the incidence of MI or recurrent angina at 30 days.

REFERENCES

1. American Heart Association data, 1997.
2. Moss AJ, Benhorin J. Prognosis and management after a first myocardial infarction. N Engl J Med 1990;322:743–753.
3. Wittels EH, Hay JW, Gotto AM. Medical costs of coronary artery disease in the United States. Am J Cardiol 1990;65:432–440.
4. DeWood MA, Spores J, Notske R, et al. Prevalence of total coronary occlusion during the early hours of transmural myocardial infarction. N Engl J Med 1980;303:897–902.
5. Fuster V, Badimon L, Badimon JJ, Chesebro JH. The pathogenesis of coronary artery disease and the acute coronary syndromes (first of two parts). N Engl J Med 1992;326:242–250.
6. Fuster V, Badimon L, Badimon JJ, Chesebro JH. The pathogenesis of coronary artery disease and the acute coronary syndromes (second of two parts). N Engl J Med 1992;326:310–318.
7. Kawai C. Pathogenesis of acute myocardial infarction. Novel regulatory systems of bioactive substances in the vessel wall. Circulation 1994;90:1033–1043.
8. Nygard O, Nordrehaug JE, Refsium H, Euland PM, Farstad M, Vollset SE. Plasma homocystein levels and mortality in patients with coronary artery disease. N Engl J Med 1997;337:230–236.
9. Abrams J. Role of endothelial dysfunction in coronary artery disease. Am J Cardiol 1997;79(12B):2–9.
10. Reimer KA, Jennings RB. The wavefront phenomenon of myocardial ischemic cell death II. Transmural progression of necrosis within the framework of ischemic bed size (myocardium at risk) and collateral flow. Lab Invest 1979;40:633–644.
11. Sabia PJ, Powers ER, Ragosta M, et al. An association between collateral blood flow and myocardial viability in patients with recent myocardial infarction. N Engl J Med 1992;327:1825–1831.
12. Charney R, Cohen M. The role of the coronary collateral circulation in limiting myocardial ischemia and infarct size. Am Heart J 1993; 126:937–945.
13. Antaloczy Z, Barcsak J, Magyar E. Correlation of electrocardiographic and pathologic findings in 100 cases of Q wave and non-Q wave myocardial infarction. J Electrocardiol 1988;23:331–335.
14. Kinch JW, Ryan TJ. Right ventricular infarction. N Engl J Med 1994; 330:1211–1217.
15. Pfeffer MA, Braunwald E. Ventricular remodeling after myocardial infarction. Experimental observations and clinical implications. Circulation 1990;81:1161–1172.
16. Gaudron P, Eilles C, Kugler I, Ertl G. Progressive left ventricular dysfunction and remodeling following myocardial infarction: Potential mechanism and early predictors. Circulation 1993;87: 755–763.
17. Gaudron P, Eilles C, Ertl G, Kochsiek K. Compensatory and noncompensatory left ventricular dilatation after myocardial infarction: Time course and hemodynamic consequences at rest and during exercise. Am Heart J 1992;123:377–385.
18. Swedberg K, Held P, Kjekshus J, et al. Effects of the early administration of enalapril on mortality in patients with acute myocardial infarction. N Engl J Med 1992;327:678–684.
19. Pfeffer MA, Braunwald E, Moye LA, et al. Effect of captopril on mortality and morbidity in patients with left ventricular dysfunction after myocardial infarction. N Engl J Med 1992;327:669–677.
20. Gruppo Italiano per lo Studio della Sopravivenza nell'Infarto Miocardico (GISSI-3): Effects of lisinopril and transdermal glyceryl trinitrate singly and together on 6-week mortality and ventricular function after acute myocardial infarction. Lancet 1994;343: 1115–1122.

21. Peterson ED, Shaw LJ, Califf RM. Risk stratification after myocardial infarction. Ann Intern Med 1997;126:561–582.
22. Kleiman NS, Terrin M, Mueller H, et al. Mechanisms of early death despite thrombolytic therapy: Experience from the thrombolysis in myocardial infarction phase II (TIMI II) study. J Am Coll Cardiol 1992;19:1129–1135.
23. The GUSTO Angiographic Investigators. The effect of tissue plasminogen activator, streptokinase, or both on coronary-artery patency, ventricular function, and survival after acute myocardial infarction. N Engl J Med 1993;329:1615–1622.
24. Lenderink T, Simoons ML, Van Es G-A, et al. Benefit of thrombolytic therapy is sustained throughout five years and is related to TIMI perfusion grade 3 but not grade 2 flow at discharge. Circulation 1995;92:1110–1116.
25. TIMI Study Group. The thrombolysis in myocardial infarction (TIMI) trial: Phase 1 findings. N Engl J Med 1985;312:932–936.
26. Stringer KA. TIMI grade flow, mortality and the GUSTO III trial. Pharmacotherapy 1998;18:699–705.
27. Ryan TJ, Anderson JL, Antman EM, et al. ACC/AHA guidelines for the management of patients with acute myocardial infarction. A report of the American College of Cardiology/American Heart Association task force on practice guidelines (Committee on Management of Acute Myocardial Infarction). J Am Coll Cardiol 1996;28: 1328–1428.
28. Ohman EM, Armstrong PW, Christenson RH, et al. Cardiac troponin T levels for risk stratification in acute myocardial ischemia. N Engl J Med 1996;335:1333–1341.
29. Hamm CW, Goldmann BU, Heeschen C, Kreymann G, Berger J, Meinertz T. Emergency room triage of patients with acute chest pain by means of rapid testing for cardiac troponin T or troponin I. N Engl J Med 1997;337:1648–1653.
30. Herlitz J, Hjalmarson A, Waagstein F. Treatment of pain in acute myocardial infarction. Br Heart J 1989;61:9–13.
31. Jugdutt BI, Warnica W. Intravenous nitroglycerin therapy to limit myocardial infarct size, expansion, and complications: Effect of timing, dosage, and infarct location. Circulation 1988;78:906–919.
32. Yusuf S, Slight P, Held P, McMahon S. Routine medical management of acute myocardial infarction. Lessons from overviews of recent randomized controlled trials. Circulation 1990;82(suppl II):117–134.
33. The Fourth International Study of Infarct Survival (ISIS-4) Collaborative Group. A randomised factorial trial assessing early oral captopril, oral mononitrate, and intravenous magnesium sulfate in 58,050 patients with suspected acute myocardial infarction. Lancet 1995; 345:669–685.
34. Teo KK, Yusuf S, Furberg CD. Effects of prophylactic antiarrhythmic drug therapy in acute myocardial infarction: An overview of results from randomized controlled trials. JAMA 1993;270:1589–1595.
35. Roberts R, Rogers WJ, Mueller HS, et al. Immediate versus deferred beta-blockade following thrombolytic therapy patients with acute myocardial infarction. Results of the Thrombolysis in Myocardial Infarction (TIMI) II-B Study. Circulation 1991;83:422–437.
36. Held PH, Yusuf S. Effects of beta-blockers and calcium channel blockers in acute myocardial infarction. Eur Heart J 1993;14(suppl F):18–25.
37. Hennekens CH, Albert CM, Godfried SL, Gaziano JM, Buring JE. Adjunctive drug therapy of acute myocardial infarction—evidence from clinical trials. N Engl J Med 1996;335:1660–1667.
38. Rogers WJ, Bowlby LJ, Chandra NC, et al. Treatment of myocardial infarction in the United States [1990 to 1993]: observations from the National Registry of Myocardial Infarction. Circulation 1994;90: 2103–2114.
39. Chadda K, Goldstein S, Byington R, Burb JD. Effect of propranolol after acute myocardial infarction in patients with congestive heart failure. Circulation 1986;73:503–510.
40. Gundersen T. Influence of heart size on mortality and reinfarction in patients treated with timolol after myocardial infarction. Br Heart J 1983;50:135–139.
41. Skolnick AE, Frishman WH. Calcium channel blockers in myocardial infarction. Arch Intern Med 1989;149:1669–1677.
42. Pashos CL, Normand S-LT, Garfinkle JB, Newhouse JP, Epstein AM, McNeil BJ. Trends in use of drug therapies in patients with acute myocardial infarction: 1988 to 1992. J Am Coll Cardiol 1994;23: 1023–1030.
43. Wong S-C, Greenberg H, Hager WD, Dwyer EM. Effects of diltiazem on recurrent myocardial infarction in patients with non-Q wave myocardial infarction. J Am Coll Cardiol 1992;19:1421–1425.
44. Gibson RS, Boden WE, Theroux P, et al. Diltiazem and reinfarction in patients with non-Q-wave myocardial infarction. N Engl J Med 1986;315:423–429.
45. Boden WE, Scheldewaert R, Walters EG, et al. Design of a placebo-controlled clinical trial of long-acting diltiazem and aspirin versus aspirin alone in patients receiving thrombolysis with a first acute myocardial infarction. Incomplete Infarction Trial of European Research Collaborators Evaluating Prognosis Post-Thrombolysis (diltiazem) (INTERCEPT) Research Group. Am J Cardiol 1995;75: 1120–1123.
46. The Multicenter Diltiazem Postinfarction Trial Research Group. The effect of diltiazem on mortality and reinfarction after myocardial infarction. N Engl J Med 1988;319:385–392.
47. The Danish Study Group on Verapamil in Myocardial Infarction. Effect of verapamil on mortality and major events after acute myocardial infarction. Am J Cardiol 1990;66:779–785.
48. Rengo F, Carbonin P, Pahor M, et al. A controlled trial of verapamil in patients after acute myocardial infarction: Results of the calcium antagonist reinfarction Italian study (CRIS). Am J Cardiol 1996;77:365–369.
49. Echt DS, Liebson PR, Mitchell B, et al. Mortality and morbidity in patients receiving encainide, flecainide, or placebo. N Engl J Med 1991;324:781–788.
50. The Cardiac Arrhythmia Suppression Trial II Investigators. Effect of the antiarrhythmic agent moricizine on survival after myocardial infarction. N Engl J Med 1992;327:227–233.
51. Cairns JA, Connolly SJ, Roberts RS, Gent M, CAMIAT Investigators. Randomised trial of outcome after myocardial infarction in patients with frequent or repetitive ventricular premature depolarisations: CAMIAT. Lancet 1997;349:675–682.
52. Julian DG, Camm AJ, Frangin G, Janse MJ, Munoz A, Schwartz PJ, Simon P, EMIAT Investigators. Randomised trial of effect of amiodarone on mortality in patients with left ventricular dysfunction after recent myocardial infarction: EMIAT. Lancet 1997;349: 667–674.
53. Amiodarone Trials Meta-Analysis Investigators. Effect of prophylactic amiodarone on mortality after acute myocardial infarction and in congestive heart failure: Meta-analysis of individual data from 6500 patients in randomised trials. Lancet 1997;350:1417–1424.
54. Teo KK, Yusuf S, Collins R, et al. Effects of intravenous magnesium in suspected acute myocardial infarction: Overview of randomized trials. Br Med J 1991;303:1499–1503.
55. Woods KL, Fletcher S, Roffe C, Haider Y. Intravenous magnesium sulphate in suspected acute myocardial infarction: Results of the second Leicester Intravenous Magnesium Intervention Trial (LIMIT-2). Lancet 1992;339:1553–1558.
56. Antman EM. Magnesium in acute MI: Timing is critical. Circulation 1995;92:2367–2372.
57. Anderson HV, Willerson JT. Thrombolysis in acute myocardial infarction. N Engl J Med 1993;329:703–709.
58. Gruppo Italiano per lo Studio Della Sopravvivenza nell'Infarto Miocardico (GISSI-2): A factorial randomised trial of alteplase versus streptokinase and heparin versus no heparin among 12,490 patients with acute myocardial infarction. Lancet 1990;336:65–71.
59. The International Study Group. In-hospital mortality and clinical course of 20,891 patients with suspected acute myocardial infarction randomised between alteplase and streptokinase with or without heparin. Lancet 1990;336:71–75.

60. Third International Study of Infarct Survival Collaborative Group (ISIS-3): A randomised comparison of streptokinase vs tissue plasminogen activator vs anistreplase and of aspirin plus heparin vs aspirin alone among 41,299 cases of suspected acute myocardial infarction. Lancet 1992;339:753–770.
61. The GUSTO Investigators. An international randomized trial comparing four thrombolytic strategies for acute myocardial infarction. N Engl J Med 1993;329:673–682.
62. Bode C, Smalling RW, Berg G, et al. Randomized comparison of coronary thrombolysis acheived with double bolus reteplase (rPA) and front-loaded "accelerated" alteplase (tPA) in patients with acute myocardial infarction. Circulation 1996;94:891–898.
63. The Global Use of Strategies to Open Occluded Coronary Arteries (GUSTO III) Investigators. A comparison of reteplase with alteplase for acute myocardial infarction. N Engl J Med 1997;337:1118–1123.
64. Weaver WD, Cerqueira M, Hallstrom AP, et al. Prehospital-initiated vs hospital-initiated thrombolytic therapy: The myocardial infarction triage and intervention trial. JAMA 1993;270:1211–1216.
65. Mark DB, Hlatky MA, Califf RM, et al. Cost effectiveness of thrombolytic therapy with tissue plasminogen activator as compared with streptokinase for acute myocardial infarction. N Engl J Med 1995;332:1418–1424.
66. Pfeffer MA, Moye LA, Braunwald E, et al. Selection bias in the use of thrombolytic therapy in acute myocardial infarction. JAMA 1991;266:528–532.
67. Sane DC, Califf RM, Topol EJ, et al. Bleeding during thrombolytic therapy for acute myocardial infarction: Mechanisms and management. Ann Intern Med 1989;111:1010–1022.
68. Stringer KA. Clinical trials in thrombolytic therapy, part 1: Outcome markers that go beyond mortality reduction. Am J Health Syst Pharm 1997;54(suppl 1):S23–S26.
69. Meyer J, Merx W, Schmitz H, et al. Percutaneous transluminal coronary angioplasty immediately after intracoronary streptolysis of transmural myocardial infarction. Circulation 1982;66:905–913.
70. Grines CL, Browne KF, Marco J, et al. A comparison of immediate angioplasty with thrombolytic therapy for acute myocardial infarction. N Engl J Med 1993;328:673–679.
71. Zijlstra F, de Boer MJ, Hoorntje JCA, et al. A comparison of immediate coronary angioplasty with intravenous streptokinase in acute myocardial infarction. N Engl J Med 1993;328:680–684.
72. Gibbons RJ, Holmes DR, Reeder GS, et al. Immediate angioplasty compared with the administration of a thrombolytic agent followed by conservative treatment for myocardial infarction. N Engl J Med 1993;328:685–691.
73. Michel KB, Yusuf S. Does PTCA in acute myocardial infarction affect mortality and reinfarction rates? Circulation 1995;91:476–485.
74. Zahn R, Koch A, Rustige J, et al. Primary angioplasty versus thrombolysis in the treatment of acute myocardial infarction. Am J Cardiol 1997;79:264–269
75. Stone GW, Grines CL, Rothbaum D, et al. for the PAMI Trial Investigators. Analysis of the relative costs and effectiveness of primary angioplasty versus tissue-type plasminogen activator: The primary angioplasty in myocardial infarction (PAMI) trial. J Am Coll Cardiol 1997;29:901–907.
76. DeBoer MJ, Hoorntje JCA, Ottervanger JP, Reffers S, Suryapranata H, Zijlstra F. Immediate coronary angioplasty versus intravenous streptokinase in acute myocardial infarction: Left ventricular ejection fraction, hospital mortality, and reinfarction. J Am Coll Cardiol 1994;23:1004–1008.
77. The Global Use of Strategies to Open Occluded Coronary Arteries in Acute Coronary Syndromes (GUSTO IIb) Angioplasty Substudy Investigators. A clinical trial comparing primary coronary angioplasty with tissue plasminogen activator for acute myocardial infarction. N Engl J Med 1997;336:1621–1628.
78. Bates ER, Topol EJ. Limitations of thrombolytic therapy for acute myocardial infarction complicated by congestive heart failure and cardiogenic shock. J Am Coll Cardiol 1991;18:1077–1084.
79. Berger PB, Holmes DR, Stebbins AL, Bates ER, Califf RM, Topol EJ for the GUSTO-I Investigators. Impact of an aggressive invasive catheterization and revascularization strategy on mortality in patients with cardiogenic shock in the Global Utilization of Streptokinase and Tissue Plasminogen Activator for Occluded Coronary Arteries (GUSTO-I) trial. Circulation 1997;96;122–127.
80. Weaver WD, Simes J, Betriu A, et al. Comparison of primary coronary angioplasty and intravenous thrombolytic therapy for acue myocardial infarction. JAMA 1997;278:2093–2098.
81. O'Neill WW, Weintraub R, Grines CL, et al. A prospective, placebo-controlled, randomized trial of intravenous streptokinase and angioplasty versus lone angioplasty therapy of acute myocardial infarction. Circulation 1992;86:1710–1717.
82. Vaitkus PT, Laskey WK. Efficacy of adjunctive thrombolytic therapy in percutaneous transluminal coronary angioplasty. J Am Coll Cardiol 1994;24:1415–1423.
83. Second International Study of Infarct Survival (ISIS-2). Randomised trial of intravenous streptokinase, oral aspirin, both, or neither among 17,187 cases of suspected acute myocardial infarction: ISIS-2. Lancet 1988;ii:349–360.
84. CAPRIE Steering Committee. A randomised, blinded, trial of clopidogrel versus aspirin in patients at risk of ischaemic events (CAPRIE). Lancet 1996;348:1329–1339.
85. Wood AJJ. Aspirin, heparin and fibrinolytic therapy in suspected acute myocardial infarction. N Engl J Med 1997;336:847–860.
86. Antiplatelet Trialists' Collaboration. Collaborative overview of randomised trials of antiplatelet therapy—I: Prevention of death, myocardial infarction, and stroke by prolonged antiplatelet therapy in various categories of patients. Br Med J 1994;308:81–106.
87. Ridker PM, Hebert PR, Fuster V, Hennekens CH. Are both aspirin and heparin justified as adjuncts to thrombolytic therapy for acute myocardial infarction? Lancet 1993;341:1574–1577.
88. Hirsh J, Raschke R, Warkentin T, Dalen JE, Deykin D, Piller L. Heparin: Mechanism of action, pharmacokinetics, dosing considerations, monitoring, efficacy, and safety. Chest 1995;108:258S–275S.
89. Collins R, MacMahon S, Flather M, et al. Clinical effects of anticoagulation in suspected acute myocardial infarction: Systemic overview of randomised trials. Br Med J 1996;313:652–659.
90. Davis MJE, Ireland MA. Effect of early anticoagulation on the frequency of left ventricular thrombi after anterior wall acute myocardial infarction. Am J Cardiol 1986;57:1244–1247.
91. Kontny F, Dale J, Abildgaard U, et al. Adverse effect of warfarin in acute MI: Increased left ventricular thrombus formation in patients not treated with high dose heparin. Eur Heart J 1993;14:1040–1043.
92. Clagett GP, Anderson FA, Heit J, Levine M, Wheeler HB. Prevention of venous thromboembolism. Chest 1995;108:312S–334S.
93. Hirsh J, Fuster V. Guide to anticoagulant therapy Part 1: Heparin. Circulation 1994;89:1449–1468.
94. Smith P, Arnesen H, Holme I. The effect of warfarin on mortality and reinfarction after myocardial infarction. N Engl J Med 1990;323: 147–152.
95. Meijer A, Verheugt FWA, Werter CJPJ, et al. Aspirin versus coumadin in the prevention of reocclusion and recurrent ischemia after successful thrombolysis: A prospective placebo-controlled angiographic study. Results of the APRICOT study. Circulation 1993; 87:1524–1530.
96. Aspect Research Group. Effect of long-term oral anticoagulant treatment on mortality and cardiovascular morbidity after myocardial infarction: Anticoagulants in the Secondary Prevention of Events in Coronary Thrombosis (ASPECT) Research Group. Lancet 1994;90: 499–503.
97. Coumadin Aspirin Reinfarction Study [CARS] Investigators. Randomised double-blind trial of fixed low-dose warfarin with aspirin after myocardial infarction. Lancet 1997;350:389–396.
98. Loh E, St. John Sutton M, Wun C-CC, et al. Ventricular dysfunction and the risk of stroke after myocardial infarction. N Engl J Med 1997;336:251–257.

99. The Acute Infarction Ramipril Efficacy [AIRE] Study Investigators. Effect of ramipril on mortality and morbidity of survivors of acute myocardial infarction with clinical evidence of heart failure. Lancet 1993;342:821–828.
100. Lastini R, Maggioni AP, Flather M, Sleight P, Tognoni G. ACE-inhibitor use in patients myocardial infarction: Summary of evidence from clinical trials. Circulation 1995;92:3132–3137.
101. The SOLVD Investigators. Effect of enalapril on survival in patients with reduced left ventricular ejection fractions and congestive heart failure. N Engl J Med 1991;325:293–302.
102. Kober L, Torp-Pedersen C, Carlsen JE, et al., for the Trandolapril Cardiac Evaluation (TRACE) Study Group. A clinical trial of the angiotensin-converting-enzyme inhibitor trandolapril in patients with left ventricular dysfunction after myocardial infarction. N Engl J Med 1995;333:1670–1676.
103. National Cholesterol Education Program. Second Report of the Expert Panel on Detection, Evaluation, and Treatment of High Blood Cholesterol in Adults (Adult Treatment Panel II). Circulation 1994; 89:1333–1345.
104. Scandinavian Simvastatin Survival Study Group. Randomised trial of cholesterol lowering in 4444 patients with coronary heart disease: The Scandinavian Simvastatin Survival Study (4S). Lancet 1994; 344:1383-1389.
105. Sacks FM, Pfeffer MA, Braunwald E, et al. for the CARE Investigators. Effect of pravastatin on coronary events after myocardial infarction in patients with average cholesterol levels. N Engl J Med 1996;335:1001–1009.
106. Baigent C, Collins R, Appleby P, Parish S, Sleight P, et al. ISIS-2: 10 year survival among patients with suspected acute myocardial infarction in randomised comparison of intravenous streptokinase, oral aspirin, both or neither. BrMJ 1998;316:1337–1343.
107. Boden WE, O'Rourke RA, Crawford MH, Blaustein AS, Deedwania PC, et al. Outcomes in patients with acute non-Q-wave myocardial infarction randomly assigned to an invasive as compared with a conservative management strategy. N Engl J Med 1998;338:1785–1792.
108. Lefkovits J, Plow EF, Topol EJ. Platelet glycoprotein IIb/IIIa receptors in cardiovascular medicine. N Engl J Med 1995;332:1553–1559.
109. Stringer KA. New Platelet inhibitors for management of acute coronary syndromes. Ann Pharmacother, in press.
110. Theroux P. Oral inhibitors of platelet membrane receptor glycoprotein IIb/IIIa in clinical cardiology: Issues and opportunities. Am Heart J 1998;135:S107–S112.
111. Willerson JT. Inhibitors of platelet glycoprotein IIb/IIIa receptors. Will they be useful when given chronically? Circulation 1996; 94:866–868.
112. Cohen M, Demers C, Gurfinkel EP, Turpie AGG, Fromell GJ, et al. A comparison of low molecular weight heparin with unfractionated heparin for unstable coronary artery disease. N Engl J Med 1997; 337:447–452.

14

Arrhythmias

Jerry L. Bauman, PharmD, BCPS, FCCP, FACC, and Marieke Dekker Schoen, PharmD, BCPS

The heart has two basic properties, namely an electrical property and a mechanical property. The synchronous interaction between these two properties is complex, precise, and relatively enduring. The study of the electrical properties of the heart has grown at a slow steady rate, interrupted by salvos of information due to paroxysmal scientific breakthroughs. Einthoven's pioneering work has allowed graphic electrical tracings of cardiac rhythm and probably represents the first of these breakthroughs. This discovery (of the surface electrocardiogram) has remained the cornerstone of diagnostic tools for cardiac rhythm disturbances. However, one must be aware that, prior to the availability of the electrocardiogram, meticulous clinical observation of venous and arterial pulsations provided a relatively sophisticated classification of many cardiac arrhythmias. More recently, intracardiac recordings and programmed cardiac stimulation have led to a wealth of both basic and clinical data. Microelectrode, voltage clamp, and patch clamping techniques have allowed considerable insight into the electrophysiologic actions and mechanisms of antiarrhythmic drugs. In terms of drug therapy, the use of digitalis and later quinidine constitutes important first steps. The 1980s led to a considerable number of new agents; the theme of drug discovery was initially to find orally absorbed lidocaine congeners and later other drugs that had extremely potent effects on conduction, that is, flecainide-like agents. Unfortunately, the initial promise of a "magic bullet" in terms of antiarrhythmic drug therapy has gone unfulfilled. It is noteworthy that many of the problems associated with these new agents became clear after they were approved and marketed. Indeed, the overall volume of antiarrhythmic drug usage in the United States has declined in the past 4 years. The reasons for this are severalfold. First is the heightened awareness of the significance of drug-related proarrhythmia. That proarrhythmia is an important side effect and has a potential effect on patient mortality was highlighted by the Cardiac Arrhythmia Suppression Trial (CAST). This study is perhaps the most important ever performed regarding the treatment of rhythm disorders and continues to have a far-reaching impact on the clinical use of drugs and drug discovery. Second is the technical advances in the development of non-drug therapies. For instance it is quite possible that interrupting reentry circuits by radiofrequency ablation could render long-term antiarrhythmic drug use obsolete in many arrhythmias. Further, refinement of internal cardioverter/defibrillators continues to advance at an impressive rate and this combined with the now-known hazards of drugs have led some to choose this form of therapy as the first-line treatment of serious, recurrent ventricular arrhythmias.

What does the future hold for the use of antiarrhythmic drugs? Certainly new knowledge and technological advances have forced investigators and clinicians to rethink the concept of traditional membrane-active drugs. The current focus of investigational antiarrhythmic drugs is the potassium-channel blockers, with sotalol being the first approved in the United States. Although considerable enthusiasm exists currently, the overall impact of these efforts has yet to be determined.

The purpose of this chapter is to review the principles involved in both normal and abnormal cardiac conduction and to address the pathophysiology and treatment of the more commonly encountered arrhythmias. Certainly, many volumes of complete text could be (and have been) devoted to basic and clinical electrophysiology. Therefore, this chapter briefly addresses those principles necessary for clinical pharmacists.

ARRHYTHMOGENESIS

NORMAL CONDUCTION

Electrical activity is initiated by the sinoatrial (SA) node and courses through cardiac tissue by a tree-like conduction network. The SA node initiates cardiac rhythm under normal circumstances because this tissue possesses the highest degree of automaticity or rate of spontaneous impulse generation. The degree of automaticity of the SA node is largely influenced by the autonomic nervous system in that both cholinergic and sympathetic innervation control sinus rate. Most tissues within the conduction system also possess varying degrees of inherent automatic properties. However, the rates of spontaneous impulse generation of these tissues are less than the rate of the SA node. Thus, these latent automatic pacemakers are continuously excited and overdriven by impulses arising from the SA node (primary pacemaker) and do not become clinically apparent.

From the SA node, electrical activity moves in a wavefront through an atrial specialized conducting system and eventually gains entrance to the ventricle via the atrioventricular (AV) node and a large bundle of conducting tissue referred to as the bundle of His. Aside from this AV nodal–Hisian pathway, the atria and ventricles are separated by a fibrous AV ring that will not permit electrical stimulation. The conducting tissues bridging the atria and ventricles are referred to as the junctional areas. Again, this area of tissue (junction) is largely influenced by autonomic input and possesses a relatively high degree of inherent automaticity (but still less than that of the SA node). From the bundle of His, the cardiac conduction system bifurcates into several (usually three) bundle branches: one right bundle and two left bundles. These bundle branches further arborize into a conduction network referred to as the Purkinje system. The conduction system as a whole innervates the mechanical myocardium and serves to initiate excitation-contraction coupling and the contractile process. When a cell or group of cells within the heart is electrically stimulated, a brief period of time follows in which those cells cannot again be excited. This time period is referred to as the refractory period. As the electrical wavefront moves down the conduction system, the impulse eventually encounters tissue refractory to stimulation (recently excited) and subsequently dies out. Then the SA node recovers, fires spontaneously, and begins the process again.

Prior to cellular excitation, an electrical gradient exists between the inside and the outside of the cell membrane. At this time the cell is said to be polarized. In atrial and ventricular conducting tissue, the intracellular space is about 80 to 90 mV negative with respect to the extracellular environment. The electrical gradient just prior to excitation is referred to as resting membrane potential (RMP) and is the result of differences in ion concentrations between the inside and the outside of the cell. At RMP, the cell is polarized primarily by the action of active membrane ion pumps, the most notable of these being the sodium–potassium pump. For example, this specific pump (in addition to other systems) attempts to maintain the intracellular sodium concentration at 5 to 15 mEq/L and the extracellular sodium at 135 to 142 Meq/L; the intracellular potassium concentration at 135 to 140 mEq/L and the extracellular potassium concentration at 3 to 5 mEq/L. RMP can be calculated by using the Nernst equation:

$$\text{RMP} = -61.5 \log \frac{[\text{ion outside}]}{[\text{ion inside}]}$$

Electrical stimulation (or depolarization) of the cell will result in changes in membrane potential over time or a characteristic action potential curve (Fig. 14–1). The action potential curve results from the transmembrane movement of specific ions and is divided into different phases. Phase 0 (rapid depolarization) of atrial and ventricular tissues is due to an abrupt increase in the permeability of the membrane to sodium influx. This rapid depolarization more than equilibrates (overshoot) the electrical potential, resulting in a brief initial repolarization or phase one. Phase one is due to a passive chloride influx, active potassium efflux, or both. Calcium begins to move into the intracellular space at about −60 mV (during phase 0), causing a slower depolarization. Calcium influx continues throughout phase 2 of the action potential (plateau phase) and is balanced to some degree by potassium efflux. Calcium entrance (only through L-channels in myocardial tissue) distinguishes cardiac conducting

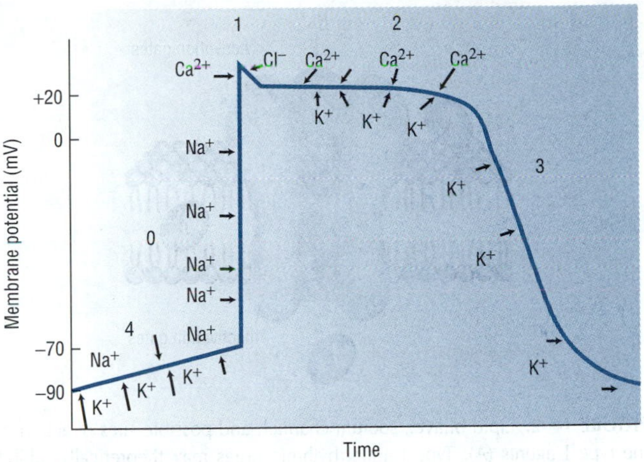

FIGURE 14–1. Purkinje fiber action potential showing specific ion flux responsible for the change in membrane potential.

cells from nerve tissue and provides the critical ionic link to excitation-contraction coupling and the mechanical properties of the heart as a pump (see Chap. 11). The membrane remains permeable to potassium efflux during phase 3, resulting in cellular repolarization. Phase 4 of the action potential is the gradual depolarization of the cell and is related to a constant sodium leak into the intracellular space balanced by a decreasing (over time) efflux of potassium. The slope of phase 4 depolarization determines, in large part, the automatic properties of the cell. As the cell is slowly depolarized during phase 4, an abrupt increase in sodium permeability is encountered, allowing the rapid cellular depolarization of phase 0. The juncture of phase 4 and phase 0, where rapid sodium influx is initiated, is referred to as the threshold potential of the cell. The level of threshold potential also regulates the degree of cellular automaticity.

Not all cells in the cardiac conduction system rely upon sodium influx for initial depolarization. Some tissues depolarize in response to a slower inward ionic current caused by calcium influx. These "calcium-dependent" tissues are found primarily in the SA and AV nodes (both L- and T-channels) and possess distinct conduction properties in comparison to "sodium-dependent" fibers. Calcium-dependent cells generally have a less negative RMP (−40 to −60 mV) and a slower conduction velocity. Furthermore, in calcium-dependent tissues, recovery of excitability outlasts full repolarization, whereas in sodium-dependent tissue, recovery is prompt after repolarization. These two types of electrical fibers also differ dramatically in how drugs modify their conduction properties (see later).

Ion conductance across the lipid bilayer of the cell membrane occurs via the formation of membrane pores or "channels" (Fig. 14–2). Selective ion channels probably form in response to specific electrical potential differences between the inside and the outside of the cell (voltage dependance). The membrane itself is composed of both organized and disorganized lipids and phospholipids in a

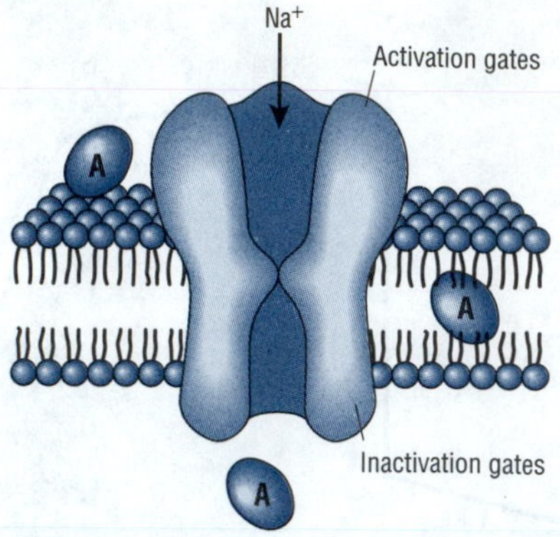

FIGURE 14–2. Lipid bilayer, sodium channel, and possible sites of action of the type I agents (A). Type I antiarrhythmic drugs may theoretically inhibit sodium influx at an extracellular, intramembrane, or intracellular receptor site. However, all approved agents appear to block sodium conductance at a single receptor site by gaining entrance to the interior of the channel from an intracellular route. Active ionized drugs block the channel predominantly during the activated or inactivated state and bind and unbind with specific time constants (described as fast on–off, slow on–off, and intermediate).

dynamic sol–gel matrix. During ion flux and electrical excitation, changes in this sol–gel equilibrium occur and permit the formation of activated ion channels. Besides channel formation and membrane composition, the transmembrane movement of ions is also regulated by intrachannel proteins or phospholipids referred to as gates. These gates are believed to be positioned strategically within the channel to modulate ion flow (Fig. 14–2). Each ion channel conceptually has two types of gates: an activation gate and an inactivation gate. The activation gate opens during depolarization to allow the ion current to enter or exit from the cell and the inactivation gate closes to stop ion movement. When the cell is in a rested state, the activation gates are closed and the inactivation gates are open. The activation gates then open to allow ion movement through the channel and the inactivation gates later close to stop ion conductance. Therefore, the cell cycles between three states: resting, activation, and inactivation. Activation of SA and AV nodal tissue is dependent upon a slow depolarizing current through calcium channels and gates, whereas the activation of atrial and ventricular tissue is dependent upon a rapid depolarizing current through sodium channels and gates.

ABNORMAL CONDUCTION

The mechanisms of tachyarrhythmias have been classically divided into two general categories: those resulting from an abnormality in impulse generation or "automatic" tachycardias and those resulting from an abnormality in impulse conduction or "reentrant" tachycardias.

Automatic tachycardias depend upon spontaneous impulse generation in latent pacemakers and may be due to several different mechanisms. Experimentally, chemicals such as digitalis glycosides or catecholamines and conditions such as hypoxemia, electrolyte abnormalities (e.g., hypokalemia), or fiber stretch (cardiac dilatation) may lead to an increased slope of phase 4 depolarization in tissues other than the SA node. These factors, which experimentally lead to abnormal automaticity, are also known to be arrhythmogenic in clinical situations. The increased slope of phase 4 causes heightened automaticity of these tissues and competition with the SA node for dominance of cardiac rhythm. If the rate of spontaneous impulse generation of the abnormally automatic tissue exceeds that of the SA node, then an automatic tachycardia may result. Automatic tachycardias have the following characteristics: (1) the onset of the tachycardia is not related to an initiating event such as a premature beat; (2) the initiating beat is usually identical to subsequent beats of the tachycardia; (3) the tachycardia cannot be initiated by programmed cardiac stimulation; (4) the tachycardia often occurs in association with digitalis toxicity, high degrees of sympathetic tone, hypokalemia, and/or severe pulmonary disease; and (5) onset of the tachycardia is usually preceded by a gradual acceleration in rate and termination by a deceleration in rate.

Triggered automaticity is also a possible mechanism for abnormal impulse generation. Briefly, triggered automaticity refers to transient membrane depolarizations that occur during repolarization (early after-depolarizations) or after repolarization (delayed after-depolarizations) but prior to phase 4 of the action potential. After-depolarizations may be related to abnormal calcium and sodium influx during or just after full cellular repolarization. Experimentally, early after-depolarizations may be precipitated by hypokalemia, type Ia antiarrhythmic drugs, or slow stimulation rates and have been implicated as a cause of torsades de pointes. Late after-depolarizations may be precipitated by digitalis or catecholamines and suppressed by calcium channel inhibitors, and have been suggested as the mechanism for multifocal atrial tachycardia and exercise-provoked ventricular tachycardia. Triggered automatic rhythms possess some of the characteristics of automatic tachycardias and some of the characteristics of reentrant tachycardias.

As previously mentioned, the impulse originating from the SA node in an individual with sinus rhythm eventually meets previously excited and thus refractory tissue. Reentry is a concept that involves indefinite propagation of the impulse and continued activation of previously refractory tissue. There are three conduction requirements for the formation of a viable reentrant focus: two pathways for impulse conduction; an area of unidirectional block (prolonged refractoriness) in one of these pathways; and slow conduction in the other pathway (Fig. 14–3). Usually a critically timed premature beat initiates reentry. This premature impulse enters both conduction pathways but encounters refractory tissue in one of the pathways at the area of unidirectional block. The impulse dies out because it is still refractory from the previous (sinus) impulse. Although it fails to propagate in one pathway, the impulse may still proceed in a forward direction (antegrade) through the other pathway

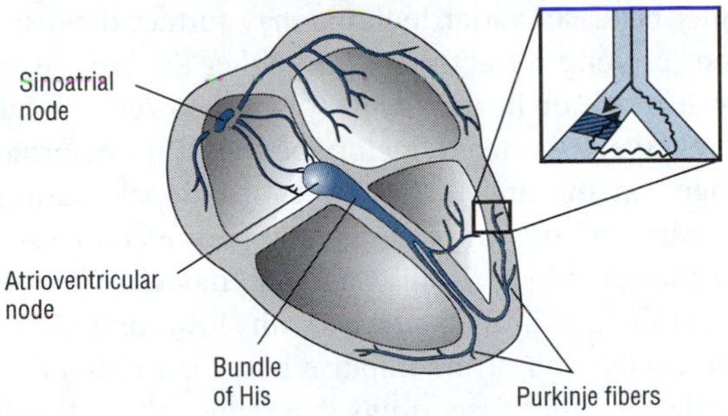

FIGURE 14–3. Conduction system of the heart. The magnified portion shows a bifurcation of a Purkinje fiber traditionally explained as the etiology of reentrant ventricular tachycardia. A premature impulse travels to the fiber, damaged by heart disease or ischemia. It encounters a zone of prolonged refractoriness (area of unidirectional block—hatched area) but fails to propagate because it remains refractory to stimulation from the previous impulse. However, the impulse may slowly travel (squiggly line) through the other portion of the Purkinje twig and will "reenter" the cross-hatched area if the refractory period is concluded and it is now excitable. Thus, the premature impulse never meets refractory tissue; circus movement ensues. If this site stimulates the surrounding ventricle repetitively, clinical reentrant ventricular tachycardia results.

because of this pathway's relatively shorter refractory period. The impulse may then proceed through a loop of tissue and "reenter" the area of unidirectional block in a backward direction (retrograde). Because the antegrade pathway has slow conduction characteristics, the area of unidirectional block has time to recover its excitability. The impulse can proceed retrogradely through this (previously refractory) tissue and continue around the loop of tissue in a circular fashion. Thus, the key to the formation of a reentrant focus is crucial conduction discrepancies in the electrophysiologic characteristics of the two pathways. The reentrant focus may excite surrounding tissue at a rate greater than that of the SA node and a clinical tachycardia results. The above model is anatomically determined in that there is only one pathway for impulse conduction with a fixed circuit length. Another model of reentry, referred to as a functional reentrant loop or leading circle model may also occur (Fig. 14–4).[1] In a functional reentrant focus, the length of the circuit may vary depending on the conduction velocity and recovery characteristics of the impulse. The area in the middle of the loop is continually kept refractory by the inwardly moving impulse. The length of the circuit is not fixed, but is the smallest circle possible such that the leading edge of the wavefront is continuously exciting tissue just as it recovers; the head of the impulse chases its tail. It differs from the anatomic model in that the leading edge of the impulse is not preceded by an excitable gap of tissue, and it does not have an obstacle in the middle nor a fixed anatomic circuit. Clinically, many reentrant foci probably have both anatomic and functional characteristics. In the figure 8 model, a zone of unidirectional block is present, allowing for two impulse loops that join and reenter the area of block in a retrograde fashion to form a pretzel-shaped reentrant circuit. This model combines functional characteristics with an excitable gap. All of these theoretical models require a critical balance of refractoriness and conduction velocity within the circuit and as such have helped to explain the effects of drugs on terminating, modifying, and causing cardiac rhythm disturbances.

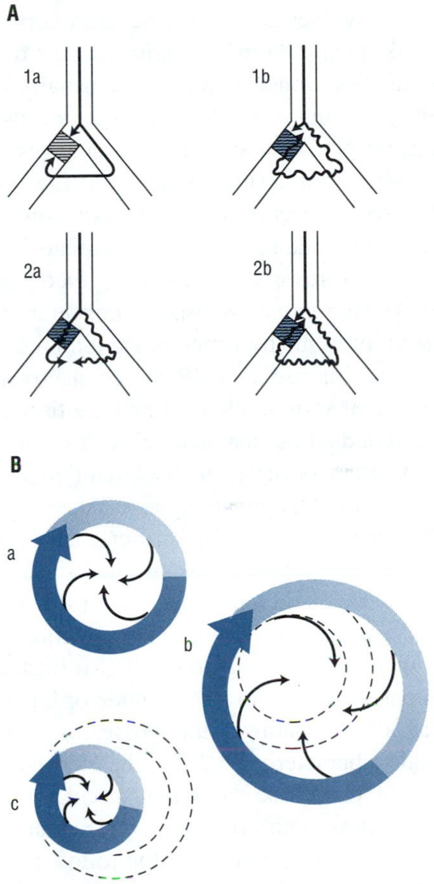

FIGURE 14–4. A. Possible mechanism of proarrhythmia in the anatomic model of reentry. (1a) Nonviable reentrant loop due to bidirectional block (shaded area). (1b) Instance where a drug slows conduction velocity without significantly prolonging the refractory period. The impulse is now able to reenter the area of unidirectional block (shaded area) because slowed conduction through the contralateral limb allows recovery of the block. A new reentrant tachycardia may result. (2a) Nonviable reentrant loop owing to a lack of a unidirectional block. (2b) Instance where a drug prolongs the refractory period without significantly slowing conduction velocity. The impulse moving antegrade meets refractory tissue (shaded area) allowing for unidirectional block. A new reentrant tachycardia may result. **B.** Mechanism of reentry and proarrhythmia. (a) Functionally determined (leading circle) reentrant circuit. This model should be contrasted with anatomic reentry: Here the circuit is not fixed (it does not necessarily move around an anatomic obstacle) and there is no excitable gap. All tissue inside is held continuously refractory. (b) Instance where a drug prolongs the refractory period without significantly slowing conduction velocity. The tachycardia may terminate or slow in rate as shown owing to a greater circuit length. The dashed lines represent the original reentrant circuit prior to drug treatment. (c) Instance where a drug slows conduction velocity without significantly prolonging the refractory period (i.e., type Ic agents) and accelerates the tachycardia. The tachycardia rate may increase (proarrhythmia) as shown owing to a shorter circuit length. The dashed lines represent the original reentrant circuit prior to drug treatment. *(From Ref. 51, with permission.)*

What causes reentry to become clinically manifest? Reentrant foci may occur at any level of the conduction system: within the branches of the specialized atrial conduction system, the Purkinje network, and even within portions of the SA and AV nodes. The anatomy of the Purkinje system is felt to provide a suitable substrate for the formation of microreentrant loops and is often used as a model to facilitate the understanding of reentry concepts (Fig. 14–3). Of course, reentry does not usually occur in normal, healthy conduction tissue and therefore various forms of heart disease or conduction abnormalities must usually be present before reentry becomes manifest. In other words, the various forms of heart disease can result in changes in conduction in the pathways of a suitable reentrant substrate. An often used example is reentry occurring as a consequence of ischemic or hypoxic damage: with inadequate cellular oxygen, cardiac tissue resorts to anaerobic glycolysis for ATP production. As high-energy phosphate concentration diminishes, the activity of the transmembrane ion pumps declines and RMP rises. This rise in RMP causes inactivation in the voltage-dependent sodium channel and the tissue begins to assume slow conduction characteristics. If changes in conduction parameters occur in a discordant manner due to varying degrees of ischemia or hypoxia, then a reentry circuit may become manifest. Furthermore, an ischemic, dying cell liberates intracellular potassium, also causing a rise in RMP. In other cases, reentry may occur due to anatomic or functional variants in the normal conduction system. In another example, patients may possess two (instead of one) conduction pathways within the AV node or have an anomalous, extranodal AV pathway that possesses different electrophysiologic characteristics from the normal AV nodal pathway. Reentry in these cases may occur within the AV node or encompass both atrial and ventricular tissue (see later). Reentrant tachycardias have the following characteristics: (1) the onset of the tachycardia is usually related to an initiating event (i.e., premature beat), (2) the initiating beat is usually different in morphology from subsequent beats of the tachycardia, (3) initiation of the tachycardia is usually possible with programmed cardiac stimulation, and (4) the initiation and termination of the tachycardia is usually abrupt, without an acceleration or deceleration phase.

MECHANISM OF ANTIARRHYTHMIC DRUGS

In a theoretical sense, drugs may have antiarrhythmic activity by directly altering conduction in several ways. First, a drug may depress the automatic properties of abnormal pacemaker cells. An agent may do this by decreasing the slope of phase 4 depolarization and/or by elevating threshold potential. If the rate of spontaneous impulse generation of the abnormally automatic foci becomes less than that of the SA node, normal cardiac rhythm can be restored. Second, drugs may alter the conduction characteristics of the pathways of a reentrant loop.[1,2] An agent may facilitate conduction (shorten refractoriness) in the area of unidirectional block, allowing antegrade conduction to proceed. On the other hand, an antiarrhythmic may further depress conduction (prolong refractoriness) in either the area of unidirectional block or in the pathway with slowed conduction and a relatively shorter refractory period. If refractoriness is prolonged in the area of unidirectional block, retrograde propagation of the impulse is not permitted, causing a "bidirectional" block. In the anatomic model, if refractoriness is prolonged in the pathway with slow conduction, antegrade conduction of the impulse is not permitted through this route. In either case, drugs that reduce the discordance and cause a uniformity in conduction properties of the two pathways may suppress the reentrant substrate. In the functionally determined model, if refractoriness is prolonged without significantly slowing conduction velocity, the tachycardia may terminate or slow in rate owing to a greater circuit length (Fig. 14–4). There are other possible ways to stop reentry: a drug may eliminate the critically timed premature impulse that triggers reentry, or a drug may slow conduction velocity to such an extent that conduction is extinguished.

Antiarrhythmic drugs have specific electrophysiologic actions that alter cardiac conduction in patients with or without heart disease. These actions form the basis of grouping antiarrhythmics into specific categories based on their electrophysiologic actions *in vitro*. The most frequently used classification system was first proposed by Vaughan Williams (Table 14–1).[2] This classification has been criticized because (1) it is incomplete and does not allow for the classification of agents such as digoxin or adenosine, (2) it is not pure and many agents have properties of more than one class of drugs, (3) it does not incorporate drug characteristics such as mechanisms of tachycardia termination/prevention, clinical indications, or side effects, and (4) agents become "labeled" within a class although they may be distinct in many regards.[3] These criticisms formed the basis for the Sicilian gambit, which was an attempt to reclassify antiarrhythmic agents based on a variety of basic and clinical characteristics. Nonetheless, the Vaughan Williams classification remains the most frequently used despite many proposed modifications and alternative systems and is important from an educational point of view. The type Ia drugs such as quinidine, procainamide, and disopyramide slow conduction velocity, prolong refractoriness, and decrease the automatic properties of sodium-dependent (normal and diseased) conduction tissue. Therefore, the type Ia agents can be effective in automatic tachycardias by decreasing the rate of spontaneous impulse generation of atrial or ventricular foci. In reentrant tachycardias, these drugs generally depress conduction and prolong refractoriness, theoretically transforming the area of unidirectional block into a bidirectional block. Clinically, type Ia drugs are broad-spectrum antiarrhythmics, being effective for both supraventricular and ventricular arrhythmias.

Historically, lidocaine and phenytoin were categorized separately from quinidine-like drugs. This was due to early

TABLE 14–1. Classification of Antiarrhythmic Drugs

Type	Drug	Conduction Velocity[a]	Refractory Period	Automaticity	Ion Block
Ia	Quinidine Procainamide Disopyramide	↓	↑	↓	Sodium (intermediate)
Ib	Lidocaine Mexiletine Tocainide	0/↓	↓	↓	Sodium (fast on–off)
Ic	Flecainide Propafenone[c] Moricizine[d]	↓↓	0	↓	Sodium (slow on–off)
II[b]	β-Blockers	↓	↑	↓	Calcium (indirect)
III	Amiodarone[c,e] Bretylium[c] Sotalol[c] Ibutilide	0	↑↑	0	Potassium
IV[b]	Verapamil Diltiazem	↓	↑	↓	Calcium

[a]Variables for normal tissue models in ventricular tissue.
[b]Variables for SA and AV nodal tissue only.
[c]Also has type II, β-blocking actions.
[d]Classification controversial.
[e]Amiodarone also blocks calcium and sodium channels (fast on–off).

work demonstrating that lidocaine had distinctly different electrophysiologic actions. In normal tissue models, lidocaine generally had facilitative actions on cardiac conduction by shortening refractoriness and having little effect on conduction velocity. Thus, it was postulated that these agents could improve antegrade conduction, eliminating the area of unidirectional block. Of course, arrhythmias do not usually arise from normal tissue, leading investigators to study the actions of lidocaine and phenytoin in ischemic and hypoxic tissue models. Interestingly, studies have shown these drugs to possess quinidine-like properties in diseased tissues. Therefore, it is probable that lidocaine acts in clinical tachycardias in a similar fashion to the type Ia drugs, that is, accentuated effects in diseased tissues lead to bidirectional block in a reentrant circuit. Lidocaine and similar agents have accentuated effects in ischemic tissue owing to the local acidosis and potassium shifts that occur during cellular hypoxia. Changes in pH alter the time that local anesthetics occupy the sodium channel receptor and therefore affect the agent's electrophysiologic actions. The type Ib agents such as lidocaine (and structural analogs such as tocainide or mexiletine) are considerably more effective in ventricular arrhythmias than supraventricular arrhythmias.

The third group of type I drugs, type Ic, includes propafenone, flecainide, and moricizine. These agents profoundly slow conduction velocity while leaving refractoriness relatively unaltered. Type Ics theoretically eliminate reentry by slowing conduction to a point where the impulse is extinguished and cannot propagate further. Although effective for both ventricular and supraventricular arrhythmias, their use for ventricular arrhythmias has been limited by the risk of proarrhythmia (see later).

Type I drugs exert their effects on a subcellular basis by inhibiting the transmembrane influx of sodium. In essence, type I agents can be referred to as sodium channel blockers. The receptor site for the antiarrhythmics is probably inside the sodium channel so that, in effect, the drug plugs the pore. The agent may gain access to the receptor either via the intracellular space through the membrane lipid bilayer or directly through the channel. There are several principles inherent in antiarrhythmic–sodium channel receptor theories, and these are listed below.[4]

1. Type I antiarrhythmics have predominant affinity for a particular state of the channel, such as during activation or inactivation. For example, lidocaine and flecainide block sodium current primarily when the cell is in the inactivated state whereas quinidine is predominantly an open (or activated)-channel blocker.
2. Type I antiarrhythmics have specific binding and unbinding characteristics to the receptor. For example, lidocaine binds to and dissociates from the channel receptor quickly (termed fast on–off) but flecainide has very "slow on–off" properties. This explains why flecainide has such potent effects on slowing ventricular conduction but lidocaine has little effect on normal tissue. In general the type Ics are slow on–off, the type Ibs fast on–off, and the Ias intermediate in their binding kinetics.

3. Type I antiarrhythmics possess rate dependance, that is, sodium channel blockade and slowed conduction are greatest at fast heart rates and least during bradycardia. For slow on-off drugs, sodium channel blockade is evident at normal rates (60 to 100 bpm) but for fast on–off agents, slowed conduction is apparent only at rapid rates of stimulation.
4. Type I antiarrhythmics (except phenytoin) are weak bases with a pK_a >7.0 and block the sodium channel in their ionized form. Therefore, pH will alter these actions: acidosis will accentuate and alkalosis diminish sodium channel blockade.
5. Type I antiarrhythmics appear to share a single receptor site in the sodium channel.

These principles are important in understanding additive drug combinations (e.g., quinidine and mexiletine), antagonistic combinations (e.g., flecainide and lidocaine), and potential antidotes to excess sodium channel blockade (sodium bicarbonate or propranolol).

The β-adrenergic antagonists are classified as type II antiarrhythmic drugs. For the most part, the clinically relevant antiarrhythmic mechanisms of the β-blockers result from their antiadrenergic actions. Because the SA and AV nodes are heavily influenced by adrenergic innervation, β-blockers would be most useful in tachycardias in which these nodal tissues are abnormally automatic or are a portion of a reentrant loop. These agents are also helpful in slowing ventricular response in atrial tachycardias (e.g., atrial fibrillation) by their effects on the AV node. Furthermore, some tachycardias are exercise related or precipitated by states of high sympathetic tone (perhaps through triggered activity), and β-blockers may be useful in these instances. β-Adrenergic stimulation results in increased conduction velocity, shortened refractoriness, and increased automaticity of the nodal tissues; β-adrenergic blockers will antagonize these effects. Propranolol is often noted to have "local anesthetic" or quinidine-like activity; however, suprapharmacologic concentrations are usually required to elicit this action. In the nodal tissues, β-blockers interfere with calcium entry into the cell by altering catecholamine-dependent channel integrity and gating kinetics. In sodium-dependent atrial and ventricular tissue, β-blockers shorten repolarization somewhat, but otherwise have little direct effect. The antiarrhythmic properties of β-blockers observed with long-term, chronic therapy in patients with heart disease are less well understood. Although it is clear that β-blockers decrease the likelihood of sudden death (presumably arrhythmic death) after myocardial infarction, why this is so remains unclear but may relate to the complex interplay of changes in sympathetic tone, damaged myocardium, and ventricular conduction.

Type III antiarrhythmics include those agents that specifically prolong refractoriness in atrial and ventricular fibers. This class includes very different drugs: bretylium, amiodarone, sotalol, and recently ibutilide; they share the common effect of delaying repolarization by blocking potassium channels. The electrophysiologic actions of bretylium are related to its multifaceted pharmacology. Bretylium is structurally similar to guanethidine and can, likewise, cause an initial increase in catecholamine release from the adrenergic neuron. This action may potentially affect arrhythmogenesis by an indirect mechanism: increase in coronary blood flow and myocardial perfusion that reverses ischemia-related arrhythmias (similar to epinephrine's action in a patient with ventricular fibrillation). After causing catecholamine release, bretylium then causes an uncoupling of autonomic nerve stimulation from the release step, resulting in antiadrenergic effects. Theoretically, bretylium may also be antiarrhythmic by these sympatholytic actions. Nonetheless, bretylium prolongs repolarization due to blockade of potassium conductance, independent of the sympathetic nervous system, and many researchers feel these direct actions account for its clinical effectiveness. Importantly, bretylium increases the ventricular fibrillation threshold and seems to have selective antifibrillatory but not antitachycardic effects. In other words, bretylium can be effective in ventricular fibrillation, whereas it is often ineffective in ventricular tachycardia.

In contrast, amiodarone and sotalol are effective in most tachycardias. Amiodarone displays electrophysiologic characteristics consistent with each class within the Vaughan Williams scheme; it is a sodium channel blocker with relatively fast on-off kinetics, has non-competitive β-blocking actions, blocks potassium channels, and also has a small degree of calcium antagonist activity. At normal heart rates, its predominant effect is to prolong repolarization. Theoretically, amiodarone, like type I agents, may interrupt the reentrant substrate by transforming an area of unidirectional block into an area of bidirectional block. However, electrophysiologic studies using programmed cardiac stimulation imply that amiodarone may leave the reentrant loop intact. Rather, it is possible that amiodarone abolishes the premature impulse that usually triggers the reentry process. On the other hand, the potent β-blocking properties of amiodarone may contribute significantly to its acute and chronic efficacy. The observed impressive effectiveness of amiodarone coupled with its low proarrhythmic potential has challenged the notion that selective ion channel blockade by antiarrhythmic agents is preferable. Amiodarone inhibits movement of sodium, calcium, and potassium in addition to its β-blocking actions. However, despite being the most highly effective agent available, amiodarone unfortunately has the most impressive adverse effect profile. Sotalol is a potent inhibitor of outward potassium movement during repolarization and also possesses β-blocking actions.

Indeed, it was first synthesized as a nonselective β-antagonist but now has evolved into the prototype type III agent on which most investigational agents are based. Recently, ibutilide has been approved for the conversion of atrial fibrillation; this agent is structurally similar to sotalol. Ibutilide possesses type III activity by activating a slow, inward sodium current (I_{Nas}) and by blocking the potassium delayed rectifier current (I_K).

There are a number of different potassium channels that function during normal conduction, but the most relevant in terms of approved and investigational antiarrhythmic drugs is the delayed rectifier current (I_K) responsible for phase 2 and 3 repolarization. Subcurrents make up I_K; the rapid component is termed I_{Kr} and the slow component is termed I_{Ks}. NAPA and dofetilide (investigational) selectively block I_{Kr} whereas amiodarone and sotalol block both I_{Kr} and I_{Ks}. The clinical relevance of selectively blocking components of the delayed rectifier current remains to be determined. Potassium current blockers display "reverse use-dependance," that is, their effects on repolarization are greatest at low heart rates. Sotalol and like drugs also appear to be much more effective in preventing ventricular fibrillation (in dog models) than the traditional sodium blockers. They also decrease defibrillation threshold, in contrast to type I agents, which tend to increase this parameter. This could be important in patients with automatic internal defibrillators because concurrent therapy with type Is may require more energy for successful cardioversion or, worse, render it ineffective in terminating the tachycardia. Although most of the excitement surrounding antiarrhythmic drug therapy currently centers around sotalol-like agents, most if not all may cause proarrhythmia in the form of torsades de pointes; more long-term data regarding safety and efficacy are necessary to ascertain their true place in therapy.

The calcium channel antagonists comprise the type IV antiarrhythmic category. At least two types of calcium channels are operative in SA and AV nodal tissues: an L-type channel and a T-type channel. Therefore, both L-channel blockers (verapamil and diltiazem) and selective T-channel blockers will slow conduction, prolong refractoriness, and decrease automaticity of the calcium-dependent tissue in the SA and AV nodes. These agents are effective in automatic or reentrant tachycardias, which arise from or use the SA or AV nodes. In atrial tachycardias these drugs can slow ventricular response (e.g., atrial fibrillation) by slowing AV nodal conduction. Furthermore, because calcium entry seems to be integral to exercise-related tachycardias and/or tachycardias due to some forms of triggered automaticity, preliminary evidence shows effectiveness in these types of arrhythmias. In all likelihood, verapamil and diltiazem work at different receptor sites because of their dissimilar chemical structures and pharmacologic actions. Nifedipine (or any of the dihydropyridine calcium antagonists) does not have significant antiarrhythmic activity because a reflex increase in sympathetic tone due to vasodilation counteracts this agent's direct negative dromotropic action. Calcium antagonists can slightly shorten repolarization in normal sodium-dependent tissue but otherwise have little effect. The pharmacokinetics of the antiarrhythmic agents are summarized in Table 14–2 and a nomogram for estimating effective dosages of the oral forms (except amiodarone) is shown in Figure 14–5.

TABLE 14–2. Pharmacokinetics of Antiarrhythmic Drugs

Drug	Bioavailability (%)	Primary Route of Elimination[a]	$V_{D,ss}$ (L/kg)	Protein Binding (%)	$t_{1/2}$	Therapeutic Range (mg/L)
Quinidine	70–80	H	2.0–3.5	80–90	5–9 h	2–6
Procainamide	75–95	H/R	1.5–3.0	10–20	2.5–5.0 h	4–15
Disopyramide	70–95	H/R	0.8–2.0	50–80	4–8 h	2–6
Lidocaine	20–40	H	1–2	65–75	60–180 min	1.5–5.0
Mexiletine	80–95	H	5–12	60–75	6–12 h	0.8–2.0
Tocainide	90–95	H	1.5–3.0	10–30	12–15 h	4–10
Moricizine	34–38	H	6–11	92–95	1–6 h	—
Flecainide	90–95	H/R	8–10	35–45	13–20 h	0.3–2.5
Propafenone[b]						
Poor	11–39	H	2.5–4.0	85–95	12–32 h	—
Extensive					2–10 h	
Amiodarone	22–88	H	70–150	95–99	15–100 d	1.0–2.5
Sotalol	90–95	R	1.2–2.4	30–40	12–20 h	—
Ibutilide	—	H	6–12	40–50	3–6 h	—
Bretylium	15–20	R	4–8	Negligible	5–10 h	0.5–2.0
Verapamil	20–40	H	1.5–5.0	95–99	4–12 h	>0.05
Diltiazem	35–50	H	3–5	70–85	4–10 h	>0.05

[a]H = hepatic; R = renal.

[b]Variables for parent compound (not 5-OH, propafenone).

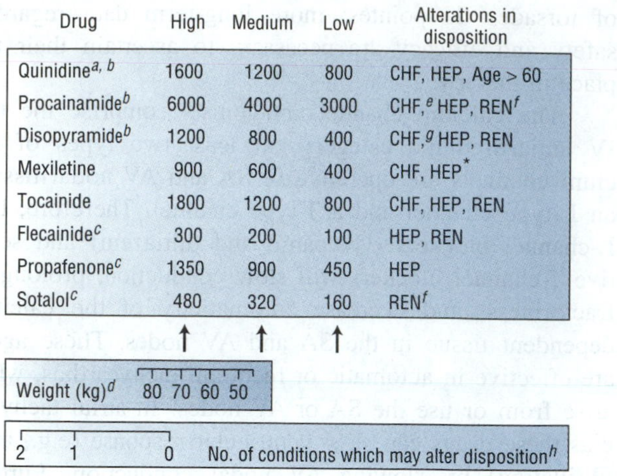
Drug
High
Medium
Low
Alterations in disposition
Quinidine[a, b] 1600 1200 800 CHF, HEP, Age > 60
Procainamide[b] 6000 4000 3000 CHF,[e] HEP, REN[f]
Disopyramide[b] 1200 800 400 CHF,[g] HEP, REN
Mexiletine 900 600 400 CHF, HEP*
Tocainide 1800 1200 800 CHF, HEP, REN
Flecainide[c] 300 200 100 HEP, REN
Propafenone[c] 1350 900 450 HEP
Sotalol[c] 480 320 160 REN[f]
Weight (kg)[d] 80 70 60 50
2 1 0 No. of conditions which may alter disposition[h]

FIGURE 14–5. Nomogram for estimating effective daily doses of commonly used oral antiarrhythmic drugs for acute efficacy testing. The dosages are grouped into high, medium, and low categories based on commonly used regimens and commercially available dosage forms. The dosages for each drug are listed as milligrams per day and are expected to result in the average steady-state concentrations shown in Table 14–2. Abbreviations: CHF = congestive heart failure; HEP = hepatic disease; REN = renal insufficiency (creatinine clearance < 50 mL/min).

Notes:

[a]Sulfate salt equivalents.

[b]Sustained-release forms may allow less fluctuation in concentrations.

[c]Best to initiate low-dose regimens in all patients and slowly escalate.

[d]Ideal body weight.

[e]Conflicting data regarding alteration in disposition.

[f]Significant accumulation of active metabolites or patent in renal disease limit use.

[g]Disopyramide not recommended in congestive heart failure.

[h]Use 1 for each suspected alteration but 2 where indicated (*).

Use of nomogram:

Step 1. Connect a straight line from the bar indicating the number of alterations in disposition, through the patient's weight to the base of the box.

Step 2. Approximate daily dosage is shown directly above the arrow. When the line connects between the arrows, use the crossbars between the arrows to choose high, medium, or low dosages or estimate an intermediate amount. Exercise caution when choosing dosages in the high range.

Example: A 70-kg patient with poor left ventricular function (e.g., CHF) and frequent paroxysmal episodes of atrial fibrillation is to be treated with oral quinidine. A straight line drawn between 1 on the conditions bar and 70 kg on the weight bar will intersect near the center arrow on the box. Directly above the point of intersection are the medium dosage ranges; quinidine sulfate can be initiated at 1200 mg/d or 300 mg every 6 hours in this patient. *(From Ref. 56, with permission.)*

SUPRAVENTRICULAR ARRHYTHMIAS

The common supraventricular tachycardias that often require drug treatment are (1) atrial fibrillation or atrial flutter, (2) paroxysmal supraventricular tachycardia, and (3) automatic atrial tachycardias. Other common supraventricular arrhythmias that usually do not require drug therapy include premature atrial complexes (PACs), wandering atrial pacemaker, sinus arrhythmia, and sinus tachycardia. As an example, PACs rarely cause symptoms and never cause hemodynamic compromise, and therefore drug therapy is usually not indicated. Likewise, sinus tachycardia is usually the result of underlying metabolic or hemodynamic disorders (such as infection, dehydration, hypotension) and therapy should be directed at the underlying cause not the tachycardia per se. Of course, there are exceptions to these suggestions. For example, sinus tachycardia may be deleterious in patients after cardiac surgery or myocardial infarction, or with an unusual rhythm termed nonparoxysmal sinus tachycardia, so that antiarrhythmic drugs may be indicated. Stated in another way, although many arrhythmias generally do not require therapy, clinical judgment and patient-specific variables play an important role in this decision. Nevertheless, for the purpose of this discussion, only the tachycardias usually requiring antiarrhythmic drug therapy as listed above will be addressed.

Supraventricular tachycardias may cause a variety of symptoms. Some patients may be totally asymptomatic or complain of only minor palpitations or irregular pulse. In contrast, severe and even life-threatening symptoms can sometimes result. Patients may experience dizziness or acute syncopal episodes associated with the onset of their tachycardia, because of an abrupt drop in cardiac output, blood pressure, and cerebral perfusion. This drop in forward cardiac output occurs owing to the rapid ventricular rate with resultant poor ventricular filling and asynchronous atrioventricular contraction. Heart failure symptoms may also occur and patients tolerate the tachycardia particularly poorly if preexisting left ventricular dysfunction is present. Furthermore, patients may experience anginal chest pain if underlying coronary obstruction is present, owing to altered coronary perfusion (low cardiac output) and elevated myocardial oxygen demand (rapid heart rate). More often, patients complain of a choking or pressure sensation during the tachycardia episode, which can be confused with angina pectoris. It also should be noted that symptoms such as palpitations and even syncope correlate rather poorly with documented recurrences of the tachycardia.

ATRIAL FIBRILLATION AND ATRIAL FLUTTER

Atrial fibrillation and atrial flutter are common supraventricular tachycardias. These tachycardias occur more often in men and those who are elderly. The overall incidence of atrial fibrillation is about 1% to 2% (independent of gender and age) and this approximately doubles in elderly men.[5] These arrhythmias may present as a chronic, established tachycardia; an acute tachycardia; or a self-terminating, paroxysmal form. Atrial fibrillation is characterized as an extremely rapid (400 to 600 atrial bpm) and disorganized atrial activation. With this disorganized atrial activity, there is a loss of the contribution of atrial contraction (atrial kick) to forward cardiac output. Supraventricular impulses penetrate the AV conduction system in variable degrees, resulting in an irregular activation of the ventricles and an irregularly irregular pulse. The AV junction will not conduct most of the supraventricular impulses, thus causing ventricular response to be considerably slower (120 to 180 bpm) than the atrial rate. Atrial flutter occurs less frequently than atrial fibrillation, but is similar in its precipitating factors, consequences, and drug therapy approach (exceptions noted below). This arrhythmia is characterized by rapid (270 to 330 atrial bpm) but regular atrial activation. The slower and regular electrical activity results in a regular ventricular response and pulse that is in approximate multiples of 300 bpm (i.e., 1:1 AV conduction = ventricular rate 300 bpm; 2:1 AV conduction = ventricular rate 150 bpm; 3:1 AV conduction = ventricular rate 100 bpm). Atrial flutter may occur in two distinct forms (type I and type II). Type I flutter is the more common classic form with atrial rates of approximately 300 bpm and the typical "saw tooth" pattern of atrial activation as shown by the surface electrocardiogram. Type II flutter tends to be faster, being somewhat of a hybrid between classic atrial flutter and atrial fibrillation. Although the ventricular response usually has a regular pattern, atrial flutter with varying degrees of AV block or that occur with episodes of atrial fibrillation ("fib-flutter") can cause an irregular ventricular rate and pulse.

It is generally accepted that the predominant mechanism of atrial fibrillation and atrial flutter is reentry. Atrial fibrillation appears to result from multiple atrial reentrant loops (or wavelets) and atrial flutter is due to a single, dominant reentrant substrate. Atrial fibrillation or flutter usually occurs in association with forms of organic heart disease that causes atrial distention. Forms of heart disease that commonly lead to atrial stretch and precipitate atrial fibrillation or flutter include ischemia or infarction, hypertensive heart disease, valvular disorders such as mitral stenosis, mitral insufficiency, congenital abnormalities such as septal defects, and primary myocardial disease such as dilated or hypertrophic cardiomyopathy. Disorders that cause right atrial stretch and are associated with atrial fibrillation or flutter include acute pulmonary embolus and chronic lung disease resulting in pulmonary hypertension and cor pulmonale. These arrhythmias may also occur in association with states of high adrenergic tone such as thyrotoxicosis, alcohol withdrawal, sepsis, or excessive physical exertion. Established or paroxysmal atrial fibrillation occurring without identifiable heart disease or known precipitating factors is termed "lone" atrial fibrillation. Other states in which patients are predisposed to episodes of atrial fibrillation are the presence of an anomalous AV pathway (Kent bundle) and sinus node dysfunction (tachy-brady or sick sinus syndrome).

Patients with atrial fibrillation or flutter may experience the entire range of symptoms associated with other supraventricular tachycardias, although syncope as a presenting symptom is uncommon. Since atrial kick is lost with the onset of atrial fibrillation, severe low output states may result in forms of heart disease that rely heavily on atrial contraction to maintain cardiac output (such as mitral stenosis or hypertrophic obstructive cardiomyopathy; see Chap. 15). An additional complication of atrial fibrillation is arterial embolization resulting from atrial stasis and poorly adherent mural thrombi. Of course, the most devastating complication in this regard is the occurrence of an embolic stroke. The overall incidence of stroke in patients with atrial fibrillation not receiving antithrombotic therapy is about 3% to 6%.[6,7] Patients with concurrent mitral stenosis or severe systolic heart failure and atrial fibrillation are at particularly high risk for cerebral embolism. Other risk factors for stroke identified from recent trials are increasing age, history of hypertension, previous transient ischemic event or stroke, and diabetes.[6] Stroke can precede the onset of documented atrial fibrillation, probably due to undetected paroxysms prior to the onset of established atrial fibrillation. In contrast, patients with atrial fibrillation in whom precipitating factors cannot be identified (e.g., lone atrial fibrillation) and those with only atrial flutter have a low risk of embolic stroke.[7]

▶ TREATMENT: Atrial Fibrillation and Atrial Flutter

The ultimate treatment goals of atrial fibrillation or flutter are the restoration of sinus rhythm, the prevention of thromboembolic complications, and the prevention of further recurrences (Fig. 14–6). However, the methods by which to attain these goals vary depending on the patient's symptom severity. First, consider the patient with new onset atrial fibrillation or flutter. If presenting symptoms are severe (see above), patients may require direct-current cardioversion (DCC) in an attempt to immediately restore sinus rhythm. Atrial flutter often requires relatively low energy levels of countershock (25 to 50 W/s), whereas atrial fibrillation often requires higher energy levels (greater than 200 W/s). On the other hand, if tolerable symptoms are present, no such emergency measures are necessary. Type Ia and III antiarrhythmic agents may restore sinus rhythm but should not be administered initially. These agents may paradoxically increase ventricular response in the absence of drugs that slow AV nodal conduction. Traditionally, this observation has been attributed to the vagolytic action of these drugs, despite the fact that only disopyramide displays major anticholinergic side effects. Therefore, a more likely alternative explanation exists: All these agents slow atrial conduction, decreasing the number of impulses reaching the AV node, and as a result, the AV node paradoxically allows more impulses to gain entrance to the ventricular conduction system (increasing ventricular rate). Because of this phenomenon and the lack of need for immediate restoration of sinus rhythm, drugs that slow conduction and increase refractoriness in the AV node should be used as initial therapy. Traditionally, loading dosages of digoxin have been used owing to time-proven effectiveness and the high incidence of concurrent heart failure. However, digoxin's place in therapy has been questioned in both the acute and chronic setting.[8,9] Digoxin is sometimes ineffective and often slow in onset; although an initial decrease in ventricular response can sometimes be observed within 1 hour of intravenous administration, full control (heart rate less than 100 bpm) is usually not achieved for 24 to 48 hours. Digoxin will not restore sinus rhythm, although spontaneous termination of atrial fibrillation

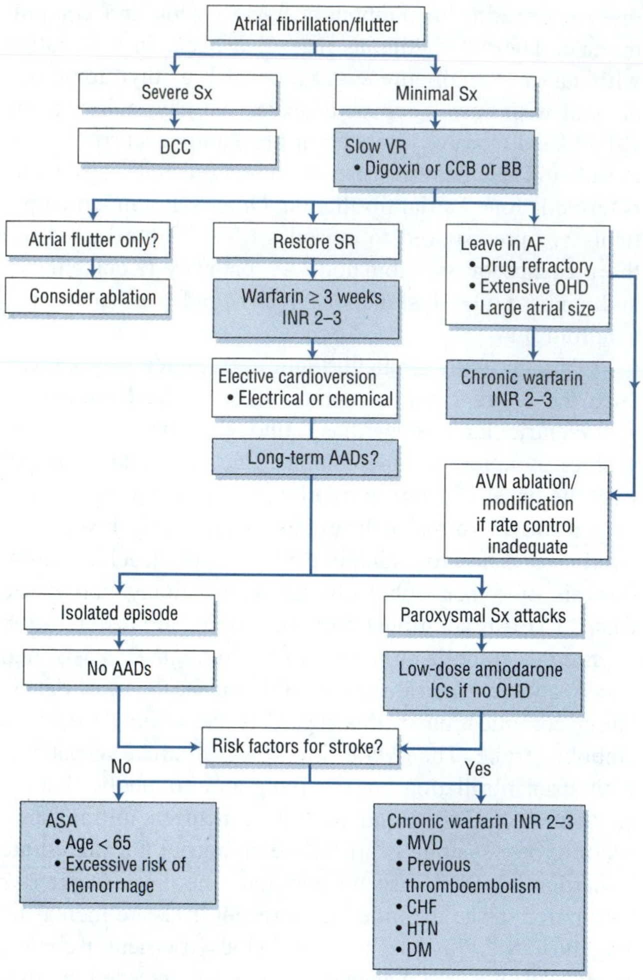

FIGURE 14–6. Algorithm for the treatment of atrial fibrillation and atrial flutter. Sx = symptoms; AVN = AV node; DCC = direct-current cardioversion; CCB = calcium channel antagonist (verapamil or diltiazem); BB = β-blocker; ASA = aspirin; OHD = organic heart disease; AADs = antiarrhythmic drugs; INR = International Normalized Ratio; MVD = mitral valve disease; CHF = congestive heart failure; HTN = hypertension; DM = diabetes mellitus.

may occur in some patients during the loading procedure. As mentioned previously, patients can present at two ends of the spectrum (either severely symptomatic or with no or mild symptoms) and often they present somewhere in between. Consequently, clinical judgment is necessary in choosing the proper treatment strategy. For example, intravenous calcium antagonists (diltiazem or verapamil) provide an alternative approach, allowing for a rapid decrease in ventricular rate and symptomatic relief without the need for DCC.[10,11] Because control of ventricular response can be transient, verapamil or diltiazem can be given as an initial intravenous bolus followed by a continuous infusion titrated to heart rate. Although digoxin has in the past been considered the drug of first choice to slow ventricular rate, many now choose calcium antagonists in most patients with atrial fibrillation or flutter. Further, atrial fibrillation or flutter precipitated by states of high adrenergic tone, such as thyrotoxicosis, is often resistant to digoxin therapy (digoxin slows AV nodal conduction primarily through vagotonic mechanisms). In these cases, intravenous β-blockers (propranolol, esmolol) can be highly effective and should be consider first.

Patients may present with a slow ventricular response (in the absence of AV nodal-blocking drugs) and thus do not require therapy with digoxin, verapamil, or esmolol. This type of presentation should alert the clinician to the possibility of preexisting SA or AV nodal conduction disease such as sick sinus syndrome. DCC should not be attempted in these patients without a temporary pacemaker in place (see later).

After treatment with AV nodal-blocking agents and a subsequent decrease in ventricular response, the patient should be evaluated for the possibility of restoring sinus rhythm. Within the context of this evaluation several factors should be considered. First, maintenance of sinus rhythm for a significant length of time is usually not feasible in patients, with a history of chronic (more than 1 year) established atrial fibrillation or with large atrial size (greater than 45 mm determined by echocardiography). Therefore, cardioversion may not be attempted and these patients can remain in atrial fibrillation, chronically treated with AV nodal-blocking agents to control ventricular response (resting rate ≈ 80 bpm). Often, long-term therapy with digoxin alone for this purpose will not control exercise-related increases in ventricular response and tachycardia symptoms. In these patients small doses of calcium antagonists or β-blockers can be added; the need for these ancillary agents can be readily evaluated by treadmill exercise testing or by simple ambulation. Occasionally, patients may be encountered who are highly refractory to AV nodal blocking agents (including combination drug therapy) and ventricular response remains rapid. Aggressive attempts to lower rate are necessary; chronic tachycardias can result in a progressive decline in left ventricular function, causing a tachycardia-induced cardiomyopathy. Hence, in drug-refractory patients, ablation modification of the AV node by a transvenous catheter delivering radiofrequency current is indicated.[12] This procedure blocks conduction from the atrium to the ventricle and may require the concurrent implantation of a permanent pacemaker with a ventricular lead.

The second consideration is that restoration of sinus rhythm itself (by pharmacologic or electrical means) is associated with an increased risk of thromboembolism. The return of sinus rhythm restores an effective contraction, which may dislodge poorly adherent thrombi. Anticoagulation prior to cardioversion prevents clot growth and the formation of new thrombi and allows those present to become organized and well adherent to the atrial wall. This form of preventive therapy has been shown to prevent stroke associated with cardioversion, but several weeks of anticoagulation is necessary. Therefore, current recommendations are to institute warfarin treatment (INR 2.0 to 3.0) for at least 3 weeks prior to cardioversion; the common clinical scenario is to discharge the patient from the hospital, monitor him or her on an ambulatory basis, and readmit for elective cardioversion after this time period.[7] After restoration of sinus rhythm, full atrial contraction does not occur immediately. Rather it returns gradually to a maximum contractible force over a 3-week period. Therefore, warfarin should be continued for about 1 month after effective cardioversion. There are several exceptions to this recommended process of anticoagulation. Because the risk of thromboembolism appears lower in general, some clinicians do not routinely anticoagulate patients with only atrial flutter (unless concurrent risks for thrombosis are present, e.g., severe left ventricular dysfunction or mitral valve disease) or lone atrial fibrillation. Also, in patients with atrial fibrillation of less than 48 hours' duration, anticoagulation prior to cardioversion is probably not necessary because there has not been sufficient time to form atrial thrombi. However, in most presentations of atrial fibrillation, the exact time of onset is unclear. Transesophageal echocardiography (TEE) is being investigated as a tool to stratify which patients may require anticoagulation prior to DCC from those who may not. If an atrial thrombus or severe stasis is not noted on TEE, then perhaps these patients can be cardioverted without the mandatory 3 weeks of warfarin pretreatment. However, conclusive data have not been published and some believe that DCC itself promotes thrombogenesis, necessitating anticoagulation anyway.

After prior anticoagulation, the methods available to restore sinus rhythm can be considered. There are two methods of restoring sinus rhythm in patients with atrial fibrillation or flutter: pharmacologic cardioversion and DCC. Which of these is the method of choice is a matter of clinical preference. With pharmacologic cardioversion, antiarrhythmic drugs such as quinidine, procainamide, flecainide, propafenone, sotalol, or ibutilide can be used. The time-honored method is to begin oral quinidine therapy; maintenance dosages are sufficient and oral loading schedules are unnecessary. In some centers, intravenous amiodarone has been used to terminate atrial fibrillation or atrial flutter. This practice should be discouraged because it is extremely expensive and has recently been shown to be of limited effectiveness.[13] Rather, intravenous procainamide, oral flecainide, propafenone, sotalol, and more recently ibutilide are all effective and suitable alternatives to quinidine. Oral loading doses of the type Ic antiarrhythmic (e.g., propafenone 600 mg as a single dose) have demonstrated effectiveness compared to placebo and provide a simple and increasingly popular regimen.[14] The newest alternative is intravenous ibutilide, which was approved for rapid conversion of new-onset atrial fibrillation and flutter late in 1995. Ibutilide appears to be more effective for atrial flutter than atrial fibrillation. Comparative trials have shown it to be somewhat more effective than sotalol and procainamide albeit with a significant risk of proarrhythmia in the form of torsades de pointes.[15,16] If after a short-term trial of antiarrhythmic drugs, atrial fibrillation or flutter persists, DCC can be used. The advantages of choosing the drug therapy approach first are that an effective agent may be determined in case long-term therapy is required and many feel there is little to lose with a short trial. The disadvantages of pharmacologic cardioversion are the risk of significant side effects such as drug-induced torsades de pointes,[17] the inconvenience of drug– drug interactions (e.g., digoxin–quinidine), and the fact that drugs are generally less effective when compared to DCC. The advantages of DCC are that it is quick and more often successful. The disadvantages of DCC are the need for prior sedation/anesthesia and a risk (albeit small) of serious complications such as sinus arrest or ventricular arrhythmias. Contrary to past beliefs, DCC carries very little risk in patients receiving digoxin without evidence of digitalis toxicity.

After sinus rhythm is successfully restored, what chronic medications should the patient receive? In many cases, maintenance digoxin therapy is continued simply because of underlying ventricular dysfunction. This common practice has been questioned; digoxin may occasionally be profibrillatory.[8] There are two other forms of therapy that the clinician must consider in each patient: long-term antithrombotic therapy to prevent stroke, and long-term antiarrhythmic drugs to prevent recurrences of atrial fibrillation. Consider the issue of antithrombotic therapy first. In the past, patients with atrial fibrillation were not routinely anticoagulated (unless there was a history of stroke or concurrent mitral valve disease) because it was felt that the risk of warfarin exceeded its potential (though unknown) benefit. In the past several years, five major randomized, placebo-controlled trials designed to evaluate this issue have been published. Four of these trials were primary prevention studies and the remaining one was secondary prevention (patients had a stroke prior to enrollment).[7] All possess very similar findings and all were terminated prematurely because of a significant effect in the treatment group (warfarin). Perhaps the best known of these trials was the Stroke Prevention in Atrial Fibrillation (SPAF) Study.[18] This study, like the other four, found warfarin to significantly reduce the incidence of stroke in patients with atrial fibrillation (not associated with prior thromboembolic episodes or mitral valve disease) with an acceptable risk of bleeding complications. In all, these studies culminated in the American College of Chest Physicians Consensus Conference[7] on antithrombotic therapy strongly recommending the following: that all patients with atrial fibrillation should receive chronic warfarin treatment (INR 2.0 to 3.0). Exceptions may include young (< 60 years) patients with "lone" atrial fibrillation, those with only atrial flutter, and unreliable/poorly compliant patients. In lieu of warfarin, these latter patients may receive daily aspirin. Indeed the use of aspirin (versus warfarin) is one of remaining controversies. The original SPAF study (SPAF I) found aspirin (325 mg/d) to be effective in preventing stroke but could not directly compare it to warfarin because of sample size and study design. The debate over aspirin use for this indication was complicated by the second SPAF trial (SPAF II).[19] In this study, warfarin tended to be more effective than aspirin (though not statistically different) but it was also associated with a higher risk of intracranial hemorrhage, particularly in elderly patients. Young patients (< 75years) had an extremely low incidence of stroke if risk factors (hypertension, heart failure, and/or prior thromboembolism) were absent. Subsequently, investigators from all five major trials pooled their findings and analyzed the results.[6] Although only two of the trials had an aspirin arm, warfarin was more effective and consistent in reducing the risk of stroke. Pharmacoeconomic analyses tend to support the use of aspirin only in those patients with atrial fibrillation without risk factors for stroke.[20] Warfarin is more cost-effective in those patients at risk for the complications of recurrent atrial fibrillation. Therefore, at this time, most patients (exceptions noted above) with atrial fibrillation and a risk factor for stroke should receive chronic warfarin treatment. Aspirin should generally be considered second-line treatment and for those without risk factors for thromboembolic complications.

The second form of chronic therapy to be considered is antiarrhythmic drugs to prevent recurrences of atrial fibrillation. With some exceptions (thyrotoxicosis, postoperative situations) atrial fibrillation usually recurs after initial cardioversion because most patients have irreversible, underlying heart disease. Historically, many clinicians would prescribe oral antiarrhythmic drugs (usually quinidine) to prevent these recurrences despite the fact that only small studies with conflicting results existed evaluating this approach. To evaluate the efficacy of quinidine in preventing atrial fibrillation, a meta-analysis of the existing literature was completed.[21] This meta-analysis demonstrated that indeed more patients remain in sinus rhythm with quinidine therapy (compared to placebo), although about 50% have recurrences of atrial fibrillation within a year despite quinidine. However, this reported effectiveness was at the cost of an associated increase in mortality (presumably due, in part, to proarrhythmia) in the quinidine-treated patients. These disturbing results (published soon after the CAST[22]) became widely quoted and highly visible, making clinicians question the wisdom of long-term prevention of recurrences of atrial fibrillation with antiarrhythmic drugs. Although the results were questioned because some of the reported causes of death in the treated patients could not be directly attributed to quinidine, a subanalysis of the SPAF Study[23] tended to support the findings of the meta-analysis.

It is possible that the newer antiarrhythmic agents such as the type Ic and the type III agents may provide alternatives to quinidine. Flecainide and propafenone tend to be better tolerated than the type Ia agents and have been shown to be highly effective in the termination and prevention of atrial fibrillation. However, the major fear with the type Ic agents is the risk of ventricular proarrhythmia. The CAST[22] and other studies demonstrate that patients being treated for ventricular arrhythmias with coexisting ischemic heart disease and poor left ventricular function are at increased risk of proarrhythmia. Patients with atrial fibrillation often possess these risks. Recent data regarding antiarrhythmic drug prescribing trends[24] show a large increase in the use of the type III agents (sotalol and amiodarone). Studies[25] indicate that low doses of amiodarone (100 to 200 mg/d) are highly effective in preventing the recurrence of atrial fibrillation, perhaps at a lower risk of serious toxicity than that associated with higher doses (400 mg/d). Another alternative, sotalol, has been shown to be at least as effective as quinidine in preventing recurrences of atrial fibrillation.[26] However, treatment with either quinidine or sotalol is associated with a similar incidence of torsades de pointes. Since this form of proarrhythmia primarily occurs with higher doses of sotalol (compared to the non-dose-related torsades de pointes caused by quinidine), it may be more easily predicted and therefore avoided. Nonetheless, sotalol may, similar to quinidine, increase mortality in patients with atrial fibrillation, and this requires further study.[27]

At this time and in view of newer studies implying increased mortality due to the time-honored approach of prescribing long-term quinidine and other agents, we suggest the following approach. Reserve chronic antiarrhythmic drugs for only those patients with documented symptomatic recurrences or symptomatic paroxysmal atrial fibrillation. Those with an isolated episode should not receive chronic preventive therapy. In terms of drug choice, we feel that low-dose amiodarone should be given preference as the agent of first choice. After appropriate oral loading doses, patients should receive 200 mg/d on a chronic basis. If this dose has successfully prevented recurrences, attempt to reduce it to 100 mg/d, although more data are required on this practice. Although the methods of oral amiodarone loading vary considerable, we use 800 mg/d for 1 week followed by 400 mg/d for 1 month before initiation of the 200 mg/d maintenance dose. The reader should also note that current studies are underway to compare the use of long-term antiarrhythmic drugs to prevent atrial fibrillation/flutter and the use of drugs that simply control ventricular rate (e.g., digoxin and/or calcium antagonists) with mortality as the primary end point. These studies should more clearly define the long-term approach to these arrhythmias. One such study (AFFIRM, Atrial Fibrillation Follow-up Investigation of Rhythm Management) began in 1996 and will randomize patients to an arm with strategies to control ventricular response (e.g., AV nodal-blocking drugs) or an arm with strategies to maintain sinus rhythm (e.g., antiarrhythmic drugs). It is possible that, in the future, most patients can be managed by strategies to control only rate (drugs, AV nodal ablation) without chronic antiarrhythmic drug therapy. Also, investigational methods using catheter ablation to create a series of linear lesions in the atria are being studied in patients with recurrent atrial fibrillation. There is one important exception to the scenario outlined above for patients with only the common form (type I) of atrial flutter. In these individuals, ablation with radiofrequency current is rapidly becoming an attractive treatment alternative and should be strongly considered. In one series, ablation was 80% successful in preventing recurrences of atrial flutter.[28]

PAROXYSMAL SUPRAVENTRICULAR TACHYCARDIA CAUSED BY REENTRY

Paroxysmal supraventricular tachycardia (PSVT) arising by reentrant mechanisms includes those arrhythmias caused by AV nodal reentry, AV reentry incorporating an anomalous AV pathway, SA nodal reentry, and intraatrial reentry. AV nodal reentry and AV reentry are by far the most common of these tachycardias.

The underlying substrate of AV nodal reentry is the functional division of the AV node into two (or more) longitudinal conduction pathways or "dual" AV nodal pathways.[29] Although there is some disagreement, most electrophysiologists now believe that there are not two distinct, anatomic pathways inside the AV node itself. Rather, it is likely that a fan-like network of perinodal fibers insert into the AV node and represents the second pathway. The two pathways possess key differences in conduction characteristics: one is a fast conducting pathway with a relatively long refractory period (fast pathway) and the other is a slower conducting pathway with a shorter refractory period (slow pathway). The presence of dual pathways does not necessarily imply that the patient will have clinical PSVT. In fact, it is estimated that between 10% and nearly 50% of patients have discernible dual pathways, but the incidence of PSVT is considerably lower.[29] Sustenance of the tachycardia depends on the critical electrophysiologic discrepancies and the ability of one pathway (usually the slow) to allow repetitive antegrade conduction and the ability of the other pathway (usually the fast) to allow repetitive retrograde conduction. During sinus rhythm, a patient with dual pathways conducts supraventricular impulses antegradely through both pathways. Electrical activity reaches the distal common pathway at the level of or above the His bundle and continues to depolarize the ventricles in an antegrade direction. Conduction proceeds via the two pathways but reaches the distal common pathway first through the fast AV nodal route (Fig. 14–7). For this reason, a short PR interval is sometimes observed during sinus rhythm.

PSVT caused by AV nodal reentry may occur by the following sequence of events. The occurrence of an appropriately timed premature impulse penetrates the AV node, but is blocked in the fast pathway, which is still refractory from the previous beat. However, the slow pathway, which has a shorter refractory period, permits antegrade conduction of the premature impulse. By the time the impulse has reached the distal common pathway, the fast pathway has recovered its excitability and now will permit retrograde conduction. The impulse reaches the common proximal pathway, preceded by an excitable gap of tissue, and reenters the slow pathway. A reentrant circuit that does not require atrial or ventricular tissue is completed within (or nearly so) the AV node, and a tachycardia is thereby initiated (Fig. 14–7). The common form of this tachycardia uses the slow pathway for antegrade conduction and the fast pathway for retrograde conduction. Lown–Ganong–Levine

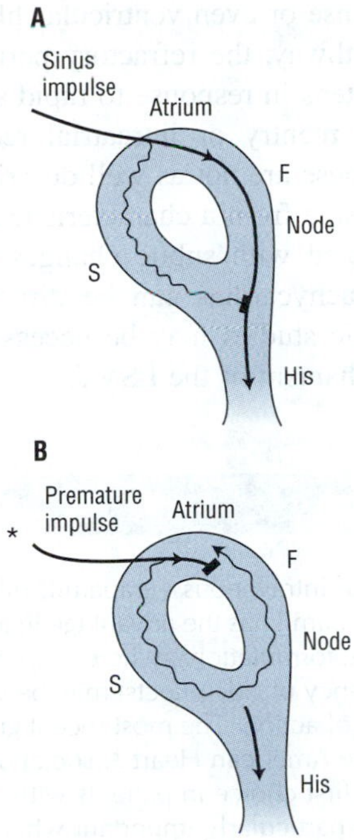

FIGURE 14–7. Reentry mechanism of dual AV nodal pathway PSVT. **(A)** Sinus rhythm: the impulse travels from the atrium through the fast pathway (F) and then to the His–Purkinje system. The impulse also travels through the slow pathway (S) but is stopped when refractory tissue is encountered. **(B)** Dual AV nodal reentry: a critically timed premature impulse (*) is stopped in the fast pathway (because of prolonged refractoriness) but is able to travel antegrade down the slow pathway and retrograde through the fast pathway.

syndrome (LGL) is defined by paroxysms of a narrow QRS tachycardia associated with a short PR interval on surface electrocardiograms (during sinus rhythm) and is commonly caused by AV nodal reentry.

AV reentrant tachycardia depends on the presence of an anomalous, or accessory, extranodal pathway that bypasses the normal AV conduction pathway. Several different types of accessory pathways have been described, depending on the specific anatomic areas they connect (atrioventricular bundles or nodoventricular tracts); some are also referred to by eponyms, such as the Kent bundle. A Kent bundle is an extranodal AV connection that is associated with the Wolff–Parkinson–White syndrome (WPW). During sinus rhythm (Fig. 14–8) patients with WPW depolarize the ventricles simultaneously through both AV pathways (AV nodal pathway and the Kent bundle), creating a fusion pattern on the early portion of the QRS complex (δ wave). The degree of ventricular "preexcitation" depends on the contribution of antegrade ventricular activation through the accessory pathway. Patients may have an accessory pathway that is not evident on surface electrocardiograms or a "concealed" Kent bundle. These concealed accessory pathways are often incapable of antegrade conduction and can accept electrical stimulation in only a retrograde fashion. The electrocardiographic expression of preexcitation (Δ wave) depends on the location of the accessory pathway, the distance from the wavefront of sinus activation, and the conduction characteristics of the various structures involved. It should be noted that (similar to patients with dual AV nodal pathways) not all patients with preexcitation owing to an accessory AV pathway are capable of having clinical PSVT.

Patients with an accessory AV pathway may have three forms of supraventricular tachycardia: orthodromic reentry, antidromic reentry, and/or atrial fibrillation or flutter. AV reentrant PSVT usually occurs by the following sequence of events. Analogous to AV nodal reentry, two pathways (the normal AV nodal pathway and the accessory AV pathway) exist that have different electrophysiologic characteristics. The AV nodal pathway usually has a relatively slower conduction velocity and shorter refractory period and the accessory pathway has a faster conduction velocity and a longer refractory period. A critically timed premature impulse may block in the accessory pathway because it is still refractory from the previous sinus beat. However, the AV nodal pathway with a relatively shorter refractory period may accept antegrade conduction of the premature impulse. Meanwhile, the accessory pathway may recover its excitability and now allow retrograde conduction. A macroreentrant tachycardia is thereby initiated in which the antegrade pathway is the AV nodal pathway; the distal common pathway is the ventricle; the retrograde pathway is the accessory pathway; and the proximal common pathway is the atrium (Fig. 14–8). This sequence of events (down node, up Kent), termed orthodromic PSVT, is the common variety of reentry in patients with an accessory AV pathway,

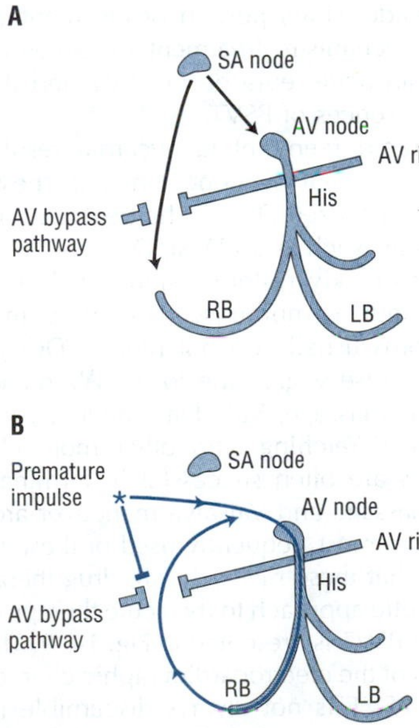

FIGURE 14–8. Reentry mechanism for AV accessory pathway PSVT in Wolff–Parkinson–White syndrome. **(A)** Sinus rhythm: the impulse travels from the atrium to the ventricle by two pathways—the AV node and an accessory bypass pathway. **(B)** AV reentry: a critically timed premature impulse (*) is stopped in the Kent bundle (because of prolonged refractoriness) but travels antegrade through the AV node and retrograde through the Kent bundle.

resulting a narrow QRS tachycardia. In the uncommon variety (down Kent, up node), conduction proceeds in the opposite direction, resulting in a wide QRS tachycardia, termed antidromic PSVT. Patients with WPW can have a third type of tachycardia, namely atrial fibrillation. The mechanism for its occurrence is unknown, but the occurrence of this arrhythmia can be very serious and sudden death is well described. Because atrial fibrillation is an extremely rapid atrial tachycardia, conduction can proceed down the accessory AV pathway, resulting in a very fast ventricular response or even ventricular fibrillation. Unlike the AV nodal pathway, the refractory period of the accessory bundle shortens in response to rapid stimulation rates.

Sinus node reentry or intraatrial reentry occur less commonly and these are not as well described as AV nodal or AV reentry. Aside from a characteristic abrupt onset and termination coupled with subtle changes in P-wave morphology, these tachycardias can be difficult to diagnose. Electrophysiologic studies may be necessary to determine the ultimate mechanism of the PSVT.

▶ TREATMENT: Paroxysmal Supraventricular Tachycardia

Both pharmacologic and nonpharmacologic methods have been used to treat patients with PSVT. Drugs used in the treatment of PSVT can be divided into three broad categories: (1) those that directly or indirectly increase vagal tone to the AV node such as edrophonium, vasopressors, and digoxin; (2) those that depress conduction through slow, calcium-dependent tissue such as adenosine, β-blockers, and calcium channel blockers; and (3) those that depress conduction through fast, sodium-dependent tissue such as quinidine, procainamide, disopyramide, and flecainide. Drugs within these categories alter the electrophysiologic characteristics of the reentrant substrate so that PSVT cannot be sustained.[30,31] In PSVT caused by AV nodal reentry, type I antiarrhythmic drugs such as procainamide act primarily on the retrograde fast pathway. Digoxin and propranolol may work on either the retrograde fast or the antegrade slow limb. Verapamil, diltiazem, and adenosine prolong conduction time and increase refractoriness primarily in the slow antegrade pathway of the reentrant loop. In PSVT due to AV reentry incorporating an extranodal pathway, type I drugs increase refractoriness in the fast accessory pathway or within the His–Purkinje system. Propranolol, digoxin, adenosine, and verapamil all act by their effects on the AV nodal (antegrade, slow) portion of the reentrant circuit. Regardless of the mechanism, treatment measures are directed at first terminating an acute episode of PSVT and then preventing symptomatic recurrences of PSVT.

As in any rapid reentrant tachycardia resulting in severe symptoms (syncope, near syncope, anginal chest pain, severe heart failure), synchronized DCC is the treatment of choice. Even at low energy levels (such as 25 W/s), DCC for PSVT is almost always effective in quickly restoring sinus rhythm and correcting severe hemodynamic compromise. Patients with only mild to moderate symptoms usually do not require DCC, and nondrug measures that increase vagal tone to the AV node can be used first. Carotid sinus massage, Valsalva maneuver, ice water facial immersion, induced retching, and other more elaborate vagomimetic measures are often successful in terminating PSVT, although carotid massage and Valsalva maneuver are the simplest, least obtrusive, and most frequently used of these techniques.

In the event that these methods fail, drug therapy is the next option. A therapeutic approach to the acute therapy of the different forms of reentrant PSVT is presented in Fig. 14–9. This approach is based on analysis of the electrocardiographic characteristics of the rhythm because PSVT is not always discernible from other arrhythmias, and some forms of PSVT require different treatment. In patients with a narrow QRS, regular arrhythmia (AV nodal reentry or orthodromic AV reentry), intravenous verapamil (5 to 10 mg), intravenous diltiazem (15 to 25 mg), or adenosine (6 to 12 mg) are all equally efficacious; any may be chosen as agents of first choice. About 80% to 90% of PSVT episodes will revert to sinus rhythm within 5 minutes of intravenous verapamil, diltiazem, or adenosine therapy.[32] Verapamil has the advantage in terms of cost, being available in generic formulations, whereas adenosine (although it has a higher frequency of side effects) may be safer because of its ultrashort duration of action. The most recent guidelines for emergency care from the American Heart Association promote adenosine as the drug of first choice in patients with PSVT.[33] These recommendations are particularly important when treating a patient who presents with a wide QRS, regular tachycardia that may be ventricular tachycardia (VT), or PSVT (antidromic AV reentry or owing to aberrancy). Because of its short duration of action (seconds), adenosine will not cause the severe and prolonged hemodynamic compromise seen in patients with VT who are mistakenly treated with verapamil and suffer from its negative inotropic effects and vasodilator properties.[34] If in fact the arrhythmia is PSVT, adenosine will likely terminate it. An alternative treatment for this type of patient is intravenous procainamide, which works on the fast, sodium-dependent extranodal pathway as well as for VT. Likewise, intravenous procainamide should be used for the patient who presents with a wide-QRS, irregular arrhythmia. This rhythm could represent atrial fibrillation with ventricular activation through an extranodal pathway. Administration of intravenous verapamil or adenosine to these patients could result in a paradoxical increase in ventricular response causing severe symptoms, requiring cardioversion. These agents (particularly long-acting AV nodal-blockers such as verapamil, diltiazem, and digoxin) are to be considered contraindicated in this specific setting.

Once the acute episode of PSVT is terminated, a decision on long-term preventive therapy must follow. Some patients may require long-term drug therapy; preventive treatment is indicated if (1) frequent episodes occur that necessitate therapeutic intervention (emergency room visits or interference with the patient's lifestyle), or (2) infrequent but severe symptoms occur. Also, effective vagal maneuvers can sometimes be taught to the patient, obviating the need for chronic drug therapy. For those patients in whom a preventive drug therapy regimen is deemed necessary, three traditional treatment strategies have been used. First, clinicians may use a trial-and-error approach on an ambulatory basis for those patients with frequently recurrent, mildly symptomatic PSVT. Ambulatory electrocardiographic recordings (Holter) or telephonic transmissions of cardiac rhythm (event monitors) can be used to objectively document the efficacy or failure of drug therapy. How should one choose empiric drug regimens? AV nodal-blockers such as digoxin, propranolol, or verapamil can be effective so that the clinician can try one of these agents first. However, maintenance digoxin or other AV nodal-blockers should be used with caution in patients with manifest preexcitation (delta wave on ECG during sinus rhythm). If atrial fibrillation occurs in such a patient, one consequence is ventricular fibrilla-

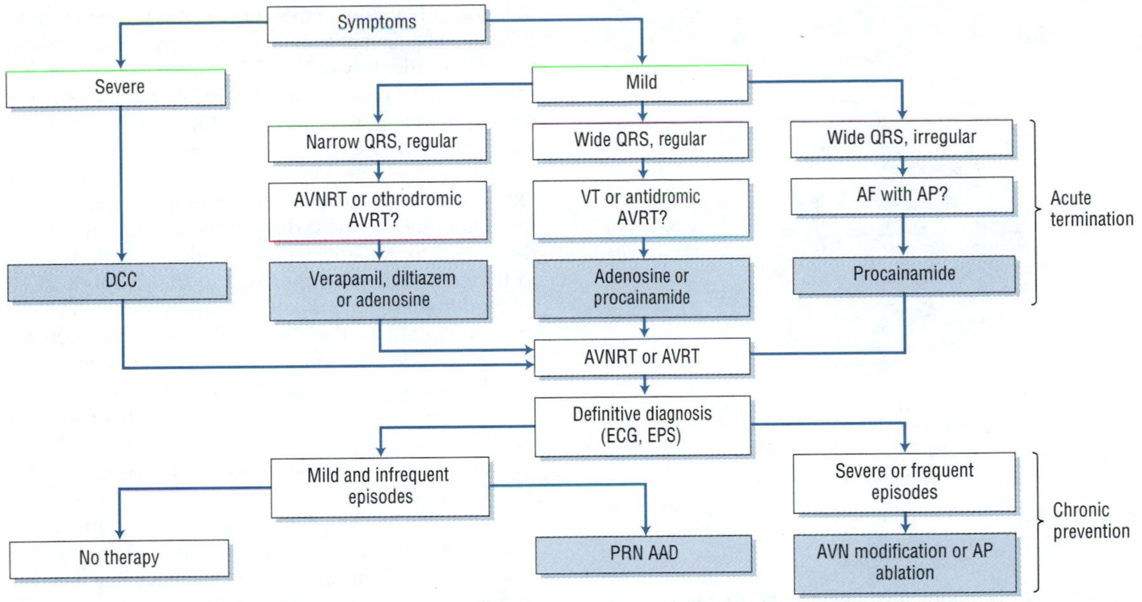

FIGURE 14–9. Algorithm for the treatment of acute (top portion) PSVT and chronic prevention of recurrences (bottom portion). DCC = direct current cardioversion; AVNRT = AV nodal reentrant tachycardia; VT = ventricular tachycardia; AF = atrial fibrillation; AP = accessory pathway; ECG = electrocardiographic monitoring; EPS = electrophysiologic studies; PRN = as needed, AAD = antiarrhythmic drugs. Note: for empiric bridge therapy prior to radiofrequency ablation procedures, calcium antagonists (or other AV nodal blockers) should not be used if the patient has AV reentry with an accessory pathway.

tion by rapid AV conduction through the accessory bundle. Digoxin is safest in patients with concealed Kent pathways or AVN reentry. Another strategy is to assume that the agent that was successful in terminating the acute episode of PSVT will also provide effective preventive therapy. However, chronic oral verapamil is often ineffective, even in those patients who responded to intravenous therapy. This is probably owing to significant pharmacodynamic and pharmacokinetic differences between the oral and intravenous dosage forms of verapamil coupled with stereoselective first-pass metabolism with the oral racemate.[35]

Bauernfeind and coworkers[36] studied the patterns of drug response in patients with AV reentrant tachycardia, which may help the clinician choose empiric therapy. These investigators found a significant concordance of responses between drugs that work on the slow antegrade limb (e.g., propranolol, digoxin), a concordance of drug responses for those agents that act on the fast retrograde limb (e.g., procainamide, quinidine), and a discordance of response between these two groups of drugs. In other words, if quinidine is effective it is likely that procainamide will also be effective but unlikely that propranolol or digoxin will be effective. These findings imply that there is a "weak link" in the reentrant pathway that is susceptible to drug therapy. The second method to find effective long-term therapy is to use the trial-and-error method during hospitalization. In this case, Holter monitoring or telemetry can be used to objectively assess drug efficacy or failure. Initially, all antiarrhythmics should be discontinued and attacks detected and quantified. Following this drug-free control period in which the frequency and characteristics of the tachycardia are defined, antiarrhythmic agents are administered in a serial fashion and evaluated for efficacy. It is crucial to determine drug efficacy (abolition of symptomatic PSVT) with consideration to the tachycardia frequency during the control period.

The trial-and-error methods for determining drug effectiveness have inherent shortcomings. If the PSVT episodes are infrequent, a considerable time period may be consumed before an effective regimen is realized. Also, if the patient has moderate to severe symptoms associated with PSVT, several troublesome episodes may be experienced by the patient before the correct agent(s) is identified. Therefore, serial testing of antiarrhythmic agents by invasive electrophysiologic techniques has been used to determine effective long-term therapy in those patients with sporadic and/or symptomatic PSVT. Basically, the patient's clinical tachycardia is replicated in the laboratory by inserting appropriately timed, premature extra stimuli via a transvenous right heart catheter. The patient is first studied off of antiarrhythmic therapy; induction of the tachycardia by premature stimuli by programmed stimulation serves as a control study. Then, over a period of several days specific drugs are administered in a serial fashion and tested for efficacy in preventing the induction of PSVT.[30,31]

Regardless of the method for choosing long-term therapy, chronic antiarrhythmic drug treatment in these often young, otherwise healthy patients is problematic. Besides the necessity of taking daily medication possibly for life, antiarrhythmic drugs are not well tolerated, sometimes precipitate severe side effects, and are commonly ineffective. For these reasons, non-drug therapies have been pioneered. One such procedure, namely transcutaneous catheter ablation using radiofrequency current on the PSVT substrate, has dramatically altered traditional treatment of these patients (Fig.14–10). Radiofrequency energy delivered through a transvenous or arterial catheter causes small, discrete lesions through thermal energy. During invasive electrophysiologic studies, portions of the reentrant circuit can be located (or "mapped") by the use of a number of catheters. Once this is completed, radiofrequency energy is applied to kill or damage the tissue necessary for reentry. In this way the substrate for reentry is destroyed, "curing" the patient of recurrent episodes of PSVT and obviating the need for chronic drug therapy. Historically, ablation procedures were reserved for drug-refractory patients because they

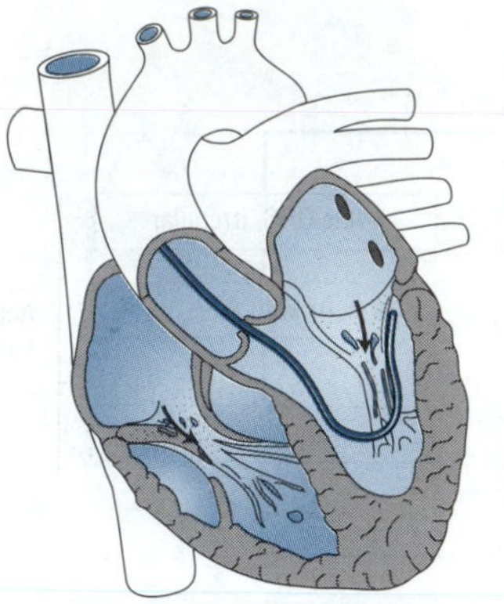

FIGURE 14–10. Drawing showing catheter placement for radiofrequency ablation of left free wall accessory pathway. Here, the retrograde arterial approach is taken although a venous (atrial) transseptal puncture has also been used.

necessitated open-heart surgery. However, breakthroughs in technology have allowed, first, transvenous catheter approaches and then, later, the use of radiofrequency (rather than direct current) energy. Complications, although unusual, include tamponade, pericarditis, valvular insufficiency, and AV block. Radiofrequency ablation is highly effective, preventing the recurrence of PSVT in 85% to 98% of patients.[37,38] The procedure was originally pioneered in patients with Wolff–Parkinson–White syndrome.[37] Here, the extranodal pathway is often located at the left lateral free wall of the left ventricle (Fig.14–10). After the pathway is located, the catheter is put as close to the site as possible and radiofrequency current applied to make small burns in the tissue. Ablation of the extranodal connection occurs promptly and evidence of preexcitation (delta waves) disappears. Later, a similar approach was developed for patients with AV nodal reentry placing the catheter in the coronary sinus, proximal to the AV node.[38] The preferred method in these individuals is to apply small amounts of radiofrequency current to the slow pathway of the reentrant circuit to modify its properties enough so that PSVT cannot recur.

Although radiofrequency catheter ablation is a relatively new technique, and long-term follow-up of potential late complications remains necessary, it has been suggested that *all* patients with symptomatic PSVT undergo the procedure.[39] This is because it is highly effective and curative, rarely resulting in complications and obviates the need for chronic antiarrhythmic drug therapy. In other words, no longer should radiofrequency ablation be reserved for only drug-refractory patients; it should be considered in *any* patient who would previously be considered for chronic antiarrhythmic drug treatment (effective or ineffective). Radiofrequency ablation is also a cost-effective approach (in the long term) because, if effective, it precludes the costs of drugs and repeated hospital visits.

AUTOMATIC ATRIAL TACHYCARDIAS

Automatic atrial tachycardias such as multifocal atrial tachycardia appear to arise from supraventricular foci that have enhanced automatic properties.[40] It is presumed that multifocal atrial tachycardia (sometimes referred to as chaotic atrial tachycardia) is the result of multiple ectopic atrial pacemakers, which account for the variable and differing P-wave morphology. In unifocal atrial tachycardia (sometimes referred to as ectopic atrial tachycardia), a single P-wave morphology different from that of sinus rhythm is recorded. In either case, the underlying, precipitating disorder present in the majority (60% to 80%) of these patients is severe pulmonary disease. Other disease states associated with these arrhythmias include acute infection (pneumonia and sepsis) and dilated congestive cardiomyopathy. It should be noted that young patients without associated precipitating factors may rarely present with rapid atrial tachycardias from unknown etiologies. In these cases, long-standing tachycardias *cause* a cardiomyopathic state. Effective treatment of the tachycardia may result in reversal of left ventricular dysfunction. Traditionally many factors (electrolyte disturbances, hypoxia, catecholamines, tissue stretch) may cause an elevated slope of phase 4 depolarization and theoretically result in abnormal heightened automaticity. Noteworthy is that many of these factors are often clinically present in patients with concurrent pulmonary disease and automatic atrial tachycardia. However, recent information implies that triggered activity is a more likely mechanism in the genesis of these tachycardias. Atrial tachycardias with AV block or a slow ventricular response should alert the clinician to the possibility of digitalis toxicity.

▶ TREATMENT: Automatic Atrial Tachycardia

The first step in the treatment of automatic atrial tachycardia is to correct the underlying, precipitating factors.[40] One should ensure proper oxygenation and ventilation and correct acid–base or electrolyte disturbances. These measures alone may result in the return of sinus rhythm, but in some cases, the tachycardia will persist. Patients with an asymptomatic atrial tachycardia and a relatively slow ventricular response usually require no drug therapy. In symptomatic patients, medical therapy can be tailored either to control ventricular response or to restore sinus rhythm. Type I antiarrhythmic drugs such as procainamide or quinidine are occasionally effective in restoring sinus rhythm, presumably by their ability to decrease the automatic properties of latent pacemakers, but these agents are usually not considered first-line therapy. Direct current cardioversion is usually ineffective in restoring sinus rhythm, and the use of programmed stimulation will not replicate the clinical tachycardia so that serial drug testing is of no value. β-Blockers, to slow ventricular response, are usually contraindicated because of the frequent coexistence of severe pulmonary disease or heart failure. Digoxin has been used but is controversial because of its ability to increase the automatic properties of atrial tissue, and the high sympathetic state of these patients frequently overrides the vagotonic effects of digoxin, rendering it ineffective. Calcium antagonists such as verapamil are most effective and may now be considered first-line drug therapy.[41] Surprisingly, verapamil seems to decrease ventricular response by altering atrial automaticity, not by slowing AV nodal conduction.[41] Recent information suggests that intravenous magnesium (independent of serum magnesium) can also be effective.[40] Both verapamil and parenteral magnesium probably act by suppressing calcium-mediated triggered activity.

VENTRICULAR ARRHYTHMIAS

The common ventricular arrhythmias include (1) ventricular premature beats (VPBs), (2) ventricular tachycardia (VT), and (3) ventricular fibrillation (VF). Again, these arrhythmias may result in a wide variety of symptoms. VPBs often cause no symptoms or only mild palpitations. VT may be a life-threatening situation associated with hemodynamic collapse or be totally asymptomatic. VF, by definition, is an acute medical emergency necessitating cardiopulmonary resuscitation.

VENTRICULAR PREMATURE BEATS

VPBs are very common ventricular rhythm disturbances that occur in patients with or without heart disease. Experimental models have shown that premature ventricular depolarizations may be elicited by abnormal automaticity, triggered activity, or reentrant mechanisms. It has become well known that VPBs can be commonly observed in apparently healthy individuals. However, VPBs occurring in overtly normal subjects without discernible heart disease seem to have little if any prognostic significance. VPBs occur more frequently and in more complex forms (see later) in patients with detectable heart disease than in healthy individuals. The prognostic meaning of VPBs has been well studied in patients with myocardial infarction (acute or remote) with several consistent themes. Less is known about the significance of VPBs occurring in association with forms of heart disease (other than ischemic heart disease) such as hypertension, mitral valve prolapse, or primary myocardial disease.

Some investigators have promoted the concept that patients in the acute phase of myocardial infarction may have types of VPBs that are predictive of VF and sudden cardiac death. These types of VPBs were referred to as "warning arrhythmias" and include frequent ectopy (more than 5 per minute), multiform configuration (different morphology), couplets (two in a row), and R-on-T phenomenon (VPBs occurring during the repolarization phase of the preceding sinus beat in the vulnerable period of ventricular recovery). However, using sophisticated monitoring techniques, it has become apparent that almost all patients have warning arrhythmias in the acute infarct setting. In those patients who experience VF, warning arrhythmias are no more common than in those without VF. Therefore, warning arrhythmias observed during acute myocardial infarction are neither a sensitive nor a specific predictive tool in determining which patients will have VF. Therefore, in patients with acute myocardial infarction, there is little need to direct drug therapy (usually lidocaine) specifically at VPB suppression. Studies have shown that effective prevention of VF in the acute infarct setting may be achieved without the abolition of VPBs. The inability of VPBs (warning arrhythmias) to predict the occurrence of VF coupled with the lack of correlation between a drug's effectiveness in preventing VF and suppressing VPBs forms the basis of suggesting antiarrhythmic drug prophylaxis (e.g., lidocaine, magnesium) for all patients with an uncomplicated acute myocardial infarction (see later).

On the other hand, data strongly imply that VPBs documented in the convalescence period of myocardial infarction do carry important long-term prognostic significance.[42] VPBs occurring after a myocardial infarction seem to be a risk factor for patient death that is independent of the degree of left ventricular dysfunction or the extent of coronary atherosclerosis. Lown and Wolf[43] have developed a grading scale for classifying different types of VPBs. The grading scale is as follows: grade 0, no ectopy; grade I, less than 30 VPBs/h of uniform morphology; grade II, more than 30 VPBs/h of uniform morphology; grade III, multiform VPBs; grade IVa, couplets; grade IVb, 3 or more consecutive VPBs (nonsustained ventricular tachycardia); grade V, R-on-T phenomenon. A common assumption is that the higher grades of VPBs within this classification system imply a higher risk of subsequent arrhythmogenic death. It should be emphasized that this assumption has never been proven. Ruberman and coworkers[42] have devised a simple alternative classification based on the significance of simple or benign (infrequent and monomorphic) versus complex or malignant (all other types in the Lown classification) forms of VPBs. These investigators found that the presence of "complex" ventricular ectopy in the setting of ischemic heart disease was associated with a higher incidence of cardiac death, but not necessarily arrhythmogenic death. One can see that within the controversy of the significance of VPBs is a basic question: Are complex forms of VPBs simply an unimportant marker of underlying structural heart disease or are VPBs an important electrical disorder that should be addressed independently?

▶ TREATMENT: Ventricular Premature Beats

Because VPBs without associated heart disease in apparently healthy individuals carry little or no risk, drug therapy is unnecessary. However, due to the prognostic significance of complex VPBs in patients with heart disease, the use of antiarrhythmic drug therapy to suppress them has been controversial. Traditionally, many supported aggressive drug therapy designed to suppress a high percentage of VPBs, based upon the Lown grading system. The underlying premise of this approach is to attempt to eliminate a risk factor for cardiac death in patients with coronary disease, namely the presence of complex VPBs. However, others have favored a more conservative approach and disregarded drug therapy in the absence of significant symptoms. The release of the CAST results[22] clearly supports the later conservative approach but it is worthwhile to review the issues and difficulties involved in this controversy.

First, the frequency of VPBs is sporadic and extremely variable, making it difficult to determine effective drug therapy. Winkle,[44] by evaluating continuous electrocardiograms and VPB frequency, found a marked spontaneous variability that often mimicked drug efficacy or drug-induced aggravation of VPBs. Morganroth and coworkers[45] analyzed the variations in VPB frequency on 24-hour Holter recordings. These investigators estimated that to attribute a reduction in VPB frequency to drug effectiveness instead of spontaneous variability, a decrease in VPB frequency of greater than 83% was necessary. Despite this finding, many clinicians and published studies judged drug efficacy by a 50% reduction in VPB frequency or simply a statistically significant reduction in the number of VPBs by serial Holter monitors. These criteria obviously do not account for the spontaneous variability in VPB frequency. Other investigators have noted an impressive discordance between the drug concentrations necessary for 83% reduction in VPBs frequency and those necessary to prevent VT or VF. In other words, a high degree of VPB suppression is not a necessary prerequisite for the successful prevention of VT or VF.

Second, all antiarrhythmic agents currently available have an impressive side-effect profile (Table 14–3). A considerable percentage of patients cannot tolerate long-term therapy with these drugs and chances are good that an agent will have to be discontinued because of side effects. In one trial,[46] over 50% of patients had to discontinue long-term procainamide (mostly due to a lupus-like syndrome) after myocardial infarction. In another study,[47] disopyramide caused anticholinergic side effects in about 70% of patients. Flecainide and disopyramide may precipitate congestive heart failure in a significant number of patients with underlying left ventricular dysfunction.[48] The type Ib agents such as tocainide and mexiletine cause neurologic and/or gastrointestinal toxicity in a high percentage of patients. Tocainide, specifically, has been reported to cause both pulmonary fibrosis and leukopenia, the significance of which came to light after FDA approval. Long-term therapy with amiodarone frequently causes multisystem toxicity including occasional cases of hepatitis and pulmonary fibrosis.[49,50] However, many adverse effects of amiodarone therapy are dose-related and may be avoided by treating patients with the lowest effective dose. Clearly the most frightening adverse effects related to antiarrhythmic drugs are the aggravation of underlying ventricular arrhythmias or the precipitation of new (and life-threatening) ventricular arrhythmias (see later).[51]

Despite these issues, the prevailing assumption among many clinicians was historically to suppress asymptomatic ectopy in

TABLE 14–3. Side Effects of Antiarrhythmic Drugs

Drug	Side Effects
Quinidine	Cinchonism, diarrhea, GI,[a] hypotension, torsades de pointes, aggravation of underlying heart failure, conduction disturbances or ventricular arrhythmias, hepatitis, thrombocytopenia, hemolytic anemia
Procainamide	Systemic lupus erythematosus, GI, torsades de pointes, aggravation of underlying heart failure, conduction disturbances or ventricular arrhythmias, agranulocytosis
Disopyramide	Anticholinergic symptoms, GI, torsades de pointes, heart failure, aggravation of underlying conduction disturbances and/or ventricular arrhythmias, hypoglycemia, hepatic cholestasis
Lidocaine	CNS,[b] seizures, psychosis, sinus arrest, aggravation of underlying conduction disturbances
Mexiletine	CNS, psychosis, GI, aggravation of underlying conduction disturbances or ventricular arrhythmias
Tocainide	CNS, psychosis, GI, aggravation of underlying conduction disturbances or ventricular arrhythmias, rash/arthralgias, pulmonary infiltrates, agranulocytosis, thrombocytopenia
Moricizine	Dizziness, headache, GI, aggravation of underlying conduction disturbances or ventricular arrhythmias
Flecainide, Propafenone	Blurred vision, dizziness, headache, GI, bronchospasm,[c] aggravation of underlying heart failure, conduction disturbances or ventricular arrhythmias
Amiodarone	CNS, corneal microdeposits/blurred vision, optic neuropathy/neuritis, GI, aggravation of underlying ventricular arrhythmias, torsades de pointes, bradycardia or AV block, bruising without thrombocytopenia, pulmonary fibrosis, hepatitis, hypothyroidism, hyperthyroidism, photosensitivity, blue-gray skin discoloration, myopathy, hypotension and phlebitis (IV use)
Sotalol	Fatigue, GI, depression, torsades de pointes, bronchospasm, aggravation of underlying heart failure, conduction disturbances or ventricular arrhythmias
Ibutilide	Torsades de pointes, hypotension
Bretylium	Hypotension, GI

[a]GI = nausea, anorexia.
[b]CNS = confusion, paresthesias, tremor, ataxia, etc.
[c]Propafenone only.

postinfarct patients with antiarrhythmic drug therapy in an effort to decrease the risk of sudden cardiac death. However, the results of the CAST indicate that although well intentioned, this approach is flawed: Ectopy was suppressed but the risk of death increased.

The CAST[22,52] was initiated by the National Institutes of Health (NIH) in 1987 to determine if suppression of ventricular ectopy with encainide, flecainide, or moricizine could decrease the incidence of death from arrhythmia in patients who had suffered a myocardial infarction. Entrance criteria included documented myocardial infarction between 6 days and 2 years prior to enrollment, and 6 or more VPBs per hour without runs of ventricular tachycardia greater than 15 beats in length. Also, patients were required to have an ejection fraction of ≤ 55% if recruited within 90 days of myocardial infarction or ≤ 40% if recruited 90 days or more after infarction. Patients with an ejection fraction < 30% were randomized only to encainide or moricizine. Patients were randomized to receive drug therapy or placebo after demonstrating VPB suppression with one of the agents. The drug and dose were determined during an open-label dose titration phase that preceded randomization.

In April 1989 a routine, preliminary review of the study by the Safety and Monitoring Board revealed alarming results, and the study was interrupted. The results show that compared to placebo, treatment with encainide or flecainide was associated with a significantly higher rate of total mortality and death due to arrhythmia, presumably due to proarrhythmia (Fig. 14–11). Analysis of the moricizine arm indicated neither harm nor benefit from this therapy; therefore only this portion of the study was allowed to continue as CAST II. However, later (July 1991) CAST II was also prematurely stopped; there was a trend toward an increase in mortality in moricizine-treated patients. This was particularly true during the initiation of moricizine therapy (dose titration phase) but not observed during the chronic treatment phase. The overall results of the two CASTs conclusively prove that patients with VPBs post-myocardial infarction do not benefit from chronic antiarrhythmic drug therapy (beyond the general use of β-blocking agents) and, in fact, most drugs are detrimental. The study also puts into perspective the risk associated with the use of antiarrhythmic therapy and the need to carefully select only those patients with a defined therapeutic benefit.

The CAST is considered one of the most important trials ever undertaken by the NIH and has had a tremendous influence on the overall approach to the treatment of tachycardias in addition to a far-reaching impact on new drug development. The results have colored the long-term use of all antiarrhythmics, causing a broad skepticism in the risk–benefit profile of this class of drugs. Pharmaceutical companies, as a result, have shifted their drug discovery and investigative efforts away from potent sodium channel blockers. As immediate fallout, encainide was pulled from the market by the pharmaceutical company, and another pharmaceutical manufacturer decided not to market the type Ic agent, indecainide, despite Food and Drug Administration (FDA) approval. These findings also provided additional fuel for the pursuit of non-drug therapies for tachycardias such as ablation and implantable devices.

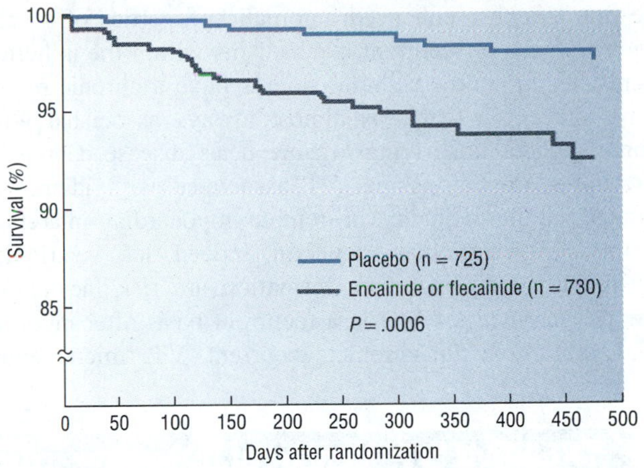

FIGURE 14–11. Life table curves from the CAST, specifically for patients receiving encainide or flecainide (lighter line) and matching placebo (darker line). Note the divergent slopes of each line implying sustained risk of death (presumed proarrhythmia). *(From Ref. 96, with permission.)*

Despite the discouraging results of the CAST, post-myocardial infarction patients with complex ventricular ectopy remain at risk for death. Other drugs, besides the type Ics, have been studied including sotalol. Sotalol is marketed as a racemic mixture of a *d* and *l* isomer: both are type III potassium blockers but the *l* isomer has β-blocking actions. Chronic therapy with *d*-sotalol was studied in patients with remote myocardial infarction complicated by complex ectopy in the SWORD (Survival With Oral *d*-Sotalol) trial.[53] Unlike the CAST, *d*-sotalol treatment was not designed to cause VPB suppression, yet (like the CAST) the trial was halted prematurely because of excessive mortality in the treatment arm. Again the presumed reason for this observation was *d*-sotalol-related proarrhythmia. The only type I or III antiarrhythmic drug that has *not* been shown to be harmful in this way is amiodarone. Two trials[54,55] have shown amiodarone to decrease the incidence of sudden (or arrhythmic) death but not total mortality in post-myocardial infarction patients with complex ventricular ectopy. It is unclear if these findings can be attributed to one property (e.g., β-blocking) or a combination of amiodarone's complex pharmacologic effects on conduction. Clearly because of its impressive adverse effect profile and its inability to improve survival, amiodarone cannot routinely be recommended in patients with heart disease such as remote myocardial infarction and complex VPBs. Taken together, VPBs should not be treated with any antiarrhythmic drug beyond the routine use of β-blockers.

VENTRICULAR TACHYCARDIA

VT is a wide QRS tachycardia that may acutely occur as a result of metabolic abnormalities, ischemia, or drug toxicity; or chronically recur as a paroxysmal form. On electrocardiographic inspection, VT may appear as either repetitive monomorphic or polymorphic ventricular complexes. The definition of VT is three or more repetitive VPBs occurring at a rate greater than 100 beats/min. An acute episode of VT may be precipitated by severe electrolyte abnormalities (hypokalemia), hypoxemia, or digitalis toxicity or (most commonly) occur during an acute myocardial infarction. In these cases, correction of the underlying precipitating factors will usually prevent further recurrences of VT. As an example, if VT occurs during an acute myocardial infarction and is effectively treated, it will probably not reappear on a chronic basis after the infarcted area has healed or ischemia resolved. This form of acute VT may be due to either enhanced automatic properties of a ventricular focus or reentrant mechanisms within the ischemic ventricle. In contrast, some patients have a chronic recurrent form of VT that is almost always associated with some type of underlying organic heart disease. Common examples are paroxysmal VT associated with idiopathic dilated cardiomyopathy or remote myocardial infarction with a left ventricular aneurysm. Indeed, left ventricular dysfunction and aneurysm formation are risk factors for the development of VT on a recurrent basis after myocardial infarction. In chronic, recurrent VT, microreentry within the distal Purkinje network is presumed to be responsible for the underlying substrate in a large majority of patients (Fig. 14–3). Theoretically, electrophysiologic discrepancies occur as a result of structural damage and heart disease within the ventricular conducting system. The reentrant circuit may possess both anatomically determined and functional properties coursing through normal, damaged (but not dead) tissue and islands of necrosed tissue. In a minority of patients, macroreentrant circuits may be responsible for recurrent ventricular tachycardia, including reentry incorporating the bundle branches.

▶ TREATMENT: Ventricular Tachycardia

Patients with acute VT associated with a precipitating factor often suffer severe symptoms requiring immediate treatment measures. Chronic recurrent VT may also cause severe hemodynamic compromise but sometimes only mild symptoms that are generally well tolerated result. Different varieties of VT may occur and require some definition. Sustained VT is that which requires therapeutic intervention to restore a stable rhythm or lasts a relatively long time (usually greater than 30 seconds). Nonsustained VT (NSVT) is that which self-terminates after a brief duration (usually less than 30 seconds). If the patient has VT more frequently than sinus rhythm (VT is the dominant rhythm), this is referred to as incessant VT. Exercise-induced VT is that which occurs during times of high sympathetic tone such as physical exertion. Monomorphic VT has a consistent QRS configuration, whereas polymorphic VT has varying QRS complexes. A characteristic type of polymorphic VT, in which the QRS complexes appear to undulate around a central axis and is associated with evidence of delayed ventricular repolarization (long QT interval or prominent U waves), is referred to as torsades de pointes (see later).

Like other rapid tachycardias, the initial management of an acute episode of VT requires a quick assessment of the patient's status and symptoms. If severe symptoms are present, then DCC should be instituted to immediately restore sinus rhythm. An investigation should be made into possible precipitating factors and these should be corrected if possible. The diagnosis of acute myocardial infarction should be entertained. If VT is felt to be an isolated electrical event associated with a transient initiating factor (such as acute myocardial ischemia or digitalis toxicity), then lidocaine should be administered and continued for 24 to 48 hours or until the patient is stable. In these cases, there is no need for long-term antiarrhythmic therapy once the precipitating factors are corrected. Nevertheless, the patient should be monitored closely for possible recurrences of VT.

Patients with mild or no symptoms during an acute episode of VT can be initially treated with antiarrhythmic drugs (DCC should be readily available). The reader is referred to the most recent Guidelines for Cardiopulmonary Resuscitation and Emergency Cardiac Care put forth by the American Heart Association.[33] Lidocaine (1 to 2 mg/kg loading dose followed by 2 mg/min infusion) is usually considered the drug of choice because of a high degree of effectiveness, quick onset, and ease of administration. In the event that lidocaine fails to terminate the tachycardia, intravenous procainamide (loading dose and infusion) can be tried next. DCC should be instituted if the patient's status deteriorates, VT degenerates to VF, or drug therapy fails. As an alternate to DCC, a transvenous pacing wire can be inserted and VT terminated by overdrive pacing methods. There is basically no reason to allow the patient to remain in VT without intervention even if symptoms are minimal.

Once an acute episode of sustained VT has been successfully terminated by electrical or pharmacologic means and an acute myocardial infarction ruled out, the possibility of paroxysmal VT reappearing on a recurrent basis should be considered. This possibility can often be confirmed by the use of invasive electrophysiologic study using programmed ventricular stimulation. The management of the patient with chronic recurrent sustained VT deserves considerable attention. Because these patients are at extremely high risk for death, trial-and-error attempts to find effective therapy is unwarranted. Two methods using surrogate end points have been used: (1) inability to induce sustained VT with programmed extrastimuli by invasive electrophysiologic studies and (2) suppression of ventricular ectopy by serial 24-hour continuous electrocardiographic (Holter) monitoring.

Electrophysiologic studies using programmed stimulation incorporate the concepts of reentry to replicate the patient's clinical tachycardia in a controlled laboratory setting. The patient is admitted to the hospital (often an intensive care setting) and strips of the clinical tachycardia carefully analyzed. All antiarrhythmic drugs are discontinued and (after the systemic elimination of these drugs) the patient is brought to the electrophysiology laboratory in the nonsedated state. Here transvenous multipolar catheters, which can both pace the heart and record electrical activity, are inserted into the right heart. Next, attempts to replicate the clinical tachycardia are made by the insertion of early beats and/or pacing methods via programmed stimulation. If replication of the clinical tachycardia is achieved, this initial study (without drug therapy) serves as a control that can be compared to subsequent studies on drug therapy. The electrophysiologist usually uses a protocol of several different grades of programmed stimulation from at least two sites (right ventricular apex and outflow tract): S1 = continuous pacing train; S1,S2 = one extra stimuli; S1,S2,S3 = two extra stimuli; S1,S2,S3,S4 = three extra stimuli; and rapid ventricular pacing (V burst) at variable rates. Induction of polymorphic VT or ventricular fibrillation with aggressive grades of stimulation (V burst, S4) in a patient with a monomorphic VT can be viewed as a "nonclinical" artifact of the test. Once VT is induced by programmed stimulation, it can be terminated by programmed stimulation, overdrive pacing, or DCC depending on the patient's status. Antiarrhythmic drugs are then serially administered and the electrophysiologic study is repeated (at presumed drug steady state). If a patient has sustained VT induced during the control study, then the inability to reproduce VT or the induction of only brief, self-terminating episodes of VT (usually less than 15 beats) generally predicts that the drug will be effective in preventing recurrent episodes on a long-term basis. When VT is rendered noninducible with drug therapy, a serum drug level should be obtained immediately. This serum level then serves as the patient's target level for chronic oral therapy

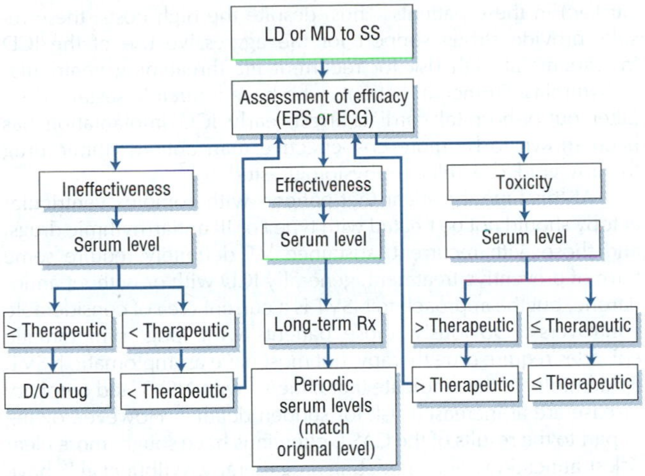

FIGURE 14–12. Algorithm for the clinical approach to therapeutic drug monitoring of antiarrhythmic drugs. EPS = electrophysiologic study; ECG = continuous electrocardiographic monitoring; D/C = discontinue drug.

(Fig. 14–12). Efforts should be directed to keep the serum level at or above this target to prevent recurrence of the arrhythmia.[56]

Although this method is efficacious in determining effective antiarrhythmic drug therapy in patients with recurrent VT, it has several drawbacks besides its invasive nature. Foremost in this regard is that the yield for finding an effective drug is low. Sustained monomorphic VT can be rendered noninducible or nonsustained in only 15% to 25% of patients. Therefore, the clinician frequently must search for other therapeutic options or settle for other treatment end points such as slower and more tolerable inducible VT. Sometimes combination therapy is tried for patients refractory to single agents. The combination of a type Ia drug with a type Ib drug (quinidine and mexiletine) is effective in some patients who are resistant to either drug used alone.[57] Amiodarone is clearly the most effective (about 50%/2 years) agent in patients with recurrent VT. Although a matter of continuing controversy, many feel that electrophysiologic drug testing does not predict the clinical efficacy of amiodarone. Patients may have continued inducibility of VT on amiodarone despite long-term success. Indeed, empiric amiodarone has been compared to therapy with other agents guided by electrophysiologic testing in patients at high risk for recurrent VT.[58] Amiodarone therapy without invasive testing was superior in preventing cardiac death and recurrences of severe ventricular arrhythmias at all time points.

Older trials that seemingly demonstrated that serial drug testing identifies effective chronic agents always lack a control group (patients rendered noninducible after treatment with an antiarrhythmic drug who are not treated chronically with that agent). This was obviously done because of ethical concerns but raises the possibility that noninducibility simply identifies low-risk patients, independent of drug treatment.

The second method used to determine therapy for patients with chronic recurrent sustained VT is the use of serial Holter monitors with drug testing. The surrogate end point in this case is the suppression of ventricular ectopy (> 83%) and total abolition of NSVT compared to control (drug-free) recordings. This method was not used routinely in the United States; initial small studies[59] demonstrated a superiority of invasive electrophysiologic testing over serial Holter recordings. Nonetheless, enough controversy was generated to initiate a large study to compare the two methods of drug testing. The ESVEM (electrophysiologic study versus electrocardiographic monitoring)[60,61] trial enrolled patients with documented clinical VT/VF, inducible ventricular tachycardia, and frequent ventricular ectopy. These patients were randomized to electrophysiologic studies or serial Holter recordings to test up to 7 antiarrhythmic drugs (imipramine, mexiletine, pirmenol, procainamide, quinidine, propafenone, or sotalol). Holter testing had a greater yield of identifying effective agents and there was no statistical difference between this method and electrophysiologic testing in terms of VT recurrence or sudden death. Although patients with poor left ventricular systolic function could not receive it in the ESVEM, sotalol proved to be the most effective drug in the trial. The study has been criticized to some extent because of the methods of using programmed stimulation and patient selection so that many invasive electrophysiologists remain unconvinced about the relative merits of serial Holter testing. Further, because there was no placebo group in ESVEM (for ethical reasons) one cannot be sure that either method is truly effective. Perhaps suppression of ectopy by Holter criteria or noninducibility during serial electrophysiologic studies in and of themselves portend an overall good prognosis, independent of any drug effect. The relatively impressive results in the ESVEM with racemic sotalol contrasted with the poor results of its *d*-isomer in the SWORD (albeit in a different population) speaks strongly for the importance of chronic treatment with β-blockers in patients with serious ventricular arrhythmias. Regardless of the methods of drug testing, recurrence rate of VT in the ESVEM was high (20% to 50% per year depending on the drug chosen). These findings and the impressive side-effect profiles of antiarrhythmic agents have again led investigators to study non-drug approaches to the treatment of recurrent VT/VF.[62]

Some centers have had excellent results with the surgical excision of the VT focus in appropriate candidates for this extensive procedure. With the aid of endocardial mapping techniques, procedures such as ventricular aneurysectomy, encircling ventriculotomy, and cryo or laser ablation can successfully abolish the arrhythmogenic substrate. Also, for some unusual forms of recurrent ventricular tachycardia, catheter ablation using radiofrequency current has been used successfully. However, the introduction and advances in the implantable automatic cardioverter defibrillator (ICD) has made it the most frequent form of current therapy for patients with recurrent, sustained VT/VF (Fig. 14–13). Early ICDs required a thoracotomy for placement and were programmed to tachycardia rate. Once the patient's rate rose to a certain level, a series of internal defibrillations were delivered. Although effective in terminating VT/VF, inappropriate shocks were sometimes delivered for SVTs or NSVT. Further, a pulse generator was placed in

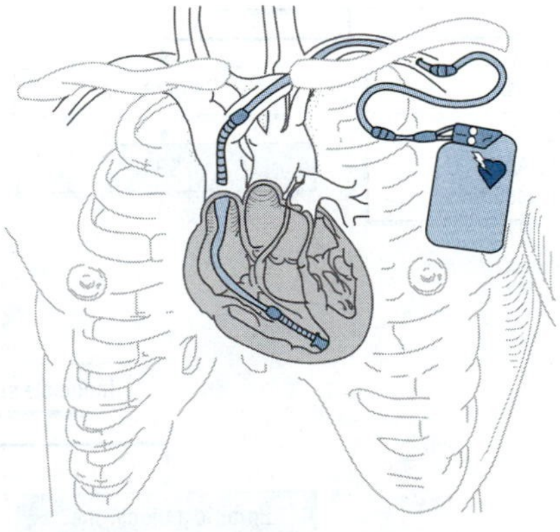

FIGURE 14–13. Drawing showing an automatic implantable cardioverter-defibrillator with newer methods of device placement. It shows an endocardial lead system where the leads are placed transvenously without the need for a thoracotomy. The generator is now small enough to be placed in the pectoral region of the chest. *(Cardiac Pacemakers, Inc. St. Paul, MN, with permission.)*

the abdomen with a relatively short battery life in these early models. ICD technology is rapidly expanding so that now the newer devices employ a "tiered therapy approach." New ICDs provide in a sequential fashion, programmed stimulation, overdrive pacing, and low-energy cardioversion before internal defibrillation is employed as a last step. In addition, backup bradycardia pacing and extended battery lives have made these devices much more attractive. Importantly, transvenous insertion techniques not requiring a thoracotomy are now being routinely used at most institutions and the pulse generator is now small enough to implant in the pectoral region of the chest (Fig. 14–13).

Most would agree that the ICD is highly effective in preventing sudden death due to recurrent VT or VF,[63] although several problems remain. First, the device and implantation are expensive. The approximate cost for the ICD device alone is $25,000. Total cost for the device, implantation procedure, electrophysiologic studies, hospitalization, and physician fees may be as much as $100,000. Second, many patients (as high as 50%) end up receiving antiarrhythmic drugs (usually amiodarone) in addition to the ICD. Here, the end point of drug therapy is different than without the ICD, that is, the drugs do not necessarily need to prevent all sustained recurrences. Antiarrhythmic drugs are prescribed in this instance to decrease the frequency of VT/VF episodes and NSVT, minimize patient discomfort, and save battery life. Some immediately couple antiarrhythmic drugs with the ICD implantation but we do not recommend this approach. Rather, each patient should be individualized and antiarrhythmic drugs administered in those with frequent VT and shocks. If antiarrhythmic drugs are added to ICD therapy, one should note that many agents alter defibrillation thresholds and therefore the device should be reprogrammed.[64] Third, it remains unclear if the ICD decreases overall mortality in patients with recurrent VT/VF.[65] Perhaps the ICD alters the cause of death without decreasing all-cause mortality. Recently, the use of the ICD in patients with remote myocardial infarction, left ventricular dysfunction, and NSVT who had inducible sustained VT during programmed stimulation was compared to chronic antiarrhythmic drug (mostly amiodarone) therapy.[66] The trial was stopped early because of a demonstrated superiority of the ICD in preventing death (mainly cardiac) in these patients. Thus, despite the high costs, these results provide strong support for the aggressive use of the ICD in patients at high risk for recurrent life-threatening ventricular arrhythmias. Further, in patients who have inducible sustained VT (after out-of-hospital cardiac arrest) early ICD implantation has been shown to be more cost-effective than antiarrhythmic drug therapy guided by electrophysiologic studies.[67]

At this time it is clear that patients with complex ventricular ectopy should not be treated with type I or III antiarrhythmic drugs, and those with recurrent, sustained VT definitely require some form of preventive treatment, generally ICD with or without amiodarone, but the approach to NSVT is a current area of considerable controversy. Obviously, those patients with long, symptomatic episodes require drug therapy, but most have asymptomatic NSVT. Epidemiologic data indicate that patients with NSVT and coronary disease are at increased risk for sudden death.[68] However, owing in part to the results of the CAST, clinicians have sought more clear risk stratification before initiating drug therapy. Wilbur et al.[69] have suggested that electrophysiologic studies may provide a useful tool to stratify patients at increased risk. These investigators found that post-MI patients with NSVT who had inducible sustained VT were at increased risk for subsequent arrhythmia or sudden death. Alternatively, those without inducible sustained tachycardias were at low risk for subsequent spontaneous sustained arrhythmias. In patients with inducible sustained VT in whom the tachycardia was rendered noninducible by drugs, the risk of death was similar to those who had no inducible arrhythmias at all. Perhaps patients with NSVT should undergo programmed stimulation and those found to have inducible sustained VT should be treated aggressively with antiarrhythmic drugs or the ICD. Those with no inducible sustained tachycardia can then be followed closely without drug therapy (Fig. 14–14).

Another approach to risk stratification involves the use of noninvasive tools. Gomes et al[70] evaluated the predictive utility of Holter monitoring, left ventricular ejection fraction assessment, and signal-averaged electrocardiogram (SAECG) for determining prognosis after myocardial infarction. The SAECG detects "late potentials" felt to be reflective of areas in the ventricle that possess slow and fragmented conduction, promoting the proper sub-

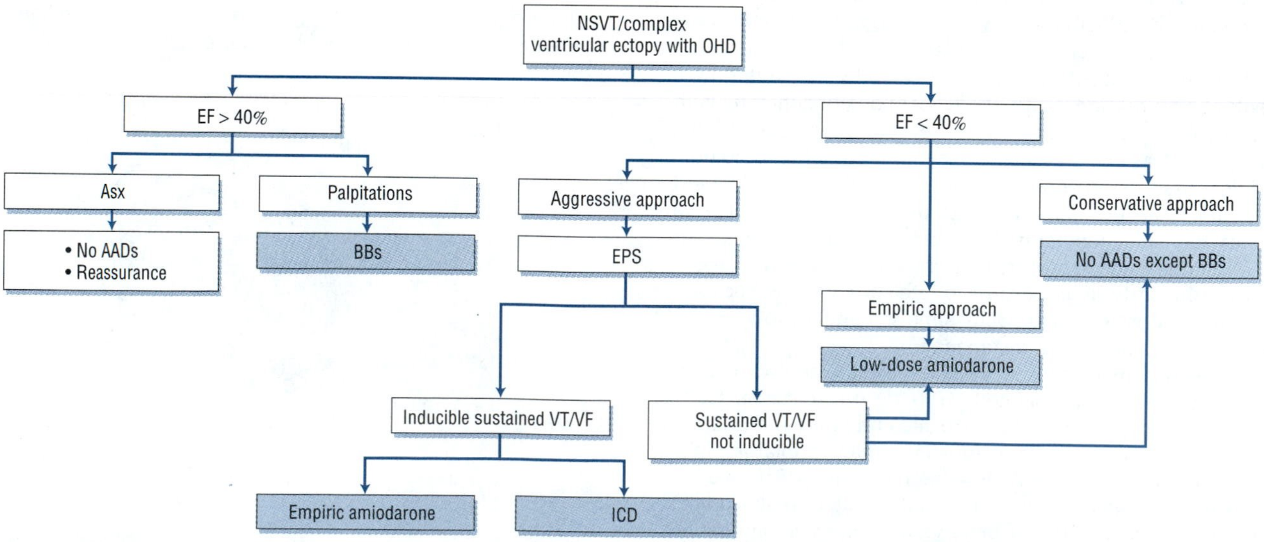

FIGURE 14–14. An algorithm for management of patients with ventricular ectopy or nonsustained ventricular tachycardia (NSVT) in patients with organic heart disease (OHD, usually after myocardial infarction). EF = ejection fraction; EPS = electrophysiologic studies; VT/VF = ventricular tachycardia/ventricular fibrillation; ICD = implantable cardioverter-defibrillator; BB = β-blockers; AADs = antiarrhythmic drugs.

strate for VT. The results indicate that the presence of complex ectopy and NSVT, decreased ejection fraction (< 40%), and abnormal SAECG are all significant risk factors for subsequent arrhythmia (sustained VT) or sudden death. Further, the more risk factors a patient has, the greater the risk. It has been proposed that those individuals with two or more risk factors undergo electrophysiologic studies for further risk stratification based on the inducibility of sustained ventricular tachycardia. It should be pointed out that this approach, with the final step being invasive programmed stimulation and possibly ICD implantation, represents an aggressive treatment strategy. Some clinical electrophysiologists choose to ignore most cases of brief (e.g., 3 beats), asymptomatic episodes of NSVT. Some use empiric amiodarone. Again there are no data to suggest that these divergent approaches alter overall mortality in patients with NSVT. Another confounding factor is the underlying form of heart disease associated with NSVT. Patients with idiopathic dilated cardiomyopathy and NSVT also appear to be a high risk for sudden death yet usually do not have inducible sustained VT with invasive studies (unlike those with coronary disease). Clearly, further large prospective trials are necessary (and currently ongoing) to discern the proper approach to NSVT. One such study referred to as the MUSTT (Multicenter UnSustained Tachycardia Trial) is in progress. This trial will compare the value of electrophysiologic-guided therapy (including the ICD) to (importantly) no therapy in patients with NSVT and coronary disease.

PROARRHYTHMIA

All antiarrhythmic agents have the potential to aggravate existing arrhythmias or to cause new arrhythmias. It is believed that antiarrhythmic drugs may cause proarrhythmia in 5% to 20% of patients.[51] Although drug-induced arrhythmias have been recognized for several years, it has only been recently that this adverse effect has gained widespread attention. Many definitions for proarrhythmia have been proposed; however, in simplest terms it indicates the development of a significant new arrhythmia (such as VT, VF, or torsades de pointes) or worsening of an existing arrhythmia (episodes are longer, faster, or more frequent). As with all arrhythmias, the consequences of proarrhythmia are varied. Some patients who develop proarrhythmia may be totally asymptomatic, and others may notice a worsening of symptoms, whereas some may die suddenly from this side effect. The development of proarrhythmia results from the same mechanisms that cause arrhythmias in general (quinidine-induced torsades de pointes owing to early after-depolarizations) or from an alteration in the underlying substrate owing to the antiarrhythmic agent (development of an accelerated tachycardia owing to flecainide, which decreases conduction velocity without significantly altering the refractory period).[51] The diagnosis of proarrhythmia is sometimes difficult to make because of the variable nature of the underlying arrhythmias. However, in all cases, the agent should be discontinued if proarrhythmia is detected or suspected.

The issue of proarrhythmia, particularly from type Ic agents, has gained considerable publicity due to the results of the CAST. Flecainide and encainide have been known to cause a rapid, sustained, monomorphic VT with a characteristic sinusoidal QRS pattern resistant to resuscitation with cardioversion or overdrive pacing. This arrhythmia was thought to occur within the first several days of drug initiation; however, the results of the CAST indicate that the risk may exist as long as the agent is continued. Patient factors that definitely predispose to this form of proarrhythmia are the presence of underlying ventricular arrhythmias, ischemic heart disease, and poor left ventricular function. Provocation of proarrhythmia owing to the type Ics is frequently reported during exercise; this is more than likely caused by augmented slowed conduction at rapid heart rates (rate-dependant sodium blockade). The incidence of proarrhythmia is greatest in patients with all three risk factors (approximately 10% to 20%) and considerably less (less than 5%) in those without risks, such as patients with good left ventricular function and supraventricular tachycardias. Other factors that have a less-defined association with proarrhythmia are elevated antiarrhythmic serum concentrations (and rapid dosage escalation) and recent therapy with a type Ia antiarrhythmic. It has been proposed that the presence of underlying ventricular conduction delays may also pose a risk. Interestingly, in this study, the incidence of death caused by proarrhythmia from encainide and flecainide was approximately the same as the chance of long-term effectiveness.[71] As mentioned earlier, this arrhythmia is resistant to resuscitation; however, some have had success with intravenous lidocaine or the administration of sodium bicarbonate.

TORSADES DE POINTES

Torsades de pointes (TdP) is a rapid form of polymorphic VT (Fig. 14–15) associated with evidence of delayed ventricular repolarization (long QT interval or prominent U waves) on surface electrocardiograms. It is important to note that polymorphic VT, occurring in the setting of a normal QT interval, is similar to monomorphic VT in terms of etiology and treatment strategies. TdP may occur in association with hereditary syndromes or as acquired forms. The underlying etiology in both cases is delayed ventricular repolarization owing to blockade of potassium conductance. Two well-described heritable forms are Romano and Ward syndrome (long QT, TdP, and high incidence of sudden death) and Jervell and Lange–Neilson syndrome (long QT, TdP, high incidence of sudden death, and congenital deafmutism). These relatively unusual syndromes are caused by genetic abnormalities in the formation of cardiac potassium channels. Recent breakthroughs in the understanding of the

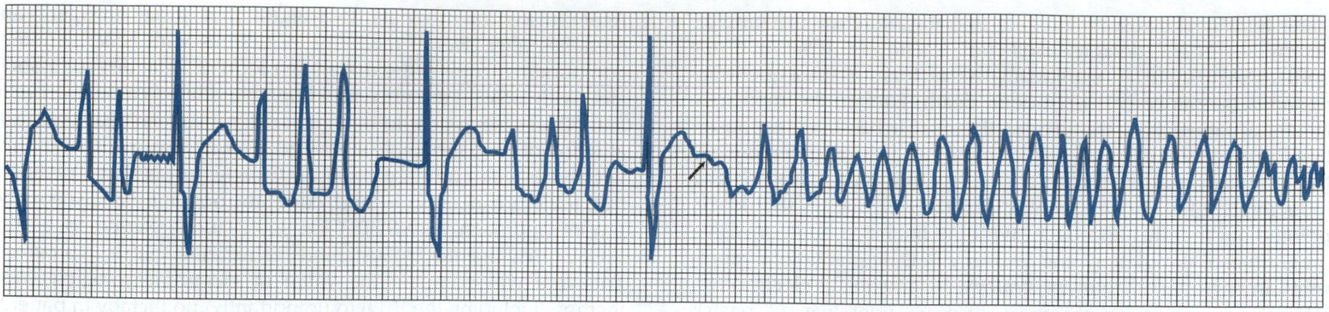

FIGURE 14–15. Torsades de pointes owing to quinidine. The reader should note a couplet and two triplets that follow each extra systolic pause. The pause gets progressively longer until it is long enough to result in an episode of sustained torsades de pointes. Also as the pause lengthens, discernible U waves (labeled ↑) (EADs?) begin to appear. The amplitude of the U wave is somewhat greater with the longest pause. *(From Ref. 97, with permission.)*

exact genetic abnormalities of these disorders have been made.[72] It is possible, however, that many individuals have a partially expressed form of these congenital syndromes but never suffer TdP unless some other external factor (drugs, diseases) further delay ventricular repolarization. Acquired forms of TdP are associated with electrolyte disturbances (hypokalemia or hypomagnesemia), subarachnoid hemorrhage, myocarditis, liquid-protein diets, arsenic poisoning, hypothyroidism, or drug therapy (notably phenothiazines, antihistamines, antidepressants, and antiarrhythmics) (Table 14–4). The type Ia drugs (especially quinidine) are most notorious for precipitating torsades de pointes but type Ibs and Ics rarely if ever cause it. The syndrome often referred to as "quinidine syncope" is, in most cases, due to drug-induced TdP. Quinidine syncope occurs in 4% to 8% of patients treated with this agent. Associated features, most of which are shared with other forms of drug-induced TdP, are as follows[17]: (1) low to "therapeutic" quinidine serum concentrations without other evidence of quinidine-related toxicity such as prolonged QRS duration; (2) concurrent organic heart disease, commonly ischemic; (3) evidence of mild delayed repolarization prior to quinidine therapy; (4) documentation usually within 1 week of initiating therapy; (5) high incidence of cross-sensitivity (recurrence of TdP) with other type Ia antiarrhythmic agents but not type Ibs, Ics, or amiodarone; (6) frequent coexisting electrolyte disturbances such as hypokalemia or hypomagnesemia; and (7) a characteristic long–short initiating sequence ("pause" dependence) of the episode of TdP (Fig. 14–15). However, none of these associations is an absolute prerequisite to the occurrence of quinidine syncope and TdP. Although generally documented early in the course of therapy, patients may suffer TdP during chronic quinidine treatment.[73] Other drug-related causes of TdP occur more frequently with high concentrations and doses, for example, sotalol, and *N*-acetylprocainamide. Amiodarone is an infrequent cause of TdP. Cisapride and terfenadine are

TABLE 14–4. Reported Causes of QT Prolongation and Torsades de Pointes

Conditions	
Congenital long QT syndromes	
Myocarditis	
Myocardial ischemia/infarction	
Severe bradycardia owing to AV block; < 50 beats per minute	
Hypokalemia	
Severe hypothermia	
Hypomagnesemia	
Hypothyroidism	
Cardiomyopathy	
Subarachnoid hemorrhage	
Drugs	
Antiarrhythmic drugs	
—quinidine	—bepridil
—procainamide	—*N*-acetylprocainamide
—disopyramide	
—amiodarone	
—sotalol	
—ibutilide	
Psychotropics	
—phenothiazines	
—tricyclic and tetracyclic antidepressants	
—haloperidol	
Toxins	
—organophosphate insecticides	
—arsenic	
Antihistamines	
—terfenadine	
—astemizole	
Antibiotics	
—pentamidine	
—erythromycin	
—trimethoprim-sulfamethoxazole	
Miscellaneous	
—liquid-protein diets[a]	—chloroquine
—corticosteroids[a]	—chloral hydrate
—diuretics[a]	—probucol
—vasopressin	—cisipride
—quinine	—tacrolimus

[a]Due, more than likely, to severe electrolyte imbalance.

potent potassium channel blockers than may also precipitate torsades de pointes. This is usually not observed because both agents are rapidly metabolized by cytochrome (CYP) P450 3A4 to active moities that are not proarrhythmic. However, in the presence of drugs that block the CYP3A4 isozyme (ketoconazole, erythromycin, diltiazem) torsades de pointes and death may occur.

It has been suggested that TdP may be owing to discrepancies in ventricular repolarization and inhomogeneous ventricular recovery, allowing the formation of multiple reentrant circuits. More likely, recent investigations have suggested that TdP is likely a result of triggered activity (early after-depolarizations) caused by a delay in ventricular repolarization. For an acute episode of TdP, most patients will require and respond to DCC. However, TdP tends to be paroxysmal in nature and often will rapidly recur after countershock. Therefore, after the initial restoration of a stable rhythm, therapy designed to prevent recurrences of TdP should be instituted. Almost all antiarrhythmics have been reported to be successful in isolated case reports, but because of the unpredictable and self-terminating nature of TdP, it is difficult to establish a cause-and-effect relationship. Drugs that further prolong repolarization such as intravenous procainamide are absolutely contraindicated. Lidocaine is usually ineffective. Intravenous magnesium sulfate, by suppressing triggered activity, is now considered the drug of choice in preventing recurrences of TdP.[74] If that is ineffective, treatment strategies designed to increase heart rate and shorten ventricular repolarization should be initiated: either temporary transvenous pacing (105 to 120 bpm) or pharmacologic pacing (isoproterenol or epinephrine infusion). All agents that prolong QT interval should be discontinued and exacerbating factors (such as hypokalemia) corrected.

In heritable long-QT syndromes propranolol has been shown to prevent recurrences of TdP and prevent sudden death. β-Blockers, although effective, may not prevent all episodes and therefore they are commonly treated with an ICD. In acquired long-QT syndromes, correction of the underlying cause is the key to long-term preventive therapy. No drug agents need be used on a chronic basis. In the case of quinidine syncope, type Ia agents should be avoided for the future treatment of the patient's underlying arrhythmias.

VENTRICULAR FIBRILLATION

VF is electrical anarchy of the ventricle resulting in no cardiac output and cardiovascular collapse. Death will ensue rapidly if effective treatment measures are not taken. In patients who died suddenly during electrocardiographic monitoring, VF often preceded by VT is the most frequently documented rhythm.[75] Sudden cardiac death accounts for about 400,000 deaths per year or 1000 deaths per day in the United States. Sudden cardiac death occurs most commonly in patients with ischemic heart disease and primary myocardial disease; less commonly in WPW, mitral valve prolapse; and occasionally those without associated heart disease. Patients who have sudden cardiac death (not associated with acute myocardial infarction) but survive because of appropriate cardiopulmonary resuscitation usually have inducible sustained VT and/or VF during electrophysiologic studies.[76] These individuals are at high risk for the recurrence of VT and/or VF.

In contrast, patients who have VF associated with acute myocardial infarction usually have little risk of recurrence. Of all patients who die from an acute MI, approximately 50% die suddenly prior to hospitalization, presumably due to VF. VF associated with acute myocardial infarction (MI) can be subdivided into two types: primary VF and complicated or secondary VF. Primary VF occurs in an uncomplicated MI not associated with heart failure; secondary VF occurs in an MI complicated by heart failure. The time course, incidence, mechanisms, treatment, and complications of these two forms of VF are different. For example, about 1% to 2% of patients with acute myocardial infarction suffer primary VF within 24 hours of chest pain but the risk of VF declines rapidly over time and is very low after the initial 24-hour period. Complicated VF does not follow such a predictable time course and may occur in the late infarction period. The premise of prophylactic antiarrhythmic drugs administered to all patients with uncomplicated MI is based on the inability to predict which patients are at risk for primary VF and the predictable time course of primary VF (in contrast to complicated VF). Of the prophylactic therapies used, lidocaine has been the most widely debated and studied. Lie and coworkers[77] performed the classic study showing the effectiveness of lidocaine in preventing primary VF. Although lidocaine significantly reduced the incidence of VF compared to placebo, there was not a decrease in mortality due to VF between the groups. This fact and the effectiveness of rapidly instituted DCC in modern coronary care units with sophisticated monitoring techniques have caused most to reject the notion of prophylactic lidocaine administration for all patients with uncomplicated myocardial infarction. Two meta-analyses[78,79] also conclude against the routine use of prophylactic lidocaine owing to a possible increase in mortality in lidocaine-treated patients[78] and the declining incidence of primary VF documented in recent years.[79]

More recently, the use of intravenous magnesium sulfate has been entertained for the prevention of VF during the acute infarct period. Small trials implying effectiveness were subsequently incorporated into a meta-analysis.[80] This meta-analysis found a decrease in the incidence of VT/VF and a reduction in total mortality with magnesium therapy. A subsequent large multicenter trial[81] found similar results, although most of the decrease in mortality was (surprisingly) attributed to heart failure deaths rather than deaths due to ventricular arrhythmias. These results would

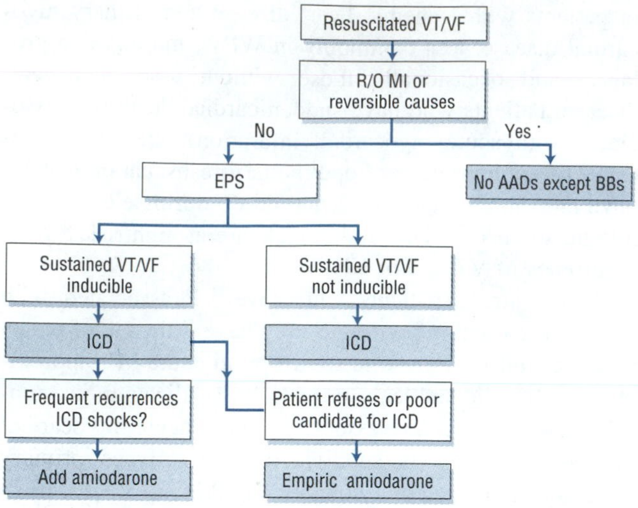

FIGURE 14–16. Example of an approach to the management of survivors of cardiac arrest (resuscitated VT/VF). Reversible causes of cardiac arrest (e.g., electrolyte abnormalities, acute phase of MI) should be treated with specific therapy. AADs = antiarrhythmic drugs; BBs = β-blockers; EPS = invasive electrophysiologic studies; ICD = implantable cardioverter-defibrillator; VT/VF = ventricular tachycardia/ventricular fibrillation; MI = myocardial infarction.

lead one to conclude that magnesium sulfate should be routinely administered to patients with suspected MI because of its ease of administration and safety. However, data from another large trial (ISIS-IV) have verified no such effectiveness of magnesium therapy in this setting.[82] Hence, prophylactic magnesium cannot be recommended at this time; indeed, no therapies (lidocaine, magnesium, or other antiarrhythmic drugs) have shown a conclusive benefit to prevent VF in the acute infarct period (at least for now).

A patient with VF (with or without associated myocardial ischemia) should be managed according to the American Heart Association's recommendations for advanced cardiac life support.[33] Summarizing, DCC should be immediately instituted and repeated twice (if unsuccessful) prior to drug therapy. If DCC does not restore a stable rhythm, epinephrine (intravenous or intratracheal if a line is not established) should be administered prior to the next DCC. It has been debated whether the standard dose of epinephrine (1.0 mg) is sufficient (see Chap. 9). A large multicenter trial[83] found that "high-dose" epinephrine (0.2 mg/kg) did not affect success or survival (compared to 0.02 mg/kg) of patients with cardiac arrest (including VF). Nevertheless, if epinephrine (coupled with DCC) is unsuccessful, lidocaine then bretylium should be given and DCC repeated as necessary. Bear in mind that the onset of action of bretylium can be delayed (10 to 20 minutes), presumably owing to slow distribution to the myocardium. Treatment guidelines for VF have not been revised since the approval of intravenous amiodarone for this indication but preliminary information implies that it is effective as the first drug administered after countershock. Unlike its oral counterpart, intravenous amiodarone has a quick onset of action and may be effective in 40% to 60% of patients with VT or VF refractory to lidocaine. In one trial[84] amiodarone was as effective as bretylium but caused less postconversion hypotension. At this time, amiodarone can be used in lieu of (or after) bretylium in patients with VF (or VT) refractory to DCC and lidocaine. With more research and clinical experience, it would not be surprising to see intravenous amiodarone become a first-line drug for VF in the future.

Once the patient is successfully resuscitated, antiarrhythmics should be continued until the patient's rhythm and overall status are stable. If the episode of VF was associated with acute ischemia, long-term antiarrhythmic drugs are probably unnecessary but the patient should be monitored closely for recurrence of VT and/or VF. If, on the other hand, VF was not associated with acute MI (or a known precipitating factor), the patient should undergo invasive electrophysiologic studies and (depending upon the results) probably ICD implantation (Fig. 14–16).

BRADYARRHYTHMIAS

The previous sections reviewed the pathophysiology and treatment of tachyarrhythmias, and this section serves to briefly consider the bradyarrhythmias. For the most part, the symptoms of bradyarrhythmias result from a decline in cardiac output. Because cardiac output increases as heart rate increases (to a point), patients experience symptoms in association with hypotension such as dizziness, syncope, fatigue, and confusion. If left ventricular dysfunction exists, patients may have an exacerbation of congestive heart failure symptoms. Except in the case of recurrent syncope, these symptoms are often subtle and nonspecific.

SINUS NODE DYSFUNCTION

Sinus bradyarrhythmias (heart rate less than 60 bpm) is a common finding especially in young, athletically active individuals and usually is neither symptomatic nor requires therapeutic intervention. On the other hand, some patients, particularly the elderly, have sinus node dysfunction. This may be the result of underlying organic heart disease and the normal aging process which, over time, attenuates SA nodal function. Sick sinus syndrome refers to this process resulting in symptomatic sinus bradycardia and/or periods of sinus arrest.[85] Sinus node dysfunction is usually representative of diffuse conduction disease, and accompanying AV block is not uncommon. Furthermore, symptomatic bradyarrhythmias may be accompanied by paroxysmal tachycardias such as atrial fibrillation. Because of diffuse conduction disease, atrial fibrillation sometimes presents with a rather slow ventricular response (in the absence of AV nodal-blocking drugs). The occurrence of alternating bradyarrhythmias and tachyarrhythmias are referred to as the "tachy-brady syndrome." The occurrence of paroxysmal atrial fibrillation in a patient with sinus node dysfunction may be a result of underlying heart disease with atrial dysfunction or to atrial escape in response to reduced sinus node automaticity. In fact, because the rate of impulse generation by the sinus node is generally depressed or may fail altogether, other automatic pacemakers within the conduction system may "rescue" the sinus node. These rescue rhythms may present as paroxysmal atrial rhythms or as a junctional escape rhythm.

The treatment of sinus node dysfunction involves the elimination of symptomatic bradycardia and the possibility of managing alternating tachycardias such as atrial fibrillation. In general, the long-term therapy of choice is a permanent ventricular pacemaker. Pacemaker therapy, however, should be reserved for patients with significant symptoms. In other words, the aim of pacing is not to correct electrocardiographic findings but to improve the patient's symptoms and quality of life.

Drugs that are commonly employed to treat supraventricular tachycardias should be used with caution, if at all, in the absence of a functioning pacemaker.[85] Type I agents such as quinidine can suppress the escape or rescue rhythms that appear in severe sinus bradycardia or sinus arrest. In this way they may transform an asymptomatic patient with bradycardia into a symptomatic one. It is also important to remember that the addition of type I antiarrhythmic agents can affect pacemaker threshold and result in loss of capture if the pacemaker is not appropriately interrogated and adjusted.[64] Other drugs that depress SA or AV nodal function such as β-blockers or calcium channel antagonists may significantly exacerbate bradycardia. Even agents with indirect sympatholytic actions such as α-methyldopa or clonidine may worsen sinus node dysfunction. Digitalis use in these patients is controversial, but in most cases, it can be used safely.

Another reason for paroxysmal bradycardia and sinus arrest that is not due directly to sinus node dysfunction is carotid-sinus hypersensitivity.[86,87] Again, this syndrome occurs commonly in the aged with underlying heart disease. Symptoms occur when the carotid sinus is stimulated, resulting in an accentuated baroreceptor reflex. Thus, the patient may experience paroxysmal episodes of dizziness or syncope because of sinus arrest due to increased vagal tone and sympathetic withdrawal (cardioinhibitory type), drop in systemic blood pressure due to sympathetic withdrawal (vasodepressor type), or both (mixed cardioinhibitory and vasodepressor types). The diagnosis can be confirmed by performing carotid sinus massage with electrocardiographic and blood pressure monitoring in controlled conditions.

Carotid-sinus hypersensitivity can also be treated with permanent pacemaker therapy.[86] However, some patients, particularly those with a significant vasodepressor component, still experience syncope or dizziness. In these cases, α-adrenergic stimulants such as ephedrine, sometimes in combination with β-blockers to achieve maximal α-sympathetic stimulation, can be tried in addition to the pacemaker.[87]

Another syndrome, vasovagal syncope, is believed to be the cause of syncope in many patients who present with recurrent syncope of unknown origin.[88,89] This reaction is presumed to be a neurally mediated, paradoxical reaction involving stimulation of cardiac mechanoreceptors (Bezold–Jarisch reflex). Forceful contraction of the ventricle coupled with low ventricular volumes provides a powerful stimulus for cardiac mechanoreceptors. Syncope results from the spontaneous development of transient hypotension (sympathetic withdrawal) and bradycardia (vagotonia). Patients believed to have frequent episodes of vasovagal syncope have been evaluated and diagnosed using the upright body tilt test, a potent stimulus for the development of vasovagal symptoms. Although commonly used, the sensitivity and reproducibility of this test have been questioned.

Vasovagal syncope can usually be successfully treated with oral β-blockers. Although these agents may seem inappropriate to treat a syndrome resulting from vasodilation and bradycardia, the therapeutic approach is designed to block an inappropriate vasovagal reaction. β-Blockers act by inhibiting the sympathetic surge that causes forceful ventricular contraction and precedes the onset of hypotension and bradycardia. Drug testing with IV esmolol or metoprolol during repeat head-up tilt tests has been used to predict the long-term response of oral β-blockers.[90] Other drugs that have been used successfully (with or without β-blockers) include scopolamine patches, α-adrenergic agonists, theophylline, dipyridamole, and disopyramide. More information is required, particularly comparative trials with effective agents, to make definitive conclusions regarding the place of these alternatives to β-blockers in this disorder.

ATRIOVENTRICULAR BLOCK

Conduction delay or block may occur in any area of the AV conduction system: the AV node, the His bundle, or the bundle branches. AV block is usually categorized into three different types based on surface electrocardiographic findings (Table 14–5). First-degree AV block is 1:1 AV conduction with a prolonged PR interval. Second-degree AV block is divided into two forms: Mobitz I AV block (Wenkebach periodicity) is less than 1:1 AV conduction with progressively lengthening PR intervals until a ventricular complex is dropped; Mobitz II AV block is intermittently dropped ventricular beats in a random fashion without progressive PR lengthening. Third-degree AV block is complete heart block where AV conduction is totally absent (AV dissociation). By using intracardiac His bundle electrocardiograms, the actual site of conduction delay/block can be correlated to the above diagnosis. First-degree AV block usually represents prolonged conduction in the AV node. Mobitz I, second-degree AV block is also usually a result of prolonged conduction in the AV node. Indeed, Wenkebach periodicity is a normal AV nodal response to rapid supraventricular stimulation or high vagal tone. In contrast, Mobitz II AV block is usually a result of conduction disease below the AV node (i.e., His bundle). Third-degree AV block may be caused by disease at any level of the AV conduction system: complete AV nodal block, His bundle block, or trifasicular block. The ventricle will beat independently of the atria (AV dissociation), and the rate of ventricular activation and QRS configuration are determined by the site of AV block. The usual degree of automaticity of ventricular pacemakers progressively declines as impulses move down the conduction system. Therefore, the ventricular escape rate in cases of trifasicular block will be significantly less than complete AV nodal block.

AV block may be found in patients without underlying heart disease such as trained athletes or during sleep when vagal tone is high. Also, AV block may be transient where the underlying etiology is reversible such as in myocarditis, myocardial ischemia, after cardiovascular surgery, or during drug therapy. β-Blockers, digitalis, or calcium antagonists may cause AV block, primarily in the AV nodal area. Type I antiarrhythmic agents may exacerbate conduction delays below the level of the AV node (sodium-dependant tissue). In other cases, AV block may be irreversible such as that due to acute myocardial infarction, rare degenerative diseases, primary myocardial disease, or congenital forms.

TABLE 14–5. Forms of Atrioventricular Block

Type	Criteria
First-degree block	Prolonged PR interval (> 0.2 s), 1:1 AV conduction
Second-degree block	
Mobitz I	Progressive PR prolongation until QRS is dropped, < 1:1 AV conduction
Mobitz II	Random nonconducted beats (absence of QRS), < 1:1 AV conduction
Third-degree block	AV dissociation, absence of AV conduction

▶ TREATMENT: Atrioventricular Block

The cornerstone to the acute treatment of acute, symptomatic bradycardia or AV block is temporary, transvenous pacing.[33] However, since it takes time for the insertion of a right ventricular lead, bridge therapy with transcutaneous pacing devices or drugs that improve sinus and AV nodal conduction (atropine, epinephrine infusion) should be used in the meantime. In the past, isoproterenol infusion was frequently chosen for this purpose but is now not recommended because of its vasodilating properties and its ability to increase myocardial oxygen consumption (particularly during acute infarction). Pharmacologic therapies such as atropine or sympathomimetics may improve symptoms and conduction in sinus bradycardia/arrest and AV nodal block. These agents will not help when the site of AV block is below the AV node (Mobitz II or trifasicular AV block).

Patients with chronic symptomatic AV block should be treated with the insertion of a permanent pacemaker. Patients without symptoms can usually be followed closely without the need for a pacemaker. Because symptoms often correlate with the ventricular rate and the ventricular rate corresponds to the site of block, pacemaker therapy is usually necessary in distal AV blocks such as those occurring in the His bundle or the bundle branches. Patients with acute myocardial infarction and evidence of new AV block or conduction disturbances will often require the insertion of a temporary transvenous pacemaker. AV block more commonly occurs as a complication of inferior wall infarcts because of high vagal innervation at this site, and the coronary blood flow to the nodal areas usually supplies the inferior wall. However, the AV block may be only transient, obviating the need for permanent pacing. In patients with chronic AV conduction disturbances, intracardiac recordings (His bundle electrocardiograms) are sometimes used to document the actual site of block and define the potential need for and specific type of pacemaker therapy.

EVALUATION OF THERAPEUTIC AND ECONOMIC OUTCOMES

Generally, patients who suffer from tachyarrhythmias can be monitored for one or several possible therapeutic outcomes. Obviously, the presence or recurrence of any arrhythmia can be documented by electrocardiographic means: surface ECG, Holter monitor, or event monitor. Furthermore, patients may experience a decrease in blood pressure that may result in symptoms from lightheadedness to abrupt syncope depending on the rate of the arrhythmia and the status of the underlying heart disease. For some patients, the potential alteration in hemodynamics may result in death if the arrhythmia is not detected and treated immediately. Besides these clinical outcomes, many patients with tachyarrhythmias experience alterations in quality of life owing to recurrent symptoms of the arrhythmia or from side effects of therapy. And, finally, there are the economic considerations of medical or surgical intervention, continued medical care, and chronic drug or non-drug treatment. In comparison to the treatment of other forms of cardiovascular disease, there are relatively few pharmacoeconomic analyses available. What exists has been comprehensively reviewed by Kupersmith et al[91,92] and is limited to the use of non-drug therapies such as the ICD or radiofrequency ablation. Since that technology is rapidly evolving, what is not cost-effective now may indeed be so in the next several years. For example, original cost-effectiveness analysis of the ICD showed it to be highly sensitive to the life of the generator, yet newer generation devices have made significant advances not only in the size but

TABLE 14–6. Outcomes—Arrhythmias

Mortality
Total, all-cause
Arrhythmic death (i.e., sudden)
Recurrences documented by ECG
Time to recurrence
Frequency of recurrences
Tolerance
Symptoms
Blood pressure
Rate of tachycardia
Necessity of non-drug interventions (e.g., ICD)
ICD shocks
Side effects of drugs/treatment complications
Quality of life
Economics
Outcomes specific to tachycardia (e.g., ventricular rate, systemic embolism in atrial fibrillation)

also with regard to battery life. Therefore, these data may not be relevant today.

Some therapeutic outcomes are unique to certain arrhythmias. For instance, patients with atrial fibrillation or flutter need to be monitored for thromboembolism and for complications of anticoagulation therapy (bleeding, drug interactions) prescribed to prevent it. However, the most important monitoring parameters for most patients fall into the following categories: (1) mortality (total and arrhythmic); (2) arrhythmia recurrence (duration, frequency, symptoms); (3) hemodynamic consequences (rate, blood pressure, symptoms); and (4) treatment complications (need for alternative or additional drugs, devices, surgery) (Table 14–6). Care should be taken when evaluating the arrhythmia literature to consider real outcomes. For example, total mortality is more meaningful than only sudden death rates; it is possible an intervention prevents arrhythmic death but patients die from other causes, leaving all-cause mortality unaltered. Likewise, surrogate markers of drug efficacy (noninducible tachycardia, suppression of minor arrhythmias) should be judged with some degree of skepticism. One should ask: Did the treatment make patients live longer (improve mortality)? Did it make them feel better (improve humanistic outcomes or quality of life)? And/or was it economically worth it (cost-effective)?

▶ PRINCIPLES OF PHARMACOTHERAPY

- Clinical tachycardias are most often caused by reentry; available drugs used in these disorders work by altering transmembrane ion movement affecting electrical conduction within the reentrant circuit.
- The use of antiarrhythmic drugs in the United States is declining because of major trials that show increased mortality with their use in several clinical situations, the realization of proarrhythmia as a significant side effect, and the advancing technology of non-drug therapies such as ablation and the internal cardioverter-defibrillator.
- Antiarrhythmic drugs frequently cause side effects and are complex in their pharmacokinetic characteristics. The therapeutic range of these agents provides only a rough guide to modifying treatment; it is preferable to attempt to define an individual's effective (or target) concentration and match that during long-term therapy.
- In patients with atrial fibrillation, therapy is aimed at controlling ventricular response (digoxin, calcium antagonists, β-blockers), preventing thromboembolic complications (warfarin, aspirin), and restoring and maintaining sinus rhythm (antiarrhythmic drugs, direct current cardioversion).
- Paroxysmal supraventricular tachycardia is usually a result of reentry in or proximal to the AV node or AV reentry incorporating an extra nodal pathway; common tachycardias can be terminated acutely with AV nodal-blocking agents such as adenosine and recurrences can be prevented by ablation with radiofrequency current.
- Patients with Wolff–Parkinson–White syndrome may have several different tachycardias that are acutely treated by different strategies: orthodromic reentry (adenosine or calcium antagonists), antidromic reentry (adenosine or procainamide), and atrial fibrillation (procainamide). AV nodal-blocking drugs are contraindicated with WPW and atrial fibrillation.
- Because of the Cardiac Arrhythmia Suppression Trials (type I agents) and Survival With Oral *d*-Sotalol Study (type III agent) that demonstrated increased mortality with antiarrhythmic drugs in patients with complex ectopy after myocardial infarction, antiarrhythmic drugs (except β-blockers) should not be used in these patients.
- Life-threatening proarrhythmia generally takes two forms: sinusoidal or incessant monomorphic ventricular tachycardia (type Ic agents) and torsades de pointes (quinidine-like agents, sotalol-like agents, and others such as select antihistamines).
- The clinical approach to patients with left ventricular dysfunction and nonsustained ventricular tachycardia is a major remaining controversy with three divergent strategies: invasive electrophysiologic studies with possible internal cardioverter-defibrillator implantation, empiric amiodarone therapy, and conservative (no treatment beyond β-blockers) management.
- Patients with hemodynamically significant ventricular tachycardia or ventricular fibrillation not associated with an acute myocardial infarction who are successfully resuscitated (lidocaine, amiodarone, bretylium) are at high risk for death and should receive implantation of an internal cardioverter-defibrillator.

REFERENCES

1. Allessie MA, Bonke FIM, Schopman FJG. Circus movement in rabbit atrial muscle as a mechanism of tachycardia. III. The "leading circle" concept: A new model of circus movement in cardiac tissue without the involvement of an anatomic obstacle. Circ Res 1977; 41:9–18.
2. Vaughan Williams EM. A classification of antiarrhythmic actions reassessed after a decade of new drugs. J Clin Pharmacol 1984; 24: 129–147.
3. Working Group on Arrhythmias of the European Society of Cardiology. The Sicilian Gambit. A new approach to the classification of antiarrhythmic drugs based upon their actions on arrhythmogenic mechanisms. Circulation 1991;84:1831–1851.
4. Hondeghem LM, Katzung BG. Antiarrhythmic agents: The modulated receptor mechanism of action of sodium and calcium channel-blocking drugs. Ann Rev Pharmacol Toxicol 1984;24:387–423.
5. Prystowsky EN, Benson W, Fuster V, et al. Management of patients with atrial fibrillation. A statement for healthcare professionals from the Subcommittee in Electrocardiography and Electrophysiology, American Heart Association. Circulation 1996;93:1262–1277.
6. Atrial Fibrillation Investigators. Risk factors for stroke and efficacy of antithrombotic therapy in atrial fibrillation. Analysis of pooled data from five randomized controlled trials. Arch Intern Med 1994; 154:1449–1457.
7. Laupacia A, Albers G, Dunn M, Feinberg W. Antithrombotic therapy in atrial fibrillation. Chest 1995;108:352S–359S.
8. Falk RH, Leavitt JI. Digoxin for atrial fibrillation: A drug whose time has gone? Ann Intern Med 1991;114:573–575.
9. Roberts SA, Diaz C, Nolan PE, et al. Effectiveness and costs of digoxin treatment for atrial fibrillation and flutter. Am J Cardiol 1993;72:567–573.
10. Ellenbogen KA, Dias VC, Plumb VJ, et al. A placebo-controlled trial of continuous intravenous diltiazem infusion for 24-hour heart rate control during atrial fibrillation and atrial flutter. A multicenter study. J Am Coll Cardiol 1991;18:891–897.
11. Barbarash R, Bauman JL, Srebro J, et al. Verapamil infusions in the treatment of atrial tachyarrhythmias. Crit Care Med 1986;14:886–888.
12. Feld GK, Fleck P, Fujimura O, et al. Control of rapid ventricular response by radiofrequency catheter modification of the atrioventricular node in patients with medically refractory atrial fibrillation. Circulation 1994;90:2299–2307.
13. Galve E, Ruis T, Ballester R, et al. Intravenous amiodarone in the treatment of recent-onset atrial fibrillation: Results of a randomized controlled study. J Am Coll Cardiol 196;27:1079–1082.
14. Boriani G, Biffi M, Alessandro C, et al. Oral propafenone to convert recent-onset atrial fibrillation in patients with and without underlying heart disease. A randomized, controlled trial. Ann Intern Med 1997;126:621–625.
15. Murray KT. Ibutilide. Circulation 1998;97:493–497.
16. Cropp JS, Antal EG, Talbert RL. Ibutilide: A new class III antiarrhythmic agent. Pharmacotherapy 1997;17:1–9.
17. Bauman JL, Bauernfeind RA, Hoff JV, et al. Torsades de pointes due to quinidine: Observations in 31 patients. Am Heart J 1984; 107:425–430.
18. The Stroke Prevention in Atrial Fibrillation Investigators. Stroke prevention in atrial fibrillation: Final results. Circulation 1991; 84: 527–539.
19. The Stroke Prevention in Atrial Fibrillation Investigators. Warfarin versus aspirin for prevention of thromboembolism in atrial fibrillation: Stroke Prevention in Atrial Fibrillation II Study. Lancet 1994; 343:687–691.
20. Gage BF, Cardinally AB, Abers GW, Owens DR. Cost-effectiveness of warfarin and aspirin for prophylaxis of stroke in patients with nonvalvular atrial fibrillation. JAMA 1995;274:1839–1845.
21. Coplen SE, Antman EM, Berlin JA, et al. Efficacy and safety of quinidine therapy for maintenance of sinus rhythm after cardioversion: A meta-analysis of randomized control trials. Circulation 1990; 82: 1106–1116.
22. Echt DS, Liebson PR, Mitchell B, et al. Mortality and morbidity in patients receiving encainide, flecainide, or placebo. The cardiac arrhythmia suppression trial. N Engl J Med 1991;324:781–788.
23. Flaker GC, Blackshear JL, McBride R, et al. Antiarrhythmic drug therapy and cardiac mortality in atrial fibrillation. J Am Coll Cardiol 1992;20:527–532.
24. Phillips BG, Bauman JL. Prescribing trends and pharmacoeconomic considerations of antiarrhythmic drugs; a focus on atrial fibrillation and flutter. Pharmacoeconomics 1995;7:521–533.
25. Gosselink ATM, Crijns HJM, VanGelder IC, et al. Low-dose amiodarone for maintenance of sinus rhythm after cardioversion of atrial fibrillation or flutter. JAMA 1992;267:3289–3292.
26. Juül-Moller S, Edvardsson N, Rehnqvist-Ahlberg N. Sotalol versus quinidine for the maintenance of sinus rhythm after direct current conversion of atrial fibrillation. Circulation 1990;82:1932–1939.
27. Nattel S. Newer developments in the management of atrial fibrillation. Am Heart J 1995;130:1094–1106.
28. Fischer B, Haissaguerre M, Garrigues S, et al. Radiofrequency catheter ablation of common atrial flutter in 80 patients. J Am Coll Cardiol 1995;25:1365–1372.
29. Sung RJ, Lauer MR, Chun H. Atrioventricular node reentry: Current concepts and new perspectives. Pacing Clin Electrophysiol 1994; 17:1413–1430.
30. Bauernfeind RA, Wyndham CR, Dhingra RC, et al. Serial electrophysiologic testing of multiple drugs in patients with atrioventricular nodal reentrant paroxysmal tachycardia. Circulation 1980; 62: 1341–1349.
31. Wu D, Amat-Y-Leon F, Simpson R, et al. Electrophysiological studies with multiple drugs in patients with atrioventricular reentrant tachycardias utilizing an extra nodal pathway. Circulation 1977; 56:727–736.
32. DiMarco JP, Miles W, Akhtar M, et al. Adenosine for paroxysmal supraventricular tachycardia: Dose ranging and comparison with verapamil. Assessment in placebo-controlled, multicenter trials. Ann Intern Med 1990;1113:104–110.
33. Cummins RO, ed. Advanced Cardiac Life Support. Dallas, TX, American Heart Association, 1997.
34. Rankin AC, McGovern BA. Adenosine or verapamil for the acute treatment of supraventricular tachycardia? Ann Intern Med 1991; 114:513–515.
35. Hoon TJ, Bauman JL, Rodvold KA, et al. The pharmacodynamic and pharmacokinetic differences of the *d*- and *l*- somers of verapamil: Implications in the treatment of PSVT. Am Heart J 1986;112: 396–403.
36. Bauernfeind RA, Swiryn S, Petropolous AT, et al. Concordance and discordance of drug responses in atrioventricular reentrant tachycardia. J Am Coll Cardiol 1983;2:345–350.
37. Jackman WM, Wang Z, Friday KJ, et al. Catheter ablation of accessory atrioventricular pathways (Wolff–Parkinson–White syndrome) by radiofrequency current. N Engl J Med 1991;324:1605–1611.
38. Jackman WM, Beckman KJ, McClelland JH, et al. Treatment of supraventricular tachycardia due to atrioventricular nodal reentry by radiofrequency catheter ablation of slow pathway conduction. N Engl J Med 1992;327:313–318.
39. Scheinman MM. Radiofrequency catheter ablation for patients with supraventricular tachycardia. Pacing Clin Electrophysiol 1993;16: 671–679.
40. Kastor JA. Multifocal atrial tachycardia. N Engl J Med 1990; 322:1713–1717.
41. Levine JH, Michael JR, Guarnier T. Treatment of multifocal atrial tachycardia with verapamil. N Engl J Med 1985;312:21–25.
42. Ruberman W, Weinblatt E, Goldberg JD, et al. Ventricular premature beats and mortality after myocardial infarction. N Engl J Med 1977; 297:750–757.
43. Lown B, Wolf M. Approaches to sudden death from coronary heart disease. Circulation 1971;44:130–142.

44. Winkle RA. Antiarrhythmic drug effect mimicked by spontaneous variability of ventricular ectopy. Circulation 1978;57:1116–1121.
45. Morganroth J, Michelson EL, Horowitz LN, et al. Limitations of routine electrocardiographic monitoring to assess ventricular ectopic frequency. Circulation 1978;58:408–414.
46. Kosowsky BD, Taylor J, Lown B, et al. Long-term procaine amide following acute myocardial infarction. Circulation 1973;47:1204–1210.
47. Bauman JL, Gallastegui J, Strasberg B, et al. Long-term therapy with disopyramide phosphate: Side effects and effectiveness. Am Heart J 1986;111:654–660.
48. Podrid PJ, Schoeneburger A, Lown B. Congestive heart failure caused by oral disopyramide. N Engl J Med 1980;302:614–617.
49. Dusman RE, Stanton MS, Miles WM, et al. Clinical features of amiodarone-induced pulmonary toxicity. Circulation 1990;82:51–59.
50. Podrid PJ. Amiodarone: Reevaluation of an old drug. Ann Intern Med 1995;122:689–700.
51. McCollam PL, Parker RB, Beckman KJ, et al. Proarrhythmia: A paradoxic response to antiarrhythmic agents. Pharmacotherapy 1989; 9:144–153.
52. The Cardiac Arrhythmia Suppression Trial II Investigators. Effect of the antiarrhythmic agent moricizine on survival after myocardial infarction. N Engl J Med 1992;327:227–233.
53. Waldo AL, Camm AJ, deRuyter H, et al. Effect of *d*-sotalol on mortality in patients with left ventricular dysfunction and remote myocardial infarction. Lancet 1996;348:7–12.
54. Julian DG, Camm AJ, Frangin G, et al. Randomised trial of effect of amiodarone on mortality in patients with left ventricular dysfunction after recent myocardial infarction: EMIAT. Lancet 1997;349:667–674.
55. Cairns JA, Connolly SJ, Roberts R, et al. Randomised trial of outcome after myocardial infarction in patients with frequent or repetitive ventricular premature depolarisations: CAMIAT. Lancet 1997;349: 675–682.
56. Bauman JL, Schoen MD, Hoon TJ. Practical optimization of antiarrhythmic drug therapy using pharmacokinetic principles. Clin Pharmacokinet 1991;20:151–166.
57. Greenspan AM, Spielman SR, Webb CR, et al. Efficacy of combination therapy with mexiletine and a type Ia agent for inducible ventricular tachyarrhythmias secondary to coronary artery disease. Am J Cardiol 1985;56:277–284.
58. The Cascade Investigators. Randomized antiarrhythmic drug therapy in survivors of cardiac arrest (the CASCADE Study). Am J Cardiol 1993;72:280–287.
59. Mitchell LB, Duff HJ, Manyari DE, et al. A randomized clinical trial of the noninvasive and invasive approaches to drug therapy of ventricular tachycardia. N Engl J Med 1987;317:1681–1687.
60. Mason JW and the Electrophysiologic Study versus Electrocardiographic Monitoring Investigators. A comparison of electrophysiologic testing with Holter monitoring to predict antiarrhythmic drug efficacy for ventricular tachyarrhythmias. N Engl J Med 1993; 329:445–451.
61. Mason JW and the Electrophysiologic Study versus Electrocardiographic Monitoring Investigators. A comparison of seven antiarrhythmic drugs in patients with ventricular tachyarrhythmias. N Engl J Med 1993;329:452–458.
62. Zipes DP. Cardiac electrophysiology: Promises and contributions. J Am Coll Cardiol 1989;13:1329–1352.
63. Powell AC, Fuchs T, Finklestein DM, et al. Influence of implantable cardioverter-defibrillators on long-term prognosis of survivors of out-of-hospital cardiac arrest. Circulation 1993;88:1083–1092.
64. Tworek DA, Nazari J, Ezri M, Bauman JL. Interference by antiarrhythmic agents with the function of electrical cardiac devices. Clin Pharm 1992;11:48–56.
65. Kim SG, Fisher JD, Furman S, et al. Benefits of implantable defibrillators are overestimated by sudden death rates and better represented by the total arrhythmic death rate. J Am Coll Cardiol 1991; 17: 1587–1592.
66. Moss AJ, Hall WJ, Cannom DS, et al. Improved survival with an implanted defibrillator in patients with coronary disease at high risk for ventricular arrhythmia. N Engl J Med 1996;335:1933–1940.
67. Wever EFD, Hauer RNW, Schrijvers G, et al. Cost-effectiveness of implantable defibrillator as first-choice therapy versus electrophysiologically guided tiered strategy in post infarct sudden death survivors. A randomized study. Circulation 1996;93:489–496.
68. Mitra RI, Buxton AE. The clinical significance of nonsustained ventricular tachycardia. J Cardiovasc Electrophysiol 1993;4:490–496.
69. Wilber DJ, Olshansky B, Moran JF, et al. Electrophysiological testing and nonsustained ventricular tachycardia. Use and limitations in patients with coronary artery disease and impaired ventricular function. Circulation 1990;82:350–358.
70. Gomes JA, Winters SL, Stewart D, et al. A new noninvasive index to predict sustained ventricular tachycardia and sudden death in the first year after myocardial infarction: Based on signal-averaged electrocardiogram, radionuclide ejection fraction and Holter monitoring. J Am Coll Cardiol 1987;10:349–357.
71. Herre JM, Titus C, Oeff M, et al. Inefficacy and proarrhythmic effects of flecainide and encainide for sustained ventricular tachycardia and ventricular fibrillation. Ann Intern Med 1990;113:671–676.
72. Ackerman MJ, Clapham DE. Ion channels—Basic science and clinical disease. N Engl J Med 1997;336:1575–1586.
73. Oberg KC, O'Toole MF, Gallastegui JL, Bauman JL. "Late" proarrhythmia due to quinidine. Am J Cardiol 1994;74:192–194.
74. Tzivoni D, Banai S, Schuger C, et al. Treatment of torsades de pointes with magnesium sulfate. Circulation 1987;77:392–397.
75. Zipes DP, Heger JJ, Prystowsky EN. Sudden cardiac death. Am J Med 1981;70:1151–1153.
76. Ruskin JN, DiMarco JP, Garan H. Out-of-hospital cardiac arrest. Electrophysiologic observation and selection of long-term antiarrhythmic therapy. N Engl J Med 1980;303:607–613.
77. Lie KI, Wellens HJJ, Van Capelle FJ. Lidocaine in the prevention of primary ventricular fibrillation. N Engl J Med 1974;291:1324–1326.
78. MacMahon S, Collin R, Peto R, et al. Effects of prophylactic lidocaine in suspected acute myocardial infarction. An overview of results from the randomized controlled trials. JAMA 1988;260: 1910–1916.
79. Antman EM, Berlin JA. Declining incidence of ventricular fibrillation in myocardial infarction. Implications for the prophylactic use of lidocaine. Circulation 1992;86:764–773.
80. Horner SM. Efficacy of intravenous magnesium in acute myocardial infarction in reducing arrhythmias and mortality. Meta-analysis of magnesium in acute myocardial infarction. Circulation 1992;86: 774–779.
81. Woods KL, Fletcher S, Roffe C, Haider Y. A randomized trial of intravenous magnesium sulfate in suspected acute myocardial infarction: Results of the second Leicester Intravenous Magnesium Intervention Trial (LIMIT-2). Lancet 1992;339:1553–1558.
82. Sleight P. Vasodilators after myocardial infarction—ISIS IV. Am J Hypertens 1994;7:1025–1055.
83. Brown CG, Martin DR, Pepe PE, et al. A comparison of standard-dose and high dose epinephrine in cardiac arrest outside the hospital. N Engl J Med 1992;327:1051–1055.
84. Kowey PR, Levine JH, Herre JM, et al. Randomized, double-blind comparison of intravenous amiodarone and bretylium in the treatment of patients with recurrent, hemodynamically destabilizing ventricular tachycardia or fibrillation. Circulation 1995;92:3255–3263.
85. Talano JV, Euler D, Randall WC, et al. Sinus node dysfunction. An overview with emphasis on autonomic and pharmacologic consideration. Am J Med 1978;64:773–781.
86. Sugrue DD, Gersh BJ, Holmes DR, et al. Symptomatic "isolated" carotid sinus hypersensitivity: Natural history and results of treatment with anticholinergic drugs or pacemaker. J Am Coll Cardiol 1986; 7:158–162.
87. Strasberg B, Sagie A, Erdman S, et al. Carotid sinus hypersensitivity and the carotid sinus syndrome. Prog Cardiovasc Dis 1989;31:379–391.

88. Milstein S, Reyes WJ, Benditt DG. Upright body tilt for evaluation of patients with recurrent, unexplained syncope. Pacing Clin Electrophysiol 1989;12:117–124.
89. Almquist A, Goldenberg I, Milstein S. Provocation of bradycardia and hypotension by isoproterenol and upright posture in patients with unexplained syncope. N Engl J Med 1990;320:346–351.
90. Sra JS, Vishnubhakta S, Murthy S, et al. Use of intravenous esmolol to predict efficacy of oral beta-adrenergic blocker therapy in patients with neurocardiogenic syncope. J Am Coll Cardiol 1992;19: 402–408.
91. Kupersmith J, Holmes-Novner M, Hogan A, et al. Cost-effectiveness analysis in heart disease, Part I: General principles. Prog Cardiovasc Dis 1994;37:161-184.
92. Kupersmith J, Holmes-Novner M, Hogan A, et al. Cost-effectiveness analysis in heart disease, Part III: Ischemia, congestive heart failure, and arrhythmias. Prog Cardiovasc Dis 1995;37:307–346.
93. Bauman JL. Understanding and treating supraventricular arrhythmias. Clin Pharm 1983;2:314.
94. Bauman JL, et al. Tachycardias. In Carter B, et al, eds. Pharmacotherapy Self-Assessment Program, 2nd ed. Kansas City, ACCP, 1995.
95. Scheinman MM. Catheter ablation. Present role and projected impact on health care for patients with cardiac arrhythmias. Circulation 1991; 83:1489–1498.
96. The CAST Investigators. Preliminary report: Effect of ecainide and flecainide on mortality in a randomized trial of arrhythmia suppression after myocardial infarction. N Engl J Med 1989;321:406–412.
97. Bauman JL. Drug Safety: Cardiac arrhythmias. Antihistamine update symposium. Hosp Med 1995;31:24.

15

CARDIOMYOPATHIES

Jean Nappi, PharmD, FCCP, BCPS

The cardiomyopathies represent a variety of diseases affecting the myocardium in either a diffuse or multifocal manner that frequently results in heart failure. The terminology and classification used for the cardiomyopathies is confusing due to overlap among the diseases and classification schemes. Cardiomyopathies are sometimes defined according to etiology or as primary or secondary forms. Primary cardiomyopathies are disorders where either the structure or function of the myocardium is affected in the *absence* of other known causes of heart disease or systemic diseases known to affect the heart. Secondary forms of cardiomyopathy are conditions where the myocardial abnormality is due to a recognized factor. Infectious agents, inflammation, metabolic disorders, infiltrative diseases, and toxins are a few of the causative factors of secondary cardiomyopathy.[1,2]

Many times a specific etiology is not evident. Therefore, another commonly used categorization of the cardiomyopathies is made on the basis of the structural or functional abnormalities present. The three groups of cardiomyopathies are usually described as dilated (congestive), hypertrophic, and restrictive. An understanding of the pathophysiologic basis for each type of cardiomyopathy leads to a rational selection of drug therapy or other treatment modality. The characteristics for each of the types of cardiomyopathy are presented in Table 15–1. The distinction among the cardiomyopathies is not absolute, and there is some overlap in the functional abnormalities.

In *dilated cardiomyopathy* (DCM), the cardinal feature is dilatation of the ventricles. Systolic function is abnormal, leading to a decreased cardiac output. In those patients with *hypertrophic cardiomyopathy* (HCM), the ventricular cavity is not dilated, and the ventricular muscle mass is increased. Ventricular cavity size is normal or decreased and systolic function is often preserved. Patients with HCM may have an obstructive or nonobstructive form. Patients with *restrictive cardiomyopathy* have inadequate ventricular compliance, causing diastolic dysfunction due to endocardial and/or myocardial disease. The clinical presentation is similar to constrictive pericarditis.

Other terms are frequently encountered in discussions of patients with cardiomyopathy. "Familial cardiomyopathy" is used to denote a condition found in more than one family member. Genetic predisposition may occur in all three functional types. "Ischemic cardiomyopathy" is another frequently used term. Patients with occlusive atherosclerotic coronary artery disease and left ventricular dysfunction are said to have ischemic cardiomyopathy. Ischemic cardiomyopathy is not a true cardiomyopathy, because there is an identifiable cause of the ventricular muscle dysfunction.

Myocardial hypertrophy is one of the most important adaptive measures that the failing heart uses to compensate for pressure and volume overload conditions. However, these hypertrophied cells are not normal, and this "cardiomyopathy of overload" may eventually lead to myocardial cell deterioration and death.[3] The role of altered gene expression in the hypertrophied myocardium is an area of extensive research. It appears that the phenotype of the hypertrophied heart differs from the normal heart. The expression of genes that encode the proteins responsible for contraction (myosin and actin) and relaxation (calcium–adenosine triphosphatase and phospholamban) appears to be of primary importance.[4]

DILATED CARDIOMYOPATHY

EPIDEMIOLOGY AND ETIOLOGY

Dilated cardiomyopathy is the most common of the cardiomyopathies. There are approximately 20,000 new cases of DCM diagnosed each year in the United States.[5] DCM occurs in people of all ages worldwide, but it is more frequent in African Americans and men, particularly those of middle age.[6] In the majority of patients, the cause is unknown; however, there are over 75 specific diseases of the heart muscle that can lead to DCM. DCM is characterized by systolic pump failure (ejection fraction < 0.4) and dilatation of the ventricles. Mural thrombi frequently occur in the left ventricle or atrial appendages. When there is no known cause, the term *idiopathic dilated cardiomyopathy* (IDC) is used.

The natural history of DCM is quite variable. Survival data from tertiary referral centers estimated that 25% to 30% of patients die within 1 year, whereas stabilization or even improvement may be seen in 20% to 50% of patients. More recent data suggests a 5-year mortality rate closer to 20%.[6] The usual course for DCM is steadily downhill, with death from progressive pump failure, ventricular tachycardia, or fibrillation. The prognosis depends primarily on the severity of left ventricular dysfunction at the time of diagnosis. Left bundle branch block has been found to be an adverse prognostic indicator by some investigators. Ventricular arrhythmias are common in patients with DCM, but their significance is unclear. The severity of left ventricular

TABLE 15–1. Characteristics of the Cardiomyopathies

	Dilated	Hypertrophic	Restrictive
Myocardial mass	↑ → ↑↑	↑↑↑	nl → ↑
Ventricular cavity size	↑↑ → ↑↑↑↑	↓↓ → nl	nl → ↓
Contractile function	↓↓↓	↑↑ → ↓	nl → ↓
LV filling pressure	↑↑	nl → ↑	↑
Chest x-ray	Moderate to marked cardiac enlargement	Mild to moderate cardiac enlargement	Mild cardiac enlargement
Electrocardiogram	ST and T-wave abnormalities	ST and T-wave abnormalities, left ventricular hypertrophy	Low voltage, conduction defects
Echocardiogram	LV dilatation and dysfunction	Asymmetric septal hypertrophy systolic anterior motion of the mitral valve	Increased LV wall thickness possible
Radionuclide studies	LV dilatation and dysfunction	Vigorous systolic function	Normal systolic function

↑ = increased; ↓ = decreased; nl = normal; LV = left ventricular.

dysfunction seems to be a more accurate and consistent predictor of sudden cardiac death than studies using ambulatory electrocardiographic recordings (Holter monitoring), programmed electrical stimulation (electrophysiologic testing), or signal-averaged electrocardiograms.[5,7]

There are many conditions associated with the development of DCM, including chronic alcoholism (alcoholic cardiomyopathy), pregnancy or the postpartum period (peripartum or postpartum cardiomyopathy), administration of anthracyclines (anthracycline cardiomyopathy), selenium deficiency (Keshan disease), and occlusive coronary artery disease (ischemic cardiomyopathy).

PATHOPHYSIOLOGY

In addition to dilatation of the ventricles and poor ventricular contractility, patients with DCM have an increase in myocardial mass and elevated left (and sometimes right) ventricular pressures. The pathophysiologic changes seen in patients with DCM are the same as those in patients with heart failure from other known causes (Chap. 11). There are short-term and long-term compensatory responses to the decrease in cardiac performance. What may be beneficial to sustain cardiac output for a short period of time is detrimental when sustained over a prolonged period.

Patients with cardiomyopathy undergo a progressive process that involves ventricular enlargement, eccentric hypertrophy, mechanical inefficiency, and depressed ventricular performance. The initial insult may be due to ischemic insufficiency (infarction), inflammation (myocarditis), hemodynamic overload (hypertension or valvular disease), or genetic causes (inherited disorders of metabolism or abnormalities of contractile and structural proteins). Many times a cause is never identified.[8]

Compensatory mechanisms are thought to be triggered by tissue hypoperfusion and central venous congestion. Pump performance is enhanced by increasing heart rate and contractility, increasing preload, and increasing the mass of the contractile elements (hypertrophy). An increase in the autonomic (adrenergic) and the renin–angiotensin systems is primarily responsible for activating and sustaining the compensatory mechanisms. These two systems cross-regulate each other such that activation of one increases the activity of the other.[8] Initially these mechanisms stabilize blood pressure and redistribute cardiac output to the brain and heart. However, eventually the increase in peripheral resistance and left ventricular wall stress leads to a decrease in ventricular performance. Because of this, there is also activation of several counterregulatory mechanisms (atrial naturetic peptide and vasodilatory prostaglandins) that enhance vasodilatation and minimize the vasoconstrictive effects of α-adrenergic and angiotensin II vasoconstriction.

The progression of left ventricular dysfunction is due to continued myocyte dysfunction and cell loss. There are several proposed mechanisms whereby the compensatory responses may ultimately cause harm. The failing heart requires more oxygen due to the increases in heart rate, contractility, and wall stress, but structural changes make coronary perfusion less efficient; therefore the heart becomes "energy-starved." The β-adrenergic system mediates the release of angiotensin II and norepinephrine, both of which are thought to be directly cardiotoxic to the myocyte. In addition, through the process of ventricular hypertrophy, alterations in gene expression affect calcium handling and changes in the contractile proteins, leading to inefficient contraction. Some of these changes are thought to be due to an up-regulation in gene expression of atrial naturetic peptide and down-regulation in the expression of sarcoplasmic reticulum calcium ATPase and α-myosin heavy chain.[8]

The failing heart also loses its ability to respond to sympathetic neurotransmitters. This is partially explained by the decrease in total β-adrenergic receptor density (also known as down-regulation).[5] The human heart contains both β_1- and β_2-receptors in a ratio of approximately 80 to 20 (β_1 to β_2). The β_1-adrenergic receptor density is decreased by approximately 60% to 70% in the failing heart, changing the β_1 to β_2 ratio to 60 to 40. Although the density of the β_2-receptor is unchanged, the receptor is partially "uncoupled" from the adenylate cyclase enzyme. Although desensitization of the β-adrenergic system blunts the response of the failing heart to sympathetic stimulation, other biochemical processes leading to increased inotropy are intact. It is not clear whether the desensitization of the β-adrenergic receptors is beneficial or harmful in patients with heart failure.

Although it was thought that the adaptive mechanism of hypertrophy was intended to preserve myocardial function, it is ultimately detrimental. The hypertrophy that occurs in response to heart failure can exacerbate the energy production/expenditure imbalance. The distance between the capillaries and the impaired diffusion of substrates is problematic. Myofibrils, which are energy consumers, take up a larger portion of the cell relative to the energy-providing mitochondria. This further leads to the chronic energy deprivation of the myocardium. Myocyte necrosis stimulates the proliferation of fibroblasts, which replace myocardial tissue with connective tissue. Patients with DCM have an increase in intramyocardial fibrillar collegen that may adversely affect ventricular compliance.[9]

In addition to myocyte dysfunction, patients with cardiomyopathy suffer from the loss of myocytes. Myocyte loss occurs via two general mechanisms: apoptosis and necrosis.[10] Necrosis is due to the cytotoxic effects of norepinephrine and angiotensin II. Apoptosis (or programmed cell death) is a result of cell cycle dysfunction, where the myocyte is responding to stimuli that usually promote growth. Angiotensin II and tumor necrosis factor-α (TNF-α) are both stimulators of growth and may enhance apoptosis.[8]

Up to 20% of the cases of idiopathic DCM may be familial. Autosomal dominant, autosomal recessive, and X-linked transmission have been reported.[11] DCM is also commonly seen in patients with Duchenne's muscular dystrophy and may be related to specific mutations of the Xp21 locus of the dystrophin gene. Others have shown an increased frequency of HLA-DR4 in patients with IDC, so that a linkage of DCM to the HLA locus is possible. In addition, the synthesis of the myosin heavy chains, which determine ATPase activity, is altered.

It has been noted that there is a 30% to 40% increase in the activity of the inhibitory guanine nucleotide-binding protein (G_i proteins) in myocardial cells in failing hearts. The change in the G_i protein blunts the response of the failing heart to sympathetic stimulation.[8] Furthermore, there is evidence for the existence of anti-β-receptor antibodies that inhibit adenylate cyclase activity in some patients with DCM.[12] The presence of these antibodies may be linked to specific human leukocyte antigen (HLA) phenotypes.

Alcohol consumption causes an acute depressant effect on myocardial contractility, even in normal subjects. Impaired early filling of the left ventricle due to delayed relaxation has been noted in asymptomatic alcoholics.[13] This diastolic dysfunction may be one of the earliest signs of alcoholic cardiomyopathy. Although a direct causal relation between alcohol ingestion and heart disease is well supported, the mechanism by which chronic alcohol consumption may cause progressive cardiomyopathy is not known. Alcoholic cardiomyopathy is indistinguishable from IDC except that it may be reversible if alcohol consumption is completely stopped.[1] The amount of alcohol necessary to cause permanent damage is highly variable. Nutritional deficiencies may also play a role. The presence of skeletal muscle weakness in an alcoholic should trigger an evaluation of cardiac function.[14]

Selenium deficiency has caused cardiomyopathy (Keshan disease) in China and may also be a cause of increased platelet aggregation. Selenium appears to be required for normal immune function in some species. In the United States, selenium deficiency might occur in the setting of prolonged total parenteral nutrition. Hypophosphatemia, hypocalcemia, beriberi, pellagra, scurvy, and carnitine deficiency have also been identified as affecting cardiac function.[1,2]

Myocarditis is defined as inflammation and injury of the myocardium in the absence of ischemia.[15] The clinical presentation of myocarditis varies from an asymptomatic state to acute heart failure or sudden cardiac death. Animal models suggest that myocardial damage occurs in two phases. The acute phase involves cellular destruction due to replication of an organism and the subsequent reaction to cellular or humoral defense mechanisms. The second phase involves myocardial infiltration by inflammatory cells and the production of cardiotropic antibodies. Others have suggested that repeated episodes of microvascular spasm, secondary to endothelial cell infection, may lead to cellular damage. Serologic studies have shown that patients with myocarditis or DCM have a higher incidence of antibodies to a variety of viruses, particularly Coxsackie B3. Some patients with myocarditis may also have antibodies against myosin.[16] Many viral, bacterial, protozoal, and fungal organisms have been identified as potential causes of myocarditis.[17] The incidence of DCM following biopsy-proven myocarditis has been estimated to be as high as 25% to 50%. However, this incidence may be overestimated, because many cases of myocarditis are asymptomatic and never diagnosed. The true natural history of myocarditis is poorly defined. It has been suggested that there are immunoregulatory defects (abnormalities in suppressor T-cell function and reduction in natural killer cells) in patients with DCM or myocarditis. These defects could lead to an exaggerated immune response and unchecked myocardial inflammation.

Three types of anthracycline-induced cardiotoxicity have been described.[18] There is an acute injury that occurs immediately after treatment and manifests as a transient arrhythmia, pericarditis-myocarditis syndrome, or acute failure. This acute type of toxicity is rare. The more common toxicity is known as "chronic cardiotoxicity." Chronic cardiotoxicity presents as cardiomyopathy within 1 year of completion of anthracycline treatment. The third type of cardiotoxicity is of late-onset (years to decades after treatment), and presents as cardiomyopathy and/or arrhythmias.

The chronic cardiomyopathy is caused by an anthracycline-induced selective inhibition of cardiac muscle gene expression for α-actin, troponin, myosin light-chain 2, and the M isoform of creatine kinase.[18] The proposed mechanisms of action at the cellular level that cause myofibrillar loss include free-radical-mediated injury, damage from calcium overload, disturbances in adrenergic function, release of vasoactive amines or proinflammatory cytokines, and cellular toxicity from metabolites of doxorubicin.

It is well known that there is a relationship between anthracycline doses and the development of cardiomyopathy. Heart failure rarely occurs at cumulative doxorubicin doses below 450 mg/m^2, but, the incidence of cardiomyopathy is 7% at cumulative doses of 550 mg/m^2. There is a considerable amount of variability among patients with regard to the damage done and the dose received. In addition to the cumulative anthracycline dose, radiation to the mediastinal area will also predispose the patient to cardiomyopathy. The degree of myocardial cell damage found with biopsy is proportional to the dose received, but myocardial function is preserved until a threshold dose or critical amount of damage occurs. This means that a certain amount of myocardial damage must occur before cardiac function is affected. Once this deterioration process begins, it will proceed quite rapidly.

Evaluations of left ventricular ejection fraction should be performed routinely in order to assess risk for anthracycline cardiomyopathy. Serial gated equilibrium radionuclide measures of left ventricular ejection fraction are sensitive measures to detect subclinical cardiac contractile dysfunction and are commonly used.[19] In addition to measuring left ventricular ejection fraction, the analysis of peak filling rate (the peak slope of the cardiac filling curve) provides insight to diastolic function and improves the sensitivity of the test. Abnormalities in diastolic function have been found to precede a decrease in systolic function in many patients with doxorubicin-induced cardiomyopathy.

There are a number of methods available that attempt to decrease the incidence of anthracycline cardiotoxicity. Alterations in dosing schedules have increased the cumulative amount of anthracycline that patients can tolerate. Although the optimal dosing schedule of doxorubicin has yet to be established, it is thought that prolonged continuous infusions will decrease cardiotoxicity without compromising the antitumor effect of the drug.[18] Liposomal drug delivery systems are also being investigated and may be less cardiotoxic.

Doxorubicin is able to chelate iron, and the resulting iron complex can bind to DNA and cell membranes and catalyze the cleavage of hydrogen peroxide to the hydroxyl radical. Dexrazoxane (Zinecard), an iron chelator, appears to reduce free-radical generation and thus offer protection against the cardiotoxicity of doxorubicin. Dexrazoxane has permitted breast cancer patients to receive more cycles and higher cumulative doses of doxorubicin while protecting them from cardiotoxicity.[20] Dexrazoxane is currently approved for use in patients with metastatic breast cancer after a cumulative doxorubicin dose of 300 mg/m^2 has been given. Concerns have been raised regarding the interference of dexrazoxane with the efficacy of doxorubicin, and further study is needed.

Those patients with ischemic cardiomyopathy may have a form of DCM that is characterized by discrete but multifocal sites of myocardial damage. Necrosis due to infarction places a demand on the surviving tissue to sustain cardiac function. This is done through the process of hypertrophy of the myocytes and hyperplasia of the interstitial fibroblasts and endothelial cells.[21] Unfortunately, there is usually inadequate growth of the vascular beds to sustain this hypertrophied tissue, leading to continued ischemia and necrosis. Pump function is reduced in direct proportion to the amount of necrosed myocardium. Persistent left ventricular dysfunction in the absence of tissue necrosis is referred to as “hibernating myocardium.”[22] Improvement in ventricular function is possible, even after years of impairment, if revascularization is successful.

The cardiomyopathy associated with pregnancy usually develops during the latter part of pregnancy or within the first few months after delivery. Some women spontaneously recover, whereas others will have a rapidly fatal course. In one study of 26 matched female patients, significant differences between patients with IDC and patients with peripartum cardiomyopathy were described.[23] Both groups had high elevated filling pressures. Right-sided filling pressures tended to be higher in the IDC group, but the difference was not statistically significant. The patients with peripartum cardiomyopathy had a higher mean cardiac index, with 3 patients having a cardiac index level above the upper limit of normal. The patients with peripartum cardiomyopathy had a significantly lower mean systemic vascular resistance and lower right ventricular stroke work index when compared to the women with IDC. It would appear that peripartum cardiomyopathy does not have a homogenous hemodynamic presentation. There is a subset of patients with peripartum cardiomyopathy who have high output cardiac failure. Prior myocarditis may play a role in some patients. Women who recover should be encouraged to avoid further pregnancies, especially if cardiomegaly persists.[1]

CLINICAL PRESENTATION

The diagnosis of DCM is usually one of exclusion. The differential diagnosis includes other causes of congestive heart failure, specifically atherosclerotic heart disease, hypertensive heart disease, valvular disease, and heart muscle disease secondary to other systemic disease. The signs and symptoms of DCM are similar to those seen in patients with congestive heart failure, (see Chap. 11). The onset of heart failure is frequently insidious and commonly manifests initially as dyspnea. Fatigue, orthopnea, paroxysmal nocturnal dyspnea, peripheral edema, tachycardia, and palpitations gradually appear in most patients. Chest pain occurs in one-fourth to one-half of patients, consistent with myocardial ischemia despite normal coronary arteries.[4] Typical auscultatory findings include systolic murmurs secondary to mitral regurgitation and a third heart sound or a summation gallop. Although the heart is increased in weight, the thickness of the left ventricular free wall is diminished due to the ventricular dilatation.

Ischemic cardiomyopathy is more commonly seen than IDC in the United States. The opposite is true in the underdeveloped nations of the world, where an infectious agent may be the cause. Viral, bacterial, rickettsial, mycobacterial fungal, parasitic, and spirochetal organisms have been implicated as causative agents.[1]

Blood gases show a reduced oxygen saturation of the mixed venous blood sample, resulting in a high arteriovenous oxygen difference. Elevated pulmonary artery pressure may ultimately lead to right-sided heart failure. Patients may suffer from thromboembolic complications as a result of the mural thrombi that form in either the left or right side of the heart.

The chest roentgenogram demonstrates cardiac enlargement due to dilatation of both ventricles. The atria may also be enlarged. There may be pulmonary vascular redistribution changes and pleural and pericardial effusions. The electrocardiogram may have nonspecific ST-T wave changes. Sinus tachycardia is frequently present. Atrial fibrillation is common, as is left bundle branch block. Frequent ventricular ectopy and nonsustained ventricular tachycardia have been noted.[4] Gated blood pool scans (radionuclide angiography) will show that the ventricles have a global or homogeneous reduction in wall motion. The ejection fraction may be as low as 10%.

Echocardiography is the most useful initial diagnostic tool.[6] Left ventricular dilatation and global hypokinesis are common. An ejection fraction below 45% is generally required for diagnosis. Hemodynamic studies will reveal a reduced cardiac output that does not increase normally with exercise. Left ventricular end-diastolic, left atrial, and pulmonary capillary wedge pressures are usually elevated. When right-sided heart failure is present, the right ventricular end-diastolic, right atrial, and central venous pressures will be elevated. Coronary angiography may be necessary to differentiate IDC from ischemic cardiomyopathy.[4]

The results of an endomyocardial biopsy tend to be nonspecific in most cases of DCM. Biopsy may be helpful if there is a suspicion of active myocarditis and specific inflammatory changes are seen. Other indications for endomyocardial biopsy are for the detection of cardiac involvement in systemic diseases like amyloidosis and sarcoidosis and for the diagnosis of rejection following cardiac transplantation.[17]

▶ TREATMENT: Dilated Cardiomyopathy

When a patient first presents with the signs and symptoms of cardiomyopathy, other causes or conditions associated with cardiomyopathy should first be excluded. A systemic disorder with myocardial involvement can usually be excluded by a thorough history and physical examination with appropriate laboratory studies. Pericardial disease can be identified by echocardiography or other cardiac imaging studies. Ischemic cardiomyopathy is determined by performing a coronary angiogram. It may be more appropriate to treat the underlying cause or condition rather than the patient's symptoms.

Patients with DCM are generally treated in the same manner as those with congestive heart failure (see Chap. 11). Therapy is aimed at improving the signs and symptoms of heart failure and prolonging survival. Strategies include sodium restriction, diuretics, angiotensin-converting enzyme inhibitors, or other vasodilators and inotropic agents, which will not be discussed in detail in this chapter. Nonpharmacologic therapy includes avoiding strenuous activity. Patients with ischemic cardiomyopathy may benefit from revascularization. Alcohol should be completely avoided (particularly in the case of alcoholic cardiomyopathy). Pregnancy is not advised in women with a history of peripartal cardiomyopathy.[1]

NONPHARMACOLOGIC THERAPY

Just as short-term responses to drug therapy do not always predict long-term effects, improvements in hemodynamic measurements and exercise capacity do not always translate into improved survival. Other nonpharmacologic modes of therapy are also being investigated. Improvements in both symptoms and hemodynamic variables have been reported with dual chamber pacing.[24] The mechanism by which pacing improves cardiomyopathy is probably related to factors influencing preload or afterload rather than heart rate or myocardial contractility. Ventricular filling may be improved by a controlled atrioventricular delay leading to an improved "atrial kick." As more data become available, the role of pacemakers in the setting of DCM will be evaluated.

SURGICAL THERAPY

For the patient with ischemic cardiomyopathy, a coronary artery bypass graft (CABG) may offer improvement in myocardial function. However, this procedure would not be helpful in patients with ischemic cardiomyopathy whose lesions are diffuse. Cardiomyoplasty is a procedure where skeletal muscle (latissimus dorsi) is wrapped around the heart and then stimulated to contract in synchrony with the heart. This is a relatively new procedure with limited results. Some investigators have reported increases in left ventricular ejection fraction, but long-term increases in peak exercise did not occur.[25]

Lastly, cardiac transplantation is an option. The survival rate following cardiac transplantation has improved dramatically with the advent of improved immunosuppression (see Chap. 16). However, due to the limited supply of donors, relatively few patients with cardiomyopathy will be able to receive a new heart.

Implantable left ventricular assist devices (LVADs) are being used as long-term bridges to cardiac transplantation.

PHARMACOLOGIC THERAPY

IMMUNOSUPPRESSION

When a patient presents with the recent onset of the signs and symptoms of heart failure and no apparent cause, the differential diagnosis is frequently between myocarditis and the early phase of DCM. This distinction is important if one believes that treating myocarditis with immunosuppression could be beneficial. The exact relationship between myocarditis and DCM has yet to be established. However, endomyocardial biopsy findings consistent with the diagnosis of myocarditis can be found in some patients (ranging from 0% to 67%) with recent onset of symptoms suggesting DCM.[17] The large range among studies may be due to different diagnostic criteria used and the length of time from the onset of symptoms to the time of biopsy. Although specific criteria for endomyocardial biopsy (Dallas classification system) have been established for making the diagnosis of myocarditis, the true incidence of the disease is difficult to assess. There is a possibility that patchy or focal myocarditis may exist and that due to sampling error, the diagnosis is missed when performing endomyocardial biopsy. The natural history of viral myocarditis is ill defined. Persistent inflammation following myocardial infection has been thought to be a common cause of DCM. Patients with myocarditis are usually younger, and the left ventricular dysfunction less severe, when compared to those with DCM. In the majority of cases, the clinical course is benign and complete recovery without sequelae is expected. In those patients with residual left ventricular dysfunction after the acute illness, 50% will show gradual improvement.[26]

The results of studies using immunosuppressives in patients with biopsy-proven myocarditis have varied greatly. This is not surprising given the difficulty in making the diagnosis and the variability in the clinical course of the disease. In addition, many of the studies published have not been randomized and/or controlled. The results of a randomized, multicenter study of patients with myocarditis sponsored by the National Institutes of Health (myocarditis treatment trial) did not demonstrate any difference in outcome measurements between patients with biopsy-proven myocarditis who were randomized to either conventional therapy for heart failure or conventional therapy plus immunosuppression with cyclosporin and/or prednisone.[27] Although overall there was no demonstrable benefit from immunosuppression, there may be some subsets of patients who respond favorably. It is not known if antiviral therapy would be beneficial in patients with documented viral cardiomyopathy.

β-BLOCKADE

As described earlier, cardiac contractility is regulated in part by the autonomic nervous system. Sympathetic nerves innervate the ventricles, resulting in a potent inotropic effect. Although there are other receptors in the myocardium, the β-adrenergic pathway is the most potent in terms of stimulating cardiac contractility. Both β_1- and β_2-adrenergic receptors are coupled to adenylate cyclase stimulation and myocardial contractility. Norepinephrine, by virtue of its higher affinity for β_1-receptors, acts as a relatively selective β_1-agonist.[5] In the setting of heart failure, circulating levels of norepinephrine are increased and correlate with the severity of the disease. Patients with a high plasma norepinephrine level have a less favorable prognosis. Norepinephrine is a potent vasoconstrictor and increased levels lead to an increase in systemic vascular resistance. The failing heart already has an imbalance between energy expenditure and energy production, and excessive sympathetic stimulation may lead to a further imbalance. Increased sympathetic stimulation may contribute to arrhythmogenesis and sudden cardiac death. Excessive catecholamines may also have a direct toxic effect on the myocardium, resulting in intracellular calcium overload. Clinical trials with the inotropes milrinone and intermittent dobutamine were stopped prematurely due to the higher mortality rate in treated patients. Therefore it has been proposed that the β_1-adrenergic receptors are "down-regulated" as a protective mechanism from overstimulation by the sympathetic nervous system in the failing heart.

TABLE 15–2. Classification of β-blockers

First generation	Nonselective with no ancillary properties (propranolol, timolol)
Second generation	Selective for subtypes of β-receptors with no ancillary properties (metoprolol, atenolol, bisoprolol)
Third generation	Nonselective with ancillary properties (carvedilol, labetalol, bucindolol)

For years, clinicians were taught that β-blocking agents were contraindicated in patients with heart failure. It was believed that the heart required the increase in sympathetic activity in order to compensate for the decrease in myocardial function. This concept was first questioned in the 1970s, when β-blockers were used clinically in patients with heart failure and tachycardia, and reported to have beneficial effects.

In the last two decades, β-blockers have been shown to improve ventricular function, energy utilization, and clinical symptoms of patients with systolic dysfunction. Some trials have suggested that β-blockers may improve survival in patients with heart failure.[28] Recently, carvedilol was the first β-blocker approved for use in patients with heart failure.

There are three "generations" of β-blockers, (Table 15–2). Carvedilol and labetalol have a moderate α-receptor antagonist property, thus providing vasodilator activity; whereas bucindolol's vasodilatory effect is thought to be mediated by a cyclic guanosine monophosphate-dependent mechanism. Carvedilol and its metabolite also have antioxidant properties, which may contribute to its beneficial effect. Beta-blockers with vasodilatory properties (that offset the negative inotropic effects) are better tolerated in patients with systolic dysfunction, but there are no studies to date that compare β-blockers to each other, and there are no conclusive data to suggest that there is a difference in effect on survival.[28]

Several characteristics have been noted in those trials where patients receiving β-blockade have shown improvement. The initial dose of the β-blocker has been very small and increased in a gradual fashion over 1 to 2 months. In addition, the hemodynamic or functional improvement occurred over a period of months in most patients. Several of the studies showing a poor response to β-blockade evaluated the patients after a short duration

TABLE 15–3. Dosing Regimens for Commonly Used β-blockers in Heart Failure

Drug	Starting Dose	Maximal Dose
Metoprolol	6.25 mg po BID	75 mg po BID
Labetalol	5 mg po BID	100 mg po BID
Bisoprolol	1.25 mg po QD	10 mg po QD
Carvedilol	3.125 mg po BID	50 mg po BID
Bucindolol	3 mg po BID	100 mg po BID

TABLE 15–4. Therapeutic Approaches to Decompensation During Titration with β-Blockers

Problem	Strategy
Fluid retention that responds to increased diuretic or ACE inhibitor	Treat as an outpatient with increased diuretic or ACE inhibitor. Reduce or slow titration of β-blocker.
Recurrent fluid retention unresponsive to diuresis	Consider intermittent short courses of low-dose inotropic therapy (milrinone) or intravenous vasodilator. If patient cannot be maintained on β-blocker, reduce gradually.
Cardiogenic shock	Discontinue β-blocker and administer inotrope. Restart β-blocker when patient is well compensated.

From Ref. 32.

of treatment (e.g., 1 month) or started therapy with a "usual" maintenance dose of the drug instead of a gradual titration. Table 15–3 lists the most commonly used dosing regimens of β-blocker therapy for patients with heart failure. Increases in doses should occur on a weekly basis by doubling the previous dose.[28] Up-titration is most difficult in the early weeks of the initiation of therapy, and may have to go more slowly early in the course of treatment. Table 15–4 provides approaches on how to treat patients who decompensate during titrations with β-blockade.

VASODILATORS

Patients with heart failure due to various types of cardiomyopathy are frequently included in clinical heart failure trials using a variety of treatment modalities. The use of vasodilators, including calcium channel blockers, nitrates, angiotensin-converting enzyme (ACE) inhibitors, and angiotensin II receptor antagonists in the treatment of heart failure are discussed in detail in Chapter 11.

The rationale for the use of calcium channel blockers in patients with heart failure includes their vasodilatory and anti-ischemic effects and their ability to reduce diastolic dysfunction.[29] By decreasing systemic vascular resistance, which results in afterload reduction, cardiac output is often enhanced. However, some calcium channel blockers also have the propensity to cause a decrease in myocardial contractility. This negative inotropic property may offset any potential benefit from the vasodilatation. More recent and ongoing trials in patients with heart failure are using the second-generation dihydropyridine calcium channel blockers (amlodipine, felodipine, and nisoldipine).[30] These newer agents have fewer direct effects on myocardial contractility and are sometimes referred to as being vasoselective.

Amlodipine was compared to placebo in a double-blind fashion to over 1100 patients with ejection fractions less than 30% despite treatment with digoxin, diuretics, and ACE inhibitors in the PRAISE (prospective randomized amlodipine survival evaluation) trial.[31] There was no significant difference in survival in patients with ischemic heart disease. In patients with nonischemic cardiomyopathy, amlodipine was associated with a better outcome. In the PRAISE II trial, the use of amlodipine is being evaluated in patients with nonischemic causes of cardiomyopathy. The V-HeFT III trial evaluated the use of felodipine in a similar manner.[32] In V-HeFT III, felodipine was shown to be safe and well tolerated, but was no different than placebo when looking at the end points of mortality or hospitalizations. Combination therapy with ACE inhibitors and verapamil is possible; small trials have shown beneficial effects. Calcium channel blockers are appropriate for use in those patients with ongoing ischemia.

Nitrates have been used in patients with heart failure for many years. Nitrates act by reducing systemic and coronary vascular resistance and by minimizing left ventricular dilation through their effects on the venous capacitance vessels. Additionally, coronary blood flow is shifted to enhance endocardial perfusion. Their use results in a reduction in mitral regurgitation, improvement in exercise tolerance, and prevention of remodeling.[33] Nitrates have been shown to prolong survival when used in conjunction with hydralazine for CHF. Large clinical trials specifically designed to evaluate the effectiveness of nitrate therapy alone do not exist. Concern has been raised regarding the tolerance known to develop to some of the hemodynamic effects of nitrates, although it is not clear whether tolerance to the effect on the venous or arterial vasculature predominates.[34] In addition, most of the studies examining nitrate tolerance have been done in patients with angina, not heart failure. How the concurrent use of ACE inhibitors and diuretics affects nitrate tolerance is unclear at this time. Until definitive studies are done in this patient population, a nitrate-free interval should be recommended.

One of the most significant advances in the therapy of heart failure has been the demonstration of a decrease in mortality and morbidity secondary to the use of ACE inhibitors (see Chap. 11 for a detailed discussion). In most studies with symptomatic patients, an ACE inhibitor has been added to a regimen of digoxin and diuretic. It is interesting to note that angiotensin II is not only a vasoconstrictor but also a mitogen, whereas bradykinin is a vasodilator and an inhibitor of cell growth. The effects that the ACE inhibitors have on cell growth may contribute in an important way to the beneficial effects seen in clinical trials.[3] As mentioned previously, combination therapy with calcium channel blockers that have negative inotropic effects is also under investigation. It is not known at this time whether there are significant differences among the different ACE inhibitors in terms of patient outcomes.

INOTROPIC AGENTS

In addition to digoxin, which will not be discussed in this chapter, investigations with β-adrenergic agonists and phosphodiesterase inhibitors have been carried out in patients with cardiomyopathy. The β-adrenergic agonists enhance contractility by stimulating either β_1- or β_2-receptors, which in turn stimulate adenylate cyclase to produce cyclic AMP. Cyclic AMP is active until it is destroyed by cytoplasmic phosphodiesterase. The use of β-adrenergic agonist agents such as pirbuterol, albuterol, and prenaterol was disappointing. Down-regulation of β-adrenergic receptors was exacerbated with chronic dosing of these agents, and despite initial beneficial hemodynamic effects, chronic dosing led to tachyphylaxis and loss of effectiveness.[35] Intermittent intravenous infusions of dobutamine have been tried, but the enthusiasm for such regimens was tempered when a controlled trial was halted due to a high mortality rate. Intravenous infusions of dobutamine cause a transient hypokalemia, which could contribute to proarrhythmia.

The phosphodiesterase inhibitors amrinone, milrinone, and vesnarinone increase myocardial contractility by inhibiting the phosphodiesterase enzyme, which is responsible for the breakdown of cyclic AMP. Short-term beneficial hemodynamic effects have been observed with the phosphodiesterase inhibitors. Increases in cardiac output and ejection fraction, along with decreases in systemic vascular resistance and left- and right-sided filling pressures, have been noted. Unfortunately, proarrhythmia is associated with the use of these agents. It is possible that excess mortality may be due to using doses that were too high; however, a dosing regimen that exerts a beneficial hemodynamic effect without adverse effects has not been identified.

Patients refractory to oral therapy may require inotropic support as a bridge to transplantation or for symptomatic relief. Both intermittent and continuous infusions of dobutamine and milrinone can be used (occasionally in combination), although the long-term safety of such regimens is unproven.[36]

ANTIARRHYTHMIC AGENTS

Sudden cardiac death occurs in a significant number of patients with hypertrophic and dilated cardiomyopathy. Although the presence of complex ventricular arrhythmias in patients with DCM is a poor prognostic indicator, it has not been shown that suppression of ventricular ectopy with antiarrhythmic agents will alter mortality rates. In patients with cardiomyopathy, the exact relationship between nonsustained ventricular tachycardia and sudden cardiac death is controversial, as is the use of antiarrhythmic drugs.[37] It is also unclear which is the best way to assess drug efficacy in cardiomyopathy patients. Electrophysiologic studies have been less useful in patients with cardiomyopathy when compared to patients with arrhythmias in the presence of coronary artery disease.[38] The predictive value of ambulatory electrocardiographic monitoring and signal-averaged electrocardiography is also debated.

There are many factors that should be considered in evaluating a patient with cardiomyopathy and arrhythmias. These include whether the sympathetic stimulation known to occur in heart failure can be attenuated, a problem with ongoing ischemia, or if the patient is receiving a drug known to have proarrhythmic effects or to adversely affect electrolyte balance. Before initiating therapy with an antiarrhythmic agent, any reversible factor known to cause an arrhythmia or heart failure should first be corrected. Treatment with an ACE inhibitor and/or a β-blocker should be considered. If antiarrhythmic agents are used, those that decrease contractility should be avoided. Patients with DCM and *symptomatic* ventricular arrhythmias should be evaluated and treated with conventional methods. Empiric use of type I antiarrhythmic agents (quinidine-like) should be avoided. Results with amiodarone in patients with heart failure have been inconsistent. In the GESICA study, low-dose amiodarone (300 mg/d) reduced mortality and hospitalizations in patients with severe heart failure, and particularly in those with an elevated baseline heart rate.[39,40] Amiodarone was compared to placebo in a randomized, placebo-controlled trial of 674 patients (STAT-CHF).[41] In this trial, amiodarone did not reduce the incidence of sudden death or prolong survival, but a trend toward improved survival was observed in patients with nonischemic cardiomyopathy. Early cardiac transplantation or implantation of an automatic defibrillator are other options to be considered. Patient selection criteria have not yet been well defined.

ANTITHROMBOTIC THERAPY

Systemic embolization is a possible complication of DCM. It has been noted that patients with DCM exhibit hypercoagulability, but it is unknown whether high levels of markers for coagulation put patients at greater risk for thromboembolism.[42] The presence of a left ventricular mural thrombus has been associated with a greater risk of thromboembolism and as a predictor of increased mortality.[43] There may be important differences between the mural thrombus formation found after myocardial infarction and DCM. For example, the risk of embolization is high in the early weeks after myocardial infarction and lessens after 3 to 6 months, whereas the risk in patients with DCM is fairly constant over time.[44] Furthermore, the thrombi found in cardiomyopathy patients may have a smaller area of attachment to the endomyocardial surface. Some clinicians use anticoagulation in patients with ejection fractions of 20% or less, unless a contraindication exists.[5] Lower than normal doses may be adequate for patients with cardiomyopathy, because hepatic clearance of the drug may be compromised. In a retrospective evaluation of the SOLVD (studies of left ventricular dysfunction) data, antiplatelet therapy and anticoagulant monotherapy were each associated with a reduction in the risk of sudden cardiac death.[45] A large, randomized controlled trial of anticoagulation versus placebo would be useful in determining the risk–benefit ratio of warfarin in this patient population.

HYPERTROPHIC CARDIOMYOPATHY

Hypertrophic cardiomyopathy (HCM) is a primary myocardial disorder characterized by a hypertrophied and nondilated left ventricle, existing in the absence of known causes of left ventricular hypertrophy. The distribution of the hypertrophy is usually asymmetric, meaning segments of the left ventricle are thickened to varying degrees. There may also be enlargement of the atria, thickening of the mitral valve leaflets, and fibrotic areas within the ventricular wall. Hypertrophic cardiomyopathy has also been termed idiopathic hypertrophic subaortic stenosis (IHSS) and hypertrophic obstructive cardiomyopathy. These latter terms are used less frequently now because they overemphasize the obstructive component of the disease, which is present in a minority of patients.[46] Treatment strategies are aimed at improving symptoms and preventing sudden cardiac death.

PATHOPHYSIOLOGY

The genetic predisposition to HCM is thought to be an autosomal dominant trait with variable penetrance. Due to the wide variability of presentation, not all cases in a family may be detected. HCM is usually caused by mutations in the genes for β-myosin heavy chain, α-tropomyosin, myosin-binding protein C, or cardiac troponin T.[47,48] HCM appears to have several different pathophysiologic mechanisms leading to similar clinical manifestations, although the prognoses for patients will vary. Overall, HCM has an estimated prevalence in the United States of 1 in 500.

The pathophysiology of HCM is a complex relationship among several factors including: (1) asymmetric left ventricular hypertrophy, (2) diastolic dysfunction, (3) dynamic obstruction of the outflow tract, and (4) myocardial ischemia. Each of these components contributes to the overall presentation of the patient to a varying degree.

LEFT VENTRICULAR HYPERTROPHY

The hypertrophy seen in HCM is usually diffuse and involves the septum and left ventricular anterolateral free wall to a greater degree than the posterior segment. Asymmetric septal hypertrophy (ASH) is a sensitive marker for HCM but is not specific for this disorder. In patients with outflow obstruction, the basal septum is usually markedly thickened at the level of the mitral valve. In patients with nonobstructive HCM, the outflow tract is larger and the septal hypertrophy that occurs has a more distal or apical distribution.

Cellular disorganization is a common histologic finding of HCM. Morphologic abnormalities are found at the gross, microscopic, and ultrastructural levels. The disarray of myocytes may contribute to diastolic and systolic dysfunction as well as serving as a nidus for ventricular arrhythmias. It appears that the degree of left ventricular hypertrophy is associated with a worse clinical course. Patients with severe and diffuse hypertrophy are predisposed to symptoms of heart failure, lethal arrhythmias, and sudden death.

DIASTOLIC DYSFUNCTION

Diastolic dysfunction is the most common abnormality found in patients with HCM. Approximately 80% of patients will exhibit symptoms associated with diastolic dysfunction. Studies of the left ventricle led to the realization that diastolic dysfunction is the result of abnormalities in relaxation, distensibility (compliance), and filling. The abnormalities of diastolic function can be both regional and global and lead to an incoordination of contraction and relaxation. Abnormal relaxation is manifested by a prolonged isovolumic relaxation period and a reduced rate of decline in left ventricular pressure. Filling of the left ventricle is prolonged in most patients. The presence of mitral regurgitation tends to normalize these abnormalities. β-adrenergic stimulation can aggravate these abnormalities, whereas β-blockade may diminish them.[46,49]

Myocardial relaxation is an energy-dependent process sensitive to episodes of ischemia. Calcium ions are inactivated by being taken up by the sarcoplasmic reticulum. In the event of ischemia, the sequestration of calcium is inhibited, allowing the calcium to continue its interaction with the myofibrillar contractile proteins. Calcium channel blocking drugs have been used with some success in patients with diastolic dysfunction.[46]

Abnormalities in filling are also related to the chamber stiffness that occurs in HCM. This stiffness may be the result of myocardial fibrosis, cellular disorganization, or the increase in myocardial mass. The decreased distensibility leads to an abnormally steep slope of the diastolic pressure–volume curve, such that an increase in left ventricular volume results in a disproportionate increase in diastolic pressure.[46]

SYSTOLIC FUNCTION AND OUTFLOW TRACT OBSTRUCTION

Abnormalities of systolic function also occur in patients with HCM. The hypertrophied left ventricle may cause a powerful but sometimes uncoordinated contraction presumably due to the abnormal architecture of the myocardium. The increase seen in the left ventricular wall thickness results in decreased wall stress during systole. Therefore, the left ventricle contracts against a decreased afterload, so that the left ventricle is described as being hyperdynamic rather than hypercontractile.[46] Ejection fraction is often increased.

Considerable controversy has surrounded the issue of the importance of outflow tract obstruction in conjunction with HCM. The presence of a gradient (the diastolic pressure difference between the atrium and ventricle) is indicative of a dynamic obstruction of the left ventricular outflow tract. Outflow tract gradients occur in about 25% of patients with HCM.[49] The obstruction that occurs usually shows spontaneous variability, and may be reduced by interventions that decrease myocardial contractility. The gradient can be augmented by factors that increase contractility (Table 15–5).[46]

Factors that may contribute to the production of a systolic pressure gradient include enhanced contraction; apposition of the anterior mitral leaflet to the hypertrophied septum, impeding aortic flow; large papillary muscles; and reduced left ventricular cavity size. The importance of the pressure gradient remains controversial because there is a poor correlation between the presence of a gradient and the clinical symptoms or prognosis of a patient.

MYOCARDIAL ISCHEMIA

Chest pain, in the absence of coronary artery disease, is a common symptom of patients with HCM. There are several mechanisms proposed for the myocardial ischemia seen in this patient population. There may be inadequate capillary density in relation to the increased left ventricular muscle mass. The small intramural coronary arteries may be abnormally narrowed or excessively compressed during systole. Impaired relaxation during diastole may inhibit blood flow

TABLE 15–5. Factors Known to Affect Gradients

Factors That Diminish Gradients
Decreasing myocardial contractility
β-blocking drugs
Verapamil
Increasing ventricular volume
Increasing arterial pressure
Factors That Enhance Gradients
Increasing myocardial contractility
Exercise
Inotropic agents
Decreasing ventricular volume
Decreasing arterial pressure

to the subendocardium. Once myocardial ischemia develops, further increases in left ventricular filling pressure may occur, which in turn leads to more ischemia. Repeated episodes of ischemia may be responsible for progressive myocyte loss and fibrosis. The subendocardium is at greatest risk for ischemic damage due to the lower capillary density and higher oxygen demand secondary to wall tension.[49]

CLINICAL PRESENTATION

The natural history of HCM is quite variable, ranging from an asymptomatic form to a severe life-threatening illness. There is no relation between the presence or absence of an outflow tract gradient and clinical presentation or prognosis. The clinical presentation of patients varies widely, ranging from no symptoms to severe symptoms of angina, heart failure, or sudden cardiac death. The most common symptoms are chest pain, dyspnea, fatigue, palpitations, presyncope, and syncope. In general, the severity of symptoms corresponds to the degree of left ventricular hypertrophy, but this relationship is not absolute. Some patients with mild or localized hypertrophy will have severe symptoms, whereas other patients with marked hypertrophy will have minimal symptoms. Furthermore, the presence or absence of a dynamic obstruction does not seem to play a role in the patient's presentation.

The symptoms of fatigue, orthopnea, and dyspnea are usually due to the elevated pressures secondary to diastolic dysfunction. However, some patients may develop dyspnea due to systolic dysfunction secondary to myocardial ischemia and fibrosis. Chest pain is seen in as many as 75% of patients even though the incidence of atherosclerotic coronary artery disease is much less. The chest pain may have atypical features including a prolonged duration, occurrence at rest, and limited relief from nitrates.[49]

The development or increase of a murmur suggests progression of disease, but disappearance of a murmur does not imply improvement. In fact, disappearance of a murmur may herald further impairment of systolic function. Some patients will progress to congestive heart failure due to atrial fibrillation, mitral regurgitation, or myocardial infarction. If heart failure develops, the patient has a poor prognosis.

Of major concern is the incidence of sudden cardiac death among patients with HCM. Sudden cardiac death occurs more commonly in younger patients (10 to 35 years of age). Sometimes the first manifestation of HCM is sudden death. The mechanisms responsible for sudden cardiac death are ill defined. Younger age, marked left ventricular hypertrophy, family history of sudden death, and the presence of nonsustained ventricular tachycardia on ambulatory electrocardiograms have been identified as risk factors for sudden death in patients with HCM.[46]

In one long-term study of 314 patients with HCM and 82 patients with DCM, 68% of the deaths that occurred in the HCM patients were sudden.[50] Age less than 30 years, fractional shortening less than 35%, and left ventricular end-diastolic pressures greater than 20 mm Hg were factors associated with sudden cardiac death. Patients who were less than 30 years of age rarely (5%) had ventricular tachycardia on Holter monitoring. It was suggested that young patients with hypertrophic cardiomyopathy may die suddenly as a result of exercise-induced ischemia rather than ventricular arrhythmias.

A variety of other rhythm abnormalities may be seen, including supraventricular and ventricular tachyarrhythmias, bradyarrhythmias, aberrant atrioventricular nodal pathways, and complete heart block. In 25 children with HCM, 6 (24%) were found to have a prolonged QT interval.[51] Either DCM or HCM may be a cause of QT prolongation.

Less often, sudden death may be the result of hemodynamic changes. The onset of atrial fibrillation, in the face of severe left ventricular diastolic dysfunction, may result in a significant decrease in stroke volume. This decrease in cardiac output could lead acute left ventricular failure, myocardial infarction, or sudden death.

The diagnosis of HCM may be difficult as it is confused with coronary artery disease, mitral regurgitation, and aortic stenosis. Patients with HCM are often physically active. The physical signs of the cardiac examination depend on the presence of a systolic pressure gradient (the rate of pressure change) within the left ventricle. If a gradient is present, a late-onset systolic murmur is often heard. The murmur is intensified by standing and the Valsalva maneuver and lessened with squatting or handgrip. Some patients develop an end-stage left ventricular dilatation and a declining left ventricular ejection fraction, which is often confused with IDC.[49]

Doppler echocardiography is used to confirm the diagnosis. In the past, findings consistent with HCM include a low normal or decreased end-diastolic dimension, a septal wall thickness of 15 mm or more, and a septal to posterior wall thickness ratio of at least 1.3 to 1. The presence of a hyperdynamic left ventricle and systolic anterior motion (SAM) of the anterior mitral leaflet increased the likelihood of the diagnosis. More recently, the classic echocardiographic criteria have been called into question, because there is overlap between left ventricular wall thickness of genetically affected and unaffected persons.[52]

Presentation of HCM in the latter decades of life is common. Patients who present with HCM at an advanced age (> 65 yr) in general have a prognosis no different than age- and gender-matched controls.[53] It is not clear whether this elderly patient subgroup had a better prognosis as compared to patients presenting at a younger age as a result of a different pathophysiologic process. Elderly patients presenting with New York Heart Association functional class III dyspnea had a higher mortality rate when compared to a control group. Increased left atrial size was associated with reduced survival.

Sudden death can be a complication, especially in young athletes with HCM. It is recommended that young patients with HCM refrain from competitive athletics.

▶ TREATMENT: Hypertrophic Cardiomyopathy

NONPHARMACOLOGIC THERAPY

Surgical treatment is generally reserved for those patients who are refractory to medical management, have an outflow gradient of 50 mm Hg or more, a very thick ventricular septum, and high left ventricular pressures. Surgical intervention is designed to relieve the outflow obstruction and the elevated left ventricular pressures. This is accomplished by performing a partial septal resection and/or incision (ventricular myotomy–myectomy). One can expect an overall early mortality rate following surgery of approximately 5%. However, significant improvement can be expected in patients with symptoms of dyspnea, angina, near-syncope, and syncope.[54] Complications may include septal perforation and late occurrence of congestive heart failure. Mitral valve replacement has been used to abolish the subaortic gradient that occurs due to the anterior motion of the mitral leaflets during systole. This procedure is generally reserved for patients with severe mitral regurgitation or those with mild ventricular septal hypertrophy where myotomy–myectomy may cause perforation.[46,47,49] Dual chamber pacing has been shown to be helpful to some patients with obstructive cardiomyopathy who have failed pharmacologic approaches.[24]

PHARMACOLOGIC THERAPY

Because there are no known means available to prevent HCM, methods to minimize the consequences of disease prevail. The treatment of HCM is designed to reduce symptoms, improve exercise tolerance, retard disease progression, and improve prognosis. Agents that decrease contractility, improve diastolic dysfunction, reduce ischemia, and suppress arrhythmias have been used with some success.

β-BLOCKING AGENTS

β-Blocking agents have been used in obstructive and nonobstructive forms of HCM since the 1960s. Approximately one-third to one-half of patients with angina, dyspnea, light-headedness, or syncope will have a favorable response to these agents. Most patients require doses of 320 mg/d of propranolol or its equivalent, and it is recommended that maximally tolerated doses be used.[49] Standing heart rate should be 60 beats/min, and the maximum exercise heart rate should be less than 130 beats/min. The mechanism by which β-blockade is beneficial is by inhibiting sympathetic stimulation of the heart. Myocardial oxygen demand is reduced by decreasing heart rate, left ventricular contractility, and myocardial wall stress during systole. Outflow tract obstruction may be minimized with β-blockade, especially under conditions of stress or exercise, when sympathetic stimulation is high. Furthermore, consequences of a decreased resting and exercise heart rate include an increase in left ventricular diastolic filling time, reduction of the abnormally prolonged isovolumic relaxation period, and lengthening of early rapid filling. Cardioselective β-blocking drugs are thought to be less desirable because their effect on outflow tract gradient is less. It has been suggested that they should be reserved for those patients with chronic obstructive pulmonary disease. Furthermore, β-blocking agents with intrinsic sympathomimetic activity (ISA) may not reduce resting heart rate sufficiently.[49]

CALCIUM CHANNEL BLOCKING AGENTS

Patients who have no response to β-blockade may respond to verapamil.[47] There are a number of reasons why calcium channel blocking agents may be of benefit to patients with HCM. Increased calcium concentrations have been shown to play a role in prolonging the ventricular action potential and the duration of isometric contraction and relaxation. Patients with HCM have a hyperdynamic ventricle in systole and delayed relaxation and decreased compliance during diastole. Calcium channel blocking drugs decrease the myocardial oxygen determinants, resulting in an improved balance between oxygen supply and demand; therefore diastolic function may be improved.

Most patients with HCM who have been treated with a calcium channel blocker have received verapamil, although others have also been used. In one study of 101 patients, 85% of previously symptomatic patients reported improvement or complete relief of symptoms when treated with a calcium channel blocker.[55] Intravenous verapamil has been noted to reduce the outflow tract gradient in those patients with obstructive HCM. The mechanism may be a decrease in systolic function as well as an increase in left ventricular volumes due to enhanced left ventricular diastolic filling.

The adverse effects associated with the use of verapamil include sinus node dysfunction, prolongation of the PR interval, atrioventricular dissociation, hypotension, and pulmonary congestion.[52] The risks may outweigh the benefits in those patients with (1) a pulmonary capillary wedge pressure greater than 20 mm Hg, (2) a history of paroxysmal nocturnal dyspnea or orthopnea, (3) sick sinus syndrome or significant atrioventricular nodal disease in the absence of a permanent pacemaker, (4) low systolic blood pressure, and (5) a substantial outflow gradient.[47]

Studies using other calcium channel blockers are limited. Improvement in diastolic dysfunction may occur; however, the dihydropyridines may cause a reflex increase in heart rate, cause hypotension, or worsen the outflow tract gradient. It has been suggested that a combination of a β-blocker with a calcium channel blocker may be useful. In that situation, a β-blocker should be initiated prior to starting a dihydropyridine.[49] If verapamil has been used first, additional benefit has been reported with the addition of pindolol.[56] Trials using combination therapy are extremely limited.

There is no evidence that either β-blockade or verapamil protects the patient from sudden cardiac death.

ANTIARRHYTHMIC AGENTS

The incidence of sudden cardiac death in patients with HCM is a cause of great concern. Sudden death is thought to be related to ventricular arrhythmias as a primary event or secondary to myocardial ischemia, diastolic dysfunction, outflow obstruction, systemic hypotension, or supraventricular tachyarrhythmias.[47] Patients who are identified to be at high risk for sudden death should be treated aggressively (Table 15–6). It is less clear whether other patients with nonsustained ventricular tachycardia benefit from antiarrhythmic agents. Unfortunately, electrophysiologic testing has not been shown to be helpful in identifying patients at high risk. Patients with characteristics known to be associated with a

TABLE 15–6. Patients with HCM at High Risk for Sudden Death

Survivors of cardiac arrest with documented ventricular fibrillation
Episodes of recurrent sustained ventricular tachycardia
Young patients with a family history (2 or more family members) of sudden death

low risk of sudden death should be reassured and do not warrant therapy with antiarrhythmic agents nor restriction of activities.

Patients with HCM at high risk for sudden death should be considered eligible for treatment with amiodarone or an implantable cardioverter-defibrillator (ICD). Amiodarone is a complex agent with α, β, and calcium blocking effects. As a result, it has negative chronotropic, inotropic, and coronary vasodilating properties. Amiodarone may relieve symptoms and prolong exercise duration in some patients, independent of its antiarrhythmic actions.[57] In one trial where 35 patients with HCM were assessed by electrophysiologic study, amiodarone prevented or made it more difficult to induce ventricular tachycardia in 31% of patients who were inducible off drug.[58] Ventricular tachycardia was easier to induce or inducible only while the patient was taking amiodarone in 51% of patients. During a follow-up period, 4 of 18 patients in whom amiodarone facilitated ventricular tachycardia died or received appropriate electrical shocks from ICDs. None of the 17 patients taking amiodarone in whom ventricular tachycardia was rendered more difficult to induce, died. Amiodarone may be proarrhythmic in some patients, and electrophysiologic studies may help identify those patients who will do poorly if placed on amiodarone for long-term therapy.

Disopyramide has been used in treating both the supraventricular and ventricular arrhythmias occurring in patients with HCM. In addition, disopyramide's negative inotropic effect and ability to increase peripheral vascular resistance has been used to reduce outflow tract obstruction.[55] The number of patients receiving disopyramide is small and there are few controlled trials available. The anticholinergic side effects (blurred vision, dry mouth, and urinary retention) make disopyramide a less desirable agent for long-term therapy.

A significant portion of patients with HCM develop atrial fibrillation. Amiodarone is one of the most effective agents available used to maintain normal sinus rhythm for these patients. For those patients requiring rate control, β-blockade or verapamil may be used. Anticoagulation should be considered, because these patients are at a risk for systemic embolization and stroke. If amiodarone is added to a patient already receiving warfarin, the prothrombin time or INR should be closely monitored.[47]

NEW TYPES OF PHARMACOLOGIC TREATMENT

Because growth factors have been shown to be associated with primary HCM, approaches to treatment through interruption of growth stimulation are being investigated. Octreotide is a somatostatin analog that can prevent the stimulating effect of growth factors. Octreotide has been given to small numbers of patients with HCM and has demonstrated hemodynamic improvement.[59] Approaches with this type of therapy may hold promise for the future.

RESTRICTIVE CARDIOMYOPATHY

Restrictive cardiomyopathy is the cardiomyopathy encountered least frequently. Restrictive cardiomyopathy is defined as heart muscle disease that results in impaired filling, with normal or decreased diastolic volume. It is associated with normal systolic function early in the course of the disease. Restrictive cardiomyopathy is one type of diastolic dysfunction, resulting from increased stiffness of the myocardium causing ventricular pressure to rise dramatically with only small increases in volume.[60] Either one or both of the ventricles may be affected; therefore restrictive cardiomyopathy may present as either left- or right-sided heart failure.

EPIDEMIOLOGY AND ETIOLOGY

Because of the rare occurrence of restrictive cardiomyopathy, the natural course of the disease is not well characterized and reports on prognosis have been highly variable. Restrictive cardiomyopathies may be classified as either myocardial or endomyocardial. The myocardial types may be noninfiltrative, infiltrative, or storage diseases. The endomyocardial types are due to endomyocardial fibrosis, hypereosinophilic syndrome, carcinoid heart disease, metastatic cancers, radiation, anthracycline toxicity, or secondary to drugs known to cause fibrosis.[60]

The most common cause in the industrialized world is amyloidosis, whereas endomyocardial fibrosis is a common cause in tropical areas of the world. There is a genetic predisposition to idiopathic restrictive cardiomyopathy.[60]

The cause of the disease, the severity of heart failure symptoms, and the presence of cardiac thrombi and arrhythmias are factors that affect long-term survival. Children diagnosed with restrictive cardiomyopathy have a worse prognosis than adults and should be considered for early cardiac transplantation.[61]

PATHOPHYSIOLOGY

The major hemodynamic abnormality in restrictive cardiomyopathy is a limitation of ventricular filling leading to increased filling pressures. Thrombi are frequently found in the cardiac chambers. Patients have signs and symptoms consistent with congestive heart failure. The abnormality is similar to what is seen in pericardial disease causing constriction or tamponade. Atrial dimensions are often increased.

Restrictive myocardial disease may result from several local or systemic disorders. Amyloidosis, hemochromatosis, scleroderma, carcinoid, sarcoidosis, diabetes, pseudoxanthoma elasticum, and endomyocardial fibrosis have been known to cause restrictive cardiomyopathy.[62]

CLINICAL PRESENTATION

Patients present with dyspnea, orthopnea, fatigue, edema, ascites, and at times, chest pain. The heart is either normal in size or has atrial enlargement. Significant jugular venous distention is quite common. Mitral and/or tricuspid regurgitant murmurs may be heard. The electrocardiogram may show atrial arrhythmias, tachy-brady syndrome, or conduction abnormalities. Recordings of ventricular pressure may show a characteristic dip and plateau (square root sign). This is a result of rapid completion of ventricular filling early in diastole. The square root sign is not always present, as it can be affected by heart rate, degree of hydration, and the severity of disease.

The diagnosis of restrictive cardiomyopathy should be considered in the patient who presents with signs and symptoms of congestive heart failure but has only mild cardiomegaly. Differentiation from constrictive pericarditis is important, because pericardectomy is an effective form of treatment for constrictive pericarditis.

▶ TREATMENT: Restrictive Cardiomyopathy

The treatment of restrictive cardiomyopathy is complex because of the heterogeneity of the pathophysiologic abnormalities. Diuretics and vasodilators are used for the symptoms of congestive heart failure in the presence of restrictive cardiomyopathy, but caution is advised because these patients require high filling pressures to maintain an adequate stroke volume and cardiac output. Hypotension and hypoperfusion may occur as a result of the use of diuretics. Because systolic function is often normal, digoxin is of little or no benefit. Amiodarone is used to maintain normal sinus rhythm in patients who have atrial fibrillation. Anticoagulation is needed to decrease the risk of systemic embolization, particularly in those patients with atrial fibrillation, valvular regurgitation, and low cardiac output. In the case of hemachromatosis, chelation therapy and/or repeated phlebotomy may be of benefit. Corticosteroids and cytotoxic drugs have been used with some success in the early phase of endomyocardial fibrosis and eosinophilic cardiomyopathy.[60]

EVALUATION OF THERAPEUTIC OUTCOMES

Patients with DCM should be treated no differently than patients with known causes of congestive heart failure (see Chap. 11). Therapy should include an ACE inhibitor and a diuretic for those patients with congestive symptoms. Blood pressure should be closely monitored to ensure that the patient has adequate perfusion yet at the same time trying to minimize systemic vascular resistance. Some basilar rales or mild pedal edema may be tolerated in order to ensure an adequate filling pressure. Generally loop diuretics are necessary to achieve an adequate diuresis. Patients should be instructed to weigh themselves on a regular basis and to contact their health care provider if their weight increases by 5 or more pounds or if their symptoms worsen. Potassium and magnesium serum concentrations should be monitored and supplements administered if needed. Digoxin should be added if the patient remains symptomatic. Finally, carvedilol may be gradually titrated over a period of several weeks with the heart rate, blood pressure, and patient's symptoms carefully monitored.

If the patient has an ejection fraction below 20% or if a mural thrombus is suspected, a trial of anticoagulation may be warranted if the benefit is thought to outweigh the risk. If the patient has experienced an episode of sudden death or has sustained ventricular tachycardia, an antiarrhythmic agent is usually prescribed. Selection of the agent may be based on the results of an electrophysiologic study (EPS) or amiodarone may be empirically prescribed. If the patient continues to deteriorate, cardiac transplantation may be a viable alternative.

The goal of treatment for patients with HCM is primarily to reduce their symptoms of dyspnea and exercise intolerance. Either β-blockers or calcium channel blockers may be used. If a β-blocker is chosen, it is best to use an agent that does not have intrinsic sympathomimetic activity. The dose should be maximized. If the patient does not tolerate a β-blocker or has a contraindication to the use of a β-blocker, then a rate-lowering calcium channel blocker may be tried. The most commonly used calcium channel blocker is verapamil. Patients should be monitored for resolution of symptoms and an increase in exercise tolerance. Resolution of symptoms may take months. In addition, both β-blockers and calcium channel blockers may cause hypotension and conduction abnormalities. β-blockers may worsen pulmonary function. Combination therapy with a β-blocker and calcium channel blocker may be tried if the desired therapeutic response is not achieved with either agent alone. If dyspnea continues with maximal doses of a β-blocker and calcium channel blocker, a diuretic agent or a nitrate may be added. Those patients who are at high risk for sudden cardiac death should be considered candidates for amiodarone or an ICD.

For those patients with a significant obstruction to left ventricular outflow that do not respond to medical management, a surgical approach may be necessary. Septal myotomy–myectomy has been employed. Surgical therapy is generally reserved for those patients who have a outflow gradient of 50 mm Hg or more and/or severe symptoms and who have failed an adequate trial of medical therapy.

The first step in assessing and treating a patient with restrictive cardiomyopathy is to rule out constrictive pericarditis because the two conditions have a similar presentation. Constrictive pericarditis is easily treated with surgery, whereas patients with restrictive cardiomyopathy have a varied approach to therapy dependent upon the etiology of their disorder. The treatment is aimed at relieving the symptoms associated with high filling pressures. This is generally achieved through the use of diuretics. Diuretic therapy should be initiated with low doses. Normalization of filling pressures is not possible or desirable. Patients symptoms should be monitored for improvement. Overdiuresis will result in an inadequate cardiac output. Chelation therapy has been advocated for patients with hemochromatosis. Prednisone has been suggested for patients with sarcoidosis. There is no curative treatment for restrictive cardiomyopathy.

▶ PRINCIPLES OF PHARMACOTHERAPY

- There are three types of cardiomyopathy that may manifest with similar symptoms.
- Patients with diastolic dysfunction are treated differently than those with systolic dysfunction.
- Patients with dilated cardiomyopathy should follow the heart failure guidelines: ACE inhibitors or hydralazine and nitrates, with diuretics and digoxin when needed.
- Patients with persistent symptoms of heart failure who are maximized on ACE inhibitors, diuretics, and digoxin may benefit from the addition of a β-blocker.
- Patients with NYHA class IV symptoms may require intravenous inotropic support.
- Anticoagulation should be considered in patients with DCM and HCM who are at risk for thromboembolic complications.
- Patients with DCM or HCM who are at high risk for sudden cardiac death should receive amiodarone or an ICD.
- Patients with HCM who are symptomatic may benefit from β-blockade or verapamil.

REFERENCES

1. Wynne J, Braunwald E. The cardiomyopathies and myocarditidies. In: Braunwald E, ed. Heart Disease. A Textbook of Cardiovascular Medicine, 5th ed. Philadelphia, Saunders, 1997:1404–1463.
2. Mason JW. Classification of cardiomyopathy. In: Schlant RC, Alexander RW, eds. Hurst's The Heart, 8th ed. New York, McGraw-Hill, 1994:1585–1590.
3. Katz AM. Cardiomyopathy of overload: An unnatural growth response in the hypertrophied heart. Ann Intern Med 1994;121:363–371.
4. Schwartz K, Chassagne C, Boheler K. The molecular biology of heart failure. J Am Coll Cardiol 1993;22(suppl A):30A–33A.
5. Gilbert EM, Bristow MR. Idiopathic dilated cardiomyopathy. In: Schlant RC, Alexander RW, eds. Hurst's The Heart, 8th ed. New York, McGraw-Hill, 1994:1609–1619.
6. Dec GW, Fuster V. Idiopathic dilated cardiomyopathy. N Engl J Med 1994;331:1564–1575.
7. Middlekauff HR, Stevenson WG, Woo MA, et al. Comparison of frequency of late potentials in idiopathic dilated cardiomyopathy and ischemic cardiomyopathy with advanced congestive heart failure and their usefulness in predicting sudden death. Am J Cardiol 1990; 66:1113–1117.
8. Eichhorn EJ, Bristow MR. Medical therapy can improve the biological properties of the chronically failing heart. Circulation 1996; 94:2285–2296.
9. Marijianowski MMH, Teeling P, Mann J, et al. Dilated cardiomyopathy is associated with an increase in the type I/type III collagen ratio: A quantitative assessment. J Am Coll Cardiol 1995;25:1263–1272.
10. Olivetti G, Abbi, R, Quaini F, et al. Apoptosis in the failing human heart. N Engl J Med 1997;336:1131–1141.
11 Marian AJ, Roberts R. Molecular basis of hypertrophic and dilated cardiomyopathy. Texas Heart Inst J 1994;21:6–15.
12. Limas C, Limas CJ, Boudoulas H, et al. Anti-β-receptor antibodies in familial cardiomyopathy: Correlation with HLA-DR and HLA-DQ gene polymorphisms. Am Heart J 1994;127:382–386.
13. Kupari M, Koshkinen P, Suokas A, Ventila M. Left ventricular filling impairment in asymptomatic chronic alcoholics. Am J Cardiol 1990; 66:1473–1477.
14. Fernandez-Sola J, Estrauch R, Grau JM, et al. The relation of alcoholic myopathy to cardiomyopathy. Ann Intern Med 1994;120:529–536.
15. Brown CA, O'Connell JB. Myocarditis and idiopathic dilated cardiomyopathy. Am J Med 1995;99:309–314.
16. Lauer B, Padberg K, Schultheiss H, Strauer B. Autoantibodies against human ventricular myosin in sera of patients with acute and chronic myocarditis. J Am Coll Cardiol 1994;23:146–153.
17. O'Connell JB, Renlund DG. Myocarditis and specific myocardial diseases. In: Schlant RC, Alexander RW, eds. Hurst's The Heart, 8th ed. New York, McGraw-Hill, 1994:1591–1607.
18. Shan K, Lincoff M, Young JB. Anthracycline-induced cardiotoxicity. Ann Intern Med 1996;125:47–58.
19. Ganz WI, Sridhar KS, Ganz SS et al. Review of tests for monitoring doxorubicin-induced cardiomyopathy. Oncology 1996;53:461–470.
20. Swain SM, Whaley FS, Gerber MC et al. Cardioprotection with dexrazoxane for doxorubicin-containing therapy in advanced breast cancer. J Clin Oncol 1997;15:1318–1332.
21. Anversa P, Sonnenblick EH. Ischemic cardiomyopathy: Pathophysiologic mechanisms. Prog Cardiovasc Dis 1990;33:49–70.
22. Vlay SC. Innovations in the management of ischemic cardiomyopathy. Am Heart J 1994;127;235–242.
23. Marin-Neto JA, Maciel BC, Urbanetz LLT, Gallo L, Almeida-Filho OC, Amorim DS. High output failure in patients with peripartum cardiomyopathy: A comparative study with dilated cardiomyopathy. Am Heart J 1991;121:134–140.
24. Nishimura RA, Symanski JD, Hurrell DG, et al. Dual-chamber pacing for cardiomyopathies: A 1996 clinical perspective. Mayo Clin Proc 1996;71:1077–1087.
25. Cohen-Solal A, Choussat R, Chachques JC, et al. Serial assessment of cardiopulmonary exercise capacity after cardiomyoplasty for either ischemic or idiopathic dilated cardiomyopathy. Am J Cardiol 1996; 77:623–627.
26. Maze SS, Adolph RJ. Myocarditis: Unresolved issues in diagnosis and treatment. Clin Cardiol 1990;13:69–79.
27. Mason JW, O'Connell JB, Herskowitz A, et al. A clinical trial of immunosuppressive therapy for myocarditis. N Engl J Med 1995; 333:269–275.
28. Eichhorn EJ, Bristow MR. Practical guidelines for initiation of beta-adrenergic blockade in patients with heart failure. Am J Cardiol 1997;79:794–798.
29. Elkayam U, Shotan A, Mehra A, Ostrzega E. Calcium channel blockers in heart failure. J Am Coll Cardiol 1993;22(suppl A):139A–144A.
30. Garg R, Yusuf S. Current and ongoing randomized trials in heart failure and left ventricular dysfunction. J Am Coll Cardiol 1993;22(suppl A):194A–207A.
31. Packer M, O'Connor CM, Ghali JK, et al. Effect of amlodipine on morbidity and mortality in severe chronic heart failure. N Engl J Med 1996;335:1107–1114.

32. Cohn JN, Ziesche S, Smith R, et al. Effect of the calcium antagonist felodipine as supplementary vasodilator therapy in patients with chronic heart failure treated with enalapril. V-HeFT III. Circulation 1997;96:856–863.
33. Elkayam U. Nitrates in the treatment of heart failure. Am J Cardiol 1996;77(suppl):41C–51C.
34. Kelly RA, Smith TW. Nitric oxide and nitrovasodilators: Similarities, differences and interactions. Am J Cardiol 1996;77(suppl):2C–7C.
35. Packer M. The development of positive inotropic agents for chronic heart failure: How have we gone astray? J Am Coll Cardiol 1993; 22(suppl A):119A–126A.
36. Mehra MR, Ventura HO, Kapoor C, et al. Safety and clinical utility of long-term intravenous milrinone in advanced heart failure. Am J Cardiol 1997;80:61–64.
37. Podrid PJ, Wilson JS. Should asymptomatic ventricular arrhythmia in patients with congestive heart failure be treated? An antagonist's viewpoint. Am J Cardiol 1990;66:451–457.
38. Das SK, Morady F, DiCarlo L, et al. Prognostic usefulness of programmed ventricular stimulation in idiopathic dilated cardiomyopathy without symptomatic ventricular arrhythmias. Am J Cardiol 1986; 58:998–1000.
39. Doval HC, Nul DR, Grancelli HO, et al. Randomised trial of low dose amiodarone in severe congestive heart failure. Lancet 1994: 344:493–498.
40. Nul Dr, Doval HC, Grancelli HO, et al. Heart rate is a marker of amiodarone mortality reduction in severe heart failure. The GESICA-GEMA investigators. Grupo de estudio de la sobrevida en la insuficiencia cardiaca en Argentina–grupo de estudios multicentreicos en Argentina. J Am Coll Cardiol 1997;29:1199–1205.
41. Singh SN, Fletcher RD, Fisher SG, et al. Amiodarone in patients with congestive heart failure and asymptomatic ventricular arrhythmia. N Engl J Med 1995;333:77–82.
42. Yamamoto K, Ikeda U, Furuhashi K, et al. The coagulation system is activated in idiopathic cardiomyopathy. J Am Coll Cardiol 1995; 25:1634–1640.
43. Katz SD, Marantz PR, Biasucci L, et al. Low incidence of stroke in ambulatory patients with heart failure: A prospective study. Am Heart J 1993;126:141–146.
44. Falk RH. A plea for a clinical trial of anticoagulation in dilated cardiomyopathy. Am J Cardiol 1990;65:914–915.
45. Dries DL, Domanski MJ, Waclawiw MA, Gersh BJ. Effect of antithrombotic therapy on risk of sudden coronary death in patients with congestive heart failure. Am J Cardiol 1997;79:909–913.
46. Maron BJ, Roberts WC. Hypertrophic cardiomyopathy. In: Schlant RC, Alexander RW, eds. Hurst's The Heart, 8th ed. New York, McGraw-Hill, 1994:1621–1635.
47. Spirito P, Seidman CE, McKenna WJ, Maron BJ. The management of hypertrophic cardiomyopathy. N Engl J Med 1997;336:775–785.
48. Watkins H, McKenna WJ, Thierfelder L, et al. Mutations in the genes for cardiac troponin T and α-tropomyosin in hypertrophic cardiomyopathy. N Engl J Med 1995;332:1058–1064.
49. von Dohlen TW, Frank MJ. Current perspectives in hypertrophic cardiomyopathy: Diagnosis, clinical management and prevention of disability and sudden cardiac death. Clin Cardiol 1990;13:247–252.
50. Koga Y, Ogata M, Kihara K, et al. Sudden death in hypertrophic and dilated cardiomyopathy. Jpn Circ J 1989;53:1546–1556
51. Martin AB, Garson A, Perry JC. Prolonged QT interval in hypertrophic and dilated cardiomyopathy in children. Am Heart J 1994; 127:64–70.
52. Posma JL, van der Wall EE, Blanksma PK, et al. New diagnostic options in hypertrophic cardiomyopathy. Am Heart J 1996; 132:1031–1041.
53. Fay WP, Talierco CP, Ilstrup DM, et al. Natural history of hypertrophic cardiomyopathy in the elderly. J Am Coll Cardiol 1990; 16:821–826.
54. McCully RB, Nishimura RA, Tajik AJ, et al. Extent of clinical improvement after surgical treatment of hypertrophic obstructive cardiomyopathy. Circulation 1996;94:467–471.
55. Hopf R, Kaltenbach M. Management of hypertrophic cardiomyopathy. Annu Rev Med 1990;41:75–83.
56. Dimitrow PP, Dubiel JS. Effects on left ventricular function of pindolol added to verapamil in hypertrophic cardiomyopathy. Am J Cardiol 1993;71:313–316.
57. Fananapazir L, Leon MB, Bonow RO, et al. Sudden death during empiric amiodarone therapy in symptomatic hypertrophic cardiomyopathy. Am J Cardiol 1991;67:169–174.
58. Fananapazir L, Epstein SE. Value of electrophysiologic studies in hypertrophic cardiomyopathy treated with amiodarone. Am J Cardiol 1991;67:175–182.
59. Gunal AI, Isik A, Celiker H, et al. Short term reduction of left ventricular mass in primary hypertrophic cardiomyopathy by octreotide injections. Heart 1996;76:418–421.
60. Kushwaha S, Fallon JT, Fuster V. Restrictive cardiomyopathy. N Engl J Med 1997;336:267–276.
61. Lewis AB. Clinical profile and outcome of restrictive cardiomyopathy in children. Am Heart J 1992;123:1589–1593.
62. Shabetai R. Restrictive cardiomyopathy. In: Schlant RC, Alexander RW, eds. Hurst's The Heart, 8th ed. New York, McGraw-Hill, 1994: 1637–1646.

16

CARDIAC TRANSPLANTATION

Kathleen D. Lake, PharmD, FCCP, BCPS, and Maria-Teresa Olivari, MD, FACC

Despite advances in heart failure management, cardiac transplantation remains the mainline therapeutic modality for selected patients with end-stage cardiac disease. The use of refined donor and recipient selection criteria; improved donor organ preservation; endomyocardial biopsy surveillance for rejection; improved diagnostic, prophylactic, and treatment strategies for infections in immunocompromised recipients; as well as the introduction of new immunosuppressive agents have all contributed to the dramatic improvements in survival. Actuarial survival rates following cardiac transplantation in excess of 82% and 77% at 1 and 2 years, respectively, point to the considerable progress made over the last 2 decades.[1] Long-term survival is now limited primarily by the development of late-stage problems including cardiac allograft vasculopathy (CAV) (also known as chronic rejection, transplant coronary artery disease, accelerated graft atherosclerosis) and complications related to chronic maintenance immunosuppression (e.g., infections, malignancy, hypertension, and nephrotoxicity).[2–6]

The number of transplant centers and number of transplanted patients rose progressively over time until 1994 when, due to a shortage of donors, the number of transplants plateaued. In 1996, 2342 heart transplants were performed in the United States. More than 41,000 heart and heart/lung transplants have been performed worldwide to date.[1]

CONDITIONS LEADING TO THE NEED FOR CARDIAC TRANSPLANTATION

It is estimated that there are 15,000 to 25,000 patients, 55 years of age and younger, with end-stage cardiac disease for whom survival and quality of life may be improved through cardiac transplantation.[7] This number could increase to 40,000 if patients up to age 65 are included and if the current progression rate to end-stage heart failure were to remain unchanged. In addition, this number is expected to grow as 400,000 new cases of heart failure are diagnosed each year. In the United States, more than $34 billion are spent annually for care of patients with heart failure.[8]

Although demand for cardiac donors continues to grow, the number of potential organ donors, according to current brain death criteria, remains relatively fixed at 14,000 per year. Of these 14,000 patients, only 4500 become organ donors, and of these, only slightly more than 2000 are suitable cardiac donors. Currently, there are more than 4500 patients on the national organ network waiting list for cardiothoracic transplantation.[9] Procurement of donor hearts with longer ischemic times, the use of older donors, and even the use of donors with borderline left ventricular function are being considered in an effort to increase donor supply.[10] This inequity between donor supply and recipient demand has resulted in a dramatic increase in waiting time from 6 weeks in 1988 to 6 months in 1990 to more than 1 year in 1993. Individual waiting times vary considerably based on recipient blood type, body size, clinical condition, and geographic location. As a result of this prolonged waiting time, 1 out of every 5 patients accepted for transplantation dies while waiting for a donor.

Optimal recipient management in the pretransplantation period has been shown to reduce the morbidity and mortality associated with end-stage heart failure. The timing for selection of the heart failure patient to become a transplant candidate is often difficult.[11] Optimal medical therapy includes the use of digoxin, angiotensin-converting enzyme (ACE) inhibitors, β-blockers, diuretics, and potassium and magnesium supplements.[12,13] Intermittent inotropic infusion therapy (e.g., dopamine, dobutamine, milrinone) may also be required. Frequent patient follow-up with careful attention to weight gain, nutrition, and electrolyte surveillance appears to reduce morbidity and the necessity for hospital admission. The high mortality rate of patients on the transplant waiting list will be altered only by improved methods of treating congestive heart failure or by possible alternatives to cardiac transplantation (e.g., ventricular reduction, cardiomyoplasty, mechanical devices).[14] Clinical testing of two implantable chronic cardiac replacement systems is underway. The devices consist of a permanently implanted pump coupled to a rechargeable power supply. The Novacor wearable left ventricular assist system (LVAS) has been in use in Europe since 1994, for patients in and out of the hospital,[15] and is currently in clinical trials in the United States (Fig. 16–1). In 1995, the HeartMate implantable left ventricle assist device was approved by the FDA as a "bridge" to transplant[16] (Fig. 16–2).

The major etiologies of heart failure in potential recipients include idiopathic cardiomyopathy in 51% and ischemic heart disease in 40%.[1] Other less common etiologies include valvular disease 4%, retransplantation for graft atherosclerosis or dysfunction 2.3%, and congenital heart disease 1.8%. The majority of recipients have been males between 30 and 55 years of age (mean 45 years).[17] However, the percentage of pediatric patients and patients greater than 55 years of age has continued to increase.

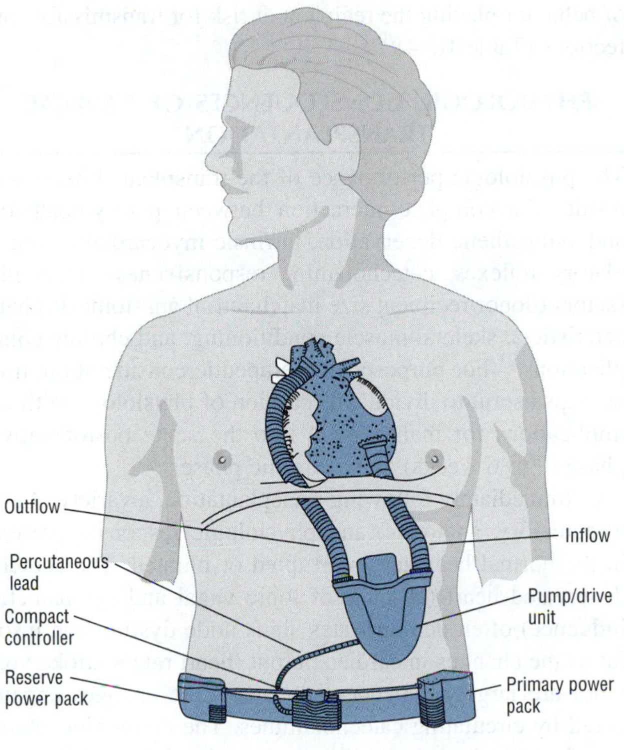

FIGURE 16–1. Wearable Novacor LVAS.

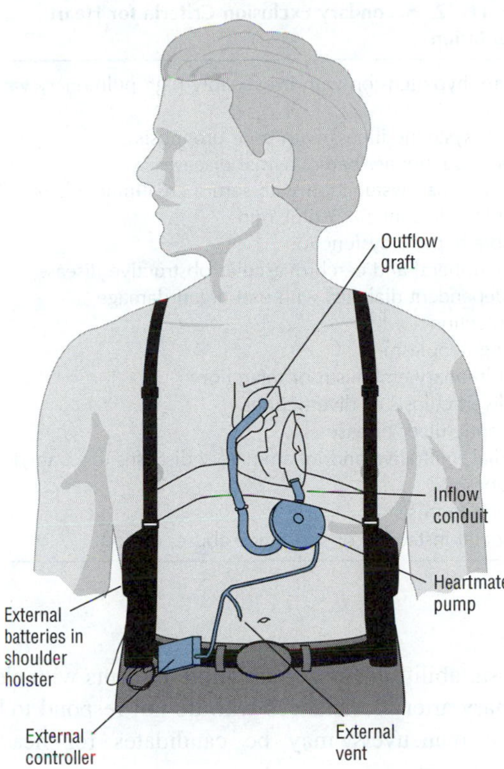

FIGURE 16–2. The vented electric HeartMate left ventricular assist device is battery powered and portable. Electrical wires and an air vent exit the skin to connect with the external controller. The pump also can be pneumatically actuated via the vent.

Cardiac transplant candidates typically are patients with end-stage heart failure who have New York Heart Association (NYHA) class III or IV symptoms, who are refractory to maximal medical management, and who have a life expectancy of less than 1 year. Based on the large number of patients who currently meet these general criteria, more objective methods of identifying patients with the poorest prognosis as candidates for cardiac transplant are needed (Table 16–1).[11] Peak V_{O_2} measured during maximal exercise testing provides an objective assessment of functional capacity and an indirect assessment of cardiovascular reserve; however, a variety of factors including age, gender, conditioning status, muscle mass, and angina can limit peak V_{O_2}.[18] Other predictors of poor survival include presence of sustained ventricular arrhythmias, right ventricular failure, hyponatremia, and elevated serum catecholamines.

Absolute contraindications to orthotopic cardiac transplantation include the presence of an active infection or the presence of other diseases (i.e., malignancy) that may limit survival and/or rehabilitation. Severe, irreversible pulmonary hypertension (defined as pulmonary vascular resistance [PVR] > 4 Wood units or a transpulmonary gradient [difference in mean pulmonary artery pressure and capillary wedge pressure > 15 mm Hg]), is also a contraindication because it could cause posttransplantation right ventricular failure. Candidates with borderline elevations in pulmonary resistance should be assessed to determine reversibility of pulmonary hypertension with vasodilatory agents such as nitroprusside, PGE_1, prostacyclin, or nitric oxide.[19] A patient with reversible pulmonary hypertension may be an acceptable candidate if pulmonary hypertension does not progress. The patient needs to be reassessed periodically to

TABLE 16–1. Criteria for Transplantation

I. Accepted Indications for Transplantation
1. Maximal V_{O_2} < 10 mL/kg/min with achievement of anaerobic metabolism
2. Severe ischemia consistently limiting routine activity not amenable to bypass surgery or angioplasty
3. Recurrent symptomatic ventricular arrhythmias refractory to all accepted therapeutic modalities, including AICD

II. Probable Indications for Cardiac Transplantation
1. Maximal V_{O_2} < 14 mL/kg/min and major limitation of patient's daily activities
2. Recurrent unstable ischemia not amenable to bypass surgery or angioplasty
3. Instability of fluid balance/renal function not owing to patient noncompliance with regimen of weight monitoring, flexible use of diuretic drugs, and salt restriction

III. Inadequate Indications for Transplantation
1. Ejection fraction < 20% in an asymptomatic or mildly symptomatic patient
2. History of Class III or IV symptoms of heart failure
3. Previous ventricular arrhythmias
4. Maximal V_{O_2} > 15 mL/kg/min without other indications

From Ref. 11.

TABLE 16–2. Secondary Exclusion Criteria for Heart Transplantation

Pulmonary hypertension with irreversibly high pulmonary vascular resistance
Coexistent systemic illness with poor prognosis
Irreversible pulmonary parenchymal disease
Irreversible renal dysfunction with serum creatinine > 2 mg/dL or creatinine clearance < 50 mL/min
Irreversible hepatic dysfunction
Severe peripheral and cerebrovascular obstructive disease
Insulin-dependent diabetes with end-organ damage
Active infection
Coexisting neoplasm
Acute pulmonary embolism or infarction
Active diverticulosis or diverticulitis
Active peptic ulcer disease
Myocardial infiltrative and inflammatory diseases (e.g., amyloidosis)
Severe obesity
Severe osteoporosis
Psychosocial instability or substance abuse, or both

From Ref. 11.

ensure suitability for transplantation. Patients with elevated pulmonary artery resistances who do not respond to hemodynamic maneuvers may be candidates for heart–lung transplantation.

Other exclusion criteria are listed in Table 16–2. Reversible renal and hepatic dysfunction may be the sequelae of chronic heart failure and should not necessarily disqualify the candidate.[11]

MECHANICS OF CARDIAC TRANSPLANTATION

DONOR SELECTION

Patients with irreversible neurologic damage become candidates for organ donation following a declaration of brain death.[20] Conventional cardiac donor criteria (Table 16–3), such as age, have been expanded considerably over the past several years in response to the continuing imbalance between donor supply and recipient demand. However, according to the International Society for Heart & Lung Transplantation (ISHLT), the use of donors older than 45 years is associated with a higher risk for 1-year mortality.[1] Several principles remain standard in donor selection. There should be ABO blood group compatibility with the prospective heart recipient, because mismatching in this system will result in hyperacute rejection. Human leukocyte antigen (HLA) tissue matching of the donor organ and recipient is not performed routinely pre-heart transplant unless the potential recipient is reactive against a panel of random donor antigens (i.e., positive crossmatch), in which case a negative T-cell crossmatch is required prior to transplantation. The donor should be hemodynamically stable, requiring only mild to moderate vasopressor support following volume replacement and have a normal echocardiogram. The donor should have no active infection or history of behavior placing the recipient at risk for transmissible infections (Table 16–4)[20]

PHYSIOLOGIC CONSEQUENCES OF CARDIAC TRANSPLANTATION

The physiologic performance of the transplanted heart is a result of a complex interaction between parasympathetic and sympathetic denervation, intrinsic myocardial autoregulatory reflexes, catecholamine responsiveness, anatomic factors (donor/recipient size match, atrial anastomosis characteristics), skeletal muscle conditioning, and chronic complications.[21] For purposes of therapeutic consideration, it is perhaps useful to divide a discussion of physiology with its implications for management into the acute postoperative phase (0 to 6 weeks) and a chronic phase.

Immediately following transplantation, a variety of autoregulatory, anatomic, and physiologic responses present in the normal heart are interrupted or blunted. The acutely denervated heart (absence of tonic vagal and sympathetic influence) often demonstrates sinus node dysfunction insofar as the changes in cardiac output (heart rate × stroke volume) are largely dependent on heart rate changes engendered by circulating catecholamines. The donor sinus node function may be impaired by preservation injury, direct surgical trauma at excision, the presence of long acting antiarrhythmics (e.g., amiodarone) taken prior to transplant by the recipient,[22] as well as by a lack of "conditioning" responsiveness to catecholamines. Therefore, the transplanted heart generally requires chronotropic support with either isoproterenol or pacing in the early posttransplant period to maintain a heart rate of 90 to 110 bpm and satisfactory hemodynamics (blood pressure, urine output, and tissue perfusion). Approximately 10% of transplant patients will have persistent chronotropic incompetence and require either extended (permanent) cardiac pacing or pharmacologic manipulation of the heart with isoproterenol, theophylline, or terbutaline.[23] Transplant with the bicaval anastamosis instead of the classical Shumway's donor–recipient atrial anastomosis has been reported to decrease the incidence of sinus node dysfunction and permanent pacer requirements.

In the early posttransplant period, anatomic variables may further compromise optimal hemodynamic function

TABLE 16–3. Criteria for Cardiac Donation

ABO blood type compatibility
Negative T-cell crossmatch if PRA[a] ≥ 5%
Age ≤ 60 years (older organs may be used in older recipients)
Size within 30% of recipient
Negative cardiac history
Normal electrocardiogram
Normal echocardiogram
Minimal pressor support (e.g., < 10 μg/kg/min dopamine or equivalent)
Central venous pressure ≤ 12 mm Hg

[a]PRA = panel reactive antibody.
From Ref. 20.

TABLE 16–4. Absolute and Relative Contraindications to Cardiac Donation

Absolute contraindications include:
1. Death from carbon monoxide poisoning, with blood carboxyhemoglobin level > 20%
2. Intractable ventricular arrhythmia
3. Inadequate oxygenation, with arterial saturation < 80% on ventilatory support
4. Documented previous myocardial infarction
5. Clinically significant structural heart disease, intracardiac tumor, or severe global hypokinesia with ejection fraction < 30% as determined by echocardiogram
6. Severe occlusive coronary artery disease on arteriography

Relative contraindications include:
1. Hepatitis B surface antigen positivity (? except in cases of surface-antigen-positive recipients)
2. Bacterial sepsis
3. Hepatitis C positivity
4. History of metastatic cancer
5. Extensive chest wall trauma with evidence of cardiac contusion by ECG or echocardiography
6. Prolonged hypotension, defined as a systolic blood pressure < 60 mm Hg for > 6h
7. Recurrent supraventricular and ventricular arrhythmias
8. Prolonged need for inotropic support, defined as a dopamine dosage > 20 μg/kg/min for > 24 h or comparable dosage of other β-agonist or epinephrine, norepinephrine, or dobutamine for the same period
9. Prolonged resuscitation time after cardiopulmonary arrest, defined as attempted cardiopulmonary resuscitation for > 30 min performed within 24 h of organ harvest or multiple episodes of attempted cardiopulmonary resuscitation
10. Severe left ventricular hypertrophy on electrocardiogram or echocardiogram
11. Echocardiogram revealing moderate hypokinesia
12. Noncritical coronary disease on arteriogram
13. History of carbon monoxide inhalation, with blood carboxyhemoglobin < 20%
14. History of intravenous drug abuse

From Ref. 20.

and complicate hemodynamic assessment of the patient. Right ventricular function is frequently impaired, presumably as a result of "preservation injury," and elevated pulmonary resistance. A "restrictive" hemodynamic pattern may be present initially, but it usually improves over 6 weeks following transplantation. Also, donor–recipient size mismatch may contribute to early posttransplantation hemodynamic abnormalities characterized by higher right and left ventricular end-diastolic pressures.

The chronically transplanted heart has been studied extensively both at rest and in response to exercise, which may unmask physiologic abnormalities not seen in the resting state.[24] Persistent abnormalities of diastolic function are noted in the chronically transplanted heart such that intracardiac pressures increase in an exaggerated fashion with response to exercise and/or volume infusion. These abnormalities of diastolic function may be due to acute rejection or to the scarring secondary to previously treated rejection episodes, hypertension, cardiac allograft vasculopathy, or most likely denervation.

The peculiar physiology of the transplanted heart has several implications for pharmacologic therapy. Drugs such as digoxin and atropine, whose mechanism of action is mediated by the parasympathetic nervous system, will have little effect in the transplanted heart. Augmentation of cardiac output is usually mediated via heart rate increases and, to a lesser extent, inotropic responses. Thus, drugs such as epinephrine and isoproterenol with their marked β-adrenergic effect are particularly useful in increasing cardiac output in transplant patients, whereas β-blocking agents may precipitate catastrophic cardiovascular collapse. The sinus node of the denervated heart is particularly sensitive to the negative chronotropic effects of acetylcholine or adenosine and caution must be used if these agents are given. Wilson has suggested that reinnervation may occur over time in the denervated heart, thereby facilitating more normal physiologic and pharmacologic responses.[25,26] Supraventricular arrhythmias are not uncommon in the early posttransplant period, but are usually transient. They are often related to acute rejection and do not usually mandate chronic antiarrhythmic therapy.

QUALITY OF LIFE AFTER TRANSPLANTATION

Quality of life indicators have been studied in cardiac transplant recipients as researchers and society seek to objectify and justify the rewards of transplantation.[21] Although cynics would maintain that heart transplantation involves the trading of one disease (heart failure) with a poor prognosis for another disease with a less dismal prognosis (posttransplantation status), most recipients self-assess themselves positively when compared with both their prior health status and in comparison to normals.[27]

CARE OF THE CARDIAC TRANSPLANT PATIENT

POSTOPERATIVE MANAGEMENT

Immediate postoperative care is similar to that provided for other patients undergoing cardiac surgery. Patients are generally extubated on the first postoperative day. Early ambulation, vigorous pulmonary toilet, and early removal of all central lines, catheters, and chest tubes are of considerable importance in minimizing infectious complications. The uncomplicated patient is transferred out of the intensive care unit within 48 to 72 hours and discharged from the hospital after 10 to 14 days.

Many early postoperative complications in the heart transplant recipient can be avoided by carefully screening donors (see Tables 16–3 and 16–4) and recipients prior to transplantation (see Tables 16–1 and 16–2). Primary graft failure and/or myocardial depression resulting from a combination of poor preservation, myocardial ischemia, catecholamines, and high energy phosphate depletion may occur and require inotropic support and often transient mechanical support. Commonly used inotropic agents are dopamine and epinephrine. Cardiac output in the transplanted heart is largely rate-dependent; therefore, isoproterenol (0.005 to 0.01 μg/kg/min) may be required to maintain the heart rate in the range of 110 to 130 beats/min to optimize cardiac output. The incidence of right ventricular failure secondary to high pulmonary vascular resistances can be decreased by carefully screening recipients. On occasion, intra- or postoperative administration of prostaglandins, vasodilators, including nitric oxide, and inotropic agents may be necessary to treat right-sided failure in the transplant patient. Cardiac function generally returns to normal within 3 to 4 days, during which time most patients can be weaned from chronotropic and inotropic support.

Hypertension may occur following surgery and may be caused by pain, hypothermia, stress, or the presence of preoperative hypertension. Systolic blood pressure is maintained at less than 140 mm Hg using afterload reduction with nitroprusside or nitroglycerin, thereby further augmenting cardiac function.

Because the incidence of acute rejection is highest during the first 6 months following transplantation, endomyocardial biopsies are performed at regularly scheduled intervals following transplantation: (weekly for the first month, every 2 weeks months 2 and 3, every 4 to 6 weeks months 4 through 6, every 3 months in months 7 through 12; then during the second year posttransplant, biopsies are performed only every 6 months, and beyond 2 years biopsies are performed yearly and as needed according to the clinical status of the patient.

IMMUNOSUPPRESSION PROTOCOLS

The implementation of triple-drug therapy regimens (cyclosporine, azathioprine, and prednisone) by Bolman and associates in 1983 resulted in improved survival rates and reduced nephrotoxicity, infection, and hypertension.[28] This regimen remains the cornerstone of many immunosuppressive protocols in use today,[29] even if modifications (e.g., early withdrawl of corticosteroids) have been introduced to improve complication rates and long-term results.

Current preoperative regimens consist primarily of azathioprine (2 to 4 mg/kg orally or intravenously) or mycophenolate mofetil (3.0 g orally) and varying dosages of cyclosporine (CsA) (0 to 10 mg/kg) administered orally 2 to 6 hours prior to surgery. All patients receive methylprednisolone 500 mg intravenously immediately after discontinuation of cardiopulmonary bypass and 125 mg intravenously every 12 hours for the first 36 hours after surgery.

The administration of lower doses of CsA is often employed until day 3 or 4 to decrease potential nephrotoxicity in the immediate postoperative period. CsA is usually titrated to achieve whole-blood levels as assayed by high-performance liquid chromatography in the range of 175 to 250 ng/mL, or plasma levels by radioimmunoassay of 180 to 250 ng/mL. Intravenous cyclosporine may be used in patients with absorption problems; however, controversy exists as to what steady-state concentrations are desirable. The advent of microemulsion cyclosporine with improved absorptive characteristics has decreased the need for intravenous administration.[30] Azathioprine is initiated at 2 mg/kg/d and the dose is adjusted to maintain a peripheral white blood cell count of 3500 to 6000 cells/mm^3. As an alternative to azathioprine, mycophenolate mofetil 1 to 1.5 g bid may be used. Prednisone is tapered from an initial dose of 1 to 1.5 mg/kg/d to 5 to 10 mg/d. Many programs are currently trying to withdraw prednisone by 6 to 12 months after transplant.[31,32] Potential benefits of steroid withdrawal include a lower incidence of osteoporosis, hypertension, hyperlipidemia, obesity, and diabetes. However, no multicenter studies have been conducted to assess the full impact of early steroid withdrawal on the incidence of cardiac allograft vasculopathy and long-term survival.

Tacrolimus (formerly FK506) was approved in 1994 and has been used as an alternative agent for cyclosporine in double and triple drug regimens.[33] The majority of experience with this agent in cardiac transplant recipients comes from a nonrandomized, open-label trial[34] and two unpublished randomized, multicenter comparisons between tacrolimus- and cyclosporine-based protocols.[35,36] The overall incidence of rejection during the first year appears similar to that with CsA; however, the incidence of side effects varies according to agent. With mechanisms of action, pharmacokinetic profiles, analytical difficulties, and toxicity profiles similar to those of cyclosporine, the major advantages of tacrolimus have been its efficacy as a "rescue" agent in patients with recalcitrant rejection, its steroid-sparing effects, and its lower propensity to cause hypertension, hyperlipidemia, gingival hyperplasia, and hirsutism.[34–40] The lower incidence of hypertension may be more related to its steroid-sparing effects, as it appears to be equally nephrotoxic as CsA.[39,40]

The usual starting dosage for cardiac transplant patients of tacrolimus is 0.1 to 0.2 mg/kg/d administered orally as a twice-daily dosage, or 0.025 to 0.075 mg/kg/d as a continuous intravenous infusion. Initially, tacrolimus concentrations are titrated to achieve whole-blood levels of 10 to 20 ng/mL or plasma levels of 0.5 to 2 ng/mL and lower concentrations (5 to 10 ng/mL) are used after 6 months if there are no rejection episodes.[34–37] Drug concentrations need to be monitored whenever the patient's condition changes, toxicity is suspected, or other drugs metabolized by CYP4503A are administered concomitantly (Table 16–5)

TABLE 16–5. Substrates, Inducers, and Inhibitors of Cytochrome P450 Enzymes

CYP1A	CYP2C	CYP2D6		CYP3A	
Substrates	***Substrates***	***Substrates***		***Substrates***	
Acetaminophen	Amitriptyline	Amitripyline	Nelfinavir	ABT-378	Flutamide
Amitriptyline	Benzphetamine	Bufuralol	Nortriptyline	Alfentanil	Indinavir
Antipyrine	Clomipramine	Captopril	Omeprazole	Alprazolam	Itraconazole
Caffeine	Cyclophosphamide	Citalopram	Ondansetron	Amiodarone	Ketoconazole
Chlorotrianisene	Dapsone	Chlorpromazine	Phenformin	Amiodipine	Lidocaine
Chlorzoxazone	Diazepam	Clomipramine	Propafenone	Antipyrine	Loratadine
Clarithromycin	Diclofenac	Clozapine	Propranolol	Astemizole	Lovastatin
Clomipramine	Ethosuximide	Codeine	Quinidine	Benzphetamine	Mephenytoin
Clozapine	Hexobarbital	Debrisoquine	Retinoic acid	Carbamazepine	Miconazole
Dantrolene	Ibuprofen	Desipramine	Risperidone	Cisapride	Midazolam
Diethylstilbestrol	Lansoprazole	Dextromethorphan	Ritonavir	Chlorpromazine	Nefazodone
Estradiol	Mephenytoin	Doxepin	RU486	Clarithromycin	Melfinavir
Flutamide	Naproxen	Encainide	Sparteine	Cocaine	Nevirapine
Fluvoxamine	Nelfinavir	Ethylmorphine	Tamoxifen	Cortisol	Nicardipine
Haloperidol	Nifedipine	Flecainide	Taxol	Cyclophosphamide	Nifedipine
Imipramine	Omeprazole	Fluoxetine (40%)	Teniposide	Cyclosporine	Omeprazole
Lidocaine	Phenylbutazone	Fluphenazine	Testosterone	Dantrolene	Paclitaxel
Methadone	Phenytoin	Haloperidol (small %)	Thioridazine	Dapsone	Paracetamol
Ondansetron	Piroxicam	Imipramine	Timolol	Delavirdine	Prednisone
Paracetamol	Progesterone	Indoramin	Tramadol	Dextromethorphan (min %)	Propafenone
Paraxathine	Proguanil	Labetolol	Trazadone	Diazepam	Progasterone
Phenacetin	Propranolol	Lidocaine	Triazolam	Digitoxin	Quindine
Procarbazine	Ritonavir	Maprotiline	Trifluperidol	Diltiazem	R-warfarin (minor)
Propafenone	S,R-warfarin	(R)-methadone (active isomer)	Trimipramine	Disopyramide	Ritonavir
Prostaglandins	Sulfinpyrazone	Metoprolol	Venlafaxine	Enalapril	Saquinavir
R-warfarin	Sulfaphenazole	Mexiletine	Vinblastine	Erythromycin	Sertraline
Ritonavir	Sulfonamides	Morphine	Zonisamide	Estradiol	Tacrolimus
Tacrine	Tamoxifen			Estrogen	Tamoxifen
Tamoxifen	Taxol			Ethosuccimide	Taxol
Theobromine	Tenoxicam			Ethylmorphine	Terfenadine
Theophylline	Testosterone			Etoposide	Testosterone
Toltrazuril	Tetrahydrocannabinol			Felodipine	Triazolam
Verapamil	Tolbutamide			FK506	Verapamil
	Tricyclics				Vinblastine
	Trimethadione				
	Valproic acid				
Inducers	***Inducers***	***Inducers***		***Inducers***	
Charbroiled food	For CYP2C9/10:	None identified		Carbamazepine	
Cigarette smoke	rifampicin			Dexamethasone	
Cruciferous vegetables	dexamethasone			DMP-266	
Omeprazole	phenobarbital			Isoniazid	
Phenobarbital	For CYP2C19:			Nevirapine	
Phenytoin	none identified			Phenobarbital	
				Phenytoin	
				Prednisone	
				Rifabutin/rifampicin	
Inhibitors	***Inhibitors***	***Inhibitors***		***Inhibitors***	
Cimetidine	Amiodarone (2C9/10)	Cimetidine	Norfluoxetine	Cimetidine	Miconazole
Ciprofloxacin	Cimetidine	Clomipramine	Paroxetine	Clarithromycin	Nefazodone
Enoxacin	Disulfiram	Desipramine	Perphenazine	Clotrimazole	Nelfinavir
Fluvoxamine	Fluconazole	Fluoxetine	Quinidine	Delavirdine	Nifedipine
Naldixic acid	Fluoxetine	Fluvoxamine (weak)	Ritonavir	Diltiazem	Norfloxacin
Norfloxacin	Fluvoxamine	Haloperidol	Sertraline	Erythromycin	Omeprazole
	Ketoconazole (2C9/10)	Methadone	Thioridazine	Fluoxetine	Paroxetine
	Omeprazole (2C9/10)	Moclobemide		Fluvoxamine	Propoxyphene
	Ritonavir			Grapefruit juice (6′, 7′-dihydroxybergamottin)	Ritonavir
	Sertraline			Indinavir	Saquinavir
				Itra / flu / ketoconazole	Sertraline
					Verapamil

TABLE 16–6. Drug Interactions of CsA and Tacrolimus

CsA Levels		Tacrolimus Levels	
Increase	*Decrease*	*Increase*	*Decrease*
Ketoconazole	Rifampicin	Ketoconazole	Rifampicin
Fluconazole	Phenytoin	Fluconazole	Dexamethasone
Itraconazole	Phenobarbital	Itraconazole	Phenytoin
Erythromycin	Carbamazepine	Erythromycin	
Diltiazem	Sulphadimine	Diltiazem	
Verapamil	Trimethoprim	Verapamil	
Danazol		Danazol	
Nicardipine		Cimetidine	
Metoclopramide		Clotrimazole	
Methylprednisolone		CsA	
Norethisterone			
Tacrolimus			

From Ref. 38.

The propensity for drug interactions for tacrolimus appears to be similar or greater than that with CsA. Until clinical data document the contrary, drugs known to interact with CsA should be assumed to interact with tacrolimus (Table 16–6).[41] Because tacrolimus is a macrolide, it may possibly interact with other drugs (e.g., theophylline) known to interact with erythromycin.[42]

Mycophenolate mofetil (MMF; formerly RS61443) was approved for use in renal transplant patients in 1995 and heart transplant patients in 1998 as an alternative to azathioprine. This drug is a prodrug that is rapidly hydrolyzed to the active ingredient mycophenolic acid, which is an anti-T and B cell agent that has less bone marrow toxicity than azathioprine.[43] It has demonstrated efficacy both as maintenance immunosuppression and "rescue" therapy for rejection episodes.[44–46] Its exact role in cardiac transplant patients remains to be identified. An international, multicenter, randomized, blinded 3-year comparison of MMF (3 g/d) and azathioprine (1.5 to 3.0 mg/kg/d) in combination with cyclosporine and oral corticosteroids recently completed enrollment of 650 primary heart transplant recipients.[47] In treated patients (MMF, n = 289; azathioprine, n = 289), the MMF group compared with the azathioprine group was associated with significant reduction in mortality at 1 year (6.2% versus 11.4%; $P = 0.031$) and a significant reduction in the requirement for rejection treatment (65.7% versus 73.7%; $P = 0.026$). Opportunistic infections, mostly herpes simplex, were more common in the MMF group (53.3% versus 43.6%; $P = 0.025$).

Because mycophenolic acid (MPA) is primarily eliminated by the kidneys and is also highly protein bound to albumin, therapeutic drug monitoring may prove useful in optimizing efficacy and/or minimizing toxicity. However, no clear association between prevention of rejection and toxicity and drug concentrations has been demonstrated to date, but this may be related more to analytical problems or measurement of total rather than free concentrations. Drug interactions have resulted in decreased absorption of MMF in combination with cholestyramine or antacids containing magnesium and aluminum, increased acyclovir and MPA's glucuronide metabolite concentrations secondary to competition for renal tubular secretion, and an increase in MPA trough concentrations when administered with tacrolimus, however, the exact mechanism is not known.[43]

Some centers have used monoclonal or polyclonal cytolytic agents (e.g., muromonab-CD3, OKT3, antilymphocyte globulin, or antithymocyte globulin) as "induction" therapy during the first 7 to 14 postoperative days to minimize the adverse side effects observed with the other agents.[48–50] To date, pooled data series show no clear-cut survival advantages with induction therapy, though it appears that a higher percentage of patients may be weaned from prednisone, thereby reducing the incidence of steroid-associated complications.[48,50,51] Controversy exists as to whether prophylactic therapy with these cytolytic agents confers any added benefit. In addition, cytolytic therapy is very expensive, is inconvenient to administer, possibly alters the incidence and character of infectious complications, and may result in a higher incidence of malignancy. With the recent introduction of less expensive and potentially less toxic immunosuppressants, the monoclonal and polyclonal agents are usually reserved for selective use in patients at high risk for toxicity from the other immunosuppressive agents and/or those who are more immunoreactive (e.g., treatment of steroid-resistant rejection). Daclizumab, the first humanized monoclonal antibody, was FDA approved in 1997 for prophylaxis of acute organ rejection in renal transplant recipients but has not been used extensively in heart recipients.[51] All of these medications are reviewed in greater detail in Chapter 43.

COMPLICATIONS AFTER CARDIAC TRANSPLANTATION

MORTALITY

Mortality in the early posttransplant period (first 3 months) occurs as a result of early graft failure usually owing to poor graft preservation, RV failure caused by pulmonary hypertension, or as a result of rejection or infection. Risk factors for death within the first postoperative year include prior transplantation, the use of a ventricular assist device or ventilator, very young or old recipient (< 5 years or > 60 years), older donor, and prolonged ischemic time.[17] In addition to infection and acute graft rejection, late mortality (> 12 months) occurs as a result of cardiac allograft vasculopathy, malignancy, cerebrovascular accident, or renal and/or hepatic failure.[3]

IMMUNOSUPPRESSION-RELATED COMPLICATIONS

ACUTE REJECTION

Despite advances in immunosuppression and refinement of postoperative care, acute cardiac allograft rejection remains a major determinant of survival following cardiac transplantation. Acute rejection continues to account for approximately 17% of all deaths.[52] The incidence of rejection is substantially higher during the early months following transplantation, with 90% of all rejections occurring within the first 6 months. In addition, the severity of rejection tends to be greater when it occurs early in the postoperative period. Although a minority of patients (37%) remain rejection-free, most will experience at least one episode of rejection during the first year (cumulative number of rejection episodes is 1.3 ± 0.7/patient).[52]

Clinical manifestations of rejection may include low-grade fever, malaise, heart failure (S_3), or atrial arrhythmias; however, most patients remain entirely asymptomatic. Although in the precyclosporine era, ECG changes (decrease in QRS voltage) served as an indicator of rejection, currently, the reliability of ECG monitoring to detect rejection has diminished owing to the more subtle presentation. The gold standard for detection of rejection is histologic confirmation using endomyocardial specimens obtained by transvenous biopsy. Biopsy specimens are examined for evidence of rejection and graded, based on histologic severity of the rejection.[53] Because endomyocardial biopsies are an invasive, expensive, and labor-intensive procedure, great efforts have been expended to identify an accurate and reproducible noninvasive method/marker to detect or predict acute rejection.[54] Unfortunately, none of the methods studied thus far, except for echo-Doppler, has the reliability of the endomyocardial biopsy.

The treatment of rejection is based on a number of factors including type, histologic grade, clinical symptoms, hemodynamic changes, noninvasive findings, and time after transplantation.

Mild degrees of acute cellular rejection (ISHLT Grade 1) are not usually treated unless the patient is symptomatic, whereas the presence of moderate to severe rejection (Grades 3 and 4) with or without necrosis, generally mandates treatment. Treatment of Grade 2 rejection is still a subject of debate. Acute rejection is usually treated with daily doses of methylprednisolone 500 to 1000 mg administered intravenously for 3 days. Lower doses (250 mg) may be equally effective[55] and in some situations, an oral prednisone taper (1.5 mg/kg/d tapered to ≤ 0.15 mg/kg/d over 7 to 14 days), either alone or in addition to intravenous therapy, may be used.[56] An endomyocardial biopsy is usually repeated within 7 days. If there is evidence of continuing or worsening rejection, the steroid therapy may be repeated and/or cytolytic therapy (ATG or OKT3) may be employed. Other innovative forms of therapy for persistent or intractable rejection have been investigated, including mycophenolate mofetil,[44,46] tacrolimus,[40] low-dose methotrexate,[57,58] sirolimus (formerly rapamycin),[59,60] total lymphoid irradiation,[58] and photopheresis.[61]

The majority of rejection episodes are histologically characterized by lymphocytic infiltrates with or without myocyte degeneration; however, in approximately 20% of those episodes, myocyte damage and lymphocytic infiltrates are absent. In contrast, extensive vascular damage is present and characterized by endothelial cell swelling, hemorrhages, interstitial edema, and occlusion of small capillaries. Immunofluorescence staining has shown deposition of immunoglobulins (IgG), complement, and fibrinogen at the level of the capillaries. This form of rejection is called humoral or vascular rejection and is usually preceded by the appearance of circulating immunocomplexes and the deposition of immunoglobulins and improves with their removal by plasmapheresis. It typically occurs early after transplant, is more frequent in female, younger recipients, and usually leads to severe, often irreversible, graft dysfunction; the mortality remains elevated.[62,63]

INFECTION

Both the severity and incidence of infections and deaths due to infections have decreased dramatically since the introduction of cyclosporine and use of lower steroid dosages. Nonetheless, infection and rejection remain the most frequently encountered complications associated with immunosuppression in the first year posttransplant.[64] The risk of infection is directly related to the overall level of immunosuppression and is greatest during the first 3 postoperative months, as well as following treatment of rejection episodes.[65] Laboratory or clinical evidence of an evolving infectious process necessitates the institution of aggressive diagnostic and frequently empiric therapeutic strategies. Infections in the transplant recipient can be categorized as nosocomial (catheter or wound related or pneumonia with staphylococcus or gram negatives), donor related (toxoplasmosis, hepatitis, cytomegalovirus [CMV]), or opportunistic

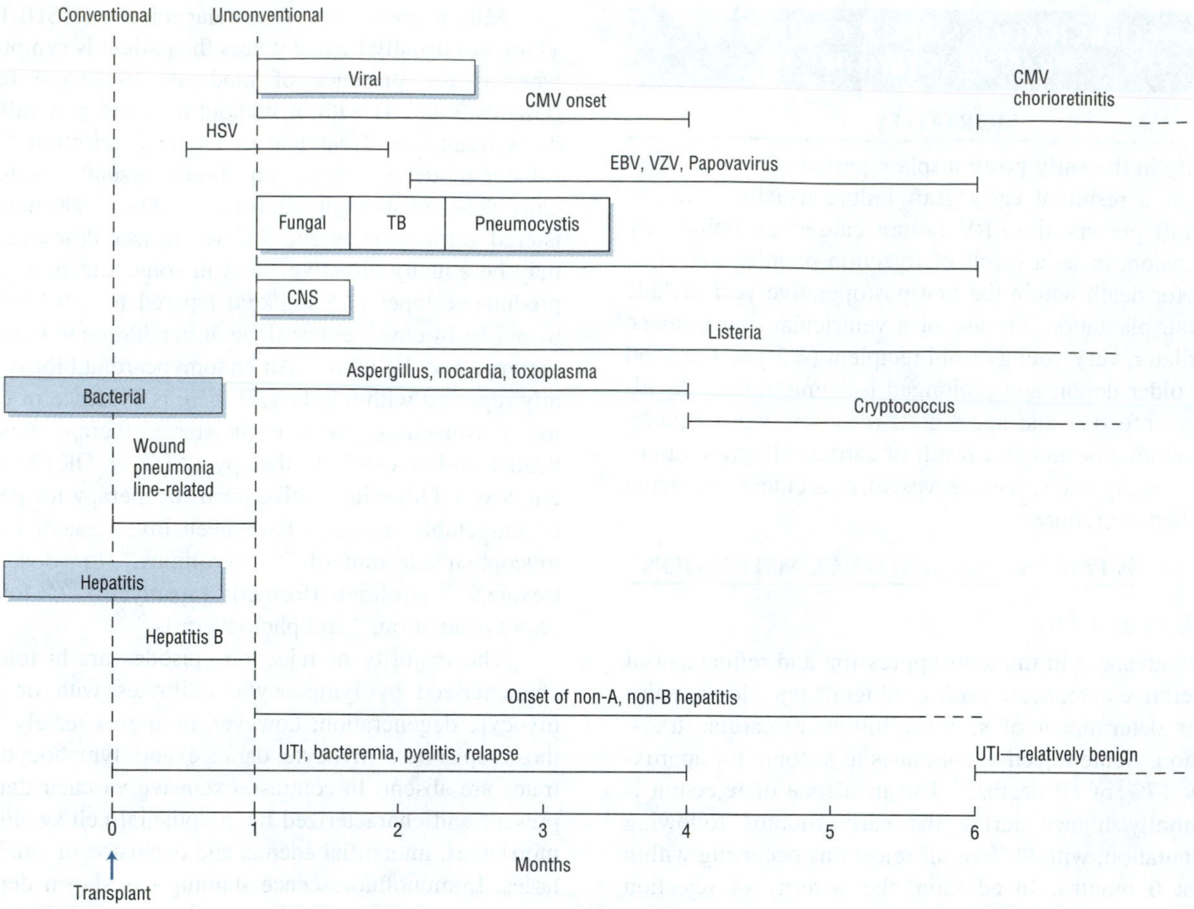

FIGURE 16–3. Timetable of infection for organ transplantation.

(CMV, pneumocystis, nocardia, fungal).[65,66] The infections usually present in a characteristic time course (Fig. 16–3) following transplant.[66] The most common sites of infection include lung, blood, urine, gastrointestinal tract, and sternal wound.[2] The latter accounts for only 7% of infections but represents 25% of the deaths; therefore, mediastinitis in an immunosuppressed patient can be devastating.[64] A number of preventive strategies are employed routinely in the transplant recipient and include trimethoprim–sulfamethoxazole (pneumocystis, toxoplasma, and nocardia prophylaxis), miconazole (candida), and antiviral agents (acyclovir, ganciclovir, immune globulin, CMV hyperimmune globulin) for CMV, herpes simplex virus (HSV), and Epstein Barr virus (EBV).[66–70]

CMV can cause direct damage (infection) or indirect damage such as stimulating antigen expression, inhibiting immune responses resulting in rejection, or allowing opportunistic infections and possibly chronic rejection.[71] Based on the premise that preventing CMV infection is preferable to treating CMV disease, most centers have adopted some type of preventive regimen.[70] The major limitation is that the anti-CMV agents appear to be most efficacious in preventing reactivation (secondary infection) but have had little impact on the incidence of primary infection in the highest risk group (seronegative recipients of seropositive allografts).[67,68] The added benefit of acyclovir and ganciclovir prophylaxis is that they have significant activity against the other herpes viruses, including EBV, which may provide a protective effect against posttransplant lymphoproliferative disease. Based on the current literature, there is no ideal regimen for CMV prevention. More aggressive strategies including intravenous ganciclovir ± CMV hyperimmune globulin followed by high-dose acyclovir or oral ganciclovir may be most appropriate for the highest risk patients (CMV-negative recipients of seropositive organs or those receiving antilymphocyte therapy with OKT3 or ATG), whereas selective preemptive therapy with ganciclovir (treating the infection once it manifests itself rather than administering prophylaxis to all patients) may be used in those seropositive recipients at risk for reactivation.[68]

CARDIAC ALLOGRAFT VASCULOPATHY

Cardiac allograft vasculopathy (CAV), also referred to as transplant coronary artery disease or chronic rejection, has been defined as the occurrence of an accelerated atherosclerosis in the coronary arteries of the graft. Numerous reports have suggested that the average incidence of this disease is approximately 10% per year or approximately 40% to 50%

of angiographically defined CAV by year 5 following transplantation.[72] This entity is thought to be similar to the "chronic rejection" processes also seen in renal, lung (obliterative bronchiolitis), and liver (vanishing bile duct syndrome) allografts. Achieving an understanding of and treatment for CAV remains the single major obstacle to improving long-term survival in cardiac transplant recipients.[73] Despite improvements in immunosuppression and consequently in overall survival, the incidence of the disease has not changed over the past 20 years.

Manifestations of CAV may include arrhythmias, impaired left ventricular function, congestive heart failure, acute myocardial infarction, and sudden cardiac death. Most heart transplant recipients with graft atherosclerosis do not experience "classic" angina because the allograft is denervated (true silent ischemia); however, angina should not be ignored, because reinnervation has been reported.[25,26] Accelerated graft atherosclerosis is characterized by a diffuse, concentric, intimal proliferation, which in contrast to traditional atherosclerosis, is not usually focal but involves the entire vessel length, frequently resulting in obliteration of the small vessels of both epimyocardial and intramyocardial coronary branches. To aid in the diagnosis of CAV, most centers perform annual cardiac evaluations including cardiac catheterization, thallium stress testing, and echocardiography. Because of the concentric, diffuse pattern of graft atherosclerosis, quantitive and serial assessment of coronary angiography must be compared to appreciate the concentric reduction in luminal diameter or obliteration of second- and third-order vessels. Intravascular ultrasound has been shown to be more sensitive than angiography in determining extent and degree of coronary intimal thickening and to better correlate with outcome.[74–76] By virtue of its diffuse nature, this type of graft atherosclerosis is rarely amenable to angioplasty or coronary artery bypass surgery. Focal atherosclerotic involvement, as seen in nontransplant ischemic heart disease, may also be found in the transplanted allograft. This latter process tends to occur in the proximal portions of the extramural coronary vessels and may be amenable to percutaneous balloon dilation.

The pathogenesis of CAV has not yet been delineated, but the frequent observation of intimal thickening and a mononuclear cell inflammatory reaction within the intima suggest that it may in part be caused by rejection, possibly as a result of a reaction to immunologic markers carried on vascular endothelial cells. It has been reported that CMV infection and subsequent rejection episodes are associated with the development of atherosclerosis in the transplanted heart.[77] It is possible the CMV contributes to an initial injury to the coronary endothelium, perhaps on an immunologic basis, that progresses to coronary artery disease. Another theory is that CMV expresses a protein that inhibits the beneficial function of a tumor suppression gene, thus promoting angiogenesis and accelerated atherosclerosis.[78] The potential long-term benefit of ganciclovir prophylaxis and treatment of CMV infections and its association with CAV remain to be assessed.

Conventional preventive measures used to decrease the incidence of graft atherosclerosis in the transplant recipient include maintenance of ideal body weight, control of blood pressure, and implementation of dietary and drug therapy for lipid disorders.[79] Other therapies including angiopeptin, low-molecular-weight heparin, calcium channel blockers, L-arginine, and estrogen are being studied.[80–83]

As previously mentioned, percutaneous transluminal coronary angioplasty and coronary bypass surgery are not usual options for treatment of diffuse graft atherosclerosis, even if both have been used, leaving retransplantation as the only potential therapy. The prognosis following retransplantation is suboptimal, as reflected by a 1-year actuarial survival rate of 49%.[17] In addition, the extensive incidence of graft atherosclerosis potentially necessitating retransplantation introduces several additional ethical considerations regarding the allocation of scarce donor organs.

MALIGNANCY

Therapy with potent immunosuppressive agents may engender diminished immune surveillance and direct carcinogenic or mutagenic action, chronic antigenic stimulation, or activation of oncogenic viruses resulting in an increased potential for tumor development.[84] Malignant neoplasms are an unfortunate consequence of chronic immunosuppression and may be an unavoidable complication of modifying the normal immune process.

The prevalence of cancers that occur most frequently in the general population (carcinomas of the lung, prostate, breast, and colon and invasive carcinomas of the uterine cervix) is not increased among transplant recipients. However, a variety of cancers that are uncommon in the general population often occur with a higher prevalence in transplant recipients: lymphomas (21% of cancers in transplant recipients are lymphomas, 93% of which are non-Hodgkin's or lymphoproliferative disorders), squamous-cell carcinomas of the lip and skin, Kaposi's sarcoma, other sarcomas, carcinomas of the vulva and perineum, carcinomas of the kidney, and hepatobiliary tumors.

The incidence of lymphoma appears to correlate with the intensity of immunosuppression. The use of more intensive immunosuppression in extrarenal transplant recipients is particularly common and is reflected in the higher incidence of lymphomas seen in cardiac recipients when compared to renal recipients.[85]

The incidence, time to occurrence, and features of the tumors appear to vary with use of various immunosuppressive agents. Azathioprine-based immunosuppressive regimens have been associated with a high incidence (40% of all malignancies) of cutaneous malignancies. One possible mechanism to explain this unusually high incidence of skin cancer involves azathioprine's metabolite, nitroimidazole, which causes significant photosensitivity resulting in subsequent skin cancer.[86] Azathioprine therapy is associated with a 2:1 predominance of squamous over basal cell carcinomas, whereas basal cell carcinoma occurs more frequently in the general population. Azathioprine-induced cutaneous squamous cell carcinoma is also associated with more metastatic disease and accounts for 6% of all deaths in comparison to less than 1% with cyclosporine.

With the introduction of CsA, the incidence of non-Hodgkin's lymphoma or lymphoproliferative disorder (LPD) increased to 29% as compared to 11% with regimens based on azathioprine or cyclophosphamide. The tumors tended to occur earlier (15 months after transplantation in the CsA group versus 48 months in the azathioprine or cyclophosphamide group); and 32% occurred within 4 months postoperatively in the CsA group versus 11% for older non-CsA-based regimens. Among patients treated with OKT3 and other monoclonal antibodies, lymphomas account for 64% of all tumors. These lymphomas frequently develop soon after transplantation (average, 7 months).[85] In one report, LPD developed in 1.3% of patients receiving triple-drug immunosuppression as compared to 11.4% in patients receiving the monoclonal antibody OKT3. A statistically significant increase in incidence was noted in patients receiving cumulative OKT3 dose of greater than 75 mg.[87] This report demonstrates the contribution of overall immunosuppressive load in comparison to centers using lower doses.[88] Similarly, the use of ATG was found to increase the risk of LPD.[85] T-cell-specific agents (CsA, OKT3, ATG) that directly impair T-cell function may produce a reduction in host response to viral infections, particularly EBV and CMV. EBV has been shown to have infectious as well as oncogenic properties and may play a causal role in the development of mononucleosis, Burkitt's lymphoma, and nasal pharyngeal carcinoma. Reduction in immunosuppression intensity and concomitant therapy with acyclovir have resolved some forms of LPD.[89]

The clinical presentation of LPD may vary from a flu-like syndrome to multisystem organ failure. A higher proportion of patients receiving conventional immunosuppression have extranodal involvement as compared with CsA-based regimens. Extranodal involvement occurs in 69% of cases in transplant recipients versus 24% to 48% in the general population. Central nervous system involvement occurs more frequently in patients with conventional immunosuppression (39%) as compared with CsA-based regimens (14%).

The diagnosis of LPD is made by a tissue biopsy. The histologic types of LPD are described in Chapter 12. Treatment depends on symptoms, presentation, and extent of involvement. In general, reduction of immunosuppression and concomitant therapy with acyclovir have been often associated with resolution and remission of LPD.[86,87] Radiotherapy, chemotherapy, and surgical excision may be necessary in certain situations as palliative therapy but are rarely curative. Optimal preventive therapy is to avoid overimmunosuppression in transplant recipients. A 5-year mortality rate of 37% has been reported in patients with LPD.[85]

IMMUNOSUPPRESSANT-RELATED ADVERSE EFFECTS

HYPERTENSION

Arterial hypertension is the most common posttransplantation medical problem, which, despite intensive investigation, remains poorly understood. The incidence of posttransplantation hypertension in cardiac recipients has increased from less than 20% in the conventional immunosuppression era to greater than 90% in the current era using cyclosporine-based regimens.[90] In the conventional era, hypertension was felt to be a result of mineralocorticoid excess engendered by immunosuppressive regimens heavily based on prednisone. Paradoxically, with the introduction of cyclosporine-based regimens allowing for steroid dosage reduction or discontinuation, hypertension has become more prevalent.[90]

The primary mechanism of CsA-associated hypertension in heart transplant recipients may be related to the CsA-induced stimulation of intact renal sympathetic nerves and the absence of reflex cardiac inhibition of the sympathetic nervous system,[90] but a variety of other mechanisms including decreased prostacyclin and NO production have also been proposed.[91,92] In addition to CsA's propensity to cause peripheral vasoconstriction, it promotes sodium retention by increasing proximal tubular sodium retention, resulting in extracellular fluid volume expansion. Thus, diuretics and dietary sodium restriction are used routinely in heart transplant recipients. Because CsA and diuretics also induce renal magnesium wasting, hypomagnesemia may contribute to the hypertension as magnesium is purported to be a vasorelaxant. Magnesium supplementation is usually necessary in CsA-treated patients unless they have renal insufficiency. Diuretics, although effective, may aggravate lipid abnormalities in these patients.[93]

No single antihypertensive agent has been found to be uniformly effective in controlling CsA-associated hypertension. Currently, the use of calcium channel antagonists (e.g., diltiazem), inhibitors of central sympathetic outflow (clonidine), and ACE inhibitors have all been found to be effective in the treatment of this form of hypertension.[94] Calcium channel blockers, particularly diltiazem, are often considered drugs of choice because they have other purported benefits on the development of graft atherosclerosis and may also be renal protective.[95] Polydrug regimens are often necessary. Additional hypertension control is seen as a salutary effect of current immunosuppressive protocols that eliminate prednisone after transplantation.

NEPHROTOXICITY

One of the most common side effects observed in heart transplant recipients receiving maintenance cyclosporine or tacrolimus therapy is nephrotoxicity.[96] Two types of toxicity occur: Acute nephrotoxicity is often seen early and is dose dependent and reversible, but chronic nephropathy is more common. Clinical manifestations of cyclosporine nephrotoxicity include elevated serum creatinine and BUN, hyperkalemia, hyperuricemia, mild proteinuria, and a decreased fractional excretion of sodium.

The predominant mechanism for cyclosporine nephrotoxicity is renal vasoconstriction, primarily of the afferent arteriole, resulting in increased renal vascular resistance, decreased renal blood flow by up to 40%, reduced GFR by up to 30%, and increased proximal tubular sodium reabsorption with a reduction in urinary sodium and potassium excretion.[92] A number of other mechanisms have been implicated including changes in the renin–angiotensin–aldosterone system, prostaglandin synthesis, NO production, sympathetic nervous system activation, and alterations in calcium handling.[92]

Measures to reduce CsA nephrotoxicity include delaying its administration immediately postop in patients at high risk for nephrotoxicity (using alternative induction protocols including OKT3 or ATG), monitoring CsA trough blood levels and reducing the cyclosporine dosage if the vasoconstrictive effects present, and cautiously using other nephrotoxins (e.g., aminoglycosides, amphotericin B, nonsteroidal anti-inflammatory agents). When using these agents, drug concentrations of CsA and those of the other drugs, if available, should be monitored closely. In addition, the concomitant administration of drugs (e.g., azole antifungals, especially ketoconazole and to a lesser extent fluconazole and itraconazole, the macrolide antibiotics [erythromycin, clarithromycin, tacrolimus], the calcium antagonists [diltiazem, nicardipine, verapamil], and antidepressants [nefazadone, fluvoxamine]) known to elevate cyclosporine levels requires intentional dosage reductions to avoid unnecessary renal and other toxicity.[97] Similar management strategies are useful when dealing with tacrolimus (FK506) because it is at least as nephrotoxic as CsA.[38,42] Other drugs may also increase CsA and tacrolimus concentrations (Table 16–6). Some centers take advantage of these interactions by routinely using "CsA-sparing agents" to reduce the dosage and cost of therapy while maintaining the same therapeutic concentrations.[98]

Currently, no proven therapies consistently prevent or reverse the nephrotoxic effects of cyclosporine; however, a number of agents have been studied including prostaglandin analogs, pentoxyphylline, fish oils, and so on. Based on their effects on calcium flux and on endothelin production (vasoconstrictive substance), the calcium channel blockers appear to be the most promising.[95]

HYPERLIPIDEMIA

Although hypercholesterolemia is a known risk factor for the development of coronary artery disease and reduction of serum cholesterol levels decreases cardiac morbidity and mortality in the general population, conflicting evidence exists regarding the relationship between the hyperlipidemia commonly seen in heart recipients and the development of CAV.[99] A progressive rise in serum cholesterol and triglyceride occurs in a time-dependent fashion following cardiac transplantation. Both steroids and cyclosporine are known to increase serum cholesterol and triglyceride levels.[93] Other drugs, including diuretics, β-blockers, ethanol, may aggravate hyperlipidemia in transplant patients.[93] Drug therapy to reduce cholesterol and triglycerides may be used but dosage reduction of lovastatin and monitoring for myositis are necessary to avoid rhabdomyolysis if it is used concomitantly with CsA.[100] The other "statins" (pravastatin, simvastatin) are preferred because of a lower interactive potential with CsA and may have a salutory immunosuppressive effect as well.[99] Management of hyperlipidemia in the heart transplant recipient is reviewed elsewhere.[100]

FUTURE PROSPECTS FOR CARDIAC TRANSPLANTATION AND TREATMENT

A variety of factors, including refined selection criteria, improvements in immunosuppressive regimens, diagnostic techniques for rejection, donor organ preservation, and treatment of infectious complications, have contributed to the overall success of cardiothoracic transplantation. The majority of patients return to NYHA functional class I and are able to achieve a desirable quality of life following transplantation. Despite the tremendous progress made in cardiothoracic transplantation over the last decade, much remains to be done.

The therapeutic-to-toxic ratio of currently used immunosuppressive agents remains narrow, mandating lifelong monitoring of patients. The identification of more specific immunosuppressive agents, with a higher therapeutic-to-toxic index or one capable of inducing tolerance to the grafted organ, remains a desirable, though elusive goal at this time. Similarly, the development of noninvasive techniques for the diagnosis of graft rejection would substantially reduce the inconvenience, cost, and morbidity associated with long-term surveillance.

Chronic graft atherosclerosis remains to be understood, and until the pathogenesis and appropriate treatment are defined, graft dysfunction secondary to this form of atherosclerosis will remain the leading impediment to long-term survival.

Although ideally legislative and public awareness programs will have an impact on resolving the chronic shortage of suitable donors, the rapidly increasing number of patients afflicted with congestive heart failure will necessitate developing alternative options for patients with end-stage disease. The role of long-term mechanical circulatory assistance, xenotransplantation, ventricular reduction surgery (Batista procedure), and dynamic cardiomyoplasty remain to be defined. It is likely that the coming decade will witness enhanced therapeutic and laboratory research designed to evaluate and refine the clinical, immunologic, and socioeconomic impact of using these alternative options.

▶ PRINCIPLES OF PHARMACOTHERAPY

- Survival and quality of life after heart transplantation are limited by posttransplant events, such as infection and acute and chronic rejection.
- Patients require lifelong immunosuppression to maintain the stability of their grafts.
- Overimmunosuppression predisposes patients to infection, malignancy, and drug toxicity, whereas underimmunosuppression increases the risk of rejection.
- Combinations of two or three immunosuppressants are usually necessary to maximize immunosuppressive efficacy while minimizing the toxicity of the individual agents.
- Immunosuppressant-induced side effects, including nephrotoxicity, hypertension, hyperlipidemia, and diabetes, occur frequently and usually require additional drug therapy.
- Antimicrobial prophylaxis is necessary to decrease the risk of bacterial, viral (e.g., CMV, HSV, EBV), fungal (e.g., candida, aspergillus), and other opportunistic infections (e.g., PCP, nocardia).
- Heart transplant patients receive multiple medications and both pharmacokinetic and pharmacodynamic interactions are very common.
- The consequences of drug interactions (e.g., over- or underimmunosuppression) can be life-threatening, and heart transplant patients must be monitored closely whenever new drugs are added or existing medications are discontinued from their drug therapy regimens.
- As more immunosuppressive agents are introduced to the marketplace, drug therapy regimens in heart transplant patients need to be individualized based on each patient's immunologic status and toxicity-risk profile.
- Cardiac allograft vasculopathy remains the number one cause of long-term morbidity and mortality, and the incidence has been minimally affected by the advent of new immunosuppressants.

REFERENCES

1. Hosenpud JD, Bennet LE, Keck BM, et al. The Registry of the International Society for Heart and Lung Transplantation: Fourteenth Official Report—1997. J Heart Lung Transplant 1997;16:691–712.
2. Miller LW, Schlant RC, Kobashigawa JA, et al. 24th Bethesda conference: Cardiac Transplantation Task Force 5: Complications. J Am Coll Cardiol 1993;22:41–54.
3. Gallo P, Agozzino L, Angelini A, et al. Causes of late failure after heart transplantation: A ten-year survey. J Heart Lung Transplant 1997;16:1113–1121.
4. Costanzo MR, Augustine S, Bourge R, et al. Selection and treatment of candidates for heart transplantation. A statement for health professionals from the Committee on Heart Failure and Cardiac Transplantation of the Council of Clinical Cardiology, American Heart Association. Circulation 1995;92:3593–3612.
5. Shaw LM, Kaplan B, Kaufman D. Toxic effects of immunosuppressive drugs: Mechanisms and strategies for controlling them. Clin Chem 1996;42:1316–1321.
6. Rossi SJ, Schroeder TJ, Hariharan S, First MR. Prevention and management of the adverse effects associated with immunosuppressive therapy. Drug Saf 1993;9:104–131.
7. Evans RW, Manninen DL, Dong F, et al. The National Cooperative Transplantation Study. Seattle, WA, Battelle Research Center, 1991.
8. O'Connell JB, Bristow MR. Economic impact of heart failure in the United States: Time for a different approach. J Heart Lung Transplant 1994;13:S107–S111.
9. UNOS Scientific Registry, Richmond, VA. December 10, 1997.
10. O'Connell JB, Gunnar RM, Evans RW, et al. 24th Bethesda conference: Cardiac Transplantation Task Force 1: Organization of heart transplantation in the U.S. J Am Coll Cardiol 1993;22:8–14.
11. Mudge GH, Goldstein S, Addonizio LJ, et al. 24th Bethesda conference: Cardiac Transplantation Task Force 3: Recipient guidelines/prioritization. J Am Coll Cardiol 1993;22:21–31.
12. Stevenson LW. Selection and management of candidates for heart transplantation. Curr Opin Cardiol 1996;11:166–173.
13. Packer M, Bristow MR, Cohn JN, et al. The effect of carvedilol on morbidity and mortality in patients with chronic heart failure. U.S. Carvedilol Heart Failure Study Group. N Engl J Med 1996;334: 1349–1355.
14. Costanzo-Nordin MR, Cooper DKC, Jessup M, et al. 24th Bethesda conference: Cardiac Transplantation Task Force 6: Future developments. J Am Coll Cardiol 1993;22:54–64.
15. Vetter HO, Kaulbach HG, Schmitz C, et al. Experience with the Novacor left ventricular assist system as a bridge to cardiac transplantation, including the new wearable system. J Thorac Cardiovasc Surg 1995;109:74–80.
16. McCarthy PM. HeartMate implantable left ventricular assist device: Bridge to transplantation and future applications. Ann Thorac Surg 1995;59:S46–S51.
17. Kaye MP. The Registry of the International Society for Heart and Lung Transplantation: Tenth Official Report—1993. J Heart Transplant 1993;12:541–548.
18. Mancini DM, Eisen H, Kussmaul W, et al. Value of peak exercise oxygen consumption for optimal timing of cardiac transplantation in ambulatory patients with heart failure. Circulation 1991;83:778–786.
19. Costard-Jackle A, Fowler MB. Influence of pre-operative pulmonary artery pressure on mortality after heart transplantation: Testing of potential reversibility of pulmonary hypertension with nitroprusside is useful in defining a high risk group. J Am Coll Cardiol 1992; 19:48–54.
20. Baldwin JC, Anderson JL, Boucek MM, et al. 24th Bethesda conference: Cardiac Transplantation Task Force 2: Donor guidelines. J Am Coll Cardiol 1993;22:15–20.
21. Young JB, Winters WL, Bourge R, Uretsky BF. 24th Bethesda conference: Cardiac Transplantation Task Force 4: Function of the heart transplant recipient. J Am Coll Cardiol 1993;22:31–41.
22. Chelimsky-Fallick C, Middlekauff H, Stevenson W, et al. Amiodarone therapy does not compromise subsequent heart transplantation. J Am Coll Cardiol 1992;20:1556–1561.
23. Redmond JM, Zehr KJ, Gillinov MA, et al. Use of theophylline for treatment of prolonged sinus node dysfunction in human orthotopic heart transplantation. J Heart Lung Transplant 1993;12:133–139.
24. Kao AC, Van Trigt P, Shaeffer-McCall GS, et al. Central and peripheral limitations to upright exercise in untrained cardiac transplant recipients. Circulation 1994;89:2605–2615.
25. Wilson RF, Christensen BV, Olivari MT, et al. Evidence for structural sympathetic reinnervation after orthotopic cardiac transplantation in humans. Circulation 1991;83:1210–1220.
26. Wilson RF. Reinnervation reexamination. J Heart Lung Transplant 1998;17:137–139.
27. Hershberger RE. Clinical outcomes, quality of life, and cost outcomes after cardiac transplantation. Am J Med Sci 1997;314:129–138.

28. Bolman RM, Elick B, Olivari MT, et al. Improved immunosuppression for heart transplantation. J Heart Transplant 1985;11:315–318.
29. Olivari MT, Kubo SH, Braunlin EA, et al. Five-year experience with triple-drug immunosuppression therapy in cardiac transplantation. Circulation 1990;82(suppl):IV276–280.
30. Friman S, Backman L. A new microemulsion formulation of cyclosporin: Pharmacokinetic and clinical features. Clin Pharmacokinet 1996;30:181–193.
31. Olivari MT, Jessen ME, Baldwin BJ, et al. Triple-drug immunosuppression with steroid discontinuation by six months after heart transplantation. J Heart Lung Transplant 1995;14:127–135.
32. Taylor DO, Bristow MR, O'Connell JB, et al. Improved long-term survival after heart transplantation predicted by successful early withdrawal from maintenance corticosteroid therapy. J Heart Lung Transplant 1996;15:1039–1046.
33. Kelly PA, Burckart GJ, Venkataramanan R. Tacrolimus: A new immunosuppressive agent. Am J Health Syst Pharm 1995;52:1521–1535.
34. Pham SM, Kormos RL, Hattler BG, et al. A prospective trial of tacrolimus (FK506) in clinical heart transplantation: Intermediate-term results. J Thorac Cardiovasc Surg 1996;111:764–772.
35. Reichart B, Meiser B, Vigano M, et al. Tacrolimus (FK506) vs cyclosporin in heart transplantation: Results from a randomized, European, multicentre pilot study. J Heart Lung Transplant 1997;16:43.
36. Taylor DO, Marr BL, Radovanic B, et al. A comparison of tacrolimus- and cyclosporine-based immunosuppression in cardiac transplantation. J Heart Lung Transplant 1997;16:72.
37. Taylor DO. The use of tacrolimus and mycophenolate mofetil after cardiac transplantation. Curr Opin Cardiol 1997;12:161–165.
38. Meiser BM, Uberfuhr P, Fuchs A, et al. Tacrolimus: A superior agent to OKT3 for treating cases of persistent rejection after intrathoracic transplantation. J Heart Lung Transplant 1997;16:795–800.
39. Pratschke J, Neuhaus R, Tullius SG, et al. Treatment of cyclosporine-related adverse effects by conversion to tacrolimus after liver transplantation. Transplantation 1997;64:938–940.
40. Bennett WM. The nephrotoxicity of immunosuppressive drugs. Clin Nephrol 1995;43(suppl 1):S3–7.
41. Mignat C. Clinically significant drug interactions with new immunosuppressive agents. Drug Saf 1997;16:267–278.
42. Ludden TM. Pharmacokinetic interactions of the macrolide antibiotics. Clin Pharmacokinet 1985;10:63–79.
43. Sievers TM, Rossi SJ, Ghobrial RM, et al. Mycophenolate mofetil. Pharmacotherapy 1997;17:1178–1197.
44. Renlund DG, Gopinathan SK, Kfoury AG, Taylor DO. Mycophenolate mofetil (MMF) in heart transplantation: Rejection prevention and treatment. Clin Transplant 1996;10:136–139.
45. Taylor DO, Ensley RD, Olsen SL, et al. Mycophenolate mofetil (RS-61443): Preclinical, clinical, and three-year experience in heart transplantation. J Heart Lung Transplant 1994;13:571–582.
46. Kirklin JK, Bourge RC, Naftel DC, et al. Treatment of recurrent heart rejection with mycophenolate mofetil (RS-61443): Initial clinical experience. J Heart Lung Transplant 1994;13:444–450.
47. Kobashigawa J, Miller L, Renlund D, et al. A randomized active-controlled trial of mycophenolate mofetil in heart transplant recipients. Mycophenolate Mofetil Investigators. Transplantation 1998;66:507–515.
48. Prieto M, Lake KD, Pritzker MR, et al. OKT3 induction and steroid-free maintenance immunosuppression for treatment of high-risk heart transplant recipients. J Heart Lung Transplant 1991;10: 901–911.
49. Costanzo-Nordin MR, O'Sullivan JE, Johnson MR, et al. Prospective randomized trial of OKT3 versus horse antithymocyte globulin-based immunosuppressive prophylaxis in heart transplantation. J Heart Transplant 1990;9:306–315.
50. Wilde MI, Goa KL. Muromonab CD3: A reappraisal of its pharmacology and use as prophylaxis of solid organ transplant rejection. Drugs 1996;51:865–894. Review.
51. Vincenti F, Kirkman R, Light S, et al. Interleukin-2 receptor blockade with daclizumab to prevent acute rejection in renal transplantation. N Engl J Med 1998;338:161–165.
52. Kobashigawa JA, Kirklin JK, Naftel DC, et al. Pre-transplantation risk factors for acute rejection after heart transplantation: A multi-institutional study. J Heart Lung Transplant 1993;12:355–366.
53. Billingham ME, Cary NRB, Hammond ME, et al. A working formulation for the standardization of nomenclature in the diagnosis of heart and lung rejection: Heart rejection study group. J Heart Transplant 1990;9:587–593.
54. Tugulea S, Ciubotariu R, Colovai AI, et al. New strategies for early diagnosis of heart allograft rejection. Transplantation 1997;64:842–847.
55. Wahlers T, Heublein B, Cremer J, et al. Treatment of rejection after heart transplantation: What dosage of pulsed steroids is necessary? J Heart Transplant 1990;9:568–574.
56. Hosenpud JD, Norman DJ, Pantely GA. Low dose oral prednisone in the treatment of acute cardiac allograft rejection not associated with hemodynamic compromise. J Heart Transplant 1990;9:292–296.
57. Costanzo MR, Koch DM, Fisher SG, et al. Effects of methotrexate on acute rejection and cardiac allograft vasculopathy in heart transplant recipients. J Heart Lung Transplant 1997;16:169–178.
58. Ross HJ, Gullestad L, Pak J, et al. Methotrexate or total lymphoid radiation for treatment of persistent or recurrent allograft cellular rejection: A comparative study. J Heart Lung Transplant 1997;16:179–189.
59. Miller L, Brozena S, Valantine H, for the Rapamycin Investigators. Treatment of acute cardiac allograft rejection with rapamycin: A multicenter dose ranging study. J Heart Lung Transplant 1997;16:44.
60. Kelly PA, Gruber SA, Behbod F, Kahan BD. Sirolimus, a new potent immunosuppressive agent. Pharmacotherapy 1997;17:1148–1156.
61. Barr ML. Immunomodulation in transplantation with photopheresis. Artif Organs 1996;20:971–973.
62. Olivari MT, May CB, Johnson NA, et al. Treatment of acute vascular rejection with immunoadsorption. Circulation 1994;90:II70–II73.
63. Hammond EH, Yowell RL, Nunoda S, et al. Vascular (humoral) rejection in heart transplantation: Pathologic observations and clinical implications. J Heart Transplant 1989;8:430–443.
64. Miller LW, Naftel DC, Bourge RC, et al, and the Cardiac Transplant Research Database Group. Infection after heart transplantation: A multiinstitutional study. J Heart Lung Transplant. 1994;13:381–393.
65. Thaler SJ, Rubin RH. Opportunistic infections in the cardiac transplant patient. Curr Opin Cardiol 1996;11:191–203.
66. Rubin RH, Tolkoff-Rubin NE. Antimicrobial strategies in the care of organ transplant recipients. Antimicrob Agents Chemother 1993;37:619–624.
67. Merigan TC, Renlund DG, Keay S, et al. A controlled trial of ganciclovir to prevent cytomegalovirus disease after heart transplantation. N Engl J Med 1992;326:1182–1186.
68. Griffiths PD. Prophylaxis against CMV infection in transplant patients. J Antimicrob Chemother 1997;39:299–301.
69. Ross H, Gamberg P, Hunt SA, et al. Sequelae of cytomegalovirus infection in the era of ganciclovir prophylaxis: Is ganciclovir enough? J Heart Lung Transplant 1997;16:110.
70. Couchoud C, Cucherat M, Haugh M, Pouteil-Noble C. Cytomegalovirus prophylaxis with antiviral agents in solid organ transplantation. Transplantation 1998;65:641–647.
71. McCarthy JM, Karim MA, Krueger H, et al. The cost impact of cytomegalovirus disease in renal transplant recipients. Transplantation 1993;55:1277–1282.
72. Weis M, von Scheidt W. Cardiac allograft vasculopathy: A review. Circulation 1997;96:2069–2077. Review.
73. Libby P, Tanaka H. The pathogenesis of coronary arteriosclerosis ("chronic rejection") in transplanted hearts. Clin Transplant 1994;8:313–318.
74. Buszman P, Zembala M, Wojarski J, et al. Comparison of intravascular ultrasound and quantitative angiography for evaluation of

coronary artery disease in the transplanted heart. Transplant Proc 1996;28:3535–3537.
75. Liang DH, Gao SZ, Botas J, et al. Prediction of angiographic disease by intracoronary ultrasonographic findings in heart transplant recipients. J Heart Lung Transplant 1996;15:980–987.
76. Mehra MR, Ventura HO, Jain SP, et al. Heterogeneity of cardiac allograft vasculopathy: Clinical insights from coronary angioscopy. J Am Coll Cardiol 1997;29:1339–1344.
77. McDonald K, Rector TJ, Braunlin EA, et al. Association of coronary artery disease in cardiac transplant recipients with cytomegalovirus infection. Am J Cardiol 1989;64:359–362.
78. Speir E, Modali R, Huang E-S, et al. Potential role of human cytomegalovirus and p53 interaction in coronary restenosis. Science 1994;265:391–394.
79. Summary of the second report of the National Cholesterol Education Program (NCEP) Expert Panel on Detection, Evaluation, and Treatment of High Blood Cholesterol in Adults (Adult Treatment Panel II). JAMA 1993;269:3015–3023.
80. Schroeder JS, Gao SZ, Alderman EL, et al. A preliminary study of diltiazem in the prevention of coronary artery disease in heart transplant recipients. N Engl J Med 1993;328:164–170.
81. Lou H, Kodama T, Wang YN, et al. L-Arginine prevents heart transplant arteriosclerosis by modulating the vascular cell proliferative response to insulin-like growth factor-1 and interleukin-6. J Heart Lung Transplant 1996;15:1248–1257.
82. Wahlers T, Mugge A, Oppelt P, et al. Preventive treatment of coronary vasculopathy in heart transplantation by inhibition of smooth muscle cell proliferation with angiopeptin. J Heart Lung Transplant 1995;14:143–150.
83. Foegh ML, Zhao Y, Lou H, et al. Estrogen and prevention of transplant atherosclerosis. J Heart Lung Transplant 1995;14:S170–172.
84. Penn I. Incidence and treatment of neoplasia after transplantation. J Heart Lung Transplant 1993;12:S328–336.
85. Penn I. Tumors after renal and cardiac transplantation. Hematol Oncol Clin North Am 1993;7:431–445.
86. Penn I. Cancers in cyclosporine-treated vs azathioprine-treated patients. Transplant Proc 1996;28:876–878.
87. Swinnen LJ, Costanzo-Nordin MR, Fisher SG, et al. Increased incidence of lymphoproliferative disorder after immunosuppression with the monoclonal antibody OKT3 in cardiac transplant recipients. N Engl J Med 1990;323:1723–1728.
88. Emery RW, Lake KD. Post-transplantation lymphoproliferative disorder and OKT3. N Engl J Med 1991;324:1437. Letter.
89. Walker RC, Paya CV, Marshall WF, et al. Pretransplantation seronegative Epstein-Barr virus status is the primary risk factor for post-transplantation lymphoproliferative disorder in adult heart, lung, and other solid organ transplantations. J Heart Lung Transplant 1995; 14:214–221.
90. Textor SC, Taler SJ, Canzanello VJ, Schwartz L. Cyclosporine, blood pressure and atherosclerosis. Cardiol Rev 1997;5:141–151.
91. Ventura HO, Malik FS, Mehra MR, et al. Mechanisms of hypertension in cardiac transplantation and the role of cyclosporine. Curr Opin Cardiol 1997;12:375–381. Review.
92. Sturrock ND, Struthers AD. Hormonal and other mechanisms involved in the pathogenesis of cyclosporin-induced nephrotoxicity and hypertension in man. Clin Sci 1994;86:1–9.
93. Henkin Y, Como JA, Oberman A. Secondary dyslipidemia inadvertent effects of drugs in clinical practice. JAMA 1992;267:961–968.
94. Brozena SC, Johnson MR, Ventura H, et al. Effectiveness and safety of diltiazem or lisinopril in treatment of hypertension after heart transplantation. Results of a prospective, randomized multicenter trial. J Am Coll Cardiol 1996;27:1707–1712.
95. Epstein M. Calcium antagonists and the kidney. Implications for renal protection. Am J Hypertension 1993;6:251S–259S.
96. Goldstein DJ, Zuech N, Sehgal X, et al. Cyclosporine-associated end-stage nephropathy after cardiac transplantation: Incidence and progression. Transplantation 1997;63:664–668.
97. Lake KD. Drug interactions in transplant patients. In: Emery RW, Miller LW, eds. Handbook of Cardiac Transplantation. Philadelphia, Hanley & Belfus, 1995;173–200.
98. Jones TE. The use of other drugs to allow a lower dosage of cyclosporin to be used. Therapeutic and pharmacoeconomic considerations. Clin Pharmacokin 1997;32:357–367. Review.
99. Kobashigawa JA, Kasiske BL. Hyperlipidemia in solid organ transplantation. Transplantation 1997;63:331–338. Review.
100. Lake, KD. Management of post-transplant obesity and hyperlipidemia. In: Emery RW, Miller L, eds. Handbook of Cardiac Transplantation. Philadelphia, Hanley & Belfus, 1995:147–164.

17

THROMBOEMBOLIC DISORDERS

Sharon M. Erdman, PharmD, Susan K. Chuck, PharmD, and Keith A. Rodvold, PharmD, FCCP, BCPS

Venous thromboembolism, which includes both venous thrombosis and its most feared complication, pulmonary embolism, is a serious and potentially fatal disorder that can occur in bedridden hospitalized patients as well as in healthy ambulatory individuals. It is estimated that there are approximately 600,000 cases of pulmonary embolism in the United States each year, with about 10% (60,000) of these cases resulting in death.[1] In one-third of these patients, death can occur within the first few hours of onset, making rapid diagnosis and early, effective treatment critical determinants in patient outcome.[2]

A pulmonary embolism (PE) is a thrombus or foreign substance that arises from the systemic circulation and lodges in the pulmonary artery or one of its branches, causing complete or partial obstruction of pulmonary blood flow. It is estimated that greater than 95% of pulmonary emboli originate as thrombi in the deep-venous system of the lower extremities.[2,3] A deep vein thrombosis (DVT) is a thrombus composed of cellular material (red and white blood cells, and platelets) bound together with fibrin strands, which form in the venous portion of the vasculature.[3] Venous thrombosis can involve any vein in the body, but most often occurs in the lower limbs involving the superficial large veins, the deep veins of the calf, and the deep veins above the knee (including the popliteal and proximal veins). Thrombi of the larger leg veins (those above the knee) are the most common source of PE that reach clinical attention. Thrombi of the deep calf veins are often small in size and generally pose only a small risk of developing subsequent PE and long-term clinical disability.[1] In addition, a small number of patients develop PE secondary to pelvic, renal, or upper extremity vein thrombosis, or by the injection of a foreign substance (as in intravenous drug abusers).

Pulmonary embolism has often been called the "great masquerader" due to its multiple clinical presentations as well as the lack of specificity of associated signs and symptoms. In addition, the clinical diagnosis of venous thrombosis and PE is notoriously unreliable. Treatment is often initiated before a firm diagnosis has been made owing to the seriousness of the condition in addition to the uncertainty associated with the clinical diagnosis of venous thrombosis.

ETIOLOGY

A number of factors, either inherited or acquired, may place a patient at risk for the development of venous thromboembolism. A comprehensive list of risk factors is presented in Table 17–1. Thrombosis may be caused by resistance to activated protein C (APC resistance) in as many as 33% of patients who do not have an obvious predisposition to thromboembolic diseases.[4] It is not known if age itself is an independent risk factor for the development of venous thromboembolism but the prevalence of many risk factors increases with age.

The incidence or risk of developing venous thromboembolism also appears to differ depending on the surgical procedure being performed, the clinical situation (emergent versus elective), the duration of general anesthesia (increased risk with duration >30 minutes), and the age of the patient (clinically important by 40 years). In general, the overall incidence of either DVT or PE in patients who undergo major surgery is 30% to 35%. In addition, elective hip surgery patients are at a 0.3% to 1.7% risk of developing fatal PE, which increases to 4% to 7% in patients who undergo emergent hip surgery.

PATHOPHYSIOLOGY

Three primary components—venous stasis, vascular injury, and hypercoagulability (Virchow's triad)—play a role in the development of a thrombus.[1] In addition, the fibrinolytic state of the patient is also a key component. Venous stasis is characterized by altered or decreased blood flow in the deep veins of the lower limbs and is a critical determinant in the formation of thrombi in many patients. Ineffective venous emptying can lead to local endothelial damage to venous valves secondary to hypoxia, as well as the local concentration of activated clotting factors in the area of stasis. Venostasis may result from a number of conditions including immobility, prolonged bedrest, massive obesity, venous obstruction, congestive heart failure, hypovolemia, varicose veins, late-stage pregnancy, shock, and severe myocardial infarction.

Vascular wall injury or endothelial damage occurs secondary to mechanical or chemical trauma that evokes an inflammatory response (phlebitis). Mechanical injury to the intima of vessel walls may result from venipuncture, indwelling cannulas and catheters, fractured bones, and direct trauma as with surgery. Chemical irritation may result from the infusion or injection of agents such as potassium or hypertonic glucose. As a result of the exposure of collagen, the coagulation cascade is activated locally, leading to platelet aggregation and the formation of an intraluminal thrombus.

The coagulation process is regulated by a number of feedback mechanisms that normally limit thrombus

TABLE 17–1. Risk Factors Predisposing to Thromboembolism

Inherited Risk Factors	
	Activated protein C resistance
	Antithrombin III deficiency
	Protein C deficiency
	Protein S deficiency
	Dysfibrinogenemia
	Sickle cell anemia
	Polycythemia vera
	Leiden factor V abnormalities
Acquired Risk Factors	
	Immobility (bedridden, debilitated) or paralysis (stroke, spinal cord injury)
	Trauma/surgery of lower extremity, pelvis, hip, abdomen
	Peripartum period
	Obesity
	Malignancy, especially pancreatic, gastrointestinal, bronchogenic, genitourinary, breast
	Estrogen use: oral contraceptives, hormonal replacement
	History of DVT or PE
	Lupus anticoagulant
	Antiphospholipid antibodies
	History of varicose veins
	Chronic venous insufficiency
	Chronic lung disease
	Heart disease: congestive heart failure, atrial fibrillation, acute myocardial infarction, dilated cardiomyopathy
	Inflammatory bowel disease
	Myeloproliferative disorders
	Renal transplantation
	Splenectomy

Compiled from Refs. 101, 102.

formation. However, there are circumstances (hypercoagulable states) when the activation of the coagulation cascade exceeds the ability of the body's natural fibrinolytic system to prevent thrombus formation. APC resistance, deficiencies of protein C, protein S, or antithrombin III, and certain types of malignancy are conditions in which there is an increased activation of the blood coagulation system, which predisposes to the development of a thrombus.[4]

The coagulation process is activated by a number of factors including tissue or vascular trauma and inflammation. Venous stasis appears to augment the coagulation process by concentrating activated clotting factors locally. The coagulation cascade (see Fig. 92–1) can be triggered through either the intrinsic or extrinsic pathways. The intrinsic pathway is activated by the contact of factor XII with exposed collagen from damaged subendothelial vessels, or by contact with a foreign substance such as a prosthetic surface. All of the clotting factors necessary for the activation of the intrinsic system are present in the circulating blood. The extrinsic pathway is activated by the exposure of blood to tissue thromboplastin, a tissue factor released after vascular wall damage, which combines with and activates factor VII to form a complex that activates factor X. It is at this point that the intrinsic and extrinsic pathways meet to continue along a common pathway ultimately leading to the activation of factor XII, which stabilizes the fibrin clot. In addition, tissue factor has been shown to activate factor IX, thus providing an alternative pathway of blood coagulation. Tissue factor pathway inhibitor appears to play a role in regulating this alternative pathway.

NATURAL HISTORY OF DEEP VEIN THROMBOSIS AND PULMONARY EMBOLISM

Most venous thrombi involve the veins of the lower extremities, where they develop behind venous valve cusps or at bifurcations in the intramuscular veins of the calf. The major consequences of DVT include venous valvular damage (postphlebitic syndrome), compromised venous blood flow return from the lower extremities or chronic venous insufficiency (leading to tissue hypoxia), and embolization of thrombus to the lungs. In most patients, venous thrombi and PE are broken up by the endogenous lytic system, with complete clot resolution occurring over several weeks. Subsequently, clinically apparent thrombotic disease is observed in patients in whom this mechanism fails.

As mentioned before, most pulmonary emboli originate as thrombi in the deep venous system, which dislodge and produce complete or partial interruption of blood flow to a portion of the lungs. It is estimated that 15% to 20% of untreated proximal deep venous thrombi embolize to the lungs. Upper extremity thrombosis may lead to a PE, especially in the presence of a central indwelling catheter.

Pulmonary emboli may be generally classified into two groups: (1) submassive, in which less than 50% of the pulmonary vascular bed is occluded, and (2) massive, in which greater than 50% of the pulmonary vascular bed is occluded. The severity of the pulmonary and hemodynamic effects of a PE depends on several factors including the extent of anatomic obstruction and the underlying cardiopulmonary status of the patient.

The pulmonary effects of a PE may include the formation of an alveolar dead space (an area ventilated in excess of perfusion), pneumoconstriction (a decrease in the functional size of the area not being perfused), and arterial hypoxemia; loss of pulmonary surfactant (which occurs after 24 hours) leading to atelectasis and transudation of alveolar fluid into alveolar spaces; and pulmonary infarction (< 10%).[1,2]

Hemodynamically, a PE causes a decrease in the cross-sectional area of the pulmonary bed, which increases pulmonary vascular resistance and subsequently right ventricular afterload. If these changes become marked, they may lead to tricuspid regurgitation, pulmonary hypertension, right ventricular failure, and low cardiac output, especially in patients who have underlying cardiopulmonary disease.[1,2] In addition, chronic pulmonary hypertension and cor pulmonale may develop in a small number of patients who experience recurrent pulmonary emboli.

CLINICAL PRESENTATION

Frequently, venous thrombi are clinically silent.[1–3,5] Signs and symptoms develop as a consequence of venous outflow obstruction, inflammation of the vessel wall or perivascular tissue, or embolization of the thrombus to the pulmonary vascular bed. The most common clinical symptoms include pain, tenderness, swelling, and discoloration. The pain and tenderness are usually localized to the calf in patients with calf vein thrombosis, and tend to be more diffuse and intense in patients with proximal vein thrombosis. The severity of the pain and tenderness, however, does not appear to correlate with the size or extent of the thrombus. Edema secondary to proximal vein obstruction or vascular inflammation is most often responsible for the swelling and ranges in severity. The swelling is typically localized or unilateral and can occur with or without pain.

The signs and symptoms of venous thrombosis are neither sensitive nor specific. The differential diagnosis of lower extremity pain and/or tenderness includes muscle strain/trauma/tear, spontaneous muscle hematoma, arterial insufficiency, neurogenic pain, ruptured Baker's cyst, arthritis of the knee or ankle joint, Achilles tendonitis, varicose veins, pregnancy, or oral contraceptive use. Other conditions that may cause leg swelling include compression of the iliac vein, postphlebitic syndrome, leg immobilization/inflammation, lymphedema, or lipedema.

Patients with DVT may exhibit a discolored lower extremity, which is manifested as cyanosis because of a large venous obstruction; paleness secondary to reflex arterial vasospasm; or a reddish color from perivascular inflammation which at times may be indistinguishable from cellulitis.

Other signs and symptoms that may be present include a palpable cord and a positive Homan's sign (discomfort in the calf upon dorsiflexion of the foot).[6] The Homan's sign, however, is nonspecific and insensitive, with a positive result in 50% of patients who do not have DVT, and in only 30% of patients with objectively documented DVT.[3]

After a sufficient period of chronic venous obstruction, postphlebitic syndrome may occur. Symptoms may range from chronic pain and swelling in the lower extremities to the formation of stasis ulcers and the development of infection.

The signs and symptoms of PE are also nonspecific and insensitive and also may result from a number of other medical conditions, as presented in Table 17–2. While most pulmonary emboli are clinically silent, some patients may present with a variety of symptoms depending on the size and number of the emboli, the arteries involved, and the patient's underlying disease states. The most common signs and symptoms include a sudden onset of unexplained dyspnea, cough, tachypnea, tachycardia, pleuritic chest pain, and anxiety or a feeling of impending doom. Occasionally, a patient may experience diaphoresis or substernal chest pain. Hemoptysis, although infrequently present, is usually an indicator of pulmonary infarction or congestive atelectasis. In addition, patients with massive PE often present with signs of circulatory collapse, such as syncope or shock, secondary to a reduced cardiac output, or with evidence of acute cor pulmonale or right ventricular failure. However, a normal PaO_2 or a normal alveolar–arterial oxygen difference does not exclude PE.

TABLE 17–2. Differential Diagnosis of the Clinical Features of Pulmonary Embolism

Dyspnea	**Hemoptysis**
Atelectasis	Pneumonia
Pneumonia	Bronchial neoplasm
Pneumothorax	Bronchiectasis
Acute pulmonary edema	Acute bronchitis
Acute bronchitis	Mitral stenosis
Acute bronchiolitis	Tuberculosis
Acute bronchial obstruction (asthma)	**Acute Right Heart Failure**
	Myocardial failure
Hyperventilation	Myocarditis
Metabolic acidosis	Cardiac tamponade
Pleuritic Chest Pain	Acute respiratory infection complicating chronic lung disease
Pneumonia	
Pneumothorax	
Pericarditis	**Cardiovascular Collapse**
Pulmonary neoplasm	Myocardial infarction
Bronchiectasis	Acute massive hemorrhage
Subdiaphragmatic inflammation	Gram-negative hemorrhage
Myositis	Cardiac tamponade
Muscle strain	Spontaneous pneumothorax
Rib fracture	

From Ref. 103, with permission.

DIAGNOSIS

The diagnosis of DVT or PE should be suspected in any patient with suggestive clinical signs and symptoms. Because none of the signs or symptoms is specific for DVT or PE, the diagnosis cannot be made on the basis of clinical judgment alone, and objective testing methods are necessary to aid in the diagnosis.

In any patient suspected of having a DVT or PE, empiric therapy (e.g., heparin) is started to decrease the risk of further embolic events while waiting for the results of diagnostic tests. The initial steps in the evaluation of any patient with suspected thromboembolic disease should include a medical history, a medication history, and a thorough physical exam. All of these are important in identifying underlying risk factors that may have led to the development of the thrombus. As previously mentioned, objective testing is necessary for the diagnosis of either DVT or PE because of the nonspecificity of associated signs and symptoms.

Several studies have evaluated D-dimer as a negative predictor of DVT and PE.[7,8] Normal D-dimer concentrations (< 500 ng/mL) have been shown to be strongly predictive of a normal pulmonary angiogram.[9] Combining D-dimer concentrations (< 500 ng/mL to rule out PE) and real time B-mode ultrasonography (to diagnose DVT) resulted in a definitive noninvasive diagnosis in 62% of patients in whom the ventilation–perfusion (V/Q) radionuclide scan was nondiagnostic. At the 6-month follow-up, of those patients initially ruled out for PE there was only a 1% incidence of PE or DVT noted.[10] According to the ACCP Consensus Committee on PE, data are insufficient to allow complete reliance on D-dimer as a diagnostic tool for PE.[7]

There are a number of invasive and noninvasive diagnostic techniques that may be useful for the detection of DVT (Table 17–3).[11] Some techniques visualize the thrombus (contrast venography, ultrasound, magnetic resonance imaging); some measure obstructions to venous outflow (impedance plethysmography [IPG], Doppler ultrasound); and others detect the incorporation of radiolabeled proteins into the developing thrombus (^{125}I-fibrinogen scan, monoclonal antibodies). The clinical usefulness of any of these tests depends on whether the patient has clinically suspected DVT, or whether a high-risk patient is being screened for DVT.

When venous thrombosis is suspected clinically, initiating heparin in those patients without any contraindications should be considered. A noninvasive diagnostic test (IPG, Doppler ultrasound, or real-time ultrasound) should be the first step in diagnosing DVT. If the test is positive, in the absence of clinical conditions known to produce a false-positive result, then anticoagulant therapy should be initiated. However, if the test is negative then serial exams are obtained on days 5 to 7, and again on days 10 to 14. Impedance plethysmography, Doppler ultrasound, and real-time ultrasound all have the limitation of being insensitive to calf vein thrombosis. Serial testing is required based on the observation that a calf vein thrombosis is clinically important only when it extends into the proximal veins, at which point the noninvasive tests would be useful in de-

TABLE 17–3. Diagnostic Tests for Deep Vein Thrombosis

Diagnostic Test	Description	Comments
Noninvasive		
^{125}I-fibrinogen leg scanning	Radioiodine-labeled fibrinogen scanning depends on the incorporation of circulating labeled fibrinogen as fibrin into the thrombus, which is then detected by an isotope detector.	—Not available; transmission of blood-borne pathogens is a concern —Screening tool or adjunctive test to IPG —Never used as the only diagnostic tool for suspected DVT because it fails to detect many high proximal vein thrombi
Impedance plethysmography (IPG)	Using a pneumatic cuff on the midthigh and calf, electrode changes in electrical resistance which accompany changes of blood volume in legs are measured. The cuff is inflated to 50 mm Hg to occlude venous return, and then as the cuff is deflated alterations in blood flow are detected.	—Sensitive and specific for thrombosis of the proximal veins, but is less sensitive for thrombosis of the calf veins —Cannot distinguish between thrombotic and nonthrombotic obstruction to venous outflow
Doppler ultrasonography	Venous flow patterns are detected using a transducer with acoustic gel to emit and measure sound waves reflected off red blood cells. Loss of sound fluctuation, usually found with respiration, indicates partial obstruction caused by a DVT. DVT may also present as an absence of spontaneous venous flow.	—Highly sensitive to proximal vein thrombi, but less sensitive to nonocclusive or calf vein thrombi —Test accuracy dependent on operator experience —Advantages over IPG: convenience, low cost, increased sensitivity for calf vein thrombi, and use in patients with arterial insufficiency or plaster casts
Real-time B-mode ultrasonography	Three-dimensional pictures of the deep veins are produced by using high-frequency sound waves emitted from a transducer. Lack of vein compressibility with light pressure from the transducer is diagnostic for DVT.	—Useful test to detect acute and chronic thrombi in the lower extremities —Very accurate and sensitive for the diagnosis of proximal vein thrombosis, but less accurate in detecting calf vein thrombi
Duplex ultrasonography	Real-time B-mode ultrasonography is combined with Doppler ultrasonography to allow venous circulation imaging with venous flow information.	—As above
Invasive		
Venography	Radiopaque contrast dye is injected, guided by fluoroscopy, into a dorsal foot vein or the femoral vein, and oblique and lateral X-rays are made of the calf, knee, thigh, and pelvis. This procedure provides visualization of the entire venous system of the leg. DVT is diagnosed based on the presence of intraluminal filling defects on at least two different viewing angles.	—Reference standard for the diagnosis of DVT; most accurate and reliable —Experienced personnel required for operation and interpretation —Expensive and with possible complications of immediate or delayed foot pain, superficial phlebitis, or hypersensitivity reaction to contrast dye —Used in morbidly obese or patients with edema in whom ultrasonic techniques are not useful

Adapted with permission from Ref. 11.

tecting the thrombus. If the test becomes positive during the serial testing, the patient is diagnosed with DVT and anticoagulant therapy is initiated. A positive test in the presence of conditions known to produce false positives (e.g., congestive heart failure) should be confirmed by venography. The use of follow-up noninvasive tests at the end of anticoagulant therapy has been used to better assess future DVT. However, follow-up testing has been found to be cost effective only in patients with a continuing predisposition to PE and DVT.[7]

If a patient with signs and symptoms suggestive of PE has a finding of proximal vein thrombosis of the legs, invasive studies that might be used to confirm the diagnosis of PE can be avoided since the same therapies would be employed (Fig. 17–1). In contrast, PE cannot be excluded in patients with negative findings on leg examination so that further tests may be necessary to make the diagnosis in a patient with a compatible clinical picture.

In addition to the initial medical history and physical examination, an electrocardiogram (ECG), chest x-ray, and arterial blood gas should be obtained in any patient with suspected PE. Evidence of right heart strain caused by elevated pulmonary artery pressures may be seen on the ECG of patients with PE. Patterns may include nonspecific ST-segment elevations or depression, T-wave inversion, right axis deviation, new incomplete right bundle-branch block, or evidence of right ventricular hypertrophy.[2] The radiographic patterns in patients with PE may include effusions, infiltrates, enlargement of right descending pulmonary artery, Westermark's sign (avascular lung zones), and elevation of the diaphragm. An arterial blood gas may be useful in assessing the patient's degree of ventilation; however, approximately 10% to 20% of patients with PE have pO_2 values of > 80 mm Hg. Although these tests are nonspecific for PE, they may be used to exclude other causes for the patient's condition, in addition to assisting in the interpretation of other diagnostic tests.

Ventilation–perfusion (V/Q) radionuclide scans are one of the objective testing methods used initially for the diagnosis of PE. The V/Q scan estimates the probability of PE in a given patient based on the anatomic patterns of injected and inhaled radioactive materials. Technetium-99-labeled macroaggregates of albumin are injected intravenously for the assessment of pulmonary perfusion. The distribution of these macroaggregates as they are trapped in the pulmonary capillary bed is detected radiographically and reflects the blood flow within the lungs. Because it cannot distinguish between pulmonary perfusion defects from PE and those from other causes, it is nonspecific. Therefore, the assessment of ventilation is also used to help in the diagnosis. In the ventilation phase of the test, the patient inhales and exhales radioactive inert xenon, which permits imaging of the pattern of distribution of air in the alveolar gas-exchange units. Because an embolus obstructs arterial blood flow in one of the pulmonary arteries but does not affect ventilation, this scan can detect areas that are being ventilated but not perfused (a V/Q mismatch). Repeat V/Q scans may be required 3 months after an acute PE to serve

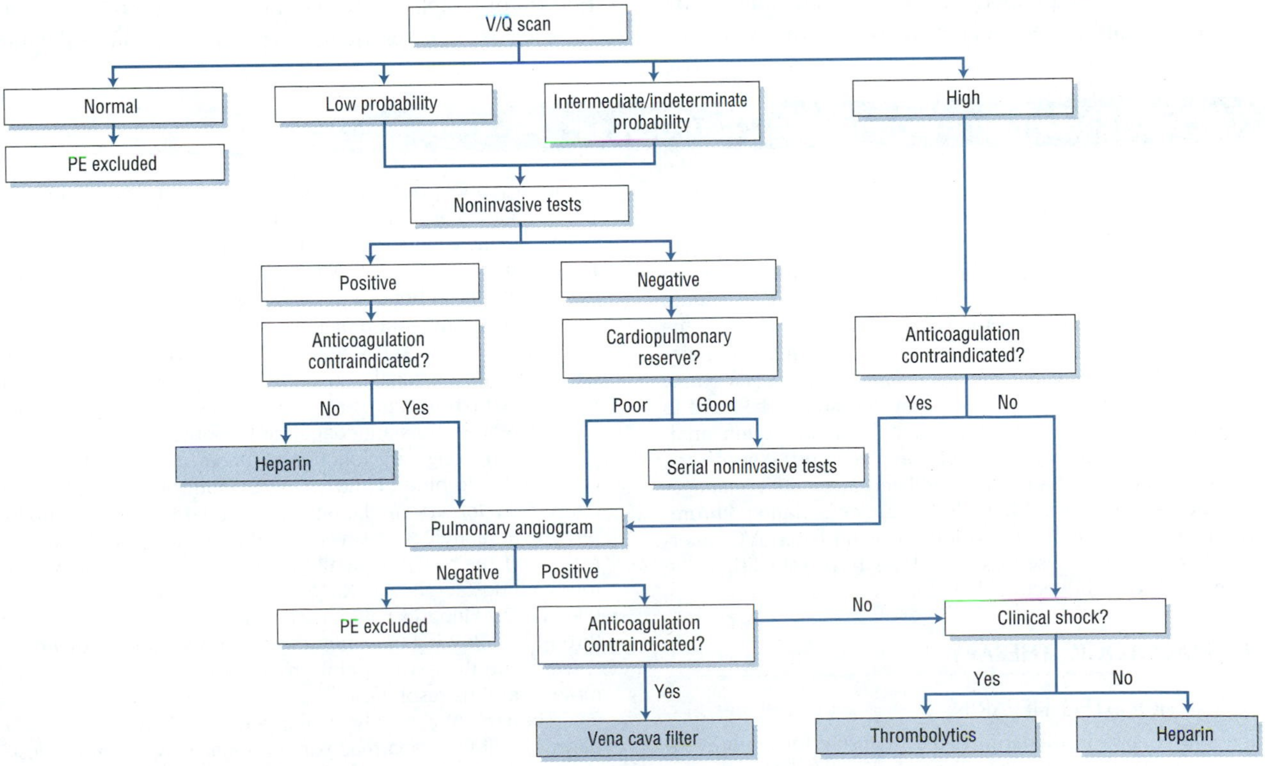

FIGURE 17–1. Diagnostic algorithm for patients with suspected pulmonary embolism. V/Q = ventilation–perfusion.

as a baseline in patients at high risk of recurrence (e.g., with coagulopathy, malignancy, continuing predisposition to DVT, or a history of PE recurrence).[7]

Results of this test are expressed in terms of the probability that a particular patient has a PE. A normal V/Q scan reliably excludes the diagnosis of PE, whereas a high-probability V/Q scan supports the diagnosis of a PE.[12,13] If the results are interpreted as low or intermediate/indeterminate probabilities, diagnosing PE is more difficult. It is estimated that the prevalence of PE by pulmonary angiogram was 16% in patients with low-probability lung scans, and 32% in patients with intermediate- or indeterminate-probability lung scans, although all of these emboli detected may not be clinically significant.[13] The prospective investigation of PE diagnosis (PIOPED) study demonstrated that clinical assessment combined with V/Q scan improves the likelihood of correctly determining which patients may be left untreated. However, the diagnostic certainty was limited to a minority of patients.[13] Therefore, in this subset of patients with inconclusive results from V/Q scans, further objective testing is necessary to confirm the diagnosis of PE.

As mentioned earlier, a number of patients with PE also have venographically detectable DVT, making IPG or Doppler ultrasonography possibly useful as a predictor of thromboembolism. It is estimated that approximately 70% of patients with angiographically proven PE have concurrent DVT by venography. If DVT is detected by venography testing, the patient should be treated with anticoagulant therapy, circumventing the need for pulmonary angiography. If the results of the above tests are negative or inconclusive, pulmonary angiography is then indicated to establish the diagnosis of PE. Alternatively, serial noninvasive tests for DVT can be used as an effective alternative to pulmonary angiogram in patients with nondiagnostic V/Q scans and normal cardiorespiratory reserve. Of 711 patients, 84 (11.8%) developed positive results on serial testing and 1.9% of the remaining patients had a thromboembolic event with one death.[14]

Pulmonary angiography is the accepted diagnostic standard for PE to which all other tests are compared. In terms of diagnosing PE, it has the greatest diagnostic certainty, and can identify emboli as small as 0.5 mm. The procedure involves the injection of contrast media into the right and left pulmonary arteries, and radiographically detecting any filling defects on multiple magnification views. Some indications for pulmonary angiography include a nondiagnostic V/Q scan with or without a normal IPG in a patient with a picture suggestive of PE; a disagreement between V/Q scan interpretation and clinical impression; a contraindication to anticoagulation; and anticipation of thrombolytic therapy, inferior vena cava interruption, or embolectomy. Risks or complications of the pulmonary angiography include cardiac arrhythmias, cardiac perforation, hypotension, and reaction to contrast media. Recently, modified pulmonary angiography techniques have improved diagnostic accuracy and reduced the risks of this procedure.[13]

Newer imaging techniques that are less invasive than pulmonary angiography are currently being investigated as diagnostic tools for PE.[15] These techniques include magnetic resonance imaging (MRI); computed tomography (CT) with contrast; radiolabeled platelets; intravascular pulmonary ultrasound; fiberoptic pulmonary ultrasound; and digital subtraction angiography, which is simpler and faster and does not require catheterization of the pulmonary artery.[1,2] Echocardiography is an ancillary test that provides clues of PE such as right ventricular hypokinesis and/or dilatation.[7]

▶ TREATMENT: Thromboembolic Disorders

The main objectives of treating venous thrombosis are (1) to prevent the development of pulmonary embolism, (2) to prevent the postphlebitic syndrome, (3) to reduce morbidity from the acute event, and (4) to achieve these objectives with a minimum of adverse effects and cost. Thus, successful treatment of DVT should prevent extension of the thrombus, prevent embolism to the lungs, and restore patency to the venous circulation while maintaining normal venous valve function. General management of DVT includes bedrest with the heels elevated above the heart to enhance venous return, and administration of nonaspirin analgesics for pain. For PE, oxygen should be given and, if necessary, patients should be mechanically ventilated. Definitive management of acute DVT and PE includes anticoagulation, thrombolytic therapy, embolectomy, or inferior vena cava (IVC) interruption. Practice and consensus guidelines have established the provisions of safe and effective therapy.[16–18]

PHARMACOLOGIC THERAPY

UNFRACTIONATED HEPARIN

Unfractionated heparin (heparin) is the mainstay for the prevention and treatment of venous thromboembolism.[1,6,18] Heparin is a complex mucopolysaccharide that is extracted either from porcine gastrointestinal (GI) sources or from beef lung. Commercially available heparin is a heterogeneous mixture of polymers ranging from 3000 to 30,000 Daltons in molecular weight, with varying antithrombotic activity.[19] Apparently, a small and distinct fraction of the heparin molecule is responsible for most of its anticoagulant effect. Anticoagulant therapy with heparin is complicated by the chemical and pharmacologic heterogeneity of the product, which accounts for some of the inter- and intraindividual differences in its anticoagulant response.

The anticoagulant function of heparin is thought to depend on its ability to bind to and catalyze antithrombin III (ATIII) or heparin cofactor, a circulating anticoagulant that neutralizes the proteolytic activities of several clotting factors that have a serine residue at their enzymatically active site.[19] These activated factors include factors XII, XI, X, and IX, kallikrein, and thrombin (Fig. 17–2). Heparin halts further growth and propagation of the thrombus, allowing the patient's endogenous thrombolytic system to eradicate the existing clot. In addition, heparin may also promote thrombus resolution.[19]

The lack of a readily available direct chemical assay for heparin has limited pharmacokinetic data. Few carefully designed prospective evaluations of the disposition of heparin in patients

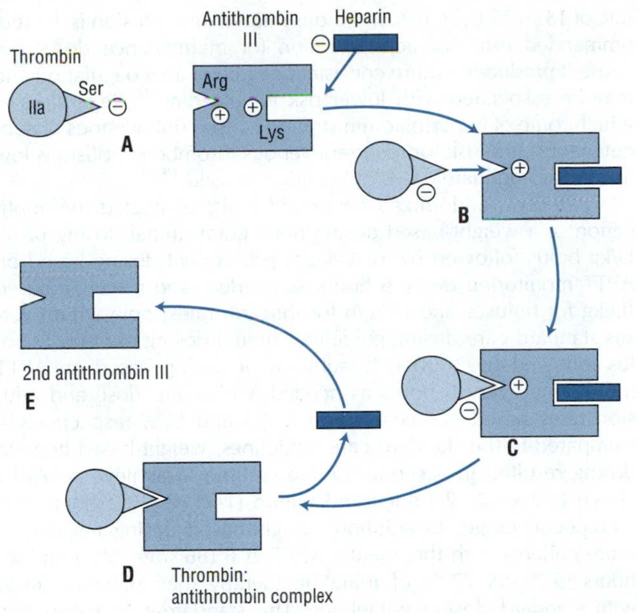

FIGURE 17–2. Mechanism of action of heparin. Heparin interacts with antithrombin III (A, B, C, E), which catalyzes the formation of thrombin: antithrombin complexes (D). Heparin and antithrombin also inactivate factors XIIa, XIa, and Xa by a similar mechanism. *(Adapted from Ref. 104, with permission.)*

are available. Data are not available on the rate and extent of absorption of heparin after oral administration. The total amount of heparin required to achieve the same degree of anticoagulant effect over the same time period does not appear to differ whether the agent is administered by intravenous, subcutaneous, or intrapulmonary routes.[19] Some studies have demonstrated significantly lower peak plasma heparin concentrations or decreased anticoagulant effects from the calcium salts; other investigators have failed to find significant differences between sodium and calcium salts.[20]

Heparin is distributed primarily throughout the vascular system, and the apparent volume of distribution (V_D) quantitatively resembles that of plasma or blood volume (mean $V_D = 60$ mL/kg; range: 40 to 100).[20] The V_D is directly related to body weight. However, there is no consensus as to whether ideal body weight or total body weight should be used when dosing heparin. The majority of data suggests that total body weight and estimations of blood volume should be used to dose heparin, especially in morbidly obese patients.[20]

The metabolism and excretion of heparin are complex, but involve primarily the metabolic processes of depolymerization and desulfation. Enzymes likely involved in heparin degradation include heparinases and desulfatases.[19,20]

The anticoagulant activity of heparin in plasma decreases exponentially with time after intravenous administration; however, the half-life increases with increasing dose. The biologic half-life of heparin in humans after a single intravenous injection has been reported to range from 0.4 to 2.5 hours.[20] Up to a 10-fold range in heparin half-life has been reported within individual studies involving the administration of large doses. Heparin clearance ranges from 0.25 to 2 mL/min/kg and has been found to be related to both total body weight and ideal body weight as well as circadian variation.[20] The interpatient variability in heparin clearance is reported to be 6- to 12-fold. The disappearance of the anticoagulant activity follows nonlinear pharmacokinetics, and has been described by a combination of a saturable and a linear mechanism.[20] The elimination of heparin is thought to be influenced by both renal and hepatic dysfunction.

Patients with PE have shorter heparin elimination half-lives and more rapid total clearances of heparin than patients treated for venous thrombosis.[20] This observation was supported by investigators who have recommended larger heparin doses for patients with pulmonary emboli. However, several other investigators have reported no significant differences in heparin dosage requirements between patients with PE and DVT.[20] Clinical observational studies have suggested that patients with verified thromboembolic diseases required significantly larger mean heparin doses (25 U/kg/h) than did patients without thromboembolic disease (15 U/kg/h). These data indicate that patients with acute thromboembolic disorders have rapid clearance rates and require larger heparin doses to ensure adequate anticoagulant activity.

Therapeutic Indications

Anticoagulation with heparin is indicated in patients with a thrombus extending above the popliteal vein because of the high risk of PE and postphlebitic syndrome in these patients.[1,3,18,19] Patients with symptomatic calf vein thrombosis should receive heparin, because recent studies have shown a higher incidence of recurrent DVT in proximal veins in nonanticoagulated patients compared with anticoagulated patients. However, there are no definitive recommendations in patients with asymptomatic calf vein thrombosis detected by routine postoperative leg scanning. Patients with superficial thrombophlebitis should not receive anticoagulation. Heparin is clearly indicated for patients with documented PE. Heparin is also used for the prevention of venous thromboembolism.[6]

Heparin therapy is contraindicated in patients who are hypersensitive to the drug, who are actively bleeding or who have hemophilia, thrombocytopenia, intracranial hemorrhage, bacterial endocarditis, active tuberculosis, ulcerative lesions of the GI tract, severe hypertension, threatened abortion, or visceral carcinoma. Heparin should be withheld during and after surgery of the brain, eye, or spinal cord, and should not be administered to patients undergoing lumbar puncture or regional anesthetic block. The drug should be used only when clearly indicated in pregnant women, despite its apparent lack of transfer across the placenta.[21]

Clinical Efficacy

The pharmacodynamic goals of heparin therapy are the prevention of thrombosis as well as hemorrhagic episodes, which may be caused by excessive anticoagulation. The evidence that heparin is effective as an anticoagulant is well documented.[17,18] Several studies have documented a reduced mortality rate in patients with venous thromboembolic disease or PE when given heparin compared to patients in whom anticoagulants were withheld.[18,19]

Zero percent to 5% of patients treated with adequate doses of intravenous heparin develop clinical evidence of recurrence, and the likelihood of fatal embolism during treatment is very low.[1–3,5,19,20] Raschke et al.[22] demonstrated that recurrent venous thromboembolism occurred less often (5% vs 25%) in patients who had achieved therapeutic activated partial thromboplastin time (APTT) values with dosing by a weight-based heparin nomogram than patients receiving standard heparin doses (5000 U bolus followed by 1000 U/h). Hull et al.[23] recently reaffirmed that the risk of recurrent venous thromboembolism for DVT is associated with achievement of therapeutic APTT within 24 to 48 hours of starting heparin therapy. For both adjusted-dose subcutaneous heparin and continuous intravenous heparin therapy, several contemporary studies have demonstrated the relationship between clinical effectiveness and maintaining the APTT at least 1.5 times the control value.[24,25]

Administration/Monitoring of Intravenous Heparin

Heparin has traditionally been initiated with an intravenous bolus injection (5000 to 10,000 U) followed by either an intravenous continuous infusion (starting at 1000 U/h) or intermittent intravenous injections (5000 U every 4 to 6 hours). However, the most efficient method for providing patients with rapid and effective heparin anticoagulation is for the clinician to consider individual heparin pharmacokinetic and pharmacodynamic data to determine initial dosages, systematically monitor anticoagulation tests, and make subsequent dosage adjustments as indicated. These points have been exemplified in studies that have found that the most common practices that led to delays and/or less than adequate anticoagulation (APTT less than 1.5 times control) are (1) failure to start heparin therapy at the time of clinical presentation, (2) suboptimal dosages, (3) delay in measuring APTT, (4) inadequate response to an APTT less than 1.5 times the control, and (5) excessive and prolonged reductions in heparin dosing when APTT is greater than 3 times the control.[20]

Weight-based and dose-titration heparin nomograms (Table 17–4) have improved heparin dosing and established the provisions for safe and effective anticoagulant therapy.[5,18,19,22,25–29] Figure 17–3 is an algorithm intended for the acute management of DVT or PE with heparin therapy as well as how to manage excessive anticoagulation. Doses should be based on total body weight: a loading dose of 70 to 100 U/kg followed by an initial infusion rate of 15 to 25 U/kg/h. Continuous intravenous infusion is the recommended route of administration for maintenance doses because it produces a more consistent degree of anticoagulation and may be associated with lower risk for bleeding.[18] Regardless of which route of heparin administration is used (intravenous or subcutaneous), the risk for recurrent venous thromboembolism is low as long as adequate doses of heparin are used.[18,23]

A recent randomized controlled trial[22] evaluated the application of a weight-based dosing nomogram (initial dosing of 80 U/kg bolus followed by 18 U/kg/h; subsequent dosing based on APTT monitoring every 6 hours as needed, and a weight-based [U/kg for boluses and U/kg/h for infusion rates] nomogram) versus standard care dosing guidelines (initial dosing of 5000 U bolus followed by 1000 U/h; subsequent dosing based on APTT monitoring every 6 hours as needed, with bolus dose and infusion rates based on fixed amounts [U and U/h, respectively]). Compared to the standard care guidelines, weight-based heparin dosing resulted in a shorter period of time to achieve an APTT above (8.2 vs 20.2 hours) and within (14.1 vs 20.2 hours) the therapeutic range. In addition, weight-based dosing resulted in more patients with therapeutic APTT at 6 (86% vs 32%) and 24 hours (97% vs 77%) of initiating therapy than patients dosed with standard dosing guidelines. The standard-care group had one major bleeding complication. Long-term follow-up demonstrated that recurrent venous thromboembolism occurred less often (5% vs 25%) in patients who received weight-based dosing. This study, as well as others,[25–29] supports the use of weight-based or dose-titration nomograms to provide effective and safe

TABLE 17–4. Three Heparin Dosing Nomograms

Weight-Based Nomogram[22]	
Initial Dosing: 80 U/kg IV bolus followed by 18 U/kg/h continuous IV infusion. APTT is measured in 6 h, and then:	
Subsequent Dosing Based on APTT:	
Measured Value	*Adjustment*
APTT <35 s (<1.2 × control value)	80 U/kg IV bolus, and increase IV infusion rate by 4 U/kg/h
APTT 35–45 s (1.2–1.5 × control value)	40 U/kg IV bolus, and increase IV infusion rate by 2 U/kg/h
APTT 46–70 s (>1.5–2.3 × control value)	No change
APTT 71–90 s (>2.3–3 × control value)	Decrease IV infusion rate by 2 U/kg/h
APTT >90 s (>3 × control value)	Stop infusion for 1 h, then decrease IV infusion rate by 3 U/kg/h
Heparin Nomogram[26]	
Initial Dosing: 5000 U IV bolus followed by 1280 U/h continuous IV infusion. APTT is measured in 6 h, and then:	
Subsequent Dosing Based on APTT:	
Measured Value	*Adjustment*
APTT <50 s	5000 U IV bolus, and increase IV infusion rate by 120 U/h
APTT 50–59 s	Increase IV infusion rate by 120 U/h
APTT 60–85 s	No change
APTT 86–95 s	Decrease IV infusion rate by 120 U/h
APTT 96–120 s	Stop infusion for 30 min, then decrease IV infusion rate by 80 U/h
APTT >90 s	Stop infusion for 1 h, then decrease IV infusion rate by 160 U/h
Heparin Dose-Titration Nomogram[25]	
Initial Dosing: 5000 U IV bolus followed by a continuous IV infusion of 1667 U/h (if patient has a low risk of bleeding) or 1250 U/h (if patient has a high risk of bleeding). APTT is measured in 6 h, and then:	
Subsequent Dosing Based on APTT:	
Measured Value	*Adjustment*
APTT ≤45 s	Increase IV infusion rate by 240 U/h
APTT 46–54 s	Increase IV infusion rate by 120 U/h
APTT 55–85 s	No change
APTT 86–110 s	Stop infusion for 1 h; then decrease IV infusion rate by 120 U/h
APTT >110 s	Stop infusion for 1 h; then decrease IV infusion rate by 240 U/h

Adapted from Ref. 5 with permission.

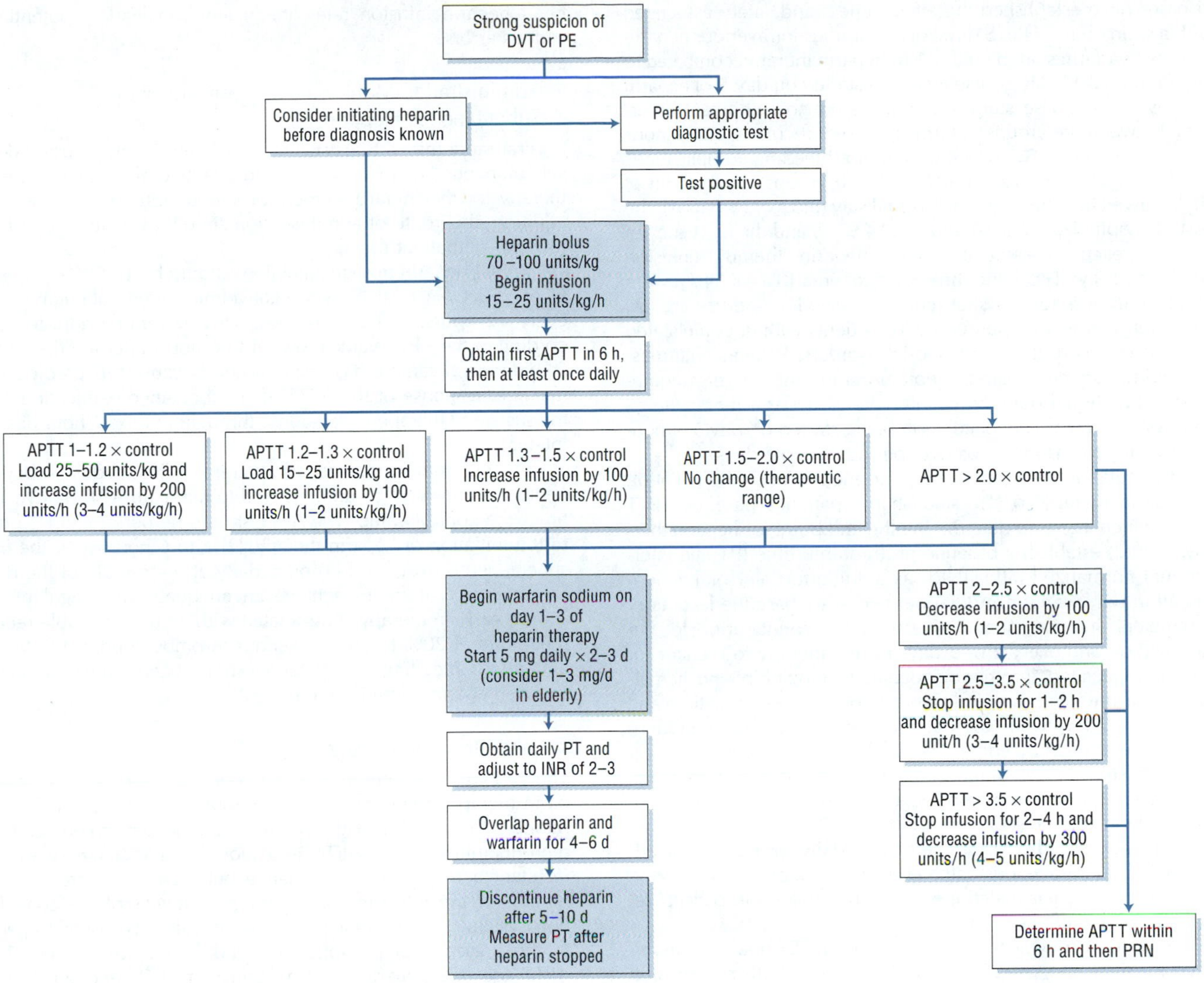

FIGURE 17–3. Algorithm for acute management of DVT or PE with heparin. *(Adapted from Ref. 105, with permission.)*

heparin therapy, and appears to avoid long periods of under- or overanticoagulation.

It is imperative that blood samples for coagulation tests (APTT) for monitoring heparin therapy be carefully timed. After beginning the heparin infusion or after any dosage change, the clinician should wait at least 6 hours to draw samples for coagulation tests to assess the effect of the heparin dose. Samples collected too early are often misleading, may result in inappropriate dosage alteration, and frequently start a costly cycle of "dosage change–coagulation test" in a clinically stable patient. It is often most efficient to wait until steady-state conditions exist to monitor the degree of anticoagulation and make dosage alterations. The risk of bleeding is minimal during the first 48 hours of heparin therapy (in patients without identified risk factors), and coagulation tests are helpful primarily to ensure adequate heparinization. In addition, there is no association between bleeding complications and APTT values considered above the therapeutic range during the first 4 days of therapy.[25]

When a continuous infusion is not feasible, heparin can be administered by intravenous intermittent injections. The half-life of heparin ranges from 0.4 to 2.5 hours; therefore, an every-4-hour dosing interval is appropriate for most patients. Coagulation tests are best performed 3.5 to 4 hours after the heparin injection. It is imperative to schedule and document the times of heparin injections and blood sampling for coagulation tests. The heparin dosage is considered adequate when the coagulation test collected 3.5 hours after an intravenous injection is in the therapeutic range for the test (APTT 1.5 to 2.0 times baseline).

Once a heparin dose has been determined that produces the desired degree of anticoagulation, daily monitoring of coagulation tests is indicated for minor dosing adjustments. Laboratory monitoring should be performed at the same time of the day (e.g., every morning) to minimize the influence of circadian variation.[20] Large variations in subsequent coagulation tests necessitate investigation to ensure that the patient's condition has not dramatically changed (e.g., extension or recurrence of the thromboembolic event), that the prescribed heparin dose is being administered accurately, and that blood samples are being collected and assayed appropriately. If substantial changes in heparin dosage are made, the modified dosage regimen needs to be monitored in a manner similar to the initial heparin therapy.

The optimal duration of anticoagulation with heparin therapy for the treatment of thromboembolic diseases continues to be evaluated.[18] Several studies in patients with acute thromboembolic diseases have established the effectiveness and safety associated with a short course (4 to 5 days) of continuous intravenous heparin therapy (warfarin started on day 1 of heparin therapy) compared to the traditional 10-day course (warfarin started on day 5 of heparin therapy).[1,30,31] These studies demonstrated no significant difference between the groups in terms of rate of recurrence of venous thromboembolism (3.7% vs 4.6%), major bleeding complications (3.7% vs 3.2%), or fatal PE (0% for both groups). Mohiuddin et al.[31] showed that the length of hospital stay (8.62 vs 13.0 days), the cost of hospitalization ($10,485 vs $14,987), and the frequency of adverse reactions associated with heparin therapy (infusion phlebitis [2% vs 18%] and thrombocytopenia [0% vs 14%]) were significantly less for the short-course versus long-course groups. This approach seems appropriate for patients with uncomplicated and less extensive thromboembolic disorders. Patients with massive pulmonary embolism or ileofemoral thrombosis may require a more traditional duration of intravenous heparin therapy (e.g., 10 days), with oral anticoagulation being started on day 5 of heparin therapy to ensure a crossover period of 4 to 5 days.[18]

Coagulation tests should be performed prior to the initiation of heparin therapy to (1) establish the patient's baseline APTT value, which assists in determining the end point for heparin therapy, and (2) establish a baseline prothrombin time (PT and international normalized ratio [INR]) as a guide for later oral anticoagulation with warfarin. Additional necessary baseline laboratory parameters include quantitative platelet count prior to heparinization and every 2 or 3 days during therapy to monitor for heparin-associated thrombocytopenia. Hemoglobin and hematocrit measurements are indicated prior to heparinization and every 1 to 2 days while the patient is receiving heparin to identify the presence of bleeding. These laboratory parameters are especially useful in determining the existence of occult bleeding, such as retroperitoneal hemorrhage. The stool should be examined daily for the presence of blood.

Patients should be examined twice daily for signs of bleeding including intravenous catheter sites, hematomas, and ecchymosis. Intramuscular injections should be avoided in patients receiving therapeutic heparin.

Patients receiving heparin for DVT or PE should be monitored for signs and symptoms of pulmonary embolism every shift for 1 to 2 days, followed by daily monitoring for the occurence or changes in dyspnea, apprehension, cough, pleuritic chest pain, and hemoptysis. In addition, repeat arterial blood gases and lung scans and/or perfusion–ventilation studies may be indicated to assess progress of antithrombotic therapy in patients being treated for PE.[7] Similarly, patients being treated for venous thrombosis should be initially monitored twice daily and then daily for changes in pain, limb circumference, swelling, and tenderness, as well as for signs of PE.

In addition to the laboratory and clinical monitoring parameters just mentioned, clinicians must be aware of other practical concerns in patients receiving heparin. Four of the most common errors associated with heparin therapy have been the (1) lack of precision of pumps being used to infuse heparin, (2) interruption in the continuous infusion, (3) errors in preparation of solution containing the heparin dose, and (4) errors in charting the dose administered.[20] For the intravenous administration of continuous infusion heparin, reliable infusion pumps should be used. Every effort should be made not to interrupt the continuous infusions. During a 1-hour interruption, the APTT can fall from 60 seconds (therapeutic) to less than 40 seconds; hence, interruptions in the infusion longer than 60 minutes may require an additional bolus injection in addition to restarting the infusion (Fig. 17–3).

To interpret a coagulation test properly, it is essential to know the actual rate of heparin infusion. Failure to document and chart heparin infusion rates adequately can lead to potentially serious errors.

Administration/Monitoring of Dose-Adjusted Subcutaneous Heparin

Several randomized trials suggest that intermittent, adjusted-dose subcutaneous heparin is a safe and effective alternative route of therapy for the initial treatment of venous thrombosis.[18–20,25] In addition, this route of administration simplifies treatment and allows for outpatient therapy.

Initial heparin dosage guidelines should be 15,000 to 17,500 U or 250 U/kg total body weight administered subcutaneously every 12 hours.[19] The initial dose can be rapidly adjusted according to the APTT value drawn 4 to 6 hours after the first dose. A midinterval sample has been chosen because this predicts the maximal response of the APTT after subcutaneous injection and the sustained therapeutic response throughout the 12-hour dosing interval.

As with intravenous heparin therapy, adjusted-dose subcutaneous heparin must be administered to maintain APTT above 1.5 times the control value. The APTT should be performed (1) prior to the initiation of heparin therapy, (2) 4 to 6 hours after the first subcutaneous dose, and (3) once daily at the middle of the dosing interval. Failure to achieve an adequate anticoagulant response early in therapy is associated with an unacceptable recurrence rate of 20% to 25% of venous thromboembolism.[19] Major and minor bleeding complications have been similar to intravenous heparin administration.

Laboratory Monitoring

The APTT has become the most popular test for monitoring heparin therapy largely because of its routine use by clinical laboratories, the rapidity with which it can be performed, and its reproducibility.[20] The APTT is a global test that measures the resultant activity from the balance between activators and inhibitors of the intrinsic and common pathways of the coagulation system. Platelet-poor plasma is activated by contact agents in the presence of phospholipids and is then recalcified. The APTT uses the generation of a fibrin clot as its end point. The APTT reacts similarly with heparin derived from bovine lung and porcine mucosa. The three major disadvantages to using APTT to monitor heparin therapy are that (1) it is unable to distinguish between the anticoagulant activity of heparin and several clotting factor deficiencies, (2) the instrumentation used requires that the APTT be performed in a laboratory, and (3) the heparin sensitivity of different commercial APTT reagents is variable.[19,32,33] This last point emphasizes the need for each clinical laboratory to use a standardized procedure in the reporting of APTT values.[33]

The goal of therapy is to balance the prevention of unwanted clotting and increased risk of hemorrhage by keeping the degree of anticoagulation within the therapeutic range (APTT between 1.5 and 2.5 times control or baseline).[18,19] Normal adult control values vary among laboratories and range from about 28 to 42 seconds. The association between subtherapeutic APTT values and recurrent thrombosis is firmly established.[18–20,22,23] However, in the absence of randomized studies, evidence of a correlation between elevated APTT and risk of hemorrhage is suggestive but not conclusive.[18,19]

A recent study has suggested that an antifactor Xa assay (target range: 0.4 to 0.7 U/mL) may be more useful for monitoring heparin therapy than APTT in patients who require large daily doses (e.g., > 35,000 U/d).[34] Bleeding complications occurred in only 1 of 65 (1.5%) patients monitored by the antifactor Xa assay compared to 4 of 66 (6.1%) patients monitored by APTT values;

recurrent thromboembolic complications were similar for the two groups (4.6% vs 6.1%, respectively). The antifactor Xa assay is not influenced by coagulation factors and is more specific for the effect of heparin to neutralize factor Xa or thrombin. In this select group of patients, the antifactor Xa assay avoids excessive heparin doses and the increased risk of bleeding complications encountered when the APTT is monitored.

Adverse Effects

Hemorrhage is the adverse effect of greatest concern with anticoagulant therapy. The risk of major bleeding (bleeding requiring blood transfusion and/or discontinuation of the anticoagulant) with therapeutic doses of heparin for the treatment of thromboembolic disease has been reported to range from 1% to 33%, although most studies have reported a frequency of 2% to 5%.[1,18–20,35,36] The frequency of fatal, major, and major plus minor bleeding during heparin therapy has been estimated to be 0.05%, 0.8%, and 2.0%, respectively.[36] These frequencies are approximately twice the expected values in patients not receiving heparin therapy.

The most common sites of bleeding with heparin therapy are from the GI tract, the urinary tract, soft tissues, and the oropharynx.[36] The most frequently encountered bleeding episodes include melena, hematomas, and hematuria, which occur in 2% to 3% of patients. Less common are ecchymosis, epistaxis, and hematemesis, which occur in 0.5% to 1.2% of patients.

The frequency of bleeding complications has been related to several treatment-related factors (dose, route, and duration of therapy) and patient-related factors (age, gender, past history of GI bleeding or peptic ulcer diseases, comorbid diseases, concurrent medications). Several studies have shown that the risk of bleeding greatly increases as the dose increases and with the administration of heparin by intermittent bolus as compared with continuous infusion. Exceeding the normal values of "therapeutic" coagulation tests has been suggested to be predictive of these hemorrhagic complications.

In general, the risk of bleeding not only varies with the dose but also increases with the length of heparin therapy. The 7-day cumulative risk of bleeding during heparin therapy is 3.4% to 9.1%.[20] Also, this cumulative risk increases with the length of therapy, and by 3 weeks of continuous heparin therapy, bleeding occurs in nearly 20% of patients.

The risk of bleeding is also influenced by several patient-related factors. Risk factors associated with both major and minor bleeding episodes in nonsurgical patients have included gender, age, dose, concurrent aspirin use, and heavy alcohol use.[20] Other predictive factors of major bleeding in hospitalized patients receiving anticoagulant (warfarin or heparin) therapy are (1) comorbid conditions such as heart, liver, or kidney failure, cancer, and severe anemia; (2) age greater than 60 years in patients receiving heparin; (3) the intensity of anticoagulation; and (4) liver failure that worsened during therapy. The risk of bleeding increased as the number of comorbid conditions increased, and was more likely in patients who received intravenous heparin than warfarin.[36]

When bleeding occurs during heparin therapy, it is often related to preexisting hemostatic defects (uremia, drug-related defects in platelet aggregation, thrombocytopenia, liver disease), invasive procedures (venous cutdowns, arterial punctures, thoracentesis), or patient factors such as gender and age. Women have approximately a twofold greater risk of bleeding than men. This gender difference is further exaggerated when advanced age is examined as an additional risk factor. Overall, prophylactic low-dose heparin (5000 U subcutaneously every 12 hours) is not associated with an increased risk of major hemorrhage, and the risk of minor bleeding is also very low.

Minor bleeding from an excess of heparin can usually be controlled by discontinuing the drug. For major bleeding or the threat of significant hemorrhage, specific therapy is warranted. Blood transfusion will correct massive blood loss, but it is not a specific antidote. Protamine sulfate remains the drug of choice for the reversal of heparin effect. Protamine combines quickly with heparin to form salts that are devoid of anticoagulant effect. One milligram of protamine sulfate neutralizes approximately 90 USP units of beef lung heparin or 115 USP units of porcine mucosal heparin. For patients receiving heparin as a continuous infusion, 1 mg of protamine should be administered for each 100 U of heparin delivered during the past 4 hours. Protamine should be administered by slow intravenous infusion (up to 50 mg over 10 minutes) to decrease the frequency and severity of adverse reactions (hypotension, vasodilation, bradycardia, dyspnea). Excessive doses of protamine can also be associated with bleeding complications.

Other important adverse effects of heparin therapy are thrombocytopenia with thrombosis and osteoporosis.[19] Although the reported incidence of thrombocytopenia has varied from less than 1% to 30%, the probable frequency is 1% to 5%.[5,20,37] Thrombocytopenia seems to be more frequent with beef lung heparin; however, switching to porcine mucosa heparin is not recommended because of the high incidence of cross-sensitivity between products. Two distinct platelet phenomena are associated with the administration of heparin and can be seen in patients who receive therapeutic doses of heparin, as well as in patients who receive low-dose subcutaneous heparin and heparin flushes. An early, slight decrease in circulating platelets is almost universal. The effect is mild and transient, with platelet counts seldom dropping below 100,000/mm^3, and usually does not require discontinuation of heparin therapy. It is most likely caused by a temporary sequestration of platelets, secondary to heparin's mild platelet aggregating effect. The patients are usually asymptomatic, and it appears to be of no clinical importance.

The second effect is a rare but severe thrombocytopenia that occurs between 5 and 14 days after the initiation of heparin therapy. The effect is independent of dose or route, and most likely has an immunologic basis, which increases platelet consumption. Platelet counts may fall below 100,000/mm^3 and will remain low until the heparin is discontinued. In addition, thromboembolic complications may occur in arteries (white clot) as well as veins (myocardial infarction, DVT, PE) with this type of thrombocytopenia. Careful monitoring of platelet counts (every 2 to 3 days) to evaluate the decline of platelet count (greater than 30%) as well as the absolute number (less than 100,000/mm^3) can minimize the risk of heparin-associated thrombocytopenia.[20]

A limited number of reports have described osteoporosis secondary to heparin therapy.[5,18,19] This adverse effect has been rarely reported and is generally found in patients receiving in excess of 20,000 U/d for 6 months or longer.

Other rare complications of heparin therapy include skin necrosis, local urticaria, hypoaldosteronism, and hypersensitivity reactions.[38]

LOW-MOLECULAR-WEIGHT HEPARIN

Like unfractionated heparin, low-molecular-weight heparins (LMWH) belong to a class of anticoagulants termed glycosaminoglycans. Overall, LMWHs differ from unfractionated heparin in their molecular size and weight, method of preparation, and anticoagulant properties, as depicted in Table 17–5. Although unfractionated heparin is a heterogeneous mixture of polysaccharide chains ranging in molecular weight from 3000 to 30,000 Daltons (mean 15,000), LMWHs are derived from unfractionated heparin by various manufacturing methods to elaborate compounds with smaller, less variable molecular weights (mean

TABLE 17–5. Characteristics of Low-Molecular-Weight Heparins (LMWH)

LMWH Manufacturer	Method of Preparation	Average Molecular Weight (Mean; Da)	Bioavailabilitiy (%)	Half-Life (h)	Anti-Xa Potency (U/mg)	Anti-IIa Potency (U/mg)
FDA-Approved						
Enoxaparin (Lovenox) Rhone Poulenc Rorer	Benzylation followed by alkaline hydrolysis	3500–5500 (4371)	91	4.5	100–110	25–30
Dalteparin (Fragmin) Kabi Pharmacia	Controlled nitrous acid depolymerization	4000–6000 (5819)	87	2.4–4	140–150	60
Ardeparin (Normiflo) Wyeth Ayerst	Peroxidative cleavage	5500–6500 (6000)	90	3.5	100	48
Not FDA-Approved						
Nadroparin (Fraxiparine) Sanofi	Optimized nitrous acid depolymerization	4855	99	2–5	90–100	25–30
Certoparin (Sandoparin) Novartis/Sandoz	Isoamyl nitrite digestion	4849		4.3	80–95	30–35
Tinzaparin (Logiparin) Nova-Nordisk	Heparinase digestion	4900	90	1.5	80–85	45
Reviparin (Clivarin) Knoll	Nitrous acid degradation	4653			130	40
Parnaparin (Fluxum) Opocrin	Peroxidative cleavage	4500–5500	90	3.8–5.9	85–90	<30
Bemiparin Rovi	Nitrous acid digestion					
Miniparin Syntex	Nitrous acid digestion					

5000).[37,39] Like unfractionated heparin, LMWHs also bind to antithrombin III and produce a conformational change in antithrombin III to expedite its natural function, as explained earlier in this chapter. LMWHs exhibit a preferential effect on activated factor X with fewer effects on platelets than standard heparin.[39,40] However, unlike standard heparin, LMWHs are less able to inhibit thrombin formation because fewer than half of the polysaccharide chains of LMWHs are of sufficient length to bind to both antithrombin III and thrombin.[37,39] This preferential effect on factor Xa of LMWHs along with fewer effects on thrombin and platelets were thought to be properties that might lead to less bleeding while still retaining anticoagulant effects. Overall, the LMWHs are comparable but their biologic properties and anti-factor Xa potency vary widely so that each agent should be considered a separate drug, especially when evaluating clinical trials.

When comparing the pharmacokinetic characteristics of standard heparin and LMWHs, the LMWHs again exhibit some distinct advantages. Standard heparin binds nonspecifically to a variety of plasma proteins and endothelial cells, thus limiting the amount available to interact with antithrombin III. This is thought to account for the unpredictable dose–response relationship that is frequently observed with heparin administration as well as for the low bioavailability seen after subcutaneous administration. LMWHs display less nonspecific binding to plasma proteins and endothelial cells, which, in addition to their smaller size, may account for the excellent bioavailability of LMWHs after subcutaneous administration.[37,40] The decreased binding of LMWHs to plasma proteins may also account for the more predictable anticoagulant response and less interpatient variability observed with LMWHs. LMWHs also have a longer duration of anti-factor Xa activity than unfractionated heparin so that they can be administered either once or twice daily depending on the LMWH and the indication. Most of the LMWHs are eliminated primarily by the kidney so that dosage adjustments are necessary in patients with renal insufficiency. Table 17–5 lists some of the pharmacokinetic characteristics of the LMWHs.

There are limited data on the use of LMWHs in children so that data obtained in adults should not be extrapolated to children. Variations in response and unpredictable efficacy have made the use of LMWHs in children problematic.[40] One small study has demonstrated that the dose of LMWH is age-dependent (higher doses are needed to achieve the same anticoagulant effect), possibly reflecting an increased clearance or larger volume of distribution in children < 2 months of age.[41] More studies are needed to evaluate the use of LMWHs in children before firm recommendations can be made. Finally, LMWHs do not appear to cross the placenta and have been used in a number of pregnant patients without any adverse effects to the fetus.[37,39,42] Currently, there is insufficient evidence to recommend them for routine use in pregnant patients.

The adverse effects associated with the LMWHs are similar to those observed with standard heparin, namely bleeding and thrombocytopenia. Although the incidence of bleeding complications was postulated to be less with LMWHs because of their preferential effects on factor Xa with fewer effects on thrombin and platelets, this has not been conclusively proven in the clinical trials to date that evaluated LMWHs for the prophylaxis or treatment of venous thromboembolism. When evaluating LMWHs as prophylaxis against venous thromboembolism, the incidence of major bleeding is greater than placebo, comparable to low-dose unfractionated heparin, and comparable to or less than warfarin. When LMWHs are used for the treatment of established venous thromboembolism, the risk of major bleeding is slightly less than that observed with standard heparin or warfarin. The overall incidence of minor bleeding episodes and wound hematoma with LMWHs is comparable to standard heparin, and less than warfarin (wound hematomas greater with LMWHs).

The overall incidence of thrombocytopenia (of any kind) is less than 2% with LMWHs.[42–45] It has been shown in a recent study that LMWHs are associated with a lower risk of immune sensitization in addition to a lower risk of heparin-induced thrombocytopenia (HIT) and associated thrombotic effects when compared with standard heparin.[45] Although LMWHs appear to *cause* less HIT, in patients with documented HIT, the risk of cross-reactivity between LMWHs and heparin-induced antibodies ranges from 20% to 100%.[46] There have been a few successful reports of the use of LMWHs in patients with documented HIT; however, LMWHs are not indicated for the treatment of HIT because of the high rate of cross-reactivity between the two forms of heparin.[39] It is recommended that plasma from patients with HIT who are being considered for treatment with any LMWH undergo extensive *in vitro* testing to determine if the LMWH will cross-react with the heparin-induced antibodies of the patient and cause platelet aggregation.[45]

LMWHs have been associated with the development of delayed hypersensitivity skin reactions; skin necrosis; and eczematous, pruritic plaques either at the injection site or at a site distant from the injection site. These reactions appear to display cross-reactivity with other LMWHs or heparin so that these agents should be used with caution in a patient with a history of a skin reaction to a LMWH or heparin.[42,43] The incidence of osteoporosis may be less with LMWHs than standard heparin;[37,39] however more studies are needed to confirm this observation. In addition, LMWHs have been associated with elevated serum transaminase levels.

Currently, there is only one test available to monitor the anticoagulant effects of LMWHs because the APTT or other common bleeding tests are not altered during LMWH therapy. During therapy with LMWHs, the plasma anti-Xa activity may be measured to monitor the anticoagulant effect. For the prevention of DVT, routine monitoring is not required. However, when using LMWHs for the treatment of established venous thromboembolism, it is recommended that anti-Xa levels be measured at least once at the beginning of therapy to assure that an adequate level of anticoagulation is achieved in addition to assessing the risk of hemorrhage.[40]

Although the LMWHs are not currently FDA-approved in the United States for the treatment of DVT or PE, there have been a number of open label and comparative studies evaluating the efficacy and safety of some of the LMWHs for the treatment of thromboembolic disease. The LMWHs are attractive alternatives to heparin and warfarin for the treatment of venous thromboembolism because they exhibit a predictable dose–response relationship, which promotes standard dosing once or twice daily (fixed or weight-adjusted) and negates the need for routine laboratory monitoring and dosage adjustment; and they are absorbed well after subcutaneous administration, making them easy to administer on an outpatient basis and resulting in a decrease in the number of inpatient hospital days. LMWHs have been evaluated as initial treatment for acute venous thromboembolism in comparison with heparin (Tables 17–6 and 17–7) or as secondary

TABLE 17–6. Comparative Trials of LMWHs as Initial Treatment for DVT

Reference	Regimens Compared	No. of Patients	Recurrent VTE: *During Tx*	Recurrent VTE: *Within 3 mo*	Bleeding: *Major*	Bleeding: *Minor*	Death	Comments
47	Enoxaparin 1 mg/kg SC bid	247	7	13	5	6	11	Acute proximal DVT All patients given warfarin on day 2 (INR 2–3) for 3 months
	IV heparin (APTT 60–85 s)	253	12	17	3	6	17	Length of hospitalization significantly shorter in LMWH group
48	Dalteparin 5000 IU bolus; 200 anti-Xa U/kg SC qd	96	1	4			5	All patients given oral anticoagulant on day of or day after initiation into study
	IV heparin (APTT 1.5–3 × control)	103	1	2	2		4	6-month follow-up
49	Dalteparin 5000 IU bolus; 200 anti-Xa U/kg SC qd	92	2	3		6	1	All patients started oral anticoagulants immediately
	IV heparin (APTT 1.5–3 × control)	98	2	1	5	4		
50	Reviparin SC bid weight-adjusted	510	16	27	10		39	Oral anticoagulation started on first or second day for 3 months
	IV heparin (APTT 1.5–2.5 × control)	511	15	25	8		36	Overall death rates reported Equally effective and safe LMWH: shorter hospital stay

LMWH = low-molecular-weight heparin; DVT = deep vein thrombosis; VTE = venous thromboembolic events; Tx = treatment; SC = subcutaneous; IV = intravenous; bid = twice daily; qd = once daily.

TABLE 17–7. Comparative Trials of LMWH as Initial Treatment for Nonmassive Pulmonary Embolism

Reference	Regimens Compared	No. of Patients	Recurrent VTE		Bleeding		Death	Comments
			During Tx	*Within 3 mo*	*Major*	*Minor*		
51	Dalteparin 120 anti-Xa U/kg SC bid	29	0	0	0	1	0	Patients received 10 days of either drug
	IV heparin (APTT 2–3 × control)	31	1		0	4	0	Oral anticoagulation started on day 7 of therapy (INR 2–3) for 3 months
52	Tinzaparin 175 anti-Xa U/kg SC qd	304	3	2	4	17	12	Oral anticoagulation started between days 1 and 3; continued for 3 months
	IV heparin (APTT 2–3 × control)	308	2	4	6	8	14	Similar efficacy and safety rates

LMWH = low-molecular-weight heparin; VTE = venous thromboembolic events; Tx = treatment; SC = subcutaneous; IV = intravenous; bid = twice daily; qd = once daily.

treatment to prevent recurrences of DVT or PE in comparison with warfarin (Table 17–8).[47–54] To date, there have been no clinical trials published directly comparing different LMWH preparations in terms of safety or efficacy in the treatment of venous thromboembolism.

Most of the initial treatment studies evaluated the effects of the LMWH preparation in comparison with adjusted dose intravenous or subcutaneous heparin on thrombus size and progression, recurrent thromboembolism, bleeding complications, and death. These studies have been reviewed elsewhere[18,39,55,56] and evaluated in meta-analysis.[57–59] When evaluating the change in thrombus size, earlier studies demonstrated a significant reduction in thrombus size with LMWHs when compared to standard heparin.[18,56] However, the clinical significance of decreased thrombus size is unknown, so that more objective criteria such as recurrence of venous thromboembolism, incidence of bleeding, and death then became the primary clinical outcome measures. Overall, the results from the individual studies have demonstrated that LMWHs are at least as safe and effective as unfractionated heparin for the initial treatment of DVT or nonmassive PE, and as safe and effective as adjusted-dose warfarin for the prevention of recurrent venous thromboembolism. In the majority of studies, however, there was no significant difference between the LMWH and heparin or warfarin in the rate of recurrent venous thromboembolism, bleeding, or death. Meta-analysis[57–59] evaluating initial treatment studies has shown a significant risk reduction for symptomatic thromboembolic complications, clinically important bleeding, and mortality. However, each of the meta-analyses included several different LMWH preparations, which, as alluded to earlier, are not interchangeable and should not be grouped together. Therefore, the results of the meta-analyses may not be applicable to all LMWHs.

One of the clear therapeutic advantages of LMWH over unfractionated heparin is the ability to administer initial treatment for DVT at home without the need for laboratory monitoring. Pharmacy-managed programs for outpatient treatment of uncomplicated acute proximal vein thrombosis with subcutaneous enoxaparin followed by warfarin have been implemented with promising results.[60] However, further large-scale studies are needed to clearly define the role of the individual LMWHs for the initial treatment of venous thromboembolism or for the prevention of recurrent thromboembolic events (and until they are approved by the FDA for these indications).[15] Unfractionated heparin and warfarin remain the respective drugs of choice.

WARFARIN

The coumarin derivative warfarin was synthesized at the University of Wisconsin in 1948 (the name warfarin being derived from the Wisconsin Alumni Research Foundation). Warfarin is the

TABLE 17–8. LMWHs Versus Warfarin for the Prevention of Recurrent Venous Thromboembolism

Reference	Regimens Compared	No. of Patients	Recurrent VTE	Bleeding		Death	Comments
				Major	*Minor*		
53	Enoxaparin 40 mg SC qd	93	6	3	1	11	Patients initially treated with SC heparin for 10 days (APTT 1.5–2.5 × control)
	Warfarin (INR 2.7) adjusted dose	94	4	3	9	8	Duration of therapy 3 months 1-year follow-up
54	Dalteparin 5000 anti-Xa units SC qd	50	3	0	6	1	Patients initially treated with 10 days of SC heparin
	Warfarin (INR 2–3) adjusted dose	55	1	0	5	3	Both therapies started on day 8 of heparin therapy Duration of therapy 3 months Patients discharged home on average 3 days sooner in LMWH group

LMWH = low-molecular-weight heparin; VTE = venous thromboembolic events; SC = subcutaneous; qd = once daily.

most useful of the vitamin K antagonists because of its predictable clinical effects, including onset of action and long duration of effect. The indications for warfarin therapy include the treatment of venous thromboembolism, the prevention of recurrent venous thromboembolism, the prevention of thromboembolism in patients with prosthetic heart valves or chronic atrial fibrillation, the prophylaxis against venous thrombosis in patients undergoing moderate- to high-risk surgical procedures, or as an adjunct in the treatment of coronary artery occlusion.[61,62] Because the risk of recurrent thromboembolic disease is significant in the first 3 months after DVT or PE, and moderate for 6 months or greater, warfarin administration is indicated after the initial course of heparin therapy to prevent further thromboembolic complications.[18,62]

The pharmacologic effects of warfarin include anticoagulation and antithrombotic action. The mechanisms by which warfarin accomplishes these effects include prevention of the formation of γ-carboxyglutamic acid residues (by blocking the carboxylation system) and release of certain proteins that are deficient in γ-carboxyglutamic acid (Fig. 17–4). Six vitamin K-dependent proteins are involved in the coagulation system (factors II, VII, IX, X, and proteins C and S), whose synthesis is inhibited by warfarin.

The inhibition of coagulation factors and the indirect anticoagulation of warfarin occurs 12 to 24 hours after oral administration. This is at the same time that depression of protein C and factor VII occurs. In contrast, antithrombotic effects of warfarin may not occur until 2 to 7 days following the initiation of therapy. The *in vivo* antithrombotic effect occurs after a steady state has been achieved between the decrease in the rate of synthesis and the rate of disappearance of existing clotting factors in plasma. The average half-lives of the vitamin K-dependent clotting factors are 6, 24, 40, and 60 hours for factors VII, IX, X, and II, respectively. Factor VII concentrations decrease first and account for the initial change in the PT.

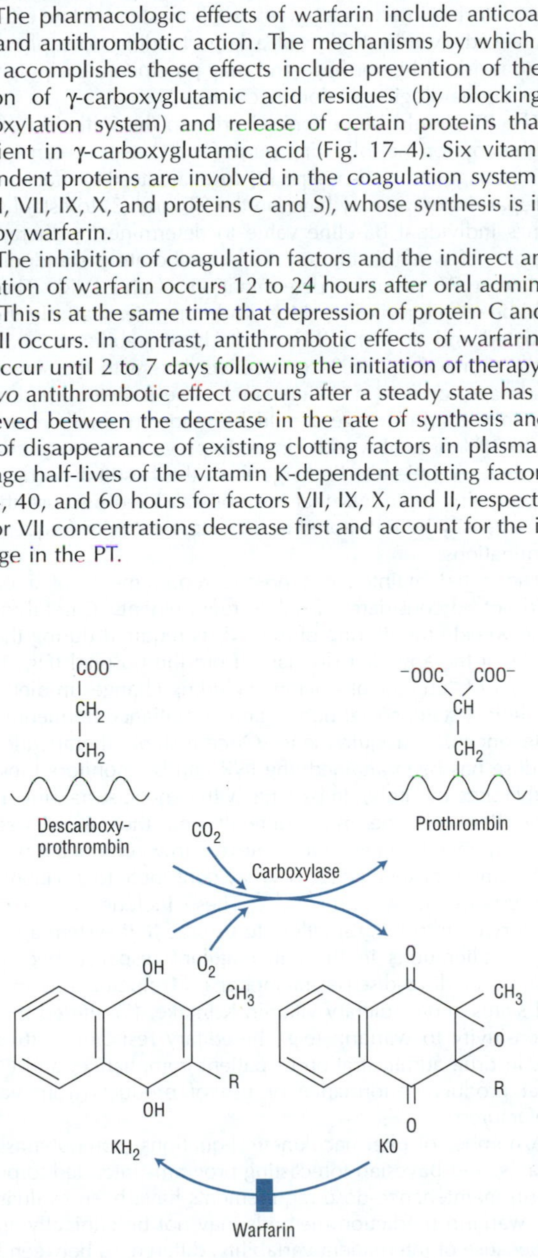

FIGURE 17–4. Interactions between vitamin K and warfarin. Warfarin and other vitamin K antagonists inhibit the reduction of vitamin K epoxide to vitamin K by the enzyme vitamin K-epoxide reductase. The oxidation–reduction cycle between the two forms of vitamin K is linked in some unknown way to the γ-carboxylation of glutamic acid residues on vitamin K-dependent coagulation factors II, VII, IX, and X.

Pharmacokinetics

Warfarin is commercially available as a racemic mixture of the enantiomers *R*- and *S*-warfarin that exhibit differing pharmacokinetic and pharmacodynamic characteristics.[61–64] After oral administration, warfarin is well absorbed, with peak plasma concentrations occurring from 0.3 to 8 hours (mean 90 minutes) after a dose.[64] The bioavailability of warfarin is 100%, with minimal differences among the various commercial warfarin products. However, difficulties may arise in controlling a patient's anticoagulant therapy when products are interchanged.[65]

Warfarin is extensively protein bound (97.4% to 99.9%), principally to albumin, with the *R*-enantiomer having greater binding affinity than *S*-warfarin. When protein binding is taken into account, the *S*-enantiomer has an inherent potency approximately eight times greater than the *R*-enantiomer. Warfarin is stereoselectively oxidized by hepatic microsomal enzyme systems to hydroxy metabolites, and then reduced to alcohols that are renally excreted.

Warfarin is a capacity-limited binding-sensitive drug, which has a low intrinsic clearance and a low unbound fraction. Protein binding determines the unbound drug fraction available for metabolism and explains the linear relationship observed between total body clearance of warfarin and the unbound fraction in plasma. In addition, isomers of warfarin have different rates of elimination. Mean (range) half-lives for the *R*- and *S*-isomers are 45.4 (37.4 to 88.6) and 33 (21.2 to 42.6) hours, respectively. These differences in half-life of the isomers influence the contribution of the *R*-isomer to the anticoagulant effects of warfarin and have implications on drug interactions.

Plasma clearance of warfarin is increased in patients with renal insufficiency. More unbound fraction of warfarin is available for metabolism in patients with renal failure. In addition, there is the potential for the renally excreted active alcohol metabolites to accumulate. However, these alterations have not increased pharmacologic responsiveness of warfarin in patients with renal failure.

Therapeutic Indications/Clinical Efficacy

Warfarin effectively prevents recurrent thromboembolic events following the acute treatment of DVT or PE with heparin therapy. The rationale for warfarin after initial heparin therapy was derived from studies that showed a protective effect of anticoagulant therapy for the first 6 months after hospital discharge.[1,5,18,37] Beyond this time, the potential beneficial effects of anticoagulation must be weighed against the risk of bleeding complications. The incidence of serious bleeding complications while receiving warfarin ranges from 2.4% to 10% in most series.[35,36,62,63] The risk of recurrent thromboembolic disease is highest in those patients with previous episodes of the same phenomenon. Thus, warfarin administration is indicated for at least 3 months after an initial episode of DVT and indefinitely for long-term anticoagulation in patients with recurrent venous thromboembolism.[18,66]

Several studies have searched for a suitable alternative strategy for managing patients with long-term anticoagulation.[18,62] The clinical efficacy of fixed-low-dose subcutaneous heparin, dose-adjusted subcutaneous heparin, and "less intensive" warfarin therapy (prothrombin times ranging from 1.2 to 1.8 times control or baseline values) has been evaluated in patients initially treated with a continuous intravenous infusion of heparin for 10 to 14 days. These studies demonstrate that adjusted-dose heparin and less intense warfarin therapy are as effective as conventional warfarin therapy for treating proximal-vein thrombosis, with risk of hemorrhage significantly greater with conventional warfarin therapy. Fixed-low-dose heparin is not effective for treating proximal vein thrombosis. A cost-effectiveness analysis was performed for the various approaches to long-term treatment of proximal venous thrombosis. It was concluded that the less intense warfarin therapy was the most cost effective and that oral therapy was preferred by the majority of patients. However, dose-adjusted subcutaneous heparin is an acceptable alternative to warfarin therapy, particularly in patients who cannot take warfarin (e.g., in pregnancy) and in those patients who cannot have their coagulation tests (PT) monitored on a continual basis.

All of the contraindications listed above for heparin apply to warfarin as well. Relative contraindications for warfarin therapy include severe hepatic or renal disease, vitamin K deficiency, chronic alcoholism, a requirement for intensive acetaminophen, salicylate or nonsteroidal anti-inflammatory drug therapy, and the inability of the patient to comply with the regimen.

Laboratory Monitoring

The international normalized ratio (INR) is now considered the standard of practice for monitoring warfarin therapy.[18,61,67] The INR takes into account the sensitivity of the thromboplastin used in determining the PT for each specific laboratory.[67] The World Health Organization (WHO) has prepared a thromboplastin standard to promote standardization of oral anticoagulation therapy by allowing any commercial thromboplastin reagent to be calibrated against this reference standard.

The calculation of the INR is represented by the following equation demonstrating the relationship between the INR and the observed PT ratio:

$$\text{INR} = (\text{observed PT ratio})^{\text{ISI}}$$

where ISI is the international sensitivity index, which is calibrated based on the type of thromboplastin used. The sensitivity of the thromboplastin reagent can dramatically influence the INR value. For example, if a patient has a PT of 17 seconds using a more responsive thromboplastin with a low ISI value of 1.2, and the laboratory mean normal value for the PT is 12.6 seconds, the INR for this patient would be 1.43. However, the INR would be 1.99 in the same patient if the thromboplastin used was less sensitive and had an ISI value of 2.3. The different values in thromboplastin reagents illustrates the limitation of monitoring warfarin with only PT ratios, which have been associated with significant errors when monitoring warfarin therapy.[67,68]

The current recommendation for monitoring most indications of warfarin therapy is an INR of 2.0 to 3.0.[18,61,67] The exceptions to this range include patients with mechanical prosthetic heart valves (recommended INR of 2.5 to 3.5) and the management of thrombosis in antiphospholipid-antibody syndrome (recommended INR of greater than 3.0).

It is important to recognize the effect that heparin has on the PT when heparin and warfarin therapies are "overlapped." It has been shown that heparin increases PT results. However, the effects are minimal and the PT will decrease once heparin therapy is discontinued, which may require further adjustment of warfarin maintenance doses.

Warfarin Administration/Monitoring

Warfarin can be initiated at any time during heparin treatment and should be initiated as soon as it becomes apparent that oral anticoagulation will be used. Initiation of warfarin should occur before intravenous heparin is discontinued to prevent a break in the level of anticoagulation. The "overlapping period" of heparin and warfarin should be 4 to 5 days because of the delayed onset of warfarin's effect and the hypercoagulable state occurring after heparin is discontinued.[18,19,61,62] Heparin can usually be discontinued once the INR is within the desired range for 2 consecutive days.

The risk of recurrent venous thromboembolism approaches 0% if warfarin therapy is initiated during a 5- to 14-day course of heparin therapy.[19] In addition, several studies have demonstrated that the number of hospitalization days, days of heparin therapy, adverse effects of heparin, and cost of hospitalization are decreased when warfarin is administered within the first 24 to 48 hours of heparin therapy.[30,31]

It must be emphasized that warfarin dosages must be individualized by monitoring the INR closely and examining the patient for signs of bleeding. The initiation of oral warfarin therapy with small doses of approximately 5 mg/d for 2 to 4 days is generally agreed to be less toxic than administration of large loading doses (50–75 mg).[62,63,69] In elderly patients (age > 65 years), initial doses may need to be lower (1 to 3 mg/d) as well as laboratory monitoring intervals ≥1 week to allow steady-state effects to be achieved. Administration of a large loading dose places the patient at risk of hemorrhage and may precipitate the potentially serious dermatologic reaction (necrosis).[64]

The PT should be performed prior to the initiation of warfarin therapy for the following purposes: (1) as a screen for preexisting coagulation disorders; (2) to evaluate the effect, if any, that heparin therapy may have on the PT; and (3) to establish the patient's individual baseline value to determine the therapeutic end point of warfarin therapy from a laboratory standpoint (to calculate a PT ratio for determination of the INR). The INR should be monitored every 24 to 48 hours after warfarin therapy is initiated and until the INR results have stabilized (i.e., INRs that are similar for 2 or 3 consecutive days with the same warfarin dosage) or until a maintenance dose is determined. Alterations in warfarin dosage should be made in small increments (10% to 20% of total weekly doses) to prevent excessive changes in the INR. A patient's discharge from the hospital need not be delayed owing to an INR that has not stabilized because the patient can easily be monitored as an outpatient with frequent INR determinations.

The initial maintenance dosage requirements of a patient should not be considered absolute requirements. Careful follow-up and weekly monitoring of the INR is required during the first 4 weeks of therapy after discharge from the hospital (Fig. 17–5). A number of "outpatient" factors including changes in diet, exercise, clinical state, social habits, and compliance frequently alter maintenance-dose requirements. Once a stable therapeutic warfarin dose has been attained, the INR can be monitored less frequently (once monthly). In patients with cancer, sustaining a therapeutic INR may be more difficult and thus more frequent monitoring may be needed to achieve a low complication rate.[70]

A number of specific factors may contribute to a patient's unusual response to warfarin.[62,64,65] These include (1) inaccurate laboratory monitoring, (2) failure to use the INR system appropriately, (3) alterations in the anticoagulant response because of drug–drug or drug–disease interactions, (4) fluctuations in nutritional status and/or dietary vitamin K intake, (5) altered receptor site sensitivity to warfarin (e.g., hereditary resistance), (6) alterations in drug administration or patient compliance, and (7) abnormal product performance or use of products from various manufacturers.

A number of pharmacokinetic equations, computer-assisted programs, and Bayesian forecasting programs intended to predict warfarin maintenance-dose requirements have been evaluated.[64] These warfarin prediction methods may not be clinically applicable because of interpatient variability, differences between laboratory techniques, and use of a therapeutic PT ratio of 1.5 to 2.5, making further evaluations necessary.

A guideline-based consultation service that used specific practice guidelines (Antithrombotic Consensus Conference[18]) has been shown to be an effective method of decreasing major (from 13% to 4%) and minor (from 18% to 9%) bleeding episodes in

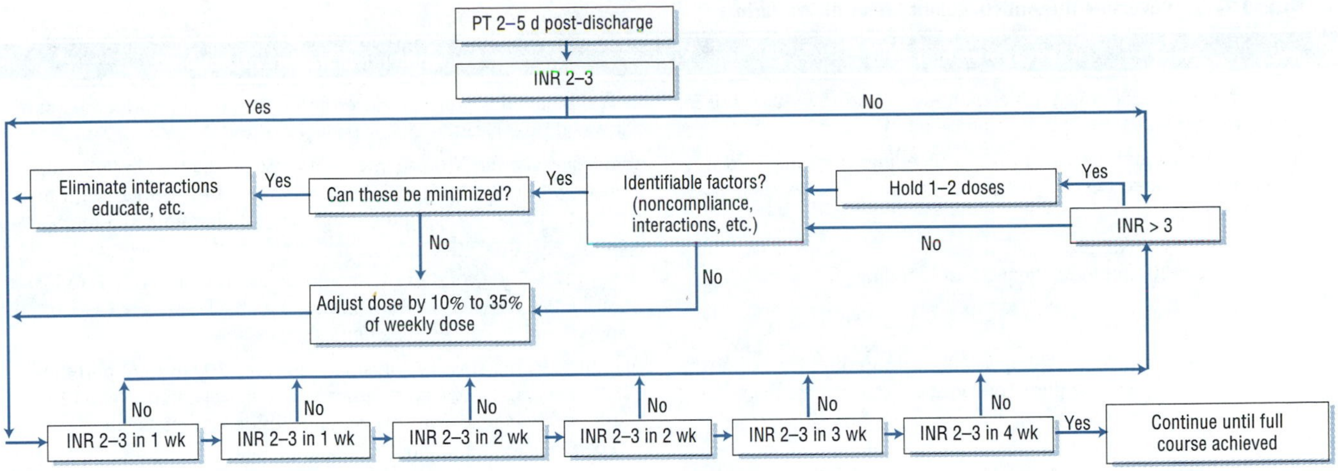

FIGURE 17–5. Algorithm for management of long-term warfarin therapy after hospital discharge.

medium- to high-risk hospitalized patients receiving heparin and warfarin therapy.[71] This type of service, as well as pharmacy-managed warfarin-monitoring services for inpatient and outpatient therapy,[17,63,72] provides an excellent way of (1) introducing standard of care guidelines, (2) evaluating risks and benefits of therapy, (3) assessing alternative treatments, (4) providing dosing recommendations, (5) monitoring efficacy and safety of therapy, and (6) improving patient compliance.

The optimal duration of anticoagulation treatment after the first episode of PE or DVT has not been determined. Several randomized trials attempted to address this issue.[73] In patients without a continuing risk factor for thrombosis (e.g., surgical patients), a 4- to 6-week anticoagulation course may be as effective as a longer course of 3 to 6 months. Patients at high risk of recurrence (e.g., presence of continuing risk factors; idiopathic venous thrombosis, previous DVT, or malignancy) with a low bleeding risk should be on anticoagulation for up to 6 months. After a second episode of DVT or PE, indefinite anticoagulation therapy may be required based on dramatic reductions in recurrences compared to a 6-month course.[73,74]

Adverse Effects

As with heparin, the major toxic effect of warfarin is hemorrhage. Bleeding during anticoagulation does not always correlate with the INR; however, the risk of bleeding episodes increases when the INR is excessively elevated.[1,35,61,62] The overall frequency of hemorrhagic complications has ranged from 2.5% to 27%.[35,71] The frequency of fatal, major, and major plus minor bleeding during warfarin therapy has been estimated to be 0.6%, 3.0%, and 9.6%, respectively.[36] These frequencies are approximately five times the values expected in patients not receiving warfarin therapy.

Bleeding complications are increased with high-intensity anticoagulation (INR 2.5 to 4.5), during the first year of therapy (highest in the first month), and increased by the presence of risk factors. These risk factors include age greater than 65 years (controversial), past GI bleeding, indication for therapy, history of stroke, deviation of the prothrombin time, and comorbid diseases (treated hypertension, ischemic cerebral vascular disease, serious heart disease, renal insufficiency, liver disease, and alcoholism).[35,36] Treatment of bleeding in patients on warfarin depends on (1) the clinical severity of bleeding, including the rate of hemorrhage and the location; (2) the extent to which the INR is prolonged; (3) the expected duration of anticoagulant therapy; and (4) the initial indication for anticoagulation.

Table 17–9 outlines the recent guidelines for reversing the anticoagulant effect of warfarin according to the INR and the clinical situation (e.g., presence of bleeding).[67] Minor bleeding episodes with a prolonged INR may merely require interruption of warfarin therapy until the INR has returned to the therapeutic range. Major life-threatening bleeding requires discontinuation of therapy, immediate treatment with coagulation factors (e.g., fresh frozen plasma), and the administration of vitamin K (phytonadione) to correct the INR to normal. If the risk of hemorrhage outweighs the need for long-term anticoagulation with warfarin, vitamin K may be administered parenterally. Vitamin K administered orally, subcutaneously, or via slow intravenous infusion will usually reverse the effects of warfarin in 6 to 12 hours. The appropriate dose and/or route of administration of vitamin K remains controversial. However, intramuscular administration of vitamin K should be avoided because of the risk of hematoma formation. Patients who will be resumed on warfarin therapy should receive lower doses of vitamin K (less than 1 mg) to avoid full normalization of the INR and subsequent "warfarin resistance" that may occur with larger doses.

Warfarin-induced skin necrosis and purple-toe syndrome are rare side effects of warfarin.[5,38,62,63] Both side effects are unrelated to the intensity of anticoagulation and may be the result of protein C deficiency or a direct toxic effect. The most commonly involved sites of warfarin-induced skin necrosis are the thigh, breast, and buttocks. It usually occurs within the first 10 days of therapy, and women are more likely to experience this effect than men. Of 57 reported cases of warfarin-induced skin necrosis, seven patients have resumed therapy without adverse effects. If the clinical condition absolutely requires prolonged anticoagulation, then resume with intravenous heparin and small doses of warfarin (2 to 5 mg/day).[75]

Purple-toe syndrome usually occurs 3 to 8 weeks after warfarin is begun and causes pain in the toe; the color blanches with pressure and fades with elevation.[38] It is recommended that warfarin be discontinued for this adverse reaction; however, discoloration may persist for weeks to months.

Anticoagulants During Pregnancy

Table 17–10 outlines the most recent recommendations for the use of antithrombotic agents during pregnancy.[21] Anticoagulants are indicated for the prevention and treatment of venous thromboembolism, the prevention of systemic embolism associated with valvular heart disease or prosthetic valves, and in pregnant women with antiphospholipid antibodies (APLA). There is a lack of prospective, randomized trials that have included pregnant women.

TABLE 17–9. Reversing the Anticoagulant Effect of Warfarin

Clinical Situation	Recommended Treatment Action
INR > 3 but < 6, patient is not bleeding, and rapid reversal is not indicated for reasons of surgical intervention	Omit the next few warfarin doses and resume warfarin therapy at a lower dose when the INR is between 2 and 3.
INR ≥ 6 but < 10 and the patient is not bleeding, or more rapid reversal is required because the patient requires elective surgery	Administer vitamin K 0.5–1 mg, oral or SC; reduction in INR will occur within 8 h; INR may be in the range of 2–3 in 24 h. If the INR at 24 h is still high, a second dose of vitamin K 0.5 mg SC can be given. Warfarin can then be restarted at a lower dose.
INR ≥ 10 but < 20 and the patient is not bleeding	Vitamin K 3–5 mg, oral or SC should be given with the INR reduced substantially at 6 h. The INR should be checked every 6–12 h, and vitamin K can be repeated as necessary.
Major warfarin overdose (e.g., INR > 20) or a rapid reversal of an anticoagulant effect is required because of serious bleeding	Vitamin K 10 mg slow IV infusion (e.g., over 20–30 min) and the INR checked every 6 h. Vitamin K may be repeated every 12 h and supplemented with plasma transfusion or factor concentrate depending on the urgency of the situation.
Life-threatening bleeding or serious warfarin overdose	Replacement with factor concentrates as indicated supplemented with vitamin K 10 mg slow IV infusion (e.g., over 20–30 min). Vitamin K may be repeated as necessary depending on the INR.

Adapted from Ref. 67, with permission.

Heparin is currently the anticoagulant of choice in pregnant females (FDA Pregnancy Category C) because it does not cross the placenta and does not cause fetal complications.[1,5,19,21] Maternal effects of anticoagulation include hemorrhage and osteoporosis. Hemorrhage is a possible adverse effect of treatment with heparin, and it must be used judiciously with careful monitoring. Long-term use of high doses of heparin (20,000 U/day for greater than 5 months) during pregnancy has been associated with maternal osteoporosis. Heparin associated thrombocytopenia may also occur.

Warfarin should be avoided in pregnant patients (FDA Pregnancy Category X) because it crosses the placenta and causes fetal malformation at *any* time during pregnancy.[1,21,62] During the sixth and twelfth weeks of pregnancy, "warfarin embryopathy" may occur, which is associated with skeletal abnormalities. Exposure during any trimester carries the risk of central nervous system abnormalities. Fetal cerebral hemorrhage may occur owing to the greater anticoagulation effect observed in the fetus compared to the mother. This is a result of the diminished production of vitamin K-dependent clotting factors by the immature liver and inability of maternal procoagulants to cross the placental barrier. All women of childbearing age should be counseled to use contraceptive methods to avoid becoming pregnant while on warfarin therapy. If the mother's condition requires anticoagulation, heparin should be used from at least the start of the sixth gestational week and until the end of the twelfth gestational week, and again at term to lessen the risks to the fetus.

TABLE 17–10. Recommendation of Antithrombotic Agents During Pregnancy

Condition	Recommendation
Previous venous thrombosis or pulmonary embolism prior to current pregnancy	Heparin 5000 U SC q12h throughout pregnancy, then 4–6 wk of postpartum warfarin or clinical surveillance combined with periodic IPG **or** CUS followed by 4–6 wk of postpartum warfarin
Venous thrombosis or pulmonary embolism during current pregnancy	Heparin in full IV doses for 5–10 days, followed by q12h SC injection to prolong 6-h postinjection APTT to 1.5 times control until delivery. Warfarin can then be used postpartum
Planning pregnancy in patients requiring long-term anticoagulation	Either heparin q12h SC to prolong 6-h postinjection APTT to 1.5 times control, **or** Frequent pregnancy tests and substitute heparin (as above) for warfarin when pregnancy achieved
Mechanical prosthetic heart valves	Either heparin q12h SC to prolong 6-h postinjection APTT to 1.5 times control, **or** Adjusted-dose SC heparin until the 13th week, warfarin (INR 2.5–3.0) until the middle of the third trimester, then adjusted-dose SC heparin until delivery
APLA and >1 previous pregnancy loss	Either aspirin plus prednisone, **or** aspirin plus heparin, **or** aspirin
APLA and 0 or 1 previous pregnancy loss	Low-dose aspirin during the second and third trimester
APLA and previous venous thrombosis	Heparin q12h SC to prolong 6-h postinjection APTT to 1.5–2.5 times control
APLA without previous venous thrombosis	Either clinical surveillance combined with IPG or CUS, **or** heparin 5000 U q12h throughout pregnancy

APLA = antiphospholipid antibodies; IPG = impedance plethysmography; CUS = compression ultrasonography.
Adapted from Ref. 21, with permission.

During lactation, heparin is not secreted in breast milk and can be safely administered to nursing mothers. Warfarin has not been detected in breast milk and has not produced an anticoagulant effect in infants; however, further studies are needed before routine use of warfarin during lactation is recommended.

Low-molecular-weight heparin (LMWH) appear to be a safe alternative to unfractionated heparin for obstetric thromboprophylaxis since LMWHs do not cross the placenta.[21] As well, only once-daily subcutaneous administration is required. Clinical experience remains limited to a small number of pregnant patients. In these small studies LMWH appear effective; however, the optimal dosage, safety profile, and bone demineralization effects require further investigation.

Food and Drug–Drug Interactions

There are more food and drug–drug interactions reported with warfarin than for any other drug.[61–63] Current use of warfarin with alcohol and prescription or over-the-counter medications must routinely be considered as a cause of increased or decreased anticoagulant effect. Mechanisms responsible for these interactions involve (1) altered vitamin K availability, (2) reduced warfarin absorption, (3) changes in warfarin protein binding, (4) effects on warfarin's metabolism, (5) changes in receptor affinity for warfarin, (6) reduction in vitamin K-dependent clotting factor levels, and (7) independent effect on hemostatic metabolism. The clinician must be aware of the high probability of drug–drug and drug–food interactions.[61–63,76] Each patient's response needs to be closely monitored and additional INR determinations may be indicated whenever other medications are initiated or discontinued or when an alternation in consumption of vitamin K-containing foods (brussel sprouts, broccoli, cabbage, lettuce, spinach, chick peas, turnip greens) is noted.[76]

Patient Education

Safe and efficient warfarin therapy requires careful patient selection, cooperation of the patient, and patient education. Areas that need to be included in patient education are outlined in Table 17–11. It is also important that patients inform other health care professionals (physician, dentist, nurse) that they are taking warfarin. It may be useful for patients to carry an identification card or a MEDALERT bracelet stating that they are receiving warfarin. Providing a calendar to the patient will assist the patient in documenting the prescribed dosing schedule, which can sometimes be complicated. The calendar can also serve as a compliance aid to minimize missed doses and double dosing when the patient cannot remember if the dose was taken.

THROMBOLYTIC THERAPY

The principal aim of thrombolytic therapy in the treatment of acute PE and DVT is to restore circulation through a previously occluded vessel by the rapid and complete removal of a pathologic intraluminal thrombus or embolus that has not been dissolved by the endogenous fibrinolytic system.[18,77–79] The potential benefits of thrombolytic therapy for the treatment of PE include prompt dissolution of physiologically compromising pulmonary emboli, faster recovery, prevention of recurrent thrombus formation, and rapid restoration of hemodynamic disturbances.[18,77,79–82] For DVT, lysis of thrombus can prevent PE and permanent pathologic changes such as venous valvular dysfunction and postphlebitic syndrome.[18,77,78,83,84] However, thrombolytic agents have not been generally accepted as a standard form of therapy for DVT or PE because of the possible bleeding complications, the lack of mortality differences and adequate long-term follow-up among studies performed, the amount of patient monitoring required once therapy is initiated, and the substantial cost of these agents.

Currently, four thrombolytic agents are available: streptokinase (SK), urokinase (UK), recombinant alteplase (rt-PA, recombinant human tissue-type plasminogen activator), and acylated plasminogen streptokinase activator complex (APSAC).[18,77,81,85] All thrombolytics are plasminogen activators and act either directly (UK, rt-PA) or indirectly (SK, APSAC) (Fig. 17–6). Plasminogen, an inactive proteolytic enzyme, is converted to plasmin, which has the ability to lyse fibrin, as well as to hydrolyze fibrinogen and other coagulation factors, leading to a systemic lytic state. The agents differ with respect to their mechanism of plasminogen activation, their specificity for fibrin, their half-lives, source, and cost (Table 17–12).

Streptokinase is a nonenzymatic protein derived from strains of β-hemolytic streptococci. It is an indirect plasminogen activator in that it must first form a complex with plasminogen, which then converts other plasminogen molecules to be activated to plasmin. Because streptokinase is a bacterial protein, it is antigenic and can lead to the production of antibodies as well as allergic reactions. Antibodies from previous streptococcus or streptokinase exposure can bind to streptokinase, rendering it biologically inactive. Part of the rationale for using a loading dose is to overcome the antibody binding and still achieve some therapeutic activity.

Urokinase is a direct plasminogen activator isolated from human fetal kidney cells grown in culture. The advantage of this agent is that it is nonantigenic; however, it is considerably more expensive than streptokinase, which limits its use. Neither urokinase nor streptokinase is specific for thrombi, making either agent prone to lysing any fresh platelet–fibrin hemostatic plug, which is

TABLE 17–11. Information for the Patient on Warfarin

1. *Need for strict compliance.* The importance of taking warfarin and other medications as directed and of following instructions regarding INR and follow-up office visits must be stressed.
2. *Side effects.* The sites and signs of bleeding as well as instructions on when and where to call if bleeding occurs should be reviewed.
3. *Dietary instruction.* The patient should be told that no major dietary restrictions are necessary; however, no abrupt changes in dietary habits should be made. Rarely, diets with excessive quantities of vitamin K have interfered with warfarin therapy.
4. *Frequent INR.* The patient needs to be aware of the required monitoring of INR and why this is necessary. Some patients question the need for continued monitoring of warfarin, and this issue is best addressed early in the course of treatment.
5. *Drug interactions.* The patient should be informed that other drugs can greatly influence the effect of warfarin and should be told not to start or stop medications without first asking the physician. It may be useful to make specific recommendations regarding the use of common nonprescription drugs (e.g., antacids, analgesics, and cold products).
6. *Physical activity instructions:* Limitations on physical activities (e.g., contact sports) should be reviewed.
7. *Pregnancy avoidance:* The risks of warfarin during conception and the first trimester of pregnancy should be discussed. Alternatives should be presented to those patients who want to conceive. Methods of contraception should be reviewed with female patients.

Adapted from Ref. 106, with permission.

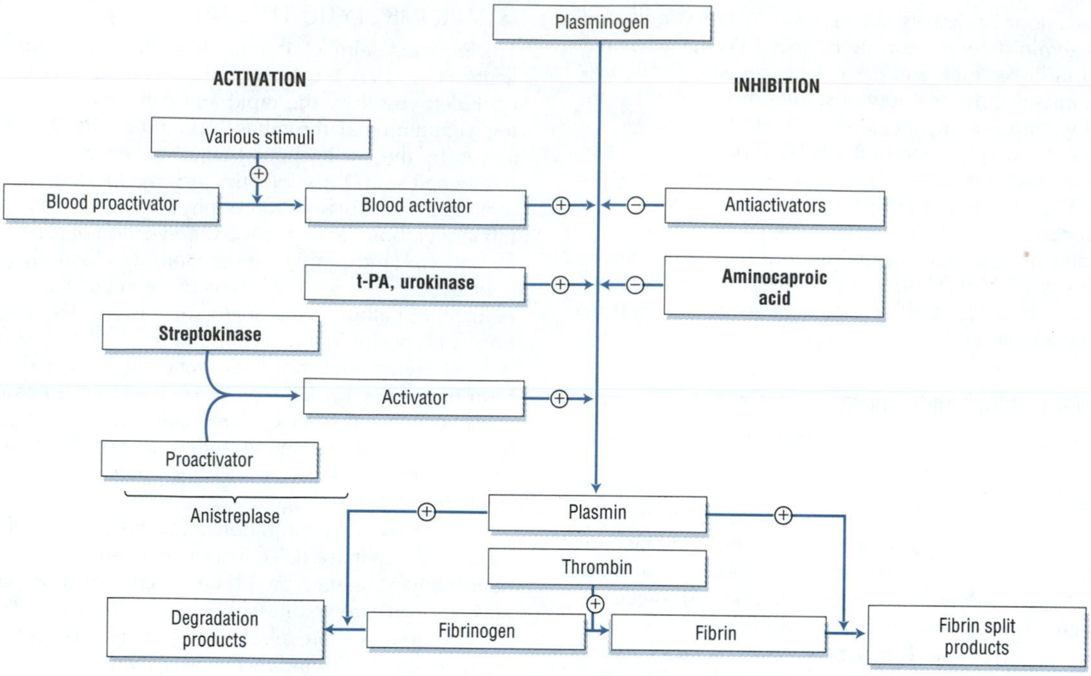

FIGURE 17–6. Fibrinolysis during thrombolytic therapy. Urokinase and streptokinase activate the fibrinolytic system and convert plasminogen to the active enzyme plasmin, which then lyses a fresh fibrin clot.

thought to be responsible for the observed hemorrhagic complications. However, bleeding complications are associated with fibrin-specific and nonspecific thrombolytic agents.

Alteplase (rt-PA) is a recombinant, second-generation thrombolytic agent that has relative fibrin specificity and is a direct activator of plasminogen. It is described as being more fibrin specific in that it activates plasminogen associated with thrombi or hemostatic plugs in preference to circulating plasminogen. It seems that systemic activation of the fibrinolytic system may be dependent on the dose and rate of administration of rt-PA. However, there is no evidence to date that this agent is associated with a lower incidence of bleeding.[18,80,85]

TABLE 17–12. Properties of Thrombolytic Agents

	Streptokinase	Urokinase	rt-PA	APSAC
Source	Streptococcal culture	Heterologous mammalian tissue culture	Heterologous mammalian tissue culture	Streptococcal culture
Molecular weight	47,000	32,000–54,000	70,000	131,000
Type of agent	Bacterial proactivator	Tissue plasminogen activator	Tissue plasminogen activator	Bacterial proactivator
Plasma half-life (min)	12–18	15–20	2–6	40–60
Fibrinolytic activation	Systemic	Systemic	Systemic	Systemic
Antigenic	Yes	No	No	Yes
Cost[a]	$804–2260[b]	$5231[c]	$2641[d]	$2234[e]
Loading dose	250,000 U over 30 min	4400 U/kg over 30 min	100 mg over 2 h	[f]
Maintenance dose	100,000 U/h	4400 U/kg/h	None	[f]
Duration of therapy	12–48 h for PE 24–72 h for DVT	12–48 h for PE 24–72 h for DVT	None	[f]

[a]Represents drug cost to the pharmacy, not actual cost to the patient.
[b]Based on a dosage of 250,000 U (bolus) and an infusion of 100,000 U/h for 24 h.
[c]Based on a dosage for a 154-lb patient, bolus of 4400 U/kg and an infusion of 4400 U/kg/h for 12 h.
[d]Based on 100-mg dose.
[e]A 30-unit dose.
[f]No approved dosage regimen for PE or DVT.
Adapted from Ref. 107, with permission.

APSAC is an equimolar complex of streptokinase and plasminogen, which can be given as an intravenous bolus injection. It is chemically inert and relies on deacylation under physiologic conditions to become active. This agent has mainly been used for the treatment of evolving acute myocardial infarction.

Therapeutic Indications

Streptokinase is FDA approved for the treatment of acute PE and DVT; urokinase and rt-PA are FDA approved for the treatment of acute PE. All of the agents are approved for use in acute myocardial infarction. Although these agents have been investigated in numerous other thromboembolic disorders including arterial occlusions, the lack of randomized, control trials does not permit any conclusions to be drawn, and therefore no clinical recommendation can be made.[86]

The proposed indications for the use of thrombolytic therapy in patients with thromboembolic disease include massive/submassive PE with hemodynamic compromise, massive PE without hemodynamic compromise, submassive PE in patients who cannot tolerate further cardiopulmonary compromise, heparin treatment failures, and extensive proximal DVT. At present, thrombolytic agents offer the greatest benefit to PE patients suffering from acute decompensation with hypotension and low cardiac output; their role in patients with less severe episodes remains to be defined.[18,80]

Guidelines for selection of patients for systemic thrombolytic therapy should be based on the presence of clinical indications. This should include a documented diagnosis of thromboembolism and evidence that the thrombus is of recent origin (within the last 7 days). Recent origin of thrombus seems particularly important in the treatment of DVT. However, Goldhaber[79] suggests that effective thrombolytic therapy can be administered up to 14 days after the signs and symptoms of PE commence.

The selection of patients must also include the absence of contraindications for the use in thrombolytic therapy. Relative contraindications and precautions for the use of thrombolytic agents are summarized in Table 17–13.

TABLE 17–13. Contraindications to Thrombolytic Therapy

Major Contraindications
Recent surgery/internal organ biopsy (7–10 days)
Cerebrovascular vascular process or neurosurgical procedure (within prior 2 months)
Recent needle puncture of noncompressible vessels (i.e., jugular/subclavian, aorta, femoral vessel)
Active bleeding: gastrointestinal or genitourinary
Uncontrolled hypertension
Intracranial malignancy
Pregnancy
Recent trauma with possibility of internal injury
CPR with rib fractures
Minor Contraindications
Paracentesis
Thoracentesis (repeated attempts are a major contraindication)
Prolonged cardiopulmonary resuscitation (CPR)
Septic thrombophlebitis (with appropriate antimicrobial therapy)
Other conditions deemed potential bleeding risks

From Ref. 77, with permission.

Clinical Efficacy

A rapid decline in the signs and symptoms of DVT and a reduced risk of PE have been demonstrated with successful resolution of the thrombus. Streptokinase achieves thrombolysis 3.7 times more often than does heparin therapy in patients being treated for DVT.[78,83,84] Pooled results of short-term venographic studies suggest that either substantial or partial improvement occurs in 61% of streptokinase-treated patients compared to only 25% of heparin-treated patients. In studies with long-term evaluation of DVT, streptokinase resulted in normal venographic evaluations (57% vs 7%), less chronic postthrombotic changes (43% vs 93%), and less clinically symptomatic patients (19% vs 75%) than heparin therapy. However, not all studies with long-term follow-up have demonstrated these results favoring thrombolytic therapy. Urokinase and rt-PA have also been reported to have results similar to streptokinase in the treatment of DVT.[18,78,84]

It is suggested that thrombolytic therapy may be associated with a reduction in the incidence of the postphlebitic syndrome, particularly if treatment is given soon after the development of symptoms.[79,83,84,87] Successful clot resolution on venogram has been reported to occur in more than 65% of patients treated within 5 days of symptom onset, compared to 33% if treatment is initiated between 6 and 9 days and 0% if after 9 days.[78] In addition, predictive factors that appear to influence the effectiveness of streptokinase in patients treated for DVT include the following: (1) nonocclusive clots are more easily lysed than occlusive clots; (2) among nonocclusive clots, proximal are more easily lysed than popliteal; and (3) long-term venous sequelae later than 2 years after therapy occur less frequently when a normal phlebogram (compared residual occlusion) is observed at time of discharge.[87]

Successful resolution of pulmonary thromboemboli occurs in about 80% to 90% of patients with massive and submassive PE. In controlled trials of patient with angiographically confirmed PE, urokinase and streptokinase, compared with heparin, produced (1) greater resolution of pulmonary emboli, (2) greater improvement of the abnormal hemodynamic status of the right heart and pulmonary circulation, (3) greater reperfusion of the original pulmonary perfusion defects, and (4) maximal clot resolution and general improvement in patients with the largest pulmonary emboli.[18,79] However, in these studies there was no difference in the mortality rate among patients given heparin compared with those given thrombolytic therapy, and the incidence of bleeding complications was nearly double for those who received thrombolytic therapy.

Several clinical studies have established the role of rt-PA in the treatment of PE.[18,79,80,84] Short-term hemodynamic and angiographic improvements have been demonstrated to occur more often with rt-PA and urokinase than with heparin therapy. Major bleeding complications, including intracranial bleeding, occur more frequently with thrombolytic therapy.

Drug Administration

Safe and effective administration of thrombolytic agents is best accomplished with continuous intravenous infusion in a precise manner. The commonly recommended dosage schedules were derived from the large clinical trials for the treatment of PE and DVT.[18,77,78,80,81]

For streptokinase, the initial loading dose of 250,000 units in normal saline or 5% dextrose in water is administered over 30 minutes. Maintenance therapy consists of 100,000 U/h for 24 to 72 hours. For PE, results from the major studies favor 24 hours of administration. Infusions for DVT have been continued for up to 120 hours, but have not demonstrated additional benefit when continued beyond 72 hours. Intravenous administration of a bolus followed by intravenous infusion results in a systemic lytic state (decreased fibrinogen and increased fibrin degradation products) in more than 90% of patients.

Urokinase is given in a loading dose of 4400 U/kg of body weight in normal saline over 10 minutes. Maintenance therapy consists of 4400 U/kg/h for a total of 12 hours for PE. The total volume of fluid administered should not exceed 200 mL. In one study the drug was administered for 24 hours, but no additional benefit was demonstrated after 12 hours.[18]

The approved dose of rt-PA for treatment of PE is 100 mg administered by intravenous infusion over 2 hours. Other studies have been conducted that employed lower doses and/or shorter infusion rates of rt-PA and urokinase in the treatment of PE.[18,79] Although these alternative delivery modalities are more convenient to administer and potentially less expensive, the frequency of therapeutic efficacy and bleeding complications has not changed compared to traditional dosing recommendations.

Thrombolytic therapy should not be considered a substitute for anticoagulant therapy. Once thrombolytic therapy is discontinued and the thrombin time or APTT has fallen to less than twice the normal values (usually in 2 to 4 hours), continuous intravenous heparin should be started followed by oral warfarin therapy.

Laboratory Monitoring/Treatment Guidelines

Laboratory monitoring of thrombolytic therapy is used simply to determine whether some degree of systemic fibrinolysis has been achieved.[18,88] As long as some degree of lysis is established, vigorous dissolution of clots can be expected, provided that the fibrin clots are fresh. Simple but adequate laboratory monitoring for safe and effective administration of thrombolytic therapy has more recently been recommended.

Thrombin time or APTT can be used. Whatever test is selected, it should be performed prior to the administration of thrombolytic therapy and 3 to 4 hours after the initiation of thrombolytic treatment. As long as the test values during thrombolytic infusion are prolonged beyond the control value, it can be assumed that a systemic lytic state has been established.[18,88]

The following treatment guidelines should be established to minimize local and major hemorrhage of patients receiving thrombolytic therapy: (1) minimize physical handing of patient; (2) minimize invasive procedures, including needle punctures and parenteral (subcutaneous or intramuscular) drug administration; (3) apply compression bandages at puncture sites; and (4) avoid concurrent anticoagulation therapy or use of platelet-active drugs (aspirin-containing products, antiplatelet agents).

Adverse Effects

Hemorrhage, allergy, and fever are the three major types of adverse reactions that have been reported with thrombolytic agents.[77,78,89] The most disturbing and common side effect is bleeding, causing thrombolytic therapy to be discontinued in 5% to 25% of patients. Thrombolytic therapy is associated with a 6% to 30% frequency of major bleeding complications in patients treated for DVT, and approximately 20% for patients being treated for PE. The relative risk of major bleeding during thrombolytic therapy is approximately threefold higher than with heparin therapy.

A literature review of the most recent trials with rt-PA therapy for the treatment of PE estimated the incidence of major hemorrhage as 8.4%, with fatal hemorrhage occurring at 2.2%.[80] The incidence of intracranial bleeding in 559 patients treated with rt-PA was 2.1%. This incidence was greater than seen with rt-PA in patients treated for acute myocardial infarction (0.5%) or with heparin in patients treated for DVT (0.2%).[80,89]

Minor bleeding or oozing at cutaneous puncture sites can be controlled locally with pressure dressings. In cases of serious bleeding, thrombolytic therapy should be quickly discontinued. Because of the very short half-life of these agents, the lytic activity stops promptly. If blood replacement is indicated, whole blood or blood products (packed red cells, fresh-frozen plasma, or cryoprecipitate) may be given and should rapidly reverse the hemostatic alterations. In situations where bleeding unresponsive to blood replacement therapy must be rapidly corrected, ε-aminocaproic acid (EACA) may be administered in 5-g doses.

A decision analysis evaluated the preference of patients based on possible outcomes (postphlebitic syndrome, PE, major bleeding, death) in choosing therapy of streptokinase plus heparin or heparin therapy alone for the treatment of DVT.[90] The preferred choice of all patients evaluated (n = 36) was heparin alone. Patients did not feel that the avoidance of the postphlebitic syndrome with thrombolytic therapy was worth the risk of death. This study emphasizes the need to consider the patient's preference in addition to the risks and benefits of thrombolytic therapy.

Allergic or hypersensitivity reactions associated with streptokinase include urticaria, itching, flushing, nausea, headache, and transient elevation or decrease of systolic blood pressure. Anaphylaxis (1.3% to 2.5%) has ranged in severity from minor breathing difficulties to bronchospasm, periorbital swelling, or angioneurotic edema. Although urokinase and rt-PA are considered to be nonantigenic, relatively mild allergic reactions have been reported (0.9% to 4.5%).

With streptokinase, the frequency of temperature increase greater than 1.5°F is 30%, but only 3.5% of patients have temperatures greater than 104°F. Fever, which is more common with streptokinase therapy, can also occur with the administration of rt-PA and urokinase (15%). Both allergic and febrile reactions may be treated with antihistamines at the time of detection, and acetaminophen is very effective for treating temperature increases. Corticosteroids have also been used for the prophylaxis of these adverse reactions.

Hypotension (10% to 20%) can occur with rapid infusions of streptokinase. Hypotensive reactions have also been reported for high-dose intravenous infusions of urokinase (14% to 24%) and rt-PA (10% to 16%). The hypotension can often be prevented by slowing the rate of administration.

Thrombocytopenia has been reported in approximately 10% of patients receiving rt-PA, and therapy should be discontinued if the platelet counts fall below 75,000/mm^3.

SURGICAL THERAPY

Surgical interventions are additional options usually reserved for situations in which anticoagulation and thrombolytic therapy have an absolute contraindication, cannot be safely administered, or have failed.[18] Surgical therapy for acute DVT remains controversial and thrombectomy is reserved for patients with severe limb ischemia (phlegmasia cerulea dolens).[3] Pulmonary embolectomy and venous interruption are the most common procedures considered for PE. The placement of percutaneous transvenous filters (Greenfield filter) and umbrellas (Mobin–Uddin) have replaced older surgical techniques to prevent recurrence of thromboembolism from the lower extremities. These procedures have replaced the use of caval ligation, a procedure indicated only for severe septic pelvic thrombophlebitis unresponsive to conventional therapy. In life-threatening situations, pulmonary embolectomy (Trendelenburg's procedure) can be considered; however, it is associated with an extremely high mortality rate.

PREVENTION OF VENOUS THROMBOEMBOLISM

The key to reducing the morbidity and mortality of venous thromboembolism is the prevention of DVT and subsequent PE.[3] The strategies for preventing DVT are aimed at preventing stasis as well as reversing coagulability changes that allow thrombi to form in patients at risk for developing venous thromboembolism. The choice of a particular prophylactic modality for each patient will depend on the degree of risk of developing thromboembolism and/or bleeding complications from therapy.

Several patient populations have been identified as being at risk for developing DVT or PE and were discussed earlier in this chapter. All medical and surgical patients admitted to the hospital should be evaluated for the presence of these risk factors. Among surgical patients, those having procedures that require general anesthesia for longer than 30 minutes, those having procedures that involve prolonged immobility, and those having procedures that involve injury or surgery to the lower extremities or pelvis have the highest risk of developing DVT or PE.[2,6] In addition, the period of risk of developing DVT for surgical patients appears to extend from the time of surgery for up to 30 days after surgery. Because the risk for developing DVT or PE is longer than the immediate postoperative period, some patients may require prolonged prophylaxis after hospital discharge.

A task force of leading experts is currently evaluating the issue of which patients may require prolonged prophylaxis after hospital discharge in addition to the length of therapy they should receive. One study has evaluated the duration of prophylaxis in patients undergoing hip replacement surgery.[91] After receiving standard enoxaparin prophylaxis during hospitalization for the surgical procedure, patients were randomized to receive enoxaparin (40 mg daily) versus placebo as continued prophylaxis for a total of one month after surgery (n = 131 in each group). The incidence of all thromboembolic events was 18% in the enoxaparin groups and 39% in the placebo group ($P < .001$). In addition, the incidence of proximal vein thrombosis was also significantly less in the group who received prolonged enoxaparin prophylaxis. The authors concluded that prolonged prophylaxis significantly decreased the incidence of postoperative deep vein thrombosis. However, more studies are needed to definitively determine the appropriate length of prophylaxis.[3]

General prophylactic guidelines against DVT and PE in patients at risk have been developed through careful literature search and evaluation.[3,6] A consensus panel of the National Heart, Lung and Blood Institute and the NIH Office of Medical Application of Research concluded that none of the preventive measures are ideal but that most are relatively simple to use, the complications are generally minor, and the need for laboratory monitoring is minimal. The need for prophylaxis against DVT and PE in patients at risk is well recognized, and primary prophylaxis seems to be the most effective means of preventing death from venous thromboembolism. However, not all patients at risk receive the appropriate prophylaxis because of physician concerns regarding adverse effects (such as bleeding or heparin-induced thrombocytopenia) with therapeutic modalities, the misconception that the actual risk of venous thromboembolism may be low in their patient population, and the cost associated with prophylaxis. Therefore, clinicians should make the recognition of patients at high risk for developing thromboembolism a high priority as well as assuring that the appropriate prophylaxis is used for the appropriate length of time. Educational programs may be necessary to increase the awareness of the actual risk of venous thromboembolism in patients at risk in addition to which prophylactic measures have been found to be most effective.

The prophylactic guidelines (Table 17–14) have been developed based on the age of the patient, the underlying risk factors for the development of thromboembolism, underlying characteristics of the patient, and the type of surgery or indication for prophylaxis. In addition, any patient who is at high risk of developing thromboembolism should be monitored routinely for signs of DVT and/or PE through the use of careful clinical evaluation as well as objective tests such as impedance plethysmography or Doppler ultrasonography.

Because the pharmacologic agents used to prevent DVT and PE have potentially serious side effects, many studies have been performed evaluating nonpharmacologic methods to decrease stasis and subsequently thromboembolic disease without the added risk or cost of pharmacologic therapy. Some nonpharmacologic techniques include early ambulation, leg elevation, leg exercises, elastic compression or thromboembolic deterrent (TED) stockings, intermittent calf compression, electrical stimulation of calf muscles during surgery, and inferior vena cava (IVC) interruption. Because these methods do not increase the risk of bleeding, they are especially useful in patients at increased risk of bleeding from anticoagulation.

One of the best nonpharmacologic techniques for the prevention of DVT in the postoperative period is early ambulation. However, because this may not be feasible in every patient, other techniques have been employed. Standard elastic compression stockings (graduated compression stockings, GCS) are the simplest of prophylactic approaches behind early ambulation. They are relatively inexpensive, easy to use, and generally free of adverse effects. GCS have a graduated compression that is highest at the ankle and decreases as it approaches the thigh, thus increasing blood flow to the proximal vein (decreases stasis). The stockings should be placed on the patient before surgery and worn until the patient is fully ambulatory. In a recent meta-analysis, they have been shown to provide a clinically important risk reduction in the incidence of postoperative DVT in moderate-risk surgical patients, and may produce a decrease in the risk in the development of PE.[92] However,

TABLE 17–14. Guidelines for Prophylaxis of Thromboembolism

Type of Surgery/Indication	Recommended Prophylaxis
General Surgery	
Low risk (minor surgery, < 40 years old, no risk factors)	Early ambulation
Moderate risk (major surgery, > 40 years old, no additional risk factors)	GCS, LDUH (every 12 h), or IPC[a]
High risk (major surgery, > 40 years old, with additional risk factors)	LDUH (every 8 h) or LMWH
Above but prone to wound complications (hematoma)	IPC
Very high risk (above with multiple risk factors)	LDUH (every 8 h), LMWH, or dextran **with** IPC[b] Warfarin (INR 2.0–3.0) may be used in select patients
Total hip replacement	LMWH, low-intensity warfarin (INR 2.0–3.0), or ADUH; GCS or IPC may be additive[c]
Hip fracture surgery	LMWH or low-intensity warfarin (INR 2.0–3.0); IPC may be additive[d]
Total knee replacement	LMWH or IPC[e]
Multiple trauma patients (especially patients with hip and lower extremity fractures)	IPC, warfarin, or LMWH
High-risk orthopedic and multiple-trauma patients, other prophylaxis contraindicated	IVC filter
Neurosurgery-intracranial	IPC and/or GCS; LDUH (alternative); LDUH and IPC may be additive in high-risk patients
Acute spinal cord injury with paralysis[f]	ADUH or LMWH; warfarin (alternative) GCS or IPC may be additive
Myocardial infarction	LDUH or full-dose heparin; IPC and/or GCS useful if heparin contraindicated
Ischemic stroke with lower extremity paralysis	LDUH or LMWH; IPC and GCS also effective
General medicine patients with VTE risk factors	LDUH or LMWH
Long-term indwelling central venous catheters	Warfarin 1 mg daily

[a]LDUH should be started 2 h preoperatively and given every 12 h postoperatively. GCS and IPC should be applied during surgery, if possible, and throughout the postoperative period.
[b]LDUH and LMWH should be started preoperatively; dextran should be started intraoperatively; IPC should be applied intraoperatively.
[c]LMWH should begin postoperatively; warfarin should be started preoperatively or immediately postoperatively; ADUH should be started postoperatively. Duration of prophylaxis is **at least** 7–10 d postoperatively regardless of the duration of hospital stay; risk may be as long as 2 months.
[d]LMWH should be started preoperatively.
[e]LMWH should be started postoperatively; IPC should be started intraoperatively or immediately postoperatively and should be worn continuously except during ambulation.
[f]Greatest risk is during the first 2 wk after injury; prophylaxis should be continued for a minimum of 3 months in patients unable to ambulate.
GCS = graduated compression stockings; LDUH = low-dose unfractionated heparin at a dose of 5000 units; IPC = intermittent pneumatic compression; LMWH = low-molecular-weight heparin; ADUH = adjusted-dose unfractionated heparin; IVC = inferior vena cava; VTE = venous thromboembolism.

GCS should not be used as sole prophylaxis in high-risk patients. If used, they must be properly fitted to achieve the greatest benefit of reducing stasis in the legs; however, 15% to 20% of patients cannot wear these stockings because of unusual leg shape or size.[6]

Intermittent pneumatic leg compression (IPC) employs an inflatable cuff to the ankles, calves, and/or thighs of the patient to increase venous flow to the proximal femoral vein. This technique prevents stasis by periodically emptying the deep veins of the legs as well as activating the fibrinolytic system. This method is usually initiated at the time of surgery and is continued throughout the entire period of immobilization; the cuff should be worn continually for best results because fibrinolytic activity declines rapidly once the device has been removed. IPC is effective in reducing the incidence of DVT in moderate-risk general surgery patients, in patients undergoing neurosurgical procedures, in multiple-trauma patients, and in patients who have had a myocardial infarction or ischemic stroke.[6] IPC devices are a cost-effective approach with no risk of hemorrhage, and when combined with GCS or pharmacologic modalities may prove more effective in some patients. However, IPC devices are somewhat cumbersome and inconvenient to use and cannot be used in patients with lower extremity fractures or trauma.

Electrical stimulation of the calf muscles is occasionally employed as a prophylactic measure used primarily during the surgical procedure. It is used to induce muscle contractions and subsequently enhance venous blood return. The overall use of this method of prophylaxis is limited owing to poor patient acceptance because of discomfort associated with its use.

Inferior vena cava interruption, such as with a Greenfield filter, is useful in patients in whom the use of anticoagulant therapy is contraindicated or a complication to anticoagulant therapy is present; in patients at high risk for proximal vein thrombosis of the lower extremity; in patients who experience recurrent thromboembolism despite adequate anticoagulation; and in patients with chronic recurrent embolism.[18] It is important to note that the IVC filter does not prevent the formation of DVT but is used to prevent PE from a DVT. IVC filters cannot be used in up to 33% of trauma patients due to the presence of lower extremity fractures, casts, or bandages. In patients who receive a filter secondary to anticoagulant treatment failure, anticoagulant therapy with heparin followed by warfarin should continue to prevent recurrence or extension of the thrombus in the leg, as well as thrombosis of the filter.

Pharmacologic approaches for the prophylaxis against DVT include low-dose unfractionated heparin (LDUH), adjusted-dose unfractionated heparin (ADUH), warfarin, low-molecular-weight heparins (LMWH), and dextran.[18] In general, prophylaxis has conclusively been shown to decrease the risk of venous thromboembolism with an acceptably low risk of bleeding. Platelet inhibitors such as aspirin only affect thrombus formation that is dependent on prostaglandins such as thromboxane A_2. When compared to other forms of prophylaxis, aspirin has limited efficacy in preventing venous thromboembolism in general surgery patients, patients undergoing total hip or knee replacement surgery, patients undergoing hip fracture surgery, and patients with acute spinal cord injury.[6]

The most widely applicable and carefully studied method of DVT prophylaxis is LDUH.[6] A less intense anticoagulant effect is required for the prevention of venous thromboembolism than is required for the treatment of established thrombosis. Therefore, low doses of heparin given subcutaneously have been shown to be highly effective in reducing the incidence of postoperative DVT and fatal PE in general, abdominal, thoracic, urologic, gynecologic, and limited orthopedic surgery patients, as well as in bedridden patients after myocardial infarction and stroke, and in immobilized medical patients.[6] Low-dose unfractionated heparin also has the added advantage of not requiring any laboratory monitoring. A cost–benefit study of LDUH as prophylaxis against postoperative venous thromboembolism has shown it to be cost-effective by decreasing postoperative morbidity and mortality.[93] However, LDUH has been shown to be ineffective in preventing DVT in high-risk surgical patients (total hip or knee replacement, hip fracture surgery), so that other methods of prophylaxis such as ADUH, LMWH, or warfarin should be used.[6]

LDUH therapy involves the subcutaneous administration of 5000 units every 8 to 12 hours. When administered subcutaneously, the bioavailability is only 30%, and the anticoagulant effect is delayed for 1 to 2 hours.[37] In general, the "every 8 hours" schedule (15,000 U/d) is not more effective than the "every 12 hours" schedule, except for very high-risk general surgery patients as outlined in Table 17–14. In addition, the higher dose regimen may be associated with a slightly higher rate of bleeding episodes. Because of the delayed anticoagulant effect, the first dose of heparin should be administered 2 hours before the procedure and then every 8 to 12 hours thereafter for the duration of risk when used as prophylaxis for surgery patients.

ADUH has been shown to be effective in high-risk patients in whom LDUH is not effective or has limited effectiveness (hip replacement patients or patients with acute spinal cord injury).[6,37] The average daily heparin dose is 15,000 to 18,000 units, with the dose being administered subcutaneously every 12 hours. The heparin dose is adjusted to slightly prolong the APTT (APTT ratio 1.1 to 1.2).[37] For dosage adjustment, the APTT should be drawn 4 to 6 hours after the first dose and at the midpoint of the dosing interval thereafter. This regimen is limited by the need for careful and frequent laboratory monitoring.

Warfarin is an effective agent for the prophylaxis of venous thromboembolism in patients undergoing total hip replacement or hip fracture surgery; patients undergoing major gynecologic surgery; high-risk general surgery patients; patients with multiple trauma or acute spinal cord injury; or cancer patients with long-term indwelling central venous catheters.[6,61] It can be administered either as a fixed low dose of 1 to 2 mg daily (long-term central venous catheter) or an adjusted dose to slightly prolong the prothrombin time to an INR of 2.0 to 3.0 (general surgery, hip surgery, trauma). Both methods usually require preoperative treatment with repeated laboratory monitoring. It has been suggested that therapy may be initiated to prolong the INR to 1.5 at the time of surgery, and then increased postoperatively to achieve an INR of 2.0 to 3.0. Benefit of warfarin therapy has also been demonstrated when therapy is initiated on the first postoperative day. The risk of bleeding with low-intensity warfarin therapy is less than that observed with full anticoagulation, but hemorrhagic episodes still occur. Because of this risk and the fact that warfarin therapy is complicated to use requiring repeated laboratory monitoring, warfarin should be reserved for high-risk patients such as those undergoing major orthopedic procedures or those with a history of recurrent venous thrombosis.

Dextran is a partially hydrolyzed glucose polymer with a molecular weight of 40,000 to 70,000 Daltons. It works by impairing platelet function and decreasing their ability to aggregate.[6] Dextran is not as effective as other prophylactic modalities in the prevention of DVT after surgery, but it does appear to reduce the incidence of PE. The main use of dextran as a prophylactic agent appears to be in high-risk general surgery patients who cannot receive heparin owing to adverse effects or bleeding.[6] Use of dextran is also limited because it must be administered intravenously; it is relatively expensive; and it is associated with fluid overload, bleeding, and allergic reactions.

The pharmacologic and pharmacokinetic characteristics of LMWHs are listed in Table 17–5. The favorable properties of LMWHs over standard heparin include greater bioavailability after subcutaneous administration, less nonspecific protein binding, longer elimination half-life, possibly fewer adverse effects, and the lack of required routine laboratory monitoring, as mentioned earlier. Data from clinical trials have demonstrated the efficacy of LMWHs in terms of DVT prevention in high-risk general surgery patients, in patients undergoing elective hip or knee replacement, in patients undergoing elective hip fracture repair, in acute spinal cord injury patients with paralysis, in multiple trauma patients, in patients with ischemic stroke and lower limb paralysis, and in general medicine patients.[3,18,42,44,56] In addition, LMWHs have other potential uses and are being studied as prophylaxis against venous thromboembolism in patients with plaster cast immobilization of the legs, emergency abdominal surgery patients, cancer patients with long-term venous access devices (upper extremity); in addition to maintaining the late patency of peripheral arterial grafts, reduction of restenosis after interventional cardiologic procedures, and during maintenance hemodialysis as an anticoagulant.[3,18,42,44,56]

Each LMWH should be evaluated separately for a specific indication. Currently, there are three LMWH preparations as well as danaparoid with FDA-approved indications for prophylactic use in the United States (Table 17–15). Each of these agents is approved for use for different indications, and the doses and instructions for use are drug-specific.

THROMBOPROPHYLACTIC AGENTS

ENOXAPARIN

Enoxaparin (Lovenox, Rhone Poulenc Rorer) was the first LMWH to be approved in the United States, in 1993. It is currently FDA-approved for the prevention of DVT in patients undergoing hip or knee replacement surgery and the prevention of ischemic complications of unstable angina and non-Q-wave myocardial infarction.

Enoxaparin is derived from standard heparin by benzylation and alkaline depolymerization, and has an average molecular weight of 3500 to 5500 Daltons. Following subcutaneous administration, the bioavailability is 91% and is linear within the dosage range of 20 to 80 mg.[44] The time to maximal anti-Xa activity is 3 to 5 hours after subcutaneous injection, and the volume of distribution in healthy volunteers is approximately 7 L. Enoxaparin is excreted primarily as unchanged drug in the urine, mainly by glomerular filtration.[44] Following subcutaneous administration, the elimination half-life of enoxaparin is 4.5 hours, and may be prolonged as much as twofold in patients with renal failure.[44] Enoxaparin is classified as FDA Pregnancy Category B.

The major adverse effects associated with enoxaparin therapy include bleeding and thrombocytopenia. A decrease in the incidence of bleeding over unfractionated heparin has not been convincingly shown in clinical trials, and the incidence of bleeding appears to increase with increasing dose. Bleeding episodes may be partially controlled with protamine sulfate. The incidence of thrombocytopenia with enoxaparin therapy is less than 2%. Because of the risk of cross-reactivity between unfractionated heparin and LMWHs, enoxaparin should not be used in patients with documented heparin-induced thrombocytopenia without extensive *in vitro* evaluation to demonstrate if enoxaparin will also cause platelet aggregation. Other adverse effects of enoxaparin include urticaria, pain, local irritation or hematoma at the injection site, and elevated serum transaminases.

Numerous studies have evaluated enoxaparin for the prevention of DVT following orthopedic, general, gynecologic, urologic, and thoracic surgery.[14,44,56] Enoxaparin has

TABLE 17–15. Indications, Doses, Instructions for Use, and Availability of FDA-Approved LMWHs

LMWH	Indication	Dose	Instructions for Use	Availability and Cost
Enoxaparin	Prevention of DVT in patients undergoing hip or knee replacement surgery who are at risk for thromboembolic complications and the prevention of ischemic complications of unstable angina and non-Q-wave myocardial infarction	30 mg SC bid	First dose should be given as soon as possible after surgery but not more than 24 hours postop; duration is at least for 7–10 d	Prefilled single-use syringe: 30 mg—AWP $13.44 40 mg—AWP $17.92
Dalteparin	Prevention of DVT in patients requiring abdominal surgery who are at risk for thromboembolic complications	2500 anti-Xa units SC qd (5000 anti-Xa units in high-risk patients)	First dose should be given 1–2 h preop and then qd for 5 d postop	Prefilled single-use syringes: 2500 anti-Xa units—AWP $11.16 5000 anti-Xa units—AWP $18.97
Ardeparin	Prevention of DVT in patients undergoing knee replacement surgery who are at risk for thromboembolic complications	50 anti-Xa units/kg of actual weight SC bid	First dose should be given on the evening of the day of surgery and continued for 14 d or until the patient is fully ambulatory	Prefilled single-use syringes: 5000 anti-Xa units—AWP $12.36 10,000 anti-Xa units—AWP $19.60

been shown to significantly reduce the incidence of DVT in patients undergoing hip replacement or knee replacement surgery when compared to placebo, dextran, heparin, and warfarin.[18,44,56,94] A recent meta-analysis that evaluated methods to prevent venous thromboembolism following total hip replacement surgery demonstrated that LMWHs were superior to most other treatments and that only LMWH and graduated compression stockings reduced the risk of PE.[95] Overall, LMWH and warfarin were found to be equally effective and more effective than all other treatments in preventing proximal venous thrombosis in this subset of patients.[95] In terms of bleeding, enoxaparin has not been associated with a significant decrease in major bleeding, minor bleeding, or transfusion requirements when compared to unfractionated heparin or warfarin.

In conclusion, although enoxaparin is currently only FDA-approved for the prophylaxis of DVT in patients undergoing hip or knee replacement surgery, it appears to be effective prophylaxis for other surgical patients.

DALTEPARIN

Dalteparin (Fragmin, Pharmacia) was approved by the FDA in 1994 for the prevention of DVT in patients undergoing abdominal surgery who are at risk for thromboembolic complications.

Dalteparin is derived from standard heparin by nitrous acid depolymerization and has an average molecular weight of 4000 to 6000 daltons. After subcutaneous administration, dalteparin is almost completely absorbed, with a bioavailability of 87%.[96] Peak plasma anti-Xa activity occurs approximately 4 hours after a subcutaneous injection. The volume of distribution of dalteparin correlates with plasma volume and is 40 to 60 mL/kg in healthy volunteers.[96] Dalteparin is excreted primarily by the kidneys. Following subcutaneous administration, the elimination half-life of dalteparin is 2.4 to 4 hours. Patients with renal insufficiency may require dosage adjustment. Dalteparin is classified as FDA Pregnancy Category B.

The major adverse effects associated with dalteparin therapy include bleeding, thrombocytopenia, and hematoma and pain at the site of injection. A decrease in the incidence of major and minor bleeding complications has not been observed with dalteparin when compared to standard heparin therapy, and appears to be dose-related.[96] The bleeding effects may be reversed with the administration of protamine sulfate. The incidence of thrombocytopenia was less than 1% during clinical trials; however, the rate of cross-reactivity of LMWHs with heparin-induced antibodies precludes the use of dalteparin in a patient with HIT unless *in vitro* testing has determined that it is safe. Other adverse effects associated with dalteparin therapy include pain and hematoma formation at the site of injection, allergic reactions, skin necrosis, and elevated transaminases.

There have been numerous prospective, randomized, double-blind trials evaluating the safety and efficacy of various dosages of dalteparin with placebo or low-dose unfractionated heparin as thromboprophylaxis in patients undergoing general abdominal surgery.[18,56,96] In general, dalteparin has been found to be more effective at preventing DVT when compared to placebo and equal in efficacy when compared to standard heparin. Different dosage regimens of dalteparin (2500 units qd vs bid; 2500 units qd vs 5000 units qd) have been compared as DVT prophylaxis. In all studies, the higher daily dose of dalteparin was associated with a similar rate of efficacy than the lower daily dose, but was associated with a higher rate of bleeding (in some cases significantly).[96] Dalteparin has also been studied as thromboprophylaxis in orthopedic surgery patients, in patients with acute ischemic stroke and lower limb paralysis, and in general medicine patients; for the prevention of early restenosis after PTCA; in intracoronary stenting; and as an anticoagulant in hemodialysis patients.[96] In conclusion, when used at the appropriate doses, dalteparin is as safe and effective as LDUH as thromboprophylaxis in general surgery patients, but its role as thromboprophylaxis in patients undergoing other surgical procedures requires further study before routine use is recommended.

ARDEPARIN

Ardeparin (Normiflo, Wyeth-Ayerst) is a newly FDA-approved LMWH for the prevention of DVT potentially leading to PE in patients undergoing knee replacement surgery.

Ardeparin is derived from standard heparin by peroxidative depolymerization. It has a mean molecular weight of 5500 to 6500 Daltons. After subcutaneous administration, the bioavailability of ardeparin is 90%, and the time to maximal anti-Xa activity is approximately 3 hours.[97] The volume of distribution of ardeparin is 190 mL/kg after subcutaneous dosing.[97] Ardeparin is primarily excreted renally as unchanged drug; however, ardeparin clearance decreases as the dose increases, suggesting saturable elimination.[97] The elimination half-life of ardeparin is 3.5 hours with normal renal function and may be prolonged in patients with renal insufficiency. Ardeparin is classified as FDA Pregnancy Category C.

The major adverse effects associated with ardeparin therapy include bleeding, thrombocytopenia, and dermatologic effects. The incidence of bleeding complications with ardeparin in controlled clinical trials is approximately 5% and does not appear to be significantly less than that observed with heparin. Thrombocytopenia occurred in 2% of patients in early trials, and because of the risk of cross-reactivity, ardeparin should not be used in a patient with documented heparin-induced thrombocytopenia unless *in vitro* aggregation tests have determined it to be safe. Other adverse effects of ardeparin include pruritus and rash at the injection site, allergic reactions, and asymptomatic elevations in serum transaminases.

Ardeparin has been evaluated in only a limited number of comparative trials as prophylaxis against DVT in patients undergoing knee or hip replacement surgery.[18] For patients undergoing knee replacement surgery, ardeparin was associated with a nonsignificant decrease in the incidence of proximal vein thrombosis as well as the overall incidence of DVT when compared to adjusted-dose warfarin.[18] The incidence of bleeding was similar in both groups. When compared to adjusted-dose warfarin for the prevention of venous thrombosis in patients undergoing hip replacement surgery, ardeparin was as safe and effective as warfarin.[18] At this time, ardeparin has limited clinical applications. More well-controlled, comparative prophylaxis and treatment studies are needed to better define the role of ardeparin in the treatment or prophylaxis of thromboembolism.

DANAPAROID

Danaparoid (Orgaran) is a new anticoagulant that was approved by the FDA in December 1996 for the prophylaxis of postoperative DVT that may lead to PE in patients undergoing elective hip replacement. Danaparoid is a low-molecular-weight glycosaminoglycan (mean MW = 6000 Da) derived from porcine intestinal mucosa like heparin and LMWHs; however, the extraction process removes heparin and heparin-like fragments, yielding a mixture of heparan sulfate (84%), dermatan sulfate (12%), and chondroitin sulfate (4%).[46] This difference in structure results in a low degree of cross-reactivity (0% to 20%) between danaparoid and heparin or LMWH, so that danaparoid is an alternative anticoagulant in patients with HIT.

Like heparin and LMWH, danaparoid accelerates the inactivation of factor Xa and thrombin by binding to antithrombin III. Danaparoid exerts selective inhibition of factor Xa over thrombin (like LMWHs), in addition to preventing thrombus formation by inhibiting fibrin formation and deposition.[46] Danaparoid produces minimal effects on the PT, APTT, or thrombin time so that routine laboratory monitoring is not required.

After subcutaneous administration, danaparoid is well absorbed with a bioavailability of 89% to 100%.[46] The volume of distribution of danaparoid is 8 to 9 L, and is confined to the vasculature.[46] It is excreted primarily by the kidneys and has an elimination half-life (based on anti-Xa activity) of 17 to 28 hours,[46] whereas the anti-IIa activity is much shorter (2 to 4 hours). Due to the differences in the rate of elimination of the various components of danaparoid, it is typically administered twice daily to maintain adequate anti-Xa and anti-IIa activity for prophylaxis against thrombosis. Dosage adjustments are recommended in patients with renal insufficiency.

The major adverse effects of danaparoid include pain at the injection site, bleeding, fever, rash, and nausea. The major and minor bleeding observed with danaparoid therapy is similar in occurrence to adjusted-dose warfarin or low-dose subcutaneous heparin and is more frequent with higher doses. Protamine cannot be used to neutralize the anticoagulant effects of danaparoid.[46] In addition, danaparoid should not be used in patients who are allergic to sulfites or in children. Based on animal reproductive studies, danaparoid is Pregnancy Category B. It has been used successfully in pregnant women with heparin-associated thrombocytopenia who require continued anticoagulation and has become a preferred agent in this setting.

Danaparoid has been evaluated for the prophylaxis of DVT in six randomized, prospective studies of patients undergoing elective hip replacement or hip fracture surgery in comparison with placebo, aspirin, dextran, heparin with dihydroergotamine, or adjusted-dose warfarin.[46] In the two studies that compared danaparoid with adjusted-dose warfarin as prophylaxis (the only truly appropriate comparison), danaparoid was significantly more effective in decreasing the overall incidence of DVT.[46] In addition, danaparoid also decreased the incidence of proximal vein and calf vein thrombosis when compared with adjusted-dose warfarin. The incidence of major and minor bleeding was similar between the two groups. Unfortunately, studies comparing danaparoid with LMWHs are lacking.

The dose of danaparoid for the prophylaxis of DVT in hip surgery patients is 750 anti-Xa units subcutaneously administered twice daily. The first dose should be administered 1 to 4 hours preoperatively, and subsequently at least 2 hours postoperatively. It should be continued throughout the postoperative period for 7 to 10 days, or until the risk of DVT is diminished. The drug should be injected in alternating sites. Danaparoid is available as ampules or prefilled syringes that contain 750 anti-Xa units in 0.6 mL

COST-EFFECTIVENESS OF THROMBOPROPHYLAXIS

The key to reducing the morbidity and mortality of venous thromboembolism is to prevent DVT and subsequent PE from occurring in the first place. It is well recognized that some form of prophylaxis should be used against venous thromboembolism in patients who are at high risk for their development, such as hip fracture patients. All cost-effectiveness studies to date have documented that it is far less expensive to employ routine prophylaxis than to pay for the treatment of a clinically documented DVT or PE. When evaluating the cost-effectiveness of a particular regimen, one must take into account the cost of the agent, the cost of administration, the cost of required laboratory tests for monitoring, the efficacy of the particular modality, and the risk of complications (such as bleeding) and their subsequent costs. Some potential cost-effective properties of the LMWHs are the ease of administration which can be done by the patient at home if necessary, the lack of required laboratory monitoring during therapy, and their relative safety and efficacy in the prevention of DVT. The major drawback of therapy with LMWHs is that they cost more than low-dose unfractionated heparin or oral warfarin when looking at drug costs alone (Table 17–15).

Cost-effectiveness studies have emerged with conflicting results as to the cost-effectiveness of LMWHs. In two cost-effectiveness studies comparing the cost-effectiveness of enoxaparin with adjusted-dose warfarin in hip or knee replacement patients, both studies projected that enoxaparin would decrease the overall number of DVT occurrences and the number of deaths, but would do so at an increased cost of care (up to $50.00 per patient).[98,99] In a retrospective, decision analysis study comparing the cost-effectiveness of low-dose heparin, dalteparin, and intermittent pneumatic compression as thromboembolic prophylaxis in moderate-risk general surgery patients undergoing abdominal surgery, low-dose unfractionated heparin was found to be the most cost-effective prophylactic modality.[100] It is clear that routine thromboprophylaxis is more cost-effective than treatment of documented DVT or PE, but more cost-effectiveness studies are needed to define which agents prove to be most cost-effective for each situation where thromboprophylaxis is necessary.

EVALUATION OF THERAPEUTIC OUTCOMES

Venous thromboembolism is a potentially fatal disorder that employs either prophylactic therapy to prevent high-risk patients from developing a DVT or PE, or treatment of an existing thrombus. The overall pharmaceutical care plan, which includes the therapeutic goals, choice of a particular agent, and monitoring parameters, differs depending on whether prophylactic therapy or treatment against DVT or PE is being employed.

Because DVT and PE are potentially preventable diseases, health care professionals (including pharmacists) can play a major role in identifying which patients are at risk for developing venous thromboembolism, deciding which prophylactic modality would be most suitable based on the patient's degree of risk of developing DVT or PE and the potential for adverse effects from the therapy, and monitoring the patient for signs of DVT, PE, or adverse drug effects.

The therapeutic goals in the treatment of DVT or PE include (1) inhibiting the growth of the thrombus or embolus, (2) preventing recurrent embolic episodes, (3) restoring normal hemodynamics and oxygenation in the case of PE, and (4) minimizing the symptoms of the postphlebitic syndrome. The choice of a particular therapeutic agent will depend on the urgency of the case; the presence of contraindications to anticoagulants or thrombolytics; the relative safety, efficacy, and cost of the treatment; and the availability of resources necessary to carry out the treatment. Patients in this group should be monitored not only for adverse effects from treatment but also for the resolution of symptoms, the development of recurrent thrombosis, and symptoms of the postphlebitic syndrome.

CONCLUSIONS

Venous thromboembolism continues to be the target of intensive clinical research. The disorder is an important source of morbidity and mortality owing to complicating PE in patients on both medical and surgical wards. A major problem in the care of these patients has always been diagnosis. Many patients are asymptomatic, and both false-positive and false-negative diagnoses are common. Significant progress has been made in recent years in diagnostic procedures, identification of high-risk groups, and therapeutic management, although studies are needed to better define the role of thrombolytic therapy in acute DVT and PE. Most clinicians agree, however, that management of venous thromboembolism is ideally achieved through prophylactic approaches rather than by allowing thromboembolism to occur.

▶ PRINCIPLES OF PHARMACOTHERAPY

- Most venous thrombi involve the veins of the lower extremities (DVT). If not broken up by the endogenous lytic system, the thrombi may dislodge and produce complete or partial interruption of blood flow to a portion of the lungs (PE).
- Diagnosis of DVT involves noninvasive and invasive techniques; venography is usually limited to those patients in whom noninvasive techniques were inconclusive or ultrasonic techniques are not useful (morbidly obese patient, edema).
- Main objectives of treating venous thrombosis include prevention of the development of PE and postphlebitic syndrome, reducing morbidity from the acute event, and maximizing efficacy while minimizing adverse effects and cost.
- Weight-based unfractionated heparin nomograms and guidelines provide safe and effective anticoagulant therapy.
- The duration of anticoagulant therapy has not been well established but should be at least 3 months, and may be indefinite in those patients with recurrent PE/DVT or continuing risk factors.
- The frequency of bleeding complications is associated with several treatment factors (dose, route, and duration of therapy) and patient-related factors (age, comorbid diseases, concurrent medications).
- International normalized ratio (INR) is the standard of practice for monitoring warfarin therapy.
- Since warfarin is associated with fetal abnormalities, heparin and low-molecular-weight heparins are the preferred anticoagulant agents in pregnant patients.
- The key to reducing the morbidity and mortality of venous thromboembolism is the prevention of DVT and subsequent PE by using effective and safe prophylactic modalities for each patient.

REFERENCES

1. Hirsh J, Hoak J. Management of deep vein thrombosis and pulmonary embolism: A statement for healthcare professionals. Circulation 1996;93:2212–2245.
2. Stein PD. Acute pulmonary embolism. Dis Mon 1994;40:467–523.

3. Weinmann EE, Salzman EW. Deep-vein thrombosis. N Engl J Med 1994;331:1630–1641.
4. Dahlback B. Inherited thrombophilia: Resistance to activated protein C as a pathogenic factor of venous thromboembolism. Blood 1995; 85:607–614.
5. Ginsbury JS. Management of venous thromboembolism. N Engl J Med 1996;335:1816–1828.
6. Clagett GP, Anderson FA, Heit J, et al. Prevention of venous thromboembolism. Chest 1995;108(suppl):313S–334S.
7. ACCP Consensus Committee on Pulmonary Embolism. Opinions regarding the diagnosis and management of venous thromboembolic disease. Chest 1996;109:233–237.
8. Becker DM, et al. D-dimer testing and acute venous thromboembolism. Arch Intern Med 1996;156:939–946.
9. Bounameaux H, Cirafici P, de Moerloose P, et al. Measurement of D-dimer in plasma as diagnostic aid in suspected pulmonary embolism. Lancet 1991;1:196–200.
10. Perrier A, et al. Diagnosis of PE by decision analysis-based strategy including clinical probability, D-dimer, and ultrasonography. Arch Intern Med 1996;156:531–536.
11. Haines ST, Bussey HI. Diagnosis of deep vein thrombosis. Am J Health Sys Pharm 1997;54:66–74.
12. Hull RD, Raskob GE, Coates G, Panju AA. Clinical validity of a normal perfusion lung scan in patients with suspected pulmonary embolism. Chest 1990;97:23–26.
13. PIOPED Investigators. Value of the ventilation/perfusion scan in acute pulmonary embolism: Results of the prospective investigation of pulmonary embolism diagnosis (PIOPED). JAMA 1990; 263:2753–2759.
14. Hull RD, Raskob GE, Ginsberg JS, et al. Noninvasive strategy for the treatment of patients with suspected PE. Arch Intern Med 1994; 154:289–297.
15. ACCP Consensus Committee on Pulmonary Embolism. Opinions regarding the diagnosis and management of venous thromboembolic disease. Chest 1998;113:499–504.
16. Pearson JD, Lee TH, McCage-Sassan S, et al. Critical pathway to treatment of proximal lower-extremities DVT. Am J Med 1996; 100:283–289.
17. Ansell JE, Buttaro ML, Thomas OV, et al. Consensus guidelines for coordinated outpatient oral anticoagulation therapy management. Ann Pharmacother 1997;31:604–615.
18. Hyers TM, Hull RD, Weg JG. Antithrombotic therapy for venous thromboembolic disease. Chest 1995;108(suppl):335S–351S.
19. Hirsh J, Fuster V. Guide to anticoagulant therapy part 1: Heparin. Circulation 1994;89:1449–1468.
20. Cipolle RJ, Rodvold KA. Heparin. In: Evans WE, Schentag JJ, Jusko WJ, eds. Applied Pharmacokinetics, Principles of Therapeutic Drug Monitoring, 3rd ed. Vancouver, WA, Applied Therapeutics, 1992: Chap 30:1–39.
21. Ginsberg JS, Hirsh J. Use of antithrombotic agents during pregnancy. Chest 1995;108(suppl):305S–311S.
22. Raschke RA, Reilly BM, Guidry JR, et al. The weight-based heparin dosing nomogram compared with a "standard care" nomogram: A randomized controlled trial. Ann Intern Med 1993;119:874–881.
23. Hull RD, Raskob GE, Brant RF, et al. Relation between the time to achieve the lower limit of the APTT therapeutic range and recurrent venous thromboembolism during heparin treatment for deep vein thrombosis. Arch Intern Med 1997;157:2563–2568.
24. Hommes DW, Bura A, Mazzolai L, et al. Subcutaneous heparin compared with continuous intravenous heparin administration in the initial treatment of deep vein thrombosis: A meta-analysis. Ann Intern Med 1992;116:279–284.
25. Hull RD, Raskob GE, Rosenbloom D, et al. Optimal therapeutic level of heparin therapy in patients with venous thrombosis. Arch Intern Med 1992;152:1589–1595.
26. Cruickshank MK, Levine MN, Hirsh J, et al. A standard heparin nomogram for the management of heparin therapy. Arch Intern Med 1991;151:333–337.
27. Hollingsworth JA, Rowe BH, Brisebois FJ, et al. The successful application of a heparin nomogram in a community hospital. Arch Intern Med 1995;155:2095–2100.
28. Gunnarsson PS, Sawyer WT, Montague D, et al. Appropriate use of heparin: Empiric vs nomogram-based dosing. Arch Intern Med 1995;155:526–532.
29. Raschke RA, Gollihare B, Peirce JC. The effectiveness of implementing the weight-based heparin nomogram as a practice guideline. Arch Intern Med 1996;156:1645–1649.
30. Hull RD, Raskob GE, Rosenbloom D, et al. Heparin for 5 days as compared with 10 days in the initial treatment of proximal venous thrombosis. N Engl J Med 1990;322:1260–1264.
31. Mohiuddin SM, Hilleman DE, Destache CJ, et al. Efficacy and safety of early versus late initiation of warfarin during heparin therapy in acute thromboembolism. Am Heart J 1992;123:729–732.
32. Breddin HK, Radziwon P, Bocakowska-Radziwon B. Laboratory monitoring of new antithrombotic drugs. Clin Lab Med 1994; 14:825–846.
33. Brill-Edwards P, Ginsberg JS, Johnston M, Hirsh J. Establishing a therapeutic range for heparin therapy. Ann Intern Med 1993;119: 104–109.
34. Levine MN, Hirsh J, Gent M, et al. A randomized trial comparing activated thromboplastin time with heparin assay in patients with acute venous thromboembolism requiring large daily doses of heparin. Arch Intern Med 1994;154:49–56.
35. Levine MN, Raskob G, Landefeld S, Hirsh J. Hemorrhagic complications of anticoagulant treatment. Chest 1995;108(suppl): 276S–290S.
36. Landefeld CS, Beyth RJ. Anticoagulant-related bleeding: Clinical epidemiology, prediction, and prevention. Am J Med 1993; 95:315–328.
37. Hirsh J, Raschke R, Warkentin TE, et al. Heparin: Mechanism of action, pharmacokinetics, dosing considerations, monitoring, efficacy, and safety. Chest 1995;108(suppl):258S–275S.
38. Sallah S, Thomas DP, Roberts HR. Warfarin and heparin-induced skin necrosis and the purple toe syndrome: Infrequent complications of anticoagulant treatment. Thromb Haemost 1997;78: 785–790.
39. Weitz JI. Low molecular weight heparins. N Engl J Med 1997; 337:688–698.
40. Fareed J, Hoppensteadt D, Jeske W, et al. Low molecular weight heparins: A developmental perspective. Exp Opin Invest Drugs 1997; 6:705–733.
41. Massicotte P, Adams M, Marzinotto V, et al. Low molecular weight heparin in pediatric patients with thrombotic disease: A dose finding study. J Pediatr 1996;128:313-318.
42. Dunn CJ, Sorkin EM. Dalteparin sodium: A review of its pharmacology and clinical use in the prevention and treatment of thromboembolic disorders. Drugs 1996;52:277–305.
43. Schiele F, Vuillemenot A, Kramarz P, et al. Use of recombinant hirudin as antithrombotic treatment in patients with heparin-induced thrombocytopenia. Am J Hematol 1995;50:20–25.
44. Buckley MM, Sorkin EM. Enoxaparin: A review of its pharmacology and clinical applications in the prevention and treatment of thromboembolic disorders. Drugs 1992;44:465–497.
45. Warkentin TE, Levine MN, Hirsh J, et al. Heparin-induced thrombocytopenia in patients treated with low-molecular-weight heparin or unfractionated heparin. N Engl J Med 1995;332:1330–1335.
46. Skoutakis VA. Danaparoid in the prevention of thromboembolic complications. Ann Pharmacother 1997;31:876–887.
47. Levine M, Gent M, Hirsh J, et al. A comparison of low-molecular-weight heparin administered primarily at home with unfractionated heparin administered in the hospital for proximal vein thrombosis. N Engl J Med 1996;334:677–681.
48. Fiessinger JN, Lopez-Fernandez M, Gatterer E, et al. Once-daily subcutaneous dalteparin, a low molecular weight heparin, for the initial treatment of acute deep vein thrombosis. Thromb Haemost 1996; 76:195–199.

49. Luomanmaki K, Grankvist S, Hallert C, et al. A multicentre comparison of once-daily subcutaneous dalteparin (low molecular weight heparin) and continuous intravenous heparin in the treatment of deep vein thrombosis. J Intern Med 1996;240:85–92.
50. The Columbus Investigators. Low molecular weight heparin in the treatment of patients with thromboembolism. N Engl J Med 1997; 337:657–662.
51. Meyer G, Brenot F, Pacouret G, et al. Subcutaneous low-molecular-weight heparin Fragmin versus intravenous unfractionated heparin in the treatment of acute non massive pulmonary embolism: An open randomized pilot study. Thromb Haemost 1995;74:1432–1435.
52. Simonneau G, Sors H, Charbonnier B, et al. A comparison of low-molecular-weight heparin with unfractionated heparin for acute pulmonary embolism. N Engl J Med 1997;337:663–669.
53. Pini M, Aiello S, Manotti C, et al. Low molecular weight heparin versus warfarin in the prevention of recurrences after deep vein thrombosis. Thromb Haemost 1994;72:191–197.
54. Das SK, Cohen AT, Edmondson RA, et al. Low-molecular-weight heparin versus warfarin for prevention of recurrent venous thromboembolism: A randomized trial. World J Surg 1996;20:521–527.
55. Chaffee BJ. Low-molecular-weight heparins for the treatment of deep vein thrombosis. Am J Health Syst Pharm 1997;54: 1995–1999.
56. Green D, Hirsh J, Heit J, et al. Low molecular weight heparin: A critical analysis of clinical trials. Pharmacol Rev 1994;46:89–109.
57. Leizorovicz A, Simonneau G, Decousus H, Boissel JP. Comparison of efficacy and safety of low molecular weight heparins and unfractionated heparin in initial treatment of deep vein thrombosis: A meta-analysis. Br Med J 1994;309:299–304.
58. Hirsh J, Siragusa S, Cosmi B, Ginsberg JS. Low molecular weight heparins (LMWH) in the treatment of patients with acute venous thromboembolism. Thromb Haemost 1995;74:360–363.
59. Lensing AWA, Prins MH, Davidson BL, Hirsh J. Treatment of deep venous thrombosis with low-molecular-weight heparins: A meta-analysis. Arch Intern Med 1995;155:601–607.
60. Dedden P, Chang B, Nagel D. Pharmacy-managed program for home treatment of deep vein thrombosis with enoxaparin. Am J Health Syst Pharm 1997;54:1968–1972.
61. Hirsh J, Dalen JE, Deykin D, Poller L. Oral anticoagulants: Mechanism of action, clinical effectiveness, and optimal therapeutic range. Chest 1995;108(suppl):231S–246S.
62. Hirsh J, Fuster V. Guide to anticoagulant therapy part 2: Oral anticoagulants. Circulation 1994;89:1469–1480.
63. Ansell JE. Oral anticoagulant therapy: 50 years later. Arch Intern Med 1993;153:586–596.
64. Porter RS, Sawyer WT. Warfarin. In: Evans WE, Schentag JJ, Jusko WJ, eds. Applied Pharmacokinetics, Principles of Therapeutic Drug Monitoring, Vol 31, 3rd ed. Vancouver, WA, Applied Therapeutics, 1992:1–46.
65. DeCara JM, Croze S, Falk RH. Generic warfarin: A cost-effective alternative to brand-name drug or a clinical wild card? Chest 1998; 113:261–263.
66. Schulman S, Rhedin AS, Lindmarker P, et al. A comparison of six weeks with six months of oral anticoagulant therapy after a first episode of venous thromboembolism. N Engl J Med 1995; 332: 1661–1665.
67. Hirsh J, Poller L. The international normalized ratio: A guide to understanding and correcting its problems. Arch Intern Med 1994; 154:282–288.
68. Bussey HI, Force RW, Bianco TM, Leonard AD. Reliance on prothrombin time ratios causes significant errors in anticoagulation therapy. Arch Intern Med 1992;152:278–282.
69. Harrison L, Johnston M, Massicotte MP, et al. Comparison of 5-mg and 10-mg loading doses in initiation of warfarin therapy. Ann Intern Med 1997;126:133–135.
70. Bona RD, Hickey AD, Wallace DM. Efficacy and safety of oral anticoagulation in patients with cancer. Thromb Haemost 1997;78: 137–140.
71. Landefeld CS, Anderson PA. Guideline-based consultation to prevent anticoagulant-related bleeding: A randomized, controlled trial in a teaching hospital. Ann Intern Med 1992;116:829–837.
72. Ellis RF, Stephens MA, Sharp GB. Evaluation of a pharmacy-managed warfarin-monitoring service to coordinate inpatient and outpatient therapy. Am J Hosp Pharm 1992;49:387–394.
73. Schulman S. Optimal duration of oral anticoagulant therapy in venous thromboembolism. Thromb Haemost 1997;78:693–698.
74. Schulman S, Granqvist S, Holmstrom M, et al. Duration of oral anticoagulation therapy after a second episode of venous thromboembolism (DURAC II). N Engl J Med 1997;336:393–398.
75. Jillella AP, Lutcher CL. Reinstituting warfarin in patients who develop warfarin skin necrosis. Am J Hematol 1996;52;1117–1119.
76. Wells PS, Holbrook AM, Crowther NR, Hirsh J. Interactions of warfarin with drugs and food. Ann Intern Med 1994;121:676–683.
77. Sasahara AA, St Martin CC, Henkin J, Barker WM. Approach to the patient with venous thromboembolism: Treatment with thrombolytic therapy. Hematol Oncol Clin North Am 1992;6:1141–1159.
78. Francis CW, Marder VJ. Fibrinolytic therapy for venous thrombosis. Prog Cardiovasc Dis 1991;34:193–204.
79. Goldhaber SZ. Contemporary pulmonary embolism thrombolysis. Chest 1995;107(suppl):45S–51S.
80. Dalen JE, Alpert JS, Hirsh J. Thrombolytic therapy for pulmonary embolism: Is it effective? Is it safe? When is it indicated? Arch Intern Med 1997;157:2250–2256.
81. Ludlam CA, Bennett B, Fox FAA, et al. Guidelines for the use of thrombolytic therapy. Blood Coagl Fibrinolysis 1995;6:273–285.
82. Goldhaber SZ. Thrombolytic therapy in venous thromboembolism: Clinical trials and current indications. Clin Chest Med 1995;16: 307–320.
83. Rogers LQ, Lutcher CL. Streptokinase therapy for deep vein thrombosis: A comprehensive review of the English literature. Am J Med 1990;88:389–395.
84. Comerota AJ, Aldridge SC. Thrombolytic therapy for deep venous thrombosis: A clinical review. Can J Surg 1993;36:359–364.
85. Wagstaff AJ, Gillis JC, Goa KL. Alteplase: A reappraisal of its pharmacology and therapeutic use in vascular disorders other than acute myocardial infarction. Drugs 1995;50:289–316.
86. Weitz JI, Byrne J, Clagett P, et al. Diagnosis and treatment of chronic arterial insufficiency of the lower extremities: A critical review. Circulation 1996;94:3026–3049.
87. Thery C, Bauchart JJ, Lesenne M, et al. Predictive factors of effectiveness of streptokinase in deep venous thrombosis. Am J Cardiol 1992; 69:117–122.
88. Bell WR. Laboratory monitoring of thrombolytic therapy. Clin Lab Med 1995;15:165–178.
89. Levine MN, Goldhaber SZ, Gore JM, et al. Hemorrhagic complications of thrombolytic therapy in the treatment of myocardial infarction and venous thromboembolism. Chest 1995;108(suppl):291S–301S.
90. O'Meara JJ, McNutt RA, Evans AT, et al. A decision analysis of streptokinase plus heparin as compared with heparin alone for deep-vein thrombosis. N Engl J Med 1994;330:1864–1869.
91. Bergquist D, Benoni G, Bjorgell O, et al. Low-molecular-weight heparin (enoxaparin) as prophylaxis against venous thromboembolism after total hip replacement. N Engl J Med 1996;335:696–700.
92. Wells PS, Lensing AWA, Hirsh J. Graduated compression stockings in the prevention of postoperative venous thromboembolism: A meta analysis. Arch Intern Med 1994;154:67–72.
93. Hauch O, Khatter SC, Jorgensen LN. Cost-benefit analysis of prophylaxis against deep vein thrombosis in surgery. Semin Thromb Hemost 1991;17:280–283.
94. Hull R, Raskob G, Pineo G, et al. A comparison of subcutaneous low-molecular weight heparin with warfarin sodium for prophylaxis against deep-vein thrombosis after hip or knee implantation. N Engl J Med 1993;329:1370–1376.
95. Imperiale TF, Speroff T. A meta-analysis of methods to prevent venous thromboembolism following total hip replacement. JAMA 1994;271:1780–1785.

96. Howard PA. Dalteparin: A low molecular weight heparin. Ann Pharmacother 1997;31:192–203.
97. Troy S, Fruncillo R, Ozawa T, et al. The dose proportionality of the pharmacokinetics of ardeparin, a low molecular weight heparin, in healthy volunteers. J Clin Pharmacol 1995;35:1194–1199.
98. Menzin J, Colditz GA, Regan MM, et al. Cost-effectiveness of enoxaparin vs. low-dose warfarin in the prevention of deep-vein thromboisis after total hip replacement surgery. Arch Intern Med 1995;155:757–764.
99. Hull RD, Raskob GE, Pineo GF, et al. Subcutaneous low-molecular-weight heparin vs. warfarin for prophylaxis of deep vein thrombosis after hip or knee implantation. Arch Intern Med 1997; 157:298–303.
100. Mamdani MM, Weingarten CM, Stevenson JG. Thromboembolic prophylaxis in moderate-risk patients undergoing elective abdominal surgery: Decision and cost-effectiveness analysis. Pharmacotherapy 1996;16:1111–1127.
101. Goldhaber SZ, Morpurgo M. Diagnosis, treatment, and prevention of pulmonary embolism. JAMA 1992;141:1727–1729.
102. Nielsen HK. Pathophysiology of venous thromboembolism. Semin Thromb Hemost 1991;17(suppl 3):250–253.
103. Hirsh J, Hull RD, Raskob GE. Diagnosis of pulmonary embolism. J Am Coll Cardiol 1986;8(6 suppl B):128B–136B.
104. Stead RB. Clinical pharmacology. In: Goldhaber SZ, ed. Pulmonary Embolism and Deep Venous Thrombosis. Philadelphia, Saunders, 1985:99–119.
105. Carter BL. Therapy of acute thromboembolism with heparin and warfarin. Clin Pharm 1991;10:503–518.
106. Carter BL, Jones ME, Waickman LA. Pathophysiology and treatment of deep vein thrombosis and pulmonary embolism. Clin Pharm 1985; 4:279–297.
107. Bell WR. Fibrinolytic therapy: Indications and management. In: Hoffman R, Benz EJ, Shattil SJ, eds. Hematology: Basic Principles and Practice, 2nd ed. New York, Churchill Livingstone, 1995:1814–1829.

18

STROKE

J. Chris Bradberry, PharmD

Stroke, or brain attack, is a syndrome and is a major manifestation of cerebrovascular disease. Stroke refers to the sudden onset of a focal neurologic deficit. Cerebrovascular disease refers to any type of pathophysiologic vascular disease of the brain. This vascular pathology can include any abnormality of the vessel, blood flow, or quality of the blood. Abnormalities of the vessel include many processes such as developmental defects, arteritis, aneurysm, hypertensive disease, vasoconstriction, and atherosclerosis. Blood flow can be affected by disease of the vessel and also by thrombotic or embolic processes. The changes in the brain that these abnormalities can produce are either a decrease in blood flow, termed ischemia, or bleeding. Ischemia can be present with or without brain tissue infarction. When a stroke occurs, the neurologic manifestations produced are the result of the location of insult in the brain and the extent of ischemia, infarct, or hemorrhage. A stroke may show varied manifestations, reversible and irreversible, ranging from hemiplegia to sensory deficits. Hemiplegia may or may not be accompanied by other manifestations.

It is a challenge for the clinician to accurately diagnose a particular lesion because of these variations in presentation; however, a good clinical examination can aid in locating a lesion as well as in helping to determine if the stroke is ischemic or hemorrhagic in nature. The advent of imaging studies such as computed tomography (CT) and magnetic resonance imaging (MRI) has been of tremendous importance in the diagnosis and assessment of stroke. Results of the CT scan must be known prior to therapy of certain stroke syndromes with anticoagulants, thrombolytics, or platelet antiaggregating agents.

Although the causes of stroke are many, this chapter centers on the most common types of stroke, with further emphasis on ischemic cerebrovascular disease and cardiogenic embolic stroke. Hemorrhagic and other more unusual forms are de-emphasized.

EPIDEMIOLOGY AND ETIOLOGY

Figure 18–1 outlines the classification by mechanism of stroke. Since the 1940s, cerebrovascular disease death rates have declined in the United States.[1] In 1971, the American Heart Association (AHA) issued a special statement on risk factors. At that time, major risk factors for ischemic stroke were identified as transient ischemic attacks, cerebral infarction, hypertension, cardiac abnormalities, and other consequences of atherosclerosis and diabetes mellitus.

Since that statement, mortality from stroke has continued to decline,[2] although we may be seeing a leveling off over the last few years. In fact, during the mid-1970s, the rate of decline in mortality from cerebrovascular disease was far greater than that from cardiovascular disease. The reasons for this decline are not clear, but evidence would suggest that this decline in mortality from cerebrovascular disease, and ischemic stroke in particular, may be related to more effective treatment of hypertension and life-style changes.

General population studies show that atherothrombotic infarction is the most common type of stroke, representing almost 65% of the reported cases of the 85% caused by ischemia. Therefore, the majority of strokes are caused by ischemia and infarction secondary to disease of the large, small, and medium-size arteries supplying the brain. Cerebral embolism causes stroke about 20% of the time. Hemorrhage into the brain tissue (cerebral or intraparenchymal hemorrhage) and subarachnoid hemorrhages account for about 15% of all strokes. In 1995, the AHA estimated that in the United States more than 157,991 people (1 of every 15 deaths) died from a stroke, and that cumulatively 4,000,000 people survived a stroke.[2] Stroke remains the third leading cause of death in the United States even though mortality has declined. It is estimated that 600,000 people per year have a new or recurrent stroke.

One of the major impacts of stroke is the resultant disability in up to 50% of patients hospitalized for cerebrovascular disease. The overall direct and indirect economic impact is estimated to be as high as $43.3 billion annually and is expected to increase further.[2,3] Obviously, with this impact, both economically and emotionally, stroke is one of the most devastating diseases. Prevention is of primary importance, and proper prevention requires correction of risk factors in persons at highest risk.[4] As noted earlier, there is good evidence to show that improved treatment, specifically of hypertension, may decrease death from stroke. The risk factors for ischemic stroke are shown in Table 18–1 divided into groups on the basis of their relationship to stroke prevention.[2,3]

SINGLE RISK FACTORS

It is clear that stroke incidence is related to increasing age, with doubling of stroke rates each decade after age 55 where most stroke victims are 65 years or older.[2] Stroke generally has a 19% higher incidence in men than women. There is a higher death rate in blacks, Asian-Pacific Islanders, and Hispanics than whites. In blacks, this may be a

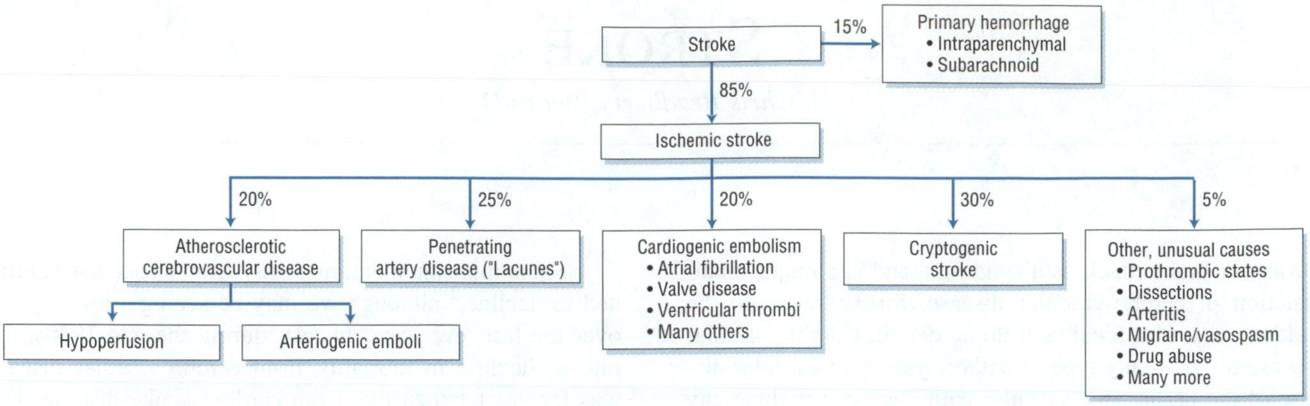

FIGURE 18–1. A classification of stroke by mechanism with estimates of the frequency of various categories of abnormalities. About 30% of ischemic strokes are cryptogenic. *(From Fourth ACCP Consensus Conference on Anti-thrombotic Therapy.)*

result of the increased incidence of hypertension and environmental factors, such as a high-sodium diet. Diabetes mellitus contributes independently to atherothrombotic brain infarction and the risk is greater in women than men. An individual with a prior stroke has a high risk of developing a recurrent stroke. Carotid bruits are evidence of increased risk of stroke; however, asymptomatic carotid bruits have been a controversial topic with regard to treatment. In asymptomatic individuals, a carotid bruit is an indication of a generalized atherosclerotic disease and does not necessarily indicate that a cerebral infarction will occur in the cerebral territory supplied by the affected carotid.

Of the single risk factors identified, hypertension is the major predisposing factor for stroke and is strongly related to atherothrombotic brain infarction as well as cerebral hemorrhage. Hypertension is a factor in almost 70% of all strokes. The Framingham study indicated that there is a direct relationship between elevation of blood pressure and stroke risk.[5] There does not seem to be a gender difference in the risk for hypertensive patients, and elevated blood pressure appears to be closely associated with stroke. The risk does not decrease with age; however, with effective treatment, the elderly hypertensive patients have a reduction in stroke as great as or greater than that of the younger

TABLE 18–1. Risk Factors in Ischemic Stroke

Single risk factors
- Nonmodifiable risk factors or risk markers
  - Age
  - Gender
  - Race
  - Ethnicity
  - Heredity
- Potentially modifiable
  - Hypertension—single most important risk factor for ischemic stroke
  - Cardiac disease
    - Atrial fibrillation—most important and treatable cardiac cause of stroke
    - Mitral stenosis
    - Mitral annular calcification
    - Left atrial enlargement
    - Structural abnormalities such as atrial-septal aneurysm
    - Myocardial disease
      - 1% to 6% of myocardial infarction patients develop a stroke
  - Transient ischemic attacks—major independent risk factor
  - Diabetes—independent risk factor
  - Hypercholesterolemia—positive risk factor for extracranial atherosclerosis but link still under study for ischemic stroke
  - Cigarette smoking
  - Alcohol
  - Illicit drug use—cocaine, heroin, amphetamines, LSD, PCP and others linked with stroke
  - Life-style factors—associated with stroke risk
    - Obesity
    - Physical inactivity
    - Diet
    - Acute triggers—emotional stress
  - Oral contraceptives—positive only with estrogen content >50 μg
  - Migraine—risk not clear
  - Hemostatic and inflammatory factors—fibrinogen linked to increased risk; elevated hematocrit and sickle cell disease are positive risk factors
  - Homocysteine—still under study, but hyperhomocysteinemia may be related to increased stroke risk
  - Asymptomatic carotid stenosis
  - Subclinical disease—aortic arch atheromas

Multiple risk factors—stroke is increased by the presence of multiple risk factors
- Framingham profile
  - Elevated systolic blood pressure
  - Elevated serum cholesterol
  - Glucose intolerance
  - Cigarette smoking
  - Left ventricular hypertrophy

Adapted from Ref 4.

population. Impaired cardiac function is the next most important single treatable risk factor for stroke. Individuals with cardiac diseases such as coronary heart disease, congestive heart failure, left ventricular hypertrophy, and arrhythmias—and specifically atrial fibrillation—have more than twice the stroke risk compared to those with normal cardiac function. Cardiovascular risk reduction must be implemented in order to reduce the risk of coronary heart disease (CHD) and, in turn, stroke risk. Atrial fibrillation is strongly correlated with embolic stroke, and those patients with nonrheumatic atrial fibrillation have a sixfold increase in stroke frequency over those without fibrillation.[6–8]

Transient ischemic attacks (TIAs) are defined as episodes of focal ischemic neurologic deficit lasting less than 24 hours. The neurologic deficit depends on the thrombotic or embolic activity in the particular arterial supply to the brain. TIAs precede an ischemic stroke in about 60% of cases, and 35% of untreated patients will develop a stroke within 5 years of a TIA. TIAs precede 10% of strokes from all causes. The greatest risk for stroke is early, within the first few weeks of the TIA, with about 20% occurring within the first month after the TIA and 50% within the first year after the TIA. The more frequently TIAs occur, the higher the probability of stroke, and a previous stroke is a greater risk factor for subsequent stroke than a TIA alone.[9] TIAs as risk factors are also influenced by other stroke risk factors; therefore, treatment of other risk factors may influence the occurrence of stroke in patients with TIAs.

Another risk factor is elevated hematocrit. Stroke in patients with elevated hematocrits has been attributed to decreased collateral flow caused by increased blood viscosity. Sickle cell disease patients also appear to have an increased incidence of stroke. Stroke in middle-age men has been shown to correlate significantly with a maternal history of stroke.

Hyperlipidemia and hypercholesterolemia are risk factors for atherosclerosis and CHD and stroke. It has been clearly established that lipoproteins play a primary role in atherogenesis, and lowering plasma cholesterol concentration reduces arterial cholesterol accumulation.[10] A recent review of published studies involving 29,000 patients treated with 3-hydroxy-3-methylglutaryl coenzyme a reductase inhibitors (statins) showed that lowering cholesterol for primary and secondary prevention of coronary heart disease reduced the risk of stroke 29% and total mortality 22%, thus clearly emphasizing the importance of elevated cholesterol as a risk factor for stroke.[11,12]

Cigarette smoking is a major risk factor for ischemic and hemorrhagic strokes. Causative factors may be increased blood concentration of fibrinogen, increased platelet aggregability, decreased HDL-C, damage to the vascular endothelium, and increasing the hematocrit. Smokers had two to three times the risk of stroke compared with nonsmokers, and a fourfold to sixfold increase in stroke risk compared with those who had never smoked.[13] It was also shown that cessation of smoking had significant benefits in reducing stroke risk. The risk of stroke for women smokers is higher than that for men smokers; however, the risk for all smokers decreases to that of nonsmokers 2 to 5 years after cessation.

Low levels of alcohol consumption and ischemic stroke are inversely related, and risk in men increases with heavy consumption (>300 g/wk). Alcohol should not be construed as a preventative measure for stroke.

The association between oral contraceptives as an independent risk factor and the incidence of stroke is dose dependent. Higher dose formulations have been shown to increase stroke risk in subgroups of women, such as those greater than 35 years of age, smokers, hypertensives, those with hyperlipidemia, and those with histories of migraine. Newer products contain much lower doses of estrogen (< 50 μg) and progestin, and more recent studies have not shown an association between low-dose oral contraceptive use and stroke. A definitive statement about risk of stroke cannot be made at this time and caution is recommended in the use of oral contraceptives in women at high risk for stroke.

The use of estrogen replacement therapy in postmenopausal women is well-documented to reduce the risk of coronary heart disease; however, there is some concern about stroke in these women. Data are limited and more research is needed.[14]

MULTIPLE RISK FACTORS

The Framingham study determined five factors: elevated systolic blood pressure, elevated serum cholesterol, glucose intolerance, cigarette smoking, and left ventricular hypertrophy by electrocardiogram (ECG). These factors, if present, can be used to identify the 10% of the population who will have one-third of the strokes. Interestingly, various combinations of factors have been studied, including low ponderal index (height in inches/cube root of weight in pounds), and risk can vary fourfold to eightfold depending on the number of multiple risk factors present. The most important single factor, however, was found to be elevated blood pressure. In addition, certain risk factors have been identified that can help to determine those at high risk for ischemic stroke. Table 18–2 shows these high risk factors and stroke rates.

TABLE 18–2. High-Risk Factors for Ischemic Stroke

High-Risk Factor	Ischemic Stroke Rate per Year (%)
Asymptomatic bruit	1.5
Prior myocaridal infarction	1.5
Asymptomatic carotid stenosis	2.0
NVAF	5.0
TIA (varies with territory involved)	6
Prior ischemic stroke	10

Stroke rate for the general population 70 years of age = 0.6%.

The treatable single risk factors should be vigorously addressed. When risk factors occur in combination, therapy should be initiated aggressively, with particular emphasis on hypertension and life-style changes.

PATHOPHYSIOLOGY OF ACUTE STROKE

The vascular anatomy of the brain with blood flow from the heart is shown in Fig. 18–2. The reader may also refer to the diagrams of the brain territory supplied by the middle cerebral artery (Fig. 18–3), the anterior cerebral artery (Fig. 18–4), and the vertebral-basilar system (Fig. 18–5).

The large majority of acute strokes result either from ischemic infarction or from inadequate blood flow, while only 15% result from primary intracranial hemorrhage. Exact pathophysiologic mechanisms remain controversial. Figure 18–5 describes the anatomic basis of stroke syndromes.

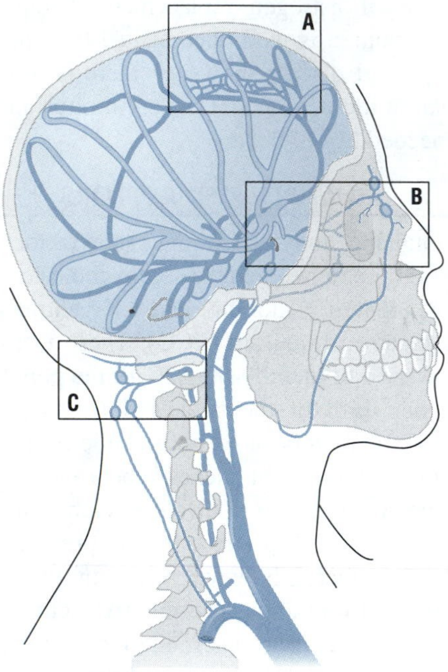

FIGURE 18–2. Arrangement of the major arteries of the right side carrying blood from the heart to the brain. Also shown are vessels of collateral circulation that may modify the effects of cerebral ischemia *(A–C)*. Not shown is the circle of Willis, which also provides a source for collateral circulation. *(A)* The anastomotic channels between the distal branches of the anterior and middle cerebral artery, termed *borderzone* or *watershed anastomotic channels*. Note that they also occur between the posterior and middle cerebral arteries and the arterior and posterior cerebral arteries. *(B)* Anastomotic channels occurring through the orbit between branches of the external carotid artery and the ophthalmic branch of the internal carotid artery. *(C)* Wholly extracranial anastomotic channels between the muscular branches of the ascending cervical arteries and the muscular branches of the occipital artery that anastomose with the distal vertebral artery. Note that the occipital artery arises from the external carotid artery, thereby allowing reconstitution of flow in the vertebral artery from the carotid circulation. *(From Braunwald E. Isselbacher KJ, et al, eds. Harrison's Principles of Internal Medicine, 11th ed. New York, McGraw-Hill, 1987: 1931, with permission.)*

CEREBROVASCULAR DISEASE

ATHEROTHROMBOTIC DISEASE

Atherosclerosis of brain arteries is a process similar to that found in other extracranial vessels. It is generally held that the atherosclerotic process occurs in parallel fashion throughout the body, although the severity may be slightly less in arteries of the brain than in such arteries as the aorta, the arteries of the extremities, and the coronary arteries. Atherosclerosis and subsequent plaque formation result in arterial narrowing or occlusion and constitute the most common cause of aortacranial stenosis. The process of atherosclerosis results in plaque formation, which stimulates platelet aggregation. Atherosclerosis itself is initially seen as a fatty streak on the vascular wall. This fatty streak starts as a deposition of lipids in the endothelial cells of the vessel wall. This process may regress, remain stable, or progress. If the process continues, yellow fatty, fibrous plaques are formed. Again, if there is progression, an atheromatous lesion may form secondary to the interaction of a number of atherogenic substances including LDL-C and others, and hemorrhage into the plaque, and subintimal necrosis, loss of intimal integrity, ulcer formation, or calcification may occur.[15,16] Thrombosis may be more likely to occur in areas where plaque has caused the greatest narrowing of the vessel. Formation of a blood clot superimposed on atherosclerotic plaque may cause significant stenosis of large extracranial arteries of the deep penetrating intracerebral arteries. Additional factors such as blood hypercoagulability and increased platelet counts and hematocrit may also contribute to clotting and sludging of blood flow.

Embolism can produce a stroke when a clot, plaque, or platelet aggregate breaks off into the circulation and blocks an artery. When atherosclerotic plaque ulcerates and pieces embolize distally, the emboli are called artery-to-artery emboli. Other embolic phenomena are discussed in the "Cerebral Embolism and Cardiogenic Embolism" section under "Clinical Presentation and Diagnosis" later in the chapter. Platelets play an important role in thrombosis and loss of integrity of the endothelial surface of the arterial wall, even if the defect is minor, and resultant platelet activation can lead to formation of a thrombus. This endothelial damage can result from trauma or from diseases such as atherosclerosis, and when this occurs, vessel collagen can be exposed to the blood. This exposed collagen acts as a trigger mechanism to activate the platelets. This activation results in release of adenine diphosphate (ADP) from the platelets, which in turn causes platelets to aggregate. Aggregation is consolidated by coagulation factors, red and white blood cells, and formation of a fibrin network. Other factors are also produced including thromboxane A_2, which promotes platelet aggregation and vasoconstriction. Various other substances, such as cytokines, can also affect the function of vascular endothial cells. This is balanced by the production of prostacyclin (PGI_2) by the vessel endothelium.

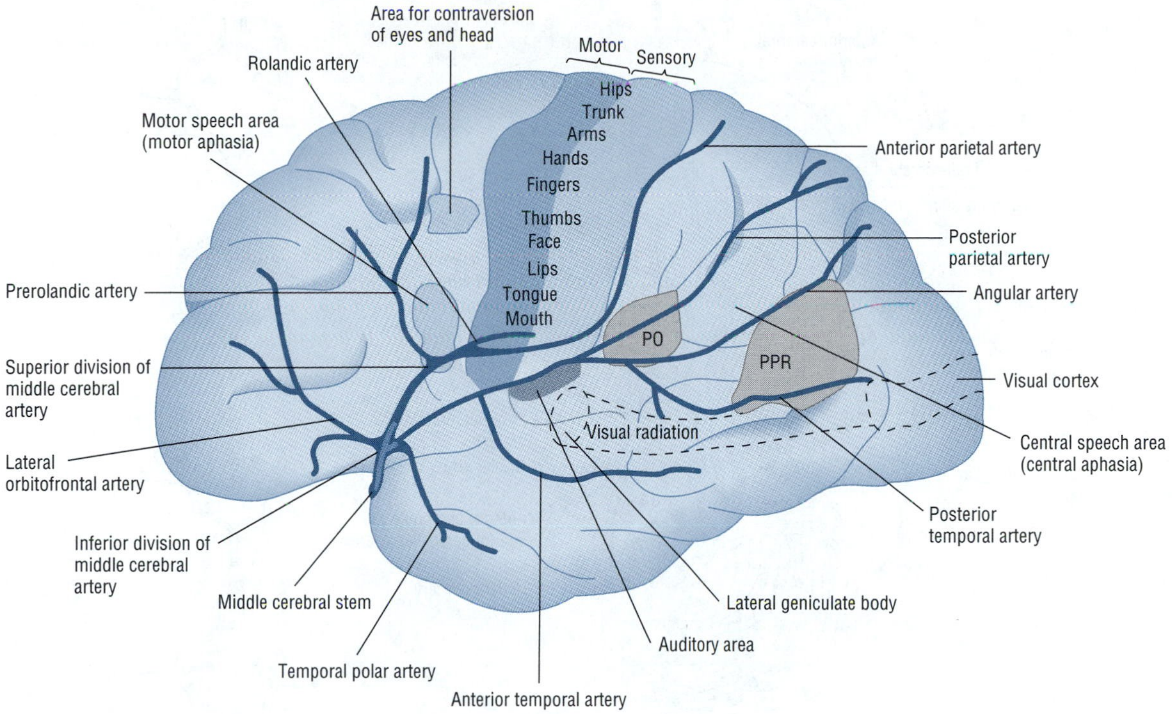

FIGURE 18–3. Diagram of a cerebral hemisphere, lateral aspect, showing the branches and distribution of the middle cerebral artery and the principal regions of cerebral localization. Note the bifurcation of the middle cerebral artery into a superior and an inferior division. *(From Braunwald E, Isselbacher KJ, et al, eds. Harrison's Principles of Internal Medicine, 11th ed. New York, McGraw-Hill, 1987:1936, with permission.)*

Prostacyclin is a vasodilator and inhibitor of platelet aggregation. This thrombus may continue to increase in size until the entire lumen of the vessel is blocked, or pieces of the thrombus may break off and embolize into more distal areas. The atherosclerotic process is variable and the ischemic consequences resulting from this process depend on (1) adequacy of blood flow and collateral circulation and (2) embolism. These factors determine the outcome of any individual ischemic event. To produce a low-blood-flow state leading to ischemia, the blood pressure must be reduced distal to the stenosis or occlusion and, usually, the carotid lumen must be reduced 75% in diameter.[17] Impaired collateral circulation to the affected area is also critical. The collateral circulation is composed of a network of arteries on the surface of the brain and those of the circle of Willis.

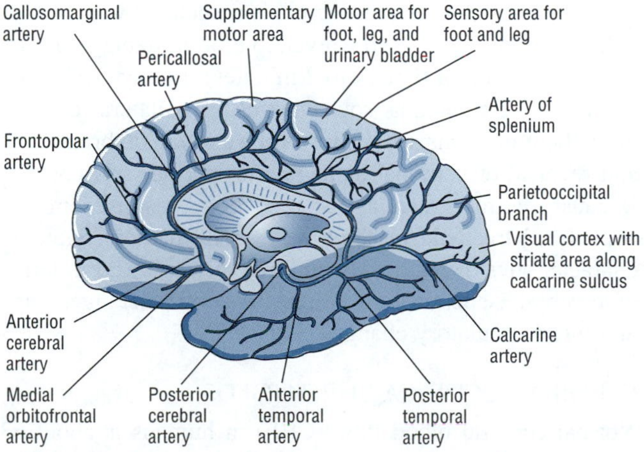

FIGURE 18–4. Diagram of a cerebral hemisphere, medial aspect, showing the branches and distribution of the anterior cerebral artery and the principal regions of cerebral localization. *(From Braunwald E, Isselbacher KJ, et al, eds. Harrison's Principles of Internal Medicine, 11th ed. New York, McGraw-Hill, 1987:1937, with permission.)*

The most common sites for the atherosclerotic process to occur are at the bifurcation of the common carotid siphon, the origin of the common carotid artery from the aorta and occasionally in the aortic arch; at the bifurcation of the internal carotid artery into the anterior and middle cerebral arteries; and in the circle of Willis at the proximal segments of the anterior, middle, and posterior cerebral arteries (Fig. 18–6). The process of atherogenesis may also be stimulated by vascular endothelial damage caused by the increased expression of cell adhesion molecules in patients with dyslipidemia. Adhesion molecules such as vascular cell adhesion molecule (VCAM-1), which is specific for monocytes, promote atherogenesis by binding monocytes on the endothelium and increasing their numbers in the atherosclerotic lesion. Additionally, intracellular adhesion molecule (ICAM-1) can contribute to neutrophil adhesion and movement into endothelial cells.[18–20]

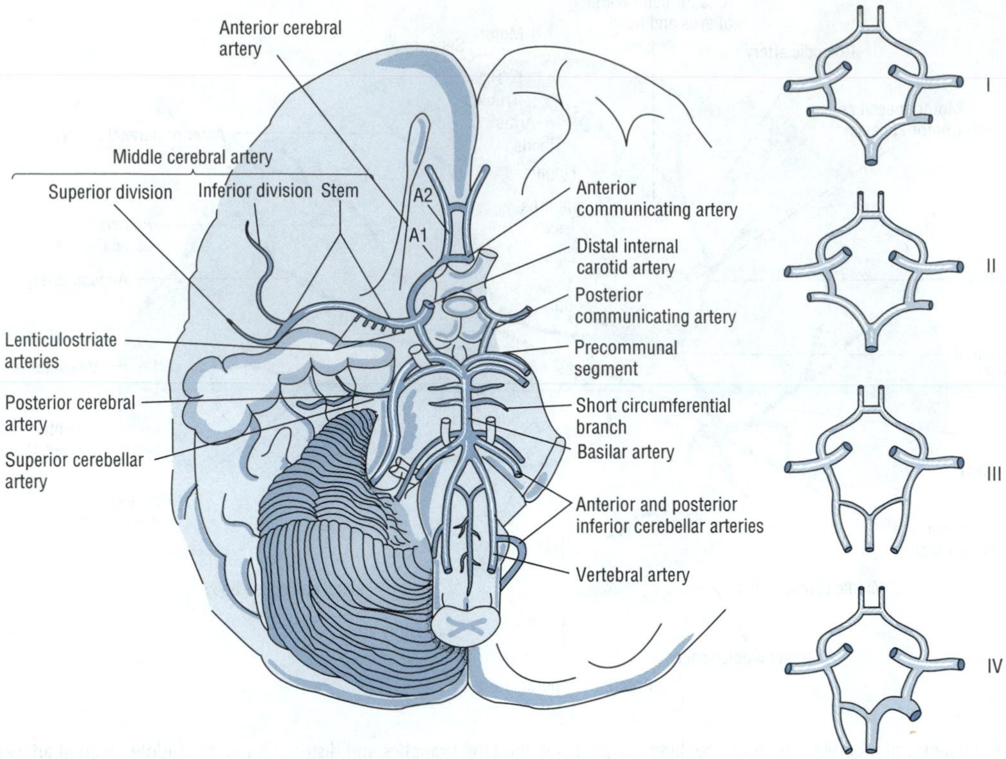

FIGURE 18–5. Diagram of the brain stem, cerebellum, inferior right frontal lobe, and temporal lobe transected. Principal branches of the vertebrobasilar arterial system are pictured. Small branches of the vertebral and basilar arteries that penetrate the medulla and pons are not pictured. The stem of the middle cerebral artery with its small, deep penetrating lenticulostriate arteries and the circle of Willis with its small, deep penetrating branches are pictured. Roman numerals I, II, III, and IV represent some of the possible variations of the circle of Willis resulting from atresia of one or more of its arterial components. Great variability in infarct size and location occurs when the basilar or vertebral arteries, or one of their penetrating branches, occlude because of variation in arterial anatomic location and available collateral circulation. Thus the stroke syndromes produced are often atypical or incomplete, or merge with one another. *(From Braunwald E, Isselbacher KJ, et al, eds. Harrison's Principles of Internal Medicine, 11th ed. New York, McGraw-Hill, 1987:1932, with permission.)*

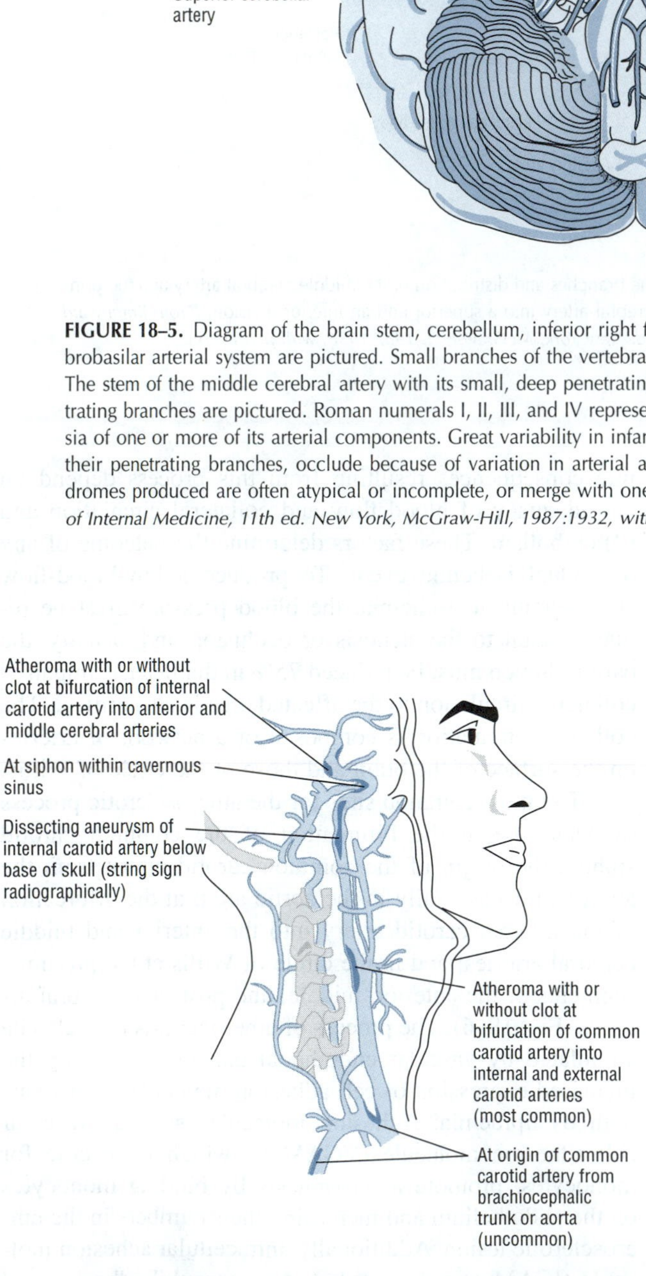

FIGURE 18–6. Common sites of atherosclerotic disease in the aortocranial circulation. *(From Ciba Collection of Medical Illustrations. Ciba Foundation, 1982, vol I pt II, p 55, with permission.)*

CEREBRAL ISCHEMIA

Cerebral ischemia can be divided into focal and general (or global) ischemia. Global ischemia is associated with lack of collateral blood flow, and irreversible brain damage occurs in a short period of time (4 to 8 minutes). In focal ischemia, however, there remains some degree of collateral circulation; therefore, this may allow for survival of brain cells and reversal of neuronal damage after periods of ischemia. Because of this potential for recovery, focal ischemia is considered treatable in some cases. The pathophysiologic characteristics of focal ischemia may be reviewed in terms of cerebral ischemia thresholds, metabolic derangements, and microcirculatory changes.[17,21]

CEREBRAL ISCHEMIA THRESHOLDS

Normal cerebral blood flow (CBF) in humans is about 53 mL/100 g of brain tissue per minute. Reductions in CBF to the range 15 to 18 mL/100 g/min result in abnormal brain electrical activity. At a flow of 10 mL/100 g/min, alterations in intracellular calcium and extracellular potassium homeostasis occur. Also, free fatty acids are released, and adenosine triphosphate (ATP) is depleted. A severe intracellular acidosis ensues in cells in the ischemic area. A CBF of 10 mL/100 g/min results in failure of ionic regulation and is thought to result in rapid irreversible damage to neurons. The CBF range between electrical failure and ionic failure is thought to be enough to maintain cell function for a time, possibly up to 4 hours, and recovery might be possible in acute focal ischemia, provided adequate collateral flow could supply basic energy requirements. Clinical outcome, as noted earlier, is dependent on the severity and duration of the decreased CBF.

METABOLIC DERANGEMENTS

When the CBF decreases to 10 mL/100 g/min, accumulation of lactic acid, depletion of ATP, and an increase in intracellular calcium and sodium may be seen. Extracellular potassium increases because of a failure of the ATP-dependent sodium-potassium pump. This rise in extracellular K^+ and sodium depolarizes the neuronal membrane, which in turn stimulates the opening of the voltage-dependent calcium channels, and an influx of calcium into the intracellular space occurs. Calcium cannot be pumped out normally because of the failure of the ATP-dependent calcium transport system and, in addition, calcium is not taken up normally by the endoplasmic reticulum. This unbalanced intracellular increase in calcium is thought to result in production of free fatty acids from membrane phospholipids. This loss of phospholipid decreases the integrity of the cell, and the permeability of the cell membranes increases and further impairs calcium homeostasis. Excitatory substances, such as amino acids, glutamate, and aspartate are released from the neuron as a result of depolarization. Glutamate activates the NMDA receptor (*N*-methyl-D-asparate) as well as other receptors that increase metabolic activity. Activation of these receptors allows further influxes of calcium and sodium into the cell, thereby enhancing depolarization.[21]

Accumulation of free fatty acids, including arachidonic acid, results in oxidation via cyclooxygenase and lipoxygenase pathways, producing prostaglandins, leukotrienes, and free radicals. Thromboxane A_2 is a potent vasoconstrictor, leukotrienes affect membrane permeability, and free radicals can attack cell membranes. Free radical production during ischemia overwhelms the endogenous methods for scavenging, and these free radicals can further disrupt cell membranes and produce vasoconstriction. All of these actions can lead to further intracellular acidosis and increasingly impair cell function. Ischemia and the subsequent production of intracellular acidosis can have devastating effects on the brain cell. These effects include glial edema and denaturation of proteins. Focal ischemia is associated with preserved but marginal CBF, and continued glucose delivery in the face of ischemia promotes anaerobic glycolysis with production of lactic acidosis. This continues to worsen the intracellular acidosis.

MICROCIRCULATORY CHANGES AND EDEMA

At the time of occlusion, blood viscosity and resistance to flow are increased, and blood flow is further slowed as ischemia develops. Soon after this, an ischemia-induced arterial spasm occurs, possibly as a result of the increased extracellular potassium and intracellular calcium, free radical accumulation, or a combination. It is not entirely clear why vasospasm of the microcirculation occurs, and it is also not clear if this impaired vascular filling is the primary determinant of neuronal damage. In any case, damage to the endothelium of the vessels occurs.

ISCHEMIA EDEMA

Swelling is one of the primary responses of brain tissue to acute injury. An early or intracellular phase and a late or extracellular phase occur. The early phase primarily involves the glial cells surrounding the vessel itself, suggesting a defect in vascular permeability, possibly enhanced by lactic acidosis. The primary difficulty caused by the glial edema is that collateral flow is decreased as a result of the "squeezing down" on the collateral circulation. The late phase, or extracellular phase, occurs hours to days after vessel occlusion and is probably a result of ischemic damage to vessel endothelial tissue. Movement of plasma into the extracellular space results in increased intracranial pressure. Brain herniation can result from the increased pressure. In animals, there are regional differences in brain tissue vulnerability to ischemia, and some tissues may be more or less resistant to ischemic damage than other tissues[21]. Some investigators postulate that these differences may result from the greater number of calcium channels in those tissues that are most vulnerable.

LACUNAR INFARCTS

Occlusion of the small arterial branches of the circle of Willis and of the anterior, middle, and posterior cerebral and basilar arteries can result in infarcts deep in the cerebral hemispheres (subcortical) and brainstem. These are small arteries with diameters in the range of 100 to 400 mm, and their occlusion results in small infarcts 2 to 15 mm in diameter. The term "lacunar" or "lacune" refers to the small cavity left after necrotic tissue has been removed. The pathophysiology of these infarcts is somewhat different from that of infarcts closer to the surface of the brain. About 25% of all strokes are a result of lacunar infarcts. Arterial hypertension is closely related to the occurrence of lacunar infarcts and is the major risk factor for lacunar disease. The pathophysiology of the small arteries has been described as being a degenerative process in the media of the artery (lipohyalinosis), leading to vessel occlusion. The degenerative occlusive process may be, on occasion, histologically different in appearance compared with the atherosclerotic process affecting extracranial and other larger intracranial arteries, and may in fact circumscribe portions of the involved artery. Microatheroma (plaque) may also be found in the proximal portions of the arterial branches. These different occlusive processes probably account for the multiple types of clinical presentations of lacunar infarcts. The patient's clinical presentation will reflect which small arterial branches are involved in the occlusive process. For example, the lenticulostriate artery is often involved, and the most common lacunar syndrome results from an infarct in the internal capsule of the brain and a pure motor hemiparesis is seen.

TRANSIENT ISCHEMIC ATTACKS

TIAs of cerebral origin are episodes of temporary focal cerebral dysfunction of vascular origin in which the onset is rapid, is of variable duration, and lasts from a few seconds up to 24 hours. The most common duration is a few seconds up to 5 to 10 minutes, depending on the territory of the brain where the event occurs. Between attacks there may be no neurologic abnormality. The clinical manifestation reflects the territory of the artery involved and usually occurs in the carotid system, the vertebrobasilar system, or both. TIAs have great significance in that they herald an impending stroke. Threatened stroke is a term used to describe any prestroke syndrome, such as TIAs, or patients who have had small or minor strokes or progressing or evolving stroke, and are at further risk for a major stroke.

The pathophysiology of TIAs involves the atherosclerotic process of thrombus formation in cerebrovascular arteries and low CBF. It is from the cerebral thrombus that small microemboli, in the form of platelet aggregates and cholesterol crystals, break off and travel to distal areas and lodge, producing the ischemic attack. Cerebral or cerebellar artery thrombosis is most commonly responsible for TIAs. Low flow will also result in a TIA when the CBF is sufficiently reduced in stenosed arteries. Other causes include emboli from the heart caused by valvular disease or endocardial damage and increased blood viscosity from conditions such as polycythemia. Polycythemia is an uncommon cause of TIA. Transient monocular blindness (TMB), although not a TIA, is a focal retinal deficit caused by localized retinal ischemia.

CEREBRAL EMBOLISM

Any region of the brain can be affected by embolism; however, the area or territory of the middle cerebral artery is commonly involved. Embolism may result from pieces or fragments of an arterial thrombus that have broken off or from a heart valve vegetation. Occasionally, an embolus may form from an ulcerated atheromatous plaque. Other forms of embolism such as air, fat, or tumor cells occur only rarely. Cerebral embolism from bacterial sepsis occurs frequently, but bacterial emboli large enough to produce a stroke are infrequent. After breaking off from a thrombus or heart valve vegetation, an embolism usually circulates until it is too large to traverse the arterial lumen. The point of occlusion may be at a bifurcation or other narrowed area. Both hemispheres of the brain appear to be equally affected. Hemorrhagic transformation frequently occurs in the embolic process because of the reperfusion of blood into the ischemic tissue, causing hemorrhage, and the area of the middle cerebral artery is often the involved site. The size of the embolus may vary from large to very small; in fact, the embolus may be so small that it produces no infarct or produces an infarct so small that it cannot be detected.

Cerebral embolism secondary to thrombotic disease usually has a rapid onset and it is not preceded by a TIA. This rapid onset is problematic because there is less time for collateral circulation to develop as in cerebral thrombosis. As a result, embolic strokes are often functionally devastating. Cerebral embolism may result from heart disease. It is currently recognized that cardiogenic embolism accounts for 20% of all ischemic strokes. Embolism has been associated with many types of heart disease, and the following discussion focuses on the most common types (Table 18–3).

CARDIOGENIC EMBOLISM AND ATRIAL FIBRILLATION

Chronic atrial fibrillation (AF) is the most common cause of cardiogenic embolism and is the most common sustained dysrhythmia. The incidence of AF increases with age, such that 2% to 5% of patients older than 60 years of age have AF, and more than half of AF-associated strokes occur in individuals older than 75 years.[22]

Patients with nonvalvular atrial fibrillation have about the same stroke risk as patients who experience a TIA. Atrial fibrillation enhances the development of left atrial thrombi and arterial embolism. The most common site (75%) in which left atrial thrombi form in patients with nonvalvular AF (NVAF) is the atrial appendage rather than the atrial wall. Patients with AF and valvular disease have thrombi both on the atrial wall and on the appendage in equal incidence. Factors involved in the pathogenesis of atrial thrombus formation in patients with AF include increased left atrial pressure and outflow obstruction. Mitral valve obstruction, such as stenosis, can enhance left atrial stasis similar to that seen in AF alone. Enlargement of the

TABLE 18–3. Major Causes of Cardiogenic Cerebral Embolism

Nonvalvular atrial fibrillation	50%
Coronary heart disease	20%
Myocardial infarction	
Rheumatic heart disease	15%
Mitral stenosis ± atrial fibrillation	
Prosthetic cardiac valves	10%
Other	5%
Cardiomyopathy	
Cardiac tumors	
Septic endocarditis	
Nonbacterial thrombotic endocarditis (marantic)	
Congenital heart disease	
Venous clots/intracardiac shunt (paradoxic emboli)	
Mitral annulus calcification	
Calcific aortic stenosis	
Mitral valve prolapse	

From Easton JD, Hart RG, Sherman DG, et al. Diagnosis and management of ischemic stroke. Part 1. Threatened stroke and its management. Curr Prob Cardiol 1983;8:20.

left atrium occurs in AF, and the incidence of thrombus formation increases with left atrial enlargement. Damage to the endothelial surface could also induce thrombus formation and initiate AF. Such disorders as rheumatic heart disease, myocardial infarction, and pericarditis can also initiate AF by involvement of the sinoatrial node and change the atrial endothelial surface such that thrombus formation is enhanced. The risk of stroke in patients with AF is high, and 20% to 35% of all patients with AF will have an embolic stroke of clinical significance.[22] The risk of stroke in those with AF is five to six times that of the general population and averages about 5% per year. Those at greatest risk are those patients with AF and rheumatic valvular disease. The risk for development of systemic embolism for these individuals is 17 times that of the general population. The largest group of patients comprises those with NVAF; their rate of systemic embolism is around 35% and their stroke risk is six times that of the general population.[22]

Predictors of stroke risk in AF include history of hypertension, prior stroke or transient ischemic attack, diabetes, and recent (within 3 months) heart failure. Risk factors have been identified by various authors and groups and are summarized in the literature.[23] The clinical utility of this risk stratification will be discussed under treatment. Even those patients with idiopathic AF have an increased rate of embolism of 7% in the first year, and up to 14% at 5 years of AF. The presence of carotid stenosis may also help to identify a subgroup of NVAF who are at higher risk of stroke.[24] Patients who develop AF have a high rate of embolus formation soon after the onset of AF. Recurrence of embolism is frequent. Up to 50% of patients who develop one embolus develop another. In addition, changing the rhythm by cardioversion increases the rate of embolus occurrence, and about 2% of these patients may develop an embolus the first few days after cardioversion of AF to normal sinus rhythm. Generally, anticoagulation should be used 3 weeks before conversion and continued 4 weeks postconversion.[25–27] Studies are ongoing concerning the need for reversion to normal sinus rhythm versus ventricular rate control in AF.[28]

Ischemic heart disease and ischemic stroke share the same risk factors, and most younger patients with TIAs and stroke die from myocardial infarction. In myocardial infarction, the primary cause of emboli is mural thrombus formation in the left ventricle. Thrombus formation is thought to be started by platelet adherence to and deposition on the damaged (infarcted) akinetic or dyskinetic endocardial surface. There is also an inflammatory white cell response in the damaged area secondary to the tissue infarction. Additionally, the infarcted area may develop into an aneurysmal region where fibrin accumulation can occur. Mural thrombus formation depends on the size and location of the infarct. Thrombus formation and the presence of apical akinesis or dyskinesis are seen almost exclusively in anterior myocardial infarctions. Aneurysms occur most frequently in the apex region of the heart. About 50% to 60% of patients with aneurysm formation in the left ventricle develop a mural thrombus. Most of these mural thrombi develop within the first week of the acute myocardial infarction (AMI), and patients who have mural thrombi as evidenced by echocardiography after anterior AMI are most probably those patients at risk for eventual embolization.[29] The overall incidence of systemic emboli in patients who suffer an anterior AMI is around 5% to 6% and is similar to the incidence in those patients who develop a left ventricular aneurysm. Therefore, of the 50% to 60% of patients with an aneurysm who develop a mural thrombus, only 5% to 6% develop a systemic embolus. In patients surviving AMI who develop congestive heart failure, the risk of stroke is approximately 2% per year, and it is increased during the first 3 months after AMI.[30–34] Risk factors for stroke in patients surviving AMI are advanced age, presence of AF, prior stroke, previous MI, and left ventricular dysfunction as shown by echocardiography. Therefore, cardiogenic embolism may be likely if there is severe impairment of left ventricular function or if there is a left ventricular thrombus that is mobile or protruding.

VALVULAR HEART DISEASE

Thromboembolism is commonly found in patients with valvular heart disease, such as rheumatic mitral disease, and in those with prosthetic heart valves. Mitral stenosis is also associated with an increased risk of thromboembolism. Thrombus formation in patients with valvular disease or prosthetic valves most often occurs in the left ventricle or on the prosthetic valve. Thrombi can also form, but with a lower incidence, in the left atrium.

In valvular heart disease, those patients with mitral stenosis and those with mitral stenosis combined with incompetence of the mitral valve have a thromboembolic prevalance of 15% to 20%. Up to 16% of these events may be fatal. Patients with only mitral incompetence are at less risk than those with mitral stenosis and the embolic rate is approximately 3%, although this rate may be higher in patients with a severe form of mitral incompetence. Prolapse of the mitral valve appears to carry a very low risk of embolism. The risk of embolism also appears to be low in patients with aortic valve disease. Additional factors that increase risk for systemic embolism in patients with valvular disease are atrial fibrillation, increased left atrial size, increased age, and history of a previous embolic event. Atrial fibrillation is the most important single risk factor and, as noted previously, thrombus formation is rare in patients with a normal sinus rhythm. Atrial fibrillation is closely associated with mitral valve disease and emboli may develop shortly after fibrillation develops. Enlargement of the left atrium usually occurs with mitral valve disease, and left atrial enlargement predisposes to atrial fibrillation; therefore, there is an indirect relationship between left atrial enlargement and embolism. Recurrent embolic events can occur in up to 20% of mitral stenosis patients with previous embolic history. The mortality rate is quite high in this group of patients and may reach 42%.

PROSTHETIC CARDIAC VALVES

Thrombus formation on prosthetic cardiac valves (PCVs), whether aortic or mitral valves, is related to the production of turbulence in blood flow by the valve and the thrombogenic potential of the valve material. Patients who have had PCV replacement are at long-term risk of arterial thrombolism. Examples of mechanical valves currently used are the Starr–Edwards ball valve, Bjork–Shiley disk valve, St. Jude Medical, and others. The early Starr–Edwards valve used in the 1960s may have a higher embolic rate than those used in recent years. This may be a result of improved operative procedures and valve factors, as well as less severe disease and better atrial and ventricular function. The embolism rate with the Bjork–Shiley valve is similar to that with the Starr–Edwards valve; however, a newer material, pyrolytic carbon, in the disk of the valve is less thrombogenic and the embolism rate is lower. The bioprosthetic valves, such as the Hancock, Carpentier–Edwards, and Lonescu–Shiley, have a different, central flow design. This design produces less turbulence in blood flow, and the biologic material (porcine valve) is less thrombogenic, and thromboembolism occurs less frequently than with the other valves. Other risk factors include atrial fibrillation, large left atrium, valve placement in the mitral position, inadequate anticoagulation, multiple PCVs, and a previous embolic event.

The overall risk of neurologic deficit with mechanical prosthetic valve-induced embolism is high. For instance, data from follow-up of the older Starr–Edwards ball valve show that 85% of systemic emboli entered the cerebral circulation and 50% of these emboli resulted in a neurologic deficit, with 10% of all embolic events being fatal. Overall, the rate of embolism in anticoagulated patients with mechanical PCVs averages 3% per year for mitral valves and 1.5% per year for aortic valves.[34] Embolic rates for nonanticoagulated patients with bioprosthetic valves are 2% to 4% per year. A new stentless porcine tissue aortic valve from St. Jude Medical has recently received FDA approval. This valve does not have the plastic or metal support structure that other tissue valves have, and it may be more similar to the natural heart valve. Postmarketing follow-up is necessary to determine the place in treatment of this valve. There is general agreement that all adults with any type of mechanical valve should be on long-term anticoagulation, and that bioprosthetic valves also require treatment with short-term anticoagulation and optional long-term antiplatelet therapy.[35]

INFECTIVE ENDOCARDITIS

Emboli may result from bacterial vegetations that can form in infective endocarditis. Arterial emboli are one of the most frequent complications of this disease. Major cerebral emboli have been observed in nearly one-third of patients with endocarditis, with the middle cerebral artery and its branches being most frequently involved. The highest frequency of major embolic events occurs in association with infections on the left side of the heart that produce large, mobile vegetations from *Haemophilus parainfluenzae,* or slow-growing fastidious, gram-negative bacilli, fungi *(Aspergillus),* and *Streptococcus viridans.* Emboli from the right side of the heart, as seen in intravenous drug abusers, are often caused by staphylococcal organisms and can produce clinical manifestations of pulmonary emboli. Cerebral emboli from right-sided endocarditis can also occur if the patient has a patent foramen ovale (PFO). About 15% of adults have PFO. There is another type of endocarditis, called nonbacterial, thrombotic endocarditis (NBTE), in which sterile thrombi are present on the valves. This condition is seen most often in patients with mucin-secreting adenocarcinomas and other debilitating diseases. This process is nonbacterial and the vegetations are composed mainly of platelets and fibrin thrombi. Formation of systemic emboli has an average incidence of 42%.[36]

UNUSUAL AND OTHER CAUSES OF INFARCTION

Other causes of cerebral infarction are listed in Table 18–4.

INTRACRANIAL HEMORRHAGE

Hemorrhage is the third most frequent cause of stroke. Approximately 15% of cases of stroke are due to intracranial hemorrhage. The more frequent causes of stroke from intracranial hemorrhage are hypertensive intracerebral hemorrhage, ruptured saccular aneurysms, hemorrhage associated with bleeding disorders, anticoagulation, and arteriovenous malformations (AVMs).

Hypertensive intracerebral hemorrhage occurs generally when the blood pressure is significantly elevated. The bleeding occurs in the brain tissue as a result of the rupture of an artery. This allows for an extravasation of blood into the brain tissue, which forms a mass. This mass damages the tissue and continues to enlarge as bleeding continues. Brain tissue is pushed, displaced, and compressed and brain functions may be impaired. The larger the hemorrhage, the greater the displacement of tissue. Escape of blood into the ventricles of the brain can occur, and when this happens, the spinal fluid becomes bloody. The cerebrospinal fluid may remain clear if the hemorrhage is small or at a distance from the ventricular system. The extravascular blood un-

TABLE 18–4. Unusual Causes of Infarction

Venous thrombosis	Contraceptive steroid use
Systemic hypotension	Polycythemia
Arteriography	Idiopathic thrombocytosis
Carotid occlusion	Dissecting aortic aneurysm
Arteritis	Hypercoagulable states
Moyamoya disease	

TABLE 18–5. Causes of Intracranial Hemorrhage

Hypertensive intracerebral hemorrhage
Lobar hemorrhage of undetermined cause and intracerebral hemorrhage associated with congophilic angiopathy (analyzed)
Ruptured saccular aneurysm, giant aneurysm, or mycotic aneurysm
Ruptured angioma
Hemorrhagic disorders: leukemia, aplastic anemia, thrombocytopenic purpura, liver disease, complication of anticoagulant therapy, hyperfibrinolysis, hypofibrinogenemia, hemophilia, Christmas disease
Trauma, including posttraumatic apoplexy
Hemorrhage into primary and secondary brain tissue
Hemorrhagic infarction, arterial or venous
Inflammatory disease of the arteries and veins
Miscellaneous rare types: after vasopressor drugs, upon exertion, during arteriography, during painful urologic examination, as a late complication of early-life carotid occlusion, complication of carotid–cavernous arteriovenous fistula, with anoxemia, migraine, teratomatous malformations (acute inclusion body encephalitis produces xanthochromia and up to 2000 red blood cells or more in the cerebrospinal fluid; acute necrotizing hemorrhagic encephalopathy may be associated with up to 100 red blood cells in the cerebrospinal fluid; tularemia and snake venom poisoning may cause bloody cerebrospinal fluid)

From Braunwald E, Isselbacher KJ, et al, eds. Harrison's Principles of Internal Medicine, 11th ed. New York, McGraw-Hill, 1987:1952, with permission.

dergoes changes such as phagocytosis, and the mass gradually shrinks; after 2 to 6 months, only discoloration is left at the site. Hemorrhagic infarcts, discussed earlier, are due primarily to the reflow or reperfusion of ischemic tissue, with resultant bleeding into the tissue. In hypertensive hemorrhage, the vessels most often involved are the penetrating arteries in the putamen and internal capsule and parts of the white matter, including the frontal lobe, thalamus, pons, and cerebellar hemisphere. Causes of intracranial hemorrhage are listed in Table 18–5.

CLINICAL PRESENTATION AND DIAGNOSIS

ATHEROTHROMBOTIC DISEASE

Thrombosis of cerebral vessels produces variable clinical manifestations as compared to embolic disease or intracranial hemorrhage. In a large percentage of cases (> 50%), the stroke is preceded by one or more transient ischemic attacks. If the evolving thrombosis involves the internal carotid and middle cerebral arteries, then such focal symptoms as mono- or hemiplegia, mono- or hemiparesthesia, blindness in one eye, and speech disturbance may occur. If the vertebrobasilar system is involved, such symptoms as dizziness, diplopia, numbness, impaired vision, and dysarthria may occur. Usually these attacks are short-lived and resolve in less than 10 minutes. The stroke itself most often develops suddenly as a single attack, or it may show an intermittent or stuttering progression pattern over hours to days. Additionally, a patient may suffer a partial stroke, improve for several hours, then develop full paralysis of one or more parts of the body; other parts become paralyzed in a stepwise manner until the stroke is completed. When the thrombosis produces a developing involvement over hours, days, or weeks, it is called stroke in evolution or progressing stroke. Interestingly, the majority of cerebral thrombotic strokes occur at rest while sleeping or after arising. Headache may occur, but is often absent; when present, it may occur several days prior to the other symptoms of the stroke.

Diagnosis consists of evaluation of the clinical presentation and laboratory findings. Laboratory evaluation can include tests such as cerebral arteriography, imaging studies such as CT with or without contrast enhancement, MRI, radioactive brain scan study (such as a technetium scan), x-rays of the head, electroencephalogram, ECG, transcranial Doppler studies, digital subtraction angiogram, and lumbar puncture (LP). The definitive test for arterial occlusion or narrowing is the arteriogram; however, the procedure carries a neurologic risk itself and should only be used if the diagnosis of vascular disease is not clear or if vascular surgery is a possibility, such as in carotid TIA patients. Complications from cerebral angiography occur in 2% to 12% of patients and consist primarily of aortic or carotid dissection and embolic stroke. Hydration may reduce these risks. Because of the risks of arteriography, brain imaging is the most important test after a stroke has occurred. When it is performed, transfemoral angiography is usually the procedure of choice as compared with the direct carotid puncture procedure. The CT scan in cerebral thrombosis usually shows an area of decreased attenuation or hypodense lesion in the infarcted area. The CT scan is often normal, however, during the first 48 hours after the thrombotic infarction. The CT scan is extremely useful in excluding tumors and identifying intracranial hemorrhage, both of which dictate different treatment modalities. CT scans, however, may not show small ischemic strokes, especially on the cortical surface, and bone may cause difficulty in interpretation. MRI can adequately detect small infarcts in the cortical surface and elsewhere usually within 1 hour of occurrence. MRI is a noninvasive imaging technique that, unlike CT, does not require x-rays or isotopes. MRI uses magnetic fields to generate images and it takes longer to perform than a CT scan.

Radioisotopic brain scans can be helpful and show infarcts earlier than CT scans. Skull x-rays are usually not helpful, and the electroencephalogram and LP are of limited value, because they are usually normal. Noninvasive techniques like Doppler flow studies and Doppler scanning have been developed but have some disadvantages with consistent differentiation of stenosis from occlusion and detection of distal atherosclerosis.

Digital subtraction angiography (DSA) is a recent addition that holds promise as a diagnostic tool. Arterial injection of contrast medium in DSA currently provides better imaging of the cerebral vasculature than does intravenous administration, which gives imperfect detail.

Other new diagnostic imaging techniques include transesophageal echocardiography (TEE); xenon blood flow; positron-emission tomography (PET); single-photon emission computed tomography (SPECT), which can give an image of dynamic physiology after injection of positron-emitting isotopes; and MRI angiography (MRA). TEE is more sensitive than transthoracic echocardiography (TTE) in detection of left atrial thrombi, atrial septal aneurysms, and aortic atheromas.[37] These techniques are very promising advances, and as they become more refined their place in diagnosis will become clear.

Recommendations for imaging of the brain in suspected hemispheric TIA are as follows:

1. CT scan, without contrast, to exclude other lesions that may produce TIA-like manifestations, such as a tumor.
2. MRI is not routinely recommended over CT unless CT is a failure.
3. Routine use of MRI in vertebrobasilar TIA is not recommended.[38]

Recommendations for imaging of the brain in acute stroke are as follows:

1. CT of the head, without contrast, can detect almost 100% of hemorrhages.
2. Follow-up CT without contrast 2 to 7 days after the acute event if the initial CT was negative, in order to document potential hemorrhagic transformation or to determine the location of the infarction.
3. MRI is not recommended for routine evaluation in acute stroke.[38]

LACUNAR INFARCTS

The clinical presentation varies depending on the perforating cerebral arteries involved. The most frequently occurring lacunar syndrome is pure motor hemiparesis, which is due to an infarct in the posterior portion of the internal capsule. This infarct results from occlusion of a middle or posterior cerebral perforating artery. The manifestations of the pure motor hemiparesis syndrome are hemiparesis or hemiplegia of the arm, leg, face, and trunk. In addition, a mild dysarthria occurs without sensory or consciousness alterations or visual field defects. The different parts of the body involved in the stroke display the same degree of weakness. This is in contrast to a stroke in the cortical region involving the middle or anterior cerebral artery, where there is usually an unequal degree of weakness of the affected parts of the body.

Diagnosis is usually based on clinical evaluation of the patient after careful neurologic examination. A CT or MRI scan can provide evidence of the infarction if performed within about 7 to 10 days of the event; however, infarcts smaller than 2 mm may be missed. Treatment after lacunar strokes requires control of hypertension to help in the prevention of progression of the degenerative occlusive process.

TRANSIENT ISCHEMIC ATTACKS

Most TIAs last 5 to 10 minutes, and those lasting 1 or more hours may be a result of embolism rather than ischemia or atherosclerosis. An ischemic event that lasts longer than 24 hours but completely resolves in a short period (up to 3 weeks) is termed a reversible ischemic neurologic defect (RIND). A TIA resulting from a carotid system lesion and anterior cerebral artery involvement manifests as weakness in the opposite leg and shoulder. If the anterior cortical branches of the middle cerebral artery are involved, a sensory and motor loss results in the contralateral face, arm, and hand. If the ischemia is in the dominant hemisphere, a nonfluent (Broca's) aphasia usually is present. Ischemia occurring in the posterior portions of the middle cerebral artery often produces contralateral sensory loss and homonymous hemianopia (defective vision or blindness affecting the right halves or the left halves of the visual fields of the two eyes). If there is posterior middle cerebral artery involvement in the dominant hemisphere, a fluent aphasia is likely to occur. Ischemia of the lenticulostriate arteries may result in findings that involve motor and sensory defects in the arms, legs, face, and trunk as noted in the discussion of lacunar infarcts. Clinical manifestations of TIAs arising from ischemia in the vertebrobasilar circulation are numerous. Vertigo and ataxia are seen in ischemia affecting cerebellar and vestibular areas. Bilateral weakness of the extremities indicates that the corticospinal nerve tracts are involved as they cross the brainstem.

Diagnosis of a TIA is difficult because the episode is usually over before the patient can be examined. Therefore, the diagnosis is really made on the basis of the patient's recollection of the symptoms. Table 18–6 shows the symptoms of TIAs. There are many singular symptoms or events that can be confused with TIAs and usually are not TIAs. Some of these events are fainting, convulsions, loss of consciousness, dizziness, spots before the eyes, dysarthria, imbalance and falling, and headache. Diagnostic studies may indicate the presence of vascular disease; however, history is a key to the diagnosis of a TIA. Proper attention to the history is important because treatment of TIAs is important in stroke prevention.

Laboratory studies in the diagnosis of TIA should rule out blood or other disorders that may produce decreased cerebral blood flow. Routine studies include erythrocyte sedimentation rate, complete blood count, platelet count, blood chemistry, urinalysis, coagulation profile, and syphilis (serology). To reveal systemic disease in selected patients, serum protein electrophoresis, antinuclear antibody titers, blood and plasma viscosities, plasma fibrinogen, and cerebrospinal fluid (CSF) examination may be performed. Embolism of cardiac origin should be a consideration in every patient with a single TIA. In these cases, a 12-lead ECG should be performed to test for recent myocardial infarction

TABLE 18–6. Symptoms of Transient Ischemic Attacks

Carotid system TIAs
- Unilateral weakness—usually hemiparesis
- Unilateral sensory complaints—numbness, paresthesia
- Aphasia—language comprehension, output, or both
- Monocular visual loss (amaurosis fugax)

Vertebrobasilar system TIAs
- Motor deficit—especially if bilateral
- Sensory complaints—especially if bilateral
- Simultaneous, bilateral visual complaints
- Diplopia, Vertigo, Dysarthria[a], Ataxia without weakness, Dysphagia — Only in combination, not as isolated symptoms

Either carotid or vertebral TIAs
- Severe dysarthria[a]
- Homonymous visual complaints

Isolated symptoms rarely resulting from TIAs
- Vertigo, dizziness
- Diplopia
- Loss of consciousness
- Confusion
- Bilateral leg weakness, falling spells

[a]Often difficult to distinguish from nonfluent dysphasia on the basis of history.
From Easton JD, Hart RG, Sherman DG, et al. Diagnosis and management of ischemic stroke. Part 1. Threatened stroke and its management. Curr Prob Cardiol 1983;8:13, with permission.

and/or dysrhythmias such as atrial fibrillation. Other laboratory tests include a chest x-ray to exclude heart enlargement or disease of the valves. In patients suspected of having TIAs of embolic origin, echocardiography is an important diagnostic tool. Two-dimensional echocardiography is indicated in patients with cerebral ischemia who have evidence of cardiac disease such as AF, enlarged heart, and mitral valve prolapse. The yield of thrombus detection in the hearts of these patients is 10% to 20%. The lower limit of clot size that is detected accurately by echocardiography is 2 to 3 mm. In addition, results from the Stroke Prevention in Atrial Fibrillation Investigators (SPAF) studies indicate that echocardiography in NVAF can serve as a clinical predictor of thromboembolism by detecting increased left atrial size and left ventricular dysfunction.[23,31] Left atrial size and left ventricular size are strong independent predictors of later thromboembolism. Therefore, the echocardiogram can add to the clinical variables for risk stratification. If TTE detects an embolic source, TEE is generally not necessary. As mentioned earlier, cerebral angiography should be performed only in selected patients, and patients who have had a carotid TIA should be studied with angiography as soon as reasonably possible because of the high risk of cerebral infarction in these patients.

CEREBRAL EMBOLISM AND CARDIOGENIC EMBOLISM

Cardiogenic brain embolism is the major cause of cerebral embolism. The brain is involved in approximately 70% of all emboli from the heart, whereas systemic or noncerebral nervous system emboli often go unrecognized. Cardiogenic brain embolism accounts for 20% of all ischemic strokes. The clinical diagnosis is based on a variety of findings (Table 18–7). The onset is characteristically abrupt, often occurring in an awake patient.

TABLE 18–7. Clinical Features Suggestive of Cardiogenic Brain Embolism

Primary Features
- Abrupt onset of maximal deficit
- Presence of a potential embolic source
- Infarct involving the cerebral cortex or cerebellum
- Previous ischemic events in other vascular territories

Secondary Evidence
- Hemorrhagic infarct by CAT
- Absence of occlusive cerebrovascular disease by cerebral angiography or reliable noninvasive imaging
- Angiographic evidence of vanishing occlusions
- Evidence of embolism to other organs
- Cardiac thrombi demonstrated by echocardiography, catheterization, cardiac CAT, or MRI

From Sherman DG, Dyken ML, Fisher M, et al. Cerebral embolism. Chest 1986;89(suppl 2):845, Table 2, with permission.

A stuttering course may be seen in about 10% of patients. This represents a distal lodging of emboli. Most cardiogenic emboli that go to the brain lodge in the middle cerebral artery (MCA) or one of its branches. Vertebrobasilar or anterior cerebral artery emboli occur less frequently (< 10%) than MCA emboli. Cardiogenic embolism may be suspected when there are multifocal neurologic findings. Seizure or headache at the onset of the stroke is not as useful an indicator as once thought. Cardiogenic embolism should be considered when the following conditions are present: age over 60, sudden onset of maximal neurologic deficit, prior cortical infarct, past history of valvular heart disease or left ventricular myocardial infarct, and atrial fibrillation or congestive heart failure. Laboratory studies in those with suspected cardiogenic brain embolism may include two-dimensional echocardiography to assess the presence of left ventricular thrombi and mitral valve dysfunction, and M-mode echocardiography for the presence of left ventricular dysfunction. Echocardiography does not reliably indicate atrial thrombi, although transesophogeal echocardiography (TEE) may be better at detection than two-dimensional echocardiography. The ECG may indicate a dysrhythmia such as AF. MRI and CT are currently being evaluated for their clinical usefulness in detecting cardiogenic emboli.

INTRACRANIAL HEMORRHAGE

Usually the clinical manifestations of intracranial hemorrhage have an abrupt onset, and changes generally occur over minutes to hours (up to 24 hours). This gradual evolution depends primarily on the bleeding rate and accounts for the time range for the neurologic deficit to become maximal. The neurologic physical findings vary with the site of bleeding and the size of the bleed. The majority of patients lose consciousness, and many die without recovering awareness.

Typically, the patient with spontaneous intracerebral hemorrhage may experience head pain and dizziness prior to losing consciousness. In the case of hypertension-related external capsule (putaminal) hemorrhage, the patient quickly develops signs of hemiplegia and loss of consciousness. Hypertensive intracerebral hemorrhages are most often associated with prolonged and sustained hypertension and frequently occur while the patient is awake.

Conjugate deviation of the eyes to the side opposite the affected limbs is commonly seen. If the lesion becomes larger, compression of the upper brainstem produces deepening coma and the patient has dilated and fixed pupils, Babinski signs, bilateral motor hypertonus, and irregular respirations.

In the case of internal capsule (thalamic) hemorrhage, the onset is similar to that for putamenal hemorrhage; however, if the patient is still alert, a homonymous hemianopia may be seen because of optic nerve involvement in the internal capsule. The location of this hemorrhage produces a variety of gaze disturbances including defective vertical and lateral gaze, fixed downward deviation of the eyes, and unequal pupils. The reader is referred to other sources for discussion of other types of intracranial hemorrhage.

In the diagnosis of hypertensive intracerebral hemorrhage the sudden onset and quick evolution of the physical findings are important. Headache occurs at the onset in approximately 50% of the cases, whereas the occurrence of headaches in thromboembolism is less than 25%. Neck rigidity is common and the funduscopic examination of the eye may reveal periarteriolar hemorrhages and decreased arteriolar size. Ocular signs are very helpful in localizing hemorrhages of putaminal and thalamic origin. Convulsions are common, as is vomiting, and a history of hypertension is an important clue. Generally, the immediate prognosis for intracerebral hemorrhage is extremely poor, with up to 70% of patients dying in a few days.

Important laboratory findings include evidence of bleeding on the CT scan. CT, without contrast, is the diagnostic procedure of choice in assessing intracranial and subarachnoid hemorrhage. It is extremely sensitive in detection of blood in very small amounts, as noted earlier, and is extremely useful in the differential diagnosis of hemorrhage versus infarction. Lumbar puncture, if performed, is usually done after CT, because LP may induce intracranial hypertension and brain herniation.

▶ TREATMENT: Stroke

GENERAL THERAPEUTIC CONSIDERATIONS

The therapeutic approach to patients with cerebrovascular disease involves multiple phases, including preventive measures against stroke and vascular disease in general, supportive and medical management during the acute phase of a stroke, measures necessary to mitigate the pathologic or atherothrombotic process, and appropriate rehabilitative and physical therapy programs during the poststroke period. Importantly, significant public attention has been focused on stroke (brain attack). The development of practice guidelines, stroke teams, and stroke care units in hospitals have greatly improved the awareness and care of patients with acute stroke.

Prevention of cerebrovascular disease is the most important aspect of therapeutic management, and elimination and/or management of the risk factors discussed earlier in the section on epidemiology and etiology is required. Control of hypertension, hyperlipidemia, obesity, cigarette smoking and other tobacco use, and alcohol use, as well as other risk factors for atherothrombotic disease is essential to the overall care of the patient with cerebrovascular disease. In the patient with hypertension who has atherosclerotic cerebrovascular disease or who has developed an ischemic infarction, care must be taken to avoid drug-induced or other hypotensive episodes. In general, preservation of the systemic circulation in acute stroke, and avoidance of orthostatic changes, are also advised.

SPECIFIC THERAPEUTIC CONSIDERATIONS

As indicated earlier, the focus of this chapter is on ischemic stroke, and the following discussion emphasizes this condition; however, therapeutic management of some of the other types of cerebrovascular disease covered in this chapter is discussed briefly.

ISCHEMIC CEREBROVASCULAR DISEASE

The major goals of treatment for patients with acute ischemic stroke are to (1) remove or limit the obstruction to flow in the vessel and (2) protect brain cells distal to the obstruction or blockage from suffering hypoxic changes. It is currently possible to attain the first goal with thrombolytic and anticoagulation therapy; however, neuroprotective therapy is still under study.

ANTICOAGULATION THERAPY

Anticoagulation therapy was the first to gain acceptance in ischemic cerebrovascular disease, and because this therapy has been used for some time, some conclusions can be drawn about the usefulness of anticoagulation in various types of ischemic cerebrovascular disease. A number of studies have been performed with heparin and coumarin derivatives since the 1970s; however, criticisms of poor design, wrong diagnosis, and inadequate number of patients for comparative purposes have limited the acceptance of these studies.

The following is a brief review of anticoagulation therapy in TIA, progressing stroke, and completed stroke.[39–42]

Transient Ischemic Attacks.

Four randomized prospective studies comparing patients on anticoagulation therapy to control subjects showed no significant difference in the occurrence of stroke or death. Only one of the four studies was a double-blind study; all had small numbers of patients, and three studies had short follow-up periods. Although weak, data from these studies indicate that the rate of recurrence of TIAs is reduced. Definite conclusions regarding anticoagulation cannot be stated on the basis of these studies. Six nonrandomized studies have been reported and no reduction was shown in mortality; however, one study did show a decreased incidence of TIAs and one showed a decrease in recurrence of TIAs. It appears from the literature that anticoagulation does not decrease mortality in TIA patients, but it may reduce the rate of recurrence of TIAs and subsequent ischemic infarction.

Progressing Stroke (Stroke-in-Evolution)

Three randomized and three nonrandomized studies strongly suggest that anticoagulation is of benefit in this condition. Although these studies are strongly suggestive, they are not conclusive because of flaws in study design. There were only slight differences in mortality in the treated groups (most patients were heparinized); however, there were favorable trends reported in the prevention of stroke progression. Other more recent data point out the variability of patient response to the heparin anticoagulation of acute brain ischemia and the problem of intracerebral hemorrhage in stroke patients. It appears that although conclusive statements cannot be made because efficacy is unproven, heparin anticoagulation is still an anecdotal therapy, and if it is to be used at all in the acute phase of a progressing stroke it must be made certain that cerebral hemorrhage has not occurred.

Completed Stroke

Seven randomized studies have addressed anticoagulation therapy in completed stroke. These studies showed no difference between treatment and control groups in the incidence of recurrent stroke or death. There is also a risk of major bleeding in patients treated for several months with anticoagulation therapy. Therefore, the risk of anticoagulation therapy in completed stroke outweighs any benefits obtained, and based on the best studies to date, anticoagulation generally should not be used.

The risk of hemorrhage is highest in patients with ischemic cerebrovascular disease when anticoagulation therapy lasts longer than 4 weeks. Compared with other indications for anticoagulation, anticoagulation for stroke is associated with a greater risk of hemorrhagic complications. Although intensity of therapy and type of reagents used in laboratory testing were the source of some of the differences in European and North American studies, hemorrhagic complications are still the major risk in anticoagulated patients with ischemic cerebrovascular disease.

Recommendations and Monitoring

It is recommended that anticoagulation not be routinely used in patients with TIAs and not be used at all in patients with completed stroke. Prophylaxis of thromboembolism is important in patients with completed stroke since prior stroke is a risk factor for another stroke. Aspirin 325 mg/d can be recommended. Alternatively, ticlopidine 250 mg twice daily or clopidogrel 75 mg/d can be used. The use of anticoagulation in progressing stroke is still controversial; however, individual judgment must be used in this situation when intracerebral hemorrhage has been ruled out by CT scan. Short-term anticoagulation may be useful in TIA patients who refuse surgery for a surgically correctable lesion, who are not surgical candidates for whatever reason, or who are awaiting surgery. Patients who remain symptomatic with TIAs and on aspirin therapy who do not have surgical disease may be candidates for anticoagulation. Some would use a combination of aspirin and ticlopidine or clopidogrel if aspirin alone fails; however, there are no data to support this approach. If anticoagulation is used, careful monitoring is required, and heparin should be administered acutely by continuous infusion to a target partial thromboplastin time of 1.5 times control value. In general, if warfarin is to be used to continue chronic anticoagulation, it should overlap with heparin for approximately 5 days to obtain warfarin antithrombotic activity. By maintaining an international normalized ratio of 2.0 to 3.0, a slightly less intensive anticoagulation effect is obtained with a decreased incidence of bleeding without a decrease in efficacy.[43] Continuous monitoring for minor and major bleeding is required. The use of special anticoagulation services can be of significant assistance in the therapy and monitoring of patients on warfarin therapy and is recommended whenever possible.

PHARMACOLOGIC THERAPY

ANTIPLATELET THERAPY

Antiplatelet agents have been studied for use in ischemic cerebrovascular disease for a number of years; the proposed mechanism of action is an alteration in blood platelet aggregation, thus inhibiting the formation of thrombi in arterial vessels. Several antiplatelet agents have been used; however, aspirin and triclopidine are the only agents currently commercially available with convincing clinical effects.

Aspirin

The antiplatelet effects of aspirin are theoretically responsible for aspirin's beneficial antithrombotic effects in TIAs. Aspirin inhibits platelet aggregation by irreversible inactivation of the enzyme cyclooxygenase which, in platelets, prevents conversion of arachidonic acid to thromboxane A_2 (TXA_2), which is a powerful vasoconstrictor and stimulator of platelet aggregation. Platelets remain impaired for their life span (5 to 7 days) after exposure to aspirin. Aspirin also inhibits prostacyclin activity in the smooth muscle of vascular walls. PGI_2 inhibits platelet aggregation, and the vascular endothelium can synthesize prostacyclin such that the platelet antiaggregating effect is maintained. The suppression of PGI_2 production by aspirin has been found to be dose and duration related; the higher the dose, the longer the cyclooxygenase production is suppressed. Therefore, the lower the aspirin dose, the less effect on prostacyclin. The optimal dose of aspirin is still under study, but it should be the dose that inhibits TXA_2 with the least amount of prostacyclin inhibition. It has been shown that an aspirin dose of 325 mg/d will inhibit TXA_2 but will not significantly inhibit PGI_2 production. There is probably a point at which lower doses of aspirin do not completely block TXA_2, and recent studies indicate the lowest effective dose may be in the range of 30 to 40 mg/d.

Aspirin (acetylsalicylic acid) was found in the early 1970s to prevent amaurosis fugax (monocular visual loss) and to decrease the number of TIAs without affecting the death rate. The Canadian Cooperative Study Group was published in 1978.[44] This study involved treatment of 585 patients with one or more cerebral or retinal ischemic attacks. These patients were randomized to aspirin, sulfinpyrazone, and placebo. The average follow-up was 26 months and the aspirin dose was 325 mg four times daily and sulfinpyrazone 200 mg four times daily. For the overall study group, aspirin reduced the risk of TIA, stroke, or death by 19%. If only stroke or death was considered, aspirin reduced the risk of these by 31%. Interestingly, there was no significant benefit shown for women in this study, however, this sex difference was not confirmed in later studies.[45] Sulfinpyrazone did not show any risk reduction for TIA. Other randomized trials have been done and all show statistically significant differences between aspirin and placebo for some ischemic events.

The doses of aspirin used in ischemic cerebrovascular disease studies have ranged from 30 mg/d to 1.5 g/d. A controversy still exists over the appropriate dose of aspirin. Although low doses of aspirin (325 mg/d) have been shown to be effective in other conditions such as protection against myocardial infarction in unstable angina patients, prevention of coronary bypass shunt thrombosis, and prevention of thrombosis in arteriovenous shunts of chronic hemodialysis patients, the effectiveness of low doses in preventing stroke is still controversial. One of the recent studies to address the low-dose issue is the United Kingdom Transient Ischemic Attack/Aspirin Trial (UKTIA).[46] This is the first large study to evaluate low versus high dose (300 versus 1200 mg/d). Between July 1979 and September 1985, 2435 patients were enrolled in the study. All patients had experienced at least one TIA or mild ischemic stroke within 3 months of entry. The mean age was 60, and 75% of patients were male. Patients were randomly assigned to three groups. One group received 600 mg aspirin twice daily, the second group received 300 mg daily, and the third group received placebo. The dose ranges were selected somewhat arbitrarily, and patients were followed an average of 4 years. Results that have been reported indicate that the incidence of stroke, myocardial infarction, or sudden death was the same in both aspirin-treated groups and 20% lower (statistically significant) than the incidence in the placebo-treated groups. The risk of cerebral infarction alone was 11% higher in the placebo group, although this was not statistically significant. When women were considered separately in the study, no significant differences were found between aspirin and placebo in risk for cerebral infarction or other major vascular event. The investigators note, however, that the number of women in the study was small. Side effects were less frequent with the lower dose of aspirin (29%) as compared with the 1200-mg dose (39%) and were least frequent in the placebo group (24%). Therefore, the lower dose of aspirin in this study was just as effective as the higher dose and had fewer side effects. Although this study showed that aspirin had less effect on fatal events than on nonfatal events, antiplatelet treatment conclusively reduces the risk of nonfatal vascular events.

Another recent study to address the low-dose aspirin issue is the Dutch TIA Trial.[47] This study was a double-blind trial in patients with TIAs or nondisabling stroke. This particular study had a different twist in that two main hypotheses were tested; first was the question of the effectiveness of 30 mg/d of aspirin versus 300 mg/d in preventing vascular death and disability; second was the question of whether 50 mg of atenolol was more effective than placebo in preventing vascular death and disability. A double randomization technique was used to compare these two different therapeutic modalities. A total of 3131 patients were enrolled and follow-up was 2.6 years. It was found that 30 mg/d of aspirin was no less effective than 300 mg/d in the prevention of the composite outcome event of death from vascular causes, nonfatal stroke, or nonfatal myocardial infarction. There were also fewer adverse effects in the 30 mg/d group. Therefore, a dose of 30 mg/d of aspirin was effective in TIA prevention.

Meta-analysis of 29,000 patients with histories of TIAs, minor strokes, unstable angina, or myocardial infarction was reported by the Antiplatelet Trialists' Collaboration. This analysis represented 25 trials. All antiplatelet agents and regimens were evaluated. Results of the analysis showed an overall 25% odds reduction (similar to relative risk reduction) for vascular events (stroke, myocardial infarction, or death from a vascular cause) and a 27% odds reduction in nonfatal stroke. A second meta-analysis from this group evaluated more than 100,000 patients in 145 trials.[48] A 25% overall odds reduction was shown for vascular events and 22% for patients with previous minor stroke or TIAs.

Pharmacodynamically, as aspirin is converted to salicylate during the normal metabolic process, the ratio of salicylate to aspirin may be important because salicylate may prevent aspirin inhibition of PGI_2. Excessive salicylate concentrations may displace or prevent aspirin from binding to platelets, thereby potentially minimizing the antiplatelet effect of aspirin. Whether or not this proves to be clinically relevant remains to be shown in clinical studies. The interaction can be minimized by using low doses and sustained-release preparations. There is also some suggestion that a specific dose of aspirin in a specific patient may work at one point in time but at a later time may be ineffective.

Dipyridamole

Dipyridamole has weak inhibiting properties *in vitro* on platelet aggregation and also inhibits platelet phosphodiesterase. Clinical studies have not yielded supportive data for the use of this drug in ischemic cerebrovascular disease, and dipyridamole alone has no role in stroke prevention.[49]

Sulfinpyrazone

Sulfinpyrazone has been studied in several trials for ischemic cerebrovascular disease. Sulfinpyrazone, like aspirin, produces an inhibition of cyclooxygenase; however, this inhibition is reversible, whereas the aspirin inhibition is not. The drug has metabolites that also have inhibitory effects on cyclooxygenase. Clinical studies have found no beneficial effect for sulfinpyrazone in the treatment of ischemic cerebrovascular disease.[44]

Ticlopidine

Ticlopidine has unique platelet antiaggregatory effects in that it is an inhibitor of the adenosine diphosphate pathway of platelet aggregation and inhibits known stimuli to platelet aggregation.[50–52] This effect causes an alteration of the platelet membrane and interference with the membrane–fibrinogenic interaction, leading to a blocking of the platelet glycoprotein IIb/IIIa receptor. A time lag of 8 to 11 days before the antiplatelet effect is maximal should be expected. The bleeding time is prolonged up to fivefold and will return to normal in 14 days after discontinuation. Ticlopidine, a thienopyridine, has been evaluated in two large clinical trials, and the results in stroke prevention have been beneficial in both men and women. In the TASS trial, the relative-risk reduction for fatal or nonfatal stroke at 3 years was 21% greater with ticlopidine as compared to aspirin. The CATS trial showed a 30% relative-risk reduction as compared to placebo.[51] Ticlopidine does possess a significant side-effect profile and is costly. Side effects include suppression of bone marrow, rash, diarrhea, and elevation of serum cholesterol. Neutropenia may occur in up to 2% of patients but is reversible on discontinuation of therapy. Monitoring is required because of these side effects, and it is recommended that patients have CBCs with differential every 2 weeks for 3 months. More than 50% of patients report at least one side effect, with gastrointestinal complaints being the most common. Drug interactions may occur with digoxin, theophylline, and antacids and these effects should be monitored. Ticlopidine (500 mg/d) in divided doses of 250 mg/d can be recommended as an alternative to aspirin in those patients who cannot tolerate aspirin or in whom aspirin treatment has not been effective.[52] A new thienopyridine, clopidogrel, is 50 to 100 times as potent as ticlopidine in inhibiting thrombosis and prolonging bleeding time. Clinical effectiveness and tolerability appear similar in preliminary studies using a dose of 75 mg/d. A large international trial has recently been completed (CAPRIE trial) comparing 75 mg/d of clopidogrel to 325 mg/d aspirin in secondary prevention of ischemic disease in 19,000 patients with atherosclerotic disease.[53] The atherosclerotic processes evaluated were ischemic stroke, myocardial infarction, or vascular death. Patients were followed for 1 to 3 years, and intention-to-treat analysis on the first events showed that clopidogrel had an annual 5.32% risk of ischemic stroke, myocardial infarction, or vascular death compared to 5.83% with aspirin. This represents a relative risk reduction of 8.7% (P = .043) in favor of clopidogrel. On-treatment analysis showed a relative risk reduction of 9.4%. Importantly, the safety profile was at least as good as aspirin with regard to bleeding, with no difference as compared to aspirin in neutrophil reduction and no requirement for monitoring for neutropenia. CAPRIE concluded that long-term administration of clopidogrel in patients with the atherosclerotic diseases studied is slightly more effective than aspirin and at least as safe. Clopidogrel can be used in place of ticlopidine but not as a substitute for aspirin.

Recommendations and Monitoring

Clinical trials have shown the beneficial effects of aspirin in men in prevention of secondary TIAs as well as in producing a decrease in major vascular events. A dose of 325 to 1300 mg/d can be recommended in preventing TIAs and stroke.[27] The effectiveness of doses lower than 300 mg/d for TIA or minor strokes of arterial origin is still not resolved and additional study is required to adequately answer the dose questions. Other potential mechanisms of antithrombotic action of aspirin are currently under investigation. An enteric-coated product may be better tolerated by some individuals and may be used if needed. Patients should be monitored for gastrointestinal bleeding because the risk for bleeding is slightly increased. Triclopidine is effective for the secondary prevention of stroke. It is slightly superior to aspirin in patients with TIAs; however, ticlopidine is less tolerable and more costly than aspirin. Ticlopidine 250 mg twice daily should be used if aspirin has failed to decrease or eliminate TIAs or if the patient cannot tolerate or has an allergy to aspirin. Patients require careful monitoring while on ticlopidine as noted previously, particularly during the first 3 months of therapy. Clopidogrel has similar efficacy to ticlopidine and appears to have a better safety profile and could serve as an alternative to ticlopidine.

THROMBOLYTIC THERAPY

Thrombolytic therapy for acute ischemic stroke was first proposed in the 1950s; however, intracranial hemorrhage was such a limiting factor that use of thrombolysis as a therapy became dormant until just recently, when better understanding about brain hemorrhage, use of plasminogen activators, and better imaging techniques have shed new light upon this type of therapy in acute ischemic stroke.[54] The therapeutic effect of tissue plasminogen activators is to activate plasmin and thereby lyse fresh thromboemboli. Agents include streptokinase, anisoylated plasminogen streptokinase activator complex (APSAC), and tissue plasminogen activator (t-PA) single chain (alteplase). Results of major clinical trials using streptokinase have been recently reported.[55,56] In all of these trials, treatment with streptokinase (SK) resulted in increased mortality and morbidity from intracranial hemorrhage and SK cannot be recommended in stroke therapy. Recently, two major trials have been reported using alteplase in acute ischemic stroke, the European Cooperative Acute Stroke Study (ECASS) and the National Institute of Neurological Disorders and Stroke t-PA Trial (NINDS).[57,58] The ECASS trial was established to assess the safety and efficacy of alteplase in acute ischemic stroke. The study was a double-blind, placebo-controlled, randomized, prospective multicenter trial. A total of 620 patients were randomized to alteplase or placebo 6 hours or less of ischemic stroke after CT ruled out hemorrhage. Alteplase was infused at a rate of 1.1 mg/kg over 60 minutes, after a bolus of 10% of total dose. Primary end points measured were the Barthel Index and modified Rankin scale at 30 and 90 days and 30-day mortality and secondary end points using the Scandanavian Stroke Scale at 30 days. These stroke scales quantify neurologic functioning and overall functional disability. Because of protocol violations (IV heparin) and difficulty in interpreting the results, the conclusion reached was that alteplase improves some functional measures and neurologic outcomes in patients without extended infarcts; however, t-PA should not be used in the general stroke population.

The NINDS trial had the same objective as ECASS, but the design of the study was quite different in that it was in two parts. The study consisted of two sequential randomized trials comparing t-PA with placebo in which 624 patients were randomized to one of two treatment groups within 3 hours poststroke. Alteplase was infused at a rate of 0.9 mg/kg (maximum 90 mg) over 1 hour after a bolus of 10% of the total dose over 1 minute. Careful review of the CT scan, before treatment, for evidence of hemorrhage; exclusion of patients with hypertension; good blood pressure control; and no heparin or aspirin use in the first 24 hours were significant parameters used to select the most appropriate patients. Part 1 evaluated 291 patients and showed that a favorable clinical improvement at 24 hours was evident; 47% improvement with alteplase versus 39% with placebo ($P = .18$). Part 2 of the study was the same as part 1, except it evaluated outcomes of 333 randomly assigned patients on four stroke scales at 3 months. Part 2 is considered to be a pivotal study and the investigators were blinded to the outcomes of part 1. Results of part 2 show sustained clinical benefit that was statistically significant on all four stroke scales (Barthel Index, modified Rankin, Glasgow outcome, and NIHSS). The global statistic for improvement on all four stroke scales was significant at $P = .0008$, thereby denoting the clinical improvement seen in these study patients. A subgroup analysis of the study showed the benefit was across all subtypes of stroke and patient groups. There was, however, a significant increase in the occurrence of cerebral hemorrhage (6.4% of all t-PA patients versus 1% in placebo group) within 36 hours of treatment. Most of these hemorrhages were in patients with large strokes. Even with the increased rate of hemorrhage, t-PA did not cause a significant increase in early or late mortality. The conclusion is that alteplase, when administered within 3 hours of acute ischemic stroke onset, improves 3-month clinical outcome. These findings represent a most significant advance in the acute treatment of ischemic stroke. Table 18–8 shows the combined results of parts 1 and 2.

Recommendations and Monitoring

The development of t-PA therapy is indeed an exciting advance in the treatment of acute ischemic stroke, but caution must be exercised in using this mode of therapy and adherence to clinical protocol is a necessity.[59] The recommended alteplase treatment protocol is (1) stroke team activation; (2) onset of symptoms must be within 3 hours; (3) cranial CT scan to rule out hemorrhage; (4) intravenous administration of alteplase at 0.9 mg/kg (maximum, 90 mg) over 1 hour after a bolus of 10% of the total dose given over 1 minute; and (5) monitoring the patient for response and hemorrhage. Alteplase should be used only with the same inclusion and exclusion criteria used in NINDS as noted in the clinical protocol. It is essential that patients not receive any antiplatelet agents or anticoagulants for 24 hours after the use of alteplase. Table 18–9 summarizes the inclusion and exclusion criteria for use of alteplase in acute ischemic stroke.

SURGICAL THERAPY

The purpose of surgery in ischemic cerebrovascular disease is to prevent the occurrence of cerebral infarctions and TIAs. Generally, the goal of a surgical procedure is to remove the source of occlusion and/or embolus and, hopefully, to increase cerebral blood flow to an ischemic area.

Carotid endarterectomy (CEA) is the most common surgical procedure used for occlusive cerebrovascular disease. This procedure has been popular since its introduction over 30 years ago. CEA involves exposing the carotid artery in the neck and removing the occlusive atheromatous plaque usually at the carotid

TABLE 18–8. NINDS Combined Results of Part 1 and Part 2

End Points	TPA	Placebo	RR (95% CI)	*P* Value
NIHSS at 24 h (% with improvement)	47	39	1.2 (1.0–1.4)	.06
0–90 min (% with favorable outcome)				
Global test			1.9 (1.2–2.9)	.005
Barthel index	53	38	1.8 (1.2–2.9)	.010
Modified Rankin scale	40	28	1.7 (1.0–2.6)	.035
Glasgow outcome scale	43	32	1.6 (1.0-2.5)	.057
NIHSS	34	20	2.0 (1.2-3.4)	.008
91–180 min (% with favorable outcome)				
Global test			1.9 (1.3–2.9)	.002
Barthel index	51	38	1.6 (1.1–2.5)	.026
Modified Rankin scale	45	25	2.4 (1.5–3.7)	< .001
Glasgow outcome scale	47	30	2.0 (1.3–3.2)	.002
NIHSS	34	21	2.0 (1.2–3.2)	.008
Mortality at 90 days (%)	17	21		NS

NIHSS = NIH Stroke Scale; RR = risk reduction.

bifurcation. The indications have generally been considered to be TIAs and mild completed stroke in the presence of ulcerated or highly stenotic (> 75%) plaque. Two recent multicenter studies of CEA in symptomatic carotid artery disease have been reported: the North American Symptomatic Carotid Endarterectomy Trial Collaborators (NASCET), which is still ongoing[60]; and the European Carotid Surgery Trial (ECST).[61] In both of these trials, analysis showed that for symptomatic patients with stenosis of 70% or greater, CEA was superior to medical treatment alone at 2 to 3 years. In both studies, surgery was not beneficial in patients with less than 70% stenosis; however, results are still awaited from the NASCET trial group with stenosis of 30% to 69%. The rate of complications such as stroke or death of CEA for an institution should be equal to or better than NASCET (< 5%) in order to have an acceptable risk-to-benefit ratio. Additionally, in symptomatic carotid artery stenosis, the number-needed-to-treat analysis indicates that six endarterectomies would need to be performed to prevent one stroke over a 2-year span. Other indications, such as asymptomatic bruits and progressing stroke, are controversial; however, results from the Asymptomatic Cartoid Atherosclerosis Study (ACAS) show that symptom-free patients with 60% to 99% carotid artery stenosis had a 55% relative risk reduction for ipsilateral stroke or any stroke or death after carotid endarectomy compared to medical therapy. Number-needed-to-treat analysis has shown that in patients with asymptomatic carotid artery stenosis, 67 endarterectomies would have to be performed to prevent one stroke over a 2-year period. CEA is not indicated in patients with permanent deficits from moderate to severe completed strokes. For patients with a complete occlusion of an extracranial vessel, CEA is usually unsuccessful, and these patients may be considered for an extracranial–intracranial (EC-IC) bypass procedure. The most common EC-IC bypass procedure is anastomosis of the superficial temporal artery to a branch of the middle cerebral artery. This can augment blood flow to the brain by bypassing the stenotic or occluded artery. The clinical efficacy of this procedure has been disputed and further well-controlled studies are needed to clarify this point.

TABLE 18–9. Inclusion and Exclusion Criteria for Alteplase Use in Acute Ischemic Stroke

Inclusion Criteria (all YES boxes must be checked before treatment)

YES

- ☐ Age 18 years of older
- ☐ Clinical diagnosis of ischemic stroke causing a measurable neurological deficit
- ☐ Time of symptom onset well established to be less than 180 minutes before treatment would begin

Exclusion Criteria (all NO boxes must be checked before treatment)

NO

- ☐ Evidence of intracranial hemorrhage on noncontrast head CT
- ☐ Only minor or rapidly improving stroke symptoms
- ☐ High clinical suspicion of subarachnoid hemorrhage even with normal CT
- ☐ Active internal bleeding (e.g., GI/GU bleeding within 21 days)
- ☐ Known bleeding diathesis, including but not limited to platelet count < 100,000/mm^3
- ☐ Patient has received heparin within 48 hours and had an elevated APTT
- ☐ Recent use of anticoagulant (e.g., warfarin) and elevated PT (>15 sec)/INR
- ☐ Intracranial surgery, serious head trauma, or previous stroke within 3 months
- ☐ Major surgery or serious trauma within 14 days
- ☐ Recent arterial puncture at noncompressible site
- ☐ Lumbar puncture within 7 days
- ☐ History intracranial hemorrhage, arteriovenous malformation, or aneurysm
- ☐ Witnessed seizure at stroke onset
- ☐ Recent acute myocardial infarction
- ☐ SBP > 185 mm Hg or DBP > 110 mm Hg at time of treatment

INVESTIGATIONAL THERAPY

Investigational therapy for prevention of TIAs and stroke includes a number of new and emerging interventions.[62] Therapy to improve or reverse the effects of an acute stroke is being actively pursued and includes prostacyclin and the calcium channel blocking agents nimodipine and nicardipine. These agents are currently being tested in clinical trials; however, calcium channel blockers have not shown convincing evidence in reducing infarct size, although nimodipine may have a potential benefit if given within 12 hours of stroke onset. Early use of aspirin as well as the combination of aspirin and calcium channel blockers have been used very early after ischemic stroke (during hospitalization), and initial results are encouraging due to fewer deaths and stroke protection.[63] Another agent, naloxone, has been studied in ischemic cerebrovascular disease; however, controlled trials have failed to show beneficial effects. However, other opioid antagonists such as nalmafene, which is a derivative of naltrexone, are currently being tested. Other therapies with steroids, vasoactive agents, and barbiturates have shown no benefit. Low-molecular-weight heparins and heparinoids are currently under study in ischemic stroke. They appear to have a decreased bleeding tendency, and the potential of these compounds is promising.[64] Aspirin given in a single oral dose of 325 mg may have usefulness in acute stroke similar to its effectiveness as a platelet antiaggregating agent in treating AMI. Other antiaggregating agents such as anti-ICAM-1 (intracellular adhesion molecule) are being studied in the hope that microvascular activity will be clinically important in embolic stroke prevention. Intra-arterial thrombolysis is under investigation, and direct delivery of the t-PA may prove to be superior to intravenous delivery. Ancrod (pit viper venom extract) is still experimental. Research with glutamate receptor antagonists, such as the NMDA receptor subtype, is ongoing and with the hope that infarct size reduction can be attained; however, there is a high rate of side effects with these compounds in humans. Neuroprotective drugs are under study, but currently none has been shown to reduce infarct size or improve outcome. Sodium channel blocking agents and glycine antagonists that can inhibit presynaptic glutamate release may have potential therapeutic value. Antioxidants and free radical scavengers have not shown efficacy, but, higher-dose studies are underway. Extracranial cerebral vessel angioplasty and stenting are being studied for feasibility as alternatives to carotid endarterectomy, and intracranial angioplasty is also being investigated.

CEREBRAL EMBOLISM OF CARDIAC ORIGIN

In patients with cardiogenic brain embolism, immediate anticoagulation should be considered, because approximately 12% of such patients have a second embolic stroke within 2 weeks. In nonhypertensive patients with small to moderate stroke, heparin should be given 24 hours after stroke onset without a loading dose so that a less intensive anticoagulation effect is obtained. The partial thromboplastin time (PTT) should be no greater than 1.5 times the control value using rabbit brain thromboplastin. Before heparin is started, however, a CT scan should document the absence of spontaneous hemorrhagic transformation. Anticoagulation should be maintained with warfarin at an INR of 2.0 to 3.0. In patients who develop hemorrhagic transformation shortly after embolic stroke, anticoagulation should be postponed 8 to 10 days.

The role of platelet antiaggregating agents in this situation is not clear; however, antiplatelet agents are generally not recognized to have therapeutic value in those instances where red thrombi can develop, as in patients with cardiac mural thrombi, venous thrombosis, or large thrombi in any artery. In general, anticoagulation with warfarin is recommended in these situations. Obviously, prevention of the embolic event is the best therapy, and those patients at high risk for cardiogenic embolism, such as patients with atrial fibrillation or mechanical or prosthetic valves, should be treated with prophylactic chronic anticoagulation with warfarin. Six recent studies looking at preventative therapy in patients with nonvalvular atrial fibrillation (NVAF) have been completed. Five were primary intervention trials and one (EAFT) was for secondary intervention. Table 18–10 summarizes the studies of antithrombotic therapy in patients with AF.[25]

TABLE 18–10. Antithrombotic Therapy in Patients with AF

Study	Type[a]	*n*	Target INR or Aspirin Dosage	Relative Risk Reduction % (*P*)[b]	Absolute Risk Reduction (%/yr)	NNT
Warfarin Versus Placebo						
AFASAK	1°	671	2.8–4.2	58 (<.05)	2.6	39
SPAF I	1°	421	2.0–4.58[c]	65 (.01)	4.7	22
BAATAF	1°	420	1.5–3.0[c]	86 (.002)	2.6	39
CAFA	1°	378	2.0–3.0	33 (>.05)	2.5	40
SPINAF	1°	571	1.5–3.0[c]	79 (.001)	3.4	30
EAFT	2°	439	2.5–4.0	66 (.001)	8.4	12
Aggregate[d]				68 (<.001)		
Aspirin Versus Placebo						
AFASAK	1°	672	75 mg/d	18 (>.05)	0.7	143
SPAF I	1°	1120	325 mg/d	44 (.01)	2.5	40
EAFT	2°	782	300 mg/d	15 (>.05)	1.3	77
Aggregate				21 (<.05)		
Warfarin Versus Aspirin						
SPAF II	1°	1100	325 mg/d	31 (<.05)	0.8	125
AFASAK	1°	671	2.8–4.2, 75 mg/d	50 (.05)	1.9	53
SPAF III	1°	1044	325 mg/d[e]	76 (.001)	6.0	17
EAFT	2°	455	2.5–4.0, 300 mg/d	62 (.001)	6.4	16
Aggregate				55 (<.01)		

INR = International Normalized Ratio; NNT = number needed to treat or prevent one ischemic stroke per year; AFASAK = Atrial Fibrillation Aspirin Study of Anticoagulation from Kopenhaven; SPAF = Stroke Prevention in Atrial Fibrillation; BAATAF = Boston Area Anticoagulation Trial for Atrial Fibrillation; CAFA = Candadian Atrial Fibrillation Anticoagulation; SPINAF = Stroke Prevention in Nonrheumatic Atrial Fibrillation; EAFT = European Atrial Fibrillation Trial.

[a]1° = Primary prevention (in several studies, 5% to 10% of patients had remote thromboembolism); 2° = secondary intervention (previous transient ischemic attack or stroke).

[b]Reduction compared with control (active treatment or placebo) by intention-to-treat analysis.

[c]INR estimated for BAATAF, SPAF I, and SPINAF, which used prothrombin time ratios.

[d]Average of all studies cited.

[e]Aspirin 325 mg/d plus warfarin given to achieve an INR in the range of 1.2–1.5.

Adapted from Ref. 25.

In summary, these studies indicate that patients with NVAF can be effectively and safely treated with either warfarin or aspirin. The overall reduction of the relative risk of stroke in AF patients treated with warfarin was 68% compared to placebo, and aspirin was 21% compared to placebo. In all studies, the aggregate relative risk reduction of 68% is impressive; however, when the absolute risk reduction is calculated, it is about 1.5% per year. Therefore, in order to gain maximum therapeutic benefit, the risk of intracranial bleeding must be less than the benefit of stroke prevention. In addition, warfarin may be the agent of choice in the stasis-related thromboembolism seen in patients with NVAF and heart failure.

RECOMMENDATIONS

Because of the potential of intracerebral hemorrhage in elderly patients and the probability of lifetime treatment with warfarin, identification of subgroups of AF patients with high and low rates of stroke has been studied in two large trials (SPAF I and SPAF II).[23,31] AF patients with certain risk factors are more likely to develop stroke than those without these factors. Data from SPAF II indicate that the risk of thromboembolism in AF patients 75 years or younger given aspirin is low, less than 3%/yr, and that younger low-risk AF patients can be treated with 325 mg/d aspirin for stroke prevention. High-risk patients 75 years or younger in whom anticoagulation is judged to be safe can be treated with warfarin to an INR of 2.0 to 3.0. High-risk patients older than 75 years may be treated with lower-intensity warfarin at an INR of 1.5 to 2.5. Higher INRs can be used as an alternative. In those AF patients who have had an ischemic stroke or TIA, anticoagulation will be necessary for most patients. Lone AF should be managed with no therapy or aspirin.

Patients who have had prosthetic cardiac valve replacement have a clinically significant and long-term risk of thromboembolism. The pathophysiologic events that precede arterial thromboembolism actually begin as soon as the device is sewn in place and blood flows across the PCV. Generally, patients who have undergone aortic valve replacement are at a lower risk of thromboembolism than those with mitral PCV. Patients with both aortic and mitral valve replacement are usually considered to have the highest risk of thromboembolism. Other risk factors for thromboembolism include presence of atrial fibrillation, a large left atrium, previous thromboembolism, left ventricular dysfunction, and valve type and design.

Treatment recommendations for patients with mechanical PCVs are based on prospective randomized trials of anticoagulant therapy with and without a platelet inhibitor. These trials indicate that oral anticoagulation plus dipyridamole decreased the incidence of thromboembolism when compared to anticoagulation alone. Aspirin plus anticoagulation was found to produce excessive major bleeding (primarily gastrointestinal) when compared to warfarin plus dipyridamole. Oral anticoagulation plus dipyridamole for prevention of mechanical PCV-induced thromboembolism is a Food and Drug Administration-approved therapy. Thromboembolism is less frequent after bioprosthetic valve replacement. Even though the thrombogenicity of bioprosthetic valves is lower than that of mechanical valves, specific therapy is still required. The current recommendations for antithrombotic therapy for PCV replacement are presented next for mechanical and bioprosthetic valves.[35]

MECHANICAL PCVS

Therapy should begin with intravenous heparin 6 hours after surgery to maintain the activated partial thromboplastin time at 1.5 to 2 times control followed by subcutaneous heparin, 10,000 U every 12 hours after chest tube removal continuing until discharge. Warfarin should be started as soon as possible after operation and dosed to maintain the prothrombin time at an INR of 2.5 to 3.5. Aspirin 80 to 100 mg/d can be added to warfarin and may offer additional protection in those who have systemic embolism despite adequate oral anticoagulation. Dipyridamole 5 to 6 mg/kg divided every 6 hours may be added to warfarin as as alternative to the warfarin–aspirin combination. For those patients who cannot take oral anticoagulants, dipyridamole plus sulfinpyrazone 800 mg/d may be tried empirically.

BIOPROSTHETIC PCVS

Initial therapy with heparin is similar to mechanical PCVs as previously described. In those patients with aortic valve replacement who are in sinus rhythm, anticoagulation is optional. Aspirin 325 mg/d can be used empirically. For patients who have mitral valve replacement, initiate warfarin therapy as soon as possible after operation and for 3 months thereafter, at a less intense INR of 2.0 to 3.0. Aspirin 325 mg/d long term is optional. For patients who have atrial fibrillation, an enlarged left atrium, or previous thromboembolism, warfarin should be continued indefinitely at an INR of 2.0 to 3.0.

INTRACRANIAL HEMORRHAGE

General medical management and supportive therapy are indicated in the patient with intracranial hemorrhage. This condition, as noted earlier, has a generally poor prognosis. Preventive therapy of intracranial bleeding is possible in the case of hypertension, where blood pressure can be controlled by diet and/or medication. Surgical management in the acute or early stage of the event is removal of the clot by aspiration or evacuation; this treatment is usually beneficial only in those patients whose hemorrhage is near the surface of the brain and who are not comatose. Cerebellar hemorrhage, on the other hand, is often amenable to surgery within the first 2 days of onset.

Corticosteroids and, more recently, dexamethasone have been used in the treatment of cerebral edema resulting from primary intracerebral hemorrhage. A recent study has shown no beneficial effect; in fact, a harmful effect (infection and diabetic complications) was seen.[65] Therefore, the use of dexamethasone in this condition should be reconsidered. The use of mannitol and other osmotic agents to reduce edema around the hemorrhage is appropriate, provided systemic hypotensive and hypertensive episodes are avoided. The use of mannitol is well established and is guided by maintaining the serum osmolality and arterial pressure. Generally, 0.25 to 2 g/kg mannitol intravenously can be administered every 4 to 8 hours until the serum osmolality is raised between 300 and 310 mOsm/L. Cerebral edema is rarely a problem in ischemic stroke unless a very large MCA territory infarction occurs. Treatment is the same as noted earlier for intracranial hemorrhage. Cerebral vasospasm in subarachnoid hemorrhage can be severe, and therapeutic efforts to prevent or treat the vasospasm have been disappointing. Reserpine, kanamycin, isoproterenol, aminophylline, and nitroprusside have all failed in this condition. Recently, dopamine (3 to 6 mg/kg/min) has been used, but there is a risk of rebleeding. Percutaneous intra-arterial angioplasty, although not recommended, may be considered when vasospasm persists in spite of optimal medical treatment. However, data from well-designed trials are lacking. Barbiturate coma has been used to reduce intracranial pressure resulting from intracerebral hemorrhage when pressure reduction with dopamine or mannitol has not been successful.[66] Further research is needed in the treatment of cerebral vasospasm and the resulting increased intracranial pressure.

PHARMACOECONOMIC CONSIDERATIONS

Cost-effectiveness of therapy in acute ischemic stroke has been examined in only a few studies. In antithrombotic prophylaxis for atrial fibrillation, warfarin therapy was evaluated using quality-adjusted life year (QALY) saved. It was found that in patients with AF and one additional risk factor, warfarin therapy cost $8000 per quality-adjusted life year saved. In high-risk patients, those with AF and two or more risk factors, warfarin use was estimated to save $6200 in costs from stroke and TIA. Costs of monitoring and hemorrhages from warfarin were estimated to be $5500, thus showing a positive savings from warfarin use. Those without risk factors were much more costly to treat at an estimated $370,000 per quality-adjusted life saved when compared to aspirin treatment.[67] Warfarin is cost effective in high-risk patients, particularly if the hemorrhagic side effects are lower relative to the stroke risk. For comparison purposes, hypertension screening is estimated to cost $10,000 to 50,000 per quality-adjusted life year saved. A Swedish study reported the cost-effectiveness of primary stroke prevention in AF patients with oral anticoagulants or aspirin based on four published clinical trials.[68] The authors found that the total cost per stroke prevented was a $16 savings if the intracerebral bleeding was 0.3% and a cost of $43 if the bleeding rate was 2%. At a bleeding complication rate of 1.3%, warfarin would prevent 1000 strokes per year and save about $29 million. Unpublished cost-analysis data on the NINDS trial with t-PA estimates total health care costs (including acute and long-term costs) could be reduced by almost $5 million for every 1000 patients treated with t-PA. Although t-PA is expensive, when the total health care costs are factored in, savings can accrue to the health care system as a direct result of appropriate t-PA therapy. Primary prevention strategies that address the risk factors for ischemic stroke can be powerful in reducing the costs of stroke. Many of the stroke risk factors can be modified and some eliminated at very low costs (life-style changes), therefore developing risk factor reduction strategies may be the most cost-effective measure of all. More research is needed in identifying the cost-effectiveness of other forms of acute stroke treatment.

▶ PRINCIPLES OF PHARMACOTHERAPY

- Prevention of cerebrovascular disease is most important. Heart and brain healthy life-style changes and control of modifiable risk factors are key steps in prevention of ischemic stroke.
- Anticoagulation for TIA is not routinely recommended.
- Antiplatelet therapy is the therapy of choice for secondary prevention of TIA; 325 mg/d aspirin is recommended.
- Aspirin 325 mg/d is recommended for secondary stroke prevention, if the stroke is not due to atrial fibrillation. A study is ongoing to see if warfarin is superior to aspirin.[69]
- Ticlopidine 250 mg twice daily orally or clopidogrel 75 mg/d orally, are the currently recommended alternatives to aspirin in cases where aspirin intolerance or failure occurs.
- Aspirin 325 mg/d is recommended in patients with nonvalvular atrial fibrillation (NVAF) who are at low risk for stroke.
- NVAF patients at high risk for stroke should receive warfarin, dosing dependent upon age. Age less than 75 years requires an INR of 2.0 to 3.0. Age 75 or greater can be dosed at a lower intensity INR of 1.5 to 2.5. Monitor patient closely for bleeding.
- Mechanical PCVs require warfarin therapy indefinitely, dosed to an INR of 2.5 to 3.5. Bioprosthetic PCVs in the mitral position require warfarin dosed to an INR of 2.0 to 3.0 for the first 3 months after placement followed optionally by aspirin 325 mg/d indefinitely.
- Alteplase 0.9 mg/kg infused over 1 hour after a bolus of 10% total dose is recommended as emergency therapy in acute ischemic stroke if CT scan is negative for intracranial hemorrhage and if therapy can be initiated within 3 hours of the acute event. Patient selection is critical and strict adherence to the AHA guidelines is mandatory in order to avoid bleeding complications. Monitor patient closely for bleeding.[59]

REFERENCES

1. Abbott RD, Yin Y, Reed DM, et al. Risk of stroke in male cigarette smokers. N Engl J Med 1986;315:717–720.
2. Heart and Stroke Facts: 1998 Statistical Supplement. Dallas, American Heart Association, 1997.
3. Taylor TN, Davis PH, Torner JC, et al. Lifetime cost of stroke in the United States. Stroke 1996;27:1459–1466.
4. Helgason CM, Wolf PA. American Heart Association Prevention Conference IV: Prevention and rehabilitation of stroke. Circulation 1997; 96:701–707.
5. Bronner LL, Kanter DS, Manson JE. Primary prevention of stroke. N Engl J Med 1995;333:1392–1400.
6. Wolf PA, Abbott RD, Kannel WB. Atrial fibrillation as an independent risk factor for stroke: The Framingham study. Stroke 1991; 22:983–988.
7. Hart RG, Halperin JL. Atrial fibrillation and stroke. Revisiting the dilemmas. Stroke 1994;25:1337–1341.
8. Chesebro JH, Fuster V, Halperin JL. Atrial fibrillation—Risk marker for stroke. N Engl J Med 1990;323:1556–1558.
9. WHO task force on stroke and other cerebrovascular disorders. Recommendations on stroke prevention, diagnosis, and therapy. Stroke 1989;20:1407–1431.
10. Adult treatment panel II. National cholesterol education program: Second report of the expert panel on detection, evaluation, and treatment of high blood cholesterol in adults. Circulation 1994;89; 1333–1445.
11. Hebert PR, Gaziano JM, Chan KS, Hennekens CH. Cholesterol lowering with statin drugs, risk of stroke, and total mortality—An overview of randomized trials. JAMA 1997;278:313–321.
12. Scandinavian simvastatin survival study group. Randomized trial of cholesterol lowering in 4444 patients with coronary heart disease: The Scandinavian simvastatin survival study (4S). Lancet 1994; 344:1383–1389.
13. Donnan GA, McNeil JJ, Adena MA, et al. Smoking as a risk factor for cerebral ischemia. Lancet 1989;II:643–647.

14. Cotton P. Women's health initiative leads way as research begins to fill gender gaps. JAMA 1992;267:469–470.
15. O'Brien KD, Chait A. The biology of the artery wall in atherogenesis. Med Clin North Am 1994;78:41–67.
16. Ross R. The pathogenesis of atherosclerosis: An update. N Engl J Med. 1986;314:488–500.
17. Fisher M, Garcia JH. Evolving stroke and the ischemic penumbra. Neurology 1996;47:884–888.
18. Schiter W, Pietersma A, Lamers JM, Koster JT. Leukocyte adhesion molecules on the vascular endothelium: Their role in the pathogenesis of cardiovascular disease and the mechanisms underlying their expression. J Cardiovasc Pharmacol 1993;22(suppl 4):S37–S44.
19. Hackman A, Abe Y, Insull W, et al. Levels of soluble cell adhesion molecules in patients with dyslipidemia. Circulation 1996;93: 1334–1338.
20. Libby P, Sukhova G, Lee RT, Galis ZS. Cytokines regulate vascular function related to stability of the atherosclerotic plaque. J Cardiovasc Pharmacol 1995;25(suppl 2):S9–S12.
21. Meyer FB, Sundt TM, Yanagihara T, et al. Focal cerebral ischemia: Pathophysiologic mechanisms and rationale for future avenues of treatment. Mayo Clin Proc 1987;62:35–55.
22. Feinberg WM, Blackshear JL, Laupacis A, et al. Prevalence, age distribution, and gender of patients with atrial fibrillation. Arch Intern Med 1995;155:469–473.
23. Stroke prevention in atrial fibrillation investigators. Predictors of thromboembolism in atrial fibrillation, I. Clinical features of patients at risk. Ann Intern Med 1992;116:1–5.
24. Tegeler C. Carotid stenosis in atrial fibrillation. Neurology 1989; 39(suppl):159. Abstract.
25. Nelson KM, Talbert RL. Preventing stroke in patients with nonrheumatic atrial fibrillation. Am J Hosp Pharm 1994;51:1175–1183.
26. American Society of Health-System Pharmacists. ASHP therapeutics position statement on antithrombotic therapy in chronic atrial fibrillation. Am J Health Syst Pharm 1998;55:376–381.
27. Sherman DG, Dyken ML, Gent M, et al. Antithrombotic therapy for cerebrovascular disorders. An update. Chest 1995;108(suppl): 444S–456S.
28. National Heart, Lung, and Blood Institute [NHLBI] AFFIRM investigators. Atrial fibrillation follow-up investigation of rhythm management—The AFFIRM study design. The planning and steering committee of the AFFIRM study for the NHLBI AFFIRM investigators. Am J Cardiol 1997;79:1198–2202.
29. Chesebro JH, Ezekowitz M, Badimon L, et al. Intracardiac thrombi and systemic thromboembolism: Detection, incidence, and treatment. Annu Rev Med 1985;36:579–605.
30. Laupacis A, Albern G, Daley J, Dunnar, et al. Antithrombotic therapy in atrial fibrillation. Chest 1995;108(suppl):3528–3595.
31. Stroke prevention in atrial fibrillation investigators. Predictors of thromboembolism in atrial fibrillation, II. Echocardiographic features of patients at risk. Ann Intern Med 1992;116:6–12.
32. Tanne D, Goldbourt U, Zion M, et al. Frequency and prognosis of stroke/TIA among 4808 survivors of acute myocardial infarction. Stroke 1993;24:1490–1495
33. Loh E, St. John Suton M, Wren CC, et al. Ventricular dysfunction predicts cerebrovascular and arterial thromboembolic events following myocardial infarction. Circulation 1995;92(suppl):1–483.
34. Dunnbman WB, Johnson GR, Carson PE, et al. Incidence of thromboembolic events in congestive heart failure. Circulation. 1993; 87(suppl 1):94–101.
35. Stein PD, Alpert JS, Copeland J, et al. Antithrombotic therapy in patients with mechanical and prosthetic heart valves. Chest 1995; 108(suppl):371S–379S.
36. Lopez, JA, Ross RS, Fishbein MC, et al. Non-bacterial thrombotic endocarditis: A review. Am Heart J 1987;113:773–784.
37. Cheitlin MD, Alpert JJ, Armstrong WF, et al. ACC/AHA guidelines for the clinical application of echocardiography: Executive summary. A report of the American College of Cardiology/American Heart Association task force on practice guidelines. J Am Coll Cardiol 1997; 29:862–879.
38. Culebras A, Kase CS, Masdeu JC, et al. Practice guidelines for the use of imaging in transient ischemic attacks and acute stroke. Stroke 1997;28:1480–1497.
39. Miller VT, Hart RG. Heparin anticoagulation in acute brain ischemia. Stroke 1988;19:403–406.
40. Slivka A, Levy D. Natural history of progressive ischemic stroke in a population treated with heparin. Stroke 1990;21:1657–1662.
41. Babikian VL, Kase CS, Pessin MS, et al. Intracerebral hemorrhage in stroke patients anticoagulated with heparin. Stroke 1989;20: 1500–1503.
42. Estol CJ, Pessin MS. Anticoagulation: Is there still a role in atherothrombotic stroke? Stroke 1990;21:820–824.
43. Hirsh J, Dalen JE, Deykin D, et al. Oral anticoagulants: Mechanism of action, clinical effectiveness, and optimal therapeutic range. Chest 1995;108(suppl):231S–246S.
44. Canadian cooperative study group. A randomized trial of aspirin and sulfinpyrazone in threatened stroke. N Engl J Med 1978;299: 53–59.
45. Kelton JG, Hirsh J, Carter CJ, et al. Sex differences in the antithrombotic effects of aspirin. Blood 1978;52:1073–1076.
46. UK-TIA study group. United Kingdom transient ischaemic attack (UK-TIA) aspirin trial: Interim results. Br Med J 1988;296:316–320.
47. Dutch TIA study group. The Dutch TIA trial: Protective effects of low-dose aspirin and atenolol in patients with transient ischemic attacks or nondisabling stroke. Stroke 1988;19:512–517.
48. Antiplatelet trialists' collaboration. Collaborative overview of randomized trials of antiplatelet therapy, I. Prevention of death, myocardial infarction, and stroke by prolonged antiplatelet therapy in various categories of patients. BMJ 1994;308:81–106.
49. The American–Canadian cooperative study group. Persantine aspirin trial in cerebral ischemia, part II. Endpoint results. Stroke 1985; 16:406–415.
50. Saltiel E, Ward A. Ticlopidine: A review of its pharmacodynamic and pharmacokinetic properties, and therapeutic efficacy in platelet-dependent disease states. Drugs 1987;34:222–262.
51. Gent M, Blakely JA, Easton JD, et al. The Canadian American ticlopidine study (CATS) in thromboembolic stroke. Design, organization, and baseline results. Stroke 1988;19:1203–1210.
52. Robert S, Miller AJ, Fagan SC. Ticlopidine: A new antiplatelet agent for cerebrovascular disease. Pharmacotherapy 1991;11:317–325.
53. CAPRIE steering committee. A randomized blinded, trial of clopidogrel versus aspirin in patients at risk of ischaemic events (CAPRIE). Lancet 1996;348:1329–1339.
54. Dumo P, Fagan SL, Carhuapoma J. Thrombolysis in acute ischemic stroke. Am J Health Syst Pharm 1997;54:2213–2217.
55. Multicentre acute stroke trial—Italy. Randomised controlled trial of streptokinase, aspirin, and combination of both in treatment of acute ischaemic stroke. Lancet 1995;346:1509–1514.
56. Multicentre acute stroke trial–Europe study group. Thrombolytic therapy with streptokinase in acute ischaemic stroke. N Engl J Med 1996; 335:145–150.
57. Hacke W, Kaste M, Fieschi C, et al. Intravenous thrombolysis with recombinant tissue plasminogen activator for acute hemispheric stroke: the European cooperative acute stroke study (ECASS). JAMA 1995; 274:1017–1025.
58. The National Institute of Neurological Disorders and Stroke rt-PA stroke study group. Tissue plasminogen activator for acute ischemic stroke. N Engl J Med 1995;333:1581–1587.
59. Adams HP Jr, Brott TG, Furlan AJ, et al. Guidelines for thrombolytic therapy for acute stroke: A supplement to the guidelines for the management of patients with acute ischemic stroke. A statement for healthcare professionals from a special writing group of the Stroke Council, American Heart Association. Circulation 1996; 94:1167–1174.

60. North American symptomatic carotid endarterectomy trial collaborators. Beneficial effect of carotid endartecrectomy in symptomatic patients with high-grade carotid stenosis. N Engl J Med 1991;325: 445–453.
61. Rothwell PM, Gibson RJ, Slattery J, et al. Risk of stroke in the distribution of an asymtomatic carotid artery. The European carotid surgery trialists' collaborative group. Lancet 1995;345:209–212.
62. Ryan M, Rhoney DH, Luer MS, Hatton J. New and investigational treatment options for ischemic stroke. Pharmacotherapy 1997; 17: 959–969.
63. Chinese acute stroke trial collaborative group. CAST: Randomized placebo-controlled trial of early aspirin use in 20,000 patients with acute ischemic stroke. Lancet 1997;349:1641–1642.
64. Massey EW, Biller J, Davis JN, et al. Large-dose infusion of heparinoid ORG 10172 in ischemic stroke. Stroke 1990;21:1289–1292.
65. Poungvarin N, Bhoopat W, Viriyavejakul A, et al. Effects of dexamethasone in primary supratentorial intracerebral hemorrhage. N Engl J Med 1987;316:1229–1233.
66. Woster PS, LeBlanc KL. Management of elevated intracranial pressure. Clin Pharm 1990;9:762–772.
67. Gage BF, Cardinalli AB, Albers GW, Owens DK. Cost-effectiveness of warfarin and aspirin for prophylaxis of stroke in patients with nonvalvular artrial fibrillation. JAMA 1995;274:1839–1845.
68. Gustafsson C, Asplund K, Britton M, et al. Cost effectiveness of stroke prevention in atrial fibrillation. Br Med J 1992;305:1457–1460.
69. Chimowitz MI, Kobbinos J, Strong J, et al. The warfarin-aspirin symptomatic intracranial disease study. Neurology 1995;45:1488–1493.

19

HYPERLIPIDEMIA

Robert L. Talbert, PharmD, FCCP, BCPS

Cholesterol, triglycerides, and phospholipids are the major lipids in the body and they are transported as complexes of lipid and specialized proteins (apolipoproteins) known as lipoproteins. Plasma lipoproteins are spherical particles with a surface that consists largely of phospholipid, free cholesterol, and protein, and a core that consists mostly of triglyceride and cholesterol ester (Fig. 19–1). Abnormalities of plasma lipoproteins can result in a predisposition to coronary artery disease, pancreatitis, xanthomas, or neurologic disease. Accumulating evidence over the last decades had linked elevated total and low-density lipoprotein cholesterol (LDL-C) and reduced high-density lipoprotein cholesterol (HDL-C) to the development of coronary heart disease. Premature coronary atherosclerosis, leading to the manifestations of ischemic heart disease (see Chap. 12), is the most common and significant consequence of hyperlipidemia. In 1994, the National Cholesterol Education Program (NCEP) adult treatment panel II (ATP II) published their second report summarizing these data and giving recommendations for the management of hypercholesterolemia in adults.[1]

EPIDEMIOLOGY

Total cholesterol and LDL-C increase throughout life in men and women, representing an atherogenic pattern characteristic of Westernized society diet (Fig. 19–2). Based on the National Health and Nutrition Examination Survey (NHANES 1988 to 1991) and ATP II guidelines, 40% of all adults aged 20 to 74 years would require fasting lipoprotein analysis and 29% (52 million Americans) would be candidates for dietary therapy. Assuming that dietary intervention would reduce LDL cholesterol by about 10%, then about 7% (approximately 12.7 million Americans) might be candidates for lipid-lowering drugs. This reflects about 4 million Americans with known coronary heart disease (CHD) and about 8.7 million adults without established CHD. Of the latter group, up to 3.1 million are aged 65 years and older.[2] Although these numbers seem staggering in their enormity, substantial progress had been made, and the number of Americans with a desirable blood cholesterol level (< 200 mg/dL) has risen to 49% from 45% from the earlier survey (1976 to 1980), while the average total cholesterol in this country has fallen from 220 mg/dL in 1960 to 1962 to 203 mg/dL in 1988 to 1994.[3]

Data from the Framingham study and other studies demonstrate that the risk for developing cardiovascular disease is related to the degree of total cholesterol and LDL-C elevation in a graded, continuous fashion.[4,5] Hypercholesterolemia is additive to the other nonlipid risk factors for coronary heart disease including cigarette smoking, hypertension, diabetes, low HDL-C levels, and electrocardiographic abnormalities. The presence of established CHD or prior myocardial infarction increases the risk of myocardial infarction five to seven times that seen in men or women without CHD, and LDL-C is a significant predictor of subsequent morbidity and mortality.[6] About 50% of all myocardial infarctions and at least 70% of CHD deaths occur in patients with known CHD, and these patients should therefore be a target for screening, identification, and treatment. Unfortunately, the identification of patients at high risk due to hypercholesterolemia or other lipid disorders is too frequently overlooked, because blood lipid levels are not always evaluated in this population even after an event such as myocardial infarction.[6,7]

Comparison of the United States to other countries has shown similar relationships between total cholesterol, LDL-C, and an inverse relationship with HDL-C to coronary artery disease mortality.[5] On a positive note, the U.S. mortality rate is midway among the countries studied, and this country has had the greatest decline in coronary artery disease mortality (35% to 40%) in men and women over the last 10 years compared with other countries. A decline in the prevalence of hypercholesterolemia in certain segments of the U.S. population parallels these trends in mortality.[8] LDL-C and the ratio of LDL-C to HDL-C have also been used to assess risk, but their use adds little information to total cholesterol alone unless HDL-C is abnormally high or low. HDL-C has been shown to be protective for the occurrence of coronary heart disease, and an inverse relationship exists between coronary heart disease and HDL-C levels.

Two fractions of HDL-C occur, HDL_2-C and HDL_3-C, and it is thought that HDL_2 is more important for prevention of cardiovascular disease. HDL transports cholesterol from lipid-laden foam cells to the liver. In general, for every 1 mg/dL decline in HDL, CHD risk is increased by 2% to 3%. Elevated triglycerides may cause pancreatitis, but their relationship to coronary heart disease is much weaker than cholesterol, and studies of unselected patients have not found a significant relationship between triglycerides and the prevalence of coronary heart disease. Very-low-density lipoprotein (VLDL), which is enriched with cholesterol esters, is smaller, more dense, and more atherogenic than less dense VLDL. Routine measurement of

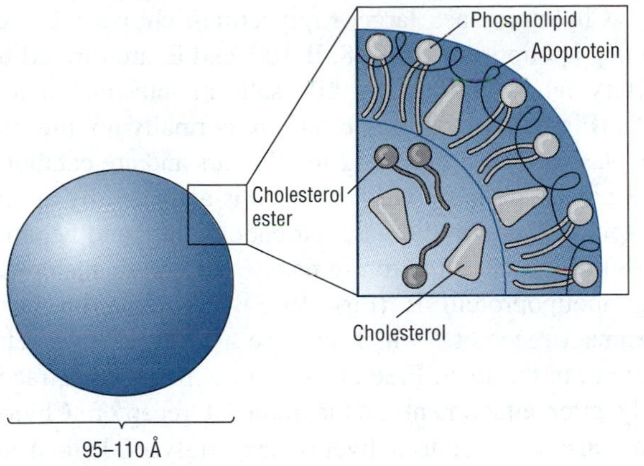

FIGURE 19–1. Schematic of a high-density-lipoprotein particle. The protein is represented as having a helical structure and forming the outer 110-Å shell of the particle. The polar head groups of phospholipids are shown interacting with the helices of the protein. Cholesteryl esters are drawn such that the cholesterol moiety interacts with the fatty acyl chains of the phospholipids.

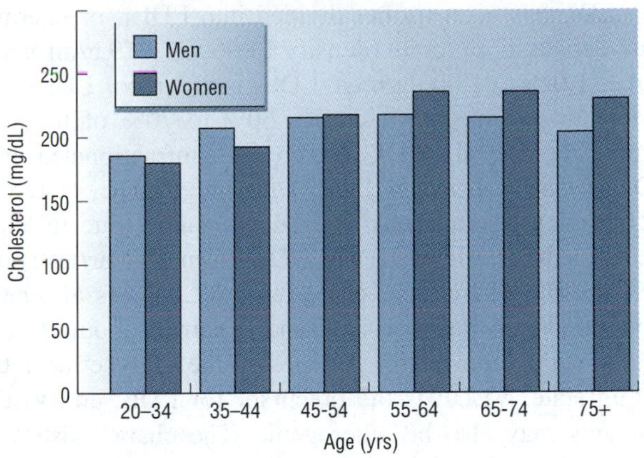

FIGURE 19–2. Serum cholesterol levels in men and women 20 years of age and over from 1988 to 1994. *(Based on data from the Third National Health and Nutrition Examination survey. Health, United States, 1996–97. Hyattsville, MD, National Center for Health Statistics, 1997:1–345.)*

triglycerides cannot distinguish between the types of VLDL present in plasma. Elevation of triglyceride-rich lipoproteins is associated with low HDL, and this ratio predicts increased risk. The 8-year follow-up of the Copenhagen male study found a clear gradient of risk of ischemic heart disease (IHD) with increasing triglyceride levels within each level of HDL cholesterol and that compared to the lowest one-third of triglyceride concentrations; the highest one-third had 2.2 relative risk for IHD; the relationship extended across all concentrations of HDL-C.[9] The Helsinki heart study has shown hypertriglyceridemia and low HDL-C are associated with obesity (BMI > 26 kg/m^2), smoking, sedentary life-style, blood pressure of 140/90 mm Hg or more, and blood glucose above 4.4 mmol/L, and that the benefit of gemfibrozil (risk reduction 68%, P = .03) was largely confined to overweight subjects.[10] The Stockholm ischemic heart disease study using niacin and clofibrate found the greatest reduction in CHD in patients with elevated triglycerides.[9] Hypertriglyceridemia in certain instances—for example, diabetes mellitus, nephrotic syndrome, chronic renal disease, and perhaps in women—is associated with increased cardiovascular risk. This is thought to be due to the presence of atherogenic lipoproteins and hypertriglyceridemia being a marker for them, as triglycerides are usually not independently predictive for coronary heart disease.[11]

LIPOPROTEIN METABOLISM AND TRANSPORT

Cholesterol and triglycerides, as the major plasma lipids, are essential substrates for cell membrane formation and hormone synthesis, and provide a source of free fatty acids.[12,13] Hyperlipidemia is defined as an elevation of one or more of the following: cholesterol, cholesterol esters, phospholipids, or triglycerides. Lipids, being water immesible, are not present in free form in the plasma, but rather circulate as lipoproteins. Hyperlipoproteinemia describes an increased concentration of the lipoprotein macromolecules that transport lipids in the plasma. The density of plasma lipoproteins is determined by their relative content of protein and lipid. Density, composition, and electrophoretic mobility have been used to divide lipoproteins into four classes (Table 19–1).

TABLE 19–1. Composition of Lipoprotein Isolated from Normal Subjects

Lipoprotein Class[a]	Density range (g/mL)	Electrophoretic Mobility	Composition (Weight %)				
					Cholesterol		
			Protein	*Triglyceride*	*Free*	*Ester*	*Phospholipid*
Chylomicrons	<0.94	Origin	1–2	85–95	1–3	2–4	3–6
VLDL	0.94–1.006	Prebeta	6–10	50–65	4–8	16–22	15–20
LDL	1.006–1.063	Beta	18–22	4–8	6–8	45–50	18–24
HDL	1.063–1.21	Alpha	45–55	2–7	3–5	15–20	26–32

[a]VLDL = very-low-density lipoprotein; LDL = low-density lipoprotein; and HDL = high-density lipoprotein.
From Schaefer EJ, Levy RI. Pathogenesis and management of lipoprotein disorders. N Engl J Med *1985;312:1300–1310, with permission.*

LDL has been further divided into LDL_1, or intermediate-density lipoprotein (density 1.006 to 1.019 g/mL); and LDL_2 (1.019 to 1.063 g/mL). LDL_2 is the major LDL component in plasma and it carries 60% to 70% of the total serum cholesterol. HDL has been subfractionated into HDL_2 (density 1.063 to 1.125 g/mL) and HDL_3 (1.125 to 1.21 g/mL). Fluctuations in HDL is usually due to alterations in the levels of HDL_2. HDL normally carries about 20% to 30% of the total cholesterol. VLDL has also been subdivided into three classes, and it carries about 10% to 15% of serum cholesterol and most of the triglyceride in the fasting state. VLDL is the precursor for LDL, and VLDL remnants may also be atherogenic. The characteristics of the protein constituent of lipoproteins, known as apolipoproteins, are shown in Table 19–2.

Chylomicrons, large triglyceride-rich particles containing apolipoprotein B-48, B-100, and E, are formed from dietary fat solubilized by bile salts in intestinal mucosal cells (Fig. 19–3). Chylomicrons are normally not present in the plasma after a fast of 12 to 14 hours and are catabolized by lipoprotein lipase (LPL), which is activated by apolipoprotein C-II and in the vascular endothelium and hepatic lipase to form chylomicron remnants. The remnants containing apolipoprotein E (Fig. 19–3) are taken up by the "remnant receptor," which may be a LDL receptor-related protein, in the liver. Free cholesterol is liberated intracellularly after attachment to the remnant receptor. Chylomicrons also function to deliver dietary triglyceride to skeletal muscle and adipose tissue. During the catabolism of nascent chylomicrons to remnants, triglyceride is converted

TABLE 19–2. Characteristics and Functions of Apolipoproteins

Apolipoprotein	Lipoprotein Density Class	Approximate Plasma Concentration (mg/dL)	Approximate Molecular Weight (kd)	Reported Functions	Major Site of Synthesis
A-I	Chylomicrons, HDL	120	28	Cofactor with LCAT, structural protein on HDL, ligand for HDL receptor	Liver, intestine
A-II	Chylomicrons, HDL	35	18	Structural protein for HDL, ligand for HDL receptor	Liver
A-IV	Chylomicrons, 1.21B	15	45	?	Intestine
ApoLp(a)	LDL, HDL	10	500±	Bound to B-100, high homology with plasminogen, may prevent LDL uptake by B, E receptor	Liver
B-100	VLDL, LDL	100	500	Structural protein on intestinal chylomicrons and hepatic VLDL, ligand for LDL receptor	Liver
B-48	Chylomicrons	Trace	250	Structural protein on intestinal chylomicrons	Intestine
C-I	Chylomicrons, VLDL, HDL	7	7	Cofactor with LCAT	Liver
C-II	Chylomicrons, VLDL, HDL	4	10	Cofactor with LPL	Liver
C-III	Chylomicrons, VLDL, HDL	13	9	Inhibitor with LPL	Liver
D	HDL	6	32	?	?
E2-E4	Chylomicrons, VLDL, HDL	5	34	Ligand for several cell receptors	Liver

LCAT = lecithin-cholesterol acyltransferase; HL = hepatic lipase.

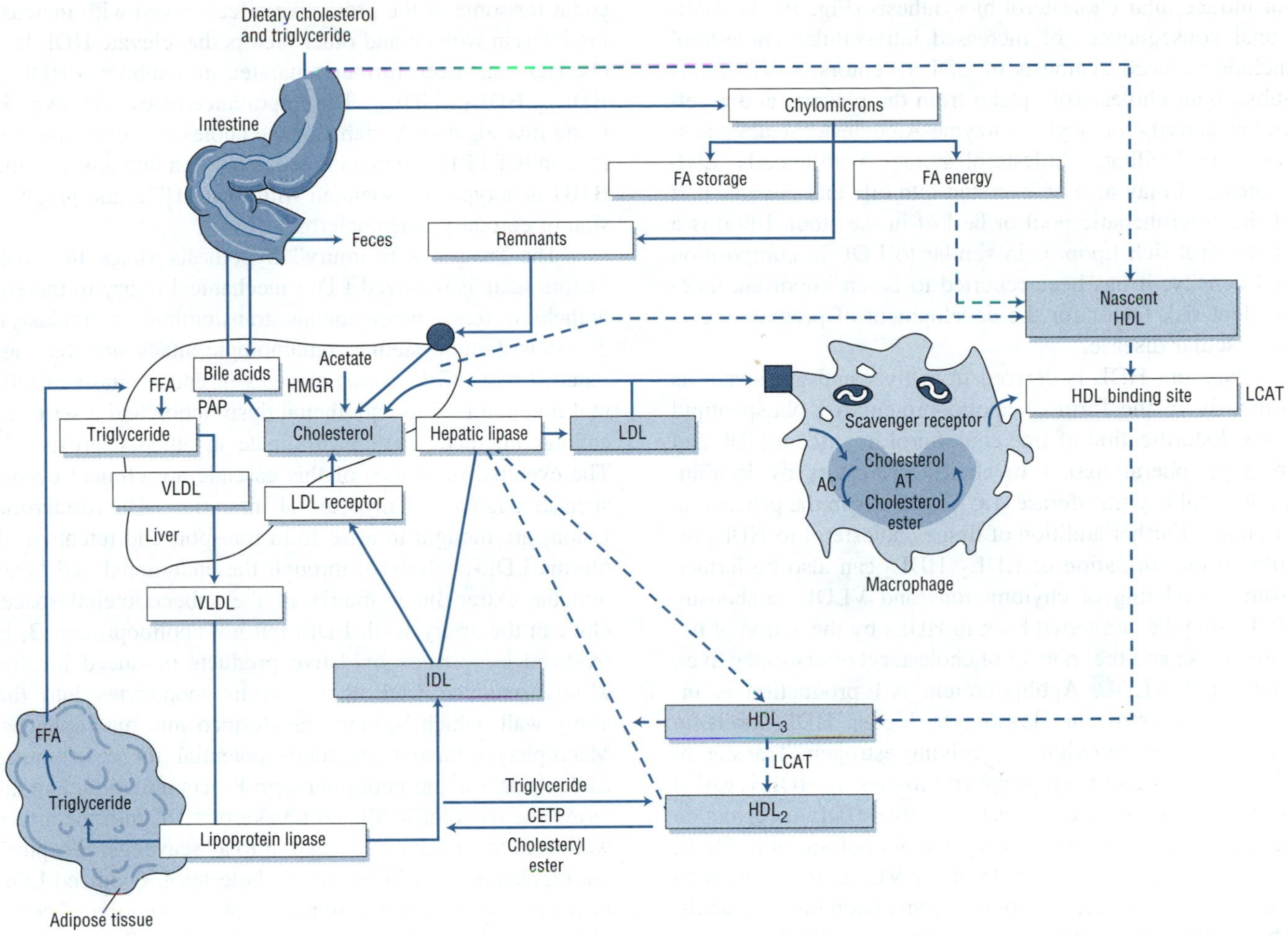

FIGURE 19–3. Overview of lipoprotein metabolism. (ACAT = acyl CoA:cholesterol acyltransferase; LCAT = lecithin:cholesterol acyltransferase; HMGR = HMG CoA reductase; PAP = phosphatidic acid phosphatase; CETP = cholesteryl ester transfer protein; FFA = free fatty acid.) *(From Ref. 12, with permission.)*

to free fatty acids and apolipoproteins A-I, A-II, A-IV (free in plasma), C-I, C-II, and C-III, and phospholipids are transferred to HDL. Apolipoprotein E and apolipoprotein C-II are transferred to chylomicrons from HDL and eventually back through these metabolic events. Hepatic VLDL synthesis is regulated in part by diet and hormones, and is inhibited by uptake of chylomicron remnants in the liver. VLDL is secreted from the liver and serially converted via LPL to intermediate-density lipoprotein (IDL), and finally LDL. VLDL receptors are found in adipose tissue and muscle and bear close homology to the structure of LDL receptors.

LDL, the major cholesterol transport lipoprotein and having virtually only apolipoprotein B-100, is mostly derived from VLDL catabolism and cellular synthesis. When fasted and on low fat intake in normal subjects, most cholesterol is synthesized and used in the extrahepatic organs, while most of the cholesterol carried by LDL is taken up by the liver for catabolism.[13] In patients with homozygous familial hypercholesterolemia, enhanced synthesis of LDL may occur, because LDL clearance is reduced due to the lack of LDL receptors. LDL is catabolized through interaction of cell surface receptors found on liver, adrenal, and peripheral cells (including fibroblasts and smooth muscle cells). These cells recognize apolipoprotein B-100 on LDL, and after binding to a receptor on the cell membrane, LDL is internalized and degraded. In the normal fasting state, approximately 70% of LDL is cleared through receptor-dependent mechanism, although this is highly dependent on the availability and type of saturated and mono- or polyunsaturated fat from dietary sources. Ingestion of cholesterol and saturated fatty acids such as C12:0, 14:0, and 16:0 are associated with reduction in LDL receptor activity, increased LDL production rate, and elevation in LDL plasma concentration. Receptor-independent mechanisms are also involved to a lesser extent in the catabolism of LDL, and these receptors are present in many tissues but are most active in animals in the adrenals and ovary.[13] Increased intracellular cholesterol resulting from LDL catabolism inhibits the activity of 3-hydroxy-3-methylglutaryl coenzyme A reductase (HMG-CoA reductase), the rate limiting enzyme for intracellular cholesterol biosynthesis (Fig. 19–4). Additional consequences of increased intracellular cholesterol include reduced synthesis of LDL receptors, which limits subsequent cholesterol uptake from the plasma; and accelerated activity of acyl coenzyme-A:cholesterol acyltransferase to facilitate cholesterol storage within cells. LDL cholesterol may also be excreted into bile and become part of the enterohepatic pool or be lost in the stool. Lp(a) is a cholesterol-rich lipoprotein similar to LDL in composition and density; it has been reported to be an important independent risk factor for the development of premature cardiovascular disease.[14]

Nascent HDL is derived from liver and gut synthesis primarily in the form of apolipoprotein A-I phospholipid discs. Esterification of free cholesterol in nascent HDL and from peripheral tissues to cholesteryl esters by lecithin: cholesterol acyltransferase (LCAT) results in the production of HDL_3. Further addition of tissue cholesterol to HDL_3 results in the formation of HDL_2. HDL_2 can also be formed from remodeling of chylomicrons and VLDL catabolism. HDL_2 may be converted back to HDL_3 by the action of hepatic lipase and the transfer of cholesteryl esters to the liver, LDL, and VLDL. Apolipoprotein A-I production is increased by estrogens, leading to higher HDL levels in women and in individuals receiving estrogen. Transfer of excess cholesterol from peripheral tissues by HDL is called *reverse cholesterol transport.* Putative HDL receptors in peripheral cells facilitate the uptake of cholesterol by HDL, which transfers cholesterol to either VLDL and LDL or to the liver for secretion into bile or conversion into bile acids. These processes serve to rid peripheral tissue (e.g., coronary arteries) of excessive amounts of cholesterol, and account for some of the protective effects noted with increasing HDL in women and other factors that elevate HDL levels. HDL has been further separated into subtypes HDL_{2a}, HDL_{2b}, HDL_{3a}, HDL_{3c}. The importance of each subtype is being investigated. Variants of the cholesterol ester transfer protein (CETP) have been demonstrated in humans, and the B1B1 genotype is associated with lower HDL and progression of coronary atherosclerosis.[15]

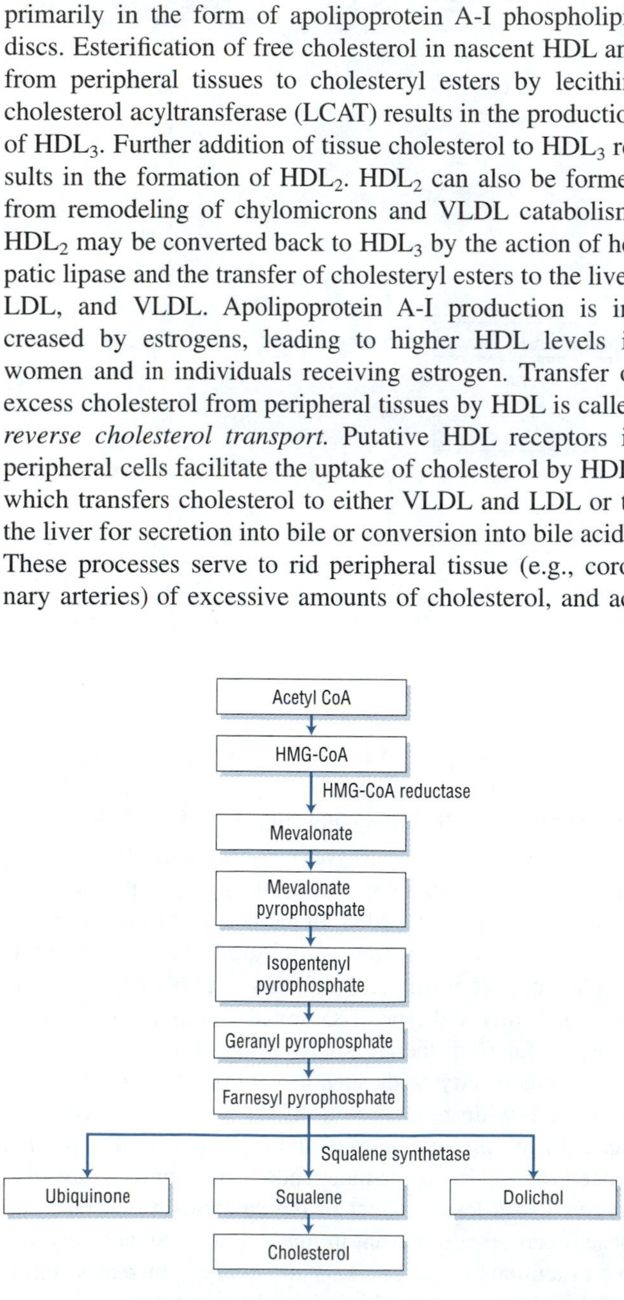

FIGURE 19–4. Biosynthetic pathway for cholesterol. The rate-limiting enzyme in this pathway is 3-hydroxy-3-methylglutaryl coenzyme A reductase (HMG-CoA reductase).

The "response-to-injury" hypothesis states that risk factors such as oxidized LDL, mechanical injury to the endothelium (e.g., percutaneous transluminal angioplasty), excessive homocysteine, immunologic attack or infection-induced (e.g., *Chlamydia*) changes in endothelial and intimal function lead to endothelial dysfunction and a series of cellular interactions that culminate in atherosclerosis.[16,17] The eventual outcomes of this cascade are clinical events such as angina and myocardial infarction. Atherosclerotic lesions are thought to arise from transport and retention of plasma LDL-cholesterol through the endothelial cell layer into the extracellular matrix of the subendothelial space. Once in the artery wall, LDL, but not apolipoprotein B, is oxidized by various oxidative products produced locally. Mildly oxidized LDL then recruits monocytes into the artery wall, which become transformed into macrophages. Macrophages have tremendous potential for accelerating LDL oxidation and apolipoprotein B accumulation, and altering the receptor-mediated uptake of LDL into the artery wall from the usual LDL-receptor to a "scavenger receptor" not regulated by cell content of cholesterol. Oxidized LDL increases plasminogen inhibitor levels (promotion of coagulation), induces the expression of endothelin (vasoconstrictive substance), inhibits the expression of nitric oxide (a vasodilator and platelet inhibitor), and is toxic to macrophages if highly oxidized. As oxidation of biologically active lipids proceeds, other lipids such as lysophosphatidylcholine and oxysterol are formed, which continue the reaction within the tissue. These events lead to a massive accumulation of cholesterol. The cholesterol-laden cells are called foam cells; foam cells are the earliest recognized cell of the arterial fatty streak.

Oxidized LDL provokes an inflammatory response, which is mediated by a number of chemoattractants and cytokines. Examples of each that appear to be involved at different stages of lesion development include monocyte chemoattractant protein 1 (MCP-1), monocyte colony stimulating factor (M-CSF), *gro,* vascular cell adhesion molecule (VCAM-1), E-selectin (ELAM-1), intercellular adhesion molecule (ICAM-1), platelet-derived growth factor (PDGF), vascular endothelial growth factor (VEGF), transforming growth factors (TGF_α and TGF_β), interleukin-1 and interleukin-6 (IL-1, IL-6), and the ratio of interleukins-10 and -12 (IL-10, IL-12). It appears that some of these factors (e.g., MCP-1 and M-CSF) participate early in the process of monocyte–macrophage attachment and transmigration across the endothelium, while others (PDGF and VCAM-1) promote later lesion growth.[18] The extent of ox-

TABLE 19–3. Fredrickson–Levy–Lees Classification of Hyperlipoproteinemia

Type	Lipoprotein Elevation	Approximate Mean Lipid Elevation	
		Cholesterol (mg/dL)	*Triglycerides (mg/dL)*
I	Chylomicrons	324	3316
IIa	LDL[a]	368	148
IIb	LDL + VLDL	354	135
III	IDL (LDL_1)	441	694
IV	VLDL	251	438
V	VLDL + chylomicrons	373	2071

[a]Heterozygotes for familial hypercholesterolemia.
Adapted from Schafer EJ, Levy RI. Pathogenesis and management of lipoprotein disorders. N Engl J Med 1985;312:1302.

idation and the inflammatory response is under genetic control of a major gene termed *Ath*-1 based on murine model studies. Two proteins associated with HDL—apolipoprotein J (apoJ) and paraoxonase (PON)—appear to play an important role.[19] Increased recognition of the role of these growth-regulatory molecules provides the possibility of future directions for antagonists to regulatory molecules such as PDGF, TGF_β, and the interleukins.

Lipoprotein disorders have been classified into six categories commonly used today for phenotypical description of hyperlipidemia. (Table 19–3). More recently, it has become apparent that specific genetic defects with disrupted protein, cell, and organ function give rise to several disorders within each family of lipoproteins (Table 19–4). In other words, an elevated cholesterol level does not necessarily equate with familial hypercholesterolemia or type IIa, as cholesterol may also be elevated in other lipoprotein disorders and the lipoprotein pattern does not describe the underlying genetic defect. The preceding discussion has focused on primary or genetic hyperlipoproteinemia, it should be remembered that secondary forms exist and several drugs may also elevate lipid levels (Table 19–5). These secondary forms of hyperlipidemia should be initially managed by correcting the underlying abnormality, including modification of drug therapy when appropriate.

TABLE 19–4. Lipoprotein Disorders

Increased Chylomicrons (Types I and V HLP)	Increased VLDL (Type IV HLP)	Increased Beta VLDL (Type III HLP)	Increased LDL (Type II HLP)	Abnormal LDL	Chylomicron, VLDL, and LDL Deficiency	HDL Deficiency
Familial hypertriglyceridemia[a]	Familial hypertriglyceridemia[a]	Apolipoprotein E2 phenotype[b]	Familial hypercholesterolemia[c]	Betasitosterolemia[a]	Abetalipoproteinemia[e]	Hypoalphalipoproteinemia[a]
Familial combined hyperlipidemia[a]	Familial combined hyperlipidemia[a]	Apolipoprotein E variants[b]	Familial combined hyperlipidemia[a]	Hyperapobetalipoproteinemia[a]	Hypobetalipoproteinemia[e]	Apolipoprotein A-I variants[b]
Lipoprotein lipase deficiency[d]	Apolipoprotein C-III DNA polymorphism[b]	Apolipoprotein E deficiency[e]		Cerebrotendinous xanthomatosis[d]	Normotriglycceridemic abetalipoproteinemia[e]	Tangier disease[b]
Lipoprotein lipase inhibitor[d]		Hepatic lipase deficiency[d]				HDL deficiency with planar xanthomas[a]
Apolipoprotein C-II deficiency[e]						Apolipoprotein A-I and C-III deficiency[e]
Abnormal apolipoprotein C-III sialylation[b]						LCAT deficiency[d]
Apolipoprotein E4 phenytype[b]						Fish eye disease[a]

HLP = hyperlipoproteinemia.
[a]Unknown defect.
[b]Apolipoprotein abnormality.
[c]Receptor abnormality.
[d]Enzyme abnormality.
[e]Apolipoprotein deficiency.
From Schaefer EJ, Levy RI. Pathogenesis and management of lipoprotein disorders. N Engl J Med *1985;312:1300–1310.*

TABLE 19–5. Secondary Forms of Hyperlipoproteinemia

Disease Induced	Drug Induced
Endocrine/Metabolic	Alcohol
Diabetes mellitus	Progestins
Von Gierke's disease	Thiazide diuretics
Lipodystrophies	β-Blockers
Cushing's syndrome	Glucocorticoids
Sexual ateliotic dwarfism	Isotretinoin
Acromegaly	Protease inhibitors
Hypothyroidism	
Anorexia nervosa	
Werner's syndrome	
Acute intermittent porphyria	
Renal	
Uremia	
Nephrotic syndrome	
Hepatic	
Primary biliary cirrhosis	
Acute hepatitis	
Hepatoma	
Immunologic	
Systemic lupus erythematosus	
Monoclonal gammapathies	
Stress Induced	

Familial hypercholesterolemia is the best understood of the primary hyperlipoproteinemia disorders due to the Nobel prize-winning work of Goldstein and Brown in their characterization of the LDL receptor (LDL-R) function and importance. Familial hypercholesterolemia is characterized by (1) a selective elevation in the plasma level of LDL, (2) deposition of LDL-derived cholesterol in tendons (xanthomas) and arteries (atheromas), and (3) inheritance as an autosomal dominant trait with homozygotes more severely affected than heterozygotes. Homozygotes (prevalence 1 in 1,000,000) have severe hypercholesterolemia (650 to 1000 mg/dL), with the early appearance of cutaneous xanthomas and fatal coronary heart disease (CHD) generally before the age of 20. The primary defect in familial hypercholesterolemia is the inability to bind LDL to the LDL-R or, rarely, a defect of internalizing the LDL-R complex into the cell after normal binding. This leads to lack of LDL degradation by cells and unregulated biosynthesis of cholesterol, with total cholesterol and LDL-C being inversely proportional to the deficit in LDL receptors. Heterozygotes have only about one-half of the normal number of LDL receptors. Homozygotes have essentially no functional LDL receptors.

Familial lipoprotein lipase deficiency is a rare, autosomal recessive trait characterized by a massive accumulation of chylomicrons and corresponding increase in plasma triglycerides or a type I lipoprotein pattern. VLDL concentration is normal. The presenting manifestations include repeated attacks of pancreatitis and abdominal pain, eruptive cutaneous xanthomatosis, and hepatosplenomegaly beginning in childhood. Symptom severity is proportional to dietary fat intake, and consequently to the elevation of chylomicrons. LPL is normally released from vascular endothelium or by heparin and hydrolyzes chylomicrons and VLDL (Fig. 19–3). Diagnosis is based on low or absent enzyme activity with normal human plasma or apolipoprotein C-II, a cofactor of the enzyme.[20] Accelerated atherosclerosis is not associated with this disease. Type V (VLDL and chylomicrons) is characterized by abdominal pain, pancreatitis, eruptive xanthomas, and peripheral polyneuropathy. Symptoms may occur in childhood but usually the disorder is expressed at a later age. The risk of atherosclerosis is increased with this disorder. These patients are commonly obese, hyperuricemic, and diabetic; while alcohol intake, exogenous estrogens, and renal insufficiency tend to be exacerbating factors.

Patients with familial type III hyperlipoproteinemia (also called dysbetalipoproteinemia, broad-band or beta VLDL) develop the following clinical features after age 20: xanthoma striata palmaris (yellow discolorations of the palmar and digital creases); tuberous or tuberoeruptive xanthomas (bulbous cutaneous xanthomas); and severe atherosclerosis involving the coronary arteries, internal carotids, and abdominal aorta. A defective structure of apolipoprotein E does not allow normal hepatic surface receptor binding of remnant particles derived from chylomicrons and VLDL (known as IDL); aggravating factors such as obesity, diabetes, or pregnancy may promote overproduction of apo B-containing lipoproteins. Although homozygosity for the defective allele (E_2/E_2) is common (1 in 100), only 1 in 10,000 express the full-blown picture, and interaction with other genetic or environmental factors or both is needed to produce clinical disease.

Type IV hyperlipoproteinemia is common and occurs in adulthood primarily in patients who are obese, diabetic, and hyperuricemic and do not have xanthomas. It may be secondary to alcohol ingestion and can be aggravated by stress, progestins, oral contraceptives, thiazides, or β-blockers. Two genetic patterns occur in type IV hyperlipoproteinemia: familial hypertriglyceridemia, which does not carry a great risk for premature coronary artery disease; and familial combined hyperlipidemia, which is associated with increased risk of cardiovascular disease.

Rare forms of lipoprotein disorders may include abnormal LDL or deficiencies in chylomicrons, VLDL, LDL, and HDL (Table 19–4). Most of these rare lipoprotein disorders do not result in premature atherosclerosis, with the exceptions of familial lecithin:cholesterol acyltransferase (LCAT) deficiency, cerebrotendinous xanthomatosis (CTX), and sitosterolemia with xanthomatosis. Their treatment consists of dietary restriction of plant sterols (sitosterolemia with xanthomatosis), chenodeoxycholic acid (CTX), or, potentially, blood transfusion (LCAT deficiency).

PATIENT EVALUATION

Total cholesterol and HDL should be measured in all adults 20 years of age or older at least once every 5 years. Once hyperlipidemia is suspected, major components of the evaluation are the history (including age, gender, and, if female, menstrual and estrogen replacement status), physical examination, and laboratory investigations. A complete history and physical exam should assess the following: (1) presence or absence of cardiovascular risk factors or definite cardiovascular disease in the individual; (2) family history of premature cardiovascular disease or lipid disorders; (3) presence or absence of secondary causes of hyperlipidemia, including concurrent medications (Table 19–5); and (4) presence or absence of xanthomas or abdominal pain, or history of pancreatitis, renal or liver disease, peripheral vascular disease or cerebral vascular disease (carotid bruits, stroke, or transient ischemic attack). This approach for a single patient is referred to as case finding or patient-based; whereas large-scale screening and recommendations for the general populace, health care providers, and the food industry are called a population-based approach.

Measurement of plasma cholesterol (which is about 3% lower than serum determinations), triglyceride, and HDL-C levels after a 12-hour or longer fast is important, as triglycerides may be elevated in nonfasted individuals; total cholesterol is only modestly affected by fasting. Analytic and biologic variability can have a major impact on the measurement and interpretation of cholesterol (or any other laboratory test). Analytic variability can be minimized through the use of adequate quality-control procedures including internal training, routine calibration and monitoring, and external proficiency testing. Even with these measures, the coefficient of variability in the best procedures can acceptably be up to 5%, and when combined with average biologic variability, total variability may be as high as about 22%. Analytic variability with desktop equipment generally is greater in the finger-stick capillary blood methods (e.g., Reflotron, Vision, and DT-60), usually yielding measurements less than those from a clinical laboratory, and this technology should be considered for use only as a screening method.[22,23] Reliance on desktop methods can result in misclassification of 7% to 14% of patients if capillary blood is used. Two determinations, 1 to 8 weeks apart, with the patient on a stable diet and weight, and in the absence of acute illness, are recommended to minimize variability and to obtain a reliable baseline.[1] If the total cholesterol is greater than 200 mg/dL, a second determination is recommended, and if the values are more than 30 mg/dL apart, the average of three values should be used. Familiarity with the method and quality control procedures employed by local laboratories is essential for interpretation of reported values. If the physical examination and history are insufficient to diagnose a familial disorder, then agarose-gel lipoprotein electrophoresis is useful to determine which class of lipoproteins is affected. If the triglyceride levels are below 400 mg/dL and neither type III hyperlipidemia nor chylomicrons are detected by electrophoresis, then one can calculate VLDL-C and LDL-C concentrations: VLDL-C = triglyceride/5; LDL-C = total cholesterol − (VLDL-C + HDL-C). Initial testing uses total cholesterol for case finding, but subsequent management decisions should be based on LDL-C.

Because total cholesterol is comprised of cholesterol derived from LDL, VLDL, and HDL, determination of HDL-C is useful when total plasma cholesterol is elevated. Although HDL-C may be elevated by moderate alcohol ingestion (less than 2 drinks per day), physical exercise, smoking cessation, weight loss, oral contraceptives, phenytoin, and terbutaline, smoking, obesity, a sedentary lifestyle, and drugs such as β-blockers lower HDL. Of these, only exercise and smoking cessation could be recommended as interventions for low HDL-C concentrations. The lipid-lowering agents niacin and gemfibrozil also increase HDL concentrations, but they are not Food and Drug Administration (FDA) approved for this use.

The range of lipid concentrations represents a population mean plus or minus two standard deviations and does not define the risk of disease. Reference values for plasma total, LDL, and HDL cholesterol concentrations for men and women as well as various ethnic groups are available from the National Health and Nutritional Survey (NHANES III).[3] Cholesterol and triglycerides increase throughout life until about the seventh decade for men and women. At that point, total cholesterol and LDL plateau and fall slightly in men but continue to rise in women. HDL tends to fall slightly with time and more rapidly after menopause in women. Institution of a population-based approach for cholesterol reduction should shift the entire curve to the left, and the potential reduction in cardiovascular mortality would be proportional to mean reductions at any cholesterol concentration.

TREATMENT RECOMMENDATIONS

Based on a careful review of the experimental pathologic, genetic, and epidemiologic evidence relating to the relationship between blood cholesterol levels and CHD, the adult treatment panel II of the National Cholesterol Education Program (NCEP) has recommended that total cholesterol determinations and risk factor assessment be used in the initial classification of adults.[1] If total cholesterol is less than 200 mg/dL, the patient has a *desirable blood cholesterol level* Table 19–6).[1] Cholesterol levels between 200 and 239 mg/dL are classified as *borderline-high blood cholesterol levels,* and assessment of risk factors (Table 19–7) is needed to more clearly define disease risk. Blood cholesterol levels of 240 mg/dL and above are classified as *high blood cholesterol levels.* If the total cholesterol is below 200 mg/dL and the HDL is above 35 mg/dL, no further follow-up is recommended for patients without known CHD and less

TABLE 19–6. Initial Classification of Cholesterol and Triglycerides

Classification	Total Cholesterol (mg/dL)	LDL Cholesterol (mg/dL)	HDL Cholesterol (mg/dL)	Triglycerides (mg/dL)
Desirable/normal	< 200	< 130	—	< 200
Borderline-high	200 to 239	130 to 159	—	200 to 400
High	≥ 240	> 160	> 60	400 to 1000
Very high	—	—	—	> 1000
Low	—	—	< 35	—

than two risk factors. When the serum total cholesterol is 200 mg/dL or more or the HDL cholesterol is below 35 mg/dL, or when there are borderline-high levels with two or more risk factors, a lipoprotein analysis (two measurements 1 to 8 weeks apart) to measure total and HDL cholesterol and triglycerides so that LDL-C may be estimated is recommended. In patients with evidence of CHD or other clinical atherosclerotic disease, the LDL goal is less than 100 mg/dL and most patients will require diet and/or drug intervention. Decisions regarding classification and management are based on the LDL-C levels as outlined in Table 19–8.

Screening of children and adolescents for elevated cholesterol remains a controversial issue; however, the Expert Panel on Children and Adolescents of the NCEP has recommended screening and dietary intervention in higher-risk children.[21] The rationale, in part, for this approach is based on the recognition that atherosclerosis begins in the childhood and adolescent years as documented in the pathobiological determinants of atherosclerosis in youth (PDAY) and the Bogalusa studies.[22,23] Likewise, if children with high blood lipids or lipoproteins levels are identified, and the levels in the parents are not known, the parents should be screened as well, as they are likely to be at high risk. Racial and gender differences do exist in the determination of lipoprotein fractions, and these factors should be considered in screening. Use of the serum cholesterol level alone may not be of sufficient specificity or sensitivity depending on the cut points used in screening, and other discretionary factors such as hypertension, smoking, obesity, high-fat diet, and use of cholesterol-raising medication may be needed to correctly identify children at risk. These recommendations are presented in Table 19–9. Presently, children over the age of 10 years are candidates for drug therapy if a trial of diet (6 months to 1 year) proves to be inadequate and LDL-C remains above 190 mg/dL, or above 160 mg/dL if two or more risk factors or CHD are present. Bile acid sequestrants are the recommended drugs for this population.[24] The long-term consequences of drug therapy in this population are unknown. In special instances, familial hypercholesterolemia (particularly the homozygous form), or the existence of CHD or two or more risk factors in the child, would prompt the earlier institution on drug therapy after a trial of dietary intervention.[25]

The goals of therapy expressed as LDL-C levels and the level of initiation of diet and drug therapy are provided in Tables 19–8 and 19–9 for adults and children, respectively. Ideally, dietary means should be used to attain even lower LDL-C, if possible, to achieve further reductions in CHD

TABLE 19–7. Risk Status Based on Presence of CHD Risk Factors Other Than LDL Cholesterol[a]

Positive Risk Factors

Age
- Men: ≥ 45 years
- Women: ≥ 55 years or premature menopause without estrogen replacement therapy

Family history of premature CHD (definite myocardial infarction or sudden death before 55 years of age in father or other male first-degree relative, or before 65 years of age in mother or other female first-degree relative)

Current cigarette smoking

Hypertension (≥ 140/90 mm Hg or on antihypertensive medication)

Low HDL cholesterol (< 35 mg/dL)

Diabetes mellitus

Negative Risk Factor[b]

High HDL cholesterol (≥ 60 mg/dL)

[a]High risk is defined as a net of two or more CHD risk factors or the presence of coronary or peripheral atherosclerosis.

[b]If the HDL cholesterol level is ≥ 60 mg/dL, subtract one risk factor, because high HDL cholesterol levels decrease CHD risk.

TABLE 19–8. Treatment Decisions Based on LDL Cholesterol

	Initiation Level (mg/dL)	LDL Goal (mg/dL)
Dietary Therapy		
Without CHD and < 2 risk factors	≥ 160	< 160
Without CHD and ≥ 2 risk factors	≥ 130	< 130
With CHD	> 100	≤ 100
	Consideration Level (mg/dL)	**LDL Goal (mg/dL)**
Drug Treatment		
Without CHD and < 2 risk factors	≥ 190[a]	< 160
Without CHD and ≥ 2 risk factors	≥ 160	< 130
With CHD	≥ 130[b]	≤ 100

[a]In men less than 35 years old and premenopausal woment with LDL cholesterol levels of 190 to 219 mg/dL, drug therapy should be delayed except in high-risk patients such as those with diabetes.

[b]In patients with CHD and LDL cholesterol levels of 100 to 129 mg/dL, the clinician should excercise clinical judgment in deciding whether to initiate drug treatment.

TABLE 19–9. Classification of Total and LDL Cholesterol in Children and Adolescents from Families with Hypercholesterolemia or Premature Cardiovascular Disease[a]

Category	Total Cholesterol (mg/dL)	LDL Cholesterol (mg/dL)	Dietary Intervention
Acceptable	< 170	< 110	Recommended population eating pattern
Borderline	170–199	110–129	Step1 diet prescribed and other risk factor intervention
High	≥ 200	≥ 130	Step 1 diet prescribed and then step 2 diet if necessary

[a]For use in children with a definite family history of premature (< 50 yr in females; < 60 yr in males) coronary heart disease including diagnostic coronary arteriography, angioplasty, coronary artery bypass grafting, myocardial infarction, angina pectoris, peripheral vascular disease, or cerebrovascular disease before age 55 yr. Screening should also be done in the offspring of a parent or sibling with blood cholesterol of ≥ 240 mg/dL or, in the absence of family history, the presence of other risk factors (corticosteroid use, juvenile diabetes mellitus, hypothyroidism, or other renal, endocrine, or hepatic disease known to affect cholesterol level).

From Expert panel, National Cholesterol Education Program. Report of the expert panel on blood cholesterol levels in children and adolescents. Pediatrics 1992;89 (suppl 2):525–584.

risk. Based on angiographic studies, aggressive reduction in total and LDL cholesterol is beneficial to prevent the development of atheromatous lesions in vascular beds and to induce the regression of existing lesions. Furthermore, data from trials of secondary and primary intervention also provide evidence that CHD morbidity and mortality as well as total mortality can be reduced with diet and drug therapy. The extent of lipid reduction is related to CHD risk reduction, and the goals outlined in the tables should be considered as *minimal* goals. Hypertriglyceridemia is classified as normal, borderline, high, or very high, as outlined in Table 19–6.

▶ TREATMENT: Hyperlipidemia

NONPHARMACOLOGIC THERAPY

Many clinicians believe that reduction of elevated levels of cholesterol in patients with hypercholesterolemia should lessen the risk for CHD. Results form numerous epidemiologic studies are consistent with this concept. Without doubt, hypercholesterolemia increases the risk for CHD. However, proof of the lipid hypothesis (that reduction of elevated cholesterol would reduce risk) was lacking until the publication of the Lipid Research Clinics coronary primary prevention trial (LRC-CPPT) unequivocally demonstrated a reduction in CHD death and nonfatal myocardial infarction in a large number of asymptomatic men with primary hypercholesterolemia.[26,27] The investigators found that for every 1% reduction in cholesterol, approximately a 2% reduction in CHD was seen. More recently the Scandinavian simvastatin survival study (4S), a secondary intervention trial, demonstrates that intervention with diet and simvastatin reduces CHD mortality and total mortality compared to diet and placebo treatment.[28] Results from angiographic studies demonstrate halting of progression of established lesions, prevention of new lesion formation, and, to a lesser extent, regression of existing atherosclerotic plaques in coronary arteries. This has been shown in native vessels or venous bypass grafts in patients who have undergone coronary artery bypass grafting. Of interest, these angiographic trials, which typically cause animalculine changes in luminal diameter (e.g., about 0.04 mm difference in change between placebo and active treatment), result in fewer clinical events such as myocardial infarction or the need for revascularization.[29] This unexpected finding suggests that plaque size and luminal encroachment by plaque may be less important that the effects that cholesterol lowering may have on the activity in the plaque and endothelial dysfunction.[30] These studies provide a strong rationale for attempting to lower plasma cholesterol and LDL in patients with hypercholesterolemia. Present evidence clearly demonstrates the benefit of cholesterol lowering in patients with known CHD and in patients with multiple risk factors. Many more patients without established CHD or risk factors must be treated to show a reduction in cardiovascular end points; however, the LRC-CPPT[26,27] and the West of Scotland[31] trials provide convincing evidence that primary intervention is also effective.

DIETARY THERAPY

The objectives of dietary therapy are to progressively decrease the intake of total fat, saturated fatty acids (i.e., saturated fat), and cholesterol and to achieve a desirable body weight. Typical American diets now include 13% to 20% of total calories from saturated fat and a cholesterol intake of 350 to 450 mg/d, both in excess of a "heart healthy" diet for normal Americans, let alone patients with a lipid disorder. The targeted saturated fatty acids have carbon chain lengths of 12 (lauric acid), 14 (myritisc acid), and 16 (palmitic acid). The rationale for using a nutritionally balanced low-fat, low-cholesterol diet for the treatment of hypercholesterolemia is based on the following principles: (1) it represents a reasonable extension of the diet recommended for the general public, (2) it progressively decreases the major cholesterol-raising constituent of the diet, (3) it precludes large intakes of polyunsaturated fats, and (4) it facilitates weight reduction by removing foods of high caloric density.[1] Dietary modification, weight control, and increased physical activity are essential first steps in the treatment of most lipid disorders. The dietary approach recommended by the NCEP ATP II for treating high blood cholesterol is outlined in Table 19–10.

Many patients with hyperlipidemia may be managed with dietary therapy alone, obviating the need for drugs. Diet is a cost-effective form of intervention.[1] Diet is considered to be the cornerstone for most forms of hyperlipidemia, and the use of a dietitian for patient counseling is recommended. Several cookbooks with recipes generally suitable for implementing an alternate diet as part of the stepped diet approach have been published. The basic rationale for reducing dietary cholesterol, saturated fat, and excessive calories is based on the overproduction of VLDL and subsequently, LDL. Excessive dietary intake of cholesterol and saturated fatty acids leads to decreased hepatic clearance of LDL and deposition of LDL and oxidized LDL in

TABLE 19–10. Dietary Therapy of High Blood Cholesterol

Nutrient[a]	Step I Diet	Recommended Intake	Step II Diet
Total fat		≤ 30% of total calories	
Saturated fatty acids	8–10% of total calories		< 7% of total calories
Polyunsaturated fatty acids		Up to 10% of total calories	
Monounsaturated fatty acids		Up to 15% of total calories	
Carbohydrates		≥ 55% of total calories	
Cholesterol	< 300 mg/d		< 200 mg/d
Total calories		To achieve and maintain desirable body weight	

[a]Calories from alcohol not included.

peripheral tissues.[32] The predicted reduction in total serum cholesterol following institution of the step 1 diet would be reduction of 3% to 14%, with average reductions of about 5% to 7% in men consuming 13% to 14% of their calories as saturated fat.[1] Progressing to step 2 diet therapy should provide an additional reduction of about 3% to 7%. Considering the baseline LDL-C concentration, the percentage of patients who were prescribed diet was 26%, 30%, and 40% for patients with less than two risk factors, two or more risk factors, and known coronary heart disease, respectively, based on the NHANES III survey data.[3] Some individuals are more responsive to dietary therapy than others and deviation from the predictions can be expected. Assessment of response to dietary therapy can be done with a dietary assessment instrument as described in the NCEP report.[1] Depending on the response to diet, the patient may be advanced until the target total or LDL-C level is reached. Each phase of the diet should be maintained for a minimum of 4 to 6 weeks for the minimal goal; however, the optimal response may not be seen for 3 to 6 months or more. In general, drug therapy should not be instituted until the trial of diet has continued for 6 months in primary prevention. Exceptions to these suggestions include patients with severe forms of hyperlipidemia or the presence of two or more risk factors or definite CHD. Long-term counseling of the patient and family to encourage diet compliance, and education about the risks and benefits that can be derived from diet modification and life-style changes, are important. Overall, reduction of cholesterol and saturated fat intake provides a reduction of coronary heart risk. This seems to be true regardless of the time of intervention (primary versus secondary), and diet modification works adjunctively with other risk factor interventions, such as cessation of smoking and treating hypertension. Continuation of diet therapy is imperative if drug therapy is to be optimal.

Adherence to diet therapy may be improved by presenting the changes in diet in a positive perspective and making changes over a reasonable time frame. The entire family, including the preparer of meals, should be included in diet counseling, considering that the step I diet is recommended for all Americans. Realistic goals should be set, and monitoring of response to diet intervention with feedback to the patient and family will improve compliance. A registered dietitian is an important member of the team. His or her expertise in providing a wide range of options and suggestions in preparation of food can make the difference between a good or an inadequate response to diet. Information concerning how one can eat out in a healthy fashion and advice in shopping are also important factors for success in diet therapy. An example is being aware of products with misleading labels such as coffee creamers that state they contain "no cholesterol," when they may contain hydrogenated (saturated) fats or oils (e.g., palmitic acid, palm kernel oil, or coconut oil), which makes them undesirable because of their saturated fat content. Variations in polyunsaturated and saturated fat and cholesterol intake influence the LDL concentration, but the amount of cholesterol has been found to have a greater effect than the proportion of polyunsaturated or saturated fat.[33] There were also ethnic differences in elevation of LDL with high saturated fat diets being greater in Caucasians than other groups. The isomeric form of fatty acids is also important. Fatty acids with the cis configuration are the preferred substrate for the ACAT reaction and significantly increase hepatic LDL receptor clearance while reducing LDL cholesterol production rate. The *trans* isomeric form cannot be used by ACAT and is biologically inactive with no effect on LDL concentration.[32] In addition to the commercial publications mentioned earlier, the NCEP also has publications available that assist in diet therapy.

Other dietary interventions or diet supplements may be useful in certain patients with lipid disorders. Increased intake of soluble fiber in the form of oat bran, pectins, certain gums, and psyllium products can result in useful adjunctive reductions in total and LDL cholesterol, but these dietary alterations or supplements should not be substituted for more active forms of treatment. Total daily fiber intake should be about 20 to 30 g/d, with about 25% or 6 g/day being soluble fiber.[1] Studies with psyllium seed in doses of 10 to 15 g/d have shown reductions in total and LDL cholesterol ranging from about 5% to 20%.[34,35] They have little or no effect on HDL-C or triglyceride concentrations. These products may also be useful in managing constipation associated with the bile acid sequestrants. Psyllium binds cholesterol in the gut but also reduces hepatic production and clearance.[35] Fish oil supplementation provides an increased amount of the omega-3 polyunsaturated fatty acids such as eicospentaenoic acid and docosahexaenoic acid. In epidemiologic studies from Scandinavia, ingestion of large amounts of cold water fish is associated with a reduction in CHD risk, but it is unclear if the same advantage is conferred with commercially prepared fish oil products. Fish oil supplementation has a fairly large effect in reducing triglycerides and VLDL-C, but it either has no effect on total and LDL cholesterol or may cause elevations in these fractions.[36] Other actions of fish oil may account for their protective effects. These effects include quantitative and qualitative alterations in the synthesis of prostanoid substances, changes in immune function and cellular proliferation, and potential antioxidative actions.[37,38] Responses noted with fish oil are further discussed under drug therapy.

Fat substitutes such as Olestra (Olean, sucrose polyester, Proctor and Gamble), a mixture of hexa-, hepta-, and octa-esters formed from the reaction of sucrose with long-chain fatty acids, have been approved by the FDA as a nondigestible, nonabsorable, noncaloric fat substitute for snack foods. Olestra is heat stable, an advantage over several other fat substitutes, allowing it to be used in the preparation of fried and baked foods. It is similar in composition to triglycerides, but Olestra is not hydrolyzed in the gastrointestinal tract by pancreatic lipase, and consequently not taken up by the intestinal mucosa. The principal adverse effects associated with Olestra use are bloating, flatulence, diarrhea, and "anal leakage." Because of the ability of Olestra to solubilize lipophilic substances, there has been concern over potential drug interactions in which lipophilic drugs (e.g., digitoxin, cyclosporin, or colchicine) or vitamins (vitamins A, D, E, and K) are solubilized in Olestra and excreted in the feces.[39]

Drug therapy is indicated following an adequate trial of diet therapy when LDL-C is greater than or equal to 190 mg/dL in patients without definite CHD or two other risk factors. In patients with CHD or two or more risk factors, drug therapy should be considered when LDL-C is greater than or equal to 160 mg/dL.[1] Drug therapy in patients with established CHD is indicated if LDL-C exceeds 130 mg/dL after dietary therapy (Table 19–8). Other guidelines have used a greater than 20% risk of coronary event at 10 years or a greater than 1.5% risk of coronary death per year as indications for treatment.[40]

PHARMACOLOGIC THERAPY

Several excellent reviews on the treatment of hyperlipidemia and the adverse effects of the drugs used have been published.[12,41,42] Although many efficacious lipid-lowering drugs exist, none is effective in all lipoprotein disorders, and all such agents are associated with some adverse effects.[43] Lipid-lowering drugs can be broadly divided into agents that decrease the synthesis of VLDL and LDL, agents that enhance VLDL clearance, agents that enhance LDL catabolism, agents that decrease cholesterol absorption, agents that elevate HDL, or some combination of these characteristics (Table 19–11). Recommended drugs of choice for each lipoprotein phenotype and alternate agents are given in Table 19–12. Products that are available and their doses are provided in Table 19–13.

Treatment of type I hyperlipoproteinemia is directed toward reduction of chylomicrons derived from dietary fat with the subsequent reduction in plasma triglycerides. Total daily fat intake should be no more than 10 to 25 g/d or approximately 15% of total calories. Secondary causes of hypertriglyceridemia (Table 19–5) should be excluded or, if present, the underlying disorder should be treated appropriately. Type V hyperlipoproteinemia also requires a stringent restriction of the fat component of dietary intake; in addition, drug therapy is indicated, as outlined in Table 19–12, if the response to diet alone is inadequate. Medium-chain triglycerides, which are absorbed without chylomicron formation, may be used as a dietary supplement for caloric intake if needed for types I and V. Hepatic fibrosis has been reported with medium-chain triglycerides. Omega-3 fatty acids may be useful in lipoprotein lipase deficiency in some patients. In patients with apolipoprotein C-II deficiency, infusion of plasma may normalize plasma triglyceride levels.

Primary hypercholesterolemia (familial hypercholesterolemia, familial combined hyperlipidemia, type IIa hyperlipoproteinemia) is treated with the bile acid sequestrants (BAR, colestipol and cholystramine), HMG Co-A reductase inhibitors (statins), or niacin. The primary action of BAR is to bind bile acids in the intestinal lumen, with a concurrent interruption of enterohepatic circulation of bile acids and a markedly increased excretion of acidic steroids in the feces. This decreases the bile acid pool size and stimulates hepatic synthesis of bile acids from cholesterol. Depletion of the hepatic pool of cholesterol results in an increase in cholesterol biosynthesis and an increase in the number of LDL receptors on the hepatocyte membrane. The increased number of receptors stimulates an enhanced rate of catabolism from plasma and lowers LDL levels. Cholesteryl ester transfer protein (CETP), which is correlated with total and LDL cholesterol concentrations, is also reduced by BAR perhaps by interfering with hepatic microsomal cholesterol content.[44] Patients with homozygous familial hypercholesterolemia (FH) genetically lack the ability to increase synthesis of LDL receptors and bile acid resins are generally ineffective. The increase in hepatic cholesterol biosynthesis may be paralleled by increased hepatic VLDL production and, consequently, bile acid resins may aggravate hypertriglyceridemia in patients with combined hyperlipidemia. Gastrointestinal complaints of constipation, bloating, epigastric fullness, nausea, and flatulence are most commonly reported.[43] With intensive education, patients can learn to tolerate resins on a long-term basis as evidenced by adherence in clinical trials to active drug regimens but in routine clinical practice 40% or more

TABLE 19–11. Effects of Drug Therapy on Lipids and Lipoproteins

Drug	Mechanism of Action	Effects on Lipids	Effects on Lipoproteins	Comment
Cholestyramine and colestipol	↑ LDL catabolism, cholesterol absorption	↓ Cholesterol	↓ LDL, ↑ VLDL	Problem with compliance; binds many coadministered drugs
Niacin	↓ LDL and VLDL synthesis	↓ Triglyceride and cholesterol	↓ VLDL, ↓ LDL, ↑ HDL	Problems with patient acceptance; good in combination with bile acid resins
Probucol	↑ LDL clearance	↓ Cholesterol	↓ LDL and HDL	Lowers HDL; modest efficacy but inhibits LDL oxidation and facilitates reverse cholesterol transport
Fibric acids Clofibrate Gemfibrozil Fenofibrate	↑ VLDL clearance, ↓ VLDL synthesis	↓ Triglyercide and cholesterol	↓ VLDL, ↑ ↓ LDL, ↑ HDL	Long-term toxicity of gemfibrozil may be less than clofibrate; raises HDL
Lovastatin, pravastatin, simvastatin, fluvastatin, atorvastatin, cerivastatin	↑ LDL catabolism, inhibit LDL synthesis	↓ Cholesterol	↓ LDL	Highly effective in heterozygotous familial hypercholesterolemia and in combination with other agents

TABLE 19–12. Lipoprotein Phenotype and Recommended Drug Treatment

Lipoprotein Type	Drug of Choice	Combination Therapy
I	Not indicated	—
IIa	HMG Co-ARI (statins)	Niacin or BAR
	Cholestyramine or colestipol	Statins or niacin
	Niacin	Statins or BAR ERT/HRT[a]
IIb	Statins	BAR, gemfibrozil or niacin
	Fibric acids	Statins, niacin, or BAR[b]
	Niacin	Statins or fibric acids
III	Fibric acids	Statins or niacin
	Niacin	Statins or fibric acids
IV	Fibric acids	Niacin
	Niacin	Fibric acids
V	Fibric acids	Niacin
	Niacin	Fish oils

HMG Co-ARI = hydroxymethylglutaryl coenzyme-A reductase inhibitor; BAR = bile acid resin; ERT/HRT = estrogen replacement therapy or hormone replacement therapy.
[a]In selected women, ERT may be first-line therapy and may be adequeate to reach LDL-C and HDL-C targets.
[b]BAR is not used as first-line therapy if triglycerides are elevated at baseline, because hypertriglyceridemia may be worsen with BAR alone.

of patients will discontinue therapy within 1 year.[45–47] These adverse effects can be managed by increasing the fluid intake, modifying the diet to increase bulk, and using stool softeners.[48] The other major limiting complaint is the gritty texture and bulk; these problems may be minimized by mixing the powder with orange drink or juice. Tablet forms of bile acid sequestrants should help in improving compliance with this form of therapy, whereas the bar does not improve compliance.[24] Other potential adverse effects include impaired absorption of fat-soluble vitamins A, D, E, and K; hypernatremia and hyperchloremia; gastrointestinal obstruction; and reduced bioavailability of acidic drugs such as coumarin anticoagulants, digitoxin, nicotinic acid, thyroxine, acetaminophen, hydrocortisone, hydrochlorothiazide, loperamide, and possibly iron.[43] Hyperchloremic metabolic acidosis, hypernatremia, and gastrointestinal obstruction have been reported almost exclusively in children, and malabsorption of fat-soluble vitamins is probably most common with high doses (e.g., 30 g/d of cholestyramine) of the bile acid resins. Drug interactions may be avoided by alternating administration times with an interval of 6 hours or greater between the bile acid resin and other drugs. Colestipol and cholestyramine have comparable side effects; however, colestipol may have better palatability because it is odorless and tasteless.

Niacin (nicotinic acid) may also be used in primary hypercholesterolemia in combination with bile acid sequestrants or as monotherapy for this disorder and others (Table 19–12). Niacin reduces the hepatic synthesis of VLDL, which in turn leads to a reduction in the synthesis of LDL. Factors responsible for decreased production of VLDL include inhibition of lipolysis with a decrease in free fatty acids in plasma, decreased hepatic esterification of triglycerides, and a possible direct effect on the hepatic production of apolipoprotein B. The complementary action of niacin and bile acid sequestrants to increase catabolism and decrease synthesis of LDL may account for the additive effects of this combination in hyperlipidemia. Niacin also increases HDL by reducing its catabolism. Niacin selectively decreases hepatic removal of HDL apoA-I but not cholesterol esters, thereby increasing the capacity of retained apoA-I to augment reverse cholesterol transport in isolated hepatic cells.[49] The principle use of niacin is for mixed hyperlipemia or as a second-line agent in combination therapy for hypercholesterolemia. It is also considered to be the first-line agent or an alternative for the treatment of hypertriglyceridemia.[50–52] There are numerous smaller trials suggesting that lower doses of niacin may be combined with statins

TABLE 19–13. Comparison of Drugs Used in the Treatment of Hyperlipidemia

Drug	Manufacturer	Dosage Forms	Usual Daily Dose	Maximum Daily Dose
Cholestyramine (Questran)	Bristol-Myers Squibb	Bulk powder/4-g packets	8 g tid	32 g
Cholestyramine (Questran Light)	Bristol-Myers Squibb	Bulk powder/4-g packets		
Cholestyramine (Cholybar)	Parke-Davis	4-g resin per bar		
Colestipol hydrochloride (Colestid)	Upjohn	Bulk powder/5-g packets	10 g bid	30 g
Niacin	Various	50-, 100-, 250-, and 500-mg tablets; 125-, 250-, and 500-mg capsules	2 g tid	9 g
Fenofibrate (Tricor)	Abbott	67-mg tablets	20 mg bid	20 mg
Clofibrate (Atromid-S)	Ayerst	500-mg capsules	1 g bid	2 g
Gemfibrozil (Lopid)	Parke-Davis	300-mg capsules	600 mg bid	1.5 g
Lovastatin (Mevacor)	MSD	20- and 40-mg tablets	20–40 mg	80 mg
Pravastatin (Pravachol)	Bristol-Myers Squibb	10- and 20-mg tablets	10–20 mg	40 mg
Simvastatin (Zocor)	MSD	5-, 10-, 20-, and 40-mg tablets	10–20 mg	80 mg
Atorvastatin (Lipitor)	Parke-Davis	10-mg tablets	10 mg	80 mg
Cervistatin (Baycol)	Bayer	0.2- and 0.3-mg tablets	0.3 mg	0.3 mg

or gemfibrozil to minimize adverse effects and maximize response. These combinations require careful monitoring because interactions do occur.

Niacin has many adverse drug reactions that occur commonly; fortunately, most of the symptoms and biochemical abnormalities seen do not require discontinuation of therapy. Cutaneous flushing and itching appear to be prostaglandin mediated and can be reduced by aspirin 325 mg given shortly before niacin ingestion.[53] Flushing seems to be related to rising plasma concentrations of niacin; taking the dose with meals and slowly titrating the dose upward may minimize these effects. Gastrointestinal intolerance and flushing are common problems. Sustained-release products may minimize these complaints in some patients, but controlled trials with regular-release products do not demonstrate much of a difference between sustained- and regular-release products. Potentially important laboratory abnormalities occurring with niacin therapy include elevated liver function tests, hyperuricemia, and hyperglycemia. With less than 3 g/d, the degree of liver function test elevation is generally not marked and often transient, and a temporary reduction in dosage frequently corrects the problem. Niacin-associated hepatitis is more common with sustained-release preparations, and their use should be restricted to patients intolerant of regular-release products.[54] Sustained-release products are often more expensive and given the lack of data for reduced adverse effects and increased incidence of hepatitis, regular-release products should always be used first. Preexisting gout and diabetes may be exacerbated by niacin; these patients should be monitored more closely and their medication titrated appropriately. Niacin is contraindicated in patients with active liver disease. Dry eyes and other ophthalmologic complaints are also occasionally noted. Concomitant alcohol and hot drinks may magnify flushing and pruritus with niacin and they should be avoided at the time of ingestion. Nicotinamide should not be used in the treatment of hyperlipidemia, as it does not effectively lower cholesterol or triglyceride levels.

Probucol, neomycin, and dextrothyroxine have also been used as alternative drugs for primary hypercholesterolemia; however, their utility is limited by detrimental changes in lipoproteins, adverse effects, and lack of efficacy. Fractional catabolism of LDL and increased biliary excretion of cholesterol reduces both LDL and HDL with probucol.[55] The decrease in HDL levels seen with probucol is due to a decreased synthesis of apolipoprotein A-I and decreased lipoprotein lipase activity.[56] VLDL levels are unaffected with probucol. Probucol reduces total and LDL cholesterol by 8% to 21% while *reducing* HDL concentrations by up to 26%. Probucol inhibits the oxidation of LDL and it also facilitates reverse cholesterol transport.[57] HDL levels may drop during reverse cholesterol transport, and this may explain this lipoprotein change seen in probucol therapy. The undesirable effect of probucol on HDL, its propensity to increase the QT interval, and lack of regression in the femoral vascular bed (discussed later) has led the manufacturer to remove this drug from the market. Neomycin and dextrothyroxine have been used in lowering cholesterol, but the advent of more potent and safer agents such as the statins has further reduced their potential role in therapy.

Statins interrupt the conversion of HMG-CoA to mevalonate, the rate-limiting step in de novo cholesterol biosynthesis, by inhibiting 3-hydroxy-3-methylglutaryl coenzyme A (HMG-CoA) reductase (Fig. 19–4). Currently available products include lovastatin, pravastatin, simvastatin, fluvastatin, atorvastatin, and cervastatin. The pharmacokinetic properties of the statins are given in Table 19–14.[58,59] The plasma half-lives for all the statins have been reported to be short except for atorvastatin, and this may account for its potency.[60] In CURVES, the largest head-to-head comparison of statins, atorvastatin was found to the most potent drug for lowering total cholesterol and LDL-C, with reductions in LDL-C of 38%, 46%, 51%, and 54% for the 10, 20, 40, and 80-mg doses, respectively.[61] Metabolic studies with statins in normal volunteers and patients with hypercholesterolemia suggest reduced synthesis of LDL-C as well as enhanced catabolism of LDL mediated through LDL receptors as the principle mechanisms for lipid-lowering effects.[1] Total and LDL cholesterol are reduced in a dose-related fashion by 30% or more on average when added to dietary therapy, with the effects being more pronounced in nonfamilial than in familial hypercholesterolemia. Combination therapy with bile acid sequestrants and lovastatin is rational as LDL receptor numbers are increased, leading to greater degradation of LDL-C; intracellular synthesis of cholesterol is inhibited, and enterohepatic recycling of bile acids is interrupted. In the expanded clinical evaluation of lovastatin (EXCEL) study of over 8000 patients, lovastatin reduced LDL-C by 24% to 40% when given in doses ranging from 20 mg once daily to 40 mg twice daily.[62] Constipation in placebo-treated patients occurred in 4.7% of patients, while lovastatin was associated with 4.2% to 7.7% (20 mg twice a day). Other adverse events related to lovastatin use were noted. Elevation of serum transaminase levels (primarily alanine aminotransferase) to above three times the upper limit of normal and associated muscle symptoms (myopathy) were most common at higher doses, 40 mg given twice a day; 1.5% compared with placebo of 0.1%. Creatine kinase (CK) greater than 10 times the upper limit of normal and muscle symptoms occurred in 0% of the placebo group versus 0.2% of the lovastatin group, and any elevation of CK was highest at 40 mg given twice a day, 3.5% versus 1.6% for placebo. Lens opacities have been reported with lovastatin; however, in the age groups studied, these abnormalities are common and tend to wax and wane with time irrespective of drug therapy, and no statistical association is known to exist. As a category of monotherapy, the HMG-CoA reductase inhibitors are the most potent total and LDL cholesterol-lowering agents and among the best tolerated.[28,31,63–65]

Combined hyperlipoproteinemia (type IIb) may be treated with statins, niacin, or gemfibrozil to lower LDL cholesterol without elevating VLDL and triglycerides. Niacin is the most effective agent and may be combined with a bile acid sequestrant. Cholestyramine or colestipol alone in this disorder may elevate

TABLE 19–14. Pharmacokinetics of the Statins[a]

Parameter	Lovastatin	Simvastatin	Pravastatin	Fluvastatin	Atorvastatin	Cerivastatin
Isoenzyme[b]	3A4	3A4	None	2C9	3A4	3A4
Lipophilic	Yes	Yes	No	Yes	Yes	Yes
Protein binding (%)	>95	95–98	~50	>90	96	>99
Active metabolites	Yes	Yes	No	No	Yes	Yes
Elimination half-life (h)	3	2	1.8	1.2	14	2

[a]Pharmacokinetic parameters in this table are based on studies and reviews presented in the literature.
[b]Isoenzyme refers to the specific isoenzyme in the cytochrome P450 system responsible for the metabolism of each drug.

VLDL and triglycerides, and their use as single agents for treating combined hyperlipoproteinemia should be avoided. Gemfibrozil as a single agent is effective in reducing VLDL, but a reciprocal rise in LDL may occur and total cholesterol values may remain relatively unchanged. Gemfibrozil reduces the synthesis of VLDL and, to a lesser extent, apolipoprotein B, with a concurrent increase in the rate of removal of triglyceride-rich lipoproteins from plasma. Plasma HDL concentrations may rise 10% to 15% or more with gemfibrozil. As a fibric acid derivative of clofibrate, there has been concern that detrimental and adverse effects similar to those observed with clofibrate would occur; however, evidence from the Helsinki Heart Study has shown no significant differences between gemfibrozil and placebo.[66,67] Gastrointestinal complaints occur in 3% to 5% of patients, rash in 2%, dizziness in 2.4%, and transient elevations in transaminase levels and alkaline phosphatase in 4.5% and 1.3%, respectively. Similar to clofibrate, gemfibrozil may enhance the formation of gallstones associated with an increase in the lithogenic index; however, the rate is low (0.6%) and similar to that seen with placebo in the Helsinki heart study. Gemfibrozil may potentiate the effects of oral anticoagulants as seen with clofibrate, but this is not well documented.

Type III hyperlipoproteinemia may be treated with clofibrate, gemfibrozil, fenofibrate, or niacin. Although clofibrate has been suggested as the drug of choice for this disorder, given the lack of data supporting its efficacy in altering cardiovascular mortality in the major studies on hypercholesterolemia, and numerous, well-documented and serious adverse effects, it is reasonable to consider niacin or gemfibrozil prior to the use of clofibrate. Clofibrate increases the activity of lipoprotein lipase and reduces to a lesser extent the synthesis or secretion of VLDL from the liver into the plasma. Clofibrate is less effective than gemfibrozil or niacin in reducing VLDL production. The most disturbing aspects of clofibrate adverse effects are its potential to induce gallstones (4.7%, clofibrate; 0.54%, placebo), promote ventricular ectopy, and potentially cause gastrointestinal malignancy, causing a greater overall mortality than placebo alone (WHO).[68,69] A myositis syndrome of myalgia, weakness, stiffness, malaise, and elevations in creatinine phosphokinase and asparate aminotransaminase is seen with clofibrate, and it seems to be more common in patients with renal insufficiency. Enhanced hypoprothrombinemic and hypoglycemic effects are reported to occur when clofibrate is given to patients on coumarin anticoagulants and sulfonylurea compounds, but the mechanisms for these interactions are not well understood. Rifampin, an hepatic enzyme inducer of oxidative pathways, may induce the metabolism of clofibrate but the long-term consequences are unknown.

Three fibric acid derivatives (clofibrate, gemfibrozil, and fenofibrate) are approved in the United States; however, several others are under development or are being used in Europe, including benzafibrate and ciprofibrate.[70,71] Fenofibrate appears to be the most useful. All reduce LDL-C by 20% to 25% in heterozygous familial hypercholesterolemia. The response of LDL-C, HDL-C, and triglycerides to this category of drug is very dependent on the specific lipoprotein type (e.g., type IIa versus IIb) and the baseline triglyceride concentration.[71]

As a potential alternative therapy, for this phenotype, numerous epidemiologic and normal volunteer studies have found that diets high in omega-3 polyunsaturated fatty acids (from fish oil), mostly commonly eicosapentaenoic acid, reduce cholesterol, triglycerides, LDL-C, and VLDL-C, and may elevate HDL-C.[36,72] The effects of fish oil on lipoprotein metabolism are mediated through a reduction in VLDL production and suppression of VLDL apolipoprotein B. In patients with hypertriglyceridemia, either phenotypes type IIb or type V, a diet high in omega-3 fatty acids given for 4 weeks reduced cholesterol 27% and 45%, and triglyceride 64% and 79%, in the type IIb and type V patients, respectively.[73] A diet high in eicosapentaenoic acid (EPA) given to hyperlipidemic hemodialysis patients resulted in significant decreases in cholesterol and triglycerides for up to 13 weeks. Fish oil supplementation may be most useful in patients with hypertriglyceridemia; however, its role in treatment is not well defined. Potential complications of fish oil supplementation, such as thrombocytopenia and bleeding disorders, have been noted, especially with high doses (EPA 15 to 30 g/d), and well-controlled trials are needed to determine if fish oils are safe and effective doses before their use may be broadly recommended.

Combination drug therapy may be considered after adequate trials of monotherapy and in patients documented compliant to the prescribed regimen. Two to three monthly lipoprotein determinations should confirm lack of response prior to initiation of combination therapy. Cholestyramine may be added in patients with fasting hypertriglyceridemia, but it should not be used as the initial drug, because triglycerides are likely to increase. Contraindications to and drug interactions with combined therapy should be carefully screened, as well as consideration of the extra cost of drug product and monitoring that may be required. In general, a statin and a BAR or niacin with a BAR provide the greatest reduction in total and LDL cholesterol. Regimens intended to increase HDL levels should include either gemfibrozil or niacin, and it should be remembered that statins combined with either of these drugs may result in a greater incidence of hepatoxicity or myositis. Familial combined hyperlipidemia may respond better to a fibric acid and a statin than fibric acids and BAR.[74,75]

Severe forms of hypercholesterolemia—such as familial hypercholesterolemia (FH), familial defective apolipoprotein B-100, severe polygenic hypercholesterolemia, familial combined hyperlipidemia, and familial dysbetalipoproteinemia (type III)—may require more intensive therapy. In particular, FH patients often require combination therapy (2 or 3 drugs) and have been managed with surgical therapy (partial ileal bypass), plasmapheresis (LDL-apheresis), and liver transplantation (to replace LDL receptors).

HYPERTRIGLYCERIDEMIA

It is important to remember that lipoprotein pattern types I, III, IV, and V are associated with hypertriglyceridemia, and these primary lipoprotein disorders and underlying diseases should be excluded prior to implementing therapy. A positive family history of CHD is important in identifying patients at risk for premature atherosclerosis. If a patient with CHD has elevated triglycerides, the associated abnormality is probably a contributing factor to CHD and should be treated.[52]

High serum triglycerides (Tables 19–6 and 19–12) should be treated by achieving desirable body weight, consumption of a low saturated fat and cholesterol diet, regular exercise, smoking cessation, and restriction of alcohol (in selected patients). In patients with borderline-high triglycerides but with accompanying risk factors of established CHD disease, family history of premature CHD, concomitant LDL elevation or low HDL, and genetic forms of hypertriglyceridemia associated with CHD (familial dysbetalipoproteinemia, familial combined hyperlipidemia), drug therapy with niacin should be considered. Niacin should not be used in diabetics because of the risk of worsening glycemic control. Alternative therapies include gemfibrozil, statins, and fish oil.[76] Fibrates may increase LDL, and their use in borderline-high triglyceridemia requires careful monitoring to detect this deleterious change in lipid profile. Statins may also be used, because they provide modest reductions in triglycerides and modest elevations in HDL.[77,78] Atorvastatin, in the currently approved doses, has the greatest triglyceride-lowering effects of the available statins.[79] The goal of therapy in this situation is to lower triglycerides and VLDL particles that may be atherogenic, increase HDL, and reduce LDL.

Very high triglycerides are associated with pancreatitis and other consequences of the chylomicron syndrome. At this level of elevation of triglycerides, a genetic form of hypertriglyceridemia often coexists with other causes of elevated triglycerides such as diabetes. Dietary fat restriction (10% to 20% of calories as fat), weight loss, alcohol restriction, and treatment of the coexisting disorder are the basic elements of management. Drugs useful in hypertriglyceridemia include gemfibrozil, niacin, and certain statins (atorvastatin and simvastatin). Gemfibrozil is the preferred drug in diabetics due to the effect of niacin on glycemic control. Success in treatment is defined as a reduction in triglycerides below 500 mg/dL.[1]

SPECIAL CONSIDERATIONS

ELDERLY

Hypercholesterolemia is an independent risk factor for CHD in the elderly, as it is in the younger patient. The attributable risk, which is the difference in absolute rates of CHD between segments of the population with higher or lower serum cholesterol levels, increases with age. Older patients potentially benefit to a greater extent from cholesterol lowering than younger populations. Data from studies of elderly men in a variety of settings are consistent with a relative risk of at least 1.5 in the highest compared to lower quartile of cholesterol levels.[80] Treatment of hypercholesterolemia in the elderly may bring about a comparable reduction in absolute risk to that obtained in younger persons.[1] Subgroup analyses of the West of Scotland (primary) and 4S (secondary) intervention studies show that elderly patients have lower CHD risk reduction (relative risk reduction of 27% and 29%, respectively) compared with younger patients (relative risk reduction of 40% and 39%, respectively).[28,31] The Framingham study suggests that elderly women are at higher risk due to high blood cholesterol levels, but no other large studies have included women and their risks or benefits from cholesterol reduction are not well defined. Primary prevention in younger patients requires about 2 years before reduction in CHD risk is apparent, and this lag time should be taken into consideration in patient selection for therapy. Nonlipid CHD risk factors do not decline in relative risk with aging, and aggressive management of the modifiable nonlipid risk factors is important in the older patient. Because most women with CHD are elderly and also at risk for osteoporosis, they are logical candidates for diet therapy with consideration of calcium intake consistent with osteoporosis prevention, exercise, and estrogen replacement therapy.

Step I diet can be recommended for most elderly patients with hypercholesterolemia, but step II diets may not be advisable given potential malnutrition and concurrent disease in the elderly. Drug therapy in principle differs little from younger patients, and older patients' respond to lipid-lowering drugs as well as younger patients based on the 4S trial and smaller studies.[31] Predicted reductions in CHD morbidity and mortality suggest that elderly patients with hypercholesterolemia should benefit from treatment; however, the gain in life expectancy may be small depending on the age at the start of treatment and the magnitude of cholesterol reduction.[81,82] Changes in body composition, renal function, and other physiologic changes of aging may make older patients more susceptible to adverse effects of lipid-lowering drug therapy. In particular, older patients are more likely to have constipation (bile acid resins), skin and eye changes (niacin), gout (niacin), gallstones (fibric acid derivatives), conduction abnormalities (probucol), and bone/joint disorders (fibric acid derivatives, reductase inhibitors). Therapy should be started with lower doses and titrated up slowly to minimize adverse effects.

WOMEN

Cholesterol is an important determinant of CHD in women, but the relationship is not as strong as that seen in men. HDL may be a more important predictor of disease in women.[6] LDL and HDL genetic regulation in women and men does not appear to be different. Based on the Nurses' Health Study, obesity is an important determinant of CHD in women, with the relative risk being 3.3 in the highest Quetelet index (weight in kilograms divided by the square of the height in meters) compared to the lowest category (i.e., < 21 versus ≥ 29); low HDL levels usually accompany obesity. No major differences exist in the influence of exercise, alcohol ingestion, and smoking on lipid levels between men and women. Women in the highest tertile of cholesterol appear to be more responsive to dietary therapy than those in the lower tertiles, and more responsive than formulas based on men predict. Oral contraceptives adversely influence LDL and HDL, and the products containing the lowest estrogen dose and the strongest antiestrogenic progestin produce the largest changes. Unopposed estrogen replacement for menopausal therapy increases HDL by 9% to 13% and decreases LDL by 4% to 10%, which is enough to influence CHD risk. Cyclic therapy with estrogen–progestin therapy may offset the beneficial effect of estrogen alone, depending on the particular estrogen–progestin combination and the doses used. The relative risk reduction of CHD in women was greater than men in AFCAPS/TexCAPS (54% versus 34%),[63] CARE (46% versus 20%),[64] and 4S (35% versus 34%),[28] but less in LIPID (7% versus 25%).[83] Regression of coronary atherosclerosis in women can be induced with aggressive therapy and, based on one study, the mean percent change in area of stenosis was greater in women than men when LDL was reduced by about 38% and HDL was increased by 28%.[84]

Cholesterol and triglyceride levels rise progressively throughout pregnancy, with an average increment in cholesterol of 30 to 40 mg/dL occurring around 36th to 39th weeks. Triglyceride levels may go up by as much as 150 mg/dL. Drug therapy is not instituted nor is it usually continued during pregnancy. Dietary therapy is the mainstay of treatment, with emphasis on maintaining a nutritionally balanced diet as per the needs of pregnancy.

CHILDREN

Drug therapy in children is not recommended until the age of 10 years or older, and the guidelines for institution of therapy and the goals of therapy are different from those in adults (Table 19–9). Younger children are generally managed with dietary therapy following the NCEP step I and II diets after the age of 2 years. Bile acid sequestrants are used in children because they minimize the risks of systemic toxicity.[85] Some literature does exist suggesting that resins are safe and effective in children.[25,86] Severe forms of hypercholesterolemia (e.g., familial hypercholesterolemia) may require more aggressive treatment.

CONCURRENT DISEASE STATES

Diabetes mellitus, nephrotic syndrome, end-stage renal disease and nephrotic syndrome, and hypertension compound the risk of dyslipemia and may present difficult-to-treat lipid abnormalities. Diabetic dyslipemia leads to threefold increased risk of CHD (women > men) and macrovascular complications associated with hyperinsulinemia and/or insulin resistance that may precede the onset of clinical diabetes during the prediabetic phase. Hyperinsulinemia may contribute to dyslipemia and hypertension and have direct atherogenic effects on the arterial wall (syndrome X); it is an independent predictor of future cardiovascular disease in a number of studies. Diabetics also have enhanced oxidation and glycation of LDL, making their LDL more atherogenic; and have a pattern of smaller, more dense LDL (pattern B), considered to be more atherogenic. The characteristic pattern in type II diabetes is hypertriglyceridemia, low HDL, and, less commonly, elevated total and LDL cholesterol. In the diabetic, hypertriglyceridemia is a stronger predictor of CHD risk than are cholesterol levels. Although the target LDL concentration in all diabetics is less than 130 mg/dL, because of the tremendous synergy between diabetes and the associated dyslipemic state, many feel that LDL cholesterol should be reduced to less than 100 mg/dL when possible. The relative risk reduction for CHD in diabetics versus nondiabetics is greater in the West of Scotland trial (37% versus 20%),[31] AFCAPS/TexCAPS (43% versus 36%),[63] CARE (25% versus 23%),[64] and 4S (55% versus 32%).[28] Diet and weight reduction, if the patient is obese (particularly type II patients), and good glycemic control should be instituted prior to drug therapy. The availability of metformin and troglitzaone should prove useful in dyslipemic diabetics because both have little effect on weight (tendency for weight loss) and improve lipid levels slightly. Cholestyramine in diabetic patients may result in lower LDL levels, but VLDL and triglyceride levels, which are commonly elevated in diabetes, may be further increased in this population. Resins may aggravate constipation, which is common in diabetics. Niacin is very effective in lowering total and LDL cholesterol and raising HDL concentrations, but it is associated with worsened glycemic control.[50,87,88] Fibric acids principally lower VLDL and triglycerides while increasing HDL with only modest lowering of total and LDL cholesterol; on occasion, fibric acid derivatives may increase LDL levels. Fibric acid derivatives tend to improve glucose tolerance, in contrast to niacin; the greatest effect has been seen with bezafibrate. Data from the Helsinki Heart Study suggest that gemfibrozil should be an effective drug in diabetic patients as it corrects the common lipid defects that are seen.[8] Although the effect of statins on triglycerides and HDL-C abnormalities commonly seen in diabetes is less than with fibric acids, the subgroup analyses cited earlier suggest that they reduce CHD risk significantly.[89] The diabetes atherosclerosis intervention study (DAIS) is an angiographic study underway investigating fenofibrate for CHD in diabetics.[90]

Abnormalities of lipoprotein metabolism in the nephrotic syndrome include elevated total and LDL cholesterol, Lp(a), VLDL, and triglycerides. The apolipoprotein C-III to C-II ratio is elevated, consistent with greater lipoprotein lipase inhibitor activity, and the extent of hypoalbuminemia is correlated with dyslipemia. The basic abnormality appears to be one of overproduction of LDL-apoB from VLDL rather than reduced clearance of LDL-C and related proteins.[91,92] Protein restriction and a "vegan" diet corrects lipid abnormalities to some extent.[93] Statins have been shown to be effective in reducing elevated total and LDL cholesterol in the nephrotic syndrome, although the levels do not usually return to normal.[94] Clofibrate should not be used if renal insufficiency exists, whereas the pharmacokinetics of gemfibrozil are apparently not altered by renal insufficiency and it is effective in lowering total cholesterol by about 15% for this disorder.[66]

Renal insufficiency without proteinuria leads to hypertriglyceridemia, slightly elevated total and LDL cholesterol (particularly with chronic ambulatory peritoneal dialysis), and low HDL levels (especially during hemodialysis). These abnormalities are thought to be due to a deficiency in apolipoprotein C-II, perhaps due to sustained use of heparin during hemodialysis and depletion of lipoprotein lipase, carbohydrate-induced obesity and hypertriglyceridemia, loss of carnitine during hemodialysis, use of acetate buffer (acetate is a precursor to fatty acid synthesis) during hemodialysis, and decreased lecithin-cholesterol acyltransferase (LCAT) activity during hemodialysis. Dialysis does not correct the lipid abnormalities. Renal transplantation may correct lipid abnormalities in some patients; however, in others the use of transplantation-related medications such as corticosteroids, cyclosporine, and certain antihypertensive agents (see Chap. 43 on renal transplantation and Chap. 10 on hypertension) may aggravate the lipid abnormalities. Cyclosporine interferes with the metabolism of reductase inhibitors, and patients need to be observed closely for myositis and worsening renal function. Of interest, correction of lipid abnormalities may improve renal hemodynamics.[95] Small, short-term studies have suggested that fluvastatin may be safer than other reductase inhibitors, but this needs to be validated in larger, long-term trials. Diet will modify lipoprotein levels and polyunsaturated fatty acids may have a role in impeding the progression of renal disease as well as the cardiovascular complications. Bile acid sequestrants do not correct the lipid abnormalities seen in renal insufficiency. Lovastatin or its active metabolite may accumulate in renal insufficiency, and lower doses of reductase inhibitors should be used to avoid adverse effects. Gemfibrozil may be used with caution as its pharmacokinetics are unchanged and it lowers triglycerides and increases HDL.[96] Statins and fibric acid derivatives may increase the risk of severe myopathy, and attention to symptoms of myositis is needed. Niacin may also be useful in nondiabetic patients with renal insufficiency.

Hypertensive patients have a greater than expected prevalence of high blood cholesterol levels, and conversely, patients with hypercholesterolemia have a higher than expected prevalence of hypertension. Recommendations for the management of hypertension in patients with hypercholesterolemia include avoiding the use of drugs that elevate cholesterol such as diuretics and β-blockers and using agents that are either lipid-neutral or may reduce cholesterol slightly (see Chap. 10).[1] Bile acid sequestrants may bind to thiazide diuretics and some β-blockers and interfere with their absorption. This interaction may be avoided by giving the antihypertensive 1 hour before or 4 hours after the resin. Niacin may magnify the hypotensive effects of vasodilators.

COST-EFFECTIVENESS OF ANTIHYPERLIPEMIC THERAPY

The clinical benefits of lipid-lowering therapy for primary and secondary intervention are now well established based on the results of the AFCAPS/TexCAPS, 4S, and other studies showing a reduction in CHD morbidity and mortality. The balance of benefits and costs has been examined in a few studies.[82,97] The cost per year of life saved has been estimated to range from less than $10,000 to over $1 million dollars depending on the presence or absence of CHD, age of the patient, baseline total or LDL-C level and reduction in cholesterol, and number of risk factors present. In general, intervention in patients with known CHD or secondary intervention are cost effective with statin therapy, while other types of therapy may be cost effective if certain assumptions concerning compliance, efficacy, and so forth, are met. The range for secondary intervention based on the 4S study is $3800 for a 70-year-old man with a high cholesterol level to $27,400 per year of life gained for a middle-aged woman with an average cholesterol level.[82] In contrast, primary prevention in men based on the West of Scotland trial averages about $35,000 per year of life gained.[97] These studies demonstrate that primary and secondary intervention are well within the accepted boundry of less than $50,000 for a medical intervention to be considered to be cost effective. Based on the specific lipoprotein phenotype, fibric acid derivatives, niacin, or combination therapy of statins plus BAR may be cost effective.[98–100] Cost-effectiveness is maximized by treating high-risk patients and those with established CHD.

Specialty lipid clinics have become increasingly popular and many use pharmacists to provide direct patient care in this setting. An interesting recent analysis shows that a specialty clinic may be more expensive ($659 ± $43 versus $477 ± $42 per patient, $P < .001$) than usual care. However, the overall cost-effectiveness is improved when expressed as program costs per unit (mmol/L) reduction in the LDL-C, a measure of cost-effectiveness, which was significantly lower for specialized care ($758 ± $58 versus $1058 ± $70, $P = .002$) because more patients achieve their targeted goal.[101]

OTHER THERAPIES

Partial ileal bypass has been used in severe heterozygous and homozygous familial hypercholesterolemia; however, it is ineffective in the latter case. Ileal bypass removes the site of bile acid reabsorption, depleting the bile acid pool and increasing the catabolism of cholesterol. A randomized trial of diet versus surgery, program on the surgical control of the hyperlipidemias (POSCH), reported that total and LDL cholesterol were decreased (23.3% and 37.7%, respectively) and HDL increased (4.3%) in patients who had undergone ileal bypass for hypercholesterolemia.[102–104] Overall death was delayed by nearly 3 years ($P = .032$) and CHD mortality was delayed by nearly 4 years ($P = .046$) by surgery compared to the control group. Revascularization procedures were delayed by an average of 7 years ($P < .001$). Postsurgery diarrhea was more common in the surgical group, as was the rate of kidney stones (4% versus 0.4%), gallstones (10% versus 2%), and bowel obstruction (13.5% versus 3.6%).

Portacaval shunts have been used to decrease the formation of LDL-C and reductions of 10% to 20% have been reported.[105] Plasma exchange combined with niacin was found to reduce plasma cholesterol levels by about 50% in homozygous familial hypercholesterolemia over 5 years, and coronary atherosclerosis did not progress as documented by angiography. LDL-apheresis, selective removal of LDL-C via a filtering system, plus statin therapy is effective in LDL-C and appears to affect the progression of vascular disease.[106–109] Combined liver and heart transplantation in homozygous familial hypercholesterolemia reduces total and LDL cholesterol concentrations from about 1100 and 900 mg/dL to about 300 and 185 mg/dL, prior to and after surgery, respectively. Liver transplantation replaced the missing LDL receptors, enhanced catabolism, and reduced lipoprotein synthesis in this patient.[105]

SUMMARY OF MAJOR STUDIES

Primary and secondary prevention diet and drug trials have been performed to determine if lowering of cholesterol will prevent CHD; these are summarized in Tables 19–15 and 19–16. A number of angiographic studies have also been performed that demonstrate that cholesterol reduction leads to regression of atherosclerosis. Most of the primary and secondary studies were double blinded, randomized, and placebo controlled, lasting for 5 years or longer, and most had sufficient patient numbers to be meaningful. Exceptions to these qualifications were seen in the early studies such as the Newcastle and Edinburgh trials, which were small; and the CDP using dextrothyroxine, which was terminated early due to adverse effects on CHD mortality.[69,110,111] In the Edinburgh study, 180 patients were also given warfarin, and the patients remained blinded while the physicians were aware of the treatment group allocation. The Helsinki heart study, using gemfibrozil, resulted in a reduction in nonfatal myocardial infarction, which was the primary contributor to reduced CHD incidence (Table 19–15).[66,67,112]

Total and LDL cholesterol were reduced an average of 13.4% and 20.3%, respectively, by cholestyramine in the LRC-CPPT, and the reduction of lipid levels was related to the amount of drug ingested[26,27] (e.g., 1 to 2 packets, 5.4% reduction in total cholesterol, versus 5 or more packets, 19.0% reduction). The prescribed dose of cholestyramine was 24 g or 6 packets per day. The cholestyramine group experienced a 19% reduction in risk ($P < .05$) of the primary end point—definite CHD death and/or definite nonfatal myocardial infarction—reflecting a 24% reduction in definite CHD death and a 19% reduction in nonfatal

TABLE 19–15. Primary Prevention Trials with Lipid-Lowering Drugs

Trial	Treatment	No.	Baseline Cholesterol (mg/dL)	CHD Mortality	Total Mortality
Helsinki Heart Study[67]	Placebo	2030	290	1.13	2.07
	Gemfibrozil	2050		1.07	2.19
World Health Organization[68]	Placebo	5296	247	0.12	0.38
	Clofibrate	5331		0.13	0.49
LRC-CPPT[26]	Placebo	1900	290	2.3	3.7
	Cholesytramine	1906		1.7	3.6
WOSCOPS[31]	Placebo	3293	272	2.3	4.1
	Pravastatin	3302		1.6	3.2
AFCAPS/TexCAPS[63]	Placebo	3304	221	0.9	2.3
	Lovastatin	3301		0.6	2.4
ALLHAT	Usual care	40,000+	NA		
	Pravastatin				
WHI	Usual care	27,500	NA		
	Diet, HRT				

LRC-CPPT = Lipid Research Clinics coronary primary prevention trial; WOSCOPS = West of Scotland coronary prevention study; ALLHAT = antihypertensive and lipid-lowering treatment to prevent heart attack trial; WHI = women's health initiative; AFCAPS/TexCAPS = Air Force coronary/Texas atherosclerosis prevention study.

TABLE 19–16. Secondary Prevention Trials with Lipid-Lowering Drugs

Trial	Treatment	No.	CHD Mortality	Total Mortality
CDP[69,110,114]	Placebo	2789	22.7	25.4
	Clofibrate	1103	21.8	25.5
	Niacin	1119	21.3	24.4
Newcastle[111]	Placebo	253	NA	20.2
	Clofibrate	244		12.7
Edinburg[110]	Placebo	367	NA	11.7
	Clofibrate	350		12.3
Stockholm[28]	Placebo	276	27.2	29.7
	Clofibrate + niacin	279	19.4	21.9
4S	Placebo	2223	9.3	11.5
	Simvastatin	2221	6.1	8.3
LIPID[83]	Placebo	9014	8.3	14.1
	Pravastatin		6.4	11.0
CARE[64]	Placebo	2078	5.7	9.4
	Pravastatin	2081	4.6	8.6
GISSI Prevention	Usual care	6000	NA	NA
	Pravastatin			
BIP	Placebo	3122	NA	NA
	Bezafibrate			
HIT	Placebo	2500	NA	NA
	Gemfibrozil			

BIP = Benzafibrate Infarction Prevention; CARE = Cholesterol and Recurrent Events; CDP = Coronary Drug Project; GISSI = Gruppo Italiano per lo Studio della Sopravivenza nell'Infarto miocardico; HIT = High-density Lipoprotein Cholesterol Intervention Trial; LIPID = Long-term intervention with Provastatin in Ischemic Disease; NA = not available; 4S = Scandinavian Simvastatin Survival Study.

myocardial infarction. Other end points were reduced by 25%, 20%, and 21% for new positive exercise tests, angina, and coronary bypass surgery, respectively. Death from all causes was not significantly reduced by cholestyramine secondary to more accidents and violence in this group. The mean falls in total and LDL cholesterol in the cholestyramine group were 8% and 12% relative to levels in placebo-treated men, providing evidence that for every 1% reduction in cholesterol, a 2% decline in CHD mortality can be realized.

The cooperative trial sponsored by WHO used clofibrate 1.6 g/d in high-risk males (upper third of cholesterol distribution) and compared to a similar high-risk group given placebo and a low-risk group (lower third of cholesterol distribution).[113] Cholesterol was reduced an average of 9%, but ranged from 7% to 11% from the three study centers in the clofibrate-treated group. Clofibrate reduced nonfatal myocardial infarcts by 25% and CHD was reduced by 20%, primarily due to nonfatal myocardial infarction reductions. Fatal myocardial infarction was similar in the two high-cholesterol groups, and all-cause mortality was higher ($P < .05$) in the clofibrate-treated group. Mortality from gastrointestinal malignancy was seen more commonly with clofibrate, and the cholecystectomy rate for gallstones was also significantly higher. AFCAPS/TexCAPS is the most recent primary prevention trial. In this study, conducted in 6605 men and women aged 57 to 63 years with average total cholesterol and LDL (< 221 mg/dL and < 150 mg/dL, respectively) treated with lovastatin 20 to 40 mg/d for 5.2 years, a 37% reduction ($P < .001$) was shown in the risk for first acute major coronary event (fatal or nonfatal MI, unstable angina, or sudden cardiac death).[63] The need for revascularization procedures was also reduced by 33% ($P < .001$). The implications of this trial are enormous; potentially millions of "normal" people could benefit from lipid-lowering with statins based on these results. How this trial will impact public policy remains to be seen.

In the secondary intervention trials, clofibrate (1.5 g/d) in the Newcastle study significantly reduced mortality (11.1% versus 19.0%) from sudden deaths (9 versus 21 patients in clofibrate and placebo groups, respectively) but not from myocardial infarction or congestive heart failure.[111] Nonfatal infarcts were 11.9% with clofibrate versus 18.2% in the placebo group ($P < .055$). Clofibrate (1.6 to 2 g/d) in the Edinburgh trial was less impressive, with no significant effect on the occurrence of fatal or nonfatal myocardial infarction or overall mortality seen.[110]

Niacin in the CDP significantly reduced definite, nonfatal myocardial infarction compared to placebo (10.1% versus 13.9%), whereas clofibrate did not reduce death from any cause or nonfatal or fatal myocardial infarction at the 5-year follow-up period.[114] Clofibrate did increase the rate of definite or suspected fatal or nonfatal pulmonary embolism or thrombophlebitis compared to placebo (5.8% versus 3.6%) after adjusting for baseline characteristics for total follow-up.[69] Other findings with clofibrate that occurred more frequently than with placebo included intermittent claudication, arrhythmias, palpable spleen, cholelithiasis (including cholecystectomy), and more frequent use of anticoagulants. Skin reactions, gastrointestinal complaints, and the use of gout medication were more common with niacin than with placebo. The 5-year total mortalities were 20.0% for clofibrate and 20.9% for placebo. The 5-year total mortality for niacin was 21.2%. Long-term follow-up of the CDP has shown a reduction in total mortality with niacin which occurred 9 years after the drug had been stopped.[114] The mechanism for this effect is unclear.

One of the most important studies published in the last few years has been the 4S trial, a secondary intervention trial in a large number of patients.[28] Simvastatin, 20 to 40 mg/d, reduced LDL cholesterol by 35% and reduced the risk of death from any cause by 30%. Coronary deaths were also reduced with simvastatin (relative risk, 0.58; confidence interval, 0.46 to 0.73). Therapy was also shown to be effective in women (18% to 19% of patients enrolled) and in the elderly (≥ 60 yr). Indeed, the relative risk of death or major coronary event was reduced to a greater extent in the elderly than in younger patients. Death from noncardiovascular causes was similar for simvastatin and placebo (2.1% and 2.2%, respectively). The survival curves for simvastatin and placebo began to separate at 1 year and became more divergent with additional follow-up. The 4S study clearly demonstrates the benefit in cholesterol lowering and placates long-held fears of death from non-CHD causes. The long-term intervention with pravastatin in ischemic disease (LIPID) study (N = 7498 men and 1516 women) has investigated the effect of pravastatin on CHD mortality in patients with prior MI or unstable angina and mean cholesterol level of 219 mg/dL over 6 years.[83] Pravastatin reduced the risk of CHD mortality by 24% (8.3% versus 6.4%, P = .0004) and total mortality by 23% (14.1% versus 11.0%, P = .00002); stroke was also reduced by 20% (4.3% versus 3.5%, P = .22) as well as reduction in the need for CABG (11.3% versus 8.9%, P = .0001) or PTCA (5.3% versus 4.4%, P = .04) based on the abstract presented in 1997.

Regression of atherosclerosis and atheromatous plaques in various arterial systems has been demonstrated in numerous studies. Intensive dietary and drug therapy has been used in these trials, and the duration of therapy required for regression to be seen is about 2 years. Regression has been noted in native vessels as well as in grafted vessels in coronary artery bypass grafts. Regression has been seen in the carotid as well as the coronary system. Presumably, regression can be induced in other vascular beds as well, and these effects appear to be independent of the drug therapy used to induce regression. Based on meta-analysis and pooling project analysis of angiographic trial data, clinical outcomes such as MI and the need for interventions are reduced in a time frame not consistent with regression of plaque.[115–120] This interesting observation suggests that alteration in plaque activity, so-called plaque stabilization, may play an important role favoring aggressive lipid lowering that has not been previously recognized.

EVALUATION OF THERAPEUTIC OUTCOMES

Short-term evaluation of therapy for hyperlipidemia is based on response to diet and drug treatment as measured in the clinical laboratory by total cholesterol, LDL cholesterol, HDL cholesterol, and triglycerides for patients being treated for primary intervention as well as secondary intervention. The interval for follow-up is dependent on the severity of illness, and patients with known CAD or multiple risk factors should be monitoring more closely. Less commonly used laboratory measurements would include apolipoprotein B and Lp(a) levels. Because many patients being treated for primary hyperlipidemia have no symptoms and may not have any clinical manifestations of a genetic lipid disorder such as xanthomas or eruptions, then monitoring and outcome are solely laboratory based. In patients treated for secondary intervention, symptoms of atherosclerotic cardiovascular disease, such as angina or intermittent claudication, may improve over months to years. If patients have xanthomas or other external manifestations of hyperlipidemia, these lesions should regress with therapy. Lipid measurements should be obtained in the fasted state to minimize interference from chylomicrons, and once the patient is stable, monitoring is needed at intervals of 6 months to 1 year. The goals for LDL and HDL cholesterol are provided in Tables 19–8 and 19–9.

Patients with multiple risk factors and established CHD should also be monitored and evaluated for progress in managing their other risk factors such as hypertension, smoking cessation, exercise and weight control, and glycemic control if diabetic. The goals would be to maintain a blood pressure of below 140/90 mm Hg or less (presence of diabetes or renal insufficiency), stop smoking, maintain an ideal body weight, exercise for at least 20 minutes for three or more times per week, and keep plasma glucose below 126 mg/dL. Invasive evaluation such as cardiac catheterization is useful in patients with established CHD and is typically used for planning revascularization rather than monitoring of lipid-lowering therapy.

Evaluation of dietary therapy is part of the outcome evaluation for treating hyperlipidemia and the assistance of a dietitian is recommended. Use of diet diaries and recall survey instruments allow information about diet to be collected in a systemic fashion and may improve patient adherence to dietary recommendations.

▶ PRINCIPLES OF PHARMACOTHERAPY

- Hypercholesterolemia, elevated LDL-C, and low HDL-C are unequivocally linked to increased risk for CHD and cerebrovascular morbidity and mortality.
- Reductions in elevated total cholesterol and LDL-C reduce CHD mortality and total mortality. Aggressive treatment of hypercholesterolemia results in fewer patients progressing to myocardial infarction, angina, and stroke, and reduces the need for interventions such as CABG and PTCA.
- Initial therapy for any lipoprotein disorder is dietary restriction (step I, then step II) of total and saturated fat and cholesterol and a modest increase in polyunsaturated fat intake along with a program of regular exercise.
- Recent clinical trials in primary and secondary intervention with the statins have shown a 25% to 35% reduction in CHD risk, and patients with high to moderate LDL-C concentrations benefit from treatment.
- Considering compliance, adverse effects and effectiveness, statins are the drugs of choice for patients with hypercholesterolemia because they are the

most potent form of monotherapy and have been shown to be cost-effective in patients with known CAD or multiple risk factors and in high-risk primary prevention patients.

- Gemfibrozil, cholestyramine, and niacin reduce nonfatal MI and niacin may also reduce total mortality.
- Patients not responding to statin monotherapy may be treated with combination therapy for hypercholesterolemia, but should be monitored closely due to an increased risk for adverse effects and drug interactions.
- Hypertriglyceridemia usually responds well to niacin, gemfibrozil, or high-dose/potency statins (atorvastatin, simvastatin); niacin should be avoided in diabetics due to worsening glycemic control.
- Low HDL-C is addressed with life-style modifications such as smoking cessation and increased exercise; niacin and gemfibrozil can significantly increase HDL-C as well.

REFERENCES

1. National Cholesterol Education Program. Second report of the National Cholesterol Education Program (NCEP) expert panel on detection, evaluation, and treatment of high blood cholesterol in adults (adult treatment panel II). Circulation 1994;89:1329–1445.
2. Sempos CT, Cleeman JI, Carroll MD, Johnson CL, et al. Prevalence of high blood cholesterol among US adults. An update based on guidelines from the second report of the National Cholesterol Education Program adult treatment panel. JAMA 1993;269:3009–3014.
3. Fingerhut LA, Warner M. Health, United States, 1996–97 and Injury Chartbook. Hyattsville, MD: National Center for Health Statistics, 1997.
4. Kannel WB, Wilson PW. Comparison of risk profiles for cardiovascular events: Implications for prevention. Adv Internal Med 1997; 42:39–66.
5. Menotti A, Keys A, Blackburn H, et al. Comparison of multivariate predictive power of major risk factors for coronary heart diseases in different countries: Results from eight nations of the seven countries study, 25-year follow-up. J Cardiovasc Risk 1996;3:69–75.
6. Kannel WB. Range of serum cholesterol values in the population developing coronary artery disease. Am J Cardiol 1995;76:69C–77C.
7. Rossouw JE, Lewis B, Rifkind BM. The value of lowering cholesterol after myocardial infarction. N Engl J Med 1990;323:1112–1119.
8. Sytkowski PA, D'Agostino RB, Belanger A, Kannel WB. Sex and time trends in cardiovascular disease incidence and mortality: The Framingham heart study, 1950–1989. Am J Epidemiol 1996;143:338–350.
9. Jeppesen J, Hein HO, Suadicani P, Gyntelberg F. Triglyceride concentration and ischemic heart disease: An eight-year follow-up in the Copenhagen male study. Circulation 1998;97:1029–1036.
10. Tenkanen L, Manttari M, Manninen V. Some coronary risk factors related to the insulin resistance syndrome and treatment with gemfibrozil. Experience from the Helsinki heart study. Circulation 1995; 92:1779–1785.
11. NIH consensus conference. Triglyceride, high-density lipoprotein, and coronary heart disease. NIH consensus development panel on triglyceride, high-density lipoprotein, and coronary heart disease. JAMA 1993;269:505–510.
12. Shepherd J. Lipoprotein metabolism. Drugs 1994;47:1–10.
13. Dietschy JM. Theoretical considerations of what regulates low-density-lipoprotein and high-density-lipoprotein cholesterol. Am J Clin Nutr 1997;65:1581S–1589S.
14. Kannel WB. Hazards, risks, and threats of heart disease from the early stages to symptomatic coronary heart disease and cardiac failure. Cardiovasc Drugs Ther 1997;11:199–212.
15. Kuivenhoven JA, Jukema JW, Zwinderman AH, et al. The role of a common variant of the cholesteryl ester transfer protein gene in the progression of coronary atherosclerosis. The regression growth evaluation statin study group [see comments]. N Engl J Med 1998; 338:86–93.
16. Ross R. Cell biology of atherosclerosis. Annu Rev Physiol 1995; 57:791–804.
17. Kuo CC, Grayston JT, Campbell LA, et al. Chlamydia pneumoniae (TWAR) in coronary arteries of young adults (15–34 years old). Proc Natl Acad Sci USA 1995;92:6911–6914.
18. Libby P, Schoenbeck U, Mach F, et al. Current concepts in cardiovascular pathology: The role of LDL cholesterol in plaque rupture and stabilization. Am J Med 1998;104:14S–18S.
19. Navab M, Hama-Levy S, Van Lenten BJ, et al. Mildly oxidized LDL induces an increased apolipoprotein J/paraoxonase ratio. J Clin Invest 1997;99:2005–2019. Erratum appears in J Clin Invest 1997;99:3043.
20. Jukema JW, van Boven AJ, Groenemeijer B, et al. The Asp9 Asn mutation in the lipoprotein lipase gene is associated with increased progression of coronary atherosclerosis. REGRESS study group, Interuniversity Cardiology Institute, Utrecht, The Netherlands. Regression growth evaluation statin study. Circulation 1996;94:1913–1918.
21. Diller PM, Huster GA, Leach AD. Definition and application of the discretionary screening indicators according to the National Education Program for Children and Adolescents. J Pediatr 1994; 126:345–352.
22. Berenson GS, Srinivasan SR, Bao W, et al. Association between multiple cardiovascular risk factors and atherosclerosis in children and young adults. N Engl J Med 1998;338:1650–1656.
23. Strong JP, Malcom GT, Oalmann MC, Wissler RW. The PDAY Study: Natural history, risk factors, and pathobiology. Pathobiological determinants of atherosclerosis in youth. Ann NY Acad Sci 1997;811:226–237.
24. McCrindle BW, O'Neill MB, Cullen-Dean G, Helden E. Acceptability and compliance with two forms of cholestyramine in the treatment of hypercholesterolemia in children: A randomized, crossover trial. J Pediatr 1997;130:266–273.
25. Lambert M, Lupien PJ, Gagne C, et al. Treatment of familial hypercholesterolemia in children and adolescents: Effect of lovastatin. Canadian lovastatin in children study group. Pediatrics 1996; 97:619–628.
26. The lipid research clinics coronary primary prevention trial results. II. The relationship of reduction in incidence of coronary heart disease to cholesterol lowering. JAMA 1984;251:365–374.
27. The Lipid Research Clinics coronary primary prevention trial results. I. Reduction in incidence of coronary heart disease. JAMA 1984; 251:351–364.
28. Randomised trial of cholesterol lowering in 4444 patients with coronary heart disease: The Scandinavian simvastatin survival study (4S). Lancet 1994;344:1383–1389.
29. Blankenhorn DH, Azen SP, Crawford DW, et al. Effects of colestipol–niacin therapy on human femoral atherosclerosis. Circulation 1991; 83:438–447.
30. Anderson TJ, Meredith IT, Yeung AC, et al. The effect of cholesterol-lowering and antioxidant therapy on endothelium-dependent coronary vasomotion. N Engl J Med 1995;332:488–493.
31. Shepherd J, Cobbe SM, Ford I, et al. Prevention of coronary heart disease with pravastatin in men with hypercholesterolemia. West of Scotland coronary prevention study group. N Engl J Med 1995;333: 1301–1307.

32. Dietschy JM. Dietary fatty acids and the regulation of plasma low density lipoprotein cholesterol concentrations. J Nutr 1998; 128: 444S–448S.
33. Fielding CJ. Response of low density lipoprotein cholesterol levels to dietary change: Contributions of different mechanisms. Curr Opin Lipidol 1997;8:39–42.
34. Spence JD, Huff MW, Heidenheim P, et al. Combination therapy with colestipol and psyllium mucilloid in patients with hyperlipidemia. Ann Intern Med 1995;123:493–499.
35. Turley SD, Dietschy JM. Mechanisms of LDL-cholesterol lowering action of psyllium hydrophillic mucilloid in the hamster. Biochim Biophys Acta 1995;1255:177–184.
36. Connor SL, Connor WE. Are fish oils beneficial in the prevention and treatment of coronary artery disease? Am J Clin Nutr 1997; 66:1020S–1031S.
37. Harris WS. N-3 fatty acids and serum lipoproteins: human studies. Am J Clin Nutr 1997;65:1645S–1654S.
38. Berrettini M, Parise P, Ricotta S, et al. Increased plasma levels of tissue factor pathway inhibitor (TFPI) after n-3 polyunsaturated fatty acids supplementation in patients with chronic atherosclerotic disease. Thromb Haemost 1996;75:395–400.
39. Talbert RL, Hatfield C. Olestra: Fatuous fad or fat phenomenon? Fat Facts 1996;4:1–3.
40. Simon A, Megnien JL, Levenson J. Coronary risk estimation and treatment of hypercholesterolemia. Circulation 1997;96:2449–2452.
41. Rackley CE. Advances in treatment of cholesterol abnormalities. The role of HMG-CoA reductase inhibitors. Postgrad Med 1996; 100:61–65, 70–72.
42. Shepherd J. Statin therapy in clinical practice: New developments. Curr Opin Lipidol 1995;6:254–255.
43. Steiner A, Weisser B, Vetter W. A comparative review of the adverse effects of treatments for hyperlipidaemia. Drug Saf 1991;6:118–130.
44. Carrilho AJ, Medina WL, Nakandakare ER, Quintao EC. Plasma cholesteryl ester transfer protein is lowered by treatment of hypercholesterolemia with cholestyramine. Clin Pharmacol Ther 1997;62:82–88.
45. Schectman G, Hiatt J, Hartz A. Evaluation of the effectiveness of lipid-lowering therapy (bile acid sequestrants, niacin, psyllium and lovastatin) for treating hypercholesterolemia in veterans. Am J Cardiol 1993;71:759–765.
46. Andrade SE, Walker AM, Gottlieb LK, et al. Discontinuation of antihyperlipidemic drugs—Do rates reported in clinical trials reflect rates in primary care settings? N Engl J Med 1995;332:1125–1131.
47. Konzem SL, Gray DR, Kashyap ML. Effect of pharmaceutical care on optimum colestipol treatment in elderly hypercholesterolemic veterans. Pharmacotherapy 1997;17:576–583.
48. Maciejko JJ, Brazg R, Shah A, et al. Psyllium for the reduction of cholestyramine-associated gastrointestinal symptoms in the treatment of primary hypercholesterolemia. Arch Fam Med 1994;3:955–960.
49. Jin FY, Kamanna VS, Kashyap ML. Niacin decreases removal of high-density lipoprotein apolipoprotein A-I but not cholesterol ester by Hep G2 cells. Implication for reverse cholesterol transport. Arterioscler Thromb Vasc Biol 1997;17:2020–2028.
50. Crouse JR III. New developments in the use of niacin for treatment of hyperlipidemia: New considerations in the use of an old drug. Coron Artery Dis 1996;7:321–326.
51. American Society of Health System Pharmacists. ASHP therapeutic position statement on the safe use of niacin in the management of dyslipidemia. Am J Health Syst Pharm 1997;54:2815–2819.
52. Grundy SM. Consensus statement: Role of therapy with "statins" in patients with hypertriglyceridemia. Am J Cardiol 1998;81:1B–6B.
53. Whelan AM, Price SO, Fowler SF, Hainer BL. The effect of aspirin on niacin-induced cutaneous reactions. J Fam Pract 1992;34: 165–168.
54. McKenney JM, Proctor JD, Harris S, Chinchili VM. A comparison of the efficacy and toxic effects of sustained- vs immediate-release niacin in hypercholesterolemic patients. JAMA 1994;271:672–677.
55. Homma Y, Kobayashi T, Yamaguchi H, et al. Decrease of plasma large, light LDL (LDL1), HDL2 and HDL3 levels with concomitant increase of cholesteryl ester transfer protein (CETP) activity by probucol in type II hyperlipoproteinemia. Artery 1993;20:1–18.
56. Okubo M, Horii A, Kamata K, et al. Effect of probucol on serum lipoprotein and apoprotein profiles in renal transplant patients. Am J Kidney Dis 1998;31:356–359.
57. Regnstrom J, Walldius G, Nilsson S, et al. The effect of probucol on low density lipoprotein oxidation and femoral atherosclerosis. Atherosclerosis 1996;125:217–229.
58. Lennernas H, Fager G. Pharmacodynamics and pharmacokinetics of the HMG-CoA reductase inhibitors. Similarities and differences. Clin Pharmacokinet 1997;32:403–425.
59. Desager JP, Horsmans Y. Clinical pharmacokinetics of 3-hydroxy-3-methylglutaryl-coenzyme A reductase inhibitors. Clin Pharmacokinet 1996;31:348–371.
60. Naoumova RP, Dunn S, Rallidis L, et al. Prolonged inhibition of cholesterol synthesis explains the efficacy of atorvastatin. J Lipid Res 1997;38:1496–1500.
61. Jones P, Kafonek S, Laurora I, et al. Comparative dose efficacy study of atorvastatin versus simvastatin, pravastatin, lovastatin, and fluvastatin in patients with hypercholesterolemia. (The CURVES study.) Am J Cardiol 1998;81:582–587.
62. Bradford RH, Shear CL, Chremos AN, et al. Expanded clinical evaluation of lovastatin (EXCEL) study results: Two-year efficacy and safety follow-up. Am J Cardiol 1994;74:667–673.
63. Downs JR, Clearfield M, Weis S, et al. Primary prevention of acute coronary events with lovastatin in men and women with average cholesterol levels. JAMA 1998;279:1615–1622.
64. Sacks FM, Pfeffer MA, Moye LA, et al. The effect of pravastatin on coronary events after myocardial infarction in patients with average cholesterol levels. Cholesterol and recurrent events trial investigators. N Engl J Med 1996;335:1001–1009.
65. Post coronary artery bypass graft trial investigators. The effect of aggressive lowering of low-density lipoprotein cholesterol levels and low-dose anticoagulation on obstructive changes in saphenous-vein coronary-artery bypass grafts. N Engl J Med 1997;336:153–162.
66. Spencer CM, Barradell LB. Gemfibrozil. A reappraisal of its pharmacological properties and place in the management of dyslipidaemia. Drugs 1996;51:982–1018.
67. Frick MH, Elo O, Haapa K, et al. Helsinki heart study: Primary-prevention trial with gemfibrozil in middle-aged men with dyslipidemia. Safety of treatment, changes in risk factors, and incidence of coronary heart disease. N Engl J Med 1987;317:1237–1245.
68. A co-operative trial in the primary prevention of ischaemic heart disease using clofibrate. Report from the committee of principal investigators. Br Heart J 1978;40:1069–1118.
69. Coronary Drug Project report on clofibrate and niacin. Atherosclerosis 1978;30:239–240.
70. Adkins JC, Faulds D. Micronised fenofibrate: A review of its pharmacodynamic properties and clinical efficacy in the management of dyslipidaemia. Drugs 1997;54:615–633.
71. Steinmetz A, Schwartz T, Hehnke U, Kaffarnik H. Multicenter comparison of micronized fenofibrate and simvastatin in patients with primary type IIA or IIB hyperlipoproteinemia. J Cardiovasc Pharmacol 1996;27:563–570.
72. Fasching P, Rohac M, Liener K, et al. Fish oil supplementation versus gemfibrozil treatment in hyperlipidemic NIDDM. A randomized crossover study. Horm Metab Res 1996;28:230–236.
73. Connor WE, DeFrancesco CA, Connor SL. N-3 fatty acids from fish oil. Effects on plasma lipoproteins and hypertriglyceridemic patients. Ann NY Acad Sci 1993;683:16–34.
74. Athyros VG, Papageorgiou AA, Hatzikonstandinou HA, et al. Safety and efficacy of long-term statin-fibrate combinations in patients with refractory familial combined hyperlipidemia. Am J Cardiol 1997; 80:608–613.

75. Guerin M, Bruckert E, Dolphin PJ, et al. Fenofibrate reduces plasma cholesteryl ester transfer from HDL to VLDL and normalizes the atherogenic, dense LDL profile in combined hyperlipidemia. Arterioscler Thromb Vasc Biol 1996;16:763–772.
76. Yang CY, Gu ZW, Xie YH, et al. Effects of gemfibrozil on very-low-density lipoprotein composition and low-density lipoprotein size in patients with hypertriglyceridemia or combined hyperlipidemia. Atherosclerosis 1996;126:105–116.
77. Bell DS. A comparison of lovastatin, an HMG-CoA reductase inhibitor, with gemfibrozil, a fibrinic acid derivative, in the treatment of patients with diabetic dyslipidemia. Clin Ther 1995;17:901–910.
78. Franceschini G, Paoletti R. Pharmacological control of hypertriglyceridemia. Cardiovasc Drugs Ther 1993;7:297–302.
79. Bakker-Arkema RG, Davidson MH, Goldstein RJ, et al. Efficacy and safety of a new HMG-CoA reductase inhibitor, atorvastatin, in patients with hypertriglyceridemia. JAMA 1996;275:128–133.
80. Kannel WB. Cardiovascular risk factors in the elderly. Coron Artery Dis 1997;8:565–575.
81. Hamilton VH, Racicot FE, Zowall H, et al. The cost-effectiveness of HMG-CoA reductase inhibitors to prevent coronary heart disease. Estimating the benefits of increasing HDL-C. JAMA 1995;273:1032–1038.
82. Johannesson M, Jonsson B, Kjekshus J, et al. Cost effectiveness of simvastatin treatment to lower cholesterol levels in patients with coronary heart disease. Scandinavian simvastatin survival study group. N Engl J Med 1997;336:332–336.
83. Tonkin AM. Management of the long-term intervention with pravastatin in ischaemic disease (LIPID) study after the Scandinavian simvastatin survival study (4S). Am J Cardiol 1995;76:107C–112C.
84. Kane JP, Malloy MJ, Ports TA, et al. Regression of coronary atherosclerosis during treatment of familial hypercholesterolemia with combined drug regimens. JAMA 1990;264:3007–3012.
85. Tonstad S. A rational approach to treating hypercholesterolaemia in children. Weighing the risks and benefits. Drug Saf 1997;16:330–341.
86. Knipscheer HC, Boelen CC, Kastelein JJ, et al. Short-term efficacy and safety of pravastatin in 72 children with familial hypercholesterolemia. Pediatr Res 1996;39:867–871.
87. Garg A, Grundy SM. Nicotinic acid as therapy for dyslipidemia in non-insulin-dependent diabetes mellitus. JAMA 1990;264:723–726.
88. Gray DR, Morgan T, Chretien SD, Kashyap ML. Efficacy and safety of controlled-release niacin in dyslipoproteinemic veterans. Ann Intern Med 1994;121:252–258.
89. Laakso M. Dyslipidemia, morbidity, and mortality in non-insulin-dependent diabetes mellitus. Lipoproteins and coronary heart disease in non-insulin-dependent diabetes mellitus. J Diabetes Complications 1997;11:137–141.
90. Steiner G. The diabetes atherosclerosis intervention study (DAIS): A study conducted in cooperation with the World Health Organization. The DAIS project group. Diabetologia 1996;39:1655–1661.
91. D'Amico G, Gentile MG. Pharmacological and dietary treatment of lipid abnormalities in nephrotic patients. Kidney Int Suppl 1991;31:S65–S69.
92. Aguilar-Salinas CA, Barrett PH, Kelber J, et al. Physiologic mechanisms of action of lovastatin in nephrotic syndrome. J Lipid Res 1995;36:188–199.
93. Gentile MG, Fellin G, Cofano F, et al. Treatment of proteinuric patients with a vegetarian soy diet and fish oil. Clin Nephrol 1993;40:315–320.
94. Thomas ME, Harris KP, Ramaswamy C, et al. Simvastatin therapy for hypercholesterolemic patients with nephrotic syndrome or significant proteinuria. Kidney Int 1993;44:1124–1129.
95. Fuiano G, Esposito C, Sepe V, et al. Effects of hypercholesterolemia of renal hemodynamics: Study in patients with nephrotic syndrome. Nephron 1996;73:430–435.
96. Samuelsson O, Attman PO, Knight-Gibson C, et al. Effect of gemfibrozil on lipoprotein abnormalities in chronic renal insufficiency: A controlled study in human chronic renal disease. Nephron 1997;75:286–294.
97. Caro J, Klittich W, McGuire A, et al. The West of Scotland coronary prevention study: Economic benefit analysis of primary prevention with pravastatin [see comments]. BMJ 1997;315:1577–1182.
98. Perreault S, Hamilton VH, Lavoie F, Grover S. A head-to-head comparison of the cost effectiveness of HMG-CoA reductase inhibitors and fibrates in different types of primary hyperlipidemia. Cardiovasc Drugs Ther 1997;10:787–794.
99. Brown WV. Niacin for lipid disorders. Indications, effectiveness, and safety. Postgrad Med 1995;98:185–189, 192–193.
100. Heudebert GR, Van Ruiswyk J, Hiatt J, Schectman G. Combination drug therapy for hypercholesterolemia. The trade-off between cost and simplicity. Arch Intern Med 1993;153:1828–1837.
101. Schectman G, Wolff N, Byrd JC, et al. Physician extenders for cost-effective management of hypercholesterolemia. J Gen Intern Med 1996;11:277–286.
102. Buchwald H, Campos CT, Boen JR, et al. Disease-free intervals after partial ileal bypass in patients with coronary heart disease and hypercholesterolemia: Report from the program on the surgical control of the hyperlipidemias (POSCH). J Am Coll Cardiol 1995;26:351–357.
103. Buchwald H, Bourdages HR, Campos CT, et al. Impact of cholesterol reduction on peripheral arterial disease in the program on the surgical control of the hyperlipidemias (POSCH). Surgery 1996;120:672–679.
104. Matts JP, Buchwald H, Fitch LL, et al. Subgroup analyses of the major clinical endpoints in the program on the surgical control of the hyperlipidemias (POSCH): Overall mortality, atherosclerotic coronary heart disease (ACHD) mortality, and ACHD mortality or myocardial infarction. J Clin Epidemiol 1995;48:389–405.
105. Hoeg JM. Pharmacologic and surgical treatment of dyslipidemic children and adolescents. Ann NY Acad Sci 1991;623:275–284.
106. Kroon AA, van Asten WN, Stalenhoef AF. Effect of apheresis of low-density lipoprotein on peripheral vascular disease in hypercholesterolemic patients with coronary artery disease. Ann Intern Med 1996;125:945–954.
107. Kroon AA, Aengevaeren WR, van der Werf T, et al. LDL apheresis atherosclerosis regression study (LAARS). Effect of aggressive versus conventional lipid lowering treatment on coronary atherosclerosis. Circulation 1996;93:1826–1835.
108. Donner MG, Richter WO, Schwandt P. Long term effect of LDL apheresis on coronary heart disease. Eur J Med Res 1997;2:270–274.
109. Thompson GR, Maher VM, Matthews S, et al. Familial hypercholesterolaemia regression study: A randomised trial of low-density-lipoprotein apheresis. Lancet 1995;345:811–816.
110. Dewar HA, Oliver MF. Secondary prevention trials using clofibrate: a joint commentary on the Newcastle and Scottish trials. Br Med J 1971;790:784–786.
111. Trial of clofibrate in the treatment of ischaemic heart disease. Five-year study by a group of physicians of the Newcastle upon Tyne region. Br Med J 1971;790:767–775.
112. Huttunen JK, Manninen V, Manttari M, et al. The Helsinki heart study: Central findings and clinical implications. Ann Med 1991;23:155–159.
113. (WHO) CoPI. A co-operative trial in the primary prevention of ischaemic heart disease using clofibrate. Br Heart J 1978;40:1069–1118.
114. Canner PL, Berge KG, Wenger NK, et al. Fifteen year mortality in coronary drug project patients: Long-term benefit with niacin. J Am Coll Cardiol 1986;8:1245–1255.
115. Byington RP, Jukema JW, Salonen JT, et al. Reduction in cardiovascular events during pravastatin therapy. Pooled analysis of clinical events of the pravastatin atherosclerosis intervention program. Circulation 1995;92:2419–2425.

116. Byington RP, Furberg CD, Crouse JR III, et al. Pravastatin, lipids, and atherosclerosis in the carotid arteries (PLAC-II). Am J Cardiol 1995;76:54C–59C.
117. Watts GF, Lewis B, Brunt JN, et al. Effects on coronary artery disease of lipid-lowering diet, or diet plus cholestyramine, in the St Thomas' atherosclerosis regression study (STARS). Lancet. 1992; 339:563–569.
118. Pitt B, Mancini GB, Ellis SG, et al. Pravastatin limitation of atherosclerosis in the coronary arteries (PLAC I): Reduction in atherosclerosis progression and clinical events. PLAC I investigation. J Am Coll Cardiol 1995;26:1133–1139.
119. Sacks FM, Pasternak RC, Gibson CM, et al. Effect on coronary atherosclerosis of decrease in plasma cholesterol concentrations in normocholesterolaemic patients. Harvard atherosclerosis reversibility project (HARP) group. Lancet 1994;344: 1182–1186.
120. Watts GF, Burke V. Lipid-lowering trials in the primary and secondary prevention of coronary heart disease: New evidence, implications and outstanding issues. Cur Opin Lipidol 1996;7:341–355.

20

Peripheral Vascular Disease

Robert L. Talbert, PharmD, FCCP, BCPS

The term *peripheral vascular disease* (PVD), in its broadest sense, applies to disease of any of the blood vessels outside the heart and thoracic aorta and to disease of the lymph vessels. Although this term includes cerebrovascular and hypertensive vascular disease, these two topics are discussed in Chapters 10 and 18. The other major area included in this term is peripheral vascular disease of the extremities, which can be divided into two distinct systems: (1) venous disorders, such as acute deep vein thrombosis and its complications of pulmonary embolism and postthrombotic syndrome (Chap. 17); and (2) peripheral arterial disease, resulting from occlusion and arterial vasospasm.[1] This chapter will focus on peripheral vascular disease. Because there are several distinct peripheral vascular diseases, the epidemiology, pathophysiology, clinical presentation, and treatment are oriented to the particular disease. A general review of the structure and function of the normal vascular system and its reactive changes is presented first to aid in the understanding of the specific peripheral vascular disorders.[2–4]

STRUCTURE AND FUNCTION OF THE NORMAL VASCULAR SYSTEM

The vascular system consists of varying histologic portions of five component parts: endothelium, basement membrane, elastic tissue, collagen, and smooth muscle (Fig. 20–1).[4,5] The endothelium is the monolayer lining of the luminal surface of the entire vascular system, and functions to regulate the flow of blood in and out of the vessel lumen. Endothelial cells have several important functions including the active transport of circulating substances through their cytoplasm. Endothelium-derived relaxing factor (EDRF), which is thought to be nitric oxide or a mixture of *S*-nitrosothiol and nitric oxide, is synthesized through three pathways by the endothelium from L-arginine in response to a host of neurochemical and mechanical stimuli including wall and shear stress, endothelin-1, platelet activation, thrombin, serotonin, adenosine diphosphate (ADP), arachidonic acid, catecholamines, vasopressin, histamine, and acetylcholine.[6–8] EDRF diffuses from endothelial cells to adjacent smooth muscle cells, and relaxes vascular smooth muscle and counteracts the action of numerous vasoconstrictor substances on smooth muscle as well as inhibiting platelet aggregation. The effects of EDRF seem to be most pronounced in the basal state and contribute to dilator tone of the skin and extremities; less of an effect is seen during reflex symptathetic vasoconstriction.[9] Vasorelaxation and inhibition of platelet aggregation derived from the actions of EDRF stem from stimulation of the formation of cyclic guanosine monophosphate (cGMP) from guanosine triphosphate (GTP) and elevated cytosolic concentrations of cGMP, which stimulates intracellular binding of free calcium. Endothelin-1, the arachidonic acid metabolites prostacyclin H_2 and thromboxane A_2, and angiotension II are vasconstricting substances derived from the endothelium, which are counter-balanced by the vaodilating properties of nitric oxide when endothelial function is normal.[2,10] Down-regulation of the endothelin receptor (ETA) may reflect overactivity of this system.[7] Loss of endothelium from atherosclerotic plaque formation, percutaneous transluminal angioplasty, or other means of disruption of this monolayer of cells such as smoking reduces synthesis of EDRF and the protective homeostatic function of this paracrine substance (Fig. 20–2). Disease states that facilitate this process or are worsened because of it include hypertension, diabetes mellitus, dyslipemia (hypercholesterolemia, hypertriglyceridemia, and low HDL cholesterol), atherosclerosis, and coronary artery disease.[11,12]

Basement membrane is a dense sheath adjacent to the external surface of endothelial cells and serves as a transport barrier and support structure. The basement membrane contains a ground substance that is a mixture of mucopolysaccharides, protein–polysaccharide complexes, and glycoproteins, which retain large amounts of water and provide a gelatinous medium for transport of materials. Elastic tissue encircles the wall just outside the endothelium and basement membrane. It is also found in the media and adventitia of all vessels except the terminal arterioles, capillaries, and small venules, and allows for expansion of the vessel. The internal elastic lamella is prominently affected by nearly all pathologic changes that involve the vascular system.

Another important component of vessel walls is collagen. In normal vessels it is present in the media and adventitia and is involved in all reactions of vessels to injury.[4] Collagen is highly resistant to stretching and functions to prevent overdistension of the vessels. The fifth component is smooth muscle, which is the actively contracting element of the vascular system. Arterial metabolism is dependent mainly on smooth muscle cells. These are the major connective tissue-forming cells of the vascular wall, producing elastic tissue, collagen, mucopolysaccharides, and myosin. Smooth muscle cells can metabolize glucose; synthesize fatty acids, cholesterol, phospholipids, and triglycerides;

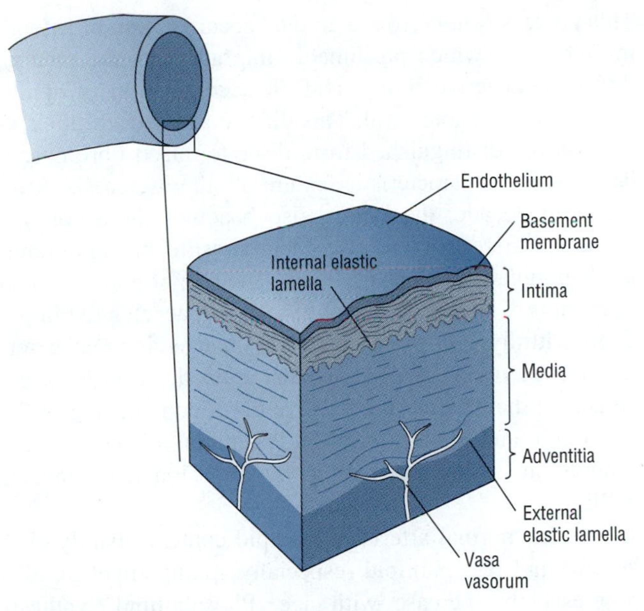

FIGURE 20–1. Schematic drawing of structural organization of the vascular wall. *(From Lie JR. The structure of the normal vascular system and its reactive changes. In: Juergens JL, Spittell JA, Fairbairn JF, eds. Peripheral Vascular Diseases. Philadelphia, Saunders, 1980: 57, with permission.)*

and facilitate the entry of lipoproteins into the cell. Several catabolic enzymes are also present, including mixed-function oxidases, fibrinolysins, and lysosomal hydrolases. This function and the proliferative nature of smooth muscle cells are important factors in the reaction of arterial walls to injury and atherogenesis.[13] In contrast to the differentiated, contractile type of smooth muscle cell usually seen in adults, smooth muscle cells lose their contractility and instead gain the ability to secrete extracellular matrix components and divide, which is thought to be an early step in the development of atherogenesis.

The structural organization of the vessel wall consists of three well-defined layers: the intima, media, and adventitia (Fig. 20–1). The intima is a single continuous layer of endothelial cells and associated basement membrane. It is delineated on its outer surface by a perforated tube of elastic tissue, the internal elastic lamella. This structure is especially prominent in the large elastic arteries and medium-caliber muscular arteries, but is not seen in capillaries. The media consists of only one cell type, the smooth muscle cell. These cells are surrounded by small amounts of collagen and elastic tissue. The media is delineated on the luminal side by internal elastic lamina, and on the abluminal side by a less continuous sheet of elastic tissue, the

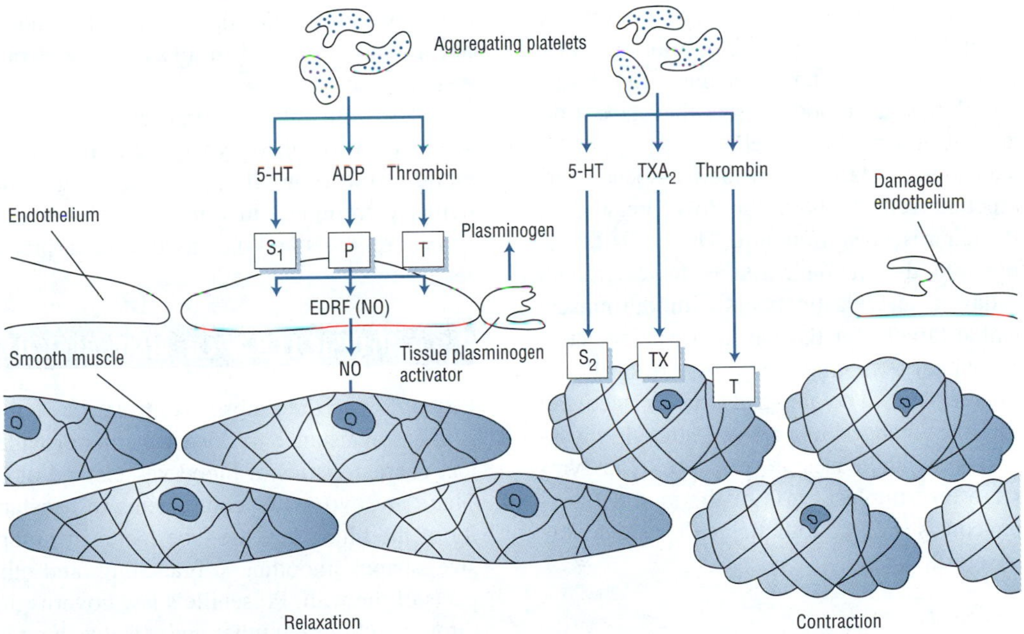

FIGURE 20–2. Mechanisms of vasospasm in atherosclerotic arteries. *Left:* normal endothelium. If platelets were to aggegate and release 5-hydroxytryptamine (5-HT; serotonin) and adenosine diphosphate (ADP), these would act on specific receptors on the endothelial cells (S_1, serotoninergic receptor; P, purinergic receptor) to release endothelium-derived relaxing factor (EDRF). EDRF is nitric oxide (NO) or a nitrosothiol. Also, if any thrombin were formed, this would act on a specific receptor (T) to enhance the release of relaxing factor. Also, tissue plasminogen activator would be stimulated to form plasminogen. *Right:* If the endothelium is damaged, platelets aggregate because of the loss of the inhibitory action of NO and prostacyclin. The resultant release of 5-HT and thromboxane A_2 (TXA_2) and the formation of thrombin cause vasoconstriction or vasopasm by acting directly on receptors on the smooth muscle cells. Not shown is the fact that some of the 5-HT can be taken up by the sympathetic nerve endings and released again as a false transmitter to enhance the contraction. Also the resultant tissue hypoxia–anoxia releases a contracting factor from the vessel wall, which further aggravates and prolongs the vasospasm.

external elastic lamella. The outer portion is nourished by small blood vessels (vasa vasorum) in the adventitia, and the inner layers receive nutrients from the lumen. The outer layer of the vascular wall is the adventitia. This layer contains a mixture of collagen, elastic fibers, smooth muscle fibers, and fibroblasts. The outer layer also contains nerve fibers, the vasa vasorum, and lymphatics that nourish the vessel wall and remove metabolic waste products.

The vascular system can be divided into elastic arteries, muscular arteries, arterioles, capillaries, veins, and lymphatics. Elastic arteries, such as the aorta and major pulmonary arteries, contain large amounts of elastic tissue. The walls of these arteries distend and increase their elastic tension with systole. During diastole, the elastic fibers recoil, which helps propel the blood distally and maintain flow (see Chap. 10).

Smooth muscle cells predominate in muscular arteries such as the renal, superior mesenteric, and femoral arteries. These arteries regulate peripheral flow and supply organs that require a specific blood supply based on the amount of work they are preforming. These arteries can vary their caliber by contracting (vasoconstriction) and relaxing (vasodilation), so that a given cardiac output can be allocated to various tissues depending on their current needs. Thus, muscular arteries function as resistance vessels and are major regulators of systemic blood pressure.

Arterioles are branches of the muscular arteries that differ structurally and functionally from small arteries only by their size. Because of their large number, arterioles form the most important class of resistance channels in the vascular system. Capillaries are blood vessels that have a diameter similar to that of a red blood cell.

Veins are considerably larger than their associated arteries. Their structure reflects both the low pressure of this system and their reservoir function. The walls of the veins are thinner and the media contains fewer smooth muscle cells, collagen, and elastic fibers. Smooth muscle cells are responsible largely for the vasoconstrictive activity of the veins, which is seen mainly in the small peripheral veins in the skin. The larger veins can actively constrict during acute changes in pressure, but they passively dilate with slow increases in pressure. The lymphatic channels are the simplest parts of the vascular system. The intima consists of endothelial cells and a few collagen and muscle fibers.

REACTIVE CHANGES OF THE VASCULAR SYSTEM

The arteries are not static structures, but rather they change in response to various physical and chemical stimuli, react to injury, and undergo structural alterations throughout growth and aging.[5] The major change that occurs with normal aging is a slow, continuous symmetric increase in the intimal thickness, especially in the large elastic arteries. This process results from a gradual accumulation of smooth muscle cells (which presumably migrate from the media), diffuse connective tissue, and an accumulation of sphingomyelin and cholesterol. This diffuse age-related thickening is to be distinguished from discrete raised fibromuscular plaques, a characteristic feature of atherosclerosis. After the sixth decade, the intima also becomes more collagenized and there is a loss of cellular constituents and granular degranulation of elastic fibers. The rate of aortic intimal thickening is more prominent in men and accelerated in patients with hypertension. Structural changes in small arteries and arterioles differ somewhat from those in systemic vessels in that there is progressive fibrotic thickening of the adventitia and media, with little intimal change. These changes are closely linked to hypertension and diabetes mellitus.

In the normal arterial wall, lipid content, mainly cholesterol and phospholipid (especially sphingomyelin), also progressively increase with age. Phospholipid synthesis rises with age followed by a compensatory increase in all phospholipases except sphingomyelinase. Accumulations of cholesterol and low-density lipoprotein (LDL) appear to be derived from plasma. Functionally, these changes result in increased rigidity of arteries and loss of endothelial function. Endothelial dysfunction leads to vasoconstriction, thrombosis, and greater involvement of the inflammatory response, promoting atherosclerosis. The larger arteries may become dilated, elongated, and tortuous, and aneurysms may form in areas of degenerating arteriosclerotic plaques.

The veins also undergo age-related changes. Phlebosclerosis, also called hyperplastic phlebitis, refers to thickening of the veins. It appears to be age related and is particularly prominent in veins of the lower extremity that are subject to stasis and increased luminal pressure.

PHYSIOLOGY OF LIMB BLOOD FLOW

Blood flow to the limbs is controlled by arterial blood pressure and resistance to flow, which is provided by the physical characteristics of blood vessels and of the blood itself. There are two major components to resistance: the viscosity of the blood and the tube factor or hindrance, based on size, shape, smoothness, branching, and other physical aspects of the wall. Poiseuille's law governs the flow of fluids through cylindrical tubes and it states that resistance to flow is proportional to the fourth power of the radius. Viscosity is usually fairly constant, but exceptions to this would be the presence of abnormal or abnormally high numbers of red or white blood cells such as in chronic obstructive airways disease, sickle cell disease, high circulating levels of fibrinogen, or certain types of leukemia.[14] Active changes in the radius of the resistance vessels in the limbs are caused by local and neurogenic mechanisms.[5]

LOCAL CONTROL

Local control of limb blood flow includes intrinsic, metabolic, humoral, and physical factors. The relative importance of each of these varies for different tissues and for different vessels within the same tissue. Intrinsic smooth muscle tone appears to be directly influenced by changes in wall tension, which in turn is determined by intravascular pressure. A decrease in intravascular pressure and wall tension would result in spontaneous activity of the smooth muscle cells, and an increase in intravascular pressure would have the opposite effect.

The intrinsic myogenic activity is modified by chemical changes in the resistance vessels, which adjust blood flow to the limbs (active hyperemia). Similar increases are seen after temporary arrest of circulation to the limbs (reactive hyperemia). Metabolic factors play an important role in controlling blood flow to skeletal muscles. The accumulation of metabolic products such as carbon dioxide, potassium, phosphate, and adenosine during exercise, an increase in the osmolality of venous effluent, or a change in pH cause direct vasodilation of peripheral vessels (Fig. 20–3). The humoral factors that cause dilation of skeletal muscle vessels include epinephrine, acetylcholine, histamine, prostaglandins, and serotonin. As described previously, many of the effects of these substances are mediated via the endothelial release of EDRF. Norepinephrine, angiotensin, and vasopressin cause vasoconstriction. In skin, epinephrine causes vasoconstriction because there is a preponderance of α-adrenergic receptors in cutaneous vessels, in contrast to skeletal muscle vessels, which have both α- and β-receptors. Epinephrine has a greater affinity for β_2-receptors in skeletal muscle resistance vessels, and thus causes vasodilation.

Such physical factors as local temperature also control blood flow to extremities. Low temperatures can cause vasoconstriction or vasodilation depending on the thermal state of the body. Application of heat to an extremity dilates the blood vessels. This vasodilation is enhanced by increasing the temperature of the body as a whole.

NEURAL CONTROL

The skin of the hands and feet is innervated by sympathetic fibers that mediate reflex changes in vessel tone. Alterations in activity of these fibers under central control cause large fluctuations in the flow to all fingers simultaneously. Skin vasoconstrictive sympathetic reflex is preserved in chronically ischemic limbs with PVD, suggesting that sympathetic nerve fibers are relatively resistant to chronic ischemia; however, diabetics do not have preserved sympathetic reflexes.[15] Temperature changes alter the sympathetic outflow to the skin. Exposure of the body to cold augments the vasoconstrictor tone, whereas an increase in body temperature decreases tone. The circulation in the skin also plays an essential role in thermal homeostasis. Arteriovenous anastomoses, which are numerous in fingers and toes, favor heat dissipation. Sweat glands cause local production of bradykinin, and consequently vasodilation, when stimulated by sympathetic cholinergic nerves.

Changes in the diameter of resistance vessels in skeletal muscle are influenced by sympathetic adrenergic nerves, which are abundant in small arteries and arterioles. Sympathetic nerve fibers to muscle are of two types: vasoconstrictor

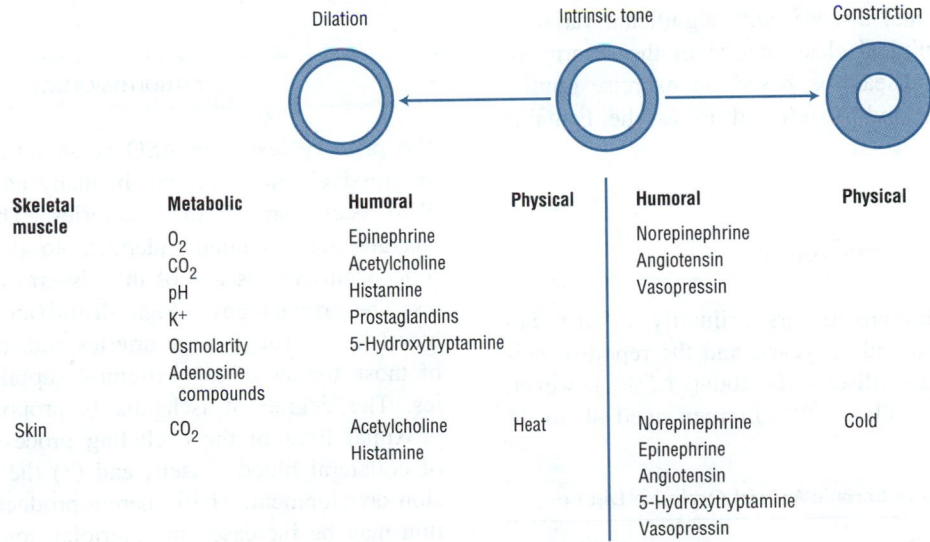

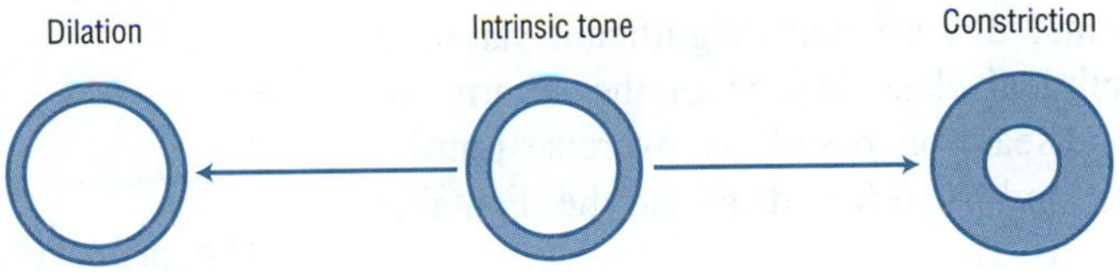

	Metabolic	Humoral	Physical	Humoral	Physical
Skeletal muscle	O_2 CO_2 pH K^+ Osmolarity Adenosine compounds	Epinephrine Acetylcholine Histamine Prostaglandins 5-Hydroxytryptamine		Norepinephrine Angiotensin Vasopressin	
Skin	CO_2	Acetylcholine Histamine	Heat	Norepinephrine Epinephrine Angiotensin 5-Hydroxytryptamine Vasopressin	Cold

FIGURE 20–3. Active changes in vascular diameter are caused by local and nervous mechanisms. Local control includes intrinsic, metabolic, humoral, and physical factors, and the relative importance of each of these varies for different tissues and for different vessels within the same tissue. This figure identifies actions of local factors that can alter arterial diameter in skeletal muscle and skin. *(From McGrath MA, Verhaeghe RH, Shepherd JT. The physiology of limb blood flow. In: Juergens JL, Spittell JA, Fairbairn JF, eds. Peripheral Vascular Diseases. Philadelphia, Saunders, 1980: 84, with permission.)*

fibers, whose activity is mediated by the release of norepinephrine; and vasodilator fibers, whose activity is mediated through the release of acetylcholine. Although vessels in both the skin and muscles are innervated by sympathetic fibers, the vasomotor centers controlling these vessels can function independently. In reflex control of body temperature, only the vessels to the skin are involved, whereas with alterations in position, the reflex changes are confined to the vessels in the muscles.

PERIPHERAL ARTERIAL DISORDERS

Peripheral vascular disease of the arteries can be generally classified as obstructive and vasospastic. Examples of an obstructive abnormality include arteriosclerosis obliterans and thromboangiitis obliterans (Buerger's disease). Raynaud's disease is the most common example of a vasospastic disorder.

ARTERIOSCLEROSIS OBLITERANS

Arteriosclerosis obliterans, also called atherosclerosis obliterans (ASO), is a chronic occlusive arterial disease of the aorta, particularly their terminal portion of the abdominal aorta and its major branches to the extremities. It is one of several types of chronic arterial occlusive disease (Table 20–1). This disease also involves the large and medium-sized arteries of the extremities, especially the iliofemoral and popliteal arteries and, in the lower leg, the posterior tibial artery at the ankle and the anterior tibial artery at its origin. Arteriosclerosis obliterans is considered a segmental disease, with significant variation in its extent. The clinical classification of the severity of peripheral vascular disease is based on exercise limitiation and symptoms and is referred to as the Fontaine classification (Table 20–2).

EPIDEMIOLOGY

Arteriosclerosis obliterans occurs primarily in men between the ages of 50 and 70 years, and the reported incidence of symptomatic disease is about 1.5%; however, the incidence is age related.[2,4,16] In men aged 40 to 44 years, 50 to 54 years, and 60 to 64 years, the reported incidence is 0.9%, 3.6%, and 7.5%, respectively. The disease affects women less commonly, about 0.07%, usually after the age of 60 years, perhaps in part because of a menopausal loss of the protective effect of estrogens and an increased incidence of diabetes in women of this age.[17] If noninvasive testing is performed, the incidence of large leg artery disease is 11.7% and small artery disease is 16% while only about 10% report symptoms.[18] Asymptomatic arterial insufficiency may be detected using the ankle–brachial index (ABI, described later), and the incidence is about 10% when the ABI is below 0.9.[19] As in the case of atherosclerosis, hypercholesterolemia plays an important role in the development of this disease. Arteriosclerotic lesions in the lower extremities are commonly associated with coronary and cerebrovascular disease, as noted in the coronary artery surgery study and others.[20] Diabetes mellitus significantly increases the prevalence (11-fold) and severity of ASO (10 years later than if diabetes is not present). Other risk factors important for the pathogenesis of ASO include age, hypertension, hypercholesterolemia, and smoking.[21,22]

TABLE 20–1. Causes of Chronic Arterial Occlusive Disease

Arteriosclerosis obliterans
Thromboangiitis obliterans (Buerger's disease)
Arteritis
Trauma
Congenital arterial narrowing

From Anonymous. Lancet 1996;348:1329–1339, with permission.

TABLE 20–2. Fontaine Classification for Claudication

Stage	Symptoms
I	Asymptomatic
II	Intermittent claudication
IIa	Pain-free, claudication walking > 200 m
IIb	Pain-free, claudication walking < 200 m
III	Rest/nocturnal pain
IV	Necrosis/gangrene

From Ref. 57.

PATHOPHYSIOLOGY

The primary lesion in ASO is an intimal plaque, which progressively narrows and, in many cases, leads to complete occlusion of these arteries. The histopathologic changes are essentially identical to those of arteriosclerotic occlusive disease of the visceral and cerebral arteries. The primary physiologic disturbance is obstruction of blood flow through large arteries and, therefore, ischemia of those tissues of the extremity supplied by these arteries. The degree of ischemia is proportional to (1) the proximal limit of the occluding process, (2) the patency of collateral blood vessels, and (3) the rapidity of occlusion development. The ischemia produced by the obstruction may be increased by arteriolar constriction from any cause. If the occlusion is not too extensive, dilation may improve circulation. Obstruction of the large arteries decreases pressure and blood flow in smaller arteries distal to the obstruction, and thrombosis and gangrene may result. Peripheral occlusive arterial disease is often associated with increased blood viscosity, hyperfibrinogenemia, and a relatively high hematocrit.

Clinical Presentation

Unless there is an acute arterial occlusion such as a thrombosis, the signs and symptoms of ASO have a gradual onset. The most common is intermittent claudication, which is described as pain, cramping, numbness, or weakness in certain muscles that develops only during exercise. The distress is quickly relieved by rest without change in position. About one third of patients do not have symptoms of intermittent claudication or any other ischemic symptoms. Intermittent claudication is caused by inadequate blood supply to muscles(s) stressed by exercise. The distance a person is able to walk before the pain develops varies with the extent and severity of arterial occlusion. It is usually unilateral at first, may become bilateral with time, and is often worse in one of the extremities if both are involved. The location of the involved muscle group may predict the most proximal level of occlusion. For example, claudication of the calf muscles suggests occlusion of the popliteal artery or higher; claudication of the hip indicates disease low in the aorta or in the iliac artery. Edema of disuse and dependency may occur if a limb is kept in the dependent position for long periods of time in the attempt to relieve symptoms.

Another important group of symptoms includes pain at rest, paresthesias, and numbness. These symptoms are usually the result of more severe ischemia of tissues and a more advanced form of the disease resulting from multiple levels of occlusion or obstruction of collateral vessels. It is usually felt in the digits but may be noted in the foot and lower leg as well. Ulceration and gangrene are common when the disease reaches this stage. Pain caused by ischemic neuropathy is another clinical feature of ASO, especially in diabetic patients. Peripheral nervous tissue has a low metabolism and requires very little blood to keep it healthy; this ischemic neuropathy, regardless of symptoms, is consistent with advanced disease. This pain may be continuous or paroxysmal and may be described as a series of sharp pains or the sensation of electrical shocks. A sensation of numbness, coldness, or burning may also occur. When diabetics with a neuropathy develop ulcers, the lesions are often painless.

The physical findings in arteriosclerosis of the extremities are for the most part indistinguishable from those seen in other occlusive arterial diseases. Impairment of arterial pulsations, often noted by palpation, is the most important and consistent finding. Others include systolic bruits over the involved arteries; color (waxy, pale, and dry appearance) and temperature changes in the skin of the extremity; edema; and hypoesthesia and hyporeflexia in patients with severe neuropathy.

Diagnosis

The diagnosis of ASO is often made on the basis of a good history and physical examination. Sophisticated laboratory studies and diagnostic tests are rarely necessary to establish the diagnosis; however, routine laboratory tests such as blood chemistry, electrocardiogram, and x-ray studies may be needed to determine the extent of associated disease as well as prognosis and therapy. The magnitude of arterial occlusion can be assessed simply by measuring the extremity blood pressure at rest and after exercise to the point of claudication. Another easily obtained measure of disease severity is the ankle–brachial index (ABI). This can be done using a Doppler ultrasonic probe or by a variety of plethysmographs. The ABI (sometimes called the arm–ankle index, AAI) is abnormal if the ratio of the arm (right or left) to dorsalis pedis (DP) or posterior tibial (PT) blood pressure is below 0.8. If both DP and PT are abnormal, the extent of disease is more severe and atherosclerosis is likely to be widespread.[23] ABI is inversely related to cardiovascular risk factor as well as subclinical and clinical cardiovascular disease in older adults. The lower the ABI, the greater the increase in CVD risk; even those with asymptomatic reductions in the ABI (0.8 to 1.0) appear to be at increased risk of cardiovascular disease.[24] The 6-minute walk or accelerometer and pedometer may also be used as reproducible measures of disability due to occlusive arterial disease and they correlate fairly well with the ABI and rating scales of physical activity.[25,26] Arteriography is rarely necessary to establish the diagnosis, but is usually used prior to surgery to precisely locate the disease. Traditional or digital subtraction arteriography are considered to be the "gold standard" diagnostic tests for peripheral vascular disease. Other techniques include vascular sonography (standard and color Doppler ultrasound), magnetic resonance imaging, computed axial tomography, and angioscopy, which uses a thin, flexible fiber-optic scope to directly visualize the vessel lumen. A triple-lumen probe to detect skin surface Po_2 has been developed and correlates well with laser Doppler flowmetry (LDF).[27] After physical examination and ABI determination, the next diagnostic test is usually sonography.[28] The sensitivity and specificity of duplex ultrasonography are greater than 80% unless adjacent segments have more than 50% stenosis; color duplex sonongraphy improves the sensitivity and specificity.[29–31]

Noninvasive methods available for evaluating skin microcirculation include transcutaneous oxygen tension measurements ($tcPo_2$), laser Dopper fluxmetry (LDF), and vital capillaroscopy (VC).[2] These methods differ in the amount of skin area and depth of microcirculation that can be evaluated. They are all highly variable in assessing the blood flow. The clinical differentiation of ASO from other types of occlusive peripheral arterial diseases is given in Table 20–3.

TABLE 20–3. Factors in Differential Diagnosis of Peripheral Vascular Disease

Factor	Arteriosclerosis Obliterans	Thromboangiitis Obliterans	Raynaud's Phenomenon
Gender distribution	Predominantly male	98% male	90% female
Age at onset of symptoms	Usually over 50 yr Earlier in diabetes	<35 yr	Usually 11–45 yr
Symmetry	Often asymmetrical	Generally asymmetrical	Symmetrical
Onset	Insidious	Acute and preceded by migratory phlebitis (30–70%)	Often in cold climate and after stress
Intermittent claudication	Common	Common	Absent
Vasospasm	Not remarkable	Almost invariable in involved limb	Invariably symmetrical
Absent pulses	Infrequent in upper and common in lower extremities	Common in upper and lower extremities	Occurs only in late and extreme cases
Skin (if involved)	Thin, often hairless	Thin, atrophic, and red or cyanotic	Normal except during spasm
Ulcers (if any)	Dry and usually superficial	Moist, deep, inflamed, and invasive	Dry, fingertip
Plain radiograms	Calcification of artery	Normal	Often atrophy of phalanges
Cholesterol	High	Borderline	Normal
Presence of coronary or cerebral disease	Common	Rare early in disease	Coincidental

Modified from McCombs PR, Horwitz O. Diseases of the arteries of extremities. In: Horwitz O, McCombs PR, Roberts B, eds. Diseases of Blood Vessels. Philadelphia, Lea & Febiger, 1985:210–211.

▶ TREATMENT: Arteriosclerosis Obliterans

DESIRED OUTCOME AND NONPHARMACOLOGIC THERAPY

The goals of therapy in patients with ASO are to arrest progression of the disease, improve blood flow, relieve pain, and prevent and treat ulceration and gangrene. Progression of the disease may be prevented by control of hyperlipoproteinemia, control of any associated diseases such as diabetes and hypertension, and tobacco abstinence. (Regression of atherosclerosis with lipid lowering is described in Chap. 19.) Normalizing cholesterol serum levels through diet and drug therapy as well as LDL-apheresis in patients with peripheral atherosclerosis improves both endothelium-dependent and endothelium-independent relaxation in human peripheral small arteries.[32] For patients who have severe ischemia manifested by rest pain, ulceration, and gangrene, rest of the extremity is an important adjunct of treatment. If the pain is severe, narcotics and other pain medications may be necessary as well as either angioplasty or surgery. It is important to take meticulous care of the extremities and avoid even minor trauma as it may lead to ulceration. In these patients, ulceration is usually treated with local care, medical management including antibiotics if necessary, and surgical amputation if required.

Another effective method of improving blood flow to the extremities is to increase collateral flow. This can be accomplished by a warm environmental temperature; avoidance of vasoconstriction caused by drugs, cold, and tobacco; elevation of the head of the bed 12 to 16 inches; and exercise. A daily exercise training program is very effective in patients with mild to moderate intermittent claudication. Important features of a successful program are (1) repetitive daily walks to 75% of the claudication distance with intermittent periods of rest (1 to 2 minutes); (2) weekly increase in walking time and distance; and (3) continuation of this program, as cessation results in loss of improvement. In general, the exercise program needs to be 20 minutes per session or more three times per week for at least 6 months.[33] Controlled studies have shown a 25% to 30% increase in walking distance with an average of about 1000 feet, although 40% of patients may show increases of nearly a mile even though the ABI may not be significantly increased.[33,34] Compared to strength training, treadmill training provides more improvement in exercise time and maximum oxygen uptake.[34] A consistent exercise training program will prevent abrupt deterioration and the need for amputation and may reduce mortality compared to patients with claudiation not on an exercise program.[1,35,36] The mechanism by which exercise improves functionality and symptoms is not clear.[1]

Cigarette smoking is one of the most important risk factors for chronic peripheral vascular disease. Continued smoking is associated with a greater risk for disabling claudication, limb-threatening ischemia, amputation, and need for intervention. Although smoking cessation is universally recommended in patients with PVD, there are few data suggesting improvement in PVD with cessation other than improved postoperative graft patency rates and reduced complications of peripheral arterial disease.[1,36,37] Smoking cessation should be attempted to improve coronary artery disease end points and this alone justifies this intervention.[38]

PHARMACOLOGIC THERAPY

Various vasodilating drugs (e.g., tolazoline, nylidrin, isoxsuprine, niacin derivatives, cyclandelate, and papaverine) have been used in ASO, but none have been shown to be consistently effective. Ischemia is one of the most potent stimuli for vasodilation and drug therapy does not augment the physiologic response to ischemia. Vasodilators are of no value in treating ASO.[1]

Controversy surrounds the use of β-adrenergic blocking agents in PVD patients with concurrent coronary artery disease or hypertension. A number of case reports have been published indicating that these agents can cause or worsen intermittent claudication. By reducing systemic blood pressure, these agents could decrease blood flow through stenotic arteries or collateral vessels. A nonselective β-blocker may attenuate epinephrine-induced vasodilation during exercise by blocking β_2-receptors in peripheral vessels. Controlled trials using both selective and nonselective agents have produced mixed results in patients with PVD. A few studies have demonstrated an increase in muscle blood flow and symptomatic improvement when β-blockers were withdrawn, or no affect on either blood flow or claudication. A meta-analysis of six trials found that β-blockers do not adversely affect walking capacity or symptoms of intermittent claudication in patients with mild to moderate peripheral arterial disease.[39] Beta-adrenergic blocking agents, if used, should probably be cardioselective agents, but because other drugs are available for hypertension and angina, β-blocker use should be minimized.[40,41]

Pentoxifylline (Trental) has been shown to be of benefit in patients with chronic occlusive arterial disease, but the results have been inconsistent due in part to placebo responses.[1,42] Pentoxifylline increases red blood cell deformibility, and decreases platelet adhesiveness, blood fibrinogen, and neutrophil elastase/α_1 proteinase inhibitor complex levels, which are thought to lead to a reduction in blood viscosity and improved blood flow.[43] The average increase in walking distance was about one-half of a city block and pentoxifylline has been shown to be effective in moderately severe chronic obstructive arterial disease if the resting AAI is less than 0.8 and if symptoms of intermittent claudication have been present for longer than 1 year.[44] Patients more likely to improve with pentoxifylline are those with moderately severe ischemia and without rest pain, ischemic ulcers, or severe claudication.[45] In contrast to the unpredictable and less than impressive effects with oral pentoxifylline for chronic therapy, intravenous pentoxifylline (400 mg bid) given for 21 days improved the symptoms of critical limb ischemia.[46] Pentoxifylline has been used to prevent postoperative rethrombosis after vascular surgery for arterial occlusive disease, but worldwide, aspirin and anticoagulation are more commonly used to prevent graft occlusion depending on the graft site.[47,48] Pentoxifylline has been evaluated in various diabetic complications including PVD; the effects are inconsisent and only marginally better than placebo. A cost-effectiveness analysis suggests that pentoxifylline may reduce the risk of vascular surgery while not increasing the total cost of PAD care.[49] Modification of risk factors such as hypertension, tobacco use, and hyperlipidemia are also considered to be cost effective.[50,51]

Antiplatelet therapy with aspirin (325 mg qod) reduced the relative risk (RR) of peripheral artery surgery (RR, 0.54, 95% confidence interval 0.30 to 0.95, $P = .03$) in the U.S. physician's health study.[52] Aspirin (80 to 325 mg/d) is recommended by the American College of Chest Physicians consensus conference because patients with PVD are at high risk for MI and stroke.[53] Several small studies have used dipyridamole in combination with aspirin, but the effects of dipyridamole alone are unclear. The Swedish ticlopidine multicenter study, a large randomized, placebo-controlled trial with ticlopidine, found no significant improvement in walking distance or ABI with ticlopidine.[54] EMATAP, a randomized, stratified, placebo-controlled double-blind multicenter trial with ticlopidine, did find a significant reduction in first events (sudden deaths, myocardial infarctions, and strokes) compared to placebo.[55] Aspirin (80 to 325 mg/d) is also recommended for patients undergoing saphenous vein or prosthetic femoropopliteral bypass operation.[53] More recently, a French trial assessed the utility of ticlopidine 250 mg twice daily in patients with femoropopliteal or femorotibial saphenous–venous bypass grafts for 2 years. Cumulative graft patency with ticlopidine was 82%, while 63% of the grafts in the placebo group were patent.[56] A randomized, blinded, trial of clopidogrel versus aspirin (CAPRIE) found that clopidogrel had an annual 5.32% risk of ischemic stroke, myocardial infarction, or vascular death compared with 5.83% for aspirin, a small but significant difference (relative risk reduction of 8.7%) between the two drugs. Most of the benefit from clopidogrel was restricted to patients entering the study with peripheral arterial disease.[57] Prostaglandin E_1 (PGE_1) and I_2 (PGI_2, prostacyclin) are potent vasodilators and inhibitors of platelet aggregation that have been shown to improve claudication, relieve pain, and promote ulcer healing in short-term studies.[58] More recent studies have confirmed the earlier findings and suggest that the effects of infusions of PGE_1 and PGI_2 have persisting effects on blood flow and exercise capacity that may last for weeks to months after treatment.[59,60] The major drawback to prostaglandin therapy is the need for intravenous infusion of the drugs due to their short half-lives; however, oral analogs are under development.[61] Other antiplatelet drugs undergoing clinical evaluation include trapidil, cilostazol, and picotamide.[62–64]

Short-term studies with calcium channel blockers have also shown some promise, but interest has recently focused on the potential for antiatherosclerosis effects of calcium blockers.[65–67] This approach to therapy presently is only theoretical, although there is some hope that calcium channel blockers may limit or delay the progression of atherosclerosis. Defibrotide, an investigational agent, has been shown in open-label trials to improve symptoms and treadmill exercise time in about 50% of treated patients.[68] Defibrotide increases tissue plasminogen activator production and release and PGI_2 formation, and inhibits platelet activation.

Based on results from the prevention of atherosclerosis complications with ketanserin (PACK) trial, ketanserin has no significant effect in reducing the symptoms of intermittent claudication.[69,70] Another approach, based on improved muscle metabolism with L-carnitine (2 g twice a day for 3 weeks), was shown to improve walking distance.[71,72] Carnitine skeletal muscle stores are reduced in animal models and when replenished, muscle performance is improved. At this point, an appropriate reminder would be that many trials in the treatment of peripheral vascular disease and intermittent claudication are either poorly controlled or have significant design flaws, and that an inverse correlation exists between the sample size and the number of studies reporting positive results.

Intra-arterial thrombolysis should be considered (1) in an attempt to, time permitting, convert an emergent surgical procedure into an elective one; (2) to convert a major surgical procedure into a less extensive one; (3) to restore the patency of any acutely occluded vessel that is inaccessible to mechanical thrombectomy; (4) to identify the underlying cause of thrombosis so that it can be corrected with salvage of native artery or bypass graft; (5) to prevent arterial intimal damage from balloon thrombectomy; and (6) to reduce the level of amputation when clot retrivial is incomplete.[1] The success rate for acute native arterial occlusion ranges from 58% to 100% and the need for adjunctive revascularization procedures is comparable to bypass grafting, thrombectomy, or PTA. Ouriel and colleagues, in a randomized, multicenter trial (thrombolysis or peripheral arterial surgery, TOPAS) compared intra-arterial urokinase (4000 IU/h for 4 hours and then 2000 IU/h until lysis was complete) to vascular surgery in patients ($N = 272$ in each group) with acute occlusion of native or bypass grafts (45% and 55%, respectively), and found that the amputation-free survival was similar (65.0% and 69.6%,

$P = .23$) while the need for operative procedures was greater in the surgery group.[73] Major hemorrhage was more significantly common with urokinase (12.5% versus 5.5%). Tissue plasminogen activator (TPA), urokinase, and streptokinase have all been used for acute arterial occlusion and none are clearly superior. Passage of a guidewire through the thrombus predicts success and is the most common method of thrombolytic delivery; however, the exact method of delivering thrombolytics (e.g., pulse-spray, slow infusion), the relative efficacy among available agents, optimal patients to be treated, and duration of response remain to be determined.[1,74] An economic analysis of thrombolysis versus vascular surgery showed no difference for initial intervention for urokinase versus surgery, with both costing about $40,000 for acute arterial occlusion treatment.[75] In chronic native arterial thrombosis, the duration of occlusion (< 7 days versus > 6 months) has a large effect of the success of clot lysis (72% versus 24%, respectively).

When medical management with exercise, control of risk factors, and vasodilator or antithrombotic therapy is inadequate, interventional therapeutic technology is useful. The indications for revascularization are patients truely incapacitated by exercise limitations or critical limb ischemia. The types of technology that exist include atherectomy, atheroablation, percutaneous transluminal angioplasty (PTA), endovascular stents, angioscopy, laser angioplasty, and direct open arterial surgery using endarterectomy. Prosthetic bypass grafts or vein-patch arterioplasty may be effective in bypassing or removing areas of stenosis but should be reserved for patients with severe and disabling symptoms (Fontaine class IIb and above). Indications for surgery include relief of symptoms of limb-threatening ischemia, including ischemic pain at rest, ischemic ulcers, and gangrene. Intermittant claudication is only a relative indication for surgery and only after an adequate trial of nonsurgical therapy.[1] Patients most likely to have complete relief of symptoms and normalization of pressure gradients are those with smaller, more focal segments involved (about 2 to 5 cm, depending on the vascular bed), those without calcification, and those with less than total occlusion. Revascularization through angioplasty or surgery has been shown to be more cost effective than amputation of a limb due to rehabiliation costs; angioplasty is more cost effective than surgery if the 5-year patency rate with angioplasty is 30% or less.[76,77] Intravascular stents (e.g., Palmaz) may improve long-term patency, but no well-controlled trials are currently available. Vein grafts are preferred for infrainguinal bypass because of a lower incidence of thrombosis and occlusion compared with synthetic materials (e.g., 68% versus 38%).[1] Aortic bifurcation prosthesis appears to provide the same outcome as aortofemoral bypass for aortoiliac disease.[1] For patients with venous insufficiency, sclerotherapy with hypertonic saline or dextrose of sodium morrhuate, sodium tetradecyl sulfate, or polidocanol and others may be useful in controlling telangiectasias and varicosities.

As with atherectomy, atheroablation, and angioplasty procedures for coronary revascularization, these revascularization procedures for peripheral artery occlusion are associated with primary failure and restenosis, hematomas at the site of device insertion, dissection, and pseudoaneurysms at the site of catheter entry.[78–80] Acute closure occurs in 1% to 4% of peripheral angioplasties and antithrombotic therapy with urokinase or other thrombolytics, and heparin may be used to reopen a vessel occluded with thrombus.[78] Spasm postprocedure is managed with nitroglycerin and calcium channel blockers. Longer-term antithrombotic therapy may be continued with aspirin. Minar and colleagues found aspirin 100 mg/d was as effective as 1000 mg/d to prevent restenosis, but 30% of patients in either group still developed closure.[81] Neither antiplatelet agents nor anticoagulation with warfarin have been shown to be very effective in preventing restenosis; however, omega-3 polyunsaturated fatty acid supplementation with fish oil shows some promise.[79] Longer-term patency rates following angioplasy typically have ranged from about 60% to 75% at 1 year depending on the site of intervention, and this compares favorably with surgery. Human gene therapy is being attempted in PVD to prevent restenosis by percutaneous catheter-based delivery of a plasmid carrying the gene encoding vascular endothelial growth factor (VEGF) to promote therapeutic angiogenesis.[82]

Percutaneous lumbar neurolytic sympathetic blockade (NSB) using 1.5 mL ethanol 95% has been shown to improve walking distance and muscle metabolic activity in a small trial.[83] Lumbar sympathectomy may be useful in patients with mild ischemia rest pain, but temporary sympathectomy with local anesthetics should be performed first to ensure benefit from the procedure. Sympathectomy does alter the long-term course of ASO.

THROMBOANGIITIS OBLITERANS (BUERGER'S OR VON WINIWARTER'S DISEASE)

Thromboangiitis obliterans (TAO) is a disease involving segmental inflammatory and proliferative nonartheromatous lesions of the medium and small arteries, veins, and nerves that usually occurs in young males and frequently leads to nonhealing ulcers and gangrene (see Table 20–3). The cause of thromboangiitis obliterans is unknown but virtually all patients are heavy smokers of cigarettes or use other forms of tobacco. Many patients show cutaneous sensitivity to tobacco and there is a high prevalence of the human leukocyte antigens (HLAs) A9 and B5 in affected persons, which suggests a genetic basis for the disease. Lymphocyte sensitivity to type I and III collagens has been shown for 77% of patients and about 50% have anticollagen antibodies.[59]

Common presenting complaints include a superficial, migratory, nodular phlebitis, associated with cutaneous erythema, and tenderness. TAO may present with intermittent claudication, most commonly in the arch of the foot (relieved by rest), or less commonly in the calf and occasionally on both sides. Rest pain may present as a severe ache, or numb, gnawing pain that may worsen by elevation of the limb. Cold sensitivity of the hands occurs in about 50% of TAO patients. Pulsations in the posterior tibial and dorsalis pedis arteries may be impaired or absent, and affected extremities may be abnormally red. Segmental thrombophlebitis occurs in about 40% of the patients.

Goals of therapy in TAO include arresting progression of the disease, producing vasodilation, relieving pain, and treating ulcers and gangrene. All patients with TAO should abstain completely and permanently from tobacco of any type. Failure to abstain from tobacco results in disease progression, severe rest pain, ulceration, and amputation. Other measures that have been suggested but do not work well include anticoagulants, sympathectomy, vascular surgery, and vasodilating drugs. Iloprost has shown some benefit, and an oral preparation provides similar plasma concentrations to the intravenous form in TAO.[58,84] None of these measures can be recommended at the present time. Patients should be advised to avoid cold exposure and vasoconstricting drugs.

RAYNAUD'S DISEASE

In 1862 Maurice Raynaud described episodes of discoloration of the skin of the digits on exposure to cold and he thought this was due to increased sensitivity of the sympathetic nervous system. This condition, which is limited to the skin, usually accompanied by cyanosis, rubor, pain, or parethesias, and associated gangrene, came to be termed Raynaud's disease. More than a century later, the pathogenesis, diagnosis, and treatment are still unclear.[85] Raynaud's disease may be classified as primary, in which the cause is unknown, or secondary in which an associated condition exists (Table 20–4).[85–89]

EPIDEMIOLOGY

The prevalence of Raynaud's disease in the general population is unknown, but the gender ratio is 4 or 5 to 1 female to male, and most cases occur prior to age 40 years (Table 20–3). Men with Raynaud's disease generally present at an older age, and have a much higher incidence of associated atherosclerosis, which accounts for their symptoms when compared with women.

One interesting group of patients with Raynaud's symptoms comprises those whose occupations involve routine use of vibratory equipment or frequent exposure to cold temperature. From 40% to 90% of loggers and 50% of miners using vibratory equipment have been diagnosed with Raynaud's disease. Heredity may also play a role in the development of this disease.[85]

TABLE 20–4. Classification of Raynaud's Phenomenon

I. Primary Raynaud's syndrome or phenomenon—no known association or contributing condition
   A. Raynaud's disease
II. Secondary Raynaud's phenomenon
   A. After trauma—pneumatic hammer, pianists, typists
   B. Neurogenic lesions—carpal tunnel syndrome, thoracic outlet syndrome
   C. Occlusive arterial disease—ASO, TAO, thrombotic arterial occlusion
   D. Miscellaneous diseases and conditions
      1. Common causes—connective tissue diseases
      2. Uncommon causes—cryoproteinemias, polycythemia, vinyl chloride, hepatitis B antigenemia, hypothyrodism, renal disease
   E. Drugs
      1. β-andrenergic receptor blocking drugs
      2. Ergot preparations
      3. Methysergide
      4. Vinblastine and bleomycin
      5. Amphetamines
      6. Imipramine
      7. Bromocriptine
      8. Clonidine
      9. Cyclosporin
      10. Cocaine

Adapted from Coffman JD. Raynaud's phenomenon. An update. Hypertension 1991;17:593–602, and Spittell JA Jr. Raynaud's phenomenon and allied vasopastic disorders. In: Juergens JL, Spittell JA, Fairbairn F, eds. Peripheral Vascular Diseases. Philadelphia, Saunders, 1980: 554–583.

PATHOPHYSIOLOGY

The two theories of the cause of digital artery vasospasm in primary Raynaud's disease are (1) an increased activity of the sympathetic nervous system and (2) a local fault in the digital arteries.[87] Although several lines of evidence favoring increased sympathetic activity exist, evidence against this mechanism includes lack of increased cutaneous nervous system activity, the fact that local cooling of one hand does not lead to reflex vasoconstriction in the opposite hand, and normal plasma and urinary catecholamine concentrations in primary Raynaud's disease. In contrast, the local fault theory is supported by the induction of vasospastic attacks in sympathetically denervated fingers, the induction of attacks in single fingers, an enhancement of reflex sympathetic vasoconstriction by local hand cooling, and a loss of digital systolic blood pressure with a local ischemia and cold stimulus. One of the mechanisms to explain these observations focuses on the activity of α_2-adrenergic receptors in patients with primary Raynaud's disease and the sensitivity of the receptor to cold exposure. Patients with primary Raynaud's disease have a greater sensitivity of the α_2-receptor with exposure to cold, and specific agonists and antagonists for α_1- and α_2-receptors point to altered α_2 activity as one of the defects in this syndrome. Reflex sympathetic stimulation also leads to greater S_2-sertonergic receptor activity even in the presence of α_1- and α_2-blockade, suggesting a pathophysiologic role for serotonin (5-hydroxytryptamine) in vasospasm of Raynaud's disease. Coffman and Cohen studied Raynaud's patients and could not document a role for sertontin in these patients.[90] It is still possible that serotonin is produced at the local level and contributes to the disease, but this remains to be further clarified. Young women with primary Raynaud's disease usually exhibit the purest form of vasospasm. These patients have lower digital, artery, and arteriolar systolic blood pressure than normal subjects.[91] Older male patients usually have secondary Raynaud's disease involving both a vasospastic and obstructive disease. In these patients a normal vasoconstrictive stimulus acting on an arterial bed with reduced intraluminal pressure is sufficient to cause arterial closure. Initially these patients may demonstrate pure vasospasm, but later they develop obstruction as underlying autoimmune processes cause damage to the arterial wall.

Additional factors that may contribute to the pathogenetic mechanisms of Raynaud's disease include increased blood viscosity, platelet abnormalities, low systemic blood pressure, abnormal secretion of prostacyclin and thromboxane B_2, and abnormal endothelial function. Evidence does exist of increased factor VIII/von Willebrand factor antigen and factor activity along with elevated fibrinogen levels that promote hyperviscosity (especially in connective tissue disorders) and thrombosis, but the importance of these factors as well as the others described remains to be determined.

Clinical Presentation

Digital color changes are a common manifestation of this disease. A classic attack begins with a sudden loss of arterial blood flow, causing blanching. Next, a small quantity of blood enters the capillary and venous system and desaturates, and the digits become cyanotic. The third phase of the attack involves vasodilation, causing rubor. Not all patients exhibit a triphasic color change; many demonstrate only pallor or cyanosis, during which the digits turn absolutely white. At first only the tips of the fingers of both hands are involved; later the more proximal parts of the fingers are affected. In the late stage the color change may extend back to involve the rest of the hands. Symptoms are worse in the cold season and less severe in warm weather. Pain is not a prominent symptom during the attack or in the interval between attacks. Paresthesias are common during the attack and consist of numbness, tingling, burning, or a feeling of tightness. Slight swelling of the involved fingers may occur, but only during attacks.

Diagnosis

Primary Raynaud's disease usually includes the following features:

1. Vasospastic attack induced by cold exposure.
2. Bilateral involvement of the extremities.
3. Absence of gangrene or involvement of only the skin of the fingertips.
4. History of symptoms for at least 2 years.
5. No evidence of underlying disease including absence of antinuclear antibodies, a normal erythrocyte sedimentation rate, and normal nailfold capillaroscopy and esophageal motility studies.[91]

All patients should have a complete history and physical examination, with special emphasis on signs and symptoms of connective tissue disease. Routine laboratory tests should include a complete blood count, erythrocyte sedimentation rate, chemistry profile, antinuclear antibody, rheumatoid factor, cryoglobulins, urinalysis, and hand radiography. Digital plethysmography (pulse volume recordings) is often used to follow the course of the disease or to evaluate the response to therapy. Digital systolic blood pressure and its response to cold stress and ischemia has also been used to aid in diagnosis. Hand arteriography may sometimes be used in assessing the relative roles of vasospastic and occlusive disease, but is rarely used to establish a diagnosis.

▶ TREATMENT: Raynaud's Disease

NONPHARMACOLOGIC THERAPY

Conservative measures will suffice for the majority of patients with primary or secondary Raynaud's disease. General considerations for treatment include avoidance of cold temperatures, tobacco, emotional situations, and certain drugs (Table 20–4). These patients should dress warmly, wear lined gloves, and use Styrofoam coasters when handling iced drinks. Large meals and long periods of standing should be avoided as they both reduce peripheral circulation.[87,88,91,92]

Therapy for Raynaud's disease is aimed at increasing digital blood flow and consists of behavioral therapy or biofeedback and drug therapy. Biofeedback is of benefit in some patients and it is used to lessen the severity of the attacks.[91] The goal with these techniques is to self-regulate the nervous system and reduce vasoconstrictive autonomic tone. Biofeedback is accomplished with the use of a thermoprobe or thermistor attached to the person's finger or hand, which relays skin temperature information back to the patient. The patient can then concentrate further on raising the peripheral temperature. One of the more successful regimens has been immersing the hands in 43°C water while the body is exposed to 0°C temperatures. After 3 weeks of daily sessions, improvement has been noted for several months. When attacks interfere with the patient's ability to function normally, drug therapy should be tried. Drug therapy is associated with significant adverse effects, and objective changes in blood flow do not always correlate with symptom improvement; only about two-thirds of patients can be expected to respond to drug therapy.

PHARMACOLOGIC THERAPY

Drug therapy for Raynaud's disease is directed toward vasodilation and involves several classes of drugs toward this end, including sympatholytics, α-adrenergic antagonists, direct-acting vasodilators, calcium channel antagonists, serotonin receptor antagonists, angiotensin-converting enzyme inhibitors, prostaglandins, and thyroid hormones.

SYMPATHOLYTIC AGENTS

Reserpine and other drugs have been used for years in the treatment of Raynaud's disease; unfortunately there are few controlled trials with these agents to suggest that any benefit is derived from their use.[91] Reserpine in oral doses of 0.25 to 0.75 mg daily may increase capillary blood flow in short-term studies, but long-term improvement is doubtful. Reserpine in higher doses causes several unpleasant adverse effects including nasal congestion, bradycardia, postural hypotension, dyspepsia, fluid retention, lethargy, and depression. Intra-arterial reserpine has been shown to be no better than placebo. Guanethidine in doses of 10 to 50 mg daily produces postural hypotension, explosive diarrhea, fatigue, and impotence, and is generally not well tolerated. It may increase capillary blood flow during cooling in patients with Raynaud's disease resulting from scleroderma. Methyldopa has been shown to offer subjective improvement in uncontrolled studies, but no objective benefit has been observed in comparisons with other drugs. Adverse effects seen with methyldopa include drowsiness, headache, dry mouth, postural hypotension, nasal congestion, edema, and diarrhea.

ALPHA-ADRENERGIC ANTAGONISTS

Prazosin and terazosin have been studied in Raynaud's disease but the trials have mixed results. Although prazosin produces about a 60% response rate, larger doses of prazosin lead to an unacceptable number of adverse effects, and a dose of 1 mg three times a day is best tolerated and improves symptoms, finger skin blood flow, and temperature. The early response to prazosin may dissipate in a few weeks; increasing to maximum tolerated doses leads to multiple adverse effects such as headache, dizziness, fatigue, edema, dyspnea, rash, or diarrhea.

Other nonselective α-adrenergic antagonists such as phentolamine and phenoxybenzamine provide inconsistent improvement in blood flow and symptoms. Their use is further limited by difficulties in oral dosing as well as frequent and bothersome adverse effects. Intra-arterial phentolamine infused at 50 to 150 μg/min, or as a single brachial artery injection of 0.05 to 10 mg, improves finger blood flow, digital pulse volume amplitude, and forearm blood flow, and this route is useful for unrelenting vasospasm and ischemia when the sympathetic nervous system is the cause.[93]

DIRECT-ACTING VASODILATORS

Nitroglycerin, nitroprusside, niacin and its derivatives, papaverine, isoxsuprine, griseofulvin, cyclandelate, and hydralazine fall into this category.[91] With the exception of nitroglycerin, none of these agents can be recommended because of the lack of controlled studies to support their use and the frequency of adverse effects. Nitroglycerin ointment usually improves the symptoms, and at times, objective measures of effectiveness have been shown in patients with primary and secondary Raynaud's disease. Nitroglycerin transdermal patches reduced the number and seveity of attacks but headache symptoms limited patient acceptance.[94] Headaches, dizziness and postural hypotension are the most frequent reasons for failure with nitroglycerin.

CALCIUM CHANNEL ANTAGONISTS

Numerous studies with calcium channel antagonists, particularly nifedipine, have been performed in patients with Raynaud's disease. As the name implies, these drugs block the entry of calcium ions through the slow channel that reduces the availability of cytosolic calcium and decreases smooth muscle contractility. Additionally, they may inhibit vascular responses evoked by α_2-adrenergic receptors, which are activated predominantly during reflex sympathetic stimulation of body cooling.[91] Subjective and objective improvements have been demonstrated with drugs in this category. Table 20–5 summarizes clinical trials of calcium channel antagonists for Raynaud's disease. Nifedipine is more effective in primary Raynaud's disease and its effects are more pronounced early in therapy. Chronic therapy may result in loss of response as determined by objective measures, as reported by Gush and associates and Wollersheim (Table 20–5). Nifedipine may also be used as prophylactic therapy prior to cold exposure.

Diltiazem has been reported to reduce the number, severity, and duration of attacks in doses of 30 to 120 mg given three times a day.[61] Objective measures of effect have not demonstrated benefit with diltiazem. Verapamil has been reported to improve the symptoms in one small study, but diary data and objective measures did not confirm any beneficial effect.

Newer calcium blockers such as nicardipine, isradipine, and nisoldipine have also been used with varying degrees of success for Raynaud's disease. Nicardipine provides subjective improvement in about one-half of the patients receiving it, and the frequency and severity of attacks are significantly reduced with its use. It is more effective in primary Raynaud's disease than secondary, and subjective, symptomatic improvement is seen more often than objective improvement. Other studies (Table 20–5) have shown no benefit, either subjective or objective, from nicardipine, even though the drug was shown to inhibit platelet aggregation. Nifedipine was compared with misoprostol 200 μg q 12 hours for 10 days and both drugs caused similar effects on attack severity and blood flow (Table 20–5).[95]

RECEPTOR ANTAGONISTS

Serotonin (5-hydroxytryptamine, 5-HT) has been shown to induce vasospasm and platelet aggregation in animals and humans through the 5-HT_2 receptor. Ketanserin is a selective antagonist of the 5-HT_2 receptor, and it may also have some α_1-adrenoreceptor blocking activity. It increases finger blood flow with intra-arterial and intravenous injection during sympathetic vasoconstriction induced by body cooling, and its effects are evident in the presence of α-blockade.[96] The largest study (n = 222) with oral use found that ketanserin (40 mg three times a day) decreased the duration and frequency of attacks (34% reduction versus 18%) and was preferred by both patients and investigators over placebo.[69] About 50% to 70% of the patients experienced subjective mild to moderate improvement. Ketanserin had no effect on total finger blood flow in warm or cold environments. There was no difference in response between primary and secondary Raynaud's disease. Headache, asthenia, dizziness, and gastrointestinal complaints were the most common symptoms seen with ketanserin; respiratory infections were also more common with ketanserin than placebo. Ketanserin may also prolong the QT interval, and it should be used cautiously in patients with hypokalemia, second- or third-degree heart block, ventricular arrhythmias, prolonged QT interval at baseline, or in combination with potassium-losing diuretics or antiarrhythmics.[70] Part of the variability in response to ketanserin may be due to the frequency in dosing, as some evidence exists that its effects on platelet aggregation are minimal at 12 hours after dosing. When compared with other drugs such as nifedipine or pentoxiphylline, ketanserin may provide better subjective improvement and perhaps better objective improvement as illustrated in small studies to date.[97] Ketanserin may also be effective in combination therapy with prostacyclin derivatives.[98]

ANGIOTENSIN-CONVERTING ENZYME INHIBITORS

The proposed mechanism for improvement of Raynaud's disease with angiotensin-converting enzyme (ACE) inhibitors is the inhibition of the breakdown of bradykinin and vasodilation resulting from its accumulation. Early studies showed improved blood flow and some improvement in symptoms. Double-blinded, placebo-controlled trials have not documented any improvement with enalapril 20 mg/d; as up to one-third of patients with PVD have renal artery stenosis, ACE inhibitors would be a logical choice.[99–101]

PROSTANOIDS

Prostacyclin and prostaglandins E_1 and E_2 have been studied in Raynaud's disease because of their properties of vasodilation and inhibition of platelet aggregation. Iloprost, an intravenous synthetic analog of prostacyclin, and oral analogs such as beraprost,

TABLE 20–5. Effect of Calcium Channel Antagonists in the Treatment of Raynaud's Disease

Reference	No. Patients	Study Duration (wk)	Additional Assessment	Results
Nifedipine				
Aldoori et al. Cardiovasc Res 1986;20:446	30p + 10s	3	Digital blood flow	9/13 patients had improved clinical symptoms
Belcaro et al. Panminerva Med 1987;29:223	34p	3	Digital blood flow	N improved digital blood flow
Challenor et al. Angiology 1989;40:122	22	3	Vibrotactile thresholds	40% reduction in mean number of attacks; better response at lower thresholds
Corbin et al. Eur Heart J 1986;7:165	23p	4	Digital blood pressure	N significantly reduced the number of attacks
Finch et al. Clin Rheum 1986;5:493	16s	4	Digital blood pressure	N produced "better" clinical results than placebo
Fisher et al. Zeit Kardiol 1985;74:298	6 PAH		Hemodynamic testing	Raynaud's patients more responsive to nifedipine than other PAH patients
Gjorup et al. Am Heart J 1986;3:742	19p	4		N significantly reduced frequency of attacks and attack severity
Gush et al. J Cardiovasc Pharmocol 1987;9:628	9p	5 d	Peripheral blood flow	Tendency for N to offer some protection against reductions in blood flow
Hawkins et al. Rhem Int 1986;6:85	20p + 37s	3	Mitogenic activity	Overall, N reduced both frequency and severity of attacks, but large individual variations in response. N inhibited mitogen-induced lymphocyte proliferation but only in patients who responded to the drug clinically
Kallenberg et al. J Rheum 1987;14:284	8p + 8s	4	Digital blood flow	N reduced frequency and severity of attacks and improved digital blood flow
Lewis et al. Eur Heart J 1987;8 (suppl): 83	20	OD	Radial artery blood flow	N prevented reduction in blood flow by cooling
Meyrick et al. Br J Derm 1987;117:237	10	6	Digital blood flow	Reduction in number and severity of attacks but no change in blood flow or red blood cell deformability or white blood cell CL
Nilsson et al. Acta Med Scand 1987;221:53	28p	2	Digital blood pressure	17 patients showed symptomatic improvement with N versus 5 with placebo; digital blood pressure improved significantly with N
Riccio et al. Clin Ther 1987;9:232	6p + 7s	5 d	Thermography	More marked increases of hand tissue temperature in patients with secondary disease (progressive systemic sclerosis) than primary disease
Sarkozi et al. J Rheum 1986;13:331	39p	10		N significantly reduced frequency and severity of attacks compared with placebo
Waller et al. Br J Clin Pharm 1986;22:449	34p	4	Rheology	N produced a 25% reduction in mean number of attacks; no difference versus placebo in red cell deformability
White et al. Am J Med 1986;80:623	6p + 5s	1	Digital skin temperature recovery time	9/11 patients reported symptomatic improvement; N significantly improved skin temperature recovery time
Wollersheim. J Clin Pharmacol 1987;27:907	16	4	Digital blood flow	Open label, no correlation between sublingual acute use and oral long term; lack of objective long-term benefit
Dompeling and Smit. Vasa Suppl 1992;34:34–37	14p	1d	Photoelectric plethysmography	Single-dose study; N better than placebo and a potassium channel opener, pinacidil
Varela-Aguila Rev Clin Esp 1997;197:77	205	10d	Doppler duplex	

TABLE 20–5. Effect of Calcium Channel Antagonists in the Treatment of Raynaud's Disease (cont.)

Reference	No. Patients	Study Duration (wk)	Additional Assessment	Results
Nicardipine				
French Cooperative Multicenter Group. Am Heart J 1991;122:352-355	69p		Symptomatic	Double-blind, placebo-controlled study; 21% symptomatic improvement; no improvement in cold-reactive hyperemia test
Ferri et al. Clin Rheumatol 1992; 11(1):76–80	21p + s	3	Peak flow after postischemic reactive hyperaemia	18/21 completed study; subjective improvement noted with fewer episodes and improved hand disability score
Wollersheim et al. J Cardiovasc Pharmacol 1991;18:813–818	16p + 9s	3	Finger skin temperature and laser Doppler flux	Double-blind, placebo-controlled study; NS between nicardipine and placebo for number, duration, or severity of vasospastic attacks or for any of the microcirculatory parameters
Felodipine				
Kallenberg et al. Eur J Clin Pharmacol 1991;40:313–315	10p	6	Symptomatic and finger plethysmography	Single blind; subjective improvement in the number and intensity of attacks; blood flow improved only at certain temperatures
Flunarizine				
Centonze et al. Clin Ter 1991;137:77–82	28	4	Symptomatic	Flunarizine caused NS clinical improvement; adverse effects were common

p = primary Raynaud's disease; s = secondary Raynaud's disease; N = nifedipine; PAH = pulmonary arterial hypertension; CL = clearance; OD = one dose; NS = not significant.

improve blood flow and walking distance acutely but do not seem to have long-term benefit.[102,103] An intravenous prodrug of prostaglandin E_1 (AS-013) incorporated into lipid microspheres provided modest improvement in walking distance for up to 8 weeks in early trials.[104] Use of intravenous iloprost did not improve vein or prosthetic graft patency at 1 year.[105] Oral and intravenous misoprostol improved blood flow and walking distance in small, short-term trials.[95,106]

THYROID HORMONES

Triiodothyronine (T_3) 80 μg/d has been shown in one small (n = 18), double-blind controlled crossover trial to reduce the frequency, duration, and severity of attacks as well as increase skin temperatures and promote ulcer healing.[107] The proposed mechanisms for this effect are activation of heat-dissipating mechanisms and enhanced β_2-adrenoreceptor activity in vascular smooth muscle. T_3 significantly elevated T_3 and T_4 concentrations and reduced thyroid-stimulating hormone concentrations to less than 0.1 mIU/L in 14 of 18 patients. Palpitations, headaches, and weight loss were reported by about one-third of patients. The overall attack rate reduction was approximately 75%, somewhat higher than that reported for other types of treatment. The authors suggest follow-up studies using a lower dose of 60 μg/d of triiodothyronine to minimize adverse effects and chemical hyperthyroidism. Other case reports suggest similar findings.[107,108]

Other approaches to therapy have included β-adrenergic blocking agents and pentoxiphylline. Atenolol and propranolol have been reported to benefit some patients with Raynaud's disease based on diary data of attack frequency.[91] The premise for their use is that presynaptic blockade of β_2-receptors should prevent postsynaptic activation of adrenergic receptors; few data support this concept at the present time. Pentoxifylline, in a study of 11 patients, was reported to improve symptoms in 7 patients and to improve red cell filtration.[109] Improved skin temperatures to cold challenge have been noted with pentoxiphylline as well.[92]

Calcitonin gene-related peptide is an endogenous vasodilator that seems to be specific for skin blood flow and it may be deficient in Raynaud's disease.[110,111] Trials giving this substance intravenously for up to 5 days have shown improved hand warming and skin temperature, improved hand and digital blood flow, and ulcer healing in small groups of patients, and it seems to be better tolerated than prostacyclin.[112,113] Another drug with some promise is piracetam, an antiplatelet agent that also increases the synthesis of PGI_2.[114]

Cervicothoracic sympathectomy may produce temporary relief from symptoms, but they usually return within 6 months to 2 years.[115] Several complications may occur because of the surgery and the success rate is considered to be no better than conservative management.[92]

EVALUATION OF THERAPEUTIC OUTCOMES

Drug therapy responses in peripheral vascular disease may be evaluated using patient symptoms, presence or absence of peripheral at various sites, the ABI index, exercise capacity, angiographic documentation of improved flow, and need for subsequent procedures and surgery. Using the Fontaine classification system (see Table 20–2) or other rating scales that are available,[1,79] semiquantative assessments of symptomatic clinical improvement can be obtained. For example, a patient might move from class IIb to IIa or I as a measure of improvement following pharmacotherapeutic or interventional therapy. The ABI index provides an estimate of the restoration of blood flow to an extremity, and this index can easily be obtained by measuring blood pressures at different points of the circulatory system. Exercise capacity can be evaluated using the Fontaine classification or through other estimates made by the patient or clinician of exercise duration or effort. This could be expressed as the time to cover a set distance (e.g., one block), or the total amount of distance covered without a time restriction. Angiographic studies to document improved blood flow are usually not necessary and are more often used for research purposes to objectively assess outcome of some intervention. The need for a revascularization procedure as primary or secondary intervention, or the need for vascular surgery after pharmacotherapy or interventional technologies, could also be used as an outcome measure. This would be more important for groups of patients than individual patients but need for revascularization certainly would suggest failure of the primary mode of therapy.

Symptom remission is the primary method of evaluating therapy for Raynaud's disease. Digital plethysmography and finger blood pressure would be used for a more objective method of assessment or for research purposes. Patients with TAO should be evaluated for symptom response, but smoking cessation is important as well. This may be evaluated through history, but a more objective means would be serum cotinine concentrations.

▶ PRINCIPLES OF PHARMACOTHERAPY

- All patients 55 years and older should have pedal pulses evaluated, and if nonpalpable, the ABI or other examination should be used to evaluate the patient for arterial insufficiency.
- The cornerstone of therapy for arterial insufficiency is risk factor modification including an exercise program, smoking cessation, and diabetic and dyslipidemia management.
- Aspirin 80–325 mg/day should be given to most patients with PVD to reduce the risk of future cardiovascular events (i.e., stroke, MI, or vascular death); aspirin does not affect the development of atherosclerosis.
- Pentoxifylline is not recommended for intermittant claudication since the trial results are inconsisent and show only marginal benefit over exercise alone.
- PTA and surgery are effective treatments for intermittant claudication and are recommended after an adequate trial of nonoperative therapy.
- Intra-arterial thrombolytic therapy is recommended for acute thrombotic or embolic occlusion of a native artery or prosthetic graft and may delay or prevent vascular surgery. No particular agent has documented superiority.
- Conservative management of Raynaud's disease, including avoiding cold, emotional stress, tobacco, and certain drugs, should be tried before trials of drug therapy.
- Calcium channnel blockers, in particular nifedipine, are the best studied form of pharmacotherapy for Raynaud's disease and they provide at least symptomatic relief; evidence for efficacy with other vasodilating drugs (e.g., nitroglycerin) is available in a limited number of studies.
- Although still investigational, ketanserin, a serotonin antagonist, improves the symptoms of Raynaud's disease.
- Other approaches for Raynaud's disease such as prostacyclin and its analogs, thyroid hormones and calcitonin gene related protein are under development.

REFERENCES

1. Weitz JI, Byrne J, Clagett GP, et al. Diagnosis and treatment of chronic arterial insufficiency of the lower extremities: A critical review. Circulation 1996;94:3026–3049.
2. Clement DL, Shepherd JT. Vascular Diseases in the Limbs. Mechanisms and Principles of Treatment. St. Louis, Mosby-Year Book, 1993.
3. Young JR, Olin JW, Bartholomew JR. Peripheral Vascular Disease. St. Louis, Mosby-Year Book, 1996.
4. Loscalzo J, Creager MA, Dzau VJ. Vascular Medicine. A Textbook of Vascular Biology and Diseases. Boston, Little, Brown, 1996.
5. Lie JR. The structure of the normal vascular system and its reactive changes. In: Juergens JL, Spittell JA, Fairbairn JF, eds. Peripheral Vascular Diseases. Philadelphia, Saunders, 1980:51–81.
6. Bell DM, Johns TE, Lopez LM. Endothelial dysfunction: Implications for therapy of cardiovascular diseases. Ann Pharmacother 1998;32:459–470.
7. Newby DE, Flint LL, Fox KA, et al. Reduced responsiveness to endothelin-1 in peripheral resistance vessels of patients with syndrome X. J Am Coll Cardiol 1998;31:1585–1590.
8. Schellong SM, Boger RH, Burchert W, et al. Dose-related effect of intravenous L-arginine on muscular blood flow of the calf in patients with peripheral vascular disease: A H215O positron emission tomography study. Clin Sci 1997;93:159–165.
9. Coffman JD. Effects of endothelium-derived nitric oxide on skin and digital blood flow in humans. Am J Physiol 1994;267:H2087–2090.
10. Berkenboom G, Crasset V, Giot C, et al. Endothelial function of internal mammary artery in patients with coronary artery disease and in cardiac transplant recipients. Am Heart J 1998;135:488–494.
11. Curb JD, Masaki K, Rodriguez BL, et al. Peripheral artery disease and cardiovascular risk factors in the elderly. The Honolulu heart program. Arterioscler Thromb Vasc Biol 1996;16:1495–1500.
12. Violi F, Criqui M, Longoni A, Castiglioni C. Relation between risk factors and cardiovascular complications in patients with peripheral vascular disease. Results from the A.D.E.P. study. Atherosclerosis 1996;120:25–35.
13. Libby P, Tanaka H. The molecular bases of restenosis. Prog Cardiovasc Dis 1997;40:97–106.
14. Lowe GD, Fowkes FG, Dawes J, et al. Blood viscosity, fibrinogen, and activation of coagulation and leukocytes in peripheral arterial disease and the normal population in the Edinburgh artery study. Circulation 1993;87:1915–1920.
15. Nukada H, van Rij AM, Packer SG, Patterson A. Preservation of skin vasoconstrictor responses in chronic atherosclerotic peripheral vascular disease. Angiology 1998;49:181–188.
16. Ouriel KE. Lower Extremity Vascular Disease. Philadelphia, Saunders, 1995.

17. Gerhard M, Baum P, Raby KE. Peripheral arterial-vascular disease in women: Prevalence, prognosis, and treatment. Cardiology 1995; 86:349–355.
18. Shepherd JT, Bergan JJ, Cohen RA, et al. Report of the task force on vascular medicine. Circulation 1994;89:532–535.
19. Fowkes FG, Housley E, Cawood EH, et al. Edinburgh artery study: Prevalence of asymptomatic and symptomatic peripheral arterial disease in the general population. Int J Epidemiol 1991; 20:384–392.
20. Rihal CS, Eagle KA, Mickel MC, et al. Surgical therapy for coronary artery disease among patients with combined coronary artery and peripheral vascular disease. Circulation 1995;91:46–53.
21. Criqui MH, Denenberg JO, Langer RD, Fronek A. The epidemiology of peripheral arterial disease: Importance of identifying the population at risk. Vasc Med 1997;2:221–226.
22. Landi A, Keller L, Kiss K, et al. Relation of angiographic changes to clinical data and risk factors in patients with arteriosclerosis obliterans. Orvosi Hetilap 1993;134:2579–2584.
23. Hiatt WR, Hoag S, Hamman RF. Effect of diagnostic criteria on the prevalence of peripheral arterial disease. The San Luis Valley diabetes study. Circulation 1995;91:1472–1479.
24. Newman AB, Siscovick DS, Manolio TA, et al. Ankle-arm index as a marker of atherosclerosis in the cardiovascular health study. Cardiovascular heart study (CHS) collaborative research group. Circulation 1993;88:837–845.
25. Montgomery PS, Gardner AW. The clinical utility of a six-minute walk test in peripheral arterial occlusive disease patients. J Am Geriatr Soc 1998;46:706–711.
26. Sieminski DJ, Cowell LL, Montgomery PS, et al. Physical activity monitoring in patients with peripheral arterial occlusive disease. J Cardiopulm Rehabil 1997;17:43–47.
27. Franzeck UK, Huch A, Zimmermann AR, et al. A triple electrode for simultaneous investigations of transcutaneous oxygen tension, laser-Doppler flowmetry and dynamic fluorescence video microscopy. Int J Microcirc Clin Exp 1994;14:269–273.
28. Androulakis AE, Giannoukas AD, Labropoulos N, et al. The impact of duplex scanning on vascular practice. Int Angiol 1996;15:283–290.
29. Allard L, Cloutier G, Durand LG, et al. Limitations of ultrasonic duplex scanning for diagnosing lower limb arterial stenoses in the presence of adjacent segment disease. J Vasc Surg 1994;19:650–657.
30. De Vries SO, Hunink MG, Polak JF. Summary receiver operating characteristic curves as a technique for meta-analysis of the diagnostic performance of duplex ultrasonography in peripheral arterial disease. Acad Radiol 1996;3:361–369.
31. Koelemay MJ, den Hartog D, Prins MH, et al. Diagnosis of arterial disease of the lower extremities with duplex ultrasonography [see comments]. Br J Surg 1996;83:404–409.
32. Kroon AA, van Asten WN, Stalenhoef AF. Effect of apheresis of low-density lipoprotein on peripheral vascular disease in hypercholesterolemic patients with coronary artery disease. Ann Intern Med 1996;125:945–954.
33. Gardner AW, Poehlman ET. Exercise rehabilitation programs for the treatment of claudication pain. A meta-analysis [see comments]. JAMA 1995;274:975–980.
34. Regensteiner JG, Hiatt WR. Exercise rehabilitation for patients with peripheral arterial disease. Exerc Sport Sci Rev 1995;23:1–24.
35. Ernst E, Fialka V. A review of the clinical effectiveness of exercise therapy for intermittent claudication. Arch Intern Med 1993; 153:2357–2360.
36. Radack K, Wyderski RJ. Conservative management of intermittent claudication. Ann Intern Med 1990;113:135–146.
37. Smith I, Franks PJ, Greenhalgh RM, et al. The influence of smoking cessation and hypertriglyceridaemia on the progression of peripheral arterial disease and the onset of critical ischaemia. Eur J Vasc Endovasc Surg 1996;11:402–408.
38. Lakier JB. Smoking and cardiovascular disease. Am J Med 1992; 93:8S–12S.
39. Radack K, Deck C. Beta-adrenergic blocker therapy does not worsen intermittent claudication in subjects with peripheral arterial disease. A meta-analysis of randomized controlled trials. Arch Intern Med 1991;151:1769–1776.
40. Solomon SA, Ramsay LE, Yeo WW, et al. Beta blockade and intermittent claudication: Placebo controlled trial of atenolol and nifedipine and their combination. BMJ 1991;303:1100–1104.
41. Heintzen MP, Strauer BE. Peripheral vascular effects of beta-blockers. Eur Heart J 1994;15:2–7.
42. Frampton JE, Brogden RN. Pentoxifylline (oxpentifylline). A review of its therapeutic efficacy in the management of peripheral vascular and cerebrovascular disorders. Drugs Aging 1995;7:480–503.
43. Currie MS, Simel DL, Christenson RH, et al. Anti-inflammatory effects of pentoxifylline in claudication. Am J Med Sci 1991;301:85–90.
44. Lindgarde F, Labs KH, Rossner M. The pentoxifylline experience: Exercise testing reconsidered. Vasc Med 1996;1:145–154.
45. AbuRahma AF, Woodruff BA. Effects and limitations of pentoxifylline therapy in various stages of peripheral vascular disease of the lower extremity. Am J Surg 1990;160:266–270.
46. European study group. Intravenous pentoxifylline for the treatment of chronic critical limb ischaemia. Eur J Vasc Endovasc Surg 1995; 9:426–436.
47. Lucas MA. Prevention of post-operative thrombosis in peripheral arteriopathies. Pentoxifylline vs. conventional antiaggregants: A six-month randomized follow-up study. Angiology 1984;35:443–450.
48. Lindblad B, Wakefield TW, Stanley TJ, et al. Pharmacological prophylaxis against postoperative graft occlusion after peripheral vascular surgery: A world-wide survey. Eur J Vasc Endovasc Surg 1995; 9:267–271.
49. Stergachis D, Sheingold S, Luce BR, et al. Medical care and cost outcomes after pentoxifylline for peripheral arterial disease. Arch Intern Med 1992;152:1220–1224.
50. West JA. Cost-effective strategies for the management of vascular disease. Vasc Med 1997;2:25–29.
51. Hirsch AT, Treat-Jacobson D, Lando HA, Hatsukami DK. The role of tobacco cessation, antiplatelet and lipid-lowering therapies in the treatment of peripheral arterial disease. Vasc Med 1997;2:243–251.
52. Goldhaber SZ, Manson JE, Stampfer MJ, et al. Low-dose aspirin and subsequent peripheral arterial surgery in the physicians' health study. Lancet 1992;340:143–145.
53. Clagett PG, Krupski WC. Antithrombotic therapy in peripheral arterial occlusive disease. Chest 1995;108:431S–443S.
54. Fagher B. Long-term effects of ticlopidine on lower limb blood flow, ankle/brachial index and symptoms in peripheral arteriosclerosis. A double-blind study. The STIMS group in Lund. Swedish ticlopidine multicenter study. Angiology 1994;45:777–788.
55. Blanchard J, Carreras LO, Kindermans M. Results of EMATAP: A double-blind placebo-controlled multicentre trial of ticlopidine in patients with peripheral arterial disease. Nouv Rev Fr Hematol 1994; 35:523–528.
56. Becquemin JP. Effect of ticlopidine on the long-term patency of saphenous-vein bypass grafts in the legs. Etude de la ticlopidine apres pontage femoro-poplite and the Association Universitaire de Recherche en Chirurgie. N Engl J Med 1997;337:1726–1731.
57. CAPRIE steering committee. A randomised, blinded, trial of clopidogrel versus aspirin in patients at risk of ischaemic events (CAPRIE). Lancet 1996;348:1329–1339.
58. Grant SM, Goa KL. Iloprost. A review of its pharmacodynamic and pharmacokinetic properties, and therapeutic potential in peripheral vascular disease, myocardial ischaemia and extracorporeal circulation procedures. Drugs 1992;43:889–924.
59. Wolf DL, Metzler CM, Froeschke MO, Luderer JR. Continuous intravenous dosing with ciprostene using a portable pump in ambulatory patients. J Clin Pharmacol 1993;33:150–153.
60. Loosemore TM, Chalmers TC, Dormandy JA. A meta-analysis of randomized placebo control trials in Fontaine stages III and IV peripheral occlusive arterial disease. Int Angiol 1994;13:133–142.

61. Nony P, Ffrench P, Girard P, et al. Platelet-aggregation inhibition and hemodynamic effects of beraprost sodium, a new oral prostacyclin derivative: A study in healthy male subjects. Can J Physiol Pharmacol 1996;74:887–893.
62. Money SR, Herd JA, Isaacsohn JL, et al. Effect of cilostazol on walking distances in patients with intermittent claudication caused by peripheral vascular disease. J Vasc Surg 1998;27:267–275.
63. Milani M, Longoni A, Maderna M. Effects of picotamide, an antiplatelet agent, on cardiovascular events in 438 claudicant patients with diabetes: A retrospective analysis of the ADEP study. Br J Clin Pharmacol 1996;42:782–785.
64. Hiatt WR. Current and future drug therapies for claudication. Vasc Med 1997;2:257–262.
65. Schachter M. Calcium antagonists and atherosclerosis. Int J Cardiol 1997;62:S9–S15.
66. Schroeder JS, Gao SZ. Calcium blockers and atherosclerosis: Lessons from the Stanford transplant coronary artery disease/diltiazem trial. Can J Cardiol 1995;11:710–715.
67. Paoletti R, Corsini A, Soma MR, Bernini F. Calcium, calcium antagonists and experimental atherosclerosis. Blood Press. Suppl 1996; 4:12–15.
68. Cimminiello C. Clinical trials with defibrotide in vascular disorders. Semin Thromb Hemost 1996;22:29–34.
69. Coffman JD, Clement DL, Creager MA, et al. International study of ketanserin in Raynaud's phenomenon. Am J Med 1989;87:264–268.
70. Verstraete M. The PACK trial: Morbidity and mortality effects of ketanserin. Prevention of atherosclerotic complications. Vasc Med 1996;1:135–140.
71. Brevetti G, Perna S, Sabba C, et al. Effect of propionyl-*L*-carnitine on quality of life in intermittent claudication. Am J Cardiol 1997; 79:777–780.
72. Bolognesi M, Amodio P, Merkel C, et al. Effect of 8-day therapy with propionyl-*L*-carnitine on muscular and subcutaneous blood flow of the lower limbs in patients with peripheral arterial disease. Clin Physiol 1995;15:417–423.
73. Ouriel K, Veith FJ, Sasahara AA, ToPAST investigators. A comparison of recombinant urokinase with vascular surgery as initial treatment for acute peripheral arterial occlusion of the legs. N Engl J Med 1998;338:1105–1111.
74. Comerota AJ, Cohen GS. Thrombolytic therapy in peripheral arterial occlusive disease: Mechanisms of action and drugs available. Can J Surg 1993;36:342–348.
75. Ouriel K, Kolassa M, DeWeese JA, Green RM. Economic implications of thrombolysis or operation as the initial treatment modality in acute peripheral arterial occlusion. Surgery 1995;118:810–814.
76. Singh S, Evans L, Datta D, et al. The costs of managing lower limb-threatening ischaemia. Eur J Vasc Endovasc Surg 1996; 12:359–362.
77. Hunink MG, Wong JB, Donaldson MC, et al. Revascularization for femoropopliteal disease. A decision and cost-effectiveness analysis. JAMA 1995;274:165–171.
78. Lowe GD, Reid AW, Leiberman DP. Management of thrombosis in peripheral arterial disease. Br Med Bull 1994;50:923–935.
79. Pentecost MJ, Criqui MH, Dorros G, et al. Guidelines for peripheral percutaneous transluminal angioplasty of the abdominal aorta and lower extremity vessels. A statement for health professionals from a special writing group of the Councils on Cardiovascular Radiology, Arteriosclerosis, Cardio-Thoracic and Vascular Surgery, Clinical Cardiology, and Epidemiology and Prevention, the American Heart Association. Circulation 1994;89:511–531.
80. Isner JM, Rosenfield K. Redefining the treatment of peripheral artery disease. Role of percutaneous revascularization. Circulation 1993; 88:1534–1557.
81. Minar E, Ahmadi A, Koppensteiner R, et al. Comparison of effects of high-dose and low-dose aspirin on restenosis after femoropopliteal percutaneous transluminal angioplasty. Circulation 1995; 91:2167–2173.
82. Isner JM, Walsh K, Symes J, et al. Arterial gene transfer for therapeutic angiogenesis in patients with peripheral artery disease. Hum Gene Ther 1996;7:959–988.
83. Gleim M, Maier C, Melchert U. Lumbar neurolytic sympathetic blockades provide immediate and long-lasting improvement of painless walking distance and muscle metabolism in patients with severe peripheral vascular disease. J Pain Symptom Manage 1995; 10:98–104.
84. Hildebrand M. Pharmacokinetics and tolerability of oral iloprost in thromboangiitis obliterans patients. Eur J Clin Pharmacol 1997; 53:51–56.
85. Coffman JD. The diagnosis of Raynaud's phenomenon. Clin Dermatol 1994;12:283–289.
86. Belch J. Raynaud's phenomenon. Cardiovasc Res 1997;33:25–30.
87. Cerinic MM, Generini S, Pignone A. New approaches to the treatment of Raynaud's phenomenon. Curr Opin Rheumatol 1997; 9:544–556.
88. Wigley FM, Flavahan NA. Raynaud's phenomenon. Rheum Dis Clin North Am 1996;22:765–781.
89. Isenberg DA, Black C. ABC of rheumatology. Raynaud's phenomenon, scleroderma, and overlap syndromes. BMJ 1995;310:795–798.
90. Coffman JD, Cohen RA. Plasma levels of 5-hydroxytryptamine during sympathetic stimulation and in Raynaud's phenomenon. Clin Sci 1994;86:269–273.
91. Coffman JD. Raynaud's phenomenon. An update. Hypertension 1991;17:593–602.
92. Belch JJ, Ho M. Pharmacotherapy of Raynaud's phenomenon. Drugs 1996;52:682–695.
93. Sylaidis P, Logan A. Local injection of phentolamine to treat digital ischaemic necrosis in Raynaud's syndrome. J Wound Care 1997; 6:356–357.
94. Teh LS, Manning J, Moore T, et al. Sustained-release transdermal glyceryl trinitrate patches as a treatment for primary and secondary Raynaud's phenomenon. B J Rheumatol 1995;34:636–641.
95. Varela-Aguilar JM, Sanchez-Roman J, Talegon Melendez A, Castillo Palma MJ. Comparative study of misoprostol and nifedipine in the treatment of Raynaud's phenomenon secondary to systemic diseases. Hemodynamic assessment with Doppler duplex. Rev Clin Esp 1997; 197:77–83.
96. Frishman WH, Huberfeld S, Okin S, et al. Serotonin and serotonin antagonism in cardiovascular and non-cardiovascular disease. J Clin Pharmacol 1995;35:541–572.
97. Arosio E, Montesi G, Zannoni M, et al. Comparative efficacy of ketanserin and pentoxiphylline in treatment of Raynaud's phenomenon. Angiology 1989;40:633–638.
98. De Cree J, Geukens H, Gutwirth P, et al. The effect of a combined administration of ridogrel and ketanserin in patients with intermittent claudication. Int Angiol 1993;12:59–68.
99. Challenor VF. Angiotensin converting enzyme inhibitors in Raynaud's phenomenon. Drugs 1994;48:864–867.
100. Challenor VF, Waller DG, Hayward RA, et al. Subjective and objective assessment of enalapril in primary Raynaud's phenomenon. Br J Clin Pharmacol 1991;31:477–480.
101. Wachtell K, Ibsen H, Olsen MH, et al. Prevalence of renal artery stenosis in patients with peripheral vascular disease and hypertension. J Hum Hypertens 1996;10:83–85.
102. Vayssairat M. Controlled multicenter double blind trial of an oral analog of prostacyclin in the treatment of primary Raynaud's phenomenon. French Microcirculation Society Multicentre Group for the Study of Vascular Acrosyndromes. J Rheumatol 1996; 23:1917–1920.
103. Belch JJ, Capell HA, Cooke ED, et al. Oral iloprost as a treatment for Raynaud's syndrome: A double blind multicentre placebo controlled study. Ann Rheum Dis 1995;54:197–200.
104. Belch JJ, Bell PR, Creissen D, et al. Randomized, double-blind, placebo-controlled study evaluating the efficacy and safety of AS-

013, a prostaglandin E1 prodrug, in patients with intermittent claudication. Circulation 1997;95:2298–2302.
105. Iloprost bypass international study group. Effects of perioperative iloprost on patency of femorodistal bypass grafts. Eur J Vasc Endovasc Surg 1996;12:363–371.
106. Goszcz A, Grodzinska L, Kostka-Trabka E, et al. Misoprostol—oral prostanoid—the first clinical trial for use in patients with peripheral vascular disease. Przeglad Lekarski 1997;54:505–509.
107. Dessein PH, Morrison RC, Lamparelli RD, van der Merwe CA. Triiodothyronine treatment for Raynaud's phenomenon: A controlled trial. J Rheumatol 1990;17:1025–1028.
108. Gledhill RF, Dessein PH, Van der Merwe CA. Treatment of Raynaud's phenomenon with triiodothyronine corrects co-existent autonomic dysfunction: Preliminary findings. Postgrad Med J 1992; 68:263–267.
109. Neirotti M, Longo F, Molaschi M, et al. Functional vascular disorders: Treatment with pentoxifylline. Angiology 1987;38:575–580.
110. Wigley FM. Raynaud's phenomenon and other features of scleroderma, including pulmonary hypertension. Curr Opin Rheumatol 1996;8:561–568.
111. Bunker CB, Goldsmith PC, Leslie TA, et al. Calcitonin gene-related peptide, endothelin-1, the cutaneous microvasculature and Raynaud's phenomenon. Br J Dermatol 1996;134:399–406.
112. Shawket S, Dickerson C, Hazleman B, Brown MJ. Prolonged effect of CGRP in Raynaud's patients: A double-blind randomised comparison with prostacyclin. Br J Clin Pharmacol 1991;32:209–213.
113. Bunker CB, Reavley C, O'Shaughnessy DJ, Dowd PM. Calcitonin gene-related peptide in treatment of severe peripheral vascular insufficiency in Raynaud's phenomenon. Lancet 1993;342:80–83.
114. Moriau M, Lavenne-Pardonge E, Crasborn L, et al. Treatment of the Raynaud's phenomenon with piracetam. Arzneimittel forschung 1993;43:526–535.
115. Beretta L, Bortolani EM, Tolva V, et al. Long-term results of radical lumbar ganglionectomy. Minerva Chir 1998; 53:173–177.

21

USE OF VASOPRESSORS AND INOTROPES IN THE PHARMACOTHERAPY OF SHOCK

Maria I. Rudis, PharmD, ABAT, BCPS, Bertil Wagner, PharmD, FCCM, and Joseph F. Dasta, MS, FCCM

Shock is an acute, generalized, state of inadequate perfusion of critical organs that can produce serious pathophysiologic consequences, including death. Thirty years ago, mortality from septic or cardiogenic shock exceeded 70%.[1] Currently, approximately 10% of patients are admitted to hospitals with severe sepsis or experience cardiogenic shock following a myocardial infarction, with mortality rates of at least 50% despite enhanced treatment modalities and sophisticated monitoring techniques.[1,2] This chapter will review the theory and current status of hemodynamic monitoring and will present an update on the optimal use of inotropes and vasopressor drugs in shock states.

Hemodynamic and perfusion monitoring can be categorized into two broad areas: global and regional monitoring. Global parameters, such as systemic blood pressure and pulse oximetry, assess perfusion and oxygen utilization of the entire body. Regional monitoring techniques, such as gastrointestinal tonometry, focus on flow and subsequent changes in metabolism of individual organs and tissues. Normal values for commonly monitored parameters are lised in Table 21–1.

GLOBAL PERFUSION MONITORING

ARTERIAL BLOOD PRESSURE MEASUREMENT

Arterial blood pressure is the product of cardiac output and systemic vascular resistance. Conditions that may lower blood pressure in the critically ill include cardiac failure or hypovolemia (by lowering of cardiac output) and vasodilation (by sepsis, drugs, or neurotrauma). Arterial blood pressure can be determined by noninvasive and invasive methods. All noninvasive blood pressure monitoring techniques depend on the use of an occluding cuff. Systolic and diastolic blood pressure are further determined by auscultation, palpation (systolic pressure only), oscillometry, or Doppler technique (systolic pressures most reliable). Auscultation is the most commonly used method outside the intensive care unit (ICU). Its use, however, is limited in patients with hypovolemia, hypothermia, or cardiogenic shock when pulses or Korotkoff sounds may be difficult to hear. Similar constraints exist for the palpation and oscillometric methods. However, oscillometry is preferred in edematous patients. Oscillometry measures blood pressure by sensing arterial blood pressure changes, or oscillations, against an inflated cuff. Rapid changes in oscillation amplitude correspond to systolic and diastolic pressure. It is the only noninvasive method to measure mean arterial pressure even in low flow states and lends itself to automatic cycling and serial measurements (every 1 to 3 minutes) that do not require operator intervention, a key component in ICU monitoring. The use of narrow cuffs or cuffs applied too loosely can result in falsely high readings, whereas wide cuffs may produce falsely low readings.[3] Fingertip devices offer another avenue for continuous indirect blood pressure measurement, but their accuracy in ICU patients may be significantly diminished by concurrent administration of vasoactive drugs.[4]

The use of invasive arterial catheters makes it possible to continuously measure arterial blood pressures as well as to obtain blood samples for blood gas monitoring. The radial artery is the most commonly used vessel, but the dorsalis pedis, femoral, brachial, and axillary arteries and the umbilical artery in the newborn can also be accessed. This method of blood pressure monitoring is a standard technique against which all other methods are compared. Major complications of peripheral artery catheterization include infection and distal ischemia. Acute distal ischemia and catheter-related bacteremia occur in less than 1% of catheter insertions. Ischemia is most common in patients with multiple or prolonged arterial cannulations, hypertension, or vasopressor therapy.[3] Invasive techniques are labor intensive, require aseptic techniques, and offer potential sources of equipment errors, such as length and quality of tubing, air bubbles, stopcocks, thrombus formation, tube kinking, and placement of transducer. Hypertension, advanced age, and atherosclerosis may also affect the accuracy of invasive blood pressure readings.[5]

CENTRAL VENOUS CATHETER

The central venous catheter is used to measure the central venous blood pressure (CVP), to obtain venous blood gas samples, and to administer drugs or fluids directly to the central circulation. A triple-lumen catheter is often used whereby drugs with known incompatibility can be administered. Blood volume, venous wall compliance, right cardiac function, intra-abdominal and intra-thoracic pressure, and vasopressor therapy affect central venous pressure. The CVP is not a reliable estimate of blood volume but can be used to qualitatively assess blood volume changes in patients during the early phases of fluid resuscitation. Sustained elevated pressures are indicative of fluid overloading.[6] There

TABLE 21–1. Hemodynamic and Oxygen Transport Monitoring Parameters

Parameter	Normal Value
Blood pressure (systolic/diastolic)	100–130/70–85 mm Hg
Mean arterial pressure (MAP)	80–100 mm Hg
Pulmonary artery pressure (PAP)	25/10 mm Hg
Mean pulmonary artery pressure (MPAP)	12–15 mm Hg
Central venous pressure (CVP)	2–6 mm Hg
Pulmonary capillary wedge pressure (PCWP)	8–12 (normal), 15–18 (ICU) mm Hg
Heart rate (HR)	60–80 beats/min
Cardiac output (CO)	4–7 L/min
Cardiac index (CI)	2.8–3.6 L/min/m^2
Stroke volume index (SVI)	30–50 mL/m^2
Systemic vascular resistance index (SVRI)	1300–2100 dyne·sec/m^{2}cm^5
Pulmonary vascular resistance index (PVRI)	45–225 dyne·sec/m^{2}cm^5
Arterial oxygen saturation (Sao_2)	97% (range, 95% to 100%)
Mixed venous oxygen saturation (Svo_2)	75% (range, 60% to 80%)
Arterial oxygen content (Cao_2)	20.1 vol % (range, 19–21)
Venous oxygen content (Cvo_2)	15.5 vol % (range, 11.5–16.5)
Oxygen content difference ($C(a\text{-}v)o_2$)	5 vol % (range, 4–6)
Oxygen consumption index (Vo_2)	131 mL/min/m^2 (range, 100–180)
Oxygen delivery index (Do_2)	578 mL/min/m^2 (range, 370–730)
Oxygen extraction ratio (O_2 ER)	25% (range, 22% to 30%)
Mucosal pH (pHi)	7.40 (range, 7.35–7.45)
Index	Parameter indexed to body surface area

are few data supporting the use of CVP monitoring in the ICU. However, initial reports in septic patients suggest that CVP monitoring of fluid therapy during shock was associated with an over 50% reduction in mortality.

PULMONARY ARTERY CATHETER

Pulmonary artery catheterization, introduced in 1970, is a routinely performed bedside procedure in many ICUs. With this catheter, also known as the Swan–Ganz catheter, the practitioner can obtain multiple cardiovascular parameters, including central venous, pulmonary artery, and pulmonary capillary wedge pressures, and cardiac output. Mixed-venous blood samples from the pulmonary artery may also be obtained. Most importantly, inflation of the balloon at the catheter tip occludes the pulmonary artery, isolates the distal catheter tip from the right side of the heart, and allows the user to measure the pulmonary capillary "wedge" pressure (PCWP), an approximate measure of the left ventricular end-diastolic volume and a major determinant of left ventricular preload. Ideally, the pulmonary artery catheter should be fluoroscopically positioned; however, satisfactory placement may also be obtained by observing pulmonary artery pressure readings during catheter advancement. Proper positioning in the lower lung (zone 3) is essential to measure PCWP and to prevent distal pulmonary artery collapse. Poor wedging may be caused by catheter migration, patient movement, mechanical ventilation, or eccentric balloon inflation. Pulmonary artery catheters equipped with a distal thermistor also allow measurement of cardiac output by thermodilution. Rapid injection of saline solutions via the right atrial port allows complete mixing of blood with injectate and the resultant change in blood temperature is measured in the pulmonary artery. From the temperature change, the patient's cardiac output can be calculated. Newer pulmonary artery catheters contain a temperature coil that intermittently warms the blood in the right ventricle for near-continuous cardiac output measurement.[7] Significant tricuspid regurgitation, an intracardiac shunt, and significant positive-end-expiratory pressure (PEEP) decrease the validity of cardiac output measurements. The most common complications of pulmonary artery catheterization include mural thrombus formation (14% to 91%), transient ventricular tachydysrhythmias (11% to 63%), pulmonary infarction (1% to 7%), pulmonary artery rupture (0.06% to 2.0%), and sepsis (0.3% to 0.5%).[8]

Despite its ubiquitous use, much controversy surrounds the utility and safety of the pulmonary artery catheter. Tuman and colleagues found that pulmonary artery catheterization did not affect outcome in 1094 patients who underwent coronary artery surgery.[9] In fact, Connors and associates observed in a multicenter, retrospective, matched-case study of 5735 critically ill patients that pulmonary artery catheter use was associated with an increase in mortality and resource utilization.[10] In a subsequent consensus statement, a panel of experts found few studies investigating the device's impact on patient outcome. The catheter was, however, found useful in the diagnosis of cardiovascular alterations and in guidance of cardiovascular drug therapy, especially in those with high-risk procedures or in severely ill patients.[11] Studies in both Europe and the United States have found that one out of two physicians incorrectly interpreted a tracing from the right heart catheter.[12] These findings could explain some of the results of studies concluding no benefit to right heart catheterization.

OXYGEN PRESSURE AND SATURATION MONITORING

Arterial oxygen pressure (Pao_2) and saturation (Sao_2) may be measured invasively by obtaining an arterial blood sample. Arterial blood gases measured by conventional arterial sampling are considered standard, but their accuracy and usefulness are affected by poor sampling techniques, transportation and analysis delays, analyzer accuracy, sample cellular metabolism, and inability to trend results. Indwelling fiber-optic and electrochemical systems allow continuous monitoring and trend analysis of blood pH, Pao_2, and $Paco_2$ while decreasing patient blood loss due to frequent sampling. Unfortunately, studies evaluating the *in-vitro* accuracy of these devices may not apply to the ICU environment. The indwelling sensors may exhibit lower Pa_{O_2}, higher Pa_{CO_2}, and lower pH than central arterial blood when peripheral flow is diminished. Furthermore, sensor contact with blood vessel wall and vigorous arterial line flushing will also diminish sensor accuracy.[13]

Subcutaneous tissue oxygenation (Psq_{O_2}) is linked to tissue perfusion and, by extension, total body hemodynamic status. The main limitation to subcutaneous tissue oximetry is its sensitivity to peripheral flow changes induced by catecholamines. Transcutaneous oximetry, a similar noninvasive method, is currently used in some neonatal ICUs. This method may, unlike invasive subcutaneous tissue oximetry, artificially elevate tissue oxygen values and is less sensitive to changes in perfusion. Both methods, however, provide continuous measurement of Psq_{O_2}.[14] Pulse oximetry is based on the principles of the Lambert–Beer law, which states that light transmission is inversely proportional to the density of a substance (hemoglobin). The concentrations of different types of hemoglobin (oxygenated, deoxygenated, carboxy, and methemoglobin) can thus be measured at different wavelengths. Pulse oximeters measure oxygen saturation by determining the ratio of oxygenated hemoglobin to total hemoglobin in a finger or toe. Increased concentrations of carboxyhemoglobin (resulting from carbon monoxide toxicity) may elevate Sa_{O_2} readings. In contrast, increased levels of methemoglobin (methemoglobinemia), and methylene blue (a methemoglobinemia antidote) may decrease Sa_{O_2}. Nail polish, onychomycosis, dark skin pigmentation, strong light sources, patient motion, and peripheral vasoconstriction may also affect Sa_{O_2} readings. These effects are more pronounced when saturations are decreased. The incidence of equipment malfunction is approximately 1% to 2%.[15]

Pulse oximetry is very commonly used in the perioperative arena or ICU. Despite this use, few studies have investigated its usefulness. The false-positive alarm rate for pulse oximeters used in the ICU may be in excess of 80%.[16] In a large study of 20,802 patients, pulse oximetry was not shown to alter outcome following general surgery.[17] However, Cullen and coworkers, in a retrospective review of 17,093 surgical patients, concluded that pulse oximetry reduced the rate of unintended intensive care unit admissions from the recovery area.[18]

OXYGEN DELIVERY AND CONSUMPTION

The concept of tissue oxygen debt as a determinant of organ damage in critical illness was proposed over 10 years ago. In normal individuals, oxygen consumption (V_{O_2}) is dependent on oxygen delivery (D_{O_2}) up to a certain critical level (V_{O_2} flow dependency). At this point, tissue oxygen requirements have apparently been satisfied and further increases in D_{O_2} will not alter V_{O_2} (V_{O_2} flow independency) (Fig. 21–1).

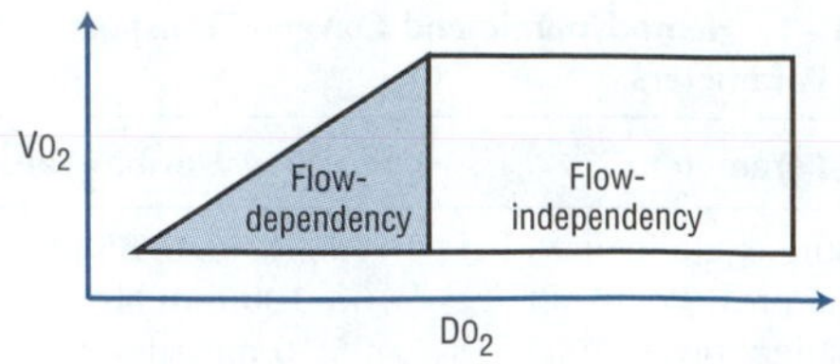

FIGURE 21–1. Relationship between oxygen consumption (V_{O_2}) and oxygen delivery (D_{O_2}).

Although animal models of sepsis have substantiated this relationship, studies in critically ill humans show a continuous, pathologic dependence relationship of V_{O_2} on D_{O_2}. Furthermore, ICU survivors exhibited higher D_{O_2} and V_{O_2} levels than nonsurvivors. This became the basis for targeting supranormal levels of oxygen delivery and consumption parameters in the treatment of ICU patients.[19] However, a recent meta-analysis of randomized clinical trials involving 1016 adult ICU patients failed to show that achievement of this goal improved patient mortality.[20] This may, in part, have been due to the heterogeneous nature of ICU patients studied, lack of study blinding, crossover patients (control patients who achieve supranormal D_{O_2} and V_{O_2} levels by themselves), or lack of adequate control of cointerventions. Furthermore, the apparent linear relationship between D_{O_2} and V_{O_2} has been questioned as both share variables, and this so-called "mathematical coupling" can produce artifactual relationships between variables. The D_{O_2} and V_{O_2} indexed parameters are calculated as follows:

$$D_{O_2} = CI \times Ca_{O_2}$$

$$V_{O_2} = CI \times (Ca_{O_2} - Cv_{O_2})$$

where CI = cardiac index, Ca_{O_2} = arterial oxygen content, and Cv_{O_2} = mixed-venous oxygen content.

However, variable relationships between D_{O_2} and V_{O_2} have been observed when V_{O_2} was measured independently by indirect calorimetry. A linear relationship between D_{O_2} and V_{O_2} may therefore be the result of mathematical coupling or flow-dependent V_{O_2}. Currently available data do not support the concept that patient outcome or survival may be altered by treatment measures directed to achieve supranormal levels of D_{O_2} and V_{O_2}.[20] Furthermore, achievement of supranormal D_{O_2} does not assure parallel improvements in regional organ blood flow and oxygenation.[21] The V_{O_2}/D_{O_2} ratio (oxygen extraction ratio, or O_2ER) can be used to assess adequacy of perfusion and metabolic response. Patients who are able to increase V_{O_2} when D_{O_2} is increased show improved survival. However, low V_{O_2} and O_2ER values are indicative of poor oxygen utilization and lead to greater mortality.[22] Another approach that may decrease the effect of mathematical coupling and provide individualized therapy may lie in titrated therapy, with sequential measurements of D_{O_2} and V_{O_2} to achieve V_{O_2} flow independency, along with normalization of blood lactate and hemodynamic parameters.[23,24]

SERUM LACTATE

The use of serum lactate concentrations as an alternate or complimentary measure of tissue oxygenation and function has been suggested, as Do_2 and Vo_2 may change independently of blood lactate levels.[19] Lactate concentrations may in some patients show better correlation with outcome than oxygen transport parameters,[25] and may be superior to hemodynamic markers in determining adequacy of systemic oxygenation restoration.[26] Lactate is a metabolic product of pyruvate and its production is increased under anaerobic conditions, as may occur during shock. However, lactate may also accumulate in patients with significant liver dysfunction who are not in shock and in patients with the acute respiratory distress syndrome and endotoxin-inactivated pyruvate dehydrogenase.[27] Interestingly, the intestines and kidneys may take up lactate during near-zero flow states.[28] Furthermore, both well-perfused and poorly perfused tissues contribute to arterial and mixed-venous lactate concentrations and are therefore not reflective of regional perfusion. Increased lactate concentrations have been correlated with increased mortality,[29] but the utility of blood lactate measurements in guiding therapy has not been clearly demonstrated.

REGIONAL PERFUSION MONITORING

GASTROINTESTINAL TONOMETRY

Blood pressures, cardiac output, serum lactate, and global oxygen homeostasis parameters do not offer information as to individual organ function. Gastric tonometry measures gut luminal Pco_2 at equilibrium by placing a saline-filled gas-permeable balloon in the gastric lumen. Assuming that CO_2 permeates freely among tissues and that the arterial bicarbonate concentration $[HCO_3^-]$ is equal to that of the gut mucosa, the intramucosal pH (pHi) may be calculated using the Henderson–Hasselbach equation:

$$pHi = 6.1 + \log [HCO_3^-]0.03 \times Pco_2$$

Increases in mucosal Pco_2 and calculated decreases in pHi are associated with mucosal hypoperfusion and perhaps increased mortality.[30] The calculation of pHi can be confounded by increases in luminal Pco_2 as may occur when buffering antacids are used. Histamine-2-receptor antagonists may be used instead. The presence of respiratory acid–base disorders, systemic bicarbonate administration, arterial blood gas measurement errors, enteral feeding solutions, or stool in the gut may confound pHi determinations.[31] The time delay associated with this measurement (30 minutes) makes this method inconvenient for routine bedside monitoring. Recent investigations suggest that an air-filled balloon may require a shorter equilibrium time, be simpler to use, and be equally accurate.[32] A randomized, prospective, multicenter trial of pHi-directed therapy was not able to show that the use of pHi reduced mortality in critically ill patients.[33] However, patients with a normal pHi (> 7.35) upon admission, who subsequently received pHi-guided treatment to increase Do_2, experienced a 38% reduction in mortality. In a smaller trial of 57 patients, Ivatury and associates compared pHi-directed therapy (end point pHi > 7.3) to Do_2-directed therapy (end point Do_2 > 600 $mL/min/m^2$).[34] The incidence of multiple organ failure and mortality were not statistically different between the groups. Some clinicians believe that gastric mucosal Pco_2 may be more accurate than pHi. Furthermore, because mucosal Pco_2 is influenced by arterial Pco_2, one suggestion is that using the mucosal–arterial Pco_2 difference (Pco_2 gap) may be the optimum measurement. Additional trials are clearly needed to define the role of tonometry and other measures of organ-specific function on guiding therapy and predicting outcomes in critically ill patients.

VASOPRESSORS AND INOTROPES

Vasopressors and inotropes in septic shock are required when volume resuscitation fails to maintain adequate blood pressure and organ and tissue perfusion. The clinician must decide on the choice of agent, therapeutic end points, and the safe and effective doses of vasopressors and inotropes to be used. This section reviews adrenergic receptor pharmacology, exogenous catecholamine use, and alterations in receptor function in the critically ill. It will also provide guidelines for the clinical use of adrenergic agents, optimization of pharmacotherapeutic outcomes, and minimization of adverse effects in critically ill patients with septic shock.

It should be noted that agents other than catecholamines have been used as inotropes and vasopressors in shock states. These include phosphodiesterase III inhibitors, naloxone, nitric oxide synthase inhibitors, and vasopressin. However, the focus of this chapter is on catecholamines.

RECEPTOR PHARMACOLOGY

Comparative receptor activity of endogenous and exogenously administered catecholamines are summarized in Table 21–2. Endogenous catecholamines are responsible for regulation of vascular and bronchiolar smooth muscle tone and myocardial contractility.[35] These effects are mediated by sympathetic adrenergic receptors of the autonomic system located in the vasculature, myocardium, and bronchioles. Postsynaptic adrenoceptors are located at or near the synaptic junction. These receptors can be activated by naturally circulating or exogenous catecholamines (e.g., norepinephrine, epinephrine, phenylephrine), whereas presynaptic adrenoceptors are stimulated by locally released neurotransmitters (e.g., norepinephrine) and are controlled by a negative feedback mechanism.

Figure 21–2 depicts adrenoceptor–G protein interaction. Beta and DA_1–adrenoceptor agonists activate the

TABLE 21–2. Adrenergic and Dopaminergic Receptor Pharmacology and Organ Distribution

Effector Organ	Receptor Subtype	Physiologic Response
Heart		
SA node	β_1, β_2	Increased heart rate
Atria	β_1, β_2	Increased contractility Increased conduction velocity
AV node	β_1, β_2	Increased automaticity Increased conduction velocity
His–Purkinje system	β_1, β_2	Increased automaticity Increased conduction velocity
Ventricles	β_1, β_2, α_1	Increased contractility Increased conduction velocity Increased automaticity Increased rate idioventricular pacemaker cells
Arterioles		
Coronary	α_1, α_2; β_2, DA_1	Constriction, dilatation
Skin and mucosa	α_1, α_2	Constriction
Skeletal muscle	α_1; β_2	Constriction, dilatation
Cerebral	α_1	Constriction (slight)
Pulmonary	α_1; β_2	Constriction, dilatation
Abdominal viscera (mesentery)	α_1; β_2, DA_1	Constriction, dilatation
Renal	α_1, α_2; β_1, β_2, DA_1	Constriction, dilatation
Veins (systemic)	α_1, α_2; β_2	Constriction, dilatation
Lungs		
Trachial/bronchial smooth muscle	β_2	Relaxation
Bronchial glands	α_1; β_2	Decrease, increase secretion
Stomach		
Motility and tone	α_1, α_2; β_2	Decrease (usually)
Sphincter	α_1	Contraction (usually)
Intestine		
Motility and tone	α_1, α_2; β_1, β_2	Decrease
Sphincters	α_1	Contraction
Secretions	α_2	Inhibition (?)
Kidney		
Renin secretion	α_1	Decrease
Skeletal muscle	β_2	Increased contractility, glyconeogenesis, K^+ uptake
Liver	α_1, β_2	Glycogenolysis and gluconeogenesis

Compiled from Refs. 35 and 36.

stimulatory G protein, Gs, which dissociates from the receptor and activates membrane-bound adenyl cyclase (AC). $Alpha_2$ and DA_2 agonists activate the inhibitory G protein, Gi, which dissociates from the receptor and blocks adenyl cyclase. Adenyl cyclase converts ATP to cAMP, which stimulates protein kinases, resulting in alterations in cellular functions.

The heart contains primarily postsynaptic β_1-receptors, which cause increased rate and force of contraction when stimulated. This effect appears to be mediated by activation of adenylate cyclase and subsequent generation and accumulation of cyclic AMP (cAMP). Stimulation of postsynaptic cardiac α_1-receptors causes a significant increase in contractility without an increase in the rate, an effect apparently not mediated by cAMP. The increased contractility is more pronounced at lower heart rates, and has a slower onset and longer duration in comparison with β_1-mediated inotropic response. Presynaptic α_2-adrenoceptors are also found in the heart and appear to be activated by norepinephrine released by the sympathetic nerve itself. Their activation inhibits further norepinephrine release from the nerve terminal.

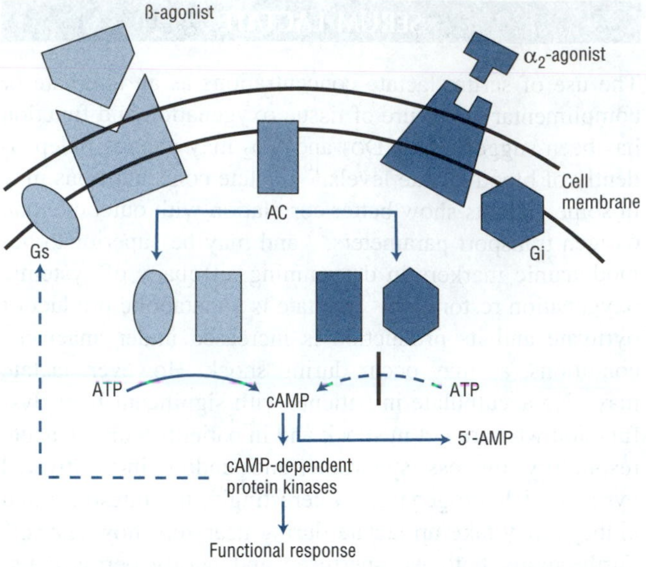

FIGURE 21–2. Adrenoceptor–G protein interaction. *(Adapted with permission from Ref. 37.)*

Both presynaptic and postsynaptic adrenoceptors are present in the vasculature. Postsynaptic α_1- and α_2-receptors mediate vasoconstriction, whereas postsynaptic β_2-receptors induce vasodilation. Presynaptic α_2-receptors inhibit norepinephrine release in the vasculature as well. Presynaptic β_1-adrenoceptors promote neurotransmitter release. Stimulation of peripheral DA_1 receptors produces renal, coronary, and mesenteric vasodilation and a natriuretic response. Stimulation of DA_2 receptors inhibits norepinephrine release from sympathetic nerve endings and prolactin release, and may induce nausea and vomiting.[38] DA_1 and DA_2 receptor stimulation also suppresses peristalsis and may precipitate ileus.[38] Cloning techniques have identified novel DA_1- and DA_2-like receptors, but their function beyond positive and negative adenyl cyclase coupling to the α-subunit of the G proteins has yet to be determined.[39]

ALTERED ADRENOCEPTOR FUNCTION: IMPLICATIONS FOR THE CRITICALLY ILL

The majority of the work describing receptor function and associated clinical pharmacology has been done either in animal models or human volunteers and not in critically ill patients with bacteremia or septic shock. Derangements in adrenergic receptor activity may result in resistance to exogenous catecholamine administration in the critically ill.[37] This "desensitization" is frequently characterized by myocardial and vascular hyporesponsiveness to high dosages of inotropes and vasopressor agents. Prolonged exposure of vascular endothelial tissue to vasopressor drugs (α-adrenergic agonists) or hormones (catecholamines) may produce this attenuation in response.[40,41] Increased endogenous catecholamine concentrations have been reported in endotoxemic and other critically ill patients, suggesting an acquired β-adrenergic receptor defect and desensitization of β-adrenergic receptors.[42] Although the problem in critically ill patients may lie in decreased β-receptor activity, in septic shock patients, the catecholamine concentrations are even higher, and thus abnormalities in β-adrenergic receptor function may be greater.[42] The worsened receptor abnormality may be explained by defects distal to the receptor site, such as an uncoupling of the β-adrenergic receptor from adenylate cyclase, or a dysfunction in the regulatory (G)-protein unit of the adenylate cyclase system.

Mediators other than catecholamines (e.g., circulating cytokines) may be responsible for these distal alterations. Macrophage-derived interleukin-1 and TNF-α produce impaired coupling of β-adrenergic receptors to adenylate cyclase in rat cardiac myocytes.[41] Septic shock patients have exhibited impaired β-adrenergic receptor stimulation of cAMP associated with myocardial hyporesponsiveness to dobutamine and reduced myocardial performance when compared to normal volunteers, nonbacteremic critically ill, and septic patients not in shock.[41] However, increased chronotropic sensitivity to β-adrenergic stimulation with hypersensitivity of the adenylate cyclase system to isoproterenol stimulation has also been reported in animal models of bacteremia and endotoxemia. In the presence of intrinsic myocardial dysfunction and increased metabolic demands, this dysfunctional adrenergic system is incapable of mobilizing functional cardiac reserve to maintain adequate myocardial performance.[41] These conflicting findings were observed in early stages of sepsis, and thus adrenergic receptor sensitivity may be time dependent. In fact, in an *in vivo* rodent model of sustained endotoxemia (48 hours) and continuous parenteral nutrition simulating advanced critical illness, Dickerson and colleagues showed no difference in α_1-adrenergic maximal responsiveness (in MAP) to phenylephrine.[40] Time-dependent different alterations in the production of endothelium-derived nitric oxide, a potent vasodilator, may explain the apparent differences in vascular reactivity to phenylephrine during the phases of endotoxemia.[40] These findings suggest that the clinical response to vasopressor and inotropic agents is variable during different stages of the hemodynamic, myocardial and peripheral vascular derangements of septic shock. These derangements vary among patients and during each bacteremic insult, and therefore doses of catecholamines vary during the actual insult and from patient to patient. For these reasons, these drugs should be dosed to clinical end points and not arbitrary maximal doses.

CLINICAL PHARMACOLOGY OF CATECHOLAMINES

The receptor selectivity of clinically used vasopressors and inotropes and hemodynamic effects are listed in Table 21–3. In general, these drugs are rapidly acting with short durations of action.[43] As such these drugs are given as continuous infusions. Careful monitoring and calculation of infusion rates is advised because dosing adjustments are made frequently and varying admixtures concentrations are used in volume-restricted patients.

TABLE 21–3. Receptor Pharmacology of Selected Inotropic and Vasopressor Agents Used in Septic Shock[a]

Agent	α_1	α_2	β_1	β_2	DA[b]
Dobutamine (500 mg/250 mL D_5W or NS)					
2–10 μg/kg/min	+	0	++++	++	0
>10–20 μg/kg/min	++	0	++++	+++	0
Dopamine (800 mg/250 mL D_5W or NS)					
1–3 μg/kg/min	0	0	+	0	++++
3–10 μg/kg/min	0/+	0	++++	++	++++
>10–20 μg/kg/min	+++	0	++++	+	0
Dopexamine (investigational)					
0.5–4.0 μg/kg/min	0	0	++[c]	+++	++++
Epinephrine (2 mg/250 mL D_5W or NS)					
0.01–0.05 μg/kg/min	++	++	++++	+++	0
>0.05 μg/kg/min	++++	++++	+++	+	
Norepinephrine (4 mg/250 mL D_5W or NS)					
0.02–3.0 μg/kg/min (2–20 μg/min)	+++	+++	+++	+/++	0
Phenylephrine (50 mg/250 mL D_5W or NS)					
0.5–9 μg/kg/min	+++	+	?	0	0

[a]Activity ranges from no activity (0) to maximal (++++) activity or ? when activity is not known.
[b]DA = dopaminergic.
[c]Dopexamine inhibits neuronal reuptake of norepinephrine.
Compiled from Refs. 43–45.

Dopamine is often recommended as the initial catecholamine in sepsis because it increases blood pressure by increasing myocardial contractility and vasoconstriction. Dopamine has been described to have dose-related receptor activity at DA_1, β_1- and α_1-receptors. Unfortunately, this dose–response relationship has not been confirmed in critically ill patients. In patients with septic shock, there is a great overlap of hemodynamic effects even at doses as low as 3 μg/kg/min.[46] Tachydysrhythmias are common due to the release of endogenous norepinephrine by dopamine entering the sympathetic nerve terminal. Dopamine may increase the PCWP through pulmonary vasoconstriction.[46–49] This drug may also depress ventilation and worsen hypoxemia in patients dependent on the hypoxic ventilatory drive.

Dobutamine, a synthetic catecholamine, is primarily a selective β_1-agonist with mild β_2- and vascular α_1-activity, resulting in strong positive inotropic activity without concomitant vasoconstriction. In comparison with dopamine, dobutamine produces a larger increase in CO and is less arrhythmogenic.[37] Ruffolo and colleagues showed that α_1-adrenoceptors in the heart are directly stimulated by the (–) isomer of dobutamine, and the β_1- and β_2-agonist activity resides in the (+) isomer.[38] This suggests that the strong inotropic action of dobutamine is a function of its structure, the additive effect of the cardiac α_1- and β_1-agonist activity, and a relatively weak chronotropic effect limited to the (+) isomer action on the β-receptors. Clinically, the increased myocardial contractility and subsequent reflex reduction in sympathetic tone leads to a decrease in SVR. Even though dobutamine is optimally used for low CO states with high filling pressures, or in cardiogenic shock, vasopressors may be needed to counteract arterial vasodilation.

Norepinephrine is a combined α- and β-agonist, but mainly produces vasoconstriction primarily via its more α-effects on all vascular beds, thus increasing SVR.[36,50,51] Norepinephrine administration generally produces either no change or a slight decrease in CO.

Phenylephrine is a pure α_1-agonist and is believed to increase blood pressure through vasoconstriction. Given the presence of cardiac α_1-receptors, phenylephrine may also increase contractility and CO.[52]

Epinephrine exerts combined α- and β-agonist effects and has traditionally been reserved as the vasopressor of last resort because of reports of peripheral vasoconstriction, particularly in the splanchnic and renal beds. At the high epinephrine infusion rates used in septic shock, predominantly α-adrenergic effects are seen, and SVR and MAP are increased.[53]

Dopexamine is an investigational synthetic catecholamine with marked intrinsic agonist activity at β_2-receptors with less activity at dopaminergic (DA_1 and DA_2) receptors. Direct stimulation of cardiac β_2-receptors may result in a reflex baroceptor stimulation and mild inotropic activity. Dopexamine has no clinically significant direct β_1-agonist activity and no α-effects. Cardiac β_1-receptors are indirectly stimulated due to inhibition of neuronal reuptake of catecholamines.[44,54]

CLINICAL USE OF VASOPRESSORS AND INOTROPES

Traditionally, there have been few vasopressors and inotropes used for hemodynamic support: dopamine, dobutamine, epinephrine, norepinephrine, and phenylephrine. Optimizing mean arterial pressure (MAP) as the goal of vasopressor therapy does not uniformly correlate with a decrease in mortality in septic shock.[45] Historically, significant concerns about the adverse effects of the vasopressors limited their use. The recent focus on goal-directed therapy, with optimization of oxygen transport variables to supranormal values has also yielded poor results in patients with septic shock.[20,45] In fact, normalization of systemic Do_2 and Vo_2, whether spontaneously or by design, is associated with improved outcome and is not dependent on administration of vasopressor agents. Part of our inability to detect an improvement with vasopressor or inotrope therapy may result from our limited ability to quantify regional tissue perfusion.

ADVERSE EFFECTS

Catecholamine vasopressors may result in adverse peripheral vasoconstrictive, metabolic, and dysrhythmogenic effects that limit or outweigh their positive effects on the central circulation.[55] Norepinephrine, phenylephrine, and epinephrine can produce a lactic acidosis secondary to excessive constriction in peripheral arterioles, enhanced glycogenolysis, or as a result of mobilization of lactate from peripheral tissues as a result of improved oxygenation.[55,56] Additionally, excessive peripheral vasoconstriction may cause ischemia or necrosis of already poorly perfused areas such as the skin, mesenteric, and splanchnic circulations.[37,57] Some of these profound vasoconstrictive effects have been compounded by the use of epinephrine and phenylephrine in septic shock patients, who are significantly hypovolemic. These agents are used in the context of late septic shock, where hypotension is refractory to less selective vasoconstrictors (e.g., norepinephrine, dopamine) such that very large doses of epinephrine or phenylephrine are required, with little or no benefit. Myocardial ischemia and dysrhythmias may occur in patients with coronary artery disease, atherosclerosis, cardiomyopathies, left ventricular hypertrophy, congestive heart failure, and underlying dysrhythmias due to their inability to tolerate β_1-cardiac stimulation that mediates increases in CO. The effect is usually the opposite, however, in healthy myocardium and in young patients. Beta-1 cardiac stimulation is well tolerated, ventricular filling pressures decrease, and CO and Do_2 increase, with a resulting increase in peripheral perfusion. An extensive review of the dysrhythmogenic potential of the catecholamine vasopressors reveals a variety of resulting atrial and ventricular arrhythmias.[58] Sympathomimetic vasopressors have also been found to occupy neutrophil β_2-receptors (e.g., epinephrine) and directly scavenge oxygen free radicals (e.g., dopamine, dobutamine).[59] These effects may be either beneficial or deleterious, by dampening harmful effects of oxygen free radicals mediated tissue injury, or by reducing neutrophilic defense against bacteria. At clinically relevant concentrations, dopamine inhibits *in vitro* endothelial adhesion molecule expression of E-selectin.[60] This and other adhesion molecules mediate leukocyte interaction with and adherence to endothelial cells, which is implicated in enhancing sepsis-induced multiple organ failure and lung injury in many animal models.[59,60] Epinephrine, dopamine, and other β-adrenergic agonists can inhibit production of TNF-α by neutrophils or expression of cellular adhesion molecules such as E-selectin by increasing cAMP, but the mechanism is more complex than previously thought.[60,61]

Vasopressor catecholamines have the potential to cause extravasation-associated tissue damage if infusions infiltrate during peripheral administration. In the event of infiltration, an α-receptor antagonist such as phentolamine (10 mg in 10 mL-saline) should be injected intradermally to reverse local vasoconstriction. As such, it is recommended to administer vasopressor drugs into a large central vein.

EPINEPHRINE

By convention, epinephrine has been reserved as a last-line agent in hemodynamic support of sepsis. There are very few objective data evaluating its comparative efficacy in early sepsis, with most studies examining the effects of epinephrine in refractory septic shock.[45] Despite this, epinephrine is an acceptable choice as a single agent due to its combined vasoconstrictor and inotropic effects. Epinephrine infusion rates of 0.04 to 1.0 μg/kg/min alone increase hemodynamic and oxygen transport variables to "supranormal" values without adverse effects in patients without CAD. In 69 patients evaluated in 5 studies, epinephrine alone or combined with either dobutamine or low doses of dopamine, achieved the desired outcomes.[41,56,62–64] Large doses (0.5 to 1.0 μg/kg/min) are required when epinephrine is added to other agents.[56] Smaller doses (0.10 to 0.50 μg/kg/min) are effective if dobutamine and dopamine infusions are kept constant, potentially due to exposure to less β-receptor stimulation and thus less receptor desensitization.[64] The same holds true when epinephrine is used as a first-line agent, and when used in younger patients.[41,62,63] A linear dose–response curve is seen, with a rapid improvement of hemodynamic variables and oxygen delivery. Although Do_2 increases mainly as a function of consistent increases in CI, and a more variable increase in SVR, Vo_2 may not increase and O_2ER may fall. A transient fall in pHi may be seen during the epinephrine administration, and this impairment in gastric mucosal perfusion can be counteracted by dobutamine. Furthermore, lactate concentrations may rise during the first few hours of epinephrine therapy; however, it normalizes over the ensuing 24 hours in survivors.[56,65] An increase in venous pool of lactic acid may precede its clearance, although an increase secondary to an increase in glycogenolysis cannot be definitively excluded. There is recent evidence, however, to suggest that epinephrine, in contrast to dopamine, may increase the proportion of total CO delivered to the splanchnic circulation, although Vo_2 is not increased sufficiently to increase O_2ER.[66] In contrast, when epinephrine is compared to a short infusion (2 hours) of a combination of norepinephrine and dobutamine, it preferentially decreases splanchnic oxygen delivery, worsens pHi, and increases systemic lactate concentration without increasing Vo_2.[67] It is important to note that despite large doses used in these studies, no clinically important ventricular or supraventricular dysrhythmias have been reported in the young, in older patients, or in those with long-standing underlying cardiac disease states.[41,62,63] Nevertheless, caution must be exercised before considering epinephrine in managing hypoperfusion in hypodynamic patients with coronary artery disease where ischemia, chest pain, and myocardial infarction may result. Factors that may influence successful therapy with epinephrine may include the time from the onset of septic shock to effective therapy, its use as a primary or initial agent, and the age of the population.

PHENYLEPHRINE

Despite its purported use in refractory septic shock, very little information is published regarding the clinical efficacy of phenylephrine. Nevertheless, it is an attractive agent for use in sepsis due to its selective α-agonism and its rapid onset, short duration, and primary vascular effects. It is generally initiated at dosages of 0.5 μg/kg/min, and may be titrated quickly to desired effect.

There are three clinical trials using phenylephrine in septic shock evaluating 38 patients. Phenylephrine (0.5 to 9 μg/kg/min), when used alone or in combination with dobutamine or low doses of dopamine, improves blood pressure and myocardial performance in fluid resuscitated septic patients.[68] Incremental doses of phenylephrine over 3 hours result in linear dose-related increases in MAP, SVRI, HR, and SI, when administered as a single agent in stable, nonhypotensive but hyperdynamic, volume-resuscitated SICU patients. In septic shock, phenylephrine does not impair CI, PCWP, or peripheral perfusion.[52,69] Yamazaki showed that although its administration resulted in improved myocardial performance in hyperdynamic, normotensive septic patients,[68] phenylephrine worsened it in cardiac controls.[68] At a dosage of 70 μg/min, phenylephrine improved CI and MAP by increasing venous return to the heart (increase in CVP and SI) and by acting as a positive inotrope because SVR did not change. There was a clinically insignificant decrease in HR (3 beats/min). However, in cardiac patients, myocardial performance worsened as a result of an increase in MAP and SVR, and a decrease in CI with no change in HR. Although these results suggest caution, it is noteworthy that the cardiac indices of the two groups were not comparable at baseline.

In septic shock, phenylephrine appears to increase global tissue oxygen use, although there is conflicting information regarding the relationship of the oxygen transport variables with increases in MAP and CI.[52,69] Increases in Vo_2 appear to be dissociated from Do_2, representing an increase in O_2ER because CI remains unchanged. Increases in Vo_2 may result from redistribution of blood flow to previously underperfused areas, improving oxygen use due to changes in MAP and SVRI. With phenylephrine administration, no organ dysfunction was documented and evidence of globally improved peripheral tissue perfusion was seen as the lactic acid fell or remained unchanged, and urine output increased significantly at increased or maximal Vo_2. An increased O_2ER may contribute to improved tissue use.[52,69] In one small study, measured Do_2 and Vo_2 values paralleled MAP in most patients.[69] As with epinephrine, phenylephrine doses (1.3 to 3.7 μg/kg/min) required to achieve goals of therapy were significantly higher than those traditionally recommended for use. When phenylephrine (0.5 μg/kg/min) was titrated to a plateau in Vo_2 or the appearance of adverse cardiac effects, there was greater than a 15% increase in Do_2 and Vo_2. When combined with dobutamine, phenylephrine resulted in a more consistent and statistically significant increase in both Do_2 and Vo_2. However, these observations may be biased, because baseline Do_2 and Vo_2 values were somewhat higher in patients who did not require dobutamine (5 of 11). In a second study, Flancbaum and colleagues evaluated the use of phenylephrine as a single agent, without another cardiotonic agent, in ten septic, hyperdynamic SICU patients.[52] Eight of ten had a clinically significant increase (> 15%) in Vo_2 with variable doses of phenylephrine, while Do_2 increased in only three patients. Phenylephrine predictably increased MAP but not the Vo_2 in a dose-dependent fashion in the surgical patient population. In a similar group of high-risk surgical patients, Shoemaker and colleagues demonstrated that an increase in survival was associated with goal-directed therapy to supranormal oxygen transport variables. Since then, however, several studies have demonstrated that patients' intrinsic ability to achieve supranormal oxygen transport parameters is associated with increased survival, and is not a function of any pharmacologic intervention.[45,70]

The available data on hemodynamics, oxygen transport variables, and mortality with phenylephrine in septic shock may not be generalizable due to small numbers of patients evaluated. Adverse effects such as tachydysrhythmias are notably infrequent with phenylephrine, particularly when used as a single agent or with higher doses. It is unclear, however, how sustained the beneficial effects may be with longer administration of phenylephrine.[52] It also remains unclear what the optimal duration of therapy with phenylephrine is in septic shock. Like other vasopressors, phenylephrine is continued until resolution of the hemodynamic instability associated with the septic episode, and weaned when patients are clinically stable.

NOREPINEPHRINE

Norepinephrine was first used three decades ago for the treatment of hypotensive states prior to the development of the newer synthetic catecholamines dopamine and dobutamine. Traditionally, norepinephrine was viewed as causing significant peripheral tissue vasoconstriction, which could selectively impair regional flow and thus Do_2, to the renal and splanchnic beds. Norepinephrine is used to induce renal failure in animals; this may be a reason why clinicians may be reluctant to use it in septic shock. However, recent clinical studies of norepinephrine support the use of norepinephrine to restore blood pressure in septic shock.[45,50]

In clinical practice, norepinephrine is frequently initiated after vasopressor doses of dopamine (4.0 to 20 μg/kg/min) and/or combined use with dobutamine (2.0 to 40.0 μg/kg/min) fail to achieve desired goals.[45,50,51,71] Doses of dopamine and dobutamine are kept constant, stopped altogether, or in some instances, dopamine is kept at low doses for purported renal protection.[45,57,72] Norepinephrine infusions have been titrated to establish preset goals of MAP above 70 mm Hg, improved peripheral perfusion (improved urine output or mentation), and/or achievement of desired oxygen transport variables. Norepinephrine 0.01 to 2.0 μg/kg/min reliably and predictably improves hemodynamic parameters to "normal" or "supranormal" values in the majority of patients with septic shock. Doses that exceed those recommended by the manufacturer are needed in critically ill patients with septic shock to achieve predetermined goals. A significant increase in MAP is generally accompanied by an increase in the SVR. Heart rate either decreases or remains unchanged, although insignificant increases have been reported.[45] Cardiac index is either increased or does not change with few exceptions,[45,50] and there is no change in PCWP.[45,50,51,69]

Whereas the effects on MAP, SVRI, CI, and HR appear to be desirable and more predictable, the effect of norepinephrine on urine output is variable[45,46] and may depend on concurrently administered vasoactive agents.[46,51] Concurrent inotropic support with dobutamine and dopamine, or low doses of dopamine, preclude attributing any beneficial effects to norepinephrine alone.[45] An increase in urine output may be due to increased renal perfusion pressure secondary to the increases in MAP and SVRI, especially given that norepinephrine has a greater vasoconstrictive effect on the efferent arteriole of the kidney than on the afferent arteriole.[50]

The effect of norepinephrine on oxygen transport parameters is variable and depends on baseline values and concurrently administered vasoactive agents. In the majority of the studies, either an increase or no change in Do_2 is seen with no change in O_2ER, particularly when mean Do_2 values were "supranormal" prior to therapy.[45,72,73] In all but one study,[74] patients had received dobutamine and/or dopamine prior to initiation of goal-directed therapy with norepinephrine. Martin and associates[74] found norepinephrine alone to be superior to dopamine in achieving and maintaining for at least 6 hours, preset hemodynamic and oxygen transport variables (93% versus 31% of patients, $P < .001$). The authors suggested that differences between the two agents resulted from norepinephrine's combined increase in V_{O_2} and decrease in lactate concentrations due to correction of splanchnic ischemia and efficient hepatic clearance of lactate, or due to a preferential increase in D_{O_2} to areas of greatest oxygen demand, thus optimizing O_2ER.

DOBUTAMINE

Dobutamine is an inotrope with vasodilatory properties (so-called "inodilator"), and is used in the treatment of septic and cardiogenic shock to increase CI. In septic shock, LVEF and right ventricular function are depressed despite a high CI, while ventricular volumes and compliance are increased. Stroke index is maintained by an increased heart rate and ventricular dilatation. In survivors, the myocardial depression is reversible and normalizes at 5 to 10 days after the onset of sepsis.[75] Dobutamine has been shown to increase SI, LVSWI, and thus CI and D_{O_2} without increasing PCWP in septic shock in animals, human volunteers, or in controlled studies of human septic shock.[45,76,77] As a direct result of its effects on increased CI, dobutamine also nonpreferentially increases splanchnic blood flow.[78] The addition of dobutamine to epinephrine-treated patients has been shown to improve gastric mucosal perfusion, as measured by improvements in pHi, arterial lactate concentrations, and pCO_2 gap. Recent evidence suggests that redistribution of blood flow results from dobutamine's β_2-activity.[79]

Most prospective, randomized, controlled studies of goal-directed therapy with dobutamine were performed in human septic shock in surgical and medical critically ill patients refractory to concurrently administered vasopressors (dopamine and/or norepinephrine).[45,80–83] Dobutamine appears to help increase D_{O_2} and CI when given concurrently with or after volume resuscitation, and causes parallel proportional increases in the splanchnic circulation.[80] If, however, dobutamine is given to patients who are intravascularly depleted, dobutamine will result in hypotension and a reflexive tachycardia. The oxygen transport effects may not be significant, or may be transient, particularly during prolonged infusions. It appears that achievement of supranormal oxygen transport values with dobutamine in hyperdynamic septic shock refractory to fluid resuscitation and vasopressors is of little value as compared to treatment to normal values. In addition, administration of dobutamine to achieve these high values has resulted in an unchanged or an increased mortality and a greater incidence of adverse effects.[83] Results in medical and surgical patients may differ due to differences in time of starting dobutamine infusion, the duration of the infusion, and dosages administered. Subgroups of patients with septic shock (6% to 34%) among critically ill, high-risk, trauma and surgical patients have small and insignificant changes in D_{O_2}, V_{O_2}, O_2ER, and CI.[45,82] The lack of response may be related to late treatment (> 72 hours after surgery) resulting in irreversible changes due to hypoperfusion and hypoxia. In a group of medical patients, the lack of sustained effect may have been attributed to the fact that very large doses were needed to achieve the desired effects over a longer treatment period (72 hours). The requirement for vasopressor support with dopamine may have decreased oxygen extraction ratio (O_2ER) and negated beneficial effects of increased delivery. Oxygen extraction ratio, mixed venous oxygen tension, and relative changes in SVR were not reported. In populations of medical[81] and surgical patients,[80,83] dobutamine did not increase the likelihood of patients achieving supranormal oxygen transport variables. Continuation of dobutamine until death or resolution of acute illness resulted in an increased mortality despite an increase in the mean area under the D_{O_2} curve. This is partially explained by the fact that no change in V_{O_2} was seen, and thus O_2ER decreased. Also, much higher doses of dobutamine were used in this study as compared to the previous study (5 to 200 versus 5–20 μg/kg/min).[83] Seventeen of the 50 patients in the experimental group received 50 μg/kg/min or more of dobutamine at some time during the study. Despite these high doses, 35 of 50 patients (70%) were unable to achieve the predetermined goals. In fact, dose increments of dobutamine were limited by complications in half of the dobutamine patients in the treatment group, with tachycardia, ischemic changes on ECG, hypertension, and tachydysrhythmias, despite the absence of preexisting cardiac abnormalities.

Dobutamine should be started with doses ranging 2.5 to 5.0 μg/kg/min. Although generally a dose response may be seen, recent evidence suggests that doses in excess of 5.0 μg/kg/min may provide limited beneficial effects on oxygen transport values and hemodynamics, and may increase adverse cardiac effects.[84] Klem and associates found significant inter- and intrapatient variability in the pharmacokinetics of dobutamine in unstable critically ill patients.[85] Pathophysiologic factors influence dosing requirements and pharmacokinetic parameters over the time course of the illness and the duration of the infusion. Thus, infusion rates should be guided by clinical end points. Decreases in Pa_{O_2} and increases in Pv_{O_2}, as well as myocardial adverse effects such as tachycardia, ischemic changes on ECG, tachydysrhythmias, and hypotension, are seen.[83] Dobutamine, like other inotropes, is usually given until there is an improvement in myocardial function with resolution of the septic episode or when dose-limiting side effects are seen.[80,81]

DOPAMINE

Dopamine is frequently the initial vasopressor used in septic shock. Doses of 5 to 10 μg/kg/min are initiated to improve MAP. Most studies in patients with septic shock have shown that dopamine at these doses increases cardiac index by improving ventricular contractility and heart rate, resulting primarily from its β_1-effects. It increases arterial pressure and systemic vascular resistance as a result of both the increased cardiac output and, at higher doses (> 10 μg/kg/min), as a result of the α_1-effects.

Oxygen transport variables parallel the hemodynamic effects. Dopamine improves global Do_2 in septic patients, but compromises tissue oxygen extraction in the splanchnic or mesenteric circulation by α_1-mediated vasoconstriction. Indeed, despite increasing systemic Do_2 and Vo_2, large doses of dopamine decrease gastric intramucosal pH (pHi). This is reflected by a decrease or lack of change in regional Vo_2 and decrease in tissue O_2ER.

The clinical utility of dopamine in the setting of septic shock is limited, because large doses are frequently necessary to maintain CO and BP. At doses exceeding 20 μg/kg/min, there is limited further improvement in cardiac performance and regional hemodynamics. Its clinical use is frequently hampered by tachycardia and tachydysrhythmias. Although the latter should theoretically not be expected to occur until 5 to 10 μg/kg/min of dopamine, these β_1-effects may occur with doses as low as 3 μg/kg/min. They seem to be more prevalent in patients who are elderly, who have preexisting or concurrent cardiac ischemia or dysrhythmias, or in those currently receiving other dysrhythmogenic agents including other vasopressors and inotropes.

Other adverse effects that may limit the use of dopamine in septic shock are increases in PCWP, pulmonary shunt, and decreases in Pao_2.[47] The increase in PCWP may be due to changes in diastolic volumes from decreased cardiac compliance or increased venous return to the heart by α-adrenergic receptor-mediated venoconstriction. This may affect gas exchange and decrease Pao_2. The increase in pulmonary shunt may also result from acute enhancement of pulmonary blood flow to nonhomogeneous lung regions. Thus dopamine should be used with caution in patients with elevated preload, as the drug may worsen pulmonary edema. In the instance of high filling pressures, tachycardia or tachydysrhythmias in the presence of absence of refractory hypotension, dopamine should be substituted with another vasopressor or inotrope such as norepinephrine, dobutamine, phenylephrine, or epinephrine, depending on the desired effect.

Low doses (1 to 3 μg/kg/min) of dopamine are clinically used in the critically ill in the setting of septic shock with vasopressors or in oliguric patients. The goal of therapy in both situations is to preserve or increase urine output by way of dopamine's dopaminergic (DA_1-agonist) activity at low doses. When other vasopressors or inotropes are used for pressor or inotropic support, low doses of dopamine may be started concurrently. More commonly, however, dopamine is found to be ineffective (or is not tolerated) in pressor doses and another agent is added. At this point, the dopamine dose is titrated down to improve mesenteric and renal blood flow, in an attempt to prevent renal ischemia and renal failure. In the setting of oliguria, either with or without bacteremia/septic shock, low-dose dopamine is initiated in an attempt to convert oliguric renal failure to nonoliguric renal failure. Although low doses of dopamine are frequently employed, evidence supporting its ability to preserve kidney function in any of these situations is lacking.[86] Dopamine has been shown to increase renal blood flow, either due to its dopaminergic effect at low doses or as a result of an increase in CI. In normal volunteers, the addition of dopamine to incremental doses of norepinephrine may blunt norepinephrine-induced renal vasoconstriction, thereby maintaining renal blood flow, natriuresis, urine output,[46,87] and in one study, glomerular filtration.[87] In oliguric patients, dopamine may increase fractional excretion of sodium and increase urine output. These effects have also been observed during the course of dopamine administration in oliguric patients,[88] as well as in oliguric[89] and nonoliguric[90] patients with septic shock.

Studies in septic shock patients stabilized with norepinephrine to whom low-dose dopamine is added have shown variable results. In these studies, splanchnic blood flow and Do_2 may increase, but there is no preferential increase in the splanchnic perfusion as a fraction of cardiac output and systemic increases in Do_2.[89,90] An increase in urine output was not associated with an increase in glomerular filtration rate. The potentially beneficial effects of dopamine may be obscured in septic shock studies by the large variability in baseline fractional splanchnic flow found in this population compared to nonseptic controls. One study[89] found an inverse relationship between fractional splanchnic flow at baseline and the change in fractional splanchnic blood flow, such that dopamine was effective in increasing the fractional splanchnic blood flow in those where it was normal, but worsened it in those patients with high baseline values, such as occurs with redistribution of regional blood flow in septic shock. Clinically, it is difficult to prospectively distinguish either subset of patients. Recently, Lherm and coworkers demonstrated a differential response to low-dose dopamine in septic shock patients on catecholamines and nonoliguric patients with sepsis syndrome.[91] The latter group showed an increase in creatinine clearance and diuresis but the former did not. Furthermore, tolerance to the vasodilatory effects of dopamine after 24 to 48 hours was evident in the nonoliguric patients with sepsis syndrome and has been reported in others.[91] The lack of response to dopamine in septic shock patients on vasopressors and the tolerance that develops in responders to low-dose dopamine may be partly explained by time- and disease-dependent desensitization of dopamine receptors; this may not occur in those with sepsis syndrome or normal volunteers.[46,91] Furthermore, differences in the extent of preexisting vasodilation and pathophysiology of renal dysfunction in oliguric and septic shock may also contribute to differential responses seen to the administration of low doses of dopamine. Currently, there is insufficient evidence to promote the use of low-dose dopamine, as regional hemodynamics, oxygen use, and functional parameters of improved organ perfusion such as creatinine clearance and pHi, are not improved in a sustained manner.[88,90]

EXPERIMENTAL THERAPIES

DOPEXAMINE

Dopexamine is an investigational synthetic catecholamine used in low cardiac output states with coexisting elevated systemic or pulmonary vascular resistance. Dopexamine has been used in acute heart failure, impaired left ventricular function after surgery and in septic shock. As is the case with dobutamine in septic shock, dopexamine is most frequently used in combination with a vasopressor agent such as norepinephrine or dopamine, due to coexisting refractory hypotension.

Dopexamine improves cardiac performance by a marked vasodilation and a mild inotropic activity. In two studies of septic shock in predominantly surgical patients (n = 39), dopexamine produced a dose-related (range, 2 to 6 μg/kg/min) increase in CI, SV, HR, and a decrease in SVR over the course of the infusion (0.5 to 1 hr).[44,54] Epinephrine[54] or norepinephrine and dobutamine[44] dosages were kept constant during the study period. There appears to be less of an increase in myocardial oxygen demand than with dopamine, although tachycardia and tachydysrhythmias may lead to myocardial ischemia, particularly in patients with ischemic heart disease.[44,54]

Global oxygen transport variables are similar to those of dopamine. Oxygen delivery increases significantly, but Vo_2 increases insufficiently and thus O_2ER decreases. Dopexamine's combined β_2-adrenergic and DA_1 agonist activities theoretically should be advantageous in improving distribution of blood flow in septic shock. Only one study evaluated the regional effects of dopexamine.[45] During dopexamine infusion, pHi increased (n = 7/10) and remained high an hour after discontinuation of the drug. The improvements in pHi, however, did not parallel changes in CO and Do_2. The authors suggest that this may represent a preferential effect on gastric mucosal blood flow. Further studies in greater numbers of patients with septic shock are required to determine whether improvements in regional flow in the cerebral, mesenteric, splanchnic, and renal vasculature will be demonstrated.

NITRIC OXIDE SYNTHASE INHIBITORS

Nitric oxide (NO) is a short-acting, potent vasodilator derived from the enzymatic oxidation of arginine. Its production is under control of nitric oxide synthase (NOS). This enzyme is present (expressed) in two forms: a constitutive form (ecNOS) and an inducible form (iNOS). Small amounts of NO are normally produced by the vascular endothelium under the control of ecNOS for the physiologic control of vascular tone and blood flow distribution. Under pathophysiologic conditions such as stimulation by lipopolysaccharide or cytokines, iNOS becomes diffusely expressed, producing large amounts of NO. The latter has been implicated in the cardiovascular failure of septic shock.[92,93]

Pharmacologic inhibition of NO production has been investigated as an adjunct to standard therapies of septic shock. L-arginine analogs such as monomethyl-L-arginine (L-NMMA) or L-arginine-methylester (L-NAME) are competitive inhibitors of NOS and have been shown to increase blood pressure and partially restore vascular reactivity in experimental and human septic shock.[94] However, because these arginine analogs nonselectively block ecNOS and iNOS, their use has been associated with extensive vasoconstriction, decreased cardiac output, and regional hypoperfusion, and thus organ failure and mortality. Currently, there is increased focus on identification of selective inhibitors of iNOS.[92,93] Some S-substituted thiourea derivatives have demonstrated both *in vitro* and *in vivo* (rodent) dose-dependent selectivity for iNOS inhibition. Recently, Rosselet and associates demonstrated that low doses (0.1 mg/kg/h) of S-methyl-isothiourea (SMT) were superior to norepinephrine in the treatment of rat endotoxic shock. These doses of SMT prevented hypotension by maintaining CI, without increasing SVRI, as did norepinephrine. However, only low doses of SMT limited the development of lactic acidosis.[92]

VASOPRESSIN

Recently, vasopressin has been used anecdotally in a series of patients with vasodilatory septic shock who remain hypotensive on vasopressors.[95,96] Arginine vasopressin has little pressor activity in normal subjects but markedly increases blood pressure when sympathetic nerve function is impaired, including in an experimental animal model of septic shock. When administered in low doses (0.01 to 0.05 U/min) to patients with vasodilatory septic shock receiving high doses and long courses of norepinephrine, vasopressin successfully increased arterial blood pressure and SVRI, with cardiac output remaining stable. Urine flow rates increased significantly in 3 of 5 patients, most likely due to increased renal perfusion and arterial pressure. In 4 of 5 patients, norepinephrine therapy was successfully tapered and discontinued within 15 minutes. No clinical or laboratory signs of cardiac or mesenteric ischemia were observed, nor was PCWP or oxygenation adversely affected.[95] Vasopressin should not be used in patients with hypovolemia, cardiogenic shock, or septic shock with myocardial depression as it may decrease cardiac output and cause profound cutaneous vasoconstriction and necrosis.[96]

GENERAL CONCLUSIONS AND RECOMMENDATIONS

The choice of vasopressor or inotropic agent in septic shock should be made according to the needs of the patient (Fig. 21–3). The traditional algorithm suggests a stepwise approach first using dopamine, then norepinephrine; dobutamine is added for low cardiac output states, and occasionally epinephrine and phenylephrine are used when necessary.

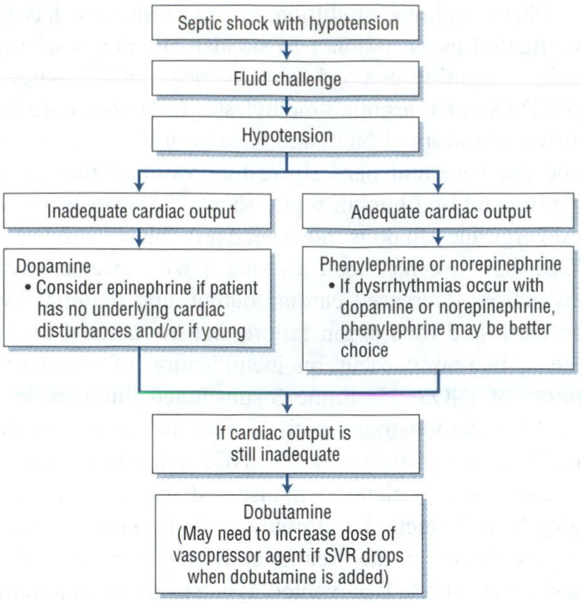

FIGURE 21–3. Algorithmic approach to the use of vasopressors and inotropes in septic shock. Approach is intended to be used in conjunction with clinical judgment, hemodynamic monitoring parameters, and therapeutic end points. *(Modified from Ref. 97.)*

Although this approach is empirical, it is broadly used in clinical practice, and has been justified by a desire to avoid strong vasoconstriction and by the sense of safety with graded doses of dopamine. This dose–response relationship, however, has never been established in the critically ill. In addition, recent observations of decreased regional perfusion are calling into question the use of dopamine as a first-line agent.

For all catecholamine vasopressors larger doses than those traditionally recommended are required for goal-directed therapy to MAP and for normalization of oxygen transport variables, DO_2 and VO_2. Attainment of supranormal DO_2 and VO_2 values is difficult in the majority of patients, even if large doses are used. Patients who develop supranormal DO_2 and VO_2 have a lower mortality, but whether this is achieved intrinsically or with exogenous administration of vasopressors/inotropes appears inconsequential. Goal-directed therapy cannot therefore be recommended, as little or no benefit has been demonstrated to date. Further work is required to better elucidate the differential effects of vasopressors on regional hemodynamic and oxygen transport values, as measures of local tissue perfusion.

Although difficult to demonstrate, there may be true differences in pharmacologic activity of vasopressors and inotropes. For example, recent evidence suggests that when used appropriately with fluid replenishment, epinephrine is safe and effective in large doses. It may be particularly useful when used earlier in the course of septic shock in young patients and those who do not have any known cardiac abnormalities. Although epinephrine may cause a short-lived increase in lactic acid, this resolves in 24 hours and there is no difference in outcome. Unlike epinephrine, dopamine does not preferentially increase the proportion of CO that preferentially goes to the splanchnic circulation. The ability of dopamine to increase CO by no more than 35% and accompanied by a tachycardia or tachydysrhythmias limits its utility. Dopamine, as opposed to norepinephrine, has been shown to worsen splanchnic VO_2 and O_2ER and to be of limited value in improving urine output. Low doses of dopamine have not been shown to consistently increase the glomerular filtration rate, and indeed worsen splanchnic tissue oxygen use. Routine use of concurrently administered dopamine with vasopressors is not recommended. Phenylephrine should be used when a pure vasoconstrictor is desired in patients who may not require or do not tolerate the beta effects of dopamine with or without dobutamine. In patients with high filling pressure and hypotension, the combination of phenylephrine and dobutamine may be useful.

However, shortcomings of study methodology prevent the establishment of definitive conclusions. Short infusions (not exceeding 2 hours) during studies may show differences that are not clinically significant at 24 hours or more, as demonstrated for epinephrine and dobutamine. Clinically, vasopressors and inotropes are used for hours to days. Also, variable times at which a study is initiated with respect to the stage of sepsis or septic shock, the inherent differences in circulating catecholamine levels, and changes in receptor activity all may be confounding factors, as may be the prestudy duration and type of exogenous catecholamine administration.

Further pharmacotherapeutic and outcome studies are still required to elucidate the place in therapy that individual vasopressors and inotropes or their combinations occupy in the supportive care of patients with bacteremia or septic shock. Once this is accomplished, then we will need to direct our efforts to pharmacoeconomics and cost-effectiveness of these therapies.

▶ PRINCIPLES OF PHARMACOTHERAPY

- Continuous and invasive hemodynamic monitoring with a pulmonary artery catheter should be used early and throughout the course of septic shock to assess intravascular fluid status and ventricular filling pressures and monitor arterial and venous oxygenation. It should also be used for monitoring the response to drug therapy and guide dosage titration.
- Derangements in adrenergic receptor sensitivity or activity frequently result in resistance to vasopressor and inotropic therapy in critically ill patients. These changes may be a function of endogenous catecholamine concentrations, dose/duration of exposure to and type of exogenously administered vasopressors, stage of septic shock, preexisting illness, as well as other factors.
- In refractory septic shock, the rational use of vasopressor or inotropic agents should be guided by re-

ceptor activity, pharmacologic characteristics, and regional and systemic hemodynamic effects of the drug, and should be tailored to the patient's physiologic needs. Pharmacologically sound combinations of agents should be initiated early to optimize response.

- Goals of therapy with vasopressors and inotropes should be predetermined and should optimize regional perfusion to tissues (e.g., cardiac, renal, mesenteric, periphery). Goal-directed therapy with vasopressors and inotropes to supranormal global oxygen transport variables cannot be recommended, as there is no clear benefit and morbidity may be increased. However, achievement of supranormal DO_2 and VO_2, whether intrinsically or pharmacologically, is associated with decreased mortality in septic shock.
- Much higher dosages of all vasopressors and inotropes than traditionally recommended are required in order to improve the hemodynamic and oxygen transport variables in septic shock.
- Dose titration and monitoring of vasopressor and inotropic therapy should be guided by the "best clinical response," while observing for and minimizing evidence of myocardial ischemia (e.g., tachydysrhythmias, ECG changes); renal (decreased glomerular filtration rate and/or urine output), splanchnic/gastric (low pHi, bowel ischemia), or peripheral (cold extremities) hypoperfusion; and worsening of PaO_2, PCWP, and other hemodynamic variables.
- Dopamine is typically used as an initial vasopressor agent for hemodynamic support but is limited by its ability to increase cardiac output (35%). Its use is frequently complicated by tachycardia and tachydysrhythmias, and occasionally by an increase in PCWP. In contrast to norepinephrine, it decreases splanchnic oxygen use. Although commonly used, low-dose dopamine either with norepinephrine or other agents has not been proven to be of any benefit in oliguric patients in septic shock.
- Phenylephrine may be a particularly useful alternative in those who cannot tolerate tachycardia or tachydysrhythmias with dopamine or norepinephrine, or those patients with known underlying myocardial dysfunction.
- Epinephrine appears to be safe and effective as a single agent and as an add-on agent. It is particularly useful in the young, in patients with otherwise healthy myocardia, and when used early in the course of treatment. It causes a significant increase in lactate, which gradually resolves; and it appears to cause little cardiac disturbance in patients with no known cardiac abnormalities. It should be used cautiously in patients with a history of coronary artery disease or underlying cardiac disturbances.
- Therapy with vasopressors and inotropes is continued until the myocardial depression and vascular hyporesponsiveness of septic shock improves, usually measured in hours to days. Discontinuation of vasopressor or inotropic therapy should be executed slowly; therapy should be "weaned" to avoid a precipitous worsening in regional and systemic hemodynamics.

REFERENCES

1. Parrillo JE. Pathogenetic mechanisms of septic shock. New Engl J Med 1993;328:1471–1477.
2. Califf RM, Bengtson JR. Cardiogenic shock. New Engl J Med 1994; 330:1724–1730.
3. Gorny DA. Arterial blood pressure measurement technique. AACN Clin Issues Crit Care Nurs 1993;4:66–80.
4. Lal SKL, Henderson RJ, Cejnar M, et al. Physiological influences on continuous finger and simultaneous intra-arterial blood pressure. Hypertension 1995;26:307–314.
5. Keckeisen M, Monsein S. Techniques for measuring arterial pressure in the postoperative cardiac surgery patient. Crit Care Nurs Clin N Am. 1991;3:699–708.
6. Shoemaker WC, Parsa MH. Invasive and noninvasive physiologic monitoring. In: Ayres SM, Grenvik A, Holbrook PR, et al. Textbook of Critical Care, 3rd ed. Philadephia, Saunders, 1995;252–266.
7. Burchell SA, Yu M, Takiguchi SA, et al. Evaluation of a continuous cardiac output and mixed venous oxygen saturation catheter in critically ill surgical patients. Crit Care Med 1997;25:388–391.
8. Ermakov S, Hoyt JW. Pulmonary artery catheterization. Crit Care Clin 1992;8:773–806.
9. Tuman KJ, McCarthy RJ, Spiess BD, et al. Effect of pulmonary artery catheterization on outcome in patients undergoing coronary artery surgery. Anesthesiology 1989;70:199–206.
10. Connors AF, Speroff T, Dawson NV, et al. The effectiveness of right heart catheterization in the initial care of critically ill patients. JAMA 1996;18:889–897.
11. Pulmonary artery catheter consensus conference. Consensus statement. Crit Care Med 1997;25:910–925.
12. Ginosar Y, Thijs LG, Sprung CL. Raising the standard of hemodynamic monitoring: Targeting the practice or the practitioner. Crit Care Med 1997;25:209–211.
13. Venkatesh B, Hendry SP. Continuous intra-arterial blood gas monitoring. Intens Care Med 1996;22:818–828.
14. Wipke-Tevis DD. Subcutaneous tissue oximetry. Crit Care Nurs Clin N Am 1995;7:275–285.
15. Wahr JA, Tremper KK. Noninvasive oxygen monitoring techniques. Crit Care Clin 1995;11:199–217.
16. Tsien CL, Fackler JC. Poor prognosis for existing monitors in the intensive care unit. Crit Care Med 1997;25:614–619.
17. Moller JT, Pedersen T, Rasmussen LS, et al. Randomized evaluation of pulse oximetry in 20,802 patients: II. perioperative events and postoperative complications. Anesthesiology 1993;78:445–453.
18. Cullen DJ, Nemeskal AR, Cooper JB, et al. Effect of pulse oximetry, age, and ASA physical status on the frequency of patients admitted unexpectedly to a postoperative intensive care unit and the severity of their anesthesia-related complications. Anesth Analg 1992;74:181–188.
19. Vincent JL, De Backer D. Oxygen uptake/oxygen supply dependency: Fact or fiction? Acta Anaesthesiol Scand 1995;39(suppl 107):229–237.
20. Heyland DK, Cook DJ, King D, et al. Maximizing oxygen delivery in critically ill patients: A methodologic appraisal of the evidence. Crit Care Med 1996;24:517–524.
21. Meier-Hellmann A, Reinhart K, Bredle DL, et al. Epinephrine impairs splanchnic perfusion in septic shock. Crit Care Med 1997;25: 399–404.

22. Kelly KM. Does increasing oxygen delivery improve outcome? Yes. Crit Care Med 1996;12:635–644.
23. Erstad BL. Oxygen transport goals in the resuscitation of critically ill patients. Ann Pharmacother 1994;28:1273–1284.
24. Dasta JF, Brackett CC. Defining and achieving optimum therapeutic goals in critically ill patients. Pharmacotherapy 1994;14:678–688.
25. Tuchschmidt JA, Mecher CE. Predictors of outcome from critical illness. Crit Care Clin 1994;10:179–195.
26. Rady MY, Rivers EP, Nowak RM. Resuscitation of the critically ill in the ED: Responses of blood pressure, heart rate, shock index, central venous oxygen saturation, and lactate. Am J Emerg Med 1996; 14:218–225.
27. Brown SD, Clark C, Gutierrez G. Pulmonary lactate release in patients with sepsis and the adult respiratory distress syndrome. J Crit Care 1996;11:2–8.
28. Schlichtig R, Tønnessen TI, Nemoto EM. Detecting dysoxia in "silent" organs. Critical Care State of the Art, Society of Critical Care Medicine 1993;14:239–273.
29. Bakker JM, Coffernils M, Leon P, et al. Blood lactate levels are superior to oxygen-derived variables in predicting outcome in human septic shock. Chest 1991;99:956–962.
30. Pastores SM, Katz DP, Kvetan V. Splanchnic ischemia and gut mucosal injury in sepsis and multiple organ dysfunction syndrome. Am J Gastroenterol 1996;91:1697–1710.
31. Benjamin E, Oropello JM. Does gastric tonometry work? No. Crit Care Clin 1996;12:587–601.
32. Creteur J, DeBacker K, Vincent JL. Monitoring gastric mucosal carbon dioxide pressure using gas tonometry. Anesthesiology 1997; 87:504–510.
33. Gutierrez G, Palizas F, Doglio G, et al. Gastric intramucosal pH as a therapeutic index of tissue oxygenation in critically ill patients. Lancet 1992;339:195–199.
34. Ivatury RR, Simon RJ, Islam S, et al. A prospective randomized study of end points of resuscitation after major trauma-global oxygen transport indices versus organ-specific gastric mucosal pH. J Am Coll Surg 1996;183:145–154.
35. Lefkowitz RJ, Hoffman BB, Taylor P. The autonomic and somatic motor nervous system. In: Hardman JG, Gilman AG, Limbird LE, et al., eds. Goodman & Gilman's The Pharmacological Basis of Therapeutics. 9th ed. New York, McGraw-Hill, 1996:110–111.
36. Hoffman BB, Lefkowitz RJ. Catecholamines, sympathomimetic drugs and adrenergic receptor antagonists. In: Hardman JG, Gilman AG, Limbird LE, et al., eds. Goodman & Gilman's The Pharmacological Basis of Therapeutics. 9th ed. New York, McGraw-Hill, 1996: 199–248.
37. Zaritsky AL. Catecholamines, inotropic medications, and vasopressor agents. In: Chernow B, Brater DC, Holaday JW, et al., eds. The Pharmacological Approach to the Critically Ill Patient. 3rd ed. Baltimore, MD: Williams & Wilkins, 1994:387–404.
38. Ruffolo RR. Cardiovascular adrenoceptors: Physiology and critical care implications. In: Chernow B, Brater DC, Holaday JW, et al., eds. The Pharmacological Approach to the Critically Ill Patient. 3rd ed. Baltimore, MD: Williams & Wilkins, 1994:167–181.
39. Sokoloff P, Schwartz JC. Novel dopamine receptors half a decade later. Trends Pharmacol Sci 1995;16:270–275.
40. Dickerson RN, Lima JJ, Kuhl DA, et al. Effect of sustained endotoxemia on-α1-adrenergic responsiveness in parenterally fed rats. Pharmacotherapy 1998;18:170–174.
41. Silverman HJ, Penaranda R, Orens JB, Lee NH. Impaired β-adrenergic receptor stimulation of cyclic adenosine monophosphate in human septic shock: Association with myocardial hyporesponsiveness to catecholamines. Crit Care Med 1993;21:31–39.
42. Hahn PY, Wang P, Tait SM, et al. Sustained elevation in circulating catecholamine levels during polymicrobial sepsis. Shock 1995; 4:269–273.
43. Sypniewski E. Hypovolemic and cardiogenic shock. In: DiPiro JT, Talbert RL, Yee GC, et al., eds. Pharmacotherapy: A Pathophysiologic Approach, 3rd ed. Stamford, CT, Appleton & Lange, 1993:509–531.
44. Hannemann L, Reinhart K, Meier-Hellmann A, et al. Dopexamine hydrochloride in septic shock. Chest 1996;109:756–760.
45. Rudis MI, Basha MA, Zarowitz BJ. Is it time to reposition vasopressors and inotropes in sepsis? Crit Care Med 1996;24:525–537.
46. Richer M, Robert S, Lebel M. Renal hemodynamics during norepinephrine and low-dose dopamine infusions in man. Crit Care Med 1996;24:1150–1156.
47. Hanneman L, Reinhart K, Grenzer O, et al. Comparison of dopamine to dobutamine and norepinephrine for oxygen delivery and uptake in septic shock. Crit Care Med 1995;23:1962–1970.
48. Gordon IL, Wesley R, Wong DH, et al. Effect of dopamine on renal blood flow and cardiac output. Arch Surg 1995;130:864–868.
49. Sabol SJ, Ward DS. Effect of dopamine on hypoxic-hypercapnic interaction in humans. Anesth Analg 1987;66:619–624.
50. Dasta JF. Norepinephrine in septic shock: Renewed interest in an old drug. Drug Intell Clin Pharm 1990;24:153–156.
51. Redl-Wenzl EM, Armbruster C, Edelmann G, et al. The effects of norepinephrine on hemodynamics and renal function in severe septic shock states. Intensive Care Med 1993;19:151–154.
52. Flancbaum L, Dick M, Dasta J, et al. A dose-response study of phenylephrine in critically ill, septic surgical patients. Eur J Clin Pharmacol 1997;51:461–465.
53. Wilson W, Lipman J, Scribante J, et al. Septic shock: Does adrenaline have a role as a first line inotropic agent? Anaesth Intens Care 1992;20:470–474.
54. Smithies M, Yee TH, Jackson L, et al. Protecting the gut and the liver in the critically ill: Effects of dopexamine. Crit Care Med 1994; 22:789–795.
55. Marino PL. Oxygen transport. In: Marino PL, ed. The ICU Book. Philadelphia, Lea & Febiger, 1991:14–24.
56. Bollaert PE, Bauer P, Audibert G, et al. Effects of epinephrine on hemodynamics and oxygen metabolism in dopamine-resistant septic shock. Chest 1990;98:9–53.
57. Hayes MA, Yau EHS, Hinds CJ, et al. Symmetrical peripheral gangrene: Association with noradrenaline administration. Intensive Care Med 1992;18:433–436.
58. Tisdale JE. Patel R. Webb CR. et al. Electrophysiologic and proarrhythmic effects of intravenous inotropic agents. Progr Cardiovasc Dis 1995;38:167–180.
59. Weiss M, Schneider EM, Tarnow J, et al. Is inhibition of oxygen radical production of neutrophils by sympathomimetics mediated via β-2 adrenoceptors. J Pharmacol Exp Ther 1996;278:1105–1113.
60. Fortenberry JD, Huber AR, Owens ML. Inotropes inhibit endothelial cell surface adhesion molecules induced by interleukin-1. Crit Care Med 1997;25:303–308.
61. Van der Poll T, Calvano SE, Kumar A, et al. Epinephrine attenuates down-regulation of monocyte tumor necrosis factor receptors during human endotoxemia. J Leukoc Biol 1997;61:156–160.
62. Mackenzie SJ, Kapadia F, Nimmo GR, et al. Adrenaline in treatment of septic shock: Effects on haemodynamics and oxygen transport. Intensive Care Med 1991:17:36–39.
63. Moran JL, O'Fathartaigh, Peisach AR, et al. Epinephrine as an inotropic agent in septic shock: A dose-profile analysis. Crit Care Med 1993;21:70–77.
64. Lipman J, Roux A, Kraus P. Vasoconstrictor effects of adrenaline in human septic shock. Anaesth Intens Care 1991;19:61–65.
65. Levy B, Bollaert PE, Charpentier C, et al. Comparison of norepinephrine and dobutamine to epinephrine for haemodynamics, lactate metabolism, and gastric tonometric variables in septic shock: A prospective, randomized study. Intensive Care Med 1997;23:282–287.
66. Day NPJ, Phu NH, Bethell DP, et al. The effects of dopamine and adrenaline infusions on acid–base balance and systemic haemodynamics in severe infection. Lancet 1996;348:219–223.
67. Meier-Hellmann A, Reinhart K, Bredle DL, et al. Epinephrine impairs splanchnic perfusion in septic shock. Crit Care Med 1997;25:399–404.
68. Yamazaki T, Shimada Y, Taenaka N, et al. Circulatory responses to afterloading with phenylephrine in hyperdynamic sepsis. Crit Care Med 1982;10:432–435.

69. Gregory JS, Bonfiglio MF, Dasta JF, et al. Experience with phenylephrine as a component of the pharmacologic support of septic shock. Crit Care Med 1991;19:1395–1400.
70. Shoemaker WC, Appel PL, Kram HB. Hemodynamic and oxygen transport responses in survivors and nonsurvivors of high-risk surgery. Crit Care Med 1993;21:977–990.
71. Marik PE, Mohedin M. The contrasting effects of dopamine and norepinephrine on systemic and splanchnic oxygen utilization in hyperdynamic sepsis. JAMA 1994;272:1354–1357.
72. Lucas CE. A new look at dopamine and norepinephrine for hyperdynamic septic shock. Chest 1994;105:7–8.
73. Ruokonen E, Takala J, Kari A, et al. Regional blood flow and oxygen transport in septic shock. Crit Care Med 1993;21:1296–1303.
74. Martin C, Papazian L, Perrin G, et al. Norepinephrine or dopamine for the treatment of hyperdynamic septic shock? Chest 1993; 103:1826–1831.
75. Parillo JE. Myocardial depression during septic shock in humans. Crit Care Med 1990;18:1183–1184.
76. Bhatt SB, Hutchinson RC, Tomlinson B, et al. Effect of dobutamine on oxygen supply and uptake in healthy volunteers. Br J Anaesthesia 1992;69:298–303.
77. Haywood GA, Tighe D, Moss R, et al. Goal directed therapy with dobutamine in a porcine model septic shock: Effects on systemic and renal oxygen. Postgrad Med J 1991;67(suppl 1):S36–S39.
78. Reinelt H, Radernacher P, Fischer G, et al. Effects of a dobutamine-induced increase in splanchnic blood flow on hepatic metabolic activity in patients with septic shock. Anesthesiology 1997;86:818–824.
79. Levy B, Bollaert PE, Lucchelli JP, et al. Dobutamine improves the adequacy of gastric mucosal perfusion in epinephrine-treated septic shock. Crit Care Med 1997;25:1649–1654.
80. Yu M, Levy MM, Smith P, et al. Effect of maximizing oxygen delivery on morbidity and mortality rates in critically ill patients: A prospective, randomized, controlled study. Crit Care Med 1993; 21:830–838.
81. Tuchschmidt J, Fried J, Astiz M, et al. Elevation of cardiac output and oxygen delivery improves outcome in septic shock. Chest 1992; 102:216–220.
82. Shoemaker WC, Appel PL, Kram HB. Oxygen transport measurements to evaluate tissue perfusion and titrate therapy: Dobutamine and dopamine effects. Crit Care Med 1991;19:672–688.
83. Hayes MA, Timmins AC, Yau EHS, et al. Elevation of systemic oxygen delivery in the treatment of critically ill patients. N Engl J Med 1994;330:1717–1722.
84. De Backer D, Moraine JJ, Berre J, et al. Effects of dobutamine on oxygen consumption in septic patients. Am J Respir Crit Care Med 1994;150:95–100.
85. Klem C, Dasta JF, Reilley TE, Flancbaum LJ. Variability in dobutamine pharmacokinetics in unstable critically ill surgical patients. Crit Care Med 1994;22:1926–1932.
86. Klahr S, Miller SB. Acute oliguria. N Engl J Med 1998;338:671–675.
87. Hoogenberg K, Smith AJ, Girbes ARJ. Effect of low-dose dopamine on renal and systemic hemodynamics during incremental norepinephrine infusion in healthy volunteers. Crit Care Med 1998;26:260–265.
88. Rudis MI, Zarowitz BJ. Low-dose dopamine in acute oliguric renal failure. Am J Med 1997;102:320–321.
89. Meier-Hellman A, Bredle DL, Specht M, et al. The effects of low-dose dopamine on splanchnic blood flow and oxygen uptake in patients with septic shock. Intensive Care Med 1997;23:31–37.
90. Olson D, Pohlman A, Hall JB. Administration of low-dose dopamine to nonoliguric patients with sepsis syndrome does not raise intramucosal gastric pH nor improve creatinine clearance. Am J Resp Crit Care Med 1996;154:1664–1670.
91. Lherm T, Troche G, Rossignol M, et al. Renal effects of low-dose dopamine in patients with sepsis syndrome or septic shock treated with catecholamines. Intensive Care Med 1996;22:213–219.
92. Rosselet A, Feihl F, Market M, et al. Selective iNOS inhibition is superior to norepinephrine in the treatment of rat endotoxic shock. Am J Resp Crit Care Med 1998;157:162–170.
93. Griffiths MJD, Messent M, Curzen NP, Evans TW. Aminoguanidine selectively decreases cyclic GMP levels produced by inducible nitric oxide synthase. Am J Respir Crit Care Med 1995;152:1599–1604.
94. Grover R, Bakker J, McLuckie A, et al. for the international 546C88 septic shock group. Crit Care Med 1998;26(suppl):A29.
95. Landry DW, Levin HR, Gallant EM, et al. Vasopressin deficiency contributes to the vasodilation of septic shock. Circulation 1997; 95:1122–1125.
96. Landry DW, Levin HR, Gallant EM, et al. Vasopressin pressor hypersensitivity in vasodilatory septic shock. Circulation 1997; 25:1279–1282.
97. Society of Critical Care Medicine (SCCM). Practice parameters on adult hemodynamic support of sepsis. Crit Care Med. In press.

22
HYPOVOLEMIC SHOCK

Brian L. Erstad, PharmD

This chapter discusses the assessment and management of hypovolemic shock. Depending on the classification scheme being used for shock, spinal and anaphylactic shock may be considered separately from hypovolemic shock since fluid loss from the body is not necessary for their occurrence. Spinal shock results from loss of sympathetic tone with resultant vasodilatation, and anaphylactic shock results from increased vascular permeability due to antigen–antibody interaction.[1] Although these forms of shock will not be discussed in detail, it is important to note that the initial therapy for both is the same as for hypovolemic shock (i.e., adequate volume replacement), because *circulating* volume is decreased. In this regard, adequate fluid resuscitation to maintain circulating blood volume is a common principle in managing all forms of shock.

EPIDEMIOLOGY

It has been estimated that approximately one million deaths a year in the United States occur in patients with shock.[2] The number is much higher when one considers that all causes of death ultimately result in circulatory failure (i.e., the last stage of shock). It is much more difficult to estimate the number of patients with reversible organ dysfunction or patients with end-organ damage who survived an episode of hypovolemic shock. Part of the problem is defining when progressive circulatory insufficiency results in the loss of normal compensatory responses by the body, which could reverse the processes leading to irreversible organ dysfunction. This loss of appropriate compensation varies from patient to patient and is not always readily apparent during the initial patient presentation.

ETIOLOGY

Hypovolemic shock may result from a number problems including blood loss, sequestered fluid within the body (e.g., third-spacing), thermal injury, and various forms of dehydration. In some cases, such as in postoperative patients, a number of these problems may occur at the same time. For example, a patient may have had blood loss secondary to trauma or surgery with additional fluid being third-spaced postoperatively. As the example of third-spaced fluid indicates, fluid (i.e., plasma) does not have to be lost from the body for a person to develop hypovolemic shock.

Dehydration may result from primary water deficiency, usually due to decreased intake, but in some instances (e.g., diabetes insipidus) due to increased losses. In general, the term *dehydration* implies intracellular and interstitial fluid depletion, in contrast to *volume depletion,* which implies extracellular, and particularly intravascular, depletion or hypovolemia. In the case of a primary water deficit, cell dehydration occurs, with delayed circulatory failure from decreased circulatory volume with ongoing losses.[3] Initially the patient may be thirsty and possibly have some mental status changes such as confusion. If the cellular dehydration occurs slowly, intracellular substances referred to as idiogenic osmols will develop, which limit progressive complications (e.g., coma). With combined water and salt deficiencies as might occur with gastrointestinal losses (e.g., diarrhea), interstitial and intravascular depletion are an early occurrence. Fortunately, dehydration is relatively easy to prevent with routine vigilance and water replacement compared to some of the other causes of shock.

PATHOPHYSIOLOGY

Hypovolemic shock is often described in terms of its clinical manifestations such as lowered blood pressure, but patients with shock have died with "normal physiological, hematological, fluid, and electrolyte balance."[4] Therefore, an appropriate definition should mention the underlying problem, which is inadequate tissue perfusion resulting from circulatory failure. In the case of hypovolemic shock, the cause of the altered perfusion is fluid (or volume) depletion resulting from trauma, surgery, thermal injury, or some form of dehydration. Figure 22–1 provides a simplified version of the pathophysiology of circulatory insufficiency. Cell damage and death may occur from the primary insult or from reperfusion injury. The latter problem is most frequently associated with trauma and blood loss that cause the release of a multitude of mediators of inflammation and injury that have complex interactions.[5] Cells have varying responses to hypoxia, ranging from astrocytes that quit functioning almost immediately to hepatic cells that may function for several hours postinjury.[3] Left unmitigated, cell death will occur.

The body attempts to compensate for volume depletion beginning with autoregulatory changes involving smaller blood vessels. When the cause of circulatory insufficiency continues unabated, local mechanisms eventually fail to provide adequate compensation and macrocirculatory changes ensue. Approximately 75% of blood volume is contained in venous capacitance vessels, with gravity being

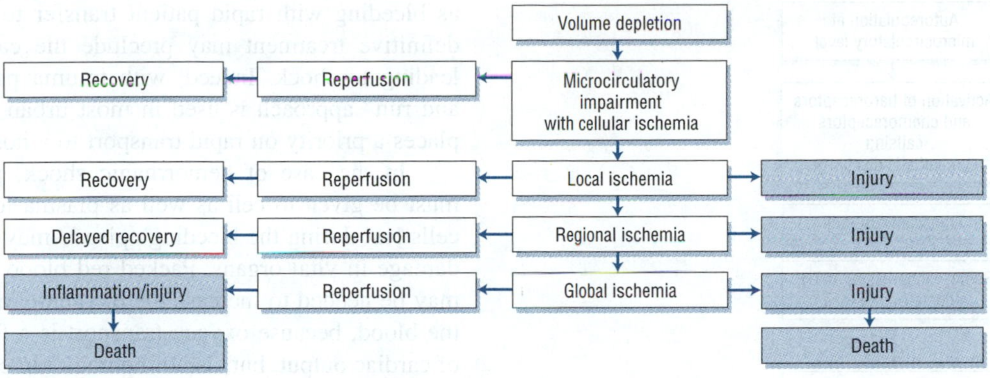

FIGURE 22–1. Pathophysiology of circulatory insufficiency.

the major impedance to flow back to the heart.[3] With increasing volume depletion, blood flow to the heart (preload) is decreased, with subsequent activation of baroreceptors and chemoreceptors leading to sympathetic discharge. Also, fluid shifting from the interstitial space to the intravascular space occurs through a phenomenon known as transcapillary refill, and hormones (adrenocorticotrophic hormone, angiotensin, catecholamines, vasopressin) are released that cause sodium and water retention by the kidneys. The phenomenon of transcapillary refill means that the body can have fluid losses exceeding normal plasma volume. These responses cause alterations in stroke volume, heart rate, and peripheral vascular resistance so that blood pressure and hence tissue perfusion can be maintained.

The microcirculatory changes associated with shock are complex and difficult to study. Although some mediators such as endothelin-1 cause vasoconstriction, others such as adenosine and nitric oxide yield vasodilatation.[6] These changes result in hypoperfusion or hyperperfusion depending on the area. As these microcirculatory changes fail to maintain adequate organ perfusion, more widespread sympathetic nervous system activation and vasoconstriction ensue.

The factors involved in fluid shifting between the intravascular and interstitial spaces are described by the modified Starling equation:

$$J_V = K_{f,c}\,[(P_c - P_t) - \sigma(\pi_c - \pi_t)]$$

where

J_V = net transvascular flow rate; cannot be measured in clinical setting.

$K_{f,c}$ = capillary filtration coefficient for fluids; cannot be measured in clinical setting.

P_c = capillary hydrostatic pressure; indirectly estimated in clinical setting (e.g., pulmonary artery occlusive pressure).

P_t = tissue hydrostatic pressure; cannot be measured in clinical setting.

σ = reflection coefficient for proteins; cannot be measured in clinical setting.

π_c = plasma colloid osmotic pressure; not usually measured in clinical setting, but technology is available.

π_t = tissue colloid osmotic pressure; cannot be measured in clinical setting.

Proteins act as osmotic (or oncotic) agents in each of these spaces to attract fluid, while hydrostatic forces push fluid into or out of the vessels. The equation has distinct permeability values for water and protein, since each crosses the vascular membrane at a different rate. Although the Starling equation is useful to the practitioner in terms of understanding the factors involved in fluid shifting between compartments, the rate and direction of transvascular flow cannot be accurately calculated in the clinical setting since the majority of factors cannot be measured directly.

The body's compensatory mechanisms may have beneficial and harmful consequences. For example, if preload is not substantially decreased, cardiac output can be increased approximately fivefold by increases in stroke volume or heart rate.[1] Though this may be useful for providing blood flow to inadequately perfused tissues, it may cause large (e.g., fourfold) increases in oxygen consumption by the heart that could aggravate preexisting ischemia in patients with underlying coronary artery disease. Another example is the sympathetic-nervous-system–mediated vasoconstriction that causes blood to shift from the skin, skeletal muscle, and some internal organs such as the kidneys and gastrointestinal tract to organs (e.g., heart, brain) that are less tolerant of inadequate flow. If the vasoconstriction continues unabated, the hypoperfused organs eventually become damaged. Figure 22–2 provides an overview of the compensatory changes that occur with a loss of circulating blood volume.

In addition to the more acute implications of hypovolemia and attendant complications, reperfusion damage is likely to occur particularly after prolonged resuscitation attempts. In addition to oxygen free-radical damage of cell membranes, a number of cellular (e.g., white blood cells, platelets) and humoral (e.g., procoagulants, anticoagulants, complement, kinins) components are activated, causing the release of other inflammatory mediators.[6] The

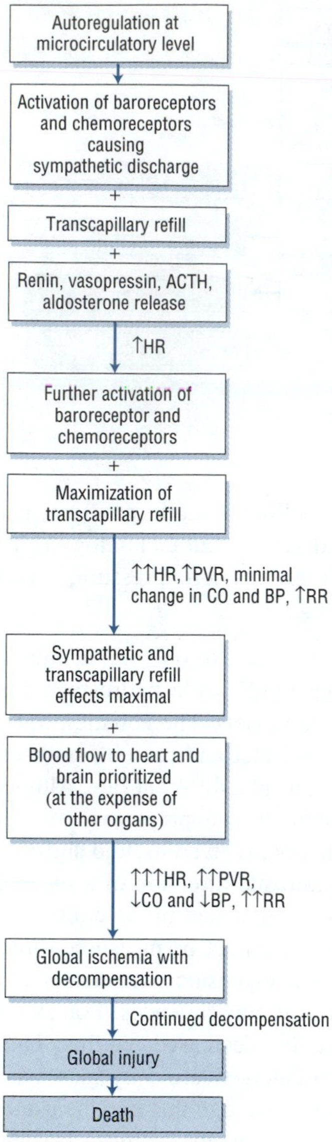

FIGURE 22–2. Activation of compensatory mechanisms with loss of circulatory volume. Certain stages may be absent depending on a number of factors such as age, preexisting disease states, and cause of circulatory insufficiency. HR = heart rate; PVR = peripheral vascular resistance; CO = cardiac output; BP = blood pressure; RR = respiratory rate.

resulting reperfusion injury may range from readily reversible organ dysfunction to multiple organ failure and death.

Although the basic pathophysiology is similar for the various causes of hypovolemic shock, there are unique considerations relative to each. For example, whereas isolated head injuries associated with trauma typically do not result in substantial blood loss or shock, pelvic fractures may sequester several liters of blood as hematoma formation.[7] Patients with traumatic or thermal injuries, as well as postoperative patients, may have substantial fluid accumulation in sites where it cannot be readily transferred back into blood vessels (i.e., third-spaced fluid) for maintaining pressure. With these types of injures, early control of problems such as bleeding with rapid patient transfer to the hospital for definitive treatment may preclude the cascade of events leading to shock. Indeed, with trauma patients, a "scoop and run" approach is used in most urban hospitals, which places a priority on rapid transport to a hospital.[8]

In the case of hemorrhagic shock, prompt attention must be given to cell as well as plasma losses. Red blood cells lost during the bleeding episode may lead to ischemic damage in vital organs. Packed red blood cell transfusions may be needed to increase the oxygen-carrying capacity of the blood, because oxygen transport is a function not only of cardiac output, but also of hemoglobin concentration and saturation and of hemoglobin affinity for oxygen.

Clotting factors and platelets are also lost in hemorrhage. The resulting bleeding problems may be aggravated by the dilutional effect of fluid resuscitation on clotting factor activity. Fresh frozen plasma that contains necessary clotting factors and platelets is often needed in massive blood loss to restore adequate coagulation. Somewhat paradoxically, trauma patients are at increased risk for deep venous thrombosis and pulmonary embolism due to multiple factors including vessel damage, abnormal blood flow patterns, and the hypercoagulable state associated with injury. Therefore, some form of venous thromboembolism prophylaxis is usually indicated in multiple-trauma patients or patients with severe single-system injuries (e.g., spinal cord damage).

The pathophysiology becomes more complicated if the severity of shock is sufficient to require admission to the intensive care unit (ICU) after initial resuscitation or surgery. The majority of patients admitted to the ICU have a systemic inflammatory response syndrome (SIRS), which is the body's response to injury.[9] This syndrome is defined by a number of hypermetabolic changes reflected in the patient's temperature, white blood cell count and differential, and respiratory and heart rates. When SIRS and infection are combined, the patient has sepsis. The stress response involves complex interactions between the nervous system and immunomodulating substances and has similar (if not the same) harmful and helpful consequences described with reperfusion following shock.[10] If the underlying problems are left untreated, the patient with SIRS may develop multiple organ dysfunction syndrome (MODS) during the final stages of illness.

CLINICAL PRESENTATION

The initial presentation of patients with suspected volume depletion can vary markedly depending on factors such as age, concomitant disease states and medications, and the etiology and rapidity of depletion. In contrast to simple dehydration, volume depletion is signified by orthostatic blood pressure changes, and such measurements should be performed. Other signs and symptoms (e.g., mental status changes) of dehydration and intravascular depletion are relatively nonspecific and may occur with either condition.

TABLE 22–1. Acute Circulatory Insufficiency: Initial Presentation and Therapy[a]

	Mild	Severe
Plasma/blood loss	10 mL/kg adult 20 mL/kg child	30 mL/kg adult 35 mL/kg child
Mental status/level of consciousness	None—small changes (e.g., anxious, irritable)	Marked changes (e.g., confusion to unconscious)
Vital signs/orthostatic changes	Minor changes	Marked changes
Therapy	20 mL/kg lactated Ringer's over 10–15 min Unlikely to need blood cell replacement even if hemorrhagic loss	Lactated Ringer's as rapidly as possible until response in adult, then decrease rate of infusion 20 mL/kg lactated Ringer's in child (repeat quickly if minimal response), likely to need blood cell replacement and surgery if hemorrhagic

[a]Patients may have intermediate degrees of volume loss in addition to those listed, but the amount of loss is often difficult to quantify. The presentations may also vary greatly in patients with similar amounts of loss (young athlete vs sedentary, elderly person). Refer to text for a more in-depth discussion of some of the guidelines in this table.

Plasma volume losses of less than 10 mL/kg of body weight are usually associated with minor signs and symptoms of distress. For example, in most patients, the heart and respiratory rates would be less than 100 beats per minute and 20 breaths per minute, respectively, and the blood pressure and urine output would be normal, but the person would appear somewhat anxious. Larger losses are not likely to be well tolerated (Table 22–1), particularly in the elderly. Such patients would have marked increases in heart rate (e.g., > 120 beats/min) and respiratory rate (e.g., > 30 breaths/min) assuming no concurrent diseases or drugs that alter these rates, and substantial decreases in blood pressure (e.g., systolic blood pressure < 90 mm Hg) and urine output (e.g., < 0.5 mL/kg/h). A young athlete and an elderly, sedentary individual are likely to have much different responses to a similar amount of fluid loss. The young patient may lose one-fourth of her circulating blood volume with minimal changes in arterial blood pressure and a relatively low heart rate. However, the elderly patient may have orthostatic changes in blood pressure that are not well tolerated by organs such as the kidneys.[3] Unfortunately, this same elderly patient may not have "classic" signs and symptoms of volume depletion such as skin turgor changes or thirst, but instead have more subtle changes (e.g., mental status alterations).[11] Regardless of patient age or preexisting conditions, the initial monitoring of a patient with suspected volume depletion should include the following noninvasive parameters: vital signs, urine output, mental status, and physical examination (Fig. 22–3).

While the presenting signs and symptoms of circulatory insufficiency are variable, patients will usually have decreased blood pressure, increased heart and respiratory rates, and a normal or low-normal temperature (e.g., 36 to 37°C) in the absence of infection or exposure to extremes of temperature. As mentioned earlier, blood pressure and heart rate recordings must be interpreted in light of known or suspected baseline conditions. For example, medications such as β-blockers and calcium channel blockers may alter resting blood pressure and heart rate, as well as the subsequent response to therapeutic manipulations. Similarly, while a blood pressure reading of 110/70 (systolic/diastolic) may be acceptable in many patients, it may be inadequate for a patient with preexisting hypertension who normally has a blood pressure of 170/105. On the other extreme, patients with very low blood pressure may have inaudible or inaccurate determinations with cuff (sphygmomanometric) measurements. See Chap. 10 on Hypertension for details of blood pressure measurement (e.g., cuff size, position). In this case, intraarterial monitoring is indicated. As a noninvasive tool, the respiratory rate may correlate better with volume loss than the heart rate, but is often not used.[3] The respiratory rate may be elevated due to anxiety or as a compensatory mechanism for the metabolic acidosis associated with poor tissue perfusion.

Although urine is continually produced by the kidneys, it is stored in the bladder for intermittent elimination. For the initial diagnosis and management of acute circulatory insufficiency, a catheter can be inserted into the bladder for measuring urine output. In contrast to thirst, which is a relatively insensitive indicator of volume depletion, urine output is generally diminished with inadequate fluid administration and increases with appropriate resuscitation. This presumes of course that acute renal failure or medications such as diuretics are not altering the expected response. Adults should produce at least 0.5 to 1 mL/kg/h of

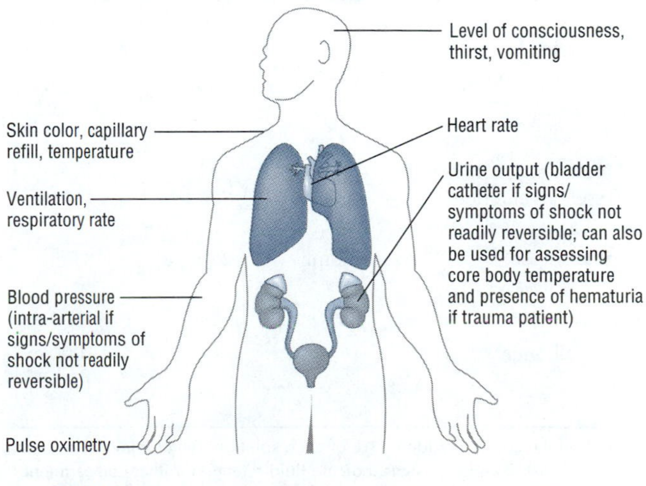
Level of consciousness, thirst, vomiting
Skin color, capillary refill, temperature
Heart rate
Ventilation, respiratory rate
Urine output (bladder catheter if signs/symptoms of shock not readily reversible; can also be used for assessing core body temperature and presence of hematuria if trauma patient)
Blood pressure (intra-arterial if signs/symptoms of shock not readily reversible)
Pulse oximetry

FIGURE 22–3. Noninvasive assessment of circulatory insufficiency.

urine, whereas children should produce at least 1 mL/kg/h (2 mL/kg/h if less than 1 year of age).[7]

Mental status changes associated with volume depletion, if present, may range from subtle fluctuations in mood to unconsciousness. Although the latter finding is typically indicative of more severe depletion, less dramatic findings should not be interpreted as indicating mild fluid deficits. Losses of 4 L of plasma volume may be associated only with lassitude in an otherwise healthy adult patient.[3] Similar interpretation difficulties must be considered when performing the initial physical examination. An orderly progression from warm, reddish skin with appropriate capillary refill to cold, cyanotic discoloration with impaired refill may not occur. Also, dry mucous membranes in elderly patients may be due to mouth breathing or anticholinergic medications and not fluid depletion.[11]

▶ TREATMENT: Hypovolemic Shock

DESIRED OUTCOME

The desired outcomes of therapy for circulatory insufficiency that has led to hypovolemic shock are to prevent further progression of the disease with subsequent organ damage and, to the extent that it is possible, reverse organ dysfunction that has already taken place.

GENERAL APPROACH TO TREATMENT

Milder forms of volume depletion may be managed in outpatient settings. For example, supplemental fluids can be added to the usual estimated daily requirements of 30 mL/kg in elderly patients with dehydration. Commercially available carbohydrate/electrolyte drinks are generally more palatable than water and may promote earlier recovery.[11] When the dehydration involves substantial losses of salt, as well as water, additional sodium may need to be added to these drinks since they usually contain ≤50 mEq/L of sodium. This is less than the amounts of sodium (e.g., 90 to 120 mEq/L) generally recommended for rehydration.[12] The additional sodium will increase osmolarity, but this does not appear to delay gastric emptying.[13] Also, guidelines for oral rehydration of children with acute diarrhea are available, which if used appropriately may prevent future hospitalization.[14] Intravenous rehydration of children in outpatient settings has been accomplished, but patients must be carefully selected.[15,16] Outpatient rehydration of children generally should be limited to those with uncomplicated (e.g., vomiting < 48 hours) acute gastroenteritis and relatively mild dehydration, after the exclusion of more severe illnesses such as bowel obstruction.

Hospitalization is indicated in more severe forms of circulatory insufficiency. If access to the circulatory system for fluids and medication administration was not obtained prior to hospitalization, this should be a priority. Venous access is generally obtained during the preliminary examination process that includes the "ABCs" of life support (i.e., airway, breathing, and circulation), assessment of vital signs and mental status, and urine output after catheterization. Whenever large-volume fluid resuscitation is expected, as in hemorrhagic shock, it is desirable to have at least two IV catheters. Because flow is a function of tubing length and catheter diameter, large-bore peripheral IVs are preferred over longer central lines. Unfortunately, vascular access in children may be problematic and other routes (e.g., intraosseous) may be necessary.[7]

PHARMACOLOGIC THERAPY

Although dextrose-in-water solutions may be appropriate for uncomplicated dehydration caused by water deprivation, crystalloid (sodium-containing) solutions should be used for forms of circulatory insufficiency that are associated with hemodynamic instability. In the latter situation, IV solutions with sodium concentrations approximating normal serum sodium values are usually indicated since they cause more expansion of the intravascular and interstitial spaces compared to dextrose solutions (Table 22–2). Lactated Ringer's and normal saline solutions are examples of such

TABLE 22–2. Fluid Distribution and Major Indications[a]

Fluid	Intracellular	Interstitial	Intravascular	Major Indication
Normal saline or lactated Ringer's	None	750 mL	250 mL	Intravascular repletion in symptomatic patients
3% sodium chloride	→	750 mL +	250 mL +	Small amounts (e.g., 250 mL) have been used in conjunction with normal saline or lactated Ringer's for severe intravascular depletion in adults
5% dextrose/0.45% sodium chloride	333 mL	500 mL	167 mL	Maintenance fluid in euvolemic or dehydrated (sodium and water loss) patients with mild signs/symptoms of volume depletion
5% dextrose	667 mL	250 mL	83 mL	Dehydration (primarily water loss) in patients with mild signs/symptoms of volume depletion
5% albumin	None	None	1000 mL[b]	Intravascular repletion in symptomatic patients
25% albumin	→	→	1000 mL +[b]	Smaller amounts (e.g., 50–100 mL or by continuous infusion in adults) titrated to response in hypovolemic patients with excess total body water

[a]Based on the administration of 1 L of each solution (*which may not be an appropriate amount for clinical use*); numbers are approximations; arrows indicate direction of fluid shift and plus signs indicate fluid retention in that compartment.
[b]After distribution, 60% of albumin (and associated fluid) is in interstitial compartment and 40% is in intravascular compartment.

TABLE 22–3. Adverse Effects of Plasma Expanders: Crystalloids

Normal saline
Primarily extensions of pharmacologic actions (e.g., fluid overload; dilutional coagulopathy)
Hyperchloremic metabolic acidosis (has 154 mEq/L of chloride)
Hypernatremia (has 154 mEq/L of sodium)
Lactated Ringer's
Primarily extensions of pharmacologic actions (e.g., fluid overload; dilutional coagulopathy)
Hyponatremia (has 130 mEq/L of sodium)
Aggravation of preexisting hyperkalemia (has 4 mEq/L potassium)
Hypertonic saline
Primarily extensions of pharmacologic actions (e.g., fluid overload; dilutional coagulopathy; intracellular volume depletion)
Hypernatremia (has 513 mEq/L of sodium)
Hyperchloremia (has 513 mEq/L of chloride)

crystalloid solutions, although lactated Ringer's is the preferred solution according to some published guidelines (see *Advanced Trauma Life Support Guidelines*) because it is unlikely to cause the hyperchloremic metabolic acidosis seen with infusion of large amounts of normal saline (Table 22–3).[7] A "large" amount of fluid does not mean the typical bolus volumes used as fluid challenges in critically ill patients. Isolated boluses (e.g., 500 mL in adults) are unlikely to cause substantial changes in blood pressure or acid–base balance.[17]

Although lactated Ringer's solution does contain lactate, it does not cause substantial elevations in circulating lactate concentrations when used as a resuscitation solution.[18] However, blood samples for lactate determinations drawn through catheters (arterial and venous) that have not been flushed appropriately may have spurious increases or decreases in lactate concentrations due to retained lactated Ringer's and nonlactated solutions (e.g., varying concentrations of dextrose-in-water or sodium chloride), respectively.[19] Therefore, blood samples for lactate concentrations should be drawn from a catheter that has been adequately cleared (e.g., 5 mL) of infusate after temporarily stopping the fluid infusion.

Larger-molecular-weight solutions (i.e., > 30,000) known as colloids have been recommended in conjunction with, or as replacements for, crystalloid solutions. Examples of colloids used as plasma expanders include albumin, hetastarch, and dextran. Albumin is known as a monodisperse colloid because all of its molecules are of the same molecular weight, whereas hetastarch and dextran solutions are polydisperse compounds with molecules of varying molecular weights. This has important implications for the distribution of the products, because lower-molecular-weight substances are retained in the intravascular space for a shorter period of time due to more rapid leakage across the vessel membrane. The theoretical usefulness of colloids is based on their increased molecular weight (average molecular weight in the case of hetastarch and dextran) that corresponds to increased intravascular retention time in the absence of increased capillary permeability. Even in patients with intact capillary permeability, the colloid molecules will eventually leak through the membrane. In the case of albumin, approximately 60% of the albumin molecules (and associated fluid) will be contained in the interstitial space within 5 days of exogenous administration. In patients with altered permeability (e.g., acute respiratory distress syndrome), the leakage of albumin from the intravascular to the interstitial space may occur within hours, not days.

Albumin is available in a 5% and a 25% concentration. Plasma protein fraction has oncotic actions similar to a 5% albumin solution, which is not surprising since albumin is the predominant protein in this product. It takes approximately three to four times as much lactated Ringer's or normal saline solution to yield the same volume expansion as 5% albumin solution, but even when given in equipotent amounts, albumin is much more costly than crystalloid solutions. Additionally, the 5% and 25% albumin solutions are typically priced in such a way that there is no cost savings associated with dilution of the 25% product to make a 5% concentration. The 5% albumin solution is relatively iso-oncotic, which means that it does not pull fluid into the compartment in which it is contained. In contrast, 25% albumin is referred to as hyperoncotic albumin since it tends to pull fluid into the compartment containing the albumin molecules. In general, the 5% albumin solution is used for hypovolemic states. The 25% solution should probably not be used for acute circulatory insufficiency unless diluted with other fluids, or unless it is being used in patients with excess total body water but intravascular depletion, as a means of pulling fluid into the intravascular space. This presumes that there is evidence of adverse effects associated with this excess water such as interstitial fluid accumulation in the lungs. Although theoretically appealing, this indication has not been well documented by randomized controlled trials. Additionally, the effect is temporary since the albumin will cross the vascular membrane over time.

Hetastarch 6% has comparable plasma expansion to a 5% albumin solution, but is usually less expensive, which accounts for much of its use. The majority of trials comparing albumin to hetastarch for volume expansion have found no significant differences in clinically important outcomes (e.g., mortality). Few trials have compared directly hetastarch to crystalloid solutions for intravascular expansion. Although hetastarch is often stated as being contraindicated in severe bleeding disorders, it has been most-studied in patients with blood loss (e.g., trauma and perioperative patients). Because the definition of severe bleeding is somewhat nebulous, hetastarch is best avoided in conditions such as intracranial bleeding; it may aggravate bleeding through mechanisms specific to this colloid (e.g., decreased factor VIII activity). These mechanisms have not been well elucidated and are often difficult to distinguish from the dilutional effects on clotting factors caused by all plasma expanders. Hetastarch may also cause elevations in serum amylase concentrations that may be misinterpreted as pancreatitis, which it does not cause.

Dextran 40, dextran 70, and dextran 75 are available for use as plasma expanders in the United States. The numbers refer to the average molecular weight of the solutions. In general, dextran solutions are not used as often as albumin or hetastarch solutions for plasma expansion, possibly due to concerns related to aggravation of bleeding (i.e., anticoagulant actions related to inhibiting stasis of microcirculation) and anaphylaxis that is more likely to occur with the higher-molecular-weight solutions. However, both of these concerns are probably overstated and can be limited if proper attention is paid to patient selection and, in the case of bleeding, published dosing guidelines. There are few comparative trials involving the dextran solutions, but the intravascular expansion within hours after infusion is approximately equal to the amount of dextran infused.

Twenty-six trials (1315 patients) comparing resuscitative solutions were reviewed recently with particular emphasis on discovering possible differences in mortality related to crystalloid versus colloid administration. Nineteen trials had published information concerning mortality and no additional information was gained through direct contacts with investigators. The trials involved patients with various types of injuries and diseases. Hypovolemic shock appeared to be the most common explanation for giving fluids, since the majority of patients were stratified into groups commonly associated with plasma losses from the body (i.e., trauma, surgery, or thermal injury). The study found a

4% absolute increase in the risk of death associated with colloid administration (95% confidence interval = 0% to 8%).[19A] The presumed comparability of studies and interventions needed to perform such analyses does raise questions concerning extrapolation of the results to specific patient populations. With this caution in mind, these trials provide additional evidence that crystalloid solutions should be considered first-line therapy in patients with hypovolemic shock. Similar results were found in a subsequent review of 30 randomized trials in 1419 patients (relative risk of death with albumin 1.68, 95% confidence interval = 1.26–2.23).[19B] For hypovolemia specifically, the risk of death associated with albumin administration was not quite statistically significant (relative risk 1.46, 95% confidence interval 0.97–2.22).

SPECIAL POPULATIONS

Trauma/Perioperative Patients

The immediate treatment of hemorrhagic circulatory insufficiency with plasma expanders (i.e., crystalloids or colloids) seems obvious and has widespread acceptance, but no large, well-controlled trials in humans have been conducted that support this practice.[20] One prospective study involving 598 adult patients with gunshot or stab wound injuries to the torso and systolic blood pressure measurements ≤ 90 mm Hg found that delayed fluid resuscitation until operation was associated with increased survival and discharge from the hospital ($P = .04$).[21] However, concerns were expressed about comparability of the immediate and delayed resuscitation groups, particularly since true randomization did not take place.[22] Additionally, the study was conducted in a populated urban area with approximately 2 hours from time of injury to operation. Therefore, the results are not applicable to rural areas with extended transport times. While the applicability of this study to other populations and settings is debatable, the *presumption* of benefits from immediate plasma expansion in all perioperative patients with circulatory insufficiency is no longer valid.

The latter study has dampened interest in other solutions being investigated primarily for prehospital utilization.[23] For example, hypertonic solutions have several characteristics that make them attractive for acute resuscitation. The intravascular and interstitial expansion resulting from the administration of these solutions is much greater than the volume infused by emergency personnel. By causing redistribution (i.e., pulling fluid) from the intracellular space, hypertonic solutions cause rapid expansion of the intravascular compartment, which is essential for vital organ perfusion. In head-injured patients, this redistribution should decrease intracranial pressure since the vessels of the brain are more impermeable to sodium ions than vessels in other areas of the body.[23] Additionally, hypertonic saline solutions have beneficial immunomodulating actions when compared to more isotonic solutions in experiments with animals.[24,25]

Potential adverse effects associated with hypertonic fluid administration for circulatory insufficiency include cellular crenation and damage caused by the dramatic fluid shifts, as well as peripheral vein destruction from their high osmolality. Also, in the case of hypertonic sodium chloride solutions, there are the possibilities of neurologic damage from hypernatremia and hyperchloremic metabolic acidosis from hyperchloremia. In the limited number of studies conducted in humans to date, such adverse effects have been uncommon and apparently of little clinical importance.[26–28]

Unfortunately, beneficial outcome data attributable to administration of these hypertonic solutions have also been lacking. Most of these studies were conducted in prehospital and emergency department settings using 250 mL of 7.5% sodium chloride with or without 6% dextran 70. A meta-analysis of randomized controlled trials found no statistical difference between the survival rates of patients receiving the hypertonic saline solutions and those receiving standard isotonic crystalloid solutions.[29] Part of the explanation for this finding may be related to supplemental crystalloid fluids that were routinely given to patients in both the treatment and control groups, which would probably increase the number of patients needed to demonstrate a statistically significant difference in mortality. Until the concerns regarding efficacy and toxicity of these solutions have been resolved, normal saline could be considered as an alternative for head-injured patients when a hypertonic solution is desirable since it contains 154 mmol/L of both sodium and chloride. Hypotonic solutions are best avoided in this population given their relatively poor intravascular expansion and association with poor outcome in animal models of closed head injury.[30]

In addition to crystalloid solutions, colloids have been used for plasma expansion in patients with hemorrhagic circulatory insufficiency. In the United States, albumin and starch (i.e., hetastarch) derivatives are most commonly used, although dextran solutions are also commercially available. The theoretical advantage to these compounds is their prolonged intravascular retention time compared to crystalloid solutions. In contrast to isotonic crystalloid solutions that have substantial interstitial distribution within minutes of intravenous administration, colloids remain in the intravascular space for hours or days depending on factors such as capillary permeability.

The colloids, in particular albumin, are expensive solutions. Therefore, it is difficult to justify the additional cost of colloidal products unless the benefit-to-risk ratio is substantially greater than that associated with inexpensive crystalloid solutions. This does not appear to be the case based on four randomized controlled studies comparing colloid and crystalloid solutions for acute circulatory insufficiency. In one study involving 94 patients being resuscitated by an emergency surgical service, albumin administration was titrated based on albumin levels.[31] All patients were given crystalloids and blood products in addition to the supplemental albumin. There were statistically significant increases in length of stay and pulmonary shunting in patients randomized to receive albumin, albeit the clinical significance of the calculated shunting differences is questionable. Pulmonary shunting refers to blood that is diverted through the lungs without being oxygenated. It is an indirect indicator of impaired oxygenation and is estimated by calculations that use various measured arterial and venous respiratory parameters (and hemoglobin concentration). Values greater than 20% are usually considered substantial impairment. Three additional studies titrated albumin to achieve hemodynamic stabilization. In the two larger studies (141 and 36 patients) involving patients undergoing exploratory laparotomy, there were no significant differences in ventilatory support, pulmonary shunting, or alveolar–arterial oxygen difference between groups receiving crystalloids or albumin.[32,33] The third study randomized 26 elderly patients (mean age 79 years) to receive albumin, hetastarch, or normal saline for hypovolemic shock.[34] Despite the small number of patients in each group, the incidence of pulmonary edema was 22% in patients receiving the colloids, but 87.5% in the patients receiving the saline ($P < .05$). In addition to the small number of patients enrolled in this investigation, another concern was the radiographic definition of pulmonary edema at 24 hours postresuscitation without supporting clinical data. In summary, of the four randomized studies comparing colloids to crystalloids for acute circulatory insufficiency, there is no obvious benefit to using colloid products for resuscitation with the possible exception of elderly patients in shock.

Because other colloids such as hetastarch have almost always been compared to albumin and not crystalloid solutions in published clinical studies (with no clinically important differences being found), there is no reason to suspect these other colloids have any unique advantages as volume expanders. Adverse effects associated with colloids appear to be uncommon and are generally extensions of their pharmacologic activity (Table 22–4), but this is

TABLE 22–4. Adverse Effects of Plasma Expanders: Colloids

Albumin
Primarily extensions of pharmacologic actions (e.g., fluid overload; dilutional coagulopathy; crystalloids are usually needed with 25% albumin in hypovolemic states to prevent intracellular volume depletion and renal failure)
Amino acid profile and catabolism alterations (clinical significance?); potential protein overload if given with exogenous protein (e.g., parenteral nutrition)
Anaphylactoid/anaphylaxis (life-threatening reactions rare; higher in patients with IgA deficiency)
Infectious complications (all reported cases have been associated with improper handling by manufacturer or institution; no reported cases of HIV or hepatitis transmission)
Interactions with medications and nutrients (clinical significance varies)
Metal loading, particularly aluminum (long-term administration in patients with renal failure)
Negative inotropic effect, reductions in ionized calcium concentrations?
Pyrogenic reactions?
Hetastarch
Primarily extensions of pharmacologic actions (e.g., fluid overload; dilutional coagulopathy)
Bleeding (decreases factor VIII/C activity; not recommended in patients with severe bleeding conditions such as subarachnoid hemorrhage)
Macroamylase formation may cause elevation in blood amylase that leads to inaccurate diagnosis of pancreatitis
Dextrans
Primarily extensions of pharmacologic actions (e.g., fluid overload; dilutional coagulopathy)
Anaphylaxis (increased incidence with increased molecular weight)
Bleeding (sometimes used for anticoagulant activity so not recommended in patients with severe bleeding)

also true of crystalloids. The benefit-to-risk ratio appears to be similar for colloids and crystalloids, so based on cost, crystalloids are preferred for initial treatment of circulatory insufficiency.

Another consideration in the patient with injuries or surgery is the potential need for blood-product administration (Table 22–5) to replace oxygen-carrying and clotting functions. Although a small group of trauma patients respond to the initial fluid bolus and remain stable, most patients respond initially and then deteriorate.[7] The latter patients, as well as patients undergoing blood loss associated with surgery, frequently need blood components such as packed red blood cells. In the case of the latter component, red blood cells contain hemoglobin that delivers oxygen to tissues. Neither crystalloids nor colloids perform this function.

Blood products are not without risk. For example, there is the rare, but important risk of virus transmission. The administration of blood products has its own risks. For example, citrate that is added to stored blood to ensure its anticoagulation properties may bind to calcium, resulting in hypocalcemia. In contrast, potassium and phosphate concentrations are often elevated in stored blood, particularly when hemolysis has taken place during storage. Additionally, administration of excessive blood products may lead to counterproductive results. In the case of red blood cells, attempts to raise the hematocrit to high normal or supranormal concentrations may decrease oxygen delivery by increasing blood viscosity.[3] Although there is no optimal hematocrit value for all patients, higher concentrations (e.g., ≥ 30%) are indicated for patients at particular risk for ischemia such as those with coronary artery disease. Other issues that must be considered with blood-product administration include monitoring for transfusion-related reactions and attention to appropriate warming, particularly when large volumes are given to pediatric patients, because hypothermia is associated with increased fluid requirements and mortality.[35]

TABLE 22–5. General Indications for Blood Products in Acute Circulatory Insufficiency Due to Hemorrhage[a]

Packed red blood cells
Increase oxygen-carrying capacity of blood—usually indicated in patients with continued deterioration after volume replacement or obvious exsanguination; needs to be warmed, particularly when used in children
Fresh frozen plasma
Replacement of clotting factors—generally overused; indicated if ongoing hemorrhage in patients with PT/PTT > 1.5 times normal, severe hepatic disease, or other bleeding diathesis
Platelets
Used for bleeding due to severe thrombocytopenia (i.e., platelet count < 10,000 μL) or rapidly dropping platelet counts as would occur with massive bleeding
Other products
Components such as cryoprecipitate and factor VIII are generally not indicated in acute hemorrhage, but rather are used once specific deficiencies have been identified

[a]Although whole blood could be used for large-volume blood loss, most hospitals use component therapy, with crystalloids or colloids used for plasma expansion.

Patients with Thermal Injuries

There are a wide variety of formulas for estimating fluid requirements in thermally injured patients, but there is little reason to choose one over another based on well-controlled studies. In general, the amount of loss corresponds to the size of the thermal injury.[3] Approximately 3 mL/kg of isotonic fluid (lactated Ringer's) for each percent burn can be used for calculating the expected fluid requirements for the first 24 hours postburn. For example, a 60-kg person with 30% body-surface-area burns would be expected to require 5400 mL of fluid over the initial 24 hours. Regardless of the calculated deficit, fluids should be administered until adequate tissue perfusion has been documented or adverse effects (e.g., pulmonary edema) occur. While the choice of plasma expander is based primarily on cost considerations for blood loss due to trauma or surgery, crystalloids are preferred as initial therapy for burn victims because they are less likely to cause interstitial fluid accumulation. Only one randomized trial has been conducted in which patients were given either albumin or lactated Ringer's solution to maintain urine output and vital signs during the first 24 hours after occurrence of the burn.[36] Lung water accumulation was significantly higher ($P < .0001$) in the albumin-treated patients, and there were trends toward increased pulmonary edema and death in the albumin group. In another study conducted immediately after the first 24-hour resuscitation period, infusion of albumin reduced glomerular filtration rate ($P < .05$) despite increasing plasma volume by 37%.[37]

In a more recent randomized trial involving 70 patients less than 19 years of age with more than 20% body-surface-area thermal injuries, patients were given albumin based on albumin concentrations.[38] Both groups received conventional resuscitation with crystalloid solutions. In one group, albumin was given if the concentration decreased to less than 2.5 g/dL, whereas patients in the other group were given albumin only if the concentration was less than 1.5 g/dL. No statistically significant differences were found in any of the resuscitation or nutritional parameters.

Some novel therapies for thermal resuscitation are currently under study. For example, in guinea pigs with 70% body-surface-area burns, antioxidant therapy with high-dose vitamin C (340 mg/kg/24 h) has been shown to decrease the amount of resuscitation fluid needed for maintaining cardiac output.[39] The proposed mechanism is reduction in free-radical–induced increases in capillary permeability.

ONGOING MONITORING

Although the monitoring of patients in the emergency room setting is relatively straightforward, it becomes much more controversial in the perioperative period. This is particularly true concerning the value of right heart catheterization (a.k.a. pulmonary artery or Swan–Ganz catheter). However, most clinicians would agree that certain forms of monitoring are important, since patients in the postresuscitation phase of management are at risk for various complications secondary to ischemia. A more complete discussion of invasive and noninvasive hemodynamic monitoring is found in Chapter 21.

One form of monitoring that may take place in the emergency and operating rooms, as well as in the intensive care unit, requires placement of a central venous pressure (CVP) line. Monitoring of CVP provides the clinician with an indirect and insensitive, yet useful estimate of the relationship between increased right atrial pressure and cardiac output.[7]

A number of laboratory tests are indicated for the subacute monitoring of shock. These include a renal battery for assessing possible electrolyte alterations and kidney perfusion (blood urea nitrogen, creatinine). Among other things, a complete blood count will allow for assessment of possible infection (white blood cell count), oxygen-carrying capacity of the blood (hemoglobin, hematocrit), and ongoing bleeding (hemoglobin, hematocrit, platelet count). The prothrombin time (PT) and partial thromboplastin time (PTT) will give an indication of the ability of the blood to clot, since in the case of hemorrhagic shock, clotting factors are lost and diluted. An increasing lactate concentration (arterial, mixed venous, or central venous)[40] and base deficit are consistent with inadequate perfusion, leading to anaerobic metabolism with accumulation of lactic acid. Other tests may be indicated if organ dysfunction is likely. For example, the transaminases on a liver panel may be markedly elevated in the first couple of days after marked hypotension, although the concentrations should decrease over time.[3] Along with laboratory testing, a more extensive history can be obtained during the subacute monitoring period.

The value of pulmonary artery catheters has been hotly debated since its introduction. The debate was intensified when early studies by Shoemaker and associates suggested improved outcomes when cardiac output and oxygen transport variables were raised to supranormal levels, the monitoring of which required placement of a pulmonary artery catheter.[41] Subsequent studies using similar monitoring parameters associated with pulmonary artery catheterization gave conflicting results.[42]

A resolution to this controversy involving supranormal therapeutic goals seemed possible with a study involving the largest number of patients to date.[43] This study randomized 762 patients to a control group in which traditional therapies were titrated to normal physiologic values, a treatment group in which therapies were titrated to achieve a supranormal cardiac index of > 4.5 L/min/m^2, and a treatment group in which therapies were titrated to achieve a normal mixed venous oxygen saturation of ≥ 70%. Morbidity, mortality, and length of stay were similar for all three groups. This study did not prove that supranormal goals are not desirable in any patient, however, because it included a heterogeneous group of patients most of whom were studied postoperatively. In contrast, three studies that have shown value in titrating therapies to supranormal goals were all conducted in high-risk surgery or trauma patients with early (preoperative or intraoperative) initiation of monitoring by pulmonary artery catheterization.[41,44,45] It would be expected that most of these patients would have a hypovolemic form of shock. It is important to realize that most clinicians would agree that *conservative* management of patients with circulatory insufficiency is not appropriate.[46]

The titration of therapies to supranormal therapeutic goals requires placement of a pulmonary artery catheter, but the controversy surrounding this type of catheterization extends beyond this particular issue. A large observational study involving 5735 critically ill patients found that placement of a pulmonary artery catheter for a variety of reasons resulted in increased mortality, as well as increased costs.[47] An editorial accompanying the published study was more controversial than the study itself because the authors recommended a moratorium on pulmonary artery catheter placement *if* a multicenter, randomized trial was not initiated.[48] At least one organization condemned the suggestion of a moratorium on catheter placement and made plans for a consensus conference to address the issue of pulmonary artery catheterization.[49] Results of the consensus conference, which was endorsed by five major health professional organizations, were subsequently published.[50] The consensus participants concluded that while a randomized controlled trial would be ethical, a moratorium on pulmonary artery catheter placement should not be enacted pending such a trial.

Part of the concern regarding pulmonary artery catheterization relates to the interpretation of its results by inexperienced practitioners. Studies in both Europe and the United States have found that one out of two physicians incorrectly interpreted a tracing from a pulmonary artery catheter.[51] This could explain some of the results of studies finding no benefits to pulmonary artery catheterization or, in some cases, worse outcomes in the pulmonary artery catheterization group by actions taken as a result of inaccurate measurements or misinterpretation of information obtained from the monitoring process. Data from one nonrandomized study conducted in shock patients without evidence of myocardial infarction suggest that treatment alterations based on pulmonary artery catheter measurements are most effective in patients who have failed to respond to fluids and vasopressor therapy.[52]

Complications related to pulmonary artery catheterization insertion, maintenance, and removal include damage to vessels and organs during insertion, arrhythmias, infections, and thromboembolic damage.[53] To avoid the complications associated with pulmonary artery catheterization, other less invasive tools have been developed to obtain similar information. For example, cardiac output determinations have been made by Doppler, bioimpedance, dye, and ionic dilution techniques, although such measurements would not provide other data routinely obtained with pulmonary artery catheters (e.g., left heart-filling pressure).[54] Additionally, advances in pulmonary artery catheter technology are being investigated that expand the information obtained from such monitoring (e.g., mixed venous oxyhemoglobin).[55] However, given the lack of well-defined outcome data associated with pulmonary artery catheterization, its use is best reserved for complicated cases of shock not responding to conventional fluid and medication therapies.

Commonly measured and calculated hemodynamic and oxygen transport indices associated with invasive monitoring are primarily global indicators of tissue perfusion. There have been attempts to find regional and local indicators of hypoperfusion so that circulatory insufficiency can be treated before overt shock occurs. One focus of recent research has been monitoring modalities involving the gastrointestinal tract.

It has been demonstrated that intramucosal stomach pH (pHi) determinations < 7.35 are associated with very high mortality ($> 65\%$), which may not be altered by standard interventions. For example, one study used a protocol (normal saline boluses followed by a dobutamine infusion if the pHi remained < 7.35) aimed at increasing oxygen transport and reducing oxygen demand in patients with initial pHi determinations < 7.35 or ≥ 7.35 after "conventional" therapy had been used to stabilize all patients.[56] Survival in the protocol group was not improved when compared to a control group for patients with pHi values < 7.35 on admission. However, mortality was significantly decreased in the protocol compared to the control group in patients with relatively normal pHi values (i.e., initial pHi values ≥ 7.35) on admission. Interestingly, pulmonary artery catheterization was not used in this study, but there were limits placed on the dose of dobutamine (e.g., no more than 10 μg/kg/min) to try to decrease the incidence of drug toxicity. Though the literature is fairly consistent concerning low pHi values being predictive of death,[57,58] pHi-guided therapy to decrease mortality has demonstrated mixed results.[59] Additionally, there are a number of technical considerations that remain to be resolved when using pHi for monitoring and therapy.[60]

In addition to regional monitoring of tissue perfusion, local methods of monitoring are also being studied. For example, subcutaneous measurement of tissue oxygen pressure has shown promise in preliminary investigations. It is unlikely that regional and local measurements will replace more global indicators of perfusion, but rather the methods should complement each other.

ONGOING MANAGEMENT

Proper attention to plasma expansion must be continued into the intraoperative and postoperative periods. A number of neurohormonal changes take place that affect urine output,[61] and patients may have substantial third-spacing of fluid depending on the operation and the preexisting condition of the patient. Furthermore, postoperative patients are prone to hyponatremia from renal generation of electrolyte-free water and from antidiuretic hormone release.[62] As in acute resuscitation, the administration of hypotonic solutions in the perioperative period does not prevent the decrease in extracellular volume that often occurs.[63] Therefore, although excess fluid administration is to be avoided in the perioperative setting, isotonic crystalloid solutions should be used when fluids are indicated to prevent intravascular depletion and circulatory insufficiency.

Of the randomized studies comparing albumin to crystalloid solutions in the perioperative period, the majority found no statistically significant differences between groups.[64] The significant differences that did occur involved isolated hemodynamic or respiratory variables with no obvious clinical correlates (e.g., duration of mechanical ventilation).[65,66] This similarity in efficacy has been substantiated by meta-analyses comparing albumin to crystalloid solutions.[67,68] Therefore, albumin (and other colloids) cannot be recommended for the prevention or initial treatment of circulatory insufficiency, although their use may be appropriate in patients who are not responding to crystalloids and are developing problems such as interstitial fluid accumulation. Practice guidelines published by a consortium of academic medical centers reflect this recommendation,[69] but colloids continue to be widely used.[70]

In general, medications are not indicated in the initial therapy of hypovolemic shock. With hypovolemia, the body's natural response is to increase cardiac output and constrict blood vessels to maintain blood pressure. There is no reason why most patients should need inotropic or vasoactive agents assuming fluid therapy is adequate. For that matter, there is no evidence that these medications improve outcome in patients with hypovolemic shock. However, once the cause of acute circulatory insufficiency has been stopped or treated and fluids have been optimized, some patients continue to have signs and symptoms of inadequate tissue perfusion. This may be due to reperfusion injury. Although the search for a cryptogenic source (e.g., intraabdominal bleeding in a trauma patient) should continue, the clinician may need to administer medications to improve perfusion.

Pressor agents such as norepinephrine and high-dose dopamine are to be avoided, if at all possible, because they may increase blood pressure at the expense of peripheral tissue ischemia. Some sources use stronger language and state that vasopressors are contraindicated in certain forms of shock (e.g., hemorrhagic).[7] This does not help the clinician who is treating a patient with unstable blood pressure despite massive fluid replacement and increasing interstitial fluid accumulation. In such situations, inotropic agents such as dobutamine are preferred if blood pressure is adequate (e.g., systolic blood pressure ≥ 90 mm Hg), because they should not aggravate the existing vasoconstriction. The inotropes are justified by presumed inadequate cardiac output for the specific situation, although the measured values may be in the normal range.[3]

When pressure cannot be maintained with inotropes, or when inotropes with vasodilatory properties cannot be used due to inadequate blood pressure concerns, pressors may be required as a last resort. Although the response to pressor agents may be variable in hypovolemic shock, there does not appear to be resistance due to altered receptor response sometimes seen in patients with septic shock.[3] Potent vasoconstrictors such as norepinephrine and phenylephrine should be given through central veins due to the possibility of extravasation and necrosis with peripheral administration.

A number of interesting treatments for shock are under investigation, including autotransfusion for removing harmful cytokines from the body. Various alternatives to conventional blood components are also being studied, such as stroma-free hemoglobin and perfluorocarbon compounds, as virus-free alternatives to red blood cell transfusion. Hopefully these will be useful adjuncts to adequate volume replacement, which is the primary therapeutic intervention in managing acute circulatory insufficiency due to volume depletion.

PHARMACOECONOMIC CONSIDERATIONS

The primary therapy for hypovolemic shock is fluid replacement. The institutional cost of 1 L of most crystalloid solutions is less than $1. Assuming such fluids are used, it is the associated costs of personnel and equipment that become the primary economic considerations in the resuscitation of patients with hypovolemic shock. However, as mentioned, many clinicians have recommended that colloid plasma expanders (e.g., albumin, hetastarch, dextrans) be used to replace some or all of the standard crystalloid solutions. While the costs of these solutions vary, depending on contractual arrangements as might occur with purchasing groups, in general, albumin solutions are more expensive than hetastarch and dextran products. All of these are markedly more costly than crystalloid solutions; in some cases there are 50- to 100-fold differences even when used in equipotent amounts.

The only recent trial that investigated albumin use on a large-scale basis was an observational study involving 15 academic medical centers in the United States.[69] Based on previously published guidelines,[70] 62% of albumin use was defined as inappropriate at a cost of $124,939. Presuming equal efficacy and toxicity (as available studies indicate) between crystalloid and colloid solutions, cost minimization analysis clearly indicates the economic advantages of the crystalloids.

Because medications are not simply alternatives to crystalloids, but rather are used when crystalloid therapy has been optimized, there is little reason to compare medication and fluid therapies from an economic perspective. Furthermore, there are no economic comparisons of the various inotropic and vasopressor medications used in the treatment of hypovolemic shock.

CONCLUSIONS

Figure 22–4 is an algorithm that summarizes many of the treatment principles discussed in this chapter. The algorithm is intended to be used as an example of one approach to the adult patient presenting with hypovolemic shock. It presumes that initial rehydration attempts (i.e., outpatient or pre-hospital) have been unsuccessful in restoring circulation. Obviously, modifications may be needed for patient-specific forms of hypovolemic shock. Other limitations of the algorithm should be recognized, particularly the decisions to add or substitute colloid or medication therapies when crystalloid solutions are not yielding desired results and when to perform pulmonary artery catheterization for more invasive monitoring. Medications become more important for the ongoing management of hypovolemic shock,

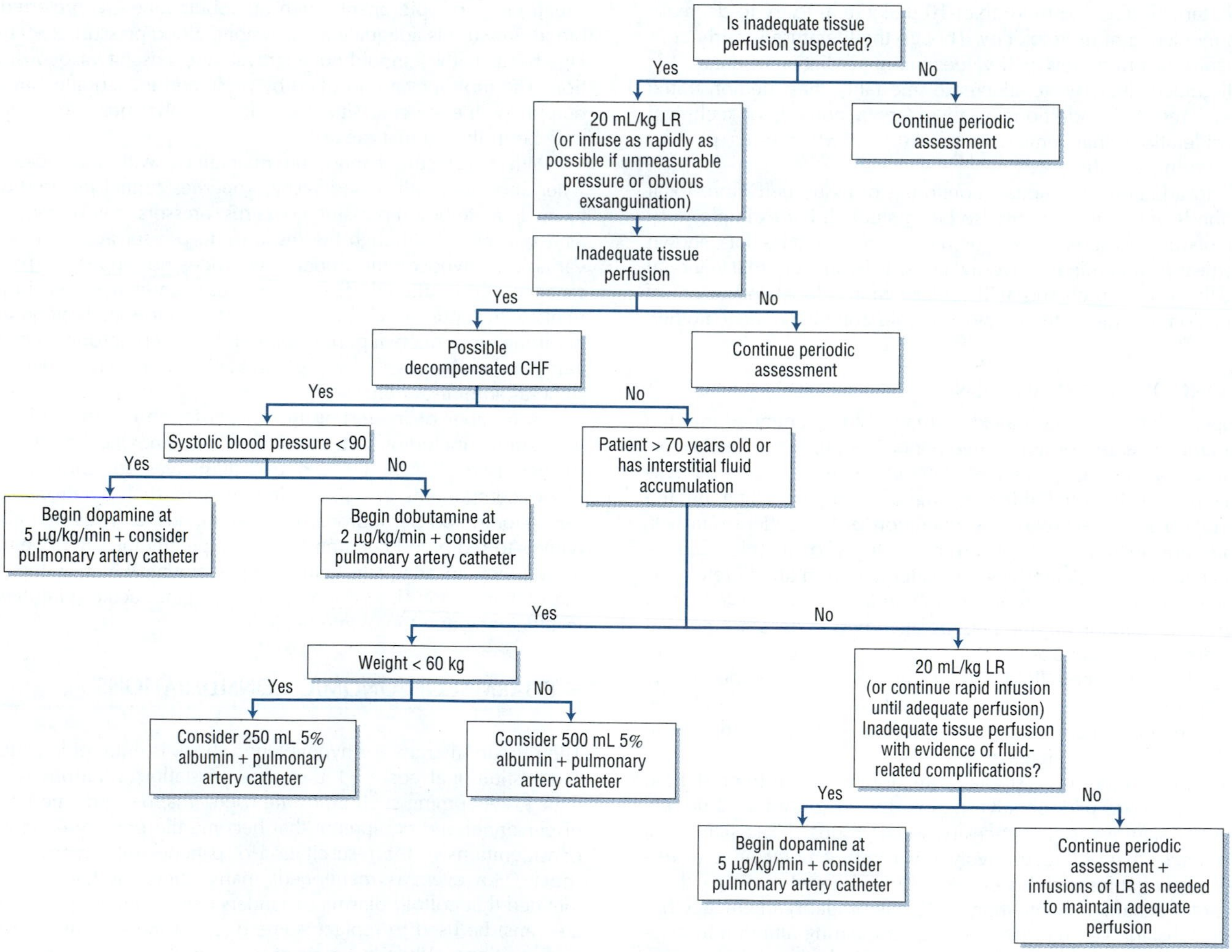

FIGURE 22–4. Hypovolemia protocol for adults. This protocol is not intended to replace or delay therapies such as surgical intervention or blood products for restoring oxygen-carrying capacity or hemostasis. If available, some measurements may be used in addition to those listed in the algorithm, such as mean arterial pressure or pulmonary artery catheter recordings. The latter may be used to assist in medication choices (e.g., agents with primary pressor effects may be desirable in patients with normal cardiac outputs, whereas dopamine or dobutamine may be indicated in patients with suboptimal cardiac outputs). Lower maximal doses of the medications in this algorithm should be considered when pulmonary artery catheterization is not available. LR = lactated Ringer's solution; CHF = congestive heart failure. Colloids that may be substituted for albumin are hetastarch 6% and dextran 40. See text for an in-depth discussion of these and other issues involved in this protocol.

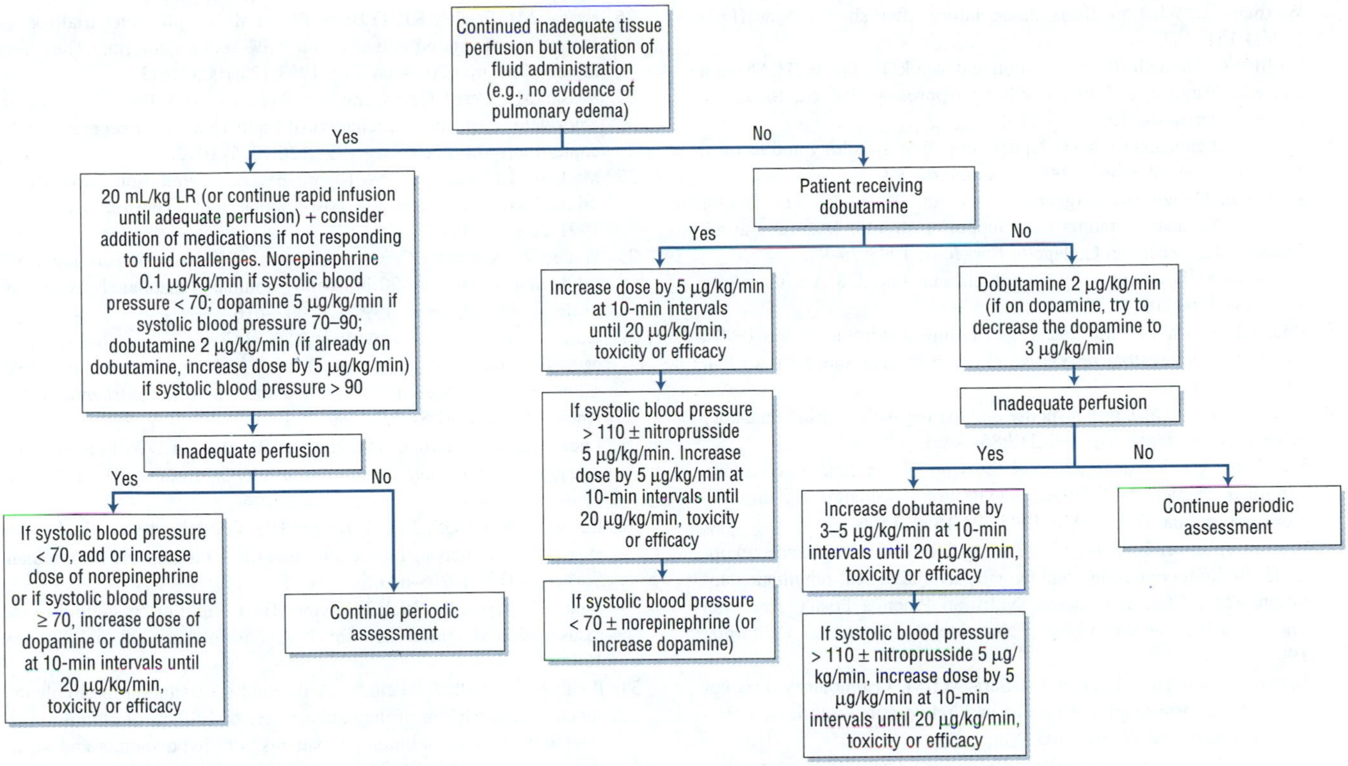

FIGURE 22–5. Ongoing management of inadequate tissue perfusion. LR = lactated Ringer's solution; CHF = congestive heart failure.

particularly when the patient is unresponsive to fluids (see Fig. 22–5). Additionally, it is hoped that the options for more complicated cases of hypovolemic shock do not detract from the primary effective resuscitative measure for most patients: fluid.

▶ PRINCIPLES OF PHARMACOTHERAPY

- Restoring circulating blood volume is a common goal in managing all forms of shock.
- Tissue injury and death may result from inadequate tissue perfusion during the primary shock event or from reperfusion injury associated with subsequent compensatory changes.
- The presentation of patients with acute circulatory insufficiency can vary markedly depending on the cause, as well as patient-specific considerations such as age, concomitant disease states, and medications.
- All patients with suspected circulatory insufficiency should be assessed and monitored by vital signs, urine output, mental status, physical examination, and history.
- In patients with hemodynamic instability due to circulatory insufficiency, isotonic crystalloid solutions such as lactated Ringer's are preferred over dextrose-based solutions.
- Colloids such as albumin have theoretical advantages compared to crystalloid solutions when treating patients with hypovolemic shock, but no substantial differences in efficacy have been demonstrated in published clinical investigations.
- The prehospital administration of fluids in patients with circulatory insufficiency due to blood loss should not be performed if it is likely to cause substantial delays in transportation to a medical facility.
- In patients with hemorrhagic shock, blood products may be needed to restore the oxygen-carrying and clotting functions of blood, because neither crystalloids nor colloids have these properties.
- The value of pulmonary artery catheterization for monitoring patients with hypovolemic shock is controversial.
- Vasopressor medications should not be used in the initial stages of hypovolemic shock, because they may increase blood pressure at the expense of peripheral flow.

REFERENCES

1. Cowley RA, Attar S, LaBrosse E, et al. Some significant biochemical parameters found in 300 shock patients. J Trauma 1969;9:926–938.
2. Shoemaker WC. Temporal physiologic patterns of shock and circulatory dysfunction based on early descriptions by invasive and noninvasive monitoring. New Horiz 1996;4:300–318.
3. Ramsay G, Boom S. Pathophysiology and management of shock. In: Cuschieri A, Giles GR, Moossa AR, eds. Essential Surgical Practice, 3rd ed. Oxford, Butterworth-Heinemann, 1995:72–89.

4. Waxman K. What mediates tissue injury after shock? New Horiz 1996;4:151–152.
5. Cioffi WG, Gamelli RL. Circulation and shock. In: Davis JH, Sheldon GF, eds. Surgery: A Problem-solving Approach, 2nd ed. St. Louis, Mosby–Year Book, 1995:126–165.
6. Marzi I. Hemorrhagic shock: Update in pathophysiology and therapy. Acta Anaesthesiol Scand 1997;111(suppl):42–44.
7. American College of Surgeons. Shock. In: Alexander RH, Proctor HJ, eds. Advanced Trauma Life Support Instructor Manual, 5th ed. Chicago, IL, American College of Surgeons, 1993:76–94.
8. Richardson JD. What's new in trauma and burns. J Am Coll Surg 1997;184:210–216.
9. Beal AL, Cerra FB. Multiple organ failure syndrome in the 1990s: Systemic inflammatory response and organ dysfunction. JAMA 1994; 271:226–233.
10. Sternberg EM. The stress response and the regulation of inflammatory disease. Ann Intern Med 1992;117:854–866.
11. Weinberg AD, Minaker KL, and the Council on Scientific Affairs, American Medical Association. Dehydration: Evaluation and management in older patients. JAMA 1995;274:1552–1556.
12. Tarrosa V, Stoner G, George L, Fleming CR. Alterations needed to optimize sodium content in commercially available oral rehydration solutions. 21st Clinical Congress Nutrition Practice Poster. American Society of Parenteral and Enteral Nutrition. San Francisco, California, 1997 January.
13. Brouns F, Senden J, Beckers EJ, Saris WHM. Osomolarity does not affect the gastric emptying rate of oral rehydration solutions. J Parenter Erenter Nutr 1995;19:403–406.
14. Duggan C, Santosham M, Glass RI. The management of acute diarrhea in children: Oral rehydration, maintenance, and nutritional therapy. MMWR 1992;41:1–20.
15. Reid SR, Bonadio WA. Outpatient rapid intravenous rehydration to correct dehydration and resolve vomiting in children with acute gastroenteritis. Ann Emerg Med 1996;28:318–323.
16. Luten RC. Rapid rehydration of pediatric patients. Ann Emerg Med 1996;28:353–355.
17. Axler OA, Tousiganant C, Thompson CR, et al. Small hemodynamic effect of typical rapid volume infusions in critically ill patients. Crit Care Med 1997;25:965–970.
18. Didwania A, Miller J, Kassel D, et al. Effect of intravenous lactated Ringer's solution infusion on the circulating lactate concentration: Results of a prospective, randomized, double-blind, placebo-controlled trial. Crit Care Med 1997;25:1851–1854.
19. Jackson EV, Wiese J, Sigal B, et al. Effects of crystalloid solutions on circulating lactate concentrations: Part 1. Implications for the proper handling of blood specimens obtained in critically ill patients. Crit Care Med 1996;24:1840–1846.
19A. Schierhout G, Roberts I. Fluid resuscitation with colloid or crystalloid solutions in critically ill patients: A systematic review of randomised trials. BMJ 1998;316:961–964.
19B. Cochrane Injuries Group Albumin Reviewers. Human albumin administration in critically ill patients: Systematic review of randomized controlled trials. BMJ 1998;317:235–240.
20. Bickell WH. Are victims of injury sometimes victimized by attempts at fluid resuscitation? Ann Emerg Med 1993;22:225–226.
21. Bickell WH, Wall MJ, Pepe PE, et al. Immediate versus delayed fluid resuscitation for hypotensive patients with penetrating torso injuries. N Engl J Med 1994;331:1105–1109.
22. Jacobs LM. Timing of fluid resuscitation in trauma. N Engl J Med 1994;331:1153–1154.
23. Prough DS, Zornow MH. Solutions in search of problems. Crit Care Med 1996;24:1104–1105.
24. Saetzler Rk, Badellino MM, Buckman RF, et al. Hypertonic saline attenuates leukocyte/endothelium and leukocyte/platelet interactions following hemorrhagic shock. Surg Forum 1996;47:41–43.
25. Angle N, Coimbra R, Hoyt DB, et al. Hypertonic saline resuscitation prevents lung injury following hemorrhagic shock. Surg Forum 1996; 47:43–45.
26. Vassar MJ, Fischer RP, O'Brien PE, et al. A multicenter trial for resuscitation of injured patients with 7.5% sodium chloride: The effect of added dextran 70. Arch Surg 1993;128:1003–1013.
27. Vassar MJ, Perry CA, Gannaway WL, Holcraft JW. 7.5% sodium chloride/dextran for resuscitation of trauma patients undergoing helicopter transport. Arch Surg 1991;126:1065–1072.
28. Mattox KL, Maningas PA, Moore EE, et al. Prehospital hypertonic saline/dextran infusion for post-traumatic hypotension. Ann Surg 1991;213:482–491.
29. Wade CE, Kramer GC, Grady JJ, et al. Efficay of hypertonic 7.5% saline and 6% dextran-70 in treating trauma: A meta-analysis of controlled studies. Surgery 1997;122:609–616.
30. Gurevich B, Talmore D, Artru AA, et al. Brain edema, hemorrhagic necrosis volume, and neurological status with rapid infusion of 0.45% saline or 5% dextrose in 0.9% saline after closed head trauma in rats. Anesth Analg 1997;84:554–559.
31. Lucas CE, Ledgerwood AM, Higgins RF, Weaver DW. Impaired pulmonary function after albumin resuscitation from shock. J Trauma 1980:20;446–451.
32. Lowe RJ, Moss GS, Jilek J, Levine HD. Crystalloid vs colloid in the etiology of pulmonary failure after trauma: A randomized trial in man. Surgery 1977;81:676–683.
33. Moss GS, Lowe RJ, Jilek J, Levine HD. Colloid or crystalloid in the resuscitation of hemorrhagic shock: A controlled clinical trial. Surgery 1981;89:434–438.
34. Rackow EC, Falk JL, Fein A, et al. Fluid resuscitation in circulatory shock: A comparison of the cardiorespiratory effects of albumin, hetastarch, and saline solutions in patients with hypovolemia and septic shock. Crit Care Med 1983;11:839–850.
35. Gentileilo LM, Jurkovich GJ, Stark MS, et al. Is hypothermia in the victim of major trauma protective or harmful: A randomized, prospective study. Ann Surg 1997;226:439–449.
36. Goodwin CW, Dorethy J, Lam V, Pruitt BA. Randomized trial of efficacy of crystalloid and colloid resuscitation on hemodynamic response and lung water following thermal injury. Ann Surg 1983; 197:520–531.
37. Gore DC, Dalton JM, Gehr TWB. Colloid infusions reduce glomerular filtration in resuscitated burn victims. J Trauma 1996;40:356–360.
38. Greenhalgh DG, Housinger TA, Kagan RJ, et al. Maintenance of serum albumin levels in pediatric burn patients: A prospective, randomized trial. J Trauma 1995;39:67–74.
39. Tanaka H, Matsuda H, Shimazaki S, et al. Reduced resuscitation fluid volume for second-degree burns with delayed initiation of ascorbic acid therapy. Arch Surg 1997;132:158–161.
40. Gallagher EJ, Rodriguez K, Touger M. Agreement between peripheral venous and arterial lactate levels. Ann Emerg Med 1997; 29:479–483.
41. Shoemaker WC, Appel PL, Kram HB, et al. Prospective trial of supranormal values of survivors as therapeutic goals in high-risk surgical patients. Chest 1988;94:1176–1186.
42. Erstad BL. Oxygen transport goals in the resuscitation of critically ill patients. Ann Pharmacother 1994;28:1273–1284.
43. Gattinoni L, Brazzi L, Pelosi P, et al. A trial of goal-oriented hemodynamic therapy in critically ill patients. N Engl J Med 1995; 333:1025–1032.
44. Fleming A, Bishop M, Shoemaker W, et al. Prospective trial of supranormal values as goals of resuscitation in severe trauma. Arch Surg 1992;127:1175–1181.
45. Boyd O, Grounds RM, Bennett ED. A randomized clinical trial of the effect of deliberate perioperative increase of oxygen delivery on mortality in high-risk surgical patients. JAMA 1993;270: 2699–2707.
46. Hinds C, Watson D. Manipulating hemodynamics and oxygen transport in critically ill patients. N Engl J Med 1995;333:1074–1075.
47. Connors AF, Speroff T, Dawson NV, et al. The effectiveness of right heart catheterization in the initial care of critically ill patients. JAMA 1996;276:889–897.
48. Dalen JE, Bone RC. Is it time to pull the pulmonary artery catheter? JAMA 1996;276:916–918.

49. Dobb GJ. The pulmonary artery catheter: Too early for its swan song? Intensive Care World 1996;13:139–140.
50. Taylor RW, Ahrens T, Beilin Y, et al. Pulmonary artery consensus conference: Consensus statement. Crit Care Med 1997;25:190–200.
51. Ginosar Y, Thijs LG, Sprung CL. Raising the standard of hemodynamic monitoring: Targeting the practice or the practitioner? Crit Care Med 1997;25:209–211.
52. Mimoz O, Rauss A, Rekik N, et al. Pulmonary artery catheterization in critically ill patients: A prospective analysis of outcome changes associated with catheter-prompted changes in therapy. Crit Care Med 1994;22:573–579.
53. Connors AF. Right heart catheterization: Is it effective? New Horiz 1997;5:195–200.
54. Peruzzi WT. Hemodynamic monitoring: Does the end justify the means? Crit Care Med 1997;25:1767–1768.
55. Burchell SA, Yu M, Takiguchi SA, Ohta RM. Evaluation of a continuous cardiac output and mixed venous oxygen saturation catheter in critically ill surgery patients. Crit Care Med 1997;2:388–391.
56. Gutierrez G, Palizas F, Doglio G, et al. Gastric intramucosal pH as a therapeutic index of tissue oxygenation in critically ill patients. Lancet 1992;339:195–199.
57. Maynard N, Bihari D, Beale R, et al. Assessment of splanchnic oxygenation by gastric tonometry in patients with acute circulatory failure. JAMA 1993;270:1203–1210.
58. Ivatury RR, Simon RJ, Islam S, et al. A prospective randomized study of end points of resuscitation after major trauma: Global oxygen transport indices verses organ-specific gastric mucosal pH. J Am Coll Surg 1996;183:145–154.
59. Gomersall CD, Joynt GM, Freebairn RC, et al. Does pHi guided therapy reduce mortality in the critically ill? Intensive Care Med 1996; 22(suppl 3):S438.
60. Garrett SA, Pearl RG. Improved gastric tonometry for monitoring tissue perfusion: The canary sings louder. Anesth Analg 1996;83:1–3.
61. Quesne LP, Cochrane JPS, Fieldman NR. Fluid and electrolyte disturbances after trauma: The role of adrenocortical and pituitary hormones. Br Med Bull 1985;41:212–217.
62. Steele A, Gowrishankar M, Abrahamson S, et al. Postoperative hyponatremia despite near-isotonic saline infusion: A phenomenon of desalination. Ann Intern Med 1997;126:20–25.
63. Roberts JP, Roberts JD, Skinner C, et al. Extracellular fluid deficit following operation and its correction with Ringer's lactate. Ann Surg 1985;202:1–8.
64. Erstad BL, Gales BJ, Rappaport WD. The use of albumin in clinical practice. Arch Intern Med 1991;151:901–911.
65. Boutros AR, Ruess R, Olson L, et al. Comparison of hemodynamic, pulmonary, and renal effects of use of three types of fluids after major surgical procedures on the abdominal aorta. Crit Care Med 1979; 7:9–13.
66. Zetterstrom H, Hedstrand U. Albumin treatment following major surgery. I. Effects on plasma oncotic pressure, renal function and peripheral oedema. Acta Anaesth Scand 1981;25:125–132.
67. Velanovich V. Crystalloid versus colloid fluid resuscitation: A meta-analysis of mortality. Surgery 1989;105:65–71.
68. Bisonni AS, Holtgrave DR, Lawler F, Marley DS. Colloids versus crystalloids in fluid resuscitation: An analysis of randomized controlled trials. J Fam Pract 1991;32:387–390.
69. Vermeulen LC, Ratko TA, Erstad BL, et al. A paradigm for consensus: The University Hospital Consortium guidelines for the use of albumin, nonprotein colloid, and crystalloid solutions. Arch Intern Med 1995;155:373–379.
70. Yim JM, Vermeulen LC, Erstad BL, et al. Albumin and nonprotein colloid solution use in US academic health centers. Arch Intern Med 1995;155:2450–2455.

23
PULMONARY FUNCTION TESTING

Jay I. Peters, MD, and David C. Shelledy, PhD

GENERAL CONCEPTS

The primary function of the respiratory system is to maintain Pa_{O_2} and Pa_{CO_2} (the arterial pressure of oxygen and carbon dioxide) within the normal range. To accomplish this task, several processes must be accomplished, including alveolar ventilation, pulmonary perfusion, ventilation–perfusion matching, and gas transfer across the alveolar–capillary membrane.

Alveolar ventilation is achieved by the cyclic process of air movement into and out of the lung. During inspiration, the inspiratory muscle contracts and generates negative pressure in the pleural space. This pressure gradient between the mouth and the alveoli draws fresh air (tidal volume) into the lung. Approximately one-third of the inspired gas stays in the conducting airways (dead space) while two-thirds reaches the alveoli.

The human lung contains a series of branching, progressively tapering airways that originate at the glottis and terminate in a matrix of thin-walled alveoli. Coursing through this matrix of alveoli is a rich network of capillaries that originates from the pulmonary arterioles and terminates in the pulmonary venules. The adequacy of respiration in each gas-exchange unit depends on the opposition of a thin film of mixed venous blood with just the right amount of fresh alveolar gas. During "ideal" gas exchange, there is uniform blood flow and uniform ventilation; accordingly, there is no alveolar–aterial P_{O_2} difference (P_{A-aO_2} gradient, sometimes called the A–a gradient). Gas exchange is not perfect, however, even in the normal lung. Normally, there is less alveolar ventilation than pulmonary blood flow, and the overall ventilation-to-perfusion ratio is 0.8 (not 1.0).

Normal expiration is a passive process, and when the inspiratory muscles end their contraction, the elastic recoil of the lung pulls the lung back to its original size and shape. This process makes the alveolar pressure positive relative to the pressure at the mouth, and air flows out of the lung. During inspiration, the respiratory muscles must overcome the elastic properties of the lung (elastic recoil) and the resistance to airflow by the airways. During expiration, the flow of air is primarily determined by the elastic recoil and airway resistance.

Different pulmonary function tests (PFTs) are used to evaluate the physiologic process of the respiratory system. Physiologic abnormalities that can be measured by pulmonary function testing include obstruction to airflow, restriction of lung size, and decrease in the transfer of gas across the alveolar–capillary membrane. Abnormal values on pulmonary function tests are those outside the range of values obtained from a group of normal individuals matched according to age, height, gender, and race. A pulmonary function test is labeled abnormal when the results fall outside the range in which 95% of people the same age, height, and gender would be found (95% confidence interval). This definition is arbitrary and may misclassify a small percentage of normals as having lung dysfunction. Therefore, clinical correlation and serial pulmonary function testing may be necessary for optimal interpretation of PFTs.

Potential uses of PFTs include the evaluation of patients with known or suspected lung disease; the evaluation of symptoms such as chronic cough, dyspnea, or chest tightness; monitoring the effects of exposure to dust, chemicals, or pulmonary toxic drugs; risk stratification prior to surgery; monitoring the effectiveness of therapeutic interventions; and objective assessment of impairment or disability.[1]

Summary of Abbreviations

COPD	Chronic obstructive pulmonary disease
DL	Lung diffusing capacity
DLCO	Carbon monoxide diffusing capacity
ERV	Expiratory reserve volume
$FEF_{25\%-75\%}$	Forced expiratory flow during 25% to 75% FVC
FEV_1	Forced expiratory volume in one second
FIF	Forced inspiratory flow
FRC	Functional residual capacity
FVC	Forced vital capacity
IC	Inspiratory capacity
IRV	Inspiratory reserve volume
MIP	Maximum inspiratory pressure
MMEF	Maximum midexpiratory flow
MVV	Maximum voluntary ventilation
Pa_{O_2}	Arterial partial pressure of oxygen
P_{A-aO_2}	Alveolar – arterial P_{O_2} difference in partial pressure of oxygen
Pa_{CO_2}	Arterial partial pressure of carbon dioxide
PEF	Peak expiratory flow
PFT	Pulmonary function test
RV	Residual volume

Sa_{O_2}	Arterial oxygen saturation
Sp_{O_2}	Arterial oxygen saturation estimated from pulse oximetry
SVC	Slow vital capacity
TLC	Total lung capacity
V_A	Alveolar volume
VC	Vital capacity
$\dot{V}CO_2$	Carbon dioxide production
$\dot{V}O_2$	Oxygen consumption
$\dot{V}_E$	Expired minute volume
V_T	Tidal volume

DEFINITIONS OF LUNG VOLUMES AND EXPIRATORY VALUES

The air within the lung at the end of a forced inspiration can be divided into four compartments or lung volumes (Fig. 23–1). The volume of air exhaled during normal quiet breathing is termed "tidal volume" (V_T). The maximum volume of air inhaled above tidal volume is called the inspiratory reserve volume (IRV) and the maximum air exhaled below tidal volume is called the expiratory reserve volume (ERV). The residual volume (RV) is the amount of air remaining in the lungs after a maximum exhalation.

The combinations or sums of two or more lung volumes are termed *capacities* (Fig. 23–1). Vital capacity (VC) is the maximum amount of air that can be exhaled after a maximum inspiration. It is equal to the sum of the IRV, V_T, and ERV. When measured on a forced expiration, it is called the forced vital capacity (FVC). When measured over an exhalation of at least 30 seconds, it is called the slow vital capacity (SVC, VC). The VC is approximately 75% of the total lung capacity (TLC), and when the SVC is within the normal range, a significant restrictive disorder is unlikely. Normally, the value for SVC and FVC are very similar unless airway obstruction is present.

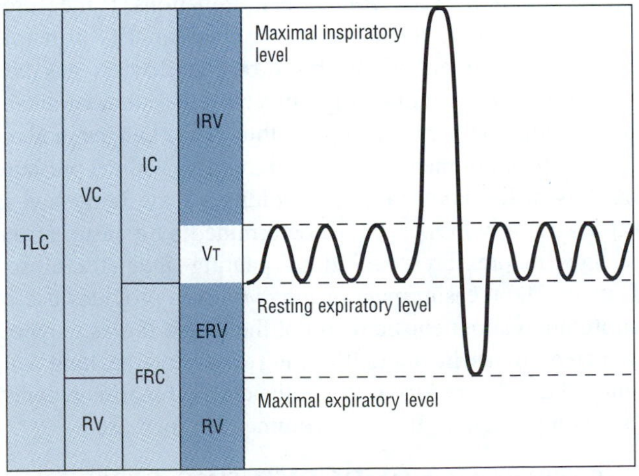

FIGURE 23–1. Lung volumes and capacities. V_T = tidal volume; IRV = inspiratory reserve volume; ERV = expiratory reserve volume; RV = residual volume; IC = inspiratory capacity; FRC = functional residual capacity; VC = vital capacity; TLC = total lung capacity. *(Adapted from Ref. 12.)*

The TLC is the volume of air in the lung after the maximum inspiration and is the sum of the four primary lung volumes (IRV, V_T, ERV, RV). Its measurement is difficult because the amount of air remaining in the chest after maximum exhalation (RV) must be measured by indirect methods. The definition of restrictive lung disease is based on a reduction in TLC (i.e., inability to get air into the lung or restriction to air movement on inhalation).

The functional residual capacity (FRC) is the volume of air remaining in the lungs at the end of a quiet expiration. FRC is the normal resting position of the lung and occurs when there is no contraction of either inspiratory or expiratory muscles and is normally 40% of TLC. Inspiratory capacity (IC) is the maximum volume of air that can be inhaled from the end of a quiet expiration and represents the sum of V_T and IRV.

The FVC, which represents the total amount of air than can be exhaled, can be expressed as a series of timed volumes. The forced expiratory volume in 1 second (FEV_1) is the volume of air exhaled during the first second of the FVC maneuver. Although the FEV_1 is a volume, it conveys information on obstruction because it is measured over a known time interval. The FEV_1 is dependent on the volume of air within the lung and the effort during exhalation; therefore, it can be diminished by a decrease in TLC or by a lack of effort. A more sensitive way to measure obstruction is to express the FEV_1 as a ratio of FVC. This ratio is independent of the patient's size or the TLC; therefore, the FEV_1/FVC is a specific measure of airway obstruction with or without restriction. Normally, this ratio is 75% or greater and any value below 70% to 75% suggests obstruction.

Because flow is defined as the change in volume with time, forced expiratory flow (FEF) may be determined graphically by dividing the volume change by the time change. The FEF during 25% to 75% of FVC ($FEF_{25\%-75\%}$) represents the mean flow during the middle half of the FVC. The $FEF_{25\%-75\%}$, formerly called the maximum midexpiratory flow (MMEF), is frequently reported to assess small airways. The 95% confidence limit is so wide that the $FEF_{25\%-75\%}$ has limited utility in the early diagnosis of small-airways disease in an individual subject. The peak expiratory flow (PEF), also called maximum forced expiratory flow (FEF_{max}) is the maximum flow obtained during the FVC. This measurement is often used in the outpatient management of asthma because it can be measured with inexpensive peak flow meters.

SPIROMETRY/FLOW–VOLUME LOOP

Spirometry is the most widely available and useful PFT. It takes only 15 to 20 minutes, carries no risks, and provides information about obstructive and restrictive disease. Spirometry allows for the measurement of all lung volumes and capacities except RV, FRC, and TLC and allows

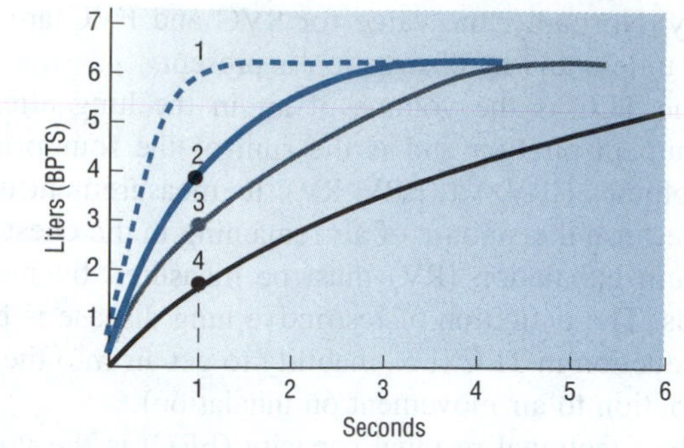

FIGURE 23–2. Standard spirometry. Curve (1) is a normal subject with a normal FEV_1; (2) FEV_1 in a patient with mild airways obstruction; (3) a patient with moderate airways obstruction; (4) a patient with severe airways obstruction. BPTS = body temperature saturated with water vapor.

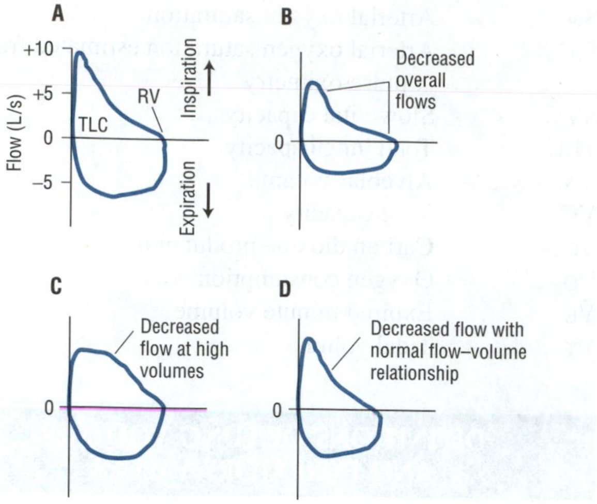

FIGURE 23–4. Flow–volume loops depicting (A) mild obstruction characterized by decreased flow at low lung volumes, (B) moderate airflow obstruction characterized by a more concave curve, (C) variable intrathoracic obstruction in which peak flow is decreased at higher lung volume with normalization of curve at lower lung volumes, and (D) restrictive lung disease with a curve that is decreased in height and width but with a normal shape. *(From George RB, Light RW, Mathay MA, Mathay RA. Chest Medicine, 3rd ed. Baltimore, Williams & Wilkins, 1995, with permission.)*

the assessment of FEV_1 and $FEF_{25\%-75\%}$. Spirometry measurements can be reported in two different formats: standard spirometry (Fig. 23–2) and the flow–volume loop (Fig. 23–3). In standard spirometry, the volumes are recorded on the vertical (*y*) axis and the time on the horizontal (*x*) axis. In flow–volume loops, volume is plotted on the horizontal (*x*) axis and flow (derived from volume/time) is plotted on the vertical (*y*) axis. The shape of the flow–volume loop can be helpful in differentiating obstructive and restrictive defects (Fig. 23–4) and in the diagnosis of upper-airway obstruction. This curve gives a visual representation of obstruction because the expiratory descent becomes more concave with worsening obstruction.

LUNG VOLUMES

Spirometry measures three of the four basic lung volumes but cannot measure RV. RV must be measured to determine the TLC. TLC should be measured anytime there is a reduced VC. In the setting of chronic obstructive pulmonary disease (COPD) with a low VC, measurement of TLC can help determine if there is a superimposed restrictive disorder. There are four methods to measure TLC: helium dilution, nitrogen washout, body plethysmography, and chest x-ray measurement (planimetry). The first two methods are called dilution techniques and measure only lung volumes in communication with the upper airway. In patients with airway obstruction who have trapped air, dilution techniques will underestimate the actual volume of the lungs. Planimetry measures the circumference of the lungs on the posterior–anterior view and lateral view of a chest x-ray and estimates the total lung volume.

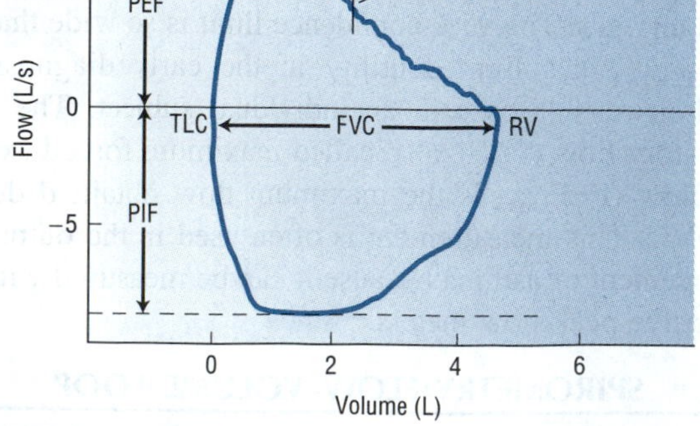

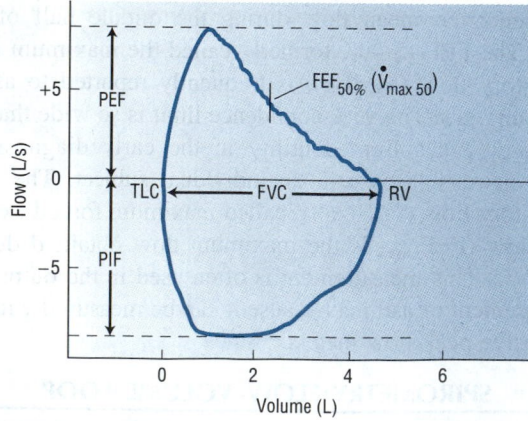

FIGURE 23–3. Normal flow–volume loop. Flows measured on the vertical (*y*) axis and lung volumes measured on the horizontal (*x*) axis. FVC can be read from the tracing as the maximal horizontal deflection. Instantaneous flow (V_{max}) at any point in FVC can also be measured directly. FVC = forced vital capacity. *(Adapted from Ref. 12, with permission.)*

Body plethysmography or body box is the most accurate technique for lung volume determinations. It measures all the air in the lungs, including trapped air. The principle of the measurement of the body box is Boyle's gas law ($P_1V_1 = P_2V_2$): a volume of gas in a closed system varies inversely with the pressure applied to it. The changes in alveolar pressure are measured at the mouth as well as pressure changes in the body box. The volume of the body box is known. Lung volumes can be determined by measuring the changes in pressures caused by panting against a closed shutter.[2] The measurement of lung volumes provides useful information about elastic recoil of the lungs. If elastic recoil is increased (as in interstitial lung disease), the lung volumes (TLC) are reduced. When the elastic recoil is reduced (as in emphysema), the lung volumes are increased.

CARBON MONOXIDE DIFFUSING CAPACITY

The diffusing capacity of the lungs (DL) is a measurement of the ability of a gas to diffuse across the alveolar–capillary membrane. Carbon monoxide is the usual test gas because it is not normally present in the lungs and is much more soluble in blood than in lung tissue. When the diffusing capacity is determined with carbon monoxide, the test is called the carbon monoxide diffusing capacity (DLCO). Because the DLCO is directly related to the alveolar volume (VA), it is frequently normalized to this value (DL/VA), which allows for its interpretation in the presence of abnormal lung volumes (e.g., after surgical lung resection).

The DL will be reduced in all clinical situations in which there is impairment of gas transfer from the alveoli to capillary blood.[2,3] Common conditions that reduce the DLCO include lung resection, emphysema (loss of functioning alveolar–capillary units), and interstitial lung disease (thickening of the alveolar–capillary membrane). Normal PFTs with a reduced DLCO should suggest the possibility of pulmonary vascular disease (e.g., pulmonary embolus) but can also be seen with anemia, early interstitial lung disease, and mild pneumocystic carinii (PCP) infection in AIDS patients.

OBSTRUCTIVE LUNG DISEASE

Obstructive lung disease implies a reduced capacity to get air through the conducting airways and out of the lungs. This reduction in airflow may be caused by a decrease in the diameter of the airways (bronchospasm), a loss of their integrity (bronchomalacia), or a reduction in the elastic recoil (emphysema) with a resultant decrease in the driving pressure. The most common diseases associated with obstructive pulmonary functions are asthma, emphysema, and chronic bronchitis; however, bronchiectasis, infiltration of the bronchial wall by tumor or granuloma, aspiration of a foreign body, and bronchiolitis also cause obstructive pulmonary function tests. The standard test used to evaluate airway obstruction is the forced expiratory spirogram.

Standard spirometry and flow–volume loop measurements include many variables; however, according to the ATS guidelines, the diagnosis of obstructive and restrictive ventilatory defects should be made using the basic measurements of spirometry.[3] A reduction in FEV_1 (with a normal FVC) establishes the diagnosis of obstruction. When both the FEV_1 and FVC are reduced, the FEV_1 cannot be used to assess airway obstruction because such patients may have either obstruction or restriction. In restrictive lung disease, the patient has an inability to get air into the lung, which results in a reduction of all expiratory volumes (FEV_1, FVC, SVC). In obstructive patients, a better measurement is the ratio of the FEV_1 to FVC. Patients with restrictive lung disease have a reduced FEV_1 and a reduced FVC, but the FEV_1/FVC ratio remains normal. Although a normal FEV_1/FVC% is above 70% to 75%, the ratio is age dependent and slightly lower values may be normal in older patients. Caution should be used in interpreting obstruction when the ratio of FEV_1/FVC is below normal but the FEV_1 and FVC are both within the normal range because this pattern can be seen with healthy, athletic subjects. The measurement of $FEF_{25\%-75\%}$ will also be abnormal in patients with obstructive airways disease. In general, this test has so much variability that it adds little to the measurement of FEV_1 and the FEV_1/FVC ratio. $FEF_{25\%-75\%}$ has been of value in monitoring lung transplant patients for graft rejection[4] and may be seen in bone marrow transplant recipients with graft-versus-host disease.

Although there is no standardization for interpretation of severity of obstruction, most pulmonary laboratories state that an FEV_1/FVC ratio of less than 75% of the predicted value is mild obstruction, less than 60% of the predicted value is moderate obstruction, and less than 40% of the predicted value is severe obstruction. In patients with obstruction, a dose of a bronchodilator (e.g., isoproterenol) by metered-dose inhaler is given during the initial exam. If patients have angina or a history of cardiac arrhythmias, a selective β_{-2} agonist (e.g., albuterol) is used. An increase in the FEV_1 of more than 12% and greater than 0.2 L suggests an acute bronchodilator response.[3] Because bronchodilator responsiveness is variable over time, the lack of an acute bronchodilator response should not preclude a 6- to 8-week trial of bronchodilators and/or corticosteroids.

Although all patients with obstructive lung disease of any etiology will have reduced flow rates on forced exhalation, the pattern on pulmonary function tests may be helpful in differentiating among the various etiologies (see Table 23–1). Asthma is characterized by variable obstruction that often improves or resolves with appropriate therapy. Because asthma is an inflammatory disorder of the airways (predominately large airways), the DLCO is normal. Most patients with acute asthma have a bronchodilator response of over 15% to 20%; however, this response is also seen in 20% of patients with COPD. These patients are said to have *asthmatic bronchitis*. Chronic bronchitis may be limited to the airways, but the vast majority of patients with chronic bronchitis and airway obstruction have a mixture of bronchitis and emphysema and have a reduction in DLCO. Therefore, DLCO is the best pulmonary function test in separating asthma from COPD.

TABLE 23–1. Specific Patterns of Pulmonary Function in Patients With Chronic Obstructive Pulmonary Disease (COPD)

	COPD		
	Asthma	*Chronic Bronchitis*	*Emphysema*
Decrease FEV_1	++++	++++	++++
Decrease FEV_1/FVC	++++	++++	++++
Increase airway resistance	++++	++++	+
Decrease DLCO	–	–/++[a]	++++
Response to bronchodilators	++++	+[a]	–[b]

FEV_1 = forced expiratory volume after 1 second; FVC = forced vital capacity; DLCO = diffusing capacity of carbon monoxide.

[a]Most smokers with chronic bronchitis have reduced DLCO.

[b]Twenty percent of patients with COPD have large (++++) bronchodilator response.

Once the diagnosis of obstructive airways disease is established, the course and response to therapy are best followed by serial spirometry. The multicenter Lung Health Study demonstrated an abnormally rapid decline in the FEV_1 (90 to 150 mL/yr) in patients with COPD who continue to smoke.[5] Smoking cessation often resulted in an increase in FEV_1 during the first year and a near-normal rate of decline (30 to 50 mL/yr) in subsequent years.

AIRWAY HYPERREACTIVITY

Airway hyperreactivity or hyperresponsiveness is defined as an exaggerated bronchoconstrictor response to physical, chemical, or pharmacologic stimuli. Individuals with asthma by definition have hyperresponsive airways. Recently, the Lung Health Study Research Group[6] observed nonspecific hyperresponsiveness in a significant number of patients with COPD. This group of patients with airway hyperreactivity appears to have a worse prognosis and an accelerated rate of decline in FEV_1.

Some patients with asthma (especially cough-variant asthma) present with no history of wheezing and normal pulmonary function tests. The diagnosis of asthma can still be established by demonstrating hyperresponsiveness to provocative agents. The two agents most widely used in clinical practice are methacholine and histamine. Other agents used for bronchial provocation include distilled water, cold air, and exercise. During a typical bronchoprovocation test, a baseline FEV_1 is measured after the inhalation of isotonic saline, and then increasing doses of methacholine are given at set intervals. Hyperresponsiveness is defined by a decline in FEV_1 of 20% or greater and by reversibility of obstruction to bronchodilators. The result can best be expressed as the provocative concentration necessary to cause a fall in FEV_1 of 20% (PC_{20}). A test is considered positive if either methacholine or histamine demonstrate a PC_{20} for FEV_1 at 8 mg/mL or less, or fewer than 60 to 80 cumulative breath units.[7] This test is most frequently used to establish a diagnosis of asthma in patients with normal PFTs but may be useful in following patients with occupational asthma, establishing the severity of asthma, and assessing the response to treatment.

UPPER-AIRWAY OBSTRUCTION

Obstruction of airflow by abnormalities in the upper airway often go undiagnosed or misdiagnosed because of improper interpretation of the pulmonary function tests. The patients have obstructive physiology and often are misclassified as having asthma or COPD. The shape of the flow–volume loop, which includes inspiratory and expiratory flow–volume curves, and ratio of the expiratory and inspiratory flow at 50% of vital capacity ($FEF_{50\%}$/forced inspiratory flow $[FIF]_{50\%}$) may be useful in the diagnosis of upper-airway obstruction.[8]

The shape of the flow–volume curve differs depending on whether the obstruction is fixed or variable. Fixed lesions, as in strictures from previous intubation or tracheostomy, cause a uniform caliber of the airway during inspiration and expiration. With variable lesions, however, the airway caliber changes with changes in intrathoracic pressure. Variable lesions are subclassified into variable intrathoracic and variable extrathoracic. If the lesion is intrathoracic, as with tumors of the trachea, the negative pressure generated during inspiration opens the obstruction, whereas the positive pressure during expiration worsens the obstruction. If there is variable extrathoracic obstruction, as with vocal cord dysfunction, the negative pressure within the airways will pull the vocal cord toward the midline and potentiate the obstruction. In this case, there will be a plateau on the inspiratory limb on the flow–volume loop and the $FEF_{50\%}/FIF_{50\%}$ will be greater than one. Typical flow–volume curves from upper-airway obstruction can be seen in Fig. 23–5.

Another test used to distinguish upper-airway obstruction from COPD and asthma is the $FEV_1/FEV_{0.5}$ (forced expiratory volume at 1 second/forced expiratory volume at 0.5 second). This ratio is usually greater than 1.5 in patients with upper-airway obstruction.[9] This is because the $FEV_{0.5}$ is proportionately more reduced in upper-airway obstruction because forced expiration measured at 0.5 second better reflects obstruction at high lung volumes. The abnormality seen on the flow–volume loop has been referred to as "straightening" of the curve during early expiration.

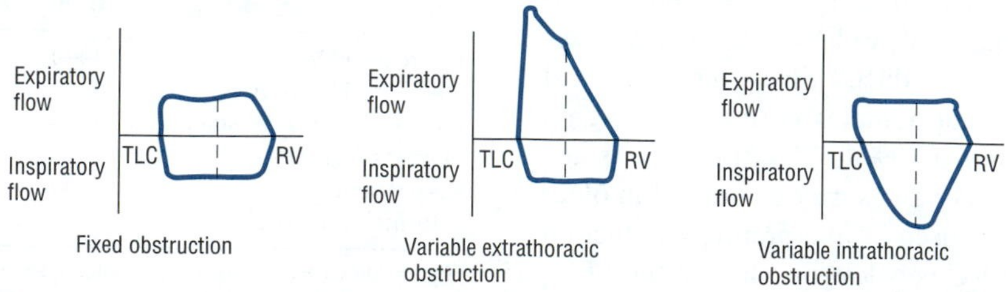

FIGURE 23–5. Maximum expiratory flow volume curves from patients with fixed obstruction, variable extrathoracic obstruction, and variable intrathoracic obstruction. TLC = total lung capacity; RV = residual volume.

RESTRICTIVE LUNG DISEASE

Restrictive lung disease is defined as an inability to get air into the lungs and maintain normal lung volumes. Restrictive lung disease reduces all the subdivisions of lung volumes (IRV, VT, ERV, RV) without reduction in airflow. These patients have normal airway resistance, and their FEV_1/FVC ratio is greater than 75%.

Although restriction could be defined as a reduction in vital capacity (VC or FVC) with a normal FEV_1/FVC ratio, poor effort will also reduce FVC with a normal FEV_1/FVC ratio. A reduction in the TLC is the most accurate measurement of restrictive lung function. As mentioned previously, TLC can be measured by various techniques. The gas dilution methods (helium dilution, nitrogen washout) are unable to measure gas trapped in cysts or bullae and may underestimate the true lung volume. Therefore, TLC is best measured by plethysmography. Most restrictive lung disease is associated with impairment or destruction of the alveolar–capillary membrane, and therefore the DLCO is reduced in most patients with restrictive lung disease. The measurement of DLCO may occur prior to reduction in lung volumes and is used as a marker of early interstitial (restrictive) lung disease. The DLCO may be abnormal even with a normal chest x-ray, and thin-cut computed tomography scans of the chest may be required to diagnose early interstitial lung disease. Since peribronchiolar inflammation and fibrosis occurs in patients with restrictive parenchymal lung disease, the $FEF_{25\%-75\%}$ may be reduced and fails to respond to bronchodilators.

The severity of restrictive disease has not been standardized; however, many laboratories classify patients with a reduced TLC into mild (TLC ≤ 80%), moderate (TLC ≤ 65%), and severe (TLC ≤ 50%). These definitions are completely arbitrary because a patient with obstructive lung disease may start with a TLC of 120% and subsequently develop a moderately severe restrictive lung disease while maintaining a TLC within the normal range. On flow–volume loop, patients with restrictive disease have normal-shaped curves with a reduction in the height and width of the curve because the peak expiratory flow rate (PEFR) and VC are both dependent on the amount of air within the lung prior to performing expiratory maneuvers (see Fig. 23–4).

Restrictive lung function can be produced by increased elastic recoil of the lung parenchyma (interstitial lung disease), respiratory muscle weakness, mechanical restrictions (chest wall deformities), and/or poor effort. A list of common causes of restrictive lung disease is given in Table 23–2.

Restrictive lung function from parenchymal lung disease can usually be differentiated from processes causing mechanical restriction caused by chest bellows malfunction (Table 23–3). Restrictive parenchymal diseases are associated with a reduction in alveolar volume and an increase in lung elastic recoil. All lung volumes are reduced as well as the DLCO. The RV/TLC ratio (normal = 30%) and measurements of maximum inspiratory pressure (MIP; normal = −75 cm H_2O males, −50 cm H_2O females) remain normal. In addition, these patients exhibit mild resting hypoxemia that worsens with exercise. Monitoring gas exchange during exercise may be the most sensitive test for detecting progression of interstitial lung disease.[10]

Mechanical restriction caused by chest bellows malfunction may result from chest wall or skeletal deformity, loss of neuromuscular function, fibrosis of the pleural space, or abdominal overdistention causing upward displacement of the diaphragm as well as decreased diaphragm movement. The most common pulmonary function pattern seen in these patients is a decrease in TLC and VC with only a slight decrease in RV. The RV is maintained in these diseases because lung compliance remains normal. The DLCO

TABLE 23–2. Causes of Restrictive Lung Disease

- Interstitial lung diseases
  - Idiopathic pulmonary fibrosis
  - Sarcoidosis
  - Collagen vascular disease
  - Pneumoconiosis
  - Drug-induced lung disease
  - Pulmonary edema
- Infiltrative lung diseases
  - Granulomatosis
  - Tumor
- Pleural diseases
  - Pleural effusion
  - Fibrothorax
  - Pneumothorax
- Chest wall diseases
  - Kyphoscoliosis
  - Ankylosing spondilitis
  - Neuromuscular disease
- Miscellaneous causes
  - Obesity
  - Pregnancy
  - Ascites
  - Paralyzed diaphragm
- Lung resection

TABLE 23–3. Patterns of Pulmonary Function

	Obstructive Lung Disease		Restrictive Lung Disease	
	Asthma	*COPD*	*Parenchymal Disease*	*Chest Bellows Disease*
FVC	N1 or I	N1 or I	D	D
FEV_1	D	D	D	D
FEV_1/FVC	< 75%	< 75%	> 75%	> 75%
TLC	N1 or I	N1 or I	D	D
RV/TLC	N1 or I	N1 or I	N1	I
Airway resistance	I	I	N1	N1 or D
DLCO	N1	D	D	N1

N1 = normal; I = increased; D = decreased.

is normal or only minimally reduced and the DLCO/VA (corrected for alveolar volume) is normal. The RV/TLC ratio is often increased in patients with restrictive chest bellows disease. Patients with neuromuscular disease also have reduced respiratory muscle function with a reduction in their maximum inspiratory pressure (MIP).

PULMONARY GAS EXCHANGE

The essential function of the lungs is to maintain blood-gas homeostasis. Arterial blood-gas measurement plays an important role in the diagnosis and management of patients with pulmonary disease and should be ordered whenever hypoxemia, hypercapnia (CO_2 retention), and/or acid-base disorders are clinically suspected. Every time arterial blood gases are ordered, the A–a gradient (the difference of the partial pressure of oxygen in the alveolus minus the partial pressure of oxygen in arterial blood) should be calculated. This is done by computer on all automated blood-gas machines and a normal $PA–aO_2$ can be approximated for sea-level breathing room air by multiplying the age by 0.3. The presence of hypoxemia with a normal A–a gradient usually implies alveolar hypoventilation (e.g., sedative overdose). Most patients develop hypoxemia secondary to mismatching of ventilation and perfusion and the $PA–aO_2$ will be significantly elevated.

Pulse oximetry (SpO_2) is widely used in clinical practice to monitor arterial saturation. Although very useful clinically, SpO_2 is only an estimate of the arterial saturation and the actual SaO_2 can be ± 4% of the oximetry reading. The error may be even greater with a saturation of less than 88%. Pulse oximeters do not measure carboxyhemoglobin and the SpO_2 may be significantly overestimated in patients with smoke inhalation or recent smokers. An initial validation of pulse oximetry with direct measurement of SaO_2 is recommended in any critically ill patient.

EXERCISE TESTING

The major indications for exercise testing are dyspnea upon exertion, evaluation of exercise-induced bronchospasm, and suspected arterial desaturation during exercise.[11,12] Exercise testing can also be useful in the evaluation of ventilatory or cardiovascular limitations to work, assessment of general fitness or conditioning, evaluation of disability, establishment of safe levels for exercise, evaluation of drug therapy, determining the need and liter flow for supplemental oxygen therapy during exercise, and assessment of the effects of a rehabilitation program.[12,13]

Tests for general fitness include the 12-minute walking distance and the Harvard step test.[13] For the 12-minute walking distance, the subject simply walks as fast as possible a predetermined route or circuit for 12 minutes. The greater the distance covered, the better the patient's general fitness and exercise tolerance. For the Harvard step test, the subject steps up and down on a 20-inch step at a set rate for 5 minutes. A 1-minute rest period is followed by measurement of the subject's recovery heart rate. The lower the recovery heart rate, the better the subject's general fitness.

Exercise testing is sometimes done to determine if exercise results in arterial oxygen desaturation ($SaO_2 < 90\%$).[12,13] This may be useful to quantify the level of exertion the patient can perform during the activities of daily living, as well as determining appropriate levels of supplemental oxygen therapy. Typically, this test is done using a treadmill or cycle ergometer. A baseline measurement of arterial blood-gas values is followed by up to 6 minutes of exercise, during which time the patient is monitored for oxygen desaturation using pulse oximetry. If significant desaturation occurs, the test is terminated. In the event of oxygen desaturation, the test may be repeated to determine the level of supplemental oxygen therapy needed to compensate for the desaturation that would otherwise occur.

Exercise tolerance tests or cardiopulmonary stress testing may include the measurement of oxygen consumption ($\dot{V}O_2$), carbon dioxide production ($\dot{V}CO_2$), minute volume ($\dot{V}E$), oxygen saturation via pulse oximeter (SpO_2), heart rate, and blood pressure, and recording or monitoring the subject's electrocardiogram (ECG). During exercise, $\dot{V}O_2$ increases with workload in a linear fashion, until a maximum oxygen consumption level is reached ($\dot{V}O_{2max}$). Consequently, $\dot{V}O_{2max}$ is a measure of an individual's muscular work capacity.[12,13] Normal $\dot{V}O_{2max}$ is about 1700 mL/min for a sedentary person and up to 5800 mL/min in a trained athlete.[13] This compares to a resting VO_2 of about 250 mL/min. Ventilatory equivalents for oxygen and carbon dioxide and O_2 pulse are often calculated. Ventilatory equivalent for oxygen is a measure of the efficiency of the ventilatory pump at various workloads[12] and is calculated as follows:

$$\text{Ventilatory equivalent for } O_2 = \dot{V}E/\dot{V}O_2$$

A normal ventilatory equivalent for oxygen is 20 to 30 L/L $\dot{V}O_2$.[12]

O_2 pulse is an estimate of oxygen consumption per cardiac cycle and may be decreased with cardiac problems. O_2 pulse can be calculated as follows:

$$O_2 \text{ pulse} = (\dot{V}O_2 \times 1000)/\text{heart rate}$$

A normal O_2 pulse is 2.5 to 4.0 mL/beat at rest, increasing to 10 to 15 mL/beat during strenuous exercise.[12]

The anaerobic threshold is the point during strenuous exercise at which anaerobic metabolism and lactic acid production begin.[12,13] Carbon dioxide production ($\dot{V}CO_2$) increases with exercise at about the same rate as $\dot{V}O_2$, until the subject's anaerobic threshold is reached. From that point on, $\dot{V}CO_2$ increases faster than $\dot{V}O_2$ and this change can be used to estimate the anaerobic threshold. A breath-by-breath plot of the ventilatory equivalents for O_2 and CO_2 can also be used to determine the anaerobic threshold. Anaerobic threshold is a measure of fitness in normal subjects, and aerobic training can delay the anaerobic threshold.[12]

For exercise tolerance testing, the subject is typically subjected to either a constant workload (steady-state tests) or an increasing workload (progressive multistage tests) using a cycle ergometer or treadmill.[12,13] With the progressive multistage tests, the subject is exercised until exhaustion or the occurrence of an adverse reaction, at which point the test is stopped. Safety during exercise testing is of major importance, and rigorous guidelines for the termination of the test should be followed. Both types of tests can be used to determine VO_{2max}. A limit to exercise, as indicated by a decrease in VO_{2max}, can be a result of (1) poor conditioning, (2) a pulmonary limitation, or (3) a cardiac limitation. In the case of poor conditioning, SpO_2 and O_2 pulse will be normal. With a pulmonary limitation to exercise, SpO_2 will be reduced and O_2 pulse will be normal. With a cardiac limitation to exercise, SpO_2 will be normal and O_2 pulse reduced. Indications and contraindications for exercise testing are summarized in Table 23–4. Table 23–5 summarizes the findings during maximum exercise associated with poor conditioning, pulmonary limitations to exercise, and cardiac limitations to exercise.

TABLE 23–4. Indications and Contraindications for Exercise Testing

Indications

Dyspnea on exertion
Exercise-induced bronchospasm
Suspected arterial desaturation with exercise
Evaluation of ventilatory limitations to exercise
Evaluation of cardiac limitations to exercise
Assessment of general fitness or conditioning
Evaluation of cardiopulmonary disability
Establishment of safe levels for exercise
Evaluation of drug therapy
Determining appropriate use of supplemental oxygen therapy
Assessment of the effect of a rehabilitation program
Evaluation of specific disease states or conditions (e.g., asthma, COPD, interstitial lung disease, pulmonary vascular disorders, coronary artery disease, other vascular disorders, neuromuscular disorders, obesity, anxiety-induced hyperventilation)

Contraindications

PaO_2 less than 40 mm Hg on room air
$PaCO_2$ greater than 70 mm Hg
FEV_1 less than 30% of predicted
Recent (within 4 weeks) myocardial infarction
Unstable angina pectoris
Second- or third-degree heart block
Rapid ventricular/atrial arrhythmias
Orthopedic impairment
Severe aortic stenosis
Congestive heart failure
Uncontrolled hypertension
Limiting neurologic disorders
Dissecting/ventricular aneurysms
Severe pulmonary hypertension
Thrombophlebitis or intracardiac thrombi
Recent systemic or pulmonary embolus
Acute pericarditis

TABLE 23–5. Typical Findings During Maximum Exercise With Poor Conditioning, Pulmonary Limitations to Exercise, and Cardiac Limitations to Exercise

Test Parameter	Poor Conditioning	Pulmonary Limitation	Cardiac Limitation
VO_{2max}	↓	↓↓	↓
SpO_2	N	↓	N
O_2 pulse	N	N or ↓	↓
Anaerobic threshold	↓ or N	Variable	↓ or N
Ventilatory reserve[a] ($MVV - VE_{max}$)	N or ↓	↓	N or ↓

[a]Ventilatory reserve = Maximum voluntary ventilation (MVV) − minute volume during maximum exercise (VE_{max}).
Adapted from Ref. 13.

REFERENCES

1. Zibrak JD, O'Donnell CR, Marton K. Indications for preoperative pulmonary function testing. Ann Intern Med 1990;112;763.
2. Crapo RO. Pulmonary function testing. N Engl J Med 1994;331:25.
3. American Thoracic Society. Lung function testing: Selection of reference values and interpretive strategies. Am Rev Respir Dis 1991; 144:1202.
4. Tillis W, Levine SM, Anzueto A, et al. Clinical predictors of graft dysfunction following single lung transplantation. Chest 1992;102:73S.
5. Anthonisen NR, Connett JE, Kiley JP, et al. Effects of smoking intervention and the use of an inhaled anticholinergic bronchodilator on the rate of decline of FEV_1: The Lung Health Study. JAMA 1994; 272:1497–1505.
6. Tashkin DP, Altose MD, Bleeker ER, Connett JE, Kanner RE, Lee WW, Wise R, and the Lung Health Study Research Group. The Lung Health Study: Airway responsiveness to inhaled methacholine in smokers with mild to moderate airflow limitation. Am Rev Respir Dis 1992;145:301–310.
7. Rijcken B, Schouten JP, Mensinga TT, et al. Factors associated with bronchial responsiveness to histamine in a population sample of adults. Am Rev Respir Dis 1993;147:1447–1453.
8. Acres JC, Kryger MH. Upper airway obstruction. Chest 1981;80: 207–211.
9. Rotman HH, Liss HP, Weg JG. Diagnosis of upper airway obstruction by pulmonary function testing. Chest 1975;68:796–799.
10. Keogh BA, Crystal RG. Pulmonary function testing in interstitial pulmonary disease. Chest 1980;78:856–865.
11. Wasserman K, Hansen JE, Sue DY, Whipp BJ. Principles of Exercise Testing and Interpretation. Philadelphia, Lea & Febiger, 1986.
12. Ruppel GE. Manual of Pulmonary Function Testing, 6th ed. St. Louis, Mosby, 1994.
13. Madama VC. Pulmonary Function Testing and Cardiopulmonary Stress Testing. Albany, Delmar, 1993.

24

ASTHMA

H. William Kelly, PharmD, FCCP, BCPS, and Alan K. Kamada, PharmD

Asthma has been known since antiquity, yet it is a disease that still defies precise definition. The word *asthma* is of Greek origin and means "panting." More than 2000 years ago, Hippocrates used the word *asthma* to describe episodic shortness of breath; however, the first detailed clinical description of the asthmatic patient was made by Aretaeus in the second century.[1] Since that time *asthma* has been used to describe any disorder with episodic shortness of breath or dyspnea. However, *asthma* now refers to a disorder of the respiratory system characterized by episodes of difficulty in breathing. An Expert Panel of the National Institutes of Health, National Asthma Education and Prevention Program (NAEPP) has provided the following working definition of asthma[2]:

> Asthma is a chronic inflammatory disorder of the airways in which many cells and cellular elements play a role, in particular, mast cells, eosinophils, T lymphocytes, macrophages, neutrophils, and epithelial cells. In susceptible individuals, this inflammation causes recurrent episodes of wheezing, breathlessness, chest tightness, and coughing, particularly at night or in the early morning. These episodes are usually associated with widespread but variable airflow obstruction that is often reversible either spontaneously or with treatment. The inflammation also causes an associated increase in the existing bronchial hyperresponsiveness to a variety of stimuli.

This descriptive definition for asthma is attributed to our lack of knowledge of the precise pathogenic defect that results in the clinical syndrome we recognize as asthma. The current definition does allow for the important heterogeneity of the clinical presentation of asthma. New technologies have added substantially to our understanding of the interrelationships of immunology, biochemistry, and physiology to the clinical presentation of asthma, and further research may yet uncover a specific genetic defect in asthma. Until such time, asthma will continue to defy exact definition.

EPIDEMIOLOGY

An estimated 14 to 15 million persons in the United States have asthma (about 5% of the population).[2] Asthma is the most common chronic disease of children, affecting 4.8 million (6.9%).[2] Minorities, particularly in the inner cities, disproportionately share the burden of asthma.[3,4] African-Americans have a 19% higher incidence of asthma than whites and are twice as likely to be hospitalized. The estimated cost of asthma in the United States in 1990 was $6.2 billion.[3] Asthma accounted for 13.7 million ambulatory care visits (53.4 per 1000 persons) in 1993 to 1994, according to the National Ambulatory Medical Care Survey, and results in more than 470,000 hospitalizations per year.[5]

Asthma continues to be a significant cause of missed school days in children with over 10 million school days missed in 1990. This resulted in an estimated cost of $900 million dollars lost to parents to stay home and care for their children.[3] Between 1980 and 1993 the age-specific death rate from asthma increased 118%. Asthma mortality is consistently highest among African-Americans, who are four times more likely to die from asthma than other groups. Hospitalization rates have also increased 28% over the same period. For all physician visits, asthma was the sixth most frequently reported principal diagnosis and the 11th most frequent diagnosis in emergency departments in 1993 to 1994.[5]

The prevalence of asthma has been increasing worldwide. Although the precise reason for this increase is unknown, early exposure to allergens and airway irritants such as tobacco smoke in infancy increases the risk of developing asthma.[2] Worsening air quality has also been promoted as a cause of the increased asthma prevalence and morbidity. However, in some large inner cities morbidity and mortality have increased despite improvement in air quality.[6]

NATURAL HISTORY

The natural history of asthma is still not well defined. Between 30% and 70% of children with asthma will markedly improve or become symptom free by early adulthood; chronic disease persists in about 30% of patients. Although asthmatic patients who develop the disease in childhood are more likely to have remissions, patients who present at an early age have a poor prognosis. Ongoing airway obstruction may persist undetected in asthmatic children who are clinically well if objective measures are not made. Weiss et al[7] reported that females developing asthma by age 7 could expect a 7% reduction in lung function by age 15. These findings and others raise the question of whether ongoing asthma may produce fixed airways obstruction and whether therapy may be able to change the natural history of childhood asthma. Approximately 60% of patients who are symptom free as adults continue to exhibit bronchial hyperreactivity to inhaled histamine challenges. In general, subjects with less-frequent attacks and normal pulmonary function on initial assessment have higher remission rates, whereas smokers have the lowest remission and highest relapse rates.

Both the morbidity and mortality from asthma are increasing. Although death from asthma is still relatively rare, in the United States more than 5000 deaths occur yearly.[2] This is consistent with the increase in death rates found worldwide. Among children 5 to 14 years and young adults 15 to 24 years of age the death rate has approximately doubled from 1980 to 1993, with African-Americans six times more likely to die from asthma than whites. Hospitalizations for asthma among children 0 to 17 years have increased 4.5% per annum while total hospitalizations for all causes actually decreased.[3] In a study in New York City, the highest annual rate of hospitalizations for asthma was in Hispanics (62.9 per 10,000) followed by African-Americans at 59.9 per 10,000 and non-Hispanic whites at 12.2 per 10,000.[8] Interestingly, Hispanics in rural areas do not have an increased prevalence or morbidity from asthma.[4] Recent evidence supports the notion that the increased prevalence and morbidity from asthma is associated with poor economic status regardless of race.[3,6,8]

Studies of the cause and prevention of death from asthma indicate that 80% to 90% of the deaths are preventable.[2] Most deaths from asthma occur outside of the hospital, and death is rare after hospitalization. The most common causes of death from asthma are inadequate assessment of the severity of airway obstruction by the patient or physician and inadequate therapy.[2] Because poor, inner-city, minority populations have a disproportionate share of deaths from asthma, inadequate access to the health care system is believed to play a significant role.[8] The most common cause of death in the hospitalized patient is also inadequate or innappropriate therapy. Thus, the key to prevention of death from asthma as advocated by NAEPP is education.[2] This includes education of the patients as well as the clinicians caring for them.

ETIOLOGY

The heterogeneity of asthma appears most obvious when listing the diverse triggers of bronchospasm in asthmatic subjects (Table 24–1). In the past, a good deal of the confusion concerning the definition and etiology of asthma centered on the inclusion of the various triggering events as the etiology. Thus, asthma has been variously defined as an allergic or atopic, emotional, and infectious disease. However, it has become clear that asthma is first a lung disease, and specific triggering events have relative degrees of importance from patient to patient.

Epidemiologic studies strongly support the concept of a genetic predisposition to the development of asthma. Twin studies suggest that genetic factors account for 50% of the susceptibility.[9] Asthma represents a complex genetic disorder in that the asthma phenotype is likely a result of polygenic inheritance or different combinations of genes. Currently genome-wide searches to establish links between atopy (genetically determined state of hypersensitivity to environmental allergens) or bronchial hyperresponsiveness (BHR)[9] are being carried out. BHR is uniform increased responsiveness to challenge with a variety of stimuli, including methacholine, histamine, and exercise, and is often used to define and diagnose asthma.

TABLE 24–1. List of Agents and Events Triggering Asthma

Respiratory infection	Respiratory syncytial virus (RSV), rhinovirus, influenza, parainfluenza, *Mycoplasma pneumonia*
Allergens	Airborne pollens (grass, trees, weeds), house-dust mites, animal danders, cockroaches, fungal spores
Environment	Cold air, fog, ozone, sulfur dioxide, nitrogen dioxide, tobacco smoke, wood smoke
Emotions	Anxiety, stress, laughter
Exercise	Particularly in cold, dry climate
Drugs/preservatives	Aspirin, NSAIDs (cyclooxygenase inhibitors), sulfites, benzalkonium chloride, β-blockers
Occupational stimuli	Bakers (flour dust); farmers (hay mold); spice and enzyme workers; printers (arabic gum); chemical workers (azo dyes, anthraqui none, ethylenediamine, toluene diisocyanates, polyvinyl chloride); plastics, rubber, and wood workers (formaldehyde, western cedar, dimethylethanolamine, anhydrides)

Studies of occupational asthma and the induction of BHR in healthy individuals emphasize the effect of environment on the development of asthma. Early exposure of infants to house-dust mites and tobacco smoke is associated with increased incidence of asthma in children.[2] Atopy or a family history of atopy is strongly associated with continuing asthma in those infants who have wheezing with viral infections.[2] So genetic predisposition to atopy is a significant risk factor for devloping asthma, although not all atopic individuals develop asthma nor do all asthmatics exhibit atopy.

PATHOPHYSIOLOGY

BRONCHIAL HYPERRESPONSIVENESS

Hyperresponsiveness of the airways to physical, chemical, and pharmacologic stimuli is a hallmark of asthma.[2,8,9] BHR also occurs in some patients with chronic bronchitis and allergic rhinitis.[2,8] Normal healthy subjects may also develop a transient BHR after viral respiratory infections or exposure to ozone.[8] However, the degree of BHR is quantitatively greater in asthmatic patients than in other groups. Bronchial responsiveness of the general population fits a unimodal distribution that is skewed toward increased reactivity.[7] Patients with clinical asthma represent the extreme end of the distribution. The degree of BHR within asthmatics correlates with the clinical course of their disease and medication requirement necessary to control symptoms.[2] Patients with mild symptoms or in remission demonstrate lower levels of responsiveness, though still greater than the normal population.

Our current understanding recognizes that the increased BHR seen in asthma is at least in part owing to an inflammatory response within the airway.[8] Early investigations found correlations with inflammatory cells in bronchoalveolar lavage fluids and degree of BHR.[2] New evidence suggests that airways remodeling, subepithelial fibrosis, or collagen deposition correlates with BHR.[10] Although the precise link is not known, BHR is in part related to the extent of inflammation in the airways.

HISTOLOGIC CHANGES IN THE LINING OF THE AIRWAYS

Histologic studies performed on patients with mild to moderate chronic asthma have shown marked inflammatory changes within the airway along with extensive epithelial damage.[8,10,11] Similar but more severe changes have also been seen in patients who have died from acute asthma attacks.[2,8] The intact lungs of patients at autopsy are hyperinflated because of air trapping from widespread mucus plugging. The histologic examination is characterized by (1) marked hypertrophy and hyperplasia of the airway smooth muscle, (2) increased airway wall thickness with an exudative inflammatory reaction, epithelial desquammation, and edema, and (3) mucous gland hypertrophy and mucus hypersecretion (Fig. 24–1). Studies in mild asthmatics have found correlations between the degree of epithelial denudation and BHR.[2]

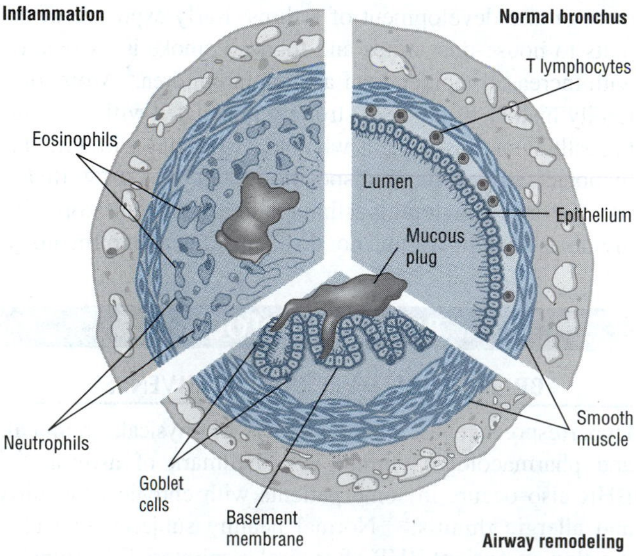

FIGURE 24–1. Representative illustration of the pathology found in the asthmatic bronchus compared with a normal bronchus (upper right). Each section demonstrates how the lumen is narrowed. Hypertrophy of the basement membrane, mucous plugging, smooth muscle hypertrophy, and constriction contribute (lower section). Inflammatory cells infiltrate, producing submucosal edema, and epithelial desquammation fills the airway lumen with cellular debris and exposes the airway smooth muscle to other mediators (upper left).

Structural changes in the airway, so-called airway remodeling, including subepithelial fibrosis, and increased ratio of goblet to ciliated epithelial cells have also been described in the bronchi of patients with chronic asthma.[2,10,11] This finding is not surprising considering that fibrosis occurs as a result of other chronic inflammatory diseases. It is not known whether the airway remodeling precedes the development of reactive airways or if these features occur simultaneously.[10] Airway remodeling is of concern because it may represent an irreversible process that can have more serious sequelae such as the development of chronic obstructive pulmonary disease.[2]

CELLULAR AND BIOCHEMICAL FEATURES

INFLAMMATORY PROCESSES

Inflammation of the airways and the release of mediators of inflammation contributes significantly to the development and maintenance of BHR.[8] Asthmatic inflammation is associated with epithelial cell damage and increased mucosal permeability. This improves access of noxious stimuli from the lumen to the airway smooth muscle, submucosal mast cells, and the cholinergic irritant receptors located in the junction between cells.[11] Inflammation can also account for mucus hypersecretion.[11] Figure 24–2 provides a schematic of inflammatory mediators, their origin, and pathophysiologic processes with which they are associated.[11] Although our understanding of the complex interactions and origin of the inflammatory process is still incomplete, the role of inflammation in producing or increasing BHR in asthma appears central. Attempting to minimize inflammation is an important aspect of asthma therapy.

INFLAMMATORY CELLS

Numerous types of leukocytes are present in the circulation, lung tissues, and lumen of airways. The involvement of mast cells, eosinophils, alveolar macrophages, lymphocytes, and neutrophils within the airways and surrounding tissues are important in asthma. Future therapeutic strategies aimed specifically at decreasing the number of inflammatory cells or removing their effect on asthma pathogenesis are being developed.

MAST CELLS

Mast-cell degranulation is important in the initiation of immediate responses following exposure to allergens.[2] Mast cells are found throughout the walls of the respiratory tract, and increased numbers of these cells (threefold to fivefold) have been described in the airways of asthmatics with an allergic component.[12] Once binding of allergen to cell-bound immunoglobulin E (IgE) occurs, mediators such as histamine; eosinophil and neutrophil chemotactic factors; leukotrienes C_4, D_4, and E_4; prostaglandins; platelet-activating factor; and others are released from mast cells (Fig. 24–2).

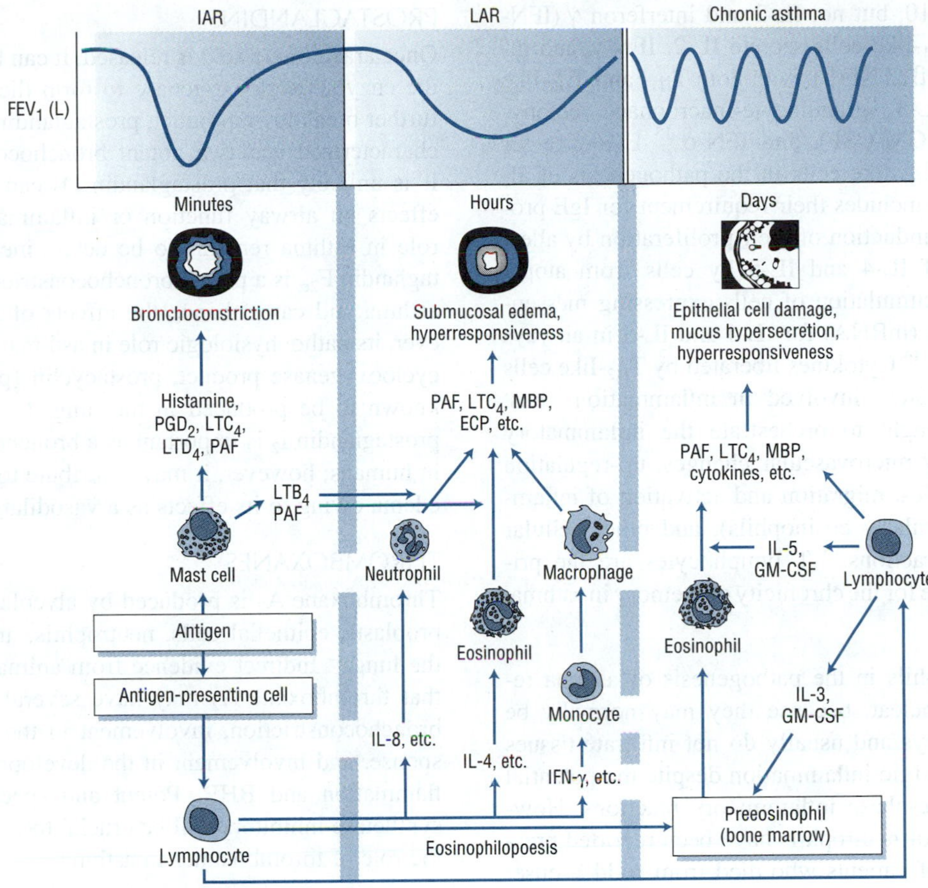

FIGURE 24–2. Diagrammatic presentation of the relationship between inflammatory cells, lipid and preformed mediators, inflammatory cytokines, and proposed pathogenesis and clinical presentation in asthma. See text for details. PG = prostaglandin; LT = leukotriene; PAF = platelet-activating factor; IL = interleukin; MBP = major basic protein; GM-CSF = granulocyte-macrophage colony-stimulating factor.

Histologic examination has revealed decreased numbers of granulated mast cells in the airways of patients who have died from acute asthma attacks, suggesting that mast-cell degranulation is a contributing factor in the progression of the disease.[12] Mast-cell degranulation is believed to be an integral cause of exercise-induced bronchospasm (EIB) following either drying or cooling of the airways.[13]

EOSINOPHILS

Eosinophils have long been linked to asthma, primarily owing to the association between asthma and peripheral blood eosinophilia.[2] They are the primary effector cells in the airway inflammation of asthma. The degree of BHR has been related to the number of eosinophils in peripheral blood and bronchoalveolar lavage fluid.[14] Major basic protein (MBP), a constituent of the granules present in the eosinophil, is responsible for damage to airway epithelium and has been found in very high quantities in the sputum of patients with asthma.[14] The damage to airway epithelium contributes to development of the BHR characteristic of asthma.

ALVEOLAR MACROPHAGES

The primary function of alveolar macrophages in the normal airway is to serve as "scavengers," engulfing and digesting bacteria and other foreign materials.[8] They are found in large and small airways, ideally located for affecting the asthmatic response. A number of mediators produced and released by macrophages have been identified, and their roles in initiating and amplifying inflammation in allergic asthma have been determined. A partial list of mediators produced by these cells includes platelet-activating factor, leukotriene B_4, leukotriene C_4, and leukotriene D_4.[8] Additionally, alveolar macrophages are able to produce neutrophil chemotactic factor and eosinophil chemotactic factor, which in turn further the inflammatory process.

T LYMPHOCYTES

In recent years much emphasis has been placed on the role of T lymphocytes in the pathogenesis of asthma, specifically the regulation of inflammation. Several studies have demonstrated increased numbers of T lymphocytes in bronchoalveolar lavage fluid and airway biopsy specimens of asthmatics,[12,15] even in mild and newly diagnosed cases.[11] The presence of T lymphocytes has been correlated to BHR.[14] The T_{H2}-like T lymphocytes have received particular attention owing to the profile of cytokines produced and released by these cells, which includes interleukin (IL)-4,

IL-5, IL-6, and IL-10, but not IL-2 and interferon γ (IFN-γ).[8] Conversely, T_{H1}-like cells secrete IL-2, IFN-γ, and tumor necrosis factor β (TNF-β), with both T_{H1}- and T_{H2}-like cells producing IL-3, granulocyte-macrophage colony-stimulating factor (GM-CSF), and IFN-α.[15] Evidence for the importance of T_{H2}-like cells in the pathogenesis of allergic inflammation includes their requirement for IgE production by B cells, induction of their proliferation by allergens, production of IL-4 and IL-5 by cells from atopic individuals, and accumulation of cells expressing messenger ribonucleic acid (mRNA) for IL-4 and IL-5 in airways of atopic asthmatics.[14] Cytokines liberated by T_{H2}-like cells appear to be intimately involved in inflammation; thus, these cells are thought to orchestrate the inflammatory process, particularly microvascular changes, up-regulation of adhesion molecules, migration and activation of inflammatory cells (particularly eosinophils), and other cellular and molecular interactions.[15] T lymphocytes are the primary cell responsible for the chronicity or memory in asthma.

NEUTROPHILS

The role of neutrophils in the pathogenesis of asthma remains somewhat unclear, because they may normally be present in the airways and usually do not infiltrate tissues showing chronic allergic inflammation despite the potential to participate in late-phase inflammatory reactions. However, high numbers of neutrophils have been reported present in the airways of patients who died from sudden-onset fatal asthma.[16] This suggests that neutrophils may play a pivotal role in the disease process, at least in the sudden-onset fatal cases, with a lesser role in the chronic inflammation of asthma. The neutrophil can also be a source for a variety of mediators platelet-activating factor, prostaglandins, thromboxanes, and leukotrienes, which contribute to BHR and airway inflammation.

MEDIATORS

HISTAMINE

Associated with asthma for many years, histamine is capable of inducing smooth-muscle constriction and bronchospasm and is thought to play a role in mucosal edema and mucus secretion.[8,17] Lung mast cells are an important source of histamine. The release of histamine can be stimulated by exposure of the airway to a variety of factors including physical stimuli (such as exercise) and exposure to relevant allergens.[2,8,13] Histamine is involved in acute bronchospasm following allergen exposure; however, other mediators such as leukotrienes are also involved.[18] Antihistamines have only a small benefit in asthma.

Besides histamine release mast-cell degranulation releases interleukins, proteases, and other enzymes that activate the production of other mediators of inflammation. Several classes of important mediators, including arachidonic acid and its metabolites (i.e., prostaglandins, leukotrienes, and platelet-activating factor) are derived from cell membrane phospholipids.

PROSTAGLANDINS

Once arachidonic acid is released, it can be broken down by the enzyme cyclooxygenase to form the prostaglandins. A further breakdown product, prostaglandin D_2, has been well characterized and is a potent bronchoconstricting agent.[17] It is unlikely that prostaglandin D_2 can produce sustained effects on airway function or inflammation; however, its role in asthma remains to be determined. Similarly, prostaglandin $F_{2\alpha}$ is a potent bronchoconstrictor in patients with asthma and can enhance the effects of histamine.[17] However, its pathophysiologic role in asthma is unclear. Another cyclooxygenase product, prostacyclin (prostaglandin I_2) is known to be produced in the lung. It is unclear whether prostaglandin I_2 is important as a bronchoconstricting agent in humans; however, it may contribute to inflammation and edema owing to its effects as a vasodilator.[12]

THROMBOXANES

Thromboxane A_2 is produced by alveolar macrophages, fibroblasts, epithelial cells, neutrophils, and platelets within the lung.[12] Indirect evidence from animal models suggests that thromboxane A_2 may have several effects, including bronchoconstriction, involvement in the late asthmatic response, and involvement in the development of airway inflammation and BHR. Potent and specific thromboxane-synthetase inhibitors will be crucial tools for understanding the role of thromboxanes in asthma.

LEUKOTRIENES

The 5-lipoxygenase pathway of arachidonic acid breakdown is responsible for production of the class of compounds called leukotrienes (LTs).[18] Leukotrienes C_4, D_4, and E_4 (cysteinyl LTs) constitute the slow-reacting substance of anaphylaxis (SRS-A).[19] These leukotrienes are liberated during inflammatory processes in the lung. Leukotriene D_4 and E_4 share a common receptor (LTD_4 receptor) that when stimulated produces bronchospasm, mucus secretion, microvascular permeability, and airway edema.[19] Potent LTD_4 receptor antagonists can produce improvement in symptoms and lung function in patients with chronic asthma. Specific LTD_4 receptor antagonists and 5-lipoxygenase inhibitors have recently gained FDA approval for the treatment of asthma.

PLATELET-ACTIVATING FACTOR

Thought to be produced by macrophages, eosinophils, and neutrophils within the lung, platelet-activating factor (PAF) is involved in the mediation of bronchospasm, sustained induction of BHR, edema formation, and chemotaxis of eosinophils.[8,12] Selective and potent PAF-receptor antagonists have been developed but have so far been disappointing in clinical trials of asthma.

ADHESION MOLECULES

An important step in the inflammatory process is the adhesion of the various cells to each other and the tissue matrix to facilitate infiltration and migration of these cells to the site of inflammation. To promote this, cell membranes express a number of glycoproteins, or adhesion molecules. Adhesion molecules have additional functions involved in the inflammatory process aside from promoting cell adhesion, including activation of cells and cell-to-cell communication, and promoting cellular migration and infiltration.[17] The many adhesion molecules are divided into families on the basis of their chemical structure. These families are the integrins, cadherins, immunoglobulin supergene family, selectins, vascular adressins, and carbohydrate ligands.[20] Those thought to be important in inflammation include the integrins, immunoglobulin supergene family, selectins, and carbohydrate ligands including intercellular adhesion molecule 1 (ICAM-1) and vascular cell adhesion molecule 1 (VCAM-1).[21]

Adhesion molecules are found on a variety of cells, such as neutrophils, monocytes, lymphocytes, basophils, eosinophils, granulocytes, platelets, endothelial cells, and epithelial cells,[21] and can be expressed or activated by the many inflammatory mediators present in asthma.[20] Thus, complex interactions occur whereby mediators affect expression of adhesion molecules, and adhesion molecules can produce mediators. In addition to these interactions, a major role of adhesion molecules is in the recruitment of leukocytes from the vascular lumen to tissues. The initial step involved in this leukocyte–endothelial cell adhesion cascade is transient and reversible binding of the adhesion molecule to specific ligands on endothelial cells, which results in slowing or rolling of the circulating leukocyte along the surface of the vasculature. Activation of the leukocyte or endothelial cell follows in response to a mediator or the initial adhesion event. Finally, firm adhesion (anchoring) of the leukocyte to the endothelial cell surface allows for diapedesis between endothelial cells and migration of the leukocyte into the extracellular matrix.[21] For instance, ICAM-1 and VCAM-1 are involved in the migration of lymphocytes and eosinophils.[17]

Although the role of adhesion molecules in the pathogenesis of asthma remains undefined, studies have begun to address the mechanisms of leukocyte infiltration into the airways. The availability of monoclonal antibodies to the functional epitopes of adhesion molecules will facilitate our understanding of their role in inflammation. In addition, specific blocking of adhesion molecules by monoclonal antibodies appears promising as a novel therapeutic approach or complement to existing anti-inflammatory therapy.

MUCUS PRODUCTION

The mucociliary system is the lung's primary defense mechanism against irritants and infectious agents. Mucus, composed of 95% water and 5% glycoproteins, is produced by bronchial epithelial glands and goblet cells.[22] The lining of the airway consists of a continuous aqueous layer controlled by active ion transport across the epithelium where water moves toward the lumen along the concentration gradient. Catecholamines and vagal stimulation enhance the ion transport and fluid movement.[22] Mucus transport is dependent on the viscoelastic properties of the mucus. Mucus that is either too watery or too viscous will not be optimally transported. The exudative inflammatory process and sloughing of epithelial cells into the airway lumen impairs mucociliary transport. The bronchial glands are increased in size and the goblet cells are increased in size and number in asthma.[11] Expectorated mucus from patients with asthma tends to have a high viscosity. The mucus plugs in the airways of patients who died in status asthmaticus are tenacious and tend to be connected by mucous strands to the goblet cells.[22] Asthmatic airways may also become plugged with casts consisting of epithelial and inflammatory cells. Although it is tempting to speculate that death from asthma attacks is a result of the mucus plugging resulting in irreversible obstruction, there is no direct evidence for this. Autopsies of asthmatics who died from other causes have shown similar pathology.[8] In addition, some subjects who have died of sudden severe asthma did not show the characteristic mucus plugging on necropsy.[16,22]

AIRWAY SMOOTH MUSCLE

The smooth muscle of the airways does not form a uniform coat around the airways but is wrapped around in a connecting network best described as a spiral arrangement.[22] The muscle contraction displays a sphincteric action that is capable of completely occluding the airway lumen. The airway smooth muscle extends from the trachea through the respiratory bronchioles. When expressed as percentage of wall thickness, the smooth muscle represents 5% of the large central airways and up to 20% of the wall thickness in the bronchioles.[22] Total smooth muscle mass decreases rapidly past the terminal bronchioles to the alveoli, and so the contribution of smooth muscle tone to airway diameter in this region is relatively small. In the large airways of asthmatics, smooth muscle may account for 11% of the wall thickness.[22] Airway smooth muscle contraction *in vivo* is measured indirectly by determining the flow of air into and out of the patient. The difficulties in using changes in airflow as a measurement of smooth muscle contraction have been delineated elsewhere.[22] The relationship between airway diameter and flow is dictated by Poiseuille's law[11]:

$$P = 8nl/r^4$$

where n = viscosity of the air, l = length of the tube, r = radius of the tube, and P = drop in pressure. Because resistance is equal to P divided by airflow, a twofold change in airway diameter would produce a 16-fold change in airflow resistance. It is possible that the increased smooth muscle mass of the asthmatic airways is important in magnifying and maintaining BHR in chronic asthma.[22] However, it appears that the hypertrophy and hyperplasia are secondary processes caused by chronic inflammation and are not the primary cause of BHR.[8,22]

NEURAL CONTROL

The airway is innervated by parasympathetic, sympathetic, and nonadrenergic inhibitory nerves.[17] Parasympathetic innervation of the smooth muscle consists of efferent motor fibers contained in the vagus nerves and sensory afferent fibers in the vagus and other nerves.[22] The normal resting tone of human airway smooth muscle is maintained by vagal efferent activity.[22] Maximum bronchoconstriction mediated by vagal stimulation occurs in the small bronchi and is absent in the small bronchioles. The nonmyelinated C fibers of the afferent system lie immediately beneath the tight junctions between epithelial cells lining the airway lumen.[22] These endings probably represent the irritant receptors of the airways. Stimulation of these irritant receptors by mechanical stimulation, chemical and particulate irritants, and pharmacologic agents such as histamine produces reflex bronchoconstriction.[22]

The sympathetic innervation of the airway smooth muscle is sparse and does not directly control airway smooth muscle tone.[22] All airway smooth muscle contains noninnervated β_2-adrenergic receptors that produce bronchodilation.[22] Circulating catecholamines play an important role in regulating bronchial tone. The major resistance airways contain α-adrenergic receptors whose stimulation produces bronchoconstriction that is enhanced by pretreatment with histamine.[22] The importance of these receptors in asthma is unknown; however, specific α-adrenergic blockers have minimal effect on asthma.[11] One theory on the pathogenesis of BHR is that asthma represents a relative β-adrenergic blockade. The demonstration of a β-adrenergic defect in asthmatic patients has been inconsistent, and the production of β-blockade in normal subjects is insufficient, by itself, to cause bronchial hyperreactivity.[8]

The nonadrenergic, noncholinergic (NANC) nervous system has been described in the trachea and bronchi. Substance P, neurokinin A, neurokinin B, and vasoactive intestinal peptide (VIP) are the best characterized neurotransmitters in the NANC nervous system.[17] VIP is an inhibitory neurotransmitter in the system. Inflammatory cells in asthma can release peptidases that can degrade VIP, producing exaggerated reflex cholinergic bronchoconstriction.[17] NANC excitatory neuropeptides such as substance P and neurokinin A are released by stimulation of C-fiber sensory nerve endings.[17] The NANC system may play an important role in amplifying inflammation in asthma by releasing nitric oxide.

NITRIC OXIDE

Nitric oxide (NO) is produced by cells within the respiratory tract. It has been thought to be a neurotransmitter of the NANC system.[17] Endogenous NO is generated from the amino acid L-arginine by the enzyme NO synthase.[23] There are three isoforms of NO synthase. One isoform is induced in response to pro-inflammatory cytokines, inducible NO synthase (iNOS), in airway epithelial cells and inflammatory cells of asthmatic airways.[23] NO produces smooth muscle relaxation in the vasculature and bronchials; however, it appears to amplify the inflammatory process and is unlikely to be of therapeutic benefit.[17] Recent investigations measuring exhaled NO concentrations have suggested it may be a useful measure of ongoing lower airway inflammation in patients with asthma and for measuring effectiveness of therapy.[24]

CLINICAL PRESENTATION

CHRONIC ASTHMA

Classic asthma is characterized by episodic dyspnea associated with wheezing; however, the clinical presentation of asthma is as diverse as the number of triggering events.[8,25] Although wheezing is the characteristic symptom of asthma, the medical literature is replete with the warning that "not all that wheezes is asthma." A wheeze is a high-pitched, whistling sound created by turbulent airflow through an obstructed airway so that any condition that produces significant obstruction can result in wheezing as a symptom. In addition, "all of asthma does not wheeze" is an equally justifiable warning. Patients may present with a chronic persistent cough as their only symptom.[8]

The diagnosis of asthma is based primarily on a good history of recurrent episodes of dyspnea and/or wheezing (Table 24–2).[2,17] The patient may complain of a feeling of tightness in the chest or sometimes a burning sensation. The patient may have a family history of allergy or asthma or have symptoms of allergic rhinitis.[2,17] A history of exercise or cold air precipitating the dyspnea or an association of increased symptoms during specific allergen seasons would also point to asthma.

TABLE 24–2. Sample Questions[a] for the Diagnosis and Initial Assessment of Asthma

A "yes" answer to any question suggests that asthma diagnosis is likely. In the past 12 months, . . .

- Have you had a sudden severe episode or recurrent episodes of coughing, wheezing (high-pitched whistling sounds when breathing out), or shortness of breath?
- Have you had colds that "go to the chest" or take more than 10 days to get over?
- Have you had coughing, wheezing, or shortness of breath during a particular season or time of the year?
- Have you had coughing, wheezing, or shortness of breath in certain places or when exposed to certain things (e.g., animals, tobacco smoke, perfumes)?
- Have you used any medications that help you breathe better? How often?
- Are the symptoms relieved when the medications are used?

In the past 4 weeks, have you had coughing, wheezing, or shortness of breath . . .

- At night that has awakened you?
- In the early morning?
- After running, moderate exercise, or other physical activity?

[a]*These questions are recommended by the NAEPP but have not been formally validated.*

Asthma has a widely variable presentation from chronic daily symptoms to only intermittent symptoms. The intervals between symptoms could be weeks, months, or years. It is a disease characterized by recurrent exacerbations and remissions. The next variable is severity. The NAEPP has provided a means of classifying asthma presented in Table 24–3.[2] The intermittent and/or chronic nature of symptoms does not necessarily determine the severity of symptoms during exacerbations. The severity is by lung function and symptoms prior to therapy as well as by the amount of medication required to adequately control the patients' symptoms. Patients can present with mild intermittent symptoms that require no medications or only occasional use of inhaled bronchodilators to severe chronic asthma symptoms despite receiving multiple medications.

ACUTE SEVERE ASTHMA

Uncontrolled asthma, with its inherent variability, can progress to an acute state where inflammation, airway edema, excessive accumulation of mucus, and severe bronchospasm result in a profound airway narrowing that is poorly responsive to usual bronchodilator therapy.[2,17] Although this progression is the most common scenario, some patients experience rapid onset or hyperacute attacks.[2,16] Recently, investigators reported that hyperacute attacks may be associated with an increased risk of near fatality in acute severe asthma.[16] Hyperacute attacks resolve rapidly with bronchodilator therapy, suggesting that smooth muscle spasm is the major pathogenic mechanism.[14] In many cases, emergency department visits for acute severe asthma represent the failure of an adequate therapeutic regimen for chronic asthma. Patients present with severe dyspnea, inspiratory as well as expiratory wheezing, anxiety, tachypnea, tachycardia, and, in severe cases, cyanosis. They exhibit supraclavicular and intercostal retractions, a hyperinflated chest, and coughing. In severe obstruction, air movement into and out of the lungs is substantially decreased so that wheezing may actually decrease.[2]

ALLERGIC ASTHMA

An allergic component can be demonstrated in 35% to 55% of asthmatic patients, and this may be higher in childhood asthma.[2,8,25] The allergens (see Table 24–1) that provoke asthma are airborne and evoke the asthmatic response through the classic allergic pathway. Although the allergic reaction plays an important role in the atopic asthmatic patient, atopy is not necessary for the development of asthma and not all atopic individuals develop asthma.[8] Many patients with hay fever will develop some BHR (though less than asthmatics) during their allergen season. However, the study of the response to allergen has improved our understanding of the role of inflamation in asthma.

When allergic asthmatics are given an inhalational challenge with an allergen to which they are sensitized, the patients demonstrate an immediate asthmatic reaction (EAR) (Fig. 24–3). The reaction is characterized by a drop in pulmonary function that reaches maximum intensity in 10 to 20 minutes and reverses spontaneously by 60 to 120 minutes.[25] In addition, many subjects experience a late asthmatic reaction that begins 4 hours after the challenge, reaches maximum intensity in 6 to 8 hours, is often more severe than the EAR, and may last as long as 24 hours. The late asthmatic reaction (LAR) may be the pathogenetic mechanism for inducing and maintaining BHR in atopic asthmatics.[25] Patients who experience an LAR demonstrate increased BHR that may last up to 6 weeks, whereas subjects who experience only the EAR demonstrate no increased BHR.[25] The degree of BHR and its duration

TABLE 24–3. Classification of Asthma Severity: Clinical Features Before Treatment

	Symptoms	Lung Function[a]
Step 1 Mild Intermittent	Daytime ≤ 2 times/wk Asymptomatic between exacerbations Exacerbations brief (from a few hours to a few days); intensity may vary Nocturnal ≤ 2 times/mo	FEV_1 or PEF ≥ 80% PEF variability < 20%
Step 2 Mild Persistent	Daytime > 2 times/wk but < 1 time/d Exacerbations may affect activity Nocturnal > 2 times/mo	FEV_1 or PEF ≥ 80% PEF variability 20% to 30%
Step 3 Moderate Persistent	Daily symptoms Daily use of inhaled, short-acting β_2-agonists Exacerbations affect activity Exacerbations ≥ 2 times/wk; may last days Nocturnal > 1 time/wk	FEV_1 or PEF > 60% to < 80% PEF variability > 30%
Step 4 Severe Persistent	Continual symptoms Limited physical activity Frequent exacerbations Nocturnal frequent	FEV_1 or PEF ≤ 60% PEF variability > 30%

[a]The presence of one of the features of severity is sufficient to place a patient in that category. An individual should be assigned to the most severe grade in which any feature occurs. The characteristics noted are general and may overlap because asthma is highly variable. Furthermore, an individual's classification may change over time. Patients at any level of severity can have mild, moderate, or severe exacerbations. Some patients with intermittent asthma experience severe and life-threatening exacerbations separated by long periods of normal lung function and no symptoms.

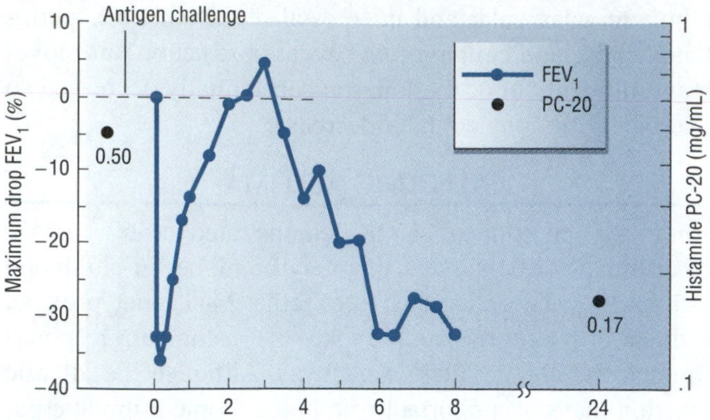

FIGURE 24–3. Biphasic response to allergen exposure in a sensitive patient with asthma. The immediate response occurs within 10 to 30 minutes following exposure and may revert to baseline without intervention. The late asthmatic response occurs within 2 to 8 hours following exposure. The provocative concentration of inhaled histamine, which produces a 20% decrease in forced expiratory volume in 1 second (FEV_1) (PC-20), an index of airways reactivity, also shows a marked decrease following development of a late asthmatic response. This is suggestive of an increase in the propensity of the airways to constrict to nonspecific stimuli.

correlate with the intensity of the LAR. The LAR is associated with increased serum concentrations of neutrophil and eosinophil chemotactic factors and the influx of neutrophils and eosinophils into the tissue as well as the degranulation of mast cells.[25] The LAR is associated with greater degrees of obstruction in small airways and air trapping than occur with the EAR.

The measurement of BHR is made by having the patient breath increasing log concentrations or doubling doses of histamine or methacholine. Following each increment the patient performs spirometric measurement until the forced expiratory volume in 1 second (FEV_1) drops at least 20% from the baseline value. Then either a provocative dose (PD) or provocative concentration (PC) that produces the 20% drop is calculated (the PC20 in Fig. 24–3).[26] Most patients with asthma will have a $PC20FEV_1$ of 8 mg/L methacholine. The usual variation over time without change in therapy usually does not exceed one dose step or one doubling dose so that a clinically significant change is considered to be at least 1.5 to 2 doubling doses.[26] The NAEPP considers drugs to be anti-inflammatory if they reduce markers of airway inflammation and decrease BHR.[2]

The EAR is easily blocked or reversed with inhaled β_2-agonists.[27] Theophylline, anticholinergics, and oral β_2-agonists blunt the response but are inconsistently effective.[2,19] The LAR is not prevented by pretreatment with any of these bronchodilators, although the bronchospastic component may be attenuated if therapeutic doses are administered at the time of the LAR.[19,26] Glucocorticoid pretreatment does not alter the EAR but prevents the LAR, whereas pretreatment with cromolyn sodium or nedocromil blocks both responses.[2,17] Long-term treatment with glucocorticoids can attenuate the immediate response by decreasing overall BHR.[19]

Clinically, allergic asthmatics develop increased BHR with increased exposure to allergens during a pollen season.[28] Avoidance of the pollen or prophylaxis with cromolyn sodium prevents the increased bronchial hyperreactivity.[26,28] Studies have shown that long-term therapy with cromolyn, nedocromil, and glucocorticoids reduces BHR.[26,28] In contrast, long-term therapy with β_2-agonists and theophylline has not been associated with similar decreases in bronchial hyperreactivity.[2,27] The leukotriene modifiers have not demonstrated a reduction in BHR.[19]

EXERCISE-INDUCED ASTHMA

During vigorous exercise, pulmonary function in asthmatic patients (as measured by forced expiratory maneuvers) increases during the first few minutes but then begins to decrease after 6 to 8 minutes (Fig. 24–4).[13] Exercise-induced bronchospasm (EIB) is defined as a drop in FEV_1 of greater than 15% to 20% of baseline (preexercise value).[2,13] Most studies suggest that 70% to 90% of asthmatics experience EIB.[2] The exact pathogenesis of EIB is unknown; however, heat loss and/or water loss from the central airways appear to play an important role.[13] EIB is more easily provoked in cold, dry air, and warm, humid air can blunt or block it.[13]

Studies using isocapnic hyperventilation of cold air and inhalation of hypertonic saline have demonstrated similar degrees of bronchospasm as seen in EIB.[13] A number of studies have demonstrated increased plasma histamine and tryptase concentrations during EIB, suggesting a role for mast-cell degranulation. In addition, pretreatment with cromolyn sodium, a drug that stabilizes mast cells, inhibits EIB and inhibits the associated rise in neutrophil chemotactic factor.[13] A small number of patients with EIB will have a late response similar to the LAR and associated with a secondary rise in neutrophil chemotactic factor.

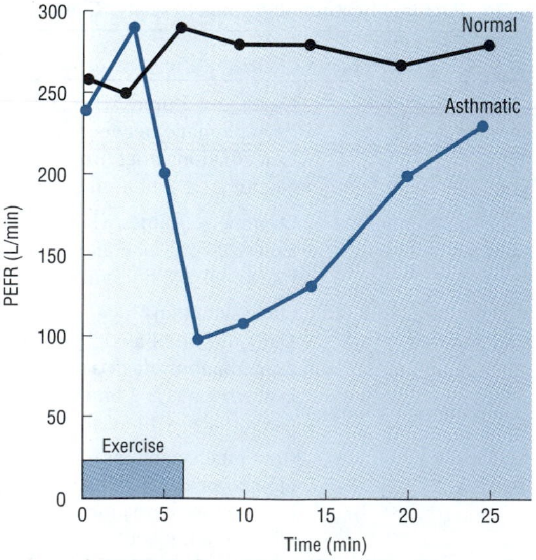

FIGURE 24–4. Typical responses to exercise in a normal subject and an asthmatic subject. Note the initial bronchodilation. PEFR = peak expiratory flow rate.

A refractory period following EIB lasts up to 3 hours after exercise. During this period, repeat exercise of the same intensity produces either no decrease in pulmonary function or a drop less than 50% of the initial response.[13,22] The refractory period is thought to be caused by an acute depletion of mast-cell mediators and time required for their repletion. Patients with known refractoriness to exercise will still respond to histamine so that acute hyporesponsiveness of airway smooth muscle does not appear to be a factor.[13,22]

EIB is believed to be a reflection of the increased BHR of asthmatics. A correlation, though not perfect, exists between EIB and reactivity to histamine and methacholine.[22,26] Other patient groups with BHR (postviral infection, cystic fibrosis, hay fever) show bronchoconstriction after exercise to a lesser degree (5% to 10%) than asthmatics (20% to 40%).[13] Asthmatics will not always demonstrate the same sensitivity. During periods of remission, they often have a decreased sensitivity to the same degree of exercise. Finally, a number of children and adults with EIB are otherwise normal, without symptoms or abnormal pulmonary function.

NOCTURNAL ASTHMA

Worsening of asthma during sleep is referred to as nocturnal asthma. Patients with nocturnal asthma exhibit significant falls in pulmonary function between bedtime and awakening.[2,29] Although the pathogenesis of this phenomenon is unknown, it has been associated with diurnal patterns of endogenous cortisol secretion and circulating epinephrine.[29] Direct evidence for an inflammatory component to nocturnal asthma includes increased circulating histamine and activated eosinophils at night associated with increased hyperresponsiveness to methacholine.[29] It has been postulated that the decrease in endogenous hormones results in enhanced pulmonary T-cell release of pro-inflammatory cytokines, which then activate the airway inflammatory cells at night. Increased urinary leukotriene excretion has been found in patients with nocturnal asthma.[19]

Numerous other factors that may affect nocturnal worsening of asthma, including allergies and improper environmental control, gastroesophageal reflux, and sinusitis, must also be considered when evaluating these patients.[2,22] Although nocturnal asthma can often be controlled with long-acting bronchodilators, most experts consider it a symptom of inadequately treated chronic asthma and advocate increased anti-inflammatory therapy.[2,17]

FACTORS CONTRIBUTING TO ASTHMA SEVERITY

RESPIRATORY INFECTIONS

Viral infections and not bacteria are primarily responsible for exacerbations of asthma.[2,17] Viral upper respiratory tract infections are a major precipitant of acute asthma in children, being involved in up to 20% to 40% of acute episodes.[2] Infants are particularly susceptible to airway obstruction and wheezing with viral infections because of their small airways. The most common cause of exacerbations in both children and adults is the common rhinovirus.[2] Other viruses isolated include respiratory syncytial virus (RSV), parainfluenza virus, coronavirus, and influenza viruses.[17] The inflammatory response to viral infection is thought to be directly associated with the increasing BHR. Certain viruses (RSV and parainfluenza) are capable of inducing specific IgE antibodies, and rhinovirus can directly activate eosinophils in asthmatics.[17] The increase in asthma symptoms and BHR that occurs may last for days or weeks following resolution of the symptoms of the viral infection. The NAEPP recommends annual influenza vaccinations for patients with asthma.[2]

ENVIRONMENTAL AND OCCUPATIONAL FACTORS

Agents and events and the mechanisms that are known to trigger asthma are listed in Table 24–1.[17] The general mechanisms are unknown, but are presumably caused by epithelial damage and inflammation in the airway mucosa. Ozone and sulfur dioxide, common components of air pollution, have been used to induce BHR in animals. Exposure to ozone 0.2 ppm for 2 to 3 hours can induce bronchoconstriction and increase BHR in asthmatics.[22] Sulfur dioxide in the ambient atmosphere is highly irritating, but it is not known how it induces bronchoconstriction. Pretreatment with cromolyn sodium will block the obstruction, implicating mast-cell or irritant-receptor involvement.[22] Asthma produced by repeated prolonged exposure to industrial inhalants is a significant health problem. It has been estimated that occupational asthma accounts for 2% of all asthmatic persons.[2] Persons with occupational asthma have the typical symptoms of asthma with cough, dyspnea, and wheeze. Typically, the symptoms are related to work with improvement on weekends and vacations.[2] In some instances, symptoms may persist even after termination of exposure.[2]

PSYCHOLOGICAL FACTORS

Emotions and stress can rarely precipitate attacks of asthma, but more commonly worsen an attack in progress.[2] Bronchoconstriction from psychological factors appear to be primarily mediated through excess parasympathetic input.[22] Atropine has been shown to block experimental psychogenic bronchoconstriction.[22] It is most important to emphasize to patients and to parents of asthmatic children that asthma is not an emotional disease; however, calming influences and relaxation techniques may benefit the patient who becomes severely emotionally distraught during asthma attacks.

SINUSITIS AND/OR RHINITIS

Disorders of the upper respiratory tract, particularly sinusitis and rhinitis, have been linked with asthma for many years. As many as 40% to 50% of asthmatics have abnormal sinus radiographs.[22] However, chronic sinusitis may just represent a nonbacterial coexistent condition with allergic asthmatics because the histologic changes in the paranasal sinuses are similar to those seen in the lung and nose.[2] Some studies have shown that asthma symptoms improve with treatment of sinusitis.[17] The mechanism by which sinusitis aggravates asthma is unknown. The treatment of allergic rhinitis with inhaled corticosteroids and cromolyn but not antihistamines will reduce BHR in asthmatic patients.[2] It has been postulated that transport of mucus chemotactic factors and inflammatory mediators from nasal passages during allergic rhinitis into the lung may accentuate BHR.

GASTROESOPHAGEAL REFLUX

Gastroesophageal reflux has been associated with asthma for many years.[2,17] Nocturnal asthma may be associated with nighttime reflux.[29] Reflux of acidic gastric contents into the esophagus is thought to initiate a vagally mediated reflex bronchoconstriction.[22] Also of concern is that most medications that decrease airways smooth muscle tone have a relaxant effect on gastroesophageal sphincter tone as well. The therapeutic approach most commonly taken for patients with gastroesophageal reflux and asthma is to initiate standard antireflux therapy and observe the asthma symptoms.

PREMENSTRUAL ASTHMA

Premenstrual worsening of asthma has been reported in as many as 30% to 40% of women in some studies.[30] Others have noted worsening of pulmonary functions associated with menstruation even in women not aware of worsening of symptoms.[30] One study reported that 50% of exacerbations in adult nonpregnant females requiring emergency department treatment occurred within 2 days before to 4 days into menses.[30] Recent evidence suggests there may be an abnormal regulation of β_2-adrenergic receptors in women who experience premenstrual asthma. In addition to premenstrual asthma, asthma in pregnancy has been a poorly studied phenomenon.[31] Studies would indicate that, in general, BHR and symptoms improve in asthmatics during pregnancy.[22,31]

FOODS, DRUGS, AND ADDITIVES

Documentation in the literature of food allergens as triggers for asthma is not available.[17] However, additives, specifically sulfites used as preservatives, can trigger life-threatening asthma exacerbations. Beer, wine, dried fruit, and open salad bars in particular have high concentrations of metabisulfites.[2] Severe oral steroid-dependent patients should be warned about ingesting foods processed with sulfites. Another additive producing bronchospasm is benzalkonium chloride found as a preservative in some nebulizer solutions of antiasthmatic drugs.[32]

Aspirin and other nonsteroidal anti-inflammatory drugs can precipitate asthma in up to 20% of adults with asthma.[17] The mechanism is related to cyclooxygenase inhibition, and 5-lipoxygenase inhibition can prevent the symptoms.[19] The prevalence increases with increasing age. The greatest frequency occurs in severe steroid-dependent asthmatics in their fourth and fifth decades who also have perennial rhinitis and nasal polyposis (presence of several polyps).[22] Other drugs that do not precipitate bronchospasm but that prevent its reversal are the β-blocking agents.[2]

DIAGNOSTIC TESTS

The diagnosis of asthma is primarily made by history and confirmatory spirometry.[2,17] The NAEPP has provided a list of questions that would lead to the diagnosis of asthma (see Table 24–2). In the older child and adult patient in whom spirometric evaluations can be performed, abnormal pulmonary functions that improve 15% or more following bronchodilator administration help confirm the diagnosis.[2] Failure of pulmonary functions to improve acutely does not necessarily rule out asthma. Patients with long-standing disease or substantial inflammation may require an intensive, prolonged course of bronchodilators and glucocorticoids before reversibility is detected.[2,17] If baseline spirometry is normal, challenge testing with exercise, histamine, or methacholine can be used to elicit BHR.[2] Patients with significant symptoms and/or an $FEV_1 < 65\%$ of predicted normal should not be challenged. Spirometry and bronchoprovocation have been shown to be more reliable indicators of BHR than a history of wheezing and physical exam.[22] Studies for atopy such as serum IgE and sputum and blood eosinophils are not necessary to make the diagnosis of asthma, but they may help differentiate asthma from chronic bronchitis in adults. Clinically, this distinction is often difficult to make. Some patients with chronic bronchitis may have a reversible component and some patients with long-standing severe chronic asthma may have significant irreversible damage and obstruction. Very high peripheral blood eosinophil counts may point to the diagnosis of aspergillosis or other hypereosinophilic syndromes.[22] Skin testing is of no value in diagnosing asthma, but may be useful in identifying triggers.[2,17] In small infants unable to perform spirometry, the diagnosis is more difficult. They may demonstrate hyperinflation on the chest roentgenogram.[2] Radiologic exam is helpful in ruling out other causes of wheezing (e.g., foreign body aspiration, parenchymal lung disease, cardiac disease, and congenital anomalies).[2] In place of pulmonary functions, the parents should be given a diary card to record symptoms and precipitating events.

BLOOD-GAS MEASUREMENT

Gas exchange at the alveoli–capillary interface is dependent on ventilation (V_a), or the mechanical properties of the lung, perfusion (Q), the flow of blood, and diffusion of the gases across the membrane. Blood–gas abnormalities are not found in chronic asthma. In acute severe asthma, diffusion capacity is slightly increased or unchanged.[22] Arterial hypoxemia is common during acute asthma attacks and is caused by V_a/Q mismatch.[22] The airway narrowing during asthma attacks, though diffuse, results in large abnormalities in the distribution of ventilation. The normal response to alveolar hypoxia is active vasoconstriction to shunt blood flow to better ventilated areas.[22] Unfortunately, the V_a and Q are not perfectly matched in acute asthma. This may in part be caused by the increased vascular resistance produced by the lung hyperinflation.[22]

When lungs initially become obstructed, patients demonstrate a marked respiratory drive thought to be caused by the stimulation of the irritant receptors because it is not obliterated by correcting the hypoxemia.[22] As a result, the asthmatic tends to "blow off" carbon dioxide (CO_2) and the arterial carbon dioxide concentration decreases. Unfortunately, the patient is forced to breath at higher lung volumes because of air trapping. This requires the use of accessory respiratory muscles. When obstruction worsens ($FEV_1 < 20\%$ of predicted) and the accessory respiratory muscles begin to fatigue, the patient will retain CO_2, and this may signal impending respiratory failure.[22]

Most patients who present with severe asthma in the emergency department will present with a mild metabolic acidosis (lactic acidosis from hypoxic metabolism in accessory respiratory muscles) and a low Pa_{O_2} and Pa_{CO_2}. More severely obstructed patients may have "normal" or elevated Pa_{CO_2}.

▶ TREATMENT: Asthma

DESIRED OUTCOMES

The NAEPP has provided the following goals for asthma management:

> 1) Maintain normal activity levels (including exercise and other physical activity); 2) Maintain (near) "normal" pulmonary function; 3) Prevent chronic and troublesome symptoms (e.g., coughing or breathlessness in the night, in the early morning, or after exertion); 4) Prevent recurrent exacerbations of asthma and minimize the need for emergency department visits or hospitalizations; 5) Provide optimal pharmacotherapy with minimal or no adverse effects; and 6) Meet patients' and families' expectations of satisfaction with asthma care.[2]

Toward these goals, every effort should be made to decrease the patient's baseline BHR and prevent it from increasing.

GENERAL APPROACH TO TREATMENT

Although the mainstay of the management of asthma is pharmacologic therapy, it is likely to fail without attending to the nonpharmacologic therapy issues. Figure 24–5 depicts the stepwise approach to asthma therapy recommended by the NAEPP.[2] It is important to see that the nonpharmacologic aspects of therapy are incorporated into the steps. The guidelines were designed to give primary health care providers a framework from which to develop the proper approach to the individualized therapy of patients. The heterogeneity of asthma demands an individualized approach to therapy with the basic goals of therapy as primary outcome measures.[2]

The knowledge that inflammation plays a primary role in the pathogenesis of asthma has led to the conviction that the focus of therapy is the prevention and suppression of the underlying inflammation.[2,17] Thus, current therapeutic options in asthma consist of acute reliever medications used for acute exacerbations, and long-term control medications used for the prevention of symptoms and the suppression of inflammation.[2] The currently accepted approach is to use drugs that suppress the inflammatory response as primary long-term control therapy thereby reducing the degree of BHR and improving long-term control and outcome in asthma by preventing airway remodeling.[2]

NONPHARMACOLOGIC THERAPY

The development of a partnership in care through patient education and the teaching of patient self-management skills should be the cornerstone of any treatment program.[2] There are a number of published self-management programs for children and adults available through local American Lung Association chapters as well as asthma treatment centers and nationally through the NAEPP and the Asthma and Allergy Foundation of America.[2] Asthma self-management programs have been shown to improve patient adherence to medication regimens, improve self-management skills, and improve use of health care services.[2] The object of these programs is to develop a partnership relationship between the patient and the health care provider. Table 24–4 lists the key educational messages recommended by the NAEPP.[2]

Self-management programs instruct patients in the pathogenesis of asthma and the appropriate use of their medications but principally focus on teaching patients to recognize triggers for their asthma and how to recognize early signs of deterioration.

TABLE 24–4. Key Educational Messages for Patients

Basic Facts About Asthma
• The contrast between asthmatic and normal airways
• What happens to the airways in an asthma attack
Roles of Medications
• How medications work
Long-term control: medications that prevent symptoms, often by reducing inflammation
Quick relief: short-acting bronchodilator relaxes muscles around airways
• Stress importance of long-term-control medications and not to expect quick relief from them
Skills
• Inhaler use (patient demonstrate)
• Spacer and holding chamber use
• Symptom monitoring, peak flow monitoring, and recognizing early signs of deterioration
Environmental Control Measures
• Identifying and avoiding environmental precipitants or exposures
When and How to Take Rescue Actions
• Responding to changes in asthma severity (daily self-management plan and action plan)

Treatment			Preferred treatments are in bold print.
	Long-term control	Quick relief	Education
STEP 4 Severe Persistent	Daily medications: • **Anti-inflammatory: inhaled corticosteroid (high dose)** AND • Long-acting bronchodilator: either **long-acting inhaled β_2-agonist,** sustained-release theophylline, or long-acting β_2-agonist tablets AND • Corticosteroid tablets or syrup long term (2 mg/kg/d, generally do not exceed 60 mg/d/).	• Short-acting bronchodilator: **inhaled β_2-agonists** as needed for symptoms. • Intensity of treatment will depend on severity of exacerbation; see component 3–Managing Exacerbations. • Use of short-acting inhaled β_2-agonists on a daily basis, or increasing use, indicates the need for additional long-term–control therapy.	Steps 2 and 3 actions plus: • Refer to individual education/counseling
STEP 3 Moderate Persistent	Daily medication: • Either **Anti-inflammatory: inhaled corticosteroid (medium dose)** OR **Inhaled corticosteroid (low-medium dose)** and add a long-acting bronchodilator, especially for nighttime symptoms: either **long-acting inhaled β_2-agonist,** sustained-release theophylline, or long-acting β_2-agonist tablets. • If needed Anti-inflammatory: **inhaled corticosteroids (medium-high dose)** AND **Long-acting bronchodilator**, especially for nighttime symptoms; either **long-acting inhaled β_2-agonist,** sustained-release theophylline, or long-acting β_2-agonist tablets.	• Short-acting bronchodilator: **inhaled β_2-agonists** as needed for symptoms. • Intensity of treatment will depend on severity of exacerbation; see component 3—Managing Exacerbations. • Use of short-acting inhaled β_2-agonists on a daily basis, or increasing use, indicates the need for additional long-term–control therapy.	Step 1 actions plus: • Teach self-monitoring • Refer to group education if available • Review and update self-management plan
STEP 2 Mild Persistent	One daily indication: • **Anti-inflammatory:** either **inhaled corticosteroid** (low doses) or **cromolyn or nedocromil** (children usually begin with a trial of cromolyn or nedocromil). • Sustained-release theophylline to serum concentration of 5–15 mg/mL is an alternative, but not preferred, therapy. Zafirlukast or zileuton may also be considered for patients ≥ 12 years of age, although their position in therapy is not fully established.	• Short-acting bronchodilator: **inhaled β_2-agonists** as needed for symptoms. • Intensity of treatment will depend on severity of exacerbation; see component 3—Managing Exacerbations. • Use of short-acting inhaled β_2-agonists on a daily basis, or increasing use, indicates the need for additional long-term–control therapy.	
STEP 1 Mild Intermittent	• No daily medication needed.	• Short-acting bronchodilator: **inhaled β_2-agonists** as needed for symptoms. • Intensity of treatment will depend on severity of exacerbation; see component 3–Managing Exacerbations. • Use of short-acting inhaled β_2-agonists more than 2 times a week may indicate the need to initiate long-term–control therapy.	• Teach basic facts about asthma • Teach inhaler/spacer/holding chamber technique • Discuss roles of medications • Develop self-management plan • Develop action plan for when and how to take rescue actions, especially for patients with a history of severe exacerbations • Discuss appropriate environmental control measures to avoid exposure to known allergens and irritants (See component 4.)

↓ Step down
Review treatment every 1–6 months; a gradual stepwise reduction in treatment may be possible.

↑ Step up
If control is not maintained, consider step up. First, review patient medication technique, adherence, and environmental control (avoidance of allergens or other factors that contribute to asthma severity).

Note:
- **The stepwise approach presents general guidelines to assist clinical decision making; it is not intended to be specific prescription. Asthma is highly variable; clinicians should tailor specific medication plans to the needs and circumstances of the individual patients.**
- Gain control as quickly as possible; then decrease treatment to the least medication necessary to maintain control. Gaining control may be accomplished by either starting treatment at the step most appropriate to the initial severity of the condition or starting at higher level of therapy (e.g., a course of systemic corticosteroids or higher dose of inhaled corticosteroids).
- A rescue course of systemic corticosteroids may be needed at any time and at any step.
- Some patients with intermittent asthma experience severe and life-threatening exacerbations separated by long periods of normal lung function and no symptoms. This may be especially common with exacerbations provoked by respiratory infections. A short course of systemic corticosteriods is recommended.
- At each step, patients should control their environment to avoid or control factors that make their asthma worse (e.g., allergens, irritants); this requires specific diagnosis and education.
- Referral to an asthma specialist for consultation or comanagement is *recommended* if there are difficulties achieving or maintaining control of asthma or if the patient requires step 4 care. Referral may be *considered* if the patient requires step 3 care.

FIGURE 24–5. Stepwise approach for managing asthma in adults and children older than 5 years of age. *(From Ref. 2.)*

Use of objective measurement of airflow obstruction with a home peak-flow meter is integral to many of the programs.[2] However, following a review of the literature, the NAEPP suggests that routine peak-flow monitoring in and of itself does not improve patient outcomes.[2]

The NAEPP now advocates the routine use of peak-flow meters for only those patients with moderate and severe persistent asthma.[2] They have recommended a system based on a traffic light scenario (based on percentage of normal predicted values or personal best values): Green Zone is equal to 80% to 100%; yellow zone is equal to 50% to 79%; red zone is less than 50%. The yellow zone is cautionary and requires increasing as needed bronchodilator use and either increasing the anti-inflammatory dose or beginning prednisone if not improved, whereas the red zone warrants contacting the patient's health care provider.[2] This approach can assist the patient and health professional determine the next level of therapy.

Patient education is essential before monitoring can be effective. Patient education has proven successful regardless of the health professional who provided the information (physician, nurse, or pharmacist). The NAEPP advocates significant involvement of the primary health care provider in the educational process. The provision of written treatment plans enhances the success of education and peak-flow monitoring and is considered an essential component of care.[2] Samples of clinically tested written action plans are available from the NAEPP Expert Panel Report 2.[2]

In patients with known allergenic triggers for their asthma, allergen avoidance has resulted in an improvement in symptoms, a reduction in medication use, and a decrease in BHR.[2,17,28] Relatively simple environmental controls for patients with house-dust-mite allergy such as removing carpeting from bedrooms, washing sheets in hot water (≥ 130°F), and using plastic pillow and mattress covers can reduce symptoms and need for medications.[2,17] Obvious environmental triggers (i.e., warm-blooded animals, cockroaches), if the patient is sensitive, should be avoided; however, there is very little evidence that extensive environmental controls (i.e., home air-filtering systems, chemicals for killing house-dust mites) are of any value.[2,28] Patients who smoke should be encouraged to stop. Parents of asthmatic children should stop or at least not smoke around their children.[33]

The role of immunotherapy (allergy shots) in asthma, although a proven and accepted therapy for allergic rhinitis, is still controversial.[2,28] Some studies have shown that immunotherapy of patients with very specific allergy reduces the number of late asthmatic responses and decreases BHR to the allergen whereas others have shown no effect.[26] A recent meta-analysis of immunotherapy trials suggested a positive benefit for specific immunotherapy against known allergens; however, the benefit was small in comparison to placebo.[34] A recent trial demonstrating an initial response to immunotherapy in the first year failed to find a continued effect in the second year.[35] Studies comparing immunotherapy to pharmacotherapy are warranted to determine the role for immunotherapy in asthma treatment.[28]

Oxygen therapy is indicated in patients requiring emergency therapy for acute severe asthma.[2,22] Oxygen reverses bronchial hyperreactivity induced by hypoxemia, as well as the hemoglobin desaturation produced by V_a/Q mismatching. Patients hospitalized with acute severe asthma should be given adequate maintenance hydration to mobilize secretions; however, excessive hydration should be avoided to prevent excessive lung fluid at a time when patients have inflammation and bronchial edema.[24]

PHARMACOLOGIC THERAPY

The current NAEPP recommendations for therapy of chronic asthma and acute exacerbations are illustrated in Figs. 24–5 to 24–7.[2] For persistent asthma the preferred therapies are listed in boldface. Regardless of the long-term control therapy all patients need to have quick relief-medication available for acute symptoms. The short-acting inhaled β_2-agonists are the drugs of first choice for quick relief. Alternatives would include oral short-acting β_2-agonists in infants and small children and inhaled anticholinergics in those patients intolerant to β_2-agonists. The preferred long-term controllers for moderate and severe persistent asthma are the inhaled corticosteroids. Cromolyn or nedocromil are acceptable alternatives in mild persistent asthma, particularly in young children. Alternatives that are *not preferred* in mild persistent asthma include theophylline and the leukotriene-modifying drugs. The current drug of choice as a second (additional) long-term controller in moderate and severe persistent asthma is salmeterol. Sustained-release theophylline (SRT) or long-acting oral β_2-agonists are alternative drugs.

β_2-AGONISTS

The β_2-agonists are the most effective bronchodilators available. β_2-Adrenergic receptor stimulation activates adenyl cyclase, which produces an increase in intracellular cyclic AMP.[27] This in turn decreases unbound intracellular calcium, producing smooth muscle relaxation, mast-cell membrane stabilization, and skeletal muscle stimulation.[27] β_2-Adrenergic stimulation also activates $Na^+ \rightarrow K^+$ ATPase, produces gluconeogenesis, and enhances insulin secretion, producing a mild to moderate decrease in serum potassium concentration by driving potassium intracellularly.[27] The chronotropic response to β_2-agonists is mediated in part by baroreceptor reflex mechanisms as a result of the drop in blood pressure from vascular smooth muscle relaxation, as well as by direct stimulation of cardiac β_2-receptors and some β_1 stimulation at high concentrations.[22,27] Table 24–5 lists the pharmacologic effects of adrenergic receptor stimulation. Because the excessive cardiac stimulation produces cardiac arrhythmias and the inotropic effect enhancing myocardial oxygen consumption leads to myocardial necrosis, there is no rationale for using non–β_2-selective agonists in the treatment of asthma.[22,27]

Table 24–6 compares the various β-adrenergic agonists in terms of selectivity, potency, oral activity, and duration of action. The β_2-agonists are functional or physiologic antagonists in that they relax airway smooth muscle regardless of the mechanism for constriction.[22,27] When administered in equipotent doses, all the short-acting drugs will produce the same intensity of response; the only differences will be in duration of action and cardiac toxicity.[2] All of the β-agonists are more bronchoselective when administered by the aerosol route.[22,27] Differences in myocardial effects are discernible between selective and nonselective agents even when administered as aerosols, particularly at the higher doses used for acute severe asthma.

The aerosol administration of β_2-agonists not only enhances bronchoselectivity but provides a greater degree of protection against provocations that induce bronchospasm such as exercise and allergen challenges than does systemic administration. Currently, the only disadvantage to aerosol administration of β_2-agonists is the relative complexity of administration. The two new long-acting β_2-agonists, formoterol and salmeterol, provide long-lasting protection (12 or more hours) when administered as aerosols.[27] Salmeterol is more β_2-selective than albuterol and more bronchoselective by virtue of its property of remaining in the lung, which produces its longer duration.

The dose–response relationship for β_2-agonist-induced bronchodilation has been extensively studied, and two aspects have significant clinical relevance. Both the intensity and duration of response are dose dependent, and more importantly the dose–response relationship is dynamic. At increasing levels of baseline bronchoconstriction (irrespective of the stimulus), the

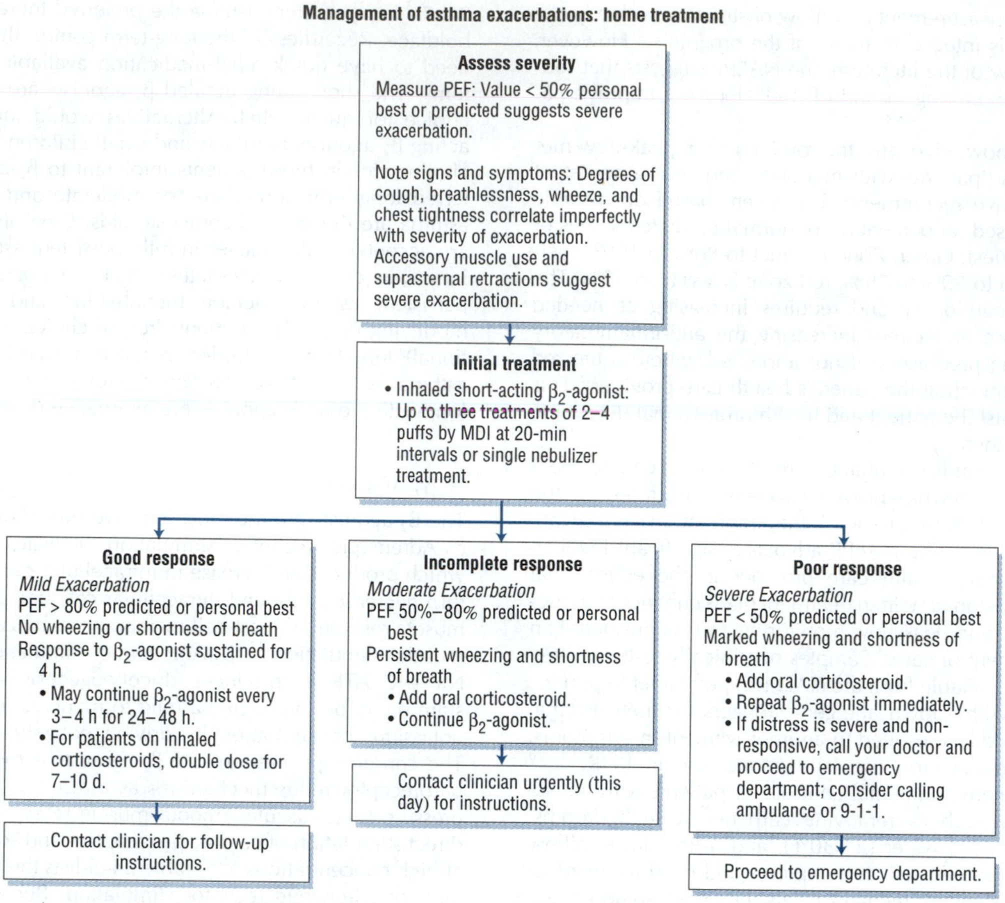
Management of asthma exacerbations: home treatment
Assess severity
Measure PEF: Value < 50% personal best or predicted suggests severe exacerbation.
Note signs and symptoms: Degrees of cough, breathlessness, wheeze, and chest tightness correlate imperfectly with severity of exacerbation. Accessory muscle use and suprasternal retractions suggest severe exacerbation.
Initial treatment
• Inhaled short-acting β2-agonist: Up to three treatments of 2–4 puffs by MDI at 20-min intervals or single nebulizer treatment.
Good response
Mild Exacerbation
PEF > 80% predicted or personal best
No wheezing or shortness of breath
Response to β2-agonist sustained for 4 h
• May continue β2-agonist every 3–4 h for 24–48 h.
• For patients on inhaled corticosteroids, double dose for 7–10 d.
Contact clinician for follow-up instructions.
Incomplete response
Moderate Exacerbation
PEF 50%–80% predicted or personal best
Persistent wheezing and shortness of breath
• Add oral corticosteroid.
• Continue β2-agonist.
Contact clinician urgently (this day) for instructions.
Poor response
Severe Exacerbation
PEF < 50% predicted or personal best
Marked wheezing and shortness of breath
• Add oral corticosteroid.
• Repeat β2-agonist immediately.
• If distress is severe and non-responsive, call your doctor and proceed to emergency department; consider calling ambulance or 9-1-1.
Proceed to emergency department.

FIGURE 24–6. Home management of acute asthma exacerbation. Patients at risk of asthma-related death should receive immediate clinical attention after initial treatment. Additional therapy may be required. *(From Ref. 2.)*

dose–response curve is shifted to the right and the duration of bronchodilation is decreased.[22,36] This is reflected in the need for higher, more frequent doses in acute asthma exacerbations[36] as well as by the fact that the duration of protection against significant provocation is much less than the duration of bronchodilation in chronic stable asthma (see Table 24–3).[27] The ability to increase the dose of the short-acting aerosolized β_2-agonists by as much as fivefold to 10-fold over those doses producing adequate bronchodilation in chronic stable asthmatics is what contributes to their efficacy in reversing the bronchospasm of acute severe asthma.[38]

Despite the fact that β_2-agonists are potent inhibitors of mast-cell degranulation, they do not inhibit the late asthmatic response to allergen challenge or the subsequent bronchial hyperresponsiveness.[2,27] Long-term administration of β_2-agonists does not reduce BHR, confirming a lack of significant anti-inflammatory activity.[27] Chronic administration of β_2-agonists can lead to a down-regulation (decreased number of β_2-receptors) and a decreased binding affinity for these receptors.[22,27] Glucocorticoid therapy can both prevent and partially reverse this phenomenon.[2,27] A significantly greater tolerance develops in all other β_2-receptors (lymphocyte, cardiac and skeletal muscle) compared with respiratory smooth muscle β_2-receptors.[22] Thus, the development of tolerance to the extrapulmonary effects (cardiac stimulation and hypokalemia) may account for a lack of significant cardiac effects with retention of the bronchodilator response despite chronic inhaled β_2-agonist therapy, whereas tolerance to mast-cell stabilization may be a drawback to chronic use.[22,27] The body of literature suggests that chronic β_2-agonist administration may produce a small degree of tolerance of minimal clinical significance that is easily overcome by increasing the dose or by administering glucocorticoids.[2,27] Tolerance also develops to the long-acting β_2-agonists when assessed with bronchoprovocation as would be expected from a receptor phenomenon.[27]

The β_2-Agonist Controversy

The potential for chronic use of inhaled β_2-agonists to worsen asthma and for excessive use to increase the risk of dying from asthma has been a concern for over 20 years, since the first publication of the association between increased asthma deaths and isoproterenol metered-dose inhalers (MDIs). A complete review is beyond the scope of this chapter. Only one study has reported significantly worsening asthma from regular use of short-acting β_2-agonists.[37] Reanalysis of that report[38] and subsequent double-blind, placebo-controlled trials in large numbers of patients have not confirmed that regular administration short-acting inhaled β_2-agonists worsens asthma.[39,40] However, regular use of short-acting inhaled β_2-agonists provides little if any benefit over as needed use[40] and therefore is not recommended.[2,27]

A case-control epidemiologic study suggested an increased risk of asthma death and near-death episodes associated with excessive use of both fenoterol and albuterol by MDI that correlated with the number of canisters used.[41] Follow-up cohort analysis demonstrated that the increased risk of death occurred primarily after usage exceeded 2 canisters per month, which was in excess of recommended limits.[2,27] The final analysis found that the increased risk appeared primarily if the increased use of the

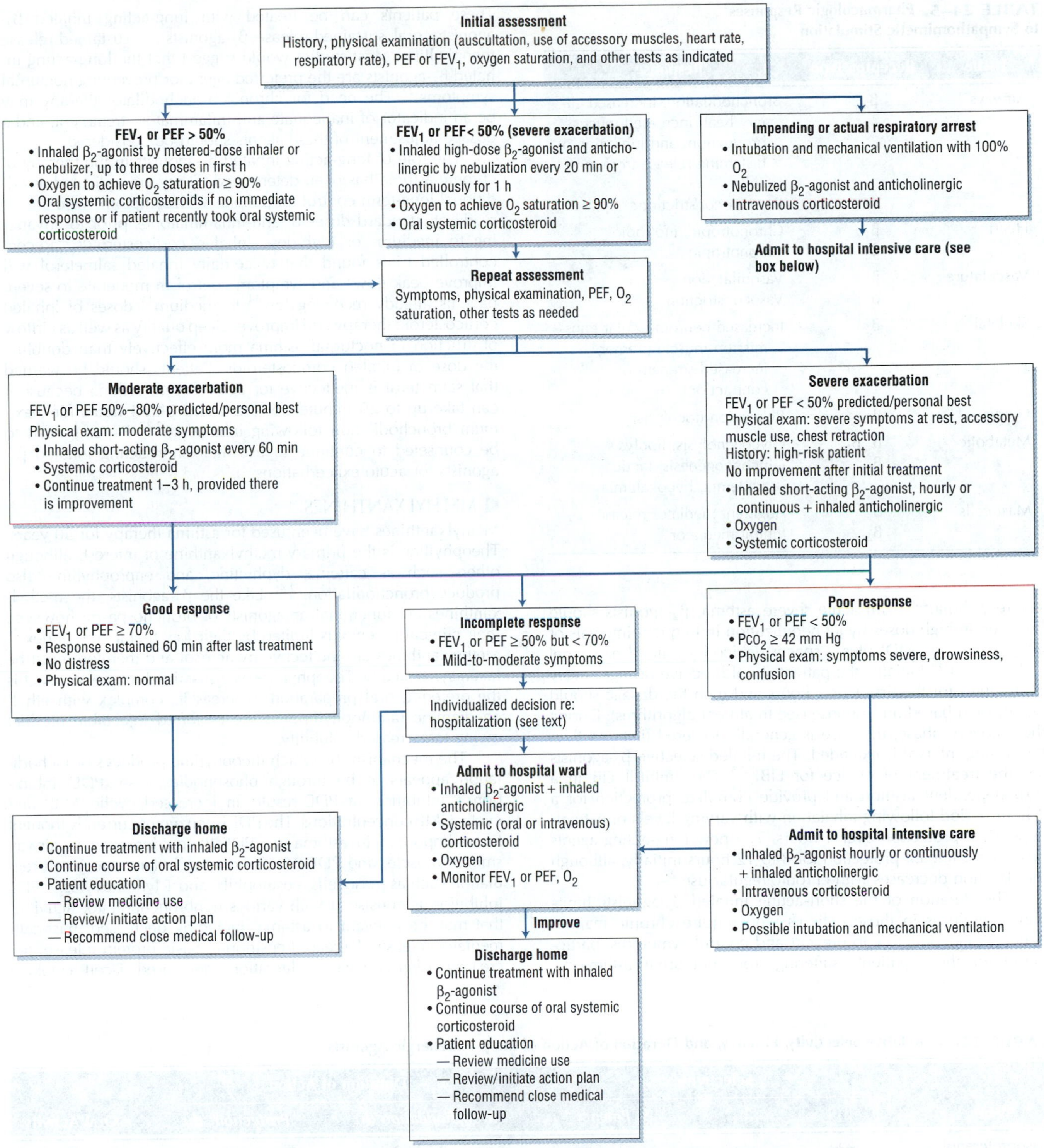

FIGURE 24–7. Emergency department and hospital care of acute asthma exacerbations. *(From Ref. 2.)*

β_2-agonists occurred in the 2 months prior to the event, suggesting that the increased use was a marker for asthma deterioration as opposed to a causative factor.[42] A meta-analysis of all case-control trials evaluating the role of inhaled β_2-agonists and asthma deaths demonstrated only a weak association with nebulized β_2-agonists.[43] Because the more severe patients receive home nebulizers, this again suggests that asthma severity is the strongest link to death from asthma. No convincing evidence exists for either increased risk of death or worsening asthma from regular use of the long-acting inhaled β_2-agonists.[2,27]

Clinical Use

Inhaled short-acting selective β_2-agonists are indicated for the treatment of intermittent episodes of bronchospasm and are the bronchodilator as well as the first treatment of choice for acute

TABLE 24–5. Pharmacologic Responses to Sympathomimetic Stimulation

Tissue	Receptor Type	Response
Airways	β_2	Bronchodilation, increased ciliary beat, increased mucus production, and inhibition of histamine release from mast cells
	α	Bronchoconstriction?
Heart	β_1	Chronotropic, inotropic
	β_2	Chronotropic
Vasculature	β_2	Vasodilatation
	α	Vasoconstriction
Skeletal	β_2	Increased neuromuscular transmission muscle (tremor, increased strength of contraction)
Uterus	β_2	Relaxation (tocolysis)
Metabolic	α, β_1	Glycogenolysis, lipolysis
	β_2	Gluconeogenesis, lactic acidemia, hypokalemia
Mast cells	α	Augment mediator release
	β_2	Inhibit mediator

severe asthma.[2,22,36] In acute severe asthma, β_2-agonists should be given in high doses by jet nebulization in frequent intervals or alternatively via MDI plus a spacer device by trained personnel (Table 24–7).[36] Initially, the patient should receive dosages every 20 minutes for the first 1 or 2 hours and then the dosage should be adjusted based on response (see treatment algorithms). During the recovery phase, the dose is generally lowered first and then the dosing interval is extended. The inhaled selective β_2-agonists are the treatment of choice for EIB.[2,13] They inhibit EIB in a dose-dependent fashion and provide complete protection for a 2-hour period following inhalation with varying levels of patient-dependent protection over 4 hours. The new long-acting agents provide significant protection for 8 to 12 hours initially, although the duration decreases with chronic regular use.[27]

The duration of the short-acting inhaled β_2-agonists limits their usefulness in those patients who require chronic maintenance bronchodilators to prevent and control symptoms, particularly for those patients suffering from nocturnal asthma.[2,27] These patients can be treated with long-acting inhaled β_2-agonists, oral sustained-release β_2-agonists, or sustained-release theophylline. Most studies would suggest that the long-acting inhaled β_2-agonists are the preferred agent for preventing nocturnal symptoms.[27] The need for chronic bronchodilator therapy may be an indicator of inadequate anti-inflammatory treatment, and a dosage adjustment of these agents should be considered.

The role of long-acting inhaled β_2-agonists in the therapy of chronic asthma has been determined.[2] They are indicated as additional long-term control for patients with symptoms who are already on standard doses of anti-inflammatories prior to advancing to medium- or high-dose inhaled corticosteroids.[2] Recent controlled trials found that twice-daily inhaled salmeterol will improve peak flows and symptom control in moderate to severe patients already receiving low[44] to medium[45] doses of inhaled corticosteroid therapy and improves sleep quality as well as airflow obstruction in nocturnal asthma more effectively than doubling the dose of inhaled corticosteroids. Patients should be warned that salmeterol is ineffective for acute severe asthma because it can take up to 20 minutes for onset and 1 to 4 hours for maximum bronchodilation following inhalation.[2,27] Patients need to be counseled to continue to use their short-acting inhaled β_2-agonists for acute exacerbations.

METHYLXANTHINES

Methylxanthines have been used for asthma therapy for 50 years. Theophylline is the primary methylxanthine of interest, although others such as caffeine, dyphylline, and enprophylline also produce bronchodilation.[22,46] Like the β_2-agonists, the methylxanthines are functional antagonists of bronchospasm; however, their clinical potency is limited by their low therapeutic index.[22] Methylxanthines are ineffective by aerosol and therefore must be taken systemically. Theophylline as a sustained-release product is the preferred oral preparation, whereas its complex with ethylenediamine (aminophylline) is the preferred injectable product owing to increased solubility.

The mechanism by which theophylline produces bronchodilation appears to be through phosphodiesterase (PDE) inhibition.[47] Inhibition of PDE results in increased cyclic AMP and cyclic GMP concentrations. The PDE isoenzymes currently thought to be important in asthma are PDE III, predominant in airway smooth muscle, and PDE IV, important in inflammatory cell regulation such as mast cells, eosinophils, and T lymphocytes.[47] PDE inhibition is consistent with various nonbronchodilator activities that may be relevant to asthma, including decreased mast-cell-mediator release, decreased eosinophil basic-protein release, decreased T-lymphocyte proliferation, decreased T-cell cytokine

TABLE 24–6. Relative Selectivity, Potency, and Duration of Action of the β-Adrenergic Agonists

Agent	Selectivity			Duration of Action		Oral Activity
	β_1	β_2	β_2 *Potency*[a]	*Bronchodilation (h)*	*Protection*[b] *(h)*	
Isoproterenol	++++	++++	1	0.5–2.0	0.5–1.0	No
Metaproterenol	+++	+++	15	3–4	1–2	Yes
Isoetharine	++	+++	6	0.5–2.0	0.5–1.0	No
Albuterol	+	++++	2	4–8	2–4	Yes
Bitolterol	+	++++	5	4–8	2–4	No
Pirbuterol	+	++++	5	4–8	2–4	Yes
Terbutaline	+	++++	4	4–8	2–4	Yes
Formoterol	+	++++	0.24	> 12	> 12	Yes
Salmeterol	+	++++	0.50	> 12	> 12	UK[c]

[a]Relative molar potency: 1 = most potent.
[b]Protection refers to the duration of time that bronchoconstriction may be prevented.
[c]UK = unknown.

TABLE 24–7. Dosages of Drugs for Acute Severe Exacerbations of Asthma in the Emergency Department or Hospital

Medications	Dosages: Adults	Dosages: Children	Comments
Inhaled β_2-agonists			
Albuterol Nebulizer Soln (5 mg/mL)	2.5–5 mg every 20 min for 3 doses, then 2.5–10 mg every 1–4 has needed, or 10–15 mg/h continuously.	0.15 mg/kg (minimum dose 2.5 mg) every 20 min for 3 doses, then 0.15–0.3 mg/kg up to 10 mg every 1–4 h as needed, or 0.5 mg/kg/h by continuous nebulization.	Only selective β_2-agonists are recommended. For optimal delivery, dilute aerosols to minimum of 4 mL at gas flow of 6–8 L/min.
MDI 90 μg/puff	4–8 puffs every 30 min up to 4 h then every 1–4 h as needed.	4–8 puffs every 20 min for 3 doses, then every 1–4 h as needed.	In patients in severe distress, nebulization is preferred; use holding-chamber–type spacer.
Bitolterol Nebulizer Soln (2 mg/mL)	See albuterol dose.	See albuterol dose. Thought to be as potent to one-half as potent as albuterol on an mg basis.	Has not been studied in acute severe asthma. Do not mix with other drugs.
MDI 370 μg/puff	See albuterol dose.	See albuterol dose.	Has not been studied in acute severe asthma.
Pirbuterol MDI 200 μg/puff	See albuterol dose.	See albuterol dose. One-half as potent as albuterol on an mg basis.	Has not been studied in acute severe asthma.
Systemic β-agonists			
Epinephrine 1:1000 (1 mg/mL)	0.3–0.5 mg every 20 min for 3 doses SQ.	0.01 mg/kg up to 0.5 mg every 20 min for 3 doses SQ.	No proven advantage of systemic therapy over aerosol.
Terbutaline (1 mg/mL)	0.25 mg every 20 min for 3 doses SQ.	0.01 mg/kg every 20 min for 3 doses, then every 2–6 h as needed SQ.	Not recommended.
Anticholinergics			
Ipratropium Br-Nebulizer Soln (0.25 mg/mL)	500 μg every 30 min for 3 doses, then every 2–4 h as needed.	250 μg every 20 min for 3 doses, then 250 μg every 2–4 h.	May mix in same nebulizer with albuterol. Do not use as first-line therapy, only add to β_2-agonist therapy.
MDI 18 μg/puff	4–8 puffs as needed.	4–8 puffs as needed.	Not recommended as dose in inhaler is low and has not been studied in acute asthma.
Corticosteroids			
Prednisone Methylprednisolone Prednisolone	120–180 mg in 3 or 4 divided doses for 48 h, then 60–80 mg/d until PEF reaches 70% of personal best.	1 mg/kg every 6 h for 48 h, then 1–2 mg/kg/d in 2 divided doses until PEF reaches 70% of normal predicted.	For outpatient "burst" use 1–2 mg/kg/d max 60 mg for 3–7 d. It is unnecessary to taper following the course.

No advantage has been found for very–high-dose corticosteroids in acute severe asthma, nor is there any advantage for intravenous administration over oral therapy. The usual regimen is to continue the frequent multiple daily dosing until the patient achieves an FEV_1 or PEF of 50% of personal best or normal predicted value and then lower the dose to twice-daily dosing. This usually occurs within 48 hours. The final duration of therapy following a hospitalization or emergency department visit may be from 7 to 14 days. If patients are then started on inhaled corticosteroids, studies indicate that there is no need to taper the systemic steroid dose. If the follow-up therapy is to be given once daily, studies indicate that there may be an advantage to giving the single daily dose in the afternoon at around 3:00 PM.

release, and decreased plasma exudation.[46] Selective PDE isoenzyme inhibitors are currently being evaluated for possible treatment of asthma. Theophylline is a nonselective PDE inhibitor.[47] Some clinical trials indicate that theophylline may provide anti-inflammatory activity in asthma.[46] However, studies have failed to demonstrate an effect on BHR except when the drug is present as a functional antagonist to the provocative agent.[2,22] Theophylline is a competitive antagonist of adenosine; however, this property is not shared by enprofylline, a more potent bronchodilator than theophylline.[22] Theophylline also stimulates endogenous catecholamine release.[46] These latter two effects are important determinants of toxic symptoms of excess theophylline.[2,46]

Both bronchodilation and protection against bronchoprovocation challenges are concentration dependent. Theophylline produces linear increases in bronchodilation with logarithmic increments in serum drug concentrations.[46] The majority of chronic stable asthmatics will obtain significant bronchodilation when the serum theophylline concentration reaches 5 μg/mL and most patients will have no toxic symptoms with serum concentrations less than 15 μg/mL.[2,48] The percentage of patients experiencing adverse effects is approximately 18% at serum concentrations between 15 and 20 μg/mL.[48] This increases sharply to 60% at concentrations between 20 and 30 μg/mL, and 80% at concentrations greater than 30 μg/mL.[48]

As with the β_2-agonists, the dose–response curves for smooth muscle relaxation by theophylline are dynamic and shifted to the right in the face of increasing contractile stimuli.[48] This probably explains theophylline's relative lack of bronchodilatory effect in acute severe asthma.[2] The severity of theophylline's toxicity precludes even doubling the usual dosage.

Theophylline has other effects that may be important to its antiasthmatic action. Theophylline inhibits pulmonary edema by decreasing vascular permeability, enhances mucociliary clearance, and strengthens contraction of a fatigued diaphragm.[46] *In vitro* theophylline inhibits the release of histamine in sensitized human lung fragments but has provided an inconsistent protection against the early asthmatic response to allergens.[46] When present in therapeutic concentrations, theophylline attenuates the bronchospasm of the late asthmatic response,[46] but has no apparent effect on the subsequent increase in BHR.[2]

Other Effects

Theophylline stimulates the central nervous system through its adenosine antagonism and produces cerebral vasoconstriction.[46] Both effects contribute to the neurotoxicities seen with theophylline. Theophylline acts as a respiratory stimulant by enhancing the hypoxic ventilatory drive, decreases the lower esophageal sphincter pressure and increases gastric acid secretion, and has both inotropic and chronotropic cardiac effects.[22] Acutely theophylline acts as a diuretic but tolerance develops rapidly.

Pharmacokinetics

An understanding of the pharmacokinetics combined with routine monitoring of serum concentrations is essential for the safe and effective use of theophylline.[2,46] Theophylline is primarily eliminated by metabolism via the hepatic cytochrome P450 mixed-function oxidase microsomal enzymes (primarily the CYP1A2 and CYP3A3 isozymes) with 10% or less excreted unchanged in the kidney.[46,49] Each of the major metabolic pathways for theophylline is saturable within the usual therapeutic concentration so that theophylline frequently, though not always, exhibits nonlinear pharmacokinetics.[46,49] This may partially explain the relatively large intrapatient variability in theophylline clearance (often as great as 30%) over time.[49] Part of the intrapatient variability in clearance is age dependent with 1- to 9-year-olds having the greatest clearance rates, and therefore requiring the largest dosages (on a weight basis) for theophylline. However, even within the same age groups theophylline clearance can vary twofold to threefold so that no patient should be treated with theophylline without routine monitoring of serum theophylline concentrations.[2] Figure 24–8 gives a dosing and monitoring schedule for theophylline.

The hepatic cytochrome P450 enzymes are susceptible to induction and inhibition by various environmental factors and drugs. These are listed in Table 24–8. Only those drugs or diseases that produce a 20% or greater inhibition or 50% or greater induction of theophylline metabolism are likely to result in clinically significant interactions.[49] Also, significant interpatient susceptibility to developing an interaction exists even with potent P450 inhibitors such as cimetidine. However, the clinician needs to be aware of drugs that have been proven to alter theophylline metabolism, or could potentially do so, to provide appropriate alternatives and monitor the patient appropriately.

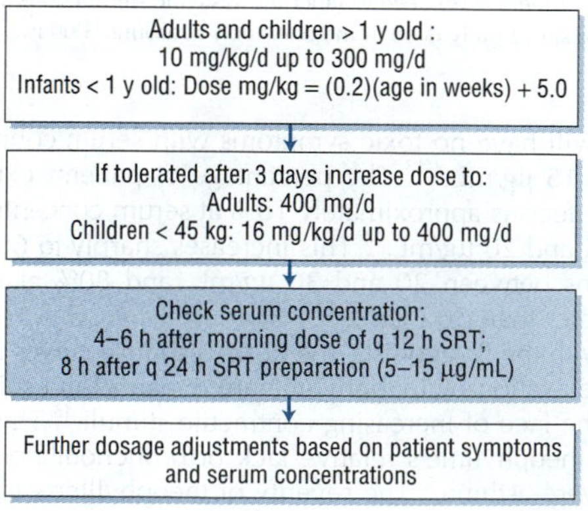

FIGURE 24–8. Algorithm for slow titration of theophylline dosage and guide for final dosage adjusment based on serum theophylline concentration measurement. For infants < 1 year of age, the initial daily dosage can be calculated by the following regression equation: Dose (mg/kg) = (0.2) (age in weeks) + 5.0. *Whenever side effects occur, dosage should be reduced to a previously tolerated lower dose.*

TABLE 24–8. Factors Affecting Theophylline Clearance

Decreased Clearance	Percent Decrease (%)	Increased Clearance	Percent Increase (%)
Cimetidine	−25 to −60	Rifampin	+53
Macrolides: Erythromycin, TAO, clarithromycin	−25 to −50	Carbamazepine	+50
Allopurinol	−20	Phenobarbital	+34
Propranolol	−30	Phenytoin	+70
Qinolones: Ciprofloxacin, enoxacin, pefloxacin	−20 to −50	Charcoal-broiled meat	+30
Thiabendazole	−65	High-protein diet	+25
Ticlopidine	−25	Smoking	+40
Zileuton	−35	Sulfinpyrazone	+22
Systemic viral illness	−10 to −50		

Owing to the relatively short elimination half-life of theophylline (3 to 5 hours in children and 6 to 12 hours in adults), sustained-release oral preparations are favored for outpatient therapy.[2,49] These preparations can be administered every 8 to 24 hours and maintain relatively constant therapeutic serum concentrations in patients, and the decreased dosing frequency improves compliance.[46,49] The degree of serum theophylline concentration fluctuation over the dosing interval is dependent on the release characteristics of the products as well as the elimination rate characteristics of the patients.[46] Thus, patients with rapid clearances for theophylline will experience greater fluctuations than patients with slow clearances, given the same product over the same dosing interval. Neither an optimal nor an acceptable maximum fluctuation has been absolutely established for theophylline serum concentrations, but it seems reasonable that it should not exceed the usual therapeutic range. That is, it should not exceed 100% for twice-daily dosing or 150% for once-daily dosing where percent fluctuation = $(Cp_{max} - Cp_{min})/Cp_{min}$. Each of the sustained-release theophylline products has different release characteristics, and the products are variably susceptible to altered absorption from food or gastric pH changes.[46] Preparations with slower release characteristically exhibit a significant diurnal variation in absorption, with the rate significantly slower at night in the recumbent patient.[49] As a result of these differences, it is best not to consider the sustained-release preparations interchangeable. In general, preparations unaffected by food that can be administered a minimum of every 12 hours in most patients are preferable.

Clinical Use

Theophylline has not been shown to add to the efficacy of aerosolized β_2-agonists in acute severe exacerbations of asthma and is no longer recommended.[2] In the outpatient setting chronic theophylline administration can reduce asthma symptoms, reduce the amount of as-needed inhaled β_2-agonists used, and reduce the oral steroid requirement in steroid-dependent asthmatics.[46] Sustained-release theophylline once nightly is effective for nocturnal asthma.[46] Comparative studies between sustained-release theophylline and oral sustained-release β_2-agonists have not shown any advantage for theophylline.[50] Significant disadvantages to chronic theophylline therapy include theophylline's lack of effect on BHR and the dangers inherent in giving a drug that can produce severe neurologic toxicity, including seizures, permanent neurologic deficit, and death at serum concentrations only twofold greater than optimal therapeutic concentrations. Death has occurred in children receiving their usual doses of theophylline during acute systemic viral illnesses.[48] Studies comparing cromolyn and theophylline as first-line therapy for chronic asthma have failed to demonstrate an advantage for theophylline over cromolyn.[51]

Serum theophylline concentrations must be routinely monitored for the safe and effective use of theophylline. The therapeutic range of 5 to 15 μg/mL is not an absolute but a statistical concept.[49] This therapeutic range has been recommended by the NAEPP as an effective and safe range of steady-state concentrations for most patients. Owing to the log-linear nature of the concentration–response curve, there is little to gain in terms of bronchodilation by going from 15 μg/mL to 20 μg/mL.[35] Patients whose theophylline concentrations are maintained near 20 μg/mL are more susceptible to developing serious adverse effects when confronted with an environmental exposure that inhibits theophylline metabolism. Owing to its high risk–benefit ratio theophylline is considered a second- or third-line drug in the therapy of asthma.

ANTICHOLINERGICS

The anticholinergic agents have been used for centuries in the form of stramonium herbal treatments for asthma.[22] However, their systemic effects, particularly involving the central nervous system, limited their usefulness. The introduction of quaternary ammonium derivatives such as ipratropium bromide has renewed interest in these compounds. Anticholinergic bronchodilators are competitive inhibitors of muscarinic receptors. Unlike β_2-agonists and theophylline, they are not functional antagonists; they produce bronchodilation only in cholinergic-mediated bronchoconstriction. Normal bronchial tone is maintained through parasympathetic innervation of the airways via the vagus nerve. A number of the triggers and mediators of asthma (histamine, prostaglandins, sulfur dioxide, exercise, allergens) produce bronchoconstriction in part through vagal reflex mechanisms.[22] Studies of asthmatics consistently demonstrate that anticholinergics are effective bronchodilators though not as potent as β_2-agonists. Anticholinergics attenuate but do not block allergen- or exercise-induced asthma in a dose-dependent fashion and have no effect on the LAR or BHR.[22] Ipratropium bromide consistently produces a 10% to 20% improvement in FEV_1 over β_2-agonists alone in acute severe asthma.[52] However, a significant interpatient variability exists, with some patients obtaining significantly greater (40% to 80%) improvements and others minimal improvement.[53] Regular administration of ipratropium bromide has not improved outcomes in chronic asthma over β_2-agonists alone.[2]

Currently available anticholinergics are nonselective muscarinic receptor blockers, and blockade of inhibitory muscarinic receptors could theoretically result in an increased release of acetylcholine and overcome the block on the smooth muscle receptors (M3).[22] This mechanism may explain why some patients have experienced paradoxical bronchoconstriction from nebulized anticholinergics. Only the quaternary ammonium derivatives (ipratropium bromide) should be used because they have the advantage of poor absorption across mucosae and the blood–brain barrier. This results in negligible systemic effects with a prolonged local effect (i.e., bronchodilation). In addition, the quaternary compounds do not appear to produce a decrease in mucociliary clearance.[22] Ipratropium bromide has a duration of action of 4 to 8 hours. Both intensity and duration of action are dose dependent. Time to reach maximum bronchodilation is considerably slower than from aerosolized short-acting β_2-agonists (2 hours vs 30 minutes). However, this is of little clinical consequence because some bronchodilation is seen within 30 seconds, 50% of maximum response occurs within 3 minutes, and 80% of maximum is reached within 30 minutes.[22,52] A recent trial using aggressive dosing of nebulized ipratropium bromide in the emergency department reported a decrease in the number of children admitted to the hospital.[54]

Clinical Use

The role of anticholinergics in the treatment of asthma is limited. They are not indicated for the long-term control of asthma. Ipratropium bromide is indicated only as adjunctive therapy in acute severe asthma not completely responsive to β_2-agonists alone.[2,53,54]

CROMOLYN SODIUM AND NEDOCROMIL SODIUM

Cromolyn sodium has been available for the prophylactic treatment of asthma for over 20 years, whereas nedocromil sodium, a pyranoquinoline dicarboxylic acid that is pharmacologically similar, has just recently been released in the United States.[2] The exact mechanism of action for these agents is still unknown. Although minor differences in activity do exist, the principal difference appears to be potency, with 4 mg of nedocromil by MDI equivalent to 20 mg of cromolyn sodium by Spinhaler.[55] These drugs produce mast-cell-membrane stabilization inhibiting the EAR to allergen challenge as well as EIB.[51,55] Unlike the β_2-agonists and other experimental mast-cell-membrane stabilizers, cromolyn and nedocromil also inhibit the LAR and prevent the subsequent increased BHR.[51,55] Long-term treatment with cromolyn prevents the usual rise in BHR associated with specific pollen seasons and may produce a modest decrease in baseline BHR.[2] Both cromolyn and nedocromil inhibit *in vitro* activation of human neutrophils, macrophages, and eosinophils.[22,55] Each agent also inhibits neurally mediated bronchoconstriction through C-fiber sensory nerve stimulation in the airways.[55] Neither drug has a bronchodilatory effect.

Cromolyn and nedocromil are effective by inhalation only and are available as MDIs, whereas cromolyn also comes as a nebulizer solution. The pharmacokinetics of both drugs are also very similar. They are not bioavailable orally but the portion of the dose that reaches the lung is completely absorbed.[22] Absorption from the airway is significantly slower than elimination (hours vs minutes). Both the intensity and duration of protection against various challenges is dose dependent.[22,55] Higher doses produce greater and more-prolonged protection.

Both drugs are remarkably nontoxic. No evidence of mutagenesis or teratogenesis has been found for cromolyn and less than 0.1% of an intravenous dose crosses the placenta or enters breast milk.[51] Cough and wheeze have been reported following inhalation of each and bad taste and headache following nedocromil. The taste from nedocromil is sufficiently bad for some patients (approximately 20%) to preclude them from taking the drug. Cromolyn is undoubtedly the least toxic drug used to treat asthma, with significant adverse effects occurring in less than 1 in 10,000 patients.[51] Tolerance to cromolyn or nedocromil has not been demonstrated.

Approximately 60% to 75% of patients (adults and children) with mild persistent asthma will be adequately controlled with cromolyn.[51] Comparative studies between cromolyn and theophylline do not demonstrate a significant advantage for either agent in controlling symptoms of asthma or improving baseline pulmonary functions.[51] However, theophylline therapy may produce more side effects and require more patient visits for monitoring.[51] Neither is as effective as inhaled corticosteroids.

Clinical Use

Cromolyn and nedocromil are indicated for the prophylaxis of mild persistent asthma in both children and adults regardless of etiology. They are particularly effective for allergic asthmatics on a seasonal basis or just prior to an acute exposure (i.e., animals or mowing the lawn).[2] Cromolyn is the second drug of choice for the prevention of EIB and may be used in conjunction with a β_2-agonist in more severe cases not completely responding to either agent alone.[13] The NAEPP has suggested that cromolyn and nedocromil be the anti-inflammatories of first choice for childhood asthma owing to their efficacy and safety.[2,17] Nedocromil therapy may allow the patient to decrease inhaled steroid dosage.[2,55]

The efficacy of each drug is directly related to its degree of deposition in the lung, so when beginning therapy it is important that the airways be patent. A short course of systemic glucocorticoids and around-the-clock inhaled β_2-agonists may initially be required in patients with significant obstruction. Most patients will experience an improvement in 1 to 2 weeks but it may take longer to achieve maximum benefit. Patients should initially receive cromolyn or nedocromil four times daily, and then only after stabilization of symptoms may the frequency be reduced to two to three times daily.

GLUCOCORTICOID THERAPY

The inhaled corticosteroids are the most effective anti-inflammatories available to treat asthma.[2,56] The mechanism of action and use of glucocorticoids in asthma have been recently reviewed.[57,58] Actions useful in treating asthma include (1) increasing the number of β_2-adrenergic receptors and improving the receptor responsiveness to β_2-adrenergic stimulation; (2) reducing mucus production and hypersecretion; and (3) inhibiting the inflammatory response at all levels.[57] The anti-inflammatory effects of possible benefit in asthma include decreasing the synthesis and release of several pro-inflammatory cytokines such as IL-1, GM-CSF, IL-3, IL-4, IL-5, IL-6, and IL-8; reducing inflammatory cell activation, recruitment, and infiltration; and decreasing vascular permeability.[57,58]

Cortisol and its synthetic derivatives all have beneficial effects in the treatment of asthma related to the prevention or suppression of airway inflammation. Suppressing the ongoing airway inflammation results in reduction of BHR and prevention and reversal of airway remodeling.[2,59]

Time Course of Response

Glucocorticoids act through binding to specific sites on nuclear DNA to modify gene expression, messenger RNA, and protein synthesis such as increasing the synthesis of lipocortin and β_2-adrenergic receptors; therefore, the time required to see the particular effect is dependent on the time required for new protein synthesis, decreased formation of the particular mediator, and resolution of the response.[56] Generally, the cellular and biochemical effects are immediate, but varying amounts of time are required to produce a clinical response. β_2-receptor density increases within 4 hours of glucocorticoid administration.[56] Improved responsiveness to β_2-agonists occurs within 2 hours.[22] In acute severe asthma, 4 to 12 hours may be required before any clinical response is noted.[60] Reversal of seasonal increased BHR requires at least 1 week of therapy.[56,58] Sensitivity to EIB decreases after 4 weeks of therapy.[13] Although single doses do not inhibit the immediate asthmatic response to antigen challenge, continued therapy for 1 week partially suppresses the response. These two latter effects are likely owing to a reduction in mucosal mast cells.[56,58]

The response to inhaled corticosteroids is somewhat more delayed. Most patients' symptoms will improve in the first 1 to 2 weeks of therapy and reach maximum improvement in 4 to 8 weeks. Improvement in baseline FEV_1 and PEFs requires 3 to 6 weeks for maximum improvement,[61,62] whereas improvement in BHR requires 1 to 3 months and may continue to improve over 1 year.[56] No evidence indicates that the use of glucocorticoids in the persistent asthmatic will induce a state of steroid dependence. In fact, most of the evidence demonstrating a decrease in BHR with steroid therapy implies just the opposite.

Systemic Glucocorticoid Therapy

Acute severe asthma, status asthmaticus, is treated with high-dose systemic glucocorticoids combined with frequent administration of inhaled β_2-agonists.[2,22] Glucocorticoids can be administered by the parenteral route (methylprednisolone sodium succinate, hydrocortisone sodium succinate) or alternatively by the oral route (prednisone, methylprednisolone), either of which provides a rapid onset of action and a systemic effect.[60] The glucocorticoids used in asthma are compared in Table 24–9. Recommended dosages for acute asthma are listed in Table 24–7. No difference in response between intravenous and oral administration has been shown.[60] Although the duration of action has been poorly studied, evidence suggests that divided doses should be used initially. Following resolution of severe obstruction (achievement of > 50% of predicted normal FEV_1, which generally occurs in the first 48 hours), the steroid dose is reduced as one or two doses orally.[60] The duration of treatment is dependent on the patient's response and past history. Tapering the steroid dosage after hospitalization does not affect outcome in terms of recovery or reexacerbation rate and, therefore, is unnecessary.[2]

TABLE 24–9. Glucocorticoid Comparison Chart

Systemic	Relative Anti-Inflammatory Potency	Relative Sodium-Retaining Potency	Duration Biologic Activity (h)	Plasma Elimination Half-Life (h)
Hydrocortisone	1	1.0	8–12	1.5–2.0
Prednisone	4	0.8	12–36	2.5–3.5
Methylprednisolone	5	0.5	12–36	3.3
Dexamethasone	25	0	36–54	3.4–4.0
Aerosol	**Topical Potency (Skin Blanching)**	**Receptor-Binding Affinity**	**Receptor Complex Half-Life (h)**	**Oral Bioavailability (%)**
Flunisolide (FLU)	330	1.8	3.5	21
Triamcinolone acetonide (TAA)	330	3.6	3.9	10.6
Beclomethasone dipropionate (BDP)	600	13.5	7.5	20
Budesonide (BUD)	980	9.4	5.1	11
Fluticasone propionate (FP)	1200	18	10.5	< 1

TABLE 24–10. Adverse Effects of Chronic Systemic Glucocorticoid Administration

Hypothalamic–pitutitary–adrenal suppression	Hypertension
Growth retardation	Skin striae
Skeletal muscle myopathy	Impaired wound healing
Osteoporosis/fractures	Inhibition of leukocyte and monocyte function
Aseptic necrosis of bone	Subcutaneous tissue atrophy
Pancreatitis	Glaucoma
Pseudotumor cerebri	Posterior subcapsular cataracts
Psychiatric disturbances	Moon facies
Sodium and water retention	Central redistribution of fat
Hypokalemia/hyperglycemia	

Systemic glucocorticoids are also recommended for the treatment of impending episodes of severe asthma unresponsive to bronchodilator therapy.[2,60] Prednisone, approximately 1 to 2 mg/kg/d (up to 40 to 60 mg/d), is administered orally in two divided doses for 3 to 10 days.[2] If an adequate response is not achieved, administration of prednisone three times daily may be worthwhile. The dose and duration of treatment are based on the patient's response and past history. The effects of glucocorticoids in asthma are dose and duration dependent. This is true for the adverse effects as well (Table 24–10).[57] The clinician is continually forced to balance the toxicity of chronic systemic glucocorticoid therapy versus control of asthma symptoms. Because short-term (1 to 2 weeks) high-dose steroids (1 to 2 mg/kg/d prednisone) do not produce serious toxicities, the ideal use is to administer the glucocorticoids in a short "burst" and then maintain the patient on appropriate long-term control therapy with long periods between systemic glucocorticoid treatment.[2] In general, therapy for more than 5 days at doses that exceed the usual physiologic endogenous cortisol production will cause temporary aberration in adrenal cortisol release. However, hypothalamic–pituitary–adrenal (HPA) axis suppression is short lived (1 to 3 days) and readily reversible following short bursts (10 days or less) of pharmacologic doses.[60] A maximum number of short bursts a patient can receive probably exists after which chronic steroid side effects occur. Patients receiving at least eight bursts were shown to have a similar decrease in trabecular bone density as those patients on daily or alternate-day steroids over 1 year.[60] Children who received four or more bursts of prednisone exhibited a subnormal response to hypoglycemic stress or adrenocorticotropic hormone (ACTH) administration.[60] Very short courses (3 to 5 days) have been effective in reducing hospitalization from acute exacerbations. Short-burst steroid therapy is often effective in reducing hospitalizations in moderate asthmatics.[60]

In patients who require chronic systemic glucocorticoids for control of asthma, the lowest possible dose required to control symptoms should be used. Physicians will often sacrifice complete control of the patient's symptoms to avoid toxicity. Two methods of decreasing the toxicity are to use alternate-day therapy or to use topical inhaled glucocorticoids. Studies have suggested that administering a single daily dose at 3:00 to 5:00 PM provides increased efficacy.[2,29] Once control is achieved, the prednisone dose is tapered and replaced by inhaled glucocorticoids.

Inhaled Glucocorticoids

The inhaled glucocorticoids are considered first-line therapy for persistent asthma in adults and children.[2] The glucocorticoids currently available for inhaled use are compared and listed in Table 24–9. Existing evidence suggests the the inhaled corticosteroids differ significantly in topical potency and that the pharmacokinetic differences may result in differences in topical: systemic activity.[61–63] As a result the NAEPP has provided a table of clinically comparable doses to be used by clinicians (Table 24–11).[2] In low to moderate doses, risk of systemic toxicity is low, whereas in high doses, systemic effects are more likely to occur. Thus, HPA axis, growth in prepubertal children, and bone density should be monitored.[2] The inhaled glucocorticoids demonstrate a favorable topical:systemic potency ratio, but should not be considered benign. The "ideal" glucocorticoid for inhaled use should have a high degree of topical potency, minimal systemic absorption of active drug, and minimal local or systemic side effects. None of the available inhaled glucocorticoids are considered ideal, and ongoing investigation into topical: systemic potency ratios will reveal important and much needed information.[62]

The inhaled glucocorticoids have high topical anti-inflammatory effects and are either poorly absorbed or metabolized to less-active substances when absorbed.[56] As with systemic glucocorticoid therapy, the lowest dose required to control symptoms is the appropriate dose. The inhaled glucocorticoids produce dose-dependent systemic effects (Table 24–10), but much less than systemic glucocorticoids.[56,57] Although differences in oral absorption and first-pass metabolism produce differences in oral bioavailability, essentially all of the drug that reaches the lung is systemically absorbed.[2,61] Aerosol delivery of the preparations varies from 10% to 30% which can make a difference in both apparent topical potency and systemic activity.[61,63] Thus, the delivery system can make a significant difference in the relative comparable dose.[2] The potential advantage of the drugs with low oral

TABLE 24–11. Comparative Dosages for Adults (≥ 12 Years) and Children[a]

Drug	Low Dose	Medium Dose	High Dose
Beclomethasone dipropionate MDI 42 µg/puff; 84 µg/puff	≥ 12 yr: 168–504 µg < 12 yr: 84–336 µg	≥ 12 yr: 504–840 µg < 12 yr: 336–672 µg	≥ 12 yr: > 840 µg < 12 yr: > 672 µg
Budesonide Turbuhaler DPI 200 µg/dose	≥ 12 yr: 200–400 µg < 12 yr: 100–200 µg	≥ 12 yr: 400–600 µg < 12 yr: 200–400 µg	≥ 12 yr: > 600 µg < 12 yr: > 400 µg
Flunisolide MDI 250 µg/puff	≥ 12 yr: 500–1000 µg < 12 yr: 500–750 µg	≥ 12 yr: 1000–2000 µg < 12 yr: 750–1500 µg	≥ 12 yr: > 2000 µg < 12 yr: > 1500 µg
Triamcinolone acetonide MDI 100 µg/puff	≥ 12 yr: 400–1000 µg < 12 yr: 400–600 µg	≥ 12 yr: 1000–2000 µg < 12 yr: 600–1200 µg	≥ 12 yr: > 2000 µg < 12 yr: > 1200 µg
Fluticasone propionate MDI 44, 110, 220 µg/puff; DPI 50, 100, 250 µg/dose	≥ 12 yr: 88–264 µg < 12 yr: 88–176 µg	≥ 12 yr: 264–660 µg < 12 yr: 176–440 µg	≥ 12 yr: > 660 µg < 12 yr: > 440 µg

[a]Based on dosages recommended for mild, moderate, and severe persistent asthma from the guidelines.[2]

bioavailability is obviated by using a spacer device with the drugs with higher oral bioavailability because appropriate holding-chamber–style spacers reduce the oral dose by 80%.[61] Mouth rinsing and spitting will also reduce the oral availability and is particularly useful for dry-powder inhaler (DPI) devices.[2]

Local adverse effects of inhaled steroids include oropharyngeal candidiasis and dysphonia that are dose dependent. The dysphonia appears to be a result of local steroid-induced myopathy of the vocal cords.[56] The use of a spacer device can decrease oropharyngeal deposition and decrease the incidence and severity of local side effects.[56]

Optimal dosing of inhaled steroids has not been thoroughly investigated. Most patients may be controlled with bid dosing; however, investigations have demonstrated an improved asthma response with decreased systemic effects by giving the same total daily dose four times daily as opposed to twice daily.[61] This may be due to dosing at 3:00 to 5:00 PM, which improves efficacy as with oral glucocorticoid dosing.[29,64] Twice-daily dosing produces less thrush. The inflammatory response of asthma has been shown to inhibit steroid receptor binding.[65] This provides strong theoretical evidence for initially beginning patients on higher doses and then tapering down once control has been achieved. Many specialists have used this approach and it is now advocated by the NAEPP.[2] Regardless of the type of glucocorticoid therapy, bronchodilator therapy may be needed for breakthrough symptoms.[2] This strategy may allow a significantly lower glucocorticoid dose with equivalent to superior asthma control.[44,45]

Well-controlled, prospective, long-term studies to compare the safety and efficacy of the various inhaled glucocorticoids are sorely needed. In addition more studies are required in children, particularly in regard to growth and development, bone metabolism, and other adverse effects as well as the potential for altering the natural history of the disease.[2,56,61]

Spacer Devices and Inhaled Glucocorticoids

The bioavailability of the inhaled glucocorticoids is influenced by the method of delivery and systemic absorption from the gastrointestinal tract and lung.[2,63] Deposition to the site of drug action within the airways can be substantially increased by application of spacer devices available from various manufacturers. This enhanced deposition will decrease asthma symptoms and improve spirometry in patients with moderate to severe asthma.[63,66] However, some spacers may also decrease delivery of certain preparations.[66] Most spacers are effective in reducing oropharyngeal deposition, which will decrease the frequency of topical adverse effects, dysphonia, and colonization of the oropharynx with candida.[2]

LEUKOTRIENE MODIFIERS

Three asthma treatments approved since 1996 represent entirely new therapeutic modalities. These medications, zafirlukast (Accolate), montelukast (Singulair), and zileuton (Zyflo), act by inhibiting the action of cysteinyl leukotrienes (LTC_4, LTD_4, and LTE_4).[19] Zafirlukast is a leukotriene-receptor antagonist. By blocking the leukotriene receptor the pro-inflammatory effects of leukotrienes (increasing microvascular permeability and airways edema) and their bronchoconstriction may be reduced. At doses of 20 mg twice daily, zafirlukast has been shown to reduce airway responses to inhaled allergen, platelet-activating factor, and exercise.[19] Zafirlukast has also improved pulmonary function and reduced symptoms and bronchodilator requirements in patients with asthma.[67] Adverse effects are minimal, although experience with this medication is somewhat limited at the present time. Rare cases of hepatotoxicity and eosinophilic vasculitis have been reported. Food impairs its absorption, and zafirlukast interacts with warfarin, resulting in prolonged prothrombin time or International Normalized Ratio (INR). Montelukast, 10 mg in the evening (5 mg chewable tablet for children 6 to 14 years of age), provides a modest improvement in mild chronic asthma or EIB. Other LTD_4-receptor antagonists are undergoing development.

Zileuton directly inhibits 5-lipoxygenase whereas other investigational–agents bind to and prevent translocation of 5-lipoxygenase–activating protein (FLAP).[19] Zileuton reduces bronchoconstriction caused by allergen, exercise, aspirin (in aspirin-sensitive asthmatics), and cold, dry air.[19] Doses of 600 mg four times daily reduce symptoms and bronchodilator requirements and improve pulmonary function.[68] Zileuton produces elevated liver enzymes, which more likely occur in the first few months of treatment. It also inhibits the hepatic CYP3A4 isozymes, increasing concentrations of terfenadine, theophylline, and warfarin.[2]

Clinical Uses

Neither zafirlukast nor zileuton completely attenuated induced bronchospasm in the various challenge models mentioned. Also, neither improves BHR.[19] These are new medications and thus clinical experience with these agents is limited. Their place in the scheme of asthma management is not clearly defined. The NAEPP guidelines suggest that these drugs may be alternatives to low-dose inhaled steroids in mild persistent asthmatics;[2] however, the appropriate use may be as adjuncts to inhaled steroids in patients with more severe asthma. Because they are oral medications, adherence may be improved as compared to inhaled medications; this should be considered when choosing treatment alternatives. It is recommended that when zileuton therapy is initiated in patients receiving theophylline, theophylline doses be reduced by 50% in addition to blood-level monitoring. Prothrombin times of patients receiving warfarin should be monitored when either zileuton and zafirlukast is begun. Liver enzymes must be monitored when zileuton is begun. It is recommended that ALT be evaluated when zileuton is begun, monthly for the first 3 months, every 2 to 3 months for the remainder of the first year, and periodically thereafter. Caution should be used in patients with existing hepatic dysfunction.

MISCELLANEOUS THERAPIES

Antihistamines

Antihistamines are of little value in asthma therapy.[2,18] However, the theoretical (but unproven) grounds that antihistamines through their anticholinergic effect could produce harmful drying of mucus in asthma has now been refuted and should be finally put to rest.[69] Thus, though antihistamines are generally not indicated for asthma, they are not contraindicated. Indeed, most studies of chronic and acute administration of antihistamines in asthma have demonstrated small improvement of symptoms and pulmonary functions or no effect.[22,69] Some of the newer agents have been touted to have other anti-inflammatory effects on bronchodilation but have not been proven to have significant efficacy in asthma.[22] Currently, antihistamines are useful adjunctive therapy for the patient with allergic rhinitis.

Methotrexate

Low-dose methotrexate (15 mg/wk) used for inflammatory diseases, psoriatic and rheumatoid arthritis, and polymyositis has been used to reduce the systemic steroid dose in patients with severe steroid-dependent asthma.[22] Double-blind, placebo-controlled trials have given decidedly mixed results, with one-half of the studies showing no effect.[70] A recent meta-analysis determined that a statistically significant reduction (mean 4.37 mg/d prednisone or 23% of original dose) can be achieved.[70] The mechanism of action is unknown but may be anti-inflammatory or immunomodulatory effects. Methotrexate inhibits chemotaxis of neutrophils, inhibits leukotriene B_4-induced adherence to endothelium, and inhibits the pro-inflammatory activity of interleukin-1.[22] Low-dose weekly methotrexate is not without hazard. Both hepatotoxicity and pulmonary fibrosis have been reported in patients receiving similar therapy for psoriasis and rheumatoid arthritis.[22] At least one trial had a subject expire from pneumocystis carinii pneumonia following methotrexate.[69] No evidence for induction of asthma remission exists because patients' steroid requirement returns upon discontinuation of the methotrexate. Methotrexate should still be considered experimental and reserved for only severe steroid-dependent asthmatics under the care of specialists. Patients require careful monitoring including periodic liver biopsies.[69] Owing to the marginal effect of methotrexate the risk–benefit should be carefully evaluated prior to institution.

Macrolides

The macrolide antibiotics troleandomycin (TAO) and erythromycin produce a steroid-sparing effect.[22,69] This was initially thought to be primarily a result of their ability to inhibit methylprednisolone metabolism.[69] However, the macrolides inhibit activation and chemotaxis of neutrophils and reduce asthmatic BHR in trials.[69] Three open trials and two double-blind crossover trials of TAO in a total 125 patients have documented a positive steroid-sparing effect and/or improvement in symptoms.[22] The potential for hepatotoxicity limits their usefulness. They also inhibit the metabolism of a number of drugs used by asthmatics, most notably theophylline, terfenadine, and astemizole, producing life-threatening cardiac arrhythmias (torsades de pointes) with the latter two drugs.[22] The aggressive use of inhaled corticosteroids has limited the usefulness of macrolides.

Other Agents

As a result of the inflammatory nature of asthma and the risk of toxicities from corticosteroids, a number of the drugs with anti-inflammatory or immunomodulatory activity such as hydroxychloroquine, dapsone, gold, intravenous γ-globulin, cyclosporine, and colchicine have been studied in severe steroid-dependent asthma, with mixed results.[2,22,69]

Gold therapy has been used as a standard therapy in Japan for the past 50 years.[22] However, the studies have been poorly controlled and better well-controlled trials are essential prior to subjecting patients to the potential serious toxicities associated with gold therapy. The nonsteroidal anti-inflammatory agents are ineffective in asthma but up to 25% may have their asthma aggravated. Double-blind, placebo-controlled trials have shown colchicine to be ineffective.[2] The other agents have been evaluated only in open-label trials and anecdotal reports.[69] Inhaled heparin through its inactivation of histamine and other mast-cell mediators and inhaled furosemide by possibly blocking specific chloride channels inhibit EIB.[22,69] Furosemide also inhibits allergen, adenosine, and metabisulfite challenges but is not active orally.[69]

The use of expectorants has not been demonstrated to be beneficial in asthma, although mucolytic therapy to assist removal of impacted mucus plugs in a large bronchus has been life saving in a few instances. Adequate hydration is usually all that is required. In acute asthma, the large negative intrathoracic pressures coupled with mediator-induced capillary permeability may predispose to pulmonary edema that will worsen oxygenation so that excessive hydration should be avoided.[22]

Therapies for Recalcitrant Acute Severe Asthma

Intravenous magnesium sulfate ($MgSO_4$) has been advocated for patients with acute severe asthma who exhibit a suboptimal response to inhaled β_2-agonists.[22] However, the initial trials often used inadequate doses of inhaled β_2-agonists and the bronchodilation from the $MgSO_4$ was modest and did not exceed the β_2-agonist response. Placebo-controlled trials of intravenous $MgSO_4$ in emergency department patients failed to detect any significant bronchodilation or outcome difference from $MgSO_4$ added to optimal inhaled β_2-agonists.[2] Numerous other therapies have been reported on an anecdotal basis only; these include ketamine infusion, halothane and isoflurane anesthesia, as well as ventilating patients with a helium/oxygen mixture.[22] The NAEPP considers these therapies experimental.[2]

FUTURE THERAPIES

OTHER IMMUNOMODULATORS

Much of the research is evaluating ways of inhibiting the airways inflammatory response. Thus, selective phosphodiesterase inhibitors may have anti-inflammatory activity. Investigations of monoclonal antibodies to specific cytokines and intercellular adhesion molecules (ICAM-1) are in preclinical investigation as well as platelet-activating-factor and neurokinin antagonists.[22,71]

AEROSOL THERAPY FOR ASTHMA

Aerosol delivery of drugs for asthma has the advantage of being site specific, thus enhancing the therapeutic ratio.[2,17] Inhalation of short-acting β_2-agonists provides more-rapid bronchodilation than either parenteral or oral administration as well as a greater degree of protection against EIB and other challenges.[13,22] Inhalation of glucocorticoids appears to have a greater effect on BHR than systemic administration;[56] other agents (cromolyn, nedocromil, salmeterol, and ipratropium) are effective only by inhalation.[2] Therefore, an understanding of aerosol drug delivery is essential to optimal asthma therapy. Table 24–12 lists the factors determining lung deposition of therapeutic aerosols.

The various devices used to generate therapeutic aerosols include MDIs, jet nebulizers (JNs), ultrasonic nebulizers, and dry-powder inhalers (DPIs). The single most important device factor determining the site of aerosol deposition is particle size.[72] Devices for delivering therapeutic aerosols generate particles with aerodynamic diameters from 0.5 to 35 μm.[72] Particles greater than 10 μm deposit in the oropharynx, particles between 5 and 10 μm deposit in the trachea and large bronchi, particles

TABLE 24–12. Factors Determining Lung Deposition of Aerosols

Device	Device Factors	Patient Factors
Metered-dose inhaler	Canister held inverted	Inspiratory rate (slow, deep)
	Formulation	Breath-holding
	Actuator cleanliness	Coordinating actuation and inhalation
	Addition of spacer device	Shaking device
Jet nebulizer	Volume fill (4–6 mL)	Inspiratory rate (slow, deep)
	Gas flow (6–12 L/min)	Breath-holding
	Open vs closed system	Tapping nebulizer
	Dead-space volume	
	Thumb-activating valve	
Ultrasonic nebulizer	Volume fill	Inspiratory rate (slow, deep)
		Breath-holding
		Tapping nebulizer
Dry-powder inhaler	Device cleanliness	Inspiratory rate (rapid, deep)
		Breath-holding
		Tilting head back

1 to 5 μm reach the lower airways, and particles smaller than 0.5 μm act as a gas and are exhaled. Respirable particles are deposited in the airway by three mechanisms: (1) inertial impaction, (2) gravitational sedimentation, and (3) Brownian diffusion.[72] The first two are the most important for therapeutic aerosols and are probably the only factors that can be manipulated by patients.

The most important patient factor determining aerosol deposition is inspiratory rate.[72,73] High inspiratory flow rates increase the degree of deposition owing to impaction of all sizes of particles, thereby increasing deposition centrally (i.e., large airways) and decreasing peripheral deposition.

Besides the two major factors, there are a number of other factors that can be altered to improve delivery and efficacy of clinical aerosols. Most of these factors tend to be device specific and will be discussed under the individual device. Patient factors that cannot be controlled include interpatient variability in airway geometry (particularly the differences between children and adults), the effect of bronchospasm, edema, and mucus hypersecretion. Mild obstruction actually increases aerosol deposition; however, severe obstruction probably leads to increased central deposition from impaction.[72]

Metered-Dose Inhaler

Metered-dose inhalers are the most popular form of aerosol delivery owing to their convenience (easy portability) and efficacy. They consist of a pressurized canister with a metering valve containing active drug; low-vapor-pressure propellants, chlorofluorocarbon (CFC) or hydrofluoralkane (HFA); cosolvents; and/or surfactants.[72] The drug is either in solution or in a suspended micronized powder. To disperse the suspension for accurate delivery, the canister must be shaken. The metering chamber measures a liquid volume, and therefore the device must be held with the valve stem downward so that the chamber is covered with liquid.[17,72] The canister is placed inverted in an actuator and when pressed, the device releases the propellant and drug in a forceful spray whose particles are large (mass median aerodynamic diameter [MMAD] 45 μm) with an initial velocity of 100 mph.[72] As evaporation occurs, the particle size is reduced to a final MMAD of 2.8 to 5.5 μm, depending on the MDI. The aerosol cloud extends at least 10 inches beyond the MDI at the lowest MMAD (Fig. 24–9).[72] Although CFCs can produce cardiac arrhythmias at high doses, investigations have failed to detect adverse effects from the dose delivered via MDIs in recommended dosages. However, as a result of the Montreal Protocol, which phases out the production and use of CFCs, newer propellants such as the HFAs are being developed.[73] Surfactants, particularly oleates, can produce lung irritation and coughing at excessive doses.[73]

Appropriate technique is required to achieve optimal drug delivery and therapeutic effect from an MDI (see Table 24–12).[74] With optimal technique, about 10% to 30% of the metered dose

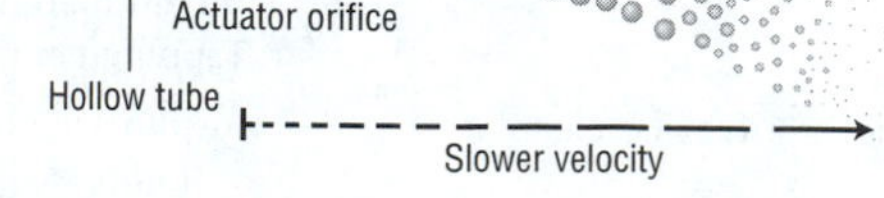

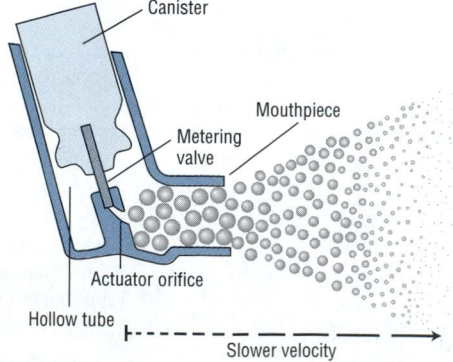

FIGURE 24–9. Illustration of a metered-dose inhaler demonstrating the particle size difference as the aerosol cloud extends outward.

is deposited in the lung depending on the device.[66,75] Approximately 80% impacts on the oropharynx owing to the initial high velocity, and this portion is then swallowed; the rest is either left in the actuator or exhaled.[74] It is important that actuation occur during inhalation, although the time during inspiration is unimportant provided the inspiratory rate is slow (30 L/min or 5 to 10 seconds for entire inspiration).[2,74] A number of authors advocate holding the actuator 2 to 3 cm in front of an open mouth to allow more evaporation and less impaction. Although radiolabeled studies indicate improved delivery, physiologic studies with bronchodilators have failed to document an advantage for this method.[74] A large number of studies have shown that many patients do not use their MDIs optimally and also that patient instruction with demonstration is the most effective means of improving inhaler technique.[2,17,74] Even with instruction, up to 30% of patients, particularly young children and the elderly, cannot master the use of an MDI. For these patients the attachment of auxiliary devices or spacers to the MDI or use of a breath-activated MDI can significantly improve efficacy.[66,74]

Holding Chamber and Spacer Devices. Advantages to the use of spacers with an MDI are decreased oropharyngeal deposition and enhanced lung delivery.[2,66] However, not all spacer devices produce similar effects. The design of spacers varies from simple open-ended tubes that maintain the MDI away from the mouth to holding chambers with one-way valves that open during inhalation. The purpose of a spacer is to allow evaporation of the propellant prior to inhalation. This allows inhalation after actuation of the device, obviating the need for good hand–lung coordination and for a greater number of drug particles to achieve a respirable droplet size.[73,75] Additionally, most of the large particles that would normally deposit in the oropharynx rain out in the spacer.[66] All of the available spacers significantly reduce oropharyngeal deposition of aerosols, with the holding-chamber devices superior to the open-ended tubes.[66] This is an important factor in reducing local adverse effects (hoarseness, thrush), may decrease HPA-axis suppression from orally absorbed inhaled glucocorticoids,[61] and may have clinical importance for bronchodilators delivered by MDI in acute severe asthma.[74] The use of spacers significantly enhances the clinical effect from bronchodilators in ambulatory patients with poor hand–lung coordination but offers no advantage in those patients who can optimally use an MDI alone, despite the fact that radiolabeled studies show an increased lung deposition.[74,75] Either the increased amount of bronchodilator drug deposited in the lung is clinically insignificant or these patients reside at the top of the dose–response curve. The inconsistent result may also be due to the use of different spacers.[66] The lung delivery is dependent on both the MDI and the device, where one device may enhance delivery with one MDI preparation and decrease delivery with others.[66,75] In general, the larger volume holding chambers (> 600 mL) consistently enhance delivery.

Breath-Actuated MDIs. The breath-actuated MDI (Autohaler) is cocked with a lever to "load" the dose of medication, a baffle is opened by inspiratory pressure and the dose is expelled from the canister metering chamber.[2,17] Although the need for hand–lung coordination for proper actuation is significantly reduced with breath-actuated MDI, these devices do not allow the use of a spacer and still use CFC propellants (although the Autohaler releases 60% less CFC than conventional MDIs).[73] Also, use of these devices improves pulmonary drug deposition only in patients unable to adequately coordinate the use of conventional metered-dose inhalers.[74] These devices may be particularly helpful in the elderly who have difficulty actuating the conventional MDIs.[73]

Jet Nebulizers

Jet nebulizers are primarily used to deliver aerosols to hospitalized patients or patients with acute asthma exacerbations presenting to the clinic or emergency room. They have the advantage of not requiring significant patient coordination or cooperation other than tidal breathing. Jet nebulizers produce an aerosol from a liquid solution placed in a cup. A tube connected to a stream of compressed air or oxygen flows up through the bottom and draws the liquid up an adjacent open-ended tube. The air and liquid strike a baffle, creating a droplet cloud that is then inhaled.[72] Large droplets adhere to the sides of the nebulizer and baffles, coalesce, and drip to the bottom to be renebulized. The aerosol output and lung delivery vary among the commercially available nebulizers even when operated in the same manner.[75] This is because of differing dead-space volumes and baffle systems. Altering the operating parameters can also significantly affect lung delivery. Because dead space (the volume left behind after nebulization stops) remains constant, increasing fill volume will increase total amount of drug delivered; however, it will also take longer to nebulize the dose.[75] A total fill volume of 4 to 6 mL is considered optimal but will take 10 to 15 minutes to complete.[75] Though this length of time may be an inconvenience to the outpatient, the slower nebulization is probably an advantage in the patient experiencing an acute exacerbation. Tapping the side of the nebulizer during operation induces the droplets on the sides to fall back into the reservoir, minimizing loss. The MMAD of the droplets is directly related to the gas flow rate, with flow rates of 5 to 12 L/min providing an aerosol cloud with MMAD of 4 to 8 μm for most nebulizers.[72] Putting a hole in the gas-supply tube so nebulization will occur only during inhalation when the patients close their thumb over the hole also decreases aerosol loss. Quiet tidal breathing through a mouthpiece or face mask is the usual method of aerosol delivery from a nebulizer; however, slow deep inhalation and breath-holding will also improve delivery from this device as well as from an MDI.

Approximately 10% (5% to 15%) of the dose placed in a nebulizer is delivered to the patient's lungs with 60% to 80% lost in the apparatus, up to 20% exhaled, and 2% deposited in the mouth under usual operating conditions.[72] Ultrasonic nebulizers that produce an aerosol by vibrating liquid lying above a transducer at speeds of about 1 mHz produce degrees of lung deposition similar to jet nebulizers.[72] It is easy to see why patients not responding to multiple doses of bronchodilator via MDI during acute attacks respond to the usual doses administered via a nebulizer. For example, 2.5 mg of albuterol via a nebulizer should deliver approximately 0.25 mg into the airways, whereas 10 puffs from an MDI would be expected to deliver only 0.1 mg to the airways. This is without the increased risk of poor MDI technique during the attack. However, this should not be interpreted as meaning that jet nebulizers are superior to MDIs, for even in acute asthma when β_2-agonists are given in the same dosage by MDI plus spacer or nebulizer over the same time period, they have been shown to be equally effective.[73]

Dry Powder Inhalers (DPIs)

Dry micronized powders can be inhaled directly into the lungs. Cromolyn was first introduced for administration in this fashion via a Spinhaler. Because of the impending ban on CFC propellants, a number of other DPI devices have been developed. These include the Rotahaler, Turbuhaler (Fig. 24–10), and Diskhaler (Fig. 24–11), with other devices undergoing development. The Rotahaler requires that a capsule of medication be placed in the back of the device, and then the device is twisted to break open the capsule and release the medication for inhalation. The Turbuhaler and Diskhaler are multidose devices that require "loading" a dose prior to inhalation by twisting the grip and puncturing a blister of medication, respectively.

An advantage of DPIs is that they are breath actuated and require minimal hand–lung coordination.[73] DPIs require higher inspiratory flow rates (≈ 60 L/min) and a change in inhalation technique (deep, forceful inspiration) for optimal actuation as

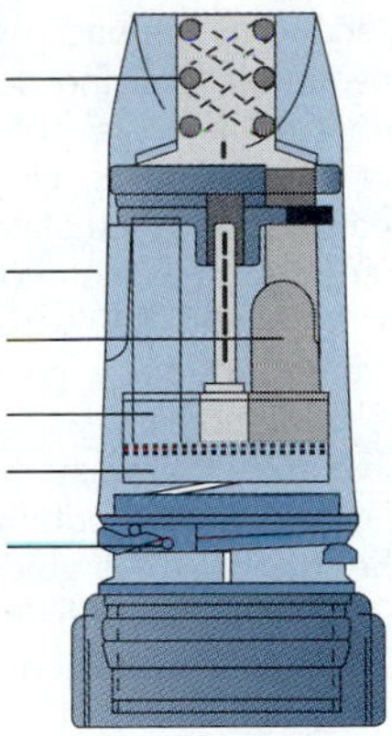

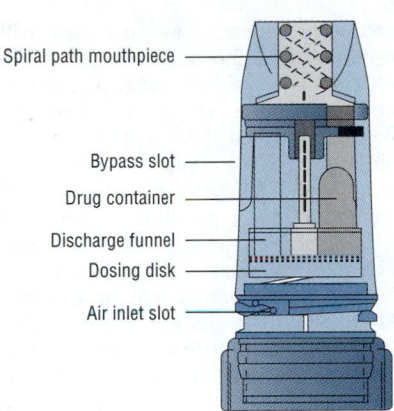

FIGURE 24–10. Illustration of the newer breath-activated DPI, the Turbuhaler.

compared to conventional MDI, which in turn increases the amount of drug impacted into the oropharynx.[73] Thus, mouth-rinsing following treatment with glucocorticoids will be important to minimize local effects and oral absorption.[73] The higher inspiratory flow rates required and the inherent inhaler resistance of DPIs have increased concern that patients in acute distress will be unable to adequately actuate the devices for symptomatic relief. However, preliminary studies in acutely obstructed asthmatics have shown that adequate (equivalent to or better than with conventional MDIs) relief can be achieved when bronchodilator medications are administered via DPIs. The Turbuhaler only requires an inspiratory flow of 30 L/min; however, children less than 5 years of age are usually unable to generate a sufficient inspiratory flow for optimal delivery.[2,75] Another concern is that the powder may be irritating and may produce cough; however, this has not been widely reported.[22] The Turbuhaler device delivers twice the drug to the lungs as compared to the counterpart MDIs.[2,73] This has produced clinically significant differences for budesonide and terbutaline.[61] The Diskhaler appears to deliver the same as its counterpart MDIs.[73]

PHARMACOECONOMIC CONSIDERATIONS

Of the estimated $6.2 billion cost of asthma in the United States in 1990, the largest single direct medical expenditure was inpatient hospital services (emergency care), reaching almost $1.5 billion, followed by prescription medications ($1.1 billion).[3] In total,

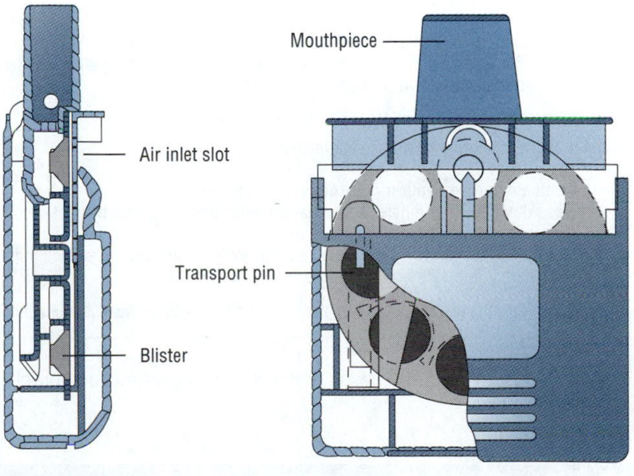

FIGURE 24–11. Illustration of the newer breath-activated DPI, the Diskhaler.

43% of the economic impact was associated with emergency room use, hospitalization, and death. A cost-of-illness approach takes in all measurable costs, both indirect costs or costs to society and direct medical costs. Using this approach the costs per patient per year in the United States was $640.[3] Two-thirds of this was indirect costs such as lost work and death.

Between 1988 and 1992 the total number of asthma prescriptions increased 8% yet expenditures increased 16% to $1.64 billion.[19] The cost increase was primarily a result of a shift to more-expensive anti-inflammatory drugs, which increased in cost by 60%. The change in prescribing may have been a result of the release of the first NAEPP guidelines[19] (Fig. 24–12). Asthma severity obviously has an impact on cost of care. Studies from health maintenance organizations suggest that up to 45% of the cost of asthma is accrued by 10% of the patients, primarily as a result of emergency care.

Numerous studies have demonstrated the cost effectiveness of patient-education programs for asthma.[3] One study has shown that for $28 per person an educational program significantly improved adherence. Others who targeted patients coming to an emergency department showed that the $82 per person cost was offset by an estimated $628 per person reduction in emergency department charges.[3] Several studies have reported positive results from pharmacist interventions, reducing overall cost of care. Similar studies have demonstrated the cost effectiveness of specialist care compared to generalist care.

Few trials have evaluated the cost effectiveness of pharmaceutical interventions. A study of inhaled corticosteroids in children has shown a reduction of $9.45 per symptom-free day gained.[3] Others evaluating a mixed group of adults with asthma and COPD found the addition of inhaled corticosteroids to β_2-agonists to provide an incremental cost-effectiveness ratio of $5.00 per symptom-free day. The difference between the studies is that the latter included only direct medical costs, which will underestimate the benefit.[3] In a retrospective cost comparison of the addition of cromolyn in a large group practice, the cost of medicine in the cromolyn group was higher ($2.79/mo) but emergency department and hospitalization costs declined significantly. Thus, despite the higher costs of anti-inflammatory medication, studies suggest that they may reap a cost savings. Obviously many more studies are needed.

Steps for Using Your Inhaler

Please demonstrate your inhaler technique at every visit.

1. Remove the cap and hold inhaler upright.
2. Shake the inhaler.
3. Tilt your head back slightly and breathe out slowly.
4. Position the inhaler in one of the following ways (A or B is optimal, but C is acceptable for those who have difficulty with A or B. C is required for breath-activated inhalers):

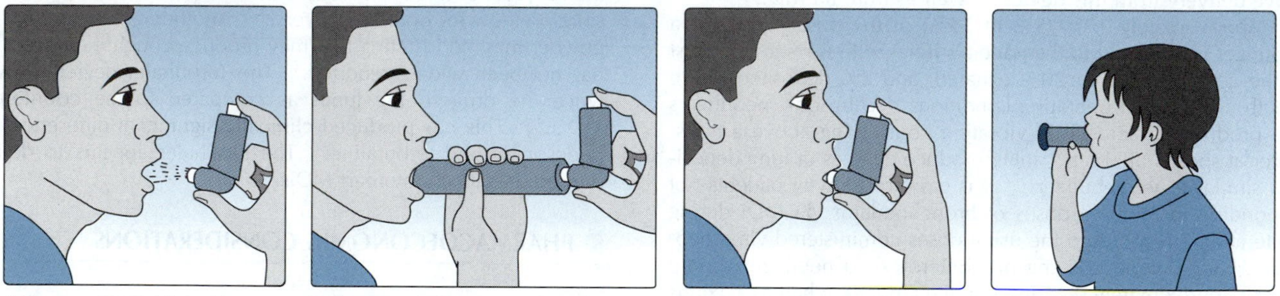

A Open mouth with inhaler 1 to 2 inches away.

B Use spacer/holding chamber (that is recommended especially for young children and for people using corticosteroids).

C In the mouth. Do not use for corticosteroids.

D NOTE: Inhaled dry powder capsules require a different inhalation technique. To use a dry powder inhaler, it is important to close the mouth tightly around the mouthpiece of the inhaler and to inhale rapidly.

5. Press down on the inhaler to release medication as you start to breathe in slowly.
6. Breathe in slowly (3 to 5 seconds).
7. Hold your breath for 10 seconds to allow the medicine to reach deeply into your lungs.
8. Repeat puff as directed. Waiting 1 minute between puffs may permit second puff to penetrate your lungs better.
9. Spacers/holding chambers are useful for all patients. They are particularly recommended for young children and older adults and for use with corticosteroids.

Avoid common inhaler mistakes. Follow these inhaler tips:

- Breathe out *before* pressing your inhaler.
- Inhale *slowly.*
- Breathe in through your mouth, not your nose.
- Press down on your inhaler at the *start* of inhalation (or within the first second of inhalation).
- Keep inhaling as you press down on inhaler.
- Press your inhaler only *once* while you are inhaling (one breath for each puff).
- Make sure you breathe in evenly and deeply.

NOTE: Other inhalers are becoming available in addition to those illustrated above. Different types of inhalers require different techniques.

FIGURE 24–12. Instructions for inhaler use from the NAEPP Expert Panel Report 2.[2]

EVALUATION OF THERAPEUTIC OUTCOMES

CHRONIC ASTHMA

The desired outcomes have been previously described. Control of asthma is defined as achieving a minimal need for as-needed short-acting β_2-agonists (ideally none), no acute episodes, no limitations on activity, no emergency care visits, no nocturnal symptoms, normal pulmonary functions (FEV_1 and PEF), minimal to no medication side effects, and satisfaction of the patient and family with the care. Depending on the severity of the patient's asthma, compromises from the ideal control are made, and the best possible outcome balancing between disease and posssible adverse effects from the drugs is attempted.

Monitoring consists of quantitating the use of inhaled short-acting β_2-agonists, days of limited activity, and number of symptoms; the NAEPP also recommends yearly spirometric studies. In moderate to severe persistent patients, once daily, upon awakening peak-flow monitoring is recommended. Patients should also be asked about exercise tolerance and nocturnal symptoms. All patients on inhaled drugs should have their inhalation technique evaluated periodically—monthly initially and then every 3 to 6 months.

Following initiation of anti-inflammatory therapy or an increase in dosage, most patients should begin experiencing a decrease in symptoms in 1 to 2 weeks and achieve maximum symptomatic improvement within 4 to 8 weeks. The use of higher doses or more potent agents may accelerate the process. Improvement in FEV_1 and PEF should follow a similar time frame; however, a decrease in BHR as measured by morning PEF and exercise tolerance may take longer and improve over 1 to 3 months.[2,17] Patients should be informed that following a viral respiratory infection they may experience increased exercise intolerance for up to 4 weeks.

Initial visits with the patient should focus on the patient's concerns, expectations, and goals of treatment. Basic education should focus on asthma as a chronic lung disease and the type of medications and how they are to be used. Inhaler technique is taught and when to seek medical advice is explained. *Written* action plans should be given. The first follow-up visit should be in 2 to 4 weeks. At this time the educational messages of the first visit should be repeated as well as answering questions about the patient's current medications and any difficulties with therapy the patient may be having.

ACUTE SEVERE ASTHMA

The goals of therapy for an acute asthma exacerbation are to

- Relieve airway obstruction as quickly as possible (within minutes).
- Relieve hypoxemia immediately.
- Restore lung function to normal as soon as possible (within hours).
- Plan avoidance of future exacerbations.
- Develop a written action plan for treating future exacerbations.

Patients at risk for severe exacerbations should be taught how to use a peak-flow meter and monitor morning peak flows at home. In young children unable to perform peak flows, supraclavicular retractions, increased respiratory rate, increased heart rate, and inability to speak more than one or two words between breaths are signs of severe obstruction. Oxygen saturation by pulse oximetry and peak flow should be measured in all patients not completely responding to initial intensive inhaled β_2-agonists therapy. Upon admission peak flow or clinical symptoms should be monitored every 2 to 4 hours. Prior to discharge from the emergency department or hospital, the patient should be given sufficient prednisone to finish the course, taught the purpose of the medications and how to use inhalers correctly, and given a written action plan and an appointment for a follow-up visit.

▶ PRINCIPLES OF PHARMACOTHERAPY

- Asthma is a chronic inflammatory disease of the lung characterized by intermittent symptoms of airway obstruction and reactivity to numerous stimuli that may also progress to irreversible changes.
- Therapeutic agents are classified by how they are used as either quick-relief or long-term control medication in asthma.
- Drugs with anti-inflammatory activity (inhaled corticosteroids, cromolyn, and nedocromil) are preferred for long-term control therapy in asthma.
- A stepwise approach to asthma therapy is preferred, but it is recommended that patients be started at a higher step initially to gain control and then step down.
- The preferred quick-relief medication for asthma is short-acting inhaled β_2-agonists.
- Regular use of β_2-agonists does not worsen asthma, but short-acting agents should be used as needed so the frequency of use can be monitored to assess appropriateness of long-term control therapy.
- Education and development of a partnership in the care of patients with asthma are essential to the success of any pharmacotherapy plan.
- Written action plans are considered essential for all asthma patients to assist in self-management.

REFERENCES

1. Rosenblatt MB. History of bronchial asthma. In: Weiss EB, Segal MS, Stein M, eds. Bronchial Asthma: Mechanisms and Therapeutics, 2nd ed. Boston, Little, Brown, 1976:5–17.
2. NHLBI, National Asthma Education and Prevention Program, Expert Panel Report 2. Guidelines for the diagnosis and management of

asthma. NIH Publication No. 97-4051. Bethesda, MD: US Department of Health and Human Services, 1997.
3. National Asthma Education and Prevention Program Task Force. Report on the cost effectiveness, quality of care, and financing of asthma care. Am J Respir Crit Care Med 1996;154(suppl):S81–S130.
4. Coultas DB, Gong H Jr, Grad R, et al. Respiratory diseases in minorities of the United States. Am J Respir Crit Care Med 1993; 149:S93–S131.
5. Burt CW, Knapp DE. Ambulatory Care Visits for Asthma: United States, 1993–94. Advance data from vital and health statistics, No. 277. Hyattsville, MD: National Center for Health Statistics; 1996.
6. Lang DM, Polansky M. Patterns of asthma mortality in Philadelphia from 1969 to 1991. N Engl J Med 1994;331:1542–1546.
7. Weiss ST, Tosteson TD, Segal MR, et al. Effects of asthma on pulmonary function in children. A longitudinal population-based study. Am Rev Respir Dis 1992;145:58–64.
8. McFadden ER, Gilbert IA. Asthma. N Engl J Med 1992;327: 1928–1937.
9. Sandford A, Weir T, Pare P. The genetics of asthma. Am J Respir Crit Care Med 1996;153;1749–1765.
10. Boulet L-P, Laviolette M, Turcotte H, et al. Bronchial subepithelial fibrosis correlates with airway responsiveness to methacholine. Chest 1997;112:45–52.
11. Laitinen LA, Laitinen A, Haahtela T. Airway mucosal inflammation even in patients with newly diagnosed asthma. Am Rev Respir Dis 1993;147:697–704.
12. Kay AB. Asthma and inflammation. J Allergy Clin Immunol 1991; 87:893–910.
13. McFadden ER, Gilbert IA. Exercise-induced asthma. N Engl J Med 1994;330:1362–1367.
14. Smith H. Asthma, inflammation, eosinophils and bronchial hyperresponsiveness. Clin Exp Allergy 1992;22:187–197.
15. Ricci M, Rossi O, Bertoni M, Matucci A. The importance of Th2-like cells in the pathogenesis of airway allergic inflammation. Clin Exp Allergy 1993;23:360–369.
16. Sur S, Crotty TB, Kephart GM, et al. Sudden-onset fatal asthma. A distinct entity with few eosinophils and relatively more neutrophils in the airway submucosa? Am Rev Respir Dis 1993;148:713–719.
17. Global Initiative for Asthma. Global strategy for asthma management and prevention NHLBI/WHO workshop report. National Institutes of Health, National Heart, Lung and Blood Institute publication No. 95-3659, 1995.
18. Roquet A, Dahlen B, Kumlin M, et al. Combined antagonism of leukotrienes and histamine produces predominant inhibition of allergen-induced early and late phase airway obstruction in asthmatics. Am J Respir Crit Care Med 1997;155:1848–1863.
19. Hendeles L, Scheife RT, eds. New frontiers in asthma therapy: Leukotriene receptor antagonists and 5-lipoxygenase inhibitors. Pharmacotherapy 1997;17(suppl):1S–54S.
20. Calderón E, Lockey RF. A possible role for adhesion molecules in asthma. J Allergy Clin Immunol 1992;90:852–865.
21. Corrigan CJ. Immunological aspects of asthma: Implications for future treatment. Clin Immunother 1994;1:31–42.
22. Weiss EB, Stein M, eds. Bronchial Asthma: Mechanisms and Therapeutics, 3rd ed. Boston, Little, Brown, 1993.
23. Barnes PJ. NO or no NO in asthma? Thorax 1996;51:218-220.
24. Barnes PJ, Kharitonov SA. Exhaled nitric oxide: A new lung function test. Thorax 1996;51:233–237.
25. Larsen GL. Asthma in children. N Engl J Med 1992;326:1540–1545.
26. Kelly HW, Murphy S. Assessment of inflammation and its suppression in lung disease. J Biopharm Sci 1992;3:155–161.
27. Nelson HS. β-Adrenergic bronchodilators. N Engl J Med 1995; 333:499–506.
28. Duff AL, Platts-Mills TAE. Allergens and asthma. Pediatr Clin North Am 1992;39:1277–1291.
29. Martin RJ. Nocturnal asthma: Circadian rhythms and therapeutic interventions. Am Rev Respir Dis 1993;147(suppl):S25–S28.
30. Alberts WM. "Circa menstrual" rhythmicity and asthma. Chest 1997; 111:840–842.
31. National Heart, Lung and Blood Institute. Executive Summary: Management of Asthma During Pregnancy. NIH publication No. 92-3279a. Bethesda, MD, 1992.
32. Beasley R, Rafferty P, Holgate ST. Adverse reactions to the non-drug constituents on nebuliser solutions. Br J Clin Pharmacol 1988;25: 283–287.
33. Murray AB, Morrison BJ. The decrease in severity of asthma in children of parents who smoke since the parents have been exposing them to less cigarette smoke. J Allergy Clin Immunol 1993;91:102–110.
34. Abramson MJ, Puy RM, Weiner JM. Is allergen immunotherapy effective in asthma? A meta-analysis of randomized controlled trials. Am J Respir Crit Care Med 1995;151:969–974.
35. Creticos PS, Reed CE, Norman PS, et al. Ragweed immunotherapy in adult asthma. N Engl J Med 1996;334:501–506.
36. Kelly HW, Murphy S. Beta-adrenergic agonists for acute, severe asthma. Ann Pharmacother 1992;26:81–91.
37. Sears MR, Taylor DR, Print CG, et al. Regular inhaled beta-agonist treatment in bronchial asthma. Lancet 1990;336:1391–1396.
38. Taylor DR, Sears MR, Herbison GP, et al. Regular inhaled β agonist in asthma: Effects on exacerbations and lung function. Thorax 1993; 48:134–138.
39. Chapman KR, Kesten S, Szalai JP. Regular vs as-needed inhaled salbutamol in asthma control. Lancet 1994;343:1379–1382.
40. Drazen JM, Israel E, Boushey HA, et al. Comparison of regularly scheduled with as needed use of albuterol in mild asthma. N Engl J Med 1996;335:841–847.
41. Spitzer WO, Suissa S, Ernst P, et al. The use of β-agonists and the risk of death and near death from asthma. N Engl J Med 1992; 326:501–506.
42. Suissa S, Blais L, Ernst P. Patterns of increasing beta-agonist use and the risk of fatal or near-fatal asthma. Eur Respir J 1994;7:1602–1609.
43. Mullen M, Mullen B, Carey M. The association between β-agonist use and death from asthma: A meta-analytic integration of case-control studies. JAMA 1993;270:1842–1845.
44. Greening AP, Wind P, Northfield M, Shaw G. Added salmeterol versus higher-dose corticosteroid in asthma patients with symptoms on existing inhaled corticosteroid. Lancet 1994;344:219–224.
45. Woolcock A, Lundback B, Ringdal N, Jacques LA. Comparison of addition of salmeterol to inhaled steroids with doubling of the dose of inhaled steroid. Am J Respir Crit Care Med 1996;153:1481–1488.
46. Weinberger M, Hendeles L. Theophylline in asthma. N Engl J Med 1996;334:1380–1388.
47. Barnes PJ. Theophylline in the management of asthma: Time for a reappraisal? Eur Respir J 1994;7:579–591.
48. Kelly HW. Theophylline toxicity. In: Jenne JS, Murphy SA, eds. Drug Therapy for Asthma: Research and Clinical Practice. New York, Dekker, 1987:925–951.
49. Edwards D, Zarowitz BJ, Slaughter RL. Theophylline. In: Evans WE, Schentag JJ, Jusko WJ, eds. Applied Pharmacokinetics: Principles of Therapeutic Drug Monitoring, 3rd ed. Vancouver, Applied Therapeutics, 1992:13-1–13-38.
50. Pierson WE, LaForce CF, Bell TD, et al. Long-term, double-blind comparison of controlled-release albuterol versus sustained-release theophylline in adolescents and adults with asthma. J Allergy Clin Immunol 1990;85:618–626.
51. Murphy S, Kelly HW. Cromolyn sodium: A review of mechanisms and clinical use in asthma. Drug Intell Clin Pharm 1987;21:22–35.
52. Kelly HW, Murphy S. Should anticholinergics be used in acute severe asthma? Ann Pharmacother 1990;24:409–416.
53. Osmond MH, Klassen TP. Efficacy of ipratropium bromide in acute childhood asthma: A meta-analysis. Acad Emerg Med 1995;2: 651–656.
54. Schuh S, Johnson DW, Callahan S, et al. Efficacy of frequent nebulized ipratropium bromide added to frequent high-dose albuterol therapy in severe childhood asthma. J Pediatr 1995;126:639–645.

55. Wasserman SI, ed. Nedocromil sodium: A pyranoquinoline antiinflammatory agent for the treatment of asthma. J Allergy Clin Immunol 1993;92(suppl):143–216.
56. Barnes PJ. Inhaled glucocorticoids for asthma. N Engl J Med 1995; 332:868–875.
57. Baraniuk JN, ed. Steroids in asthma: Molecular mechanisms of glucocorticoid actions. J Allergy Clin Immunol 1996;97(suppl):141–182.
58. Lee TH, Brattsand R, Leung D, eds. Corticosteroid action and resistance in asthma. Am J Respir Crit Care Med 1996;154(suppl):S1–S79.
59. Olivieri D, Chetta A, Del Dono M, et al. Effect of short-term treatment with low-dose inhaled fluticasone propionate on airway inflammation and remodeling in mild asthma: A placebo-controlled study. Am J Respir Crit Care Med 1997;155:1864–1871.
60. Kelly HW, Murphy S. Corticosteroids for acute severe asthma. Ann Pharmacother 1991;25:72–79.
61. Kamada A, Szefler SJ, Martin RJ, et al. Issues in the use of inhaled glucocorticoids. Am J Respir Crit Care Med 1996;153:1739–1748.
62. Lipworth BJ. Airway and systemic effects of inhaled corticosteroids in asthma: Dose response relationship. Pulm Pharmacol 1996;9:19–27.
63. Kelly HW. Comparison of inhaled corticosteroids. Ann Pharmacother 1998;32:220–232.
64. Pincus DJ, Szefler SJ, Ackerson LM, Martin RJ. Chronotherapy of asthma with inhaled steroids: The effect of dosage timing on drug efficacy. J Allergy Clin Immunol 1995;95:1172–1178.
65. Spahn JD, Leung DYM, Surs W, et al. Reduced glucocorticoid binding affinity in asthma is related to ongoing allergic inflammation. Am J Respir Crit Care Med 1995;151:1709–1714.
66. Ahrens R, Lux C, Bahl T, Han S-H. Choosing the metered-dose inhaler spacer or holding chamber that matches the patient's need: Evidence that the specific drug being delivered is an important consideration. J Allergy Clin Immunol 1995;96:288–294.
67. Spector SL, Smith LJ, Glass M. Effects of 6 weeks of therapy with oral doses of ICI 204,219, a leukotriene D_4 receptor antagonist, in subjects with bronchial asthma. Am J Respir Crit Care Med 1994; 150:618–623.
68. Israel E, Rubin P, Kemp JP, et al. The effect of inhibition of 5-lipoxygenase by zileuton in mild-to-moderate asthma. Ann Intern Med 1993;119:1059–1066.
69. Spector SL, Nicklas RA, eds. Practice parameters for the diagnosis and treatment of asthma. J Allergy Clin Immunol 1995;96(suppl): 707–870.
70. Marin MG. Low-dose methotrexate spares steroid usage in steroid-dependent asthmatic patients: A meta-analysis. Chest 1997;112:29–33.
71. Barnes PJ. New drugs for asthma. Eur Respir J 1992;1126–1136.
72. MacIntyre NR, Brougher P, Hess D, et al. Aerosol consensus statement. Chest 1991;100:1106–1109.
73. Kamada AK. Therapeutic controversies in the treatment of asthma. Ann Pharmacother 1994;28:904–914.
74 McFadden ER Jr. Improper patient techniques with metered dose inhalers: Clinical consequences and solutions to misuse. J Allergy Clin Immunol 1995;96:278–283.
75. Matthys H. Inhalation delivery of asthma drugs. Lung 1990;(suppl): 645–652.

25

CHRONIC OBSTRUCTIVE LUNG DISEASE

Sherri L. Konzem, PharmD, and Mark A. Stratton, PharmD, BCPS, FASHP

Chronic obstructive lung disease (COLD) is defined as a disease state characterized by the presence of airflow obstruction owing to chronic bronchitis or emphysema; the airflow obstruction is generally progressive, may be accompanied by airway hyperreactivity, and may be partially reversible.[1] The definition provided here is the one adopted by the American Thoracic Society in the 1995 statement of the Standards for the Diagnosis and Care of Patients with Chronic Obstructive Pulmonary Disease and serves to distinguish COLD from asthma or other potentially reversible causes of lung dysfunction such as tuberculosis or tumors.[1] The terms *chronic obstructive airway disease* (COAD) and *chronic obstructive pulmonary disease* (COPD) are synonymous with COLD.

COLD has conventionally included the subsets of chronic bronchitis and emphysema, although one should note that COLD may exist before evidence of airflow obstruction is demonstrated.[2] Recently, two additional subsets have been made, one from a pathologic perspective, peripheral airway disease, and the other from a clinical perspective, asthmatic bronchitis. Although the pathology and clinical characteristics of these subsets differ, most patients with COLD show characteristics of most of these subsets.

Chronic bronchitis, as reaffirmed by the American Thoracic Society in 1995, is a condition with chronic or recurrent excess mucus secretion into the bronchial tree with cough that occurs on most days during a period of at least 3 months of the year for at least 2 consecutive years in a patient in whom other causes of chronic cough have been excluded.[1] Patients with predominant chronic bronchitis may have an associated asthmatic bronchitis, which implies some degree of reversibility to their disorder. Bronchitis is defined in clinical terms, but emphysema in terms of anatomic pathology. Emphysema classically was defined on histologic examination at autopsy. Because this definition is of no clinical value, it has been defined as a condition of the lung characterized by abnormal, permanent enlargement of the air spaces distal to the terminal bronchiole, accompanied by destruction of their walls, yet without obvious fibrosis.[1] Peripheral airway disease is a condition that includes inflammation of the terminal and respiratory bronchioles, fibrosis with narrowing of airway walls, and goblet cell metaplasia of the bronchiolar epithelium. These changes appear before clinically detectable emphysema is present and are consistent with the pathology traditionally associated with chronic bronchitis.

EPIDEMIOLOGY

Approximately 14 million Americans suffer from COLD—about 12.5 million from chronic bronchitis and about 1.65 million from emphysema.[3,4] The estimated number of those with COLD has increased 41.5% since 1982.[3] It is the fourth most common cause of death in the United States. This is notable because COLD is the only leading cause of death other than congestive heart failure that is increasing in prevalence.[5] The group with the highest increase in deaths from COLD most recently has been white women. Data from the National Center for Health Statistics indicate that in a 13-year period, the age-adjusted mortality rate from COLD increased approximately 5.8% in men and 100% in women.[4,5] Rates of death from COLD increase with age, and are 1.8 times higher in males than females and 2.8 times higher in whites than in blacks. In 1995, 102,899 people in the United States died from COLD. This represented a 32.9% increase in COLD mortality since 1979 even though the prevalence of smoking has decreased since 1965.[1,6] This probably reflects the long latency period between smoking exposure and death from COLD. Cigarette smoking is clearly recognized as the principal risk factor for the development of COLD and is implicated in 90% of cases.[7]

According to the National Health Interview Survey, in 1985, nearly 5.5 million Americans 55 years of age and over were estimated to have COLD. This same survey revealed that, from the period 1979 to 1985, prevalence rates for COLD for the age group 65 to 74 years were 136 per 1000 for men and 118 per 1000 for women.[6] This striking increase from earlier data may reflect a broadening acceptance of the definition of COLD rather than an increased incidence of the disease.

Although the mortality associated with COLD is impressive, the disability associated with it is also of concern. COLD is the second leading cause of disability in the United States.[3,8] The prevalence rate of chronic bronchitis and emphysema increases with age and is higher in men than women and in whites than non-whites.[4,5] However, the ratio of men to women is higher for emphysema than for chronic bronchitis. The prevalence rate of chronic bronchitis increased from 1982 to 1992 from 33.9 per 1000 to 53.7 per 1000 persons.[4,5] In 1992, the prevalence rate of emphysema was 7.6 per 1000 persons, a 25% decrease over that reported in 1982.[4,5]

Assessing the use of medical resources can provide an estimate of the impact of COLD on society. Data indicate that from 1979 to 1985, physician office visits for COLD increased 15% for men and 8% for women. In addition, individuals with COLD have approximately double the number of hospital stays, days of restricted activity, and days of being confined to bed than do individuals without COLD.[2]

Of the numerous risk factors (Table 25–1) associated with the development of chronic bronchitis and emphysema, clearly cigarette smoking is the most common. The median risk ratio for smokers versus nonsmokers to develop chronic bronchitis is 5.3 for men and 4.2 for women. Of concern is that the incidence of women with chronic bronchitis or emphysema has increased because of the increased number of women smokers.

Only 15% of smokers go on to develop COLD.[9] Note, however, that in 1986, 82% of COLD mortality was a result of smoking.[10] Although the risk is lower in pipe and cigar smokers, it is still higher than for nonsmokers. Age of starting, total pack-years, and current smoking status are predictive of COLD mortality. However, not all smokers who have equivalent smoking histories develop the same degree of pulmonary impairment, suggesting that other physiologic or environmental factors contribute to the degree of lung dysfunction in smokers.[11] Nevertheless, the rate of loss of lung function is above all determined by smoking status and history.[12] Children and spouses of smokers are also at increased risk of developing significant pulmonary dysfunction by passive smoking also known as environmental tobacco smoke or "secondhand smoke."

Increasing age, male gender, and existing impaired lung function have also been identified as risk factors for the development of COLD. Individuals with existing impairment experience a greater decline in lung function over time than their counterparts with normal pulmonary function. Other increasingly identified familial factors are genetic and environmental.

Occupational hazards are difficult to identify, because they primarily affect blue-collar workers, who also have a higher incidence of cigarette smoking and may live in areas of higher air pollution. Reduced lung function and deaths from COLD are higher for individuals engaged in occupations such as gold and coal mining, working in glass or ceramic industries with exposure to silica dust, and in jobs that expose workers to cotton dust or grain dust, toluene diisocyanate, or asbestos. Cigarette smokers have a higher incidence of pulmonary dysfunction than their nonsmoking counterparts in jobs with this type of exposure.[11,13] Numerous other possible occupational risk factors also exist.

TABLE 25–1. Risk Factors for the Development of COLD

Major	Minor
Smoking	Air pollution
Age	Alcohol
Male gender	Race
Existing impaired lung function	Nutritional status
Occupation	Family history
α_1-Antitrypsin deficiency	Socioeconomic status
	Respiratory tract infections
	Bronchial reactivity

It is unclear whether or not air pollution alone is a significant risk factor for the development of COLD. However, in individuals with existing pulmonary dysfunction, significant air pollution worsens symptoms. Studies have shown an association between intensity of air pollution and number of emergency room admissions for COLD.[14] There are as yet insufficient data to suggest that air pollution contributes to the development of COLD in individuals with normal pulmonary function, whether smokers or not.

α_1-Antitrypsin (AAT) deficiency has been clearly defined as a genetic disorder that contributes to the risk of developing COLD, specifically emphysema. True AAT deficiency accounts for less than 1% of COLD cases.[1] AAT is a protease inhibitor that normally inhibits trypsin and other proteases from destroying normal lung tissue. The protease inhibitor (Pi) phenotypes with the highest incidence of COLD are the homozygous PiZZ (because they have the lowest level of AAT) and, to a lesser extent, PiSZ and Pi-null phenotypes.[1] PiMZ heterozygotes have lower levels of AAT than normal, but there is as yet an unclear association with an increased risk of COLD from smoking.

PATHOPHYSIOLOGY

The pathophysiology of COLD can best be understood by examining chronic bronchitis and emphysema separately. Peripheral airway disease is a major component of both conditions contributing to obstruction. In the majority of patients, evidence of each condition is present.

CHRONIC BRONCHITIS

As described earlier, chronic bronchitis is characterized by excessive tracheobronchial mucus secretion with cough. This excessive production of mucus results from hyperplasia and hypertrophy of mucus-producing glands and goblet cells owing to continued bronchial irritation. Additional morphologic changes occur in the bronchi, including increased smooth muscle, cartilage atrophy, inflammation characterized by neutrophil and lymphocyte infiltration, and loss of cilia. These bronchial changes do not contribute significantly to obstruction.[15]

In the COLD patient with predominant chronic bronchitis, changes in the peripheral airways contribute most to obstruction. Inflammation exists with mucus production and narrowing of the lumen in the more distal noncartilagenous or membranous bronchioles. In addition, there is fibrosis, tortuosity, and irregularity of these smaller airways. Autopsies have shown that individuals with chronic bronchitis have more airways smaller than 0.4 mm in diameter when compared with nonbronchitic patients.

Many chronic bronchitis patients will show minimal improvement with bronchodilators. Some display much more improvement in obstruction after bronchodilator therapy and would be more appropriately referred to as patients with asthmatic bronchitis. There may be a significant component of atopy in these patients.[15] Ventilatory impairment is unrelated to atopic status in individuals without a history of asthma, according to the literature,[16] further supporting the theory that nonallergic inflammation is important in the pathogenesis of chronic airflow obstruction.

The lung damage produced by smoking or exposure to other chronic irritants has long been considered to begin in the small airways. Airways less than 2 mm in diameter contribute only 10% to 20% of normal resistance to airflow, because their total cross-sectional diameter is much greater than that of larger airways. Thus, by the time obstruction is detected by pulmonary function tests, extensive damage has occurred. The best predictor of moderate disease has been suggested to be the presence of diminished breath sounds on physical examination, especially when combined with a clinical history consistent with COLD.[17] As chronic bronchitis progresses over several years, the changes in small airways begin to impair ventilation (V), while perfusion (Q) remains fairly adequate, resulting in a V/Q imbalance and hypoxemia. The hypoxemia leads to pulmonary hypertension with subsequent right ventricular failure (cor pulmonale). Autopsy data indicate that patients with pulmonary hypertension have markedly increased percentages of the intima and media in the musculature of the pulmonary arteries, specifically the larger vessels. These alterations do not, however, correlate with either the severity of the pulmonary hypertension or the ability of the vasculature to respond to oxygen.[18] The persistent hypoxemia stimulates erythropoiesis with resultant secondary polycythemia and increased blood viscosity, with its attendant complications of mental confusion and thrombotic stroke.

An additional component of chronic bronchitis is repeated respiratory infections. Patients are predisposed to repeated infections owing to mucus stagnation and plugging as well as lack of cilia or ciliary movement to clear mucus. The signs of infection usually consist of sputum changes, such as an increase in volume, thickening, and a change in color. Fever or other objective evidence of infection need not be present. Repeated respiratory infections in the chronic bronchitis patient can cause severe acute exacerbations in pulmonary status and can contribute significantly to accelerating the decline in pulmonary function tests resulting from the inflammation-induced fibrosis of bronchi and bronchioles. The most frequent respiratory pathogens are viral, although bacterial infection may follow a viral infection. The respiratory syncytial virus is considered the most common overall pathogen, whereas *Streptococcus pneumoniae* and *Haemophilus influenzae* are the most common bacterial pathogens. Because these are not the only bacteria that act as pathogens, the host's condition and environment must be considered when searching for a pathogen in a patient with chronic bronchitis with a suspected respiratory infection.

EMPHYSEMA

Emphysema refers specifically to involvement of the acinus, which is the unit of the lung responsible for gas exchange. It consists of three levels—respiratory bronchioles, alveolar ducts, and alveolar sacs—proceeding distally. In a simplistic sense, emphysema is a condition in which there is destruction of walls within the acinus such that the surface area for gas exchange is diminished. Intrinsic damage to the small airways is the major cause of airflow limitation and not emphysema.[19]

Several types of emphysema have been described and deserve comment:

1. *Proximal acinar emphysema.* This type includes the centrilobular emphysema (i.e., central lobes of acinus) characteristically seen in cigarette smokers, especially in the upper lobes, and simple pneumoconiosis of coal workers. This type of emphysema is confined largely to the proximal portion of the acinus, with the respiratory bronchioles being particularly affected.
2. *Panacinar emphysema.* The entire acinus is involved in this type. It is found in those genetically susceptible individuals who possess the homozygous PiZZ phenotype. These patients have a deficiency of protease inhibitors (AAT) such that proteases are allowed to destroy the alveolar walls of the acinus. This type usually involves the entire lung field.
3. *Distal (paraseptal) emphysema.* As the term suggests, this type of emphysema is associated with the distal portion of the acinus. It is seen as a consequence of spontaneous pneumothorax in young adults.
4. *Irregular emphysema.* This type of emphysema is produced as a consequence of trauma to lung tissue.

Our understanding of the pathogenesis of centrilobular emphysema (the most common type) extends from an understanding of the panacinar emphysema associated with protease inhibitor deficiency states. In centrilobular emphysema specifically caused by smoking, an imbalance develops between the protective protein inhibitors and proteases from activated neutrophils and mast cells. Women are less likely to experience this imbalance, possibly because of a protective effect of estrogens that may stimulate synthesis of protease inhibitors. Damage occurs because cigarette smoke causes a macrophage alveolitis and a respiratory bronchiolitis. These macrophages are chemotactic for neutrophils. Both the macrophages and neutrophils release a greater amount of elastase (which breaks down elastin, a protein integral to the structural integrity of alveolar walls) in response to smoke in smokers than in nonsmokers. Cigarette smoke is also thought to impair the synthesis of elastin.[20] Alveolar inflammatory cells in smokers with emphysema have been shown to spontaneously inactivate α_1-proteinase inhibitor, suggesting that the progressive lung damage is related to an ongoing inflammation in peripheral airways.[21]

The destruction of the surface area for gas exchange within the acinus results in a loss of elastic recoil. This loss permits compression of distal airways during expiration, contributing to the significant obstructive pattern that is seen in pulmonary function tests. The exact changes in pulmonary function are described later in this chapter. In cigarette smokers with centrilobular emphysema, the respiratory bronchiolitis leads to narrowing of the terminal bronchioles.[22,23]

In addition to a reduction in elastic recoil, loss of alveolar walls results in a loss of the capillary network essential to adequate perfusion. This results in not only a decrease in ventilation (V) but also a loss in perfusion (Q); thus, the V/Q ratio is maintained better than in chronic bronchitis.[22,23] Therefore, although predominant emphysematous patients experience greater dyspnea than predominant chronic bronchitis patients, the former are better able to preserve gas exchange because their respiratory centers are more responsive to hypoxia. The net result of this on other physiologic systems is less cor pulmonale and less polycythemia than seen in the predominant chronic bronchitic.

CLINICAL PRESENTATION

By the time a patient presents with obstructive airway disease, the diagnosis can be rapidly made often by simply observing the patient's breathing pattern. The clinical features are presented in Table 25–2. As described previously, though the majority of patients with COLD will have components of both chronic bronchitis and emphysema, it is best to describe the physical examination of each predominant constituent condition separately.

CHRONIC BRONCHITIS

The patient presenting with predominant chronic bronchitis is often overweight and has an impressive history of productive cough and increasing dyspnea on exertion. By history the cough has been increasing in frequency and duration. Predominant chronic bronchitis patients are referred to classically as "blue bloaters" (type B) because they tend to retain carbon dioxide because of a decreased responsiveness of the respiratory center to hypoxemia and ultimately hypercarbia. They will commonly have peripheral edema from cor pulmonale and usually have a normal or only slightly increased respiratory rate at rest. With advanced disease, the anteroposterior diameter of the chest is often increased, resulting in the classical "barrel chest" appearance. This does not always indicate advanced disease, because it is also a normal part of the aging process. Percussion of the chest is resonant, and the breath sounds are distant on auscultation. Rhonchi and wheezes are frequently heard and change in location as the patient breathes deeply or coughs. A rapid assessment of obstruction can be done by placing the stethoscope over the trachea and instructing the patient to forcefully expire. Forced expiration lasting greater than 4 seconds correlates with obstruction in pulmonary function tests. The use of the scalene or sternocleidomastoid muscles of the neck to assist respiration may not be apparent unless severe obstruction is present.

As the degree of obstruction worsens and the arterial oxygen tension (Pao_2) continues to drop, pulmonary hypertension from vasoconstriction ensues. This leads to right ventricular strain and ultimately cor pulmonale. On physical examination, this is manifested by jugular venous

TABLE 25–2. Clinical Features of COLD

	Predominant Emphysema	Predominant Chronic Bronchitis
Age (yr)	60±	50±
Dyspnea	Severe	Mild
Cough	After dyspnea starts	Before dyspnea starts
Sputum	Scanty, mucoid	Copious, purulent
Bronchial infection	Less frequent	More frequent
Respiratory insufficiency episode	Often terminal	Repeated
Chest film markings	Increased diameter Flattened diaphragms	Increased bronchovascular Large heart
$Paco_2$ (mm Hg)	35–40	50–60
Pao_2 (mm Hg)	65–75	45–60
Hematocrit (%)	35–45	50–60
Pulmonary hypertension		
Rest	None to mild	Moderate to severe
Exercise	Moderate	Worsens
Cor pulmonale	Rare	Common
Diffusion capacity	Decreased	None to slightly decreased

(Adapted from Ref. 32.)

distention, hepatomegaly, hepatojugular reflux, and peripheral edema. Conventional cardiac examination may be difficult if a barrel chest is present; however, by palpating the epigastric area, a heave may be felt or even seen in thin patients and auscultation of the area may reveal a gallop rhythm suggestive of right ventricular hypertrophy.

In the face of chronic hypoxemia, cyanosis of the lips, mucous membranes, or extremities may be seen. The cyanosis worsens during the night, frequently because of chronic oxygen desaturation secondary to sleep apnea. Clubbing of the fingers is rarely seen in chronic bronchitis. Sleep apnea has recently become an area of increasing study in patients with COLD and may play a much greater role than previously understood in the pathogenesis of disease, especially with respect to cor pulmonale. Individuals with sleep apnea are at greater risk for developing respiratory insufficiency and cor pulmonale.[24]

EMPHYSEMA

The patient presenting with predominant emphysema is characteristically older than the chronic bronchitis patient. The chief complaint is often increasing dyspnea, even at rest, with minimal cough. These patients have been classically termed "pink puffers" (type A) because of their obvious tachypnea and flushed appearance, which is a result of their respiratory centers being quite responsive to hypoxemia as a stimulus to breathe.

These patients are frequently thin in physical stature and will present with "pursed lip" breathing. This maneuver compensates for loss of elastic recoil so that exhalation of a larger volume of air is possible. They also are tachypneic at rest and often sit with their chests forward and hands resting on their knees; this position requires the least energy for breathing. Frequently, the patient uses accessory muscles of the chest and neck to assist in the work of breathing. Percussion of the chest is hyperresonant and auscultation reveals diminished breath sounds with rhonchi and minimal wheezes. Excursion of the diaphragms is limited because of persistent hyperinflation of the lungs.

Hypoxemia is not a significant problem in the predominant emphysema patient until late in the disease state. As a result, cor pulmonale is not as common a problem as seen in the predominant chronic bronchitic until the terminal stages.

DIAGNOSTIC TESTS

PULMONARY FUNCTION TESTS

Measurements of pulmonary function by objective means are considered essential in any patient with COLD to determine the severity of the disease, responsiveness to therapeutic agents, and prognosis. Several tests of small-airway function are available, including the single-breath nitrogen test and mid- and end-expiratory flows from spirometry. Spirometry has been extensively used and is preferred owing to its cost, technical ease, and clinical applicability.[25]

In both chronic bronchitis and emphysema, the vital capacity (VC) is decreased, the residual volume (RV) is increased, and the total lung capacity (TLC) is often normal or increased.

In patients with chronic bronchitis and/or emphysema leading to COLD, there are reductions in forced expiratory volume after 1 second (FEV_1), forced vital capacity (FVC), FEV_1/FVC%, and forced expiratory flow ($FEF_{25\%-75\%}$). The FEV_1/FVC ratio expressed as a percentage is helpful in determining the degree of obstruction. If it is less than 80%, obstruction is present. The FEF over the middle 50% of the expiratory curve (maximum midexpiratory flow rate [MMFR], $FEF_{25\%-75\%}$, or $FEF_{50\%}$) is helpful specifically in the predominant emphysema patient because it represents the elastic recoil of the lung. In predominant chronic bronchitis, flow rates are decreased. It is now understood that in addition to loss of elastic recoil (i.e., elasticity of the lung parenchyma) in the emphysema patient, there is also a significant component of peripheral airway disease, also referred to as bronchiolitis, which contributes to the obstructive picture.

The majority of patients with mixed disease will usually experience exertional dyspnea when the FEV_1 is less than 50% of predicted and will have dyspnea at rest when the FEV_1 is less than 25% of predicted. Patients with predominant chronic bronchitis experience carbon dioxide retention and cor pulmonale when the FEV_1 is greater than 25% of predicted values, but the predominantly emphysematous patient does not experience these complications until the FEV_1 is less than 25% of predicted.

Measurement of diffusion capacity using carbon monoxide (DCO) can help distinguish predominant bronchitis from emphysema. In emphysema, the diffusion capacity is diminished because of loss of surface area available for gas diffusion. In bronchitis, the diffusion capacity is normal or only slightly decreased.

ARTERIAL BLOOD GASES

Just as pulmonary function tests are essential for determining the severity and prognosis of patients with COLD, so are arterial blood gases. Arterial blood gases should be determined at rest and after exercise. The predominant chronic bronchitis patient is characterized as having a low arterial oxygen tension (PaO_2 = 45 to 60 mm Hg) and an elevated arterial carbon dioxide tension ($PaCO_2$ = 50 to 60 mm Hg). The predominantly emphysematous patient has by comparison a higher PaO_2 and usually normal $PaCO_2$ with similar degrees of pulmonary dysfunction. In the predominant chronic bronchitis patient, the initial abnormality is a decrease in the PaO_2. The major cause of this hypoxemia is an underventilation (V) of acini relative to the perfusion (Q) of the area. This low V/Q ratio will progress over a period of several years, resulting in a consistent decline in the PaO_2. For reasons that are not entirely understood, the predominant chronic bronchitic loses the ability to increase the rate or depth of respiration in response to persistent hypoxemia. This decreased ventilatory drive may have its origin in either abnormal peripheral or central respiratory receptors. This relative hypoventilation subsequently leads to hypercapnia. The respiratory centers again do not respond to the persistently increasing $Paco_2$.

These changes in Pao_2 and $Paco_2$ are subtle and progress over a period of many years; as a result, the pH is usually near normal because the kidneys compensate by retaining bicarbonate. If an acute change occurs such as might be seen in an acute pneumonia with impending respiratory failure, the $Paco_2$ may rise sharply, temporarily resulting in a primary respiratory acidosis until the kidneys can compensate (24 to 72 hours later) or the acid–base defect is corrected by mechanical ventilation.

The persistent hypoxemia leads to pulmonary vascular constriction and cor pulmonale. The hypoxemia and hypercarbia lead to an increase in 2,3-diphosphoglyceric acid (2,3-DPG) and a shift of the oxyhemoglobin dissociation curve to the right. This results in a decrease in the affinity of hemoglobin for oxygen, allowing more oxygen to be released to tissues in which the Pao_2 is lowest. Hypoxemia also stimulates erythropoiesis, which leads to the secondary polycythemia common in the predominant chronic bronchitic.

Compared to the predominant chronic bronchitic, the predominant emphysematous patient can maintain a near-normal Pao_2 in the face of declining pulmonary function, until the terminal stages, because ventilation and perfusion decrease proportionately. These individuals have normal or excess responsiveness of peripheral and central respiratory receptors to hypoxemia or hypercarbia. This explains why the predominant emphysematous patient does not develop cor pulmonale, cyanosis, or polycythemia until the end stages of the disease process.

CHEST ROENTGENOGRAM

A chest roentgenogram (posteroanterior and lateral views) is most useful in the diagnosis of the predominant emphysema patient. Characteristic findings include flattened diaphragms that move less than 3 cm between inspiration and expiration, loss of peripheral vascular markings, bullous lesions, and increased retrosternal air space. All these findings indicate extensive air trapping consistent with severe emphysema. Whether or not the dimensions of the thoracic cage itself are truly increased is a matter of controversy; it may be that the cage appears large because of the loss of physical mass in the rest of the body. In the predominant chronic bronchitic, the only changes are increased bronchovascular markings in the lower lung field and an increased cardiac silhouette in the presence of right ventricular failure with prominent pulmonary arteries.

ELECTROCARDIOGRAM

The electrocardiogram is helpful in COLD patients only when cor pulmonale develops. Common findings are right-axis deviation, prominent R waves in V_1 and V_2, S wave in V_5 or $V_6 \geq 7$ mm, and tall peaked P waves in lead II.

OTHER LABORATORY TESTS

HEMATOLOGY

In the predominant chronic bronchitic patient, the hemoglobin and hematocrit will be elevated secondary to erythropoiesis caused by hypoxemia. In exacerbations of chronic bronchitis, the white cell count may or may not rise and a left shift may or may not be present.

SPUTUM

Examination of sputum (e.g., Gram stain) is helpful in exacerbations of chronic bronchitis to identify potential bacterial pathogens that may have precipitated the exacerbation and aid in the selection of antimicrobial therapy. It is important to ensure that what is examined microscopically is truly sputum and not saliva. Sputum is identified by the presence of alveolar macrophages; saliva is identified by squamous epithelial cells. Many laboratories have developed scoring systems to help clinicians assess the adequacy of the sputum sample being examined. Sputum should also be examined for eosinophils to rule out an allergic component that would be consistent with asthmatic bronchitis.

α_1-ANTITRYPSIN ASSAY

This test is particularly useful in patients younger than 40 years of age who present with emphysema and obstructive lung disease. Markedly low levels may indicate a PiZZ phenotype. Moderately low levels may indicate other Pi phenotypes who may be more predisposed to emphysema caused by smoking than the general population.

COURSE AND PROGNOSIS

The clinical course and prognosis of patients having chronic bronchitis and/or emphysema with obstructive pulmonary disease are marked by variable morbidity and mortality. Little is known of the early natural history of COLD, but it is probably characterized by slowly deteriorating pulmonary function for several years before clinical illness is appreciated by patients. Much more is known of the prognosis and clinical course once symptomatology has become evident. Delay in recognition of the true impact of COLD may occur because the disease develops at a time of life when people generally begin to modify activities to less stressful pursuits. There may also be a process of physical detraining that obscures the fact that dyspnea is the underlying cause of their reduced exercise tolerance. This may result in a loss of cardiopulmonary fitness and some disuse atrophy of leg muscles. This is of interest and importance because patients with lung disease may cease exercise because of leg fatigue rather than dyspnea and patients with COLD have relatively poor work efficiency.[26]

The predominant emphysema patient's pattern is characterized by progressive dyspnea without exacerbations precipitated by increased sputum production, as is characteristic of the predominant chronic bronchitic patient. The predominant emphysema patient's terminal event is often characterized by rapidly progressive cor pulmonale and intractable hypercapnia leading to respiratory arrest. The usual course of a patient with predominant bronchitis is characterized by increasing frequency of exacerbations of acute pulmonary insufficiency precipitated by bronchitis. This is accompanied by progressive decline in pulmonary function, with the chronic complications (previously described) of cor pulmonale, hypercapnia, and polycythemia. Exacerbations of bronchitis are characterized by increased mucopurulent sputum and frequently lead to acute respiratory failure from which the patient rapidly recovers with appropriate antibiotics and other therapies. These episodes tend to increase in severity and frequency until intractable cor pulmonale and hypercapnia occur.

Mean rate of decline of FEV_1 appears to be the most useful objective tool to assess the course of COLD. The rates of decline in prospective follow-up studies of patients with initially abnormal FEV_1s or FEV_1/FVC ratios followed for 3 to 16 years revealed a decline in the FEV_1 of 44 to 75 mL/yr; however, there was considerable variability. The rate of decline in FEV_1 for normal patients from age alone was 24 mL/yr.[27,28] In any study assessing rate of decline, an appropriate observation period is essential. In the study reporting the rate of decline in FEV_1 of 44 mL/yr, the observation period was only 3 years.[27] This may be too short to project rate of decline throughout the life of the patient, because during the first year many patients improve their pulmonary function with pharmacologic agents. In longer studies the rate of decline of FEV_1 is greater and linear.[28,29] Rate of decline of blood gases has not been shown to be a useful parameter to assess progression of the disease.

In terms of functional capacity, the predominant chronic bronchitic patient will show more physical impairment at a higher FEV_1 than the predominant emphysema patient because of the comparatively worse arterial blood gases. Most people with mixed disease are not able to perform extremely vigorous activity once the FEV_1 falls below 1.5 L, but they can work. Once the FEV_1 falls below 1.0 L their ability to perform usual daily activities becomes impaired.

The survival rate in patients with COLD is related to the initial level of impairment in the FEV_1 and age. Other less important factors include degree of reversibility with bronchodilators, resting pulse, perceived physical disability, diffusing capacity, cor pulmonale, and blood-gas abnormalities.[30]

A rapid decline in pulmonary function tests indicates a poor prognosis. People living at high altitudes also have a reduced survival rate.[29] Median survival is approximately 10 years when the FEV_1 is 1.4 L, 4 years when the FEV_1 is 1.0 L, and about 2 years when the FEV_1 is 0.5 L.[29]

As yet it is not clear that treatment with pharmacologic agents improves survival; however, they do improve the quality of life, probably reduce hospitalizations, and may prevent some premature deaths. In recent years, several disease-specific quality-of-life measures have been developed to assess the overall efficacies of therapies for COPD including the Chronic Respiratory Questionnaire (CRQ) and the St. George's Respiratory Questionnaire (SGRQ).[31] These questionnaires measure the impact of various therapies on disease variables such as severity of dyspnea and level of activity; they do not measure impact of therapies on survival. Currently, they have been used only to a limited degree to quantify short-term health gain obtained from bronchodilators[31]; however, there appears to be a trend toward greater use of these disease-specific quality-of-life measures. The only intervention shown to improve survival rate is oxygen therapy.[29] Smoking cessation leads to decreased symptomatology and slows the rate of decline of pulmonary function even after significant abnormality in pulmonary function tests have been detected (FEV_1/FVC < 60%).[12,28]

ACUTE RESPIRATORY FAILURE IN COLD

The diagnosis of acute respiratory failure in COLD is definitively made on the basis of an acute change in the arterial blood gases. Defining acute respiratory failure as a Pa_{O_2} less than 50 mm Hg or a Pa_{CO_2} of greater than 50 mm Hg may often be incorrect and inadequate because these values may not represent a significant change from a patient's baseline values. A more precise definition is an acute drop in Pa_{O_2} of 10 to 15 mm Hg or any acute increase in Pa_{CO_2} that decreases the serum pH to 7.3 or less.[32] Additional acute clinical manifestations of respiratory failure include restlessness, confusion, tachycardia, diaphoresis, cyanosis, hypotension, irregular breathing, miosis, and unconsciousness.[32]

The most common cause of acute respiratory failure in COLD is acute exacerbation of bronchitis with an increase in the volume and viscosity of sputum. This serves to worsen obstruction and further impair alveolar ventilation, resulting in worsening hypoxemia and hypercapnia. Additional causes of acute respiratory failure in COLD are pneumonia, pulmonary embolism, left ventricular failure, pneumothorax, and central nervous system depressants.

▶ TREATMENT: Chronic Obstructive Lung Disease

DESIRED OUTCOME AND NONPHARMACOLOGIC THERAPY

Therapy of the patient with COLD is multifaceted. The goals of therapy are presented in Table 25–3. The importance of smoking cessation cannot be overemphasized—it is the obvious and first step in the secondary prevention plan. Smoking cessation will slow the rate of decline in pulmonary function tests, decrease symptoms,[33] and improve the patient's quality of life. The use of nicotine gum, patch, or clonidine may be helpful in assisting the smoker to quit. Behavioral modification techniques or other forms of psychotherapy may also be helpful. Programs that address the many issues associated with smoking (i.e., learned be-

TABLE 25–3. Goals of Therapy

Smoking cessation
Improvement of the chronic obstructive status
Treatment and prevention of acute exacerbations
Reduction of the rate of progression of the disease
Improvement of physical and psychologic well-being of the patient so that daily activities can be resumed or maintained
Reduction in days lost from work
Reduction in hospitalizations
Reduction in mortality

haviors, environmental influences, chemical dependence) using a team approach are more likely to be successful.[34]

Comprehensive pulmonary rehabilitation programs should include exercise training along with smoking cessation, breathing exercises, optimal medical treatment, psychosocial support, and health education. High-intensity training (70% maximal workload) is possible even in advanced COLD, and the level of intensity improves peripheral muscle and ventilatory function. An inexpensive, comprehensive outpatient rehabilitation program can produce long-term improvement in activities of daily living, quality of life, and exercise tolerance in patients with moderate to severe chronic obstructive pulmonary disease. Supplemental oxygen and adequate nutrition are important adjuncts in a training program.

PHARMACOLOGIC THERAPY

There was a long-standing opinion that COLD was associated with irreversible obstruction. This reasoning allowed pharmacotherapy to be chosen empirically. This opinion, however, has been challenged by the Intermittent Positive Pressure Breathing Group.[35] The data reported from their studies suggest that many individuals with COLD do obtain some degree of improvement in their obstruction from bronchodilators. This group may include many patients who would now be described as having asthmatic bronchitis. In addition, COLD patients with the greatest bronchodilatory response have the lowest annual decline in FEV_1 and the greatest 5-year survival.[2] It also appears that a single test of reversibility using an inhaled sympathomimetic followed by pulmonary function tests is not adequate to assess whether patients with COLD will benefit from bronchodilators. Even if a positive response is not detected, these patients deserve an adequate therapeutic trial of pharmacologic agents for the following reasons: (1) Although objective tests may not reveal a response, possibly because of sensitivity of equipment, a subjective improvement may occur; (2) some patients may respond to inhaled sympathomimetics on one occasion and not on another; (3) the response to bronchodilators may require prolonged administration; (4) patients may respond to pharmacologic agents via mechanisms besides bronchodilation; (5) patients not responding in initial tests with sympathomimetics may respond to anticholinergics or methylxanthines; and (6) some parameters may be improved (e.g., exercise capacity) while others are not (e.g., FEV_1). The hypothesis that regular bronchodilation may slow the deterioration of lung function is being studied.[2]

There is no clear answer to the question of which of the bronchodilator classes to initiate first (e.g., anticholinergics, sympathomimetics, methylxanthines). Patients whose disease is primarily caused by bronchial wall inflammation accompanied by bronchospasm as seen in the chronic bronchitic respond better to bronchodilator therapy than the patient suffering primarily from irreversible emphysematous damage. The decision of drug therapy selection should be based on patient compliance, individual response, and side effects. For the purposes of this chapter, agents will be presented in the sequence indicated by trends in therapy currently. These are anticholinergics, sympathomimetics, methylxanthines, and corticosteroids.

ANTICHOLINERGICS

In the past decade, anticholinergic agents have emerged as first-line therapy for the stable COLD patient. The only agents currently available in the United States are atropine and ipratropium bromide (Atrovent). When given by inhalation, anticholinergics produce bronchodilation by competitively inhibiting cholinergic receptors in bronchial smooth muscle. This activity blocks acetylcholine, with the net effect being a reduction in cyclic guanosine monophosphate (GMP), which normally acts to constrict bronchial smooth muscle. These agents maintain their effectiveness during years of regular continuous use.[35–37] Ipratropium bromide has been shown to decrease the effectiveness of voluntary cough on clearing mucus from the airways, which may affect its role in the treatment of patients who have excessive mucus production.[38] The clinical significance of this effect is unknown.

The inhaled anticholinergics have been well demonstrated in the literature to be effective bronchodilators in COLD.[35–38] However, data from the Lung Health Study demonstrate that the rate of decline of lung function in smokers with mild to moderate COPD can be significantly slowed by smoking cessation, but not by ipratropium.[39] Anticholinergic agents have been compared to inhaled sympathomimetic agents and been found to produce greater improvement in pulmonary function tests than the sympathomimetic agents with fewer systemic side effects such as tachycardia.[40,41] This is likely because patients with COLD do not exhibit dramatic responsiveness to adrenergic compounds, unlike patients with asthma. Moreover, with aging, the sensitivity of the adrenergic system decreases, making the cholinergic system the more readily manipulated for purposes of achieving bronchodilation.[42] Ipratropium has a slower onset of action and a more prolonged bronchodilator effect compared to standard β-agonists and has been considered to be less suitable for use on an "as-needed" basis for immediate relief of bronchospasm.[1,43] However, it has recently been demonstrated that in acute exacerbations of COLD in the critically ill patient, anticholinergics may be valuable as additive agents or as single agents for patients intolerant to β-agonist side effects.

Atropine can be administered via either a hand-held or a jet nebulizer using the parenteral or ophthalmic solution, which is diluted with 2 to 4 mL of saline for administration. The dose of atropine is initiated at 0.025 to 0.05 mg/kg. The duration of effect is approximately 4 hours. Atropine is used in both the inhaled and nebulized forms for COLD; however, it does not have a Food and Drug Administration (FDA)-approved indication for this use. Atropine has a tertiary structure and is readily absorbed across the oral and respiratory mucosa, whereas ipratropium has a quaternary structure that is poorly absorbed.[44] The lack of systemic absorption of ipratropium greatly diminishes the anticholinergic side effects such as blurred vision, urinary retention, nausea, and tachycardia associated with atropine.[43,44] Thus, ipratropium is considered the anticholinergic agent of choice for COLD. An alternative to ipratropium and atropine with minimal systemic side effects owing to its quaternary structure is glycopyrrolate.

Ipratropium bromide is available as a metered-dose inhaler (MDI) and a solution for inhalation. It is three to five times more potent on muscarinic receptors than atropine.[36] It provides a peak effect in 1.5 to 2 hours and has a duration of 4 to 6 hours.[36] Although the recommended dose is 2 puffs four times a day, many clinicians prescribe two to three times that dose to produce maximal bronchodilation. The results of a recent trial demonstrate that ipratropium increases maximum exercise performance in stable COLD patients with doses of 8 to 12 puffs prior to exercise but not with doses of 4 puffs or less.[45] Side effects of ipratropium appear to be limited to dry mouth and an occasional metallic taste. Oxitropium bromide and Ba679Br are long-acting agents being studied in Europe that appear to be even more potent.[46]

The objective in therapy with inhaled bronchodilators is to provide relatively small doses to the affected airways and to achieve the desired pharmacologic effect with minimal systemic toxicity. The remaining issue is to determine which method of inhaling bronchodilators best achieves this objective: (1) use of an MDI; (2) use of an MDI with a spacer; or (3) use of a powered nebulizer to deliver the medication. Regardless of which method is used, the most critical factor is proper technique. Although usual doses and dosing intervals may be obtained from several sources, a patient's dose and frequency should be adjusted based on needs and tolerance.

MDIs are convenient for the mobile patient and are quite adequate when used appropriately. (A description of appropriate administration technique is provided in Chapter 24, Asthma.) The greatest problems are inappropriate technique and overuse; therefore, patient education and reinforcement are critical. Spacer devices improve aerosol delivery from MDIs in patients who are unable to adequately coordinate MDI actuation with inhalation (e.g., elderly COLD patients). The wet nebulization method should be reserved for those with the most debilitated lung function. When a wet nebulizer is used, the bronchodilator is diluted with 2 to 3 mL of normal saline or water, which is sufficient to provide a treatment for approximately 10 minutes. A T-tube is necessary to prevent excessive loss of drug and diluent. As when using the MDI, inspiration must be slow and deep. The patient should try to hold each inspiration for 3 to 5 seconds. Exhalation should be through the nose. It may be desirable to use more diluent to further moisten secretions and promote their expectoration, but this will alter the delivered dose because the dead volume (the volume of liquid left in the nebulizer following treatment) remains the same but will contain less drug.

SYMPATHOMIMETICS

Sympathomimetics have traditionally been the cornerstone of pharmacotherapy for COLD but have now fallen behind anticholinergics as preferred chronic therapy in stable patients. Most authorities recommend that sympathomimetics be used as second-line therapy, either to supplement or to replace ipratropium for patients who do not obtain satisfactory clinical benefit from ipratropium alone.[43] However, in acute exacerbations sympathomimetics remain the initial treatment of choice owing to their rapid onset of action. The issue of continuous and "as-needed" sympathomimetics in COLD is currently controversial. The clinical situations in which sympathomimetics are used other than acute exacerbations include (1) as-needed use for monotherapy for mild, episodic symptomatic COLD, (2) as-needed use for chronically stable symptomatic COLD in combination with anticholinergics, and (3) as a fixed schedule plus as needed for chronically stable symptomatic COLD.

Numerous sympathomimetics are currently available in the U.S. market; however, it is more desirable to use the newer agents with greater β_2 selectivity and longer duration of action. These agents include albuterol, bitolterol, pirbuterol, salmeterol, and terbutaline. β_2-Selective sympathomimetics cause bronchodilation by stimulating the enzyme adenyl cyclase to increase the formation of adenosine 3′,5′-monophosphate (3′,5′-cAMP).[37] In addition, they are thought to improve mucociliary clearance. Although shorter-acting and less selective β-agonists are still widely used (metaproterenol, isoetharine, isoproterenol), it is difficult to advocate their continued use because of the shorter duration of action and increased cardiostimulatory effects. Note that salmeterol, which has the longest onset and duration of action of the β-agonists, is used for chronic, not acute, therapy.

In contrast to asthma, there is little evidence to suggest that the regular use of a β-agonist is deleterious in COLD. However, some studies suggest that it may result in a slow decline of FEV_1 beyond that which is disease related.[47,48] There is no evidence to suggest that prolonged use of β-agonists significantly decreases survival in patients with COLD. The peak response tends to be preserved over the course of long-term therapy with a β-agonist, but a slight decline in the duration of the bronchodilation may develop.[49] The reader is referred to Chapter 24, Asthma, for a comparative table of these agents.

Sympathomimetics are available in inhaled, oral, and parenteral dosage forms. The preferred route of administration is by inhalation. The use of oral and parenteral β-agonists in COLD is discouraged because they are no more effective than a properly used MDI and the incidence of systemic adverse effects (tachycardia and hand tremor) is greater.[43] The inhalation route minimizes the intracellular shift of potassium and resultant hypokalemia, which is augmented by theophylline.[37] Administration of β-agonists via MDIs is as effective as nebulization therapy and usually favored for reasons of cost and convenience.[50,51]

If response to ipratropium alone is unsatisfactory, all patients with COLD should receive a trial of an inhaled β_2-selective agonist even if their FEV_1 is not changed because mechanisms other than bronchodilation may be helpful (e.g., increase in mucociliary clearance). An individual's perceived benefit from these agents may significantly affect their usefulness.[52] The dose of the β-agonist can be increased in an acute exacerbation, although the limiting factor is an excessive increase in heart rate.

COMBINATION ANTICHOLINERGICS AND SYMPATHOMIMETICS

The body of evidence indicates that combination inhaled anticholinergic and sympathomimetic regimens are more effective than either as monotherapy.[33,53–55] Before the combination is used, the dose of the anticholinergic should first be titrated. Combination of a β-agonist and an anticholinergic agent has been shown to be more effective than using either agent alone.[53–55] Recently, a combination sympathomimetic and anticholinergic MDI (Combivent) has been released by the FDA for use in the United States.

METHYLXANTHINES

Methylxanthines have been available for the treatment of COLD for at least five decades and at one time were considered first-line therapy for the treatment of COLD. However, in the past 20 years with the advent of long-acting inhaled β-agonists and inhaled anticholinergics, they have been relegated as third-line agents. Theophylline, the most common methylxanthine used in clinical practice, can be an effective bronchodilator in many patients with chronic, stable disease.[53] The methylxanthines may produce bronchodilation through numerous mechanisms, including (1) inhibition of phosphodiesterase, thus increasing cyclic adenosine monophosphate levels, (2) inhibition of calcium ion influx into smooth muscle, (3) prostaglandin antagonism, (4) stimulation of endogenous catecholamines, (5) adenosine receptor antagonism, and (6) inhibition of release of mediators from mast cells and leukocytes.[37] However, there is no certainty about these mechanisms. Long-term theophylline use in patients with COLD has been demonstrated to exert improvements in lung function, including VC, FEV, minute ventilation, and gas exchange.[54] Subjectively, theophylline has been shown to lessen dyspnea and enhance exercise tolerance in the COLD patient.[55,56] Other nonpulmonary effects of theophylline that may contribute to improved overall functional capacity in patients with COLD include improved cardiac function and decreased pulmonary artery pressure.[54]

Numerous reliably absorbed sustained-release theophylline (1,3-dimethylxanthine) preparations are currently available. These have the advantages of improving patient compliance and achieving more consistent serum concentrations over rapid-release theophylline and aminophylline preparations; however, caution must be used in switching from one sustained-release preparation to another, because there are considerable variations in sustained-release characteristics.[57] Aside from aminophylline, there is no need to use any of the various other theophylline complexes. There is no indication for rectal suppositories of theophylline or aminophylline or intramuscular administration of these drugs. Dissolution from rectal suppositories is inconsistent, absorption from intramuscular injections is unreliable, and the injections are painful. Aminophylline and theophylline with 5% dextrose are available as intravenous preparations. Oral and intravenous theophylline are equivalent in terms of dosage strength. Aminophylline is 80% anhydrous theophylline. Aminophylline can be converted to intravenous or oral theophylline by using 80% of the aminophylline dose.

Theophylline has been shown to be of value in exacerbations of COLD.[58,59] In acute exacerbations, loading doses of theophylline or aminophylline should be administered to achieve therapeutic serum theophylline concentrations rapidly. Without a loading dose, COLD patients would require 40 to 60 hours (five half-lives, using the usual elimination half-life of 8 to 12 hours) before steady-state serum concentrations would be reached with maintenance dosing only. Loading doses may be administered orally or intravenously. Oral theophylline is well absorbed from the intestines and is effective for loading when gastrointestinal function is thought to be intact. Intravenous therapy should be reserved for severe acute decompensation in patients unable to take oral medication. The loading dose is based on actual body weight.[60] Recommended loading doses are 5 mg/kg (theophylline) and 6 mg/kg (aminophylline) for patients who have not taken any theophylline in the previous 24 hours. Each 0.5 mg/kg (theophylline) or 0.6 mg/kg (aminophylline) will raise the serum theophylline concentration by approximately 1 μg/mL. Ideally, for patients currently taking theophylline, the loading dose should be deferred until a theophylline concentration can be obtained rapidly. However, if this is not possible, then it is recommended to administer a partial loading dose of 2.5 mg/kg (theophylline) or 3 mg/kg (aminophylline) if the patient has taken sustained-release theophylline within the past 24 hours or immediate-release theophylline within the past 12 hours.

The intravenous administration rate of aminophylline and theophylline with dextrose should not exceed 25 mg/min to avoid cardiac arrhythmias or cardiovascular collapse. A controlling device is recommended when infusing aminophylline or theophylline.

The desired therapeutic range of theophylline is 10 to 20 μg/mL. Because most COLD patients are elderly and often have a rapidly changing clinical picture that may affect theophylline clearance, it is prudent to aim for levels in the range of 10 to 15 μg/mL to minimize the likelihood of toxicity. Factors in COLD patients that decrease theophylline clearance leading to reduced maintenance-dose requirements include advanced age, bacterial or viral pneumonia, left or right ventricular failure, liver dysfunction, hypoxemia from the acute decompensation, and use of drugs such as cimetidine, macrolide, and fluoroquinolone antibiotics. Factors that may enhance theophylline clearance, resulting in the need for higher maintenance doses, include tobacco and cannabis smoking, hyperthyroidism, and the use of such drugs as phenytoin, phenobarbital, and rifampin. Maintenance-dose recommendations for intravenous aminophylline for these conditions have been proposed (Table 25–4). Again, when using oral or intravenous theophylline, 80% of the aminophylline dose should be used. These recommendations should be considered as starting points, because serum theophylline concentrations must be obtained to guide and individualize therapy. The conditions described are dynamic, and as they fluctuate so will the clearance of theophylline.

TABLE 25–4. Maintenance Doses of Parenteral Aminophylline in Exacerbations of COLD

Usual loading dose, mg/kg	6
Maintenance dose, mg/kg/h	
Smokers	0.8
Nonsmokers	0.5
Elderly	0.3
Cor pulmonale	0.3
Congestive heart failure	0.1–0.2
Liver disease	0.1–0.2

Oral therapy should be substituted for intravenous once the patient is stabilized, serum concentrations are reasonably consistent, and the patient is able to take oral medications. The oral sustained-release preparation can be initiated at the time the intravenous solution is stopped. The oral dose is calculated from the 24-hour intravenous theophylline dose. The total 24-hour dose may then be divided in thirds or in halves depending on the desired interval and strength of preparation available.

In the severely decompensated patient, serum concentrations should be obtained 12 to 24 hours after administration of the loading dose and every 24 hours thereafter until the patient is stable. The reason for evaluating concentrations early is that, should the patient have a clearance much lower than anticipated, the dose can be reduced before the patient becomes toxic, and should the clearance be much higher than anticipated, modest elevations in dose can be made. Maintenance therapy in the non-acutely ill patient can be initiated at 400 to 900 mg/d of the sustained-release preparation. Trough serum levels should be evaluated in 1 to 2 weeks after initiation of therapy or with any dose adjustment. Once a dose is established, it should not be necessary to routinely monitor serum concentrations unless the patient's disease worsens or toxicity is suspected.

Another regimen used clinically is to administer long-acting theophylline preparations at bedtime. This has been demonstrated to reduce overnight declines in FEV_1 and morning respiratory symptoms.[61]

Attempting to make adjustments in dose to attain a desired concentration using first-order pharmacokinetic equations is fraught with error. Theophylline is metabolized by microsomal enzymes to three major metabolites: 1,3-dimethyluric acid, 1-methyluric acid, and 3-methylxanthine. Each metabolic pathway is potentially saturable. This results in the nonlinear kinetics of theophylline that are witnessed in acute overdoses. Apparent nonlinearity may occur because of physiologic changes that happen during therapy of acute exacerbations. Diminished hemodynamics due to either right or left ventricular failure may result in hepatic congestion, which affects theophylline clearance. Acutely ill and hypoalbuminemic patients may have increased free (as opposed to protein-bound) theophylline concentrations while their total serum theophylline concentrations are in the "therapeutic range."[62] This perhaps explains why toxicity develops at low serum concentrations in some patients. Each patient's physiologic character should be carefully monitored, with serum theophylline concentrations obtained if any significant changes are noted. Because there are other pharmacologic interventions for COLD, it is unnecessary to push the theophylline dose to toxicity.

Serum theophylline concentrations above 20 μg/mL are associated with nausea and vomiting and those above 35 to 40 μg/mL with arrhythmias and seizures. In the elderly with exacerbations of COLD, these values should not be used to judge the likelihood of toxicity, because this population exhibits these catastrophic side effects at lower serum concentrations. Nausea is a common complication in elderly patients with concentrations greater than 15 μg/mL, and seizures and atrial tachyarrhythmias have been reported with serum concentrations of 20 to 30 μg/mL. These seizures and arrhythmias are quite refractory to conventional treatment.

There has been considerable debate as to the relative risk–benefit ratio of methylxanthines in COLD patients.[2] Regular use of methylxanthines has not been shown to have either a beneficial or a detrimental effect on the course of COLD. Because of the uncertainty regarding their role, they are now placed after anticholinergics and sympathomimetics when listing preferred therapies. Methylxanthines should be added to the treatment plan of patients who have not achieved an optimal clinical response to an inhaled β-agonist and ipratropium. Recent information suggests that adding theophylline to the combination of albuterol and ipratropium can result in maximum benefit in stable COLD, supporting the hypothesis that there is a synergistic bronchodilatory effect.[61,63,64] When methylxanthines are used to treat COLD patients, parameters other than objective measurements, such as FEV_1, should be monitored to assess efficacy. Subjective parameters, such as perceived exercise tolerance, become increasingly important in assessing the acceptability of methylxanthines for the COLD patient. Note that although objective improvement may be minimal, clinical benefit to the individual may be meaningful.[61,63–66]

CORTICOSTEROIDS

The use of corticosteroids in COLD remains controversial. Corticosteroids may be used in COLD in many different clinical scenarios, including (1) systemic use for acute exacerbations, (2) systemic use for chronic stable COLD, and (3) inhalation for chronic stable COLD.

The literature evaluating the use of corticosteroids in exacerbations of COLD is sparse and debatable. Three randomized, placebo-controlled studies have evaluated the use of systemic steroids during exacerbations of COLD.[67–69] In 1980, Albert and colleagues demonstrated that patients receiving IV methylprednisolone at 0.5 mg/kg every 6 hours for 72 hours showed greater improvement in pulmonary function tests than patients who received placebo.[67] Emerman and colleagues studied the effect of one dose of IV methylprednisolone (100 mg) in patients presenting to the emergency department for exacerbations of COLD.[68] No differences were found between the steroid- and placebo-treated groups in spirometry over a several-hour observation period, need for hospital admission, or future emergency department visits in the ensuing 48 hours. More recently, Thompson and colleagues found oral prednisone to be more effective than placebo using a 9-day tapering dose resulting in a more rapid improvement in arterial Po_2 (Pao_2) (1.12 mm Hg/d vs −0.03 mm Hg/d; $P = .002$), alveolar–arterial oxygen gradient ($PAO_2 - Pao_2$) (−1.16 mm Hg/d vs −0.03 mm Hg/d; $P = .04$), FEV_1 (0.05 L/d vs 0.00 L/d; $P = .006$), and peak expiratory flow (PEF) (0.15 L/s/d vs 0.04 L/s/d; $P = .009$). Prednisone also resulted in fewer treatment failures ($P = .002$).[69]

Despite the lack of compelling evidence supporting the use of corticosteroids in acute exacerbations of COLD, it is currently considered the standard of care by many health care professionals to administer large doses of intravenous corticosteroids during the first few days of illness, followed by tapering oral regimens over subsequent days or weeks. Less severely ill patients frequently receive oral therapy on an outpatient basis.

The role of steroids in chronic stable COLD patients was clarified in a review by Callahan and associates.[70] In this meta-analysis, 33 original studies of oral steroids in COLD published since 1951 were evaluated. The authors concluded that COLD patients treated with steroids showed clinically significant improvement in baseline FEV_1 (increase of 20%) 10% more often than similar patients who received placebo. It therefore appears that the number of stable COLD patients who will benefit from steroids is modest. Attempts to determine patient characteristics that may be helpful in assessing which patients would most likely benefit from steroid administration appear to show that either a significant eosinophilia (> 300/mm^3), eosinophils on sputum examination, or significant response on pulmonary function tests to sympathomimetics are the best predictors. A 25% or greater response of the FEV_1 has been reported to be the best predictor of responsiveness.[2]

Corticosteroids produce significant side effects; therefore, many clinicians follow the axiom that as soon as a decision is made to initiate therapy, a similar plan should be made to discontinue therapy as soon as is possible. Objective parameters should be followed to substantiate drug use. The anti-inflammatory mechanisms whereby corticosteroids exert their beneficial effect in COLD include (1) reduction in capillary permeability to decrease mucus, (2) inhibition of release of proteolytic enzymes from leukocytes, and (3) inhibition of prostaglandins. These desired effects occur because of the ability of steroids to be transported into the nucleus of the cell and stimulate RNA synthesis.

The decision to use corticosteroids is usually initiated during an acute exacerbation when the patient is deteriorating or not improving as expected despite adequate anticholinergic and/or sympathomimetic therapy and possibly methylxanthines. Patients taking chronic oral steroids who present in acute distress are commonly started on parenteral steroids. Therapy is initiated with methylprednisolone or its equivalent 0.5 to 1.0 mg/kg intravenously every 6 hours. It generally requires 3 to 6 hours or longer for a beneficial pharmacologic effect to be observed.

As soon as the patient's symptoms have stabilized, he or she may be switched to 40 to 60 mg of prednisone daily. The oral dose is largely empiric. A short- to intermediate-acting corticosteroid is preferred to minimize suppression of the hypothalamic–pituitary–adrenal (HPA) axis. If possible, steroids should be stopped in 7 to 14 days, because extending beyond 2 to 4 weeks with supraphysiologic doses suppresses the HPA axis. If therapy needs to be prolonged, the ideal is to achieve the lowest possible effective dose with a minimal likelihood of HPA axis suppression (e.g., prednisone 7.5 mg/d). The dose should be given once per day in the morning to mimic the normal diurnal variation of endogenous cortisol secretion. If possible, the patient should be moved to an alternate-day schedule. This is accomplished by raising one day's dose, while decreasing the alternate day's dose. If a patient requires continuous steroid therapy, giving short bursts of higher doses of oral prednisone during periods of worsening clinical status may be effective at decreasing hospitalizations.

The role of inhaled corticosteroids in COLD has not been completely clarified. Previously, they were thought to be of no benefit in patients with COLD. Current studies, including a prospective 4-year trial from Europe, indicate that inhaled corticosteroids have a positive effect on the annual decline of FEV_1.[71–74] In a prospective study by Dompeling and colleagues,[71] adding inhaled beclomethasone to bronchodilator therapy was found to slow the unfavorable course of COLD, but the effect was not as positive as that exhibited by the asthmatic patients who were studied. The results of another multicenter trial indicate that while younger, nonsmoking individuals had the greatest response when inhaled corticosteroids were added to maintenance regimens of β-agonists, all groups showed benefit from the combination in terms of reduction in morbidity, hyperresponsiveness, and airway obstruction.[73] A recent trial with fluticasone propionate 500 mg ($n = 142$) or placebo ($n = 139$) twice daily via an MDI for 6 months found that fluticasone reduced severe exacerbations of

COLD, increased FEV_1 and FVC, and increased walking times compared with placebo.[74] Evidence from these and other studies gives strength to the use of inhaled corticosteroids in COLD; however, the data indicate that asthmatic patients gain greater benefit from these agents than do COLD patients.

Studies are currently under way reevaluating the use of corticosteroids as systemic treatment for acute exacerbations of COLD and as inhaled treatment for chronic stable COLD. One such study is the Veteran Affairs Systemic Corticosteroids in COLD Exacerbations (SCCOPE) clinical trial, which is attempting to determine whether the withholding of systemic corticosteroids in patients who are hospitalized for COLD exacerbations and treated with other usual therapy results in a clinically significant increase in the rate of treatment failures.[75]

LONG-TERM OXYGEN

Although long-term oxygen has been used for many years in patients with advanced COLD, it was not until 1980 that data became available documenting its benefits. At that time, the Nocturnal Oxygen Therapy Trial Group published their data comparing nocturnal oxygen therapy (NOT) (12 h/d) with continuous oxygen therapy (COT) (average of 20 h/d).[76] The patients were followed for at least 12 months. The results revealed a mortality rate in the NOT group nearly double that of the COT group, 41 in 80 versus 23 in 87. Statistical estimates of the COT group suggest that COT may have added 3.25 years to a COLD patient's life.[77] The decline in mortality with oxygen therapy was further substantiated in 1981 in a study by the British Medical Research Council, which compared 15 h/d of oxygen versus no supplemental oxygen in COLD patients.[78] Additional data from the Nocturnal Oxygen Therapy Trial Group revealed that COT patients had fewer (but statistically insignificant) hospitalizations, improved quality of life and neuropsychological function, reduced hematocrits, and decreased pulmonary vascular resistance. Recent analyses have shown that long-term oxygen therapy provides even more benefit in terms of survival after at least 5 years of use, and it improves the quality of life of these patients by increasing walking distance and neuropsychological condition, and reducing time spent in the hospital.[79] Once stable on oxygen for 6 months, patients do not need to be reevaluated more often than every 6 months. Whether oxygen therapy consistently improves exercise tolerance or sleep remains controversial.

Before patients are considered for long-term oxygen therapy, they should be stabilized in the outpatient setting for 1 month and pharmacotherapy should be optimized. Once this is accomplished, long-term oxygen therapy should be instituted if either of two conditions exists:

1. A resting Pa_{O_2} of less than 55 mm Hg.
2. Evidence of right heart failure, polycythemia, or impaired neuropsychiatric function with a Pa_{O_2} of less than 60 mm Hg.

Oxygen therapy may also be used in patients who develop hypoxemia during exercise or at night. The possible benefits of long-term oxygen in borderline hypoxemic patients is currently under study in a large multicenter trial.[80]

The most practical means of administering long-term oxygen is with the nasal cannula, which provides 24% to 28% oxygen. The goal is to raise the Pa_{O_2} above 60 mm Hg. Patients known to retain carbon dioxide should be cautioned to not raise the Pa_{O_2} so high that they depress their respiratory drive. Patient education about flow rates and avoidance of flames is of the utmost importance.

There are three different ways of delivering oxygen, including (1) in liquid reservoirs, (2) compressed into a cylinder, and (3) via an oxygen concentrator. Though the conventional liquid oxygen and compressed oxygen are quite bulky, smaller, portable tanks are available to permit the patient more mobility. Oxygen concentrator devices separate the nitrogen from room air and concentrate the oxygen. These may prove the most convenient and ultimately the least expensive method of oxygen delivery. Disadvantages of these devices are that they currently require a continuous electrical supply, thus necessitating a backup system, and are somewhat noisy. Oxygen conservation devices are available that allow oxygen to flow only during inspiration, making the supply last longer. These may be particularly useful to prolong the oxygen supply for mobile patients using portable cylinders. However, the devices are bulky and subject to failure.[81] Controversy exists concerning the efficacy and tolerability of nasal nocturnal positive pressure ventilation for COLD, and many patients may be unwilling to accept this form of oxygen therapy.

The cost of oxygen therapy may be substantial. In 1993, there were approximately 616,000 persons receiving home oxygen in the United States at a cost of $1.4 billion.[81] The use of an oxygen concentrator may cost between $200 and $400 per month. Portable oxygen tanks may cost $300 per month. It is therefore important to discuss the economic issues of therapy with the patient and family before initiating oxygen.

ANTIBIOTICS

Acute bacterial exacerbations in COLD can cause considerable morbidity and mortality, particularly in the elderly. Effective antibiotic therapy results in fewer hospitalizations and better resolution in symptoms. However, the emergence of drug-resistant organisms has mandated that antibiotic regimens be chosen judiciously. Antibiotics are not of proven value in the prevention or treatment of COLD exacerbations unless there is evidence of infection, such as fever, leukocytosis, change in sputum quantity, viscosity, or color, and/or change in chest radiograph. Sputum Gram stain may be helpful in determining the need for oral antibiotic therapy; however, given the difficulty of obtaining an appropriate sputum in the outpatient setting, this may not always be practical. Early in the stage of infectious exacerbations, patients do not always have fever, chills, or leukocytosis. Sputum cultures, initially, are of little practical value and were shown to be of less benefit at identifying the organism than Gram stain.

Although the majority of infections are viral, bacterial infection may follow the initial viral infection. Therapy should be initiated within 24 hours of symptoms to prevent unnecessary hospitalization. It is also important to prevent an accelerated rate of decline in pulmonary function from irritation and mucus plugging owing to the infectious process. In a large double-blind placebo-controlled study, higher success rates were shown with antibiotic therapy, but it should be noted that those patients with less severe exacerbations did not show benefit.[82] Saint and colleagues performed a meta-analysis on six studies evaluating the effectiveness of antibiotics in treating exacerbations of COLD. They summarized that patients receiving antibiotics had a greater improvement in PEF rate than those who were not.[83]

The bacterial organisms usually responsible for exacerbations are *S. pneumoniae*, *H. influenzae*, and *Moraxella catarrhalis*. The penicillins (amoxicillin and amoxicillin/clavulanate) are the antibiotics used most frequently for treatment of COLD exacerbations in patients not allergic to penicillin. The principal concern of amoxicillin is the increasing rate of resistance by β-lactamase–producing organisms. Resistance rates of 30% for encapsulated strains and 16% for nonencapsulated strains of *H. influenzae* have been reported. Resistance rates greater than 90% have been reported for *M. catarrhalis* in some geographic areas.[84] An increased number of prior antibiotic courses and hospital admissions have been correlated with a higher incidence of β-lactamase–producing bacteria in patients with COLD.[85]

Amoxicillin/clavulanate is stable against β-lactamases and should be the preferred agent of the two in areas of high amoxicillin resistance. Other acceptable oral alternatives include tetracyclines, cephalosporins, cotrimoxazole, the macrolides, and the fluoroquinolones. The newer fluoroquinolones (e.g., levofloxacin) have greater activity against gram-positive organisms compared to ciprofloxacin and are the preferred fluoroquinolones for treatment of COLD exacerbations. Therapy should generally be continued for at least 7 to 10 days. Certain regimens of shorter duration are as effective (e.g., azithromycin 3- or 5-day regimens). If the patient deteriorates or does not improve as anticipated, hospitalization may be necessary and more aggressive attempts should be made to identify potential pathogens responsible for the exacerbation. Parenteral antibiotics may be required.

IMMUNOTHERAPY

Because influenza is a common complication in COLD that can lead to respiratory failure, an annual influenza vaccine is recommended to protect those individuals who are not allergic to eggs. Amantadine can be considered for patients with COLD who have not received the vaccination and who are at risk for influenza A or for patients with early influenza A infection. The dose should be decreased from 100 mg twice daily to 100 mg once daily in those older than 65 years of age owing to reduced renal clearance.

The polyvalent pneumococcal vaccination, administered one time, is widely recommended for people from 2 to 64 years of age who have chronic lung disease. Although the recommendation of the pneumococcal vaccine has been questioned, the argument for continued use of the vaccine is that the current vaccine has 23 antigens and now provides coverage for 85% of pneumococcal disease. Currently, administering the vaccine remains the standard of practice and is recommended by the Centers for Disease Control and Prevention (Morbidity & Mortality Weekly Report, 1997, RR-8) and the American Lung Association. Repeated vaccination with the 23-valent product is not recommended for patients aged 2 to 64 years with chronic lung disease; however, revaccination is recommended for patients over 65 years if the first vaccination was more than 5 years earlier and the patient was younger than 65 years. Individuals who received the original 18-valent product should receive the 23-valent vaccine.

RESPIRATORY STIMULANTS

The role of respiratory stimulants in COLD patients is controversial. Agents that have been used as respiratory stimulants include acetazolamide, progesterone, protriptyline, almitrine bimesylate, and doxapram. These agents, with the exception of doxapram, are not FDA approved as respiratory stimulants and almitrine is available only in Europe. Acetazolamide and progesterone have not been widely used as respiratory stimulants owing to side effects. Protriptyline has been shown in one study to improve diurnal and nocturnal hypoxemia.[86] However, nortriptyline has been reported to depress ventilatory control, although exercise tolerance increased.[87] Almitrine, demonstrated to be useful in managing hypoxemia in patients with COLD, has limited usefulness owing to its potential to impair peripheral motor nerve function and cause increase in ventilatory drive and dyspnea.[88] Doxapram produces respiratory stimulation by activating the peripheral carotid chemoreceptors. It is available intravenously only and in hospitalized patients is no better than nasal intermittent positive pressure ventilation.

CHOICE OF THERAPY

An algorithm to provide guidance in the choice of therapy for a patient with COLD is shown in Fig. 25–1. It cannot be stressed enough that individualized treatment regimens are necessary to optimize outcome because patients differ in their compliance with medication, technique in using inhalers and equipment, and values in terms of quality of life.

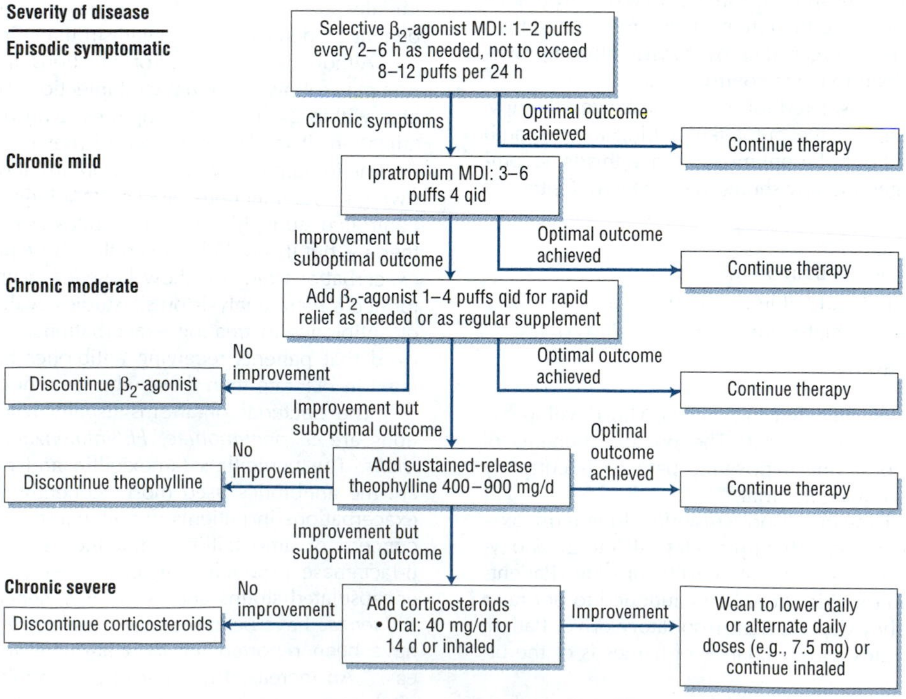

FIGURE 25–1. COLD treatment algorithm.

COMPLICATIONS

COR PULMONALE

Diuretics have been the mainstay of therapy for cor pulmonale. The greatest concern with using diuretics is hypokalemic metabolic alkalosis. The hypokalemia may be exacerbated by concomitant use of β-agonists or corticosteroids. Therefore, the decision to use diuretics must be based on a risk–benefit ratio. If only peripheral edema exists without hepatic congestion, the risk of diuretics may exceed potential benefit. If hepatic congestion is evident, judicious use of diuretics is certainly indicated because other modes of therapy may be compromised by the congestion. Digitalis glycosides have no role in the treatment of cor pulmonale.

Recently, research into the treatment of cor pulmonale has been directed at reducing the force against which the right ventricle has to work by dilating the pulmonary vasculature. One method of doing this is to remove a primary cause of pulmonary hypertension (e.g., hypoxia). This can be improved by raising the Pa_{O_2} higher than 60 mm Hg. Hydralazine and nifedipine have been the most extensively examined pharmacologic agents. Other agents that show promise include angiotensin-converting enzyme inhibitors, angiotensin II antagonists (e.g., losartan), and other calcium antagonists (e.g., felodipine).[89,90] Data are currently insufficient to offer guidelines for the role of these agents on COLD patients with cor pulmonale.

POLYCYTHEMIA

Polycythemia secondary to chronic hypoxemia in COLD patients can be improved by either oxygen therapy or periodic phlebotomy if oxygen is not sufficient. Continuous oxygen therapy was shown by the Nocturnal Oxygen Therapy Trial Group to reduce hematocrits.[76] Acute phlebotomy is indicated if the hematocrit is above 55% to 60% and the patient is experiencing central nervous system effects suggestive of sludging from high blood viscosity. Long-term oxygen can then be used to maintain a lower hematocrit.

α_1-PROTEINASE INHIBITOR (α_1-ANTITRYPSIN)

This genetically engineered compound is indicated for those patients with panacinar emphysema who have the PiZZ and Pi-null phenotypes. Its use should not be considered in patients with emphysema who are other Pi phenotypes. The therapeutic objective is to maintain ATT serum concentrations higher than 80 mg/dL to have sufficient antielastase activity in the lung epithelial lining fluid. The recommended dosing regimen is 60 mg/kg administered intravenously once a week, at a rate of 0.08 mL/kg/min (adjusted to patient tolerance). It has been estimated that this form of augmentation therapy will have an annual cost of $20,000 to $30,000 per patient.[91]

ACUTE RESPIRATORY FAILURE

Acute respiratory failure is an emergency situation. When it occurs in a patient with COLD, all pharmacologic maneuvers should be optimized initially and low-flow oxygen delivered. If these agents fail to stabilize or improve the patient's condition, intubation and mechanical ventilation must be considered. This is an extremely difficult decision. Ideally, all severe COLD patients should be involved in the decision to intubate. Preferably, this decision should be made before an acute event occurs. If a decision is made to mechanically ventilate because of impending respiratory failure, it is important that ventilator settings not be adjusted to return the patient to normal values; rather, settings should be adjusted to achieve the patient's baseline values in a stable state. This will facilitate weaning from the ventilator. Maintaining the physical strength and nutritional status of the patient is vital in aiding the weaning procedure. Recent data indicate that a systematic multiparameter approach to assessing nutritional status is critical for COLD patients requiring mechanical ventilation, because malnutrition is common and has a deleterious effect on the weaning process.[92] Physical therapy and a nutritional intake of 3000 kcal/d with a relatively high proportion of protein are advised that may improve airflow. Unfortunately, most patients remain in negative nitrogen balance, and muscle wasting is strongly correlated with the dose of corticosteroid used. If mechanical ventilation persists beyond 5 to 7 days, the patient should be switched to a tracheostomy to prevent tracheal erosion and to facilitate feeding.

Many patients requiring mechanical ventilation for COLD are able to undergo extubation without weaning. However, some require gradual weaning. The most important factors that determine the ability of patients to wean from prolonged mechanical ventilation are neuromuscular reserve capacity relative to respiratory load, cardiovascular performance, oxygenation, and psychological factors.[1] A variety of objective indices (e.g., maximum inspiratory pressure, VC, respiratory frequency/tidal volume) are designed to evaluate patients for extubation. Weaning values are institution specific and no clear physiologic indices assist the selection of patients for weaning, determination of the rapidity of weaning, or identification of the ideal weaning method. For example, for patients with an Fi_{O_2} of 40% or less and a tidal volume of 400 mL or less, extubation can be considered. Methods that can assist in weaning include T-piece trials, intermittent mandatory ventilation (IMV), and pressure support ventilation (PSV).[93] IMV and PSV are preferred because they provide partial support when the patient is connected to the ventilator and they provide less opportunity for barotrauma.[1]

CONTROVERSIES

EXPECTORANTS AND MUCOLYTICS

Water has been, and continues to be, the expectorant of choice in COLD patients. Adequate hydration is safe and effective when compared to saturated solution of potassium iodide, ammonium chloride, or guaifenesin. Although these agents may promote expectoration, the doses required are so large that they are frequently associated with undesirable side effects.

Use of the mucolytic agent acetylcysteine to aid the clearance of mucus has been a matter of controversy for some time. There is no question that it is effective as a mucolytic. However, it causes irritation when administered via nebulization, which may cause further narrowing of the airways. For this reason, use of inhaled acetylcysteine has fallen into disfavor. It should always be preceded by an inhaled sympathomimetic if this route is chosen. Another mucolytic, iodinated glycerol, was compared to placebo at a dose of 60 mg four times a day and was found to be superior in terms of cough frequency, cough severity, and chest discomfort, but no improvement in blood oxygenation or pulmonary function was reported.[94] However, objective evidence of benefit was deemed insufficient, and the FDA required that marketing of the drug be discontinued.

ANTIOXIDANTS

In the past decade, use of nonenzymatic antioxidants, including vitamins E, C, and β-carotene, has increased dramatically. They have been indicated for a variety of disease states and are associated with reduced mortality in lung and heart disease.[95] It is postulated that their benefit in COLD may be a result of an imbalance between oxidants and antioxidants that has been considered in the pathogenesis of smoking-induced lung disease.[95] Increased ascorbic acid concentrations in the serum has been associated with improvement in pulmonary function, and vitamin

E supplementation has been reported to diminish markers of oxidant stress, such as the levels of lipid peroxides, in the plasma of smokers. Data are currently insufficient to offer guidelines pertaining to their dosage or duration of treatment in patients with COLD.

OTHER ASPECTS OF MANAGEMENT

The standard of practice for many years was to avoid administering narcotics and benzodiazepines to patients with COLD. These drugs can further depress respiration, especially when given parenterally. Recent work in this area suggests that this issue is not yet settled. The current debate is over the risk of loss of sleep versus the risk of sedatives. As yet there is no clear resolution to this issue. Some have found diphenhydramine useful as an anxiolytic or sedative, but there has not been an objective analysis of its effectiveness or safety in patients with COLD. Opiates alone or with phenothiazines have been used to increase exercise tolerance in individuals in whom dyspnea is severely disabling; however, the results from various trials do not show consistent results. Inhaled morphine does not appear to decrease breathlessness in patients with COLD.[96]

The importance of psychological variables cannot be ignored in determining the functional status of the patient with COLD. Recent studies indicate that exercise capacity and depression are the best predictors of functional status.[97]

A substantial number of COLD patients have nutritional abnormalities. The association between weight loss and COLD, especially emphysema, is well established. Weight loss adversely impacts the progression of COLD; however, whether it is a marker for more severe disease or represents the pathogenesis of deterioration of pulmonary function is unclear. Recent data indicate that body mass index (BMI) is a simple and accurate indicator of nutritional status that correlates with several pulmonary function tests.[98] Although these topics are beyond the scope of this chapter, the role of chest physiotherapy, breathing retraining, and nutrition cannot be overlooked.

PHARMACOECONOMIC CONSIDERATIONS

The overall cost of therapy is an important consideration in contemporary medical practice. Meaningful cost analysis goes beyond the cost of the medication itself and incorporates the impact of a given therapeutic agent on overall health care cost. Pharmacoeconomic analyses in COLD are limited at this time; however, outcome information is available regarding acute hospitalized exacerbations of COLD and the use of theophylline versus ipratropium.

Connors and colleagues evaluated the outcomes of patients hospitalized with severe acute exacerbations of COLD. Outcomes were evaluated for 1016 patients over a 6-month period. Median length of hospital stay was 9 days and median cost of hospital stay was $7100. Of the total, 11% of patients died during the original hospital stay; however, the mortality at 60 days, 180 days, 1 year, and 2 years was 20%, 33%, 43%, and 49%, respectively. At 6 months, only 26% of patients were both alive and able to report a good, very good, or excellent quality of life. The authors demonstrate that poor outcomes related to cost and quality of life are associated with hospitalization for exacerbations of COLD, reinforcing the importance of prevention through pharmacologic or other means.[99]

Jubran and associates performed a Markov analysis comparing the strategies of treatment with theophylline or ipratropium and found that ipratropium was only marginally better than theophylline in terms of efficacy. However, the total cost per year (e.g., hospitalization for toxic events, monitoring of blood levels) was significantly higher for patients using theophylline despite the fact that ipratropium costs more on formularies. This study reinforces the concept that the total cost of therapy and not simply the cost of drug must be taken into account when determining the cost effectiveness of a given therapeutic regimen.[100]

▶ PRINCIPLES OF PHARMACOTHERAPY

- COLD includes the terms *chronic bronchitis* and *emphysema*. Bronchitis is defined in clinical terms, whereas emphysema is defined in terms of anatomic pathology. Most patients have a combination of chronic bronchitis and emphysema.
- The most common cause of COLD is cigarette smoking. The first and most important step in the treatment of COLD is smoking cessation. Exercise rehabilitation also plays an important role in improving daily function in most patients.
- The main classes of drug treatment for COLD include anticholinergics, sympathomimetics, methylxanthines, and corticosteroids. Current clinical trends indicate use in that order.
- The foregoing therapies have demonstrated improvement in subjective and objective symptoms. However, it is unknown whether morbidity and mortality associated with COLD are decreased. The only treatment shown to increase survival is oxygen administered for most of the hours of the day.
- The treatment of COLD is not an exact science and is very patient dependent. For instance, some patients may respond better to one bronchodilator than another or may respond to pharmacologic agents via mechanisms other than bronchodilation.
- In COLD, combination treatments (e.g., anticholinergics and sympathomimetics) have been found to be more effective than either treatment alone.
- There continues to be great controversy regarding the most beneficial treatment of COLD, particularly regarding the use of corticosteroids and antibiotics for acute exacerbations.
- Many agents, particularly corticosteroids and methylxanthines, are not without considerable potential toxicity. Therefore, embarking on a pharmacologic plan for the treatment of COLD requires weighing the risk–benefit ratio carefully and having a comprehensive plan to assess subjectively and objectively the efficacy and toxicity of the chosen therapy.

REFERENCES

1. American Thoracic Society. Standards for the diagnosis and care of patients with chronic obstructive pulmonary disease. Am J Respir Crit Care Med 1995;152:S77–S120.
2. Edelman NH, Kaplan RM, Buist AS, et al. Chronic obstructive pulmonary disease. Chest 1992;102(suppl 3):243–256.
3. Higgins MW, Thorn T. Incidence, prevalence, and mortality: Intra- and inter-county differences. In: Hensley MJ, Saunders NA, eds. Clinical Epidemiology of Chronic Obstructive Pulmonary Disease. New York, Dekker, 1989:23–43.
4. National Center for Health Statistics. Current Estimates from the National Health Interview Survey, United States, Selected Years 1971–1994.
5. National Center for Health Statistics. Advanced Report of Final Mortality Statistics, 1973–1994.
6. Fingerhut LA, Warner M. Injury Chartbook. Health, United States, 1996–97. Hyattsville, MD, National Center for Health Statistics, 1997:117.
7. Anon. Deaths from chronic obstructive pulmonary disease in the United States, 1987. Stat Bull 1990;July–Sept:20–26.
8. Buist SA. Smoking and other risk factors. In: Murray JF, Nadel JA, eds. Textbook of Respiratory Medicine, 2nd ed. Philadelphia, Sanders, 1994:1259–1287.
9. Pauwels RA, Lofdahl CG, Pride NB, et al. European Respiratory Society study on chronic obstructive pulmonary disease (EUROSCOP): Hypothesis and design. Eur Respir J 1992;5:1254–1261.
10. Chronic Disease Reports. Chronic obstructive pulmonary disease mortality—United States, 1986. MMWR 1989;38:549–552.
11. Coultas DB, Samet JM. Cigarette smoking. In: Hensley MJ, Saunders NA, eds. Clinical Epidemiology of Chronic Obstructive Pulmonary Disease. New York, Dekker, 1989:109–138.
12. Kerstjens H, Brand P, Postma D. Risk factors for accelerated decline among patients with chronic obstructive pulmonary disease. Am J Respir Crit Care Med 1996;154:S266–S272.
13. Oxman AD, Muir DC, Shannon HS, et al. Occupational dust exposure and chronic obstructive pulmonary disease. A systemic overview of the evidence. Am Rev Respir Dis 1993;148:38–48.
14. Sunyer J, Saez M, Murillo C, et al. Air pollution and emergency room admissions for chronic obstructive pulmonary disease: A 5-year study. Am J Epidemiol 1993;137:701–705.
15. Petty TL. Definitions in chronic obstructive pulmonary disease. Clin Chest Med 1990;11:363–373.
16. O'Connor GT, Sparrow D, Segal M, Weiss ST. Risk factors for ventilatory impairment among middle-aged and elderly men. Chest 1993;103:376–382.
17. Badgett RG, Tanaka DJ, Hunt DK, et al. Can moderate chronic obstructive pulmonary disease be diagnosed by historical and physical findings alone? Am J Med 1993;94:188–195.
18. Wright JL, Petty T, Thurlbeck WM. Analysis of the structure of the muscular pulmonary arteries in patients with pulmonary hypertension and COPD: National Institutes of Health Nocturnal Oxygen Therapy Trial. Lung 1992;170:109–124.
19. Gelb AF, Schein M, Kuie J, et al. Limited contribution of emphysema in advanced chronic obstructive pulmonary disease. Am Rev Respir Dis 1993;147:1157–1161.
20. Shapiro SD. The pathogenesis of emphysema: The elastase:antielastase hypothesis 30 years later. Pro Asso Am Physicians 1995;107: 346–352.
21. Wallaert B, Gressier B, Hugo C, et al. Inactivation of α_1-proteinase inhibitor by alveolar inflammatory cells from smoking patients with or without emphysema. Am Rev Respir Dis 1993;147:1537–1543.
22. Snider GL. Chronic obstructive pulmonary disease: Risk factors, pathophysiology and pathogenesis. Ann Rev Med 1989;40: 411–429.
23. Lamb D. Chronic bronchitis, emphysema, and the pathological basis of chronic obstructive pulmonary disease. In: Hasleton PS, ed. Spencer's Pathology of the Lung, 5th ed. New York, McGraw-Hill, 1996:597–629.
24. Weitzenblum E, Krieger J, Oswald M, et al. Chronic obstructive pulmonary disease and sleep apnea syndrome. Sleep 1992;15: S33–S35.
25. Hayes GB, Christiani DC. Measures of small airways disease as predictors of chronic obstructive pulmonary disease. Occup Med State Art Rev 1993;8:375–395.
26. Killian KF, Leblance P, Martin DH, et al. Exercise capacity and ventilatory, circulatory and symptom limitation in patients with chronic airflow limitation. Am Rev Respir Dis 1992;146:835–840.
27. Anthonisen NR, Wright SC, Hodgkin JE. Prognosis in chronic obstructive pulmonary disease. Am Rev Respir Dis 1986;133:14–20.
28. Petty TL, Good JT, White DP. Long-term follow-up of a random population observed for the prevalence and outcome of COPD. In: Petty TL, ed. Chronic Obstructive Pulmonary Disease. New York, Dekker, 1985:93–103.
29. Burrows B. Cause and prognosis in advanced disease. In: Petty TL, ed. Chronic Obstructive Pulmonary Disease. New York, Dekker, 1985:31–42.
30. Anthonisen NR. Prognosis in chronic obstructive pulmonary disease: Results from multicenter clinical trials. Am Rev Respir Dis 1989; 140:S95–S99.
31. Jones PW. Issues concerning health-related quality of life in COPD. Chest 1995;107:187S–193S.
32. Ingram RH. Chronic bronchitis, emphysema, and airways obstruction. In: Wilson JD, Braunwald E, Isselbacher KJ, et al, eds. Harrison's Textbook of Internal Medicine. New York, McGraw-Hill, 1994:1197–1206.
33. Leader WG, Wolf KM, Cooper TM, Chandler MHH. Symptomatology, pulmonary function and response, and T lymphocyte β_2-receptors during smoking cessation in patients with chronic obstructive pulmonary disease. Pharmacotherapy 1994;14:162–172.
34. Chapman KR. Therapeutic algorithm for chronic obstructive pulmonary disease. Am J Med 1991;91(suppl 4A):17–23.
35. Anthonisen NR, Wright EC, IPPB Trial Group. Response to inhaled bronchodilators in COPD. Chest 1987;91:36S–39S.
36. Gross NJ. Ipratropium bromide. N Engl J Med 1989;319:486–494.
37. Skorodin MS. Pharmacotherapy for asthma and chronic obstructive pulmonary disease. Arch Intern Med 1993;153:814–828.
38. Bennett WD, Chapman WF, Mascarella JM. The acute effect of ipratropium bromide bronchodilator therapy on cough clearance in COPD. Chest 1993;103:488–495.
39. Anthonisen NR, Connett JE, Kiley JP, et al. Effects of smoking intervention and the use of an inhaled anticholinergic bronchodilator on the rate of decline of FEV1: The Lung Health Story. JAMA 1994;272:1497–1505.
40. Friedman M. A multicenter study of nebulized bronchodilator solutions in chronic obstructive pulmonary disease. Am J Med 1996; 100(suppl 1A):30S–39S.
41. Wiggins J. The role of anticholinergics in "stable" chronic obstructive pulmonary disease: Unanswered questions. Respiration 1994;61: 303–304.
42. Chapman KR. The role of anticholinergic bronchodilators in adult asthma and chronic obstructive pulmonary disease. Lung 1990;168: S295–S303.
43. Schapira RM, Reinke LF. The outpatient diagnosis and management of chronic obstructive pulmonary disease: Pharmacotherapy, administration of supplemental oxygen, and smoking cessation techniques. J Gen Intern Med 1995;10:40–55.
44. Siefkin AD. Optimal pharmacologic treatment of the critically ill patient with obstructive airways disease. Am J Med 1996;100(suppl 1A):54S–61S.
45. Ikeda A, Nishimura K, Koyama H, et al. Dose response study of ipratropium bromide aerosol on maximum exercise performance in stable patients with chronic obstructive pulmonary disease. Thorax 1996;51:48–53.

46. Maesen FPV, Smeets JJ, Costongs MAL, et al. Ba 679 Br, a new long-acting antimuscarinic bronchodilator: A pilot dose-escalation study in COPD. Eur Respir J 1993;6:1031–1036.
47. Friedman M. A multicenter study of nebulized bronchodilator solutions in chronic obstructive pulmonary disease. Am J Med 1996; 100:30S–39S.
48. Van Schayck CP, Dompeling E, van Herwaarden LA, et al. Bronchodilator treatment in moderate asthma or chronic bronchitis: Continuous or on demand? A randomized controlled study. BMJ 1991; 303(6815):1426–1431.
49. Georgopoulos D, Wong D, Anthonisen NR. Tolerance to β_2-agonists in patients with chronic obstructive pulmonary disease. Chest 1990; 97:280–284.
50. Fromm RE, Varon J. Acute exacerbations of obstructive lung disease. Postgrad Med 1994;95:101–106.
51. Berry RB, Shinto RA, Wong FH, et al. Nebulizer vs spacer for bronchodilator delivery in patients hospitalized for acute exacerbations of COPD. Chest 1989;96:1241–1246.
52. Noseda A, Schmerber J, Prigogine T, Yernault JC. Perceived effect on shortness of breath of an acute inhalation of saline or terbutaline: Variability and sensitivity of a visual analogue scale in patients with asthma or COPD. Eur Respir J 1992;5:1043–1053.
53. Imhof E, Elasasser S, Karrer W, et al. Comparison of bronchodilator effects of fenoterol/ipratropium and salbutamol in patients with chronic obstructive pulmonary lung disease. Respiration 1993;60: 84–88.
54. Wesseling G, Mostert R, Wouters EFM. A comparison of the effects of anticholinergic and β_2-agonist and combination therapy on respiratory impedance in COPD. Chest 1992;101:166–173.
55. Combivent Inhalation Aerosol Study Group. In chronic obstructive pulmonary disease, a combination of ipratropium and albuterol is more effective than either agent alone. Chest 1994;105:1411–1419.
56. Vaz Fragoso CA, Miller MA. Review of the clinical efficacy of theophylline in the treatment of chronic obstructive pulmonary disease. Am Rev Respir Dis 1993;147:S40–S47.
57. Ramsdell J. Use of theophylline in the treatment of COPD. Chest 1995;107:206S–209S.
58. Fink G, Kaye C, Sulkes J, et al. Effect of theophylline on exercise performance in patients with severe chronic obstructive pulmonary disease. Thorax 1994;49:332–334.
59. Miller WF, Geumei AM. Respiratory and pharmacological therapy in COPD. In: Petty TL, ed. Chronic Obstructive Pulmonary Disease. New York, Dekker, 1985:205–238.
60. McKay SE, Howie CA, Thomson AH, et al. Value of theophylline treatment inpatients handicapped by chronic obstructive lung disease. Thorax 1993;48:227–232.
61. Man GC, Champman KR, Ali SH, Darke AC. Sleep quality and nocturnal respiratory function with once-daily theophylline (Uniphyl) and inhaled salbutamol in patients with COPD. Chest 1996;110: 648–653.
62. Zarowitz B, Shlom J, Eichenhorn MS, Popovich J. Alterations in therapy protein binding in acutely ill patients with COPD. Chest 1985;87:766–769.
63. Wrenn K, Slovis CM, Murphy F, Greenberg RS. Aminophylline therapy for acute bronchospastic disease in the emergency room. Ann Intern Med 1991;115:241–247.
64. Nesse RE. COPD pharmacotherapy. Postgrad Med 1992;91:76–84.
65. Nishimura K, Koyama H, Ikeda A, et al. The additive effect of theophylline on a high-dose combination of inhaled salbutamol and ipratropium bromide in stable COPD. Chest 1995;107:718–723.
66. Karpel JP, Kotch A, Zinny M, et al. A comparison of inhaled ipratropium, oral theophylline plus inhaled beta agonist, and the combination of all three in patients with COPD. Chest 1994;105: 1089–1094.
67. Albert RK, Martin TR, Lewis SW. Controlled clinical trial of methylprednisolone in patients with chronic bronchitis and acute respiratory insufficiency. Ann Intern Med 1980;92:753–758.
68. Emerman CL, Connors AF, Lukens TW, et al. A randomized controlled trial of methylprednisolone in the treatment of acute exacerbations of COPD. Chest 1989;95:563-567.
69. Thompson WH, Nielson CP, Carvalho P, et al. Controlled trial of oral prednisone in outpatients with acute COPD exacerbation. Am J Respir Crit Care Med 1996;154:407–412.
70. Callahan CM, Dittus RS, Katz BP. Oral corticosteroid therapy for patients with stable chronic obstructive pulmonary disease: A meta-analysis. Ann Intern Med 1991;114:216–223.
71. Dompeling E, Van Schayck CP, Van Grunsven PM, et al. Slowing the deterioration of asthma and chronic obstructive pulmonary disease observed during bronchodilator therapy by adding inhaled corticosteroids. Ann Intern Med 1993;118:770–778.
72. Thompson AB, Mueller MB, Heires AJ, et al. Aerosolized beclomethasone in chronic bronchitis. Am Rev Respir Dis 1992; 146:389–395.
73. Kerstjens HAM, Brand PLP, Hughes MD, et al. A comparison of bronchodilator therapy with or without inhaled corticosteroid therapy for obstructive airways disease. N Engl J Med 1992; 327:1413–1419.
74. Paggiaro PL, Dahle R, Bakran I, et al. Multicentre randomised placebo-controlled trial of inhaled fluticasone propionate in patients with chronic obstructive pulmonary disease. International COPD Study Group. Lancet 1998;351:773–780.
75. Niewoehner DE. Systemic corticosteroids in COPD: An unresolved dilemma. Chest 1996;110:867–869. Editorial.
76. Nocturnal Oxygen Therapy Trial Group. Continuous or nocturnal oxygen therapy in hypoxemic chronic obstructive lung disease. Ann Intern Med 1980;93:391–398.
77. Petty TL. Long-term outpatient oxygen therapy. In: Petty TL, ed. Chronic Obstructive Pulmonary Disease. New York, Dekker, 1985: 375–388.
78. Medical Research Council Working Party. Long-term domiciliary oxygen therapy in chronic hypoxic cor pulmonale complicating chronic bronchitis and emphysema. Lancet 1981;1:681–685.
79. Weitzenblum E, Apprill M, Oswald M. Benefit from long-term O_2 therapy in chronic obstructive pulmonary disease patients. Respiration 1992:59(suppl 2):14–17.
80. Mitlehner W. Effects of long-term oxygen therapy due to portable liquid oxygen tanks in disabled malnourished chronic obstructive pulmonary disease patients with borderline hypoxemia. Respiration 1992;59(suppl 2):40–45.
81. O'Donohue WJ. Home oxygen therapy. Med Clin North Am 1996; 80:611–622.
82. Staley H, McDade HB, Paes D. Is an objective assessment of antibiotic therapy in exacerbations of chronic bronchitis possible? J Antimicrob Chemother 1993;31:193–197.
83. Saint S, Brent S, Vittinghoff E, Grady D. Antibiotics in chronic obstructive pulmonary disease exacerbations: A meta-analysis. JAMA 1995;273:957–960.
84. Verghese A, Ismail HM. Acute exacerbations of chronic bronchitis: Preventing treatment failures and early reinfection. Postgrad Med 1994;96:75–89.
85. Sportel JH, Koeter GH, van Altena R, et al. Relation between beta-lactamase producing bacteria and patient characteristics in chronic obstructive pulmonary disease (COPD). Thorax 1995; 50:249–325.
86. Series F, Cormier Y. Effects of protriptyline on diurnal and nocturnal oxygenation in patients with chronic obstructive pulmonary disease. Ann Intern Med 1990;113:507–511.
87. Greenberg HE, Scharf SM, Green H. Nortriptyline-induced depression of ventilatory control in a patient with chronic obstructive pulmonary disease. Am Rev Respir Dis 1993;147:1303–1305.
88. Winkelmann BR, Kullmer TH, Kneissl DG, et al. Low-dose almitrine bismesylate in the treatment of hypoxemia due to chronic obstructive pulmonary disease. Chest 1994;105:1383–1391.

89. Sajkov D, Wang T, Frith PA, et al. A comparison of two long-acting vasoselective calcium antagonists in pulmonary hypertension secondary to COPD. Chest 1997;111:1622–1630.
90. Kiely DG, Cargill RI, Wheeldon NM, et al. Haemodynamic and endocrine effects of type 1 angiotensin II receptor blockade in patients with hypoxaemic cor pulmonale. Cardiovasc Res 1997;33:201–208.
91. MacDonald JL, Johnson CE. Pathophysiology and treatment of α_1-antitrypsin deficiency. Am J Health Syst Pharm 1995;52:481–489.
92. Laaban JP, Kouchakji B, Dor MF, et al. Nutritional status of patients with chronic obstructive pulmonary disease acute respiratory failure. Chest 1993;103:1362–1368.
93. Curtis JR, Hudson LD. Emergent assessment and management of acute respiratory failure in COPD. Clin Chest Med 1994;15:481–500.
94. Morgan EJ, Petty TL. Summary of the national mucolytic study. Chest 1990;97:24S–27S.
95. Rahman I, MacNee W. Role of oxidants/antioxidants in smoking induced lung diseases. Free Radic Biol Med 1996;21:669–681.
96. Ferguson GT, Cherniack RM. Management of chronic obstructive pulmonary disease. N Engl J Med 1993;328:1017–1022.
97. Weaver TE, Narsavage GL. Physiological and psychological variables related to functional status in chronic obstructive pulmonary disease. Nurs Res 1992;41(5):286–291.
98. Sahebjami H, Doers JT, Render ML, Bond TL. Anthropometric and pulmonary function test profiles of outpatients with stable chronic obstructive pulmonary disease. Am J Med 1993;94:469–474.
99. Connors AF, Dawson NV, Thomas C, et al. Outcomes following acute exacerbation of severe chronic obstructive lung disease. The SUPPORT investigators. Am J Respir Crit Care Med 1996;154:959–967.
100. Jubran A, Gross N, Ramsdell J, et al. Comparative cost-effectiveness analysis of theophylline and ipratropium bromide in chronic obstructive pulmonary disease three-center study. Chest 1993;103:678–684.

26

Respiratory Distress Syndrome

Peter Gal, PharmD, BCPS, FCCP, FASHP, Sharon M. Watling, PharmD, BCPS, and Christopher L. Shaffer, PharmD

This chapter addresses the problems of acute respiratory distress syndromes in neonates and adults. Abbreviations are used throughout the text, and a glossary for physiology, diseases, and drugs is presented in Table 26–1. Descriptions of ventilator-related terms are provided in Table 26–2. Because the physiology of neonatal respiratory distress syndrome (RDS) and acute RDS have some differences, these diseases will be discussed separately.

NEONATAL RESPIRATORY DISTRESS SYNDROME

RDS, historically known as hyaline membrane disease (HMD), is more appropriately termed surfactant deficiency RDS. RDS is associated with considerable morbidity and mortality. Before 35 weeks' gestation, the risk of RDS and the severity of disease increase with greater degree of prematurity, occurring in over 50% of newborns ≤30 weeks' gestation.[1]

RDS is primarily due to insufficient formation and differentiation of type II pneumocytes with consequent impaired production and release of surfactant. Pulmonary surfactant contains phospholipids that function at the air–liquid interface in the alveolus to lower surface tension, thus preventing alveolar collapse. In the face of surfactant deficiency, atelectasis and impaired gas exchange occur. Additionally, alveolar transudation of protein-rich fluid forms a hyaline membrane, giving rise to the term HMD.[1] Epithelial sodium channel (ENaC) maturation also appears important in RDS. In utero, fluid is actively secreted into lungs via chloride channels. At birth, ENaC takes over and fluid is actively reabsorbed from lungs. In premature infants, immaturity of ENaC results in failure to reabsorb lung fluid, with consequent pulmonary edema.[2] In term infants, this conversion occurs at birth in response to circulating catecholamines. Failure of the conversion to occur in preterm infants results in an inability to clear alveolar fluid and consequent pulmonary edema.[3]

Measurement of lung maturation in amniotic fluid using biochemical markers of surfactant deficiency is an important consideration in preventive and therapeutic interventions, as well as predicting the likelihood of developing RDS. Measurement of surfactant components in amniotic fluid using either the ratio of lecithin to sphingomyelin (L/S ratio), or phosphatidylglycerol (PG), has been particularly useful for confirming lung maturity. PG is the better test because, unlike the L/S ratio, it is reliable in the presence of blood, meconium, or maternal diabetes. Also, turnaround time for PG is more rapid.[4] A positive PG test or L/S ratio is associated with a sensitivity of 95% to 99% and a positive predictive value of 97% to 98%. Both tests suffer from limited specificity (50% to 70%) and limited negative predictive value (54% to 56%). Thus, a test result indicating immaturity does not ensure development of RDS; but a test indicating maturity makes RDS very unlikely.[4]

RDS severity and risk are made worse by a variety of perinatal factors (Table 26–3). These factors may further compromise pulmonary blood supply, consequently causing death of an already limited number of type II alveolar cells and limiting surfactant production. Chronic intrauterine stress, on the contrary, lowers the risk of RDS by promoting lung maturation, perhaps by increasing endogenous glucocorticoid concentrations.[1]

CLINICAL PRESENTATION

A premature infant with RDS may appear normal at birth, although evidence of intrapartum depression or asphyxia is often present. During the first few hours after birth, these newborns develop early signs of respiratory failure (forceful intercostal retractions, the use of accessory neck muscles, expiratory grunting, paradoxical seesaw respirations, gradual increase in oxygen requirements, and tachycardia). Pallor or cyanosis may also develop. Fluid retention, edema, and oliguria are common in the first 48 hours.

A characteristic chest x-ray film (Fig. 26–1) shows a reticulogranular (ground-glass) pattern to the peripheral lung fields, along with clearly defined large airways (air bronchograms) resulting from the presence of air in the large airways and the collapse of small air spaces around the large airways.[1]

A number of neonatal disorders may mimic and be indistinguishable from RDS (Table 26–4), the most important being sepsis caused by group B β-hemolytic streptococcus, pneumococcus, or gram-negative bacilli. Sepsis accounted for 8% of consecutively admitted infants with RDS during a 1-year study.[5] All neonates with suspected RDS should be evaluated for sepsis. Antibiotics should be used until sepsis can be ruled out or a full therapeutic course is completed.

PREVENTION

Several perinatal/antenatal interventions can be adopted to prevent or minimize the severity of RDS. These include optimizing care at labor and delivery and control of maternal diseases to avoid factors listed in Table 26–3. Additionally, drug therapy to delay premature delivery (tocolytics), or to

TABLE 26–1. Glossary of Terms and Abbreviations

ENaC	epithelial sodium channel	ALI	acute lung injury
L/S ratio	lecithin to sphingomyelin ratio	PCWP	pulmonary capillary wedge pressure
PG	phosphatidylglycerol	CO	cardiac output
CXR	chest x-ray	TRH	thyrotropin-releasing hormone
RDS	(neonatal) respiratory distress syndrome	SRT	surfactant replacement therapy
HMD	hyaline membrane disease	PFC	perfluorocarbon
PIE	pulmonary interstitial emphysema	NO	nitric oxide
BPD	bronchopulmonary dysplasia	ABG	arterial blood gas
IVH	intraventricular hemorrhage	Pa_{O_2}	partial pressure of oxygen in arterial blood
PVL	periventricular leukomalacia	Pa_{CO_2}	partial pressure of carbon dioxide in arterial blood
PDA	patent ductus arteriosus	Sa_{O_2}	oxygen saturation
NEC	necrotizing enterocolitis	M_{VO_2}	mixed venous oxygenation
ARDS	acute (adult) respiratory distress syndrome	ECMO	extracorporeal membrane oxygenation

TABLE 26–2. Glossary of Terms for Ventilator Management

Ventilator Setting	
Et	Expiratory time; in the ventilatory cycle, the amount of time devoted to exhalation.
It	Inspiratory time; in the ventilatory cycle, the amount of time devoted to inspiration.
I:E	Ratio of inspiratory time to expiratory time; in a normal, spontaneously breathing patient this is 1:1.5.
Pa_{O_2}	Partial pressure of oxygen present in arterial blood; normal level for adults is 80–100 mm Hg; normal level for premature babies is 50–70 mm Hg.
Pa_{CO_2}	Paritial pressure of carbon dioxide present in arterial blood; normal is 35–45 mm Hg, but higher levels are acceptable to minimize ventilator support.
PEEP	Positive end-expiratory pressure; positive pressure at the end of exhalation designed to prevent alveoli from collapsing during expiration.
PIP	Peak inspiratory pressure; the maximum level of pressure achieved by the ventilator during inspiration.
IMV	Intermittent mandatory ventilation; a mode of ventilation designed to deliver a preset inspiratory rate; continuous flow of gas is available for patient's spontaneous breaths.
Fi_{O_2}	Fraction (percentage) of inspired oxygen.
TV	Tidal volume; volume of gas delivered during a single inspiration.
MAP	Mean airway pressure; a constant distending pressure.
Hz	Hertz; normally described as cycles per second; this is the number of breaths per minute.
FRC	Functional residual capacity; the volume of air remaining in the lung after normal expiration.
Amp	Amplitude; a wave-like change in pressure centered around a mean airway pressure.
Sigh	A breath that recruits and maintains alveolar patency; used in HFJV. Similar to pressure provided with PIP.
CWF	Chest wiggle factor; a clinical observation ensuring appropriate chest wall movement with HFOV.
BPM	Breaths per minute.
Types of Mechanical Ventilations	
CMV	Controlled mechanical ventilation; a ventilator mode in which RR + TV are under machine rather than patient control.
AC	Assist control; mode in which patient receives a full TV if the patient breathes over the ventilator.
PC	Pressure control; ventilator delivers a TV until a certain pressure is achieved.
SIMV	Synchronized intermittent mandatory ventilation; a ventilator breath "synchronized" with patient's inspiratory effort.
PS	Pressure support; pressure on inspiration designed to assist generation of tidal volume.
IRV	Inverse ratio ventilation; ventilator mode in which inspiratory time is prolonged in comparison to expiration time. Used to decrease plateau pressure and improve oxygenation.
HFOV	High-frequency oscillatory ventilation; a mechanical diaphragm produces oscillations superimposed on a constant gas flow.
HFJV	High-frequency jet ventilation; small volumes of air are released in a pulsating fashion and directed down the airway in a patient simultaneously receiving conventional ventilation.
HFFI	High-frequency flow interruption; similar to HFJV but air pulses are delivered at lower pressures and volumes.
HFPPV	High-frequency positive-pressure ventilation; conventional mechanical ventilation at faster-than-usual rates.
PPAV	Patient proportional assist ventilation; a collective term describing ventilators using patient-controlled rates and tidal volumes.
OH	Oxygen hood; a clear plastic enclosure placed over a nonintubated infant to allow humidification of room air (21% Fi_{O_2} or increased Fi_{O_2}).

TABLE 26–3. Factors Worsening the Severity and Increasing the Incidence of Respiratory Distress Syndrome

Perinatal asphyxia or hypoxia
Cold stress
Prematurity
Failure of closure of the patent ductus arteriosus
Diabetes mellitus in mother
Acidosis

assist with lung maturation (steroids), can be instituted (Fig. 26–2). Early initiation of antibiotics to treat bacterial vaginosis and trichomoniasis has also been associated with significant reduction in preterm births.[6]

Delaying delivery with tocolysis (usually a β-sympathomimetic) is feasible for only a few days in most cases. However, this may provide sufficient time to resolve a reversible etiology or promote lung maturation. Tocolysis is generally started when frequent contractions are noted. Although preterm labor may be overdiagnosed in up to 70% of cases using this approach, waiting for cervical changes will reduce the likelihood of successful inhibition of labor.[7] The contribution of tocolysis should not be underestimated. For example, around 25 weeks' gestation, even a 2-day increase in length of gestation could increase survival by 10% (from 15% to 25%).[3] Contraindications to tocolytic therapy include fetal death or lethal abnormality, eclampsia, abruptio placenta, and proven chorioamnionitis. Relative contraindications are preeclampsia, severe chronic hypertension, renal disease, heart disease, fetal distress, and fetal growth retardation.

Fetal lung maturation can be accelerated with antenatal corticosteroids. Contrary to previous beliefs, glucocorticoid

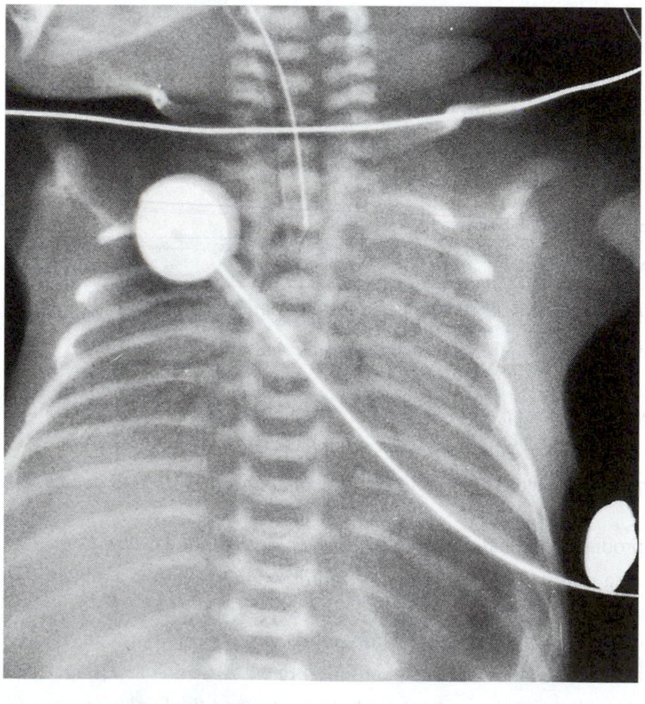

FIGURE 26–1. Chest radiograph demonstrating hyaline membrane disease with ground-glass appearance and air bronchograms.

TABLE 26–4. Differential Diagnosis of Hyaline Membrane Disease

Pneumonia, especially group B streptococcus
Spontaneous pneumothorax
Transient tachypnea of the newborn
Congenital cyanotic heart disease
Hypoplastic lungs
Diaphragmatic hernia

benefits are seen at all gestational ages below 35 weeks' gestation.[8–10] The mechanisms by which corticosteroids enhance lung maturation include acceleration of the normal rise in the antioxidant enzymes—for example, superoxide dismutase, catalase, and glutathione peroxidase—that protect lungs against damage from O_2 free radicals,[9,10] increased production of surfactant,[9,10] and up-regulation of ENaC to promote alveolar fluid absorption.[3] The NIH consensus conference published in 1995 concluded that all fetuses between 24 and 34 weeks' gestation at risk for preterm delivery should receive corticosteroids regardless of gender, race, maternal infection, and availability of surfactant.[9] Failure to treat all appropriate candidates is common as noted by the observation that corticosteroids were given to 12% to 18% of women delivering infants weighing 500 to 1500 g.[9] Antenatal steroid therapy is relatively devoid of toxicity but markedly affects neonatal morbidity. The odds ratio (95% confidence interval [CI]) for developing RDS is reduced to 0.49 (CI 0.41 to 0.6) if steroids are started 24 hours to 7 days before delivery. Even if treatment is started < 24 hours or > 7 days from delivery, risk is still reduced (odds ratio 0.69, CI 0.50 to 0.94). Antenatal steroids also reduced the risk of intraventricular hemorrhage (odds ratio 0.5, CI 0.3 to 0.9), necrotizing enterocolitis (odds ratio 0.35, CI 0.18 to 0.68), and neonatal mortality (odds ratio 0.6, CI 0.5 to 0.8).[8,9] An estimated "number of patients needed to treat" (NNT) to prevent RDS in one preterm infant ≤ 30 weeks' gestation, where RDS occurs in 50% of untreated cases, is six patients.[9] One report estimated that over $3000 was saved per treated neonate, and that if treatment rates increased to 60%, annual savings in health care costs from initial hospitalization alone would exceed $157 million.[9]

Use of thyrotropin-releasing hormone (TRH) as an adjunct to antenatal corticosteroids was thought to further accelerate fetal lung maturation.[9] However, the ACTOBAT study failed to show additional benefits from TRH 200 μg every 12 hours. The frequencies of RDS (relative risk 1.17, CI 1.00 to 1.36) and need for ventilation (relative risk 1.15, CI 1.01 to 1.31) were not reduced, and treatment was associated with maternal nausea, vomiting, and lightheadedness.[11] Of more concern was the 12-month follow-up report in which TRH treatment was associated with motor delays (odds ratio 1.51, CI 1.11 to 2.05), sensory impairment (odds ratio 2.00, CI 1.06 to 3.74), social delays (odds ratio 1.41, CI 1.01 to 1.95), and severe impairment (odds ratio 1.75, CI 1.07 to 2.87).[12] At this point, antenatal TRH treatment cannot be advised.

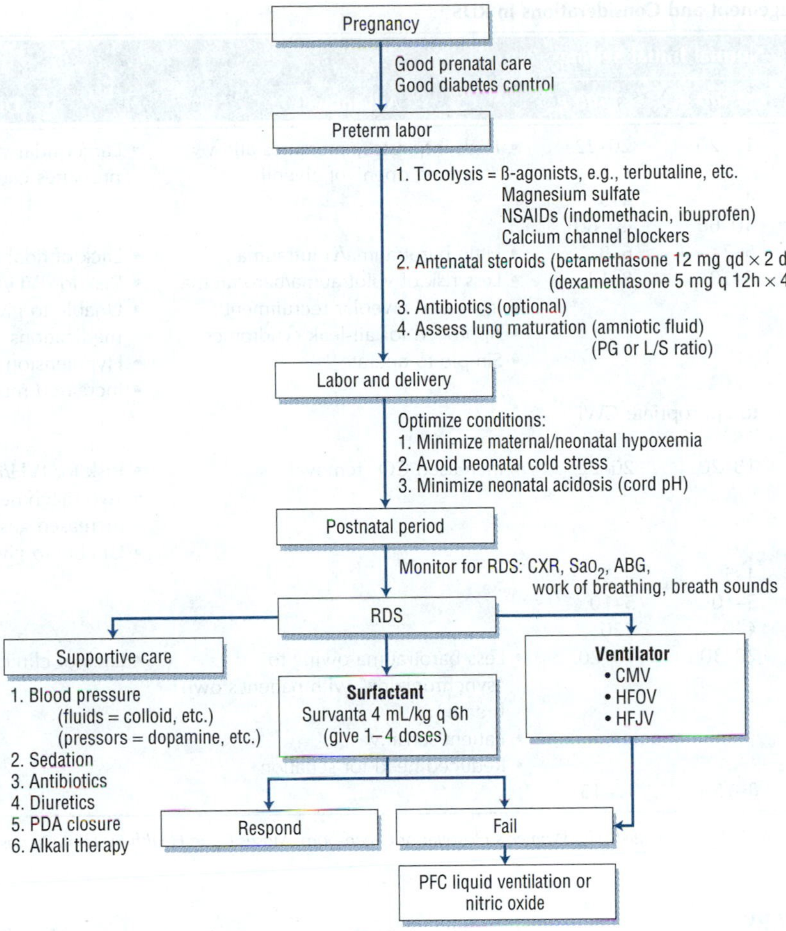

FIGURE 26–2. Algorithm for selective interventions to prevent and treat neonatal RDS.

▶ TREATMENT: Neonatal Respiratory Distress Syndrome

GENERAL APPROACH TO TREATMENT

Recently, treatment options for RDS have significantly advanced. Drug therapies include surfactant, perfluorocarbons (PFCs), and nitric oxide (NO) (Fig. 26–2). Supportive therapies such as mechanical ventilation, management of acidosis, and diuresis are also important.

NONPHARMACOLOGIC THERAPY

VENTILATOR THERAPY

Positive pressure ventilation (PPV) provides vital support to maintain adequate ventilation and oxygenation during the acute phase of RDS. Effective PPV is accomplished by generating a pressure that exceeds the "closing" pressure of the lung. Ventilation modes delivering this positive pressure are conventional mechanical ventilation (CV), high-frequency ventilation (HFV), patient proportional assist ventilation (PPAV), synchronized intermittent mandatory ventilation (SIMV), and continuous positive airway pressure (CPAP). A comprehensive review describing these modes of ventilation is beyond the scope of this chapter and the authors recommend the reader to an excellent review.[13]

The increased neonatal survival seen today can be credited, in part, to the extensive technologic advances in respiratory care, including mechanical ventilation. Conventional ventilation (CV), employed since the early 1970s, is based on delivering a volume of air (TV) by using inspiratory and expiratory pressures (PIP/PEEP) at a specific rate (IMV).[13] Although successful, the CV-induced lung morbidity has required continual assessment of new ventilatory modes that decrease baro- and volutrauma. A summary of these new ventilation modes is described in Table 26–5 with the average initial settings listed.

The improved outcomes in premature infants can also be attributed to better understanding of oxygen–hemoglobin dissociation curves, resulting in target Pa_{O_2} values of 50 to 75 mm Hg and $Sa_{O_2} > 90\%$. In addition, improved ventilator technologies and strategies allow for greater selection of the appropriate fit for the circumstance. For example, though CV is currently the best choice for many neonates, those with pulmonary air leaks are probably more safely managed with high-frequency oscillatory ventilation (HFOV).

The goals of CV are to achieve appropriate ABG parameters (Pa_{O_2} 50 to 75 mm Hg, Pa_{CO_2} 35 to 50 mm Hg, pH 7.28 to 7.40), chest expansion (diaphragm on an inspiratory film at 8 to 9 ribs), and avoidance of toxicities. Often a trade-off of either higher Fi_{O_2} or higher PIP must be made. Such decisions involve clinician bias and the "art" of medicine rather than being based on a strong scientific basis.

TABLE 26–5. Ventilator Management and Considerations in RDS

Ventilator Type	Setting	Normal Initial Settings < 1500 g	Normal Initial Settings > 1500 g	Advantages	Disadvantages
CMV	PIP (cm H_2O)	18–20	20–22	• High inspiratory pressures allow "popping open" of alveoli	• Larger tidal volumes and inspiratory pressures causing lung injury
	PEEP (cm H_2O)	4	4–5		
	IMV (BPM)	40–60	40–60		
CPAP	(cm H_2O)	5–7	6–8	• Little barotrauma/volutrauma	• Lack of tidal volume
HFOV	MAP (cm H_2O)	7–10	8–12	• Less risk of volutrauma/barotrauma • Increased alveolar recruitment • Approved for air-leak syndromes • Simple to operate	• Risk for IVH/PVL? • Unable to give aerosolized respiratory medications • Hypotension • Increased mucostasis?
	Amplitude	to appropriate CWF			
	Hz	15	15		
HFJV	PIP (cm H_2O)	18–20	20–22	• Increased CO_2 removal	• Risk for IVH/PVL? • Two machines • Increased gas trapping • Unable to give respiratory medicines
	PEEP (cm H_2O)	4–5	4–5		
	Sigh rate (BPM)	5–10	5–10		
	Rate (BPM)	420	420		
PPAV SIMV	Rate (BPM)	20–30	10–20	• Less barotrauma owing to "synchronizing" with patient's own breath • Patient sensitive • Reduced need for sedation	• Lack of clinical experience
	Volume (mL/kg)	8–15	10–15		

Assistance provided by Andrew Davey, MD, Neonatalogist, The Women's Hospital of Greensboro, Moses Cone Health System, Greensboro, North Carolina.

PHARMACOLOGIC THERAPY

SURFACTANT THERAPY

Surfactant replacement therapy (SRT) is widely accepted as the most clinically and cost-effective approach to treatment of RDS. Clinical trials have been carried out worldwide using an array of artificial, modified natural, and natural surfactants. The differences in key components are summarized in Table 26–6.

Natural human surfactant contains 85% phospholipids, 10% neutral lipids, and 5% surfactant proteins or apolipoproteins. Animal surfactants have similar protein and lipid content. Most exogenous surfactants incorporate dipalmitoyl phosphotidylcholine (DPPC) that constitutes 45% to 70% of endogenous lung surfactant and is the major phospholipid causing the low surface tension of surfactant. Other phospholipids, mainly phosphatidyl ethanolamine, phosphatidyl glycerol, phosphatidylinositol, and sphingomyelin, are responsible for adsorbing to the air–liquid interface. Four surfactant proteins (SP-A, SP-B, SP-C, and SP-D) comprise 2% to 5% of the weight of surfactant.[14,15] SP-A appears to regulate pulmonary surfactant turnover, formation of tubular myelin, and immune regulation. SP-B appears to be involved in formation of tubular myelin and in the surface activity of surfac-

TABLE 26–6. Exogenous Surfactants Used for the Treatment of Neonates With RDS

	Source	Components
Artificial Surfactants		
ALEC (Pumactant)	Synthetic	DPPC, unsaturated phosphatidylglycerol
Colfosceril palmitate (Exosurf)	Synthetic	DPPC, hexadecanol, tyloxapol
Human Surfactants		
Human	Amniotic fluid	Surfactant lipids, SP-A, SP-B, SP-C, SP-D
Animal Surfactants		
Infasurf	Lipid extract of calf lung lavage	Surfactant lipids, SP-B, SP-C
CLSE	Lipid extract of calf lung lavage	
Alveofact	Lipid extract of cow lung lavage	Surfactant lipids, SP-B, SP-C
Curosurf	Organic solvent of pig lung purified by chromatography	Lung phospholipids, SP-B, SP-C
Surfactant-TA (Surfacten)	Lipid extract of cow lung + added synthetic lipids	Lung lipids + DPPC, tripalmitin, palmitic acid
Survanta	Lipid extract of cow lung + synthetic lipids	Lung lipids + DPPC, tripalmitin, palmitic acid, SP-B, SP-C

Key: ALEC = artificial lung-expanding compound; CLSE = calf lung surfactant extract; DPPC = dipalmitoyl phosphatidylcholine; SP-A = surfactant protein A; SP-B = surfactant protein B; SP-C = surfactant protein C; SP-D = surfactant protein D.

Adapted from Hallman M, Merritt TA, Bry K. The fate of exogenous surfactant in neonates with respiratory distress syndrome. Clin Pharmacokinet 1994;26:215–232.

TABLE 26–7. Dosing Comparison Studies for Different Surfactants: Effects of Higher Doses Compared to Lower Doses

Ref.	Surfactant	Doses	Short Term	Long Term
20	Exosurf	5 mL/kg ≤ 4 vs ≤ 2 doses	Not stated	28 days: no differences
21	Exosurf	2.5 vs 5 mL 2.5 vs 7.5 mL 5 vs 7.5 mL	↓ FiO_2, ↓ vent (MAP) ↓ FiO_2, ↓ vent (MAP) No difference	14 days: no differences
22	Infasurf	100 mg/kg 1 vs ≤ 4 doses	↓ FiO_2, ↓ vent (PIP × IMV)	28 days: ↓ O_2 suppl (0% vs 8.3%) ↓ pneumothorax (11.1% vs 16.7%)
23	Surfactant-TA	30 mg/mL 2 vs 4 mL/kg	↓ FiO_2	30 days: ↓ O_2 suppl (13% vs 43.5%) ↓ vent (4.3% vs 30.4%)
24	Curosurf	200 mg/kg × 1 vs 200 mg/kg × 1 + 100 mg/kg (x ≤ 2)	↓ FiO_2, ↓ vent (MAP)	28 days: ↓ death (13% vs 21%) ↓ pneumothorax (9% vs 18%)
25	Curosurf	100 mg/kg × ≤ 3 vs 200 mg/kg + 100 mg/kg (x ≤ 4)	↓ FiO_2	28 days: no differences
26	Alveofact	100 mg/kg vs 50 mg/kg (repeat doses to max 200 mg/kg)	↓ FiO_2	28 days: ↓ pulmonary air leak (14% vs 33%)

tant, perhaps by increasing the lateral stability of the phospholipid layer. SP-C is speculated to be involved in the spreadability and surface activity of surfactant, although its exact function is unknown. SP-D function is unknown at this time.[14] Surfactant is synthesized in type II pneumocytes in the alveoli. After secretion, the major route of clearance is via reuptake by type II cells. Small quantities are removed by absorption into the lymphatics and clearance by alveolar macrophages. After reuptake into the type II cells, the phospholipids are either recycled for secretion or degraded and reused to synthesize new phospholipids.[14]

Surfactant is best administered via a sideport in the endotracheal adapter in two bolus fractional doses at a 45° upward tilt angled to the right then left.[16] Animal studies confirm that this technique delivers and distributes surfactant evenly. Use of the slow infusion technique delivered surfactant primarily to the upper lobes,[17] and nebulized surfactant concentrated in select pockets of each lobe, resulting in areas of hypo- and hyperinflation.[18] The optimum dose of exogenous surfactant remains uncertain. Controlled trials comparing single and multiple doses of surfactant have shown multiple doses to significantly reduce the incidence of pneumothorax and neonatal mortality.[15,19] This makes physiologic sense because animal studies suggest that much of the initial surfactant dose is inhibited by soluble proteins and other factors in the small airways and alveoli. Multiple doses may overcome this initial inactivation. The OSIRIS study showed that limiting therapy to two doses of Exosurf was as effective as allowing two to four doses depending on clinical need.[20] Many clinicians use up to four doses of Survanta based on clinical need. A summary of trials comparing surfactant doses is shown in Table 26–7. A requirement of four doses of Survanta to treat RDS may be a valuable predictor of increasing oxygen requirements around day 10, with the subsequent development of bronchopulmonary dysplasia (BPD.)[27]

SRT can be initiated as prophylaxis in the delivery room or as rescue therapy after clinical signs of RDS appear. Although some argue advantages to prophylaxis,[28,29] this may result in unnecessary treatment and costs. In recent trials using surfactant rescue[30,31] in newborns weighing 501 to 1500 g, only 45% of over 5000 patients were eligible for treatment. Also, meta-analyses do not support superior response rates for rescue therapy rather than prophylaxis (Table 26–8).[14,15] If an argument can be made for prophylaxis, it is in neonates delivered at 26 weeks' gestation or earlier.[29]

Outcome measures examined during surfactant trials include oxygen and ventilator requirements, severity of RDS, RDS mortality, total mortality, pneumothorax and other air-leak syndromes, pulmonary interstitial emphysema (PIE), BPD, and complications some investigators associate with surfactant therapy, such as IVH, pulmonary hemorrhage, and PDA (Table 26–9). In general, the primary benefits are more rapid resolution and milder course of RDS, and lower risk of pneumothorax, death, or chronic lung disease. These benefits are seen with natural and synthetic surfactants and are markedly enhanced when antenatal glucocorticoids were also used.[9,15] Despite the high success rates, 20% of neonates fail to respond to treatment. Factors associated with poor response include sepsis, pneumonia, PDA, congenital heart disease, and pulmonary hypoplasia.[15] Whether retreatment of RDS with surfactant after resolution of these factors is useful is currently unknown.

Although surfactant appears to be generally well tolerated, some possible toxicities and associated problems include brady-

TABLE 26–8. Relative Risks for Potential Beneficial and Adverse Effects of Synthetic and Natural Surfactants

	Synthetic				Surfactant			
Outcome	No.	*Prophylaxis*	No.	*Rescue*	No.	*Prophylaxis*	No.	*Rescue*
Pneumothorax	5	0.64 (0.49–0.89)	3	0.52 (0.42–0.65)	9	0.31 (0.22–0.44)	12	0.34 (0.27–0.44)
BPD	5	1.09 (0.80–1.47)	3	0.68 (0.46–0.99)	7	0.88 (0.67–1.17)	10	1.01 (0.81–1.27)
Death	7	0.67 (0.52–0.88)	3	0.47 (0.30–0.74)	9	0.60 (0.42–0.85)	11	0.59 (0.47–0.74)
Death + BPD	3	0.82 (0.63–1.08)	2	0.65 (0.50–0.82)	7	0.64 (0.49–0.84)	10	0.66 (0.53–0.82)
All IVH	4	0.94 (0.73–1.21)	2	0.77 (0.62–0.97)	8	0.95 (0.73–1.24)	10	0.94 (0.76–1.15)
Severe IVH						1.05 (0.86–1.18)		0.91 (0.72–1.14)
PDA	5	1.27 (1.03–1.57)	3	0.73 (0.60–0.88)	9	1.16 (0.89–1.50)	12	0.96 (0.79–1.18)
Pulmonary bleed	4	3.12 (1.54–6.32)	3	1.49 (0.57–3.79)	2	0.73 (0.31–1.69)	2	1.25 (0.74–2.13)

TABLE 26–9. Comparison of Rescue SRT on Outcomes in Neonates < 1750 g Expressed as NNT

Adverse Outcomes % Events Controls Mean (range) NNT	Air Leaks 23 (15–31)	PIE 38 (33–44)	Died 2° RDS 24 (18–29)	Died +/or DPD 57 (44–67)	Severe IVH	PVL
Exosurf vs control[a]	+11 (6,100)[c]	+4 (3,5)[c]	+14 (8,100)[c]	+5 (3,14)[c]		
Survanta vs control[a]	+8 (6,20)[c]	+4 (3,5)[c]	+10 (7,25)[c]	+5 (3,14)[c]		
Infasurf vs control[a]	+8 (6,20)[c]	+3 (3,4)[c]	+9 (6,20)[c]	+4 (3,9)[c]		
Survanta vs Exosurf[b]	+17[c]	NA	+50	+33		
Infasurf vs Exosurf[b]	+20[c]	+17[c]	+25	I = E	−29	−31[c]
Infasurf vs Survanta[b]	+33	+25	−20[c]	+25	−100	

[a]Compared to data from separate studies.
[b]Direct comparison of treatments.
[c]Indicates statistically significant difference ($P < .05$).
NA = Information not available; NNT = the number of neonates needed to be treated with the test surfactant (listed first) compared with second listed treatment to avoid (+) or cause (–) one adverse outcome in one patient.
Untreated controls data from Refs. 15 and 30. SRT data from Refs. 28, 35, and 37.

cardia, airway obstruction, and oxygen desaturation during administration; pulmonary hemorrhage; IVH; and the theoretical risk of allergy to natural surfactants,[30] though antibodies were absent in over 1400 Survanta-treated neonates.[31] Surfactant treatment is also associated with higher likelihood of clinically significant PDA. The pulmonary edema associated with PDA is thought to cause a hemorrhagic pulmonary edema rather than serious pulmonary hemorrhage,[19] as was the case in 10% to 45% of neonates with RDS in the presurfactant era. Furthermore, this pulmonary hemorrhage seems primarily to be a risk for prophylaxis with Exosurf (Table 26–9).[32] Early closure of the PDA may minimize the risk of hemorrhagic pulmonary edema as well as optimize surfactant response. While the relationship of IVH to surfactant use is controversial, cerebral blood flow velocity has been shown to be altered in some studies.[19] The risks of surfactants causing periventricular leukomalacia (PVL), a marker of hypoxic–ischemic brain injury, is poorly understood, but two recent trials[28,33] comparing Infasurf and Exosurf found increased risk with Infasurf (odds ratio 2.03, CI 1.09 to 3.80).[28] A theoretical basis for this is the hypocarbia noted with Infasurf, as this is associated with decreased cerebral blood flow. This trend needs to be assessed for all surfactants in additional studies that better measure this important end point.

Selection of surfactant products will require measuring positive and toxic outcomes in direct comparisons and meta-analyses with sufficient study numbers to document small differences in clinically important end points, because sample sizes cannot readily be achieved in individual clinical trials. Studies comparing Exosurf with natural surfactants (Survanta[34,35] and Infasurf[33,34]), found that the natural surfactant groups have a more rapid onset and lower requirements for oxygen supplementation and positive-pressure ventilation. Natural surfactant treatment resulted in fewer air leaks (e.g., pneumothorax).[28,33–35] Although survival trends favored natural surfactants (2% to 4% lower mortality rates), a statistically significant reduction in death was not shown and would require a study of at least 9000 patients to demonstrate statistical significance.[36]

Comparisons of natural surfactants show Infasurf[37] and Curosurf[38] to have a more rapid onset of pulmonary benefits (decreased oxygen supplementation and ventilator pressures) and longer duration of action[36] than the modified natural surfactant, Survanta. However, no clinically significant findings were statistically different, except the counterintuitive finding that fewer RDS-related deaths occurred with Survanta prophylaxis than Infasurf prophylaxis. Because studies are limited, natural surfactants should be considered equivalent at this time, although the problems of hypocarbia and PVL documented with Infasurf[28,33] must be studied for all surfactants for the true risk to be clarified. If problems with increased PVL risk are unique to Infasurf, it would place this surfactant product at a disadvantage.

Pharmacoeconomics of SRT

The pharmacoeconomic impact of SRT is documented in several reports.[39–41] SRT has lowered RDS mortality by at least 30%. From 1989 to 1990 (when Exosurf was introduced), 80% of the decline in infant mortality nationwide was attributable directly to SRT.[39] The reduction in resource use resulted in projected savings (using 1991 dollars) of $5800 in survivors and $4400 in infants who died.[39] Survanta use was projected to save $3300 in hospital resources for infants surviving to 28 days.[40] Savings as high as $18,000 in total hospital charges per surviving infant were projected in one analysis.[41] Each RDS- or treatment-related adverse outcome confers cost to health care. Although data are limited, the relative number of neonates with RDS treated with SRT to avoid or cause an event is estimated in Table 26–9. All surfactants are clinically and cost-effective for RDS.

LIQUID VENTILATION WITH PERFLUOROCHEMICALS

An investigational, but highly promising, approach to treating refractory RDS is the use of partial liquid ventilation, also called perfluorocarbon-associated gas exchange (PAGE).[42] Studies with perflubron, a perfluorocarbon (PFC), have reported dramatic increase in partial pressure of oxygen in arterial blood (PaO_2) and dynamic lung compliance within 1 hour of starting therapy and treatment resulted in prevention of RDS-associated deaths.[43] PFCs are inert liquids in which oxygen and carbon dioxide are highly soluble. PFCs have low surface tension and are evenly distributed throughout the lung at low inflation pressures. The surface tension with PFCs at the alveolar air–liquid interface is markedly lower than seen with air ventilation, allowing for markedly lower ventilator pressures and a reduced risk of barotrauma.[42] Clinically, PFC has been dosed by instillation into the endotracheal tube through the sideport at a rate of 1 mL/kg/min without interrupting mechanical gas ventilation, until a column of fluid is welled up in the endotracheal tube. This volume of PFC is felt to represent the infant's liquid functional residual capacity (FRC). Fluid that evaporates is replaced hourly to maintain this liquid FRC.[43] In animal studies, PFCs also offered a vehicle for improved drug delivery via the lungs.[44] Addition of exogenous surfactant to PFC ventilation appears to improve surfactant delivery and enhance response to PFC and surfactant in animals,[44,45] although studies in humans are unavailable. Adverse events associated with PFC use are mild and manageable, although long-term studies are lacking. Problems include endotracheal tube obstruction, hypoxic episodes, pneumo- or fluorothorax, and pulmonary hemorrhage.[43] These are not necessarily causal relationships and, overall, PFCs have been remarkably toxicity-free. The limited experience with PFCs and PAGE requires that this therapy be viewed as a promising, but investigational option in RDS unresponsive to surfactant.

NITRIC OXIDE

Nitric oxide (NO) is a natural endothelium-derived relaxing factor that is important in regulating vascular tone, especially the pulmonary vasculature.[46] Under normal physiologic conditions, NO is synthesized in endothelial cells and released into the vascular smooth muscle, where it stimulates cyclic GMP for vascular dilatation. At birth, NO helps in the transition from the markedly elevated pulmonary pressures in utero to normal pulmonary pressures and respiratory function.[47] Clinical studies are currently in progress to evaluate the role of NO in persistent pulmonary hypertension of the newborn, meconium aspiration syndrome, and RDS. Exogenous NO delivery is achieved by either premixing or "blending" with oxygen and other gases to achieve an NO concentration defined in parts per million (ppm).[47]

The potential benefit of NO in RDS is reduction of the ventilation–perfusion (V/Q) mismatch that occurs in RDS. Since the premature pulmonary vascular bed fails to uniformly dilate with the onset of ventilation, areas of V/Q mismatch result in decreased oxygen delivery, requiring higher ventilatory pressures and oxygen concentrations. NO has been shown to improve RDS and V/Q mismatch at doses of 5 to 20 ppm.[47] Thus, it would appear that the combination of surfactant and NO could result in more uniform pulmonary recruitment, thereby lowering ventilatory pressure and limiting the risk for BPD. Potential toxicities are few but include methemoglobinemia, inhibited platelet aggregation, and severe acute pulmonary edema secondary to the NO_2 oxidant metabolite. Future studies need to examine the clinical impact of this adjunctive therapy and the cost–benefit ratio as well.

SUPPORTIVE PHARMACOTHERAPY

Supportive pharmacotherapy in RDS is aimed at alleviating pain and discomfort, minimizing ventilator complications, and correcting any metabolic and/or fluid imbalance.

Narcotics/Benzodiazepines

Appropriate pharmacologic treatment is effective in alleviating pain and discomfort that neonates experience. Many ventilator-induced complications are secondary to asynchrony between ventilator rates and patient-driven respirations, resulting in pneumothorax and increased cerebral pressures that may promote IVH. Avoidance of these serious adverse effects can be accomplished by nonpharmacologic methods (e.g., PPAV) or through the use of sedative and paralytic agents. A comprehensive review of sedation in neonates is available[48]; therefore, the following discussion will be limited. The most commonly used sedative agents are morphine, fentanyl, and lorazepam. Studies have shown a significantly greater percentage of ventilator time in synchrony and a decrease in catecholamine levels in neonates who routinely receive morphine.[49] Intuitively, it is assumed that fentanyl produces the same results. However, studies examining fentanyl have shown an increase in ventilator support, tolerance, and addictive effects with long-term use.[50] The most common side effects demonstrated with both agents include decreased GI motility and risk of hypotension. Lorazepam is the preferred sedative agent in the absence of pain owing to its fast onset of action, its lack of hemodynamic toxicities, and its low risk of metabolite accumulation in comparison to diazepam. Muscle paralysis has been used to reduce ventilator fighting and the consequent complications. However, its role in RDS has diminished owing to adverse effects (edema, hypoventilation). If paralysis is induced, assessment of sedation and seizures is confounded; therefore, concurrent phenobarbital serum concentrations above 40 mg/L are recommended. Independent of agent use, it is imperative to establish target sedation scores to guide the clinical team in optimizing sedation. The use of sedation scores provides a mechanism to titrate drug to effect, which maximizes effectiveness while limiting complications.

Acidosis

Acidosis is associated with a number of physiologic effects that increase the severity of RDS, including increased pulmonary vascular resistance, impaired synthesis of surfactant, reduced cardiac output, and depressed ventilation. Consequently, measures that reduce the risk of acidosis, such as prevention of hypoxemia, hypotension, and excessive blood loss through venipuncture and minimizing oxygen consumption through careful temperature control, are critical. Correction of metabolic acidosis with sodium bicarbonate or 0.3 M tromethamine (THAM) is recommended when blood pH falls below 7.28 and base excess is –5 or less. Patients should not receive sodium bicarbonate in congestive heart failure or any other conditions where sodium administration worsens the clinical condition. Patients receiving THAM should be monitored for episodes of apnea and bradycardia, which may worsen following administration.

Diuretics

Pulmonary edema is a prominent feature of RDS. The severity of RDS is correlated with the presence of factors that cause pulmonary edema. This is not unexpected since excess fluid in the alveolar and interstitial spaces impairs pulmonary gas exchange, lowers lung compliance, and reduces FRC. Prevention of fluid overload and pulmonary edema is critical to minimize the risk of opening the ductus arteriosus and the need for high ventilatory pressures. Pulmonary edema can benefit from PEEP because of redistribution of fluid from air spaces to interstitial tissue and improvement in gas exchange. Oliguria is well recognized during the early stages of RDS. The routine use of a diuretic, furosemide, to correct this oliguria remains questionable.[51] The potential benefits of furosemide must be weighed against its risks, which include electrolyte imbalances and prostaglandin synthesis, which may increase the risk of a PDA.

CONCLUSIONS

Advances in prevention and reversal of RDS have had considerable impact on morbidity and mortality from RDS. Nevertheless, chronic lung disease, although less severe, continues to occur in about 35% to 45% of neonates. The challenge for the future is to manage effectively the 20% of neonates with RDS responding poorly to surfactant and to add therapies that will further reduce long-term pulmonary sequelae associated with RDS. This is a valuable area for future research.

TABLE 26–10. American–European Consensus Criteria Defining ARDS

Timing	Oxygenation	Chest Radiograph	Pulmonary Capillary Wedge Pressure
Acute onset	$Pa_{O_2}/Fi_{O_2} \le 200$ mm Hg (ALI ≤ 300 mm Hg)	Bilateral infiltrates	≤ 18 mm Hg (without pulmonary hypertension)

ACUTE RESPIRATORY DISTRESS SYNDROME

"Adult" respiratory distress syndrome (ARDS), now referred to as "acute" respiratory distress syndrome, was first described as a syndrome including diffuse bilateral lung infiltrates on chest x-ray, a high oxygen requirement, high ventilatory inflation pressures, and an improvement in oxygenation after the addition of PEEP.[52] In all cases the syndrome occurred 1 to 96 hours after an acute insult such as trauma, pancreatitis, pneumonia, or drug overdose. Controversy continues in regard to defining the syndrome, eliciting causes, and developing treatment strategies for this often fatal disease.

EPIDEMIOLOGY

Controversy concerning the definition of ARDS makes it difficult to determine the incidence and mortality of ARDS. The American–European ARDS Consensus Conference recommended the criteria listed in Table 26–10 to define ARDS (including chest x-ray patterns, pulmonary artery catheter pressures, and onset).[53] Unfortunately, these criteria inadequately describe the ARDS population.[54]

The incidence of ARDS ranges between 1.5 and 71 cases/100,000 population/year with 38% to 58% mortality depending on the diagnostic criteria used.[55,56] ARDS survival depends on the avoidance of concomitant end-organ damage and infection.[56] Uninfected patients and patients with an identifiable infection source survive more often than do their counterparts.[57] The incidence of end-organ failure increases with infection. Acidemic and uremic patients are less likely to survive.[58] In ARDS survivors, 44% are not back to normal work activities by 1 year.[59] Pulmonary function tests are abnormal at the time of extubation, improving significantly by 3 months. Improvement in pulmonary function tests and self-health assessment scores plateau at 6 months.[59]

ETIOLOGY

ARDS risk factors as determined by the most stringent studies are sepsis, multiple transfusions, aspiration, and trauma.[55,60] Organisms associated with ARDS include gram-negative bacilli, gram-positive cocci, and atypical organisms such as fungi, viruses, *Pneumocystis carinii,* and *Legionella* spp. Most commonly, an abdominal infection is the source causing ARDS secondary to sepsis. Sepsis occurring after an initial episode of ARDS is usually caused by a pulmonary source.[61]

PATHOPHYSIOLOGY

Understanding the pathophysiology of ARDS is important to evaluate therapeutic modalities. It is described by the Starling equation of fluid movement across cellular membranes (Fig. 26–3).

$$Q_T = K_f[(P_{mv} - P_{is}) - \sigma(p_{mv} - p_{is})] \quad (1)$$

where Q_T is the amount of fluid filtered per unit time; K_f is the vessel permeability to fluid; $(P_{mv} - P_{is})$ is the hydrostatic pressure gradient across the membrane separating the pulmonary microvasculature (mv) from the interstitium (is); $(p_{mv} - p_{is})$ is the osmotic gradient between the pulmonary microvasculature (mv) and interstitium (is); and σ is the membrane permeability to protein.

ARDS describes the situation in which σ approaches zero, that is, the membrane allows protein and fluid to freely cross into the pulmonary interstitium. Clinicians call this "leak." This differs from congestive heart failure, in which σ is normal (approximately 1) and the membrane is relatively impermeable to fluid and protein movement. In CHF the hydrostatic pressure increases, forcing fluid across

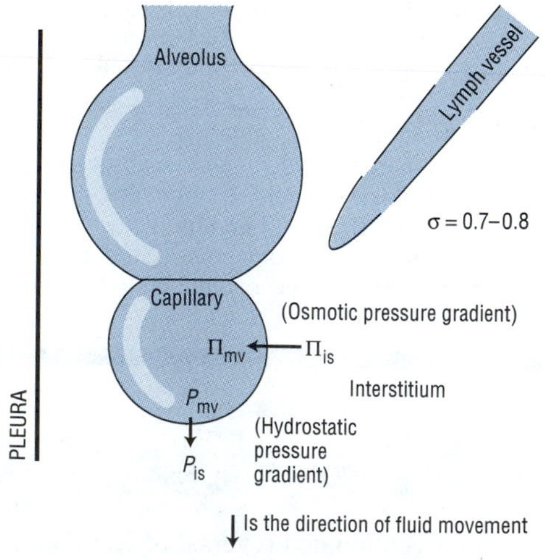

FIGURE 26–3. Fluid movement in the normal lung. σ = permeability of the membrane between the pulmonary vessels and interstitium to protein. *(From Ref. 61, with permission.)*

the membrane. Because formation of lung edema differs, the therapeutic end points of ARDS and CHF differ[61] (Table 26–11).

TABLE 26–11. Differences Between Cardiogenic and Noncardiogenic (ARDS) Causes of Pulmonary Edema

Cause Parameter	Hydrostatic Gradient ($P_{mv} - P_{is}$)	Membrane Permeability (σ)
Protein in fluid	↓	↑
Resolution	Fast	Slow
Pulmonary capillary wedge pressure	↑	↓
Left ventricular dysfunction	Yes	No

CLINICAL PRESENTATION

Clinically, lung injury allowing membrane permeability (σ) to approach zero occurs after a variety of insults, including trauma, sepsis, and other diseases causing tissue inflammation. This lung injury (altered membrane permeability) causes an increase in lung water. Increased lung water increases shunt, areas that are perfused, but not ventilated. This shunt leads to the clinical hallmark of ARDS, severe hypoxemia requiring mechanical ventilation. A fall in pulmonary compliance ensues, all with normal microvascular pressure (P_{mv}) and normal pulmonary capillary wedge pressures (PCWPs). The clinical vernacular describing decreased compliance is "stiff lung." The increase in lung water appears on chest x-ray as bilateral symmetrical infiltrates.

▶ TREATMENT: Adult Respiratory Distress Syndrome

DESIRED OUTCOME

No effective therapy is available to treat the underlying cause of ARDS.[61] Therapy is primarily supportive with a primary goal of perfusion; that is, to improve cardiopulmonary status to deliver adequate oxygen to tissues. Equally important is the prevention of ARDS-associated complications (end-organ disease and infection) while the underlying lung injury heals. Mortality approaches 100% when three or more organs fail.[62] Patients with multisystem organ failure are also more likely to be infected.[57]

GENERAL APPROACH TO TREATMENT

Drug therapy is an integral part of the supportive therapy of ARDS. Supportive therapy issues will be discussed initially with few specific drug therapy guidelines, because they can be obtained from other chapters. Drug therapy specific to treatment of ARDS will be discussed in the pharmacologic treatment section (Fig. 26–4).

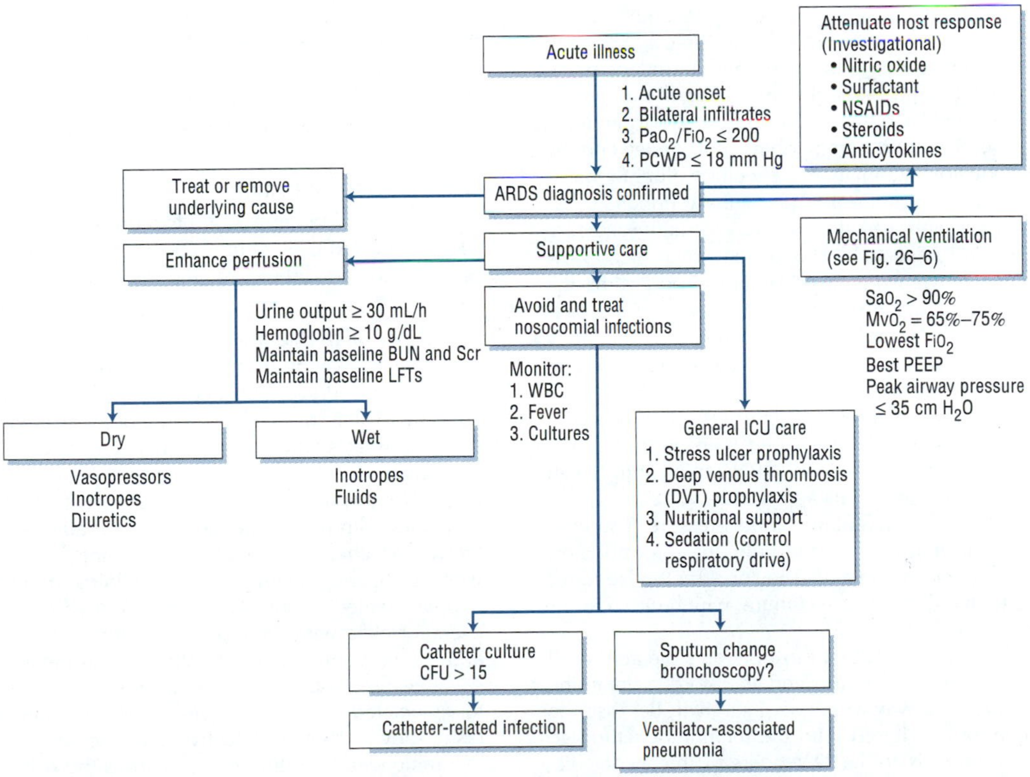

FIGURE 26–4. Algorithm for the treatment of ARDS and prevention of complications associated with ARDS and its management. BUN = blood urea nitrogen; CFU = colony-forming unit; LFT = liver function test; NSAID = nonsteroidal anti-inflammatory agent; Scr = serum creatinine; WBC = white blood cell count.

SUPPORTIVE PHARMACOTHERAPY

PERFUSION/PREVENTION OF END-ORGAN DAMAGE

Adequate perfusion supplies necessary nutrients (oxygen, glucose, and electrolytes) and disposes of metabolic by-products. Monitoring perfusion consists of two basic approaches. The first is to assess end-organ function, such as central nervous system or renal function. ARDS patients are usually sedated, and therefore central nervous system function is difficult to assess. Urine output as a marker of renal function rapidly becomes the most available measure of perfusion.

The second approach equates adequate oxygen delivery with perfusion. The goal of therapy is to optimize oxygen delivery. Remember, hypoxemia is the predominant effect of ARDS; therefore, this latter approach addresses the most abnormal aspect of organ perfusion. Oxygen saturation, mixed venous oxygenation (Mv_{O_2}), Pa_{O_2}, and serum lactate are usually followed. Maintaining an Mv_{O_2} in the normal range (65% to 75%) assumes adequate delivery, if oxygen extraction is not deranged by sepsis. Lactate production occurs during anaerobic metabolism. Monitoring serum lactate is less than ideal because lactate clearance is abnormal in renal and hepatic dysfunction and lactate metabolism is altered by endotoxin.[63]

Hemodynamic and Fluid Management

Theoretically, improving the oxygen supply should improve oxygen delivery to the tissues. A classic and often cited study in ARDS patients showed a linear relationship between oxygen supply and uptake.[64] Unfortunately, the methods used to calculate supply and uptake both incorporate cardiac output, and therefore a linear relationship is to be expected. Rigorous evaluations of oxygen supply and utilization using respiratory gas analysis refutes the linear relationship.[72] Regardless, most clinicians optimize cardiac output in ARDS patients to assure adequate perfusion by using fluids, red cell transfusions, inotropic agents, and afterload-reducing agents. Pa_{O_2}, urine output, blood pressure, PCWP, CO, Sa_{O_2} >90%, and hemoglobin (> 10 g/dL) are monitored to determine which agent is most appropriate to improve perfusion. Other than Sa_{O_2} and hemoglobin, goals depend on the patient's overall perfusion rather than a specific value. Monitoring arterial oxygen (and saturation) is particularly important because inotropic agents and vasodilators may actually decrease Pa_{O_2} by increasing V/Q mismatch. This occurs when blood flow to flooded alveoli increases from vasodilatation produced by the inotropic agent, overcoming the increase in mixed venous oxygenation produced by the increased cardiac output. Fortunately the net effect usually is an increase in Pa_{O_2} and improved organ perfusion.[61]

Fluid management is an important component of hemodynamic monitoring. Two hotly debated fluid management strategies exist. The "dry" theorists lower PCWP, keeping it just high enough to maintain perfusion.[66] This approach requires vasopressors and inotropic agents to maintain blood pressure. Theoretically, although all fluid leaks across the pulmonary membranes, the amount of leak will be minimized. The "dry" method requires extreme vigilance to avoid acute renal failure, which often causes death in ARDS patients.

The other strategy contends that most patients die from end-organ disease, not from hypoxemia, and therefore maintaining organ perfusion is the only way to improve survival. Because the amount of leak cannot be altered until the membrane returns to normal,[67] fluid restriction is futile. Defenders of this theory discuss data showing only 16% of deaths owing to an inability to oxygenate the patient.[68]

Data support both viewpoints. Many clinicians blend both views and limit fluids whenever adequacy of perfusion permits. As discussed previously, this requires monitoring of CO, PCWP, urine output, hemoglobin, blood pressure, BUN, and creatinine.

Limiting Oxygen Utilization

ARDS management includes limiting oxygen utilization by aggressively managing fever, seizures, respiratory drive, and other causes of increased metabolism. Sedation is critical to patient survival because increased oxygen usage can be detrimental. Nonphysiologic ventilatory modes require obliteration of the respiratory drive. Typically, patients receive a benzodiazepine/opiate combination. Neuromuscular blockage use is undergoing heated debate,[69] but single doses are often needed to gain acute control during titration of other sedatives.

Stress Ulcerations

Stress-induced gastrointestinal bleeding complicates ARDS therapy. Mechanical ventilation and coagulopathy are indications for stress ulcer prophylaxis.[70] Drug choice is based on patient-specific factors rather than advantages of a particular agent,[70] because gastric pH has not been shown to correlate with the development of ventilator-associated pneumonia.[71]

Nutritional Support

Nutritional support does not affect the outcome of ICU patients, but most clinicians nevertheless initiate this therapy.[72] Parenteral nutrition is often necessary in seriously ill ARDS patients because blood flow to the gastrointestinal tract is limited. Enteral nutrition is preferred if the patient can tolerate enteral feedings, even if in small amounts. The advantages of enteral feeding include decreased central access, increased gastrointestinal blood flow perhaps decreasing the risk of bacterial transport across the gut, and decreased risk of stress ulceration. Lipid administration in ARDS is controversial, although withholding lipids from ARDS patients is not clearly supported nor recommended in the literature. Hypercarbia solely owing to excessive calorie and/or dextrose administration should be avoided.

Nosocomial Infections

Prevention and treatment of infection is also critical to improving survival in ARDS patients. Specific issues include nosocomial pneumonia and catheter-related infections.

Nosocomial Pneumonia. Nosocomial pneumonia in ARDS patients causes mortality in 67% versus 23% of patients without pneumonia.[57] Prevention and early treatment are critical to decreasing ARDS mortality. Ventilator-associated pneumonia directly correlates with length of mechanical ventilation.[73]

Diagnosis of ventilator-associated pneumonia is difficult because no diagnostic method, even protected specimen brush, correlates with microbiologic results on autopsy[74] or affects mortality.[75] Mechanically ventilated patients are always colonized with pathogenic organisms. When clinical findings suggest ventilator-associated pneumonia, the causative organism does, however, correlate with the organism colonizing the upper airways[76] and should be the target of antimicrobial therapy.

Because gastric colonization does not correlate with ventilator-associated pneumonia and mortality differences have not been shown, routine selective gut decontamination cannot be recommended.[72] Antibiotic use carries the risk of acquiring multiresistant organisms, which increase mortality.[77] Unit-specific monitoring of pathogenic organisms and resistance patterns may be important for decreasing the development of multiresistant organisms.[78]

Catheter-Related Infection. ARDS patients are also at risk for the development of catheter-related infections, especially bacteremia, which is life threatening.[79]

Attention to aseptic placement and follow-up care is extremely important to avoid infection. Catheter alterations such as antibiotic impregnation, cuffs, and the like do not decrease the risk of infection.[80,81] Decreasing the use and/or number of central lines may be preventive. Attention to alternate methods of drug delivery and compatibility issues can limit central intravenous line use.

Diagnosis of catheter-related infection is relatively difficult, although most clinicians agree that semiquantitative cultures of the removed catheters are helpful. Organisms are usually gram-positive bacteria, with methicillin-resistant *Staphylococcus* being relatively common in ICU patients. Catheter removal and antimicrobial therapy are cornerstones of treatment.

NONPHARMACOLOGIC THERAPY

VENTILATOR MANAGEMENT OF ARDS

Mechanical Ventilation

A cornerstone of supportive care in fulminate respiratory failure is mechanical ventilation. Mechanical ventilation can be lifesaving, yet attention to detail is critical to avoid and manage the life-threatening complications associated with it. Clinicians caring for the critically ill must have a rudimentary understanding of the technical aspects of mechanical ventilation to optimize drug therapy. Also important are the postulated effects of mechanical ventilation on the disposition of drugs.[82] Mechanical ventilation is as much an art as a science, and proper use cannot be simplified in

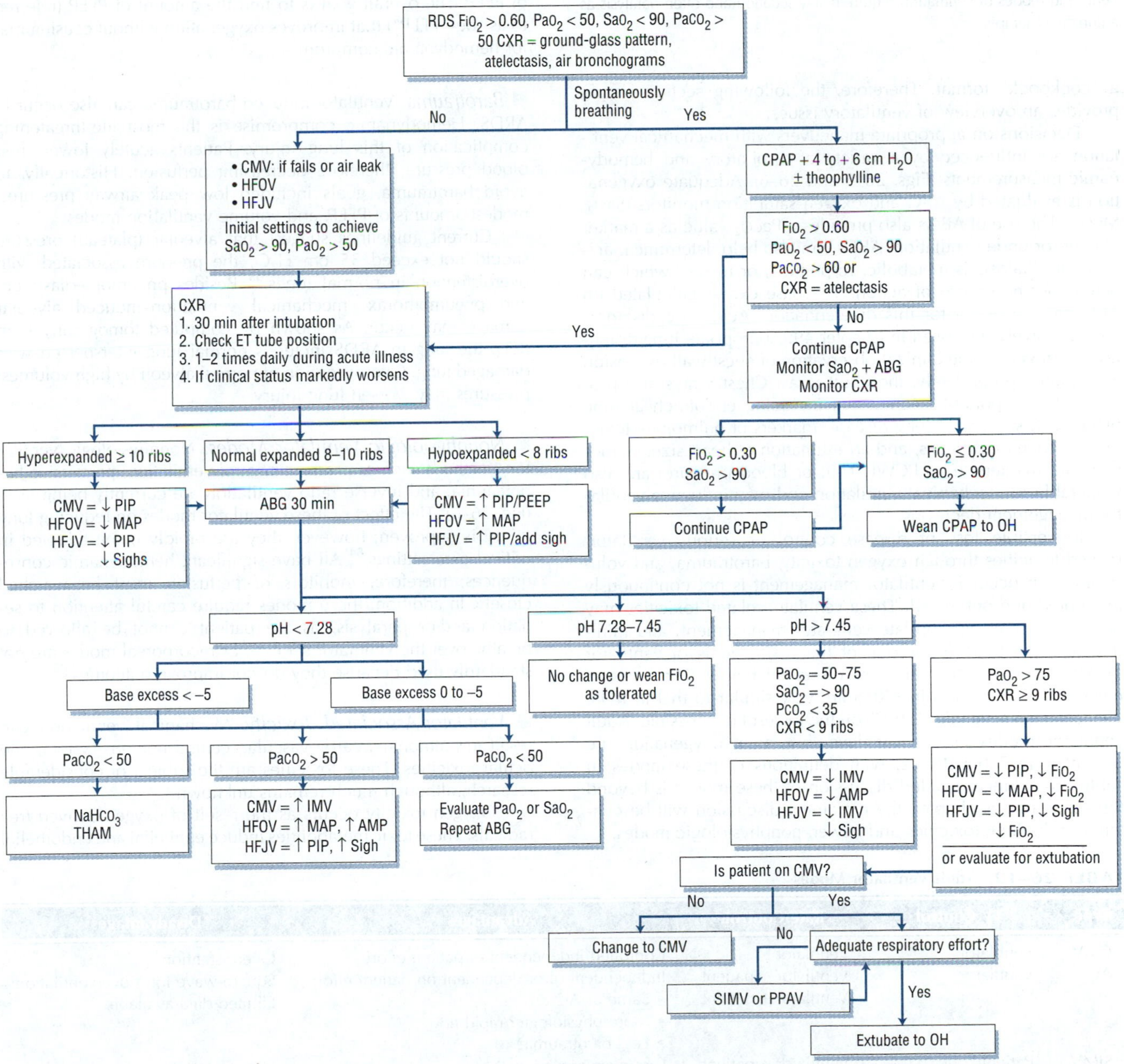

FIGURE 26–5. Algorithm for ventilator management of neonatal RDS.

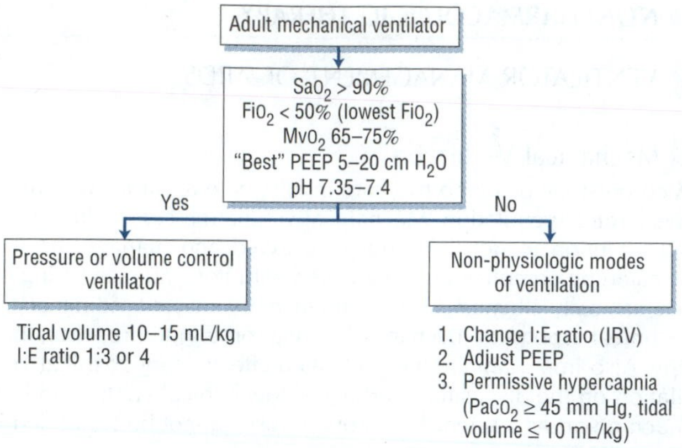

FIGURE 26–6. Algorithm for ventilator management of ARDS. *Note:* All patients and modes of ventilation require heavy sedation and often paralysis as adjunctive therapy.

a "cookbook" format. Therefore, the following section simply provides an overview of ventilatory issues.

Decisions on appropriate maneuvers with mechanical ventilation are influenced by a variety of respiratory and hemodynamic measurements (Figs. 26–5 and 26–6). Adequate oxygenation is evaluated by ABG and oxygen saturation monitors (SaO_2, MvO_2). The use of ABGs also provides a $PaCO_2$ value as a marker of over- or underventilation. ABGs can also help determine if acidosis or alkalosis is metabolic, respiratory, or mixed, which can determine the course of action. The base excess calculated on ABG can be useful for this differentiation. Acid–base disorders are extensively discussed in Chapter 49. Appropriate lung distention is gauged by the clinical observation of chest wall expansion and, more appropriately, the chest x-ray. Chest x-rays also provide other important information, including endotracheal tube placement, severity of lung disease, markers of pulmonary toxicity, presence of air leaks, and an estimation of heart size. Hemodynamic markers (e.g., PCWP, CO, or blood pressure) are also vulnerable to mechanical ventilation and may influence ventilator management decisions.

Irreversible loss of disease control or serious ventilator-related toxicities through oxygen toxicity, barotrauma, and volutrauma can occur if ventilator management is not continuously monitored and optimized. These ventilator-related toxicities may occur even with appropriate ventilator management, and minimizing these toxicities is one of the major goals of ventilator management. The toxicities are discussed below. The goals of mechanical ventilation in ARDS are very similar to that in RDS. The target SaO_2 remains ≥ 90% on the lowest FiO_2 possible. Adult ventilator modes used to achieve this target oxygenation are presented in Table 26–12, with definitions of these modes in Table 26–2. Since detailed discussion of these modes is beyond the scope of this chapter, the remaining discussion will be centered on limiting toxicities and newer, nonphysiologic modes.

Positive End-Expiratory Pressure. PEEP can limit the FiO_2 needed for adequate oxygen saturation. PEEP is a pressure applied by the ventilator that prevents complete lung emptying at end expiration, increasing lung volume. This improves gas exchange and redistributes (but does not decrease) lung water. PEEP reduces hypoxemia by reducing V/Q mismatch.[61] Early use of PEEP does not decrease atelectasis, pneumonia, barotrauma, or mortality.[83]

PEEP has variable effects on oxygenation, because the lung injury in ARDS is heterogeneous. PEEP reaching normal lung regions causes overdistension, sending blood from normal to abnormal areas, and therefore worsening shunt and hypoxemia. PEEP effects on PaO_2, SaO_2, and MvO_2 are monitored closely.[61] PEEP also can decrease cardiac output, primarily by decreasing venous return, affecting oxygenation. Because of this, hemodynamic parameters such as cardiac output and PCWP are monitored to assess and correct any problems induced by high levels of PEEP. The overall goal is to find the amount of PEEP (referred to as "best PEEP") that improves oxygenation without causing major hemodynamic compromise.

Barotrauma. Ventilator-induced barotrauma can also occur in ARDS. Hemodynamic compromise is the most life-threatening complication of this lung injury. Patients acutely lower their blood pressure, therefore decreasing perfusion. Historically, to avoid barotrauma, goals included low peak airway pressures, modest amounts of PEEP, and volume ventilation modes.

Current guidelines suggest that alveolar (plateau) pressure should not exceed 35 cm H_2O, the pressure associated with overdistention in normal lungs.[53] Besides pneumomediastinum and pneumothorax, mechanical ventilation–induced alveolar damage may occur. As shown by computed tomography scan (CT), the lung in ARDS includes normal lung interspersed with damaged lung. Overdistention of normal alveoli by high volumes/pressures may worsen lung injury.

Nonphysiologic Ventilator Modes. Nonphysiologic ventilatory methods such as pressure-control ventilation, permissive hypercapnia, and inverse ratio ventilation are currently being used (Fig. 26–6). The effect of these ventilator modes on reducing lung injury is unproven; however, they are rapidly being adopted in critical care settings.[84] All have significant hemodynamic consequences; therefore, monitors of perfusion must be watched closely. In addition, these modes require careful attention to sedation and/or paralysis, as the patient cannot be allowed to breathe over the ventilator set rate. Extracorporeal modes are not standardly used because they do not improve outcomes.[85]

Ventilator-Associated Toxicity. Mechanical ventilation can result in pulmonary, cardiovascular, central nervous system, and ocular toxicities. These toxicities are the subject of considerable research, although much remains unknown.

Oxygen toxicity occurs as the result of oxygen-derived free radicals. These toxic metabolities induce epithelial and endothelial

TABLE 26–12. Adult Ventilator Modes

Type	TV Control	Rate Control	Advantages	Disadvantages
CMV	Ventilator	Ventilator	Contolled independent of patient effort	Overdistention
AC	Ventilator	Ventilator + patient	Independent of or dependent on patient effort	Square-wave form overventilation
PC	Ventilator	Ventilator + patient	• Same as AC • More physiologic?/rapid flow • Less barotrauma?	Limited data available
SIMV	Patient	Ventilator + patient	Less overventilation	Not for ARDS
PS	Ventilator + patient	Patient	Patient controls	Not for ARDS

cell damage, surfactant inactivation, and inflammatory changes that result in BPD.[86] Neonates are particularly susceptible to oxygen toxicity owing to a deficiency in antioxidant enzymes, such as superoxide dismutase (SOD) and catalase, which normally inactivate oxygen free radicals. Neonatal studies examining the role of intratracheal SOD within 3 hours after surfactant use demonstrated decreased markers of acute lung injury but no change in long-term outcome.[87] Future SOD studies need to consider optimal doses, timing, and duration. Oxygen toxicity in neonates has also been associated with a serious ocular complication called retinopathy of prematurity (ROP), which is associated with retinal detachment and severe visual impairment.[13]

Positive pressure ventilation can result in "barotrauma" owing to high inspiratory pressures and "volutrauma" owing to large TVs. These positive pressures cause a cascade of physiologic responses and mediator release, which may result in inflammation, edema, surfactant inactivation, V/Q mismatch, and lung rupture with consequent air leak.[13] Further, high distending pressures designed to prevent alveolar collapse (PEEP) may decrease cardiac output to the point of hemodynamic compromise. ARDS patients appear particularly vulnerable to these hemodynamic effects.

Overventilation in neonates may also result in hypocarbia ($Paco_2 < 30$). This has been associated with reduced cerebral blood flow and consequent toxicity of PVL.[88] PVL is associated with development of cerebral palsy. Therefore, episodes of hypocarbia in premature infants should be minimized.

PHARMACOLOGIC THERAPY

SURFACTANT

Unlike neonatal respiratory distress syndromes caused by a primary surfactant deficiency, the injury associated with ARDS is more complex. Malfunction of the surfactant system is probably a secondary effect of the underlying disease process. A randomized, placebo-controlled trial showed no effect of surfactant on 30-day mortality, ICU stay, duration of mechanical ventilation, or physiology.[89] A dose–response relationship may exist, but requires further study.[90]

NITRIC OXIDE

As ARDS progresses to fibrosis, pulmonary vascular resistance increases and hypoxemia worsens. Systemic vasodilators decrease pulmonary vascular resistance and increase perfusion to ventilated areas. Unfortunately most patients with ARDS cannot tolerate the associated hypotension. Inhaled nitric oxide offers a means to vasodilate the ventilated lung areas, yet not worsen shunt while minimizing systemic effects.[91]

Animal studies and small uncontrolled studies in humans suggest an ability of NO to decrease pulmonary vascular resistance and improve oxygenation; however, mortality has not been affected.[92] Not all patients respond, perhaps a predictor of mortality.[93]

Nitric oxide is difficult to deliver and its toxicity is worth mention. In combination with high concentrations of oxygen, it may be cytotoxic.[92] Controlled, multicentered trials are currently underway and, until completed, routine nitric oxide use cannot be recommended.

ANTI-INFLAMMATORY/ANTICYTOKINE MEDIATORS

Sepsis mediators (e.g., interleukin-1, tumor necrosis factor α) are associated with the protein and fluid leak across the alveolar–vascular membrane in ARDS. Blocking the sepsis mediators should decrease the incidence and mortality of ARDS. Unfortunately, blockers of sepsis mediators do not influence mortality.[94] In some instances, our worst fears were realized as patients with less severe illness actually had an increased mortality rate when treated with active drug. Attenuating the inflammatory process may actually be harmful rather than helpful to patients with sepsis and ARDS. There are phase III studies underway and/or needed with soluble TNF receptor, the antioxidant L-2-oxothiazolidine-4-carboxylate (OTC), and C1 (complement) inhibitor. More importantly, significantly more research regarding mechanism, timing, and dosing is needed before these agents find a place in ARDS treatment.

General Anti-Inflammatory Agents

Ketoconazole, prostaglandin E_1, ibuprofen, pentoxyfylline, and fibronectin showed benefit in animal or small human studies. They have either failed or not been studied in larger phase III trials and therefore cannot be recommended at this time.[94]

Corticosteroids

Since the pathogenesis of ARDS is an acute inflammatory lung process, corticosteroid anti-inflammatory effects were initially thought to ameliorate this process. A multicentered trial showed that corticosteroid treatment of ARDS patients did not affect outcome.[53] Furthermore, early corticosteroid administration in septic patients did not prevent ARDS development. In fact, the time to ARDS resolution was shorter in the placebo group.[95]

Several uncontrolled, open-label studies have investigated corticosteroid use in patients with persistent ARDS. The theory is that this group progresses from acute inflammation to fibrosis, and therefore corticosteroids should ameliorate this process. Until a controlled trial is completed, use of corticosteroids to prevent the fibroproliferative stage of ARDS is extremely controversial, perhaps dangerous, and is not recommended.[94]

EVALUATION OF OUTCOMES AND MONITORING PLAN

Mortality, ICU stay, and duration of mechanical ventilation are common outcome measures used in ARDS studies. There is considerable debate about the usefulness of these or other surrogate markers in determining efficacy of ARDS therapies.

Specific patient monitoring is complex and requires intimate knowledge of and attention to details. Monitoring for the usual signs of infection and culture data is critical, albeit difficult in ICU patients. End-organ function must be monitored. All drug doses must be carefully assessed especially if the drug causes or is eliminated by critical end organs.

Monitoring ventilatory parameters, arterial blood gases, and oxygen saturation assists in the determination of illness severity as well as provides rudimentary end points of perfusion. For example, most clinicians agree that maintaining an oxygen saturation ($Sao_2 \geq 90\%$ is an important end point. Effects of inotropic agents, blood products, and vasopressors must be monitored in light of all of these measures to determine if oxygenation is improved or worsened.

Some centers try to manage ARDS patients without a pulmonary artery catheter, although very few patients are

TABLE 26–13. Monitoring Parameters in ARDS

Hemodynamic	Ventilator Status	Infection	End-Organ Damage
PCWP	FiO_2	White blood cells/differential	BUN
Cardiac output/index	PaO_2	Chest x-ray findings	Creatinine
Oxygen saturation (SaO_2)	SaO_2	Temperature	Urine output
Mixed venous oxygenation (MvO_2)	MvO_2	Cultures	Liver function tests
Hemoglobin/hematocrit	Plateau pressure	Change in color/quantity sputum	PT/PTT
Urine output	Respiratory effort/rate	New-onset hypotension	
		Abdominal examination	
		Number of central catheter days	

managed in this way. The diagnosis of ARDS is dependent on measuring pulmonary capillary wedge pressure (PCWP), which can be obtained only by a pulmonary artery catheter. Radiographically, noncardiogenic pulmonary edema (ARDS) cannot be distinguished from cardiogenic pulmonary edema;[96] therefore a pulmonary artery catheter is almost essential. High-pressure ventilation interferes with cardiac function, which must be measured and managed to improve perfusion. Unfortunately these ventilatory pressures also interfere with measurements obtained with pulmonary artery catheters.

Many centers use pulmonary artery catheters that include an oxygen saturation monitor to directly measure SaO_2 and MvO_2. This catheter eliminates the need for pulse oximetry, especially in poorly perfused patients. Table 26–13 lists monitoring parameters to be followed in patients with ARDS.

CONCLUSIONS

ARDS-related mortality plagues the modern ICU. Therapy is supportive, with vigilant attention to detail perhaps providing the only means to decrease mortality. In particular, the search for and avoidance of nosocomial infection is critical to survival. Improving perfusion and avoiding end-organ damage is also critical. Research is ongoing for pharmacologic therapy directed at the underlying disease process.

▶ PRINCIPLES OF PHARMACOTHERAPY

- Neonatal RDS is predominantly a disease of surfactant deficiency.
- Surfactant availability can be affected antenatally with maternal glucocorticoids to promote production and postnatally with surfactant replacement therapy.
- Surfactant replacement therapy markedly reduces neonatal pulmonary morbidity and mortality. Modified natural and natural surfactants appear superior to synthetic surfactant in these effects.
- ARDS is a syndrome characterized by bilateral pulmonary infiltrates, high oxygen requirements, and noncardiogenic pulmonary edema that occurs secondary to an inflammatory insult such as sepsis.
- No therapeutic modality has been shown to improve outcome in ARDS. Supportive therapy is necessary while the lung injury heals.
- Infection and end-organ damage are the usual causes of ARDS mortality.
- Ventilator management is essential to manage the respiratory failure associated with RDS and ARDS.
- Selection of ventilator maneuvers is based on a combination of clinical experience and scientific merits.
- Mechanical ventilation is not without toxicities; therefore, every effort should be made to limit duration of ventilation.
- Positive pressure ventilation can impair cardiac output, resulting in diminished organ perfusion and drug elimination.

REFERENCES

1. Farrell PM, Avery ME. Hyaline membrane disease. Am Rev Respir Dis 1975;111:657–668.
2. Barker PM, Gowen CW, Lawson EE, Knowles MR. Decreased sodium ion absorption across nasal epithelium of very premature infants with respiratory distress syndrome. J Pediatr 1997;130:373–377.
3. O'Bradovich HM. The role of active Na^+ transport by lung epithelium in the clearance of airspace fluid. New Horiz 1995;3:240–247.
4. Gerdes JS. Assessment of lung maturity. In: Spitzer AR, ed. Intensive Care of the Fetus and Newborn. St. Louis, Mosby-Year Book, 1996: 130–134.
5. Boyle RJ, Oh W. Respiratory distress syndrome. Clin Perinatol 1978;5:287–297.
6. Novy MJ, McGregor JA, Iams JD. New perspectives on the prevention of extreme prematurity. Clin Obstet Gynecol 1995;38:790–808.
7. Leonardi MR, Hankins GDV. What's new in tocolytics. Clin Perinatol 1992:19:367–384.
8. Kierse MJ. New perspectives for the effective treatment of preterm labor. Am J Obstet Gynecol 1995;173:618–628.
9. NH Consensus Panel. Effect of corticosteroids for fetal maturation on perinatal outcomes. JAMA 1995;273;413–418.
10. Gardner MO, Goldenberg RL. The clinical use of antenatal corticosteroids. Clin Obstet Gynecol 1995;38:746–754.
11. ACTOBAT Study Group. Australian Collaborative Trial of Antenatal Thyrotropin-Releasing Hormone (ACTOBAT) for prevention of neonatal respiratory disease. Lancet 1995;345:877–882.
12. Crowther CA, Hiller JE, Studs DS, et al. Australian Collaborative Trial of Antenatal Thyrotropin-Releasing Hormone: Adverse effects at 12-month follow-up. Pediatrics 1997;99:311–317.

13. Goldsmith JP, Karotkin EH. Assisted Ventilation of the Neonate, 3rd ed. Philadelphia, Saunders, 1996.
14. Kresch MJ, Lin WH, Thrall RS. Surfactant replacement therapy. Thorax 1996;51:1137–1154.
15. Jobe AH. Pulmonary surfactant therapy. N Engl J Med 1993;328: 861–868.
16. Zola EM, Gunkel JH, Chan RK, et al. Comparison of three dosing procedures for administration of bovine surfactant to neonates with respiratory distress syndrome. J Pediatr 1993;122:453–459.
17. Veda T, Ikegami M, Rider ED, Jobe AH. Distribution of surfactant and ventilation in surfactant-treated preterm lambs. J Appl Physiol 1994; 76:45–55.
18. Lewis JF, Tabor B, Ikegami M, et al. Lung function and surfactant distribution in saleine-lavaged sheep given instilled vs. nebulized surfactant. J Appl Physiol 1993;74:1256–1264.
19. Pramanik AK, Holtzman RB, Merritt TA. Surfactant replacement therapy for pulmonary diseases. Pediatr Clin North Am 1993;40: 913–936.
20. OSIRIS. Early v. delayed neonatal administration of a synthetic surfactant—the judgment of OSIRIS. Lancet 1992;340:1363–1369.
21. Berry DD, Pramanik AK, Phillips JB, et al. Comparison of the effect of three doses of a synthetic surfactant on the alveolar–arterial oxygen gradient in infants weighing ≥ 1250 grams with respiratory distress syndrome. J Pediatr 1994;124:294–301.
22. Dunn MS, Shennan AT, Possmayer F. Single- versus multiple-dose surfactant replacement therapy in neonates of 30 to 36 weeks gestation with respiratory distress syndrome. Pediatrics 1990;86:564–570.
23. Konishi M, Fujiwara T, Naito T, et al. Surfactant replacement therapy in neonatal respiratory distress syndrome. A multicentre randomized clinical trial: Comparison of high- versus low-dose of surfactant-TA. Eur J Pediatr 1988;147:20–25.
24. Speer CP, Robertson B, Curstedt T, et al. Randomized European Multicenter Trial of Surfactant Replacement Therapy for Severe Neonatal Respiratory Distress Syndrome: Single versus multiple doses of Curosurf. Pediatrics 1992;89:13–20.
25. Halliday HL, Tarnow-Mordi WO, Corcoran JD, Paterson CC. Multicentre randomized trial comparing high and low dose surfactant regimens for the treatment of respiratory distress syndrome (the Curosurf 4 trial). Arch Dis Child 1993;69:276–280.
26. Gotner L, Pohlandt F, Bartmann P, et al. High-dose versus low-dose bovine surfactant treatment in very premature infants. Acta Paediatr 1994;83:135–141.
27. Sobel DB, Carroll A. Postsurfactant slump: Early prediction of neonatal chronic lung disease? J Perinatol 1994;14:268–274.
28. Hudak ML, Martin DJ, Egan EA, et al. A multicenter randomized, masked comparison trial of natural versus synthetic surfactant for the treatment of respiratory distress syndrome. Pediatrics 1997;100: 39–50.
29. Kendig JW, Natter RH, Cox C, et al. A comparison of surfactant as immediate prophylaxis and as rescue therapy in newborns of less than 30 weeks gestation. N Engl J Med 1991;324:865–871.
30. Survanta® (beractant) Package Insert, April 1995 (Ross Products Division, Abbott Laboratories).
31. Spafford PS, Kendig JW, Maniscalco WM. Use of natural surfactants to prevent and treat respiratory distress syndrome. Semin Perinatol 1993;17:285–294.
32. Rajo TNK, Langenberg P. Pulmonary hemorrhage and exogenous surfactant therapy: A meta-analysis. J Pediatr 1995;123:603–610.
33. Hudak ML, Martin DJ, Egan EA, et al. A multicenter randomized masked comparison trial of synthetic surfactant versus calf lung surfactant extract in the prevention of neonatal respiratory distress syndrome. J Pediatr 1996;128:396–406.
34. Harbor JD, Wright LL, Soll RF, et al. A multicenter randomized trial comparing two surfactants for the treatment of neonatal respiratory distress syndrome. J Pediatr 1993;123:757–766.
35. Vermont-Oxford Neonatal Network. A multicenter, randomized trial comparing synthetic surfactant with modified bovine surfactant extract in the treatment of neonatal respiratory distress syndrome. Pediatrics 1996;97:1–6.
36. Tarnow-Mardi WO, Soll RF. Artificial versus natural surfactant—Can we base clinical practice on a firm scientific footing? Eur J Pediatr 1994;153(suppl):17–21.
37. Bloom BT, Kattwinkel J, Hall RT, et al. Comparison of Infasurf (calf lung surfactant extract) to Survanta (beractant) in the treatment of respiratory distress syndrome. Pediatrics 1997;100:31–38.
38. Speer CP, Gofeller O, Groneck P, et al. Randomized clinical trial of two treatment regimens of natural surfactant preparations in neonatal respiratory distress syndrome. Arch Dis Child 1995;72:8–13.
39. Schwartz RM, Luby AM, Scalon JW, et al. Effect of surfactant on morbidity, mortality, and resource use in newborn infants weighing 500 to 1500 g. N Engl J Med 1994;330:913–936.
40. Soll RF, Jacobs J, Pashko S, Thomas R. Cost effectiveness of beractant in the prevention of respiratory distress syndrome. Pharmaco Economics 1993;4:278–286.
41. Maniscalco WM, Kendig JW, Shapiro DL. Surfactant replacement therapy: Impact on hospital charges for premature infants with respiratory distress syndrome. Pediatrics 1989;83:1–6.
42. Gal P, Reed MD, Nahata MC. Recent advances in pediatrics. Ann Pharmacother 1995;29:66–70.
43. Leach CL, Greenspan JS, Rubenstein SD. Partial liquid ventilation with perflubron in premature infants with severe respiratory distress syndrome. N Engl J Med 1996;335:761–767.
44. Wolfson MR, Greenspan JS, Shaffer TH. Pulmonary administration of vasoactive substances by perfluorochemical ventilation. Pediatrics 1996;97:449–455.
45. Tarczy-Hornoch P, Hildebrandt J, Mates EA. Effects of exogenous surfactant on lung pressure–volume characteristics during liquid ventilation. J Appl Physiol 1996;80:1764–1771.
46. Anderson TJ, Meredith IT, Ganz P, et al. Nitric oxide and nitrovasocilators: Similarities, differences and potential interactions. J Am Coll Cardiol 1994;24:555–566.
47. Skimming JW, Bender KA, Hutchison AA, Drummond WH. Nitric oxide inhalation in infants with respiratory distress syndrome. J Pediatr 1997;130:225–30.
48. Jacqz-Aigrain E, Burtin P. Clinical pharmacokinetics of sedatives in neonates. Clin Pharmacokinet 1996;31:423–443.
49. Quinn MVV, Wild J, Dean HG, et al. Randomised double-blind controlled trial of effect of morphine on catecholamine concentrations in ventilated pre-term babies. Lancet 1993;342:324–327.
50. Orsini AJ, Leef KH, Costarino A, et al. Routine use of fentanyl infusions for pain and stress reduction in infants with respiratory distress syndrome. J Pediatr 1996;129:140–145.
51. Green T. The use of diuretics in infants with respiratory distress syndrome. Semin Perinatol 1982;6:172–180.
52. Ashbaugh DG, Bigelow DB, Petty TL, Levine B. Acute respiratory distress in adults. Lancet 1967;2:319–23.
53. Bernard GR, Artigas A, Brigham KL, et al. The American–European Consensus Conference on ARDS. Am J Respir Crit Care Med 1994; 149:818–824.
54. Knaus WA, Sun X, Hakim RB, Wagner DP. Evaluation of definitions for adult respiratory distress syndrome. Am J Respir Crit Care Med 1994;150:311–317.
55. Garber BG, Hebert PC, Yelle JD, et al. Adult respiratory distress syndrome: A systematic overview of incidence and risk factors. Crit Care Med 1996;24:687–695.
56. Doyle RL, Szaflarski N, Modin GW, et al. Indentification of patients with acute lung injury. Am J Respir Crit Care Med 1995;152: 1818–1824.
57. Bell R, Coalson JJ, Smith JD, Johanson WG. Multiple organ system failure and infection in adult respiratory distress syndrome. Ann Intern Med 1983;99:293–8.
58. Fowler AA, Hamman RF, Zerbe GO, et al. Adult respiratory distress syndrome: Prognosis after onset. Am Rev Respir Dis 1985;98: 472–478.

59. McHugh LG, Milberg JA, Whitcomb ME, et al. Recovery of function in survivors of the acute respiratory distress syndrome. Am J Respir Crit Care Med 1994;150:90–94.
60. Hudson LD, Milberg JA, Anardi D, Maunder RJ. Clinical risks for development of the acute respiratory distress syndrome. Am J Respir Crit Care Med 1995;151:293–301.
61. Watling SM, Yanos J. Acute respiratory distress syndrome. Ann Pharmacother 1995;29:1002–1009.
62. Knaus WA, Wagner DP. Multiple systems organ failure: Epidemiology and prognosis. Crit Care Clin 1989;5:221–232.
63. Curtis S, Cain S. Regional and systemic oxygen delivery/uptake relations and lactate flux in hyperdynamic endotoxin-treated dogs. Am Rev Respir Dis 1992;145:348–354.
64. Danek SJ, Lynch JP, Weg JG, Dantzker DR. The dependence of oxygen uptake on oxygen delivery in the adult respiratory distress syndrome. Am Rev Respir Dis 1980;122:387–395.
65. Phang PT, Cunningham KF, Ronco JJ, et al. Mathematical coupling explains dependence of oxygen consumption on oxygen delivery in ARDS. Am Rev Respir Crit Care Med 1994; 150:318–323.
66. Simmons RS, Berdine GG, Seidenfeld JJ, et al. Fluid balance and the adult respiratory distress syndrome. Am Rev Respir Dis 1987; 135:924–929.
67. Matthay MA, Wiener-Kronish JP. Intact epithelial barrier function is critical for the resolution of alveolar edema in humans. Am Rev Respir Dis 1990;142:1250–1257.
68. Montgomery AB, Stagber MA, Carrico CJ, Hudson LD. Causes of mortality in patients with the adult respiratory distress syndrome. Am Rev Respir Dis 1985;132:485–489.
69. Watling SM, Dasta JF. Prolonged paralysis in intensive care unit patients after the use of neuromuscular blocking agents: A review of the literature. Crit Care Med 1994;22:884–893.
70. Smythe MA, Zarowitz BJ. Changing perspectives of stress gastritis prophylaxis. Ann Pharmacother 1994;28:1073–1085.
71. Bonten MJM, Gaillard CA, Geest SVD, et al. The role of intragastric acidity and stress ulcer prophylaxis on colonization and infection in mechanically ventilated ICU patients. Am J Respir Crit Care Med 1995;152:1825–1834.
72. Koretz RL. Nutritional supplementation in the ICU. Am J Respir Crit Care Med 1995;151:570–573.
73. Bonten MJM, Bergmans DC, Ambergen AW, et al. Risk factors for pneumonia and colonization of respiratory tract and stomach in mechanically ventilated ICU patients. Am J Respir Crit Care Med 1996;154:1339–1346.
74. Torres A, El-Ebiary M, Padro L, et al. Validation of different techniques for the diagnosis of ventilator-associated pneumonia. Am J Crit Care Med 1994;149:324–331.
75. Timsit JF, Chevret S, Valcke J, et al. Mortality of nosocomial pneumonia in ventilated patients: Influence of diagnostic tools. Am J Respir Crit Care Med 1996;154:116–123.
76. deLatorre FJ, Pont T, Ferrer A, et al. Pattern of tracheal colonization during mechanical ventilation. Am J Respir Crit Care Med 1995; 152:1028–1033.
77. Fagon J, Chastre J, Domart Y, Trouillet J, Gibert C. Mortality due to ventilator-associated pneumonia or colonization with pseudomonas or acinetobacter species: Assessment by quantitative culture of samples obtained by a protected specimen brush. Clin Infect Dis 1996;23: 538–542.
78. Bryce E, Smith J. Focused microbiological surveillance and gram-negative beta-lactamase mediated resistance in an intensive care unit. Infect Control Hosp Epidemiol 1995;16:331–334.
79. Mermel LA, Maki DG. Infectious complications of Swan-Ganz pulmonary artery catheters. Am Rev Respir Crit Care Med 1994;149: 1020–1036.
80. Pemberton LB, Ross V, Cuddy P, et al. No difference in catheter sepsis between standard and antiseptic central venous catheters. Arch Surg 1996;131:986–989.
81. Hasaniya NWA, Angelis M, Brown MR, Yu M. Efficacy of subcutaneous silver-impregnanted cuffs in preventing central venous catheter infections. Chest 1996;109:1030–1032.
82. Perkins MW, Dasta JF, DeHaven B. Physiologic implications of mechanical ventilation on pharmacokinetics. Ann Pharmacother 1989; 23:316–323.
83. Pepe PE, Hudson LD, Carrico CJ. Early application of positive end-expiratory pressure in patients at risk for the adult respiratory-distress syndrome. N Engl J Med 1984;311:281–286.
84. Marini JJ, Kelsen SG. Re-targeting ventilatory objectives in adult respiratory distress syndrome. Am Rev Respir Dis 1992;146:2–3.
85. Donahoe MP, Rogers RM. An anecdote is an anecdote. Am J Respir Crit Care Med 1994;149:293–294.
86. Moores RR, Abman SH. Bronchopulmonary dysplasia: Persistent cardiopulmonary sequelae of neonatal respiratory distress and its treatment. Semin Respir Med 1990;11:140–151.
87. Davis JM, Rosenfield WN, Richter SE, et al. Safety and pharmacokinetics of multiple doses of recombinant human CuZn superoxide dismutase administered intratracheally to premature neonates with respiratory distress syndrome. Pediatrics 1997;100:24–30.
88. Jackson JC, Truog WE, Standaert TA, et al. Reduction in lung injury after combined surfactant and high-frequency ventilation. Am J Respir Crit Care Med 1994;150:534–539.
89. Anzueto A, Baughman RP, Guntupali KK, et al. Aerosolized surfactant in adults with sepsis-induced acute respiratory distress syndrome. N Engl J Med 1996;334:1417–1421.
90. Gregory TJ, Steinberg KP, Spragg R, et al. Bovine surfactant therapy for patients with acute respiratory distress syndrome. Am J Respir Crit Care Med 1997;155:1309–1315.
91. Zapol WM, Rimar S, Gillis N, et al. Nitric oxide and the lung. Am Rev Respir Crit Care Med 1994;149:1375–1380.
92. Brett SJ, Evans TW. Inhaled vasodilator therapy in acute lung injury: First, do NO harm? Thorax 1995;50:821–823.
93. Krafft P, Fridrich P, Fitzgerald RD, et al. Effectiveness of nitric oxide inhalation in septic ARDS. Chest 1996;109:486–493.
94. Hudson LD. New therapies for ARDS. Chest 1995;108:79S–91S.
95. Putterman C. Use of corticosteroids in the adult respiratory distress syndrome: A clinical review. J Crit Care 1990;5:241–251.
96. Aberle DR, Wiener-Kronish JP, Webb WR, Matthay MA. Hydrostatic versus increased permeability pulmonary edema: Diagnosis based on radiographic criteria in critically ill patients. Radiology 1988;168: 73–79.

27

DRUG-INDUCED PULMONARY DISEASES

Patricia L. Marshik, PharmD, and H. William Kelly, PharmD, FCCP, BCPS

The manifestations of drug-induced pulmonary diseases span the entire spectrum of pathophysiologic conditions of the respiratory tract. As with most drug-induced diseases, the pathologic changes are nonspecific. Therefore, the diagnosis is often difficult and, in most cases, is based on exclusion of all other possible causes. In addition, the true incidence of drug-induced pulmonary disease is difficult to assess as a result of the pathologic nonspecificity and the interaction between the underlying disease state and the drugs.

Considering the physiologic and metabolic capacity of the lung, it is surprising that drug-induced pulmonary disease is not more common. The lung is the only organ of the body that receives the entire circulation. In addition, the lung contains a heterogeneous population of cells capable of various metabolic functions, including *N*-alkylation, *N*-dialkylation, *N*-oxidation, reduction of *N*-oxides, and *C*-hydroxylation.

Evaluation of epidemiologic studies on adverse drug reactions provides a perspective of the importance of drug-induced pulmonary disease. In a 2-year prospective survey of a community-based general practice, 41% of 817 patients experienced adverse drug reactions.[1] Four patients, or 0.5% of the total respondents, experienced adverse respiratory symptoms. Respiratory symptoms occurred in 1.2% of patients experiencing adverse drug reactions. A surveillance study of 3181 general pediatric outpatients receiving 4244 courses of drug therapy reported adverse reactions in 473 (11.1%) of the courses.[2] Of these, only 200 were considered definite or probably related to the drug. Gastrointestinal symptoms, skin reactions, and central nervous system (CNS) symptoms made up 96.5% of the reactions, with respiratory symptoms included with all other reactions.

Adverse pulmonary reactions are uncommon in the general population, but are among the most serious reactions, often requiring intervention. In a study of 270 adverse reactions leading to hospitalization from two populations, 3.0% were respiratory in nature.[3] Of the reactions considered to be life threatening, 12.3% were respiratory. An early report on death caused by drug reactions from the Boston Collaborative Drug Surveillance Program indicated that 7 of 27 drug-induced deaths were respiratory in nature.[4] This was confirmed in a follow-up study in which 6 of 24 drug-induced deaths were respiratory in nature.[5]

DRUG-INDUCED APNEA

Apnea may be induced by CNS depression or respiratory neuromuscular blockade (Table 27–1). Patients with chronic obstructive airway disease, alveolar hypoventilation, and chronic carbon dioxide retention have an exaggerated respiratory depressant response to narcotic analgesics and sedatives. In addition, the injudicious administration of oxygen in patients with carbon dioxide retention can remove their hypoxic ventilatory drive, producing apnea.[6] Although the benzodiazepines are touted as causing less respiratory depression than barbiturates, they may produce a profound additive or synergistic effect when taken in combination with other respiratory depressants. Combining intravenous diazepam with phenobarbital to stop seizures in an emergency department frequently results in admissions to an intensive care unit (ICU) for a short period of assisted mechanical ventilation, regardless of the drug administration rate. Too rapid intravenous administration of any of the benzodiazepines, even without coadministration of other respiratory depressants, will result in apnea. The risk appears to be the same for the various available agents (diazepam, lorazepam, midazolam). Respiratory depression and arrests resulting in death and hypoxic encephalopathy have occurred following rapid intravenous administration of midazolam for conscious sedation prior to medical procedures. This has been reported more commonly in the elderly and the chronically debilitated or in combination with opioid analgesics.

Prolonged apnea may follow administration of any of the neuromuscular blocking agents for surgery, particularly in patients with hepatic or renal dysfunction. In addition, persistent neuromuscular blockade and muscle weakness has been reported in critically ill patients receiving neuromuscular blockers continuously for more than 2 days to facilitate mechanical ventilation.[7] This has resulted in delayed weaning from mechanical ventilation and prolonged ICU stays. The prolonged neuromuscular blockade has been principally confined to pancuronium and vecuronium in patients with renal disease. Both agents have pharmacologic active metabolites that are renally excreted. The persistent muscular weakness is less well defined but appears to represent an acute myopathy.[7] High-dose corticosteroids appear to produce a synergistic effect, supported by animal studies showing that corticosteroids at dosages greater than or equal to 2 mg/kg/d prednisone produce atrophy in denervated muscle. The fluorinated corticosteroids (e.g., triamcinolone) appear to be more myopathic. Dose-dependent respiratory muscle weakness has been reported in chronic obstructive pulmonary disease (COPD) and asthma patients receiving repeated short courses of oral prednisone in the previous 6 months.

TABLE 27–1. Drugs That Induce Apnea

Central Nervous System Depression	
Narcotic analgesics	F[a]
Barbiturates	F
Benzodiazepines	F
Other sedative and hypnotics	I
Tricyclic antidepressants	R
Phenothiazines	R
Ketamine	R
Promazine	R
Anesthetics	R
Antihistamines	R
Alcohol	I
Fenfluramine	R
L-Dopa	R
Oxygen	R
Respiratory Muscle Dysfunction	
Aminoglycoside antibiotics	I
Polymyxin antibiotics	I
Neuromuscular blockers	I
Quinine	R
Digitalis	R
Myopathy	
Corticosteroids	F
Diuretics	I
Aminocaproic acid	R
Clofibrate	R

[a]Relative frequency of reactions: F = frequent; I = infrequent; R = rare.

Respiratory failure has been known to occur following local spinal anesthesia. Apnea from respiratory paralysis and rapid respiratory muscle fatigue has followed the administration of polymyxin and aminoglycoside antibiotics.[6] The mechanism appears to be related to the complexation of calcium and its depletion at the myoneural junction. Intravenous calcium chloride has been variably effective in reversing the paralysis.[6] The aminoglycosides competitively block neuromuscular junctions. This has resulted in life-threatening apnea when neomycin, gentamicin, streptomycin, or bacitracin have been administered into the peritoneal and pleural cavities.[6] The aminoglycosides will produce an additive blockade and ventilatory paralysis with curare or succinylcholine and in patients with myasthenia gravis or myasthenic syndromes.[6] Intravenous administration of aminoglycosides has resulted in respiratory failure in babies with infantile botulism. The treatment consists of ventilatory support and administration of an anticholinesterase agent (neostigmine or edrophonium).[6]

DRUG-INDUCED BRONCHOSPASM

Bronchoconstriction is the most common drug-induced respiratory problem. Bronchospasm can be induced by a wide variety of drugs through a number of disparate pathophysiologic mechanisms (Table 27–2). Regardless of the pathophysiologic mechanism, drug-induced bronchospasm is almost exclusively a problem of patients with preexisting bronchial hyperreactivity (e.g., asthma, chronic obstructive lung disease).[8] By definition, all patients with nonspecific bronchial hyperreactivity will experience bronchospasm if given sufficiently high doses of cholinergic or anticholinesterase agents. Severe asthmatics with a high degree of bronchial reactivity may wheeze following the inhalation of a number of particulate substances, such as the lactose in cromolyn (by Spinhaler) or corticosteroids, presumably through direct stimulation of the central airway irritant receptors. Other pharmacologic mechanisms for inducing bronchospasm include β_2-receptor blockade and nonimmunologic histamine release from mast cells and basophils.[8] A wide variety of agents are capable of producing bronchospasm through immunoglobulin (IgE)–mediated reactions.[8] These drugs can become a significant occupational hazard for pharmacists, nurses, and pharmaceutical industry workers.[8]

ASPIRIN-INDUCED BRONCHOSPASM

Aspirin sensitivity or intolerance occurs in 4% to 20% of all asthmatics.[9] The frequency of aspirin-induced bronchospasm increases with age. Patients older than 40 years have a frequency approximately four times that of patients younger than 20 years.[9] The frequency increases to 14% to 23% in patients with nasal polyps.[9] Women predominate over men, and there is no evidence for a genetic or familial predisposition.[10]

TABLE 27–2. Drugs That Induce Bronchospasm

Anaphylaxis (IgE-Mediated)		**Anaphylactoid Mast-Cell Degranulation**	
Penicillins	F[a]	Narcotic analgesics	I
Sulfonamides	F	Ethylenediamine	R
Serum	F	Iodinated-radiocontrast media	F
Cephalosporins	F	Platinum	R
Bromelin	R	Local anesthetics	I
Cimetidine	R	Steroidal anesthetics	I
Papain	F	Iron–dextran complex	I
Pancreatic extract	I	Pancuronium bromide	R
Psyllium	I	Benzalkonium chloride	I
Subtilase	I	**Pharmacologic Effect**	
Tetracyclines	I	β-Adrenergic receptor blockers	I–F
Allergen extracts	I	Cholinergic stimulants	I
L-Aspariginase	F	Anticholinesterases	R
Pyrazolone analgesics	I	α-Adrenergic agonists	R
Direct Airway Irritation		Ethylenediamine tetraacetic acid (EDTA)	R
Acetate	R	**Unknown Mechanisms**	
Bisulfite	F	ACE inhibitors	I
Cromolyn	R	Anticholinergics	R
Smoke	F	Hydrocortisone	R
N-Acetylcysteine	F	Isoproterenol	R
Inhaled steroids	I	Monosodium glutamate	I
Precipitating IgG Antibodies		Piperazine	R
α-Methyldopa	R	Tartrazine	R
Carbamazepine	R	Sulfinpyrazone	R
Spiramycin	R	Zinostatin	R
Cyclooxygenase Inhibition		Losartan	R
Aspirin/NSAIDs	F		
Phenylbutazone	I		
Acetaminophen	R		

[a]Relative frequency of reactions: F = frequent; I = infrequent; R = rare.

The classic description of the aspirin-intolerant asthmatic includes the triad of severe asthma, nasal polyps, and aspirin intolerance. The typical patient experiences intense vasomotor rhinitis, which may or may not be associated with aspirin exposure, beginning during the third or fouth decade of life.[11] Over a period of months, nasal polyps begin to appear, followed by severe asthma exacerbated by aspirin. Bronchospasm typically begins within minutes to hours following ingestion of aspirin and is associated with rhinnorhea, flushing of the head and neck, and conjunctivitis.[11] The reactions are severe and often life threatening.

All aspirin-sensitive asthmatics do not fit the classic "aspirin triad" picture and not all patients with asthma and nasal polyps develop sensitivity to aspirin.[10] In most cases, aspirin-sensitive asthmatics are clinically indistinguishable from the general population of asthmatics except for their intolerance to aspirin and other nonsteroidal anti-inflammatory drugs (NSAIDs).

PATHOGENESIS

Aspirin-induced asthma is correctly classified as an idiosyncratic reaction in that the pathogenesis is still unknown. Patients with aspirin intolerance have increased plasma histamine concentrations after ingestion of aspirin and elevated peripheral eosinophil counts.[10,11] All attempts to define an immunologic mechanism have been unsuccessful. Chemically similar drugs such as salicylamide and choline salicylate do not cross-react, whereas a large number of chemically dissimilar NSAIDs do produce reactions.[10,11] Table 27–3 lists the analgesics that do and do not cross-react with aspirin.

The currently accepted hypothesis of aspirin-induced asthma is that aspirin intolerance is integrally related to inhibition of cyclooxygenase. This is supported by the following evidence: (1) All NSAIDs that inhibit cyclooxygenase produce reactions; (2) the degree of cross-reactivity is proportional to the potency of cyclooxygenase inhibition; and (3) each patient with aspirin sensitivity has a threshold dose for precipitating bronchospasm that is specific for the degree of cyclooxygenase inhibition produced and, once established, the dose of another cyclooxygenase inhibitor needed to induce bronchospasm can be estimated.[11]

The mechanism by which cyclooxygenase inhibition produces bronchospasm in susceptible individuals is unknown. Arachidonic acid metabolism through the 5-lipoxygenase pathway may lead to the excess production of leukotrienes (LTs) C_4 and D_4.[12] LTC_4, LTD_4, and LTE_4 produce bronchospasm and promote histamine release from mast cells,[11] whereas the administration of leukotriene receptor antagonists and 5-lipoxygenase inhibitors ablate the pulmonary and nonpulmonary responses to aspirin in aspirin-sensitive asthmatics.[12] The precise mechanism by which augmented leukotriene production occurs is unknown, and available hypotheses do not explain why only a small number of asthmatic patients react to aspirin and NSAIDs.

TABLE 27–3. Tolerance of Anti-Inflammatory and Analgesic Drugs in Aspirin-Induced Asthma

Cross-Reactive Drugs	Drugs With No Cross-Reactivity
Diclofenac	Acetaminophen[a]
Diflunisal	Benzydamine
Fenoprofen	Chloroquine
Flufenamic acid	Choline salicylate
Flurbiprofen	Corticosteroids
Hydrocortisone hemisuccinate	Dextropropoxyphene
Ibuprofen	Phenacetin[a]
Indomethacin	Salicylamide
Ketoprofen	Sodium salicylate
Mefenamic acid	
Naproxen	
Noramidopyrine	
Oxyphenbutazone	
Phenylbutazone	
Piroxicam	
Sulindac	
Sulphinpyrazone	
Tartrazine	
Tolmetin	

[a]A very small percentage (5%) of aspirin-sensitive patients react to acetaminophen and phenacetin.

DESENSITIZATION

Patients with aspirin sensitivity can be desensitized. The ease of desensitization correlates with the sensitivity of the patient.[11] Highly sensitive patients who initially react to less than 100 mg of aspirin require multiple rechallenges to produce desensitization.[10] Desensitization usually persists for 2 to 5 days following discontinuance, with full sensitivity reestablished within 7 days.[10] Cross-desensitization has been established between aspirin and all NSAIDs tested to date. Because patients may experience life-threatening reactions, desensitization should be attempted only in a controlled environment by personnel with expertise in handling these patients. In addition, there have been reports of patients who have failed to maintain a desensitized state despite continued aspirin administration.[10] The chronic asthma symptoms have markedly improved in a number of aspirin-sensitive asthmatics who have undergone desensitization.[10]

CROSS-SENSITIVITY WITH FOOD AND DRUG ADDITIVES

Up to 80% of aspirin-sensitive asthmatics will have an adverse reaction to the yellow azo dye tartrazine (FD&C Yellow No. 5), which is widely used for coloring foods, drinks, drugs, and cosmetics.[9] However, those studies reporting high cross-reactivity were poorly controlled and often used only subjective criteria.[9,13] In double-blind placebo-controlled trials using pulmonary-function testing, sensitivity to tartrazine has proven to be a rare event.[13] Tartrazine sensitivity appears to occur only in aspirin-intolerant patients at a prevalence of 2%.[13]

Reactions to other azo dyes, monosodium glutamate (MSG), parabens, and non–azo dyes have been reported much less frequently than reactions to tartrazine and have been equally difficult to confirm with controlled challenges.[13] Positive reactions to sodium benzoate, a food preservative, have been reported in as many as 23% of aspirin-sensitive individuals.[9] Acetaminophen is a weak inhibitor of cyclooxygenase. As such, approximately 5% of aspirin-sensitive asthmatics will experience reactions to acetaminophen.[9] Most aspirin-sensitive asthmatics can use acetaminophen as a safe alternative to aspirin. Sporadic cases of worsening bronchospasm and anaphylaxis have been reported in aspirin-sensitive asthmatics receiving intravenous hydrocortisone succinate but have not been reported with the use of other corticosteroids.[10] It is not known whether it is the hydrocortisone or the succinate that is the problem.

▶ TREATMENT: Aspirin-Sensitive Asthma

Therapy of aspirin-sensitive asthmatics takes one of two general approaches: desensitization or avoidance. Avoidance of triggering substances seldom alters the clinical course of patients' asthma. The therapy of asthma has been nonspecific; however, the availability of 5-lipoxygenase inhibitors such as zileuton or leukotriene antagonists should provide specific therapy. Many of these patients require chronic steroid therapy to control the asthma. The respiratory symptoms can be decreased but not prevented by pretreatment with antihistamines and cromolyn.[10]

β-BLOCKERS

β-Adrenergic receptor blockers comprise the other large class of drugs that can be hazardous to the asthmatic. Even the more cardioselective agents such as acebutolol, atenolol, and metoprolol have been reported to cause asthma attacks.[8] Asthmatics may take nonselective and β_1-selective blockers without incident for long periods; however, the occasional reports of fatal asthma attacks resistant to therapy with β-agonists should provide ample warning of the dangers inherent in β-blocker therapy.[8]

If a patient with bronchial hyperreactivity requires β-blocker therapy, one of the relatively selective β_1-blockers (acebutolol, atenolol, metoprolol, or pindolol) should be used at the lowest possible dose. Two newer agents, celiprolol and betaxolol, appear to possess greater cardioselectivity than currently marketed drugs.[14] Fatal status asthmaticus has occurred with the topical administration of the nonselective timolol maleate ophthalmic solution for the treatment of open-angle glaucoma.[15] Early investigations with ophthalmic betaxolol suggest that it is well tolerated even in timolol-sensitive asthmatics.[16]

SULFITES

Severe, life-threatening asthmatic reactions following restaurant meals and wine have occurred secondary to ingestion of the food preservative potassium metabisulfite.[13] Sulfites have been used for centuries as preservatives in wine and food. As antioxidants, they prevent fermentation of wine and discoloration of fruits and vegetables caused by contaminating bacteria.[17] Previously sulfites had been given generally-recognized-as-safe (GRAS) status by the Food and Drug Administration (FDA). Sensitive patients react to concentrations ranging from 5 to 100 mg, amounts that are routinely consumed by anyone eating in restaurants. Consumption of sulfites in U.S. diets is estimated to be 2 to 3 mg/d in the home with 5 to 10 mg per 30 mL of beer or wine consumed.[13] Anaphylactic or anaphylactoid reactions to sulfites in nonasthmatics is extremely rare. In the general asthmatic population, reactions to sulfites are uncommon. Approximately 5% of steroid-dependent asthmatics demonstrate a sensitivity to sulfiting agents, but the prevalence is only around 1% in non–steroid-dependent asthmatic patients.[17]

Mechanism

The mechanism by which sulfites induce asthma is still unknown. The inhalation of 1 to 5 ppm (parts per million) sulfur dioxide produces bronchoconstriction in all asthmatics through direct stimulation of afferent parasympathetic irritant receptors.[17] When So_2 comes in contact with water, it forms H_2So_3, which dissociates to H and HSo_3. It is unknown whether So_2 or HSo_3 is the asthmagenic stimulus. On oral ingestion of metabisulfites, less than 10% of all asthmatics will develop bronchospasm. It has been postulated that sulfite-sensitive asthmatics have an inability to clear a sulfite load normally and therefore the sulfite accumulates.[13,17] At the air–fluid surface of the bronchial mucosa, HSo_3 ions associate with water to form H_2So_3 and So_2. A reduced concentration of sulfite oxidase enzyme (the enzyme that catalyzes oxidation of sulfites to sulfates) compared with normals has been demonstrated in a group of sulfite-sensitive asthmatics.[13] There has been no correlation between sulfite sensitivity and sensitivity to cyclooxygenase inhibitors.

A number of pharmacologic agents contain sulfites as preservatives and antioxidants. The FDA now requires warning labels on drugs containing sulfites. Most manufacturers of drugs for the treatment of asthma have discontinued the use of sulfites. In addition, labeling is required on packaged foods that contain sulfites at 10 ppm or more, and sulfiting agents are no longer allowed on fresh fruits and vegetables (excluding potatoes) intended for sale.

Pretreatment with cromolyn, anticholinergics, and cyanocobalamin have protected sulfite-sensitive patients.[18] Presumably, pharmacologic doses of vitamin B_{12} catalyze the nonenzymatic oxidation of sulfite to sulfate.

OTHER PRESERVATIVES

Both ethylenediamine tetraacetic acid (EDTA) and benzalkonium chloride used as bacteriostatic and stabilizing agents, respectively, can produce bronchoconstriction.[19] In addition to producing bronchoconstriction, EDTA potentiates the bronchial responsiveness to histamine.[19] These effects are presumably mediated through calcium chelation by EDTA. Benzalkonium chloride is more potent than EDTA and its mechanism appears to be a result of mast-cell degranulation and stimulation of irritant C fibers in the airways.[19]

The bronchoconstriction from benzalkonium chloride can be blocked by cromolyn but not the anticholinergic ipratropium bromide.[20] Benzalkonium chloride is found in the commercial multiple-dose nebulizer preparations of ipratropium bromide and beclomethasone diproprionate found in the United Kingdom and Europe and is presumed to be in part responsible for paradoxical wheezing following administration of these agents.[19,20] Benzalkonium chloride is also found in albuterol nebulizer solutions marketed in the United States and has been implicated as a possible cause of paradoxical wheezing in infants receiving this preparation.[19] However, β_2-agonists are potent mast-cell stabilizers, and the anecdotal reports have not yet been confirmed with controlled investigations.[19,20]

CONTRAST MEDIA

Iodinated-radiocontrast materials are the most common cause of anaphylactoid reactions producing bronchospasm.[21] The reader is referred to Chapter 81, Allergic and Pseudoallergic Drug Reactions, for a discussion of this topic.

ANGIOTENSIN-CONVERTING ENZYME INHIBITOR–INDUCED COUGH

Cough has become a well-recognized side effect of angiotensin-converting enzyme (ACE) inhibitor therapy. According to spontaneous reporting by patients, cough occurs in 1% to 10% of patients receiving ACE inhibitors, with a preponderance of females. Studies specifically evaluating cough caused by ACE inhibitors have reported prevalences of 19% to 25%.[22,23] Patients receiving ACE inhibitors had a 2.3 times greater likelihood of developing cough than a similar group of patients receiving diuretics.[22] Patients with hyperreactive airways do not appear to be at greater risk.[24] Cough occurs with all ACE inhibitors.[24]

The cough typically is dry and nonproductive, persistent, and not paroxysmal.[24] The cough can begin within 3 days or have a delayed onset of up to 12 months following initiation of ACE inhibitor therapy.[24] The cough remits within 1 to 4 days of discontinuing therapy but, rarely, can last up to 4 weeks and recur with rechallenge.[24] The chest x-ray is normal as are pulmonary function tests (spirometry and diffusing capacity). Bronchial hyperreactivity, as measured by histamine and methacholine provocation, may be worsened in patients with underlying bronchial hyperreactivity such as asthma and chronic bronchitis. However, bronchial hyperreactivity is not induced in others.[24,25] The cough reflex to capsaicin is enhanced but not to nebulized distilled water or citric acid.[24]

The mechanism of ACE inhibitor–induced cough is still unknown. ACE is a nonspecific enzyme that also catalyzes the hydrolysis of bradykinin and substance P (see Chap. 24) that produce or facilitate inflammation and stimulate lung irritant receptors.[24] ACE inhibitors may also induce cyclooxygenase to cause the production of prostaglandins. NSAIDs, benzonatate, inhaled bupivacaine, theophylline, and cromolyn sodium have all been used to suppress or inhibit ACE inhibitor–induced cough.[24,26] The cough is generally not responsive to cough suppressants or bronchodilator therapy. Patients should be given a 4-day withdrawal to determine if the cough is ACE inhibitor induced. The preferred therapy is withdrawal of the ACE inhibitor and replacement with an alternative antihypertensive agent. Owing to its decrease in ACE inhibitor–induced side effects, losartan, an AT_1 receptor antagonist, is often recommended in place of an ACE inhibitor; however, there are rare reports of this agent inducing bronchospasm.[27] The use of alternative therapies to treat ACE inhibitor–induced cough is not generally recommended.[24]

PULMONARY EDEMA

Pulmonary edema may result from the failure of any of a number of homeostatic mechanisms. The most common cause of pulmonary edema is an increase in capillary hydrostatic pressure because of left ventricular failure. Excessive fluid administration in compromised and noncompromised cardiovascular patients is the most frequent cause of iatrogenic pulmonary edema. Besides hydrostatic forces, other homeostatic mechanisms that may be disrupted include the osmotic and oncotic pressures in the vasculature, the integrity of alveolar epithelium, interstitial pulmonary pressure, and the interstitial lymph flow.[6] The edema fluid in cardiogenic pulmonary edema contains a low amount of protein, whereas noncardiogenic pulmonary edema fluid has a high protein concentration.[6] This indicates that noncardiogenic pulmonary edema results primarily from disruption of the alveolar epithelium.

The clinical presentation of pulmonary edema includes persistent cough, tachypnea, dyspnea, tachycardia, rales on auscultation, hypoxemia from ventilation–perfusion imbalance and intrapulmonary shunting, widespread fluffy infiltrates on chest roentgenogram, and decreased lung compliance (stiff lungs). Noncardiogenic pulmonary edema may progress to hemorrhage; cellular debris collects in the alveoli followed by hyperplasia and fibrosis with a residual restrictive mechanical defect.[6]

NARCOTIC-INDUCED PULMONARY EDEMA

The most common drug-induced noncardiogenic pulmonary edema is produced by the narcotic analgesics (Table 27–4).[6] Narcotic-induced pulmonary edema is most commonly associated with intravenous heroin use but has also occurred with morphine, methadone, meperidine, and propoxyphene use.[6,28] There have also been two reported cases associated with the use of the opiate agonist naloxone.[26] The mechanism is unknown but may be related to hypoxemia similar to the neurogenic pulmonary edema associated with cerebral tumors or trauma, or a direct toxic effect on the alveolar capillary membrane.[28] Initially thought to occur only with overdoses, most evidence now supports the theory that narcotic-induced pulmonary edema is an idiosyncratic reaction to moderate as well as high narcotic doses.[28]

TABLE 27–4. Drugs That Induce Pulmonary Edema

Cardiogenic Pulmonary Edema	
Excessive intravenous fluids	F[a]
Blood and plasma transfusions	F
Corticosteroids	F
Phenylbutazone	R
Sodium diatrizoate	R
Hypertonic intrathecal saline	R
β_2-Adrenergic agonists	I
Noncardiogenic Pulmonary Edema	
Heroin	F
Methadone	I
Morphine	I
Oxygen	I
Propoxyphene	R
Ethchlorvynol	R
Chlordiazepoxide	R
Salicylate	R
Hydrochlorothiazide	R
Triamterene + hydrochlorothiazide	R
Leukoagglutinin reactions	R
Iron–dextran complex	R
Methotrexate	R
Cytosine arabinoside	R
Nitrofurantoin	R
Dextran 40	R
Fluorescein	R
Amitriptyline	R
Colchicine	R
Nitrogen mustard	R
Epinephrine	R
Metaraminol	R
Bleomycin	R
Iodide	R
Cyclophosphamide	R
VM-26	R

[a]Relative frequency of reactions: F = frequent; I = infrequent; R = rare.

Patients with pulmonary edema may be comatose with depressed respirations or dyspnea and tachypnea. They may or may not have other signs of narcotic overdose. Symptomology varies from cough and mild crepitations on auscultation with characteristic radiologic findings to severe cyanosis and hypoxemia even with supplemental oxygen. Symptoms may appear within minutes of intravenous administration, but may take up to 2 hours to occur, particularly following oral methadone.[28] Hemodynamic studies in the first 24 hours have demonstrated normal pulmonary capillary wedge pressures in the presence of pulmonary edema.

Clinical symptoms generally improve within 24 to 48 hours and radiologic clearing occurs in 2 to 5 days, but abnormalities in pulmonary-function tests may persist for 10 to 12 weeks. Therapy consists of naloxone administration, supplemental oxygen, and ventilatory support if required. Mortality is less than 1%.[28]

OTHER DRUGS THAT CAUSE PULMONARY EDEMA

Noncardiogenic pulmonary edema has also been associated with the oral and intravenous administration of ethchlorvynol.[28] A parodoxical pulmonary edema has been reported in a few patients following hydrochlorothiazide ingestion but not any other benzothiazide diuretic.[6] Acute pulmonary edema has rarely followed the injection of high concentrations of contrast medium into the pulmonary circulation during angiocardiography.[6] Rare occurrences of pulmonary edema have followed the intravenous administration of bleomycin, cyclophosphamide, and vinblastine.[6]

The selective β_2-adrenergic agonists terbutaline and ritodrine have been reported to induce pulmonary edema when used as tocolytics.[6] This has never occurred with their use in asthma patients, even in inadvertent overdosage. This reaction may result from excess fluid administration used to prevent the hypotension from β_2-mediated vasodilation or the particular hemodynamics of pregnancy.

Pulmonary edema has occasionally occurred with salicylate overdoses. The serum salicylate concentrations are often greater than 45 mg/dL and the patients have other signs of toxicity, although some cases have been associated with concentrations in the usual therapeutic range.[28]

PULMONARY EOSINOPHILIA

Pulmonary infiltrates with eosinophilia (Loeffler's syndrome) have been associated with nitrofurantoin, para-aminosalicylic acid, methotrexate, sulfonamides, tetracycline, chlorpropamide, phenytoin, NSAIDs, and imipramine (Table 27–5).[6,29] The disorder is characterized by fever, nonproductive cough, dyspnea, cyanosis, bilateral pulmonary infiltrates, and eosinophilia in the blood.[6] Lung biopsy has revealed perivasculitis with infiltration of

TABLE 27–5. Drugs That Induce Pulmonary Infiltrates With Eosinophilia (Loeffler's Syndrome)

Nitrofurantoin	F[a]	Tetracycline	R
para-Aminosalicylic acid	F	Procarbazine	R
Sulfonamides	I	Cromolyn	R
Penicillins	I	Niridazole	R
Methotrexate	I	Gold salts	R
Imipramine	I	Chlorpromazine	R
Chlorpropamide	R	Naproxen	R
Carbamazepine	R	Sulindac	R
Phenytoin	R	Ibuprofen	R
Mephenesin	R		

[a]Relative frequency of reactions: F = frequent; I = infrequent; R = rare.

eosinophils, macrophages, and proteinaceous edema fluid in the alveoli. The symptoms and eosinophilia generally respond rapidly to withdrawal of the offending drug.

Sulfonamides were first reported as causative agents in users of sulfanilamide vaginal cream.[6] Para-aminosalicylic acid frequently produced the syndrome in tuberculosis patients being treated with this agent.[6] There have been nine reported cases associated with sulfasalazine use in inflammatory bowel disease.[29] The drug most frequently associated with this syndrome is nitrofurantoin.[6,28] Nitrofurantoin-induced lung disorders appear to be more common in postmenopausal women.[28] Lung reactions made up 43% of 921 adverse reactions to nitrofurantoin reported to the Swedish Adverse Drug Reaction Committee between 1966 and 1976.[29] No apparent correlation exists between duration of drug exposure and severity or reversibility of the reaction.[29] Most cases occur within 1 month of therapy. Typical symptoms include fever, tachypnea, dyspnea, dry cough, and, less commonly, pleuritic chest pain. Radiographic findings include bilateral interstitial infiltrates, predominant in the bases and pleural effusions 25% of the time. Although there are anecdotal reports that steroids are beneficial, the usual rapid improvement following discontinuation of the drugs brings their utility into question. Complete recovery usually occurs within 15 days of withdrawal.

A few cases of pulmonary eosinophilia have been reported in asthmatics treated with cromolyn.[6,29] The significance of this is unknown in light of the occasional spontaneous occurrence of pulmonary eosinophilia in asthmatic patients. Cases of acute pneumonitis and eosinophilia have been reported to occur with phenytoin and carbamazepine therapy.[29] Patients have had other symptoms of hypersensitivity including fever and rashes. The symptoms of dyspnea and cough subside following discontinuation of the drug.

OXYGEN TOXICITY

Because of the similarity to pulmonary fibrosis, oxygen-induced lung toxicity is briefly reviewed. More extensive reviews on this topic have been published.[30,31]

The earliest manifestation of oxygen toxicity is substernal pleuritic pain from tracheobronchitis.[31] The onset of toxicity follows an asymptomatic period and presents as cough, chest pain, and dyspnea. Early symptoms are usually masked in ventilator-dependent patients. The first noted physiologic change is a decrease in pulmonary compliance caused by reversible atelectasis. Then decreases in vital capacity occur, followed by progressive abnormalities in carbon monoxide–diffusing capacity (DLCO).[31] Decreased inspiratory flow rates, reflected in the need for high inspiratory pressures in ventilator-dependent patients, occur as the fractional concentration of inspired oxygen (FiO_2) requirement increases. The lungs become progressively stiffer as the ability to oxygenate becomes more compromised.

The FiO_2 and duration of exposure are both important determinants of the severity of lung damage. Normal human volunteers can tolerate 100% oxygen at sea level for 24 to 48 hours with minimal to no damage.[30] Oxygen concentrations of less than 50% are well tolerated even for extended periods. Inspired oxygen concentrations between 50% and 100% carry a substantial risk of lung damage and the duration required is inversely proportional to the FiO_2.[29] Underlying disease states may alter this relationship.

Oxygen-induced lung damage is generally separated into the acute exudative phase and the subacute or chronic proliferative phase. The acute phase consists of perivascular, peribronchiolar, interstitial, and alveolar edema with alveolar hemorrhage and necrosis of pulmonary endothelium and type I epithelial cells.[30] The proliferative phase consists of resorption of the exudates and hyperplasia of interstitial and type II alveolar lining cells. Collagen and elastin deposition in the interstitium of alveolar walls then leads to thickening of the gas-exchange area and the fibrosis.[30]

The biochemical mechanism of the tissue damage during hyperoxia is the increased production of highly reactive, partially reduced oxygen metabolites (Fig. 27–1).[31] These

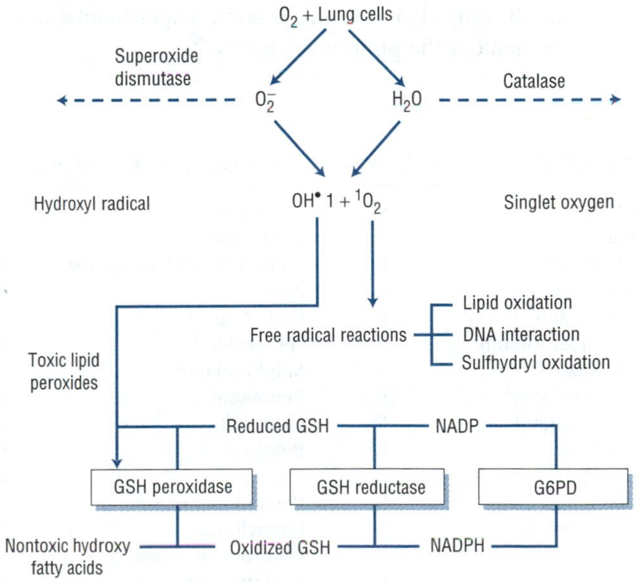

FIGURE 27–1. Schematic of the interaction of oxygen radicals and the antioxidant system. GSH, glutathione; G6PD, glucose-6-phosphate dehydrogenase; NADP = nicotinamide-adenine dinucleotide phosphate; NADPH = reduced NADP.

oxidants are normally produced in small quantities during cellular respiration and include the superoxide anion (O_2), hydrogen peroxide (H_2O_2), the hydroxyl radical (OH^-), singlet oxygen ($^1O_2$), and hypochlorous acid (HOCl).[31] Oxygen free radicals are normally formed in phagocytic cells to kill invading microorganisms, but they are also toxic to normal cell components. The oxidants produce toxicity through destructive redox reactions with protein sulfhydryl groups, membrane lipids, and nucleic acids.[31]

The oxidants are products of normal cellular respiration that are normally counterbalanced by an antioxidant defense system that prevents tissue destruction. The antioxidants include superoxide dismutase, catalase, glutathione peroxidase, ceruloplasmin, and α-tocopherol (vitamin E). Antioxidants are ubiquitous in the body. Hyperoxia produces toxicity by overwhelming the antioxidant system. There is experimental evidence that a number of drugs and chemicals produce lung toxicity through increasing production of oxidants (e.g., bleomycin, cyclophosphamide, nitrofurantoin, paraquat) and/or by inhibiting the antioxidant system (e.g., carmustine, cyclophosphamide, nitrofurantoin).[32,33]

PULMONARY FIBROSIS

A large variety of drugs have been associated with chronic pulmonary fibrosis with or without a preceding acute pneumonitis (Table 27–6). The cancer chemotherapeutic agents make up the largest group and have been the subject of numerous reviews.[32,33] Although the mechanisms by which all of the drugs produce pneumonitis and/or fibrosis are not known, the clinical syndrome, pulmonary function abnormalities, and histopathology present a relatively homogeneous pattern.[32] The histopathologic picture closely resembles oxidant lung damage and in some experimental cases oxygen enhances the pulmonary injury.[32]

TABLE 27–6. Drugs That Induce Pneumonitis and/or Fibrosis

Oxygen	F[a]	Chlorambucil	R
Radiation	F	Melphalan	R
Bleomycin	F	Lomustine and semustine	R
Busulfan	F	Zinostatin	R
Carmustine	F	Procarbazine	R
Hexamethonium	F	Teniposide	R
Paraquat	F	Sulphasalazine	R
Amiodarone	F	Phenytoin	R
Mecamylamine	I	Gold salts	R
Pentolinium	I	Pindolol	R
Cyclophosphamide	I	Imipramine	R
Practolol	I	Penicillamine	R
Methotrexate	I	Phenylbutazone	R
Mitomycin	I	Chlorphentermine	R
Nitrofurantoin	I	Fenfluramine	R
Methysergide	I		
Azathioprine, 6-mercaptopurine	R		

[a]Relative frequency of reactions: F = frequent; I = infrequent; R = rare.

TABLE 27–7. Possible Causes of Pulmonary Fibrosis

Idiopathic pulmonary fibrosis (fibrosing alveolitis)
Pneumoconiosis (asbestosis, silicosis, coal dust, talc berylliosis)
Hypersensitivity pneumonitis (molds, bacteria, animal proteins, toluene diisocyanate, epoxy resins)
Smoking
Sarcoidosis
Tuberculosis
Lipoid pneumonia
Systemic lupus erythematosus
Rheumatoid arthritis
Systemic sclerosis
Polymyositis/dermatomyositis
Sjögren's syndrome
Polyarteritis nodosa
Wegener's granuloma
Byssinosis (cotton workers)
Siderosis (arc welders' lung)
Radiation
Oxygen
Chemicals (thioureas, trialkylphosphorothioates, furans)
Drugs (see Tables 27–5, 27–6, and 27–8)

The lung damage following ingestion of the contact herbicide paraquat classically resembles hyperoxic lung damage. Hyperoxia accelerates the lung damage induced by paraquat. Lung toxicity from paraquat occurs following oral administration in man and aerosol administration and inhalation in experimental animals.[33] The pulmonary specificity of paraquat results in part from its active uptake into lung tissue. Paraquat readily accepts an electron from reduced nicotinamide-adenine dinucleotide phosphate (NADPH) and is then rapidly reoxidized, forming superoxide and other oxygen radicals.[33] The toxicity may be a result of NADPH depletion (see Fig. 27–1) and/or excess oxygen free radical generation with lipid peroxidation. Treatment with exogenous superoxide dismutase has had limited and conflicting results.[33]

A number of furans have been shown to produce oxidant injury to lungs.[33] Occasionally, patients with acute nitrofurantoin lung toxicity will progress to a chronic reaction leading to fibrosis, and rarely, a patient may develop chronic toxicity without an antecedent acute reaction. Like paraquat, nitrofurantoin undergoes cyclic reduction and reoxidation that may produce superoxide radicals or deplete NADPH. In addition, nitrofurantoin inhibits glutathione reductase, an enzyme involved in the glutathione antioxidant system (see Fig. 27–1). Table 27–7 provides a list of possible nondrug causes of pulmonary fibrosis.

DRUGS ASSOCIATED WITH PULMONARY FIBROSIS

ANTINEOPLASTICS

A number of cancer chemotherapeutic agents produce pulmonary fibrosis. In an excellent review,[32] six predisposing factors for the development of cytotoxic drug-induced pulmonary disease were described: (1) cumulative dose, (2) increased age, (3) concurrent or previous radiotherapy,

(4) oxygen therapy, (5) other cytotoxic drug therapy, and (6) preexisting pulmonary disease. Drugs that are directly toxic to the lung would be expected to show a dose–response relationship. Dose–response relationships have been established for bleomycin, busulfan, and carmustine (BCNU).[32] Bleomycin and busulfan exhibit threshold-cumulative doses below which a very small percentage of patients exhibit toxicity, but carmustine shows a more linear relationship.[33] Older patients appear to be more susceptible, possibly as a result of a decrease in the antioxidant defense system.

Excessive irradiation produces a pneumonitis and fibrosis thought to be caused by oxygen-radical formation.[32] Evidence for synergistic toxicity with radiation exists for bleomycin, busulfan, and mitomycin.[32] Hyperoxia has shown synergistic toxicity with bleomycin, cyclophosphamide, and mitomycin.[32] Carmustine, mitomycin, cyclophosphamide, bleomycin, and methotrexate all appear to show increased lung toxicity when they are part of multiple-drug regimens.

NITROSOUREAS

BCNU is associated with the highest incidence of pulmonary toxicity (20% to 30%).[32] The lung pathology generally resembles that produced by bleomycin and busulfan. Unique to BCNU is the finding of fibrosis in the absence of inflammatory infiltrates. BCNU preferentially inhibits glutathione reductase, the enzyme required to regenerate glutathione, thus reducing glutathione tissue stores.[32,33] The patients present with dyspnea, tachypnea, and nonproductive cough that may begin within a month of initiation of therapy but may not develop for as long as 3 years.[32] A more recent report suggested that most patients receiving BCNU develop fibrosis that may remain asymptomatic or become symptomatic any time up to 17 years after therapy.[34] The cumulative dose has ranged from 580 to 2100 mg/m^2.[30] The disease is usually slowly progressive with a mortality rate from 15% to greater than 90% depending on the study and period of follow-up. Rapid progression and death within a few days occur in a small percentage of patients.[32] Corticosteroids do not appear to be effective in reducing damage.[32] Other nitrosoureas, lomustine and semustine, have also been reported to produce lung damage in patients receiving unusually high doses.[32]

BLEOMYCIN

Bleomycin is the best studied cytotoxic pulmonary toxin. Because of its lack of bone marrow suppression, pulmonary toxicity is the dose-limiting toxicity of bleomycin therapy. The cumulative dose above which the incidence of toxicity significantly increases is 450 to 500 units.[32] However, rapidly fatal pulmonary toxicity has occurred with doses as low as 100 units.[32]

Experimentally, bleomycin generates superoxide anions, and the lung toxicity is increased by radiation and hyperoxia.[32] Pretreatment with superoxide dismutase and catalase reduces toxicity in experimental animals.[32] Bleomycin also oxidizes arachidonic acid, which may account for the marked inflammation. Bleomycin may also affect collagen deposition by its stimulation of fibroblast growth.[32] Combination of bleomycin with other cytotoxic agents, particularly regimens containing cyclophosphamide, may predispose patients to pulmonary damage.

There are two distinct clinical patterns of bleomycin pulmonary toxicity. Chronic progressive fibrosis is the most common; acute hypersensitivity reactions occur infrequently. Patients present with cough and dyspnea. The first physiologic abnormality seen is a decreased DLco.[32] Chest radiographs show a bibasilar reticular pattern, and gallium scans show marked uptake in the involved lung.[32] Chest radiographic changes lag behind pulmonary function abnormalities. Spirometry tests before each bleomycin dose are not predictive of toxicity. The single-breath DLco is the most sensitive indicator of bleomycin-induced lung disease. Although it is not absolutely predictive, a drop of 20% or greater in the DLco is an indication for using alternative therapies.[32] Corticosteroid therapy appears to be helpful in patients with acute pneumonitis, although there have been no controlled trials. Patients with chronic fibrosis would be less likely to respond. Although corticosteroids have been used for a number of drug-induced pulmonary problems, a study in mice showing a potential for worsening of lung damage when administered early during the repair stage should sound a word of caution against their indiscriminate use.[35]

MITOMYCIN

Mitomycin is an alkylating antibiotic that produces pulmonary fibrosis at a frequency of 3% to 12%.[32] The mechanism is unknown, but oxygen and radiation therapy appear to enhance the development of toxicity.[32] The clinical presentation and symptoms are the same as for bleomycin. The mortality rate is about 50%. Early withdrawal of the drug and administration of corticosteroids appear to significantly improve the outcome.

ALKYLATING AGENTS

A number of alkylating agents have been associated with pulmonary fibrosis (see Table 27–5). The incidence of clinical toxicity is around 4%, although subclinical damage is apparent in up to 46% of patients at autopsy. The mechanism of toxicity is unknown; however, epithelial-cell damage that triggers the arachidonic acid inflammatory cascade may be the initiating event.[32] The clinical presentation is insidious, with 4 years being the average duration of therapy before the onset of symptoms.[32] Patients present with low-grade fever, weight loss, weakness, dyspnea, cough, and rales.[32] Pulmonary-function tests initially show abnormal diffusion capacity followed by a restrictive pattern (low vital capacity). The histopathologic findings are nonspecific. The prognosis is one of slow progression with a mean survival of 5 months following diagnosis.[32] Although there is no direct dose-dependent correlation, patients receiving less than 500 mg do not develop the syndrome without concomitant radiation or use of other pulmonary-toxic chemotherapeutic agents.[32] There are anecdotal reports of beneficial responses to corticosteroids, but no controlled studies have been done.

Cyclophosphamide infrequently produces pulmonary toxicity. More than 20 well-documented cases have been reported to date. In animal models, cyclophosphamide produces reactive oxygen radicals. High oxygen concentrations produce synergistic toxicity with cyclophosphamide. The duration of therapy before the onset of symptoms is highly variable, and there may be a delay of several months between the onset of symptoms and discontinuation of the drug.[32] Cyclophosphamide may potentiate carmustine lung toxicity.[32] Clinical symptoms usually consist of dyspnea on exertion, cough, and fever. Inspiratory crackles and the bibasilar reticular pattern typical of cytotoxic drug-induced radiographic changes are present. Histopathologic changes are also nonspecific. Approximately 60% of patients recover. Corticosteroid therapy has been reported to be beneficial; however, death despite corticosteroid administration has also been reported.

Chlorambucil, melphalan, and uracil mustard have also been associated with pulmonary fibrosis. Of the alkylating agents, only nitrogen mustard and thiotepa have not been reported to cause fibrotic pulmonary toxicity.[32]

ANTIMETABOLITES

Methotrexate was first reported to induce pulmonary toxicity in 1969.[32] The pulmonary toxicity to methotrexate is unique in that discontinuation is not always necessary and reinstitution of the drug may not produce recurrence of symptoms.[6] Methotrexate pulmonary toxicity most commonly appears to result from hypersensitivity.[29] Pulmonary edema and eosinophilia are common, and fibrosis occurs in only 10% of the patients who develop acute pneumonitis.[32] Systemic symptoms of chills, fever, and malaise are common before the onset of dyspnea, cough, and acute pleuritic chest pain. Methotrexate has also been associated with granuloma formation.[32]

The prognosis of methotrexate-induced pulmonary toxicity is good with a 1% or less mortality rate.[29] Pulmonary toxicity has followed intrathecal as well as oral administration, and has occurred after single doses as well as long-term daily and intermittent administration.[32] Pneumonitis has been reported to occur up to 4 weeks following discontinuation of therapy.[32] Numerous anecdotal reports have claimed dramatic benefit from corticosteroid therapy. It is unknown whether intermittent (weekly) dosing as is done for rheumatoid arthritis decreases the risk of methotrexate-induced pulmonary toxicity, and pneumonitis has occurred with this form of dosing.

Rarely, azathioprine and its major metabolite 6-mercaptopurine have been reported to produce an acute restrictive lung disease. Procarbazine, a methylhydrazine more commonly associated with Loeffler's syndrome, has rarely been associated with pulmonary fibrosis.[29] The vinca alkaloids, vinblastine and vindesine, have been reported to produce severe respiratory toxicity in association with mitomycin. The incidence with the combination is 39% and may represent a true synergistic effect between these agents.[32]

NONCYTOTOXIC DRUGS

Pulmonary fibrosis associated with the ganglionic-blocking agent hexamethonium was first reported in 1954 (see Table 27–6).[6] Patients developed extreme dyspnea after several months on the drug. Pathologic findings were consistent with bronchiectasis, bronchiolectasis, and fibrosis.[6] This phenomenon has occasionally occurred with the use of the other ganglionic blockers, mecamylamine and pentolinium.[6]

In 1959, radiographic changes characteristic of diffuse pulmonary fibrosis were reported in 87% of 31 patients who had taken phenytoin for 2 years or more.[28] Since then studies have been conflicting. If phenytoin does produce chronic fibrosis, it would appear to be a relatively rare event.

Gold salts (sodium aurothiomalate) used in the treatment of rheumatoid arthritis have produced pulmonary fibrosis with cough, dyspnea, and pleuritic pain 5 to 16 weeks following institution of therapy.[28] Pulmonary function tests show a restrictive defect, and patients generally have an eosinophilia. The reactions improve on discontinuation of the gold therapy and promptly recur on reexposure. The pulmonary deficit may not completely improve.

AMIODARONE

Amiodarone, a benzofuran derivative, produces pulmonary fibrosis when used for supraventricular and ventricular arrhythmias (see Table 27–6).[36] The duration of amiodarone therapy before the onset of symptoms has ranged from 4 weeks to 6 years.[28,36] The estimated incidence is 1 in 1000 to 2000 treated patients per year. The clinical course is variable, ranging from acute onset of dyspnea with rapid progression into severe respiratory failure and death caused by slowly developing exertional dyspnea over a few months. Patients generally improve on discontinuation of the drug.[36] The majority of patients develop reactions while taking maintenance doses greater than 400 mg daily.[36] Routine spirometry does not appear to be predictive for identifying patients at risk.[37] Carbon monoxide–diffusing capacity studies are sensitive indicators of amiodarone pulmonary toxicity but have only a 21% positive predictive value.[37] Clinical findings include exertional dyspnea, nonproductive cough, weight loss, and occasionally low-grade fever.[28,36] Radiographic changes are nondiagnostic and consist of diffuse bilateral interstitial changes consistent with a pneumonitis. Pulmonary function abnormalities include hypoxia, restrictive changes, and diffusion abnormalities.

The mechanism of amiodarone-induced pulmonary toxicity is unknown. Amiodarone is an amphiphilic molecule that contains both a highly apolar aromatic ring system and a polar side chain with a positively charged nitrogen atom.[36] Amphiphilic drugs characteristically produce a phospholipid storage disorder in the lungs of experimental animals and man.[33] Chlorphentermine, an anorectic, is the prototype amphiphilic compound. The mechanism is currently believed to be the inhibition of lysosomal phospholipases.[33] The inflammation and fibrosis are thought to be a late finding resulting from nonspecific inflammation following the breakdown of phospholipid-laden macrophages.[36]

In a review of 39 cases, 9 patients died and the remaining 30 patients had resolution of abnormalities after withdrawal of the drug.[36] Some patients have had resolution with lowering of the dosage, and therapy has been reinstituted at lower doses without problems in others. Of the patients who died, one-half received corticosteroids. There have been reports of a protective effect with prophylactic corticosteroids and other reports of patients developing amiodarone lung toxicity while on corticosteroids.[24] At this time, any benefit of corticosteroids is unclear because most patients improve on stopping the drug.

PULMONARY HYPERTENSION

Primary pulmonary hypertension (PPH) is a rare disorder, occurring with an approximate incidence of one to two cases per million in the general population.[38] With progression of the disease, right ventricular afterload increases and the ability to increase cardiac output with activity decreases. This progresses to right heart failure and death.[39]

Patients with PPH often complain of exertional dyspnea, chest pain, and syncope. Owing to the nonspecific nature of these symptoms and lack of a noninvasive diagnostic test for detecting PPH, there are often delays in the diagnosis of the disease, many times up to a year after the onset of symptoms.[39]

The factors leading to the development of PPH are unclear, although associations with portal hypertension and pregnancy have been detected. Additionally, the use of cocaine, oral contraceptives, infection with human immunodeficiency virus, and the use of anorexic agents[40] have also been implicated.

The first reports of the association between PPH and the use of anorexic agents occurred in the late 1960s and early 1970s[41,42] in Western Europe when the drug aminorex was used for weight reduction. The incidence of PPH returned to baseline after the drug was removed from the market. In the early 1990s, an association between fenfluramine use and PPH was established.[43] Shortly thereafter, the International Primary Pulmonary Hypertension Study Group investigated the potential role of anorexic agents in causing PPH.[40] Included in this multinational, case-control study were 95 patients with pulmonary hypertension and 355 controls from general practices, matched for gender and age. The use of anorexic agents, primarily fenfluramine and dexfenfluramine, within the last year was associated with an increased risk of PPH with an odds ratio of 10:1. When anorexic drugs were used for a total of more than 3 months, the odds ratio increased to 23:1.

The mechanism by which anorexic agents cause PPH is unknown. Studies have shown that fenfluramine, dexfenfluramine, and aminorex inhibit potassium channels in isolated pulmonary artery smooth muscle cells in rats, which results in vasoconstriction. Potassium channel activity is altered in pulmonary artery smooth muscle cells obtained from patients with PPH, leading to speculation that anorexic agents may cause vasoconstriction followed by vascular growth and remodeling.[39] Another potential mechanism involves serotonin, a pulmonary vasoconstrictor that has been found in increased levels in patients with PPH.[39]

Patients with PPH associated with anorexic use may experience a considerable improvement in their condition or possibly even remission following discontinuation of the drug.[44] Pharmacologic agents used in the treatment of PPH include vasodilators and anticoagulants.[38] Additionally, lung and heart–lung transplantations have played a role in the treatment of PPH.

In September 1997, the FDA requested the manufacturers of fenfluramine and dexfenfluramine to voluntarily withdraw their products from the market. This was done following case reports of valvular heart disease in patients taking either medication as monotherapy or in combination with another anorexic agent, phentermine. Because no association has been found between phentermine alone and valvular heart disease, it is still available. Isolated case reports of PPH and phentermine monotherapy have been reported[45,46]; however, present data do not support an association.

MISCELLANEOUS PULMONARY TOXICITY

Drugs may produce serious pulmonary toxicity as part of a more generalized disorder. The pleural thickening, effusions, and fibrosis that occur as an extension of the retroperitoneal fibrotic reactions of methysergide and practolol or as part of a drug-induced lupus syndrome are the most common examples (Table 27–8).

Methysergide therapy for prophylaxis of poorly controlled migraine headache occasionally results in pulmonary toxicity associated with pleural effusions. The patients develop pleural pain, dyspnea, and fever. Chest radiography reveals a uniform hazy shadowing over the lower lung fields, and a loud pleural rub is heard on auscultation.[6] The mechanism is unknown and most patients improve with discontinuation of the drug. Pleural and pulmonary fibrosis has been reported in one patient taking pindolol, a β-blocker structurally similar to practolol, an agent known to produce fibrosis.[28] Acute pleuritis with pleural effusions and fibrosis is a prominent manifestation of drug-induced lupus syndrome. Procainamide is associated with the largest number of pulmonary reactions, with 46% of patients with the lupus syndrome developing pulmonary complications.[6] Symptoms include pleuritic pain and fever with muscle and joint

TABLE 27–8. Drugs That May Induce Pleural Effusions and Fibrosis

Idiopathic	
Methysergide	F[a]
Practolol	F
Pindolol	R
Methotrexate	R
Nitrofurantoin	R
Owing to Drug-Induced Lupus Syndrome	
Procainamide	F
Hydralazine	F
Isoniazid	R
Phenytoin	R
Mephenytoin	R
Griseofulvin	R
Trimethadione	R
Sulfonamides	R
Phenylbutazone	R
Streptomycin	R
Ethosuximide	R
Tetracycline	R
Pseudolymphoma Syndrome	
Cyclosporine	R
Phenytoin	R

[a]Relative frequency of reactions: F = frequent; I = infrequent; R = rare.

pain. Chest radiographs show bilateral pleural effusions and linear atelectasis. Patients have a positive antinuclear antibody (ANA) test. Symptoms usually resolve within 6 weeks of drug withdrawal.[6]

Hydralazine is the next most common cause of lupus syndrome. Most patients who develop pleuropulmonary manifestations have antecedent symptoms of generalized lupus.[6] Other drugs that produce the lupus syndrome include isoniazid and phenytoin. Phenytoin can also produce hilar lymphadenopathy as part of a generalized pseudolymphoma or lymphadenopathy syndrome.[6]

MONITORING THERAPEUTIC OUTCOMES

Monitoring for drug-induced pulmonary diseases consists primarily of having a high index of suspicion that a particular syndrome may be drug induced. Most hypersensitivity or allergic reactions (bronchospasm) occur rapidly, within the first 2 weeks of therapy with the offending agent and reverse rapidly with appropriate therapy (e.g., withdrawal of the offending agent, administration of corticosteroids and bronchodilators). Loeffler's syndrome and acute pulmonary edema syndromes also improve rapidly in 1 to 2 days for the dyspnea. However, some residual defect in diffusion capacity and roentgenogram may persist for a few weeks. It is probably unnecessary to do follow-up spirometry or diffusion capacity in these patients unless there is some concern that the syndrome will progress to pulmonary fibrosis (through use of bleomycin or nitrofurantoin).

The routine monitoring of patients receiving known pulmonary toxins with dose-dependent toxicity such as amiodarone, bleomycin, or carmustine is still controversial. For chronic fibrosis the DLco is the most sensitive test and may be useful in patients receiving bleomycin for detecting and preventing further deterioration of lung function with continued administration. Carmustine lung toxicity may be delayed up to 10 years following administration, and routine monitoring has not proven preventive. Monitoring patients every 4 to 6 months receiving amiodarone in doses greater than 400 mg daily may prove useful in detecting early disease that requires lowering the amiodarone dose or stopping the drug. Because there is no evidence of a cumulative dose effect once it has been established that the patient can tolerate the elevated dose, continued routine monitoring past the first year is unnecessary.

REFERENCES

1. Martys CR. Adverse reactions to drugs in general practice. Br Med J 1979;2:1194–1197.
2. Kramer MS, Hutchinson TA, Flegel KM, et al. Adverse drug reactions in general pediatric outpatients. J Pediatr 1985;106:305–310.
3. Levy M, Kewitz H, Altwein W, et al. Hospital admissions due to adverse drug reactions: A comparative study from Jerusalem and Berlin. Eur J Clin Pharmacol 1980;17:25–31.
4. Shapiro S, Slone D, Lewis GP, et al. Fatal drug reactions among medical inpatients. JAMA 1971;216:467–472.
5. Porter J, Jick H. Drug-related deaths among medical inpatients. JAMA 1977;237:879–881.
6. Brewis RAL. Respiratory disorders. In: Davies DM, ed. Textbook of Adverse Drug Reactions, 2nd ed. New York, Oxford University Press, 1981:154–178.
7. Hansen-Flaschen J, Cowen J, Raps EC. Neuromuscular blockade in the intensive care unit: More than we bargained for. Am Rev Respir Dis 1993;147:234–236.
8. Fisher HK. Drug-induced asthma syndromes. In: Weiss EB, Segal MS, Stein M, eds. Bronchial Asthma: Mechanisms and Therapeutics, 2nd ed. Boston, Little, Brown, 1985:938–949.
9. Settipane GA. Aspirin and allergic diseases: A review. Am J Med 1983;74(suppl 6a):102–109.
10. Stevenson DD. Diagnosis, prevention, and treatment of adverse reactions to aspirin and nonsteroidal antiinflammatory drugs. J Allergy Clin Immunol 1984;74:617–622.
11. Szczeklik A, Gryglewski RJ. Asthma and antiinflammatory drugs: Mechanisms and clinical patterns. Drugs 1983;25:533–543.
12. Lee TH. Mechanism of bronchospasm in aspirin-sensitive asthma. Am Rev Respir Dis 1993;148:1442–1443.
13. Mathison DA, Stevenson DD, Simon RA. Precipitating factors in asthma: Aspirin, sulfites, and other drugs and chemicals. Chest 1985; 87(suppl):50–54.
14. Riddell JG, Shanks RG. Effects of betaxolol, propranolol, and atenolol on isoproterenol-induced β-adrenoceptor responses. Clin Pharmacol Ther 1985;38:554–559.
15. Fraunfeder FT, Barker AF. Respiratory effects of timolol. N Engl J Med 1984;311:1441.
16. Dunn TL, Gerber MJ, Shen AS, et al. The effect of topical ophthalmic instillation of timolol and betaxolol on lung function in asthmatic subjects. Am Rev Respir Dis 1986;133:264–268.
17. Bush RK, Taylor SL, Busse W. A critical evaluation of clinical trials in reactions to sulfites. J Allergy Clin Immunol 1986;78:191–202.
18. Anibarro B, Caballero T, Garcia-Ara C, et al. Asthma with sulfite intolerance in children: A blocking study with cyanocobalamin. J Allergy Clin Immunol 1992;90:103–109.
19. Beasley R, Rafferty P, Holgate ST. Adverse reactions to the nondrug constituents of nebulizer solutions. Br J Clin Pharmacol 1988;25: 283–287.

20. Zhang YG, Wright WJ, Tam WK, et al. Effect of inhaled preservatives on asthmatic subjects II. Benzalkonium chloride. Am Rev Respir Dis 1990;141:1405–1408.
21. Greenberger PA. Contrast media reactions. J Allergy Clin Immunol 1984;74:600–605.
22. Sebastian JL, McKinney WP, Kaufman J, et al. Angiotensin-converting enzyme inhibitors and cough: Prevalence in an outpatient medical clinic population. Chest 1991;99:36–39.
23. Simon SR, Black HR, Moser M, Berland WE. Cough and ACE inhibitors. Arch Intern Med 1992;152:1698–1700.
24. Israili ZH, Hall WD. Cough and angioneurotic edema associated with angiotensin-converting enzyme inhibitor therapy: A review of the literature and pathophysiology. Ann Intern Med 1992;117:234–242.
25. Kaufman J, Casanova JE, Riendl P, et al. Bronchial hyperreactivity and cough due to angiotensin-converting enzyme inhibitors. Chest 1989;95:544–548.
26. Allen TL, Gora-Harper ML. Cromolyn sodium for ACE inhibitor–induced cough. Ann Pharmacother 1997;31:773–775.
27. Dicpinigaitis PV, Thomas SA, Sherman MB, et al. Losartan-induced bronchospasm. J Allergy Clin Immunol 1996; 98:1128–1130.
28. Cooper JAD, White DA, Matthay RA. Drug-induced pulmonary disease. Part 2: Noncytotoxic drugs. Am Rev Respir Dis 1986;133: 488–505.
29. Obermiller T, Lakshminarayan S. Drug-induced hypersensitivity reactions in the lung. Immunol Allergy Clin North Am 1991;11: 575–594.
30. Frank L, Massaro D. Oxygen toxicity. Am J Med 1980;69:117–126.
31. Jackson RM. Pulmonary oxygen toxicity. Chest 1985;88:900–905.
32. Cooper JAD, White DA, Matthay RA. State of the art: Drug-induced pulmonary disease. Part 1: Cytotoxic drugs. Am Rev Respir Dis 1986; 133:321–340.
33. Kehrer JP, Kacew S. Systematically applied chemicals that damage lung tissue. Toxicology 1985;35:251–293.
34. O'Driscoll BR, Hasleton PS, Taylor PM, et al. Active lung fibrosis up to 17 years after chemotherapy with carmustine (BCNU) in childhood. N Engl J Med 1990;323:378–382.
35. Kehrer JP, Klein-Szanto AJP, Sorensen EMB, et al. Enhanced acute lung damage following corticosteroid treatment. Am Rev Respir Dis 1984;130:256–261.
36. Rakita L, Sobol SM, Mostow N, et al. Amiodarone pulmonary toxicity. Am Heart J 1983;106:906–914.
37. Gleadhill IC, Wise RA, Schonfeld SA, et al. Serial lung-function testing in patients treated with amiodarone: A prospective study. Am J Med 1989;86:4–10.
38. Rubin LJ. Primary pulmonary hypertension. N Engl J Med 1997; 336:111–117.
39. McCann UD, Seiden LS, Rubin LJ, Ricaurte GA. Brain serotonin neurotoxicity and primary pulmonary hypertension from fenfluramine and dexfenfluramine. A systematic review of the evidence. JAMA 1997; 278;666–672.
40. Abenhaim L, Moride Y, Brenot F, et al. Appetite-suppressant drugs and the risk of primary pulmonary hypertension. N Engl J Med 1996; 335:609–616.
41. Gurtner HP. Aminorex and pulmonary hypertension. A review. Cor Vasa 1985;27:160–171.
42. Follath F, Burkart F, Schweizer W. Drug-induced pulmonary hypertension. BMJ 1971;1:265–266.
43. Brenot F, Herve P, Petitpretz P, et al. Primary pulmonary hypertension and fenfluaramine use. Br Heart J 1993;70:537–541.
44. Nall KC, Rubin LJ, Lipskind S, Sennesh JD. Reversible pulmonary hypertension associated with anorexigen use. Am J Med 1991; 91:97–99.
45. Heuer L, Benoit W, Heydrich D. Diagnostic error: Pulmonary hypertension caused by an appetite suppressant (Mirapront). Chir Praxis 1978;23:497–504.
46. Schnabel KF, Schultz V, Busch S, Just H. Drug-induced primary vascular pulmonary hypertension. Medizinische Welt (Stuttgart) 1976; 27:1300–1303.

28

Cystic Fibrosis

John A. Bosso, PharmD, FCCP, BCPS

Cystic fibrosis is the most common lethal, genetically inherited disease affecting the Caucasian population. It is a disease mainly involving the exocrine glands and thus affects a number of organs or organ systems (Table 28–1). The more common manifestations of the disease involve the gastrointestinal and pulmonary systems, with most of the observed morbidity and mortality associated with the latter. Most pathology is a result of production of viscous secretions. The underlying disorder leading to this pathophysiology is a chloride transport channel defect at the secretory epithelial-cell level. The protean nature of the disease dictates that care be multidisciplinary with a wide variety of therapeutic interventions.

EPIDEMIOLOGY

Cystic fibrosis is inherited through an autosomal (Mendelian) recessive genetic mode. This implies that each parent must be at least a carrier (heterozygous) for the trait and, with such a couple, each child would have a one-in-four chance of having the disease, a one-in-two chance of being a carrier, and a one-in-four chance of being normal (having neither the disease nor the trait). The incidence of cystic fibrosis is greatest in the Caucasian population, with a rate of 1 in 2000 live births in the United States.[1] The incidence of the trait (carrier state) in this group is about 5%. The frequency of the disease is considerably less in other races, occurring in 1 in 17,000 Blacks and about 1 in 90,000 Asians.[2]

After years of intensive research, the cystic fibrosis gene was discovered and cloned.[3–5] The protein (cystic fibrosis transmembrane regulator, or CFTR) encoded by this gene, which is on the long arm of chromosome 7, is a membrane protein that represents a channel involved in the transport of electrolytes and water. The most common genetic mutation associated with cystic fibrosis involves a 3-base pair deletion at position 508,[3–5] but over 700 cystic fibrosis–associated mutations within the gene have been described. The common mutation is referred to as the ΔF_{508} allele and is present in about 70% of patients. The possible mutations have been divided into four classes: I—defective protein production, II—defective protein processing, III—defective regulation, and IV—defective conduction.[6] Patients who are homozygous for the ΔF_{508} mutation, which falls into class II, tend to be diagnosed at an earlier age, owing to earlier onset of airway disease, and have a greater frequency of pancreatic insufficiency (99% vs 72% in heterozygotes and 36% in patients with other genotypes).[7,8]

PATHOPHYSIOLOGY

Cystic fibrosis is a disease of secretory epithelial cells or tissues involved with the transport of chloride, sodium, and water into and out of the blood. In the normal state, there is a net chloride transport out of blood, with sodium and water following this flux. This net secretion is activated or affected by hormones or neurotransmitters such as protein kinases and further involves intracellular second messengers such as cyclic adenosine 3′,5′-monophosphate (cAMP) or calcium.[9] It is an apical membrane cAMP-stimulated chloride channel where activity is apparently affected in cystic fibrosis, leading to a decrease in secretion of chloride and water and increased absorption of sodium (Fig. 28–1). ΔF_{508}-homozygous individuals have this abnormal chloride channel in the cells of several exocrine organs including pancreatic and hepatobiliary ducts, microvilli of the gastrointestinal tract, and the lungs. In pulmonary epithelial cells, there also appears to be excessive absorption of sodium. These phenomena then lead to the thick, dehydrated secretions or mucus, depending on the organ. These secretions can block pancreatic and hepatobiliary exocrine outflow and also accumulate in and obstruct the airways.

GASTROINTESTINAL TRACT

Involvement of the gastrointestinal tract in cystic fibrosis is a result of both the increased viscosity of mucus secretions and a relative deficiency of pancreatic digestive enzymes. In 10% to 16% of cystic fibrosis patients, the first gastrointestinal manifestation of the disease is an intestinal obstruction evident shortly after birth and is known as meconium ileus. Again, the basic electrolyte transport defect is involved, and this complication is caused by an inability of these patients to evacuate the abnormally viscid meconium. A similar condition, known as distal intestinal obstruction syndrome or meconium ileus equivalent, occurs in older cystic fibrosis patients; it is also thought to result from abnormally viscous gastrointestinal secretions and fecal impaction often following ingestion of fatty meals or nonadherence with pancreatic enzyme therapy. Other intestinal complications include intussusception, volvulus, gastroesophageal reflux, atresia, perforation, giant cystic meconium peritonitis, and rectal prolapse.

A deficiency of pancreatic digestive enzymes (pancreatic achylia) is present with most genotypes and thus is present in 85% of patients. Pancreatic lesions including fibrosis, fatty replacement, and cyst formation are secondary to obstruction of small pancreatic ducts by thickened

TABLE 28–1. Organ Involvement in Cystic Fibrosis

Organ System/Organ	Abnormality	Consequence
Gastrointestinal		
Pancreas	Digestive enzyme deficiency	Maldigestion Malnutrition
	Insulin deficiency	Glucose intolerance
Intestines	Viscous secretions	Obstruction
Liver	Biliary cirrhosis/fatty infiltration	Portal hypertension/esophageal varices
Pulmonary	Viscous secretions Infection	Chronic obstructive Endobronchial infection
Sweat glands	Failure to reabsorb sodium	Hyponatremia
Reproductive	Obstruction of epididymis, vas deferens, and seminal vesicles	Aspermia
	Viscous cervical mucus	Decreased fertility
Hematologic	Chronic disease?	Anemia
Bone and joint	Unknown	Arthritis, osteopenia

secretions and cellular debris. Inspissated eosinophilic material is also present in acini and ductules. As a result, pancreatic secretions are viscous and low in volume and in concentrations of pancreatic enzymes and bicarbonate. Affected enzyme concentrations include trypsin, chymotrypsin, carboxypeptidase, amylase, and lipase. This leads to a maldigestion of ingested nutrients, including fats and protein. Increased fecal loses of bile acids (binding to undigested fecal fat decreases enterohepatic recycling) also contributes to fat maldigestion.

Because of the lipase deficiency, fat-soluble vitamin (A, D, E, and K) deficiencies sometimes occur. Whether lipase is involved in fat-soluble vitamin absorption directly (e.g., in micelle formation) or indirectly, with continuing steatorrhea resulting in abnormally high losses of these nutrients in the feces, is unclear. Vitamin B_{12} and zinc deficiencies can also occur as a result of the pancreatic enzyme deficiency. Although pancreatic involvement is predominantly exocrine in nature, insulin deficiency/glucose intolerance occurs in many older cystic fibrosis patients. The carbohydrate intolerance observed is characterized by low insulin concentrations and enhanced peripheral sensitivity to insulin but not the presence of islet cell or anti-insulin antibodies nor by ketosis common to type 1 diabetes. This complication involves an increase in the number of insulin receptors with decreased affinity for insulin. Despite a concomitantly increased tissue affinity for insulin, 8% of cystic fibrosis children over 12 years of age require insulin therapy.

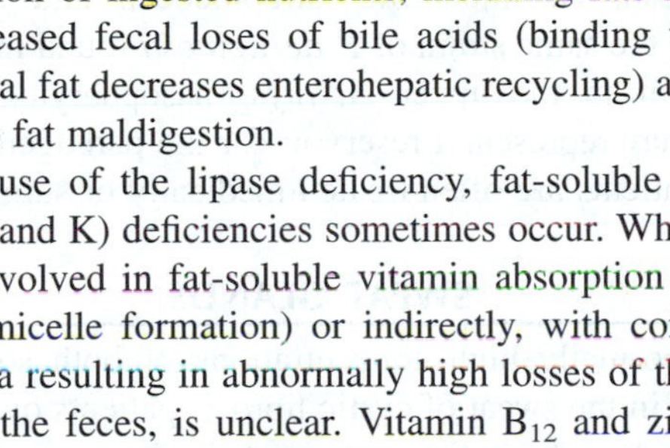

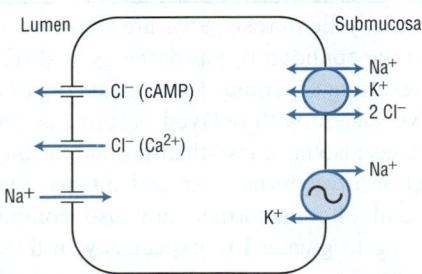

FIGURE 28–1. Electrolyte transport in the airway epithelial cell. CFTR is the cyclic-3′,5′-AMP (cAMP)-dependent chloride channel.

The liver is sometimes involved in cystic fibrosis. Biliary cirrhosis secondary to bile duct obstruction occurs in as many as 18% of patients, whereas fatty infiltration occurs in about 30% of patients in a pattern unrelated to nutritional status. Bile duct obstruction occurs with inspissated mucus and may lead to focal or multilobar cirrhosis.[10] Such hepatic involvement, which can occur at any age, is more common as the cystic fibrosis life span increases and can lead to portal hypertension and thus bleeding esophageal varices and hypersplenism. The most common laboratory abnormality associated with hepatic involvement is elevated serum alkaline phosphatase (hepatic isoenzyme).

PULMONARY SYSTEM

Manifestations within this organ system result from the accumulation of viscous mucus in the small airways. There are two important consequences of this pulmonary condition: obstruction and infection/inflammation. Obstruction of both small and large airways by thick mucus results in air trapping, bronchiectasis, and atelectasis resulting in a chronic obstructive pulmonary disease–like phenomenon. Thus, a progression of lung disease from small airway obstruction to large airway or generalized obstruction and finally to a restrictive lung disease component is evident. Hyperinflation or dilation of the air spaces is the common lesion. Further, the persistence of this same mucus is an excellent growth medium for microorganisms, and pulmonary infections are commonplace. Although systemic host defenses appear normal in cystic fibrosis, recent evidence suggests that local defenses in the airways (i.e., human β-defensin) are inhibited by the high salt concentrations present in respiratory secretions of affected patients[11] and that abnormal CFTR itself may contribute to susceptibility to infection with *Pseudomonas aeruginosa*.[12] Though bacterial infection is thought to be the major factor in this aspect of the respiratory disease, it is clear that viruses and other nonbacterial pathogens play an important pathologic role as well.[13–15] Environmental factors, such as exposure to tobacco smoke, also contribute.[16] The three most common bacterial pathogens isolated from the respiratory secretions (sputum) of cystic fibrosis patients are *Staphylococcus aureus, P. aeruginosa,* and *Haemophilus influenzae,* with *P. aeruginosa* predominating throughout life. *Proteus* and *Klebsiella* species and *Stenotrophomonas maltophilia* are observed much less frequently. Mucoid strains (alginate producers) of *P. aeruginosa* commonly observed in cystic fibrosis may be particularly resistant to antibiotics,[17] as are nonmotile forms. The isolation of *Burkholderia cepacia* from the sputum of cystic fibrosis patients has become more common at some cystic fibrosis centers. The significance of the presence of this highly contagious organism varies from one patient to the next. Three fairly distinct syndromes associated with this *B. cepacia* have been described, these being asymptomatic colonization, chronic deterioration with intermittent fever and weight loss, and rapid, usually fatal, deterioration.[18] The nature of the initially cultured oropharyngeal flora in patients less than 2 years of age has prognostic significance. The finding of *P. aeruginosa* or *P. aeruginosa* plus *S. aureus* in initial cultures appears related to increased morbidity and mortality, respectively.[19]

The presence of the above bacteria is responsible for a portion of the destructive changes to the lungs in cystic fibrosis owing to both direct damage from bacterial toxins and the body's immune reaction to the presence of these same bacteria. For example, *P. aeruginosa,* which elaborates a number of extracellular toxins, proteases, hemolysins, and exopolysaccharides, may be responsible for direct or indirect pulmonary damage, increases mucin production in respiratory epithelium, and stimulates the production of immune complexes (IgG and IgM), which may also contribute to local damage. Elevated levels of such mediators as granulocyte elastase, tumor necrosis factor-α, interleukin-1 and -2, and related complexes with associated inhibitors have been well documented in cystic fibrosis patients. One inflammatory mediator that clearly contributes to pulmonary pathophysiology is neutrophil elastase. Present in excess, it overwhelms and neutralizes native antiproteases (α_1-antitrypsin and secretory leukocyte protease inhibitor [SLPI]), destroys structural fibers, and inhibits complement-mediated phagocytosis and antipseudomonal antibodies. Combined with other inflammatory mediators, a self-sustaining, vicious cycle leading to progressive and often permanent tissue damage is established. The neutrophil influx that is part of this cycle results in release of neutrophil-derived DNA, which is thought to contribute to sputum viscosity. The occasional presence of *Aspergillus fumagatus* in the sputum of these patients may also contribute to the pulmonary pathology because it can induce a steroid-responsive, allergic reaction.

The major consequence of these pulmonary processes is a decrease in gas exchange by the lungs. The challenge of moving air into and out of such congested airways often requires the use of accessory muscles, resulting in an increased anterior–posterior chest diameter (also referred to as "barrel chest"), a flattened diaphragm, and pulmonary hypertension. The increased work of breathing in these patients produces a relative exercise intolerance and increased resting energy expenditure. Hemoptysis secondary to bronchiectasis occurs but is seldom massive. Other respiratory complications include gastroesophageal reflux, pneumothorax, and right-sided heart failure (cor pulmonale), secondary to the pulmonary hypertension. Although seldom overt clinically, findings such as right ventricular hypertrophy, increased heart weight, and right atrial and right ventricular chamber dilation are usually present at autopsy. Digital clubbing, a common finding in cystic fibrosis as well as other chronic pulmonary conditions, may be related to chronic hypoxia.

The upper respiratory tract is also involved and chronic rhinitis is common. Sinusitis and nasal polyposis occur in 90% and 50% of patients, respectively.[20] Sinusitis is chronic in character and acute symptoms are unusual. Although its etiology is not entirely clear, sinusitis may result from obstruction of the sinus ducts, thus preventing drainage. The bacteria generally isolated in these cases include *P. aeruginosa, H. influenzae,* streptococci, and anaerobes. Usually, the same strain of *P. aeruginosa* found in the lungs is present in the upper airways (nasopharynx, sinuses), which may represent a reservoir for the pathogen. Symptomatic patients are often treated medically or surgically.

SWEAT GLANDS

The abnormally high concentrations of both sodium and chloride in the sweat of cystic fibrosis patients owing to defective salt reabsorption can result in the need for supplementary dietary intake of these electrolytes and forms the basis for the diagnosis of the disease. Sodium and chloride are not excreted in abnormally high concentrations by the sweat glands. Instead, there is a failure of the sweat ducts to reabsorb these electrolytes in a normal fashion, again owing to the chloride impermeability in the epithelial cells of the sweat ducts. Similar abnormalities are seen in the excretions of the salivary glands.

REPRODUCTIVE SYSTEM

Of males with cystic fibrosis, 95% are sterile because of obstruction of the epididymis, vas deferens, and seminal vesicles, with resulting aspermia. There is late maturation of the reproductive system with delayed onset of puberty in both sexes. Females also have less-than-normal fertility owing to the production of abnormal cervical mucus. Menstrual irregularity and oligomenorrhea are also common. Nonetheless, owing to greater life expectancy in these patients, increasing numbers are becoming mothers. In these individuals, the course and tolerance of pregnancy are related to pregravid nutritional and pulmonary status.

HEMATOLOGIC SYSTEM

Anemia is observed in some cystic fibrosis patients despite chronic hypoxia. The apparent deficient erythroid response occurs, at least in part, from disturbances in erythropoietin regulation and iron availability (impaired gastrointestinal absorption). Despite the chronic hypoxia characteristic of cystic fibrosis, erythropoietin concentrations are normal or low. The condition is characterized by decreased hematocrit and serum ferritin, increased carboxyhemoglobin, and normal or low hemoglobin. Vitamin E concentrations are usually normal. Many patients have documentable iron deficiency, the causes of which appear to include decreased dietary intake, malabsorption, and blood loss.

BONE AND JOINT

Arthritis occurs in cystic fibrosis patients and can take one of several forms.[21] This arthritis may be either mono- or polyarticular and is usually nondestructive. An episodic form is most common and may be due to immune complexes formed in response to the chronic pulmonary infections. Hypertrophic osteoarthropathy occurs in cystic fibrosis as it does in association with other pulmonary diseases. The incidence of arthritis may be increasing as median survival age increases. Osteopenia and osteoporosis also occur with abnormally high frequency in adult cystic fibrosis patients. The causes of the resultant bone demineralization are multifactorial and include vitamin D malabsorption and decreased vitamin conversion (via sunlight), delayed puberty and endocrine development, poor nutrition, limited physical activity, and chronic acidosis.

CLINICAL PRESENTATION

The clinical findings of cystic fibrosis occur as direct consequences of the pathophysiologic processes described above. Thus, the clinical findings can be conveniently subdivided by organ system.

GASTROINTESTINAL SYSTEM

Intestinal symptomatology is secondary to obstruction and maldigestion of nutrients. Obstruction, manifested as meconium ileus or distal intestinal obstruction syndrome, causes symptoms such as vomiting of bile-stained material, abdominal distention, and pain. Pain may be an especially prominent feature when obstruction results in intussusception.

The more frequent gastrointestinal clinical presentation is caused by maldigestion of ingested food, resulting in steatorrhea and malnutrition. Stools are characterized by their foul smell, bulk, greasy nature, and abnormally high number per day; they may precipitate rectal prolapse. The stool's high fat content results from the relative lipase deficiency. Perhaps the most significant consequence of maldigestion is malnutrition; cystic fibrosis children characteristically fall below age-related norms for both weight and height.

PULMONARY SYSTEM

The respiratory symptoms of cystic fibrosis are those of obstructive disease and pneumonia. Hypoxia with resultant cyanosis and digital clubbing are common. Likewise, labored breathing with retractions and resultant increased anterior–posterior chest diameter, flattened diaphragm, and overaeration observed on chest roentgenogram are frequent findings.

A patient's respiratory status follows a cyclical pattern, from a state of relative well-being to one of acute pulmonary deterioration theoretically paralleling the course of the infectious process. Marked declines in pulmonary status (presumably secondary to infection) are referred to as acute respiratory exacerbations and are generally associated with symptoms of acute bacterial endobronchial infection. Thus, fever, increased coughing, increased sputum production, change in sputum character (e.g., thicker, change in color), increased respiratory rate, dyspnea on exertion, increased oxygen requirements, and decreased exercise tolerance are commonly described. Symptoms of chronic sinusitis and nasal polyposis may include rhinorrhea, nasal obstruction, pain over affected sinuses, and disturbances of smell.

Concomitantly, laboratory tests of peripheral blood reveal an increased white blood count with increased polymorphonuclear leukocytes and immature forms consistent with acute infection. Tests of pulmonary function often demonstrate both acute and long-term changes in forced vital capacity (FVC), forced expiratory volume (FEV), and residual volume. Tests reflective of small airway function are more markedly affected as the pulmonary disease progresses. Arterial blood gases typically reveal hypoxia and hypercapnia.

OTHER SIGNS AND SYMPTOMS

The relative insulin deficiency observed in older cystic fibrosis patients is often asymptomatic and only detected on laboratory analysis of serum performed for other reasons. Symptomatic patients present as untreated cases of diabetes mellitus type 2. Cases of cor pulmonale are not usually clinically evident until signs of left-sided heart failure ensue. An enlargement of cardiac size is often noted on routine chest roentgenogram prior to that time, however. Signs and symptoms of anemia and arthritis with cystic fibrosis patients do not differ from those in other patients.

Although the abnormal loss of sodium and chloride in the sweat of cystic fibrosis patients seldom results in profound symptoms such as those of heat prostration, this phenomenon has formed the basis of some large-scale public awareness/screening programs owing to the resultant "salty" taste on the skin of affected patients.

DIAGNOSIS

Cystic fibrosis is normally diagnosed on the basis of an abnormal sweat test. Although diagnosis through chromosomal analysis is now possible, this test as well as others such as nasal cell potential difference are currently reserved for cases in which results of sweat testing are unclear.[22] With the former, a sample of sweat is collected (usually with the use of pilocarpine iontophoresis) and the concentration of chloride is determined. A chloride concentration of 60 mEq/L or more is considered diagnostic, although values up to 80 mEq/L may be observed in non-cystic fibrosis adults. A number of other disorders, such as adrenal insufficiency and hypothyroidism, may be inconsistently associated with elevated sweat chloride concentrations but do not generally present a problem in the differential diagnosis of cystic fibrosis. Ninety-eight percent of cystic fibrosis patients will have a sweat chloride concentration 60 mEq/L or greater. The remaining 2% will have sweat chloride concentrations between 50 and 60 mEq/L and the test may have to be repeated one or more times to obtain definitive results. Nonetheless, the results of a sweat test are not necessarily proof-positive of the presence or absence of cystic fibrosis. The presence of chronic obstructive respiratory disease, exocrine pancreatic insufficiency, and/or a positive family history of the disease help to confirm the diagnosis. The diagnosis is established in most patients by 7 months of life. Genetic (DNA) analysis may be used to diagnose the disease in utero or to detect heterozygotes (carriers) with obvious implications for genetic counseling. Although newborn screening is possible, more study of its potential benefits on long-term outcomes is needed before it receives an unqualified recommendation.[23]

COURSE

Cystic fibrosis is a heterogeneous disease in terms of initial presentation, organ involvement, and clinical course. Most patients are not diagnosed at birth. Only 16% of affected patients have meconium ileus, the value of neonatal screening programs have not been proven, and prenatal diagnosis is early in its implementation. Therefore, the average patient is diagnosed later in life based on a history of recurrent respiratory infections, steatorrhea, and/or failure to thrive. The median age at diagnosis is 7 months and most patients are diagnosed by 12 years of age.[24]

The course of the disease after diagnosis varies markedly from one patient to the next. Some patients have a rapid downhill course based on early pulmonary involvement, whereas others suffer only from gastrointestinal complaints for many years. Although the expected life span of cystic fibrosis patients has increased to 25 to 30 years of age in the last two decades, some patients still die early in life secondary to a fulminant pulmonary process. Others, owing to minimal involvement and mild course, are not diagnosed until their second decade of life. The increased longevity now realized with early diagnosis and aggressive treatment has led to an increase in formerly unusual complications such as diabetes and hepatic disease. Two-year mortality rates above 50% are associated with FEV_1 less than 30% of predicted, Pao_2 less than 50 mm Hg, or Pco_2 greater than 50 mm Hg.[25]

▶ TREATMENT: Cystic Fibrosis

DESIRED OUTCOME

The desired pharmacotherapeutic outcomes for cystic fibrosis are both long and short term. In the long term, one obviously wants to slow or halt the progression of the disease to allow normal growth and development. In the short term, acute problems must be dealt with. The ultimate goal of pharmacotherapy for the gastrointestinal involvement of cystic fibrosis is optimal nutrition. On a day-to-day basis, normal bowel habits and continued weight gain are desirable. Acute goals of therapy for the pulmonary component center around air movement and gas exchange. Thus, antibiotic and bronchodilator/mucolytic therapy are geared toward treating the complications that compromise these functions. For an acute pulmonary exacerbation, return of pulmonary function to preexacerbation status is the central goal of therapy.

GENERAL APPROACH TO TREATMENT

The Cystic Fibrosis Foundation has published clinical guidelines for the diagnosis and care of cystic fibrosis patients, including applicable pharmacotherapy.[26] The following information is generally in agreement with those guidelines except that it may contain more current information. The interested reader is referred to that publication for more detail on the drug treatment of cystic fibrosis and its various complications.

GASTROINTESTINAL SYSTEM

The treatment of gastrointestinal involvement is ultimately aimed at correcting the nutritional deficit present in so many patients.[27] In addition to the pancreatic enzyme replacement and other drug therapy described below, nutritional supplementation is frequently employed. Nutritional interventions range from behavioral modification to nocturnal feedings via gastrostomies.[28]

Pancreatic Enzyme Supplementation

The backbone of gastrointestinal therapy in cystic fibrosis is pancreatic enzyme replacement or supplementation. The preferred products are microencapsulated pancreatic enzymes, although powders are marketed and are useful in patients unable to swallow capsules or to otherwise use the microencapsulated beads they contain. Microencapsulated products protect the contained enzymes from destruction by gastric acid and may be given in much lower doses than their predecessors, which were susceptible to acid breakdown. Most contemporary enzyme replacement products vary mainly in enzyme content per capsule, with lipase content being the chief variable. Representative products and their contents are presented in Table 28–2. Infants are normally given 2000 to 4000 lipase units per 120 mL of formula or breast milk, which provides 450 to 900 lipase units per gram of ingested fat. In general, patients require 500 to 4000 lipase units per gram of ingested fat with the average pediatric or adult patient requiring 1800 units per gram of fat. Enzymes may also be dosed based on weight, with an initial dose of 1000 lipase units being

TABLE 28–2. Pancreatic Enzyme Products

Trade Name	Manufacturer	Enzyme Content (Units)			
		Lipase	Protease	Amylase	Form[a]
Cotazym	Organon	8000	30,000	30,000	C
Cotazym-S		5000	20,000	20,000	ECM
Creon	Reid-Rowell	8000	13,000	30,000	ECM
Ilozyme	Adria	11,000	30,000	30,000	T
Ku-Zyme	Schwarz Pharma	8000	30,000	30,000	C
Pancrease	McNeil	4000	25,000	20,000	ECM
Pancrease MT4		4000	12,000	12,000	ECM
Pancrease MT10		10,000	30,000	30,000	ECM
Pancrease MT16		16,000	48,000	48,000	ECM
Pancrelipase	Geneva	4000	25,000	20,000	ECM
Protilase	Rugby	4000	25,000	20,000	ECM
Ultrase MT12	Scandipharm	12,000	39,000	39,000	ECM
Ultrase MT20		20,000	65,000	65,000	ECM
Ultrase MT24		24,000	78,000	78,000	ECM
Viokase	Robins	8000	30,000	30,000	T
Viokase		16,800	70,000	70,000	P[b]
Zymase	Organon	12,000	24,000	24,000	ECM

[a]Dosage form: C = capsule; ECM = enteric-coated microspheres or beads; T = tablet; P = powder.
[b]Viokase powder, units of enzymes per 700 mg.

administered per kilogram of body weight per meal. One-half that amount is administered with snacks.

Before the introduction of microencapsulated enzyme products, various maneuvers were used to circumvent or overcome the problem of acid breakdown. The most obvious of these was to administer large quantities of enzyme product. Enteric-coated (microencapsulated) pancreatic enzymes have largely solved this problem. The occasional patient may yet require large quantities of even the microencapsulated enzyme product. Whether such difficulties are caused by residual acid breakdown or perhaps low pH in the upper small intestine (secondary to deficient bicarbonate excretion by the pancreas) resulting in a failure to dissolve the coating of the microencapsulated beads is unknown. Defective enteric coating on some generic brands has also been described and led to FDA reclassification of these products, requiring bioequivalence data. Histamine H_2-receptor antagonists and omeprazole have been used to reduce the enzyme dose when residual acid breakdown of enzymes is suspected. Another possible maneuver is to administer both microencapulated and non–enteric-coated enzyme products (e.g., powder) concomitantly.

For patients who are unable to swallow capsules, the contents may be emptied into applesauce, jelly, or some other nonalkaline vehicle provided that the patient does not chew the microencapsulated beads. Side effects of pancreatic enzyme products are uncommon. Perianal irritation resembling diaper rash may occur in infants fed excess quantities of enzyme powders. Hyperuricosuria has also been reported to occur secondary to pancreatic enzyme use, apparently related to their high purine content. Proximal colonic stricture (fibrosing colonopathy) is a dose-related side effect associated with lipase doses in excess of 24,000 units/kg/d.[29]

Vitamin Supplementation

Patients should receive two multivitamin tablets per day, which will provide adequate water-soluble vitamins along with reasonable amounts of vitamins D and K. While clinically evident fat-soluble vitamin deficiencies are unusual in those patients taking adequate pancreatic enzymes and receiving a balanced diet, obvious vitamin K deficiency, manifested as bleeding diathesis, can occur. Demineralization of bone has also been described and vitamin E deficiency has been related to neurologic dysfunction. Further, appropriate laboratory tests (serum carotene, vitamin E, and cholecalciferol concentrations) will often help document other deficiencies, leading to recommendations for additional supplementation of these vitamins. Water-miscibilized vitamin A, 4000 international units (IU)/d, and vitamin E, 100 to 400 IU/d should also be administered either singly or in the form of a water-miscibilized combination product (containing vitamins A, D, E, and K). Vitamin K, in a dose of 5 mg twice weekly, should be given to those patients with prolonged prothrombin times. It should also be noted that appropriately adjusted doses of fat-soluble preparations may be more cost effective than their water-miscible counterparts (e.g., 800 IU fat- soluble vitamin E vs 200 IU water-miscible vitamin E).[30]

Treating Meconium Ileus and Distal Intestinal Obstruction Syndrome

The treatment of meconium ileus or distal intestinal obstruction syndrome can sometimes be limited to the use of enemas with iso-osmolar contrast. Unfortunately, surgery (bowel resection and primary anastomosis) is sometimes necessary to treat this condition and prevent its complications. Distal intestinal obstruction syndrome usually responds to management by oral administration of electrolyte lavage solutions. The adequacy of enzyme dosage should be reassessed in the face of distal intestinal obstruction.

Prevention and Treatment of Cirrhosis

Ursodeoxycholic acid, a bile acid with choleretic properties, has been shown to produce morphologic and functional improvement in affected patients with long-term treatment. The effects are dose related and 15 to 20 mg/kg/d has been used, sometimes in combination with taurine supplementation.[31] The potential of administering this agent prophylactically to patients at risk for liver disease, if feasible, has been speculatively proposed.[32]

CARDIOVASCULAR SYSTEM

Various modalities have been used in attempts to treat the pulmonary hypertension and secondary cor pulmonale of cystic fibrosis. These treatments, which include the use of vasodilators, inotropic agents, and diuretics, have all resulted in limited and transient effects. This is most likely due to the fact that none of these modes of therapy address the underlying cause of the cor pulmonale, hypoxia. Likewise, supplemental (often nocturnal) oxygen treatment has also failed to affect mortality rates or disease progression, although it does appear to prevent exercise-induced oxygen desaturation as well as that occurring with sleep. Thus, the most beneficial approach may be to attempt to improve oxygenation with aggressive pulmonary therapy.

PULMONARY SYSTEM

Management of the pulmonary component of cystic fibrosis can be broken down into two areas: respiratory therapy, including anti-inflammatory therapy, and anti-infective therapy.[33]

Respiratory Therapy

The cornerstone of pulmonary therapy is percussion and postural drainage, which aids in the clearance of pulmonary mucus and is performed once or twice daily in "healthy" patients and as often as five times daily or more during an acute pulmonary exacerbation. New flutter devices also appear to be useful adjuncts in this regard. Percussion is often preceded by nebulizer therapy during which nebulized sterile water or 0.9% sodium chloride solution is breathed to liquefy pulmonary secretions. Bronchodilators and/or mucolytic agents (e.g., *N*-acetylcysteine; Mucomyst, Mead Johnson) may be added to the nebulizer solution to prevent bronchospasm and further liquefy pulmonary secretions, respectively. Although the effects of bronchodilators administered by inhalation are readily demonstrated with pulmonary function tests, those of mucolytic agents are not as obvious, and a number of attempts to demonstrate the effects of inhaled *N*-acetylcysteine have been unsuccessful. Moreover, many patients prefer not to use *N*-acetylcysteine because of its unpleasant taste and odor and because it often induces bronchospasm. Normal saline and sodium bicarbonate solution are also commonly administered by aerosol as aids to sputum expectoration, but again, documentation of efficacy is elusive.

Recombinant human DNase has been approved for use in cystic fibrosis. When given by inhalation (2.5 mg once or twice daily), rhDNase reduces the viscosity of cystic fibrosis sputum and leads to statistically significant, though modest, improvement in indices of pulmonary function.[34] Importantly, rhDNase use may lower the incidence (or lengthen the time between) respiratory exacerbations and thus improve quality of life and may indirectly decrease the overall costs of care in patients with mild to moderate disease. Should these outcomes be borne out in further long-term studies, the cost of this therapy may well be justified for some patients.

In attempts to block the consequences of the inflammatory component of the disease, corticosteroid therapy has been evaluated. Although results of preliminary trials were encouraging, a large, multicenter, placebo-controlled trial found alternate-day prednisone treatment at 2mg/kg to have positive effects on pulmonary function but had negative consequences on growth and glucose metabolism.[35] Reanalysis of the data from this same study suggested that the benefits of a 1 mg/kg dose might outweigh the risks.[36] The efficacy of short-term systemic corticosteroid use, as well as inhalation of these agents, will continue to be evaluated. Although data concerning inhaled corticosteroids are scant, a long-term trial of oral ibuprofen indicates a positive effect in slowing pulmonary deterioration.[37] Unfortunately, therapeutic drug monitoring (periodic determination of ibuprofen serum concentrations) is required.

Because many cystic fibrosis patients have a reactive airway component to their pulmonary disease, systemic bronchodilators such as theophylline and β-agonists may be of benefit. Wheezing and responsiveness to bronchodilators represent legitimate indications. Responsiveness to such agents (> 15% improvement in FEV_1) should be documented, however, before a protracted course is begun. Normal antiasthmatic doses of most bronchodilators should be appropriate for cystic fibrosis patients. However, theophylline clearance may be different in cystic fibrosis patients, and bioavailability of some products may be decreased, sometimes necessitating the use of higher-than-usual doses.[38] Because of the necessity of pharmacokinetic monitoring and its involvement in a number of common drug interactions, theophylline should be considered second-line bronchodilator therapy at most in these patients. Because cystic fibrosis patients are at high risk to develop the complications of influenza, influenza vaccine should be administered on a yearly basis, and amantadine prophylaxis or treatment may be indicated as well.

Antibiotic Therapy

Antibiotics are used for two purposes in cystic fibrosis, these being for chronic suppressive therapy and for treatment of acute exacerbations. The use of antibiotics in cystic fibrosis patients is somewhat controversial and certainly challenging. Controversy exists because of the observation that during treatment for an acute pulmonary exacerbation, clinical improvement occurs despite failure to eradicate bacterial pathogens from the sputum. This suggests to some that the bacteria present are colonizers rather than pathogens, which would argue against the use of antibiotics. The results of one published study comparing antibiotic therapy to placebo indicated that antibiotics may not always contribute to recovery from an acute exacerbation.[39] However, this small study only evaluated patients with mild to moderate disease and therefore is not convincing. At the same time, these results do emphasize the fact that not all exacerbations of pulmonary disease in cystic fibrosis are caused by bacteria. It is logical that other factors such as viral infection and air pollutants could at least contribute to such episodes. Clearly, bacteria such as *P. aeruginosa* are pathogenic both by virtue of inherent properties such as exotoxin release and the body's immune response to their presence and products. Moreover, it is apparent that sublethal effects of antibiotics on *P. aeruginosa* (e.g., decreased exoenzyme production) contribute to clinical improvement.[40] Therefore, the routine presence of known bacterial pathogens dictates antibiotic use, and most if not all clinicians caring for cystic fibrosis patients regularly employ antibiotic therapy. Suppressive or prophylactic therapy is given with the intention of prolonging the time between acute exacerbations. Although intuitively attractive, the practice is not supported by well-designed clinical trials.[41] Moreover, the practice of routine, quarterly administration of intravenous courses of antibiotics used at some European centers is also lacking in proof of efficacy.[42]

Once one is committed to antibiotic therapy, a number of other important, and sometimes perplexing, issues emerge. These include the selection of the best antibiotic(s) for the individual patient, the best dosage and dosage regimen given altered pharmacokinetics, the optimal route of administration, emergence of antibiotic-resistant bacteria, and identification of appropriate end points of therapy.

Selection of Antibiotic. Suppressive therapy is usually accomplished with the use of common orally administered antibiotics such as trimethoprim-sulfamethoxazole, amoxicillin/clavulanic acid, or one of the many oral cephalosporins. Specific therapy for acute exacerbations is directed at proven or likely pathogens such as *P. aeruginosa* and *S. aureus* and usually includes an aminoglycoside and an extended-spectrum penicillin. As most *S. aureus* encountered are β-lactamase producers, use of an extended-spectrum penicillin/β-lactamase inhibitor combination (e.g., ticarcillin/clavulanate) will help avoid the necessity of triple-drug therapy. Single-agent therapy with newer antibiotics, especially on an outpatient basis, is frequently employed at some centers where significant resistance to these agents has not yet emerged. Such agents would include ceftazidime, aztreonam, and ciprofloxacin . However, the evidence supporting the clinical superiority of two-drug combinations over single-agent therapy leads many clinicians to only treat with combinations.[43–46] The fact that such combinations are sometimes synergistic *in vitro* and the possibility that they may act to suppress or delay the emergence of resistance provide attractive rationales for their use. Further, *in vitro* synergism has been reported to persist even in the face of resistance to one of the single agents in a given combination.[47] Last, monodrug therapy has been met with rapid emergence of resistance.[48]

Unlike other cases of lower respiratory tract infection, organism-specific drug treatment may be based on results from sputum cultures in cystic fibrosis patients because good agreement between sputum and thoracotomy cultures has been demonstrated.[49] Typically, such results will lead one to prescribe or recommend aminoglycoside/extended-spectrum penicillin combinations, although other antibiotics such as ciprofloxacin and older agents such as colistin may also play a role. While the complete eradication of *S. aureus* and *H. influenzae* are practical goals or end points of antibiotic therapy, the total eradication of *Pseudomonas* species is infrequent and transient. Thus, once a patient has been colonized/infected with *P. aeruginosa,* it is prudent to assume that it is always present regardless of culture results. Consistent with these infectious phenomena, the complete resolution of pulmonary signs and symptoms becomes less and less likely as the disease progresses. *B. cepacia* and *S. maltophilia* are generally resistant to most antibiotics. These bacteria may be susceptible to trimethoprim-sulfamethoxazole or chloramphenicol. *B. cepacia* from cystic fibrosis patients is frequently susceptible to ceftazidime, whereas some strains of *S. maltophilia* may be susceptible to other agents such as doxycycline and piperacillin.

Selection of Dose-Altered Pharmacokinetics. Although altered pharmacokinetics in cystic fibrosis are not limited to antibiotics (Table 28–3), this drug class has been the most extensively studied.[50] As is true for theophylline, many cystic fibrosis patients have increased total body clearance for many antibiotics, including the aminoglycosides, some of the β-lactams, and trimethoprim-sulfamethoxazole. Thus, higher doses of these agents may be necessary to produce therapeutic concentrations (Table 28–4). Unfortunately, these alterations in pharmacokinetics are neither consistent nor predictable. Why the pharmacokinetics of these antibiotics are different in cystic fibrosis patients is unknown. It appears that for many β-lactam antibiotics, increased total body clearance could be accounted for by increased renal clearance. However, it should be pointed out that renal function, as reflected by glomerular filtration rate and renal blood flow, is not different in cystic fibrosis patients as compared to non-cystic fibrosis controls.[51] Moreover, a concomitant increase in renal clearance does not completely explain the increase in total body clearance of aminoglycosides, leading some to speculate about extrarenal pathways for elimination. In any event, increased total body clearance dictates higher doses in many but not all patients. However, a range of dosage requirements should be expected, consistent with a range in the variation of pharmacokinetics in these patients. For example, experience with netilmicin revealed a dosage requirement range of 7 to 17 mg/kg/d to achieve peak concentrations (one-half hour after the end of a drug infusion) of 8 μg/mL or greater.[52] The mean dosage requirement in this study was approximately 12 mg/kg/d. Peak concentrations of this magnitude are felt to be necessary to adequately treat pneumonia caused by gram-negative bacteria.[53,54] Variations in hepatic metabolic activity or in phenotypic distribution of metabolic polymorphisms may explain some pharmacokinetic differences in cystic fibrosis.[55,56]

TABLE 28–3. Changes in Pharmacokinetics in Cystic Fibrosis[38,50]

Agent	$\beta t_{1/2}$	V_d	Cl_B	Cl_R
Antibiotics				
Methicillin	NC	I	I	I
Cloxacillin	D	I	I	I
Dicloxacillin	I	NR	NR	I
Azlocillin	D	I	I	NR
Piperacillin	D	I	I	NR
Ticarcillin	D	NC	I	I
Aztreonam	D	I	I	I
Ceftazidime	D	I	I	I
Imipenem	NC	I	I	NR
Trimethoprim-sulfamethoxazole	D/D	NC/NC	I/I	I/NC
Gentamicin	NC	I	I	NR
Tobramycin	NC	I	I	NC
Amikacin	NC	I	I	I
Netilmicin	NC	I	I	NR
Fleroxacin	D	D	I	D
Other				
Theophylline	D	I	I	I
Furosemide	NC	NC	I	NC
Acetaminophen	NC	NR	I	NR

$\beta t_{1/2}$ = elimination half-life; V_d = apparent volume of distribution; Cl_B = total body clearance, Cl_R = renal clearance; D = decreased; I = increased; NC = no change; NR = not reported. *From Refs. 38 and 50.*

Although the pharmacokinetics of antibiotics may correlate with the severity of pulmonary disease,[57,58] it is not possible to predict changes in antibiotic pharmacokinetics in cystic fibrosis patients based on markers of clinical status or disease progression. Attempts to correlate antibiotic pharmacokinetics with Shwachman score (a gross method for quantitation of disease status) have been unsuccessful.[59,60] Attempts to guide aminoglycoside dosing are often based on measured serum concentrations during a course of therapy. However, this method may also meet with mixed success owing to changing pharmacokinetics of this family of antibiotics during an acute pulmonary exacerbation.[61] This observation should not, however, deter one from attempts to adjust doses to desirable concentrations based on serum concentration determinations and subsequent pharmacokinetic calculations.

Alternate Routes of Administration. An additional route of antibiotic administration that is intuitively attractive in patients with cystic fibrosis is by inhalation of aerosolized solution. Such a route of administration should, theoretically, deliver the drug to the actual site of infection and perhaps avoid systemic toxicity. Certainly, many classes of antibiotics including β-lactams, aminoglycosides, and polymyxins have been administered to cystic fibrosis patients in this fashion, often in conjunction with systemic antibiotics. However, until recently, no clear effect or advantage had been consistently demonstrated. Early studies suffered from lack of controls, small sample size, and a failure to ensure that the respiratory equipment used would, in fact, guarantee that drug is delivered to the small airways. In a subsequent, placebo-controlled, multicenter trial, 600 mg tobramycin administered by aerosol three times daily was found to produce a small but statistically significant improvement in FEV_1, FVC, $FEF_{25\%-75\%}$, *P. aeruginosa* density in sputum, and peripheral white blood cell count.[62]

TABLE 28–4. Antibiotic Doses in Cystic Fibrosis

Antibiotic	Dose (mg/kg/d)	Regimen	Adult Maximum Dose (g/d)
Parenteral Antibiotics			
Tobramycin,[a] gentamicin,[a] or netilmicin[a]	6–9	q8h	NA
Amikacin[a]	20–30	q8h	NA
Azlocillin	400	q4–6h	24
Aztreonam	200	q6h	8
Ceftazidime	150	q8h	6
Colistin	2.5–6.0	q6–8h	NA
Imipenem	45–100	q6h	4
Nafcillin	100	q4–6h	6
Ticarcillin or ticarcillin/clavulanate	400	q4–6h	18
Piperacillin	400	q4–6h	18
Oral Antibiotics			
Amoxicillin	20	q8h	
Amoxicillin/clavulanate	20	q6h	
Ciprofloxacin[b]	1500 mg/d	q12h	1.5
Cephalexin	50–100	q6–8h	6
Dicloxacillin	80–100	q6h	6
Trimethoprim-sulfamethoxazole	10–15[c]	q12h	0.64[c]
Inhaled Antibiotics			
Colistin	150 mg/d	q6–12h	NA
Gentamicin or tobramycin	600–1800 mg/d	q12h	NA
Polymixin B	250 mg/d	q6–12h	NA

[a]Starting doses; adjust to desired serum concentrations based on dose/serum concentration relationship.
[b]Adult dose.
[c]Based on trimethoprim.

This being recognized, appropriate clinical circumstances for this form of therapy (type and condition of patient), length of therapy, and frequency of therapy remain to be clarified. One-half of this dose is apparently also effective and a 300-mg dose is the current norm. If such doses are to be used, preservative-free antibiotic preparations should be used. The efficacy of smaller doses of inhaled aminoglycosides remains unproven.

Bacterial Resistance. As already noted, emergence of antimicrobial resistance seems to follow the introduction and use of a new antibiotic.[48] *P. aeruginosa* can exhibit many resistance mechanisms revealed as resistance to quinolones (altered DNA gyrase target site), β-lactams (production of Bush group 1 β-lactamase), aminoglycosides (decreased permeability and modifying enzymes), and carbapenems (decreased permeability). *B. cepacia* is inherently resistant to most antibiotics. Methicillin-resistant staphylococci are increasingly common in institutional settings and will become a more pervasive problem in cystic fibrosis populations. These phenomena require close attention to susceptibility reports in selecting therapy and the avoidance of unnecessary or unnecessarily protracted courses of antibiotic therapy.

Recommendations for Antibiotic Therapy. Despite these inherent difficulties, a number of recommendations regarding the use of systemic antibiotics in cystic fibrosis can be made. The selection of antibiotics should be based on specific culture and susceptibility results. When instituting empiric therapy in the absence of culture results, the clinician can be guided by the most recent laboratory data or institute therapy based on likely pathogens in the patient's age group. Aminoglycosides should be initially dosed at the upper end of the normal dosage range (e.g., 6 to 7.5 mg/kg/d for tobramycin), and serum concentrations should be determined so that dosage can be appropriately adjusted to achieve peak concentrations of at least 8 μg/mL. It should be kept in mind that aminoglycoside serum half-lives may lengthen during the course of treatment so that a constant relationship between dose and serum concentration may not exist. Upward adjustments in dosage should therefore be made with some degree of caution and should be followed with further determination of serum concentrations. Once-daily administration of aminoglycosides is gaining popularity as in other settings. Obviously, such a dosing practice would result in much larger peak concentrations than those mentioned above. Comparative efficacy and safety of such dosing regimens in cystic fibrosis patients have not yet been fully elucidated, but this practice is likely to be increasingly employed as cystic fibrosis-specific data are generated.

β-Lactam antibiotics such as extended-spectrum pencillins should be prescribed with aminoglycosides to take advantage of their frequent synergy and prevent the emergence of resistance. These agents should be prescribed in large doses to delay stepwise resistance. Ticarcillin, azlocillin, and piperacillin should be prescribed in a dose of at least 350 mg/kg/d divided into four to six doses. For patients with *P. aeruginosa* and *S. aureus,* the combination of an aminoglycoside and ticarcillin/clavulanate or piperacillin/tazobactam is appropriate. Selection among these agents should be based on local susceptibility patterns and cost considerations. The possible increased incidence of fever and exanthema with the newer pencillins should be kept in mind.[63] Aztreonam would be a safe and effective β-lactam to use in patients experiencing these serum sickness–like reactions to the penicillins.[64] In older patients with *P. aeruginosa* isolates with broad resistance patterns, the clinician should work closely with the microbiology laboratory to identify effective agents or combinations. The potential use of older agents with unique mechanisms of action, such as colistin, should not be overlooked.

Oral antibiotics may be prescribed in symptomatic outpatients with susceptible pathogens in their sputum. Agents with activity against common pathogens such as *S. aureus* and *H. influenzae* are useful in this setting. These typically include such antibiotics as first-generation cephalosporins, trimethoprim-sulfamethoxazole, and amoxicillin/clavulanic acid. The use of such agents on a "prophylactic" basis is discouraged because the data available at present suggest that a beneficial effect does not outweigh the risk of development of resistance among the common bacterial pathogens of cystic fibrosis.[65] The 4-fluoroquinolone antibiotic ciprofloxacin possesses potent activity against most cystic fibrosis pathogens and has been evaluated in adult patients undergoing pulmonary exacerbations. Although not conclusive because of shortcomings in the studies, available data suggest that this oral agent is as effective as standard intravenous therapy.[66] The availability of a potent, oral antipseudomonal agent poses a number of potential uses in the cystic fibrosis population. However, it should be kept in mind that repeated or long-term use will likely lead to resistance and that antibiotics play only a supportive role in the treatment of these patients. Thus, oral antibiotic therapy, regardless of efficacy, does not negate the need for other forms of therapy which are often best administered in the hospital setting. It should also be pointed out that although ciprofloxacin appears to be safe in patients less than 18 years of age with little evidence of joint or cartilage toxicity,[67] this agent should be used with caution in the younger population.

Treatment of Other Pulmonary Complications

The drug and/or nondrug treatment of the most serious of pulmonary complications including pulmonary hypertension, right-sided heart failure, respiratory failure, pneumothorax, and hemoptysis are beyond the scope of this chapter. In general, the therapeutic approach does not vary substantively from that in other patients.

EVALUATION OF THERAPEUTIC OUTCOMES

GASTROINTESTINAL

The patient's nutritional status should be closely monitored on both short-term and long-term bases. Height and weight should be followed with time; anthropometric measurements give more precise information. The adequacy of pancreatic enzyme replacement can be grossly assessed by following stool patterns with the goal of normal number per day and normal consistency. Any evidence of steatorrhea may indicate suboptimal enzyme therapy. A more precise method would involve assessment of fat quantities in the stool. If a patient does not respond to normal doses of enzyme supplement, other factors that can cause similar symptoms (bloating, abdominal pain, symptomatic steatorrhea) should be considered. These would include lack of adherence with directions for taking the enzymes, outdated enzymes, dietary factors such as excessive fruit juice consumption, high-fat meals, and concomitant gastrointestinal disease (e.g., enteric bacterial or parasitic infection, celiac disease, inflammatory bowel disease). Vitamin status can be assessed though serum monitoring of fat-soluble vitamin concentrations.

PULMONARY

Pulmonary status can be monitored with a combination of clinical observation and examination and a variety of laboratory tests. Over the long run, pulmonary function is usually followed with spirometry along with assessment of lung volume and oxygenation. Physical examination should focus on signs and symptoms of upper and lower respiratory tract infection. In addition, exercise tolerance, recent character of sputum production, and oxygen requirements are key to long-term and short-term assessment. With antibiotic and bronchodilator treatment of acute respiratory exacerbations, a return to preexacerbation clinical status, based on physical examination or pulmonary function testing, becomes a practical end point for antimicrobial treatment. Although the goal of bacterial eradication is desirable, other attainable end points may be more reasonable, as discussed earlier. Bacterial density in sputum, sputum DNA and protein content, and C-reactive protein all have proven value as monitoring parameters but may not be available at many centers. Of the objective parameters, pulmonary function tests correlate best with clinical observations and scoring systems.[68] Response to intravenous antibiotics and aggressive chest physiotherapy, as measured by FEV_1 at the end of 1 week of treatment, has been used to predict total length of therapy necessary. In patients whose FEV had recovered more than 40% at the end of 1 week, a total of 2 weeks of therapy was generally sufficient.[69] Little has been done by way of pharmacodynamic studies in treating cystic fibrosis. Therefore, symptomatic improvement is largely relied on to assess the relative success of antibiotic therapy. Oral antibiotic therapy should also be limited in length with specific end points, such as decreased cough and/or improved pulmonary function, identified as treatment commences.

NEW DIRECTIONS IN THERAPY

Now that the gene and gene product of cystic fibrosis have been identified, gene therapy becomes an obvious potential for treatment.[70] Research to date has centered on introduction of the correct gene into affected tissues. Viral vectors, chiefly adenovirus, have been studied in animal models, and human trials are under way. Liposomes may represent another useful delivery mode to introduce the correct gene.

Other, novel approaches to therapy are currently being investigated and, for the most part, are directed at the inflammatory component of the disease or the basic cellular defect. Protease inhibitors hold potential in this condition for reasons cited earlier. α_1-Antitrypsin administered by aerosol shows promise, as does secretory leukocyte protease inhibitor (SLPI) and other antiproteases.[71–73] Pentoxifylline, which is known to inhibit tumor necrosis factor-α-transcription and its stimulatory effect on polymorphonuclear leukocytes, also shows promise.[74] In an attempt to directly approach the cellular defect in cystic fibrosis, the diuretic amiloride had been shown to possess positive activity in improving respiratory secretion rheology and clearance,[75] presumably by blocking excessive sodium reabsorption, but was found to be no more effective than placebo in a large-scale, controlled trial. At a similar level, the secretagogues adenosine and uridine triphosphate (ATP and UTP) have been shown to increase chloride excretion in epithelial cells of cystic fibrosis patients.[76] The combination of amiloride and UTP (thereby both blocking sodium absorption and stimulating chloride secretion) may also promote clearance of airway secretions.[77] Other experimental therapies interact with the defects in CFTR production or processing. Studies with phenylbutyrate (which increases the amount of functional protein that reaches the cell surface), 8-cyclopentyl-1,3-dipropylxanthine (CPX), milrinone (a phosphodiesterase inhibitor), and genistein (a tyrosine-kinase inhibitor), each of which activate mutant CFTR, and low concentration gentamicin, which suppresses certain premature stop mutations in CFTR, are all active.

It is hoped that some, if not all, of these approaches will provide viable additions to our pharmacologic armamentarium for this disease. For older, more severely affected patients who may not be able to benefit from such advances, organ transplants (single lung, double lung, heart–lung) are more widely available and reasonably successful.[78]

CONCLUSIONS

Pharmacotherapeutic intervention plays an important role in the management of these patients but is complex. The clinician is, as yet, faced with many unresolved issues in attempting to apply sound therapeutic principles in this population. Although close attention should be paid to pharmacologic treatment, the approach to these patients should be multifaceted and multidisciplinary in character. In addition to the involvement of such pediatric subspecialties as pulmonology, gastroenterology, pharmacology, and infectious diseases, contributions from such areas as nutrition support and social work should be a regular and ongoing part of the management effort.

▶ PRINCIPLES OF PHARMACOTHERAPY

- Cystic fibrosis is a genetic disorder of chloride ion secretion from epithelial cells ultimately causing thickened secretions and affects cells in the lungs, pancreas, intestines, and other exocrine glands/organs.
- Thickened secretions in airways lead to obstruction, infection, and finally, inflammation, leading to most of the morbidity and mortality observed with this disease.
- Pulmonary infections are mainly caused by *P. aeruginosa,* and antibiotic therapy is usually directed at that organism.
- Use of antibiotics and other pharmacologic agents must account for the altered pharmacokinetics often observed in cystic fibrosis patients.
- Maneuvers to aid in airway clearance of thickened sections include respiratory therapy and use of bronchodilators and mucolytic agents.
- Thickened secretions in the pancreas lead to deficiencies in pancreatic digestive enzymes and bicarbonate, which leads to maldigestion, malnutrition, and fat-soluble–vitamin deficiency.
- Treatment of the gastrointestinal component of cystic fibrosis includes pancreatic enzyme and vitamin supplementation.
- Complications of cystic fibrosis are mainly secondary to the pulmonary component.
- Experimental therapies are directed at the chloride secretion abnormality and the responsible dysfunctional protein.
- Corrective gene therapy will be the ultimate treatment for this disease.

REFERENCES

1. Steinberg AG, Brown DC. On the incidence of cystic fibrosis of the pancreas. Am J Hum Genet 1960;12:416–424.
2. Wright SE, Morton NE. Genetic studies on cystic fibrosis in Hawaii. Am J Hum Genet 1968;20:157–169.
3. Rommens JM, Iannuzzi MC, Kerem B, et al. Identification of the cystic fibrosis gene: Chromosome walking and jumping. Science 1989; 245:1059–1065.
4. Riordan JR, Rommens JM, Kerem B, et al. Identification of the cystic fibrosis gene: Cloning and characterization of complementary DNA. Science 1989;245:1066–1073.
5. Kerem B, Rommens JM, Buchanan JA, et al. Identification of the cystic fibrosis gene: Genetic analysis. Science 1989;245:1073–1080.
6. Welsh MJ, Smith AE. Molecular mechanisms of CFTR chloride channel dysfunction in cystic fibrosis. Cell 1993;73:1251–1254.
7. Kerem E, Corey M, Kerem B, et al. The relationship between genotype and phenotype in cystic fibrosis—Analysis of the most common mutation (ΔF_{508}). N Engl J Med 1991;323:1517–1522.
8. Mohon RT, Wagener JS, Abman SH, et al. Relationship of genotype to early pulmonary function in infants with cystic fibrosis identified through neonatal screening. J Pediatr 1993;122:550–555.
9. Collins FC. Cystic fibrosis: Molecular biology and therapeutic implications. Science 1992;256:774–779.
10. Feigelson J, Anagnostopoulos C, Poquet M, et al. Liver cirrhosis—Therapeutic implications and long term follow up. Arch Dis Child 1993;68:653–657.
11. Goldman, MJ, Anderson GM, Stolzenberg ED, et al. Human β-defensin-1 is a salt-sensitive antibiotic in lung that is inactivated in cystic fibrosis. Cell 1997;88:553–560.
12. Pier GB, Grout M, Zaida TS, et al. Role of mutant CFTR in hypersusceptibility of cystic fibrosis patients to lung infections. Science 1996;271:64–67.
13. Wang EEL, Prober CG, Manson B, et al. Association of respiratory viral infections with pulmonary deterioration in patients with cystic fibrosis. N Engl J Med 1984;311:1653–1658.
14. Abman SH, Ogle JW, Butler-Simon N, et al. Role of respiratory syncytial virus in early hospitalizations for respiratory distress of young infants with cystic fibrosis. J Pediatr 1988;113:826–830.

15. Pribble CG, Black PG, Bosso JA, et al. Clinical manifestations of exacerbations of cystic fibrosis associated with nonbacterial infections. J Pediatr 1990;117:200–204.
16. Campbell PW, Parker RA, Roberts BT, et al. Association of poor clinical status and heavy exposure to tobacco smoke in patients with cystic fibrosis who are homozygous for the F_{508} deletion. J Pediatr 1992; 120:261–264.
17. May TB, Shinabarger D, Maharaj R, et al. Alginate synthesis by *Pseudomonas aeruginosa:* A key pathogenic factor in chronic pulmonary infections of cystic fibrosis patents. Clin Microbiol Rev 1991;4:191–206.
18. Isles A, Maclusky I, Corey M, et al. *Pseudomonas cepacia* infection in cystic fibrosis: An emerging problem. J Pediatr 1984;104:206–210.
19. Hudson VL, Wielinski CL, Regelmann WE. Prognostic implications of initial oropharyngeal bacterial flora in patients with cystic fibrosis diagnosed before the age of two years. J Pediatr 1993;122:854–860.
20. Triglia JM, Belus JF, Dessi P, et al. Rhinonasal manifestations of cystic fibrosis. Ann Otolaryngol Chir Cervicofac 1993;110:98–102.
21. Lawrence JM, Moore TL, Madson KL, et al. Arthropathies of cystic fibrosis: Case reports and review of the literature. J Rheumatol 1993; 20(suppl 38):12–15.
22. Rosenstein BJ, Cutting GR. The diagnosis of cystic fibrosis: A consensus statement. J Pediatr 1998;132:589–595.
23. Newborn screening for cystic fibrosis: A paradigm for public health genetics policy development. Proceeding of a 1997 workshop. MMWR 1997;46(RR-16):1–24
24. FitzSimmons SC. The changing epidemiology of cystic fibrosis. J Pediatr 1993;122:1–9.
25. Kerem E, Reisman J, Corey M, et al. Prediction of mortality in patients with cystic fibrosis. N Engl J Med 1992;326:1187–1191.
26. Clinical Practice Guidelines for Cystic Fibrosis Committee. Clinical practice guidelines for cystic fibrosis. Bethesda, MD, Cystic Fibrosis Foundation, 1997.
27. Riedel BD. Gastrointestinal manifestations of cystic fibrosis. Pediatr Ann 1997;26;235–241.
28. Ramsey BW, Farrell PM, Pencharz P, et al. Nutritional assessment and management in cystic fibrosis. Am J Clin Nutr 1992;55:108–116.
29. FitzSimmons SC, Burkhart GA, Borowitz D, et al. High-dose pancreatic-enzyme supplements and fibrosing colonopathy in children with cystic fibrosis. N Engl J Med 1997;336:1283–1289.
30. Nasr SZ, O'Leary MH, Hillerman C. Correction of vitamin E deficiency with fat-soluble versus water-miscible preparations of vitamin E in patients with cystic fibrosis. J Pediatr 1993;122:810–812.
31. Colombo C, Battezzati PM, Podda M, et al. Ursodeoxycholic acid for liver disease associated with cystic fibrosis: A double-blind multicenter trial. Hepatology 1996;23:1484–1490.
32. Columbo C, Grazia M, Ferrari M, et al. Analysis of risk factors for the development of liver disease associated with cystic fibrosis. J Pediatr 1994;124:393–399.
33. Ramsey BW. Management of pulmonary disease in patients with cystic fibrosis. N Engl J Med 1996;335:179–188.
34. Fuchs HJ, Borwitz DS, Christainsen DH, et al. Effect of aerosolized recombinant human DNase on exacerbations of respiratory symptoms and on pulmonary function in patients with cystic fibrosis. N Engl J Med 1994:331:637–642.
35. Rosenstein BJ, Eigen H. Risks of alternate-day prednisone in patients with cystic fibrosis. Pediatrics 1991;87:245–246.
36. Eigen H, Rosenstein BJ, FitzSimmons S, et al. A multicenter study of alternate-day prednisone therapy in patients with cystic fibrosis. J Pediatr 1995;126:515–523.
37. Konstan MW, Byard PJ, Hoppel CL, et al. Effect of high-dose ibuprofen in patients with cystic fibrosis. N Engl J Med 1995;332:848–854.
38. Spino M. Pharmacokinetics of drugs in cystic fibrosis. Clin Rev Allergy 1991;9:169–210.
39. Gold R, Carpenter S, Heurter H, et al. Randomized trial of ceftazidime versus placebo in the management of acute respiratory exacerbations in patients with cystic fibrosis. J Pediatr 1987;111:907–913.
40. Grimwood K, Semple RA, Rabin HR, et al. Elevated exoenzyme expression by *Pseudomonas aeruginosa* is correlated with exacerbations of lung disease in cystic fibrosis. Pediatr Pulmonol 1993;15:135–139.
41. Beardsmore CS, Thompson JR, Williams A, et al. Pulmonary function in infants with cystic fibrosis: The effect of antibiotic treatment. Arch Dis Child 1994;71:133–137.
42. Jensen T, Pedersen SS, Høiby N, et al. Use of antibiotics in cystic fibrosis: The Danish approach. Antibiot Chemother 1989;42:237–246.
43. Parry MF, Neu HC, Merlino M, et al. Treatment of pulmonary infections in patients with cystic fibrosis: A comparative study of ticarcillin and gentamicin. J Pediatr 1977;90:144–148.
44. Møller NE, Høiby N. Antibiotic treatment of chronic *Pseudomonas aeruginosa* infection in cystic fibrosis patients. Scand J Infect Dis 1981;24(suppl):87–91.
45. Friis B. Chemotherapy of chronic infections with mucoid *Pseudomonas aeruginosa* in lower airways of patients with cystic fibrosis. Scand J Infect Dis 1979;11:211–217.
46. Krause PJ, Young LS, Cherry JD, et al. The treatment of exacerbations of pulmonary disease in cystic fibrosis: Netilmicin compared with netilmicin and carbenicillin. Curr Ther Res 1979;25:609–617.
47. Aronoff SC, Klinger JD. *In vitro* activities of aztreonam, piperacillin and ticarcillin combined with amikacin against amikacin-resistant *Pseudomonas aeruginosa* and *P. cepacia* isolates from children with cystic fibrosis. Antimicrob Agents Chemother 1984;25:279–280.
48. Bosso JA, Allen JE, Matsen JM. Changing susceptibility of *Pseudomonas aeruginosa* isolates from cystic fibrosis patients with the clinical use of newer antibiotics. Antimicrob Agents Chemother 1989; 33:526–528.
49. Thomassen MJ, Klinger JD, Badger SJ, et al. Cultures of thoracotomy specimens confirm usefulness of sputum cultures in cystic fibrosis. J Pediatr 1984;104:352–356.
50. Lindsay CA, Bosso JA. Optimization of antibiotic therapy in cystic fibrosis patients. Clin Pharmacokinet 1993;24:496–506.
51. Spino M, Chai RP, Isles AF, et al. Assessment of glomerular filtration rate and effective renal plasma flow in cystic fibrosis. J Pediatr 1985; 107:64–70.
52. Bosso JA, Townsend PL, Herbst JJ, et al. Pharmacokinetics and dosage requirements of netilmicin in cystic fibrosis patients. Antimicrob Agents Chemother 1985;28:829–831.
53. Moore RD, Smith CR, Lietman PS. Association of aminoglycoside plasma levels with therapeutic outcome in gram-negative pneumonia. Am J Med 1984;77:657–662.
54. Noone P, Parsons MC, Pattison JR, et al. Experience in monitoring gentamicin therapy during treatment of serious gram negative sepsis. Br J Med 1974;1:477–481.
55. Kearns GL. Hepatic drug metabolism in cystic fibrosis: Recent developments and future directions. Ann Pharmacother 1993;27:74–79.
56. Bosso JA, Liu Q, Evans WE, et al. CYP2D6, *N*-acetylation, and xanthine oxidase activity in cystic fibrosis. Pharmacotherapy 1996; 16:749–753.
57. MacDonald NE, Anas NG, Peterson RG, et al. Renal clearance of gentamicin in cystic fibrosis. J Pediatr 1983;103:985–990.
58. Nahata MC, Lubion AH, Visconti JA. Cephalexin pharmacokinetics in patients with cystic fibrosis. Dev Pharmacol Ther 1984;7:221–228.
59. Spino M, Chai RP, Isles AF, et al. Cloxacillin absorption and disposition in cystic fibrosis. J Pediatr 1984;105:829–835.
60. Jacobs RF, Trang JM, Kearns GL, et al. Ticarcillin/clavulanic acid pharmacokinetics in children and young adults with cystic fibrosis. J Pediatr 1985;106:1001–1007.
61. Bosso JA, Relling MV, Townsend PL, et al. Intrapatient variations in aminoglycoside disposition in cystic fibrosis. Clin Pharm 1987; 6:54–58.
62. Ramsey BW, Dorkin HL, Eisenberg JD, et al. Efficacy of aerosolized tobramycin in patients with cystic fibrosis. N Engl J Med 1993; 328:1740–1746.
63. Møller NE, Eriksen KR, Feddersen C, et al. Chemotherapy against *Pseudomonas aeruginosa* in cystic fibrosis. A study of carbenicillin,

azlocillin or piperacillin in combination with tobramycin. Eur J Respir Dis 1982;63:130–139.
64. Jensen T, Koch C, Pedersen SS, et al. Aztreonam for cystic fibrosis patients who are hypersensitive to other β-lactams. Lancet 1987;1: 1319–1320.
65. Beardsmore CS, Thompson JR, Williams A, et al. Pulmonary function in infants with cystic fibrosis. Arch Dis Child 1994;71:133–137.
66. Bosso JA. Use of ciprofloxacin in cystic fibrosis patients. Am J Med 1989;87(suppl 5A):123S–127S.
67. Høiby N, Pedersen SS, Jensen T, et al. Fluoroquinolones in the treatment of cystic fibrosis. Drugs 1993;45(suppl 3):98–101.
68. Bosso JA, Walker KB. Lack of correlation between objective indicators and clinical-response scores during antimicrobial therapy for acute pulmonary exacerbations of cystic fibrosis. Clin Pharm 1988; 7:897–901.
69. Rosenberg SM, Schramm CM. Predictive value of pulmonary function testing during pulmonary exacerbations in cystic fibrosis. Pediatr Pulmonol 1993;16:227–235.
70. Rosenfeld MA, Collins FS. Gene therapy for cystic fibrosis. Chest 1996;109:241–252.
71. McElvaney NG, Hubbard RC, Birrer P, et al. Aerosol α_1-antitrypsin treatment for cystic fibrosis. Lancet 1991;337:392–394.
72. McElvaney NG, Nakamura H, Birrer P, et al. Modulation of airway inflammation in cystic fibrosis: *In vivo* suppression of interleukin-8 levels on the respiratory epithelial surface by aerosolization of recombinant secretory leukoprotease inhibitor. J Clin Invest 1992;90:296–301.
73. Meyer KC, Kewandeski JR, Zimmerman JJ, et al. Human neutrophil elastase and elastase/alpha 1-antiprotease complex in cystic fibrosis. Am Rev Respir Dis 1991;144:580–585.
74. Aronoff SC, Quinn FJ, Carpenter LS, et al. Effects of pentoxifylline on sputum neutrophil elastase and pulmonary function in patients with cystic fibrosis: Preliminary observations. J Pediatr 1994;125:992–997.
75. Knowles MR, Church NL, Waltner WE, et al. A pilot study of aerosolized amiloride for the treatment of lung disease in cystic fibrosis. N Engl J Med 1990;322:1189–1194.
76. Knowles MR, Clarke LL, Boucher RC. Activation by extracellular nucleotides of chloride secretion in the airway epithelia of patients with cystic fibrosis. N Engl J Med 1991;325:533–538.
77. Bennett WD, Olivier KN, Zeman KL, et al. Effect of uridine 5′-triphosphate plus amiloride on mucociliary clearance in adult cystic fibrosis. Am J Respir Crit Care Med 1996;153:1796–1801.
78. Yankaskas JR, Westerman JH, Thompson JT, et al. Improved results of lung transplantation for patients with cystic fibrosis. J Thorac Cardiovasc Surg 1995;109:224–234.

29
Evaluation of the Gastrointestinal Tract

Marie A. Chisholm, PharmD, and Mark W. Jackson, MD

The gastrointestinal (GI) tract encompasses organs and tissues that have diverse forms and functions. It includes the esophagus, stomach, small intestine, large intestine, colon, rectum, biliary tract, gallbladder, liver, and pancreas. Despite the rapid proliferation of technology for the diagnosis of digestive diseases, the patient history and physical examination still hold dominant roles. Combined with a thorough patient history and physical examination, diagnostic procedures are extremely useful in the evaluation of GI disorders. This chapter describes the most commonly used tools available in clinical practice to evaluate patients with GI diseases.

SYMPTOMS OF GASTROINTESTINAL DYSFUNCTION

There are various symptoms arising from GI dysfunction. Common GI symptoms include heartburn, abdominal pain, dyspepsia, nausea, vomiting, diarrhea, constipation, and gastrointestinal bleeding. Signs and symptoms of malabsorption, hepatitis, and GI infection are also commonly seen. The next sections describe methods commonly used to assess patients with GI complaints. For specific details concerning each GI disease state, please consult that particular chapter in this book.

PATIENT HISTORY

A comprehensive patient history is the cornerstone in the evaluation of a patient with digestive complaints. A clear, detailed, chronological account of the patient's problems should be ascertained. This account should include the onset of the problem, the setting in which it developed, and its manifestations. The onset of the problem often provides important information helping to confirm diagnosis. For example, biliary pain, such as that encountered with symptomatic gallstone disease, typically evolves over minutes and lasts for hours; but pain due to pancreatitis evolves over hours and lasts for days. The setting is always relevant as it provides clues to the possibilities of origin. For example, is the patient an alcoholic (liver disease, esophageal varices, pancreatitis)? Does the patient have severe atherosclerosis (mesenteric ischemia)? Is the patient a transplant recipient on immunosuppressant drugs (opportunistic infection)? Also aiding in the differential diagnosis is identification of factors that alleviate or exacerbate the principle symptom. For instance, ingesting a meal often relieves the pain of duodenal ulcer but worsens that of gastric ulcer. Asking questions that address the potential etiologic possibilities including motility disorders, structural diseases, malignancies, infections, psychosocial factors, dietary factors, and travel-associated diseases.[1,2] Questions concerning past medical and family history detailing illnesses, surgeries, injuries, and habits are extremely valuable (Table 29–1). Because many drugs have been reported to cause GI injury, a patient's medication history is vital (Table 29–2).

PHYSICAL EXAMINATION

A complete physical examination is necessary to evaluate patients with GI complaints.[3] A patient's appearance and vital signs may suggest clues to their overall condition and stability. Inspection of the abdomen may disclose signs of abdominal inflammation, scars, abdominal bulges, or hernias. Abdominal auscultation permits an appraisal of bowel sounds and other noises such as abdominal bruits. The liver and spleen are measured, and air in the stomach and bowel is identified by abdominal percussion. Marked tenderness, involuntary rigidity, or muscle spasm detected by palpating the abdomen may indicate peritoneal inflammation. Digital rectal examinations are used to detect rectal cancers and other lesions.[1,3] The hemoccult slide is a fecal occult blood test that is used to screen for colon cancer.

LABORATORY AND MICROBIOLOGIC TESTS

Laboratory and microbiologic tests may be used to (1) assess organ function, (2) screen for certain GI diseases, and (3) evaluate the effectiveness of therapy.

To achieve an accurate diagnosis and provide the best care, it is important to assess the patient's fluid and electrolyte status, nutritional status, and abdominal organ function. A serum chemistry panel provides clinicians with valuable information. For example, serum creatinine (SCr) and blood urea nitrogen (BUN) are often used as a measure

TABLE 29–1. General Questions in a GI History

1. Tell me about the problem that you are experiencing? When did it start?
2. Where is your pain located? Please point to the area where you feel pain. What were you doing when the pain occurred? How rapidly did the pain come on? Is your pain constant or intermittent? What factors exacerbate or alleviate your pain? Does the pain awaken you at night?
3. What medications are you taking to help the pain? How much do you take? Do these medications work?
4. What other medications are you currently taking? Why are you taking them?
5. Have you recently had a change in dietary intake? If so, please describe. Can you draw any correlation between the foods that you eat and your GI complaint?
6. Have you recently had a change in bowel habits? Have you experienced any diarrhea or constipation lately? Do you experience painful bowel movements?
7. Have you experienced any nausea or vomiting lately? If so, please describe conditions centered around this event.
8. Have you experienced any recent change in weight? Was this intentional? How many pounds have you gained or lost and over what time period did this occur? How has your appetite been?
9. Have you passed any blood from your rectum or vomitted blood? Have you noticed any dark, tarry stools?
10. Have you had any acid indigestion?
11. Do you have difficulty swallowing?
12. Has anyone in your family experienced similar GI complaints? If so, please describe. Does anyone in your family have a history of GI disorders, including cancer of the GI tract?
13. Describe your past medical history, including illnesses and surgeries.
14. Please describe any past injuries that you have experienced.
15. Have you recently traveled outside of the United States? If so, where? When? How long did you stay? What kind of living conditions did you experience? What foods and drinks did you ingest?

of hydration status as well as serve as indicators for renal function. Elevations in SCr and BUN may be indicative of renal dysfunction or dehydration, and bleeding from the GI tract may lead to elevations in BUN. Albumin levels can be used to assess the patient's nutritional and hydration status and provide information concerning hepatic and renal function. Specifically, a high albumin measurement may be indicative of dehydration, whereas low albumin may be indicative of hepatic dysfunction or nephrotic syndromes. Low albumin may also be seen in patients experiencing protein-losing enteropathies such as Crohn's disease and ulcerative colitis. Serum measurements of sodium, chloride, and potassium are useful to determine electrolyte abnormalities associated with diarrheal illnesses. A complete blood count (CBC) helps to provide information concerning infection, malignancy, bone marrow suppression, anemia, and blood loss.[4]

Specific laboratory blood tests are used as a screening tool for certain GI disorders. For example, measurements of serum aspartate transaminase (AST) and alanine transaminase (ALT) are elevated in most diseases of the liver, and serum alkaline phosphatase and bilirubin are often elevated in hepatobiliary disorders. Because prothrombin time is related to hepatocyte synthesis of vitamin K-dependent clotting factors, it serves as an indirect measure of hepatic function. When evaluating patients with suspected pancreatitis, serum and urine measurements of amylase and lipase are important, because most patients with acute pancreatitis will have elevated concentrations of amylase and lipase.

Microbiologic studies are useful in evaluating patients with unexplained diarrhea, abdominal pain, and suspected GI infections. Microbiologic studies of the stool may be used to detect the presence of bacteria and parasites. Pathogens most often responsible for infectious diarrhea and enteritis include bacteria such as *Shigella, Salmonella, Escherichia coli,* and *Yersinia;* viruses such as *cytomegalovirus,* especially in AIDS patients; and parasites such as *Entamoeba histolytica* and *Giardia lambia.*[5]

Because *Helicobacter pylori* is a significant factor associated with peptic ulcer disease and gastritis, identification of this organism is critical in evaluating patients experiencing dyspepsia. Serologic or saliva-based tests are capable of determining the presence of *H. pylori* antibodies in patients. Although serologic *H. pylori* antibody testing can determine whether a patient has been exposed to the organism,

TABLE 29–2. Drugs that May Commonly Cause GI Injury

Gastrointestinal Mucosal Injury	**Pancreatitis (continued)**
Aspirin	Metronidazole
Chemotherapeutic agents	Opiates
Corticosteroids	Sulindac
Ethacrynic acid	Sulfonamides
Ethanol	Tetracycline
Gentian violet	Thiazides
Isoproterenol	**Liver Damage**
Nonsteroidal anti-inflammatory agents	Acetaminophen
Pancrease supplementation	Allopurinol
Potassium chloride	Aminosalicylic acid
Reserpine	Dapsone
Warfarin	Erythromycin
Jaundice	Ethanol
Acetohexamide	Glyburide
Androgens	Isoniazid
Chlorpropamide	Ketoconazole
Corticosteroids	Methotrexate
Erythomycin	Methyldopa
Estrogens	Monamine oxidase inhibitors
Ethanol	Niacin
Gold salts	Nifedipine
Nitrofurantoin	Nitrofurantoin
Phenothiazines	Phenytoin
Warfarin	Propylthiouracil
Pancreatitis	Pyridium
Azathioprine	Rifampin
Corticosteroids	Salicytates
Estrogens	Sulfonamides
Ethacrynic acid	Tetracycline
Ethanol	Verapamil
Furosemide	Warfarin
	Zidovudine

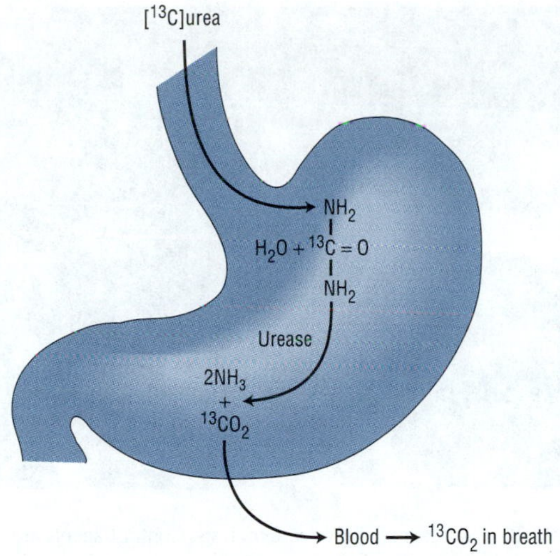

FIGURE 29–1. If urease is present in the stomach during testing with urease carbon 13 breath test, urea will be hydrolyzed to form ammonia and labeled carbon dioxide. The labeled carbon dioxide is absorbed into the bloodstream and is detected in expired air.

it is unable to indicate active infection. The unique capability of *H. pylori* to produce urease enzyme is exploited in certain direct tests of active *H. pylori* infection. At the time of endoscopy, biopsies of the stomach may be used to detect urease activity; for example, the CLO test uses a colored pH indicator that changes when ammonia is generated by *H. pylori.* Carbon[13] and carbon[14] breath tests involve the indirect measurement of urease activity by measuring labeled carbon dioxide in expired air (Fig. 29–1).[6] Tests that detect active *H. pylori* infection may be considered after antibiotic eradication medication use to determine effectiveness of therapy.

DIAGNOSIS

The patient history, physical examination, and routine laboratory tests are extremely useful in establishing a GI diagnosis, but frequently a more specific study is required to confirm or deny a clinical suspicion. The most appropriate diagnostic test depends on the anatomic region involved, the suspected abnormality, patient preferences, patient's overall condition, and clinical manifestation of the patient. The next sections outline the most frequently used diagnostic studies and procedures and their role in evaluating the GI tract.

RADIOLOGY

Radiologic procedures rely on the differential absorption of radiation between adjacent tissues to highlight anatomy and pathology. Radiologic procedures important in evaluating the GI tract include plain radiography, upper GI series, lower GI series, and enteroclysis.[7,8]

PLAIN RADIOGRAPHY OF GI SYSTEM

Radiographic evaluation of the GI tract often starts with plain films of the abdomen, which are straightforward, uncontrasted radiographs.[8] Specific abdominal structures that may be identified include the kidney, ureters, and bladder (KUB); esophagus; stomach; intestine; stones; and vessels. Plain films are often used to evaluate abdominal pain.[9] Clinicians frequently employ plain radiographic fluoroscopy to guide and position other instruments used to evaluate and treat GI disorders; an example is the manipulation of dilation devices to treat esophageal strictures. Bowel obstruction and perforation are especially well identified by this technique.

CONTRAST AGENTS

Many different types of contrast agents are available. Two types of contrast agents commonly used to enhance visualization of the GI tract are barium sulfate and iodinated aqueous compounds. Barium sulfate is the contrast agent of choice for studying the esophagus, stomach, and intestine except in special clinical situations.[8] Barium sulfate is not generally absorbed, and constipation is the most frequent adverse effect reported with its use. Two widely used iodinated contrast agents for visualizing the GI tract are diatrizoate meglumine and diatrizoate sodium. Unlike barium, these agents are relatively nontoxic if inadvertently introduced into the peritoneal cavity; therefore, the main indications for iodinated agents in GI radiologic films are for suspected bowel perforations. Because iodinated contrast agents are hyperosmolar, they possess the potential to cause severe diarrhea, dehydration, and electrolyte imbalances. Nephrotoxicity associated with iodinated contrast agents may occur and is generally self-limited.[8,10] Allergies and hypersensitivity reactions such as rashes associated with contrast agents are possible and should be monitored and treated accordingly.

UPPER GI SERIES

The upper GI series refers to the radiographic visualization of the esophagus, stomach, and small intestine. Patient preparation for an upper GI usually consists of instructing patients to refrain from eating or drinking 8 to 12 hours prior to testing, thereby allowing the upper GI tract to empty. A contrast agent such as barium sulfate is administered to the patient at the beginning of the study. The observed swallowing of the contrast agent permits visualization and monitoring of esophageal structural and motor functions. This phase of the procedure is most often referred to as a barium swallow. As the contrast medium flows into the stomach and small intestine, several regional radiographic films are taken in order to inspect these areas. This tracking of contrast agents through the small intestine is referred to as the small bowel follow-through. The upper GI series with the small bowel follow-through includes the examination of the esophagus to the distal end of the small intestine and is useful to evaluate and detect obstructions, tumors, ulcers, and abnormal intestinal loops. The upper GI series with small bowel follow-through commonly uncovers gastric cancer, peptic ulcer disease, esophagitis, gastric outlet obstruction, and Crohn's disease (Fig. 29–2).

LOWER GI SERIES

Patients complaining of lower abdominal pain, constipation, or diarrhea are often referred for a lower GI series. Before the procedure the colon is prepared by instructing the patient to refrain from eating or drinking 8 to 12 hours before the procedure and by administering bowel cleansing agents such as bisacodyl, magnesium citrate, magnesium hydroxide, and polyethylene glycol-electrolyte solution. During a lower GI series a barium sulfate enema is given to contrast the terminal large intestine and rectum. The lower GI series is useful to detect and evaluate enterocolitis, obstructions, volvulus, and mucosal and structural lesions.[8] The lower GI series is commonly used to diagnose Crohn's disease, ulcerative colitis, colon cancers, and diverticulitis.

SMALL BOWEL ENTEROCLYSIS

Enteroclysis or small bowel enema refers to the technique of direct small bowel introduction of a contrast agent through a tube inserted through the patient's mouth or nose. Intermittent radiographic films are taken of the small bowel as the contrast agent flows distally (Fig. 29–3). Because enteroclysis provides detailed imaging, it is the most

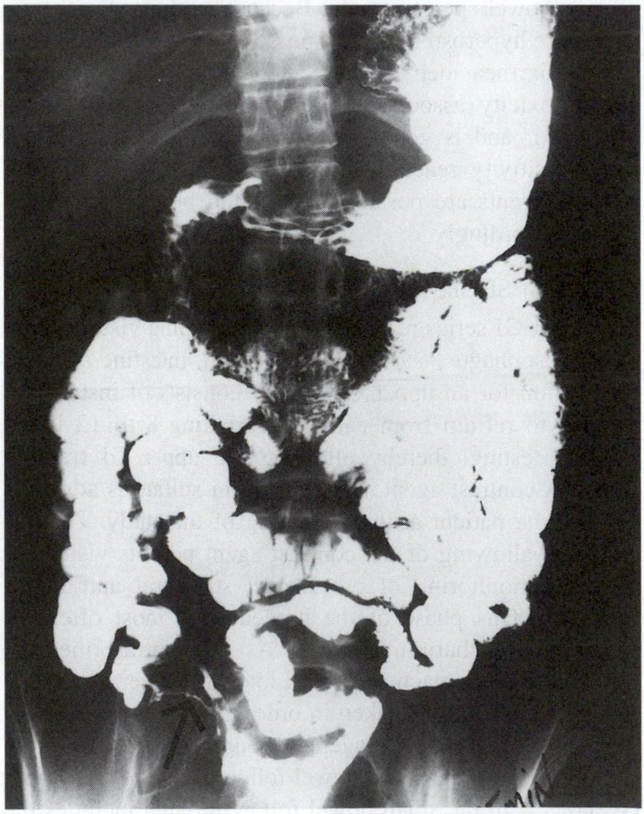

FIGURE 29–2. Upper GI series with small bowel follow-through demonstrating narrowed distal terminal ileum and separation of small bowel loops. These findings are consistent with Crohn's disease.

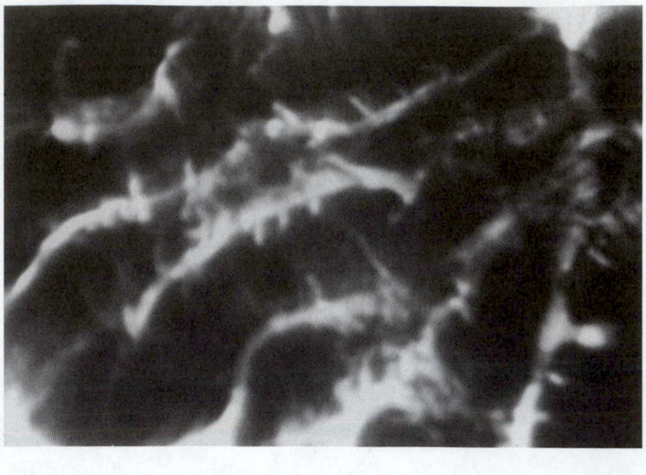

FIGURE 29–3. Normal small bowel enteroclysis. Contrast agents are instilled into the small bowel to highlight tumors, strictures, or other lesions. In this image, one can identify the normal circular folds.

accurate method for evaluating the small bowel and detecting small mucosal lesions that have been overlooked on the traditional small bowel follow-through.[11] Methylcellulose is used to enhance the detail of the small intestine in enteroclysis, thereby improving visualization. Patient preparation for this procedure involves instructing patients to refrain from eating or drinking 8 to 12 hours before testing and administering bowel cleansing agents. The most frequent disorder evaluated by enteroclysis is obscure GI bleeding.

IMAGING STUDIES

Through computer-assisted techniques, it is possible to generate cross-sectional radiographic images through the body. Ultrasonography, computed tomography, radionuclide scanning, and magnetic resonance imaging are frequently used imaging procedures for evaluating digestive disorders.

ULTRASONOGRAPHY

Ultrasonography provides images of deeper structures such as the gallbladder, pancreas, and abdominal wall. The clinician is able to image slices of the GI tract by directing a narrow beam of high-energy sound waves into the body and recording the reflections from the various organs and structures. Because ultrasonography is noninvasive, relatively inexpensive, requires no ionizing radiation, and can be performed with a portable unit, it is a well-accepted and useful technology. It accurately detects gallstones and gallbladder, hepatobiliary, and pancreatic diseases (Fig. 29–4). When combined with Doppler technologies, ultrasonography may image GI vascularity. Ultrasonography is limited by the presence of bowel gas and excessive amounts of body fat.[12,13]

COMPUTED TOMOGRAPHY

Computed tomography (CT) or computed axial tomography (CAT) scans provide detailed images of the GI system in which transverse planes of tissue are swept by a radi-

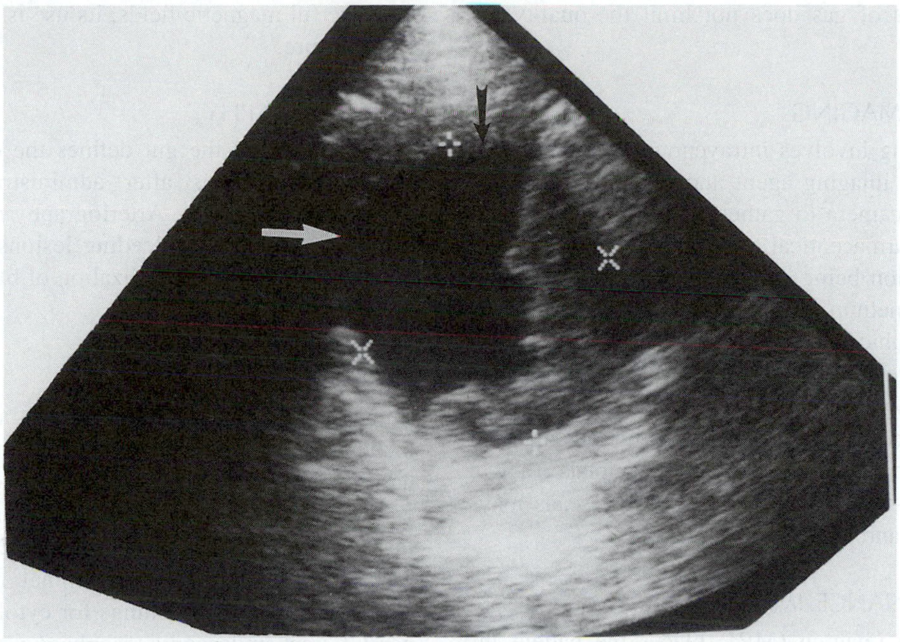

FIGURE 29–4. Abdominal ultrasound demonstrating a chronic pancreatic pseudocyst *(arrows)*.

ographic beam and a computer analysis of the variance in absorption produces a precise reconstructed image of that area.[7,12] Contrast agents may be added in a CT procedure to illuminate specific hollow structures and vascularity of the GI tract. The abdominal CT displays organs from the diaphragm down to the pelvic brim and is especially valuable for detecting GI diseases of the liver, pancreas, spleen, and colon. Patient preparation for CT includes refraining from eating or drinking for a minimum of 4 hours before the test. The remarkable detail that CT offers in imaging organs and tissues adds to its popularity for evaluation of the GI system. CT is useful in the identification of liver cancer, pancreatitis, pancreatic cancer, intra-abdominal abscesses, and cysts (Fig. 29–5).[12] Unlike ultrasonography, patient body

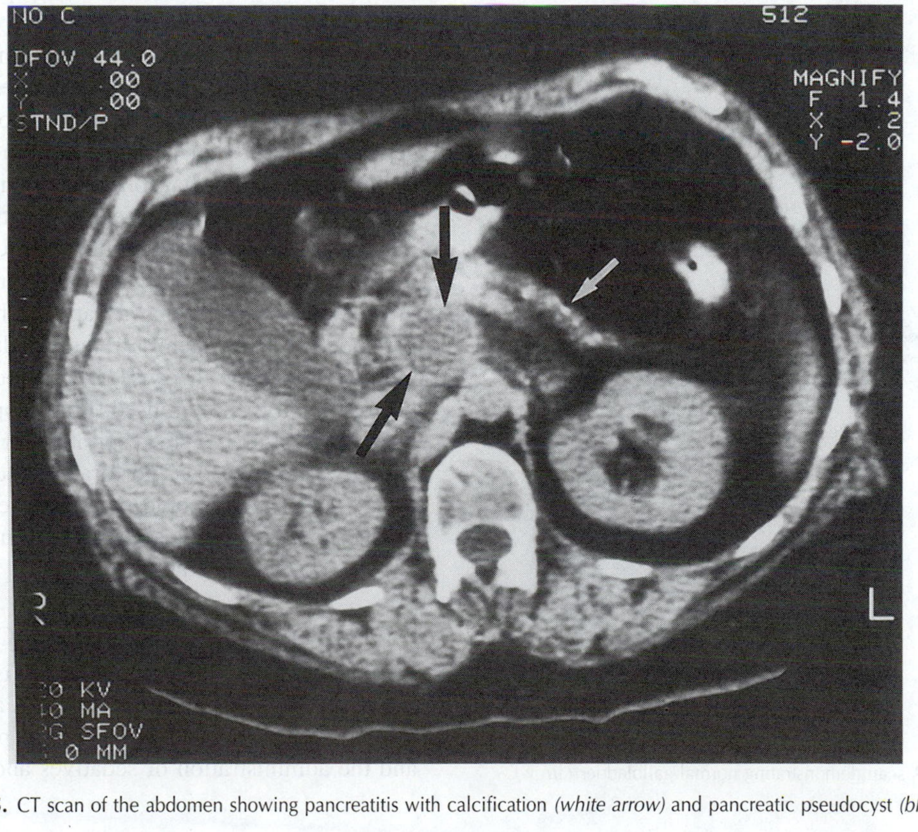

FIGURE 29–5. CT scan of the abdomen showing pancreatitis with calcification *(white arrow)* and pancreatic pseudocyst *(black arrows)*.

size or the presence of gas does not limit the quality of imaging with CT.

RADIONUCLIDE IMAGING

Radionuclide imaging involves intravenous injections of a radiopharmaceutical imaging agent and the use of a computerized detection camera to gather images. Although the choice of a radiopharmaceutical agent depends on the specific organ or function being studied, the most commonly used agent is technetium (Tc-99m) tagged to a carrier molecule. Radiographic imaging is useful to visualize the liver and spleen (liver-spleen scan), bile ducts, gallbladder (HIDA [hepato-iminodiacetic acid] scan), and gut (bleeding scan).[12] Cysts, abscesses, tumors, and obstructions are detected and displayed as areas of differential uptake of radioactivity (Fig. 29–6).[7] Radionuclide bleeding scans may detect hemorrhages and assist in localization.

MAGNETIC RESONANCE IMAGING

Magnetic resonance imaging (MRI) places the patient in close proximity to a high-strength magnetic field through which pulses of radiofrequency irradiation are projected, thereby exciting the nuclei of hydrogen, phosphorus, oxygen, and other elements. The radiofrequency signals are manipulated and recorded by computer and a two-dimensional picture representing a section of the patient is produced.[12] MRI has greater sensitivity to identify liver tumors than ultrasonography, CT, or radionuclide imaging. Although the current use of MRI is not as popular as other imaging techniques due to limited availability, expense, slow scanning time, and problems associated with the use of powerful magnetic fields, its use is predicted to increase in the future.[13]

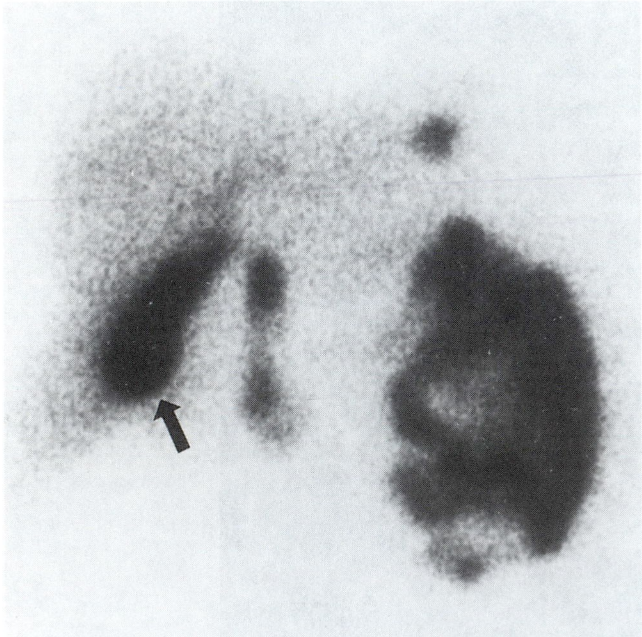

FIGURE 29–6. HIDA scan demonstrating normal gallbladder *(arrow)*.

ARTERIOGRAPHY

Arteriography of the gut defines the configuration of visceral blood vessels after administration of a contrast medium intravenously. Arteriography may be employed for detecting tumors and bleeding lesions and therapeutic applications including embolization of bleeding vessels, fistulas, and inoperable tumors.[12]

ENDOSCOPY

Refinement in optical engineering and fiber optics has made possible the development of the endoscope, which has revolutionized the management of GI disorders. An endoscope is an illuminated optical instrument designed to inspect the interior of the GI tract. Endoscopes allow the practitioner to inspect intraluminal mucosal lesions and obtain biopsies and washings for cytology studies. The upper GI tract endoscopy (esophagogastroduodenoscopy) is capable of inspecting the esophagus, stomach, and proximal small bowel. The lower GI tract endoscopy of the rectum and colon may be accomplished by colonoscopy or sigmoidoscopy.

Preparation for endoscopic examinations includes instructing patients to refrain from eating or drinking 8 to 12 hours prior to the endoscopic procedures. Bowel cleansing is necessary for colonoscopy and sigmoidoscopy. Topical pharyngeal anesthetics such as viscous lidocaine or benzocaine usually improve patient acceptance of the upper endoscopic tube. Intravenous sedating agents such as meperidine hydrochloride, diazepam, lorazepam, and midazolam hydrochloride are among the most common agents used to induce "conscious sedation" minutes prior to the endoscopy. These sedating agents tend to improve patient acceptance and ease of procedure. With the development of flumazenil, a benzodiazepine antagonist, the popularity of benzodiazepines for mild sedation with GI procedures has increased. In addition, antimuscuranic agents such as atropine sulfate are used occasionally for their cardiovascular effects such as increasing a patient's heart rate or its antispasmodic effects such as reducing duodenal and colonic motility. Glucagon, because of its effectiveness at reducing bowel motility, is often used. Endoscopy is contraindicated for patients with severe respiratory or cardiac failure, and patients with suspected perforated viscera. The most commonly used endoscopic studies are upper endoscopy, colonoscopy, sigmoidoscopy, and endoscopic retrograde cholangiopancreatography.

ESOPHAGOGASTRODUODENOSCOPY

Esophagogastroduodenoscopy (EGD) is used to examine the esophagus, stomach, and duodenum. Patient preparation for EGD includes fasting for 6 to 8 hours prior to the procedure and the administration of sedatives and topical anesthetics.

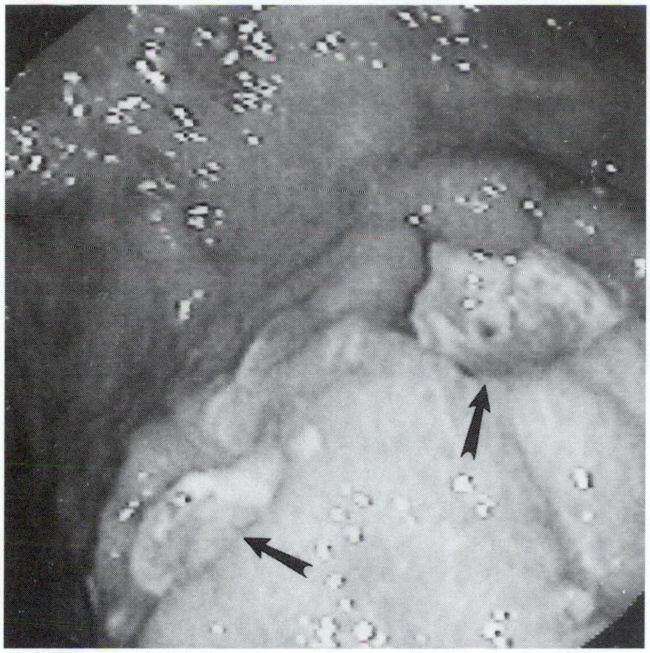

FIGURE 29–7. Deep "punched out" gastric ulcers *(arrows)* seen by EGD.

Common indications may be either diagnostic or therapeutic in nature and include evaluating suspected upper GI bleeding, obstructions, upper abdominal pain, persistent vomiting, and radiographic abnormalities.[14] EGD commonly uncovers peptic ulcers and other lesions (Fig. 29–7).

COLONOSCOPY

Colonoscopy permits direct examination of the large intestine and rectum. To prepare for colonoscopy, the patient should fast for about 8 hours prior to the examination and bowel cleansing should be completed. Agents such as midazolam and meperidine are usually given to produce conscious sedation. Similar to upper GI endoscopy, indications for lower GI endoscopy can be either diagnostic or therapeutic in nature and include evaluation and detection of abnormalities indicated on radiographic film, GI hemorrhaging, colonic lesions, volvulus, ulcerative colitis, Crohn's disease, diverticulitis, and excision of colonic polyps.[15]

SIGMOIDOSCOPY

Sigmoidoscopy is used to evaluate the sigmoid colon and rectum. Flexible sigmoidoscopy has virtually replaced the rigid sigmoidoscopy because of increased patient comfort and superior examining. The major indication for this examination is to evaluate symptoms related to the colon or rectum and to conduct screening of asymptomatic patients for colon polyps or cancer. Patient preparation involves instructing patients to abstain from eating or drinking 8 to 12 hours prior to the procedure and administering bowel cleansing agents. Anoscopy is especially useful in evaluating the anus. The major indications for the anoscopic examination include symptoms related to the anus and rectum such as bleeding, protrusions or swelling, pain, and severe itching. Patients undergoing sigmoidoscopy or anoscopy generally do not require sedation.

ENDOSCOPIC RETROGRADE CHOLANGIOPANCREATOGRAPHY

Endoscopic retrograde cholangiopancreatography (ERCP) is an important procedure used to evaluate and treat diseases of the biliary tree and pancreas. By injecting contrast agents through a catheter placed in the pancreaticobiliary ducts during ERCP, abnormalities such as obstructions, calculi, and strictures can be examined. Preparation for ERCP consists of conscious sedation and glucagon to relax gut motility. Common reasons for ERCP include detection and evaluation of pancreatic malignancy, pancreatitis, biliary obstruction, bile duct stones, jaundice, and patients whose clinical presentation suggests biliary disease (Fig. 29–8).

MISCELLANEOUS TESTS

ESOPHAGEAL MANOMETRY

Esophageal manometry is used to evaluate esophageal motor functions. Common indications for this procedure include dysphagia and obscure chest pain. A special catheter equipped with pressure transducers is placed into the esophagus to measure esophageal pressures and peristalsis. Provocative testing with pharmacologic agents such as edrophonium chloride, a cholinergic muscle stimulant, may be used to precipitate esophageal pain during this procedure.[16] Typical reasons for esophageal manometry include evaluating esophageal dysmotility, nonobstructive dysphagia, obscure chest pain, scleroderma, intestinal pseudoobstruction, achalasia, and aiding in positioning instruments such as pH probes.

AMBULATORY pH MONITORING

Gastric fluid pH monitoring in patients who complain of gastroesophageal reflux may be necessary. Indications for pH monitoring include evaluating atypical chest pain and severe or unusual reflux disorders. Ambulatory 24-hour pH monitoring is an elegant way to link esophageal acid exposure, as defined by a probe in the esophagus, with patient's symptoms. The pH probe is placed approximately 5 cm above the distal esophagus. Since intraesophageal pH is normally higher ($pH \geq 6$) than that of the stomach (pH approximately 1 to 3), the pH probe will record a decrease in pH if gastroesophageal reflux occurs.

The Bernstein test, another procedure used to measure gastric fluid pH, is less expensive than ambulatory pH monitoring. This procedure requires inserting a nasogastric (NG) tube and administrating alternating dripped solutions of normal saline and 0.1 N hydrochloric acid (HCl) into the esophagus via the NG tube. If patient symptoms are reproduced by the acid perfusion and not the saline, the study is considered abnormal and indicative of acid hypersensitivity.[17]

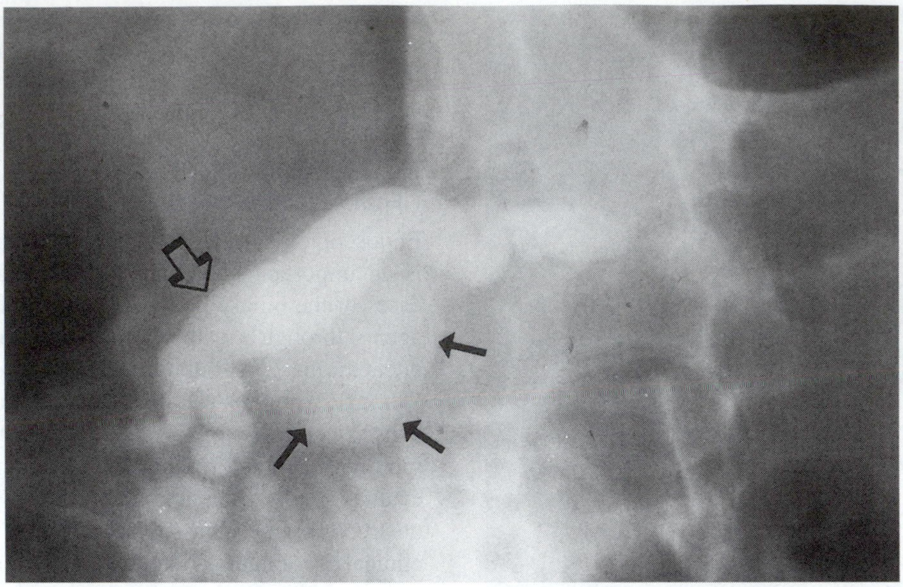

FIGURE 29–8. ERCP demonstrating a dilated, irregular pancreatic duct with areas of stricturing *(large arrow)*. A pancreatic pseudocyst is visible immediately adjacent to the spine *(small arrows)*.

LAPAROSCOPY

Laparoscopy uses a tubelike device with an elaborate optical system that permits distinct visualization of the peritoneal cavity. General anesthesia is often done and a surgical incision is made in the abdomen to allow the passage of the laparoscopic instrument. The exterior of the liver, gallbladder, spleen, peritoneum, diaphragm, and pelvic organs may be clearly examined during the laparoscopic examination. Similar to the other endoscopic techniques mentioned, biopsies and therapeutic interventions may occur during the laparoscopy. Reasons for doing laparoscopy include evaluating patients with ascites, abdominal masses, chronic abdominal pain, abnormalities indicated on liver-spleen scan, liver diseases, obstructive jaundice, and hepatic malignancy.

CLINICAL APPLICATIONS OF GI STUDIES

Gastrointestinal evaluations are largely driven by patient's dominant symptoms. Therefore, a brief evaluation overview is given for some common symptom complexes. The most common GI symptoms can be classified in the following sections: (1) heartburn, dysphagia, and dynophagia; (2) abdominal pain and dyspepsia; (3) nausea and vomiting; (4) diarrhea and constipation; (5) malabsorption; (6) gastrointestinal bleeding; and (7) hepatitis and jaundice.

HEARTBURN, DYSPHAGIA, AND ODYNOPHAGIA

The patient's history is especially useful in evaluating esophageal disease. Cardinal symptoms of the esophagus are heartburn, dysphagia (difficulty in swallowing), and odynophagia (painful swallowing). Heartburn is the most common esophageal complaint and when present is often sufficient to make the diagnosis of gastroesophageal reflux disease (GERD). The ambulatory 24-hour pH study may convincingly link the patient's symptom to an acid event (Fig. 29–9). The role of endoscopy in reflux disease is to evaluate severe or atypical cases and to uncover complications of reflux including esophageal stricture, bleeding, ulcers, and Barrett's esophagus. Dysphagia prompts concern for structural diseases that may be either benign such as peptic strictures or malignant such as esophageal carcinomas. When dysphagia is the dominant symptom, the patient is appropriately referred for a barium swallow. Upper endoscopy offers the ability to inspect the mucosa of the esophagus and take biopsies.

Esophageal manometry may prove useful in documenting abnormal motility as a basis for dysphagia in those patients who lack evidence for structural disease. Achalasia, also diagnosed with manometry, is an unusual

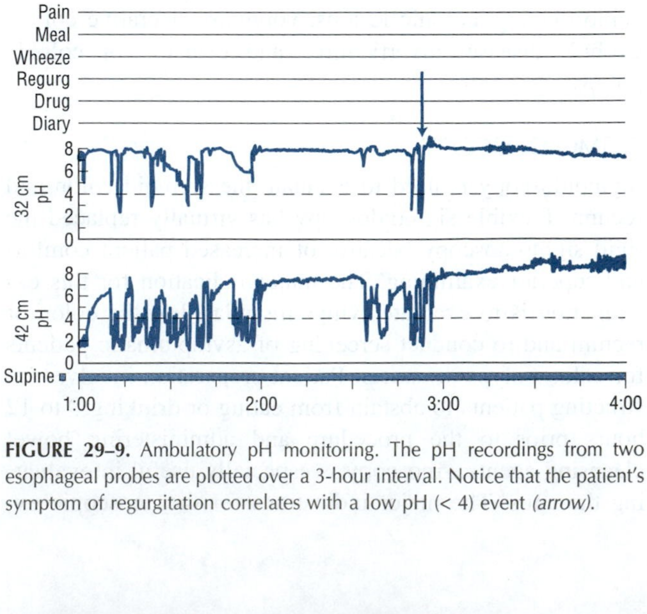

FIGURE 29–9. Ambulatory pH monitoring. The pH recordings from two esophageal probes are plotted over a 3-hour interval. Notice that the patient's symptom of regurgitation correlates with a low pH (< 4) event *(arrow)*.

cause of dysphagia due to absent peristalsis in the esophagus. Odynophagia often results from infection and requires biopsy for confirmation.

ABDOMINAL PAIN AND DYSPEPSIA

Abdominal pain is a common reason for patients to seek medical care. A rapid onset of acute pain accompanied by signs of peritonitis, fever, and leukocytosis suggests the possibility of a severe intra-abdominal infection or inflammation. An upright abdominal film may reveal evidence of free peritoneal air under the diaphragm, suggesting a perforated bowel. A serum amylase confirms or denies the possibility of acute pancreatitis. The evaluation may include ultrasonography or CT scans that may be helpful in demonstrating inflammatory or structural diseases such as appendicitis, cholecystitis, diverticulitis, abscesses, or aneurysm.

Patients with long-standing, chronic abdominal pain should undergo a more deliberate evaluation depending on the location and the temporal patterns of their abdominal pain. For example, nocturnal pain relieved by antacids may suggest peptic ulcer disease. A patient with abdominal pain, early satiety, and weight loss may have gastric cancer, and upper endoscopy and biopsy are particularly useful in diagnosing and evaluating this condition. Persistent attacks of pain radiating to the back may be due to pancreatic diseases, and abdominal imaging with ultrasonography or CT scans is generally indicated for confirmation.

Patients experiencing abdominal pain associated with nausea, vomiting, and abdominal distention may have a small bowel obstruction. An upper GI with small bowel follow-through may demonstrate a mechanical obstruction due to adhesions and hernias. Postprandial bloating and right lower quadrant pain occurs with Crohn's disease of the terminal ileum that may be detected with a small bowel follow-through as well. Left lower quadrant pain may reflect diverticulitis; although not always necessary, this may be detected by flexible sigmoidoscopy or barium enema. Patients with anemia or GI blood loss should undergo an evaluation by colonoscopy.

Dyspepsia generally refers to a variety of symptoms associated with the ingestion of food and can include such symptoms as belching, burning, epigastric pain, and bloating. Dyspepsia may be the presenting symptom for a variety of disorders including gastric and pancreatic carcinoma, cholelithiasis, intestinal obstruction, and functional disorders. An upper endoscopy can provide visual and histologic information that greatly aids in the differential diagnosis of patients with dyspepsia. An upper GI tract barium series is reasonably accurate in making a diagnosis although it is unable to define mucosal disease. Tests detecting *Helicobacter pylori* should be employed in patients complaining of dyspepsia.

NAUSEA AND VOMITING

As usual, evaluation of nausea and vomiting begins with a careful history. Is the patient pregnant? Is the patient undergoing chemotherapy? Does the patient have a central nervous system disease? Is the patient experiencing an adverse or toxic effect from a drug such as theophylline, digoxin, or an antibiotic? After ruling out the more common causes for persistent nausea and vomiting such as food-borne or viral gastroenteritis, it is advantageous to consider "working up" the patient to detect bowel obstructions. A plain abdominal film may detect bowel obstruction. An upper GI series or an upper endoscopy may show structural lesions or obstructions of the GI tract as well. If an obstruction is not found, serum amylase and lipase should be measured to evaluate the diagnosis of acute pancreatitis. Timing of vomiting relative to meals provides important information. Nausea and vomiting on awakening suggest alcoholic gastritis; vomiting after meals suggests peptic ulcer disease and gastric cancer; and vomiting 3 to 8 hours after meals suggests an obstruction in the upper gastrointestinal tract.

DIARRHEA AND CONSTIPATION

Patient history may be useful in identifying diarrhea associated with recent travel, male homosexuality, antibiotics, or food-borne gastroenteritis. It is helpful to quantify the average number of stools per day, presence of blood and mucus, and color. Many patients experience mild abdominal discomfort and diarrhea when taking antibiotics. Other patients may continue to have diarrhea after discontinuing the antibiotics and experience fever and abdominal tenderness, suggesting antibiotic-associated colitis. This diagnosis can be achieved through sigmoidoscopy by observing yellow adherent plaques or "pseudomembranes" (Fig. 29–10). A stool sample may also be examined to detect *Clostridium difficile* toxins. A patient with acute diarrhea who appears

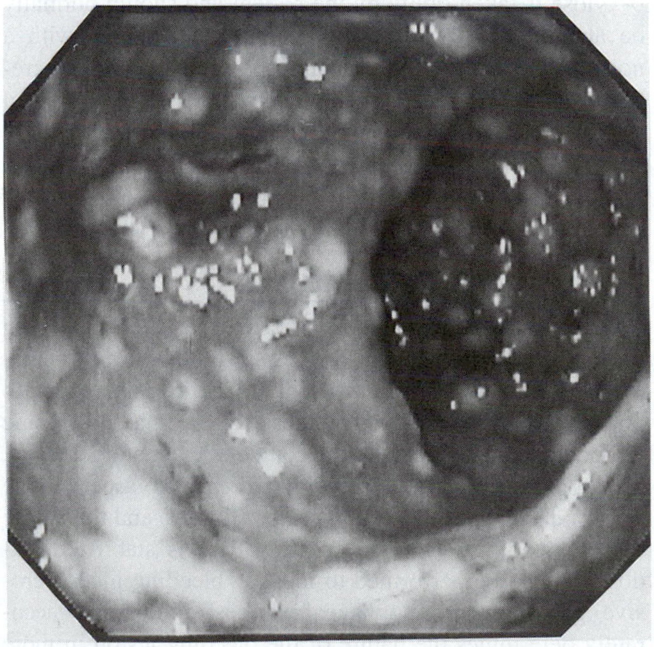

FIGURE 29–10. Sigmoidoscopic photograph revealing the light raised lesions of antibiotic-associated pseudomembranous colitis.

feverish and dehydrated or has bloody diarrhea may have an infection and should undergo stool cultures to detect *C. difficile,* ova, and parasites. In addition, evaluation of diarrhea for leukocytes is useful to determine if inflammation is present.

The history and physical examination may provide important clues to direct evaluation of chronic diarrhea. Sigmoidoscopy is reliable for excluding colitis and obstruction due to cancer or diverticula. A patient with a normal sigmoidoscopy may have the remainder of his or her colon evaluated with an air-contrast barium enema to rule out inflammatory bowel disease or obstruction. A patient with a negative evaluation probably has irritable bowel syndrome ("spastic colon").

Constipation is an imprecise term that implies either infrequent or difficult defecation. It is important for clinicians to obtain a detailed dietary, laxative, and medication history because these may play a role. Appropriate laboratory tests should be performed to exclude metabolic disorders such as hypothyroidism, hypokalemia, hypercalcemia, and hypomagnesemia. If a metabolic disorder cannot be found, an underlying structural abnormality should be sought. Sigmoidoscopy and an air-contrast barium enema are usually the best approaches for evaluation.

MALABSORPTION

Malabsorption is classically manifested by steatorrhea (fat in the stool) and weight loss. Steatorrhea is evaluated by first examining the stool for the presence of fat and, once established, tests are performed to differentiate pancreatic insufficiency from small bowel disease. The D-xylose test is a measure of small bowel absorption that is nearly always abnormal in small bowel malabsorption. A 5-g dose of D-xylose is taken orally by the patient and should normally be absorbed and secreted in the urine. A patient with a normal D-xylose test and steatorrhea probably has pancreatic insufficiency. However, a patient with an abnormal D-xylose test and steatorrhea favors small bowel disease. An upper GI with small bowel follow-through or small bowel biopsies may prove useful to show the presence of celiac sprue, Whipple disease, lymphoma, or other lesions.

GI BLEEDING

Gastrointestinal bleeding may occur as a life-threatening emergency marked by hematemesis (bloody vomit), hematochezia (bloody stool), or melena (black, tarry stool due to upper GI bleeding); or at the other extreme, may be chronic or occult and discovered in the course of evaluating anemia. The goal in evaluating a bleeding patient is to ascertain the site of bleeding (upper versus lower GI tract) and the nature of the bleeding lesion. After the patient is stabilized, endoscopy can be performed to identify bleeding ulcers, erosive gastritis, and esophageal varices. Endoscopy accurately determines the nature of the bleeding lesion in more than 90% of presenting patients and is often the vehicle for the delivery of therapy (sclerosis injections or cautery). In cases where endoscopy has technically failed to identify or treat the source of the bleeding or in cases of rapid bleeding, arteriography (angiography) may be advisable. Under these circumstances, arteriography can be used to localize the bleeding site and afford treatment of the bleeding vessel. Barium studies have no role in the management of acute GI bleeding.

HEPATITIS AND JAUNDICE

When the history and physical examination identify active or chronic liver disease, a detailed medication history is critical because numerous agents are known to induce these disorders. When transaminases are 10 times normal, viral hepatitis or acute cholangitis is considered and should prompt further specific diagnostic efforts including viral markers. Milder elevation of the transaminases is a nonspecific finding and considerations should include alcohol liver disease. In a symptomatic patient with hepatomegaly or clinical signs of liver disease, liver ultrasonography or CT scans may help exclude cancer. The function of the liver may be measured indirectly by measuring serum albumin and performing coagulation studies.

When hepatocellular disease is suspected, ultrasonography or CT scans of the liver are performed to exclude focal defects such as tumors, abscesses, and vascular lesions prior to performing a percutaneous liver biopsy (Fig. 29–11). Often a liver biopsy is the best way to resolve questions as to the reason for underlying hepatocellular injury. When alkaline phosphatase is elevated, especially in conjunction with transaminases, one considers cholestatic

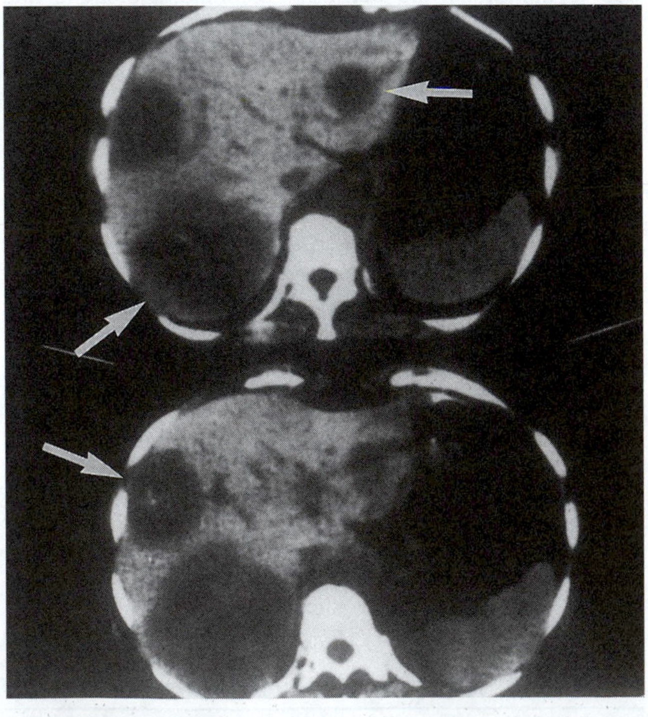

FIGURE 29–11. CT scans of the abdomen showing metastatic cancer of the liver *(arrows).*

liver diseases. In suspected biliary disease, an abdominal ultrasound is usually done with special attention to the interhepatic ducts. If the ducts are dilated, one considers an obstructive pancreas, bile duct cancer, bile duct strictures, or common bile duct stones. "Cholestatic" patients without dilated bile ducts may have primary biliary cirrhosis, diagnosed by liver biopsy; or primary sclerosing cholangitis, diagnosed by characteristic bile duct changes on ERCP. Cholestasis may occur with or without jaundice.

Jaundice often, but not always, reflects underlying liver disease. The clinician is commonly faced with the question as to whether the patient's jaundice is due to an extrahepatic process or an intrahepatic parenchymal liver disease. An extrahepatic lesion is suggested by a disproportionate elevation in alkaline phosphatase and may be confirmed by observing dilated intrahepatic ducts on ultrasonography or CT scan. Often an ERCP is necessary to visualize the biliary tree and pancreatic ducts to identify the precise location and character of the obstructing lesion. Liver biopsy plays a role in determining the parenchymal role in the cholestatic process.

Hepatomegaly found on physical exam suggests chronic disease. Hepatitis might be the culprit under these circumstances and is easily detected by measurement of serum transaminases. Ultrasonography or CT scans are used to determine if there is focal or diffuse liver disease and obstruction of the biliary tree. A patient with abdominal pain and an enlarged liver may have an abscess, hematoma, or tumor that may be best demonstrated by a CT scan.

CONCLUSIONS

A comprehensive history and physical examination play a critical role in evaluating patients with digestive diseases. Laboratory and microbiologic tests, radiography, ultrasonography, computed tomography, radionuclide scanning, magnetic resonance imaging, arteriography, endoscopy, esophageal manometry, pH monitoring, and laparoscopy have definite roles in diagnosing and evaluating GI disorders. These tests should be used in combination with the patient's history and physical examination to facilitate diagnosis and effective disease state management of the GI disorder at nominal cost and risk to the patient.

REFERENCES

1. Isselbacher KJ, Podolsky DK. Approach to the patient with gastrointestinal disease. In: Wilson JD, Braunwald E, et al, eds. Harrison's Principles of Internal Medicine. New York, McGraw-Hill, 1991: 1213–1216.
2. Janowitz HD. Approach to the patient with gastrointestinal symptoms. In: Sachar DB, Waye JD, et al, eds. Pocket Guide to Gastroenterology. Baltimore, Williams & Wilkins, 1989:1–7.
3. Bates B. A Guide to Physical Examination. Philadelphia, Lippincott, 1994.
4. Jacobs DS, Demott WR, Finley PR, et al. Laboratory Test Handbook. Cleveland, Lexi-Comp, 1994.
5. Guerrant RL. Principles and syndromes of enteric infection. In: Mandell GL, Douglas RG, et al, eds. Principles and Practice of Infectious Diseases. New York, Churchill Livingstone, 1990:837–851.
6. Walsh JH, Peterson WL. The treatment of *Helicobacter pylori* infection in the management of ulcer disease. N Engl J Med 1995;333: 984–991.
7. Novelline RA. Squire's Fundamentals of Radiology. Cambridge, Harvard University Press, 1997.
8. Cohen AJ. Radiologic general diagnostic and imaging studies of the small and large bowel. In: Gitnick G, ed. Principles and Practice of Gastroenterology and Hepatology. Stamford, CT, Appleton & Lange, 1994:441–432.
9. Eisenberg RL, Heineken P, Hedgcock MW, et al. Evaluation of plain abdominal radiographs in the diagnosis of abdominal pain. Ann Intern Med 1982;97:257–261.
10. Smith CR, Petty BG. Specific complications of medical management. In: Harvey AM, Johns RT, et al, eds. The Principles and Practice of Medicine. Stamford, CT, Appleton & Lange, 1988:1155–1162.
11. Miller RE, Sellink JL. Enteroclysis: The small bowel enema. How to succeed and how to fail. Gastrointest Radiol 1979;4:269–283.
12. Friedman LS, Needleman L. Hepatobiliary imaging. In: Wilson JD, Braunwald E, et al, eds. Harrison's Principles of Internal Medicine. New York, McGraw-Hill, 1991:1303–1308.
13. Wall SD. Diagnostic imaging procedures in gastro-enterology. In: Bennet JC, Plum F, eds. Cecil Textbook of Medicine. Philadelphia, Saunders, 1996:630–635.
14. Sartor RB. Upper gastrointestinal endoscopy. In: Drossman DA, ed. Manual of Gastroenterologic Procedures. New York, Raven, 1993: 131–139.
15. Shinya H, Wolf WI. Colonoscopy. Surg Ann 1976;8:257–295.
16. Benjamin SB, Richter JE, Cordova CM, et al. Prospective manometric evaluation with pharmacologic provocation of patients with suspected esophageal motility dysfunction. Gastroenterology 1983;84: 893–901.
17. Sandler RS. Bernstein (acid perfusion) test. In: Drossman DA, ed. Manual of Gastroenterologic Procedures. New York, Raven, 1993: 56–60.

30

Gastroesophageal Reflux Disease

Dianne B. Williams, PharmD

Gastroesophageal reflux disease (GERD) is a common medical disorder seen by health care practitioners of all specialties. Although mortality associated with GERD is very low (1 death per 100,000 patients), it reportedly has a greater impact on quality of life than duodenal ulcers, untreated hypertension, mild congestive heart failure, angina, or menopause.[1,2] GERD refers to any symptomatic clinical condition or histologic alteration that results from episodes of gastroesophageal reflux. Gastroesophageal reflux refers to the retrograde movement of gastric contents from the stomach into the esophagus. When the esophagus is repeatedly exposed to refluxed material for prolonged periods of time, inflammation of the esophagus (reflux esophagitis) can occur, and in some cases it can progress to erosion of the esophagus (erosive esophagitis). Gastroesophageal reflux may also be associated with disease processes in organs other than the esophagus, such as the lungs. This is referred to as extraesophageal GERD.[3] Many patients suffering from mild GERD do not go on to develop erosive esophagitis and are often managed with life-style changes, antacids, and over-the-counter (OTC) histamine (H_2)-receptor antagonists. Patients who present with erosive esophagitis predictably follow a course of relapsing disease requiring more intensive treatment with acid-suppressive therapy followed by long-term maintenance therapy.[4] Laparoscopic antireflux surgery offers an alternative to medical management for those patients who fail therapy or for those patients where medical management is undesirable.

EPIDEMIOLOGY

Gastroesophageal reflux disease occurs in both adults and children. The prevalence of GERD is dependent on the geographic region and is noted to be highest in Western countries.[1] In general, the prevalence increases in adults over the age of 40 years. Except for pregnant women, there does not appear to be a major difference in incidence between men and women. Heartburn is a common complaint during pregnancy, with as many as 25% of women experiencing heartburn on a daily basis.[5] Although gender does not play a major role in the development of GERD, it is an important factor in the development of Barrett's esophagus, a complication of GERD where the normal squamous epithelium is replaced with columnar epithelium. Barrett's esophagus affects males more than females by a ratio of 6 to 1.[6] The true prevalence and incidence of GERD is difficult to assess due to several factors: (1) many patients do not seek medical treatment, (2) symptoms do not always correlate well with severity of disease, and (3) there is no standardized definition or universal gold standard method for diagnosing the disease.[1]

Approximately 10% of Americans suffer from heartburn daily and more than one-third have intermittent symptoms.[5] Yet many of these patients choose not to seek medical help from a physician and self-treat with OTC medications. Interestingly, as many as 46% of patients with mild disease will heal spontaneously with self-medication and another 31% will show significant improvement, indicating a relatively benign process in patients with minimal symptoms.[7,8] Conversely, the presence of symptoms in patients who do seek medical advice does not always correlate well with the presence of esophageal inflammation or erosion, making it extremely difficult to identify which patients will have severe esophageal damage as opposed to those with merely symptoms. Of the 20% to 40% of patients who experience heartburn, approximately 30% to 79% of these patients will have evidence of esophagitis.[9] Luckily, fewer than 15% of patients suffer severe esophagitis, indicating that most patients only suffer from mild to moderate degrees of esophagitis. On the other hand, many patients with esophageal damage may not experience symptoms or they may present with atypical symptoms.[10]

Finally, the lack of a standardized definition and universal gold standard for diagnosing GERD presents another obstacle in assessing epidemiologic data.

PATHOPHYSIOLOGY

The key factor in the development of GERD is the movement of acid or other noxious substances from the stomach into the esophagus.[11] In many patients with GERD, the problem is not that they produce too much acid, but that the acid produced spends too much time in contact with the esophageal mucosa. A prolonged acid clearance is seen in many patients with gastroesophageal reflux.

In many cases, gastroesophageal reflux is due to a defective lower esophageal sphincter pressure. Patients may have decreased gastroesophageal sphincter pressures related to (1) spontaneous transient lower esophageal sphincter relaxations, (2) transient increases in intra-abdominal pressure, or (3) atonic lower esophageal sphincter—all of which may lead to the development of gastroesophageal reflux. Problems with other normal mucosal "defense mechanisms" such as anatomic factors, mucosal resistance, and gastric emptying may also contribute to the development of GERD. "Aggressive factors" that may promote esophageal damage upon reflux into the esophagus include gastric acid, pepsin, bile acids, and pancreatic enzymes. Thus, the composition and volume of the refluxate are the most important aggressive factors in determining the consequences of gastroesophageal reflux.

Gastroesophageal reflux may lead to many severe complications, including esophagitis, strictures, and Barrett's esophagus.[11] Strictures are common in the distal esophagus and are generally 1 to 2 cm in length. The use of nonsteroidal anti-inflammatory drugs (NSAIDs) or aspirin has been implicated as an additional risk factor that may contribute to the development or worsening of esophageal strictures. In one study, 31% of patients undergoing initial dilation for benign esophageal strictures used NSAIDs compared with only 14% in control subjects.[12] Although GERD may lead to esophageal bleeding, the blood loss is usually chronic and low grade in nature. However, anemia can occur. In some patients the reparative process leads to the replacement of the squamous epithelial lining of the esophagus by columnar-type epithelium. This condition, known as Barrett's esophagus, is more likely to occur in those patients with a long history (years) of reflux that, in many cases, improves without intervention.[13] It is found in 4.5% to 12.4% of patients undergoing endoscopy for reflux symptoms and is associated with a 5% to 10% incidence of adenocarcinoma and a 30% to 80% incidence of esophageal stricture formation.[14]

Rational therapeutic regimens in the treatment of gastroesophageal reflux are designed to maximize normal mucosal defense mechanisms and/or attenuate the aggressive factors.

LOWER ESOPHAGEAL SPHINCTER PRESSURE

The lower esophageal sphincter is a manometrically defined zone of high resting pressure. The sphincter is normally in a tonic state, preventing the reflux of gastric material from the stomach, but relaxes on swallowing to permit the free passage of food into the stomach. Typically, patients with more severe gastroesophageal disease have resting lower esophageal sphincter pressures below 5 mm Hg. Mechanisms by which defective lower esophageal sphincter pressure may cause gastroesophageal reflux are threefold. First, and probably most important, reflux may occur following spontaneous transient lower esophageal sphincter relaxations that are not associated with swallowing.[15] Although the exact mechanism is unknown, esophageal distention, vomiting, belching, and retching have all been shown to cause relaxation of the lower esophageal sphincter. Although not thought to contribute significantly to erosive esophagitis, these transient relaxations, which are normal postprandially, may play an important role in intermittent nonerosive reflux.[4] Transient decreases in sphincter pressure are responsible for approximately 65% of the reflux episodes in patients with GERD. The propensity to develop gastroesophageal reflux secondary to transient decreases in lower esophageal sphincter pressure is probably dependent on numerous factors, including degree of sphincter relaxation, efficacy of esophageal clearance, patient position (more common in recumbent position), gastric volume, and intragastric pressure.

Second, reflux may occur following transient increases in intra-abdominal pressure (stress reflux).[11] An increase in intra-abdominal pressure such as that occurring during straining, bending over, coughing, eating, or a Valsalva maneuver may overcome a weak lower esophageal sphincter, and thus may lead to reflux. Third, the lower esophageal sphincter may be atonic, thus permitting free reflux.

Although transient relaxations are more likely to occur when there is substantial lower esophageal sphincter pressure, the latter two mechanisms are more likely to occur when the lower esophageal sphincter pressure is decreased by such factors as fatty foods, gastric distention, smoking, or certain medications.[11] Table 30–1 lists factors and conditions that affect lower esophageal sphincter pressures.[16] Factors that decrease lower esophageal sphincter pressure

TABLE 30–1. Factors That Affect Lower Esophageal Sphincter Pressure

Decrease Lower Esophageal Sphincter Pressure	Increase Lower Esophageal Sphincter Pressure
Foods	
Carminatives (peppermint, spearmint)	Protein meal
Chocolate	
Fatty meal	
Coffee, cola, tea, citrus juices	
Tomato juice	
Onions, garlic	
Drugs	
Anticholinergics	Prokinetic agents (bethanechol cisapride, metoclopramide)
Barbiturates	Edrophonium
Benzodiazepines (diazepam)	Methacholine
Caffeine	Norepinephrine
Calcium channel blockers	Pentagastrin
Dopamine	Phenylephrine
Estrogen	
Ethanol	
Isoproterenol	
Narcotics (meperidine, morphine)	
Nicotine (smoking)	
Nitrates	
Phentolamine	
Progesterone	
Theophylline	
Hormones/Physiologic Factors	
Cholecytokinin	Gastric alkalinization
Estrogen	Gastrin
Gastric acidification	Prostaglandin F_2
Glucagon	
Progesterone	
Prostaglandins (E_1, E_2, A_2)	
Secretin	
Vasoactive intestinal peptide (VIP)	

Adapted from Ref. 16.

predispose patients to gastroesophageal reflux. Various foods aggravate esophageal reflux. Some of these foods cause a decrease in lower esophageal sphincter pressure. Other foods, such as spicy foods, orange juice, tomato juice, and coffee, may precipitate symptomatic reflux by direct mucosal irritation.[5] Pregnancy, achalasia, and scleroderma are conditions in which reflux is common. There are many postulated reasons for the increased incidence of heartburn during pregnancy including hormonal effects on esophageal muscle, lower esophageal sphincter tone, and physical factors (increased intra-abdominal pressure) resulting from an enlarging uterus.[17]

A decrease in lower esophageal sphincter pressure resulting from any of the previously mentioned causes is not always associated with gastroesophageal reflux. Likewise, individuals who experience decreases in sphincter pressures and subsequently reflux do not always develop GERD. The other natural defense mechanisms (anatomic factors, esophageal clearance, mucosal resistance, and gastric factors) must be evoked to explain this phenomenon.

ANATOMIC FACTORS

Proposed anatomic factors can be categorized into valvular mechanisms, extrinsic compression, intra-abdominal esophageal segment, mucosal choke, and spiral stretch mechanisms. Disruption of the normal anatomic barriers by a hiatal hernia was once thought to be a primary etiology of gastroesophageal reflux and esophagitis. Now it appears a more important factor related to the presence or absence of symptoms in patients with hiatal hernias is the lower esophageal sphincter pressure. Patients with hypotensive lower esophageal sphincter pressures and large hiatal hernias are more likely to experience gastroesophageal reflux following abrupt increases in intra-abdominal pressure as compared to patients with hypotensive lower esophageal sphincter and no hiatal hernia.[18] The combination of these two conditions (hypotensive lower esophageal sphincter pressures and hiatal hernia) has a more than additive effect, resulting in an incompetent gastroesophageal junction.[18] Although anatomic factors are still considered significant by some, the diagnosis of hiatal hernia is currently considered a separate entity with which gastroesophageal reflux may or may not simultaneously occur.

ESOPHAGEAL CLEARANCE

Approximately 50% of GERD patients with esophagitis will have a prolonged acid clearance time.[11] This is not surprising, because the symptoms and/or severity of damage produced by gastroesophageal reflux are partially dependent on the duration of contact between the gastric contents and the esophageal mucosa.[19] This contact time is in turn dependent on the rate at which the esophagus clears the noxious material and the frequency of reflux. The esophagus is cleared by primary peristalsis in response to swallowing, secondary peristalsis in response to esophageal distention, and gravitational effects. Swallowing contributes to esophageal clearance by increasing salivary flow. Saliva contains bicarbonate that buffers the residual gastric material on the surface of the esophagus. The production of saliva decreases with increasing age, making it more difficult to maintain a neutral intraesophageal pH. Therefore, esophageal damage due to reflux occurs more often in the elderly and, similarly, in those patients with Sjögren's syndrome.[20]

Defective esophageal clearance may be a primary event or a secondary consequence in gastroesophageal reflux. The decreased esophageal clearance seen in patients with symptomatic gastroesophageal reflux may be marked by a defect in esophageal emptying, which may be worse in the presence of a hiatal hernia, and/or a decrease in the amplitude of esophageal peristalsis.[19] Up to 50% of patients with severe esophagitis have peristaltic dysfunction compared with 25% of patients with mild esophagitis.[21] Gastroesophageal reflux may also contribute to decreased clearing and decreased lower esophageal sphincter pressures, both of which may further worsen reflux.

Notably, acid clearance times improve when a patient is in an upright position or when the head of the bed is elevated due to gravitational effects on esophageal clearance. Individuals who have symptomatic reflux while upright experience excessive acid exposure secondary to an increased frequency of reflux episodes. Because esophageal clearance is impaired during sleep, excessive acid exposure in symptomatic patients in the supine position is primarily due to an increase in the duration of the reflux episodes (decreased clearance). The patient's awareness of heartburn during sleep may be impaired, and this may contribute to the extended duration of acid exposure while recumbent.

MUCOSAL RESISTANCE

Within the esophageal mucosa and submucosa there are mucus-secreting glands. The mucus secreted by these glands may contribute to the protection of the esophagus.[22] Bicarbonate moving from the blood to the lumen can neutralize acidic refluxate in the esophagus. When the mucosa is repeatedly exposed to the refluxate in GERD or if there is a defect in the normal mucosal defenses, hydrogen ions diffuse into the mucosa, leading to the cellular acidification and necrosis that ultimately cause esophagitis.[11] In theory, mucosal resistance may be related not only to esophageal mucus but also to tight epithelial junctions, epithelial cell turnover, nitrogen balance, mucosal blood flow, tissue prostaglandins, and the acid–base status of the tissue.[22]

COMPOSITION OF REFLUXATE

The composition and volume of the refluxate are the most important aggressive factors in determining the consequences of gastroesophageal reflux. In animals, acid has two primary effects when it is refluxed into the esophagus. First, if the pH of the refluxate is less than 2, esophagitis may develop secondary to protein denaturation. In addition, pepsin is activated at this pH and may also cause esophagitis. Alkaline esophagitis refers to esophagitis induced by the reflux of bilious and pancreatic fluid. The term "alkaline esophagitis" may be a misnomer in that the refluxate may be either weakly alkaline or acidic in nature. Pure alkaline reflux is relatively rare.[23] An increase in gastric bile concentrations may be due to increased duodenogastric reflux because of a generalized motility disorder or slower clearance of the refluxate.[24] Although bile acids have both a direct irritant effect on the esophageal mucosa and an indirect effect of increasing hydrogen ion permeability of the mucosa, symptoms are more often related to acid reflux than bile reflux. Esophageal pH monitoring has demonstrated that severity of disease is related to degree of esophageal acid exposure and not so much to bile exposure. Specifically, the percentage of time that esophageal pH is below 4 is greater for patients with severe disease as compared to mild disease.[25,26] However, esophageal pH monitoring in conjunction with 24-hour bile monitoring has demonstrated a higher incidence of Barrett's esophagus in patients with both acid and alkaline reflux.[24] More study is needed to substantiate this finding. Nevertheless, the combination of acid, pepsin, and bile is a potent refluxate in producing esophageal damage.

GASTRIC EMPTYING

Delayed gastric emptying can also contribute to gastroesophageal reflux. An increase in gastric volume may increase both the frequency of reflux and the amount of gastric fluid available to be refluxed. Gastric volume is related to the volume of material ingested, rate of gastric secretion, rate of gastric emptying, and amount and frequency of duodenal reflux into the stomach. Patients with Barrett's esophagus may have a hypersecretory condition that is unresponsive to standard doses of H_2 antagonists. Factors that increase gastric volume and/or decrease gastric emptying, such as smoking and high fatty meals, are often associated with gastroesophageal reflux. This in part explains the prevalence of postprandial gastroesophageal reflux. Fatty foods may increase postprandial gastroesophageal reflux by increasing gastric volume, delaying the gastric emptying rate, and decreasing the lower esophageal sphincter pressure. Delayed gastric emptying of liquid–solid meals has been shown to occur in approximately 41% of patients with symptoms of gastroesophageal reflux.[27] Patients with gastroesophageal reflux may have a defect in antral motility.[28] This is commonly seen in infants. The delay in emptying may promote regurgitation of feedings, which may in turn contribute to the development of the two most common complications of gastroesophageal reflux disease in infants (i.e., failure to thrive and pulmonary aspiration).[29]

The pathophysiology of gastroesophageal reflux is a complex, cyclic process. It is difficult, if not impossible, to determine which event occurred first in a given patient. For example, did gastroesophageal reflux lead to a defective peristalsis with delayed clearing, or did an incompetent lower esophageal sphincter pressure lead to gastroesophageal reflux? Understanding the factors associated with the development of GERD provides insight into the treatment modalities currently used to manage a patient who suffers from the disease.

CLINICAL PRESENTATION

Patients with GERD may display symptoms that can be described as (1) typical, (2) atypical, or (3) complicated. The hallmark symptom of gastroesophageal reflux and esophagitis is heartburn (i.e., pyrosis), classically described as a substernal sensation of warmth or burning that may radiate to the neck. It is waxing and waning in character, and is often aggravated by activities that worsen gastroesophageal reflux such as supine position, bending over, or eating a meal high in fat. Heartburn is a common complaint of both healthy individuals and patients with GERD, and is most commonly reported when the gastric pH falls below 4. Other symptoms include water brash (hypersalivation), belching, and regurgitation, which usually occur after eating a large meal (especially a large fatty meal), lying down shortly after eating, or bending over.[30] Regurgitation, which refers to the effortless movement of food or liquid from the esophagus into the mouth, is frequently associated with reflux (especially in infants). Typical symptoms generally improve, at least temporarily, with the use of antacids.

Atypical symptoms include nonallergic asthma, chronic cough, hoarseness, pharyngitis, and chest pain that mimics angina.[30] Dental erosions have also been reported in patients with gastroesophageal reflux.[31] Further follow-up is necessary in patients presenting with chest pain to distinguish it from chest pain that is cardiac in nature. In some cases, these "extraesophageal" symptoms are the only symptoms present, making it more difficult to recognize GERD as the cause, especially when endoscopic studies and x-rays are normal.[13] Patients presenting with asthma poorly responsive to standard medical therapies should be evaluated for GERD as a possible cause for their symptoms.[13] Pulmonary symptoms result from either direct irritation of the vagus nerve when refluxed acid comes in contact with the esophageal mucosa yielding bronchospasm (reflex theory) or, less commonly, from aspiration of the refluxate into the lungs causing chemical irritation that manifests as pneumonia or pulmonary fibrosis (reflux theory).[14,32] The severity of the symptoms of gastroesophageal reflux does not usually correlate with the degree of esophagitis, but it does correlate with the duration of reflux.

Patients presenting with continual pain, dysphagia, or odynophagia indicate complicated disease, which usually occurs in patients with more severe esophagitis.[30] Esophageal strictures may be present in patients presenting with dysphagia. However, these symptoms may occur in other esophageal disorders such as esophageal diverticulum, achalasia, obstruction, esophageal spasm, esophageal infections, scleroderma, and malignancy. The presence of complicated symptoms should be further investigated to differentiate other diseases as the cause.

DIAGNOSIS

The most useful tool in the diagnosis of gastroesophageal reflux is the clinical history, including both presenting symptomology and associated risk factors. Patients presenting with typical symptoms of reflux (heartburn, regurgitation) do not usually require invasive esophageal evaluation. These patients will generally benefit from empiric treatment consisting of life-style modifications and H_2-receptor antagonists. Patients presenting with atypical symptoms (chest pain, chronic cough, hoarseness, asthma) should first be evaluated to exclude other cardiac or respiratory causes for their symptoms. If cardiac and respiratory systems are normal, esophageal studies are needed to confirm the diagnosis of gastroesophageal reflux. Diagnostic evaluation is also important in patients failing empiric therapy, in patients presenting with recurrent disease, and in patients presenting with complicated symptoms (dysphagia, odynophagia, bleeding, and weight loss).[7]

The primary esophageal studies used to diagnose GERD can be categorized on the basis of their ability to detect (1) mucosal injury and esophagitis (endoscopy), (2) presence of reflux (24-hour ambulatory esophageal pH monitoring), and (3) peristaltic dysfunction or decreased lower esophageal sphincter pressure (manometry). Each of the tests currently available has some limitation associated with it; some lack specificity or sensitivity, some are difficult to perform, some are invasive, and some are expensive. Choosing which test to use depends on which of the three problems listed you are trying to detect and the diagnostic facilities available at your institution.

In patients who fail empiric therapy or who present with complicated symptoms, it is important to evaluate the esophagus for the presence of mucosal injury.[7] This can be accomplished by using endoscopy or an air-contrast barium esophagogram. Endoscopy, which is the primary technique used to assess the severity of esophageal injury, allows visualization and biopsy of the esophageal mucosa. Histologic changes, which can be the only finding in as many as 40% of patients, can only be diagnosed by endoscopy with biopsy.[7] Several systems have been used to classify severity of disease; a common grading scale is shown in Table 30–2.[33] Although endoscopy is a highly specific test, it is not extremely sensitive. In mild cases of GERD the esophageal mucosa may appear relatively normal; however, diagnostic yield may be increased by obtaining mucosal biopsies. In addition, noninflammatory GERD and major motor disorders may be missed by endoscopy, and it is significantly more costly than a barium esophagogram.

Although more cost effective than endoscopy, barium esophagograms lack the sensitivity and specificity needed to accurately determine the presence of mucosal injury.[7] This test is even more limited in its ability to distinguish between Barrett's esophagus and esophagitis. Barrett's esophagus requires histologic confirmation that can only be obtained by endoscopy with biopsy. However, in patients presenting with dysphagia, barium esophagograms are the most sensitive test for detecting esophageal strictures or obstruction. They can also detect the presence of hiatal hernia and esophageal motor function.[30] Endoscopy, although less sensitive, is also useful in detecting esophageal strictures or hiatal hernia and may be preferred by many patients.[11]

TABLE 30–2. Endoscopic Classification of Esophagitis

Grade 0	Normal esophageal mucosa
Grade 1	Erythema or diffusely red mucosa, edema causing accentuated folds
Grade 2	Isolated round or linear erosions extending from the gastroesophageal junction upward, not involving entire circumference
Grade 3	Confluent erosions extending around entire circumference or superficial ulceration without stenosis
Grade 4	Complicated cases; erosions as in grade 3 plus deep ulcerations, strictures, or columnar epithelium-lined esophagus

From Ref. 33.

Provocative tests such as the acid perfusion (Bernstein) test, gastrointestinal scinti-scanning, or maneuvers to induce reflux during barium esophagograms or with the standard acid reflux test are used to establish a causal relationship between patient symptoms and abnormal acid exposure, especially when esophagitis is not present.[7] In general, provocative tests have limited utility in the diagnosis of routine GERD.

Twenty-four-hour ambulatory pH monitoring is most useful in diagnosing gastroesophageal reflux in (1) patients who continue to have symptoms without evidence of esophageal damage, (2) patients who are refractory to standard treatment, or (3) patients who present with atypical symptoms (chest pain or pulmonary symptoms).[7] In patients with atypical symptoms, 24-hour ambulatory pH monitoring may be the only way to objectively prove the symptoms are reflux related. Ambulatory pH monitoring documents the percentage of time the intraesophageal pH is low.[20] It is very effective at determining the frequency and severity of reflux. It is also useful in identifying patients with supine or supine/upright reflux, which is prognostic for more severe esophagitis.[7] Evaluation of "alkaline reflux" with ambulatory pH monitoring is currently being investigated.[34]

Continuous pH monitoring can be performed by passing a small-electrode pH probe intranasally and placing it approximately 5 cm above the lower esophageal sphincter.[20] Patients keep a diary of symptoms and these can be correlated with the pH measurement corresponding to the time the symptom was reported. Problems with esophageal pH monitoring arise when different methods are used to perform the test or a patient's baseline differs significantly from the standard. Recently, ambulatory pH monitoring for less than 24 hours has been evaluated and may be useful in some cases.[35]

Esophageal manometry is useful in excluding motility disorders and should be performed in any patient who is a candidate for antireflux surgery.[20] To perform manometry, a multilumen tube is passed into the stomach and the pressures are measured as the tube is pulled back across the lower esophageal sphincter, esophagus, and pharynx. Although the exact role of impaired peristalsis in the development of GERD is not known, up to 50% of patients with severe esophagitis have peristaltic dysfunction compared with 25% of patients with mild esophagitis, suggesting more severe disease in those with impaired peristalsis.[21] Evaluation of peristaltic function with manometry is important in any patient undergoing antireflux surgery to determine the appropriate procedure to perform to avoid dysphagia or gas-bloat syndrome (inability to belch or vomit).[21]

▶ TREATMENT: Gastroesophageal Reflux Disease

DESIRED OUTCOME

Therapeutic modalities used in the treatment of gastroesophageal reflux are targeted at reversing the various pathophysiologic abnormalities. The goals of treatment are to (1) alleviate or eliminate the patient's symptoms, (2) decrease the frequency or recurrence and duration of gastroesophageal reflux, (3) promote healing of the injured mucosa, and (4) prevent the development of complications. Therapy is directed at augmenting defense mechanisms that may prevent reflux and/or decreasing the aggressive factors that worsen reflux or mucosal damage (Fig. 30–1). Specifically, therapy is directed at (1) increasing lower esophageal sphincter pressure, (2) enhancing esophageal acid clearance, (3) improving gastric emptying, (4) protecting the esophageal mucosa, (5) decreasing the acidity of the refluxate, and (6) decreasing the gastric volume available to be refluxed.[36]

GENERAL APPROACH TO TREATMENT

The treatment of GERD is categorized into the following modalities: life-style changes, including the use of antacids and/or OTC H_2-receptor antagonists (phase I); pharmacologic intervention primarily with standard or high-dose antisecretory agents (phase II); and surgical intervention (phase III). The initial therapeutic modality used is in part dependent on the patient's condition (degree of esophagitis, presence of complications).[37] Historically, a stepwise approach has been used, starting with noninvasive life-style modifications (phase I) and progressing up to pharmacologic management (phase II) or surgical intervention (phase III) (Table 30–3).[7,10,11,30,37–39] Dietary and life-style modifications and education about factors that may worsen GERD symptoms should be the cornerstone of initial GERD therapy.[7] Table 30–4 lists many of the life-style changes that are included in phase I therapy.[10,40] Although most patients do not respond to life-style changes alone, the importance of maintaining these life-style changes should be stressed to the patient on a routine basis, no matter what other therapeutic modality is used.

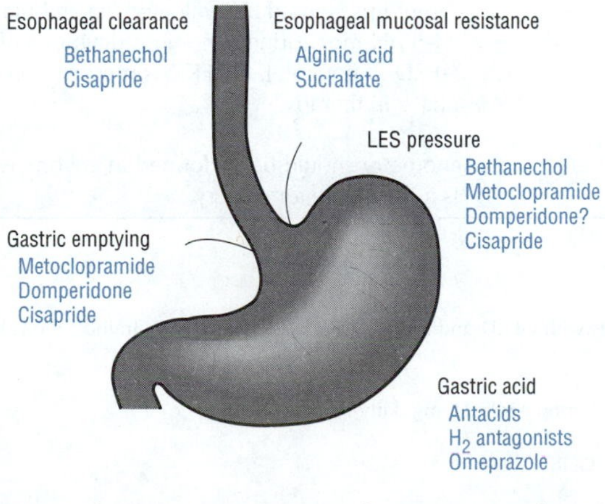

FIGURE 30–1. Therapeutic interventions in the management of gastroesophageal reflux disease. Pharmacologic interventions are targeted at improving defense mechanisms or decreasing aggressive factors. (LES = lower esophageal sphincter.)

Patients not responding to life-style changes alone are generally started on a pharmacologic treatment regimen consisting of an acid-suppressing agent. Patients with mild symptoms may see improvement with the inexpensive over-the-counter H_2-receptor antagonists, antacids, or alginic acid. However, the mainstay of therapy in patients with moderate symptoms and nonerosive disease is an H_2-receptor antagonist given in divided daily doses. Patients not responding to standard doses of H_2-receptor antagonists or those with more severe disease may require higher doses and/or more frequent dosing, because improvement correlates with the extent and duration of acid suppression.[13] In some cases, standard H_2-receptor antagonist doses may be increased to two to four times the normal dose. Another alternative in patients not responding to standard doses of an H_2-receptor antagonist is the use of a more potent acid-suppressive agent such as the proton pump inhibitors. Patients presenting with more complicated symptoms or with erosive esophagitis should be started on a proton pump inhibitor as initial therapy, because it provides the most rapid symptomatic relief and healing of esophagitis in the highest percent of patients.[7] Prokinetic agents (e.g., cisapride) offer an alternative to standard doses of H_2-receptor antagonists in mild to moderate, nonerosive GERD, but may not be as effective as acid-suppressing agents in some cases and can be more expensive. These agents are effective in improving defects related to esophagogastric motility such as decreased lower esophageal sphincter pressure, decreased esophageal clearance, or decreased gastric emptying, and can be used as an adjunct to acid-suppressing therapy if one of these motility problems is noted in a patient with GERD. This combination may also be useful in the rare patient who fails high-dose proton pump inhibitor therapy. These are generally the only scenarios where combination therapy is indicated in the management of GERD. In general, combination therapy offers only modest improvements in symptoms over standard doses of H_2-receptor antagonists and should not be routinely recommended.

Maintenance therapy is generally necessary to prevent relapse, especially in those patients with esophagitis. In patients with nonerosive disease, standard doses of H_2-receptor antagonists or prokinetic agents are generally effective.[11] However, in patients with more severe disease, especially those with erosive esophagitis or other complications, maintenance therapy with a proton pump inhibitor is most effective. Routine use of combination therapy has no role in maintenance therapy of GERD.

TABLE 30–3. Therapeutic Approach To Gastroesophageal Reflux Disease

Patient Presentation	Recommended Treatment Regimen	Comments
Phase I Intermittant, mild heartburn	A. Life-style changes **PLUS** B. Antacids (Maalox TC 1–2 tsp 20 min–1h PC & HS; Gaviscon 2 tabs [PC & HS]; calcium carbonate 0.5–1 g as needed) **AND/OR** C. Low-dose, OTC H_2-receptor antagonists (each taken up to bid) • Cimetidine 200 mg[a] • Famotidine 10 mg[a] • Nizatidine 75 mg • Rantidine 75 mg	Life-style changes should be started initially and continued throughout the course of treatment. If symptoms are unrelieved with phase I therapy, then begin phase IIa therapy.
Phase IIa Mild to moderate, typical symptoms not relieved by phase I therapy **OR** Atypical symptoms with nonerosive GERD (per endoscopy)	A. Life-style modifications **PLUS** B. Standard doses of H_2-receptor antagonists for 6–12 wk • Cimetidine 400 mg bid • Famotidine[b] 20 mg bid • Nizatidine[c] 150 mg bid • Ranitidine[c] 150 mg bid **OR** C. Prokinetic agent[d] cisapride 10 mg qid OR 20 mg bid (up to 20 mg qid)	For typical symptoms, treat empirically with phase IIa therapy. If symptoms are relieved, treat recurrences on as-needed basis. If symptoms recur frequently, consider maintenance therapy (MT) with lowest effective dose of ranitidine,[e] cisapride, or a proton pump inhibitor (PPI).[f] *Note:* Most patients will require standard doses for MT. For atypical symptoms, obtain endoscopy (if possible) to evaluate mucosa. If nonerosive GERD present, give a trial of H_2-receptor antagonist therapy. If symptoms are relieved, consider MT. (May require a PPI for MT.) For patients with typical OR atypical symptoms resistant to phase IIa therapy, or for patients with erosive disease per endoscopy, begin phase IIb therapy.
Phase IIb Moderate to severe symptoms not relieved by phase I or IIa therapy **OR** "Erosive disease," or other complication such as strictures or Barrett's esophagus, noted on endoscopy	A. Titrate to higher, more frequent dose of H_2-receptor antagonist for 8–12 wk • Cimetidine[g] 400 mg qid OR 800 mg bid • Famotidine[g] 40 mg bid • Nizatidine 150 mg qid • Ranitidine[g] 150 mg qid **OR** B. Proton pump inhibitor • Omeprazole[h] 20 mg qd (up to bid) × 8 wk • Lansoprazole[i] 30 mg qd (up to bid) × 8 wk	If symptoms relieved with phase IIb therapy, consider MT with the lowest effective dose. A PPI is the drug of choice for both treatment and MT in patients with "erosive disease" or in patients with other complications. PPIs are also preferred for patients with atypical symptoms not responding to standard doses of H_2-receptor antagonists. Patients not responding to phase IIb therapy, including those with persistent atypical symptoms, should be evaluated via ambulatory 24-h pH monitoring to confirm diagnosis of GERD (if possible). If GERD is present, consider phase III therapy.
Phase III Surgery		Manometry should be performed in anyone who is a candidate for surgery.

[a]FDA labeled indication: Heartburn, acid indigestion, and sour stomach (OTC).
[b]FDA labeled indication: GERD (for up to 6 wk).
[c]FDA labeled indication: GERD.
[d]Concurrent use of an H_2-receptor antagonist plus a prokinetic agent may be useful in patients with GERD and motor dysfunction. Review contraindications before using cisapride.
[e]FDA labeled indication: Maintenance of healing erosive esophagitis (150 mg bid).
[f]FDA labeled indication: To maintain healing of erosive esophagitis (omeprazole 20 mg daily, lansoprazole 15 mg daily).
[g]FDA labeled indication: Erosive esophagitis up to 12 wk.
[h]FDA labeled indication: Erosive esophagitis (up to 8 wk) and poorly responsive symptomatic GERD.
[i]FDA labeled indication: Erosive esophagitis (up to 8 wk).

TABLE 30–4. Nonpharmacologic Treatment of GERD With Life-style Modifications

- Elevate the head of the bed (increases esophageal clearance)
  - Use 6–8 inch blocks under the head of the bed
  - Sleep on a foam wedge
- Dietary changes
  - Avoid foods that may decrease lower esophageal sphincter pressure (fats, chocolate, alcohol, peppermint, and spearmint)
  - Avoid foods that have a direct irritant effect on the esophageal mucosa (spicy foods, orange juice, tomato juice, and coffee)
  - Include protein-rich meals in diet (augments lower esophageal sphincter pressure)
  - Eat small meals and avoid eating immediately prior to sleeping (within 3 h if possible) (decreases gastric volume)
  - Weight reduction (reduces symptoms)
- Stop smoking (decreases spontaneous esophageal sphincter relaxation)
- Avoid alcohol (increases amplitude of the lower esophageal sphincter, peristaltic waves, and frequency of contraction)
- Avoid tight-fitting clothes
- Discontinue, if possible, drugs that may promote reflux (calcium channel blockers, beta blockers, nitrates, theophylline)
- Take drugs that have a direct irritant effect on the esophageal mucosa with plenty of liquid if they cannot be avoided (tetracyclines, quinidine, and KCl, iron salts, aspirin, nonsteroidal anti-inflammatory drugs)

Compiled from Refs. 10 and 40.

Antireflux surgery should be considered in patients (1) with esophagitis who fail to respond to pharmacologic treatment, (2) who have strictures, (3) with bleeding from refractory esophagitis, (3) who are very young and face long-term expensive therapy, and (4) who have pulmonary complications.[13]

NONPHARMACOLOGIC THERAPY

Nonpharmacologic treatment of GERD includes life-style modifications, which should be started initially and continued as an adjuvant even when pharmacologic intervention becomes necessary, and surgical intervention, which is reserved for patients with refractory disease or in those where pharmacologic management is undesirable.

LIFE-STYLE MODIFICATIONS

The most common life-style changes that a patient should be educated about include (1) weight loss, (2) smoking cessation, (3) avoidance of alcohol, (4) elevation of the head of the bed, (5) avoidance of foods or medications that exacerbate GERD, and (6) eating smaller meals and avoidance of eating immediately prior to sleeping. These and other recommended life-style modifications are listed in Table 30–4. Although there are no clear data indicating that reflux occurs more often with obesity, it would seem logical that the increased intra-abdominal pressure and dietary habits of obese patients would predispose them to reflux.[4] Therefore, weight loss is recommended despite the lack of data showing that it decreases the symptoms of GERD. Smoking can cause aerophagia, which leads to increased belching and regurgitation.[4] However, data are lacking to show that symptoms improve in patients who quit smoking. Nevertheless, patients with GERD should be encouraged to quit smoking. Alcohol, although not thought to play a role in severe disease, decreases lower esophageal sphincter pressure and may exacerbate symptoms such as heartburn.[4] Elevating the head of the bed (not just elevating the head with pillows) decreases nocturnal esophageal acid contact time and should also be recommended.[11]

An important thing we can do as pharmacists is to evaluate patient profiles and identify potential medications that may exacerbate GERD symptoms. Certain medications decrease lower esophageal sphincter pressure, such as anticholinergics, barbiturates, calcium channel blockers, and theophylline. Other medications act as a direct irritant to the esophageal mucosa, including aspirin, iron, NSAIDs, quinidine, potassium chloride, and the newer agent, alendronate. Patients taking alendronate should be instructed to drink 6 to 8 ounces of plain tapwater and remain upright for at least 30 minutes following administration. Proper patient education can help prevent dysphagia or esophageal ulceration. These agents should be avoided if at all possible, especially in patients with more severe disease. However, the clinician must weigh the risks and benefits of continuing a drug known to worsen GERD and esophagitis.

The major obstacle associated with life-style modifications is that many patients are noncompliant, and even those who do comply generally continue to have symptoms requiring acid-suppression therapy. Nonetheless, it is important to regularly stress the value of life-style modification.

SURGICAL INTERVENTION

Surgical intervention is the other nonpharmacologic intervention that is used in the management of GERD. It should be considered in patients (1) with esophagitis who fail to respond to pharmacologic treatment, (2) who have strictures, (3) with bleeding from refractory esophagitis, (3) who are very young and face long-term expensive therapy, and (4) who have pulmonary complications.[13] Surgical procedures include Nissen, Belsey, Mark IV, and Hill operations. Due to the diminished surgical complications with the newer laparoscopic surgical procedures (Nissen fundoplication being one of the most commonly used procedures), the role of surgery in the long-term management of GERD has become controversial.[17] The goal of this surgical procedure is to reduce the size of a hiatal hernia and to construct a valve mechanism to reestablish the competency of the gastroesophageal junction.[3] Antireflux surgery has been found to be superior to medical management (with an H_2-receptor antagonist or prokinetic agent). However, similar comparisons with proton pump inhibitors are lacking. The major complications that have been reported with antireflux surgery include gasbloat syndrome (inability to belch or vomit), dysphagia, vagal denervation, splenic trauma, and very rarely, death.[3]

PHARMACOLOGIC THERAPY

ANTACIDS AND ANTACID–ALGINIC ACID PRODUCTS

Patients should be educated that antacids are an appropriate component of treating mild GERD, even though documentation of their efficacy in placebo-controlled clinical trials is lacking.[7] Although the literature is somewhat controversial on the superiority of antacids to placebo, physicians and patients clearly consider antacids to be effective for immediate, symptomatic relief, and antacids are often used concurrently with other acid-suppressing therapies. Antacids increase the pH of gastric contents through their acid-neutralizing ability. Maintaining the intragastric pH above 4 decreases the activation of pepsin from pepsinogen. Also, neutralization of gastric fluid leads to an increased lower esophageal sphincter pressure.

An antacid product combined with alginic acid (Gaviscon) is not a potent neutralizing agent and does not enhance lower esophageal sphincter pressure; however, it does form a highly viscous solution that floats on the surface of the gastric contents.

This viscous solution may act by mechanically impairing reflux or by coating the esophagus, thus preventing mucosal contact of the irritants in refluxate.[41] Several studies have compared the efficacy of the combination product (antacid–alginic acid) with that of antacids alone.[41–43] Overall, these studies demonstrate that the combination product (Gaviscon) usually relieves symptoms associated with reflux. Efficacy data indicating endoscopic healing are lacking.

Antacid or antacid combination products may cause gastrointestinal adverse effects (diarrhea or constipation depending on the product), alterations in mineral metabolism, and possible acid–base disturbances. Aluminum-containing antacids may bind to phosphate in the gut and lead to bone damage. In addition, antacids interact with a variety of drugs by altering gastric pH, increasing urinary pH, absorbing medications to their surfaces, providing a physical barrier to absorption, or forming insoluble complexes with other medications.[44] Clinically significant antacid–drug interactions include those with tetracycline, ferrous sulfate, isoniazid, and quinolone antibiotics. Antacid–drug interactions are influenced by composition, dose, and dosage schedule of the antacid, as well as by the formulation of the drug.

The dosage recommendations for antacids in the management of GERD are somewhat difficult to derive from the literature (see Table 30–3 for general dosing guidelines). Doses have ranged from hourly to only on an as-needed basis. In general, antacids have a short duration of action, which necessitates frequent administration throughout the day to provide continuous neutralization of acid. Typical doses are two tablets four times daily after meals and at bedtime. Taking antacids after meals can increase the duration of action from about 1 hour to about 3 hours; however, night-time acid suppression cannot be maintained with bedtime doses of antacids.

ACID SUPPRESSION WITH H_2-RECEPTOR ANTAGONISTS

The H_2-receptor antagonists (cimetidine, famotidine, nizatidine, and ranitidine) in divided doses are the mainstay of treatment of GERD.[7] Because all of the H_2-receptor antagonists are equally efficacious, selection of the specific agent to use in the management of GERD should be based on other factors such as differences in pharmacokinetics, safety profile, and cost. For symptomatic relief of mild GERD, low-dose, over-the-counter H_2-receptor antagonists may be beneficial. For nonerosive disease, H_2-receptor antagonists are generally given at standard doses twice daily. Patients not responding to standard doses may be hypersecreters of gastric acid and require higher doses.[7] For these patients and those with erosive disease, higher doses and/or four times daily dosing (cimetidine 800 mg bid, famotidine 40 mg bid, nizatidine 150 mg qid, or ranitidine 150 mg qid) provides better acid control, especially after mealtime acid surges.[4] However, proton pump inhibitors are generally considered the drug of choice in patients with erosive disease.

Extensive literature exists regarding the efficacy of the H_2-receptor antagonists in the treatment of GERD.[45–54] The clinical trials clearly indicate that the efficacy of H_2-receptor antagonists in the management of GERD is extremely variable and is frequently lower than desired. Response to the H_2-receptor antagonists appears to be dependent on the (1) severity of disease, (2) duration of therapy, and (3) dosage regimen used. These factors are important to keep in mind when comparing various clinical trials and/or assessing a patient's response to therapy.

Severity of Disease

The severity of esophagitis at baseline has a profound impact on the patient's response to H_2-receptor antagonists. In one study, patients with severe esophagitis (grade 3) had dramatically lower healing rates compared with those with less severe disease independent of the dosage regimen used.[55] Following 12 weeks of cimetidine therapy (400 mg four times daily), endoscopic healing was observed in 80% of patients with mild esophagitis (grade 1) and in only 46% of patients with severe disease (grade 3). Clearly, the more severe the esophageal damage, the poorer the response to H_2-receptor antagonists.

Duration of Therapy

Unlike duodenal ulcer disease, in which the duration of therapy is relatively short (e.g., 4 to 6 weeks), prolonged courses (8 weeks or more) of H_2-receptor antagonists are frequently required in the treatment of GERD. In an open-label trial of famotidine 40 mg daily, endoscopic healing increased as the duration of therapy increased.[56] After 4 weeks of therapy, healing was observed in 50% of patients. The healing rate increased with continued therapy to yield healing rates of 82% and 83% after 12 and 16 weeks of therapy, respectively. Similar results were observed with cimetidine.[55]

Dosage Regimen Used

H_2-receptor antagonists can be given in low-dose (over-the-counter) regimens, which may give symptomatic relief to patients with mild, typical symptoms of GERD. They can be given in standard doses, usually twice daily, in patients with nonerosive, mild to moderate GERD; or they can be given in higher doses (usually given more frequently) for patients not responding to standard doses or for patients with more severe disease.

Low-dose (over-the-counter) H_2-receptor antagonists have been shown to be effective in treating intermittent heartburn and in preventing meal-provoked heartburn in patients with mild disease (without evidence of esophagitis).[46,57] In one study, 41%, 59%, 70%, 69%, and 62% of heartburn episodes were relieved following as-needed treatment with placebo, famotidine 5 mg, 10 mg, 20 mg, or antacids, respectively.[57]

Standard doses of H_2-receptor antagonists (cimetidine 400 mg four times daily or 800 mg twice daily, ranitidine 150 mg twice daily, famotidine 20 mg twice daily, or nizatidine 150 mg twice daily) are effective in providing symptomatic relief and endoscopic healing in patients with GERD. The majority of the trials assessing the efficacy of standard doses of H_2-receptor antagonists indicate that symptomatic improvement is achieved in approximately 30% to 80% (average, 60%) of patients.[7] However, endoscopic healing rates tend to be much lower (average 48%).[7]

Although data identifying the ideal H_2-receptor antagonists dosage regimen to use in the treatment of GERD are lacking, it is thought that dosage regimens that achieve profound acid suppression may lead to increased healing rates. Thus, the efficacy of higher dosage regimens of H_2-receptor antagonists has been evaluated in many recent studies.[48–52,54] The theory that higher doses (usually given more often) increase healing rates is based on four observations. First, gastroesophageal reflux occurs during both daytime and night-time hours. Thus, acid suppression for only part of the day may not be sufficient to prevent the refluxate from injuring the esophageal mucosa, especially postprandially and during the night-time hours. H_2-receptor antagonists do not easily overcome the stimulus for acid secretion following a meal, and thus postprandial acid secretion may be inadequately suppressed.[26] Dividing the H_2-receptor antagonist dose may provide coverage for both daytime and night-time acid reflux and may theoretically improve symptom control and esophageal healing. However, studies have yielded conflicting results.[26,53]

Second, high-dose ranitidine (> 300 mg daily) provides a greater degree of acid suppression compared with the standard-dose regimen of 300 mg daily or placebo and is also associated with higher healing rates.[47,49] Studies evaluating higher doses of other H_2-receptor antagonists also exist.[50–52,54] Endoscopic healing was shown to be superior following famotidine 40 mg twice daily as compared to famotidine 20 mg twice daily; with healing rates of 58% versus 43% at 6 weeks and 76% versus 67% at 12 weeks, respectively.[51] Higher dosage regimens of nizatidine have been shown to provide higher healing rates.[54] Specifically, endoscopic healing rates of 81.3%, 79.2%, and 67% have been reported for patients receiving nizatidine 150 mg three times daily; 150 mg + 150 mg + 300 mg; or 300 mg twice daily, respectively.

Third, a subset of patients with GERD has been reported to have hypersecretion of gastric acid and may therefore require higher doses of antisecretory agents.[58] Finally, a relationship between the 8-week healing rate of esophagitis and the time duration that the gastric pH is above 4 has been demonstrated.[26] Similarly, an inverse relationship between healing rate and esophageal acid exposure was also found. Based on these findings, one may be able to predict responses to antisecretory regimens based on their ability to maintain intragastric pH levels above 4.

Although higher doses of H_2-receptor antagonists may provide higher symptomatic and endoscopic healing rates, limited information exists regarding the safety of these regimens. Therefore, the higher doses of H_2-receptor antagonists should be reserved for patients who do not respond to standard doses or for patients with more severe disease. In general the H_2-receptor antagonists are well tolerated. The most common adverse effects are headache, somnolence, fatigue, dizziness, and either constipation or diarrhea. Patients should be monitored for the presence of adverse effects, as well as potential drug interactions, especially when on cimetidine.

ACID SUPPRESSION WITH PROTON PUMP INHIBITORS

Proton pump inhibitors (omeprazole and lansoprazole) are the drugs of choice in patients with moderate to severe erosive esophagitis, in patients with GERD not responding to H_2-receptor antagonist therapy, and in patients with complicated symptoms (Barrett's esophagus, strictures). In these patient populations, relapse is common and long-term maintenance therapy is generally indicated.

Omeprazole and lansoprazole inhibit gastric acid secretion by inhibiting gastric H^+/K^+-adenoside triphosphate.[59] This produces a profound, long-lasting antisecretory effect capable of maintaining the gastric pH above 4, even during acid surges seen postprandially.[4,11] Clinical trials clearly indicate that proton pump inhibitors are superior to H_2-receptor antagonists in their ability to control symptoms and heal esophagitis in a significant percentage of patients with severe GERD.[59-65] They are also more cost effective in patients with severe disease. In general, 71% to 96% of patients receiving omeprazole for 4 to 8 weeks reported symptomatic relief, while healing rates were reported in 62% to 94% of patients.[7] Rarely, a patient may continue to secrete acid even on high doses of omeprazole (40 mg twice daily).[66] Lansoprazole has also been shown to provide superior symptom relief and endoscopic healing rates (92%) compared with standard doses of ranitidine (70%).[65] The results from two comparative studies demonstrate that healing rates after 8 weeks of treatment with lansoprazole 30 mg daily are similar to those observed following 8 weeks of omeprazole 20 mg daily.[67,68]

The proton pump inhibitors have also been shown to be efficacious in patients who are refractory to H_2-receptor antagonists.[69–71] The efficacy of lansoprazole 30 mg daily and ranitidine 150 mg twice daily was evaluated for the treatment of erosive esophagitis that was resistant to H_2-receptor antagonists.[69] Following 8 weeks of treatment, the healing rate was significantly higher for patients receiving lansoprazole compared to those who continued receiving ranitidine (89% and 38%, respectively). In another study, 80% of patients previously resistant to H_2-receptor antagonist therapy responded to omeprazole 40 mg daily within 12 weeks.[70]

Omeprazole (40 to 60 mg daily) and lansoprazole (30 to 60 mg daily) also appear to be effective in healing esophagitis and esophageal ulcers in patients with gastroesophageal reflux complications.[72,73] In one study, patients with complications of GERD (Barrett's esophagus, strictures, or failed antireflux surgery) who were refractory to high-dose H_2-receptor antagonist therapy received omeprazole 40 mg daily. All patients were healed during 20 weeks of therapy.[72]

The proton pump inhibitors degrade in acidic environments and are therefore formulated in a delayed-release capsule containing enteric-coated (pH-sensitive) granules. In patients unable to swallow the capsule, the contents of the capsule can be mixed in applesauce. If a patient has a nasogastric tube, the contents should be mixed in an acidic fruit juice such as apple or orange juice. However, in patients with a feeding tube going directly into the duodenum, the contents of the capsules should be mixed in a basic solution such as sodium bicarbonate. Patients should be instructed to take their proton pump inhibitor in the morning before breakfast to maximize efficacy.[4]

The proton pump inhibitors are usually well tolerated; however, potential adverse effects include headache, dizziness, somnolence, diarrhea, constipation, and nausea. The frequency of adverse events appears to be similar to that seen with the H_2-receptor antagonists. Concern and controversy regarding the safety of therapy with a proton pump inhibitor are based on their ability to produce hypergastrinemia and gastric carcinoid tumors in rats. After nearly a decade of experience with the proton pump inhibitors, gastric carcinoid tumors have not been directly linked to omeprazole use.[7] An excellent review of this controversy is available.[59]

PROKINETIC AGENTS

The efficacy of the prokinetic agents cisapride, metoclopramide, and bethanechol has been evaluated in the treatment of GERD. The poorer efficacy and side effect profiles associated with metoclopramide and bethanechol compared with cisapride limit their use in the treatment of GERD. Cisapride, on the other hand, has been shown to have comparable efficacy to H_2-receptor antagonists in treating patients with mild esophagitis; however, it is less effective than acid suppression in more severe disease.[74] Prokinetic agents have also been used as adjunctive therapy with an H_2-receptor antagonist. The only scenario where this combination is appropriate is in a patient with GERD who has a known or suspected motility disorder or in a patient who has failed high-dose proton pump inhibitor therapy.

Cisapride

Cisapride is a synthetic, substituted piperidinyl benzamide chemically related to metoclopramide.[75] It is thought to increase lower esophageal sphincter pressure and accelerate gastric emptying through the facilitation of acetylcholine release at the myenteric plexus.[75] Cisapride also increases the amplitude of esophageal contractions and is effective in improving esophageal clearance in some selected patient populations.[75] Cisapride is currently indicated for treatment of nocturnal heartburn.

The efficacy of cisapride appears similar to that of the H_2-receptor antagonists in patients with mild esophagitis and may be used as an alternative to H_2-receptor antagonists in these patients. However, cisapride generally costs more than the H_2-receptor antagonists and offers no real advantage, especially in patients with normal GI motility.[11] The efficacy of cisapride 10 mg four times daily has been shown to be similar to that of cimetidine 400 mg four times daily and ranitidine 150 mg twice daily.[76,77] Cisapride 10 mg twice daily or 20 mg four times daily was compared with cimetidine 400 mg twice daily or 400 mg four times daily.[78] All patients showed improvement in severity of diurnal and nocturnal heartburn and regurgitation. Endoscopic healing rates were similar with 69%, 64%, 55%, and 55% for cisapride 10 mg twice daily, 20 mg four times daily, cimetidine 400 mg twice daily, and 400 mg four times daily, respectively. Cisapride appears to be a potential agent for the treatment of infants with gastroesophageal reflux. One study demonstrated the superiority of cisapride (0.15 to 0.3 mg/kg given three times daily) as compared with placebo in the management of GERD in infants.[79]

Unlike metoclopramide, cisapride is devoid of antidopaminergic effects and, therefore, does not cause extrapyramidal side effects or prolactin secretion.[74] The most commonly reported adverse effects are gastrointestinal in nature and include transient abdominal cramping, borborygmi, diarrhea, and loose stools. Other reactions that have been reported through postmarketing studies include: allergic reactions (bronchospasm, urticaria, and angioedema), exacerbation of asthma, confusion, depression, hallucinations, urinary incontinence, and hyperprolactinemia. Cisapride is extensively metabolized via oxidative *N*-dealkylation and -hydroxylation pathways. Therefore, cisapride use should be avoided in patients taking other drugs that inhibit cytochrome P450 3A4, such as fluconazole, ketoconazole, miconazole, itraconazole, clarithromycin, erythromycin, indavir, ritanovir, or nefazodone because concurrent use may cause prolongation of the QT interval, leading to ventricular arrhythmias. Cisapride should also be avoided in patients with a history of prolonged QT intervals, renal failure, history of ventricular arrhythmias, ischemic heart disease, congestive heart failure, uncorrected electrolyte disorders (potassium and magnesium), repiratory failure, and concomitant medications known to prolong the QT interval, including quinidine, procainamide, sotalol, tricyclic antidepressants, maprotiline, sparfloxacin, terodiline, bepridil, certain phenothiazines, and sertindole. These conditions predispose the patient to arrhythmias and increase the risk for QT prolongation, torsades de points, cardiac arrest, and even death. Special caution should be taken in pediatric patients. Cisapride is not FDA approved for pediatric use and several pediatric deaths have been reported in the package insert. Other adverse effects reported in pediatric patients include anemia, methemoglobinemia, hyperglycemia with acidosis, confusion, apathy, and photosensitivity reactions.

Evidence suggests that cisapride can be dosed 20 mg twice daily instead of 10 mg four times daily for treating GERD due to its long half-life.[80] Twice-daily dosing would increase compliance.

Metoclopramide

Metoclopramide, a dopamine antagonist, increases lower esophageal sphincter pressure in a dose-related manner and has also been shown to accelerate gastric emptying in gastroesophageal reflux patients.[81] However, unlike cisapride, metoclopramide does not improve esophageal clearance. Metoclopramide has been shown to provide symptomatic improvement for some patients with gastroesophageal reflux disease; however substantial data indicating that metoclopramide provides endoscopic healing are lacking.[82]

In addition, metoclopramide's side effect profile and the incidence of tachyphylaxis with continued use limits its usefulness in treating many patients with GERD. Forty-eight percent of patients experienced adverse effects in one study with doses ranging from 10 to 50 mg daily.[83] Seventeen percent of the population withdrew from the study because of adverse effects. The most commonly reported adverse reactions were somnolence, nervousness, fatigue, dizziness, weakness, depression, diarrhea, and rash. Anxiety, insomnia, extrapyramidal effects, and increased prolactin levels (gynecomastia, galactorrhea, menstrual irregularity) have also been reported. The risk of adverse effects is much greater in patients with renal dysfunction because the drug is primarily eliminated by the kidneys. Contraindications include Parkinson's disease, mechanical obstruction, concomitant use of other dopamine antagonists, anticholinergic agents, and pheochromocytoma.

Bethanechol

Although bethanechol has been shown to increase lower esophageal sphincter pressure, improve esophageal clearance, and have some efficacy in providing symptomatic and endoscopic improvements in patients with GERD, its side effect profile severely limits its use. Oral bethanechol can cause abdominal cramps, urinary frequency, malaise, blurred vision, and diarrhea. In addition, bethanechol may increase gastric acid secretion. Because bethanechol is a cholinergic agonist, relative contraindications for its use include asthma, chronic obstructive pulmonary disease, and peptic ulcer disease.

MUCOSAL PROTECTANTS

Sucralfate, a nonabsorbable aluminum salt of sucrose octasulfate, has very limited value in the treatment of GERD. Limited comparative trials have shown that sucralfate has similar healing rates as compared with H_2-receptor antagonists for patients with mild esophagitis.[84–88] However, sucralfate is less effective than higher doses of H_2-receptor antagonists in patients with refractory esophagitis.[88] Overall, the efficacy of sucralfate varies greatly among the studies. The wide range of response rates may in part be related to patient population, baseline degree of esophagitis, duration of treatment, dose used, or sucralfate formulation used. More studies are needed before sucralfate can be routinely used in the treatment of anything but the mildest cases of GERD.

Sucralfate is generally well tolerated; however, constipation, dry mouth, nausea, and abdominal discomfort may occur. Caution should be used when sucralfate is administered to a patient with renal dysfunction, because the aluminum may accumulate. Sucralfate may also lead to hypophosphatemia, presumably due to binding with phosphate in the gut. Sucralfate may also interact with several medications, leading to a decrease in drug absorption.[44]

COMBINATION THERAPY

Combination therapy with an acid-suppressing agent and a prokinetic agent or a mucosal protectant agent would seem logical given the multifactorial nature of the disease, particularly in light of the disappointing results seen with many monotherapy regimens. However, sufficient data to support combination therapy are limited, and this approach should not be routinely recommended unless a patient has esophagitis plus motor dysfunction occurring concurrently or if the patient has failed high-dose proton pump inhibitor therapy. In this case, cisapride is the prokinetic agent of choice. Most studies suggest that combination therapy offers only modest improvements over standard doses of H_2-receptor antagonists alone. Therefore, patients not responding to standard doses of H_2-receptor antagonists should have their dose of H_2-receptor antagonists increased or switched to a proton pump inhibitor instead of adding a prokinetic agent. Monotherapy with a proton pump inhibitor is not only more efficacious in patients not responding to an H_2-receptor antagonist or prokinetic agent alone, but it also improves compliance with once-daily dosing and is ultimately more cost effective.

Data with other drug combinations for the treatment of GERD are even more limited. One study demonstrated benefit from the combination of cimetidine 300 mg four times daily plus sucralfate 1 g after meals and 2 g at bedtime compared with cimetidine alone.[8] Although patients receiving combination therapy showed greater endoscopic improvement of esophagitis when compared with those patients receiving monotherapy, healing rates were not significantly different. Until studies show a true benefit resulting from an H_2-receptor antagonist combined with sucralfate, this combination cannot be recommended.

MAINTENANCE THERAPY

Although healing and/or symptomatic improvement may be achieved via many different therapeutic modalities, a large percentage of patients with gastroesophageal reflux will relapse following discontinuation of therapy, especially those with more severe disease.[90] Follow-up studies indicate that 70% to 90% of patients will relapse within 1 year of discontinuation of therapy regardless of what therapeutic regimen is used.[90] Patients who have symptomatic relapse following discontinuation of therapy or lowering of dose, including patients with complications such as Barrett's esophagus, strictures, or hemorrhage, should be considered for long-term maintenance therapy to prevent complications or worsening of esophageal function.[11] The goal of maintenance therapy is to improve quality of life by controlling the patient's symptoms and preventing complications.[7] These goals cannot generally be achieved by decreasing the dose of the therapeutic modality used for initial healing or switching to a less potent acid-suppressing agent. Most patients will require standard doses to prevent relapses.[72, 91, 92] Patients should be counseled on the importance of complying with life-style changes and long-term maintenance therapy in order to prevent recurrence or worsening of disease.[7]

H_2-receptor antagonists or cisapride may be effective maintenance therapy for patients with mild disease.[4] However, the proton pump inhibitors are the drug of choice for maintenance treatment of moderate to severe esophagitis.[93] Lower doses of a proton pump inhibitor or alternate day dosing may be effective in some patients with less severe disease—allowing titration in some cases.[4] However, patients with more severe disease and/or complications should be started on omeprazole 20 mg daily or lansoprazole 30 mg daily.

Maintenance Therapy With Proton Pump Inhibitors

In a comparison of maintenance regimens, omeprazole (20 mg daily) alone or in combination with cisapride (10 mg three times daily) was found to be significantly more effective in preventing recurrence than ranitidine (150 mg three times daily) alone or cisapride (10 mg three times daily) alone.[93] Omeprazole was also effective in patients with complicated forms (grades 4 and 5) of esophagitis.

Omeprazole and lansoprazole in doses of 20 mg and 30 mg daily, respectively, have been shown to decrease relapse rates significantly.[92,93] At 1 year, relapse rates were 15% and 10%, respectively. In another study, omeprazole 20 mg (given on the weekend) was compared to omeprazole 20 mg daily and ranitidine 150 mg twice daily. The relapse rate at 12 months was 68%, 11%, and 75%, respectively, indicating that weekend regimens are not effective in preventing recurrence.[91] Alternate-day regimens may be beneficial in patients with mild disease.[94] Omeprazole 10 mg daily prevented relapse in 79% of patients. Lansoprazole 15 mg daily was compared to lansoprazole 30 mg daily or placebo in preventing recurrence of erosive esophagitis. At 12 months, relapse rates were 21%, 10%, and 65% for lansoprazole 15 mg, 30 mg, and placebo, respectively. Lansoprazole 15 mg and 30 mg daily were found to be comparable in maintaining remission of erosive esophagitis.

Long-term use of the proton pump inhibitors indicates that they are safe, with no evidence of carcinoid tumors directly linked to their use. However, there is a propensity for patients treated with a proton pump inhibitor to develop atrophic gastritis while on therapy. Atrophic gastritis may increase the risk of gastric cancer.[3] In one study, 30% of patients treated with omeprazole over an average of 5 years developed atrophy, whereas none of a cohort group that received antireflux surgery developed atrophy within the same time frame.[95] Most of the patients who developed atrophic gastritis were found to have concomitant *Helicobacter pylori* infection. Therefore, it may be prudent to test patients for the presence of *H. pylori* and eradicate the organism if long-term maintenance therapy with a proton pump inhibitor is indicated.

Maintenance Therapy With H_2-Receptor Antagonists

The studies evaluating the efficacy of the H_2-receptor antagonists in maintaining GERD patients in remission have been somewhat disappointing. Currently, ranitidine 150 mg twice daily is the only H_2-receptor antagonist regimen FDA approved for maintenance of healing of erosive esophagitis. The recurrence rates of esophagitis have been shown to be significantly less in patients receiving ranitidine 150 mg twice daily as compared to placebo.[96]

Maintenance Therapy With Cisapride

Emerging data suggest that cisapride may be effective in preventing relapse in certain patients. Patients with endoscopically diagnosed reflux esophagitis received cisapride 10 mg four times daily for 8 to 16 weeks (phase I).[97] Healing was seen in 69% and symptoms decreased by 67%. Eighty patients from phase I who were healed on cisapride 10 mg four times daily received cisapride 10 mg twice daily or placebo as maintenance therapy. Patients in the cisapride group had a 20% relapse rate compared to 39% in the placebo group. Patients with less severe disease remained in remission longer than patients with more severe disease.

PHARMACOECONOMIC CONSIDERATIONS

In addition to the traditional clinical end points that demonstrate a certain therapy is effective, we must also evaluate the cost effectiveness of the therapy in relation to predicted outcomes and its effects on quality of life.[4] For GERD, one must consider the primary goals of treatment: to relieve symptoms, to prevent recurrence, and to prevent complications. These factors must be evaluated separately, because different costs will be associated with achieving each end point. For example, patients with complications associated with GERD, such as strictures, would be more likely to use medical resources due to revisits and diagnostic tests.[4] Although effects on quality of life may be difficult to evaluate when your goal is preventing recurrence,[4] untreated GERD has been shown to have a more negative impact on psychological well-being than untreated hypertension, mild heart failure, angina pectoris, or menopause.[2] Improving a patient's quality of life is a measure of treatment success and may help decide which therapy a patient receives.[4]

As far as direct drug cost, the proton pump inhibitors are generally more expensive than the H_2-receptor antagonists or prokinetic agents. However, the most expensive therapy is the one that is ineffective.[4] This means that if the H_2-receptor antagonist does not accomplish the treatment goals then it costs more because the patient must be retreated.

Patient compliance is another factor that will affect the outcome of drug therapy. Drug regimens that are easily managed will improve compliance and therefore outcome for the patient. This can especially be a problem in patients who require high-dose therapy with H_2-receptor antagonists. Not only is the patient required to take the drug more often in higher doses, but there is also increased expense associated with such regimens. The same holds true for combination therapy with an H_2-receptor antagonist plus cisapride. This regimen is generally more expensive than monotherapy with a proton pump inhibitor. The patient may be unable to afford the drug. Choosing a drug that is the least expensive and provides the greatest benefit related to dosing interval and number of tablets taken is the optimal regimen. Studies comparing the cost effectiveness of the various treatment strategies for GERD are limited.[98, 99] Decision analysis has been used to evaluate the cost effectiveness of phase I therapy or phase I therapy combined with omeprazole 20 mg daily or ranitidine 150 mg twice daily for patients with persistent symptomatic gastroesophageal reflux disease who failed phase I therapy. A complex model that evaluated the influence of empiric versus definitive therapy, compliance, and efficacy of the three treatment regimens was employed. Although the retail cost of omeprazole was highest among the treatments evaluated, it was the most cost-effective strategy and was associated with the lowest overall cost. Additional studies are needed evaluating the cost effectiveness of various treatment regimens as well as assessing the impact of these treatments on quality-of-life issues.

EVALUATION OF THERAPEUTIC OUTCOMES

Evaluation of the long-term benefits of treatment are difficult to assess due to the limited information known about the epidemiology and natural history of GERD. Therefore, successful outcomes are generally measured in terms of three separate end points: (1) relieving symptoms, (2) healing the injured mucosa, and (3) preventing complications.

The short-term goal of therapy is to relieve symptoms, such as heartburn and regurgitation, to the point where they do not impair the patient's quality of life. Patients should be educated regarding life-style modifications that should be adhered to throughout the course of therapy including smoking cessation, weight loss, raising the head of the bed, eating smaller meals, and avoiding eating prior to bedtime. Patients should also be instructed to avoid foods that aggravate GERD symptoms, such as fat and chocolate. In addition, the patient's drug profile should be reviewed to identify medications that may contribute to GERD symptoms. These agents should be avoided if possible.

The pharmacist or other health care provider should take an active role in educating the patient about potential adverse effects and drug interactions that may occur with drug therapy. The frequency and severity of symptoms should be monitored and patients should be counseled on symptoms that may suggest the presence of complications requiring immediate medical attention, such as dysphagia or odynophagia. Patients with persistent symptoms should be evaluated for the presence of strictures or other complications. Patients should also be monitored for the presence of atypical symptoms such as cough, nonallergic asthma, or chest pain. These symptoms require further diagnostic evaluation. Long-term maintenance treatment is indicated in patients who have strictures because they commonly recur if esophagitis is not treated.[100]

The second goal is to heal the injured mucosa. Again, life-style modifications and the importance of complying with the therapeutic regimen chosen to heal the mucosa should be stressed. Patients should be educated about the risk of relapse and the need for long-term maintenance therapy to prevent recurrence or complications.

The final, more long-term goal of therapy is to decrease the risk of complications (esophagitis, strictures, and Barrett's esophagus). A small subset of patients may continue to fail treatment, despite therapy with high doses of H_2-receptor antagonists or omeprazole. Maintenance therapy with standard to higher doses of antisecretory agents may be indicated in these acid hypersecretors, because severe esophagitis that is not adequately treated may lead to Barrett's esophagus and its associated risk of adenocarcinoma. Unfortunately, data are lacking that show that effective treatment of esophagitis decreases the risk of developing adenocarcinoma in patients with Barrett's esophagus. Patients should be monitored for the presence of continual pain, dysphagia, or odynophagia.

CONCLUSIONS

Gastroesophageal reflux disease is a common entity that classically presents as heartburn. The pathophysiology of reflux is complex, involving both aggressive factors (acid, pepsin, bile acids, pancreatic enzymes, and prostaglandins) and defense mechanisms (anatomic factors, lower esophageal sphincter pressure, esophageal clearance, and gastric emptying). Therapeutic modalities are designed to minimize the aggressive factors and/or augment defense mechanisms. The pharmacologic critical elements outlined should be considered when evaluating and treating a patient with GERD.

▶ PRINCIPLES OF PHARMACOTHERAPY

- The goals of treatment are to alleviate or eliminate symptoms, decrease the frequency or recurrence and duration of gastroesophageal reflux, promote healing of mucosa, and prevent complications.
- Treatment of GERD often involves a stepwise approach depending on severity of disease and includes phase I, life-style changes; phase II, pharmacologic treatment; and phase III, surgical intervention.
- Patients presenting with typical symptoms should be treated with life-style modifications and trial of empiric acid-suppression therapy.
- The importance of life-style modifications should be stressed throughout a patient's treatment course. Patients not responding to empiric therapy or who have more complicated symptoms should receive diagnostic tests.
- Endoscopy or barium esophagogram is used to evaluate for mucosal damage, 24-hour ambulatory pH testing is useful in patients with persistent symptoms or atypical symptoms, and manometry

is useful in evaluating motility and before antireflux surgery.

- Acid suppression is the mainstay of GERD treatment. H_2-receptor antagonists in divided doses are routinely used. Cisapride, a prokinetic agent, provides comparable efficacy to standard doses of H_2-receptor antagonists. Proton pump inhibitors show the greatest relief of symptoms and healing, especially in patients with erosive disease.
- Patients who fail H_2-receptor therapy can have their dose and frequency of H_2-receptor antagonist increased or they can be switched to a proton pump inhibitor.
- Many patients will relapse and require long-term maintenance therapy with an H_2-receptor antagonist, cisapride, or a proton pump inhibitor. A proton pump inhibitor is the drug of choice for maintenance of moderate to severe erosive disease.
- Antireflux surgery offers an alternative for refractory GERD or when pharmacologic management is undesirable.
- Patients should be assessed for relief of symptoms, such as heartburn, and for signs and symptoms of complications that require immediate medical attention, such as dysphagia or bleeding. Patient profiles should also be reviewed for other medications that may aggravate GERD, and these medications should be avoided if possible. Patients should be monitored for adverse drug reactions and potential drug–drug interactions, especially when cimetidine or cisapride are used. Finally, patients should be assessed for compliance to both treatment and maintenance regimens, as well as life-style modifications.

REFERENCES

1. Spechler SJ. Epidemiology and natural history of gastro-oesophageal reflux disease. Digestion 1992;51(suppl 1):24–29.
2. Dimenas E. Methodological aspects of evaluation of quality of life in upper gastrointestinal diseases. Scand J Gastroenterol 1993;28:18–21.
3. Kahrilas PJ. Gastroesophageal reflux disease. JAMA 1996;276: 983–988.
4. Johnson DA. Medical therapy of GERD: Current state of the art. Hosp Prac 1996;31:135–148.
5. Nebel OT, Fornes MF, Castell DO. Symptomatic gastroesophageal reflux: Incidence and precipitating factors. Dig Dis 1976;21:953–956.
6. Spechler SJ, Goyal RK. Barrett's esophagus. N Engl J Med 1986; 315:362–371.
7. DeVault KR, Castell DO (for the Practice Parameters Committee of the American College of Gastroenterology). Guidelines for the diagnosis and treatment of gastroesophageal reflux disease. Arch Intern Med 1995;155:2165–2173.
8. Ollyo JB, Monnier P, Fontolliet C, Savary M. The natural history, prevalence and incidence of reflux oesophagitis. Gullet 1993; 3(suppl):1–10.
9. Richter JE. Severe reflux esophagitis. Gastrointest Endosc Clin North Am 1994;4:677–698.
10. Kitchin LI, Castell DO. Rationale and efficacy of conservative therapy for gastroesophageal reflux disease. Arch Intern Med 1991;151: 448–454.
11. Fennerty MB, Castell D, Fendrick AM, et al. The diagnosis and treatment of gastroesophageal reflux disease in a managed care environment. Suggested disease management guidelines. Arch Intern Med 1996;156:477–484.
12. Orenstein SR. Gastroesophageal reflux disease. Semin Gastrointest Dis 1994;5:2–14.
13. Krueger KJ. Changing clinical perspectives toward gastroesophageal reflux. South Med J 1996;89:548–550. Editorial.
14. Kozarek RA. Complications of reflux esophagitis and their medical management. Gastroenterol Clin North Am 1990;19:713–731.
15. Holloway RH, Dent J. Pathophysiology of gastroesophageal reflux: Lower esophageal sphincter dysfunction in gastroesophageal reflux disease. Gastroenterol Clin North Am 1990;19:517–535.
16. Weinberg DS, Kadish SL. The diagnosis and management of gastroesophageal reflux disease. Med Clin North Am 1996;80:411–429.
17. Castell DO. Long-term management of GERD: The pill, the knife or the endoscope? Gastrointest Endosc 1994;40:252–253.
18. Sloan S, Rademaker AW, Kahrilas PJ. Determinants of gastroesophageal junction incompetence: Hiatal hernia, lower esophageal sphincter, or both? Ann Intern Med 1992;117:977–982.
19. Kahrilas PJ. Esophageal motor activity and acid clearance. Gastroenterol Clin North Am 1990;19:537–550.
20. Bozymski EM. Pathophysiology and diagnosis of gastroesophageal reflux disease. Am J Hosp Pharm 1993;50(suppl 1):S4–S6.
21. Kahrilas PJ, Dodds WJ, Hogan WJ, et al. Esophageal peristaltic dysfunction in peptic esophagitis. Gastroenterology 1986;91:897–904.
22. Goldstein JL, Schlesinger PK, Mozwecz HL, et al. Esophageal mucosal resistance: A factor in esophagitis. Gastroenterol Clin North Am 1990;19:565–585.
23. Fiorucci S, Santucci L, Chiucchiu S, Morelli A. Gastric acidity and gastroesophageal reflux patterns in patients with esophagitis. Gastroenterology 1992;103:855–861.
24. Fein M. Duodenogastroesophageal reflux parallels acid and not alkaline exposure in the esophagus and contributes to complications of reflux disease. Am J Gastroenterol 1996;91:1662–1663.
25. Dent J. Roles of gastric acid and pH in the pathogenesis of gastro-oesophageal reflux disease. Scand J Gastroenterol 1994;29(suppl 201):55–61.
26. Bell NJV, Burger D, Howden CW, et al. Appropriate acid suppression for the management of gastro-oesophageal reflux disease. Digestion 1992;51(suppl 1):59–67.
27. McCallum RW, Berkowitz DM, Lerner E. Gastric emptying in patients with gastroesophageal reflux. Gastroenterology 1981;80: 285–291.
28. Behar J, Ramsby G. Gastric emptying and antral motility in reflux esophagitis: Effect of oral metoclopramide. Gastroenterology 1978; 74:253–256.
29. McCallum RW. Gastric emptying in gastroesophageal reflux and the therapeutic role of prokinetic agents. Gastroenterol Clin North Am 1990;19:551–564.
30. Larsen RR. Gastroesophageal reflux disease—Gaining control over heartburn. Postgrad Med 1997;101:181–187.
31. Taylor G, Taylor S, Abrams R, Mueller W. Dental erosion associated with asymptomatic gastroesophageal reflux. ASDC J Dent Child 1992;49:182–185.
32. Simpson WG. Gastroesophageal reflux disease and asthma. Diagnosis and management. Arch Intern Med 1995;155:798–803.
33. Savary M, Miller G. The esophagus. In: Gassmann SA, ed. Handbook and Atlas of Endoscopy. Solothurn, Switzerland, 1978.
34. Waring JP, LeGrand J, Chinichian A, et al. Duodenogastric reflux in patients with Barrett's esophagus. Dig Dis Sci 1990;35:759–762.
35. Dobhan R, Castell DO. Prolonged intraesophageal pH monitoring compared with 16-hour overnight recording. Dig Dis Sci 1992;37: 857–864.

36. Tytgat GNJ, Nio CY, Schotborgh RH. Reflux esophagitis. Scand J Gastroenterol 1990;25(suppl 175):1–12.
37. Hogan WJ. Gastroesophageal reflux disease: An update on management. J Clin Gastroenterol 1990;12(suppl 2):S21–S28.
38. Morton LS, Fromkes JJ. Gastroesophageal reflux disease: Diagnosis and medical therapy. Geriatrics 1993;48:60–66.
39. Hixson LJ, Kelley CL, Jones WN, Tuohy CD. Current trends in the pharmacotherapy for gastroesophageal reflux disease. Arch Intern Med 1992;152:717–723.
40. Richter JE, Castell DO. Drugs, foods and other substances in the cause and treatment of reflux esophagitis. Med Clin North Am 1981; 65:1223–1234.
41. Bamardo DE, Lancaster-Smith M, Strickland ID, et al. A double-blind controlled trial of "Gaviscon" in patients with symptomatic gastro-oesophageal reflux. Curr Med Res Opin 1975;3:388–391.
42. Chevrel B. A comparative crossover study on the treatment of heartburn and epigastric pain: Liquid Gaviscon and a magnesium-aluminum antacid gel. J Med Res 1980;8:300–302.
43. Graham DY, Lanza F, Dorsch ER. Symptomatic reflux esophagitis: A double-blind controlled comparison of antacids and alginate. Curr Ther Res 1977;22:653–658.
44. Welage LS, Berardi RB. Drug interactions with antiulcer agents: Considerations in the treatment of acid-peptic disease. J Pharm Prac 1994;7:177–195.
45. Farup PG, Weberg R, Berstad A, et al. Low-dose antacids versus 40 mg cimetidine twice daily for reflux oesophagitis. Scand J Gastroenterol 1990;25:315–320.
46. Gottlieb S, Decktor DL, Eckert JM, et al. Efficacy and tolerability of famotidine in preventing heartburn and related symptoms of upper gastrointestinal discomfort. Am J Ther 1995;2:314–319.
47. Johnson NJ, Boyd EJS, Mills JG, et al. Acute treatment of reflux oesophagitis: A multicentre trial to compare 150 mg ranitidine b.d. with 300 mg ranitidine q.d.s. Aliment Pharmacol Ther 1989;3:259–266.
48. Castell DO. Rationale for high-dose H_2 blockade in the treatment of gastroesophageal reflux disease. Aliment Pharmacol Ther 1991; 5(suppl):59–67.
49. Euler AR, Murdock RH, Wilson TH, et al. Ranitidine is effective therapy for erosive esophagitis. Am J Gastroenterol 1993;88:520–524.
50. Edge DP. High-dose famotidine in ranitidine-resistant severe oesophagitis: A pilot study. NZ Med J 1990;103:150–152.
51. Wesdorp ICE, Dekker W, Festen HPM. Efficacy of famotidine 20 mg twice a day versus 40 mg twice a day in the treatment of erosive or ulcerative reflux esophagitis. Dig Dis Sci 1993;38:2287–2293.
52. Festen HPM, Wesdorp ICE, Dekker W. The efficacy of famotidine 20 mg bid vs 40 mg bid in the treatment of erosive/ulcerative esophagitis: Significance of severity of esophagitis and duration of therapy. Gastroenterology 1991;100(part 2, suppl):A63.
53. Cloud ML, Offen WW, Robinson M. Nizatidine versus placebo in gastroesophageal reflux disease: A 12-week, multicenter, randomized, double-blind study. Am J Gastroenterol 1991;86:1735–1742.
54. Baldi F, Longanesi A, Ferrarini F, et al. Nizatidine in gastroesophageal reflux disease: A review. Gastrointest Res 1991;20:5–6.
55. Tytgat GNJ, Nicolai JJ, Reman FC. Efficacy of different doses of cimetidine in the treatment of reflux esophagitis. Gastroenterology 1990;99:629–634.
56. Sekiguchi T, Nishioka T, Kogure M, et al. Once-daily administration of famotidine for reflux esophagitis. Scand J Gastroenterol 1987; 22(suppl 134):51–54.
57. Simon TJ, Berlin RG, Gardner AH, et al. Self-directed treatment of intermittent heartburn: A randomized, multicenter, double-blind, placebo-controlled evaluation of antacid and low doses of an H_2-receptor antagonist (famotidine). Am J Ther 1995;2:304–313.
58. Collen MJ, Johnson DA, Sheridan MJ. Basal acid output and gastric acid hypersecretion in gastroesophageal reflux disease. Dig Dis Sci 1994;39:410–417.
59. Maton PN. Drug therapy: Omeprazole. N Engl J Med 1991;324: 965–975.
60. Berardi RR, Dunn-Kucharski VA. Omeprazole: Defining its role in gastroesophageal reflux disease. Hosp Formulary 1995;30: 216–225.
61. Spencer CM, Faulds D. Lansoprazole: A reappraisal of its pharmacodynamic and pharmacokinetic properties, and its therapeutic efficacy in acid related disorders. Drugs 1994;48:404–430.
62. Dehn TCB, Shepherd HA, Colin-Jones D, et al. Double-blind comparison of omeprazole (40 mg od) versus cimetidine (400 mg qd) in the treatment of symptomatic erosive reflux oesophagitis, assessed endoscopically, histologically and by 24-h pH monitoring. Gut 1990;31:509–513.
63. Bardhan KD, Long R, Hawkey CJ, et al. Lansoprazole, a new proton pump inhibitor vs ranitidine in the treatment of reflux erosive esophagitis. Gastroenterology 1991;100:A30. Abstract.
64. Benhaim MC, Evreux M, Salduccci J, et al. Lansoprazole and ranitidine in treatment of reflux oesophagitis: Double blind comparative trial. Gastroenterology 1990;98:A20. Abstract
65. Robinson M, Sahba B, Avner D, et al. A comparison of lansoprazole and ranitidine in the treatment of erosive oesophagitis. Aliment Pharmacol Ther 1995;9:25–31.
66. Klinkenberg-Knol EC, Meuwissen SGM. Combined gastric and oesophageal pH-metry in patients with reflux disease resistant to omeprazole. Aliment Pharmacol Ther 1990;4:485–489.
67. Corallo J, Vicari F, Forestier S, et al. Lansoprazole in acute treatment of reflux esophagitis. Gastroenterology 1003;104(suppl):A58. Abstract.
68. Hatlebakk JG, Berstad A, Carling L, et al. Lansoprazole versus omeprazole in short-term treatment of reflux oesophagitis. Results of a Scandinavian multicentre trial. Scand J Gastroenterol 1993;28: 224–228.
69. Feldman M, Harford WV, Fisher RS, et al. Treatment of reflux esophagitis resistant to H_2-receptor antagonists with lansoprazole, a new H^+/K^+-ATPase inhibitor: A controlled, double-blind study. Am J Gastroenterol 1993;88:1212–1217.
70. Sontag SJ. Gastroesophageal reflux disease. Aliment Pharmacol Ther 1993;7:293–312.
71. Robinson M, Campbell DR, Sontag S, et al. Treatment of erosive esophagitis resistant to H_2-receptor antagonist therapy. Dig Dis Sci 1995;40:590–597.
72. Klinkenberg-Knol EC, Festen HPM, Jansen JBMJ, et al. Long-term treatment with omeprazole for refractory reflux esophagitis: Efficacy and safety. Ann Intern Med 1994;121:161–167.
73. Sampliner RE. Effect of up to 3 years of high dose lansoprazole on Barrett's esophagus. Am J Gastroenterol 1994;89:1844–1848.
74. Reynolds JC. Prokinetic agents: A key in the future of gastroenterology. Gastroenterol Clin North Am 1989;18:437–456.
75. McCallum RW. Cisapride: A new class of prokinetic agent. Am J Gastroenterol 1991;86:135–149.
76. Galmiche JP, Fraitag B, Filoche B, et al. Double-blind comparison of cisapride and cimetidine in treatment of reflux esophagitis. Dig Dis Sci 1990;35:649–655.
77. Janisch HD, Huttemann W, Bouzo MH. Cisapride versus ranitidine in the treatment of reflux esophagitis. Hepatogastroenterology 1988; 35:125–127.
78. Maleev A, Mendizova A, Popov P, et al. Cisapride and cimetidine in the treatment of erosive esophagitis. Hepatogastroenterology 1990; 37:403–407.
79. Cucchiara S, Staiano A, Boccieri A, et al. Effects of cisapride on parameters of oesophageal motility and on the prolonged intraoesophageal pH test in infants with gastro-oesophageal reflux disease. Gut 1990;31:21–25.
80. Geldof H, Hazelhoff B, Otten MH. Two different dose regimens of cisapride in the treatment of reflux oesophagitis: A double-blind comparison with ranitidine. Aliment Pharmacol Ther 1993;7:409–415.
81. Fink SM, Lange RC, McCallum RW. Effect of metoclopramide on normal and delayed gastric emptying in gastroesophageal reflux patients. Dig Dis Sci 1983;28:1057–1061.

82. Ramirez B, Richter JE. Review article: Promotility drugs and the treatment of gastro-oesophageal reflux disease. Aliment Pharmacol Ther 1993;7:5–20.
83. Taylor DM. Evaluation of the safety of metoclopramide in patients with gastroesophageal reflux disease. Clin Ther 1984;7:28–32.
84. Ross E, Toledo-Pimentel V, Bordas JM, et al. Healing of erosive esophagitis with sucralfate and cimetidine: influence of pretreatment lower esophageal sphincter pressure and serum pepsinogen I levels. Am J Med 1991;91(suppl 2A):107S–113S.
85. Bremner CG, Marks IN, Segal I, Simjee A. Reflux esophagitis therapy: Sucralfate versus ranitidine in a double-blind multicenter trial. Am J Med 1991;91(suppl 2A):119S–122S.
86. Elsborg L, Jorgensen F. Sucralfate vs. cimetidine in reflux esophagitis: A double-blind clinical study. Scand J Gastroenterol 1991; 26:146–150.
87. Jorgensen F, Elsborg L. Sucralfate vs. cimetidine in treatment of reflux esophagitis with special reference to the esophageal motor function. Am J Med 1991;91(suppl 2A):114–117.
88. Pace F, Lazzaroni M, Bianchi-Porro G. Failure of sucralfate in the treatment of refractory esophagitis vs. high dose famotidine: An endoscopic study. Scand J Gastroenterol 1991;26:491–494.
89. Herrera JL, Shay SS, McCabe M, et al. Sucralfate used as adjunctive therapy in patients with severe erosive peptic esophagitis resulting from gastro-esophageal reflux. Am J Gastroenterol 1990;85:1335–1338.
90. Hetzel DJ, Dent J, Reed WD, et al. Healing and relapse of severe peptic esophagitis after treatment with omeprazole. Gastroenterology 1988;95:903–912.
91. Dent J, Yeomans ND, Mackinnon M, et al. Omeprazole v ranitidine for prevention of relapse in reflux oesophagitis: A controlled double blind trial of their efficacy and safety. Gut 1994;35:590–598.
92. Robinson M, Lanza F, Avner D, Haber M. Effective maintenance therapy of reflux esophagitis with low dose lansoprazole: A randomized, double blind placebo-controlled trial. Ann Intern Med 1996; 124:859–867.
93. Vigneri S, Termini R, Leandro G, et al. A comparison of five maintenance therapies for reflux esophagitis. N Engl J Med 1995; 333:1106–1110.
94. Isal JP, Zeitoun P, Barbier P, et al. Comparison of two dosage regimens of omeprazole—10 mg once daily and 20 mg weekends. Gastroenterology 1990;98:A63. Abstract.
95. Kuipers EJ, Lundell L, Klinkenberg-Knol EC, et al. Atrophic gastritis and *Helicobacter pylori* infection in patients with reflux esophagitis treated with omeprazole or fundoplication. N Engl J Med 1996; 334:1018–1022.
96. Euler AR, Murdock RH, Brotherton BJ, et al. Ranitidine 150 mg b.i.d. prevents erosive esophagitis. Gastroenterology 1992;102:A65. Abstract.
97. Toussaint J, Gossuin A, Deruyttere M, et al. Healing and prevention of relapse of reflux oesophagitis by cisapride. Gut 1991;32:1280–1285.
98. Hillman AL, Bloom BS, Fendrick AM, et al. Cost and quality effects of alternative treatments for persistent gastroesophageal reflux disease. Arch Intern Med 1992;152:1467–1472.
99. Marks RD, Richter JE, Rizzo J, et al. Omeprazole versus H_2 receptor antagonists in treating patients with peptic stricture and esophagitis. Gastroenterology 1994;106:907–915.
100. Dent J. Long-term aims of treatment of reflux disease, and the role of non-drug measures. Digestion 1992;51(suppl 1):30–34.

31

PEPTIC ULCER DISEASE

Rosemary R. Berardi, PharmD, FASHP

Acid-related diseases (gastritis, erosions, and peptic ulcer) of the upper gastrointestinal (GI) tract require gastric acid for their formation. Peptic ulcer disease (PUD) differs from gastritis and erosions in that ulcers typically extend deeper into the muscularis mucosa. There are three common forms of peptic ulcers: *Helicobacter pylori* (HP)-associated, nonsteroidal anti-inflammatory drug (NSAID)-induced, and stress ulcers (Table 31–1). The term "stress-related mucosal damage" (SRMD) is preferred to stress ulcer, because the mucosal lesions range from superficial gastritis and erosions to deep ulcers. Nonulcer dyspepsia (NUD) is distinguished from PUD in that ulcer symptoms are present and an ulcer is suspected, but an ulcer crater cannot be confirmed upon endoscopy.

Peptic ulcers vary in etiology, clinical presentation, and tendency to recur. Acute ulcers (SRMD) develop in critically ill hospitalized patients whereas chronic ulcers (HP and NSAID-associated) occur primarily in ambulatory patients. Chronic duodenal ulcer (DU) and gastric ulcer (GU) occur most often, but occasionally, ulcers develop in the esophagus, jejunum, ileum, or colon. Uncommonly, ulcers are associated with Zollinger-Ellison syndrome, radiation, chemotherapy, and vascular insufficiency (Table 31–2). This chapter will focus on HP-associated and NSAID-induced ulcers. A brief discussion of SRMD and Zollinger-Ellison-associated ulcers is included.

Chronic PUD is characterized by frequent ulcer recurrence. Approximately 50% to 90% of ulcers recur within 1 year of initial ulcer healing with conventional antiulcer regimens.[1] A number of factors influence the tendency for ulcers to recur. These include the presence of HP, cigarette smoking, NSAID use, gastric acid hypersecretion, patient noncompliance, incomplete ulcer healing, a long duration of PUD, and a history of ulcer-related complications.[1–3] The cause of ulcer recurrence, like that of the initial ulcer, is probably multifactorial.

EPIDEMIOLOGY

Approximately 10% of Americans will develop chronic PUD during their lifetime.[1] The incidence varies with ulcer type, age, gender, and geographical location. Racial, occupational, and societal variables require reevaluation in light of differences in HP infection rates. In the United States, the overall prevalence of PUD has shifted from predominance in men to nearly comparable prevalence of DU and GU in men and women. Recent trends suggest a declining rate for younger men and an increasing rate for older women.[1] Factors that have influenced these trends include the increasing prevalence of HP infection with age, NSAID-induced ulcers in the elderly, and the declining smoking rates, especially in younger men. Stress associated with increased social, occupational, and family responsibilities may also be related to recent changes observed in the male-to-female ratio.

A number of genetic, environmental, and therapeutic factors have been implicated in the changing patterns of PUD over time. Since 1960, ulcer-related hospitalizations, operations, and deaths in the United States have declined, suggesting a decrease in the incidence of PUD.[1] The decline in hospitalizations for ulcers has resulted primarily from a reduction in hospital admissions for uncomplicated DU, with a less dramatic decrease in GU. It is uncertain whether this decline reflects an actual decrease in the incidence of PUD or the combined influences of changes in diagnostic practices, more effective treatment, hospitalization criteria, and a shift to ambulatory care. Mortality from PUD has declined among persons of all ages, but declining death rates for men are in contrast to increasing rates for women. Despite these changes, PUD is one of the most common GI diseases, resulting in work loss, disability, and high-cost medical care.

ETIOLOGY AND RISK FACTORS

Most peptic ulcers occur in the presence of acid and pepsin when HP, NSAIDs, or other possible factors (Table 31–2) disrupt normal mucosal defense and healing mechanisms (Fig. 31–1).[1–4] Hypersecretion of acid is the primary pathogenic mechanism in hypersecretory states such as Zollinger-Ellison syndrome.[1,4] The pathogenesis of DU and GU is multifactorial and most likely reflects a combination of pathophysiologic abnormalities and environmental and genetic factors. Ulcer location appears to be related to a number of etiologic factors. Most DU occur in the first part of the duodenum (duodenal bulb). Benign GU can occur anywhere in the stomach, although most are located on the lesser curvature, just distal to the junction of the antral and acid-secreting mucosa.

HELICOBACTER PYLORI

A strong association exists between *Helicobacter pylori* (formerly *Campylobacter pylori*) and PUD (Fig. 31–2).[2,5,6] Most patients with DU and GU who are not taking NSAIDs have evidence of HP infection and antral gastritis.[2,6] Although a causal relationship between HP and chronic superficial gastritis is well established, a similar relationship

TABLE 31–1. Comparison of Common Forms of Peptic Ulcers

Characteristic	*Helicobacter pylori*	NSAID	SRMD
Site of damage	Duodenum > stomach	Stomach > dodenum	Stomach > duodenum
Intragastric pH	More dependent	Less dependent	Less dependent
Symptoms	Usually epigastric pain	Often asymptomatic	Asymptomatic
Ulcer depth	Superficial	Deep	Most superficial
GI bleeding	Less severe	More severe	More severe

between HP and PUD has been difficult to confirm because only 15% of individuals infected with HP actually develop clinical manifestations of an ulcer.[2,6] Support for a causal role in PUD is based on the fact that most non-NSAID ulcers are infected with HP, and that HP eradication markedly decreases ulcer recurrence.[2,6,7] It is likely that host-specific cofactors and HP strain variability play an important role in the pathogenesis of PUD.[8,9]

Evidence suggests that over 50% of the world's population is colonized by HP.[5] The prevalence of HP is higher in underdeveloped countries, where the socioeconomic and sanitary conditions are low and acquisition occurs during childhood.[2] In developed countries, there is an age-related increase in the prevalence of HP in adults, but the overall frequency is lower as successive generations have been less likely to acquire the infection as children.[2,8] In the United States, prevalence varies among different ethnic groups of similar socioeconomic status, with infection more common in African Americans and Hispanics than in Caucasians.[2] One explanation may be that improvement in socioeconomic status in African Americans and Hispanics has lagged behind other groups. Infection rates do not appear to differ with gender or smoking status.

The exact mode of transmission of HP is not known. However, transmission of the organism in Western countries is thought to be person to person by the fecal–oral and oral–oral routes, as humans are the only reservoir of infection.[2,10] Members of the same household are more likely to become infected, when someone in the same household is infected, than are members of an uninfected household.[2] Transmission of HP can also occur iatrogenically when infected instruments such as endoscopes are used.[10] Recent data suggest that the housefly has the potential to mechanically transmit HP from human waste to food or children.[10]

Epidemiologic data provide strong evidence that, in some individuals, asymptomatic HP infection is associated with chronic atrophic gastritis (CAG), gastric mucosa-associated lymphoid tissue (MALT) lymphoma, and gastric adenocarcinoma (Fig. 31–2).[2,6,11–13] In addition, serologic studies have shown an association between HP and gastric cancer.[2,11] The development of atrophic gastritis and gastric carcinoma is generally a slow process that occurs over 20 to 40 years. As with PUD, host-specific cofactors and conditions that influence the severity of gastritis are likely to influence the development of CAG. A highly specific type of atrophic gastritis (with intestinal metaplasia) is considered to be a precursor of gastric cancer.[6,11] In 1994, the World Health Organization concluded that HP infection is carcinogenic to humans (group I carcinogen).[6,11] The relationship between HP and NUD is controversial.[14,15] The most recent data suggest that HP does not appear to cause NUD.[15]

TABLE 31–2. Potential Causes of Peptic Ulcers

Helicobacter pylori
Nonsteroidal anti-inflammatory drugs
Stress-related mucosal damage (stress ulcer)
Hypersecretion of gastric acid (e.g., Zollinger-Ellison syndrome)
Viral infections (e.g., cytomegalovirus)
Vascular insufficiency (crack cocaine-associated)
Radiation
Chemotherapy (e.g., hepatic artery infusions)
Rare genetic subtypes
Idiopathic

NONSTEROIDAL ANTI-INFLAMMATORY DRUGS

Nonsteroidal anti-inflammatory drugs are one of the most widely prescribed classes of medications in the United States, particularly in patients 65 years of age and older. The availability of over-the-counter NSAIDs has contributed to their widespread use and associated complications. There is overwhelming evidence linking chronic NSAID (including aspirin) use to a wide variety of GI tract injuries.[3,16–23] Hemorrhagic gastric erosions are most common. These lesions heal within a few days and tend to occur less frequently with continued NSAID use. Gastric ulcers occur primarily in the antrum and are of greater importance than erosions because of their potential to bleed or perforate. Duodenum ulcers occur less often and may be produced by a different mechanism. Evidence suggests that

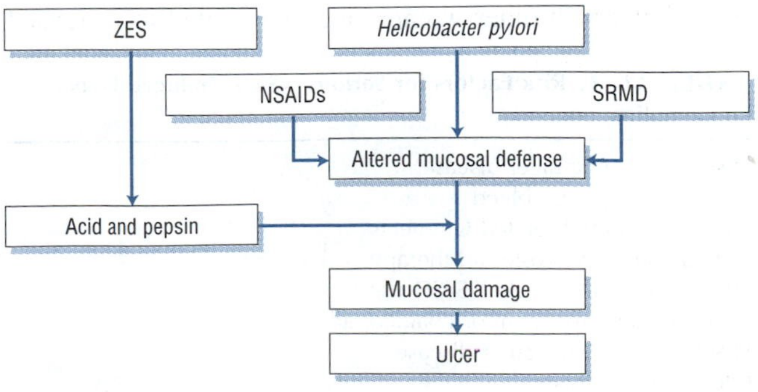

FIGURE 31–1. Pathogenesis of peptic ulcer disease. Acid and pepsin cause ulcers when mucosal defense mechanisms are altered by NSAIDs, *H. pylori*, or stress-related mucosal damage (SRMD). Hypersecretion of gastric acid causes ulcers in Zollinger-Ellison syndrome (ZES).

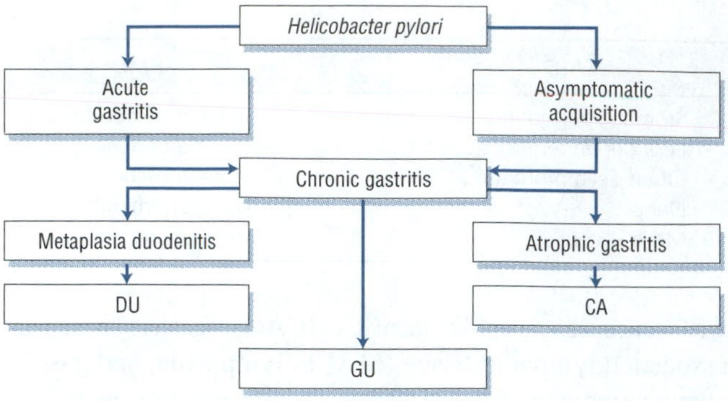

FIGURE 31–2. The natural history of *H. pylori* infection in the pathogenesis of gastric ulcer (GU), duodenal ulcer (DU), and gastric cancer (CA).

NSAIDs can exacerbate quiescent inflammatory bowel disease or cause colonic ulcers.[3,16]

Hospitalizations, complications, and mortality are dramatically increased in chronic NSAID users.[17–19] Each year, NSAIDs account for 7600 deaths and 76,000 hospitalizations in the United States.[20] Approximately 1% to 3% of NSAID users will have a GI bleed and will be prescribed antiulcer therapy. Ulcer bleeding and perforation occur with prescription and over-the-counter NSAIDs, and account for almost all of the NSAID-associated GI mortalities.[3,17,18] Ulcers have been reported with low doses of aspirin (10 to 100 mg/d) or nonaspirin NSAIDs, and complications have occurred following a few days of treatment. Patients with a history of PUD, upper GI bleeding, NSAID-related GI complications, or those taking concurrent corticosteroids, high-dose NSAIDs, or anticoagulants, are at greatest risk for serious GI complications (Table 31–3).[21,22] Asymptomatic patients taking antacids or H_2-receptor antagonists were reported to be at increased risk for serious GI complications when compared to patients not taking these medications.[21,22] It has been hypothesized that, although these antiulcer agents may not have prevented GI bleeding, they masked the symptoms associated with GI complications. Cigarette smoking and ethanol ingestion contribute to increased risk but do not appear to be independent factors. The high incidence of NSAID-related ulcer complications in individuals 65 years of age or older, and the increased risk of ulcers in older women, may be related to increased consumption.[20–23] It is likely that NSAIDs induce ulcers through a mechanism that does not require HP.[24] Conversely, NSAID-induced ulcers do not seem to increase susceptibility to HP infection.

TABLE 31–3. Risk Factors for Serious NSAID-Induced Upper GI Complications

History of peptic ulcer disease
History of upper GI bleed
History of NSAID-related GI effects
Concomitant corticosteroid therapy
High-dose and multiple NSAID use
Anticoagulant treatment or coagulopathy
History of cardiovascular disease
Older age patients
Smoking or alcoholism
Poor general health
Asymptomatic patients taking H_2-receptor antagonists or antacids

Compiled from Refs 21–23.

CORTICOSTEROIDS

The association between corticosteroids and PUD remains controversial.[1] Although it is possible that corticosteroids induce ulcers because of their ability to increase gastric acid secretion and inhibit prostaglandin synthesis, sufficient evidence is lacking to support a causal relationship. Discrepant findings among early retrospective studies may have been due in part to differences in the use of NSAIDs among study participants. One study suggests that elderly patients on concurrent oral corticosteroids and NSAIDs are at a much higher risk for PUD than those receiving either of these agents alone, and that ulcer risk is related to the dose and duration of the corticosteroid.[25] It is possible that corticosteroids either delay or inhibit the healing of ulcers caused by aspirin and other NSAIDs. Patients receiving concurrent corticosteroids and NSAIDs are at increased risk of developing an NSAID-induced ulcer.

UNCOMMON FORMS OF PEPTIC ULCERS

Peptic ulcers have been reported in individuals using crack cocaine, in patients with viral infections, and in those receiving abdominal radiation or undergoing chemotherapy administered through a hepatic artery pump, such as with 5-fluorouracil (Table 31–2).[1]

CIGARETTE SMOKING

There is strong epidemiologic evidence that links cigarette smoking to PUD; however, smoking appears to be a risk only before, not after, HP eradication.[1] Cigarette smoking increases the risk for both DU and GU, and the risk appears to be proportional to the amount smoked. When conventional antiulcer medications are used to heal or prevent ulcers, smoking impairs ulcer healing and promotes recurrence. The risk of recurrence and impaired healing is modest when fewer than 10 cigarettes are smoked per day; however, recurrences in 3 months can approach 100% when more than 30 cigarettes are smoked daily.[1] Ulcer healing is markedly impaired, as evidenced by the need for longer treatment periods or higher antisecretory doses. Smoking increases the likelihood of complications and the need for surgery. Death rates are higher among patients who smoke than among nonsmokers, although it is not known whether the increase in mortality reflects PUD or the cardiac and pulmonary sequelae of smoking.

How cigarette smoking influences ulcer incidence, recurrence, healing, and complications remains unclear. Possible mechanisms include accelerated gastric emptying of liquids, inhibition of pancreatic bicarbonate secretion, promotion of duodenogastric reflux, and reduction in mucosal PG production. Although smoking has been reported to increase gastric acid, it appears to have no consistent effect on acid secretion. It is uncertain whether nicotine or other components of smoke are responsible for these physiologic alterations.

GENETIC FACTORS

A number of genetic factors have been proposed to explain familial aggregation of PUD. However, recent data suggest that HP, and its association with hypergastrinemia and hyperpepsinogenemia I, offers a more plausible explanation for family clustering than inherited autosomal dominance.[1] Blood group O and increased risk for DU may be related to a recent finding that blood group O antigens constitute apical receptors for HP in the parietal cell.[1] Certain rare genetic syndromes are associated with peptic ulcers.

PSYCHOLOGICAL STRESS

The importance of psychological factors in the genesis of PUD is controversial.[1] Clinical observation supports the belief that ulcer patients are adversely affected by stressful life events. However, controlled studies have failed to document a cause-and-effect relationship. Alternatively, psychological factors may predispose selected patients to PUD or alter the degree of pain or disability that results from an ulcer. Major psychological stress is reported to substantially increase the basal acid secretion and, independent of acid secretion, predispose to gastric and duodenal mucosal injury. It is possible that emotional stress also induces behavioral risks such as smoking and the use of NSAIDs or alters the inflammatory response or resistance to HP infection. The role of stress in the pathogenesis of chronic PUD is complex and probably multifactorial.

DIETARY FACTORS

The role of diet and nutrition in PUD is uncertain, but may explain regional variations.[1] Coffee, tea, cola beverages, beer, milk, and spices may cause dyspepsia, but do not increase the risk for PUD. In addition, beverage restrictions and bland diets do not alter the frequency of ulcer recurrence. Although caffeine is a gastric acid stimulant, other constituents in decaffeinated coffee or tea, caffeine-free carbonated beverages, beer, and wine are responsible for increasing gastric acid. Ethanol, in high concentrations, is associated with acute gastric mucosal damage and upper GI bleeding; however, there is insufficient evidence to confirm that ethanol causes ulcers.

DISEASES ASSOCIATED WITH PEPTIC ULCERS

A few diseases have been associated with peptic ulcers, but many apparent associations have been based on inconclusive evidence.[1] Duodenal ulcers are commonly associated with reflux esophagitis and Barrett's esophagus. Peptic ulcers occur in up to 30% of patients with chronic pulmonary disease, but cigarette smoking appears to fully account for this association. The increased incidence of ulcers in patients with rheumatoid arthritis is probably related to the use of aspirin, NSAIDs, and corticosteroids. The incidence and prevalence of DU and GU are increased in cirrhosis, but a relationship has not been confirmed. The association between PUD and renal failure in patients on hemodialysis and after transplant is controversial. A recent decline in risk of ulcers is attributed to improved medical and psychological care of the patient. Ulcers in renal transplant patients may be caused by viruses related to immunosuppression (see Table 31–2). Patients with atrophic gastritis and pernicious anemia, Addison's disease, autoimmune thyroid disease, and hypoparathyroidism appear to have a low incidence of peptic ulcers.

PATHOPHYSIOLOGY

GASTRIC ACID SECRETION

A minimal level of gastric acid secretion is necessary for the formation of peptic ulcers. Thus, gastric acid serves as a cofactor with HP infection or NSAID use (see Fig. 31–1).[1] About 30% to 50% of patients with DU are hypersecretors of gastric acid.[26] Factors responsible for acid hypersecretion include increased parietal cell mass, increased basal secretory drive, and increased postprandial secretory drive. Mechanisms that underlie basal and postprandial hypersecretion include enhanced sensitivity of the parietal cell to secretogogues or vagal stimulation as well as impaired acid inhibitory mechanisms. Acid hypersecretion may also be a consequence of HP infection.[27] Patients with Zollinger-Ellison syndrome (described later in the chapter) have basal acid hypersecretion resulting from a gastrin-producing tumor. In contrast to DU, patients with GU have normal or reduced rates of acid secretion, reflecting a low-normal parietal cell mass. Decreased acid secretion (hypochlorhydria) or an absence of acid secretion (achlorhydria) has been reported in the elderly.

Acid secretion is usually expressed as the amount of acid secreted under basal or fasting conditions, as with basal acid output (BAO); after maximal stimulation, as with maximal acid output (MAO); or in response to a meal. Basal, maximal, and meal-stimulated acid secretion varies according to time of day, psychological state, age, gender, and health status. The lowest acid secretory rates occur between 5 AM and 11 AM, while the highest rates occur between 2 PM and 11 PM.[26] The reason why circadian variations occur is unknown. The BAO is usually higher in men than in women. An increase in the BAO/MAO ratio suggests a basal hypersecretory state such as Zollinger-Ellison syndrome. A comprehensive review of gastric acid secretion and its regulation can be found elsewhere.[26]

PEPSIN

Pepsin appears to play a critical role in the proteolytic activity involved in ulcer formation.[1] Gastric mucosal cells secrete two types of proteolytic proenzymes. Pepsinogen I (PI) is produced only in the chief and mucous neck cells of the acid-secreting mucosa, whereas pepsinogen II (PII) is found in gastric acid-secreting and antral mucosa. Pepsin is activated by acid pH (optimal pH of 1.8 to 3.5), inactivated reversibly at pH 4, and irreversibly destroyed at pH 7. Pepsinogen I secretion is directly proportional to the rate of acid secretion. Hypergastrinemia and HP infection are associated with increased serum PI concentrations, although HP itself may induce hypergastrinemia.[1] Eradication of HP is reported to decrease serum PI concentrations.

ALTERED MUCOSAL DEFENSE AND HEALING

Several mechanisms protect the GI mucosa from endogenous and exogenous noxious substances. These defensive mechanisms include mucus and bicarbonate secretion, intrinsic epithelial cell defense, and mucosal blood flow.[1,26] Mucosal repair after injury is related to epithelial cell restitution, growth, and acute wound healing. The maintenance of mucosal integrity and repair is mediated by the production of endogenous prostaglandins. The term "cytoprotection" is often used to describe this process, but "mucosal defense" or "mucosal protection" are more accurate terms, as prostaglandins prevent deep mucosal injury and not superficial damage to individual cells. Adaptive cytoprotection, the short-term adaptation of mucosal cells to mild topical irritants, is characterized by gastric hyperemia and increased PG synthesis. This phenomenon allows the stomach to initially withstand the damaging effects of irritants. Alterations in mucosal defense, induced by HP or NSAIDs, appear to be important cofactors in the formation of peptic ulcers (see Fig. 31–1).

ABNORMALITIES IN GASTRIC MOTILITY

Gastric motility determines the rate of delivery of stomach contents to the duodenum, whereas duodenal motility affects the clearance of gastric, biliary, and pancreatic secretions from the duodenum. In a subset of DU patients, accelerated gastric emptying may contribute to a relative increase in the acidity of the proximal duodenum. Abnormal antral–pylorus–duodenal motility patterns permit duodenal contents containing bile salts and pancreatic enzymes to reflux into the stomach. Delayed gastric emptying increases exposure of the stomach to acid, pepsin, and refluxed duodenal contents. It is possible that in a subset of patients, gastric stasis and duodenal reflux may influence the severity of gastric injury induced by HP or NSAIDs.[1]

HELICOBACTER PYLORI

Helicobacter pylori is a spiral-shaped, pH-sensitive, gram-negative, microaerophilic bacterium that resides between the mucous layer and surface epithelial cells in the stomach or any location where gastric-type epithelium is found.[1,2,28] The combination of its spiral shape and flagella permits it to move from the lumen of the stomach, where the pH is low, to the mucous layer, where the local pH is neutral. The acute infection is accompanied by transient hypochlorhydria, which permits the organism to survive in the acidic gastric juice. The exact method by which HP initially induces hypochlorhydria is unknown. One theory is that HP produces large amounts of urease, which hydrolyzes urea in the gastric juice and converts it to ammonia and carbon dioxide.[2] It is possible that local neutralization by ammonia protects the organism from the lethal effect of acid. Another possible mechanism includes the production of mediators such as acid-inhibitory proteins. *Helicobacter pylori* attaches to gastric-type epithelium by adherence pedestals, which prevent the organism from being shed during cell turnover and mucus secretion. Antral organisms colonize gastric metaplastic tissue in the duodenum, which is thought to arise secondary to changes in acid or bicarbonate secretion, products of HP, or host inflammatory responses (see Fig. 31–2).[2]

A number of bacterial and host factors are thought to play a role in the pathogenesis of GI mucosal damage caused by HP infection. Evidence suggests that HP contributes to gastric mucosal injury by (1) direct mechanisms, (2) alterations in the immune/inflammatory response, and (3) hypergastrinemia leading to increased acid secretion.[27–30] In addition, HP appears to enhance the carcinogenic conversion of susceptible gastric epithelial cells.

Direct mucosal damage is produced by elaborating bacterial enzymes (lipases, proteases, and urease); virulence factors (vacuolating cytotoxin, cytotoxin-associated gene protein, and growth-inhibitory factor); and adherence.[29] Lipases and proteases degrade gastric mucus, ammonia produced by urease may be toxic to gastric epithelial cells, and bacterial adherence enhances the uptake of toxins into gastric epithelial cells. About 50% of HP strains produce a protein toxin (Vac A) that is responsible for cellular vacuole formation. Strains with cytotoxin-associated gene (cagA) protein have been associated with DU, atrophic gastritis, and adenocarcinoma, but this association remains controversial.[2,29] *Helicobacter pylori* infection alters the inflammatory response and damages epithelial cells directly by cell-mediated immune mechanisms or indirectly by activated neutrophils or macrophages attempting to phagocytose bacteria or bacterial products.[30] *Helicobacter pylori* infection may increase gastric acid secretion in patients with DU, or diminish acid output in patients with gastric cancer.[27] Infection of the gastric antrum leads to postprandial hypergastrinemia and hypersecretion of gastric acid. Responsible mechanisms include cytokines, such as tumor necrosis factor (TNF)-α released in HP gastritis; products of HP, such as ammonia; and diminished expression of somatostatin. The reason why somatostatin is diminished remains unclear, but cytokines might be involved.[27] Corpus gastritis promotes gastric atrophy and leads to a decrease in acid output.

NONSTEROIDAL ANTI-INFLAMMATORY DRUGS

The exact mechanism by which chronic NSAID therapy causes GUs is not known. However, there are two major components to their ulcerogenic effects in the stomach: (1) direct or topical irritation of the gastric epithelium and (2) systemic

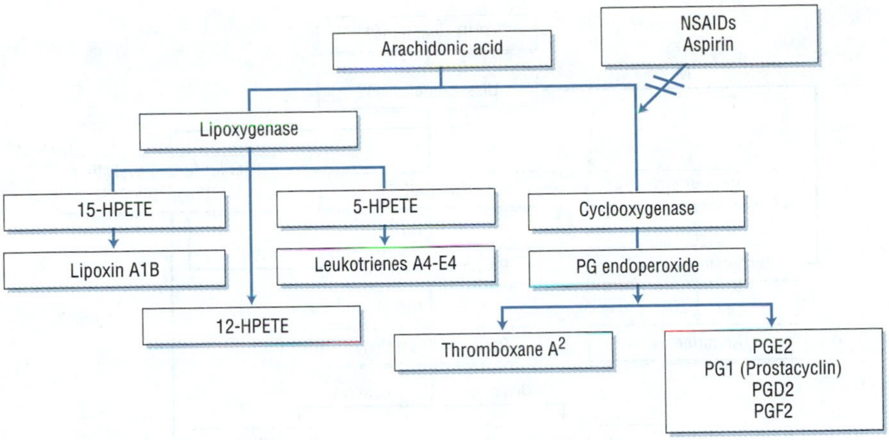

FIGURE 31–3. Metabolism of arachidonic acid after its release from membrane phospholipids. HPETE = hydroperoxyeicosatetraenoic acid; HETE = hydroxyeicosatetraenoic acid; PG = prostaglandin; NSAIDs = nonsteroidal anti-inflammatory drugs; ASA = aspirin.

inhibition of endogenous GI mucosal prostaglandin synthesis (Fig. 31–3).[3,16] Although the initial injury occurs because of local toxicity, systemic inhibition of prostaglandins appears to be the most important factor and correlates with the ability of an NSAID to cause gastric damage.[16] Cyclooxygenase (COX), the rate-limiting enzyme in the conversion of arachidonic acid to prostaglandin, is inhibited by NSAIDs (Fig. 31–3). Two similar COX isoforms exist in mammalian cells: cyclooxygenase-1 (COX-1) is found in body tissue such as the stomach, kidney, intestine, and platelets; cyclooxygenase-2 (COX-2) is undetectable in most tissues under normal physiologic conditions, but its expression is increased during acute inflammation and arthritis (Fig. 31–4).[3,16] Cyclooxygenase-1 plays an important role in producing protective prostaglandins that regulate physiologic processes such as GI cytoprotection, vascular homeostasis, and renal function. Cyclooxygenase-2 is induced (upregulated) by inflammatory stimuli such as cytokines and produces prostaglandins involved with inflammation and pain. Evidence suggests that the adverse effects (e.g., gastrointestinal effects, renal toxicity) of NSAIDs result from the inhibition of COX-1, whereas the anti-inflammatory actions of NSAIDs result from the inhibition of COX-2.[3,16] It is hypothesized that all of the available NSAIDs inhibit both COX-1 and COX-2 to varying degrees (Table 31–4).

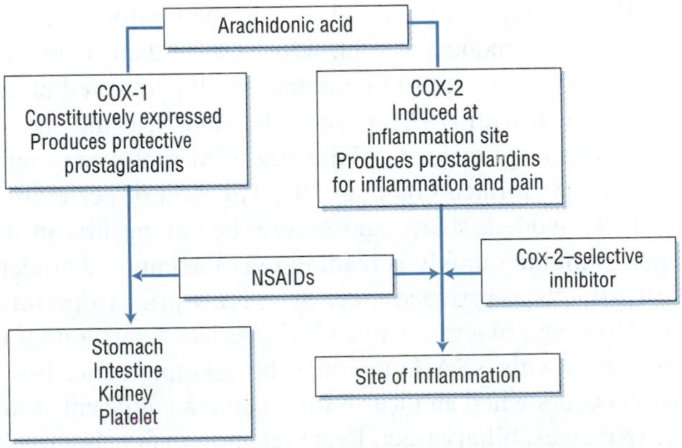

FIGURE 31–4. Synthesis of prostaglandins from arachidonic acid. Currently available NSAIDs inhibit cyclooxygenase-1 (COX-1) and cyclooxygenase-2 (COX-2) to varying degrees.

In addition to prostaglandin inhibition, a number of other mechanisms probably contribute to the development of NSAID-induced mucosal injury. There is experimental evidence that TNF-α may be an important signal for NSAID-induced neutrophil adherence within the gastric microcirculation.[16] Adherence of neutrophils may (1) damage the vascular endothelium and lead to a reduction in mucosal blood flow or (2) liberate oxygen-derived free radicals and proteases. Leukotrienes, products of lipoxygenase metabolism, are inflammatory substances that may contribute to mucosal injury through stimulatory effects on neutrophil adherence (see Fig. 31–3). Topical irritant properties are predominately associated with acidic NSAIDs (e.g., aspirin) and the ability of the NSAID to decrease the hydrophobicity of the mucous gel layer in the stomach.[3,16] Although most nonaspirin NSAIDs have topical irritant effects, aspirin appears to be the most ulcerogenic. Prodrugs, enteric-coated aspirin tablets or capsules, salicylate derivatives, and

TABLE 31–4. Selectivity of NSAIDs for Cyclooxygenase-1 Versus Cyclooxygenase-2

NSAID	COX-2/COX-1[a]	Selectivity
Aspirin	166	↑
Indomethacin	60	
Ibuprofen	15	Greater selectivity for COX-1
Diclofenac	0.7	
Naproxen	0.6	Greater selectivity for COX-2
Nabumetone	0.2	
Entodolac	0.1	
L745,337[b]	0.0025	↓

[a]Ratio of mean inhibitory concentration of drug required to inhibit COX-2 by 50% divided by concentration of drug required to inhibit COX-1 by 50%; data obtained from *in vitro* studies.
[b]Selective COX-2 inhibitor.
Adapted from Ref. 16.

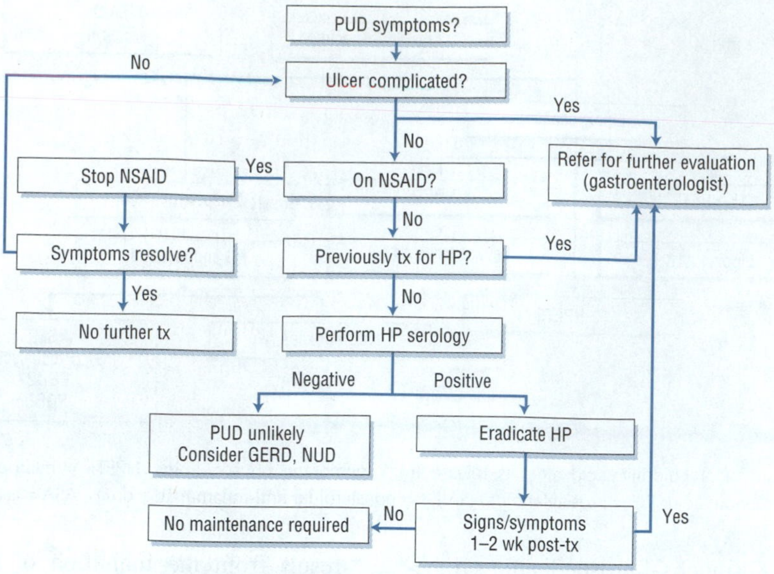

FIGURE 31–5. Algorithm for the evaluation and treatment (tx) of chronic peptic ulcer disease (PUD). HP = *Helicobacter pylori;* NSAIDs = nonsteroidal anti-inflammatory drugs; GERD = gastroesophageal reflux disease; NUD = nonulcer dyspepsia.

parenteral or rectal preparations may cause less acute superficial gastric erosions than conventional oral aspirin or NSAID formulations. However, they can cause peptic ulcers and related life-threatening complications presumably as a result of systemic prostaglandin inhibition.

NSAIDs (including aspirin) cause de novo ulcers and can also interfere with the healing of preexisting lesions by interfering with the process of restitution.[16] NSAIDs probably contribute to GI bleeding from current or preexisting ulcers by inhibiting platelet aggregation that results from suppression of thromboxane synthesis. The pathogenesis of small intestinal damage (e.g., duodenal ulcer) and colonic damage is not as well understood as the pathogenesis of NSAID-induced gastropathy. Enteric bacteria and enterohepatic recirculation of NSAIDs appear to play a more important role in the pathogenesis of NSAID-induced injury to the small intestine than does prostaglandin inhibition. The mechanisms by which NSAIDs cause or exacerbate preexisting colonic ulcerations and inflammatory bowel disease have been attributed to inhibition of colonic prostaglandins, but experimental data are conflicting. A more detailed discussion of the pathogenesis of NSAID-induced small intestinal and colonic injury can be found elsewhere.[16]

COMPLICATIONS

Gastrointestinal bleeding, perforation, and obstruction occur with HP and NSAID ulcers and constitute the most serious, life-threatening complications of chronic PUD. Bleeding is caused by the erosion of an ulcer into an artery and is reported to occur in approximately 15% to 20% of patients.[31] The bleeding may be insidious or may present as melena or hematemesis. Peptic ulcers account for about one-half of all patients who have an upper GI bleed.[32] Patients are more likely to bleed from a DU than a GU, but the use of NSAIDs (especially in the elderly) is the most important risk factor for GI bleeding. The mortality rate with bleeding GU is 7% to 16% and with DU is 1% to 7%.[32] Deaths occur primarily in patients who continue to bleed after hospitalization or in those who rebleed after the initial bleeding has stopped. In about 90% of patients, bleeding responds satisfactorily to gastric lavage and supportive therapy. In most controlled trials, treatment with H_2-receptor antagonists, sucralfate, antacids, proton pump inhibitors (PPIs), and somatostatin, or drug combinations, appears to offer no advantage when compared to placebo. Although the prevalence of HP infection in bleeding peptic ulcers is uncertain, clinical trials comparing HP eradication to maintenance antisecretory therapy in HP-positive patients have reported lower or no rebleeding rates in the 12 months following HP eradication.[32]

Perforation of a peptic ulcer into the peritoneal cavity occurs more frequently with DU (60%) than with GU (40%).[32] About one-third to one-half of all perforated ulcers are associated with NSAID use in the elderly, while HP accounts for a large majority of the others. Mortality is usually higher for perforated GU than DU. The pain of perforation is usually sudden, sharp, and severe, beginning first in the epigastrium but quickly spreading over the entire abdomen. Most patients experience ulcer symptoms prior to perforation. However, older patients who experience perforation in association with NSAID use may be asymptomatic. Penetration occurs when an ulcer burrows into an adjacent structure (pancreas, biliary tract, liver) rather than opening freely into a cavity.

Gastric outlet obstruction occurs in less than 5% of hospitalized patients with peptic ulcers.[32] Mechanical obstruction is caused by scarring or edema of the duodenal bulb or pyloric channel and can lead to delayed gastric emptying. Symptoms usually occur over several months and include early satiety, bloating, anorexia, nausea, vomiting, and weight loss. As with perforation and penetration, gastric outlet obstruction usually occurs in patients with long-standing ulcer disease.

Medical therapy has improved so dramatically over the last few years that even the most virulent ulcers can be managed medically. Although there are limited data, it is reasonable to assume that eradicating HP or discontinuing NSAID therapy should prevent ulcer recurrence and decrease ulcer-related complications (Fig. 31–5). Intractability to medical therapy is now an infrequent manifestation of PUD and an infrequent indication for surgery.

CLINICAL PRESENTATION

SIGNS AND SYMPTOMS

Epigastric pain is the classic and most frequent symptom of DU and GU (Table 31–5).[1] The pain is often described as burning but can present as a vague discomfort, abdominal fullness, or cramping. Many patients with DU describe a typical nocturnal pain that awakens them at night. Ulcer-related pain in DU often occurs 1 to 3 hours after meals and is usually relieved by food, but this is variable. In GU, food may precipitate or accentuate ulcer pain. Antacids usually provide immediate pain relief in most patients with DU or GU. Epigastric pain usually diminishes or disappears during treatment; however, recurrence of pain after healing usually indicates a recurrent ulcer.

The severity of ulcer pain varies from patient to patient, and in some patients may be seasonal, occurring more frequently in the spring or fall. Episodes of discomfort usually occur in clusters lasting up to a few weeks followed by a pain-free period or remission lasting from weeks to years. Epigastric pain does not always correlate with the presence or absence of acid or an ulcer crater. Asymptomatic patients may have an ulcer at endoscopy, and patients with endoscopically proven healed ulcers may have persistent symptoms. Changes in the character of the pain may suggest the presence of complications. Patients, particularly the elderly, with NSAID-induced ulcers are less likely to have symptoms (silent ulcer). As many as 40% of patients with NSAID ulcers and 60% with bleeding are asymptomatic. The reasons for this are unclear, but may relate to differences in which the elderly perceive pain or result from the analgesic effect of the NSAID.

Patients with PUD often present with other dyspeptic symptoms including heartburn, belching, and bloating. Dyspepsia in itself is of little clinical value when trying to identify subsets of patients most likely to have an ulcer. Nausea, vomiting, anorexia, and weight loss are more common in patients with GU. Unusual findings may be present when ulcers are associated with hypersecretory states such as Zollinger-Ellison syndrome. Ulcer-like symptoms may occur in the absence of peptic ulceration (nonulcer dyspepsia) and in association with HP gastritis (Table 31–5). It is currently unclear whether HP infection plays a role in causing symptoms in patients with NUD.[14]

TABLE 31–5. Clinical Features of Duodenal Ulcer (DU), Gastric Ulcer (GU), and Nonulcer Dyspepsia (NUD)[a]

Feature	DU	GU	NUD
Pain	++++	++++	++++
Primary pain is epigastric pain	++++	+++	+++
Frequently severe	+++	+++	++
Occurs in clusters (episodic)	+++	+	++
Occurs at night (nocturnal)	++++	++	++
Radiates to back	++	++	++
Relieved by antacids	++++	++++	+++
Increased by food	++	+	++
Relieved by food	+++	++	++
Heartburn	+++	+	++
Bloating	+++	+++	+++
Belching	+++	+++	+++
Nausea	++	+++	++
Vomiting	++	+++	+
Anorexia	+	++	+
Weight loss	++	++	+

[a]Frequencies represent estimates and are categorized as being consistent (++++), frequent (+++), infrequent (++), or rare (+). None of the features are always present or always absent.

DIAGNOSIS

LABORATORY EVALUATION

Routine laboratory tests are not helpful in establishing the diagnosis of uncomplicated PUD.[1] Acid secretory studies and a fasting serum gastrin concentration are only recommended for patients unresponsive to therapy or those in whom hypersecretory diseases are suspected. The hematocrit, hemoglobin, and stool hemoccult tests are used to detect bleeding. An elevated serum PI may provide indirect evidence of HP, but the test is not widely available.

TESTS FOR *HELICOBACTER PYLORI*

The diagnosis of HP can be made using invasive or noninvasive tests (Table 31–6).[2,33–35] The invasive methods require upper GI endoscopy with a mucosal biopsy taken for histology, culture, or detection of urease activity. Recommendations to maximize the diagnostic yield include taking at least three tissue samples from specific areas of the stomach. Histologic identification has a sensitivity and specificity greater than 95% and allows classification of gastritis that may be present. Culture has a specificity of 100% and enables susceptibility testing of antimicrobial agents to detect resistance and permit appropriate treatment. The sensitivity and specificity of the rapid urease test, which detects HP urease enzyme activity, are above 90%.

TABLE 31–6. Tests for Detection of *Helicobacter pylori*

Test	Description	Advantages	Disadvantages
Serology	Detects antibodies to HP in blood	Endoscopy not required Inexpensive Office based, immediate results	Lower specificity than endoscopic tests or urea breath tests Not possible to determine if antibody is related to active or cured infection
Urea breath test	HP urease breaks down ingested labeled C-urea, patient exhales labeled CO_2	Endoscopy not required Less expensive than endoscopy Nonendoscopic method to confirm HP eradication Avoids biopsy sampling errors	Potential for false-negative results after antibiotics, bismuth, PPIs Results are not immediate (2 days)
Histology	Microbiologic examination (Warthin–Starry stain)	Gold standard High specificity and sensitivity	Requires endoscopy, patient discomfort Expensive (includes endoscopy) Patchy distribution of HP can cause false-negative results
Culture	Culture of biopsy	Used to test for antibiotic resistance High specificity	Requires endoscopy, patient discomfort Expensive (includes endoscopy) Patchy distribution of HP can cause false-negative results Results are not immediate
Rapid urease	Urease of HP generates ammonia, which causes a color change	Test of choice at endoscopy High specificity and sensitivity Easily performed, rapid results	Requires endoscopy, patient discomfort Expensive (includes endoscopy) Antibiotics, bismuth, and PPIs can cause false-negative results Patchy distribution of HP can cause false-negative results

Compiled from Refs. 2, 33–36, and 45.

This test provides information on the presence of HP, but does not determine the status of the mucosa or the susceptibility to antibiotics.

The noninvasive tests (Table 31–6) do not require a mucosal biopsy and include the urea breath test (UBT) and serology. These tests are simpler and less expensive than endoscopic tests for HP. The UBT is based on urease production by HP. The carbon 13 (nonradioactive isotope) and carbon 14 (radioactive isotope) tests require that the patient ingest the labeled urea, which is broken down in the stomach to ammonia and labeled bicarbonate. The labeled bicarbonate is absorbed in the blood and excreted in the breath. A mass spectrometer is needed to detect carbon 13, whereas carbon 14 can be measured using a scintillation counter.

Serologic tests are useful to detect circulating immunoglobulin (Ig) G or IgA directed against HP. Serology performed in the laboratory, the enzyme-linked immunosorbent assay (ELISA), has a sensitivity and specificity in the range of 90%. Rapid whole blood tests (in-office) appear to be less accurate than the laboratory tests.[35] Serologic tests are not useful to assess HP eradication, as antibody titers to HP vary markedly between individuals and take 6 months to 2 years or more to return to the uninfected range.[34] Proportional reductions from pretreatment levels may predict treatment success or failure. With the exception of serology, tests for HP may produce false-negative results if antibiotics or bismuth are taken within the previous 4 weeks or if a proton pump inhibitor is taken within the previous 2 weeks.[33–35] These agents appear to temporarily suppress HP and cause falsely negative results. One report suggests that the falsely negative effect is resolved within 5 days after stopping the PPI and that it parallels gastric acid suppression.[35] The UBT and serology, as opposed to biopsy-based tests, evaluate the whole stomach without the potential of sampling error.

The selection of a specific test depends on the clinical situation of the patient. Serologic tests are the initial screening test of choice as they are quick, inexpensive, and reliable. The UBT may be used if there is concern regarding a positive serologic test. When endoscopy is indicated, the primary diagnosis should be established using the rapid urease test. Patients with GU should have extra biopsy samples taken to rule out malignancy. Culturing for antibiotic sensitivity is not practical at this time. Posttreatment assessment, to confirm eradication, is not required in most patients unless they have a complicated ulcer, MALT lymphoma, or gastric cancer. The UBT is the best noninvasive method to verify HP eradication after treatment. In order to avoid confusing bacterial suppression with eradication, the UBT must be delayed at least 4 weeks after the completion of HP eradication therapy. Serology should not be used for patient follow-up because antibody titers remain elevated after successful treatment.

IMAGING AND ENDOSCOPY

Peptic ulcers should be differentiated from other acid-related disorders of the upper abdomen, and DU should be distinguished from GU. The diagnosis of PUD depends on visualizing the ulcer crater either by upper GI radiography or endoscopy.[1] Routine single barium contrast techniques can detect 30% of peptic ulcers, whereas it is possible to detect 60% to 80% of ulcers using optimal double-contrast radiography. Fiber-optic endoscopy detects more than 90% of peptic ulcers and permits direct inspection, biopsy, visualization of superficial erosions, and sites of active bleeding. Because of its lower cost, greater availability, and perhaps greater safety, many physicians believe that radiography should remain the initial diagnostic procedure in evaluating patients with suspected uncomplicated peptic ulcers. If complications are thought to exist or if an accurate diagnosis of PUD is warranted, endoscopy is the diagnostic procedure of choice. If a GU is found on radiography, malignancy should be excluded by direct endoscopic visualization and biopsy for histologic examination.

CLINICAL COURSE AND PROGNOSIS

The natural history of PUD is characterized by periods of exacerbations and remissions.[1] Ulcer pain is usually recognizable and episodic, but symptoms are variable, especially in the elderly and in patients taking NSAIDs. Conventional antiulcer medications, such as H_2-receptor antagonists, PPIs, and sucralfate, relieve symptoms, accelerate ulcer healing, and prevent ulcers from recurring, but they do not cure the disease. Both DU and GU recur unless the underlying cause (HP or NSAID) is removed. Eradication of HP infection alters the natural history of the disease, thereby markedly decreasing ulcer recurrence and complications. Nonsteroidal anti-inflammatory drugs increase the risk for ulcers and ulcer-related complications, especially in the elderly. About 20% of all patients with chronic PUD will experience GI bleeding, perforation, or obstruction. Mortality in patients with GU is slightly higher than in DU and the general population. The lifetime risk of gastric adenocarcinoma in HP-infected patients is about 1%. Symptomatic MALT occurs less frequenty.[11–13]

▶ TREATMENT: Peptic Ulcer Disease

DESIRED OUTCOME

The treatment of chronic PUD varies depending on the etiology of the ulcer (HP or NSAID), whether the ulcer is initial or recurrent, and whether complications have occurred. Overall treatment is aimed at relieving ulcer pain, healing the ulcer, preventing ulcer recurrence, and reducing ulcer-related complications. The goal of therapy in HP-positive patients with an active ulcer, with a history of ulcer-related complications, or receiving conventional maintenance therapy is to eradicate HP and cure the disease with a cost-effective drug regimen.

GENERAL APPROACH TO TREATMENT

Patients with PUD should eliminate or reduce psychological stress, cigarette smoking, and the use of NSAIDs (including aspirin). If possible, alternative agents such as acetaminophen or nonacetylated salicylates (e.g., salsalate) should be used for analgesia. In those patients in whom NSAIDs cannot be discontinued, lowering the NSAID dose or using a less damaging agent (see Table 31–4), coadministered with food or antacids, may decrease symptoms and mucosal damage. Although there is no "ulcer diet," the patient should avoid foods and beverages (e.g., spicy foods, caffeine, alcohol) that cause dyspepsia or exacerbate ulcer symptoms. Antacids may be used in conjunction with other antiulcer medications to relieve occasional ulcer symptoms. An algorithm for the evaluation and treatment of chronic PUD is presented in Figure 31–5.

Eradication is recommended for all HP-infected PUD patients (1) with an active ulcer, (2) with a history of ulcer-related complications, or (3) who require maintenance therapy.[2,5,36–39] There are no definitive recommendations regarding HP eradication in patients with dyspepsia or NUD as results from clinical trials are conflicting.[2,5,14,15,39] Therefore, testing for HP is only recommended if eradication therapy is planned. Although data are limited, treatment of HP is recommended for HP-positive patients with low-grade MALT lymphoma and after resection of gastric cancer.[5,12,13,39] Asymptomatic patients should not be tested for HP; however, if a positive test results, HP eradication should be offered after discussing the benefits and risks of therapy.[5,39]

The selection of an HP eradication regimen should be individualized and based on efficacy, tolerability, drug interaction potential, antibiotic resistance, cost, and the likelihood of compliance (Tables 31–7 and 31–8). In most patients, treatment should be initiated with a PPI-based three-drug regimen, as these regimens are more efficacious, better tolerated, simpler, and associated with better compliance. The efficacy of two-drug regimens is inferior to PPI-based three-drug regimens (Table 31–7). In addition, the inclusion of only one antibiotic may lead to antimicrobial resistance. Bismuth-based four-drug regimens, although effective, involve a more complicated dosing schedule than the PPI-based three-drug regimens and are associated with a higher incidence of adverse effects. Patients with an active ulcer should receive cotherapy with an antisecretory drug, such as a PPI or H_2-receptor antagonist, to facilitate the relief of ulcer symptoms. If a second course of eradication therapy is necessary, treatment should be instituted using a different antibiotic regimen. Patients who may not warrant HP eradication include those who are intolerant or will not comply with the drug regimen, those with HP-free NSAID ulcers, or patients with Zollinger-Ellison syndrome.

Treatment with a conventional antiulcer drug, such as an H_2-receptor antagonist, PPI, or sucralfate, may be an alternative (Table 31–9) to HP eradication, but is discouraged because of the high rate of ulcer recurrence and ulcer-related complications.[1,36] Combination therapy using conventional antiulcer medications (such as H_2-receptor antagonist plus sucralfate) usually adds to drug treatment costs without enhancing efficacy.[36] There is no rationale for combining an H_2-receptor antagonist with a PPI. Maintenance therapy with a low-dose H_2-receptor antagonist or PPI (Table 31–9) should be limited to high-risk patients who fail HP eradication, patients with severe complications, or those with HP-negative ulcers.[36]

Most uncomplicated NSAID-induced ulcers will heal with standard regimens of either an H_2-receptor antagonist, PPI, or

TABLE 31–7. Comparison of Therapeutic Strategies Used to Eradicate *Helicobacter pylori*

Strategy	Efficacy[a]	Adverse Effects[b]	Compliance[c]
Two-drug Regimens			
Amoxicillin + PPI	Poor–fair	Low–medium	Likely
Clarithromycin + PPI	Fair–good	Low–medium	Likely
Clarithromycin + RBC	Fair–good	Low–medium	Likely
Three-drug Regimens			
Clarithromycin + metronidazole + PPI	Good–Excellent	Medium	Likely
Clarithromycin + amoxicillin + PPI	Good–Excellent	Low–medium	Likely
Amoxicillin + metronidazole + PPI	Good	Medium	Likely
Clarithromycin + metronidazole + RBC	Good	Medium	Unlikely
Tetracycline + metronidazole + sucralfate	Good	Medium	Unlikely
Four-drug Regimens			
BSS + metronidazole + tetracycline + H_2-receptor antagonist[d]	Good–excellent	Medium–high	Unlikely
BSS + metronidazole + amoxicillin + H_2-receptor antagonist[d]	Fair–good	Medium–high	Unlikely
BSS + metronidazole + tetracycline + PPI	Good–excellent	Medium–high	Unlikely
BSS + metronidazole + clarithromycin + PPI	Good–excellent	Medium–high	Unlikely

PPI = proton pump inhibitor; RBC = ranitidine bismuth citrate; BSS = bismuth subsalicylate.
[a]Efficacy (eradication rate) = excellent (> 90%); good (> 80%–90%); fair (> 70%–80%); poor (< 70%).
[b]Safety (frequency of clinically important adverse effects) = high; medium; low.
[c]Compliance (estimate based on total number of tablets/capsules, frequency of administration, and clinically important adverse effects) = likely; unlikely.
[d]H2-receptor antagonist indicated when used in patients with an active ulcer.

TABLE 31–8. Drug Treatment Regimens Used to Eradicate *Helicobacter pylori*

Drug	Dose	Frequency	Duration
1. Clarithromycin[a]	500 mg	tid	14 days
Omeprazole[b]	40 mg	qd	14 days
2. Amoxicillin[d]	1 g	tid	14 days
Lansoprazole[b,c]	30 mg	tid	14 days
3. Amoxicillin	1 g	bid–tid	14 days
Omeprazole[b,c]	20 mg	bid	14 days
4. Clarithromycin[a]	500 mg	tid	14 days
Ranitidine bismuth citrate	400 mg	bid	28 days
5. Clarithromycin[a]	500 mg	bid	10–14 days
Amoxicillin	1 g	bid	10–14 days
Lansoprazole[b,c]	30 mg	bid	10–14 days
6. Clarithromycin	500 mg	bid	10–14 days
Metronidazole	500 mg	bid	10–14 days
Omeprazole[b,c]	20 mg	bid	10–14 days
7. Clarithromycin	500 mg	bid	14 days
Metronidazole	500 mg	bid	14 days
Ranitidine bismuth citrate	400 mg	bid	14–28 days
8. Bismuth subsalicylate[e]	525 mg	qid	14 days
Metronidazole	250 mg	qid	14 days
Tetracycline	500 mg	qid	14 days
H_2-receptor antagonist[e]	As directed using conventional ulcer-healing dosage regimen		28 days
9. Bismuth subsalicylate	525 mg	qid	14 days
Metronidazole	250 mg	qid	14 days
Amoxicillin	500 mg	qid	14 days
H_2-receptor antagonist[e]	As directed using conventional ulcer-healing dosage regimen		28 days
10. Bismuth subsalicylate	525 mg	qid	7–10 days
Metronidazole	500 mg	qid	7–10 days
Tetracycline	500 mg	qid	7–10 days
Omeprazole[b,c]	20 mg	bid	7–10 days
11. Bismuth subsalicylate	525 mg	qid	7–10 days
Metronidazole	500 mg	qid	7–10 days
Clarithromycin	500 mg	bid	7–10 days
Omeprazole[b,c]	20 mg	bid	7–10 days
12. Tetracycline	500 mg	qid	14 days
Metronidazole	500 mg	qid	14 days
Sucralfate	1 g	qid	14–28 days

[a]Approved by the Food and Drug Administration (FDA).
[b]When eradicating *Helicobacter pylori,* only proton pump inhibitor may be used in its recommended eradication dosage.
[c]In patients with an ulcer at the time of initiation of therapy, the proton pump inhibitor may be extended to 28 days using conventional anti-ulcer dosages.
[d]Approved by the FDA for patients unable to tolerate clarithromycin.
[e]When treating an ulcer, any H_2-receptor antagonist may be used in its conventional ulcer-healing dosage regimen.

TABLE 31–9. Oral Drug Treatment Regimens Used to Heal Ulcers or Maintain Ulcer Healing

	Ulcer Healing		Maintenance of Ulcer Healing	
Drug	*Duodenal Ulcer (mg/dose)*	*Gastric Ulcer (mg/dose)*	*Duodenal Ulcer (mg/dose)*	*Gastric Ulcer (mg/dose)*
H2-Receptor Antagonists				
Cimetidine	300 qid[a] 400 bid[a] 800 hs[a]	300 qid[a] 800 hs[a]	400 hs[a]	400–800 hs
Famotidine	20 bid[a] 40 hs[a]	20 bid 40 hs[a]	20 hs[a]	20 hs
Nizatidine	150 bid[a] 300 hs[a]	150 bid[a] 300 hs[a]	150 hs[a]	150–300 hs
Ranitidine	150 bid[a] 300 hs[a]	150 bid[a] 300 hs	150 hs[a]	150[a]–300 hs
Proton Pump Inhibitors				
Omeprazole	20 qd[a]	40 qd[a]	20	20–40 qd
Lansoprazole	15 qd[a]	30 qd[a]	15[a]	15–30 qd
Mucosal Defense				
Sucralfate (g/dose)	1 qid[a] 2 bid	1 qid 2 bid	1 bid	1 qid

[a]Approved by the Food and Drug Administration (FDA).

sucralfate (Table 31–9) if the NSAID is discontinued.[3,16,36,40] If the NSAID must be continued, or if there is a large ulcer, PPIs are the drugs of choice because they accelerate ulcer healing.[3,16,36] If HP is present, treatment should be initiated with an eradication regimen that contains a PPI.[36] Prophylactic cotherapy is indicated for patients who are at increased risk of developing serious ulcer-related complications (see Table 31–3).[3,16,36] Although H_2-receptor antagonists or PPIs may be useful in relieving dyspeptic symptoms and may prevent ulcers, misoprostol remains the treatment of choice for preventing NSAID-induced GU and DU.[3,16,21,36,40]

Patients with a complicated ulcer (signs or symptoms of bleeding, obstruction, perforation, or penetration) may require endoscopic or surgical treatment. A definitive diagnosis should be made in these patients as malignancy may be present. Empiric ulcer therapy should not be used in this setting. Figure 31–6 displays an algorithm for the long-term treatment of a bleeding ulcer based on etiology.

NONPHARMACOLOGIC THERAPY

Advances in the medical management of PUD have led to a steady decline in operations.[41] A subset of patients, however, will require emergency surgery for bleeding, perforation, or obstruction. Classically, surgical procedures performed for PUD included vagotomy with pyloroplasty or vagotomy with antrectomy. Vagotomy (truncal, selective, or parietal cell) inhibits vagal stimulation of gastric acid. A truncal or selective vagotomy frequently results in postoperative gastric dysfunction and requires a pyloroplasty

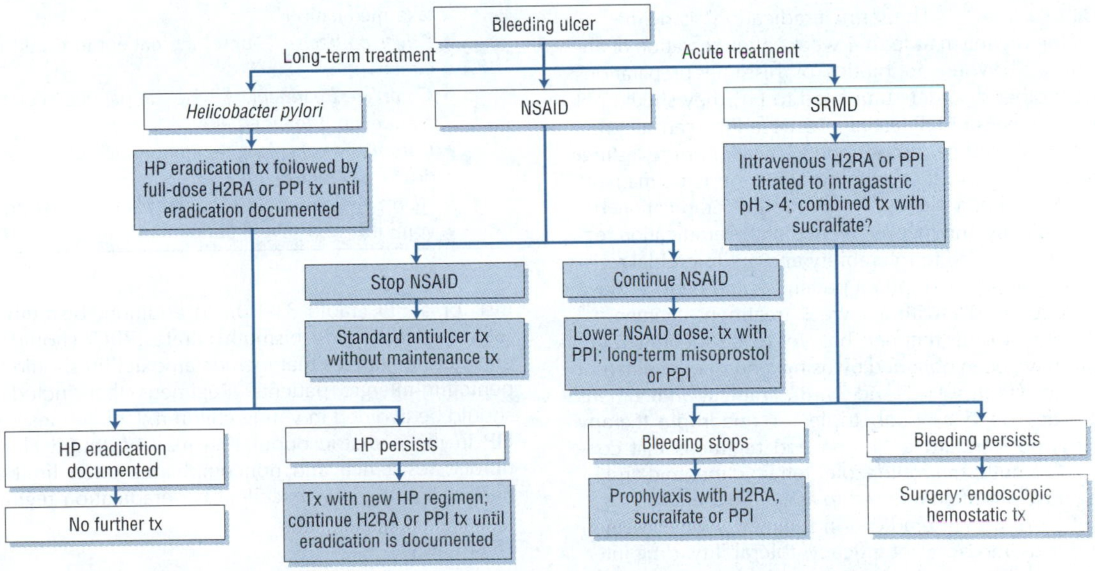

FIGURE 31–6. Algorithm for the long-term treatment (tx) of a bleeding *H. pylori* (HP)-associated or NSAID-induced ulcer and the acute treatment of bleeding associated with stress-related mucosal damage (SRMD). If NSAID ulcer is HP positive, then bleeding should be treated with HP eradication, as shown in the algorithm. H2RA = H_2-receptor antagonist; PPI = proton pump inhibitor; tx = treatment.

or antrectomy to facilitate gastric drainage. When an antrectomy is performed, the remaining stomach is anastomosed with the duodenum (Billroth I) or with the jejunum (Billroth II). A vagotomy is not necessary when an antrectomy is performed for GU. Although surgery for PUD is effective, postoperative consequences (e.g., recurrent ulceration, postvagotomy diarrhea, dumping syndrome, and anemia) occur and alter quality of life.

PHARMACOLOGIC THERAPY

RECOMMENDATIONS

Patients should eliminate or reduce psychological stress, cigarette smoking, and NSAID use. Foods and beverages that cause dyspepsia or exacerbate ulcer symptoms should be avoided. Eradication of HP is recommended for HP-positive patients with active DU or GU, or HP-positive patients with PUD who require maintenance therapy or have a history of ulcer-related complications. Treatment should be initiated with a PPI-based three-drug regimen, as they have the highest HP eradication rates and best safety profile, and are associated with better compliance. Recommendations will change, however, as more data from controlled trials become available to clarify optimal drug combinations, dosages, and treatment periods. If a second course of therapy is required, the regimen should contain different antibiotics. Maintenance therapy with an H_2-receptor antagonist or PPI is recommended for high-risk patients who fail HP eradication, patients with severe complications, or those with HP-negative ulcers.

Standard H_2-receptor antagonist, PPI, or sucralfate regimens heal uncomplicated NSAID-induced ulcers if the NSAID is discontinued. A PPI is recommended if the NSAID cannot be discontinued or if the ulcer is large. If HP is present, the ulcer should be healed and the HP eradicated using antibiotics and a PPI. Cotherapy with Misoprostol or a PPI is recommended for patients who are at increased risk of developing serious ulcer-related complications from NSAIDs. The long-term treatment of a bleeding ulcer depends on the etiology of the ulcer.

TREATMENT OF *HELICOBACTER PYLORI*–ASSOCIATED ULCERS

The eradication of HP infection heals ulcers, alters the natural history of HP-positive PUD, and reduces the risk of recurrence to less than 10% in 1 year.[2,36] The term "eradication" is defined as the absence of the organism at least 4 weeks after cessation of antibiotic therapy.[2,5,36] When antibiotics or bismuth preparations are used to treat other disorders unrelated to HP, they should not be taken within 4 weeks of HP testing. Because PPIs can suppress the infection, they should be discontinued 1 week prior to testing. An HP-associated ulcer is *cured* when eradication is permanent.

Clinicians have been slow to embrace HP eradication because of the complexity and inconvenience of the eradication regimens and concerns related to tolerability and antimicrobial resistance. A realistic goal in a compliant patient would be to achieve an eradication rate of 90% with a 1-week treatment regimen.[2,36] Although the optimal drug regimen has yet to be identified, acceptable results have been obtained by using a number of different drug combinations (Tables 31–7 and 31–8). Eradication regimens should not be described as dual, triple, or quadruple therapy because there is no standard definition and regimens that contain four drugs (bismuth, metronidazole, tetracycline, and an H_2-receptor antagonist) are often referred to as "triple therapy."

The selection of an HP eradication regimen should be individualized and take into account efficacy, tolerability, drug interaction potential, antibiotic resistance, cost, and compliance. Until studies prove otherwise, the following drugs should not be substituted: ampicillin for amoxicillin, doxycycline for tetracycline, azithromycin for clarithromycin, or an H_2-receptor antagonist for a PPI (Table 31–10). In addition, bismuth subsalicylate (BSS) and ranitidine bismuth citrate (RBC) should not be interchanged. Regimens that include amoxicillin should be avoided in penicillin-allergic patients. Regimens that include tetracycline should be avoided in young children. Guidlelines for treatment of HP in the pediatric population may be found elsewhere.[42] Antibiotic resistance and noncompliance often limit the effectiveness of an otherwise excellent HP eradication regimen.

TABLE 31–10. Recommendations for Providing Pharmaceutical Care to Ulcer Patients Receiving HP Eradication Therapy

1. Recommend drug treatment as presented in the chapter text and Principles of Pharmacotherapy.
2. Counsel patients to discontinue or reduce psychological stress, cigarette smoking, and NSAIDs, and to avoid foods or beverages that cause dyspepsia or exacerbate ulcer symptoms.
3. Assess likelihood of patient compliance and advocate most effective, but simplest drug regimen.
4. Assess patient allergies to determine if allergic to penicillin (or other antibiotics) so that drug regimens that contain penicillin (or other antibiotics) can be avoided. Avoid regimens that contain tetracycline in children.
5. Assess patient use of ethanol or ethanol-containing products and counsel appropriately when metronidazole is included in the eradication regimen.
6. Assess patient use of oral birth control medications and counsel appropriately when antibiotics are used in the drug regimen.
7. Inform patient of change in stool color when regimens containing bismuth subsalicylate or ranitidine bismuth citrate are included in an HP eradication regimen.
8. Assess and monitor patients for potential adverse effects, especially those associated with metronidazole, claithromycin, and amoxicillin.
9. Assess and monitor patients for potential drug interactions, especially those receiving metronidazole, clarithromcyin, and cimetidine.
10. Assess and monitor patients for potential salicylate toxicity, especially in patients receiving cotherapy with other salicylates or anticoagulants, or in patients with renal failure.
11. Assess noncompliance and the possibility of antibiotic resistance to either metronidazole or clarithromycin when a patient fails HP eradication.
12. Provide patient education to patients with PUD who are receiving HP eradication. Information should include:
    - *Cause.* Explain that ulcers are associated with bacteria.
    - *Treatment.* Explain that treatment consists of antibiotics and antiulcer medications.
    - *Administration.* Instruct the patient on when and how to take medications.
    - *Adverse effects.* Counsel the patient to report intolerable effects.
    - *Complete treatment.* Advise the patient to complete treatment even if feeling better.
    - *Compliance.* Explain the importance of compliance to the drug treatment regimen.
    - *Alarm symptoms.* Instruct the patient to report bleeding, vomiting, and severe abdominal pain.

Efficacy

Numerous clinical trials of multiple drugs, drug combinations, and dosage regimens have been conducted in an attempt to eradicate HP and cure PUD.[2,5,36–39,43–47] The effectiveness of a specific regimen varies with the method used to analyze results (intention-to-treat versus per protocol), the method used to test for HP eradication (endoscopy with biopsy versus UBT), and the inclusion of patients from different geographic locations (North America versus Europe).[37] In addition, there are only a few head-to-head trials and many of the studies include an insufficient number of patients.

None of the conventional antiulcer agents (including bismuth preparations) have any clinically important effect on HP eradication.[2,37,48] Although HP is sensitive to most antibiotics *in vitro,* monotherapy with antibiotics including amoxicillin, metronidazole, tetracycline, azithromycin, erythromycin, or the fluoroquinolones *in vivo* is disappointing.[2,37,39] Clarithromycin is the most effective single antibiotic *in vivo* with an eradication rate of 40% to 70%. A discrepancy between high *in vitro* and low *in vivo* efficacy may be explained in part by the degradation of the antimicrobial in the acidic environment of the stomach or by insufficient penetration into the gastric mucus.[2,38] Because of the poor results with monotherapy and the emergence of resistance to single antibiotic therapy, a remarkable number of combined drug regimens have been investigated. Explanations as to why PPIs, in particular, enhance the efficacy of antibiotics include possible PPI-induced suppression of HP, better activity or stability of the antibiotic in the hypoacidic stomach, or a higher topical antibiotic concentration due to decreased gastric secretions.[49]

Two-drug Regimens. Several two-drug regimens have evolved in response to concerns (complicated dosing schedules, high incidence of adverse effects, noncompliance) with the early bismuth-based four-drug regimens (Tables 31–7 and 31–8). The most widely studied two-drug regimen has been the 2-week combination of amoxicillin (1 to 3 g/d) and omeprazole (40 mg/d). Initial clinical trials in Europe suggested that HP was eradicated in over 80% of patients when various dosage regimens were evaluated; however, a wide variation in eradication rates (0% to 90%) was observed.[37,50] When similar clinical trials were conducted in the United States, eradication rates were less than 60%.[37,50] Although there is no one factor that explains these variable and low eradication rates, theories include differences in the timing of the course of amoxicillin relative to omeprazole and the timing of the amoxicillin and omeprazole dose in relationship to meals, and different strains of HP.[50] Larger daily doses (Table 31–8) of amoxicillin and the PPI may increase HP eradication, but these regimens should not be considered first-line therapy.

More favorable and consistent HP eradication has been reported when clarithromycin is combined with either a PPI or RBC.[37,43,51] Although these regimens were among the first to be approved by the FDA (Table 31–8), their use as a first-line regimen should be discouraged as they contain only one antibiotic and are associated with antimicrobial resistance. Continuation of the PPI or RBC for an additional 2 weeks is recommended by the FDA but is probably unnecessary unless the patient has a complicated ulcer or gastroesophageal reflux disease.

Three-drug Regimens. The search for drug treatment regimens with higher eradication rates and less chance for antibiotic resistance led to studies that combine a PPI plus two antibiotics (Tables 31–7 and 31–8). Two-week regimens with clarithromycin, metronidazole, and a PPI or clarithromycin, amoxicillin, and a PPI provide eradication rates of greater than 90% (Table 31–8). No significant difference in eradication rates has been observed between these two regimens. The simplicity of therapy (three tablets twice a day) and the possibility of a shorter treatment course (7 days or 10 days versus 14 days) is attractive as adverse effects are minimized and compliance is increased.[45,46] The ideal duration of therapy, however, is under investigation as there are limited data to support 7-day therapy. The optimal dose of clarithromycin is also uncertain when it is combined with metronidazole and a PPI. It is possible that a lower dose of 250 mg twice daily is sufficient.[44]

Proton pump inhibitor-based regimens that combine amoxicillin and metronidazole tend to have lower eradication rates than those that combine clarithromycin with either metronidazole or amoxicillin.[36] Three-drug combinations that contain either sucralfate or RBC (instead of a PPI) do not reveal a superior additive effect, but data are limited (Table 31–8). A number of three-drug regimens containing azithromycin are under investigation, but early reports are unclear as to the most effective drug combination, dosage regimen, and duration of treatment.[44,52] An H_2-receptor antagonist has been combined with two antibiotics (amoxicillin with metronidazole or clarithromycin), but it remains uncertain as to whether a standard dosage regimen enhances HP eradication similar to a PPI.[38,49]

Four-drug Regimens. The first and most widely studied HP eradication regimens contained bismuth and two antibiotics. The fourth drug, an H_2-receptor antagonist, is added to the regimen of patients with an active ulcer to facilitate the relief of ulcer symptoms. The addition of the H_2-receptor antagonist appears to modestly accelerate ulcer healing. The HP eradication rates for a 2-week regimen containing BSS, metronidazole, tetracycline, and an H_2-receptor antagonist (Tables 31–7 and 31–8) range from 80% to 90%. Of interest is the fact that the FDA approved this regimen (Table 31–9) based on clinical trials previously reported in the literature. When amoxicillin is substituted for tetracycline, eradication rates decline to about 75%. Increasing the duration of treatment to 1 month does not substantially increase eradication. The efficacy of a 1-week regimen containing BSS, higher metronidazole doses (500 mg four times daily), tetracycline, and a PPI (Table 31–8) suggests that eradication rates may exceed 90%. However, additional studies are required to confirm these results.

Tolerability

There are few data comparing the tolerability of various HP eradication regimens. Adverse effects have been reported in up to 70% of patients receiving bismuth-based four-drug regimens, in 15% to 65% receiving two-drug regimens, and in fewer than 30% of patients treated with a PPI-based three-drug regimen.[47,53] Although data are limited, it appears that PPI-based three-drug regimens have the best safety profiles. Metronidazole-containing regimens increase the frequency of adverse effects and may contribute to a disulfiram-like reaction with alcohol. Common adverse effects include abnormal taste (metronidazole and clarithromycin), nausea, vomiting, abdominal pain, and diarrhea.[38] Diarrhea has been reported in up to 30% of patient receiving bismuth-based four-drug regimens; antibiotic-associated colitis occurs occasionally.

Antimicrobial Resistance

There is increasing concern regarding the emergence of resistant strains of bacteria to antimicrobials. Resistance of HP to antibiotics included in eradication regimens is an important reason for therapeutic failure. Resistance has been linked to noncompliance resulting from the large number of tablets or capsules that have to be taken each day and the intolerable adverse effects.[54,55] Resistance to metronidazole is most common (10% to 50%), but varies depending on prior antibiotic exposure and geographical region.[2,36,54] Metronidazole resistance appears to be higher in women, possibly because of the use of the drug in treating genital infections.[54] The clinical relevance of metronidazole resistance, when used with PPI-based three-drug regimens or bismuth-based four-drug regimens, remains unclear. Resistance to clarithromycin is lower (less than 10%) than with metronidazole and its clinical relevance is not questioned.[54] In addition, acquired resistance occurs in up to two-thirds of treatment failures. When clarithromycin was used with amoxicillin (and omeprazole), the HP eradication rate was greater than 90% in patients infected with a clarithromycin susceptible strain compared to 50% for those infected with a resistant strain.[54] Thus, clarithromycin resistance may be more likely to predict treatment failure. When fluoroquinolones were used as single agents to eradicate HP, a high secondary resistance was found. These agents, however, are not included in current regimens. Resistance to tetracycline and amoxicillin has been reported, but is uncommon.

Drug Administration

The administration of the HP regimen should be based on how the drugs were given in clinical trials and not how they should be taken when used as single agents for other indications. In addition, multiple drugs and multiple doses taken at multiple times during the day foster noncompliance. Patients should be instructed to take all of their medications (except PPIs) with meals and at bedtime (if necessary).[36] The PPI should be taken 30 to 60 minutes before meals (see section on PPIs).

Compliance

Compliance with drug treatment has a significant impact on HP eradication and is an important factor in determining therapeutic efficacy. Compliance in published studies is often substantially greater than that observed in clinical practice. Compliance decreases with multiple medications, increased frequency of administration, increased length of treatment, and intolerable adverse effects.[55–57] Noncompliance has been reported to decrease the efficacy of an HP eradication regimen containing bismuth, metronidazole, and tetracycline.[56,57] When a 14-day PPI-based three-drug regimen was studied, compliance at 14 days was significantly less than at 7 or 10 days; however, efficacy was maintained.[46] It is possible that there is a threshold below which efficacy is compromised. The patient should be able to comply with at least 80% to 90% of all medication doses over the treatment period.

Immunization

Helicobacter pylori resides in the human mucosa of the gastric antrum. To protect against virulent bacteria, the mucosal tissues possess many types of natural immune components (e.g., pH, macrophages, mucus). To protect against bacterial infection, mucosal surfaces can generate an adaptive immune response, leading to the production of IgA. Vaccines that are administered parenterally usually result in production of IgM and IgG. Therefore, most research has been directed at oral immunization to control HP infection. In the mouse model, both preventative and therapeutic oral vaccinations have shown to be effective against HP. If progress continues, there will be a vaccine in the near future. A more detailed discussion of HP and vaccines can be found elsewhere.[58]

CONVENTIONAL TREATMENT OF ACTIVE DUODENAL AND GASTRIC ULCERS

Conventional treatment with an H_2-receptor antagonist, sucralfate, or antacid alleviates ulcer symptoms and heals approximately 70%, 80%, or 90% of DU at 4, 6, or 8 weeks, respectively.[1,36,59–63] Increasing acid suppression with a PPI or a high-dose H_2-receptor antagonist provides comparable DU healing rates over a shorter treatment period (4 weeks).[1,36,64–67] A higher daily dose (Table 31–9) or a longer duration of treatment is often required to heal GU, because the average ulcer size is larger and healing does not correlate as strongly with gastric acid suppression. The efficacy of sucralfate is well established in DU, but is less so in GU.[1,61,62] Antacids, although effective, are not used as single agents to heal ulcers because of their high and frequent doses (100 to 144 mEq of acid-neutralizing capacity 1 and 3 hours after meals and at bedtime) and associated adverse effects.[1] When conventional antiulcer drugs are discontinued, most HP-positive patients develop a recurrent ulcer within 1 year.[1,7]

TREATMENT OF REFRACTORY ULCERS

Ulcers are usually considered refractory to therapy when symptoms, ulcers, or both persist beyond 12 weeks despite conventional treatment or when several courses of HP eradication fail.[1] Poor patient compliance, antimicrobial resistance, cigarette smoking, NSAID use, or a gastrinoma may contribute to refractory PUD. The exact role of HP infection is uncertain; however, in patients not previously treated with antibiotic therapy, HP eradication is appropriate. A number of patients will respond to markedly suppressed gastric acid, which possibly destroys pepsin.[1] A higher PPI dose (e.g., omeprazole 40 mg/d) heals the majority of ulcers proven refractory to standard PPI doses (e.g., omeprazole 20 mg/d) as well as conventional or high-dose H_2-receptor antagonists.[1,64–66] However, ulcers usually recur when therapy is discontinued or reduced to lower levels. Switching from one H_2-receptor antagonist or PPI to another is not beneficial. Combination therapy with an antisecretory agent plus sucralfate or misoprostol may appear rational because of the different mechanisms by which these drugs act, but it is without established benefit. Combined treatment with an H_2-receptor antagonist and a PPI is irrational. Patients with refractory GU will usually require surgery because of the fear of malignancy.

PREVENTION OF ULCER RECURRENCE AND COMPLICATIONS

In patients that are HP positive, antibiotic therapy should be the first step in preventing ulcer recurrence and complications.[36,37] Eradication should reduce ulcer recurrence to less than 10% and thereby cure the disease. Several clinical trials have also shown that patients with ulcer-related bleeding, who were treated with HP eradication, had no episodes of rebleeding when compared to about 30% of patients who healed their ulcer with an antisecretory drug.[32,68–70] In a high-risk subgroup of patients with frequent recurrences, refractory ulcers, or complications, maintenance therapy should be continued until HP eradication has been confirmed. Conventional maintenance therapy is indicated for high-risk patients who fail HP eradication or who have HP-negative ulcers.

Maintenance therapy with low-dose H_2-receptor antagonists, PPIs, or sucralfate (see Table 31–9) reduces symptomatic DU recurrence to 20% to 25% within 1 year.[1,59–62,64–66] Prevention lasts only as long as maintenance therapy is continued. Up to 90% of ulcers recur after conventional maintenance therapy is withdrawn.[1,7,36] When a reduced dose of an H_2-receptor antagonist is given at bedtime, all four H_2-receptor antagonists provide comparable efficacy.[1,36] Maintenance therapy with omeprazole 20 mg or lansoprazole 15 mg is comparable. Although low-dose H_2-receptor antagonists, PPIs, and sucralfate are effective in preventing DU, most patients with GU require continuation of the full ulcer-healing dose. Long-term maintenance therapy with an H_2-receptor antagonist, PPI, or sucralfate appears to be safe and effective, although sucralfate should be avoided in patients with renal impairment. Ulcer recurrence while on maintenance therapy suggests heavy smoking, noncompliance with the drug regimen, NSAIDs, persistent HP infection, or Zollinger-Ellison syndrome.

TREATMENT OF NSAID-INDUCED ULCERS

When an NSAID-induced ulcer is confirmed, the NSAID should be discontinued or the dose reduced. If the NSAID is discontinued, most uncomplicated ulcers will heal with standard regimens of an H_2-receptor antagonist, PPI, or sucralfate (see Table 31–9).[3,16,36,41,67] Large GU or DU may require prolonged therapy with a PPI. If the NSAID must be continued, a higher PPI dose (e.g., omeprazole 40 mg/d) should be used, as the ulcer tends to heal at a slower rate.[3,16,36] If HP is present, treatment should be initiated with an eradication regimen that contains a PPI.[36]

PREVENTION OF NSAID-INDUCED ULCERS

The most effective way to prevent an NSAID-induced ulcer is to avoid the use of the NSAID. However, this is an impractical alternative for many arthritic patients. Strategies aimed at reducing the topical irritant effects of NSAIDs—prodrugs, slow-release formulations, enteric-coated products—are ineffective in reducing the incidence of clinically important adverse effects such as bleeding or perforation. Cotherapy with misoprostol, an H_2-receptor antagonist or a PPI is used to diminish NSAID-induced ulcers in high-risk patients (see Table 31–3).[1,16,67,71–76] A number of newer NSAIDs that may spare GI complications are under investigation.[16,75,76]

Misoprostol

Prophylactic treatment with misoprostol is aimed at replenishing mucosal prostaglandins that have been depleted by the NSAID. In a dose of 200 μg four times per day, misoprostol markedly reduces the incidence of NSAID-induced GU and DU.[1,16,71,72] Unfortunately, the use of the drug at the recommended dose is associated with adverse effects (e.g., diarrhea, abdominal cramping) that often limit its usefulness. Evidence now confirms that a lower misoprostol dose of 200 μg two or three times a day offers adequate protection against GU and DU, and that these doses are better tolerated.[71] However, the GU preventing effects, as with the GI adverse effects, appear to be dose dependent. Because misoprostol's protective effect plateaus between 200 μg twice daily and 200 μg three times daily, 200 μg four times daily does not appear to offer any additional protection for most patients. Whether misoprostol prevents serious adverse effects (e.g., upper GI bleeding, perforation, gastric outlet obstruction) is a subject of great controversy. In a study of about 9000 rheumatoid arthritis patients, misoprostol reduced the incidence, but did not prevent about 60% of the adverse GI events.[21] Fixed combinations of misoprostol and an NSAID (e.g., diclofenac) may enhance compliance in some patients, but the flexibility to individualize drug dosage is lost.[73]

Conventional Antiulcer Agents

An H_2-receptor antagonist, PPI, or sucralfate is often used in conjunction with NSAID therapy to reduce dyspeptic symptoms or to prevent NSAID-induced ulcers. Although H_2-receptor antagonists and PPIs may be effective in relieving symptoms, their use in preventing NSAID ulcers (especially GU) remains uncertain. Indeed, these agents, may place the patient at increased risk of a serious complication by masking symptoms related to the complication (see Table 31–3).[22] A number of studies have documented a beneficial effect of standard-dose H_2-receptor antagonists in preventing NSAID-induced DU, but their protective effect against NSAID-induced GU has not been shown until recently.[16,74,75]

High-dose H2RAs (e.g., famotidine 40 mg twice a day) may prevent DU and GU in arthritic patients; however, conventional daily doses (e.g., famotidine 40 mg/d) do not appear effective in preventing GU.[16,67,74] In a similar study, arthritic patients, who initially received famotidine 40 mg twice daily to heal an NSAID-induced DU or GU were then continued on the same famotidine dosage regimen after the ulcer was healed.[75] In patients who continued their NSAIDs, high-dose famotidine, when compared to placebo, reduced the cumulative incidence of gastroduodenal ulcer recurrence over 6 months. The PPIs have also been shown to reduce the incidence of NSAID-induced DU and GU.[16,64,67] Omeprazole 20mg/d is associated with a lower relapse rate than misoprostol 200 μg bid or ranitidine 150 mg bid and is better tolerated than misoprostol.[67]

There are potential concerns regarding the use of high-dose antisecretory drugs to prevent NSAID ulcers. An observation in rats suggests that, while reducing NSAID-induced gastric damage, these agents significantly reduced the anti-inflammatory and analgesic effects of the nonsteroidal drug.[16] The efficacy of sucralfate in preventing NSAID-induced ulcers is disappointing and the drug should not be used for this purpose.

New NSAIDs That Spare the GI Tract

The association of GI damage with NSAIDs remains the major limitation to their use. Although a number of approaches have been taken to reduce GI toxicity, few have reduced the incidence of clinically important complications. Several novel strategies for developing NSAIDs that spare GI injury are under investigation. These include highly selective inhibitors of COX-2, nitric oxide-releasing NSAIDs, pure enantiomers of chiral NSAIDs, and NSAIDs preassociated with zwitterionic phospholipids.[16,75,76] Of these, the selective COX-2 inhibitors are most likely to be the first to be approved for use in the United States (see Table 31–4). Studies to date suggest that these agents are as effective as nonspecific NSAIDs in treating the inflammatory aspect of arthritis and that they are associated with fewer GI and possibly fewer renal toxicities. Questions remain, however, about their long-term efficacy and safety in clinical practice.

ANTIULCER AGENTS

Proton Pump Inhibitors

The PPIs (omeprazole, lansoprazole, pantoprazole, and rabeprazole) dose-dependently inhibit basal and stimulated gastric acid secretion.[1,64–66,77–79] Under acidic conditions in the parietal cell, the parent compound is protonated and converted to active metabolites, which react covalently with H^+/K^+-ATPase (the proton pump). A sulfhydryl bond is formed that noncompetitively and irreversibly inhibits activity of the enzyme. Full restoration of acid secretion after discontinuing the PPI takes about 3 to 5 days. Because PPIs are concentrated and activated in acidified compartments, they inhibit only those proton pumps that are actively secreting acid. Thus, PPIs are most effective when taken shortly before meals.

The PPIs are formulated as a gelatin capsule containing enteric-coated pH-sensitive granules that prevent degradation and premature protonation of the drug in acid. Upon dissolution of the capsule in the stomach, the intact granules pass into the duodenum, where the drug is released and absorbed. The granules may be removed from the capsule and (1) administered with orange or apple juice by mouth, nasogastric tube, or gastrostomy tube; (2) sprinkled on applesauce; or (3) a suspension can be prepared for nasoduodenal administration by dissolving the PPI granules in a 8.4% solution of sodium bicarbonate.[79]

Omeprazole, lansoprazole, pantoprazole, and rabeprazole provide similar DU and GU healing rates and symptomatic relief when used in recommended dosage regimens. When higher doses are indicated, the daily dose should be divided in order to enhance 24-hour control of acid secretion. A dosage reduction for both omeprazole and lansoprazole should be considered in patients with severe hepatic disease and in Asians.[80] A dosage reduction in renal impairment or in the elderly is usually not necessary.

Adverse effects related to the short-term (< 12 weeks) use of PPIs are well established and similar to those observed with the H_2-receptor antagonists, although clinical experience with omeprazole and lansoprazole is much more extensive than with pantoprazole and rebeprazole.[1,64–66,77–79,81] In general, the adverse effects observed with long-term (> 12 weeks) PPI treatment are similar to those reported with short-term use.[81] A dose-dependent decrease in protein-bound cyanocobalamin absorption has been observed in patients receiving long-term omeprazole therapy. The PPIs profoundly inhibit gastric acid secretion and may alter the bioavailability of orally administered drugs, such as ketoconazole, digoxin, iron, or pH-dependent dosage forms.[1,82,83] Omeprazole selectively inhibits hepatic P450 isoenzymes and decreases the elimination of phenytoin, diazepam, R-warfarin, and cyclosporine.[82,83] Lansoprazole does not appear to interact with these drugs but has been reported to increase theophylline clearance by 10%.[83] Clinically important interactions with either omeprazole or lansoprazole are uncommon. Pantoprazole and rebeprazole do not appear to interact with hepatic P450 enzymes.[77,78,83]

Consequences of Prolonged Hypochlorhydria. The PPIs increase fasting and postprandial serum gastrin concentrations as a function of their acid-inhibitory effect.[81] Low intragastric pH serves as a feedback mechanism to inhibit gastrin secretion from the antral G cells. Sustained hypo- or achlorhydria causes gastrin to be released into the circulation proportional to the degree of acid inhibition. Although drug-induced hypergastrinemia may be of no direct clinical concern, an important consequence is its trophic effect on enterochromaffin-like (ECL) cells in the gastric epithelium, which has led to the formation of gastric carcinoid tumors in female rats (Fig. 31–7).[81]

There is no evidence to indicate that hypergastrinemia and the subsequent development of ECL hyperplasia has resulted in dysplastic lesions in patients taking omeprazole for as long as 10 years. The degree and duration of hypergastrinemia needed to produce ECL hyperplasia or carcinoid formation in humans is unknown. It is possible that, in humans, progression of ECL hyperplasia to carcinoid tumor requires the presence of unknown factors in addition to hypergastrinemia. Alternatively, ECL hyperplasia may be related to underlying HP gastritis rather than to the PPI.[6,27,81] Experimental evidence does not support an association between hypergastrinemia and the presence of colonic polyps or colonic adenocarcinoma.[81] Although bacterial overgrowth occurs in the stomach as a consequence of hypochlorhydria and may lead to the formation of carcinogenic *N*-nitroso compounds in animals, it is unlikely to result in significant gastric nitrosation in humans.[81]

H_2-Receptor Antagonists

The H_2-receptor antagonists (cimetidine, famotidine, nizatidine, and ranitidine) competitively and reversibly bind H_2 receptors on the parietal cell, diminishing cytosolic cyclic AMP production and the secretion of histamine-stimulated gastric acid.[1,59,60] In most patients, DU and GU healing is comparable with multiple daily doses or a single full dose given after dinner or at bedtime (Table 31–9). Twice-daily administration suppresses daytime acid and benefits patients with daytime ulcer pain. Cigarette smokers may require higher doses or a longer duration of treatment. A reduction in H_2-receptor antagonist daily dose is recommended in patients with moderate to severe renal failure.

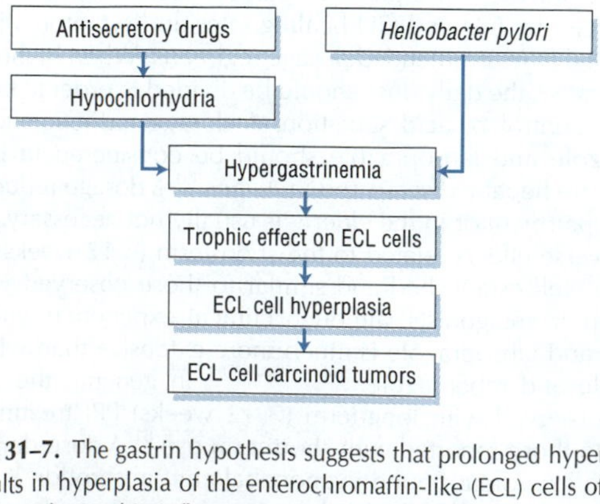

FIGURE 31–7. The gastrin hypothesis suggests that prolonged hypergastrinemia results in hyperplasia of the enterochromaffin-like (ECL) cells of the gastric fundus. The trophic influence of gastrin may be a risk factor for ECL cell carcinoid tumor formation.

In general, H_2-receptor antagonists are safe and well tolerated.[1,59,60] When used in recommended doses for the treatment of PUD, their short- and long-term safety profiles are similar.[1,59,60] Gastrointestinal disturbances occur most frequently. Central nervous system effects, particularly drowsiness and headache, occur most often in ambulatory patients and have been reported with all of the H_2-receptor antagonists. These drugs are associated with reversible adverse hematologic reactions; thrombocytopenia is the most common, regardless of the H_2-receptor antagonist implicated.[1,59,60] Gynecomastia and impotence can occur in men receiving prolonged or high doses of cimetidine and is thought to be a dose-related antiandrogen effect.[1,59,60] The cardiovascular effects and changes in gastric emptying associated with the oral H_2-receptor antagonists are probably of minimal clinical consequence in most patients. Cimetidine interferes with the renal tubular secretion of creatinine, but increases in serum creatinine do not represent renal toxicity. Numerous metabolic drug interactions have been reported, especially with cimetidine (theophylline, phenytoin, warfarin), but the majority do not lead to a pharmacodynamic effect.[82] Famotidine and nizatidine do not interact with drugs metabolized by hepatic P450 isoenzymes. The clinical relevance of the interaction of ethanol with H_2-receptor antagonists remains uncertain.[82]

Sucralfate

Sucralfate is an aluminum salt of a sulfated disaccharide that, when exposed to gastric acid, forms a viscous adhesive that binds electrostatically to positively charged protein molecules in the ulcer crater, forming a protective barrier that inhibits back-diffusion of hydrogen ions.[1,61] Attachment to the ulcer crater lasts for up to 6 hours following oral administration. Sucralfate inhibits pepsin, adsorbs bile salts, stimulates endogenous prostaglandins, and may suppress HP.[1,61] Although aluminum appears to mediate some of these actions, the sucrose moiety may also play a role in ulcer healing. Sucralfate does not have an important effect on acid secretion. The majority of the dose is excreted unchanged in the feces with 3% to 5% excreted in the urine. Because the drug is minimally absorbed, it may be preferred in pregnancy.

Sucralfate should be taken on an empty stomach to prevent binding to dietary protein and phosphate. Deterrents to its use include a multiple-dosing regimen, large tablet size, and the need to separate the drug from meals and other potentially interacting medications. Adverse effects to sucralfate are usually minor and occur in less than 5% of patients. Constipation is most common and develops in about 2% of patients.[1,61] Nausea, indigestion, dry mouth, dizziness, and a metallic taste occur infrequently. Seizures have been reported in dialysis patients who were also receiving aluminum-containing antacids.[1] Hypophosphotemia may develop in patients on prolonged sucralfate therapy (see the section on antacids later in the chapter). Gastric bezoar formation has been reported.[61] The concomitant use of sucralfate with fluoroquinolones, phenytoin, digoxin, theophylline, quinidine, amitriptyline, warfarin, ketoconazole, and L-thyroxine may reduce their bioavailability and effectiveness.[82,84] In most instances, the interaction can be minimized by giving the interacting drug at least 2 hours before sucralfate.[82] Alternative antiulcer therapy may be warranted in patients taking oral fluoroquinolones.

Prostaglandins

Misoprostol, a synthetic PGE_1 analog, moderately inhibits acid secretion and enhances mucosal defense.[1] Antisecretory effects are dose dependent over the range of 50 to 200 μg; cytoprotective effects occur in humans at doses of at least 200 μg. Because protective effects occur at higher doses, it is difficult to establish the protective effect independent of the antisecretory action. Although not recommended for the treatment of PUD in the United States, a dose of 200 μg four times daily or 400 μg twice daily heals DU and GU comparable to conventional H_2-receptor antagonist or sucralfate regimens.

The most common adverse effects reported with misoprostol are crampy abdominal pain and diarrhea. Diarrhea develops in about 11% of patients within 1 to 2 weeks of initiating therapy.[1,16] Life-threatening diarrhea has been reported in a patient with inflammatory bowel disease.[85] Nausea, flatulence, headache, and dyspepsia often accompany the diarrhea, but usually resolve with continued treatment. Antacids (other than magnesium) may be taken with misoprostol when needed for abdominal pain. Taking the drug with or after meals and at bedtime may minimize the diarrhea.

Misoprostol is uterotrophic and produces contractions that may endanger pregnancy; therefore, the drug is contraindicated in pregnant women. If misoprostol is prescribed to women in their childbearing years, use of adequate contraceptive measures should be confirmed and a negative serum pregnancy test should be documented within 2 weeks of initiating treatment. Patients should be counseled regarding the potential GI effects and the need to avoid magnesium antacids. Young women should be warned about the importance of adequate contraception. Misoprostol does not interfere with the beneficial effects of NSAIDs in patients with rheumatoid arthritis.

Bismuth Preparations

The most commonly used bismuth salts in the United States are bismuth subsalicylate (BSS or Pepto-Bismol) and ranitidine bismuth citrate (RBC).[1,48,63] Bismuth subsalicylate is an insoluble complex that, at a pH below 3.5, reacts with acid to form bismuth oxide and salicylic acid, which is readily absorbed. In the colon, bismuth oxide reacts with hydrogen sulfide to form bismuth sulfide, which blackens the stool. Although the precise method by which bismuth acts to heal ulcers remains uncertain, possible mechanisms include its local gastroprotective effect, its ability to stimulate endogenous prostaglandins, and its ability to suppress HP.[1,48,63] Bismuth salts do not inhibit or neutralize acid.

Bismuth absorption varies with the bismuth salt. The bismuth salts (BSS and RBC) used in the United States are safe and have few adverse effects.[48] Although prolonged treatment with bismuth subgallate has been associated with neurologic toxicity, clinical trials with intermittent use of BSS or RBC have not reported significant neurologic effects. Renal failure decreases bismuth elimination and may result in an increased bismuth load. Bismuth subsalicylate should be used with caution in the elderly or patients with renal failure, salicylate sensitivity, or bleeding disorders, or in combination with high-dose salicylate therapy. Patients should be advised that bismuth preparations may impart a black color to their stool (Table 31–10).

Antacids

Antacids neutralize gastric acid, inactivate pepsin, and bind bile salts. Aluminum-containing antacids also suppress HP and enhance mucosal defense.[1,63] These later effects probably contribute to ulcer healing at lower doses. When taken on an empty stomach, the antacid-neutralizing effect lasts for about 15 to 30 minutes. When taken 1 hour after a meal, food acts as a buffer for about an hour and prolongs the antacid-neutralizing effect for an additional 2 hours.[63] Magnesium/aluminum-containing antacids are used most widely.[63] Magnesium hydroxide has a more prolonged neutralizing effect than either sodium bicarbonate or calcium carbonate. The effects of magnesium oxide and carbonate are similar to magnesium hydroxide. Aluminum hydroxide possesses a low neutralizing capacity; aluminum phosphate has little antacid activity. Magaldrate (hydroxymagnesium aluminate) is transformed to magnesium and aluminum ions in gastric acid. Its effects resemble those of other magnesium/aluminum-containing antacids, but it contains less magnesium per unit of weight. Most antacids have been reformulated to contain only small amounts of sodium.[63]

Gastrointestinal effects occur most often with antacids and are dose dependent.[63] Magnesium salts cause an osmotic diarrhea, whereas aluminum salts cause constipation. Diarrhea usually predominates with magnesium/aluminum preparations. Antacids that are similar in potency, but contain less magnesium, may cause less diarrhea. Aluminum-containing antacids (except aluminum phosphate) form insoluble salts with dietary phosphorus and interfere with phosphorus absorption.[63] Hypophosphotemia may occur in patients with low dietary phosphate intake (e.g., malnutrition, alcoholism). Combined treatment with sucralfate may amplify the hypophosphotemia and the potential for aluminum toxicity (see the section on sucralfate earlier in the chapter).

Magnesium-containing antacids should not be used in patients with a creatinine clearance of less than 30 mL/min because magnesium excretion is impaired. Although calcium stimulates gastrin, acid rebound is of questionable clinical importance. Hypercalcemia may occur in patients with normal renal function taking more than 20 g/d of calcium carbonate and in renal failure patients taking more than 4 g/d. The milk-alkali syndrome (hypercalcemia, alkalosis, renal stones, increased blood urea nitrogen, increased creatinine concentration) occurs with high calcium intake in patients with systemic alkalosis.[63] The alkalosis may be produced by absorbable antacids (sodium bicarbonate) or by prolonged vomiting. Antacids may alter the absorption and excretion of drugs when administered concomitantly.[63,82] Clinically important interactions may occur when antacids are administered with tetracycline, warfarin, digoxin, quinidine, isoniazid, ketoconazole, or the fluoroquinolones.[63,82] Most interactions can be avoided by separating the antacid from the oral drug by 2 hours.

PHARMACOECONOMIC CONSIDERATIONS

HELICOBACTER PYLORI-ASSOCIATED ULCERS

Peptic ulcer disease is a chronic disease that results in a considerable economic burden on the health care system. The therapeutic advantage of HP eradication over conventional management strategies is acknowledged as clinical trials have confirmed a significant decrease in ulcer recurrence and ulcer-related complications. A number of theoretical cost-effectiveness analyses suggest that for patients with uncomplicated DU, HP eradication is superior to conventional treatment with H_2-receptor antagonists.[86–88] In addition, preliminary reports of prospective "real patients" confirm short-term cost savings. Thus, it appears that the costs of continued treatment and recurrence far outweigh the cost of HP drug regimens. Additional studies are required to evaluate the overall cost effectiveness of HP eradication in patients with complicated ulcer disease. Although the optimal drug regimen is unknown, it is likely that high efficacy and minimal adverse effects will be major determinants of the relative cost effectiveness of a specific drug regimen.

NONSTEROIDAL ANTI-INFLAMMATORY-INDUCED ULCERS

The economic implications of NSAIDs and the costs associated with complications and prophylaxis, particularly in the elderly, are of great concern. There are limited and conflicting data regarding the cost effectiveness of misoprostol in the prevention of NSAID-induced complications.[89] Several studies suggest that misoprostol cotherapy is not cost effective as a primary prophylaxis for NSAID-induced GI bleeding, and that it may confer greater costs without an increase in quality of life.[89] Other studies indicate disparate results. Whether the prophylaxis of NSAID ulcers with misoprostol, high-dose H_2-receptor antagonists, or PPIs is cost effective remains to be determined.

ZOLLINGER–ELLISON SYNDROME

Zollinger-Ellison syndrome is characterized by gastric acid hypersecretion (see Fig. 31–1) and recurrent peptic ulceration that results from a gastrin-producing tumor (gastrinoma).[4,90,91] In the United States, Zollinger-Ellison syndrome accounts for 0.1% of patients with DU. At surgery, more than 90% of gastrinomas are located in the region of the pancreas, the most common site being the duodenum. Malignant gastrinomas occur in 30% to 50% of patients, with metastases to regional lymph nodes, liver, spleen, and bone.

The most frequent clinical manifestation is severe and recurrent peptic ulceration typically accompanied by epigastric pain and often associated with esophagitis, GI bleeding, or perforation. Ulcers occur most often in the duodenum, but may involve the stomach or jejunum. Diarrhea occurs in 30% to 50% of patients and results from high concentrations of acid that overwhelm the duodenum's buffering capacity and damage the mucosa. Intraluminal acid causes steatorrhea by inactivating pancreatic lipase and precipitating bile acids. Vitamin B_{12} malabsorption may result from reduced intrinsic factor activity. Patients may have other symptoms when the parathyroid, pituitary, thyroid, or adrenal glands are involved. The diagnosis is established in patients with a BAO greater than 15 mEq/h (without prior gastric surgery) and when the fasting serum gastrin is higher than 1000 pg/mL.[4,90] Location of the tumor is essential as surgical resection is curative.

Treatment is based on the presence or absence of peptic ulcers, esophagitis, diarrhea, and a gastrinoma, which may be malignant. The PPIs are the oral drugs of choice for managing acid hypersecretion, although most experience has been obtained with omeprazole. Treatment should be instituted with either omeprazole or lansoprazole at a dose of 60 mg/d and should be adjusted to individual patient response.[4,90,91] Dividing the daily dose and giving the drug every 8 to 12 hours is most effective in controlling acid output and relieving symptoms. Although doses as high as 360 mg/d of omeprazole have been administered, an average dose of 60 to 80 mg/d reduces basal acid output to target levels. In a subset of patients, acid hypersecretion can be adequately controlled with 20 to 40 mg/d of omeprazole. An average dose of 60 to 90 mg/d of lansoprazole appears to provide adequate control of acid secretion in most patients. The PPIs appear to be safe and well tolerated in patients with Zollinger-Ellison syndrome. Octreotide decreases acid secretion both by directly inhibiting gastric acid and by release of gastrin.[4] A subcutaneous dose of 100 to 250 μg three times a day has been reported to substantially reduce serum gastrin and acid secretion.[4] Octreotide may also reduce the formation of gastric carcinoid by reducing the serum gastrin concentration. Patients with metastatic gastrinoma require tumor resection or treatment with chemotherapeutic agents.

STRESS-RELATED MUCOSAL DAMAGE

Stress-related mucosal damage (SRMD) occurs in critically ill patients with serious trauma, burns, and intracranial disease or severe medical problems (coagulopathy, ventilator dependency).[92,93] When accompanied by acute upper GI bleeding, it is a cause of significant morbidity and mortality. In contrast to chronic peptic ulcers, these lesions are characteristically asymptomatic, multiple, located in the proximal stomach, unlikely to perforate, and associated with bleeding from superficial mucosal capillaries (see Table 31–1). The damage is progressive and can result in overt bleeding severe enough to require blood transfusions. The primary pathogenic factor is most likely mucosal ischemia resulting from reduced gastric blood flow (see Fig. 31–1). Gastric acid appears necessary for the lesions to occur, but acid hypersecretion is not usually present.[92,93]

Endoscopic evidence of SRMD is present in most critically ill patients within 24 hours of admission to an intensive care unit (ICU). Prophylactic therapy to prevent bleeding is most effective if initiated early in the patient's course. However, controversies exist as to the need for prophylaxis, the relative importance of risk factors, the optimal drug regimen, and whether sucralfate is less likely to contribute to nosocomial pneumonia than antacids or H_2-receptor antagonists. Important considerations in the selection of a prophylactic agent include (1) risk factors, (2) type of ICU patient, (e.g., medical versus surgical), (3) comparative efficacy of the drug regimen, (4) adverse effects and potential drug interactions, (5) overall cost of treatment, and (6) ease of administration.

The need to initiate prophylactic drug therapy in a critically ill patient remains controversial and depends on the number and severity of the risk factors and whether the patient is a medical or surgical ICU patient.[92,94,95] One group of investigators concluded that the routine prophylaxis of medical ICU patients with either cimetidine or sucralfate offers no advantage over no treatment and is therefore not warranted.[95]

Medications used to prevent stress-related mucosal bleeding (SRMB) include antacids (titrated to an intragastric pH above 4), intravenous H_2-receptor antagonists administered intermittently or by continuous infusion, sucralfate (usually given by nasogastric or nasoduodenal tube), and oral PPIs (given by nasoduodenal tube) or IV PPIs. Numerous clinical trials have documented the efficacy of antacids, IV H_2-receptor antagonists (cimetidine, ranitidine, famotidine), and sucralfate.[92,96] The use of PPIs has been reported, but their efficacy is not well documented. Antacids, although effective, require high doses, frequent administration, and pH monitoring, and are associated with increased adverse effects.

Intravenous H_2-receptor antagonists remain the cornerstone of therapy in most ICUs. When given in recommended doses, either intermittently or by continuous infusion, they provide similar efficacy.[92] Although maintenance of intragastric pH above 4 is often recommended, especially in high-risk patients, pH control is not the sole factor in determining drug efficacy. Sucralfate does not requiring pH monitoring or intravenous access, and may decrease the risk of nosocomial pneumonia (when compared to antacids and possibly H_2-receptor antagonists) in patients requiring ventilation.[92,97,98] Ranitidine was found to result in a lower rate of clinically important GI bleeding with a similar rate of pneumonia when compared with sucralfate in mechanically ventilated patients.[99] When a decision analysis model was used to estimate the cost of cimetidine compared to sucralfate in patients at low risk of bleeding, the cost per bleeding episode averted was 6.5-fold greater with cimetidine than the cost per bleeding episode averted with sucralfate.[100] The value of parenteral and enteral nutrition in preventing SRMB remains controversial and requires further investigation.

Improvement in the patient's overall medication condition (discharge from the ICU, extubation, oral intake) suggests that the prophylactic agent can be discontinued. If a patient develops clinically significant bleeding, endoscopic evaluation of the GI tract is indicated along with aggressive medical treatment. The efficacy of drug therapy with an IV H_2-receptor antagonist, sucralfate, or a combined regimen of an H_2-receptor antagonist and sucralfate has not been shown to be superior to placebo in most well-controlled trials; however, it is utilized until bleeding stops or surgery is indicated (see Fig. 31–6).

EVALUATION OF THERAPEUTIC OUTCOMES

Relief of epigastric pain should be monitored throughout the course of treatment in patients with either HP or NSAID-induced ulcers. Ulcer pain typically resolves in a few days when NSAIDs are the cause of the symptoms and within 7 days upon initiation of antiulcer therapy (see Fig. 31–5). Most patients with uncomplicated PUD will be rendered symptom-free after treatment with any one of the recommended antiulcer regimens. The persistence, or redevelopment, of symptoms after 14 days of treatment suggests failure of ulcer healing or an alternative diagnosis such as cancer. The majority of patients with uncomplicated HP-positive ulcers do not require confirmation of ulcer healing or HP eradication. When endoscopy is not indicated, the UBT is the best test to confirm HP eradication. Assess patient compliance and the possibility of antibiotic resistance in patients who fail therapy.

Ulcer patients, especially the elderly or other high-risk patients on NSAIDs, should be closely monitored for signs or symptoms of bleeding, obstruction, penetration, or perforation. Patients that remain symptomatic, have recurrent attacks, or who appear to have ulcer-related complications should be referred for further evaluation. Follow-up endoscopy to determine if ulcers or HP are present can be justified in patients with frequent symptomatic recurrence, refractory disease, complications, or suspected hypersecretory states.

CONCLUSIONS

The discovery of HP has revolutionized the way in which chronic PUD is treated and, for the most part, cured. Fundamental questions about the organism, including methods of transmission, virulence, and specific pathogenic mechanisms, require answers. Important issues related to who to treat and who to test require further clarification. In the meantime, the search continues for the optimal and most cost-effective drug regimen. Future research will surely provide us with less complicated and safer antimicrobial regimens and perhaps a vaccine. The widespread use of NSAIDs and their associated GI complications is of major concern, especially in the elderly. Although prophylaxis with misoprostol reduces GI complications, its cost effectiveness remains uncertain. Future research should lead to drugs that spare the GI tract and also decrease NSAID-related morbidity and mortality. The pharmacist has an important role to play in the successful management of patients with either HP-associated or NSAID-induced ulcers (see Table 31–10).

▶ PRINCIPLES OF PHARMACOTHERAPY

- Patients with chronic PUD should eliminate or reduce psychological stress, cigarette smoking, and NSAID use and avoid foods and beverages that exacerbate ulcer symptoms.
- Eradication of HP is recommended for HP-positive patients with active DU or GU and HP-positive patients with PUD who require maintenance therapy or have a history of ulcer-related complications. There are no definitive recommendations regarding HP eradication in patients with dyspepsia or nonulcer dyspepsia. Treatment of HP is recommended for HP-positive patients with low-grade MALT lymphoma and after resection of gastric cancer.
- The selection of a HP eradication regimen should be based on efficacy, safety, antibiotic resistance, cost, and the likelihood of compliance. Treatment with a PPI-based three-drug regimen is generally preferred to two- or four-drug regimens. If a second course of HP therapy is required, the regimen should contain different antibiotics.
- When eradicating HP, ampicillin should not be substituted for amoxicillin, doxycycline should not be substituted for tetracycline, azithromycin should not be substituted for clarithromycin, an H_2-receptor antagonist should not be substituted for a PPI, and bismuth salts should not be interchanged.
- Treatment with a conventional antiulcer drug (H_2-receptor antagonist, PPI, or sucralfate) may be an alternative to HP eradication, but is discouraged

because of the high rate of ulcer recurrence and ulcer-related complications. Combination therapy using conventional antiulcer medications adds to drug treatment costs without enhancing efficacy.

- Conventional maintenance therapy with a low-dose H_2-receptor antagonist or PPI is only indicated for high-risk patients who fail HP eradication, patients with severe complications, or those with HP-negative ulcers.
- Prophylactic cotherapy with an antiulcer drug is indicated for patients at increased risk of developing NSAID ulcer complications. Although H_2-receptor antagonists or PPIs may be useful in relieving dyspeptic symptoms and may prevent ulcers, cotherapy with misoprostol remains the treatment of choice for preventing NSAID-induced GU and DU.
- Patients with PUD, especially those receiving HP eradication or misoprostol cotherapy, require patient education regarding their disease and drug treatment in order to successfully achieve a positive therapeutic outcome.
- Patients with PUD, who develop recurrent ulcer symptoms or signs or symptoms of GI bleeding or perforation, should be referred for further evaluation. Assess possible reasons for therapeutic failure, including noncompliance to the drug regimen, antibiotic resistance (HP eradication), heavy smoking, NSAID ingestion, and the need for HP eradication in a patient on conventional antiulcer medications.
- Remember that the determinants of drug treatment costs in clinical practice are often based on the acquisition cost of medications, but this may be erroneous as the overall cost of the treatment strategy is dependent on its success. Ultimately, the most expensive treatment is one that does not work.

REFERENCES

1. Soll AH. Peptic ulcer and its complications. In: Feldman M, Scharschmidt BF, Sleisenger MH, eds. Sleisinger and Fordtran's Gastrointestinal and Liver Disease: Pathophysiology/Diagnosis/Management, 6th ed. Philadelphia, Saunders, 1998:620–678.
2. Peterson WL, Graham DY. *Helicobacter pylori.* In: Feldman M, Scharschmidt BF, Sleisenger MH, eds. Sleisinger and Fordtran's Gastrointestinal and Liver Disease: Pathophysiology/Diagnosis/Management, 6th ed. Philadelphia, Saunders, 1998:604–619.
3. Cryer B. Nonsteroidal anti-inflammatory drugs and gastrointestinal disease. In: Feldman M, Scharschmidt BF, Sleisenger MH, eds. Sleisinger and Fordtran's Gastrointestinal and Liver Disease: Pathophysiology/Diagnosis/Management, 6th ed. Philadelphia, Saunders, 1998:343–357.
4. McGuigan JE. Zollinger-Ellison syndrome and other hypersecretory states. In: Feldman M, Scharschmidt BF, Sleisenger MH, eds. Sleisinger and Fordtran's Gastrointestinal and Liver Disease: Pathophysiology/Diagnosis/Management, 6th ed. Philadelphia, Saunders, 1998:679–695.
5. The Report of the Digestive Health Initiative International Update Conference on *Helicobacter pylori.* Gastroenterology 1997;113(suppl): S4–S8.
6. Kuipers EJ. *Helicobacter pylori* and the risk and management of associated diseases: Gastritis, ulcer disease, atrophic gastritis and gastric cancer. Aliment Pharmacol Ther 1997;11:(suppl 1):71–88.
7. Graham DY, Lew GM, Klein PD, et al. Effect of treatment of *Helicobacter pylori* infection on the long-term recurrence of gastric or duodenal ulcer: A randomized, controlled study. Ann Intern Med 1992;116:705–708.
8. Go MF. What are the host factors that place an individual at risk for *Helicobacter pylori*-associated disease? Gastroenterology 1997;113 (suppl):S15–S20.
9. Mobley HLT. *Helicobacter pylori* factors associated with disease development. Gastroenterology 1997;113(suppl):S21–S28.
10. Cave DR. How is *Helicobacter pylori* transmitted? Gastroenterology 1997;113(suppl):S9–S14.
11. Asaka M, Takeda H, Sugiyama T, et al. What role does *Helicobacter pylori* play in gastric cancer? Gastroenterology 1997;113(suppl): S56–S60.
12. Bayerdorffer E, Miehlke S, Neubauer A, et al. Gastric MALT-lymphoma and *Helicobacter pylori* infection. Aliment Pharmacol Ther 1997;11:(suppl 1):89–94.
13. Thiede C, Morgner A, Alpen B, et al. What role does *Helicobacter pylori* eradication play in gastric MALT and gastric MALT lymphoma? Gastroenterology 1997;113(suppl):S61–S64.
14. Veldhuyzen SJO, Van Zanten V. The role of *Helicobacter pylori* in non-ulcer dyspepsia. Aliment Pharmacol Ther 1997;11:(suppl 1): 63–69.
15. Talley NJ, Hunt RH. What role does *Helicobacter pylori* play in dyspepsia and nonulcer dyspepsia? Arguments for and against *H. pylori* being associated with dyspeptic symptoms. Gastroenterology 1997; 113(suppl):S67–S77.
16. Wallace JL. Nonsteroidal anti-inflammatory drugs and gastroenteropathy; the second hundred years. Gastroenterology 1997;112:1000–1016.
17. Blower AL, Brooks A, Fenn GC, et al. Emergency admissions for upper gastrointestinal disease and their relation to NSAID use. Aliment Pharmacol Ther 1997;11:281–291.
18. Peura DA, Lanza FL, Gostout CJ. The American College of Gastroenterology Bleeding Registry: Preliminary findings. Am J Gastroenterol 1997;92:924–928.
19. Hawkey CJ, Cullen DJ, Greenwood DC, et al. Prescribing of nonsteroidal anti-inflammatory drugs in general practice; determinants and consequences. Aliment Pharmacol Ther 1997;11:293–298.
20. Tamblyn R, Berkson L, Dauphinee WD. Unnecessary prescribing of NSAIDs and the management of NSAID-related gastropathy in medical practice. Ann Intern Med 1997;127:429–438.
21. Silverstein FE, Graham DY, Senior FR, et al. Misoprostol reduces serious gastrointestinal complications in patients with rheumatoid arthritis receiving nonsteroidal anti-inflammatory drugs. Ann Intern Med 1995;123:241–249.
22. Singh G, Rosen DR, Morfield D, et al. Gastrointestinal tract complications of nonsteroidal anti-inflammatory drug treatment in rheumatoid arthritis. Arch Intern Med 1996;156:1530–1536.
23. Talley NJ, Evans JM, Fleming KC, et al. Nonsteroidal anti-inflammatory drugs and dyspepsia in the elderly. Dig Dis Sci 1995; 40:1345–1350.
24. Wilcox CM. Relationship between nonsteroidal anti-inflammatory drug use, *Helicobacter pylori,* and gastroduodenal mucosal injury. Gastroenterology 1997;113(suppl):S85.
25. Piper JM, Ray WA, Daugherty JR, et al. Corticosteroid use and peptic ulcer disease; role of nonsteroidal anti-inflammatory drugs. Ann Intern Med 1991;114:735–740.
26. Feldman M. Gastric secretion: Normal and abnormal. In: Feldman M, Scharschmidt BF, Sleisenger MH, eds. Sleisinger and Fordtran's Gastrointestinal and Liver Disease: Pathophysiology/Diagnosis/Management, 6th ed. Philadelphia, Saunders, 1998:587–603.
27. Calam J, Gibbons A, Zoe V, et al. How is *Helicobacter pylori* cause mucosal damage? Its effect on acid and gastrin physiology. Gastroenterology 1997;113(suppl):S43–S49.

28. Peura DA. Ulcerogenesis: Integrating the roles of *Helicobacter pylori* and acid secretion in duodenal ulcer. Am J Gastroenterol 1997; 92(suppl):8S–16S.
29. Smoot DT. How does *Helicobacter pylori* cause mucosal damage? Direct mechanisms. Gastroenterology 1997;113(suppl):S31–S34.
30. Ernst PB, Crowe SE, Reyes VE. How does *Helicobacter pylori* cause mucosal damage? The inflammatory response. Gastroenterology 1997;113(suppl):S35–S42.
31. Laine L. Acute and chronic gastrointestinal bleeding. In: Feldman M, Scharschmidt BF, Sleisenger MH, eds. Sleisinger and Fordtran's Gastrointestinal and Liver Disease: Pathophysiology/Diagnosis/Management, 6th ed. Philadelphia, Saunders, 1998:198–219.
32. Vaira D, Menegatti M, Miglioli M. What is the role of *Helicobacter pylori* in complicated ulcer disease? Gastroenterology 1997; 113(suppl):S78–S84.
33. Cohen H, Laine L. Endoscopic methods for the diagnosis of *Helicobacter pylori.* Aliment Pharmacol Ther 1997:11(suppl 1):3–9.
34. Atherton JC. Non-endoscopic tests in the diagnosis of *Helicobacter pylori.* Aliment Pharmacol Ther 1997:11(suppl 1):11–20.
35. Megraud F. How should *Helicobacter pylori* infection be diagnosed? Gastroenterology 1997;113(suppl):S93–S98.
36. Soll AH. Medical treatment of peptic ulcer disease: Practice guidelines. JAMA 1996;275:622–629.
37. Pounder RE, Williams MP. The treatment of *Helicobacter pylori* infection. Aliment Pharmacol Ther 1997;11(suppl 1):35–41.
38. Hunt RG. Peptic ulcer disease: defining the treatment strategies in the era of *Helicobacter pylori.* Am J Gastroenterol 1997;92(suppl): 36S–43S.
39. Lee J, O'Morain C. Who should be treated for *Helicobacter pylori* infection? A review of consensus conferences and guidelines. Gastroenterology 1997;113(suppl):S99–S106.
40. Hawkey CJ, Hudson N. Healing and prevention of NSAID-induced peptic ulcers. Scand J Gastroenterol 1994;29(suppl 201):42–44.
41. Seymour NE. Operations for peptic ulcer and their complications. In: Feldman M, Scharschmidt BF, Sleisenger MH, eds. Sleisinger and Fordtran's Gastrointestinal and Liver Disease: Pathophysiology/Diagnosis/Management, 6th ed. Philadelphia, Saunders, 1998: 696–710.
42. Robinson DH, Abdel-Rahman SM, Nahata MC, et al. Guidelines for the treatment of *Helicobacter pylori* in the pediatric patient. Ann Pharmacother 1997;31:1247–1249.
43. Hopkins RJ. Current FDA-approved treatments for *Helicobacter pylori* and the FDA approval process. Gastroenterology 1997;113(suppl): S126–S130.
44. Unge P. What other regimens are under investigation to treat *Helicobacter pylori* infection? Gastroenterology 1997;113(suppl): S131–S148.
45. Fennerty MB, Melnyk CS. Helicobacter pylori: Review of triple, dual, 7-day and other treatment strategies. Formulary 1995;30: 682–688.
46. Laine L, Estrada R, Trujillo M, et al. Randomized comparison of differing periods of twice-a-day triple therapy for the eradication of *Helicobacter pylori.* Aliment Pharmacol Ther 1996;10:1029–1033.
47. Fennerty MB. What are the treatment goals for *Helicobacter pylori* infection? Gastroenterology 1997;113(suppl):S120–S125.
48. Lambert JR, Midolo P. The actions of bismuth in the treatment of *Helicobacter pylori* infection. Aliment Pharmacol Ther 1997;11 (suppl):27–33.
49. Peterson WL. The role of antisecretory drugs in the treatment of *Helicobacter pylori* infection. Aliment Pharmacol Ther 1997;11(suppl 1): 21–25.
50. Graham KS, Malaty H, El-Zimaity HMT, et al. Variability with omeprazole-amoxicillin combinations for treatment of *Helicobacter pylori* infection. Am J Gastroenterol 1995;90:1415–1417.
51. Markham A, McTavish D. Clarithromycin and omeprazole as *Helicobacter pylori* eradication therapy in patients with *H. pylori*-associated gastric disorders. Drugs 1996;51:161–178.
52. Al-Assi MT, Genta RM, Karttunen TJ, et al. Azithromycin triple therapy for *Helicobacter pylori* infection: Azithromycin, tetracycline, and bismuth. Am J Gastroenterol 1995;90:403–405.
53. Hackelsberger A, Malfertheimer P. A risk-benefit assessment of drugs used in the eradication of *Helicobacter pylori* infection. Drug Saf 1996;15:30–52.
54. Megraud F. Resistance of *Helicobacter pylori* to antibiotics. Aliment Pharmacol Ther 1997;11(suppl 1):43–53.
55. Malfertheiner P. Compliance, adverse events and antibiotic resistance in *Helicobacter pylori* treatment. Scand J Gastroenterol 1993;28(suppl 196):34–37.
56. Graham DY, Lew GM, Malaty HM, et al. Factors influencing the eradication of *Helicobacter pylori* with triple therapy. Gastroenterology 1992;102:493–496.
57. Cutler A, Schubert T. Patient factors affecting *Helicobacter pylori* eradication with triple therapy. Am J Gastroenterol 1993;88:505–509.
58. Czinn SJ. What is the role for vaccination in *Helicobacter pylori?* Gastroenterology 1997;113(suppl):S149–S153.
59. Feldman M, Burton ME. Histamine$_2$-receptor antagonists: Standard therapy for acid-peptic diseases, I. N Engl J Med 1990;323: 1672–1680.
60. Feldman M, Burton ME. Histamine$_2$-receptor antagonists: Standard therapy for acid-peptic diseases, II. N Engl J Med 1990;323: 1749–1755.
61. McCarthy DM. Sucralfate. N Engl J Med 1991;325:1017–1025.
62. Jensen SL, Jensen PF. Role of sucralfate in peptic disease. Dig Dis 1992;10:153–161.
63. Pinson JB, Weart CW. Acid-peptic products. In: Covington TR, Berardi RR, Young LY, et al, eds. Handbook of Nonprescription Drugs, 9th ed. Washington, DC, American Pharmaceutical Association, 1996:193–224.
64. Blum RA. Lanoprazole and omeprazole in the treatment of acid peptic disorders. Am J Health Syst Pharm 1996;53:1–15.
65. Langtry HD, Wilde MI. Lansoprazole: An update of its pharmacological properties and clinical efficacy in the management of acid-related disorders. Drugs 1997;54:473–500.
66. Zimmermann AE, Katona BG. Lansoprazole; a comprehensive review. Pharmacotherapy 1997;17:308–326.
67. Langtry HD, Wilde MI. Omeprazole: A review of its use in *Helicobacter pylori* infection, gastroesophageal reflux disease and peptic ulcer induced by nonsteroidal antiinflammatory drugs. Drugs 1998; 56:447–486.
68. Rokkas T, Karameris A, Mavrogeorgis A, et al. Eradication of *Helicobacter pylori* reduces the possibility of rebleeding in peptic ulcer disease. Gastrointest Endosc 1995;41:1–4.
69. Jaspersen D, Koerner T, Schorr W, et al. *Helicobacter pylori* eradication reduces the rate of rebleeding in ulcer hemorrhage. Gastrointest Endosc 1995;41:5.
70. Howden CW. For what conditions is there evidence-based justification for treatment of *Helicobacter pylori* infection? Gastroenterology 1997;113(suppl):S107–S112.
71. Raskin JB, White RH, Jackson JE, et al. Misoprostol dosage in the prevention of nonsteroidal anti-inflammatory drug-induced gastric and duodenal ulcers: a comparison of three regimens. Ann Intern Med 1995;123:344–350.
72. Koch M, Dezi A, Ferrario F, et al. Prevention of nonsteroidal anti-inflammatory drug-induced gastrointestinal mucosal injury: A meta-analysis of randomized controlled clinical trials. Arch Intern Med 1996;156:2321–2332.
73. Isdale A, Wright V. Misoprostol/NSAID fixed conbinations: Help or hindrance in clinical practice? Drug Saf 1995;12:291–298.
74. Hudson N, Taha AS, Russell RI, et al. Famotidine for healing and maintenance in nonsteroidal anti-inflammatory drug-associated gastroduodenal ulceration. Gastroenterology 1997;112:1817–1822.
75. Donnelley MT, Hawkey CJ. Review article: COX II inhibitors—A new generation of safer NSAIDs? Aliment Pharmacol Ther 1997; 11:227–236.

76. Jouzeau JY, Terlain B, Abid A, et al. Cyclo-oxygenase isoenzymes: How recent finds affect thinking about nonsteroidal antiinflammatory drugs. Drugs 1997;53:563–582.
77. Fitton A, Wiseman L. Pantoprazole: A review of its pharmacologic properties and therapeutic use in acid-related disorders. Drugs 1998; 51:460–482.
78. Prakash A, Faulds D. Rabeprazole. Drugs 1998;55:261–267.
79. Berardi RR, Welage LS. Proton pump inhibitors in acid-related disease. Am J Health Syst Pharm. 1998;55:2289–2298.
80. Caraco Y, Wilkinson GR, Wood AJJ. Differences between white subjects and Chinese subjects in the *in vivo* inhibition of cytochrome P450s 2C19, 2D6, and 3A by omeprazole. Clin Pharmacol Ther 1996;60:396–404.
81. Freston JW. Long-term acid control and proton pump inhibitors: Interactions and safety issues in perspective. Am J Gastroenterol 1997;92:51S–57S.
82. Welage LS, Berardi RR. Drug interactions with antiulcer agents: Considerations in the treatment of peptic ulcer disease. J Pharm Pract 1994;7:177–195.
83. Anderson T. Pharmacokinetics, metabolism and interactions of acid pump inhibitors; focus on omeprazole, lansoprazole, and pantoprazole. Clin Pharmacokinet 1996;31:9–28.
84. Sherman SI, Tielens ET, Ladeson PW. Sucralfate causes malabsorption of L-thyroxine. Am J Med 1994;96:531–535.
85. Kornbluth A. Life-threatening diarrhea after short-term misoprostol use in a patient with Crohn's ileocolitis. Ann Intern Med 1990; 113:474–475.
86. Bodger K, Daly MJ, Heatley RV. Clinical economics review: *Helicobacter pylori*-associated peptic ulcer disease. Aliment Pharmacol Ther 1997;11:273–282.
87. Taylor JL, Zagari M, Murphy, et al. Pharmacoeconomic comparison of treatments for the eradication of *Helicobacter pylori.* Arch Intern Med 1997;157:87–97.
88. Vakil N, Fennerty MB. Cost effectiveness of treatment regimens for the eradication of *Helicobacter pylori* in duodenal ulcer. Am J Gastroenterol 1996;91:239–245.
89. Phillips AC, Polisson RP, Simon LS. NSAIDs and the elderly: Toxicity and economic implications. Drugs Aging 1997;10:119–130.
90. Hirschowitz BI. Zollinger-Ellison syndrome: Pathogenesis, diagnosis, and management. Am J Gastroenterol 1997;92(suppl):44S–50S.
91. Maton PN. Zollinger-Ellison syndrome: Recognition and management of acid hypersecretion. Drugs 1996;1:33–44.
92. Smythe MA, Zarowitz BJ. Changing perspectives of stress gastritis prophylaxis. Ann Pharmacother 1994;28:1073–1085.
93. Fisher RL, Pipkin GA, Wood JR. Stress-related mucosal disease: Pathophysiology, prevention, and treatment. Crit Care Clin 1995; 11:323–345.
94. Navab F, Steingrub J. Stress ulcer: Is routine prophylaxis necessary? Am J Gastroenterol 1995;90:708–712.
95. Ben-Menachem T, Fogel R, Patel RV, et al. Prophylaxis for stress-related gastric hemorrhage in the medical intensive care unit: A randomized, controlled, single-blind study. Ann Intern Med 1994; 121:568–575.
96. O'Keefe G, Maier RV. Current management of patients with stress ulceration. Adv Surg 1996;30:155–157.
97. Prod'hom G, Leuenberger P, Koerfer J, et al. Nosocomial pneumonia in mechanically ventilated patients receiving antacid, ranitidine, or sucralfate: A randomized controlled trial. Ann Intern Med 1994; 120:653–662.
98. Cook DJ, Reeve BK, Guyatt GH, et al. Stress ulcer prophylaxis in critically ill patients; resolving discordant meta-analyses. JAMA 1996;275:308–314.
99. Cook D, Guyatt G, Marshall J, et al. Comparison of sucralfate and ranitidine for the prevention of upper gastronintestinal bleeding in patients requiring mechanical ventilation. N Engl J Med 1998;338: 791–797.
100. Ben-Menachem T, McCarthy BD, Fogel R, et al. Prophylaxis for stress-related gastrointestinal hemorrhage: A cost effective analysis. Crit Care Med 1996;24:338–345.

32
INFLAMMATORY BOWEL DISEASE

Joseph T. DiPiro, PharmD, FCCP, and Robert R. Schade, MD

There are two forms of idiopathic inflammatory bowel disease (IBD): (1) ulcerative colitis, a mucosal inflammatory condition confined to the rectum and colon; and (2) Crohn's disease, a transmural inflammation of the gastrointestinal tract that can affect any part, from the mouth to the anus. The etiologies of both conditions are unknown, but they may have some common pathogenetic mechanisms.

EPIDEMIOLOGY

At least 1 million Americans are believed to have IBD, with 15,000 to 30,000 new cases diagnosed annually.[1] Crohn's disease has a reported incidence of 4.3 to 6.8 in the United States and a prevalence of 20 to 40 per 100,000 people.[2] The rates of IBD are highest in Scandanavia, Great Britain, and North America. The incidence of Crohn's disease varies considerably among studies but has clearly increased dramatically over the last 3 or 4 decades.[3] Ulcerative colitis has a reported incidence of 3.7 to 15 and a prevalence of 37 to 212 per 100,000.[3] The incidence of ulcerative colitis has remained relatively constant over many years.[3] Although most epidemiologic studies combine ulcerative proctitis with ulcerative colitis, from 17% to 49% of cases are proctitis. The incidence of ulcerative proctitis ranges from 1.1 to 7.1 per 100,000.[3]

Both sexes are affected equally with inflammatory bowel disease,[1,2] although some studies have shown slightly greater numbers of women with Crohn's disease and males with ulcerative colitis.[4,5] Ulcerative colitis and Crohn's disease have bimodal distributions in age of initial presentation. The peak incidence occurs in the second or third decades of life with a second peak occurring between 50 and 80 years.[3] Significantly increased incidence of ulcerative colitis (four to five times normal) has been observed in Ashkenazi Jews, while Blacks and Asians have a relatively low incidence of occurrence.[2]

ETIOLOGY

Although the exact etiology of ulcerative colitis and Crohn's disease is unknown, similar factors are believed responsible for each condition (Table 32–1). The major theories of the cause of IBD involve infectious or immunologic etiologies.[6] The infectious theory assumes that the body is reacting normally to an as-yet-unrecognized pathogen, whereas the immunologic theory posits that the immune system is responding inappropriately to antigens to which most people are exposed, leading to an autoimmune reaction.[7]

INFECTIOUS THEORIES

Microorganisms have been suspected of being involved in the pathogenesis of IBD, including viruses, protozoans, mycoplasmas, and other bacteria.[8] However, no definitive infectious cause of IBD has been found even though the presentation is similar to that caused by some invasive microbial pathogens. Also, certain strains of bacteria produce toxins (necrotoxins, hemolysins, and enterotoxins) that cause mucosal damage. Bacteria elaborate peptides (e.g., formyl-methionyl-leucyl-phenylalanine [FMLP]) that have chemotactic properties and cause an influx of inflammatory cells with subsequent release of inflammatory mediators and tissue destruction. Microbes may elaborate super antigens, which are capable of global T-lymphocyte stimulation and subsequent inflammatory response.[8] Through lumenal exposure to potent nonspecific stimulatory bacterial products, the state of activation of the immune system pathways may be upregulated.[9]

Investigators have examined the difference in bowel flora of IBD patients and normal individuals.[10] In up to one-third of patients with Crohn's disease, abnormal flora (increased anaerobes) were observed in the upper small bowel. However, diarrhea alone can cause changes in bowel flora.

GENETIC FACTORS

Genetic factors are believed to predispose patients to inflammatory bowel diseases, particularly Crohn's disease. In studies of monozygotic twins, there has been a high concordance rate, with both individuals of the pair having an IBD (particularly Crohn's disease). Also, first-degree relatives of patients with IBD had a 10-fold increase in the risk of disease. Other investigators have observed genetic markers that are found more frequently in those with IBD (particularly major histocompatability complex class II genes). A number of genes have been associated with IBDs; however, the nature of the gene products has not been established.

IMMUNOLOGIC MECHANISMS

The immunologic basis of IBD is supported by a number of observations.[7] First is the pathology of the lesions. With Crohn's disease, the bowel wall has been observed to be infiltrated with lymphocytes, plasma cells, mast cells, macrophages, and neutrophils. Similar infiltration has been observed in the mucosal layer of the colon in patients with ulcerative colitis. Second, many of the systemic manifestations of IBD have an immunologic etiology (e.g., arthritis or uveitis). Finally, IBD is responsive to immunosuppressive drugs (e.g., corticosteroids and azathioprine).

TABLE 32–1. Proposed Etiologies for Inflammatory Bowel Disease

Infectious Agents	
	Viruses
	L-forms of bacteria
	Mycobacteria
	Chlamydia
Genetics	
	Metabolic defects
	Connective tissue disorders
Environmental Factors	
	Diet
Immune Defects	
	Altered host susceptibility
	Immune-mediated mucosal damage
Psychological Factors	
	Stress
	Emotional or physical trauma
	Occupation

As previously stated, the immune theory of IBD assumes that IBD is caused by an "inappropriate" reaction of the immune system. This may involve an immunodeficiency, such as a defect in cell-mediated immunity or of macrophages or neutrophils. Autoimmunity may be involved. Also, oxidant injury in colon epithelial crypt cells can be demonstrated from inflamed mucosa of patients with inflammatory bowel disease.[11]

Potential immunologic mechanisms include both autoimmune and nonautoimmune phenomena.[8,12] Autoimmunity may be directed against mucosal epithelial cells or against neutrophil cytoplasmic elements. Some patients with IBD have abnormal structural features for colonic epithelial cells even in the absence of active disease. Autoantibodies to these structures have been reported. Also, antineutrophil cytoplasmic antibodies are found in a high percentage of patients with ulcerative colitis (70%) and much less frequently with other forms of colitis (6% with Crohn's disease).[13] Presence of antineutrophil cytoplasmic antibodies in left-sided ulcerative colitis has been associated with resistance to medical therapy.[14]

Dysregulation of cytokines is a component of inflammatory bowel disease. Specifically, Th_1 cytokine activity (which enhances cell-mediated immunity and inhibits humoral immunity) is enhanced, and Th_2 cytokine activity (which inhibits cell-mediated immunity and enhances humoral immunity) is impaired with disease. Expression of interferon-γ (a Th_1 cytokine) in intestinal mucosa of diseased patients is reported to be increased while interleukin-4 (a Th_2 cytokine) is reduced.[15–17] The activity of the proinflammatory cytokine, tumor necrosis factor α, is increased in the stool of patients with relapsing ulcerative colitis or active Crohn's disease.[18]

A number of nonautoimmune phenomena have been reported with IBD. Patients with IBD have increased numbers of IgG-bearing cells and altered production of IgG subtypes. Mucosal injury with IBD may result from mucosal T-cell activation. These cells may have cytotoxic effects directly or through the actions of cytokines. Inflammatory cytokines such as interleukin-1 and interleukin-6 are reported to be increased with IBD. Also, eicosanoids such as leukotriene B_4 (LTB4) are increased in rectal dialysates and tissues of IBD patients and are related to disease activity. LTB4 enhances neutrophil adherence to vascular endothelium and acts as a neutrophil chemoattractant. These findings have led to the consideration of anticytokine and leukotriene inhibitor stategies for therapy.

PSYCHOLOGICAL FACTORS

Mental health changes appear to correlate with remissions and exacerbations, especially of ulcerative colitis, but psychological factors overall are not thought to be an etiologic factor. Most rigorous studies have concluded that no connection can be made between stress-inducing events and disease symptoms.[19]

DIET AND SMOKING

Changes in diet by people in industrialized countries where Crohn's disease is more common have not been consistently associated with the disease. Studies of increased intake of refined sugars or chemical food additives and reduced fiber intake have been conflicting regarding risk for Crohn's disease.

Smoking plays an important but contrasting role in ulcerative colitis and Crohn's disease. The incidence of ulcerative colitis is inversely associated with smoking.[20,21] Ulcerative colitis primarily occurs in nonsmokers. Clinical relapses have been associated with smoking cessation, and nicotine transdermal administration has been effective in improving symptoms in patients with ulcerative colitis.[22] In contrast, Crohn's disease has been directly associated with smoking.[20]

PATHOPHYSIOLOGY

Ulcerative colitis and Crohn's disease differ in two general respects: anatomic sites and depth of involvement within the bowel wall. There is, however, overlap between the two conditions, with a small fraction of patients showing features of both diseases. Confusion can occur, particularly when the inflammatory process is limited to the colon. Table 32–2 compares pathologic and clinical findings of the two diseases.[23]

ULCERATIVE COLITIS

Ulcerative colitis is confined to the rectum and colon, and affects the mucosa and the submucosa. In some instances, a short segment of terminal ileum may be inflamed; this is referred to as backwash ileitis. Unlike Crohn's disease, the deeper longitudinal muscular layers, serosa, and regional lymph nodes are not usually involved.[4] Because inflammation is usually confined to the mucosa and submucosa, fistulas, perforation, or obstruction are uncommon.

TABLE 32–2. Comparison of Clinical and Pathologic Features of Crohn's Granulomatous Colitis and Ulcerative Colitis

Feature	Crohn's Colitis	Ulcerative Colitis
Intestinal		
Malaise, fever	Common	Uncommon
Rectal bleeding	Intermittent, about 50%	Common
Abdominal tenderness	Common	May be present
Abdominal mass	Very common (especially with ileocolitis)	Not present
Abdominal pain	Very common	Unusual
Abdominal wall and internal fistulas	Very common	Rare
Endoscopic		
Rectal disease	About 20%	Almost 100%
Diffuse, continuous symmetric involvement	Uncommon	Very common
Aphthous or linear ulcers	Common	Rare
Pathologic		
Continuous disease	Rare	Very common
Rectal involvement	Rare	Common
Ileal involvement	Very common	Nonexistent
Strictures	Common	Rare
Fistulas	Common	Rare
Transmural involvement	Common	Rare
Crypt abscesses	Rare	Very common
Granulomas	Common	Rare
Linear clefts	Common	Rare

The primary lesion of ulcerative colitis occurs in the crypts of the mucosa (crypts of Lieberkuhn) in the form of a crypt abscess. Here, frank necrosis of the epithelium occurs; it is usually visible only with microscopy but may be seen grossly when coalescence of ulcers occurs. Extension and coalescence ulcers may surround areas of uninvolved mucosa. These islands of mucosa are called pseudopolyps. Other typical ulceration patterns include a "collar-button ulcer," which results from extensive submucosal undermining at the ulcer edge.[4,24] The extensive mucosal damage seen in ulcerative colitis can result in significant diarrhea and bleeding, although a small percentage of patients experience constipation.

Ulcerative colitis can be accompanied by complications that may be local (involving the colon or rectum) or systemic (not directly associated with the colon). With either type the complications may be mild, serious, or even life threatening.

Local complications occur in the majority of ulcerative colitis patients. Relatively minor complications include hemorrhoids, anal fissures, or perirectal abscesses. These complications are more likely to be present during active colitis. Enteroenteric fistulas are rare.

A major complication is toxic megacolon, a severe condition that occurs in 1% to 3% of patients with active ulcerative colitis or Crohn's disease. With toxic megacolon, ulceration extends below the submucosa, sometimes even reaching the serosa. Vasculitis, swelling of the vascular endothelium, and thrombosis of small arteries occurs; involvement of the muscularis propria causes loss of colonic tone, which leads to dilatation and potential perforation.[4] The patient with toxic megacolon usually has a high fever, tachycardia, distended abdomen, and elevated white blood cell count, and a dilated colon is observed on x-ray. Colonic perforation, however, may occur with or without toxic megacolon and is a greater risk with the first attack.

Another infrequent major local complication is massive colonic hemorrhage. Colonic stricture, sometimes with clinical obstruction, may also complicate ulcerative colitis. Finally, the risk of colonic carcinoma is much greater in patients with ulcerative colitis as compared to the general population. The risk of colon cancer begins to increase 10 to 15 years after the diagnosis of ulcerative colitis. The absolute risk may be as high as 30% 35 years after diagnosis, and 49% for patients who have a long history of disease and were less than 15 years of age at the time of diagnosis.[12]

The inflammatory response seen in IBD has also been blamed for the "systemic" complications seen in both Crohn's disease and ulcerative colitis. The systemic extraintestinal complications of ulcerative colitis are summarized in the next section.

HEPATOBILIARY COMPLICATIONS

Approximately 11% of patients with ulcerative colitis have been reported to have hepatobiliary complications.[25] However, the reported frequency ranges from 5% to 95% in IBD patients overall.[26] Hepatic complications include fatty liver, pericholangitis, chronic active hepatitis, and cirrhosis. Biliary complications include sclerosing cholangitis, cholangiocarcinoma, and gallstones.

Fatty infiltration of the liver may be due to malabsorption, protein-losing enteropathy, or concomitant steroid use. The most common hepatic complication is pericholangitis (acute inflammation surrounding the intrahepatic portal venules, bile ducts, and lymphatics), which occurs in up to one-third of ulcerative colitis patients. This is believed to be associated with progressive fibrosis of intrahepatic and extrahepatic bile ducts in a few percent of ulcerative colitis patients, referred to as primary sclerosing cholangitis. Cirrhosis may be a sequela of cholangitis or chronic active hepatitis. Often the severity of hepatic disease does not correlate with GI disease.

Gallstones occur more commonly in patients with Crohn's disease (particularly with terminal ileal disease) and may be related to bile salt malabsorption. Also, cholangiocarcinoma occurs 10 to 20 times more frequently in IBD patients compared with the general population.[25]

JOINT COMPLICATIONS

Arthritis was found to be present in 4.9% of patients.[25] Arthritis is typically migratory and involves one or a few, usually large joints. The joints most often affected, in decreasing frequency, are the knees, hips, ankles, wrists, and elbows. Sacroiliitis also occurs commonly. Arthritis associated with ulcerative colitis is generally related to the severity of colonic disease, and resolution without recurrence is seen with proctocolectomy. Also, arthritis in this setting is different from rheumatoid arthritis in that rheumatoid factors are generally not detected. Also, it is nondeforming and nondestructive, even after multiple episodes.

Another potential joint complication is ankylosing spondylitis, which is often unresponsive to treatment. The incidence of ankylosing spondylitis in patients with ulcerative colitis is 30 times that of the general population and occurs most commonly in patients with the HLA-B27 phenotype.

OCULAR COMPLICATIONS

Ocular complications, including iritis, uveitis, episcleritis, and conjunctivitis, occur in up to 10% of patients with IBD. The most commonly reported symptoms with iritis and uveitis include blurred vision, eye pain, and photophobia. Episcleritis is associated with scleral injection, burning, and increased secretions. These complications may parallel the severity of intestinal disease, and recurrence after colectomy with ulcerative colitis is uncommon.

DERMATOLOGIC AND MUCOSAL COMPLICATIONS

Skin and mucosal lesions associated with IBD include erythema nodosum, pyoderma gangrenosum, and aphthous ulceration. Most studies report that 5% to 10% of IBD patients experience dermatologic or mucosal complications.[27]

Erythema nodosum is manifested by raised, red, tender nodules that vary in size from 1 to several cm. They are typically found on the tibial surfaces of the legs and arms. These lesions are more commonly observed in Crohn's disease patients and are noted to correlate with disease severity.

Pyoderma gangrenosum occurs more commonly in patients with ulcerative colitis (1% to 5% incidence) and is characterized by discrete skin ulcerations that have a necrotic center and a violaceous color of the surrounding skin.[27] They can be seen on any part of the body but are more commonly found on the lower extremities.

Oral lesions are found in 6% to 20% of patients with Crohn's disease and 8% of patients with ulcerative colitis.[27] The most common lesion is aphthous stomatitis, which is most often seen with Crohn's disease. The severity of these lesions tends to parallel GI disease.

CROHN'S DISEASE

Crohn's disease is best characterized as a transmural inflammatory process. The terminal ileum is the most common site of the disorder (14% to 30%), but it may occur in any part of the GI tract. About two-thirds of patients have some colonic involvement, and 15% to 25% of patients have only colonic disease.[8] Patients often have normal bowel separating segments of diseased bowel; that is, the disease is often discontinuous.

Regardless of the site, bowel wall injury is extensive and the intestinal lumen is often narrowed. The mesentery becomes first thickened and edematous and then fibrotic. Ulcers tend to be deep and elongated and extend along the longitudinal axis of the bowel, at least into the submucosa. The "cobblestone" appearance of the bowel wall results from deep mucosal ulceration intermingled with nodular submucosal thickening.

Complications of Crohn's disease may involve the intestinal tract or organs unrelated to it. Small bowel stricture and subsequent obstruction is a complication that may require surgery. Fistula formation is common and occurs much more frequently than with ulcerative colitis.[8] Fistulas often occur in the areas of worst inflammation, where loops of bowel have become matted together by fibrous adhesions. Fistulas may connect a segment of the GI tract to skin (enterocutaneous fistula), two segments of the GI tract (enteroenteric fistula), or the intestinal tract with the bladder (enterovesicular fistula) or vagina. Crohn's disease fistulas or abscesses associated with them frequently require surgical treatment.

Bleeding with Crohn's disease is usually not as severe as with ulcerative colitis, although patients with Crohn's disease may have hypochromic anemia. Also, as with ulcerative colitis, the risk of carcinoma is increased but not as great as with ulcerative colitis.

Systemic complications of Crohn's disease are common, and similar to those found with ulcerative colitis. Arthritis, iritis, skin lesions, and liver disease often accompany Crohn's disease. Renal stones occur in up to 10% of patients with Crohn's disease (less frequently with ulcerative colitis) due to fat malabsorption, which allows for greater oxalate absorption. Gallstones also occur with greater frequency in patients with ileitis, possibly due to bile acid malabsorption at the terminal ileum.

Nutritional deficiencies are common with Crohn's disease.[28] Reported frequencies of various nutritional parameters are as follows: weight loss, 40% to 80%; growth failure in children, 15% to 88%; iron deficiency anemia, 25% to 50%; vitamin B_{12} deficiency, 20% to 37%; folate deficiency, 13% to 37%; hypoalbuminemia, 25% to 76%; hypokalemia, 33%; and osteomalacia, 36%. There are usually decreased fat stores and lean tissue. Growth failure in children may be associated with hypozincemia.

CLINICAL PRESENTATION

The patterns of clinical presentation of IBD can vary widely. Patients may have a single acute episode that resolves and does not recur, but most patients experience acute exacerbations after periods of remission. With more severe disease, prolonged illness may occur.

ULCERATIVE COLITIS

Although a typical clinical picture of ulcerative colitis can be described, there is a very wide range of presentation. Symptoms may range from mild abdominal cramping with frequent, small-volume bowel movements to profuse diarrhea. Most patients with ulcerative colitis experience intermittent bouts of illness after varying intervals with no symptoms. Only a small percentage of patients have continuous unremitting symptoms or have a single acute attack with no subsequent symptoms.

Complex disease classifications are generally not used in clinical practice for ulcerative colitis. The arbitrarily determined distinctions of mild, moderate, and severe disease activity are generally used, and these are determined largely by clinical signs and symptoms. Mild disease has been defined as fewer than 4 stools daily without anemia, tachycardia, weight loss, or hypoalbuminemia; and severe disease as more than 6 stools daily with the signs just listed (Table 32–3).[7] It is also important to determine disease extent; that is, what part of the colon is involved—rectum, descending colon only, or the entire colon.

Two-thirds of patients with ulcerative colitis have mild disease, which almost always starts in the rectum. Occasionally, the mild form may progress to severe disease, which may be called "fulminant" if it occurs acutely. Systemic signs and symptoms of the disease (e.g., arthritis, uveitis, pyoderma gangrenosum) may be present in these patients and, in fact, may be the reason the patient seeks medical attention. Patients with mild disease are believed to be at lower risk of colon cancer. Moderate disease is observed in one-fourth of patients. These patients have more prominent abdominal discomfort and usually present with diarrhea and bleeding as the major complaints. They may be noted to have a low-grade fever.

With severe disease the patient is usually found to be in acute distress, has profuse bloody diarrhea, and often has a high fever with leukocytosis and hypoalbuminemia. Often the patient is dehydrated and therefore may be tachycardic and hypotensive. This presentation may have a sudden onset with rapid progression.

The diagnosis of ulcerative colitis is made on clinical suspicion and confirmed by biopsy, stool examinations, sigmoidoscopy or colonoscopy, or barium radiographic contrast studies. The presence of extracolonic manifestations such as arthritis, uveitis, and pyoderma gangrenosum may also aid in establishing the diagnosis.

CROHN'S DISEASE

As with ulcerative colitis, the presentation of Crohn's disease is highly variable. A single episode may not be followed by further episodes, or the patient may experience continuous, unremitting disease. An average of 3 years between the onset of complaints and the initial diagnosis has been reported. The patient typically presents with diarrhea and abdominal pain. Hematochezia occurs in about one-half of the patients with colonic involvement and much less frequently when there is no colonic involvement. Commonly, a patient may first present with a perirectal or perianal lesion. The diagnosis should also be suspected in children with growth retardation, especially with abdominal complaints.

The course of Crohn's disease is characterized by periods of remission and exacerbation. Some patients may be free of symptoms for years, while others experience chronic problems in spite of medical therapy. Nearly all patients have a recurrence of Crohn's disease within 10 years of the initial episode.[12] As with ulcerative colitis, the diagnosis of Crohn's disease involves a thorough evaluation using laboratory, endoscopic, and radiologic testing to detect the extent and characteristic features of the disease. Because of similarities that may exist between ulcerative colitis and Crohn's disease confined to the colon, a definitive diagnosis cannot be made in up to 15% of cases, even with pathologic specimens in hand. Small bowel involvement and strictures detected on radiographs are characteristic of Crohn's disease.

TABLE 32–3. Severity Criteria for Ulcerative Colitis

Variables	Mild	Severe	Fulminant
Bowel movement frequency	< 4/d	> 6/d	> 10/d
Blood in stool	+/–	++	Continuous
Fever	Normal	> 37.5°C	> 37.5°C
Pulse	Normal	> 90/mm	< 90/mm
Hemoglobin	Normal	< 75% normal	Transfusion required
ESR	< 30 mm/h	> 30 mm/h	> 30 mm/h
Colon		Colonic air	Dilated colon
Radiography		Edematous wall, thumbprinting	–
Clinical sign		Abdominal tenderness	Abdominal distension and tenderness

ESR = erythrocyte sedimentation rate.
From Ref. 4.

▶ TREATMENT: Inflammatory Bowel Disease

DESIRED OUTCOME

To treat IBD properly, the clinician must have a clear concept of realistic therapeutic goals for each patient. These goals may relate to resolution of acute inflammatory processes; resolution of attendant complications (e.g., fistulas, abscesses); alleviation of systemic manifestations (e.g., arthritis); maintenance of remission from acute inflammation; or surgical palliation or cure. The approach to the therapeutic regimen differs considerably with varying goals as well as with the two diseases, ulcerative colitis and Crohn's disease.

When determining goals of therapy and selecting therapeutic regimens it is important to understand the natural history of IBD.[29] Some cases of acute ulcerative colitis are self-limited. With mild to moderate acute colitis, without systemic symptoms, 20% of patients may experience spontaneous improvement in their disease within a few weeks; however, a small percentage of patients may go on to experience more serious disease. With severe colitis, improvement without treatment cannot be expected. For instance, the response to medical management of toxic megacolon is variable and emergent colectomy may be required. When remission of ulcerative colitis is achieved, it is likely to last at least 1 year with medical therapy. In the absence of medical therapy, one-half to two-thirds of patients are likely to relapse within 9 months.[29] In some reports, remission rates with placebo have approached those with active treatment.

A considerable number of patients with active Crohn's disease may achieve at least temporary remission without drug therapy. In two large trials, 26% and 42% of ambulatory patients on placebo achieved remission.[30,31] Once remission is achieved, two-thirds to three-fourths of patients remain in remission up to 2 years without drug therapy.[29] The implication of these data is that up to 40% of patients with active Crohn's disease improve in 3 to 4 months with observation alone, and that most patients remain in remission for prolonged periods without medical intervention. These observations apply more to mild or moderate disease than to severe disease.

GENERAL APPROACH TO TREATMENT

Treatment of IBD centers on agents used to relieve the inflammatory process. Salicylates, corticosteroids, antimicrobials, and immunosuppressive agents such as azathioprine and 6-mercaptopurine are commonly used to treat active disease and, for some agents, to lengthen the time of disease remission.

In addition to the use of drugs, surgical procedures are sometimes performed when active disease is not adequately controlled or when the required drug dosages pose an unacceptable risk of adverse effects. For most patients with IBD, nutritional considerations are also important, because these patients are often malnourished. Finally, a variety of therapies may be used to address complications or symptoms of IBD. For example, antidiarrheals may be used in some patients, although these are generally to be avoided in ulcerative colitis because they may contribute to the development of toxic colonic dilatation. Antimicrobial agents may be used in conjunction with drainage when abscesses are present. Iron may be required, particularly with ulcerative colitis, where blood loss from the colon can be significant.

NONPHARMACOLOGIC THERAPY

NUTRITIONAL SUPPORT

Proper nutritional support is an important aspect of the treatment of patients with IBD, not because specific types of diets are useful in alleviating the inflammatory conditions but because patients with moderate to severe disease are often malnourished. The patient with IBD may be malnourished because of decreased nutrient intake (anorexia or when eating causes exacerbation of symptoms), because the inflammatory process results in significant malabsorption or maldigestion, or because of the catabolic effects of the disease process. Malabsorption may occur in the patient with Crohn's disease with inflammatory involvement of the small bowel, where many nutrients are absorbed, and also in patients who have undergone multiple small bowel resections with subsequent reduction in absorptive surface ("short gut"). Maldigestion can occur if there is a bile salt deficiency in the gut.

A number of specific diets have been tried in attempts to improve the condition of patients with IBD, but none has gained widespread acceptance. With each individual it is helpful to eliminate specific foods that exacerbate symptoms. This elimination process must be conducted cautiously, as patients have been known to exclude a wide range of nutritious products without adequate justification. Many patients with IBD, although not the majority, have lactase deficiency; therefore, diarrhea may be associated with milk intake. In these patients, avoidance of milk or supplementation with lactase generally improves the patient's symptoms.

Dietary supplementation with fish oil has been proposed to treat IBD. In one placebo-controlled trial, patients with active ulcerative colitis were treated with fish oil supplementation for 4 months and had significant improvements in histologic findings and weight gain.[32] In another trial, 2.7 g/d of fish oil was effective in reducing the rate of relapse in Crohn's disease.[33] Fish oil contains eicosapentaenoic acid, which is metabolized by lipoxygenase and cyclooxygenase (similar to arachidonic acid), and results in lower production of leukotriene B_4 and prostaglandin E_2, which are believed to be important mediators in IBD.

The nutritional needs of the majority of patients can be adequately addressed with enteral supplementation.[34] Patients who have severe disease may require a course of parenteral nutrition to attain a reasonable nutritional status or in preparation for surgery. In one report of patients with severe acute ulcerative colitis, enteral nutrition resulted in a significantly greater increase in serum albumin, fewer adverse effects related to the nutritional regimen, and fewer postoperative infections, compared with isocaloric, isonitrogenous parenteral nutrition. The regimens were similar with regard to remission rate and the need for colectomy.[35] Consideration should be given to lipid administration, not only for caloric value but also in recognition of depleted peripheral fat stores in many IBD patients and the greater potential for fatty acid deficiency.

Parenteral nutrition is an important component of the treatment of severe Crohn's disease or ulcerative colitis. The use of parenteral nutrition allows complete bowel rest in patients with severe ulcerative colitis, which may alter the need for proctocolectomy. Parenteral nutrition has also been valuable in Crohn's disease, because remission may be achieved with parenteral nutrition in about one-half of patients.[36] In some patients, the disease may worsen when parenteral nutrition is stopped. Patients with enterocutaneous fistulas of various etiologies have been reported to benefit from parenteral nutrition.[36] Parenteral nutrition may also be valuable in children or adolescents with growth retardation associated with Crohn's disease, but surgery is often necessary with severe disease. Finally, when possible, home parenteral nutrition should be used for patients requiring long-term therapy, particularly those with "short gut" due to surgical resection.

SURGERY

Surgical procedures have an established place in the treatment of IBD. Although surgery (proctocolectomy) is curative for ulcerative

TABLE 32–4. Mesalamine Derivatives for Treatment of Inflammatory Bowel Disease

Product	Trade Name(s)	Formulation	Dose/Day	Site of Action
Sulfasalazine	Azulfidine	Tablet	4–6 g	Colon
Mesalamine	Rowasa, Salofalk, Claversal, Pentasa	Enema	1–4 g	Rectum, terminal colon
	Rowasa	Suppository	1 g	Rectum
	Asacol	Mesalamine coated with Eudragit-S (delayed-release acrylic resin)	2.4–4.8 g	Distal ileum, colon
	Pentasa	Mesalamine coated in ethylcellulose microgranules (oral tablet)	2–4 g	Small bowel, colon
Olsalazine	Dipentum	Dimer of mesalamine oral capsule	1.5–3 g	Colon
Balsalazide	Colazide	Capsule	2 - 6 g	Colon

colitis, this is not the case for Crohn's disease. Surgical procedures involve resection of segments of intestine that are affected, as well as correction of complications (e.g., fistulas) or drainage of abscesses.

For ulcerative colitis, colectomy may be performed when the patient has disease uncontrolled by maximum medical therapy or when there are complications of the disease such as colonic perforation, toxic dilatation (megacolon), uncontrolled colonic hemorrhage, or colonic strictures. Colectomy may be indicated in patients with long-standing disease (greater than 8 to 10 years), as a prophylactic measure against the development of cancer, and in patients with premalignant changes (severe dysplasia) on surveillance mucosal biopsies. The most common surgical procedures include proctocolectomy, after which the patient is left with a permanent ileostomy, and abdominal colectomy, with removal of the mucosa of the rectum and anastomosis of an ileal pouch to the anus (ileoanal pull-through). The risk from surgery in these patients is relatively low if the operations are performed on a nonemergent basis.

The indications for surgery with Crohn's disease are not as well established as for ulcerative colitis, and surgery is usually reserved for the complications of the disease. A recognized problem with intestinal resection for Crohn's disease is the high recurrence rate. Surgery may be appropriate in well-selected patients who are documented to continue to have severe or incapacitating disease or obstruction in spite of aggressive medical management. The surgical procedures performed include resections of the major intestinal areas of involvement. In some patients with severe rectal or perineal disease, diversion of the fecal stream is performed with a colostomy. Other indications for surgery include the finding of colon cancer, an inflammatory mass, or intestinal perforations.

PHARMACOLOGIC THERAPY

Drug therapy plays an integral part in the overall treatment of IBD. None of the drugs used for IBD is curative; at best they serve to control the disease process. Therefore, a reasonable goal of drug therapy is resolution of disease symptoms such that the patient can carry on normal daily functions. The major types of drug therapy used in IBD include aminosalicylates; corticosteroids; immunosuppressives (azathioprine, 6-mercaptopurine, cyclosporine, and methotrexate); antimicrobials (metronidazole); and other agents used investigationally such as immune enhancers (e.g., levamisole or bacillus Calmette-Guérin [BCG]), mast cell stabilizers (cromolyn sodium), antibodies against tumor necrosis factor α, and leukotriene inhibitors.

Sulfasalazine, an agent that combines a sulfonamide (sulfapyridine) antibiotic and mesalamine (5-ASA) in the same molecule, has been used for many years to treat IBD but was originally intended to treat arthritis. Sulfasalazine is cleaved by gut bacteria in the colon to sulfapyridine (which is mostly reabsorbed and excreted in the urine) and mesalamine (which mostly remains in the colon and is excreted in stool).[37]

The active component of sulfasalazine is mesalamine.[37] The mechanism of action of mesalamine is not well understood. Cyclooxygenase or lipoxygenase inhibition alone do not account for the agent's effects. Aminosalicylates may inhibit macrophage production of cyclooxygenase, thromboxane synthetase, platelet-activating factor synthetase, and interleukin-1.[38] An alternative theory suggests that mesalamine acts as a superoxide-free radical scavenger.[39]

As the mechanism of action of sulfasalazine is not related to the sulfapyridine component and as sulfapyridine is believed responsible for many of the adverse reactions to sulfasalazine, mesalamine alone can be used. Mesalamine has been used topically as an enema or suppository for the treatment of proctitis. Oral derivatives of mesalamine were also developed. Olsalazine is a dimer of two 5-aminosalicylate molecules linked by an azo bond. With this product, there is minimal GI absorption. Mesalamine is released in the colon after olsalazine is cleaved by colonic bacteria. Other products have used inert, pH-dependent coatings to delay 5-aminosalicylate release until the tablet reaches the small bowel (Table 32–4; Fig. 32–1). The recommended daily doses of the oral mesalamine derivatives are intended to approximate the molar equivalent of mesalamine present in 4 g of sulfasalazine. At present, sulfasalazine is used in preference to oral mesalamine derivatives, mainly because it costs much less. However, it is often less well tolerated than the mesalamine alternatives.

Corticosteroids and adrenocorticotropic hormone (ACTH) have been widely used for the treatment of ulcerative colitis and Crohn's disease. There has been a long-standing controversy as to the relative merits of corticosteroids versus ACTH; however, most clinicians prefer corticosteroids. ACTH may be more effective in patients who have not previously received steroids (steroid-naive patients).[40] Although ACTH is administered parenterally, corticosteroids may be given parenterally, orally, or rectally. The exact

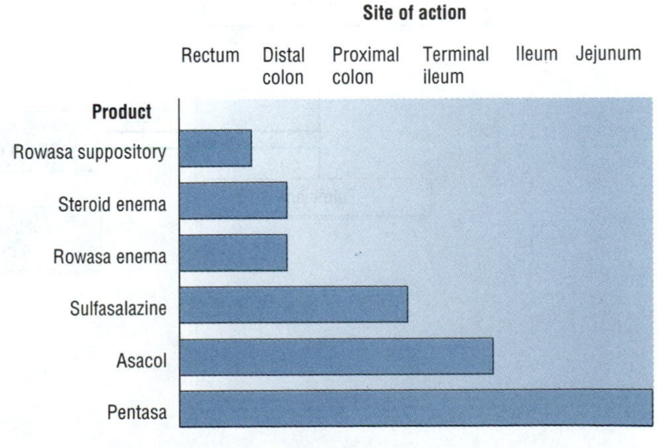

FIGURE 32–1. Site of activity of various agents to treat inflammatory bowel disease.

mechanism of action of corticosteroids is not known but is believed to involve modulation of the immune system and inhibition of production of cytokines and mediators. It is not clear if the most important steroid effects are systemic or local (mucosal).

Immunosuppressive agents such as azathioprine and 6-mercaptopurine (a metabolite of azathioprine) or cyclosporine are sometimes used for the treatment of IBD.[41] Azathioprine and 6-mercaptopurine are effective for long-term treatment of Crohn's disease and ulcerative colitis.[42] These agents are generally reserved for patients who are refractory to steroids, and they may be associated with serious adverse effects such as lymphomas, pancreatitis, or nephrotoxicity. The agents are usually used in conjunction with mesalamine derivatives and/or steroids, and must be used for long periods of time (up to 6 months) before benefits may be observed.[43] Remission can be prolonged by azathioprine in steroid-dependent patients with ulcerative colitis.[44] Cyclosporine has also been of short-term benefit in treatment of acute, severe ulcerative colitis when used in a continuous intravenous infusion. Oral doses have not been effective. The agent poses risk of nephrotoxicity and neurotoxicity.

Antimicrobial agents, particularly metronidazole, are frequently used in attempts to control Crohn's disease. Metronidazole has been demonstrated to be of value in some patients with active Crohn's disease, particularly that involving the perineal area or fistulas.[45] The mechanism of metronidazole's effect on Crohn's disease has not been determined but is theorized to relate to interruption of a bacterial role in the inflammatory process. Although other antimicrobial agents have been studied, none has gained as much attention as metronidazole.

ULCERATIVE COLITIS

Mild to Moderate Disease

The majority of patients with active ulcerative colitis have mild to moderate disease and do not require parenteral medications (Fig. 32–2). The first line of drug therapy for these patients is oral sulfasalazine or an oral mesalamine derivative. For proctitis the preferred therapy is rectally administered steroids or mesalamine. When given orally, usually 4 g/d, and up to 8 g/d, of sulfasalazine is required to attain control of active inflammation. There does not appear to be an increased rate of response with increased dosage over 4 g/d, although side effects increase. Even with the use of adequate doses, patient improvement usually takes 2 to 3 weeks and sometimes longer. The dosage of sulfasalazine that can be given is usually limited by the patient's tolerance of the agent; most adverse effects of sulfasalazine are dose related (GI disturbances, headache, arthralgia).[43] Sulfasalazine therapy should be instituted at 500 mg/d and increased every few days up to 4 g or the maximum tolerated. It should not be used in patients with allergy to sulfa drugs.

Oral mesalamine derivatives (such as those listed in Table 32–4) are reasonable alternatives to sulfasalazine for treatment of ulcerative colitis. Most of these agents have been demonstrated to be effective for ulcerative colitis but no more effective than sulfasalazine.[46] The majority of patients intolerant to sulfasalazine should tolerate one of the other oral mesalamine derivatives.

Olsalazine (a dimer of 5-ASA, given orally) has been demonstrated effective for treatment of mild to moderate ulcerative colitis. Of patients taking olsalazine, however, 15% to 25% experience se-

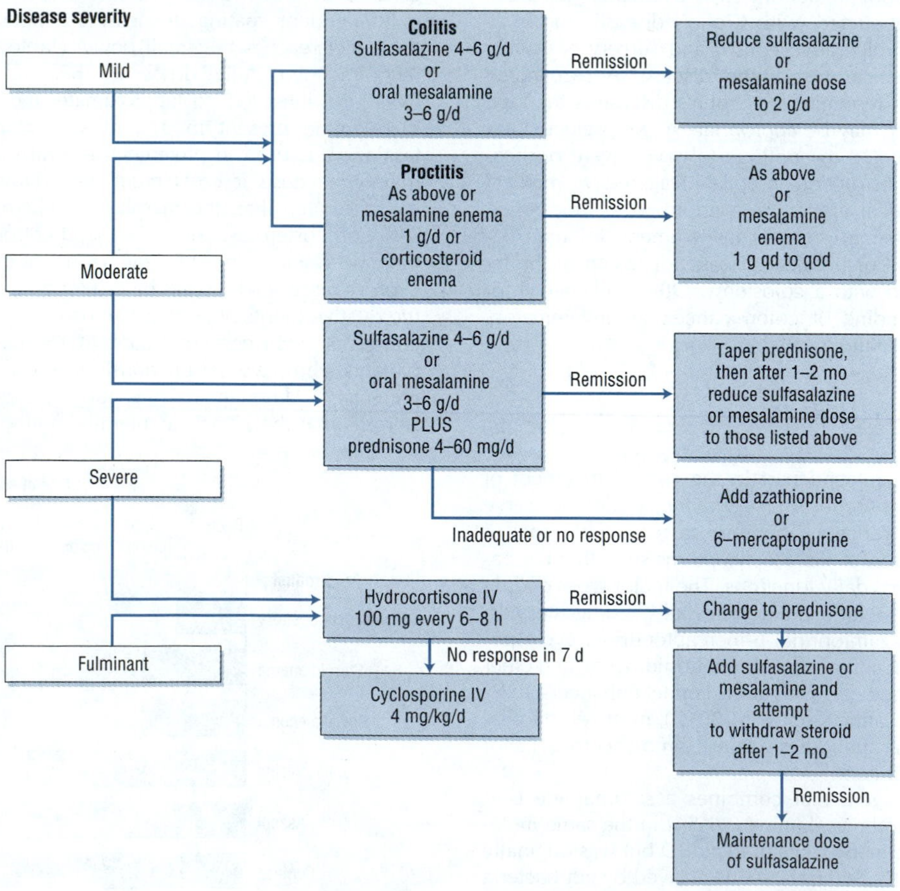

FIGURE 32–2. Treatment approaches for ulcerative colitis. *(Reprinted with permission from the American College of Clinical Pharmacy.)*

vere diarrhea, often necessitating discontinuation of the drug. This results from a direct effect of the drug to induce small bowel fluid secretion. For this reason it is not the drug of first choice. In some patients, combined use of oral sulfasalazine, Pentasa, or olsalazine and rectal steroids or rectal 5-ASA may provide advantages.[47]

Steroids have a place in the treatment of moderate to severe ulcerative colitis. Oral steroids (usually up to 1 mg/kg per day of prednisone equivalent) may be used for patients who do not have an adequate response to sulfasalazine or mesalamine. Prednisone dosages in the range of 40 mg/d to 60 mg/d have been superior to regimens of 20 mg/d in inducing remission.[48] Overall, steroids and sulfasalazine appear to be equally efficacious; however, the response to steroids may be evident sooner. The use of oral steroids as initial therapy for mild to moderate ulcerative colitis should be avoided, mainly because of the known risks of steroid use. If steroids are used to attain remission, tapered drug withdrawal should be accomplished to minimize long-term steroid exposure.

Rectally administered steroids or mesalamine can be used as initial therapy for patients with ulcerative proctitis or distal colitis. Rectal agents are also beneficial for treatment of tenesmus. With these agents, local actions are believed to be responsible for drug effects. Rectal steroids are effective in the treatment of active, distal ulcerative colitis. However, rectal mesalamine was more effective than rectal steroids for inducing remission.[49,50]

The choice of rectally administered steroid has been a subject of debate as there is varying potential for systemic steroid absorption with different products. Although many steroids have been administered rectally, certain agents such as betamethasone-17-valerate, beclomethasone dipropionate, prednisolone metasulfobenzoate, prednisolone-21-phosphate, and budesonide have been used in attempts to reduce systemic steroid effects. Systemic side effects may be the least severe with beclomethasone dipropionate, because this agent is rapidly metabolized by the gut wall and liver.[49] Most patients do not experience adrenal suppression from rectal steroids. The use of rectal steroids may often result in reduction of the required oral dose.

Nicotine has been proposed as a treatment for ulcerative colitis (but not Crohn's disease) based on the observation of the onset of a flare of ulcerative colitis after smoking cessation in some individuals. Transdermal nicotine, when used in the highest tolerated dose, improved symptoms of patients with mild to moderate, active ulcerative colitis.[51]

Severe or Intractable Disease

Patients with uncontrolled severe colitis or incapacitating symptoms require hospitalization for effective management. Under these conditions, patients generally receive nothing by mouth to put the bowel at rest; however, one study has demonstrated the benefit of enteral nutrition in these patients.[35] Most medication is given by the parenteral route. With severe colitis, there is a much greater reliance on parenteral steroids and surgical procedures. Sulfasalazine or mesalamine derivatives have not been proven beneficial for treatment of severe colitis. The reason for this may relate to rapid elimination of these agents from the colon with diarrhea, thereby not allowing sufficient time for gut bacteria to cleave the molecules. Overall, it is difficult to evaluate drugs in this setting, because patients with severe disease almost always receive additional medications including steroids.

Steroids have been valuable in the treatment of severe disease because the use of these agents may allow some patients to avoid colectomy. A trial of steroids is warranted in most patients before proceeding to colectomy, unless the condition is grave or rapidly deteriorating. The dose of steroid generally used is 1 mg/kg of prednisone equivalent daily (up to 60 mg/day), although some patients may require much less or much more for satisfactory control. With higher doses, however, steroid side effects may limit drug benefits. The length of the medical trial before consideration of surgery is open to debate. Steroids increase surgical risk, particularly infectious risk, if an operation is required later. After a colectomy is performed, steroids should no longer be required for the disease; however, they must be withdrawn gradually (usually over 3 to 4 weeks) to avoid hypoadrenal crisis from adrenal suppression.

A major development in the treatment of severe ulcerative colitis refractory to steroids has been intravenous cyclosporine.[52–54] Continuous intravenous infusion of cyclosporine (4 mg/kg/per day) was rapidly effective in steroid-resistant, acute, severe ulcerative colitis and reduced the need for emergent colectomy.[55] Intravenous cyclosporine has been recommended for all patients with acute, severe, active ulcerative colitis refractory to steroids.[56]

Maintenance of Remission

Once remission from active disease has been achieved, the goal of therapy is to maintain remission. The major agents used for maintenance of remission are sulfasalazine and the mesalamine derivatives; steroids usually do not have a role. The value of sulfasalazine in preventing recurrences has been documented in placebo-controlled trials. One-fourth of patients taking sulfasalazine (2 g/d) had a relapse within 1 year, while three-fourths of patients taking placebo had a relapse.[57]

Olsalazine, Pentasa (a slow-release oral form of mesalamine), and mesalamine enema have also been demonstrated effective for maintaining remission in patients with ulcerative colitis. Pentasa, given 500 mg three times daily, was as effective as sulfasalazine, given 1 g three times daily, in maintaining remission (54% versus 46% in remission at 12 months, respectively).[58] Mesalamine (Asacol), 0.8 or 1.6 g daily, was found effective for prevention of relapses over a 6-month period.[59]

A major question about the use of sulfasalazine for maintenance of remission with ulcerative colitis is the duration of the preventive regimen. Maintenance of remission has been well documented up to 1 year and may last as long as 3 years. The efficacy of sulfasalazine appears to be related to dose administered, up to a point. Although 4 g/day has a lower recurrence rate than 2 g or 1 g, a 4-g dose will result in intolerable side effects in about one-fourth of patients. Therefore 2 g/d is recommended.

Steroids do not have a role in the maintenance of remission with ulcerative colitis because they are ineffective.[43] Steroids should be gradually withdrawn after remission is induced (over 3 to 4 weeks). If they are continued, the patient will be exposed to steroid side effects without likelihood of benefits. For patients who require chronic steroid use (> 20 mg/d), there is a strong justification for alternative therapies or colectomy. Azathioprine is effective in preventing relapse of ulcerative colitis for periods of up to 2 years.[60] However, 3 to 6 months may be required for beneficial effect. Oral azathioprine has also been shown to maintain long-term remission after IV cyclosporine induction.[61]

CROHN'S DISEASE

Management of Crohn's disease often proves more difficult than that of ulcerative colitis, partly because of the greater complexity of presentation with Crohn's disease (Fig. 32–3). The disease may be found to involve any segment of the GI tract, from mouth to anus, and may involve other visceral structures and soft tissues through fistulization. There is a greater reliance on drug therapy with Crohn's disease, because resection of all involved intestine may not be possible and disease recurrence after surgery is common.

Active Crohn's Disease

The goal of treatment for active Crohn's disease is to achieve remission; however, in many patients, reduction of symptoms so that the patient may carry out normal activities, or reduction of the steroid dose required for control, is a significant accomplishment.

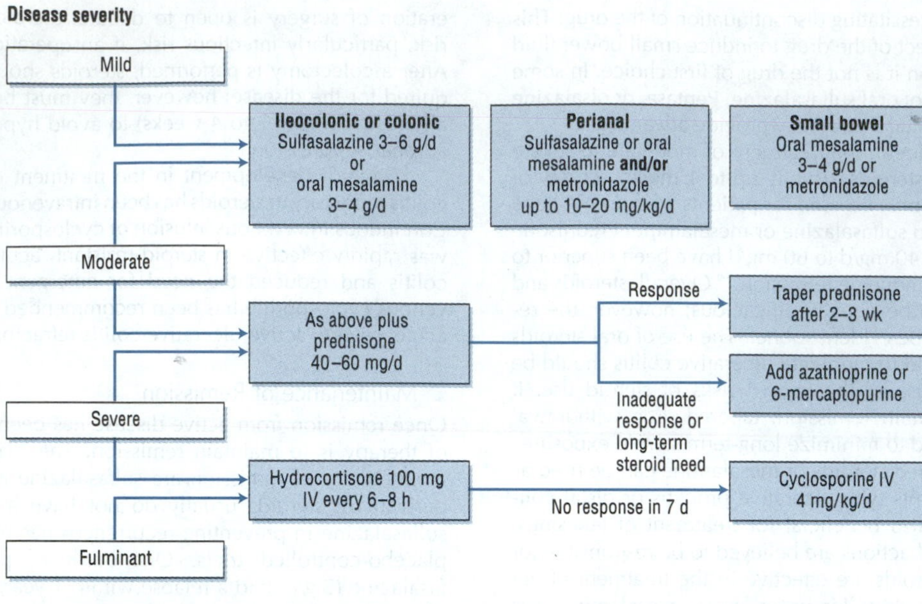

FIGURE 32–3. Treatment approaches for Crohn's disease. *(Reprinted with permission from the American College of Clinical Pharmacy.)*

In the majority of patients, active Crohn's disease is treated with sulfasalazine, mesalamine derivatives, or steroids, although azathioprine, 6-mercaptopurine, methotrexate, or metronidazole are frequently used.

The role of sulfasalazine in the treatment of active Crohn's disease is accepted but not as well established as its role in the treatment of ulcerative colitis. Sulfasalazine is more effective when Crohn's disease involves the colon.[30] In these circumstances, sulfasalazine has been reported to be as effective as prednisone.[30,62] It appears reasonable to initiate a trial of sulfasalazine or oral mesalamine derivative in patients with mild to moderate Crohn's disease, particularly when the colon is involved.

There is limited information also suggesting the benefit of sulfasalazine in ileal Crohn's disease.[63] Other mesalamine derivatives (such as Pentasa or Asacol) that release mesalamine in the small bowel may be more effective than sulfasalazine for ileal involvement. In a trial of 310 patients with active Crohn's disease, Pentasa alone was more effective than placebo in achieving remission in a 16-week trial (43% versus 18%, respectively).[64] This beneficial effect was dose dependent and greatest with a dose of 4 g/d. A course of steroids would be appropriate in patients who then cannot be controlled. When a patient is maintained on steroids, however, there appears to be no benefit from the addition of sulfasalazine.

Steroids are frequently used for the treatment of active Crohn's disease, particularly with more severe presentations. In the National Cooperative Crohn's Disease Study,[30] prednisone was more effective than placebo in achieving remission. In this trial, the prednisone doses were 0.25 mg/kg per day for mild disease, 0.5 mg/kg per day for moderate disease, and 0.75 mg/kg per day for severe disease. Prednisone was found to be effective for disease limited to the small bowel. The major limitation of steroids is the risk of adverse effects with long-term use.

Steroids are preferred for treatment of severe Crohn's disease, mainly because these agents can be given parenterally and response to therapy may occur sooner than with other agents. Once remission is achieved, however, it may prove difficult to reduce steroid dosage without a flare of active disease.[38]

Metronidazole (given orally up to 20 mg/kg per day in divided doses) may be useful in some patients with Crohn's disease, particularly in patients with colonic involvement or those with perineal disease.[45] For most patients, metronidazole would be added to sulfasalazine, a mesalamine derivative, or steroid therapy when those agents alone are not effective. The role for metronidazole is not fully defined. It may deserve a trial as adjunctive therapy for patients with colonic or perineal disease, where satisfactory control is not gained with first-line agents, or in attempts to reduce steroid dosage.[38,65]

The immunosuppressive agents (azathioprine and 6-mercaptopurine) are generally limited to use in patients not achieving adequate response to standard medical therapy, or to reduce steroid doses when high steroid doses are required. Azathioprine and 6-mercaptopurine demonstrated long-term benefits in patients with Crohn's disease.[42] The usual doses of azathioprine are 2 to 2.5 mg/kg per day, and for 6-mercaptopurine 1 to 1.5 mg/kg per day. They are begun at 50 mg/day and increased at 2-week intervals while monitoring white blood cell and platelet counts. Treatment with azathioprine may need to be continued for up to 6 months to observe a response.[43] In one trial of patients already receiving sulfasalazine or prednisone, 6-mercaptopurine decreased steroid requirement and healed fistulas. One problem noted with 6-mercaptopurine was that more than 3 months was required to observe a response in 32% of patients. In a report of 20 years of experience with 148 patients, 6-mercaptopurine (50 mg/d for mean 34 months) was judged effective for reduction of steroid dosage or elimination of the need for steroids, healing of fistulas and abscesses, and healing of Crohn's disease of the stomach and duodenum.[66] Some investigators have suggested that azathioprine or 6-mercaptopurine should be started earlier in the course of treatment than has been traditional.

Cyclosporine has also demonstrated benefit in active Crohn's disease.[52,53] Improvement was noted with cyclosporine in patients who were resistant or intolerant to corticosteroids.[67] The dose of cyclosporine is important in determining efficacy. An oral dose of 5 mg/kg per day was not effective,[68] whereas 7.9 mg/kg per day was effective.[67] However, toxic effects limit application of the higher dosage. At present, the therapeutic blood or plasma concentration range for cyclosporine has not been established. When using cyclosporine, however, clinicians should recognize the accompanying long-term risk of renal toxicity. Methotrexate given as a weekly injection of 25 mg has demonstrated corticosteroid-sparing effects.[69,70] It is not clear if the benefit of methotrexate surpasses the risks (bone marrow suppression, hepatotoxicity, pulmonary toxicity).

Maintenance of Remission

Prevention of recurrence of disease is clearly more difficult with Crohn's disease than with ulcerative colitis. There is evidence that some agents, particularly sulfasalazine and oral mesalamine derivatives, are effective in preventing acute recurrences in quiescent Crohn's disease.[71] The support for sulfasalazine has been largely anecdotal[71]; however, a trial of 232 patients demonstrated a lower relapse rate compared with placebo for up to 2 years when given 3 g/d.[72]

There is support for the use of oral mesalamine derivatives for maintenance of symptomatic remission. On average, oral mesalamine derivatives decrease recurrence rates by 40% compared with placebo in long-term studies.[68] In one trial of 161 patients in remission, 2 g/d of mesalamine (Pentasa) for 2 years resulted in a significantly reduced relapse rate when begun within 3 months of achieving remission.[73] In another trial of mesalamine (Asacol), 125 patients received 2.4 g/d or placebo for 12 months, resulting in a significantly reduced relapse rate with Asacol.[74] Steroids also have no place in the prevention of recurrence of Crohn's disease; these agents do not appear to alter the long-term course of the disease. However, a study of oral budesonide 6 mg/day demonstrated prolongation of time to relapse in ileal and ileocecal disease.[75]

Azathioprine has been studied as an adjunctive agent for the treatment and prevention of Crohn's disease. Although the published data are not consistent, there is evidence to suggest that azathioprine and 6-mercaptopurine are effective in maintaining remission in Crohn's disease.[43,44] This agent should be reserved for patients who cannot tolerate dosages of steroids required to control their disease and who are not good surgical candidates.

Many new agents are under investigation for treatment of inflammatory bowel diseases. Among the most exciting are monoclonal antibodies that bind to inflammatory mediators. In a small trial, a single infusion of an antitumor necrosis factor α antibody (cA2) induced remission and endoscopic healing in patients with active Crohn's disease.[76] Lipoxygenase inhibitors have also gained attention as possible treatments for inflammatory bowel disease.

SELECTED COMPLICATIONS

TOXIC MEGACOLON

Toxic megacolon or "toxic colonic dilatation" is a serious complication of IBD that occurs in about 1% or 2% of patients with IBDs, particularly ulcerative colitis. As previously described, the patient with toxic megacolon is usually severely ill with fever, abdominal pain and distention, and decreased bowel sounds; has bloody diarrhea; and is often dehydrated. Immediate and aggressive measures are required to minimize mortality.

The treatment required for toxic megacolon includes general supportive measures to maintain vital functions, consideration for early surgical intervention, and drugs (steroids, cyclosporine, and antimicrobials). Aggressive fluid and electrolyte management is required for dehydration. Fluids and electrolytes may be lost through vomiting, diarrhea, and nasogastric intubation, as well as through fluid accumulation in the bowel. When the patient has lost significant amounts of blood (through the rectum), blood replacement is also necessary. Opiates and anticholinergics should be discontinued because these agents enhance colonic dilatation, thereby increasing the risk of bowel perforation. Broad-spectrum antimicrobials should be used that include coverage for gram-negative bacilli and intestinal anaerobes.

Steroids in high dosages should be administered intravenously to reduce acute inflammation. Doses as high as 2 mg/kg per day of prednisone equivalent have been recommended (generally administered as hydrocortisone).[4] The duration of steroid administration is not certain; however, most clinicians continue the high-dose steroids for up to 2 weeks after improvement is observed and then reduce the dosages (approximately 0.5 to 1 mg/kg per day) for a few additional weeks. Antimicrobial regimens that are effective against enteric aerobes and anaerobes (e.g., aminoglycoside with clindamycin or metronidazole, imipenem, or extended-spectrum penicillin with β-lactamase inhibitor) should be administered from the time of diagnosis and continued until patient improvement is assured. The duration of the antimicrobial regimen (often 2 to 3 weeks) should be determined with consideration that there may be significant intra-abdominal contamination with signs and symptoms hidden by steroid effects.

Surgical intervention, mainly an abdominal colectomy with formation of an ileostomy, is an important consideration in patients with toxic megacolon and prevents death in some patients. Early surgical intervention in these patients may result in a reduced mortality rate. In most cases in which colectomy is performed in the face of toxic megacolon, there is a significant risk of operative complications, including postoperative infection.

SYSTEMIC MANIFESTATIONS

The common systemic manifestations of IBD include arthritis, anemia, skin manifestations such as erythema nodosum and pyoderma gangrenosum, uveitis, and liver disease. These problems may be related to the inflammatory process. For some of these manifestations, specific therapies can be instituted, while for others, treatment that is used for the GI inflammatory process also addresses the systemic manifestations.

Anemia occurs when there is significant blood loss from the GI tract. If the patient can consume oral medication, ferrous sulfate should be administered. If the patient is not able to take oral medication and the patient's hematocrit is sufficiently low, blood transfusions may be required. Anemia may also be related to malabsorption of vitamin B_{12} or folic acid, so these may also be required.

There are no consistently recommended therapies for liver disease, skin manifestations, or uveitis associated with IBD. Some reports suggest that these manifestations are worse during exacerbations of the intestinal disease and that measures improving intestinal disease will improve these systemic manifestations. Unfortunately, this association has not been demonstrated consistently. Liver transplantation is being used more frequently for definitive treatment of sclerosing cholangitis. For arthritis associated with IBD, aspirin or another NSAID may be beneficial, as would be steroids.

SPECIAL CONSIDERATIONS

PREGNANCY

Either the occurrence or consideration of pregnancy may cause significant concerns in the patient with IBD. Questions arise as to fertility in patients with IBD, the effect of pregnancy on the disease course, the effect of the disease on the outcome of pregnancy, and the effects of the drugs used in IBD on the fetus.[77]

Patients with IBD do not appear to be less fertile than women in general.[4,78] The rate of normal childbirth is similar to that for healthy populations. Some studies have noted, however, a greater risk of spontaneous abortions in patients with IBD. Also, there is a greater incidence of low-birthweight infants of mothers with chronic idiopathic ulcerative colitis.[79] Pregnancy does not affect the course of IBD. Patients who are pregnant experience recurrence rates similar to those of nonpregnant females. Also, there is no justification for therapeutic abortion with IBD because termination of the pregnancy has not been observed to improve the disease. There is also unfounded concern that the drugs required to treat IBD may be teratogenic.

Steroids and sulfasalazine should be administered during pregnancy with the same guidelines that would be applied to the nonpregnant patient.[4,78] Steroids given systemically do not appear to be detrimental to the fetus. Sulfasalazine is generally well tolerated; however, there has been suggestion of increased frequency of congenital abnormalities when it is given during pregnancy.[80] Interestingly, sulfasalazine has also been reported to cause decreased sperm counts and reduced fertility in males.[81] This effect is reversible on discontinuation of the drug and it is not reported with mesalamine. Immunosuppressive drugs (azathioprine and 6-mercaptopurine) may be associated with fetal deformities in humans; however, they have been used without detriment in some patients.[78] Metronidazole should not be used in those contemplating pregnancy as it may be teratogenic.

Overall, drug therapy for IBD is not a contraindication for pregnancy, and most pregnancies are well managed in patients with these diseases. The indications for medical and surgical treatment are similar to those in the nonpregnant patient. If a patient has an initial bout of IBD during pregnancy, a standard approach to treatment should be initiated.

Recommendations for use of drugs in nursing mothers vary. Although prednisone and prednisolone can be detected in breast milk, breast feeding is believed to be safe for the infant when low doses of prednisone are used.[82] Sulfasalazine does not pose a risk of kernicterus, as levels of sulfapyridine in breast milk are low or undetectable. Metronidazole should not be given to nursing mothers because it is excreted into breast milk.[82]

ADVERSE EFFECTS

Drug intolerance often limits the usefulness of agents used to treat IBD. Many patients receiving sulfasalazine, mesalamine, corticosteroids, metronidazole, azathioprine, or 6-mercaptopurine experience some undesired effects. In some cases, these adverse effects can be significant and require discontinuation of the therapy. Knowledge of the common or important adverse reactions will assist in avoiding or minimizing their effects.

Sulfasalazine is often associated with adverse drug effects and these effects may be classified as either dose related or idiosyncratic. Dose-related side effects usually include GI disturbances such as nausea, vomiting, diarrhea, or anorexia, but may also include headache and arthralgia.[38] These adverse reactions tend to occur more commonly on initiation of therapy and decrease in frequency as therapy is continued. Patients may experience these adverse effects at the commonly used dosages. One approach to the management of these reactions is to discontinue the agent for a short period and then reinstitute therapy at a reduced dosage. Some have suggested that the rate of adverse effects may be related to the concentration of free sulfapyridine in serum, suggesting that the sulfa portion of the molecule is responsible for the adverse effects.[83] Folic acid absorption is impaired by sulfasalazine, which may lead to anemia. Patients receiving sulfasalazine should receive oral folic acid supplementation.

Adverse effects that are not dose related include rash, fever, or hepatotoxicity most commonly, as well as relatively uncommon but serious reactions such as bone marrow suppression, thrombocytopenia, pancreatitis, and hepatitis.[38] For most patients with idiosyncratic reactions, sulfasalazine must be discontinued. In some patients who have experienced allergic reactions to sulfasalazine, a desensitization procedure can be instituted. By gradually increasing sulfasalazine dosage over weeks to months, patient tolerance has been improved.[84] Most of the idiosyncratic reactions observed with sulfasalazine are similar to those with the class of sulfonamides in general.

Oral mesalamine derivatives may impose a lower frequency of adverse effects compared with sulfasalazine. Many patients who are intolerant to sulfasalazine will tolerate oral mesalamine derivatives.[85] Olsalazine, however, may frequently (up to 25%) cause watery diarrhea, sometimes requiring drug discontinuation.[86,87]

Adverse reactions to corticosteroids have been well recognized and may occur when corticosteroids are used for any indication. There is a greater potential for adverse effects when corticosteroids are used for the treatment of IBD, however, because high doses must often be used for extended periods. In the National Cooperative Crohn's Disease Study, 50% of patients receiving high-dose steroid therapy experienced side effects, as did one-third of the patients on the lower-dose regimens for prophylaxis.[88] The well-appreciated adverse effects of corticosteroids include hyperglycemia, hypertension, osteoporosis, acne, fluid retention, electrolyte disturbances, myopathies, muscle wasting, increased appetite, psychosis, and reduced resistance to infection. In addition, corticosteroid use may cause adrenocortical suppression. Specific regimens for withdrawal of corticosteroid therapy have been suggested.[89] To minimize corticosteroid effects, clinicians have used alternate-day steroid therapy; however, some patients do not do well on the days when no steroid is given. For most patients, a single daily corticosteroid dose suffices, and divided daily doses are unnecessary.

Immunosuppressants such as azathioprine and 6-mercaptopurine have a significant potential for adverse reactions. Azathioprine causes bone marrow suppression and has been associated with lymphomas (in renal transplant patients), skin cancer, and pancreatitis (about 3% of patients). 6-Mercaptopurine causes adverse reactions similar to azathioprine; however, there are fewer reports of lymphomas with this agent. With 6-mercaptopurine, pancreatitis usually occurs within 1 month of initiating therapy and recurs if the patient is rechallenged.[89] In one trial, 10% of patients who received azathioprine or 6-mercaptopurine required discontinuation of treatment due to adverse effects.[90] Allopurinal inhibits the metabolism of 6-mercaptopurine, and a dosage reduction of the latter is required when the two are used in combination.

Most patients receiving metronidazole for Crohn's disease tolerate the agent fairly well; however, mild adverse effects occur frequently. They commonly include paresthesias and reversible peripheral neuropathy, metallic taste, urticaria, and glossitis.[45,91] Other effects include a disulfiram-like reaction if alcohol is ingested in conjunction.

EVALUATION OF THERAPEUTIC OUTCOMES

The success of therapeutic regimens to treat IBD can be measured by patient-reported complaints, signs, and symptoms; direct physician examination (including endoscopy); history and physical examination; selected laboratory tests; and quality-of-life measures. Evaluation of IBD severity is difficult, because much of the assessment is subjective. To create more objective measures, disease rating scales or indices have been created. The Crohn's Disease Activity Index (CDAI) is a commonly used scale, particularly for evaluation of patients during clinical trials.[92] The scale incorporates eight elements: (1) number of stools in the past 7 days, (2) sum of abdominal pain ratings from the past 7 days, (3) rating of general well-being in the past 7 days, (4) use of antidiarrheals, (5) body weight, (6) hematocrit, (7) finding of abdominal mass, and (8) a sum of symptoms present in the past week. Elements of this index provide a guide for those measures that may be useful in assessing the effectiveness of treatment regimens.

Standardized assessment tools have also been constructed for ulcerative colitis.[22,93] Elements in these scales include (1) stool frequency, (2) presence of blood in the stool, (3) mucosal appearance (from endoscopy), and (4) physician's global assessment based on physical examination, endoscopy, and laboratory data.

Additional studies that are often useful include direct endoscopic examination of affected areas and/or radiocontrast studies. For patients with acute disease, assessment of fluid and electrolyte status is important, because these may be lost during diarrheal episodes. Other laboratory tests, such as serum albumin, transferrin, or other markers of visceral protein status, as well as markers of inflammation (erythrocyte sedimentation rate) may be used.

Assessment of the IBD patient must include consideration of adverse drug effects. Given that many of the agents used have a relatively high probability of causing adverse effects, particularly corticosteroids and other immunosuppressive agents, patient assessment should include collection of history and physical and laboratory data that are necessary to prevent or recognize adverse drug effects.

Finally, a patient quality-of-life assessment should be performed regularly.[94] Agents that appear clinically equivalent may differ substantially in resulting quality of life. Inquiry should be made regarding general well-being, emotional function, and social function. The latter may include assessment of the ability to perform routine daily functions, maintain occupational activities, sexual function, and recreation.

▶ PRINCIPLES OF PHARMACOTHERAPY

- The exact cause of inflammatory bowel disease is unknown, although there are components that appear to be infectious and others that suggest immune dysregulation.
- Ulcerative colitis is confined to the rectum and colon, causes continuous lesions, and affects primarily the mucosa and the submucosa. Crohn's disease can involve any part of the GI tract, often causes discontinuous (skip) lesions, and is a transmural process that can result in fistulas, perforations, or strictures.
- Common complications of IBD include rectal fissures, fistulas (Crohn's disease), perirectal abscess (ulcerative colitis), and colon cancer, in addition to hepatobiliary complications, arthritis, uveitis, skin lesions (including erythema nodosum and pyoderma gangrenosum), and aphthous ulcerations of the mouth.
- The severity of ulcerative colitis may be assessed by factors such as stool frequency, presence of blood in stool, fever, pulse, hemoglobin, erythrocyte sedimentation rate, abdominal tenderness, and radiologic or endoscopic findings. The severity of Crohn's disease can be assessed by the Crohn's Disease Activity Index, which includes stool frequency, presence of blood in stool, endoscopic appearance, and physician's global assessment.
- The goals of treatment of IBD are resolution of acute inflammation and complications, alleviation of systemic manifestations, maintenance of remission, and, in some patients, surgical palliation or cure.
- The first line of treatment for mild to moderate ulcerative colitis or Crohn's colitis consists of oral sulfasalazine or mesalamine, while mesalamine or steroid enemas may be used for rectosigmoid disease. Delayed-release oral formulations of mesalamine (Pentasa or Asacol) may be used for Crohn's ileitis.
- Corticosteroids are often required for acute ulcerative colitis or Crohn's disease. The duration of steroid use should be minimized and the dose tapered gradually over 3 to 4 weeks.
- Intravenous continuous infusion cyclosporine is effective in treating severe colitis refractory to steroids.
- Sulfasalazine and mesalamine derivatives can prevent recurrence of acute disease in many patients, while steroids are not effective for this purpose.
- Other drugs that are useful for treatment of Crohn's disease include metronidazole (for perineal disease), azathioprine or 6-mercaptopurine (for inadequate response or to reduce steroid dosage), or cyclosporine (for refractory disease).

REFERENCES

1. Kraft SC. Modern clinical aspects of inflammatory bowel disease. Radiol Clin North Am 1987;25:213–224.
2. Whelan G. Epidemiology of inflammatory bowel disease. Med Clin North Am 1990;74:1–12.
3. Sandler RS. Epidemiology of inflammatory bowel disease. In: Targan SR, Shanahan F, eds. Inflammatory Bowel Disease, from Bench to Bedside. Baltimore, Williams & Wilkins, 1994:5–30.
4. Cello JP. Ulcerative colitis. In: Sleisenger MH, Fordtran JS, eds. Gastrointestinal Disease, 5th ed. Philadelphia, Saunders, 1993: 1122–1168.
5. Russel MG, Stockbtugger RW. Epidemiology of inflammatory bowel disease. Scand J Gastroenterol 1996;31:417–427.
6. Pavli P, Cavanaugh J, Grimm M. Inflammatory bowel disease: Germs or genes? Lancet 1996;347:1198.
7. Elson CO. The immunology of inflammatory bowel disease. In: Kirsner JB, Sorter RG, eds. Inflammatory Bowel Disease. Philadelphia, Lea & Febiger, 1988:97–164.

8. Shanahan F. Pathogenesis of ulcerative colitis. Lancet 1993:342: 407–411.
9. MacDermott RP. Alterations of the mucosal immune system in inflammatory bowel disease. J Gastroenterol 1996;31:907–916.
10. Gorbach SI. Intestinal microflora in inflammatory bowel disease—Implications for etiology. In: Kirsner JB, Shorter RG, eds. Inflammatory Bowel Disease. Philadelphia, Lea & Febiger, 1988: 51–64.
11. McKenzie SJ, Baker MS, Buffington GD, Doe WF. Evidence of oxidant-induced injury to epithelial cells during inflammatory bowel disease. J Clin Invest 1996;98:136–141.
12. Podolsky DK. Inflammatory bowel disease. Second of two parts. N Engl J Med 1991;325:1008–1015.
13. Yang H, Rotter JI. Genetics of inflammatory bowel disease. In: Targan SR, Shanahan F, eds. Inflammatory Bowel Disease, from Bench to Bedside. Baltimore, Williams & Wilkins, 1994:32–64.
14. Sandborn WJ, Landers CJ, Tremaine WJ, Targan BR. Association of antineutrophil cytoplasmic antibodies with resistance to treatment of left-sided ulcerative colitis: Results of a pilot study. Mayo Clin Proc 1996;71:431–436.
15. Nielsen OH, Koppen T, Rudiger N, et al. Involvement of interleukin-4 and -10 in inflammatory bowel disease. Dig Dis Sci 1996;41: 1786–1793.
16. Parronchi P, Romagnani P, Annunziato F, et al. Type 1 T-helper cell predominance and interleukin-12 expression in the gut of patients with Crohn's disease. Am J Pathol 1997;150:823–832.
17. Niesser M, Volk BA. Altered Th1/Th2 cytokine profiles in the intestinal mucosa of patients with inflammatory bowel disease as assessed by quantitative reversed transcribed polymerase chain reaction (RT-PCR). Clin Exp Immunol 1995;101:428–435.
18. Braegger CP, Nicholls S, Murch SH, et al. Tumour necrosis factor alpha in stool as a marker of intestinal inflammation. Lancet 1992; 339:89–91.
19. Talala AH, Drossman DP. Psycosocial factors in inflammatory bowel disease. Gastroenterol Clin North Am 1995;24:699–716.
20. Podolsky DK. Inflammatory bowel disease. First of two parts. N Engl J Med 1991;325:928–937.
21. Boyko ES, Koesell TD, Perera DR, Inui TS. Risk of ulcerative colitis among former and current cigarette smokers. N Engl J Med 1987; 316:707–710.
22. Pullan RD, Rhodes J, Ganesh S, et al. Transdermal nicotine for active ulcerative colitis. N Engl J Med 1994;330:811–815.
23. Ramming KP. Diseases of the rectum and colin. In: Sabiston DC, ed. Essentials of Surgery. Philadelphia, Saunders, 1987:483.
24. Lichenstein JE. Radiologic-pathologic correlation of inflammatory bowel disease. Radiol Clin North Am 1987;25:3–24.
25. Monsen V, Sorstad J, Hellers G, et al. Extracolonic diagnosis in ulcerative colitis: An epidemiologic study. Am J Gastroenterol 1990; 85:711–716.
26. Harmatz A. Hepatobiliary manifestations of inflammatory bowel disease. Med Clin North Am 1994;78:1387–1398.
27. Rankin GB. Extraintestinal and systemic manifestations of inflammatory bowel disease. Med Clin North Am 1990;74:39–50.
28. O'Keefe SJD, Rosser BG. Nutrition and inflammatory bowel disease. In: Targan SR, Shanahan F, eds. Inflammatory Bowel Disease, from Bench to Bedside. Baltimore, Williams & Wilkins, 1994: 461–477.
29. Janowicz HD. The "natural history" of inflammatory bowel disease and therapeutic decisions. Am J Gastroenterol 1987;82:498–503.
30. Summers RW, Switz DM, Sessions JT, et al. National Cooperative Crohn's Disease Study: Results of drug treatment. Gastroenterology 1979;77:847–869.
31. Malchow H, Ewe K, Brandes JW, et al. European Cooperative Crohn's Disease Study (ECCDS): Results of drug treatment. Gastroenterology 1984;86:249–266.
32. Stenson WF, Cort D, Rogers J, et al. Dietary supplementation with fish oil in ulcerative colitis. Ann Intern Med 1992;116:609–614.
33. Belluzzi A, Brignola C, Campieri M, et al. Effect of an enteric-coated fish-oil preparation on relapses in Crohn's disease. N Engl J Med 1996;334:1557–1560.
34. Wu S, Craig RM. Intense nutritional support in inflammatory bowel disease. Dig Dis Sci 1995;40:843–852.
35. Gonzalez-Huix F, Fernandez-Banares F, Esteve-Comas M, et al. Enteral versus parenteral nutrition as adjunct therapy in acute ulcerative colitis. Am J Gastroenterol 1993;88:227–232.
36. Lewis JD, Fisher RL. Nutritional support in inflammatory bowel disease. Med Clin North Am 1994;78:1443–1456.
37. Klotz U, Maier K, Fischer C, et al. Therapeutic efficacy of sulfasalazine and its metabolites in patients with ulcerative colitis and Crohn's disease. N Engl J Med 1980;303:1499–1502.
38. Hanauer SB. Inflammatory bowel disease. N Engl J Med 1996;334: 841–848.
39. Ruderman WB. Newer pharmacologic agents for therapy of inflammatory bowel disease. Med Clin North Am 1990;74:133–153.
40. Meyers S, Sachar DB, Goldberg JD, Janowitz HD. Corticotropin versus hydrocortisone in the intravenous treatment of ulcerative colitis. A prospective, randomized, double-blind trial. Gastroenterology 1983;85:351–357.
41. Sandborn WJ. A review of immune modifier therapy for inflammatory bowel disease: Azathioprine, 6-mercaptopurine, cyclosporine. Am J Gastroenterol 1996;91:423–433.
42. Pearson DC, May GR, Fick GH, et al. Azathioprine and 6-mercaptopurine in Crohn's disease: A meta analysis. Ann Intern Med 1995;123:134–142.
43. Hanauer SB, Baert F. Medical therapy of inflammatory bowel disease. Med Clin North Am 1994;78:1413–1426.
44. Hawthorne AB, Logan RFA, Hawkey CJ, et al. Randomized controlled trial of azathioprine withdrawal in ulcerative colitis. BMJ 1992; 305:20–22.
45. Sutherland L, Singleton J, Sessions J, et al. Double-blind, placebo controlled trial of metronidazole in Crohn's disease. Gut 1991;32: 1071–1075.
46. Sutherland LR, May GR, Shaffer EA. Sulfasalazine revisited: A meta-analysis of 5-aminosalicylic acid in the treatment of ulcerative colitis. Ann Intern Med 1993;118:540–549.
47. D'Albasio G, Pacini F, Camarri E, et al. Combined therapy with 5-aminosalicylic acid tablets and enemas for maintaining remission in ulcerative colitis: A randomized double-blind study. Am J Gastroenterol 1997;92:1143–1147.
48. Powell-Tuck J, Brown RL, Lennard-Jones JE. A comparison of oral prednisone given as single or multiple daily doses for active proctocolitis. Scand J Gastroenterol 1975;13:833–837.
49. Marshall JK, Irvine EJ. Rectal corticosteroids versus alternative treatments in ulcerative colitis: A meta-analysis. Gut 1997;40: 775–781.
50. Lee FI, Jewell DP, Mani V, et al. A randomized trial comparing mesalamine and prednisone foam enemas in patients with acute distal ulcerative colitis. Gut 1996;38:229–233.
51. Sandborn WJ, Tremaine WJ, Offord KP, et al. Transdermal nicotine for mild to moderately active ulcerative colitis. A randomized, double-blind, placebo controlled trial. Ann Intern Med 1997;126:364–371.
52. Sandborn WJ, Tremaine WJ. Cyclosporine treatment of inflammatory bowel disease. Mayo Clin Proc 1992;67:981–990.
53. Present DH, Lichtiger S. Efficacy of cyclosporine in treatment of fistula of Crohn's disease. Dig Dis Sci 1994;39:374–380.
54. Carbonnel F, Boruchowicz A, Duclos B, et al. Intravenous cyclosporine in attacks of ulcerative colitis: Short term and long term responses. Dig Dis Sci 1996;41:2471–2476.
55. Lichtiger S, Present DH, Kornbluth A, et al. Cyclosporine in severe ulcerative colitis refractory to steroid therapy. N Engl J Med 1994; 330:1841–1845.
56. Present DH. Cyclosporine and other immunosuppressive agents: Current and future role in the treatment of inflammatory bowel disease. Am J Gastroenterol 1993;88:627–630.

57. Misiewicz JJ, Lennard-Jones JE, Connell AM, et al. Controlled trial of sulphasalazine in maintenance therapy for ulcerative colitis. Lancet 1965;1:185–188.
58. Mulder CJ, Tytgat GNJ, Weterman IT, et al. Double-blind comparison of slow-release 5-aminosalicylate and sulfasalazine in remission maintenance in ulcerative colitis. Gastroenterology 1988;95:1449–1453.
59. Mesalamine Study Group. An oral preparation of mesalamine therapy for ulcerative colitis. A randomized, placebo controlled trial. Ann Intern Med 1996;124:204–211.
60. Hawthorne AB, Logan RFA, Hawkey CJ. Randomized controlled trial of azathioprine withdrawal in ulcerative colitis. Br Med J 1992; 305:20–22.
61. Fernandez-Banares F, Bertran X, Esteve-Comas M, et al. Azathioprine is useful in maintaining long-term remission induced by intravenous cyclosporine in steroid-refractory severe ulcerative colitis. Am J Gastroenterol 1996;91:2498–2499.
62. Salomon P, Kornbluth A, Aisenberg J, et al. How effective are current therapies for Crohn's disease? A meta-analysis. Am J Gastroenterol 1992;14:211–215.
63. Goldstein F, Farquhar S, Thornton JJ, et al. Favorable effects of sulfasalazine on small-bowel Crohn's disease. A long-term study. Am J Gastroenterol 1987;82:848–853.
64. Singleton JW, Hanauer SB, Gitnick GL, et al. Mesalamine capsules for the treatment of active Crohn's disease: Results of a 16-week trial. Gastroenterology 1993;104:1293–1301.
65. Ewe K, Press AG, Singe CC, et al. Azathioprine combined with prednisolone or monotherapy with prednisolone in active Crohn's disease. Gastroenterology 1993;105:367–372.
66. Korelitz BI, Adler DJ, Mendelsohn RA, Sacknoff AL. Long-term experience with 6-mercaptopurine in the treatment of Crohn's disease. Am J Gastroenterol 1993;88:1198–1205.
67. Brynskov J, Freund L, Rasmussen SN, et al. A placebo-controlled, double-blind, randomized trial of cyclosporine therapy in active chronic Crohn's disease. N Engl J Med 1989;321:845–850.
68. Stark ME, Tremaine WJ. Maintenance of symptomatic remission in patients with Crohn's disease. Mayo Clin Proc 1993;68:1183–1190.
69. Feagan BG, Rochon J, Fedorak RN, et al. Methotrexate for the treatment of Crohn's disease. N Engl J Med 1995;332:292–297.
70. Egan LJ, Sandborn WJ. Methotrexate for inflammatory bowel disease: Pharmacology and preliminary results. Mayo Clin Proc 1996; 71:69–80.
71. Goldstein F. Maintenance treatment for Crohn's disease: Has the time arrived? Am J Gastroenterol 1992;87:551–556.
72. Ewe K, Herfarth C, Malchow H, Jesdinsky HJ. Postoperative recurrence of Crohn's disease in relation to radicality of operation and sulfasalazine prophylaxis: A multicenter trial. Digestion 1989;42: 224–232.
73. Gendre JP, Mary JY, Florent C, et al. Oral mesalamine (Pentasa) as maintenance treatment in Crohn's disease: A multicenter placebo-controlled study. Gastroenterology 1993;104:435–439.
74. Prantera C, Pallone F, Brunetti G, et al. Oral 5-aminosalicylic acid (Asacol) in the maintenance treatment of Crohn's disease. Gastroenterology 1992;103:363–368.
75. Lofberg R, Rutgeerts P, Malchow H. Budesonide prolongs time to relapse in ileal and ileocecal Crohn's disease. A placebo controlled, one year study. Gut 1996;39:82–86.
76. Van Dulleman, van Deventer SJH, Hommes DW, et al. Treatment of Crohn's disease with anti-tumor necrosis factor chimeric monoclonal antibody (cA2). Gastroenterology 1995;109:129–135.
77. Brostrom O. Prognosis in ulcerative colitis. Med Clin North Am 1990;74:201–218.
78. Hanan IM. Inflammatory bowel disease in the pregnant woman. Compr Ther 1993;19:91–95.
79. Schade RR, Van Thiel DH, Gavaler JS. Chronic idiopathic ulcerative colitis: Pregnancy and fetal outcome. Dig Dis Sci 1984;29:614–619.
80. Willoughby JMT, Truelove SC. Ulcerative colitis and pregnancy. Gut 1980;21:469.
81. Toovey S, Hudson E, Hendry WF, et al. Sulfasalazine and male infertility: Reversibility and possible mechanism. Gut 1981;22: 445–451.
82. Farraye FA. Pregnancy and nursing. In: Peppercorn MA, ed. Therapy of Inflammatory Bowel Disease. New York, Marcel Dekker, 1990.
83. Das KM, Eastwood MA, McManus JPA, et al. Adverse reactions during salicylazosulfapyridine therapy and the relation with drug metabolism and acetylator phenotype. N Engl J Med 1973;289: 491–495.
84. Korelitz BI, Present DH, Rubin PH, et al. Desensitization to sulfasalazine after hypersensitivity reactions in patients with inflammatory bowel disease. J Clin Gastroenterol 1984;6:27–31.
85. Linn FV, Peppercorn MA. Drug therapy for inflammatory bowel disease, I. Am J Surg 1992;164:85–89.
86. Feurle GE, Theuer D, Velasco S, et al. Olsalazine versus placebo in the treatment of mild to moderate ulcerative colitis: A randomized double-blind trial. Gut 1989;30:1354–1361.
87. Zinberg J, Molinas S, Das KM. Double-blind placebo-controlled study of olsalazine in the treatment of ulcerative colitis. Am J Gastroenterol 1990;85:562–566.
88. Azad Khan AK, Truelove SC. Circulating levels of sulphasalazine and its metabolites and their relation to the clinical efficacy of the drug in ulcerstive colitis. Gut 1980;21:706–710.
89. Haber CJ, Meltzer SJ, Present DH, et al. Nature and course of pancreatitis caused by 6-mercaptopurine in the treatment of inflammatory bowel disease. Gastroenterology 1986;91:982–986.
90. O'Brien JJ, Bayless TM, Bayless JA. Use of azathioprine or 6-mercaptopurine in the treatment of Crohn's disease. Gastroenterology 1991;101:39–46.
91. Duffy LF, Daum F, Fisher SE, et al. Peripheral neuropathy in Crohn's disease patients treated with metronidazole. Gastroenterology 1984; 88:681–684.
92. Best WR, Becktel JM, Singleton JW, et al. Development of a Crohn's disease activity index. Gastroenterology 1976;70:439–444.
93. Sanborn WJ, Tremaine WJ, Schroeder KW, et al. Cyclosporine enemas for treatment-resistant, mildly to moderately active, left sided ulcerative colitis. Am J Gastroenterol 1993;88:640–645.
94. Irvine EJ, Zhou Q, Thompson AK. The short inflammatory bowel disease questionaire: A quality of life instrument for community physicians managing inflammatory bowel disease. CERPT investigators. Canadian Crohn's relapse prevention trial. Am J Gasroenterol 1996;91:1571–1578.

33

NAUSEA AND VOMITING

A. Thomas Taylor, PharmD

Nausea and vomiting are common complaints among many individuals with gastrointestinal (GI) disorders. However, because of the variable etiologies of these problems, management may be quite simple or detailed and complex, essentially innocuous or associated with therapy-induced adverse reactions. This chapter provides an overview of nausea and vomiting, two multifaceted problems.

Nausea is usually defined as the inclination to vomit or as a feeling in the throat or epigastric region alerting an individual that vomiting is imminent. Vomiting is defined as the ejection or expulsion of gastric contents through the mouth and is often a forceful event. Either condition may occur transiently with no other associated signs or symptoms; however, these conditions also may be only part of a more complex clinical presentation.

ETIOLOGY

Nausea and vomiting may be associated with a variety of clinical presentations. In addition to GI diseases, either or both may accompany cardiovascular, infectious, neurologic, or metabolic disease processes. Nausea and vomiting may be a feature of such conditions as pregnancy or may follow operative procedures or administration of certain medications such as those used in cancer chemotherapy. Psychogenic etiologies of these symptoms may be present, especially in young women with an underlying emotional disturbance. Anticipatory etiologies may be involved, such as in patients who have previously received cytotoxic chemotherapy. Specific etiologies associated with nausea and vomiting are presented in Table 33–1.[1]

In addition to identifying conditions associated with nausea and vomiting, it is important to address the specific causative medical problems. For example, nausea and vomiting may occur in as many as 70% of patients with inferior myocardial infarction or diabetic ketoacidosis. As many as 80% to 90% of patients with an Addisonian crisis, acute pancreatitis, or acute appendicitis may present with nausea and vomiting.

The etiology of nausea and vomiting may vary with the age of the patient. For example, vomiting in the newborn during the first day of life suggests upper digestive tract obstruction or an increase in intracranial pressure. Other illnesses associated with vomiting in children include pyloric stenosis, duodenal ulcer, stress ulcer, adrenal insufficiency, septicemia, or diseases of the pancreas, liver, or biliary tree. Also, the hepatocellular failure seen in Reye's syndrome may lead to profound cerebral edema followed by persistent emesis. One of the most common etiologies of vomiting in children, however, is viral gastroenteritis caused by rotavirus. Vomiting in infants may be associated with something as simple as overfeeding, rapid feeding, inadequate burping, or lying down too soon after feeding. It should be recognized that these types of vomiting are usually indicative of minor problems and may be altered by changing the approach to feeding.

Drug-induced nausea and vomiting are of particular concern, especially with the increasing number of patients receiving cytotoxic treatment and the number of agents implicated. Included in Table 33–2 are specific cytotoxic agents categorized by their emetogenic potential. Although some agents may have greater emetogenic potential than others, combinations of agents, high doses, clinical settings, psychological conditions, prior treatment experiences, and unusual stimuli to sight, smell, or taste may alter a patient's response to drug treatment. In this setting, nausea and vomiting may be unavoidable and potentially devastating to the patient's desire to continue treatment. Indeed, some patients experience these problems so intensely that chemotherapy is postponed or discontinued. In addition to the emetogenic potential of various cytotoxic regimens, a variety of other common etiologies have been proposed for the development of nausea and vomiting in cancer patients. These are presented in Table 33–3.[2]

PATHOPHYSIOLOGY

The three consecutive phases of emesis include nausea, retching, and vomiting. Nausea, the imminent need to vomit, is associated with gastric stasis and may be considered a separate and singular symptom. Retching is the labored movement of abdominal and thoracic muscles before vomiting. The final phase of emesis is vomiting, the forceful expulsion of gastric contents due to GI retroperistalsis. The act of vomiting requires the coordinated contractions of the abdominal muscles, pylorus, and antrum, a raised gastric cardia, diminished lower esophageal sphincter pressure, and esophageal dilatation.[3] Vomiting should not be confused with regurgitation, an act in which the gastric or esophageal contents rise to the pharynx because of pressure differences due to, for example, an incompetent lower esophageal sphincter. Accompanying autonomic symptoms of pallor, tachycardia, and diaphoresis account for many of the distressing feelings associated with emesis.

Vomiting is triggered by afferent impulses to the vomiting center, a nucleus of cells in the medulla. Impulses are re-

TABLE 33–1. Specific Etiologies of Nausea and Vomiting

Gastrointestinal Mechanisms
Mechanical gastric outlet obstruction
- Peptic ulcer disease
- Gastric carcinoma
- Pancreatic disease

Motility disorders
- Gastroparesis
- Drug-induced gastric stasis
- Chronic intestinal pseudo-obstruction
- Postviral gastroenteritis
- Irritable bowel syndrome
- Postgastric surgery
- Idiopathic gastric stasis
- Anorexia nervosa

Intra-abdominal emergencies
- Intestinal obstruction
- Acute pancreatitis
- Acute pyelonephritis
- Acute cholecystitis
- Acute cholangitis
- Acute viral hepatitis

Acute gastroenteritis
- Viral gastroenteritis
- Salmonellosis
- Shigellosis
- Staphylococcal gastroenteritis (enterotoxins)

Cardiovascular Diseases
- Acute myocardial infarction
- Congestive heart failure
- Shock and circulatory collapse

Neurologic Processes
- Midline cerebellar hemorrhage
- Increased intracranial pressure
- Migraine headache
- Vestibular disorders
- Head trauma

Metabolic Disorders
- Diabetes mellitus (diabetic ketoacidosis)
- Addison's disease
- Renal disease (uremia)

Psychogenic Causes
- Self-induced
- Anticipatory

Therapy-induced Causes
- Cytotoxic chemotherapy
- Radiation therapy
- Theophylline preparations (intolerance, toxic)
- Anticonvulsant preparations (toxic)
- Digitalis preparations (toxic)
- Opiates
- Amphotericin
- Antibiotics

Drug Withdrawal
- Opiates
- Benzodiazepines

Miscellaneous Causes
- Pregnancy
- Any swallowed irritant (foods, drugs)
- Noxious odors
- Operative procedures

Partially adapted from Ref. 1, with permission.

ceived from sensory centers, such as the chemoreceptor trigger zone (CTZ), cerebral cortex, and visceral afferents from the pharynx and GI tract. When excited, afferent impulses are integrated by the vomiting center, resulting in efferent impulses to the salivation center, respiratory center, and the pharyngeal, GI, and abdominal muscles, leading to vomiting.

The CTZ, located in the area postrema of the fourth ventricle of the brain, is a major chemosensory organ for emesis and is usually associated with chemically induced vomiting. Due to its location, blood-borne and cerebrospinal fluid toxins have easy access to the CTZ. Therefore, cytotoxic agents stimulate primarily this area rather than the cerebral cortex and visceral afferents. Similarly, pregnancy-associated vomiting probably occurs through stimulation of the CTZ.

TABLE 33–2. Emetogenic Potential of Cytotoxic Chemotherapy

Most Emetogenic	Moderate	Least Emetogenic
Amsacrine	Azacytidine	Asparaginase
Cisplatin	Etoposide	Bleomycin
Cyclophosphamide	Mitomycin C	Busulfan
Dacarbazine	Procarbazine	Chlorambucil
Dactinomycin	Thiotepa	Cytarabine
Daunorubicin		Diaziquone
Doxorubicin		Estramustine
Hexamethylmethamine		Floxuridine
Mechlorethamine		Fluorouracil
Mitoxantrone		Hydroxyurea
Nitrosoureas		Melphalan
Streptozocin		Mercaptopurine
		Methotrexate
		Teniposide
		Thioguanine
		Vinca alkaloids

Numerous neurotransmitter receptors are located in the vomiting center, CTZ, and GI tract. Examples of such receptors include cholinergic and histaminic, dopaminergic, opiate, serotonergic, and benzodiazepine receptors. It is theorized that chemotherapeutic agents, their metabolites, or other emetic compounds trigger the process of emesis through stimulation of one or more of these receptors. Effective antiemetics are able to antagonize or block the emetogenic receptors.

Anticipatory nausea and vomiting may be elicited either by specific stimuli associated with the administration of noxious, often cytotoxic, agents or by the anxiety associated with these treatments. Many patients demonstrate both types. The most often accepted theory for this pattern of conditioning is that by repeated pairing of chemotherapy and its aftereffects, previously neutral stimuli such as odors, sounds, and settings acquire the ability to elicit nausea and vomiting.[4,5] These types of stimuli should be expected to be most troublesome in patients receiving agents with the greatest inherent emetogenic potential.

TABLE 33–3. Nonchemotherapy Etiologies of Nausea and Vomiting in Cancer Patients

Fluid and electrolyte abnormalities
Hypercalcemia
Volume depletion
Water intoxication
Adrenocortical insufficiency
Drug induced
Opiates
Antibiotics
Gastrointestinal obstruction
Increased intracranial pressure
Peritonitis
Metastases
Brain
Meninges
Hepatic
Uremia
Infections (septicemia, local)
Radiation therapy

Adapted from Ref. 2. Copyright 1981, American Medical Association, with permission.

CLINICAL PRESENTATION

Because it is impossible to discuss all clinical settings in which the presence of nausea and vomiting might be a pertinent finding, these processes are presented as they might occur together and also as *simple* or *complex* in presentation. Defined here, the term *simple* applies to those episodes of nausea and/or vomiting that (1) occur occasionally and are self-limiting or relieved by the minimal use of antiemetic methods or medications; (2) account for little patient deterioration such as fluid–electrolyte imbalances, pain, or noncompliance with prescribed therapies; or (3) are not related to the administration of or exposure to noxious agents. Conversely, the term *complex* is used when describing a patient's clinical course as including symptoms that (1) are not adequately or readily relieved by the administration of a single antiemetic method or medication; (2) lead to progressive patient deterioration secondary to fluid-electrolyte imbalances, pain, or noncompliance with prescribed therapies; or (3) are caused by noxious agents or psychogenic events. Psychogenic vomiting is often related to sexual or marital disturbances, health problems of friends or family members, or deeper emotional strains. Pertinent features of this condition may include a positive family history of this condition. Episodes may be induced by meals, are recurrent, are generally not accompanied by nausea, and may be suppressed by the patient. Often these events are not noted to be important by the patient. Unless associated with anorexia nervosa, appetite is usually normal. Many of these conditions subside with reductions in stress.

Most episodes of nausea and vomiting decrease in frequency, duration, and severity as the underlying process resolves. However, during the recovery period, it may be desirable to combat the specific symptoms of nausea and vomiting. Most cases of nausea and vomiting are self-limiting, resolve spontaneously, and only require symptomatic therapy. Antiemetic therapy is indicated in patients with electrolyte disturbances secondary to vomiting, severe anorexia or weight loss, or progression of disease either due to refusal of continued therapy or poor nutritional status.

Included in the GI etiologies of nausea and vomiting are a variety of specific disorders associated with mechanical obstruction, motility changes, and infectious diseases of the vital organs within the abdominal cavity. Although each of these conditions may vary in onset, duration, and severity of symptoms, each is nevertheless a potential source of nausea and vomiting that may need to be addressed. In this regard, attention to simultaneous signs and symptoms is helpful in making an accurate diagnosis and evaluation of a specific patient. Additional knowledge of a patient's GI history, with particular emphasis on the presence of abdominal pain or discomfort, diarrhea, and blood from the upper or lower GI tract, should always be sought. Knowledge of the patient's tolerance of food is important. Also, the timing of these symptoms in relation to meals as well as the consistency, content, odor, and frequency of the vomitus may be characteristic findings for specific conditions. Further information that may be helpful in understanding a specific clinical presentation includes concomitant findings such as fever or weight loss, a description of precipitating factors, a complete history of recent medication use, and the history or presence of myalgias, behavioral or visual changes, headache, or pain outside the abdomen.

▶ TREATMENT: Nausea and Vomiting

DESIRED OUTCOME

The overall goal of antiemetic therapy is to prevent or eliminate nausea and vomiting with clinically acceptable adverse effects for each patient. Although this goal may be accomplished easily in patients with simple nausea and vomiting, patients with more complex problems require greater assistance. In addition to these clinical goals, appropriate cost issues should be considered, particularly in the management of chemotherapy-induced and postoperative nausea and vomiting.

GENERAL APPROACH TO TREATMENT

The treatment of nausea and vomiting is quite varied depending on the associated medical situation. Even though a number of potentially effective measures are available, most patients receive a medication at some point in their care. For simple nausea and vomiting, patients may choose to do nothing or to select from a variety of over-the-counter drugs. As symptoms become worse or are associated with more serious medical problems, patients are more likely to benefit from proven prescription antiemetic drugs.

When prescribed according to reliable clinical information, these agents often provide acceptable relief. However, some patients will never be totally free of symptoms. This lack of relief is most disabling to the patient when it is associated with an unresolving medical problem or when the necessary therapy for this condition is the cause, as in the case of patients receiving emetogenic chemotherapy.

NONPHARMACOLOGIC MANAGEMENT

Nonpharmacologic management of nausea and vomiting may include a variety of dietary, physical, or psychological changes consistent with the etiology of symptoms. For patients with simple complaints, perhaps resulting from excessive or disagreeable food or beverage consumption, avoidance or moderation in dietary intake may be preferable. Patients suffering symptoms of systemic illness may improve dramatically as their underlying condition resolves. Finally, patients in whom these symptoms result from labyrinthine changes produced by motion may benefit quickly by assuming a stable physical position.

The variables associated with the development of anticipatory nausea and vomiting have been studied. These variables include the use of cisplatin, the severity of postchemotherapy vomiting, and the duration of the patient's worst nausea.[6] Although anxiolytic and antiemetic agents offer the most successful treatment for these patients, various relaxation techniques have been reported, including hypnosis, behavior modification, and guided mental imagery.[7–9] However, the efficacy of these nonpharmacologic approaches requires further evaluation. Nevertheless, prevention of these symptoms is extremely important. This may be accomplished through supportive care coupled with potent prophylactic antiemetic regimens prior to chemotherapy treatment.

The management of psychogenic vomiting is greatly dependent on psychological intervention. However, because the underlying problems are so complex and intertwined in personal relationships, psychological therapy may require lengthy, in-depth follow-up. Pharmacologic therapy offers only minimal benefit in these patients. Surgery, such as gastroenterostomy, is of no value.

PHARMACOLOGIC THERAPY

Although many approaches to the treatment of nausea and vomiting have been suggested, antiemetic drugs (over-the-counter [OTC] and prescription) are most often recommended. These agents represent a variety of pharmacologic and chemical classes as well as dosage regimens and routes of administration. With so many treatment possibilities available, factors that enable the clinician to discriminate among various choices must be recognized. These factors include (1) the suspected etiology of the symptoms; (2) the frequency, duration, and severity of the episodes; (3) the ability of the patient to use oral, rectal, injectable, or transdermal topical medications; and (4) the success of previous antiemetic medications. For example, many antiemetics are commercially available as oral agents. Provided a patient can and will adhere to oral dosing, a suitable and effective agent can often be selected; however, for certain other situations, oral medications may be inappropriate because of the patient's inability to retain any appreciable oral ingestions. In these patients, rectal or injectable routes of administration might be preferred. Information concerning commonly available antiemetic preparations is given in Table 33–4.

Some individuals initially experience nausea and vomiting at home or outside formal medical settings. For these symptoms, patients may choose from a lengthy list of OTC products. Although suitable for occasional simple nausea and vomiting, OTC agents are often abandoned by the patient as symptoms continue or become progressively worse. As the patient's condition warrants, prescription medications may be chosen, either as single-agent therapy or in combination. For most conditions, a single antiemetic agent is preferred; however, for those patients not responding to such therapy and those receiving highly emetogenic chemotherapy, multiple-agent regimens are usually required. Numerous combinations have been employed through clinical investigation and practice.

The treatment of simple nausea and vomiting usually requires minimal therapy. Products available for self-medication include antacids; histamine$_2$ antagonists such as cimetidine, famotidine, and ranitidine; antihistamine–anticholinergic agents such as cyclizine, dimenhydrinate, diphenhydramine, and meclizine; and phosphorated carbohydrate solutions. Agents requiring physician prescription include some antihistaminic–anticholinergic drugs and phenothiazine agents. The latter agents include benzquinamide, buclizine, parenteral dimenhydrinate and diphenhydramine, hydroxyzine, prochlorperazine, promethazine, and trimethobenzamide. Both OTC and prescription drugs useful in the treatment of simple nausea and vomiting are usually effective in small, infrequently administered doses. Side effects and toxic effects in these settings are also usually minimal.

The management of complex nausea and vomiting may require aggressive drug therapy, often with more than one antiemetic agent. For patients with complex symptoms, effective combinations may include two of the following drugs: benzquinamide, chlorpromazine, dimenhydrinate, droperidol, hydroxyzine, prochlorperazine, promethazine, thiethylperazine, or trimethobenzamide. In combination, each of these drugs is prescribed in small to moderate dosages, achieving symptomatic control through different pharmacologic mechanisms while avoiding the untoward effects caused by high doses. For patients receiving highly emetogenic chemotherapy, antiemetic regimens may include one or more of the following agents: prochlorperazine, metoclopramide, ondansetron, granisetron, dolasetron, dexamethasone, or lorazepam (see "Chemotherapy-induced Nausea and Vomiting" later in the chapter).

In general, the clinician should evaluate the patient's condition and determine the need for antiemetic treatment of an existing condition or prophylactic therapy to prevent or lessen anticipated nausea and vomiting episodes, as is seen in patients requiring cytotoxic drugs or operative procedures. Once this decision has been made, along with the complete and overall medical evaluation, the antiemetic selection process may proceed. Common antiemetic preparations are listed in Table 33–4.

ANTACIDS

Various antacids may be sought by patients experiencing simple nausea and vomiting. In this setting, single or combination OTC antacid products, especially those containing magnesium hydroxide, aluminum hydroxide, and/or calcium carbonate, may provide sufficient relief, primarily through gastric acid neutralization. Likewise, patients may seek histamine$_2$ antagonists for these symptoms, particularly in the presence of heartburn or brief episodes of gastroesophageal reflux. Patients responding to small, occasional doses of these agents probably do not have significant pathology. However, it is not uncommon for patients with significant GI disease to self-medicate with larger and more frequent doses of antacids with or without a trial of histamine$_2$ antagonist prior to seeking medical care.

Common antacid regimens for the relief of nausea and vomiting include one or more small doses of single- or multiple-agent products. Although antacid therapy may be aggressively applied for the treatment of known ulcer disease, OTC products sought by patients are usually taken in response to acute and sporadic

TABLE 33–4. Common Antiemetic Preparations and Adult Dosage Regimens

Drug	Adult Dosage Regimen	Dosage Form/Route	Availability
Antacids			
Antacids (various)	15–30 mL every 2–4 h prn	Liquid	OTC
Histamine H_2 Antagonists			
Cimetidine (Tagament HB)	200 mg bid prn	Tab	OTC
Famotidine (Pepcid AC)	10 mg bid prn	Tab	OTC
Nizatidine (Axid AR)	75 mg bid prn	Tab	OTC
Ranitidine (Zantac 75)	75 mg bid prn	Tab	OTC
Antihistaminic–Anticholinergic Agents			
Benzquinamide (Emete-Con)	25–50 mg every 3–4 h prn	IM, IV	Rx
Buclizine (Bucladin-S)	50 mg twice daily	Tab	Rx
Cyclizine (Marezine)	50 mg every 4–6 h prn	Tab, IM	Rx/OTC
Dimenhydrinate (Dramamine)	50–100 mg every 4–6 h prn	Tab, chew tab, cap, liquid, IM, IV	Rx/OTC
Diphenhydramine (Benadryl)	10–50 mg every 4–6 h prn	Tab, cap, liquid, IM, IV	Rx/OTC
Hydroxyzine (Vistril, Atarax)	25–100 mg every 6 h prn	Tab, cap, liquid, IM	Rx
Meclizine (Bonine, Antivert)	25–50 mg every 24 h prn	Tab, chew tab, cap	Rx/OTC
Promethazine (Phenergan)	12.5–25 mg every 4–6 h prn	Tab, liquid, IM, IV, supp	Rx
Pyrilamine (Nisaval)	25–50 mg 3 to 4 times daily	Tab	Rx/OTC
Scopolamine (Transderm Scop)	0.5 mg every 72 h prn	Transdermal patch	Rx
Trimethobenzamide (Tigan)	200–250 mg 3 to 4 times daily prn	Cap, IM, supp	Rx
Phenothiazines			
Chlorpromazine (Thorazine)	10–25 mg every 4–6 h prn	SR, cap, tab, liquid, IM, IV	Rx
	50–100 mg every 6–8 h prn	Supp	Rx
Fluphenazine (Prolixin)	1.25–2.5 mg every 6–8 h prn	Tab, liquid, IM	Rx
Perphenazine (Trilafon)	8–30 mg/d divided prn	Tab, liquid, IM, IV	Rx
Prochlorperazine (Compazine)	5–10 mg 3 to 4 times daily prn	SR, cap, tab, liquid IM, IV	Rx
	25 mg twice daily prn	Supp	Rx
Promazine (Sparine)	25–50 mg every 4–6 h prn	Tab, IM	Rx
Thiethylperazine (Torecan)	10 mg 3 times daily	Tab, IM, supp	Rx
Cannabinoids			
Dronabinol (Marinol)	5–7.5 mg/m^2 every 2–4 h prn	Cap	Rx (C-II)
Nabilone (Cesamet)	1–2 mg 2 to 3 times daily prn	Cap	Rx (C-II)
Butyrophenones			
Haloperidol (Haldol)	1–5 mg every 12 h prn	Tab, liquid, IM, IV	Rx
Droperidol (Inapsine)	2.5–5.0 mg every 4–6 h prn	IM, IV	Rx
Corticosteroids			
Dexamethasone (Decadron)	10 mg prior to chemotherapy, repeat with 4–8 mg every 6 h for total of 4 doses	IV	Rx
Methylprednisolone (Solu-Medrol)	125–500 mg every 6 h for total of 4 doses	IV	Rx
Benzodiazepines			
Lorazepam (Ativan)	0.5–4.0 mg prior to chemotherapy	IV	Rx (C-IV)
Diazepam (Valium)	2–5 mg every 3 h	Tab	Rx (C-IV)

episodes of nausea and vomiting. Depending on dose, common commercial products usually supply sufficient ingredients to allow a range of approximately 40 to 180 mEq of acid-neutralizing capacity.[10–12] Potential adverse effects from antacids are usually related to the presence of magnesium, aluminum, or calcium salts. Specifically, osmotic diarrhea from magnesium and constipation from aluminum or calcium salts may be of concern to patients, particularly those self-medicating with high or frequently administered antacid doses. Generally, however, when used occasionally for acute episodic relief of nausea and vomiting, antacids do not produce serious toxicities.

HISTAMINE$_2$ ANTAGONISTS

Histamine$_2$ antagonists may be used by patients in low doses for the management of simple nausea and vomiting associated with heartburn. Individual dosages of cimetidine 200 mg, famotidine 10 mg, nizatidine 75 mg, or ranitidine 75 mg may be used for brief periods. Except for potential drug interactions with cimetidine, these agents should be expected to cause few side effects when used for episodic relief.

ANTIHISTAMINE–ANTICHOLINERGIC DRUGS

Antiemetic drugs from the antihistaminic–anticholinergic category appear to interrupt various visceral afferent pathways that stimulate nausea and vomiting and may be appropriate in the treatment of simple symptomology. However, when used alone, each provides little efficacy in patients with more complex complaints such as those caused by cytotoxic chemotherapy. Adverse reactions that may be apparent with the use of the antihistaminic–anticholinergic agents primarily include drowsi-

TABLE 33–4. (Continued)

Drug	Adult Dosage Regimen	Dosage Form/Route	Availability
Selective Serotonin Antagonists			
Dolasetron (Anzemet), for CINV	1.8 mg/kg 30 min prior to chemotherapy (undiluted, up to 100 mg over 30 min, or diluted, over 30 min	IV	Rx
	OR		
	100 mg within 1 h before chemotherapy	Tab	Rx
Dolasetron (Anzemet), for PONV undiluted as single injection	12.5 mg 15 min before the cessation of anesthesia	IV	Rx
	OR		
	100 mg within 2 h before surgery	Tab	Rx
Granisetron (Kytril), for CINV	10 µg/kg prior to chemotherapy (diluted, infuse, over 5 min or undiluted over 30 s)	IV	Rx
Granisetron (Kytril) for PONV	20–40 µg/kg 30 min before end of anesthesia	IV	Rx
Ondansetron (Zofran), for CINV	32 mg prior to chemotherapy as a single dose (diluted, give over 15 min), or 0.15 mg/kg prior to chemotherapy, repeat at 4 and 8 h	IV	Rx
	OR		
	8 mg 30 min prior to chemotherapy, repeat at 4 and 8 h and every 12 h for 1–2 d after chemotherapy completion	Tab	Rx
Ondansetron (Zofran), for PONV	4 mg prior to induction of anesthesia or postoperatively (undiluted, give over 2–5 min)	IV	Rx
	OR		
	16 mg given 1 h before anesthesia	Tab	Rx
Miscellaneous Agents			
Dextrose, fructose, phosphoric acid (Emetrol)	15–30 mL every 1–3 h prn	Liquid	OTC
Diphenidol (Vontrol)	25–50 mg every 4 h prn	Tab	Rx
Metoclopramide (Reglan), for CINV	1–2 mg/kg every 2 h × 2, then every 3 h × 3	IV	Rx
Metoclopramide (Reglan), for PONV	10–20 mg about 10 min prior to anesthesia	IV	Rx
Metoclopramide (Reglan), for delayed CINV	0.5 mg/kg or 20 mg every 6 h prn, days 2 to 4	Tab	Rx

Rx = prescription; OTC = over the counter; cap = capsule; chew tab = chewable tablet; IM = intramuscular; IV = intravenous; liquid = oral syrup, concentrate, suspension; SR cap = sustained-release capsule; supp = rectal suppository; tab = tablet; CINV = chemotherapy-induced nausea and vomiting; PONV = postoperative nausea and vomiting.

ness, confusion, blurred vision, dry mouth, urinary retention, and possibly tachycardia, particularly in elderly patients. Also, as doses are increased or are more frequently administered, patients with narrow-angle glaucoma, prostatic hyperplasia, or asthma are at greater risk of complications from the anticholinergic effects of these drugs.

PHENOTHIAZINES

Historically, phenothiazines have been the most widely prescribed antiemetic agents. These agents appear to block dopamine receptors, most likely in the CTZ. Some investigators have found phenothiazines to demonstrate greatest efficacy when compared with placebo and less efficacy when compared with other more potent antiemetics.[13–15] Phenothiazines are marketed in an array of dosage forms, none of which appears to be more efficacious than another; however, there are perhaps some important generalizations concerning their use in overall clinical practice. These agents may be most practical for long-term treatment and are inexpensive in comparison with newer drugs, with the exception of sustained-release products of chlorpromazine or prochlorperazine that may be too costly and of no established clinical advantage. Little distinguishing information is available in the present literature concerning the efficacy of rectal preparations. Rectal administration is most preferred in patients in whom parenteral administration is impractical or in whom oral medications cannot be retained and are therefore ineffective. In many patients, low doses of phenothiazine drugs may not be effective, while larger doses may produce unacceptable risks.[2] Phenothiazines are most useful in patients with simple nausea and vomiting or in those receiving mildly emetogenic doses of chemotherapy. Problems associated with these drugs include troublesome and potentially dangerous side effects, including extrapyramidal reactions, hypersensitivity reactions with possible liver dysfunction, marrow aplasia, and excessive sedation.

BUTYROPHENONES

Two butyrophenone compounds that have antiemetic activity are haloperidol and its congener droperidol. Each agent blocks dopaminergic stimulation of the CTZ. Although each agent is effective in relieving nausea and vomiting, droperidol has been used most often. Depending on its specific indication, the optimal dosage range may vary considerably. For example, preoperative doses of droperidol may range from 2.5 to 10 mg, while dosage regimens during cytotoxic chemotherapy have been documented as low as 0.5 to 2.5 mg by intermittent injection to as high as 1.0 to 1.5 mg/h by intravenous infusion.[16–19] Adverse reactions resulting from the use of the butyrophenone compounds primarily include sedation and the possibility of dystonic reactions. Although dystonia may occur after the initial dose, some patients may experience this problem later in therapy. Injectable diphenhydramine usually rapidly resolves these extrapyramidal reactions.[17]

CORTICOSTEROIDS

Corticosteroids have demonstrated antiemetic efficacy since the initial recognition that patients receiving prednisone as part of their Hodgkin's disease protocol appeared to develop less nausea and vomiting than those treated with protocols excluding this agent. Other corticosteroids showing efficacy include methylprednisolone and dexamethasone. Although the exact mechanism of action for corticosteroids is unknown, the inhibition of prostaglandin synthesis may explain their antiemetic activity.[20] Such an explanation is most appealing in light of the known high emetogenic potential of prostaglandins themselves. However, because of their numerous metabolic effects, a single site of steroid antiemetic activity may be difficult to locate or assess. In addition to the antiemetic benefits of corticosteroids, other desirable effects include increased appetite and an elevation of mood or feelings of well-being. Depending on the patient and the drug regimen, these effects may provide the primary benefit of corticosteroid therapy.

Corticosteroids have been used successfully in the management of chemotherapy-induced nausea and vomiting with few problems. However, reported adverse effects have included mood changes ranging from anxiety to euphoria as well as headache, metallic taste, abdominal discomfort, hyperglycemia, and itchy throat.[20] For patients with simple nausea and vomiting, steroids are not indicated and may be associated with unacceptable risks. As with other conditions, steroids should be employed only when the benefit-to-risk ratio is sufficient to warrant a medication with such complex and potentially deleterious effects.

METOCLOPRAMIDE

Metoclopramide, procainamide's congener, provides significant antiemetic effects by blocking the dopaminergic receptors centrally in the CTZ. Peripherally, metoclopramide increases lower esophageal sphincter tone, aids gastric emptying, and accelerates transit through the small bowel, possibly through the release of acetylcholine. Because the adverse reactions of metoclopramide include extrapyramidal effects, IV diphenhydramine 25 to 50 mg should be prophylactically administered or provided on-call for its anticipated need. Other adverse effects may include restlessness, drowsiness, fatigue, nausea, and diarrhea.[21,22]

OTHER AGENTS

Serotonin-receptor antagonists have become increasingly important to antiemetic therapy in recent years, particularly in the management of chemotherapy-induced and postoperative nausea and vomiting. Issues involved in the use of ondansetron, granisetron, and dolasetron are reviewed in detail in the sections that follow.

A final group of antiemetic preparations available to patients experiencing nausea and vomiting necessitates some mention. First, the phosphorated carbohydrate solutions (mixtures of fructose, dextrose, and phosphoric acid) are available OTC and may be administered in 15- to 30-mL doses as often as every 3 hours or as needed. As might be predicted, this mixture is intended only for mild and infrequent symptoms. Because of the inability of these agents to relieve significant symptoms, the solution should not be used in patients with complex problems, especially those receiving chemotherapy. However, this combination is safe and effective in patients with morning sickness. Adverse reactions to these solutions may include abdominal pain or diarrhea as a consequence of large doses of fructose, or lack of control in diabetic patients because of the dextrose included in the formulations. With the use of small doses, most patients experience little benefit or adversity.

An agent that has received comparatively little attention in the antiemetic literature is diphenidol. Although this agent inhibits the CTZ as well as conduction in vestibular–cerebellar pathways and is indicated for the management of nausea and vomiting associated with surgery, malignant neoplasms, antineoplastic chemotherapy, radiation sickness, infectious diseases, and labyrinthine disturbances, it should be used extremely cautiously. Diphenidol should be used only when there is a clear and unquestionable benefit potential. Even though it is an oral agent, this product should be used only in a hospital or under comparable conditions. The primary reason for these measures required for the use of diphenidol is its adverse reaction profile. Auditory and visual hallucinations, disorientation, and confusion have been reported and are the usual warnings against its use. These problems may be even more pronounced in elderly patients or those with declining renal function, because approximately 90% of diphenidol is excreted in the urine. Last, diphenidol should be avoided during pregnancy or lactation and in children weighing less than 50 pounds.

Pyridoxine has also been cited as an antiemetic agent; however, its efficacy has not been accepted beyond that of a placebo and it probably has little place in the approach to simple or complex symptoms. Its beneficial mechanism has been suggested to be restoration of depleted pyridoxine body stores.

COMBINATION REGIMENS

The management of nausea and vomiting may require combinations of antiemetic drugs. Most combination protocols are reserved for patients with complex symptoms, especially those receiving cytotoxic chemotherapy. Such combinations may include as few as two or as many as five antiemetic agents, each in moderate to high doses. These multiagent regimens should be carefully administered by experienced personnel in a hospital or specialty clinic setting. Although oral agents may be used, most regimens are administered intravenously and require continuous patient assessment and feedback for evaluation of efficacy and side effects. Because an increasing number of patients may require such regimens, careful monitoring should be developed and employed to eliminate possibly severe adverse reactions.

The primary goal of combination antiemetic regimens is to select beneficial agents that have different pharmacologic mechanisms as well as toxic effects that are not considered additive or synergistic. These protocols may affect the vomiting center, the CTZ, the cerebral cortex, and/or the peripheral mechanisms that mediate nausea and vomiting.[23] Combinations often include metoclopramide, diphenhydramine, and dexamethasone. Other agents that may be added to the regimen include droperidol, diazepam, thiethylperazine, secobarbital, pentobarbital, chlorpromazine, or prochlorperazine. Dexamethasone may be combined with ondansetron, granisetron or dolasetron. From this list of possible combinations, it should be apparent that the ideal multiagent antiemetic protocol has not been established. Nevertheless, protocols using injectable metoclopramide or a setotonin antagonist appear to have a high degree of efficacy in preventing nausea and vomiting, even in patients receiving cisplatin.[23–25]

CHEMOTHERAPY-INDUCED NAUSEA AND VOMITING

Information concerning antiemetic drug selection for patients with chemotherapy-induced nausea and vomiting (CINV) is changing rapidly. Although newer agents may be readily acceptable in clinical practice, older agents may be appropriately prescribed. For example, prior to the use of metoclopramide, phenothiazine antiemetics were frequently chosen in patients with chemotherapy-induced nausea and vomiting. Even with newer therapies, if relief of symptoms is provided and side effects are absent or acceptable, these drugs may be continued. Conversely, failure to achieve adequate antiemetic efficacy during the first course of chemotherapy should prompt the clinician to search for more acceptable agents, possibly combination therapies.[14,15,26] Because of the complexities of chemotherapy-induced nausea and vomiting and the variable patient response, many patients require two or more antiemetic agents, particularly when the cytotoxic regimen includes high-dose cisplatin.

Droperidol, usually given intravenously, has been documented as safe and effective, even in ambulatory cancer patients.[16] Although the optimal antiemetic dose of droperidol for patients receiving chemotherapy may vary, many patients benefit from small doses, particularly when combined with other antiemetic drugs.

A variety of study protocols have been employed in corticosteroid antiemetic clinical trials with variations in drug, dosage regimen, and route of administration. Although studies using steroids in both single- and multiple-agent protocols have demonstrated acceptable efficacy, their exact ranking among antiemetic alternatives is not clear for patients receiving cytotoxic chemotherapy.

Benefits from corticosteroids have been quite variable. Of the corticosteroids studied, the use of dexamethasone has been best defined. During therapy with mildly to moderately emetogenic agents, dexamethasone appeared to be comparable to metoclopramide and superior to prochlorperazine when each was used alone; however, metoclopramide has shown greater efficacy when studied in patients receiving highly emetogenic regimens, especially those including cisplatin.[27–29] Methylprednisolone has been compared with metoclopramide and thiethylperazine. Benefit appeared to be greater for methylprednisolone than thiethylperazine and comparable to typical metoclopramide doses of less than 2 mg/kg.[30–33] Dosage regimens vary widely among steroid antiemetic protocols. When used alone, dexamethasone has often been administered parenterally as a single dose of 8 to 20 mg prior to chemotherapy, followed by oral doses of 4 to 12 mg up to 24 hours after completion of chemotherapy. Methylprednisolone has been administered prior to chemotherapy in a dose of 250 mg. After chemotherapy, up to four subsequent doses have been given. Dexamethasone is effective in patients with delayed nausea and vomiting, particularly when given with metoclopramide and lorazepam.

Metoclopramide is most often prescribed for the prevention and treatment of complex nausea and vomiting in response to chemotherapy administration, particularly cisplatin. For such patients, it has been employed in multiagent combination protocols; however, it has shown efficacy as a single therapy. Alone or in combination, metoclopramide has demonstrated significant efficacy in high doses (1 to 2 mg/kg IV), with one dose administered approximately 30 minutes prior to chemotherapy. Up to four subsequent doses are given at 2-hour intervals after chemotherapy. Although cisapride, an agent similar to metoclopramide, may provide relief in select patients with nausea and vomiting, this agent is at present indicated primarily for the management of acid-reflux disorders.[34]

Three selective 5-HT_3 serotonin antagonists—ondansetron, granisetron, and dolasetron—are effective in the management of chemotherapy-induced nausea and vomiting.[35] By blocking serotonin receptors located in the area postrema and possibly vagal afferent fibers in the upper GI tract, these agents inhibit emesis.[36] Because these agents do not affect dopamine receptors, they are not associated with akathisia or acute dystonia.[37–39]

Ondansetron is usually administered intravenously 30 minutes prior to chemotherapy at a dose of 0.15 mg/kg over 15 minutes. Similar subsequent doses are given 4 and 8 hours after the first dose. As an alternative, a single 32-mg dose may be used intravenously in adults. Oral doses of 8 mg for adults and 4 mg for children may also be used. Little information is known concerning the dosage in children under the age of 2 years. Although ondansetron is generally well tolerated, reported side effects include diarrhea, headache, fever, constipation, dizziness, and drowsiness.

In adults and children at least 2 years of age, granisetron should be intravenously infused in a dose of 10 μg/kg over 5 minutes, beginning within 30 minutes before the initiation of chemotherapy, only on the day(s) chemotherapy is given. Oral doses of 1 mg may be used in adults. Children under the age of 2 years have not been adequately studied. Reported side effects of granisetron include headache, asthenia, somnolence, diarrhea, and constipation.

Dolasetron, the most recently marketed 5-HT_3 serotonin antagonist, may be administered as a single dose of 1.8 mg/kg or a fixed dose of 100 mg intravenously over 30 seconds or diluted in a compatible solution and infused over a period of 15 minutes. With each method, the dose should be given approximately 30 minutes prior to chemotherapy. For children 2 to 16 years of age, dolasetron may be given as a single dose of 1.8 mg/kg up to a maximum of 100 mg. However, safety and efficacy for patients under 2 years of age have not been established. Side effects most commonly noted in clinical trials include headache, diarrhea, and dizziness.

Although the availability of serotonin antagonists has made a significant impact on the management of patients receiving cytotoxic chemotherapy, these agents have not been effective in adequately controlling delayed emesis in many patients. Furthermore, some patients have experienced a reduction of efficacy with multiple-day chemotherapy or after several cycles of chemotherapy.[40] Due to these problems, most clinicians recommend the addition of dexamethasone or methylprednisolone to the regimen to improve response rates.

The cannabinoids are effective antiemetic agents, even in patients in whom other regimens have failed.[41,42] Dronabinol, Δ-9-tetrahydrocannabinol (THC), is the major psychoactive substance present in marijuana. Cannabinoids are only indicated for nausea and vomiting associated with cancer chemotherapy. Pharmacologic effects on opiate receptors and the cortical and vomiting centers of the brain may explain the beneficial effects of cannabinoids.[41–43] Cannabinoids may be associated with potentially undesirable features and are not equally effective against all stimuli or all doses of the same stimuli. As expected, a number of CNS effects are common, including mood changes, anxiety, memory loss, fear, confusion, motor incoordination, time distortion, hallucinations, euphoria, relaxation, and hunger. Depending on the severity of these effects, doses should be lowered or discontinued. However, there is a strong correlation between a subjective "high" and antiemetic efficacy. Nabilone has been associated with less euphoric effects than dronabinol. Other potential side effects of the cannabinoids include sedation, blurred vision, hypotension, tachycardia, and paranoid ideation. Tolerance usually develops to most of the side effects, but not to the antiemetic activity.[44,45] Both increased effectiveness and improved tolerance of the cannabinoids may be observed in younger patients. Administration of the cannabinoids should be initiated the night before chemotherapy, because failure to achieve adequate blood concentrations will likely result in vomiting.

Anticipatory nausea and vomiting is a somewhat unique problem sometimes associated with cytotoxic chemotherapy. As many as one in four cancer patients may experience this condition during repeated courses of therapy. According to one study, patients with four or more of the following characteristics may be more likely to develop anticipatory symptoms by their fourth chemotherapy treatment: nausea and/or vomiting experienced after first treatment; nausea after treatment described as "moderate, severe, or intolerable"; vomiting after treatment described as "moderate, severe, or intolerable"; less than 50 years of age; a susceptibility to motion sickness; feeling warm or hot all over after treatment; sweating following treatment; or feelings of generalized weakness following treatment.[46]

Benzodiazepines represent the best of the therapeutic alternatives in the treatment of anticipatory nausea and vomiting. The most often prescribed agent in this pharmacologic class is lorazepam, administered orally or intravenously for its amnestic effects. Dosage regimens include one dose before and multiple doses after each treatment with cytotoxic chemotherapy. Although some patients appreciate their lack of recall of having received chemotherapy, others find it uncomfortable and unacceptable. The latter patients may refuse lorazepam for subsequent treatments; however, acceptability of this feature of one's care may be highly dependent on the overall severity of symptoms. Similar to other benzodiazepines, lorazepam may display an array of pharmacologic activities including sedation, hypnosis, anxiolysis, and muscle relaxation in doses of 0.5 to 4.0 mg, with little change in a patient's respiratory or cardiovascular function. Other CNS effects such as disorientation, hallucinations, incontinence, and amnesia appear directly related to dose escalation.[47,48]

POSTOPERATIVE NAUSEA AND VOMITING

Nausea and vomiting associated with operative procedures are common problems for some patients. However, not all operative procedures produce these problems to the same degree. Specifically, procedures of the abdomen, eye, ear, nose, and throat are generally associated with higher incidences of nausea and vomiting than other procedures. Women, perhaps related to high gonadotropin levels, appear more susceptible to postoperative problems and experience a threefold higher incidence of nausea and vomiting compared to men, independent of the type of operation or anesthetic.[49] Children are about twice as susceptible as adults.[49] Other risk factors that may be associated with an increase in postoperative symptoms include patient variables such as obesity, increased age, a history of motion sickness, or prior postoperative emesis. The choice of premedication or general anesthetic agent is also important. For example, inhalational anesthetics such as cyclopropane and nitrous oxide are particularly emetogenic, whereas agents such as isoflurane, enflurane, and halothane cause less, but still significant, postoperative nausea and vomiting. Of the intravenous anesthetics, propofol may be less emetogenic than some agents previously used.[50]

Most patients do not require preoperative prophylactic antiemetic therapy. In 70% to 90% of cases, patients either do not experience these symptoms or may have incomplete resolution when they occur. Simple premedication with atropine may decrease the potential occurrence of these symptoms in some patients. Other anticholinergic agents that may be effective include promethazine, scopolamine, cyclizine, and possibly glycopyrrolate. Although each of these agents has been effective in the prevention of nausea and vomiting in some clinical settings, sedation, dry mouth, and disorientation may limit their usefulness. Few patients will require the administration of additional preoperatively administered therapy.

The use of antiemetic therapy immediately following an operative procedure has been much more aggressively evaluated and applied, either as prophylaxis for potential postoperative symptoms or as acute management of actual nausea and vomiting. A variety of pharmacologic approaches are available and should be prescribed as single or combination therapy in their minimally effective dosage regimens. In doing so, patients will experience fewer adverse effects, some of which may otherwise be very troublesome for the overall recovery of the patient. Among the commonly prescribed antiemetic therapies in the postoperative setting, droperidol has been effective, particularly in patients undergoing obstetric and gynecologic procedures. Limiting effects, however, may include sedation, hypotension, and extrapyramidal signs.

Studies of metoclopramide have provided conflicting results, with some clinical trials documenting control of symptoms and others having concluded little value. Such findings perhaps have been due to metoclopramide's short duration of action, particularly when compared in settings in which patients had received morphine, a known emetogenic analgesic. Metoclopramide in intravenous doses of 10 to 20 mg administered 10 minutes prior to the induction of anesthesia may be used. Adverse effects of metoclopramide by such regimens include sedation and infrequently extrapyramidal signs. Although possible, extrapyramidal effects appear to be much less likely with the low doses most often prescribed in this setting. Intravenous droperidol in a single dose of 0.625 to 1.25 mg may be prescribed with or without metoclopramide.

Selective serotonin antagonists are very effective in the prevention of postoperative nausea and vomiting. To date, ondansetron, granisetron, and dolasetron have provided favorable outcomes when compared to placebo, metoclopramide, or droperidol. Ondansetron in oral regimens of 0.15 mg/kg up to a total of 8 mg or IV regimens of 0.1 mg/kg up to a total of 8 mg may be effective when given prophylactically prior to surgery. Intravenous granisetron in doses of 20 to 40 μg/kg given 30 minutes before the end of anesthesia have also been successfully used as postoperative prophylaxis. Similarly, oral doses of dolasetron of 25 to 100 mg given 1 to 2 hours before surgery or IV doses of 12.5 mg given 15 minutes before the cessation of anesthesia also may be effective. A single IV dexamethasone dose of 8 to 20 mg may be combined with one of the selective serotonin antagonists to enhance antiemetic efficacy.

Regardless of which drug or regimen is chosen, one of the most often cited reasons for selecting a serotonin antagonist in the postoperative period appears to be the reduction of extrapyramidal effects noted with these agents, particularly compared to droperidol and metoclopramide. Even so, the true role of serotonin antagonists is controversial. In fact, many clinicians prefer the use of older, more traditional, and less expensive antiemetic therapy. Unlike the more clearly defined etiologies of CINV, the unpredictable occurrence and severity of nausea and vomiting for surgical patients depends on the type of surgery, anesthesia, and patient. Therefore, serotonin antagonists are perhaps best reserved for patients who have failed to respond to traditional therapy, or for patients in whom drug allergies or other specific risk factors exist.

Other antiemetic medications with value in the management of postoperative nausea and vomiting include promethazine, prochlorperazine, scopolamine, diphenhydramine, lorazepam, and ephedrine. These latter medications may be prescribed in doses similar to those used in other settings and produce similar beneficial and adverse effects. With or without antiemetic therapy, certain nonpharmacologic methods may be effective in reducing the potential for emesis and should be applied universally. These include assisting patients with movement and providing particularly close attention to adequate hydration and pain management.

DISORDERS OF BALANCE

A variety of clinical conditions may be associated with vertigo and dizziness. The etiology of these complaints may include diseases that are infectious, postinfectious, demyelinative, vascular, neoplastic, degenerative, traumatic, toxic, psychogenic, or idiopathic. Therefore, symptoms of imbalance or perceived imbalance by the patient present a particular clinical challenge. Whether associated with a minor or complex disorder, motion sickness may be associated with nausea and vomiting.

Although much progress has been made in the management of other illnesses associated with emesis, motion sickness represents an area in which newer agents have provided little benefit. Studies of serotonin antagonists in motion sickness suggest that the 5-HT_3 receptor is not involved in the neural pathways that bring about motion sickness.[51] In fact, 5-HT_3 serotonin receptor antagonists have provided no beneficial effects in reducing motion sickness when compared with placebo.[52] Interestingly, vertigo has been documented among the adverse reactions of these agents. Therefore, beneficial therapy for patients in this setting can most reliably be found among the antihistaminic–anticholinergic agents. However, their precise mechanisms of action are unknown to date. Neither the antihistaminic nor the anticholinergic potency appears to correlate well with the ability of these agents to prevent or treat the nausea and vomiting associated with motion sickness.

When used for their depressant effects on labyrinth excitability, these agents have been shown to produce variable efficacy and safety profiles. The most useful antiemetic agent for motion sickness prophylaxis appears to be scopolamine, particularly when used 1 to 2 hours prior to symptom-producing exposures.[53] When using the transdermal scopolamine system, the patch should be applied to the hairless area behind one ear at least 4 hours before the antiemetic effect is needed. By delivering a total dose of 1.0 mg of scopolamine, beneficial effects may be recognized for up to 3 days. Oral regimens of antihistaminic–anticholinergic agents given one to several times each day may be effective, especially when the first dose is administered prior to motion.

ANTIEMETIC USE DURING PREGNANCY

More than one-half of pregnant women experience nausea and vomiting or hyperemesis gravidarum. Because drugs may influence embryonic development most during the first 2 months of pregnancy, there has been much interest in the potential maternal and fetal benefits and risks of the antiemetic agents during this early phase.[54–62] Included among the commonly prescribed agents are the phenothiazines (prochlorperazine and promethazine); the antihistaminic–anticholinergic agents (dimenhydrinate, diphenhydramine, meclizine, and scopolamine); metoclopramide; and pyridoxine.

Although many women experience nausea and vomiting during pregnancy, the etiology of hyperemesis gravidarum is not well understood. Numerous mechanisms have been proposed. In addition, the severity of symptoms may vary greatly. In its most severe state, hyperemesis gravidarum may result in volume contraction, starvation, and electrolyte abnormalities; however, as a mild condition, it may be self-limiting and intermittent and may respond favorably to placebo. Other clinical strategies include attention to fluid and electrolyte management, the use of vitamin supplements, reduced intake of dietary fats with increased intake of carbohydrates, and methods aimed at reducing psychosomatic complaints.[58]

Evaluation of teratogenicity of drugs administered during the first trimester of pregnancy is of great importance, particularly in patients with a condition with such variability in its presentation. However, proof of teratogenicity varies among animals and humans. In animals, tests of this nature are performed in the laboratory, may vary with animal strain and breed, and may not be good predictors of human experience. Conversely, the clinical laboratory of patient care is the testing ground for agents used in humans. From this setting, case reports and retrospective epidemiologic reports document the outcome of these human experiences.

Teratogenicity is a major consideration for the use of antiemetic drugs during pregnancy and is the primary factor that dictates this condition's drug of choice. Therefore, both the benefit and side effect profiles for the mother as well as potential fetal risks are important. Of the agents commonly used, those that have demonstrated teratogenicity in animals include diphenhydramine, meclizine, prochlorperazine, and thiethylperazine.[57–61] In humans, however, meclizine has not been shown to have these same effects. Most authors currently do not recommend metoclopramide because its use during pregnancy requires further study. Also, its primary benefit in nonpregnant patients with nausea and vomiting has been in association with cancer, chemotherapy, and high intravenous doses. In addition, serotonin antagonists cannot be recommended in this setting, even though animal studies to date have revealed no harm. Presently, cyclizine and meclizine are considered the drugs of choice for the treatment of nausea and vomiting during pregnancy.[62] Promethazine should be considered as a third choice and prescribed only if symptoms are severe and cannot be controlled by adequate trials of one of the first two agents.

ANTIEMETIC USE IN CHILDREN

Most studies of antiemetic drugs have primarily included adult patients. Appropriate drug and dosage selection as well as the use of combination regimens lead to unique clinical questions in the management of children. For example, children may not require or tolerate the same mg/kg doses of drugs commonly used in adults. This finding is particularly true for metoclopramide. During the 1960s and 1970s this drug was given as an antiemetic to European children with gastroenteritis. From these populations came numerous reports citing extrapyramidal reactions at cumulative daily doses less than 2.0 mg/kg.[63,64] It is now appreciated that these side effects should be anticipated in children and may occur at intravenous doses as low as 0.5 mg/kg given as repeated doses four times per day. Interestingly, differences in drug disposition, including plasma metoclopramide concentrations, probably do not explain the occurrence of dystonia.[65]

Dosage regimens and anticipated outcome of other antiemetic drugs in children are also unique compared to adults. Phenothiazines appear more likely to produce neuromuscular reactions, particularly dystonias, in children, especially when administered during acute viral illnesses such as chickenpox, measles, and gastroenteritis. Therefore, phenothiazines should be reserved for patients with prolonged vomiting in whom the benefit-to-risk ratio has been examined carefully. Promethazine may be the best agent in this class because its activity is most like that of the antihistamines rather than the phenothiazines.

Antihistaminic–anticholinergic agents may present some difficulty in selection depending on the exact age of the child. For example, the use of benzquinamide, buclizine, cyclizine, and scopolamine is not recommended in children under the age of 12 years. Dimenhydrinate, however, has been used in children at doses that differ by age for those less than 2 years, those 2 to 6 years, and children 6 to 12 years. Interestingly, trimethobenzamide may be used in children orally or rectally but is not recommended for injection. When chosen, it should be prescribed according to weight. Trimethobenzamide is also not recommended by any route for premature or newborn infants. The butyrophenones, haloperidol and droperidol, have been used in children but not usually in those younger than 2 to 3 years. In children older than 3 years of age, most patients studied have received droperidol in the preoperative setting as an adjunct to general anesthesia. Fewer children, comparatively, have received droperidol during chemotherapy. Diphenidol, an agent associated with significant adverse effects, is usually not prescribed in children and is not recommended in patients weighing less than 50 pounds. Parenteral lorazepam, although perhaps useful in adults, is not generally recommended for patients younger than 18 years. Likewise, dronabinol is not indicated for children because it has been studied most in patients older than 12 years. Corticosteroids are often included in the anticancer regimens received by children and may be prescribed as antiemetics in this age group, particularly in combination with serotonin antagonists. Finally, serotonin antagonists have been evaluated in children of various ages and have been shown to be both safe and effective, particularly in patients receiving cytotoxic chemotherapy or those in the postoperative period. These agents have been shown to provide a significant reduction in nausea and vomiting in the absence of extrapyramidal effects.[66–68] However, consistent dosage information is primarily available for children 4 to 18 years of age. Comparatively little information is available for children 3 years of age and younger.

PHARMACOECONOMIC CONSIDERATIONS

As new drugs become accepted into clinical practice, the pharmacoeconomic issues associated with these drugs become increasingly important. Most pharmacoeconomic issues for the antiemetic drugs have concerned the use of 5-HT_3 antagonists in patients with chemotherapy-induced or postoperative nausea and vomiting. However, regardless of the medical reason associated with these symptoms, the use of expensive medications will always come under scrutiny, particularly because there are numerous potentially effective antiemetic therapies. For example, the routine use of 5-HT_3 antagonists in surgical patients has been questioned because so many procedures produce minimal risk of nausea or vomiting. Depending upon the variables previously reviewed, some patients are at much higher risk of developing these symptoms than others. Clearly, studies are needed that evaluate the pharmacoeconomic issues involved in all common medical situations in which nausea and vomiting pose a clinically significant problem.

There are many important variables to consider when attempting to document the overall costs of using a medication in a particular medical situation. Medication costs alone cannot begin to explain the true pharmacoeconomic outcome associated with the use of antiemetic drugs. For example, the costs associated with an unexpected hospital admission due to vomiting in an outpatient undergoing a surgical procedure quickly offsets the savings related to the selection of an inexpensive antiemetic drug. In this and other similar situations, it is economically and clinically important to develop antiemetic protocols based upon appropriate decision-analysis and clinical outcomes so that certain patients appropriately receive an expensive drug while other patients appropriately receive a less expensive agent. In developing such protocols, all issues related to nausea and vomiting must be taken into account. As the number of patients who receive outpatient chemotherapy and surgery increases, the need to prevent subsequent hospitalizations from potentially unsuccessful antiemetic therapy will become increasingly important. However, as the cost of serotonin antagonists declines due to the availability of generic substitutes, greater acceptance of these agents as first-line therapy is more likely.

EVALUATION OF THERAPEUTIC OUTCOMES

In accordance with the information presented concerning age and clinical condition, individualized therapy may be possible through drug selection and dosage adjustment. Monitoring criteria for drug therapy should include the subjective assessment of the patient's severity of nausea as well as objective parameters such as the number of vomiting episodes each day, the volume of vomitus lost, and evaluation of fluid, acid–base balance, and electrolyte status, with particular attention to serum sodium, potassium, and chloride concentrations. In addition, evaluation of renal function may become important, particularly in patients with volume contraction and progressive electrolyte disturbances. Specific parameters include daily urine volume, urine specific gravity, and urine electrolyte concentrations. Physical assessment of patients should include evaluation of mucous membranes and skin turgor, because dryness of these tissues may be indicative of significant volume loss.

▶ PRINCIPLES OF PHARMACOTHERAPY

- Nausea and vomiting may be a part of the symptom complex for a variety of gastrointestinal, cardiovascular, infectious, neurologic, metabolic, or psychogenic processes.
- Nausea and vomiting may be caused by a variety of medications or other noxious agents, including cytotoxic chemotherapy, analgesics, general anesthetics, antibiotics, theophylline, digitalis, and amphotericin.
- The overall goal of treatment should be to prevent or eliminate nausea and vomiting regardless of etiology.
- Nondrug treatment of nausea and vomiting may include dietary, physical, or psychological management. In each case, the simplest effective therapy should be employed.
- Drug treatment options for the management of nausea and vomiting may be as simple as the use of

antacids or as complex as the combination of two or more potent antiemetic drugs.

- Common antiemetic regimens used in patients with cancer should usually include medication prior to chemotherapy, with one or more possible doses after chemotherapy. Common regimens include (1) prochlorperazine with or without lorazepam; (2) ondansetron, granisetron, or dolasetron alone; (3) ondansetron, granisetron, or dolasetron plus dexamethasone or methylprednisolone; and (4) any of the preceding regimens plus dexamethasone or lorazepam as needed.
- Common antiemetic regimens used in patients undergoing surgical procedures may include (1) ondansetron, granisetron, or dolasetron alone; (2) metoclopramide alone; (3) droperidol alone; or (4) ondansetron or granisetron plus dexamethasone or methylprednisolone.
- The therapeutic end point for antiemetic therapy is an acceptable reduction or absence of nausea and vomiting before and after surgery, chemotherapy, or other symptom-inducing activities.
- Evaluation of adverse reactions from antiemetic therapy includes attention to sedation and extrapyramidal effects.
- The total costs associated with antiemetic therapy should be considered, especially in settings involving the management of complex symptoms or other uses of serotonin antagonists.

REFERENCES

1. Hanson JS, McCallum RW. The diagnosis and management of nausea and vomiting: A review. Am J Gastroenterol 1985;80:210–218.
2. Frytak S, Moertel CG. Management of nausea and vomiting in the cancer patient. JAMA 1981;245:393–396.
3. Feldman M. Nausea and vomiting. In: Sleisenger MH, Fordtran JS, eds. Gastrointestinal Disease. Philadelphia, Saunders, 1983:160–177.
4. Redd WH. Control of nausea and vomiting in chemotherapy patients: Four effective behavioral methods. Postgrad Med 1984;75:105–113.
5. Eyre HJ, Ward JH. Control of cancer chemotherapy-induced nausea and vomiting. Cancer 1984;54:2642–2648.
6. Morrow GR. Prevalence and correlation of anticipatory nausea and vomiting in chemotherapy patients. J Natl Cancer Inst 1982;68: 585–588.
7. Lyles JN, Burish TG, Knozely MG, et al. Efficacy of relaxation training and guided imagery in reducing the aversiveness of cancer chemotherapy. J Consult Clin Psychol 1982;50:509–524.
8. Morrow GR, Morrell C. Behavioral treatment for the anticipatory nausea and vomiting induced by cancer chemotherapy. N Engl J Med 1982;307:1476–1480.
9. Redd WH, Andresen GV, Minagawa RY. Hypnotic control of anticipatory emesis in patients receiving cancer chemotherapy. J Consult Clin Psychol 1982;50:14-19.
10. Dutro MP, Ammerson AB. Comparison of liquid antacids. N Engl J Med 1980;302:967.
11. Fordtran JS, Morawski S, Richardson C. *In vitro* and *in vivo* evaluation of antacids. N Engl J Med 1973;288:923.
12. Seipler JK, Mahakian K, Trudeau WT. Current concepts in clinical therapeutics: Peptic ulcer disease. Clin Pharm 1986;5:128–142.
13. Edmunds SJ, Prys RC. Pharmacology of drugs used in neuroleptanalgesia. Br J Anaesth 1970;42:207–216.
14. Wampler G. The pharmacology and clinical effectiveness of phenothiazines and related drugs for managing chemotherapy-induced emesis. Drugs 1983;25(suppl):35–51.
15. Lucas VS. Phenothiazines as antiemetics. In: Lazlo J, ed. Antiemetics and Cancer Chemotherapy. Baltimore, Williams & Wilkins, 1983: 93–107.
16. Jacobs AJ, Deppe G, Cohen CJ. A comparison of the antiemetic effects of droperidol and prochlorperazine in chemotherapy with cisplatinum. Gynecol Oncol 1980;10:55–57.
17. Cersosimo RJ, Bromer R, Hoffer S, et al. The antiemetic activity of droperidol administered by intramuscular injection during cisplatin chemotherapy: A pilot study. Drug Intell Clin Pharm 1985;19: 118–121.
18. Paladine W, Price L, Sokol G, et al. Antiemetic trial of droperidol. Proc Am Soc Clin Oncol 1980;21:381.
19. Brown RE, Gregg RE, Hood JC. Droperidol treatment of streptozotocin-induced nausea and vomiting. Drug Intell Clin Pharm 1982; 16:775–776.
20. Cersosimo RJ, Karp DD. Adrenal corticosteroids as antiemetics during cancer chemotherapy. Pharmacotherapy 1986;6:118–127.
21. Gralla RJ. Metoclopramide: A review of antiemetic trials. Drugs 1983;25(suppl):63–73.
22. Schyulze-Delriev K. Metoclopramide. Gastroenterology 1979;77: 768–779.
23. Strum SB, McDermed JE, Lauer D, et al. Control of acute-onset and delayed-onset chemotherapy-induced nausea and emesis with metoclopramide-based regimens. Intern Med Specialist 1985;6: 104–112.
24. Fortner CL, Finley RS, Grove WR. Combination antiemetic therapy in the control of chemotherapy-induced emesis. Drug Intell Clin Pharm 1985;19:21–24.
25. Plezia PM, Alberts DS, Kessler J, et al. Immediate termination of intractable vomiting induced by cisplatin combination chemotherapy using an intensive five-drug antiemetic regimen. Cancer Treat Rep 1984;68:1493–1495.
26. Stoudemire A, Cotanch P, Lazlo J. Recent advances in the pharmacologic and behavioral management of chemotherapy-induced emesis. Arch Intern Med 1984;144:1029–1033.
27. Cognetti F, Pinnaro P, Carlini P, et al. Randomized open crossover trial between metoclopramide and dexamethasone for the prevention of cisplatin-induced nausea and vomiting. Eur J Cancer Clin Oncol 1984;20:183–187.
28. Aapro MS, Plezia PM, Albert DS, et al. Double-blind crossover study of the antiemetic efficacy of high-dose dexamethasone versus high-dose metoclopramide. J Clin Oncol 1984;2:466–471.
29. Markman M, Sheidler V, Ettinger DS, et al. Antiemetic efficacy of dexamethasone. Randomized, double-blind, crossover study with prochlorperazine in patients receiving cancer chemotherapy. N Engl J Med 1984;311:549–552.
30. Kolaric K, Roth A. Methylprednisolone as an antiemetic in patients on cis-platinum chemotherapy. Results of a controlled randomized study. Tumori 1983;69:43–46.
31. Giaconne G, Donadio M, Musella R, et al. Comparison of methylprednisolone and metoclopramide in the prophylactic treatment of cisplatin-induced nausea and vomiting. Tumori 1984;70:237–241.
32. Schallier D, Van Belle S, De Greve J, et al. Methylprednisolone as an antiemetic drug. A randomized double-blind study. Cancer Chemother Pharmacol 1985;14:235–237.
33. Ell C, Konig HJ, Brockmann P, et al. Antiemetic efficacy of moderately high-dose metoclopramide in patients receiving varying doses of cisplatin. Controlled comparison with combination of methylprednisolone and metoclopramide. Oncology 1985;42:354– 357.

34. Pope CE II. Acid-reflux disorders. N Engl J Med 1994;331:656–660.
35. Marty M, Pouillart P, Scholl S, et al. Comparison of the 5-hydroxytryptamine$_3$ (serotonin) antagonist ondansetron (GR 38032F) with high-dose metoclopramide in the control of cisplatin-induced emesis. N Engl J Med 1990;322:816–821.
36. Tyers MB, Bunce KT, Humphrey PPA. Pharmacological and antiemetic properties of ondansetron. Eur J Cancer Clin Oncol 1989; 25(suppl):S15–S19.
37. Bryson JC, Finn AL, Plagge PB, et al. The safety profile of IV ondansetron from clinical trials. Proc ASCL 1990;9:328. Abstract.
38. Smith RN. Safety of ondansetron. Eur J Cancer Clin Oncol 1989; 25(suppl):S47–S50.
39. Chaffee BJ, Tankanow RM. Ondansetron—The first of a new class of antiemetic agents. Clin Pharm 1991;10:430–446.
40. Aapro MS. Review of experience with ondansetron and granisetron. Ann Oncol 1993;4(suppl 3):S9–S14.
41. Lazlo J, Lucas VS. Synthetic cannabinoids. In: Lazlo J, ed. Antiemetics and Cancer Chemotherapy. Baltimore, Williams & Wilkins, 1983: 116–128.
42. Herman TS, Einhorn LH, Jones SE, et al. Superiority of nabilone over prochlorperazine as an antiemetic in patients receiving cancer chemotherapy. N Engl J Med 1979;300:1295–1297.
43. Tortorice PV, O'Connell MB. Management of chemotherapy-induced nausea and vomiting. Pharmacotherapy 1990;10:129–145.
44. Anderson PO, McGuire GG. Δ-9-Tetrahydrocannabinol as an antiemetic. Am J Hosp Pharm 1981;38:639–646.
45. Neidhart JA, Gagen M. Experimental antiemetic agents (other than cannabinoids and metoclopramide): In: Lazlo J, ed. Antiemetics and Cancer Chemotherapy. Baltimore, Williams & Wilkins, 1983: 142–163.
46. Morrow FR, Lindke J, Black PM. Predicting development of anticipatory nausea in cancer patients: Prospective examination of eight clinical characteristics. J Pain Symptom Manage 1991;6:215–223.
47. Lazlo J. Oral lorazepam to improve tolerance of cytotoxic therapy. Lancet 1981;1:1316–1317.
48. Meyer M, Long AM, Natale RB, et al. Phase I, II and III trials of a new antiemetic agent—lorazepam. Proc Am Soc Clin Oncol 1983; 2:88.
49. Mitchelson F. Pharmacological agents affecting emesis: A review. Drugs 1992;43:443–463.
50. Kenny GN. Risk factors for postoperative nausea and vomiting. Anaesthesia 1994;49(suppl):6–10.
51. Scott JR, Barnes GR, Wright RJ, Ruddock CJ. The effect on motion sickness and oculomotor function of GR 38032F, a 5-HT$_3$-receptor antagonist with anti-emetic properties. Br J Clin Pharmacol 1989; 27:147–157.
52. Stott JR, Barnes GR, Wright RJ, et al. The effect on motion sickness and oculomotor function of GR 38032F, a 5-HT$_3$-receptor antagonist with antiemetic properties. Br J Clin Pharmacol 1989;27:147–157.
53. Wood CD. Antimotion sickness and antiemetic drugs. Drugs 1979; 17:471–479.
54. Jarnfelt-Samsioe A, Samsioe G, Velinder GM. Nausea and vomiting in pregnancy—A contribution to its epidemiology. Gynecol Obstet Invest 1983;16:221–229.
55. Tuchmann-Duplessis H. Drugs and xenobiotics as teratogens. Pharmacol Ther 1984;26:273–344.
56. Leathem AM. Safety and efficacy of antiemetics used to treat nausea and vomiting in pregnancy. Clin Pharm 1986;5:660–668.
57. Fairweather DV. Nausea and vomiting during pregnancy. Obstet Gynecol Annu 1978;7:91–105.
58. Kousen M. Treatment of nausea and vomiting in pregnancy. Am Fam Physician 1993;48:1279–1284.
59. Schardein JL. Drugs as Teratogens. Cleveland, CRC Press, 1976: 5, 130.
60. Shepard TH. Catalog of Teratogenic Agents, 4th ed. Baltimore, Johns Hopkins University Press, 1983.
61. Nishimura H, Tanimura T. Clinical Aspects of Teratogenicity of Drugs. New York, Elsevier, 1976:212, 241.
62. American Medical Association Department of Drugs. AMA Drug Evaluations Annual. Chicago, AMA, 1995:471
63. Low LCK, Goel KM. Metoclopramide poisoning in children. Arch Dis Child 1980;55:310–312.
64. Casteels-Van Daele M, Jaeken J, Van Der Schueren P, et al. Dystonic reactions in children caused by metoclopramide. Arch Dis Child 1970;45:130–133.
65. Bateman DN, Craft AW, Nicholson E, et al. Dystonic reactions and the pharmacokinetics of metoclopramide in children. Br J Clin Pharmacol 1983;15:557–559.
66. Furst SR, Rodarte A, Demars P. Ondansetron reduces postoperative vomiting in children undergoing tonsillectomy. Anesthesiology 1993;79:A1197. Abstract.
67. Lawhorn CD, Brown RE, Jr., Schmitz ML, et al. Prevention of postoperative vomiting in pediatric outpatient strabismus surgery. Anesthesiology 1993;79:A1196. Abstract.
68. Stevens RF. The role of ondansetron in paediatric patients: A review of three studies. Eur J Cancer 1991;27(suppl 1):S20–S22.

34

Diarrhea and Constipation

R. Leon Longe, PharmD, and Joseph T. DiPiro, PharmD, FCCP

DIARRHEA

In the United States, diarrhea is a troublesome discomfort that is sometimes fatal. Usually, diarrheal episodes begin abruptly and subside within 1 or 2 days without treatment. This chapter focuses primarily on noninfectious diarrhea, with only minor reference to infectious diarrhea (see Chap. 103). Diarrhea is often a symptom of a systemic disease and not all possible causes are covered. This chapter presents a basic understanding of management.

To understand diarrhea, one must have a reasonable definition of the condition, but the literature is extremely variable on this. Simply, diarrhea is abnormal frequency and liquidity of fecal discharge compared with the patient's normal stools. Frequency and consistency are variable within and between individuals. For example, some individuals defecate as many as three times per day, while others defecate only two or three times per week. A Western diet usually produces a daily stool weighing between 100 and 300 g, depending on nonabsorbable materials (mainly carbohydrates). Patients with serious diarrhea have a stool of more than 300 g/d; however, a subset of patients have frequent small, watery passages. Another exception is the vegetable fiber-rich diet (eaten in some Eastern cultures such as African), which normally produces stools weighing more than 300 g/d.

Diarrhea may be associated with a specific disease of the intestines or secondary to a disease outside the intestines. For instance, bacillary dysentery directly affects the gut, while diabetes mellitus causes neuropathic diarrheal episodes. Furthermore, we divide diarrhea into acute or chronic forms. Infectious diarrhea is often acute; diabetic diarrhea is chronic. Whether acute or chronic, diarrhea has the same pathophysiologic causes that help identification of specific treatments.

EPIDEMIOLOGY

The epidemiology of diarrhea is different in developed versus developing countries.[1] In the United States, diarrheal illnesses are usually not reported to the Centers for Disease Control and Prevention (CDC) unless associated with an outbreak or an unusual organism or condition. For example, AIDS has been identified with protracted diarrheal illness. Some populations are particularly affected and generate a public health concern. Diarrhea is a major problem in day care centers and nursing homes, probably because early childhood and senescence plus environmental conditions are risk factors. However, an exact epidemiologic profile in the United States is not available through the CDC or published literature.

In the United States, viral and bacterial organisms account for most of the infectious diarrhea. Common bacterial organisms are *Shigella, Salmonella, Campylobacter, Staphylococcus,* and *Escherichia coli*. Food-borne bacterial infection has become a major concern as the result of several major food poisoning episodes that were traced to poor sanitary conditions in meat processing plants. Acute viral infections are attributed mostly to Norwalk and rotavirus groups.

In developing cultures, acute diarrhea kills 5 million children annually.[2] The World Health Organization (WHO) estimates that 744 million to 1 billion diarrheal attacks occur annually in the world's children. These findings are associated with poor sanitation, poor nutrition, and age less than 5 years, especially infancy. The leading cause is an invasion by infectious organisms. In the United States about 3 million children are stricken annually, with 500,000 children needing medical care and 55,000 being hospitalized. Usually the children recover without ill effects, but some deaths occur each year. The estimated direct medical cost is about $400 million annually.

PATHOPHYSIOLOGY

In the fasting state, 9 L of intestinal fluid enters the proximal small intestine each day. Of this fluid, we ingest 2 L with the diet; the remainder comes from internal secretions. Because of meal content, duodenal chyme is usually hypertonic. When chyme reaches the ileum, osmolality adjusts to equal that of plasma, with most dietary fat, carbohydrate, and protein absorbed. Ileal chyme reduces to about 1 L/d entering the colon. The electrolyte profile of ileal chyme per liter is normally sodium 140 mEq, potassium 8 mEq, chloride 60 mEq, and bicarbonate 70 mEq. In the normal state, the colon absorbs 900 mL, reducing chyme to 100 mL water loss daily. Fecal electrolyte content (mEq/L) is sodium 40, chloride 15, potassium 90, and bicarbonate 30.

From the preceding description, one visualizes diarrhea as an imbalance in absorption and secretion of water and electrolytes. In normal volunteers, small intestine water has a maximum rate of absorption. If the small intestine absorption capacity is exceeded, chyme overloads the colon, resulting in diarrhea. In humans, the colon absorptive capacity is about 5 L daily. Colonic fluid transport is critical to water and electrolyte balance. In simplistic terms, diarrhea is a seesaw with absorption on one end and secretion on the other. If these processes are equally weighed, one has a normal bowel movement. If absorption decreases or secretion increases beyond normal, diarrhea results. Normally, the absorption of water and electrolytes exceeds secretory fluxes. One should understand the mechanisms at work controlling water, electrolyte, and glucose movements.

Absorption through the intestines occurs by three mechanisms: active transport, diffusion, and solvent drag. Active transport means the expenditure of energy is required to move a substrate against a concentration gradient across a membrane. Diffusion, a nonenergy-dependent means for moving substrates, transports substances through a membrane along a concentration gradient. A solvent can "drag" a substrate across a membrane.

Water moves across the gut after the movement of solutes such as sodium and by diffusion.[3] Diffusion obeys the principle of osmosis. For example, when chyme is dilute, water diffuses from the gut into the blood. Also, as ions (e.g., sodium) or nutrients (e.g., glucose) cross a membrane, water quickly "follows" to maintain an isosmotic state. The intestinal mucosa is semipermeable and allows selective solute and solvent movements. For instance, the proximal intestine rapidly makes meal content isosmotic. In the colon, chyme may be hypertonic; bacterial metabolism of carbohydrates partly explains hypertonic colonic state. Unabsorbed carbohydrates metabolize into volatile fatty acids and are absorbed across the colon.

Active transport and diffusion handle sodium transport. Because of the high luminal sodium concentration (142 mEq/L), sodium diffuses from the sodium-rich gut into the epithelial cell. Inside the epithelial cell, sodium is actively pumped from a lower concentration (50 mEq/L) to a higher concentration (142 mEq/L) in the blood by an active sodium-potassium–activated ATPase.

To keep an isoelectric condition across the epithelial membrane, chloride moves from the lumen into the epithelial cell. The absorption of sodium through the epithelial cells creates an electronegativity in the chyme. To reestablish electric neutrality, positively charged sodium ions pull negatively charged chloride ions into the epithelial cell. In the epithelial cell chloride channels opened by cyclic adenosine monophosphate (AMP) permit movement of chloride into the intestinal lumen.

Hydrogen ions are handled by an indirect mechanism in the upper small intestine. As sodium is absorbed, hydrogen ions are secreted into the gut. Once in the gut, hydrogen ions combine with bicarbonate ions to form carbonic acid, which then dissociates into carbon dioxide and water. The carbon dioxide readily diffuses into the blood for expiration through the lung. The water remains in the chyme.

Paracellular pathways are major routes of ion movement. As ions, monosaccharides, and amino acids are actively transported, they create an osmotic pressure, drawing water and electrolytes across the intestinal wall. This pathway accounts for very large amounts of ion transport, especially sodium.

Sodium plays an important role in stimulating glucose absorption. Glucose absorption happens with active transport of sodium from the epithelial cell into the blood. For active sodium absorption, glucose combines with the transport protein carrying sodium into the blood. This phenomenon is called cotransport. This biologic mechanism is extremely important in dietary management of diarrhea. Another glucose absorption mechanism is diffusion, which is concentration dependent and accounts for a major mechanism.

Sodium cotransport of amino acids happens as described for sodium-glucose cotransport. Amino acids are transported into most cells against large concentration gradients. When an amino acid combines with extracelluar sodium to specific transport protein, both substrates move from the lumen to the blood. Cotransport absorption mechanisms of glucose-sodium and amino acid-sodium are extremely important for treating diarrhea.

Gut motility influences absorption and secretion. Time in which luminal content is in contact with the epithelium is under neural and hormonal control. Neurohormonal substances and neurotransmitters also regulate ion transport. Some are circulating hormones like angiotensin, vasopressin, glucocorticoid, and aldosterone. For instance, in the kidney, aldosterone strongly conserves sodium from the gut along with water, chloride, and other electrolytes.

MECHANISMS

Four general pathophysiologic mechanisms disrupt water and electrolyte balance, leading to diarrhea, and are the basis of diagnosis and therapy. These are (1) a change in active ion transport by either decreased sodium absorption or increased chloride secretion, (2) change in intestinal motility, (3) increase in luminal osmolarity, and (4) increase in tissue hydrostatic pressure. These mechanisms have been related to four broad clinical diarrheal groups: secretory, osmotic, exudative, and altered intestinal transit.

Secretory diarrhea occurs when a stimulating substance either increases secretion or decreases absorption of large amounts of water and electrolytes. Substances that cause excess secretions include vasoactive intestinal peptide (VIP) from a pancreatic tumor, unabsorbed dietary fat in steatorrhea, laxatives, hormones (such as secretin), bacterial toxins, and excessive bile salts. Many of these agents stimulate intracellular cyclic AMP and inhibit Na^+/K^+-ATPase, leading to increased secretion. Also, many of these mediators inhibit ion absorption simultaneously. Clinically, secretory diarrhea is recognized by large stool volumes (> 1 L/d) with normal ionic contents and osmolality about equal to plasma. Fasting does not change the stool volume.

Poorly absorbed substances retain intestinal fluids, making osmotic diarrhea. This mechanism occurs with malabsorption, lactose intolerance, divalent ions (e.g., antacids), or poorly soluble carbohydrate (e.g., lactulose). As a poorly soluble solute is transported, the gut adjusts the osmolality to plasma; in so doing, water and electrolytes flux into the lumen. The loss of sodium and water is less than with some diarrheal mechanisms. Clinically, osmotic diarrhea is distinguishable from other types because it stops when the patient fasts.

Inflammatory gut diseases discharge mucus, serum proteins, and blood into the gut. Sometimes bowel movements consist only of mucus, exudate, and blood. Exudative diarrhea probably affects other absorptive, secretory, or motility functions to account for the large stool volume.

Changed intestinal motility causes diarrhea by three mechanisms: reduction of contact time in the small intestine, premature emptying of the colon, and bacterial overgrowth. Chyme must be exposed long enough for normal absorption and secretion. If contact time decreases, diarrhea occurs. Intestinal resection or bypass surgery and drugs (such as metoclopramide) cause this type of diarrhea. Increased exposure time also allows fecal bacteria overgrowth. A characteristic small intestine diarrheal pattern is rapid, small, coupling bursts of waves. These waves are inefficient, do not allow absorption, and rapidly dump chyme into the colon. Once in the colon, chyme exceeds the colonic capabilities to absorb water or a diseased colon does not function properly.

CLINICAL PRESENTATION

Diarrhea is divided into acute and chronic disorders. Usually, acute diarrheal episodes subside with 72 hours of onset. Chronic diarrhea involves frequent attacks over two to three extended periods. If diarrhea persists or gross blood is present, the patient needs an extensive evaluation.

HISTORY AND PHYSICAL EXAMINATION

Onset and duration differentiate acute and chronic diarrhea. The leading cause of acute diarrhea is viral gastroenteritis. With acute diarrhea, the patient complains of an abrupt onset of nausea, vomiting, abdominal pain, headache, fever, chills, and malaise. Bowel movements are frequent and never bloody, and diarrhea lasts 12 to 60 hours. Abdominal pain is evaluated for duration, location, and character. Intermittent periumbilical or lower right quadrant pain with cramps and audible bowel sounds is characteristic of small intestinal disease. When pain is present in large intestinal diarrhea, it is a gripping, aching sensation with tenesmus (straining ineffective and painful stooling). Pain localizes to the hypogastric region, right or left lower quadrant, or sacral region. In chronic diarrhea, history of previous bouts, weight loss, anorexia, and chronic weakness are important findings. Certain diarrheal diseases are associated with specific ages. For example, diarrhea from colon cancer is common with advancing age while diarrhea from viral gastroenteritis is largely a childhood condition.

Americans traveling abroad may have traveler's or parasitic diarrhea. Environmental conditions such as the recent ingestion of bacteria-contaminated foods identify

TABLE 34–1. Drugs Causing Diarrhea

Laxatives
Antacids (magnesium containing)
Antibiotics
Clindamycin
Tetracyclines
Sulfonamides
Any broad-spectrum antibiotic
Antihypertensives
Reserpine
Guanethidine
Methyldopa
Guanabenz
Guanadrel
Cholinergics
Bethanechol
Metaclopramide
Neostigmine
Cardiac agents
Quinidine
Digitalis
Digoxin

"food poisoning" as a possible etiology. An attentive dietary history identifies offending foods (e.g., dairy products with lactose intolerance). With AIDS, we cannot overlook a history that focuses on high-risk situations. Recent gastrointestinal surgery may cause a "dumping syndrome."

A medication history is extremely important in identifying drug-induced diarrhea (Table 34–1). For example, many agents, including antibiotics and other drugs, cause pseudomembranous colitis. Self-inflicted laxative abuse for weight loss is popular. Neurotic or psychotic behavior leads to laxative abuse. Drug side effects (e.g., quinidine) often present as diarrhea.

Stool characteristics are important. A description of the frequency, volume, consistency, and color provides diagnostic clues. For instance, diarrhea starting in the small intestine produces a copious, watery or fatty (greasy), and foul-smelling stool; contains undigested food particles; and is usually free from gross blood. Colonic diarrhea appears as small, pasty, and sometimes bloody or mucoid movements. Rectal tenesmus with flatus accompanies large intestine diarrhea.

In diarrhea, physical examination of the abdomen shows hyperperistalsis with borborygmi (growling stomach sounds) and generalized or local tenderness. A rectal examination detects masses or possibly fecal impaction, a common cause of diarrhea in the elderly. Checking skin turgor and degree of oral saliva assesses hydration. We should identify physical signs of systemic disease (e.g., diabetic neuropathy). If the patient has hypotension, tachycardia, weak radial pulse, or stupor, severe dehydration is present. Fever strongly suggests an infectious cause.

LABORATORY AND ENDOSCOPIC TESTS

Special tests are used for diagnosing unexplained diarrhea, especially in chronic situations.[4,5] Stool studies include examination for parasites and ova, blood, mucus, fat, osmolality, pH, electrolyte analysis, and cultures. Stool test kits are useful for detecting gastrointestinal viruses, particularly rotavirus. Antibody serologic testing shows rising titer over a 3- to 6-day period, but the test is not practical and nonspecific. Occasionally total daily stool volume is also determined. Besides stool studies, direct endoscopic visualization and biopsy are used to diagnose certain conditions such as colitis or cancer. Radiographic studies are helpful in neoplastic and inflammatory conditions.

PROGNOSIS

Most acute diarrhea is self-limiting, subsiding within 72 hours. However, infants, young children, the elderly, and debilitated persons are at risk for morbid and mortal events in prolonged or voluminous diarrhea. These groups are at risk for water, electrolyte, and acid–base disturbances, and potentially cardiovascular collapse and death. The prognosis for chronic diarrhea depends on the cause; for example, diarrhea secondary to diabetes mellitus waxes and wanes throughout life.

PREVENTION

Acute viral diarrheal illness often occurs in day care centers and nursing homes. Because person-to-person route is the mechanism of spreading viral gastroenteritis, isolation techniques prevent spread between these populations and health care workers. For bacterial, parasite, and protozoal infections, strict food handling, sanitation, water, and other environmental hygiene practices prevent and control their transmission. Patients should identify and avoid hidden dietary sources, such as sorbitol in dietetic products or "Chinese food dumping" syndrome; a milk allergy is also a cause. If diarrhea is secondary to another illness, controlling the primary condition is necessary. Antibiotics and bismuth subsalicylate are advocated for preventing traveler's diarrhea, along with special care with drinking water and fresh vegetables.

▶ TREATMENT: Diarrhea

DESIRED OUTCOME

If prevention is not successful and diarrhea occurs, the therapeutic goals are to (1) manage diet; (2) prevent excessive water, electrolyte, and acid–base disturbances; (3) provide symptomatic relief; (4) treat curable causes; and (5) manage secondary disorders causing diarrhea (Figs. 34–1 and 34–2). Clinicians must clearly understand that diarrhea, like a cough, may be a body defense mechanism for ridding itself of harmful substances or pathogens. The correct therapeutic response is not necessarily to stop diarrhea at all costs!

NONPHARMACOLOGIC MANAGEMENT

Management of the diet is a first priority. Most clinicians continue to recommend stopping solid foods for 24 hours and avoiding dairy products. However, fasting is questionable because the assumptions have not been studied. In osmotic diarrhea, these maneuvers control the problem. If the mechanism is secretory, the diarrhea persists. When the patient is nauseated or vomiting, a mild, digestible low-residue diet is administered for 24 hours. If vomiting is present and uncontrollable with antiemetics (see Chap. 33), nothing is taken by mouth. As bowel movements de-

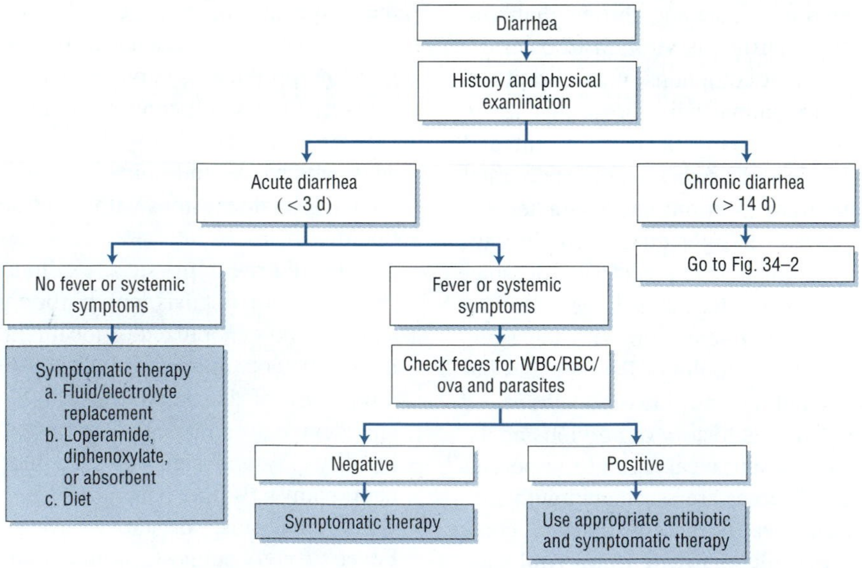

FIGURE 34–1. Recommendations for treating acute diarrhea. Follow these steps: (1) Perform a complete history and physical examination. (2) Is the diarrhea acute or chronic? If chronic diarrhea, go to Fig. 34–2. (3) If acute diarrhea, check for fever and/or systemic signs and symptoms (i.e., toxic patient). If systemic illness (fever, anorexia, volume depletion), check for infectious source. If positive for infectious diarrhea, use appropriate antibiotic/anthelminthic drug, and symptomatic therapy. If negative for infectious cause, use only symptomatic treatment. (4) If no systemic findings, then use symptomatic therapy, based on severity of volume depletion, oral or parenteral fluid/electrolytes, antidiarrheal agents (see Table 34–3), and diet.

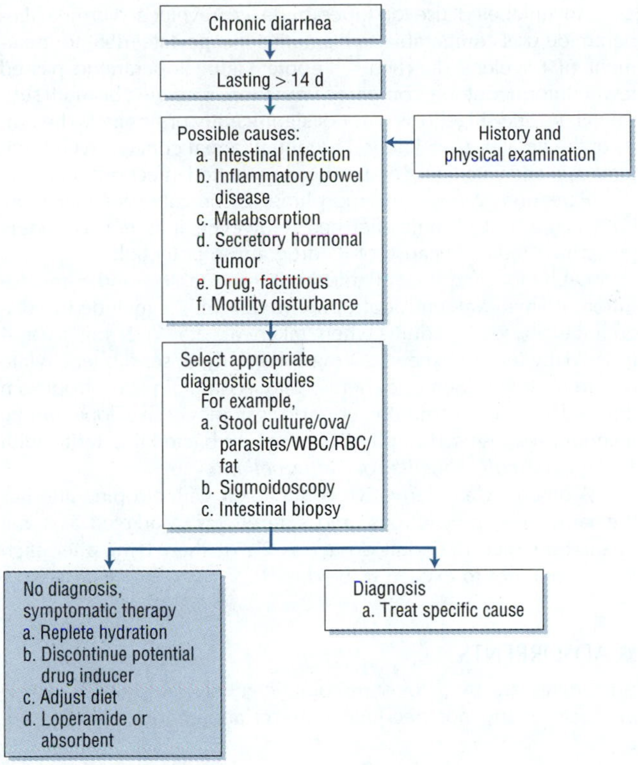

FIGURE 34–2. Recommendations for treating chronic diarrhea. Follow these steps: (1) Perform a careful history and physical examination. (2) The possible causes of chronic diarrhea are many. These can be classified into intestinal infections (bacterial, protozoal), inflammatory disease (Crohn's disease, ulcerative colitis), malabsorption (lactose intolerance), secretory hormonal tumor (intestinal carcinoid tumor, VIPoma), drug (antacid), factitious (laxative abuse), or motility disturbance (diabetes mellitus, irritable bowel syndrome, hyperthyroidism). (3) If the diagnosis is uncertain, selected appropriate diagnostic studies should be ordered. (4) Once diagnosed, treatment is planned for the underlying cause with symptomatic antidiarrheal therapy. (5) If no specific cause can be identified, symptomatic therapy is prescribed.

crease, a bland diet is begun. Research shows that feeding should continue in children with acute bacterial diarrhea.[6] Fed children have less morbidity and mortality, whether or not they receive oral rehydration fluids. Studies are not available in the elderly or other risk groups to decide the value of continued feeding in bacterial diarrhea.

WATER AND ELECTROLYTES

Rehydration and maintenance of water and electrolytes are the primary goals until the diarrheal episode ends. If the patient is volume depleted, rehydration replaces water and electrolytes to normal body composition. Then water and electrolytes losses are maintained by replacing volume losses. Many patients are not volume depleted and only need maintenance therapy. Parenteral and enteral routes supply water and electrolytes. If vomiting and dehydration are not severe, enteral feeding is the less costly and preferred method. In the United States, many commercial oral rehydration preparations are available (Table 34–2). Because of concerns about hypernatremia, American physicians continue to hospitalize and intravenously correct these deficits for severe dehydration. Oral solutions have been strongly recommended.[7] In developing countries, the World Health Organization Oral Rehydration Solution (WHO-ORS) saves the lives of millions of children (Table 34–2).

During diarrhea, the small intestine retains its ability to actively transport monosaccharides such as glucose. Glucose actively carries sodium with water and other electrolytes. Because the WHO-ORS has a high sodium concentration, U.S. physicians have been reluctant to use it in well-nourished children. This attitude could be changing as controlled comparative studies describe more favorable results with WHO-ORS than with parenteral fluids.[8] Amino acids promote sodium transport and act as an antisecretory agent. Researchers have added glycine to ORS in an attempt to create a "super-ORS." Reports, however, are disappointing, because glycine causes an osmotic diarrhea and diuresis in experimental concentrations.[9] Rice-based oral solution is a hyposmotically active substrate. Rice supplies long-chain molecules and elutes glucose without increasing stool or urine outflows. Pizarro and associates[10] reported effective rehydration of infants with acute diarrhea using a rice-based solution. They also reported decreased stool output and greater absorption and retention of fluid and electrolytes. In summary, oral rehydration solution is a life-saving treatment for millions afflicted in developing countries. Acceptance in the developed countries is less enthusiastic, but preventing hospitalization may win endorsement as a cost-effective alternative, saving millions of dollars.

TABLE 34–2. Oral Rehydration Solutions

	WHO–ORS[a]	Pedialyte[b] (Ross)	Rehydralyte[b] (Ross)	Infalyte (Mead Johnson)	Resol[b] (Wyeth)
Osmolality (mOsm/L)	333	249	304	200	269
Carbohydrates[b] (g/L)	20	25	25	30[c]	20
Calories (cal/L)	85	100	100	126	80
Electrolytes (mEq/L)					
Sodium	90	45	75	50	50
Potassium	20	20	20	25	20
Chloride	80	35	65	45	50
Citrate	—	30	30	34	34
Bicarbonate	30	—	—	—	—
Calcium	—	—	—	—	4
Magnesium	—	—	—	—	4
Sulfate	—	—	—	—	—
Phosphate	—	—	—	—	5

[a]World Health Organization Oral Rehydration Solution.
[b]Carbohydrate is glucose.
[c]Rice syrup solids are carbohydrate source.

PHARMACOLOGIC THERAPY

Various drugs have been used to treat diarrheal attacks (Table 34–3). These drugs are grouped into several categories: antimotility, adsorbents, antisecretory compounds, antibiotics, enzymes, and intestinal microflora. Usually, these drugs are not curative but palliative.

OPIATES AND THEIR DERIVATIVES

Opiates and opioid derivatives (1) delay the transit of intraluminal content or (2) increase gut capacity, prolonging contact and absorption. Enkephalins, endogenous opioid substances, regulate fluid movement across the mucosa by stimulating absorptive processes. Most opiates act through peripheral and central mechanisms, except loperamide, which acts peripherally. Loperamide is antisecretory; it inhibits the calcium-binding protein calmodulin, controlling chloride secretion.

Loperamide, available as 2-mg capsules or 1 mg/5 mL solution (both are nonprescription products), is suggested for managing acute and chronic diarrhea. The usual adult dose is initially 4 mg orally, followed by 2 mg after each loose stool, up to 16 mg/d. Used correctly, the drug has rare side effects such as dizziness and constipation. If the diarrhea is concurrent with a high fever or bloody stool, the patient should be referred to a physician. Also, diarrhea lasting beyond 48 hours after starting loperamide warrants medical attention.

An unlabeled use of loperamide is traveler's diarrhea. Loperamide was comparable to bismuth subsalicylate (BSS) for treatment of traveler's diarrhea.[11] People taking loperamide passed fewer unformed stools compared with those receiving bismuth subsalicylate, and shigellosis was not significantly prolonged. The limits of the opiates are addiction potential (a real concern with long-term use) and worsening of diarrhea in selected infectious diarrhea.

Paregoric, 2 mg/5 mL morphine, is indicated for managing both acute and chronic diarrhea. However, it is not as widely prescribed today, because of its drug abuse potential.

Diphenoxylate is available as 2.5-mg tablets and 5-mL solution. A small amount of atropine (0.025 mg) is included to discourage abuse. In adults when taken as 2.5 to 5 mg 3 or 4 times daily, not to exceed 20 mg total daily dose, diphenoxylate is rarely toxic. Some patients may complain of atropinism (blurred vision, dry mouth, urinary hesitancy). Like loperamide, it should not be used in patients at risk of bacterial enteritis with *Escherichia coli, Shigella,* or *Salmonella.*

A dipehoxylate derivative is difenoxin with atropine and has the same uses, precautions, and side effects. Marketed as 1 mg difenoxin tablet, the adult dosage is 2 mg, then 1 mg after each loose stool, not to exceed 8 mg/d.

ADSORBENTS

Adsorbents are used for symptomatic relief (Table 34–3). These products, many not needing a prescription, are nontoxic, but

TABLE 34–3. Selected Antidiarrheal Preparations

	Dose Form	Adult Dose
Antimotility		
Diphenoxylate	2.5 mg/tablet 2.5 mg/5 mL	5 mg qid; do not exceed 20 mg/d
Loperamide	2 mg/capsule 1 mg/5 mL	Initially 4 mg, then 2 mg after each loose stool; do not exceed 16 mg/d
Paregoric	2 mg/5 mL (morphine)	5–10 mL 1–4 times daily
Opium tincture	5 mg/mL (morphine)	0.6 mL qid
Difenoxin	1 mg/tablet	Two tablets, then one tablet after each loose stool; up to 8 tablets/d
Adsorbents		
Kaolin–pectin mixture	5.7 g kaolin + 130.2 mg pectin/30 mL	30–120 mL after each loose stool
Polycarbophil	500 mg/tablet	Chew 2 tablets qid or after each loose stool; do not exceed 12 tablets/d
Attapulgite	750 mg/15 mL 300 mg/7.5 mL 750 mg/tablet 600 mg/tablet 300 mg/tablet	1200–1500 mg after each loose bowel movement or every 2 hours; up to 9000 mg/d
Antisecretory		
Bismuth subsalicylate	1050 mg/30 mL 262 mg/15 mL 524 mg/15 mL 262 mg/tablet	Two tablets or 30 mL every 30 min to 1 h as needed up to 8 doses/d
Enzymes (lactase)	1250 neutral lactase units/4 drops 3300 FCC lactase units per tablet	3–4 drops taken with milk or dairy product 1 or 2 tablets as above
Bacterial replacement (*Lactobacillus acidophilus, Lactobacillus bulgaricus*)		2 tablets or 1 granule packet 3 to 4 times daily; give with milk, juice, or water
Octreotide	0.05 mg/mL 0.1 mg/mL 0.5 mg/mL	Initial: 50 µg subcutaneously 1–2 times per day and titrate dose based on indication up to 600 µg/d in 2–4 divided doses

their effectiveness remains unproven. Adsorbents are nonspecific in their action; they adsorb nutrients, toxins, drugs, and digestive juices. Coadministration with other drugs reduces their bioavailability. The Food and Drug Administration over-the-counter review panel recommends only polycarbophil as an effective adsorbent.

Polycarbophil absorbs 60 times its weight in water and treats both diarrhea and constipation. Polycarbophil, a nonprescripton product, is sold as 500-mg chewable tablets. This hydrophilic, nonabsorbable product is safe and may be taken four times daily up to 6 g in adults.

ANTISECRETORY AGENTS

Bismuth subsalicylate (BSS) appears to have antisecretory, anti-inflammatory, and antibacterial effects. As a nonprescription product, it is marketed for indigestion, relieving abdominal cramps, and controlling diarrhea, including traveler's diarrhea. BSS dosage strengths are 262-mg chewable tablets, 262 mg/5 mL liquid, and 524 mg/15 mL liquid. The usual adult dose is 2 tablets or 30 mL every 30 minutes to 1 hour up to 8 doses per day.

Bismuth subsalicylate contains multiple components that might be toxic if given excessively to prevent or treat diarrhea. For instance, an active ingredient is salicylate, which may interact with anticoagulants or cause effects of salicylism (tinnitus, nausea, and vomiting). Bismuth can interfere with tetracycline intestinal absorption and interfere with some gastrointestinal radiographic studies. Patients may complain of darkening tongue and stools with repeat administration. Salicylate can induce gout attacks in susceptible individuals.

Infectious agents cause many acute diarrheas, which have a strong secretory component. Agents blocking copious fluid flow are highly desirable in secretory diarrheas, so bismuth subsalicylate suspension has been studied. When 30 mL of this suspension was given every 30 minutes for eight doses, unformed stools decreased in the first 24 hours in active infection. Bismuth subsalicylate has also been studied to prevent traveler's diarrhea.

Octreotide (Sandostatin), a synthetic octapeptide analog of endogenous somatostatin, is prescribed for the symptomatic treatment of carcinoid tumors and vasoactive intestinal peptide-secreting tumors (VIPomas).[12,13] Metastatic intestinal carcinoid tumors secrete excessive amounts of vasoactive substances, including histamine, bradykinin, serotonin, and prostaglandins. Primary carcinoid tumors are located throughout the GI tract, with most in the ileum. The predominant clinical signs and symptoms are attributable to excessive 5-hydroxytryptophan and serotonin. The collection of their clinical effects is termed the *carcinoid syndrome.* Paroxysmal vasomotor attacks characterize carcinoid syndrome, most notably sudden red to purple flushing of the face and neck. These attacks are often caused by emotional outbursts or by ingestion of food or alcohol. Some patients have a violent, watery diarrhea with cramping. Initially, diarrhea might be managed with various agents such as codeine, diphenoxylate, cyproheptadine, methysergide, phenoxybenzamine, or methyldopa. Recently, octreotide has become the drug of choice.

Octreotide blocks the release of serotonin and many other active peptides and has been effective in controlling diarrhea and flushing. It is reported to have direct inhibitory effects on intestinal secretion and stimulatory effects on intestinal absorption. Nongastrin-secreting adenomas of the pancreas are tumors associated with profuse watery diarrhea. This condition is termed by various names including Verner-Morrison syndrome; WDHA (watery diarrhea, hypokalemia, achlorhydria) syndrome; pancreatic cholera; watery diarrhea syndrome; and VIPoma. Excessive secretion of VIP from a retroperitoneal or pancreatic tumor causes most of the clinical features. Excessive VIP is isolated in about half of patients along with numerous other peptide hormones (peptide histidine methionine [PHM], serotonin, somatostatin, gastrin, glucagon). Surgical tumor dissection is the treatment of choice. In nonsurgical candidates, however, the profuse watery diarrhea and other symptoms are managed with octreotide.

Octreotide, a parenteral drug, is packaged in vials of 0.05, 0.1, and 0.5 mg/mL. The dosage varies with the indication, disease severity, and variable patient response.[15] For managing diarrhea and flushing associated with carcinoid tumors in adults, the dosage range is 100 to 600 μg/d in two to four divided doses subcutaneously. In so-called carcinoid crisis, octreotide is given as an IV infusion at 50 μg/h for 8 to 24 hours. For controlling secretory diarrhea of VIPomas, the dosage range is 200 to 300 μg/d in two to four divided doses for 2 weeks. Some patients may need higher doses. Because octreotide inhibits many other gastrointestinal hormones, it has a variety of intestinal side effects. With prolonged use, gallbladder and biliary tract complications, like cholelithiasis, have been reported. About 5% to 10% of patients complain about nausea, diarrhea, and abdominal pain. Local injection pain occurs with about an 8% incidence. With high doses, octreotide may reduce dietary fat absorption, leading to steatorrhea.

Octreotide has a very brief half-life, 60 to 110 minutes, that has stimulated the search for longer-acting compounds or dosage formulations. Currently two other somatostatin analogs, lanreotide and vapreotide, are in clinical trials.[14–16] Two long-acting octreotide formulations are currently being tested: Sandostatin LAR and OncoLAR. Sandostatin LAR is a formulation of microspheres for subcutaneous injection. OncoLAR is a microencapsulated polymer microsphere product for intramuscular injection. Both formulations are for once monthly injection.

MISCELLANEOUS PRODUCTS

Lactobacillus preparations replace colonic microflora. A controversial treatment is seeding the gut with this organism. This supposedly restores intestinal functions and suppresses the growth of pathogenic microorganisms. However, a dairy product diet containing 200 to 400 g of lactose or dextrin is equally effective in recolonization. Again, clinical studies are lacking. The dosage varies depending on the brand and is given with milk, juice, water, or cereal. Intestinal flatus is the primary patient complaint.

Anticholinergic drugs, such as atropine, block vagal tone and prolong gut transit time (Table 34–3). They are available in combination in many nonprescription products and as single entities. Their value in controlling diarrhea is questionable and limited by side effects. To stop diarrhea, clinicians have been falsely taught to dose anticholinergics until they decrease salivary and sweat secretion. Angle closure glaucoma, selected heart diseases, and obstructive uropathies are relative contraindications to use of anticholinergic agents.

Lactase enzyme products are helpful for patients with lactose intolerance. Lactase is needed for carbohydrate digestion. When a patient lacks this enzyme, eating dairy products causes an osmotic diarrhea. Several products are available for current use each time a dairy product, especially milk or ice cream, is eaten.

EVALUATION OF THERAPEUTIC OUTCOMES

ACUTE DIARRHEA

Most patients have mild to moderate distress with acute diarrhea. Without moderate to severe dehydration, high fever, and blood or mucus in their stool, the illness is usually self-limiting within 3 to 7 days. Mild to moderate acute diarrhea is usually managed without hospitalization using oral rehydration, symptomatic treatment, and diet. Elderly persons with chronic illness and infants may need hospitalization for parenteral rehydration and close monitoring.

With the urgency/emergency situation, evaluation of the patient's volume status is the most important outcome. Toxic patients (fever, dehydration, hematochezia, hypotension) require hospitalization; they need IV electrolyte solutions and empiric antibiotics while awaiting cultures. With quick management, they usually recover within a few days.

Therapeutic outcomes are directed to key symptoms, signs, and laboratory studies. The constitutional symptoms usually improve within 24 to 72 hours. One should check the frequency and character of bowel movements each day along with the vital signs and improving appetite. Also, the clinician needs to monitor body weight, serum osmolality, serum electrolytes, complete blood cell count, urinalysis, and cultures (if appropriate).

CONTROVERSIES IN DRUG MANAGEMENT

Many experimental drugs have been used to control diarrhea. Phenothiazines, β-blockers, nonsteroidal anti-inflammatory drugs (NSAIDs), calcium channel blockers, and α-adrenergic agonists are only a few agents under investigation in either animals or humans.

Nifalatide is an enkephalin analog that delays the onset of castor oil-induced diarrhea and decreases stool frequency. Dizziness and dry mouth are frequent side effects.[17] Enkephalinase inhibitors (e.g., acetorphan) offer another therapeutic choice.[18] In the search for proabsorption/antisecretory drugs, lidamidine, a prototype α_2-adrenergic agonist, was compared with loperamide and found to counter diarrhea by either promoting absorption or preventing secretion.[20] With lidamidine, a clonidine analog, hypotension is a limiting dose-related problem. Prostaglandin inhibitors, aspirin and its analogs, and indomethacin are safe and effective in childhood gastroenteritis; studies in animals support indomethacin in enteropathogen secretory states such as with *Vibrio cholerae*.[19,20]

Vaccines are a new therapeutic frontier in controlling infectious diarrheas, especially in developing countries.[2] Cholera vaccine yields some protection but is not totally effective and does not prevent transmission. Oral *Shigella* vaccine was effective under field conditions, but calls for five doses with repeat booster doses, limiting its practicality in developing nations. With about 1500 serotypes for *Salmonella*, a vaccine still is not available. In the United States, rotavirus vaccine would protect many infants and children, and a new vaccine is being reviewed by the FDA. If approved, the rotavirus vaccine is given as a three oral dose sequence.[21]

CONSTIPATION

Constipation is a common problem, as evidenced by the tremendous dollar volumes spent on laxatives and the prominence they have gained in the advertising media and on the shelves of retail outlets. Most treatments for constipation are initiated by the patient, often without consultation from a health care professional. One reason constipation continues to be a frequent problem in the United States is the inadequate diets of many people. Another unfortunate problem is that many people have misconceptions about normal bowel function, and think that daily bowel movements are required for health and well-being. Others believe that the lack of a daily bowel movement contributes to the accumulation of toxic substances or is associated with various somatic complaints. These misconceptions lead to the inappropriate use of laxatives by the general public.

Constipation does not have one consistently used definition. When using the term, the lay public or health care professional may be referring to several difficult-to-quantify variables: bowel movement frequency, stool size or consistency, and such symptoms as a feeling of incomplete defecation. Stool frequency is most often used to describe constipation; however, the frequency of bowel movements used to define constipation is not well established. Normal subjects pass at least three stools per week.

Some of the definitions of constipation used in clinical studies include (1) less than three stools per week for women and five for men despite a high-residue diet, or a period of greater than 3 days without a bowel movement; (2) straining at stool greater than 25% of the time and/or two or fewer stools per week; or (3) straining at defecation and less than one stool daily with minimal effort. These varying definitions demonstrate the difficulty in characterizing this problem.

An international committee defined and classified constipation on the basis of stool frequency, consistency, and difficulty of defecation.[24,25] Functional constipation is defined as two or more of the following complaints present for at least 12 months when patients are not taking laxatives: (1) straining at least 25% of the time, (2) lumpy or hard stools at least 25% of the time, (3) feeling of incomplete evacuation at least 25% of the time, or (4) two or less bowel movements in a week. Rectal outlet delay was defined as anal blockage more than 25% of the time and prolonged defecation or manual disimpaction (when necessary).

EPIDEMIOLOGY

Up to 40% of patients over age 65 years report symptoms of constipation.[26] The results from 42,375 participants of the National Health Interview Survey on Digestive Disorders demonstrated that there is not an age-related increase in infrequent bowel movements; however, there was an age-related increase in laxative use.[27] The frequency of subjects reporting two or less bowel movements per week was 5.9% for those less than 40 years, 3.8% for 60 to 69 years, and 6.3% for those over age 80 years. In a prospective study of 3166 people over the age of 65 in a Florida community,[28] 26% of women and 15.8% of men reported recurrent constipation. Factors found to correlate with self-reported constipation were age, sex (higher frequency in females), total number of drugs taken, abdominal pain, and hemorrhoids.

ETIOLOGY AND PATHOPHYSIOLOGY

Constipation is not a disease but a symptom of an underlying disease or problem. Approaches to treatment of constipation should begin with attempts to determine its cause. Disorders of the GI tract (irritable bowel syndrome or diverticulitis), metabolic disorders (diabetes), or endocrine disorders (hypothyroidism) may be involved. Constipation commonly results from a diet low in fiber or from use of constipating drugs such as opiates. Finally, it is believed that constipation may sometimes be psychogenic in origin. Each of these causes is discussed.

Constipation is a frequent problem in the elderly, probably the result of improper diets (low in fiber and liquids), diminished abdominal wall muscular strength, and possibly diminished physical activity. However, the frequency of bowel movements is not decreased with normal aging.[25] In addition, diseases that may cause constipation, such as colon cancers and diverticulitis, are more common with increasing age.

GASTROINTESTINAL DISORDERS

Gastrointestinal disorders are a common cause of constipation. The most frequent GI-related causes of constipation are disorders of the large bowel (irritable bowel syndrome, diverticulitis), but diseases of the upper GI tract (gastroduodenal obstruction from ulceration or cancer) may also be responsible. Irritable bowel syndrome may be associated with constipation, diarrhea, or both. In these patients, objective findings of disease are often absent, but colonic motility is usually abnormal.

Anal and rectal diseases associated with pain on defecation may cause constipation. Hemorrhoids, anal fissures, or ulcerative proctitis may all result in painful elimination and inhibition of the urge to defecate. The result may be a decreased frequency of bowel movements.

Constipation may be an indication of obstruction from tumors that originate in the lumen of the colon or from organs or structures adjacent to the colon. Also, constipation may result from hernias, volvulus of the bowel (torsion or twisting of a loop of intestine), or a variety of diseases (syphilis, tuberculosis, helminthic infections, or lymphogranuloma venereum), all of which may cause stricture of the lumen of the colon.

Neurologic disorders of the GI tract may be a cause of constipation. The most prominent neurologic disorder of the GI tract resulting in constipation is Hirschsprung's disease, also called aganglionosis (congenital absence of neurons to the terminal segments of the bowel).

METABOLIC AND ENDOCRINE DISORDERS

Many metabolic and endocrine disorders affect bowel function. Examples include diabetes mellitus with associated neuropathy, which may affect multiple segments of the GI tract and result in an atonic colon, uremia, and hypokalemia. Hypothyroidism and panhypopituitarism may result in inhibited bowel function. In fact, for some cases of hypothyroidism the presenting symptom is constipation or bowel obstruction. Other disorders such as pheochromocytoma may cause constipation, because catecholamines inhibit GI smooth muscle activity. Hypercalcemia (from any cause) and enteric glucagon excess may also result in inhibited bowel function.

PREGNANCY

Constipation is a frequent problem during pregnancy, possibly resulting from complex factors that include depressed gut motility, increased fluid absorption from the colon, decreased physical activity, and dietary changes.[29] Predisposing dietary factors include inadequate fluid intake, low dietary fiber, and the use of iron salts.

NEUROGENIC CONSTIPATION

In addition to peripheral neurologic disorders that may cause constipation, central nervous system (CNS) disorders also may be responsible. The CNS is an important component in GI regulation, either through reflexes or coordination of other organs. In addition, the CNS modifies GI function in response to conscious effort or emotional stimuli. Many diseases of the CNS can therefore affect GI function. Trauma to the brain (particularly the medulla) or spinal cord may result in inhibited bowel function, as may CNS tumors. Also, cerebrovascular accidents and Parkinson's disease may cause inhibited bowel function.

PSYCHOGENIC CONSTIPATION

The term *psychogenic constipation* has variable acceptance among experts in the field because objective evidence for its existence is slim; however, bowel habits, particularly those developed early in life, may relate to chronic constipation. Ignoring or postponing the urge to defecate may cause blunting of the colonic and rectal response and may possibly lead to prolonged stool retention. People in certain occupations, such as truck drivers, may be particularly predisposed to this problem. Finally, patients with psychiatric diseases often have constipation. In many instances, improvement in constipation is observed with the onset of psychotherapy.

DRUG-INDUCED CONSTIPATION

Drugs that inhibit the neurologic or muscular function of the GI tract, particularly the colon, may result in constipation (Table 34–4). The majority of cases of drug-induced constipation are caused by opiates, various agents with anticholinergic properties, and antacids containing aluminum or calcium. With most of the agents listed, the inhibitory bowel effects are dose dependent, with larger doses clearly causing constipation more frequently.

Opiates have effects on all segments of the bowel, but effects are most pronounced on the colon. The major mechanism of opiate action has been proposed to be prolongation of intestinal transit time by causing spastic, nonpropulsive contractions.[30] An additional contributory mechanism of action may be an increase in electrolyte absorption.[31]

All opiate derivatives are associated with constipation, but the degree of intestinal inhibitory effects seems to differ between agents. Orally administered opiates appear to have greater inhibitory effects than parenterally administered agents; oral codeine is well known as a potent antimotility agent. Orally administered enkephalins (endogenous opiate-like polypeptides) are recognized to have antimotility properties.

Agents with anticholinergic properties inhibit bowel function by parasympatholytic actions on innervation to many regions of the GI tract, particularly the colon and rectum. Many types of drugs possess anticholinergic action (Table 34–4), and these agents are used commonly in hospitalized and nonhospitalized patients. One study demonstrated that amitriptyline, diphenhydramine, and thioridazine were associated with laxative use in 800 nursing home patients.[32]

In patients over age 65, the drugs that correlated with constipation were anticholinergics, aspirin, furosemide, nitroglycerin, and amitriptyline.[28] Serum chloride and aspartate aminotransferase, as well as alcohol consumption, were found to be negatively related to constipation. The most important predictors of constipation were age and the total number of medications taken.

TABLE 34–4. Drugs Causing Constipation

Analgesics
Inhibitors of prostaglandin synthesis
Opiates
Anticholinergics
Antihistamines
Antiparkinsonian agents (e.g., benztropine or trihexaphenidyl)
Phenothiazines
Tricyclic antidepressants
Antacids containing calcium carbonate or aluminum hydroxide
Barium sulfate
Calcium channel blockers
Clonidine
Diuretics (non–potassium sparing)
Ganglionic blockers
Iron preparations
Muscle blockers (D-tubocurarine, succinylcholine)
Nonsteroidal anti-inflammatory agents
Polystyrene sodium sulfonate

CLINICAL PRESENTATION

Constipation may vary from a minor discomfort in an otherwise healthy adult to a symptom of colon cancer or other serious diseases. A basis for evaluation and treatment should be a thorough history including questions about the nature of the "constipation." It is important to ascertain whether the patient perceives the problem as infrequent bowel movements, stools of insufficient size, a feeling of fullness, or difficulty and pain on passing stool. The patient should be asked about the frequency of bowel movements and the chronicity of constipation. Constipation occurring recently in an adult may indicate significant colon pathology such as malignancy; constipation present since early infancy may be indicative of neurologic disorders. The patient also should be carefully questioned about usual diet and laxative regimens. Does the patient have a diet consistently deficient in high-fiber items and containing mainly highly refined foods? What laxatives or cathartics has the patient used to attempt relief of constipation? Finally, the patient should be questioned about other concurrent medications, with interest toward agents that might cause constipation.

For most patients complaining of constipation, a thorough physical examination is not required once it is established that constipation (1) is not a chronic problem, (2) is not accompanied by signs of significant GI disease (e.g., rectal bleeding or anemia), and (3) does not cause severe discomfort. In these circumstances the patient may be referred directly to the first-line therapies for constipation described in the next section (mainly bulk-forming laxatives and dietary fiber with occasional use of saline or stimulant laxatives). Certain patients, however, require a full examination by a physician to determine the cause of constipation. Patients may then have a series of examinations, proctoscopy, sigmoidoscopy, colonoscopy, or barium enema to determine the presence of colorectal pathology. Also, tests such as thyroid function studies may be performed to determine the presence of metabolic or endocrine disorders.

Chronic constipation can result in a more complex picture. Patients may have long-standing complaints of GI irregularities with a variety of symptoms. The laxative abuser may present with contradictory findings, sometimes diarrhea or weight loss. Laxative abusers may deny laxative use and present with vomiting, abdominal pain, lassitude, thirst, edema, and bone pain (due to osteomalacia). With prolonged abuse patients may have fluid and electrolyte imbalances (most commonly hypokalemia), protein-losing gastroenteropathy with hypoalbuminemia, and syndromes resembling colitis.

TREATMENT: Constipation

DESIRED OUTCOME

The ultimate goal of treatment for constipation is alteration of life-style (particularly diet) to prevent further episodes of constipation. Short-term goals include alleviation of acute constipation with relief from symptoms. For patients with chronic constipation, the goals will be more long term and include use of proper diet and decreased reliance on laxatives. Effective treatment of constipation requires the patient to become more knowledgeable about the causes of constipation, proper diet, and appropriate use of laxatives.

GENERAL APPROACH TO TREATMENT

The proper management of constipation requires a number of different modalities; however, the basis for therapy should be dietary modification. The major dietary change should be an increase in the amount of fiber consumed daily. In addition to dietary management, patients should be encouraged to alter other aspects of their life-styles to some extent if necessary. Important considerations would be to encourage patients to exercise (achieved even by brisk walking after dinner) and to adjust bowel habits so that a regular and adequate time is made to respond to the urge to defecate. Another general measure is to increase fluid intake. This is generally recommended and believed beneficial, although there is little objective evidence of benefit.

If an underlying disease is recognized as the cause of constipation, attempts should be made to correct it. GI malignancies may be removed through a surgical resection. Endocrine and metabolic derangements should be corrected by the appropriate methods. For example, when hypothyroidism is the cause of constipation, cautious institution of thyroid-replacement therapy is the most important treatment measure.

As discussed earlier, many drug substances may cause constipation. After determination of a patient's prescription and nonprescription drug therapy, potential drug causes of constipation should be identified. If the patient is consuming medications well known to cause constipation, consideration should be given to alternative agents. For some medications (e.g., antacids), nonconstipating alternatives exist. If no reasonable alternatives exist to the medication thought to be responsible for constipation, consideration should be given to lowering the dose. If a patient must remain on constipating medications, then more attention must be paid to general measures for prevention of constipation, as discussed next.

NONPHARMACOLOGIC THERAPY

DIETARY MODIFICATION AND BULK-FORMING AGENTS

The most important aspect of the therapy for constipation for the majority of patients is dietary modification to increase the amount of fiber consumed. Fiber, the portion of vegetable matter not digested in the human GI tract, increases stool bulk, retention of stool water, and rate of transit of stool through the intestine.[33] The result of fiber therapy is an increased frequency of defecation. Also, fiber has been shown to decrease intraluminal pressures in the colon and rectum, which is thought to be beneficial for diverticular disease and irritable bowel syndrome. The specific physiologic effects of fiber are not well understood.

Patients should be advised to include at least 10 g of crude fiber in their daily diets.[25] Fruits, vegetables, and cereals have the highest fiber content. Bran, a byproduct of milling of wheat, is often added to foods to increase fiber content. Raw bran is generally 40% fiber. Medicinal products, often called "bulk-forming agents," such as psyllium hydrophillic colloids (Effersyllium), methylcellulose (Cologel), or polycarbophil (Mitrolan), have properties similar to those of dietary fiber and may be taken as tablets, powders, or granules (Table 34–5).

A trial of dietary modification with high-fiber content should be continued for at least 1 month before effects on bowel function are determined. Most patients begin to notice effects on bowel function 3 to 5 days after beginning a high-fiber diet, but some patients may require a considerably longer time. Patients should be cautioned that abdominal distention and flatus may be particularly troublesome in the first few weeks of fiber therapy, particularly with high bran consumption. In most patients, these problems resolve with continued use.

Bulk-forming laxatives have few side effects and minimal systemic effects. The only major caution in the use of bulk-forming laxatives is that obstruction of the esophagus, stomach, small intestine, and colon has been reported when the agents have been consumed without fluid, so these products should not be used without adequate fluids or in patients with intestinal stenosis.

SURGERY

In a small percentage of patients presenting with complaints of constipation, surgical procedures are necessary (with most colonic malignancies and with GI obstruction from a number of

TABLE 34–5. Dosage Recommendations for Laxatives and Cathartics

Agent	Recommended Dose
Agents That Cause Softening of Feces in 1–3 d	
Bulk-forming agents	
Methylcellulose	4–6 g/d
Polycarbophil	4–6 g/d
Psyllium	Varies with product
Emollients	
Docusate sodium	50–360 mg/d
Docusate calcium	50–360 mg/d
Docusate potassium	100–300 mg/d
Lactulose	15–30 mL orally
Sorbitol	30–50 g/d orally
Mineral oil	15–30 mL orally
Agents That Result in Soft or Semifluid Stool in 6–12 h	
Bisacodyl (oral)	5–15 mg orally
Phenolphthalein	30–270 mg orally
Cascara sagrada	Dose varies with formulation
Senna	Dose varies with formulation
Magnesium sulfate (low dose)	< 10 g orally
Agents That Cause Watery Evacuation in 1–6 h	
Magnesium citrate	18 g 300 mL water
Magnesium hydroxide	2.4–4.8 g orally
Magnesium sulfate (high dose)	10–30 g orally
Sodium phosphates	Varies with salt used
Bisacodyl	10 mg rectally
Polyethylene glycol–electrolyte preparations	4 L

causes). In each case, the involved segment of intestine may be resected or revised to allow flow of GI contents through an enterostomy or through the anus. Surgery may be required in some endocrine disorders causing constipation, such as pheochromocytoma, which requires removal of a tumor.

BIOFEEDBACK

The majority of patients with constipation related to pelvic floor dysfunction can benefit from electromyogram-guided biofeedback therapy.[34] The value of biofeedback in children with chronic constipation has not been well demonstrated.[35]

PHARMACOLOGIC THERAPY

DRUG REGIMENS OF CHOICE

Treatment and prevention of constipation should consist of bulk-forming agents in addition to dietary modifications that increase dietary fiber.[36] A variety of products are available that provide adequate bulk. Whichever agent is chosen, it should be used daily and continued indefinitely in most patients, particularly those with chronic constipation. Bulk-forming agents available in combination with diphenylmethane or anthraquinone derivatives should be avoided because the added agents should not be used routinely.

For most nonhospitalized persons with acute constipation, the infrequent use (less than every few weeks) of most laxative products is acceptable; however, before more potent laxative/cathartics are used, relatively simple measures may be tried. For example, acute constipation may be relieved by the use of a tap-water enema or a glycerin suppository; if neither is effective, the use of oral sorbitol, low doses of diphenylmethane or anthraquinone laxatives, or saline laxatives (e.g., milk of magnesia) may provide relief. If laxative treatment is required for longer than 1 week, the person should be advised to consult a physician to determine if there is an underlying cause of constipation that requires treatment with agents other than laxatives.

For some bedridden or geriatric patients, or others with chronic constipation, bulk-forming laxatives remain the first line of treatment, but the use of more potent laxatives may be required relatively frequently. Fiber should be avoided in bedridden patients who are cognitively impaired.[25] When other than bulk-forming laxatives are used, they should be administered in the lowest effective dose and as infrequently as possible to maintain regular bowel function (more than three stools per week). Agents that may be used in these situations include diphenylmethane and anthraquinone derivatives, milk of magnesia, and sorbitol or lactulose. Mineral oil should be avoided, particularly in bedridden patients, because of the risk of aspiration and lipoid pneumonia. Some patients with chronic constipation may present with fecal impactions. Before vigorous oral laxatives can be used, the impaction needs to be removed using mechanical methods, including tap-water or saline enemas and digital extraction.

In the hospitalized patient without GI disease, constipation may be related to the use of general anesthesia and/or opiate substances. Most orally or rectally administered laxatives may be used. For prompt initiation of a bowel movement, a tap-water enema or glycerin suppository is recommended, or oral milk of magnesia.

With infants and children, constipation may occur commonly. The approach to the treatment of constipation in young persons should consider neurologic, metabolic, or anatomic abnormalities when constipation is a persistent problem. When not related to an underlying disease, the approach to constipation is similar to that in an adult. Dietary modification should be considered, emphasizing high-fiber food. For acute constipation in most age groups, a tap-water enema or glycerin suppository may be helpful. Occasional use of milk of magnesia or anthraquinone laxatives in low doses is justified for acute constipation.

Prokinetic agents (such as cisapride) have been used in patients with neurologic disorders such as Parkinson's disease or chronic idiopathic constipation.[37] Cisapride doses have varied from 5 mg orally tid to 20 mg twice daily. The duration of cisapride effectiveness, however, is limited to about 6 months.[38]

DRUG CLASSES

The traditional classification system for laxatives and cathartics, by suspected mode of action, has not been very useful; the mode of action of many products is not clearly understood.[39,40] In general, most agents work by promoting some of the mechanisms involved in diarrhea, including active electrolyte secretion, decreased water and electrolyte absorption, increased intraluminal osmolarity, and increased hydrostatic pressure in the gut. Laxatives convert the intestine from primarily an organ that absorbs water and electrolytes to an organ that secretes water and electrolytes.[40] The various classes of laxatives are discussed in this section. The agents are divided into three general classifications: (1) those causing softening of feces in 1 to 3 days (bulk-forming laxatives, docusates, and lactulose); (2) those that result in soft or semifluid stool in 6 to 12 hours (diphenylmethane derivatives and anthraquinone derivatives); and (3) those causing water evacuation in 1 to 6 hours (saline cathartics, castor oil, and polyethylene glycol–electrolyte lavage solution).[41]

EMOLLIENT LAXATIVES

Emollient laxatives are surfactant agents, docusate in their various salts, which work by facilitating mixing of aqueous and fatty materials within the intestinal tract. They may increase water and electrolyte secretion in the small and large bowel.[42] These products are generally given orally, although docusate potassium has also been used rectally. These products result in a softening of stools within 1 to 3 days.

Emollient laxatives are not effective in treating constipation but are used mainly to prevent constipation. They may be helpful in situations where straining at stool should be avoided, such as after recovery from myocardial infarction, with acute perianal disease, or after rectal surgery. It is unlikely that these agents would be very effective in preventing constipation if major causative factors (e.g., heavy opiate use, uncorrected pathology, inadequate dietary fiber) are not concurrently addressed.

Although docusates are generally safe, a few adverse effects have been noted. They may increase the intestinal absorption of agents administered concurrently and alter toxic potential.

LUBRICANTS

Mineral oil is the only lubricant laxative in routine use. This agent, obtained from petroleum refining, acts by coating stool and allowing easier passage. It inhibits colonic absorption of water, thereby increasing stool weight and decreasing stool transit time. Mineral oil may be given orally or rectally in a dose of 15 to 45 mL. Generally, the effect on bowel function is noted after 2 or 3 days of use.

Mineral oil is helpful in situations similar to those suggested for docusates: to maintain a soft stool and avoid straining for relatively short periods of time (a few days to 2 weeks); however, it possesses a much greater potential for adverse effects and its routine use should be discouraged. Mineral oil may be absorbed systemically and cause a foreign-body reaction in lymphoid tissue. Also, in debilitated or recumbent patients, mineral oil may be aspirated, causing lipoid pneumonia.[43] For this reason it should not be used just before bedtime or when a patient is recumbent.

Mineral oil has been reported to decrease the absorption of fat-soluble vitamins (A, D, E, and K) with chronic use by causing retention in the GI tract. Finally, even when given orally, mineral oil may leak from the anal sphincter, causing pruritus and soiling of clothing.

LACTULOSE AND SORBITOL

Lactulose is a disaccharide used orally or rectally. It is metabolized by colonic bacteria to low-molecular-weight acids, resulting in an osmotic effect whereby fluid is retained in the colon.[29] The fluid retained in the colon lowers the pH and increases colonic peristalsis. Lactulose is generally not recommended as a first-line agent for the treatment of constipation because it is costly and not necessarily more effective than such agents as sorbitol or milk of magnesia. It may be justified as an alternative for acute constipation, and has been useful particularly in elderly patients. Occasionally, the use of lactulose may result in flatulence, cramps, diarrhea, and electrolyte imbalances.[44] Sorbitol, a monosaccharide, exerts its effect by osmotic action and has been recommended as a primary agent in the treatment of functional constipation in cognitively intact patients.[25] It is as effective as lactulose and much less expensive.[45]

DIPHENYLMETHANE DERIVATIVES

The two commonly used diphenylmethane derivatives are bisacodyl and phenolphthalein. The actions of these agents are believed to be primarily on the colon. Bisacodyl stimulates the mucosal nerve plexus of the colon; the mechanism of action of phenolphthalein is poorly understood (possibly it inhibits active glucose absorption and sodium absorption, resulting in fluid accumulation in the colon by osmotic action). The dose of these agents effective in various individuals appears to vary greatly. A dose that causes no effects in one patient may result in excessive cramping and fluid evacuation in others. With phenolphthalein, a small portion of the dose undergoes enterohepatic recirculation, which may result in a prolonged laxative action.

These agents are not recommended for regular daily use. Their use is acceptable intermittently (every few weeks) to treat constipation or as a bowel preparation before diagnostic procedures in which cleansing of the colon is necessary. These agents may sometimes cause severe abdominal cramping as well as significant fluid and electrolyte imbalances with chronic use. They should not be used for patients in whom appendicitis is a possibility (perforation of the appendix may result) or during pregnancy or lactation. Finally, the patient taking phenolphthalein-containing laxatives should be cautioned that it may turn urine pink.

ANTHRAQUINONE DERIVATIVES

Anthraquinone derivatives include cascara sagrada, sennosides, and casanthrol. These agents are metabolized by gut bacteria to their active compounds, but the exact mechanisms of action are not understood. Effects are limited to the colon, and stimulation of Auerbach's plexus may be involved. Recommendations for the use of these agents are similar to those for the diphenylmethane derivatives. In most cases, intermittent use is acceptable; daily use should be strongly discouraged.

Most of the concerns with the use of diphenylmethane derivatives (bisacodyl and phenolphthalein) apply to the anthraquinone derivatives. In addition, the anthraquinone derivatives may cause melanosis coli, an accumulation of dark pigment, mainly in the cecum and rectum, that is evident after 4 to 13 months of use. A pathologic effect of melanosis coli has not been demonstrated, and it appears reversible after anthraquinones have been discontinued for 3 to 6 months.

SALINE CATHARTICS

Saline cathartics are composed of relatively poorly absorbed ions such as magnesium, sulfate, phosphate, and citrate, which produce their effects primarily by osmotic action to retain fluid in the GI tract. Magnesium has been shown to stimulate the secretion of cholecystokinin, a hormone that causes stimulation of bowel motility and fluid secretion. These agents may be given orally or rectally. A bowel movement may result within a few hours after oral doses and in 1 hour or less after rectal administration.

These agents should be used primarily for acute evacuation of the bowel, which may be necessary before diagnostic examinations, after poisonings, and in conjunction with some anthelmintics to eliminate parasites. Such agents as milk of magnesia (an 8% suspension of magnesium hydroxide) may be used occasionally (every few weeks) to treat constipation in otherwise healthy adults. Saline cathartics should not be used on a routine basis to treat constipation. With fecal impactions the enema formulations of these agents may be helpful.

As with most laxatives, these agents may cause fluid and electrolyte depletion. Also, magnesium or sodium accumulation may occur when magnesium-containing cathartics are used in patients with renal dysfunction or when sodium phosphate is used in patients with congestive heart failure.

CASTOR OIL

Castor oil is metabolized in the GI tract to an active compound, ricinoleic acid, which stimulates secretory processes, decreases glucose absorption, and promotes intestinal motility, primarily in the small intestine. Castor oil usually results in a bowel movement within 1 to 3 hours of administration. Because the agent has such a strong purgative action, it should not be used for the routine treatment of constipation.

GLYCERIN

Glycerin is usually administered as a 3-g suppository and exerts its effect by osmotic action in the rectum. As with most agents given as suppositories, the onset of action is usually less than 30 minutes. Glycerin is considered a very safe laxative, although it may occasionally cause rectal irritation. Its use is acceptable on an intermittent basis for constipation, particularly in children.

POLYETHYLENE GLYCOL–ELECTROLYTE LAVAGE SOLUTION

Whole-bowel irrigation with polyethylene glycol–electrolyte lavage solution (PEG–ELS) has become popular for colon cleansing before diagnostic procedures or colorectal operations.[46] Four liters of this solution is administered over 3 hours to obtain complete evacuation of the GI tract. The solution is not recommended for the routine treatment of constipation and its use should be avoided in patients with intestinal obstruction.

OTHER AGENTS

Tap-water enemas may be used to treat simple constipation. The administration of 200 mL of water by enema to an adult often results in a bowel movement within one-half hour. Soapsuds are no longer recommended for use in enemas because their use may result in proctitis or colitis.

Cisapride is a GI prokinetic agent that is used in motility disorders. It is effective in relieving acute and chronic constipation in both adults and children.[47] The agent is considerably more expensive than most alternatives. Erythromycin has also been studied for patients with idiopathic constipation.[48]

PREVENTION

For certain groups of patients, such as those recovering from myocardial infarction or rectal surgery, straining at defecation is to be avoided. For these patients, the basis of preventive therapy should be the use of bulk-forming laxatives. In addition to these products, the use of docusate has become popular, although its effectiveness is debated. In pregnant patients, constipation may result because of alterations in anatomy or iron supplementation. As described earlier, bulk-forming laxatives and docusates should be the first line of prevention.

LAXATIVE ABUSE SYNDROME

Misconceptions about normal bowel patterns and the effect of laxatives have contributed to a syndrome of laxative abuse that is relatively common in the United States. The availability of laxatives as chocolates or gums conveys to the public that the use of these agents is without adverse consequences. Abuse of laxatives has occurred traditionally in persons trying to maintain daily bowel function, but more recently has extended to others who use laxatives for the purpose of controlling weight. In either case, the consistent abuse of strong laxatives and cathartics may lead to serious illness.

Laxative abuse for the purpose of maintaining daily bowel function begins with misconceptions about the frequency, quantity, or consistency of stools. With the use of strong purgatives, the colon may be so thoroughly cleansed that a bowel movement may not occur normally until a few days later. This delay reinforces the need for more purgatives and the cycle of laxative dependence is begun. Eventually the patient may require daily laxatives to maintain bowel function.

The laxative abuser may present with contradictory findings of diarrhea and weight loss.[49,50] In addition, long-term abusers of laxatives tend to have vomiting, abdominal pain, lassitude, weakness, thirst, edema, and bone pain (caused by osteomalacia). With prolonged use of laxatives a number of serious illnesses may arise. These include fluid and electrolyte imbalances (including acid–base imbalances and hypokalemia), protein-losing gastroenteropathy with hypoalbuminemia, and syndromes resembling colitis.

The determination of laxative abuse syndrome can be difficult because many laxative abusers vigorously deny laxative use. Middle-aged women tend to be the most common laxative abusers. The chronic laxative abuse problem should be addressed by a combination of measures, including psychiatric evaluation, dietary modification with reliance on bulk-forming laxatives, and specific guidelines to the patient for the withdrawal of stimulant laxatives.

A variation of laxative abuse is seen in persons who use them as a method of weight loss.[51] It appears from the medical literature and daily news sources that this type of abuse is on the increase. Treatment of patients who abuse laxatives in this way has proven very difficult.

▶ PRINCIPLES OF PHARMACOTHERAPY

Diarrhea

Diarrhea is most often a minor discomfort, not life threatening, and usually self-limited.

- Children, AIDS patients, and the elderly are groups at high risk for severe complications of acute diarrhea. Usually, a diagnosis is based on the history and physical examination, with extensive diagnostic tests reserved for chronic diarrhea.
- Management focuses on preventing excessive water and electrolyte losses, dietary care, relieving symptoms, treating curable causes, and treating secondary disorders.
- The foundation of treatment for diarrhea is fluid and electrolyte replacement, usually by the oral route. A variety of oral rehydration solutions may be used for this purpose.
- Medical referral is indicated when any of these are detected: children less then 3 years old, pregnant, frail elderly, moderate to severe (5% to 10% body weight loss) volume depletion, chronic heart, renal or liver disease, AIDS, moderate to severe abdominal pain, high fever, bloody or mucoid stool, or chronic diarrhea.
- Patients should be taught the proper use of antidiarrheal medications.

Constipation

Potential drug causes of constipation should be identified and the regimen altered if possible.

- The foundation of treatment of constipation is dietary fiber or bulk-forming laxatives that provide 10 to 15 g/d of raw fiber.
- Underlying causes of constipation should be identified when possible and corrective measures taken (e.g., alteration of diet or treatment of diseases such as hypothyroidism).
- Acute constipation may be treated with a tap-water enema or glycerin suppository. If neither is effective, the use of oral sorbitol, low doses of diphenylmethane, or anthraquinone laxatives may provide relief.
- Laxative abuse is a common problem that results from GI complaints or the desire to lose weight. Laxative abusers may deny their condition and may present with constipation or diarrhea.

REFERENCES

1. Nelson JD. Etiology and epidemiology of diarrheal diseases in the United States. Am J Med 1985;78(suppl 6B):78–80.
2. Rohde JE. Selective primary health care: Strategies for control of disease in the developing world. XV. Acute diarrhea. Rev Infect Dis 1984;6:840–854.
3. Field M, Ras MC, Chang EB. Intestinal electrolyte transport and diarrheal disease. N Engl J Med 1989;321:879–883.
4. Johnson DA, Cattau EL. Stool chemistries in patients with unexplained diarrhea. Am Fam Physician 1986;33:131–134.
5. Shiau YF, Feldman GM, Resnick MA, et al. Stool electrolyte and osmolality measurements in the evaluation of diarrheal disorders. Ann Intern Med 1985;102:773–775.
6. Anonymous. Feeding during diarrhea. Nutr Rev 1986;44:102.
7. Avery ME, Snyder JD. Oral therapy for acute diarrhea. N Eng J Med 1990;323:891–894.
8. Mahalanabis D. Current status of oral rehydration as a strategy for the control of diarrheal diseases. Indian J Med Res 1996;104:115–124.
9. Vesikari T, Isolauri E. Glycine supplemented oral rehydration solutions for diarrhoea. Arch Dis Child 1986;61:372–376.
10. Pizarro D, Posada G, Sandi L, et al. Rice-based electrolyte solutions for the management of infantile diarrhea. N Engl J Med 1991;324: 518–521.
11. Johnson PC, Ericsson CD, DuPont HL, et al. Comparison of loperamide with bismuth subsalicylate for the treatment of acute travelers' diarrhea. JAMA 1986;255:757–760.
12. Portnoy BL, DuPont HL, Pruitt D, et al. Antidiarrheal agents in the treatment of acute diarrhea in children. JAMA 1976;236:844–846.
13. Gordon P, Comi RJ, Maton PN, et al. NIH conference: Somatostatin and somatostain analogue (SMS 201-995) in treatment of hormone-secreting tumors of the pituitary and gastrointestinal tract and non-neoplastic diseases of the gut. Ann Intern Med 1989;110:35–50.
14. Grosman I, Simon D. Potential gastrointestinal uses of somatostatin and its synthetic analogue octreotide. Am J Gastroenterol 1990;85: 1061–1072.
15. Harris AG, O'Dorisio TM, Woltering EA, et al. Consensus statement: Octreotide dose titration in secretory diarrhea. Diarrhea Management Conference. Digestive Dis Sci 1995;40:1464–1473.
16. Ruszniewski P, Ducreux M, Chayvialle J, et al. Treatment of the carcinoid syndrome with a long acting somatstatin analogue lanreotide: A prospective study of 39 patients. Gut 1996;39:279–283.
17. Viollet C, Prevost G, Maubert E, et al. Molecular pharmacology of somatostatin receptors. Fundam Clin Pharmacol 1995;9:107–113.
18. Ryan J, Leighton J, Kirksey D, et al. Evaluation of an enkephalin analog in men with castor oil-induced diarrhea. Clin Pharmacol Ther 1986;39:40–42.
19. Lecomte JM, Costentin J, Vlaiculescu A, et al. Pharmacologic properties of acetorphan, a parenterally active "enkephalinase" inhibitor. J Pharmacol Exp Ther 1986;237:937–944.
20. Sninsky CA, Davis RH, Clench MH, et al. Effect of lidamidine hydrochloride and loperamide on gastric emptying and transit of the small intestine. Gastroenterology 1986;90:68–73.
21. Gots RE, Formal SB, Giannella RA. Indomethacin inhibition of *Salmonella typhimurium, Shigella flexneri,* and cholera-mediated rabbit ileal secretion. J Infect Dis 1974;130:280–284.
22. Burke V, Gracey M. Reduction by aspirin of intestinal fluid-loss in acute childhood gastroenteritis. Lancet 1980;1:1329–1330.
23. Rennels MB, Glass RI, Dennehy PH, et al. Safety and efficacy of high-dose rhesus-human reassortant rotavirus vaccines—Report of the national multicenter trial. Pediatrics 1996;97:7–13.
24. Whitehead WE, Chaussade S, Corazziari E. Report of an international workshop on management of constipation. Gastroenterol Int 1991;4: 99–113.
25. Romero Y, Evans J, Fleming KC, Phillips SF. Constipation and fecal incontinence in the elderly population. Mayo Clin Proc 1996;71:81–92.
26. Talley NJ, Fleming KC, Evans JM, et al. Constipation in an elderly community. A study of prevalance and potential risk factors. Am J Gastroenterol 1996;91:19–25.
27. Harari D, Gurwith JH, Avorn J, et al. Bowel habit in relation to age and gender. Findings from the National Health Survey and clinical implications. Arch Intern Med 1996;156:315–320.
28. Stewart RB, Moore MT, Marks RG, Hale WE. Correlates of constipation in an ambulatory elderly population. Am J Gastroenterol 1992; 87:859–864.
29. Clausen MR, Mortensen PB. Lactulose, disaccharides and colonic flora. Clinical consequences. Drugs 1997;53:930–942.
30. Sandgren JE, McPhee MS, Greenberger NJ. Narcotic bowel syndrome treated with clonidine. Ann Intern Med 1984;101:331–334.
31. Schiller LR, Davis GR, Santa Ana CA, et al. Mechanism of antidiarrheal action of codeine. Gastroenterology 1981;80:1275.
32. Monane M, Avorn J, Beers MH, Everitt DE. Anticholinergic drug use and bowel function in nursing home patients. Arch Intern Med 1993; 153:633–638.
33. Dwyer JT, Goldin B, Gorbach S, et al. Drug therapy reviews: Dietary fiber and fiber supplements in the therapy of gastrointestinal disorders. Am J Hosp Pharm 1978;35:278–287.
34. Ko CY, Tong J, Lehman RE, et al. Biofeedback is effective for fecal incontinence and constipation. Arch Surg 1997;132:829–833.
35. Van der Plas RN, Benninga MA, Buller HA, et al. Biofeedback training in treatment of childhood constipation: A randomised controlled study. Lancet 1996;348:766–767.
36. Tedesco FJ, DiPiro JT. Laxative use in constipation. Am J Gastroenterol 1985;80:303–309.
37. Gardner VY, Beckwith JV, Heyneman CA. Cisapride for the treatment of chronic idiopathic constipation. Ann Pharmacother 1995;29:1161–1163.
38. Jost WH, Schimrigk K. Long-term results with cisapride in Parkinson's disease. Mov Disord 1997;12:423–425.
39. Donowitz M. Current concepts of laxative action: Mechanisms by which laxatives increase stool water. Clin Gastroenterol 1979;1: 77–84.
40. Binder HJ, Donowitz M. A new look at laxative action. Gastroenterology 1975;69:1001–1005.
41. Brunton LL. Laxatives. In: Goodman LS, Gilman AG, eds. The Pharmacologic Basis of Therapeutics, 7th ed. New York, Macmillan, 1985: 994–1003.
42. Moriarity KJ, Kelly MJ, Beetham R, et al. Studies on the mechanism of action of dioctyl sodium sulphosuccinate in the human jejunum. Gut 1985;26:1008–1013.
43. Gattuso JM, Kamm MA. Adverse effects of drugs used in the management of constipation and diarrhoea. Drug Saf 1994;10:47–65.
44. Gattuso JM, Kamm A. Adverse effects of drugs used in the management of constipation and diarrhea. Drug Saf 1994;10:47–65.
45. Lederle FA, Busch DL, Mattox KM, et al. Cost-effective treatment of constipation in the elderly: A randomized double-blind comparison of sorbitol and lactulose. Am J Med 1990;89:597–601.
46. Michael KA, DiPiro JT, Bowden TA, et al. Whole-bowel irrigation for mechanical colon cleansing. Clin Pharm 1985;4:414–424.
47. Staiano A, Cucchiara S, Andreotti MR, et al. Effect of cisapride on chronic idiopathic constipation in children. Dig Dis Sci 1991;36: 733–736.
48. Sharma SS, Bhargava N, Mathur SC. Effect of oral erythromycin on colonic transit in patients with idiopathic constipation. A pilot study. Dig Dis Sci 1995;40:2446–2449.
49. Scully RE, Mark EJ, McNeely BU. Case records of the Massachusetts General Hospital. N Engl J Med 1985;313:1341–1346.
50. Oster JR, Materson BJ, Rogers A. Laxative abuse syndrome. Am J Gastroenterol 1980;74:451–458.
51. Beumont PJV, George GCW, Smart DE. "Dieters" and "vomiters and purgers" in anorexia nervosa. Psychological Med 1976;6:617–622.

35

PORTAL HYPERTENSION AND CIRRHOSIS

Mark A. Gill, PharmD, and William R. Kirchain, PharmD, CDE

Chronic disease of the liver may progress to a state of diffuse destruction and regeneration of liver parenchymal cells that results in deposition of connective tissue. This latter fibrotic tissue disrupts the lobular and vascular structures of the liver and is termed cirrhosis. The leading sequela of cirrhosis that forms the basis for this chapter is portal hypertension. Following from this vascular change are the complications of esophageal varices and ascites. While alcoholic liver disease (ALD) is the predominant cause of cirrhosis, there are many other causes (Table 35–1).[1]

EPIDEMIOLOGY

Chronic liver disease and cirrhosis as a single category has been a frequent cause of death in the US.[2] As recently as 1995, this category was the tenth most likely cause of death. In contrast to the leading cause of death (diseases of the heart), chronic liver disease and cirrhosis result in 30-fold fewer deaths nationally. There has been a downward trend over the past 20 years in the age-adjusted death rates and a 4% decline from 1996 to 1997 for chronic liver disease and cirrhosis. Speculation as to the reason for this decline has centered on the trend for reduced per capita consumption of alcohol in the United States.

PATHOPHYSIOLOGY

Alcoholic liver disease is associated with chronic ingestion of 60 to 80 g of ethanol daily for long periods of time (e.g., over 10 years).[3] The type of ethanol does not appear to be important. A person's susceptibility is dependent on individual host factors, leading to a 1 in 12 risk of cirrhosis from chronic ethanol abuse. Other factors related to the increased risk of developing ALD include nutritional status and female sex.[4] The increased risk for female alcoholics seems to derive from reduced first-pass metabolism of ethanol by alcohol dehydrogenase in gastric mucosal cells. Even accounting for weight, females have higher blood ethanol concentrations than males. This disparity can be accounted for by the decreased enzyme activity in females and even lower activity in female alcoholics.[5]

Although some controversy still remains, ALD can be viewed as a progressive, chronic condition with four basic stages. The initial lesion, steatosis or fatty metamorphosis, may begin as early as the first drink.[6] If the pattern of heavy alcohol use is continued, these lesions become necrotic, inducing a mild inflammatory reaction called alcoholic hepatitis or steatonecrosis.[6] In some cases, these lesions lead to a third stage involving fibrotic changes of cirrhosis. The end point of the disease is hepatic failure and death.

Many theories have been put forth to explain the toxic effect of alcohol on the liver. Originally, a great deal of attention was paid to possible adulterants or contaminants in the alcohol consumed by those with liver disease. Another popular theory held that ALD is primarily a nutritional deficit.[7] Most alcoholics do have serious nutritional deficits, and the treatment of ALD often includes nutritional replacement or supplementation. It has been postulated that virtually 100% of patients with ALD have malnutrition.[8] Estimates of typical patients with chronic liver disease suggest an intake of 47 g protein and 1320 kcal daily,[9] compared with roughly 50 g of protein and 1800 kcal for an average healthy adult. A nutritional deficit does not predict the development of ALD. Yet patients with a nutritional deficit do suffer the highest mortality rate.[10]

The best explanation of ALD comes from an understanding of how alcohol is metabolized in the liver. When alcohol is ingested, it is metabolized in the liver, intestinal lumen, and pancreas via alcohol dehydrogenase to acetaldehyde, which in turn is broken down to acetic acid by the mixed-function oxidase system. This simple reaction series has tremendous cellular consequences. Both the conversion of alcohol to acetaldehyde and the mixed-function oxidase system require NADH to NAD^+or NADPH to $NADP^+$conversions. This increases the ratio of NADH to NAD^+, which increases fatty acid synthesis and triglyceride accumulation within the cell. Concurrently, the production of lactic acid increases, which can lead to increased collagen production. The increase in lactic acid can also decrease the pH slightly, decreasing uric acid excretion. This then is an intermediate stage where synthetic and metabolic capacities are normal to slightly impaired.

Continued use of alcohol appears to induce the mixed-function oxidase system. This increase in lipid synthesis, along with a decrease in oxidation of fatty acids perhaps caused by acetaldehyde, leads directly to steatosis, the first lesion of ALD.

Steatosis is a lesion characteristic of, although not exclusive to, ALD. When seen at biopsy, the hepatocytes are filled with large lipid-containing vesicles. The pattern of steatosis induced by alcohol is largely centrilobular (now often referred to as perivenular—the lobule immediately surrounding the central vein). This pathologic change is easily reversed by abstinence from alcohol, and little functional impairment is usually encountered.[7]

TABLE 35–1. Causes of Cirrhosis

Alcohol abuse	Primary biliary cirrhosis
Autoimmune hepatitis	Primary sclerosing cholangitis
Viral hepatitis	Drugs, chemicals, and toxins
Hemochromatosis	Schistosomiasis
Wilson's disease	Hepatic vein obstruction
α_1-antitrypsin deficiency	Cryptogenic

The next major pathologic event in the progression of ALD is steatonecrosis or alcoholic hepatitis. Lysis and necrosis of the fat-filled hepatocytes provoke an immune response. In susceptible persons, there is an apparent alteration of cell-mediated immunity, leading to an increased rate of damage. The most obvious changes of alcoholic hepatitis seen histologically occur in zone 3 of the hepatic acinus. This is the part furthest from oxygenated blood entering the liver. Alcohol may lead to cell necrosis by increasing the metabolic rate of cells that are already relatively hypoxic. Alcoholic hepatitis is also marked by the development of the alcoholic hyaline or Mallory bodies. These are intracellular eosinophilic perinuclear inclusion bodies. Although not diagnostic, Mallory bodies portend a more severe form of alcoholic hepatitis. Besides alcohol, griseofulvin and amiodarone may induce Mallory bodies. The fibrosis that occurs in alcoholic hepatitis often obliterates the central veins, leading to portal vein hypertension even before the patient has progressed to cirrhosis. Even at the alcoholic hepatitis stage of the disease, many patients can avoid the eventual sequelae by abstinence, although the cellular structure may never return to normal. Surprisingly, 18% of patients at this stage of ALD will continue to develop cirrhosis despite abstinence from alcohol.[11] If there is no continued insult to the liver, a resolution of symptoms can be anticipated in 3 to 8 months. The 7-year survival rate for abstainers is 80%, whereas for those continuing to drink the rate is only 50%.[12]

Cirrhosis leading to hepatic failure and its complications is the terminal event in ALD. Cirrhosis is primarily the result of fibrotic changes that distort the architectural integrity of the liver. This is generally accompanied by a loss of parenchymal mass and a concurrent loss of liver function. It is these changes in structure and decreases in function that result in the signs and symptoms of alcoholic cirrhosis, such as portal hypertension or bleeding abnormalities. The fibrosis may compress the hepatic veins, decreasing hepatic outflow and thus leading to portal hypertension.[12]

CLINICAL PRESENTATION

LABORATORY TESTS

A valuable laboratory test to evaluate several aspects of liver function is the serum bilirubin test. Bilirubin is a breakdown product of hemoglobin. This breakdown occurs in the spleen and bone marrow. The bilirubin released is an insoluble form of bilirubin (called indirect bilirubin) that is bound to plasma proteins and delivered to the liver parenchymal cells, which conjugate bilirubin with glucuronide; this is measured as direct bilirubin. Most of the bilirubin glucuronide is excreted into the bile and then converted by gut bacteria to urobilinogen, which gives stool its characteristic brown color. With advancing liver disease, less bilirubin gets conjugated, leading to increases in indirect bilirubin. Liver cell death leads to release of conjugated bilirubin from the liver into the systemic circulation, which then leads to increases in direct bilirubin. Excess conjugated bilirubin may be filtered by the kidneys, giving urine the characteristic "cola" color. Excess bilirubin leads to accumulation in the epidermis and sclera. Termed jaundice or icterus, it is characterized by a yellow tinge to the skin or eye that is noticeable when total bilirubin levels exceed 3 to 5 mg%. Another useful test is the serum alkaline phosphatase test. This enzyme is made in cells lining the biliary tract and in bone tissue. In processes that disrupt bile flow, alkaline phosphatase will increase in serum.

Once jaundice is evident, it is helpful to analyze the relative incremental increases in serum bilirubin versus alkaline phosphatase. In alcoholic liver disease the ratio of patient to normal bilirubin is much greater than that ratio for alkaline phosphatase. Serum transaminase measurements are also valuable in assessing liver damage from alcohol. The transaminases are alanine aminotransferase (ALT) and aspartate aminotransferase (AST), which have a typical normal range of 5 to 40 IU/dL. Typically, the AST increases beyond the ALT (about two-fold difference). The highest increase in AST or ALT is seen with alcoholic hepatitis and may reach into the hundreds. As the liver disease progresses into cirrhosis, the transaminases may actually fall despite worsening liver function. Another enzyme that may be useful is γ-glutamyltranspeptidase (GGTP), with a typical normal range of 0 to 65 IU/dL. GGTP is a biliary excretory enzyme that is more specific for liver disease than alkaline phosphatase (the former will not be elevated in bone disease while the latter may). Generally, GGTP and alkaline phosphatase rise in concert with cholestasis; however, with ALD a disproportionate increase in GGTP can be expected and is a useful diagnostic clue. An elevation in GGTP in ALD may reflect microsomal enzyme induction rather than cellular toxicity.[13] Whereas in viral hepatitis the enzyme elevation correlates with the extent of cellular destruction, this is not the case in ALD. As liver damage progresses, protein synthesis decreases, which will affect plasma protein concentrations of albumin and clotting factors. Combined with the malnutrition of ALD patients, the decreased hepatic protein synthesis results in serious abnormalities in serum oncotic pressure and hemostasis. Prolongation of clotting tests such as prothrombin time and activated partial thromboplastin time can be expected. The serum albumin may fall as low as 2 g/dL (normal 4.5 to 5.5 g/dL). The value of monitoring all of these lab tests has been questioned. Several of these tests used individually (GGTP, AST, or ALT) had no prognostic value in relative

TABLE 35–2. Child–Pugh Grading of Liver Disease

Clinical and Biochemical Measurements	Points Scored for Increasing Abnormality[a]		
	1	*2*	*3*
Encephalopathy (grade)	None	1 and 2	3 and 4
Ascites	Absent	Slight	Moderate
Bilirubin (mg/dL)	1–2	2–3	> 3
Albumin (g/dL)	3.5	2.8–3.5	< 2.8
Prothrombin time (increased seconds)	1–4	4–6	> 6

[a]Each row is given a point value of 1, 2, or 3. The sum of each row's score provides the overall score that is converted to a "grade" of A, B, or C.

risk estimates of 1-year mortality from ALD.[14] However, albumin, serum bilirubin, hemoglobin, or prothrombin time had very significant predictive ability.

A classification system for the severity of liver disease has been developed that incorporates several laboratory tests. The Child–Pugh classification is frequently used to stratify patients into categories for selection of various therapies. The system may be useful in monitoring the response to therapies. Patients are labeled grade A for point scores of 5 to 6, grade B for scores of 7 to 9, and grade C with scores above 10 using the point system given in Table 35–2.[15] Another schema is the Maddrey score or Maddrey discriminant function, which is a simple calculation using the sum of the prothrombin time in seconds multipled by 4.6 plus the total bilirubin (in mg/dL). Those patients with discriminant function scores over 93 are at severe risk of death.[16] Some clinicians use a modified discriminant function, which is the sum of the patient's prothrombin time minus control times 4.6 plus the serum bilirubin (in μmol/L) divided by 17, where patients with scores over 32 are at severe risk of death.[17]

In the typical patient, it will be difficult to distinguish fatty liver, alcoholic hepatitis, or cirrhosis using clinical features or common laboratory tests. Rather, the definitive diagnosis relies upon biopsy and microscopic interpretation. Cirrhotics tend to have higher serum bilirubin, lower serum albumin, more frequent encephalopathy, more frequent ascites, and lower transaminases. However, due to considerable overlap in the three populations, these variables are not diagnostic.[18]

COMPLICATIONS

PORTAL HYPERTENSION AND ASCITES

Portal hypertension in cirrhosis is the direct result of increased mechanical resistance to blood flow through the liver. In individuals with no cirrhosis, the normal liver blood flow is roughly 1 to 1.5 L/min at a pressure of only 4 to 6 mm Hg. As the flow is inhibited by the distorted liver architecture in cirrhotic patients, the pressure rises not only in the liver but also along the gastrointestinal tract and in the spleen as well. The manifestations, then, of portal hypertension are primarily the result of low-pressure vessels handling high-pressure loads. To cope with this pressure, blood is diverted into a large number of minor small collateral vessels. This collateral flow is very prominent in the azygous and subclavian veins through the lower esophagus, the abdominal wall, and between the spleen and the left renal vein. Esophageal and abdominal varices often develop; these can rupture and sometimes lead to life-threatening hemorrhage. Mortality from variceal bleeding is very high; estimates range from 30% to 50%.[19] Most deaths occur within the first two weeks following the initial bleeding episodes. There is a minimum pressure of 12 mm Hg that appears to be necessary for varices to form, then bleed.[20] There are other risk factors for bleeding, which include severity of liver dysfunction, continued alcohol abuse, and coagulopathies. Splenomegaly is also a common feature, occasionally requiring splenectomy.

Another significant complication of portal hypertension is ascites (Fig. 35–1). Ascites results from the higher pressures of portal hypertension coupled with an increased porosity in the liver sinusoids, and an increase in intrahep-

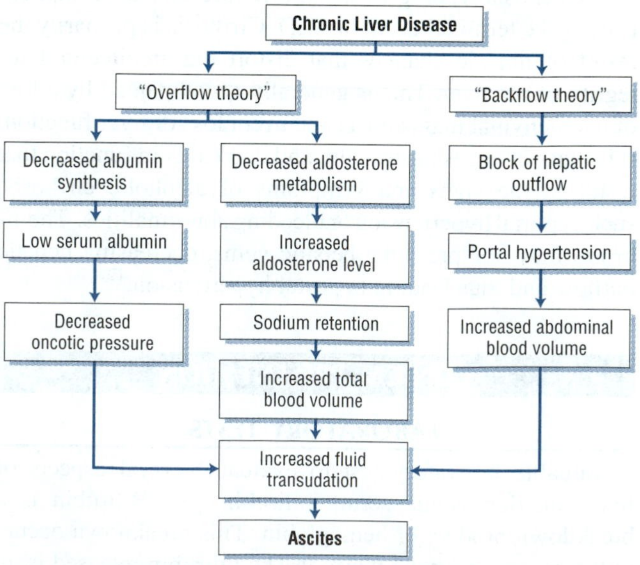

FIGURE 35–1. Theories for the development of ascites.

atic interstitial fluid. The lymphatic system of the liver is able to handle a great deal of excess fluid, but some leakage into the peritoneal cavity still occurs. The amount of fluid leaked into the peritoneal cavity can become quite large over time, leading to mechanical problems with many body systems. The increased intra-abdominal pressure acting on the diaphragm can, by affecting thoracic pressure, decrease transmural filling pressure of the heart, increase right atrial pressure, and decrease venous return to the right ventricle. The increased pooling of blood associated with portal hypertension leads to a sequestration of blood in the spleen, which along with the sequestration of fluid in the peritoneum, leads to a relative decrease in renal arteriolar perfusion. This induces the release of renin, which may lead to the increased reabsorbtion of sodium (and water). Renin levels are higher in cirrhotic patients. Because cirrhosis is often accompanied by a decrease in the hepatic production of albumin, the serum oncotic pressure is also decreased, thus reducing the ability of the body to retain fluid in the vascular space.

ESOPHAGEAL AND GASTRIC VARICES

Portal hypertension causes pooling of blood in both the spleen and the mesenteric veins and arteries. This causes engorgement of the small capillaries along the entire GI tract. These overfilled blood vessels are much easier to rupture than normal vessels. Concurrently there is a breakdown in the gastric mucosa, leading to increased damage from acid and pepsin in the stomach and esophagus caused by an apparent direct toxic effect of alcohol on the mucosal surface. It has been observed that many episodes of hemorrhage from varices occur at night. There appear to be nocturnal increases in portal pressure and blood flow, peaking at midnight.[21]

DECREASED LIVER FUNCTION

Along with the effects of the mechanical problems of cirrhosis there is a progressive loss of basic hepatocyte function because of an overall loss of parenchymal mass. There is generally a decrease in protein synthesis and use of available substrates. A loss of enzymes leads to a decrease in the liver's ability to handle both drugs and endogenous toxins, which begin to accumulate. A decrease in serum albumin leads to a decrease in the protein binding of certain drugs and a decrease in the serum oncotic pressure. Vitamin K-dependent coagulation factors (II, VII, IX, and X) synthesized by the liver slowly diminish, resulting in an increased frequency of bleeding problems. The ability of the hepatic transaminases to detoxify ammonia is decreased. Ammonia, octopamine, mercaptans, phenols, methanethiols, and other byproducts of metabolism begin to accumulate. There is some evidence that benzodiazepine-receptor reactivity is increased, and that an endogenous benzodiazepine-receptor ligand accumulates in liver disease.[22] This ligand is known to be produced in very small amounts by plants.

Along with this decrease in transamination there is an apparent increase in ammonia production in the gut. The catabolism induced by the decrease in albumin leads to an increase in aromatic amino acids (AAAs) at a rate 24 times the production of branched-chain amino acids (BCAAs).

HEPATIC ENCEPHALOPATHY

Methinks sometime I have no more wit than a Christian or an ordinary man has; but I am a great eater of beef, and I believe that does harm to my wit.

Sir Andrew in Shakespeare's "Twelfth Night" (Act 1, scene 3)

Hepatic encephalopathy (HE) is a syndrome of altered mental status associated with liver impairment characterized by impaired cognitive skills, worsened motor abilities, and steadily depressed levels of consciousness beginning with somnolence and ending with coma. The spectrum of impairment is broad and may be classified in stages as the syndrome progresses (Table 35–3). Alternative scales are in use. One, summarized in Table 35–4, may be useful in assessing the progression of the disease or response to therapies. The incidence of HE may be much greater than generally perceived. In one study, only 15% of patients with chronic liver disease but without a diagnosis of encephalopathy could pass standardized psychometric tests.[23] The cause of HE is not known; several factors, such as increased blood levels of ammonia and AAAs, have been associated with the development of HE (Table 35–5). Elevated ammonia levels have long been associated with HE. It is unclear if this elevation is the actual cause of the encephalopathic symptomatology. Ammonia metabolites (glutamine, α-ketoglutaramate) rather than ammonia in cerebrospinal fluid (CSF) correlate well with the grade of encephalopathy.[24] Mechanisms for the accumulation of ammonia and other nitrogenous compounds include reduced metabolic clearance of ammonia by the liver and bypass of the liver via collateral blood vessels because of intrahepatic outflow blockade.

TABLE 35–3. Scale for Assessing the Depth of Hepatic Encephalopathy

Grade	Cognitive/Motor	Behavior
1	Mild tremor, altered handwriting	Anxiety, insomnia, mild confusion
2	Dysarthria, ataxia asterixis	Lethargy, disorientation
3	Seizures, muscle twitching	Delirium, bizarre behavior
4	Posturing	Coma

From Ref. 83, with permission. Copyright 1984 American Society of Health-System Pharmacists, Inc. All rights reserved.

TABLE 35–4. Hepatic Encephalopathy Scores

I. Verbal response	1. None 2. Incomprehensible 3. Confused 4. Normal
II. Eye opening	1. None 2. Noxious stimuli only 3. Verbal stimuli 4. Spontaneous
III. Pupils	1. Nonreactive 2. Sluggish 3. Brisk
IV. Oculocephalic/oculovestibular	1. No reaction 2. Partial or dysconjugate 3. Full 4. Normal
V. Best motor response	1. None 2. Abnormal extensor 3. Abnormal flexor 4. Withdrawal or localizes 5. Obeys commands
VI. Respiration	1. Nil on ventilator 2. Irregular 3. Regular > 22/min 4. Regular < 22/min

From Ref. 83, with permission.

As stated earlier, there is also a tremendous change in the relative levels of aromatic amino acids in the encephalopathic patient. Increased levels of blood glucagon and/or insulin in liver impairment lead to muscle breakdown of BCAAs, gluconeogenesis, and possibly hyperammonemia. The BCAAs normally compete for central nervous system entry with AAAs. Thus, the abnormal ratio of BCAA to AAA in liver disease allows for enhanced CNS entry of tryptophan, tyrosine, and phenylalanine. Free fatty acids have been implicated in HE. Long-chain fatty acids are elevated in cirrhotic patients secondary to decreased hepatic oxidation and increased absorption. They are thought to displace neuroactive chemicals from serum albumin (e.g., tryptophan, benzodiazepines). There is evidence of increased brain concentrations of 1,4-benzodiazepines in some patients with hepatic encephalopathy due to fulminant hepatic failure.[25] γ-Aminobutyric acid (GABA) is a product of intestinal flora and intestinal mucosa. With hepatic failure, blood and CNS levels rise, allowing for its CNS depression. Evident is decreased catabolism of GABA by the impaired liver and lowered blood–brain barrier to GABA.

TABLE 35–5. Theories for the Development of Hepatic Encephalopathy

Toxin	Description
Ammonia	Direct neurotoxin
Multiple synergistic neurotoxins	Mercaptans (produced by neurotoxins dietary methionine), elevated free fatty acids
False neurotransmitters	Elevated aromatic amino acids lead to increased serotonin, octopamine, and phenylethylamine (depressants) while decreasing dopamine and noradrenaline (stimulants)
γ-Aminobutyric acid neurotransmission	Endogenous and/or exogenous benzodiazepine-like compounds

There are a variety of precipitating events for HE that may be preventable or reversible (Table 35–6). Every effort should be made to identify these factors before initiating drug therapy to reverse the encephalopathy.

PHARMACOKINETIC AND PHARMACODYNAMIC CHANGES ASSOCIATED WITH LIVER FAILURE

There is currently no exact mathematical approach to adjusting drug doses during liver failure. Drugs that are primarily excreted by the liver or extensively metabolized before renal excretion are the most affected by changes in hepatic function. As stated earlier, liver disease is a complex process that involves changes in blood flow, blood pressure, metabolic capacity, and protein binding. These changes will occur at different rates and to varying degrees, depending on the patient. The most important parameter when adjusting drug doses for liver impairment is the clinical response. Frequent close observation of an individual's response to a dose is the best way to meet the needs of the liver-disabled patient. There is value in pharmacokinetic assessment of the patient as well, but it is difficult to be exact with these assessments. Table 35–7 lists a few drugs and the known pharmacokinetic changes associated with liver impairment. Note that one of the most important considerations is the extraction ratio of a drug. Highly extracted drugs tend to be affected more by changes in hepatic blood flow than by changes in metabolic rate. The opposite is true of low extraction ratio drugs. Cirrhosis would then have a greater impact on a drug such as labetalol than would an inflammatory process such as hepatitis. Beyond the observed changes in clearance, half-life, and volume of distribution, it is important to note the impact of disease and extraction ratio. Changes during acute hepatitis are often transitory and new changes in drug dosage must be made as the disease subsides. Many drugs have FDA-approved labeling that indicates dosage adjustment may be required with impaired liver function. Lidocaine and theophylline are examples of drugs requiring dosage adjustment in liver impairment. Unfortunately, precise adjustments are not described in these package inserts.

Another important pharmacokinetic change associated with liver failure relates to protein binding. There is a slow but steady decrease in serum albumin that occurs with decreasing liver function. The free fraction of highly protein-bound drugs increases as albumin decreases, and can cause increased drug effect, usually seen as increased toxicity. An increased free fraction also means that there is more drug available to be metabolized by the still functioning hepatic enzymes. Thus until these enzymes become saturated, the clearance of a highly protein-bound drug during liver impairment can increase and the half-life can shorten. Patients

TABLE 35–6. Precipitating Causes of Hepatic Encephalopathy

Cause	Management	Mechanism
Infection	Increased tissue catabolism leads to more nitrogen load; hypotension-induced azotemia	Treat infection
Constipation	Increased ammonia from longer contact time for bacteria and substrates	Prophylactic use of stool softeners or laxatives
Metabolic alkalosis	Leads to diffusion of unionized ammonia across blood–brain barrier	KCl treatment in moderate cases; 0.1 N HCl infusion in severe cases
Excess dietary protein	Substrate for bacterial production of ammonia or other nitrogenous toxins	Limit total protein intake or restrict red meat protein
Gastrointestinal bleeding	Hypovolemia may decrease perfusion to liver/brain/kidneys; blood provides 15–20 g protein/100 mL as an ammonia substrate	Evacuate bowel
Drugs: sedative/hypnotics, opiates	Direct CNS depression	Avoid use; otherwise select short-acting nonliver metabolized or adjust dose
Azotemia	Sedative effect of uremia	Use diuretics gently

with high GGTP and alkaline phosphatase levels may experience a decrease in biliary excretion. Drugs that are excreted through the bile will accumulate in these patients.

The third-spacing of fluid associated with chronic liver disease may also alter pharmacokinetics and pharmacodynamics. Dramatic shifts in fluid can be expected in ALD, thus increasing the distribution volume of drugs with low protein binding. The fluid shift into the peritoneum from ascites has also been shown to increase the distribution volume of drugs such as the aminoglycosides, oftentimes necessitating larger drug dosages.[26]

The clinical components of liver disease also can change the dose–response relationships of drugs. Encephalopathic patients will be much more sensitive to CNS depressants. Varices, particularly bleeding varices, may increase the absorption of drugs that would normally exhibit poor absorption. Diarrhea associated with hepatitis will decrease the absorption of many drugs. Besides the hepatic components, most end-stage liver disease patients have some mild to moderate renal impairment that will further decrease drug elimination.

Once the individual factors are accounted for, it is important when dosing drugs in the hepatically impaired patient to account for the multiorgan-system nature of liver disease. One bedside method for assessing the extent of liver disease is Pugh's score. Originally developed for comparing the survival of mild versus severely diseased patients after surgical procedures, this system allows one to estimate total hepatic function.[27] Encephalopathy, ascites, bilirubin levels, serum albumin, and the prothrombin time combine to give a score that increases with increasing disease. As seen in Table 35–2, this technique accounts for the differing presentations of liver impairment by allowing each element to increase the score. Scores of 6 or less are associated with highly survivable liver disease. Scores between 7 to 9 suggest moderate disease and loss of function. Scores greater than 10 represent end-stage disease. The use of this system can give clues to the extent that drug dosage should be changed or monitored more closely. Antipyrine and other hepatic function markers, such as indocyanine green, can also be used to assess hepatic function. The administration of these agents in the clinical setting of severe liver disease is uncommon. Preprandial and postprandial bile acid levels with galactose clearance studies have also been used to assess liver function. Caffeine is also used for the study of hepatic function because of its widespread acceptance as a benign agent in low doses. Caffeine clearance studies, however, have difficulty differentiating patients at or near the end stages of the disease.[28,29]

TABLE 35–7. Selected Examples of Pharmacokinetic Changes During Liver Failure

Drug	Extraction	Disease	Plasma Clearance	Volume of Distribution	Terminal Half-life
Diazepam	Low	Cirrhosis	Decreases 30%–50%	May increase slightly	Increases 40%–50%
Diazepam	Low	Acute hepatitis	Decreases	May increase slightly	Increases 20%–40%
Oxazepam	Low	Cirrhosis	Increases slightly	Increases 10%–20%	Increases slightly
Phenobarbital	Low	Cirrhosis			Increases 10%–30%
Phenobarbital	Low	Acute hepatitis			Increases 10%–40%
Propranolol	High	Cirrhosis	Decreases 33%–50%	Increases 50%	Increases 100%–200%
Labetalol	High	Cirrhosis	Decreases 25%–60%	Decreases 20%–40%	Increases slightly
Lidocaine	High	Cirrhosis	Decreases 35%–40%		
Clindamycin	Low	Cirrhosis	Decreases 60%	Decreases 40%	Increases slightly
Theophylline	High	Cirrhosis	Decreases 33%–50%	Increases 30%–40%	Increases 100%–300%

▶ TREATMENT: Portal Hypertension and Cirrhosis

GENERAL APPROACH TO TREATMENT

The most important treatment for drug-induced liver disease is the discontinuance of drug exposure. It cannot be overemphasized that patients with alcoholic liver disease must stop drinking. With discontinuation of alcohol exposure, many patients improve dramatically. Steatosis often resolves within weeks, and alcohol hepatitis within a few months, of the last drink. Otherwise, management of cirrhosis includes treatments to inhibit the inflammatory process (corticosteroids), drugs to reverse associated problems (vitamins and calories), prophylaxis against morbid events (β-blockers), or symptomatic relief (paracentesis).

ALCOHOLIC HEPATITIS

After the discontinuation of alcohol, the therapy for ALD is primarily symptomatic. See Figure 35–2 for an algorithm useful in the management of patients with alcoholic hepatitis. In alcoholic hepatitis, glucocorticoids are sometimes used during the acute phase; the rationale is to decrease the inflammatory response to the alcoholic hyaline and other antigenic substances present. There are increased class 1 major histocompatibility complex antigens that have been found on the plasma membranes of hepatocytes in patients with alcoholic hepatitis. Subsequently, effector T cells attack the liver cells. Glucocorticoids may act by decreasing T-cell-mediated cytotoxicity.[30] There is conflicting evidence regarding glucocorticoid effect on reducing the overall morbidity of alcoholic hepatitis patients. Improvement in short-term mortality was demonstrated with methylprednisolone in very sick patients.[31] The steroid reduced mortality from 35% seen with placebo to 6%.[32] Prior studies with negative results may not have randomized subjects who were ill enough. When studies have been combined in a meta-analysis, the positive effects of glucocorticoids become more apparent.[33] The analysis revealed a particular benefit in those patients with hepatic encephalopathy. Another meta-analysis also showed a reduction in mortality with corticosteroids.[34] This analysis also found that encephalopathy was a predictor for success and additionally that the presence of GI bleeding would reverse the positive effects of glucocorticoids. Generally, prednisolone or methylprednisolone are the preferred steroids, because they do not require liver metabolism to an active compound such as prednisone does. The typical starting dose is 40 mg daily for a month, and then 20 mg daily for a week, 10 mg daily for another week, and then stopped. The long-term prognosis with glucocorticoids still remains uncertain, particularly if alcohol is still ingested. Regardless of treatment, many patients do not survive severe bouts of the disease (survival rate, 22% to 45%). Those who do survive often develop cirrhosis in 3 to 5 years. In selecting patients who might benefit from steroids, the Maddrey discriminant function calculation may be used.[35] When severely ill patients with modified Maddrey scores in excess of 32 were given prednisolone or placebo, steroid therapy significantly prolonged survival and normalized hepatic function, as evidenced by serum albumin, prothrombin time, and serum bilirubin.[17]

CIRRHOSIS

The treatment of cirrhosis is again symptomatic, directed at the particular manifestations in the particular patient. If the patient shows signs of nutritional deficiency, it should be corrected. Deficiencies in folate, thiamine, and vitamin C are very common and often severe. Replacement regimens are the following: folic acid 1 mg daily, thiamine 15 mg daily (unless beriberi exists, where parenteral doses of 50 mg tid are suggested), and vitamin C 500 mg daily. In addition, potassium, phosphorus, magnesium, and iron can be quite low in these patients. Replacement of iron should be done with particular caution in cirrhotic patients, because liver iron stores are often higher than normal despite low serum concentrations, and hemochromatosis can develop. Vitamin K injections (typical dose is 10 mg slow IVP) can sometimes help regenerate clotting factors, but as cirrhosis worsens, the response to vitamin K lessens. Treatment of the coagulopathy may require fresh whole blood or fresh frozen plasma transfusions. Replenishment of serum protein can be very difficult in cirrhotic patients, who often require protein restriction, but adequate calories should be given.

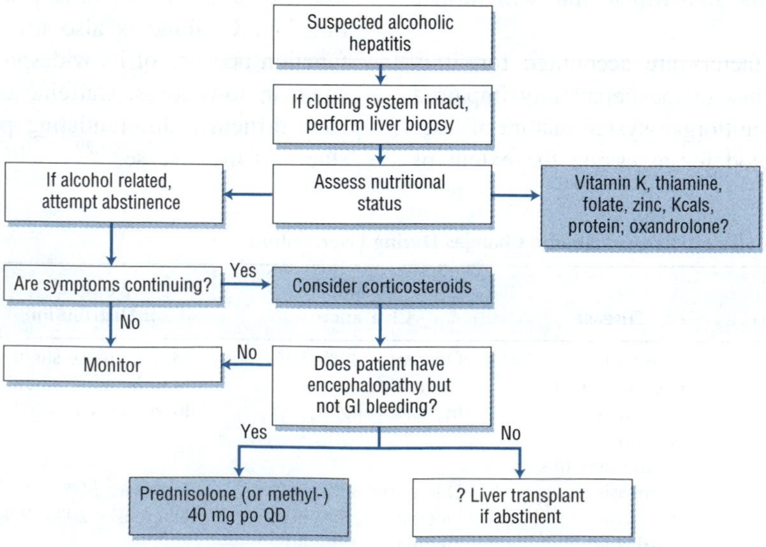

FIGURE 35–2. Treatment algorithm for alcoholic hepatitis.

Liver transplantation is a consideration for end-stage liver disease. Alcoholics have not been viewed as optimal candidates because the high rates of recidivism and poor compliance to immunosuppressive agents might result in unacceptably high rejection rates. However, in a series of 73 alcoholic patients receiving liver transplants, 71% were alive after a mean of 25 months, which was felt to be comparable to a nonalcoholic population receiving transplants.[36]

PROPYLTHIOURACIL

An experimental treatment for ALD with propylthiouracil (PTU) has been shown to reduce mortality compared to placebo.[37] Response to PTU was dependent on a reduced intake of alcohol. PTU may reduce the hypoxic conditions in the liver produced by alcohol. PTU was given in a dose of 150 mg bid with changes in thyroid function tests but no clinical hypothyroidism. These results, however, need confirmation before PTU can be recommended for alcoholics.

COLCHICINE

Also considered experimental is the use of colchicine for cirrhosis. Colchicine has antifibrotic and anti-inflammatory effects. It has *not* been found to be useful in existing cirrhosis from hepatitis B virus infection[38]; however, if colchicine is given before the viral disease results in cirrhosis, the drug may prevent the firbrotic changes.[39]

ANDROGENIC STEROIDS

Androgenic steroids have been considered in alcoholic hepatitis. A hallmark of ALD is hypogonadism as evidenced by gynecomastia and azoospermia. Additional benefits beyond reversal of low testosterone levels were expected, such as hepatic regeneration. Oxandrolone 80 mg daily was compared to prednisone and placebo. Even though the androgen was only given for 30 days, it improved survival at 6 months.[40] Androgens must still be viewed as experimental because their use beyond 30 days has not been studied and the impact on long-term morbidity or mortality is not known. Androgens seem to lower mortality in malnourished patients that are given the steroid and adequate caloric intake.[41]

ASCITES

Ascites is primarily an accumulation of fluid; therefore, the objective in treating ascites should be removal of fluid. In practice, this is often not an easy task. Figure 35–3 summarizes the stepwise treatment of ascites. The increase in fluid in the peritoneal cavity causes a relative decrease in intravascular volume. The kidney responds by retaining sodium; sodium restriction is then the first step in treating ascites.[42] Most patients with ascites can tolerate 1 g of sodium per day, which essentially means no added salt and no salted foods. The diuresis observed from this approach, though, is very slow, often taking as long as 30 days for obvious loss of ascites volume.[43] Salt restriction is generally accompanied by a concurrent restriction of fluid intake to a few hundred mL/d. Patients who are not hospitalized generally find this a difficult regimen. As the ascites begins to resolve, the amount of sodium can sometimes be increased to a more tolerable 2 to 3 g, and the amount of fluid intake increased upward to 1 L/d. The overall fluid loss per day should not exceed 1 to 2 L.[44] Patients with peripheral edema seem to tolerate faster mobilization of ascites than patients who have no edema. Nonedematous patients transfer water from the peritoneal cavity to the vascular space at a rate of 200 to 400 mL/d and should not be diuresed beyond a weight loss of about 0.5 kg/d. Because maximal ascitic

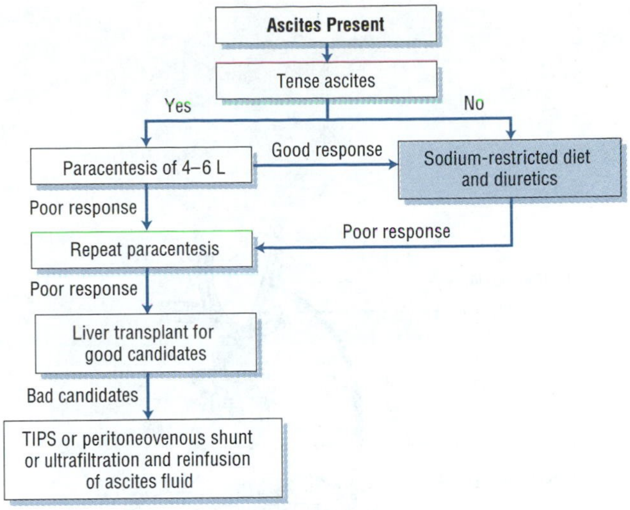

FIGURE 35–3. Treatment algorithm for ascites.

fluid mobilization occurs at a rate of only 1 to 2 L/d, diuresis that is too brisk can lead to problems of relative dehydration and a potentially fatal hepatorenal syndrome. Hepatorenal syndrome is a progressive, fatal loss of renal function in the face of severe hepatic dysfunction. The onset of hepatorenal syndrome is insidious and often unrecognized. A slow but continuous rise in serum creatinine and blood urea nitrogen eventually progresses to complete failure of the kidneys. The patient must then deal not only with a failed liver but also with all the problems associated with acute renal failure. Drug dosing can become extremely difficult in these patients, often requiring extensive use of blood levels and sophisticated pharmacokinetic methods. Ultimately, however, hepatorenal syndrome is almost uniformly fatal.

Paracentesis or diuretic therapy can be used to deplete the volume of ascites when sodium and fluid restriction fail to produce adequate diuresis. Paracentesis as a palliative measure designed to relieve pressure, respiratory insufficiency from a displaced diaphragm, and/or umbilical hernia has been employed for centuries. It is said that the composer Beethoven was "tapped" toward the end of his life. The result was reported to be a loss of 25 pounds worth of fluid and that he was symptomatically improved.[45] Paracentesis of large volumes of fluid usually results in immediate resorption of water from the vascular space into the peritoneal space that may be complete in as little as 4 days.[44] This rapid shift may lead to vascular volume depletion. To avoid these shifts, recent studies employed simultaneous administration of parenteral albumin in order to increase plasma oncotic pressure and prevent movement of substantial volumes of fluid. Paracentesis without albumin was reported to produce hyponatremia, increased plasma renin activity, and renal insufficiency more frequently than paracentesis with albumin.[46] In a randomized trial of paracentesis/albumin versus spironolactone/furosemide, diuretics were more likely to cause hyponatremia, encephalopathy, and renal impairment.[47] In addition, a satisfactory response to treatment was more common for paracentesis/albumin (96.5%) than for diuretics (72.8%). Perhaps more startling was the shorter hospital stay and lower mortality rate observed for the paracentesis group. Paracentesis should be used before diuretics when the patient is uncomfortable and requests immediate relief or where the fluid is needed for diagnostic or therapeutic reasons.

Many patients who continue to develop ascites and those who do not respond to diuretics or paracentesis may be eligible to receive a LeVeen or peritoneovenous shunt (Fig.35–4), which

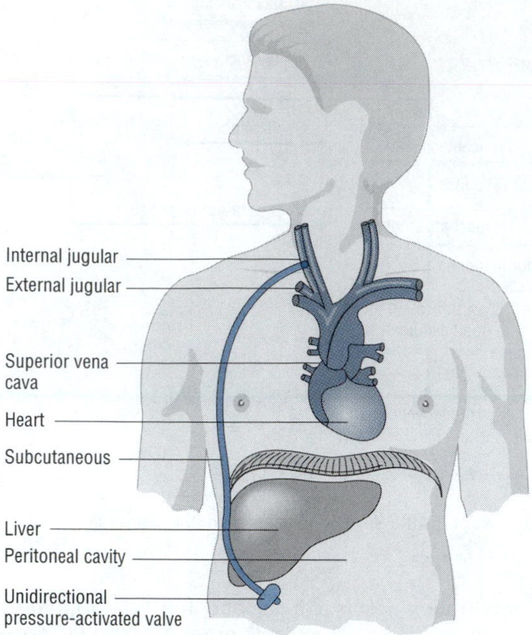

FIGURE 35–4. Representation of placement of a LeVeen shunt to reduce portal pressure and ascites.

is a catheter tunneled between the peritoneal space and a central vein such as a jugular vein. Even this does not always prevent ascites from recurring; 30% to 40% of patients with a LeVeen shunt in place may develop ascites again later.[48,49] However, a large-scale trial in veterans demonstrated delayed recurrence, shorter hospital stays, and faster ascites removal with shunting as opposed to medical treatment.[50] Encephalopathy was more common with medical treatment in certain subgroups of patients. Shunts may lead to postoperative disseminated intravascular coagulopathy, intravascular platelet agglutination, or fibrinolysis. Approaches to reduce the risk of coagulopathy include completely draining the ascites at the time the shunt is placed, preoperative aspirin, heparin, or aminocaproic acid (EACA). Nonetheless, mortality rate is not improved with shunts relative to medical treatment. A recently popular and less invasive technique than the LaVeen shunt is the transjugular intrahepatic portosystemic shunt (TIPS). This procedure involves passing a catheter through an exposed jugular vein, down the inferior vena cava through the hepatic vein, puncturing the portal vein. Then a stent is placed as a permanent communication between the two vessels (as in Fig. 35–5), which greatly reduces portal pressure. Although the portal pressure drop is rapid, natriuresis is not immediate and may take a month. Ascites and the likelihood of bleeding varices can be reduced. Where ascites and varices recur, it is likely that the stent thrombosed. Other stent complications include encephalopathy (which may respond to medical therapy, but if not, requires occlusion or reduction of the stent), sepsis, and bleeding at the catheterization site.[51–54]

Diuretic therapy with salt restriction for ascites is effective in 90% or more of patients,[55] yet the process is slow. Patients may require as long as 35 to 40 days of continuous therapy before the ascites has resolved.[42] The drugs most frequently used are the potassium-sparing diuretics, because of the ability of spironolactone, in particular, to inhibit the action of aldosterone in the kidney tubule. It is believed that ascites causes a relative decrease in intravascular volume that stimulates the aldosterone-mediated retention of sodium and water in the kidney. The dose of spironolactone required ranges from 100 to 800 mg/d and is usually not effective without concurrent sodium restriction. Because the half-life of spironolactone and its active metabolites is prolonged in patients with liver disease, single daily doses should be used to improve compliance.[56] The onset of the diuretic effect with spironolactone is slow, 2 weeks in some cases, and loop diuretics such as furosemide are often added to increase the rate of weight loss. Spironolactone is a competitive inhibitor of aldosterone in the distal segment of the renal tubule. Aldosterone causes the reabsorption of sodium from the peritubular fluid and the concurrent excretion of potassium. The amount normally presented to the distal tubule is small, and inhibiting this reabsorption produces only a mild increase in sodium and water excretion. Again, the rate of weight loss should not exceed 1 to 2 kg/d. The relative efficacy of diuretics has been examined and revealed that spironolactone produces a positive response more often than furosemide.[57] Regardless of the diuretic selected, serum electrolytes must be monitored carefully during therapy, and signs of dehydration (orthostatic blood pressure changes, changes in heart rate, decreased urine output) must be carefully monitored. When rapid diuresis is sought (e.g., for a hospitalized patient in order to reduce length of stay), furosemide in a dose of 40 mg should be started at the same time as 100 mg of spironolactone. Doses of each drug can be doubled at 3-day intervals if weight loss is inadequate. Amiloride (10 mg up to 40 mg daily) has been an alternative to spironolactone where a faster onset of diuresis is indicated or painful gynecomastia occurs.[55]

PORTAL HYPERTENSION

The therapy for portal hypertension is directed at reducing flow to the portal bed. Operative procedures such as splenectomy, portacaval shunts, or stents attempt to do this mechanically. Drug therapy with various β-blockers has also been used with some success. Use of β-blockers can be categorized into two general indications: (1) prophylaxis against the initial hemorrhage in existent varices (sometimes called *primary prevention*) and (2) prevention of rebleeding after an episode of hemorrhage (or *secondary prevention*). Several controversies exist regarding the efficacy of drug therapy, selection of useful pharmacodynamic end points, and identification of appropriate candidates. Some trials used a β-blocker dose sufficient to decrease the blood pressure by 25 mm Hg. In many trials, the dose of β-blocker was adjusted to reduce the heart rate by 20% to 25%, while others used fixed dosages.

A recent meta-analysis of β-blockers revealed improvements in likelihood of rebleeding and 2-year survival rates in cirrhotics after initial variceal bleeding.[58] Those that benefit the most seem

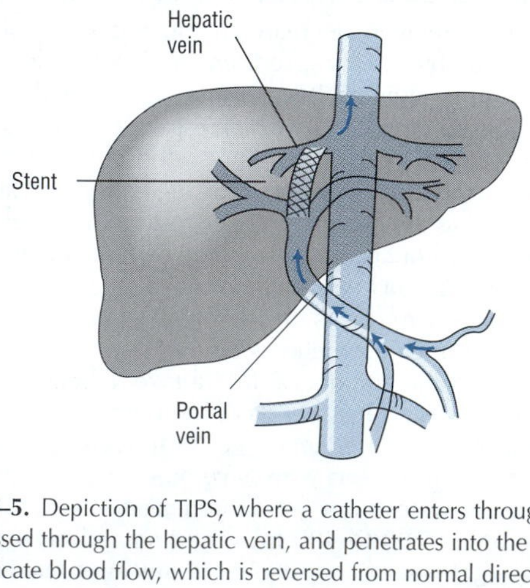

FIGURE 35–5. Depiction of TIPS, where a catheter enters through the jugular vein passed through the hepatic vein, and penetrates into the portal vein. Arrows indicate blood flow, which is reversed from normal direction.

to be patients with the greatest risk for bleeding—those with more severe liver disease using Child–Pugh scores.

Selective β-blockade (with atenolol) that is given in a fixed dose may not be as effective as pharmacodynamically adjusted propranolol in preventing rebleeding.[59] However, propranolol produces desirable (decreased portal vein pressure) and undesirable effects (decreased liver blood flow). A selective β_1-blocker (metoprolol) may reduce portal hypertension without reducing hepatic blood flow like the nonselective β-blocker propranolol.[60] One result of the reduced hepatic blood flow has been the demonstration that propranolol increases arterial blood ammonia and may precipitate hepatic encephalopathy.[61]

Given wide interpatient variability in bioavailability for propranolol, many investigators chose physiologic end points that were surrogates for hepatic venous pressure gradient (HVPG).[62–64] Pulse and systemic arterial blood pressure correlate relatively poorly with HVPG, and thus have proven somewhat unreliable in predicting response and anticipating patients most likely to benefit. An alternative, noninvasive measurement is Doppler estimate of femoral blood flow, which correlates well with HVPG.[65]

Propranolol has been used more often than other β-blockers. It can be used when sclerotherapy is contraindicated or refused. The starting dose is commonly 40 mg daily in divided doses and titrated to heart rate response. Thirty to fifty percent of patients will not have adequate reduction of portal pressure from β-blockers. To enhance the pressure reduction, isosorbide dinitrate may be added. The nitrate combined with nadolol has been shown to decrease the frequency of rebleeding by 50% compared to the β-blocker alone.[66]

SCLEROTHERAPY

Sclerotherapy is the direct application of a chemical with necroinflammatory or thrombotic properties. Sclerosants are typically introduced via a fiber-optic endoscope and injected into the bleeding varix. Figure 35–6 shows the local process of injection directly to the bleeding vessel. Injections may also be made into the side of the erosion. Ethanolamine, sodium tetradecyl sulfate, and sodium morrhuate have been used to treat esophageal varices. Sclerosants may be used to manage the acute bleeding episode and, when used prophylactically, to prevent relapse. Ulcers that develop after therapy are a serious complication of this procedure. In addition, esophageal perforation, strictures, and pleural effusions may result from sclerotherapy. There is no consensus regarding the sclerosant of choice. Efficacy varies from 70% to 100% in stopping blood loss from varices depending on the agent, site of injection, dose, and frequency.[67]

Medical therapy with propranolol has been compared with sclerotherapy, with some studies showing no difference, while others favor sclerotherapy. One factor to consider in favor of repeated sclerotherapy is the potential for noncompliance with propranolol. Some clinicians avoid this compliance risk by only using sustained-release β-blockers. There may be an advantage to using propranolol for secondary prevention after initial treatment of the bleeding with sclerotherapy. Nadolol continues to be pursued in place of propranolol as the former can be given once daily. Nadolol combined with isosorbide mononitrate were compared to sclerotherapy for secondary prophylaxis. The medication group had significantly fewer rebleeding episodes and a trend for higher survival than the sclerotherapy group.[68]

An intravenous infusion of vasopressin at 0.2 to 0.6 U/min can be used to treat acutely bleeding varices. Vasopressin increases the contractility of smooth muscles, particularly the small arterioles of the splanchnic, coronary, pancreatic, and mesenteric beds. Patients must then be monitored for adverse effects resulting from the decreased perfusion of these areas. Coronary and venous thrombosis can occur along with arrhythmias secondary to ischemia. Increases in blood pressure are possible, as are severe vascular headaches and angina. It is prudent to have any patient treated with vasopressin monitored by electrocardiogram. Nitroglycerin has been advocated as an adjunct to vasopressin to limit the coronary vasospasm. In addition, vasopressin and nitroglycerin appear to be additive in their effects on the portal bed. Vasopressin can also be administered intra-arterially into the superior mesenteric artery. This technique is usually reserved for varices that do not respond to intravenous infusions.

Ice-water lavage can also be used to slow bleeding. Figure 35–7 shows the use of direct pressure on the bleeding vessels where a tube is passed through the nose or throat and esophagus into the stomach. The balloon is inflated and the tube pulled taut, which applies the direct compression.

Surgery is often required in severe cases of bleeding. Portocaval shunting has been compared to sclerotherapy for acute variceal bleeding. Initially sclerotherapy appeared superior with shorter hospital stays, fewer transfusions, and equivalent survival

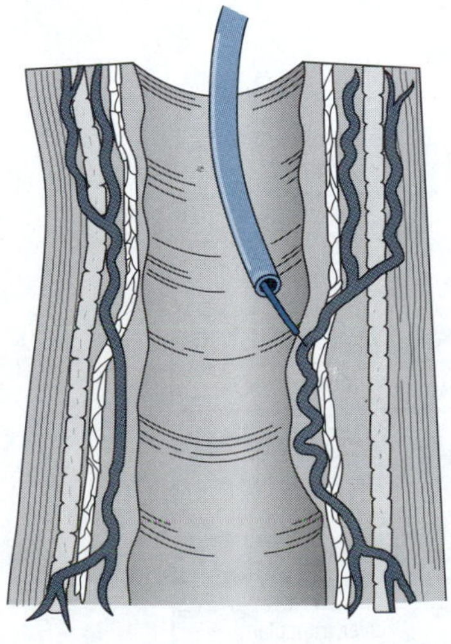

FIGURE 35–6. An example of sclerotherapy in which the sclerosant is injected within a variceal vessel.

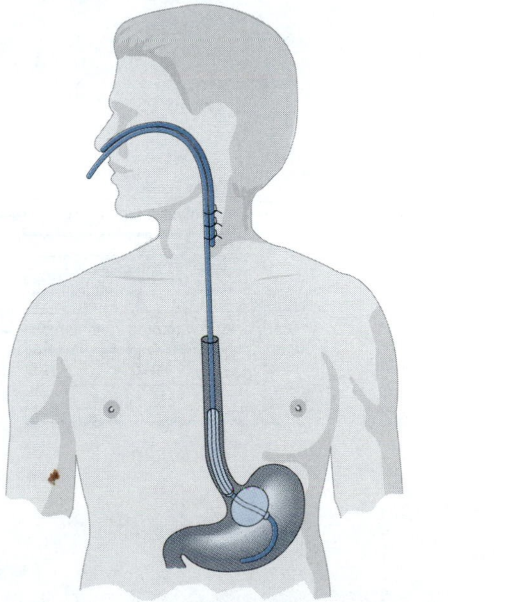

FIGURE 35–7. Placement of a tube for tamponade of bleeding varices.

compared to surgery. Yet follow-up revealed that sclerotherapy had more frequent rebleeding episodes, more rehospitalizations, and higher use of transfusions than surgery. Overall mortality and therapy costs were similar for both treatments. At this time, sclerotherapy is recommended as the initial treatment, with shunt surgery indicated for failures to sclerosants.[69]

HEPATIC ENCEPHALOPATHY

The end point of therapies directed at HE is an overall increase in the cognitive ability of the patient from baseline. If the patient is comatose, a return to consciousness is the goal. It is sometimes difficult in patients with milder forms of HE to detect changes resulting from therapy. In these patients, improvements in the mental status exam, electroencephalogram, and asterixis are sometimes used. Simple bedside psychomotor exams, such as serial signatures, nine-number connection tests, or drawing a familiar simple figure (a star, a house), can also be of assistance. Most patients with HE respond to some type of protein restriction. Care must be exercised, because nearly all patients with ALD have varying degrees of protein malnutrition and would require at least 60 g of protein daily to maintain positive nitrogen balance.[8] To further complicate the issue, much of the elevations in aromatic amino acids present in liver failure derive from endogenous protein breakdown rather than exogenous intake. Fully 5 to 12 times as much of the former compared to the latter suggests that dietary restriction would not be as effective as suppressing protein catabolism.[9] The source and types of amino acids in the diet may also be important, because aromatic amino acids (AAAs), already higher than normal cirrhotics, can be used in the CNS to produce false neurotransmitters. This ratio of AAAs to branched chain amino acids (BCAAs) can be reversed by the use of feedings high in BCAAs. Vegetable sources of protein that are high in BCAAs can often aid in this therapy by increasing the amount of fiber in the diet. This increase in fiber can also decrease total urea production in the colon and increase fecal urea excretion. Further, dairy products are less likely to precipitate HE than meat protein.[70] The classic management has been to restrict intake to about 20 g of protein per day; this was increased as the patient's symptoms improved. This approach is refuted by the false neurotransmitter theory for HE, which suggests quality of protein rather than quantity, especially in light of the protein malnutrition and anorexia present in this population.

SPECIALIZED PROTEIN DIET

Branched-chain amino acid solutions have had variable effectiveness for the management of HE. Many of the trials producing equivocal results suffer from small sample sizes and limited power. It is useful to categorize HE into acute, chronic, latent (i.e., subclinical), and fulminant phases. In latent HE, oral BCAA improves psychomotor disturbances and automobile driving capacity compared to placebo.[71] The status of BCAA in acute HE is more uncertain. In addition, most studies do not show deterioration of HE despite standard parenteral amino acid solutions or even lipid solutions. Meta-analysis did not reveal a preference of standard versus BCAA for parenteral nutrition in HE.[72] In contrast, oral BCAA has improved some measures in chronic HE including liver function tests (increased serum albumin), nutritional measures (amino acid profile, nitrogen balance), and in some studies mortality.[73] Given the years of anticipated treatment, oral BCAA for chronic use may be cost prohibitive for widespread use. Overall, to prevent negative nitrogen balance, stable cirrhotic patients may require 0.5 to 1 g/kg of protein. However, catabolic states such as alcoholic hepatitis require intakes of 1.0 g/kg of protein.

ANTIAMMONIA

Therapies that reduce the blood ammonia level appear to be effective in the management of HE that does not respond to protein restriction alone (Fig. 35–8). Cirrhotic patients have a higher rate of urea breakdown in the GI tract than do normal individuals. Lactulose, a nonabsorbed disaccharide, decreases this rate of urea breakdown and thus decreases the ammonia in the blood derived from the gut. The exact mechanism is unclear, but an increased frequency of stools per day appears to be necessary for efficacy and may rely on less contact time of protein with gut bacteria for breakdown into ammonia. Unfortunately, use of lactulose has not been shown to increase overall fecal ammonia discharge. Rather, lactulose may increase ammonia incorporation into colonic bacteria. Optimally, the lactulose dose should be titrated to produce two to three stools per day. Lactulose is broken down in the colon to acetic, lactic, and formic acids and to carbon dioxide. It has been shown to increase relative concentrations of *Lactobacillus* and other fermentative bacteria in the

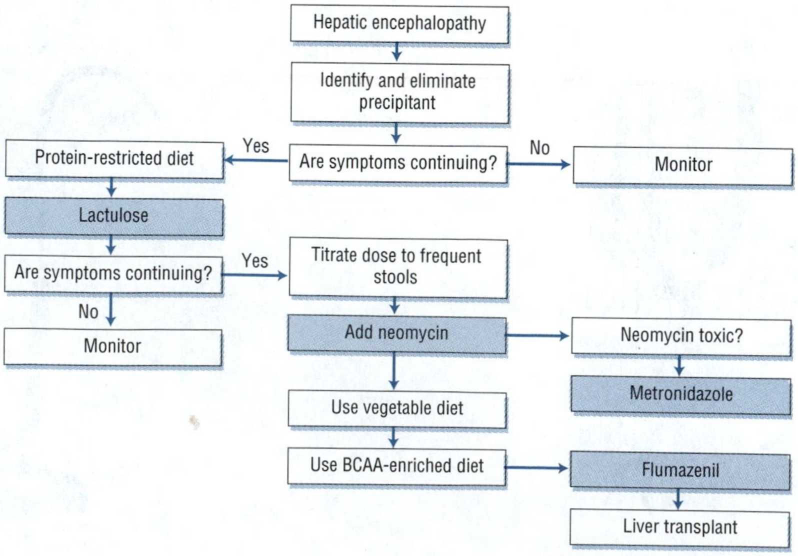

FIGURE 35–8. Treatment algorithm for the management of hepatic encephalopathy.

colon and to inhibit the proteolytic enzymes of many bacteria. By decreasing the pH in the colon, lactulose also reduces the ability of ammonia to diffuse across the gut wall. Another mechanism may well be to reduce bacterial production and systemic absorption of GABA.[74] Lactulose should be started at 50 mL every hour until catharsis occurs. The dose is then titrated to maintain two to three stools per day. Lactulose can be administered orally or rectally. It can reduce symptoms of encephalopathy in over 90% of patients.[75] Adverse effects include flatulence, diarrhea, abdominal pain, and hyperglycemia.

Neomycin given orally is also used to change colonic flora and decrease blood ammonia. Another mechanism may well be to reduce bacterial production and systemic absorption of GABA. The optimal dosing regimen is not known; however, a starting dose of 0.5 g four times daily may be used up to 4 to 6 g/d. The disadvantage with neomycin is that it is partially absorbed, causing ototoxicity and nephrotoxicity. If either agent alone does not work, neomycin and lactulose may be given together with additive effects.[76] Neomycin was first released in 1957. Despite decades of neomycin use for HE, there is some question concerning the product's efficacy. A double-blinded trial versus placebo did not reveal a statistical difference in regression to grade zero symptoms between neomycin and placebo for the acute management of hospitalized subjects.[75]

FLUMAZENIL

Small numbers of patients have been treated with the benzodiazepine antagonist, flumazenil. On occasion, rapid and startling clinical response has been seen with doses of 0.2 to 15 mg IV in uncontrolled studies. Controlled studies versus placebo show improvement in 40% to 70% treated with flumazenil and no response to placebo.[77–80] Thus, flumazenil may be an alternative when conventional treatment of HE has failed. The parenteral route and short half-life of flumazenil (about 4 hours) preclude its use in chronic HE.

Zinc replacement may have a role in hepatic encephalopathy.[81] Some of the enzymes necessary for the metabolism of ammonia to urea are zinc dependent. Patients with cirrhosis have increased urinary loss of zinc, and isolated case reports describe improved psychometric tests and lowered blood ammonia levels from zinc sulfate orally 600 mg daily.[82]

PHARMACOECONOMIC CONSIDERATIONS

Application of economic principles to the management of liver disease has not been prolific. This clearly is an area where cost–benefit analysis is needed. For example, some procedures such as peritoneovenous shunts or TIPS are invasive techniques requiring hospitalization. Are these procedures less costly than medical management? No economic analyses have been reported to answer this question. Varices and ascites can be reduced or eliminated if the liver is transplanted. Is early transplanting more cost effective than nontransplant management? Although the question is intriguing and unanswered, the rate-limiting step is organ procurement and not necessarily expense.

EVALUATION OF THERAPEUTIC OUTCOMES

When a patient with ALD is first evaluated, a careful drug history is indicated with the intent to avoid hepatotoxins and to adjust dosages where appropriate for hepatic function. Consideration should be given to vaccination against hepatitis viruses in patients with ALD, as they are more likely to have morbid events if infected with these viruses when not immune. Next, a nutritional assessment should be performed, and appropriate intake of protein, calories, and vitamin supplements recommended. Baseline lab tests for transaminases, bilirubin, albumin, protime, electrolytes, and creatinine should be obtained. Simple measures such as weight, vital signs, and abdominal circumference are necessary. Most patients will need periodic liver biopsies. A baseline mental status exam may indicate encephalopathic changes. Goals of therapy that are reasonable include patient comfort and the ability to maintain self-care. Drug therapy may prolong life but not to the extent of organ transplantation. Responses to drug therapy in ALD are typically seen in weeks to months. Thus, compliance can be problematic as the patient does not see immediate benefits. Encouragement and counseling by pharmacists may be valuable in this regard.

CONCLUSIONS

Cirrhosis is often a frustrating disease for the clinician. There are few direct therapies, and symptomatic treatment often does not work or works poorly. The overall success of therapy depends oftentimes on the patient. If associated with ALD and the patient can stop drinking, there is a chance of recovery. If the patient does not stop drinking, the disease is usually fatal.

▶ PRINCIPLES OF PHARMACOTHERAPY

- Common complications of ALD include ascites, esophageal and gastric varices, coagulopathy, and hepatic encephalopathy.
- Poor nutritional status and female gender are risk factors for developing ALD.
- Combined with the malnutrition of ALD patients, the decreased hepatic protein synthesis results in serious abnormalities in serum oncotic pressure and hemostasis.
- The most important treatment for ALD is avoidance of alcohol.
- There are a variety of precipitating events for HE that may be preventable or reversible. Every effort should be made to identify these factors before initiating drug therapy to reverse the encephalopathy.
- Lactulose is a safe and effective treatment for encephalopathy. Neomycin is an effective alternative that may be used in combination with lactulose.
- There is currently no exact mathematical approach to adjusting drug doses during liver failure. Drugs that are primarily excreted by the liver or extensively

metabolized before renal excretion are the most affected by changes in hepatic function.

- Encephalopathic patients will be much more sensitive to CNS depressants.
- The overall fluid loss per day in patients with ascites should not exceed 1 to 2 L. Patients with peripheral edema seem to tolerate faster mobilization of ascites than patients who have no edema. Nonedematous patients transfer water from the peritoneal cavity to the vascular space at a rate of 200 to 400 mL/d and should not be diuresed beyond a weight loss of about 0.5 kg/d.
- Glucocorticoids may be beneficial for severely ill patients with alcoholic hepatitis.

REFERENCE

1. Jaffe DL, Chung RT, Friedman LS. Management of portal hypertension and its complications. Med Clin North Am 1996;80:1021–1034.
2. Ventura SJ, Martin AJ, Smith BL. Births and deaths: Preliminary data for 1997. Natl Vit Stat Rep 1998;1–42.
3. Maddrey WC. Alcoholic hepatitis: Clinicopathologic features and therapy. Semin Liver Dis 1988;8:91–101.
4. Johnson RD, Williams R. Genetic and environmental factors in the individual susceptibility to the development of alcoholic liver disease. Alcohol 1985;20:137–160.
5. Frezza M, di Padova C, Pozzato G, et al. High blood alcohol levels in women. The role of decreased gastric alcohol dehydrogenase activity and first-pass metabolism. N Engl J Med 1990;322:95–99.
6. Morgan MY. The prognosis and outcome of alcoholic liver disease. Alcohol Alcohol 1994;2 (supp):335–343.
7. Klatskin G. Alcohol and its relationship to the liver. Gastroenterology 1961;41:443–451.
8. Marsano L, McClain CJ. Nutrition and alcoholic liver disease. JPEN J Parenter Enteral Nutr 1991;15:337–344.
9. Silk DB, O'Keefe SJD, Wicks C. Nutritional support in liver disease. Gut 1991;(suppl):S29–S33.
10. Cabre E, Gonzalez-Huix F, Abad-Lacruz A, et al. Effect of total enteral nutrition on the short term outcome of severely malnourished cirrhotics. Gastroenterology 1990;98:715–720.
11. Ezzell JH, Werkman RF, Dean P. Treatment of alcoholic hepatitis. Am J Gastroenterol 1989;84:1217–1221.
12. Lieber CS, Guadagnini KS. The spectrum of alcoholic liver disease. Hosp Pract 1990;25:51–69.
13. Wrona SA, Tankanow RM. Corticosteroids in the management of alcoholic hepatitis. Am J Hosp Pharm 1994;51:347–353.
14. Blake J, Orrego H. Monitoring treatment of alcoholic liver disease: Evaluation of various severity indices. Clin Chem 1991;37:5–13.
15. Pugh RNH, Murray-Lyon IM, Dawson JL, et al. Transection of the oesophagus for bleeding oesophageal varices. Br J Surg 1973;60:646–649.
16. Maddrey WC, Boitnott JK, Bedine MS, et al. Corticosteroid therapy of alcoholic hepatitis. Gastroenterology 1978;75:193–199.
17. Ramond MJ, Poynard T, Rueff B, et al. A randomized trial of prednisolone in patients with severe alcoholic hepatitis. N Engl J Med 1992;326:507–512.
18. Chedid A, Mendenhall CL, Gartside P, et al. Prognostic factors in alcoholic liver disease. Am J Gastroenterol 1991;86:210–216.
19. Bay MK, Schenker S. Beta-blockers revisited: Picking patients with alcoholic cirrhosis who will benefit. Alcohol Clin Exp Res 1996; 20:788–790.
20. Bass NM. Preventing hemorrhage from esophageal varices. N Engl J Med 1987;317:893–895.
21. Alvarez D, de las Heras, Terg R, et al. Daily variation in portal blood flow and the effect of propranolol administration in a randomized study of patients with cirrhosis. Hepatology 1997;25:548–550.
22. Butterworth RF, Layrargues GO. Benzodiazepine receptors and hepatic encephalopathy. Hepatology 1990;11:499–501.
23. Crossley IR, Williams R. Progress in the treatment of chronic portasystemic encephalopathy. Gut 1984;25:85–98.
24. Hourani BT, Hamlin EM, Reynolds TB. Cerebrospinal fluid glutamine as a measure of hepatic encephalopathy. Arch Intern Med 1971; 127:1033–1036.
25. Basile AS, Hughes RD, Harrison PM, et al. Elevated brain concentrations of 1,4-benzodiazepines in fulminant hepatic failure. N Engl J Med 1991;374:473–478.
26. Gill MA, Kern JW. Altered gentamicin distribution in ascitic patients. Am J Hosp Pharm 1979;36:1704–1706.
27. Goode HF, Kellelher J, Walker BE. Relation between zinc status and hepatic functional reserve in patients with liver disease. Gut 1990; 34:694–697.
28. Scott NR, Stambuck D, Chakraborty J, et al. The pharmacokinetics of caffeine in patients with chronic liver disease. Br J Clin Pharmacol 1989;27:205–213.
29. Juhl RP, Van Thiel DH, Dittert LW. Alprazolam pharmacokinetics in alcoholic liver disease. J Clin Pharmacol 1984;24:113–119.
30. Black M, Tavill AS. Corticosteroids in severe alcoholic hepatitis. Ann Intern Med 1989;110:677–680.
31. Carithers RL, Herlong HF, Diehl AM, et al. Methylprednisolone therapy in patients with severe alcoholic hepatitis. A randomized multicenter trial. Ann Intern Med 1989;110:685–690.
32. Theodossi A, Eddleston ALWF, Williams R. Controlled trial of methylprednisolone therapy in severe acute alcoholic hepatitis. Gut 1982;23:75–79.
33. Reynolds TB, Benhamou JP, Blake J, et al. Treatment of acute alcoholic hepatitis. Gastroenterol Int 1989;2:208–216.
34. Imperiale TF, McCullough AJ. Do corticosteroids reduce mortality from alcoholic hepatitis? A meta-analysis of the randomized trials. Ann Intern Med 1990;113:299–307.
35. Maddrey WC. Alcoholic hepatitis: Pathogenesis and approaches to treatment. Scand J Gastroenterol 1990;25:118–130.
36. Kumar S, Stauber RE, Gavaler JS. Orthotopic liver transplantation for alcoholic liver disease. Hepatology 1990;11:159–164.
37. Orrego H, Blake J, Blendis LM, et al. Long-term treatment of alcoholic liver disease with propylthiouracil. N Engl J Med 1987;317: 1421–1427.
38. Wang YJ, Lee SD, Hsieh MC, et al. A double-blind randomized controlled trial of colchicine in patients with hepatitis B virus-related postnecrotic cirrhosis. J Hepatol 1994;21:872–877.
39. Lin DY, Sheen IS, Chu CM, Liaw YF. A prospective randomized trial of colchicine in prevention of liver cirrhosis in chronic hepatitis B patients. Aliment Pharmacol Ther 1996;10:961–966.
40. Mendenhall CL, Anderson S, Garci-Pont P, et al. Short-term and long term survival in patients with alcoholic hepatitis treated with oxandrolone and prednisolone. N Engl J Med 1984;311:1464–1479.
41. Mendenhall CL, Moritz T, Roselle GA, et al. A study of oral nutritional support with oxandrolone in malnourished patients with alcoholic hepatitis. Hepatology 1993;17:564–576.
42. Quintero E, Arroyo V, Bory F, et al. Paracentesis versus diuretics in the treatment of cirrhotics with tense ascites. Lancet 1985;2:611–612.
43. Gauthier A, Levy VG, Quinton A, et al. Salt or no salt in the treatment of cirrhotic ascites. Gut 1986;27:705–709.
44. Shear L, Ching S, Gabuzda GJ. Compartmentalization of ascites and edema in patients with hepatic cirrhosis. N Engl J Med 1970;282: 1391–1396.
45. Correia JP, Conn HO. Spontaneous bacterial peritonitis in cirrhosis: Endemic or epidemic? Med Clin North Am 1975;59:963–981.
46. Gines P, Arroyo V, Quintero E, et al. Comparison of paracentesis and diuretics in the treatment of cirrhotics with tense ascites. Gastroenterology 1987;93:234–241.

47. Gines P, Tito L, Arroyo V, et al. Randomized comparative study of therapeutic paracentesis with and without intravenous albumin in cirrhosis. Gastroenterology 1988;94:1493–1502.
48. Smadja C, Franco D. The LeVeen shunt in the elective treatment of intractable ascites in cirrhosis. Ann Surg 1985;201:488–493.
49. Ring-Larsen H, Siemssen O, Krintel JJ, et al. Denver shunt in the treatment of refractory ascites in cirrhosis: A randomized controlled trial. J Hepatol 1989;9:77. Abstract.
50. Stanley MM, Ochi S, Lee KK, et al. Peritoneovenous shunting as compared with medical treatment in patients with alcoholic cirrhosis and massive ascites. N Engl J Med 1989;321:1632–1638.
51. Stanley AJ, Jalan R, Forrest EH, Redhead DN. Longterm follow up of transjugular intrahepatic portosystemic stent shunt (TIPSS) for the treatment of portal hypertension: Results in 130 patients. Gut 1996; 39:479–485.
52. Conn HO. Transjugular intrahepatic portosystemic shunts versus sclerotherapy: A discussion of discordant results. Ann Intern Med 1997;126:907–910.
53. Cello JP, Ring EJ, Olcott EW, et al. Endoscopic sclerotherapy compared with percutaneous transjugular intrahepatic portosystemic shunt after initial sclerotherapy in patients with acute variceal hemorrhage. A randomized, controlled trial. Ann Intern Med 1997;126: 858–865.
54. Sanyal AJ, Freedman AM, Luketic VA, et al. Transjugular intrahepatic portosystemic shunts compared with endoscopic sclerotherapy for the prevention of recurrent variceal hemorrhage. A randomized, controlled trial. Ann Intern Med 1997;126:849–857.
55. Runyon BA. Care of patients with ascites. N Engl J Med 1994; 330:337–342.
56. Sungaila I, Bartle WR, Walker SE, et al. Spironolactone pharmacokinetics and pharmacodynamics in patients with cirrhotic ascites. Gastroenterology 1992;102:1680–1685.
57. Perez-Ayuso RM, Arroyo V, Planas R, et al. Randomized comparative study of efficacy of furosemide versus spironolactone in nonazotemic cirrhosis with ascites. Gastroenterology 1983;84:961–968.
58. Bernard B, Lebrec D, Mathurin P, et al. Beta-adrenergic antagonists in the prevention of gastrointestinal bleeding in patients with cirrhosis: A meta-analysis. Hepatology 1997;25:63–70.
59. Colombo M, Franchis RD, Tommasini M, et al. Beta-blockade prevents recurrent gastrointestinal bleeding in well-compensated patients with alcoholic cirrhosis: A multicenter randomized controlled trial. Hepatology 1989;9:433–438.
60. Westaby D, Bihari DJ, Gimson AES, et al. Selective and non-selective beta receptor blockade in the reduction of portal pressure in patients with cirrhosis and portal hypertension. Gut 1984;25:121–124.
61. Snady H, Lieber CS. Venous, arterial, and arterialized-venous blood ammonia levels and their relationship to hepatic encephalopathy after propranolol. Am J Gastroenterol 1988;83:249–255.
62. Zimmerer J, Haubitz I, Mainos D, et al. Survival in alcoholic liver cirrhosis: Prognostic value of portal pressure, size of esophageal varices and biochemical data. Comparison with Child classification. J Gastroenterol 1996;34:421–427.
63. Sandford NL, Kerlin P. Current management of oesophageal varices. Aust NZ J Med 1995;25:528–534.
64. Feu F, Garcia Pagan JC, Bosch J, et al. Relation between portal pressure response to pharmacotherapy and risk of recurrent variceal haemorrhage in patients with cirrhosis. Lancet 1995;346:1056–1059.
65. Kimura M, Sato M, Kawai N, et al. Efficacy of Doppler ultrasonography for assessment of transjugular intrahepatic portosystemic shunt patency. Cardiovasc Intervent Radiol 1996;19:397–400.
66. Merkel C, Marin R, Enzo E, et al. Randomised trial of nadolol alone or with isosorbide mononitrate for primary prophylaxis of variceal bleeding in cirrhosis. Lancet 1996;348:1677–1681.
67. Sarin SK, Kumar A. Sclerosants for variceal sclerotherapy: A critical appraisal. Am J Gastroenterol 1990;85:641–649.
68. Villanueva C, Balanzo J, Novella MT, et al. Nadolol plus isosorbide mononitrate compared with sclerotherapy for prevention of variceal bleeding. N Engl J Med 1996;334:1624–1629.
69. Cello JP, Grendell JH, Crass RA, et al. Endoscopic sclerotherapy versus portacaval shunt in patients with severe cirrhosis and acute variceal hemorrhage. N Engl J Med 1987;316:11–15.
70. Mullen KD, Weber FL. Role of nutrition in hepatic encephalopathy. Semin Liver Dis 1991;11:292–304.
71. Plauth M, Egberts EH, Hamster W, et al. Long-term treatment of latent portosystemic encephalopathy with branched-chain amino acids. A double-blind placebo controlled crossover study. J Hepatol 1993; 17:308–314.
72. Ericksson LS, Conn HO. Branched chain amino acids in the management of hepatic encephalopathy: An analysis of variance. Hepatology 1989;10:228–246.
73. Fabbri A, Magrini N, Bianchi G, et al. Overview of randomized clinical trials of oral branched-chain amino acid treatment in chronic hepatic encephalopathy. J Parent Ent Nutr 1996;20:159–164.
74. Groeneweg M, Gyr K, Amrein R, et al. Effect of flumazenil on the electroencephalogram of patients with portosystemic encephalopathy. Results of a double blind, randomised, placebo-controlled multicentre trial. Electroencephalogr Clin Neurophysiol 1996;98:29–34.
75. Strauss E, Tramote R, Silva EPS, et al. Double-blinded randomized clinical trial comparing neomycin and placebo in the treatment of exogenous hepatic encephalopathy. Hepatogastroenterology 1992;39: 542–545.
76. Pirotte J, Guffens JM, Devos J. Comparative study of basal arterial ammonia and of orally induced hyperammonemia in chronic portal systemic encephalopathy, treated with neomycin, lacutulose, and an association of neomycin and lactulose. Digestion 1974;10:435–444.
77. Gyr K, Meier R, Haussler J, et al. Evaluation of the efficacy and safety of flumazenil in the treatment of portal systemic encephalopathy: A double blind, randomised, placebo controlled multicentre study. Gut 1996;39:319–324.
78. Van der Rijt CC, Schalm SW, Meulstee J, Stijnen T. Flumazenil therapy for hepatic encephalopathy. A double-blind crossover study. Gastroenterol Clin Biol 1995;19:572–580.
79. Cadranel JF, el Younsi M, Pidoux B, et al. Flumazenil therapy for hepatic encephalopathy in cirrhotic patients: A double-blind pragmatic randomized, placebo study. Eur J Gastroenterol Hepatol 1995;7: 325–329.
80. Devictor D, Tahiri C, Lanchier C, et al. Flumazenil in the treatment of hepatic encephalopathy in children with fulminant liver failure. Intensive Care Med 1995;21:253–256.
81. Riordan SM, Williams R. Treatment of hepatic encephalopathy. N Engl J Med 1997;337:473–479.
82. Marchesini G, Fabbri A, Bianchi G, Brizi M. Zinc supplementation and amino acid-nitrogen metabolism in patients with advanced cirrhosis. Hepatology 1996;23:1084–1092.
83. Barber JR, Teasley KM. Nutritional support of patients with severe hepatic failure. Clin Pharm 1984;3:245–253.
84. Berk PD, Hopper H. Fulminant hepatic failure. Am J Gastroenterol 1978;69:349–400.

36

DRUG-INDUCED LIVER DISEASE

William R. Kirchain, PharmD, CDE, and Mark A. Gill, PharmD

The number of drugs associated with adverse reactions involving the liver is extensive. The overall incidence of human liver injury from most drugs is fortunately very low. Chronic liver disease and cirrhosis collectively account for approximately 1% of annual mortality in the United States. Alcohol-induced liver disease accounts for most of these deaths.[1] Still, for an individual patient, drug-indcued liver disease is usually a profound, life-changing disease. The liver's function affects almost every other organ system in the body. It is important to know the patterns of drug-related pathology and to assess adverse reactions when they occur. It is also important to understand how and when to monitor for these reactions.

PATTERNS OF DRUG-INDUCED LIVER DISEASE

IDIOSYNCRATIC REACTIONS

For some drugs, a genetic or acquired abnormality must exist in a particular metabolic pathway for a toxic reaction to take place. In other cases, the reactions are typically associated with a drug concentration and often respond to simply lowering the dose of the offending drug. Idiosyncratic reactions tend to occur without association to particular blood concentrations or specifically identified metabolic abnormalities. For example, glyburide and ofloxacin have caused severe liver disease, resulting in the need for transplantation in a very small group of patients.[2,3] Idiosyncratic reactions are rare and are sometimes described as a type of liver hypersensitivity to a drug. Hypersensitivity here does not mean that allergic or autoimmune vectors are at work.

ALLERGIC HEPATITIS

Allergic reactions in the liver can be caused by many drugs and result in many different kinds of hepatic damage. The sulfonamides, including trimethoprin–sulfamethoxazole, induce a reaction typical of hepatic hypersensitivity in a few patients.[4,5] The reaction usually develops within 4 weeks of the start of therapy. It is marked by fever, pruritis, rash, eosinophilia, arthritis, and hemolytic anemia. The formation of granulomas within the liver is often seen on biopsy.[6] The reaction reverses with discontinued therapy and reappears upon rechallenge. Many other anti-infectives—erythromycin, troleandomycin, penicillin, cloxacillin, oxacillin, and amoxicillin–clavulinic acid—have been associated with this type of reaction.[4,7,8]

Allopurinol also has been associated with a number of reports of hypersensitivity reactions involving the liver. The onset of symptoms is 1 to 6 weeks after initiation of therapy. The incidence, like all the allergic liver reactions, is low, estimated at less than 1%. The clinical presentation includes eosinophilia, fever, rash, and arthritis, as previously mentioned. The biopsy may show a pattern of fibrin-ring granulomas similar to those seen in Q fever.[9]

TOXIC HEPATITIS

Toxic reactions are predictable, often dose-related effects in the liver due to specific agents. Acetaminophen, when taken in overdose, becomes bioactivated to a toxic intermediate, known as *N*-acetyl-*p*-bensoquinoneimine (NAPQI). NAPQI is very reactive, with a high affinity for sulfhydral groups. The amino acid glutathione provides a ready source of available suflhydral groups within the hepatocyte. When the liver's glutathione stores are depleted and there are no longer sulfhydral groups available to detoxify this metabolite, it begins to react directly with the hepatocyte.[10] Acetaminophen's toxicity occurs in four stages.[11] During the first hours after ingestion, some patients report mild symptoms of nausea and vomiting, but no elevations of the commonly measured liver enzymes are seen. Not for 40 to 50 hours after ingestion do elevations in the liver enzymes begin.[7]

Reye's syndrome is an aggressive form of toxic hepatitis often associated with aspirin use in children. Valproate toxicity can also present in this pattern. Early in the process of Reye's syndrome, mitochondrial dysfunction leads to the depletion of acyl coenzyme A (CoA) and carnitine. Fatty acids accumulate and gluconeogenesis is impaired, resulting in hypoglycemia. A concurrent disruption of the urea cycle occurs, leading to decrease in the removal of ammonia and a slowing of protein use. A threefold or greater rise in the blood ammonia level and an increase in the prothrombin time are common findings. In advanced stages of Reye's syndrome, many patients develop intracranial hypertension that can be life threatening and refractory to therapy.

CHRONIC ACTIVE TOXIC HEPATITIS

Methyldopa, dantrolene, isoniazid, phenytoin, nitrofurantoin, and trazadone have been reported in association with a type of autoimmune-mediated disease in the liver.[12] Patients experience periods of very symptomatic hepatitis followed by periods of convalescence, only to repeat the experience months later. It is a progressive disease with a high mortality rate. It is more common in females than males. Antinuclear antibodies appear in most patients. Methyldopa appears to form a methyldopa–antigen complex. These antiorganelle antibodies have been identified for many drugs associated with this reaction.[13,14] The exact identification of a causative agent is sometimes difficult, because diagnosis requires multiple episodes occuring long after exposure to the offending drug.

TOXIC CIRRHOSIS

The scaring affect of hepatitis in the liver leads to the development of cirrhosis. Some drugs tend to cause such a mild case of hepatitis that it may not be detected. Mild hepatitis can be easily mistaken for a more routine generalized viral infeciton. If the offending drug or agent is not discontinued, this damage will continue to progress. The patient eventually presents not with hepatitis but with cirrhosis. Methotrexate causes periportal fibrosis in most patients. The lesion results from the action of a bioactivated metabolite produced by cytochrome P450. This process has most commonly been noted in patients treated for psoriasis and arthritis.[15] The extent of damage can be reduced or controlled by increasing the dosage interval to once weekly.[16] Vitamin A, which is normally stored in liver cells, can cause significant hypertrophy and fibrosis when taken for long periods in high doses. Hepatomegaly is a common finding along with other signs of advanced liver disease including ascites and portal hypertension. In patients with vitamin A toxicity, gingivitis and dry skin are also very common.[17]

LIVER VASCULAR DISORDERS

Focal lesions in hepatic venules, sinusoids, and portal veins occur with various drugs. The most commonly associated drugs are the cytotoxic agents used to treat cancer, the pyrrolizidine alkaloids, and the sex hormones. A centralized necrosis often follows and can result in cirrhosis, usually with a significant amount of concurrent congestion. Azathioprine and herbal teas that contain comfrey (a source of pyrrolizidine alkaloids) have been reported in association with the development of veno-occlusive disease. The exact incidence is rare and may be, for the pyrrolizidine alkaloids, dose related.[18]

Peliosis hepatitis is an unusual type of hepatic vascular lesion that can be seen as both an acute and a chronic disease. The liver develops large, blood-filled lacunae within the parenchyma. Rupture of the lacunae can lead to severe peritoneal hemorrhage. Peliosis hepatitis has been associated with exposure of the liver to androgens, estrogens, tamoxifen, azathioprine, and danazol. Androgens with a 17, α-testosterone structure are the most frequently reported agents to cause peliosis hepatitis, usually after at least 6 months of therapy. The actual incidence of this reaction is rare, with less than 40 cases reported in the literature between 1943 and 1983.[19]

MECHANISMS OF DRUG-INDUCED LIVER DISEASE

CENTROLOBULAR NECROSIS

Centrolobular necrosis is often a dose-related, predictable reaction secondary to drugs such as acetaminophen; however, it also can be associated with idiosyncratic reactions, such as those caused by halothane. Also called *direct* or *metabolite-related hepatotoxicity,* centrolobular necrosis is usually the result of the production of a toxic metabolite. The damage spreads outward from the middle of a lobe of the liver.

Patients suffering from centrolobular necrosis tend to present in one of two ways, depending on the extent of necrosis. Mild drug reactions, involving only small amounts of parenchymal tissue, may be detected as asymptomatic elevations in the serum transaminases. If the reaction is diagnosed at this stage, most of these patients will recover with minimal cirrhosis and thus minimal chronic liver impairment. More severe forms of centrolobular necrosis, as documented in cases with diclofenac, trazadone, and piroxicam, are accompanied by nausea, vomiting, upper abdominal pain, and jaundice.[20–22]

STEATONECROSIS

Steatonecrosis is a specialized type of acute necrosis resulting from the accumulation of fatty acids in the hepatocyte. Drugs or their metabolites that cause steatonecrosis do so by affecting fatty-acid oxidation within the mitochondria of the hepatocyte. Hepatic vesicles become engorged with fatty acids, eventually disrupting the homeostasis of the hepatocyte. Alcohol is the most common drug that produces steatonecrotic changes in the liver. When alcohol converts into acetaldehyde, the synthesis of fatty acids is increased.[23] When the hepatocyte has become completely engorged with microvesicular fat, it often breaks open spilling into the blood. If enough hepatocytes break open, an inflammatory response begins. If the offending agent is withdrawn before significant numbers of hepatocytes become necrotic, the process is completely reversible without long-term sequelae.

Tetracycline has produced steatonecrosis and steatosis.[24] The lesions are characterized by large vesicles of fat found diffused throughout the liver. The development of this reaction is related to the high concentrations achieved when tetracycline is given intravenously and in doses greater than 1.5 g/d. The mortality of tetracycline steatonecrosis is very high (70% to 80%), and those that do survive often develop cirrhosis. Sodium valproate also can produce steatonecrosis through the process of bioactivation. Cytochrome P450 converts valproate to Δ-4-valproic acid, a potent inducer of microvesicular fat accumulation.[25]

Patients experiencing steatonecrosis may present with abdominal fullness or pain as their only complaint. Patients with more severe steatonecrosis will present with all the symptoms characteristic of alcoholic hepatitis such as nausea, vomiting, steatorrhea, abdominal pain, pruritis, and fatigue.

PHOSPHOLIPIDOSIS

Phospholipidosis is the accumulation of phospholipids instead of fatty acids. The phospholipids usually engorge the lysosomal bodies of the hepatocyte.[26] Amiodarone has been associated with this reaction. Patients treated with amiodarone who develop overt hepatic disease tend to have received higher doses of the drug. These patients also have higher amiodarone to *N*-desethyl-amiodarone ratios, indicating a greater accumulation of the parent compound. Amiodarone and its major metabolite *N*-desethyl-amiodarone remain in the liver of all patients for several months after therapy is stopped. Usually the phospholipidosis develops in patients treated for more than a year. The patient can present with either elevated transaminases or hepatomegaly; jaundice is rare.[27,28]

GENERALIZED HEPATOCELLULAR NECROSIS

Generalized hepatocellular necrosis mimics the changes associated with the more common viral hepatitis. The onset of symptoms is usually delayed as much as a week or more after exposure to toxin. Bioactivation is often important for toxic hepatitis to develop, but may not be the immediate cause of damage.[29] Many drugs that have been associated with toxic hepatitis produce metabolites that are not inherently toxic to the liver. Instead they act as haptens, binding to specific cell proteins and inducing an autoimmune reaction.[30,31] The need for bioactivation by a drug can lead to differences in the incidence of the reaction between males and females. The subspecies of cytochrome P450, *N*-acetyltransferase, and xanthine oxidase have been demonstrated to vary in abundance and affinities as a function of gender.[32–34]

The long-term administration of isoniazid can lead to hepatic dysfunction in 10% to 20% of those receiving the drug. Yet severe toxic hepatitis develops in only 1% or less of this population.[35,36] Although the exact mechanism is still controversial, patients who are rapid acetylators have a greater susceptibility.[37,38] Isoniazid is metabolized by several pathways, acetylation being the major pathway. It is acetylated to acetylisoniazid, which in turn is hydrolyzed to acetylhydrazine.[39] The acetylhydrazine and, to a lesser extent, the acetylisoniazid are directly toxic to the cellular proteins in the hepatocyte. Rapid acetylators also detoxify acetylhydrazine very rapidly, converting it to diacetylhydrazine. It may be the relative rates of reaction and affinities of the various pathways that determine susceptibility to hepatotoxicity.[40]

Ketoconazole produces generalized hepatocellular necrosis or milder forms of hepatic dysfunction in 1% to 2% of patients treated for fungal infections. This reaction has been reported to be fatal in high numbers of HIV-infected patients. The onset is usually early in therapy, although it can be delayed until several months into therapy. In immune-compromised patients where ketoconazole is used for long periods of time, special care should be taken to watch for changes in liver function.[41,42] Phenelzine has caused fulminant generalized heptocellular necrosis in a reported cases as well.[43]

CHOLESTATIC JAUNDICE

Cholestatic jaundice or cholestasis can be classified by the area of the bile canalicular or ductal system that is impaired. Canalicular cholestasis is very often associated with long-term estrogen therapy. The actual incidence is very low, and is decreasing as the estrogen doses in oral contraceptives decrease. Clinically, these patients are often asymptomatic and present with mild to moderate elevations of serum bilirubin.[44,45] An intravenous form of vitamin E, α-tocopherol acetate, causes cholestatic jaundice, primarily involving the canaliculi, in premature infants. The incidence of this reaction was very high (> 10%) and the mortality even higher (> 50%).[46]

Hepatocellular cholestasis is a much more serious form of cholestatic jaundice that involves both the parenchyma and bile canalicular cells. Chlorpromazine can precipitate bile salts and decrease total bile flow.[47,48] The administration of total parenteral nutrition for periods greater than 1 week induces cholestatic changes and nonspecific enzyme elevations in some patients. Patients with low serum albumin concentrations may be at greater risk than patients with normal serum albumin concentrations.[49] This reaction also has been reported to occur rarely with sulfonamides, sulfonylureas, erythromycin estolate and ethylsuccinate, captopril, lisinopril, toclopidine, and other phenothiazines.[8,50–54]

MIXED HEPATOCELLULAR NECROSIS AND CHOLESTATIC DISEASE

Many times patients present not with a purely hepatocellular necrosis or cholestatic damage, but rather with a mixed picture of damage. Flutamide causes a mix of lesions that appear at or about the 48th week of treatment.[55,56] Niacin in doses greater than 3 g/d, or doses greater than 1 g/d of sustained-release formulations, causes the same mixed pattern of damage.[57] These patients often present with only a few signs or symptoms at first but can progress rapidly to fulminant hepatic failure.

NEOPLASTIC DISEASE

A large body of the current literature on adverse reactions and the liver addresses the development of neoplasms following drug therapy. Both carcinoma- and sarcoma-like lesions have been identified. Fortunately, hepatic tumors associated with drug therapy are usually benign and remit when drug therapy is discontinued. Except in rare instances, these lesions are associated with long-term exposure to the offending agent.[58] Androgens, estrogens, and other hormonal-related agents are the most frequently associated causes of neoplastic disease. The model for drug-induced hepatic cancer is polyvinyl chloride exposure. Used in the production of many types of plastic products, polyvinyl chloride induces angiosarcoma in exposed workers after as few as 3 years of exposure.[34,59]

ASSESSMENT

The best and most important technique for assessing and monitoring drug-induced liver disease is the patient's history. Questions addressing the patient's drug usage along with a thorough review of systems are essential (Table 36–1). The use of drugs for recreational purposes must not be overlooked. Cocaine has been directly linked to liver disease.[60] Ecstasy, the street name of an amphetamine, has induced fulminant hepatitis leading to death in some cases.[61] The more pervasive impact of street drugs on the incidence of hepatic disease is the concomittant injection or ingestion of adulterants. Many of these adulterants are either directly toxic or serve to enhance the toxicity of the drug.

It is also good to try to determine nondrug hepatic disease risk. Arsenic, for example, is known to induce both acute and chronic hepatic reactions. Arsenic in low concentrations is found in most rot- and insect-resistant lumber.[8] Following Occupational Safety and Health Agency guidelines should decrease the danger of using these products, but not eliminate it. Even if exposure to an environmental toxin in and of itself does not produce a hepatic reaction, it may predispose a patient to a hepatic reaction when a drug is added. Table 36–2 lists some of the more common hepatic toxins from occupational or environmental exposure that can add to a patient's risk for developing a hepatic lesion.[62] It is important to keep in mind that even very common products around a house, such as the weed-killer 2,4-D, can be a cause of profound liver disease.[63]

Additionally, a person's use of alternative medicine must be solicited. Many herbal remedies were once wisely abandoned because of their common adverse reactions. Comfrey tea is a common cause of hepatocellular damage.[64,65] As in the case of the Chinese remedy *jin bu huan* or the more elegantly presented chaparral capsules containing grease wood leaves, the end of therapy with these types of agents is occasionally severe disability or death from fulminant hepatic failure.[66–68] Table 36–3 lists many of the more common herbal remedies that are associated with significant liver disease.[69]

The nutritional status of a patient can be as important to the development of a drug-induced liver disease as the hepatotoxin itself.[70] Patients who are malnourished due to illness or long-term alcohol abuse make up the most troublesome group.[71] These patients tend to react at lower doses in dose-related reactions and more severely in all types of reactions. Bioactivation can sometimes be induced by a diet heavy in charcoal-grilled meats and vegetables. A patient may also directly poison himself or herself through the ingestion of poisonous mushrooms of the deadly nightshade family.[72]

TABLE 36–1. An Approach to Evaluating a Suspected Hepatotoxic Reaction

Step 1	Does the sex or age of the patient increase his or her risk? Does the patient's occupation increase his or her risk? Does the patient's recreational drug use increase his or her risk? Is the patient using any herbal remedies, tonics, or teas that increase risk? Is the patient's diet deficient in vitamins or micronutrients? Is the patient's diet excessive in vitamins or micronutrients? Is the patient pregnant? Does the patient have diabetes mellitus?
Step 2	Is there a temporal relationship between the drug and the onset of disease?
Step 3	Is there supporting literature for this type of reaction? Is the clinical evidence consistent with the presentations in the literature? What is the statistical risk for the reaction, and for progression to fulminant failure?
Step 4	Is this a common reaction associated with this drug? Have all more common causes (viruses, alcohol) been ruled out?
Step 5	What happended when the drug was discontinued?
Step 6	Is rechallenge with the drug possible? If so, what happened?
Classifying a Lesion Established as a Case of Hepatotoxicity	
Step 7	What are the biopsy results? What are the CT, MRI, and/or ultrasound results? What is the pattern of enzyme elevation? Is there evidence of recovery or is cirrhosis dominating the clinical outcome?

TABLE 36–2. Environmental Hepatic Toxins[a]

Toxin	Group Associated With Exposure
Arsenic	Chemical, construction, agricultural workers
Carbon tetrachloride	Chemical plant workers, laboratory technicians
Copper	Plumbers, copper foundry workers
Dimethylformanide	Chemical plant workers, laboratory technicians
2,4-Dichlorophenoxyacetic acid	Horiculturalists, gardening enthusiasts
Fluorine	Chemical plant workers, laboratory technicians
Toluene	Chemical and agricultural workers, laboratory technicians
Trichloroethylene	Printers, dye workers, cleaners, laboratory technicians
Vinyl chloride	Plastics plant workers

[a]A partial list of environmental toxins that can cause liver injury. At lower exposure rates, these compounds may also predispose the patient to liver injury from a drug.

TABLE 36–3. Herbal Remedies Associated With a Relatively High Incidence of Hepatotoxicty

Aminita
Comfrey
Germander
Gordolobo
Grease wood
Margosa oil
Mistletoe
Pennyroyal (squawmint)
Skullcap
Yerba

TABLE 36–4. Relative Patterns of Hepatic Enzyme Elevation Versus Type of Hepatic Lesion

Enzyme	Abreviation(s)	Necrotic	Cholestatic	Chronic
Alkaline phosphatase	Alk Phos, AP	↑	↑↑↑	↑
5′-Nucleotidase	5-NC, 5NC	↑	↑↑↑	↑
γ-Glutamyltransferase	GGT, GGTP	↑	↑↑↑	↑↑
Aspartamine transferase	AST, SGOT	↑↑↑	↑	↑↑
Alanine transferase	ALT, SGPT	↑↑↑	↑	↑↑
Lactate dehydrogenase	LDH	↑↑↑	↑	↑

↑ = < 100% of normal; ↑↑ = > 100% of normal; ↑↑↑ = > 200% above normal.

All potential drug reactions should be judged as to the timing of the reaction versus drug administration, pharmacokinetic considerations, the literature records of previous reactions, the inclusion of alternative nondrug causes, and close clinical observation when the drug in question is stopped.[73]

Often there is no good clinical test available to determine the exact type of hepatic lesion, short of biopsy. There are still certain patterns of enzyme elevation that have been identified and can be helpful (Table 36–4).[74] The specificity of any serum enzyme depends on the distribution of that enzyme in the body. Alkaline phosphatase is found in the bile duct epithelium, bone, and intestinal and kidney cells.[75] 5′-Nucleotidase is more specific for hepatic disease than alkaline phosphatase, because most of the body's store of 5′-nucleotidase is in the liver. Glutamate dehydrogenase is a good indicator of centrolobular necrosis because it is found primarily in centrolobular mitochondria. Most hepatic cells have extremely high concentrations of transaminases. Aspartamine transferase (AST or SGOT) and alanine transferase (ALT or SGPT) are commonly measured. Because of their high concentrations and easy liberation from the hepatocyte cytoplasm, AST and ALT are very sensitive indicators of necrotic lesions within the liver. Once an acute hepatic lesion is established, it may take weeks for these concentrations to return to normal.[46]

Serum bilirubin concentration is a sensitive indicator of most hepatic lesions and has significant prognostic value.[47,76] High peak bilirubin concentrations are associated with poor survival. Other important findings that indicate poor survival are a peak prothrombin time greater than 40 seconds, elevated serum creatinine, and low aterial pH. The presence of encephalopathy or prolonged jaundice are not good signs for the survival of the patient without transplantation.[48]

Bilirubin concentrations and serum enzyme elevations give a static picture of the liver's condition. They do not indicate hepatic function. Clinically available tests to predict hepatic function include measurement of serum proteins (albumin or transferin). As hepatic function decreases, serum protein concentrations in the body decrease at a rate determined by each protein's own elimination rate. Overhydration and starvation can also decrease serum protein concentrations. Changes in the prothrombin time often occur earlier than the changes in albumin or transferrin. The response of the prothrombin time to the administration of 10 mg of parenteral vitamin K is often used to differentiate between hepatic and extrahepatic disease.

A good compound for a liver function test would theoretically be (1) nontoxic, lacking any pharmacologic effect; (2) either rapidly and completely absorbed orally or easily administered via a peripheral vein; (3) eliminated only by the liver; and (4) easily measured (drug and its metabolite) in blood, saliva, or urine.[77]

Several tests are used in research settings and in liver transplant patients to indicate liver function. Carbon-14-labeled aminopyrine measures the capacity of the mixed-function oxidase system via the production of $^{14}CO_2$.[78] Other tests, such as sulfobromophthalein excretion or indocyanine green excretion, measure qualities of hepatic clearance. Sulfobromophthalein is intravenously injected, absorbed by liver cells, conjugated to glutathione, and then excreted in the bile. Sulfobromophthalein is irritating at the injection site and has been associated with anaphylactic reactions. Indocyanine green follows a similar pathway except for conjugation.[79] There are also a few drugs that have been used to test liver function. Sorbitol is administered by intravenous infusion. Sorbitol's advantage over indocyanine green is a much lower incidence of allergic reactions. It is partially cleared by the kidney, and urine levels must also be determined during the test.[49,80] Oxpurinol production (allopurinol's metabolite) can be used to determine purine metabolism and hepatic blood flow.[81] The conversion of lidocaine to its metabolite monoethylglycinexyline (MEGX) is used before and after liver transplantation as an indicator of liver blood flow.[82] Caffeine given in very low doses is used to measure demethylation and hepatic blood flow. Caffeine is a good test to differentiate patients with mild to moderate disease as rated by Pugh's score (see Chap. 35), but is not useful in patients with Pugh's scores much above 10.[83] The administration of various benzodiazepines has also been studied. A good estimate of hepatic clearance can be obtained by serial blood levels of these drugs if an assay is locally available.[84,85]

Ultrasound pictures and CT scans can be used on a periodic basis to monitor for the development of fibrosis or vascular lesion in the liver and for hepatocellular carcinomas.[86] Hepatobiliary scanning using Tc-99m-labeled carriers also can be useful in quantifying the location and extent of obstruction or damage.[48]

If there is a liver biopsy available, the injury should be classified by the histologic findings. In cases where there is no biopsy, the pattern of liver enzyme elevation can estimate the type of injury. Hepatocellular injuries are marked by elevations in transaminase—at least two times normal. If the alkaline phosphatase is also elevated, then a hepatocellular lesion is still suspected when the elevation of ALT is notably higher than the elevation of alkaline phosphatase. If the magnitude of elevation is nearly equal between ALT and alkaline phosphatase, then the lesion is likely cholestatic.

A liver injury is acute if it lasts less than 3 months. It is considered chronic after 3 months of consistent symptoms or enzyme elevation. A liver injury is severe if the patient has marked jaundice, if the prothrombin time does not improve by more than 50% after the administration of vitamin K, or if encephalopathy is detectable. If an acute liver injury progresses from normal to severe in a matter of a few days or weeks, it is considered fulminant.[87]

In all cases, titers of serum antibodies to hepatitis A, B, and C should be drawn. Even in cases where the drug is absolutely targeted as the cause, viral hepatitis may be a complication. Some drugs may even be a facilitator of a viral infection. Cladribine has been noted to reactivate a hepatitis B infection, predisposing the patient to prolonged convalescence.[88]

MONITORING

The serum transaminases AST and ALT (SGOT and SGPT), are the most commonly used in the clinical setting. Concentrations of these enzymes should be obtained about every 4 weeks depending on the reported characteristics of the reaction in question. Methotrexate should be monitored every 4 weeks, because toxicity usually develops over a period of several weeks to months.[89,90] In addition, some recommend that sulfobromophthalein or indocyanine green excretion studies be performed on a regular basis and that patients treated for very long periods of time should have a liver biopsy performed every 12 months.

REFERENCES

1. National Center for Health Statistics. Advance report of final mortality statistics 1990, Monthly Vital Stat Rep 1993;41:7.
2. Meadow P, Tullio CJ. Glyburide-induced hepatitis. Clin Pharm 1989; 8:470.
3. Blum A. Ofloxacin-induced acute severe hepatitis. South Med J 1991;84:1158.
4. Dujovne CA, Chan CH, Zimmerman HJ. Sulfonamide hepatic injury. N Engl J Med 1967;277:785–788.
5. Alberti-Flor JJ, Hernandez ME, Ferrer JP, et al. Fulminant liver failure and pancreatitis associated with the use of sulfamethoxazole-trimethoprim. Am J Gastroenterol 1989;84:1577–1579.
6. Pohl LR. Drug-induced allergic hepatitis. Semin Liv Dis 1990;10: 305–315.
7. Valdiva-Barriga V, Feldman A, Orellana J. Generalized hypersensitivity with hepatitis and jaundice after the use of penicillin and streptomicin. Gastroenterology 1963;45:114–117.
8. Larrey D, Vital T, Micaleff A, et al. Hepatitis associated with amoxycillin–clavulinic acid combination: Report of 15 cases. Gut 1992;156: 285–286.
9. Vanderstigel M, Zafrani ES, Deyone JL, et al. Allopurinol hypersensitivity syndrome as a cause of heaptic fibrin granulomas. Gastroenterology 1986;90:188–190.
10. Simlkstein MJ, Knapp GL, Kulig KW, Rumack BH. Efficacy or oral *N*-acetylcysteine in the treatment of acetaminophen overdose: Analysis of the national multicenter study (1976 to 1985). 1988;319: 1557–1562.
11. Black M. Acetaminophen hepatoxicity. Gastroenterology 1980;78: 382–392.
12. Lee WM. Drug-induced hepatotoxicity. N Engl J Med 1995;333: 1118–1127.
13. Neuberger J, Kenna JG, Nouri Aria K, et al. Antibody-mediated hepatocyte injury in methyldopa-induced hepatotoxicity. Gut 1985;26: 1233–1239.
14. Beane PH, Bourdi M. Autoantibodies against cytochrome P_{450} in drug-induced autoimmune hepatitis. Ann NY Acad Sci 1993;685: 641–645.
15. Bjorkman DJ, Hammond EH, Lee RG, et al. Hepatic ultrastructure after methotrexate therapy for rheumatoid arthritis. Arthritis Rheum 1988;31:1465–1472.
16. Leonard PA, Clegg DO, CC, et al. Low-dose methotrexate in rheumatoid arthritis: An 8-year experience with hepatotoxicity. Clin Rheumatol 1987;6:575–582.
17. Geubal AP, Galocsy C; Alves N, et al. Liver damage caused by therapeutic vitamin A administration: Estimate of dose-related toxicity in 41 cases. Gastroenterology 1991;100:1701–1709.
18. Kumara CR, Ng M, Lin JH, et al. Herbal tea-induced hepatic venoocclusive disease: Quantification of toxic alkaloid exposure in adults. Gut 1985;26:101–104.
19. Haupt HA, Rovere GD. Anabolic steroids: A review of the literature. Am J Sports Med 1984;12:469–479.
20. Ramakrishna B, Viswanath N. Diclofenac-induced hepatitis: Case report and literature review. Liver 1994;345:555–556.
21. Hull M, Jones R, Bendall M. Fatal hepatic necrosis associated with trazodone and neuroleptic drugs. Br Med J 1994;309:378.
22. Planas R, DeLeon R, Quer JC, et al. Fatal submassive necrosis of the liver associated with piroxicam. Am J Gastroenterol 1990;85: 468–470.
23. Rubin E, Cederbaum AT. Organelle pathology of alcohol-induced hepatic injury. In: Fischer MM, Ramkin JG, eds. Alcohol and the Liver. New York, Plenium, 1977:167–193.
24. Lee WM. Acute hepatic failure. N Engl J Med 1993;329:1862–1872.
25. Rettie AE, Rettenmeier AW, Howald WN, et al. Cytochrome P-450-catalyzed formation of Δ-4-VPA, a toxic metabolite of valproic acid. Science 1987;235:890–893.
26. Lullman H, Lullman R, Wasserman O. Drug-induced phospholipodosis, II. Tissue distribution of the amphiphillic drug chlorphentermine. CRC Crit Drug Rev Toxicol 1975;4:185–218.
27. Guigul B, Perrot S, Berry JP, et al. Amiodarone-induced hepatic phospholipodosis: A morphological alteration independent of pseudoalcoholic liver disease. Hepatology 1988;8:1063–1068.
28. Pollak PT, Sharma AD, Carruthers SG. Relation of amiodarone hepatic and pulmonary toxicity to serum drug concentrations and superoxide dimutase activity. Am J Cardiol 1990;65:1185–1191.
29. Watkins PB. Drug metabolism by cytochromes P_{450} in the liver and small bowel. Gastroenterol Clin North Am 1992;21:511–526.
30. Neuberger J, Kenna JG, Nouri Aria K, et al. Anti-body mediated hepatocyte injury in methyldopa-induced hepatotoxicity. Gut 1985;26: 1233–1239.
31. Beaune PH, Bourdi M. Autoantibodies against cytochrome P_{450} in drug-induced autoimmune hepatitis. Ann NY Acad Sci 1993;685: 641–645.
32. Hunt CM, Westerkam WR, Stave GM. Effect of age and gender on the activity of human hepatic CYP3A. Biochem Pharmcol 1992;44: 275–283.
33. Relling MV, Lin JS, Ayers GD, et al. Racial and gender differences in *N*-acetyltransferase, xanthine oxidase and CYP1A2 activities. Clin Pharmacol Ther 1992;52:643–658.
34. Lew KH, Ludwig EA, Milad MA, et al. Gender-based effects on methylprednisolone pharmacokinetics and pharmacodynamics. Clin Pharmacol Ther 1993;54:402–414.

35. Maddrey WC. Isoniazid-induced liver disease. Semin Liv Dis 1981; 1:129–131.
36. Tsagaropoou-Stinga H, Mataki-Emmanouilidon T, Karida-Kavalioti S, et al. Hepatotoxic reactions in children with severe tuberculosis treated with isoniazid-rifampin. Pediatr Infect Dis 1985;4:270–273.
37. Ylitalo P, Rousteenoja R, Les Kinen O, et al. Significance of acetylator phenotype in pharmacokinetics and adverse effects of procainamide. Eur J Clin Pharm 1983;25:791–795.
38. Garibaldi RA, Drusin RE, Ferebee SH, Gregg MB. Isoniazid-associated hepatitis: Report of an outbreak. Am Rev Respir Dis 1972;106: 357–365.
39. Kergueris MF, Bourin M, Larousse C. Pharmacokinetics of isoniazid: influence of age. Eur J Clin Pharm 1986;30:335–340.
40. Mitchell I, Wendon J, Fitt S, Williams R. Anti-tuberculosis therapy and acute liver failure. Lancet 1995;345:555–556.
41. Lake-Bakaar G, Scheuer PJ, Sherlock S. Hepatic reactions associated with ketoconazole use in the United Kingdom. Br Med J 1987; 294:813–820.
42. Knight TE, Shikuma CY, Knight J. Ketoconazole-induced fulminant hepatitis necessitating liver transplantion. J Am Acad Dermatol 1991;25:398–400.
43. Gomez-Gil E, Salmerón JM, Mas A. Phenelzine-induced fulminant hepatic failure. Ann Intern Med 1996;124:692–693.
44. Boelsteri UA, Rakhit G, Balazas T. Modulation of *S*-adenosyl-*L*-methionate, hepatic Na^+, K^+-ATPase, membrane fluidity and bile flow in rats with ethinyl estradiol-induced cholestasis. Hepatology 1983; 3:12–17.
45. Foitl DR, Hyman G, Leftowitch JH. Jaundice and intrahepatic cholestasis following high-dose megestrol acetate for breast cancer. Cancer 1989;63:438–439.
46. Lorch V, Murphy D, Hoersten L, et al. Unusual syndrome among premature infants: Associated with a new intravenous vitamin E product. Pediatrics 1985;75:598–601.
47. Carey MC, Hiram PC, Small DM. A study of the physiochemical interactions between biliary lipids and chlorpromazine-HCl. Biochem J 1976;153:519–531.
48. Reichel J, Goldberg SB, Ellenberg M, et al. Intrahepatic cholestasis following administration of chlorpropamide. Am J Med 1960;28: 654–660.
49. Naji AA, Anderson FH. Relationship between serum albumin and parenteral nutrition-associated cholestasis. J Pediatr Enter Nutr 1984; 8:438.
50. Rahmat J, Gelfand RL, Gelfand MC, et al. Captopril-associated cholestatic jaundice. Ann Intern Med 1985;102:56–58.
51. Dujovne CA, Chan CH, Zimmerman HJ. Sulfonamide hepatic injury. N Engl J Med 1967;277:785–788.
52. Larrey D, Babany G, Bernuau J, et al. Fulmimant hepatitis after lisinopril administration. Gastroenterology 1990;99:1832–1833.
53. Bachman BA, Boyd WP, Brady PG. Erythromycin ethylsuccinate-induced cholestasis. Am J Gastroenterol 1982;77:397–400.
54. Grimm IS, Litynski JJ. Severe cholestasis associated with ticlopidine. Am J Gastroenterol 1994;89:279–280.
55. Gomez JL, Dupont A, Casan L, et al. Incidence of liver toxicity associated with the use of flutamide in prostate cancer patients. Am J Med 1992;92:465–470.
56. Wysowski DK, Freiman JP, Tourlelot JB, Horton ML III. Fatal and nonfatal hepatotoxicity associated with flutamide. Ann Intern Med 1993;118:860–864.
57. Rader JI, Calvert RJ, Hathcock JN. Hepatic toxicity of unmodified and time-release preparations of niacin. Am J Med 1992;92:77–81.
58. Lee FI, Smith PM, Bennett B, Williams DMJ. Occupationally related angiosarcoma of the liver in the United Kingdom 1972–1994. Gut 1996;39:312–318.
59. Epidemiologic notes and reports angiosarcoma of the liver among polyvinyl chloride workers—Kentucky. MMWR 1997;46:99–101.
60. VanThiel DH, Perper JA. Hepatotoxicity associated with cocaine abuse. Recent Dev Alcohol 1992;10:335–341.
61. Henry JA, Jeffreys KJ, Daawling S. Toxicity and deaths from 3,4-methylenedioxymethamphetamine ("ecstasy"). Lancet 1992;340: 384–387.
62. Recknagel RO, Glende EA Jr. Carbon tetrachloride hepatotoxicity: An example of lethal clevage. CRC Crit Rev Toxicol 1973;2: 263–297.
63. Leonard C, Burke CM, O'Keane C, Doyle JS. "Golf ball liver": Agent orange hepatitis. Gut 1997;40:687–688.
64. MacGregor FB, Abernathy VE, Dahabra S, et al. Hepatotoxicity of herbal remedies. Br Med J 1989;299:1156–1157.
65. Koff RS. Herbal hepatotoxicity: Revisiting a dangerous alternative. JAMA 1995;273:502.
66. Wolf GM, Petrovic LM, Rojter SE, et al. Acute hepatitis associated with the Chinese herbal product *jin bu huan.* Ann Intern Med 1994;121:729–735.
67. Gordon D, Rosenthal G, Hart J, et al. Chaparral ingestion the broadening spectrum of liver injury caused by herbal medications. JAMA 1995;273:489–490.
68. Al-Qahtani MS. Hepatic and renal toxicity among patients ingesting sheep bile as an unconventional remedy for diabetes mellitus—Saudi Arabia, 1995. MMWR 1996;46:941–943.
69. Larrey D, Vital T, Pauwels A, et al. Hepatitis after germander (tecrium chamaedrys) administration: Another instance of herbal medicine hepatotoxicity. Ann Intern Med 1992;117:129–132.
70. Wolf T, Strecker M. Endogenous and exogenous factors modifying the activity of human liver cytochrome P-450 enzymes. Exp Toxicol Pathol 1992;44:263–271.
71. Seef LB, Cuccherin BA, Zimmerman HJ, et al. Acetaminophen hepatotoxicity in alcoholics: A therapeutic misadventure. Ann Intern Med 1986;104:399–404.
72. Klein AS. Amanita poisoning: Treatment and the role of liver transplantation. Am J Med 1987;86:187–193.
73. Berkovitch M, Pope E, Philips J, Koren G. Pemoline-associated fulminant liver failure: Testing the evidence for causation. Clin Pharmacol Ther 1995;57:696–698.
74. Zimmerman JH. Chemical hepatic injury and its detection. In: Plaa G, Hewitt GG, eds. Toxicology of the Liver. Target Organ Series. Philadelphia, Raven, 1981:1–46.
75. Choppa S, Griffin PH. Laboratory tests and diagnostic procedures in evaluation of liver disease. Am J Med 1985;79:221–230.
76. O'Grady JG, Alexander GJM, Hayllar KM, Williams R. Early indicators of prognosis in fulminant hepatic failure. Gastroenterology 1989;97:439–445.
77. Barstow L, Smith RE. Liver function assessment by drug metabolism. Pharmacotherapy 1990;10:280–288.
78. Williams CN, McCauley D, Malatjalian DA, et al. The aminopyrine breath test: An inadequate early indicator of methorexate-induced liver disease in patients with psoriasis. Clin Invest Med 1987;10: 54–58.
79. Kawasaki S, Sugiyama Y, Iga T, et al. Pharmacokinetic study on the hepatic uptake of indocyanine green in cirrotic patients. Am J Gastroenterol 1985;80:801–806.
80. Zech J, Lange H, Bosch J, et al. Steady-state extrarenal sorbitol clearance as a measure of hepatic plasma flow. Gastroenterology 1988;95: 749–759.
81. VanWaeg G, Groth T, Nikiasson F, et al. Allopurinol kinetics in humans as a means to assess liver function: Comparison of different models. Am J Physiol 1987;253:R352–R360.
82. Potter Jm, Hickman PE, Lynch SV, et al. Use of monothylglycinexyline as a liver function test in liver transplant recipient. Transplantation 1993;56:1385–1388.
83. Scott NR, Stambuck D, Chakraborty J, et al. The pharmacokinetics of caffeine and its dimethylxanthine metabolites in patient with chronic liver disease. Br Clin Pharmacol 1989;27:205–213.
84. Crom WR, Webster SL, Bobo L, et al. Simultaneous administration of multiple-model substrates to asscess hepatic drug clearance. Clin Pharm Ther 1987;41:645–650.

85. Juhl RP, VanThiel DH, Dittert LW. Alprazolam pharmacokinetics in alcoholic liver disease. J Clin Pharmacol 1984;24:113–119.

86. Sekiyama K, Yoshiba M, Inoue K, et al. Prognostic value of hepatic volumetry in fulminant hepatic failure. Dig Dis Sci 1994;39: 240–244.

87. Standardization of definitions and criteria of causality assessment of adverse drug reactions, drug-induced liver disorders: Report of an international consensus meeting. Int J Clin Pharmacol Ther Toxicol 1990;28:317–322.

88. Busuttil DP, Chasty RC, Fraser M. Delayed reactivation of hepatitis B infection after cladribine. Lancet 1996;348:129.

89. Newman M, Auerbach R, Feiner H, et al. The role of liver biopsies in psoriatic patients receiving long-term methotrexate treatment: Improvement in liver abnormalities after cessation of treatment. Arch Dermatol 1989;125:1218–1224.

90. O'Connor GT, Olmstead EM, Sug K, et al. Detection of hepatotoxicity associated with methotrexate therapy for psoriasis. Arch Dermatol 1989;125:1209–1217.

37

PANCREATITIS

Rosemary R. Berardi, PharmD, FASHP, and Patricia A. Montgomery, PharmD

Pancreatitis represents either an acute or chronic inflammatory process of the pancreas with variable involvement of regional tissues and remote organs. Acute pancreatitis (AP) is characterized by severe pain in the upper abdomen and increased blood concentrations of pancreatic lipase and amylase. In most instances, mild AP involves minimal organ damage and complete recovery. Severe AP is associated with local complications such as acute fluid collection, pancreatic necrosis, abscess, and pseudocyst. Multiple organ failure—including shock, pulmonary insufficiency, metabolic and cardiac complications, and renal failure—contributes to an unfavorable prognosis. Exocrine and endocrine pancreatic function may remain impaired for variable periods after the acute attack; however, the disease rarely progresses to chronic pancreatitis.[1,2]

Chronic pancreatitis (CP) is characterized by fibrosis and destruction of exocrine and endocrine tissue. Histologic and functional changes are irreversible, but not invariably progressive.[1,3] Improvement may occur in a subset of patients when obstruction of the main pancreatic duct is relieved (Fig. 37–1). In the acutely ill, symptomatic exacerbations closely resemble attacks of AP and may not be distinguishable. Patients with AP and CP suffer from many of the same complications.[1]

The prevalence of pancreatitis varies in different geographic areas and depends on etiologic factors. The incidence of AP in the United States is less than 1%, while the number of patients with CP is undefined. The overall male-to-female ratio of AP is equal; however, there is an increased incidence of alcoholic pancreatitis in younger men and of gallstone-related disease in older women.[1,2] Alcoholic CP is more common in men and has a peak incidence between 35 and 45 years of age.[1,3]

PHYSIOLOGY OF EXOCRINE PANCREATIC SECRETION

The pancreas possesses both endocrine and exocrine functions. The islets of Langerhans, that contain the cells of the endocrine pancreas, secrete insulin, glucagon, somatostatin, and other polypeptide hormones. The exocrine pancreas is composed of acini that secrete about 1 to 2 L/d of isotonic fluid that contains water, electrolytes, and pancreatic enzymes necessary for digestion. Bicarbonate is secreted primarily by the centroacinar (ductular) cells, and is the principal ion of physiologic importance. Pancreatic juice is delivered to the duodenum via the pancreatic ducts (Fig. 37–1), where the alkaline secretion (pH about 8.3) neutralizes gastric acid and provides an appropriate pH for maintaining the activity of pancreatic enzymes.[4]

The major pancreatic exocrine enzyme groups are identified in Table 37–1. The proteolytic enzymes are secreted as inactive proenzymes, which are activated in the lumen of the duodenum. Enterokinase, secreted by the duodenal mucosa, converts trypsinogen to trypsin, which then activates all other proteolytic proenzymes. Two important mechanisms protect the pancreas from the potential degradative action of its own digestive enzymes. The synthesis of proteolytic enzymes as proenzymes requires extrapancreatic trigger enzymes for activation. In addition, pancreatic juice contains a low concentration of trypsin inhibitor, which inactivates trypsin and partially inhibits chymotrypsin. Proteolytic activity in the intestinal lumen is not inhibited because the concentration is minimal. Lipase, amylase, and nucleases are secreted in their active form by the acinar cells. Colipase facilitates the action of lipase by binding to the bile salt–lipid surface and by lowering the optimum pH of lipase from 8.5 to 6.5, the normal luminal pH in the duodenum.[4]

The regulation of exocrine pancreatic secretion depends on stimulatory and inhibitory factors exerted through hormonal and neuronal mechanisms. Two hormones, secretin (SC) and cholecystokinin (CCK), play an important role in mediating pancreatic secretions and have synergistic effects: SC stimulates ductular cells to increase water and bicarbonate; CCK stimulates acinar cells to secrete a juice that is low in volume and bicarbonate but rich in enzyme content. The release of SC from the intestinal mucosa is pH dependent and occurs when the duodenal pH is approximately 4.5. Below this pH, titratable acid in the duodenum governs pancreatic bicarbonate output. Although the postprandial release of SC is small, nonacid factors such as products of fat digestion and bile can also stimulate SC release. The release of CCK from the small intestine is largely dependent on the presence of fatty acids and amino acids in the duodenum. Vasoactive intestinal polypeptide (VIP) is structurally similar to SC and exhibits weak secretin-like effects on exocrine pancreatic secretion. Gastrointestinal peptides such as somatostatin inhibit pancreatic enzyme secretion, in part by modulating cholinergic transmission.[4]

Pancreatic exocrine secretion is divided into three phases: cephalic, gastric, and intestinal. In the fasted state, basal pancreatic secretion occurs at a low rate; output fluctuates in cycles with the interdigestive migrating myoelectric complex (IMMC), so that peak secretions occur during phase III of the IMMC.[4] The cephalic phase is stimulated by the

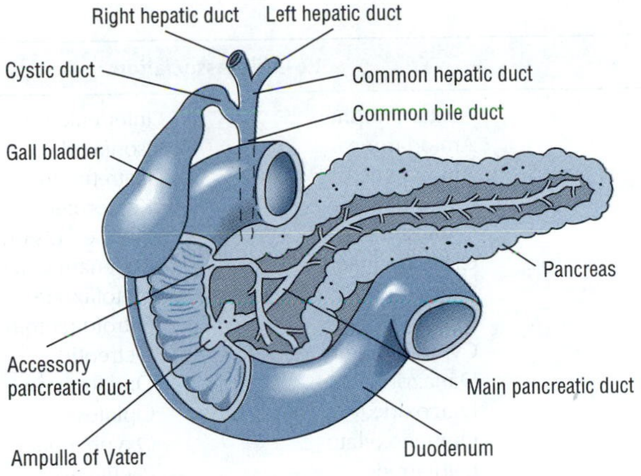

FIGURE 37–1. Anatomic structure of pancreas and biliary tract.

sight and smell of food and is thought to be mediated by vagal pathways. Gastric distention and the rate of gastric emptying stimulate an increase in enzyme-rich pancreatic fluid. In the intestinal phase, chyme and acid stimulate pancreatic secretion, largely through the release of SC and CCK. A comprehensive discussion of pancreatic physiology and the role of pancreatic enzymes in digestion can be found elsewhere.[4]

ACUTE PANCREATITIS

AP results from premature activation of proteolytic enzymes within the pancreas. The spectrum of the disease varies from mild, which is usually self-limiting, to severe, in which the severity of the attack correlates with the degree of pancreatic involvement and complications. The morphologic appearance of the pancreas and surrounding tissue ranges from interstitial edema and inflammatory cells (interstitial pancreatitis) to fat necrosis (necrotizing pancreatitis), which has a higher risk of pancreatic infection, organ failure, and mortality.[1] The rupture of blood vessels within or around the pancreas may lead to a collection of blood in the retroperitoneal spaces.

ETIOLOGY

The etiologic factors associated with AP are presented in Table 37–2. Gallstone-associated biliary tract disease (30% to 70%) and ethanol use (30%) account for most cases of AP in the United States.[1] The risk of AP after endoscopic retrograde cholangiopancreatography (ERCP) is at least 5%. About 10% to 15% have *idiopathic* pancreatitis, as a cause cannot be determined.[1,2] Pregnancy is not considered a cause of AP because pregnant women develop pancreatitis as a result of coincident processes, most commonly cholelithiasis. Because of the great functional reserve of the pancreas and the insidious loss of pancreatic function, it is possible that many patients who experience attacks of ethanol-related AP actually have CP.

TABLE 37–1. Major Pancreatic Enzymes

Proteolytic	
	Trypsinogen, chymotrypsinogen, proelastase
Amylolytic	
	Amylase
Lipolytic	
	Lipase, prophospholipase A_2, carboxylesterase lipase
Other	
	Nucleases, procolipase, trypsin inhibitor

TABLE 37–2. Etiology of Acute Pancreatitis

Structural	
	Gallstones, pancreatic tumors, sphincter of Oddi dysfunction
Toxins	
	Ethanol consumption, scorpion venom, organophosphorous insecticides
Infectious	
	Bacterial, viral, parasitic
Metabolic	
	Hyperlipidemia, hypercalcemia
Medications	
	See Table 37–3 for specific drugs
Trauma	
	Accidental pancreatic trauma, postoperative pancreatitis, ERCP (endoscopic retrograde cholangiopancreatography)
Vascular	
	Vasculitis, atherosclerosis, coronary bypass surgery
Miscellaneous	
	Congenital, idiopathic, cystic fibrosis, Crohn's disease

Compiled from Refs. 1 and 2.

MEDICATIONS

A number of medications have been implicated in AP, but a causal association is difficult to confirm because ethical and practical considerations prevent rechallenge with the suspected agent.[1,2,5–17] Table 37–3 lists medications according to their certainty of causing AP. A "definite" association implies a temporal relationship of drug administration to abdominal pain and hyperamylasemia or a positive response to rechallenge with the offending agent. Suggestive evidence exists for medications with a "probable" association, while evidence is inadequate or contradictory for drugs having a "possible" association. Allergic reactions (e.g., urticaria) usually do not accompany drug-induced AP.

The pathogenesis of drug-induced pancreatitis does not appear to differ from other causes of AP. Exactly how medications induce AP is unknown, but postulated mechanisms include immune-mediated inflammatory response, direct cellular toxicity, pancreatic duct constriction, arteriolar thrombosis, and metabolic effects. It is possible that thiazide diuretics lead to hypotension and pancreatic ischemia.[1] Combination therapy with several medications has also been reported to cause AP.[18,19] Although AP is an infrequent complication of drug therapy, it is prudent to withdraw medication when an association is suspected. A

TABLE 37–3. Medications Associated With Acute Pancreatitis

Definite Association	Probable Association	Possible Association	
5-Aminosalicylic acid	Ampicillin	Acetaminophen	Interleukin-2
Asparaginase	Bumetamide	Amiodarone	Isoniazid
Azathioprine	Calcium	Amoxapine	Isotretinoin
Didanosine	Cimetidine	Carbamazepine	Ketoprofen
Estrogens	Chlorthalidone	Cholestyramine	Lipid emulsion
Furosemide	Cisplatin	Clarithromycin	Mefenamic acid
Pentamidine	Clozapine	Clonidine	Metolazone
6-Mercaptopurine	Corticosteroids	Cyclosporine	Nitrofunantoin
Methyldopa	Cytarbine	Cyproheptadine	Octreotide
Metronidazole	Enalapril	Danazol	Ondansetron
Sulfonamides	Ethacrynic acid	Diazoxide	Opiates
Sulindac	Ifosfamide	Diphenoxylate	Oxyphenbutazone
Tetracycline	Lisinopril	Ergotamine	Paclitaxel
Thiazide diuretics	Meglumine antimoniate	Erythromycin	Phenolphthalein
Valproic acid	Phenformin	Famciclovir	Propoxyphene
	Piroxicam	Gold therapy	Rifampicin
	Procainamide	Granisetron	Ranitidine
	Salicylates	Ibuprofen	Tryptophan
	Sodium stibogluconate	Indomethacin	Warfarin
	Zalcitabine	Interferon-α	

Compiled from Refs. 1, 2, and 5–17.

discussion of the specific medications associated with AP can be found elsewhere.[5–19]

PATHOPHYSIOLOGY

The pathophysiology of AP has been related to autodigestion of the pancreas. Specific mechanisms include the reflux of duodenal contents containing enterokinase, activated pancreatic enzymes, and bile salts into the pancreatic duct; disruption of the pancreatic ducts and extravasation of juice as a result of gallstone-induced ductal hypertension; and premature intracellular activation of intrapancreatic proteases by lysosomal enzymes.[1,2] Activation of trypsin digests cell membranes and leads to the activation of other enzymes within the pancreas. After initial acinar cell injury, pancreatic enzymes leak into the interstitium, causing edema and inflammation. Lipase damages the fat cells producing noxious substances that cause further pancreatic and peripancreatic injury.

There is increasing evidence to suggest that the severity of AP and its complications are most likely mediated by polymorphonuclear leukocytes and their secretions.[1] Injured acinar cells liberate chemoattractants that attract neutrophils, macrophages, and other cells to the area of inflammation. For reasons that are unknown, leukocyte stimulation in AP is excessive and results in the release of a wide variety of destructive mediators such as elastase, platelet activating factor, reactive oxygen species, and cytokines. Elastase and other granulocyte proteases may activate the kinin, coagulation, complement, and fibrinolytic systems. Prostaglandins, histamine, and kinins are released from the inflamed pancreas into the circulation causing increased vascular permeability, vasodilation, and tissue edema. Pancreatic infection may result from increased intestinal permeability and translocation of colonic bacteria. Experimental evidence suggests that the harmful effects of leukocyte secretion impairs pancreatic microcirculation and contributes to the transition of interstitial to necrotizing pancreatitis.[1] When digestive enzymes and toxic products of leukocyte secretion enter the circulation, they combine to produce widespread injury of extra-abdominal organs.

COMPLICATIONS

Local complications—including acute fluid collection, pancreatic necrosis, abscess, and pseudocyst (collection of pancreatic juice and tissue debris enclosed by a wall of fibrous or granulation tissue)—develop about 4 weeks after the initial attack. Mortality after a pseudocyst rupture may be as high as 50%.[1] Gastrointestinal bleeding occurs secondary to numerous causes including rupture of a pseudocyst. Pancreatic abscess is usually a secondary infection of necrotic tissue or pseudocysts and correlates with the severity of the pancreatitis. Most deaths in patients with AP result from sepsis. Pancreatic ascites occurs when pancreatic secretions spread throughout the peritoneal cavity.

Systemic complications include pulmonary, cardiovascular, hematologic, renal, metabolic, and central nervous system abnormalities.[1,2] Of the early complications, shock is the main cause of death. Hypotension results from hypovolemia, hypoalbuminemia, the release of kinins, and sepsis. Renal complications are usually caused by hypovolemia. Pulmonary complications develop in approximately 10% to 20% of patients. Of the respiratory complications, hypoxia occurs in more than 50% of patients; pleural effusions occur more frequently on the left. The most serious respiratory complication is acute respiratory distress syndrome (ARDS), which usually occurs within a week after the onset of AP. Approximately 50% of patients with hypoxemia and pulmonary infiltrates die.[1]

CLINICAL PRESENTATION

SIGNS AND SYMPTOMS

The clinical presentation of AP varies depending on the severity of the inflammatory process and whether damage is confined to the pancreas or involves contiguous organs. Typical signs and symptoms are listed in Table 37–4. The initial presentation ranges from moderate abdominal discomfort to excruciating pain, shock, and respiratory distress. Abdominal pain, the major symptom of nearly all patients, is usually epigastric, often radiating to either of the upper quadrants or the back. The onset is usually sudden and the intensity is often described as "knife-like" or "boring." Generally, the pain of AP tends to be steady and usually persists for several days. Repositioning the patient relieves very little of the pain. Nausea and vomiting usually follow the onset of pain. Marked epigastric tenderness, abdominal distention, hypotension, and low-grade fever are often observed with widespread pancreatic inflammation and necrosis. In severe disease, bowel sounds are usually diminished or absent; dyspnea and tachypnea are signs of acute respiratory complications.[1]

DIAGNOSIS

The gold standard for diagnosis of AP is surgical examination of the pancreas or pancreatic histology. In the absence of these procedures, the diagnosis depends on the recognition of an etiologic factor, the clinical signs and symptoms, abnormal laboratory tests, and imaging techniques that predict the severity and course of the disease.

LABORATORY TESTS

Acute pancreatitis and its complications may be associated with leukocytosis, hyperglycemia, hypoalbuminemia, and mild hyperbilirubinemia. Elevations in serum alkaline phosphatase and liver transaminases are common. Dehydration may lead to hemoconcentration with elevated hemoglobin, hematocrit, blood urea nitrogen (BUN), and serum creatinine concentration. The total serum calcium is usually normal initially, but hypocalcemia out of proportion to the hypoalbuminemia may develop. Marked hypocalcemia is an indication of severe necrosis and a poor prognostic sign. Some patients with severe AP develop thrombocytopenia and a prolongation in the prothrombin time.

TABLE 37–4. Clinical Findings in Acute Pancreatitis

Observation	Incidence (%)
Abdominal pain	95
Radiation of pain to back	50
Abdominal distention	75
Nausea and vomiting	80
Low-grade fever	75
Hypotension	30
Mental aberrations	25
Jaundice	20

PANCREATIC ENZYMES

A number of laboratory tests are used to detect pancreatic enzymes in the blood and urine. Many of these tests do not provide sufficiently reliable information to be of clinical value. The serum amylase concentration usually rises within 24 hours of the onset of symptoms and returns to normal over the next 3 to 5 days. Persistent elevations suggest extensive pancreatic necrosis and/or related complications; however, serum amylase elevations do not correlate with either the etiology or severity of the disease. In addition, many nonpancreatic diseases may be associated with hyperamylasemia, including salivary, renal, hepatobiliary, metabolic, female reproductive tract, and neoplastic diseases.[1] Pancreatic isoamylase studies assist in determining the origin of elevated serum amylase concentrations, but are not useful for the diagnosis of AP because the diseases that simulate pancreatitis cause pancreatic rather than nonpancreatic amylase concentration to rise.

Serum lipase is specific to the pancreas and concentrations are usually elevated in AP. Serum lipase persists longer than serum amylase elevations and can be detected in the serum after the amylase has returned to normal. Urine amylase is increased in AP and may be elevated for 7 to 10 days after serum values have returned to normal. Urinary amylase concentrations are of little value, because they reflect the hydration and renal status of the patient. The amylase-to-creatinine clearance ratio is not widely used because it is associated with high false-negative and false-positive rates. The diagnosis of AP is often based on the clinical presentation and an elevated serum amylase or lipase.

IMAGING

A number of radiologic imaging techniques reveal pancreatic abnormalities during the disease course. None, however, provide a positive diagnosis of AP. The plain film of the abdomen radiograph often suggests AP. Abdominal ultrasonography is indicated in patients with suspected biliary involvement. Computed tomography (CT) is extremely useful in most patients with AP. Contrast-enhanced CT distinguishes interstitial from necrotizing pancreatitis but does not distinguish between fat necrosis and acute fluid collection. ERCP is used to visualize and remove bile duct stones in patients with gallstone pancreatitis.

CLINICAL COURSE AND PROGNOSIS

The majority of patients with AP recover uneventfully. Mortality rates appear to be influenced by the etiology of the disease and whether the acute attack is an initial or recurrent episode. Mortality is higher during the first attack of AP than during recurrent acute attacks. The severity of an acute attack may be predicted using criteria obtained upon admission and during the initial 48 hours of hospitalization (Table 37–5).[1,2] Patients with less than three criteria have a mortality rate of less than 1%, while those with six or more criteria have a 100% mortality rate.[2] Early recognition of severe AP requires aggressive clinical monitoring and therapy. The Acute Physiology and Chronic Health Evaluation (APACHE-II) score is more sensitive and specific than Ranson's criteria and can be calculated on admission.[1] Death during the first few days or weeks often results from systemic complications. When death occurs after this period, it is usually associated with local complications.

TABLE 37–5. Prognostic Factors in Severe Acute Pancreatitis—Ranson's Criteria

	Nongallstone Pancreatitis	Gallstone Pancreatitis
On Admission		
Age (yr)	> 55	> 70
White-cell count/mm^3	> 16,000	> 18,000
Glucose (mg/dL)	> 200	> 220
Lactic dehydrogenase (IU/L)	> 350	> 400
Aspartate aminotransferase (U/L)	> 250	> 250
Within 48 Hours		
Decrease in hematocrit (% points)	> 10	> 10
Increase in blood urea nitrogen (mg/dL)	> 5	> 2
Calcium (mg/dL)	< 8	< 8
Partial pressure of oxygen (mm Hg)	< 60	< 60
Base deficit (mmol/L)	> 4	> 5
Fluid deficit (L)	> 6	> 4

From Ref. 2.

▶ TREATMENT: Acute Pancreatitis

DESIRED OUTCOME

The treatment of AP varies depending on the severity of the attack (Fig. 37–2). Treatment is aimed at relieving abdominal pain, replacing fluids, minimizing systemic complications, and preventing pancreatic necrosis and infection. In most patients, mild AP is self-limiting and subsides spontaneously within 2 to 7 days of the initiation of supportive care and the reduction of pancreatic secretions. However, the disease takes a fulminant course in about 10% to 15% of patients. Patients with severe AP should be treated aggressively and monitored closely.

GENERAL APPROACH TO TREATMENT

Most patients are initially treated by withholding food or liquids in order to minimize exocrine stimulation of the pancreas. The use of nasogastric (NG) aspiration offers no clear advantage in patients with mild AP; however, it is beneficial in patients with profound pain, severe disease, paralytic ileus, and intractable vomiting.[1]

Fluid resuscitation is essential to correct intravascular volume. The prognosis of the patient often depends on the rapidity and adequacy of volume restoration. In severe disease, large quantities of fluid are sequestered within the peritoneal and retroperitoneal

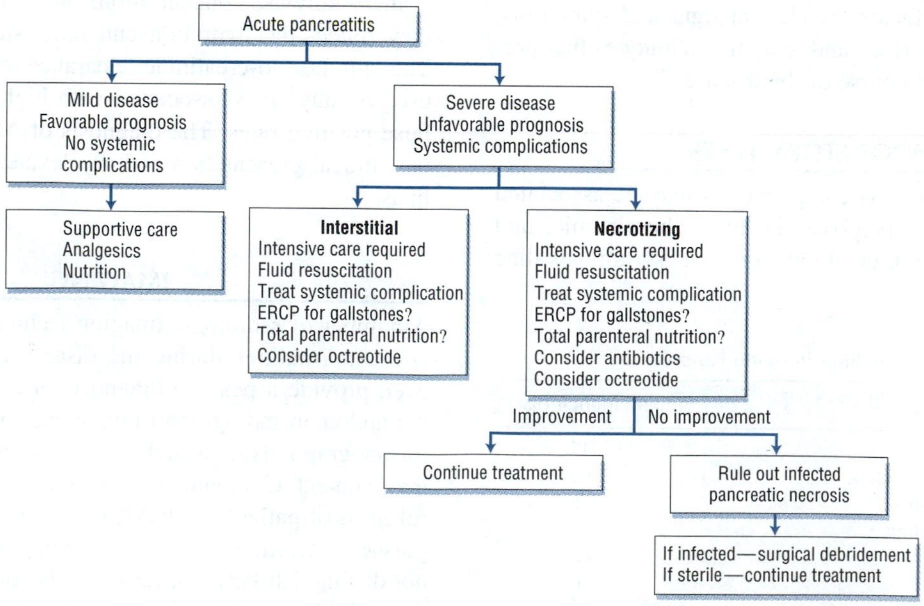

FIGURE 37–2. Algorithm for evaluation and treatment of acute pancreatitis.

spaces. Vomiting and NG suction contribute to fluid and electrolyte losses. Intravenous colloids may be required to maintain intravascular volume and blood pressure in severe disease, because fluid losses are rich in protein. Patients with severe AP will require aggressive monitoring and treatment of cardiovascular, respiratory, renal, and metabolic complications. Intravenous potassium, calcium, and magnesium should be used to correct deficiency states. Insulin may be needed to treat hyperglycemia. Local complications resolve as the inflammatory process subsides; however, patients with necrotizing pancreatitis may require antibiotics and surgical intervention.

NONPHARMACOLOGIC THERAPY

Nutritional deficits develop rapidly in patients with severe AP complicated by tissue necrosis, organ failure, and surgery. In addition, a number of factors including ileus may preclude oral nourishment for at least 3 to 6 weeks. Total parenteral nutrition (TPN) should be implemented before protein and calorie depletion becomes advanced. Intravenous lipids should not be withheld unless the serum triglyceride concentration is greater than 500 mg/dL.[1,20] Although TPN as a primary therapeutic modality does not alter the course of AP, it should be regarded as a useful adjunct in restoring and maintaining nutritional status.[1,20]

Removal of an underlying biliary tract gallstone with ERCP or surgery usually resolves AP and reduces the risk of recurrence. Surgical correction of biliary tract disease may also reduce the risk of recurrent episodes. Surgery may be indicated in AP to treat pseudocyst, pancreatic abscess, and to drain the pancreatic bed if hemorrhagic or necrotic material is present. Lavage of the peritoneal cavity is associated with numerous risks and is of questionable value.[21] Although removal of toxic pancreatic exudate may assist in the treatment of early cardiovascular and respiratory complications, it does not prevent necrosis or late abscess formation.

PHARMACOLOGIC THERAPY

RECOMMENDATIONS

Whenever possible, discontinue medications listed in Table 37–3. Administer analgesics to control abdominal pain. Inhibition of gastric acid secretion does not appear to be of benefit, but antisecretory drugs may be used to prevent stress bleeding. Octreotide may be tried in severe AP, but its efficacy remains uncertain (Fig. 37–2). Antibiotics should not be used in the absence of signs of infection except in patients with biliary tract gallstones or in severe AP when pancreatic necrosis or abscess is likely. Patients with life-threatening complications require additional intensive medical therapy or surgery.

RELIEF OF ABDOMINAL PAIN

Analgesics are administered to reduce the severity of abdominal pain. Although the administration of narcotics has been associated with mild and transient increases in serum amylase and lipase, these effects do not appear to be deleterious to the patient. A traditional approach is to begin with parenteral meperidine (50 to 100 mg) every 4 hours, because theoretically it causes less spasm of the sphincter of Oddi than other narcotic medications.[1,22] Although increased pancreatic duct pressure may correlate with the severity of pain, the difference in the degree of spasm produced by meperidine and equipotent doses of morphine is of questionable clinical importance. The primary basis for drug selection is analgesic efficacy. Morphine should be used in patients who require frequent (e.g., every 2 to 3 hours) parenteral doses of meperidine, whose pain is unresponsive to large doses of meperidine, or whose renal function precludes use of meperidine. Patient-controlled analgesia often achieves adequate pain control. However, it is important to evaluate the need for narcotic medication daily in order to prevent overuse.

LIMITATION OF SYSTEMIC COMPLICATIONS AND PREVENTION OF PANCREATIC NECROSIS

Medical therapy is aimed at limiting systemic complications and preventing pancreatic necrosis by either directly or indirectly reducing pancreatic secretion, inhibiting the action of circulating inflammatory mediators, or increasing pancreatic microcirulation (Table 37–6). Although a number of medications have been investigated, most are not effective. In mild AP, the use of intravenous H_2- receptor antagonists is no more effective than NG suction or withholding food when these modalities are used to diminish exocrine secretion.[1,23] Alternatively, an IV H_2-receptor antagonist is often used to prevent stress bleeding in the critically ill patient.

Oral pancreatic enzyme supplementation does not appear to relieve pain, decrease analgesic requirements, or decrease the incidence of complications.[24,25] Conflicting or inconclusive data exist regarding the efficacy of glucagon, calcitonin, atropine, ε-aminocaproic acid, 5-fluorouracil, corticosteroids, and indomethacin.[1,21,23] Studies have failed to confirm the value of antiprotease inhibitors such as aprotinin and gabexate mesilate.[1,21,26] Early studies with drugs such as lexipafant that block circulating inflammatory mediators produced by platelets and white blood cells suggest that they may have a beneficial effect.[1,27] The administration of low molecular weight dextran may increase pancreatic microcirculation in experimental animal models of AP, but its efficacy in preventing pancreatic necrosis in humans requires further study.[21,28]

Somatostatin and Octreotide

The efficacy of somatostatin and its analog octreotide in AP is unclear. Although these agents inhibit pancreatic enzyme secretion, experimental animal models indicate that basal and stimulated pancreatic secretion is reduced in AP.[29] Other potential benefits of somatostatin include a possible cytoprotective effect on pancreatic acinus cells and improved intestinal absorption of water and electrolytes. When all patients with pancreatitis are included in studies, octreotide does not appear to be beneficial.[29,30] However, in severe AP (patients meeting three or more Ranson's criteria), octreotide 0.1 mg subcutaneously every 8 hours decreased sepsis and length of hospital stay.[31] Preliminary reports of this ongoing trial indicate a trend in reduction of mortality. A case-controlled

TABLE 37–6. Measures Used to Limit Systemic Complications or Prevent Pancreatic Necrosis

Medications	Procedures
ε-Aminocaproic acid	Endoscopic retrograde cholangiopancreatography
Aprotinin	Hypothermia
Atropine	Nasogastric suction
Calcitonin	Pancreatic irradiation
Corticosteroids	Peritoneal lavage
Dextran	Thoracic duct drainage
5-Fluorouracil	
Gabexate mesilate	
Glucagon	
H_2-receptor antagonists	
Indomethacin	
Lexipafant	
Octreotide	
Pancreatic enzymes	

Compiled from Refs. 1, 2, 21, and 23–28.

trial in patients with necrotizing pancreatitis reported a decrease in mortality when octreotide 0.1 mg was given IV three times a day.[32] Final results of large randomized clinical trials should clarify the role of octreotide in AP. In the mean time, octreotide should be considered in patients with severe AP, as it may decrease mortality and possibly the length of hospital stay.

PREVENTION OF INFECTION

The use of prophylactic antibiotics does not offer any therapeutic advantage in patients with mild ethanol-induced AP who do not have necrosis.[1,23] Antibiotics may be warranted in patients with biliary or pancreatic duct obstruction, necrotizing pancreatitis, and those with likely pancreatic abscess. However, prophylactic antibiotic use in severe AP remains controversial. Early clinical trials found no benefit, but studies were flawed as they included patients with all degrees of disease severity and did not have a sufficient number of patients with severe necrotizing AP.[33,34] In addition, the antibiotics employed (including ampicillin) did not penetrate well into pancreatic tissue. The importance of antibiotic penetration into pancreatic tissue has been debated, however, as it is the peripancreatic retroperitoneal necrotic fat and debris, not the pancreas itself, that becomes infected.[33] Recent randomized trials in patients with severe AP have yielded conflicting results.[35–37] Cefuroxime prophylaxis lowered mortality, length of hospital stay, and the overall infection rate, but a decrease in the total number of infections was attributed to fewer urinary tract infections in the antibiotic group.[35] In contrast, prophylaxis with either ceftazidime, amikacin, and metronidazole or imipenem/cilastatin decreased the incidence of sepsis and reduced length of stay, but had no effect on mortality.[36,37] Although confounding variables could have accounted for the differences observed in these three studies, the data are compelling.

Antibiotic prophylaxis is not routinely recommended for all patients with severe AP because of conflicting mortality data and concerns regarding antibiotic resistance. Patients targeted for antibiotic prophylaxis are those with severe necrotic AP or disruption of the pancreatic ductal system (Fig. 37–2). Because the source of bacterial contamination is most likely the colon, the choice of antibiotic should be broad spectrum, covering the range of enteric aerobic gram-negative bacilli and anaerobic microorganisms. The antibiotics selected should be able to penetrate pancreatic tissue and peripancreatic necrotic tissue: for example, metronidazole, imipenem/ cilastatin, mezlocillin, and certain fluoroquinolones; penetration of aminoglycosides is poor.[38] Antibiotics should be started as soon as possible. The duration of treatment remains uncertain, although a 4-week course has been recommended.[34] Selective gut decontamination may be of benefit, but randomized controlled trials are needed to evaluate its efficacy compared to parenteral antibiotics.

CHRONIC PANCREATITS

Chronic pancreatitis is an inflammatory condition that usually results in functional and structural damage to the pancreas. In most individuals, CP is progressive and loss of pancreatic function is irreversible. Permanent destruction of pancreatic tissue usually leads to exocrine and endocrine insufficiency. Three subgroups of CP are recognized. Chronic calcified pancreatitis is related to ethanol ingestion, and characterized by fibrosis caused by intraductal protein plugs and ductal injury. Chronic obstructive pancreatitis results most often from obstruction of the main pancreatic duct by an intraductal tumor, and is characterized by fibrosis and ductal dilation. Chronic inflammatory pancreatitis is associated with autoimmune diseases and is characterized by fibrosis, mononuclear cell infiltration, and atrophy.[1] Cystic fibrosis may be associated with pancreatic exocrine insufficiency in children and is discussed in Chapter 28.

ETIOLOGY

Prolonged ethanol consumption is the most common cause of CP in the United States, accounting for approximately 70% of all cases, while half of the remaining 30% of nonethanol cases are idiopathic.[3] Infrequent causes of CP include hyperparathyroidism (and other chronic hypercalcemic states), protein–calorie malnutrition, heredity, trauma, pancreatic divisum, and obstruction of the main pancreatic duct by tumors, scars, stenosis, and pseudocysts. Although cholelithiasis may coexist with CP, gallstones rarely lead to chronic disease.

PATHOPHYSIOLOGY

The pathophysiology of ethanol-induced CP is related to ethanol-induced changes in the composition of pancreatic secretion, which lead to the precipitation of protein within the pancreatic ducts.[1,3] The precipitates form "protein plugs," which occlude the secondary pancreatic ducts, causing duct dilation and increased intraductal pressure, inflammation, acinar cell atrophy, fibrosis, scarring, and eventual calcification. It is also possible that chronic ethanol ingestion has a direct toxic effect on the pancreas, which initiates conditions conducive to autodigestion or produces products of ethanol metabolism that injure the pancreas. Other theories have been hypothesized, all of which lead to varying degrees of pancreatic destruction and insufficiency.[1,3]

The pathogenesis of the abdominal pain associated with CP is multifactorial and related, in part, to increased intraductal pressure secondary to continued pancreatic secretion, pancreatic inflammation, and neural abnormalities involving pancreatic nerves. A minority of patients develop complications including pancreatic pseudocyst, abscess, and ascites or common bile duct obstruction leading to cholangitis or secondary biliary cirrhosis. Bleeding is associated with a variety of causes.

CLINIAL PRESENTATION

SIGNS AND SYMPTOMS

The classic features of CP are abdominal pain, malabsorption, weight loss, and diabetes.[1,3] Jaundice occurs in about 10% of patients and results from extrahepatic biliary tract obstruction secondary to fibrosis of the head of the pancreas or stenosis of the common bile duct. Complications, including pancreatic pseudocysts, pleural effusions, and ascites, may be detected on physical examination.

Abdominal pain, either consistent or episodic, is the most prominent clinical feature and is described as dull, epigastric, and radiating to the back. Characteristically, the pain is deep-seated, positional, frequently nocturnal, and unresponsive to medication. The intensity of the pain varies from mild to severe, and does not usually correlate directly with the inflammatory process or other physical findings. Severe attacks last from several days to several weeks and may be aggravated by eating. The majority of alcoholic patients have chronic pain, while others have intermittent attacks or painless pancreatitis. Nausea, vomiting, and weight loss often accompany the pain. Abstinence from ethanol provides relief from pain, but may not prevent continuous exocrine dysfunction.[1,3] The course of pain is unpredictable, but frequently lessens as pancreatic insufficiency progresses.

When more than 90% of the secretory capacity of the pancreas is lost, malabsorption of protein and fat occurs.[1,3] Steatorrhea (excessive loss of fat in the feces) and azotorrhea (excessive loss of protein in the feces) are seen in the majority of patients. Because lipase secretion decreases sooner than proteolytic enzymes, steatorrhea—often associated with diarrhea and bloating—occurs earlier and is troublesome. At least 50% of patients with advanced pancreatic insufficiency present with vitamin B_{12} malabsorption.

Nausea, vomiting, anorexia, and weight loss are often seen in CP patients. Weight loss occurs primarily from avoidance of food due to fear of a painful response to eating. Pancreatic diabetes is usually a late manifestation commonly associated with pancreatic calcification. Malabsorption or poorly controlled diabetes may contribute to a reduction in weight. Neuropathy is common and may result from the additive effects of prolonged ethanol ingestion and malnutrition. Ketoacidosis, vascular complications, and nephropathy are uncommon with this form of diabetes.

DIAGNOSIS

Most patients with CP have a history of heavy alcohol use and attacks of recurrent upper abdominal pain. The classic triad of calcification, steatorrhea, and diabetes usually confirms the diagnosis.[1,3] Serum amylase and lipase concentrations usually remain normal unless the pancreatic duct is blocked or a pseudocyst is present. The white blood cell count, fluids, and electrolytes usually remain normal unless fluids and electrolytes are lost due to vomiting and diarrhea. Malabsorption of fat can be detected by Sudan staining of the feces or a 72-hour quantitative measurement of fecal fat.

Direct tests of pancreatic exocrine function involve the collection of pancreatic juice after stimulation with exogenous hormones such as secretin or cholecystokinin, and serve as the best indicators for detecting CP.[1,3] Because these tests are complicated and require intubation and special collection techniques, they are performed infrequently. Imaging techniques are helpful in detecting calcification of the pancreas, other causes of pain (ductal obstruction secondary to stones, strictures, or pseudocysts), and in differentiating CP from pancreatic cancer. ERCP is the gold standard imaging procedure for diagnosing CP and permits identification of surgically correctable lesions.[1,3]

CLINICAL COURSE AND PROGNOSIS

Patients with alcoholic CP usually present with an initial acute attack followed by successive attacks that are slower to resolve. Continued ethanol use leads to chronic abdominal pain and progressive exocrine and endocrine insufficiency. In about 50% of patients, the pain diminishes in about 5 to 10 years after the onset of symptoms. Steatorrhea, calcification, and diabetes usually develop after 10 to 20 years of heavy ethanol ingestion. Most patients present with varying degrees of pain, malnutrition, and glucose intolerance. The mortality rate of CP is approximately 50% within 20 to 25 years.[3] About 15% to 20% actually die of complications associated with acute attacks. Most deaths occur as a consequence of malnutrition, infection, or ethanol, narcotic, and tobacco use. In general, the clinical course of idiopathic CP appears to be more favorable than alcoholic pancreatitis.[1]

▶ TREATMENT: Chronic Pancreatitis

■ DESIRED OUTCOME

The treatment of uncomplicated CP is aimed primarily at the control of chronic abdominal pain (Fig. 37–3) and the correction of malabsorption with pancreatic enzymes (Fig. 37–4). Diabetes associated with CP may require exogenous insulin.

■ GENERAL APPROACH TO TREATMENT

The majority of patients with ethanol-related CP require pain control and pancreatic enzyme supplementation.[1,3,39–47] Avoidance of alcohol usually decreases pain, but analgesics remain the cornerstone of therapy. Nonnarcotic analgesics such as acetaminophen

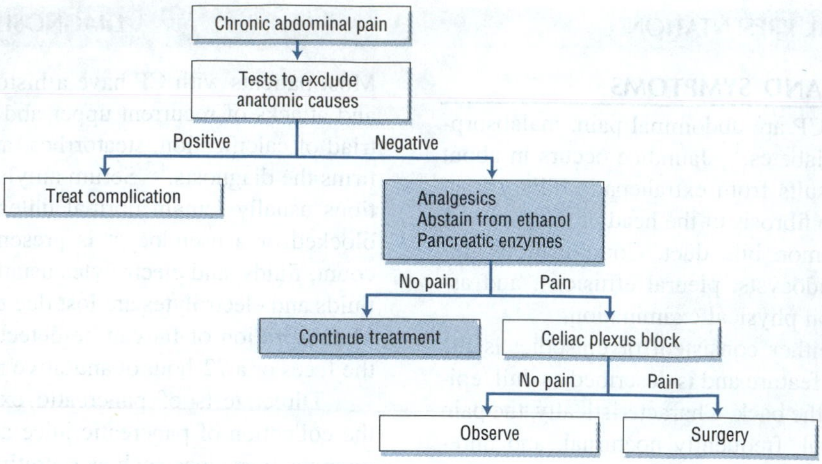

FIGURE 37–3. Algorithm for treatment of chronic abdominal pain.

or salicylates should be tried initially. The dose and frequency of administration should be increased before the patient is switched to a narcotic. Patients with nonalcoholic CP should be given a trial of pancreatic enzymes prior to using narcotics. Narcotics will be required in patients with severe pain. Celiac plexus block, or various surgical and endoscopic procedures, may be necessary in patients refractory to drug therapy. Patients with malabsorption will require pancreatic enzymes to reduce azotorrhea and steatorrhea. Most patients will achieve satisfactory results with standard dosage regimens. In patients who remain symptomatic, dietary fat should be reduced. Consideration may also be given to increasing the pancreatic enzyme dose or switching from an uncoated table to a microencapsulated enteric-coated dosage form. The addition of an antisecretory drug should be reserved for those patients who do not respond to these maneuvers or who have documented low duodenal pH levels.

NONPHARMACOLOGIC THERAPY

Abstinence from alcohol is the most important factor in preventing abdominal pain in the early stages of ethanol-induced CP.[1,3] Small and frequent meals (six meals per day) and a diet restricted in fat (50 to 75 g/d) is recommended to minimize postprandial pancreatic secretion and resulting pain. Parenteral or enteral nutrition (elemental diets) may be necessary, especially if the patient is chronically debilitated. Recent evidence suggests that the parenteral administration of nutrients is unlikely to stimulate pancreatic secretion.[20] When weight loss is refractory to diet and exogenous enzymes, supplementation with medium-chain triglycerides (MCTs) should be considered.

Nonsurgical treatment modalities have been advocated for abdominal pain relief, but none are completely effective.[1,3] In some patients, pain may be associated with pseudocysts, peptic ulcer, cholelithiasis, biliary or duodenal obstruction, or pancreatic cancer, and if detected may be amenable to other forms of treatment (Fig. 37–3). The most common indication for surgery is abdominal pain refractory to medical therapy. Surgical procedures that alleviate pain include a subtotal pancreatectomy, decompression of the main pancreatic duct, or interruption of the splanchnic nerves.[1,3] Although the pain may "burn out" as the gland deteriorates, it is unreasonable that a patient wait years for spontaneous relief. Alternatively, a percutaneous corticosteroid injection into the celiac ganglion (celiac plexus block) may be attempted. Unfortunately, pain relief obtained by this procedure may last for only 3 to 6 months, and repeated treatments are usually not as effective. A number of new endoscopic procedures (sphincterotomy, pancreatic duct stenting, and lithotriptic destruc-

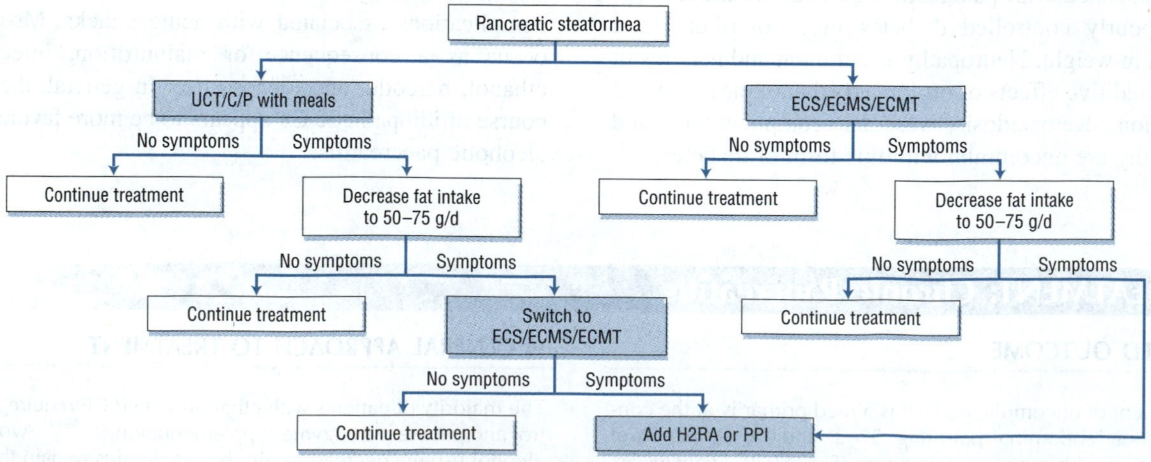

FIGURE 37–4. Algorithm for treatment of pancreatic steatorrhea. (UCT = uncoated tablet; C = capsule; P = powder; ECS = enteric-coated sphere; ECMS = enteric-coated microsphere; ECMT = enteric-coated microtablet; H2RA = H_2-receptor antagonist; PPI = proton pump inhibitor.)

tion of pancreatic calculi) are available, but are of questionable benefit to the patient.[1,3] As a last resort, the epidural administration of opiates via an epidural catheter may provide pain control.

PHARMACOLOGIC THERAPY

RECOMMENDATIONS

Pain management should begin with analgesics such as aspirin or acetaminophen (Fig. 37–3). If pain persists, the response to exogenous pancreatic enzymes should be evaluated in patients with mild to moderate nonalcoholic CP. If these measures fail, the administration of an oral narcotic should be added to the drug regimen. Parenteral narcotics should be reserved for patients with severe pain unresponsive to oral analgesics. In each case, the lowest effective analgesic dose should be used and scheduled around the clock.

Most patients with malabsorption will require pancreatic enzyme supplemention and a reduction in dietary fat in order to achieve satisfactory nutritional status and become relatively asymptomatic. An initial prandial dose of 30,000 IU of lipase (uncoated table, capsule, or powder) is recommended to be given with each meal (Fig. 37–4). Alternatively, the use of microencapsulated enteric-coated dosage forms may be used. The total daily lipase dose should be titrated to a reduction in steatorrhea. In some patients, a reduction in dietary fat may be necessary. The addition of an antisecretory drug should be reserved for patients resistant to enzyme therapy (Fig. 37–4). If these measures are ineffective, documentation of the diagnosis and exclusion of other diseases must be undertaken.

RELIEF OF CHRONIC ABDOMINAL PAIN

Analgesics

Nonnarcotic analgesics such as aspirin or acetaminophen should be tried initially, preferably before meals to prevent postprandial exacerbation of pain.[1,3,39] Treatment should be individualized and should begin with the lowest effective dose. The dosage regimen should be maximized before switching to narcotic alternatives. Analgesics should be scheduled around the clock, because they may be more effective and the total amount of medication required over 24 hours may be less. Frequently, severe pain relief necessitates the use of opiate analgesics. Narcotics should not be withheld because of the risk of inducing addiction. Oral agents (e.g., codeine derivatives) should be added to the nonnarcotic drug regimen before parenteral narcotics are administered.

Pancreatic Enzymes

The administration of large doses of pancreatic enzymes early in the course of the disease may afford pain relief by suppressing pancreatic enzyme secretion through a negative feedback mechanism involving proteases present in the duodenum. However, results from clinical trials have been variable.[1,3,39–43] Possible reasons for failure of enzyme therapy to relieve abdominal pain include insufficient concentrations of trypsin content within the pancreatic enzyme preparation, or a delayed release of trypsin from pH-dependent dosage forms,[40–43] and gastric acid inactivation or proteolytic destruction of lipase.[1,3,40–42] Beneficial effects seem to occur primarily in women with mild to moderate disease (without steatorrhea), and treatment appears to be useful in patients with a nonethanol etiology.

TREATMENT OF MALABSORPTION

Malabsorption requires treatment when steatorrhea (greater than 7 g of fat in the feces per 24 hours while on a diet of 100 g/d of fat) is documented and persistent weight loss occurs in spite of efforts to correct it. The combination of pancreatic enzymes (lipase, amylase, and protease) and a reduction in dietary fat (to less than 25 g/meal) enhances the patient's nutritional status and reduces (but does not totally correct) steatorrhea.

The success of pancreatic enzyme supplementation depends on a number of factors.[1,3,44–48] A critical amount of enzymes must be delivered to the duodenum in sufficient concentrations for digestion to occur. The maximal delivery of pancreatic lipase following a meal is approximately 140,000 IU/h for 4 hours.[23,46] Malabsorption is minimized if the concentration of enzymes delivered to the duodenum is at least 5% of normal maximal enzyme output. This requires that approximately 30,000 IU of lipase and 10,000 IU of trypsin be delivered during a 4-hour postprandial period.[1,23,46]

Another important factor to consider is that most exogenous lipase is probably rapidly and irreversibly destroyed at a intragastric pH below 4 or by proteases contained within the pancreatic formulations.[1,3,44,46] Factors other than lipase may play a role in the failure of enzymes to normalize fat absorption in pancreatic insufficiency. Microencapsulated enteric-coated preparations are more likely to empty from the stomach in synchrony with food and should mix with intestinal chyme more thoroughly.[1,23,46] Large enteric-coated tablets do not empty with partially digested stomach contents and are ineffective in treating pancreatic enzyme insufficiency.

Pancreatic Enzyme Supplements

Oral pancreatic enzyme supplements are available as a powder, uncoated or coated tablet, capsule, enteric-coated sphere (ECS) and microsphere (ECMS), or enteric-coated microtablet (ECMT) encased in a cellulose capsule (Table 37–7). Pancreatic enzyme supplements differ in enzyme content and activity, bioavailability, clinical efficacy, patient acceptance, and cost. Compliance is often a problem because of the number of tablets or capsules required per dose, the need to take them with each meal or snack, and the cost of pancreatic enzyme therapy. Consideration should be given to selecting a product that contains higher lipase activity (Table 37–7) so that fewer tablets or capsules are required.

Gastric inactivation of pancreatic enzymes and the inability to correct steatorrhea has led to the development of dosage formulations that consist of a cellulose capsule that contains pancreatic enzyme granules within an acid-resistant ECS, ECMS, or ECMT.[23,44,46] The polymer used to coat each granule is pH-dependent and dissolves in the duodenum (pH > 5), where the enzymes are released.[23,44] If a low (< 4) gastric pH prevails, the enteric-coating should remain intact and the enzymes will be released in the upper portion of the small intestine. A low (< 5) duodenal pH may prolong dissolution of the enteric coating and release of the enzymes. Microencapsulated enteric-coated products do not appear to be superior to standard doses of conventional nonenteric-coated enzyme preparations such as Viokase.[23] Perhaps this is because a lesser quantity of lipase is sometimes administered when an ECS, ECMS, or ECMT is prescribed. The quantity of active lipase delivered to the duodenum appears to be a more important determinant in pancreatic replacement therapy than the actual dosage form.[23,46]

Pancreatic enzymes contain nucleic acids and, when given in high therapeutic doses, have been associated with hyperuricosuria, hyperuricemia, and kidney stones.[23] Impaired folic acid absorption by oral pancreatic enzymes may lead to folic acid deficiency.[23] GI side effects appear to be dose-related, but occur less frequently with the enteric-coated products. Reports of colonic strictures and intestinal obstruction in cystic fibrosis patients taking high-dose pancreatic enzymes (> 20,000 IU lipase/capsule) have lead to their withdrawal from the market in the United States.[1,49,50] Sensitization and allergic reactions are uncommon but may occur in patients taking the powder.

TABLE 37–7. Enzyme Content of Selected Pancreatic Enzyme Preparations

		Enzyme Content (Units)[a]		
Product	Dosage Form[b]	*Lipase*	*Amylase*	*Protease*
Cotazym	C	8,000	30,000	30,000
Cotazym-S	ECS	5,000	20,000	20,000
Creon-5	ECMS	5,000	16,600	18,750
Creon-10	ECMS	10,000	33,200	37,500
Creon-20	ECMS	20,000	66,400	75,000
Ku-Zyme HP	C	8,000	30,000	30,000
Pancrease	ECMS	4,500	20,000	25,000
Pancrease MT-4	ECMT	4,500	12,000	12,000
Pancrease MT-10	ECMT	10,000	30,000	30,000
Pancrease MT-16	ECMT	16,000	48,000	48,000
Pancrease MT-20	ECMT	20,000	56,000	44,000
Pancrezyme 4X[c]	UCT	12,000	60,000	60,000
Ultrase MT-12	ECMT	12,000	39,000	39,000
Ultrase MT-18	ECMT	18,000	58,500	58,500
Ultrase MT-20	ECMT	20,000	65,000	65,000
Viokase	UCT	8,000	30,000	30,000
Viokase[d]	P	16,800	70,000	70,000
Zymase	ECS	12,000	24,000	24,000

[a]All listed products contain pancrealipase. Pancrealipase contains not less than 24 USP units of lipase activity, not less than 100 USP units of amylase activity, and not less than 100 USP units of protease activity per mg.
[b]C = powder encased in a cellulose capsule; ECS = enteric-coated sphere encased in a cellulose capsule; ECMS = enteric-coated microspheres encased in a cellulose capsule; ECMT = enteric-coated microtablets encased in a cellulose capsule; UCT = uncoated tablet; P = powder.
[c]Vegetable origin (suitable for vegetarians or those with allergies to beef and pork).
[d]Units of 0.7 g of powder.

Adjuncts to Enzyme Therapy

The use of antacids or antisecretory drugs as adjuncts to pancreatic enzyme supplementation does not unequivocally improve their efficacy.[23,46] Theoretically, the use of these agents in conjunction with oral pancreatic enzymes should maintain luminal gastric and duodenal pH above 4 and enhance lipase activity. Increased duodenal pH also prevents bile acid precipitation and thus increases fatty acid solubility. In most studies, antacids appear to have little or no added effect in reducing steatorrhea. The beneficial effects of an H_2-receptor antagonist or a proton pump inhibitor (PPI) result from both an increase in pH and a decrease in intragastric volume. Divergent results reported with the use of H_2-receptor antagonists in pancreatic steatorrhea may result from differences in the acid secretory status of subjects.[46] Symptomatic patients whose steatorrhea is not corrected by enzyme replacement therapy and a reduction in dietary fat, may benefit from the addition of an H_2-receptor antagonist or a PPI.[1,23,51] The additional cost of therapy and the potential for adverse effects and drug interactions should be considered.

PHARMACOECONOMIC CONSIDERATIONS

The pharmacoeconomic issues associated with the medical treatment of AP and CP have not been extensively examined. Aggressive medical and surgical care decreases mortality in AP, but the overall cost effectiveness of a specific treatment is unknown. The relief of abdominal pain in AP and CP, as well as pancreatic enzyme supplementation in patients with CP, improves quality of life and nutritional status. Although the efficacy of octreotide in AP remains uncertain, its use in severe AP is reasonable and potentially cost effective. There is evidence to suggest that antibiotic prophylaxis of targeted patients may reduce mortality and length of hospital stay, but pharmacoeconomic studies have not confirmed this suspicion. A reduction in the length of stay, however, could offset the cost of antibiotic therapy.

In some cases, medications that cost more may be more cost effective. This is particularly true with pancreatic enzymes and the microencapsulated enteric-coated dosage forms. These products may cost more, but they offer greater patient acceptance and compliance when compared to uncoated tablets. In addition, when cost is based on the number of tablets or capsules per day, rather than the cost of a single tablet or capsule, the high-potency preparations are usually similar in price. The additional cost of adding an H_2-receptor antagonist or PPI to pancreatic enzyme therapy may also result in more cost-effective treatment in patients who are not adequately controlled on maximal enzyme therapy.

EVALUATION OF THERAPEUTIC OUTCOMES

ACUTE PANCREATITIS

In patients with mild AP, pain control, fluid and electrolyte status, and nutrition should be assessed periodically depending on the degree of abdominal pain and fluid loss. Patients with severe AP should be transferred to an intensive care unit for close monitoring of vital signs, prothrombin time, fluid and electrolyte status, white blood cell count, blood glucose, lactic dehydrogenase, aspartate aminotransferase, serum albumin, hematocrit, blood urea nitrogen, and serum creatitine. Continuous hemodynamic and arterial blood gas monitoring is essential. Serum lipase, amylase, and bilirubin require less frequent monitoring. The clinician should also monitor the patient for signs of infection, relief of abdominal pain, and adequate nutritional status. Therapeutic outcome depends on the severity of the acute attack, medical mangement (which is primarily supportive), and prevention or treatment of infection. Despite appropriate supportive therapy, deterioration of respiratory, renal, and cardiovascular function may lead to death.

CHRONIC PANCREATITIS

The severity and frequency of abdominal pain should be assessed periodically in order to determine the efficacy of the patient's pain control regimen. Most patients with abdominal pain can be adequately controlled on acetaminophen or aspirin; however, patients with severe pain may require narcotics. In these patients, pain should be monitored daily and medications adjusted accordingly. Some patients will require celiac plexus block, surgery, or endoscoscopic procedures.

The effectiveness of pancreatic enzyme supplementation is measured by improvement in body weight and stool consistency or frequency. The 72-hour stool test for fecal fat may be used when there is concern regarding the adequacy of treatment. Serum uric acid and folic acid concentrations should be monitored yearly in patients prone to hyperuricemia or folic acid deficiency. Blood glucose must be carefully monitored in the diabetic patient. Therapeutic outcome depends in part on the ability of the patient to discontinue alcohol and tobacco and to maintain adequate nutriton. Pain control and pancreatic enzyme supplemention are important therapeutic measures that contribute to the patient's quality of life. Unfortunately, a small number of patients die from complications associated with an acute attack.

CONCLUSIONS

Despite modern medical knowledge, much of what we know about the pathophysiologic mechanisms, diagnosis, and treatment of AP and CP remains incomplete. Current research is directed at ways to limit the systemic complications of AP and to elminate steatorrhea in CP. In the future, answers to the many questions surrounding the mysteries of these diseases will become known. Until then, our role as pharmacists is largely supportive, but should include the provision of pharmaceutical care to patients with pancreatitis, and information to the public regarding the complications and consequences of ethanol-related diseases such as pancreatitis.

▶ PRINCIPLES OF PHARMACOTHERAPY

Acute Pancreatitis

- Discontinue medications that may potentially cause pancreatitis.
- Patients with severe AP require early and aggressive IV fluids and electrolytes.
- Use parenteral meperidine to control abdominal pain; morphine should be used in patients with renal impairment or those with an inadequate response to high or frequent meperidine doses.
- Octreotide may be used in severe AP, but its efficacy remains uncertain.
- Antibiotics should not be used in the absence of signs of infection except in patients with biliary tract gallstones or in severe AP when pancreatic necrosis or abscess is likely.

Chronic Pancreatitis

- Abstinence from alcohol is the most important factor in preventing abdominal pain in the early stages of ethanol-induced CP.
- Pain control should begin with nonnarcotic analgesics such as acetaminophen or salicylates. The dose and frequency of administration should be increased before the patient is switched to a narcotic. Parenteral narcotics should be reserved for patients with severe pain unresponsive to oral analgesics. For patients with frequent or constant pain, the lowest effective analgesic dose should be used and scheduled around the clock.
- Treatment of abdominal pain with pancreatic enzymes should be reserved for patients with a nonethanol etiology and mild to moderate disease (without steatorrhea).
- Pancreatic enzyme supplementation and a reduction of dietary fat are used to treat malabsorption and steatorrhea. An initial lipase dose of about 30,000 IU should be given with each meal.
- Symptomatic patients whose steatorrhea is not corrected by pancreatic enzyme supplementation and a reduction in dietary fat may benefit from the addition of an H_2-receptor antagonist or a PPI. Because of the cost of therapy, an H_2-receptor antagonist should be considered before trying a PPI.

REFERENCES

1. Banks PA. Acute and chronic pancreatitis. In: Feldman M, Scharschmidt BF, Sleisenger MH, eds. Sleisenger and Fordtran's Gastrointestinal and Liver Disease: Pathophysiology/Diagnosis/Management, 6th ed. Philadelphia, Saunders, 1998:809–862.
2. Steinberg W, Tenner S. Acute pancreatitis. N Engl J Med 1994;330: 1198–1210.
3. Steer ML, Waxman I, Freedman S. Chronic pancreatitis. N Engl J Med 1995;332:1482–1490.
4. Pandol SJ. Pancreatic physiology and secretory testing. In: Feldman M, Scharschmidt BF, Sleisenger MH, eds. Sleisenger and Fordtran's

Gastrointestinal and Liver Disease: Pathophysiology/Diagnosis/Management, 6th ed. Philadelphia, Saunders, 1998:771–782.
5. McArthur KE. Review article: Drug-induced pancreatitis. Aliment Pharmacol Ther 1996;10:23–38.
6. Frick TW, Speiser DE, Bimmier D, Largiader F. Drug-induced acute pancreatitis: Further criticism. Dig Dis 1993;11:113–132.
7. Madsen JS, Jacobsen IA. Angiotensin converting enzyme inhibitor therapy and acute pancreatitis. Blood Pressure 1995;4:369–371.
8. Maringhini A, Termini A, Patti R, et al. Enalapril-associated acute pancreatitis: Recurrence after rechallenge. Am J Gastroenterol 1997; 92:166–167.
9. Izaeli S, Adamson PC, Blaney SM, et al. Acute pancreatitis after ifosfamide therapy. Cancer 1994;74:1627–1628.
10. Liviu L, Yair L, Yehuda S. Pancreatitis induced by clarithromycin. Ann Intern Med 1996;125:701. Letter.
11. Sotomatsu M, Shimoda M, Ogawa C, et al. Acute pancreatitis associated with interferon-α therapy for chronic myelogenous leukemia. Am J Hemotol 1995;48:211–212. Letter.
12. Goffin E, Horsmans Y, Pirson Y, et al. Acute necrotico-hemorrhagic pancreatitis after famciclovir prescription. Transplantation 1995;59: 1218–1219.
13. Hoff PM, Valero V, Holmes FA, et al. Paclitaxel-induced pancreatitis: A case report. J Natl Cancer Inst 1997;89:91–92. Letter.
14. Rodier JM, Pujade-Lauraine E, Batel-Copel L, et al. Ganisetron-induced acute pancreatitis. J Cancer Res Clin Oncol 1996;122: 132–133. Letter.
15. Balasch J, Martinez-Romain S, Carreras J, et al. Acute pancreatitis associated with danazol treatment for endometriosis. Hum Reprod 1994;9:1163–1165.
16. Domingo P, Ferrer S, Kolle S, et al. Acute pancreatitis associated with sodium stibogluconate treatment in a patient with human immunodeficiency virus. Arch Intern Med 1996;156:1029–1032. Letter.
17. Torrus D, Massa B, Boix V, et al. Meglumine antimoniate-induced pancreatitis. Am J Gastroenterol 1996;91:820–821. Letter.
18. Abdul-Ghaffar N, El-Sonbaty MR. Pancreatitis and rhabdomyolysis associated with lovastatin-gemfibrozil therapy. J Clin Gastroenterol 1995;21:340–341.
19. Stricker RB, Man KM, Bouvier DB, et al. Pancreatorenal syndrome associated with combination antiretroviral therapy in HIV infection. Lancet 1997;349:1745–1746.
20. McClave SA, Snider H, Owens N, et al. Clinical nutrition in pancreatitis. Dig Dis Sci 1997;42:2035–2044.
21. Marshall SB. Acute pancreatitis: Review with an emphasis on new developments. Arch Intern Med 1993;153:1185–1198.
22. Isenhower HL, Mueller BA. Selection of narcotic analgesics for pain associated with pancreatitis. Am J Health Syst Pharm 1998;55:480–486.
23. Tenner S, Levine RS, Steinberg WM. Drug treatment of acute and chronic pancreatitis. In: Lewis JH, ed. A Pharmacologic Approach to Gastrointestinal Disorders. Baltimore, Williams & Wilkins, 1994: 311–323.
24. McMahon MJ. Acute pancreatitis: When is enzyme treatment indicated? Digestion 1993;54(suppl 2):40–42.
25. Patankar RV, Chaund R, Johnson CD. Pancreatic enzyme supplementation in acute pancreatitis. HPB Surg 1995;8:159–162.
26. Messori A, Rampazzo R, Scroccaro G, et al. Effectiveness of gabexate mesilate in acute pancreatitis: A metaanalysis. Dig Dis Sci 1995; 40:734–738.
27. Mckay C, Curran FJ, Sharples CE, et al. The use of lexipafant in the treatment of acute pancreatitis. Adv Exp Med Biol 1996;416: 365–370.
28. Holtz HG, Schmidt J, Ryschich EW, et al. Isovolemic hemodilution with dextran prevents contrast medium induced impairment of pancreatic microcirculation in necrotizing pancreatitis of the rat. Am J Surg 1995;169:161.
29. Buchler MW, Binder M, Friess H, Malfertheimer P. Potential role of somatostatin and octreotide in the management of acute pancreatitis. Digestion 1994;44(suppl 1):16–19.
30. Jenkins SA, Berein A. Review article: The relative effectiveness of somatostatin and octreotide therapy in pancreatic disease. Aliment Pharmacol Ther 1995;9:349.
31. Paran H, Neufeld D, Mayo A, et al. Preliminary report of a prospective randomized study of octreotide in the treatment of severe acute pancreatitis. J Am Coll Surg 1995;181:121–124.
32. Fiedler F, Jauernig G, Keim V, et al. Octreotide treatment in patients with necrotizing pancreatitis and pulmonary failure. Intensive Care Med 1996;22:909–915.
33. Barie PS. A critical review of antibiotic prophylaxis in severe acute pancreatitis. Am J Surg 1996;172(suppl 6a):38S–43S.
34. Ho HS, Frey CF. The role of antibiotic prophylaxis in severe acute pancreatitis. Arch Surg 1997;132:487–493.
35. Sainio V, Kemppainen P, Poulallainen P, et al. Early antibiotic treatment in acute necrotizing pancreatitis. Lancet 1995;346:663–667.
36. Pederzoli P, Bassi C, Vesentini S, et al. A randomized multicenter clinical trial of antibiotic prophylaxis with imipenem. Surg Gynecol Obstet 1993;176:480–483.
37. Delcenserie R, Yzet T, Ducroix JP. Prophylactic antibiotics in treatment of severe acute alcoholic pancreatitis. Pancreas 1996;13: 198–201.
38. Bassi C, Pederzoli P, Vesentini S, et al. Behavior of antibiotics during human necrotizing pancreatitis. Antimicrob Agents Chemother 1994;38:830–836.
39. Malfertheiner P, Dominguez-Munoz JE, Buchler MW. Chronic pancreatitis: Management of pain. Digestion 1994;55(suppl 1):29–34.
40. Mossner J. Is there a place for pancreatic enzymes in the treatment of pain in chronic pancreatitis? Digestion 1993;54(suppl 2):35–39.
41. Malesci A, Gaia E, Fioretta A, et al. No effect of long-term treatment with pancreatic extract on recurrent abdominal pain in patients with chronic pancreatitis. Scand J Gastroenterol 1995;30:392–398.
42. Mossner J, Secknus R, Meyer J, et al. Treatment of pain with pancreatic extracts in chronic pancreatitis: Results of a prospective placebo-controlled multicenter trial. Digestion 1992;53:54–66.
43. Malfertheiner P, Dominguez-Munoz JE. Effect of exogenous pancreatic enzymes on gastrointestinal and pancreatic hormone release and gastrointestinal motility. Digestion 1993;54(suppl 2):15–20.
44. Layer P, Groger G. Fate of pancreatic enzymes in the human intestinal lumen in health and pancreatic insufficiency. Digestion 1993;54(suppl 2):10–14.
45. Layer P, Holtmann G. Pancreatic enzymes in chronic pancreatitis. Int J Pancreatol 1994;15:1–11.
46. Lankisch PG. Enzyme treatment of exocrine pancreatic insufficiency in chronic pancreatitis. Digestion 1993;54(suppl 2):21–29.
47. Lebenthal E, Rolston DDK, Holsclaw DS. Enzyme therapy for pancreatic insufficiency: Present status and future needs. Pancreas 1994; 9:1–12.
48. Van Hoozen CM, Peeke PG, Taubeneck M, et al. Efficacy of enzyme supplementation after surgery for chronic pancreatitis. Pancreas 1997;14:174–180.
49. FDC Report. High-dose pancreatic enzymes may require clinical trials to return to market following removal due to safety concerns: Cystic fibrosis patient registry suggested. The Pink Sheet, February 21, 1994:13–14.
50. Smyth RL, Ashby D, O'Hare U, et al. Fibrosing colonopathy in cystic fibrosis: Results of a controlled trial. Lancet 1995;348:1247.
51. Bruno MJ, Rauws EAJ, Hoek FJ, et al. Comparative effects of adjuvant cimetidine and omeprazole during pancreatic enzyme replacement therapy. Dig Dis Sci 1994;39:988.

38

VIRAL HEPATITIS

Marsha A. Raebel, PharmD, FCCP, BCPS, and Shirley M. Palmer, PharmD

Viral hepatitis is a major cause of morbidity and mortality in the United States. Viral hepatitis refers to the clinically important hepatotrophic viruses responsible for hepatitis A (HAV), hepatitis B (HBV), delta hepatitis (HDV), hepatitis C (HCV), and hepatitis E (HEV). A hepatitis G virus (HGV) has also been described. However, its role in clinical illness is still not clear.

About 56,000 cases of hepatitis are reported yearly in the United States.[1] Reporting is incomplete, however, and the actual number of patients infected is closer to 600,000.[2] Hepatitis A causes an estimated 130,000 infections yearly, while hepatitis B is responsible for 300,000 cases.[1,3] About 150,000 new cases of hepatitis C occur annually, resulting in almost 4 million Americans (1.8% of the population) being infected with hepatitis C. Nine to 14 percent of all patients infected with hepatitis B develop chronic hepatitis, while chronic disease develops in about 80% of patients infected with hepatitis C.[4] Many of these patients ultimately die of complications of chronic hepatitis such as cirrhosis or hepatocellular carcinoma (HCC).

Outside the United States, viral hepatitis is a major health problem. More than 300 million people are infected with hepatitis B worldwide. The World Health Organization lists hepatitis B as the ninth leading cause of death in the world.

Viral hepatitis has several clinical forms (acute, fulminant, chronic), defined by duration or severity of infection. The clinical, biochemical, immunoserologic, and histologic features of viral hepatitis follow similar patterns regardless of the virus responsible for the patient's illness. The hepatocellular response to injury and the resulting physical signs and symptoms are all nonspecific in nature.[5]

ACUTE VIRAL HEPATITIS

Acute viral hepatitis is a systemic viral infection of up to but not exceeding 6 months in duration producing inflammatory necrosis of the liver. The natural history of the infection is divided into three stages based on viral serologic markers: incubation, acute hepatitis, and convalescence. Clinical severity of illness varies widely from asymptomatic, anicteric hepatitis to fulminant hepatitis, an often rapidly fatal disease.[5]

The incubation stage begins shortly after parenteral or oral inoculation with the virus. Once access is gained to the circulation, the infective virions accumulate in hepatic sinusoids and are internalized by the hepatocytes. The internalized viral particles replicate within either the cytoplasm or the nucleus with the assistance of the host cellular apparatus. Infective viral particles are shed into blood, bile, and other body secretions during the later phases of the incubation stage. Complete virions and/or viral antigens are found in body fluids and tissues. The duration of the incubation stage is virus specific (Table 38–1).[6] The host is essentially asymptomatic during the incubation stage of the infection.[5]

The hepatotrophic viruses cause hepatic injury either because of the host immune response or from direct viral damage to hepatocytes. For example, the acute hepatitis stage in hepatitis B begins once the host recognizes the virus and initiates an active immune response against the invading virions. The resulting cellular and humoral immune response is directed against viral antigens found on the host hepatocyte membranes and/or circulating within the vascular compartment.[7] The severity of the inflammatory response and resulting liver cell damage is variable. Under conditions of viral antigen excess, antigen–antibody complexes form within the vascular compartment and may produce immune complex–related phenomena and symptoms such as arthritis, skin rash, and urticaria.[5]

This acute hepatitis stage begins with a preicteric phase (before the onset of jaundice), which parallels initiation of the host immune response and occurs before significant liver cell injury. The preicteric phase is frequently associated with nonspecific influenza-like symptoms consisting of anorexia, nausea, fatigue, and malaise.[5]

Most patients with acute viral hepatitis develop only a few mild symptoms and minimal hepatocyte damage. This mild disease is called *acute anicteric hepatitis.* The minimal degree of liver cell damage is reflected by mild elevations of serum bilirubin, gamma globulin, and hepatic transaminase (ALT, AST) values to about twice normal. A subset of patients experience enough hepatocyte destruction to produce significant liver function derangement characterized by interruption of bilirubin metabolism and flow. This results in clinical jaundice. The icteric phase is generally accompanied by fever, right upper quadrant abdominal pain, nausea, vomiting, dark urine, acholic (light colored) stools, and worsening of systemic symptoms. Clinical symptoms are accompanied by moderate to marked elevations of the serum bilirubin, gamma globulin, and hepatic transaminases (4 to 10 times normal). Viral serologic markers and host antibodies are detectable during this stage of the illness.[5]

Most patients with either acute anicteric or icteric hepatitis go through the convalescence stage to complete recovery without developing complications or chronic

TABLE 38–1. Important Features of Hepatitis Viruses

	Hepatitis A	Hepatitis B	Hepatitis C	Hepatitis D	Hepatitis E	Hepatitis G
Virus	HAV	HBV	HCV	HDV	HEV	HGBV or HGV[a]
Family	Picornavirus	Hepadnavirus	Flavivirus	Satellite	Calcivirus	Flavivirus
Size (nm)	27	42	30–60	40	32	?
Genome	ssRNA	dsDNA	ssRNA	ssRNA	ssRNA	ssRNA
Incubation (d)	14–45	40–180	35–84	40–180 coinfection 14–45 superinfection	14–60	? ?
Transmission	Fecal–oral	Parenteral Sexual Perinatal Mucous membrane	Parenteral Sexual Perinatal (?) Mucous membrane	Parenteral Sexual (?) Perinatal	Fecal–oral	Parenteral
Serologic markers						
Antigens	HAVAg	HBsAg HBcAg HBeAg	HCVAg	HDVAg	Not available	?
Antibodies	Anti-HAV	Anti-HBs Anti-HBc Anti-HBe	Anti-HCV	Anti-HDV	Not available	?
Viral markers	HAV RNA	HBV DNA DNA polymerase	HCV RNA	HDV RNA	Not available	HGBV-C RNA
Clinical illness						
Children	Anicteric	Anicteric 70%	Anicteric 75%	Not known	High % anicteric	Not determined if associated with clinical illness
Adults	Icteric	Icteric 30%	Icteric 25%	Icteric 25%	Not known	
Acute mortality (%)	0.3	0.2–1	0.2	2–20	10 (pregnancy)	?
Chronicity (%)	No	2–7 Neonates 90	70–80	2–70	No	?
Hepatocellular carcinoma	No	Yes	Yes	Yes	No	?

[a]Comprised of several RNA viruses: HGBV-A, HGBV-B, HGBV-C.

sequelae. The duration of disease stages and the risk for developing chronic sequelae are virus-specific phenomena (Table 38–1).[5]

HEPATITIS A VIRUS

Hepatitis A virus (HAV) is the primary etiologic agent of worldwide hepatitis epidemics throughout recorded history.[8] HAV, an RNA virus, remains a significant cause of clinical hepatitis worldwide, although HEV plays a role in many epidemics.

Epidemiology

Hepatitis A virus is well suited to produce epidemics given its fecal-to-oral route of transmission and its ability to resist both gastric acid and the digestive enzymes of the upper gastrointestinal tract.[8] HAV infection also occurs sporadically. Both patterns of occurrence are related to overcrowded conditions and person-to-person spread or ingestion of contaminated food or water. The incidence of HAV correlates directly with poor sanitary conditions and hygienic practices.[1] For international travelers, longer lengths of stay in a country with a high rate of hepatitis A also correlates with increased risk. In the United States, groups at increased risk of hepatitis A, in addition to travelers, include men who have sex with men, injecting-drug users, and persons working with nonhuman primates.[3]

HAV infection in the United States occurs primarily in community-wide outbreaks, in lower socioeconomic groups, or in sporadic common-source outbreaks (outbreaks where all infected patients contract the infection from a single person or source). Occasionally, HAV has been transmitted by transfusion of contaminated blood products.[3,9] Children aged 5 to 14 years are more likely to be involved in community-wide outbreaks, whereas common-source outbreaks primarily involve young adults. Both children and young adults can be infected from common-source outbreaks at day care centers.[1]

Pathogenesis

Hepatitis A viral replication occurs in the liver. Viral antigens are found in the hepatocyte cytoplasm during the incubation stage. They are subsequently shed into bile and feces. The largest concentration of viral particles is found in stool specimens during the 1 to 2 weeks preceding clinical illness. Viral shedding declines as clinical symptoms appear. Viremia is extremely short lived, thus explaining the rare occurrence of blood-borne transmission of hepatitis A.[4,9] Cases of HAV associated with parenteral drug abuse are increasing. Liver injury is immune mediated with cytolytic T cells the most likely effector cells.[7,8] Death of hepatocytes results in viral elimination and eventual resolution of the clinical illness.

The host antibody response to HAV initially appears as the viral particles begin to disappear from stool. Like most host antibody responses, antibodies of the IgM class appear first and imply recent infection. After 2 to 6 months, the IgM antibodies are replaced with IgG antibodies, which usually persist throughout life and confer immunity to HAV.[3,4]

Clinical Presentation

Clinical symptoms are age dependent, with children less than 6 years old generally displaying a mild, influenza-like illness without clinical jaundice. In contrast, more than 70% of infected adults and older children display the characteristic clinical syndrome of acute hepatitis with elevated hepatic transaminase levels and jaundice.[3,8]

HAV infection usually produces a mild, self-limited illness, lasting less than 2 months, although a minority of patients exhibit a cholestatic illness with predominant elevations of alkaline phosphatase, gamma-glutamyl transferase, and total bilirubin that lasts several months. Pruritus may be the primary complaint of this latter patient group.[10] Rarely, HAV may cause fulminant hepatitis, resulting in approximately 100 deaths each year in the United States.[3] No cases of a chronic carrier state or chronic hepatitis have been reported. However, up to 20% of patients relapse with acute hepatitis 2 to 8 weeks after the initial illness. Recurrent symptoms tend to be milder than the initial episode.[8] Rarely, a relapse is associated with cryoglobulinemia, arthritis, and vasculitis.[10]

The diagnosis of acute HAV infection depends on clinical suspicion, characteristic symptoms (if present), elevated aminotransferases and bilirubin, and a positive anti-HAV IgM (Table 38–1). Without characteristic symptoms, clinical suspicion of HAV is extremely important.[8] Patients who receive gamma globulin will have low titers of anti-HAV for several weeks after inoculation.[6] Patients who receive hepatitis A vaccine will also have anti-HAV.[6]

HEPATITIS B VIRUS

Unlike HAV, hepatitis B virus (HBV) is a DNA virus of the *Hepadnaviridae* family (Table 38–1). As the family name implies (*Hepadnaviridae* are *hepa*totrophic *DNA* *vir*uses), these DNA viruses undergo primary replication in the liver. The *Hepadnaviridae* viruses cause chronic infection resulting in chronic liver injury. These viruses also have a propensity for integration into the host genome with associated oncogenesis.[1] HBV is not cytopathic. The liver injury (like HAV infection) is immune related, and T lymphocytes are important for both the host cellular and humoral responses.[7]

Epidemiology

Hepatitis B virus infection is a public health problem worldwide because of the chronic liver disease and primary hepatocellular carcinoma (HCC) produced. There are more than 2.5 million chronic carriers of HBV in the United States alone.[11] HBV infection has extreme geographic variation in endemicity. In highly endemic areas (China, Southeast Asia, the Middle East, and parts of Africa and South America), HBV spread is predominantly by mother-to-infant perinatal transmission and child-to-child transmission.[10] High rates of chronic viral carriage and virus-associated primary HCC are seen in such areas. In parts of the world where the endemicity of HBV is relatively low (North America, Australia, Western Europe, and temperate South America), the chronic viral carriage rate is correspondingly low and mother-to-infant transmission is relatively uncommon. Rather, HBV transmission occurs either through intimate contact or by the parenteral route. High-risk groups in these areas include IV drug abusers, multitransfused patients, health care providers, male homosexuals, heterosexual partners of HBV-infected people, and heterosexual partners of human immunodeficiency virus (HIV)-infected individuals.[1] Transmission of HBV in the United States occurs predominantly through contact with infected blood products or body secretions (e.g., saliva, vaginal fluids, semen). The routine practice of screening blood donors for HBsAg has essentially eliminated hepatitis B as a cause of posttransfusion hepatitis. However, products or concentrates of blood such as clotting factors can remain infective despite prescreening for HBsAg. Excluding cases resulting from clotting factor concentrates, most blood-borne HBV transmissions are due to accidental inoculation by health care workers and to the sharing of needles by IV drug abusers (percutaneous exposure).[1]

The chief obstacles to eradication of hepatitis B include the carrier state and infections in utero, which are not preventable.

Pathogenesis

Although HBV has been completely characterized and much is known about the biologic features of HBV infection, little is known about the mechanisms responsible for virus hepatocyte uptake, induction of viral replication, hepatocyte injury, persistent infection, or HBV-associated oncogenesis.[7]

Once the HBV gains access to the vascular compartment, the virus migrates to the liver, where primary replication occurs. The incubation period of HBV of 1 to 6 months is much longer than HAV.[1] HBV replication occurs in liver cell nuclei, with HBsAg produced in the cell cytoplasm and expressed on the cell surface. These particles are also found circulating in the plasma of patients with acute HBV, the chronic carrier state, and chronic HBV infection.[1]

Antibody to HBsAg (anti-HBs) is initially detected as the concentration of HBsAg in plasma wanes. However, identification of HBsAg/anti-HBs immune complexes suggests that the surface antibody response occurs much earlier than detected by standard serologic assays.

Additional antibodies directed against other HBV antigens are found in plasma of individuals with acute HBV infection (Table 38–2). Anti-HBc, the antibody directed against the inner core viral antigen present in hepatocyte nuclei (therefore, not a circulating plasma antigen), is first detected shortly after the onset of acute cellular injury. Anti-HBc is initially of the IgM class and, when detectable, signifies acute HBV infection. IgG-class anti-HBc antibodies become detectable several months following the acute HBV infection and persist along with HBs antibody for life. Therefore, the presence of plasma anti-HBc IgG-class antibodies signifies prior infection (Table 38–2).[7]

HBe antigen is a protein subunit of the viral core detected in plasma immediately prior to or at the onset of hepatocyte injury and correlates with a high degree of infectivity. In contrast, the presence of HBe antibody correlates with a very low degree of infectivity and portends a complete recovery. The HBe antibody becomes detectable either immediately after the peak of liver injury or in early convalescence, and may persist for years.[12]

Clinical Presentation

The clinical course of HBV infection and the associated clinical features cannot be differentiated from other types of viral hepatitis based on symptoms. A wide range of disease expression from asymptomatic infection to fulminant hepatitis occurs. In the typical case of acute HBV infection, the incubation period is followed by a symptomatic prodromal phase consisting of malaise, fatigue, weakness, anorexia, myalgias, and arthralgias. Jaundice develops in about one-third of patients as liver cell destruction increases. Jaundice may persist for several weeks.[1,4]

Clinical manifestations of HBV infection are age dependent. For example, newborns infected with HBV are generally asymptomatic, while about one-third of adult patients with acute HBV infection have symptoms. Of the approximately 65% of adults with subclinical infection, most recover completely. Twenty-five percent have symptomatic illness with jaundice, and 1% to 2% (of these 25%) develop fulminant hepatic failure during the acute illness.[4] Approximately 10% of adult patients develop chronic or persistent infection. Chronicity is more likely to occur in patients with mild, anicteric forms of acute hepatitis, and is much more likely to occur when the infection is acquired as a newborn or infant.[1,4] Over a period of years, about 25% of adults with chronic HBV infection develop chronic active hepatitis (CAH), and a smaller percentage progress to cirrhosis.[10] Immunosuppression with HIV results in more severe clinical disease with HBV infection, a higher incidence of both chronic HBV carriers and chronic hepatitis B, and reactivation of HBV in late stages of HIV.[13]

Extrahepatic manifestations such as neuropathies, glomerulonephritis, pancreatitis, and hematopoietic stem cell suppression (aplastic anemia, thrombocytopenia) are occasionally seen.[4,14] In chronic hepatitis B, "essential" mixed cryoglobulinemia (presence of abnormal plasma proteins of different types that precipitate or crystallize when cooled), polyarteritis nodosa (inflammation and necrosis of segments of medium-sized or small arteries), and other vasculitis-like lesions have been described.[14] Formerly it was thought that extrahepatic disease was mediated by circulating immune complexes. However, there is evidence now that these clinical symptoms are a direct consequence of the HBV infection.[15] In addition, hemolytic uremic syndrome, thrombotic thrombocytopenic purpura, Raynaud syndrome, Schönlein–Henoch purpura (an eruption of hemorrhaging into the skin that is nonthrombocytopenic; associated with joint pains or swelling and bleeding from the GI tract, as well as other manifestations), infantile papular acrodermatitis (an inflammatory papular eruption of the skin of the extremities of infants), Guillain–Barré syn-

TABLE 38–2. Interpretation of the Laboratory Profile in Hepatitis B Infection

Pattern	Infectious Patient	HBsAg	HBeAg	Anti-HBc Total	Anti-HBc IgM	anti-HBe	anti-HBs
Not infected/early incubation	No	–	–	–	–	–	–
Early acute HBV infection	Yes	+	–	–	–	–	–
Acute HBV infection	Yes	+	+	+	+	–	–
Chronic HBV infection[a]	Yes	+	±	+	–	–	–
Resolved infection	No	–	–	+	–	+	+
"Window" period following acute HBV infection	No	–	–	+	+	+	–

[a]Patient should be evaluated for complications of chronic infection such as cirrhosis and HCC.
From Ref. 4.

drome, meningitis, myelitis, and meningoencephalomyelitis have all been reported.

HBV has four potential gene regions: the nucleocapsid region (HBcAg and HBeAg), the envelope region (HBsAg), the P region (DNA polymerase), and the poorly understood X region.[6] In typical acute HBV infection, serologic markers proceed in sequence from the development of HBsAg followed by HBeAg (30 to 60 days prior to onset of clinical symptoms) through to the appearance of anti-HBs in late convalescence (Table 38–2). The presence of anti-HBs without HBsAg usually indicates protective immunity (Table 38–2).

Acute HBV infection is diagnosed by the presence of anti-HBc IgM (Table 38–2). There are periods during the course of HBV infection when specific serologic markers are absent; the lack of such markers complicates diagnosis of the acute infection. These serologic "window" periods can be seen in the early incubation phase when HBsAg and HBeAg are not detectable despite the presence of ongoing viral replication, and early in convalescence when these two antigens are cleared prior to the appearance of anti-HBs antibody. Markers of HBV replication (HBV DNA and DNA polymerase) are sensitive indicators.

Three other antigen markers of HBV infection include pre-S1, pre-S2 for the envelope, and the functional X protein.[16] When monitored, presence of the pre-S1 antigen (pre-S1 Ag) correlates with viral replication. Pre-S1 Ag, HBV DNA, and anti-HBc IgM help guide interferon (IFN) therapy.

Anti-HBc IgG confirms current (or implies previous) HBV infection (Table 38–2). The finding of anti-HBc IgG, without other HBV markers, indicates one of four things: (1) the patient is in the window phase of acute HBV infection; (2) the duration of anti-HBc exceeds that of anti-HBs in a resolved infection; (3) the patient has chronic HBV infection in which HBsAg is produced at levels below the detectable limit; or (4) it is falsely positive.[10]

HEPATITIS C VIRUS

Hepatitis C virus (HCV) is a single-stranded RNA virus of the *Flaviviridae* family that accounts for most cases of what was previously termed non-A, non-B hepatitis (NANBH).[17,18] At least six major genotypes have been identified with considerable genetic and immunogenic variability.[19] The genotypes are identified by number (1 through 6) and subtypes by letter (1a, 1b, and so forth).[20] The most common HCV genotype in the United States is genotype 1 (approximately 70% of cases), with type 1a being more frequent than type 1b.[20] Genotypes 1a and 1b correlate with more severe liver chronic disease and lower rates of response to interferon therapy.[20]

The virus is constantly undergoing mutation. Consequently, in any one host, the virus actually is a series of "quasispecies," each being slightly different from the primary genotype (genetic heterogeneity). As a result, the mutant species escape the neutralizing antibodies the host develops. Antibodies to one genotype confer no resistance to another genotype. In this way, HCV is able to escape immune surveillance and establish persistent infection more readily. These characteristics of the hepatitis C virus contribute to poor interferon (IFN) response and complicate vaccine development.

EPIDEMIOLOGY

Hepatitis C virus is found worldwide and is transmitted primarily through contaminated blood products and less effectively through bodily secretions. The Centers for Disease Control and Prevention (CDC) estimates that 4 million Americans carry the hepatitis C virus. Patients at risk for HCV infection in the United States include those who receive blood products, intravenous drug users, and health care workers. Together these three groups account for approximately 41% to 62% of cases of HCV.[10] HCV antibodies are detected in 85% to 90% of patients with post-transfusion hepatitis, 70% of patients with a history of IV drug abuse and who test positive for HIV, 30% to 50% of patients with sporadic NANBH, 20% of patients undergoing hemodialysis, and up to 75% of patients with primary HCC.[21] Forty to 50 percent of all cases of hepatitis C report no known risk factors, and the mechanism(s) of transmission for these sporadically occurring cases is not clear.[19] However, other potential methods of transmitting HCV infection include intranasal cocaine use, tattooing, body-piercing, and contact with other instruments capable of penetrating the skin or mucous membranes, such as shared contaminated razors. Permucosal, sexual, and maternal–neonatal transmission rates of HCV are very low.[10,11] Sexual transmission rates are much less for HCV than for HBV or HIV, but transmission is facilitated by concomitant HIV infection.[10,11,19,22] Spouses of patients with HCV infection and chronic liver disease are at increased risk of acquiring HCV. The risk is proportional to the length of the marriage.[19,22]

PATHOGENESIS

The immunopathogenesis of liver damage due to HCV infection is poorly understood. Possible mechanisms of liver damage include direct cytopathic effect, the formation of immune complexes, and cytotoxic T-cell response. The liver injury with HCV infection most closely resembles that of a cytopathic virus. For example, the general histologic picture of chronic hepatitis C is predominant lobular hepatitis with scarce periportal piecemeal necrosis. There may be immune-mediated features as well.[22] Additionally, the predominant inflammatory cell type found in liver biopsies from patients with acute and chronic hepatitis are $CD8^+$ T lymphocytes.

HCV persists in the majority of infected patients, due to the ability of the virus to replicate with a high degree of mutation.[19]

Clinical Presentation

Acute hepatitis C is clinically indistinguishable from other types of viral hepatitis. The incubation period for HCV ranges from 15 to 150 days (mean, 50 days).[1,19,21] The clinical course is generally mild with less than 25% of patients developing jaundice. Major complaints are frequently limited to fatigue and malaise.[19] Similar to other types of viral hepatitis, the hepatic transaminase values in HCV hepatitis vary from mildly to markedly elevated. Unlike the other types, HCV infections characteristically demonstrate a pattern of widely fluctuating enzyme values over the course of the infection.[21] Development of fulminant disease is rare.[19,22] Infection with HIV results in more severe clinical disease with HCV infection, as does chronic alcohol consumption.[11,22]

An important feature of this form of hepatitis is that up to 90% of cases progress to persistent infection.[7,19] Of those patients who are persistently infected, 60% to 80% will eventually develop chronic hepatitis. Others can have infection without disease. Within 5 years after infection, 30% to 35% develop CAH; 20% to 33% of these patients will progress to cirrhosis.[10,22] Others will eventually develop cirrhosis and hepatic failure after 10 to 20 years (or longer) of indolent, asymptomatic infection. Chronic HCV infection-related cirrhosis is an etiologic factor in the development of HCC.[21]

In general, the extent of liver damage evident on liver biopsy is far greater than the degree of elevation of serum enzymes would lead one to believe. The disease progresses insidiously with continuing damage to the liver in those patients who develop chronic infection with the virus.

Extrahepatic manifestations occasionally occur with hepatitis C. They include polyarteritis nodosa, erythema multiforme, thrombocytopenia, serum sickness, rash, blood dyscrasias, thyroid abnormalities, cryoglobulinemia with cutaneous vasculitis, arthralgia, and glomerulonephritis.[22] Diagnosis of acute HCV depends on clinical symptoms and sequential monitoring of liver transaminase levels until the HCV antibody becomes positive. Seroconversion to anti-HCV appears from 4 to 8 weeks following initial exposure.[19,22]

Serologic testing for HCV antibodies by enzyme immunoassay (EIA or ELISA) is the primary method of diagnosis. The current immunoassay (ELISA II, Ortho Diagnostics, Raritan, NJ) contains a number of viral antigens and is both more sensitive and specific than previous serologic tests. The recombinant immunoblot assay (RIBA II) is used as a supplemental test to confirm ELISA II results because of its high specificity and positive predictive value for HCV.[10]

Two distinct techniques for HCV RNA detection are available to determine HCV RNA in serum or blood: polymerase chain reaction (PCR; Monitor, Roche; Amplicor HCV, Roche) and branched-chain DNA (bDNA; Quantiplex HCV RNA, Chiron).[23] The sensitivity of the quantitative PCR is greater than that of the bDNA assay. HCV RNA can be detected by PCR as early as 1 to 2 weeks after infection.[10,19] Although PCR is very sensitive, there is substantial variability in assays used by different testing laboratories. PCR is usually reserved as a confirmatory test in patients whose immunoassays are indeterminate, to monitor perinatal transmission, to evaluate patients with chronic hepatitis with features of autoimmunity who may have a false-positive serologic test, or to monitor response to antiviral therapy.[19]

Viral RNA remains positive and histologic progression continues in those who develop chronic infection with HCV. However, serum aminotransferase levels can fluctuate, or even normalize, confounding the diagnosis of chronic HCV infection.[19] To assess chronic HCV, liver biopsy is the only reliable indicator of disease progression. It is not uncommon for a patient to present to a physician with cirrhosis or portal hypertension secondary to HCV infection that occurred years to decades prior, yet to have had few or no clinical signs or symptoms during the intervening years.

HEPATITIS DELTA VIRUS

The hepatitis delta virus (HDV), first identified in 1977, is a defective RNA virus that requires the presence of HBV to cause infection. Infection with HDV usually worsens the course of the HBV-infected patient. HDV is composed of a single strand of RNA, an internal protein (the delta antigen), and an outer coat of HBsAg. Serologic tests for detection of serum antibodies to the delta antigen (anti-HDV) are useful in diagnosing acute hepatitis and chronic infection.[1,11]

Epidemiology

Hepatitis delta virus parallels the transmission patterns and areas of endemicity of HBV, with only a few differences. These differences include lower endemicity rates of HDV in East and Southeast Asia and lower incidence rates in homosexual males. Three forms of HDV infection have been identified and are designated acute HDV–HBV coinfection, acute HDV superinfection, and HDV chronic infection. Coinfection describes simultaneous infection with both HBV and HDV, while superinfection occurs when HDV is transmitted after the patient has been exposed to HBV.[1,11] Chronic infection and liver disease occur in approximately 5% of cases of acute HDV–HBV coinfection, but in over 90% of cases of HDV superinfection.[10,11]

HDV is primarily transmitted by exposure to infected blood. Before screening for HDV was developed, a high percentage of HBV-infected hemophiliacs acquired HDV through receipt of contaminated blood products.[11] Currently, parenteral drug use is the most common risk factor for HDV in the United States.[1,9] It has been estimated that 20% to 50% of HBV-infected IV drug users are also infected with HDV.[9] Sexual transmission of HDV occurs less frequently than with HBV, and perinatal transmission appears to be rare.[11]

Clinical Presentation

Because of the dependence of HDV on HBV for its infectivity, the natural course of HDV coinfection and superinfection differs significantly. In coinfection, the acute delta hepatitis is almost always self-limited, although fulminant hepatitis is reported to occur more frequently with HDV coinfection than with HBV alone. The clinical course may begin with an initial, relatively mild HBV phase followed by a more severe HDV phase. Similar to HBV, replication of the delta virus occurs in the liver. Unlike the typical HBV infection, a biphasic rise in liver transaminase levels may be seen, the first peak attributable to HBV and the second to HDV. The disappearance of HBsAg from serum heralds resolution of both infections and development of specific antibodies to both agents. Lasting immunity to both viruses is provided by the antibodies to HBsAg.[11]

In HDV superinfection, delta viral replication occurs rapidly due to the persistent HBV infection, providing a ready supply of HBsAg. Liver injury and clinical symptoms appear quickly and may be severe, leading to a fulminant course. Rapid clinical decompensation in a previously stable HBV carrier should raise the possibility of HDV superinfection. Over 70% of these patients develop chronic liver disease, which frequently results in progression to cirrhosis.[11,24]

The diagnosis of HDV infection depends on clinical suspicion, elevated hepatic aminotransferases, and serologic evidence of HBV and HDV infection. In acute superinfection of a chronic HBV carrier, markers for acute HBV are negative. HBsAg, anti-HBc IgG, HDVAg, and anti-HDV IgM are usually present. In acute coinfection, HDVAg, anti-HDV IgM, and anti-HBc IgM are usually present. Anti-HDV IgG follows. HDV RNA may be detected by PCR in either serum or in liver tissue. Currently, only a test for total anti-HDV is commercially available.[1]

The mortality rate in acute delta hepatitis is 2% to 20%. Patients with superinfection in whom both viruses are simultaneously replicating may rapidly develop severe liver disease and progress to liver failure within 2 years.[11]

HEPATITIS E VIRUS

During the past century, enterically transmitted, waterborne hepatitis has caused major epidemics in undeveloped countries. These epidemics, originally attributed to HAV, were later found to be serologically unrelated to HAV infection.[25] This agent was designated hepatitis E virus (HEV), in part to identify it as the agent responsible for enterically transmitted hepatitis epidemics (enterically transmitted non-A, non-B hepatitis [NANBH]).[1,21]

Epidemiology

Hepatitis E virus is endemic in Africa, Southeast and Central Asia, Mexico, and Central and South America. Many sporadic cases of acute hepatitis in areas endemic for HEV are also attributed to HEV. To date, Western travelers to endemic areas provide the reported cases of HEV in developed countries.[1,21,26]

Clinical Presentation

Although serologically distinct, HEV infection is similar to HAV infection. The similar features include enteric transmission, ability to cause epidemics, existence of areas of endemicity relating to poor sanitary conditions, occurrence of primary viral replication in hepatocyte cytoplasm, heavy shedding of viral particles into bile and feces, similarity of incubation period and clinical course, and lack of demonstrated chronic persistent viral infection.[21] HEV is spread through the fecal–oral route. Contaminated drinking water is the most common vehicle of transmission.[26] The incubation period ranges from 2 to 9 weeks, with a mean of 45 days.[26] Viremia and fecal shedding occur at onset of clinical illness, peak at the onset of transaminitis, and persist for more than 2 weeks.[7,25,27] The presence of viremia raises the possibility of parenteral transmission of HEV, though no cases have been documented.[27] Vertical transmission from mother to fetus has been reported, however. HEV acquired during pregnancy has resulted in spontaneous abortion or birth of infants with clinical markers of acute hepatitis.[25] Infection with HEV is usually self-limited and follows a benign course, except in pregnant women; women who contract HEV during the third trimester are at considerable risk for developing fulminant hepatitis, with a mortality rate exceeding 15%.[21,26]

The diagnosis is made on clinical grounds in conjunction with serologic tests. Recently, ELISA tests have been developed to detect anti-HEV IgM and IgG; in addition, virus can be detected in blood and stool using PCR.[27] Antibodies may not be detected in all patients, suggesting either that current assays are not sensitive enough to detect antibodies to variant virus or that an antibody response is not necessary for resolution of acute infection.[27] Anti-HEV IgG has been reported to persist for at least 2 years following initial infection and appears to be protective against subsequent infection with HEV.[28]

HEPATITIS F VIRUS

A virus designated as hepatitis F was isolated from the stool of a patient with hepatitis; however, this virus has not been isolated since, and its role in disease remains unclear.[29]

HEPATITIS G VIRUS

Recently, new blood-borne viruses were discovered simultaneously by two investigators and named hepatitis GB virus C (HGBV-C) and hepatitis G virus (HGV). These viruses were later determined to be two isolates of the same single-stranded RNA virus, were identified as a member of the *Flaviviridae* family, and are now referred to as HGV.[30] HGV RNA may be detected in serum using PCR. Much about this virus remains unknown. The primary route of transmission is parenteral. The virus is often present in injection drug users, hemophiliacs, and patients on hemodialysis. There is also evidence of both perinatal and sexual transmission.[31–34] The site of viral replication has not been identified.

HGV can cause persistent infection and viremia. The virus has been detected in at least 2% of blood donors in the United States, an incidence exceeding that of either HBV or HCV, and in 14% to 52% of patients with other types of hepatitis.[31,35] Infection with HGV is unaccompanied by evidence of hepatitis or hepatocellular injury. In addition, the presence of HGV does not appear to alter the clinical course of hepatitis A, B, or C.[31] The prevailing theory is that HGV does not cause clinical disease, but may be present in patients with unexplained hepatitis due to yet-unidentified non-A through E viruses.[30,35] Whether HGV actually is a hepatotrophic virus is unclear.

▶ TREATMENT: Acute Viral Hepatitis

Management of acute viral hepatitis is primarily supportive. General measures include a healthy diet, rest, maintaining fluid balance, and avoiding hepatotoxic drugs and alcohol.[14] Management includes monitoring for development of chronic liver disease and preventing disease spread. Treatments that offer no benefit include special diets, corticosteroids, and antiemetics. Vitamin K is recommended only if the patient has a prolonged prothrombin time. Hospitalization is necessary only for those who have prolonged vomiting, coagulation defects, or fulminant hepatitis.[14]

Preliminary trials and case reports of the use of IFN-α and IFN-β as therapy in acute HBV and HCV infections report promising results.[36,37] Because not all studies have demonstrated IFN to be useful, further studies are ongoing to define the place of IFN in acute hepatitis treatment. If results from these studies demonstrate that a lower rate of chronicity results when treatment is initiated during the acute phase of infection, early identification and treatment could become the primary focus. This would apply to only a few patients, however, because acute HCV infection related to blood transfusion is declining, and most cases of acute community-acquired HCV infection are asymptomatic.[19]

FULMINANT HEPATITIS

Liver injury that results in fulminant hepatic necrosis and hepatic failure is relatively rare. When it occurs, death results in a few days or weeks in nearly 80% of cases.[14,38] Any potential hepatotoxic agent can be responsible, although the most frequent cause is viral hepatitis (70%), especially HBV.[38] In the United States, fulminant hepatitis is mainly due to HBV with or without HDV, occasionally HAV, and only rarely HCV.[38] Acute hepatitis B leads to acute liver failure in up to 1% of patients.[39]

Although patients with acute HBV usually are viremic for weeks, many of those who develop liver failure become seronegative for HBsAg within a few days.[39] This rapid viral clearance is secondary to a massive immune response by the infected patient. Patients with fulminant hepatic necrosis typically develop signs and symptoms of viral hepatitis, and then rapidly develop evidence of hepatic failure. The clinical syndrome is usually a 1- to 3-week course of hepatic failure and encephalopathy with coma developing within 8 weeks of the onset of acute hepatitis.[14] Hyperexcitability, insomnia, somnolence, irritability, and impaired mental status are evidence of impending hepatic failure in patients with acute hepatitis.[14] Particularly ominous signs include a rapid decrease in liver size, a rapid decline in aminotransferase levels, prolonged prothrombin time, and hypoglycemia.[14] Manifestations of hepatic failure include metabolic encephalopathy, coma, coagulation defects, ascites, and edema. In fulminant liver failure, complications include GI hemorrhage, sepsis, cerebral edema, renal failure, lactic acidosis, and disseminated coagulopathy, with death resulting from bleeding, cerebral edema, hypoglycemia, infection, and/or multisystem organ failure.[14,38]

There is no specific treatment for fulminant hepatic failure. Management of fulminant hepatitis focuses on recognition, prevention of complications, and aggressive management of complications. Measures that improve survival of patients include intensive supportive care plus early referral for liver transplantation.[38,40] Fresh frozen plasma should be administered for bleeding, H_2-blocker therapy should be given to prevent GI bleeding, and aggressive antibiotic therapy should be used for infections. Cerebral edema occurs in the majority of cases that progress to grade IV encephalopathy, and is the leading cause of death in these patients.[39]

Management includes intracranial pressure monitoring and administration of mannitol (0.3 to 0.4 g/kg body weight as a 20% solution) to decrease intracranial pressure.[14,39] Dexamethasone and hyperventilation are of little value in cerebral edema related to acute liver failure.[39] Pentobarbital will lower intracranial pressure, but also lowers systemic blood pressure.[39] For further information on therapy and dosing of these drugs, the reader is referred to the corresponding topics in appropriate chapters of this book.

Urgent liver transplantation is the therapy of choice for most patients with fulminant hepatic failure.[40] Patients who could potentially be candidates for liver transplantation should be transferred at the first sign of altered mentation, because these patients can worsen very rapidly. Survival rates with liver transplantation for fulminant hepatitis approach 55% to 75%.[14]

Patients do not benefit from administration of corticosteroids, heparin, insulin, or glucagon.[39] Antiviral therapy would not be expected to help because viral replication in fulminant hepatitis is low (or has ceased) by the time the patient is admitted to the hospital. However, agents such as foscarnet have been tried in uncontrolled studies with apparent improvement in survival. Some investigators have postulated that the beneficial effect of foscarnet may have been due to its immunomodulatory effects and not its antiviral activity.[41] This theory is supported by a report of successful treatment of fulminant hepatitis with a combination of interferon and cyclosporine A.[42] Other treatments that do not improve survival (if liver transplantation is not done) include plasmapheresis, peritoneal dialysis, cross-circulation with nonhuman primate livers, extracorporeal liver perfusion, plasma perfusion over sorbents, and total body washout.[14]

CHRONIC VIRAL HEPATITIS

Chronic viral hepatitis is the chief cause of chronic liver disease, cirrhosis, hepatic failure and hepatocellular carcinoma (HCC) throughout the world.[43] It is also the most common reason for liver transplantation.[43]

Chronic viral hepatitis describes continuation of the hepatic necroinflammatory process 6 months or more beyond the onset of the acute illness. Failure to clear viral antigen from the serum within 6 months of acute infection indicates ongoing viral replication, persistent infection, and inflammation with resulting liver cell injury. In hepatitis B infection, subsequent clearance of serum HBsAg may occur at a rate of 1% per year. The spontaneous clearance rate of viral antigen from serum in patients with chronic HCV is extremely low. The clinical findings, course, and histologic features are similar in all patients with chronic hepatitis regardless of etiology.

EPIDEMIOLOGY

Sixty to 80% of all cases of chronic hepatitis are related to HBV or HCV infection.[5] Other causes include such varied entities as chronic biliary cirrhosis and alcoholic hepatitis. Worldwide, chronic infection with hepatitis B is the most common, while in the United States, the majority of chronic hepatitis cases are caused by HCV. Five to ten percent of the cases of chronic liver disease and cirrhosis in the United States are secondary to chronic HBV.[43]

The principal reservoir of HBV for infection of others is the chronically infected individual. HBV carriers have a relative risk of acquiring HCC that is more than 100-fold that of noncarriers. Furthermore, 40% of male HBV carriers die of causes related to their liver disease. The Centers for Disease Control and Prevention (CDC) estimates that 5000 people die yearly in the United States as a consequence of acute and chronic HBV infections.

The primary determinant of chronicity with HBV infection is age when exposed: HBV causes chronic infection in up to 90% of infected neonates, 20% to 50% of infected children under 6 years of age, and 6% to 10% of infected adults.[1,11] Persistent HBsAg is more common in males and neonates.

Chronic HBV is more likely to occur in individuals with antecedent episodes of mild, anicteric acute hepatitis, suggesting that viral clearance is the ultimate result of significant hepatic necrosis. This has been demonstrated in patients with acute fulminant hepatitis. If the patient with fulminant hepatitis survives, complete recovery without development of chronic sequelae generally occurs. Another important factor in determining chronicity is host immune competence. Persistent infection is more common in immunologically compromised individuals. No specific pattern of antibody response in acute HCV has been linked with chronic infection.[7]

Over 80% of those infected with HCV develop chronic disease. Chronic hepatitis C is often diagnosed 10 or more years after acute illness. More than 20% of those with chronic hepatitis C have a low-grade, smoldering progression to cirrhosis, with potential for end-stage liver disease and/or HCC. Cirrhosis and HCC occur more than 20 years and 25 to 30 years after diagnosis, respectively. The three factors that contribute to the role of HCV as a major cause of chronic liver disease include the high rate at which individuals develop chronic hepatitis, the high rate at which infected persons develop persistent infections (> 85%) even in the absence of biochemical evidence of liver disease, and the lack of an effective protective antibody (which prevents the development of a vaccine or adequate postexposure prophylaxis).

PATHOPHYSIOLOGY

The host immune response is responsible for the persistence of HBV infection in healthy carriers and the hepatocyte damage in CAH. A weak cell-mediated immune response is present in these patients. In healthy carriers, an absent or poor cell-mediated response results in persistent viral replication but only minimal liver damage. As previously stated, viral clearance is dependent on destruction and elimination of infected hepatocytes. Thus, a poor host immune response ensures persistent viral replication. Healthy carriers have high titers of serum HBsAg and correspondingly high HBsAg concentrations within infected hepatocytes.

Patients with chronic HBV infection are deficient in producing, or responding to, IFN, which is needed to stimulate production of HLA class I protein. This lack of HLA class I protein expression on the hepatocyte membrane results in incomplete direction of the lymphocyte to the target infected cell.

A poor immune response may also produce a smoldering inflammatory form of hepatic injury as seen in chronic active hepatitis (CAH). Although the host immune response is capable of destroying some infected hepatocytes, such a response is incapable of eliminating the virus entirely. The result is persistent viral replication and continued stimulation of the host immune system. If persistent viral replication and subsequent hepatocyte inflammatory destruction continue, the number of functioning hepatocytes gradually decreases over time, and fibrosis resulting from cellular repair mechanisms distorts the basic cellular architecture. Hepatic nodules are formed. When widespread, the hepatic fibrosis with nodule formation is termed cirrhosis. The consequences of cirrhosis do not differ with regard to initial etiologies and include portal hypertension and ascites.

In addition to cirrhosis, another long-term complication of chronic HBV, HCV, and delta hepatitis infections is primary HCC. The exact mechanism of action of these viruses in the development of HCC is not clear. Worldwide, HBV is the most important etiologic factor in the development of HCC.

CLINICAL PRESENTATION

The spectrum of clinical symptoms, course, and histologic features is broad in chronic hepatitis B. "Healthy" carriers exhibit no symptoms, have normal or near normal liver transaminase values, and minimal nonspecific histologic abnormalities. Most of these carriers are HBeAg negative and anti-HBe positive, and do not develop chronic active hepatitis or cirrhosis. In contrast to the healthy carriers, chronic HBsAg carriers with markers of ongoing viral replication (HBcAb IgM, HBeAg, and HBV DNA) display persistent hepatic injury.

Males predominate (80%) with chronic hepatitis and the mean age at presentation is greater than 30 years. Unlike acute hepatitis, physical symptoms do not correlate well with the severity of liver injury. Many patients are asymptomatic and are diagnosed only after elevated serum liver transaminases and/or serum HBsAg are found. An additional group of patients do not present for medical care until they experience a complication of chronic hepatitis or cirrhosis such as ascites or esophageal variceal bleeding.

Aminotransferase levels in patients with chronic HBV infection can be minimally elevated or normal. The extent of elevation correlates roughly with the extent of active inflammation. When a relatively asymptomatic carrier of HBV experiences an acute exacerbation of hepatitis, then several causes must be considered. These include superinfection with another virus, spontaneous reactivation of hepatitis B, or clearance of the hepatitis B e-antigen. In chronic hepatitis B, markers that are present include HBsAg, HBV DNA, pre-S1 Ag, pre-S2 Ag, and anti-HBs (see Table 38–2). HBeAg can be positive or negative, depending on the virus variant. HBeAg is lost spontaneously at the rate of 7% to 20% per year.

In chronic hepatitis C, there is frequently little clinical evidence that the disease is progressing. The patient is asymptomatic, yet liver biopsy demonstrates ongoing liver injury and progressive histologic changes. Serum enzymes can be normal or only mildly elevated. Unfortunately, the patient can be on an insidious course that progresses to complications after a period of years to decades. Extra vigilance is important in the patient with hepatitis C to assess whether "silent" progression is occurring.

In either chronic HBV or chronic HCV, if the patient is symptomatic, fatigue, malaise, anorexia, and weight loss are common. Many patients have a history of jaundice. On physical examination, hepatomegaly is usually present, but the stigmata of chronic liver disease (spider nevi, splenomegaly, palmar erythema, testicular atrophy, caput medusa, female escutcheon) are generally absent until late in the disease course. Mild but persistent elevations of the serum aminotransferases, bilirubin, and gamma globulin levels are most commonly seen.

Both chronic HBV and chronic HCV are associated with extrahepatic syndromes. These include mixed cryoglobulinemia, polyarteritis nodosa, and a sicca-like syndrome that resembles Sjögren's syndrome. HBV infection is also occasionally associated with renal failure. Whether this is also true for HCV is not known.

In a patient with a history of blood transfusion, chronically elevated aminotransferase levels, a positive ELISA II for anti-HCV and CAH on liver biopsy, the diagnosis of chronic HCV is easily made. For patients without risk factors, other potential causes must be ruled out before making the diagnosis of chronic HCV. Serum aminotransferase levels correlate poorly with the histologic extent of disease, and liver biopsy provides diagnostic and prognostic information. Most patients with positive anti-HCV will have chronic hepatitis C, even if the aminotransferase levels are normal.

In patients with chronic viral hepatitis, the presence of ongoing viral replication is the most important factor in evaluating disease progression. However, the prognosis for a patient with chronic viral hepatitis is indicated by the degree of liver damage noted on liver biopsy. The typical histologic features are the presence of chronic inflammatory cells within portal triads, hepatocellular necrosis, and a variable degree of fibrosis. The severity of these histologic features varies within regions of the involved liver and among individual patients.

In an attempt to standardize the histologic features and to provide prognostic information, a classification scheme was developed. This scheme divides chronic hepatitis into two categories: chronic persistent hepatitis (CPH, good prognosis, 97% 5-year survival) and CAH (86% 5-year survival without cirrhosis), which can proceed to further hepatic damage and eventually cirrhosis (55% 5-year survival).[10,44] CAH is divided into mild and severe forms. A third category, chronic lobular hepatitis, describes the histologic picture of persistent acute hepatitis of greater than 3 months' duration; like CPH, this histologic diagnosis carries a good prognosis.

Prognosis in chronic HCV correlates with histologic findings. Recently, investigations into the HCV genotype have suggested that the genotype has important implications for benign or severe disease. Further information on the relationship of genotype to long-term prognosis is awaited.

▶ TREATMENT: Chronic Viral Hepatitis

DESIRED OUTCOME

The goal of treatment is to prevent progression to end-stage liver disease by eradicating the HBV or HCV early in the course of disease. Effective treatment of chronic viral hepatitis should decrease morbidity and mortality and prevent infected patients from serving as reservoirs of infection. Ideal treatment of chronic hepatitis would permanently inhibit viral replication, prevent cirrhosis, avert incorporation of the viral genome (for HBV), stop progression of disease, and eliminate the virus entirely (Table 38–3).

GENERAL APPROACH TO TREATMENT

General therapeutic measures in patients with compensated chronic hepatitis include exercise as tolerated, avoidance of potentially hepatotoxic drugs and chemicals (such as alcohol), and a healthy diet. Patients should not donate blood. Serum monitoring for exacerbations of disease should be done periodically. For patients with chronic HBV, monitoring should also be done for spontaneous seroconversion. Patients with chronic HCV should be vaccinated against hepatitis A and hepatitis B. Sexual partners and children of patients with chronic HBV should be vaccinated against hepatitis B.

TABLE 38–3. Goals of Therapy in Patients With Chronic Hepatitis B and Chronic Hepatitis C

Lose HBV DNA (lose HBV replication)	X	
Lose HBeAg (low infectious potential)	X	
Lose of HBsAg (eradicate HBV)	X	
Lose HCV RNA (lose HCV replication)		X
Lose HCVAg (lose infectious potential)		X
Normalize aminotransferases (cease hepatic inflammation)	X	X
Improve symptoms	X	X
Decrease progression of liver disease	X	X
Reduce cirrhosis	X	X
Reduce hepatocellular carcinoma	X	X
Increase survival	X	X

Inhibition of replication of HBV by adenine arabinoside (ara-A) and interferon (IFN) was first reported in 1976.[45] IFN is now the treatment of choice for patients with chronic HBV, HCV, and HDV infection. Unfortunately, IFN therapy has limitations in management of chronic hepatitis: Only a proportion of patients respond favorably; considerably fewer have lasting response; very few are cured. A need remains for more effective, more widely applicable, and less costly therapy for chronic hepatitis.

PHARMACOLOGIC THERAPY

CHRONIC HBV INFECTION

The decision to treat patients with chronic hepatitis should not be made based on the presence or absence of symptoms or the degree of abnormality of biochemical tests. Activity and extent of liver disease correlate poorly with the level of serum aminotransferases or the patient's symptoms. A systematic approach to treatment should be developed.[46]

No known drug can consistently eradicate HBV. Current therapeutic options include antiviral agents and immunomodulatory agents that alter viral replication and modify the host immune response.[19] End points of therapy include normalization of serum aminotransferase levels, disappearance of HBV DNA, and improvement of liver histology. Normalization of the serum aminotransferases does not always correlate with virologic response. Measurement of serum HBV DNA levels is more reliable.

Interferons in Chronic HBV

Interferon-α is effective in relieving symptoms, halting progression, and terminating HBV replication in one-third of immunocompetent patients from Western countries.[43,47,48] Responders lose HBV DNA (disappearance of viral replication) and HBeAg, serum aminotransferases normalize, and liver histology improves.[43] In comparison, only about 12% of patients not treated with IFN have spontaneous disappearance of HBeAg from serum.[43] Clearance of HBsAg (termination of the HBV carrier state) occurs in 10% to 15% of responders during the first year after completion of therapy, but with longer follow-up, more responders lose HBsAg and develop anti-HBs.[47,48] Delayed clearance of HBeAg occurs in some patients who remain HBV DNA negative.[48] A small percentage of responders relapse, usually within 1 year of terminating therapy. (This is in direct contrast to HCV, where approximately 50% of HCV patients who are IFN responders relapse within 1 year.) Patients infected with HBV mutants that prevent HBeAg expression are less likely to respond to IFN therapy and have a higher rate of relapse upon discontinuation of IFN.[47]

Resolution of viremia is associated with a transient exacerbation of the hepatitis, marked by a rise in serum aminotransferase levels during the second or third month of therapy. This "flare" is related to an increased host immune response caused by IFN treatment (Fig. 38–1). In the patient who responds to IFN, HBV DNA levels decrease within days of starting IFN. After 8 to 12 weeks, ALT levels increase and the patient loses HBV DNA and HBeAg. ALT levels then normalize, and the patient develops anti-HBe.[48] Without the flare, loss of viral replication rarely occurs (Fig. 38–1). In many patients who respond to IFN, HBsAg is cleared from serum, occasionally up to several years later.[49]

Effective dosing regimens of IFN in clinically stable adult patients with chronic HBV are 5 million units (MU) daily or 10 MU subcutaneously three times weekly for 4 to 6 months. IFN-α administered three times weekly is better tolerated than daily administration. One FDA-approved regimen for IFN-α-2b is 5 MU 5 days per week or 10 MU every other day for 16 weeks. Patients who should be treated with IFN are those with persistent elevations in serum aminotransferases, detectable viral and antibody markers (HBsAg, HBeAg, and HBV DNA) in serum, chronic hepatitis on liver biopsy, and compensated liver disease.[43] Predictors of good response to IFN-α (sustained loss of HBeAg and HBV DNA) in chronic HBV and chronic HCV are listed in Table 38–4.[48]

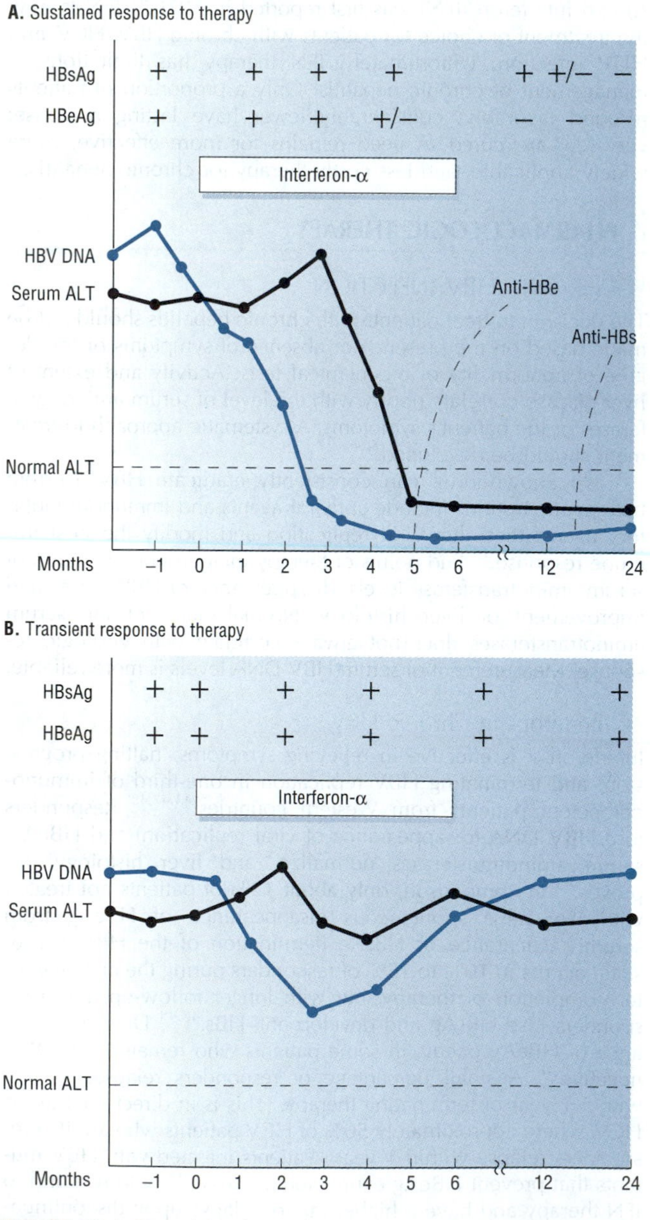

FIGURE 38–1. Typical biochemical responses to IFN-α in patients with chronic hepatitis B.

Evaluation of Therapeutic Outcomes

Vigilance for clinical and laboratory decompensation is essential. Laboratory monitoring parameters during treatment include the aminotransferases (measured at 2- to 4-week intervals), HBeAg, HBsAg, and HBV DNA (at the start of therapy, the end of therapy, and 6 months later).[43] It is important to measure the markers of chronic HBV infection (HBeAg and HBV DNA) immediately prior to initiating treatment, because a few patients with chronic HBV infection spontaneously lose HBV DNA and seroconvert each year without treatment.

The long-term effect of therapy is not well defined (probably because of the short length of time IFN has been available). Evidence is accumulating that liver disease progression is delayed or halted and HBsAg positivity and HBV DNA are lost in IFN responders.[49] In a study of 23 patients who had responded to therapy with a loss of HBsAg and improvement in serum aminotransferases, only 3 patients relapsed in 3 to 7 years of follow-up.[49] All the relapsing patients did so within the first year after discontinuing therapy. A meta-analysis of randomized, controlled trials indicated a loss of HBV DNA in 37% and a loss of HBsAg in 7.8% of IFN-treated patients.[50] Thus, termination of the HBV carrier state is possible. Data are not yet available to determine whether IFN therapy results in a decreased frequency of HCC, decreased cirrhosis, and improved survival.[48]

There is no evidence that retreating IFN nonresponders (either with the same or a higher dose) is effective. These patients should be informed of this and offered either observation or considered candidates for entry into an investigational drug trial.

Nucleoside Analogs in Chronic HBV

Lamivudine (Epivir, Glaxo Wellcome Oncology), a nucleoside analog that is a reverse transcriptase inhibitor, is not only an inhibitor of HIV-1 reverse transcriptase but also a potent inhibitor of HBV replication. Preliminary results of clinical trials show that lamivudine inhibits HBV replication in chronically HBV infected immunocompetent patients and in patients coinfected with HBV and HIV.[51,52] The mechanism of action is thought to be a specific effect of lamivudine against HBV, not an immunomodulating effect.[51]

At lamivudine doses of 100 to 300 mg/d (300 to 600 mg/d for those infected with both HBV and HIV) for 3 to 12 months, patients with chronic hepatitis B infection lose detectable levels of HBV DNA, although HBV DNA usually reappears after therapy is completed.[52,53] Less than 20% of patients have sustained suppression of HBV DNA and normalization of ALT levels, and some of these will later lose HBeAg.[52] Sustained responses are more likely in patients with low HBV DNA and high ALT levels prior to therapy. Despite the fact that lamivudine has no known direct immune system effects, lamivudine responders sometimes have elevations in ALT during or after therapy, followed by suppression of HBV DNA.[52]

Advantages of lamivudine include oral administration and a less toxic adverse effect profile than IFN. Serious side effects occur in approximately 5% of patients.[53] Adverse effects include anemia, nausea, neuropathy, elevated lipases, and increased liver enzymes.[53] Chronic lamivudine therapy has been suggested. Resistance of the hepatitis B virus to lamivudine has been reported in both HIV-infected patients and in patients given lamivudine to prevent recurrent infection after orthotopic liver transplantation.

Lamivudine could have a place in therapy for individuals who are unlikely to respond to IFN, patients with decompensated cirrhosis awaiting liver transplantation, and to prevent posttrans-

TABLE 38–4. Predictors of Good Response to Interferon Therapy

Chronic Hepatitis B	Chronic Hepatitis C
Short duration of infection[a]	Short duration of infection
Low pretreatment HBV DNA (< 100 pg/mL)	Low pretreatment HCV RNA
High pretreatment aminotransferases	Absence of cirrhosis or minimal amounts of hepatic fibrosis
Active histologic changes (inflammation and necrosis) and fibrosis	Mild inflammation; inflammation limited to portal tracts
Female gender	Genotype other than 1 or absence of a high degree of genetic heterogeneity
Wild-type (HBeAg-positive) virus	Young age
Absence of complicating illnesses (HIV infection, renal failure)	Low hepatic iron stores
	Negative for HIV

[a]Sometimes stated as age greater than 20 when infected, or of non-Asian origin because Asians typically are infected perinatally or in early childhood.
Compiled from Refs. 19 and 43.

plant graft infection.[54,55] Lamivudine will not replace IFN in treating chronic HBV unless it is demonstrated that courses of lamivudine bring about sustained remissions in 30% to 50% of patients.[54]

Results from initial studies show that famciclovir, the oral prodrug of penciclovir (alone or in combination with other agents), decreases HBV DNA levels and is well tolerated.[56] Dosages range from 125 to 750 mg three times daily for 16 weeks.[53] Famciclovir causes a rapid, dose-dependent reduction in HBV DNA levels and serum transaminases in up to 50% of patients. Famciclovir has been preliminarily assessed in patients with chronic HBV infections and in HBV reinfections after liver transplants.

The newer nucleoside analogs have the potential to change the approach to therapy of chronic HBV from that of a limited course of IFN to long-term suppressive therapy aimed at inhibiting viral replication and ameliorating disease.[43]

Combination Therapy in Chronic HBV

In chronic HBV, regimens involving combination antiviral chemotherapy or combinations of antiviral plus immunomodulating agents (e.g., prednisone and IFN) have been studied with the hope of synergy or additive effects. In most patients there is no added benefit to corticosteroid treatment plus IFN over IFN alone. Corticosteroids lead to reduced hepatic inflammation, but also result in dramatic increases in viral replication, and can contribute to decompensation in some patients. In addition, withdrawal of the steroids causes a flare in hepatitis disease activity. However, for certain patients (Chinese patients and those patients with low pretreatment ALT and low levels of HBV DNA), corticosteroids act as immunologic primers to induce clearance of HBeAg and, in some cases, HBsAg.[53] These patients can be tried on a 4- to 8-week tapering course of prednisone or prednisolone followed by IFN-α.[57] Use of corticosteroids even in these patient populations is controversial, however.[57]

Some combinations of therapeutic agents show promise for the treatment of chronic HBV, such as lamivudine plus IFN-α. Cyclooxygenase inhibitors have been studied in combination with IFN to boost the arachidonic acid pathway-mediated effects of IFN.[10] Most combinations, such as acyclovir plus IFN-α, *N*-acetyl cysteine plus lymphoblastoid IFN, prednisone plus acyclovir, and IFN-α plus ribavirin, do not yield better initial response rates than IFN-α alone.[19,49,53] Some combinations, such as levamisole plus lymphoblastoid IFN, are associated with a lower rate of response than IFN alone.[58] Nevertheless, combining therapeutic agents to treat chronic HBV is one of the most promising areas of research.

Other Therapies in Chronic HBV

Many other therapies have been studied for chronic viral hepatitis. Ribavirin demonstrates activity in chronic HBV.[53] All trials with ribavirin show a high relapse rate when therapy is discontinued.[59] A potential use for agents such as ribavirin is in combination therapy with IFN to reduce IFN dose and side effects. It is not yet clear whether relapse rates are reduced in responders.[53]

A number of agents have been used to treat HBV recurrence after transplantation. These agents range from ganciclovir and famciclovir to prostaglandin E. HBV replication usually occurs when the drug is discontinued.[53] Optimal drug therapy after liver transplantation to treat or prevent recurrent HBV infection remains to be defined.

Agents shown to have either little lasting clinical effect or unacceptable toxicity when used alone against HBV include acyclovir; ara-AMP; vidarabine; 6-deoxyacyclovir; corticosteroids (prednisone, prednisolone); suramin; zidovudine (and certain other nucleoside analogs including dideoxyinosine, dideoxyguanosine, and dideoxycytosine); levamisole; azathioprine; interleukin-2; quinacrine; cyanidanol; bacillus Calmette–Guérin (BCG) vaccine; IFN gamma; thymosin; foscarnet; levamisole; thymopentin; and fialuridine (FIAU).[10,53]

Treatment of HBV in Special Populations

Only a small proportion of cases of HBV infection in the United States are in children. The efficacy of IFN in children with chronic HBV infection is debated. As with adults, those with elevated ALT levels at initiation of therapy are more likely to respond.[57] Children who are infected perinatally (or as young children) usually have normal serum aminotransferase concentrations and respond poorly to IFN treatment.[53] One regimen of IFN for children is 6 million units per square meter of body surface area, given three times weekly for 4 to 6 months.[43]

IFN therapy alone is of little benefit in Chinese patients with HBV infection and normal ALT levels prior to therapy.[57] One reason for this is that at least 50% of Chinese HBV carriers are infected perinatally. Additionally, HBV DNA may have been integrated into the host genome. Alternatively, poor response to IFN could be related to immunologic tolerance to HBV induced by exposure to the virus early in life.

As previously mentioned, use of IFN in patients with decompensated cirrhosis is controversial. Cirrhotic patients respond to IFN at rates similar to those seen in patients with less advanced disease; however, evidence of long-term benefit of IFN in these patients is very limited. IFN side effects are more common and severe—potentially even life threatening—in those with advanced cirrhosis. Lower IFN doses should be used (1 to 3 million units three times weekly).[53] Extreme caution must be used in treating any patient with cirrhosis with IFN. It should be attempted only in those patients with mild or early decompensation. Therapy should be closely supervised.

There are several patient groups with chronic HBV in whom IFN therapy has not been adequately studied. For example, little information is available on IFN use in HBV-infected renal dialysis patients, those with malignancies receiving chemotherapy, and patients with kidney, heart, or liver transplants. Anecdotal information suggests that IFN has little effect in patients with major immune deficiencies.[53] Data are also incomplete for individuals coinfected with HIV. In general, it seems that immunocompromised individuals respond poorly to IFN, probably because immunosuppression blocks the antiviral actions of IFN.[43]

How to manage the chronic HCV patient with normal serum aminotransferase levels is a controversy. Some recommend that these patients should be monitored, but should not receive therapy with IFN.[43] These patients are unlikely to respond to IFN treatment. Optimal management of this group of patients will hopefully be better defined over the next several years.

CHRONIC DELTA HEPATITIS

In chronic delta hepatitis, high-dose IFN-α treatment (9 MU three times weekly for at least 12 months) produces clearance of HDV RNA from serum and normalization of serum aminotransferases in about 50% of patients.[60] Lower doses are ineffective. Relapse rates are high when therapy is stopped, and can occur more than 1 year after therapy is stopped.[60] Sustained improvement occurs in 15% to 25% of patients.[43] Prolonged, indefinite IFN therapy may be necessary to achieve a sustained response. No predictors of response to IFN have been identified.

IFN has not been specifically approved for use in chronic HDV. Use of IFN should be limited to those patients who have elevated aminotransferases, HBsAg, and anti-HDV in serum; HDVAg in liver; and either CAH or active cirrhosis. Little data exist on the use of other agents in chronic delta hepatitis.

CHRONIC HCV INFECTION

As with chronic HBV, the decision to pharmacologically treat patients with chronic HCV should not be made based on the presence or absence of symptoms or the degree of abnormality of biochemical tests because extent of liver disease correlates poorly with the level of serum aminotransferases or the patient's symptoms. Only a small proportion of patients develop complications of HCV infection, and therefore few patients benefit from therapy.

Interferons in Chronic HCV

Interferon (α-2a, α-2b, α-n1, β, and consensus) therapy appears to lead to complete eradication of HCV infection in long-term adult responders.[43,61] However, it will only be after an additional 10 to 20 (or more) years of further patient follow-up that we definitely know if IFN decreases cirrhosis, HCC, and death in patients with chronic hepatitis C.[53] Because the disease often does not progress for 1 to 2 decades or more, most study results to date have focused on surrogate markers of disease clearance, improvement of ALT and HCV RNA in serum.

In contrast to chronic HBV, where IFN acts as an immunostimulant, in chronic HCV, IFN inhibits HCV replication directly.[10] The pattern of response is different in HCV. No flare occurs during treatment in those who respond to IFN; rather, aminotransferase and HCV RNA levels decrease, with HCV RNA becoming undetectable 1 to 4 weeks after starting therapy (Fig. 38–2).[43] Responses occur within the first 12 weeks of therapy. If viral RNA is still detectable or serum ALT does not normalize after 3 months of therapy, the patient is unlikely to respond.[43]

Initial trials of IFN in chronic HCV used primarily IFN-α-2b. In general, it appears that other forms of IFN-α and IFN-β are similar in safety and efficacy. Optimal dosage differs between preparations. An FDA-approved regimen is IFN-α-2b, 3 MU given three times weekly for 6 to 12 months. Therapy for 12 to 24

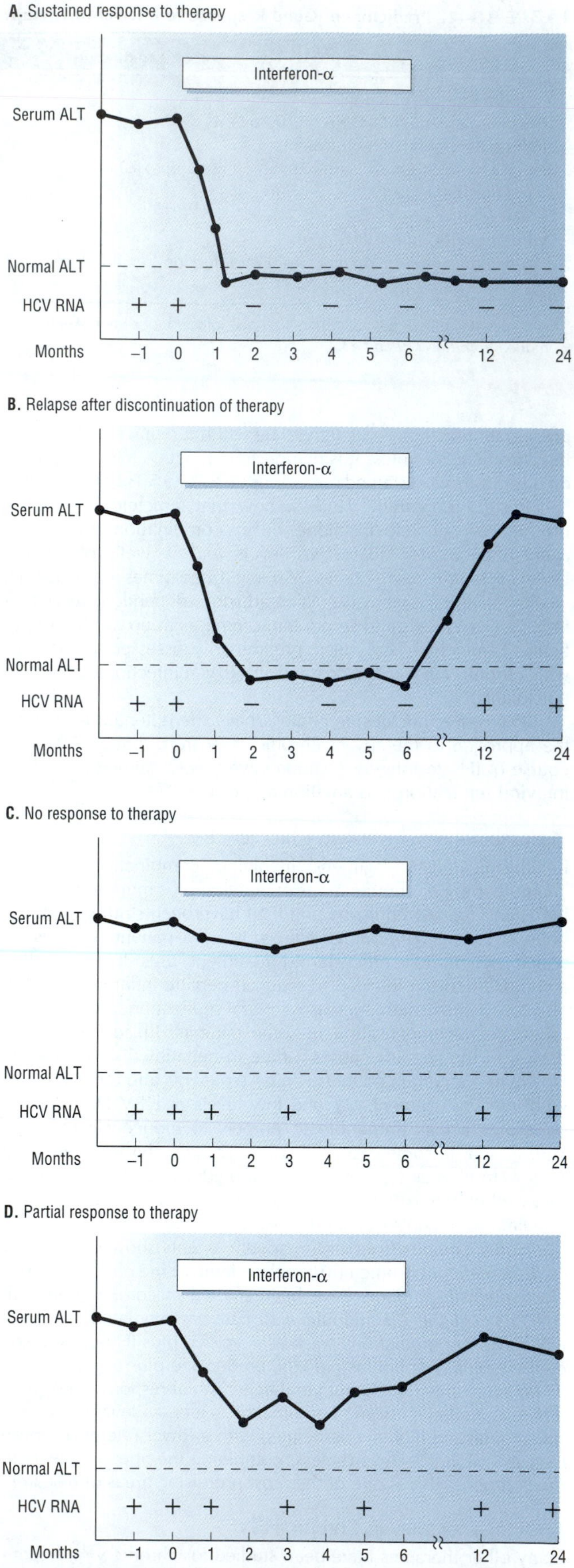

FIGURE 38–2. Typical biochemical responses to IFN-α in patients with chronic hepatitis C.

months (or longer) possibly yields a higher response rate, although data conflict.[43] With FDA-approved dosing for 6 months, one-third to one-half of treated adult patients improve (aminotransferase levels normalize, hepatic inflammation improves, HCV RNA becomes undetectable). At least one-half of these responders relapse within 6 months of stopping therapy (HCV RNA again becomes detectable in serum and aminotransferase levels rise to pretreatment values)—a higher relapse rate than in patients with HBV.[62,63] If ALT and/or HCV RNA levels are still high after 3 months of therapy, IFN should be stopped.

A long-term response is defined as one in which HCV RNA is not detectable for at least 6 months after completion of IFN therapy, and where the serum aminotransferase levels remain normal.[43] The long-term response rate is only 15% to 25%.[43] Four distinct patterns of IFN response are seen (Fig. 38–2).

There is much debate about who should be treated, for how long, and with what dose. Higher initial doses of IFN (5 or 6 MU daily or three times weekly) as well as longer durations of therapy (12 to 24 months) reduce the risk for early relapse and improve the chances of a sustained response.[19,43] At a National Institutes of Health consensus conference in March 1997, a 12-month course of therapy was recommended for most chronic HCV patients. Unfortunately, even with longer duration and higher doses, relapses still occur. Longer courses of therapy and higher doses are more expensive and less well tolerated. At the present time, a longer duration of therapy (e.g., 3 MU three times weekly for at least 12 months) should be offered to patients who respond to IFN.

Because most patients treated with IFN do not have a lasting response, it is important to identify those patients who should be offered treatment. The rate of response to IFN can be improved by careful patient selection. The two most important predictors of IFN response are low pretreatment levels of HCV RNA (low viral load) and HCV viral genotype other than type 1 (Table 38–4).[19,64] Genotype 1 patients respond poorly to IFN. Patients with genotype 1a or 1b have a less than 10% response rate, while patients with genotype 2 or 3 have response rates greater than 40%.[43] As previously stated, the majority of HCV-infected patients in the United States are infected by genotype 1a or 1b. The predictive factors for a sustained response in chronic HCV are different from those in chronic HBV, where the presence of cirrhosis is associated with a high rate of IFN response.[43] These predictive factors can help providers and patients choose appropriate therapy, using a shared decision-making model. Unfortunately, it appears that those most likely to develop complications from chronic HCV are least likely to be IFN responders.

Controversy also exists over management of partial responders. An option for the partial responder is to increase the IFN dosage to 5 MU three times weekly for 3 months, and then measure the HCV RNA to guide further treatment. If HCV RNA is still high, treatment should be stopped. If the patient is responding, IFN can be continued for 12 to 18 months.

Evaluation of Therapeutic Outcomes

Pre- and posttherapy monitoring for IFN efficacy includes liver biopsy, concentrations of serum markers (anti-HCV and HCV RNA in treatment of chronic HCV or HBeAg, HBsAg, HBV DNA, and anti-HBs in treatment of chronic HBV), and serum thyrotropin (see "Drug Class Information: Interferons" later in the chapter). Serum markers can also be followed during therapy. Other laboratory monitoring includes aminotransferases, prothrombin time, alkaline phosphatase, albumin, and bilirubin concentrations before therapy, monthly for the first 3 months of therapy, and then every 2 months.

Combination Therapy in Chronic HCV

Several small studies have shown a 6-month course of a combination of ribavirin and IFN is associated with a higher response rate than is either agent alone.[43] This response is not due to an increased initial response rate; rather the addition of ribavirin seems to decrease the rate of relapse when therapy is stopped.

Preliminary evidence suggests that prednisolone pretreatment reduces the cumulative relapse rate with IFN treatment.[58] These results require confirmation, and this combination should be considered experimental. The role of other combinations of agents has not been defined in chronic HCV.

Other Therapies in Chronic HCV

The search for new drugs to treat chronic hepatitis C has been disappointing. Because lower hepatic iron stores correlate with improved outcome for both chronic HBV and chronic HCV, phlebotomy prior to IFN treatment has been tried in an attempt to improve response rates. It is thought that increased hepatic iron facilitates viral replication of HCV, enhances hepatic injury, or decreases the host's immune system ability to clear the virus.

In two small studies, indomethacin and ketoprofen enhanced response in patients who were previously IFN resistant.[19] Nonsteroidal anti-inflammatory drugs (NSAIDs) inhibit the cyclooxygenase pathway of prostaglandin synthesis, thus blocking the production of prostaglandin E_2 and resulting in an increase in 2′,5′- oligoadenylate synthase.

Interferon gamma, corticosteroids, thymosin, ursodeoxycholic acid, and acyclovir have little or no long-term benefit in patients with chronic HCV. Ribavirin administration for 12 months yields an aminotransferase response in over one-half of treated patients but no sustained HCV RNA response. Serum aminotransferase concentrations return to pretreatment values after completion of therapy.

Treatment of Chronic HCV in Special Populations

Controversy surrounds management of many types of patients with chronic HCV, such as those with normal to minimally elevated aminotransferases. Few patients with normal serum aminotransferase levels and no symptoms of chronic liver disease will respond to IFN. However, it is not known whether treatment with IFN alters the natural history of disease in these patients. IFN therapy is not currently indicated in this population.

Some patients with chronic HCV have extrahepatic manifestations of disease, such as essential mixed cryoglobulinemia or membranoproliferative glomerulonephritis. These patients respond to IFN at similar rates, and often have improvement in the extrahepatic manifestations.[43] Relapse is frequent after therapy is stopped. Long-term maintenance IFN treatment should be considered in patients whose extrahepatic disease manifestations respond to IFN.

IFN is useful in the treatment of chronic hepatitis C in children at doses of 3 MU per square meter for a 6- to 12-month course.[43] It currently seems appropriate to treat children with chronic hepatitis C if serum aminotransferase concentrations are elevated, even if symptoms are absent and histologic features suggest mild disease. However, data are scarce in children, and treatment of HCV infection in children should be considered experimental.[65]

For the present time, IFN therapy for chronic HCV should be offered to those in whom disease symptoms are disabling, those in whom the disease is histologically advanced, patients with rapidly progressive disease, those with markedly elevated aminotransferase levels, and those with high serum HCV RNA levels.

There are patient groups with chronic HCV in whom IFN has not been adequately studied. These include patients with clinically unstable disease and immunosuppressed patients. Therapy in these patients is experimental. IFN should not be used in patients with evidence of hepatic decompensation (hepatic encephalopathy, variceal bleeding, ascites, very low serum albumin, prolonged prothrombin time, serum bilirubin concentration above 3 mg/dL, low serum albumin, leukopenia, thrombocytopenia, encephalopathy, and/or progressive jaundice). Other patients in whom IFN should be avoided include those with liver disease of other causes, patients on immunosuppressive therapy, patients actively abusing drugs, those with significant psychiatric illness, and those with significant other medical illnesses such as cardiac, renal, or thyroid disease that are not successfully treated.[50]

LIVER TRANSPLANTATION

Liver transplantation is an option for patients with end-stage chronic liver disease secondary to viral infection. Unfortunately, recurrent viral hepatitis infection in the transplanted liver is a common problem.

Transplanting HBV DNA and/or HBeAg-positive patients is not routine.[66,67] These patients are at extremely high risk of HBV recurrence and have a more aggressive postoperative course.[50] HBV patients who receive liver transplants have 1- and 5-year survival rates of 73% and 44%, respectively.[66] The following are suggested as guidelines to determine candidates for transplant: All patients with fulminant hepatitis B infection; those patients with chronic HBV and cirrhosis who do not have markers of viral replication; and patients with HDV infection.[66] Patients who are positive for HBV DNA and/or HBeAg at the time of liver transplantation should be transplanted only in the context of the controlled clinical research environment.

Cirrhosis as a result of chronic HCV disease is one of the foremost reasons for liver transplantation in the United States. Current estimates are that 15% to 30% of liver transplants are HCV related.[68] Over 90% of patients develop reinfection of the liver graft,[10,19] but cumulative survival rates for the HCV-infected patients who receive liver transplantation are similar to HCV-negative transplant recipients.[69] Approximately 40% of patients develop chronic hepatitis C with damage to the graft within 1 to 3 years after transplantation, and within 4 years after transplant, 8% have cirrhosis.[69] Graft survival is usually 5 to 10 years or longer.[19] Infection with genotype 1b is associated with more severe graft injury.[69]

The most common therapy used to prevent HBV reinfection in the transplanted liver is high doses of HBIG, usually given intravenously postoperatively.[67] HBIG does not prevent recurrence in the majority of recipients and it is very expensive.[53]

IFN has been used in an attempt to decrease HBV DNA and/or to clear HBeAg before transplantation. It is not beneficial, and is dangerous in patients with end-stage liver disease because it can induce hepatic decompensation.[66] IFN is not usually successful in the posttransplantation setting to prevent recurrence.

Both famciclovir and ganciclovir reduce HBV DNA levels posttransplant.[53] To date, the most promising therapy is pre- and posttransplant treatment with lamivudine.

FUTURE DIRECTIONS IN THERAPY

The therapeutic approach to the treatment of chronic HBV and/or HCV infection might consist of combination therapy with an immune modulator and an antiviral agent, or perhaps several antiviral drugs. There are several steps in the life cycle of HBV that could serve as targets for therapy. Cellular targeting systems are potentially more effective and less toxic. To date, however, most anti-HBV agents studied aim to inhibit viral DNA synthesis. Adjunctive therapies are also actively being researched.

For chronic HCV, the search for effective drug therapy would be helped if a cell culture or animal model for HCV infection was developed. Protease inhibitors are being researched. Effective therapies are especially important for this virus because of the frequency of infection coupled with the poor prospects for vaccine development.

DRUG CLASS INFORMATION: INTERFERONS

Several varieties of IFN-α are currently available. These include recombinant IFN-α (IFN-α-2a Roferon A, Hoffmann-LaRoche); IFN-α-2b (Intron A, Schering); natural IFN-α-n3 (Alferon N, Interferon Sciences, manufacturer; Purdue Frederick, distributor); lymphoblastoid IFN (α-n1, Wellferon, Burroughs Wellcome); and consensus IFN (CIFN, Infergen, Amgen). IFN-α-2b is the only FDA-approved drug for treatment of both chronic HBV and chronic non-A, non-B (HCV) hepatitis. IFN-α-2a and CIFN are approved for use in chronic HCV.

The side effects of IFN are frequent enough that the patient should be informed about them before treatment begins (Table 38–5). Many side effects are dose related. Premedication with a single dose of acetaminophen around the time of administering the injection will help ameliorate these flu-like symptoms. Severity decreases with subsequent injections.[48]

Because IFN therapy can exacerbate autoimmune disorders, it is important to exclude autoimmune diagnoses before initiating therapy. Thrombocytopenia and granulocytopenia are more common in patients with cirrhosis and hypersplenism. The psychiatric complications are especially severe in those with severe liver disease, occur in up to 20% of patients, and are the most common dose-limiting side effects. IFN should be discontinued if serious

TABLE 38–5. Side Effects of IFN-α

Early (first 2 wk of therapy)	Hematologic	Neuropsychiatric	Autoimmune	Miscellaneous
Fever	Neutropenia	Irritability	Development of autoantibodies	Chronic fatigue
Chills	Thrombocytopenia	Mood lability	Hepatitis	Infections
Myalgias	Anemia	Depression	Thyroid dysfunction	Increased sleep requirement
Fatigue		Tearfulness	Thyroiditis	Anorexia
Malaise		Delirium	Arthropathy	Weight loss
Nausea		Paresthesias	Type I diabetes mellitus	Myalgias
Sleep disturbance		Seizures	Exacerbation of psoriasis or lichen planus	Low-grade fevers
Abdominal pain		Psychosis	Exacerbation of other autoimmune phenomena	Decreased libido
Diarrhea				Alopecia
Headache				Hypertriglyceridemia
Appetite changes				Irritability
				Anxiety
				Depression
				Attention span deficits

complications occur. The dose of IFN must be reduced in 10% to 40% of patients. Treatment must be discontinued due to adverse effects in 5% to 10% of patients. For many patients, reassurance that the side effects are therapy related, not severe, and will disappear when therapy is stopped is sufficient. It is always important to reassure both patient and family, especially when psychiatric side effects are evident.

Ongoing monitoring of IFN toxicity includes complete blood counts weekly during the first 2 weeks of therapy and monthly thereafter. Patients should be asked about level of performance, mood changes, ability to concentrate, and symptoms. The dose of IFN should be decreased by 50% if any of the following develop: fatigue that interferes with the daily routine, serious mood changes, daily nausea with occasional vomiting, granulocytopenia (less than 750/mm^3), and/or thrombocytopenia (less than 50,000/mm^3). IFN should be immediately discontinued if fatigue is so severe that it requires bed rest, vomiting occurs more than twice daily, or if profound granulocytopenia (less than 500/mm^3) or thrombocytopenia (less than 30,000/mm^3) occur.[47,48]

Several drugs can potentially interact with IFN. Examples include theophylline (increased theophylline concentration), zidovudine (enhanced hematologic toxicity), vidarabine (vidarabine-induced neurotoxicity), and cytotoxic agents (increased myelosuppression). Careful evaluation for drug interactions with IFN is an integral part of monitoring IFN therapy.

PATIENT EDUCATION ABOUT CHRONIC HEPATITIS B AND C

Patients should be told to expect that they will have chronic HBV or HCV for life. Many will feel healthy and have no signs of liver disease. Some will develop the complications previously discussed. Patients will feel better if they lead as normal a life as possible, but encourage them to develop a life-style that allows time for short naps, frequent rest, and is low stress. Warn them to avoid giving the virus to others by not sharing personal items (such as razors), covering open wounds, and not donating blood, semen, or organs. Advise them to tell dentists, physicians, and other health care professionals that they have HBV or HCV. Safe sex should be recommended for all chronic HBV patients and for those chronic HCV patients with multiple partners.

Chronic hepatitis patients should drink alcohol rarely, if at all, and they should be warned about taking drugs like acetaminophen. Recommend vaccination against hepatitis A for all patients with chronic HCV or HBV, and vaccination against hepatitis B for those patients with chronic HCV.

Because certain alternative treatments such as herbs and vitamins can damage the liver, you should remind your patients to ask you before using any over-the-counter drug, herbal remedy, or unconventional therapy. Encourage regular medical follow-up. Offer self-help groups, such as the Hepatitis Information Network (www.hepnet.com).

For those patients who are being treated with IFN, education about self-administration of subcutaneous injections is necessary. Additionally, the patient and family members or care giver should be informed about side effects and how to identify serious adverse effects. Methods to decrease the severity of side effects should also be discussed.

ECONOMIC AND HUMANISTIC OUTCOME CONSIDERATIONS

The cost of a 6-month course of IFN-α-2b 3 MU three times weekly for chronic HCV is $2035 (based on average wholesale price).[70] For treatment of chronic HBV, at a dose of 5 MU 5 days per week for 16 weeks, the cost is $3768 (based on average wholesale price).[70] This cost must be balanced against the risk, the chance of response, and the expected consequences of untreated chronic hepatitis along with the fact that (especially for chronic HCV) the optimal dose, duration, and combination of therapy are poorly defined.

Dusheiko and Roberts estimated the long-term economic impact of treatment of chronic HBV and chronic HCV in a model—and indicated cost savings.[71] An accompanying editorial identified limitations to the model, and stated that data are insufficient to make the assumptions indicated.[72] Bennett and colleagues attempted to account for varying rates of chronic HCV disease progression and severity in a decision analysis model of IFN treatment.[73] In this model, the assumptions of treatment cost and disease progression were varied, and the estimated marginal cost per year of life gained from IFN therapy ranged from $3000 to $55,000.[73] A group of patients where data document a significant reduction in the cost of health care and an increased life expectancy with IFN treatment is the group of young chronic HCV patients without fibrosis.[74] Yet, one study that followed a cohort of mostly chronic HCV patients and control patients over an 18-year time frame showed no difference between groups in mortality from all causes.

Thus, is it cost beneficial to treat chronic HCV?[68] This question has yet to be answered. What are the additional benefits and costs associated with the increased dose/duration of IFN treatment?[68] Are these additional benefits worth the additional costs? The limited overall response coupled with the cost, dose-dependent side effects, and potential for selection of IFN-resistant mutants make universal application of IFN treatment debatable. For the time being, patient selection on the basis of predictors of response, coupled with informed patient decision making regarding benefits and risks, is appropriate until better definition is given to the cost effectiveness of IFN treatment in chronic hepatitis C. Efficient management of IFN therapy is important so that clinical maximization of response is achieved with consideration of other health care expenditures.[68] Ultimately, the clinical effectiveness—and cost effectiveness—of IFN will be dependent on the effect of therapy on the morbidity and mortality of HCV infection.

It is accepted by most that treatment of chronic HBV in patients with good predictors of response is cost effective.[71,75] The cost effectiveness of IFN in patients with chronic hepatitis B was demonstrated in a model based on increased life expectancy and quality-adjusted life years leading to decreased projected lifetime cost.[75]

Quality of life changes as a result of disease or therapy are important for chronic hepatitis. Using a quality of life (QOL) instrument based on the Medical Outcomes Study short-form health survey (SF-36), patients with chronic hepatitis C scored significantly lower than the general population on each of the eight subscales in this survey (physical function, physical disability, bodily pain, general health, vitality, social function, emotional disability, and mental health).[76] They also scored significantly lower than patients with hypertension in seven of the subscales and two additional generic scales. Patients with chronic HCV were most comparable to those with type 2 diabetes.[76] The presence of cirrhosis on liver biopsy did not correlate with differences in the perceived QOL. The presence of physical findings was associated with poorer QOL scores. The patient population in this study was fairly homogeneous. A larger study with a wider diversity of patients is ongoing.

PREVENTION OF VIRAL HEPATITIS

The goals of immunization against viral hepatitis include preventing the short-term viremia that can lead to transmission of infection, preventing the morbidity and occasional mortality associated with the disease, and avoiding chronic infection.[77,78] The mainstays of hepatitis prevention are risk reduction, education, passive immunization with immune globulins, and active immunization through vaccination programs. The spread of HAV can be controlled by cautious handling of fomites contaminated with feces coupled with good hand-washing techniques. Universal precautions are used to prevent hepatitis B and C spread within the hospital setting. HBV and HCV spread are reduced, but not eliminated, through screening of blood donors and testing for HBsAg and anti-HCV.

HEPATITIS A

Within the last few years, inactivated vaccines have been marketed that are highly effective in preexposure prophylaxis. Active immunization provides long-term protection against HAV infection. Hepatitis A vaccines provide an opportunity to substantially lower the incidence of infection, and potentially even eradicate the disease.[3] The most effective means of achieving control of HAV infection is to vaccinate all children by incorporating hepatitis A vaccination into the routine childhood immunizations. This is not currently possible because data are lacking to determine the appropriate dose and timing of vaccination for children less than 2 years of age. Until routine infant vaccination is feasible, the interim strategy in the United States is to prevent and control hepatitis A via preexposure vaccination of target groups.[3]

The importance of avoiding exposure cannot be overemphasized. The most important measures to avoid exposure include good hand-washing techniques and good personal hygiene practices. Travelers can minimize risk by avoiding uncooked shellfish, uncooked fruits and vegetables, and by avoiding drinking water (and other beverages with ice) of unknown purity.

IMMUNE GLOBULIN

Immune globulin (IG) provides protection against HAV by passive transfer of antibody against the hepatitis A virus (anti-HAV). IG is effective in modifying the course and preventing the spread of HAV in 85% or more of exposures when used within 2 weeks following the exposure.[1] IG available in the United States does not contain HBsAg, HIV, or anti-HCV. Pregnancy and lactation are not contraindications to receiving IG.

International travelers have been the major group receiving preexposure prophylaxis with IG.[1] IG is recommended for susceptible persons traveling to developing countries. The CDC publication, *Health Information for International Travel,* or the CDC web site (www.cdc.gov) can be consulted for specific recommendations. A single dose of IG of 0.02 mL/kg IM (in the deltoid or gluteus) is recommended if travel is for less than 3 months. For lengthy stays, 0.06 mL/kg IM should be given every 3 to 5 months. Dosing is the same for adults and children.

The availability of an effective hepatitis A vaccine has reduced the use of IG in travelers. IG is much less expensive than vaccination, however, and remains a reasonable alternative for the traveler who does not need long-term protection. If the interval between the first dose of the hepatitis A vaccine and travel is less than 2 weeks, administration of IG should be considered to provide passive immunity during the interval before active vaccine-induced immunity develops. In this situation, the low dose of IG should be used.

The postexposure prophylactic benefit from IG is greatest early in the incubation period and is of no benefit more than 2 weeks after exposure.[1] Serologic screening of contacts for anti-HAV is not recommended before IG administration because such screening is costly and delays prophylaxis. A single IG dose of 0.02 mL/kg IM is used for postexposure prophylaxis. Again, the dose is the same for adults and children. People who have been given one dose of hepatitis A vaccine at least 1 month before exposure do not need IG.

IG should be given to previously unvaccinated people in the following situations: Close personal contact with a person who has hepatitis A; all staff and attendees of day care centers when hepatitis A is documented; classroom contacts of patients; common-source exposures (other food handlers at locations where a food handler has hepatitis A; patrons, if the infected food handler handled food and had diarrhea or poor hygienic practices); and schools, hospitals, and work settings when close contact occurs with index patients.[3]

Serious adverse events to IG are rare. Anaphylaxis has been reported in individuals with IgA deficiency who have received repeated doses of IG.[3] People who need repeat doses while overseas should use products that meet U.S. standards for purity.

IG does not interfere with the immune response to yellow fever vaccine, oral poliovirus vaccine, or inactivated vaccines. IG can interfere with the response to live, attenuated vaccines such as measles, rubella, mumps, and varicella. Administration of live, attenuated vaccines should be delayed for at least 5 months after administration of IG. Conversely, IG should not be administered within 2 weeks after the administration of live, attenuated vaccines (3 weeks for varicella vaccine), unless the benefits of IG clearly outweigh the benefits of vaccination. If IG is administered within 2 weeks after administration of these vaccines (3 weeks for varicella vaccine), the person should be revaccinated—but not sooner than 5 months after the administration of IG.[3]

HEPATITIS A VACCINE

Inactivated HAV vaccines, Havrix (SmithKline Beecham) and Vaqta (Merck) demonstrate protective efficacy in over

TABLE 38–6. Recommended Dosing of Havrix and Vaqta

Vaccine	Vaccinee's Age (yr)	Dose	Volume (mL)	No. Doses	Schedule (mo)[a]
Havrix	2 to 18	720 ELISA U[b]	0.5	2	0, 6 to 12
	> 18	1440 ELISA U	1	2	0, 6 to 12
Vaqta	2 to 17	25 U	0.5	2	0, 6 to 18
	> 17	50 U	1	2	0, 6

[a]0 months represents the timing of the initial dose; subsequent numbers represent months after the initial dose.
[b]Havrix is also available as 360 ELISA units per dose, three-dose schedule for persons 2 to 18 years of age. The 720 ELISA units per dose, two-dose schedule is preferred.
From Ref. 3.

94% of vaccinees within 1 month after primary vaccination.[79–81] Eighty to ninety percent of adults have protective levels of antibody in 15 days after immunization. When a booster dose is given 6 or more months later, essentially 100% of recipients develop high antibody levels. Older individuals, obese individuals, and HIV-infected persons have a lower seroconversion rate.

Both vaccines are indicated for immunization of individuals 2 years of age or greater who are at increased risk of hepatitis A infection. No information is available about whether these vaccines can be substituted for each other in booster immunizations.[78]

Approved dosing for hepatitis A vaccines is given in Table 38–6. The primary vaccination is a single dose, with a booster dose 6 to 12 months later for children and adults. Both vaccines are injected intramuscularly into the deltoid muscle. The primary immunization should be given at least 2 weeks (preferably 4 weeks) prior to expected exposure to HAV. The vaccine can be given at the same time as a wide variety of other vaccines (diphtheria-tetanus-pertussis, polio, oral typhoid, cholera, Japanese encephalitis, rabies, yellow fever, and hepatitis B) without interfering with the immune responses. Each vaccine should be given with a different syringe and at a different injection site. Havrix and Vaqta can be given concomitantly with IG; however, the antibody titer ultimately obtained is likely to be lower than when the vaccine is given alone.

Antibody titers achieved after either vaccination or IG administration are 10- to 100-fold lower than those achieved after active disease.[3] Commercial assays can detect anti-HAV present after natural infection, but the titers achieved after vaccination are often below the levels detected by commercially available assays. These low antibody levels are still protective.[78]

Because the vaccines have been evaluated for less than 10 years, data are limited on long-term persistence of antibody and of immune memory. To date, the vaccines are known to have protective levels of anti-HAV for at least 4 years. Based on kinetic models of antibody decline, it is projected that protective anti-HAV levels could be present for 20 years or more.[3]

The vaccine is very safe. Side effects include local reactions at the injection site (soreness, induration, redness, and swelling), headache, malaise, fatigue, fever, and GI upset.[3,81] Any adverse event related to hepatitis A vaccination should be reported to the Vaccine Adverse Events Reporting System (1-800-822-7967). As with other inactivated vaccines, hepatitis A vaccine can be administered to immunocompromised persons.

Much controversy surrounds who should receive hepatitis A vaccine. Preexposure immunization with hepatitis A vaccine is recommended for individuals in the groups listed in Table 38–7. Additionally, preexposure vaccination can be considered for food handlers, but epidemiologic data do not support routine immunization.

Although vaccination of a person who is immune (because of prior infection) does not increase the risk of adverse effects, there are certain populations where prevaccination testing should be conducted. Such testing is cost effective in the United States in populations that are expected to have high rates of prior HAV infection. Testing of children is not indicated. For adults, the populations for whom prevaccination testing is likely to be cost effective include adults who were born or lived for an extended period in geographic areas with a high endemicity of HAV, older adolescents and adults in the population groups listed in Table 38–8, adults in certain groups with a high prevalence of infection, and "older" adults (often considered as those above 40 years of age because of higher anti-HAV

TABLE 38–7. Groups Recommended for Active Immunization Against Hepatitis A

Persons at increased risk for HAV infection or its consequences
- Travelers to countries that have high or intermediate endemicity of infection[a]
- Injecting drug users
- Men who have sex with men
- Persons who have occupational risk for infection (e.g., working with nonhuman primates)
- Persons who have chronic liver disease
- Persons with clotting factor disorders

Children living in communities that have high rates of hepatitis A (help prevent recurrent epidemics)

Children and young adults in communities that have intermediate rates of hepatitis A (help control ongoing and prevent future epidemics)

Contacts of case-patients

[a]Africa, Asia (except Japan), the Mediterranean Basin, Eastern Europe, the Middle East, Central and South America, Mexico, Greenland, and parts of the Caribbean. Essentially all countries other than Australia, Canada, Japan, New Zealand, countries in Western Europe, and Scandinavia.
From Ref. 3.

TABLE 38–8. People in the United States Who Should Be Considered for Prevaccination Serologic Testing for Susceptibility to Hepatitis A

Men who have sex with men
American Indians
Alaskan Natives
Hispanics
Older adults

prevalence, but see the next paragraph).The place of the vaccine in postexposure prophylaxis is not known.

At Kaiser Permanente Rocky Mountain Division, guidelines for the prevention of hepatitis A in travelers have been developed and implemented.[82] These guidelines have been used primarily within the International Travel Clinic (www.kaiser-co.org; or travel@henge.com). These guidelines include recommendations to screen for prior exposure to hepatitis A those individuals 55 years of age or older, individuals born in a country of high endemicity for hepatitis A, and frequent travelers. The incidence of protective antibodies against hepatitis A in these populations is such that screening is cost effective. For a patient who is traveling within 2 weeks of initially contacting the Travel Clinic, it is recommended that he or she receive IG, and the patient is counseled to contact the Travel Clinic with more advanced notice before future travel. If the traveler contacts the Travel Clinic within 2 weeks of travel and will be traveling for more than 3 months, the patient is offered both IG and the first dose of hepatitis A vaccine. Hepatitis A vaccine is offered to all travelers whose departure date is more than 2 weeks away who are traveling to an area where there is a high risk of contracting hepatitis A. Vaccination is particularly important for those individuals who travel internationally more than three times in 10 years, and for those with trip durations exceeding 6 months. In all cases, it is important to counsel the patient about receiving the booster dose 6 to 12 months after the primary vaccine dose, as well as to talk with the individual about food and water precautions.

Vaccines are needed that combine HAVAg with other antigens to integrate hepatitis A vaccine into existing childhood vaccinations schedules (hepatitis B or DPT). Vaccines combining hepatitis A and hepatitis B vaccines are being studied.[78] Additionally, we need to determine (1) the duration of protection and immunologic memory after hepatitis A immunization, (2) the most effective vaccination strategies for interrupting and preventing community-wide outbreaks, and (3) whether hepatitis A vaccine provides an adequate level of postexposure protection.

HEPATITIS B

The two products available for prevention of hepatitis B infection include hepatitis B vaccine (provides active immunity) and hepatitis B immune globulin (HBIG, provides temporary passive immunity).[1] The vaccine is used in preexposure prophylaxis, and in postexposure prophylaxis in combination with HBIG. Vaccination is the most effective method for preventing hepatitis B. (See Tables 38–9, 38–10, and 38–11.)

HBIG

Hepatitis B immune globulin is used only in postexposure prophylaxis. Postexposure prophylaxis for HBV is recommended for infants of HBV-carrier mothers (perinatal exposure), sexual exposure to HBsAg-positive persons, accidental percutaneous or permucosal exposure to HBsAg-positive blood, and exposure of an infant to a caregiver who has acute hepatitis B.[1] HBIG should be given to immunocompromised patients for the same indications and in the same doses as immunocompetent individuals.[83] The recommended dose is

TABLE 38–9. Recommended Schedule of Immunoprophylaxis to Prevent Perinatal or Sexual Transmission of HBV Infection

Vaccine Recipient	Immunoprophylaxis	Timing
Infant born to HBsAg-positive mother	Vaccine dose 1	Within 12 h of birth
	HBIG[a]	Within 12 h of birth
	Vaccine doses 2 and 3[b]	Usual schedule
Infant born to mother not screened for HBsAg	Vaccine dose 1[c]	Within 12 h of birth
	HBIG	If mother is found to be HBsAg positive, administer dose to infant as soon as possible, but no later than 1 wk after birth
	Vaccine doses 2 and 3[b]	Usual schedule
Sexual exposure	HBIG[d]	Single dose within 14 d of sexual contact
	Vaccine dose 1	At time of HBIG treatment[e]

[a]0.5 mL IM, at a site different from that used for the vaccine.
[b]The four-dose schedule for Engerix-B can also be used.
[c]The first dose of vaccine is the same as that for the infant of an HBsAg-positive mother. If the mother is found to be HBsAg-positive, that dose is continued. If the mother is found to be HBsAg-negative, the remaining vaccine doses are those appropriate for other infants and children.
[d]0.06 mL/kg IM.
[e]The first dose can be given at the same time as the HBIG dose but in a different site; subsequent doses should be given as recommended in Table 38–11.
Compiled from Refs. 84 and 87.

TABLE 38–10. Recommendations for Hepatitis B Prophylaxis Following Percutaneous or Permucosal Exposure

Vaccination Status of Exposed Person	Treatment According to HBsAg Status of Source		
	HBsAg-Positive	HBsAg-Negative	Source Not Tested or Unknown
Unvaccinated	HBIG × 1[a] and initiate vaccine[b]	Initiate vaccine[b]	Initiate vaccine[b]
Previously vaccinated, known responder	Test exposed person for anti-HBs level If adequate,[c] no treatment If inadequate or titer unknown, 1 vaccine booster dose	No treatment	No treatment
Previously vaccinated, known nonresponder	HBIG × 2 (1 mo apart) or HBIG × 1; plus 1 dose of vaccine	No treatment	If known high-risk source, may treat as if source were HBsAg-positive
Previously vaccinated, response unknown	Test exposed person for anti-HBs level If inadequate,[c] HBIG × 1, plus 1 vaccine booster dose If adequate, no treatment If titer unknown, 1 vaccine booster dose	No treatment	Test exposed person for anti-HBs level If inadequate,[c] vaccine booster dose If adequate, no treatment

[a]HBIG dose 0.06 mL/kg IM.
[b]HB vaccine dose; see Table 38–11.
[c]Adequate anti-HBs is ≥ 10 mIU/mL by radioimmunoassay or enzyme immunoassay.
From Ref. 84.

0.06 mL/kg administered intramuscularly. Guidelines for use are listed in Tables 38–9 and 38–10.[1,84]

Use of IG for prophylaxis of HBV infection is only recommended when HBIG is not available. IG contains anti-HBs in titers of 1:100 to 1:1000, in comparison to the 1:100,000 or greater anti-HBs titer found in HBIG. IG and HBIG available in the United States do not transmit HBV, HIV, or other viruses.

HEPATITIS B VACCINE

Currently there are two recombinant hepatitis B vaccine products: Recombivax HB (Merck Sharp & Dohme) and Engerix-B (SmithKline Beecham), which have comparable immune responses and safety profiles.[1] Hepatitis B vaccines contain 5 to 40 μg HBsAg protein per mL adsorbed onto aluminum, with thimerosal added as preservative.[1]

The hepatitis B vaccines available in the United States are some of the safest vaccines available.[78] Side effects of the vaccine are soreness at the injection site, headache, fatigue, irritability, and fever. The number of patients experiencing these adverse reactions decreases with each vaccine dose, and adverse reactions are less common in infants and children than in adults. There is no association between Guillain–Barré syndrome and the recombinant vaccine. The hepatitis B vaccine is contraindicated in patients with anaphylaxis to common baker's yeast. The vaccine does not transmit HIV.[85] Hepatitis B vaccines are inactivated and can be simultaneously administered with other vaccines.[1] Breast-fed infants can be vaccinated with hepatitis B vaccine, as can immunocompromised infants and children.[83,86,87] The vaccine can also be given to pregnant and lactating women.

TABLE 38–11. Recommended Doses and Schedules of Currently Licensed HB Vaccines

Group	Vaccine	
	Recombivax HB[a] dose, μg (mL)	Engerix-B[a,b] dose, μg (mL)
Infants of HBsAg-positive mothers	5 (0.5)	10 (0.5)
Other infants, children, and adolescents ≤ 19 years	5 (0.5)	10 (0.5)
Adults age 20 and greater	10 (1.0)	20 (1.0)
Dialysis patients and other immunocompromised persons	40 (1.0)[c]	40 (2.0)[d,e]

[a]Usual schedules: Infants, 3 doses given at birth, at 1 to 2 mo, and at 6 to 18 mo or, for infants, with other routine immunizations at 1 to 2 mo, 4 mo, and 6 to 18 mo. Older children and adults, 3 doses given at 0, 2 mo, and 6 mo or at 0, 2, and 4 mo. Higher titers of HBsAb are achieved with the last 2 doses of vaccine being spaced at least 4 months apart.
[b]Alternative approved schedule: 4 doses, one given at 0, 1, 2, and 12 mo.
[c]Special formulation for dialysis patients.
[d]Two 1.0-mL doses given at different sites.
[e]Four-dose schedule recommended at 0, 1, 2, and 6 months.

The dose of vaccine to induce the desired antibody response or protective effect varies between the two available vaccines (Table 38–11).[84] HBV vaccine is given as a series of three IM doses into the deltoid (anterolateral thigh in infants) over a period of months. Specific dosing guidelines for all age groups are listed in Table 38–11.[84,87] Partial protection is achieved after the second dose. The vaccination series can be started with one vaccine type and completed with another.[86,87] All dosing schedules give excellent seroconversion rates, although the postvaccination titer is lower with accelerated dosing and shorter intervals between the second and third dose.[78] The vaccination process does not need to be restarted because of missed doses.[1] In general, if the interval between doses one and two is 1 to 5 months, and/or the interval between doses two and three is 2 to 12 months, completion of the series is indicated. If the interval between vaccine doses is greater than recommended, protection is still attained in immunocompetent individuals, and the vaccine series can simply be completed. The purpose of the third vaccine dose is to boost the antibody titers and provide a more durable response.[78]

Dosing guidelines for infants born to HBsAg-positive mothers and mothers whose HBsAg status is unknown are given in Table 38–9.[84,87] All infants (premature or full term) born to HBsAg-positive women should be vaccinated within 12 hours of birth with HBV vaccine and one dose of HBIG. Infants of HBsAg-positive mothers should have anti-HBs testing done 1 to 3 months after the third dose.[88]

For premature infants with birthweights of less than 2000 g born to HBsAg-negative mothers, hepatitis B vaccination should be delayed until just before hospital discharge (or until the infant weighs at least 2000 g) or the infant reaches 2 months of age.[88] Serologic testing for response is not routinely recommended.

The three-dose vaccination series induces an adequate anti-HBs response in more than 90% of healthy adults and more than 95% of infants and children.[1] No response to the vaccine in immunocompetent adults appears to be genetically determined. An adequate response is defined as anti-HBs of 10 mIU/mL or greater, which is approximately equal to 10 sample ratio units (SRU), measured 1 to 6 months after completion of the vaccine series.[1] Low responders (10 to 100 mIU/mL), as well as those with good response (greater than or equal to 100 mIU/mL) have complete protection against clinical infection with the virus. Many factors affect the immunogenicity of hepatitis B vaccines.[1,77,85] Some factors that diminish vaccine immunogenicity include immunocompromised states, smoking, increased age, immunization into the buttock, low dose, renal insufficiency, alcoholism, and increased body mass.

Persistence of anti-HBs is directly related to the height of the antibody response.[77] Up to 50% of responders lose detectable antibody within 7 years, but immunologic memory and protection against viremia and clinical illness persists for at least 10 to 13 years in immunocompetent individuals.[4] Healthy persons respond promptly to booster doses (even if antibody is undetectable prior to the booster dose).[77] For adults and children whose immune status is normal, booster doses of vaccine are not recommended, and serologic testing for immunity is not needed.

Postvaccination testing for immunity is only important for persons at risk for poor antibody response and for those at very high risk for exposure.[1,78] Examples include hemodialysis patients, HIV-infected patients, certain public safety personnel, and the extremely obese.[1] Testing for peak anti-HBs should be conducted 1 to 3 months after completion of the vaccine series to determine if a response occurred and to evaluate the need for booster dose(s).[85]

Nonresponders and inadequate (or hyporesponders) responders (< 10 mIU/mL) should be immediately revaccinated with one or two booster dose injections of vaccine, and then every year or two thereafter.[1,77,85] Up to 50% of nonresponders will develop anti-HBs after two additional doses of vaccine,[1,78] although the level of antibody achieved is low.

It is not yet known whether an initial infant hepatitis B immunization series confers lifelong immunity; however, data from long-term studies indicate that the vast majority of vaccine responders continue to be protected from both symptomatic and chronic HBV infection.[89]

Immunocompromised adults can receive hepatitis B vaccine when indicated. Hemodialysis patients have decreased seroconversion rates, decreased antibody titers to surface antigens, and a faster rate of loss of antibody after HBV vaccination.[85] These patients require higher vaccine doses or an increased number of doses.[83] A special formulation of Recombivax HB (40 μg/mL) is available for these patients. A more rapid rise in antibody concentration is observed with a 0-, 1-, 2-, and 6-month vaccination schedule in these patients, although overall conversion rate is similar whether the final (fourth) dose is given 6 or 12 months after the series begins. Protection in this group is maintained only as long as the anti-HBs level remains above 10 mIU. Routine anti-HBs testing (at 12-month intervals) and booster doses to maintain adequate anti-HBs are recommended in hemodialysis patients.[1] Patients with renal disease who will likely need dialysis or transplantation should also receive hepatitis B vaccination—and before dialysis is initiated, if feasible.

Vaccine response is reduced to less than 70% in males infected with HIV, even in those in early stages of the infection.[85,90] Nonresponders and inadequate responders are unlikely to respond to revaccination.[90] HIV-infected patients are prone to have an impaired response to HBV infection and are more likely to become chronic carriers.[90] Testing for antibody response is recommended, with notification of nonresponders of the potential consequences (infection, carrier state, delta virus superinfection).

Other immunosuppressed groups with decreased response to HBV vaccine include alcoholics with clinical liver disease and patients with hematologic malignancies, organ transplants, diabetes, or hemophilia.[85]

The vaccine is safe in chronic carriers, but ineffective in eliminating HBsAg. Antibody acquired from HBIG or IG administration or via the placenta will not interfere with development of active immunity; for example, HBIG can be administered concomitantly with the first dose of vaccine.[1,85]

PATIENT COUNSELING

Patients with hepatitis B (acute or chronic) should be counseled that they can transmit the disease to others. They should not donate blood, body organs, semen, or other tissue. Household articles such as toothbrushes and razors should not be shared because they could be contaminated with blood. Any cuts or open lesions should be covered to prevent the accidental spread of infectious secretions. Sex partners and household contacts should be screened for susceptibility to HBV and then vaccinated if susceptible.

PREEXPOSURE VACCINATION

The comprehensive vaccination strategy being emphasized in the United States targets interruption of transmission at all age groups through routine infant immunization, continued vaccination of high-risk older adolescents and adults, routine screening of pregnant women for HBsAg, and "catch-up" vaccination of children (Table 38–12).[4] Routine infant vaccination can eliminate transmission of the virus (after several decades). There is little immediate impact on the incidence of clinical hepatitis B, but a relatively immediate impact on the number of new HBV carriers. Several states now have laws mandating hepatitis B immunization prior to entry into kindergarten or middle school.

In countries such as the United States, where the risk of hepatitis B is relatively low, determination of whom to vaccinate prior to exposure depends on the risk of infection in that group and the relative cost of pretesting versus the cost of vaccination.[1,85] Cost–benefit analyses favor vaccination for high-risk groups.[1] The groups currently recommended for preexposure vaccination are listed in Table 38–12.[1] Everyone in high-risk, low-prevalence groups (such as health care professionals in training) can be vaccinated without screening.[1,85] To comply with federal guidelines, health care workers with potential exposure to blood are offered hepatitis B vaccination at no cost by their employers.

In countries where hepatitis B is endemic, hepatitis B vaccination of infants and children has begun to impact the incidence of hepatocellular carcinoma and death related to HBV. In Taiwan, where a mass vaccination program was launched in 1984, the incidence of HCC in children dropped by 50% from 1981 to 1994.[91]

TABLE 38–12. High-Risk Groups Recommended for Preexposure Hepatitis B Vaccination

All 11- to 12-year-old children who have not previously received hepatitis B vaccine[a]
All unvaccinated children ages < 11 yr who are Pacific Islanders or who reside in households of first-generation immigrants from countries where HBV is of high or intermediate endemicity
Health care and public safety workers who have occupational exposure to blood
Injection drug users
Heterosexual individuals who have had more than one sexual partner in the previous 6 mo and/or those with a recent episode of a sexually transmitted disease
Sexually active homosexual or bisexual males
Hemodialysis patients
Recipients of certain blood products (i.e., patients with hemophilia and other clotting disorders)
Clients and staff of institutions for the developmentally disabled
Household and sexual contacts of HBsAg-positive persons
Household contacts of adoptees from countries where HBV is highly endemic
Populations where HBV is highly endemic (e.g., Alaskan Eskimos)
Inmates of long-term correctional facilities
International travelers to highly endemic HBV regions for > 6 mo and who have close contact with the local population. Also short-term travelers who have contact with blood or sexual contact with residents in high- or intermediate-risk areas
Unvaccinated infants under 12 mo exposed to acute HBV infection through primary caregiver
Household contacts with blood exposure to a patient with acute HBV infection

[a]The CDC recommends that all newborns be vaccinated against hepatitis B.
Compiled from Refs. 1 and 88.

MEASURES TO PREVENT HEPATITIS B TRANSMISSION IN THE HEALTH CARE SETTING

In addition to vaccinating health care workers against hepatitis B, other infection control practices are important in preventing transmission of the virus (not all people develop an adequate antibody response to the vaccine). The most important infection control measure is the use of universal precautions. These precautions prevent exposure to blood and blood-derived body fluids via use of a variety of barrier precautions, measures to prevent needle sticks, environmental control measures, and good hand-washing techniques. However, if a worker is exposed to material that potentially contains HBV, recommendations for percutaneous exposure to HBV should be followed (discussed in the next section).

POSTEXPOSURE PROPHYLAXIS

If an individual is infected with HBV within 72 hours of receiving the vaccine and the person responds to the vaccine, symptoms of the infection either are absent or less severe. This forms the basis for vaccination plus HBIG treatment as postexposure prophylaxis.[85] Hepatitis B vaccination is recommended for any person not previously vaccinated who is exposed to blood potentially containing HBsAg. The source should be tested for HBsAg. If positive, the exposed person should receive HBIG. Specific recommendations are in Tables 38–10 and 38–11.

One dose of HBIG prevents hepatitis B in 75% of people with sexual exposure to HBV, if given within 2 weeks of exposure.[1] Testing of sexual partners for susceptibility is recommended before treatment.[1] All sexual partners of persons with acute HBV infections or hepatitis B carriers should receive one dose of HBIG. Hepatitis B vaccination should be started if ongoing sexual contact with the infected person will occur.[1]

Perinatal transmission of HBV occurs in 70% to 90% of cases and depends on the hepatitis B e-antigen status of the mother.[1] Even with administration of three doses of HBIG, 25% of infants exposed to HBV will become carriers.[85] With one dose of HBIG given within 24 hours of birth plus the hepatitis B vaccine series started within 1 week of birth, only 5% to 15% of infants develop the carrier state.[1,85] Current recommendations therefore include administration of both HBIG and HBV vaccine to neonates with HBV exposure, although vaccination without HBIG may be effective.[85] Unfortunately, those 5% to 15% of infants infected in utero cannot be helped with treatment.[85]

Twenty to thirty percent of infants infected with HBV die of complications of the infection.[92] A higher percentage experience substantial morbidity. Therefore, pregnant women are routinely screened for HBsAg. Infants at risk of acquiring HBV receive HBIG and hepatitis B vaccine shortly after birth.[1] If the HBV status of a woman is unknown at the time she presents for delivery, HBsAg testing is done then, and the baby receives appropriate prophylaxis. Infants born to HBsAg-positive mothers should begin prophylaxis within 12 hours of birth, or as soon as possible, using the schedule in Table 38–9. These infants should be tested for HBsAg and anti-HBs at 12 to 15 months of age. Testing for anti-HBs is not useful, because the maternal antibody can persist longer than 1 year.[1] Routine childhood vaccinations can be given.

HEPATITIS C

No vaccine for hepatitis C is available. Vaccine development for HCV is difficult because of the extensive genomic variability of the virus, viral mutants, and the lack of efficacy of serum antibodies. Although universal screening of blood donors has virtually eliminated HCV transmission through blood and blood products, screening has had little effect on the number of cases of hepatitis C in the United States because only a small percentage of cases result from blood transfusion. Programs that focus on reducing HIV transmission should decrease transmission of HCV in high-risk groups (universal precautions; no blood, organ, or tissue donation by HCV-positive individuals; safe sex practices for those with multiple partners; and avoidance of sharing razors and toothbrushes in households with an HCV-positive member). It is not clear if protected sexual intercourse should be recommended to couples in monogamous relationships or whether the domestic partner of infected patients should be followed for evidence of HCV infection.[19] Likewise, no clear policy for counseling women of childbearing age exists (although pregnancy is not contraindicated in HCV-positive individuals). Prophylaxis with immunoglobulin after needle stick exposure to hepatitis C is not recommended.

Benefit associated with identification of HCV infections in health care workers is limited. However, the CDC, in collaboration with the Hospital Infection Control Practices Advisory Committee, recommends that health care institutions consider implementing policies and procedures for follow-up for HCV infection after percutaneous or permucosal exposures to blood.[93] Follow-up should include testing the source for anti-HCV; baseline and 6-month follow-up testing for anti-HCV and AST for the person exposed to an anti-HCV–positive source; confirmation by supplemental anti-HCV testing of all anti-HCV–reactive results; and education of health care workers about blood-borne infections. Postexposure prophylaxis with IG or IFN is not recommended.

DELTA HEPATITIS

The delta virus depends on HBV for replication, and thus prevention of HBV infection will prevent HDV.[1] Exposure to HBV and HDV should be treated as an exposure to HBV alone.[1] No products are available to help prevent HDV superinfection in HBsAg carriers.

HEPATITIS E

The best prevention method for hepatitis E is avoidance of potentially contaminated food or water and maintenance of good sanitary practices.[1] There is no evidence that IG or HBIG will prevent hepatitis E, and it is unlikely that immunoglobulins prepared in the United States would have high concentrations of antibody to hepatitis E, because the disease is rare in the United States. It is likely that a vaccine for HEV will be developed in the next few years.[78]

ECONOMIC CONSIDERATIONS

Vaccination against hepatitis A without prior screening will only produce cost savings for groups of young adults who are exposed to a relatively high risk of HAV infection.[94] Prior screening for HAV antibodies can only be recommended from a cost-effectiveness point of view at expected levels of natural immunity exceeding 35% (moderately endemic countries or in older travelers).[94] Passive immunization remains the most cost-effective option for occasional short-duration travel to highly endemic areas. Based on average wholesale price (AWP), the cost of hepatitis A vaccine is about $30 for a pediatric dose and about $60 for an adult dose.[70] Vaccination is cost effective for individuals who are likely to spend several or prolonged periods in highly endemic countries. On average, vaccination is not going to be cost saving, and the cost per infection prevented can be several thousands of dollars.[94]

It is not appropriate to recommend vaccination for the entire traveler population. It is preferable to tailor the advice to the specific situation of each tourist or business traveler depending on travel plans and circumstances. From the traveler's and the societal perspective, lost productivity time related to acute hepatitis A is 21 to 28 days on average. For the unfortunate individual with severe acute hepatitis A, productivity can be diminished for over 3 months.

Hepatitis A vaccination in communities with high rates of hepatitis A is cost saving.[3] Further study is needed to determine whether cost–benefit is evident with hepatitis A vaccination in communities with sporadic outbreaks.

Several investigators have examined the cost effectiveness of the United States hepatitis B vaccination strategies.[95–97] Not all studies used strong, clear methodology,[95] and thus the conclusions must be interpreted cautiously. However, nearly all studies conclude that universal vaccination of infants, combined with catch-up programs, is cost effective.[95,96] In other words, preventing hepatitis B is less expensive than treating the disease. Cost per life year saved compares favorably with programs such as smoking cessation, coronary artery bypass surgery, and pneumococcal vaccination.[96] The current cost of the vaccine is $100 to $165 per adult vaccination series (based on AWP).[70] The infant vaccination series is proportionately one-half as costly or less.

▶ PRINCIPLES OF PHARMACOTHERAPY

- Viral hepatitis causes significant morbidity and mortality. Despite breakthroughs in diagnosis and management in the last few years, acute and chronic viral hepatitis infections remain a worldwide health problem.
- Hepatitis A usually does not cause clinical illness in children, but adults with acute HAV can be clinically ill for 1 or more months. Treatment is symptomatic. Prevention with vaccine or immunoglobulin is encouraged.
- Hepatitis B virus causes acute and chronic disease, with complications that include chronic active hepatitis, cirrhosis, hepatocellular cancer, and death. Some individuals carry the virus and transmit it to others, but are not clinically ill themselves. For patients with chronic hepatitis B, IFN-α is the most effective known treatment. Dosing is 5 MU daily for 4 to 6 months. About one-third of treated patients have a sustained response.
- Chronic hepatitis C infection is a significant public health problem that has important clinical and financial consequences. The only effective treatment is IFN (3 MU three times weekly for 6 to 24 months). Unfortunately, a sustained response is seen in only approximately 15% to 25% of patients. Patients who relapse usually do so within the first few months after stopping therapy. Tailoring therapy on the basis of viral load or genotype, coupled with better patient selection, and use of combination drug regimens may improve response rates.
- Further clarification of the role of IFN in chronic HCV and HBV (dosing, evaluation parameters, optimal population for use) is needed. Additional therapeutic options and therapeutic combinations are desirable. IFN is expensive, requires administration by the subcutaneous route, and is associated with moderate to severe adverse effects. Long-term effects of IFN therapy and predictors of response to IFN therapy are two primary areas for future research.
- Persons at increased risk for HAV infection or its consequences such as frequent international travelers, should be vaccinated against hepatitis A. Children living in communities with high rates of hepatitis A as well as contacts of case-patients should also receive hepatitis A vaccination.
- More widespread use of vaccines provides the best weapon against viral hepatitis. Immunoprophylaxis of viral diseases is one of the most cost effective of medical strategies. All infants should be vaccinated against hepatitis B. Older children and adults in high-risk groups should also be vaccinated.

REFERENCES

1. Centers for Disease Control and Prevention. Protection against viral hepatitis: Recommendations of the Immunization Practices Advisory Committee (ACIP). MMWR 1990;39:1–26.
2. Purcell RH. The discovery of the hepatitis viruses. Gastroenterology 1993;104:955–963.
3. Centers for Disease Control. Prevention of hepatitis A through active or passive immunization. MMWR 1996;45:1–30.
4. Moyer LA, Mast EE. Hepatitis B: Virology, epidemiology, disease, and prevention, and an overview of viral hepatitis. Am J Prevent Med 1994;10(suppl):45–55.
5. Losowsky MS. The clinical course of viral hepatitis. Clin Gastroenterol 1980;91:3–21.
6. Hoofnagle JH, DiBisceglie AM. Serologic diagnosis of acute and chronic viral hepatitis. Semin Liver Dis 1991;11:73–83.
7. Koziel MJ. Immunology of viral hepatitis. Am J Med 1996;100: 98–109.
8. Gust ID, Feinstone SM. Hepatitis A. Prog Liver Dis 1990;9:371–378.
9. Shapiro CN. Transmission of hepatitis viruses. Ann Intern Med 1994; 120:82–84.
10. Kiyasu PK, Caldwell SH. Diagnosis and treatment of the major hepatotrophic viruses. Am J Med Sci 1993;306:248–261.
11. London WT, Evans AA. The epidemiology of hepatitis viruses B, C, and D. Clin Lab Med 1996;16:251–271.
12. Sjogren MH. Serologic diagnosis of viral hepatitis. Med Clin North Am 1996;80:929–956.
13. Bernstein BM, Gill JC. Natural history and therapy of hepatitis B and C in patients with HIV disease. AIDS Clin Rev 1993–94;129–143.
14. Carey WD, Patel G. Viral hepatitis in the 1990s, I. Current principles of management. Cleve Clin J Med 1992;59:317–325.
15. Yoffe B, Noonan CA. Hepatitis B virus. Dig Dis Sci 1992;37:1–9.
16. Trepo C, Zoulim F, Alonso C, et al. Diagnostic markers of viral hepatitis B and C. Gut 1993;34(suppl 2):S81–S86.
17. Sherlock S, Dusheiko G. Hepatitis C virus updated. Gut 1991;32: 965–967.
18. Weiland O, Schvarcz R. Hepatitis C: Virology, epidemiology, clinical course and treatment. Scand J Gastroenterol 1992;27:337–342.
19. Sharara AI, Hunt CM, Hamilton JD. Hepatitis C. Ann Intern Med 1996;125:658–668.
20. Zein NN, Rakela J, Krawitt EL, et al. Hepatitis C virus genotypes in the United States: Epidemiology, pathogenicity, and response to interferon therapy. Ann Intern Med 1996;125:634–639.
21. Alter MJ. Non-A, non-B hepatitis: Sorting through a diagnosis of exclusion. Ann Intern Med 1989;110:583–585.
22. Iwarson S, Norkrans G, Wejstal R. Hepatitis C: Natural history of a unique infection. Clin Infect Dis 1995;20:1361–1370.

23. Tedeschi V, Seeff LB. Diagnostic tests for hepatitis C: Where are we now? Ann Intern Med 1995;123:383–385.
24. Casey JL. Hepatitis delta virus. Clin Lab Med 1996;16:451–464.
25. Scharschmidt BF. Hepatitis E: A virus in waiting. Lancet 1995;346: 519–520.
26. Centers for Disease Control. Hepatitis E among U.S. travelers, 1989–1992. MMWR 1993;42:1–4.
27. Clayson ET, Myint KSA, Snitbhan R, et al. Viremia, fecal shedding, and IgM and IgG responses in patients with hepatitis E. J Infect Dis 1995;172:927–933.
28. Bryan JP, Tsarev SA, Iqbal M, et al. Epidemic hepatitis E in Pakistan: Patterns of serologic response and evidence that antibody to hepatitis E virus protects against disease. J Infect Dis 1994;170:517–521.
29. Deka N, Sharma MD, Mukerjee R. Isolation of the novel agent from human stool samples that is associated with sporadic non-A, non-B hepatitis. J Virol 1994;68:7810–7815.
30. Miyakawa Y, Mayumi M. Hepatitis G virus—A true hepatitis virus or an accidental tourist? N Engl J Med 1997;336:795–796.
31. Alter MJ, Gallagher M, Morris TT, et al. Acute non-A-E hepatitis in the United States and the role of hepatitis G virus infection. N Engl J Med 1997;336:741–746.
32. Rubio A, Rey C, Sanchez-Quijano A, et al. Is hepatitis G virus transmitted sexually? JAMA 1997;277:532–533.
33. Stark K, Bienzle U, Hess G, et al. Detection of the hepatitis G virus genome among injecting drug users, homosexual and bisexual men, and blood donors. J Infect Dis 1996;174:1320–1323.
34. Feucht HH, Zollner B, Polywka S, Laufs R. Vertical transmission of hepatitis G. Lancet 1996;347:615–616.
35. Alter HJ, Nakatsuji Y, Melpolder J, et al. The incidence of transfusion-associated hepatitis G virus infection and its relation to liver disease. N Engl J Med 1997;336:747–754.
36. Esteban R. Is there a role for interferon in viral hepatitis? Gut 1993; 34(suppl 2):S77–S80.
37. Takano S, Satomura Y, Omata M, Japan Acute Hepatitis Cooperative Study Group. Effects of interferon beta on non-A, non-B acute hepatitis: A prospective, randomized, controlled-dose study. Gastroenterology 1994;107:805–811.
38. Pappas SC. Fulminant viral hepatitis. Gastroenterol Clin North Am 1995;24:161–173.
39. Lee WM. Acute liver failure. N Engl J Med 1993;329;1862–1872.
40. Martin P, Munoz SJ, Friedman LS. Liver transplantation for viral hepatitis: Current status. Am J Gastroenterol 1992;87:409–418.
41. Hansson BG, Riesbeck K, Nordenfelt E, Weiland O. Successful treatment of fulminant hepatitis B and fulminant hepatitis B and D coinfection explained by inhibitory effect on the immune response? Prog Clin Biol Res 1991;364:421–427.
42. Yoshiba M, Sekiyama K, Inoue K, Fujita R. Interferon and cyclosporin A in the treatment of fulminant viral hepatitis. J Gastroenterol 1995;30:67–73.
43. Hoofnagle JH, DiBisceglie AM. The treatment of chronic viral hepatitis. N Engl J Med 1997;336:347–356.
44. Weissberg JI, Andres LL, Smith CI, et al. Survival in chronic hepatitis B: An analysis of 397 patients. Ann Intern Med 1984;101: 613–616.
45. Greenberg HB, Pollard RB, Lutwick LI, et al. Effect of human leukocyte IFN on hepatitis B virus infection in patients with chronic active hepatitis. N Engl J Med 1976;295:517–522.
46. Main J, Jacyna MR, Thomas HC. The diagnosis and management of viral hepatitis. Communicable Dis Rep 1992;2:R117–R120.
47. Perrillo RP. Interferon in the management of chronic hepatitis B. Digest Dis Sci 1993;38:577–593.
48. Perillo RP, Mason AL. Therapy for hepatitis B virus infection. Gastroenterol Clin North Am 1994;23:581–601.
49. Korenman J, Baker B, Waggoner J, et al. Long-term remission of chronic hepatitis B after alpha-IFN therapy. Ann Intern Med 1991; 114:629–634.
50. Wright TL, Lau JYN. Clinical aspects of hepatitis B virus infection. Lancet 1993;342:1340–1344.
51. Benhamou Y, Katlama C, Lunel R, et al. Effects of lamivudine on replication of hepatitis B virus in HIV-infected men. Ann Intern Med 1996;125:705–712.
52. Dienstag JL, Perrillo RP, Schieff ER, et al. A preliminary trial of lamivudine for chronic hepatitis B infection. N Engl J Med 1995; 333:1657–1661.
53. Dusheiko GM. New treatments for chronic viral hepatitis B and C. Clin Gastroenterol 1996:10:299–333.
54. Grimm I. Lamivudine: A magic bullet for chronic hepatitis B? Gastroenterology 1996:111:262–264.
55. Grellier L, Mutimer D, Ahmed M, et al. Lamivudine prophylaxis against reinfection in liver transplantation for hepatitis B cirrhosis. Lancet 1996;348:1212–1215.
56. Cirelli R, Herne K, McCrary M, et al. Famciclovir: Review of clinical efficacy and safety. Antiviral Res 1996:29:141–151.
57. Lok ASF. Treatment of chronic hepatitis B. J Viral Hepat 1994; 1:105–124.
58. Perillo RP. Antiviral agents in the treatment of chronic viral hepatitis. Prog Liver Dis 1992;10:283–309.
59. DiBisceglie AM, Shindo M, Fong TL, et al. A pilot study of ribavirin therapy for chronic hepatitis C. Hepatology 1992;16:649–654.
60. Farci P, Mandas A, Coiana A, et al. Treatment of chronic hepatitis D with interferon alpha-2a. N Engl J Med 1994;330:88–94.
61. Romeo R, Pol S, Berthelot P, Brechot C. Eradication of hepatitis C virus RNA after alpha-IFN therapy. Ann Intern Med 1994;121: 276–277.
62. DiBisceglie AM, Martin P, Kassianides C, et al. Recombinant IFN alpha therapy for chronic hepatitis C. A randomized, double-blind, placebo-controlled trial. N Engl J Med 1989;321:1506–1510.
63. Davis GL, Balart LA, Schiff ER, et al. Treatment of chronic hepatitis C with recombinant IFN alpha. A multicenter randomized, controlled trial. Hepatitis International Therapy Group. N Engl J Med 1989; 321:1501–1506.
64. Saracco G, Rizzetto M. Predictors of response to interferon therapy. Dig Dis Sci 1996:41:115S–120S.
65. Maggiore G. Chronic hepatitis in children. Curr Opin Pediatr 1995; 7:539–546.
66. Poterucha JJ, Wiesner RH. Liver transplantation and hepatitis B. Ann Intern Med 1997;126:805–807. Editorial.
67. Shorrock C, Neuberger J. The changing face of liver transplantation. Gut 1993;34:295–298.
68. Briggs A, Shiell A. Interferon-α in hepatitis C. Pharmacoeconomics 1996;10:205–209.
69. Gane EJ, Portmann BC, Naoumov NV, et al. Long-term outcome of hepaitis C infection after liver transplantation. N Engl J Med 1996; 334:815–820.
70. 1997 Red Book. Montvale, NJ, Medical Economics, 1997:281, 321,350,486,490,562.
71. Dusheiko GM, Roberts JA. Treatment of chronic type B and C hepatitis with interferon ala: An economic appraisal. Hepatology 1995; 22:1863–1873.
72. Koff RS, Seeff LB. Economic modeling of treatment in chronic hepatitis B and chronic hepatitis C: Promises and limitations. Hepatology 1995;22:1880–1882.
73. Bennett WG, Pauker SG, Davis GL, Wong JB. Modeling therapeutic benefit in the midst of uncertainty. Therapy for hepatitis C. Dig Dis Sci 1996;41:56S–62S.
74. Bennett WG, Inoue Y, Beck JR, et al. Estimates of the cost-effectiveness of a single course of interferon α2b in patients with histologically mild chronic hepatitis C. Ann Intern Med 1997;127:855–865.
75. Wong JB, Koff RS, Tine F, Pauker SG. Cost-effectiveness of interferon-alpha 2b treatment of hepatitis Be antigen-positive chronic hepatitis B. Ann Intern Med 1995;122:664–675.
76. Carithers RL Jr, Sugano D, Bayliss M. Health assessment for chronic HCV infection. Dig Dis Sci 1996;41:75S–80S.
77. Hollinger FB. Factors influencing the immune response to hepatitis B vaccine, booster dose guidelines, and vaccine protocol recommendations. Am J Med 1989;87(suppl 3A):36S–40S.

78. Lemon SM, Thomas DL. Vaccines to prevent viral hepatitis. N Engl J Med 1997;336:196–204.
79. Werzberger A, Mensch B, Kuter B, et al. A controlled trial of a formalin-inactivated hepatitis A vaccine in healthy children. N Engl J Med 1992;327:453–457.
80. Innis BL, Snitbhan R, Kunasol P, et al. Protection against hepatitis A by an inactivated vaccine. JAMA 1994;271:1328–1334.
81. Lee SD, Lo KJ, Chan CY, et al. Immunogenicity of inactivated hepatitis A vaccine in children. Gastroenterology 1993;104:1129–1132.
82. Kaiser Permanente of Colorado. Guidelines for the Prevention of Hepatitis A in Travelers. May 1995:1–2.
83. Centers for Disease Control and Prevention. Recommendations of the Advisory Committee on Immunization Practices: Use of vaccines and immune globulins in persons with altered immunocompetence. MMWR 1993;42:1–18.
84. Centers for Disease Control. Hepatitis B virus: A comprehensive strategy for eliminating transmission in the United States through universal childhood vaccination. MMWR 1991;40:1–25.
85. Troisi CL, Hollinger FB. Hepatitis B vaccines. Prog Liver Dis 1990; 9:405–442.
86. Centers for Disease Control and Prevention. General recommendations on immunization: Recommendations of the Advisory Committee on Immunization Practices (ACIP). MMWR 1994;43:1–38.
87. Centers for Disease Control and Prevention. Update: Recommendations to prevent hepatitis B virus transmission—United States. MMWR 1995;44:574–575.
88. Committee on Infectious Diseases, 1993 to 1994. American Academy of Pediatrics. Update on timing of hepatitis B vaccination for premature infants and for children with lapsed immunization. Pediatrics 1994;94:403–404.
89. Greenberg DP. Pediatric experience with recombinant hepatitis B vaccines and relevant safety and immunogenicity studies. Pediatr Infect Dis J 1993;12:438–445.
90. Hadler SC. Hepatitis B prevention and human immunodeficiency virus (HIV) infection. Ann Intern Med 1988;109:92–94. Editorial.
91. Chang MH, Chen CJ, Lai MS, et al. Universal hepatitis B vaccination in Taiwan and the incidence of hepatocellular carcinoma in children. N Engl J Med 1997;336:1855–1859.
92. Arevalo JA, Washington ARE. Cost-effectiveness of prenatal screening and immunization for hepatitis B virus. JAMA 1988;259:365–369.
93. Centers for Disease Control and Prevention. Recommendations for follow-up of health-care workers after occupational exposure to hepatitis C virus. MMWR 1997;46:603–606.
94. Van Doorslaer E, Tormans G, van Damme P, Beutels P. Cost effectiveness of alternative hepatitis A immunisation strategies. Pharmacoeconomics 1995;8:5–8.
95. Jefferson T, Demicheli V. Is vaccination against hepatitis B efficient? A review of world literature. Health Econ 1994;3:25–37.
96. Hollinger FB. Comprehensive control (or elimination) of hepatitis B virus transmission in the United States. Gut 1996;38(suppl 2): S24–S30.
97. Bloom BS, Hillman AL, Fendrick AM, Schwartz JS. A reappraisal of hepatitis B virus vaccination strategies using cost-effectiveness analysis. Ann Intern Med 1993;118:298–306.

39

LIVER TRANSPLANTATION

Alka Z. Somani, PharmD, and Gilbert J. Burckart, PharmD, FCCP

Liver transplantation is a life-saving procedure for patients with severe hepatic disease who have no other medical option. Approximately 120 transplant centers in the United States now perform the operation. Liver transplantation makes up about 20% of all transplant surgeries performed in the United States. The 3-month graft and patient survival rate for liver transplantation is 81.1% and 87.8%, and the 1-year graft and patient survival rate is 74.1% and 82.2%, in the United States. In 1997 a total of 4167 liver transplants were performed, of which 4099 were cadaveric and 68 were from a living donor. In spite of the number of liver transplantation procedures, about 10,000 patients are still on the waiting list for a liver transplant in the United States. The mean waiting time for a liver transplant is 366 days, and 1131 patients died in 1997 waiting for a liver transplant.[1]

ETIOLOGY

The principal indications for transplantation in adults have been postnecrotic cirrhosis and primary biliary cirrhosis, but other common indications have included alcoholic cirrhosis, primary sclerosing cholangitis, acute hepatic failure, primary liver cancer, and inborn errors of metabolism.[2] Pediatric liver transplantation has been performed primarily for biliary atresia and inborn errors of metabolism. Postnecrotic cirrhosis, biliary atresia, and primary biliary cirrhosis make up almost 60% of all liver transplant indications. Postnecrotic cirrhosis is most commonly caused by alcohol use or hepatitis B or C.

The inborn errors of metabolism that have been treated by liver transplantation are a heterogeneous group of disorders, and correction of the metabolic defect has not always occurred. Liver transplantation has corrected α_1-antitrypsin deficiency; Wilson's disease; tyrosinemia; types I, III, and IV glycogen storage disease; type I hyperoxaluria; and hemophilia A and B. Correction has been incomplete in other disorders such as familial hyperlipidemia. Timing of the transplant is critical for correction of the metabolic disease in order to prevent irreversible damage to the end organ (e.g., central nervous system in ornithine transcarbamylase deficiency) or to prevent hepatocellular carcinoma (e.g., tyrosinemia).

To justify transplantation the patient should have a reasonable life expectancy after transplantation. Age does not appear to be a barrier to liver transplantation, with good 5-year survival rates in patients older than 50 years of age. Unfortunately, hepatitis can reoccur after liver transplantation and cause hepatic failure in the transplanted liver.[3] Survival following primary orthotopic liver transplantation for hepatitis is favorable, but survival after retransplantation is poor.[4] Table 39–1 summarizes the relative contraindications for liver transplantation and management techniques.

The shortage of donor organs has stimulated work in the area of hepatocyte transplantation[5] and in the development of artificial liver support.[6] Hepatocyte transplantation, where the cells are implanted into the liver or the spleen, may be considered as a temporary bridge to provide liver function in patients with end-stage liver failure until a donor becomes available. Cellular transplantation with hepatocytes is potentially a simpler, less expensive, and less invasive procedure when compared to liver transplantation.[7] Hepatocyte transplantation can involve the use of (1) heterologous cells being transplanted into an immunosuppressed recipient, or (2) partial hepatectomy of the recipient with an *in vitro* genetic correction with a recombinant vector to reverse the genetic defect followed by retransplantation of the autologous cells into a nonimmunocompromised recipient. Studies in animals and some preliminary human data indicate that the transplanted hepatocytes seed and proliferate in organs such as the spleen and liver over an entire life span.

THE PROCEDURE

Liver transplantation is the most technically demanding of the surgical transplant procedures. This difficulty has produced a slow increase in the number of successful centers performing liver transplant procedures. Figure 39–1 shows the anatomic structures critical to liver transplantation.

The first critical step in liver transplantation is the proper procurement of the donor organ. In approximately one-third of human donors, arterial abnormalities in the liver will be encountered that would make the organ useless without special techniques. New preservation solutions have extended the preservation period for livers to up to 24 hours. This extension in preservation has dramatically affected liver procurement practices and the availability of viable organs.

The recipient operation is roughly conducted in three phases: removal of recipient liver, donor graft revascularization, and biliary reconstruction. The venous hypertension produced by clamping of the inferior vena cava and portal vein during the anhepatic phase can cause edema of the intestinal mucosa, and has been circumvented in adult patients through the use of the venovenous bypass. Graft revascularization involves performing anastomosis of the

TABLE 39–1. Relative Contraindications for Liver Transplantation

Relative Contraindication	Additional Therapy or Management
Primary liver cancer	Chemotherapy
Hepatitis B	Hyperimmune globulin (HBIG)
Hepatitis C	Interferon-γ
Multiple abdominal surgeries (adhesions)	New surgical management techniques
AIDS	Lowered doses of immunosuppressants

vena cava above and below the liver (Fig. 39–1a) followed by the portal venous anastomosis (Fig. 39–1b). Biliary reconstruction can be accomplished in several ways: by end-to-end anastomosis of the donor and recipient common bile ducts over a T-tube stent, by side-to-side choledochostomy after closure of the donor and recipient duct ends, or by anastomosing the graft's common duct to a defunctionalized limb of jejunum (Roux limb, Fig. 39–1c). The complete procedure takes many hours, often requires several teams of surgeons, and is frequently accomplished with the replacement of multiple blood volumes for the patient.

One of the most difficult problems in pediatric transplantation is the availability of size-matched allografts. A donor liver allograft has to be within about 20% of the recipient's size. Otherwise the graft can impair breathing or closure of the abdomen if too large and may not be adequate for survival if too small. In order to overcome this problem, reduced-size liver transplantation has evolved as a technique where the donor liver is surgically reduced in size to meet the needs of the recipient. This technique has been most commonly used in split-liver transplantation, where a donor graft provides livers for two recipients,[8] and in living-related donor operations where a portion of the left lobe of the healthy liver is taken for the donor graft from the parent. Although some donor morbidity has resulted, there have been no cases of donor mortality. Immunosuppressive therapy is similar to a cadaveric donor

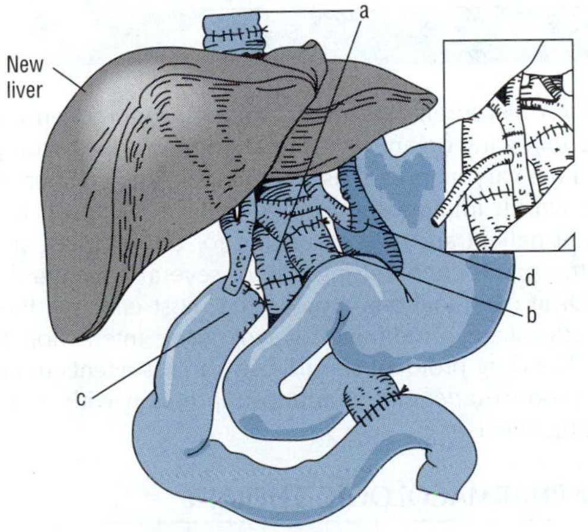

FIGURE 39–1. Orthotopic liver transplantation with (a) suprahepatic and intrahepatic inferior vena cava anastomosis, (b) portal venous anastomosis, (c) choledochojejunostomy, and (d) hepatic arterial anastomosis.

graft, but episodes of rejection that are resistant to corticosteroids appear to be less common in the recipient of a living-related donor liver allograft. Living-related donor operations may become more common at an increasing number of centers as the shortage of donor organs continues.[9]

EARLY TRANSPLANT FAILURE

Failure of the newly transplanted liver occurs in 10% to 15% of cases and can result from several different mechanisms. Early graft failure can result from preexisting disease in the donor, and even coagulation defects have been acquired through donor organs. The technical complexity of the operation can produce flaws in revascularization that also lead to graft nonfunction. Surgical complications occur in about 25% of cases and result in a doubling of the hospital expense for the patient.[10] Portal vein thrombosis, hepatic artery thrombosis, and bile duct leaks are all technical problems that have been encountered. Ischemic injury to the donor liver through preservation is difficult to predict, and can produce early graft dysfunction. Perioperative immune events rarely lead to the classic picture of hyperacute rejection in liver transplantation, but graft failure in the first 2 postoperative weeks may still indicate antibody-mediated graft destruction.

CLINICAL PRESENTATION OF THE POSTOPERATIVE LIVER TRANSPLANT PATIENT

The physiologic consequences of liver transplantation are complex, but an oversimplification can be made by combining models of rapidly changing hepatic function, postoperative patients with ileus and biliary tract dysfunction, catabolic patients on high doses of steroids, and immunocompromised patients. The liver transplant patient is represented by all of these models with each intricate component interacting with the other models in an individualized manner. The transition from poor hepatic function to normal liver processes is one that involves changes in both hepatic metabolic and synthetic function. The postoperative patient will have fluid, electrolyte, and nutritional abnormalities that will be combined with biliary tract dysfunction. Subsequently there is disruption of bile flow through removal of the gallbladder and, in some cases, temporary placement of a drainage tube (T tube) in the bile duct, which will alter the absorption of fats and fat-soluble drugs. Corticosteroids and the other immunosuppressive drugs have metabolic consequences that affect both endogenous and exogenous substrates. The immunosuppressed liver transplant patient will have the attendant risk of infection and requirement for the use of multiple anti-infective drugs.

The physiologic changes that the patient is undergoing result in alterations in the biopharmaceutical profile of any agent administered to a liver transplant patient.[11] Changes in drug absorption are quite dramatic in liver transplant patients. After a successful liver transplant operation, the absorption of lipid-soluble compounds is considerably improved. The poor absorption of the lipid-soluble drug cyclosporine A (CyA) improves after successful liver transplantation and reestablishment of bile flow. Tacrolimus (TAC) is also a fat-soluble drug, but its absorption does not appear to be bile-dependent in liver transplant patients. Vitamin E deficiency and its neurologic complications in liver failure patients are reversed after successful liver transplantation in pediatric patients. In stable adult liver transplant patients, the concentrations of retinol and tocopherol are similar to those seen in normal healthy subjects, indicating recovery of transplanted liver production and excretion of bile salts needed for fat-soluble vitamin absorption.

The protein binding of drugs in liver transplant patients is affected both by the synthetic capacity of the liver and by the pathophysiologic changes associated with the postoperative state. The serum concentration of albumin in liver transplant patients is frequently lower than that observed in normal subjects for months following surgery, resulting in a lower protein-bound fraction for drugs binding to albumin. When compared with patients with chronic liver disease, the binding of agents such as diazepam and salicylic acid is greater in liver transplant patients due to the removal of endogenous binding inhibitors. Studies in liver transplant patients indicate that the concentration of α_1-acid glycoprotein (AAG) increases after surgery and stays at an elevated level for at least 45 days. Correspondingly, the unbound fraction of lidocaine in plasma obtained from stable liver transplant patients is lower than the free fraction values observed in plasma from normal volunteers. Propranolol also binds to AAG, but no significant difference was observed in the unbound fraction of propranolol in stable liver transplant patients when compared with normal subjects. The increase in propranolol binding due to an increase in AAG concentration is offset by a reduction in albumin concentration, because albumin also contributes significantly to the binding of propranolol.

Liver metabolism is altered by a combination of factors related to physiologic changes (preservation injury or decreased effective hepatic blood flow initially), stimulation of hepatic microsomes by some immunosuppressant agents, and inhibition of microsomal drug transformation by other immunosuppressant agents. Metabolism mediated by the cytochrome P450 enzymes is generally depressed during the first month post-transplantation, and then recovers during the next few months. Clear exceptions are the cytochrome P450 isoenzyme CYP2E1, which has enhanced activity in liver transplant patients during the first month, and CYP2D6, which appears to be unaffected by the procedure. The oxidative metabolizing capacity of the liver as determined by antipyrine kinetics is similar in clinically stable liver transplant patients to that observed in normal subjects. First-pass metabolism is also expected to be altered during the transition to normal hepatic function. The conjugative processes of metabolism, as represented by the sulfation and glucuronidation of acetaminophen, normalizes in liver transplant patients, but the renal clearance of the conjugates is altered due to abnormal renal capacity to eliminate the metabolites. Altered biliary function not only affects the absorption of lipophilic compounds, but also affects the elimination of drugs and metabolites. For example, biliary dysfunction in liver transplant patients produces a high concentration of the CyA metabolites in blood. Biliary excretion of ceftriaxone is significantly decreased during the immediate postoperative period.

Renal elimination of drugs in liver transplant patients should not be considered normal in the immediate postoperative period. Earlier studies with liver transplant patients receiving CyA demonstrated that elimination of gentamicin, vancomycin, and the cephalosporin antibiotics is less than would be predicted by serum creatinine. These physiologic alterations in a liver transplant patient must be considered when developing individualized drug regimens.

▶ TREATMENT: Immunosuppressive Measures

DESIRED OUTCOME

1. Prevent acute and chronic rejection of the transplanted organ.
2. Prevent infectious complications of immunosuppression.
3. Prevent adverse drug effects and drug interactions with immunosuppressants.
4. Educate the patient on medications and promote proper medication compliance.

GENERAL APPROACH TO TREATMENT

The goal of immunomodulatory therapy in transplantation is to promote acceptance of donor tissue, while preventing rejection and maintaining the functional status of the immune system with respect to other foreign materials. Immunosuppression with medications following organ transplantation may appear complex because of the varying protocols used by transplant centers throughout the world. Immunosuppressive measures chosen for a liver transplant patient are largely specific for the protocol at an individual transplant center, using one of several effective drug regimens. Drug combinations provide the most effective therapy by taking advantage of additive or synergistic interaction between agents. The drug protocol should use various agents in combination to produce adequate immunosuppression with minimal adverse drug effects.

NONPHARMACOLOGIC THERAPY

Lymphoid irradiation was one of the earliest nonpharmacologic means of immunosuppression, and is still used in some centers for resistant rejection. Another nonpharmacologic treatment that may influence drug therapy is induction of microchimerism, or the state in which the donor cells are tolerated by the host. To accomplish this, the organ transplant recipient is administered an intravenous infusion of bone marrow from the donor. Adjusting the immunotherapy in the immediate posttransplant period so that the host is not totally suppressed may also facilitate microchimerism. Microchimerism can occur when donor cells migrate from the transplanted organ to establish mutual tolerance with the host's T cells. A small number of donor cells can be identified in the skin biopsies of long-term survivors of liver and kidney transplants .[12] A stable balance of donor cell and recipient cell interaction may be necessary for long-term graft survival. At the present time, nonpharmacologic manipulation must be supplemented with pharmacologic therapy that has been proven to be successful.

Graft versus host disease (GVHD) develops when the graft, which contains immunologically competent cells, recognizes the host as foreign and mounts an immunologic response against the host. This is a rare complication that has been observed in liver and bone marrow transplantation. GVHD clinically presents as fever, rash, and pancytopenia within 4 to 6 weeks of transplantation. The recommended management of GVHD is the aggressive administration of immunosuppressive therapy.[13]

PHARMACOLOGIC THERAPY

DRUG TREATMENTS OF FIRST CHOICE

Commercially available immunosuppressive agents for liver transplantation include the following.

Immunophilin-binding agents: Cyclosporine (CyA) or tacrolimus (TAC).
Steroids: Methylprednisolone or prednisone (PRED).
Antiproliferative agents: Azathioprine (AZA) or mycophenolate mofetil (MMF).
Anti–T-cell biologic products: Muromonab-CD3 (OKT3) or antilymphocyte (ALG) / antithymocyte globulin (ATG).
Interleukin-2 receptor monoclonal antibody: Daclizumab or basiliximab.

PUBLISHED GUIDELINES OR TREATMENT PROTOCOLS

Transplant centers use double, triple, or quadruple therapy (Table 39–2). Studies have shown that the various protocols are equally safe and effective when used by a transplant center that is familiar with medication regimens. Drug combinations should use the lowest effective dose to minimize adverse effects. Deciding which protocol to use may depend on individual patient parameters including the cause of liver failure, whether the patient has had a previous transplant, sensitization to histocompatability antigens, and side effects caused by the immunosuppressant medications. To avoid the nephrotoxic effects of CyA, initial therapy may include PRED + AZA or MMF and OKT3 or ALG. Cyclosporine therapy is then started 1 to 2 weeks after transplant.

TABLE 39–2. Examples of Immunosuppression Protocols

1.	CyA or TAC	+	PRED				
2.	CyA or TAC	+	PRED	+	AZA or MMF		
3.	CyA or TAC	+	PRED	+	AZA or MMF	+	OKT3 or ALG/ATG
4.	CyA or TAC	+	PRED			+	OKT3 or ALG/ATG
5.			PRED	+	AZA or MMF		
6.			PRED	+	AZA or MMF	+	OKT3 or ALG/ATG

PIVOTAL CLINICAL TRIALS

An open-label randomized multicenter trial comparing CyA and TAC in liver transplantation in the United States found that the actuarial survival rates for patients and grafts were similar between the two groups.[14] The TAC group did have significantly lower incidences of acute rejection and corticosteroid-resistant rejection. Nephrotoxicity and neurotoxicity required that more patients be withdrawn from TAC therapy than from CyA therapy. A European trial found similar results in that survival and adverse effects were similar with CyA and TAC in liver transplant patients, but that the incidence of acute, refractory, and chronic rejection was lower in the TAC group.[15] One of the primary uses for TAC in centers that use CyA as their primary immunosuppressant drug is as rescue therapy. Patient survival rates exceeding 80% have been reported in liver transplant patients who were converted from CyA to TAC due to failure of the conventional immunosuppressive therapy, which is considered an outstanding response rate.[16] CyA-associated side effects include nephrotoxicity, hypertension, neurologic disorders, and hyperlipidemia, which may lead to posttransplant morbidity. Conversion from CyA to TAC reduces side effects while maintaining stable graft function.[17] Another advantage of TAC is that corticosteroid therapy can frequently be eliminated in the long-term regimen, reducing the adverse effects of prolonged corticosteroid therapy.

ALTERNATIVE TREATMENTS AND OTHER DRUG TREATMENTS

Other pharmacologic agents are often required for the adequate management of a transplant patient. Anti-infective prophylaxis (antibiotic, antifungal, and antiviral) and therapy is used to prevent and treat infections in the immunocompromised patient. The balance between immunosuppression and infection control is critical in the liver transplant patient because of the constant exposure of the graft to intestinal flora. In the presence of rejection, the liver can become an open portal for entry of bacterial organisms from the GI tract. Bacterial or fungal invasion can result in local abscess formation or in general sepsis, both of which represent life-threatening infectious complications of transplantation and immunosuppression. Antibiotics also need to be given for surgical or dental prophylaxis. The most frequent cause of death after liver transplantation is severe infection.[18] Table 39–3 shows the routine medications given to a liver transplantation patient upon discharge from the University of Pittsburgh Medical Center in 1998.

Certain patient populations are more susceptible to infectious disease, such as the recipient who lacks antibodies to cytomegalovirus (CMV) but receives an organ from a CMV-positive donor. Liver transplant patients have an increased incidence of symptomatic CMV infection in comparison with renal transplant patients (32% versus 8%, respectively).[19] These infections are most frequently observed from 3 to 8 weeks following transplantation or after an intensive treatment course for rejection. As with other transplants, liver recipients who are seronegative for CMV prior to transplantation are at increased risk for symptomatic CMV infections (88% of infections) in comparison with liver recipients who were preoperatively seropositive (32% of symptomatic infections). Although prophylactic therapy with ganciclovir or acyclovir is used in some centers, a newer approach is to follow the patient's CMV leukocyte antigen concentration and to treat the patient aggressively when the antigen concentration increases.[20] The antigen level can then also be used as a measure of response to therapy in patients undergoing treatment with intravenous ganciclovir. The place of oral ganciclovir in the prophylaxis against CMV disease has not been determined in liver transplant patients. Other significant viral diseases in liver transplant patients include herpes simplex types 1 and 2, hepatitis B,

TABLE 39–3. Routine Medications Orders Upon Discharge for an Adult Liver Transplant Patient (University of Pittsburgh, 1998)

Medication	Usual Dose	Long-term Goal
Immunosuppression		
Tacrolimus	bid (to achieve level of 5–20 ng/mL)	Taper dose and level over time if no rejection and stable liver enzymes.
Prednisone	20 mg qd	Taper and discontinue by 6 mo if no rejection and stable liver enzymes.
± Mycophenolate mofetil	1 g bid	Taper and discontinue after 1 yr if no rejection and stable liver enzymes.
Anti-infective Prophylaxis		
Sulfamethoxazole/trimethoprim	SS tab	M-W-F for PCP, continue lifelong. Alternative: Pentamidine 300 mg inhalation q mo.
Acyclovir	200 mg bid	For herpes virus, discontinue after 6 mo, then use only if needed.
Nystatin	5 cc qid	For thrush, taper and discontinue within 6 mo, then use only if needed.
Gastrointestinal Prophylaxis		
Nizatidine	150 mg bid	Change to prn when prednisone dose reduced to 5 mg qd (or omeprazole 20 mg qd-bid).

adenoviral hepatitis, and Epstein–Barr viral (EBV) diseases ranging from an infectious mononucleosis syndrome to life-threatening lymphoproliferative disease. An expanded discussion of the post-transplant lymphoproliferative disease (PTLD) seen in transplant patients and associated with EBV can be found in Chapter 16.

Hypertension (Chap. 10), hypergylcemia (Chap. 70), and hyperlipidemia (Chap. 19) may also be caused or exacerbated by the immunosuppressive medications. Modifying the immunosuppressive therapy may assist in the management of these secondary conditions but may not result in the desired control. Selection of medications to treat hypertension, hyperglycemia, and hyperlipidemia follow the same guidelines used in nontransplant patients. The pharmacotherapist must be aware of the drug interactions in a liver transplant patient and their role in medication selection. Diltiazem increases CyA levels, but diltiazem is considered the drug of choice for hypertension at some transplant centers because it allows the dose of CyA to be reduced. Another drug-related problem in liver transplant patients is the development of PTLD. Lymphomas develop in 1% to 5% of posttransplant patients, which may require decreasing or stopping immunosuppressive therapy. This approach may result in complete regression of the lymphomatous changes but places the patient at higher risk for rejection of their transplanted organ.

SPECIAL POPULATIONS: WOMEN AND PREGNANCY

Many women with liver disease have menstrual irregularities and reproductive problems, and these problems are corrected by liver transplantation. Healthy infants have been delivered by mothers receiving CyA or receiving TAC, but couples should be counseled about the possible hypertension and graft dysfunction that can accompany pregnancy in a mother with a liver transplant. Medications that are potentially harmful, such as MMF, should be discontinued prior to conception. Pregnancy must be planned and managed as a high-risk situation by both an obstetrician and a surgeon.[21]

DRUG CLASS INFORMATION

Tacrolimus (Prograf, Fujisawa) inhibits the production of IL-2 in T cells, thereby inhibiting the growth and proliferation of those cells. Tacrolimus binds to the cytoplasmic immunophilin, FK-binding protein (FKBP), with subsequent inhibition of the activity of calcineurin. Following oral administration, the bioavailability of TAC ranges from 5% to 66%, with a mean of 29% in liver transplant patients. The poor bioavailability of TAC necessitates the use of 3 to 4 times higher oral doses than IV doses to obtain similar blood concentrations. The 1-year graft survival rate when taking FK is 82%, and patient survival rate is 88%.[14] Adverse effects that occur with 10% to 20% of patients taking TAC are neurologic, including insomnia, tremors, headaches, photophobia, nightmares, and hyperthesias. Major neurologic side effects occur 8% to 21% of the time, including confusion, seizures, coma, dysarthrias, psychosis, and encephalopathy. Tacrolimus is metabolized by cytochrome P450-34A, so other medications metabolized by this enzyme can alter TAC concentrations. Macrolide antibiotics, such as erythromycin, and antifungal medications, such as itraconazole and fluconazole, can increase TAC levels, while the anticonvulsants phenytoin and phenobarbital as well as rifampin can lower TAC blood concentration levels. Medications that are nephrotoxic should be used with caution because TAC can also be nephrotoxic. Because TAC decomposes in alkaline media, antacids and medications that increase the pH of the GI tract will decrease TAC absorption, and should be spaced 2 hours apart from TAC administration. Patients should take their TAC doses at a consistent time in relation to meals. Initial intravenous TAC doses range from 0.05 to 0.1 mg/kg per day, and are administered by continuous infusion. Oral doses range from 0.1 to 0.3 mg/kg per day given in two divided doses every 12 hours. Tacrolimus doses are then adjusted according to trough blood levels (5 to 20 ng/mL), clinical response, and adverse effects. Patients with hepatic dysfunction may require a reduction in dose, but no change is needed with renal dysfunction. Pediatric transplant patients clear the drug more rapidly and require 2 to 4 times higher mg/kg doses than adults to maintain equivalent therapeutic concentrations.

Cyclosporine (Sandimmune, Neoral, Novartis) also inhibits T-lymphocyte proliferation by inhibiting the production of IL-2 and other cytokines by T cells. Cyclosporine binds to a cytoplasmic immunophilin called cyclophillin, which blocks the action of calcineurin. Following oral administration, the absorption of CyA is incomplete and erratic. Neoral is a microemulsion of CyA that has a higher and more reliable absorption of the drug than the older Sandimmune product. Neoral is associated with a lower incidence of rejection compared to those on Sandimmune.[22] The 1-year liver graft survival rate when taking CyA is 79%, and the patient survival rate is 88%.[14] Adverse reactions that occur in more than 10% of patients include hypertension, nephrotoxicity, gingival hypertrophy, hirsutism, and tremor. Side effects that occur in less than 10% of patients include seizures, headache, leg cramps, acne, pancreatitis, hepatotoxicity, tachycardia, paresthesias, and sensitivity to temperature extremes. Cyclosporine is also metabolized by cytochrome P450-34A, and shares the same drug interactions as TAC. There are more drug interactions reported with CyA, including with diltiazem and verapamil, but this may be due to greater experience with CyA. The absorption of CyA is enhanced by a meal with a moderate fat content, so the patient should be advised to take CyA with meals. The normal dose range for CyA is 2 to 5 mg/kg per day as a continuous intravenous infusion, beginning before or after transplantation. The absorption of CyA in the immediate postoperative period may be very poor in a liver transplant patient, but some centers have attempted to use the oral Neoral product to avoid intravenous CyA administration. Because oral bioavailability averages 30%, initial oral doses are 8 to 17 mg/kg per day, with long-term dosage reductions to 5 mg/kg per day divided in 1 or 2 doses/d. Cyclosporine is excreted in the bile and is nephrotoxic; therefore dosage adjustments should be made when hepatic dysfunction is present. Similar to TAC, children require higher doses of CyA to maintain therapeutic drug concentrations, which are approximately 100 to 300 ng/mL.

Prednisone is converted to active prednisolone in the body and has multiple effects on the immune system. Corticosteroids block lymphocyte proliferation through inhibition of macrophage production of IL-1 and IL-6. Steroids also reduce the formation of other cytokines such as IL-2, IL-4, and interferon-α and of adhesion molecules on endothelial cells necessary for leukocytes to migrate out of the bloodstream. Prednisone is very well absorbed from the GI tract, and has a long biological half-life so it can be dosed once daily. The first-line therapy for the treatment of acute graft rejection is high-dose IV methylprednisolone (250 to 1000 mg) daily for 3 days or oral prednisone (200 mg). Doses of oral prednisone are then tapered over 5 days to 20 mg/d. Adverse effects of prednisone that occur in over 10% of patients include increased appetite, insomnia, indigestion (bitter taste), and mood changes. Side effects that occur less commonly, but are seen with high doses or prolonged therapy, include cataracts, hyperglycemia, hirsutism, bruising, acne, sodium and water retention, hypertension, bone growth suppression, and ulcerative esophagitis. Barbiturates, phenytoin, and rifampin decrease the effectiveness of prednisone, while prednisone will decrease the effectiveness of vaccines and toxoids. Prednisone should be taken with food to minimize GI upset. The dose of prednisone varies with the transplant center's protocol but usually is highest immediately following transplant and during treatment for acute rejection. It is becoming frequent practice to taper prednisone with the goal of discontinuation over a period of months. Corticosteroids should never be abruptly discontinued; tapering should be gradual due to suppression of the hypothalamic–pituitary–adrenal axis. Corticosteroids slow the growth rates in children, prompting clinicians to use alternate-day dosing or withhold steroids until rejection occurs.

Azathioprine (Imuran, Burroughs Wellcome) is an effective antiproliferative agent against both B and T lymphocytes via the inhibition of DNA and RNA synthesis. Azathioprine is metabolized to its active metabolites 6-mercaptopurine, 6-thioinosinic acid, and 6-thioguanine. The immunosuppressive effects of AZA last 12 to 24 hours, making once-daily dosing possible. Azathioprine is used to prevent rejection, but is not used to treat acute graft rejection. Adverse effects that occur in more than 10% of patients include leukopenia, anemia, fever, chills, nausea, and vomiting. Less common side effects include thrombocytopenia, hepatotoxicity, skin rash, and retinopathy. Because AZA is metabolized by xanthine oxidase, the usual AZA dose should be reduced by 25% to 33% in patients also receiving allopurinol. Azathioprine can be taken with food to minimize any gastrointestinal upset. Intravenous doses of AZA are initially 3 to 5 mg/kg per day, with maintenance IV doses 1 to 3 mg/kg per day. The oral AZA maintenance dose may be as low as 0.25 to 0.5 mg/kg per day. Doses may need downward adjustment when hepatic or renal dysfunction is present or if the WBC falls below 3000 to 4000 mm^3.

Mycophenolate mofetil (CellCept, Roche) blocks the proliferative responses to T and B lymphocytes by inhibiting antibody formation and the generation of cytotoxic T cells. The adhesion molecules that allow leukocytes to infiltrate tissues are also blocked by MMF. After oral absorption, MMF is hydrolyzed to the active metabolite, mycophenolic acid. Mycophenolic acid is metabolized to a glucuronide conjugate, which is inactive but may be converted back to the active parent drug in the blood. The drug is 97% bound to albumin in plasma, so that total plasma concentrations will vary in a liver transplant patient as plasma protein concentrations increase with normalizing hepatic synthetic function. Mycophenolate is currently only approved for the prevention of allograft rejection following renal transplantation. Limited data on the effectiveness of MMF in liver transplantation are available, and these studies are currently being conducted. Adverse effects with MMF include gastrointestinal disturbances (nausea, vomiting, diarrhea), neutropenia, thrombocytopenia, headache, weakness, dizziness, and insomnia. Antacids decrease the absorption of MMF, and administration of the two agents should be separated by 2 hours. Food will delay the absorption of MMF, but it may be necessary to take MMF with food to minimize the GI adverse effects. The dose of MMF for optimizing immunosuppression and minimizing adverse effects is 2 g/d, administered in two divided doses given every 12 hours. Pediatric doses of MMF are approximately 40 mg/kg per day in two doses. Plasma concentration monitoring has been suggested for MMF, but a good correlation with efficacy and adverse effects has not been demonstrated. Mycophenolate appears to be a more specific immunosuppressant for lymphocytes and has less adverse effects than AZA.

Muromonab-CD3 (OKT3, Ortho Biotech) is a monoclonal antibody that binds the CD3 receptor on lymphocytes. Circulating T cells become undetectable within minutes of an infusion of OKT3. OKT3 is used as induction therapy following transplantation and treatment of acute cellular rejection. Many transplant centers reserve the use of OKT3 for treating moderate to severe acute rejection unresponsive to high-dose corticosteroids. The initial dose of OKT3 may be associated with chills, fever, chest tightness, and wheezing. This first dose reaction can be minimized by premedication with antipyretics, antihistamines, and corticosteroids. Other adverse effects include fever, headache, neck stiffness, and central nervous system toxicity. The dose of OKT3 is usually 5 mg daily administered IV push for 5 to 14 days, or 2.5 mg in a child less than 30 kg in weight. A high proportion of patients treated with OKT3 form antibodies to one of the components of OKT3 and may not be able to receive or adequately respond to retreatment.[23]

Antilymphocyte (ALG)/antithymocyte (ATG) globulin (Atgam, Upjohn) is a sterile nonpyrogenic solution of immunoglobulins obtained from horses or other animals immunized with human lymphoid cells. ALG/ATG eliminates T cells and decreases the proliferation of newly formed lymphocytes. ALG/ATG is used for induction therapy and for treatment of an acute cellular rejection. Adverse effects include chills and febrile reactions following infusion that can be minimized with premedications (similar to OKT3). Phlebitis and hypotension can be avoided by administering the intravenous infusion over 4 to 6 hours. Thrombocytopenia and increased infectious risks may also occur. The dose ranges from 10 to 30 mg/kg per day for 5 to 14 days in adults. In children, the dose is reduced to 5 to 25 mg/kg per day. At the University of Pittsburgh Medical Center, ALG/ATG is used to treat mild to moderate acute rejection unresponsive to high-dose corticosteroids.

PHARMACOECONOMIC CONSIDERATIONS

Liver transplantation is the most expensive of the solid organ transplant procedures that are routinely performed in a large number of centers. The total average cost for the first year of care after liver transplantation is about $300,000, with average subsequent costs of about $20,000 per year.[24] Actual pharmacy charges make up only approximately 15% of that cost, so that the potential impact of drug therapy on the clinical course, episodes of rejection and infection, and retransplantation is a more important cost determinant than the drug cost alone in the first year following liver transplantation. Long-term maintenance costs are more heavily influenced by the cost of the drugs that are used.

Because liver transplantation is an expensive procedure, the performance of this operation will continue to come under close scrutiny in health care systems with limited resources.[25] Retransplantation of the liver more than doubles the cost of the procedure, and may not be a cost-effective use of scarce donor resources.[26] Managed care approaches to reducing the cost following liver transplantation do affect drug therapy through changes such as the outpatient administration of therapy for treating acute episodes of rejection.[27]

The U.S. FK506 Multicenter Trial has reported valuable information on the cost of liver transplantation in the United States, even if the report is not an ideal pharmacoeconomic assessment.[24] The analysis did identify a number of areas that significantly affect the cost of the liver transplant procedure, such as the increasing expense associated with steroid and with monoclonal antibody treatment of rejection, and the impact of readmission to the intensive care unit for severe rejection. The study concluded that primary immunosuppression with TAC saved $19,290 in the first year after liver transplantation in comparison with the use of CyA.

The potential for drug therapy to influence the cost of liver transplantation should not be underestimated. Even the use of prostaglandin E_1, which appears to have no impact on mortality or primary nonfunction in liver allografts and may add $5000 in drug costs, has been claimed to save $50,000 per patient by reducing the morbidity and hospital stay for these patients.[28]

EVALUATION OF THERAPEUTIC OUTCOMES

MONITORING OF THE PHARMACEUTICAL CARE PLAN

The pharmacotherapist must attempt to balance drug therapy between adequate immunosuppression to prevent rejection and over-immunosuppression with its concurrent risks. Markers of organ function are important monitoring tools to assess rejection and drug toxicity. Organ tissue biopsies are considered the gold standards in determining the presence, absence, or severity of a rejection episode. Drug concentrations are important general guidelines in preventing rejection and drug toxicity, but patients can exhibit rejection and adverse effects from medications irrespective of drug concentration.

An intensive laboratory assessment program is used to monitor the patient following liver transplantation. Table 39–4 lists the monitoring parameters for following a liver transplant patient. No one single test can be interpreted independently; an adequate assessment comes only after considering the clinical, radiologic, and laboratory examinations as

TABLE 39–4. Monitoring Parameters for a Patient Following Liver Transplantation

Measurement	Application
Serum bilirubin and liver enzymes	Assess functional status of the liver. These tests should improve rapidly unless there is delayed graft function or primary nonfunction. An increase in these values may indicate a technical complication or rejection.
Serum creatinine and BUN (blood urea nitrogen)	Assess renal function. The BUN/creatinine ratio is normally increased in a liver transplant patient. These values should stabilize to the high-normal range in a liver transplant patient; rapid increases may indicate drug toxicity or a change in the hydration status of the patient.
Serum electrolytes	Hypomagnesemia requiring supplementation has been observed. Hyperkalemia requiring fludrocortisone therapy is common. Other abnormalities related to intensive diuretic therapy are also common.
Serum prothrombin time, INR	Assess functional capacity of liver to make coagulation factors. Also important in the event of bleeding episodes due to technical complications.
Blood pressure, weight, vital signs	Prevent hypertensive encephalopathy and the other complications of hypertension. Monitor fluid status and temperature elevations that may accompany infection or graft rejection.
Leukocyte cytomegalovirus (CMV)	Assess CMV status through identification of pp65 marker on cells.
Antigenemia	Allows preemptive antiviral therapy when the level of antigenemia increases.
Physical examination	Assess graft tenderness, neurologic status, and sites of infection on skin incisions or body cavities.
Serum albumin	Assess plasma oncotic pressure and hepatic synthetic function. Albumin supplementation is occasionally prescribed to improve diuretic efficiency until synthesis can restore normal plasma proteins.
Complete blood count	Assess white cell number and differential to monitor for infection. Follow hematocrit to observe for bleeding episodes that may indicate technical complications with the graft.

a composite representation of the patient's condition. This is particularly true when attempting to assess whether an adverse event is due to drug therapy, an infection, rejection, or some technical complication of the transplant surgery.

The frequency of laboratory and physical monitoring depends on length of time posttransplantation and stability of the patient. When a transplant recipient is in the hospital, laboratory and physical monitoring should be conducted on a daily basis. As an outpatient, monitoring is performed twice weekly for the first few months after transplantation. If the patient remains stable over time, then laboratory monitoring is extended to once weekly, once every other week, and then finally monthly. The frequency of physical monitoring is based on patient-specific parameters, and usually decreases over time if the patient remains stable.

GRAFT DYSFUNCTION

The general sequence of events that underlies graft rejection is (1) recognition of the donor's histocompatibility differences by the recipient's immune system, (2) recruitment of activated lymphocytes, (3) initiation of immune effector mechanisms, and (4) destruction of the graft. These processes can take place at varying rates and may involve different mechanisms. Rejection of the transplanted liver can take place any time following surgery and is classified as hyperacute rejection, acute cellular rejection, and chronic rejection. Although these processes generally denote a temporal sequence of events, considerable overlap exists in the actual time frame of when each type is observed. The liver appears to be less immunogenic and more likely to promote immunologic tolerance than the other vascularized organs. Hyperacute rejection rarely occurs in patients receiving a liver transplant. The liver's special status for transplantation is not fully understood, but the local release of cytokines may alter the immunologic reaction taking place in the liver.

Hyperacute rejection often occurs within minutes to 2 weeks of the transplant procedure. Early graft dysfunction is treated with supportive care and retransplantation if possible. An immunologic explanation for graft dysfunction becomes more probable as time passes in a patient with an initially functioning liver graft. Initial episodes of acute cellular rejection often occur between 6 days and 6 weeks posttransplantation, but can also occur earlier or later. Other reasons for delayed graft dysfunction include defects in bile duct reconstruction, opportunistic infections, toxicity from parenteral nutrition, sepsis, or drug-induced hepatotoxicity. The clinical signs of acute cellular rejection are fever, lethargy, graft tenderness, leukocytosis, and a change in the color or quantity of bile. An increased serum bilirubin and increases in hepatic enzymes are the most common biochemical parameters monitored and are sensitive markers of rejection. The liver biopsy is used as definitive evidence of the diagnosis of rejection, but response to antirejection medication has also been used in differentiating rejection from other causes of hepatic dysfunction in a liver transplant patient.

Acute cellular rejection can be observed within days, but may occur any time after transplantation. The treatment of acute cellular rejection varies widely from center to center, but generally involves the concepts of (1) optimizing the present immunosuppressive therapy, (2) initially giving high-dose corticosteroids, and (3) the use of OKT3 monoclonal antibody or ALG/ATG for a 7- to 14-day course when steroid resistance is encountered. A typical flow diagram of the treatment for acute rejections can be seen in Figure 39–2. Increasing the dosage of CyA can be effective in mild cases of rejection, but is infrequently used because of concerns of nephrotoxicity with the drug. The TAC dosage is increased in patients with mild rejection and is effective in some patients. The administration of corticosteroids for rejection can be done as a "pulse" of one to three large doses of methylprednisolone, or can be achieved as a "recycle" of an increased dosage of methylprednisolone, prednisolone, or prednisone for 5 to 10 days. The dosages of other immunosuppressant drugs are often decreased while administering corticosteroids, OKT3, or ALG/ATG therapy. Patients who are deemed steroid resistant are treated with a 7- to 14-day course of OKT3, ALG, or ATG. Repeated courses of immunosuppressant agents for rejection will put the patient at an increased risk for infection, which is always a concern in immunocompromised patients, and at risk for the development of PTLD.

Chronic rejection may be a slow and indolent form of cellular rejection. Chronic rejection of the liver is characterized by an obliterative arteriopathy and the loss of bile ducts, which has been referred to as the vanishing bile duct syndrome. These patients experience an asymptomatic rise in the cannalicular liver enzymes (alkaline phosphatase and γ-glutamyl transpeptidase) and become jaundiced. These changes can be seen in patients who have not responded adequately to therapy for acute rejection, and are considered the result of immunologic and ischemic injury. The changes of chronic rejection are not reversible, and CMV infection has also been implicated in the initiation of the process in transplant patients.

Noncompliance with medications or follow-up care is a preventable cause of graft loss. The reported incidence of noncompliance with medication 3 months after transplantation is about 20%. Patients most likely to become noncompliant are young and in a lower socioeconomic group. In one retrospective study, 91% of patients who were noncompliant with medications or follow-up care either lost their transplanted organs or died. Noncompliance with medications and the development of chimerism has prompted studies in the weaning of immunosuppression, but withdrawal of medications must be done under the supervision of a transplant physician.[29] The pharmacist can help educate the patient on the importance of medication compliance and help simplify the medication regimen to reduce the incidence of noncompliance in transplant recipients.[30]

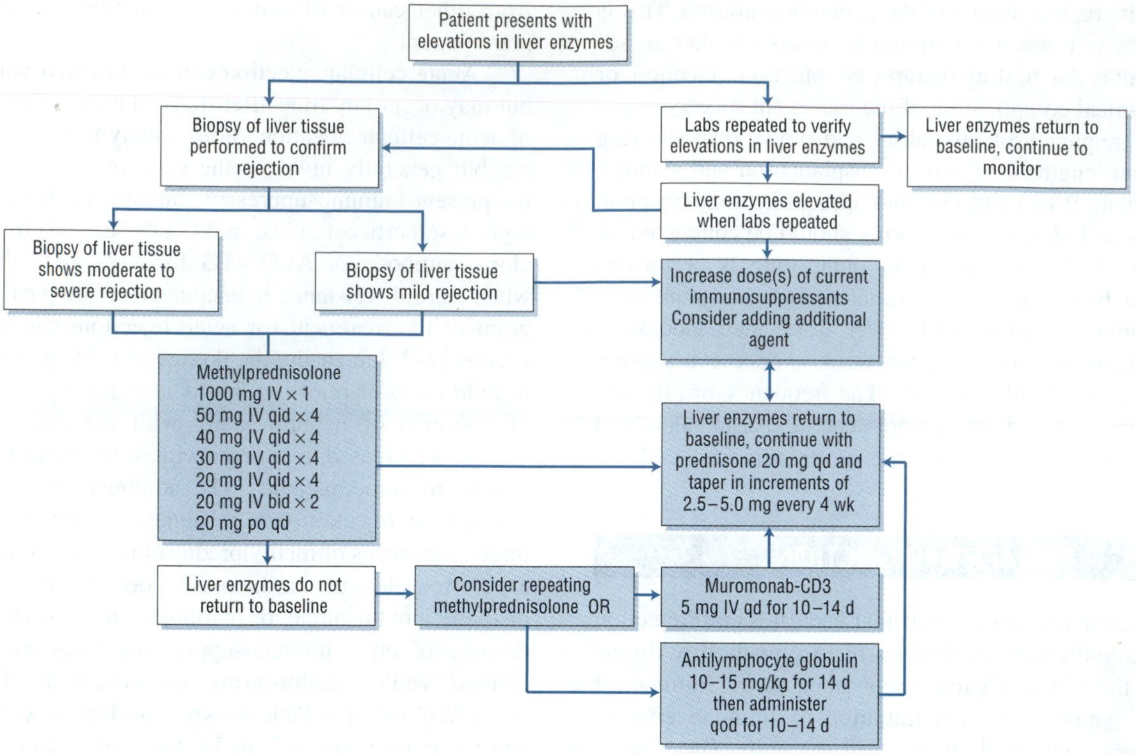

FIGURE 39–2. Flow diagram for the treatment of acute rejection in a liver transplant patient.

CONCLUSIONS

Improved organ preservation techniques have made liver transplantation a more widely available and accepted technique for an expanding list of congenital, autoimmune, and metabolic diseases. New agents such as TAC have improved the immunosuppressive management of liver transplant patients, but the absence of subtle immunologic monitoring techniques means that infection and rejection are persistent clinical problems in these patients. Drug therapy in the liver transplant patient is complicated by rapidly changing hepatic function and the need for intense immunosuppression. The immunosuppressive drug regimen is initially complex and requires intensive monitoring to optimize therapy in the presence of drug interactions and changing drug absorption, distribution, metabolism, and elimination. The pharmacotherapist can make significant contributions to the care of liver transplant patients through the management of complex drug regimens; by managing drug dosing, toxicity, and drug interactions; and by providing patient education and promoting medication compliance.

▶ PRINCIPLES OF PHARMACOTHERAPY

- Liver transplantation is the life-saving procedure in patients with severe hepatic disease and no other medical options.
- Goals of treatment include preventing organ rejection while minimizing adverse drug effects and infection.
- Nonpharmacologic treatments, such as the enhancement of chimerism, are currently being studied to potentiate immunosuppressive therapy.
- Immunosuppressive drug protocols include one to four immunosuppressants. Other medications are used to prevent infection and minimize adverse effects caused by immunosuppressants.
- Doses of certain immunosuppressants (TAC or CyA) are adjusted according to blood levels, while other immunosuppressants (MMF or AZA) are adjusted according to patient response. Doses of the immunosuppressant medications are weaned over time if the patient does not exhibit organ rejection.
- Laboratory monitoring is essential in monitoring rejection and adverse effects of immunosuppression.
- Organ rejection must be treated aggressively to prevent loss of the transplanted organ.
- The pharmacist should be knowledgeable of the management of drug interactions that can occur with the immunosuppressant medications.
- Compliance with immunosuppressive medications has been shown to decrease morbidity and mortality after liver transplantation.

REFERENCES

1. United Network for Organ Sharing. Annual Report 1997. Richmond, VA, UNOS, 1997.
2. Starzl TE, Demetris AJ. Liver Transplantation: A 31-Year Perspective. Chicago, Year Book, 1990:120.
3. Mohamed R., Hubscher SG, Darius FM, et al. Posttransplant chronic hepatitis in fulminant hepatic failure. Hepatology 1997;25:1003–1007.
4. Johnson MW, Washburn WK, Freeman RB, et al. Hepatitis C viral infection in liver transplantation. Arch Surg 1996;131:284–291.
5. Schmidt HHJ, Tietge UJF, Manns MP. Perspectives of liver transplantation: A review. Hepatogastroenterology 1997;44:1013–1018.
6. Gerlach JC. Development of a hybrid liver support system: a review. Int J Artif Organs 1996;19:645–654.
7. Mito M, Kusano M. Hepatocyte transplantation in man. Cell Transplant 1993;2:65–74.
8. Dunn SP, Haynes JH, Nicolette LA, et al. Split liver transplantation benefits the recipient of the "leftover liver." Pediatr Surg 1997;32: 252–255.
9. Whitington PF, Alonso EM, Piper JB. Pediatric liver transplantation. Semin Liver Dis 1994;14:303–317.
10. Brown RS, Ascher NL, Lake JR, et al. The impact of surgical complications after liver transplantation on resource utilization. Arch Surg 1997;132:1098–1103.
11. Venkataramanan R, Habucky K, Burckart GJ, et al. Clinical pharmacokinetics in organ transplant patients. Clin Pharmacokinet 1989; 16:134–161.
12. McDonald JC, Adamashvili I, Zibari GB, et al. Serologic allogenic chimerism. Transplantation 1997:64:865–871.
13. Sanchez-Izquierdo JA, Lumbreras C, Colina F, et al. Severe graft versus host disease following liver transplantation confirmed by PCR-HLA-B Sequencing: Report of a case and literature review. Hepatogastroenterology 1996;43:1057–1061.
14. U.S. Multicenter Tacrolimus Liver Study Group. A comparison of tacrolimus (FK-506) and cyclosporine for immunosuppression in liver transplantation. N Engl J Med 1994;331:1110–1115.
15. European Tacrolimus Multicenter Liver Study Group. Randomized trial comparing tacrolimus (FK-506) and cyclosporine in prevention of liver allograft rejection. Lancet 1994;344:423–428.
16. Sher LS, Cosenza CA, Michel J, et al. Efficacy of tacrolimus as rescue therapy for chronic rejection in orthotopic liver transplantation: A report of the U.S. Multicenter Liver Study Group. Transplantation 1997;64:258–263.
17. Pratschke J, Neuhaus R, Tullius SG, et al. Treatment of cyclosporine-related adverse effects by conversion to tacrolimus after liver transplantation. Transplantation 1997;64:938–940.
18. Platz KP, Mueller AR, Rossaint R, et al. Cytokine pattern during rejection and infection after liver transplantation—Improvements in postoperative monitoring? Transplantation 1996;62:1441–1450.
19. Dummer JS. Cytomegalovirus infection after liver transplantation: Clinical manifestations and strategies for prevention. J Infect Dis 1990;12(suppl 7):S767–S775.
20. Halwachs G, Zach R, Pogglitsch H, et al. A rapid immunocytochemical assay for CMV detection in peripheral blood of organ-transplanted patients in clinical practice. Transplantation 1993;56: 338–342.
21. Ville Y, Fernandez H, Samuel D. Pregnancy in liver transplant recipients: Course and outcome in 19 cases. Am J Obstet Gynecol 1993; 168:896–902.
22. Graziadei IW, Wiesner RH, Marotta PJ, et al. Neoral compared to Sandimmune is associated with a decrease in histologic severity of rejection in patients undergoing primary liver transplantation. Transplantation 1997;64:726–731.
23. McIntyre JA, Kincade M, Higgins NG. Detection of IGA anti-OKT3 antibodies in OKT3-treated transplant recipients. Transplantation 1996;61:1465–1469.
24. Lake JR, Gorman KJ, Esquivel CP, et al. The impact of immunosuppressive regimens on the cost of liver transplantation—Results from the U.S. FK506 multicenter trial. Transplantation 1995;60:1089–1095.
25. O'Grady JG. Clinical economics review: Liver transplantation. Aliment Pharmacol Ther 1997;11:445–451.
26. Evans RW, Manninen DL, Dong FB, McLynne DA. Is retransplantation cost effective? Transplant Proc 1993;25:1694–1696.
27. Abouljoud MS, Brown KA, May E, et al. Cost effective management of acute rejection in liver transplant recipients: A managed care perspective. Transplant Proc 1997;29:1557–1559.
28. Henley KS, Smith D. Prostaglandins in liver transplantation: A $50,000 bonus. Gastroenterology 1997;112:670–671.
29. Mazariegos GV, Reyes J, Marino IR, et al. Weaning of immunosuppression in liver transplant recipients. Transplantation 1997;63: 243–249.
30. Schweizer RT, Rovelli M, Palmeri D, et al. Noncompliance in organ transplant recipients. Transplantation 1990;49:374–377.

40
ASSESSMENT OF RENAL FUNCTION

Thomas J. Comstock, PharmD

Renal function can be assessed from both a qualitative and a quantitative perspective. Although creatinine clearance is typically considered the clinical standard for assessment of renal function, other tests, such as the urinalysis, radiographic procedures, and biopsy, are also valuable tools in the assessment of renal disease. Quantitative measures, such as clearance, are most useful in establishing the degree of kidney function, or change in function that may occur as a result of disease progression, therapeutic intervention, or toxic insult.[1] Moreover, the design of dosage regimens for drugs eliminated by the kidneys is also dependent on the quantitative measure of kidney function. Determination of the etiology of kidney disease, on the other hand, is dependent on a more qualitative assessment of the kidneys. The urinalysis, for example, may reveal red blood cells or proteinuria, suggestive of glomerular disease. Follow-up studies such as imaging procedures or kidney biopsy may then further differentiate the specific cause, thereby pointing to the appropriate therapeutic intervention.

Renal "function" includes the processes of filtration, secretion, and reabsorption, as well as endocrine and metabolic functions. Alterations of all five renal functions, whether declining or improving, have been associated primarily with glomerular filtration rate (GFR). The focus of this chapter is a critical evaluation of the various methods one can use for the quantitative assessment of kidney function (Table 40–1). Where appropriate, discussion regarding the qualitative assessment of the renal function will also be presented, including specialized tests such as kidney biopsy.

ENDOCRINE FUNCTION

Secretion of renin by the cells of the juxtaglomerular apparatus, production and metabolism of prostaglandins and kinins, and the production and secretion of erythropoietin by the interstitial cells in response to decreased oxygen tension in the blood are among the kidney's endocrine functions.[2] Since these functions are related to renal mass, decreased endocrine activity has been associated with the loss of viable cells. Hematocrit, for example, declines as a function of decreasing GFR, primarily due to a loss of erythropoietin production, leading to the complications associated with anemia, which include fatigue, dyspnea, anorexia, and the development of, or increased, angina.[3]

METABOLIC FUNCTION

The kidneys are capable of a wide variety of metabolic activities, including the activation of vitamin D_3, gluconeogenesis, and metabolism of endogenous compounds such as insulin and steroids, as well as xenobiotics. Impaired renal function results in decreased formation of activated vitamin D_3 and decreased insulin metabolism. It is common for patients with diabetes and chronic renal failure to have reduced requirements for exogenous insulin,[4] and supplemental therapy with activated vitamin D_3 (calcitriol) is often necessary in the management of renal osteodystrophy.[5] Numerous enzymes have been identified in the kidneys, primarily the cortex. These include cytochrome P450, *N*-acetyltransferase, glutathione transferase, renal peptidases, and others.[6] The cytochrome P450 system in the kidneys has been identified to be as active as that in the liver, when corrected for organ mass. Furthermore, the accumulation of uremic toxins has been associated with decreased CYP activity for selected isoenzymes. *In-vitro* studies have demonstrated impaired function of CYP3A4 and 2C9, whereas 1A2, 2C19, and 2D6 were not affected. The clinical importance of these preliminary findings is not fully understood at this time. Reversible metabolism may also be affected by renal disease when normal enzyme function is disrupted. This has been observed with clofibrate[7] and may apply to other compounds eliminated by the same route, such as ketoprofen.[8] See Chap. 47 for more detailed discussion.

EXCRETORY FUNCTION

Although endocrine and metabolic functions are important aspects of the kidney's contribution to maintenance of body homeostasis, it is the excretory function that is often perceived as the "kidney function." Through the combined processes of glomerular filtration, tubular secretion, and tubular reabsorption, the nephron, as the functional unit of the kidney, maintains balance between input and output of water and solutes from the body and is the key organ responsible for maintenance of homeostasis. This is represented as:

$$\text{Rate of excretion} = \text{Rate of filtration} + \text{Rate of secretion} - \text{Rate of reabsorption}$$

TABLE 40–1. Markers of Renal Function

Renal plasma/blood flow	*p*-Aminohippurate (PAH) ^{131}I-Orthoiodohippurate (^{131}I-OIH) ^{99m}Tc-mercaptoacetyltriglycine (^{99m}Tc-MAG3)
Glomerular filtration rate	Inulin, sinistrin Iothalamate Iohexol ^{99m}Tc-diethylenetriaminepentaacetic acid (^{99m}Tc-DTPA) ^{125}I-Iothalamate Creatinine Cystatin C
Tubular function	*p*-Aminohippurate *N*-1-Methylnicotinamide (NMN) Tetraethyl ammonium (TEA) β_2-Microglobulin Retinol-binding protein (RBP) Protein HC (α_1-microglobulin) *N*-Acetylglucosaminidase (NAG) Alanine aminopeptidase (AAP) Adenosine binding protein (ABP)

Glomerular filtration occurs through the passive diffusion of water and small-molecular-weight ions and molecules across the glomerular–capillary membrane into Bowman's capsule and the proximal tubule (Fig. 40–1). Since most proteins are too large to be substantially filtered (> 60 kDa), or their filtration is impeded by electronegative charges of the glomerulus, compounds presented to the glomerulus in the protein-bound state are not filtered and enter the peritubular circulation.[2] Secretion occurs primarily along the proximal tubule and facilitates elimination of compounds from the plasma into the tubular lumen via active transport. Anionic and cationic transport systems have been characterized and are involved in the transport of many endogenous and exogenous substances. Examples include probenecid, *p*-aminohippurate (PAH), and penicillin as anions, and creatinine, cimetidine, and procainamide as cations.[9] These systems are not mutually exclusive, as probenecid has been observed to compete with the tubular secretion of cimetidine.[10] P-glycoprotein (P-gp), a membrane glycoprotein distributed in tissues including kidney, liver, jejunum, colon, and others, has also been recognized as an important element in drug elimination by the kidneys.[11] It is located on the apical membrane of the proximal tubule and may play an important role in the elimination of cytotoxic drugs. Blockade of P-gp could result in decreased renal elimination of such compounds, leading to an increased drug exposure. Verapamil, cyclosporine, and the P-gp-specific inhibitor, PSC 833, all reduce the activity of this tubular transport mechanism.[12] Further investigations into the exact role of P-gp in drug elimination are presently underway. Reabsorption of water and solutes occurs throughout the nephron, whereas drug reabsorption occurs predominantly along the distal tubule and collecting tubules. Urine flow rate and physicochemical characteristics of the molecule influence these processes. Highly ionized compounds are not reabsorbed unless pH changes within the urine alter the fraction unionized, whereby reabsorption may be facilitated.[13]

The homeostasis afforded by the kidneys is affected by catecholamines, prostaglandins, renin, antidiuretic hormone, natriuretic hormone, and the number of functioning nephrons. The "intact nephron hypothesis" of Bricker,[14,15] which was first published over 30 years ago, proposes that "kidney function" of patients with renal disease is the net result of a reduced number of appropriately functioning nephrons. As the number of nephrons is reduced from the initial complement of 2 million, those unaffected compensate for those damaged by disease or toxic insult. The cornerstone of this hypothesis is that glomerulotubule balance is maintained, such that those nephrons capable of functioning will continue to perform in an appropriate fashion. As GFR declines, tubular reabsorption must decrease to allow for elimination of the solute load. Single nephron GFR (SNGFR) increases in the remaining nephrons, whereas the whole kidney GFR represents the sum of the SNGFR of the remaining functional nephrons. Based on this, one would presume that a measure of one component of nephron function could be used as an estimate of all renal functions. This indeed has been and remains our clinical approach.

Measurement of GFR, however, may not be an appropriate assessment for a drug that undergoes active tubular secretion, or is extensively reabsorbed. As an example, Hori et al.[16,17] demonstrated that the post-filtration renal handling of ampicillin, which is secreted, and cephalexin, which is secreted and reabsorbed, remained normal in patients with renal failure due to glomerulonephritis, but was reduced in patients with renal failure associated with tubular dysfunction. They concluded that dosage adjustment based on creatinine clearance would not be appropriate for drugs eliminated by tubular secretion. Maiza and Daley-Yates[18] have also observed glomerulotubule imbalance in experimentally induced renal failure in rats based on differential effects on inulin (an index of filtration), PAH (an index of anionic secretion), and N-1-methylnicotinamide clearance (an index of cationic secretion). Using an experimental nephrotoxic (uranyl nitrate) acute renal failure rat model, Lin and Lin[19] and Gloff and Benet[20] demonstrated differential handling of tetraethylammonium bromide (TEA) and PAH, with greater impairment of tubular secretion than of GFR. Lin and Lin[19] further studied an ischemic acute renal failure model (glycerol) and showed a parallel decline of secretion and GFR for TEA, whereas secretion of PAH decreased at a greater rate than did GFR. These results support the hypothesis that the integrity of different pathways for elimination of compounds may be dependent on the mode of injury as well as the chemical characteristics of the compound. Thus, the kidney should not be considered as a single homogeneously functioning organ, but one with several different, discrete functions. It is thus analogous to the liver in which the multiple metabolic pathways may be impaired to variable degrees dependent on the type of injury or disease.[13]

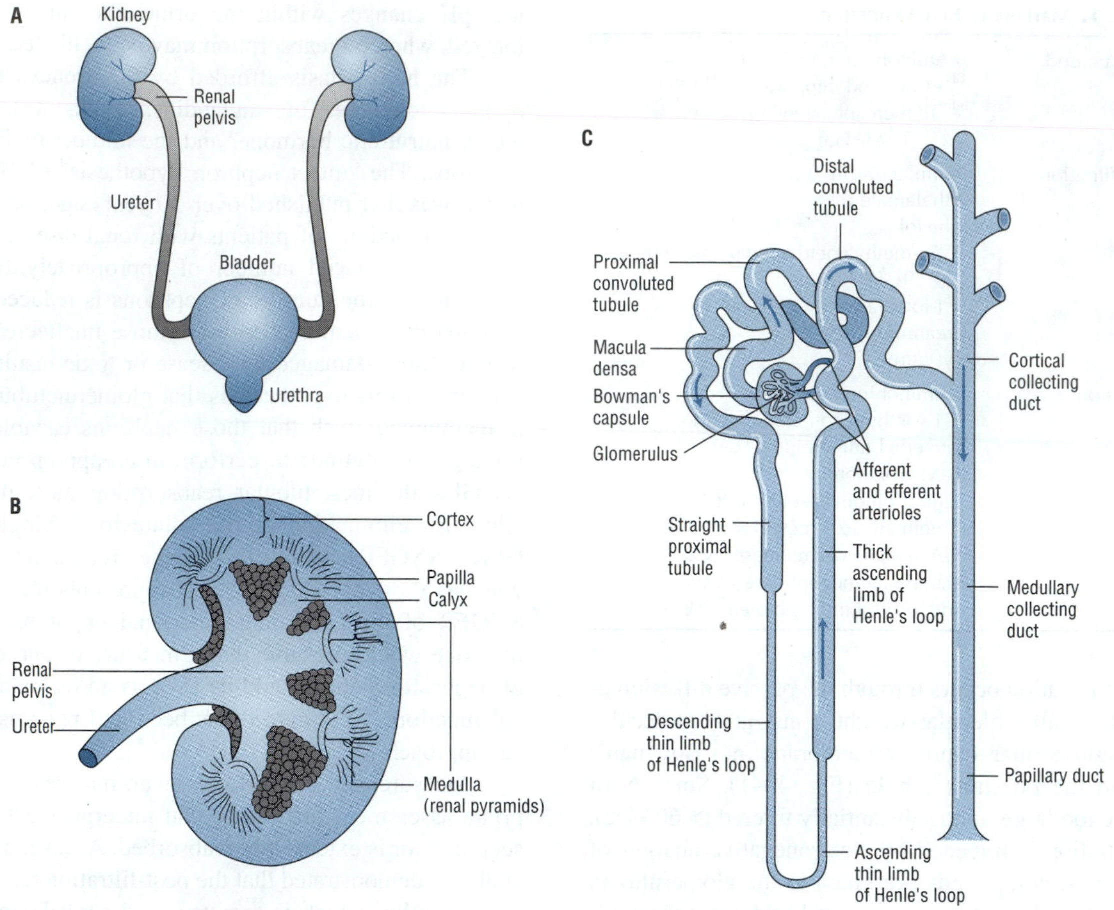

FIGURE 40–1. Structures of the **(A)** urinary system, **(B)** kidney, and **(C)** nephron, the functional unit of the kidney. The arrows in the nephron lumen indicate the route of urine flow.

The GFR as a measure of "renal function" has shifted to the issue of variability in the last few years. It has been recognized that GFR is dependent on numerous factors, one of which is protein load. Bosch[21] has suggested that an appropriate measure of renal function should reflect the "filtration capacity" of the kidney, and not the "resting GFR." Subjects with normal renal function administered an oral or intravenous protein load prior to measurement of GFR have been noted to increase their GFR by as much as 50%.[21] As renal function declines, the kidneys compensate by increasing SNGFR. The renal reserve, the maximal degree by which GFR can be increased usually declines and, thus may be a complimentary measure of renal function for these patients.

Quantification of renal function is not only an important diagnostic index, but it also serves as an important parameter for monitoring therapy directed at the etiology of the diminished function itself, thereby allowing for objective measurement of the success or failure of treatment.[22] Measurement of renal function also serves as a useful indicator of the ability of the kidneys to eliminate drugs from the body. Furthermore, alterations of drug distribution and metabolism have also been associated with the degree of renal function. See Chap. 47 for a discussion of pharmacokinetic changes in renal disease. Although several indices have been used for the quantification of renal function in the research setting, GFR, and, more specifically, creatinine clearance has been the primary marker of renal function in the clinical arena.

SIGNS AND SYMPTOMS OF RENAL DYSFUNCTION

Patients who develop renal disease remain relatively asymptomatic until impairment has progressed to the point that systemic manifestations and/or secondary complications become evident. Diabetes mellitus and hypertension are the two most common causes of end-stage renal disease (ESRD), and as renal function declines, patients may experience development or exacerbation of hypertension, edema, electrolyte abnormalities, anemia, or other complications (see Chap. 42). Urine ouput may increase as the filtration per nephron increases, resulting in a loss of urinary concentrating ability and development of an osmotic diuresis. While a mild metabolic acidosis may be present, patients will typically not demonstrate symptoms, although chronic acidosis will lead to bone demineralization. Hyperkalemia may develop as the GFR drops to 20 mL/min; this may lead to signs of muscle weakness and electrocardiographic (ECG) abnormalities. Additional monitoring of potassium is warranted in those patients also treated with angiotensin-converting enzyme inhibitors, as these agents can decrease potassium excretion. The signs and symptoms associated with the progressive loss of renal function are discussed in Chapter 42. Decreased erythropoietin production by the kidney leads to decreased red blood cell production, and the accumulation of toxins as the result of the reduction in GFR results in a decreased red cell life span. The combination of these events leads to anemia and a multitude of signs and symptoms, including weakness, fatigue, lethargy, impaired mentation, intolerance to cold, and loss of appetite, among others.[3] Occasionally, patients will present with mental confusion or severe nausea and vomiting, the result of accumulated toxins, often associated with significantly elevated urea concentrations.

Patients with glomerulonephritis, the third leading cause of ESRD, may present with hematuria, or in some cases, edema. The edema is a result of the nephrotic syndrome, a condition characterized by hypoalbuminemia, loss of more than 3 g of albumin in the urine per day, and edema[23] (see Chap. 46). Hypoalbuminemia contributes to edema formation through a decrease in plasma oncotic pressure. Presence of frothy urine may be suggestive of significant proteinuria. Nonspecific signs that may be associated with renal disease include low-grade fever, rash, arthralgias (vasculitis, interstital nephritis), auditory impairment (Alport's syndrome or aminoglycoside toxicity), or pulmonary symptoms (Goodpasture's syndrome).

ABNORMALITIES IN PHYSICAL EXAMINATION USED TO DETECT RENAL DYSFUNCTION

Findings on the physical examination are nonspecific for kidney disease, but may be present due to secondary involvement of other organ systems. Fluid overload may be manifest as dependent edema of the lower extremities, congestive heart failure with distended neck veins and presence of an S_3 gallop rhythm, and pulmonary rales. Elevation of blood pressure may also be due to volume overload, or stimulation of the renin–angiotensin–aldosterone system. Enlarged kidneys may be present with polycystic kidney disease, whereas small kidneys suggest chronic renal failure due to other causes. A palpable suprapubic mass in a patient with a distended bladder is suggestive of urinary tract obstruction.

LABORATORY EVIDENCE FOR RENAL DYSFUNCTION AND ITS INTERPRETATION

The blood urea nitrogen (BUN) and serum creatinine concentrations are the two most common clinical laboratory measurements used for the assessment of kidney function.

BLOOD UREA NITROGEN

Amino acids metabolized to ammonia are subsequently converted in the liver to form urea, the production of which is dependent on protein availability (diet) and hepatic function. Renal handling of urea includes glomerular filtration followed by reabsorption of up to 50% of the filtered load in the proximal tubule.[2] As urea is able to cross cell membranes by passive diffusion, its reabsorption rate is variable and dependent on the reabsorption of water. The excretion of urea may, therefore, be decreased under conditions of water conservation by the kidneys although the GFR may be reduced only slightly. This condition is evident when a patient exhibits prerenal azotemia, or an increase of the BUN to a greater extent than the serum creatinine. The normal BUN:creatinine ratio is 10 to 15:1, and an elevated ratio is suggestive of a decreased effective circulating volume, which stimulates increased water, and hence, urea reabsorption.[24] Creatinine is not reabsorbed to any significant extent by the kidneys. Despite these limitations, the BUN is often used as a simple screening tool for the detection of renal dysfunction, but particularly in combination with the serum creatinine concentration.

CREATININE

Creatinine is a product of creatine metabolism from muscle; therefore, its production is directly dependent on muscle mass. At steady state, the "normal" serum creatinine concentration is approximately 0.5 to 1.5 mg/dL, although numerous factors, such as age, body mass, and gender, will affect the concentration, making its interpretation alone difficult at best.[25] Creatinine is eliminated primarily by glomerular filtration, and as GFR declines, the serum creatinine concentration will rise (Fig. 40–2).

Several methods are used for the determination of the serum creatinine concentration, most of which are based on the nonspecific method using the Jaffé reaction: a colorimetric method based on the reaction of creatinine with alkaline picrate. This nonspecific method also reacts with noncreatinine chromogens in the serum, which may result in a falsely increased serum creatinine concentration.[25] The noncreatinine chromogens are not present in the urine in

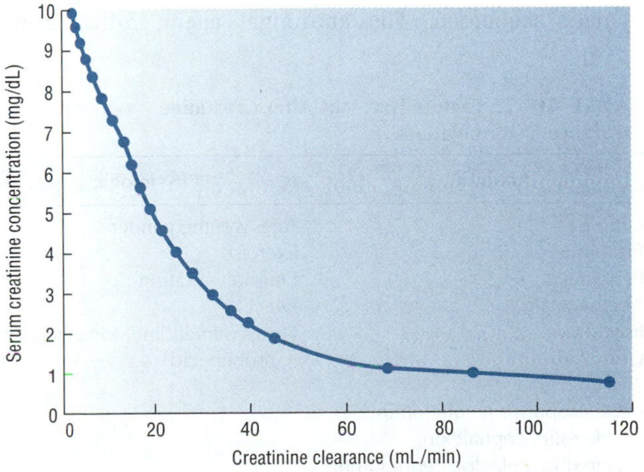

FIGURE 40–2. Relationship between serum creatinine concentration and creatinine clearance.

sufficient quantities to interfere with the creatinine measurement, which will be several-fold greater than the serum concentration. The impact of this interference is seen with the clearance calculation:

$$CrCl = (U_{cr} \times V)/(S_{cr} \times t)$$

where U_{cr} = urine creatinine concentration, V = urine volume, S_{cr} = serum creatinine concentration, and t = duration of the urine collection.

This "normal" interference results in an increase in the serum creatinine concentration of approximately 10% and thereby the creatinine clearance would underestimate the GFR by 10%. In subjects with normal renal function, this tends to counterbalance the effect of the contribution of tubular secretion of creatinine, which increases urine creatinine by nearly 10%. Thus, CrCl may serve as a good measure of GFR in subjects with normal renal function. However, this false increase in serum creatinine becomes less noticeable as the true creatinine concentration rises, due to the increasing contribution of tubular secretion to the renal clearance of creatinine.[26,27] This becomes important when kidney function is reduced to less than 50% of normal.

Diabetic ketoacidosis may produce increased concentrations of acetoacetate, which serves as a chromophore in the Jaffé reaction, thereby increasing the serum creatinine concentration.[25] Other substances that also react with this procedure in the serum include glucose, protein, pyruvate, fructose, uric acid, and ascorbic acid (Table 40–2).[25] In addition, some cephalosporin antibiotics have been associated with a false increase in the serum creatinine concentration, including cephalothin, cefazolin, cephalexin, cefoxitin, cefaclor, and cephradine,[28] whereas other antibiotics, such as the fluoroquinolones (ciprofloxacin, fleroxacin, lomafloxacin, ofloxacin, levofloxacin, sparfloxacin, and temafloxacin) have been shown not to interact.[29] The degree of interference is dependent on the serum concentration of the antibiotic, so blood samples for creatinine should be obtained when the antibiotic concentration is lowest (at the end of a dosing interval). These interferences are not observed when the serum creatinine is measured using an enzymatic technique. The antifungal agent, 5-flucytosine, causes an increase in the serum creatinine when measured using the Ektachem enzymatic system, but does not interact with the Jaffé method.[30] The Ektachem system has also been observed by Apple et al.[31] to yield serum creatinine concentrations 0.2 to 0.3 mg/dL higher than with nonenzymatic methods. These differences emphasize the need to standardize a method within the research or clinic setting, and to be aware of methods employed in the laboratory for the determination of creatinine concentrations.

TABLE 40–2. Factors That May Alter Creatinine Clearance Determinations

Analytic	Physiologic
Glucose	Age, weight, gender
Protein	Exercise
Pyruvate	Diurnal variation
Acetoacetate	Diet
Fructose	Drugs (cimetidine, trimethoprim, probenecid)
Uric acid	
Ascorbic acid	
Cephalosporins (cephalothin, cefazolin, cephalexin, cefoxitin, cefaclor, cephradine)	
5-Flucytosine	

Other compounds are known to interfere with the serum creatinine concentration, through inhibition of the active tubular secretion of creatinine. Among these are cimetidine and trimethoprim, which compete for creatinine secretion at the cationic transport system.[25] Both trimethoprim and cimetidine have demonstrated dose dependency with respect to competition with creatinine for secretion. Ranitidine, an H_2-receptor antagonist similar to cimetidine, was evaluated for its effect on creatinine clearance in 10 healthy subjects. There was no effect following single doses of 300 or 1,200 mg as determined by the ratio of CrCl to inulin Cl.[32] Cimetidine, given as a single 400-mg dose in 6 of the same subjects, resulted in a reduction of the CrCl to inulin Cl ratio from 1.30 to 1.03, without change in inulin clearance.

The serum creatinine concentration is dependent on the "input" function, or formation rate, and "output" function, or elimination rate. Its formation rate depends on the zero-order production from creatine metabolism, as well as input from other sources, such as dietary intake.[33] Creatine metabolism is directly proportional to muscle mass; therefore, individuals with larger muscle mass will have a higher serum creatinine concentration at any given degree of kidney function than an individual with less muscle mass. Exercise has been associated with an increase of approximately 10% in the serum creatinine concentration.[34] Cachectic patients, as the result of minimal muscle mass, will have very low serum creatinine concentrations, as do those with spinal cord injuries.[35] Elderly patients and those with poor nutrition may also have low serum creatinine concentrations (< 1.0 mg/dL) secondary to decreased muscle mass. Other factors that influence the serum creatinine concentration include the dietary intake of creatinine. During the cooking of meat, some creatine is converted to creatinine, which is rapidly absorbed following ingestion. Serum creatinine concentrations may rise as much as 50% within 2 hours of a meat meal and remain elevated for as long as 8 to 24 hours[33] (Fig. 40–3). This presents a problem only when a single serum creatinine concentration is used to represent the entire 24-hour collection period, which is usually the case. An alternative is to obtain multiple samples and calculate the area under the serum concentration time curve and divide this by the collection time interval to obtain the average plasma creatinine concentration. This is rarely done in clinical practice, but points out the need to question patients regarding dietary intake for the 24 hours preceding the measurement of CrCl.

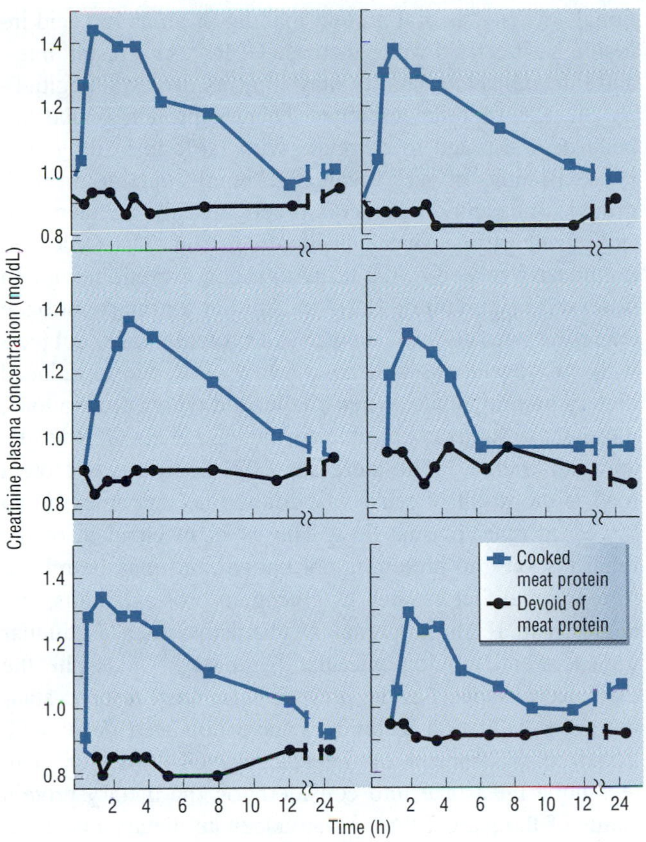

FIGURE 40–3. Creatinine plasma concentration as a function of time following a control breakfast devoid of meat protein and following the experimental breakfast of cooked meat protein. *(From Ref. 33.)*

Diurnal variation in serum creatinine concentration may also affect the accuracy of the CrCl determination. Although the fluctuation is minimal, the observed peak plasma creatinine concentration generally occurs at approximately 7:00 PM, whereas the nadir is in the morning.[36] To minimize this effect, the CrCl is usually performed over a 24-hour period with the plasma creatinine obtained in the morning, as long as the patient has stable kidney function. Collection of urine remains a limiting factor in the 24-hour CrCl due to incomplete collections. Bingham et al.[37] used *para*-amino benzoic acid as an oral marker to assess the completeness of 24-hour urine collections in 63 hospital outpatients. Twenty-nine percent were judged incomplete. Fuller and Elia[38] identified an additional complicating factor—the interconversion between creatinine and creatine that can occur if the urine is not maintained at a pH < 6.

URINALYSIS

Examination of the urine includes assessment of its chemical and physical composition, most of which can be completed with dipstick testing.

pH

The normal urine pH typically ranges from 4.5 to 7.8, and an elevation above this may suggest the presence of urea-splitting bacteria.[25]

Specific Gravity

The measure of urine weight relative to water (1.00) is its specific gravity and is dependent on water intake and urine concentrating ability. Normal values range from 1.003 to 1.030. Osmolality, which is a measure of the number of solute particles, is a more accurate measure of the kidney's ability to make a concentrated urine. Generally the two values are correlated, however, when large quantities of heavier molecules, such as glucose are in the urine, the specific gravity may be elevated relative to the osmolality. These values are used in the assessment of urine concentrating ability and are most informative when interpreted along with the hydration status of the patient and plasma osmolality.[25]

Glucose

Glucose is normally absent in the urine, since the kidney normally completely reabsorbs all the glucose filtered at the glomerulus. In patients with plasma glucose concentrations that exceed the maximum threshold for glucose reabsorption (~180 mg/dL), glucosuria will be present. In the past, patients with diabetes mellitus would use the urine glucose level as a guide to insulin therapy. However, finger-stick methods for direct blood glucose measurements have now replaced the urine tests as a guide to therapy in most clinical settings.[39] Urine glucose testing still remains a valuable tool for the detection of diabetes.

Ketones

Acetoacetate and acetone are excreted in patients with diabetic ketoacidosis. They are also produced under conditions of fasting or starvation.

Nitrite

Nitrite is formed by conversion from nitrate by urinary bacteria. The presence of nitrite may indicate that the patient has a urinary tract infection.

Leukocyte Esterase

Leukocyte esterase is released from lysed granulocytes in the urine; its presence is suggestive of urinary tract infection. If the processing of the urine sample is delayed, a false-positive leukocyte esterase may be reported if the sample is contaminated.

Heme

The heme test indicates the presence of hemoglobin or myoglobin. A positive test without the presence of red blood cells suggests either red cell hemolysis or rhabdomyolysis.[25]

Protein

Protein excretion is normally minimal in healthy individuals (< 150 mg/d). Albumin is not significantly filtered due to its size (69 kDa) and anionic character, which results in it being repelled by the negatively charged proteins of the glomerular capillary wall. Albumin excretion is thus usually < 30 mg/d in individuals without kidney disease. Smaller proteins, such as β_2-microglobulin, pass through the glomerulus but are reabsorbed in the proximal tubule. Tests for urinary protein include acid precipitation with sulfosalicylic acid, and several dipstick methods. The sulfosalicylic test provides an assessment of total protein in the urine and is performed by the addition of sulfosalicylic acid to urine supernatant in a 1:3 ratio. The resulting turbidity is a semiquantitative approach to estimate the degree of proteinuria. Most dipstick methods that detect protein are not specific for albumin, and, therefore, specific tests have been developed for the detection of microalbuminuria, 30 to 150 mg/d.[40] The 24-hour excretion of protein can be calculated as the product of the concentration of protein in the total collection and the urine volume. In an attempt to correct for the excretion rates of protein and creatinine in the urine, the ratio of urine albumin to urine creatinine is often used, and the value is an estimate of the amount of albumin excreted per day.[41] As the creatinine production per day is constant, an increased ratio indicates increased protein excretion. The normal ratio is < 0.2 (less than 200 mg/d). Further discussion of the methods for measurement of urinary protein can be found in recent reviews.[24,25,42]

Formed elements that may be detected in the urine include erythrocytes and leukocytes, casts, and crystals. An important consideration in the assessment of hematuria is whether the cells are of renal origin. More than two cells per high-power field is abnormal, and dysmorphic cells suggest renal parenchymal origin due to either damage as they pass through the glomerulus or during exposure to the varying osmotic environment of the tubular lumen. White blood cells may be present in the urine in association with infection or inflammatory conditions, such as interstitial nephritis. More than one cell per high-power field may be considered abnormal. For both red and white cells, contamination of the sample should also be considered such as during menses, or with inadequate sample collection. Casts are cylindrical forms composed of protein, with or without cells that take the shape of the collecting tubules, where they are formed. Casts without cells are labeled hyaline casts and consist of the Tamm–Horsfall mucoprotein, secreted by the renal tubules. They are nonspecific and may appear in concentrated urine. In the presence of red or white blood cells, casts may be formed that include the cells, indicating that the cells were of renal origin. Solubility of the Tamm-Horsfall protein is increased as urine pH rises; therefore, sample collection for casts should occur with the first morning void when the urine is most acidic. Otherwise, casts may dissolve and elude detection.[24,25,43]

A variety of crystals may be present in the urine, including uric acid, calcium oxalate, calcium phosphate, calcium magnesium ammonium pyrophosphate, and cystine. Many of these have a unique crystalline form, which permits them to be identified with microscopy.

PROCEDURES USED IN THE ASSESSMENT OF RENAL FUNCTION

The gold standard for the quantitative measure of kidney function is the GFR.[44,45] Recent observations, however, suggest this measure is not truly reflective of renal functional capacity, as oral protein loading or an amino acid infusion has been shown to increase GFR.[21] As a result, inter- and intrasubject variability may limit its use as a longitudinal marker of renal function. Dietary protein intake has been demonstrated to correlate with GFR in healthy subjects. Brändle et al.[46] evaluated renal function in four groups of healthy volunteers, each ingesting a diet controlled for protein over a 4-month period. The GFR was nonlinearly related to the urine nitrogen excretion, with an observed maximum of 181.7 mL/min at a urinary nitrogen excretion rate of 20 g/d, or 125 g/d protein intake. Subjects who are vegetarians will have a low GFR due to reduced dietary protein intake. When challenged with a protein load, these same subjects are able to increase their GFR to the "normal" range.[21] The increased GFR following a protein load is the result of renal vasodilation accompanied by an increased renal plasma flow. The exact mechanism of the renal response to protein is not known, but may be related to extrarenal factors such as glucagon, prostaglandins, and angiotensin II, or intrarenal mechanisms, such as tubular transport and tubuloglomerular feedback.[47,48] Despite the evidence in support of the presence of a renal reserve, standardized evaluation techniques have not been developed; therefore, assessment of the standard GFR measurement technique must take into consideration the dietary protein status of the patient through an adequate dietary history at the time of the study.

MEASUREMENT OF RENAL PLASMA AND BLOOD FLOW

Renal plasmal and blood flow are not common clinical measures of renal function but may provide insight into hemodynamic changes related to disease or drug therapy. The kidneys receive approximately 20% of cardiac output and representative values of renal blood flow in men and women of about 1,200 ± 250 and 1,000 ± 180 mL/min/1.73 m^2 have been reported, respectively.[49] Renal plasma flow (RPF) is estimated to be 60% of blood flow if one assumes that the average hematocrit is 40%, and it can be measured by the use of model compounds that are eliminated from the plasma compartment on a single pass through the kidneys. Since only 20% of the plasma is filtered at the glomerulus, the compound must undergo active tubular secretion and minimal to no reabsorption to be completely eliminated. To accurately reflect RPF, the extraction through the kidney must be nearly 100%. Aminohippurate sodium (PAH or sodium *p*-aminohippurate) is an organic anion that has been used extensively for the quantitation of renal plasma flow. PAH is approximately 17% bound to plasma proteins and is eliminated extensively by active tubular secretion. Since PAH elimination is active, saturation of the transport processes should be anticipated. Indeed, concentrations of PAH in plasma should not exceed 30 mg/L. Furthermore, PAH is metabolized, possibly within the kidney, to *N*-acetyl-PAH. The renal clearance of PAH alone has been noted by Prescott et al.[50] to decrease at low plasma concentrations while the clearance of the acetyl metabolite increases. Total PAH clearance remained unchanged. Further studies are necessary to evaluate the mechanisms and significance of these findings. The extraction ratio (ER) for PAH is 70% to 90% at plasma concentrations of 10 to 20 mg/L, hence the term "effective" renal plasma flow (ERPF) has been used when the clearance of PAH is not corrected for the extraction ratio or if it is assumed to be one.[9] Normal values are about 650 ± 160 mL/min for men and 600 ± 150 mL/min for women.[49] Children will reach normalized adult values by 3 years of age, and ERPF will begin to decline as a function of age after 30 years, reaching about one-half of its peak value by 90 years of age. The method for calculation of ERPF is based on the relationship between organ clearance, extraction ratio (ER), and flow:

$$\text{ERPF} = \text{renal PAH Cl} = \text{RPF} \times \text{ER}$$

Effective renal blood flow (ERBF) can be estimated from ERPF by assuming the extraction ratio is one and correcting for the red blood cell volume of the blood (hematocrit):

$$\text{ERBF} = \text{ERPF}/(1 - \text{Hct})$$

ERPF can also be measured using the radioisotopes ^{131}I-orthoiodohippurate or ^{99m}Tc-mercaptoacetyltriglycine (^{131}I-OIH or ^{99m}Tc-MAG3).[51] One important advantage of this method is the ability to measure ERPF in total or for each kidney independently as well as produce renal images. Russell and Dubovsky,[52] using a single-injection technique, compared clearance methods with and without urine collection and showed similar results with each method.

MEASUREMENT OF GLOMERULAR FILTRATION RATE

Normally there are approximately 1 million nephrons per kidney, and each nephron filters independently. The net effect, total GFR, is a representation of the functional renal mass, and the factors discussed above. As renal mass declines due to normal physiologic loss of nephrons secondary to the aging process or due to disease, there is a progressive decline in GFR. Thus, the total GFR represents the functional status of the kidneys.[27]

GFR is expressed as the volume of plasma filtered across the glomerulus per unit time. If one considers the normal RBF to be approximately 1.0 L/min, plasma volume to be 60% of blood volume, and filtration fraction across the glomerulus to be 20%, the normal GFR would then be approximately 120 mL/min/1.73 m^2.[2]

Accurate measurement of the GFR requires a compound that has unrestricted diffusion across the glomerulus and into Bowman's capsule without additional clearance by tubular secretion nor reduction by reabsorption. Furthermore, the solute should not be metabolized by renal tubular cells or alter renal function. Given these conditions, the GFR would be equivalent to the renal clearance of the solute marker:

$$\text{GFR} = \text{renal Cl} = (A_e)/\text{AUC}_{0-t}$$

where renal Cl is renal clearance of the marker, A_e is the amount of marker excreted in a specified period of time, t, and AUC_{0-t} is the area under the plasma concentration time curve of the marker.

Under steady-state conditions, the expression simplifies to:

$$\text{GFR} = \text{renal Cl} = (A_e)/[(C_{ss}) \times t]$$

where C_{ss} is the steady-state plasma concentration of the marker.

Several solutes have been used for the measurement of GFR and include both exogenous and endogenous compounds. Those administered as exogenous agents, such as inulin, iothalamate, iohexol, or radioisotopes, require specialized administration techniques and detection methods for the quantitation of function, but generally provide a more accurate measure of GFR. Methods that employ endogenous compounds, such as creatinine, require less technical expertise, but produce results with greater variability.[25] The marker of choice will depend on the purpose and cost of the test; research protocols will generally use a more accurate test than one used in the clinical setting (Table 40–3).

INULIN CLEARANCE

Inulin is a relatively large molecule (5200 Daltons) and has the necessary characteristics to serve as a marker for the measurement of GFR. Inulin is a fructose polysaccharide, obtained from plant tubers of the Jerusalem artichoke, dahlia, and chicory plants. It is not bound to plasma proteins, is freely filtered at the glomerulus, is not secreted or reabsorbed, and is not metabolized by the kidney.[25] The volume of distribution of inulin approximates extracellular volume, or 20% of ideal body weight. Because it is eliminated by glomerular filtration, its elimination half-life is dependent on renal function and is approximately 1.3 hours in subjects with normal renal function. For a subject with a GFR of 10 mL/min, the elimination half-life increases to approximately 16 hours. Therefore, a loading dose is essential when using the steady-state continuous infusion approach for measurement of GFR.

The most common technique for determination of GFR with inulin involves intravenous bolus administration followed by a continuous infusion of inulin.[25] The infusion

TABLE 40–3. Sensitivity and Clinical Utility of Renal Function Tests

	Accuracy	Clinical Utility	Cost
Inulin clearance	++++	+	++++
Radiolabeled markers	+++	+	+++
Nonisotopic contrast agents	+++	++	+++
Creatinine clearance	++	+++	++
Serum creatinine	+	++++	+

+ = acceptable/lowest, ++ = good/moderate, +++ = better/high, ++++ = best/very high.

dose must be adjusted in patients with diminished renal function due to the dependence of inulin elimination on GFR. A typical loading dose of 40 mg/kg is administered, followed by a maintenance infusion of 25 mg/min/1.73 $m^2 \times$ RF, where RF is the estimated fraction of normal renal function. For such situations, the maintenance infusion is reduced by the fraction of expected GFR based on an estimate of the patient's creatinine clearance. Following a 60-minute equilibration period, sequential measurements of inulin clearance are made over a period of 30 minutes for three intervals. Urine is collected, and blood samples bracket each collection period. It is necessary to maintain adequate hydration during the test because GFR is dependent on RBF and it assures adequate urine output during the procedure. A relatively constant urine flow will decrease the variability among repeated measurements and should be within the range of 1 to 10 mL/min. An initial water load of 10 to 15 mL/kg body weight will usually initiate a diuresis, and additional water equal to the urine output of each interval should be given orally or intravenously to maintain urinary output.

Inulin plasma clearance has been measured following a single-dose intravenous injection with multiple sampling of blood to estimate area under the curve. Clearance in this situation was calculated as: Cl = Dose/AUC. Continuous infusion of inulin following a bolus injection without urine collection can also provide an assessment of plasma clearance: Cl = Infusion rate/C_{ss}. Approximately 4 or more hours are needed to achieve steady state, and then the results are similar to those obtained using the traditional urine-collection method. Florijn et al.[53] compared the infusion and bolus techniques for both plasma and renal clearance in 14 patients with autosomal-dominant polycystic kidney disease. Variability was lower using plasma clearance and the bolus technique (C.V. 7.1 ± 3.1% vs 9.7 ± 5.4%), but it overestimated the renal clearance, (82.0 ± 30.5 vs 68.3 ± 27.6 mL/min/1.73 m^2). Similar observations were evident for the constant infusion method. The authors provide a regression equation to account for the overestimation; however, measurement of renal clearance will preclude the need to introduce additional variability into the assessment of renal function.

Measurement of plasma and urine inulin concentrations can be performed using a colorimetric reaction to detect fructose following acid hydrolysis of inulin, or enzymatically.[54,55] Glucose cross-reacts with the colorimetric measurement; therefore, it is necessary to correct samples with a "blank" obtained prior to infusion of the inulin. Individuals with elevated plasma glucose concentrations that change during the evaluation will show increased variability in their results.[25] A high-performance liquid chromatographic (HPLC) method using reverse-phase and UV detection has recently been described. Glucose and drugs commonly administered to patients with renal disease did not interfere with the assay, including corticosteroids, calcitriol, azathioprine, nifedipine, and atenolol.[56]

The majority of variability in the inulin clearance can be attributed to body size and is reduced if the clearance is normalized to body surface area. The normal range will decrease with increasing age, at a rate of approximately 10 mL/min/1.73 m^2 for each decade over 30 years. Gender and differences in renal function, due to physiologic conditions and/or disease state, may also contribute to the observed variability in the test. Normal inulin clearance is approximately 120 mL/min/1.73 m^2, slightly higher for men and lower for women.

Sinistrin, another polyfructosan, is handled in the same fashion as inulin in humans. It is filtered at the glomerulus and not secreted or reabsorbed to any significant extent. It is a naturally occurring substance derived from the root of the North African vegetable red squill, *Urginua maritime*. Its primary difference from inulin is water solubility. Whereas inulin must be heated prior to administration, sinistrin is soluble at room temperature. Assay methods for sinistrin have been described using enzymatic procedures, as well as HPLC with electrochemical detection.[55,57,58]

IOTHALAMATE CLEARANCE

Alternatives have been sought for inulin as a marker for GFR due to the problems of intermittent availability, high cost, sample preparation, and assay variability. Iothalamate has been commonly used in radiocontrast studies, but is also available in an unlabeled form. This agent is handled in a manner similar to that of inulin. It appears to be freely filtered at the glomerulus and does not undergo substantial tubular secretion or reabsorption.[59] Iothalamate has most commonly been employed in its radiolabeled form, ^{125}I-iothalamate, but recently has been used as a nonisotopic probe. Plasma and urine iothalamate concentrations have been measured using HPLC methods and can be analyzed simultaneously with PAH.[60] Protein binding in humans was found to be less than 1%, and iothalamate renal clearance would appear to be an excellent alternative to inulin for the measurement of GFR.[61,62]

IOHEXOL

Iohexol, a nonionic, low osmolar, iodinated contrast agent, has also been used for the determination of GFR. It is eliminated almost entirely by glomerular filtration, and plasma and renal clearance values are similar.[63,64] Brown and O'Reilly[65] performed simultaneous renal clearance studies of inulin and iohexol in 30 patients with various degrees of renal function. Clearance values were very similar: iohexol Cl is equal to 0.998 of inulin Cl plus 2.309 mL/min (r = 0.986). Detection of iohexol in plasma and urine samples was based on x-ray fluorescence analysis. Rocco et al.[66] compared iohexol plasma clearance with ^{125}I-iothalamate renal clearance and demonstrated a relationship of iohexol Cl equal to 0.90 of iothalamate Cl plus 6.8 mL/min (r = 0.95). The plasma iohexol assay was performed using a reverse-phase HPLC method. Lundqvist et al.[67] evaluated a single-sample plasma clearance calculation method using iohexol compared to ^{51}Cr-EDTA and demonstrated similar results ($r = 0.918$). These data support iohexol as a suitable alternative marker for the measurement of GFR. Following iohexol administration, a single plasma sample can be used to quantify renal function, provided sufficient time has elapsed since injection in patients with a reduced GFR—more than 24 hours if GFR is less than 20 mL/min.[64]

RADIOLABELED MARKERS

The GFR has also been evaluated using radiolabeled markers, such as ^{125}I-iothalamate (614 Daltons, radioactive half-life of 60 days), ^{99m}Tc-diethylenetriamine pentaacetic acid (DTPA, 393 Daltons, radioactive half-life of 6.03 hours), and ^{51}Cr-ethylenediaminetetraacetic acid (EDTA, 292 Daltons, radioactive half-life of 27 days).[68] They are all relatively small molecules that are minimally bound to plasma proteins and do not undergo tubular secretion or reabsorption to any significant degree.[69] ^{125}I-iothalamate and ^{99m}Tc-DTPA are used in the United States, whereas ^{51}Cr-EDTA is used extensively in Europe. Various protocols exist for the administration of the marker and subsequent determination of GFR. These protocols center on the issue of plasma clearance versus renal clearance, which requires the collection of urine during the evaluation period. The primary concern is whether the marker is cleared solely by filtration in the kidneys or if there are other significant routes of elimination. Measurement of radioactivity in plasma samples coupled with standard pharmacokinetic approaches results in plasma clearance, which will overestimate GFR if elimination occurs by other routes. The nonrenal clearance of these agents is low (3 to 8 mL/min) and thus plasma clearance should be an acceptable technique in most clinical situations. Indeed, Morton et al.[70] recently demonstrated that ^{99m}Tc-DTPA plasma clearance and ^{131}I-iothalamate renal clearance were highly correlated in patients with clearance values > 20 mL/min: DTPA Cl is equal to 0.943 of iothalamate Cl plus 1.12 mL/min ($r = 0.983$).

Simultaneous evaluation of three radiolabeled markers of GFR, ^{125}I-iothalamate, ^{169}Yb-DTPA, and ^{99m}Tc-DTPA, using renal clearance in adults, revealed that all three overestimated inulin clearance in normal subjects by approximately 5% to 10%.[71] Patients with renal impairment showed a small but significant overestimation of their inulin clearance when measured using ^{125}I-iothalamate or ^{169}Yb-DTPA. Clearance of creatinine overestimated the GFR at all levels of kidney function. Similar results have been observed with ^{99m}Tc-DTPA in children. The authors suggested that these radioisotopic filtration markers would be suitable alternatives to inulin for measurement of GFR in patients with renal insufficiency. ^{51}Cr-EDTA also yields estimates of GFR similar to inulin and in some cases slightly lower. This may be due to plasma protein binding or tubular reabsorption. As with ^{125}I-iothalamate and ^{99m}Tc-DTPA, ^{51}Cr-EDTA plasma clearance is greater than renal clearance, probably due to nonrenal routes of elimination.

Labeled markers have also been used for real-time monitoring of GFR during critical care of patients. Rabito et al.[72] studied 20 patients in an intensive care unit using an external radionuclide counting system to measure the rate of disappearance of ^{99m}Tc-DTPA from the extracellular space. Comparisons were made with short-term creatinine clearance measurements, and the rate constant for the ^{99m}Tc-DTPA disappearance predicted the renal function status in 94% of the patients. Patient outcomes were not assessed, and further studies are needed to determine its utility in the early detection of acute renal dysfunction.

An additional advantage for the determination of radiolabeled GFR is the ability to determine the individual contribution to overall renal function of each kidney. Within 2 minutes after injection, uptake of the label is proportional to GFR as measured using the gamma camera.[73]

CREATININE CLEARANCE

Despite the common use of CrCl to estimate GFR, it is a controversial measurement. Short-duration witnessed CrCl correlates with iothalamate clearance performed using the single injection technique. In a multicenter study[74] of 136 patients with type I diabetic nephropathy, GFR was assessed using (1) duplicate serum creatinine and 24-hour urine collection, (2) the mean of four iothalamate clearance periods by single injection technique during water diuresis, and (3) CrCl. Creatinine clearance was also estimated for each patient using the Cockcroft–Gault method,[75] corrected for weight and gender. The simultaneous iothalamate and CrCL were 78 ± 35 and 86 ± 35 mL/min while the separate 24-hour CrCl was 75 ± 33 mL/min. The Cockcroft–Gault estimate was 79 ± 29 mL/min. Compared to iothalamate Cl as the standard, the r^2 values for the simultaneous CrCl, 24-hour CrCl, and Cockcroft–Gault CrCl were 0.81, 0.49, and 0.67, indicating increased variability with the 24-hour clearance determinations. It was not stated whether the 24-hour CrCl measurements were performed as inpatient or ambulatory procedures.[74] In a selected group of 110 men—comprised of normals, kidney stone patients, and one nephritic—the inulin Cl was 117 ± 18 mL/min compared to 129 ± 20 mL/min for measured CrCl and 108 ± 19 for estimated CrCl using the Cockcroft–Gault method. The range of inulin clearance was approximately 80 to 160 mL/min. The relationship between the 24-hour CrCl and inulin Cl showed an r^2 of 0.74, whereas the Cockcroft–Gault CrCl was 0.41. Measurement of a 4-hour CrCl during water diuresis provided the best estimate of the GFR as determined by the iothalamate Cl, and the ratio of CrCl to iothalamate Cl did not appear to increase as the GFR decreased. These data suggest that a shorter collection period with a water diuresis may be the best method for determination of GFR when using creatinine clearance.[74]

Creatinine is eliminated by both glomerular filtration and tubular secretion. Tubular secretion augments the filtered creatinine by about 10% in subjects with normal kidney function. This, however, increases to as much as 100%

in patients with renal insufficiency.[26,27] As renal impairment develops, the remaining nephrons hypertrophy, and the degree of tubular secretion decreases disproportionately (less than) to the decrease in filtration. The result is an overestimation of creatinine clearance as a function of GFR assessed using inulin clearance (Fig. 40–4). Bauer et al.[26] assessed creatinine clearance as a function of inulin clearance in 123 subjects with various degrees of kidney function. Using a specific assay for the measurement of creatinine, the ratio of CrCl exceeded inulin Cl by 14%, thus suggesting 14% of the creatinine was eliminated by secretion. The CrCl to inulin Cl ratio in subjects with mild impairment was 1.20; for moderate impairment 1.87; and severe impairment 2.32. Thus, creatinine clearance is a poor indicator of GFR in patients with moderate to severe renal insufficiency.

Creatinine is secreted via the organic cationic pathway, which can be blocked by the coadministration of drugs that compete for the same secretory path, such as cimetidine and trimethoprim. Shemesh et al.[76] studied the effect of an infusion of cimetidine on the tubular secretion of creatinine. The ratio of CrCl to inulin Cl was reduced from 1.67 ± 0.10 to 1.16 ± 0.06 within 80 minutes of the infusion with no effect on inulin Cl. Roubenoff et al.[77] evaluated oral cimetidine as a technique to improve the accuracy and precision of creatinine clearance as an indicator of GFR. Thirteen patients with lupus nephritis and 24-hour CrCl ranging from 24 to 115.3 mL/min were given 400 mg cimetidine four times daily for 2 days before a 24-hour creatinine clearance determination. A simultaneous 4-hour ^{99m}Tc-DTPA and CrCl were also determined. Cimetidine reduced the CrCl to DTPA Cl ratio from 1.33 with placebo to 1.07 with cimetidine treatment ($P < .05$). No adverse effects were observed from the 2-day cimetidine treatment. Zaltzman et al.[78] administered cimetidine, 800 mg, as a single dose 1 hour prior to a 3-hour timed collection for creatinine and ^{125}I-iothalamate clearances. The CrCl to iothalamate Cl ratio was reduced from 1.53 ± 1.02 to 1.12 ± 0.02, and the authors suggest that this method effectively inhibited the tubular secretion of creatinine. Hilbrands et al.[79] and Van Acker et al.[80] demonstrated similar results using multiple doses, although the latter group noted a dose-dependency in the effect of cimetidine; subjects with higher renal cimetidine clearance required larger cimetidine doses for complete blockade of creatinine tubular secretion. A single oral dose of cimetidine, 800 mg, should provide adequate blockade of creatinine secretion to improve the use of the creatinine clearance measurement to estimate GFR. See Table 40–4 for the protocol used by Zaltzman et al.[78]

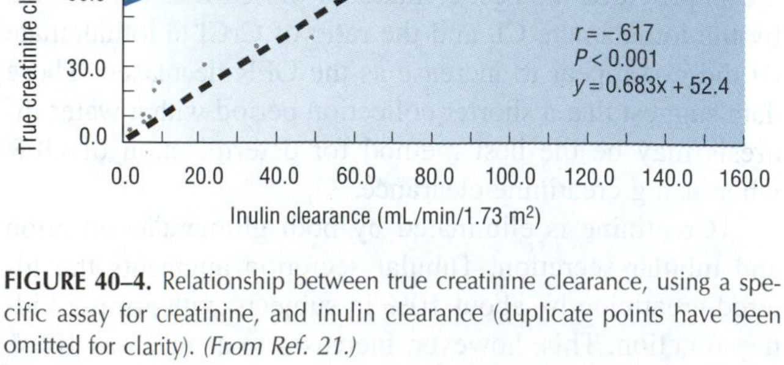

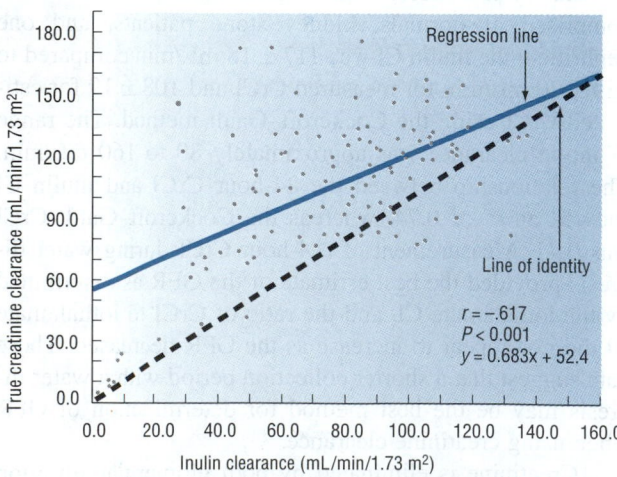

FIGURE 40–4. Relationship between true creatinine clearance, using a specific assay for creatinine, and inulin clearance (duplicate points have been omitted for clarity). *(From Ref. 21.)*

TABLE 40–4. Protocol for Cimetidine-modified Creatinine Clearance

1. Low-protein breakfast (0.2 g/kg) or fasting for morning test. Obtain height and weight.
2. 800 mg oral cimetidine with 1 L water. Void.
3. Allow 1 hour equilibration.
4. After 1 hour, complete void, ensure at least 3 mL/min (180 mL), replace urine volume with equal volume of water.
5. Begin 3-hour timed urine collection, replacing urine with water in equal volume.
6. Obtain midpoint (1.5 hour) serum creatinine.
7. Calculate timed creatinine clearance, CrCl = (Vol × U_{cr})/(S_{cr} × time). Correct for body surface area.

Derived from Ref. 78.

ESTIMATION OF CREATININE CLEARANCE

Several investigators have developed mathematical relationships (nomograms) between various patient factors and renal function to estimate CrCl when urine is not available. These factors include age, gender, weight, and serum creatinine concentration. Perhaps the most widely used of these estimators is the one developed by Cockcroft and Gault (CG),[75] which identified age and body mass as factors to incorporate in an equation to estimate CrCl. Their relationship was based on 249 male patients with stable kidney function whose 24-hour creatinine excretion was greater than 10 mg/kg, except for 23 patients who were included because their 24-hour urine volume was greater than 500 mL. Creatinine clearance ranged from 11 mL/min to normal. Creatinine excretion significantly decreases with increasing age (Fig. 40–5). Based on the usual CrCl formula and the relationship of creatinine excretion to age, they derived the following formula to estimate CrCl:

$$\text{CrCl (mL/min)} = [(140 - \text{Age}) \times \text{IBW}]/(S_{cr} \times 72)$$

where age is expressed in years, S_{cr} is the serum creatinine in mg/dL, and IBW is ideal body weight in kg. For females, the result is multiplied by 0.85.

Luke et al.[81] have evaluated the ability of the CG method and four other methods to predict CrCl (see Table 40–5), with inulin clearance being considered the standard. Simultaneous inulin and creatinine clearances, and a 24-hour ambulatory CrCl, were conducted in 109 patients. The simultaneously determined inulin and creatinine clearances correlated best, $r^2 = 0.85$, and the inulin

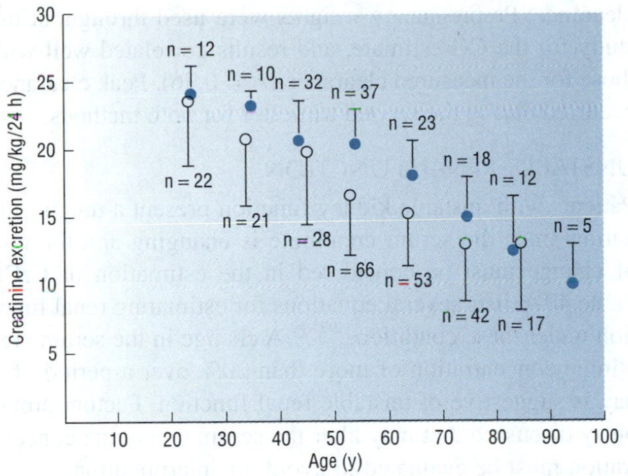

FIGURE 40–5. Creatinine excretion as a function of age. Solid circles, 149 males, age 20 to 99 years; open circles, 249 males, age 18 to 92 years. *(From Ref. 75.)*

CL was overestimated by approximately 15% due to tubular secretion of creatinine. The 24-hour ambulatory CrCl r^2 was 0.71. For the five calculated clearances, CG and Mawer et al.[82] correlated the best with inulin clearance. The CG method showed a linear relationship with inulin CL equal to 1.121 of CrCl plus 20.6 mL/min (r^2 = 0.66), whereas for Mawer the relationship was inulin CL equal to 1.051 of CrCl plus 18.3 mL/min (r^2 = 0.66). The calculated CrCl values from CG and Mawer both appeared to correlate well with the ambulatory and 4-hour CrCl, but the regressions were not reported. Based on their findings, Luke et al.[81] propose continued use of the CG or Mawer method for rapid estimation of CrCl in patients with stable kidney function. The other methods, of Jelliffe[83,84] and of Hull et al.,[85] consistently underestimated the CrCl. As kidney function declined, there was an increase in the fraction of creatinine eliminated by secretion as measured by the CrCl to inulin CL ratio, consistent with earlier reports. This limitation should be taken into consideration when attempting to use CrCl for

TABLE 40–5. Equations for the Estimation of Creatinine Clearance in Adults With Stable Renal Function

Source	Equation
Cockroft and Gault[75]	Men: CrCl = (140 – Age) IBW / (S_{cr} × 72) Women: CrCl × 0.85
Jelliffe[83]	Men: CrCl = (100/S_{cr}) – 12 Women: CrCl = (80/S_{cr}) – 7
Jelliffe[84]	Men: CrCl = 98 – [0.8 (Age – 20)]/S_{cr} Women: CrCl × 0.9
Mawer et al.[82]	Men: IBW [29.3 – (0.203 × Age)] [1 – (0.03 × S_{cr})]/(14.4 × S_{cr}) Women: IBW [25.3 – (0.175 × Age)] [1 - (0.03 × S_{cr})]/(14.4 × S_{cr})
Hull et al.[85]	Men: CrCl = [(145 – Age)/S_{cr}] – 3 Women: CrCl × 0.85

the estimation of renal function and the individualization of drug dosage regimens. Gault et al.[86] also evaluated the performance of the CG estimator of renal function compared with inulin and ^{99m}Tc-DTPA. Except for conditions of unstable kidney function, it performed similar to the 24-hour creatinine clearance method.

As demonstrated for the measured CrCl, adminstration of cimetidine has resulted in improved performance of CG to predict GFR. Ixkes et al.[87] provided 19 patients with three 800 mg doses of cimetidine for 24 hours, and measured cimetidine and creatinine plasma determinations from 3 to 7 hours following the final dose. During this 4-hour window, iothalamate Cl was determined as the measure of GFR. The CG calculations were performed with the plasma creatinine measurement 3 hours after the last dose of cimetidine. The CG Cl to iothalamate Cl ratio decreased from 1.28 ± 0.21 to 0.98 ± 0.11 in the presence of cimetidine.

LIVER DISEASE

Renal function in patients with coexisting liver disease and renal impairment has been shown to be difficult to predict by two separate investigators. Hull et al.[85] evaluated creatinine clearance prediction equations in 144 cases and showed that in patients with hepatic cirrhosis, the Mawer method[82] consistently overpredicted the measured creatinine clearance. The mean predicted clearance was 73.5 ± 11.3 compared to the measured clearance of 46.3 ± 8.3 mL/min. Echizen and Ishizaki[88] also showed an overprediction error in 142 liver cirrhosis patients of 35% and 14% in male and female patients, respectively, compared to a control population with a prediction error of 5% and 4% for male and female patients, respectively. They proposed two new equations to predict CrCl in this patient population: males, [(161 – Age) × BW]/(97 × S_{cr}); and females, [(205 – Age) × BW]/(152 × S_{cr}), where age is in years, BW is total body weight in kg, and S_{cr} is serum creatinine concentration in mg/dL. In a prospective evaluation of the new equations, the investigators reported a prediction error of 2% and –7% for males and females, respectively. The proposed reasons for these observations are: decreased excretion rate of creatinine compared to controls, increased extrahepatic creatinine metabolism or decreased synthesis of creatinine in the liver, and subsequent decreased storage in the muscle and, therefore, lowered production of creatinine.

Recent studies of renal function in patients with severe hepatic disease have confirmed the earlier observations of Hull et al.[85] and Echizen and Ishizaki.[88] Caregaro et al.[89] reported that CrCl overestimated GFR by 50% in patients with a GFR of 56 ± 19 mL/min/1.73m^2, due to increased tubular secretion of creatinine. DeSanto et al.[90] studied 19 patients with early posthepatic cirrhosis whose inulin and creatinine clearances were 90 ± 4.4 and 122 ± 7 mL/min/1.73 m^2. The overestimation of GFR by creatinine clearance was present in 18 of the patients, and inversely correlated with GFR (r = –0.452, P < .04). Measurement of renal function in patients with hepatic disease should be performed using a method specific for glomerular filtration, that is, not creatinine clearance.

OTHER SPECIAL POPULATIONS

Davis and Chandler[91] confirmed the use of the CG equation to predict CrCl in trauma patients with stable kidney function, when normalized to 72 kg, and Thakur and colleagues[92] demonstrated its successful utility in 42 paraplegic subjects. Renal transplant recipients are frequently monitored for renal function, as numerous complications may occur during the life of the allograft. Goerdt et al.[93] assessed several nomographic methods for their bias and precision in predicting iohexol clearance in 127 patients with stable kidney function. The CG method performed poorly, overestimating iohexol clearance. This is expected, as iohexol clearance provides a true measure of GFR while the CrCl is higher due to the tubular secretion of creatinine. Schück et al.[94] compared the CG method with sinistrin Cl and CrCl. Both clearance determinations were overestimated by CG, but more so for sinistrin Cl. The investigators noted significant variability and an inability of CG to reliably predict either clearance measure. Huang et al.[95] reported the inability of several CrCl equations to predict renal function in hospitalized patients with advanced HIV disease. All methods, including CG, Jelliffe, and Mawer, overestimated the measured 24-hour CrCl. The reasons for the poor predictability of these methods is unclear, although 24-hour collection methods result in increased variability, often due to inadequate collection of the sample, which could contribute to the disparity.

Renal function assessment during pregnancy is usually performed using a 24-hour creatinine clearance determination. Quadri and colleagues[96] evaluated the CG formula to estimate renal function in 34 pregnant women during each trimester, compared with the measured 24-hour creatinine clearance. Prepregnancy weights were used throughout the study for the CG estimate, and results correlated well with those for the measured clearance ($r^2 = 0.76$). Peak clearance occurred during the second trimester for both methods.

UNSTABLE RENAL FUNCTION

Patients with unstable kidney function present a unique situation since the serum creatinine is changing and the rate of change must be considered in the estimation of CrCl. Table 40–6 lists several equations for estimating renal function under these conditions.[97–99] A change in the serum creatinine concentration of more than 20% over a period of 1 day is suggestive of unstable renal function. Factors previously discussed that may alter the serum creatinine concentration must be evaluated to avoid misinterpretation.

Conclusions regarding the estimation of CrCl using nomograms are difficult. At best, these data illustrate the variability and inherent limitations of these approaches to estimate renal function.

CYSTATIN C

A relatively new marker for renal function has been identified and evaluated in small populations for its utility as a tool to assess changes in GFR. Cystatin C is a nonglycosylated 13-kDa basic protein of the cystatin superfamily of inhibitors of cysteine proteases.[63,100] It is produced by nucleated cells of the body and is present in stable concentrations, apparently not affected by infection or malignancy. It was initially recommended as a test of kidney function in 1985 and shown to correlate with GFR as well as creatinine. The recent development of an automated immunoassay technique by Newman et al.[100] and their validation of the test as a more sensitive indicator of reduced renal function than creatinine suggest that it may have future clinical

TABLE 40–6. Equations for the Estimation of Creatinine Clearance in Adults With Unstable Renal Function

Reference	Units	Equations: Males	Equations: Females
Jelliffe and Jelliffe[97]	mL/min/1.73 m²	$E^{ss} = \text{IBW}\,[29.3 - 0.203\,(\text{Age})]$ $E^{ss}_{corr} = E^{ss}\,[1.035 - 0.0337\,(S_{cr})]$ $E = E^{ss}_{corr} - \dfrac{[4\ \text{IBW}\,(S_{cr_2} - S_{cr_1})]}{\Delta t\ \text{day}}$ $\text{CrCl} = \dfrac{E}{14.4\,(S_{cr})}$	$E^{ss} = \text{IBW}\,[25.1 - 0.175\,(\text{Age})]$ $E^{ss}_{corr} = E^{ss}[1.035 - 0.0337\,(S_{cr})]$ $E = E^{ss}_{corr} - \dfrac{[4\ \text{IBW}\,(S_{cr_2} - S_{cr_1})]}{\Delta t\ \text{day}}$ $\text{CrCl} = \dfrac{E}{14.4(S_{cr})}$
Chiou et al.[98]	mL/min	$V_d = 0.6\ \text{L (IBW)}$ $\text{CrCl} = \dfrac{2\ \text{IBW}\,[28 - 0.2\,(\text{Age})]}{14.4(S_{cr_1} + S_{cr_2})} + \dfrac{2\,[V_d\text{IBW}\,(S_{cr_1} - S_{cr_2})]}{(S_{cr_1} + S_{cr_2})\Delta t\ \text{min}} - [\text{CrCl}^{NR} \times \text{IBW}]$	$V_d = 0.6\text{L (IBW)}$ $\text{CrCl} = \dfrac{2\ \text{IBW}\,[22.4 - 0.16\,(\text{Age})]}{14.4(S_{cr_1} + S_{cr_2})} + \dfrac{2\,[V_d\text{IBW}\,(S_{cr_1} - S_{cr_2})]}{(S_{cr_1} + S_{cr_2})\Delta t\ \text{min}} - [\text{CrCl}^{NR} \times \text{IBW}]$
Brater[99]	mL/min/70 kg	$\text{CrCl} = \dfrac{[293 - 2.03(\text{Age})] \times [1.035 - 0.01685(S_{cr_1} + S_{cr_2})]}{(S_{cr_1} + S_{cr_2})\Delta t\ \text{day}} + \dfrac{49(S_{cr_1} - S_{cr_2})}{(S_{cr_1} + S_{cr_2})\ \Delta t\ \text{day}}$	CrCl = Male value × 0.86

E^{ss} = steady state urinary creatinine excretion; Δt day = time in days between Scr_1 and Scr_2; Δt min = time in minutes between Scr_1 and Scr_2; CrCl^{NR} = nonrenal clearance of creatinine = 0.048 mL/min/kg.

utility in the assessment of renal function. Comparison of ^{51}Cr-labeled EDTA with 1/cystatin C and 1/creatinine for 106 measurements resulted in correlations of $r = 0.81$ and 0.50, respectively.

RENAL FUNCTION IN CHILDREN

Kidney function in the neonate is difficult to assess due to difficulty in urine and blood collection, the frequent presence of a nonsteady-state serum creatinine, and apparent disparity between development of glomerular and tubular function. A recent evaluation of GFR in preterm infants on day 3 of life, using an inulin infusion, failed to identify a relationship between patient weight and GFR. Gestational age, which ranged from 23.4 to 36.9 weeks (mean 30.2 weeks), however, correlated with both GFR and reciprocal creatinine. The inulin clearance increased from 0.67 to 0.85 mL/min in those with gestational age < 28 weeks versus 32 to 37 weeks, while S_{cr} decreased from 1.05 to 0.73 mg/dL, respectively. Creatinine was measured using a specific enzymatic method to avoid interference from bilirubin or drugs.[101] Creatinine clearance has also been evaluated in infants less than 1 week of age, and values of 17.8 mL/min/1.73 m^2 on day 1 increased to 36.4 mL/min/1.73 m^2 by day 6.[102] Preterm infants demonstrate significantly reduced GFR prior to 34 weeks, which rapidly increases and becomes similar to term infants within the first week of life.[103]

Due to difficulty in assessing GFR, Clark et al.[104] suggested monitoring the urinary ratio of retinol-binding protein to creatinine as an indicator of early tubular damage. Small-molecular-weight proteins (< 30 kDa) such as β_2-microglobulin and retinol-binding protein are normally reabsorbed through the proximal tubule following glomerular filtration. Excretion of this protein into the urine is an indication of a tubular functional defect, which usually precedes a reduction in glomerular filtration. Retinol-binding protein is more stable in an acid urine; therefore, it may be a preferred marker for tubular function. Retinol-binding protein to creatinine ratio was shown to decrease with increasing gestational age, without changes in creatinine, suggesting it may be a more sensitive indicator of tubular function.[104] It was also related to the severity of illness, whereas there were no differences for plasma creatinine alone. Kidney function expressed as GFR standardized to body surface area increases with age and stabilizes at approximately 1 year. Individual studies in older children are best assessed using standard measurement techniques for GFR. Subcutaneous administration of ^{125}I-iothalamate has been effectively used to measure GFR in children ranging in age from 1 to 20 years.[105]

Estimation of CrCl as described by Schwartz et al.[106] is dependent on the child's age and length:

$$\text{GFR} = [\text{length (cm)} \times k]/S_{cr}$$

where k is defined by age group: infant (1 to 52 weeks) = 0.45, child (1 to 13 years) = 0.55, adolescent male = 0.7, and adolescent female = 0.55.

Subsequent studies have verified these relationships in children with normal or mild renal impairment and demonstrated significant variability at clearance values < 50. The recent report of Al-Harbi and Lireman[107] from a population of 48 pediatric renal allograft recipients, aged 3 to 19 years showed a good correlation of the predicted CrCl with measured 4-hour CrCl and ^{99m}Tc-DTPA ($r = 0.75$). However, predictive performance measures of bias and precision were not reported. Fong et al.[108] evaluated the method in critically ill children (mean age 5.6 years, range 0.1 to 20.8 years), and concluded that the method significantly overestimated the measured CrCl (bias = 45%). Dose adjustments and other therapeutic decisions based on kidney function warrant appropriate measures of renal status to avoid incorrect decisions.

RENAL FUNCTION IN THE ELDERLY

Cross-sectional studies have demonstrated decreased GFR as a function of age when GFR was measured as inulin, iothalamate, or creatinine clearance.[75,109] The Baltimore Longitudinal Study on Aging,[110] an evaluation of 254 normal healthy subjects, revealed that creatinine clearance decreases at the rate of approximately 0.75 mL/min/1.73 m^2/yr beginning at the fourth decade of life. These subjects were evaluated prospectively for up to 23 years. Interestingly, approximately one-third of the subjects showed no change in renal function from their baseline value, and a small number showed an increased clearance. These changes may be due to normal physiologic changes or to subclinical insults to the kidneys initiating the events leading to chronic progressive loss of renal function.

Interpretation of the serum creatinine concentration alone is difficult in the elderly patient due to the decreased muscle mass and lower production rate of creatinine. As a result, the body load of creatinine is reduced, yet the fewer functional nephrons tend to maintain the serum creatinine within the normal range. As renal function declines, a larger fraction of creatinine is excreted by the kidneys. This perpetuates the "normal" serum creatinine. A reasonable approach to interpretation of the serum creatinine is use of the Cockcroft–Gault[75] formula to estimate the patient's CrCl. Smythe et al.[111] estimated CrCl in 23 patients > 60 years of age using seven different methods, and compared the results to a measured 24-hour CrCl determination. Estimations were performed with the actual serum creatinine concentration and also with the serum creatinine rounded to 1.0 mg/dL if the actual value was < 1.0 mg/dL. Rounding the serum creatinine to 1.0 mg/dL resulted in a significantly lower (bias = 28.8 mL/min) estimate of GFR compared with the actual clearance than when the unadjusted creatinine (bias = 2.3 mL/min) was used. These data strongly suggest that one should not arbitrarily adjust the serum creatinine concentration in elderly patients. An alternative to the estimation of GFR or a 24-hour clearance determination is a 4-hr clearance performed during water diuresis.[74] This correlates with the inulin clearance as well as the inpatient

24-hour collection, although one must be aware of the potential risk of hyponatremia in the geriatric patient who is unable to tolerate an oral water load. O'Connell et al.[112] assessed the accuracy of 2- and 8-hour urine collections compared with 24-hour creatinine clearance determinations in 45 hospitalized patients ≥ 65 years old with indwelling urethral catheters. Single, timed urine collections for CrCl showed minimal bias with the 8-hour collection compared with the 24-hour value, whereas the 2-hour determination was both biased and imprecise. Unfortunately, urinary residual was not determined, the bladder was not rinsed at each collection period, and the mean urine flow was low at 1.23 mL/min; all of these factors may have negatively affected the results of the 2-hour collection.

ASSESSMENT OF PROGRESSION

Chronic progressive kidney disease will eventually lead to end-stage renal disease (ESRD), necessitating dialysis or transplantation for survival (see Chaps. 42, 43, and 44). Attempts to slow the rate of progression through dietary and blood pressure control,[113] angiotensin-converting enzyme inhibitor therapy,[114] and improved glucose control in patients with type I diabetes mellitus[115] have recently proven successful. As a result, therapeutic intervention can now successfully decrease the incidence of ESRD. Specific therapies and their effectiveness is discussed in detail in Chapter 42. The efficacy of these and future potential interventions is optimally assessed with regular measurement of accurate and sensitive indices of renal function such as iohexol, iothalamate, or radioisotope clearances. When these are not available, alternative measures, such as reciprocal creatinine ($1/S_{cr}$), must be considered.

A linear decline in the reciprocal of the serum creatinine concentration as a function of time has been used as a simple technique to evaluate the rate of progression of renal disease and to predict the time when dialysis is necessary.[25] Fundamentally, the serum creatinine concentration is a function of input from the breakdown of creatine derived from muscle or dietary sources and its elimination, predominantly through glomerular filtration and tubular secretion. Under steady-state conditions, the formation rate of creatinine equals the elimination rate (R), and CrCl is inversely related to S_{cr} as:

$$S_{cr} = R/CrCl$$

The reciprocal relationship between S_{cr} and CrCl is then expressed as:

$$1/S_{cr} = 1/R \times CrCl$$

which demonstrates the linear relationship between the reciprocal of the S_{cr} and CrCl. This is depicted in Figure 40–6A. As renal function declines, the reciprocal of the serum creatinine concentration will decrease as a linear function of the creatinine clearance, and the slope of the relationship is the reciprocal of the elimination rate of creatinine. Under conditions of progressively decreasing kidney function, this relationship assumes that filtration clearance and secretion clearance decrease proportionately as well as any nonrenal elimination of creatinine. In addition, the rate of input is assumed constant. Based on these assumptions, clinicians can use the reciprocal serum creatinine plotted as a function of time as a prognostic tool, to predict when dialysis may be needed (when $1/S_{cr} \sim 0.1$) or as a marker for evaluating the success of therapeutic interventions to alter the rate of decline in renal function (Fig. 40–6B). If these assumptions change over time, then the linearity of the relationship will also change. Several factors such as changes in dietary intake of creatine and decreased muscle mass which are associated with a reduction in the production of creatinine may alter the utility of the relationship. Furthermore, if tubular secretion increases in response to nephron hypertrophy or disproportionately to

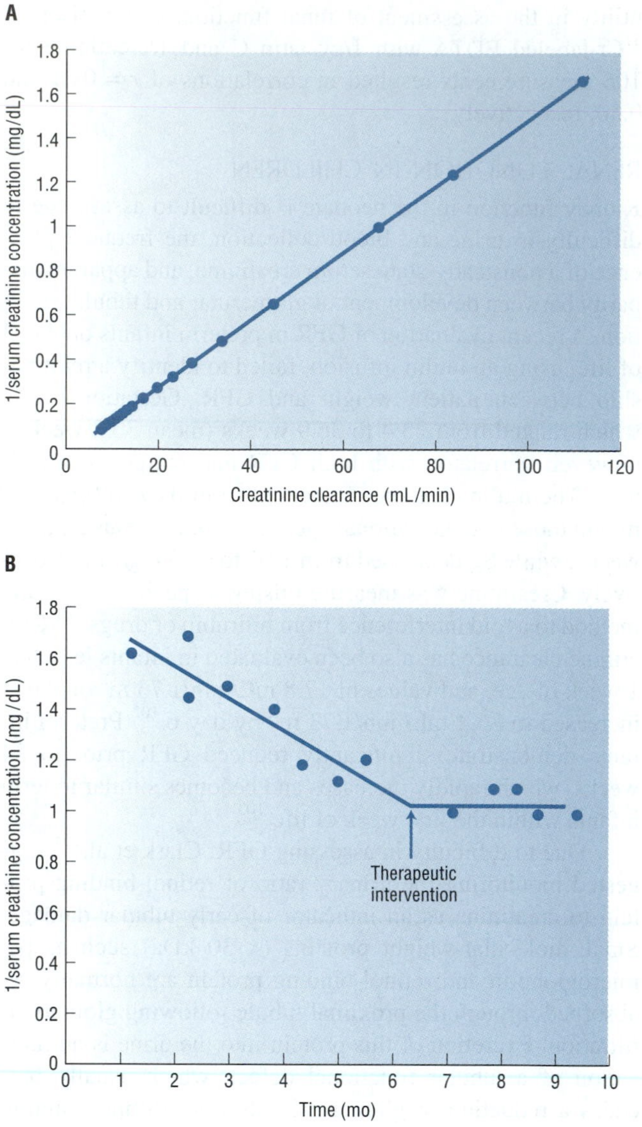

FIGURE 40–6. Linear relationship between **(A)** the reciprocal of serum creatinine concentration and creatinine clearance and **(B)** the reciprocal of serum creatinine concentration as a function of time in a hypothetical patient with progressive renal impairment. The arrow indicates a change in the rate of progression, which may be related to a therapeutic intervention.

filtration, or if nonrenal routes of elimination of creatinine, such as metabolism by intestinal bacteria, become more important, then changes in the slope of the reciprocal creatinine versus time relationship may be altered. It is most important to be aware of the limitations of serum creatinine measurement and to realize that it is not an adequate test to detect early chronic renal disease or to precisely estimate the disease's rate of progression.[22]

Although not a quantitative measure of renal function, urinary microalbuminuria has been identified as an early marker of renal disease in patients with diabetic nephropathy[116,117] and numerous other conditions, such as hypertension, and obesity.[118–120] In kidney transplant recipients, the urinary albumin to creatinine ratio was shown to accurately predict 24-hour proteinuria, a marker of renal disease. Guidelines for monitoring indicate that a urine albumin to creatinine ratio of > 30 mg/g places the patient at increased risk of developing diabetic nephropathy and is an indication for the initiation of pharmacotherapeutic intervention.[121] Microalbuminuria has also been suggested as a risk factor for renal dysfunction among patients with essential hypertension.[122] A National Institute of Diabetes, Digestive, and Kidney Diseases (NIDDK) Workshop[123] has identified microalbuminuria as the best early marker of nephropathy in patients with insulin-dependent diabetes mellitus (IDDM). Annual evaluations should be performed in patients with a 5- to 10-year history of IDDM. Patients with microalbuminuria (30 to 300 mg/day) on at least two or three occasions or overt albuminuria (> 300 mg/day) should begin to receive pharmacotherapy. For children, microalbuminuria is considered present if excretion exceeds 15 μg/kg/h, and overt albuminuria has been defined as an excretion rate that exceeds 4 mg/kg/d.

PROCEDURES USED IN THE DIAGNOSIS OF ANATOMIC ABNORMALITIES

RADIOLOGIC STUDIES

Assessment of kidney structure may be accomplished using several techniques. The standard x-ray of the kidneys, ureters, and bladder (KUB) is useful for a gross estimate of kidney size and the presence of calcifications.[68] Although an easy test to perform, the useful information achieved is minimal, and more detailed evaluations are often necessary. The intravenous urogram (IVU; formerly known as intravenous pyelogram, or IVP) involves the use of a contrast agent to facilitate visualization of the urinary collecting system. It is primarily used in the assessment of structural changes that may be associated with nonglomerular hematuria, pyuria, or flank pain, resulting from recurrent urinary tract infections, obstruction, or stone formation.[68] For patients with insufficient renal filtration, retrograde administration of dye into the ureters may be performed to facilitate visualization of the collecting system. Furthermore, local administration may avoid systemic exposure and associated adverse reactions (see Chap. 45). Contrast agents are also employed during renal angiography for the assessment of renovascular disease. As a test for the diagnosis of renovascular hypertension, the captopril (ACE inhibitor) test has shown to be a useful adjunct. Under conditions of unilateral renal artery stenosis, the affected kidney produces large quantities of angiotensin II, which vasoconstricts the efferent arteriole to maintain GFR. The administration of an ACE inhibitor will result in reduced uptake of the contrast agent since perfusion of the affected kidney will decrease. This occurs as a result of decreased efferent arteriolar vasoconstriction. For patients with bilateral disease, a decrease in uptake is observed in both kidneys.[124]

Ultrasound uses sound waves directed toward the tissue of interest and, based on the signal reflected back to the transducer, generates a two-dimensional image. The echogenicity of the kidney is compared with that of an adjacent organ—liver on the right and spleen on the left—with an increased echogenicity indicating an abnormal finding. Ultrasonography can distinguish the renal pyramids, medulla, and cortex, and abnormalities in structure, such as occurs with obstruction. Renal ultrasound is also used as a guide for site localization during percutaneous kidney biopsy.

Computerized tomography (CT) is a cross-sectional anatomic imaging procedure based on x-ray data. The procedure is frequently performed with contrast to enhance imaging. Spiral, or helical, CT, a more recent technique, provides for three-dimensional reconstruction of tissues. CT is performed as a test for the evaluation of obstructive uropathy, malignancy, and infections of the kidney.

Magnetic resonance imaging (MRI) is based on aligning hydrogen nuclei in the body with the use of a powerful magnet and applying radiofrequency pulses. The signals emitted by the H^+ during realignment on repeated pulses allows for generation of the tissue image. Realignment times can also be altered with the use of contrast agents (gadolinium, gadopentatate), leading to increased signal intensity and improved imaging. MRI is useful for the assessment of obstruction, malignancy, and renovascular lesions. Further discussions of these procedures are present in recent reviews.[68,125]

SPECIAL PROCEDURES IN THE DIAGNOSIS OF RENAL DYSFUNCTION

MEASUREMENT OF TUBULAR FUNCTION

Although GFR is perhaps the best overall indicator of renal function, it may not be reflective of tubular function, either secretory capacity[16] or cellular function.[126,127] Tubular function is best assessed by measurement of ERPF, where PAH serves as the prototype marker of the organic anion secretory system.[128] *N*-1-methylnicotinamide (NMN) and tetraethyl ammonium (TEA) are prototype compounds secreted by the cationic transport system and may be used as markers of cationic secretory capacity.[9,129] Edwards et al.[130] demonstrated delayed recovery of NMN clearance among patients with psoriasis treated with low-dose cyclosporine, compared with the recovery of GFR and renal blood flow. Earlier studies with NMN have suggested its use to assess the effects of selected renal diseases on drug handling by the kidneys.[131] It should be recognized, however, that these transport systems are not mutually exclusive. Indeed, probenecid that is secreted by the anionic pathway has been shown to inhibit the secretion of cationic compounds. Quantitative measures of tubular transport capacity are currently limited primarily to the research setting.

Other measures of tubular function are less specific and are regarded primarily as indices of damage within the nephron.[132] Schentag and Plaut[127] demonstrated a delay in the increase of serum creatinine following aminoglycoside toxicity when compared to markers for tubular damage such as the low-molecular-weight protein β_2-microglobulin (11.8 kDa) and urinary enzymes. The rise in β_2-microglobulin is related to an early functional defect in the proximal tubular cell. This is followed by a rise in the excretion of enzymes released due to structural damage of the cells and finally the formation and excretion of cellular casts. Other low-molecular-weight proteins that have been used as markers of tubular function include retinol-binding protein[133,134] (21 kDa) and protein HC (also known as α_1-microglobulin, 27 kDa).[126,132] These proteins are normally freely filtered at the glomerulus and then completely reabsorbed by the proximal tubule. Increases in their excretion are thus suggestive of tubular dysfunction but are not diagnostic, as an increased production rate or GFR less than 30 mL/min may lead to increased excretion. In both cases, the maximal reabsorptive capacity may be exceeded, leading to net excretion of the protein. Retinol-binding protein and protein HC have also been shown to be elevated with tubular damage and may be more appropriate markers than β_2-microglobulin.[126]

Numerous urinary enzymes such as *N*-acetylglucosaminidase (NAG), alanine aminopeptidase (AAP), alkaline phosphatase (AP), γ-glutamyltransferase (GGT), pyruvate kinase, glutathione transferase, lysozyme, and pancreatic ribonuclease have been used as diagnostic markers for renal disease.[126] Jung et al.[135] compared the ability of five enzymes (NAG, AAP, AP, GGT, and lysozyme) to detect early rejection episodes in kidney transplant patients. Only NAG and AAP were early predictors of rejection. NAG is an enzyme contained within the lysosome of the tubular cell and is released by damage to the lysosome, whereas AAP is an enzyme of the brush border. Both markers were increased approximately 2 days earlier than standard methods in patients with transplant rejection.

The kidney tissue protein, adenosine-binding protein (ABP), is a large, 120-kDa protein bound to the brush border of the proximal tubule and shed during damage to the tubule. It has been shown by Thompson et al.[136] to be significantly elevated in patients with acute tubular necrosis but remained near normal in patients with glomerular lesions. It has also been shown to be elevated in the urine of kidney transplant patients during acute rejection episodes. This increase often preceded elevations of the serum creatinine by 1 to 7 days. Flynn[126] has suggested that the battery of tests available for evaluation of urinary proteins and enzymes may be useful in identifying the location of injury in the kidneys and may some day provide an alternative to the renal biopsy for identification of the renal pathology.

BIOPSY

Renal biopsy is used in several conditions to facilitate diagnosis when clinical, laboratory, and imaging findings prove inconclusive. Proteinuria and hematuria are both associated with renal parenchymal disease. When less-invasive studies are unsuccessful in differentiating the cause and the possible causes have different therapeutic approaches, biopsy may be indicated. Functional status of the kidney is not assessed with biopsy, and severity of disease and progression is best measured using quantitative tests discussed above. Contraindications to renal biopsy include a solitary kidney, severe hypertension, bleeding disorder, severe anemia, cystic kidney, and hydronephrosis, among others. Complications resulting from biopsy primarily include hematuria, which may last for several days, perirenal hematoma, and arteriovenous fistulas, usually not clinically significant.[25]

▶ PRINCIPLES OF PHARMACOTHERAPY

- The glomerular filtration rate is the single best test to assess overall renal function, yet it is nonspecific regarding the site of injury.
- Measurement of the GFR is ideally performed using inulin or iothalamate as the test marker, or radioisotope techniques such as ^{99m}Tc-DTPA, when renal clearance is measured.
- Creatinine clearance is the most commonly performed test of renal function, whether measured in the ambulatory or inpatient setting or estimated using the serum creatinine along with the patient's age, gender, and weight.
- The pretreatment of patients with cimetidine prior to the creatinine clearance determination will enhance the accuracy of the GFR measurement, especially in patients with severe renal dysfunction.
- Caution should be exercised when interpreting the serum creatinine concentration as the sole measure of kidney function. Consideration should be given to patient age, lean body mass, gender, diet, concomitant diseases and drug therapy, circadian rhythm, stability of kidney function, tubular secretion, and analytic method.
- Evaluation of the reciprocal serum creatinine over time is not an acceptable alternative to the measurement of GFR for the assessment of the rate of kidney disease progression. Its use in clinical practice should be limited to those settings where more specific methods are unavailable.
- Non-GFR measures of renal function including urinalysis, x-ray, CT, MRI, sonography, and biopsy are directed toward qualitative assessment of kidney function.

REFERENCES

1. Campens D, Buntinx F. Selecting the best renal function tests. Int J Technol Assess Health Care 1997;13:343–356.
2. Vander AJ. Renal Physiology, 5th ed. New York, McGraw-Hill, 1995.
3. Valderrabano F. Erythropoietin in chronic renal failure. Kidney Int 1996;50:1373–1391.
4. Alvestrand A. Carbohydrate and insulin metabolism in renal failure. Kidney Int 1997;52(suppl 62):S48–S52.
5. Gonzalez EA, Martin KJ. Renal osteodystrophy: Pathogenesis and management. Nephrol Dial Transplant 1995;10(suppl 3):13–21.
6. Elston AC, Bayliss MK, Park GR. Effect of renal failure on drug metabolism by the liver. Br J Anaesth 1993;71:282–290.
7. Meffin PJ, Zilm DM, Veenendaal JR. Reduced clofibric acid clearance in renal dysfunction is due to a futile cycle. J Pharmacol Exp Ther 1983;227:732–738.
8. Verbeeck RK, Wallace SM, Loewen GR. Reduced elimination of ketoprofen in the elderly is not necessarily due to impairment of glucuronidation. Br J Clin Pharmacol 1984;17:783–784.
9. Sica DA, Schoolwerth AC. Renal handling of organic anions and cations and renal excretion of uric acid. In: Brenner BM, Rector FC, eds. The Kidney, 5th ed. Philadelphia, W.B. Saunders, 1996:607–626.
10. Poe-Hirr H, Gisclon LG, Hui AC, Giacomini KM. Interactions of organic anions with the organic cation transporter in renal BBMV. Am J Physiol 1988;254:F56–F61.
11. Bendayan R. Renal drug transport: A review. Pharmacotherapy 1996; 16:971–985.
12. Sikic BI. Pharmacologic approaches to reversing multidrug resistance. Semin Hematol 1997;34:40–47.
13. Rowland M, Tozer TN. Clinical Pharmacokinetics: Concepts and Applications, 3rd ed. Baltimore, Williams & Wilkins, 1995:172–173.
14. Bricker NS. On the meaning of the intact nephron hypothesis. Am J Med 1969;46:1–11.
15. Meyer TW, Baboolal K, Brenner BM. Nephron adaptation to renal injury. In: Brenner BM, Rector FC, eds. The Kidney, 5th ed. Philadelphia, W.B. Saunders, 1996:2011–2048.
16. Hori R, Okumura K, Kamiya A, et al. Ampicillin and cephalexin in renal insufficiency. Clin Pharmacol Ther 1983;34:792–798.
17. Hori R, Okumura K, Nihira H. A new dosing regimen in renal insufficiency: Application to cephalexin. Clin Pharmacol Ther 1985;38: 290–295.
18. Maiza A, Daley-Yates PT. The clearance of drugs in different types of renal disease. Renal Failure 1988;11:67. Abstract.
19. Lin JH, Lin T. Renal handling of drugs in renal failure. I. Differential effects of uranyl nitrate- and glycerol-induced acute renal failure on renal excretion of TEAB and PAH in rats. J Pharmacol Exp Ther 1988;246:896–901.
20. Gloff CA, Benet LZ. Differential effects of the degree of renal damage on *p*-aminohippuric acid and inulin clearances in rats. J Pharmacokinet Biopharm 1989;17:169–177.
21. Bosch JP. Renal reserve. A functional view of glomerular filtration rate. Semin Nephrol 1995;15:381–385.
22. Levey AS. Assessing the effectiveness of therapy to prevent the progression of renal disease. Am J Kidney Dis 1993;22:207–214.
23. Glassock RJ, Cohen AH, Adler SG. Primary glomerular disease. In: Brenner BM, Rector FC, eds. The Kidney, 5th ed. Philadelphia, W.B. Saunders, 1996:1392–1497.
24. Rose BD, Renneke HG. Renal Pathophysiology—The Essentials. Baltimore, Williams & Wilkins, 1994.
25. Kasiske BL, Keane WF. Laboratory assessment of renal disease: Clearance, urinalysis, and renal biopsy. In: Brenner BM, Rector FC, eds. The Kidney, 5th ed. Philadelphia: W.B. Saunders, 1996:1137–1173.
26. Bauer JH, Brooks CS, Burch RN. Clinical appraisal of creatinine clearance as a measurement of glomerular filtration rate. Am J Kidney Dis 1982;2:337–346.
27. Levey AS. Measurement of renal function in chronic renal disease. Kidney Int 1990;38:167–184.
28. Green AJE, Halloran SP, Mould GP, et al. Interference by newer cephalosporins in current methods for measuring creatinine. Clin Chem 1990;36:2139–2140.
29. Massoomi F, Matthews HG III, Destache CJ. Effect of seven fluoroquinolones on the determination of serum creatinine by the picric acid and enzymatic methods. Ann Pharmacother 1993;27: 586–588.
30. Young DS, ed. Effects of Drugs on Clinical Laboratory Tests, 4th ed. Washington, DC, AACC Press, 1995:3.190–3.211.
31. Apple FS, Benson P, Abraham PA, et al. Assessment of renal function by inulin clearance: Comparison with creatinine clearance as determined by enzymatic methods. Clin Chem 1989;35:312–314.
32. Van den Berg, Koopman MG, Arisz L. Ranitidine has no influence on tubular creatinine secretion. Nephron 1996;74:705–708.
33. Mayersohn M, Conrad KA, Achari R. The influence of a cooked meat meal on creatinine plasma concentration and creatinine clearance. Br J Clin Pharmacol 1983;15:227–230.
34. Statland BE, Winkel P, Bokelund H. Factors contributing to intra-individual variation of serum constituents: 2. Effects of exercise and diet on variation of serum constituents in healthy subjects. Clin Chem 1973;19:1380–1383.
35. Mirahmadi MK, Byrne C, Barton C, et al. Prediction of creatinine clearance from serum creatinine in spinal cord injury patients. Paraplegia 1983;21:23–29.
36. Pasternack A, Kuhlbäck B. Diurnal variations of serum and urine creatine and creatinine. Scand J Clin Lab Invest 1971;27:1–7.
37. Bingham SA, Murphy J, Waller E, et al. Para-amino benzoic acid in the assessment of completeness of 24-hour urine collections from hospital outpatients and the effect of impaired renal function. Eur J Clin Nutr 1992;46:131–135.
38. Fuller NJ, Elia M. Factors influencing the production of creatinine: Implications for the determination and interpretation of urinary creatine and creatinine in man. Clin Chim Acta 1988;175:199.
39. Goldstein DE, Little RR. Monitoring glycemia in diabetes. Short-term assessment. Endocrinol Metab Clin North Am 1997;26:475–486.
40. Pugia MJ, Lott JA, Clark LW, et al. Comparison of urine dipsticks with quantitative methods for microalbuminuria. Eur J Clin Chem Clin Biochem 1997;35:693–700.
41. Steinhäuslin F, Wauters J-P. Quantitation of proteinuria in kidney transplant patients: Accuracy of the urinary protein/creatinine ratio. Clin Nephrol 1995;43:110–115.
42. Anderson S. Proteinuria. In: Greenberg A, ed. Primer on Kidney Diseases, 2nd ed. San Diego, Academic Press, 1998:42–46.
43. Kashtan CE. Hematuria. In: Greenberg A, ed. Primer on Kidney Diseases, 2nd ed. San Diego, Academic Press, 1998:36–41.
44. Karlsen FM, Holstein-Rathlou N-H, Leyssac PP. A re-evaluation of the determinants of glomerular filtration rate. Acta Physiol Scand 1995;155:335–350.
45. Garwood S, Hines RL. Renal function monitoring. Int Anesthesiol Clin 1996;34:175–94.
46. Brndle E, Sieberth HG, Hautman RE. Effect of chronic dietary protein intake on the renal function in healthy subjects. Eur J Clin Nutr 1996;50:734–740.
47. Brenner BM, Lawler EV, Mackenzie HS. The hyperfiltration theory: A paradigm shift in nephrology. Kidney Int 1996;49:1774–1777.
48. Woods LL. Intrarenal mechanisms of renal reserve. Semin Nephrol 1995;15:386–395.
49. Dworkin LD, Brenner BM. The renal circulations. In: Brenner BM, Rector FC, eds. The Kidney, 5th ed. Philadelphia, W.B. Saunders, 1996:247–285.
50. Prescott LF, Freestone S, McAuslane JAN. The concentration-dependent disposition of intravenous *p*-aminohippurate in subjects with normal and impaired renal function. Br J Clin Pharmacol 1993; 35:20–29.
51. Taylor A, Manatunga A, Morton K, et al. Multicenter trial validation of a camera-based method to measure Tc-99m mercaptoacetyltriglycine, or Tc-99m MAG_3, clearance. Radiology 1997;204:47–54.

52. Russell CD, Dubovsky EV. Comparison of single-injection multi-sample renal clearance methods with and without urine collection. J Nucl Med 1995;36:603–606.
53. Florijn KW, Barendregt JNM, Lentjes EGWM, et al. Glomerular filtration rate measurement by "single-shot" injection of inulin. Kidney Int 1994;46:252–259.
54. Degenaar CP, Frenken LAM, van Hoof JP. Enzymatic method for determination of inulin. Clin Chem 1987;33:1070–1071.
55. Soper CPR, Bending MR, Barron JL. An automated enzymatic inulin assay, capable of full sinistrin hydrolysis. Eur J Clin Chem Clim Biochem 1995;33:497–501.
56. Dall'Amico R, Montini G, Pisanello L, et al. Determination of inulin in plasma and urine by reverse-phase high-performance liquid chromatography. J Chromatogr B Biomed Appl 1995;672:155–159.
57. Buclin T, Pechère-Bertschi A, Séchaud R, et al. Sinistrin clearance for determination of glomerular filtration rate: A reappraisal of various approaches using a new analytical method. J Clin Pharmacol 1997;37:679–692.
58. Ruiz R, Cordova MA, Sierra M, et al. Automated sinistrin measurement. Clin Biochem 1997;30:501–504.
59. Prueksaritanont T, Lui CY, Lee MG, et al. Renal and non-renal clearances of iothalamate. Biopharm Drug Disp 1986;7:347–355.
60. Dowling TC, Frye RF, Zemaitis MA. Simultaneous determination of P-aminohippuric acid, acetyl-*p*-aminohippuric acid and lothalamate in human plasma and urine by high-performance liquid chromatography. J Chromatogr B 1998;716(1–2):305–313.
61. Gaspari F, Masconi L, Vigano G, et al. Measurement of GFR with a single intravenous injection of nonradioactive iothalamate. Kidney Int 1992;41:1081–1084.
62. Isaka Y, Fujiwara Y, Yamamoto S, et al. Modified plasma clearance technique using nonradioactive iothalamate for measuring GFR. Kidney Int 1992;42:1006–1011.
63. Nilsson-Ehle P, Grubb A. New markers for the determination of GFR: Iohexol clearance and cystatin C serum concentration. Kidney Int 1994;46(suppl 47):S17–S19.
64. Frennby B, Sterner G, Almén, et al. The use of iohexol clearance to determine GFR in patients with severe chronic renal failure—a comparison between different clearance techniquees. Clin Nephrol 1995; 43:35–46.
65. Brown SCW, O'Reilly PH. Iohexol clearance for the determination of glomerular filtration rate in clinical practice: Evidence for a new gold standard. J Urol 1991;146:675–679.
66. Rocco MV, Buckalew VM Jr, Moore LC, Shihabi ZK. Measurement of glomerular filtration rate using nonradioactive iohexol: Comparison of two one-compartment models. Am J Nephrol 1996;16:138–143.
67. Lundqvist S, Hietala S-O, Groth S, Sjdin J-G. Evaluation of single sample clearance calculations in 903 patients. A comparison of multiple and single sample techniques. Acta Radiol 1997;38:68–72.
68. Hricak H, White SS. Radiologic assessment of the kidney. In Brenner BM, Rector FC, eds. The Kidney, 5th ed. Philadelphia: W.B. Saunders, 1996:1175–1199.
69. Taylor A. Radionuclide evaluation of renal function. Crit Rev Diagn Imaging 1991;32:1–36.
70. Morton K, Pisani DE, Whiting JH Jr, et al. Determination of glomerular filtration rate using technitium-99m-DTPA with differing degrees of renal function. J Nucl Med Technol 1997;25:110–114.
71. Perrone RD, Steinman TI, Beck GJ, et al. Utility of radioisotopic filtration markers in chronic renal insufficiency: Simultaneous comparison of ^{125}I-iothalamate, ^{169}Yb-DTPA, ^{99m}Tc-DTPA, and inulin. Am J Kidney Dis 1990;16:224–235.
72. Rabito CA, Panico F, Rubin R, et al. Noninvasive, real-time monitoring of renal function during critical care. J Am Soc Nephrol 1994; 4:1421–1428.
73. Frennby B, Almn T, Lilja B, et al. Determination of the relative glomerular filtration rate of each kidney in man. Acta Radiol 1995; 36:410–417.
74. Lemann J, Bidani AK, Bain RP, et al. Use of the serum creatinine to estimate glomerular filtration rate in health and early diabetic nephropathy. Am J Kidney Dis 1990;16:236–243.
75. Cockroft, DW, Gault MH. Prediction of creatinine clearance from serum creatinine. Nephron 1976;16:31–41.
76. Shemesh O, Golbetz H, Kriss JP, et al. Limitations of creatinine as a filtration marker in glomerulopathic patients. Kidney Int 1985; 28:830–838.
77. Roubenoff R, Drew H, Moyer M, et al. Oral cimetidine improves the accuracy and precision of creatinine clearance in lupus nephritis. Ann Intern Med 1990;113:501–506.
78. Zaltzman JS, Whiteside C, Cattran D, et al. Accurate measurement of impaired glomerular filtration using single-dose oral cimetidine. Am J Kidney Dis 1996;27:504–511.
79. Hilbrands LB, Artz MA, Wetzels JFM, et al. Cimetidine improves the reliability of creatinine as a marker of glomerular filtration. Kidney Int 1991;40:1171–1176.
80. Van Acker BAC, Koomen GCM, Koopman MG, et al. Creatinine clearance during cimetidine administration for measurement of glomerular filtration rate. Lancet 1992;340:1326–1329.
81. Luke DR, Halstenson CE, Opsahl JA, et al. Validity of creatinine clearance estimates in the assessment of renal function. Clin Pharmacol Ther 1990;48:503–508.
82. Mawer CE, Knowles BR, Lucas SB, et al. Computer-assisted prescribing of kanamycin for patients with renal insufficiency. Lancet 1972;1:12–15.
83. Jelliffe RW. Estimation of creatinine clearance when urine cannot be collected. Lancet 1971;1:975–976.
84. Jelliffe RW. Creatinine clearance: Bedside estimate. Ann Intern Med 1973;79:604–605.
85. Hull JH, Hak LJ, Koch GC, et al. Influence of range of renal function and liver disease on predictability of creatinine clearance. Clin Pharmacol Ther 1981;29:516–521.
86. Gault MH, Longerich LL, Harnett JD, et al. Predicting glomerular function from adjusted serum creatinine. Nephron 1992;62:249–256.
87. Ixkes MCJ, Koopman MG, van Acker BAC, et al. Cimetidine improves GFR-estimation by the Cockcroft–Gault formula. Clin Nephrol 1997;47:229–236.
88. Echizen H, Ishizaki T. Superiority of disease-specific over conventional formula in predicting creatinine clearance from serum creatinine in patients with liver cirrhosis. Ther Drug Monit 1988;10: 369–375.
89. Caregaro L, Menon F, Angeli P, et al. Limitations of serum creatinine level and creatinine clearance as filtration markers in cirrhosis. Arch Intern Med 1994;154:201–205.
90. DeSanto NG, Anastasio P, Loguercio C, et al. Creatinine clearance: An inadequate marker of renal filtration in patients with early posthepatitic cirrhosis (Child A) without fluid retention and muscle wasting. Nephron 1995;70:421–424.
91. Davis GA, Chandler MHH. Comparison of creatinine clearance estimation methods in patients with trauma. Am J Health Syst Pharm 1996;53:1028–1032.
92. Thakur V, Reisin E, Solomonow M, et al. Accuracy of formula-derived creatinine clearance in paraplegic subjects. Clin Nephrol 1997;47:237–242.
93. Goerdt PJ, Heim-Duthoy KL, Macres M, Swan SK. Predictive performance of renal function equations in renal allografts. Br J Clin Pharmacol 1997;44:261–265.
94. Schuck O, Teplan V, Vítko S, et al. Predicting glomerular function from adjusted serum creatinine in renal transplant patients. Int J Clin Pharmacol Ther 1997;35:33–37.
95. Huang E, Hewitt R, Shelton M, Morse GD. Comparison of measured and estimated creatinine clearance in patients with advanced HIV disease. Pharmcotherapy 1996;16:222–229.
96. Quadri KHM, Bernardini J, Greenberg A, et al. Assessment of renal function during pregnancy using a random urine protein to creatinine

ratio and Cockcroft–Gault formula. Am J Kidney Dis 1994;24:416–420.

97. Jeliffe RW, Jeliffe SM. A computer program for estimation of creatinine clearance from unstable serum creatinine concentration. Math Biosci 1972;14:17–24.
98. Chiou WL, Hsu FH. A new simple rapid method to monitor renal function based on pharmacokinetic considerations of endogenous creatinine. Res Commun Chem Pathol Pharmacol 1975;10:15.
99. Brater DC. Drug Use in Renal Disease. Balgowlah, Australia, ADIS Health Science Press, 1983:22–56.
100. Newman DJ, Thakkar H, Edwards RG, et al. Serum cystatin C measured by automated immunoassay: A more sensitive marker of changes in GFR than serum creatinine. Kidney Int 1995;47:312–318.
101. van den Anker, de Groot R, Broerse HM, et al. Assessment of glomerular filtration rate in preterm infants by serum creatinine: Comparison with inulin clearance. Pediatrics 1995;96:1156–1158.
102. Sertel H, Scopes J. Rates of creatinine clearance in babies less than one week of age. Arch Dis Child 1973;48:717–720.
103. Arant BS Jr. Developmental patterns of renal functional maturation compared in the human neonate. J Pediatr 1978;92:705–712.
104. Clark PMR, Bryant TN, Hal MA, et al. Neonatal renal function assessment. Arch Dis Child 1989;64:1264–1269.
105. Bajaj G, Alexander SR, Browne R, et al. ^{125}Iodine-iothalamate clearance in children. A simple method to measure glomerular filtration. Pediatr Nephrol 1996;10:25–28.
106. Schwartz GJ, Brion LP, Spitzer A. The use of plasma creatinine concentration for estimating glomerular filtration rate in infants, children, and adolescents. Pediatr Clin North Am 1987;34:571–590.
107. Al-Harbi N, Lireman D. Comparison of three different methods of estimating the glomerular filtration rate in children after renal transplantation. Am J Nephrol 1997;17:68–71.
108. Fong J, Johnston S, Valentino T, Notterman D. Length/serum creatinine ratio does not predict measured creatinine clearance in critically ill children. Clin Pharmacol Ther 1995;58:192–197.
109. Lindeman RD. Assessment of renal function in the old. Clin Lab Med 1993;13:269–277.
110. Lindeman RD, Tobin J, Shrock NW. Longitudinal studies on the rate of decline in renal function with age. J Am Geriatr Soc 1985;33:278–281.
111. Smythe M, Hoffman J, Kizy K, et al. Estimating creatinine clearance in elderly patients with low serum creatinine concentrations. Am J Hosp Pharm 1994;51:198–204.
112. O'Connell MB, Wong MO, Bannick-Mohrland SD, et al. Accuracy of 2- and 8-hour urine collections for measuring creatinine clearance in the hospitalized elderly. Pharmacotherapy 1993;13:135–142.
113. Porush JG. Hypertension and chronic renal failure: The use of ACE inhibitors. Am J Kidney Dis 1998;31:177–184.
114. Mackenzie HS, Brenner BM. Current strategies for retarding progression of renal disease. Am J Kidney Dis 1998;31:161–170.
115. DCCT Research Group. The effect of intensive treatment on the development and progression of long-term complications in insulin-dependent diabetes mellitus. N Engl J Med 1993;329:977–986.
116. Rossing P, Astrup A-S, Smidt UM, et al. Monitoring kidney function in diabetic nephropathy. Diabetologia 1994;37:708–712.
117. Mogensen CE, Hansen KW, Nielson S, et al. Monitoring diabetic nephropathy: Glomerular filtration rate and abnormal albuminuria in diabetic renal disease—reproducibility, progression, and efficacy of antihyptensive intervention. Am J Kidney Dis 1993;22:174–187.
118. Valensi P, Assayag M, Busby M, et al. Microalbuminuria in obese patients with or without hypertension. Int J Obes Relat Metab Disord 1996;20:574–579.
119. Halimi J-M, Ribstein J, Du Cailar G, et al. Albuminuria predicts renal functional outcome after intervention in atheromatous renovascular disease. J Hypertens 1995;13:1335–1342.
120. Berrut G, Bouhanick B, Fabbri P, et al. Microalbuminuria as a predictor of a drop in glomerular filtration rate in subjects with non-insulin-dependent diabetes mellitus and hypertension. Clin Nephrol 1997;48:92–97.
121. Bennett PH, Haffner S, Kasiske BL, et al. Screening and management of microalbuminuria in patients with diabetes mellitus: Recommendations to the scientific advisory board of the National Kidney Foundation from an ad hoc committee of the council on diabetes mellitus of the National Kidney Foundation. Am J Kidney Dis 1995;25:107–112.
122. Mimran A, Ribstein J, DuCailar G. Is microalbuminuria a marker of early intrarenal vascular dysfunction in essential hypertensin? Hypertension 1994;23:1018–1021.
123. Striker G. Report on a workshop to develop management recommendations for the prevention of progression in chronic renal disease. J Am Soc Nephrol 1995;5:1537–1540.
124. Taylor A, Nally JV. Clinical applications of renal scintigraphy. AJR 1995;164:31–41.
125. Mindell HJ, Fairbank JT. Renal imaging techniques. In: Greenberg A, ed. Primer on Kidney Diseases, 2nd ed. San Diego, Academic Press, 1998:47–53.
126. Flynn FV. Assessment of renal function: Selected developments. Clin Biochem 1990;23:49–54.
127. Schentag JJ, Plaut ME. Patterns of urinary β_2-microglobulin excretion by patients treated with aminoglycosides. Kidney Int 1980;17:654–661.
128. Gloff CA, Benet LZ. Differential effects of the degree of renal damage on *p*-aminohippuric acid and inulin clearances in rats. J Pharmacokinet Biopharm 1989;17:169–177.
129. Nassseri K, Daley-Yates PT. A comparison of *N*-1-methylnicotinamide clearance with 5 other markers of renal function in models of acute and chronic renal failure. Toxicol Lett 1990;53:243–245.
130. Edwards BD, Maiza A, Daley-Yates PT, et al. Altered clearance of *N*-1-methylnicotinamide associated with the use of low doses of cyclosporine. Am J Kidney Dis 1994;23:23–30.
131. Maiza A, Daley-Yates PT. Estimation of the renal clearance of drugs using endogenous *N*-1-methylnicotinamide. Toxicol Lett 1990;53:231–235.
132. Jung K. Urinary enzymes and low molecular weight proteins as markers of tubular dysfunction. Kidney Int 1994;46(suppl 47):S29–S33.
133. Ayatse JOI, Kwan JTC. Relative sensitivity of serum and urinary retinol binding protein and alpha-1 microglobulin in the assessment of renal function. Ann Clin Biochem 1991;28:514–516.
134. Verplanke AJW, Heber RFM, de Wit R, et al. Comparison of renal function parameters in the assessment of cis-platin induced nephrotoxicity. Nephron 1994;66:267–272.
135. Jung K, Diego J, Strobelt V, et al. Diagnostic significance of some urinary enzymes for detecting acute rejection crises in renal transplant recipients: Alanine aminopeptidase, alkaline phosphatase, gamma-glutamyl transferase, *N*-acetyl-beta-glucosaminidase, and lysozyme. Clin Chem 1986;32:1807–1811.
136. Thompson RE, Piper DJ, Galberg C, et al. Adenosine deaminase binding protein, a new diagnostic marker for kidney disease. Clin Chem 1985;31:679–683.

41
ACUTE RENAL FAILURE

Bruce A. Mueller, PharmD, FCCP, BCPS, and William L. Macias, MD, PhD

Acute renal failure is an abrupt decline in renal function characterized by the inability of the kidney to excrete metabolic waste products (nitrogenous wastes and water) and maintain acid–base balance. An elevation of the nitrogenous waste products (creatinine and urea nitrogen) is referred to as azotemia. Uremia, characterized by anorexia, nausea, vomiting, and mental status changes, is the clinical syndrome resulting from azotemia. Acute renal failure is not well defined with regard to the presence of uremic symptoms and/or changes in urea nitrogen; therefore, most clinical diagnoses are based on an elevation in the serum creatinine concentration.[1] An increase of the serum creatinine concentration of 0.5 mg/dL (when the baseline creatinine is < 3.0 mg/dL) or an increase of 1.0 mg/dL (when the baseline is ≥ 3.0 mg/dL) is one of the most commonly used definitions of acute renal failure.[2]

The use of the serum creatinine concentration to define end-stage renal disease (ESRD), although appropriate in chronic renal disease, may by itself be inadequate to define renal function in a significant number of individuals who develop acute renal failure. This inadequacy results from the finding that a large percentage of patients who develop acute renal failure are critically ill and highly catabolic. Consequently, these patients frequently accumulate noncreatinine waste products (e.g., urea nitrogen and water) out of proportion to the increase in serum creatinine. Therefore, the diagnosis of acute renal failure in critically ill patients should be made whenever the kidneys are unable to maintain acceptable control of body fluid volume, acid–base balance, and the levels of nitrogenous waste products (blood urea nitrogen [BUN]), regardless of whether the serum creatinine concentration has risen significantly. This broadened definition provides a more realistic estimate of patient outcome, anticipation of potential complications, and an increased awareness of the need for early intervention with renal replacement therapy.

EPIDEMIOLOGY

The development of acute renal failure is primarily a phenomenon of hospitalized patients, with the diagnosis appearing in their discharge or death summaries and not in their admitting history.[3] Community-acquired acute renal failure is relatively infrequent, occurring in only 1% of hospital admissions.[4] Prerenal azotemia (as a result of intravascular volume depletion) or postrenal obstruction (as a result of prostatic disease) are the most common causes of community-acquired acute renal failure. Intrinsic renal damage, although less common than pre- and postrenal causes of acute renal failure, is frequently related to infection or medications in patients presenting with acute renal failure. Most patients with community-acquired acute renal failure have a treatable cause of renal failure and their prognosis, although dependent on underlying medical conditions, is generally favorable.[1]

The incidence of hospital-acquired acute renal failure ranges between 2% and 5% of hospitalized patients, but it is difficult to quantify because of the lack of agreement on the definition of acute renal failure. The etiologies of acute renal failure in these patients can be separated by the type of patient developing renal failure. For medical/surgical patients on the general hospital ward, the etiology of acute renal failure is frequently prerenal (intravascular volume depletion or congestive heart failure) and less often related to renal injury (medications or radiocontrast agents).[5] For patients in the intensive care unit (ICU), the etiology of acute renal failure is almost always related to multiple insults to the kidney occurring as a consequence of multiple organ failure.[6,7] Risk factors for the development of acute renal failure in the intensive care unit include sepsis, bleeding, volume depletion, chronic liver disease, mechanical ventilation, and surgery.[6] The incidence of acute renal failure acquired in an ICU ranges between 6% and 23%.[1]

The prognosis for patients developing hospital-acquired acute renal failure can best be estimated by dividing the patient population into those who develop acute renal failure not requiring renal replacement therapy, those who develop acute renal failure requiring renal replacement therapy, and those who develop acute renal failure as a result of multiple organ failure (ICU-acquired acute renal failure). Patients who develop acute renal failure and do not require renal replacement therapy have the most favorable prognosis (Table 41–1). This is because they have recovered renal function, which frequently heralds recovery from the underlying medical condition. Hospitalized patients who develop acute renal failure and require renal replacement therapy have a less favorable outcome. Multiple investigators have attempted to identify those clinical and demographic factors associated with survival.[8–12] Although these analyses have been somewhat complex, certain useful trends in predicting outcome have been documented. The mortality rate of patients with acute renal failure who require renal replacement therapy and who have no other major organ system failure ranges from 10% to 25%.[13,14] As the number of failed organ systems increases, so does the

TABLE 41–1. Incidence and Outcomes of ARF Relative to Where ARF Occurs

	Community Acquired	Hospital Acquired	ICU Acquired
Incidence	Low (< 1%)	Moderate (2%–5%)	High (6%–23%)
Cause	Single	Single or multiple	Multifactorial
Overall survival rate	70%–95%	30%–50%	10%–30%
Worsened outcome if:	RRT required Poor preadmission health Other failed organ systems	RRT required Poor preadmission health Ischemic ARF cause Other failed organ systems	Intrinsic renal disease Ischemic ARF cause Septic RRT required Poor preadmission health Other failed organ systems
Better outcome if:	Nonoliguric	Nonoliguric Nephrotoxic ARF cause	Prerenal cause Postrenal cause Nonoliguric Nephrotoxic cause

RRT = renal replacement therapy.

mortality rate such that for patients with multiple organ failure (≥ 3 failed organ systems) the mortality rate exceeds 80%.[8]

The survival rates for hospitalized patients developing acute renal failure have not changed substantially during the past 2 decades. However, recent advances in our understanding of the role of nutritional support,[15] earlier intervention with renal replacement therapy, choice of renal replacement therapy (continuous versus intermittent),[16] and possibly choice of hemodialysis membrane[17] may eventually improve the dismal outcome for these patients.

ETIOLOGY

The classification of acute renal failure into broad categories based on the precipitating factors facilitates the diagnosis and management of patients presenting with this disorder (Table 41–2). Traditionally, the causes of acute renal failure have been categorized into prerenal azotemia (resulting from decreased renal perfusion), acute intrinsic renal failure (resulting from structural damage to the kidney), and postrenal obstruction (resulting from the obstruction of urine flow from the kidney out of the body). The addition of the category "functional acute renal failure" aids in the understanding of the pathophysiology of acute renal failure. This category is the result of hemodynamic changes at the level of the glomerulus without decreased perfusion of the kidney or structural damage to it.

PRERENAL AZOTEMIA

Prerenal acute renal failure results from hypoperfusion of the renal parenchyma, with or without systemic arterial hypotension.[18] Renal hypoperfusion with systemic arterial hypotension may be caused by a decline in intravascular volume (e.g., hemorrhage, dehydration) or a decline in effective blood volume (i.e., the blood volume perceived by the arterial baroreceptors). Examples of disease states in which there is a decline in effective blood volume without a decrease in intravascular volume include congestive heart failure and liver failure. Because the kidney is undamaged, at least early on, the urinalysis will be normal. Eventually, the fractional excretion of sodium will be low, reflecting an increase in the concentrations of the sodium retentive hormones; renin, angiotensin, and aldosterone. Urinary solute will be concentrated as a result of the increased circulating levels of antidiuretic hormone, which is released in response to the diminished arterial blood pressure.

Renal hypoperfusion without systemic hypotension most commonly results from bilateral renal artery occlusion, or unilateral occlusion in a patient with a single functioning kidney. In these conditions, the sodium retentive hormones are activated by the decline in renal parenchymal perfusion. However, systemic arterial blood pressure is usually elevated, leading to an inhibition of antidiuretic hormone release. Consequently, the urinary indices will reflect enhanced sodium reabsorption (a low fractional excretion of sodium), but the urinary solute may not be maximally concentrated.

FUNCTIONAL ACUTE RENAL FAILURE

Functional acute renal failure refers to those entities that result in a decline in glomerular ultrafiltrate production secondary to a reduced glomerular hydrostatic pressure without damage to the kidney itself. The decline in glomerular hydrostatic pressure is a direct consequence of changes in glomerular afferent (vasoconstriction) and efferent (vasodilation) arteriolar circumference (Fig. 41–1). These clinical conditions most commonly occur in individuals who have reduced effective blood volume (e.g., congestive heart failure, cirrhosis, severe pulmonary disease, hypoalbuminemia), or renovascular disease (e.g., renal artery stenosis) and cannot compensate for changes in afferent or efferent arteriolar tone. Examples of disorders that result in afferent arteriolar vasoconstriction (and an increase in afferent arteriolar resistance) include hypercalcemia and the administration of certain medications (e.g., cyclosporine and nonsteroidal anti-inflammatory drugs [NSAIDs]). A decrease in

TABLE 41–2. Classification of Acute Renal Failure

Category	Classification of Acute Renal Failure	Differential Diagnosis
Prerenal renal failure	With hypotension	Intravascular volume depletion Dehydration Hemorrhage
	Without hypotension	Bilateral renal artery stenosis (unilateral renal artery stenosis in solitary kidney) Emboli Cholesterol Thrombotic
Functional acute renal failure		Medications Cyclosporine ACE inhibitors NSAIDs Hypercalcemia Hepatorenal syndrome
Acute intrinsic renal failure	Vascular	Vasculitis Polyarteritis nodosa Hemolytic uremic syndrome Emboli Cholesterol Thrombotic
	Glomerular	Systemic lupus erythematosus Poststreptococcal glomerulonephritis Antiglomerular basement membrane disease
	Acute tubular necrosis	Ischemic Hypotension Vasoconstriction Exogenous toxins Contrast dye Heavy metals Drugs (amphotericin B, aminoglycosides) Endogenous toxins Myoglobin Hemoglobin
	Acute interstitial nephritis	Drugs Penicillins Ciprofloxacin Sulfonamides Infection Streptococcal
Postrenal renal failure (obstruction)	Bladder outlet obstruction	Prostatic hypertrophy Improperly placed bladder catheter
	Ureteral (bilateral or unilateral with solitary functioning kidney)	Cervical cancer Retroperitoneal fibrosis
	Renal pelvis or tubules	Crystal deposition Oxalate Sulfonamides Tumor lysis syndrome

efferent arteriolar resistance usually results from the administration of an angiotensin-converting enzyme inhibitor. With correction of the underlying pathologic process or discontinuation of the responsible medication, renal function rapidly returns to baseline. The hepatorenal syndrome is included in this classification scheme since the kidney itself is not damaged and there is intense afferent arteriolar vasoconstriction, possibly mediated by endothelin,[19] leading to a decline in glomerular filtration. In all these conditions, the urinalysis is not different from its baseline state and the urinary indices suggest prerenal azotemia. The urinary solute concentration may be variable depending on circulating levels of antidiuretic hormone.

This syndrome of functional acute renal failure is very common in individuals with congestive heart failure who receive an angiotensin-converting enzyme inhibitor in an attempt to improve left ventricular function. Although the improvement in left ventricular function resulting from the angiotensin-converting enzyme inhibitor may take weeks to be clinically significant,[20] the decline in efferent arteriolar resistance resulting from the inhibition of angiotensin II occurs rapidly.[21] Therefore, if the dose of the angiotensin-

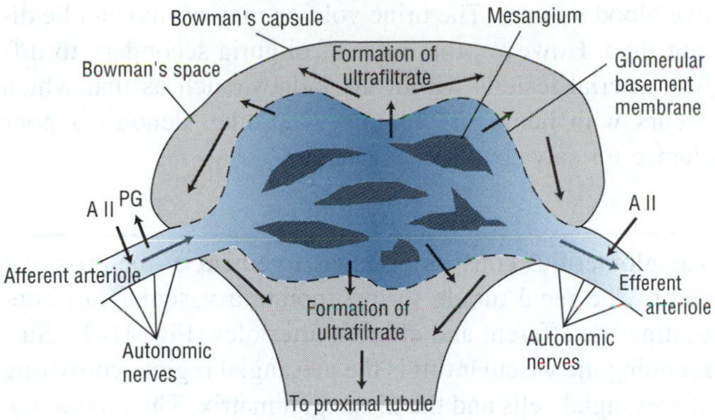

FIGURE 41–1. The formation of glomerular ultrafiltrate is dependent on the surface area of the glomerular capillaries, their permeability, and the net hydrostatic pressure across the capillary wall. As the glomerular capillary surface area increases, secondary to mesangial cell relaxation, the formation of glomerular ultrafiltrate is increased. An increase or decrease in glomerular hydrostatic pressure results in either an increase or decrease in glomerular ultrafiltrate production. Afferent arteriolar vasoconstriction (which is primarily mediated by angiotensin II) or vasodilation (which is primarily mediated by prostaglandins) can result in a decrease or increase, respectively, in hydrostatic pressure across the capillary. Efferent arteriolar vasoconstriction (which is primarily mediated by angiotensin II) results in an increase in glomerular hydrostatic pressure. Under conditions in which renal blood flow is diminished, the kidney maintains glomerular ultrafiltration by vasodilating the afferent and vasoconstricting the efferent arterioles. Medications that may interfere with these processes might result in an abrupt decline in glomerular filtration.

converting enzyme inhibitor is increased too rapidly, there will be a decline in glomerular ultrafiltrate production with a concomitant rise in the serum creatinine, leading to functional acute renal failure. If the increase in the serum creatinine is not too severe (usually < 1 mg/dL), the medication can be continued. Renal function should gradually improve as renal parenchymal perfusion pressure increases with improvement in left ventricular function.

ACUTE INTRINSIC RENAL FAILURE

Acute intrinsic renal failure results from damage to the kidney itself. Conceptually, acute intrinsic renal failure can best be organized by the structures within the kidney: the small blood vessels, glomeruli, renal tubules, and interstitium. Renal failure secondary to small vessel vasculitis (e.g., polyarteritis nodosa, hemolytic uremic syndrome, malignant hypertension) or cholesterol emboli can present with a relatively normal urinary sediment since the glomerulus and tubules, at least initially, are not damaged. When renal failure results from a small-vessel vasculitis, the vasculitic process is rarely confined to the kidney. A careful search for diagnostic clues suggesting other organ system involvement usually provides evidence of the diffuse nature of these disease processes (see Clinical Presentation, below).

Acute glomerular inflammation (acute glomerulonephritis) can result from a variety of precipitating causes (systemic lupus erythematosus, antiglomerular basement membrane disease). In these disorders, the urinalysis usually reveals the presence of heavy proteinuria (> 3 g urinary protein per 24-hour collection period) and hemoglobinuria. Microscopic analysis of the urinary sediment frequently shows numerous red blood cells and red blood cell casts, the latter being considered diagnostic for glomerulonephritis. In the early stages of the illness, the fractional excretion of sodium is less than 1 because tubular function is still intact. However, as renal failure becomes more established, the fractional excretion of sodium may increase.

The renal tubules are susceptible to a variety of insults. The tubules contained within the medulla of the kidney are particularly at risk from ischemic injury as this portion of the kidney is very metabolically active and, thereby, has a high oxygen requirement. Severe hypotension or the administration of vasoconstricting drugs preferentially affects the tubules more than any other portion of the kidney.[22] In addition, exogenous toxic substances (contrast agents, heavy metals, pharmacologic agents such as aminoglycosides, amphotericin B, foscarnet) and endogenous toxins (myoglobin, hemoglobin, uric acid) may cause tubular injury. Regardless of the etiology, tubular injury leads to a loss of urine concentrating ability, defective distal sodium reabsorption, and a reduction in the glomerular filtration rate (GFR). The etiology of acute intrinsic renal failure secondary to tubular injury (referred to as acute tubular necrosis) is usually discernible by reviewing the patient's history and medication list. The urinalysis suggests tubular injury by the presence of coarse "dirty brown" casts. Red blood cells and red blood cell casts are only rarely seen. The urinary indices suggest intrinsic renal dysfunction (i.e., high fractional excretion of sodium, isosthenuria [urine osmolality equal to plasma osmolality], and a low urine creatinine/serum creatinine ratio).

The interstitium of the kidney is also susceptible to injury from a variety of causes. Although acute interstitial nephritis is most commonly caused by medications (see Chap. 45), infections (e.g., streptococcal, Leptospirosis, Hantavirus, HIV infections) also may produce a similar syndrome. The presence of white blood cells, white blood cell casts, and coarse granular casts in the urine all suggest interstitial inflammation. The presence of eosinophilia and eosinophiluria also strongly suggest the presence of an interstitial nephritis. Interestingly, acute interstitial nephritis resulting from the administration of NSAIDs is not associated with eosinophilia and eosinophiluria. This clinical syndrome is frequently accompanied by an acute glomerulonephritis. As a consequence, the urinalysis has characteristics of both acute interstitial nephritis (white blood cells, white blood cell casts) and an acute glomerulonephritis (proteinuria, red blood cells, red blood cell casts).

POSTRENAL OBSTRUCTION

Acute renal failure resulting from obstruction may occur at any level within the urinary system from renal tubule to urethra. However, to cause acute renal failure, the obstructing process must involve both kidneys or one kidney in a patient with a single functioning kidney. Bladder outlet obstruction is the most common cause of obstructive uropathy. Crystal deposition within the tubules (e.g., secondary to uric acid, acyclovir, sulfonamide, or oxalate) and ureteral obstruction (e.g., secondary to shed renal papilla or calculi) are infrequent causes of obstructive acute renal failure. The onset of acute anuria, in the absence of a catastrophic event, should suggest acute urinary tract obstruction. However, the development of acute renal failure in a hospitalized patient admitted with normal renal function is rarely secondary to obstruction unless an indwelling urinary catheter has been misplaced. When the obstructing process (e.g., prostatic hypertrophy, cervical cancer) is gradual and incomplete, the patient may present with complaints of a decreased force of the urinary stream and polyuria.

PATHOPHYSIOLOGY

A basic knowledge of renal function facilitates the understanding of how acute renal failure manifests itself clinically. The most logical approach to understanding renal function is to divide the kidney into its four basic component parts: the vasculature, the glomeruli, the tubules, and the interstitium surrounding the other three component parts.

RENAL VASCULATURE

Blood flows to each kidney via a main renal artery, which divides in two just prior to entering the renal parenchyma. These two main branches divide into approximately five segmental branches, each of which is the sole provider of blood flow to its respective section. Consequently, arterial occlusion at the level of the segmental branch will result in complete ischemia of that portion of the kidney. In the setting of renal artery occlusion, the creatinine may or may not rise, depending on the number of segmental arteries involved. If only a few segmental arteries are occluded, the serum creatinine will remain unchanged and the urinalysis will be normal. With significant renal infarction, the urinalysis will show hematuria and proteinuria, and the urine indices will show an inability to concentrate urinary solutes.

Each segmental renal artery divides into a series of smaller arteries leading to the afferent arterioles of the glomeruli. Lesions at this level of the arterial tree (e.g., cholesterol emboli, vasculitic lesions, platelet plugs) will present as isolated decreased perfusion of the glomeruli. The serum creatinine frequently is increased, because the lesions are usually diffuse. However, the urinalysis most commonly will be normal, because the kidney itself is not ischemic and the glomeruli are not involved. The urinary indices suggest prerenal azotemia (i.e., a low urine sodium concentration and a low fractional excretion of sodium) in the absence of systemic hypotension or a decrease in effective blood volume. The urine volume may or may not be diminished. However, the onset of oliguria secondary to diffuse arterial lesions within the kidney, such as that which occurs with hemolytic uremic syndrome, denotes a poor chance for salvage of renal function.

GLOMERULUS

The glomerulus consists of an enlargement of the proximal end of the renal tubule to incorporate a vascular tuft connecting the afferent and efferent arterioles (Fig. 41–1). Surrounding the vascular tuft is the mesangial region, consisting of mesangial cells and the mesangial matrix. The production of glomerular ultrafiltrate is predominantly dependent on the transcapillary hydrostatic pressure (dictated by the afferent and efferent arteriolar resistance) and the glomerular surface area (primarily governed by the contraction and relaxation of mesangial cells that open and close glomerular capillaries). Afferent arteriolar tone is determined predominantly by the local levels of angiotensin II (which induces vasoconstriction) and prostaglandins (which induce vasodilation). Efferent arteriolar tone is predominantly determined by the local concentration of angiotensin II.

Pathophysiologic processes and medications (i.e., systemic hypotension, hypercalcemia, angiotensin-converting enzyme inhibitors, and NSAIDs) that result in alterations of the afferent and efferent arteriolar tone reduce glomerular ultrafiltrate production as a result of a decrease in glomerular hydrostatic pressure. Under these conditions, the serum creatinine will rise, the urine sediment will be normal, and the urine indices will suggest prerenal azotemia. However, the urinary solutes may or may not be maximally concentrated depending on the circulating level of antidiuretic hormone necessary to maximally concentrate the urine. Damage to the glomerular capillary tuft (e.g., acute glomerulonephritis) results in a decline in the glomerular ultrafiltrate production as a result of a decrease in glomerular capillary surface area. Under these conditions the serum creatinine rises. The urinalysis is significant for hematuria and proteinuria because of the increased permeability of the damaged glomerular capillaries. Red cell casts are found often and are considered diagnostic of glomerular capillary injury. The urine indices may suggest prerenal azotemia because the renal tubules are intact. The urinary solutes may or may not be maximally concentrated.

RENAL TUBULES

Under normal conditions, approximately 180 L of glomerular ultrafiltrate are produced per day, the vast majority of which must be reabsorbed by the renal tubules to maintain homeostasis. Clinically, the renal tubule can be divided into three major sections: the proximal tubule, Henle's loop, and the distal nephron, which includes the distal tubule, the cortical collecting tubule, and the medullary collecting ducts. In the proximal tubule, approximately 60% to 70% of the filtered load of water and solute is isovolemically reabsorbed as well as the vast majority of filtered amino acids, glucose, and bicarbonate. Isolated injury to the proximal tubule (as occurs with heavy metal poisoning or paraproteinemia) results in significant aminoaciduria, glucosuria, and bicarbonaturia. The serum creatinine may rise because of intratubular obstruction, damage to the tubular epithelial cells, or the back-leak of glomerular ultrafiltrate across the renal tubule.

In addition to its other functions, Henle's loop is responsible for a significant portion of the total reabsorption of potassium, calcium, and magnesium as well as for generating the osmotic gradient within the kidney necessary for the concentration of urinary solutes. Damage to this portion of the nephron results in wasting of potassium and magnesium by the kidney and an inability of the kidney to concentrate the urine. The medullary portions of Henle's loop are very sensitive to ischemia secondary to hypoperfusion. Consequently, in severe prerenal azotemia with renal hypoperfusion, there may be a loss of urinary concentrating ability despite the continued presence of a low urinary sodium concentration and a low fractional excretion of sodium.

Major functions of the distal nephron include the regeneration of bicarbonate, the excretion of acid (hydrogen ion), the secretion of potassium, and the reabsorption of water. Damage to this portion of the nephron may present as significant acidemia and either hypo- or hyperkalemia, depending on the mechanism of injury. For example, amphotericin B produces small pores in the lumenal membrane of distal tubular cells. These pores allow small molecules such as potassium to leak out; the molecules are then wasted in the urine. Consequently, amphotericin B nephrotoxicity is characterized by hypokalemia secondary to renal potassium wasting. Hyperkalemia may occur if the damage to the distal nephron is severe enough to cause oliguria or if the damage disrupts the renin–aldosterone axis. Defects in urine concentrating ability also are frequent. In addition to the previously mentioned findings, acute tubular necrosis as a cause of acute renal failure is associated with a urinary sediment characterized by the presence of tubular cells, coarse granular casts, and, rarely, red blood cell casts.

INTERSTITIUM

The interstitium of the kidney provides the structural support for the kidney and serves to provide the environment in which concentrating gradients can be established. In addition, the interstitium of the kidney plays a major role in urinary ammonia handling. To facilitate the regeneration of bicarbonate and the excretion of acid by the distal nephron, the kidney utilizes ammonia as a urinary buffer. When the interstitium of the kidney is damaged (e.g., in acute allergic interstitial nephritis), the concentrating gradient within the kidney may be dissipated and ammonia handling disrupted. Consequently, patients presenting with acute interstitial nephritis frequently are not able to concentrate the urinary solute. They also may have a metabolic acidosis with hyperkalemia, the degree of which is out of proportion to the rise in serum creatinine. The urinalysis may show mild proteinuria and hematuria. However, the striking finding on microscopic examination of the sediment is the presence of numerous white blood cells and white blood cell casts.

CLINICAL PRESENTATION

Rapid determination of the etiology of acute renal failure is essential. Nearly 90% of patients presenting to the hospital with community-acquired acute renal failure have a potentially reversible cause.[23] The most common cause of acute renal failure in hospitalized patients is prerenal azotemia, which may be attenuated with prompt treatment of the renal hypoperfusion. A delayed diagnosis of the acute renal failure etiology may result in a more severe nephrologic injury.

HISTORY

The diagnostic approach to the patient with acute renal failure differs depending on the clinical setting in which the kidneys fail. For patients who present to the outpatient clinic or hospital with an elevated serum creatinine, the first objective is to determine if the renal failure is acute or chronic. A past medical history of renal disease, previous laboratory data documenting the presence of proteinuria or an elevated serum creatinine, and the finding of bilateral small kidneys on renal ultrasonography all suggest the presence of chronic renal failure. The finding of an elevated parathyroid hormone concentration or evidence of renal osteodystrophy on radiographic bone survey also suggests chronicity.

For patients who do not have the above findings, their renal failure should be considered acute until proven otherwise. In these individuals, a careful review of their recent medications, including over-the-counter medications and vitamins, is mandatory. The patient's recent history can usually provide an indication of when the onset of renal dysfunction began. Frequently, patients may notice a change in their voiding habits with an increase in urinary frequency or nocturia, both suggesting a urinary concentrating defect. A decrease in the force of the urinary stream may suggest an obstructive process. The presence of cola-colored urine, indicating the presence of blood in the urine, is common in acute glomerulonephritis. If the accompanying proteinuria is severe, the patient may note excessive foaming of the urine in the toilet. The onset of bilateral flank pain may suggest swelling of the kidneys secondary to either acute glomerulonephritis or acute interstitial nephritis. The onset of severe headaches may suggest the development of hypertension as a result of acute renal failure. A recent increase in the patient's weight secondary to salt and water retention also may be helpful in defining the onset of renal failure.

For patients who develop acute renal failure while hospitalized, a review of the laboratory data is usually sufficient to define the onset of acute renal failure. However, significant renal injury can occur prior to an increase in the serum creatinine. Consequently, clinicians must pay careful attention to subtle changes in the patient's weight, blood pressure, and urine output if they are to diagnose the onset of acute renal failure. Urine output is one of the easiest parameters to measure and is one of the most useful. In the absence of obstruction, urine output directly correlates with GFR in patients with acute renal failure.[24] Changes in urine output may be helpful in diagnosing the type of renal dysfunction present. Acute anuria (< 50 mL urine production/24 hours) is secondary either to complete urinary obstruction or to a catastrophic event (shock, hemolytic uremic syndrome, acute cortical necrosis). Oli-

TABLE 41–3. Physical Examination Findings in Acute Renal Failure

Physical Examination Finding	Clinical Implication If Present	Possible Diagnoses	Category of Acute Renal Failure	Possible Confounding Factors
Vital signs				
Orthostatic hypotension	Intravascular volume status	Volume depletion	Prerenal azotemia	Antihypertensive therapy Neuropathies (diabetes mellitus)
Skin				
Tenting	Volume status	Volume depletion	Prerenal azotemia	Advanced age
Rash	Allergic reaction	Hypersensitivity reaction	Acute interstitial nephritis	Contact dermatitis
Petechiae	Platelet dysfunction	Thrombotic thrombocytopenic purpura Hemolytic uremic syndrome Sepsis	Acute intrinsic renal failure—vasculitis	Bone marrow suppression Antiplatelet drugs
Splinter hemorrhages Janeway lesions Osler's nodes	Embolic phenomenon	Endocarditis	Acute intrinsic renal failure—acute glomerulonephritis	Small vessel vasculitis
Edema	Volume status	Total body volume overload	Suggests prerenal azotemia unlikely	Right heart failure, deep venous thrombosis
HEENT				
Hollenhorst plaque	Embolic phenomenon	Cholesterol emboli	Acute intrinsic renal failure—vascular	Plaque must be in aorta to affect kidney
Roth spots	Embolic phenomenon	Endocarditis	Acute intrinsic renal failure—acute glomerulonephritis	Other systemic infection
Heart				
S_3 heart sound	Left ventricular function	Congestive heart failure	Prerenal azotemia	Preexisting compensated congestive heart failure
New murmur (particularly diastolic murmurs)	Valvular function	Endocarditis	Acute intrinsic renal failure—acute glomerulonephritis	Preexisting valvular disease Hyperdynamic state
Lung				
Rales	Pulmonary congestion	Pulmonary edema with volume overload or left ventricular dysfunction	Prerenal azotemia	Compensated CHF
Abdomen				
Renal artery bruit	Arterial integrity	Renal artery stenosis	Prerenal azotemia	Generalized atherosclerosis
Ascites	Elevated venous pressure	Liver failure or right heart failure	Prerenal azotemia Hepatorenal syndrome	Peritoneal membrane disorder (tumor)
Bladder distention	Bladder capacity	Bladder outlet obstruction	Postobstruction renal failure	
GU				
Prostatic enlargement	Prostate size	Prostatic hypertrophy or cancer	Postobstruction renal failure	Nonenlarged prostate does not exclude obstruction
GYN				
Abnormal bimanual examination	Uterine size Cervical status	Possible bilateral ureteral obstruction or cervical cancer	Postobstruction renal failure	

A variety of physical examination findings may be found in patients with acute renal failure. The first column lists the physical finding, whereas the second column is the clinical implications if these abnormal findings are present. Columns 3 and 4 list the possible diagnoses and category of acute renal failure that is likely to be present. Possible confounding factors that could also explain the physical examination findings are listed in the final column.

guria (≤ 400 mL urine production/24 hours) suggests either prerenal azotemia, functional acute renal failure, or acute intrinsic renal failure. Nonoliguric renal failure (> 400 mL urine production/24 hours) usually results from acute intrinsic renal failure or incomplete urinary obstruction. As with outpatients who present with acute renal failure, a careful review of the administered medications is also mandatory for individuals who develop acute renal failure while hospitalized.

PHYSICAL EXAMINATION AND URINALYSIS

A physical examination, including assessment of the patient's volume and hemodynamic status, is the next step in evaluating individuals with acute renal failure. Common physical findings in patients with acute renal failure are listed in Table 41–3. The urinalysis is an extremely important component of the physical examination when the clinician is attempting to classify the cause of renal failure into prerenal azotemia, functional acute renal failure, acute intrinsic renal failure, or obstruction. The finding of a high urinary specific gravity, in the absence of glucosuria or mannitol administration, suggests an intact urinary concentrating mechanism and the likely cause as prerenal azotemia or functional acute renal failure. The presence of proteinuria and hematuria indicates glomerular injury. Glucosuria, aminoaciduria, and phosphaturia are associated with acute proximal tubular dysfunction. As noted earlier, the microscopic examination of the urine also is helpful in determining the cause of acute renal failure. A benign urine sediment suggests either prerenal azotemia, functional acute renal failure, or urinary obstruction. The presence of red blood cells and red blood cell casts indicates a glomerular injury. The finding of white blood cells and white blood cell casts results from interstitial inflammation (interstitial nephritis), which can be secondary to an allergic, granulomatous, or infectious process.

LABORATORY DATA

Simultaneous measurement of serum and urinary chemistries is often helpful in determining the etiology of acute renal failure (Table 41–4). Calculation of the fractional excretion of sodium from urinary and serum creatinine and sodium concentrations can yield important information about the patient with acute renal failure. The equation for the calculation of the fractional excretion of sodium is:

$$FE_{Na} = (\text{excreted Na}/\text{filtered Na}) \cdot 100$$
$$= (U_{vol} \cdot U_{Na})/(GFR \cdot S_{Na}) \cdot 100$$

where

$$GFR = U_{vol} \cdot U_{cr}/S_{cr} \cdot \text{time}$$

Thus:

$$FE_{Na} = U_{Na} \cdot S_{cr} \cdot 100/U_{cr} \cdot S_{Na}$$

where U_{vol} = urine volume, U_{cr} = urine creatinine, U_{Na} = urine sodium, S_{cr} = serum creatinine, S_{Na} = serum sodium, GFR = glomerular filtration rate, and time = the time period over which the urine is collected.

The fractional excretion of sodium has clinical utility in differentiating prerenal azotemia and functional acute renal failure from acute intrinsic renal failure. A low urinary sodium concentration and low fractional excretion of sodium (< 1%) in a patient with oliguria suggest that there is stimulation of the sodium retentive mechanisms in the kidney and that tubular function is intact. These findings are most characteristic of prerenal azotemia or functional acute renal failure. Similarly, a fractional excretion of sodium exceeding 1% to 2% suggests acute intrinsic renal failure. However, there are a number of causes of acute intrinsic renal failure (contrast nephropathy, myoglobinuria, interstitial nephritis) that are, at least early on, associated with a low fractional excretion of sodium. Diuretic use can limit the diagnostic utility of the fractional excretion of sodium calculation by increasing natriuresis even in hypovolemic patients.

A finding of a highly concentrated urine (> 500 mOsm/L) suggests stimulation of antidiuretic hormone, indicating prerenal azotemia secondary to either hypovolemia or a decrease in effective blood volume. Under these conditions, the urine creatinine to serum creatinine ratio usually exceeds 40. On occasion, some patients may develop an extremely high blood urea nitrogen concentration while the serum creatinine remains only mildly elevated. In these instances, measurement of the urinary urea nitrogen will allow the clinician to determine if the elevated blood urea nitrogen concentration is secondary to the underexcretion of urea nitrogen or the overproduction of urea nitrogen. A critically ill patient will produce approximately 18 to 19 g of urea nitrogen per day. Excretion of a urinary urea nitrogen load substantially less than that suggests

TABLE 41–4. Diagnostic Parameters for Differentiating Causes of Acute Renal Failure

Laboratory Test	Prerenal Azotemia	Acute Intrinsic Renal Failure	Postrenal Obstruction
Urine sediment	Normal	Casts, cellular debris	Cellular debris
Urinary RBC	None	2–4+	Variable
Urinary WBC	None	2–4+	1+
Urine sodium	< 20	> 40	> 40
FE_{Na} (%)	< 1	> 1–2	Variable
Urine/serum osmolality	> 1.5	< 1.3	< 1.5
Urine/serum creatinine	> 40:1	< 20:1	< 20:1
BUN/S_{cr}	> 20	15	15

Common laboratory tests are used to classify the cause of acute renal failure. Functional acute renal failure, which is not included in this table, would have laboratory values similar to those seen in prerenal azotemia. However, the urine osmolality to plasma osmolality ratios may not exceed 1.5 depending on the circulating levels of antidiuretic hormone. The laboratory results listed under acute intrinsic renal failure are those seen in acute tubular necrosis, the most common cause of acute intrinsic renal failure.

acute renal failure. Excretion of substantially more than that suggests overproduction of urea as the cause for the increased blood urea nitrogen concentration, as might occur with gastrointestinal tract bleeding or excessive protein administration.

DIAGNOSTIC PROCEDURES

Although frequently ordered by physicians, a renal ultrasound is rarely helpful in determining the cause of acute renal failure in a hospitalized patient who previously had normal renal function. Insertion of an urinary catheter into the patient's bladder is usually adequate to exclude postrenal obstruction as the cause of acute renal failure. However, for the outpatient who presents with renal failure, the renal ultrasound is instrumental in determining whether the renal failure is acute or chronic and whether or not obstruction is present. A plain film radiograph of the abdomen may be useful in documenting the presence of two kidneys and in checking for renal stones. If the possibility of renal artery obstruction exists, a radioisotope scan or renal angiography may be required. Intravenous pyelography is rarely used in the diagnostic workup of acute renal failure. Cystoscopy with retrograde pyelography may be helpful if the possibility of obstruction exists. This last procedure may be necessary in a patient with the history of a single functioning kidney even if the ultrasound does not demonstrate hydronephrosis. If, despite a careful history, physical examination, and the above-mentioned diagnostic tests, the etiology of the acute renal failure is unclear, a percutaneous renal biopsy may be indicated. When renal biopsies are performed to determine the cause of acute renal failure, the majority of cases demonstrate acute tubular necrosis.

CLINICAL COURSE AND PROGNOSIS

The clinical course and prognosis for patients with acute renal failure depends on a number of clinical variables including: (1) the definition of acute renal failure employed; (2) the etiology of acute renal failure; (3) the presence or absence of oliguria; (4) the patient's nutritional status; (5) the presence of comorbidities; and (6) whether the patient requires renal replacement therapy. The clinical course of acute tubular necrosis can be divided into three distinct phases; an oliguric, diuretic, and recovery phase. The utility of this approach is questionable because recovery from acute tubular necrosis does not begin at a defined time from onset of renal failure. Rather, recovery from acute tubular necrosis occurs 10 to 14 days after the last insult to the kidney. Critically ill patients with acute renal failure often have recurring episodes of hypoxia and hypotension and are treated with many nephrotoxins, which may delay the recovery process.[25] Furthermore, the autoregulation of renal blood flow is deranged in acute renal failure.[26] Renal vasoconstriction results in continued reduced blood flow to the nephron even after the insult to the kidneys is removed and the tubules begin recovering from the acute injury.[27] Actual improvements in glomerular filtration rate will not be manifested until tubular cell necrosis is repaired and renal blood flow is normalized.[26]

Patients who have a mild increase in their serum creatinine concentration have an excellent renal prognosis. Their eventual outcome is almost entirely dependent on their associated illnesses[13] and procedures performed on them (e.g., cardiac catheterization). Retrospective analyses suggest that patients with mildly increased serum creatinine concentrations have increased mortality rates compared to those patients who do not have an increase in their creatinine during their hospitalization. However, it is unclear whether this is a cause-and-effect phenomenon or a selection bias.

The etiology of acute renal failure has a major influence on the eventual patient outcome. Hospitalized patients who develop acute renal failure secondary to obstruction (e.g., an improperly placed urinary catheter) have rapid recovery of renal function following relief of the obstruction. Patients with prerenal azotemia resulting from renal hypoperfusion also have rapid recovery of function following an improvement in perfusion pressure. Individuals who develop functional acute renal failure recover renal function once the effects of the offending agents resolve. In each of these three clinical conditions, the patient's prognosis is largely dependent on comorbid conditions. However, for patients developing intrinsic renal failure, the disruption in their internal milieu and the associated systemic effects of their uremia may have impact on their associated illnesses such that their acute renal failure may adversely influence their outcome.[28]

The presence or absence of oliguria has been suggested to be an independent predictor of eventual patient outcome. In multiple reports of mortality in acute renal failure, individuals with nonoliguria have significantly higher survival rates than individuals who develop oliguria or anuria.[29,30] A portion of this improved outcome may relate to selection bias, in that patients developing nonoliguric renal failure frequently have more-reversible renal insults such as obstruction or prerenal azotemia. However, the continued ability of the kidney to control volume homeostasis, even in the absence of solute control, may delay the need for renal replacement therapy and its associated risks.

Individuals who require renal replacement therapy for their acute renal failure have a more complicated clinical course and higher associated mortality rates than patients who do not require therapy. In these patients, the use of renal replacement therapy may delay the recovery of renal function,[31] activate endogenous inflammatory mediators that may promote catabolism and enhance organ injury,[17] and expose the patient to the risks related to the renal replacement therapy itself.

▶ TREATMENT: Acute Renal Failure

DESIRED OUTCOME

The treatment goals for patients with acute renal failure are driven by the cause of renal failure. In some cases, goals are more supportive in nature. In other cases, very rapid treatment decisions can change the course of the disease. A difficulty in treating these patients is quantifying their ever-changing renal function (see Chap. 40). The desired outcomes for patients with acute renal failure are to survive the insult that damaged their kidneys and to regain life-sustaining renal function.

GENERAL APPROACH TO TREATMENT

The treatment approach to the patient with acute renal failure is dependent on when, in relation to the course of acute renal failure, the patient is seen. In the case of evolving acute renal failure, efforts must be aimed at preventing further damage to the kidneys. As soon as the acute renal failure etiology is identified, the offending agent or cause must be quickly removed or reversed to minimize the damage to the kidney.[32] In the case of acute tubular necrosis, this "resuscitation" therapy is essential, particularly in the trauma or postsurgery setting, where aggressive ventilation and volume resuscitation can "rescue" hypoxic tubular cells, circumventing acute tubular necrosis. Drug-induced nephrotoxicity often can be reversed if the nephrotoxin is removed. The same is true for acute renal failure that develops secondary to renal artery disease. If detected and corrected early, renal function may return.

In the setting of established acute renal failure, the therapeutic priority becomes more supportive in nature. Often the patient with established acute renal failure is critically ill. Therefore, supportive treatment is needed to prevent further insult to the kidney. This is not always possible because the use of potentially nephrotoxic agents, like aminoglycosides, may be necessary for the patient to survive the current situation. Generally, the patient with acute renal failure does not have isolated acute renal failure, but rather acute renal failure secondary to other disease states. Consequently, these conditions must be treated aggressively, and, if necessary, the patient is supported with renal replacement therapy until renal function returns. Because the prognosis for established acute renal failure in the ICU setting is grim, early diagnosis of the cause of acute renal failure is the highest priority.

PREVENTIVE THERAPY

The treatment of established acute renal failure differs from the prevention of acute renal failure and will be discussed later in this chapter. Because the presence of acute renal failure significantly increases the mortality of hospitalized patients,[33] efforts should be focused on prevention in patients at risk for acute renal failure. One example of this strategy is the patient who requires pharmacotherapy with a known nephrotoxin or needs to undergo a potentially nephrotoxic procedure. For instance, retrospective studies have reported the characteristics of patients who are more likely to develop acute renal failure following the administration of intravenous contrast dye,[34] amphotericin B,[35] or aminoglycosides.[36] Those patients at higher risk tend to be the elderly, those with preexisting kidney or liver disease, those with diabetes mellitus, and those receiving concomitant nephrotoxins (see Chap. 45).

USING LESS-NEPHROTOXIC AGENTS

Armed with the knowledge of who is at risk for acute renal failure development, the clinician should choose the least nephrotoxic therapeutic alternative for these patients. Examples of this approach include using β-lactam antibiotics in place of aminoglycosides, fluconazole or lipid-based amphotericin B in place of the conventional amphotericin B formulation, and the substitution of low-osmolality contrast media instead of more toxic higher osmolality dyes. Alternatively, changing the methods used to administer the doses of nephrotoxins may minimize the risk of acute renal failure. Intra-arterial cisplatin has been administered during hemodialysis in patients without renal failure in an attempt to minimize cisplatin nephrotoxicity.[37] Once-daily aminoglycoside therapy has been reported to reduce the rate of nephrotoxicity compared to conventional thrice-daily dosing.[38] Meta-analysis of this question has found that once-daily dosing either is less nephrotoxic[39] or at least is not more nephrotoxic than conventional dosing.[40,41] Hospital-wide computer systems are now available that warn health care providers of nephrotoxic therapies in patients with rising serum creatinine concentrations. When these are in place, significant reductions in serious renal impairment have been observed.[42] It appears that vigilance in avoiding nephrotoxins may result in improved patient outcomes.

Frequently the acquisition cost of less nephrotoxic agents is considerably higher than conventional therapy. Examples of less nephrotoxic but more expensive alternatives include the use of lipid-based amphotericin B instead of conventional amphotericin B ($200 to $480/d versus $10/d) and low-osmolar intravenous contrast dyes instead of older, more nephrotoxic dyes (15 times greater than conventional dye). In both of these examples, the drug acquisition cost of the less nephrotoxic agent is considerably higher. Clearly, not all patients receiving these types of therapies will need the more expensive agent, because many are not at high risk for the development of nephrotoxicity. Thus, many institutions have developed guidelines for the use of low-osmolality contrast media in selecting the patient populations using risk–benefit analysis.[43] Most of these centers have found that they can reduce the overall cost of contrast media without significantly increasing their nephrotoxicity rates by reserving the more expensive therapies strictly for high-risk patients.[44,45]

Similarly, lipid-based amphotericin B formulations may cause less nephrotoxicity than the conventional agent, but they probably are not needed in all patients.[46] It may be that a "homemade" liposomal agent may work as well at a fraction of the cost.[47] The key to pharmacoeconomic analysis is to determine which patients are at highest risk for developing nephrotoxicity and reserving the more expensive agents for these patients. In selected cases, use of a more expensive, but less nephrotoxic agent may reduce overall costs by avoiding the cost of renal failure.

HYDRATION

In the situation where a nephrotoxic agent must be administered, renal-protective therapies may be used to attenuate the nephrotoxic risk. The simplest but most effective technique is simply to ensure that the patient is not volume contracted prior to nephrotoxin administration. Volume expansion allows optimal renal perfusion and reduces tubular workload because the kidney does not need to vigorously concentrate the urine. This reduction in tubular stress during nephrotoxin exposure may reduce the tubule's susceptibility to damage, but this has not been conclusively demonstrated.[18]

Volume administration prior to nephrotoxin exposure will also increase urine output, thereby helping to flush toxins from the kidney. This facet of volume administration is important in the treatment of cancer patients. Tumor lysis syndrome results from the administration of cancer chemotherapeutic agents that destroy large numbers of cells. The intracellular contents of the lysed cells are released into the blood stream, where many of them, including uric acid, are eliminated by the kidneys. The amount of uric acid present in the urine may exceed the solubility of uric acid, resulting in crystal formation in the tubules that may cause obstructive nephropathy. Attenuation or prevention of tumor lysis syndrome and uric acid crystal formation can be accomplished with vigorous hydration and urine alkalinization prior to cancer chemotherapy administration. Alkalinization is necessary in this regimen because the water solubility of uric acid is pH dependent. The goal of alkalinization in this case is to maintain a urinary pH of greater than 6. The amount of administered sodium bicarbonate in the intravenous solution is adjusted to meet the urinary pH goal. High urinary output is also desirable to dilute and eliminate the uric acid from the kidneys. This is accomplished by hydrating prior to chemotherapy administration until serum uric acid concentrations normalize. A typical hydration regimen to prevent uric acid crystallization is normal saline 1.5 to 3 $L/m^2/24$ h in a patient with normal renal function. Therapy should begin 24 to 48 hours before the administration of chemotherapy.[48] When therapy will end depends on the chemotherapy regimen and tumor burden and is guided by close monitoring of the patient's serum uric acid concentrations.

Typically, the solution used to hydrate prior to nephrotoxin exposure is normal saline, because the goal of this treatment is to expand the intravascular compartment and increase renal perfusion. Solutions like 5% dextrose are inappropriate for this purpose, because they distribute throughout the body. The rate of volume administration for the prevention of nephrotoxin-induced acute renal failure is usually 1 to 2 mL/kg/h started 3 to 6 hours before the nephrotoxin is administered. Urine output is the best indicator as to whether sufficient volume is being given and adequate hydration status has been attained. The desired urine output is usually 2 mL/kg/h. A common approach is to administer 2 L of saline prior to contrast dye administration.[49] Generally, these vigorous hydration regimens are continued for a few hours after the dye is given to help flush it out of the kidneys.

SODIUM LOADING

The use of normal saline as the volume expansion agent may yield an added benefit because of its sodium content. A technique frequently employed to mitigate the nephrotoxicity of contrast dye or amphotericin B is to "sodium load" a patient prior to giving the nephrotoxin. Sodium loading may reduce renal damage via the tubuloglomerular feedback mechanism. This regulatory mechanism for GFR is initiated when the tubule senses high urine flow or an increased delivery of sodium chloride and results in a decrease in renal blood flow, GFR, and tubular flow.[18] These actions may minimize the delivery of a nephrotoxin to the tubule and thus reduce the risk of tubular injury. Sodium depletion decreases this vasoconstrictor response whereas sodium loading enhances the vasoconstriction. Sodium loading may be helpful in attenuating amphotericin B nephrotoxicity by reducing delivery of the drug to the tubules. Dietary sodium liberalization has been shown to improve renal function during amphotericin B therapy in a small case series of patients who had already developed nephrotoxicity.[50]

Sodium loading with intravenous fluids prior to nephrotoxin administration has also shown clinical benefit. Llanos et al.[51] prospectively evaluated sodium loading in a randomized placebo-controlled trial. Prior to amphotericin B administration (50 mg three times/week for 10 weeks), one group of patients received 1 L of 5% dextrose and the other group received 1 L of 0.9% saline. The dextrose group had a significant increase in serum creatinine and a decrease in creatinine clearance compared to the saline-treated group. The results of animal studies, case reports in humans, and the findings by Llanos et al. have led some to call for sodium loading (150 mEq sodium/day) prior to amphotericin B administration as the standard of care.[52]

DRUG THERAPY FOR THE PREVENTION OF NEPHROTOXICITY

Sodium loading and vigorous hydration are simple interventions and appear to be effective in attenuating the effects of many nephrotoxins (see Table 41–5). Prevention of nephrotoxicity via pharmacotherapy has resulted in less than impressive outcomes. Studies with diuretics were a natural follow-up to the studies showing the benefits of sodium and volume pretreatment. In theory, the beneficial effects of diuretic therapy should include some of the benefits seen with hydration therapy as well as some additional benefits. Tubular obstruction from cellular debris is often associated with vasoconstriction and a reduced glomerular filtration rate, which may exacerbate acute renal failure. Diuretics increase tubule fluid flow and, therefore, may prevent tubular obstruction. Loop diuretics increase renal blood flow via their vasodilating effects, which may be beneficial in the prevention of acute renal failure. Furosemide also may be useful in preventing acute renal failure by its inhibition of the tubuloglomerular feedback mechanism. This reflex may be harmful in acute renal failure because reductions in glomerular filtration rate may worsen tubular damage. Mannitol, an osmotic diuretic, also may have some utility in preventing acute renal failure. Mannitol theoretically may reduce tubular cell damage by acting as an impermeable solvent that reduces cell swelling. While these espoused theoretical benefits of diuretic therapy appear reasonable, actual

TABLE 41–5. Evidence of Benefit for Prophylactic Therapies Aimed at Preventing Acute Renal Failure Prior to Nephrotoxin Exposure

Intervention	Evidence for Prevention of Nephrotoxicity	Situations Where Intervention Documented to Be Effective
Hydration (sodium loading)	Yes	Prior to amphotericin or contrast dye administration, tumor lysis syndrome prevention
Mannitol	No	
Loop diuretics	No	
Dopamine	No	
Calcium channel blockers	Equivocal	Prior to transplantation, recipient should receive drug, and when kidney is stored in solution containing drug Not useful for preventing contrast dye nephropathy
Pentoxifylline	No	
Theophylline	Yes	Prior to contrast dye administration
Misoprostil	No	
Atrial natriuretic peptide	No	

documentation of their value in controlled studies is nearly nonexistent.

One of these trials compared the effectiveness of diuretic and/or saline pretreatment in the prevention of nephrotoxicity of contrast dye.[53] This prospective trial was conducted in patients with chronic renal insufficiency who were considered to be at high risk for developing contrast dye nephropathy. These authors compared hydration with 1 mL/kg/h of 0.45% saline to the same hydration plus either mannitol 25 g or furosemide 80 mg. All subjects received the saline infusion for 12 hours before and after angiography. The mean increase in serum creatinine 48 hours after the dye exposure was significantly higher in the diuretic groups than in the subjects who received hydration alone. Similar results with diuretics given prior to nephrotoxins have been reported in many studies over the past few decades,[54] but a mechanism to fully explain these findings has yet to be elucidated. Diuretics do not have a beneficial effect in this setting and they should be avoided in these high-risk situations.

Similarly disappointing results have been reported with other pharmacotherapeutic drug classes.[55] Calcium channel blockers were thought possibly to play a role in preventing the development of acute renal failure because they inhibit the vasoconstrictive response of the afferent arterioles of the kidney to vasoconstrictive agonists. A subsequent increase in glomerular filtration is noted because the efferent arterioles are relatively resistant to the vasodilating effects of the calcium antagonists. Indeed, calcium channel blockers showed potential as a pretreatment for contrast dye,[56] but later studies have not confirmed this.[57]

More recent trials with other drug classes have shown promise. Theophylline has been used as a pretreatment for contrast dye. Investigators suggest that the adenosine antagonist activity of theophylline is responsible for its nephroprotective effect. The role of theophylline in preventing contrast dye nephropathy has been investigated in a randomized trial.[58] Inulin and creatinine clearances before and after contrast dye administration were unchanged in subjects receiving theophylline (5 mg/kg) prior to the dye infusion whereas clearances declined significantly in the subjects receiving placebo.[58] Similarly, Katholi et al.[59] found that oral theophylline (2.88 mg/kg every 12 hours), given prior to dye infusion, resulted in a much smaller decrement in creatinine clearance than when an oral placebo was given. The protective effect of theophylline was seen when either high-osmolality or low-osmolality dye was administered.

Other drugs have been investigated for efficacy in preventing kidney damage. Some, like pentoxifylline[60] and misoprostil,[61] have been given concurrently with a known nephrotoxin, such as maintenance cyclosporine. Unfortunately, these trials showed no beneficial effect of these therapies. Given the poor prognosis of hospital-acquired acute renal failure, prevention is key. Further studies need to clarify the role of pharmacologic preventive therapy. Until effective preventive drug therapy is found, it appears that adequate hydration with saline is the most appropriate therapy.

PHARMACOTHERAPY OF ESTABLISHED ACUTE RENAL FAILURE

In patients with established acute renal failure, the goals of therapy are to remove the primary cause of the acute renal failure, limit further nephrotoxic exposures/events, and speed up the recovery of renal function. Unfortunately, studies to date have shown that little can be done with contemporary therapy to hasten renal recovery (Table 41–6). Consequently, therapeutic measures are more supportive in nature. The first goal is to limit future nephrotoxic events until the kidney can recover on its own. Second, efforts must be aimed toward reducing the sequelae that are associated with acute renal failure itself, mainly volume, electrolyte, and azotemic control. These therapy goals are accomplished primarily by pharmacologic and renal replacement therapies (Fig. 41–2).

TABLE 41–6. Evidence for Benefit of Therapies for the Treatment of Established Acute Renal Failure

Intervention	Improved Renal Function	Improved Azotemia	Improved Mortality
Mannitol	No	Equivocal	Unknown
Loop diuretics	No	No	No
Dopamine	Equivocal	Equivocal	No
Calcium channel blockers	Equivocal	Equivocal	No
Atrial natriuretic peptide	Equivocal	Equivocal	No
Intensive dialysis	Unknown	No	No
Early dialysis	Unknown	Yes	Yes
Biocompatible hemodialyzer	Unknown	Yes	Yes
Parenteral essential amino acids	Unknown	Equivocal	Equivocal

From Ref. 54.

VOLUME CONTROL

Probably the most important patient parameter in acute renal failure is a knowledge of the patient's volume status. In the patient with oliguric prerenal azotemia, rapid fluid resuscitation can improve renal perfusion and rescue hypoxic tubules, preventing or ameliorating acute tubular necrosis. However, this same maneuver in a patient with established oliguric acute tubular necrosis would be harmful, resulting in a fluid-overloaded patient. Fluid removal from the volume-overloaded patient needs to measured in terms of net volume loss rather than simply urine output. If the volume given to the patient exceeds urine output, volume overload will worsen despite meeting urine output goals. Sources of excess exogenous fluids that can be minimized in fluid-overloaded patients include reducing the volume of fluid used to administer intravenous medications, reassessing the need for and rate of "keep-open" intravenous solutions, and using concentrated sources of enteral and parenteral feedings. Maintenance of euvolemia, tissue perfusion, and electrolyte balance should be the goals of this supportive therapy.

DIURETICS

Nonoliguric acute renal failure has a significantly better prognosis than oliguric acute renal failure.[30] It is unclear whether patients with nonoliguric acute renal failure have less extensive damage to their kidneys than their oliguric counterparts or if something is intrinsically therapeutic about having increased urine flow. It is important to remember that the finding of an improved survival with nonoliguria compared to oliguria does not necessarily mean that increasing the urine output to nonoliguria levels with diuretics will improve the oliguric patient's eventual outcome. Nonetheless, diuretics can simplify fluid management in acute renal failure patients and are a mainstay of therapy.[62]

In addition to their diuretic effect, many diuretics have other pharmacologic effects that might be beneficial for the patient with acute renal failure. Tubular obstruction from cellular debris is often associated with vasoconstriction and a reduced

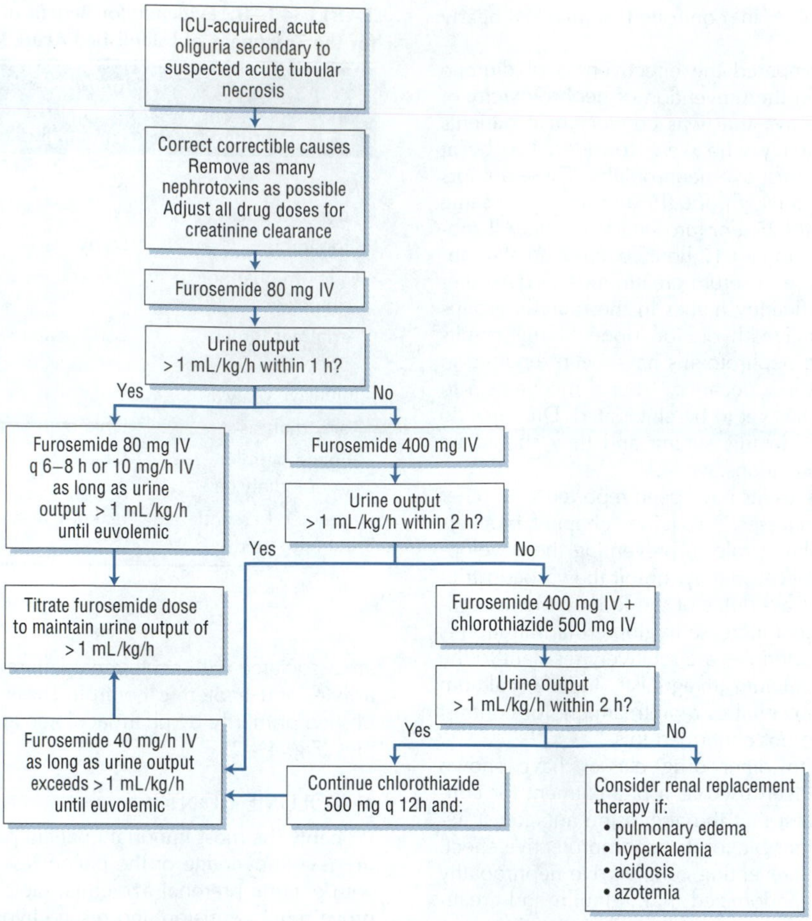

FIGURE 41–2. Treatment algorithm for ICU-acquired acute oliguria secondary to acute tubular necrosis.

GFR, which may exacerbate acute renal failure.[26] Diuretics increase tubule fluid flow and, therefore, may prevent tubular obstruction. Loop diuretics increase renal blood flow via their vasodilating effects, which may be beneficial in the prevention of acute renal failure, although clinical studies have not demonstrated this. Mannitol, an osmotic diuretic, also may have some utility in preventing acute renal failure. Mannitol theoretically may reduce tubular cell damage by acting as an impermeable solvent that reduces cell swelling. Although these espoused theoretical benefits of diuretic therapy appear reasonable, actual documentation of their value in controlled studies is nearly nonexistent.[62]

Even though diuretics have not been shown to accelerate acute renal failure recovery, most patients with acute renal failure will receive them to augment fluid management. Advantages of nonoliguric versus oliguric renal failure include easier management of fluid and electrolyte balance, the ability to administer adequate nutrition, reduced risk of developing pulmonary edema, and the reduced need for renal replacement therapies. Fluid overload can be difficult to treat with renal replacement therapy, especially in critically ill patients. Consequently, maximizing urine output should be a goal in acute renal failure, particularly in a patient at risk for fluid overload.

Because maintenance of urine output that results in net fluid loss for the fluid-overloaded patient is a primary therapeutic goal, choice of diuretic and diuretic dosing are important considerations. Typically, either mannitol or loop diuretics are used as first-line agents. The choice between these two therapies is not clear-cut since both have distinct advantages and disadvantages. Both diuretic classes have a long history of safety, and most clinicians are familiar with them. Mannitol, which works as an osmotic diuretic, can be given only parenterally. A typical starting dose is mannitol (20%) 12.5 to 25 g infused intravenously over 3 to 5 minutes. It has almost no nonrenal clearance, so when given to a patient making little urine it will remain in the patient, potentially causing a hyperosmolar state. Additionally, mannitol may itself cause acute renal failure, so its use in acute renal failure must be monitored carefully by measuring urine output and serum electrolytes and osmolality.

Furosemide, bumetanide, torsemide, and ethacrynic acid are loop diuretics. Ethacrynic acid is typically reserved for patients who are allergic to sulfa compounds. Furosemide is the most commonly used loop diuretic because of its lower cost, availability in oral and parenteral forms, and good safety and efficacy profiles. A problem with furosemide is its variable oral bioavailability in many patients. Consequently, initial doses (usually 40 to 80 mg) are usually given intravenously to assess whether the patient will respond. Torsemide and bumetanide have better oral bioavailability than furosemide. Torsemide has been documented to have an oral bioavailability of 80% to 100% in patients with congestive heart failure, a patient population known to have poor oral furosemide absorption.[63] Torsemide has a longer duration of activity than the other loop diuretics, thus allowing for less frequent administration but also possibly making it more difficult to titrate the dose. When loop diuretics are given parenterally in equipotent doses, it does not appear that there is a difference in efficacy in patients with acute renal failure.[64] Interestingly, the equipotency ratio of parenteral bumetanide:torsemide:furosemide in patients with normal renal function is 1:20:40 but in renal failure this ratio changes to 1:11:11.[64]

Continuous infusion of a loop diuretic is a relatively new administration technique. Most published studies indicate that less natriuresis occurs when equal doses of loop diuretic doses are given as a bolus instead of as a continuous infusion.[65,66] Furthermore, adverse reactions from loop diuretics (myalgias and hearing loss) occur less frequently in patients receiving continuous infusion compared to intermittent boluses, ostensibly because lower serum concentrations are obtained. The finding that the continuous infusions of loop diuretics have efficacy that is at least as good as intermittent bolus dosing, with fewer adverse effects appears to be consistent for all furosemide,[67,68] bumetanide,[69] and torsemide.[70] When continuous infusion is to be used, an initial loading dose is given (equivalent to furosemide 40 to 80 mg) prior to the initiation of the continuous infusion at a dose of 10 to 20 mg/h of furosemide or its equivalent.

One drawback of the continuous-infusion loop diuretic literature is that few carefully controlled trials in patients with acute renal failure have been conducted. Schuller et al.[68] published the first comparison of continuous-infusion and intermittent-bolus furosemide in 33 fluid-overloaded patients with chronic renal insufficiency and acute renal failure. The protocol used in this study excluded the use of other diuretics. These investigators found no difference in patient outcome or volume-removal rates between the two groups, but the study lacked sufficient statistical power to demonstrate even a 15% difference in fluid loss. Despite the paucity of evidence for diuretic use in this population, many clinicians continue to recommend diuretic use, if for no other reason than increased urine output allows for easier patient management.[62]

DIURETIC RESISTANCE

Diuretic resistance is commonly encountered in acute renal failure patients, especially in those with excessive sodium intake (Table 41–7). Patients with acute tubular necrosis have a reduced number of functioning nephrons on which the diuretic may exert its action. Other clinical states like glomerulonephritis are associated with heavy proteinuria. Intraluminal loop diuretics cannot exert their effect in the loop of Henle in this setting because they are extensively bound to the protein present in the urine. Still other patients may have reduced bioavailability of oral furosemide. Possible therapeutic options to counteract each form of diuretic resistance are presented in Table 41–7. Combination therapy of loop diuretics plus a diuretic from a different pharmacologic class can be an effective tool in the setting of acute renal failure.[71] Loop diuretics increase the delivery of sodium chloride to the distal convoluted tubule and collecting duct. With time, these areas of the nephron compensate for the activity of the loop diuretic and increase sodium and chloride reabsorption. In animals, this compensation can begin after a week of continuous furosemide infusion.[72] Whether this compensation can occur in humans with acute renal failure is unclear. Diuretics that work at the distal convoluted tubule (thiazides) or the collecting duct (amiloride, triamterene, spironolactone) may have a synergistic effect when administered with loop diuretics by blocking the compensatory increase in sodium and chloride reabsorption. The combination of loop diuretics and usual doses of thiazide diuretics may be effective in renal disease despite the accumulation of endogenous organic acids in renal disease that block the transport of loop diuretics into the lumen. If oral thiazides cannot be given to the patient, chlorothiazide can be administered parenterally.

Several drug combinations with loop diuretics have been investigated, including the addition of one or more of the following: theophylline, acetazolamide, spironolactone, thiazides, or metolazone.[71] Of these combinations, metolazone is used most frequently with furosemide. Metolazone, unlike other thiazides, produces effective diuresis at a GFR below 20 mL/min. This combination of metolazone and a loop diuretic has been used successfully in the management of fluid overload in patients with congestive heart failure, cirrhosis, and nephrotic syndrome. Additionally, this combination has been found to be efficacious in pediatric patients as well as adults.[73] Mannitol plus continuous intravenous infusion of a loop diuretic has been recommended,[62] but no convincing evidence of the effectiveness of this regimen exists.

TABLE 41–7. Common Causes of Diuretic Resistance in Patients With Acute Renal Failure and Measures Used to Counteract Them

Cause of Diuretic Resistance	Possible Therapeutic Solutions
Excessive sodium intake (sources may be dietary, IV fluids, and drugs)	Remove sodium from nutritional sources and medications
Inadequate diuretic dose or inappropriate regimen	Increase dose, use continuous infusion or combination therapy
Reduced oral bioavailability (usually furosemide)	Use parenteral therapy, switch to oral torsemide or bumetanide
Nephrotic syndrome (loop diuretic protein binding in tubule lumen)	Increase dose, switch diuretics, use combination therapy
Reduced renal blood flow	
Drugs (NSAIDs, ACE inhibitors, vasodilators)	Discontinue these drugs if possible
Hypotension	Volume and/or vasopressors
Intravascular depletion	Intravascular volume expansion
Increased sodium reabsorption	
Nephron adaptation to chronic diuretic therapy	Combination diuretic therapy, sodium restriction
NSAID use	Discontinue NSAID
Congestive heart failure (CHF)	Treat the CHF, increase diuretic dose, switch to more bioavailable loop diuretic
Cirrhosis	High-volume paracentesis
Acute tubular necrosis	Higher dose of diuretic, diuretic combination therapy, add low-dose dopamine

DOPAMINE

Low doses (0.5 to 2 μg/kg/min) of dopamine selectively dilate the renal vasculature and theoretically result in increased renal blood flow and GFR. At higher doses, the selectivity for the dopamine-1 receptor is lost as dopamine begins to bind to β-adrenergic receptors and α-adrenergic receptors. This results in renal vasoconstriction. Many clinicians attempt to take advantage of this pharmacologic finding by infusing low-dose dopamine in patients with acute renal failure.

Most published studies of low-dose dopamine show that urine output is increased in patients with established acute renal failure.[74] However, dopamine-induced increases in urine formation have not been shown to translate into improvements in creatinine clearance in acute renal failure patients. Only one report using low-dose dopamine has shown improvement in patients with stable chronic renal insufficiency and congestive heart failure.[75] Furthermore, studies using low-dose dopamine as preventive therapy prior to nephrotoxin administration have not demonstrated a protective role for dopamine.[76] Indeed, dopamine may have a deleterious effect when used in this manner in diabetic patients at risk for the development of nephrotoxicity.[76]

The commonly observed low-dose dopamine–induced improvements in urine output do not appear to have a salutary effect on overall patient outcome. Few studies have examined patient outcome of low-dose dopamine therapy. The Auriculin Anaritide Acute Renal Failure Study was designed to evaluate the effect of atrial natriuretic peptide (ANP) on the need for dialysis and mortality in patients with acute tubular necrosis.[77] In the placebo arm of the trial, the investigators examined the effect that dopamine had on these outcomes. At the discretion of the physician, approximately one-third of these 256 subjects received no dopamine, another third received low-dose dopamine (≤ 3 µg/kg/min), and the final third to high-dose dopamine (> 3 µg/kg/min). Not surprisingly, sicker patients were more likely to receive dopamine. However, when the authors statistically corrected for selection bias and confounding variables, they reported no significant differences in relative risks of death or need for dialysis among any of the treatment arms. Faced with these findings, these authors called for an end to the routine use of low-dose dopamine in acute renal failure until a prospective, randomized, placebo-controlled trial can demonstrate efficacy and safety of the therapy.[77] Furthermore, low doses of dopamine (2.5 µg/kg/min) have been documented to decrease serum prolactin concentrations by 80% in critically ill oliguric patients.[78] Prolactin is an immunomodulatory hormone involved in the endocrine response to stress. A reduction in prolactin concentrations may suppress cellular immunity and increase the risk of infectious complications in acute renal failure patients. It appears that low-dose dopamine can increase urine output, but it should be used cautiously because it has not been shown to improve patient outcome.[79]

DOBUTAMINE

Dobutamine infusions (175 µg/min), unlike low-dose dopamine, have been reported to improve creatinine clearance without increasing urine output in critically ill patients with stable creatinine clearances of ~70 to 80 mL/min.[74] The 18-mL/min increase in creatinine clearance was statistically significant compared to placebo, but probably of little clinical importance in these patients with relatively normal baseline renal function. The mechanism for the improved creatinine clearance appears to be the result of increased cardiac output and renal blood flow, because dobutamine does not possess direct effects on the renal vasculature. The effects of dobutamine in patients with oliguric acute renal failure have not been studied.

EXPERIMENTAL THERAPIES

Our understanding of the pathogenesis of acute renal failure is in its infancy. Most pharmacologic therapies that have been used to either prevent or treat established acute renal failure have been unsuccessful.[54] Atrial natriuretic peptide (ANP) is one of the latest experimental agents to be studied to pharmacologically improve ischemic acute renal failure patient outcome, with somewhat disappointing results.[80] In this trial, overall dialysis-free survival was not different between ANP and placebo-treated patients. Only a subgroup analysis of oliguric patients showed benefit of ANP. Unfortunately, nonoliguric patients actually fared significantly worse if they received ANP instead of placebo.

The development of new renal replacement techniques and our expanding understanding of the mediators of ischemic acute renal failure will hopefully lead to therapies that can alter its natural course.[81] Therapies directed toward platelet-activating factor,[82,83] integrins,[84] endothelin,[85] growth factors,[86] nitric oxide,[87] and apoptosis[88] may finally yield a breakthrough in the treatment of established acute renal failure.

THERAPIES TO AVOID IN ESTABLISHED ACUTE RENAL FAILURE

Exposure to nephrotoxins has been identified as a risk factor for acute renal failure in nearly every epidemiologic study. Avoidance of subsequent nephrotoxic therapies and procedures are essential aspects to the management of patients with established acute renal failure as well as those at risk for the development of acute renal failure.[49] Recovery from acute ischemic renal disease usually requires 14 to 21 days from the most recent insult to the kidney, not necessarily the first insult to the kidney. Consequently, repeated exposure to nephrotoxins like contrast dye, aminoglycosides, NSAIDs, vasoconstrictive agents (high-dose dopamine, norepinephrine), and others may prolong the duration of acute renal failure. Judicious use of these agents after carefully considering the risks, benefits, and alternatives is important. In many cases, no alternative exists, but all options should be explored before choosing one of these potentially nephrotoxic agents. If they are to be used, careful dosing and close monitoring of serum concentrations, where appropriate, is imperative.

Ketorolac is a parenteral NSAID commonly used in hospitalized patients. Like other NSAIDs, ketorolac may induce acute renal failure, with most case reports occurring after at least 5 days of continuous therapy.[89] Because of this and the fact that the risk of gastrointestinal bleeding increases with prolonged therapy, the manufacturer recommends that parenteral therapy be limited to 5 days. Most clinicians are aware of the importance of avoiding ketorolac in patients with acute renal failure. The incidence of acute renal failure induced by parenteral ketorolac was compared to the rate caused by opioids in a large retrospective trial conducted in 35 Philadelphia-area hospitals.[90] The multivariate adjusted relative risk of acute renal failure in those who received fewer than 5 days of ketorolac was not different from that observed in patients receiving opioids for analgesia. In both groups the incidence of acute renal failure was 1.1%. However, after 5 days of therapy, the risk of developing acute renal failure was twice as great in the ketorolac group as in the opioid group. In this same study, the risk of developing acute renal failure was more than three times higher if the patient received concomitant aminoglycoside therapy or had preexisting chronic renal disease. These data suggest that short-duration ketorolac may not be as nephrotoxic as once thought, but probably still should be avoided in patients with established acute renal failure.

COMPLICATIONS

INFECTION

The most common cause of death in patients with acute renal failure is infection.[91] Interestingly, sepsis itself is a very common cause of acute renal failure. Acute renal failure contributes somewhat to the high infection rate by altering leukocyte function and cell-mediated immunity. Other aspects in the care of the patient with acute renal failure can lead to infection. Renal replacement therapy necessitates indwelling vascular or peritoneal access, which can serve as a focus of infection. Peritoneal and vascular access site erythema or purulent drainage should be monitored routinely.

Indwelling urinary catheters also predispose patients with acute renal failure to infection. Urinary catheters should be used for no longer than necessary, but in many instances their use cannot be avoided. Frequent evaluation of urine for signs of infection is warranted.

The comorbidities found in patients with acute renal failure may play a more important role in the development of infection. Critically ill patients with acute renal failure often have failures of other organ systems. These failures predispose them to infection. Concomitant cardiopulmonary failure requiring mechanical ventilation increases the risk of pneumonia. High-dose vasopressor therapy results in reduced blood flow to the GI tract, which may cause ischemia and introduction of gut flora to the bloodstream. The management of a patient with acute renal failure requires (1) prevention of infection where possible, (2) a high index of suspicion in the recognition of infection, and (3) aggressive antibiotic therapy that has been appropriately adjusted for renal disease and renal replacement therapy.

CARDIOVASCULAR ABNORMALITIES

Patients with acute renal failure often manifest cardiovascular abnormalities. Hypertension, hypotension, heart failure, pericarditis, arrhythmias, and pulmonary edema all may be associated with acute renal failure. The causes of cardiovascular complications in these patients include electrolyte disturbances, impaired acid–base balance, uremia, and volume overload. Volume overload may cause hypertension, which may be best treated with diuretics and renal replacement therapy. Aggressive renal replacement therapy can also alleviate uremic pericarditis, electrolyte, and acid–base disorders. Swan–Ganz pressure and clinical monitoring will give an accurate assessment of the patient's volume status, which can be helpful in determining fluid replacement needs.

GASTROINTESTINAL SYMPTOMS

Critically ill patients with acute renal failure have long been recognized to be at increased risk for GI bleeding. Hypotension, the use of vasoconstrictive agents, and the high catabolic state seen in acute renal failure can contribute to stress ulceration in these patients. The uremic state also may induce bleeding by causing a defect in platelet function. Patients with acute renal failure and additional risk factors for stress-related hemorrhage (e.g., respiratory failure or high-dose corticosteroid use) are at an even higher risk for bleeding.[92] Other common GI complaints in patients with acute renal failure include nausea and vomiting associated with uremia and electrolyte imbalances.

NEUROLOGIC SYMPTOMS

Uremia more commonly affects patients with chronic renal failure. Nonetheless, the neurologic sequelae associated with uremia, altered mentation, myoclonus, and lethargy can occur in the setting of acute renal failure. Other causes of neurologic symptoms must be examined in the patient with acute renal failure before attributing them to uremia. Electrolyte disturbances common in acute renal failure frequently cause neurologic changes. Calcium, magnesium, phosphate, and sodium disorders must be ruled out in these patients. Adverse effects from improperly dosed renally eliminated drugs can also manifest as neurologic abnormalities like seizures or somnolence. Because acute renal failure often has a sudden onset, electrolyte imbalance and drug accumulation can occur rapidly in these patients. Diligent monitoring of laboratory results, renal replacement schedules, and drug dosing can help to prevent these neurologic sequelae.

RENAL REPLACEMENT THERAPY CONSIDERATIONS

Renal replacement therapy is not used in all patients presenting with acute renal failure. The usual indications for renal replacement therapy in acute renal failure patients differ somewhat from what they are in patients with end-stage renal disease (ESRD) (Table 41–8) (see Chap. 44). For many years the patient with acute renal failure who required renal replacement therapy was treated nearly the same as the patient with ESRD. This occurred despite the inherent differences in treatment goals and patient needs between these patient populations. Unlike the patient with ESRD, the patient with acute renal failure who is sick enough to require renal replacement therapy is typically an unstable patient in terms of volume, electrolyte, and azotemic control. Most patients with ESRD can be managed with a standard thrice-weekly, 4-hour hemodialysis schedule. In acute renal failure this is less likely to occur.

Recent mathematical models derived from actual protein catabolic rates measured in patients with acute renal failure have demonstrated that the renal replacement needs for critically ill patients with acute renal failure are greater than their ESRD counterparts.[93] Considerably more renal replacement therapy is required to maintain the same degree of azotemic control than is considered acceptable

TABLE 41–8. The AEIOUs That Describe the Indications for Renal Replacement Therapy

	Indications for Renal Replacement Therapy	Clinical Setting
A	Acid–base abnormalities	Metabolic acidosis resulting from the accumulation of organic and inorganic acids
E	Electrolyte imbalance	Hyperkalemia, hypermagnesemia
I	Intoxications	Salicylates, lithium, methanol, ethylene glycol, theophylline, phenobarbital
O	fluid Overload	Postoperative fluid gain
U	Uremia	High catabolism of acute renal failure

in stable patients with ESRD (prehemodialysis BUN < 100 mg/dL). The higher protein catabolic rate in acute renal failure is the main reason for this more intensive therapy. The dose of renal replacement therapy necessary to maintain azotemic control is directly related to the patient's catabolic rate and body weight. It is not unusual for critically ill patients with acute renal failure to require 4-hour hemodialysis sessions 5 to 7 times per week to maintain the pre-hemodialysis BUN < 100 mg/dL.[93]

Two consequences of this increased need for renal replacement therapy are detailed below. First, relatively new renal replacement techniques, like continuous hemofiltration and hemodiafiltration, have been developed to meet the needs of hypercatabolic patients and are now commonplace in the intensive care unit. These therapies provide new challenges in delivering effective pharmacotherapy, particularly in terms of nutritional therapy and compounding ultrafiltrate replacement solutions. Second, the optimal dosage requirement of the medications for patients receiving renal replacement therapies that are either relatively new (continuous therapies) or being used in new ways (daily intermittent hemodialysis) are poorly defined. Unfortunately, most published dosing recommendations for established therapies like hemodialysis were derived for patients receiving thrice-weekly hemodialysis (see Chap. 47). These dosing recommendations may not be applicable in a patient requiring daily hemodialysis for azotemic control.

INTERMITTENT THERAPIES

Renal replacement options for acute renal failure can be divided into two main categories: intermittent and continuous therapies. The most commonly used intermittent and continuous renal replacement therapies are listed in Table 41–9. Historically, intermittent therapies, usually hemodialysis, have been the most commonly chosen modality. Advantages of intermittent therapies are that they are technically simple, the hardware for instituting treatment is available at most institutions, and clinicians typically have expertise using them.

Intermittent hemodialysis is primarily diffusion based. Consequently, it is very efficient in removing solutes of low molecular weight (< 500 Daltons) like urea, creatinine, most electrolytes, and many drugs. Because diffusional solute removal is so dependent on molecular size and the relative pore size of the dialysis filter, conventional hemodialysis is not very effective in removing solutes of larger molecular weight (e.g., low-molecular-weight proteins and many sepsis mediators) (see Chap. 44). Newer hemodialysis membranes with larger membrane pores have been developed (high-flux membranes) to increase the clearance of some of these larger solutes. These new dialysis membranes can partially remove solutes up to approximately 15,000 Daltons, but clearances of these large molecules are still considerably lower than small-solute clearances. The most clinically relevant aspect of dialysis membrane choice to pharmacists is the differences noted in drug clearance rates with these high-permeability membranes. For example, a significantly different higher vancomycin removal rate is observed when a high-flux dialyzer is used instead of a conventional hemodialyzer.[94,95] Vancomycin's molecular weight (1450 Daltons) is such that it is not removed by conventional hemodialysis but is cleared when high-flux membranes are used. Acute renal failure patients receiving vancomycin will require more frequent dosing if high-flux hemodialyzers are used, because about 20% to 30% of the total vancomycin body load is removed with each dialysis treatment.

Higher permeability polymers are used commonly in patients with acute renal failure because they tend to be more biocompatible. As blood passes through the hemodialyzer, it comes into contact with chemicals that are found in the dialyzer fibers. Exposure to these substances results in complex humoral and cellular host responses that may include anaphylaxis, thromboembolic complications, immunosuppression, and hypercatabolism.[96] These reactions may be deleterious for patients with acute renal failure, who already have problems similar to these. Consequently, newer dialysis and hemofilter membranes are often used because they induce less of a reaction. These same dialyzers also tend to be higher flux dialyzers as well. Studies have suggested that patients with acute renal failure may have higher survival rates and renal function recovery rates when biocompatible membranes are used for renal replacement.[17]

Another drawback of intermittent hemodialysis is that it is not very well tolerated by hemodynamically unstable patients. This problem is compounded in the fluid-overloaded patient who requires extensive volume removal; often 2 to 3 L or more must occur within the 4-hour dialysis treatment. Most acute renal failure patients will not be able to maintain an adequate blood pressure with such rapid fluid removal. It has been hypothesized that these periods of hypotension during the hemodialysis session may actually prolong the duration of acute renal failure, because the recovering tubules are now subjected to a hypoxic insult.[31]

CONTINUOUS RENAL REPLACEMENT THERAPIES

PERITONEAL DIALYSIS

Peritoneal dialysis is a continuous renal replacement therapy (CRRT) usually used for ambulatory patients with chronic renal failure but can also be used in acute renal failure (see Chap. 44). Glucose-containing dialysate solutions are instilled into the patient's peritoneum. The patient's own peritoneal membrane acts as the dialysis membrane. Advantages of peritoneal dialysis in acute renal failure is that it is relatively easy to perform once the dialysis catheter is instilled into patient's peritoneum. The main disadvantage of peritoneal dialysis is that it is not very efficient for volume and solute removal. Its use in acute renal failure is generally limited to children, who tend to have a larger peritoneal membrane surface area relative to their overall body size. This anatomic difference means peritoneal dialysis

TABLE 41–9. Advantages and Disadvantages of Common Renal Replacement Therapies for Acute Renal Failure

	Intermittent Hemodialysis	Intermittent Hemofiltration	Peritoneal Dialysis	Slow Continuous Ultrafiltration (SCUF)	Continuous Arteriovenous Hemofiltration (CAVH)	Continuous Venovenous Hemofiltration (CVVH)	Continuous Arteriovenous Hemodiafiltration (CAVHDF)	Continuous Venovenous Hemodiafiltration (CVVHDF)
Solute control	Usually adequate	Inadequate	Inadequate	Inadequate	Inadequate	Adequate	Adequate	Adequate
Volume control	Variable	Adequate	Adequate	Adequate	Adequate	Adequate	Adequate	Adequate
Hemodynamic stability	Variable	Well tolerated	Well tolerated	Well tolerated	Well tolerated	Well tolerated	Well tolerated	Well tolerated
Access	Venous	Venous	Peritoneal	Arterial and venous	Arterial and venous	Venous	Arterial and venous	Venous
Anticoagulation	Short duration	Short duration	None	Continuous	Continuous high dose	Continuous low dose	Continuous high dose	Continuous low dose
Technical complexity	High	High	Low	Low	Low	Moderate	Moderate	High
Workload	Intermittent	Intermittent	Low	Low	Low	Moderate	Moderate	High
Drug dosing ease	Many published recommendations	Difficult	Difficult	Negligible drug removal	Difficult	Many published recommendations	Difficult	Difficult
Convective clearance (small and middle molecules)	Mixed	Minimal	Moderate	Moderate	Large	Large	Large	Large
Dialytic clearance (small molecules)	Large	None	Large	None	None	None	Large	Large
Common complications	Hypotension	Hypotension	Hyperglycemia, atelectasis, peritonitis	Arterial bleeding, hypotension	Arterial bleeding, filter clotting	Hypotension	Arterial bleeding, ↑ serum lactate	↑ Serum lactate, hypotension

may be able to generate enough solute removal for children to provide adequate azotemic control. Another common problem with using peritoneal dialysis in acute renal failure is that it provides a large glucose load to the patient. Patients with acute renal failure receiving rapid, frequent (30- to 90-minute dwell times) exchanges of peritoneal dialysate containing 4.25% dextrose absorbed an average of 1922 kcal/d of glucose from the dialysate, resulting in significant overfeeding.[97]

EXTRACORPOREAL THERAPIES

Several extracorporeal continuous renal replacement therapies have been developed during the past 20 years to address the unique needs of the acute renal failure patient who is hypercatabolic, hypotensive, and volume overloaded. The most commonly used continuous therapies in acute renal failure are continuous hemofiltration and hemodiafiltration. These modalities are more technically difficult and require more nursing time to operate compared to intermittent hemodialysis. However, the advantages of continuous therapies are improved fluid and metabolic control, especially in patients unable to tolerate hemodialysis. Continuous therapies generally are better tolerated because the fluid and electrolyte shifts are more gradual than with the intermittent therapies.

The continuous therapies have gone by many names over the years and only recently has consensus been reached on the nomenclature of the therapies.[98] This nomenclature helps differentiate between the many systems in place worldwide. Continuous therapies can take blood from arteries and return them to veins (arteriovenous), allowing the heart to pump blood through the system (Fig. 41–3). Alternatively, blood can be pumped through the hemofilter from a dual-lumen venous catheter (veno-venous) (Fig. 41–4). Veno-venous systems are preferred if the hardware to run these machines is available, because the cardiovascular systems of critically ill patients often do not provide adequate blood flow through the extracorporeal circuit to allow adequate solute clearance. Systems can be entirely diffusive based (continuous hemodialysis, CVVHD, where a peritoneal dialysate solution is used as a dialysate), entirely convective based with no diffusion (continuous hemofiltration, CVVH), or a combination of both (continuous hemodiafiltration, CVVHDF).

Hemofiltration employs no dialysate, but a high-flux dialyzer or hemofilter with a large pore size is usually used in the system. Solutes dissolved in the plasma water that are small enough to pass through the hemofilter pores are removed as the plasma water they are dissolved in moves across the hemofilter. This plasma water solution is called ultrafiltrate, and this type of solute removal is called "convection." Convective solute removal differs from diffusive solute removal in that the solute's molecular weight has little effect on removal. As long as the dissolved solute can fit through the hemofilter pores (< 15,000 Daltons), it will be removed by convection. Consequently, hemofiltration is more effective than dialytic therapies in the removal of larger-molecular-weight substances. Convective removal of larger-molecular-weight substances may be desirable in patients with diseases like septic shock, as many of the mediators of septic shock have molecular weights of 600 to 30,000 Daltons. Consequently, continuous hemofiltration has been proposed as an adjunctive therapy for septic shock.[99]

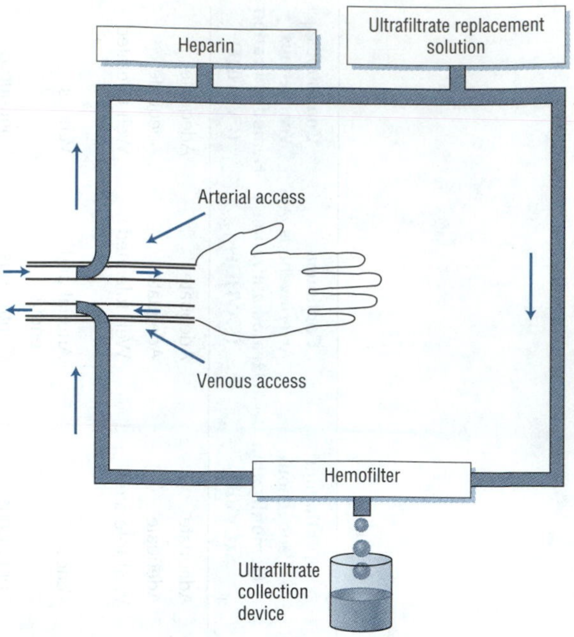

FIGURE 41–3. Schematic of continuous arteriovenous hemofiltration (CAVH). CAVH is the simplest continuous renal replacement therapy, but usually does not provide adequate solute removal for highly catabolic patients with acute renal failure. Blood enters the extracorporeal circuit from the arterial catheter and returns via a separate venous catheter. The hydrostatic force for making ultrafiltrate is provided by the patient's arterial pressure. Blood flow through the circuit and ultrafiltrate production rates are a function of the patient's cardiovascular status. Usually higher heparin doses are required to prevent filter clotting in CAVH versus venovenous systems because of the slower blood flow through the hemofilter in CAVH.

The continuous nature of these therapies gives them an advantage over intermittent therapies in the treatment of critically ill patients with acute renal failure. Solutes are continually removed as they are produced and volume can be removed slowly and consistently. Hypotensive, hypervolemic patients who could not tolerate 2 to 3 L of volume removal over a 4-hour intermittent hemodialysis treatment usually can withstand slow volume removal of 100 to 200 mL/h for 24 hours (2.4 to 4.8 L/d).

The convective aspect of continuous hemofiltration or hemodiafiltration allows for optimal volume control. Typically, 1000 mL/h of ultrafiltrate is formed and discarded and 800 to 1000 mL/h of replacement fluid is infused, depending on the fluid and cardiovascular status of the patient. This intravenous ultrafiltrate replacement solution contains physiologic concentrations of sodium, potassium, chloride, bicarbonate, and calcium. When the patient is extremely fluid overloaded, less of the volume removed will be replaced, to achieve the net desired hourly fluid loss for

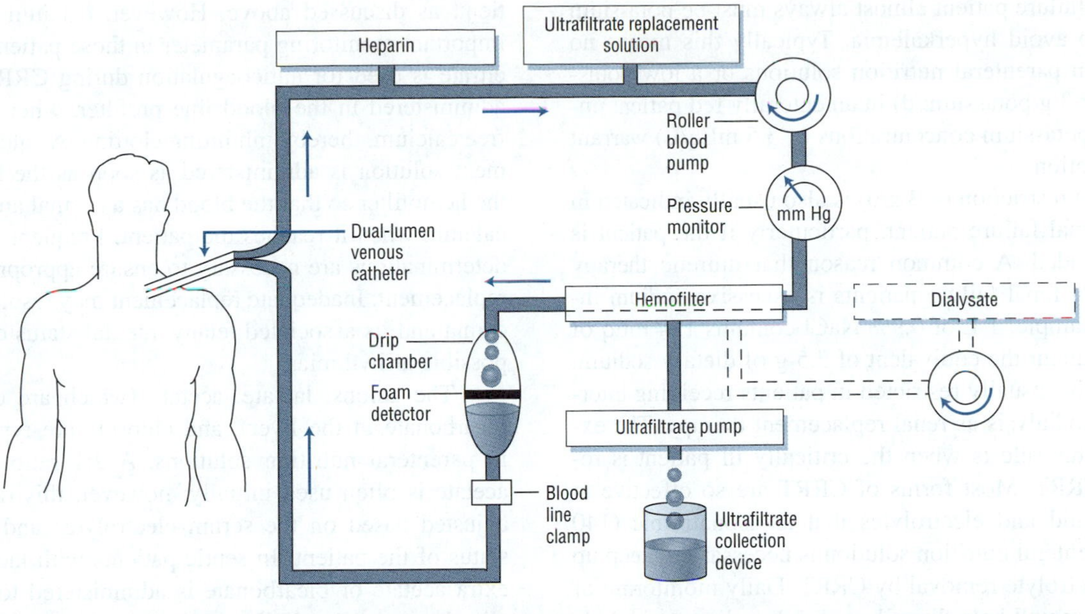

FIGURE 41–4. Schematic of the continuous venovenous renal replacement therapies. The continuous venovenous renal replacement therapies all have the same basic extracorporeal circuit. Blood is pulled into the extracorporeal circuit from a dual-lumen central catheter by a blood pump. Blood is anticoagulated prior to the hemofilter to prevent clotting of the hemofilter. Before the blood returns to the patient through the other lumen of the venous catheter, it travels through a drip chamber and foam detector to prevent accidental air embolization. In the case of continuous venovenous hemofiltration (CVVH), no dialysate is connected to the right side of the figure, and all fluid and solutes are removed convectively by the pump coming from the hemodiafilter. When continuous venovenous hemodialysis (CVVHD) is used, little or no ultrafiltrate is formed because the pump coming from the hemodiafilter is set at the same rate as the dialysate pump, resulting in mostly diffusive solute removal. Continuous venovenous hemodiafiltration (CVVHDF) occurs when the pump coming from the hemodiafilter is set at a rate much higher than the dialysate pump speed, resulting in both diffusive and convective solute removal.

the patient. Some of the ultrafiltrate replacement may be in the form of intravenous medications, blood products, and nutrition. The large hourly fluid removal and subsequent large hourly fluid replacement allows for the administration of drugs, nutrition, and blood products without concern about volume constraints. This luxury is not afforded to patients receiving intermittent hemodialysis or peritoneal dialysis. Consequently, therapies can be administered solely based on patient need instead of on how much volume they will add to the patient. Finally, the drug dosing considerations for each of these therapies will differ greatly from intermittent hemodialysis, and may vary between the different continuous therapies[98,100,101] (see Chap. 47).

BIOCOMPATIBILITY

Differences in patient outcome between those receiving intermittent versus continuous therapies have not been documented, and it is a complex issue that has not been well studied.[102,103] However, recent attention has been directed toward the actual membrane used for dialysis or hemofiltration. As blood comes into contact with the materials used in these membranes, many biochemical changes occur, including complement activation, cytokine generation, and clotting cascade activation.[104] Membranes that activate these systems are considered to be "bioincompatible," because it is postulated that these effects may be responsible for the slow recovery of renal function in acute renal failure. New synthetic, "biocompatible" membranes have been developed that do not activate these systems as much. Use of these biocompatible membranes for hemodialysis may confer an improved recovery of renal function and mortality rate in patients with acute renal failure compared to bioincompatible dialysis membranes.[17]

NUTRITIONAL NONPHARMACOLOGIC THERAPY

It is possible that no area of acute renal failure treatment is more controversial than a discussion of what constitutes the best nutritional regimen. Some have questioned whether parenteral nutrition is of any value at all in these patients.[105] While some of this discussion appears in Chap. 131, a few elements bear mention here. For example, the renal replacement therapy chosen for acute renal failure will affect electrolyte, protein, caloric, and vitamin regimens for the patient.[106]

ELECTROLYTES

About the only universally agreed-upon aspect of acute renal failure nutritional care is that of electrolyte management. Of the electrolyte abnormalities observed in acute renal failure patients, hyperkalemia is the most common and the most serious. Life-threatening arrhythmias may result from uncontrolled hyperkalemia. The treatment of hyperkalemia is discussed in Chap. 48. Vigilant monitoring of potassium serum concentrations is essential. The oliguric acute renal failure patient almost always must be potassium restricted to avoid hyperkalemia. Typically this means no potassium in parenteral nutrition solutions or a low potassium diet (< 3 g potassium/d) in an enterally fed patient unless serum potassium concentrations (< 3.5 mEq/L) warrant supplementation.

Sodium restriction (< 3 g/d) is also usually indicated in the acute renal failure patient, particularly if the patient is fluid overloaded. A common reason that diuretic therapy fails in acute renal failure patients is excessive sodium intake. For example, 1 L of 0.9% NaCl contains 154 mEq of sodium, or about the equivalent of 3.5 g of dietary sodium. Sodium is also usually restricted in patients receiving intermittent hemodialysis as renal replacement therapy. The exception to this rule is when the critically ill patient is receiving a CRRT. Most forms of CRRT are so effective at removing fluid and electrolytes that an isonatremic (140 mEq/L) parenteral nutrition solution is necessary to keep up with the electrolyte removal by CRRT. Daily monitoring of serum sodium will help direct how much sodium to include in the nutritional regimen.

Other electrolytes that must be monitored closely in this population are magnesium and phosphorus. Both are renally eliminated and are not very dialyzable. Typically they are restricted, but in acute renal failure patients with poor nutritional status or in those who receive long durations of CRRT, they may need to be supplemented. This is particularly true for phosphorus, because acute hypophosphatemia can occur as a result of refeeding syndrome in a critically ill patient who begins to receive nutritional support after a long period of having received none. More frequent is the problem of hyperphosphatemia, especially in the acute renal failure patient with concomitant tissue destruction or catabolism (trauma, rhabdomyolysis, sepsis). Serum phosphorus concentrations may rise, even when no phosphorus is administered to the patient. In these situations, phosphate-binding antacids (aluminum hydroxide, calcium carbonate, or calcium acetate) may be used, even in a patient not being enterally fed. As the antacid progresses through the gastrointestinal tract, phosphorus tightly binds to either the aluminum or calcium in the antacid and is excreted in the stool. Calcium-containing agents are considered first-line therapy, especially in patients being enterally fed. Aluminum-containing antacids are usually reserved for patients with a serum phosphate > 7 mg/dL. In these hyperphosphatemic patients, calcium is avoided to reduce the chance of precipitation of calcium and phosphate in the soft tissues. A rule of thumb is to maintain a calcium–phosphate product below 70. The calcium–phosphate product is simply calculated by multiplying the serum calcium (mg/dL) by the serum phosphorus (mg/dL). Once the serum phosphorus is reduced below 7 mg/dL, calcium antacids are again used to maintain normal serum phosphate concentrations.

In contrast to patients with ESRD, calcium balance is usually not a major problem in the patient with acute renal failure. Care must be taken in the hyperphosphatemic patient, as discussed above. However, calcium becomes an important monitoring parameter in those patients for whom citrate is used for anticoagulation during CRRT. Citrate is administered in the blood line prefilter, where it binds all free calcium, thereby inhibiting clotting. A calcium replacement solution is administered as soon as the blood leaves the hemofilter so that the blood has a normal amount of free calcium when it reaches the patient. Frequent free calcium determinations are necessary to ensure appropriate calcium replacement. Inadequate replacement may result in hypocalcemia and its associated tetany, mental status changes, and possible arrhythmias.

The anions, lactate, acetate (which are converted to bicarbonate in the liver), and chloride are typically given in parenteral nutrition solutions. A 2:1 ratio of chloride: acetate is often used initially; however, this ratio must be adjusted based on the serum electrolytes and the clinical status of the patient. In septic patients with lactic acidosis, extra acetate or bicarbonate is administered to help maintain the patient's pH. In contrast, patients receiving long-term loop diuretic therapy often develop a hypochloremic metabolic alkalosis as the diuretic removes more chloride ion than bicarbonate. Extra chloride supplementation in place of acetate, lactate, or bicarbonate as the anion in the nutritional solution will usually correct the problem when identified early.

PROTEIN

For many years, renal replacement therapies were not as readily available as they are today. Consequently, a main goal of nutritional therapy in the patient with acute renal failure was to avoid the need for dialysis. To accomplish this, protein restriction was an essential component of the nutrition prescription. Even with protein restriction, many acute renal failure patients require renal replacement therapy because of the extremely high protein catabolic rate associated with their critical illness. The stressed acute renal failure patient breaks protein down at an accelerated rate, and cells do not use amino acids efficiently.[105] The protein catabolic rate in a critically ill patient can easily approach 100 g of protein/day.[15] Early studies suggested that adequate protein administration may improve mortality in acute renal failure.[105] The administration of exogenous proteins can improve the net nitrogen balance in the patient, but it is unclear whether a positive nitrogen balance is correlated with positive patient outcome.[15]

EVALUATION OF THERAPEUTIC OUTCOMES

Key monitoring parameters for patients with acute renal failure will differ based on the patient's presentation. In early stages of suspected acute renal failure, identifying the etiology is essential so that measures to reverse the cause can be instituted. The monitoring parameters for the patient with community-acquired acute renal failure will differ from those used for ICU-acquired acute renal failure. In either case, once acute renal failure is established, monitoring becomes similar. The addition of renal replacement therapy adds to the number of monitoring parameters that must be followed. For example, the initiation of CVVHDF adds the requirements of monitoring glucose (for absorbed glucose from dialysate), anticoagulation, and ultrafiltrate and dialysate flow rates.

Clinicians formulating a care plan for a patient can follow a systematic course of action. The first step is to gather all pertinent data prior to preparing a care plan (Table 41–10). The core monitoring parameters for acute renal failure must be expanded if the patient is receiving renal replacement therapy (Table 41–11). The next step is to estimate the patient's current renal function (see Chap. 40) and find out whether renal replacement therapy is to be instituted or changed if already in place. Once this information is known, decisions about nutrition and pharmacotherapy can be made. Nutritional regimens must be adjusted to meet the patient's dynamic needs. Nutritional interventions commonly include adjustment of electrolytes and fluid restriction.

All drug doses must be evaluated in response to the assembled patient database. Diuretic doses may need to be titrated to maintain desired urine output. Most importantly, doses need to be adjusted for changes in renal function and

TABLE 41–10. Key Monitoring Parameters for Patients With Established Acute Renal Failure

Parameter	Frequency
Fluid ins/outs	Every shift
Patient weight	Daily
Vital signs	Every shift
Blood cultures and sensitivities	Check for results daily; obtain more when clinical signs of infection present
Blood chemistries	
Sodium, potassium, chloride, bicarbonate, calcium, phosphate, magnesium	Daily
BUN/S_{cr}	Daily
Albumin	Once or twice weekly
Complete blood cell count with white cell differential	Daily
Drugs and their dosing regimens	Daily
Nutritional regimen	Daily
Serum concentration data for drugs	After regimen changes and after RRT has been instituted
Times of administered doses	Daily
Doses relative to administration of RRT	Daily
Urinalysis	
Calculate measured creatinine clearance	Every time measured urine collection performed
Calculate fractional excretion of sodium	Every time measured urine collection performed
Plans for renal replacement	Daily
Invasive monitoring parameters	As indicated
Swan–Ganz readings	Every shift

TABLE 41–11. Renal Replacement Therapy-Specific Monitoring Parameters

- Hemodialysis
  - Pre- and postdialysis BUN (gives indication of delivered dose of dialysis)
  - Duration of dialysis
  - Type of dialyzer—conventional versus high-flux (especially for vancomycin therapy)
- Continuous renal replacement therapies
  - Inspection of system
    - Clotting of filter
    - Ultrafiltrate/dialysate flow rates
      - Desired rate versus actual rates
      - Nursing notes of overnight ultrafiltrate production and dialysate flow
    - Interruption of therapy for other tests
  - Vascular access (particularly if arterial line used)
    - Signs of bleeding
    - Signs of infection (redness, pus formation)
  - Anticoagulation
    - Partial thromboplastin time (PTT) and platelet count if heparin used for anticoagulation
    - Unbound calcium serum concentration and ECG if citrate used for anticoagulation
    - Signs of bleeding

renal replacement therapies. Frequent serum concentration monitoring is necessary because an assumption of a "steady-state" condition cannot be made in many of these patients with changing renal function and, occasionally, changing renal replacement therapy. Non–steady-state creatinine clearance equations and timed urine collections for direct creatinine clearance measurement are often necessary (see Chap. 40). Dosing regimens based on serum concentration results from last week in a patient with oliguria may not apply this week.

PHARMACOKINETIC CONSIDERATIONS

Typically, clinicians tend to dose renally eliminated medications in patients with acute renal failure the same as they would dose patients with ESRD. The assumption that patients with acute renal failure or ESRD have the same drug clearance is made because both groups have minimal renal function. Recent evidence suggests that although the renal elimination of drugs is the same between patients with acute renal failure and ESRD, nonrenal elimination may be quite different. The kidney metabolizes many endogenous and exogenous substances in patients with normal renal function.[107,108] The degree of renal metabolism in patients with acute renal failure has not been studied. Nonrenal clearance in patients with acute renal failure is the most difficult clearance parameter to estimate. Although most published dosing guidelines for patients with renal disease do not differentiate between acute and chronic failure, the pharmacokinetics of many agents can differ substantially in these two patient populations. Chronic renal failure is associated with derangements in the hepatic metabolism of many drugs. The mechanism(s) that slows the metabolic pathways responsible for this nonrenal clearance has not been studied extensively, but it appears that retained uremic by-products are responsible for the reduced enzymatic activity.[107] Only a few investigations have examined whether nonrenal clearance in patients with acute renal failure approximates normal values or values reported in patients with chronic renal failure. The nonrenal clearance of vancomycin and imipenem in adults with acute renal failure lies somewhere between the normal renal function values (40 and 130 mL/min, respectively) and chronic renal failure values (6 and 50 mL/min).[109–111] In theory, this may occur because uremic by-products may not have had time to accumulate and affect hepatic function. Indirect evidence from vancomycin indicates that in early acute renal failure, the nonrenal clearance is preserved but declines after 1 to 2 weeks until the nonrenal clearance approaches the values observed in patients with chronic renal failure.[109] Further studies are needed to confirm these findings and evaluate whether this pattern of change is evident with other medications. If nonrenal clearance of some antibiotics in early acute renal failure is greater than anticipated, the resultant serum concentrations would be lower than expected. This could contribute to the fact that the primary cause of death in acute renal failure is usually infection. Clearly, frequent therapeutic drug monitoring is needed in these patients to assess whether nonrenal clearance changes with time for drugs that have substantial nonrenal clearance. Because most of the published dosing guidelines in renal failure were generated from patients with chronic renal failure, future dosing guidelines for drugs with significant nonrenal clearance should specify whether they are for patients with acute or chronic renal failure if the nonrenal clearance rates differ between acute and chronic renal failure.

PHARMACOECONOMIC CONSIDERATIONS

In 1995, $13.06 billion was spent managing patients in the United States with ESRD. The economic consequences of acute renal failure are poorly defined. Pharmacoeconomic analysis suggests that instituting hemodialysis in the hospital for hospital-acquired acute renal failure costs $128,200 per quality-adjusted life year saved.[112] These costs range from $61,900 to $274,100, depending on the prognosis of the patient. These figures have been disputed[113] but highlight the high mortality rate of acute renal failure and the high expense associated with treating these patients.

Economic analyses of the use of specific agents that increase the risk of nephrotoxicity, such as aminoglycosides and intravenous contrast dyes, have been performed, as have the relative costs of various renal replacement therapies to treat acute renal failure. Typically, the costs of renal replacement therapy in the ICU range from $500 to $5500 per patient per week.[114] The least expensive therapies are the continuous arteriovenous renal replacement therapies because no pumps and fewer skilled nursing personnel are needed. Arteriovenous forms produce less ultrafiltrate and, therefore, also require less ultrafiltrate replacement solutions and dialysate. The setup costs for buying the machines that run intermittent hemodialysis or continuous venovenous renal replacement are similar; however, the day-to-day costs of continuous therapies is considerably higher.[114] Added costs come from continuous nursing supervision and the ultrafiltrate replacement solutions (usually made by the pharmacy department). A patient who has an ultrafiltrate production rate of 1000 mL/h usually requires 20 L of replacement solution that cost about $20/L.

Ancillary costs associated with CRRT have not been well described but include increased laboratory testing for urea, creatinine, electrolyte, and drug concentrations. Also, pharmacists prepare specialized enteral and parenteral nutritional products to provide adequate caloric and protein intake in minimal volume and with relatively low amounts of undesired electrolytes like potassium and phosphate. These are added costs of acute renal failure that are indirectly influenced by renal replacement therapy. Because no difference has yet been demonstrated in patient outcomes, both intermittent therapy and CRRT will be used to treat patients with acute renal failure. Until these data are available, the choice of renal replacement will be determined by availability of each of the therapies, caregiver expertise, daily cost, and physician preference.

▶ PRINCIPLES OF PHARMACOTHERAPY

- Prevention of acute renal failure is key because there is little we can do to hasten recovery from established acute renal failure.
- Early resuscitation is essential, especially in the settings of trauma and surgery. If renal perfusion can be quickly re-established, acute tubular necrosis can be attenuated.
- Find out the cause of the acute renal failure. Therapy is directed by knowing the cause. The optimal therapy for one acute renal failure etiology may complicate another.
- An understanding of the solute (drug) removal principles of the renal replacement therapy used is essential to optimize nutrition and pharmacotherapy.
- Avoid nephrotoxic therapies in at-risk patient populations whenever possible. The duration of acute renal failure may be extended with continued nephrotoxic insults.
- Fluid control is key in acute renal failure. At times you may need to administer fluid (prerenal azotemia) and at other times you will need to restrict fluid (established acute renal failure).
- Be aggressive early with diuretic dosing. Converting oliguria to nonoliguria may or may not improve outcome, but an euvolemic patient is easier to manage than a hypervolemic one. This may entail continuous infusions of diuretics or combination therapy. However, if diuretics do not work in the patient, discontinue their use and consider renal replacement therapy for azotemic and volume control.

REFERENCES

1. Elasy TA, Anderson RJ. Changing demography of acute renal failure. Semin Dial 1996;9:438–443.
2. Rose BD. Acute renal failure—prerenal disease versus acute tubular necrosis. In: Rose BD, ed. Pathophysiology of Renal Disease, 2nd ed. New York, McGraw-Hill, 1987: 63–117.
3. Kjellstrand CM, Solez K. Treatment of acute renal failure. In: Schrier RW, Gottschalk CW, eds. Diseases of the Kidney, 5th ed. Boston, Little, Brown, 1992:1371–1404.
4. Kaufman J, Dhakal M, Patel B, Hamburger R. Community acquired renal failure. Am J Kidney Dis 1991;17:191-198.
5. Shusterman N, Strom BL, Murray TG, et al. Risk factors and outcome of hospital-acquired acute renal failure. Am J Med 1987;83:65–71.
6. Jochimsen F, Schäfer JH, Maurer A, Distler A. Impairment of renal function in medical intensive care: Predictability of acute renal failure. Crit Care Med 1990;18:480–485.
7. Groeneveld ABJ, Tran DD, van der Meulen J, et al. Acute renal failure in the medical intensive care unit: Predisposing, complicating factors and outcome. Nephron 1991;59:602–610.
8. Lohr JW, McFarlane MJ, Grantham JJ. A clinical index to predict survival in acute renal failure patients requiring dialysis. Am J Kidney Dis 1988;11:254–259.
9. Corwin HL, Bonventre JV. Factors influencing survival in acute renal failure. Semin Dial 1989;4:220–225.
10. Liano F, Garcia-Martin F, Gallego A, et al. Easy and early prognosis in acute tubular necrosis: A forward analysis of 228 cases. Nephron 1989;51:307–313.
11. Smithies MN, Cameron JS. Can we predict outcome in acute renal failure? Nephron 1989;51:297–300.
12. Liano F, Gallego A, Pascual J, et al. Prognosis of acute tubular necrosis: An extended prospectively contrasted study. Nephron 1993;63: 21–31.
13. McMurray DS, Luft FC, Maxwell DR, et al. Prevailing patterns and predictor variables in patients with acute tubular necrosis. Arch Intern Med 1978;138:950–955.
14. Turney JH, Marshall DH, Brownjohn AM, Ellis CM, Parsons FM. The evolution of acute renal failure: 1956–1988. Q J Med 1990;74: 83–104.
15. Macias WL, Murphy MH, Alaka KJ, et al. Impact of the nutritional regimen on protein catabolism and nitrogen balance in patients with acute renal failure. JPEN J Parenter Enteral Nutr 1996;20:56–62.
16. Kierdorf H. Continuous versus intermittent treatment: Clinical results in acute renal failure. Contrib Nephrol 1991;93:1–12.
17. Himmelfarb J, Tolkoff Rubin N, Chandran P, et al. A multicenter comparison of dialysis membranes in the treatment of acute renal failure requiring dialysis. J Am Soc Nephrol 1998;9:257–266.
18. Blantz RC. Pathophysiology of pre-renal azotemia. Kidney Int 1998; 53:512–523.
19. Moore K, Wendon J, Frazer M, et al. Plasma endothelin immunoreactivity in liver disease and the hepatorenal syndrome. N Engl J Med 1992;327:1774–1778.
20. Parmley WW. Pathophysiology and current therapy of congestive heart failure. J Am Coll Cardiol 1989;13:771–785.
21. Dunnick NR, Sfakianakis GN. Screening for renovascular hypertension. Radiol Clin North Am 1991;29:497–510.
22. Brezis M, Rosen S, Silva P, Epstein FH. Selective vulnerability of the medullary thick ascending limb to anoxia in the isolated perfused rat kidney. J Clin Invest 1984;73:182–190.
23. Kaufman J, Dhakal M, Patel B, Hamburger R. Community-acquired acute renal failure. Am J Kidney Dis 1991;17:191–198.
24. Rahman SN, Conger JD. Glomerular and tubular factors in urine flow rates of acute renal failure. Am J Kidney Dis 1994;23:788–793.
25. Agmon Y, Brezis M. Acute renal failure: A multifactorial syndrome. In: Bourke E, Mallik NP, Pollak VE, eds. Moving Points in Nephrology. Contributions in Nephrology, vol. 102. Basel, Karger, 1993: 23–36.
26. Paller MS. Pathophysiology of acute renal failure. In: Greenberg A, ed. Primer on Kidney Diseases, 1st ed. San Diego, Academic Press, 1994:126–133.
27. Lieberthal W. Biology of acute renal failure: Therapeutic implications. Kidney Int 1997;52:1102–1115.
28. Weisberg LS, Allgren RL, Genter FC, Kurnik BRC. Cause of acute tubular necrosis affects its prognosis. Arch Intern Med 1997;157: 1833–1838.
29. Hou SH, Bushinsky DA, Wish JB, et al. Hospital-acquired renal insufficiency: A prospective study. Am J Med 1983;74:243–248.
30. Corwin HL, Teplick RS, Schreiber MJ, et al. Prediction of outcome in acute renal failure. Am J Nephrol 1987;7:8–12.
31. Conger JD. Does hemodialysis delay recovery from acute renal failure? Semin Dial 1990;3:146–148.
32. Vidt DG. Recognition and management of reversible renal failure. South Med J 1994;87:1018–1027.
33. Levy EM, Viscoli CM, Horwitz RI. The effect of acute renal failure on mortality. JAMA 1996;275;1489–1494.
34. Barrett BJ. Contrast nephrotoxicity. J Am Soc Nephrol 1994;5: 125–137.
35. Fisher MA, Talbot GH, Maislin G, et al. Risk factors for amphotericin B-associated nephrotoxicity. Am J Med 1989;87:547–552.
36. Zaske DE. Aminoglycosides. In: Evans WE, Schentag JJ, Jusko WJ, eds. Applied Pharmacokinetics, 3rd ed. Vancouver, WA, Applied Therapeutics, 1992.
37. Yura T, Badr KF, Yuasa S, et al. Alleviation of cisplatin nephrotoxicity: Efficacy of local intra-arterial injection concomitant with hemodialysis. Blood Purif 1996;14:146–156.
38. Prins JM, Buller HR, Kuijper EJ, et al. Once versus thrice daily gentamicin in patients with serious infections. Lancet 1993;341: 335–339.
39. Ferriols-Lisart R, Alos-Alminana M. Effectiveness and safety of once daily aminoglycosides: A meta-analysis. Am J Health Syst Pharm 1996;53:1141–1150.
40. Hatala R, Dinh T, Cook DJ. Once daily aminoglycoside dosing in immunocompetent adults: A meta-analysis. Ann Intern Med 1996; 124:717–725.
41. Munckhof WJ, Grayson ML, Turnidge JD. A meta-analysis of studies on the safety and efficacy of aminoglycosides given either once daily or as divided doses. J Antimicrob Chemother 1996;37: 645–663.
42. Rind DM, Safran C, Phillips RS, et al. Effect of computer-based alerts on the treatment and outcomes of hospitalized patients. Arch Intern Med 1994;154:1511–1517.
43. Ellis JH, Cohan RH, Sonnad SS, Cohan NS. Selective use of radiographic low-osmolality contrast media in the 1990's. Radiology 1996;200:297–311.
44. Levin DC, Gardiner GA Jr, Karasick S, et al. Cost containment in the use of low-osmolar contrast agents: Effect of guidelines, monitoring, and feedback mechanisms. Radiology 1993;189:753–757.
45. Hunter TB, Dye J, Duval JF. Selective use of low-osmolality contrast agents for IV urography and CT: Safety and effect on cost. Am J Roentgenol 1994;163:965–968.
46. Rapp RP, Gubbins PO, Evans ME. Amphotericin B lipid complex. Ann Pharmacother 1997;31:1174–1186.
47. Sorkine P, Nagar H, Weinbroum A, et al. Administration of amphotericin B in lipid emulsion decreases nephrotoxicity: Results of a prospective, randomized, controlled study in critically ill patients. Crit Care Med 1996;24:1311–1315.
48. Chasty RC, Lin-Yin JA. Acute tumour lysis syndrome. Br J Hosp Med 1993;49:488–492.
49. Hock R, Anderson RJ. Prevention of drug-induced nephrotoxicity in the intensive care unit. J Crit Care 1995;10:33–43.
50. Heidemann HT, Gerkens JF, Spickard WA, Jackson EK, Branch RA. Amphotericin B nephrotoxicity in humans decreased by salt repletion. Am J Med 1983;75:476–481.
51. Llanos A, Cieza J, Bernardo J, et al. Effect of salt supplementation on amphotericin B nephrotoxicity. Kidney Int 1991;40:302–308.

52. Anderson CM. Sodium chloride treatment of amphotericin B nephrotoxicity—standard of care? West J Med 1995;162:313–317.
53. Solomon R, Werner C, Mann D, D'Elia J, Silva P. Effects of saline, mannitol, and furosemide on acute decreases in renal function induced by radiocontrast agents. N Engl J Med 1994;331:1416–1420.
54. Conger JD. Interventions in clinical acute renal failure: What are the data? Am J Kidney Dis 1995;26:565–576.
55. Conger J. Prophylaxis and treatment of acute renal failure by vasoactive agents: The fact and myths. Kidney Int 1998;53(suppl 64): S23–S26.
56. Russo D, Testa A, Della Volpe L, Sansone G. Randomized prospective study on renal effects of two different contrast media in humans: Protective role of calcium channel blocker. Nephron 1990;55: 254–257.
57. Khoury Z, Schlicht JR, Como J, et al. The effect of prophylactic nifedipine on renal function in patients administered contrast media. Pharmacotherapy 1995;15:59–65.
58. Erley CM, Duda SH, Schlepckow S, et al. Adenosine antagonist theophylline prevents the reduction in glomerular filtration rate after contrast dye application. Kidney Int 1994;45:1425–1431.
59. Katholi RE, Taylor GJ, McCann WP, et al. Nephrotoxicity from contrast media: attenuation with theophylline. Radiology 1995;195: 17–22.
60. White JR, Rockwood T, Wilson D, Bettesworth L, Icenogle T. The effects of pentoxifylline on the prevention of cyclosporine-induced nephrotoxicity in cardiac transplant patients. Clin Ther 1994;16: 673–679.
61. Pouteil-Noble C, Chapiuis F, Berra N, et al. Misoprostil in renal transplant recipients: A prospective, randomized, controlled study on the prevention of acute rejection episodes and cyclosporine A nephrotoxicity. Nephrol Dial Transplant 1994;9:552–555.
62. Majumdar S, Kjellstrand CM. Why do we use diuretics in acute renal failure? Semin Dial 1996;9:454–459.
63. Vargo DL, Kramer WG, Black PK, et al. Bioavailability, pharmacokinetics, and pharmacodynamics of torsemide and furosemide in patients with congestive heart failure. Clin Pharmacol Ther 1995;57: 601–609.
64. Brater DC. Clinical pharmacology of loop diuretics. Drugs 1991;41 (suppl 3):14–22.
65. Martin SJ, Danziger LH. Continuous infusion of loop diuretics in the critically ill: A review of the literature. Crit Care Med 1994; 22:1323–1329.
66. Yelton SL, Gaylor MA, Murray KM. The role of continuous infusion loop diuretics. Ann Pharmacother 1995;29:1010–1014.
67. Dormans TPJ, van Meyel JJM, Gerlag PGG, et al. Diuretic efficacy of high dose furosemide in severe heart failure: Bolus injection versus continuous infusion. J Am Coll Cardiol 1996;28:376–382.
68. Schuller D, Lynch JP, Fine D. Protocol-guided diuretic management: Comparison of furosemide by continuous infusion and intermittent bolus. Crit Care Med 1997;25:1969–1975.
69. Rudy DW, Voelker JR, Greene PK, Esparza FA, Brater DC . Loop diuretics for chronic renal insufficiency: A continuous infusion is more efficacious than bolus therapy. Ann Intern Med 1991;115:360–366.
70. Kramer WG, Smith WB, Ferguson J, et al. Pharmacodynamics of torsemide administered as an intravenous injection and as a continuous infusion to patients with congestive heart failure. J Clin Pharmacol 1996;36:265–270.
71. Sica DA, Gehr TWB. Diuretic combinations in refractory oedema states. Clin Pharmacokinet 1996;3:229–249.
72. Ellison DH. The physiologic basis of diuretic synergism: Its role in treating diuretic resistance. Ann Intern Med 1991;114:886–894.
73. Segar JL, Chemtob S, Bell EF. Changes in body water compartments with diuretic therapy in infants with chronic lung disease. Early Hum Dev 1997;48:99–107.
74. Duke GJ, Briedis JH, Weaver RA. Renal support in critically ill patients: Low-dose dopamine or low-dose dobutamine? Crit Care Med 1994;22:1919–1925.
75. Varriale P, Mossavi A. The benefit of low-dose dopamine during vigorous diuresis for congestive heart failure associated with renal insufficiency: Does it protect renal function? Clin Cardiol 1997;20: 627–630.
76. Weisberg LS, Kurnik PS, Kurnik BR. Dopamine and renal blood flow in radiocontrast induced nephrotoxicity. Ren Fail 1993;15: 61–67.
77. Chertow GM, Sayegh MH, Allgren RL, Lazarus JM. Is the administration of dopamine associated with adverse or favorable outcomes in acute renal failure? Am J Med 1996;101:49–53.
78. Bailey AR, Burchett KR. Effect of low-dose dopamine on serum concentrations of prolactin in critically ill patients. Br J Anaesth 1997;78:97–99.
79. Harper L, Savage COS. The use of dopamine in acute renal failure. Clin Nephrol 1997;47:347–349. Letter.
80. Allgren RL, Marbury TC, Rahman SN, et al. Anaritide in acute tubular necrosis. N Engl J Med 1997;336:828–834.
81. Alkhunaizi AM, Schrier RW. Management of acute renal failure: New perspectives. Am J Kidney Dis 1996;28:315–328.
82. Grino JM. BN 52021: A platelet activating factor antagonist for preventing post-transplant renal failure. Ann Intern Med 1994;121: 345–347.
83. López-Novoa JM, Rodríguez-Barbero A, Eleno N. The role of platelet-activating factor and the effect of PAF blocking receptors on the outcome of ARF. Ren Fail 1996;18:489–499.
84. Simon EE. Potential role of integrins in acute renal failure. Nephrol Dial Transplant 1994;9(suppl 4):26–33.
85. Rabelink TJ, Kaasjager KAH, Stroes ESG, Koomans HA. Endothelin in renal pathophysiology: From experimental to therapeutic application. Kidney Int 1996;50:1827–1833.
86. Hammerman MR. Potential role of growth factors in the prophylaxis and treatment of acute renal failure. Kidney Int 1998;53(suppl 64): S19–S22.
87. Kone BC. Nitric oxide in renal health and disease. Am J Kidney Dis 1997;30:311–333.
88. Yoshimura A, Taira T, Ideura T. Expression of apoptosis-related molecules in acute renal injury. Exp Nephrol 1996;4:15–18.
89. Gillis JC, Brogden RN. Ketorolac. Drugs 1997;53:139–188.
90. Feldman HI, Kinman JL, Berlin JA, et al. Parenteral ketorolac: The risk for acute renal failure. Ann Intern Med 1997;126:193–199.
91. Woodrow G, Turney JH. Cause of death in acute renal failure. Nephrol Dial Transplant 1992;7:230–234.
92. Ben-Menachem T, Fogel R, Patel RV, et al. Prophylaxis for stress-related gastric hemorrhage in the medical intensive care unit. Ann Intern Med 1994;121:568–575.
93. Clark WR, Mueller BA, Kraus MA, Macias WL. Extracorporeal therapy requirements for patients with acute renal failure. J Am Soc Nephrol 1997;8:804–812.
94. Scott MK, Mueller BA, Kraus MA, et al. Intradialytic vancomycin administration: Dialysis membrane effects. Pharmacotherapy 1997; 17:256–262.
95. Pollard TA, Lampasona V, Akkerman S, et al. Vancomycin redistribution: Dosing recommendations following high-flux hemodialysis. Kidney Int 1994;45:232–237.
96. Ragaller M, Werner C, Bleyl J, et al. Blood compatible polymers in intensive care units: State of the art and current aspects of biomaterials research. Kidney Int 1998;53(suppl 64):S84–S90.
97. Manji N, Shikora S, McMahon M, Blackburn GL, Bistrian BR. Peritoneal dialysis for acute renal failure: Overfeeding resulting from dextrose absorbed during dialysis. Crit Care Med 1990;18: 29–31.
98. Joy MS, Matzke GR, Armstrong DK, Marx MA, Zarowitz BJ. A primer on continuous renal replacement therapy for critically ill patients. Ann Pharmacother 1998;32:362–375.
99. van Bommel EFH. Should continuous renal replacement therapy be used for "non-renal" indications in critically ill patients with shock? Resuscitation 1997;33:257–270.

100. Bressolle F, Kinowski JM, de la Coussaye JE, et al. Clinical pharmacokinetics during continuous hemofiltration. Clin Pharmacokinet 1994;26:457–471.
101. Reetze-Bonorden P, Bhler J, Keller E. Drug dosage in patients during continuous renal replacement therapy. Clin Pharmacokinet 1993; 24:362–379.
102. DuBose TD, Warnock DG, Mehta RL, et al. Acute renal failure in the 21st century: Recommendations for management and outcomes assessment. Am J Kidney Dis 1997;29:793–799.
103. Gretz N, Quintel M, Krnzlin B. Extracorporeal therapies in acute renal failure: Different therapeutic options. Kidney Int 1998;53(suppl 53):S57–S60.
104. Schulman G, Hakim R. Hemodialysis membrane biocompatibility in acute renal failure. Adv Ren Replace Ther 1994;1:75–82.
105. Sponsel H, Conger JD. Is parenteral nutrition therapy of value in acute renal failure patients? Am J Kidney Dis 1995;25:96–102.
106. Monson P, Mehta RL. Nutritional considerations in continuous renal replacement therapies. Semin Dial 1996;9:152–160.
107. Elston AC, Bayliss MK, Park GR. Effect of renal failure on drug metabolism by the liver. Br J Anaesth 1993;71:282–290.
108. Matzke GR, Frye RF. Drug administration in patients with renal insufficiency. Minimising renal and extrarenal toxicity. Drug Saf 1997;16:205–231.
109. Macias WL, Mueller BA, Scarim SK. Vancomycin pharmacokinetics in acute renal failure: Preservation of non-renal clearance. Clin Pharmacol Ther 1991;50:688–694.
110. Mueller BA, Scarim SK, Macias WL. Comparison of imipenem pharmacokinetics in patients with acute or chronic renal failure treated with continuous hemofiltration. Am J Kidney Dis 1993;21: 172–179.
111. Tegeder I, Bremer F, Oelkers R, et al. Pharmacokinetics of imipenem-cilastatin in critically ill patients undergoing continuous venovenous hemofiltration. Antimicrob Agents Chemother 1997;41: 2640–2645.
112. Hamel MB, Phillips RS, Davis RB, et al. Outcomes and cost-effectiveness of initiating dialysis and continuing aggressive care in seriously ill hospitalized adults. SUPPORT Investigators. Study to Understand Prognoses and Preferences for Outcomes and Risks of Treatments. Ann Intern Med 1997;127:195–202.
113. Chertow GM. Dialysis: Cost-effective "SUPPORT" for patients with acute renal failure. Am J Kidney Dis 1998;31:545–549.
114. Moreno L, Heyka RJ, Paganini EP. Continuous renal replacement therapy: cost considerations and reimbursement. Semin Dial 1996;9: 209–214.

42

Chronic Renal Insufficiency and End-Stage Renal Disease

Wendy L. St. Peter, PharmD, BCPS, and Matthew J. Lewis, PharmD, BCPS

The normal human kidneys contain approximately two million functionally integrated glomerulotubular units called nephrons. Under normal conditions these nephrons work in a highly organized fashion to filter, reabsorb, and excrete various solutes and fluid. In addition, the kidney plays an important role in the metabolism of various peptide hormones and in the production of renin, ammonia, erythropoietin (EPO), and 1,25-dihydroxyvitamin D_3.

Renal disease is characterized by disturbances in many of these normal functions. Evidence suggests that even as renal disease develops and adaptations take place, functioning (remnant) nephrons continue to work in a highly organized fashion. Although total kidney glomerular filtration rate (GFR) falls, the GFR of remnant nephrons rises. This adaptation blunts the drop in whole kidney glomerular filtration rate that would occur in the absence of compensatory changes. Unfortunately, this adaptive hyperfiltration process ultimately results in glomerular hypertension, which plays a significant role in glomerular injury. Indeed, in most instances when serum creatinine rises above 2 to 3 mg/dL or creatinine clearance (CrCl) falls to approximately 25 to 40 mL/min, the injury process will progress to end-stage renal failure regardless of the initial etiology of kidney disease.[1]

Solute balance is maintained in chronic renal insufficiency by increases in the fractional excretion of solutes such as sodium, potassium, creatinine, blood urea nitrogen, and phosphorus by remnant nephrons, although the adaptive mechanisms differ in each case. The urinary excretion of any substance is dependent upon the amount of solute filtered at the glomerulus plus the net contribution of tubular secretion and tubular reabsorption.

$$\text{Excretion} = \text{Filtered Load} + \text{Tubular Secretion} - \text{Tubular Reabsorption}$$

$$\text{Filtered Load} = \text{Glomerular Filtration Rate} \times \text{Plasma Concentration}$$

$$\text{Fractional Excretion} = \frac{\text{Amount Excreted}}{\text{Filtered Load}}$$

There are several ways in which remnant nephrons can adapt to maintain solute balance. Plasma concentrations of solutes that undergo minimal tubular secretion or reabsorption, such as creatinine and blood urea nitrogen, rise predictably as renal function declines. This results in an increase in the filtered load presented to each tubule, which allows remnant nephrons to increase excretion proportionally. Serum creatinine rises in proportion to the decline in GFR and can be used clinically to estimate renal function (Chap. 40). Renal tubular reabsorption is the predominant mechanism that regulates excretion for sodium and phosphorus; therefore, in chronic renal insufficiency, tubular reabsorption of these solutes decreases in order to prevent or minimize the increase in plasma concentrations. Potassium balance is maintained via further increases in distal tubular secretion, which is potassium's primary excretory pathway. Thus, the plasma concentrations of some solutes rise while the plasma concentrations of others remain relatively constant until residual renal function is quite low.

There may be "trade-offs" to many of these adaptations that actually contribute to the uremic state and its complications.[2] An understanding of these renal adaptations is crucial to an understanding of the conservative management of chronic renal insufficiency, because many therapeutic interventions follow logically from the disordered physiology. The first part of the chapter discusses chronic renal insufficiency and related treatments while the last part mainly focuses on the complications and consequences of end-stage renal disease (ESRD) and their treatment.

DEFINITIONS

For practical purposes the clinical course of progressive renal disease can be divided into four stages. The accompanying signs and symptoms and laboratory parameters of each stage are described in Figure 42–1.

- *Minimal renal insufficiency/decreased renal reserve* (CrCl 60 to 90 mL/min). The glomerular filtration rate, as measured by the CrCl, may decrease by as much as 50% before the plasma concentrations of creatinine (S_{Cr}) or urea nitrogen rise above the normal range. Adaptive increases in solute excretion in remaining nephrons compensate for the decline in functioning kidney mass.
- *Mild renal insufficiency* (CrCl 30 to 60 mL/min). A thorough evaluation to determine the etiology of the renal impairment is especially critical at this point, because the underlying disease process may reverse or stabilize with appropriate treatment.
- *Moderate renal insufficiency* (CrCl 15 to 30 mL/min). In general, patients with this degree of renal dysfunction

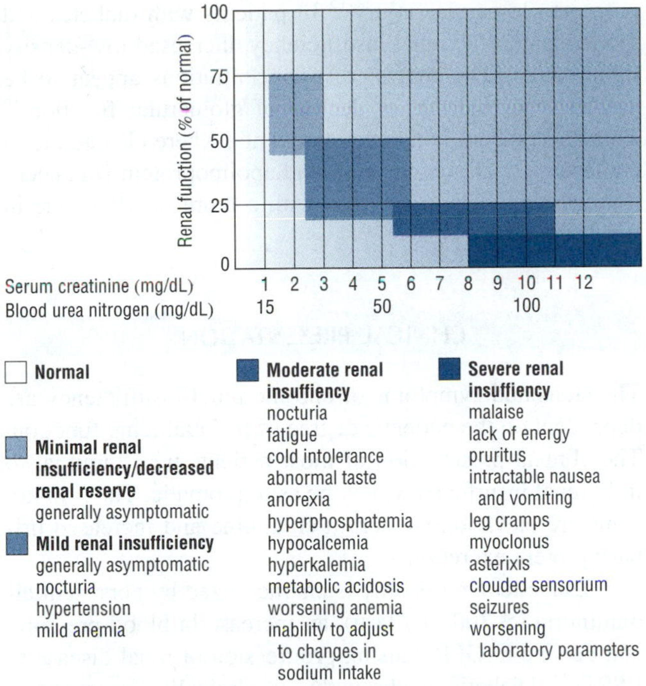

FIGURE 42–1. Staging of chronic renal disease. *(Adapted from Knochel JP. The pathophysiology of uremia. Hospital Pract 1981;16:67, with permission. Illustration by Albert Miller.)*

will progress to end-stage renal disease albeit at individual rates of decline. Nephrologists often use a plot of $1/S_{Cr}$ versus time to evaluate disease progression in individual patients. Unfortunately, the relationship between GFR and $1/S_{Cr}$ is not constant over time; changes in tubular secretion, extrarenal elimination, and rate of generation of creatinine in patients with renal insufficiency can alter the $1/S_{Cr}$ slope without a change in GFR. Therefore, misinterpretation of the rate of decline in renal function can occur if this is the only method used to estimate renal function[3] (see Chap. 40).

- *Severe renal insufficiency/uremia* (CrCl < 15 mL/min). Uremia is a clinical syndrome that develops insidiously as renal function declines. It begins with nonspecific symptoms, which become progressively worse as the creatinine clearance drops below 10 mL/min. It is at this stage that dialysis is indicated to remove the byproducts of protein metabolism, such as urea, thought to be largely responsible for this symptom complex (see Chap. 44). The patient requiring chronic dialysis or renal transplantation for relief of uremic symptoms is said to have ESRD.

EPIDEMIOLOGY OF END-STAGE RENAL DISEASE

Many diseases of the kidney, either idiopathic or secondary to systemic illness, can ultimately result in ESRD. Over 257,200 Americans were treated for ESRD in 1995.[4] Black individuals have approximately a four-fold greater rate of renal failure than white individuals. The average life expectancy of a 20- and 60-year-old ESRD patient in the United States is only 17 to 21 and 4 to 5 years, respectively, compared to 47 to 60 and 16 to 23 years, respectively, for an adult without ESRD.[4]

The incidence of ESRD has increased an average of 8.8% annually for the last several years, with the largest increase in the 65- to 79-year-old population.[4] However, the most recent data suggests that both the incidence and prevalence rates may be declining.[4] The largest increase in incidence has been in African Americans and Native Americans. Diabetes, hypertension, and primary glomerulonephritis are the three most common causes of ESRD in the United States. Even though type 1 diabetes accounts for only 5% to 10% of newly diagnosed diabetes in the U.S. population, it accounts for 41% of new ESRD patients with a primary diagnosis of diabetes.[5] Sixty-three percent of Native Americans and 38% of white ESRD patients develop renal failure as a direct result of diabetes mellitus.[4]

Hypertension is the cause of ESRD in 26% of newly diagnosed ESRD patients.[4] Patients who develop ESRD secondary to renal artery stenosis and cholesterol emboli are also categorized under hypertension. Glomerulonephritis, cystic kidney disease, and HIV nephropathy account for approximately 11%, 3%, and <1%, respectively, of new ESRD cases. In 1996, the annual cost to treat an individual with ESRD on dialytic therapy was $46,000, compared to $16,000 for an individual with a renal transplant, with 75% of the cost borne by the federal government. This translated into total expenditures of over $13 billion in 1995 for the U.S. ESRD program.[4]

PROGRESSION OF RENAL DISEASE

PATHOPHYSIOLOGY

The exact mechanisms involved in the pathogenesis of progressive renal insufficiency have not been fully elucidated, but most individuals with creatinine clearance of 25 to 40 mL/min or less progress to ESRD regardless of the underlying etiology.[1] Based on experimental animal models, hemodynamic changes at the glomerulus have been shown to exert a major influence on and/or regulate the rate of progression of renal disease.[6] Increased glomerular capillary plasma flow and glomerular capillary hydraulic pressure lead to glomerular hyperfiltration. Glomerulo hyperfiltration and hypertension lead to progressive glomerulosclerosis and development of overt proteinuria.[6] In addition, glomerular capillary hypertension contributes directly to the function of remaining intact nephrons. In experimental renal disease, pharmacologic or dietary interventions that decrease glomerular capillary pressure limit the rate and extent of overt proteinuria and glomerulosclerosis.[1] The presence of systemic hypertension is not required for the development of glomerular hyperfiltration and hypertension but, when present may amplify the pathologic effects of these intrarenal changes.[7] Early hyperfiltration is followed by persistent microalbuminuria.[8] Proteinuria may be an independent risk factor for progression of renal disease.[9] In addition, formation of advanced glycation end-products within the kidney of diabetic patients may also play a role.[10] Other risk factors considered important in the pathogenesis of progressive renal failure are summarized in Figure 42–2. A reduction of filtration area secondary to glomerular cell injury can lead to hemodynamic changes that increase glomerular capillary pressure and lead to functional and structural changes in the glomerulus. These pathologic processes lead to glomerulosclerosis, causing an elevation of systemic blood pressure, which may elicit further renal structure damage and consequent worsening of blood pressure control.[7,11,12]

The exact mechanisms involved in the development of ESRD among hypertensive individuals remains controversial. However, some of the major mechanisms include ischemia in the renal tubule causing reduction of renal mass and increased glomerular capillary pressure.[1,13]

Hyperlipidemia is a major risk factor associated with progression of renal disease.[14] Experimental studies in rats have demonstrated accelerated glomerulosclerosis when dietary cholesterol supplementation is given in the presence of various renal diseases, whereas pharmacologic therapy or low-fat diets have been shown to limit the progression of renal disease.[1] Lipid metabolism abnormalities alone in patients with normal renal function have not been shown to promote glomerular injury.[15] In patients with diabetes and moderate chronic renal insufficiency, increased low-density lipoprotein (LDL cholesterol) concentrations appear to be predictive of the rate of decline of glomerular function.[16] This differs from nondiabetic patients, where elevated total cholesterol, LDL cholesterol, and apolipoprotein B concentrations have been associated with a more rapid decline in renal function.[17]

CLINICAL PRESENTATION

The signs and symptoms of chronic renal insufficiency are dependent on the patient's degree of residual renal function. The clinical presentation of most patients with minimal to mild renal insufficiency may be asymptomatic. The primary signs are elevations in serum creatinine and increased urinary protein excretion.

Diabetic nephropathy is characterized by persistent albuminuria (> 300 mg/24 h), an increase in blood pressure, and decline in GFR causing progression of renal disease to ESRD.[18] Diabetic nephropathy is clinically diagnosed if persistent proteinuria, defined as a total protein excretion exceeding 500 mg/24 h (equivalent to urinary albumin excretion [UAE] rate of 300 mg/24 h) present in two out of three consecutive urine samples. If the UAE ranges between 30 and 300 mg/24 h, the patient is classified as having persistent microalbuminuria.[19] Clinical studies in diabetic patients have demonstrated that persistent microalbuminuria is highly predictive of progression of renal dis-

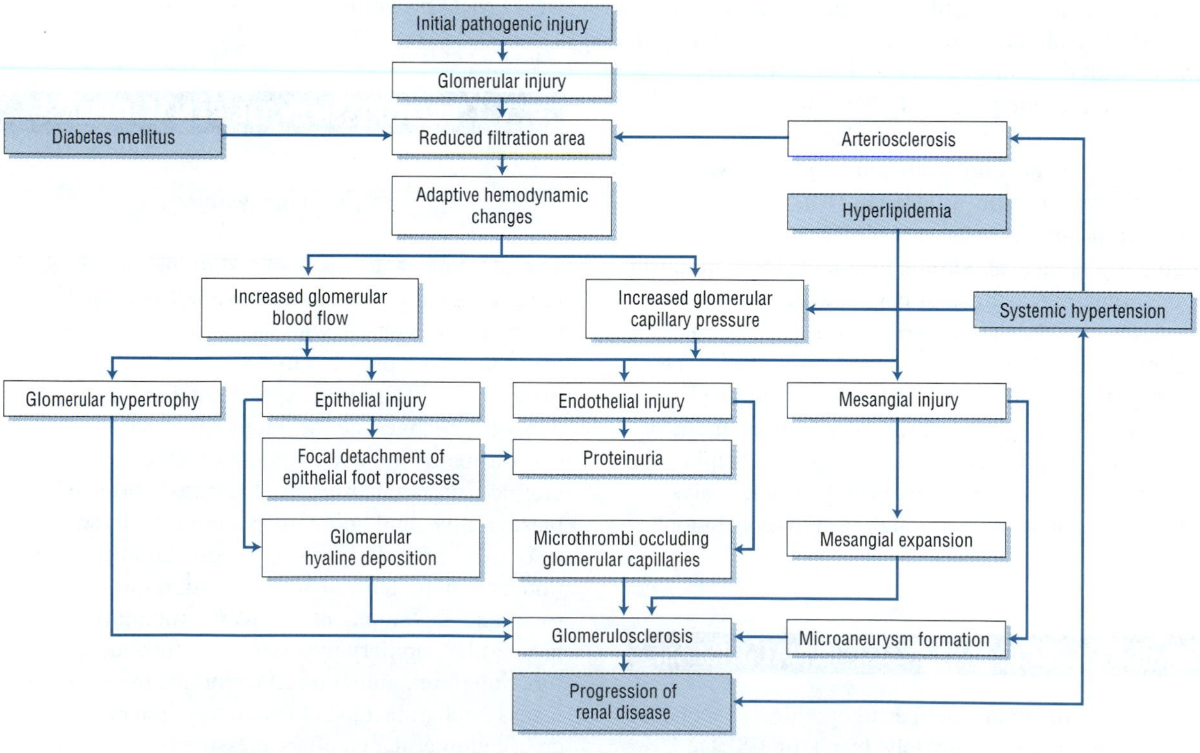

FIGURE 42–2. Proposed mechanisms for progression of renal disease.

ease and is one of the best available early predictors of diabetic nephropathy.[19]

Nondiabetic patients—those with glomerulonephritis, hypertension, polycystic kidney disease, or other causes—may also have proteinuria. Microalbuminuria occurs in approximately 30% of hypertensive patients, which is a risk factor for an increased overall mortality rate.[20] The increased UAE in hypertension may be induced by renal hemodynamic changes (Fig. 42–2), glomerular filter permeability changes, and glomerular structural changes due to nephrosclerosis. The urinary excretion of protein is generally greater than 2.5 g/d in those with glomerulonephritis. As a consequence of this, these individuals may have hyperlipidemia and edema (see Chap. 46).

▶ TREATMENT: Progressive Renal Disease

DESIRED OUTCOME

The availability of chronic dialysis and renal transplantation is limited and expensive. In addition, these treatments are associated with early morbidity and mortality and a less than optimal quality of life.[21] Recent clinical trials have focused on the use of pharmacologic and nonpharmacologic interventions to reverse or delay progressive renal injury before patients reach the point of irreversibility. Treatment and prevention programs focusing on major risk factors, such as diabetes and hypertension, that promote progression of renal disease will hopefully reduce the incidence and prevalence of ESRD. The goals of therapy include stabilizing renal function for those with a GFR above 40 mL/min and slowing the rate of progression for those in the range of 25 to 40 mL/min.

DIABETICS

GENERAL APPROACH TO TREATMENT

SCREENING MICROALBUMINURIA

Type 1 diabetic patients with elevated UAE are at high risk to develop overt nephropathy within 10 to 14 years.[19] Therefore, early detection of microalbuminuria facilitates therapeutic intervention that can slow the progression of renal disease and other vascular complications.[22] Accurate assays that can detect UAE between 30 and 300 mg/24 h have been developed.[18] Routine dipstick urinalysis does not measure UAE less than 150 mg/d and should not be used to screen for microalbuminuria. Another acceptable alternative method is measurement of the albumin–creatinine ratio in the first morning urine sample. A urinary albumin–creatinine ratio between 30 and 300 mg/g can identify patients at high risk to develop diabetic nephropathy.[23] All type 1 diabetic patients of over 5 years' duration and all type 2 diabetics should have their urine checked annually for microalbuminuria. If two out of three collections over a 3- to 6-month period demonstrate microalbuminuria, therapy is indicated.[24] It is important to note there are several factors that can acutely increase the UAE. These factors include recent heavy exercise or high-protein meal, hematuria, urinary tract infection, uncontrolled hypertension or poor glycemic control, and congestive heart failure. Initial screening or rescreening should be postponed under any of these circumstances.

NONPHARMACOLOGIC THERAPY

NUTRITIONAL MANAGEMENT

A number of clinical trials have attempted to determine whether dietary protein restriction retards the rate of chronic renal disease progression. Pedrini and colleagues examined the effect of protein restriction in diabetic renal disease using a meta-analysis. There were five trials in the analysis, which encompassed a total of only 108 patients. It was determined that a low-protein diet (range, 0.5 to 0.85 g/kg/d) reduced the risk of decline in GFR or the increase in urinary albumin excretion rate.[25] It should be noted that the analysis was done with a small number of patients and a variety of study designs and therefore may not provide definitive proof but rather a good indication that dietary restriction in diabetic patients may be beneficial.

PHARMACOLOGIC THERAPY

INTENSIVE BLOOD GLUCOSE CONTROL

Intensive blood glucose control in type 1 patients has been reported to reduce the frequency, decrease the severity, and delay the development or progression of diabetic complications including nephropathy in a number of randomized clinical trials.[26] Although most of these studies included small numbers of subjects (less than 100) and short duration of follow-up (less than 5 years), this meta-analysis of 16 clinical trials demonstrated a statistically significant benefit (decreased risk) of nephropathy in those on long-term intensive insulin therapy[26] (see Chap. 70).

The diabetes control and complications trial (DCCT) was a multicenter (1441 patients), randomized study designed with sufficient statistical power to compare intensive versus standard diabetes therapy with regard to effects on the development and progression of diabetic nephropathy, retinopathy, and neuropathy.[27] Intensive therapy either by the administration of insulin three or more times daily by injection or by external pump reduced the incidence of microalbuminuria and albuminuria when compared to conventional therapy in both a primary prevention (n = 726) and a secondary prevention (n = 715) group.[27] Unfortunately, long-term rigid glycemic control with insulin was associated with a higher incidence of hypoglycemic reactions.[27] However, decreased diabetic complications in the intensive therapy group outweighed the increased risk of hypoglycemia.[28] A longer follow-up period is needed to evaluate the degree by which intensive glucose control will prevent or delay the development of diabetic nephropathy.[28] A potential barrier to obtaining the same results as the DCCT is the feasibility of implementing these recommendations into clinical practice. Studies have shown that many poorly controlled type 1 diabetic patients are reluctant to comply with these recommendations.[29]

ANTIHYPERTENSIVE AGENTS

Elevated blood pressure is observed more often in type 1 patients with persistent microalbuminuria when compared to nonmicroalbuminuric type 1 patients. Blood pressure continues to rise or may develop at the onset of diabetic nephropathy and becomes more problematic with the progression of renal insufficiency (Fig. 42–2).

Many studies have demonstrated that adequate blood pressure control can reduce the rate of decline in GFR and albuminuria in hypertensive patients with either type 1 or type 2 diabetes.[1] A long-term study in type 1 patients with microalbuminuria demonstrated that blood pressure control with β-blocker and diuretic therapy decreased UAE.[30] Animal models of diabetic nephropathy have demonstrated that decreasing glomerular capillary pressure and volume preserves renal function.[31] Angiotensin-converting enzyme inhibitors (ACEIs) reduce both of these parameters.[32]

A meta-analysis of 100 controlled and uncontrolled clinical studies assessed the relative effect of different antihypertensive agents on proteinuria and renal function in type 1 and type 2 patients.[33] None of the antihypertensive agents or classes analyzed had a greater effect on blood pressure reduction than any other agent or class. However, only ACEIs decreased proteinuria and preserved GFR independent of the beneficial effects associated with blood pressure reduction.

Given the preliminary evidence for the potential benefit of ACEIs in diabetic nephropathy, a multicenter controlled clinical trial was designed to determine if long-term administration of captopril in type 1 patients with nephropathy (n = 409) would reduce the progression of renal failure independent of its blood pressure lowering effect.[34] This pivotal trial showed that captopril can slow the progression of renal disease. This effect was independent of blood pressure reduction and of greatest benefit in those with the lowest renal function

A 5-year double-blind trial of enalapril 10 mg every day or placebo in normotensive type 2 patients with microalbuminuria resulted in stabilization of plasma creatinine concentrations and decreased albuminuria in the enalapril group as compared to the placebo group.[35] Unfortunately, the investigators monitored renal function using $1/S_{Cr}$, which is a relatively crude way to monitor progression of renal disease.[35] Also, a large-scale clinical trial (n = 530) with lisinopril showed reductions in proteinuria in normotensive type 1 diabetic patients with microalbuminuria.[36] A variety of ACEI doses and agents have been studied and therefore a specific ACEI agent or starting dose cannot be defined. It would seem logical in normotensive patients with microalbuminuria to start with a low ACEI dose and titrate up to alleviate the microalbuminuria and yet avoid hypotension. In hypertensive patients, the obvious goal is to optimally control the blood pressure to the desired level and minimize protein losses.

Because ACEI therapy improves patient outcomes, the role of angiotensin 1 (AT-1) receptor antagonists in slowing the progression of renal disease is also being investigated. Several experimental models of chronic progressive renal disease have shown the two treatments to have similar efficacy. AT-1 receptor antagonists candesartan and lorsartan have both proven to slow the progression of glomerulopathy in diabetic rats.[37] However, there is limited data on AT-1 receptor antagonist use in humans with progressive renal disease. The Evaluation of Losartan in the Elderly (ELITE) study compared losartan versus captopril in 722 (25% diabetics) patients over 65 years old with heart failure. The study did show that there was no difference in renal dysfunction among these heart failure patients at both baseline and study completion.[38] Bradykinins may play an important role in renal hemodynamics.[39] Because ACEIs prevent the degradation of bradykinins and AT-1 receptor antagonists lack this effect, more information is necessary before the agents can be considered interchangeable. Combination therapy with ACEI and AT-1 receptor antagonists may be beneficial; however, further investigation is necessary.

Although calcium channel blockers (CCBs) mainly dilate the afferent arteriole and result in no change or an increase in glomerular capillary pressure, they have been shown to decrease glomerular injury without changing renal hemodynamics.[32] The postulated mechanisms for this decrease in renal injury include suppression of glomerular hypertrophy, inhibition of platelet aggregation, and decreased salt accumulation.[32] Three recent meta-analyses suggest that diabetic patients tended to have an increase or no reduction in albuminuria if they were treated with dihydropyridine calcium antagonists.[40,41] However, one of these meta-analyses also concluded that nondihydropyridine CCBs may have beneficial effects on proteinuria similar to ACEIs that are independent of blood pressure reductions.[40] Nondihydropyridine CCBs (verapamil SR and diltiazem SR) were compared to lisinopril and atenolol in 52 type 2 patients. The patients treated with lisinopril and the nondihydropyridine CCBs showed a similar and slower progression of renal disease compared to those treated with atenolol.[42] A few studies have looked at combination therapy with ACEIs and nondihydropyridine CCBs. The results suggest that the combination may be better than either agent alone at attenuating the progression to renal failure.[43] Overall, ACEIs and nonhydropyridine CCBs are more effective than other antihypertensive agents at decreasing albuminuria in both type 1 and type 2 diabetics.

NONDIABETICS

GENERAL APPROACH TO TREATMENT

Renal disease secondary to causes other than diabetes (nondiabetic nephropathy) includes glomerular and tubulointerstitial disease, nephrosclerosis, and polycystic kidney disease. These etiologies are frequently grouped together in large clinical trials due to the lower number of subjects with each disease. It is likely that each of these disease states progresses to ESRD and responds to therapeutic interventions differently. For instance, numerous interventions in patients with polycystic kidney disease have not been successful in slowing the progression of renal disease.[44] Therefore, it is difficult to extrapolate data from each trial to define a single optimal treatment pathway for patients with nondiabetic nephropathy, because the general approach to treatment is different.

NONPHARMACOLOGIC THERAPY

NUTRITIONAL MANAGEMENT

A meta-analysis of six randomized clinical trials concluded that patients with mild to severe renal insufficiency who followed a low-protein diet could delay the onset of ESRD.[45] Deficiencies of these clinical trials included inappropriate randomization procedures, differences in methods of assessing renal function, lack of control groups, and poor documentation of patient's compliance to dietary regimens. Some of these clinical trials failed to document if adequate nutrition and quality of life were maintained in these patients on low-protein diets.

The Modification of Diet in Renal Disease (MDRD) multicenter study was a well-designed trial that evaluated the influence of dietary restriction of protein and phosphorus on the progression of renal insufficiency in nondiabetic patients.[46] Results from a pilot study revealed a high correlation between decreased renal function and increased mean blood pressure. Consequently, the full-scale study added blood pressure control as a second independent intervention.

The full-scale MDRD study (n = 840 patients) divided the subjects into moderate (n = 585) and severe (n = 255) renal dysfunction classifications based on GFR, which was determined by the renal clearance of iothalamate. Unfortunately, 24% of the study subjects enrolled had the diagnosis of polycystic kidney disease. This may have confounded the results, because patients with polycystic kidneys may progress to renal failure regardless of the intervention. Subjects in the moderate renal function group (GFR of 25 to 55 mL/min/1.73 m^2) were randomized into one of four groups: usual or a low-protein diet (1.3 versus 0.58 g/kg/d) with a usual or low mean arterial pressure (MAP) goal (107 versus 92 mm Hg). Subjects with severe renal dysfunction (GFR 13 to 24 mL/min/1.73 m^2) were also randomized to one of four groups: a low-protein diet or very-low-protein diet (0.28 g/kg/d along with a keto acid–amino acid supplement) with a usual or low MAP goal as already described. The study concluded that no significant benefit of protein restriction was demonstrated at the end of the follow-up period in either renal disease group when all the patients with different renal disease etiologies were considered together.

However, secondary analyses of the MDRD study suggest that patients with a GFR less than 25 mL/min/1.73 m^2 should have a protein intake of 0.6 g/kg/d to retard the progression of advanced renal disease.[47] The rate of progression to ESRD was significantly reduced by 41% for each 0.2 g/kg/d reduction in dietary protein intake. The discrepancy in results can be explained by the different statistical methods used in the two studies. The original MDRD study used an intent to treat analysis, which accounted for all patients enrolled regardless of their compliance or follow-up. The secondary analyses separated out participants in the high- versus low-protein groups and then analyzed the subjects compliant with the study diet. These analyses demonstrated that if low protein intakes were actually achieved, patients with a GFR less than 25 mL/min/1.73 m^2 would benefit from a protein intake of 0.6 g/kg/d.

PHARMACOLOGIC THERAPY

ANTIHYPERTENSIVE AGENTS

All hypertensive agents do not preserve renal function to the same degree despite equal blood pressure control. It is important to realize that precipitous falls in blood pressure to normotensive levels may be acutely deleterious to renal function in patients with impaired renal function. This may be especially problematic in the patient treated for hypertensive crisis. Target blood pressure should be achieved reasonably slowly so as to allow adaptation to reduced perfusion pressures.[48] In addition, it is preferable to use antihypertensive agents that maintain renal blood flow and thus do not contribute to declining renal function. Table 42–1 outlines the effects of various antihypertensive agents on renal blood flow and glomerular filtration rate.[49,50]

Several short-term (< 12 months) and a few long-term (> 12 months) clinical trials have evaluated the effect of ACEIs on renal hemodynamics in nondiabetic patients.[51] Renal function remained stable during short-term ACEI therapy in the majority of studies. Results from two small long-term studies (1 to 2 years in duration) demonstrated reduction in the rate of progression of renal disease with ACEI therapy. A large randomized, placebo-controlled study compared ramipril to placebo in 166 nondiabetic patients with proteinuria (> 3 g/24 h). It was determined that ramipril reduced proteinuria and rate of GFR decline to a greater extent than what would have been expected from blood pressure reduction alone.[52] Both hypertensive and normotensive patients participated in the study, and all subjects received antihypertensive therapy as needed. Unfortunately, the study did not specify which antihypertensive agents were administered to study participants. Therefore, if nondihydropiridine CCBs were administered to more patients in one group, the results may have been confounded. A subsequent meta-analysis evaluated the effects of ACEIs on the progression of renal disease in 1594 nondiabetic patients from 10 studies. It concluded that ACEIs were more effective than other antihypertensive agents in reducing the progression of renal failure.[53] However, hyperkalemia can complicate their use, especially when patients are concurrently receiving nonsteroidal anti-inflammatory agents. With the exception of fosinopril, the half-lives of all ACEIs (or active metabolites) are prolonged in renal failure and lower doses may need to be given[54] (see Chap. 10).

TABLE 42–1. Effects of Antihypertensive Agents on Renal Blood Flow (RBF) and Glomerular Filtration Rate (GRF)

Antihypertensive Agent	Mechanism of Action	Effects on Renal Hemodynamics
Diuretics	Sodium and volume depletion	Decrease in GFR and RBF
	↑ Vasodilatory prostaglandin levels (IV loop diuretics)	Increase in RBF
	Renal vasoconstriction (IV thiazide diuretics)	Decrease in GFR and RBF
β-adrenergic blockers	↓ Cardiac output	Decrease in GFR and RBF
	↑ Renal vascular resistance (nonselective agents)	Decrease in GFR and RBF
	↓ Renal vascular resistance (β_1-selective agents)	No change in GFR and RBF Decrease or no change microalbuminuria
Centrally acting antiadrenergic drugs	↓ Renal vascular resistance (methyldopa)	No change in GFR and RBF
	↓ Renal perfusion pressure (clonidine, α_2–adrenergic agonist)	Decrease in GFR and RBF
Peripherally acting antiadrenergic drugs	Direct vasodilation (postsynaptic α_1–adrenoreceptor blocking agents)	No change in GFR and RBF
Direct vasodilator agents	↓ Renal vascular resistance (hydralazine, minoxidil)	Increase in RBF and no effect on GFR
	Arterial vasodilation plus dilatation of venous capacitance vessels (nitroprusside) (diazoxide—less venous dilatation)	Decrease in GFR and RBF (acute effect)
ACE inhibitors	Dilation of the efferent arteriole	Increase in RBF and GFR (only in patients with hypertension, renal insufficiency, or increased renin states)
	Dilatation of the efferent arteriole plus inhibition of angiotensin II concentration	Decrease in GFR (acute)
Calcium channel blockers	↓ Renal vascular resistance by vasodilation of afferent arterioles (hypertensive patients)	Increase in RBF and no change in GFR
	↓ Renal vasoconstriction (isolated perfused kidney)	Increase in RBF and GFR

Large controlled randomized prospective studies are needed to determine what degree of blood pressure control is most effective in delaying renal disease and which antihypertensive agents or combination of agents provide the greatest benefit. Additionally, the issue of control of systemic versus intraglomerular pressure and the potential benefit of specific agents remain to be answered. According to the National High Blood Pressure Education Program, special attention should be paid to hypertensive black patients, those with renal insufficiency, diabetics, and the elderly—groups at the highest risk of progression to ESRD if left untreated. Goal blood pressure was defined as 130/85 mm Hg, and if tolerated a lower blood pressure goal of 125/75 may be beneficial for blacks and patients with renal disease and proteinuria above 1 g/24 h.[55]

The role of AT-1 receptor blockers in the progression of nondiabetic renal disease is similar to that seen in diabetic disease. The emerging data does support similar efficacy with ACEI therapy, particularly in hemodynamically mediated renal injury.[39] One trial of 188 nondiabetic patients with stable renal insufficiency compared lisinopril (10 mg/d) to valsartan (80 mg/d) over 13 weeks. It was determined that the two agents demonstrated similar efficacy and safety for lowering blood pressure and proteinuria in subjects with a median GFR between 65 and 71 mL/min.[39]

Diuretics are commonly used to treat fluid overload and hypertension in patients with renal insufficiency. They may be particularly suited for treatment of the renally compromised older patient who tends to have salt-sensitive blood pressure.[56] Diuretic therapy is clearly indicated in the patient with volume overload, or in patients with fluid retention secondary to other antihypertensive agents. As creatinine clearance falls below 20 to 30 mL/min, the thiazide-like diuretics lose their saluretic action but still maintain a modest antihypertensive effect, possibly because of vasodilation.[57] Saluresis in these patients can be maintained through the use of potent loop diuretics such as furosemide, torsemide, or bumetanide. As creatinine clearance declines further, these agents may become ineffective saluretics as well. In such patients, a combination of a loop diuretic plus a thiazide diuretic or metolozone may prove beneficial,[58] although close clinical and laboratory monitoring should be undertaken to prevent the profound dehydration and metabolic derangements that may ensue. Potassium-sparing diuretics such as spironolactone, triamterene, and amiloride should be used with extreme caution if at all in patients with moderate renal insufficiency (< 30 mL/min) because of the risk of hyperkalemia. Triamterene should probably be avoided in renally impaired patients also receiving nonsteroidal anti-inflammatory drugs because of the potential risk of precipitating more severe renal impairment.[59]

The calcium channel blocking agents are also effective treatments for hypertension in patients with renal insufficiency and ESRD. There is some experimental data that suggest that this class of drugs (specifically the nondihydropyridines) may slow the rate of decline of renal function.[40] Dosage alterations are unnecessary in renal insufficiency and dosage should be titrated to achieve the desired degree of blood pressure reduction (see Chap. 10).

Oral and transdermal clonidine has been used with some success in patients with renal insufficiency.[60] Although the bioavailability of the transdermal system has not been evaluated in this patient population, plasma concentrations are comparable to those achieved with oral dosing.[60] Patients who respond to oral clonidine should maintain blood pressure control when switched to equivalent dosages of the transdermal patch. α_1-Adrenoceptor antagonists (prazosin, terazosin, doxazosin) are also well tolerated and reduce blood pressure in short-term clinical trials in patients with renal insufficiency.[61] There are no data available to determine if clonidine or α_1-blockers are useful in retarding renal failure progression above and beyond the benefits one would anticipate to result from blood pressure reduction alone.

Although advocated as first- or second-line therapy in the treatment of essential hypertension,[48] β-blocking agents, with the exception of nadolol and labetalol,[62,63] may reduce renal blood flow secondary to a reduction in cardiac output in patients with renal insufficiency, although a deterioration in GFR is uncommon. Hydrophilic β-blockers such as nadolol, acebutolol, and atenolol are mainly eliminated via urinary excretion of unchanged drug and may require significant dosage adjustment in renally insufficient patients.[64]

Minoxidil with concurrent β-adrenoceptor-blocking agents and diuretics (to control tachycardia and fluid retention, respectively) have been shown to effectively lower blood pressure long term in antihypertensive patients with renal insufficiency.[65] However, it is unclear if minoxidil reduces the rate of decline in renal function.

Regardless of the treatment regimen, hypertension should be controlled in the presence of underlying renal disease. If proteinuria is present, the use of ACEIs and possibly nondihydropyridine CCBs may be superior to conventional agents in decreasing proteinuria and glomerular hypertension.

PHARMACOECONOMIC CONSIDERATIONS

There have been several evaluations of the pharmacoeconomic impact of therapy aimed at preventing the progression of renal failure in type 1 diabetic patients. Siegel and colleagues evaluated the cost effectiveness of screening for microalbuminuria.[66] Four possible scenarios were analyzed using a semi-Markov model. The standard therapy approach assumed treatment with hydrochlorothiazide when hypertension was diagnosed. The new program approach assumed three different screening and treatment with ACEI strategies. Their results suggest that early screening and treatment with ACEIs when persistent microalbuminuria occurs is likely to be a very cost-effective use of health care dollars, with a cost-effectiveness ratio of $7900 to $16,500 per year of life saved. This ratio is similar to the cost effectiveness of treating hypertension in the general population.

Another group of investigators performed a similar cost-effectiveness analysis of three different strategies using the same model.[67] The model predicted that treating all patients with an ACEI 5 years after diagnosis of diabetes was as cost effective as annual screening for microalbuminuria starting 5 years after diagnosis and the initiaion of an ACEI when and if persistent microalbuminuria was detected. Finally, the DCCT research group evaluated the cost effectiveness of intensive insulin therapy compared with conventional diabetes treatment.[68] They used a Monte Carlo simulation model on a hypothetical sample of 120,000 persons in the United States meeting the eligibility criteria for enrollment in the DCCT. The analysis demonstrated that implementing intensive insulin therapy would result in a gain of 691,000 years free of ESRD along with other clinical benefits, with an incremental cost per year of life gained of $28,661. According to these authors, this ratio represents a good value to the health care system. Overall, it appears that aggressive insulin therapy as well as treatment with ACEIs when persistent microalbuminuria is identified will reduce complications, improve quality of life by preserving renal function, and ultimately increase length of life at reasonable costs to society. The results of these simulated analyses remain to be prospectively confirmed.

EVALUATION OF THERAPEUTIC OUTCOMES

DIABETICS

Based on the available clinical and experimental data, pharmacologic intervention can attenuate hemodynamic adaptations associated with progression of renal disease in diabetic patients. General approaches for the prevention of progression of renal disease in this population are summarized in Figure 42–3.[69] All patients with type 1 diabetes of more than 5 years' duration or all type 2 diabetics should be screened every year for microalbuminuria (annual UAE or urinary albumin–creatinine ratio).[24] Blood glucose should be maintained within or close to normal range either by frequent insulin injections or use of an insulin pump, while minimizing the risk of hypoglycemia with frequent blood glucose monitoring. If there are no contraindications, ACEI therapy should be initiated in normotensive or hypertensive type 1 diabetic patients with persistent microalbuminuria (30 to 300 mg/d) or overt albuminuria (> 300 mg/d). ACEIs should be titrated every 1 to 3 months to achieve a maximal reduction in UAE. Within 1 week of initiating or increasing a dose of an ACEI, serum creatinine and potassium should be evaluated to detect abrupt reductions in GFR or development of hyperkalemia (see Chap. 45). Currently, data are limited on the superiority of ACEIs in slowing the rate of renal impairment in type 2 diabetic patients who are normotensive and have microalbuminuria. However, until further data are available, ACEIs should be prescribed for type 2 patients with hypertension and/or those who demonstrate persistent albuminuria (> 300 mg/d).[69] A nondihydropyridine CCB may be an effective alternative as a single agent or in combination with an ACEI in hypertensive diabetic patients with advanced renal disease and/or proteinuria.

In animal models, use of lipid-lowering agents decreases the extent of glomerular injury when both underlying renal disease and hyperlipidemia are present.[14,16] Therefore, the correction of lipid abnormalities in patients with renal insufficiency may have a beneficial effect on the rate of progression of renal disease. Experimental data indicate that hyperlipidemia may interact with concomitant risk factors such as hypertension, diabetes, and preexisting renal damage to accelerate progression of glomerular injury. The use of a low-fat diet and/or addition of antilipidemic agents to the therapeutic regimen may be beneficial in diabetic and nondiabetic patients with renal disease and lipid abnormalities (see Chap. 19).

NONDIABETICS

Therapeutic interventions for nondiabetic patients with renal insufficiency are summarized in Figure 42–4. Nutritional management should be monitored frequently, regardless of the amount of protein intake prescribed, to avoid complications from malnutrition. Nutrition goals include maintenance of serum albumin above 4 g/dL and transferrin above 200 mg/dL. Based on the

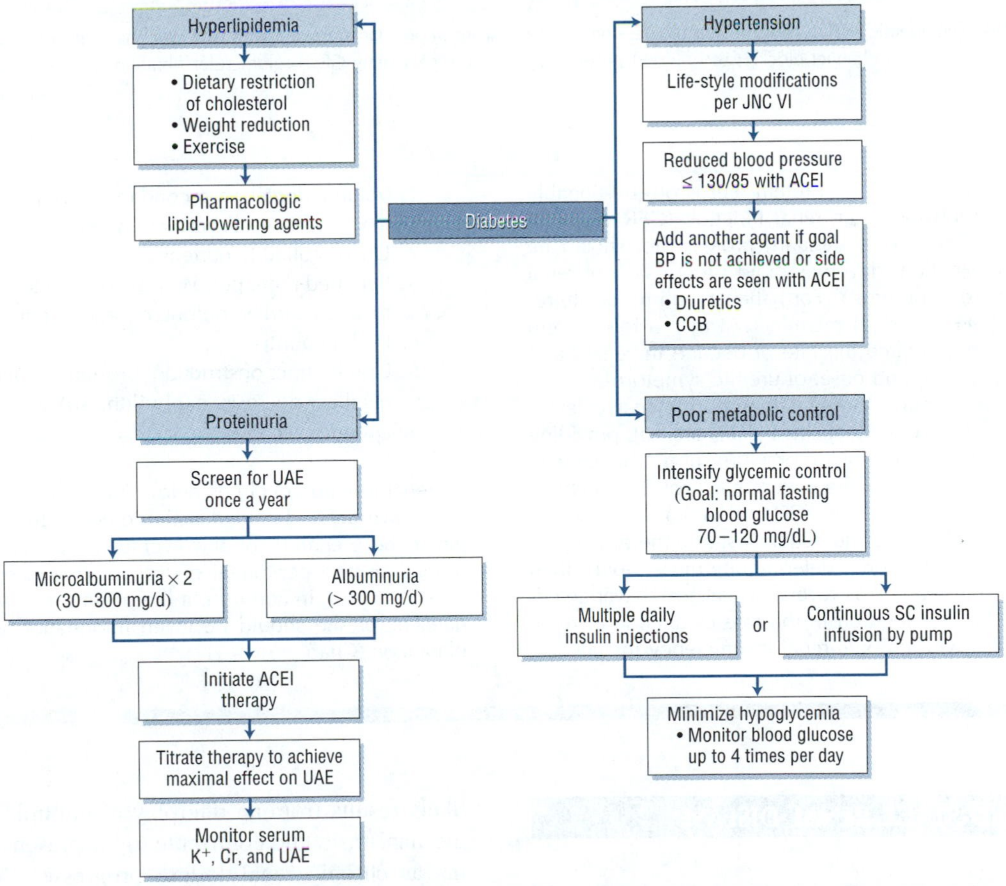

FIGURE 42–3. Therapeutic strategies to prevent progression of renal disease in diabetic individuals. (UAE = urinary albumin excretion; CCB = calcium channel blocker; SC = subcutaneous; ACEI = angiotensin-converting enzyme inhibitor; JNC VI = the sixth report of the Joint National Committee on prevention, detection, evaluation, and treatment of high blood pressure.

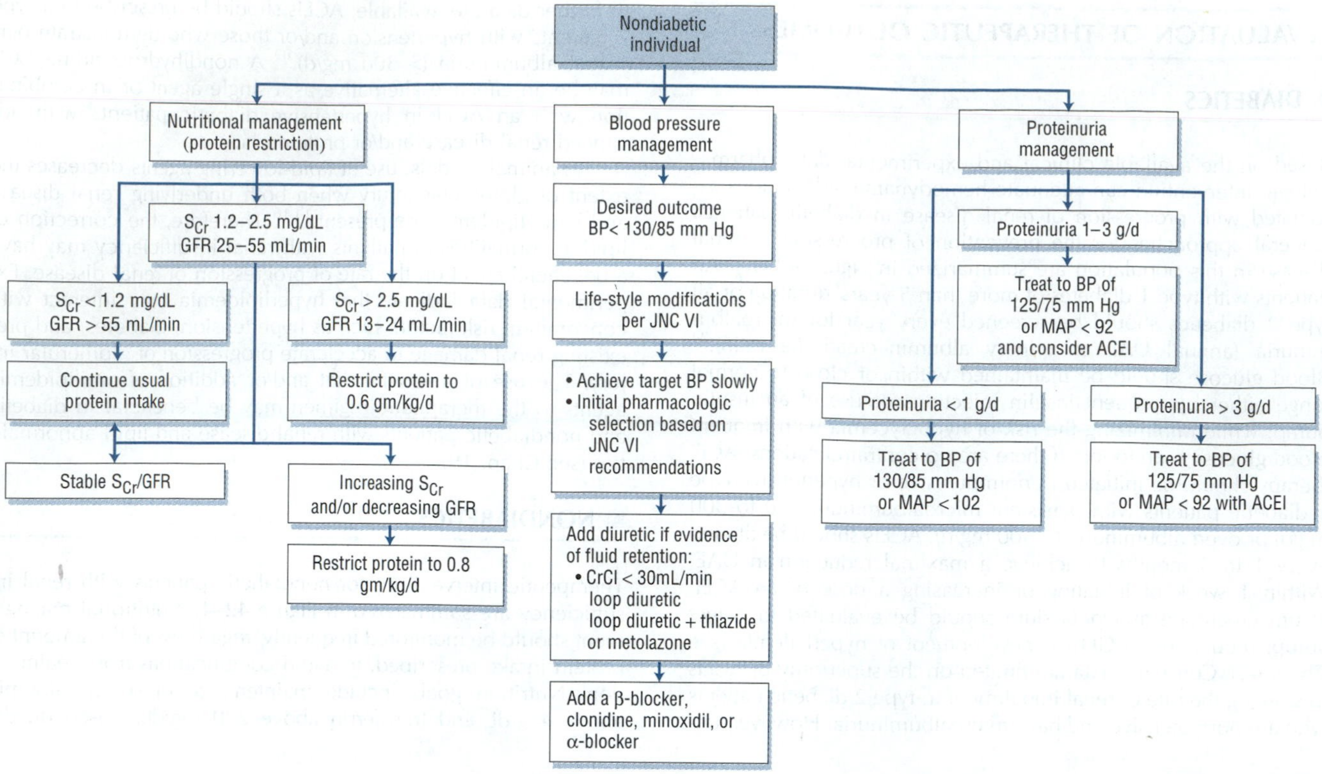

FIGURE 42–4. Therapeutic strategies to prevent progression of renal disease in nondiabetic individuals. (ACEI = angiotensin-converting enzyme inhibitor; CCB = calcium channel blocker; BP = blood pressure; S_{Cr} = serum creatinine; GFR = glomerular filtration rate; MAP = mean arterial pressure.)

results of the MDRD study, a low-protein diet is of questionable benefit in patients with moderate renal function (GFR 25 to 55 mL/min/1.73 m^2). Therefore, a standard protein diet should be followed unless the patient develops rapid progression of renal failure and/or uremic symptoms.[69] For patients with moderate renal insufficiency (GFR 13 to 24 mL/min/1.73 m^2), a low-protein diet of 0.6 g/kg/d may reduce the rate of decline in renal function, time to reach ESRD, and onset of uremic symptoms.[47]

Blood pressure control should target normotensive levels (130/85 mm Hg).[48] If proteinuria above 1 g/d is present, providing there are no contraindications, blood pressure should be reduced further (125/75 mm Hg). But if the patient has proteinuria above 3 g/d and chronic renal failure, an ACEI and perhaps a nondihydropyridine CCB should be considered as first-line therapy.[69]

If a patient's renal function is deteriorating more rapidly than predicted, a vigorous search for reversible causes is warranted. Potential reasons for acceleration in the rate of decline of renal function in a patient with chronic renal insufficiency include:

1. Volume depletion secondary to vomiting, diarrhea, or inappropriate salt restriction or diuretic therapy.
2. Uncontrolled hypertension.
3. Impaired renal perfusion secondary to hypotension, reduced cardiac output, or renovascular disease.
4. Pyelonephritis.
5. Urinary tract obstruction (prostatic hypertrophy, papillary necrosis, nephrolithiasis).
6. Drug-related effects.

As renal function declines below 20 mL/min and treatable problems have been identified and addressed, the patient should begin to be prepared for the eventuality of dialysis therapy. Hemodialysis and peritoneal dialysis options need to be discussed (see Chap. 44). In addition, if the patient is an appropriate candidate, he or she should be given information about renal transplantation (Chap. 43).

END-STAGE RENAL DISEASE

PATHOPHYSIOLOGY

No single toxin is responsible for all of the abnormalities observed in patients with ESRD, and the clinical picture likely results from an interplay of multiple factors. Several mechanisms could contribute to the presence of uremic toxins as chronic renal failure progresses. Most likely, the signs and symptoms seen in ESRD patients result from elevations in blood concentrations of various organic compounds (Table 42–2). Accumulation could be the result of increased secretion of biologically active substances such

TABLE 42–2. Potential Uremic Toxins

2,3-Butylene	Indoles
Acetoin	Indoxyl sulfate
Acids	Insulin
Aliphatic amines	Lipochromes
α_2-Glycoprotein	Lysozyme
Amino acids	Mannitol
Aromatic amines	Methylguanidine
β_1-Microglobulin	Middle molecules
β_2-Microglobulin	Myoinositol
Calcitonin	Natriuretic hormone
Chemotaxis inhibiting protein	Other guanidines
Creatinine	Oxalic acid
Cyanate	Parathyroid hormone
Cyclic AMP	P-cresol
Degranulation inhibiting proteins	Phenols
Gastric inhibitory peptide	Potassium
Gastrin	Prolactin
Glucagon	Pyridine derivatives
Glucuronic acid	Renin
Growth hormone	Retinol-binding protein
Granulocyte inhibitory proteins	Ribonuclease
Guanidines	Urea
Hippuric acid	Uric acid
Human pancreatic polypeptide	Water

as parathyroid hormone (PTH) and atrial natriuretic peptide, which are overproduced as part of the adaptation to the loss of renal mass; decreased clearance of endogenous substances normally metabolized by the kidney, including PTH, gastrin, growth hormone, glucagon, somatostatin, prolactin, calcitonin, and insulin; and/or decreased clearance of metabolic by-products of protein metabolism.

The ability of uremic toxins to produce clinical manifestations results in large part from their effects at the cellular or metabolic level, which ultimately can affect organ, immune, and other bodily functions.[70] In order to prove that a substance is a uremic toxin, investigators must show accumulation of the substance, demonstrate toxicity at a cellular or metabolic level upon administration, and show improvement by removal of the toxin by dialysis or other means.[70] Very few of these substances (with the exception of PTH and indoxyl sulfate) have been taken through the process described, so there is still much work to be done in this area.

CLINICAL PRESENTATION

Uremia can affect every major organ system. Patients usually present at the time of diagnosis with some but rarely all of the symptoms that will be outlined next.

CARDIOVASCULAR SYSTEM

Sodium retention leads to volume expansion, which can result in volume overload and pulmonary edema. Hypertension induced by volume expansion and increased systemic vascular resistance increases myocardial work and results in left ventricular hypertrophy. In addition, hypertension represents a major risk factor for cardiovascular disease, and complications of atherosclerosis are common in these patients. Hyperlipidemia may enhance atherogenesis. Some uremic toxins decrease myocardial contractility. The high cardiac output state induced by anemia may be poorly tolerated in the face of underlying heart disease. Uremic toxins can induce pericarditis, a potentially fatal complication of chronic renal failure.

PULMONARY SYSTEM

The combination of volume overload and uremic toxin-induced increases in capillary permeability can result in noncardiogenic pulmonary edema.

GASTROINTESTINAL SYSTEM

Anorexia, hiccups, and a metallic taste in the mouth are common in ESRD patients. In uremia, nausea, vomiting, diarrhea, or abdominal distention may occur. Gastric and colonic mucosal ulcerations and telangiectasias with resultant gastrointestinal bleeding are common.

NERVOUS SYSTEM

Neuromuscular irritability may be present and result in leg cramps, restless leg syndrome, and reversal of the sleep–wake cycle. The clinical manifestations of uremic encephalopathy—which include clouded sensorium, coma, seizures, myoclonic jerks, and asterixis—are now rarely seen due to the earlier initiation of dialysis.

HEMATOLOGIC SYSTEM

A normochromic, normocytic anemia secondary to decreased erythropoietin production and shortened erythrocyte survival is seen in over 90% of patients. A prolongation in the bleeding time and a bleeding diathesis can result from platelet dysfunction. Gastrointestinal bleeding is common in ESRD, which contributes to anemia. In addition, vitamin and iron deficiency can lead to mixed anemia patterns in this population.

MUSCULOSKELETAL SYSTEM

Renal osteodystrophy (bone disease) is a common manifestation of renal insufficiency and almost ubiquitously present in ESRD patients. Calcification of blood vessels or soft tissues may occur.

ENDOCRINE SYSTEM

A variety of endocrine and metabolic abnormalities are common in ESRD.[71] Most patients have symptoms of hypothyroidism (low energy, cold intolerance, constipation), but typically the levothyroxine (T_4) concentration is low and the thyroid-stimulating hormone concentration is normal. Hypothermia is common; body temperatures are approximately 1°F lower as compared to individuals with normal renal function. Hyperglycemia secondary to peripheral resistance to insulin can occur. Diabetic patients with ESRD often present with more frequent hypoglycemic episodes because the kidney is responsible, in large part, for the degradation of insulin. Insulin doses often must be adjusted downward as renal failure progresses. Primary hypogonadism as well as hypothalamic abnormalities contribute to sexual dysfunction and sterility.

DERMATOLOGIC SYSTEM

Dry, flaking skin and generalized pruritus are commonly seen in ESRD patients.

IMMUNE SYSTEM

Infectious diseases are common and result in significant morbidity and mortality in patients with ESRD. Although multiple abnormalities in host defenses and an increased susceptibility to infection have been described, the causal link between these observations remains speculative. Absolute lymphopenia and impaired cell-mediated immunity are common in ESRD patients and may be due to the presence of uremic toxins or protein–calorie malnutrition. Although plasma concentrations of IgG, IgM, and IgA are usually normal, antibody responses appear to be significantly depressed.[72]

▶ TREATMENT: End-Stage Renal Disease

GENERAL APPROACH TO TREATMENT

The therapeutic management of the patient with ESRD hinges on several important principles. First, those treatments known to slow the rate of renal disease progression should be continued to reduce cardiovascular morbidity and mortality. Second, patients must receive dietary instruction to limit protein, potassium, and phosphorus intake and maintain adequate caloric intake (see Chap. 131). Phosphate-binding medications and/or calcium supplementation should be used to control serum phosphorus and calcium concentrations in order to suppress parathyroid hormone secretion and prevent renal bone disease. Therapy with alkalinizing agents should be administered to patients with systemic acidosis. Third, renal function must be monitored closely.

INDICATIONS FOR THE INITIATION OF DIALYTIC THERAPY

In general, patients are managed conservatively until creatinine clearance drops below 10 mL/min or they become symptomatic. Criteria for the initiation of dialysis in patients with chronic renal insufficiency are largely clinical and include intractable nausea and vomiting, uremic encephalopathy, confusion, asterixis, seizures, myoclonus, uremic pericarditis, development of peripheral neuropathy, development of pruritus, and prophylactic use before major surgery. Currently, early initiation of dialysis (CrCl = 10 mL/min) is being advocated by many nephrologists to prevent symptomatology and decrease morbidity and mortality.

Once dialysis therapy is initiated, patients need further dietary instruction, because dietary protein intake can be liberalized. Adequate caloric intake and dietary phosphate restriction remain important goals of dietary management. A no-added-salt diet and fluid restriction to approximately 1000 mL/d will minimize interdialysis weight gains and hyponatremia. Vitamin D therapy is commonly prescribed to prevent renal osteodystrophy along with epoetin and iron therapy for treatment of anemia. Aggressive antihypertensive therapy remains important, because blood pressure elevation before each dialysis treatment is a strong predictor of future cardiovascular and cerebrovascular mortality.

PATHOPHYSIOLOGY AND THERAPEUTIC MANAGEMENT OF MODERATE TO SEVERE RENAL INSUFFICIENCY AND ESRD

VOLUME OVERLOAD AND EDEMA

PATHOPHYSIOLOGY

In normal subjects, sodium balance is maintained with sodium intake of 120 to 150 mEq/d. The fractional excretion of sodium (FE_{Na}) is approximately 1%. Water balance is also maintained, with a normal range of urinary osmolality of 50 to 1200 mOsm/L (see Chap. 48). In patients with chronic renal failure, sodium balance is maintained but in a volume-expanded state. FE_{Na} increases to as high as 10% to 20%. The exact mechanism whereby FE_{Na} increases is unknown but may be the result of increased concentrations of atrial natriuretic peptide (ANP).[73] The increased secretion of ANP is probably triggered by increased intravascular volume and atrial pressure.

Volume expansion results in hypertension. Increased levels of ANP may interfere with sodium and calcium transport in vascular smooth muscle, resulting in increased resting muscle tone. The resultant increase in peripheral vascular resistance probably contributes to hypertension. Elevated levels of ANP may inhibit sodium and potassium ATPase-dependent pumps in many cells of the body, resulting in altered cellular electrolyte content and membrane potentials.

Water balance is generally maintained but within a limited range. Because the fractional reabsorption of sodium is decreased secondary to ANP, free water generation by the kidney is impaired. An osmotic diuresis due to a large solute load per remnant nephron results in obligatory water losses. The ability to dilute or concentrate the urine is impaired and urine becomes isosthenuric (urinary osmolality fixed at that of plasma or approximately 300 mOsm/L).

Clinical Presentation

Nocturia is present relatively early in the course of renal insufficiency (CrCl 30 to 60 mL/min) secondary to the defect in urinary concentrating ability. Total renal sodium excretion decreases despite an increase in sodium excretion by remaining nephrons. Volume overload with pulmonary edema can result, but the most common manifestation of increased intravascular volume is systemic hypertension.[73]

▶ TREATMENT: Volume Overload and Edema

The ability of the kidney to adjust to abrupt changes in sodium intake is greatly diminished. Sodium restriction beyond a no-added-salt diet should not be recommended except in the face of hypertension or edema. The kidney maintains the ability to lower urinary sodium content to essentially zero, but this can only be accomplished by very gradual sodium restriction over a period of several days. Hospitalized patients, therefore, should not routinely be sodium restricted because they have adapted to their outpatient intake. Negative sodium balance and its resultant volume contraction can result in decreased renal perfusion and subsequent further decline in GFR. Saline-containing intravenous solutions should be used cautiously in patients with chronic renal insufficiency because the kidney's ability to excrete a salt load is impaired and such patients are prone to volume overload. Sodium retention and volume expansion contribute to hypertension in many patients with renal insufficiency and ESRD, and diuretic therapy or dialysis may be necessary for control of edema or blood pressure. Thiazide diuretics are not effective alone in patients with a CrCl below 30 mL/min. Loop diuretics, particularly when administered by continuous infusion, have been shown to increase urine volume and renal sodium excretion. A combination of a loop diuretic along with a thiazide diuretic (such as hydrochlorothiazide or metolazone) can result in a more profound excretion of sodium and water.

Fluid restriction is generally not necessary provided sodium intake is controlled. An intact thirst mechanism maintains total body water and effective plasma osmolality near normal. Because urine volume is relatively fixed at approximately 2 L/d, fluid restriction below this amount should be avoided. Large amounts of free water administered orally or as intravenous fluid may induce hyponatremia and volume overload. When the patient develops ESRD, then dialysis (specifically ultrafiltration) or a renal transplant is necessary to maintain normovolemia.

POTASSIUM HOMEOSTASIS

Pathophysiology

The kidneys normally excrete 90% to 95% of a daily potassium dietary load, predominately through distal tubular secretion (see Chap. 48). The fractional renal excretion of potassium (FE_K) is approximately 25%. Normally only 5% to 10% of ingested potassium is excreted through the gut. Potassium homeostasis is also maintained by shifting extracellular potassium to intracellular spaces, acutely, following ingestion of a potassium load.[74] In chronic renal insufficiency, potassium balance is maintained by an increase in distal tubular potassium secretion in which aldosterone plays an important role. FE_K can increase to as high as 125%. Thus the serum potassium concentration is usually maintained in the normal range until the patient reaches ESRD (GFR < 10 mL/min). A significant increase in potassium secretion by the colon also contributes to the maintenance of potassium balance, but this adaptation cannot compensate fully for the decrease in renal excretion. Although aldosterone receptors are found in the colon, it is unclear whether they play a significant role in the upregulation of colonic potassium secretion in ESRD patients.[74,75]

Clinical Presentation

The clinical consequences of hyperkalemia are similar regardless of the patient's renal function. The signs and symptoms of hyperkalemia are discussed in Chapter 48.

▶ TREATMENT: Potassium Homeostasis

Potassium-sparing diuretics are relatively contraindicated in moderate to severe renal insufficiency patients because of the high risk of hyperkalemia. Beta-blockers, predominantly via β_2-antagonistic effects, interfere with the extrarenal translocation of potassium into cells and may result in a further impairment in potassium handling and life-threatening hyperkalemia. ACEIs should be monitored closely in patients with moderate to severe renal insufficiency and ESRD because they may provoke hyperkalemia by reducing aldosterone production.

The management of hyperkalemia in ESRD can be divided into chronic and acute treatment.[74,75] The goal is to maintain prehemodialysis potassium concentrations of 4.5 to 5.5 mEq/L. The majority of patients can be managed with a dietary potassium restriction of 50 to 80 mEq/d and alterations in dialysate potassium concentrations. Constipation in dialysis patients can interfere with colonic potassium excretion; therefore, a good bowel regimen is important. Extrarenal handling of potassium is important in ESRD; therefore, discontinuing ACEI or changing to a β_1–selective β-blocker[74] may be necessary in some patients. Pharmacologic treatment is rarely necessary for the ESRD patient on dialysis. Sodium polystyrene sulfonate (with sorbitol), a potassium–sodium exchange resin, can be given orally in doses of 15 to 30 g between dialysis sessions to increase potassium excretion in the ileum and colon. Mineralocorticoids may enhance secretion of potassium into the gut by stimulating aldosterone receptors, although no clinical trials exist to support this. Finally, a short-term study showed that diltiazem 30 mg orally twice daily lessened the rate of increase in plasma potassium between dialysis sessions.[76]

The definitive treatment of severe hyperkalemia in ESRD is hemodialysis. In reality there is often a delay between diagnosis of hyperkalemia and institution of dialysis, which necessitates the use of other temporizing measures such as intravenous calcium gluconate, insulin and glucose, nebulized albuterol, and sodium polystyrene sulfonate (see Chap. 48). Unfortunately, shifting potassium into the intracellular fluid compartment with insulin and glucose or with albuterol makes dialysis removal of potassium more difficult.[77] Multiple dialysis sessions may be necessary following potassium redistribution to the extracellular space. Lastly, sodium bicarbonate therapy is no longer advocated in the treatment of ESRD hyperkalemia unless severe metabolic acidosis is also present, because the potassium-lowering effect is not reliable.[78]

METABOLIC ACIDOSIS

PATHOPHYSIOLOGY

A constant body fluid pH is maintained through the buffering of hydrogen ion by proteins, hemoglobin, phosphate, and especially bicarbonate. People with normal renal function generate enough hydrogen ion to reclaim all filtered bicarbonate and secrete approximately 1 mEq/kg/d of hydrogen ions, which are generated from the metabolism of dietary proteins (see Chap. 48). Renal ammoniagenesis and phosphate excretion buffer the urine and facilitate acid excretion. In chronic renal insufficiency, all filtered bicarbonate is reclaimed, but the ability of the kidneys to synthesize ammonia is impaired.[79] This decrease in urinary buffer results in decreased net acid excretion and continuous positive hydrogen ion balance; thus, metabolic acidosis develops. A clinically significant metabolic acidosis is commonly seen when the glomerular filtration rate drops below 20 to 30 mL/min. The plasma bicarbonate concentration tends to stabilize at 15 to 20 mEq/L.

CLINICAL PRESENTATION

Metabolic acidosis, through unknown mechanisms, contributes to renal bone disease.[80] The presence of metabolic acidosis may also cause fatigue, decreased exercise tolerance, reduced cardiac contractility, and increased ventricular irritability. Finally, metabolic acidosis appears to stimulate protein catabolism, which can worsen uremia and contribute to a negative nitrogen balance as well as growth retardation in children.[81]

▶ TREATMENT: Metabolic Acidosis

The prevention and treatment of severe metabolic acidosis in patients with chronic renal insufficiency may be important for the prevention of the sequelae of the chronic acidotic state. Generally, treatment should be instituted when plasma bicarbonate has fallen below 20 mEq/L. Metabolic acidosis in patients undergoing dialysis can almost always be managed solely by the procedure. Measures used include dialysis against acetate (a bicarbonate precursor) or bicarbonate dialysate baths.

In patients with moderate to severe renal insufficiency, the use of alkalinizing salts such as sodium bicarbonate or citrate/citric acid preparations is useful to replenish depleted body bicarbonate stores. Citrate is metabolized in the liver to bicarbonate, and citric acid is metabolized to CO_2 and water. Sodium bicarbonate tablets are manufactured in 325 and 650 mg strengths (650 mg tablet contains 7.7 mEq sodium and 7.7 mEq bicarbonate). Each mL of Shohl's solution and Bicitra contains 1 mEq sodium and the equivalent of 1 mEq bicarbonate as sodium citrate/citric acid. Polycitra, which contains potassium citrate, should not be used in patients with severe renal insufficiency or ESRD, as hyperkalemia may result. Each mL of Polycitra contains 1 mEq of sodium and potassium and 2 mEq of bicarbonate.

The first step in treatment is to calculate a replacement dose of alkali (base) that is needed to restore the serum bicarbonate concentration to normal (24 mEq/L).[80] The amount (mEq) can be approximated by multiplying the volume of distribution of bicarbonate (0.5 L/kg) by the patient's body weight (kg) and by the base deficit (difference between patient's serum bicarbonate value and 24 mEq/L). The calculated amount of bicarbonate replacement therapy should be administered over several days to prevent volume overload from excessive sodium intake.[80] If calcium acetate or calcium carbonate is also being given to the patient, decrease the amount of base administered. Once the serum bicarbonate has normalized, then reduce bicarbonate replacement therapy to that required to neutralize daily acid production (12 to 20 mEq/d) in divided doses.[80] Doses are subsequently titrated to produce normal plasma bicarbonate concentrations. Fluid balance should be monitored carefully because of the sodium content of these agents. Citrate-containing solutions should not be used in combination with aluminum-containing compounds as they can enhance aluminum absorption and increase the risk of aluminum intoxication. Excessive doses of alkalinizing agents may cause metabolic alkalosis as well as lethargy or cardiac depression secondary to a decrease in ionized serum calcium concentration. Gastrointestinal distress characterized by gastric distention and flatulence is relatively common with high doses of oral sodium bicarbonate.

Patients with renal tubular acidosis (RTA) may require higher doses of alkalinizing agents. Recommended initial doses of sodium bicarbonate for distal (type 1) and proximal (type 2) RTA are 1 to 3 mEq/kg/d and 10 to 15 mEq/kg/d, respectively in adults.[82] Suggested pediatric doses for distal and proximal RTA are up to 10 mEq/kg/d and up to 20 mEq/kg/d, respectively.[83]

RENAL OSTEODYSTROPHY AND SECONDARY HYPERPARATHYROIDISM

Metabolic bone disease is a major cause of morbidity and mortality in patients undergoing chronic dialysis treatment. Multiple types of bone lesions can be identified from bone biopsies of patients on dialysis.[84,85] When dialysis therapy was first available in the late 1960s, a high-turnover bone disease called osteitis fibrosa cystica was the only entity identified. This bone lesion is characterized histologically by areas of peritrabecular fibrosis. Dynamic measurements show a high bone formation rate, which results from high circulating concentrations of parathyroid hormone (PTH). In the 1970s, osteomalacia, characterized by a high volume of osteoid tissue, was first identified in ESRD patients. After several years, aluminum toxicity was implicated as the main cause when histologic stains revealed high levels of aluminum in patients with dialysis-associated osteomalacia. In the 1980s, an adynamic lesion was characterized. Histologically, this lesion shows low amounts of fibrosis or osteoid tissue and low bone formation rates. Initially, adynamic bone disease was also linked to aluminum toxicity as many patients exhibited high amounts of stainable aluminum in bone biopsies. Today, aluminum-containing phosphate binders are not routinely used. However, the incidence of adynamic lesions has increased dramatically over the last 10 years, and may be seen in up to 50% of dialysis patients.[85] Multiple risk factors for the development of this bone disease have been identified: aluminum toxicity, high concentrations of dialysate calcium along with high doses of calcium-containing phosphate binders, aggressive management with vitamin D therapy, diabetes, and advanced age.[84,86] Management of PTH, phosphorus and calcium balance, and minimizing patient exposure to aluminum is important in preventing the development of secondary hyperparathyroidism and slowing or preventing the progression of renal bone disease.

ETIOLOGY AND PATHOPHYSIOLOGY

Calcium and phosphorus balance is mediated through a complex interplay of hormones and their effects on bone, gastrointestinal tract, kidney, and parathyroid gland.[2,87] Phosphate retention inhibits renal activation (C_1-alpha-hydroxylation) of vitamin D, which in turn reduces gut absorption of calcium. Phosphorus retention directly decreases blood ionized (free) calcium through a physiochemical interaction. Low blood calcium concentrations provide a major stimulus for PTH secretion. Parathyroid hormone decreases proximal tubular phosphate reabsorption and restores phosphate balance until the GFR falls below 30 mL/min, at which time blood phosphorus concentrations are often noted to rise (Fig. 42–5).

The parathyroid glands release PTH in a physiologic attempt to restore normal blood calcium and phosphorus concentrations. However, as functional renal mass declines, serum calcium balance can only be maintained at the expense of increased bone resorption. Decreased production of 1,25-dihydroxyvitamin D_3 (calcitriol) results in impaired intestinal absorption of calcium, provides a stimulus for PTH release, and may contribute to defective bone mineralization.

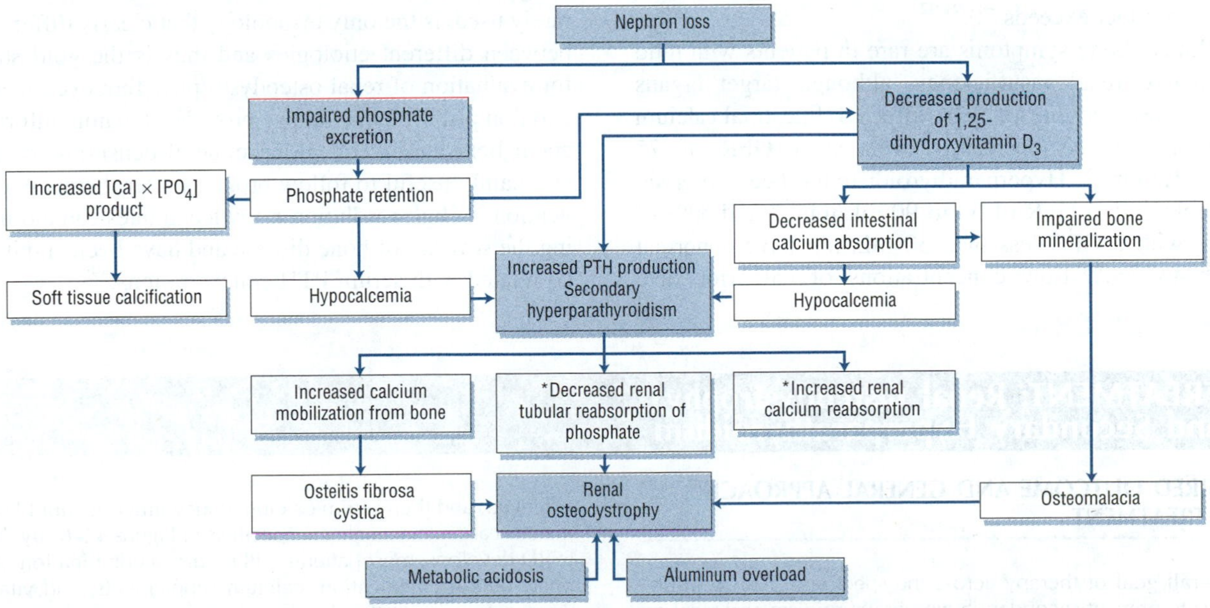

FIGURE 42–5. Pathogenesis of secondary hyperparathyroidism and renal osteodystrophy in patients with chronic renal failure. (*These adaptations are lost as renal failure progresses.)

Secondary hyperparathyroidism, a common manifestation in ESRD, can result in osteitis fibrosa cystica if left untreated. Underlying mechanisms are complex and somewhat controversial but include continued phosphorus retention and subsequent development of hypocalcemia (Fig. 42–5), which provides a stimulus for PTH secretion. Although not clearly established, high phosphorus concentrations may also directly increase secretion of PTH.[88] In addition, a new calcium-sensing receptor has been discovered on parathyroid cell membranes that may play a role in the pathogenesis of secondary hyperparathyroidism.[2,87] Parathyroid hyperplasia (nodular or diffuse) is another characteristic feature of secondary hyperparathyroidism. Nodular tissue demonstrates more rapid growth potential and appears to have lower numbers of calcitriol receptors than diffusely hyperplastic tissue.[87] Nodular hyperplasia along with low concentrations of circulating calcitriol is thought to result in an increased set point (the concentration of calcium causing half-maximal inhibition of PTH secretion).[87,89] Unfortunately, hypercalcemia may develop in the pharmacologic attempt to achieve suppression of PTH release.

Clinical Presentation

Development of secondary hyperparathyroidism and subsequent high circulating concentrations of PTH promotes progression of osteitis fibrosa cystica and may adversely affect lipid metabolism, insulin secretion, myocardial and skeletal muscle, as well as neurologic and immune functions.[90] Common signs and symptoms of secondary hyperparathyroidism include fatigue and musculoskeletal and gastrointestinal complaints. Uncontrolled hyperphosphatemia can also result in metastatic calcification of joints, vessels, and soft tissue when the calcium (mg/dL)–phosphorus (mg/dL) product exceeds 70.[91,92]

Clinical bone symptoms are rare in patients with mild to moderate renal insufficiency, although target organs (bone, kidney, and intestine) are affected. Intestinal calcium absorption can be decreased even at a GFR of 75 mL/min/1.73 m^2.[93] Hyperparathyroidism has been observed in patients with a GFR of 60 to 90 mL/min,[94] and 50% of patients with a GFR less than 50 mL/min have abnormal bone histology.[93] Low concentrations of calcitriol have been reported in patients with a CrCl of 70 mL/min or less.[2] Renal osteodystrophy progresses insidiously for several years before patients become symptomatic. When symptoms such as bone pain and skeletal fractures occur, the disease is not easily amenable to treatment. Bone marrow fibrosis and decreased hematopoiesis are also consequences of severe osteitis fibrosa. Therefore, preventative measures should be initiated in patients with mild to moderate degrees of renal insufficiency.[93]

Diagnosis

As renal osteodystrophy is heterogenic, knowledge of the underlying bone abnormality is essential to guide therapy. Serum calcium, phosphorus, PTH, alkaline phosphatase, and osteocalcin are serum biochemical markers used in the diagnostic workup and follow-up of renal osteodystrophy. New immunoradiometric and immunochemiluminescent assays for measurement of serum intact PTH, the biologically active molecule, are more sensitive in distinguishing between histologic patterns of renal osteodystrophy than older midregion and carboxy terminal PTH assays.[89,95] However, a recent study in 79 hemodialysis and peritoneal dialysis patients found that intact PTH greater than 450 pg/mL was between 95% and 100% specific for high bone turnover, but that overall, bone turnover could not be predicted in 30% of hemodialysis and 51% of peritoneal dialysis patients with intact PTH values alone.[96] Alkaline phosphatase is a nonspecific marker of ongoing bone disease. Osteocalcin, a protein synthesized by osteoblasts, is a marker for bone formation.[89] Calculation of the calcium set point following a modified calcium infusion test may be a time-intensive noninvasive method to monitor progression of hyperparathyroidism.[97] Transiliac bone biopsy, although rarely used, is the only technology that clearly differentiates between different etiologies and thus is the gold standard for evaluation of renal osteodystrophy. Tetracycline administration prior to bone biopsy provides dynamic information about bone turnover.[89] Bone mineral densitometry studies are mainly useful to follow progress after therapeutic intervention.[89] High-resolution x-ray techniques can aid in scoring the severity of bone disease and have been significantly correlated with serum PTH concentrations.[89]

▶ TREATMENT: Renal Osteodystrophy and Secondary Hyperparathyroidism

DESIRED OUTCOME AND GENERAL APPROACH TO TREATMENT

The overall goal of therapy across the spectrum of renal insufficiency is to prevent secondary hyperparathyroidism and renal osteodystrophy. First, control of serum phosphorus should be achieved, and then serum calcium concentrations should be optimized. Laboratory goals are specified in Figure 42–6. By the time ESRD develops, most patients will require a combination of phosphate-binding medication, calcium supplements, and vitamin D therapy to prevent the development of secondary hyperparathyroidism, renal osteodystrophy, and metastatic calcification.

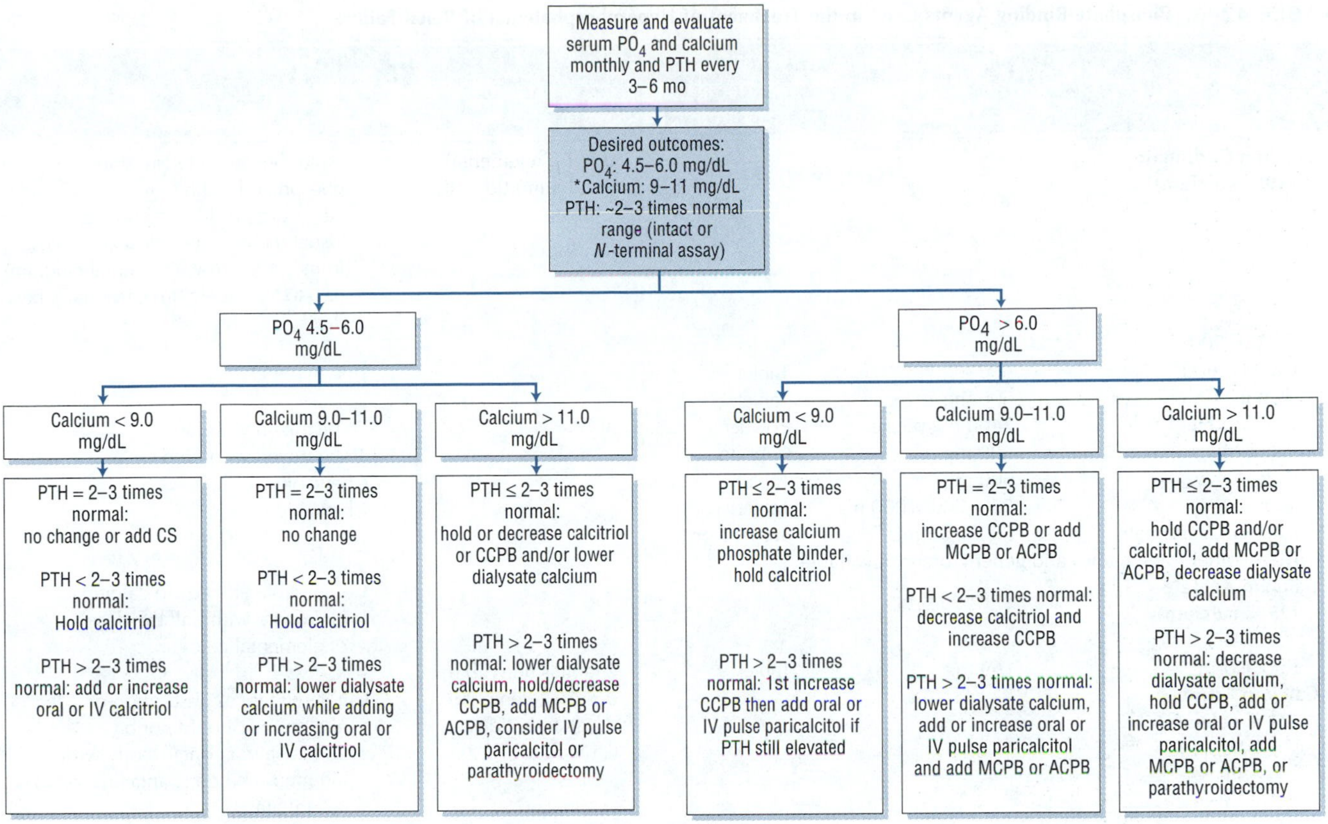

FIGURE 42–6. Approach to prevention and treatment of secondary hyperparathyroidism and renal osteodystrophy in ESRD patients. (CCPB = calcium-containing phosphate binder; MCBP = magnesium-containing phosphate binder; ACPB = aluminum-containing phosphate binder; CS = calcium supplment.) (*Corrected calcium = [(4.0 − albumin) × 0.8] + serum calcium.)

NONPHARMACOLOGIC THERAPY

Dietary phosphorus restriction (6.5 to 12.0 mg/kg/d) should be initiated in patients with a CrCl of less than 50 mL/min, to prevent early renal osteodystrophy and perhaps slow progression of renal disease.[91] This amount of phosphorus restriction is usually achievable with 0.6 to 0.8 g of protein per kg of body weight. As the number of functioning nephrons decline, dietary restriction alone is usually inadequate to control serum phosphorus, and phosphate-binding agents are instituted. Dietary phosphorus can be liberalized to 800 to 1200 mg/d (10 to 17 mg/kg/d) once dialysis is initiated as a single hemodialysis, or daily peritoneal dialysis treatment can remove up to 700 mg of phosphorus.[91] Examples of foods or beverages that contain high amounts of phosphorus per serving include meats, dairy products, dried beans, nuts, colas, peanut butter, and beer.

PHARMACOLOGIC THERAPY

PHOSPHATE-BINDING AGENTS

Currently, the ideal phosphate-binding agent does not exist. A variety of calcium-, aluminum-, and magnesium-containing phosphate-binding medications are available (Table 42–3). Phosphate-binding agents retard phosphorus absorption from the gut. These agents should be administered just before or with meals to maximize their phosphate-binding effect. The dose should be titrated to achieve normal serum phosphorus concentrations in patients with moderate to severe renal insufficiency and 4.5 to 6.0 mg/dL in ESRD patients. Pharmacist counseling is essential with phosphate-binding medications to enhance compliance, as many phosphate binders are marketed as antacids or calcium supplements and many dialysis patients do not know the indicated use.[98]

Aluminum salts were once widely used as phosphate-binding agents because of their high binding potency. However, aluminum binders can no longer be recommended as first-line therapy due to the toxicities associated with aluminum accumulation. Aluminum binders should be reserved for cases of severe hyperphosphatemia in conjunction with high serum calcium concentrations when the patient is at risk for metastatic calcification. Sucralfate, an aluminum-containing compound, has been shown to be an effective phosphate binder. However, aluminum contained in sucralfate may be more readily absorbed than with aluminum hydroxide,[99] and therefore its use should be avoided. Thus, oral calcium compounds have emerged as first-line agents for controlling both serum phosphorus and calcium concentrations.

Calcium carbonate, calcium citrate, and calcium acetate therapies have the potential advantage of partially correcting metabolic acidosis and increasing ionized calcium concentrations, thereby decreasing PTH secretion. Bone mineral content may decrease less rapidly when patients are given calcium binders as compared to aluminum binders.[100] Prevention of phosphate retention by calcium binders may also allow normal

TABLE 42–3. Phosphate-Binding Agents Used in the Treatment of Hyperphosphatemia of Renal Failure

Agents	Calcium, Aluminum, or Magnesium Content*	Dosage Form	Starting Doses	Comments
Calcium Carbonate (40% calcium)			0.5–1 g (elemental calcium) tid with meals	Dissolution characteristics and phosphate-binding effect may vary from product to product. Usual maintenance dosage ranges from 2.4 to 5.6 g (elemental calcium) or 6 to 14 g (calcium carbonate) per day.
Os-Cal 500	500 mg	Tablet		
Caltrate 600	600 mg	Tablet		
Nephro-Calci	600 mg	Tablet		
CalCarb HD	2400 mg/packet	Powder		To be mixed with food.
Calci-Mix	500 mg	Capsule		To be mixed with food.
Calci-Chew	500 mg	Tablet		Chewable.
Tums	500, 700, 1000 mg	Tablet		Chewable.
Calcium Carbonate	500 mg/5 mL	Suspension		
Many other trade names and generic brands available.				
Calcium Acetate (25% calcium)				Comparable efficacy to calcium carbonate with half the dose of elemental calcium.
Phos-Lo	169 mg	Tablet	2 tablets tid with meals	
Calcium Citrate (21% calcium)			0.5–1 g (elemental calcium) tid with meals	Citrate enhances absorption of aluminum. Should not be administered concurrently with aluminum binders, antacids, or sulcralfate.
Citracal	200 mg 500 mg	Tablet Effervescent tablet		 Contains Aspartame.
Aluminum Carbonate			400–500 mg tid with meals	Second-line agent after calcium binders. Do not use concurrently with citrate-containing products.
Basaljel	500 mg 400 mg/5 mL	Tablet, capsule Suspension		
Aluminum Hydroxide			300–600 mg tid with meals	Second-line agent after calcium binders. Do not use concurrently with citrate-containing products.
Amphogel	300, 600 mg 320 mg/5 mL	Tablet Suspension		
AlternaGel	600 mg/5 mL	Suspension		
Magnesium Carbonate				
Mag-Carb	70 mg	Capsule	70 mg tid with meals	Magnesium concentration in dialysate needs to be reduced to avoid hypermagnesemia. Serum magnesium concentration should be routinely monitored and kept within the normal range. Diarrhea is a common side effect.
Magnesium Hydroxide				
Milk of Magnesia	300,600 mg 400 mg/5 mL 800 mg/5 mL	Tablet Suspension Suspension	300–400 mg tid with meals	Magnesium concentration in dialysate needs to be reduced to avoid hypermagnesemia. Serum magnesium concentration should be routinely monitored and kept within the normal range. Diarrhea is a common side effect.

*Calcium content expressed as the amount of elemental calcium in each dosage form. The aluminum and magnesium values represent total content of the dosage form (e.g., milligrams of aluminum hydroxide).

synthesis of calcitriol until low levels of renal function are reached.[101] However, maintaining a high positive calcium balance may predispose patients to metastatic calcification.[91,92] Multiple studies have shown that calcium carbonate alone can successfully normalize phosphate concentrations in a high percentage of dialysis patients[101,102]; however, large doses (average 6 to 14 g/d of calcium carbonate) may be required.[102] Delmez and Slatopolsky showed a linear relationship between ingested dietary phosphorus and the amount of calcium carbonate (g) required to achieve goal phosphorus concentrations in ESRD patients.[92] Calcium carbonate is marketed in a variety of dosage forms (Table 42–3), and is relatively inexpensive. Unfortunately, many calcium carbonate products fall under the category of food supplements and are not required by law to meet United States Pharmacopeia (USP) disintegration and dissolution requirements. Intact calcium carbonate tablets have been detected in the stool of hemodialysis patients. In general, nationally advertised brands meet USP quality standards for disintegration and dissolution, but it is difficult to determine whether private label or house brands conform to these same standards. A home test for determining the quality of calcium carbonate tablets has been described.[103] Calcium carbonate is more soluble in an acidic medium and therefore should be administered prior to meals when stomach acidity is highest.[104] In addition, acid-suppressing agents such as ranitidine can reduce the phosphate-binding activity of calcium carbonate by increasing gastric pH.[105]

Single-meal gastrointestinal balance experiments and short-term human trials have shown that calcium acetate binds approximately twice as much phosphorus as calcium carbonate at comparable doses of elemental calcium.[106,107] Increased binding potency limits gastrointestinal calcium absorption. However, calcium acetate is more soluble, and therefore better absorbed than calcium carbonate in an alkaline pH, which may explain the similar incidence of hypercalcemia when equivalent phosphorus concentrations are achieved.[106,107] Unfortunately, calcium acetate also causes more nausea and diarrhea than does calcium carbonate, which results in poorer medication compliance.[108] A long-term pharmacoeconomic study comparing the cost effectiveness of calcium acetate versus calcium carbonate on suppression of secondary hyperparathyroidism, bone mass, and metastatic calcification is needed to definitively support calcium carbonate or acetate as the superior phosphate-binding agent.

Although the chloride and citrate salts of calcium may be used as phosphate binders, these agents exhibit several disadvantages compared to the carbonate and acetate salts. The chloride salt is very astringent and unpalatable, and absorbed chloride may contribute to systemic acidosis. The citrate salt binds phosphate poorly *in vitro,* markedly increases intestinal aluminum absorption due to the formation of soluble aluminum citrate complexes, and may contribute to aluminum intoxication.[109] Thus, citrate-containing compounds should not be combined with aluminum-containing compounds. In contrast, calcium acetate does not appear to influence the intestinal absorption of aluminum.[109] In most cases when calcium binders are used as the primary phosphate binder, a low-calcium dialysate (2.25 to 2.75 mEq/L) should be used to reduce the potential for hypercalcemia and metastatic calcification.

Magnesium-containing antacids are also fairly effective phosphate binders. Several investigators have shown that magnesium-containing phosphate binders can lessen the amount of aluminum-containing binders necessary for optimal phosphorus control,[92] although serum potassium concentrations may rise and diarrhea is a problem. Dialysate magnesium concentrations must be reduced to avoid hypermagnesemia when magnesium-binding agents are used.[92] Magnesium carbonate is less well absorbed and better tolerated than magnesium hydroxide and is now commercially available in a capsule formulation (Mag-Carb, R and D Laboratories). Magnesium and potassium serum concentrations must be closely monitored to avoid hypermagnesemia or hyperkalemia.

Finally, a nonabsorbable hydrogel phosphate-binding agent (RenaGel, GelTex Pharmaceuticals) is currently undergoing human clinical trials. This novel agent, which does not contain any aluminum, calcium, or magnesium, appears to effectively lower phosphorus, PTH, and also total and low-density lipoprotein cholesterol concentrations.[110]

In summary, patients with renal insufficiency should be initiated on calcium-containing phosphate binders to bind phosphorus and suppress PTH. If necessary, magnesium- or aluminum-containing phosphate binders can be added to optimize phosphorus control. If magnesium-containing binders are used, a reduction in dialysate magnesium is necessary to prevent hypermagnesemia. If aluminum-containing binders are used, then serum aluminum concentrations should be monitored every 3 to 6 months to prevent aluminum toxicity.

CALCIUM SUPPLEMENTATION

Once normophosphatemia has been achieved, normocalcemia should be sought using both dietary and pharmacologic means. Before calcium-containing phosphate binders were routinely used, calcium supplements were often given between meals to optimize total corrected serum calcium concentration at high-normal limits to reduce the stimulus for PTH secretion. Although dietary calcium intake is often subnormal in moderate to severe renal insufficiency patients due to the reduced intake of phosphate-containing dairy products, administration of calcium-containing phosphate binders should ensure a positive calcium balance. Therefore, calcium supplementation is no longer necessary in the majority of patients above that which is provided by the phosphate-lowering regimen.

VITAMIN D THERAPY

Vitamin D therapy should be added in patients who do not achieve normocalcemia or those with elevated parathyroid hormone and alkaline phosphatase concentrations despite the use of calcium-containing binders alone. It must be emphasized that phosphorus control must be achieved before vitamin D therapy is initiated. There is increasing evidence that hyperphosphatemia causes resistance to the PTH-suppressing effects of vitamin D analogs as well as directly stimulates PTH release and increases the risk of a high calcium–phosphorus product, which can lead to soft-tissue calcification.[111] Many vitamin D analogs are available; however, all but dihydrotachysterol, 1,25-dihydroxyvitamin D_3 (calcitriol), 19-nor-1-α-25 dihydroxy vitamin D_2 (paricalcitol), and 1-α-hydroxyvitamin D_3 (alfacalcidol, not yet available in the United States) require hydroxylation in the kidney to produce the physiologically active hormone. Although biochemical, radiologic, and histologic improvements in renal osteodystrophy have been noted in patients receiving massive doses of vitamins D_2 or D_3, use of these sterols has been rendered obsolete by more physiologically active analogs with shorter half-lives. Calcitriol has largely replaced dihydrotachysterol in the management of renal osteodystrophy in the United States, because calcitriol inhibits PTH secretion directly in addition to stimulating intestinal absorption of calcium.

Calcitriol can suppress PTH secretion by increasing serum calcium concentrations through enhanced gut absorption of calcium as well as by directly decreasing PTH synthesis and secretion by parathyroid cells.[112] Calcitriol can be administered orally as well as by intravenous injection. Controversy exists regarding the most effective route of administration, optimal dose, and dosage interval. Recent reviews nicely summarize the available literature relating to calcitriol for treatment of secondary hyperparathyroidism.[111,112]

Calcitriol directly suppresses parathyroid hormone secretion by decreasing the set point for calcium-regulated PTH production[87] and may reduce parathyroid hyperplasia.[113] High plasma levels of this sterol achievable following intermittent (pulse) intravenous dosing two or three times weekly may more effectively suppress PTH secretion than daily doses of oral calcitriol.[87] In fact, intravenous calcitriol has been safely used in the treatment of patients with hyperparathyroid bone disease in whom hypercalcemia developed during oral therapy with calcitriol.[114] Although initial uncontrolled trials suggested that intravenous pulse therapy may be more effective than oral pulse therapy, more recent controlled trials suggest that oral therapy may be just as effective with no greater risks.[115–117]

The discrepancies between studies that have evaluated parathyroid gland size and calcium set point changes probably can be explained by major differences in study population such as length of dialytic therapy, dose of calcitriol, use of aluminum versus calcium binders, presence or absence of aluminum bone disease, nodular versus diffuse parathyroid hyperplasia, and dialysate calcium concentration. It also appears that the size of the largest parathyroid gland may be a critical marker for response to calcitriol therapy. It is difficult to suppress PTH in patients with glands greater than 0.5 cm^3 in volume, while patients with smaller glands are more easily controlled with calcitriol. Larger glands are more likely to be comprised of nodular tissue, which has lesser density of vitamin D receptors and therefore is less responsive to calcitriol therapy.[118]

Unfortunately, use of calcitriol enhances phosphorus absorption from the gut and frequently leads to hyperphosphatemia.[114,116] Conventional daily oral doses of calcitriol (0.25 μg) may be more frequently associated with hypercalcemia and hyperphosphatemia, because calcitriol receptors are located in intestinal mucosa where direct stimulation can occur. Strategies to minimize hypercalcemia while maximizing PTH suppression have included use of oral or intravenous pulse doses of calcitriol and calcitriol administration at bedtime or between meals when gut calcium and phosphorus content is lowest.[112] In addition, the dialysate calcium concentrations can be lowered to 2.25 to 2.75 mEq/L to limit hypercalcemic episodes.[111] Initial dosing guidelines for calcitriol can be found in Table 42–4. Intravenous calcitriol can be administered anytime during hemodialysis, as it is highly plasma protein bound and is not removed by the procedure.[119]

Intravenous calcitriol is approximately 3 to 4 times as expensive as the oral product. However, the pattern of oral versus intravenous calcitrol use in United States dialysis units has been strongly influenced by Medicare reimbursement. Currently, intravenous calcitriol is a separately reimbursable expense item for dialysis programs. In fact, dialysis programs oftentimes profit from the intravenous administration of calcitriol to patients on dialysis. In contrast, oral calcitriol is not separately reimbursable and must be purchased by the patient. Thus, even though it appears that oral calcitriol pulse therapy is as effective as intravenous pulse therapy, and is much less expensive, most dialysis programs continue to administer intravenous calcitriol.

TABLE 42–4. Initial Calcitriol Dosing Guidelines for Prevention and Treatment of Secondary Hyperparathyroidism

Degree of Hyperparathyroidism	Range of Intact PTH (pg/mL)	Initial Calcitriol Dose
Mild to moderate	200–600	Predialysis: 0.25 μg po qd or 0.5 μg po on alternate days Dialysis: 0.5–1 μg IV or po each dialysis (B-TIW)
Moderate to severe	600–1200	Dialysis: 2–4 μg IV or po each dialysis (B-TIW)
Severe	> 1200	Dialysis: 4–6 μg IV or po each dialysis (B-TIW)

Several new vitamin D analogs have been developed that may result in less calcium and phosphorus absorption from the gut, but retain the positive physiologic actions on bone and parathyroid tissue.[120,121] 19-nor-1-α-25-dihydroxyvitamin D_2 (paricalcitol) was approved by the Federal Food and Drug Administration in 1998. Combined data from three identical double-blind, placebo-controlled human trials (n = 78) showed that paricalcitol administered intravenously three times a week after hemodialysis significantly reduced PTH over 12 weeks with a mean ending dose of 0.12 μg/kg. The mean serum calcium and phosphorus values did rise slightly during the study in the treatment group. There were 8 episodes of 401 serum calcium measurements that rose > 11 mg/dL in the treatment group as compared to 4 of 417 measurements in the placebo group. Elevations of the calcium-phosphorus product > 75 occurred in 45 of 395 determinations in the treatment group as compared to 16 of 412 determinations in the placebo group.[122] Similarly, oral 1-α-hydroxyvitamin D_2 has been tested in a 12-week trial of 24 hemodialysis patients with moderate hyperparathyroidism. PTH values were effectively suppressed in most patients with mean doses of 4.7 to 5.6 μg after each dialysis. Mean calcium and phosphorus concentrations increased slightly over the trial with 4.7 episodes of hypercalcemia (> 10.5 mg/dL) and 10.1 episodes of hyperphosphatemia (> 6.9 mg/dL) per 100 weeks of treatment as compared to 0.53 and 6.9 episodes, respectively, in the washout period.[123] The oral and IV formulations are expected to be released in 1999.

Although the efficacy and safety profiles of these two new agents look very promising in these short-term trials as compared to short-term trials with calcitriol, additional positive long-term trials and comparative trials with calcitriol will be necessary to conclude that these agents are superior to calcitriol.[121,123] Animal and preliminary clinical data are being generated for a new class of compounds, the calcimimetic agents. These compounds mimic the effect of extracellular calcium by stimulating parathyroid cell calcium receptors and may prove useful in the treatment of both primary and secondary hyperparathyroidism.[124] Investigations with bisphosphonates, which block osteoclastic bone reabsorption (etidronate also inhibits bone mineralization), have shown conflicting results; thus, along with calcitonin their place in therapy is currently confined to the acute treatment of hypercalcemia resulting from hyperparathyroidism.[102]

SURGICAL THERAPY

PARATHYROIDECTOMY

Parathyroidectomy should be undertaken as the last therapeutic option for patients with secondary hyperparathyroidism. Criteria for surgery include (1) persistent hypercalcemia (serum calcium > 11.5 mg/dL) provided aluminum toxicity has been ruled out[125]; (2) a persistently elevated calcium–phosphorus product above 70 and progressive soft-tissue calcification that persists despite vigorous dietary phosphate restriction and phosphate binder use; (3) progressive radiographic lesions of secondary hyperparathyroidism despite aggressive vitamin D therapy, particularly when associated with severe or debilitating symptoms; (4) intractable pruritus recalcitrant to other therapy; and (5) syndrome of calciphylaxis (a rare syndrome characterized by ischemic necrosis of the skin, muscles, and/or subcutaneous fat caused by vascular calcification).

Total parathyroidectomy is not recommended, as the presence of parathyroid hormone appears to be necessary for bone remodeling. Generally, approaches include either subtotal parathyroidectomy or total parathyroidectomy with transplantation of parathyroid tissue to an accessible site, such as the forearm,[126] or ablation therapy with injections of ethanol.[118] Postoperative hypocalcemia, hypophosphatemia, and hypomagnesemia may occur because of a marked increase in bone production in relation to bone absorption ("hungry bone syndrome"). The severity of the hypocalcemia depends on the degree of osteitis fibrosa, and preoperative treatment with calcitriol may prevent or minimize the risk. Treatment with supplemental calcium and calcitriol may be necessary for weeks or months. After surgery, continual efforts to prevent hyperphosphatemia and the recurrence of secondary hyperparathyroidism are necessary.

EVALUATION OF THERAPEUTIC OUTCOMES

The therapeutic goals for treatment with phosphate-binding agents and vitamin D therapy are to prevent secondary hyperparathyroidism, vitamin D deficiency, and subsequent renal osteodystrophy without inducing adynamic bone disease from oversuppression of PTH. The specific target goals for phosphorus and PTH along with suggested laboratory treatment goals are outlined in Table 42–5. In addition, the fractional reabsorption of phosphorus (FR_{phos}, normally 80% to 95%) can be monitored.

$$FR_{phos} = [1 - (U_{phos} \times S_{cr}/S_{phos} \times U_{cr})] \times 100$$

U_{phos} = urine phosphorus concentration

S_{cr} = serum creatinine concentration

S_{phos} = serum phosphorus concentration

U_{cr} = urine creatinine concentration

Elevations in PTH concentrations and a declining FR_{phos} will indicate the need for further phosphorus restriction. An algorithm approach for the treatment and evaluation of the ESRD patient on dialysis using clinically available noninvasive markers (corrected serum calcium, serum phosphorus, and intact PTH) can be found in Figure 42–6. Evidence shows higher concentrations of these substances are necessary to achieve normal bone mineralization and formation rates in dialysis patients.[121] If the patient develops hypercalcemia after several weeks of calcitriol therapy, this may indicate healing of osteitis fibrosa cystica.[125]

ALUMINUM TOXICITY

PATHOPHYSIOLOGY AND CLINICAL PRESENTATION

Although once a major problem, aluminum toxicity occurs less frequently due to use of deionizers and reverse osmosis filters for dialysate water purification and decreased use of aluminum phosphate binders.[127] Aluminum is renally excreted; thus, accumulation can occur in severe renal insufficiency when patients are exposed to various sources of aluminum. A recent study showed that the use of aluminum utensils can be a source of aluminum exposure in dialysis patients.[128] Aluminum toxicity can contribute to renal osteodystrophy (Fig. 42–5) and result in decreased hematopoiesis and encephalopathy. Impaired bone mineralization and altered bone cell proliferation from aluminum excess result in an osteomalacic or adynamic bone histologic pattern.[129] Aluminum and iron compete for the same absorption and cellular uptake pathways. Aluminum may disrupt cellular iron metabolism, causing an iron-deficiency–like pattern and decreased erythropoiesis (microcytic anemia) in the presence of normal iron stores.[129] Interestingly, patients with

TABLE 42–5. Laboratory Monitoring Parameters for Prevention and Treatment of Secondary Hyperparathyroidism

	Creatinine Clearance (mL/min/1.73 m^2)		
	> 30	*10–30*	*< 10 (ESRD)*
Calcium (mg/dL)[a,b]	9–11	9–11	9–11
Phosphorus (mg/dL)[b]	2.5–4.0	2.5–4.0	4.5–6
Ca × Phos[c]	< 70	< 70	< 70
PTH[d,e]	Normal range	1–2 × normal range	2–3 × normal range[f]

[a]Corrected calcium for albumin: Corrected calcium = [(4.0 − albumin) × 0.8] + serum calcium.
[b]Monitor once monthly in most circumstances.
[c]Calcium–phosphorus product calculated as mg^2/dL^2.
[d]Using an intact or *N*-terminal PTH assay.
[e]PTH values can be drawn as often as once monthly during dose-titration phase of phosphate binders or calcitriol to as infrequently as every 6 months once patient is stabilized.
[f]2–5 × normal range for CAPD patients.

low serum iron may be predisposed to aluminum toxicity because aluminum binds to transferrin, the major transport protein for iron.[129] Aluminum neurotoxicity can occur insidiously with speech disturbances and progress to asterixis, myoclonus, visual and auditory hallucinations, seizures, and ultimately death. Rapid manifestations of aluminum toxicity can occur under three circumstances: (1) high concentrations of aluminum in dialysate, (2) concurrent use of aluminum- and citrate-containing products, and (3) acute elevations in plasma and cerebral spinal fluid aluminum concentrations secondary to deferoxamine (DFO) administration.[130,131]

▶ PREVENTION AND TREATMENT: Aluminum Toxicity

Prevention is accomplished by (1) using water purified by deionization or reverse osmosis such that dialysate aluminum concentrations are less than 10 μg/L and (2) minimizing the use of aluminum-containing phosphate binders or medications and aluminum-containing drinks, foods, and utensils (especially in the presence of citrate). Maintaining adequate iron balance may also lessen the risk for aluminum toxicity.

The gold standard for diagnosis of aluminum-related bone disease is transiliac bone biopsy. Indirect, less invasive methods such as elevated plasma aluminum, low PTH concentrations, and positive DFO infusion test are also used to identify patients with aluminum overload, but these methods are less specific and sensitive. The DFO infusion test is based on the concept that the amount of aluminum mobilized following a single dose of DFO is representative of the total body burden of aluminum. The DFO test consists of an intravenous infusion of 5 mg/kg of DFO administered preferably after a dialysis session to minimize DFO loss through the dialyzer. Blood samples for aluminum content should be drawn before the hemodialysis session at which DFO was given and before the subsequent dialysis session.[127] The change in serum aluminum concentration is the key factor upon which therapeutic decisions are made. Although the DFO infusion test is not entirely reliable in identifying patients with aluminum overload, it continues to be widely used. A combination of a negative DFO infusion test plus high PTH concentration may be useful to rule out aluminum toxicity.[132] Although the optimal way to evaluate aluminum toxicity is controversial, Figure 42–7 outlines one approach to diagnosis.[127]

All patients with symptoms of organ dysfunction from aluminum overload should receive DFO therapy. Hemodialysis alone does not significantly remove aluminum, as it is highly bound to the plasma protein transferrin. However, hemodialysis in combination with DFO therapy can remove substantial amounts of aluminum–DFO complex. High-flux dialysis and hemofiltration (using membranes with high middle molecule clearances) are effective in removing the complex[133]; however, an investigational high-flux dialyzer with immobilized DFO appears to enhance clearance above that of a high-flux dialyzer alone.[134]

EVALUATION OF THERAPEUTIC OUTCOMES

The desired outcomes for patients with aluminum overload are to reduce the total body burden of aluminum as evidenced by a resolution of symptoms and a serum aluminum concentration less than 60 μg/L with DFO (Fig. 42–7). The use of DFO carries some risk of hypotension and ocular toxicity, and has been linked to unusual systemic infections such as mucormycosis.[135,136] Cerebrospinal fluid aluminum concentrations have been shown to rise after DFO administration,[130] and plasma concentrations greater than 500 μg/L following DFO administration have been associated with acute encephalopathy.[137] In an effort to minimize adverse reactions, once-weekly, low-dose (5 mg/kg) DFO administration has been recommended.[127] In contrast to the consensus paper,[127] which advocates administering DFO during the hemodialysis session and allowing chelation to take place over 48 to 72 hours between sessions, two recent papers suggest starting dialysis within 5 to 12 hours after DFO administration to limit toxicity and optimize removal.[138,139] However, this approach would be impractical in most outpatient dialysis centers.

ANEMIA OF CHRONIC RENAL INSUFFICIENCY

PATHOPHYSIOLOGY

The majority of patients with chronic renal insufficiency and end-stage renal disease exhibit a normochromic, normocytic anemia that progresses as renal function worsens.[140] The primary cause of anemia in patients with chronic renal insufficiency and end-stage renal disease is a relative erythropoietin (EPO) deficiency, for which therapy with recombinant human erythropoietin alpha (epoetin) has been available in the United States since 1989. Erythropoetin beta, another recombinant erythropoietin product with similar pharmacologic effects, is available in other nations. In adults, the kidneys synthesize about 90% of circulating EPO with the remainder synthesized by the liver. EPO is a glycoprotein of approximately 30,000 Daltons that is secreted in response to hypoxia.[141,142] Plasma concentrations of EPO increase to approximately 1000 mU/mL when the hematocrit drops to 20% in individuals with normal renal function. In contrast, ane-

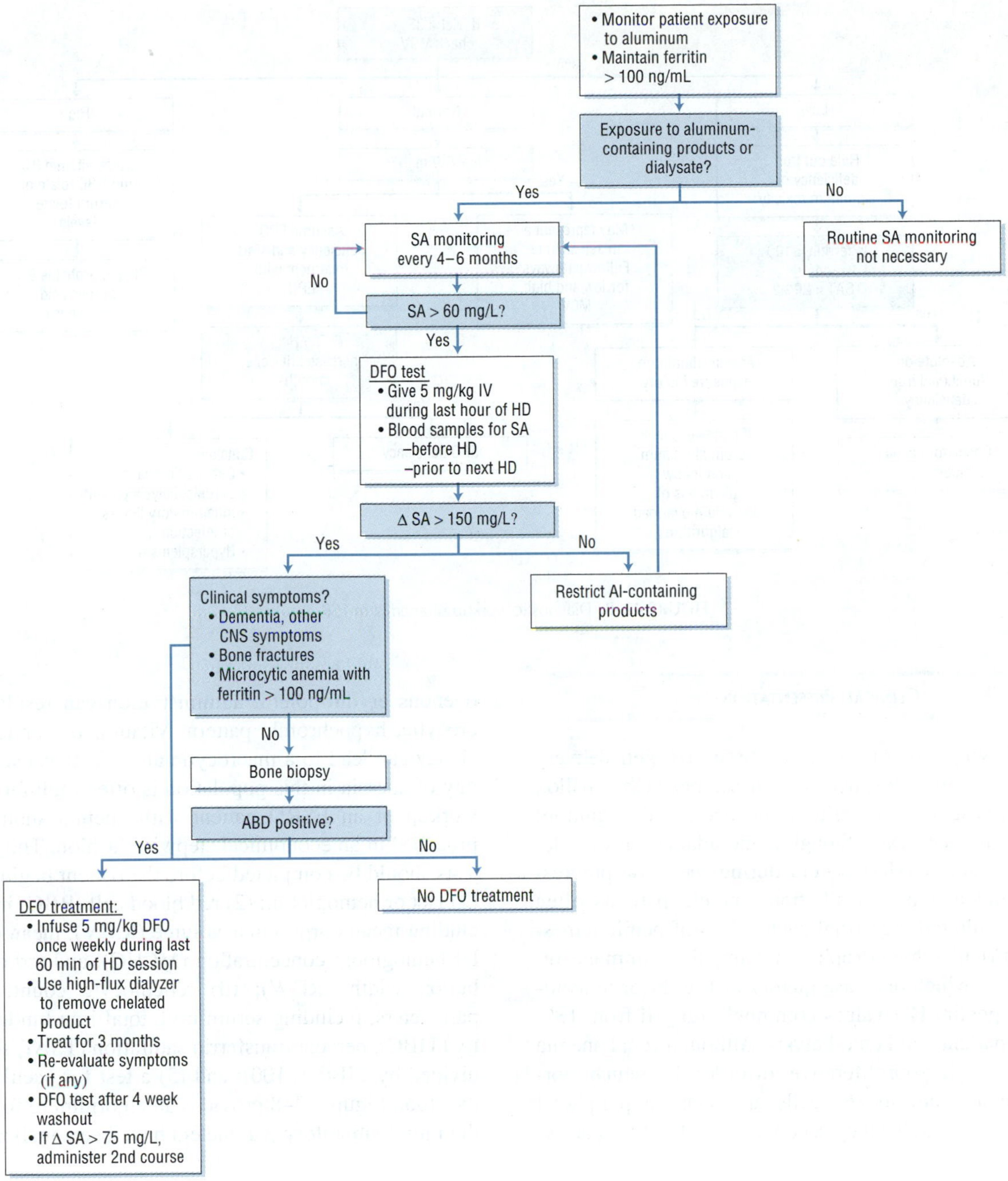

FIGURE 42–7. Diagnosis and treatment of aluminum overload in end-stage renal disease. (DFO = deferoxamine; ABD = aluminum bone disease; HD = hemodialysis; SA = serum aluminum; Δ SA = change in serum aluminum.)

mic dialysis patients produce serum EPO concentrations of about 20 mU/mL.[143] EPO stimulates the proliferation and differentiation of erythroid progenitor cells.[141] Anemia begins to develop when the GFR drops below 20 to 30 mL/min/1.73 m^2. It is of interest that patients with ESRD secondary to polycystic kidney disease can often maintain a normal hematocrit without exogenous administration of EPO. Other factors such as blood loss; iron, folic acid, or vitamin B_{12} deficiency; severe osteitis fibrosa; systemic infection or inflammatory illness; and aluminum toxicity or hypersplenism may also contribute to the anemia of CRF. Blood loss commonly occurs due to routine laboratory monitoring, dialyzer clotting, and bleeding from hemodialysis needle puncture sites. In addition, dialysis patients are prone to gastrointestinal bleeding.[144] Iron deficiency is now commonly seen due mainly to aggressive use of recombinant human erythropoietin (epoetin). Prior to epoetin availability, many patients were dependent on intermittent packed red blood cell transfusions.

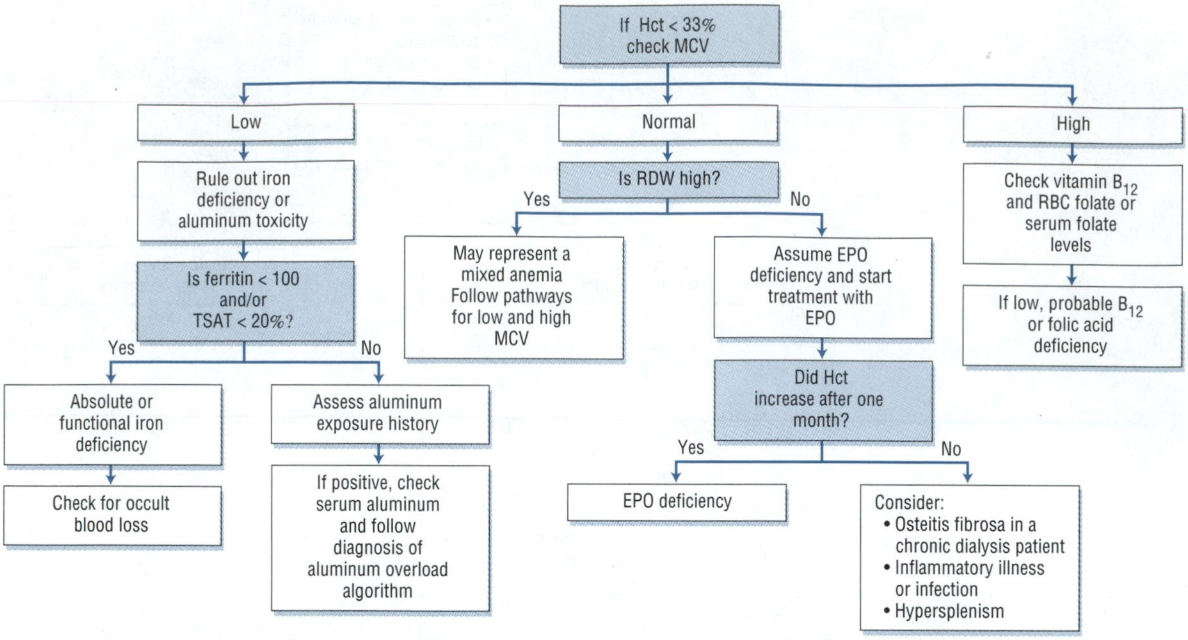

FIGURE 42–8. Diagnostic workup of anemia in ESRD.

Clinical Presentation

Signs and symptoms of decreased tissue oxygen delivery (fatigue, exertional dyspnea, dizziness, headache, pallor, angina, congestive heart failure, and decreased cognition) are commonly seen even though some adaptation to a decreased hematocrit (Hct) occurs during the slow progression of renal anemia. In addition, anemic patients often demonstrate altered menstrual cycles, loss of penile tumescence, ventricular hypertrophy, and impaired immune response, all of which decrease quality of life. Prior to availability of epoetin, Hct values commonly ranged from 18% to 25% in patients on hemodialysis. Although renal anemia is typically a hypoproliferative disorder in which normochromic and normocytic cells are seen on peripheral blood smear, iron deficiency secondary to blood loss or exogenous erythropoietin administration can result in a microcytic, hypochromic pattern. Vitamin B_{12} or folate deficiency can lead to a macrocytic anemia. Because the etiology of anemia in this population is often multifactorial, the workup of an ESRD patient with anemia should be approached in an economical stepwise fashion. The following tests should be completed before the patient begins epoetin: (1) Hct or hemoglobin; (2) red blood cell (RBC) indices, including mean corpuscular volume (MCV), mean corpuscular hemoglobin concentration (MCHC), and red cell distribution width (RDW); (3) reticulocyte count; (4) iron parameters, including serum iron, total iron-binding capacity (TIBC), percent transferrin saturation (TSAT, serum iron divided by TIBC × 100); and (5) a test for occult blood in the stool. Figure 42–8 provides an algorithm to follow once the initial laboratory parameters have been analyzed.

▶ TREATMENT: Anemia of Chronic Renal Insufficiency

In March of 1995, the National Kidney Foundation–Dialysis Outcomes Quality Initiative (NKF–DOQI) was established to improve patient outcomes by formulating recommendations for optimal clinical practices.[140] The anemia of chronic renal insufficiency was one of four clinical areas initially chosen for this structured review process because it met the following criteria: (1) significant numbers of patients affected, (2) availability of sufficient information in the literature to formulate guidelines, (3) lack of contemporary practice guidelines, (4) high variability in practice standards and high levels of controversy on how patients should be managed, and (5) associated with significant risk for patient. Several thousand literature references were reviewed and 349 references were selected as the basis for the evidence and opinion-based guidelines.[140]

DESIRED OUTCOME

The goals of therapy are to prevent or reverse the signs and symptoms of tissue oxygen deprivation and left ventricular hypertrophy, improve exercise capacity, optimize survival, and ultimately improve the quality of life of patients. Most of the physiologic and quality of life studies of epoetin that resulted in resolution of the signs and symptoms of anemia achieved Hct measurements of 36% or less, and the phase III clinical trials achieved Hct values between 33% and 38%.[140] However, when epoetin alpha was approved in 1989, the target hematocrit range recommended by the FDA (and ultimately incorporated into the package insert) was 30% to 33%. Subsequently, the FDA broadened the range to 30% to 36% in 1994. However, the latest United States Renal

Data System (USRDS) report shows that in the last quarter of 1995, the mean Hct was only 31.4%.[4] A recent study sponsored by Amgen evaluated the effects of a normal Hct (42 ± 3%) compared with a lower target Hct of 30 ± 3% in more than 1200 hemodialysis patients with documented heart disease. The study was discontinued when an interim analysis showed that the patients with the higher range experienced a higher death rate than the lower Hct group.[140] Consequently, based on this and many other clinical trials, the DOQI workgroup recommended a target Hct (hemoglobin) range of 33% to 36% (11 to 12 g/dL).

GENERAL APPROACH TO TREATMENT

Red blood cell transfusions and androgen therapy are currently second-line treatment options for treatment of renal anemia. RBC transfusions carry many undesirable risks and therefore should only be used in three situations: (1) for acute management of symptomatic anemia, (2) after significant acute blood loss, and (3) prior to surgical procedures that carry a high risk of blood loss. Androgen therapy was also used extensively before epoetin availability, but hemopoietic response was suboptimal in the majority of patients. However, androgen therapy may potentiate the effects of epoetin by increasing the sensitivity of erythroid precursors in some individuals. Although *in vitro* results have been encouraging, small human trials testing androgen effects on erythropoiesis have yielded conflicting results. A retrospective analysis of 84 patients receiving androgen therapy in Spain showed a correlation between rise in hemoglobin and increased age.[145] The authors concluded that nandrolone decanoate therapy was a less expensive alternative to epoetin and may be particularly suitable in males over 55. A recent prospective open trial, albeit small (n = 19), convincingly showed that nandrolone decanoate 100 mg intramuscularly per week along with epoetin enhanced Hct response beyond that of epoetin alone with few side effects.[146] However, the risks of liver toxicity, malignancy virilization in females, and hypertriglyceridemia outweigh the benefits of androgen therapy in most individuals.

Currently, epoetin is the therapy of choice for long-term correction and maintenance of Hct levels in predialysis and dialysis patients. It is reasonable to begin epoetin therapy in patients with hematocrit values that fall below 33%. Epoetin therapy results in dose-dependent increases in effective erythropoiesis in both predialysis and dialysis patients. Prior to initiation of epoetin, iron balance should be assessed, as iron deficiency is the most common cause of suboptimal response to epoetin.

PHARMACOLOGIC THERAPY

IRON ASSESSMENT

Iron status is usually assessed by monitoring serum iron, ferritin, TIBC, and TSAT. Plasma ferritin values tend to correlate with body stores of iron located in the liver, bone marrow, and spleen. Unfortunately, ferritin is an acute phase reactant and serum ferritin values can rise independently of body iron stores in response to inflammation, liver disease, malignancy, or infection. Circulating iron is highly bound to a protein called transferrin. Transferrin-bound iron is readily utilizable by the bone marrow for erythropoiesis. In order to prevent an absolute (low body stores) or functional (low amount of readily utilizable iron) iron deficiency in renal patients receiving epoetin, it is suggested that ferritin and TSAT values of at least 100 ng/mL and 20%, respectively, be maintained. Another test to evaluate early iron deficiency is an increase in the percentage of hypochromic red blood cells (normally less than 2.5%). This test is not routinely available in the United States but is used in Europe. Values greater than 10% are associated with functional iron deficiency. Once this methodology becomes more widely available, it should be incorporated into the workup of anemic patients with chronic renal insufficiency.[140] Finally, one other marker that may be proven to be more sensitive in predicting functional iron deficiency is reticulocyte hemoglobin content (CHr). A CHr less than 28 pg at baseline predicted functional iron deficiency and response to iron dextran better than TSAT and ferritin in one study.[147]

Ideally, iron deficiency should be corrected before epoetin therapy is initiated, which can be accomplished rapidly with intravenous iron. However, before iron therapy is initiated, several important considerations must be kept in mind: (1) blood losses, therefore iron losses, are higher in hemodialysis patients than in predialysis or peritoneal dialysis patients; (2) oral iron is not sufficient to maintain adequate iron stores in hemodialysis patients, but may be sufficient in some predialysis or peritoneal dialysis patients; (3) epoetin therapy alone will lead to functional and absolute iron deficiency by stimulating erythropoiesis; and (4) maintenance (regular) doses of iron prevent iron deficiency and promote consistent erythropoiesis.

Oral Iron

Oral iron management should begin with agents that have relatively high bioavailability and low cost. Initially, ferrous salts (sulfate, gluconate, and fumerate) should be prescribed to provide approximately 200 mg of elemental iron per day for adults (2 to 3 mg/kg for pediatric patients) (see Chap. 91). Patients should be given divided daily doses of iron and instructed to take iron on an empty stomach to maximize absorption. If patients have gastrointestinal complaints (nausea, vomiting, constipation, diarrhea), they can take oral iron with a small snack or try another dosage form or product such as ferrous sulfate solution, iron–polysaccharide complex, or sustained-release preparation. However, the two latter compounds are more expensive and bioavailability is a problem. Administration with meals reduces iron absorption due to the interactions between iron, food, and phosphate binders. Some clinicians suggest giving vitamin C concomitantly with oral iron to enhance absorption. Unfortunately, serum oxalate concentrations have been shown to rise in dialysis patients who receive more than 250 mg/d of vitamin C[148]; therefore this maneuver is not recommended.

Intravenous Iron

In order to achieve the target Hct range, most hemodialysis patients and many peritoneal and predialysis patients will require intravenous iron. There are two IV iron products currently available in the United States, both composed of iron dextran (INFeD, MW 96,000; and DexFerrum, MW 267,000). Numerous clinical trials have been conducted with iron dextran preparations as well as ferrous gluconate and iron saccharate (both available in Europe).[149] Parenteral iron has been shown to improve the responsiveness to epoetin and reduce the amount of epoetin needed to achieve and maintain a target Hct. Initially, many dialysis programs administered IV dextran either as one-time large-dose (500 to 2000 mg) infusions or as intermittent courses of therapy (100 mg given during the hemodialysis session for 10 consecutive sessions) to treat iron deficiency. Either of these approaches is reasonable to initially replete patients with an absolute iron deficiency (ferritin < 100 ng/mL),[150] but allows many hemodialysis patients to become iron deficient before the next treatment is given due to ongoing blood losses. There is mounting support for using smaller maintenance doses (25 to 100 mg/wk) particularly in hemodialysis patients to maintain iron balance. The DOQI guidelines state the following. (1) In adult hemodialysis patients with absolute iron deficiency (usually ferritin < 100 ng/mL), administer 100 mg of iron dextran during each dialysis by IV push (over 2 minutes) for 10 sessions (25 mg for pediatric patients weighing less than 10 kg, and 50 mg in those weighing 10 to 20 kg). (2) To maintain iron balance in adult hemodialysis patients with ferritin values above 100 ng/mL, administer 50 mg each week during dialysis for 10 weeks with measurement of TSAT and ferritin 2 weeks after the 10th dose. Weekly iron doses can then be adjusted (25 to 100 mg/wk) to maintain goal ferritin and TSAT values as well as optimal erythropoiesis. The weekly dose can be divided and given as one to three doses per week. (3) Predialysis or peritoneal dialysis patients who have an absolute iron deficiency or cannot maintain iron balance with oral iron alone can be given intermittent total dose infusions of 500 to 1000 mg (dilute in 250 mL of normal saline and give over 1 hour).

Iron dextran is not immediately available to the bone marrow for heme synthesis, but must be processed by the reticuloendothelial system (RES) before being released to transferrin or stored within the RES in bone marrow or splenic or hepatic tissue. The incorporation of iron into hemoglobin occurs over weeks, with a plasma disappearance half-time that is dose dependent. Serum iron, TIBC, and ferritin values should be evaluated at least 2 weeks after iron dextran has been administered to avoid errors in serum iron determination from circulating iron dextran. Total dose infusions have been associated with more delayed side effects such as arthralgias, myalgias, and serum-sickness-like symptoms. However, some investigators have reported a low incidence of problems with doses equal to or less than 500 mg.[151] Although the need for a test dose is controversial, DOQI guidelines recommend that a one-time dose of 25 mg in adults (10 to 15 mg in pediatric patients) should be administered IV before initiating iron therapy to detect the small risk (< 0.65%) of anaphylaxis. Aggressive use of intravenous iron dextran can enhance erythropoiesis, but may increase the risk of iron overload and development of hemosiderosis over time. Iron dextran should be held for at least 3 months in patients who develop a serum ferritin level above 800 ng/mL with parenteral iron.

Two other intravenous iron products (ferric gluconate and iron saccharate) have been used extensively in Europe.[149] Ferric gluconate has undergone clinical trials in the United States and is expected to be released in 1999. This product has been shown to replete iron stores effectively when given in doses of 62.5 to 125.0 mg weekly to three times weekly. European and U.S. clinical data show that allergic reactions with ferric gluconate are rare. In fact, one study showed that patients experiencing allergic reactions to iron dextran could be treated successfully with ferric gluconate.[149] There are some data to suggest that this product has the potential to oversaturate transferrin when given as a rapid infusion. Thus, it is likely that package insert guidelines will suggest a prolonged infusion in contrast to iron dextran which can be administered by rapid IV infusion when given in doses of 100 mg or less.

PHARMACOKINETIC AND PHARMACODYNAMIC PROPERTIES OF EPOETIN

Understanding the pharmacodynamic profile of epoetin is more important than the pharmacokinetics of this agent. Unlike many drugs where pharmacodynamic action is related to peak or trough concentrations or half-life can be used to predict the duration of action or time to attainment of steady state, epoetin action must be evaluated on the basis of changes in RBC production rate and the individual's RBC life span.[152] Uremic patients have a shortened RBC life span, which averages 64 days in contrast to 120 days in normal subjects.[152] The Hct response to the pharmacodynamic effect of epoetin (an increase in Hct) is illustrated in Figure 42–9. Prior to starting epoetin, the baseline Hct is constant, demonstrating that RBC production is at steady state (the rate at which RBCs are being produced equals the rate at

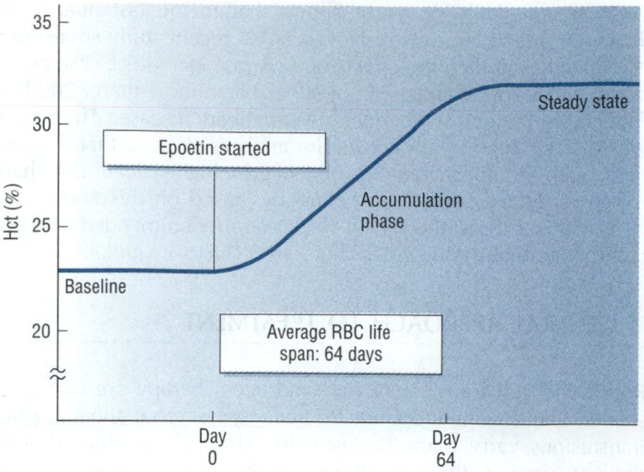

FIGURE 42–9. Pharmacodynamic effect of epoetin on hematocrit (Hct) response.

which they are dying). Although the Hct may begin to rise shortly following epoetin initiation as the result of demargination of reticulocytes, it takes approximately 10 days before erythrocyte progenitor cells mature and begin to be continuously released into the circulation at an increased rate. Gradually Hct rises as the RBC production rate exceeds daily RBC death. The Hct will continue to increase until the life span of the cells stimulated by epoetin is reached (range, 1 to 4 months) and a new steady state is achieved. Clinical trials have documented successful treatment of ESRD anemia with total weekly IV or SC doses of 80 to 180 U/kg (adults and pediatric patients > 5 years old) or up to 300 U/kg in pediatric patients less than 5 years old.

Epoetin can be administered by either the IV or subcutaneous route. Subcutaneous administration is preferable in chronic ambulatory peritoneal dialysis and prehemodialysis patients (these patients usually do not have permanent IV access), and now is being recommended in hemodialysis patients as a way to reduce expenditures for epoetin.[140] Although SC administration results in poor bioavailability (approximately 20%), low peak serum concentrations, and a prolonged half-life (approximately 22 hours as compared to 8.3 hours IV),[153] Hct response is at least as good or better than IV administration. This enhanced efficacy is presumed to be due to a more prolonged, physiologic stimulation of erythroid precursors. Although many of these comparative studies suffer from design flaws, the preponderance of data supports the use of SC epoetin, as target Hct may be maintained with lower weekly epoetin doses (15% to 50% lower) as compared to IV.[140,154] Once a week, twice a week, and three times a week subcutaneous dosing have all been shown to be effective. Currently, two formulations of epoetin alpha are available, a single-dose formulation without preservative and a multidose formulation with benzyl alcohol. A recent clinical trial compared these two formulations in terms of pain intensity after subcutaneous administration. The multiple-dose formulation caused less stinging, although several patients did not experience pain with the single-dose preparation.[155]

Resistance to Epoetin

Real or pseudoresistance to epoetin therapy can stem from multiple factors.[140] Iron deficiency is the most common cause of resistance to epoetin and develops routinely during epoetin therapy.[140] Evaluation and treatment should precede as previously outlined. Inflammation (localized or systemic infection, active inflammatory disease, surgical trauma) is associated with defective iron utilization known as reticuloendothelial (RE) block. RE block is characterized by a reduction in iron delivery from body stores to the bone marrow, and is generally refractory to iron therapy. Malignancy and autoimmune diseases can cause a resistance to epoetin by decreasing endogenous erythropoietin production, RE block, and reduced bone marrow responsiveness.[140] Cancer cells can invade the bone marrow; radiation and chemotherapy can damage erythroid progenitor cells. Epoetin therapy can be continued in the infected or postoperative patient, although increased amounts are often required to maintain or slow the rate of decline in hematocrit.

Hyperparathyroidism is known to cause resistance to epoetin. Erythropoietic response to epoetin therapy in patients with hyperparathyroidism appears to be linked to the severity of bone marrow fibrosis. Aluminum toxicity, which has been discussed previously, can reduce iron transport. Aluminum also inhibits key enzymes necessary in heme synthesis. Recognition of aluminum toxicity and appropriate chelation therapy with DFO are key steps in improving bone marrow response to epoetin. Unfortunately, DFO also chelates iron, making therapeutic management of anemia more difficult. Hemoglobinopathies are often not responsive or are poorly responsive to epoetin.[140] In patients with sickle cell anemia, epoetin can increase the release of reticulocytes containing mainly hemoglobin S with little or no increase in hemoglobin F (the more stable form). Patients with alpha-thalassemia may slowly increase their Hct with epoetin following long-term therapy with high doses. Folate and vitamin B_{12} deficiency can also cause epoetin resistance, as both of these are essential for optimal erythropoiesis. Patients on hemodialysis or peritoneal dialysis are routinely prescribed daily vitamins with folate, as this substance is water soluble and dialyzable.

One other factor that may worsen the anemia of CRF is the use of angiotensin-converting enzyme inhibitors (ACEIs). The mechanism has not been elucidated, and several brief reports have been conflicting.[140] A recent stepwise regression analysis of 108 hemodialysis patients suggested that one of the parameters associated with higher epoetin maintenance dosages was ACEI administration.[156] A prospective trial needs to be designed to clarify this issue. Patients currently receiving epoetin and initiating ACEIs should have Hct carefully assessed and epoetin dosages increased if necessary to maintain Hct within the target range. Finally, pseudoresistance can occur with occult bleeding or hemolysis. In this case, bone marrow response to epoetin is normal, but the rate of rise in hematocrit with epoetin is negatively offset by blood loss or hemolysis. Therefore, a workup of apparent epoetin resistance should always include an evaluation of potential sources of blood loss or hemolysis.

PHARMACOECONOMIC CONSIDERATIONS

Epoetin truly represents a major breakthrough in the therapy of renal anemia and relegates transfusion therapy and its attendant risks to the treatment of acute blood loss and anemia refractory to epoetin. However, this therapy is expensive, and is estimated to cost Medicare almost $1 billion per year, a significant increase in cost when compared to androgen therapy or blood transfusions. However, epoetin therapy may result in fewer days of hospitalization and rehospitalization and increased transplant success.[157,158] The use of maintenance IV iron as well as subcutaneous administration of epoetin should also reduce the per-patient Medicare cost for epoetin. Current Medicare reimbursement rates for epoetin (and IV iron) produce profits for most dialysis programs, and thus there is little incentive at this point to minimize the use of epoetin. In addition, home administration of epoetin is reimbursable for dialysis patients but not predialysis patients. In the case of iron therapy, IV iron is reimbursable by Medicare whereas oral iron is either paid for by the patient out of pocket or by secondary insurers (usually with a copayment). Managed care is rapidly infiltrating dialysis programs. Capitation of payments for medications such as epoetin and IV iron therapy will force the dialysis community to change clinical practice to provide for the economic use of both iron and epoetin therapy.

EVALUATION OF THERAPEUTIC OUTCOMES

Figure 42–10 outlines an algorithm approach to patient evaluation and treatment with epoetin and iron therapy in adults. Effective therapy with epoetin in the treatment of the anemia of CRF has been shown to decrease morbidity and increase quality of life.[140] Although the mean and median Hct have been rising in dialysis patients each year since epoetin was introduced, the mean Hct value was only 31.4% in 1995.[4] In addition, over 50% of dialysis patients had TSAT values less than 20%, and 36% of patients had ferritin concentrations less than 100 ng/mL in 1993.[140] This suggests that epoetin and iron therapy can be further optimized in a large percentage of dialysis patients.

The major side effect of epoetin is a predictable elevation in blood pressure, which occurs in approximately 23% of CRF patients.[140] The exact reason for increased blood pressure is not clear, but may be due to increased vascular reactivity and increased blood viscosity. The baseline or final levels of hemoglobin, rate of rise in hemoglobin, or uncontrolled hypertension prior to epoetin use do not appear to be risk factors for development of hypertension.[159] Increases in blood pressure should be treated aggressively and blood pressure should be stable (ideally ≤ 150/90) before epoetin initiation. Epoetin doses should only be reduced or held if aggressive ultrafiltration and antihypertensive management cannot control blood pressure or if hypertensive encephalopathy occurs. Seizures have occurred in approximately 3% of patients treated with epoetin.[140] Seizure incidence does not appear to be increased over baseline levels seen in placebo control groups. Because it is controversial whether vascular access thrombosis may be more frequent during epoetin therapy, no increased surveillance is advocated.[140]

UREMIC BLEEDING

PATHOPHYSIOLOGY

Bleeding complications are usually mild, but can result in major hemorrhagic events. The etiology of uremic bleeding is multifactorial (Table 42–6). The primary mechanisms

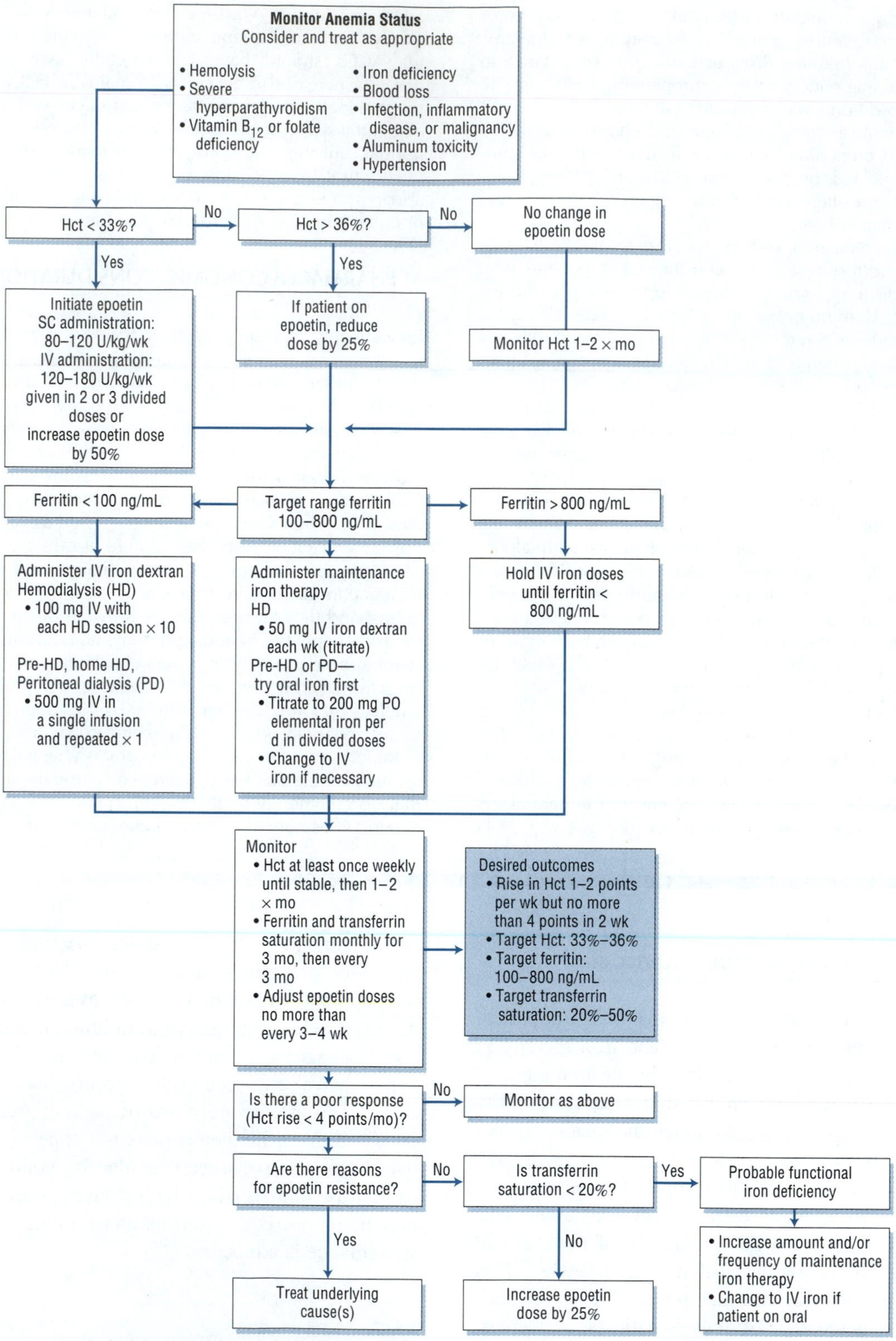

FIGURE 42–10. Approach to epoetin and iron therapy in the treatment of ESRD anemia.

TABLE 42–6. Etiology of Uremic Bleeding

Platelet Defect
Circulating toxins
Imbalance in prostacyclin/thromboxane A_2
Decrease in ADP and serotonin
Increase in parathyroid hormone
Questionable abnormal von Willebrand factor
Decreased platelet factor III
Increased platelet-derived levels of β-thromboglobulin
Anemia
Relative deficiency in erythropoietin
Shortened red blood cell life span
Blood loss
Iron, vitamin B_{12}, or folate deficiency
Antithrombotic Therapy
Heparinization during hemodialysis
Anticoagulant therapy for access clotting or other thrombotic disorder
Antiplatelet therapy for access clotting or other cardiovascular disorder

underlying the hemostatic problem are platelet biochemical abnormalities and alterations in platelet–vessel wall interactions. Decreased platelet aggregation and adhesiveness have been shown in a number of studies.[160] Additionally, there is a decreased plasma concentration and defective binding of the large multimer of von Willebrand factor (vWF), which results in abnormal platelet–blood vessel wall interactions. Normally platelets flow in a skimming pattern close to the vessel wall while RBCs occupy the center of the vessel, a situation that is ideal for platelet–vessel wall interaction. Anemia results in dispersion of platelets and red blood cells during flow through vessels, which makes it difficult for primary hemostasis to occur.[161] Heparinization during dialysis procedures also increases risk of bleeding. In addition, dialysis patients often receive systemic anticoagulation (warfarin) or antiplatelet therapy (aspirin or ticlopidine) for prevention of access clotting or other cardiovascular problems.

Clinical Presentation

Uremic patients commonly experience purpura, ecchymoses, epistaxis, and prolonged bleeding from hemodialysis venipuncture sites. Gastrointestinal bleeding occurs less commonly, but can be severe and is often related to gastrointestinal telangiectasias. Other severe hemorrhagic complications such as spontaneous retroperitoneal bleeding, hemorrhagic pericarditis, or pleural effusion occur less frequently.[144] Subdural hematoma, which may occur in up to 3% of hemodialysis patients, should be suspected with symptoms of headache, vomiting, seizures, somnolence, confusion, or coma.[144] Risk factors for a subdural bleed include head trauma or hypertension. The bleeding time is the clinical test that is most often prolonged in uremia. This test measures the time required for bleeding from a small standardized skin puncture site to cease. Filter paper is used to wipe off the blood from the incision every 30 seconds.[143] This test reflects primary hemostatic function and measures interaction between platelets and the vessel wall following injury. The normal bleeding time averages 4 to 5 minutes (range 2 to 9 minutes).[143] Unfortunately, this test has not been found to be useful in predicting the risk of bleeding in individual patients.[162]

▶ TREATMENT: Uremic Bleeding

A number of studies have shown that dialysis therapy shortens but usually does not normalize the bleeding time, and the effect is short lived (1 to 2 days).[161] Marked improvement in bleeding times have been found in patients whose Hct was corrected to above 30% with epoetin and iron therapy. The proposed mechanism is enhanced interaction between platelets and the blood vessel wall. Patients receiving coumadin anticoagulation need to be followed closely for clinical signs of bleeding; the international normalized ratio (INR) should be routinely evaluated. Patients receiving antibiotics (a common scenario in ESRD) need intensified monitoring for early detection of antibiotic-associated increases in INR.

Patients at high risk for bleeding can undergo alternative dialysis procedures rather than traditional hemodialysis with systemic heparinization (see Chap. 44). Dialytic techniques with less risk of bleeding include peritoneal dialysis; hemodialysis with minimal heparinization, regional heparinization, or regional citrate anticoagulation; or hemodialysis without heparinization.[144]

There are several nondialytic adjunctive therapies that may temporarily shorten the increased bleeding time observed in patients with renal failure.[144,160,161] Cryoprecipitate is rich in factor VIII, fibrinogen, and fibronectin and has been shown to shorten bleeding time in CRF patients. Based on positive results with cryoprecipitate, intravenous, subcutaneous, and intranasal administration of 1-deamino-8-D-arginine vasopressin (DDAVP) was evaluated. DDAVP has minimal vasoconstrictive effects as compared to vasopressin, but effectively releases autologous factor VIII (von Willebrand factor, or vWF) from the endothelial lining of vessel walls. Again, a consistent lowering of bleeding time was noted with all three routes of administration. A drawback to the use of DDAVP is tachyphylaxis with repeated doses; response may return after 3 to 4 days. This effect is felt to be due to depletion of vWF stores following the first dose. Side effects of DDAVP are minimal and include mild flushing, headache, and hyponatremia.

Based on the observation that women with von Willebrand disease improved during pregnancy, estrogens were evaluated and have been shown to reduce bleeding time in uremic subjects.[163] The mechanism of action is unknown; however, estradiol has been determined to exert the most active hemostatic effect of the conjugated mixture.[164] Five daily intravenous infusions of conjugated estrogens have been demonstrated to have a prolonged effect on bleeding time. Oral conjugated estrogens and low-dose transdermal patches have also been shown to be successful. Side effects, which are uncommon and usually mild, include hot flashes, nausea, vomiting, hypertension, gynecomastia, and loss of libido. An increased risk of thromboembolism may result from estrogen therapy, especially with chronic use. Indications and dosage of each agent can be found in Table 42–7.

TABLE 42–7. Management of Uremic Bleeding

Indication	Agent	Effect: Start	Effect: Maximum	Effect: End	Dosage
Long-term management	Adequate dialysis	—	—	—	—
	Epoetin	10 d	2–3 months	—	See section on anemia in discussion of chronic renal failure. Goal: Hct > 33%–36%
Acute bleeding episodes	Packed RBC transfusion	Immediate	—	—	Goal: Hct > 33%
	DDAVP (IV,SQ,intranasal)	1–2 h	2–4 h	6–8 h	0.3 μg/kg IV
	Conjugated estrogens	6 h	5–7 d	21–30 d	0.6 mg/kg IV each d × 5 d
Life-threatening bleeding	Cryoprecipitate	1 h	4–12 h	24–36 h	10 "bags" IV
Chronic treatment of telangiectasias	Estrogen/progestin combinations	6 h	5–7 d	—	Various products and dosages used in studies
Management of chronic bleeding tendency	Conjugated estrogens	6 h	5–7 d	—	50 mg orally each day; only studied short term (< 2 wk) 50–100 μg/24 h of transdermal estradiol

Evaluation of Therapeutic Outcomes

Preoperative and high-risk patients with uremia should have their bleeding times and other measures of coagulation (INR, aPTT, and platelet counts) assessed and normalized if possible. Abnormal bleeding times should be corrected with DDAVP and cryoprecipitate if a rapid effect is desired, and estrogens should be used in situations where prolonged bleeding risk is a consideration. Alternative dialytic procedures can be performed in patients with high bleeding risk.

HYPERLIPIDEMIA

Pathophysiology

Chronic renal failure with or without nephrotic syndrome is frequently accompanied by abnormalities in lipoprotein metabolism. In chronic renal failure without nephrotic syndrome, type IV hyperlipidemia with hypertriglyceridemia (plasma concentrations 200 to 600 mg/dL) secondary to increased plasma concentrations of very low-density lipoprotein (VLDL) is commonly seen. In addition, a normal to modest increase in total cholesterol (TC) and low density lipoprotein (LDL), and a reduction in high-density lipoprotein (HDL) concentrations as well as changes in apoproteins (reduction in apo A-I, A-II, and E and elevations in apo B and lipoprotein(a)) may accompany hypertriglyceridemia.[165] In part, lipid abnormalities in ESRD may result from reduced plasma clearance of triglyceride-rich lipoproteins secondary to inhibition of peripheral lipoprotein lipase and hepatic triglyceride lipase activity.[166] Peripheral insulin resistance, carnitine deficiency, and hyperparathyroidism may also contribute to lipid abnormalities.[166]

In the nephrotic syndrome, the major lipid abnormalities are elevation of plasma total and LDL cholesterol with variable changes in HDL cholesterol.[167,168] The proposed mechanisms involved in dyslipidemia of the nephrotic syndrome are outlined in Figure 42–11.

Clinical Presentation

"Myocardial infarction" and "other cardiac causes" are the most commonly reported causes of death in the ESRD population.[4] Whether hypertriglyceridemia or other lipoprotein changes contribute to the high incidence of cardiovascular disease in these patients is controversial. Clearly, other concomitant risk factors—such as diabetes, smoking, hypertension, and left ventricular enlargement—are often present before patients initiate dialysis therapies. In addition, hypertriglyceridemia alone has not been shown to be a strong independent risk factor for coronary heart disease in patients with

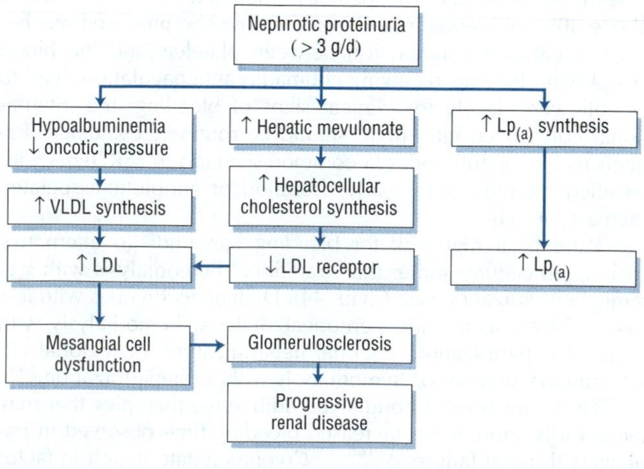

FIGURE 42–11. Potential effects of proteinuria on hyperlipidemia in the nephrotic syndrome. VLDL = very low-density lipoprotein; LDL = low-density lipoprotein; $LP_{(a)}$ = lipoprotein (a).

normal renal function following multivariate analysis of several studies.[169] However, high triglyceride concentrations are known to raise the concentrations of other lipoproteins that do promote atherogenesis, including chylomicron remnants, VLDL remnants, intermediate-density lipoproteins, and small, dense LDL.[170] Finally, hypertriglyceridemia may reduce levels of "protective" HDL, which is now classified as a major risk factor for coronary heart disease.[169] Thus, although hypertriglyceridemia itself may not be atherogenic, it may increase coronary risk through its effects on other lipoproteins.

▶ TREATMENT: Hyperlipidemia

Dietary restriction of carbohydrate and cholesterol combined with an increase in the polyunsaturated–saturated fat ratio can reduce plasma triglycerides in some patients.[171] Unfortunately, most patients with chronic renal insufficiency and those receiving dialysis have already been advised to adhere to difficult dietary regimens, which may include protein, phosphorus, sodium, potassium, and fluid restrictions as well as diabetic exchanges. Although diet therapy is a reasonable first-step approach, it is unlikely to be successful in a majority of renal disease patients due to noncompliance.

The best approach to the treatment of hyperlipidemia in patients with nephrotic syndrome is unclear. To date, clinical trials have been designed to evaluate the short-term efficacy and safety of diet and drug therapy and have not been designed to define effects on cardiac or renal end points.[168] However, if clinical experience in patients with hyperlipidemia can be extrapolated to patients with nephrotic syndrome, then patients with atherogenic lipid profiles should be treated. Reductions of 20% to 25% in total and LDL cholesterol have been reported with strict soy-based vegetarian low-cholesterol and low-fat diets,[172] but short-term use of the American Heart Association step I diet has only minimal effects.[168,173] Step II diet therapy as recommended by the National Cholesterol Education Program (NCEP) expert panel may be a reasonable first step in management.[168] However, if LDL cholesterol reduction is suboptimal after 6 months of intensive diet therapy, lipid-lowering drugs should be added.

Many nephrologists find dietary modification or use of triglyceride-lowering agents difficult to justify in hypertriglyceridemic chronic renal failure patients because (1) the specific contribution of hypertriglyceridemia to increased coronary artery disease risk in this condition is unknown, (2) a beneficial effect of drugs for reducing coronary artery disease risk in this condition has not been demonstrated, and (3) long-term drug safety has not been proven. However, it also has not been proven that patients with renal disease are more or less prone to the atherogenic effects of abnormal lipoprotein patterns. In the absence of solid data in this population, it seems prudent to follow the guidelines set forth by the NCEP panel[168] (see Chap. 19).

Five drug classes may prove useful as hypocholesterolemic therapies in patients with renal failure and nephrotic syndrome: the bile acid sequestrants, nicotinic acid, HMG-CoA reductase inhibitors, fibric acids (gemfibrozil and clofibrate), and probucol. A recent meta-regression analysis examined these medications (with the exception of nicotinic acid) along with carnitine, fish oil, low molecular weight heparins, and exercise to determine their effects in nephrotic syndrome, renal insufficiency, hemodialysis, and peritoneal dialysis.[174] Potential limitations always exist with this type of analysis; however, it does help provide a foundation for selecting initial therapy in a specific patient population with specific lipid profiles. The results of this study are summarized in Table 42–8.

The effect of *L*-carnitine supplementation on abnormal lipid metabolism in dialysis patients has been assessed in several trials, but results have been contradictory. Although *L*-carnitine supplementation cannot be advocated at this time for hyperlipidemia treatment, carnitine may prove useful for dialysis-related muscle cramps or hypotension, lack of energy, skeletal muscle weakness, cardiomyopathy, or anemia unresponsive to epoetin.[174] Interestingly, reverse flux filtration along with heparin-induced extracorporeal LDL precipitation (HELP) during hemodialysis has been successful in reducing LDL cholesterol in hemodialysis patients with type IIb hyperlipidemia.[175] Although nicotinic acid has theoretical advantages for nephrotic patients, the drug has not been systematically studied for this purpose. It also exhibits a variety of adverse effects that may mitigate its usefulness.

ADVERSE EFFECTS

Potential drug interactions and/or side effects can occur with antilipemic therapy. The nonselective binding activity of bile acid sequestrants may reduce absorption of corticosteroids, digoxin,

TABLE 42–8. Effects of Pharmacologic and Nonpharmacologic Lipid-Lowering Management in Renal Insufficiency

	Nephrotic Syndrome				Renal Insufficiency				Hemodialysis				Peritoneal Dialysis			
	Tot	*HDL*	*LDL*	*Trig*	*Tot*	*HDL*	*LDL*	*Trig*	*Tot*	*HDL*	*LDL*	*Trig*	*Tot*	*HDL*	*LDL*	*Trig*
HMG-CoA	↓↓	↑↑	↓↓	↓↓	↓↓	—	↓↓	↓	↓↓	—	↓↓	↔	↓↓	↑↑	↓↓	↓
Fibrates	↓	—	↑	↓↓	↓↓	—	↓	↓↓	↓↓	↑↑	↓↓	↓↓	↓	—	↓	↓↓
Bile seq.	↓	↑	↓	↑↑	—	—	—	—	—	—	—	—	—	—	—	—
Diet	↓↓	—	↓	↑	↑↑	—	↓	↓	↓↓	—	↓↓	↓↓	—	—	—	—
Probucol	↓↓	—	↓	↓	—	—	—	—	—	—	—	—	—	—	—	—
Exercise	—	—	—	—	—	—	—	—	↓↓	—	↑	↓	↓	—	—	↑
Carnitine	—	—	—	—	—	—	—	—	↓↓	↑↑	↓	↓↓	—	—	—	—
Fish oil	↑	—	↑	↓↓	↑↑	—	↑	↓	↓↓	↑↑	↓	↓	↑	—	↑	↓
LMWH	—	—	—	—	—	—	—	—	↓↓	—	↓	↓	—	—	—	—

Double arrows indicate a statistically significant change.

thiazide diuretics, warfarin, and other commonly used medications. Myositis and myalgias, along with increased serum creatine phosphokinase (CPK), have been reported in renal failure patients using clofibrate.[177] Determining the optimal dose of clofibrate in this patient population is difficult, as plasma protein-binding changes markedly affect free concentrations of the active metabolite, clofibric acid, which has a prolonged half-life in renal failure.[178] Gemfibrozil may be a safer alternative, as the half-life is not altered in renal dysfunction.[179] However, some investigators have reported significant increases in CPK concentrations following usual doses of gemfibrozil in dialysis patients,[180,181] which has led some authors to suggest lower doses of 300 mg bid with close monitoring of CPK levels.[180,182]

Although HMG-CoA reductase inhibitors are remarkably free of adverse effects in otherwise healthy subjects, one should be cognizant of the potential myotoxic effects of these drugs, especially during concomitant cyclosporine, gemfibrozil, and niacin administration, and in the presence of hepatic disease.[183] Large doses of omega-3 polyunsaturated fatty acids (fish oils) have been shown to lower triglyceride levels in hemodialysis patients,[165,184] but they may interfere with platelet function, predisposing to bleeding. In addition, the high doses necessary to lower triglycerides makes noncompliance more likely.

Evaluation of Therapeutic Outcomes

Nonpharmacologic treatment (weight reduction, alcohol restriction, and increased exercise) should be initiated for all patients with hypertriglyceridemia alone. Patients with triglyceride concentrations above 1000 mg/dL after 3 to 6 months of nonpharmacologic treatment should begin gemfibrozil 300 mg bid with dose titration upwards if necessary (CPK concentrations permitting) to prevent pancreatitis. Nonnephrotic patients with atherogenic concentrations of LDL cholesterol and other risk factors for coronary artery disease should be initiated on HMG-CoA reductase inhibitors. Dosages should be titrated per NCEP panel guidelines for LDL cholesterol concentrations.[169] Nephrotic patients with elevated LDL cholesterol should be initiated on a step II diet and/or drug therapy based on NCEP panel guidelines.[169] HMG-CoA reductase inhibitors appear to be a good first choice, with addition of fibric acid derivatives, bile resins, or niacin as appropriate.

HYPERTENSION IN END-STAGE RENAL DISEASE

The pathophysiology and treatment of hypertension is reviewed in detail in Chapter 10. The present discussion will focus on pathophysiology and therapeutic management of hypertension in patients with ESRD.

Pathophysiology

Hypertension can be a cause or a consequence of renal insufficiency. High blood pressure may also promote renal damage independently of the underlying mechanism of renal disease. The major pressor mechanisms are inappropriate activation of the renin–angiotensin system and an abnormal pressure–natriuresis relationship.[185] Several morphologic changes, collectively termed hypertensive nephrosclerosis, have been noted in kidneys of patients with essential hypertension. Of patients initiating dialysis, 75% to 90% are hypertensive. The pathogenesis is multifactorial but the majority of hypertensive dialysis patients have a volume component to blood pressure elevation (fluid retention promotes high blood pressure.)[185] In addition to these factors, erythropoietin use and structural changes in the arteries (e.g., metastatic calcification) may contribute to hypertension in the ESRD patient.

It has been observed that patients with moderate to severe renal insufficiency display an abnormal diurnal rhythm in their blood pressure in that blood pressure does not show a decrease during the nighttime hours.[187] It is unclear what causes this disturbance in the diurnal rhythm and also if it contributes to the progression of renal insufficiency. High blood pressure can accelerate the rate of decline in renal function as well as cause other end-organ damage.[48] In addition, hypertension is a risk factor for the severe atherosclerosis and cardiovascular disease noted in ESRD.[188] Unfortunately, hypertension may not be adequately controlled in a significant number of ESRD patients.[189]

▶ TREATMENT: Hypertension in End-Stage Renal Disease

Achievement of an individual's "dry weight" and control of total body sodium through the dialytic process results in normalization of blood pressure in 50% to 60% or more of dialysis patients.[186] The percentage of dialysis patients considered to have dialysis-resistant hypertension requiring antihypertensive medications varies considerably depending on the approach of the specific dialysis unit or physician, demographic differences, differences in the definition of hypertension in dialysis patients, and the patient's primary disease. In general, antihypertensive medications will control elevated blood pressure in the vast majority of these individuals, with bilateral nephrectomy rarely being employed today. Interestingly, the Tassin group showed that prolonged hemodialysis (8 hour sessions, 3 times per week) will help to maintain normal blood pressures.[190] However, the majority of hemodialysis programs in the United States use fast dialysis methods (3- to 4-hour sessions, 3 times per week). The J-curve phenomena may also occur in the renal failure population. This may be especially true secondary to the high incidence of ischemic cardiovascular disease in these patients. Therefore the potential complications of decreasing diastolic blood pressures to below 85 mm Hg may outweigh the benefits in some patients.[191]

The primary intervention for ESRD patients is to restrict salt (2 to 3 g/d) and water intake to reduce fluid volume accumulation between dialysis sessions. Massive doses of loop diuretics are generally ineffective in promoting diuresis and expose the patient to risks of ototoxicity, gastrointestinal upset, muscle cramps, and hyperglycemia.

Patients in whom salt and water restriction along with aggressive dialysis therapy fails to control high blood pressure may benefit from treatment with ACEIs in light of the important role of the renin–angiotensin axis in the etiology of dialysis-resistant hypertension. Because the elimination half-lives of the parent compound (captopril, lisinopril) or active metabolite (enalapril, benazepril, ramipril) are prolonged in endstage renal disease patients, downward adjustment of doses is usually necessary.[54,185] Bone marrow depression has been noted in up to 10% of renal failure subjects receiving captopril, especially those with autoimmune diseases.[186] If captopril therapy is initiated in the dialysis patient, close monitoring of white blood cell counts should be undertaken and drug doses kept as low as possible. Other ACEIs, which lack the sulfhydryl group of captopril, may be less likely to cause bone marrow depression and are probably the angiotensinconverting enzyme inhibitors of choice in these patients.

Calcium channel blockers, particularly the dihydropyridines, which selectively lower systemic vascular resistance, also appear to be effective in the treatment of hypertension in the ESRD patient. In one study, nitrendipine lowered blood pressure effectively in hemodialysis patients with large interdialytic weight gains.[192] This is similar to the observation that a high sodium intake enhances the blood pressure response to calcium channel blockade in essential hypertension. Thus, either ACEI or CCB therapy would be appropriate first-line therapy in the hypertensive endstage renal disease patient in whom achievement of the target postdialysis weight (dry weight) is inadequate to control blood pressure.

A number of other antihypertensive drugs may also be effective in patients with endstage renal disease, including drugs that interfere with renin release such as the β-blockers or the combined α- and β-blocker labetalol. Agents such as esmolol, timolol, pindolol, metoprolol, or labetalol, which are metabolized and not significantly dialyzable, may be easier to dose titrate than those agents that are both dialyzable and extensively eliminated unchanged by the kidney (atenolol, nadolol, or acebutolol).[186]

Sympathetic nervous system active agents such as prazosin, terazosin, doxazosin, clonidine, guanabenz, or guanfacine may be required in patients unresponsive to dialytic therapy plus ACEI, CCB, or α-blocker therapy. Central α_2-agonists such as clonidine appear to be the safest of these agents to use in the dialysis population. Transdermal clonidine in doses up to 1.2 mg/d (four 0.3-mg patches) has demonstrated success as monotherapy in one short-term study of hypertensive dialysis patients.[193] Postsynaptic α-blockers (e.g., prazosin) have been associated with postural hypotension following hemodialysis.[194] Guanethidine and methyldopa should also be avoided because of potential complications including severe postural hypotension, severe dialysis-related hypotension, and impotence.[186]

The addition of vasodilators such as minoxidil or hydralazine may prove useful in patients resistant to combinations of the previously mentioned agents. Hydralazine is often effective as first-line therapy for hypertension and is generally well tolerated. In addition, monotherapy with the drug is well tolerated in diabetic patients because of the underlying autonomic neuropathy that prevents reflex tachycardia. The incidence of drug-induced SLE does not appear to be increased by the presence of endstage renal disease. Minoxidil therapy may be associated with a profound reflex tachycardia, and most patients should receive a β-blocker or a central α-adenoreceptor agonist to suppress this.

PHARMACOECONOMIC CONSIDERATIONS

Other considerations in selection of antihypertensive therapy in ESRD patients should include compliance and economic factors. In general, most ESRD patients are prescribed an average of 9 to 12 medications. Choosing agents that can be administered once or twice daily may improve patient compliance. In addition, there are now many options within some antihypertensive classes such as calcium channel blockers, ACE-inhibitors, and β-blockers. In most cases, no clear therapeutic advantage has been demonstrated with any particular agent within a class. Therefore, selecting the least costly agent that can be administered once or twice daily should have a favorable economic impact over the lifetime of the patient.

EVALUATION OF THERAPEUTIC OUTCOMES

A treatment algorithm for ESRD patients with hypertension is given in Figure 42–12. Other guidelines for antihypertensive therapy selection based on other patient characteristics can be found in the JNC report.[48] The interdialytic blood pressure goal should be 130/85 mm Hg or less, although this may be difficult to achieve due to the significant interdialytic weight gains of many hemodialysis patients. The benefits of achieving this blood pressure goal need to be weighed against the harmful effects of intradialytic hypotension. Blood pressures are always obtained before, during, and after a hemodialysis session. Ambulatory blood pressure monitoring can help to identify dialysis patients with blood pressure profiles that might respond to antihypertensive therapy.[195] Prolonged antihypertensive therapies with a combination of β-blockers, ACEIs, and CCBs have clearly been shown to result in regression of left ventricular hypertrophy in hypertensive ESRD patients.[196] They also may be useful in patients with connective tissue diseases.[197]

MISCELLANEOUS THERAPEUTIC CONSIDERATIONS

PRURITUS

Despite advances in dialysis treatment, pruritus (itching) remains a vexing problem which occurs in up to 90% of ESRD patients.[198] Pruritus is a manifestation of chronic but not acute renal failure and usually occurs 6 months or so after dialysis is initiated.[198,199] The pathogenesis of uremic pruritus is poorly understood, but has been attributed to multiple factors such as poor dialysis, dialysis membranes, skin dryness, secondary hyperparathyroidism, increased vitamin A and histamine plasma concentrations, and increased

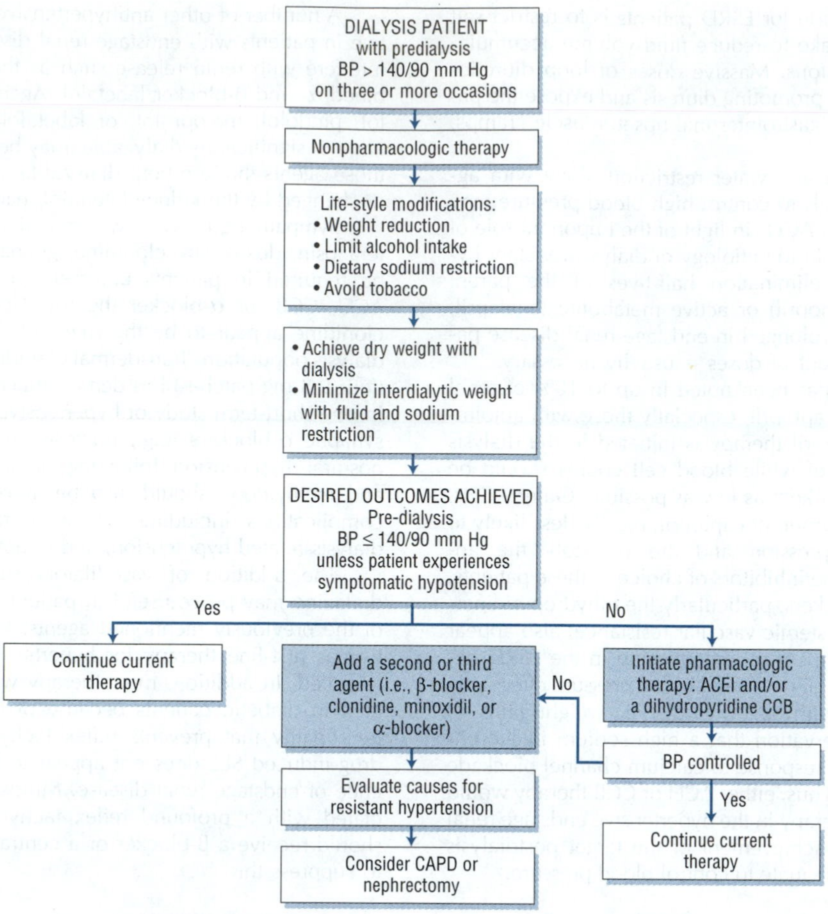

FIGURE 42–12. Treatment algorithm for ESRD patients with hypertension. (ACEI = angiotensin-converting enzyme inhibitor; CAPD = continuous ambulatory peritoneal dialysis; CCB = calcium channel blocker.)

sensitivity to histamine.[198,199] A small study in hemodialysis and peritoneal dialysis patients showed that patients with pruritus demonstrated higher numbers of degranulated mass cells as compared to patients without pruritus. In addition, higher concentrations of histamine, PTH, and middle molecular weight substances, and lower serum iron concentrations were seen in patients with pruritus.[200] ESRD patients with pruritus experience exaggerated itching sensation to exogenous administration of histamine as compared to uremic patients with no pruritus or control patients.[199]

NONPHARMACOLOGIC THERAPY

Therapy for pruritus is largely empirical. The mainstay of therapy is adequate dialysis treatment. Regular, aggressive dialysis eliminates or improves pruritus in many patients.[198] Poor tolerance to dialysis membranes and sterilants such as ethylene oxide can also cause pruritus in some patients. Thus, using a γ-irradiated membrane or noncomplement-activating membrane such as polymethylmethacrylate may be tried.[198] Other nonpharmacologic therapies include acupuncture and ultraviolet light. Acupuncture has been reported to improve pruritus for months in a small number of patients.[198] Ultraviolet B therapy has been shown to benefit a majority of patients in both controlled and uncontrolled studies. The mechanism of response has not been elucidated but may include reduction in skin content of vitamin A, divalent ions, and/or retinol; reduction in histamine-containing dermal mast cells; detoxification of unknown pathogenic substances; or desensitization of epidermal nerve endings.

PHARMACOLOGIC THERAPY

Numerous drug therapies have been evaluated for the treatment of pruritis. In fact, no single therapy has proven more effective than another in individual patients. Even though elevated plasma histamine concentrations and exaggerated responses to histamine have been noted in uremic patients with pruritus, antihistamine treatment often fails to reduce symptoms. A 2- to 3-week trial may be warranted. Some patients gain relief from topical administration of emollients, although dry skin does not appear to be a factor in pruritis. Activated charcoal and cholestyramine have also been shown to benefit some patients. However, the binding effects of these two agents on other medications, the extra fluid intake necessary to administer them, and the potential

TABLE 42–9. Recommendated Daily Allowance of Vitamins in ESRD Patients

Vitamin	Recommended Amounts
A	0
E	0
K	0
D	Individualized
B_1	1.5 mg
B_2	1.7 mg
B_6	10 mg
B_{12}	6 μg
Biotin	300 μg
Pantothenic acid	10 mg
Niacinamide	20 mg
Folic acid	0.8–1 mg
C	60 mg

for hyperchloremia with cholestyramine should be weighed against the potential benefits. The beneficial effects of lidocaine, heparin, naloxone, and ondansetron for pruritis treatment have also been described, but more clinical studies are necessary before any of these can be recommended. A stepwise process for treating uremic pruritis was recently proposed by Robertson and Mueller.[198]

VITAMIN REPLACEMENT

Vitamin requirements for ESRD patients receiving dialysis are different from those of a healthy person due to dietary modifications, renal dysfunction, and dialytic therapy.[148,201] Both vitamins A and E have been shown to be elevated in ESRD. Hypervitaminosis of vitamin A has been correlated with anemia and hypercalcemia (increased bone resorption) in hemodialysis patients. Vitamin K supplementation is probably unnecessary in most dialysis patients except for those with an elevated INR during or after a course of antibiotics. Vitamin D plays a major role in bone metabolism in ESRD; the dose of 1,25-dihyroxyvitamin D_3 (calcitriol) or other vitamin D analogs needs to be individualized. The water-soluble vitamins (B_1, B_2, B_6, B_{12}, niacin, pantothenic acid, folic acid, biotin, and vitamin C) have been shown to be low or deficient in the average Western diet. Some of the water-soluble vitamins are dialyzable; others such as vitamins C and B complex may be destroyed or the amounts reduced with cooking methods used by dialysis patients to leach out potassium. Vitamins B_6 (pyridoxine) and C (ascorbic acid) as well as folic acid are the three vitamins that have consistently been reported to be deficient in dialysis patients. Vitamin C is necessary for the normal production of oxalic acid. Higher concentrations of oxalate have been reported in hemodialysis patients receiving greater than 250 mg of vitamin C per day. Increased plasma concentrations of oxalate may lead to deposition in soft tissues, muscles, vessels, and organs. The goal for vitamin supplementation in this population should be to prevent subclinical and frank deficiency and to avoid pathology from overdosage. Table 42–9 outlines recommended allowances for ESRD patients.[201] Special vitamin supplements have been formulated for the dialysis patient, but these preparations are fairly costly. Lower-cost vitamin B with C formulations are available, although additional folic acid supplementation is then necessary.

▶ PRINCIPLES OF PHARMACOTHERAPY

- Type 1 diabetic patients with persistent microalbuminuria should be managed aggressively with intensive insulin therapy to maintain blood glucose within or close to the normal range to prevent progression of renal disease.
- Diabetic patients who demonstrate persistent microalbuminuria despite intensive insulin therapy should be initiated on an ACEI unless there is a contraindication, and the dose should be titrated to achieve maximal suppression of UAE to prevent renal failure progression.
- Blood pressure should be controlled at 130/85 mm Hg or less in all patients with renal insufficiency; patients exhibiting proteinuria above 1 g/d should have their BP reduced further to 125/75 mm Hg, preferably with an ACEI.
- Metabolic acidosis must be prevented or treated in renal insufficiency by the use of sodium bicarbonate tablets or sodium citrate-containing solutions to prevent bone demineralization, cardiac abnormalities, and growth retardation in children.
- Optimal phosphorus control using dietary phosphate restriction and phosphate binders in renal insufficiency is the primary method to reduce or halt the development of secondary hyperparathyroidism.
- Both pulse dose oral or intravenous calcitriol have been shown to be effective in suppressing PTH release; new vitamin D analogs are also effective.
- Assessment of iron balance and appropriate repletion prior to epoetin therapy and maintenance of iron balance (ferritin > 100 ng/mL and transferrin saturation > 20%) during epoetin therapy are essential to maximize erythropoietic response.
- Aggressive use of replacement and maintenance IV iron dextran in those patients who cannot tolerate or do not respond adequately to oral iron alone should optimize patient response to epoetin and reduce the total cost associated with anemia therapy.
- Blood pressure control should be attained prior to starting epoetin. Antihypertensive agents should be added as necessary to maintain a stable blood pressure.
- Epoetin should be administered subcutaneously. Doses up to 300 mg/kg/wk can be used in pediatric patients less than 5 years old. For older children and adult dosage, see Figure 42–10.
- The initial Hct response may be delayed for approximately 2 weeks, although the reticulocyte count will increase almost immediately.

- Following initiation of epoetin or any dose change, steady-state Hct levels will not be attained until one red blood cell life span has occurred (approximately 2 months). Therefore, epoetin doses should not be adjusted more often than every 3 to 4 weeks.
- The goal Hct for ESRD patients is 33% to 36%. Hct levels should be drawn prior to hemodialysis, or anytime in peritoneal dialysis patients. For consistency, Hct levels should be drawn on the same day each week.
- If the rate of rise in Hct is less than optimal (i.e., less than 4 points in one month), causes for epoetin resistance should be investigated. If no obvious reasons exist, then the dosage can be increased by approximately 25%.

REFERENCES

1. Rennke HG, Anderson S, Brenner BM. The progression of renal disease: Structural and functional correlations. In: Tisher CC, Brenner BM, eds. Renal Pathology: With Clinical and Functional Correlations. Philadelphia, Lippincott, 1994:116–139.
2. Llach F. Secondary hyperparathyroidism in renal failure: The trade-off hypothesis revisited. Am J Kidney Dis 1995;25:663–679.
3. Levey AS. Measurement of renal function in chronic renal disease. Kidney Int 1990;38:167–184.
4. U.S. Renal Data System. USRDS 1997 Annual Data Report. Bethesda, National Institutes of Health, 1997.
5. Harris MI. Summary. In: Diabetes in America. Bethesda, National Institutes of Health, 1995:1–7.
6. Neuringer JR, Brenner BM. Hemodynamic theory of progressive renal disease: A 10-year update in brief review. Am J Kidney Dis 1993;22:98–104.
7. Hostetter TH. Mechanisms of diabetic nephropathy. Am J Kidney Dis 1994;23:188–192.
8. Neuringer JR, Levey AS. Strategies to slow the progression of renal disease. Semin Nephrol 1994;14:261–273.
9. Ruggenenti P, Perna A, Mosconi L, et al. Proteinuria predicts end-stage renal failure in nondiabetic chronic nephropathies. Kidney Int 1997;52:S54–S57.
10. Makino H, Shikata K, Kushiro M, et al. Role of advanced glycation end-products in the progression of diabetic nephropathy. Nephrol Dial Transplant 1996;11:76–80.
11. Inomata S. Renal hypertrophy as a prognostic index for the progression of diabetic renal disease in non-insulin-dependent diabetes mellitus. J Diabetes Complications 1993;7:28–33.
12. Nath KA. Tubulointerstitial changes as a major determinant in the progression of renal damage. Am J Kidney Dis 1992;20:1–17.
13. Brown TER, Carter BL. Hypertension and end stage renal disease. Ann Pharmacother 1994;28:359–366.
14. Scanferla F, Landini S, Fracasso A, et al. Risk factors for the progression of diabetic nephropathy: Role of hyperlipidemia and its correction. Acta Diabetol 1992;29:268–272.
15. Keane WF, Mulcahy WS, Kasiske BL, et al. Hyperlipidemia and progressive renal disease. Kidney Int 1991;39(suppl 31):S41–S48.
16. Walker WG. Relation of lipid abnormalities to progression of renal damage in essential hypertension, insulin-dependent and non insulin-dependent diabetes mellitus. Miner Electrolyte Metab 1993;19: 137–143.
17. Samuelsson O, Mulec H, Knight-Gibson C, et al. Lipoprotein abnormalities are associated with increased rate of progression of human chronic renal insufficiency. Nephrol Dial Transplant 1997;12: 1908–1915.
18. Mathiesen ER. Prevention of diabetic nephropathy—Microalbuminuria and perspectives for intervention in insulin-dependent diabetes. Dan Med Bull 1993;40:273–285.
19. Carella MJ, Gossain VV, Rovner DR. Early diabetic nephropathy—Emerging treatment options. Arch Intern Med 1994;154:625–630.
20. Erley CM, Haefele U, Heyne N, et al. Microalbuminuria in essential hypertension—Reduction by different antihypertensive drugs. Hypertension 1993;21:810–815.
21. Whelton PK, Perneger TV, Brancati FL, Klag MJ. Epidemiology and prevention of blood pressure-related renal disease. J Hypertens 1992; 10(suppl 7):S77–S84.
22. Borch-Johnsen K, Wenzel H, Viberti GC, Mogensen CE. Is screening and intervention for microalbuminuria worthwhile in patients with insulin dependent diabetes? BMJ 1993;306:1722–1725.
23. Bennett PH, Haffner S, Kasiske BL, et al. Screening and management of microalbuminuria in patients with diabetes mellitus: Recommendations to the Scientific Advisory Board of the National Kidney Foundation from an Ad Hoc Committee of the Council on Diabetes Mellitus of the National Kidney Foundation. Am J Kidney Dis 1995; 25:107–112.
24. Expert Committee on the Diagnosis and Classification of Diabetes Mellitus, American Diabetes Association. Clinical practice recommendations 1998. Diabetes Care 1998;21:S4–S31.
25. Pedrini MT, Levey AS, Lau J, et al. The effect of dietary protein restriction on the progression of diabetic and nondiabetic renal diseases: A meta-analysis. Ann Intern Med 1996;124:627–632.
26. Wang PH, Lau J, Chalmers TC. Meta-analysis of effects of intensive blood-glucose control on late complications of type I diabetes. Lancet 1993;341:1306–1309.
27. Diabetes Control and Complication Trial Research Group. The effect of intensive treatment of diabetes on the development and progression of long-term complications in insulin-dependent diabetes mellitus. N Engl J Med 1993;329:977–986.
28. Santiago JV. Perspectives in diabetes—Lessons from the diabetes control and complications trial. Diabetes 1993;42:1549–1554.
29. Gautier JF, Beressi JP, Leblanc H, et al. Are the implications of the diabetes control and complications trial (DCCT) feasible in daily clinical practice? Diabetes Metab Rev 1996;22:415–419.
30. Parving HH. Impact of blood pressure and antihypertensive treatment on incipient and overt nephropathy, retinopathy and endothelial permeability in diabetes mellitus. Diabetes Care 1991;14: 260–269.
31. Hoelscher D, Bakris G. Antihypertensive therapy and progression of diabetic renal disease. J Cardiovasc Pharmacol 1994;23(suppl 1): S34–S38.
32. Dworkin LD, Benstein JA, Parker M, et al. Calcium antagonists and converting enzyme inhibitors reduce renal injury by different mechanisms. Kidney Int 1993;43:808–814.
33. Kasiske BL, Kalil RSN, Ma JZ, et al. Effect of antihypertensive therapy on the kidney in patients with diabetes: A meta-regression analysis. Ann Intern Med 1993;118:129–138.
34. Lewis EJ, Hunsicker LG, Bain RP, Rohde RD. The effect of angiotensin-converting-enzyme inhibition on diabetic nephropathy. N Engl J Med 1993;329:1456–1462.
35. Ravid M, Savin H, Jutrin I, et al. Long-term stabilizing effect of angiotensin-converting enzyme inhibition on plasma creatinine and on proteinuria in normotensive type II diabetic patients. Ann Intern Med 1993;118:577–581.
36. EUCLID study group. Randomised placebo-controlled trial of lisinopril in normotensive patients with insulin-dependent diabetes and normoalbuminuria or microalbuminuria. Lancet 1997;349:1787–1792.
37. Mackenzie HS, Ots M, Ziai F, et al. Angiotensin receptor antagonists in experimental models of chronic renal failure. Kidney Int 1997; 52:S140–S143.

38. Pitt B, Segal R, Martinez FA, et al. Randomized trial of losartan versus captopril in patients over 65 with heart failure (Evaluation of losartan in the elderly study, ELITE). Lancet 1997;349:747–752.
39. Tarif N, Bakris GL. Angiotensin II receptor blockade and progression of nondiabetic-mediated renal disease. Kidney Int 1997;52: S67–S70.
40. Maki DD, Ma JZ, Louis TA, Kasiske BL. Long-term effects of antihypertensive agents on proteinuria and renal function. Arch Intern Med 1995;155:1073–1080.
41. Weidmann P, Schneider M, Bohlen L. Therapeutic efficacy of different antihypertensive drugs in human diabetic nephropathy: An updated meta-analysis. Nephrol Dial Transplant 1995;10:39–45.
42. Bakris GL, Copley JB, Vicknair N, et al. Calcium channel blockers versus other antihypertensive therapies on progression of NIDDM associated nephropathy. Kidney Int 1996;50:1641–1650.
43. Epstein M. The benefits of ACE inhibitors and calcium antagonists in slowing progressive renal failure: Focus on fixed-dose combination antihypertensive therapy. Ren Fail 1996;18:813–832.
44. Klahr S, Breyer JA, Beck GJ, et al. Dietary protein restriction, blood pressure control, and the progression of polycystic kidney disease. J Am Soc Nephrol 1995;5:2037–2047.
45. Fouque D, Laville M, Boissel JP, et al. Controlled low protein diets in chronic renal insufficiency: Meta-analysis. BMJ 1992;304: 216–220.
46. Klahr S, Levey AS, Beck GJ, et al. The effects of dietary protein restriction and blood-pressure control on the progression of chronic renal disease. N Engl J Med 1994;330:877–884.
47. Levey AS, Adler S, Caggiula AW, et al. Effects of dietary protein restriction on the progression of advanced renal disease in the modification of diet in renal disease study. Am J Kidney Dis 1996;27: 652–663.
48. Joint National Committee. The Sixth Report of the Joint National Committee on Prevention, Detection, Evaluation, and Treatment of High Blood Pressure. Bethesda, National Institute of Health, 1997. NIH pub. no. 98-4080.
49. Schlueter WA, Batlle DC. Renal effects of antihypertensive drugs. Drugs 1989;37:900–925.
50. Risler T, Krämer B, Müller GA. The efficacy of diuretics in acute and chronic renal failure: Focus on torasemide. Drugs 1991;41(suppl 3):69–79.
51. Ter Wee PM, Epstein M. Angiotensin-converting enzyme inhibitors and progression of nondiabetic chronic renal disease. Arch Intern Med 1993;153:1749–1759.
52. GISEN Group. Randomised placebo-controlled trial of effect of ramipril on decline in glomerular filtration rate and risk of terminal renal failure in proteinuric, non-diabetic nephropathy. Lancet 1997; 349:1857–1863.
53. Giatras I, Lau J, Levey AS. Effect of angiotensin-converting enzyme inhibitors on the progression of nondiabetic renal disease: A meta-analysis of randomized trials. Ann Intern Med 1997;127:337–345.
54. Sica DA, Gehr TWB. The pharmacokinetics of angiotensin-converting enzyme inhibitors in end-stage renal disease. Semin Dialysis 1994;7:205–213.
55. National High Blood Pressure Education Program Working Group. 1995 update of the working group reports on chronic renal failure and renovascular hypertension. Arch Intern Med 1996;156: 1938–1947.
56. Weder AB. The renally compromised older hypertensive: Therapeutic considerations. Geriatrics 1991;46:36–48.
57. Jones B, Nanra RS. Double-blind trial of antihypertensive effect of chlorothiazide in severe renal failure. Lancet 1979;2:1258–1260.
58. Wollam GL, Tarazi RC, Bravo EL, Dustan HP. Diuretic potency of combined hydrochlorothiazide and furosemide therapy in patients with azotemia. Am J Med 1982;72:929–938.
59. Favre L, Glasson P, Vallotton MB. Reversible acute renal failure from combined triamterene and indomethacin: a study in healthy subjects. Ann Intern Med 1982;96:317-320.
60. Lowenthal DT, Saris SD, Paran E, Cristal N. The use of transdermal clonidine in the hypertensive patient with chronic renal failure. Clin Nephrol 1993;39:37–43.
61. Miura Y, Watanabe M, Yoshinaga K. An evaluation of the efficacy and safety of doxazosin in hypertension associated with renal dysfunction. Am Heart J 1991;121:381–388.
62. Innes A, Gemmell HG, Smith FW, et al. The short term effects of oral labetalol in patients with chronic renal disease and hypertension. J Hum Hypertens 1992;6:211–214.
63. Waal-Manning HJ, Hobson CH. Renal function in patients with essential hypertension receiving nadolol. BMJ 1980;281:423–424.
64. Wilkinson R. Beta-blockers and renal function. Drugs 1982;23: 195–206.
65. Pontremoli R, Robaudo C, Gaiter A, et al. Long-term minoxidil treatment in refractory hypertension and renal failure. Clin Nephrol 1991; 35:39–43.
66. Siegel JE, Krolewski AS, Warram JH, Weinstein MC. Cost-effectiveness of screening and early treatment of nephropathy in patients with insulin-dependent diabetes mellitus. J Am Soc Nephrol 1992;3: S111–S119.
67. Kiberd BA, Jindal KK. Routine treatment of insulin-dependent diabetic patients with ACE inhibitors to prevent renal failure: An economic evaluation. Am J Kidney Dis 1998;31:49–54.
68. Diabetes Control and Complications Trial Research Group. Lifetime benefits and costs of intensive therapy as practiced in the diabetes control and complications trial. JAMA 1996;276:1409–1415.
69. Jacobson HR, Striker GE. Report on a workshop to develop management recommendations for the prevention of progression in chronic renal disease. Am J Kidney Dis 1995;25:103–106.
70. Ringoir S. An update on uremic toxins. Kidney Int 1997;52(suppl 62):S2–S4.
71. Emmanouel DS, Lindheimer MD, Katz AI. Pathogenesis of endocrine abnormalities in uremia. Endocr Rev 1980;1:28–44.
72. Cohen G, Haag-Weber M, Hörl WH. Immune dysfunction in uremia. Kidney Int 1997;52(suppl 62):S79–S82.
73. Shemin D, Dworkin LD: Sodium balance in renal failure. Curr Opin Nephrol Hypertens 1997;6:128–132.
74. Allon M. Hyperkalemia in end-stage renal disease: Mechanisms and management. J Am Soc Nephrol 1995;6:1134–1142.
75. Salem MM, Rosa RM, Batlle DC. Extrarenal potassium tolerance in chronic renal failure: Implications for the treatment of acute hyperkalemia. Am J Kidney Dis 1991;18:421–440.
76. Solomon R, Dubey A. Diltiazem enhances potassium disposal in subjects with end-stage renal disease. Am J Kidney Dis 1992;19: 420–426.
77. Allon M, Shanklin N. Effect of albuterol treatment on subsequent dialytic potassium removal. Am J Kidney Dis 1995;26:607–613.
78. Allon M, Shanklin N. Effects of bicarbonate administration on plasma potassium in dialysis patients: Interactions with insulin and albuterol. Am J Kidney Dis 1996;28:508–514.
79. Giovannetti S, Cupisti A, Barsotti G. The metabolic acidosis of chronic renal failure: Pathophysiology and treatment. Contrib Nephrol 1992;100:48–57.
80. Kraut JA. The role of metabolic acidosis in the pathogenesis of renal osteodystrophy. Adv Ren Replace Ther 1995;2:40–51.
81. Ballmer PE, Imoberdorf R. Influence of acidosis on protein metabolism. Nutrition 1995;11:462–468.
82. Sharma AM. Renal tubular dysfunction and acidosis. Nephrol Dial Transplant 1995;10:1544–1545.
83. Zelikovic I. Renal tubular acidosis. Pediatr Ann 1995;24:48–54.
84. Sherrard DJ. Aplastic bone: A nondisease of medical progress. Adv Ren Replace Ther 1995;2:20–23.
85. Sherrard DJ, Hercz G, Pei Y, et al. The spectrum of bone disease in end-stage renal failure—An evolving disorder. Kidney Int 1993;43: 436–442.
86. Malberti F, Corradi B, Imbasciati E. Effect of CAPD and hemodialysis on parathyroid function. Adv Perit Dial 1996;12:239-244.

87. Slatopolsky E, Delmez J. Pathogenesis of secondary hyperparathyroidism. Miner Electrolyte Metab 1995;21:91–96.
88. Kates DM, Sherrard DJ, Andress DL. Evidence that serum phosphate is independently associated with serum PTH in patients with chronic renal failure. Am J Kidney Dis 1997;30:809–813.
89. Coen G, Mazzaferro S. Bone metabolism and its assessment in renal failure. Nephron 1994;67:383–401.
90. Bro S, Olgaard K. Effects of excess PTH on nonclassical target organs. Am J Kidney Dis 1997;30:606–620.
91. Brookhyser J, Pahre SN. Dietary and pharmacotherapeutic considerations in the management of renal ostedystrophy. Adv Ren Replace Ther 1995;2:5–13.
92. Delmez JA, Slatopolsky E. Hyperphosphatemia: Its consequences and treatment in patients with chronic renal disease. Am J Kidney Dis 1992;19:303–317.
93. Malluche HH, Monier-Faugere MC. Uremic bone disease: Current knowledge, controversial issues and new horizons. Miner Electrolyte Metab 1991;17:281–296.
94. Reichel H, Deibert B, Schmidt-Gayk H, Ritz E. Calcium metabolism in early chronic renal failure: Implications for the pathogenesis of hyperparathyroidism. Nephrol Dial Transplant 1991;6:162–169.
95. Solal MEC, Sebert JL, Boudailliez B, et al. Comparison of intact, midregion, and carboxy terminal assays of parathyroid hormone for the diagnosis of bone disease in hemodialyzed patients. J Clin Endocrinol Metab 1991;73:516–524.
96. Qi Q, Monier-Faugere MC, Geng Z, Malluche HH. Predictive value of serum parathyroid hormone levels for bone turnover in patients on chronic maintenance dialysis. Am J Kidney Dis 1995;26:622–631.
97. Ali AA, Varghese Z, Moorhead JF, et al. Calcium set point progressively worsens in hemodialysis patients despite conventional oral 1-a hydroxycholecalciferol supplementation. Clin Nephrol 1993;39:205–209.
98. Cleary DJ, Matzke GM, Alexander AM, Joy MS. Medication knowledge and compliance among patients receiving long-term dialysis. Am J Health Syst Pharm 1995;52:1895–1900.
99. Roxe DM, Mistovich M, Barch DH. Phosphate-binding effects of sulcralfate in patients with chronic renal failure. Am J Kidney Dis 1989;13:194–199.
100. Jespersen B, Jensen JD, Nielsen HK, et al. Comparison of calcium carbonate and aluminum hydroxide as phosphate binders on biochemical bone markers, PTH(1-84), and bone mineral content in dialysis patients. Nephrol Dial Transplant 1991;6:98–104.
101. Fournier A, Morinière P, Hamida FB, et al. Use of alkaline calcium salts as phosphate binder in uremic patients. Kidney Int 1992;42 (suppl 38):S50–S61.
102. Fournier A, Drüeke T, Morinière P, et al. The new treatments of hyperparathyroidism secondary to renal insufficiency. Adv Nephrol 1992;21:237–306.
103. Mason NA, Patel JD, Dressman JB, Shimp LA. Consumer vinegar test for determining calcium disintegration. Am J Hosp Pharm 1992; 49:2218–2222.
104. Janssen MJA, van der Kuy A, ter Wee PM, van Boven WPL. Aluminum hydroxide, calcium carbonate and calcium acetate in chronic intermittent hemodialysis patients. Clin Nephrol 1996;45: 111–119.
105. Tan CC, Harden PN, Rodger RSC, et al. Ranitidine reduces phosphate binding in dialysis patients receiving calcium carbonate. Nephrol Dial Transplant 1996;11:851–853.
106. Schaefer K, Scheer J, Asmus G, et al. The treatment of uraemic hyperphosphataemia with calcium acetate and calcium carbonate: A comparative study. Nephrol Dial Transplant 1991;6:170–175.
107. Morinière P, Djerad M, Boudailliez B, et al. Control of predialytic hyperphosphatemia by oral calcium acetate and calcium carbonate. Nephron 1992;60:6–11.
108. Pflanz S, Henderson IS, McElduff N, Jones MC. Calcium acetate versus calcium carbonate as phosphate-binding agents in chronic haemodialysis. Nephrol Dial Transplant 1994;9:1121–1124.
109. Nolan CR, Califano JR, Butzin CA. Influence of calcium acetate or calcium citrate on intestinal aluminum absorption. Kidney Int 1990; 38:937–941.
110. Chertow GM, Burke SK, Lazarus JM, et al. Poly[allylamine hydrochloride] (RenaGel). A noncalcemic phosphate binder for the treatment of hyperphosphatemia in chronic renal failure. Am J Kidney Dis 1997;29:66–71.
111. Fernandez E, Llach F. Guidelines for dosing of intravenous calcitriol in dialysis patients with hyperparathyroidism. Nephrol Dial Transplant 1996;11(suppl 3):96–101.
112. Daisley-Kydd RE, Mason NA. Calcitriol in the management of secondary hyperparathyroidism of renal failure. Pharmacotherapy 1996; 16:619–630.
113. Huraib S, Abu-Aisha H, Abed J, et al. Long-term effect of intravenous calcitriol on the treatment of severe hyperparathyroidism, parathyroid gland mass and bone mineral density in haemodialysis patients. Am J Nephrol 1997;17:118–123.
114. Malberti F, Surian M, Cosci P. Effect of chronic intravenous calcitriol on parathyroid function and set point of calcium in dialysis patients with refractory secondary hyperparathyroidism. Nephrol Dial Transplant 1992;7:822–828.
115. Quarles LD, Indridason OS. Calcitriol administration in end-stage renal disease: Intravenous or oral? Pediatr Nephrol 1996;10:331–336.
116. Fischer ER, Harris DCH. Comparison of intermittent oral and intravenous calcitriol in hemodialysis patients with secondary hyperparathyroidism. Clin Nephrol 1993;40:216–220.
117. Quarles LD, Yohay DA, Carroll BA, et al. Prospective trial of pulse oral versus intravenous calcitriol treatment of hyperparathyroidism in ESRD. Kidney Int 1994;45:1710–1721.
118. Fukagawa M, Kitaoka M, Kurokawa K. Resistance of the parathyroid glands to vitamin D in renal failure: Implications for medical management. Kidney Int 1997;52(suppl 62):S60–S64.
119. Ash SR, Gloeckner PJ, Barnett SL. Lack of removal of calcitriol during hemodialysis procedures. J Am Soc Nephrol 1997;8:1587–1591.
120. Brown AJ, Dusso A, Slatopolsky E. Selective vitamin D analogs and their therapeutic applications. Semin Nephrol 1994;14:156–174.
121. Fournier A, Morinière P, Oprisiu R, et al. 1-Alpha-hydoxyvitamin D_3 derivatives in the treatment of renal bone diseases: Justification and optimal modalities of administration. Nephron 1995;71:254–283.
122. Martin KJ, Gonzalez EA, Gellens M, et al. 19-nor-1-α-25-Dihydroxyvitamin D_2 (paricalcitrol) safely and effectively reduces the levels of intact parathyroid hormone in patients on hemodialysis. J Am Soc Nephrol 1998;9:1427–1432.
123. Tan AU Jr, Levine BS, Mazess RB, et al. Effective suppression of parathyroid hormone by 1-α-hydroxyvitamin D_2 in hemodialysis patients with moderate to severe secondary hyperparathyroidism. Kidney Int 1997;51:317–323.
124. Antonsen JE, Sherrard DJ, Andress DL. A calcimimetic agent acutely suppresses parathyroid hormone levels in patients with chronic renal failure. Kidney Int 1998;53:223–227.
125. Sakhaee K. Management of renal osteodystrophy. Semin Nephrol 1992;12:101–108.
126. Mallette LE, Eisenberg KL, Schwaitzberg SD, et al. Total parathyroidectomy and autogenous parathyroid graft replacement for treatment of hyperparathyroidism due to chronic renal failure. Am J Surg 1983;146:727–733.
127. Consensus Conference. Diagnosis and treatment of aluminium overload in end-stage renal failure patients. Nephrol Dial Transplant 1993;8(suppl 1):1–54.
128. Lin JL, Yang YJ, Yang SS, Leu ML. Aluminum utensils contribute to aluminum accumulation in patients with renal disease. Am J Kidney Dis 1997;30:653–658.
129. Cannata Andía JB. Aluminum toxicity: Its relationship with bone and iron metabolism. Nephrol Dial Transplant 1996;11(suppl 3): 69–73.
130. Ellenberg R, King AL, Sica DA, et al. Cerebrospinal fluid aluminium levels following deferoxamine. Am J Kidney Dis 1990;16:157–159.

131. Alfrey AC. Aluminum toxicity in patients with chronic renal failure. Ther Drug Monit 1993;15:593–597.
132. Mazzaferro S, Coen G, Ballanti P, et al. Deferoxamine test and PTH serum levels are useful not to recognize but to exclude aluminum-related bone disease. Nephron 1992;61:151–157.
133. Day JP, Ackrill P. The chemistry of desferrioxamine chelation for aluminum overload in renal dialysis patients. Ther Drug Monit 1993; 15:598–601.
134. Anthone S, Ambrus CM, Kohli R, et al. Treatment of aluminum overload using a cartridge with immobilized desferrioxamine. J Am Soc Nephrol 1995;6:1271–1277.
135. Bentur Y, McGuigan M, Koren G. Deferoxamine (desferrioxamine) new toxicities for an old drug. Drug Saf 1991;6:37–46.
136. Boelaert JR, de Locht M. Side-effects of desferrioxamine in dialysis patients. Nephrol Dial Transplant 1993;8(suppl 1):43–46.
137. McCarthy JT, Milliner DS, Johnson WJ. Clinical experience with desferrioxamine in dialysis patients with aluminum toxicity. Q J Med 1990;74:257–276.
138. Andriani M, Nordio M, Saporitti E. Estimation of statistical moments for desferrioxamine and its iron and aluminum chelates: Contribution to optimisation of therapy in uremic patients. Nephron 1996;72:218–224.
139. Barata JD, D'Haese PC, Pires C, et al. Low-dose (5 mg/kg) desferrioxamine treatment in acutely aluminum-intoxicated haemodialysis patients using two drug administration schedules. Nephrol Dial Transplant 1996;11:125–132.
140. NKF-DOQI Work Group. NKF-DOQI clinical practice guidelines for the treatment of anemia of chronic renal failure. Am J Kidney Dis 1997;30(suppl 3):S192–S237.
141. Jelkmann W. Erythropoietin: Structure, control of production, and function. Physiol Rev 1992;72:449–489.
142. Koury ST, Koury MJ. Erythropoietin production by the kidney. Semin Nephrol 1993;13:78–86.
143. Paganini EP. Hematologic abnormalities. In: Daugirdas JT, Ing TS, eds. Handbook of Dialysis. Boston, Little, Brown, 1994:445–468.
144. Lohr JW, Schwab SJ. Minimizing hemorrhagic complications in dialysis patients. J Am Soc Nephrol 1991;2:961–975.
145. Teruel JL, Aguilera A, Marcen R, et al. Androgen therapy for anaemia of chronic renal failure. Indications in the erythropoietin era. Scand J Urol Nephrol 1996;30:403–408.
146. Gaughan WJ, Liss KA, Dunn SR, et al. A 6-month study of low-dose recombinant human erythropoietin alone and in combination with androgens for the treatment of anemia in chronic hemodialysis patients. Am J Kidney Dis 1997;30:495–500.
147. Mittman N, Sreedhara R, Mushnick R, et al. Reticulocyte hemoglobin content predicts functional iron deficiency in hemodialysis patients receiving rHuEPO. Am J Kidney Dis 1997;30:912–922.
148. Makoff R. Water-soluble vitamin status in patients with renal disease treated with hemodialysis or peritoneal dialysis. J Renal Nutr 1991; 1:56–73.
149. Sunder-Plassmann G, Hörl WH. Safety aspects of parenteral iron in patients with end-stage renal disease. Drug Saf 1997;17:241–250.
150. Auerbach M, Winchester J, Wahab A, et al. A randomized trial of three iron dextran infusion methods for anemia in EPO-treated dialysis patients. Am J Kidney Dis 1998;31:81–86.
151. Rault R, Nespor S, Holley J. Safety and efficacy of 500 mg of iron-dextran as a single IV infusion in patients on chronic dialysis. ASAIO Trans 1994;23:74. Abstract.
152. Uehlinger DE, Gotch FA, Sheiner LB. A pharmacodynamic model of erythropoietin therapy for uremic anemia. Clin Pharmacol Ther 1992;51:76–89.
153. Jensen JD, Madsen JK, Jensen LW, Pedersen EB. Reduced production, absorption, and elimination of erythropoietin in uremia compared with healthy volunteers. J Am Soc Nephrol 1994;5:177–185.
154. Kaufman JS, Reda DJ, Fye CL, et al. Subcutaneous compared with intravenous epoetin in patients receiving hemodialysis. N Engl J Med 1998;339:578–583.
155. St. Peter WL, Lewis MJ, Macres MG. Pain comparison after subcutaneous administration of single-dose formulation versus multidose formulation of Epogen in hemodialysis patients. Am J Kidney Dis 1998;32:470–474.
156. Masami M, Nomura H, Koni I, Mabuchi H. Angiotensin-converting enzyme inhibitors are associated with the need for increased recombinant human erythropoietin maintenance doses in hemodialysis patients. Nephron 1997;77:164–168.
157. Sheingold S, Churchill D, Muirhead N, et al. The impact of recombinant human erythropoietin on medical care costs for hemodialysis patients in Canada. Soc Sci Med 1992;34:983–991.
158. Powe NR, Griffiths RI, Watson AJ, et al. Effect of recombinant erythropoietin on hospital admissions, readmissions, length of stay, and costs of dialysis patients. J Am Soc Nephrol 1994;4:1455–1465.
159. Abraham PA, Macres MG. Blood pressure in hemodialysis patients during amelioration of anemia with erythropoietin. J Am Soc Nephrol 1991;2:927–936.
160. Remuzzi G. Bleeding disorders in uremia: Pathophysiology and treatment. Adv Nephrol 1989;18:171–186.
161. Eberst ME, Berkowitz LR. Hemostasis in renal disease: Pathophysiology and management. Am J Med 1994;96:168–179.
162. George JN, Shattil SJ. The clinical importance of acquired abnormalities of platelet function. N Engl J Med 1991;324:27–39.
163. McCarthy ML, Stoukides CA. Estrogen therapy of uremic bleeding. Ann Pharmacother 1994;28:60–61.
164. Sloand JA. Long-term therapy for uremic bleeding. Int J Artif Organs 1996;19:439–440.
165. Beccari M. Must we treat uremic dyslipidemia? Int J Artif Organs 1993;16:235–244.
166. Wanner C, Frommherz K, Hörl WH. Hyperlipoproteinemia in chronic renal failure: Pathophysiological and therapeutic aspects. Cardiology 1991;78:202–217.
167. Olbricht CJ, Koch KM. Treatment of hyperlipidemia in nephrotic syndrome: Time for a change? Nephron 1992;62:125–129.
168. Keane WF, St. Peter JV, Kasiske BL. Is the aggressive management of hyperlipidemia in nephrotic syndrome mandatory? Kidney Int 1992;42(suppl 38):S134–S141.
169. Summary of the second report of the National Cholesterol Education Program expert panel on detection, evaluation and treatment of high blood cholesterol in adults (adult treatment panel II). JAMA 1993; 269:3015–3023.
170. Richards EG, Grundy SM, Cooper K. Influence of plasma triglycerides on lipoprotein patterns in normal subjects and in patients with coronary artery disease. Am J Cardiol 1969;63:1214–1220.
171. D'Amico G, Gentile MG. Treatment of hyperlipidemia in human renal disease. Miner Electrolyte Metab 1993;19:196–204.
172. D'Amico G, Gentile MG. Influence of diet on lipid abnormalities in human renal disease. Am J Kidney Dis 1993;22:151–157.
173. Spitalewitz S, Porush JG, Cattran D, Wright N. Treatment of hyperlipidemia in the nephrotic syndrome: The effects of pravastatin therapy. Am J Kidney Dis 1993;22:143–150.
174. Massy ZA, Ma JZ, Louis TA, Kasiske BL. Lipid-lowering therapy in patients with renal disease. Kidney Int 1995;48:188–198.
175. AAKP Carnitine Renal Dialysis Consensus Group. Role of *L*-carnitine in treating renal dialysis patients. Dial Transplant 1994;23: 177–181.
176. Bosch T, Samtleben W, Thiery J, et al. Reverse flux filtration: A new mode of therapy improving the efficacy of heparin-induced extracorporeal LDL precipitation in hyperlipidemic hemodialysis patients. Int J Artif Organs 1993;16:75–85.
177. Sherrard DJ, Goldberg AB, Haas LB, Brunzell JD: Chronic clofibrate therapy in maintenance hemodialysis patients. Nephron 1980;25: 219–221.
178. Merk W, Graben N, Hartmann H, et al. Serum levels of free non-protein bound clofibrinic acid after single dosing to patients with impaired renal function of various degrees—A multicenter study. Int J Clin Pharmacol Ther Toxicol 1987;25:59–62.

179. Evans JR, Forland SC, Cutler RE. The effect of renal function on the pharmacokinetics of gemfibrozil. J Clin Pharmacol 1987;27: 994–1000.
180. Chan MK. Gemfibrozil improves abnormalities of lipid metabolism in patients on continuous ambulatory peritoneal dialysis: The role of postheparin lipases in the metabolism of high-density lipoprotein subfractions. Metabolism 1989;38:939–945.
181. Pasternack A, Vanttinen T, Solakivi T, et al. Normalization of lipoprotein lipase and hepatic lipase by gemfibrozil results in correction of lipoprotein abnormalities in chronic renal failure. Clin Nephrol 1987;27:163–168.
182. Elisaf MS, Dardamanis MA, Papagalanis ND, Siamopoulos KC. Lipid abnormalities in chronic uremic patients—Response to treatment with gemfibrozil. Scand J Urol Nephrol 1993;27:101–108.
183. Grundy SM. HMG-CoA reductase inhibitors for treatment of hypercholesterolemia. N Engl J Med 1988;319:24–33.
184. Azar R, Dequiedt F, Awada J, et al. Effects of fish oil rich in polyunsaturated fatty acids on hyperlipidemia of hemodialysis patients. Kidney Int 1989;36(suppl 27):S239–S242.
185. Ritz E, Fliser D. Hypertension and the kidney—An overview. Am J Kidney Dis 1993;21(suppl 3):3–9.
186. Campese VM, Chervu I. Hypertension in dialysis subjects. In: Henrich WL, ed. Principles and Practice of Dialysis. Baltimore, Williams and Wilkins, 1994;148–169.
187. Farmer CKT, Goldsmith DJA, Cox J, et al. An investigation of the effect of advancing uraemia, renal replacement therapy and renal transplantation on blood pressure diurnal variability. Nephrol Dial Transplant 1997;12:2301–2307.
188. Ritz E, Koch M. Hypertension as risk factor for renal patients—Morbidity and mortality due to hypertension in patients with renal failure. Am J Kidney Dis 1993;21(suppl 2):113–118.
189. Cheigh JS, Milite C, Sullivan JF, et al. Hypertension is not adequately controlled in hemodialysis patients. Am J Kidney Dis 1992; 19:453–459.
190. Charra B, Calemard E, Ruffet M, et al. Survival as an index of adequacy of dialysis. Kidney Int 1992;41:1286–1291.
191. Rosansky SJ. Treatment of hypertension in renal failure patients: When do we overtreat? When do we undertreat? Blood Purif 1996; 14:315–320.
192. London GM, Marchais SJ, Guerin AP, et al. Salt and water retention and calcium blockade in uremia. Circulation 1990;82:105–113.
193. Rosansky SJ, Johnson KL, McConnell J. Use of transdermal clonidine in chronic hemodialysis patients. Clin Nephrol 1993;39:32–36.
194. Harter HR, Delmez JA. Effects of prazosin in the control of blood pressure in hypertensive dialysis patients. J Cardiovasc Pharmacol 1979;1(suppl):S43–S55.
195. Townsend RR, Ford V. Ambulatory blood pressure monitoring: Coming of age in nephrology. J Am Soc Nephrol 1996;7:2279–2287.
196. Cannella G, Paoletti E, Delfino R, et al. Regression of left ventricular hypertrophy in hypertensive dialyzed uremic patients on long-term antihypertensive therapy. Kidney Int 1993;44:881–886.
197. Asher JP, Murray KM. Use of angiotensin-converting-enzyme inhibitors in the management of renal disease. Clin Pharm 1991;10: 25–31.
198. Robertson KE, Mueller BA. Uremic pruritis. Am J Health Syst Pharm 1998;53:2159–2170.
199. Stahle-Bäckdahl M. Pruritis in hemodialysis patients. Skin Pharmacol 1992;5:14–20.
200. Dimkovic N, Djukanovic L, Radmilovic A, et al. Uremic pruritis and skin mast cells. Nephron 1992;61:5–9.
201. Makoff R. Vitamin supplementation in persons with renal disease. EDTNA ERCA J 1992;18:11–14.

43

RENAL TRANSPLANTATION

Heather J. Johnson, PharmD, Karen L. Heim-Duthoy, PharmD, FCCP, and Richard J. Ptachcinski, PharmD, FCCP

Each year the number of patients diagnosed with end-stage renal disease (ESRD) increases by over 50,000, reaching more than 300,000 by 1996. The primary therapeutic options for these individuals are hemodialysis (HD), peritoneal dialysis, and/or renal transplantation. HD and continuous ambulatory peritoneal dialysis (CAPD) remain options for patients with chronic, irreversible renal failure who choose not to be transplanted, are unsuitable candidates for transplantation, or who are awaiting a suitable donor. The reported causes of renal failure leading to transplantation include insulin-dependent diabetes mellitus (37.4%), hypertension (28.7%), chronic glomerulonephritis of various etiologies (13.4%), polycystic kidney disease (2.7%), interstitial nephritis (4.5%), and a number of minor causes.[1] Renal transplantation is the preferred long-term therapeutic option for most patients with ESRD because it provides patients with the greatest potential improvement in overall quality of life. Transplantation is a treatment, rather than a cure, for ESRD. Patients and clinicians are to be reminded that there are several adverse consequences/complications that have been associated with transplantation.

In spite of efforts to increase public awareness about organ donation, the waiting list continues to grow and reached 34,550 by the end of 1996.[2] The largest increase was in patients over 64 years of age. In 1995, median waiting time for an organ was 814 days. In 1996, 12,045 kidney transplants were performed in the United States; 8559 kidneys were retrieved from cadaver donors and another 3486 kidneys were transplanted from living donors. However, 1814 patients died waiting for a kidney transplant in 1996. Efforts to expand the donor pool include relaxing the absolute age limitations for organ donation and use of living-unrelated, or emotionally-related, donors. This has led to the practice of transplanting older individuals with kidneys from older donors, as well as transplanting two kidneys from a pediatric donor into adult recipients (pediatric en bloc).

Renal transplantation has several advantages over dialysis. Dialysis-catheter related infections, CAPD-associated peritonitis, and scheduled dialysis treatments are avoided, and dietary restrictions are fewer. While the analysis of quality of life is complex, patients generally report improved quality of life following transplantation as compared to patients on maintenance dialysis.[3]

Patient and graft survival rates following renal transplantation have improved significantly over the past 30 years due to advances in pharmacotherapy, surgical techniques, organ preservation, and the postoperative management of patients. Although success rates vary among transplant centers, 1-year patient survival rates range from 96% to 98% for living-related (LRT), and 92% to 94% for cadaveric renal transplantation (CRT). The 1-year graft survival rates for LRTs and CRTs range from 89% to 95% and 66% to 80%, respectively. Five-year graft survival rates currently range from 50% to 60% in most transplant centers.

Although transplantation is a less costly therapeutic option than dialysis for treating patients with chronic renal failure over the long term, the 5-year patient survival rate for each treatment is similar. The net cost–benefit ratio (or "break-even point") to Medicare from transplantation has been estimated at 3 years in patients with a functioning graft.[4]

Because of continuous improvements in clinical outcomes, cost effectiveness, and quality of life, renal transplantation is the treatment option that provides patients with renal failure the best chance of survival and return to a normal or near-normal life-style. Patients with medical conditions, such as unstable cardiac disease or recently diagnosed malignancy, for whom the risk of surgery or chronic immunosuppression would be greater than the risks associated with chronic dialysis, are excluded from renal transplantation. The most frequent reason for patient exclusion is unstable cardiac disease or recently diagnosed malignancy. Some transplant centers will also exclude patients who are human immunodeficiency virus antibody positive and patients with a history of drug abuse or noncompliance with medical regimens.

The pharmacotherapy required for the management of patients following renal transplantation, including immunosuppressive, anti-infective, and other treatments, is discussed in the remainder of the chapter.

PHYSIOLOGIC CONSEQUENCES OF RENAL TRANSPLANTATION

Based on a rapid fall in serum creatinine, the glomerular filtration rate of a successfully transplanted kidney may be near normal almost immediately after transplantation. In some patients, however, the concentration of standard biochemical indicators of renal function, such as serum creatinine and blood urea nitrogen (BUN), may remain elevated for several days. Standard formulae used to predict drug dosing rely on stable serum creatinine and may be inaccurate immediately following transplantation.

Although the allograft is able to remove uremic toxins from the body, it may take several weeks for other physiologic complications of chronic renal failure, such as anemia, calcium and phosphate imbalance, and altered lipid profiles, to resolve. The renal production of erythropoietin and 1-hydroxylation of vitamin D may return toward normal early in the postoperative period. Since the onset of physiologic effects may be delayed, continuation of pretransplant calcitriol, calcium supplementation, and/or phosphate binders may be warranted in some patients.

FACTORS AFFECTING THE SUCCESS OF RENAL TRANSPLANTATION

The success of renal transplantation can be measured in terms of length of graft and patient survival, the half-life of transplanted kidneys, or quality of life. A number of factors influence the success of renal transplantation. These factors include HLA- and DR-antigen matching between donor and recipient, donor age and serum creatinine, donor cardiac instability, and prolonged cold ischemia time. The 1-year graft survival rate was 98.1% in recipients of HLA-identical kidneys for two haplotypes, and 98.1% and 97.7%, respectively, when a parent or sibling matched for one haplotype was the donor. Long term, the estimated half-lives for kidneys is 26.9 years for HLA-identical grafts and 12.2 and 10.8 years, respectively, for grafts from a sibling or parent who are one-haplotype matches. One-year survival for cadaveric kidneys was 94.4% for HLA matched kidneys and 92% to 94% for mismatched kidneys. The estimated half-life for HLA-matched grafts was 17.3 years and 7.8 years for mismatched kidneys.[5] Recipient factors that are associated with diminished success of transplantation include age < 15 or > 50 years, retransplantation, black race, and the presence of preformed anti-HLA antibodies. Size mismatching between donor and recipient has also been implicated. Multiparous women are also at increased risk for immunologic graft loss. These factors contribute to the major determinants of graft survival/rejection and delayed graft function (Table 43–1).

DELAYED GRAFT FUNCTION

Primary nonfunction of a renal allograft or delayed graft function (DGF) may result in postoperative anuria. The primary cause is acute tubular necrosis (ATN). A number of circumstances related to the donor may affect the course of ATN. The incidence of ATN increases when kidneys have been harvested from donors following cardiac arrest, from donors who have been hypotensive or on vasopressors, or from older donors. Prolonged periods of warm and cold ischemia, greater than 40 minutes and 48 hours, respectively, have been recognized to increase a patient's risk of developing ATN. The management of patients with ATN may be difficult since serum creatinine, the major parameter used to monitor for acute rejection, remains elevated. Cyclosporine (CSA) therapy has been implicated in the prolongation of ATN, although a clear cause-and-effect relationship has not been established.

TABLE 43–1. Impact of Delayed Graft Function (DGF) and Acute Rejection (AR) on Length of Stay and Renal Allograft Survival

	I −DGF/−AR	II +DGF	III +AR	IV +DGF/+AR
Median length of stay (days)[a]	10	17	15	21
1-year graft survival (%)[b]	88	74	72	56
5-year graft survival (%)[c]	66	53	48	35

[a]ANOVA $P = .05$.
[b]I vs II, $P < .001$; I vs III, $P < .001$; IV vs I, II, III, $P < .01$.
[c]I vs II and III, $P < .001$; IV vs II and III, $P < .001$.
From Ref. 6.

Delayed graft function is defined by the need for dialysis in the postoperative period or the failure of the serum creatinine to fall below 4 mg/dL or by 30% of the pretransplant value. The incidence of DGF in primary cadaveric renal transplantation ranges from 8% to 50% and results in a slower return of the kidney's excretory, metabolic, and synthetic functions. Delayed graft function is associated with prolonged hospital stays, higher costs, difficulty in the management of immunosuppressive therapy, slower patient rehabilitation, and poor graft survival. Urinary complications such as ureteral obstruction, thrombosis or leak, or vascular complications including arterial or venous stenosis or thrombosis may also result in early graft dysfunction.

Persistently elevated serum creatinine and BUN levels confound the perioperative management of renal transplant recipients. Among the differential diagnoses are acute rejection, ATN, and/or CSA or tacrolimus (TAC) toxicity. These processes are not mutually exclusive. Definitive diagnosis is made by renal biopsy. In the presence of elevated serum creatinine, clinicians may reduce the dose of CSA or TAC to minimize the potential for drug nephrotoxicity and hasten the recovery from ATN. This practice may result in subtherapeutic immunosuppressant concentrations and hasten the occurrence of acute rejection. Delayed graft function has been shown to be a factor predisposing patients to acute rejection. Induction therapy using the strategy of delayed CSA or TAC administration may be useful in this setting.

GRAFT REJECTION

Allograft rejection depends on the activation of alloreactive T cells and antigen-presenting cells such as B lymphocytes, macrophages, and dendritic cells. Acute allograft rejection is primarily caused by the infiltration of T cells into the allograft, which triggers inflammatory and cytotoxic effects on the graft. Complex interactions between the allograft and cellular cytokines, cell-to-cell interactions, $CD4^+$ and $CD8^+$ T cells, and B cells ultimately lead to chronic rejection and graft loss if adequate immunosuppression is not maintained.[7]

The sequence of events that underlies graft rejection is (1) recognition of the donor's histocompatibility differences by the recipient's immune system, (2) recruitment of activated lymphocytes, (3) initiation of immune effector mechanisms, and (4) destruction of the graft. These processes can take place at varying rates and may involve differing effector mechanisms. Rejection of the transplanted tissue can therefore take place at anytime following surgery and is clinically classified as hyperacute rejection, acute cellular rejection, and chronic rejection. Although these processes generally denote a temporal sequence of events, considerable overlap exists in the actual time frame of when each type of rejection is observed.

HYPERACUTE REJECTION

Hyperacute rejection may occur when preformed donor-specific antibodies are present in the recipient at the time of the transplant. Hyperacute rejection often occurs within minutes of the transplant procedure, but may occur anytime within the first two postoperative weeks. Hyperacute rejection can be induced by immunoglobulin G (IgG) antibodies that bind to antigens on the vascular endothelium, such as class I major histocompatibility complex (MHC), ABO, and vascular endothelial cell antigens. Tissue damage can be mediated through antibody-dependent, cell-mediated cytotoxicity, or through the activation of the complement cascade. The ischemic damage to the microvasculature rapidly produces tissue necrosis.

Hyperacute rejection has become uncommon because transplant donors are matched for ABO blood groups and cross-match testing is done to determine the presence of donor-specific lymphocytotoxic antibodies. A positive cross-match presents a serious risk factor for graft failure even if hyperacute rejection does not occur. A negative lymphocytotoxicity cross-match does not entirely rule out the possibility of hyperacute rejection because non-MHC antigens on the vascular endothelium can serve as targets of donor-specific antibodies.

ACUTE CELLULAR REJECTION

The cellular rejection process is referred to as acute rejection. Although the earliest episodes have been observed within days postoperatively, acute rejection may occur at anytime after transplantation. Cellular rejection is mediated by alloreactive T lymphocytes that appear in the circulation and infiltrate the allograft through the vascular endothelium. Once the graft is infiltrated by lymphocytes, the cytotoxic cells can specifically kill allograft targets, whereas the local release of lymphokines will attract and stimulate macrophages to produce tissue damage through a delayed hypersensitivity-like mechanism.

Graft rejection must be differentiated from drug-induced nephrotoxicity. Acute rejection is usually accompanied by a prompt rise in serum creatinine. A specific histologic diagnosis can be obtained via biopsy of the allograft and is often used to guide therapy for rejection. A biopsy specimen with a diffuse infiltrate of lymphocytes is consistent with acute cellular rejection. After the diagnosis of rejection has been confirmed, the potential risks and benefits of specific antirejection therapies must be evaluated. Hypertension often worsens during an episode of rejection. Patients may experience edema and weight gain as a result of sodium and fluid retention. Symptomatic azotemia may also develop in severe cases. In addition, patients may experience graft tenderness, fever, and malaise. Appropriate adjustments in pharmacotherapy are warranted in the face of diminished renal function.

CHRONIC REJECTION

The prevention and treatment of chronic rejection is perhaps the most important problem to be addressed in transplantation over the next decade. Although advances have been made in the management of acute rejection, the half-life of kidney transplantation has remained largely unchanged. Chronic rejection is the most common cause of graft loss in the late posttransplant period (> 1 year). Acute rejection is a strong predictor of chronic rejection, but it is unclear why reduction in the incidence of acute rejection associated with the widespread adoption of CSA and TAC has not had an impact on the incidence of chronic rejection. The current tendency to decrease doses of CSA and TAC in the face of "good" graft function without dynamic measurement of immunologic factors may lead to subclinical rejection. Although chronic rejection may simply be a slow and indolent form of cellular rejection, the involvement of the humoral immune system and antibodies against the vascular endothelium appears to play a role. The pathogenesis of chronic rejection is difficult to dissect because of prolonged exposure to multiple drugs, and because of the presence of other abnormalities that may predispose the patient to similar pathologic changes in organ function.

Chronic rejection can occur early (within 3 to 6 months) or late (> 1 year) in the posttransplant course. Hypertension, proteinuria, and a progressive decline in renal function present as a classic triad in chronic rejection. Manifestations of chronic rejection are generally dependent on the degree of renal insufficiency and hypoalbuminemia. Classic symptoms of uremia occur as end-stage renal disease develops. These processes are very difficult to treat because their presentation is slow and indolent and the changes in renal function are usually not reversible.

▶ TREATMENT: Renal Transplantation

■ IMMUNOSUPPRESSIVE THERAPY

■ GOALS OF IMMUNOSUPPRESSION

Transplant immunosuppression must be balanced in terms of graft and patient survival (the prevention of rejection versus the risk of adverse effects associated with therapy including life-threatening infection or malignancy). A multidrug approach is rational from the immunomechanistic viewpoint since the agents may have overlapping and potentially synergistic mechanisms. Furthermore, multidrug immunosuppression may allow the use of lower doses of individual agents associated with different side effect profiles to minimize severe adverse effects.

The goals of immunosuppression vary depending on the time interval since the transplant surgery. Immediately following surgery, the primary goal of therapy is to prevent hyperacute and acute rejection. The high doses of immunosuppressants required to achieve this goal may result in serious complications (e.g., infection, thrombocytopenia, and steroid-induced diabetes) if maintained long term. Rapid tapering may minimize these effects.

During the first 1 to 3 months following transplantation, acute graft rejection affects 30% to 40% of patients. Therefore, the doses of immunosuppressants are usually kept high to prevent rejection during this high-risk period. The doses of immunosuppressants are generally reduced if the patient develops serious adverse effects such as opportunistic infections, nephrotoxicity, or hepatotoxicity. The goal of maintenance immunosuppression is to prevent acute and chronic rejection while minimizing drug-related toxicity. In the long-term management of the transplant patient, the doses of immunosuppressants are gradually reduced (over 6 to 12 months) in an effort to minimize adverse effects. Many institutions may completely withdraw specific immunosuppressives in select patients to reduce long-term toxicity as well as cost. It is important to recognize that even though the goals of transplant immunosuppression are universal, protocols for induction, maintenance, and rejection therapy vary greatly among institutions. Immunosuppressive options for induction, maintenance, and the management of acute rejection are detailed in Table 43–2. This discussion of immunosuppression includes the rationale for the most commonly used regimens and success rates generally achieved with the most popular regimens.

INDUCTION THERAPY

Induction therapy often involves the use of sequential immunosuppression. This form of immunosuppression incorporates induction with (1) a polyclonal or monoclonal antibody preparation [antilymphocyte globulin (ALG), antithymocyte globulin (ATG), or muromonab CD3 (OKT3)]; (2) azathioprine (AZA) or mycophenolate mofetil (MMF); and/or (3) glucocorticoid, followed by the delayed administration of CSA or TAC (Fig. 43–1). Induction therapy using this strategy has been based on the following rationale: (1) the newly transplanted kidney is susceptible to nephrotoxic injury from CSA or TAC; (2) CSA and TAC dosage adjustment to maintain target concentrations is difficult in the early posttransplant period; and (3) a theoretical immunologic benefit from initial, more intensive immunosuppression is added with the use of a polyclonal or monoclonal antibody preparation.[8,9]

TABLE 43–2. Options for Immunosuppression During Induction, Maintenance, and Rejection Therapy

Type of Immunosuppression	Options
Induction therapy	1. Sequential, quadruple, or triple therapy: a. ALG/ATG or OKT3 or daclizumab or basiliximab b. AZA or MMF, and/or c. glucocorticoid, followed by CSA or TAC 2. Other induction
Maintenance therapy	1. Monotherapy: immunosuppression with one drug (usually CSA or TAC) 2. Dual therapy: immunosuppression with two drugs (e.g., CSA or TAC plus corticosteroids; AZA/corticosteroids; CSA or TAC plus AZA or MMF) 3. Triple therapy: immunosuppression with three drugs (usually a glucocorticoid plus AZA or MMF, and CSA or TAC)
Rejection therapy	1. Glucocorticoid with or without MMF 2. OKT3 3. ALG/ATG 4. Radiation

The presence of nephrotoxic drugs such as CSA or TAC may exacerbate damage to the transplanted kidney that results from prolonged cold and/or warm ischemia or from the cellular damage caused by the release of oxygen free radicals, which results in reperfusion of the kidney with oxygenated blood. Therefore, immunosuppressive regimens that eliminate or minimize doses of CSA or TAC during the early postoperative period are frequently used. In addition to the nephrotoxic potential, CSA and TAC trough plasma/blood concentrations are difficult to adjust because of gastrointestinal (GI) dysfunction (i.e., postoperative ileus), which is common in the early posttransplant period. The microemulsion formulation of CSA (Neoral [Sandoz]) may minimize early CSA absorption problems.

More intense immunosuppression is often indicated in the immediate posttransplant period when the risk for organ rejection is the highest and for high-risk patients. This decreases the overall incidence and delays the onset of acute rejection, which may ultimately improve long-term graft survival. The prophylactic use of antibody preparations (ALG, ATG, or OKT3) during induction therapy is controversial. Some studies report higher graft survival with antibody prophylaxis,[10–12] whereas others report no significant improvement.[13,14] Immunosuppressive regimens that include induction therapy are preferred by about 50% of transplant centers.

Induction therapy incorporating ALG, CSA, and steroids has been compared to conventional therapy using CSA and steroids. Graft survival at 3 years posttransplant was significantly greater for the ALG group (89%) versus the conventional group (73%), $P = .041$.[11] Similarly, OKT3 induction with AZA, steroids, and delayed CSA has been compared to conventional therapy (AZA, steroids, and CSA).[10,12] OKT3 use was associated with significantly fewer rejection episodes (51% vs 66%) and a longer time to initial rejection (46 days vs 8 days).[12] Furthermore, the prophylactic use of OKT3 has resulted in improved graft survival at 18 months posttransplant (92% with OKT3 vs 79% with conventional therapy)[10] and at 5 years posttransplant (73% with OKT3 vs 64% with conventional therapy).[12]

The majority of literature on polyclonal antibody preparations was based on results with the investigational agent, Minnesota ALG (MALG), which is no longer available. Because of differences in antibody composition, potency, and preparation procedures, it is inappropriate to extrapolate results obtained with MALG to other polyclonal antibody preparations. Controversial findings resulted when MALG was compared to ATGAM (Pharmacia & Upjohn Co., Kalamazoo, MI). Sequential immunosuppression (induction with corticosteroids, AZA, and CSA) using MALG 20 mg/kg/d ($n = 33$) or ATGAM 15 mg/kg/d ($n = 14$) was evaluated by Pescovitz et al.[15] There was no difference in the number of patients experiencing rejection in the first year posttransplant (58% for MALG vs 50% for ATGAM). Lum et al. retrospectively evaluated the clinical impact of replacing MALG ($n = 323$) with ATGAM ($n = 65$); patients received 15 mg/kg/d of either MALG or ATGAM with corticosteroids, AZA, and CSA.[16] A greater incidence of rejection and steroid-resistant rejection in the first 60 days posttransplant were observed in ATGAM- (60% and 34%, respectively; $P < .0001$) versus MALG- (32% and 19%, respectively; $P = .007$) treated patients. In contrast, the efficacy of induction therapy with

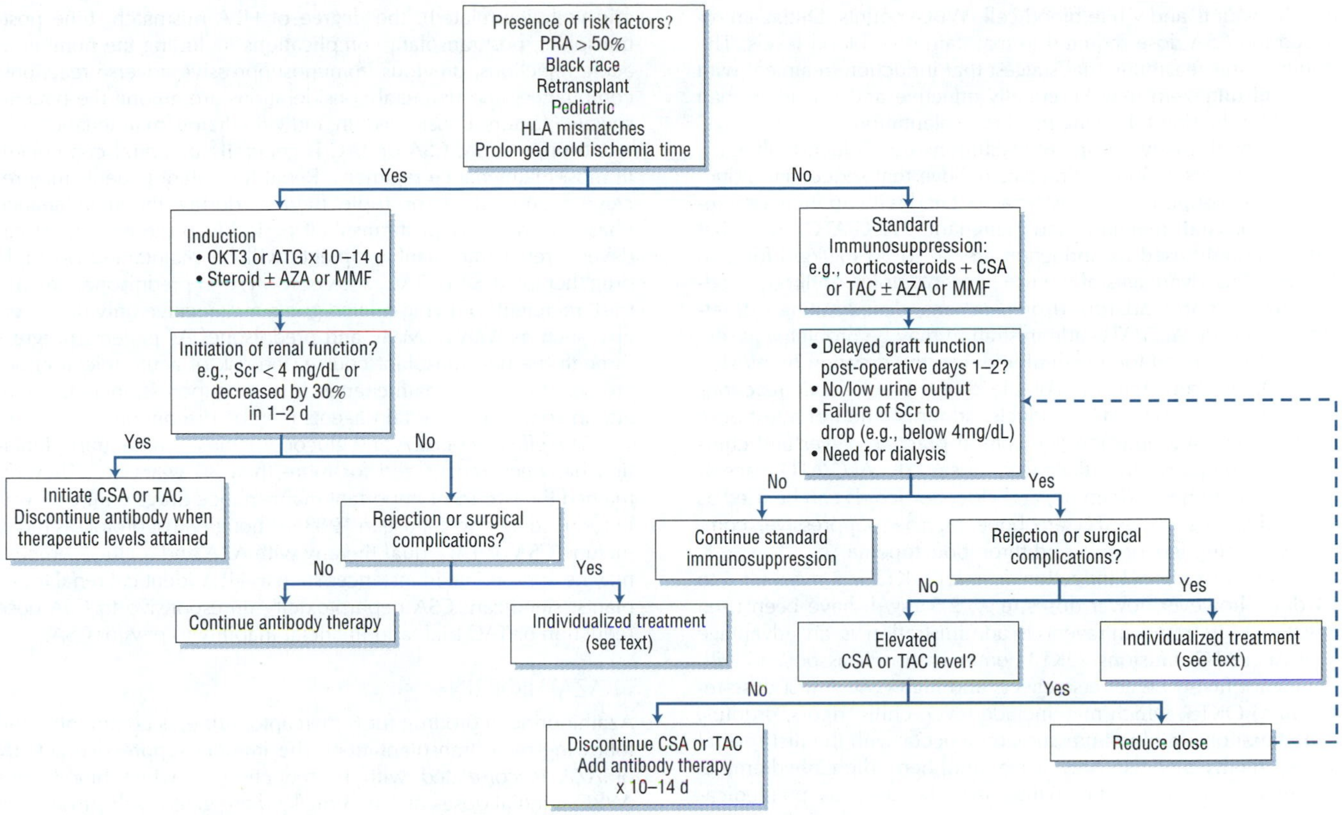

FIGURE 43–1. Decision tree for antibody induction therapy with ATG or OKT3.

polyclonal antibody preparations or OKT3 has been shown to be similar.[17,18] Sequential therapy with delayed CSA initiation using perioperative MALG or OKT3 revealed that the MALG and OKT3 groups were similar with respect to rejection, graft, and patient survival.[18,19] Hanto et al. demonstrated a reduced incidence of cytomegalovirus (CMV) infection with the use of OKT3 (10%) compared to MALG (37%) ($P = .001$).[19]

Since MALG is no longer available as an induction agent, currently available polyclonal and monoclonal antibody preparations should be the primary agents in future comparisons. MALG, ATGAM, rabbit antithymocyte serum (RATS), OKT3, and CSA induction were evaluated in 358 cadaveric renal transplant patients.[20] Although there was no significant difference in overall graft survival between the four groups, acute rejection was higher with ATGAM compared to MALG, OKT3, RATS, and CSA ($P =$ .04). In addition, the ATGAM group had higher serum creatinine concentrations at 1 and 6 months posttransplant compared to the other induction regimens.[20] The risk of rejection and decreased graft survival is increased in patients with DGF, high panel reactive antibody (PRA) titers, early rejection of a previous allograft, and prolonged ischemia times. OKT3 induction therapy appears to be particularly effective in preventing rejection in this patient population.[8,9,21]

Induction with the conventional OKT3 dose (5 mg/d for 10 to 14 days) effectively prevents rejection in renal transplant recipients.[10,12] However, there are also data demonstrating the utility of low-dose (2.5 mg) OKT3 induction therapy.[22,23] Darby et al. administered conventional or reduced doses of OKT3, based on CD3 counts, to renal allograft recipients with PRA >50%.[22] The total OKT3 doses for the conventional and low-dose groups were 64.4 ± 9.0 and 38.3 ± 8.5 mg, respectively. There were no differences in acute rejection, serum creatinine, and graft and patient survival (1 year) between the conventional and low-dose OKT3 groups.[22] Although adverse events were not directly assessed, they appear to occur less frequently with reduced OKT3 doses.[23] A sequential induction protocol using OKT3 has been shown to be more cost effective than conventional therapy in renal transplantation.[24] Furthermore, low-dose administration of OKT3 in this setting may additionally enhance cost effectiveness. The exact role of OKT3 in induction therapy needs to be further defined (i.e., high- vs low-risk patients and conventional vs reduced dosing).

Use of CSA as an induction agent is controversial. Decreased renal blood flow secondary to CSA constriction of the renal vasculature may exacerbate delayed graft function and negate some of the beneficial effects of starting CSA early after transplantation.[25] As a result, many institutions use monoclonal and polyclonal antibody preparations for induction, thus allowing CSA initiation to be postponed until graft function is established; however, antibody induction therapy is associated with substantial toxicity and expense.[26] Calcium antagonists block the renal vasoconstriction associated with CSA,[27,28] and it has been suggested that calcium antagonists could be used with CSA early after transplantation to prevent the adverse effects of CSA on delayed graft function.[29,30] In addition, calcium antagonists have been shown to increase CSA blood levels[31] and may have immunosuppressive properties of their own.[32,33]

In a randomized trial, CSA induction (combined with diltiazem) was compared to sequential therapy (ATGAM) in 100 renal transplant patients.[34] Acute rejection episodes during the first 90 days were not different with ATGAM (42%) versus CSA (28%) induction ($P = .142$). Graft failures (10% vs 16%, respectively) and the incidence of delayed graft function (28% vs 34%, respectively) were also similar with ATGAM compared with CSA. There was no difference between the two groups in serum creatinine levels within the first 90 days posttransplantation. ATGAM caused lower platelet counts and white blood cell (WBC) counts. Diltiazem reduced the CSA dose required to maintain goal blood levels. The results of this feasibility trial suggest that induction treatment with CSA and diltiazem may be equally effective and less toxic than ATGAM induction following renal transplantation.[34]

Although many transplant institutions use induction therapy, it is not universal. Some clinicians believe that sequential induction immunosuppression may be associated with an increased incidence of viral infections and malignancy. ALG/ATG doses that are commonly used for induction are 10 to 30 mg/kg/d for 5 to 14 days. Disadvantages of the use of a polyclonal antibody product include nonstandardized preparations, dose-limiting side effects, and cost. ALG/ATG administration may be problematic secondary to the need for a central line, lengthy duration of infusion (4 hour), and large infusion volume. Since anaphylactic reactions may occur with ALG/ATG products, administration of a test dose prior to the initial infusion is common practice. Fever and chills often accompany the first few doses of ALG/ATG; acetaminophen, diphenhydramine, and glucocorticoids can be used as premedications. ALG/ATG are bone marrow suppressive, commonly causing leukopenia and thrombocytopenia.

The conventional induction dose for OKT3 is 5 mg/d for 5 to 14 days; however, lower doses (e.g., 2.5 mg/d) have been used effectively. Its rapid intravenous administration is an advantage over ALG/ATG infusions. OKT3 administration is associated with significant first-dose adverse effects and high cost. A first dose reaction to OKT3, which may include fever, chills, rigors, pruritus, and alterations in blood pressure, may occur with the first several doses; methylprednisolone, acetaminophen, diphenhydramine, indomethacin, and pentoxifylline may be used as premedications. Pulmonary edema has been associated with OKT3 use in transplant patients who are significantly fluid overloaded; therefore, patients may need to be dialyzed prior to administration. Aseptic meningitis may result as a complication of OKT3 therapy. If encephalitic symptoms develop, OKT3 should be discontinued and appropriate care initiated. Finally, due to the potential development of host antibodies and inability to reuse it as an effective rejection therapy, concern existed previously regarding its use for induction. However, it has been demonstrated that OKT3 can be safely and successfully used as rejection therapy in patients that have undergone previous OKT3 induction.[12,35] Specifically, these studies have confirmed that the presence of low anti-OKT3 antibody titers ($\leq$ 1:100) does not preclude successful retreatment with OKT3 for rejection.

Daclizumab (Zenapax, Hoffman-LaRoche) is a humanized monoclonal antibody that binds to the α subunit of IL-2. In a multicenter, placebo-controlled randomized trial (n = 260), five doses of intravenous daclizumab 1 mg/kg were given every 2 weeks to patients undergoing primary cadaveric renal transplantation. Other immunosuppression included CSA, AZA,and corticosteroids. The primary end point, biopsy-proven rejection, was confirmed in 22% of daclizumab-treated patients versus 47% in the placebo group (P = .03) in the first 6 months posttransplant. Patient and graft survival were similar.[36] Similar results have been reported with basiliximab, a chimeric (mouse/human) monoclonal antibody to the IL-2 receptor, 20 mg at the time of transplant and on postoperative day 4. Patients in this study received CSA and corticosteroids.[37] Daclizumab and basiliximab have not been associated with the administration-related effects common to other antibody preparations. Neither agent has been evaluated in protocols that spare the early administration of CSA or TAC.

MAINTENANCE THERAPY

Maintenance therapy can involve numerous combinations of the various available immunosuppressives. Transplant type (cadaveric vs living-related), the degree of HLA mismatch, time posttransplant, posttransplant complications including the number of acute rejections, previous immunosuppressive adverse reactions, compliance, and financial considerations are among the patient-specific factors considered in individualizing maintenance immunosuppression. CSA or TAC is generally a central component in most maintenance regimens. Renal transplant patients may receive mono-, dual, or triple therapy during the maintenance phase. In the early posttransplant period ($\leq$ 6 months), most cadaveric renal transplant recipients will be maintained on triple drug therapy (CSA or TAC, AZA or MMF, and prednisone). In contrast, recipients of living-related grafts may receive only dual therapy, such as AZA or MMF and prednisone. As patients progress through the posttransplant course, the risk of acute rejection decreases; therefore, maintenance immunosuppression is tapered, and in some cases, certain agents may be discontinued.

The efficacy of AZA and glucocorticoids in renal transplantation has been recognized for more than 30 years.[38,39] They remained the two most important maintenance drugs until CSA was introduced for clinical use in 1983. Although most protocols today include CSA or TAC, dual therapy with AZA and a glucocorticoid may be appropriate in instances such as HLA-identical renal transplants, significant CSA nephrotoxicity unresponsive to CSA dose reduction or TAC trial, and financial inability to pay for CSA.

AZATHIOPRINE

Azathioprine, a prodrug for 6-mercaptopurine, is commonly used following renal transplantation. The immunosuppressive activity of AZA is correlated with its reduction in white blood cells (WBCs). Initial doses of 3 to 5 mg/kg/d are given with subsequent individualization (0.5 to 3 mg/kg/d) to maintain a stable serum creatinine and a WBC count of 3.5 to 5 $\times$ 10^3 cells/mm^3. Dose-limiting adverse effects of AZA are often hematologic in origin (Table 43–3). Leukopenia, anemia, and thrombocytopenia are common adverse effects and can be managed by dose reduction or discontinuation of AZA. Hepatotoxicity and pancreatitis are less common adverse effects of AZA; they are generally reversible on dose reduction or discontinuation.

GLUCOCORTICOIDS

An intravenous glucocorticoid, commonly high-dose (125 to 1000 mg/d) methylprednisolone, is given during the perioperative period. The dose of methylprednisolone is rapidly tapered and discontinued as oral prednisone (PRED) is initiated. Prednisone doses are tapered progressively over time to a baseline dose of 10 to 15 mg/d by the sixth month posttransplant. At 1-year posttransplant, maintenance doses may be less than 10 mg/d in some patients. In patients receiving TAC, PRED may be tapered even lower and eventually discontinued. As doses are tapered, it is preferable to administer steroids every other day and between 7 and 8 AM to mimic the body's diurnal release of cortisol. Although conversion to alternate-day regimens or complete withdrawal of PRED in patients with stable posttransplant courses has been used with success in some transplant centers,[40–42] steroids are often continued for the entire life of the functional graft. Long-term steroid use and its associated deleterious effects are well recognized and particularly troublesome in transplant patients.[43–45] Specific adverse effects of glucocorticoids that are commonly encountered in transplant patients are summarized in Table 43–3.

CYCLOSPORINE

Clinical Use

The introduction of CSA has significantly improved the outcomes of renal transplantation. Patient and graft survival rates have im-

TABLE 43–3. Adverse Effects of Immunosuppressive Agents and Management in the Renal Transplant Patient

Adverse Effects	Steroids	CSA	Tacrolimus	Management
Adrenal suppression	+			Taper doses slowly; administer every other day; patient identification card
Cataracts/glaucoma	+			Annual eye examinations or as indicated
Hypertension	++	++	++	Monitor blood pressure; sodium restriction and antihypertensive medications as needed
Tremor		++	++	Adjust dose as needed
Gastrointestinal abnormalities	+ GI bleeding	+	++ diarrhea, nausea, vomiting, anorexia	AZA: administer after meals; MMF: decrease or divide dose, administer with food; TAC/PRED: administer with food; ulcer prophylaxis
Respiratory abnormalities			++ includes pleural effusion, dyspnea	
Nephrotoxicity		++	++	Monitor serum creatinine/BUN; adjust dose and discontinue as needed
Headache		+	++	Check drug concentration; adjust dose
Hepatotoxicity		+	++	Monitor liver enzymes; AZA-associated toxicity is reversible and ususally occurs within the first 6 mo of therapy; adjust dose and discontinue as needed
Hyperlipidemia	++	++	+	Dietary counseling; pharmacotherapy as needed
Glucose alterations	++	+	++	Monitor glucose; adjust doses of hypoglycemics or immunosuppressants
Osteoporosis/aseptic necrosis	+/++			Annual bone examinations; weight-bearing exercise
Personality changes	++			Patient and family education
Weight gain	++			Patient education; exercise
Acne	+	+		Dose reduction; increased hygiene; topical agents (e.g., retinoic acid)
Gingival hyperplasia		++		Patient education; appropriate dental hygiene; consider TAC
Hirsutism		++		Patient education; consider TAC
Pruritis			++	Treatment when appropriate
Thrombocytopenia			+	Monitor platelets
Leukocytosis	++		++	Monitor WBCs
Leukopenia		+		Monitor WBCs; generally dose dependent and reversible with AZA/MMF
Hyperkalemia		+	++	Monitor serum electrolytes
Hypomagnesemia		+	++	Monitor serum magnesium

++ indicates > 10% risk.
+ indicates < 10% risk.

proved secondary to a lower incidence of acute rejection episodes and severe infectious complications.[46–48] Despite these improvements in survival, concerns regarding its long-term use include survival, incidence of late-rejection episodes, frequency of hypertension, drug cost, and quality of kidney function. Mono-, dual, and triple therapy with CSA are commonly employed during maintenance immunosuppression, although dual and triple therapies are most common.

In a 5-year experience with CSA monotherapy as primary immunosuppression in renal transplant recipients, actuarial patient and graft survival rates at 5 years were 89.7% and 80.0%, respectively.[49] Sixty-four percent of patients experienced rejection episodes within the first 6 months and only 3.9% of patients experienced first rejection after the first posttransplant year. The avoidance of long-term steroids is the primary advantage with CSA monotherapy, whereas the primary disadvantage is the higher incidence of rejection. Although CSA monotherapy may not jeopardize graft function, the effect of acute rejection on long-term graft survival is controversial. Maintenance glucocorticoids may be necessary in those patients initiated on CSA monotherapy who experience recurrent rejection episodes.[50,51]

CSA dual therapy usually includes a combination of CSA and glucocorticoids. Dual therapy with CSA/PRED has been compared to AZA/PRED.[52,53] With a follow-up period ranging from 3 to 6 years, Ghoneim et al. demonstrated no significant difference in the overall frequency of acute rejection episodes or graft survival between the two living-related transplant groups; however, the number of patients experiencing two or more rejection episodes was greater in the AZA/PRED group.[52] In contrast, Amend et al. observed significant differences in graft survival between CSA/PRED- and AZA/PRED-treated cadaveric renal transplant (CRT) patients. Graft survival for all study periods during the 5-year follow-up was greater for both diabetics (20% to 22%) and nondiabetics (35% to 40%) in the CSA/PRED group.[53] The different outcomes of these two studies could be attributed to the difference in study subjects and the source of the kidney, cadaveric versus living-related, since survival rates are improved following living-related transplants.

CSA triple therapy consists of CSA, glucocorticoids, and AZA. Eventual tapering and/or elimination of glucocorticoids or CSA is attempted in some patients. CSA dual therapy (CSA/PRED and CSA/AZA) has been compared to CSA triple therapy (CSA/AZA/PRED) in CRT patients. Although the CSA/AZA group had more frequent early rejection, no significant differences in 1-year patient or graft survival, morbidity, and mortality were identified.[54] The long-term (4-year follow-up) effects of CSA dual versus CSA triple immunosuppression have been evaluated.[55,56] Both studies reported no differences in graft and patient survival. However, Isoniemi et al. demonstrated other parameters of follow-up including graft function and chronic allograft damage index from renal biopsy to be significantly better in the triple therapy group,[56] whereas Lindholm et al., reported no difference in renal function determined by serum creatinine between groups.[55]

The impact of CSA on long-term (≥ 5 years) renal allograft function has been analyzed. Although patient survival did not differ between treatment groups,[57,58] Monaco et al. demonstrated a significantly greater 5-year graft survival in CSA-treated patients (triple therapy).[58] Another retrospective study demonstrated no difference in 5-year actual survival in patients who had received either (1) AZA or steroids or (2) CSA mono-, dual, or triple therapy (88% vs 90%, respectively).[59] The 5-year actual graft survival rate was not different between the AZA and CSA. In fact, 5-year graft survival after the development of chronic graft dysfunction was 34% in AZA patients and 53% in CSA patients. Similarly, Slaton et al. compared 1- and 5-year patient and graft survival in cadaveric renal transplant recipients treated with either AZA or CSA as the primary immunosuppressive agent.[60] Although patient survival rates did not differ between groups, the 5-year graft survival rate was greater in the CSA than AZA group (61% vs 29%); the mean serum creatinine concentration at 5 years was significantly greater in the CSA group (CSA 1.79 vs AZA 1.30 mg/dL, $P < .05$). In contrast, the results of a meta-analysis evaluating chronic immunosuppression in renal transplant patients refute these reports.[61] One- and 5-year graft and patient survival, rejection rate per patient, and infection rate were analyzed; no statistical differences between CSA triple therapy over dual therapy (CSA/PRED) were detected.

The results of a multicenter, long-term efficacy and safety of CSA evaluation in renal transplant patients were reported by Burke et al.[62] Graft survival was 78% after a median follow-up of 36 months. In the 1663 patients evaluated, there were 279 grafts lost. The leading cause of graft loss was acute rejection (68 patients) and chronic graft dysfunction (125 patients).[62] The optimal immunosuppressive regimen is not always clear-cut; further study in terms of longer follow-up may help determine which maintenance regimen(s) are preferred.

Formulation

CSA, a highly lipophilic cyclic polypeptide, was initially released as Sandimmune. Use of the original formulation was associated with clinically significant interpatient and intrapatient variability in pharmacokinetic parameters secondary to unpredictable bioavailability. Subsequently, CSA was reformulated using a microemulsion delivery system to improve its bioavailability. The new formulation, Neoral, is self-emulsifying and spontaneously forms a microemulsion with aqueous fluids in the GI tract.[63] Pharmacokinetic studies have been completed that compare the pharmacokinetics and tolerability of Sandimmune and Neoral.[64–66]

CSA steady-state pharmacokinetics were assessed in 55 renal transplant recipients with stable renal function receiving CSA for a minimum of 6 months.[64] Patients were converted from Sandimmune to Neoral on a 1 mg:1 mg to mg basis (no dosage adjustments were allowed). The steady-state maximum concentration (C_{max}) and area under the curve (AUC) significantly increased (59% and 30%, respectively) with conversion to Neoral. The increase in these parameters was not associated with increased adverse events. Intraindividual variability in C_{max}, T_{max}, AUC, and percent peak–trough fluctuation was significantly less with Neoral.[64]

Wahlberg et al. assessed the pharmacokinetics of CSA over a 1-year study period.[65] Renal transplant recipients were randomized (1:4) to Sandimmune (n = 12) or Neoral (n = 45). Prior to randomization, participants completed a baseline pharmacokinetic assessment. Conversion on a 1:1 mg to mg basis was completed. Subsequent pharmacokinetic assessments were performed at 8 and 12 weeks, and 1 year. With Neoral, the rate and extent of CSA absorption was significantly greater throughout the 1-year study period. With conversion, intraindividual variability in pharmacokinetic parameters was reduced, and the correlation between trough concentrations and AUC improved.[65]

In a randomized, double-blind, 12-week comparative trial, the pharmacokinetics, safety, and tolerability of Sandimmune and Neoral were evaluated in renal transplant recipients (n = 101).[66,67] With conversion, the relative bioavailability was demonstrated to significantly increase through an increase in AUC and C_{max} from 16% to 31% and 32% to 42%, respectively.[66] At baseline and at 8 and 12 weeks, the mean serum creatinine was significantly greater with Neoral than Sandimmune ($P < .05$).[67] Although the incidence of acute rejection was similar in both groups, monoclonal antibody therapy was required less often in the Neoral group. There were no significant differences in the overall incidence of adverse events including hypertension, infections, gingival hyperplasia, hirsutism, headache, tremor, and nausea.[67] Keown et al. demonstrated transient increases in neurologic and GI adverse effects as well as serum creatinine within the first month of Neoral use.[68] These adverse effects resolved either spontaneously or after a reduction in CSA dose. Long-term use of Neoral needs to be assessed for efficacy, safety, and tolerability, in particular, for its implications on renal function.

If conversion is desired, the current recommendation is to convert patients from Sandimmune to Neoral on a 1 mg:1 mg basis. Once the conversion is made, close follow-up is required to assess for changes in trough concentrations and adverse effects, including serum creatinine. Doses may need to be reduced to maintain similar goal trough concentrations. Clinical management of patients receiving Neoral may be easier as a result of less intrapa-

TABLE 43–4. Cost Comparison of Immunosuppressive Agents

Medication	Initial Dose[a]	Daily Cost	Maintenance	Daily Cost
ATGAM (ATG)	20 mg/kg/d × 7 to 10 d	$1470.00	—	
OKT3	5 mg/kg/d × 7 to 10 d	$ 585.00	—	
Zenapax (daclizumab)	1 mg/kg × 5 doses	$1040.00	—	
Simulect (basiliximab)	20 mg × 2 doses	$1020.00	—	
Methylprednisolone	500 mg/d	$ 17.86	—	
Neoral (CSA)	10 mg/kg/d	$ 37.04	5 mg/kg/d	$18.52
Sandimmune (CSA)	10 mg/kg/d	$ 43.22	6 mg/kg/d	$25.93
Prograf (TAC)	0.2 mg/kg/d	$ 31.92	0.1 mg/kg/d	$15.96
Imuran (AZA)	2 mg/kg/d	$ 3.89	1 mg/kg/d	$ 1.95
CellCept (MMF)	2 g/d	$ 15.00	2 g/d	$15.00
Deltasone (PRED)	20 mg/d	$ 0.14	7.5 mg/d	$ 0.05

[a]Doses based on starting does for 70-kg patient.
From Ref. 69.

tient variability in CSA trough concentrations. In addition, the current costs favor conversion of patients from Sandimmune to Neoral (Table 43–4).

Dosing

Initiation of oral CSA therapy generally begins with a dose of 8 to 18 mg/kg/d divided into two daily doses. Higher CSA doses are more commonly used in dual therapy regimens, while lower doses are part of triple therapy regimens. Doses are adjusted on the basis of whole blood concentrations of the drug and the clinical response of the patient. The desired blood concentration range is dependent on assay methodology and individual risk factors for rejection such as time posttransplant. As the risk for acute rejection decreases with time, oral CSA doses are reduced and may be as low as 3 mg/kg/d or less during maintenance therapy. If oral administration is not possible, CSA may be administered intravenously at one-third the oral dosage.

Therapeutic Drug Monitoring

The absorption, distribution, and metabolism of CSA are highly variable; many factors contribute to this intrapatient and interpatient variability.[70,71] As these factors change in the posttransplant course, CSA pharmacokinetic parameters change.[72] Therefore, CSA blood concentrations are routinely measured in an attempt to optimize therapy.[73] Radioimmunoassay and fluorescence polarization immunoassay are the most commonly used methods; however, high-performance liquid chromatography is recognized as the reference procedure.[74] It is important to determine which assay methodology the laboratory is using since target ranges vary between specific (which quantitates parent CSA) and nonspecific (which quantitates parent plus metabolite concentration) assays (Table 43–5). In addition, it is extremely important to interpret CSA concentrations not only in relation to goal ranges but also in the context of relevant clinical and laboratory data.

TABLE 43–5. Therapeutic CSA Concentration Ranges Are Method Dependent

Method	Sampling Medium	CSA Concentration (ng/mL)
TDx or RIA	Whole blood	375–450
TDx or RIA	Serum or plasma	175–250
HPLC	Whole blood	100–200
HPLC	Serum or plasma	75–150

TDx = a commercial fluorescence polarization assay; RIA = radioimmunoassay; HPLC = high-performance chromatography.
Modified from Ref. 74, with permission.

The most common and practical method of CSA monitoring is the measurement of trough blood concentrations.[73,75] CSA trough concentrations are measured frequently (daily or three times per week) following the initiation of the drug and during the stabilization period after transplantation. An alternative to the assessment of CSA trough concentrations is the characterization of the individual's CSA pharmacokinetic profiles.[76–78] Theoretically, a pharmacokinetic profile consisting of serial samples collected throughout a CSA dosage interval is more reflective of overall CSA exposure than are individual trough concentrations. Sequential CSA profiles provide a more comprehensive pharmacokinetic characterization, and AUC has been suggested to correlate with graft outcome.[79] However, due to the intrapatient variability in the pharmacokinetics of CSA, the usefulness of a single pharmacokinetic profile to predict long-term dosing strategies is controversial. Unlike the ease of obtaining CSA trough concentrations, measurement of CSA pharmacokinetic profiles is a more complicated procedure. The cost of additional blood samples and practicality of using these profiles for therapeutic monitoring at individual institutions must be considered. In patients receiving Neoral, the use of limited sampling strategies has resulted in an excellent correlation with drug exposure.[68,80] The relationship between trough and total exposure to CSA appears to be stronger with Neoral than with Sandimmune. This relationship may be particularly useful to minimize the potential for increased toxicity secondary to greater drug exposure.

CSA concentrations may be markedly increased as the result of drug interactions. Diltiazem[81] and ketoconazole[82] inhibit the hepatic elimination of CSA via inhibition of cytochrome P450 3A4 and thus can be used to achieve desired concentrations of CSA with lower drug doses. A complete discussion of CSA drug interactions is found elsewhere.[83]

Adverse Effects

A summary of CSA adverse effects and management in the renal transplant patient is presented in Table 43–3. The clinician is frequently required to differentiate between allograft rejection and CSA nephrotoxicity, which is generally a diagnosis of exclusion. Typically, nephrotoxicity is defined as an increase in serum creatinine of 25% over several days that reverses following a CSA dose reduction.[84] Because the clinical features of acute allograft rejection and CSA nephrotoxicity may overlap considerably, a renal biopsy continues to be the diagnostic gold standard (Table 43–6). Differentiating between CSA nephrotoxicity and chronic rejection is also difficult, because the clinical signs and symptoms may be similar. Since biopsy findings are similar in patients with CSA nephrotoxicity and chronic rejection, this is a much more difficult differential diagnosis.

TABLE 43–6. Differential Diagnosis of Acute Rejection and CSA or TAC Nephrotoxicity

	Acute Rejection	CSA or TAC Nephrotoxicity
History	Often < 4 weeks postop	Often > 6 weeks postop
Clinical	Fever	Afebrile
Presentation	Hypertension Weight gain Graft swelling/tenderness Decreased daily urine volume	Hypertension Graft nontender Good urine output
Laboratory	Rapid rise in serum Cr (0.3 mg/dL/d) Normal CSA or TAC concentration	Gradual rise in serum Cr (> 0.15 mg/dL/d) Elevated CSA or TAC concentration
Biopsy	Interstitial lymphocytic infiltrates	Intersitial fibrosis, tubular atrophy, glomerular thrombosis, arterial inflammation

CSA discontinuation in renal transplant patients may be considered in some cases of chronic nephrotoxicity or uncontrolled hypertension. In these patients, immunosuppression is generally maintained with PRED and AZA or by the addition of TAC. Improved renal function may result from such a change in therapy, but it may take several weeks for the beneficial effects to be fully realized. However, CSA discontinuation may precipitate an episode of acute graft rejection and should be completed in conjunction with careful monitoring. The financial impact of additional monitoring during the conversion period and the potential adverse effects of TAC including hyperkalemia and neurologic effects must also be considered.

TACROLIMUS

Tacrolimus (TAC), formerly FK506, was initially approved by the FDA in 1994 for patients undergoing orthotopic liver transplantation. Most of the early experience with TAC in renal transplantation was as rescue therapy for refractory rejection. Tacrolimus was approved by the FDA as primary therapy for renal transplantation in 1997. Most of the published experience with TAC comes from the University of Pittsburgh, but there is a growing body of literature from other centers. Jordan et al. converted 169 patients with biopsy-confirmed, steroid-resistant rejection from CSA-based immunosuppression to TAC in an attempt to salvage failing allografts. This practice has resulted in a success rate of 74% with a mean follow-up of 30 months.[85] In smaller series, graft survival rates ranging from 66% to 91% with follow-up ranging from 4 to 9 months have been reported.[86,87]

The early experience using TAC in renal transplantation was derived from an unblinded randomized trial comparing TAC with CSA in patients undergoing retransplantation or who had failed conventional immunosuppressive regimens. One-year actuarial patient survival for individuals receiving TAC (n = 240) was 90% versus 94% for patients receiving CSA (n = 196), whereas the 1-year graft survival for both groups was similar: 74% for TAC versus 77% for CSA. Although not statistically significant, 44% (n = 105) of TAC-treated patients were able to have steroids withdrawn as compared to no patients treated with CSA; and fewer patients treated with TAC required antihypertensive therapy as compared to CSA-treated patients (57% vs 75%). Finally, the mean serum cholesterol in TAC-treated patients was significantly lower (187 ± 51 mg/dL) than in the CSA patients (236 ± 59) ($P < .0001$).[88]

A phase III multicenter trial in the United States compared CSA (n = 207) to TAC (n = 205) in regimens consisting of antilymphocytic therapy and AZA/PRED. Although no differences were reported at 1 year in patient (95.6% vs 96.6%) or graft (91.2% vs 87.9%) survival, significantly fewer TAC-treated patients experienced biopsy-proven acute rejection (30.7% vs 46.4%, $P = .001$).[89] These similarities in patient and graft survival were maintained at 2 years.[90] In a similar European trial, TAC (n = 303) was compared to CSA (n = 145) both in combination with AZA and low-dose corticosteroids. At 1 year, TAC was associated with a reduction in acute rejection (25%) as compared to CSA (45.7%). As in the U.S. trial, there were no differences in patient or graft survival.[91]

Limited data are available with TAC in comparison to Neoral or in combination with MMF. Short-term single-center experiences give similar results for Neoral/MMF/PRED compared to TAC/MMF/PRED.[92] Whether the decreased incidence of acute rejection noted with TAC will translate into a long-term benefit remains to be determined. In an analysis of UNOS data, however, Gjertson et al. compared allograft half-lives between 544 TAC- and 35,147 CSA-treated patients, reporting a half-life of 13.8 years in TAC-treated patients as compared to 8.8 years with CSA.[93]

Dosing and Monitoring

In a 6-week trial designed to define the optimal trough blood concentrations of TAC, 120 patients were randomized to CSA-based immunosuppression or one of three TAC groups based on target trough concentrations: low (5 to 14 ng/mL), medium (15 to 25 ng/mL), or high (26 to 40 ng/mL). All patients also received AZA and PRED. Primary outcomes were biopsy-proven acute rejection or toxicity of any type. There were no differences in rejection between the three TAC groups, but patients receiving TAC had a lower incidence of rejection as compared to patients receiving CSA (14% vs 32%, $P = .048$). Neurologic and gastrointestinal side effects occurred more frequently at higher concentrations of TAC.[94] One-year follow-up of these same patients showed a similar incidence of rejection between TAC- and CSA-treated patients: 32% versus 33%. Although nephrotoxicity occurred with a similar frequency, the incidence of neurologic and gastrointestinal side effects remained higher in TAC-treated patients.[95] Data from this study suggest an oral starting dose of 0.2 mg/kg/d and target 12-hour whole-blood trough concentrations of 5 to 15 ng/mL when using TAC as primary therapy.[94] As with CSA, target concentrations vary with transplant center and time posttransplant. Early trials with TAC for treatment of refractory rejection used an aggressive approach: 0.3 mg/kg/d oral TAC and target trough concentrations of 15 to 25 ng/mL continued for 2 weeks after reversal of rejection and tapering to 5 to 7 ng/mL in the long-term (> 5 months) after rejection reversal.[87]

Tacrolimus pharmacokinetics exhibit wide variation, oral bioavailability ranging from 5% to 67% (mean 29%), and half-life of 4 to 41 hours.[96,97] Tacrolimus is metabolized by the cytochrome P450 3A enzyme system.[98] As such, there is a great potential for drug interactions with other substrates as well as inhibitors and inducers of this system. Tacrolimus is subject to pH-mediated degradation by sodium bicarbonate and magnesium oxide, whereas aluminum hydroxide gel adsorbs TAC.

Tacrolimus administration should, therefore, be separated from these compounds by at least 2 hours.[99]

Adverse Effects

The adverse effects associated with TAC in renal transplantation patients include neurologic toxicity, nephrotoxicity, and electrolyte disturbances such as hyperkalemia and hypomagnesemia.[88] Neurotoxicity including coma, tremor, headaches, paresthesias, and insomnia is more common in patients treated with > 0.3 mg/kg/d of TAC or TAC blood concentrations > 25 ng/mL. Nephrotoxicity associated with TAC varies from 18% to 42% in liver transplant recipients, but the incidence is not well defined in renal transplant recipients. In a series of 128 patients undergoing renal biopsy for the investigation of renal dysfunction, Katari et al. reported that TAC nephrotoxicity, defined primarily by the absence of rejection and a fall in serum creatinine following dose reduction, accounted for graft dysfunction in 17% of patients. Tacrolimus nephrotoxicity was accompanied by hyperglycemia, hyperkalemia, and tremors in several patients.[100] Posttransplant lymphoproliferative disorder is also associated with TAC. As observed with CSA, most adverse effects related to TAC improve with dosage reduction or discontinuation.

In comparison to CSA, TAC is associated with increased occurrence of neurologic complications including tremor, paresthesias, and anxiety. Tacrolimus is also associated with lower cholesterol levels.[89,101] Hirsutism, acne, and gingival hyperplasia are infrequently associated with TAC therapy. The incidence of posttransplant diabetes has been reported to be approximately 20%, but is often reversible when doses of TAC and/or steroids are reduced.[89,90,95]

MYCOPHENOLATE MOFETIL

Mycophenolate mofetil (MMF) is the morpholinoethyl ester of the immunosuppressant mycophenolic acid (MPA). Following oral administration, MMF is rapidly and completely converted to MPA. MPA exerts its immunosuppressive effect through noncompetitive binding to inosine monophosphate dehydrogenase, ultimately leading to a reduction in guanosine nucleotide synthesis. This eventually results in diminished DNA polymerase activity and a reduction in lymphocyte proliferation via both the de novo and salvage pathways.[102]

MMF has been studied for the prevention of acute rejection in approximately 1500 patients in three randomized controlled trials summarized in Table 43–7. These trials compared MMF (plus CSA and steroids) to regimens that included either placebo or AZA. In the European Trial, significantly fewer patients had biopsy-proven rejection or treatment failure during the first 6 months after transplantation with MMF 2 g/d (30.3%) or MMF 3 g/d (38.8%), than with placebo (56%).[103] Similar results were reported in the U.S. Trial and the Tricontinental Trial.[104,105] Among the three trials there were no differences in patient or graft survival at 1 year.[106] Pooled analysis of these trials showed a reduction in the number of patients at 1 year with biopsy-proven rejection or treatment failure in the MMF 2 g/d (36.8%) and MMF 3 g/d (39.6%) in comparison with patients who received AZA or placebo (53.8%).[107] Based on these early results, many transplant centers added MMF to or replaced AZA in existing

TABLE 43–7. Summary of Pivotal Mycophenolate Mofetil Rejection Prophylaxis Trials

	U.S. Trial			Tricontinental Trial			European Trial		
	MMF 2 g	*MMF 3 g*	*AZA*	*MMF 2 g*	*MMF 3 g*	*AZA*	*MMF 2 g*	*MMF 3 g*	*Placebo*
n	167	166	166	173	164	166	165	160	166
6-month									
Biopsy-proven rejection (%)[a]	19.8	17.5	38.0	19.7	15.9	35.5	17.0	13.8	46.4
Graft survival (%)	98.2	93.3	91.4	96.0	98.2	97.0	95.7	93.7	91.0
Patient survival (%)	96.4	94.5	97.0	99.4	98.2	98.8	97.6	97.5	98.8
Opportunistic infections (%)	44.8	45.7	47.5				38.2	34.4	27.7
Invasive CMV (%)	9.1	10.8	6.1				3.0	6.9	2.4
Malignancy (%)	3.6	0	1.2						
Lymphoma (%)	0.6	1.2	0						
Diarrhea (%)	31.5	37.3	23.8				12.7	15.6	12.7
Leukopenia (%)							10.9	13.8	4.2
12-month									
Graft survival (%)	95.8	91.0	90.2	91.2	92.0	88.8			
Patient survival (%)	94.5	94.0	95.7	96.5	95.7	95.7			
Opportunistic infections (%)				46.0	46.0	44.0			
Invasive CMV (%)				7.0	11.0	6.0			
Malignancy skin/nonskin (%)				9.0/2.0	5.0/4.0	5.0/3.0			
Lymphoma (%)	0.6	0.6	0	1.2	1.2	0.6			
Diarrhea (%)				28.0	31.0	17.0			
Leukopenia (%)				19.0	35.0	30.0			
Costs per patient ($)	27,807		29,158	29,294		28,857			
3-year									
Graft survival (%)	87.3	84.3	83.5	81.9	84.8	80.2			
Patient survival (%)	89.7	88.0	88.4	93.0	91.5	87.7			
Invasive CMV (%)	2.3	1.7	0						
Malignancy (%)				2.9	6.1	3.7			
Lymphoma (%)	0.6	1.8	0.6	1.2	1.8	0.6			
Diarrhea (%)	16.8	26.4	16.9						
Anemia (%)	16.0	20.7	12.1						

[a]MMF 2 g vs AZA, $P = .0036$; MMF 3 g vs AZA, $P = .0006$; MMF 2 g vs AZA/placebo, $P = .004$; MMF 3 g vs AZA/placebo, $P = .043$.

immunosuppression protocols. However, 3-year follow-up of the U.S. Trial failed to demonstrate a significant difference in the combined end point of graft and patient survival: MMF 2 g/d (81.2%), MMF 3 g/d (78.3%), AZA (75%).[108] Analysis of 3-year graft survival in the Tricontinental Trial produced similar results: MMF 2 g/d (81.9%), MMF 3 g/d (84.8%), AZA (80.2%).[109]

Dosing and Monitoring

Unlike other immunosuppressive agents, there is no compelling indication that MMF should be dosed in adult patients on a mg/kg basis given the weak correlation between MPA AUC and body weight.[110] In contrast to CSA and TAC, plasma appears to be the most appropriate medium for measuring MPA.[111] Therapeutic drug monitoring and pharmacodynamic monitoring are not routinely done, but are currently being evaluated for their utility in tailoring dosing regimens to achieve optimal immunosuppression.[112]

MPA AUC is unchanged in patients with renal impairment. MPAG, the inactive glucuronide metabolite, is renally eliminated and accumulates in patients with renal dysfunction. Doses should be limited to 2 g/d in patients with CrCl < 25 mL/min as this group may be more prone to adverse effects associated with MMF as demonstrated in a small number of hemodialysis-dependent patients in comparison with nondialysis patients.[113] MMF doses up to 3.5 g/d have been used for the treatment of acute rejection, but should be titrated based on efficacy and toxicity. MPA is not significantly removed by hemodialysis. Given its high degree of protein binding (97.5%), MPA is unlikely to be affected significantly by peritoneal dialysis.[110,114] Pharmacokinetic studies in renal transplant recipients showed an increase in AUC and C_{max} in patients at least 3 months posttransplant when compared to those less than 40 days posttransplant. The clinical significance of this finding remains to be determined.[115] Dose reduction in the first year posttransplant based on the pharmacokinetic and pharmacodynamic properties of MMF has not been evaluated.[114]

Numerous drug interactions have been documented with MMF. Food delays the absorption and decreases MPA C_{max} by 25% but has no effect on MPA AUC. Prescribing information indicates that MMF should be taken on an empty stomach, but MMF is often given with food in clinical practice to minimize GI effects. Administration with aluminum- and magnesium-containing antacids, however, significantly decreases both C_{max} (37%) and AUC (15%) and should be avoided.[116] It has been suggested that administration of iron may produce similar results, but this has not been tested.

Acyclovir, commonly used in renal transplant recipients for the treatment and prevention of viral infections, competes with MPAG for renal tubular secretion. AUCs of both entities are increased with concomitant acyclovir and MMF administration. Patients with severe renal insufficiency may be at increased risk of seizures and delirium due to the accumulation of acyclovir, although no cases have been reported with concomitant MMF administration.[117] Single-dose intravenous ganciclovir in combination with MMF produced no change in the disposition of ganciclovir, MPA, or MPAG.[118] Although no pharmacokinetic interaction was demonstrated, there is potential for additive pharmacodynamic effects such as bone marrow suppression.

Cyclosporine appears to have no effect on MPA pharmacokinetics, whereas concomitant administration of TAC and MMF may result in increased MPA trough levels and AUC. MPA AUC increased by greater than 50%, whereas the MPA 12-hour trough doubled in TAC-treated patients. Although studies evaluating the efficacy of different doses of MMF in combination with TAC have not been conducted, clinicians should note that patients receiving MMF and TAC may be at greater risk for MMF-associated side effects such as bone marrow suppression and GI effects. These patients may require lower doses of MMF than CSA-treated patients to achieve a similar pharmacodynamic effect. MMF does not effect the pharmacokinetics of either CSA or TAC.[119]

Adverse Effects

Unlike CSA and TAC, MMF is not associated with nephrotoxicity, neurotoxicity, or hypertension. Gastrointestinal side effects such as nausea, vomiting, diarrhea, and abdominal pain, however, occurred more frequently in MMF-treated patients compared to those receiving AZA or placebo.[103,104] Clinically, dose reduction, dividing the total daily dose into three, administration with food, and upward titration from lower doses during initial therapy may alleviate some of these GI symptoms. MMF also has hematologic effects resulting in leukopenia and anemia. Tissue invasive CMV was also more common in MMF-treated patients.[103–105] Malignancy and posttransplant lymphoproliferative disease (PTLD) are of significant concern with greater amounts of immunosuppression. At the 3-year follow-up of the U.S. Trial there was a greater prevalence of lymphoma in the MMF 3 g/d group (1.8%) compared with the MMF 2 g/d and AZA groups (each 0.6%).[108] Similar analysis of the European data showed a 1.8% prevalence of PTLD in the MMF 3 g/d group compared with 1.2% and 0.6% in the MMF 2 g/d and AZA groups, respectively. Other malignancies also occurred in more patients receiving MMF 3 g/d than in the MMF 2 g/d and AZA-treated patients, 6.1% versus 2.9% and 3.7%, respectively.[109] Given the small numbers, these findings did not reach statistical significance. Longer follow-up of patients receiving MMF is required to characterize the lifelong risk of malignancy.

Cost

The overall cost-effectiveness of any new therapy must be evaluated. The average wholesale price of MMF 2 g/d is $5475 for yearly maintenance therapy, as compared to $1277 for AZA 150 mg/d. Sullivan et al. evaluated the pharmacoeconomic impact of MMF therapy in the first year posttransplant using data from the U.S. Trial. This analysis showed a difference of approximately $1300 (4.6%) per patient per year in favor of MMF 2 g/day versus AZA.[120] In a similar analysis of the data from the Tricontinental Trial, Keown et al. reported lower costs associated with the treatment of rejection, dialysis, and graft failure in patients receiving MMF, but mean first-year costs were higher on average in the MMF patients, $29,294 versus $28,857 for AZA-treated patients. Routine use of MMF 2 g/day would be associated with a cost of $14,268 per graft year gained.[121] Given the lack of difference in patient and graft survival at 1 and 3 years discussed previously, the cost-effectiveness demonstrated by Sullivan and Keown may not persist beyond the first year. The high annual cost of MMF therapy may not translate into a pharmacoeconomic advantage given the small differences in graft loss demonstrated after the first year. The most appropriate length of therapy with this new and costly agent remains to be determined. Currently trials are underway evaluating the effect of MMF withdrawal on acute rejection in renal transplant patients.

Preliminary animal studies suggested that MPA may prevent or slow the progression of chronic rejection.[122,123] Attempts to evaluate the potential of MMF to change the course of ongoing chronic rejection in a clinical setting (as measured by a change in the slope of $1/S_{cr}$ vs time) and the 3-year follow-up of clinical trials have not produced promising results.[124]

REJECTION THERAPY

The management of transplant rejection should be individualized. A specific histologic diagnosis should be made since treatment is often individualized based on histology. Prophylactic agents such as ganciclovir, nystatin, trimethoprim/sulfamethoxazole (TMP/SMX), H_2-receptor antagonists, and/or antacids may be used to minimize adverse effects associated with intensive immunosuppression.[125]

Acute cellular rejection is the only type of rejection that responds well to therapy. High-dose steroids continue to be first-line therapy. Specific protocols vary between transplant centers; the general practice is to increase the steroid dose for 3 to 7 days, tapering down to the maintenance level or prerejection dose, whichever is higher. One option is to give 250 to 1000 mg intravenous methylprednisolone for 3 days. Another approach is to use an "oral recycle" of steroids consisting of 200 mg oral PRED, decreasing by 40 mg each day until a maintenance dose of 20 mg/d is achieved. Although no corticosteroid regimen has been show to be superior to another, oral steroid cycles are less costly and easier to administer than intravenous therapy.

MMF has also been examined for the treatment of rejection in CSA-based regimens. In an open-label trial of 75 renal transplant recipients with biopsy-proven refractory acute rejection, MMF reversed rejection in 69% of patients.[126] MMF was later assessed as rescue therapy versus intravenous corticosteroids in 150 renal transplant recipients with biopsy-proven rejection refractory to antilymphocyte therapy. Patients were randomized to methylprednisolone 5 mg/kg for 5 days or MMF 1.5 g bid, which could be increased to 3.5 g/d as needed for efficacy. The primary efficacy variable, graft loss and patient death at 6 months, was 26% in the steroid-treated patients versus 14% in the MMF group ($P = .081$). Secondary analysis at 1 year showed a difference in graft loss or death: 31.5% (steroids) versus 18% (MMF, $P = .042$). The number of patients reporting adverse events, primarily gastrointestinal (70.1% vs 33.8%) and hematologic (50.6% vs 25.5%), was significantly higher in the MMF group.[127] In patients receiving immunosuppression consisting of CSA, AZA, and PRED, Pirsch et al. evaluated conversion to MMF 1.5 g bid versus AZA 1 to 2 mg/kg/d, both in combination with intravenous corticosteroids for the treatment of first biopsy-proven acute rejection within 6 months posttransplant. Primary end points were first use of antibody therapy during 6 months and patient/graft survival at 1 year. MMF decreased the use of ATG/ALG/OKT3 (16.8% vs 41.7%, $P < .0001$) and was associated with a nonsignificant improvement in patient and graft survival (92% vs 85.2%). More patients in the MMF group, however, withdrew secondary to adverse events (17.7% vs 10.2%).[128] Given the limited data, it appears that MMF in appropriate doses with or without corticosteroids should be considered for the treatment of acute rejection in MMF-naive patients.

OKT3 therapy may also be used as a first-line treatment of acute cellular rejection. The reversal rate for acute rejection in patients treated with OKT3 is more than 80%.[129] This reversal rate compares to a reversal rate of 65% to 75% achieved with high-dose steroids.[130] In addition, it has been suggested that long-term graft survival may be higher when OKT3 is used as primary treatment for first episodes of rejection.[131] Two factors that must be considered with OKT3 use are the added potential for infectious and/or CNS toxicity and increased cost when compared to high-dose steroids. As a result of these factors and the responsiveness of acute cellular rejections to steroid treatment, OKT3 is usually reserved as a second-line agent.[132]

ALTERNATIVE STRATEGIES

STEROID WITHDRAWAL

Because of the many detrimental effects associated with chronic steroid therapy, dose minimization has been the goal of therapy. The availability of CSA and TAC has permitted complete withdrawal of corticosteroids in some patients. Steroid withdrawal protocols are now part of routine practice but must be initiated and completed with caution to avoid graft rejection and loss. There is evidence suggesting that the avoidance or discontinuation of steroids is beneficial in transplant patients receiving CSA-based immunosuppression. Six-year actual graft survival was 69% in patients withdrawn from steroids at 6 months and maintained on CSA monotherapy; reinstitution of steroids was necessary in 25% of patients secondary to rejection or graft dysfunction.[41] Hricik et al. demonstrated late steroid withdrawal (≥ 6 months posttransplant) to be successful in 79% of patients.[42] Furthermore, a meta-analysis indicated that patient and graft survival were not adversely compromised with the avoidance or withdrawal of steroids; however, the risk of acute allograft rejection was increased.[40] In contrast with previous reports, the actuarial 5-year graft survival rates were 73% and 85%, respectively ($P = 0.03$), among patients who received placebo versus low-dose PRED given on alternate days. The actuarial 5-year patient survival rates were not significantly different (≥ 92%).[133]

In 26 renal allograft recipients receiving MMF, CSA, and PRED, mean steroid withdrawal time was 17 months posttransplant; mean steroid-free follow-up time was 10 months.[134] No rejection episodes occurred following steroid withdrawal. Prospective, randomized trials are needed to further evaluate the long-term effects of steroid withdrawal in renal transplant patients, specifically addressing issues of time and protocol of steroid withdrawal as well as immunosuppressive regimen.

Special concerns exist regarding the long-term use of corticosteroids in children.[44,45] Growth rates in children receiving corticosteroid therapy are often not much better than growth rates of children with chronic renal, hepatic, or cardiac disease. Some transplant centers withhold PRED therapy in children until a first-rejection episode occurs. Alternate-day steroids may improve growth rates in patients who require corticosteroids to maintain allograft function.[44] Steroid withdrawal has been demonstrated to be beneficial by reducing blood pressure and lipids while improving growth in children maintained on CSA with or without AZA; however, acute rejection episodes following withdrawal may occur in a high percentage of patients.[43,135] Although multidrug immunosuppression regimens have resulted in improved graft and patient survival, the optimal use of corticosteroids remains unclear.

CYCLOSPORINE WITHDRAWAL

Ongoing concerns about chronic CSA nephrotoxicity and the high cost of prolonged therapy have led to the examination of different strategies for electively withdrawing CSA. Unfortunately, there have been major differences in the designs, results, and conclusions of these studies. In a meta-analysis evaluating elective CSA withdrawal in renal transplant patients, the rate of acute rejection was higher in patients undergoing CSA withdrawal than those who continued to receive CSA.[136] Although there was no evidence that the higher incidence of acute rejection following CSA withdrawal led to increased graft loss or patient mortality, it is possible that the duration of follow-up was too brief to have allowed the detection of these outcomes. When considering withdrawal for economic reasons, the cost of additional monitoring and the treatment of potential rejection episodes must be included in the analysis. Well-designed randomized controlled clinical trials are needed to compare the effects of CSA withdrawal versus continued CSA therapy on long-term graft and patient survival. Any long-term negative consequences from an increased incidence of acute rejection episodes following CSA withdrawal will need to be weighed against both the increased cost and the risk of long-term toxic effects of continued CSA therapy.

COMPLICATIONS

Infectious complications following transplantation are generally classified according to the causative organism, site of the infection, and time of appearance following surgery. Bacterial infections occur most frequently within the first month posttransplantation and generally affect the urinary tract, respiratory tract, wound, or vascular access sites. Viral infections are most commonly caused by herpes simplex (early posttransplant), herpes zoster (late posttransplant), or CMV. Other infections caused by nocardia, fungi, or protozoa occur rarely in renal transplant recipients.[137] The treatment of infection in the immunocompromised host is discussed in Chapter 111. Special considerations of therapy in renal transplant patients for CMV, herpes, and *Pneumocystis carinii* infections are described in the following sections.

Noninfectious complications following transplantation may be continuations of the conditions that led to transplantation such as diabetes and hypertension. However, some of these problems are newly diagnosed posttransplant. The treatment of anemia, diabetes, gastrointestinal disease, hyperlipidemia, hypertension, malignancy, and osteoporosis are discussed elsewhere in this text. Some of the special considerations for renal transplant recipients, however, are given in Table 43–8.

CYTOMEGALOVIRUS INFECTIONS

Cytomegalovirus is the most important viral pathogen affecting transplant patients[138]; 50% to 60% of patients have been infected with the virus. CMV is responsible for 30% of febrile episodes, 35% of leukopenia, 20% of graft failure, and 25% of mortality in kidney transplantation.[139] In individuals with a normal immune system, CMV rarely produces symptoms. However, in patients with a suppressed immune system, CMV is usually symptomatic, can be quite serious, and may be fatal. Following transplantation, patients may develop symptomatic primary or secondary CMV infections. A previously CMV-seronegative patient who receives an organ or blood product from a CMV-seropositive donor is considered to have a primary CMV infection. A secondary infection occurs in previously seropositive patients either due to reactivation of the latent virus or due to reinfection. Patients with primary infections are generally more symptomatic than patients with secondary infections.

Typically, patients with CMV infection present between 4 and 10 weeks following transplantation with general malaise, gastritis, fever, elevated liver function studies, leukopenia, thrombocytopenia, and atypical lymphocytes on a WBC differential. Deterioration in renal function may also be observed. CMV retinitis is a rare manifestation in transplant patients, whereas CMV gastritis is a common complication. The leading cause of death associated with CMV infection is pneumonia.

The incidence and severity of symptomatic CMV infections in transplant recipients are related to the intensity of immunosuppression required to prevent graft rejection. Patients treated on multiple occasions with high-dose steroids or patients receiving OKT3 or ALG/ATG are at high risk for developing symptomatic CMV disease.[138,140] Poor HLA matching, cadaveric allografts, and CMV-positive donor serology also contribute to the severity of CMV disease.[141,142]

Because many transplant patients have primary CMV infections or reinfections, it would be ideal to limit the transplantation of CMV-positive organs, but given the high prevalence of CMV in most donor pools, this is not possible. Therefore, multiple strategies have been used for the prevention of CMV. These strategies have included both prophylactic (to prevent disease) and preemptive (to prevent disease when it is likely to occur based on the detection of CMV infection without the presence of symptoms) interventions. Because of the conflicting results reported by various trials, there is controversy as to which agent(s), if any, should be used in renal transplant recipients.

PROPHYLAXIS OF CYTOMEGALOVIRUS INFECTIONS

High-dose acyclovir has been reported to reduce the incidence and severity of CMV disease in renal allograft recipients.[143] This widely quoted study was a prospective, double-blind, 12-week evaluation of 104 kidney transplant patients. Patients were randomized to receive either placebo or high-dose oral acyclovir (800 mg qid with dose adjustment based on renal function) for 12 weeks posttransplantation. There was a significant reduction in CMV isolation from blood (11% vs 41%) and disease requiring ganciclovir therapy (4% vs 13%) in patients receiving acyclovir. The greatest benefit was demonstrated in seronegative recipients of seropositive donor kidneys; however, there were only 13 patients in this subgroup.[143] Birkeland et al. demonstrated the efficacy of high-dose acyclovir prophylaxis in all patients, regardless of serology before transplant; in addition, these patients received preemptive ganciclovir during treatment with monoclonal antibodies.[144] In another case-controlled study of cadaveric kidney transplants who received high-dose acyclovir for 3 months, only seropositive patients had a significantly lower incidence of CMV disease.[145]

Other studies of prophylactic acyclovir, however, have failed to produce similar results.[55,146–148] The failure of acyclovir in these reports is consistent with *in vitro* data suggesting that CMV is unlikely to be inhibited by levels of acyclovir that are achievable *in vivo*. Some investigators have suggested that acyclovir prophylaxis is less effective in patients who receive ALA antibodies.[149,150] Discrepancies between studies may result from institutional differences in prevalence of CMV, immunosuppressive regimens, and definitions of CMV disease or infection.

Acyclovir therapy, if used, should be given for the first 12 weeks following transplantation since the risk for developing CMV is greatest during this period. Because acyclovir is primarily excreted unchanged via the kidney, the dose of acyclovir should be individualized based on renal function (Chap. 47). Oral acyclovir is well tolerated, with

TABLE 43–8. Special Pharmacotherapy Considerations in Renal Transplant Recipients

Problem	Pharmacotherapy	Special Considerations
Infection		
Perioperative prophylaxis	Cefazolin 1 g q 12 to 48 h	Donor culture results
		Penicillin allergy: vancomycin
	Bowel decontamination	
Pneumocystis carinii Pneuomonia prophylaxis	TMP/SMX 400/80 qd	Sulfa allergy
	Pentamidine 300 mg inhaled q mo OR dapsone 50–100 mg PO qd	
Fungal—Prophylaxis	Nystatin, clotrimazole	
Treatment	Fluconazole, itraconazole, ketoconazole	Inhibit P450 3A4, monitor CSA and TAC levels, decrease doses
	Amphotericin B	Consider liposomal products; decrease or stop CSA or TAC to minimize nephrotoxicity
Delayed graft function		Remember to adjust doses of renally eliminated drugs—acyclovir, ganciclovir, TMP/SMX
Prolonged uremia		
Hyperphosphatemia	Phophorus binders; restrict dietary intake	
Hypocalcemia	Calcium supplementation; calcitriol	
Metabolic acidosis	Sodium bicarbonate; Shohl's solution	
Hyperkalemia	Restrict dietary intake; dialysis	May be exacerbated by CSA or TAC or ACEIs, acidosis
Anemia	Continue erythropoietin until excretory function resumes	In patients with graft function, Hct should return to normal by 3–4 months posttransplant; if patient has good function and anemia persists, evaluate for folate, vitamin B_{12} deficiency
	Iron supplementation	
Hyperglycemia		
Pretransplant diabetes	Insulin	Insulin requirements will increase with improving renal function
	Oral hypoglycemics	Glucocorticoids, TAC, and CSA also increase hypoglycemic requirements
	Metformin	Avoid
	Troglitazone	May interact with cytochrome P450 metabolism
Posttransplant diabetes	Insulin	Risk factors: obesity, family history, African American race, cadaveric kidney, TAC > CSA
	Oral hypoglycemics	May resolve/improve as immunosuppressive doses decrease
Ulcer Prophylaxis	H_2-receptor antagonists	Renally eliminated
	Sucralfate	If DGF: caution aluminum content
		No DGF: caution hypophosphatemia
	GI symptoms?	Proton pump inhibitors ok
		Consider CMV gastritis
Hyperlipidemia	Diet	CSA > TAC, consider switch to TAC
	HMG-CoA reductase inhibitors ("statins")	CSA/TAC may increase "statin" levels; start at lowest dose
		Monitor for muscle cramps, CPK levels
		Monitor LFTs
	Gemfibrozil	Adjust for renal impairment
		Caution with concomitant "statin"
Hypertension	Calcium channel blockers	Diltiazem, verapamil inhibit CSA/TAC metabolism
		Dihydropyridines may potentiate CSA-gingival hyperplasia
	ACE inhibitors; angiotensin II receptor antagonists	May exacerbate hyperkalemia
		Monitor K^+, S_{cr} to assess for renal allograft vascular disease
		May be useful in posttransplant erythrocytosis (Hct > 55%)
Osteoporosis	Oral calcium supplementation (1000–1500 mg/d)	If daily intake < 1000 mg elemental calcium
	Oral vitamin D	Documented deficiency
	Calcifediol (1000 IU/d)	If kidney functioning
	Calcitriol (0.5 μg/d)	If kidney not functioning
	Hormone replacement therapy	Postmenopausal women without contraindications
	Calcitonin or oral bisphophonates	Documented loss in bone mineral density > 3%
		Data lacking for bisphosphonates in patients with renal insufficiency
Malignancy		
Prevention	Minimize immunosuppressant doses; avoid sun exposure (sun block, hats, clothing); routine self-examinations (skin, lymph nodes); yearly gynecologic/prostate exams	AZA particularly associated with skin cancers
		CSA/TAC may be associated with lymphoproliferative disorders (lymphomas)
Treatment	Discontinue or minimize immunosuppressants	Do not abruptly withdraw corticosteroids
	Surgical, radiologic, or antineoplastic therapy	

headache and nausea being the most commonly reported adverse effects. With high-dose therapy, adverse effects appear to be more common and include nausea, severe headaches, and neurologic toxicity, such as tremor, delirium, and paresthesias, which improve with dose reduction. High-dose oral acyclovir may cost from $300 to $1200 per 12-week course.[142] This additional cost may not produce enough benefit to warrant routine prophylaxis in all renal transplant patients.

Valacyclovir is an oral prodrug formulation of acyclovir that has increased bioavailability and, thus, results in higher systemic concentrations of acyclovir. Administration of valacyclovir 500 mg four times daily provides an AUC equal to that of 10 mg/kg of intravenous acyclovir. Trials are currently underway to examine the efficacy and safety of valacyclovir as CMV prophylaxis in renal transplant recipients.[151]

Immunoglobulins, including polyclonal (IVIG) and CMV hyperimmune (CMVIG) immunoglobulin, have demonstrated variable efficacy for preventing CMV. Polyclonal immunoglobulin preparations are not standardized with regard to CMV-antibody content.[152] As a result, high doses of polyclonal immunoglobulin preparations are generally required to deliver an effective amount of CMV antibodies. The large volumes may be especially difficult in renal transplant patients, who may not be in fluid balance.

One pediatric study demonstrated the benefit of polyclonal immunoglobulin (Gammagard) as prophylaxis in CMV-negative recipients of CMV-positive allografts.[153] Symptomatic disease developed in 17% of IVIG-treated patients versus 71% of control patients. Although results were statistically significant, the study population was small and the control group received more treatments with monoclonal antibodies (46% vs 71%, NS).[153] Conti et al. demonstrated that conventional immunoglobulin was superior to placebo and equivalent to low-dose intravenous ganciclovir for the prophylaxis of CMV disease in CMV-negative renal transplant recipients of CMV-positive organs. However, the cost of IVIG was significantly greater than that of ganciclovir ($4000/patient vs $350/patient).[154] The high cost and availability of other agents makes the use of polyclonal IVIG as a prophylactic agent for CMV uncommon.

The safety and efficacy of preventive CMVIG was evaluated in a prospective, controlled, randomized, multicenter trial in seronegative renal transplant patients receiving seropositive grafts.[155] Patients received 550 mg/kg over a 16-week period and were followed for up to 1 year. Patients who received CMVIG had significantly fewer confirmed CMV syndromes (21% vs 60%), less marked leukopenia (4% vs 37%), and fewer fungal and protozoal infections (0 vs 20%) compared to controls. Furthermore, the incidence of serious CMV disease was reduced in the CMVIG group. Adverse effects associated with CMVIG are rare but include flushing, anxiety, nausea, a metallic taste, headache, shortness of breath, palpitations, backache and muscle cramps. Currently, CMVIG is approved in the United States for attenuation of primary CMV disease in high-risk patients (donor positive/recipient negative).[156] The cost is approximately $4800 per course of therapy.[157]

Combination strategies using CMVIG and antiviral agents for CMV prevention are used in some institutions. Contrasting results have been obtained.[139,146,158,159] Carrieri et al. retrospectively compared patients who received acyclovir plus CMVIG to acyclovir alone and demonstrated a reduction in the incidence of CMV disease from 47% to 23% with the combination in high-risk patients.[160] Further evaluations need to be performed to assess the absolute benefit of combination regimens.

Ganciclovir triphosphate, the active metabolite of ganciclovir, is a potent inhibitor of the replication of human herpes viruses, including CMV. Ganciclovir has been used prophylactically and preemptively. Rondeau et al. evaluated intravenous ganciclovir 5 mg/kg initiated on day 14 posttransplantation in seronegative patients receiving seropositive grafts. Although there was no difference in incidence of CMV infection or disease between ganciclovir and control patients, ganciclovir use was associated with a delayed onset and decreased severity of CMV.[161] When used in renal transplant patients receiving monoclonal antibodies, the concurrent use of ganciclovir significantly reduced the incidence and severity of symptomatic disease.[162,163] In one of these studies, a maximum dose of 2.5 mg/kg/d was effective.[163] Other studies have suggested that the administration of ganciclovir to patients who are CMV antigen positive reduces the incidence of symptomatic disease.[164] Unfortunately, not all studies have supported this conclusion.[165]

Recently, an oral dosage form of ganciclovir has become available. Oral ganciclovir has a low mean bioavailability of 6% to 9%. One gram three times daily yields a maximum mean concentration of 1.2 μ/mL, whereas 5 mg/kg/d intravenous ganciclovir yields a concentration of 8.3 μ/mL.[166] Food increases the bioavailability of oral ganciclovir. Clinical trials describing the use of oral ganciclovir in renal transplant patients are limited.

Side effects of ganciclovir include neutropenia (50%) and thrombocytopenia (20%). Since neutropenia is frequently observed as a consequence of CMV, it is often difficult to ascertain the precise cause. In general, the adverse hematologic effects of ganciclovir are reversible within 3 to 7 days following discontinuation of therapy. Less common toxicities associated with ganciclovir therapy include CNS toxicity (headache, tremor, confusion, seizures, and hallucinations). Fever, rash, and alterations in liver function have also been reported in patients receiving ganciclovir therapy, but these side effects are uncommon and a definite cause-and-effect relationship has been difficult to establish. Future studies evaluating monotherapy as well as combination strategies will be needed to determine the optimal dose and duration for preventative therapy as well as long-term toxicity of ganciclovir.

Foscarnet prophylaxis is not advocated in renal transplant patients because of the potential additive nephrotoxicity that may occur when it is concurrently administered with agents such as CSA, TAC, and amphotericin B. Future options for the prevention of CMV disease include the use of CMV vaccines. The Towne strain of human CMV reduced the incidence of severe CMV disease in seronegative patients.[167] Such vaccines, when perfected, may prove to be less costly and more effective than current prophylactic strategies.

TREATMENT OF CYTOMEGALOVIRUS INFECTIONS

Until the development of ganciclovir, withholding immunosuppression was the mainstay of therapy for active CMV disease. Currently, ganciclovir is the therapy of choice for the treatment of CMV infections in renal transplant patients. Jordan et al. reported their experience treating 36 renal transplant patients with tissue invasive CMV disease.[168] Patients received ganciclovir (2.5 mg/kg every 12 hours) until they were asymptomatic and afebrile for 5 days. CMV disease was classified as mild in 75%, moderate in 17%, and severe in 8% of the patients. The average length of treatment was 12.2 days. Viral blood cultures were negative 7.5 days after treatment in 11/11 evaluable cases, and 9/11 urine cultures were negative in 8 days. All patients were asymptomatic after the initial course of treatment. The overall 1-year patient and graft survival rates were 100% and 56%, respectively, with a mean follow-up period of 12 months.[168] Ganciclovir was well tolerated with side effects limited to transient leukopenia, thrombocytopenia, and rash. Similar results have been reported in other centers.[169]

Foscarnet is generally reserved for the treatment of CMV infections that are unresponsive to therapy with ganciclovir. Only limited experience using the drug in renal transplant patients has been published. Andersson et al. used foscarnet as a continuous IV infusion (0.15 mg/kg/min) in eight renal transplant recipients. Seven of the patients were CMV virus culture negative 1 week after starting the foscarnet. Side effects included an increase in serum creatinine (5/8 patients), hypocalcemia (4/8 patients), and confusion (1/8 patients). All side effects were reversible after dosage reduction or discontinuation of the drug.[170] A rise in serum creatinine may be secondary to foscarnet or other clinical factors. For the present, foscarnet may be used cautiously in patients unresponsive or intolerant to therapy with ganciclovir.

CMVIG is effective in preventing CMV disease in high-risk renal transplant recipients. However, the use of CMVIG to treat CMV infections in renal transplant patients has not been evaluated. The combination of CMVIG and ganciclovir was compared to ganciclovir alone in a limited number of patients following liver transplantation. No difference in clinical outcomes was noted between the two study groups. Because of the high cost of the medication and follow-up, the use of CMVIG in the treatment of CMV disease in renal transplant patients is not justified until well-controlled studies are completed.

HERPES VIRUS INFECTIONS

Herpes simplex virus (HSV) infections in renal transplant patients are most commonly the result of reactivation of a previous infection. Symptomatic HSV infection usually presents as labial or oral lesions in the first 1 to 3 months posttransplantation, but patients may also present with reactivation of varicella zoster as "shingles." Prophylactic therapy with low-dose acyclovir has been shown to delay the development of HSV infections in patients following renal transplantation.[171] Intravenous acyclovir, as described in Chapter 111, is indicated for treatment in patients who develop disseminated HSV infections.

PNEUMOCYSTIS CARINII PNEUMONIA

The cumulative incidence of patients who develop *Pneumocystis carinii* pneumonia (PCP) within the first year post-transplantation has been reported to be 3% to 5%.[172] Low-dose TMP/SMX (400/80 mg daily) is effective in the prevention of *Pneumocystis* infections in renal transplant patients. After 3 months of therapy, it is frequently possible to reduce therapy from once daily to three times per week.[173] TMP/SMX is highly effective, relatively inexpensive, and offers protection against other susceptible bacterial pathogens.

Aerosolized pentamidine (300 mg every month) may be used alternatively in patients with allergies or intolerable adverse effects to sulfonamides.[174] Although it is generally well tolerated and has a relatively low incidence of nephrotoxicity and myelotoxicity, the prophylactic use of aerosolized pentamidine is expensive. In addition, its aerosolized administration is associated with two concerns: (1) the sensitivity of induced sputum and bronchoalveolar lavage is reduced, making the diagnosis of breakthrough PCP more difficult to establish,[175] and (2) patients cough secondary to the irritating effects, increasing the risk of spreading transmissible agents. The use of inhaled albuterol prior to aerosolized pentamidine may minimize cough and bronchospasm.[174] Dapsone may also be used as an alternative for PCP prophylaxis. Its use has been evaluated in patients with HIV and appears to be promising.[176] However, further study of dapsone in the setting of renal transplantation is needed to substantiate its role.

The duration of *Pneumocystis* prophylaxis is unclear. The risk of infection caused by *P. carinii* is likely to decrease as immunosuppression is reduced; therefore, prophylaxis is generally discontinued within 6 to 12 months following transplantation (some centers maintain lifelong PCP prophylaxis). The reinstitution of prophylaxis in patients requiring treatment for acute rejection may be appropriate. The therapy of choice for the treatment of PCP continues to be TMP/SMX. The use of TMP/SMX as well as alternative agents for PCP treatment are described in Chapter 111.

CARDIOVASCULAR DISEASE

Cardiovascular disease is a leading cause of morbidity in renal transplant patients. Hypertension, hyperlipidemia, and diabetes contribute significantly to cardiovascular disease and are common complications in transplant recipients. Impaired graft function, corticosteroids, CSA, and TAC may cause posttransplant hypertension. The treatment of hypertension is addressed in Chapter 10. Special precautions, however, are required in this population. Calcium channel blockers are considered first-line agents in this population. In addition to their ability to control blood pressure, calcium channel blockers may ameliorate the nephrotoxic effects of CSA, improve renal hemodynamics, decrease the incidence of DGF, and provide some immunosuppression.[29,177,178] Gingival hyperplasia can be a troublesome problem in patients who are also on CSA. Diltiazem, verapamil, and nicardipine inhibit CSA metabolism via the CYP450 3A4 system. This interaction may lead to CSA-induced nephrotoxicity and neurotoxicity if left unchecked. However, with proper monitoring and CSA dosage adjustments, agents like diltiazem and verapamil, can be used to decrease the daily dose of CSA.

Angiotensin-converting enzyme (ACE) inhibitors and angiotensin II (AT2) blockers may offer several benefits. ACE inhibitors have been shown to reduce proteinuria and preserve renal function in small trials in renal transplant patients.[179,180] ACE inhibitors and AT2 blockers also have a special niche in the management of posttransplant erythrocytosis. However, the combination of efferent arteriolar vasodilation caused by the ACE inhibitor or AT2 blocker and afferent vasoconstriction caused by CSA or TAC may result in a decrease in glomerular filtration when these agents are used together. Hyperkalemia caused by CSA and TAC is frequently aggravated by concomitant therapy with an ACE inhibitor. When ACE inhibitors or AT2 blockers are used in patients posttransplantation, close monitoring of serum creatinine and potassium is required.

Hyperlipidemia may be exacerbated by CSA, corticosteroids, diuretics, and β-adrenergic blockers. It is controversial whether the management of hyperlipidemia in these patients should be more aggressive than the guidelines established in the report of the second Adult Treatment Panel of the National Cholesterol Education Program, which are discussed in Chapter 19. Aggressive lipid lowering may not only arrest the progress or prevent the complications of atherosclerosis but may promote renal graft survival in this specific population. With the use of lipid-lowering agents, potential interactions with immunosuppressive regimens must be considered.[181,182]

Dietary intervention, although safe, may be relatively ineffective for the treatment of hyperlipidemia in the transplant population. Along with dietary modification, dose reduction or withdrawal of CSA and/or PRED may assist in minimizing hyperlipidemia. Bile-acid–binding resins may be used to lower cholesterol in renal transplant patients, but adequate doses are difficult to achieve without the development of GI adverse effects. Since the absorption of CSA is dependent on the presence of bile in the GI tract, patients should be instructed to separate dosing of bile-acid–binding resins and CSA by 2 hours. For those transplant patients who have hypertriglyceridemia refractory to dietary intervention, fish oil and fibric acid derivatives are well-tolerated, effective alternatives. Gemfibrozil is most effective in lowering serum triglyceride concentrations, but the dose must be reduced in patients with decreased renal function. HMG-CoA reductase inhibitors are highly effective in the treatment of hyperlipidemia, specifically increased LDL, in renal transplant patients. These agents should be used with caution because of several reports of rhabdomyolysis resulting in renal failure when lovastatin was combined with CSA. Safety measures including the use of low HMG-CoA reductase inhibitor doses and avoiding inappropriately high CSA concentrations should be taken. The concurrent use of medications known to increase the risk of myopathy (such as gemfibrozil) should be avoided. Patients should be informed of the signs and symptoms of rhabdomyolysis. Baseline and follow-up CPK measurements (every 6 months) have been used to identify patients who develop subclinical rhabdomyolysis when cholesterol-lowering therapy is used. In addition, because of the potential for hepatotoxicity from HMG-CoA reductase inhibitors, close monitoring of liver function is indicated.

Corticosteroids, CSA, and TAC can impair glucose control in previously diabetic patients as well as cause new-onset posttransplant diabetes mellitus (PTDM) in 4% to 20% of patients. Corticosteroids seem to induce insulin resistance and impair peripheral glucose uptake, whereas CSA and TAC appear to inhibit insulin production.[183] Tacrolimus seems to be more diabetogenic than CSA (20% vs 7%).[184] Patients with PTDM should be referred for nutritional counseling and advised on the merits of weight loss (if appropriate). The goals of management of diabetes are discussed in Chapter 70. There are, however, some special considerations in renal transplant patients. Up to 40% of patients with PTDM will require insulin therapy.[183] In all diabetic patients who can be managed with an oral hypoglycemic agent, glipizide, which is extensively metabolized by the liver, may be preferred over renally eliminated agents such as glyburide. Metformin should be avoided because of the risk of accumulation and lactic acidosis with renal impairment. Troglitazone may improve insulin sensitivity, but has not been evaluated in this population. Limited data indicates that troglitazone is metabolized by the cytochrome P450 3A system.[185] Its effects on CSA or TAC pharmacokinetics have not been evaluated. Regardless of therapy, frequent blood glucose monitoring is imperative in the early postoperative phase, both to improve glucose control and to identify those with PTDM. Early posttransplant, variable renal function secondary to DGF or rejection is common. Changes in renal function affect the elimination of many hypoglycemic agents, including insulin, and may result in hyper- or hypoglycemia. Patients and clinicians should also be aware that dose changes of immunosuppressant drugs also affect glycemic control. Tapering of immunosuppressive medications may result in decremental changes in insulin requirements, whereas steroid pulses for the treatment of rejection may result in increased insulin requirements.

MALIGNANCY

Advances in immunosuppression have decreased the incidence of acute rejection and increased patient survival, thus increasing the overall exposure to immunosuppression over time. While the precise mechanism is unclear, posttransplant malignancy seems to be related to the level of immunosuppression, as evidenced by a difference in the rates of malignancy associated with quadruple versus triple versus dual immunosuppressant regimens.[186] Although the introduction of CSA is associated with an increased prevalence of lymphoma in transplant patients versus AZA-based regimens, it is unclear whether this is a direct affect of CSA or is merely related to the level of immunosuppression achieved. Posttransplant malignancies are often divided into three classes: de novo malignancy, recurrent disease, and directly transmitted from donor to recipient. The overall incidence of cancer in renal transplant recipients is 6%, ranging from 4% to 18%. Malignancy increases with the length of follow-up and may affect as many as 72% of patients surviving greater than 20 years. While the risk of lung, breast, colon, and prostate cancer does not appear to be increased over the general population, Kaposi's sarcoma, squamous cell carcinoma, non-Hodgkin's lymphoma, skin cancer, and cancers of the vulva and perineum do occur more commonly in transplant recipients. In patients with a history of cancer prior to transplantation, recurrence is dependent on both the length of time since cancer treatment and the type of cancer. Most cancers recur in patients who were treated less than 2 years prior to transplantation. Malignancies that recur most frequently are renal carcinoma, malignant melanoma, sarcomas, and nonmelanoma skin cancers. The risk of transmitting a cancer from donor to recipient has decreased secondary to exclusion of donors with a history of malignancy. In the event that a donor malignancy comes to light post–renal transplant, transplant nephrectomy and return to dialysis is the most prudent course.[187]

CONCLUSIONS

Renal transplantation remains the therapy of choice for most patients with chronic renal failure. The development of new immunosuppressive agents and improved immunologic monitoring methods have reduced complications and prolonged graft survival. The importance of pharmacotherapy in the successful management of renal transplant patients has created an opportunity for pharmacists to enhance patient outcomes. Pharmacists are involved in the management of renal transplant patients along the continuum of care. Pharmacists provide patient medication counseling for pretransplant patients in the dialysis unit or pretransplant renal clinic. In the perioperative period, pharmacists assist in the early postoperative management of fluids, electrolytes, infection, hypertension, diabetes, immunosuppression, and general drug dosing in these patients with continuously changing renal function. Long term, pharmacists manage many of the complications experienced by these patients, including anemia, diabetes, GI disease, hypertension, hyperlipidemia, infection, and osteoporosis. Pharmacists provide patients and family with medication education and compliance monitoring and are frequently an invaluable source of information regarding payment and reimbursement for medication. Although there may be a direct link between these activities and improved patient outcomes, documentation is limited.

ACKNOWLEDGMENTS

The authors wish to thank Jennifer Davis, PharmD, David Lassen, BS Pharm, and Anita Goth for their assistance in the preparation of this chapter.

▶ PRINCIPLES OF PHARMACOTHERAPY

- Acute rejection and delayed graft function are the major determinants of graft survival.
- Chronic rejection, the most common cause of late graft loss, is unresponsive to currently available immunosuppressive agents.
- Patient and graft survival rates for renal transplantation have improved significantly such that it is difficult to show differences between treatment regimens. The high cost of new therapies relative to expected improvements needs to be continually evaluated.
- Given the number of immunosuppressive agents currently and soon to be available, immunosuppressive combinations can be tailored based on individual response, adverse effects, cost, and patient acceptance.
- Infection (e.g., CMV, PCP) prophylaxis should be tailored to patient and donor characteristics in addition to the degree of immunosuppression.
- Nephrotoxic agents and those with significant effect on cytochrome-P450-3A4 should be used with caution and require enhanced monitoring (e.g., S_{cr}, CSA, or TAC levels).
- In addition to immunologic complications posttransplant, renal transplant recipients are at increased risk for hypertension, hyperlipidemia, and impaired glucose metabolism, all well-associated with coronary artery disease.
- As the length of patient survival increases, malignancy becomes a significant cause of morbidity and mortality.

REFERENCES

1. US Renal Data System. USRDS 1997 Annual Data Report. Bethesda, MD, National Institutes of Health, National Institute of Diabetes and Digestive and Kidney Diseases, 1997.
2. United Network for Organ Sharing, 1996.
3. Christensen AJ, Holman JM, Turner CW, Slaughter JR. Quality of life in end-stage renal disease. Influence of renal transplantation. Clin Transplant 1989;3:46–53.
4. Effers PW. Effect of transplantation on the Medicare end-stage renal disease program. N Engl J Med 1988;318:223–229.
5. Opelz G, Wujciak T, Mytilineos J, Scherer S. Revisiting HLA matching for kidney transplantation. Transplant Proc 1993;25:173–175.
6. Ojo A, Wolfe RA, Held PJ, Port FK, Schmouder RL. Delayed graft function: Risk factors and implications for renal allograft survival. Transplantation 1997;63:968–974.
7. Suthanthiran M, Strom TB. Renal transplantation. N Engl J Med 1994;331:365–376.
8. Opelz G. Efficacy of rejection prophylaxis with OKT3 in renal transplantation. Collaborative Transplant Study. Transplantation 1995;60: 1220–1224.
9. Indudhara R, Khauli RB, Menon M, Stoff JS. Simultaneous quadruple immunosuppression with cyclosporine induction therapy in high risk renal transplant recipients. J Urol 1994;152:307–311.
10. Goldman M, Abramowicz D, De Pauw L, et al. Beneficial effects of prophylactic OKT3 in cadaver kidney transplantation: comparison with cyclosporin A in a single-center prospective randomized study. Transplant Proc 1991;23:1046–1047.
11. Grio JM, Alsina J, Sabater R, et al. Antilymphoblast globulin, cyclosporine, and steroids in cadaveric renal transplantation. Transplantation 1990;49:1114–1117.
12. Norman DJ, Kahana L, Stuart FP Jr, et al. A randomized clinical trial of induction therapy with OKT3 in kidney transplantation. Transplantation 1993;55:44–50.
13. Belitsky P, MacDonald AS, Cohen AD, et al. Comparison of antilymphocyte globulin and continuous IV cyclosporine A as induction immunosuppression for cadaver kidney transplants: a prospective randomized study. Transplant Proc 1991;23:999–1000.
14. Slakey DP, Johnson CP, Callaluce RD, et al. A prospective randomized comparison of quadruple versus triple therapy for first cadaver transplants with immediate function. Transplantation 1993; 56:827–831.
15. Pescovitz MD, Book BK, Milgrom ML, et al. Comparison of Minnesota antilymphoblast globulin and Upjohn antithymocyte globulin for induction immunosuppression of human renal allografts. Surgery 1994;116:811–818.
16. Lum CT, Umen AJ, Kasiske B, et al. Clinical impact of replacing Minnesota antilymphocyte globulin with ATGAM. Transplantation 1995;59:371–376.
17. Steinmuller DR, Hayes JM, Novick AC, et al. Comparison of OKT3 with ALG for prophylaxis for patients with acute renal failure after cadaveric renal transplantation. Transplantation 1991;52:67–71.
18. Light JA, Jonsson J, Khawand N, et al. Sequential immunosuppression: Three years' experience in 240 cadaveric renal transplants. Transplant Proc 1991;23:1032–1035.
19. Hanto DW, Jendrisak MD, So SK, et al. Induction immunosuppression with antilymphocyte globulin or OKT3 in cadaver kidney transplantation. Transplantation 1994;57:337–384.
20. Hariharan S, Alexander JW, Schroeder TJ, First MR. Outcome of cadaveric renal transplantation by induction treatment in the cyclosporine era. Clin Transplant 1996;10:186–190.
21. Abramowicz D, Norman DJ, Vereerstraeten P, et al. OKT3 prophylaxis in renal grafts with prolonged cold ischemia times: Association with improvement in long-term survival. Kidney Int 1996;49: 768–772.
22. Darby CR, Moore RH, Shrestha B, et al. Reduced dose OKT3 prophylaxis in sensitised kidney recipients. Transpl Int 1996;9:565–569.
23. Parlevliet KJ, ten Berge RJ, Raasveld MH, et al. Low-dose OKT3 induction therapy following renal transplantation: A controlled study. Nephrol Dial Transplant 1994;9:698–703.
24. Shield CF III, Jacobs RJ, Wyant S, Das A. A cost-effective analysis of OKT3 induction therapy in cadaveric kidney transplantation. Am J Kidney Dis 1996;27:855–864.
25. Michael HJ, Francos GC, Burke JF, et al. A comparison of the effects of cyclosporine versus antilymphocyte globulin on delayed graft function in cadaver renal transplant recipients. Transplantation 1989; 48:805–808.
26. Powelson JA, Cosimi AB. Antilymphocyte globulin and monoclonal antibodies. In: Morris PJ, ed. Kidney Transplantation Principles and Practice. Philadelphia, W.B. Saunders, 1994:215–232.
27. Chagnac A, Zevin D, Ori Y, et al. The effect of high-dose nifedipine on renal hemodynamics of cyclosporine-treated renal allograft recipients. Transplantation 1992;53:766–769.
28. Sorenson SS, Skovbon H, Eiskjr H, Thomsen K, Pedersen EB. Effect of felodipine on renal haemodynamics and tubular sodium handling in cyclosporin-treated renal transplant recipients. Nephrol Dial Transplant 1992;7:69–78.
29. Suthanthiran M, Haschemeyer RH, Riggio RR, et al. Excellent outcome with a calcium channel blocker—supplemented immunosuppressive regimen in cadaveric renal transplantation. Transplantation 1993;55:1008–1013.
30. Khauli RB, Wilson JM, Baker SP, et al. Triple therapy in cadaveric renal transplantation: Role of induction cyclosporine and targeted levels to avoid rejection. J Urol 1995;153:1805–1810.
31. Brockmoller J, Neumayer HH, Wagner K, et al. Pharmacokinetic interaction between cyclosporin and diltiazem. Eur J Clin Pharmacol 1990;38:237–242.
32. Weir MR, Peppler R, Gomolka D, Handwerger BS. Additive inhibition of afferent and efferent immunological responses of human peripheral blood mononuclear cells by verapamil and cyclosporine. Transplantation 1991;51:851–857.
33. Dumont L, Chen H, Daloze P, Xu D, Garceau D. Immunosuppressive properties of the benzothiazepine calcium antagonists diltiazem and clentiazem, with and without cyclosporine, in heteroptic rat heart transplantation. Transplantation 1993;56:181–184.
34. Kasiske BL, Johnson HJ, Goerdt PJ, et al. A randomized trial comparing cyclosporine induction with sequential therapy in renal transplant recipients. Am J Kidney Dis 1997;30:639–645.
35. Shield CF III. Consequences of anti-OKT3 antibody development: OKT3 reuse and long-term graft survival. Transplant Proc 1993;25 (suppl 1):81–82.
36. Vincenti F, Kirkman R, Light S, et al. Interleukin-2-receptor blockade with daclizumab to prevent acute rejection in renal transplantation. N Engl J Med 1998;338:161–165.
37. Nashan B, Moore R, Amlot P, et al. Randomised trial of basiliximab versus placebo for control of acute cellular rejection in renal allograft recipients. Lancet 1997;350:1193–1198.
38. Murray JE, Merrill JP, Harrison JH, Wilson RE, Dammin GJ. Prolonged survival of human kidney homografts by immunosuppressive therapy. N Engl J Med 1963;268:1315–1323.
39. Starzl TE, Marchioro TL, Waddell WR. The reversal of rejection in human renal homografts with subsequent development of homograft tolerance. Surg Gynecol Obstet 1963;117:385–395.
40. Hricik DE, O'Toole MA, Schulak JA, Herson J. Steroid-free immunosuppression in cyclosporine-treated renal transplant recipients: a meta-analysis. J Am Soc Nephrol 1993;4:1300–1305.
41. Hillebrand G, Schneeberger H, Schleibner S, et al. Ten years' experience with cyclosporine monotherapy after renal transplantation. Transplant Proc 1993;25:513–514.
42. Hricik DE, Whalen CC, Lautman J, et al. Withdrawal of steroids after renal transplantation—clinical predictors of outcome. Transplantation 1992;53:41–45.
43. Walker RG, Jones CL, Powell HR, Becker GJ, Francis DMA. Steroid withdrawal in paediatric renal transplant patients receiving

cyclosporine and azathioprine. Transplant Proc 1993;25:2883–2885.

44. Ettenger RB, Blifeld C, Prince H, et al. The pediatric nephrologist's dilemma: growth after renal transplantation and its interaction with age as a possible immunologic variable. J Pediatr 1987;111: 1022–1025.
45. Tejani A, Butt KMH, Rajpoot D, et al. Strategies for optimizing growth in children with kidney transplants. Transplantation 1989;47: 229–233.
46. Canadian Multicentre Transplant Study Group. A randomized clinical trial of cyclosporine in cadaveric renal transplantation. N Engl J Med 1983;309:809–815.
47. European Multicentre Trial Group. Cyclosporin in cadaveric renal transplantation: one-year follow-up of a multicentre trial. Lancet 1983;2:986–989.
48. Najarian JS, Fryd DS, Strand M, et al. A single institution, randomized, prospective trial of cyclosporine versus azathioprine-antilymphocyte globulin for immunosuppression in renal allograft recipients. Ann Surg 1985;201:142–157.
49. Andreu J, Campistol JM, Oppenheimer F, et al. Cyclosporine monotherapy as primary immunosuppression in renal transplantation—five-year experience. Transplant Proc 1994;26:337–340.
50. Griffin PJA, Gomes Da Costa CA, Salaman JR. A controlled trial of steroids in cyclosporine-treated renal transplant recipients. Transplantation 1987;43:505–508.
51. Tarantino A, Aroldi A, Stucchi L, et al. A randomized prospective trial comparing cyclosporine monotherapy with triple-drug therapy in renal transplantation. Transplantation 1991;52:53–57.
52. Ghoneim MA, Sobh MA, Shokeir AA, et al. Prospective randomized study of azathioprine versus cyclosporin in live-donor kidney transplantation. Am J Nephrol 1993;13:437–441.
53. Amend W, Soskin T, Vincenti F, et al. Long-term experience in primary cadaver renal transplants using cyclosporine. Clin Transplant 1990;4:341–346.
54. Hardie IR, Tiller DJ, Mahony JF, et al. Optimal combination of immunosuppressive agents for renal transplantation: first report of a multicentre, randomized trial comparing cyclosporine+prednisolone with cylcosporine+azathioprine and with triple therapy in cadaver renal transplantation. Transplant Proc 1993;25:583–584.
55. Lindholm A, Albrechtsen D, Tufveson G, et al. A randomized trial of cyclosporine and prednisone versus cyclosporine, azathioprine, and prednisolone in primary cadaveric renal transplantation. Transplantation 1992;54:624–631.
56. Isoniemi H, Ahonen J, Tikkanen MJ, et al. Long-term consequences of different immunosuppressive regimens for renal allografts. Transplantation 1993;55:494–499.
57. Ghoneim MA, Sobh MA, Shokeir AA, et al. Prospective randomized study of triple vs conventional immunosuppression in living donor kidney transplantation. Transplant Proc 1993;25:2243–2245.
58. Monaco AP, Sahyoun AI, Madras PN, et al. Cylcosporine in multidrug therapy in living-related kidney transplantation. Clin Transplant 1990;4:347–356.
59. Montagnino G, Colturi C, Tarantino A, et al. The impact of azathioprine and cyclosporine on long-term function in kidney transplantation. Transplantation 1991;51:772–776.
60. Slaton JW, Kropp KA, Jhunjhunwala JS, Selman SH. Cyclosporine versus azathioprine: A 5-year followup of 200 consecutive cadaver renal transplant recipients. J Urol 1994;151:582–585.
61. Helderman JH, Van Buren DH, Amend WJC Jr, Pirsch JD. Chronic immunosupression of the renal transplant patient. J Am Soc Nephrol 1994;4(suppl 1):S2–S9.
62. Burke JF, Pirsch JD, Ramos EL, et al. Long-term efficacy and safety of cyclosporine in renal-transplant recipients. N Engl J Med 1994; 331:358–363.
63. Ritschel WA. Microemulsion technology in the reformulation of cyclosporine: the reason behind the pharmacokinetic properties of Neoral. Clin Transplant 1996;10:364–373.
64. Kovarik JM, Mueller EA, van Bree JB, et al. Cyclosporine pharmacokinetics and variability from a microemulsion formulation—a multicenter investigation in kidney transplant patients. Transplantation 1994;58:658–663.
65. Wahlberg J, Wilczek HE, Fauchald P, et al. Consistent absorption of cyclosporine from a microemulsion formulation assessed in stable renal transplant recipients over a one-year study period. Transplantation 1995;60:648–652.
66. Barone G, Chang CT, Choc MG Jr, et al. The pharmacokinetics of a microemulsion formulation of cyclosporine in primary renal allograft recipients. The Neoral Study Group. Transplantation 1996;61: 875–880.
67. Barone G, Bunke CM, Choc MG Jr, et al. The safety and tolerability of cyclosporine emulsion versus cyclosporine in a randomized, double-blind comparison in primary renal allograft recipients. The Neoral Study Group. Transplantation 1996;61:968–987.
68. Keown P, Landsberg D, Halloran P, et al. A randomized, prospective multicenter pharmacoepidemiologic study of cyclosporine microemulsion in stable renal graft recipients. Report of the Canadian Neoral Renal Transplantation Study Group. Transplantation 1996;62: 1744–1752.
69. Drug Topics Redbook. Montrale, NJ, Medical Economics Data, 1997.
70. Lindholm A, Welsh M, Alton C, Kahan BD. Demographic factors influencing cyclosporine pharmacokinetic parameters in patients with uremia: Racial differences in bioavailability. Clin Pharmacol Ther 1992;52:359–371.
71. Ohlman S, Lindholm A, Hagglund H, Sawe J, Kahan BD. On the intraindividual variability and chronobiology of cyclosporine pharmacokinetics in renal transplantation. Eur J Clin Pharmacol 1993;44: 265–269.
72. Awni WM, Kasiske BL, Heim-Duthoy KL, Rao KV. Long-term cyclosporine pharmacokinetic changes in renal transplant recipients: Effects of binding and metabolism. Clin Pharmacol Ther 1989;45: 41–48.
73. Kahan BD, Shaw LM, Holt D, Grevel J, Johnston A. Consensus document: Hawk's Cay meeting on therapeutic drug monitoring of cyclosporine. Clin Chem 1990;36:1510–1516.
74. Kivisto KT. A review of assay methods for cyclosporin. Clinical implications. Clin Pharmacokinet 1992;23:173–190.
75. Rodighiero V. Therapeutic drug monitoring of cyclosporin—Practical applications and limitations. Clin Pharmacokinet 1989;16:27–37.
76. Grevel J, Welsh MS, Kahan BD. Cyclosporine monitoring in renal transplantation: Area under the curve monitoring is superior to trough-level monitoring. Ther Drug Monit 1989;11:246–248.
77. Awni WM, Heim-Duthoy K, Kasiske BL. Monitoring of cyclosporine by serial posttransplant pharmacokinetic studies in renal transplant patients. Transplant Proc 1990;22:1343–1344.
78. Grevel J, Kahan BD. Abbreviated kinetic profiles in area-under-the-curve monitoring of cyclosporine therapy. Clin Chem 1991;37: 1905–1908.
79. Lindholm A, Kahan BD. Influence of cyclosporine pharmacokinetics, trough concentrations, and AUC monitoring on outcome after kidney transplantation. Clin Pharmacol Ther 1993;54:205–218.
80. Serafinowicz A, Gaciong Z, Majchrzak J, et al. Abbreviated kinetic profiles to estimate exposure to CyA in renal allograft recipients treated with Sandimmun-Neoral. Transplant Proc 1997;29:277–279.
81. McDonald P, Keough A, Connell J, et al. Diltiazem co-administration reduces cyclosporine toxicity after heart transplantation: A prospective randomized study. Transplant Proc 1992;24:2259–2262.
82. Keough A, Spratt P, McCosker C, et al. Ketoconazole to reduce the need for cyclosporine after cardiac transplantation. N Engl J Med 1995;333:628–633.
83. Campana C, Regazzi MB, Buggia I, Molinaro M. Clinically significant drug interactions with cyclosporin; an update. Clin Pharmacokinet 1996;30:141–179.

84. Ferguson RM, Rynasiewicz JJ, Sutherland DER, Simmons RL, Najarian JS. Cyclosporin A in renal transplantation: a prospective randomized trial. Surgery 1982;92:175–182.
85. Jordan ML, Naraghi R, Shapiro R, et al. Tacrolimus rescue therapy for renal allograft rejection—five year experience. Transplantation 1997;63:223–228.
86. Scott-Douglas N, Zimmerman D, Klassen J. Treatment of acute renal transplant rejection with FK506 in patients on cyclosporine after failure of standard antirejection therapy. Transplant Proc 1996; 28:3165.
87. Woodle ES, Bruce DS, Josephson M, et al. FK 506 therapy for refractory renal allograft rejection: lessons from liver transplantation. Clin Transplant 1996;10:323–333.
88. Shapiro R, Jordan M, Scantlebury VP. Renal transplantation at the University of Pittsburgh: Impact of FK 506. In: Terasaki PI, Cecka JM, eds. Clinical Transplants. Los Angeles, UCLA Tissue Typing Laboratory, 1995:229–236.
89. Pirsch JD, Miller J, Deierhoi MH, Vincenti F, Filo RS. A comparison of tacrolimus (FK506) and cyclosporine for immunosuppression after cadaveric renal transplantation. Transplantation 1997;63: 977–983.
90. Filo RS. Tacrolimus in kidney transplantation: two-year results of the U.S. randomized, comparative, phase III study. Am Soc Transpl Physicians 1997;292. Abstract.
91. Mayer AD, Dmitrewski J, Squifflet J-P, et al. Multicenter randomized trial comparing tacrolimus (FK506) and cyclosporine in the prevention of renal allograft rejection. Transplantation 1997;64:436–443.
92. Holman MJ, Ahsan N, Dhillon S, O'Brien B, Yang HC. A randomized, prospective, comparative study of tacrolimus-mycophenolate mofetil and Neoral-mycophenolate mofetil in kidney transplantation. Am Soc Transpl Physicians 1997;173. Abstract.
93. Gjertson DW, Cecka JM, Terasaki PI. The relative effects of FK506 and cyclosporine on short- and long-term kidney graft survival. Transplantation 1995;60:1384–1388.
94. Laskow DA, Vincenti F, Neylan JF, Mendez R, Matas AJ. An open-label, concentration-ranging trial of FK506 in primary kidney transplantation. Transplantation 1996;62:900–905.
95. Vincenti F, Laskow DA, Neylan JF, Mendez R, Matas AJ. One-year follow-up of an open-label trial of FK506 for primary kidney transplantation. Transplantation 1996;61:1576–1581.
96. Venkataramanan R, Jain A, Warty V, et al. Pharmacokinetics of FK506 in transplant patients. Transplant Proc 1991;23:2736–2740.
97. Venkataramanan R, Jain A, Warty V, et al. Pharmacokinetics of FK 506 following oral administration: a comparison of FK 506 and cyclosporine. Transplant Proc 1991;23:931–933.
98. Vincent SH, Karanam BV, Painter SK, Chiu SH. *In vitro* metabolism of FK-506 in rat, rabbit, and human liver microsomes: identification of major metabolite and of cytochrome P450 3A as the major enzymes responsible for its metabolism. Arch Biochem Biophys 1992; 294:454–460.
99. Steeves M, Abdallah HY, Venkataramanan R, et al. In-vitro interaction of a novel immunosuppressant, FK506, and antacids. J Pharm Pharmacol 1991;43:574–577.
100. Katari SR, Magnone M, Shapiro R, et al. Clinical features of acute reversible tacrolimus (FK506) nephrotoxicity in kidney transplant recipients. Clin Transplant 1997;11:237–242.
101. Hohage H, Arlt M, Brückner D, et al. Effects of cyclosporin A and FK 506 on lipid metabolism and fibrinogen in kidney transplant recipients. Clin Transplant 1997;11:225–230.
102. Young CJ, Sollinger HW. Mycophenolate mofetil (RS-61443). In: Kupiec-Weglinski JW, ed. New Immunosuppressive Modalities in Organ Transplantation. Austin, R.G. Landes Co., 1994:1–13.
103. European Mycophenolate Mofetil Cooperative Study Group. Placebo-controlled study of mycophenolate mofetil combined with cyclosporin and corticosteroids for prevention of acute rejection. Lancet 1995;345:1321–1325.
104. The Tricontinental Mycophenolate Mofetil Renal Transplantation Study Group. A blinded, randomized clinical trial of mycophenolate mofetil for the prevention of acute rejection in cadaveric renal transplantation. Transplantation 1996;61:1029–1037.
105. Sollinger HW. Mycophenolate mofetil for the prevention of acute rejection in primary cadaveric renal allograft recipients. Transplantation 1995;60:225–232.
106. Gonwa TA. Mycophenolate mofetil for maintenance therapy in kidney transplantation. Clin Transplant 1996;10:128–130.
107. Halloran P, Mathew T, Tomlanovich S, et al. Mycophenolate mofetil in renal allograft recipients: A pooled efficacy analysis of three randomized, double-blind, clinical studies in prevention of rejection. Transplantation 1997;63:39–47.
108. Tomlanovich S, Cho S, Hodge E, et al. Mycophenolate mofetil in cadaveric renal transplantation: 3-year data. Am Soc Transpl Physicians 1997;361. Abstract.
109. The International Mycophenolate Mofetil Study Group. A long-term randomized multicenter study of mycophenolate mofetil (MMF) in cadaveric renal transplantation: results at 3 years. Am Soc Transpl Physicians 1997;362. Abstract.
110. Bullingham RES, Nicholls A, Hale M. Pharmacokinetics of mycophenolate mofetil (RS61443): a short review. Transplant Proc 1996;28:925–929.
111. Langman LJ, LeGatt DF, Yatscoff RW. Blood distribution of mycophenolate acid. Ther Drug Monit 1994;16:602–607.
112. Langman LJ, LeGatt DF, Halloran PF, Yatscoff RW. Pharmacodynamic assessment of mycophenolic acid-induced immunosuppression in renal transplant recipients. Transplantation 1996;62:666–672.
113. Johnson HJ, Swan SK, Heim-Duthoy KL, et al. The pharmacokinetics of a single dose of mycophenolate mofetil in patients with various degrees of renal function. Clin Pharmacol Ther 1998;63:512–518.
114. Simmons WD, Rayhill SC, Sollinger HW. Preliminary risk-benefit assessment of mycophenolate mofetil in transplant rejection. Drug Saf 1997;17:75–92.
115. Shaw LM, Nowak I. Mycophenolate acid: measurement and relationship to pharmacologic effects. Ther Drug Monit 1995;17:685–689.
116. Bullingham R, Shah J, Goldblum R, Schiff M. Effects of food and antacid on the pharmacokinetics of single doses of mycophenolate mofetil in rheumatoid arthritis patients. Br J Clin Pharmacol 1996; 41:513–516.
117. Product Information. CellCept (mycophenolate mofetil capsules). 1995.
118. Wolfe EJ, Mathur V, Tomlanovich S, et al. Pharmacokinetics of mycophenolate mofetil and intravenous ganciclovir alone and in combination in renal transplant recipients. Pharmacotherapy 1997;17: 591–598.
119. Zucker K, Rosen A, Tsaroucha A, et al. Augmentation of mycophenolate mofetil pharmacokinetics in renal transplant patients receiving Prograf and Cellcept in combination therapy. Transplant Proc 1997; 29:334–336.
120. Sullivan SD, Garrison LP Jr, Best JH, Members of the U.S. Renal Transplant Mycophenolate Mofetil Study Group. The cost effectiveness of mycophenolate mofetil in the first year after primary cadaveric transplant. J Am Soc Nephrol 1997;8:1592–1598.
121. Keown PA, Sullivan SD, Best JH, Garrison LP, Krueger H. Economic evaluation of mycophenolate mofetil (MMF) for prevention of acute graft rejection after cadaveric renal transplantation in Canada. Am Soc Transpl Physicians 1997;620. Abstract.
122. Morris RE, Wang J, Blum JR, et al. Immunosuppressive effects of the morpholinoethyl ester of mycophenolic acid (RS-61443) in rat and nonhuman primate recipients of heart allografts. Transplant Proc 1991;23(suppl 2):19.
123. Steele DM, Hullett DA, Bechstein WO, et al. Effects of immunosuppressive therapy on the rat aortic allograft model. Transplant Proc 1993;25(Pt 1):754–755.
124. Smith MT, Newby BS, Rao RN, et al. Response to MMF in patients with chronic renal allograft rejection. American Society of Transplant Physicians, Annual Meeting, May 10–14, 1997, Chicago, 1997. Abstract.

125. Rao KV. Mechanism, pathophysiology, diagnosis, and management of renal transplant rejection. Med Clin North Am 1990;74:1039–1057.
126. Sollinger HW, Belzer FO, Deierhoi MH, et al. RS-61443 (mycophenolate mofetil). A multicenter study for refractory kidney transplant rejection. Ann Surg 1992;216:513–518.
127. The Mycophenolate Mofetil Renal Refractory Rejection Study Group. Mycophenolate mofetil for the treatment of refractory, acute, cellular renal transplant rejection. Transplantation 1996;61:722–729.
128. Pirsch JD, Pescovitz MD, Ferguson R, et al. Mycophenolate mofetil for the treatment of first acute renal allograft rejection. Am Soc Transpl Physicians 1997;706. Abstract.
129. Ortho Multicenter Transplant Study Group. A randomized clinical trial of OKT3 monoclonal antibody for acute rejection of cadaveric renal transplants. N Engl J Med 1985;313:337–342.
130. Deierhoi MH, Barber WH, Curtis JJ, et al. A comparison of OKT3 monoclonal antibody and corticosteroids in the treatment of acute renal allograft rejection. Am J Kidney Dis 1988;11:86–89.
131. Tesi RJ, Elkhammas EA, Henry ML, Ferguson RM. OKT3 for primary therapy of the first rejection episode in kidney transplants. Transplantation 1993;55:1023–1029.
132. Oh C-S, Stratta RJ, Fox BC, et al. Increased infections associated with the use of OKT3 for treatment of steroid-resistant rejection in renal transplantation. Transplantation 1988;45:68–73.
133. Sinclair NR. Low-dose steroid therapy in cyclosporine-treated renal transplant recipients with well-functioning grafts. Can Med Assoc J 1992;147:645–655.
134. Grinyo JM, Gil-Vernet S, Seron D, et al. Steroid withdrawal in mycophenolate mofetil-treated renal allograft recipients. Transplantation 1997;63:1688–1690.
135. Ingulli E, Tejani A, Markell M. The benficial effects of steroid withdrawal on blood pressure and lipid profile in children posttransplantation in the cyclosporine era. Transplantation 1993;55:1029–1033.
136. Kasiske BL, Heim-Duthoy KL, Ma JZ. Elective cyclosporine withdrawal after renal transplantation: A meta-analysis. JAMA 1993;269:395–400.
137. Rubin RH, Wolfson JA, Cosimi AB, Tolkoff-Rubin NE. Infection in the renal transplant recipient. Am J Med 1981;70:405–411.
138. Farrugia E, Schwab TR. Management and prevention of cytomegalovirus infection after renal transplantation. Mayo Clin Proc 1992;67:879–890.
139. Uber L, Cofer J, Baliga P, Rajagopalan PR. Effectiveness of combination prophylaxis with cytomegalovirus hyperimmune globulin and acyclovir in the high-risk kidney transplant recipient. Transplant Proc 1995;27:42–43.
140. Snydman DR, Rubin RH, Werner BG. New developments in cytomegalovirus prevention and mangement. Am J Kidney Dis 1993;21:217–228.
141. Patel R, Snydman DR, Rubin RH, et al. Cytomegalovirus prophylaxis in solid organ transplant recipients. Transplantation 1996;61:1279–1289.
142. Dickinson BI, Gora-Harper ML, McCraney SA, Gosland M. Studies evaluating high-dose acyclovir, intravenous immune globulin, and cytomegalovirus hyperimmunoglobulin for prophylaxis against cytomegalovirus in kidney transplant recipients. Ann Pharmacother 1996;30:1452–1464.
143. Balfour HH Jr, Chace BA, Stapleton JT, Simmons RL, Fryd DS. A randomized, placebo-controlled trial of oral acyclovir for the prevention of cytomegalovirus disease in recipients of renal allografts. N Engl J Med 1989;320:1381–1387.
144. Birkeland S, Gahrn-Hansen B, Andersen H, el al. Cytomegalovirus prophylaxis in antibody-treated renal transplanted patients. Transplant Proc 1995;27:3473–3476.
145. Legendre C, Ducloux D, Ferroni A, et al. Acyclovir in preventing cyclomegalovirus infection in kidney transplant recipients: A case-controlled study. Transplant Proc 1993;25:1431–1433.
146. Bailey TC, Ettinger NA, Storch GA, et al. Failure of high-dose oral acyclovir with or without immune globulin to prevent primary cytomegalovirus disease in recipients of solid organ transplants. Am J Med 1993;95:273–278.
147. Chitwood KK, Heim-Duthoy KL, Ney AL, Kasiske BL. Questionable benefit of prophylactic acyclovir in renal transplant recipients at high risk for cytomegalovirus disease. Clin Transplant 1993;7:320–324.
148. Kletzmayr J, Kotzmann H, Popow-Kraupp T, Kovarik J, Klauser R. Impact of high-dose oral acyclovir prophylaxis on cytomegalovirus (CMV) disease in CMV high-risk renal transplant recipients. J Am Soc Nephrol 1996;7:325–330.
149. Rubin RH, Tolkoff-Rubin NE. Antimicrobial strategies in the care of organ transplant recipients. Antimicrob Agents Chemother 1993;37:624–629.
150. Snydman DR. Cytomegalovirus prophylaxis strategies in high-risk transplantation. Transplant Proc 1994;26:20–22.
151. Product Information. Valtrex (valacyclovir hydrochloride) caplets. 1997.
152. Roy DM, Grundy JE. Evaluation of neutralizing antibody titers against human cytomegalovirus in intravenous gamma globulin preparations. Transplantation 1992;54:1109–1110.
153. Flynn JT, Kaiser BA, Long SS, et al. Intravenous immunoglobulin prophylaxis of cytomegalovirus infection in pediatric renal transplant recipients. Am J Nephrol 1997;17:146–152.
154. Conti DJ, Freed BM, Gruber SA, Lempert N. Prophylaxis of primary cytomegalovirus disease in renal transplant recipients. Arch Surg 1994;129:443–447.
155. Snydman DR, Werner BG, Heinze-Lacey B, et al. Use of cytomegalovirus immune globulin to prevent cytomegalovirus disease in renal transplant recipients. N Engl J Med 1987;317:1049–1054.
156. Product Information. CytoGam (cytomegalovirus immune globulin intravenous—human). 1996.
157. Tsevat J, Snydman DR, Pauker SG, et al. Which renal transplant patients should receive cytomegalovirus immune globulin? A cost-effective analysis. Transplantation 1991;52:259–265.
158. Dunn DL, Gillingham KJ, Kramer MA, et al. A prospective randomized study of acyclovir versus ganciclovir plus human immune globulin prophylaxis of cytomegalovirus infection after solid organ transplantation. Transplantation 1994;57:876–884.
159. Nicol DL, MacDonald AS, Belitsky P, et al. Reduction by combination prophylactic therapy with CMV hyperimmune globulin and acyclovir of the risk of primary CMV disease in renal transplant recipients. Transplantation 1993;55:841–846.
160. Carrieri G, Jordan ML, Shapiro R, et al. Acyclovir/cytomegalovirus immune globulin combination therapy for CMV prophylaxis in high-risk renal allograft recipients. Transplant Proc 1995;27:961–963.
161. Rondeau E, Bourgeon B, Peraldi MN, et al. Effect of prophylactic ganciclovir on cytomegalovirus infection in renal transplant recipients. Nephrol Dial Transplant 1993;8:858–862.
162. Gomez E, de Ona M, Aguado S, et al. Cytomegalovirus preemptive therapy with ganciclovir in renal transplant patients treated with OKT3. Nephron 1996;74:367–372.
163. Hibberd PL, Tolkoff-Rubin NE, Conti D, et al. Preemptive gancyclovir therapy to prevent cytomegalovirus disease in cytomegalovirus antibody-positive renal transplant recipients—a randomized controlled trial. Ann Intern Med 1995;123:18–26.
164. Gotti E, Suter F, Baruzzo S, et al. Early ganciclovir therapy effectively controls viremia and avoids the need for cytomegalovirus (CMV) prophylaxis in renal transplant patients with cytomegalovirus antigenemia. Clin Transplant 1996;10:550–555.
165. Brennan DC, Garlock KA, Lippmann BA, et al. Control of cytomegalovirus-associated morbidity in renal transplant patients using intensive monitoring and either preemptive or deferred therapy. J Am Soc Nephrol 1997;8:118–125.
166. Paya CV. Role immunoglobulins and new antivirals in treatment of cytomegalovirus infection. Transplant Proc 1995;27:28–30.
167. Plotkin SA, Higgins RM, Kurtz JB, et al. Multicenter trial of Towne strain attenuated virus vaccine in seronegative renal transplant recipients. Transplantation 1994;58:1176–1178.

168. Jordan ML, Hrebinko RL Jr, Dummer JS, et al. Therapeutic use of ganciclovir for invasive cytomegalovirus infection in cadaveric renal allograft recipients. J Urol 1992;148:1388–1392.
169. Dunn DL, Mayoral JL, Gillingham KJ, et al. Treatment of invasive cytomegalovirus disease in solid organ transplant patients with ganciclovir. Transplantation 1991;51:98–106.
170. Andersson J, Akesson-Johansson A, Brattstrom C. Evaluation by immune scanning electron microscopy of foscarnet treatment of cytomegalovirus infection in patients with renal transplants. Scand J Infect Dis 1989;21:605–610.
171. Seale L, Jones CJ, Kathpalia S, et al. Prevention of herpesvirus infections in renal allograft recipients by low-dose oral acyclovir. JAMA 1985;254:3435–3438.
172. Higgins RM, Bloom SL, Hopkin JM, Morris PJ. The risks and benefits of low-dose cotrimoxazole prophylaxis for *Pneumocystis* pneumonia in renal transplantation. Transplantation 1989;47:558–560.
173. Hughes WT, Rivera GK, Schell MJ, Thornton D, Lott L. Successful intermittent chemoprophylaxis for *Pneumocystis carinii* pneumonitis. N Engl J Med 1987;316:1627–1632.
174. Saukkonen K, Garland R, Koziel H. Aerosolized pentamidine as alternative primary prophylaxis against *Pneumocystis carinii* pneumonia in adult hepatic and renal transplant recipients. Chest 1996;109:1250–1255.
175. Levine SJ, Masur H, Gill VJ, et al. Effect of aerosolized pentamidine prophylaxis on the diagnosis of *Pneumocystis carinii* pneumonia by induced sputum examination in patients infected with the human immunodeficiency virus. Am Rev Respir Dis 1991;144:760–764.
176. Kemper CA, Tucker RM, Lang OS, et al. Low-dose dapsone prophylaxis of *Pneumocystis carinii* pneumonia in AIDS and AIDS-related complex. AIDS 1990;4:1145–1148.
177. Weir MR. Calcium channel blockers in organ transplantation: important new therapeutic modalities. J Am Soc Nephrol 1990;1:S28–S30.
178. Shin GT, Cheigh JS, Riggio RR, et al. Effect of nifedipine on renal allograft function and survival beyond one year. Clin Nephrol 1997;47:33–36.
179. Traindl O, Falger S, Reading S, et al. The effects of lisinopril on renal function in proteinuric renal transplant recipients. Transplantation 1993;55:1309–1313.
180. Paredes D, Sola R, Guirado L, et al. Treatment of kidney transplants with chronic rejection using angiotensin-converting enzyme inhibitors. Transplant Proc 1997;29:2587–2588.
181. Kobashigawa JA, Kasiske BL. Hyperlipidemia in solid organ transplantation. Transplantation 1997;63:331–338.
182. Massy ZA, Kasiske BL. Post-transplant hyperlipidemia: mechanisms and management. J Am Soc Nephrol 1996;7:971–977.
183. Jindal RM, Sidner RA, Milgrom ML. Post-transplant diabetes mellitus: The role of immunosuppression. Drug Saf 1997;16:242–257.
184. Scantlebury V, Shapiro R, Fung J, et al. New onset of diabetes in FK 506 vs cyclosporine-treated kidney transplant recipients. Transplant Proc 1991;23:3169–3170.
185. Kaplan B, Friedman G, Jacobs M, et al. Potential interaction of troglitazone and cyclosporine. Transplantation 1998;65:1399–1400.
186. Opelz G, Schwarz V, Wujciak T, et al. Analysis of non-Hodgkin's lymphomas in organ transplant recipients. Transplant Rev 1995;9:231–240.
187. Penn I. The problem of cancer in organ transplant recipients: an overview. Transplant Sci 1994;4:23–32.

44

HEMODIALYSIS AND PERITONEAL DIALYSIS

Gary R. Matzke, PharmD, FCP, FCCP, and George R. Bailie, MS, PharmD, PhD, FCCP

Hemodialysis (HD) and peritoneal dialysis (PD) are the major treatment options for patients with end-stage renal disease (ESRD). During the 1980s, the use of PD showed a steep increase; however, since 1988, the percent increase per year for PD and HD patients is nearly the same (7% to 9% per year).[1] Thus, worldwide, there are now about 600,000 patients who chronically receive hemodialysis and over 115,000 who receive peritoneal dialysis. The ratio of peritoneal dialysis to hemodialysis patients varies enormously among countries, from 5% to 10% in Japan and Germany, to over 30% in New Zealand, Australia, and Canada.[2] There are several reasons for these differences, including the difference in costs between PD and HD, availability of equipment and trained personnel, political pressures, and physician and patient preferences.[3]

In the United States, it is projected that the number of dialysis patients will exceed 350,000 by the year 2010, assuming that the growth rate of about 7% to 9% per year observed during the 1990s continues.[4] The number of kidney transplants performed each year has remained relatively static over the last 5 to 10 years at about 8000 to 10,000, while the number of patients with end-stage renal disease awaiting transplants has increased sharply from 10,000 in 1986 to more than 30,000 in 1998.[5] The limited availability of transplantation as a treatment option for patients with ESRD has thus compounded the demand for chronic renal replacement therapy.

Although there are several major mechanical and technical differences between HD and PD, comparative mortality studies have shown inconsistent results.[6–12] Early[6,7] as well as the most recent studies[11,12] demonstrate this controversy. Bloembergen et al.[8,9] found that there was a 19% increase in the relative risk of death of U.S. peritoneal dialysis patients compared to those receiving hemodialysis, and that peritoneal dialysis patients had more deaths as a result of infections, acute myocardial infarctions, other cardiac causes, and cerebrovascular diseases. The results of two Canadian studies highlight the extent of the current controversy. Fenton et al.[11] retrospectively compared mortality rates of HD and continuous ambulatory (CAPD) or continuous cycling peritoneal dialysis (CCPD) patients who started therapy between 1990 and 1994. They reported that the mortality rate in CAPD/CCPD patients was significantly lower than that observed in HD patients; the mortality rate ratio (MRR) was 0.73 (PD/HD). This protective effect was most evident in the first 2 years of therapy, as demonstrated by the finding of similar 5-year survival probabilities of approximately 35%. Foley and colleagues[12] prospectively followed a cohort of PD and HD patients who initiated dialysis therapy between 1984 and 1991. They reported that there was no difference in mortality rate among PD patients during the first 2 years (17.8% of PD patients versus 16.5% of HD patients died during the first 2 years). However, after 2 years the mortality rate in the PD group was significantly greater than in the HD patients (MRR = 1.57). These "differences" in outcome may be related to a multiplicity of factors, such as the dose of dialysis, physician bias in selection of the initial mode of therapy, patient compliance, and unmeasured co-morbidities, such as hyperlipidemia or degree of diabetic control.[13] Thus, the selection of the optimal therapy for a given patient must be individualized. Causes of death with both treatment modalities are similar and the excess mortality among PD patients is fairly equally dispersed.[9,12] Cardiovascular events account for 25% to 40% of all deaths, whereas peritonitis is the second most common cause of mortality among peritoneal dialysis patients. Of patients leaving PD, the major reasons are death or transfer to hemodialysis because of inadequacy or frequent episodes of peritonitis.[12,14]

Irrespective of the mode of chronic renal replacement therapy, the life expectancy of U.S. dialysis patients is markedly lower than healthy subjects of the same age and gender. According to the United States Renal Data System (USRDS), age- and sex-matched ESRD patients have about 20% to 25% of the expected remaining lifetime of the general population[15] and their mortality rate is approximately 22% to 25% per year.[16] Age-adjusted mortality rates for U.S. dialysis patients are about 15% to 30% higher than for patients in Western Europe or Japan.[17] This geographic disparity is persistent irrespective of the mode of dialysis therapy the patient received. The data from the Canada–USA PD study group indicate that the 2-year survival probability was 79.7% for Canadian patients and 63.2% for U.S. patients.[18] The relative risk of death was, thus, almost twofold higher for U.S. patients. Possible reasons for these observations include the increased age, the number of comorbid conditions including cardiovascular diseases and diabetes, modality selection bias, and malnutrition among U.S. patients. The higher acceptance rate for dialysis in the United States may also be a factor, as well as the dose of the dialytic therapy.[19] The latter issue is currently being prospectively evaluated.[20]

Morbidity can be grossly assessed by the number of hospitalizations per patient-year, the number of days hospitalized, or the incidence of certain complications such as cardiovascular events.[21] Early comparative studies demonstrated more hospitalized days with PD (21.9 versus 17.3 per year), but the policy at that time was for inpatient treatment of peritonitis.[21] Because many PD infections are now treated on an outpatient basis, the number of hospital days is dramatically lower than for HD patients in some centers.[22] Hospitalizations are more frequent in whites than blacks and the frequency and duration increase with age in both groups. Vascular access problems and cardiovascular complications are now the most common reasons for hospital admission.[15] Cardiovascular morbidity (especially arrhythmias and hypotensive episodes) is significantly reduced with PD, and cardiac performance appears to be improved, as evidenced by decreases in intraventricular septum and left ventricular mass index and the lower incidence of pericarditis.[12]

In recognition of the high morbidity and mortality of dialysis patients, Health Care Finance Administration (HCFA) in 1993 developed a series of health care quality improvement programs to evaluate various aspects of dialysis care. The Core Indicators Project, which examines four markers of the quality of care (hematocrit, serum albumin, blood pressure, and adequacy of dialysis) in a sample population of about 6000 HD and PD patients, is reported annually. Although improvements in the indicators have been reported, there was still much opportunity for further improvement.[23] For example, 30% of PD patients had hematocrit values less than 30%, when the target range for hematocrit was 30% to 36%. Over 40% of PD patients had an inadequate nutritional status, defined as a serum albumin of less than 3.5 g/dL (bromcresol green [BCG] method of assay) or less than 3.2 g/dL (bromcresol purple [BCP] method). Blood pressure control was less than optimal: 26% of PD patients had systolic pressures > 150 mm Hg and 17% had diastolic pressures > 90 mm Hg. Dialysis adequacy was not assessed at all for 33% of the patients studied during 1996, in spite of recommendations that all patients have regular adequacy-of-dialysis assessments.

The pharmacotherapy regimens of ESRD patients are extremely complicated due to the multiplicity of concomitant diseases, as well as the dialysis-associated complications that develop. Although the average hemodialysis and peritoneal dialysis patient is prescribed eight scheduled and three or more as-needed medications,[24,25] the efficacy of these agents may be limited by inappropriate duplications[26] and poor compliance due to a lack of understanding by the patient of why, when, and how they should take their medication.[24,27] In the past decade, several models of pharmaceutical care have been developed and implemented to enhance the outcome of ESRD patients in the institutional and ambulatory environment.[28–31]

This chapter is a primer on the principles and practice of dialysis in which the multiple types of catheters and other accesses for HD and PD are described, and the various types of HD and PD are differentiated in light of the fact that dialysis by either route is not a generic procedure. The "optimal" dose of dialysis for each patient population is reviewed, and methodologies to quantitate what dose of dialysis an individual patient receives are described. Finally, the complications of both dialytic therapies are presented, along with pertinent nonpharmacologic and pharmacologic therapeutic alternatives.

INDICATIONS FOR DIALYSIS

Dialysis should be initiated electively rather than urgently in patients with chronic renal disease (see Chap. 42). Because of the progressive nature of the disease, the need for dialysis should begin to be planned for once the patient's creatinine clearance (CrCl) drops below 25 mL/min. Although some patients may be symptom free with this degree of renal function, many patients reduce their dietary protein intake and this reduction may result in malnutrition.[32] Beginning the preparation process at this point, if possible, should allow adequate time for proper education of the patient and family and for the creation of a suitable vascular or peritoneal access.

The primary criterion for initiation is the patient's clinical status (the presence of persistent anorexia, nausea, and vomiting, especially if accompanied by weight loss, declining serum albumin levels, uncontrolled hypertension or congestive heart failure, and neurologic deficits or pruritus). Patients are generally not started on dialysis until their serum creatinine or blood urea nitrogen (BUN) level reaches a critical value. However, if they have one or more of the signs or symptoms listed above, the National Kidney Foundation's Dialysis Outcomes Qualitative Initiative (NKF-DOQI) guidelines suggest that nondiabetic patients should be started when their CrCl is < 9 mL/min/1.73 m^2. Diabetics may need to be started earlier, that is, when CrCl is between 9 and 14 mL/min/1.73 m^2.[32] The advantages and disadvantages of hemodialysis are listed in Table 44–1, while those for peritoneal

TABLE 44–1. Advantages and Disadvantages of Hemodialysis

Advantages

1. Higher solute clearance allows intermittent treatment.
2. Parameters of adequacy of dialysis are better defined and therefore underdialysis can be detected early.
3. Technique failure rate is low.
4. Even though intermittent heparinization is required, hemostasis parameters are better corrected with hemodialysis than peritoneal dialysis.
5. In-center hemodialysis enables closer monitoring of the patient.

Disadvantages

1. Requires multiple visits each week to the hemodialysis center, which translates into loss of control by the patient.
2. Disequilibrium, dialysis hypotension, and muscle cramps are common. May require months before the patient adjusts to hemodialysis.
3. Bioincompatibility causes activation of complement, cytokines, and, perhaps, predisposes to dialysis-related amyloidosis.
4. Infections in hemodialysis patients may be related to the choice of membranes, the complement-activating membranes being more deleterious.
5. Vascular access is frequently associated with infection and thrombosis.
6. Decline of residual renal function is more rapid compared to peritoneal dialysis.

TABLE 44–2. Advantages and Disadvantages of Peritoneal Dialysis

Advantages
1. More hemodynamic stability (blood pressure) owing to slow ultrafiltration rate.
2. Increased clearance of larger solutes, which may explain good clinical status in spite of lower urea clearance.
3. Better preservation of residual renal function.
4. Convenient intraperitoneal route of administration of drugs such as antibiotics and insulin.
5. Suitable for elderly and very young patients who may not tolerate HD well.
6. Freedom from the "machine" gives the patient a sense of independence (for continuous ambulatory peritoneal dialysis).
7. Less blood loss and iron deficiency, resulting in easier management of anemia or reduced requirements for erythropoietin and parenteral iron.
8. No systemic heparinization requirement.
9. Subcutaneous versus intravenous erythropoietin is usual, which may reduce overall doses and be more physiologic.

Disadvantages
1. Protein and amino acid losses through peritoneum and reduced appetite owing to continuous glucose load and sense of abdominal fullness predispose to malnutrition.
2. Risk of peritonitis.
3. Catheter malfunction, exit site, and tunnel infection.
4. Inadequate ultrafiltration and solute dialysis in patients with a large body size, unless large volumes and frequent exchanges are employed.
5. Patient burnout and high rate of technique failure.
6. Risk of obesity with excessive glucose absorption.
7. Mechanical problems such as hernias, dialysate leaks, hemorrhoids, or back pain may occur.
8. Extensive abdominal surgery may preclude peritoneal dialysis.
9. No convenient access for intravenous iron administration.

dialysis are delineated in Table 44–2. These factors along with the patients' concomitant diseases, preferences, and support environments are the principle determinants of the dialysis mode they will receive. Finally, the initiation of dialysis in the ambulatory setting before the onset of severe complications such as pericarditis, encephalopathy, or pulmonary edema will also result in significant cost savings compared with the initiation in an acute care environment.

HEMODIALYSIS

PRINCIPLES OF HEMODIALYSIS

The basic principles of hemodialysis and peritoneal dialysis have remained unchanged since the clinical introduction of these modes of therapy almost 30 years ago.[33] Fundamentally, hemodialysis consists of the perfusion of heparinized blood and physiologic salt solution on opposite sides of a semipermeable membrane. Nitrogenous waste products such as urea and creatinine and other uremic toxins move from the blood into the dialysate by passive diffusion along concentration gradients. The rate of diffusion depends on the difference between the concentrations of solute in blood and dialysate, solute characteristics, the dialysis filter composition, and blood and dialysate flow rates. The second process that occurs during dialysis is ultrafiltration or convection; this is the primary means for removal of excess body water. Ultrafiltration (expressed as mL/h/mm Hg) can be maximized by increasing the hydrostatic pressure gradient across the dialysis membrane. Those solutes that are dissolved in plasma water will be removed along with water if the pores in the filter are large enough to allow them to pass. These two processes can be controlled independently and thus a patient's hemodialysis prescription can be individualized to attain the desired degree of solute (urea) removal and fluid balance.

VASCULAR ACCESS

Permanent access to the bloodstream for hemodialysis may be accomplished by several techniques[34] (Fig. 44–1). The native arteriovenous fistula (AV fistula) has the longest survival of all blood access devices and is associated with the lowest rate of complications. However, this access requires about 2 months or more for the venous limb of the access to "mature," that is, to dilate as the result of the increased pressure, before it can be used. This type of access is now used less frequently than in the past, especially in diabetic patients, because of peripheral vascular disease and indiscriminate use of the peripheral veins.

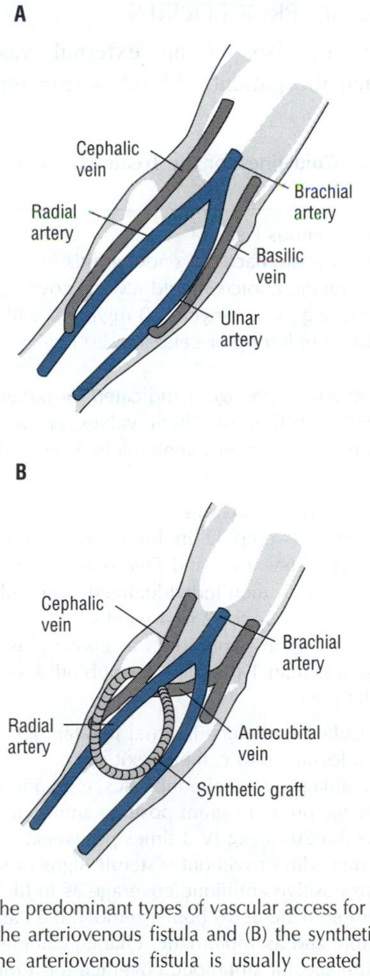

FIGURE 44–1. The predominant types of vascular access for chronic dialysis patients are (A) the arteriovenous fistula and (B) the synthetic arteriovenous forearm graft. The arteriovenous fistula is usually created by the surgical anastomosis of the end of the cephalic vein with the side of the radial artery. The anastomosis of the basilic vein to the ulnar artery is the primary alternative site.

Synthetic vascular grafts are now the chronic access initially used for most patients. Although these grafts can be made from multiple materials, polytetrafluorethylene (PTFE) has become the agent of choice and is now used as the initial access in over 60% of patients.[35] PTFE grafts require only 2 to 3 weeks to endothelialize before they can be routinely used. The primary disadvantages of this type of access are the shorter survival and the fact that they have higher rates of infection and thrombosis than native AV fistulas.

The choice of vascular access type is dependent not only on the adequacy of the patient's vasculature but also on how soon the patient will require hemodialysis.[36] Acute dialysis access can be achieved by the insertion of a dual-lumen catheter into the internal jugular, subclavian, or femoral vein or via the creation of an external AV fistula (a Scribner shunt). Once placed, these devices can be used immediately and for up to several months as the bridge between temporary and permanent access for patients with ESRD. The primary complications associated with all vascular accesses are infection, thrombosis, and stenosis.[36,37] Optimal approaches for the treatment of these complications have been proposed and the specific recommendations of the NKF-DOQI working group for the treatment of infection are outlined in Table 44–3.

HEMODIALYSIS PROCEDURES

Hemodialysis consists of an external vascular circuit through which the patient's blood is transferred in sterile polyethylene tubing to the dialysis filter (dialyzer) via a mechanical pump (Fig. 44–2). The patient's blood then passes through the dialyzer on one side of the semipermeable membrane and is returned to the patient. The dialysate solution, which consists of purified water and electrolytes, is pumped through the dialyzer countercurrent to the flow of blood on the other side of the semipermeable membrane. The dialysate circuit, unlike the vascular circuit, is not sterile and is a potential source of infection for the patient, particularly if the membrane were to rupture.

TABLE 44–3. Guidelines for the Treatment of Hemodialysis Access Infections

I. Native Arteriovenous Fistula
   A. Treat as subacute bacterial endocarditis for 6 weeks.
   B. Initial antibiotic choice should always cover gram-positive organisms, e.g., vancomycin 20 mg/kg IV with serum concentration monitoring or cefazolin 20 mg/kg IV 3 times per week.
   C. Gram-negative coverage is indicated for patients with diabetes, HIV infection, prosthetic valves, or those receiving immunosuppressive agents, gentamicin 2 mg/kg IV with serum concentration monitoring.

II. Synthetic Arteriovenous Grafts
   A. Local infection—empiric antibiotic coverage for gram-positive, gram-negative, and *Enterococcus,* e.g., gentamicin plus vancomycin then individualized once culture results available. Continue for 2 to 4 weeks.
   B. Extensive infection—antibiotics as above plus total resection.
   C. If access less than 1 month old, antibiotics as above plus remove the graft.

III. Tunneled Cuffed Catheters (Internal Jugular, Subclavians).
   A. Infection localized to catheter exit site.
      1. No drainage—topical antibiotics, e.g., mupirocin ointment.
      2. Drainage present—gram-positive antibiotic coverage, e.g., cefazolin 20 mg/kg IV 3 times per week.
   B. Bacteremia with or without systemic signs or symptoms.
      1. Gram-positive antibiotic coverage as in III A.
      2. If symptomatic at 36 hours, remove the catheter.
      3. If stable and asymptomatic, change catheter and provide culture-specific antibiotic coverage for a minimum of 3 weeks.

The use of rapid, high-efficiency dialysis (RHED) and high-flux dialysis (HFD) has gained increased acceptance since the first clinical reports over 15 years ago. These variants of hemodialysis were developed for a multiplicity of reasons, including (1) a desire to improve patient acceptance by decreasing dialysis time while maintaining the dose of dialysis; (2) to enhance patient survival and decrease morbidity by using biocompatible filters that remove higher-molecular-weight solutes; and (3) economic realities in which reimbursement per procedure was capitated and, to be fiscally responsible, dialysis units needed to find a way to deliver the desired dose of dialysis more efficiently. The higher efficiency of these two therapeutic variants has resulted in a shortening of the duration of dialysis therapy from approximately 4 to 5 hours three times per week to 2 to 3 hours three times per week.[38,39]

In conventional or standard hemodialysis, low-permeability (low-flux) membranes (Table 44–4) are used and diffusion is the primary mechanism by which uremic waste products such as urea are removed from the patient (see Fig. 44–2). The rate of blood flow through the dialyzer ranges from 200 to 350 mL/min, and the dialysate flow rate is generally fixed at 500 mL/min. Under this set of clinical conditions, the clearance of urea by the dialyzer rarely exceeds 200 mL/min, and the duration of therapy required to deliver the desired amount of dialysis is usually 4 to 5 hours per session.

The common features of RHED and HFD are procedure times usually under 3 hours, blood flow rates greater than 400 mL/min, dialysate flow rates greater than 500 mL/min, urea clearances that are usually in excess of 220 mL/min, and the use of strict controls on the rate of fluid removal. The primary difference is that cellulose-based membranes such as cuprophane, hemophan, cellulose acetate, and cuproammonium are predominantly used in RHED. These dialyzers are larger versions of the filters used in conventional dialysis and also have moderate ultrafiltration coefficients (K_{uf}) of 8 to 20 mL/h/mm Hg of transmembrane pressure (see Table 44–4). The clearance of low-molecular-weight solutes such as urea is increased dramatically in RHED as the result of the increased blood and dialysate flow rates and the contribution of convective transfer of the solute dissolved in the ultrafiltrate. However, middle- and high-molecular-weight solutes including many drugs will not be cleared at a higher rate because the major limitation to their removal is the small pore size of this type of dialyzer membrane.[40]

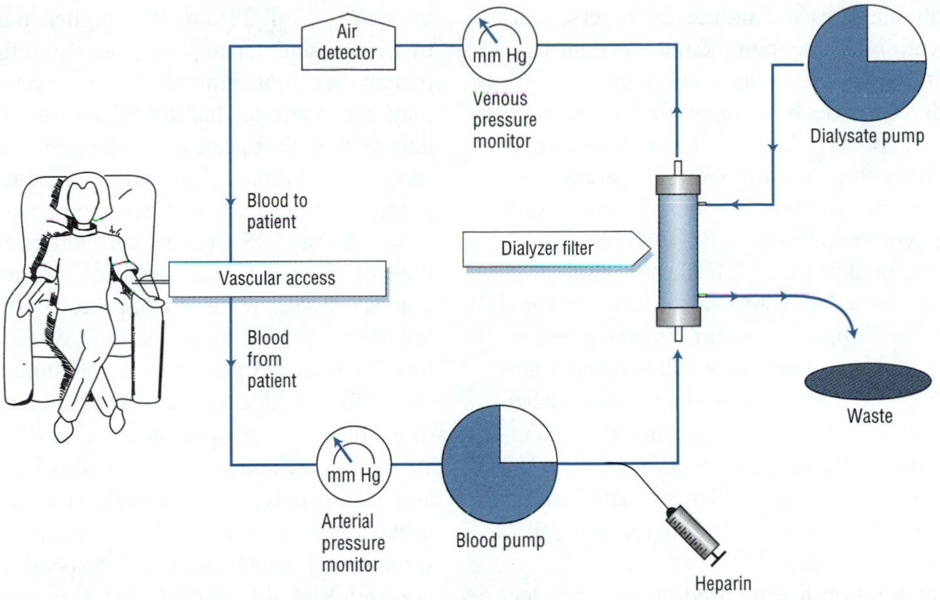

FIGURE 44–2. In conventional, rapid, high-efficiency or high-flux hemodialysis, the patient's blood is pumped to the dialyzer at a rate of 300–600 mL/min. Heparin is administered to prevent clotting in the dialyzer. The predominant dialyzers for conventional dialysis are small (0.8–1.5 m^2), low-flux filters made of cellulose acetate, cuprophane, or hemophan. The RHED dialyzer is often made of the same material but the size is larger 1.5–2.1 m^2, and the filters are usually medium flux, that is, the rate of fluid removal is 8–20 mL/h/mm Hg. High-flux hemodialysis systems incorporate a synthetic dialyzer made of polysulfone, polyacrylonitrile, polymethylmethacrylate, etc., or a high-flux cellulosic-based filter, e.g., cellulose triacetate of variable size (0.65–2.1 m^2). The dialysate, which is usually bicarbonate buffered, is pumped at a rate of 500–1000 mL/min through the dialyzer countercurrent to the flow of blood. The rate of fluid removal from the patient is controlled by adjusting the pressure in the dialysate compartment.

HFD also combines diffusion and convection; however, in contrast to RHED the dialysis filter membranes are much more open, that is, the pore sizes are larger (> 70 angstroms) and the K_{uf} is generally in the range of 20 to 60 mL/h/mm Hg. Typically, these dialyzers, which are composed of polysulfone (PS), polymethylmethacrylate (PMMA), polyamide (PA), cellulose triacetate (CTA), and polyacrylonitrile (PAN), have higher middle molecule clearances than are attainable with RHED or standard hemodialysis.[41] The other major difference between RHED and HFD is that volumetric ultrafiltration control is required with HFD due to the high K_{uf} of these filters.

There are currently more than 500 dialyzers available in the United States. The filters differ in the composition of the membrane and ultrafiltration coefficient as described above, as well as in structural design (hollow fiber versus flat plate), membrane surface area, sterilization method, and degree of biocompatibility (see Table 44–4). If the

TABLE 44–4. Characteristics of the Dialyzers Most Frequently Used in the United States

Manufacturer	Membrane	Surface Area (m^2)	K_{uf}	Biocompatibility	Urea Clearance Q_B (mL/min) 200	300	400	Vitamin B_{12} Clearance Q_B (200 mL/min)
Low Flux								
Baxter CF1511	CU	1.1	4.2	–	165	201	222	34
NMC FoCus 120	CU	1.2	4.8	–	180	229	258	61
Fresenius F6	PS	1.2	5.5	++	183	ND	ND	56
Toray B 3 1.0A	PMMA	1.0	7.0	++	175	220	240	75
Medium Flux								
Baxter CA 170	CA	1.7	8.3	+	187	244	279	70
Baxter CA 210	CA	2.1	10.1	+	192	258	299	79
Terumo T220	CR	2.2	11.1	–	195	268	317	94
High Flux								
Fresenius F60	PS	1.2	40	++	187	244	279	134
Baxter CT190G	CTA	1.9	36	++	192	257	297	157
Toray BK2.1U	PMMA	2.1	19	++	200	260	310	125

CU = cuprophane; CA = cellulose acetate; CR = cuparammonium rayon; PS = polysulfone; CTA = cellulose triacetate; PMMA = polymethylmethacrylate; ND = no data; – = bioincompatible; + = somewhat biocompatible; ++ = biocompatible.

dialysis filter membrane does not induce an adverse reaction, such as activation of the complement system (C3a and C5a) when it comes in contact with the patient's blood, it is considered to be biocompatible. In the acute setting, the incidence of hypotension, fever, bronchoconstriction, and thrombocytopenia are lower in patients dialyzed with biocompatible filters. The most biocompatible dialyzers use a synthetic membrane of PS, PAN, or PMMA, and may have a low, medium, or high ultrafiltration coefficient. In addition, these dialyzers also have minimal chronic effects on the immune system, cytokine release (interlukin-1 and -6 and tumor necrosis factor α), and production of β_2-microglobulin and, thus, have been associated with a reduced risk of morbidity and mortality.[42] Furthermore, the nutritional status of patients receiving HD with biocompatible filters may be improved[43] and residual renal function preserved relative to patients receiving dialysis with bioincompatible filters.[44,45]

Although little attention has focused on patient selection criteria for RHED or HFD versus standard hemodialysis, the best candidates for these new therapies are those with a vascular access that can deliver at least 400 mL/min, absence of severe cerebrovascular or cardiovascular disease, and weight gains of less than 5 kg between dialyses.[38,39] In addition to patient factors, the economics of the individual dialysis unit enter into the selection process. High-flux filters are three to four times as expensive as low- or medium-flux filters, plus new dialysis machines that have more precise ultrafiltration controllers are usually required and, finally, a dialyzer reprocessing system to use these expensive filters multiple times will usually be needed if this treatment modality is going to be made available. RHED, however, can be performed on standard dialysis machines and, because the filters are not nearly as costly, reprocessing is not mandatory.

THE HEMODIALYSIS PRESCRIPTION

Hemodialysis in its multiple types has been available for 10 to 25 years, but there is still no clear agreement as to the dose of dialysis that should be prescribed.[46,47] Although even a small dose will sustain life longer than no dialysis, the goal is to prescribe and deliver the "optimal" dose of dialysis for each individual patient, that is, the amount of therapy above which there is no cost-effective increment in the patient's quality-adjusted life expectancy.[48] The two key goals of the prescription are to achieve the desired dry weight (an index of optimal fluid status) and adequate removal of endogenous waste products such as urea, elevations of which have been associated with many of the complications of ESRD. Unfortunately, many nephrologists still prescribe dialysis by specifying a dialyzer manufacturer, size of the dialyzer, blood and dialysate flow rate, and the amount of weight to be removed within a certain time period with no *a priori* expectation as to the amount (dose) of dialysis being delivered.

In the past 5 years, the annual mortality rate of U.S. dialysis patients has declined from 25.2% to 22.3%[16]; however, this is still 20% to 50% higher than their counterparts in Europe and Japan.[17] Although multiple factors such as patient age, concomitant disease states, and compliance may contribute to this difference, one factor that was evident is that European patients receive approximately 30% more dialysis than U.S. patients.[49] During the past 5 to 7 years, multiple studies, mostly retrospective analyses, have reported that U.S. patient survival is improved when the dose of dialysis is increased.[19,50–54] The critical role of the dialysis dose is evident from the data of Hakim et al.[53] In this prospective trial, as the dose of dialysis was increased by 62% over a 3-year period, the annual mortality rate declined from 22.8% in 1988 to 9.1% in 1991 and the number of hospital days per patient per year decreased from 15.2 to 10.3. The key question that remains is: What is the optimal amount of dialysis that patients should receive? This issue is the primary focus of the National Institutes of Health–sponsored HEMO study, a prospective, multicenter, randomized trial of high ($Kt/V = 1.6$) versus conventional dose ($Kt/V = 1.2$) dialysis.[20]

The desired dose of dialysis can be expressed as a urea-reduction ratio (URR), which is calculated as the predialysis BUN minus the postdialysis BUN multiplied by 100, divided by the predialysis BUN,[55] or the Kt/V, which is the ratio of the dialyzer clearance of urea (K) in L/h multiplied by the duration of dialysis (t) in hours, divided by the urea distribution volume of the patient (V) in liters.[56] Kt/V is a unitless parameter that quantitates the fraction of the patient's total body water that is cleared of urea during a dialysis session. This term was developed from the prospective National Cooperative Dialysis Study (NCDS), which characterized the relationship between the delivered dialysis dose (as the time-averaged urea concentration) and patient morbidity and mortality.[56,57]

On the basis of the NCDS, a minimum Kt/V of 1.0 was deemed to be sufficient and the implication in the mid- to late 1980s was that dialysis beyond that level would not likely improve patient survival. However, we now know that patient mortality decreases as the Kt/V is increased.[19,49,52] Mortality risk from all causes is reduced by 8% for every 0.1 increase in Kt/V,[49] and no significant differences are evident among the major causes of death, that is, coronary artery disease, other cardiac causes, cerebrovascular disease, or infections.[54] This translates into a 24% decrease in mortality if the Kt/V was increased from 1.0 to 1.3 or, in other words, 18 rather than 24 deaths per 100 patient years. Thus, many nephrologists now recommend a target Kt/V of at least 1.2 for nondiabetic patients receiving standard dialysis and 1.4 to 1.5 or greater for diabetics and/or patients receiving RHED or HFD therapy.[32,39,46]

Once the desired Kt/V has been selected for a patient, the duration of each treatment (t), which is dependent on the patient's urea volume of distribution (V) and the dialyzer clearance of urea (K), can be calculated. The time on dialysis can also be impacted by the need for fluid removal owing to interdialytic weight gain and the patient's residual renal function[58] (Table 44–5).

TABLE 44–5. Considerations in Design of the Hemodialysis Prescription

Patient Variables
Urea distribution volume
Urea generation rate from protein catabolism
Residual (native kidney) urea clearance
Fluid accumulation
Procedure Variables
Dialyzer clearance
Model of dialyzer
Blood flow rate
Dialysate flow rate
Duration of dialysis
Frequency of dialysis
Desired adequacy index

CLINICAL ASSESSMENT OF THE DELIVERED DIALYSIS DOSE

The URR is an easy and frequently used measure of the delivered dialysis dose.[32] It, however, does not account for the contribution of convective removal of urea, and errors in delivered dose are difficult to detect in the target range of URR of ≥ 65% owing to the curvilinear relationship between the URR and *Kt/V*.[59] Thus, while URR is a practical tool for epidemiologic outcome studies,[32,50,60] its relative inaccuracy and incomplete characterization of key prescription variables limit its usefulness as a guide to individualize hemodialysis therapy.

Urea kinetic modeling of measured BUN levels is the optimal means to determine the delivered dose of dialysis.[32,61,62] Although simplified single-compartment models have been used and may still be applicable for patients receiving standard dialysis with the introduction of RHED and HFD, the limitations of these simplified approaches are quite evident.[61,63] When the urea clearance of the dialyzer exceeds 180 mL/min and/or blood sampling is rigorous, one can clearly see that urea kinetics are best characterized by a two-compartment model with a central compartment volume that increases during the time between dialysis treatments.[59,64] As the result of this kinetic behavior, a marked rebound in urea concentrations is seen after dialysis, as has been described for many drugs (see Chap. 47).

The easiest way to assess the dose of dialysis actually delivered to the patient is to determine the ratio of $[BUN]_{post}$ to $[BUN]_{pre}$ (R) and from it, the *Kt/V*.[63] The formula $Kt/V = \ln(R - 0.008t) + [(4 - 3.5\,R)(UF/Wt_{post})]$, where R is the ratio of post-BUN to pre-BUN, t is the duration of dialysis in hours, and UF is the predialysis weight minus the postdialysis weight, provides the best estimate of kinetically modeled *Kt/V*. This equation takes into consideration the effect of the efficiency of the treatment as a function of the treatment time, and the convective removal of urea in the ultrafiltrate (UF/Wt). Alternatively, urea kinetic modeling can be used to calculate the *Kt/V* using a two-compartment model.

Because of the two-compartment behavior of urea, the timing of the posttreatment BUN sample is critical.[46,64] If the sample is obtained immediately after the end of the treatment, equilibration between the two compartments is not complete and the sample will overestimate the magnitude of the treatment administered. The only "true" sample is the one obtained after the two compartments have reached equilibrium. In the majority of cases, an almost complete equilibration between compartments will be reached within 15 to 30 minutes after the end of the treatment. At this time, the sample is representative of the concentration of BUN in the body water. It is possible to calculate *Kt/V* using a sample immediately after the treatment if appropriate corrections are made to transform that sample into an equilibrated value (*eKt/V*).[65] This correction takes into consideration the urea clearance of the dialyzer used during the treatment owing to the fact that the magnitude of the rebound is proportional to the efficiency of the treatment. For example, if the treatment length was 240 minutes or greater, the urea reduction ratio goal should be 60% to 65%; 65% to 70% if the treatment was 180 minutes or greater; and 70% to 75% if the treatment was 120 minutes or less.[46] These are among the multiple situations that may contribute to variances between the prescribed and delivered dose of dialysis.

Unfortunately, multiple factors may result in the patient receiving less dialysis than was prescribed (Table 44–6). Sargent[66] reported several years ago that the average dialysis facility was not able to deliver the prescribed dose in more than one-third of the dialyses. The average "underdelivery" was 15%, but some treatments were up to 40% less than prescribed. USRDS data from the 1990s indicate that the mean delivered *Kt/V* in the various regions of the United States has steadily increased to values of 1.2 to 1.3.[50,67] This positive trend is encouraging; however, there are still about 40% of patients who are underdialyzed.

The deficiency in delivered hemodialysis therapy is also related to patient compliance with dialysis prescription.[68,69] Sherman et al.[68] reported that 50% of the patients they reviewed had either missed or ended their treatment early in the 3-month study period. Since compliance with the dialysis prescription is important for patient survival, different behavioral compliance styles will need to be devised and evaluated.[69]

TABLE 44–6. Situations in Which Delivered *Kt/V* May Vary From Prescribed

Less Than Prescribed
True blood flow less than marked on blood pump
Blood flow lowered during dialysis
Recirculation of blood in the patient's vascular access
Postdialysis BUN drawn late (> 5 min post) and not adjusted for equilibration
Time on dialysis reduced
Patient's urea distribution volume is larger than expected
Greater Than Prescribed
Postdialysis BUN artifactually low (drawn too early or from dialyzer outflow line)
Patient's urea distribution volume is lower than expected
Patient stayed on dialysis longer than prescribed (unusual)
Dialyzer clearance of urea is greater than expected (unusual)

BUN = blood urea nitrogen.

TABLE 44–7. Common Complications During Hemodialysis

	Incidence (%)	Etiology/Predisposing Factors
Cramps	2–50	Hypotension Idiopathic Dehydration Sodium level in dialysate too low
Headache	5	For most, mechanism unknown Acute caffeine withdrawal owing to dialytic removal Vasodilatation secondary to acetate dialysate solution
Hypotension	15–50	Excessive ultrafiltration Target weight too low Vasodilatation secondary to acetate dialysate solution Autonomic neuropathy Patient unable to compensatorily increase cardiac output
Itching	50–90	Uremic toxins Elevated calcium–phosphorus product Dry skin Allergy to heparin, plasticizers in dialysis tubing, sterilizer used, or any other medication
Nausea and vomiting	5–15	Hypotension May be an early sign of disequilibrium syndrome

Last, reuse of the dialyzer[32,70] may affect the delivery of an adequate dose of dialysis. Over 80% of dialysis facilities reuse dialyzers. Because the effective volume of the dialyzer may decrease due to the clotting of the individual fibers, DOQI guidelines recommend that they be discarded if the volume loss exceeds 20%. Despite the application of this guidance, Sherman et al.[70] recently observed that compliance with this regimen does not assure the adequate delivery of HD, and thus there is a need to routinely (every 1 to 3 months) measure the dose of dialysis patients receive. Optimal anticoagulation via heparin modeling appears to improve the urea clearance of polysulfone dialyzers (213 to 240 mL/min) and increase the delivered *Kt/V* (0.99 to 1.10) despite extensive reuse of the filters (average use: 13 to 17 with a maximum of 50).[71] Thus, dialyzer urea clearance may be preserved and patient care improved if anticoagulation is rigorously monitored.

INTRADIALYTIC COMPLICATIONS

Patients with ESRD develop several sequelae as the result of the reduction in functioning nephron mass. The pathophysiology and management of complications such as anemia, acid–base and electrolyte disorders, aluminum overload, uremic bleeding, and hyperparathyroidism are discussed in Chap. 42. In addition to these disorders, the primary pathology responsible for the patient's development of ESRD such as hypertension, diabetes mellitus, or hyperlipidemia may progress and contribute significantly to the patient's morbidity and risk of death.[72]

Intradialytic complications such as hypotension, acute hemorrhage caused by dialyzer rupture, hemolysis, cardiac arrhythmia, muscle cramps, nausea and vomiting, air embolism, chest or back pain, and pruritus are relatively frequently reported in hemodialysis patients. Despite the use of higher blood flow rates and dialyzers with increased K_{uf}, the incidence of most of these complications is lower in patients receiving RHED or HFD compared to standard hemodialysis.[38,39,73] The replacement of acetate with bicarbonate as the dialysate buffer has been a major reason for the decrease in hypotension and nausea and vomiting. The use of volumetric ultrafiltration controllers during RHED and HFD, as well as individualized dialysate sodium levels, has likely also contributed to the lower incidence of these symptoms.[39] The incidence of pruritus and headache appear to be similar among the three types of hemodialysis. The incidence and etiology or predisposing factors for the five most commonly observed intradialytic complications are delineated in Table 44–7.

▶ TREATMENT: Complications

HYPOTENSION

The incidence of symptomatic hypotension during or immediately following dialysis ranges from 15% to 50%. The etiology of these episodic events is multifactorial (see Table 44–7) and includes ingestion of antihypertensive medications or food in the hours prior to or during dialysis, as well as severe hypocalcemia and high dialysate magnesium concentrations. Acute managemant of hypotension includes placing the patient in the Trendelenburg position, decreasing the ultrafiltration rate, and/or administering normal or hypertonic saline.[74,75]

Numerous nonpharmacologic and pharmacotherapeutic interventions have been used to prevent/reduce the incidence of symptomatic dialysis hypotension (Table 44–8). Randomized, blinded prospective trials are rare and thus comparisons between therapeutic alternatives are difficult to quantify. Nonpharmacologic therapies should be the first line of therapy among patients who are unresponsive to these measures, and hematocrit should

TABLE 44–8. Management of Hypotension

Acute treatment		Trendelenburg position placement Decrease ultrafiltration rate 100–200 mL of normal saline 10–20 mL of hypertonic saline (23.4%) 12.5 g mannitol
Prevention		
	Nonpharmacologic	Accurately set "dry weight" Use steady constant UFR Increase dialysate sodium Use bicarbonate dialysate Avoid food before or during hemodialysis (HD)
	Pharmacologic	Correct anemia (i.e., erythropoietin and iron) Midodrine 5–10 mg PO ½ h before HD Caffeine 250 mg PO 2 h into dialysis session Carnitine 20 mg/kg IV during dialysis

be optimized to 33% to 36%. If they remain symptomatic, oral midodrine, an α_1-adrenergic agonist prodrug with vasoconstrictive properties and minimal direct cardiac or central nervous system effects should be considered.[76] Two recent trials indicate that this agent, when administered in doses ranging from 2.5 to 25 mg prior to dialysis, significantly increased the minimal systolic (from 93 to 96.6 to 107 to 114 mm Hg) and diastolic (from 52 to 53.2 to 58 to 59 mm Hg) blood pressures observed during dialysis.[77,78] Furthermore, the dialysis symptoms of cramps, fatigue, dizziness, and weakness were subjectively reduced.[78] Although further studies with long-term follow-up will be necessary to characterize this drug's efficacy and safety profile in dialysis patients, it appears to be the most rational and useful prophylactic pharmacologic therapy for hypotension.

The preventive use of two other pharmacologic alternatives has been associated with significant reductions in the incidence of intradialytic hypotension. The intravenous administration of carnitine (20 mg/kg at the end of each dialysis) was reported by Ahmad et al.[79] to have reduced the number of hypotensive episodes from 17 to 7 (P = .02) in a pool of 38 patients. In contrast, the placebo group (n = 44) demonstrated no significant change in the number of episodes (9 baseline versus 11 treatment). The high cost and need for intravenous administration, however, relegate this agent to a third- to fourth-line alternative.

Caffeine administration has also been reported to decrease the incidence of dialysis-associated hypotension. Shinzato et al.[80] observed a significantly lower frequency of sudden-onset (1.7 ± 1.5 times/4 weeks in the caffeine group versus 4.4 ± 1.5 times/4 weeks in the placebo group) but no effect on gradual-onset hypotension. The proposed mechanism for these differential responses is speculative, and the separation of hypotension into two types of clinical presentations makes it difficult to compare the results of this trial to other studies. Caffeine has a minimal likelihood of adverse events and can be easily administered, and thus it is a reasonable alternative to midodrine.

MUSCLE CRAMPS

Skeletal muscle cramps have been estimated to complicate as many as 1 in 2 hemodialysis treatments.[81] Although the pathogenesis of these cramps is multifactorial, plasma volume contraction caused by excessive ultrafiltration is frequently the initiating event. This perspective is supported by the fact that the incidence increases as the fractional reduction in body weight increases[81] and the fact that acute onset of cramps during hemodialysis may be relieved by an intravenous infusion of saline, hypertonic saline, or mannitol.[82] Idiopathic nocturnal cramping has frequently been reported in hemodialysis patients. Prophylactic pharmacologic therapy with several agents, as well as nonpharmacologic remedies, may provide some degree of relief.[83] Although there are no comparative data regarding the efficacy of nonpharmacologic and pharmacologic therapy, the former should be the first line of treatment because the adverse consequences are minimal (Table 44–9).

Vitamin E and quinine are the most frequently used pharmacotherapeutic interventions. Roca et al.[84] reported that both vitamin E and quinine significantly reduce the incidence of cramps (from 10.4 and 10.9 per month to 3.3 and 3.6 per month, respectively; $P < .0005$). Quinine is usually well tolerated, but occasionally it may cause temporary sight and hearing disturbances, thrombocytopenia, or gastrointestinal distress. Furthermore, it tends to increase plasma digoxin levels and may enhance the effect of warfarin. This constellation of adverse events prompted the withdrawal of OTC and prescription quinine products from the U.S. market.[85,86] Hydroquinine has recently been reported to be "safe" short-term therapy for the prevention of ordinary muscle cramps[87] and, where available, may be a reasonable therapeutic option. Prazosin also appears to significantly reduce the incidence of cramps during hemodialysis.[88] Unfortunately, its use was associated with a significant increase in the incidence of hypotension that required therapeutic intervention during and after dialysis. Thus, vitamin E appears to be the safest choice among these therapeutic options.

PRURITUS

Pruritus is one of the most common, frustrating, and potentially disabling symptoms of renal insufficiency.[89] Although it may be evident prior to the initiation of dialysis, it is more common in dialyzed patients (15% to 49% of predialysis patients versus 50% to 90% of dialysis patients). Episodic presentation after 6 or more months of dialysis is classic, with localization predominantly to the back. The severity may worsen during dialysis, and for up to 25% of patients, the itching persists after dialysis. The pathogenesis of this symptom complex is multifactorial and has been associated with dry skin, hyperphosphatemia and increased calcium phosphate deposition in the skin, inadequate dialysis, anemia, neuropathy, and hypervitaminosis A.[89] Although histamine is classically considered to be one of the mediators of the itching sensation, the poor clinical responses that patients with generalized pruritus have with antihistamine therapy suggests that it may not be the only or even the predominant one. In fact, recent data suggest that the perception of this symptom may be mediated via activation of opioid receptors.[90]

The fact that there are many therapeutic alternatives for the management of this condition is a reflection of their limited clinical utility (Table 44–10). The optimization of the delivered dose of dialysis is a logical and often useful intervention.[89] The use of

TABLE 44–9. Management of Cramps

Acute treatment		100–200 mL of normal saline 10–20 mL of hypertonic saline (23.4%)
Prevention		
	Nonpharmacologic	Hot shower or bath Ice massage Riding stationary bike before bedtime Stretching exercises
	Pharmacologic	Vitamin E 400 IU qhs Prazosin 0.25 mg PO at start of HD Quinine 200–300 mg PO qhs or as tonic water Hydroquinine 300 mg PO qd Diphenhydramine 12.5–50 mg qhs

TABLE 44–10. Therapeutic Alternatives for the Management of Pruritus in Dialysis Patients

Nonpharmacologic Therapy
1. Assure the delivery of adequate dialysis (*Kt/V* of 1.4).
2. Use biocompatible dialyzers.
3. Encourage compliance with dietary phosphate restrictions.
4. Ultraviolet B light therapy.
5. Acupuncture.

Pharmacologic Therapy
1. Initiate or optimize erythropoietin therapy to achieve hematocrit of 33%–36%.
2. Topical emollient therapy—twice a day application at a minimum.
3. Initiate a 4–6 wk trial of an oral H_1 antihistamine: hydroxyzine 25–50 mg PO q8–12h, cyproheptadine 2–4 mg PO q8–12h. If the patient has a history of drowsiness with these agents, a nonsedating agent, e.g., loratadine or fexofenadine, can be tried.
4. If no response, start cholestyramine 5 g PO bid with doses scheduled to minimize drug-absorption interactions.
5. Activated charcoal 1.0–1.5 g PO qid for 6–8 wk.
6. Combination therapy of two or more of the agents listed above.

biocompatible filters may further enhance this therapeutic option. Compliance with the patient's prescribed dietary restrictions on phosphate intake and optimization of phosphate binder therapy (see Chap. 42) may also result in marked improvement. Ultraviolet B light treatment elicits a beneficial response in many patients and is a logical option for those who are not receiving photosensitizing drug therapy.[89]

Pharmacologic alternatives range from the topical application of emollients or capsacin to the oral administration of antihistamines, cholestyramine, or activated charcoal. Although no comparative trials have been rigorously conducted, each of these has demonstrated beneficial responses relative to placebo. Dry skin is a frequent finding in hemodialysis and peritoneal dialysis patients, and the regular application of hydrating/occlusive emollients (e.g., Aquaphor, aqueous cream BP) has been shown to reduce the severity of pruritus.[91] Antihistamine therapy may also prove to be beneficial, and the choice of agent from among the myriad of options will likely depend on the patient's past history of responsiveness and sensitivity to the CNS depressant effects associated with classic agents.[92] Furthermore, the dosage regimen of some agents will need to be adjusted owing to their reduced clearance and/or drug interaction potential.[93] The therapeutic options listed in order of preference (see Table 44–10) should be evaluated for a period of 4 to 6 weeks prior to switching to another option or initiating combination therapy.

DIALYZER REACTIONS

Dialyzer reactions encompass a broad range of clinical symptoms that include anaphylactic (type A) and nonspecific (type B) events.[94] In the past, these two types of reactions were considered to be part of the "first-use" syndrome because they presented much more frequently when new as opposed to reprocessed dialyzers were used. Although reprocessing may reduce the incidence of type B events, it has little to no benefit for patients who have experienced a type A reaction.[95] The symptom complex associated with type A reactions is similar to a drug-induced anaphylactic reaction and may be a result of hypersensitivity to ethylene oxide (a common dialyzer sterilant), heparin, or formaldehyde and glutaraldehyde (common reuse sterilants). This type of reaction has also been associated with activation of the bradykinin system by some dialyzer membranes (especially the AN69), particularly in patients receiving angiotensin-converting enzyme (ACE) inhibitors, because these agents block bradykinin inactivation.[96] The dialysis procedure should be stopped immediately for those patients who experience this type of reaction. The blood in the dialyzer should not be returned to them and resuscitative therapy with epinephrine, antihistamines, and steroids will likely be required.

Type B reactions are more common than type A but less severe. Chest and back pain are the most frequently reported symptoms and they may be noted within minutes of the start of dialysis or delayed (up to 1 to 2 hours). Complement activation and subsequent anaphylatoxin formation have been associated to some degree with all dialysis membranes. Synthetic high-flux membranes have the least potential to produce this syndrome followed by modified cellulose membranes (such as hemophan and cellulose triacetate), whereas cuprophane and cellulose acetate membranes have the greatest potential to produce this syndrome. Although no specific treatment is warranted and the patient can continue with dialysis treatment, the patient should be switched to a more biocompatible dialyzer and/or put on a reprocessing program because this may minimize the occurrence of this reaction in the future.

OTHER DIALYSIS/ESRD-ASSOCIATED COMPLICATIONS

Complications associated with hemodialysis therapy that began after and/or persist include hypertension,[97] hyperlipidemia,[98] immune system dysfunction,[99] disequilibrium syndrome,[100] and amyloidosis.[101,102] ESRD patients demonstrate several abnormalities of immune function, some of which are aggravated by the mode of dialysis therapy they receive. For example, granulocyte phagocytic ability, natural killer cell functions, and lymphocyte interleukin-2 receptor density were impaired to a greater extent when dialysis was performed using bioincompatible filters relative to certain biocompatible synthetic filters.[99] Furthermore, Hornberger and colleagues[103] reported a significant reduction (almost 50%) in mortality and infection-related hospital admissions for patients treated with high-flux biocompatible membranes compared to patients treated with standard hemodialysis.

Because the dialysate-delivery circuit of hemodialysis machines is not sterile, inadequate water treatment at the municipal and/or dialysis center, poor dialysis machine design, or lack of quality control may result in acute infectious and toxic adverse effects among this population of patients.[104,105] The acuity and severity of problems like these, which are unique to hemodialysis patients, is evidenced by the fact that 81% of patients (101 of 124) who underwent hemodialysis at a Brazilian dialysis center during February 1996 had acute liver injury, and 50 died of acute liver failure secondary to exposure to the hepatotoxins (microcystins produced by algae) that were detected in the municipal water supply and the dialysate at the dialysis center.

Hypertension is present in about 70% of ESRD patients at the start of hemodialysis and is a major contributor to their high rate of cardiovascular mortality. Although excessive sodium and fluids are significant contributors to the development and maintenance of hypertension, the pathogenesis is clearly multifactorial.[94,106] In addition to an optimized dialysis prescription designed to achieve the patient's "dry weight," the vast majority of new patients (75% to 83%) will require antihypertensive therapy[24,25] (see Chaps. 10 and 42 for therapeutic alternatives). Calcium channel blockers are the most frequently used antihypertensive class; over 50% of new patients received one of these agents in 1996 to 1997.[25] ACE inhibitors were prescribed for 24% whereas β-blockers and central α_2-receptor antagonists were used by 17% and 14% of patients, respectively. Despite the extensive use of these agents alone or in combination, more than 70% of patients still have inadequately controlled blood pressure.[107] Compliance, rather than a lack of efficacious alternatives, may be the major factor limiting the attainment of the desired therapeutic goals.[27]

Hyperlipidemia is a common finding in dialysis patients. Elevated triglycerides have been noted in 30% to 70% of hemodialysis patients, wheras hypercholesterolemia is more likely to be seen in peritoneal dialysis patients. Although glucose absorption and protein losses via the peritoneum may explain the derangements of lipid metabolism in peritoneal patients, no such initiating event has been identified that would explain the findings in hemodialysis patients.[98] Therapeutic options for dialysis patients are similar to non-ESRD patients and include nonpharmacologic, such dietary, as well as pharmacologic approaches (see Chaps. 19 and 42).

Disequilibrium syndrome is characterized by a set of systemic and neurologic symptoms, as well as EEG changes that may occur during but generally soon (hours) after the end of dialysis.[100] It has been reported in the acute and chronic setting and may be caused by an acute increase in brain water content. In mild cases, one may observe only nonspecific symptoms such as nausea, vomiting, headache, or restlessness. Severe disequilibrium is characterized by the development of seizures, obtundation, or coma. Prevention is the key to the management of this syndrome. The incidence of the syndrome can be minimized by the adjustment of dialysate sodium (at least 140 mEq/L) and glucose (at least 200 mg/dL) levels and a reduction in ultrafiltration rate and the target urea-reduction ratio.

Dialysis-related amyloidosis is commonly seen in ESRD patients who have received dialysis for more than 8 to 10 years secondary to the accumulation of β_2-microglobulin.[108] The first and most prominent clinical manifestation of this syndrome is carpal tunnel syndrome. Approximately 20% to 25% of dialysis patients develop it after 5 years and the incidence increases to around 80% after 10 years.[102] Other clinical manifestations include shoulder, knee, ankle, elbow, and hip pain and stiffness with soft-tissue swelling. Radiologic lesions are usually evident before the onset of pain.

Serum β_2-microglobulin levels are significantly elevated in the presence of renal insufficiency; however, serum levels do not continuously rise, a finding that is compatible with its deposition in tissues.[101] Although the role of the dialyzer membrane is controversial, cuprophan and cellulose acetate membranes stimulate β_2-microglobulin production, and because of their small pores, the clearance of this compound is negligible. In contrast, high-flux biocompatible membranes produce little to no stimulus of β_2-microglobulin production. Furthermore, owing to their high porosity and the absorption of β_2-microglobulin to some of the membranes, postdialysis levels may be 50% lower than those prior to dialysis. Despite these beneficial effects, no progressive decrease in predialysis levels has been reported. This may be the result of the short-term nature of some of the evaluations and the massive tissue stores that would need to be removed before one could see progressive declines. The prevalence of carpal tunnel syndrome has recently been reported to be on the decline.[102,109] The confirmatory results at two centers (one in Germany and one in Japan) are encouraging and suggest that the use of high-flux membranes and/or highly purified dialysate water may reduce the risk of morbidity and mortality associated with β_2-microglobulin amyloidosis. At present, there is no adequate definitive treatment for this syndrome. Symptomatic treatment with nonsteroidal anti-inflammatory agents, systemic corticosteroids, therapeutic ultrasound, and physical therapy may be of benefit for some patients.

PERITONEAL DIALYSIS

The first patients treated with continuous ambulatory peritoneal dialysis (CAPD) were described in 1975, and the number receiving this form of dialysis increased slowly until the early 1980s. Mechanical and clinical improvements to the delivery system, such as improved catheters and dialysate bags, led to a rapid increase in the use of CAPD as a viable alternative to hemodialysis for the treatment of

ESRD in the past decade. Some patients—such as those with more hemodynamic instability (angina, hyper- or hypotension) or significant residual renal function and perhaps patients who desire to maintain a significant degree of self-care may be better suited to CAPD rather than HD as a treatment option.[110] The relative advantages and disadvantages of CAPD versus HD are shown in Table 44–2.

PRINCIPLES OF PERITONEAL DIALYSIS

The three basic components of dialysis, namely, a blood-filled compartment separated from a dialysate-filled compartment by a semipermeable membrane, are also used for peritoneal dialysis. In peritoneal dialysis, the dialysate-filled compartment is the peritoneal cavity, into which dialysate is instilled via a permanent peritoneal catheter that traverses the abdominal wall. The peritoneal cavity is surrounded by the contiguous peritoneal membrane. The cavity, which normally contains about 100 mL of lipid-rich lubricating fluid, has the ability to expand to a capacity of several liters. The peritoneal membrane that lines the cavity functions as the semipermeable membrane, across which diffusion and ultrafiltration occur. The membrane is classically described as a monocellular layer of mesothelial cells. However, in reality, the dialyzing membrane is also comprised of the basement membrane and underlying connective and interstitial tissue. The peritoneal membrane has a total area that approximates body surface area (about 1 to 2 m^2). Blood vessels supplying and draining the abdominal viscera, musculature, and mesentery constitute the blood-filled compartment.

Solutes and water to be removed from blood during PD are not in intimate contact with the dialysis membrane as they are in hemodialysis and must therefore travel a considerable distance to the dialysate-filled compartment. Unlike hemodialysis, there is no easy method to regulate blood flow to the surface of the peritoneal membrane, nor is there a countercurrent flow of blood and dialysate to increase diffusion and convection via changes in hydrostatic pressure. For these reasons, PD is a much less efficient process per unit time compared with hemodialysis and must therefore be a virtually continuous procedure to achieve acceptable goals for solute and water removal.

During most peritoneal dialysis modalities, the solute profile is markedly different from what is observed in hemodialysis patients. In intermittent hemodialysis or peritoneal dialysis, there is a "sawtooth" pattern of solute concentration over time. Since CAPD is essentially continuous, conditions similar to a steady state occur, and solute profiles are more level over time. CAPD, therefore, may represent a more physiologic process that is similar to endogenous renal function. Furthermore, the massive swings in body water content and high peak concentrations of uremic toxins in hemodialysis patients are less than optimal. CAPD may therefore be more beneficial for patients with cardiovascular instability.

The peritoneal membrane has different transport characteristics than conventional (cuprophane) or high-flux (cellulose triacetate) hemodialysis membranes (Table 44–11).[111] The peritoneal membrane permits the passage of larger-molecular-weight solutes than the older, low-flux conventional type of hemodialysis membranes. However, this difference is less marked for newer, high-flux membranes. These differences not only aid our understanding of the relative efficiency of each system in the removal of endogenous solutes but also helps us predict the dialyzability of exogenously administered drugs.

PERITONEAL ACCESS

Access to the peritoneal cavity is via the placement of an indwelling catheter. Many types are available, and a typical example is shown in Figure 44–3. Most catheters are manufactured from a silastic material, which is soft, flexible, and biocompatible. A typical adult catheter is about 40 to 45 cm long, 20 to 22 cm of which are inside the peritoneal cavity. Placement of the catheter is such that the distal end lies low in a pelvic gutter. The center section of the catheter has one or two cuffs, made of a porous material. This section is tunneled inside the anterior abdominal wall so that the cuffs provide mechanical support and stability to the catheter, a mechanical barrier to skin organisms, and prevent their migration along the catheter into the peritoneal cavity. The cuffs are placed at different sites surrounding the abdominal rectus muscle. The remainder of the central section of the catheter is tunneled subcuta-

TABLE 44–11. Comparison of Weekly Clearances of Solutes by Peritoneal and Hemodialysis Membranes

Solute	MW	Peritoneum[a] (L/wk)	Cuprophane[b] (L/wk)	Cellulose Triacetate[c] (L/wk)
Urea	60	64	119	139
Creatinine	113	57	96	126
Vitamin B_{12}	1355	37	27	86
Inulin	5200	17	14	51
β_2-Microglobulin	11,800	8	0	38

[a]Based on four 2-L exchanges daily.
[b]Based on three 3-h dialyses per week.
[c]Based on three 3-h dialyses per week.
Adapted from Ref. 111.

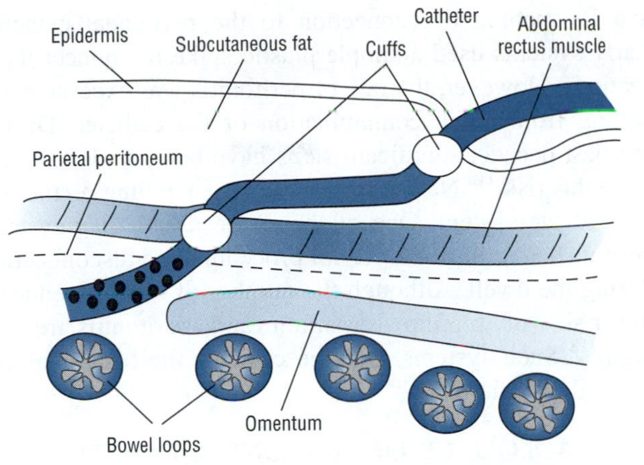

FIGURE 44–3. Schematic diagram of the placement of a peritoneal dialysis catheter through the abdominal wall into the peritoneal cavity.

neously before exiting the abdominal surface, usually midway between the umbilicus and pubis, offset to one side by a few centimeters.

The placement of the exit site of the catheter is one of the factors related to the development or prevention of exit-site infections and peritonitis. Many new catheters and surgical techniques for catheter placement have recently been developed. The driving force for this development is to enhance patient comfort and reduce infectious risk. The external section of most peritoneal catheters ends with a Luer-lock, which can be connected to a variety of administration sets.[112] These catheters can be used immediately if necessary, provided small initial volumes are instilled; however, a maturation period of 2 to 6 weeks is preferred.

PERITONEAL DIALYSIS PROCEDURES

There are several types of peritoneal dialysis, of which CAPD remains the most common. Others include a variety of automated systems, including CCPD, daily ambulatory PD (DAPD), and nightly intermittent PD (NIPD) (Fig. 44–4).[113] In recent years, there has been a substantial increase in the number of PD patients being treated with one of these automated systems, such that CCPD may soon be used to treat more patients than CAPD. In addition, a number of patients use a hybrid between CAPD and CCPD, where some of the daily exchanges (usually the overnight exchange) are completed using an automated device. All variants of PD require the placement of a dialysis solution in the peritoneal cavity, allowing it to remain *in situ* for some period of time (called the dwell time), removing the spent dialysate, and then repeating the process. All forms use the same dialysate, which is commercially available in volumes of 1 to 3 L in a flexible polyvinyl chloride plastic bag. The constituents of commercial PD solutions include sodium 132 mEq/L (132 mmol/L), chloride 102 mEq/L (102 mmol/L), lactate 35 mEq/L, and magnesium 1.5 mEq/L (0.75 mmol/L). Solutions have traditionally contained calcium 3.5 mEq/L (1.75 mmol/L), although there is a current trend to use low calcium–containing solutions of 2.5 mEq/L (1.25 mmol/L) to reduce the risk of hypercalcemia, aluminum bone disease, or metastatic calcification.[114] The osmotic load is provided by dextrose, in concentrations ranging from 1.5% to 4.25%, which provides osmolarities of 350 to 480 mOsmol, compared to that of serum, which is 280 mOsmol. Other osmotic agents have been used, including mannitol, glycerol, glucose polymers such as icodextrin, and amino acids, but are not widespread because of expense or difficulty in manufacture.[115,116] It should be recognized that dextrose is not the ideal osmotic agent for peritoneal dialysate because these solutions are not biocompatible with peritoneal mesothelial

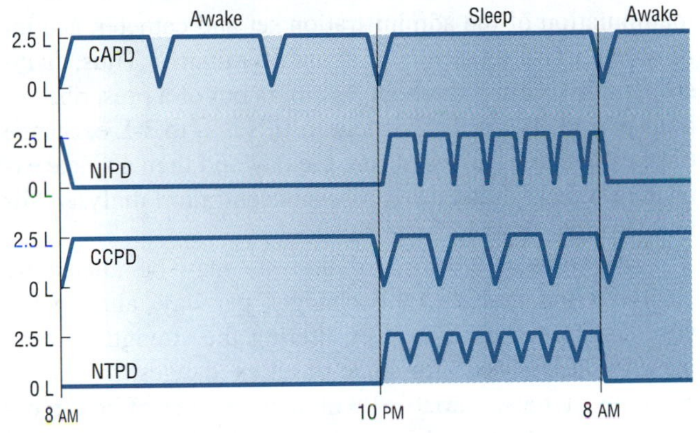

FIGURE 44–4. Comparison of peritoneal dialysis modalities. Continuous ambulatory peritoneal dialysis (CAPD). Patients perform three 2.5-L peritoneal dialysate exchanges during waking hours (8 AM to 10 PM), with each dialysate dwell lasting approximately 4 h. Before bedtime, they perform an exchange and instill 2.5 L of dialysate overnight (10 PM to 8 AM). The following morning, the patient performs an exchange and the process begins again.

Nocturnal intermittent peritoneal dialysis (NIPD). Patients are free from performing dialysate exchanges during their waking hours (8 AM to 10 PM). Prior to bedtime, they attach their Tenckhoff catheter to a cycling machine and receive six to eight 2.5-L exchanges of dialysate while they sleep. Each dialysate dwell time is approximately 2-h long. The following morning, the patients unhook their catheters from the cycler and go about normal activities with an empty peritoneum.

Continuous cyclic peritoneal dialysis (CCPD). Patients instill 2.5 L of dialysate into their peritoneal cavity upon waking and allow it to dwell for the remainder of their waking hours (8 AM to 10 PM). Prior to bedtime, they drain the daytime dwell and attach their Tenckhoff catheter to a cycling machine and receive three to five dialysate exchanges while they sleep. Each dialysate dwell time is approximately 2-h long. The following morning, a 2.5-L dwell is instilled in the peritoneal cavity and the patient carries it during waking hours (8 AM to 10 PM).

Nocturnal tidal peritoneal dialysis (NTPD). Patients are free from performing dialysate exchanges during their waking hours (8 AM to 10 PM). Prior to bedtime, they attach their Tenckhoff catheter to a cycling machine and instill a constant volume of 1200–1500 mL of dialysate into their peritoneal cavity. Over and above this constant volume, six to eight exchanges of 1250 mL (total 2.5 L of dialysate) are carried out approximately every hour. The following morning, the patients unhook their catheters from the cycler and go about normal activities with an empty peritoneum. (*Adapted from Ref. 13, with permission.*)

cells or with peritoneal leukocytes.[117] The cytotoxic effects on these cells are mediated by the osmolar load and the low pH of the solutions, as well as the peritoneal sclerosis thought to result from the leaching of a plasticizer from the dialysate container.

In a basic CAPD system, dialysate is permitted to flow into the peritoneal cavity under gravity. The dialysate is preheated to body temperature and inflow occurs over a period of about 15 minutes. A typical dwell period for daytime exchanges in CAPD is 4 to 6 hours, using one of the lower-dextrose–concentration dialysate solutions. At the end of the prescribed dwell period, the empty dialysate bag is placed in a dependent position, the administration set is unclamped, and the dialysate is permitted to flow out of the peritoneal cavity via the catheter and administration set into the original container. The bag containing the spent fluid is detached and discarded. A new bag of dialysate is attached, and the process repeated. The process of outflow, aseptic manipulation of the administration set and catheter, and inflow requires a total time of about 30 minutes. Thus, dialysis actually occurs for about 3.5 hours out of a prescribed 4-hour period. Typically a patient instills a 2- to 3-L exchange of dialysate three times during the day and then a single exchange using a higher dextrose–concentration dialysate for an overnight, 8 to 12 hour dwell.

The prescribed dose of dialysis may be altered by changing the number of exchanges per day, altering the volume of each exchange, or altering the strength of dextrose in the dialysate for some or all exchanges. Increasing any one of these variables will increase the effective osmotic gradient across the peritoneum, leading to increased ultrafiltration and diffusion (solute removal). If the dwell time is extended, an equilibrium will be reached, after which time there will be no further water or solute removal. Indeed after a critical period, reverse water movement may occur.

Alternative PD systems have been designed for patients who are unable or unwilling to perform the necessary aseptic manipulations or those who require more dialysis.[113] CCPD provides an automated cycler that performs the exchanges. The device is set up in the evening, and the patient attaches the peritoneal catheter to it at bedtime. The machine performs several short-dwell exchanges (usually 1 to 2 hours) during the night and this permits a long cycle-free daytime dwell of up to 12 to 14 hours. Thus, CCPD provides an exchange profile in reverse of that of CAPD. NIPD has a similar theme, except that the peritoneal cavity tends to be dialysate free during the day. A number of variants exist and depend largely on equipment availability, patient and prescriber preference, and whether the patient retains any residual renal function, which influences the quantity of dialysis prescribed (see Fig. 44–4).

One of the paramount factors that influence the rate of peritonitis in PD patients is the type of administration set and its method of connection to the peritoneal catheter. Early systems used a simple plastic spike to connect these sections. However, the rate of peritonitis was excessive, resulting from touch contamination of the catheter. During the past decade, significant steps have been made to minimize this risk.[112] Newer systems have a Y tubing on the bag side of the system. One of these, the double-bag system, permits both a flush-before-fill procedure and disconnection during the dwell. Although the number of steps is reduced, the risks of biofilm formation and peritonitis remain high.[118] Such systems sacrifice cost for the benefit of decreased infection risk.

ADEQUACY OF PERITONEAL DIALYSIS

Peritoneal dialysis patients may have numerous metabolic and nutritional abnormalities, such as sustained uremia (BUN levels sufficiently elevated to produce symptoms), accumulation of "middle molecule" toxins, amino acid and albumin loss into the dialysate, glucose absorption from the dialysate, loss of muscle mass and increased adipose tissue, and poor appetite.[119–121] Although the nutritional status of CAPD patients may improve for up to 1 year following the initiation of CAPD, long-term deterioration in nutritional status, as measured by serum albumin, plasma amino acid concentrations, and anthropometric parameters, is seen in over 40% of patients.[122,123] Poor nutritional status correlates with poor clinical outcome.[120,123]

Many PD patients may be malnourished when they start PD, especially if they had been receiving a low-protein diet as a means of slowing the progression of renal failure (see Chap. 42), together with the general loss of appetite that accompanies ESRD.[121] In addition, some renal diseases (such as glomerulonephritis) are treated using corticosteroids, which may increase net protein catabolism. The recommended daily protein intake for CAPD patients is > 1.2 g/kg body weight, which exceeds that for normal individuals (0.75 to 1.0 g/kg/d), because there may be a substantial loss of albumin (5 to 15 g/d) in the dialysate. The BUN concentration is the net result of both a patient's nutritional status (in terms of dietary protein intake and protein catabolic rate) and the quantity of dialysis the patient has received. For these reasons, the assessment of the adequacy of dialysis requires more than a simple examination of the BUN profile.

What constitutes "adequate" versus "optimal" dialysis is controversial. The National Kidney Foundation's Dialysis Outcomes Quality Initiative (DOQI)[32] recommends the use of two criteria to assess the dose of dialysis delivered: Kt/V_{urea} per week, and total weekly creatinine clearance (L/wk) normalized to 1.73 m^2. As in hemodialysis, Kt/V is a unitless value that correlates the patient's peritoneal membrane urea clearance (K) with the duration of dialysis (t) and the volume of distribution (V) of urea.

Several major recent studies[124,125] used multivariate analysis to assess the association between adequacy of peritoneal dialysis and survival. The largest of these, the Canada–USA cooperative study (CANUSA),[125] studied 680 PD patients in 14 centers who began dialysis between 1990 and 1992. Decreases of 0.1 in weekly Kt/V_{urea} or 5 L/1.73 m^2/wk in CrCl were associated with 5% to 7% increases in the risk for death. No plateau was observed. Thus, the greater the urea and creatinine clearances, the better is patient survival. For this reason, optimal doses of dialysis are impossible to define; rather, the more dialysis delivered, the better. The lower threshold of dialysis dose that constitutes an acceptable risk for patient outcome has been termed "adequate dialysis," and the values for the primary adequacy indices are discussed below.

Kt/V

Calculation of *Kt/V* for PD requires that the total volume of drained effluent per day be determined (this value is the volume instilled plus volume of water ultrafiltered). A dialysate to plasma (*D/P*) urea concentration is determined, and *Kt* is estimated as:

$$Kt = D/P \times \text{volume drained (L/d)}$$

The urea distribution volume (*V*) is determined from a nomogram based on height, weight, age, and gender, or is approximated as 0.6 L/kg. The *Kt/V* calculated in this way is a value per day and must be multiplied by 7 and divided by 3 to produce a value equivalent to that of intermittent, thrice-weekly hemodialysis.

Appropriate *Kt/V*s for hemodialysis per treatment range from 1.2 to 1.6, with "adequate" HD now being equated to a *Kt/V* of at least 1.2. For PD (HD equivalent treatment), *Kt/V* might range from 0.54 to 0.6. The exact requirements of *Kt/V* for PD patients remain unknown because of the lack of definitive published data.[126,127] However, the recent DOQI clinical practice guidelines recommend that, in CAPD patients, *Kt/V* values should exceed 2.0 or 0.67 in terms of HD equivalents.[32] For NIPD and CCPD, the *Kt/V* values should exceed 2.2 and 2.1, respectively. This difference may be because of the differences in efficiency of hemodialysis and different variants of PD in clearing small- and middle-sized molecules.

One problem associated with the determination of *Kt/V* for PD patients is the impracticality of 24-hour collections of dialysis effluent. Abbreviated collection periods have been used, and calculations based on the first morning exchange after an overnight dwell correlated well (r = 0.92) with a 24-hour collection.[128] It is important to note that residual renal function may provide a significant component of the total *Kt/V*. Patients may commence PD with a residual creatinine clearance of about 9 to 12 mL/min, which might equate to a Kt/V_{renal} of 0.2 to 0.4. Over a period of 1 to 2 years, residual renal function tends to progressively deteriorate to zero. Because Kt/V_{total} is the sum of Kt/V_{PD} and Kt/V_{renal}, the Kt/V_{total} will progressively diminish unless Kt/V_{PD} is increased (by increasing the prescribed dose of PD) to compensate for the reduced Kt/V_{renal}. Thus, unless Kt/V_{PD} is increased, Kt/V_{total} may diminish from 2.0 to 1.7 over this period of time.[127]

CREATININE CLEARANCE

Weekly measured creatinine clearance CrCl, normalized to 1.73 m^2, is also used to assess adequacy of PD,[129,130] because it correlates well (r = 0.71) with *Kt/V*. For CAPD patients, the total CrCl should be at least 60 L/wk/1.73 m^2, which is approximately equivalent to a weekly KT/V_{urea} of 1.96.[32] For NIPD and CCPD, the corresponding values are 66 and 63 L/wk/1.73 m^2. Such values are the sum of both peritoneal and residual renal clearance and are influenced by body muscle mass.

Patients may start PD with a significant residual CrCl, which will diminish over the following several years. This loss of residual renal function is the major cause of decreased total clearance in PD patients over time. Unfortunately, the standard regimen of four 2-L exchanges per day in CAPD may provide inadequate clearances in some patients, especially heavier patients.[127] A reevaluation of data from the CANUSA study[125] examined the influence of body surface area and residual renal function. It was suggested that clearances might be maximized by adopting larger fill volumes (2.5 to 3 L), more frequent exchanges (5 to 6/day), and the use of "wet" days in NIPD or NTPD patients. A wet day is a regimen that includes a prolonged dwell during the daytime, between the frequent, automated nighttime exchanges. Also, based on peritoneal membrane characteristics, patients with low-transport membranes should be considered for hemodialysis.

PERITONEAL EQUILIBRATION TEST

The peritoneal equilibration test (PET) is a diagnostic test designed to determine an individual PD patient's peritoneal membrane clearance and ultrafiltration characteristics.[131] It quantitates the ease with which solutes and water can transfer across the membrane. Since the peritoneal membrane permits movement of solutes in both directions, the PET simultaneously determines the passage of creatinine from blood to dialysate, glucose from dialysate to blood, and free water transfer in both directions across the peritoneal membrane. The objective of the PET is to determine which variant of PD is appropriate for an individual patient and to predict the daily dialysis requirement. Solute transport is defined as high, high average, low average, or low, and ultrafiltration rates as poor, adequate, good, or excellent. To perform a PET, a patient receives a standardized exchange, and simultaneous blood and dialysate samples are obtained at intervals throughout the exchange. Dialysate-to-plasma ratios of creatinine and glucose are plotted, and the rate and magnitude of the change

TABLE 44–12. Prognostic Value of Peritoneal Equilibration Test Results

Creatinine or Dextrose Transport	Ultrafiltration Rate	Predicted Solute Clearance	Preferred Type of PD
High	Poor	Adequate	APD, DAPD
High average	Adequate	Adequate	Standard dose PD
Low average	Good	Adequate/inadequate	Standard to high dose PD
Low	Excellent	Inadequate	High dose PD, hemodialysis

APD = automated peritoneal dialysis (PD) performed every night for 8–12 h using 10–20 L of dialysate. DAPD = daily ambulatory PD performed using 3–4 exchanges during the daytime only. Standard dose PD = CAPD with 7.5–9 L of dialysate per 24 h or standard CCPD with 6–8 L overnight and 2 L during the day. High dose = CAPD with > 9 L dialysate per 24 h or CCPD with > 8 L of dialysate overnight and > 2 L of dialysate during the day.

over 4 hours predicts the permeability of the membrane. A highly permeable membrane will allow easy passage of both creatinine and glucose. Because the glucose concentration in the dialysate is the primary force that results in ultrafiltration, it therefore follows that patients who have a high solute transport rate (in other words, a high dialysis clearance of creatinine) will also have a poor ultrafiltration rate, because there is also a high transfer of glucose to blood. The prognostic interpretation of the PET results is depicted in Table 44–12.[131]

CHANGING THE PD PRESCRIPTION

Recent DOQI clinical practice guidelines suggest that the adequacy of PD be assessed with some frequency.[32] The delivered PD dose, using measured *Kt/V* and CrCl, should be undertaken three times in the first 6 months of dialysis, that is, at months 1, 4, and 6. The reasoning behind this frequency is to accurately establish a baseline creatinine and urea excretion rate. Thereafter, the *Kt/V* and CrCl should be measured every 4 months, at months 10, 14, and so on. The rationale for this is that it is imperative to detect subtle decreases in residual renal function and noncompliance and to make the necessary alterations to the prescribed PD dose to compensate for them. In addition, every 4 months is a compromise between frequent enough to be clinically helpful, yet not so frequent as to be overly intrusive. It is recommended that the first PET be conducted within the first month of treatment.

COMPLICATIONS

Mechanical, medical, and infectious problems complicate peritoneal dialysis therapy.[110] Mechanical complications include kinking of the catheter and inflow and outflow obstruction; excessive catheter motion at the exit site leading to induration and possible infection and aggravation of tissues; pain from impingement of the catheter tip on the viscera; or inflow pain resulting from a jet effect of too rapid dialysate inflow.

The numerous medical complications are shown in Table 44–13. An average PD patient absorbs up to 60% of the dextrose in each exchange. This continuous supply of calories leads to increased adipose tissue deposition, decreased appetite, malnutrition, and altered requirements for insulin in diabetic patients. Infectious complications of PD are a major cause of morbidity and mortality and are the leading cause of technique failure and transfer from PD to hemodialysis.[132,133] The two predominant infectious complications are peritonitis and catheter-related infections, which include both exit-site and tunnel infections. Some 40% to 60% of patients develop their first episode of peritonitis within 1 year of starting PD. Peritonitis is a major cause of catheter loss in PD patients. In one series, peritonitis was responsible for the loss of 17% of all catheters in PD patients younger than 50, and for 25% of all catheters in patients older than 60 years of age.[134] Together, catheter-related infections plus peritonitis are the most common cause of catheter loss in this population, responsible for 61% and 60% of catheters lost in the < 50 and > 60 year age groups, respectively.

A statistically significant correlation between infectious complications and death rates has been reported.[135] Of patients who had more than 1 peritonitis episode per year, 0.5 to 1 episode per year, or less than 0.5 episode per

TABLE 44–13. Medical Complications of Peritoneal Dialysis

Cause	Complication	Treatment
Glucose load	Exacerbation of diabetes mellitus	IP insulin
Fluid overload	Exacerbation of CHF Edema Pulmonary congestion	Increase ultrafiltration
Electrolyte abnormalities	Hyper- and hypocalcemia	Alter dialysate content
PD additives	Chemical peritonitis	Discontinue PD additives
Malnutrition	Albumin loss Loss of amino acids Muscle wasting Increased adipose tissue	Dietary changes, parenteral nutrition, discontinue PD
Unknown	Fibrin formation in dialysate	IP heparin

PD = peritoneal dialysis; CHF = chronic heart failure; IP = intraperitoneal.

TABLE 44–14. Signs and Symptoms of Peritonitis

	% Patients
Symptoms	
Cloudy effluent	98
Abdominal pain	78
Fever	38
Nausea, vomiting	25–30
Chills	18
Signs	
Abdominal tenderness	76
Fever > 37°C	28

year, 50% died after 3, 4, and 5 years of therapy, respectively. It is important to note that these relationships are not necessarily cause and effect, because many of these patients succumb to cardiovascular events.

PERITONITIS

The incidence of peritonitis is influenced by connector technology and by the composition of patient populations. Elderly and diabetic individuals have a higher incidence of peritonitis.[133,134] The mean incidence of peritonitis for most dialysis centers in the United States is about one episode every 12 to 24 patient-months, although it may vary from as frequent as one episode every 5 to 6 patient-months, to as infrequent as one episode every 60 to 72 patient-months.

The typical signs and symptoms of peritonitis are shown in Table 44–14. Peritonitis has several imprecise definitions, but most recent guidelines suggest that an elevated dialysate white blood cell count > 100/mm^3, of which at least 50% are polymorphonuclear neutrophils, is necessary to confirm the diagnosis of peritonitis.[136] A patient who presents with abdominal pain and a cloudy effluent is usually given a provisional diagnosis of peritonitis. Inherent in this definition will be a number of false-positive and false-negative diagnoses, because 5% of patients with culture-proven peritonitis will have clear dialysate,[137] and some patients, such as menstruating females, may have cloudy PD effluent without clinical infection. Sterile culture peritonitis remains problematic; it is defined as an episode in which there is clinical suspicion of peritonitis, but for which the culture of the dialysate reveals no organism. There are several postulates for the high incidence (up to 20% of episodes) of culture-negative peritonitis. Many peritonitis-producing organisms are slime producers[118] and may adhere to the peritoneal membrane or to the catheter surface and be protected from exogenous antibiotics. Sufficient numbers of these bacteria may proliferate to cause peritoneal membrane inflammation and clinical peritonitis, but an inadequate number may seed into the peritoneal cavity to be recovered by conventional microbiologic techniques. In addition, planktonic bacteria may be rapidly phagocytosed by peritoneal WBCs, thereby rendering them unavailable for culture.

Most of the organisms producing peritonitis adhere to the peritoneal membrane, with a relatively smaller number appearing as free-floating planktonic bacteria in dialysate. There may be as few as 10^4 planktonic organisms per milliliter of effluent. Removal of a small volume of dialysate from the bag may thus result in too few organisms to culture. Contemporary methods have increased the recovery rate of organisms and decreased the culture-negative rate.[136] These methods all use some type of concentrating technique. Centrifugation is commonly employed, by which a large volume of dialysate (100 mL) is centrifuged and the resultant pellet may be cultured on plates or in broth. Filtration of a large volume through a 0.44-μm filter can be used for clear effluent, which contains few WBCs or fibrin that would otherwise clog the filter. The filter can subsequently be divided and cultured as above. Other methods that have been used for very cloudy effluent include attempts to lyse WBCs to release bacteria trapped within them using water, surfactants, and ultrasound. Blood-culturing methods also decrease the sterile culture rate.

The majority of infections (40% to 50%) are caused by gram-positive bacteria, of which *Staphylococcus epidermidis* is the predominant organism (Table 44–15).[138] There is no single predominant gram-negative organism. Together, gram-positive and gram-negative organisms account for 65% to 90% of all episodes of peritonitis and constitute the spectrum against which initial empiric therapy is directed. The ratio of gram-positive to gram-negative organisms may be decreasing, because most prophylactic measures (discussed subsequently) tend to reduce gram-positive infections with minimal effect on gram-negative infection rates.

TABLE 44–15. Organisms Causing Peritonitis

Organisms	% Episodes
Gram positive	40–50
Staphylococcus epidermidis	30–45
Staphylococcus aureus	10–20
Streptococci	10–15
Enterococci	3–5
Diphtheroids	< 5
Gram negative	25–35
Escherichia coli	5–12
Pseudomonas aeruginosa	5–8
Enterobacter	2–3
Acinetobacter	2–3
Klebsiella	2–3
Proteus	2–3
Mixed gram positive and negative	10–15
	5–10
Fungi	5–20
Sterile culture, presumed bacterial	5

▶ TREATMENT: Peritonitis

The International Society of Peritoneal Dialysis Ad Hoc Advisory Committee on Peritonitis Management evaluates the diagnostic and therapeutic data every 3 to 4 years.[136] Their most recent report includes a series of algorithms that provide excellent guidelines for diagnosis and pharmacotherapy of peritoneal dialysis–associated infections. The guidelines have changed significantly from previous versions and are now reflective of recently available information pertaining to the increasing prevalence of vancomycin-resistant enterococci and the effect of residual renal function on the pharmacokinetics of antibiotics.

Initial empiric therapy for peritonitis, regardless of whether or not a Gram stain was performed or if organisms have been identified, should include agents effective against both gram-positive and gram-negative organisms. Intraperitoneal (IP) administration is favored over the intravenous route, and combinations of a first-generation cephalosporin with an aminoglycoside are recommended. The rationale for the combination is that aminoglycosides have a synergistic activity against staplylococci and streptococci and that aminoglycosides are required for the eradication of enterococci. The dosing recommendations are shown in Figure 44–5 and, for the first time, now include the choice between intermittent (one large dose into one exchange per day) and continuous (a smaller dose into each exchange per day) therapy, as well as guidelines for dosing according to whether the patient maintains some degree of residual renal function.

The choice between these regimens requires careful consideration for several reasons. First, the dialysate and serum concentrations achieved after intermittent and continuous therapies are very different. The concentration-dependent killing characteristics of aminoglycosides are optimized by the delivery of intermittent doses, whereas the maintenance of a more continuous or steady-state concentration will optimize the response with cephalosporins because they demonstrate time-dependent killing. Care needs to be taken with the dosing of these agents, because intermittent low-dose (0.6 mg/kg) aminoglycoside regimens may produce less than optimal serum and dialysate concentrations in patients with residual renal function.[139] Higher doses (1.93 mg/kg), however, have yielded adequate serum concentrations for up to 48 hours and suggest that intermittent dosing may be feasible.[140] It should be emphasized that these guidelines are arbitrary, being based on modeling rather than upon much published clinical experience. Similarly, because there are no pharmacokinetic studies that have clearly elucidated the disposition of intermittent cephalosporins in PD patients, the guidelines are also based on modeling data.

The concept behind once-daily IP gentamicin was to employ the ideal antimicrobial characteristics of aminoglycosides, namely concentration-dependent killing, the postantibiotic effect, and saturable uptake by renal and cochlear tissue. Thus, for peritonitis, once-daily IP dosing should ideally produce dialysate concentrations at least 10 times the minimum inhibitory concentration (MIC) of susceptible bacteria and minimize the sustained, elevated serum aminoglycoside concentrations that predispose patients to ototoxicity or nephrotoxicity (an important consideration for those PD patients who have residual renal function). Unfortunately, the pharmacokinetic disposition of gentamicin following low-dose once-daily IP administration does not produce favorable serum and dialysate concentrations in many patients.[139] After a single dose of 0.6 mg/kg, mean concentrations at the end of the second, third, and fourth dwells (none of which had added gentamicin) were about 0.5 to 1.0 mg/L and 0.2 to 0.7

Cloudy fluid and/or abdominal pain and/or unexplained fever

↓

Cell count/differential Gram stain culture

↓

Initiate empiric therapy
- Cefazolin or cephalothin and aminoglycoside

↓

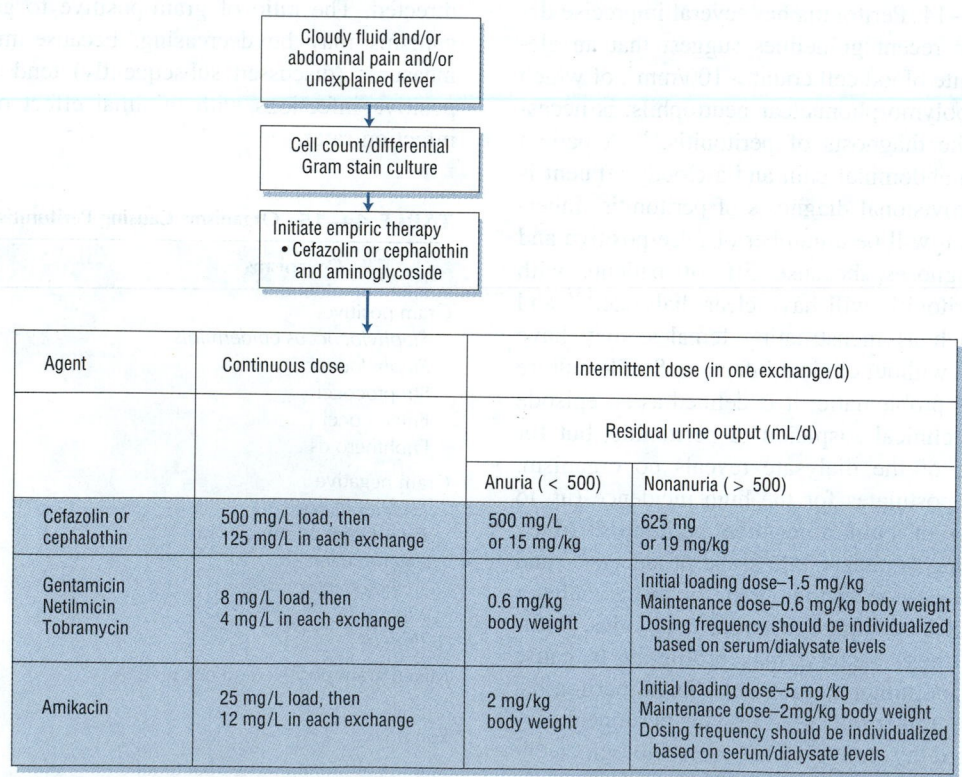

Agent	Continuous dose	Intermittent dose (in one exchange/d)	
		Residual urine output (mL/d)	
		Anuria (< 500)	Nonanuria (> 500)
Cefazolin or cephalothin	500 mg/L load, then 125 mg/L in each exchange	500 mg/L or 15 mg/kg	625 mg or 19 mg/kg
Gentamicin Netilmicin Tobramycin	8 mg/L load, then 4 mg/L in each exchange	0.6 mg/kg body weight	Initial loading dose–1.5 mg/kg Maintenance dose–0.6 mg/kg body weight Dosing frequency should be individualized based on serum/dialysate levels
Amikacin	25 mg/L load, then 12 mg/L in each exchange	2 mg/kg body weight	Initial loading dose–5 mg/kg Maintenance dose–2mg/kg body weight Dosing frequency should be individualized based on serum/dialysate levels

FIGURE 44–5. Empiric pharmacotherapy selection for peritoneal dialysis patients with suspected peritonitis. *(Adapted from Ref. 136.)*

mg/L for serum and dialysate, respectively. In addition, there may be prolonged periods of many hours during which dialysate concentrations are below the MIC of susceptible organisms. Furthermore, patients who are not yet anuric may attain even lower dialysate concentrations because of continued renal clearance. Using higher doses does seem to address this situation. In a small study, a dose of 1.93 mg/kg of tobramycin produced trough serum concentrations of about 3.5 mg/L.[140]

In the first prospective, randomized comparison of once-daily versus multiple-dose gentamicin for the treatment of CAPD peritonitis, the authors did not separately assess the differences in outcome between gram-negative and gram-positive organisms.[141] Four of sixteen (25%) gram-negative infections treated with multiple dosing resulted in treatment failure, compared with 3 of 19 (16%) treated with once-daily dosing. Furthermore, four of the failures (two in each group) resulted in relapsing infections. In another study, all CAPD patients presenting with gram-negative infections were treated with intermittent gentamicin.[142] Of the 9 episodes of peritonitis caused by 10 gram-negative species, 6 (67%) were cured and 3 (4 organisms) were treatment failures. These limited efficacy data suggest that the clinical outcomes with once-daily dosing may be unsatisfactory, because an optimal response would be a cure rate of greater than 90%. Two recent studies reported experiences with intermittent cephalosporins and aminoglycosides.[143,144] Neither was a true, prospective randomized trial. Although the reported successful outcomes of 67% and 84% of episodes are less than optimal, caution should be used in their interpretation because of vagaries in the doses used, the presence or absence of residual renal function, and the lack of information about MICs and concentrations achieved.

The Ad Hoc Advisory Committee's recommendations for treatment of a dialysate culture–positive gram-positive infection are detailed in Figure 44–6. The presence of *Enterococcus* would indicate the replacement of the cephalosporin with IP ampicillin, with the possible continuation of the aminoglycoside, depending on sensitivities. The presence of *Staphylococcus aureus* (methicillin sensitive) would warrant the discontinuation of the aminoglycoside. Oral rifampin might be added if there was an inadequate clinical response, defined as continued cloudy dialysate, abdominal pain, and elevated dialysate white blood cells. If the organism is methicillin-resistant *Staphylococcus aureus*, then the entire regimen should be changed to one of oral rifampin and IP vancomycin or clindamycin. *S. aureus* infections should be treated for 21 days. The presence of any other gram-positive species can usually be treated by the continuation of IP cephalosporins alone. *S. epidermidis* is often reported as resistant to cephalosporins. The resistance is often relative, with MICs in the 16 to 32 mg/L range. However, the recommended dosage regimens should produce peak dialysate concentrations of about 500 mg/L with trough dialysate concentrations of 50 to 100 mg/L, which usually overcomes the resistance. Enterococci and other gram positives should be treated for 14 days.

If a single gram-negative species is cultured, it is usually unnecessary to continue aminoglycosides, because monotherapy with IP cephalosporins may be sufficient. Therapy must be chosen based on organism sensitivities. However, isolation of *Pseudomonas* or *Xanthomonas* should dictate the use of two concurrent agents with activity against these organisms. In addition, in the face of limited data, but with the concerns about intermittent therapy discussed previously, the Ad Hoc Advisory Committee recommends switching patients who were on intermittent aminoglycoside to continuous therapy, together with an additional agent (Fig. 44–7).[136]

Fungal peritonitis is associated with a poor prognosis and high morbidity and mortality. One problem with prospective assessment of antifungal regimens is the infrequency with which these infections occur. This makes it difficult to design and implement comparative studies. Most literature about antifungal treatment is therefore retrospective or limited to reports of local experience.[145,146] There is controversy as to whether the PD catheter should be removed immediately upon the isolation of fungal organisms, or whether to observe the patient's response. The Ad Hoc Advisory Committee recommendations are to treat with oral flucytosine (2-g loading dose then 1 g daily) plus fluconazole 100 to 200 mg orally or IP daily.[136] Treatment should be continued for 4 to 6 weeks if the patient is responding, but the catheter should be removed in 4 to 7 days if there is inadequate clinical response.

Currently, there are few pharmacokinetic data for patients treated with automated PD systems or in children. However, the guidelines also provide some dosage recommendations for these populations.

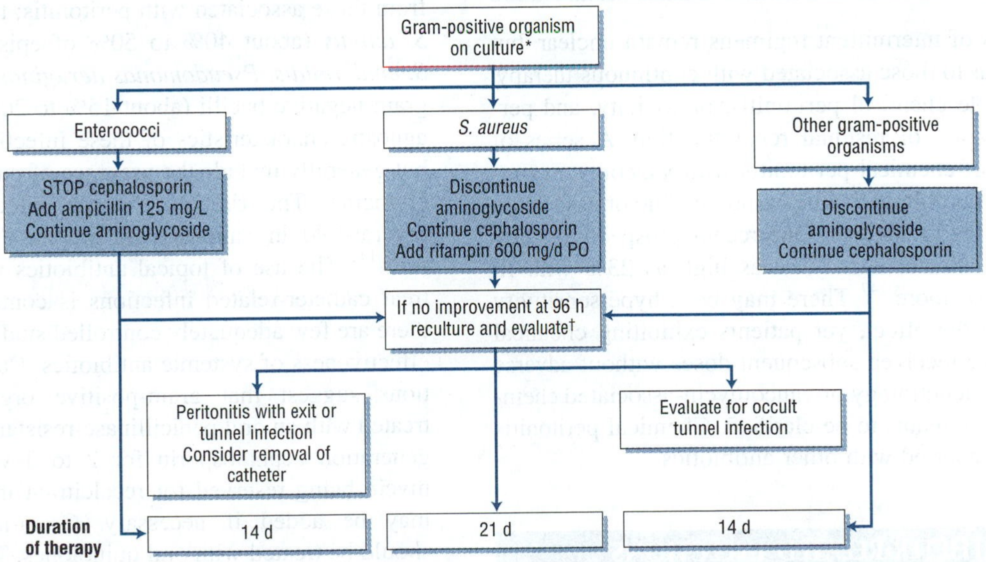

FIGURE 44–6. Pharmacotherapy recommendations for the treatment of documented gram-positive peritonitis. *Choice of therapy should always be guided by sensitivity patterns. †If as MRSA is cultured and the patient is not clinically responding, clindamycin or vancomycin should be used. *(Adapted from Ref. 136.)*

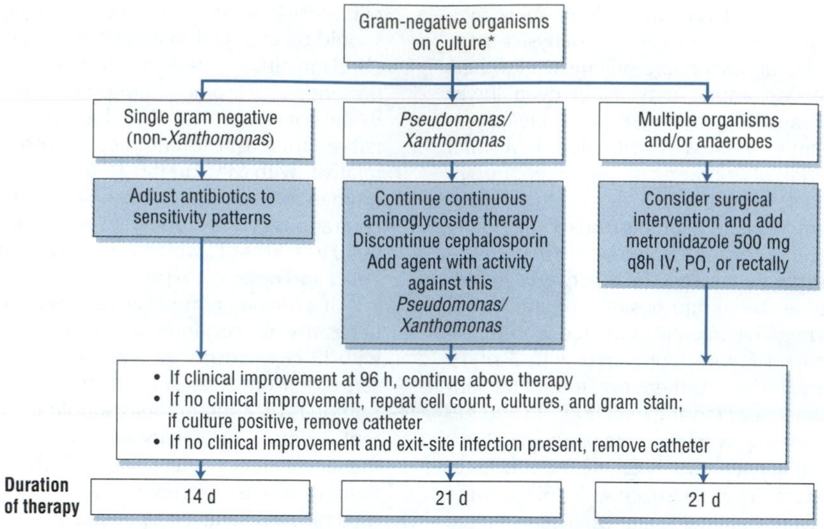

Agents with anti-*Pseudomonas* or anti-*Xanthomonas* activity

Agent	**Dosage**
Ceftazidime	125 mg/L IP
Piperacillin	4 g q12 h IV (adults) 150 mg/kg q12 h (children)
Ciprofloxacin	500 mg BID PO (avoid in children)
Aztreonam	LOAD: 1000 mg/L MAINT: 250 mg/L IP
Imipenem	LOAD: 500 mg/L MAINT: 200 mg/L IP
Sulfamethoxazole/ trimethoprim	LOAD: 1600/320 PO q1–2d MAINT: 1600/320 q1–2d PO
Aminoglycosides	Increase dose to 6–8 mg/L IP in each exchange

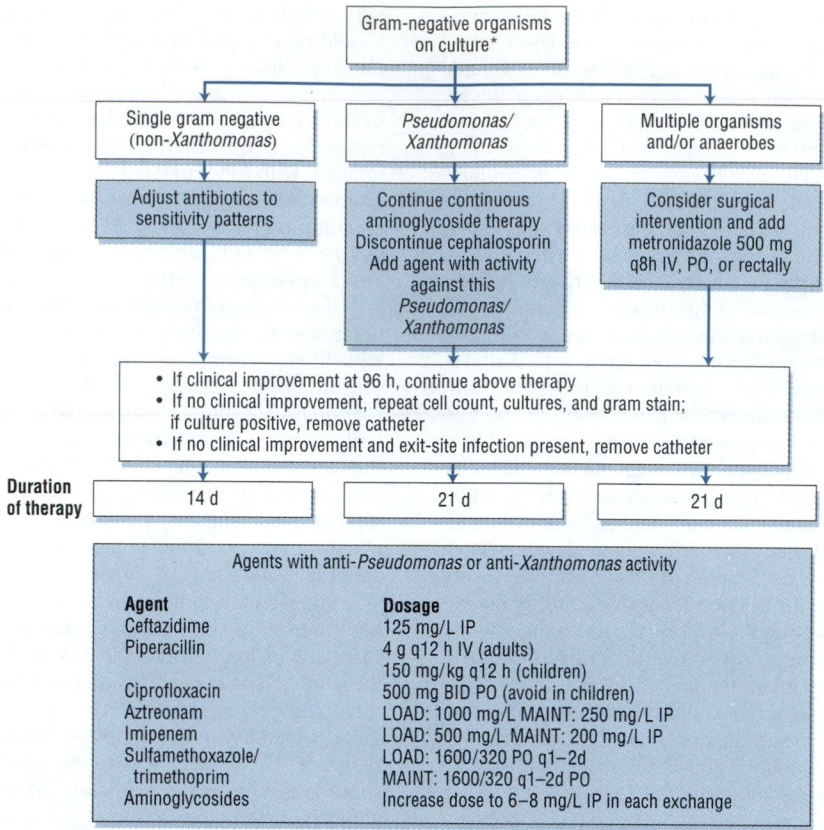

FIGURE 44–7. Pharmacotherapy recommendations for the treatment of documented gram-negative peritonitis. *Choice of treatment should always be guided by sensitivity patterns. *(Adapted from Ref. 136 with permission.)*

CHEMICAL PERITONITIS

The toxicities of intermittent regimens remain unclear, but may be similar to those associated with continuous therapy, that is, possible chemical peritonitis, ototoxicity, and perhaps deterioration of residual renal function. A series of early reports of chemical peritonitis with vancomycin suggested that the problem may be brand-specific or associated with large doses (1 to 2 g). One recent prospective study suggested the incidence may be as high as 23% with IP doses of 1 g or more.[147] There may be a hypersensitivity component to the effect, yet patients exhibiting chemical peritonitis have received subsequent doses without adverse effects. The exact etiology of vancomycin-associated chemical peritonitis remains to be clarified. Chemical peritonitis has not been reported with other antibiotics.

CATHETER-RELATED INFECTIONS

The incidence of exit-site infections is about 0.8 to 1.2 episodes per patient-year.[148] The incidence is lower in older (> 60 years) patients.[134] Causative organisms are different from those associated with peritonitis; the most common is *S. aureus* (about 40% to 50% of episodes), followed by *S. epidermidis, Pseudomonas aeruginosa,* and other enteric gram-negative bacilli (about 15% to 20% each).[138] The diagnostic characteristics of these infections are also vague but generally include the presence of purulent drainage and erythema. The risk of exit-site infections is increased several-fold in patients who are nasal carriers of *S. aureus*.[149] The use of topical antibiotics and disinfectants to treat catheter-related infections is controversial,[150,151] and there are few adequately controlled studies to determine the effectiveness of systemic antibiotics. Current recommendations suggest that gram-positive organisms should be treated with an oral penicillinase-resistant penicillin or first-generation cephalosporin for 2 to 3 weeks, with vancomycin being reserved for recalcitrant infections. Rifampin may be added if necessary. Gram-negative organisms should be treated with oral quinolones. The effectiveness of this approach may be diminished owing to the chelation drug interactions with divalent and trivalent metal ions, which are commonly taken by dialysis patients.[152]

▶ TREATMENT: Prophylaxis of Peritonitis and Catheter-Related Infections

Attempts to prevent peritonitis and catheter-related infections have included refinement of connector system technology and the use of prophylactic antibiotic regimens and vaccines. Several studies have examined the impact of antibacterial agents as prophylaxis against both peritonitis and tunnel-related infections. In one study, CAPD patients were randomized to either no treatment or to intermittent rifampin, 300 mg orally twice a day for 5 days, repeated every 3 months.[153] There was no significant change in the incidence of peritonitis; however, there was a significant decrease in the onset and number of catheter-related infections. The catheter-related infection rate per year decreased from 0.65 to 0.22 episode per patient-year for control and treated groups. The treated group had a delayed onset of the first catheter-related infection. This same regimen of rifampin was compared to topical mupirocin at the exit site.[150] Both reduced the incidence of *S. aureus* catheter infections.

There have been limited other studies of the efficacy of antibiotic prophylaxis for peritonitis and catheter-related infections. Prophylaxis with 160 mg trimethoprim, l800 mg sulfamethoxazole once daily appears to be ineffective in the prevention of peritonitis.[154] The use of staphylococcal vaccines does not alter the incidence of peritonitis or exit-site infections, or change the rate of nasal carriage of *S. aureus*.[155] However, its use continues to be considered for *Escherichia coli* and *Pseudomonas*.

Nasal carriage of *S. aureus* is associated with an increased risk of catheter-related infections and peritonitis. Current recommendations suggest that all PD patients should have a nasal culture every 2 to 4 weeks, until there is one positive culture of *S. aureus* or until there are three negative cultures.[156] Patients with a positive culture should be defined as carriers and should receive prophylactic therapy. This should include cyclic combinations of oral rifampin, intranasal mupirocin, and mupirocin at the exit site (Table 44–16). Rapid recolonization occurs after rifampin, necessitating cyclic dosing. This regimen may also reduce bacterial resistance. Unfortunately, up to 12% of patients will have nausea and vomiting, and rifampin may interact with other agents and discolor dialysate. Topical and intranasal mupirocin both have demonstrated efficacy. Intranasal mupirocin, applied thrice daily for 7 days for each positive nose culture, done monthly, reduced *S. aureus* peritonitis from 0.21 to 0.02 episode per year.[157] In spite of widespread use, there appears to have been little development of resistance to mupirocin in the dialysis population.

TABLE 44–16. Prophylaxis of Nasal Carriers of *Staphylococcus aureus* in PD Patients

Agent	Regimen
Rifampin	300 mg bid for 5 d every 3 months
Intranasal mupirocin	Bid for 5 d every month
Exit-site mupirocin	Daily

INTRAPERITONEAL DRUG THERAPY

The pharmacokinetics of intraperitoneal drug therapy have become more clearly defined in recent years.[158] Drugs may be added to dialysate to produce a local effect with limited systemic absorption. Alternatively, high systemic bioavailability may be desired for a systemic effect, or to ensure there is an adequate systemic reservoir, which would produce appropriate dialysate concentrations in subsequent drug-free exchanges (as with intermittent IP antibiotics). The primary pharmacokinetic factor that influences the bidirectional transfer of drugs is the magnitude of the ratio of systemic volume of distribution compared to the dialysate volume. The greater the ratio of the systemic volume to dialysate volume, the more readily will a drug molecule pass into the systemic circulation from the dialysate under the influence of a large concentration gradient. Conversely, drugs will more readily pass from the blood into the dialysate if the ratio of the systemic volume to the dialysate volume is small. Thus, drug regimens can be manipulated depending on whether one desires adequate clearance from dialysate into blood, or into dialysate from blood.

Over the past decade, sound pharmacokinetic information has become available for a number of drugs in CAPD patients. Significant systemic bioavailability has been reported for some agents. In addition to their local effects for the management of peritonitis, as a result of their excellent systemic bioavailability, IP antibiotics can be used to treat systemic infections.[159] Potential benefits of the IP versus IV route for the management of systemic infections include use of an already existent access for administration, ability to treat infections on an outpatient basis, avoidance of costs for intravenous lines, possible avoidance of intravenous drug–related toxicities (such as thrombophlebitis and possibly red-neck syndrome), and improved patient acceptance. The pharmacoeconomics of this strategy, however, remain to be carefully studied and reported.

Possible advantages of IP versus subcutaneous (SC) insulin include the avoidance of erratic absorption (both rate and extent of absorption), convenience, avoidance of subcutaneous injection site–related complications, and prevention of peripheral hyperinsulinemia (Table 44–17).[160] Insulin appears to be cleared into the systemic compartment by an active transport process, or via the peritoneal lymphatics. A number of studies have demonstrated the bioavailability of IP insulin to be about 25% to 30%, although none clearly compares the clinical effectiveness of IP versus subcutaneous insulin in diabetes control. Insulin requirements for PD patients may be greater than in hemodialysis patients because of the continued absorption of dextrose from the peritoneal cavity. Further, because of adsorption of insulin to the polyvinyl chloride bag and administration set, the IP dose of insulin often needs to be two to three times the SC maintenance dose.

Many PD patients secrete large quantities of fibrinogen into the peritoneal cavity, which results in fibrin formation. This can lead to intraperitoneal adhesions and outflow obstruction. IP heparin may prevent this complication as a result of its local antifibrin effect.[161] Because standard heparin has a

TABLE 44–17. Drugs Administered by the Intraperitoneal (IP) Route

Drug	Indication	IP Dose	F (%)	Reference
Insulin	Control of diabetes	Titrate	25–50	160
Heparin	Prevention of dialysate clots	500 U/L	< 1	161
Calcitriol	Secondary hyperthyroidism	60 ng/kg	66	162
Deferoxamine	Aluminum bone disease and hyperaluminism	?	?	163
Erythromycin	Diabetic gastroparesis	100 mg/2 L	?	166
Metoclopramide	Diabetic gastroparesis	15 mg/2 L	97	164
Cisapride	Diabetic gastroparesis	10 mg/2 L	?	165
Lithium	Bipolar affective disorder	0.89 mEq/L	?	167
Streptokinase/urokinase	Recurrent peritonitis	?	?	168
Amino acids	Nutrition	?	70–90	169
Erythropoietin	Anemia	400 U/kg	11–50	172
Iron dextran	Iron deficiency	?	?	171
Growth hormone	Pediatric growth retardation	0.125 mg/kg	?	170

? = unknown.

molecular weight of 12,000 to 15,000 Daltons, it is minimally absorbed and thereby has limited systemic effects.

Other drugs that have been administered by the IP route include calcitriol for the treatment of secondary hyperparathyroidism,[162] deferoxamine for the treatment of aluminum bone disease and hyperaluminemia,[163] metoclopramide, cisapride, and erythromycin for the treatment of diabetic gastroparesis,[164–166] lithium for the treatment of bipolar affective disorder,[167] streptokinase and urokinase for the treatment of recurrent peritonitis,[168] amino acids for nutritional disorders,[169] growth hormone for the management of growth retardation in children,[170] and iron dextran for the management of iron deficiency in PD patients being treated with erythropoietin.[171] The absorption of IP erythropoietin has also been studied[172] and although its bioavailability is low (F = 0.11 into a dry peritoneum), its use has been suggested as an alternative for some but not all patients, such as children.[173]

There have been relatively few stability studies of drug additives to peritoneal dialysate, and the majority of those completed have been for antibiotics.[174] It appears that most antibiotic additives are stable (usually defined as retaining at least 90% of initial activity) for about 1 week if refrigerated or 1 to 2 days at room temperature. It is important to note that some studies may not be stability indicating, that is, they may assay total concentration of an agent, some of which may be from parent-drug degradation products and which may not therefore maintain the same degree of pharmacologic activity. Thus, appropriate studies would be those that also determine the concentrations of known degradation products.

NUTRITION AND PERITONEAL DIALYSIS

For many years it has been clear that CAPD patients were protein malnourished, on the basis of biochemical, anthropometric, and subjective measurements.[120] It has been estimated that 20% to 70% of PD patients may be malnourished.[175] Data from the Core Indicators project[23] demonstrated that the mean serum albumin values for PD patients (3.5 g/dL by the bromcresol green assay [BCG], 3.2 g/dL by the bromcresol purple assay [BCP]) were lower than those of HD patients (3.8 and 3.6 g/dL, respectively). Up to 42% of PD patients had a serum albumin < 3.5 g/dL (BCG) or < 3.2 g/dL (BCP).

Malnutrition has a significant impact on patient outcome,[122] and low serum albumin concentrations may be the strongest single predictor of decreased survival.[123] The mortality in those CAPD patients who have a serum albumin of less than 3.5 g/dL is increased by 3.5-fold. There is also a strong interrelationship between nutritional status and adequacy of dialysis. As *Kt/V* increases, serum albumin increases and mortality and morbidity decrease.

Intraperitoneal nutrition (IPN) has been attempted in an effort to address the nutritional needs of PD patients.[176] IPN usually contains both amino acids and glucose and is differentiated from practices of IP administration of amino acids only (IPAA). Both are normally 1% to 1.1% solutions. Thus, assuming a 75% absorption, 2 L of 1% IPAA would provide about 15 g of amino acid to the patient (about 0.2 g/kg body weight). Unfortunately, the majority of studies are of relatively short duration (1 to 2 months), although several have examined the influence of IPN and IPAA therapy for up to 6 months.[177] The results appear equivocal, some demonstrating improvements in certain nutritional parameters, and others not. There does not appear to be a consensus that these therapies positively influence patient survival or longevity. Potential adverse effects include acidosis, exacerbation of uremia, and loss of appetite. These issues, together with the significant costs of IP amino acid–based solutions, warrant further careful, long-term study before this approach is used clinically.

TABLE 44–18. Clinical Outcome Goals for PD Patients

Parameter	Goal
PD patient survival	Unstated. Should be quantitated.
PD technique survival: peritonitis-dependent; peritonitis-independent (e.g., inadequate dialysis, motivation, membrane solute transport)	75% 2-yr technique survival.
Hospitalizations: ESRD-related; ESRD-unrelated; number of hospitalizations; number of days hospitalized	Unstated. Should be quantitated.
Quality of life: generic (e.g., Medical Outcomes Study Short Form-36 [SF-36]); disease-specific (e.g., kidney disease QOL)	Unstated. Should be conducted at baseline and at intervals.
Pediatric measures: school attendance; growth; developmental progress	Unstated. Should be measured serially.
Serum albumin	Attain the highest level possible for individual patients. Measure every 3–4 mo.
Hematocrit	75% of patients should have hematocrit between 33% and 36%.
Normalized protein nitrogen appearance	At least 0.9 g/kg/d for adults.

ESRD = End-stage renal disease; QOL = quality of life.

PATIENT OUTCOMES

During the past two decades, the renal community has focused much of its attention on technologically advancing the dialysis procedure, devising methods to quantitate the dose of dialysis delivered, and assessing the impact of the therapy on the morbidity and mortality of patients. During this time frame, the demographics of the U.S. dialysis population has changed dramatically. The median age of ESRD patients has increased from 55 to 61 years since 1980, and currently the United States has the oldest dialysis population of any industrialized nation.[178] These older patients have a larger number of coexistent medical conditions, many of which independently are associated with marked morbidity and mortality and, thereby, significantly contribute to the higher mortality seen in U.S. ESRD patients. The nutritional status of the patients at the time of dialysis initiation has also been shown to be a strong predictor of mortality.[175]

The optimal success of medical care has traditionally been defined as "curing" the disease. Recently, the paradigm has shifted in many settings to the prevention of a disease. In light of the persistent increase in the incidence of ESRD, these should remain avenues of avid research for the foreseeable future. For the patient with ESRD, however, the ultimate outcome may not be attainable, that is, decreasing annual mortality must surely have a finite limit based on the patient's concomitant disease states and life-style. Thus, a focus on quality of life (QOL)[179,180] and rehabilitation[181,182] may be a valuable and viable goal toward which the nephrology community should redirect its research resources.

Some efforts in these fields have been initiated recently, but much remains to be done. The National Kidney Foundation DOQI has suggested a series of clinical outcome goals for PD patients (Table 44–18). Although some of these are definitive statements, such as a certain hematocrit or serum albumin goal, others remain rather vague. For example, it is suggested that patient QOL and pediatric growth and development be measured, but no specific goals are cited. This is because of the lack of published literature that might indicate an appropriate goal. Under these circumstances, therefore, pharmacists along with others on the health care team need to become involved with the development, validation, and use of QOL assessments,[179,180] so that they can quantitate the contributions of their innovative interventions.

REFERENCES

1. US Renal Data System 1998 Annual Data Report. Bethesda, MD, The National Institutes of Diabetes and Digestive and Kidney Diseases, May 1998:40.
2. US Renal Data System 1998 Annual Data Report. Bethesda, MD, The National Institutes of Diabetes and Digestive and Kidney Diseases, May 1998:161.
3. Ismail N, Hakin RM, Oreopoulos DG, Patrikarea A. Renal replacement therapies in the elderly: Part 1. Hemodialysis and chronic peritoneal dialysis. In-depth review. Am J Kidney Dis 1993;22:759–782.
4. Ad Hoc Committee on Nephrology Manpower Needs. Estimating workforce and training requirements for nephrologists through the year 2010. J Am Soc Nephrol 1997;8(suppl 9):1–32.
5. US Renal Data System 1998 Annual Data Report. Bethesda, MD, The National Institutes of Diabetes and Digestive and Kidney Diseases, May 1998:43.
6. US Renal Data System 1991 Annual Data Report. Bethesda, MD, The National Institutes of Health and National Institute of Diabetes and Digestive and Kidney Diseases, August 1991.
7. Held PJ, Port FK, Turenne MN, et al. Continuous ambulatory peritoneal dialysis and hemodialysis: Comparison of patient mortality with adjustment for comorbid conditions. Kidney Int 1994;45:1163–1169.
8. Bloembergen WE, Port FK, Mauger EA, Wolfe RA. A comparison of mortality between patients treated with hemodialysis and peritoneal dialysis. J Am Soc Nephrol 1995;6:177–183.
9. Bloembergen WE, Port FK, Mauger EA, Wolfe RA. A comparison of cause of death between patients treated with hemodialysis and peritoneal dialysis. J Am Soc Nephrol 1995;6:184–191.

10. US Renal Data System 1994 Annual Data Report. Bethesda, MD, The National Institutes of Diabetes and Digestive and Kidney Diseases, July 1994:52.
11. Fenton SSA, Schaubel DE, Desmeules M, et al. Hemodialysis versus peritoneal dislysis: A comparison of adjustment mortality rates. Am J Kidney Dis 1997;30:334–342.
12. Foley RN, Parfrey PS, Harnett JD, et al. Mode of dialysis therapy and mortality in end-stage renal disease. J Am Soc Nephrol 1998; 9:267–276.
13. Wu MS, Yu CC, Yang CW, et al. Poor pre-dialysis glycaemic control is a predictor of mortality in type II diabetic patients on maintenance haemodialysis. Nephrol Dial Transplant 1997;12:2105–2110.
14. de Fijter CWH, Oe LP, Nauta JJP, et al. Clinical efficacy and morbidity associated with continuous cyclic compared with continuous ambulatory peritoneal dialysis. Ann Intern Med 1994;120:264–271.
15. US Renal Data System 1993 Annual Data Report. Bethesda, MD, The National Institutes of Diabetes and Digestive and Kidney Diseases, July 1993:13.
16. US Renal Data System 1998 Annual Data Report. Bethesda, MD, The National Institutes of Diabetes and Digestive and Kidney Diseases, May 1998:71.
17. Held PJ, Brunner F, Odaka M, et al. Five year survival for end-stage renal disease patients in the United States, Europe and Japan. Am J Kidney Dis 1990;15:451–457.
18. Churchill DN, Thorpe KE, Vonesh EF, Keshaviah PR, for the Canada–USA (CANUSA) Peritoneal Dialysis Study Group. Lower probability of patient survival with continuous peritoneal dialysis in the United States compared with Canada. J Am Soc Nephrol 1997; 8:965–971.
19. Held PJ, Port FK, Wolfe RA, et al. The dose of hemodialysis and patient mortality. Kidney Int 1996;50:550–556.
20. Eknoyan G, Levey AS, Beck GJ, et al., The hemodialysis (HEMO) study: rationale for selection of interventions. Semin Dial 1996;9: 24–33.
21. Habach G, Bloembergen WE, Mauger EA, et al. Hospitalization among United States dialysis patients: Hemodialysis versus peritoneal dialysis. J Am Soc Nephrol 1995;5:1940–1948.
22. McMurray SD, Miller J. Impact of capitation on free-standing dialysis facilities: Can you survive? Am J Kidney Dis 1997;30: 542–548.
23. Rocco MV, Flanigan MJ, Beaver S, et al. Report from the 1995 Core Indicators for Peritoneal Dialysis Study Group. Am J Kidney Dis 1997;30:165–173.
24. Cleary DJ, Matzke GR, Alexander ACM, Joy MS. Medication knowledge and prescription drug taking behavior of patients receiving chronic dialysis. Am J Health Syst Pharm 1995;52:1895–1900.
25. US Renal Data System 1998 Annual Data Report. Bethesda, MD, The National Institutes of Diabetes and Digestive and Kidney Diseases, May 1998:51–62.
26. Kaplan B, Mason NA, Shimp LA, Ascion FJ. Chronic hemodialysis patients. Part I: Characterization and drug-related problems. Ann Pharmacother 1994;28:316–319.
27. Curtin RB, Svarstad BL, Andress D, Keller T, Sacksteder P. Differences in older versus younger hemodialysis patients' noncompliance with oral medications. Geriatr Nephrol Urol 1997;7: 35–44.
28. St. Peter WL. Clinical pharmacy nephrology consultation and documentation: A comprehensive approach. J Pharm Prac 1993;6: 140–147.
29. Pahre S. Nephrology pharmacy practice in the outpatient dialysis setting. Adv Ren Replace Ther 1997;4:179–181.
30. Bailie GR. Clinical pharmacy care in continuous ambulatory peritoneal dialysis patients. J Pharm Prac 1993;6:123–132.
31. Tang I, Vrahnos D, Hatoum H, Lau A. Effectiveness of clinical pharmacists interventions in a hemodialysis unit. Clin Ther 1993;15: 459–464.
32. NKF-DOQI Clinical Practice Guidelines for Dialysis Adequacy. Am J Kidney Dis 1997;30(suppl 2):S1–S136.
33. Drukker W. Hemodialysis: A historical review. In: Maher JF, ed. Replacement of Renal Function by Dialysis, 3rd ed. Dordecht, Holland, Kluwer Academic, 1989:21–86.
34. Fan PY, Schwab SJ. Hemodialysis vascular access. In: Henrich WL, ed. Principles and Practice of Dialysis. Baltimore, Williams & Wilkins, 1994:22–37.
35. US Renal Data System 1997 Annual Data Report. Bethesda, MD, The National Institutes of Diabetes and Digestive and Kidney Diseases, April 1997:55.
36. NKF-DOQI Clincial Practice Guidelines for Vascular Access. Am J Kidney Dis 1997;30:S150–S191.
37. Albers FJ. Clinical considerations in hemodialysis access infection. Adv Ren Replace Ther 1996;3:208–217.
38. Acchiardo SR. High-flux hemodialysis. In: Bosch JP, ed. Contemporary Issues in Nephrology: Hemodialysis High-Efficiency Treatments, Vol. 27. New York, Churchill Livingstone, 1993:105–117.
39. Collins AJ. High-flux, high-efficiency procedures. In: Henrich WE, ed. Principles and Practice of Dialysis. Baltimore, Williams & Wilkins, 1994:22–37.
40. Golper TA, Vincent HH, Gleason JR, Vos MC. Drug removal during high-efficiency and high-flux hemodialysis. In: Bosch JP, ed. Contemporary Issues in Nephrology: Hemodialysis High-Efficiency Treatments, Vol. 27. New York, Churchill Livingstone, 1993:175–208.
41. Konstantin P. Newer membranes: Cuprophane versus polysulfone versus polyacrylonitrile. In: Bosch JP, ed. Contemporary Issues in Nephrology: Hemodialysis High-Efficiency Treatments, Vol. 27. New York, Churchill Livingstone, 1993:63–77.
42. van Ypersele de Strihou C. Are biocompatible membranes superior for hemodialysis therapy? Kidney Int 1997;52:S101–S104.
43. Ikizler TA. Bio-compatibility and nutrition in hemodialysis. Semin Dial 1998;11:7–9.
44. Hartman J, Fricke H, Schiffl H. Biocompatible membranes preserve residual renal function in patients undergoing regular hemodialysis. Am J Kidney Dis 1997;30:366–373.
45. McCarthy JT, Jenson BM, Squillace DP, Williams AW. Improved preservation of residual renal function in chronic hemodialysis patients using polysulfone dialyzers. Am J Kidney Dis 1997;29: 576–583.
46. Bosch JP. The prescriptions of hemodialysis. Adv Ren Replace Ther 1994;1:281–287.
47. Parker T. Hemodialysis adequacy. In: Henrich WL, ed. Principles of Practice of Dialysis. Baltimore, Williams & Wilkins, 1994:63–75.
48. Hornberger JC. The hemodialysis prescription and cost effectiveness. J Am Soc Nephrol 1993;4:1021–1027.
49. Held PJ, Carroll CE, Liska DW, et al. Hemodialysis therapy in the United States: What is the dose and does it matter? Am J Kidney Dis 1994;24:974–980.
50. Helgerson SD, McClelland WM, Frederick PR, et al. Improvement in adequacy of delivered dialysis for adults in-center hemodialysis patients in the United States, 1993 to 1995. Am J Kidney Dis 1997; 29:851–861.
51. Parker TF III. Role of dialysis dose on morbidity and mortality in maintenance hemodialysis patients. Am J Kidney Dis 1994;24: 981–989.
52. Owen WFJ, Lew NL, Liu Y, et al. The urea reduction ratio and serum albumin concentration as predictors of mortality in patients undergoing hemodialysis. N Engl J Med 1993;329:1001–1006.
53. Hakim RM, Breyer J, Ismail N, et al. Effects of dose of dialysis on morbidity and mortality. Am J Kidney Dis 1994;23:661–669.
54. Bloembergen WE, Stannard DC, Port FK, et al. Relationship of dose of hemodialysis and cause-specific mortality. Kindey Int 1996;50: 557–565.
55. Lowrie EG, Lew NL. The urea reduction ratio (URR): A simple method for evaluating hemodialysis treatment. Contemp Dial Nephrol 1991;12:11–20.
56. Gotch FA, Sargent JA. A mechanistic analysis of the National Cooperative Dialysis Study (NCDS). Kidney Int 1985;28:526–534.

57. Lowrie EG, Laird NM, Parker TF III, et al. Effect of the hemodialysis on patient morbidity: Report from the National Cooperative Dialysis Study. N Engl J Med 1981;305:1176–1181.
58. Abuelo JG. Large interdialytic weight gains: Causes, consequences, and corrective measures. Semin Dial 1998;11:25–32.
59. Depner TA. Approach to hemodialysis urea modeling. In: Henrich WL, ed. Principles of Practice of Dialysis. Baltimore, Williams & Wilkins, 1994:47–62.
60. Lowrie EG, Lew NL. Death risk in hemodialysis patients: The predictive value of commonly measured variables and an evaluation of death rate differences between facilities. Am J Kidney Dis 1990;15: 458–482.
61. Delmez JA, Windus DW, St. Louis Nephrology Study Group. Hemodialysis prescription and delivery in a metropolitan community. Kidney Int 1992;41:1023–1028.
62. Daugirdas JT, Depner TA. A nomogram approach to hemodialysis urea modeling. Am J Kidney Dis 1994;23:33–40.
63. Abramson F, Gibson S, Barlee V, et al. Urea kinetic modeling at high urea clearances: Implications for clinical practice. Adv Ren Replace Ther 1994;1:5–14.
64. Pearson P, Lew S, Abramson F, Bosch J. Measurement of kinetic parameters for urea in end-stage renal disease patients using a two compartment model. J Am Soc Nephrol 1994;4:1869–1873.
65. Daugirdas JT. Estimation of the equilibrated *Kt/V* using the unequilibrated post dialysis BUN. Semin Dial 1995;8:284.
66. Sargent J. Short falls in the delivery of dialysis. Am J Kidney Dis 1990;15:500–510.
67. US Renal Data System 1998 Annual Data Report. Bethesda, MD, The National Institutes of Diabetes and Digestive Kidney Diseases, July 1998:44.
68. Sherman RA, Cody RP, Matera JJ, et al. Deficiencies in delivered hemodialysis therapy due to missed and shortened treatments. Am J Kidney Dis 1994;24:921–923.
69. Kimmel PL, Peterson RA, Weihs KL, et al. Behavioral compliance with dialysis prescription in hemodialysis patients. J Am Soc Nephrol 1995;5:1826–1834.
70. Sherman RA, Cody RP, Rogers ME, Solanchick JC. The effect of dialyzer reuse on dialysis delivery. Am J Kidney Dis 1994;24: 924–926.
71. Wei SS, Ellis PW, Magnusson MO, Oaganini EP. Effect of heparin modeling on delivered hemodialysis therapy. Am J Kidney Dis 1994; 23:389–393.
72. Consensus Development Conference Panel. Morbidity and mortality on renal dialysis: NIH Consensus Conference Statement. Ann Intern Med 1994;121:62–70.
73. Bregman H, Daugirdas JT, Ing TS. Complications during hemodialysis. In: Daugirdas JT, Ing TS, eds. Handbook of Dialysis, 2nd ed. Boston, Little, Brown, 1994:149–168.
74. Pastan S, Bailey J. Dialysis therapy. N Eng J Med 1998;338: 1428–1437.
75. Gong R, Lindberg J, Abrams J, et al. Comparison of hypertonic saline solutions and dextran in dialysis-induced hypotension. J Am Soc Nephrol 1993;3:1808–1812.
76. Blowey DL, Balfe JW, Gupta I, Gajaria MM, Koren G. Midodrine efficacy and pharmacokinetics in a patient with recurrent intradialytic hypotension. Am J Kidney Dis 1996;28:132–136.
77. Flynn JJ, Mitchell MC, Caruso FS, McElligott MA. Midodrine treatment for patients with hemodialysis hypotension. Clin Nephrol 1996; 45:261–267.
78. Cruz DN, Mahnensmith RL, Perazella MA. Intradialytic hypotension: Is midodrine beneficial in symptomatic hemodialysis patients? Am J Kidney Dis 1997;30:772–779.
79. Ahmad SA, Robertson HT, Golper TA, et al. Multicenter trial of L-carnitine in maintenance hemodialysis patients. II. Clinical and biochemical effects. Kidney Int 1990;38:912–918.
80. Shinzato T, Miwa M, Shigeru N, et al. Role of adenosine in dialysis-induced hypotension. J Am Soc Nephrol 1994;4:1987–1994.
81. Quellhorst EA. Ultrafiltration and haemofiltration, practical applications. In: Drukker W, Parsons FM, Maher JF, eds. Replacement of Renal Function by Dialysis. Boston, Martinus Nijhoff, 1983: 265–275.
82. Sherman RA, Goodling KA, Eisinger RP. Acute therapy of hemodialysis-related muscle cramps. Am J Kidney Dis 1982;2:287–288.
83. Daniell HW. Simple cure for nocturnal leg cramps. N Engl J Med 1979;301:216.
84. Roca AO, Jarjoura D, Blend D, et al. Dialysis leg cramps. Efficacy of quinine versus vitamin E. ASAIO J 1992;38:M481–M485.
85. Federal Register Aug 22, 1994.
86. Federal Register Apr 19, 1995.
87. Jansen PH, Veenhuiezen KC, Wesseling AI, et al. Randomised controlled trial of hydroquinine in muscle cramps. Lancet 1997;349: 528–532.
88. Sidhom OA, Odeh YK, Krumlovsky FA, et al. Low-dose prazosin in patient with muscle cramps during hemodialysis. Clin Pharmacol Ther 1994;56:445–451.
89. Robertson KE, Mueller BA. Uremic pruritus. Am J Health Syst Pharm 1996;53:2159–2170.
90. Peer G, Kivity S, Agami O, et al. Randomised crossover trial of naltrexone in uraemic pruritus. Lancet 1996;348:1552.
91. Morton CA, Lafferty M, Hau C, et al. Pruritus and skin hydration during dialysis. Nephrol Dial Transplant 1996;11:2031–2036.
92. Estelle F, Simons R. H_1-receptor antagonists: Comparative tolerability and safety. Drug Saf 1994;10:350–380.
93. Estelle F, Simons R, Simons KJ. Pharmacokinetic optimisation of histamine H_1-receptor antagonist therapy. Clin Pharmacokinet 1991; 21:372–393.
94. Salem M, Ivanovich PT, Ing TS, et al. Adverse effects of dialyzers manifesting during the dialysis session. Nephrol Dial Transplant 1994;9(suppl 2):127–137.
95. Kaufman AM, Godmere RO, Levin NW. Dialyzer reuse. In: Daugirdas JT, Ing TS, eds. Handbook of Dialysis, 2nd ed. Boston, Little, Brown, 1994.
96. Pegues DA, Beck-Sague CM, Woollen SW, et al. Anaphylactoid reactions associated with reuse of hollow-fiber hemodialyzers and ACE inhibitors. Kidney Int 1992;42:1232–1237.
97. Kirchner KA. Hypertension in hemodialysis patients: More questions than answers. Am J Kidney Dis 1997;30:577–578.
98. Wheeler DC. Should hyperlipidemia in dialysis patients be treated? Nephrol Dial Transplant 1997;12:19–21.
99. Deschamps-Latscha B, Herbelin A. Long-term dialysis and cellular immunity: A critical survey. Kidney Int 1993;43(suppl 41):S135–S142.
100. Arieff AI. Dialysis disequilibrium syndrome: Current concepts on pathogenesis and prevention. Kidney Int 1994;45:629–635.
101. Hakim RM, Wingard RL, Husni L, Parker RA, Parker TF. The effect of membrane biocompatibility on plasma β_2-microglobulin levels in chronic hemodialysis patients. J Am Soc Nephrol 1996;7:472–478.
102. Schwalbe S, Holzhauer M, Schaeffer J, et al. β_2-microglobulin associated amyloidosis: A vanishing complication of long-term hemodialysis? Kidney Int 1997;52:1077–1083.
103. Hornberger JC, Chernew M, Peterson J, Garber AM. A multivariate analysis of mortality and hospital admissions with high-flux dialysis. J Am Soc Nephrol 1992;3:1227–1237.
104. Morbidity and Mortality Weekly Report. Outbreaks of gram-negative bacterial blood stream infections traced to probable contamination of hemodialysis machines—Canada 1995; United States, 1997; and Israel, 1997. MMWR 1998;47:55–59.
105. Jochimsen EM, Carmichael WW, An J, et al. Liver failure and death after exposure to microcystins at a hemodialysis center in Brazil. N Engl J Med 1998;338:873–878.
106. Rodriguez RA. Use of the medical differential diagnosis to achieve optimal end-stage renal disease outcomes. Adv Ren Replace Ther 1997;4:97–111.

107. Salem M. Hypertension in the hemodialysis population: A survey of 649 patients. Am J Kidney Dis 1995;26:461–468.
108. Gejyo F, Homma N, Arakawa M. Long-term complications of dialysis: Pathogenic factors with special reference to amyloidosis. Kidney Int 1993;43(suppl 41):S78–S82.
109. Koda Y, Nishi SI, Miyazaki S, et al. Switch from conventional to high-flux membrane reduces the risk of carpal tunnel syndrome and mortality of hemodialysis patients. Kidney Int 1997;52:1096–1101.
110. Moncrief JW, Popovich RP, Nolph KD. The history and current status of continuous ambulatory peritoneal dialysis. Am J Kidney Dis 1990;16:579–584.
111. Keshaviah P. Urea kinetic and middle molecule approaches to assessing the adequacy of hemodialysis and CAPD. Kidney Int l993; 43(suppl 40):528–538.
112. Buoncristiani U. Continuous ambulatory peritoneal dialysis connection systems. Perit Dial Int 1993;13(suppl 2):5139–5145.
113. Brophy DF, Mueller BA. Automated peritoneal dialysis: New implications for pharmacists. Ann Pharmacother 1997;31:756–764.
114. Piraino B. A review of clinical trials with 2.5 mEq/L calcium dialysate. Perit Dial Int 1993;13(suppl 2):S46–S50.
115. La Greca, Feriani M, Ronco C, et al. Proceedings of the 6th International Course on PD. Perit Dial Int 1997;17(suppl 2):S47–S83.
116. Peers E, Gokal R. Icodextrin: Overview of clinical experience. Perit Dial Int 1997;17:22–26.
117. Holmes CJ. Biocompatibility of peritoneal dialysis solutions. Perit Dial Int 1993;13:88–94. Editorial.
118. Dasgupta MX, Ward K, Noble PA, et al. Development of bacterial biofilms on silastic catheter materials in peritoneal dialysis fluid. Am J Kidney Dis 1994;23:709–716.
119. Lindholm B, Bergstrom J. Nutritional aspects on peritoneal dialysis. Kidney Int 1992;42(suppl 38):S165–S171.
120. Young GA, Kopple JD, Lindholm B, et al. Nutritional assessment of CAPD patients: An international study. Am J Kidney Dis 1991; 17:462–471.
121. Bergstrom J, Lindholm B. Nutrition and adequacy of dialysis. How do hemodialysis and CAPD compare? Kidney Int 1993:43(suppl 40): S39–S50.
122. Ikizler TA, Wingard RL, Hakim RM. Future approaches to the treatment of malnutrition. Malnutrition in peritoneal dialysis patients: Etiologic factors and treatment options. Perit Dial Int 1995: 15(suppl):S63–S66.
123. Dombros NV, Digenis GE, Oreopoulos DG. Is malnutrition a problem for the patient on peritoneal dialysis? Nutritional markers as predictors of survival in patients on CAPD. Perit Dial Int 1995: 15(suppl):S10–S19.
124. Maiorca R, Brunori G, Zubani R, et al. Predictive value of dialysis adequacy and nutritional indices for mortality and morbidity in CAPD and hemodialysis patients. A longitudinal study. Nephrol Dial Transplant 1995;10:2295–2305.
125. Churchill DN, Taylor DW, Keshaviah PR, et al. Adequacy of dialysis and nutrition in continuous peritoneal dialysis: Association with clinical outcomes. J Am Soc Nephrol 1996;7:198–207.
126. Arkouche W, Delawiri E, Laville M, et al. Which quantity of CAPD for a good clinical outcome? Perit Dial Int 1993:13(suppl l):576. Abstract.
127. Blake P, Burkhart JM, Churchill DN, et al. Recommended clinical practices for maximizing peritoneal dialysis clearances. Perit Dial Int 1996;16:448–456.
128. Dumler F, Schmidt R, Cruz C. Abbreviated method for urea kinetic modeling in continuous ambulatory peritoneal dialysis patients. Perit Dial Int 1993;13(suppl 2):S50–S52.
129. Keshaviah R. Adequacy of CAPD: A quantitative approach. Kidney Int 1992;42(suppl 38):S160–S164.
130. Tzamoloukas AR, Murata GH, Sena R. Assessing the adequacy of peritoneal dialysis. Perit Dial Int 1993;13:236–237.
131. Twardowski ZJ. Clinical value of standardized equilibration tests in CAPD patients. Blood Purif 1989;7:95–108.
132. de Fijter CWH, Oe LP, Nauta JJP, et al. Clinical efficacy and morbidity associated with continuous cyclic compared with continuous ambulatory peritoneal dialysis. Ann Intern Med 1994:120: 264–271.
133. Port FK. Risk of peritonitis and technique failure by CAPD connection technique. A national study. Kidney Int 1992:42:967–974.
134. HoIley JL, Bernardini J, Perlmutter JA, Piraino B. A comparison of infection rates among older and younger patients on continuous peritoneal dialysis. Perit Dial Int 1994;14:66–69.
135. Maiorca R, Giovanni CC, Giulio B, et al. Morbidity and mortality of CAPD and hemodialysis. Kidney Int 1993;43(suppl 40):S4–S15.
136. Keane WF, Alexander SR, Bailie GR, et al. Peritoneal dialysis-related peritonitis treatment recommendations: 1996 update. Perit Dial Int 1996;16:557–573.
137. Bunke M, Brier ME, Golper TA. CAPD peritonitis with low PD cell counts: Network #9 peritonitis study. Perit Dial Int 1994;14(suppl l): 526. Abstract.
138. Vas SI. The diagnosis of peritonitis in patients on continuous ambulatory peritoneal dialysis. Semin Dial 1995;8:232–237.
139. Low CL, Bailie GR, Evans A, Eisele G, Venezia RA. Pharmacokinetics of once-daily intraperitoneal gentamicin in CAPD patients. Perit Dial Int 1996;16:379–384.
140. Halstenson CE, Matzke GR, Comty CM. Intraperitoneal administration of tobramycin during CAPD. Kidney Int 1984;25:256. Abstract.
141. Lye WC, Wong PL, van der Straaten JC, et al. A prospective randomized comparison of single versus multidose gentamicin in the treatment of CAPD peritonitis. Adv Perit Dial 1995;11:179–181.
142. Bailie GR, Haqqie SS, Eisele G, et al. Effectiveness of once-weekly vancomycin and once-daily gentamicin, intraperitoneally, for CAPD peritonitis. Perit Dial Int 1995;15:269–271.
143. Lai MN, Kao MT, Chen CC, et al. Intraperitoneal once-daily dose of cefazolin and gentamicin for treating CAPD peritonitis. Perit Dial Int 1997;17:87–88.
144. Vas S, Bargman J, Oreopoulos DG. Treatment in PD patients of peritonitis caused by gram-positive organisms with single daily dose of antibiotics. Perit Dial Int 1997;17:91–93.
145. Nagappan R, Collins JF, Lee WT. Fungal peritonitis in continuous ambulatory peritoneal dialysis—The Auckland experience. Am J Kidney Dis 1992;20:492–496.
146. Chart TN, Chan CY, Cheung SW, et al. Treatment of fungal peritonitis complicating continuous ambulatory peritoneal dialysis with oral fluconazole: A series of 21 patients. Nephrol Dial Transplant 1994; 9:539–542.
147. Wong PN, Mak SK, Lee KF, et al. A prospective study of vancomycin- (Vacoled-) induced chemical peritonitis in CAPD patients. Perit Dial Int 1997;17:202–204.
148. Flanagan MJ, Hochstetler LA, Langholdt D, Lim VS. CAPD catheter infections: Diagnosis and management. Perit Dial Int 1995;15: 248–254.
149. Piraino B, Perlmutter JA, Holley JL, Bernardini J. *Staphylococcus aureus* peritonitis is associated with *Staphylococcus aureus* nasal carriage in peritoneal dialysis patients. Perit Dial Int 1993;13(suppl 2):5332–5334.
150. Piraino B, Bernardini J, Lutes R, et al. Randomized trial of mupirocin at exit-site vs oral rifampin to prevent *S. aureus* catheter infections. Perit Dial Int 1994;14(suppl 1):527. Abstract.
151. Waite NM, Webster N, Laurel M, et al. The efficacy of exit-site povidone–iodine ointment in the prevention of early peritoneal dialysis–related infections. Am J Kidney Dis 1997;29:763–768.
152. Lomaestro BM, Bailie GR. Absorption interactions with fluoroquinolones: 1995 update. Drug Saf 1995;12:314–333.
153. Zimmerman SW, Ahrens E, Johnson CA, et al. Randomized controlled trial of prophylactic rifampin for peritoneal dialysis–related infections. Am J Kidney Dis 1991;18:225–231.
154. Churchill DN, Taylor DW, Vas SI, et al. Peritonitis in CAPD patients: A randomized clinical trial of cotrimoxazole prophylaxis. Perit Dial Int 1988;18:125–128.

155. Poole-Warren LA, Farrell PC. The role of vaccination in the prevention of staphylococcal peritonitis in continuous ambulatory peritoneal dialysis. Perit Dial Int 1993;13:176–177.
156. Piraino B, Lu VL. Nasal mupirocin: Its role in dialysis patients. Semin Dial 1997;10:145–147.
157. Perez-Fontan M, Garcia-Falcon T, Roasales M, et al. Treatment of *Staphylococcus aureus* nasal carriers in CAPD with mupirocin: Long-term results. Am J Kidney Dis 1993;22:708–712.
158. Bailie GR, Eisele G. Pharmacokinetic issues in the treatment of CAPD-associated peritonitis. J Antimicrob Chemother 1995;35: 563–567.
159. Gorman T, Eisele G, Bailie GR. Intraperitoneal antibiotics effectively treat non-dialysis-related infections. Perit Dial Int 1995;15: 283–284.
160. Chan E, Montgomery PA. Administration of insulin via continuous ambulatory peritoneal dialysis. Pharmacotherapy 1993;13:455–460.
161. Tabata T, Shimada H, Emoto M, et al. Inhibitory effect of heparin and/or antithrombin III on intraperitoneal fibrin formation in continuous ambulatory peritoneal dialysis. Nephron 1990;56:391–395.
162. Salusky IB, Goodman WG, Horst R, et al. Pharmacokinetics of calcitriol in continuous ambulatory and cycling peritoneal dialysis. Am J Kidney Dis 1990;16:126–132.
163. Andreoli SP, Cohen M. Intraperitoneal deferrioxamine therapy for iron overload in children undergoing CAPD. Kidney Int 1989;35: 1330–1335.
164. Gora ML, Visconti JA, Seth S, Shields B, Bay W. Pharmacokinetics of intraperitoneal metoclopramide in a patient with renal failure. Clin Pharm 1992;11:174–176.
165. Lazarotivs AI, Page D. Intraperitoneal cisapride for the treatment of diabetics with gastroparesis and end-stage renal disease. Nephron 1990;56:107–109.
166. Galler P, Vigil A, Oliet A, Ortega O, Guijo G. Intraperitoneal erythromycin for diabetic gastroparesis in CAPD. Perit Dial Int 1992; 12:265–266.
167. Flynn CT, Chandran PKG, Taylor MJ, Shadtir CA. Intraperitoneal lithium administration for bipolar affective disorder in a patient on continuous ambulatory peritoneal dialysis. Int J Artif Organs 1987; 10:105–107.
168. Nankirell BJ, Lake N, Gillies A. Intracatheter streptokinase for recurrent peritonitis in CAPD. Clin Nephrol 1991;35:20–23.
169. Arfeen S, Goodship THJ, Kirkwood A, Ward MK. The nutritional/metabolic and hormonal effects of 8 weeks of continuous ambulatory peritoneal dialysis with a 1% amino acid solution. Clin Nephrol 1990;33:192–199.
170. Fine RN, Fine SE, Sherman BM. Absorption of recombinant human growth hormone (rhGH) following intraperitoneal administration. Perit Dial Int 1989;9:91–93.
171. Bastani B, Galley S. Intraperitoneal iron-dextran as a potential route of iron therapy in CAPD patients. Perit Dial Int 1996;16: 646–648.
172. Ateshkadi A, Johnson CA, Oxton LL, et al. Pharmacokinetics of intraperitoneal, intravenous, and subcutaneous recombinant human erythropoietin in patients on continuous ambulatory peritoneal dialysis. Am J Kidney Dis 1993;21:635–642.
173. Zachee P. Controversies in selection of Epoetin doses. Drugs 1995; 49:536–547.
174. Bailie GR, Kane MP. Stability of drug additives to peritoneal dialysate: A review. Perit Dial Int 1995;l5:328–335.
175. Kopple JD. Effect of nutrition on morbidity and mortality in maintenance dialysis patients. Am J Kidney Dis 1994;24:1002–1009.
176. Jones MR. Intraperitoneal amino acids: A therapy whose time has come? Perit Dial Int 1995:15(suppl):S67–S74.
177. Maurer O, Saxenhofer H, Jaeger P, et al. Six-month overnight administration of intraperitoneal amino acids does not improve lean mass. Clin Nephrol 1996;45:303–309.
178. Kurtin P, Nissenson AR. Variation in end-stage renal disease patient outcomes: What do we know, what should we know, and how do we find it out? J Am Soc Nephrol 1993;3:1738–1747.
179. Hays RD, Kallicli JD, Mapes DL, et al. Development of the kidney disease quality of life (KDQOL) instrument. Qual Life Res 1994;3: 329–338.
180. Chapman MM, Meyer KB. Assessing health status in a dialysis clinic. Am J Health Syst Pharm 1995:52(suppl 3):531–532.
181. Proceedings from Renal Rehabilitation and Health Care Reform: Strategies for a changing era. Am J Kidney Dis 1994:24(suppl 1): S1–S32.
182. Holley JL, Nespor S. An analysis of factors affecting employment of chronic dialysis patients. Am J Kidney Dis 1994;23:681–685.

45

DRUG-INDUCED RENAL DISEASE

Paul A. Abraham, MD, and Gary R. Matzke, PharmD, FCP, FCCP

Drug-induced renal disease occurs frequently in patients treated with diagnostic and therapeutic agents. The effect is most commonly a decline in the glomerular filtration rate, but may also include urine sediment abnormalities, proteinuria, pyuria, hematuria, or crystalluria. Renal insufficiency is often reversible on discontinuation of therapy, but may lead to end-stage renal failure. Water, electrolyte, and acid–base disorders may also result (see Chaps. 48 and 49).

Drug nephrotoxicity is seen in both the inpatient and outpatient settings with variable presentations depending on the drug and clinical setting. Many different mechanisms and risk factors are involved. The development of drugs with novel mechanisms of action provides the potential for the presentation and identification of new unique nephropathies. This is demonstrated by the recent recognition that some drugs that were developed to treat HIV (indinavir) and AIDS complications (foscarnet, cidofovir, acyclovir, pentamidine, trimethoprim-sulfamethoxazole, and sulfadiazine), as well as immunomodulating agents (immunoglobulin preparations, interferon-α, and OKT3), all can produce renal injury. However, if one understands the mechanisms responsible for drug-induced alterations in renal function, a nephrotoxic agent's effects can potentially result in new therapeutic indications, as demonstrated by the use of angiotensin-converting enzyme inhibitors (ACEIs) for renal hemodynamic effects to slow the progressive loss of renal function in diabetic nephropathy and to diagnose renovascular hypertension.[1,2]

INCIDENCE

Drug-induced nephrotoxicity, frequently seen in the acute care setting, accounts for nearly 7% of all drug toxicity.[3] These unintended renal effects accounted for up to one-fifth of all cases of hospital-acquired acute renal failure, with a mortality of 8%.[4] Aminoglycosides, radiographic contrast media, and cisplatin were most commonly implicated.[4] Another analysis attributed 29% of all inpatient acute renal failure to drugs: antibiotics (aminoglycosides, pentamidine, and cephalosporins), nonsteroidal anti-inflammatory drugs (NSAIDs), ACEIs, and diuretics were most frequently responsible.[5] Overall, in-hospital drug use may contribute to 35% of all cases of acute tubular necrosis (ATN) (aminoglycosides, radiocontrast agents, and cisplatin), most cases of allergic interstitial nephritis (AIN), as well as to nephropathy due to alterations in renal hemodynamics (diuretics, ACEIs, and NSAIDs) and postrenal obstruction (acyclovir, sulfonamide, and methotrexate).[6] The introduction of new NSAIDs, antihypertensives, and antibiotics as well as decreased use of aminoglycosides has changed the spectrum of commonly implicated drugs.[7] NSAIDs and ACEI, used alone or in combination, are now more commonly implicated.[7,8] Both the morbidity and mortality as well as the costs due to drug toxicity are important.

In the outpatient setting, the incidence and characteristics of drug nephrotoxicity are less well understood since mild toxicity is often unrecognized. However, the pharmacoepidemiology of these effects has become more important as care increasingly shifts to the outpatient setting. As many as 3% to 6% of hospital admissions have been attributed to adverse drug effects during outpatient therapy.[9] NSAID nephrotoxicity is most common and best defined. Prescribed and over-the-counter (OTC) NSAID therapy has been associated with a fourfold increased risk of hospitalization for acute renal failure during the first month of therapy. The predominant risk factors include males > 65 years old, high drug dose, cardiovascular disease, recent hospitalization for nonrenal disease, and concomitant use of other potentially nephrotoxic drugs.[10] Similarly, an approximate twofold increased risk for hospitalization was found for subjects more than 70 years old who were recently prescribed NSAIDs.[11] No other risk factors were identified. Despite these data the overall safety of NSAIDs has been favorable in comparison to alternative analgesics and resulted in the OTC availability of ibuprofen, naproxen, and ketoprofen in the United States.[12,13]

Other agents associated with outpatient toxicity include ACEIs, which have been associated with transient acute renal failure,[14] while long-term therapy with cyclosporine and abuse of combination analgesics have resulted in chronic interstitial nephritis. Fortunately, chronic analgesic nephropathy is slowly progressive, allowing early recognition of renal dysfunction and discontinuation of therapy to stabilize or recover renal function. Lastly, several case reports have increased our awareness that unregulated OTC health foods and nutritional supplements can cause renal failure, including interstitial nephritis from chromium picolinate,[15] L-lysine,[16] and Chinese herbal medication (aristolochic acid).[17]

COSTS OF DRUG NEPHROTOXICITY

The pharmacoeconomics of drug nephrotoxicity have not been well defined. An analysis of aminoglycoside therapy in the acute care environment for 1984 to 1985 revealed 7.3% of patients experienced nephrotoxicity. The mean additional cost for each episode of toxicity (in 1984 dollars) was $2501. The average additional cost of toxicity for each individual treated with aminoglycosides was $183.[18] Similarly, analysis of combined hospital and ambulatory care costs of radiographic contrast media use have included costs related to management of hypersensitivity reactions as well as nephropathy and have focused on the advantages of the newer nonionic contrast agents.[19] While these agents may reduce the incidence of many types of contrast reactions, routine use of nonionic contrast agents would raise the material cost for contrast procedures significantly more than the decrease in cost associated with the management of adverse effects.[20] Renal insufficiency has been proposed as a relative indication for the use of nonionic contrast agents due to the lower incidence of nephrotoxicity.[21] Obtaining a serum creatinine concentration before contrast studies to screen for risk of toxicity adds only about $15 to the procedure cost.[22] Lastly, outpatient care costs of NSAID toxicity have been evaluated. Costs for hospital care for NSAID-induced acute hemodynamically mediated renal failure and interstitial nephritis combined have been estimated at $990 million per year.[23]

RISK FACTORS

No generalizable risk factors are applicable to all drug classes and patient situations since drug toxicity develops as a result of a wide range of mechanisms, from idiosyncratic hypersensitivity reactions to direct cellular toxicity, and spans the full spectrum of age, from the newborn[24] to the very elderly. An exception is hemodynamically mediated acute renal failure due to NSAIDs and ACEIs. Their toxicity is frequently preventable by recognizing risk factors including preexisting renal insufficiency and decreased effective renal blood flow due to volume depletion, heart failure, or liver disease. The elderly arthritic patient with hypertension or heart failure may be especially sensitive to the combined use of ACEIs and NSAIDs.[8]

RECOGNITION AND ASSESSMENT OF RENAL TOXICITY

The onset of acute renal failure associated with drug use in hospitalized acutely ill patients is most often recognized by routine laboratory monitoring of serum creatinine or blood urea nitrogen (BUN) concentrations. Decreased urine output may also be an early sign of toxicity, particularly with radiographic contrast media, NSAIDs, and ACE inhibitors. In the outpatient setting, nephrotoxicity is often recognized by the symptoms of uremia (malaise, anorexia, and vomiting) or volume overload (shortness of breath or edema), which develop as the result of severe renal insufficiency. Serum creatinine or BUN concentrations and urine collection for creatinine clearance may then be measured to quantify the loss of glomerular filtration.

Nephrotoxicity may also selectively alter renal tubular function, particularly early in toxicity, without loss of glomerular filtration. In these cases, indicators of proximal tubular injury include metabolic acidosis with bicarbonaturia, glycosuria in the absence of hyperglycemia, and hypophosphatemia and hypouricemia due to increased urinary losses of phosphorus and uric acid. Indicators of distal tubular injury include polyuria from failure to maximally concentrate urine, metabolic acidosis from impaired urinary acidification, and hyperkalemia from impaired potassium excretion. Urinary excretion of enzymes and low-molecular-weight proteins, including *N*-acetyl-β-D-glucosaminidase[25] and β_2-microglobulin,[26] respectively, have been used to detect early tubular injury, particularly during aminoglycoside therapy (see Chap. 40). However, these indicators have been too sensitive to be useful clinically since drug administration can increase their excretion without causing clinically important toxicity.

CLASSIFICATION OF DRUG-INDUCED RENAL DISEASE

Drug nephropathy is highly heterogeneous with respect to the drugs involved and lesions produced. No system of classification has been satisfactory. For the student, classification based on mechanisms of toxicity is preferred but has been inadequate due to insufficient knowledge. Alternative classifications include presentation of the renal manifestations (e.g., acute or chronic renal failure, hematuria, pyuria, or proteinuria) to facilitate clinical diagnosis of nephrotoxicity; indexing of drugs by their therapeutic use or the various types of nephropathies they may produce to facilitate risk awarness; and finally awareness of the renal structural and functional alterations they induce (Table 45–1) to emphasize current knowledge of mechanisms of drug nephrotoxicity. The latter classification is used in this discussion.

MECHANISMS FOR RENAL SUSCEPTIBILITY TO DRUG TOXICITY

The kidneys are more sensitive than many other organs to drug toxicity. Both immunologic and nonimmunologic mechanisms contribute. Immune-mediated drug nephropathies include glomerulonephritis and allergic interstitial nephritis, either with or without the nephrotic syndrome. Mechanisms for immune susceptibility are not clear, but could include the large vascular surface area with exposure to circulating immune mediators as well as an intrinsic immune function of glomerular mesangial cells and renal cytokine activation. Nonimmunologic mechanisms of drug nephropathy relate to several specialized characteristics of normal renal physiology (Fig. 45–1).

HIGH BLOOD FLOW AND SPECIALIZED HEMODYNAMICS

The kidneys constitute only 0.4% of body weight, but receive 20% to 25% of resting cardiac output. This enhances

TABLE 45–1. Drug-Induced Renal Structural–Functional Alterations and Examples

Pseudo-Renal Failure
Corticosteroids
Trimethoprim
Cimetidine
Hemodynamically Mediated Renal Failure
Nonsteroidal anti-inflammatory drugs
Angiotensin-converting enzyme inhibitors
Renal Vasculitis, Thrombosis, and Cholesterol Emboli
Vasculitis and thrombosis
Mitomycin C
Methamphetamines
Cholesterol emboli
Warfarin
Thrombolytic agents
Glomerular Disease
Nephrotic syndrome
Gold
Nonsteroidal anti-inflammatory drugs
Glomerulonephritis
Hydralazine
Cytokine therapy
Tubular Epithelial Cell Damage
Osmotic nephrosis
Mannitol
Intravenous immunoglobulin
Acute tubular necrosis
Aminoglycoside antibiotics
Radiographic contrast media
Interstitial Nephritis
Acute allergic
Methicillin
Nonsteroidal anti-inflammatory drugs
Chronic
Cyclosporine
Lithium
Papillary necrosis
Combined phenacetin, aspirin, and caffeine analgesics
Obstructive Nephropathy
Intratubular
Acyclovir
Sulfadiazine
Lower urinary tract
Tricyclic antidepressants
Nephrolithiasis
Triamterene
Indinavir

the kidney's exposure to circulating drugs. Blood flow within each kidney is distributed to superficial and deep nephron units as well as the medulla and papillae. Within each nephron, blood flow and pressure are regulated by glomerular afferent and efferent arterioles to maintain capillary hydrostatic pressure and glomerular filtration. This specialized blood flow is precisely regulated by interrelations between renal prostaglandins, atrial natriuretic factor, the sympathetic nervous system, the renin–angiotensin system, and the macula densa response to distal tubular solute delivery. In this unique vascular setting, β-blockers[27] and NSAIDs may reduce total renal blood flow, radiographic contrast media may shunt intrarenal blood flow away from superficial nephrons,[28] osmotic diuresis secondary to mannitol therapy may reduce glomerular blood flow due to tubuloglomerular feedback,[29] and ACEIs may dilate glomerular efferent arterioles leading to a decrease in glomerular filtration pressure in the presence of ischemic renal vascular disease.[1] Dietary salt restriction can activate neurohumoral renal hemodynamic control systems that increase renal susceptibility to these drug nephrotoxicities.[30]

TUBULAR EPITHELIAL CELL ABSORPTIVE AND SECRETORY FUNCTIONS

Drugs or their metabolites can accumulate in renal tubular epithelial cells, particularly in the proximal tubule, as the result of active tubular transport processes involving secretion and reabsorption of organic acids and bases. Toxic drugs or metabolites that accumulate intracellularly may cause cell injury as the result of impairment of mitochondrial function and decreased adenosine triphosphate (ATP) synthesis, increased oxidative stress, depletion of reduced glutathione and other antioxidants, inhibition of phospholipid metabolism, and disruption of protein synthesis. Intracellular accumulation of nephrotoxic agents is a less operative mechanism in immature animals with undeveloped tubular transport mechanisms. Thus, toxicity data derived from animal studies may not directly correlate to findings in humans. Aminoglycosides and cyclosporine are agents that appear to mediate nephrotoxicity through intracellular accumulation.[31] In particular, gentamicin appears to increase intracellular concentrations of the superoxide ion, hydrogen peroxide, and its hydroxyl radical, while cyclosporine increases hydrogen peroxide, a reactive oxygen species that contributes to cellular oxidative stress and nephrotoxicity.[32]

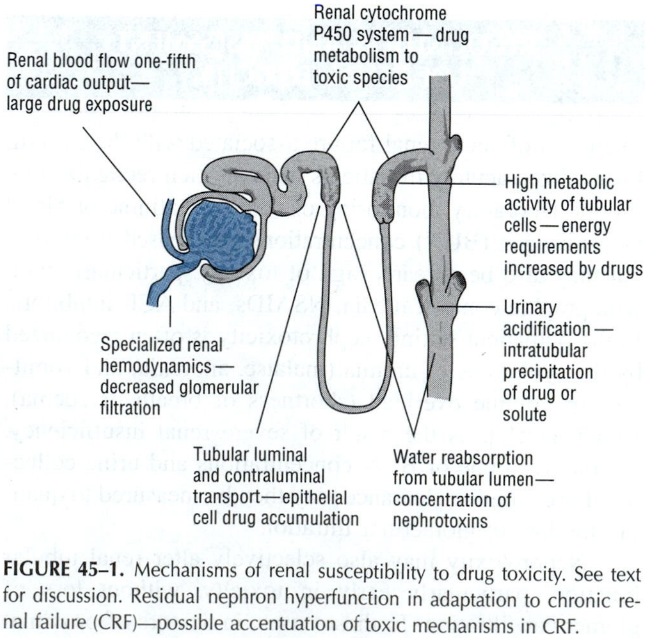

FIGURE 45–1. Mechanisms of renal susceptibility to drug toxicity. See text for discussion. Residual nephron hyperfunction in adaptation to chronic renal failure (CRF)—possible accentuation of toxic mechanisms in CRF.

DRUG METABOLISM TO TOXIC SPECIES

Multiple renal enzymes contribute to drug metabolism. These include cytochrome P450 and mixed function oxidases in proximal tubular epithelial cells which have activity similar to activity in the liver. In contrast, prostaglandin endoperoxide synthetase activity is more localized to the renal papilla and medulla. The kidney may thus transform a drug to an inactive or active metabolite, which may be nephrotoxic. As an example, acetaminophen can be oxidized to reactive species that contribute to acute tubular necrosis following acute acetaminophen overdose and to analgesic nephropathy with chronic consumption.[33]

HIGH ENERGY REQUIREMENT BY RENAL TUBULAR CELLS

Renal tubular epithelial cells have high energy requirements for active tubular transport and ongoing metabolic processes. These high energy needs are precariously supplied to medullary tubular epithelial cells, which function in a state of chronic hypoxia due to their perfusion with venous blood returning from the deep medulla. As a consequence these medullary tubular epithelial cells are especially sensitive to drugs that accentuate this hypoxia by increasing energy demands or by decreasing energy production or oxygen delivery. An example is amphotericin B–induced medullary tubular cell damage, which appears to result from an imbalance between increased cellular energy requirements and inadequate oxygen delivery.[34]

CONCENTRATION OF SOLUTE IN THE TUBULAR LUMEN

Ninety-nine percent of the water filtered by the glomerulus is reabsorbed back into the body. Normally, 50% to 85% of water reabsorption occurs in the proximal tubule while the remainder occurs in the descending loop of Henle and collecting duct. Systemic volume depletion increases the percentage of water reabsorption in the proximal tubule. As water reabsorption increases, the rate of tubular flow decreases and the concentration of solutes and toxins increases within the tubular lumen. Thus, the lumenal surfaces of cells, particularly in the proximal tubule, can be exposed to higher concentrations of potential toxins and for a longer time than most other tissues in the body. This enhances binding of drugs to tubular epithelial cells and promotes active and passive transport into cells. The enhancement of aminoglycoside nephrotoxicity by systemic volume depletion is an example.[35]

URINE ACIDIFICATION

Urine pH decreases to approximately 4.5 during maximal stimulation of renal tubular hydrogen ion secretion. Certain solutes can precipitate and obstruct the tubular lumen at this acid pH, particularly when urine is concentrated. Thus, a maximally acid urine can contribute to intratubular precipitation of methotrexate and acute renal failure during high-dose methotrexate chemotherapy.[36]

INCREASED FUNCTION OF INDIVIDUAL NEPHRONS IN ADAPTATION TO CHRONIC RENAL INSUFFICIENCY

Chronic renal insufficiency develops as the result of injury to involved glomerular and tubular units while others remain relatively intact. The remaining functional nephron units develop hyperfiltering glomeruli and hyperfunctioning tubules to compensate for the damaged nephrons. These residual nephrons are more susceptible to nephrotoxic injury due to their increased workload and accentuation of the previously described physiologic mechanisms. The nephrotoxicity of radiographic contrast media in patients with chronic renal insufficiency is such an example.[37]

AGE-RELATED DECLINE IN RENAL FUNCTION

Renal blood flow and glomerular filtration rate decline progressively, particularly in males once they have reached 40 years of age.[38] Progressive sclerosis of glomeruli occurs. Residual glomerular and tubular units increase function in compensation, similar to patients with chronic renal insufficiency. This decline in renal function is not accompanied by a rise in the serum creatinine concentration due to the age-related decline in muscle mass and decreased creatinine generation. Older individuals are also more likely to have heart failure and hepatic insufficiency, which also reduce renal blood flow and cause renal insufficiency. Together, these processes predispose the elderly to increased risk of nephrotoxicity. In addition, the doses of drugs that are primarily eliminated unchanged by the kidney, such as aminoglycosides, must be reduced to prevent toxic levels[38] (see Chap. 47).

PRINCIPLES FOR PREVENTION OF DRUG NEPHROPATHY

The basic principle for prevention of drug-induced renal disease is to avoid the use of potentially nephrotoxic agents in patients at increased risk for toxicity. However, when exposure to these drugs cannot be avoided, specific techniques may be used to reduce potential nephrotoxicity (Table 45–2).

Certain approaches to reduce drug toxicity are prudent and generally effective. These include careful and adequate hydration to establish high renal tubular flow rates and thereby permit more aggressive drug administration to maximize efficacy while minimizing toxicity. However, other measures to reduce drug toxicity are still theoretical and/or investigational. Thus, administration of oral prostaglandin analogs may reduce NSAID toxicity,[39] whereas calcium channel blockers reduce amphotericin B toxicity in animals.[40]

TABLE 45–2. Mechanisms and Principles for Prevention of Drug Nephropathy

Mechanisms of Renal Susceptibility	Principles for Prevention	Example
A. Large drug exposure due to high renal blood flow	1. Avoid systemic drug administration	1. Intraperitoneal administration of cisplatin for localized intra-peritoneal tumor[36]
	2. Limit total drug dose	2. Monitor aminoglycoside levels to maintain in therapeutic range; substitute nontoxic antibiotic based on microbial sensitivities
B. Specialized renal hemodynamics regulated by vasoactive substances	Avoid drugs that inhibit prostaglandin synthesis	Substitute acetaminophen or nonacetylated salicylates, nabumetone or sulindac for other NSAIDs
C. Tubular epithelial cell drug accumulation due to luminal and contraluminal transport	1. Inhibit drug absorption from the luminal membrane	1. Hydration with chloride anions during cisplatin therapy[36]; calcium supplementation during aminoglycoside therapy[35]
	2. Inhibit drug absorption from the contraluminal membrane	2. Cilastatin inhibition of imipenem toxicity[65]
D. Renal metabolism of drugs to toxic species	Use drugs with nontoxic renal metabolities	Renal metabolism of active sulindac sulfide to inactive sulindac sulfoxide
E. Cellular dysfunction due to drug-induced increased energy requirements	Decrease cell energy needs by reducing cell membrane transport activity	Furosemide use during amphotericin therapy to reduce ischemia and toxicity to the medullary thick ascending loop of Henle[34]
F. Water reabsorption and concentration of nephrotoxins within the tubular lumen promoting increased epithelial cell membrane contact and transport into cells	1. Prevent dehydration 2. Use of osmotic diuresis to increase luminal water volume and tubular flow rate	1. NaCl repletion to prevent amphotericin toxicity 2. Possible reduction of contrast nephropathy by mannitol diuresis
G. Urinary acidification with intratubular precipitation of drug or solute	Alkalinize urine	Urinary alkalinization to prevent uric acid and methotrexate nephropathy[36]
H. In chronic renal failure, increased toxin exposure per residual viable nephron due to nephron hyperfunction	Avoid drug use or reduce drug dose in renal failure patients	Choose alternatives to radiographic contrast agents for renal imaging: ultrasonography, computerized tomography without contrast use, radionuclide studies, magnetic resonance imaging

DRUG-INDUCED RENAL STRUCTURAL–FUNCTIONAL ALTERATIONS

Specific drug-induced renal structural–functional alterations constitute the remainder of this discussion under the eight broad headings listed in Table 45–1. The general orientation of these topics is from the systemic, hemodynamic, and renal vascular effects on renal function, through the glomerulus, the filtering surface of the kidney vasculature, into the renal tubules and surrounding interstitial support tissue of the kidney, and finally into the urinary collecting system of the kidney and lower urinary tract. Mechanisms of nephrotoxicity will be emphasized in addition to clinical findings, prevention, and management.

PSEUDO-RENAL FAILURE

Pseudo-renal failure occurs when either the blood urea nitrogen (BUN) or creatinine concentration rises suggesting a decrease in renal function, despite maintenance of the glomerular filtration rate.

The BUN concentration commonly increases without an increase in creatinine concentration during corticosteroid or tetracycline therapy. These drugs cause protein catabolism and thereby increase ureagenesis and the BUN concentration as the result of tissue breakdown. The glomerular filtration rate is unchanged and accurately reflected by the creatinine clearance and creatinine concentration.

Similarly, the serum creatinine concentration may rise while the BUN concentration remains unchanged by either of two mechanisms. First, drugs, including trimethoprim, cimetidine, or pyrimethamine, competitively inhibit secretion of creatinine into the proximal tubular lumen.[41] This effect is minimal during therapy in patients with normal renal function in whom the serum creatinine concentration usually remains in the normal range since tubular secretion of creatinine contributes only 5% to 10% to creatinine excretion.[41] In contrast, in renal-insufficient patients, the rise in serum creatinine is greater since tubular secretion of creatinine contributes a proportionately greater amount to urinary creatinine excretion.[41] Ranitidine and other H_2-receptor antagonists that are more potent than cimetidine on a molar basis and therefore have a lower molar concentration in the blood are less likely to raise the serum creatinine concentration.[42] Competitive inhibition of creatinine secretion has been considered useful in the evaluation of renal function since creatinine clearance usually overestimates true glomerular filtration rate in the presence of renal insufficiency. Administration of cimetidine during urine collection decreases creatinine secretion and provides a creatinine clearance value that more closely approximates true glomerular filtration, particularly in patients with renal disease (see Chap. 40).[43] Second, several drugs (see Table 45–3), particularly cefoxitin and other cephalosporin antibiotics, can increase the serum creatinine concentration by direct interference with the enzymatic measurement of creatinine by the Jaffé method.[41] The incidence of this effect is unknown, but it is uncommon; it is most prevalent among patients with decreased renal function. These drugs do not appear to interfere with determination of creatinine clearance.

HEMODYNAMICALLY MEDIATED RENAL FAILURE

Hemodynamically mediated renal insufficiency results from a decrease in blood flow to glomeruli, causing insufficient perfusion pressure to maintain filtration across the glomerular capillaries. Mechanisms commonly include a decrease in total renal blood flow, vasoconstriction of glomerular afferent arterioles, or vasodilation of glomerular efferent arterioles.

TABLE 45–3. Drugs That Interfere With the Jaffé Measurement of Creatinine and Can Falsely Increase the Serum Creatinine Concentration

Cefoxitin
Cephalothin
Cefazolin
Cefotaxime
Flucytosine
Methyldopa

REDUCED GLOMERULAR CAPILLARY HYDROSTATIC PRESSURE

Angiotensin II Converting Enzyme Inhibitors and Angiotension II Receptor Antagonists

Incidence. The incidence of ACEI or angiotensin II receptor antagonist nephrotoxicity has not been established. However, patients with atherosclerotic renal artery stenosis > 70%, those hospitalized with congestive heart failure or renal insufficiency with serum creatinine > 1.6 mg/dL, and those with primary renal disease, including diabetic nephropathy, and serum creatinine > 3.0 mg/dL are most likely to experience a significant decline in renal function with these agents.

Clinical Presentation. Therapy with ACEI[1] as well as losartan[44] and newly developed angiotensin II receptor antagonists can acutely reduce glomerular filtration in kidneys perfused by stenotic renal arteries. A reduction in GFR has also been reported in the absence of renal artery stenosis, when renal blood flow is reduced by a systemic disease, such as congestive heart failure or by excessive diuretic therapy, or an intrarenal vascular process, such as small vessel afferent arteriolar narrowing due to severe hypertension. In particular, nephropathy during treatment of congestive heart failure with ACEIs is now common. Urinalysis remains unchanged from baseline, with no diagnostic findings. The diagnosis is evidenced by rising serum creatinine or BUN concentrations. The rise is often minimal in renovascular disease if only one renal artery is stenotic, but is more apparent with bilateral renal artery stenosis, a single kidney with renovascular disease, or congestive heart failure, volume depletion, or bilateral renal small vessel disease. In renal artery stenosis, asymmetry of renal function on a radionuclide renogram that improves on discontinuation of ACEI is also diagnostic.[1,45]

Pathogenesis. The pathogenesis of ACEI or angiotensin II receptor antagonist nephropathy is a decrease in glomerular capillary hydrostatic pressure sufficient to reduce glomerular ultrafiltration[1] (Fig. 45–2). This occurs in settings where glomerular afferent arteriolar blood flow is reduced and the efferent arteriole is vasoconstricted by angiotensin II to maintain sufficient glomerular capillary hydrostatic pressure for ultrafiltration. ACEI or angiotensin II receptor antagonist therapy reduces angiotensin II synthesis or activity, respectively, thereby dilating the efferent arteriole and reducing glomerular capillary hydrostatic pressure. This decreases glomerular ultrafiltration and renal function.

Risk Factors. Patients at greatest risk are those dependent on angiotensin II to maintain blood pressure and renal efferent arteriolar constriction. These include patients with hemodynamically significant renal artery stenosis, particularly bilateral stenosis, and those with decreased effective arterial renal blood flow, particularly due to congestive heart failure, volume depletion from excess diuresis, hepatic cirrhosis with ascites, and the nephrotic syndrome. The fetal kidney is also sensitive to ACEI. Anuria has been

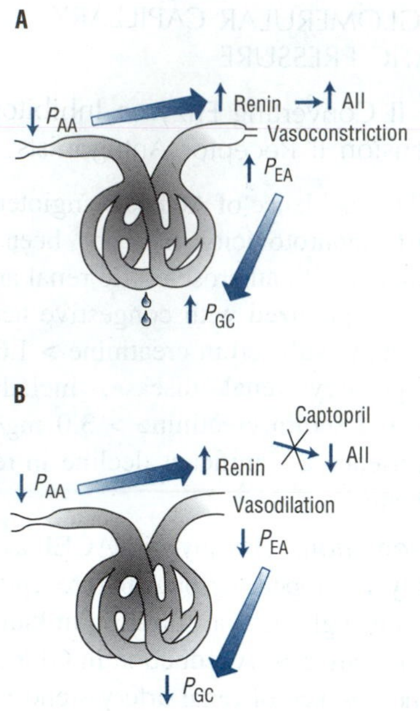

FIGURE 45–2. ACE inhibitor nephropathy occurs in the setting of reduced blood flow (involving large or small artery) to the glomerulus. In this setting **(A)**, pressure in the afferent arterioles (P_{AA}) is reduced, causing the juxtaglomerular apparatus to increase renin secretion. Increased plasma renin activity converts angiotensinogen to angiotensin I, which is converted to angiotensin II (AII) by angiotensin- converting enzyme. Increased angiotensin II constricts the efferent arteriole, increasing pressure in the efferent arteriole (P_{EA}) and thereby increases hydrostatic pressure in the glomerular capillaries (P_{GC}) to maintain glomerular filtration. When ACE inhibitor (captopril) therapy is initiated **(B)** the synthesis of angiotensin II is decreased, thereby dilating the efferent arteriole. This reduces outflow resistance from the glomerulus and decreases hydrostatic pressure in the glomerular capillaries, which alters Starling's forces across the glomerular capillaries to decrease glomerular filtration. P_{AA} = afferent arteriole pressure, P_{EA} = efferent arteriole pressure, P_{GC} = glomerular capillary pressure, AII = angiotensin II.

observed in the newborn following maternal ACEI therapy late in pregnancy.[24]

Prevention. A common strategy for at-risk hospitalized patients is to initiate therapy with very low doses of the short-acting ACEI captopril, then gradually up-titrate the dose and convert to a longer-acting agent after therapy is tolerated. This allows more rapid offset of action if hypotension or another adverse effect were to develop. Outpatients may be started on very low doses of long-acting ACEIs with gradual dose up-titration. Renal function and serum potassium levels must be monitored carefully, daily for hospitalized patients and every 2 to 3 days for outpatients, during initiation of ACEI or angiotensin II receptor antagonist therapy for patients with preexisting renal insufficiency, congestive heart failure, or suspected renovascular disease.

Management. Acute decreases in renal function and hyperkalemia usually resolve over several days after ACEI or angiotensin II receptor antagonist therapy is discontinued. Occasional patients will require management of severe hyperkalemia, usually with sodium polystyrene sulfate (see Chap. 48), but occasionally with hospitalization and intravenous glucose and insulin. ACEI or angiotensin II antagonist therapy may frequently be reattempted, particularly for patients with congestive heart failure, by correcting intravascular volume depletion and reducing diuretic doses.[46] Mild renal insufficiency (serum creatinine concentration of 2 to 3 mg/dL) or slight worsening of renal function may be an acceptable trade-off for hemodynamic improvement in certain patients with severe congestive heart failure or renovascular disease not amenable to invasive management. Congestive heart failure patients with greater renal insufficiency may be best treated by substitution of hydralazine and nitrates for afterload reduction.

Clinical Application. The pathophysiologic principles of ACEI nephropathy have now been extensively investigated and applied to diagnostic and therapeutic benefits. Diagnostically, the captopril renogram is now the most sensitive and specific screening test for the diagnosis of renovascular hypertension.[1,45] This test involves radionuclide imaging of the kidneys before and after a single dose of captopril. The renogram of the involved kidney will show a reversible decrease in function with captopril compared to without captopril in the presence of hemodynamically significant renal artery stenosis. Therapeutically, captopril, 25 mg three times daily, has received FDA approval to reduce proteinuria and slow the progressive deterioration of renal function seen in patients with diabetic nephropathy (see Chap. 42).[2]

INHIBITION OF PROSTAGLANDIN-DEPENDENT TOTAL RENAL BLOOD FLOW

Nonsteroidal Anti-inflammatory Drugs

Incidence. NSAIDs have an overall favorable safety profile resulting in OTC availability in the United States of ibuprofen, naproxen, and ketoprofen for short-term therapy. While potential adverse renal effects from OTC NSAIDs have been a concern,[12] activity of vasodilatory prostaglandins is not necessary to maintain the function of normal kidneys. NSAIDs are unlikely to impair renal function in the absence of renal ischemia or excess renal vasoconstrictor activity. Nevertheless, NSAID therapy is associated with a fourfold risk for hospitalization[10] and small reductions in glomerular filtration rate can occur in normal subjects as shown during short[47] and sustained[48] indomethacin therapy.

Clinical Presentation. Renal failure can occur within days of initiating oral therapy, particularly with a short-acting NSAID such as ibuprofen.[49,50] Serum creatinine and BUN concentrations rise proportionately. Urine volume and sodium concentration are usually low. The urine sediment is usually unchanged from baseline, but may show granular casts. Similarly, parenteral NSAID therapy with ketorolac has been associated with a transient decline in renal function, even after a single dose.[51] However, in a retrospective cohort analysis, parenteral ketorolac therapy was not identified as a risk for acute renal failure in hospitalized patients.[52] Topically administered NSAIDs can also cause nephropathy.[53]

Pathogenesis. NSAIDs inhibit cyclooxygenase and impair renal function by decreasing synthesis of vasodilatory prostaglandins from arachidonic acid. Renal prostaglandins are synthesized in the renal cortex and medulla by vascular endothelial and glomerular mesangial cells. Their effects are primarily local and result in renal vasodilation (particularly prostacyclin and PGE_2). They have limited activity in states of normal renal blood flow, but in states of decreased renal blood flow their synthesis is increased and they protect against renal ischemia and hypoxia by antagonizing renal vasoconstriction due to angiotensin II, norepinephrine, endothelin, and vasopressin. Administration of NSAIDs in the setting of renal ischemia and compensatory increased prostaglandin activity may thus alter the balance of activity between renal vasoconstrictors and vasodilators. This leaves the activity of renal vasoconstrictors unopposed and promotes renal ischemia with loss of glomerular filtration. This hemodynamically mediated acute renal failure is the most common adverse renal effect of NSAIDs, but other renal effects can occur.

Risk Factors. Persons at greatest risk for NSAID nephropathy generally have preexisting renal insufficiency, medical problems associated with high plasma renin activity (hepatic disease with ascites, decompensated congestive heart failure, or intravascular volume depletion), or systemic lupus erythematosus. Additional risk factors continue to be clarified, but include atherosclerotic cardiovascular disease and diuretic therapy. Advanced age, over 60 to 65 years, appears as a risk factor due to interaction of prevalent medical problems and multiple drug therapy with reduced renal hemodynamics,[54] although advanced age has not been an independent risk factor for toxicity in limited trials in otherwise healthy elderly subjects.[55] Combined NSAID and ACEI or cyclosporine therapy is also a concern.[8] Fetal and newborn kidneys also appear sensitive to the effects of NSAIDs administered late in pregnancy to prevent premature labor or shortly after birth to close a patent ductus arteriosus.[24]

Prevention. NSAID-induced acute renal failure can be prevented by recognizing high-risk patients and using analgesics with less prostaglandin inhibition: acetaminophen, nonacetylated salicylates, aspirin, and, possibly, sulindac or nabumetone.[56] When NSAID therapy is essential for high-risk patients, management of predisposing medical problems should be optimized and renal function monitored. Sulindac is of particular interest in high-risk patients since it is a potent NSAID that may have lesser effects on renal prostaglandin synthesis and function. The mechanism of renal prostaglandin sparing is unclear, but may involve intrarenal metabolism of the active drug, sulindac sulfide, by cytochrome P450–dependent mixed-function oxidases to an inactive metabolite, sulindac sulfoxide. However, this favorable effect of sulindac has not been consistently observed, especially at higher therapeutic doses, in patients with hepatic disease, or during prolonged therapy. The oral prostaglandin E analog, misoprostol, may be useful to prevent NSAID nephropathy.[39] Finally, cyclooxygenase-selective NSAIDs, possibly including nabumetone[56] and meloxicam in the future,[57] may selectively inhibit a cyclooxygenase isoform synthesizing prostaglandins mediating tissue inflammation (COX-2) without inhibiting activity of the cyclooxygenase isoform responsible for the synthesis of prostaglandins necessary to maintain kidney function (COX-1).[58]

Management. Acute renal failure due to NSAIDs is treated by discontinuation of therapy and supportive care. Renal failure may be severe, but recovery is usually rapid and dialysis is rarely necessary. Occasionally the hemodynamic insult is sufficiently severe to cause frank tubular necrosis, which can prolong recovery. The differential diagnosis of NSAID hemodynamically mediated acute renal failure must include NSAID-induced acute interstitial nephritis, with or without the nephrotic syndrome, because steroid therapy may benefit this lesion.

Clinical Application. The renal hemodynamic effects of NSAIDs have been applied therapeutically to reduce proteinuria in patients with nephrotic syndrome[59] (see Chap. 46). The efficacy of various NSAIDs for this purpose is directly proportional to their ability to inhibit renal prostaglandin synthesis. Renal function declines, but the decrease in proteinuria is proportionately greater than the decline in renal function.

Sulfinpyrazone. Sulfinpyrazone, a uricosuric congener of phenylbutazone used to impair platelet function following myocardial infarction or coronary artery bypass graft surgery, also causes hemodynamically mediated acute renal failure.[60] Sulfinpyrazone inhibition of renal prostaglandin synthesis or reduction of renal kallikrein–kinin activity may imbalance renal hemodynamics, causing renal ischemia. Renal insufficiency may be transient despite continued sulfinpyrazone administration or prolonged and oliguric with a low urinary sodium concentration.[60]

NONSPECIFIC RENAL VASOCONSTRICTION

Cyclosporine

Cyclosporine, a lipophilic immunosuppressive agent, has dramatically enhanced kidney, heart, liver, and pancreas transplantation and therapy of autoimmune diseases.[61,62] The mechanism is predominantly decreased T-lymphocyte lymphokine production, particularly interleukin 2. Nephrotoxicity is a major dose-limiting adverse effect of therapy causing early acute hemodynamically mediated renal insufficiency and delayed chronic interstitial nephritis (see section on Chronic Interstitial Nephritis).[62] Cyclosporine use has decreased early acute renal transplant rejection, but not later chronic rejection. Cyclosporine-induced chronic interstitial nephritis contributes to the long-term loss of renal graft function.[62]

Incidence. Historically, reversible acute renal insufficiency occurred frequently in transplant recipients during the first 6 months of cyclosporine therapy.[63] Irreversible chronic interstitial nephritis with end-stage chronic renal failure developed in 10% of heart transplant recipients following initial high-dose therapy.[62] More recently, the combined effects of lower dose therapy and use of pharmacokinetic monitoring have reduced acute renal dysfunction. Nevertheless, most patients with apparently stable renal function will experience increased renal blood flow and glomerular filtration rates following withdrawal of therapy.[62] The incidence of cyclosporine nephrotoxicity has been evaluated most accurately in patients not receiving a kidney transplant. Renal toxicity developed in 21% to 25% of patients during immunosuppression for rheumatoid arthritis, uveitis, psoriasis, and diabetes mellitus.[62,64–67]

Clinical Presentation. Acute renal toxicity may occur within days of initiating therapy. Serum creatinine concentration rises and creatinine clearance decreases. Hypertension, hyperkalemia, sodium avidity, and hypomagnesemia may occur. No urine sediment abnormalities are seen. Urinary enzyme excretions increase, but are not reliable indicators of toxicity. Renal biopsy reveals thickening of arterioles, mild focal glomerular sclerosis, proximal tubular epithelial cell vacuolization and atrophy, and interstitial fibrosis. Biopsy is useful to distinguish acute cyclosporine nephrotoxicity from acute renal allograft rejection, the latter being evidenced by acute cellular interstitial infiltrate.[61,68]

Chronic toxicity becomes apparent after 6 to 12 months of therapy as a slowly rising serum creatinine concentration and decreased creatinine clearance. However, the rise in serum creatinine concentration and decreased creatinine clearance may be delayed and not reflect the severity of histopathologic changes. Urinalysis reveals few red and white blood cells with low-range proteinuria. Renal biopsy shows progressive renal arteriolar hyalinosis, glomerular sclerosis, and a striped pattern of interstitial fibrosis. Biopsy cannot easily distinguish chronic cyclosporine toxicity from chronic rejection.[62,64,67,69]

Pathogenesis. A dose-related hemodynamic mechanism is likely during the initial months of therapy since renal function improves rapidly following dose reduction. Reversible vasoconstriction and injury to glomerular afferent arterioles occurs, possibly due to increased activity of vasoconstrictors, including thromboxane A_2, endothelin, and the sympathetic nervous system, or diminished activity of vasodilators, nitric oxide, or prostacyclin.[62,68] Vasoconstriction due to increased renin–angiotensin system activity may also contribute.[70] Infusion of renal vasodilatory doses of dopamine improves renal blood flow, glomerular filtration rate, and fractional excretion of sodium, further supporting a reversible hemodynamically mediated mechanism of acute toxicity.[71] Continuation of these effects with renal arteriolar hyalinization and chronic renal ischemia as well as increased extracellular matrix synthesis appear to contribute to cyclosporine-induced chronic renal failure.[62,68,69]

Risk Factors. Risk factors include increased age and higher initial cyclosporine dose, as well as renal graft rejection, hypotension, infection, and concomitant therapy with nephrotoxic drugs such as aminoglycosides, amphotericin B, acyclovir, NSAIDs, and radiocontrast agents, as well as drugs that inhibit cyclosporine hepatic metabolism.[61] The high incidence of acute renal insufficiency with potential progression to chronic nephropathy has decreased with current lower dose therapy, but concern remains for a slow, dose-dependent decline in glomerular filtration.[62,72]

Prevention. Because toxicity appears to be dose related, measurement of drug concentrations, and pharmacokinetic and pharmacodynamic evaluations have been used.[73,74] The new microemulsion formulation of cyclosporine, Neoral (Sandoz), which has higher, more consistent bioavailability, may result in more accurate pharmacokinetic predictions and ultimately reduce toxicity.[75] However, the persistent presence of therapeutic or low cyclosporine levels cannot preclude a nephrotoxic effect. Calcium channel blockade dilates glomerular afferent arterioles and prevents acute decreases in renal blood flow and glomerular filtration during short-term use, but these potential protective effects have not been demonstrated during prolonged therapy. Cyclosporine use may also be discontinued after initial induction of immunosuppression to prevent chronic toxicity,[76] but this strategy increases the risk of chronic rejection.[62]

Management. Acute cyclosporine renal insufficiency usually improves with withdrawal of therapy, dose reduction, and treatment of contributing illness or the discontinuation of interacting drugs. Chronic cyclosporine renal failure is usually irreversible, but progressive toxicity may be stopped by discontinuation of cyclosporine therapy or dose reduction with the continuation of prednisone and azathioprine.

Tacrolimus (FK506)

Immunosuppressive therapy with tacrolimus, an agent that inhibits T-lymphocyte interleukin-2 production, causes nephrotoxicity similar to cyclosporine.[77]

Triamterene

Triamterene, a potassium-sparing diuretic, has been associated with transient decreases in creatinine clearance and abnormal urinary sediment in normal subjects and hypertensive patients.[78] In combination with hydrochlorothiazide, triamterene has caused reversible acute renal failure in elderly patients. In combination with indomethacin, triamterene has induced acute renal failure in normal subjects and patients at risk for NSAID nephropathy. A hemodynamic mechanism is most likely as suggested by the apparent increased risk for nephrotoxicity during combined triamterene and indomethacin therapy. Presumably, triamterene causes renal vasoconstriction that is counterbalanced by increased renal synthesis of vasodilatory prostaglandins. Concomitant NSAID therapy may induce renal ischemia by preventing the compensatory increase in renal prostaglandin synthesis. The implications of these observations are unclear because triamterene and NSAIDs are frequently used together without apparent nephrotoxicity.

Propranolol

Propranolol, a nonselective β-adrenergic receptor blocker, reduces renal blood flow 10% to 20% in hypertensive patients.[27] The glomerular filtration rate is less consistently reduced.[27] In contrast, nadolol, another nonselective β-blocker, increases renal blood flow whereas other β-blockers do not appear to alter renal hemodynamics.[79] The mechanism of the propranolol-induced decrease in renal blood flow is unknown. Since renal function does not decrease with other β-blockers, the effect is unlikely to result from blockade of β-receptors or decreased cardiac output. Other postulated mechanisms include renal vasoconstriction due to unopposed α-adrenergic activity or inhibition of renal vasodilator activity, possibly mediated by the kallikrein–kinin system.[27] The clinical significance of these effects is unknown. However, it may be prudent to avoid propranolol therapy in patients with renal insufficiency.

INCREASED VASCULAR PERMEABILITY

OKT3 therapy for the prevention and treatment of acute renal and cardiac allograft rejection is often accompanied by a rise in the serum creatinine concentration that returns toward baseline after 3 to 5 days.[80] Renal biopsy findings of mild interstitial edema or no abnormalities suggest the mechanism is increased vascular permeability due to a renal capillary leak. This renal dysfunction is believed to be part of a cytokine syndrome associated with OKT3 therapy. OKT3 causes lymphocyte activation and release of cytokines, particularly tumor necrosis factor-α, interferon-γ, and interleukins-2 and -6, which may induce secretion of group II secretory phospholipase A_2 as a mediator of nephrotoxicity.[81] Renal function often improves spontaneously despite continued OKT3 therapy.

INCREASED COLLOID ONCOTIC PRESSURE AND BLOOD VISCOSITY

Drugs that alter blood rheology may have renal hemodynamic effects. Thus, intravenous dextran-40 in sufficient quantities to increase plasma oncotic pressure above plasma hydrostatic pressure may reversibly imbalance Starling's forces in the glomerular capillaries and reduce glomerular filtration.[82] Alternatively, renal insufficiency could be due to "osmotic nephrosis" with tubular obstruction from epithelial cell swelling. Dialysis and plasmapheresis can remove dextran, resulting in rapid recovery of renal function.

Epoietin therapy accelerated the loss of renal function in an animal model of progressive renal failure. The proposed mechanism is increased blood viscosity, which exacerbates systemic hypertension and raises glomerular efferent arteriolar resistance, leading to increased glomerular capillary pressure and renal damage.[83] Progressive loss of renal function, however, is not accelerated in humans with chronic renal insufficiency during epoietin therapy, providing systemic blood pressure is controlled and the hematocrit does not rise above normal.[84]

RENAL VASCULITIS, THROMBOSIS, AND CHOLESTEROL EMBOLI

Systemic polyarteritis nodosa, a vasculitis with involvement of small- and medium-sized renal arteries, has been described following methamphetamine abuse.[85] Patients may have hematuria, proteinuria, renal insufficiency, and hypertension. Renal and visceral vascular aneurysms can be demonstrated by angiography. The pathogenesis may be a toxic reaction to methamphetamine or the result of associated hepatitis B infection. Penicillin and sulfonamide therapies have also been considered as causes of polyarteritis nodosa, although these associations have been less clear.[85]

Oral contraceptive agents, cyclosporine, mitomycin C, cisplatin, and quinine can cause a thrombotic microangiopathy (hemolytic–uremic syndrome, thrombotic thrombocytopenic purpura) manifested by endothelial proliferation and thrombus formation in the renal and central nervous system vasculature.[86–88] The association with mitomycin C is notable since the pathogenesis appears to be a direct toxic effect with a predictable incidence: 1.6% in patients receiving less than 50 mg/m^2 and 27.8% in patients receiving more than 70 mg/m^2.[87] Nephrotoxicity has occurred following chemotherapy with mitomycin C alone or with 5-fluorouracil, cisplatin, bleomycin, a Vinca alkaloid, and tamoxifen.[88] Microangiopathic hemolytic anemia and thrombocytopenia are usually present. Systemic endothelial damage with multisystem organ failure has occurred.[88] Renal failure can be severe and irreversible, although corticosteroids, antiplatelet agents, vincristine sulfate, plasma exchange, plasmapheresis, and high-dose intravenous IgG have each induced clinical improvement.

Anticoagulants and thrombolytics, particularly warfarin, can systemically embolize cholesterol particles from aortic atherosclerotic plaques to small arteries and arterioles, including renal arterioles. These agents remove or prevent thrombus formation over ulcerative plaques, causing emboli.[89] Cholesterol emboli induce an inflammatory obliterative vascular response, causing renal ischemia. Purple discoloration of the toes and mottled skin over the legs are important clinical clues.

GLOMERULAR DISEASE: NEPHROTIC SYNDROME AND GLOMERULONEPHRITIS

Glomerular disease involves damage to the glomerular capillary filtration surface. More protein leaks into the urine while the glomerular filtration rate decreases. The nephrotic syndrome, proteinuria greater than 3.5 g/d with or without renal insufficiency, is common. Several different glomerula lesions may occur, mostly by immune mechanisms rather than direct toxicity. Although drug-induced glomerular disease is uncommon, a variety of agents have been implicated.

Minimal change nephrotic syndrome is characterized by normal-appearing glomeruli on light microscopy. Minimal change nephrotic syndrome due to drugs is frequently accompanied by interstitial nephritis and is most common during NSAID therapy.[90] Ampicillin, rifampin, phenytoin, and lithium have also been implicated. The pathogenesis is unknown, but nephrotic-range proteinuria due to NSAID therapy is frequently associated with a T-lymphocytic interstitial infiltrate, suggesting disordered cell-mediated immunity. These cells may release lymphokines that increase glomerular capillary permeability to proteins. Proteinuria usually resolves rapidly after discontinuation of the offending drug. Prednisone therapy, in doses ranging from 0.5 to 1 mg/kg body weight for 2 to 4 weeks, may help resolve the lesion.[91]

Focal segmental glomerulosclerosis is characterized by patchy areas of glomerular sclerosis with interstitial inflammation and fibrosis. Chronic heroin abuse is the most common drug cause of this lesion.[90] The pathogenesis is unknown but may include direct toxicity by heroin or adulterants and injury from bacterial or viral infections accompanying intravenous drug use. End-stage renal failure develops in most cases. No specific therapy is available, although discontinuation of heroin use may prevent progression. Focal segmental glomerulosclerosis is the predominant renal lesion in AIDS patients and may result from human immunodeficiency virus infection or heroin abuse. Glomerulosclerosis due to HIV infection may be distinguished from heroin nephropathy by tuboreticular structures in endothelial cells on electron microscopy and a more rapid course and poorer prognosis. Focal segmental sclerosis has also been attributed to therapy with lithium and α-interferon.[92]

Membranous nephropathy, the most common drug-induced glomerular lesion, is characterized by immune complex deposition along glomerular capillary loops. Parenteral gold is the most common cause, with an incidence of 1% to 10% in patients treated for rheumatoid arthritis.[93] Oral gold therapy has a lesser incidence. The pathogenesis may involve damage to proximal tubule epithelium with antigen release, antibody formation, and glomerular immune complex deposition. Gold has been identified in proximal tubular cells, but not in the glomerular deposits. Genetic factors appear to be important because patients with human leukocyte antigens (HLAs) DR3 or B8 have increased susceptibility. Renal function is preserved and proteinuria resolves 6 to 39 months after discontinuing gold therapy.[93] Similarly, mercury found in diuretics, topical skin preparations, and industrial vapors as well as D-penicillamine cause membranous nephropathy.[90] NSAIDs have also caused membranous nephrotic syndrome, accounting for 10% of membranous nephropathy in adults.[94] The prognosis appears favorable with resolution after discontinuing NSAID use.

Membranoproliferative glomerulonephritis is a rare consequence of drug therapy associated with hydralazine-induced systemic lupus erythematosus.[90] Rapidly progressive or crescentic glomerulonephritis may result from propylthiouracil-induced systemic lupus erythematosus, penicillamine, and combined interleukin-2 and interferon-α use.[90] Proliferative glomerulonephritis may result from chlorpropamide use. Crescentic IgA glomerulonephritis may follow recombinant interleukin-2 therapy. Glomerular amyloidosis occurs with heroin abuse, particularly by subcutaneous injection, causing immune stimulation from chronic skin inflammation.

TUBULAR EPITHELIAL CELL DAMAGE

Renal tubular epithelial cell damage may be caused by either direct toxic or ischemic effects of drugs. Damage localizes in the proximal and distal tubular epithelia. This may be seen as swelling and vacuolization of proximal tubular cells in "osmotic nephrosis" or cellular degeneration and sloughing from proximal and distal tubular basement membranes in "acute tubular necrosis" (ATN). ATN is one of the most common drug manifestations of nephrotoxicity with multiple drugs implicated (see Table 45–4). Urinalysis frequently shows red blood cells, mild proteinuria, and granular casts. Renal insufficiency is usually reversible.

OSMOTIC NEPHROSIS

Several drugs, including mannitol, low-molecular-weight dextran, and radiographic contrast media, or drug vehicles, including sucrose and propylene glycol, have been associated with vacuolization and swelling of proximal tubular epithelial cells and a decline in renal function, possibly due to pinocytosis of the involved drug.[95] Renal function decreases. This osmotic nephrosis may be due to the hypertonic and osmotically active nature of these agents. However, they have not been shown to be actually contained within cellular vacuoles and the pathogenesis is unclear. The largest experience is with mannitol, an osmotic diuretic used to reduce intracranial pressure, treat glaucoma, and prevent acute ischemic or nephrotoxic renal failure.[29] Mannitol may rarely cause oligoanuric renal failure with proximal tubular cell vacuolization on biopsy. Mechanisms include pinocytosis of mannitol into cells, causing swelling and tubular lumen obstruction.[29] Mannitol can also cause direct renal vasoconstriction or induce an osmotic diuresis with increased solute delivery to the macula densa and subsequent tubuloglomerular feedback leading to vasoconstriction of the glomerular afferent arteriole and decreased renal blood flow. Risk factors for mannitol include excessive doses, preexistent renal insufficiency, and concomitant diuretic or cyclosporine ther-

TABLE 45–4. Drugs That Cause Tubular Necrosis

Higher Incidence	Lower Incidence
Acetaminophen (overdose)	Amoxapine
Aminoglycosides	Carboplatin
Amphotericin B	Cyclosporine
Cisplatin	Low-molecular-weight dextran
Radiographic contrast agents	Mannitol
Streptozocin	Methoxyflurane anesthesia
	NSAIDs
	Tetracycline

apy.[29,96] Nephrotoxicity may be prevented by limiting the dose and avoiding dehydration and concomitant diuretic therapy. The serum mannitol concentration should be maintained < 1000 mg/dL (by maintaining the osmolal gap < 55 mOsm/kg water), although an osmolal gap of 20 mOsm/kg water is usually therapeutic.[29,96] Renal function recovers when elevated mannitol concentrations decrease following drug withdrawal or hemodialysis. Mannitol-induced osmotic diuresis and volume depletion could increase the nephrotoxicity of other drugs, particularly NSAIDs, ACE inhibitors, and cyclosporine.[97] Similar to mannitol, intravenous immunoglobulin therapy may cause osmotic nephrosis and acute renal failure, which is rapidly reversible on discontinuing therapy.[98] Immunoglobulin solutions contain hyperosmolar sucrose, which may be pinocytosed into epithelial cells. Toxicity may be prevented by diluting the solution and reducing the rate of infusion. Propylene glycol as a drug vehicle has been similarly implicated.

ACUTE TUBULAR NECROSIS

Aminoglycoside Nephrotoxicity

Incidence. Clinically significant reductions in glomerular filtration have been reported in 5% to 25% of patients during a continued course of aminoglycoside therapy, making these agents an important cause of hospital-acquired renal disease.[4,5,35] Nephrotoxicity is a major contributor to the total cost of aminoglycoside therapy.[18]

Clinical Presentation. A gradual rise in the serum creatinine concentration and decrease in creatinine clearance after 5 to 10 days of therapy are the initial clinical manifestations of toxicity. Increased renal tubular proteinuria (β_2-microglobulin) and brush border enzymuria precede the creatinine rise by several days, but are not usually detected clinically.[26,35] Urine volume less than 500 mL/day is uncommon. Renal magnesium and potassium wasting can occur. Renal failure is usually mild if aminoglycoside therapy is stopped, but may be severe and require dialysis therapy. Aminoglycoside-associated nephropathy must be evaluated carefully since not all renal failure during a course of therapy is due to the aminoglycoside. Dehydration, sepsis, and other nephrotoxic drugs frequently contribute.

Pathogenesis. The pathogenesis of reduced glomerular filtration rate in patients receiving aminoglycosides is predominantly the result of proximal tubular epithelial cell damage leading to obstruction of the tubular lumen and backleak of the glomerular filtrate across the damaged tubular epithelium.[35] The toxicity of various aminoglycosides is directly proportional to the number of their cationic charges. Neomycin, with six cationic amino groups, is the most nephrotoxic whereas streptomycin, with three groups, is least toxic. Gentamicin and tobramycin, with five amino groups, have similar and intermediate toxicity, whereas amikacin and netilmicin, with four and three amino groups, respectively, may be less toxic. Cationic charge facilitates binding of filtered aminoglycosides to renal tubular epithelial cell luminal membranes. This is followed by intracellular transport and concentration in lysosomes.[35] Phospholipids accumulate, as the result of aminoglycoside interaction with negatively charged phospholipids (phosphatidylinositol), which inhibit phospholipase activity.[35] This is seen histopathologically as myeloid bodies within lysosomes of renal tubular epithelial cells. The membrane function of mitochondria and other cell organelles is also affected.[35] Cellular dysfunction and death may result from release of lysosomal enzymes into the cytosol, generation of reactive oxygen species, altered cellular metabolism, and alterations in cell membrane fluidity leading to reduced activity of membrane-bound enzymes, including Na^+/K^+-ATPase, dipeptidyl peptidase IV, and neutral aminopeptidase.[32,35] The administration of polyaspartic acid, an investigational polyanionic peptide, reduces the interaction of aminoglycosides with anionic phospholipids and decreases cell injury.[35]

Risk Factors. Multiple potential risk factors for aminoglycoside nephrotoxicity have been identified. These relate to aminoglycoside dosing, synergistic toxicity in combination with other drugs, and predisposing conditions in the patient (Table 45–5). These risk factors have been variably identified and the reader is referred to the in-depth toxicity reviews.[35,99,100] Although combined vancomycin and aminoglycoside therapy has been considered especially nephrotoxic, a meta-analysis suggests only a 1% to 7% increased risk of toxicity with combination therapy compared to aminoglycoside therapy alone.[101]

Prevention. Nephrotoxicity can be prevented by switching to alternative antibiotics as soon as microbial sensitivities are known. Toxicity may be reduced by avoiding volume depletion, limiting the total dose administered, and avoiding concomitant therapy with other nephrotoxic drugs. The

TABLE 45–5. Potential Risk Factors for Aminoglycoside Nephrotoxicity

A. Related to aminoglycoside dosing:
   - Large total cumulative dose
   - Prolonged therapy
   - High 1-h postdose concentration
   - Trough concentration exceeding 2 mg/L
   - Recent previous aminoglycoside therapy

B. Related to synergistic nephrotoxicity. Aminoglycosides in combination with:
   - Cyclosporine
   - Amphotericin B
   - Vancomycin
   - Diuretics

C. Related to predisposing conditions in the patient:
   - Preexisting renal insufficiency
   - Increased age
   - Poor nutrition
   - Shock
   - Gram-negative bacteremia
   - Liver disease
   - Hypoalbuminemia
   - Obstructive jaundice
   - Dehydration
   - Potassium or magnesium deficiencies

role of therapeutic drug monitoring and pharmacokinetic modeling to prevent nephrotoxicity has not consistently prevented toxicity and remains controversial.[102,103] The primary value of measuring drug levels may be to improve antimicrobial efficacy. Association between elevated trough aminoglycoside levels and nephrotoxicity may be the result, rather than a cause, of toxicity. The specific aminoglycoside used does not appear to affect significantly the risk of nephrotoxicity, and therapy should be selected to optimize antimicrobial effects.

Once-daily dosing of aminoglycosides, used in combination with other antibiotics, has recently been intensively investigated as a practical cost-effective approach to maintain antimicrobial efficacy while potentially reducing nephrotoxicity and ototoxicity.[35,104] Nephrotoxicity may be reduced since proximal tubular aminoglycoside uptake may be limited during the transient, high-peak serum levels due to saturation of binding sites, whereas low aminoglycoside concentrations are then sustained for a longer period during a greater proportion of the dosing interval. Recent meta-analyses suggest greater clinical efficacy and reduced nephrotoxicity with once-daily compared to standard dosing.[104] However, these favorable results are not consistently found,[105] and this approach remains controversial. Seriously ill, immunocompromised, renal-insufficient, and elderly patients are not ideal candidates for this approach.[104] Indeed, increased nephrotoxicity was associated with accompanying high-peak gentamicin and tobramycin levels > 12.0 mg/L in elderly patients.[106]

Management. Serum creatinine concentrations should be measured frequently (every 2 to 4 days) during therapy. Aminoglycoside use should be discontinued as soon as possible once renal function declines. Other nephrotoxic drugs should be discontinued and the patient should be maintained adequately hydrated and hemodynamically stable. Dialysis may be necessary, but renal failure due solely to aminoglycoside toxicity is usually reversible.

Radiographic Contrast Media Nephrotoxicity

Incidence. Intravenous or intra-arterial administration of radiographic contrast media is one of the common causes of hospital-acquired acute renal failure.[4,5] The incidence is < 1% in patients with low risk and occurs most frequently in patients with preexistent renal insufficiency.[37,107] Hospitalized patients with a serum creatinine concentration greater than 1.5 mg/dL have up to a 30 to 40% incidence, whereas those with serum creatinine concentrations greater than 5 mg/dL may have a 70% incidence. Diabetic patients with renal insufficiency have the greatest risk.[37,107] A decrease in renal function following contrast administration may not be due to contrast toxicity since concomitant medical illness and dehydration due to fluid restriction and cathartics used for study preparation may also contribute.[107]

Clinical Presentation. Toxicity ranges from transient tubular enzymuria to irreversible oliguric (urine volume < 500 mL/d) renal failure requiring dialysis therapy.[37,107] Severe toxicity is most frequent in diabetic patients with preexistent severe renal insufficiency. The typical course is an initial transient osmotic diuresis followed by tubular proteinuria and enzymuria. The serum creatinine rises and peaks between 2 and 5 days after exposure with recovery after 4 to 10 days. Oliguria is present in about 50% of cases. No laboratory test is diagnostic and urinalysis reveals only hyaline and granular casts. The urine sodium concentration and fractional excretion of sodium are frequently low.[37,107] Few patients require dialysis therapy and toxicity has generally been considered to be mild and readily reversible. However, in a recent retrospective carefully controlled analysis, a 34% mortality was observed in 174 patients with contrast media-associated acute renal failure (rise in serum creatinine of ≥ 25% from baseline and ≥ 2.0 mg/dL) compared to 7% mortality in a cohort without acute renal failure.[108] Twelve percent required dialysis. Death was attributable to sepsis, respiratory failure, delirium, and bleeding that intensified after the onset of acute renal failure, not untreated renal failure.

Pathogenesis. Contrast nephropathy appears to be due to both direct tubular toxicity and renal ischemia.[28,37,107] Direct tubular toxicity is suggested by renal tubular enzymuria and biopsy findings of proximal tubular epithelial cell vacuolization and acute tubular necrosis. In addition to the direct toxic effects of contrast media, the nonselective proteinuria induced by contrast media may indirectly damage tubular epithelial cells. In contrast to these findings, the low urine sodium concentration and low fractional excretion of sodium frequently observed suggest preserved renal tubular function and participation of renal ischemia more than tubular toxicity. Renal ischemia may result from systemic hypotension associated with contrast injection as well as renal vasoconstriction mediated by imbalance of humoral agents including prostaglandins, adenosine, atrial natriuretic peptide, and endothelin.[37,107,109] Renal ischemia may also result from dehydration due to osmotic diuresis accompanying use of hyperosmolar agents (900 to 1780 mOsm/kg) and increased blood viscosity due to red blood cell crenation and aggregation.

Risk Factors. Preexistent renal insufficiency, particularly diabetic nephropathy with renal insufficiency, is the major risk factor. Conditions associated with decreased renal blood flow, including congestive heart failure and dehydration, also confer risk. The presence of multiple myeloma has been considered a relative contraindication for contrast use, but the risk appears to be associated with concomitant dehydration, renal insufficiency, or hypercalcemia rather than the diagnosis itself. The risk of contrast nephropathy in multiple myeloma is minimal if renal function is normal and patients are well hydrated.[110] Both larger volumes of contrast administration and use of older hyperosmolar contrast agents promote risk in susceptible patients.[37]

Prevention. High-risk patients should be identified, primarily by medical history and indication for the contrast study, but also by prestudy serum creatinine concentrations in selected patients, including older and hospitalized patients.[37] Nephrotoxicity is best prevented in these patients by using alternative imaging procedures (e.g., ultrasound, magnetic resonance imaging, and nuclear medicine scans). If contrast media must be used, the smallest adequate dose should be administered. Dose reduction proportional to the level of renal insufficiency may be protective, but may limit the adequacy of imaging.[111]

The utility of lower osmolar nonionic (iohexol and iopamidol) and ionic (ioxaglate) contrast agents to prevent nephrotoxicity remains unclear. Early studies suggested that these agents had little renal protective effect, but few truly high-risk patients were studied.[37] Subsequent larger, prospective, controlled trials[112] and a meta-analysis[113] indicated reduced nephrotoxicity when these agents are used, especially for patients with preexisting renal insufficiency. The largest prospective trial of 1196 patients revealed that a 0.5-mg/dL or greater rise in plasma creatinine occurred 55% less often in patients with preexisting renal insufficiency and 30% less often in patients with diabetic nephropathy using iohexol compared to diatrizoate.[112] However, use of these newer agents does not eliminate nephrotoxicity and caution must be continued with their use. Because lower osmolar agents are considerably more expensive than older higher osmolar ionic agents, their true cost–benefits remain controversial (Table 45–6). A cost-effective strategy may be to use newer lower osmolar contrast agents in patients with preexisting renal insufficiency, particularly those with diabetic nephropathy, and older higher osmolar contrast agents in patients with normal renal function. Additionally, the newer agents cause less histamine release and may be advantageous for hemodynamically unstable patients or those with a history of hypersensitivity to contrast media. Dialysis to remove contrast media after administration does not appear to prevent toxicity.[37]

Saline hydration for 12 hours before and after contrast administration significantly reduces the incidence of toxicity in high-risk patients.[114] Dehydration should be corrected before contrast administration, other nephrotoxic drugs discontinued, and subsequent contrast studies appropriately delayed to avoid cumulative toxicity. Use of mannitol and furosemide to prevent toxicity remains controversial. Neither mannitol nor furosemide prevented toxicity in one controlled trial,[115] whereas in another, intravenous mannitol, dopamine, or atrial natriuretic peptide ameliorated toxicity in nondiabetic, but not diabetic, patients with renal insufficiency.[116] Calcium channel blockers and intravenous theophylline may also be protective.[37,107]

TABLE 45–6. Considerations for Use of Newer, Lower Osmolar Radiocontrast Agents Compared to Older, Higher Osmolar Ionic Radiocontrast Agents

Advantages:
Less histamine release with fewer allergic or hemodynamic adverse effects
Less nephrotoxicity (30% to 50% decreased incidence in patients with preexisting nondiabetic or diabetic renal insufficiency)
Disadvantage:
Greater than 10-fold higher cost

Management. There is no specific therapy available for established contrast nephropathy. Care is supportive with dialysis as needed in selected patients. Careful attention must be given to preventing infection and bleeding and providing respiratory support in view of the high association of these complications with death in contrast nephropathy.[108]

Cisplatin Nephrotoxicity

Incidence. Cisplatin, an important chemotherapeutic agent, frequently causes renal tubular damage.[36] The incidence of nephrotoxicity during investigational multiple-course therapy was 50% to 100%. Subsequently, the incidence of toxicity decreased to 6% to 13%, primarily by limiting the total drug dose and reducing the rate of administration. However, high dose cisplatin chemotherapy, in combination with other nephrotoxins, appears to contribute to renal failure, which occurs in > 50% of patients who receive a bone marrow transplant for advanced breast cancer.[117]

Clinical Presentation. Nephrotoxicity manifests early during therapy as transient proximal tubular cell brush border and lysosomal enzymuria.[36] Peak serum creatinine concentrations occur approximately 10 to 12 days after initiation of therapy, with recovery by 21 days. However, renal damage can be cumulative with subsequent cycles of therapy and the serum creatinine concentration may continue to rise. Irreversible chronic renal insufficiency may result. Renal magnesium wasting is common and can be accompanied by hypocalcemia and hypokalemia.[36] Hypomagnesemia may be severe, causing seizures, neuromuscular irritability, or personality changes, and persist long after chemotherapy has ended. Hypomagnesemia results primarily from urinary losses due to renal tubular damage as well as magnesuric effects of saline hydration and diuretic therapy to prevent toxicity. Anorexia and diarrhea also contribute.

Pathogenesis. Renal biopsies show sparing of glomeruli with necrosis of both proximal and distal tubules and collecting ducts.[36,118] The mechanism involves cisplatin concentration in renal tissue and impairment of cell energy production, possibly by binding to proximal tubular cellular proteins and sulfhydryl groups with disruption of cell enzyme activity and uncoupling of oxidative phosphorylation.[36,118]

Risk Factors. Risk factors include increased age, dehydration, renal irradiation, and alcohol abuse.[118]

Prevention. Toxicity is best prevented by dose reduction and decreased frequency of administration, usually accomplished by using cisplatin in combination with other chemotherapeutic agents. Vigorous saline hydration is important. Protective roles for furosemide or mannitol diuresis are less clear.[36] Amifostine, an organic thiophosphate that is converted to an active metabolite, chelates cisplatin in normal cells and has been shown to reduce the nephrotoxicity, neurotoxicity, ototoxicity, and myelosuppression associated with cisplatin and carboplatin therapy.[119] Promising investigational techniques have included the use of hypertonic saline to reduce tubular cisplatin uptake, reduced renal exposure for peritoneal tumors by use of localized intraperitoneal administration in conjunction with systemic administration of sodium thiosulfate, a cisplatin neutralizer, and last, use of *N*-acetylcysteine, a sulfhydryl donor.[36,118] Carboplatin, a second-generation platinum analog, is associated with a lower incidence of nephrotoxicity.[36]

Management. Acute renal failure with cisplatin therapy is usually partially reversible with time and supportive care, including dialysis. Progressive chronic renal failure from cumulative toxicity may be less reversible and require chronic dialysis support. Serum magnesium concentrations should be monitored frequently and hypomagnesemia corrected. Hypocalcemia and hypokalemia may be difficult to reverse until hypomagnesemia is corrected.

Amphotericin B Nephrotoxicity

Incidence. The frequency of fungal infections has increased during the last decade due to therapeutic interventions leading to more immunocompromised patients. Amphotericin B remains the antifungal drug of choice for most systemic infections, but dose-dependent nephrotoxicity occurs to varying degrees in most patients.[120] Toxicity is seen initially with cumulative doses as low as 300 to 400 mg and reaches an incidence of 80% when cumulative doses approach 4 g.[121]

Clinical Presentation. Toxicity is often initially manifest by abnormalities of renal tubular function including potassium, sodium, and magnesium wasting into urine, impaired renal ability to concentrate urine, and distal renal tubular acidosis due to a leak of hydrogen ions back out of the tubular lumen.[120] Substantial potassium and magnesium replacement may be necessary. Renal blood flow and glomerular filtration rate decrease independent of or together with renal tubular abnormalities, and result in a rise in serum creatinine and blood urea nitrogen concentrations.[120]

Pathogenesis. Renal pathologic findings include focal vacuolization of small arterial and arteriolar smooth muscle cells, as well as proximal and distal tubular epithelial cell damage. The mechanisms of renal dysfunction include direct tubular epithelial cell toxicity with increased tubular permeability and necrosis, as well as arterial vasoconstriction and ischemic injury.[120] Tubular membrane permeability to solutes such as sodium and potassium increases when amphotericin binds to membranes and acts as an ionophore. Renal vasoconstriction occurs by unclear mechanisms, possibly including direct effects of amphotericin B on cellular calcium fluxes and activation of vasoconstrictor prostaglandins. Overall, the combined effects of increased cell energy and oxygen requirements due to greater cell membrane permeability and reduced cellular oxygen delivery due to renal vasoconstriction results in renal medullary tubular epithelial cell necrosis and renal failure.[34,120]

Risk Factors. Risk factors include baseline renal dysfunction, higher average daily doses, and diuretic use with volume depletion.[120,121] Rapid infusions of amphotericin B have the potential to increase toxicity. Nephrotoxicity of concomitant drug therapy, including effects of cyclosporine, aminoglycosides, and NSAIDs, may also contribute.

Prevention. Nephrotoxicity is best minimized by limiting the cumulative dose and avoiding concomitant administration of other nephrotoxins. Additionally, avoiding volume depletion and providing hydration with a full sodium diet and 1 L intravenous 0.9% sodium chloride daily appears to reduce toxicity.[120,122] Mannitol infusion to induce an osmotic diuresis has not been protective.[120] Pretreatment with a calcium channel blocker may prove useful.[42] Several liposomal amphotericin B formulations are now available and may reduce nephrotoxicity by enhancing drug delivery to sites of infection and away from mammalian cell membranes.[123] As an alternative to the high cost and limited availability of liposomal amphotericin B, investigational administration of amphotericin B in a lipid emulsion was effective and significantly reduced nephrotoxicity as well as fever, rigors, and hypotension in one study,[124] but the overall safety and efficacy remains to be unequivocally established.[125]

Management. Amphotericin nephrotoxicity is best treated by discontinuation of therapy and substitution of alternative antifungal therapy, if possible. Renal tubular dysfunction and glomerular filtration will improve gradually to some degree in most patients, but damage may be irreversible.

Pentamidine Nephrotoxicity

Pentamidine therapy for *Pneumocystis carinii* infections is also limited by nephrotoxicity.[126] Prospective studies have shown azotemia in 60% to 90% of treated patients.[127] Hyperkalemia, metabolic acidosis, hypomagnesemia, and hypocalcemia may also occur. Toxicity is more frequent in patients with AIDS than patients without this immune deficiency and may be accentuated by concomitant amphotericin B therapy.[128] The mechanism of toxicity is unknown, but tubular degeneration has been seen histopathologically. The primary alternative therapy for *P. carinii,* trimethoprim–sulfamethoxazole, may also cause renal dysfunction due to allergic interstitial nephritis and inhibition of tubular secretion of creatinine, but the incidence is lower than with pentamidine.[127]

Foscarnet Nephrotoxicity

Foscarnet, an antiviral pyrophosphate analog used in AIDS and other immunosuppressed patients to treat cytomegalovirus (CMV) retinitis and life-threatening CMV infections, appears to be highly nephrotoxic.[127] As many as 65% of patients treated with foscarnet develop renal insufficiency or electrolyte disturbances including hypokalemia, hypocalcemia, hypomagnesemia, and hypo- or hyperphosphatemia.[129] The mechanism appears to be renal tubular necrosis. Vigorous isotonic saline hydration throughout the course of therapy may prevent nephrotoxicity. In addition, cidofovir, a potent nucleotide analog administered intravenously for CMV infection in AIDS patients, has been associated with renal proximal tubular cell injury and renal failure.[130] Probenecid blocks renal tubular epithelial cell uptake of cidofovir and when combined with saline hydration can reduce the incidence of nephrotoxicity.

TUBULOINTERSTITIAL DISEASE

These diseases involve the renal tubules and their surrounding interstitial tissue. The presentation may be "acute" and reversible with interstitial inflammatory cell infiltrates, rapid loss of renal function, and systemic symptoms of fever or rash, or "chronic" and irreversible with interstitial fibrosis, slow loss of renal function, and no systemic symptoms. Papillary necrosis, a variant of chronic interstitial nephritis, originates deep in the renal medulla and papillae.

ACUTE ALLERGIC INTERSTITIAL NEPHRITIS

Incidence. Allergic interstitial nephritis (AIN) is common and the underlying cause for 3% to 14% of all cases of acute renal failure.[131] Multiple drugs have been implicated (Table 45–7).

Clinical Presentation. Methicillin allergic interstitial nephritis is the prototype for most presentations of AIN.[131] Clinical signs present 17 days (range 2 to 44 days) after initiation of therapy and include (with their approximate incidence) fever (75%), maculopapular rash (25%), eosinophilia (80%), pyuria and hematuria (90%), low-level proteinuria (90%), and oliguria (18%). Eosinophiluria, an important marker of drug-induced AIN, is frequently absent,[131] possibly due to fragility of eosinophils in urine and inadequate laboratory methodology. Anemia, leukocytosis, and elevated IgE levels may occur. Tubular dysfunction may be manifested by acidosis, hyperkalemia, salt wasting, and concentrating defects.

TABLE 45–7. Commonly Used Drugs That Cause Allergic Interstitial Nephritis

Antibiotics	**Miscellaneous**
Acyclovir	Acetaminophen
Aminoglycosides	Allopurinol
Amphotericin B	Interferon-α
Aztreonam	Aspirin
Cephalosporins	Captopril
Ciprofloxacin	Cimetidine
Erythromycin	Clofibrate
Ethambutol	Cyclosporine
Penicillins	Glyburide
Polymyxin B	Gold
Rifampin	Methyldopa
Sulfonamides	*p*-Aminosalicylic acid
Tetracyclines	Phenylpropanolamine
Trimethoprim–sulfamethoxazole	Propylthiouracil
Vancomycin	Radiographic contrast media
Neuropsychiatric	Ranitidine
Carbamazepine	Sulfinpyrazone
Lithium	Warfarin sodium
Phenobarbital	
Phenytoin	
Valproic acid	
Nonsteroidal anti-inflammatory drugs	
Diuretics	
Acetazolamide	
Amiloride	
Chlorthalidone	
Furosemide	
Triamterene	
Thiazides	

Fenoprofen-allergic interstitial nephritis, the prototype for NSAID-induced AIN, has a different clinical presentation.[91] Patients are older (reflecting NSAID use for degenerative joint disease) and the onset is delayed, a mean of 5.4 months from initiation of therapy. Systemic signs of an allergic reaction (rash, fever, and eosinophilia) are infrequent, occurring in only 19% of cases. Concomitant nephrotic syndrome (proteinuria greater than 3.5 g/d) due to minimal-change glomerulopathy is characteristic.

Cytokine therapies have caused hemodynamically mediated renal insufficiency due to a sepsis-like syndrome and systemic capillary leak.[36] Acute interstitial infiltrates have been reported during leukocyte A interferon therapy for mycosis fungoides, interleukin-2 (IL-2) and lymphokine-activated killer (LAK) cell immunotherapy for cancer and combination therapy with human alpha interferon and granulocyte colony-stimulating factor (rhG-CSF).[132]

Prompt diagnosis of allergic interstitial nephritis is important to stop the offending drug and prevent irreversible renal damage. Systemic hypersensitivity findings of fever, rash, eosinophilia, and eosinophiluria suggest the diagnosis, but these findings are not reliable since one or more are frequently absent. Renal biopsy is the most specific method for diagnosis but is usually not possible in acutely ill patients. Gallium-67 renal imaging is a sensitive diagnostic technique, but is nonspecific and of limited usefulness since acute pyelonephritis, nil lesion nephrotic syndrome, and cholesterol embolization also give positive scans.[131]

Pathogenesis. The pathology of allergic interstitial nephritis is a diffuse or focal interstitial infiltrate of lymphocytes, plasma cells, eosinophils, and occasional polymorphonuclear neutrophils.[131] Granulomas and tubular epithelial cell necrosis, are relatively common with drug-induced AIN. The pathogenesis is an allergic hypersensitivity response.[131,133] Occasionally a humoral antibody-mediated mechanism is implicated by the presence of circulating antibody to a drug hapten–tubular basement membrane complex, low serum complement levels, and deposition of IgG and complement in the tubular basement membrane. More commonly, a cell-mediated immune mechanism is suggested by the absence of these findings and the presence of a predominantly T-lymphocyte infiltrate with an increased helper to suppressor cell ratio. In particular, NSAID interstitial nephritis involves T lymphocytes, possibly in response to altered prostaglandin synthesis.

Risk Factors. No specific risk factors have been identified because these are idiosyncratic hypersensitivity reactions.

Individuals with other drug allergies may have increased risk and warrant close monitoring. Slow acetylators may be predisposed to idiosyncratic sulfonamide hypersensitivity, including AIN.[134]

Prevention. No specific prevention is known due to the idiosyncratic nature of these reactions. Patients must be monitored carefully during drug treatments to recognize adverse effects and discontinue therapy promptly.

Management. No prospective treatment trials have been reported. However, prednisone therapy in a dose of 0.5 to 1 mg/kg body weight for 1 to 4 weeks has been used and may improve the rate and extent of renal recovery.[131]

CHRONIC INTERSTITIAL NEPHRITIS

Lithium, cyclosporine, and few other drugs can cause chronic interstitial nephritis, which is usually a progressive and irreversible lesion. Streptozotocin and other antineoplastic nitrosoureas also cause dose-dependent chronic interstitial disease.[36] Lastly, mesalazine, 5-aminosalicylic acid, and ifosfamide may cause chronic interstitial nephritis, which can reverse when drug use is discontinued promptly.[36]

Lithium

Incidence. Several renal tubular lesions have been associated with lithium therapy, most common is an impaired ability to concentrate urine (nephrogenic diabetes insipidus), which has been seen in approximately 20% to 70% of patients. Acute tubular necrosis, and chronic tubulointerstitial nephritis, are less frequently noted and incomplete distal renal tubular acidosis is rarely reported.[135] The most important question for lithium use is whether long-term lithium therapy, with lithium levels maintained in the therapeutic range, causes chronic tubulointerstitial nephritis with renal insufficiency. While mild nonprogressive renal insufficiency has been reported in 10% or more of patients during long-term therapy, the role for lithium has not been established since occurrences have been infrequent and studies suggesting nephrotoxicity were frequently uncontrolled.[135] Chronic toxicity is also questioned since renal function has not declined during short- and long-term lithium therapy in studies when lithium levels have been maintained in the therapeutic range.[136]

Clinical Presentation. Patients with nephrogenic diabetes insipidus often have polydipsia and polyuria. They adapt well to their urinary-concentrating defect and these concerns are usually minimal. Acute tubular necrosis is frequent in the setting of acute lithium toxicity. The patient is generally asymptomatic. Urinalysis may show moderate proteinuria, a few red and white blood cells, and granular casts. Renal function is usually reversible after lithium levels are reduced to the therapeutic range. Chronic renal insufficiency may develop insidiously and be recognized by rising BUN or creatinine concentrations or the onset of hypertension. The urinalysis may show mild proteinuria, and a few red and white blood cells.

Pathogenesis. Impaired ability to concentrate urine is due to a dose-related decrease in collecting duct response to antidiuretic hormone. This results from impaired formation of cellular cAMP in response to antidiuretic hormone. Lithium-induced acute renal failure occurs predominantly during episodes of acute lithium intoxication.[135] The pathogenesis includes dehydration secondary to nephrogenic diabetes insipidus as well as direct proximal and distal tubular cell toxicity. Chronic tubulointerstitial nephritis attributed to lithium is evidenced by biopsy findings of interstitial fibrosis, focal tubular atrophy, and glomerular sclerosis.[135] The pathogenesis may involve cumulative damage from lithium-induced acute tubular necrosis. Alternatively, cumulative direct lithium toxicity may occur since duration of therapy has correlated with the decline in the glomerular filtration rate. Finally, some patients may have increased susceptibility to lithium toxicity. Although the reason for this is unknown, this could explain the difficulty in characterizing the nephrotoxic effects of chronic lithium therapy.

Risk Factors. The major risk factor for acute renal failure is an elevated lithium level, particularly in association with dehydration. Concomitant therapy with neuroleptic agents[135] and ACE inhibitors[137] may contribute. Chronic nephrotoxicity may result from cumulative damage due to repeated episodes of acute renal injury.

Prevention. Prevention of acute and chronic toxicity includes maintaining lithium levels as low as therapeutically possible, avoiding dehydration, and monitoring renal function. It is unknown whether progression to severe renal failure can be prevented by stopping lithium use when mild renal insufficiency is first recognized. This poses a dilemma since lithium is highly effective for affective disorders and the risks and potential benefits of discontinuing such a beneficial drug need to be carefully considered. However, if lithium therapy is continued, renal insufficiency must be monitored and therapy discontinued if renal function continues to decline.

Management. Symptomatic polyuria and polydipsia can be reversed by discontinuation of lithium therapy or ameliorated with amiloride or NSAIDs during continued lithium therapy.[138] Acute renal failure is usually reversible with supportive care, including dialysis to reduce toxic blood lithium concentrations. Progressive chronic interstitial nephritis is treated by discontinuation of lithium therapy, adequate hydration, and avoidance of other nephrotoxic agents.

Cyclosporine

Cyclosporine causes both acute hemodynamically mediated renal failure (see section on Hemodynamically Mediated Renal Failure) and chronic interstitial nephritis after 6 to 12 months of therapy. This can result in irreversible renal insufficiency and biopsy findings of arteriolar hyalinosis, glomerular sclerosis, and a striped pattern of interstitial fibrosis.[62,69] Chronic cyclosporine toxicity has become the more important of these two entities since reduced cyclosporine dosages and monitoring of drug levels has decreased acute toxicity. Chronic interstitial nephritis has been a major concern for therapy since as many as 10% of cardiac transplant patients developed end-stage renal failure with prolonged high dose therapy,[62] and most psoriasis patients developed interstitial nephritis and decreased renal function with long-term therapy.[64] The pathogenesis appears to involve sustained renal arteriolar endothelial cell injury causing chronic renal ischemia.[69] Cyclosporine may also induce synthesis and accumulation of interstitial matrix, apparently due to increased activity of cytokines, peptide growth factors, or thromboxane.[62] Nephrotoxicity has been dose-dependent in some, but not all analyses,[69] and occurs even following low-dose therapy. The risk of chronic interstitial renal disease appears to be reduced in those receiving low dose therapy.[72]

PAPILLARY NECROSIS

Analgesic Nephropathy

Incidence. "Classic" analgesic or "phenacetin" nephropathy was initially reported from Switzerland in 1953 and was subsequently recognized as a worldwide public health concern. The incidence of end-stage renal failure is quite variable, and ranges from 36% in central Europe and Australia, to 13% in North Carolina and 1% to 2% in the Northeast United States.[139] Chronic excessive consumption of combination analgesics, particularly those containing phenacetin, was believed to be the major cause and led to the removal of phenacetin and phenacetin mixtures from most world markets. Contemporary analgesics, aspirin, acetaminophen, and NSAIDs, alone or in combinations, may also potentially result in chronic tubulointerstitial disease with papillary necrosis.[140] Analgesic nephropathy is difficult to recognize and may be underdiagnosed as a cause of end-stage renal failure.

Analgesic use is the most common cause of papillary necrosis, accounting for 36% of all cases of papillary necrosis.[141] High-dose dapsone, used to treat *P. carinii* infections in AIDS patients, also causes papillary necrosis.[142]

Clinical Presentation. Analgesic nephropathy evolves insidiously over years. The most sensitive and specific diagnostic criteria include (1) a history of chronic daily "habitual" analgesic ingestion (classically this equated to a cumulative phenacetin ingestion of 3 kg or more), (2) intravenous pyelography, renal ultrasound, or renal computerized tomography imaging, which reveals decreased renal mass and bumpy renal contours, and (3) papillary calcifications.[143] Frequently, however, imaging only demonstrates "chronic pyelonephritis," small kidneys with thin renal cortices and blunted calyces. Analgesics are taken most commonly for chronic headaches.[144] Women are affected more than men. Upper gastrointestinal irritation from analgesics with blood loss leading to anemia has been characteristic. Hypertension and atherosclerotic cardiovascular disease are common. Early renal manifestations include impaired maximal urinary concentration, sterile pyuria, microscopic hematuria, and low levels of proteinuria. Urinary tract infection is common. Creatinine clearance declines slowly. Renal biopsy reveals nonspecific chronic interstitial inflammation and scarring. The incidence of lower urinary tract transitional cell carcinoma is increased with heavy phenacetin use.

Pathogenesis. Mechanisms of analgesic nephropathy remain unclear and have been difficult to study since the evolving lesion is not easily recognized in humans due to lack of diagnostic markers and since animal models have been difficult to establish. The increased risk with analgesic mixtures containing phenacetin or acetaminophen and salicylates or NSAIDs is based on the following observations.[144,145] The renal lesion begins in the papillary tip as a result of accumulated toxic metabolites, decreased blood flow, and impaired cellular energy production. The metabolism of phenacetin to acetaminophen, which is then oxidized to toxic free radicals that are concentrated in the papilla, appears to be the initiating factor that causes toxicity by mechanisms analogous to acetaminophen hepatotoxicity. Toxicity is prevented by availability of reduced glutathione. However, salicylates deplete renal glutathione and thereby facilitate phenacetin and acetaminophen toxicity. In addition, renal medullary and papillary ischemia may contribute due to decreased synthesis of vasodilatory renal prostaglandins by salicylates and NSAIDs. Evidence for nephrotoxicity from chronic ingestion of single analgesics, acetaminophen or NSAIDs alone, challenge these concepts.[146,147]

Risk Factors. The epidemiology of analgesic use and analgesic nephropathy continues to evolve.[140] The classic concept persists that risk for end-stage renal disease increases with cumulative consumption of combination analgesics, phenacetin, or acetaminophen and aspirin or NSAIDs. Caffeine contained in combination analgesics may increase risk, but the role is not clear.[145] Chronic use of therapeutic doses of NSAIDs alone, but not aspirin or salicylates alone, can cause analgesic nephropathy with end-stage renal failure.[146,148] Case-control studies have associated high-dose acetaminophen use alone with an increased risk for end-stage renal disease. However, these associations remain inconclusive due to study design flaws and since acetaminophen has been the preferentially prescribed analgesic for renal-insufficient patients.[149]

Prevention. Prevention has depended primarily on public health efforts to restrict the sale of phenacetin and combination analgesics. This has effectively reduced analgesic nephropathy in Australia and Europe. However, risk continues with continued availability of OTC combination analgesics containing aspirin, acetaminophen, and caffeine in the United States and throughout the world. The recommendations of the National Kidney Foundation have recently been summarized and reviewed.[150]

Individuals requiring chronic analgesic therapy may reduce risk by limiting the total dose, avoiding combined use of two or more analgesics, and maintaining good hydration to prevent renal ischemia and decrease the papillary concentration of toxic substances. Acetaminophen remains the preferred nonopiate analgesic for renal-insufficient patients.

Management. Treatment of established nephrotoxicity requires cessation of analgesic consumption. This can prevent progression and may improve renal function. Persistent surreptitious analgesic abuse should be considered if renal function continues to decline. Patients should also be monitored for associated transitional cell carcinoma of the renal pelvis, calyces, ureters, and bladder, which may present years after analgesic nephropathy is diagnosed.

OBSTRUCTIVE NEPHROPATHY

Obstructive nephropathy is the result of mechanical obstruction to urine flow following glomerular filtration. This may be due to intratubular obstruction from crystal precipitation within the tubules of the kidney or extrarenal obstruction of the ureters or bladder. Pain, renal failure, hematuria, and infection may result.

RENAL TUBULAR OBSTRUCTION

Drug-induced acute renal failure due to renal tubular obstruction can be caused by intratubular precipitation of tissue degradation products as well as by drugs or their metabolites. Acute uric acid nephropathy following chemotherapy, usually for hematologic malignancies, is the most common cause of renal failure due to obstruction by tissue degradation products. Acute oliguric or anuric renal failure develops rapidly. The diagnosis is supported by a urine uric acid to creatinine ratio greater than one. Uric acid precipitation can be prevented by pretreatment hydration, urinary alkalinization to pH 7.0, and allopurinol. Uric acid nephropathy was also observed at the initiation of therapy with ticrynafen, a uricosuric diuretic, and suprofen, a uricosuric NSAID, both of which share a similar chemical structure and are no longer available in the United States.[151]

Drug-induced muscle necrosis, nontraumatic rhabdomyolysis, is an important cause of acute renal failure due, in part, to intratubular precipitation of myoglobin. Drug-induced rhabdomyolysis may result from pressure necrosis during stupor or coma following alcohol or heroin abuse[152]; extreme neuromuscular stimulation and metabolic demands with abuse of phencyclidine[153] or therapy with adrenergic agents, including terbutaline[154]; and vasoconstriction and muscle ischemia due to abuse of cocaine[155] or therapeutic vasopressin infusion.[156] Rhabdomyolysis has also occurred during lovastatin therapy for hypercholesterolemia,[157] particularly in a dose-dependent association with cyclosporine therapy, but also with use of erythromycin, gemfibrozil, or niacin and other substrates for the CYP3A4 metabolic pathway. Toxicity appears to be secondary to the accumulation of myotoxic levels of lovastatin as the result of the competitive inhibition of lovastatin metabolism.

Precipitation of drugs or their metabolites in concentrated acidic urine has been an important cause of acute renal failure, particularly with previous generations of sulfonamides. Though this problem is rare with the currently used more soluble sulfonamides, it may occur during acetazolamide therapy[158] and has become more frequent with the resurgence of sulfadiazine therapy for toxoplasmosis in AIDS patients.[159] Methotrexate and its less soluble metabolite, 7-hydroxymethotrexate, also precipitate in acid urine and can cause oligoanuric renal failure during high-dose chemotherapy.[36] Intravenous and high-dose oral acyclovir therapy for acute herpes zoster has caused renal insufficiency, possibly by intratubular precipitation in dehydrated oliguric patients.[160] This can be diagnosed by the presence of birefringent needle-shaped crystals within leukocytes using polarized light microscopy. Massive administration of ascorbic acid can also result in obstruction of renal tubules with calcium oxalate crystals.[161] Oxalate, a poorly soluble ascorbic acid metabolite, can also precipitate and worsen renal function when ascorbic acid is administered to patients with acute renal failure or the congenital nephrotic syndrome. Oxalate precipitation may also contribute to renal failure induced by methoxyflurane, although proximal tubular necrosis due to fluoride toxicity is predominant in the pathogenesis.[162] Low-molecular-weight dextran therapy for volume expansion and rheologic effects has also caused renal failure, possibly by intratubular precipitation of filtered dextran.[163] Triamterene may also precipitate in renal tubules and cause renal failure.[164] Renal failure due to intratubular precipitation of most tissue-degradation products or drugs and their metabolites can be largely prevented and possibly treated by maintaining a high urine volume and urinary alkalinization.

Therapeutic agents not intended for systemic administration can cause renal failure in rare cases, apparently by intratubular or intrarenal precipitation. Severe hyperphosphatemia following administration of a hypertonic phosphate enema further reduced renal function in a renal-insufficient patient, possibly by intratubular precipitation of calcium phosphate.[165]

EXTRARENAL URINARY TRACT OBSTRUCTION

Drug therapy may also cause renal insufficiency due to lower urinary tract obstruction. Ureteral obstruction can be caused by calculi or retroperitoneal fibrosis. Bladder dysfunction with urinary outflow obstruction can result, particularly in males with prostatic hypertrophy, from anticholinergic drugs, including tricyclic antidepressants. In particular, disopyramide phosphate, an antiarrhythmic with anticholinergic effects, has caused acute renal failure due to urinary retention.[166] Bladder outlet and ureteral obstruction may result from bladder fibrosis following hemorrhagic cystitis with cyclophosphamide or ifosfamide therapy. Mesna cotherapy can prevent cystitis and this complication.

NEPHROLITHIASIS

Nephrolithiasis refers to formation of kidney stones. This is not true nephrotoxicity since renal failure does not usually occur. Nevertheless, nephrolithiasis from drug therapy represents abnormal crystal precipitation in the renal collecting system potentially causing pain, hematuria, infection, or urinary tract obstruction with renal failure.

Renal calculus formation, possibly also accompanied by intratubular precipitation of crystalline material, has been a rare complication of drug therapy. Until the AIDS era, triamterene had been the drug most frequently associated with renal calculus formation with an incidence approximating 1 in 1500 users of triamterene-hydrochlorothiazide.[78] However, it has been unclear whether triamterene or its metabolites actually cause stone formation or are passively absorbed onto the organic matrix of preexisting calculi. Currently, sulfadiazine, a poorly soluble sulfonamide used to treat *Toxoplasma gondii* infection in AIDS patients, has caused symptomatic acetylsulfadiazine crystalluria with calculus formation and flank or back pain, hematuria, or renal insufficiency in 1.9% to 7.5% of AIDS patients.[167] A high urine volume and urinary alkalinization to pH > 7.15 may be protective. Similarly, the protease inhibitor indinavir has been associated with crystalluria, dysuria, urinary frequency, back and flank pain, or nephrolithiasis in approximately 10% of AIDS patients.[168] Acute renal failure due to intratubular precipitation of crystalline indinavir and collecting system obstruction from nephrolithiasis have occurred.[169] Since indinavir is more water soluble at acid pH, urine acidification could be protective, but is not practical. Maintaining a high urine volume may be most protective. Uricosuric agents, such as streptozotocin,[170] may cause uric acid stones and renal failure due to urinary obstruction. Allopurinol may rarely cause xanthine, hypoxanthine, and oxypurinol stones during therapy for conditions having excess uric acid production: such as Lesch–Nyhan syndrome and chemotherapy of lymphosarcoma.[171] Allopurinol inhibits xanthine oxidase and increases the urinary excretion of poorly soluble xanthine, hypoxanthine, and oxypurinol. Massive ingestion of magnesium trisilicate-aluminum hydroxide for gastric symptoms has been associated with magnesium ammonium phosphate (struvite) stone formation, possibly due to hypermagnesuria and increased urinary pH.[172] Laxative abuse may lead to the unusual formation of ammonium urate stones, possibly due to increased urinary pH and ammonium concentration.[173]

▶ PRINCIPLES OF PHARMACOTHERAPY

- Know the potential nephrotoxicity of diagnostic and therapeutic pharmacologic agents.
- Compare the potential risks and expected benefits for each course of treatment.
- Consider alternative diagnostic and therapeutic approaches.
- Use the lowest dose and shortest course of therapy that is efficacious.
- Monitor appropriately for potential toxicity.
- Modify therapy if toxicity occurs.

REFERENCES

1. Hricik DE, Dunn MJ. Angiotensin-converting enzyme inhibitor-induced renal failure: Causes, consequences and diagnostic uses. J Am Soc Nephrol 1991;1:845–858.
2. Lewis EJ, Hunsicker LG, Bain RP, et al. The effect of angiotensin-converting-enzyme inhibition on diabetic nephropathy. N Engl J Med 1993;329:1456–1462.
3. Leape LL, Brennan TA, Laird N, et al. The nature of adverse events in hospitalized patients. Results of the Harvard medical practice study II. N Engl J Med 1991;324:377–384.
4. Hou SH, Bushinsky DA, Wish JB, et al. Hospital-acquired renal insufficiency: A prospective study. Am J Med 1983;74:243–248.
5. Davidman M, Olson P, Kohen J, et al. Iatrogenic renal disease. Arch Intern Med 1991;151:1809–1812.
6. Thadhani R, Pascual M, Bonventre JV. Acute renal failure. N Engl J Med 1996;334:1448–1460.
7. Hoitsma AJ, Welzels JFM, Koene AP. Drug induced nephrotoxicity. Aetiology, clinical features and management. Drug Saf 1991;6:131–147.
8. Sturrock NDC, Struthers AD. Non-steroidal anti-inflammatory drugs and angiotensin converting enzyme inhibitors: A commonly prescribed combination with variable effects on renal function. Br J Clin Pharmacol 1993;35:343–348.
9. Strom BL, Tugwell P. Pharmacoepidemiology: Current status, prospects, and problems. Ann Intern Med 1990;113:179–181.
10. Gutthan SP, Rodriguez LAG, Raiford DS, Oliart AD, Romeu JR. Nonsteroidal anti-inflammatory drugs and risk of hospitalization for acute renal failure. Arch Intern Med 1996;156:2433–2439.
11. Evans JMM, McGregor E, McMahon AD, et al. Non-steroidal anti-inflammatory drugs and hospitalization for acute renal failure. Q J Med 1995;88:551–557.
12. Mann JFE, Goerig M, Brune K, Luft FC. Ibuprofen as an over-the-counter drug: Is there a risk for renal injury? Clin Nephrol 1993;39:1–6.
13. Whelton A. Renal effects of over-the-counter analgesics. J Clin Pharmacol 1995;35:454–463.
14. Kaufman J, Dhakal M, Patel B, Hamburger R. Community-acquired acute renal failure. Am J Kidney Dis 1991;17:191–198.
15. Wasser WG, Feldman NS. Chronic renal failure after ingestion of over-the-counter chromium picolinate. Ann Intern Med 1997;126:410.
16. Lo JC, Chertow GM, Rennke H, Seifter JL. Fanconi's syndrome and tubulointerstitial nephritis in association with L-lysine ingestion. Am J Kidney Dis 1996;28:614–617.
17. Vanherweghem J-L, Abramowicz D, Tielemans C, Depierreux M. Effects of steroids on the progression of renal failure in chronic interstitial renal fibrosis: A pilot study in Chinese herbs nephropathy. Am J Kidney Dis 1996;27:209–215.
18. Eisenberg JM, Koffer H, Glick HA, et al. What is the cost of nephrotoxicity associated with aminoglycosides? Ann Intern Med 1987;107:900–909.
19. Jacobson PD, Rosenquist CJ. The introduction of low-osmolar contrast agents in radiology. Medical, economic, legal, and public policy issues. JAMA 1988;260:1586–1592.
20. Powe NR, Steinberg EP, Erickson JE, et al. Contrast medium-induced adverse reactions: Economic outcome. Radiology 1988;169:163–168.
21. Bettmann MA. Guidelines for use of low-osmolality contrast agents. Radiology 1989;172:901–903.
22. Cochran ST. Determination of serum creatinine level prior to administration of radiographic contrast media. JAMA 1997;277:517–518.
23. McGoldrick MD, Bailie GR. Nonnarcotic analgesics: Prevalence and estimated economic impact of toxicities. Ann Pharmacother 1997;31:221–227.
24. Guignard J-P. Effect of drugs on the immature kidney. Adv Nephrol Necker Hosp 1993;22:193–211.

25. Price RG. The role of NAG (*N*-acetyl-beta-D-glucosaminidase) in the diagnosis of kidney disease including the monitoring of nephrotoxicity. Clin Nephrol 1992;38(suppl 1):S14–S19.
26. Schardijn GHC, Statius van Eps LW. β_2-Microglobulin: its significance in the evaluation of renal function. Kidney Int 1987;32: 635–641.
27. Epstein M, Oster JR. Beta blockers and renal function: A reappraisal. J Clin Hypertens 1985;1:85–99.
28. Porter GA. Effects of contrast agents on renal function. Invest Radiol 1993;28(suppl 5):S1–S5.
29. Dorman HR, Sondheimer JH, Cadnapaphornchai P. Mannitol-induced acute renal failure. Medicine 1990;69:153–159.
30. Bennett WM. Drug interactions and consequences of sodium restriction. Am J Clin Nutr 1997;65(suppl):678S–681S.
31. Schnellmann RG. Pathophysiology of nephrotoxic cell injury. In: Schrier RW, Gottschalk CW, eds. Diseases of the Kidney, 6th ed. Boston, Little, Brown, 1997:1049–1067.
32. Baliga R, Ueda N, Walker PD, Shah SV. Oxidant mechanisms in toxic acute renal failure. Am J Kidney Dis 1997;29:465–477.
33. Duggin GG. Combination analgesic-induced kidney disease: The Australian experience. Am J Kidney Dis 1996;28:S39–S47.
34. Brezis M, Rosen S. Hypoxia of the renal medulla—Its implications for disease. N Engl J Med 1995;332:647–655.
35. Swan SK. Aminoglycoside nephrotoxicity. Semin Nephrol 1997;17: 27–33.
36. Berns JS, Ford PA. Renal toxicities of antineoplastic drugs and bone marrow transplantation. Semin Nephrol 1997;17:54–66.
37. Rudnick MR, Berns JS, Cohen RM, Goldfarb S. Contrast media-associated nephrotoxicity. Semin Nephrol 1997;17:15–26.
38. Ali H. Renal disease in the elderly. Postgrad Med 1996;100:44–57.
39. Antillon M, Cominelli F, Lo S, et al. Effects of oral prostaglandins on indomethacin-induced renal failure in patients with cirrhosis and ascites. J Rheumatol 1990;7(suppl 20):46–49.
40. Brouhard BH, Baetz-Greenwalt B. Calcium-channel blocking agents as therapy for amphotericin B nephrotoxicity. Cleve Clin J Med 1992;59:263–264.
41. Lafayette RA, Perrone RD, Levey AS. Laboratory evaluation of renal function. In: Schrier RW, Gottschalk CW, eds. Diseases of the Kidney, 6th ed. Boston, Little, Brown, 1997:307–354.
42. Collen MJ, Howard JM, McArthur KE, et al. Comparison of ranitidine and cimetidine in the treatment of gastric hypersecretion. Ann Intern Med 1984;100:52–58.
43. Van Acker BAC, Koomen GCM, Koopman MG, et al. Creatinine clearance during cimetidine administration for measurement of glomerular filtration rate. Lancet 1992;340:1326–1329.
44. Saine DR, Ahrens ER. Renal impairment associated with losartan. Ann Intern Med 1996;124:775.
45. Davidson RA, Wilcox CS. Newer tests for the diagnosis of renovascular disease. JAMA 1992;268:3353–3358.
46. Oster JR, Materson BJ. Renal and electrolyte complications of congestive heart failure and effects of therapy with angiotensin-converting enzyme inhibitors. Arch Intern Med 1992;152:704–710.
47. Bergamo RR, Cominelli F, Kopple JD, Zipser RD. Comparative acute effects of aspirin, diflunisal, ibuprofen and indomethacin on renal function in healthy man. Am J Nephrol 1989;9:460–463.
48. Ruilope LM, Robles RG, Paya C, et al. Effects of long-term treatment with indomethacin on renal function. Hypertension 1986;8:677–684.
49. Murray MD, Brater DC, Tierney WM, et al. Ibuprofen-associated renal impairment in a large general internal medicine practice. Am J Med Sci 1990;299:222–229.
50. Whelton A, Stout RL, Spilman PS, Klassen DK. Renal effects of ibuprofen, piroxicam, and sulindac in patients with asymptomatic renal failure: A prospective, randomized, crossover comparison. Ann Intern Med 1990;112:568–576.
51. Schoch PH, Ranno A, North DS. Acute renal failure in an elderly woman following intramuscular ketorolac administration. Ann Pharmacother 1992;26:1233–1236.
52. Feldman HI, Kinman JL, Berlin JA, et al. Parenteral ketorolac: The risk for acute renal failure. Ann Intern Med 1997;126:193–199.
53. O'Callaghan CA, Andrews PA, Ogg CS. Renal disease and use of topical non-steroidal anti-inflammatory drugs. Br Med J 1994;308: 110–111.
54. Gurwitz JH, Avorn J, Ross-Degnan D, Lipsitz LA. Nonsteroidal anti-inflammatory drug-associated azotemia in the very old. JAMA 1990; 264:471–475.
55. Solomon DH, Gurwitz JH. Toxicity of nonsteroidal anti-inflammatory drugs in the elderly: Is advanced age a risk factor? Am J Med 1997;102:208–215.
56. Aronoff GR. Therapeutic implications associated with renal studies of nabumetone. J Rheumol 1992;19(suppl 36):25–31.
57. Stichtenoth DO, Wagner B, Frolich JC. Effects of meloxicam and indomethacin on cyclooxygenase pathways in healthy volunteers. J Invest Med 1997;45:44–49.
58. DeWitt DL, Meade EA, Smith WL. PGH synthase isoenzyme selectivity: The potential for safer nonsteroidal antiinflammatory drugs. Am J Med 1993;95(suppl 2A):40S–44S.
59. Dunn MJ. The roles of angiotensin II and prostaglandins in the regulation of the glomerular filtration of albumin. J Hypertens 1990;8 (suppl 1):S47–S52.
60. Boelaert J, Lijnen P, Robbens E, et al. Impairment of renal function due to sulphinpyrazone after coronary artery bypass surgery: A prospective double-blind study. J Cardiovasc Pharmacol 1986;8: 386–391.
61. Kahan BD. Cyclosporine. N Engl J Med 1989;321:1725–1738.
62. Bennett WM, DeMattos A, Meyer MM, et al. Chronic cyclosporine nephropathy: The Achilles' heel of immunosuppressive therapy. Kidney Int 1996;50:1089–1100.
63. Puschett JB, Greenberg A, Holley J, McCauley J. The spectrum of cyclosporin nephrotoxicity. Am J Nephrol 1990;10:296–309.
64. Zachariae H, Steen Olson T. Efficacy of cyclosporin A (CyA) in psoriasis: An overview of dose/response, indications, contraindications and side-effects. Clin Nephrol 1995;43:154–158.
65. Young EW, Ellis CN, Messana JM, et al. A prospective study of renal structure and function in psoriasis patients treated with cyclosporin. Kidney Int 1994;46:1216–1222.
66. Feutren G, Mihatsch MJ, for the International Kidney Biopsy Registry of Cyclosporine in Autoimmune Diseases. Risk factors for cyclosporine-induced nephropathy in patients with autoimmune diseases. N Engl J Med 1992;326:1654–1660.
67. Cohen DJ, Appel GB. Cyclosporine: Nephrotoxic effects and guidelines for safe use in patients with rheumatoid arthritis. Semin Arthritis Rheum 1992;21(suppl 3):43–48.
68. Kopp JB, Klotman PE. Cellular and molecular mechanisms of cyclosporine nephrotoxicity. J Am Soc Nephrol 1990;1:162–179.
69. Falkenhain ME, Cosio FG, Sedmak DD. Progressive histologic injury in kidneys from heart and liver transplant recipients receiving cyclosporine. Transplantation 1996;62:364–370.
70. Lee DBN. Cyclosporine and the renin–angiotensin axis. Kidney Int 1997;52:248–260.
71. Conte G, Dal Canton A, Sabbatini M, et al. Acute cyclosporine renal dysfunction reversed by dopamine infusion in healthy subjects. Kidney Int 1989;36:1086–1092.
72. Burke JF Jr, Pirsch JD, Ramos EL, et al. Long-term efficacy and safety of cyclosporine in renal-transplant recipients. N Engl J Med 1994;331:358–363.
73. Meyer MM, Munar M, Udeaja J, Bennett W. Efficacy of area under the curve cyclosporine monitoring in renal transplantation. J Am Soc Nephrol 1993;4:1306–1315.
74. Awni WM. Pharmacodynamic monitoring of cyclosporin. Clin Pharmacokinet 1992;23:428–448.
75. Gaspari F, Anedda MF, Signorini O, Remuzzi G, Perico N. Prediction of cyclosporine area under the curve using a three-point sampling strategy after Neoral^{TM} administration. J Am Soc Nephrol 1997;8:647–652.

76. Hollander AAMJ, van Saase JLCM, Kootte AMM, et al. Beneficial effects of conversion from cyclosporin to azathioprine after kidney transplantation. Lancet 1995;345:610–614.
77. Porayko MK, Textor SC, Krom RAF, et al. Nephrotoxic effects of primary immunosuppression with FK-506 and cyclosporine regimens after liver transplantation. Mayo Clin Proc 1994;69:105–111.
78. Sica DA, Gehr TWB. Triamterene and the kidney. Nephron 1989;51: 454–461.
79. Danesh BJZ, Brunton J, Sumner DJ. Comparison between short-term renal hemodynamic effects of propranolol and nadolol in essential hypertension: A cross-over study. Clin Sci 1984;67:243–248.
80. Baiuk TD, Bennett WM, Norman DJ. Cytokine nephropathy during antilymphocyte therapy. Transplant Proc 1993;2(suppl 1):27–30.
81. Wever PC, Roest RW, Wolbink-Kamp AM, et al. OKT3-induced nephrotoxicity is associated with release of group II secretory phospholipase A_2. Eur J Clin Invest 1996;26:873–878.
82. Moran M, Kapsner C. Acute renal failure associated with elevated plasma oncotic pressure. N Engl J Med 1987;317:150–153.
83. Garcia DL, Anderson S, Rennke HG, et al. Anemia lessens and its prevention with recombinant human erythropoietin worsens glomerular injury and hypertension in rats with reduced renal mass. Proc Natl Acad Sci USA 1988;85:6142–6146.
84. Abraham PA, Opsahl JA, Rachael KM, et al. Renal function during erythropoietin therapy for anemia in predialysis chronic renal failure patients. Am J Nephrol 1990;10:128–136.
85. Porter GA, Bennett WM. Nephrotoxin-induced acute renal failure. In: Brenner BM, Stein JH, eds. Contemporary Issues in Nephrology, Vol 6. New York, Churchill Livingstone, 1980:123–162.
86. Lakkis FG, Campbell OC, Badr KF. Microvascular diseases of the kidney. In: Brenner BM, ed. Brenner and Rectors' the Kidney, 5th ed. Philadelphia, W.B. Saunders, 1996:1712–1730.
87. Valavaara R, Nordman E. Renal complications of mitomycin C therapy with special reference to the total dose. Cancer 1985;55:47–50.
88. Groff JA, Kozak M, Boehmer JP, et al. Endotheliopathy: A continuum of hemolytic uremic syndrome due to mitomycin therapy. Am J Kidney Dis 1997;29:280–284.
89. Lye WC, Cheah JS, Sinniah R. Renal cholesterol embolic disease. Case report and review of the literature. Am J Nephrol 1993;13:489–493.
90. Adler SG, Cohen AH, Glassock RJ. Secondary glomerular diseases In: Brenner BM, ed. Brenner and Rectors' the Kidney, 5th ed. Philadelphia, W.B. Saunders, 1996:1563–1566.
91. Abraham PA, Keane WF. Glomerular and interstitial disease induced by nonsteriodal anti-inflammatory drugs. Am J Nephrol 1984;4:1–6.
92. Coroneos E, Petrusevska G, Varghese F, Truong LD. Focal segmental glomerulosclerosis with acute renal failure associated with α-interferon therapy. Am J Kidney Dis 1996;28:888–892.
93. Hall CL. Gold nephropathy. Nephron 1988;50:265–272.
94. Radford MG Jr, Holley KE, Grande JP, et al. Reversible membranous nephropathy associated with the use of nonsteroidal anti-inflammatory drugs. JAMA 1996;276:466–469.
95. Yorgin PD, Theodorou AA, Al-Uzri A, et al. Propylene glycol–induced proximal renal tubular cell injury. Am J Kidney Dis 1997;30:134–139.
96. Visweswaran P, Massin EK, Dubose TD Jr. Mannitol-induced acute renal failure. J Am Soc Nephrol 1997;8:1028–1033.
97. Biesenbach G, Zazgornik J, Kaiser W, et al. Severe tubulopathy and kidney graft rupture after coadministration of mannitol and cyclosporin. Nephron 1992;62:93–96.
98. Cayco AV, Perazella MA, Hayslett JP. Renal insufficiency after intravenous immune globulin therapy: A report of two cases and an analysis of the literature. J Am Soc Nephrol 1997;8:1788–1794.
99. Smith CR, Moore RD, Lietman PS. Studies of risk factors for aminoglycoside nephrotoxicity. Am J Kidney Dis 1986;8:308–313.
100. Bertino JS Jr, Booker LA, Franck PA, et al. Incidence of and significant risk factors for aminoglycoside associated nephrotoxicity in patients dosed by using individualized pharmacokinetic monitoring. J Infect Dis 1993;167:173–179.
101. Goetz MB, Sayers J. Nephrotoxicity of vancomycin and aminoglycoside therapy separately and in combination. J Antimicrob Chemother 1993;32:325–334.
102. Bertino JS, Rodvold KA, Destache CJ. Cost considerations in therapeutic drug monitoring of aminoglycosides. Clin Pharmacokinet 1994;26:71–81.
103. Leehey DJ, Braun BI, Tholl DA, et al. Can pharmacokinetic dosing decrease nephrotoxicity associated with aminoglycoside therapy? J Am Soc Nephrol 1993;4:81–90.
104. Freeman CD, Nicolau DP, Belliveau PP, Nightingale CH. Once-daily dosing of aminoglycosides: Review and recommendations for clinical practice. J Am Antimicrob Chemother 1997;39:677–686.
105. Freeman CD, Strayer AH. Mega-analysis of meta-analysis: An examination of meta-analysis with an emphasis on once-daily aminoglycoside comparative trials. Pharmacotherapy 1996;16:1093–1102.
106. Koo J, Tight R, Rajkumar V, Hawa Z. Comparison of once-daily versus pharmacokinetic dosing of aminoglycosides in elderly patients. Am J Med 1996;101:177–183.
107. Solomon R. Contrast-medium-induced acute renal failure. Kidney Int 1998;53:230–242.
108. Levy EM, Viscoli CM, Horwitz RI. The effect of acute renal failure on mortality. A cohort analysis. JAMA 1996;275:1489–1494.
109. Clark BA, Kim D, Epstein FH. Endothelin and atrial natriuretic peptide levels following radiocontrast exposure in humans. Am J Kidney Dis 1997;30:82–86.
110. McCarthy CS, Becker JS. Multiple myeloma and contrast media. Radiology 1992;183:519–521.
111. Cigarroa RG, Lange RA, Williams RH, Hillis LD. Dosing of contrast material to prevent contrast nephropathy in patients with renal disease. Am J Med 1989;86:649–652.
112. Rudnick MR, Goldfarb S, Wexler L, et al. Nephrotoxicity of ionic and nonionic contrast media in 1196 patients: A randomized trial. Kidney Int 1995;47:254–261.
113. Barrett BJ, Carlisle EJ. Metaanalysis of the relative nephrotoxicity of high- and low-osmolality iodinated contrast media. Radiology 1993; 188:171–178.
114. Louis BM, Hoch BS, Hernandez C, et al. Protection from the nephrotoxicity of contrast dye. Ren Fail 1996;18:639–646.
115. Solomon R, Werner C, Mann D, et al. Effects of saline, mannitol, and furosemide on acute decreases in renal function induced by radiocontrast agents. N Engl J Med 1994;331:1416–1420.
116. Weisberg LS, Kurnik PB, Kurnik BRC. Risk of radiocontrast nephropathy in patients with and without diabetes mellitus. Kidney Int 1994;45:259–265.
117. Merouani A, Shpall EJ, Jones RB, Archer PG, Schrier RW. Renal function in high dose chemotherapy and autologous hematopoietic cell support treatment for breast cancer. Kidney Int 1996;50: 1026–1031.
118. Anand AJ, Bashey B. Newer insights into cisplatin nephrotoxicity. Ann Pharmacother 1993;27:1519–1525.
119. Foster-Nora JA, Siders R. Amifostine for protection from antineoplastic drug toxicity. Am J Health Syst Pharm 1997;54: 787–800.
120. Sawaya BP, Briggs JP, Schnermann J. Amphotericin B nephrotoxicity: The adverse consequences of altered membrane properties. J Am Soc Nephrol 1995;6:154–164.
121. Fisher MA, Talbot GH, Maislin G, et al. Risk factors for amphotericin B-associated nephrotoxicity. Am J Med 1989;87:547–552.
122. Anderson CM. Sodium chloride treatment of amphotericin B nephrotoxicity. Standard of care? West J Med 1995;162:313–317.
123. Leenders ACAP, de Marie S. The use of lipid formulations of amphotericin B for systemic fungal infections. Leukemia 1996;10: 1570–1575.
124. Sorkine P, Nagar H, Weinbroum A, et al. Administration of amphotericin B in lipid emulsion decreases nephrotoxicity: Results of a prospective, randomized, controlled study in critically ill patients. Crit Care Med 1996;4:1311–1315.

125. Rapp RP, Gubbins PO, Evans ME. Amphotericin B lipid complex. Ann Pharmacother 1997;31:1174–1186.
126. Lachaal M, Venuto RC. Nephrotoxicity and hyperkalemia in patients with acquired immunodeficiency syndrome treated with pentamidine. Am J Med 1989;87:260–263.
127. Peter BS, Carlin E, Weston RJ, et al. Adverse effects of drugs used in the management of opportunistic infections associated with HIV infection. Drug Saf 1994;10:439–454.
128. Antoniskis, Larsen RA. Acute, rapidly progressive renal failure with simultaneous use of amphotericin B and pentamidine. Antimicrob Agents Chemother 1990;34:470–472.
129. Smith GH. Treatment of infections in the patient with acquired immunodeficiency syndrome. Arch Intern Med 1994;154:949–973.
130. Jacobson MA. Treatment of cytomegalovirus retinitis in patients with the acquired immunodeficiency syndrome. N Engl J Med 1997; 337:105–114.
131. Toto RD. Review: Acute tubulointerstitial nephritis. Am J Med Sci 1990;299:392–410.
132. Hansen PB, Johnsen HE, Hippe E. Hypereosinophilic syndrome treated with alpha-interferon and granulocyte colony-stimulating factor but complicated by nephrotoxicity. Am J Hematol 1993;43:66–68.
133. Michel DM, Kelly CI. Acute intestinal nephritis. J Am Soc Nephrol 1998;9:506–515.
134. Shear NH, Spielberg SP, Grant DM, et al. Differences in metabolism of sulfonamides predisposing to idiosyncratic toxicity. Ann Intern Med 1986;105:179–184.
135. Walker RG. Lithium nephrotoxicity. Kidney Int 1993;44(suppl 42):S93–S98.
136. Kallner G, Petterson U. Renal, thyroid and parathyroid function during lithium treatment: Laboratory tests in 207 people treated for 1–30 years. Acta Psychiatr Scand 1995;91:48–51.
137. Lehmann K, Ritz E. Angiotensin-converting enzyme inhibitors may cause renal dysfunction in patients on long-term lithium treatment. Am J Kidney Dis 1995;25:82–87.
138. Lam SS, Kjellstrand C. Emergency treatment of lithium-induced diabetes insipidus with nonsteroidal anti-inflammatory drugs. Ren Fail 1997;19:183–188.
139. Klag MJ, Whelton PK, Perneger TV. Analgesics and chronic renal disease. Curr Opin Nephrol Hypertens 1996;5:236–241.
140. Henrich WL, Agodoa LE, Barrett B, et al. Analgesics and the kidney: Summary and recommendations to the scientific advisory board of the National Kidney Foundation from an ad hoc committee of the National Kidney Foundation. Am J Kidney Dis 1996;27:162–165.
141. Griffin MD, Larson TS, Bergstralh EJ. Renal papillary necrosis—A sixteen-year clinical experience. J Am Soc Nephrol 1995;6:248–256.
142. Hoffbrand BI. Dapsone and renal papillary necrosis. Br Med J 1978;1:78.
143. Elseviers MM, De Broe ME. Combination analgesic involvement in the pathogenesis of analgesic nephropathy: The European perspective. Am J Kidney Dis 1996;28:S48–S55.
144. Duggin GG. Combination analgesic-induced kidney disease: The Australian experience. Am J Kidney Dis 1996;28:539–547.
145. DeBroe ME, Elseviers MM. Analgesic nephropathy. N Engl J Med 1998;338:446–452.
146. Bennett WM, Henrich WL, Stoff JS. The renal effects of nonsteroidal anti-inflammatory drugs: Summary and recommendations. Am J Kidney Dis 1996;28:S56–S62.
147. Buckalew VM. Habitual use of acetaminophen as a risk factor for chronic renal failure: A comparison with phenacetin. Am J Kidney Dis 1996;28:S7–S13.
148. D'Agati V. Does aspirin cause acute or chronic renal failure in experimental animals and in humans? Am J Kidney Dis 1996;28:S24–S29.
149. Barrett BJ. Acetaminophen and adverse chronic renal outcomes: An appraisal of the epidemiologic evidence. Am J Kidney Dis 1996;28: S14–S19.
150. Matzke GR. Clinical consequences of nonnarcotic analgesic use. Ann Pharmacother 1997;31:245–248.
151. Strom BL, West SL, Sim E, Carson JL. The epidemiology of the acute flank pain syndrome from suprofen. Clin Pharmacol Ther 1989;46:693–699.
152. Cadnapaphornchai P, Taher S, McDonald FD. Acute drug-associated rhabdomyolysis: An examination of its diverse renal manifestations and complications. Am J Med Sci 1980;280:66–72.
153. Patel R, Connor G. A review of 30 cases of rhabdomyolysis-associated acute renal failure among phencyclidine users. Clin Toxicol 1985–86;23:547–556.
154. Rumpf KW, Henning HV. Rhabdomyolysis and alpha-adrenoceptor agonists. Nephron 1990;55:346-347.
155. Roth D, Alarcn FJ, Fernandez JA, et al. Acute rhabdomyolysis associated with cocaine intoxication. N Engl J Med 1988;319: 673–677.
156. Affarah HB, Mars RL, Someren A, et al. Myoglobinuria and acute renal failure associated with intravenous vasopressin infusion. South Med J 1984;77:918–921.
157. Alejandro DSJ, Peterson J. Myoglobinuric acute renal failure in a cardiac transplant patient taking lovastatin and cyclosporine. J Am Soc Nephrol 1994;5:153–160.
158. Rossert J, Rondeau E, Jondeau G, et al. Tamm-Horsfall protein accumulation in glomeruli during acetazolamide-induced acute renal failure. Am J Nephrol 1989;9:56–57.
159. Hein R, Brunkhorst R, Thon WF, et al. Symptomatic sulfadiazine crystalluria in AIDS patients: A report of two cases. Clin Nephrol 1993;39:254–256.
160. Matzke GR, Frye RF. Drug administration in patients with renal insufficiency. Drug Saf 1997;16:205–231.
161. Lawton JM, Conway LT, Crosson JT, et al. Acute oxalate nephropathy after massive ascorbic acid administration. Arch Intern Med 1985;145:950–951.
162. Coggins CH, Fang LS-T. Acute renal failure associated with antibiotics, anesthetic agents, and radiographic contrast agents. In: Brenner BM, Lazarus JM, eds. Acute Renal Failure. Philadelphia, W.B. Saunders, 1983:283–320.
163. Feest TG. Low molecular weight dextran: A continuing cause of acute renal failure. Br Med J 1976;2:1300.
164. Roy LF, Villeneuve J-P, Dumont A, et al. Irreversible renal failure associated with triamterene. Am J Nephrol 1991;11:486–488.
165. Biberstein M, Parker BA. Enema-induced hyperphosphatemia. Am J Med 1985;79:645–646.
166. Danziger LH, Horn JR. Disopyramide-induced urinary retention: Report of nine cases and review of the literature. Arch Intern Med 1983; 143:1683–1686.
167. Becker K, Jablonowski H, Haussinger D. Sulfadiazine-associated nephrotoxicity in patients with the acquired immunodeficiency syndrome. Medicine 1996;75:185–194.
168. Kopp JB, Miller KD, Mican JAM, et al. Crystalluria and urinary tract abnormalities associated with indinavir. Ann Intern Med 1997; 127:119–125.
169. Berns JS, Cohen RM, Silverman M, Turner J. Acute renal failure due to indinavir crystalluria and nephrolithiasis: Report of two cases. Am J Kidney Dis 1997;30:558–560.
170. Hricik DE, Goldsmith GH. Uric acid nephrolithiasis and acute renal failure secondary to streptozotocin nephrotoxicity. Am J Med 1988; 84:153–156.
171. Kranen S, Keough D, Gordon RB, Emerson BT. Xanthine-containing calculi during allopurinol therapy. J Urol 1985;133:658–659.
172. Millette CH, Snodgrass GL. Acute renal failure associated with chronic antacid ingestion. Am J Hosp Pharm 1981;38:1352–1355.
173. Dick WH, Lingeman JE, Preminger GM, et al. Laxative abuse as a cause for ammonium urate renal calculi. J Urol 1990;143: 244–247.

46

GLOMERULONEPHRITIS

Alan H. Lau, PharmD, FCCP

Clinical and pathologic findings associated with primary glomerular injury were first reported in the 19th century. The natural history of many glomerular diseases was not described until the 1950s, when percutaneous diagnostic kidney biopsy became available. The development of immunofluorescence microscopy and advances in immunopathology in the 1960s and 1970s further expanded our understanding of the antibody-related immune mechanisms that are responsible for the different types of glomerular injury.[1] Recent advances in cell and molecular biology afford us a plethora of new information concerning the disease processes.[2] However, the precise pathogenetic mechanisms for many glomerular diseases remain unknown and the available therapeutic regimens are still far from optimal. At present, glomerulonephritis is the third most common cause of end-stage renal disease (ESRD) and accounts for 10.7% of all new cases, or about 7000 patients each year.[3]

This chapter provides an overview of the pathophysiologic mechanisms of glomerular injury and the clinical presentations of glomerulonephritis. The specific characteristics of and the treatment approach for each of the more common forms of glomerulonephritis are also discussed. Although diabetes mellitus and amyloidosis are important secondary causes of glomerular diseases, the scope of this chapter is limited to the primary causes of glomerulonephritis.

PATHOPHYSIOLOGY

NORMAL ANATOMY AND FUNCTION

The glomerulus is a unique capillary bed that allows small nonprotein plasma constituents up to the size of inulin, which has a molecular weight of 5200 Daltons, to pass freely while excluding macromolecules equal to or larger than albumin, which has a molecular weight of 69,000 Daltons (Fig. 46–1). Both the size and charge of the molecules affect the ease of passage through the glomerular membrane.[4] For molecules with similar effective molecular radii, those that are anionic tend to experience more difficulties in passing through than molecules that are cationic.[4]

The glomerulus, which is enclosed within the Bowman's capsule, consists of two important components: the filtration barrier and the mesangium (Fig. 46–2). Blood flow in the glomerular capillary bed is supplied by the afferent arteriole while the efferent arterioles channel the flow leaving the glomerular tuft. The capillary wall, which serves as a filtration barrier, consists of three well-defined layers: fenestrated endothelium, glomerular basement membrane (GBM), and epithelial cells. The epithelial cells, also known as podocytes, have specialized foot processes embedded in the outer layer of the GBM. It is across this barrier that fluid flows and ultimately forms ultrafiltrate. Under normal conditions, the GBM appears to function as a compact hydrated gel of matrix proteins with a pore-like structure. The mesangium provides support for the glomerular capillaries and also modulates blood flow through the capillaries. It consists of mesangial cells embedded in an extracellular matrix.

Fixed, negatively charged sites are found within the glomeruli in all three layers of the capillary wall: the endothelium, the epithelium, and the GBM. Biochemical and cytochemical studies have shown that the epithelial cell coat is composed of a negatively charged glycoprotein (podocalyxin), made up largely of sialic acid. The GBM contains an abundance of negatively charged sulfated glycosaminoglycans that can affect the passage of ionic molecules through the capillary wall. The movement of negatively charged molecules is restricted more than that of neutral or positively charged molecules.[4] Different glomerular diseases affect this size- and charge-selective barrier to different extents, and glomerulopathies therefore present with varied clinical features and solute-excretion patterns.

Aside from being a barrier for solute excretion, some of the glomerular cells, such as the epithelial cells, have phagocytic function that can remove macromolecules trapped within the filtration barrier. They are also capable of synthesizing the GBM. In contrast, the mesangial cells regulate glomerular hemodynamics by responding to angiotensin II and producing prostaglandins. They also synthesize and respond to various cytokines and thus play a key role in immune-mediated glomerular diseases. There are also resident phagocytes in the mesangium. They remove macromolecules trapped in the basement membrane and move them into the urinary space. These phagocytes are involved in the development of both immune and nonimmune glomerular injury.[5]

ETIOLOGY

The etiology of most human glomerulonephritides is unknown. However, humoral and cellular immunologic mechanisms are implicated in the pathogenesis. Abnormalities in coagulation and metabolism, as well as hereditary and vascular diseases, also contribute to glomerular damage. The histopathologic manifestations vary substantially among the different types of glomerulonephritis. An overview of the primary pathogenetic mechanisms is presented in this section, and specific abnormalities for each of the primary types of glomerulonephritis are presented in subsequent sections.

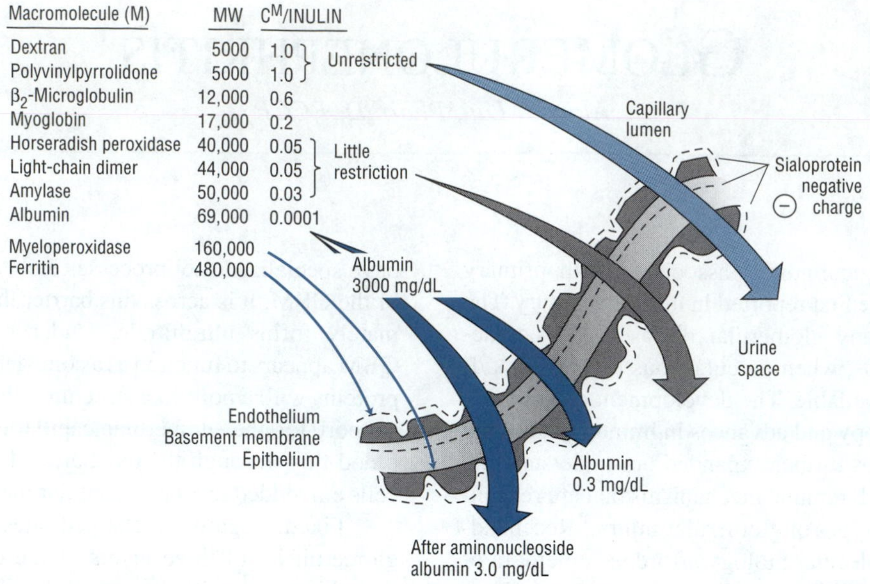

FIGURE 46–1. Movement of various macromolecules across the glomerular capillary. The thicker the arrow, the less restriction on movement. The fractional clearance of each macromolecule as compared to inulin (C^M/INULIN) decreases as molecular weight (MW) increases. The disproportionately greater restriction of albumin movement indicates importance of factors other than size, such as the negative charge of albumin. *(From Hutt MP, Kelleher SP: In Schrier RW (ed). Renal and Electrolyte Disorders, 3rd ed. Boston, Little Brown, 1986, with permission.)*

PATHOGENESIS OF GLOMERULAR INJURY AND PATHOLOGIC MANIFESTATIONS

The glomerular lesion may be diffuse (involving all glomeruli), focal (involving some but not all glomeruli), or segmental, also known as local (involving part of the individual glomeruli). The pathologic manifestations may also be described as proliferative (overgrowth of epithelium, endothelium, or mesangium), membranous (thickening of GBM), and/or sclerotic.

The glomerular capillary wall is particularly susceptible to immune-mediated injury. Antigen and antibody tend to localize in the glomerulus probably because of its high blood flow and capillary hydrostatic pressure. Parenchymal damage can be induced as a result of humoral- and cell-mediated immune reactions (Table 46–1). Antibodies and sensitized T lymphocytes are the primary mediators of glomerular injury.[6–8]

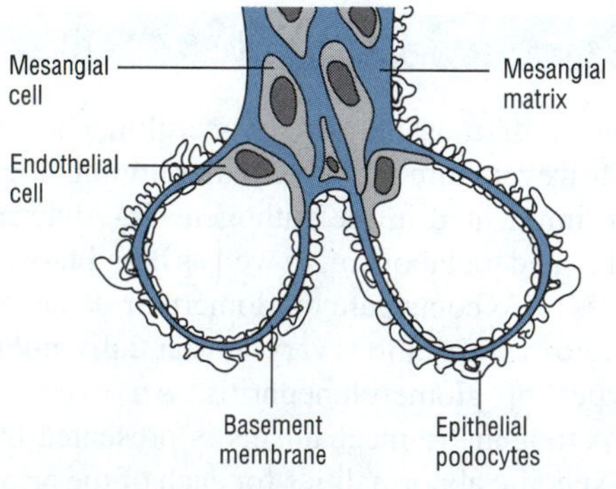

FIGURE 46–2. Schematic representation of glomerulus.

Production of antibodies to endogenous or exogenous antigens that are recognized as foreign by the host is the first step in humoral immunologic damage to the glomerulus. Endogenous antigens may be intrinsic glomerular antigens, such as Heymann's antigen on the epithelial cell or Goodpasture's antigen on the GBM, or previously sequestered antigens, such as DNA or thyroglobulin. Exogenous antigens are most often viral, bacterial, parasitic, or fungal in origin (Table 46–2). Antineutrophil cytoplasmic autoantibodies (ANCAs), autoantibodies that react to the cytoplasmic components of neutrophils and monocytes, have been found in patients with idiopathic crescentic glomerulonephritis and also in the accompanying vasculitis.[9]

Classically, it has been considered that complexes of antigens and antibodies were formed in the circulation and then passively entrapped in the glomerular capillary or mesangium. However, experimental data have shown that antibodies may combine with endogenous glomerular antigens or exogenous antigens entrapped in the glomerulus to form complexes locally, or *in situ.*[7] Regardless of the mechanism of formation, these antigen–antibody complexes are often localized along the capillary loop or the mesangium (Fig. 46–2) and can be detected by immunofluorescence microscopy. The type and extent of glomerular damage is dependent on the location of the immune complex formation

TABLE 46–1. Immunologic Mechanisms of Glomerular Injury

Circulating immune complexes
In situ antigen–antibody interaction
Intrinsic glomerular antigen; e.g., GBM antigens
Exogenous planted antigens
Cell-mediated mechanism

TABLE 46–2. Antigens Possibly Involved in Immune-Mediated Glomerular Injury

Source of Antigen	Clinical Example
Endogenous Antigens	
Released sequestered cellular antigens	DNA, thyroglobulin
Endogenous antigens modified by exogenous source	IgG modified by streptococcal neuraminidase
Tumor antigens	CEA[a] in bronchial and other solid tumors
Intrinsic glomerular antigens	Goodpasture's syndrome
Neutrophil granule constituents	ANCA[b]-associated glomerulonephritis
Exogenous	
Viral	Hepatitis B
Bacterial	Streptococcal organisms
Parasitic	Malaria
Fungal	Candida

[a]CEA = carcinoembryonic antigen.
[b]ANCA = antineutrophil cytoplasmic antibody.

and the rate at which it is removed. Impaired removal facilitates the growth of the complex and thus increases the likelihood of glomerular damage.

Subsequent to antigen–antibody formation, a series of biologic events is triggered that ultimately leads to glomerular injury. Both inflammatory and noninflammatory lesions can be induced by antibody deposition. Noninflammatory lesions can be a result of noncomplement-fixing antibody binding to the glomerular epithelial cell (mechanism 1), or activation of the complement system to form the C5b-9 membrane attack complex (mechanism 2).[7,8] Both mechanisms can damage the glomerular epithelial cell and result in capillary wall injury and proteinuria (Fig. 46–3). Inflammatory lesions are induced by glomerular infiltration of circulating inflammatory cells such as neutrophils, monocytes/macrophages, and platelets (mechanism 3), or proliferation of resident glomerular mesangial cells (mechanism 4), resulting in GBM damage[7] (Fig. 46–3). The migration of neutrophils and monocytes to the glomerular tufts is promoted by chemoattractants such as complement fragments (C3a, C5a), platelet-activating factor, interleukin-8, and monocyte chemotactic protein-1.[10] Various cytokines, chemokines, and growth factors are then released to participate in the inflammatory process.[6]

T cells sensitized to glomerular antigen, macrophages, and resident mesangial cells are important participants in cell-mediated injury. Sensitized T cells can cause glomerular hypercellularity in the absence of antibody deposition.[6–8,10] Cytotoxic T cells may bind with the target cells and destroy them. Alternatively, a delayed-type hypersensitivity reaction may be initiated by activated T cells, through the release of lymphokines, to attract, activate, and transform monocytes into macrophages.[7] These humoral and cellular mediators, in conjunction with a host of toxic molecular entities, including reactive oxygen species, proteinases, eicosanoids, and procoagulants, which are secreted by neutrophils, macrophages, platelets, and resident glomerular cells, can alter the permeability, blood flow, and function of the glomeruli. Vascular constriction and occlusion follow and result in the eventual destruction of the glomeruli.

Acute forms of glomerular injury may frequently lead to chronic and persistent renal dysfunction even though the original immune factors that induce glomerular injury have resolved. Progression to end-stage renal failure may become inevitable. Experimental and clinical investigations have suggested that a variety of factors may participate in the progression of renal injury.[11] These include systemic and glomerular hypertension,[12] high dietary protein intake, proteinuria,[13–15] glomerular hypertrophy, hyperlipidemia,[16] activation of the coagulation system,[12] abnormalities of calcium and phosphorus balance,[12] and tubulointerstitial injury.[14]

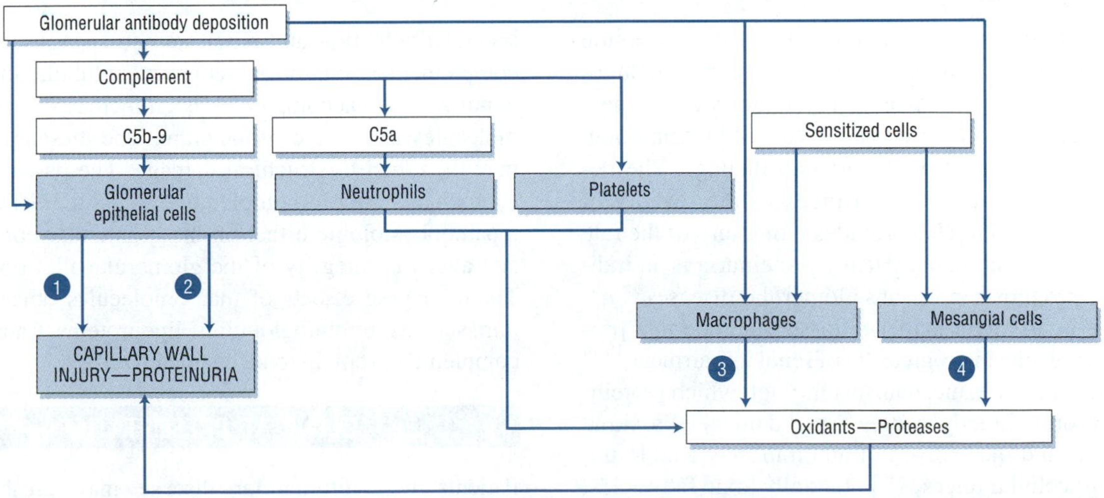

FIGURE 46–3. The major pathways of immune-mediated glomerular injury. Mechanisms 1 and 2 primarily act on the glomerular epithelial cell and result in noninflammatory lesions. Mechanisms 3 and 4 involve participation of effector cells and result in glomerular inflammation and structural damage. *(Adapted from Ref. 7, with permission.)*

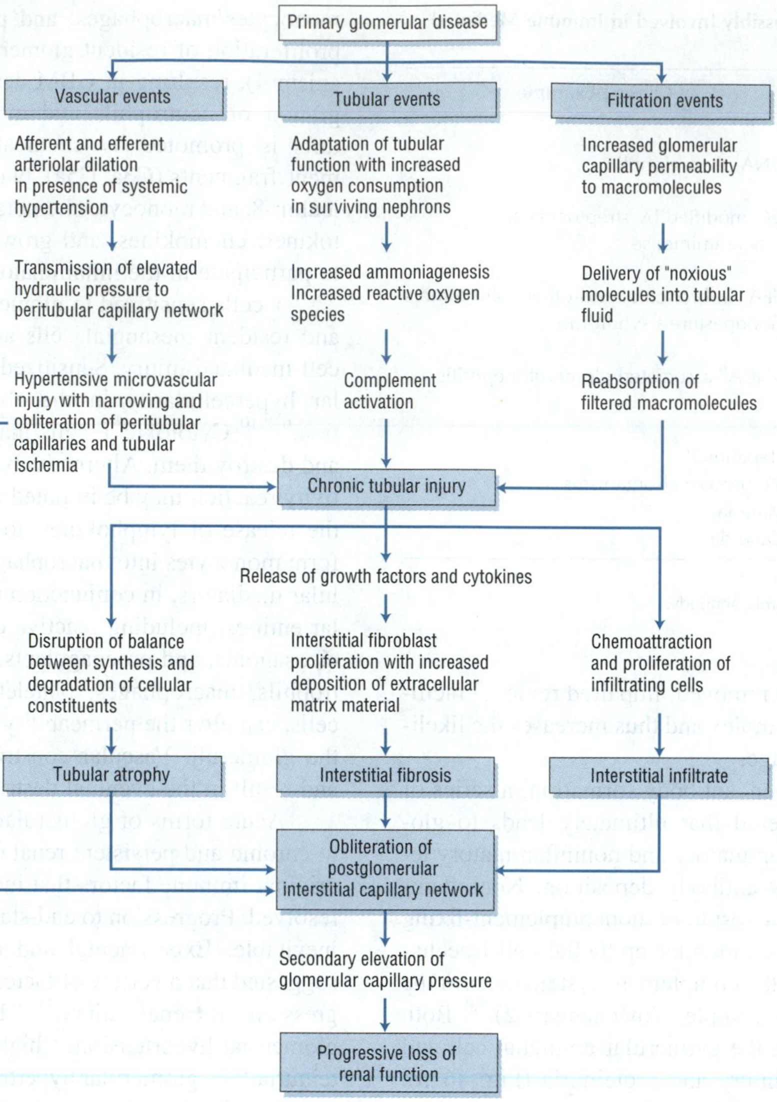

FIGURE 46–4. Proposed sequence of events leading from primary glomerular disease to progressive loss of renal function through tubulointerstitial injury. *(Modified from Ref. 14, with permission.)*

The last is considered an important factor in the progression of glomerular disease (Fig. 46–4). How these nonimmunologic factors contribute to renal injury is not well defined. Much interest has been focused on the role of proteinuria in causing glomerular and tubulointerstitial damage. The degree of proteinuria not only is an index of the severity of glomerular diseases, but also provides a measure of the rate of progression of renal injury. Heavy proteinuria is an indicator of poor prognosis in various glomerular diseases.[15] Although there is no direct evidence to substantiate that proteinuria per se results in progression of renal impairment,[13,14] there are many possible mechanisms through which proteinuria directly or indirectly causes renal damage. Proximal tubular uptake and metabolism of albumin may lead to unregulated intracellular release of potentially toxic fatty acids, which may provoke secretion of a lipid macrophage chemotactic factor, resulting in interstitial inflammation.[15] Tubular hypermetabolism may lead to increased reactive oxygen species production and renal ammoniagenesis, resulting in complement activation and consequent tubular injury.[14] Proteinuria is also accompanied by an increased flux of macromolecules across the mesangium. The mesangial overload may then lead to structural damage. The passage of serum components, such as complement, across the GBM may have a pathophysiologic effect on the glomerular epithelial cells and alter the integrity of the glomerular filtration barrier.[13] The damaging effects of macromolecules other than albumin, such as immunoglobulins, lipoproteins, transferrin, and complement, remain to be characterized.[14]

CLINICAL PRESENTATION

Patients with glomerular disease may present with a nephritic or a nephrotic syndrome (Table 46–3). Nephritic syndrome reflects glomerular inflammation and frequently results in hematuria. White cells and cellular and granular

TABLE 46–3. Tendencies of Glomerular Diseases to Manifest Nephrotic and Nephritic Features

	Nephrotic Features	Nephritic Features
Minimal-change nephropathy	++++	–
Membranous nephropathy	++++	+
Diabetic glomerulosclerosis	++++	+
Amyloidosis	++++	+
Focal segmental glomerulosclerosis	+++	++
Mesangioproliferative glomerulonephritis	++	++
Membranoproliferative glomerulonephritis	++	+++
Proliferative glomerulonephritis	++	+++
Acute poststreptococcal glomerulonephritis	+	++++
Crescentic glomerulonephritis[a]	+	++++

[a]Can be immune complex–mediated, antiglomerular basement membrane antibody–mediated, or associated with antineutrophil cytoplasmic autoantibodies.

casts are commonly found in the urine. In contrast, nephrotic syndrome reflects noninflammatory injury to the glomerular structures, and results in few cells or cellular casts in the urine. Initially, there may be limited or no reduction in renal excretory function.

Hematuria occurs when red blood cells leak through the openings of the GBM. The presence of red cell casts is highly indicative of glomerulonephritis or vasculitis. The presence of dysmorphic red blood cells in the urine is suggestive of glomerular disease. The red blood cells are damaged as they pass through the openings in the GBM or the cells may sustain osmotic injury as they travel through the different osmotic environments within the lumen of the kidney tubules.

The presence of proteinuria indicates a defect of the size- and/or charge-selective barriers within the GBM. Normal urinary protein excretion is between 40 and 80 mg/d, with a maximum of 150 mg. Fewer than 20 mg of the excreted proteins are albumin. Most of the albumin that enters the glomerular filtrate is either reabsorbed or catabolized by the tubular epithelium. The dipsticks that are commonly used to identify proteinuria detect only albumin and they become positive when protein excretion is more than 300 to 500 mg/d. The test is therefore not useful to detect early stages of renal injury secondary to diabetes mellitus or hypertension, which often result in microalbuminuria where urinary albumin excretion ranges between 30 and 300 mg/d. A simple immunoassay on a dipstick, Micral (Boehringer Mannheim Diagnostics) permits specific and semiquantitative determination of urinary albumin concentrations at five levels: 0, 10, 20, 50, and 100 mg/L. It shows no cross-reactivity with other human proteins that may possibly be present in urine. The test may be used reliably for a urine specimen that has been stored for up to 7 days at 4°C and even in the presence of bacterial contamination. Another qualitative test, Microbumintest (Ames), registers a positive reading when the urine albumin concentration is greater than 40 mg/L.[17]

Hypertension is a common feature in patients with glomerular diseases. Expansion of plasma volume as a result of renal salt retention is frequently the cause of hypertension, especially during acute disease. In contrast, increased activity of vasoconstrictors, such as angiotensin II, is often the cause in patients with chronic glomerular diseases.[18] Scarring of the glomerulus resulting in regional ischemia is thought to be responsible for the hypertension. Activation of the sympathetic nervous system and the release of vasoconstrictor substances may also contribute.

NEPHRITIC SYNDROME

Glomerular bleeding resulting in hematuria is a typical finding in nephritic syndrome. Dysmorphic red cells, especially acanthocytes, are a sensitive and specific marker of glomerular bleeding. The presence of pus and cellular and granular casts in the urine is common. The extent of proteinuria is variable, typically about 1 to 3 g/d, but it may be in the nephrotic range (> 3 g/d). Patients with severe nephritic glomerular injury have renal function impairment because of the reduced glomerular surface area available for filtration. The latter is a result of constriction of the capillary lumen by proliferating mesangial cells or inflammatory cells. As renal function declines, hypertension and edema may develop or preexisting conditions may worsen.

NEPHROTIC SYNDROME

Nephrotic syndrome is characterized by proteinuria greater than 3.5 g/d/1.73 m^2, hypoproteinemia, edema, hyperlipidemia, and, sometimes, a hypercoagulable state. The syndrome may be the result of primary diseases of the glomerulus or associated with systemic diseases such as diabetes mellitus, lupus, amyloidosis, and preeclampsia. Hypoproteinemia, especially hypoalbuminemia, results from increased urinary loss of albumin and an increased rate of catabolism of filtered albumin by proximal tubular cells. The compensatory increase in hepatic synthesis of albumin is insufficient to replenish the protein loss, probably because of malnutrition.

Edema formation in patients with nephrotic syndrome was traditionally thought to be driven by the reduced plasma oncotic pressure secondary to hypoalbuminemia. If the oncotic pressure is low, the movement of fluid from the vascular space to the interstitial compartment will result in a reduction of the plasma volume, which can cause compensatory renal sodium retention (the "underfill" mechanism). However, experimental data suggest that the plasma volume is actually normal or elevated.[19] This may be due to the fact that hypoalbuminemia has not been found to cause edema until the serum albumin concentration is less than 2 g/dL and the transcapillary oncotic pressure gradient is not as high as previously thought since increased lymphatic flow reduces the interstitial oncotic pressure by removing protein and fluid from the interstitium.[20] Thus, fluid retention is likely mediated by a primary increase in sodium reabsorption at the distal nephron, which is probably caused by tubular resistance to the action of atrial natriuretic peptide (the "overflow" mechanism).[21] At present, the sensitivity of methods for plasma volume measurements in distinguishing underfill from overfill mechanisms is still questionable. It is likely that both mechanisms may contribute to nephrotic edema in different patients.[21]

Although albuminuria below the nephrotic range appears to have a minor influence on serum cholesterol in patients with primary glomerular disease, daily urinary albumin excretion of greater than 3 g is associated with a significant increase in serum cholesterol concentrations.[22] Hyperlipidemia in nephrotic syndrome is characterized by elevated serum total cholesterol and triglyceride concentrations, with increased very-low-density lipoprotein (VLDL) and low-density lipoprotein (LDL) cholesterol concentrations. Although high-density lipoprotein (HDL) cholesterol concentrations are normally distributed, there is a maldistribution of HDL subtypes, with a reduction in HDL_2 and an increase in HDL_3.[23,24] Furthermore, lipoprotein(a) levels may also be increased. Oval fat bodies and fatty casts are also found in the urine. The mechanisms for nephrotic hyperlipidemia are not well defined. A reduction in plasma oncotic pressure as a result of hypoalbuminemia may stimulate hepatic synthesis of lipids and lipoproteins. The increased VLDL production and increased liver cholesterol synthesis along with a decrease in LDL receptor activity can then lead to an increase in LDL cholesterol concentrations. In addition, reduced serum albumin or the loss of a liporegulatory substance may result in reduced VLDL clearance[23,24] (see Fig. 42–11). Nephrotic patients with hyperlipidemia, especially those with concomitant hypertension, are presumed to have an increased risk for atherosclerotic vascular disease. Hyperlipidemia has also been shown to promote the progression of glomerular injury, as evidenced by glomerulosclerosis, mesangial expansion, and hyalinosis.[16,23,24]

Many patients with nephrotic syndrome have a hypercoagulable state due to defects of several control proteins in the coagulation cascade. Antithrombin III concentration is reduced because of increased loss in the urine.[25] A reduced amount of the coagulation inhibitors protein C and S, abnormal concentrations of clotting factors, increased fibrinogen concentrations, and abnormal platelet function may also contribute to the hypercoagulable state.[25] The net result of these alterations in coagulation is an increased risk for arterial and venous thrombosis, especially in the deep veins and renal veins.

DIAGNOSIS

Patients with suspected glomerular disease should first be evaluated for a potential systemic cause. An extensive medical history should be obtained to identify symptoms of diabetes mellitus, amyloidosis, systemic lupus erythematosus (SLE), and other familial conditions associated with renal disease. Reduced appetite, fatigue, weight gain, and edema are all suggestive of nephrotic syndrome. Thorough medication, environmental, and occupation histories should be obtained to identify possible exposure to drugs, toxins, or chemicals that are known to be nephrotoxic. A carefully conducted physical examination may reveal signs and symptoms associated with systemic diseases, such as hypertension, rash, arthritis, retinopathy, neuropathy, lymphadenopathy, and hepatomegaly, as well as evidence of malignancy.

Examination of urine for active sediments, such as red blood cells, white blood cells, and casts, can differentiate the nephrotic and nephritic nature of the disease. The patient may present with normal urinalysis, isolated hematuria, or proteinuria, or significant abnormalities, such as nephrotic-range proteinuria, hematuria, pyuria, lipiduria, and the presence of different casts. Nephrotic sediment is characterized by heavy proteinuria (usually more than 3 g/d) and lipiduria. The patient's total urinary protein excretion can be quantified by a 24-hour urine collection or estimated by measuring the total protein:creatinine ratio in a random daytime urine specimen. This ratio correlates closely with the total urinary protein excretion. A ratio of 250 mg/dL:100 mg/dL repre-

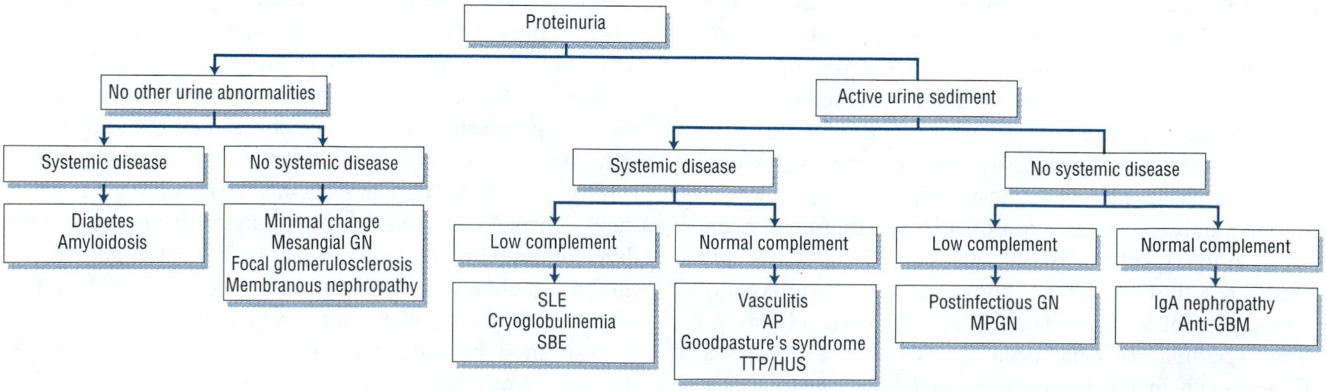

FIGURE 46–5. Clinical presentations of glomerulonephritis. GN = glomerulonephritis; MPGN = membranoproliferative glomerulonephritis; SLE = systemic lupus erythematosus; SBE = subacute bacterial endocarditis; GBM = glomerular basement membrane; TTP = thrombotic thrombocytopenic purpura; HUS = hemolytic–uremic syndrome; AP = anaphylactoid purpura.

TABLE 46–4. Diagnostic Considerations of Renal Diseases Based on Serum Complement Levels

Low Serum Complement Level	Normal Serum Complement Level
Systemic Diseases	**Systemic Diseases**
Systemic lupus erythematosus	Vasculitis group
Infection-related glomerulonephritis	Polyarteritis nodosa
Subacute bacterial endocarditis	Hypersensitivity vasculitis
"Shunt" nephritis	Wegener's granulomatosis
Cryoglobulinemia	Henoch–Schönlein purpura
	Goodpasture's syndrome
Primary Renal Diseases	**Primary Renal Diseases**
Acute poststreptococcal glomerulonephritis	IgA nephropathy
Membranoproliferative glomerulonephritis	Idiopathic rapidly progressive glomerulonephritis
	Idiopathic nephrotic syndrome

sents 2.5 g of protein excreted a day per 1.73 m^2 of body surface area.[26] In contrast, nephritic sediment includes hematuria, pyuria, cellular and granular casts, and variable degrees of proteinuria. When glomerular diseases progress to advanced renal insufficiency and result in a significant reduction in the glomerular filtration rate (GFR), urinalysis may show less proteinuria and hematuria. In patients with chronic glomerular disease, broad waxy casts may be present in the urinary sediment.

GFR in patients with glomerular disease may be variable. In the early stages of the disease, the GFR may remain normal. Initial injury to the glomerulus primarily lowers the permeability coefficient (K_f) of the GBM, by reducing the surface area available for filtration and/or the unit permeability of the membrane. The reduced permeability is compensated by an elevation in the glomerular capillary hydrostatic pressure through afferent arteriolar dilation and efferent arteriolar constriction. Extensive glomerular damage may therefore be present before a substantial reduction of total GFR is evident.

Patients who present with glomerulonephritis may be categorized according to the presence or absence of evidence for systemic disease (Fig. 46–5). Determination of the serum complement concentration is frequently helpful in defining the specific type of glomerular disease (Table 46–4). Measurement of antinuclear and anti-DNA antibodies, antistreptolysin antibodies, circulating anti-GBM antibodies, and cryoglobulins is useful in identifying the etiology (Fig. 46–6).

The patient's age is often helpful in pinpointing the specific type of glomerular disease. Many of the conditions are more prevalent in certain age groups, though they may occur at any age. Benign hematuria, for example, is primarily a disease of children. Lupus and idiopathic membranoproliferative glomerulonephritis (MPGN) are seen primarily in 15 to 40 year-old patients, and primary amyloidosis affects adults over the age of 40. Figure 46–7 indicates the distribution of the different causes of nephrotic-range proteinuria relative to the age of patients undergoing renal biopsy.

Although the cause of proteinuria and glomerular disease may be established from clinical and laboratory evaluation, more often uncertainty persists. Specific treatment of

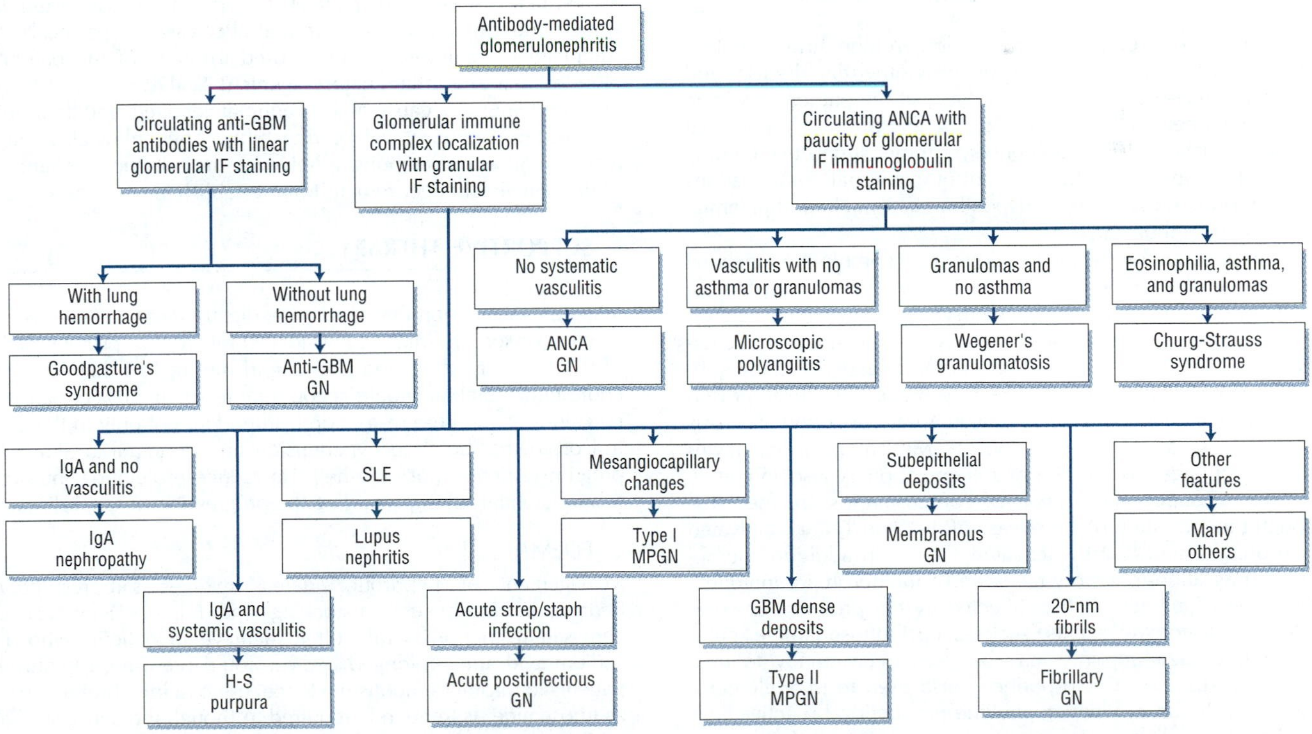

FIGURE 46–6. Features that distinguish different immunopathologic categories of antibody-mediated glomerulonephritis. GBM = glomerular basement membrane; IF = immunofluorescence microscopy; ANCA = antineutrophil cytopolasmic autoantibodies; GN = glomerulonephritis; H-S = Henoch–Schönlein; MPGN = membranoproliferative glumerulonephritis. *(From Ref. 168.)*

FIGURE 46–7. Frequency of various causes for nephrotic-range proteinuria (> 3 g/d) relative to age in patients undergoing renal biopsy evaluation at the University of North Carolina Nephropathology Laboratory. The full vertical height of the bar represents 100% of the patients. The patients with proliferative glomerulonephritis generally presented with nephritic features in addition to the proteinuria and included patients with lupus nephritis, IgA nephropathy, and postinfectious glomerulonephritis. *(From Ref. 49.)*

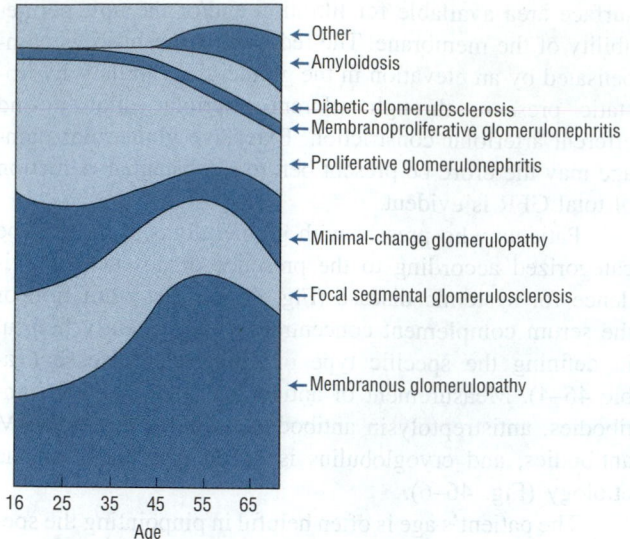

the glomerular disease depends on the underlying pathology. Percutaneous renal biopsy is, therefore, often needed to provide a definitive diagnosis. One notable exception is minimal-change disease (lipoid nephrosis), which is the most common etiology for nephrotic syndrome in children between 1 and 6 years of age. An empiric trial of corticosteroids is indicated for these patients without the need for histologic diagnosis. Biopsy is indicated only for those who fail to respond to a therapeutic course of corticosteroids.

The decision to perform a biopsy should be based on an evaluation of the potential risks of the procedure against the anticipated benefits of knowing the underlying pathology as the basis for rational therapy. The most common complication of biopsy is bleeding, which may present as hematuria or perinephric hematoma. About 10% of the patients will have gross hematuria, which usually resolves in several days. However, blood transfusion may be needed in up to 1.0% of patients and nephrectomy or therapeutic embolic infarction may be necessary in 0.1% of the patients because of severe bleeding. Mortality from renal biopsy is probably less than 0.1%. Biopsy is contraindicated in patients with a solitary kidney, polycystic kidney disease, uncontrolled hypertension, coagulation defects, or poor cooperation. Morphologic diagnosis can usually be made if tissue is examined with light, immunofluorescence, and electron microscopic techniques.

▶ TREATMENT: Glomerulonephritis

GENERAL APPROACH TO TREATMENT

The management of patients with glomerulonephritis involves specific pharmacologic therapy for the glomerular disease, and supportive measures to prevent and/or treat the pathophysiologic sequelae, namely, hypertension, edema, and progression of renal disease. In patients with nephrotic syndrome, supportive therapy should also address the management of extrarenal complications of heavy proteinuria, namely, hypoalbuminemia, hyperlipidemia, and thromboembolism.

Immunosuppressive agents, alone or in combination, may be used to alter the different immune processes that are responsible for the glomerulonephritides. Corticosteroids, in addition to their immunosuppressive effect, also possess anti-inflammatory activities. They reduce the production and/or release of many substances that mediate the inflammatory process, such as prostaglandins, leukotrienes, platelet-activating factors, tumor necrosis factors (TNFs), and interleukin-1 (IL-1). Movement of leukocytes and macrophages to the site of inflammation is also inhibited. The immunosuppressive effects of corticosteroids are mediated through the inhibition of the release of IL-1 and TNF by activated macrophages, and IL-2 by activated T cells. In addition, the actions of migration-inhibitory factor and γ-interferon are inhibited. Processing of antigens is thus affected by the presence of corticosteroids. Cytotoxic agents, such as cyclophosphamide, chlorambucil, or azathioprine, may be used occasionally to treat glomerular diseases. Cyclosporine is also used to treat glomerulonephritis. It can reduce lymphokine production by activated T lymphocytes and decrease proteinuria by improving the permselectivity of the GBM.

Since many immune factors are implicated in the pathogenesis of glomerulonephritis, plasmapheresis is used to remove these mediators. Platelets have been shown to be activated in glomerular disease and platelet factors can cause arteriolar smooth muscle cell proliferation and alter vascular permeability. Antiplatelet agents are therefore used in some of the patients. Nonsteroidal anti-inflammatory agents (NSAIDs) are used to reduce proteinuria because of their antiplatelet effect and their ability to alter capillary wall permeability. They may also affect arachidonic acid metabolism; however, the specific mechanisms of the beneficial effect remain to be established.

SUPPORTIVE THERAPY

In patients with nephrotic syndrome, dietary measures involve restriction of sodium intake to 50 to 100 mEq/d,[20,27] protein intake of 0.8 to 1.0 g/d,[27,28] and a low-lipid diet of less than 200 mg cholesterol. Total fat should account for less than 30% of daily total calories.[27] Sodium restriction is important not only in the control of edema, but also hypertension and proteinuria. Similarly, protein restriction not only helps to reduce proteinuria, but also has a potential role in retarding the progression of renal disease.

EDEMA

Management of nephrotic edema involves salt restriction, bedrest, and use of support stockings and diuretics. However, severe salt restriction is difficult to achieve in patients who are sodium-avid and prolonged bedrest could predispose nephrotic patients to thromboembolism. Hence, use of a loop diuretic, such as furosemide, is frequently required. Although the delivery of diuretic to the kidney tubules is normal, the presence of large amounts of protein in the urine promotes drug binding and thereby reduces the availability of the diuretic to the luminal receptor sites. In addition, reduced sodium delivery to the distal tubule secondary to decreased glomerular perfusion may also alter diuretic effectiveness. Large doses of the loop diuretic, such as 160 to 480 mg of furosemide, may be needed for patients with moderate edema. In some patients, a thiazide diuretic or metolazone, may be added to enhance natriuresis.[27,29] Alternatively, continuous intravenous infusion of a loop diuretic, such as furosemide 160 to 480 mg/day, may be employed and is more effective than intermittent bolus injections in inducing urinary sodium excretion.[30] In patients with morbid edema, albumin infusion may be used to expand plasma volume and to increase diuretic delivery to the renal tubules, thus enhancing diuretic effect. However, it may precipitate congestive heart failure and may also reduce therapeutic response to steroid in minimal change nephropathy.

HYPERTENSION

Optimal control of hypertension in patients with glomerular disease is important in reducing both the progression of renal disease and the risk for cardiovascular disease[28,31] (see Chaps. 42 and 19). The target blood pressure is suggested to be 130/ 80 to 85 mm Hg. In patients with chronic renal insufficiency and proteinuria greater than 1 g/d, the mean arterial pressure should be reduced further to 92 mm Hg, which is equivalent to 125/75 mm Hg.[31] However, aggressive blood pressure reduction may result in stroke and myocardial infarction in susceptible patients. Thiazide or loop diuretics with salt restriction are often used for initial blood pressure control. Angiotensin-converting enzyme (ACE) inhibitors or angiotensin II receptor antagonists may be added if blood pressure control is not adequate. The ACE inhibitors and possibly the angiotensin II receptor antagonists may reduce renal protein excretion, have renoprotective effects, and are well tolerated and effective.[32] Alternatively, nondihydropyridine calcium channel blockers (e.g., diltiazem) may have proteinuria-reduction properties and could be used as an additional agent. The dihydropyridine calcium channel blockers (e.g., nifedipine, amlodipine, nisoldipine) can also be used to lower blood pressure but without the benefit of urinary protein reduction.[33]

Dietary protein restriction reduces proteinuria and may retard renal function deterioration. Data from the Modification of Diet in Renal Disease (MDRD) study in patients with a moderate loss of renal function—GFR of 25 to 55 mL/min/1.73 m^2—did not prove the efficacy of a low-protein diet in slowing renal disease progression. However, secondary analysis revealed that protein intake of 0.65 g/kg/d reduced the rate of GFR deterioration.[34] In view of the lack of definitive proof about the benefit of protein restriction on disease progression, a standard protein diet—greater than 0.8 g/kg/d—is recommended for patients with moderate renal insufficiency. However, the patients should be made aware of the potential benefits of reducing protein intake to 0.6 g/kg/d. Decreasing dietary protein will also reduce the intake of phosphorus and potassium. For those nondialyzed patients who have GFRs of less than 13 to 25 mL/min/1.73 m^2, dietary protein intake should be reduced to 0.6 g/kg/d since it can retard the rate of renal function loss and also the time to reach end-stage renal disease.[28]

Since heavy proteinuria is the underlying cause for hypoalbuminemia and other complications of nephrotic syndrome, various strategies including protein restriction to 0.8 to 1.0 g/kg/d, plus an additional gram of protein for each gram of protein lost in the urine,[28] ACE inhibitors,[35,36] and NSAIDs,[37] are used to reduce proteinuria. An additive antiproteinuric effect has been shown by combining a low-protein diet with ACE inhibition,[36] as well as combined therapy with ACE inhibitors and NSAIDs.[38] Serum albumin concentrations were also improved during treatment.[35,36] ACE inhibition may also allow the use of a high-protein diet without risks of decreased albumin synthesis.[39] A reduction in proteinuria is usually apparent within the first few weeks of therapy while the maximal effect is attained after 8 to 12 weeks.[40] The initial antiproteinuric effect of ACE inhibitors is associated with a fall in filtration fraction, suggesting a reduction in intraglomerular pressure. However, an improvement of GBM permselectivity may be responsible for the long-term effect of ACE inhibitors.[40]

NSAIDs probably reduce proteinuria through an alteration of intrarenal hemodynamics, a decrease in GFR, and also the restoration of the barrier size-selectivity of the GBM.[27,40] Indomethacin and meclofenamate are the two NSAIDs that have been evaluated the most. Their antiproteinuric effect occurs within 1 to 2 weeks of the initiation of therapy.[27,41] NSAID therapy is indicated for patients with severe steroid-resistant nephrotic syndrome who have greater than 50% residual renal function.[41] The agents should be avoided in those with poor renal function because of their potential detrimental effect on kidney function and also the increased susceptibility of these patients to nephrotoxicity.[27,41] Long-term treatment is indicated for those who have greater than 40% reduction in urinary protein excretion and/or those whose serum albumin concentrations are doubled during therapy.[41] In conjunction with dietary sodium restriction, the antiproteinuric efficacy of protein restriction, ACE inhibition, and NSAIDs is enhanced.[40]

HYPERLIPIDEMIA

The abnormal lipoprotein profile seen in nephrotic patients may increase the risk of atherosclerosis. Even though the clinical sequelae of the dyslipidemia of nephrotic syndrome are unknown, it is prudent to treat patients with persistent nephrotic syndrome and sustained dyslipidemia—those with high VLDL and LDL cholesterol levels in the presence of a normal or low HDL cholesterol level. Therapy is especially needed for those with concurrent atherosclerotic cardiovascular disease, or with additional risk factors for atherosclerosis, such as smoking and hypertension.[23] Whether correction of lipoprotein abnormalities will slow the progression of renal disease as demonstrated in animal studies requires clinical confirmation.[23,24]

A low-fat diet is usually not sufficient to correct hyperlipoproteinemia.[17,27,42] Lipid-lowering agents are usually required. Probucol, bile acid resins, fibric acid derivatives, and hydroxymethylglutaryl coenzyme A (HMG CoA) reductase inhibitors have all been evaluated in patients with nephrotic syndrome.[23] HMG CoA reductase inhibitors, such as lovastatin, pravastatin, simvastatin, and fluvastatin, are considered the treatment of choice.[17,23,27] These agents inhibit the rate-limiting step in cholesterol biosynthesis, namely, the conversion of HMG CoA to mevalonate.[24] In short-term studies, they reduce total plasma cholesterol concentration by 22% to 36%, LDL cholesterol by 27% to 45%, and total plasma triglyceride concentration by 19% to 40%.[23] The increase in HDL cholesterol and/or decrease in atherogenic lipoprotein(a) is variable.[40,43,44] Meta-analysis showed that use of HMG CoA reductase inhibitors resulted in the greatest and most consistent decrease in LDL cholesterol levels.[42] Interestingly, the reduction in proteinuria with ACE inhibitors is accompanied by a reduction in total plasma cholesterol and the lipoprotein(a) level.[34,45] Combined use of an ACE inhibitor with an HMG CoA reductase inhibitor may therefore be more effective in controlling nephrotic hyperlipidemia. In all the patients, consistent use of a prudent diet, modest exercise, cessation of smoking, and adequate blood pressure control should be the cornerstone of hyperlipidemia management. They may offer as much or more benefit than the lowering of cholesterol levels by pharmacologic means.

ANTICOAGULATION

Intravascular thrombosis is a serious and common complication of nephrotic syndrome, particularly in membranous nephropathy. Patients are at risk for developing renal vein thrombosis, pulmonary emboli, or other thromboembolic events. While it is generally agreed that patients who have documented thromboembolic episodes should be anticoagulated with warfarin until remission of nephrotic syndrome, the use of prophylactic anticoagulation is controversial. A decision analysis study suggested that prophylactic anticoagulation is beneficial in patients with membranous nephropathy.[46] However, prospective controlled studies should be conducted to confirm these findings. Anticoagulation should also be considered in patients with increased risks for thrombosis, such as prolonged bedrest, surgery, episodes of dehydration, or use of high-dose intravenous steroids.[27] As an example, low-dose, subcutaneous heparin may be given prophylactically for a limited duration in patients with severe nephrotic syndrome who are placed on bedrest. For patients with a history of thromboembolic episode, warfarin should be given, after an initial course of standard or low-molecular-weight heparin, for as long as heavy proteinuria and hypoalbuminemia are present. The role of low-molecular-weight heparin in preventing thromboembolism is uncertain but preliminary results are encouraging.[47]

DISEASE PROGRESSION, TREATMENT EVALUATION, AND ECONOMIC CONSIDERATIONS

DISEASE PROGRESSION AND TREATMENT CONSIDERATIONS

The course and prognosis of the different glomerular diseases are extremely variable and depend on the underlying etiology. In glomerular diseases with a secondary cause, such as poststreptococcal glomerulonephritis, once the initiating factor is removed, the prognosis of the renal disease is often good. In contrast, the rates of renal function deterioration among the primary glomerulonephritides vary according to the form of glomerulonephritis. Most patients with minimal-change disease, IgA nephropathy, and membranous nephropathy have a fairly good prognosis. However, those with focal segmental glomerulosclerosis who are resistant to therapy as well as those with rapidly progressive glomerulonephritis who are untreated are likely to experience a rapid loss of renal function. Some of these patients may have half of their renal function lost within a 3-month period. Certain glomerulonephritides, such as minimal-change nephropathy, is very responsive to treatment, whereas consistently effective therapy is yet to be found for other types of glomerulonephritis, such as membranous proliferative glomerulonephritis.

The variable courses exhibited by the different glomerulonephritides require that specific treatment approaches be developed for each disease. The natural history of each type of glomerulonephritis has to be well delineated before a promising regimen can be evaluated, from both therapeutic and economic perspectives. Otherwise, patients will be exposed to unnecessary treatment-related toxicities if they have a type of glomerulonephritis that is likely to undergo spontaneous remission. Many of the drugs that are used to treat glomerular diseases are potentially toxic. The many adverse effects associated with steroids are well known, and cytotoxic agents have potentially serious toxicities. Long-term use of cyclosporine may compromise renal function and nullify the renoprotection derived from treatment. The potential therapeutic effects of treatment regimens should always be weighed against the risks that the patients are being exposed to. It is therefore imperative to identify patients who are most likely to benefit from treatment, especially those who have other risk factors that may contribute to the deterioration of their renal function. In those instances where satisfactory regimens are not available to treat the primary disease, appropriate supportive measures should be identified. Optimization of systemic and glomerular pressure, reducing proteinuria, and possibly controlling hyperlipidemia may all improve the long-term outcome and the quality of life of these patients.

TREATMENT MONITORING

Patients should be monitored closely for therapeutic response as well as the appearance of treatment-related toxicities. While the rate of renal function deterioration is an important indicator of the long-term success of the treatment, resolution of nephrotic and nephritic signs and symptoms associated with the glomerulopathies should be assessed regularly.

Serum creatinine concentration as well as creatinine clearance ought to be evaluated prior to and during treatment; 24-hour urine outflow should be collected to determine the extent of proteinuria. Alternatively, the daily urine protein excretion may be estimated by the urinary total protein:creatinine concentration ratio. After establishing the correlation between the 24-hour urinary protein excretion with the protein:creatinine ratio, single random urine specimens may be used in place of a 24-hour urine collection. Blood pressure should be monitored periodically to assess the need for and also the adequacy of antihypertensive therapy. The pressures should also be evaluated in conjunction with clinical signs and symptoms of edema and fluid overload to gauge the need for volume control as well as diuretic use. For patients with nephrotic syndrome, serum lipid concentrations should be monitored. If the patient has hematuria, urinalysis and complete blood count ought to be obtained. The clinician should also be aware of the patient's appetite and energy level since these are indicators of the patient's overall state of well-being. At times, renal biopsy is needed to assess response to treatment and disease progression, to determine future treatment strategy and to confirm the initial diagnosis.

Patients receiving cytotoxic drug treatment ought to be evaluated for drug-related toxicities every week during the initial treatment period. After 1 month of treatment, the frequency of monitoring may be reduced. When the patient is on long-term steroid treatment, monthly visits are often required for assessment of both efficacy and toxicities. If a favorable response is obtained after a course of treatment, the patient may be evaluated every 3 to 4 months. The patient's renal function, proteinuria, urinalysis, blood pressure, lipid profile, and the overall state of health should be assessed during these regular follow-up visits.

OUTCOME AND ECONOMIC EVALUATION

Prospective, randomized, controlled comparative trials need to be conducted in a sizable patient population before the efficacy and economic implications of a new regimen can be established. This type of large-scale study is quite feasible for the more common forms of glomerulonephritis such as minimal-change disease, IgA nephropathy, and membranous nephropathy. In contrast, prospective, controlled trials are difficult to conduct for the relatively uncommon glomerulonephritides such as membranous proliferative glomerulonephritis. Since the optimal approaches for treating most types of glomerulonephritis have not been identified, the economic implications of the individual treatment regimens are yet to be established.

PATHOPHYSIOLOGY AND PHARMACOTHERAPY OF INDIVIDUAL GLOMERULOPATHIES

MINIMAL-CHANGE NEPHROPATHY

Minimal-change nephropathy (also termed minimal-change disease) is commonly found in children between 3 months and 6 years of age. It is in fact one of the most common chronic diseases in childhood. In children between 1 and 4 years of age, minimal-change disease accounts for more than 90% of all cases of nephrotic syndrome. The percentage drops gradually to less than 50% after 10 years old and only accounts for 10% to 15% of all cases of idiopathic nephrotic syndrome in adults.

PATHOPHYSIOLOGY

Minimal-change disease is also known as "nil" disease primarily because of the absence of definitive pathologic changes observed under light microscopy. The characteristic lesion in patients with minimal-change disease is the spreading and fusion of the foot processes of epithelial cells over an unchanged GBM. *Lipoid nephrosis* is another term that has been used to describe this type of glomerular disease because lipids, as well as renal tubular cells, are found in the urine. The pathogenesis of minimal-change disease is still unknown. Altered cell-mediated immunologic response, specifically T-cell dysfunction, is suspected to be responsible. The activated lymphocytes are thought to secrete lymphokines that reduce the production of anions in the GBM. The permeability of the GBM to plasma albumin is therefore increased through a reduction of electrostatic repulsion. The loss of anionic charges also results in fusion of the foot processes of the epithelial cells. Other conditions that involve T-cell abnormalities, such as Hodgkin's disease, T-cell lymphoma, and nephritis induced by NSAIDs, are also associated with minimal-change disease.

CLINICAL PRESENTATION

Most patients present initially with edema, frequently acute in onset, following a nonspecific upper respiratory tract infection, allergic reaction, or vaccinations, which might have activated the T lymphocytes. Nephrotic syndrome with massive proteinuria (substantially more than 40 $mg/m^2/h$ for children and 3 g/d for adults), edema, hypoalbuminemia, and hyperlipidemia is common. The patient's weight may be increased dramatically because of sodium and fluid retention. Nephrotic features, such as gross hematuria, are uncommon. However, microscopic hematuria may be seen in up to 20% to 25% of patients. Hypertension and decreased renal function are uncommon in children but are more common in older adults.[48] In some patients, volume depletion may result in mild to moderate azotemia.

▶ TREATMENT: Minimal-Change Nephropathy

PHARMACOLOGIC THERAPY

STEROIDS

Among all the causes of nephrotic syndrome, minimal-change disease is the most responsive to corticosteroid treatment. In children, steroid therapy is expected to reduce proteinuria in about 90% of the patients. The 10-year renal survival is greater than 95%.[49] Because of the excellent response to initial therapy with steroids and the prevalence of this glomerular disease in children, reduction of proteinuria secondary to steroid treatment is considered diagnostic for minimal-change disease without the need for biopsy. In the International Study of Kidney Disease in Children (ISKDC), remission was induced, as evidenced by diuresis, loss of edema, and resolution in proteinuria, within 8 weeks of therapy in over 93% of the 363 children.[50] Prednisone was administered at a dose of 60 $mg/m^2/d$, with a maximum of 80 to 100 mg daily, in divided doses during the first 4 weeks. The dose was then reduced to 40 $mg/m^2/d$, or a maximum of 60 mg daily, in divided doses for 3 consecutive days every 7 days for another 4 weeks. An alternate-day dosage regimen can be used instead in the second 4 weeks, after which the prednisone dosage is tapered over several months.[49] Single daily doses of prednisone, instead of multiple daily doses, may result in faster and more sustained response with less frequent and less severe side effects.[49] Proteinuria will disappear in 50% of the patients after 1 week and 90% after 4 weeks of treatment. Studies were later conducted to evaluate the effectiveness of longer and shorter courses of steroid therapy for initial treatment as well as recurrences.[51] Longer therapy (6 weeks of daily prednisone followed by 6 weeks of alternate-day treatment) results in lower incidence of relapse (36%) than both standard course (4 weeks; 61%) and short course (3 weeks; 81%). It is therefore appropriate to use long-term therapy during the initial episode and short-course treatment for relapses.[52]

For adults, the dose of prednisone is 1 mg/kg/d during the initial 4 weeks with a reduction to 0.75 mg/kg/d every other day for the next 4 weeks. Proteinuria will disappear in 50% to 60% of patients after 8 weeks of treatment, and complete remission will be attained in 80% of patients after 28 weeks of therapy.[48] In some patients, 16 weeks of therapy may be needed before remission is induced.[48,50]

As many as 75% to 85% of the patients who respond to initial steroid therapy (steroid sensitive) will experience a relapse of proteinuria, mostly within 6 to 12 months after disease onset. However, some patients may not have the first relapse until 24 to 30 months later.[53] The risk of relapse is affected by the duration of initial steroid therapy.[27,51] Children who were asymptomatic with proteinuria diagnosed on a urinary screening program tend to have less frequent relapses and a more favorable clinical course.[54] In those who relapse, 50% to 65% may have steroid-responsive relapse episodes over the subsequent 3- to 5-year period.[53] The dose and duration of steroid treatment for the relapse do not influence the subsequent rate of relapse.[27] The remaining patients become steroid-dependent, requiring continuous low-dose alternate-day prednisone to maintain an extended relapse-free period. A small number of patients will eventually develop resistance to steroids and a biopsy done at that time often reveals another pathology such as focal segmental glomerular sclerosis. It is controversial whether minimal-change disease progresses into focal segmental glomerular sclerosis or whether the glomerulosclerosis that was present at the time of initial diagnosis was inadvertently diagnosed as minimal-change nephropathy because of a tissue sampling error during the renal biopsy.

For patients who are steroid resistant as well as those who require large doses of steroids to sustain remission (steroid dependent), alternative therapy should be considered. Furthermore, in pediatric patients, the growth inhibition associated with long-term steroid use often necessitates the use of alternative agents. Cyclophosphamide at 2.0 to 2.5 mg/kg/d for 8 to 12 weeks given alone or with prednisone (50 to 75 mg/m^2) is very effective in inducing remission and restoring steroid responsiveness in patients who were previously steroid dependent and then became steroid resistant. Alternatively, chlorambucil at 0.1 to 0.2 mg/kg/d may be used. This agent, however, has been associated with more adverse effects than cyclophosphamide. Azathioprine has also been used; however, favorable response is often not seen until therapy is continued for more than 6 to 12 months.[55] The use of these cytotoxic agents should thus be reserved for patients who are clearly steroid resistant, or steroid dependent (relapse within 14 days after termination of steroid treatment or dosage reduction) with significant adverse effects, or those who have two or more relapses within 6 months after the first episode or three or more relapses within 12 months.[27] The immunosuppressive effect of these agents, with or without the concurrent use of steroids, can result in serious infections, which are the primary cause of death in patients with minimal-change nephropathy.[56] Other toxicities associated with cyclophosphamide include gonadal fibrosis, which results in sterility, hemorrhagic cystitis, alopecia, and a potential to develop malignancy in those on long-term treatment.

CYCLOSPORINE

Cyclosporine has been used in adult and pediatric patients. The drug decreases lymphokine production by activated T lymphocytes and thus reduces proteinuria by reversing the lymphokine-induced alterations in the anionic charge and permeability of the GBM to albumin. Cyclosporine can also reduce proteinuria by improving the permselectivity of the GBM. In patients with steroid-sensitive or steroid-dependent minimal-change disease, cyclosporine induces remission in 80% to 85% of the patients. However, the disease-free period is frequently not sustained, and relapse, which is usually not as responsive to cyclosporine retreatment, may occur as soon as the drug is tapered or discontinued.[57] Patients with high IL-2 concentrations tend to have more sustained remission.[58] The rate of relapse is also reduced when the dose tapering is gradual or when the cyclosporine treatment period is prolonged.[59] Although only 10% to 20% of patients who have steroid-resistant disease respond to cyclosporine, combination treatment with low-dose steroid increases the effectiveness in some patients.[57,60] Use of low-dose steroid with cyclosporine may be needed in about 40% of the patients to maintain remission.[61] A 2-month trial treatment with cyclosporine may therefore be warranted in steroid-resistant patients. The steroid-sparing effect of cyclosporine is also useful in steroid-dependent patients, especially those who have experienced significant adverse effects. The usual starting daily dose of cyclosporine for remission induction is 5 mg/kg for adults and 100 to 150 mg/m^2 for children. Similar dosages are used to maintain remission long term. The need to monitor cyclosporine blood concentrations is controversial. No correlation has been found between the severity of the cyclosporine-induced tubulointerstitial lesions with either the mean dose or trough drug concentration.[57] However, the incidence of these lesions increases with the duration of treatment and cyclosporine should therefore not be given for more than 4 months in the absence of any beneficial effect.[57] Other nonrenal adverse effects associated with cyclosporine treatment include hypertrichosis, gingival hyperplasia, gastrointestinal symptoms, and hypertension.

LEVAMISOLE

Levamisole, an immunostimulant, has also been evaluated for the treatment of patients with steroid-dependent nephrotic syndrome. The agent can promote the maturation of young T cells and restore the function of T cells and phagocytes when the immune system is depressed. It may also inhibit the production of an immunosuppressive lymphokine that is associated with minimal-change nephrotic syndrome. However, its precise mechanisms of action in immunocompetent patients with glomerulonephritis remain to be identified. Levamisole was found in a placebo-controlled study to have a steroid-sparing effect in children who had steroid-responsive and steroid-dependent nephrotic syndrome.[62] About half of the 31 children in the levamisole group remained in remission 16 weeks into therapy while prednisolone was tapered in the initial 8 weeks. Two controlled studies with a longer period of follow-up did not reveal any significant beneficial effect.[63,64] The most serious adverse effect of levamisole is neutropenia, which is generally reversible. Rarely, agranulocytosis has been reported in patients with connective tissue or neoplastic diseases. Levamisole has also been shown to have a favorable effect when used in conjunction with BCG and dipyridamole in adult patients with different types of primary glomerulonephritis.[65] At present, further controlled studies are needed to define precisely the benefit of this agent in the treatment of glomerulonephritis.

THERAPEUTIC OUTCOMES

The long-term prognosis of most patients with minimal-change disease is good. The majority of pediatric patients will not experience any relapse of the disease 10 years after the initial onset, and most will be free of the proteinuria after puberty.[53] In adults, an

85% to 90% survival rate is seen 10 years after the disease onset.[53] Spontaneous remission may be present in up to 70% of untreated adults.[66] Development of renal failure is uncommon in both adult and pediatric patients. Significant deterioration of renal function is observed only in those patients who are steroid resistant or steroid dependent. Because of the overall favorable outcome of the disease and the relatively uncommon progression into chronic renal failure, aggressive use of cytotoxic agents is not indicated even in most patients with frequent relapses. Toxicities associated with aggressive therapy do not justify the need to induce remission in those patients who fail to respond to steroids and the nonaggressive use of cytotoxic agents. Symptomatic therapy with diuretics to control edema, in conjunction with a low-salt diet and albumin infusion as needed for acute development of anasarca, is often a more rewarding therapeutic approach. NSAIDs and ACE inhibitors may also be used to reduce the proteinuria.

FOCAL SEGMENTAL GLOMERULOSCLEROSIS

Focal segmental glomerulosclerosis (FSGS) is a histologic lesion that can be idiopathic (primary) or secondary to a variety of causes. Conditions such as sickle cell disease, cyanotic congenital heart disease, and morbid obesity can induce hemodynamic stress on an initially normal nephron population and result in FSGS.[67] Severe glomerular injury can also be seen in patients with nephropathy associated with heroin abuse and human immunodeficiency virus (HIV) infection.[67,68] The primary and secondary sclerotic lesions may be morphologically similar, but they represent diseases with different courses and responses to therapy.

PATHOPHYSIOLOGY

Sclerotic lesions are characteristically found in some of the glomeruli (focal) and usually involve only a portion of the glomeruli (segmental).[69] Similar to the minimal-change disease, fusion of foot processes is commonly seen in those glomeruli that are not sclerotic. It is thought that both minimal-change disease and FSGS share similar pathogenetic mechanisms, with FSGS resulting in severe injury to the glomerular epithelial cells. During the early stage of FSGS, only a small number of glomeruli may have the segmental sclerotic lesion and the disease may be confined to the juxtamedullary region. If an inadequate number of glomeruli are sampled during renal biopsy, the diagnosis of FSGS may be missed or the patient may be thought to have minimal-change disease. Resistance to steroid therapy may thus be one of the first clues that the patient indeed has FSGS rather than minimal-change disease. Alternatively, a patient may have the steroid-sensitive minimal-change disease initially, which subsequently progresses to steroid-resistant FSGS.

CLINICAL PRESENTATION

FSGS accounts for less than 15% of the cases of idiopathic nephrotic syndrome in children and about 15% to 20% in adults. Almost all the patients present with proteinuria, and many of them have all the features of nephrotic syndrome.[70] The proteinuria is nonselective, containing albumin and other higher-molecular-weight proteins, and is usually less severe when compared to patients who have minimal-change disease. Hypertension, microscopic hematuria, and renal dysfunction may be seen in up to half of the patients. The reduced renal function becomes more prevalent as the disease progresses. FSGS is more common in black patients who tend to present with proteinuria more frequently in the nephrotic range. They are also more likely to have a rapid decline in renal function.

▶ TREATMENT: Focal Segmental Glomerulosclerosis

■ PHARMACOLOGIC THERAPY

■ STEROIDS

Since the pathophysiology of primary FSGS is unknown, it is not possible to direct pharmacologic treatment against any specific pathologic processes. Furthermore, the treatment of FSGS remains controversial due to the lack of data from randomized, prospective, controlled trials. A course of prednisone (1 to 2 mg/kg/d) with tapering after 3 to 4 months of treatment may be used for nephrotic patients.[69] Urinary protein excretion and serum albumin concentration should be monitored to assess efficacy. The average time to induce complete remission is 3 to 4 months and up to 6 months may be needed in some patients.[70] A longer duration of treatment (6 months or more) has resulted in complete remission in more than 40% of patients; older studies reported a response rate of less than 20% using regimens of a shorter duration.[70,71] For patients who are not nephrotic, the relative favorable prognosis does not support the use of steroid or other immunosuppressive agents. However, close follow-up and good blood pressure control with ACE inhibitors are necessary to minimize disease progression.[69]

■ CYTOTOXIC AGENTS

Cytotoxic agents such as cyclophosphamide, chlorambucil, and azathioprine have not been found effective in the treatment of FSGS. However, combining prednisone therapy with cyclophosphamide and/or azathioprine over an extended period of time has been reported to result in complete or partial remission in 60% of 59 adult patients in one study.[71] Using an aggressive regimen incorporating pulse methylprednisolone infusions with long-term immunosuppression using oral alternate-day prednisone and an alkylating agent, a remission rate of 65% was observed in children with steroid-resistant FSGS.[52,72]

CYCLOSPORINE

Short-term cyclosporine may reduce proteinuria in some patients who have FSGS resistant to corticosteroid and cytotoxic agents.[70] However, relapse of proteinuria is frequent, especially if treatment is withdrawn abruptly.[73] The relapse may occur within 2 months of tapering or drug discontinuation.[70] A prolonged period of treatment with slow tapering may result in longer periods of remission.[59] A recent study was conducted to evaluate long-term cyclosporine therapy in 21 black and Hispanic children who had steroid-resistant FSGS.[74] These patients tend to have more rapid renal function deterioration than white children. The cyclosporine dosage was titrated to the serum cholesterol concentration. Higher doses were given to patients with severe hypercholesterolemia.[74,75] This aggressive regimen (4 to 20 mg/kg/d for 3 to 97 months) produced a reduction in proteinuria from 6.2 to 2.0 g/day and in the percentage of patients who developed ESRD (78% in the historical controls to 24% in these treated patients).[74] Although histologic evidence of cyclosporine nephrotoxicity was not seen in this study, the drug was found to be more nephrotoxic in steroid-resistant than in steroid-responsive disease.[52] Combination with low-dose or alternate-day steroids may increase the efficacy of cyclosporine in steroid-resistant patients.[52]

SYMPTOMATIC THERAPY

Due to the lack of a consistently effective regimen for primary FSGS, many patients with mild disease are treated conservatively for symptomatic control. ACE inhibitors have been found to be effective in reducing proteinuria and stabilizing renal function in patients with primary or secondary FSGS.[67,76] The constriction of afferent arterioles by these agents reduces intraglomerular pressure, which may diminish the potential effect of glomerular hypertension in promoting the development of FSGS.[76] The driving force for proteinuria may also be reduced without necessarily correcting the primary defect in glomerular wall permselectivity.[67] The NSAID meclofenamate has been found to be effective in reducing proteinuria in patients with steroid-resistant FSGS.[41] These favorable results have, however, not been confirmed in studies using a larger number of patients. Thus, their role in the overall scheme of therapy remains to be defined. For patients with more severe disease, corticosteroids with or without immunosuppressive agents should be considered. Treatment should not be continued for more than 3 to 4 months unless the patient experiences a remission. In this case, therapy may be continued for 12 to 24 months to maintain the therapeutic response.[71]

THERAPEUTIC OUTCOME

Patients with primary FSGS are at risk for developing ESRD. For the 30% to 50% of adults and children who had attained complete remission, ESRD develops in about 10% at 10 years.[70] For those patients who are resistant to therapy, the rate of renal function deterioration to ESRD may be rapid, within 1 year, or slow, over as long as 10 to 20 years. About 50% of them develop ESRD in 10 years. Those patients with severe proteinuria (> 10 to 15 g/d), high serum creatinine concentration at diagnosis, initial steroid resistance, or interstitial fibrosis on renal biopsy are likely to have a more rapid decline in renal function. Kidney transplantation is often indicated for those patients who develop ESRD; however, FSGS has recurred in 20% to 50% of the renal allografts soon after transplantation. Children and those with severe disease or rapid progression to ESRD prior to transplantation are more likely to experience a recurrence. The proteinuria may reappear within hours after transplantation and graft failure may occur in one-third to one-half of the patients. The median time to recurrence was reported to be 14 days in one study.[77] Although cyclosporine is not effective in preventing the recurrence of nephrotic syndrome after transplantation, a high dose of the agent (up to 35 mg/kg/d) has been shown to induce a remission of the recurrent disease.[78] ACE inhibitors and plasmapheresis have also been used to prolong graft survival. The effectiveness of these therapies and the rapid recurrence of the disease in the transplanted kidney substantiate the possibility that a circulating humoral mediator is responsible for the nephropathy.[79]

MEMBRANOUS NEPHROPATHY

Membranous nephropathy is the most common disorder responsible for idiopathic nephrotic syndrome in adults, accounting for about 20% to 25% of cases.[80] The hallmark histologic features of membranous nephropathy are glomerular capillary wall thickening with subepithelial deposits under light and electron microscopy. Most cases are idiopathic, but about 25% of adults and 80% of children have secondary causes.[80,81] In the United States, the most common etiologies are autoimmune diseases (e.g., lupus), infection (e.g., hepatitis B), syphilis, neoplasm (e.g., carcinoma of the lung, breast, gastrointestinal tract, or kidney),[82] and medications (e.g., organic gold, penicillamine, mercury, or captopril). Malaria and schistosomiasis are common causes in other parts of the world. De novo membranous nephropathy can also occur in the allografts of renal transplant patients.[83] It is important to identify any potential underlying causes because the treatment and prognosis of patients with idiopathic or secondary membranous nephropathy are different. Although this glomerular disease can occur at any age, the peak incidence is between 30 and 50 years and is especially likely in patients over 50 years old who present with nephrotic syndrome.[80]

PATHOPHYSIOLOGY

Examination of kidney tissue under light microscopy reveals normal mesangium and normocellularity. The glomerular capillary wall may be thickened in well-developed lesions. Trichome stain shows subepithelial deposits, and silver stain reveals spike-like projections between deposits. These projections gradually fuse to engulf the deposits such that, in the advanced stage, the capillary wall is markedly thickened and intramembranous deposits are found. Progressive changes in capillary lumen patency parallel those in the GBM, resulting in glomerulosclerosis with capillary collapse, and tubular atrophy in end-stage membranous nephropathy. Immunofluorescence microscopy shows strong capillary wall staining of IgG and C3 on the epithelial side of the basement membrane. Secondary membranous nephropathy exhibits similar lesions except for the additional presence of mesangial expansion and hypercellularity with fewer deposits. In patients with membranous nephropathy induced by lupus, subendothelial and extraglomerular deposition can also be seen.

Antibody-mediated immune injury appears to be the main pathogenetic mechanism. Animal models of membranous nephropathy, particularly Heymenn's nephritis in rats, provide evidence that it is an autoimmune disease with immune complex deposition in the subepithelium of the GBM.[84] The immune complex can be formed *in situ* or deposited from circulating immune complexes. In Heymenn's nephritis, the intrinsic antigen is megalin (formerly gp330), a glycoprotein produced by the visceral epithelial cells. The antimegalin antibodies traverse the glomerular basement membrane to form immune complexes in the coated pits of the glomerular epithelial cells. These antimegalin immune complexes then become anchored to the glomerular basement membrane and detached from the podocyte cell membrane. These processes repeat themselves, resulting in accumulation of more immune complexes in the GBM until they become morphologically apparent.[84] Although the antigen responsible for primary human membranous nephropathy is not known, the mechanism for disease progression is thought to be similar.

Clinical Presentation

The majority of patients with membranous nephropathy present with heavy proteinuria exceeding 3.5 g/d. The signs and symptoms are usually insidious in onset and consist of anorexia, malaise, edema, occasionally anasarca, ascites, and pericardial and pleural effusions. As a result of a hypercoagulable state, pulmonary embolism may be found, but rarely results in death.[85] The incidence of renal vein thrombosis varies from 5% to 62%,[25,81,85] and it should be suspected when there is a sudden onset of hematuria, loin pain, pulmonary embolus, fluctuating or worsening proteinuria or glomerular filtration rate, renal tubular acidosis, or an increase in leg edema. Hypertension is found in about 30% of patients and is more common in the presence of renal insufficiency or until the disease is advanced.

In addition to heavy proteinuria, urinalysis often reveals lipiduria and oval fat bodies. Microhematuria is seen in fewer than 25% of patients, and gross hematuria and red cell casts are rare. In idiopathic membranous nephropathy, the serum complement concentrations are normal. Low levels of complement should alert one to search for secondary causes, such as lupus, hepatitis B infection, or an alternative diagnosis. Similarly, antinuclear antibodies, anti-DNA antibodies, rheumatoid factor, hepatitis B serologies, and serum cryoglobulins are generally negative in idiopathic membranous nephropathy. Occult malignancy has been found in up to 10% of elderly patients with membranous nephropathy.[82]

The natural course of idiopathic membranous nephropathy is variable. About 25% of patients experience spontaneous remission of the disease over a mean of 5.5 years.[81] Less than 10% of the nonnephrotic patients and about one-third to one-half of the nephrotic patients will progress to end-stage renal failure over 10 to 15 years.[80] Some other patients have various degrees of renal insufficiency and persistent proteinuria. Heavy proteinuria (> 10 g/d), male gender, elevated serum creatinine concentration at the time of presentation, poorly controlled hypertension, old age at onset of disease, non-Asian race, certain HLA antigens, and tubulointerstitial fibrosis on initial renal biopsy are associated with progressive renal disease.[80,81] Overall, patients with idiopathic membranous nephropathy have a relatively benign course. The mean 10-year survival is about 70%.[86] Those who present with persistent nonnephrotic proteinuria seldom develop renal insufficiency and have a normal life expectancy. Fewer than 10% of patients develop a remitting and relapsing course.[81] The prognosis for secondary membranous nephropathy depends on the underlying cause. Remission occurs when the infection resolves or when the causative medication is withdrawn.

▶ TREATMENT: Membranous Nephropathy

The treatment of idiopathic membranous nephropathy has been controversial and has ranged from supportive therapy to immunosuppression with steroids alone, or in combination with alkylating agents. Conservative management of membranous nephropathy includes control of edema with salt restriction and diuretics[20] and reduction of proteinuria with protein restriction and ACE inhibitors.[87] Management of hypertension and hyperlipidemia will be required for most, while long-term anticoagulation is usually necessary only for patients with renal vein thrombosis or a documented pulmonary embolus.[81,88]

PHARMACOLOGIC THERAPY

STEROIDS

Remission of proteinuria, whether spontaneously or treatment related, may confer a good prognosis.[81,89] Most available studies have focused on treatment in patients with nephrosis and normal or stable renal function. Many uncontrolled and controlled studies have yielded conflicting results regarding the efficacy of corticosteroids.[73] The U.S. prospective randomized collaborative trial demonstrated a beneficial effect of high-dose oral prednisone 120 mg given every other day for 8 weeks in 72 patients with idiopathic membranous nephropathy.[90] Advanced renal failure occurred in only 1 of the treated patients, but 10 of 38 control patients progressed to ESRD. However, the unusually poor prognosis of the placebo group casts doubts on the favorable results of the study. Indeed, the British Medical Research Council, using the same steroid protocol, did not demonstrate a reduction in the incidence of ESRD.[91] The benefits of steroids were also not shown in a Canadian study, which used moderate doses of prednisone, 40 mg/m^2 daily for 6 months.[92] In contrast, high doses of intravenous steroids may improve renal function, particularly in patients with superimposed crescentic glomerulonephritis.[94]

However, results of a meta-analysis did not reveal any beneficial effect of steroids over symptomatic therapy in terms of remission or 5-year renal survival.[94]

CYTOTOXIC AGENTS

Different results have been reported with the use of alkylating agents alone or in combination with steroids. In a retrospective study of 36 patients with idiopathic membranous nephropathy, oral prednisolone 60 mg daily for 8 to 10 weeks and subsequent taper was compared with combination therapy of the same steroid regimen and oral cyclophosphamide (1.5 to 2.0 mg/kg/d) for a mean period of 3.6 months. No differences were noted with respect to the induction of complete or partial remission, or the percentage of patients who developed ESRD.[95] Similarly, a randomized, controlled trial of oral cyclophosphamide 1.5 to 2.5 mg/kg/d for 1 year did not show benefits over supportive therapy.[96] Nonetheless, a 2-year randomized, controlled trial with daily oral cyclophosphamide for 6 months with dipyridamole and warfarin for 2 years showed significant improvement in proteinuria with no significant change in renal function in either group.[97] The most impressive results to date were reported by Ponticelli and colleagues who administered intravenous methylprednisolone 1 g/d for 3 days, followed by 0.5 mg/kg/d orally for 27 days, and then alternated every other month with chlorambucil 0.2 mg/kg/d for a total of 6 months.[98] This immunosuppressive regimen resulted in remissions in 67% of the treated patients, compared to only 23% of those receiving supportive care alone.[98] Only 10% of the treated patients had elevated serum creatinine concentrations, compared to 49% of those in the supportive care group. After a 10-year follow-up, 92% of the surviving treated patients did not have ESRD, compared with 60% of the control.[99] Treatment also resulted in a slower decline of renal function and increased probability of complete or partial remission and period of time free from nephrotic syndrome.[99]

When the data from the prospective trials with steroids and those with cytotoxic agents were evaluated by meta-analysis, treatment with cytotoxic agents but not steroids was associated with an increased likelihood of complete or partial remission.[94,100] However, cytotoxic agents were associated with adverse events in 12% of the patients, compared with only 3% in steroid-treated patients.[94]

THERAPEUTIC OUTCOME

Because only about 25% of patients with new-onset idiopathic membranous nephropathy ultimately develop ESRD over a 20- to 30-year period, it is prudent not to treat all patients with new-onset membranous nephropathy.[101–103] Patients who have a low likelihood for renal disease progression can be managed with observation and symptomatic therapy. These include children 2 to 16 years of age, adult males with proteinuria less than 2 g/d, or adult females with proteinuria less than 5 g/d and normal renal function.[101,104] Patients who have a high risk of developing renal failure, including those with proteinuria greater than 10 g/d with or without impaired renal function, and patients with symptomatic nephrotic syndrome with a plasma albumin of less than 2 g/dL, should be aggressively treated to induce remission.[82,101,103] Alkylating agents, chlorambucil or cyclophosphamide, combined with steroids[103,104] or the high-dose steroid regimen used in an Italian study[99] can be used to induce remission after considering the benefits and risks of treatment.[27,104]

In patients with deteriorating renal function, several trials using either cyclophosphamide[105,106] or chlorambucil[107,108] in conjunction with steroids have shown variable effects. While some patients' proteinuria decreased and renal function stabilized,[105-107] but others did not.[108,109] In addition, the rate of complications appeared higher.[106,108] Therefore, cytotoxic therapy should be avoided in patients whose serum creatinine concentration at diagnosis is greater than 3 mg/dL.[86,102,104] Doses of cytotoxic agents should also be adjusted downward in patients with mild renal impairment to reduce side effects.

Patients with severe nephrotic syndrome who did not respond to cytotoxic therapy should be considered for treatment with cyclosporine.[80] Cyclosporine may offer some benefits to these patients; however, the potential of cyclosporine nephrotoxicity, especially during long-term therapy, is of concern. A 12-month course of cyclosporine (mean dose of 3.8 mg/kg/d) may reduce proteinuria as well as the rate of renal deterioration.[110] However, for many patients, hypertension may be exacerbated and/or result in a transient rise in serum creatinine concentration. It is also common that proteinuria will recur as cyclosporine treatment is stopped.

The treatment of secondary membranous nephropathy is directed at removing the underlying cause. For instance, membranous nephropathy secondary to syphilis can be treated with penicillin. α-Interferon has been shown to be beneficial in the management of hepatitis B–induced membranous nephropathy.[111] Corticosteroids are of no benefit in this setting and have been shown to induce transient viral replication with increased serum concentrations of hepatitis B virus antigen and hepatitis B virus DNA.[112]

Both de novo[83] and recurrent membranous nephropathy may occur in the renal allograft. The incidence of membranous nephropathy in the allograft appears to be three times greater in patients for whom membranous nephropathy was the original primary cause of renal failure. The frequency of recurrence ranges from 2% to 7%.[113] Recurrence is typically associated with nephrotic syndrome and a high risk of allograft failure from disease and/or rejection.

MEMBRANOPROLIFERATIVE GLOMERULONEPHRITIS

Membranoproliferative glomerulonephritis (MPGN) is a morphologic entity that occurs in older children and adults. Although Caucasians are more frequently affected, there is no gender difference in incidence. Many diseases and disorders, such as infections and neoplasms, may result in secondary MPGN. The several types of MPGN are classified according to the pathologic features. Type I MPGN, also known as mesangiocapillary glomerulonephritis, is characterized by diffuse thickening of glomerular capillary walls and mesangial hypercellularity. Subendothelial dense deposits that frequently contain immunoglobulins and C3 of the complement system are responsible for the capillary wall thickening. Immune complexes are therefore presumed to have a major role in the pathogenesis of type I MPGN, which is the most common type of primary, idiopathic MPGN. Type I MPGN may also be secondary to systemic immune complex-mediated disease (lupus), chronic infection (infected ventriculoatrial shunt, endocarditis, malaria), chronic liver disease (hepatitis B or C, cirrhosis), and malignancy (leukemia, lymphoma).[114]

Type II MPGN is also known as dense-deposit disease because of the presence of dense deposits of C3 within the glomerular basement membrane, which gives rise to a ribbon-like appearance. The deposit contains C3, but without immunoglobulins. Other variants of the disease include type III MPGN, which is seen rarely and consists of subendothelial and subepithelial deposits with lamination and disruption of the lamina densa of the GBM.[115]

Type I MPGN is a slowly progressive disease that accounts for 80% of all cases of MPGN, but only 5% to 15% of all cases of nephrotic syndrome seen in pediatric and adult patients. It occurs most frequently in patients between 5 and 30 years of age, and since remissions are rare, many patients develop ESRD in 9 to 12 years. Type II MPGN is a more aggressive disease that constitutes about 15% of all patients with MPGN. Only 20% of patients remain stable for more than a few years and the median time before the development of ESRD is 7 years. There is an impression that the incidence of idiopathic MPGN has declined recently worldwide.

Nephrotic syndrome is the most common presenting condition and some patients may also have a nephritic component (hematuria), hypertension, and renal insufficiency. Hypocomplementemia is commonly seen.

▶ TREATMENT: Membranoproliferative Glomerulonephritis

The efficacy of corticosteroids, cyclophosphamide, antiplatelet drugs, and anticoagulants has been evaluated in patients with MPGN. Five prospective, randomized clinical trials, using prednisone and different combinations of cyclophosphamide, dipyridamole, warfarin, and aspirin did not reveal any long-term improvement in renal function or reduction in proteinuria.[116] Two additional multicenter trials, involving more than 200 patients each, likewise did not demonstrate any consistent beneficial effects of steroids, cyclophosphamide, and azathioprine.[117,118] Cyclosporine has been evaluated in only a limited number of patients with MPGN. Some beneficial effect was suggested; however, the trials were not controlled or randomized.[119] In addition, the risks for developing adverse effects were high.

It is difficult to conduct large-scale controlled trials for MPGN due to the low incidence of the disease. Based on the available studies, none of the drugs evaluated have been shown to have any consistent, beneficial effect on renal function and proteinuria. Besides symptomatic therapy, combined use of aspirin and dipyridamole or use of alternate-day steroids may be considered for patients with type I and III diseases. Renal transplantation is another alternative; however, recurrence rate is close to 100% for type II MPGN and is about 20% to 30% for type I MPGN. Nonetheless, fewer than 10% of the transplanted patients have graft failure due to recurrence.

IMMUNOGLOBULIN A NEPHROPATHY

Immunoglobulin A nephropathy, also known as Berger's disease, was first described by Berger in France in 1968. It is now recognized to be the most common glomerulonephritis in the world and accounts for 10% of patients with ESRD in many countries. The prevalence varies around the world from as high as 50% in Japan to 10% to 30% in Europe. In the United States, the overall prevalence is about 5% but is as high as 35% among Native Americans.[120] The disease has a male predominance (two to three times that of females) and is more frequently seen in younger adults. It is uncommon in blacks both in the United States and in Africa.[120] IgA nephropathy was once thought to be a benign disease presenting with asymptomatic hematuria. It is now recognized that IgA nephropathy can present with any clinical syndrome associated with glomerular disease.

PATHOPHYSIOLOGY

Henoch–Schönlein purpura (HSP) is a systemic disease that is believed to be closely linked to IgA nephropathy because they share similar immunohistologic features. HSP may therefore be the systemic form of the disease process causing IgA nephropathy in which only the joints, skin, and gastrointestinal tract are involved rather than the kidneys. Mesangial deposition of IgA immune complex is also seen in patients with celiac disease and dermatitis herpetiformis, possibly due to an increased exposure to antigens. Patients with chronic liver disease may have IgA nephropathy because of reduced clearance of IgA immune complexes. Secondary IgA nephropathy may also be present in patients with different connective tissue diseases, carcinomas, and HIV infection.

The diagnosis of IgA nephropathy can be established by immunofluorescence examination of the kidney biopsy. The hallmark feature is the dominance or codominance of IgA deposition in the mesangium. IgG and/or IgM as well as C3 may also be present. The IgA immune complex is presumed to be deposited from the systemic circulation or formed in situ. However, the precise pathogenetic mechanisms for IgA nephropathy remain unknown. Conditions that stimulate the release of IgA are believed to cause IgA deposition in the mesangium. In fact, infections of the upper respiratory tract or intestinal mucosa are known to correlate with the onset or exacerbation of IgA nephropathy. IgA production is likely to be increased through antigenic stimulation of IgA-producing mucosal lymphoid tissue by microorganisms as well as ingested or inhaled substances.

Clinical Presentation

IgA nephropathy frequently presents as gross hematuria concurrent with an infection, most commonly pharyngitis or tonsillitis and less often pneumonia, gastroenteritis, or urinary tract infection.[120] In contrast to the 10- to 14-day delay after the pharyngitis in poststreptococcal glomerulonephritis, the hematuria of IgA nephropathy occurs 1 to 2 days after the onset of infection symptoms. The hematuria lasts from 24 hours to a few days and it may recur with a febrile illness months or years later. Frequently, there is persistent microscopic hematuria between episodes of gross hematuria. Proteinuria is common and sometimes it can be in the nephrotic range. In contrast, hypertension and edema that are frequent in poststreptococcal glomerulonephritis are infrequent in IgA nephropathy. Renal dysfunction is uncommon at the initial presentation. However, about 10% to 20% of the patients will develop ESRD within 10 years after diagnosis.[121] Hypertension, severe proteinuria, renal function impairment, old age, and the severity of histologic lesions are all predictive factors for poor long-term outcome.[122,123] The alternative but less common clinical presentations are asymptomatic, microscopic hematuria with variable degrees of proteinuria or nephrotic syndrome.

► TREATMENT: Immunoglobulin A Nephropathy

No therapy is known to be consistently effective for the treatment of IgA nephropathy. Due to the slow progression of the disease to ESRD, it is very difficult to conduct trials to evaluate the long-term effectiveness of specific treatments. The lack of understanding of the pathogenetic mechanisms and the unavailability of appropriate animal models have severely limited the development of rational treatment regimens.[123] Several different therapeutic approaches have been taken. The first is to prevent the formation of the IgA immune complex or to increase its elimination. Restriction of dietary gluten is effective in patients with celiac disease but not in patients with no identifiable nephritogenic antigens. Phenytoin was evaluated because of its ability to reduce the amount of polymeric IgA in the circulation.[124] Although phenytoin resulted in a reduction in serum IgA concentrations and in the frequency of macroscopic hematuria, the glomerular lesions deteriorated in some of the patients despite treatment. Removal of the tonsils, which produce IgA_1 and may contribute to IgA nephropathy, should be considered for patients with recurrent infections.[125]

The second approach is to reduce IgA production. Corticosteroids with or without immunosuppressive agents have been used in several studies. Prednisone does not appear to preserve renal functions, although a modest amelioration of proteinuria has been reported.[120] A meta-analysis of randomized trials reveals that heavy proteinuria (greater than 3 g/d) may be reduced by steroids and/or cytotoxic drugs in 66.7% of the patients.[126] In contrast, such an effect was not seen in patients with moderate proteinuria.

The third approach is to reduce glomerular inflammation induced by IgA deposits. Anti-inflammatory agents, antiplatelet drugs, and anticoagulants have been tried without success to decrease the production or action of mediators responsible for IgA immune complex–induced glomerular damage. However, the *n*-3 fatty acids in fish oil, which limit the production or action of cytokines and eicosanoids, have been shown to delay the progression of renal failure and to reduce proteinuria slightly in patients with marked proteinuria and serum creatinine concentrations less than 3 mg/dL prior to study enrollment.[127] A meta-analysis of five controlled studies indicated that a minor, but not statistically significant, beneficial effect on renal function may be observed.[128] Since the majority of patients with IgA nephropathy do not have severe proteinuria, the efficacy of fish oil in these patients remains to be determined.[129]

ACE inhibitors can reduce proteinuria in patients with IgA nephropathy through their effect on the filtration barrier in the glomerular membrane.[130] In addition, they have been shown to be superior to other antihypertensive agents, including β-adrenergic antagonists, in reducing the progression of renal failure as well as proteinuria in both normotensive and hypertensive patients with IgA nephropathy.[130,131] Interestingly, the reduction in proteinuria is seen only in patients with a deletion polymorphism in the ACE gene, the DD genotype.[133]

Patients with IgA nephropathy have abnormal production of IgA and several different immunoglobulins. High-dose immunoglobulins, initially administered intravenously, followed by the intramuscular route, for over 9 months arrested the decline of renal function and reduced hematuria and proteinuria in all of the 11 patients evaluated.[134] The efficacy of this regimen must be confirmed in a larger number of patients before it is used as primary therapy.

Urokinase, danazol, dapsone, sodium cromoglycate, and plasma exchange have also been evaluated but none is consistently effective.[120,136] Cyclosporine treatment for 12 weeks was evaluated in nine patients. Proteinuria was reduced and plasma albumin concentrations increased. However, the creatinine clearance decreased during treatment and did not return to baseline after termination of cyclosporine therapy.[137] Cyclosporine is therefore not indicated for patients with IgA nephropathy.

There is no regimen that is consistently effective for IgA nephropathy. Since corticosteroids have been found to reduce proteinuria, a course of alternate-day prednisone is indicated for patients with proteinuria greater than 1 g/d.[121] If the patient experiences rapid GFR decline of more than 2 mL/min/month, immunoglobulin therapy should be considered despite the fact that only limited data are available.[120] If the patient is hypertensive, ACE inhibitors, instead of other antihypertensive agents, ought to be used to control the blood pressure as well as the proteinuria.

For those patients who develop end-stage renal failure secondary to IgA nephropathy, transplantation is an effective alternative with excellent allograft survival. Patients with IgA nephropathy who had IgA antibodies to HLA antigens actually have better graft survival when compared with those without the antibodies.[136] It is hypothesized that the improved graft survival might be related to the blockade of IgG antibodies or inhibition of cellular immune response by the autoantibodies to the HLA class I molecules.

LUPUS NEPHRITIS

Glomerulonephritis is one of the most serious complications of systemic lupus erythematosus (SLE) and accounts for much of the morbidity and mortality of patients afflicted with the disease.[137] The renal manifestations of lupus nephritis are variable and encompass a wide spectrum of histopathologic lesions.[137,138] The underlying histopathology has been associated with different prognosis and response to therapy, which cannot be predicted solely based on clinical manifestations. A renal biopsy is therefore required to assess the severity of the disease and to predict the short-term and long-term outcomes associated with therapy.

PATHOPHYSIOLOGY

Lupus nephritis is the prototype of all immune complex–mediated glomerulonephritis. It is characterized by the pleomorphic histologic presentations. Immune complex deposits can be found in the mesangial, subendothelial, and subepithelial regions of the glomerulus, as well as the peritubular interstitium and vasculature outside the glomerulus.[138] Based on light, immunofluorescence, and electron microscopy findings, lupus nephritis can be categorized into five classes: I—normal; II—mesangial; III—focal proliferative; IV—diffuse proliferative; and V—membranous.[80,138,139] Semiquantitative assessment of active lesions and sclerotic changes is incorporated into an activity index and chronicity index, respectively, in an attempt to enhance the predictive values of the histologic findings.[138] However, the usefulness of these indices is still controversial.[140]

The hallmark feature in the pathogenesis of SLE is the dysregulated production of antibodies against multiple antigens in the body.[137] Circulating immune complexes can be deposited in the glomerulus or formed in situ. The size and location of the immune complexes in the glomerulus correlate with the nature and severity of renal injury.[138] Deposition of small numbers of stable immune complexes of intermediate size in the mesangium tends to produce less severe inflammation in the glomerulus. The sequestration of the immune complexes in the mesangium prevents them from activating inflammatory mediators. Hence, the lesion is noninflammatory in nature. In contrast, large numbers of intermediate-sized or large immune complexes can overload the mesangial clearing system. The eventual accumulation of these complexes in the subendothelial region allows them access to plasma inflammatory mediators, resulting in infiltration of inflammatory cells and release of necrotizing enzymes. Since subepithelial deposits are denied access to circulating inflammatory mediators, there is disproportionately more disturbance of glomerular capillary permeability than inflammatory response. Heavy proteinuria is therefore the primary clinical picture in lupus-induced membranous nephropathy.[138]

CLINICAL PRESENTATION

The onset of nephritis is usually seen within the first 4 years of diagnosis of SLE but may also be the first manifestation of the disease. The clinical presentation ranges from minimal hematuria and proteinuria to severe, rapidly progressive diffuse glomerulonephritis. Proteinuria is common and most patients with the membranous lesion also present with the nephrotic syndrome. An active urinary sediment (red cell casts, dysmorphic red cells, hematuria) is suggestive of the diffuse proliferative lesion. However, the urinary sediments are not a reliable indicator of the underlying glomerular lesion.[137] Hypertension is present in 25% to 45% of patients and is associated with a worse prognosis.[141] Most patients have hypocomplementemia and increased antibody titers for anti-double-stranded DNA. Particularly those with focal or diffuse proliferative lesions.[80] Serum creatinine concentration at the time of diagnosis is most predictive of short-term outcome.[138]

▶ TREATMENT: Lupus Nephritis

The treatment of lupus nephritis has evolved over the past several decades.[142] The choice of therapy depends on the underlying lesion, and the activity as well as the chronicity indices. Corticosteroids have been the cornerstone of therapy. However, for severe lupus nephritis, primarily the diffuse proliferative type, alkylating agents may be needed to reduce or prevent the progression to ESRD.[139,143]

Patients with normal renal function and less than 2 g of proteinuria usually do not require therapy, except for the management of extrarenal lupus manifestations. Renal biopsy can be delayed in these patients. However, close follow-up of renal function and urinalysis is required. Those with more than 2 g of proteinuria, deteriorating renal function, and/or an active urinary sediment require a renal biopsy to define the underlying lesion and determine the activity and chronicity of disease. Most patients with classes I, II, III, and V lesions can be treated with oral steroids 1 mg/kg/d for 8 weeks with subsequent tapering to maintain remission. Patients with class IV lesions, and those with class III lesions associated with subendothelial deposits and signs of severe disease activity, should be treated with a cytotoxic agent, either azathioprine and cyclophosphamide, and steroids.

In a long-term randomized NIH study of 107 patients with active lupus nephritis, the likelihood of renal failure in patients taking oral prednisone alone was found to increase substantially after 5 years of observation.[143] Renal function was more frequently preserved in patients who received cytotoxic drugs, but a statistically significant difference was only found for the group receiving both intravenous cyclophosphamide (0.5 to 1.0 g/m^2)

quarterly and low-dose oral prednisone. The benefit of therapy was particularly evident in the subgroup with chronic histologic changes on renal biopsy. Furthermore, hemorrhagic cystitis or malignancy was not reported among patients receiving intravenous cyclophosphamide. However, the small number of at-risk patients in each treatment group at the 5-year follow-up period raises doubts as to the superiority of intravenous cyclophosphamide over other cytotoxic agents.[142]

Favorable effects also have been reported when the intravenous cyclophosphamide regimen was modified from quarterly administration to monthly administration for 6 months.[144] Two regimens of pulse cyclophosphamide (monthly for 6 months versus monthly for 6 months followed by quarterly pulses for 2 additional years) were compared to pulse methylprednisolone in 65 patients with severe lupus nephritis.[145] Patients treated with the short-course cyclophosphamide had a higher probability of exacerbation than those treated with the prolonged regimen. Both regimens, however, were associated with a lower risk of doubling of serum creatinine concentration than those treated with pulse methylprednisolone alone.[146] Black Americans tend to have significantly worse renal survival than white patients.[146] It should be noted that combination therapy with steroids and cytotoxic agents is associated with increased morbidity, including major infections, malignancies (azathioprine- and cyclophosphamide-treated groups), herpes zoster, hemorrhagic cystitis (oral cyclophosphamide group), and secondary amenorrhea (particularly patients treated with cyclophosphamide).[142–145] Indeed, the longer course of cyclophosphamide treatment has been associated with a higher incidence of secondary amenorrhea, particularly in females over 25 years old.[147]

In patients who do not respond to cyclophosphamide and steroid therapy, cyclosporine has produced favorable results in some.[148] However, the number of patients studied was small and the follow-up period was short. Treatment with plasmapheresis in addition to a standard regimen consisting of a short course of oral cyclophosphamide and oral prednisone did not improve the clinical outcome of patients with severe lupus nephritis when compared to standard regimen alone.[149]

Lupus nephropathy with a membranous lesion (type V) generally carries a good prognosis, and a trial of steroids may be used to obtain remission of nephrotic syndrome. If treatment is unsuccessful after 6 months, it should be stopped to avoid infectious complications.[81] If progressive renal dysfunction occurs, or steroid therapy is not tolerated, oral cyclophosphamide 2 to 3 mg/kg/d can be used. In 10 patients with lupus membranous nephropathy, cyclosporine, 4 to 6 mg/kg/d, given alone or in combination with low-dose steroids for a period of 6 to 43 months, has been shown to decrease proteinuria and induce remission of nephrotic syndrome.[150]

The survival of patients with lupus nephritis has improved during the last 2 to 3 decades, and now ranges from 74% to 80% at 10 years.[141] This improvement cannot be explained solely by the use of cytotoxic agents. The lower steroid dosage and better management of complications such as hypertension, infections, hyperlipidemia, and other metabolic complications of the disease also likely have contributed to the more favorable long-term outcome.[142] Lupus patients with ESRD on dialysis fare as well as those with non–lupus-related renal disease. In those patients who received a renal transplant, the allograft outcome of patients with lupus nephritis is favorable.[151] Recurrence of lupus in the renal allograft can occur but is usually of minor clinical importance.

RAPIDLY PROGRESSIVE GLOMERULONEPHRITIS

Rapidly progressive glomerulonephritis (RPGN) describes a clinicopathologic syndrome of rapid loss of renal function, usually over 50% decrement of the glomerular filtration rate within 3 months. The predominant histologic finding of RPGN is extensive crescent formation, usually in more than 50% of the glomeruli. Hence, it is also known as crescentic glomerulonephritis. RPGN accounts for 2% to 7% of all renal biopsy findings and is responsible for up to 5% of patients with ESRD. Though a rare disease, RPGN usually leads to renal demise within weeks or months if left untreated.

RPGN is not a single disease entity. A variety of glomerulonephritides with or without systemic diseases may present as RPGN, including anti-GBM glomerulonephritis, Goodpasture's syndrome, lupus nephritis, poststreptococcal glomerulonephritis, membranoproliferative glomerulonephritis, IgA nephropathy, polyarteritis nodosa, Wegener's granulomatosis, and idiopathic crescentic glomerulonephritis.[152] RPGN may also be found superimposed on an underlying primary glomerulopathy such as membranous nephropathy.

Besides the hallmark feature of extensive crescents, severe endocapillary proliferation and segmental necrosis can also be seen on light microscopy. Based on immunofluorescence microscopic findings, three types of primary RPGN can be identified. Type I RPGN is characterized by the linear localization of immunoglobulins, mainly IgG, along the GBM, signifying anti-GBM antibody–induced injury. Type II is defined by the coarse granular deposition of immunoglobulins and complement within the capillary walls and mesangium, denoting immune complex–mediated injury. Type III is characterized by scanty or lack of immune complex deposits; therefore, it is also known as pauci-immune RPGN. Circulating ANCA is often detected in type III RPGN. This immunohistologic classification of RPGN reflects the immunopathogenesis of the different types of crescentic glomerulonephritis.

PATHOPHYSIOLOGY

Though the causal relationships are not firmly established, several etiologic factors have been implicated in RPGN, including toxins, drugs, viral and bacterial infections, neoplasm, autoimmune mechanisms, and various immunogenetic factors.[152,153]

Irrespective of the etiology and type of RPGN, the disruption in the glomerular capillary wall seems to be the common lesion in crescentic glomerulonephritis.[152] Various mechanisms have been proposed to account for the severe damage to the capillary wall. Both humoral and cellular pathways of inflammation are involved. Activation of the terminal C5b-9 (membrane-attacking complex) of the complement system produces severe capillary wall injury. Both neutrophils and macrophages release proteinases and reactive oxygen species and may thereby produce severe glomerular injury. Platelets and the coagulation system are activated and result in capillary thrombosis.[154] Fibrinogen and procoagulants that are released from ruptured capillaries may come into contact with thrombogenic tissue debris and lead to fibrinoid changes.[154] In anti-GBM glomerulonephritis, the direct attack of the anti-GBM antibody on the noncollagenous region of the type IV collagen molecule of the GBM is responsible for the capillary wall injury.[152] ANCAs may also play an important role in mediating the vascular injury in patients with ANCA-associated disease.[9] The interaction of ANCAs with neutrophils and monocytes, which have been primed by concurrent infections or inflammatory processes, can lead to activation of these leukocytes and release of toxic oxygen species and lytic enzymes, resulting in vascular injury.[9,155]

The disruption of the capillary wall allows movement of macrophages and other plasma constituents into Bowman's space and stimulates the formation of crescents, which are composed mainly of parietal epithelial cells, as well as macrophages and fibroblasts. Crescent formation indicates the severity of the glomerular capillary disease but not its pathogenesis. The age of crescents can serve as a marker for disease duration and the likelihood of successful therapeutic intervention.[152]

Clinical Presentation

Among the crescentic glomerulonephritides, the pauci-immune RPGN is the most frequent, accounting for over 50% of cases, whereas the anti-GBM antibody–mediated RPGN is the least frequent, occurring in roughly 10% of patients. Sixty to seventy percent of patients with type I RPGN may have concurrent pulmonary hemorrhage and Goodpasture's syndrome.[154] Most patients with immune complex–mediated RPGN have collagen vascular disease, systemic infections, or a severe form of primary glomerular disease. Approximately 70% of patients with type III RPGN also present with evidence of systemic vasculitis, such as Wegener's granulomatosis and polyarteritis nodosa, but some have only renal manifestations, and the terms idiopathic crescentic glomerulonephritis or renal vasculitis have been used.[152,154,156]

The clinical presentation is dominated by progressive renal insufficiency with complaints of tea-colored urine, malaise, anorexia, low-grade fever, and migratory polyarthropathy. Mild hypertension is usually present. Uremic signs and symptoms may develop as renal function worsens. Type I RPGN is more commonly found in the third and sixth decades of life. Patients with ANCA-mediated disease tend to be older, with peak incidence occurring between 50 to 60 years of age. The age-related incidence varies among the immune complex–mediated RPGN; for example, poststreptococcal glomerulonephritis and Henoch–Schönlein purpura nephritis are more common in young children, whereas membranoproliferative glomerulonephritis is more common in older children.[154] Urinalysis shows a nephritic sediment with hematuria, erythrocyte casts, and proteinuria. Overt nephrotic syndrome is rare, however.

Serologic analysis is very useful in distinguishing the different types of RPGN. The detection of serum anti-GBM antibodies with the appropriate clinical presentation confirms the diagnosis of anti-GBM glomerulonephritis. Over 80% of patients with pauci-immune or idiopathic crescentic glomerulonephritis have circulating ANCAs.[9,154] ANCAs are autoantibodies specific for the cytoplasmic constituents of neutrophil granules and monocyte lysosomes. Patients with ANCA-associated disease limited to renal involvement often have P-ANCA (perinuclear staining), while patients with Wegener's granulomatoses tend to have C-ANCA (cytoplasmic staining).[9,154] Both the anti-GBM antibody and the ANCAs are absent in patients with type II RPGN. Measurements of circulating immune complexes are not useful for making a specific diagnosis, but detection of specific serum antibodies known to mediate immune complex–associated nephritis is helpful: anti-DNA antibody as a marker for lupus nephritis, and elevated anti-streptolysin-O titers for poststreptococcal glomerulonephritis. The serum complement levels are normal in RPGN, although they can be low in the immune complex–mediated category.

▶ TREATMENT: Rapidly Progressive Glomerulonephritis

Early aggressive therapy has improved the renal prognosis of patients with crescentic glomerulonephritis.[157] Though no controlled prospective studies have been performed, types II and III RPGN appear to respond well to high-dose steroid therapy. Immunosuppressive therapy alone appears to be ineffective in type I RPGN.[152,158,159] Irrespective of the type of RPGN, poor response to therapy and an ominous renal survival are expected if the patient presents with oliguria, has a serum creatinine concentration greater than 6 or 7 mg/dL, is dialysis dependent, or has a renal biopsy showing advanced chronic parenchymal disease.[154]

■ ANTI-GBM GLOMERULONEPHRITIS (TYPE I)

The data on the treatment of anti-GBM glomerulonephritis are limited. Pulse intravenous administration of corticosteroids has been used successfully to alleviate pulmonary hemorrhage, but the results are not as convincing for the treatment of glomerulonephritis.[152,158,159] Plasmapheresis, in combination with steroids and cytotoxic agents, may be more beneficial than immunosuppression alone. Plasmapheresis may confer its benefits by removing the circulating pathogenetic anti-GBM antibody.[160] Compared to historical controls, an improved outcome is observed with addition of plasmapheresis to immunosuppressive therapy. Plasma exchange is usually continued for at least 2 weeks or until the circulating anti-GBM antibody concentrations decrease to undetectable levels. The immunosuppression should be maintained for 8 weeks to prevent antibody rebound.[152] Plasmapheresis has been useful in treating pulmonary hemorrhage. However, the long-term benefits on renal function are not known. Treatment should be started early. When the serum creatinine concentration is 6 mg/dL or above, or the patient is oliguric or requires dialysis, the response to therapy is usually poor and patients should therefore be treated conservatively.[152]

IMMUNE COMPLEX–MEDIATED GLOMERULONEPHRITIS (TYPE II)

The treatment of this category of RPGN varies with the underlying glomerulonephritis. Patients with postinfectious RPGN generally have a favorable prognosis even without treatment. Complete spontaneous recovery occurs in 50% of cases, whereas chronic renal failure develops in 32%.[152] Pulse doses of methylprednisolone have been shown to be beneficial in type II RPGN,[158,159] with an overall response rate of 50% to 60%.[153] Plasmapheresis does not appear to provide any additional benefit.[158]

ANTINEUTROPHIL CYTOPLASMIC AUTOANTIBODY (ANCA)–ASSOCIATED GLOMERULONEPHRITIS (TYPE III)

Type III RPGN has been treated successfully with pulse doses of steroids.[152,156,158,159] The effectiveness of cyclophosphamide in systemic vasculitis, the detection of ANCAs, and the recognition that pauci-immune necrotizing crescentic glomerulonephritis is part of the spectrum of necrotizing vasculitides have led to the use of cyclophosphamide combined with steroids in ANCA-mediated RPGN.[9,160,161] Both oral (2 to 3 mg/kg/d) and intravenous (500 to 1000 mg/m^2) cyclophosphamide have been used. In a prospective study of 70 patients with ANCA-associated disease, no difference in renal or patient survival was detected between the oral and intravenous cyclophosphamide regimens. Similarly, there was no difference in response between the steroid-treated and the cyclophosphamide-treated groups.[162] The serum ANCA levels can be monitored to determine the efficacy of therapy. To date, plasmapheresis has not been demonstrated in prospective trials to be of additional benefit in type III RPGN.[160,163]

Anti-GBM nephritis has been reported to recur in up to 55% of patients who received a renal transplant. However, only 25% of these patients showed clinical disease activity, with rare allograft failure. Since the frequency of recurrence and its severity are related to the presence of circulating anti-GBM antibody, it is recommended that transplantation should not be performed until the anti-GBM antibody is undetectable for at least 6 to 12 months.[113] The recurrence rate in idiopathic crescentic glomerulonephritis, including ANCA-associated nephritis, is unknown and is thought to be low. The outcome of the renal allograft appears favorable.

POSTSTREPTOCOCCAL GLOMERULONEPHRITIS

Poststreptococcal glomerulonephritis (PSGN) and glomerulonephritis caused by other infectious agents, such as bacteria, viruses, and parasites, were once common. Improved sanitation, personal hygiene, medical care, and public health measures helped to decrease the incidence of group A streptococcal infection in the United States and other developed countries, and led to a decline in PSGN. However, it is still frequently seen in developing countries. In contrast, glomerulonephritis secondary to other infectious agents, such as hepatitis C and HIV viruses, is seen with increasing frequency in developed countries.

It was more than two hundred years ago when hematuria and proteinuria were found to be associated with epidemics of scarlet fever. Certain strains of group A streptococci were identified in the 1950s to be responsible for the glomerular disease. PSGN is now the most common form of glomerulonephritis in children, but is less common than the other types of glomerulonephritis in adults. It normally follows pharyngeal or skin infection caused by the nephritogenic strains of group A streptococci; however, other strains of streptococci, such as group C and G, have also been reported to cause PSGN. Streptococcal pharyngitis is more common in winter and early spring, whereas skin infection is frequently found in the summer. The risk for developing acute glomerulonephritis secondary to the nephritogenic strains of bacteria is about 10% to 15% in infected patients. However, three to four times more patients may experience a subclinical form of the disease.

Pathophysiology

Despite decades of research, the characteristics of the antigens responsible for the production of the nephritogenic immune complexes remain unclear. It has been postulated that the streptococcal antigens may induce changes in the glomerular components so that they become immunogenic or that autologous IgG may be altered to become antigenic. Alternately, the streptococcal antigens may induce antibodies that react with glomerular antigens. *In situ* immune complexes are then formed and result in a complement-mediated inflammatory response. The kinin and coagulation cascades are then activated and chemotactic factors are released to recruit neutrophils and monocytes, resulting in acute glomerular lesions.

Examination of the acute PSGN kidneys reveals hypercellular glomerulus with proliferation of mesangial and endothelial cells with infiltration by neutrophils, monocytes and eosinophils, within the capillary lumen and also in the mesangial areas. Crescent formation may be seen in patients with severe disease, and if found in more than 30% of the glomeruli, RPGN may be present concurrently.[164] The prognosis is generally poor for these patients and complete recovery is not likely. When the tissue is examined under electron microscope, "humps," which are multiple large, discrete, electron-dense, dome-shaped deposits, can be found beneath the epithelial foot processes. Immunofluorescence examination reveals diffuse granular deposits of IgG and C3 along the glomerular basement membrane and also in the mesangium.

Clinical Presentation

PSGN is seen mostly in children between 5 and 15 years old, with a peak incidence between 6 and 7 years. It is uncommon under 2 years of age and also in adults over 50 years old. Males are twice as likely to be affected as females. The nephritis is preceded by a latent period following a streptococcal infection. The latent period is commonly 7 to 14 days for pharyngitis and 14 to 28 days for skin infection. In patients with preexisting nephritis such as IgA nephropathy and membranoproliferative glomerulonephritis, the streptococcal infection may exacerbate the nephritis and result in hematuria.

Following the latent period, an acute nephritic syndrome develops with hematuria and edema being the most common characteristics. Gross hematuria is seen in 70% of patients, and microscopic hematuria can be found in all patients. Edema, which is often worse in the morning, is found commonly in the periorbital area and around the eyelids. Hypertension is usually mild to moderate and results from sodium and water retention; however, it may be severe enough to cause hypertensive encephalopathy. Many patients have signs and symptoms associated with volume overload, which include dyspnea, orthopnea, and cough; it may progress to overt congestive heart failure. Neurologic abnormalities may be present secondary to severe hypertension.

Urinalysis of patients with PSGN reveals hematuria, dysmorphic red blood cells, and red cell casts. Proteinuria is common, but often not in the nephrotic range. Renal function is frequently mildly impaired, and serum creatinine concentration is often normal. However, blood urea concentration may be disproportionately high.

Throat or skin culture may be positive for group A streptococci, despite the latent period following the initial infection. However, antibiotic therapy may render the culture result negative. Serologic measurements of antibodies to different streptococcal antigens can confirm recent exposure to the infection. Titers that can be measured include the antistreptolysin (ASO), antistreptokinase, antihyaluronidase (AHase), antideoxyribonuclease B (ADNase B), and antinicotyladenine dinucleotidase (NADase). In most patients with streptococcal pharyngitis, the ASO titers begin to rise about 10 to 14 days later, peak at 3 to 4 weeks, and persist for several months before decreasing. The rise in ASO titers can be reduced by antibiotic treatment and also in patients with streptococcal skin infection where the streptolysin may bind to skin lipids. ADNase B and AHase titers should therefore be used instead because they are specific and are positive in the majority of patients. The Streptozyme test is a combined assay for ASO, ADNase B, NADase, and AHase. It has a high rate of false-positive and false-negative results, and the antibody levels do not correlate with nephritogenicity or disease severity.

Serum complements may also be measured in patients with PSGN. Hemolytic complement activity (CH_{50}) and C3 levels are reduced in more than 90% of the patients for 4 to 6 weeks. If the C3 level is depressed for more than 6 to 8 weeks, MPGN, lupus nephritis, or glomerulonephritis related to endocarditis or occult visceral abscess should be suspected.

Renal biopsy is not normally indicated for PSGN unless the patient has severe renal dysfunction, severe proteinuria, significant hypertension, and/or prolonged oliguria, which are not typical for PSGN. If the hematuria is prolonged or proteinuria or depressed C3 level persists, renal biopsy is needed to detect other types of glomerulonephritis such as lupus, RPGN, or MPGN.

▶ TREATMENT: Poststreptococcal Glomerulonephritis

The treatment of PSGN is mainly supportive and symptomatic. Early antibiotic therapy does not prevent subsequent PSGN, but it may reduce the severity of the disease.[165] It can, however, prevent the spread of the streptococcal infection to other family members. Antibiotic prophylaxis is not recommended since infected patients will develop long-lasting, often lifelong immunity against the strain of streptococci. Exposure to another nephritogenic strain of streptococci is possible, but unlikely.

Supportive measures, as discussed earlier in this chapter, should be used to control fluid volume and blood pressure. Since the hypertension is of the low-renin type, ACE inhibitors and β-blockers are expected to be not as useful. If the patient has crescentic disease, use of pulse steroids and/or immunosuppressive agents can be considered[152]; however, the efficacy and safety of these agents have not been established for this condition.

The acute manifestations of PSGN are normally self-limited, and more than 95% of the patients have renal function restored within 3 to 6 weeks. Diuresis usually begins 7 to 10 days after onset of the acute episode, whereas hypertension and azotemia resolve in 1 to 2 weeks. Gross hematuria lasts for 1 to 2 weeks and proteinuria usually resolves within 6 months in more than 90% of children. However, microscopic hematuria may persist for up to 2 years. Children, in general, have more rapid recovery than adults. Prognosis is often better when PSGN occurs during an epidemic than in those found sporadically. Most of the children will recover fully and be free from chronic complications of PSGN if they have no preexisting renal disorder, heavy proteinuria, or crescentic glomerular lesions or did not require hospitalization during the acute episode.[166] In contrast, adult patients have a less favorable long-term outcome. In one study, up to 50% of the patients had persistent proteinuria, hypertension, and renal insufficiency.[167] Some patients may develop end-stage renal failure.

CONCLUSIONS

A better understanding of the pathogenetic mechanisms leading to glomerular injury has improved the management of glomerulonephritis. However, the glomerulonephritides are a heterogeneous group of immune disorders with different clinical courses, prognoses, and responses to current immunologic and nonimmunologic therapies. The clinician should understand the natural history and prognosis of each subgroup of glomerulonephritis, the efficacy of different immunomodulating regimens in inducing disease remission and preserving renal function, and the characteristics of at-risk patients who warrant aggressive therapy. Judicious use of immunosuppressive agents with careful monitoring of their adverse effects cannot be overemphasized. In addition, treatment of the disease complications and control of factors that lead to progression of renal disease are important in reducing the morbidity and mortality of patients with glomerulonephritis.

▶ PRINCIPLES OF PHARMACOTHERAPY

- The etiology for most glomerulonephritides is unknown; thus, corticosteroid, cytotoxic, and immunomodulating agents are used to reduce the glomerular injury caused by the different immunologic mechanisms.
- Since the course and prognosis of individual glomerulonephritides are different, a specific treatment strategy has to be developed for the specific disease that the patient has.
- Supportive measures are used to reduce systemic signs and symptoms associated with the pathophysiologic sequelae of the glomerular disease, such as hypertension, edema, and renal function deterioration.
- If the patient has nephrotic syndrome, supportive measures ought to be used to treat the proteinuria, hypoalbuminemia, hyperlipidemia, and thromboembolic abnormalities associated with the syndrome.

ACKNOWLEDGMENTS

The contribution of Ignatius Y. S. Tang, PharmD, BCPS, towards the updating of this chapter is acknowledged.

REFERENCES

1. Couser WG. Research opportunities and future directions in glomerular disease. Semin Nephrol 1993;13:457–471.
2. Miller DE, Noble NA, Yu X, Border WA. Molecular and cellular biological techniques in the study of glomerular diseases. Semin Nephrol 1992;12:506–515.
3. US Renal Data System 1997 Annual Data Report. National Institutes of Health and National Institute of Diabetes and Digestive and Kidney Diseases.
4. Bohrer MP, Baylis C, Humes HD, et al. Permselectivity of the glomerular capillary wall: Facilitated filtration of circulating polycations. J Clin Invest 1978;61:72–78.
5. Schreiner GF. The mesangial phagocyte and its regulation of contractile cell biology. J Am Soc Nephrol 1992;2:S74–S82.
6. Schena FP, Gesualdo L, Grandaliano G, Montinaro V. Progression of renal damage in human glomerulonephritides: Is there sleight of hand in winning the game? Kidney Int 1997;52:1439–1457.
7. Couser WG. Mediation of immune glomerular injury. J Am Soc Nephrol 1990;1:13–29.
8. Makker SP. Mediators of immune glomerular injury. Am J Nephrol 1993;13:324–336.
9. Jennette JC, Falk RJ. Antineutrophil cytoplasmic autoantibodies and associated diseases: A review. Am J Kidney Dis 1990;15:517–529.
10. Remuzzi G, Zoji C, Perico N. Proinflammatory mediators of glomerular injury and mechanisms of activation of autoreactive T cells. Kidney Int 1994;45(suppl 44):S8–S16.
11. Klahr S, Schreiner G, Ichikawa I. The progression of renal disease. N Engl J Med 1988;318:1657–1666.
12. Ritz E, Orth S, Wennich T, et al. Systemic hypertension versus intraglomerular hypertension in progression. Kidney Int 1994;45:438–442.
13. Williams JD, Coles GA. Proteinuria: A direct cause of renal injury morbidity? Kidney Int 1994;45:443–450.
14. Ong ACM, Fine LG. Loss of glomerular function and tubulointerstitial fibrosis: Cause or effect? Kidney Int 1994;45:345–351.
15. Thomas ME, Schreiner F. Contribution of proteinuria to progressive renal injury: Consequences of tubular uptake of fatty acid bearing albumin. Am J Nephrol 1993;13:385–398.
16. Keane WF. Lipids and the kidney. Kidney Int 1994;46:910–920.
17. Kasiske BL, Keene WF. Laboratory assessment of renal disease: Clearance, urinalysis and renal biopsy. In: Brenner BM, ed. The Kidney, 5th ed. Philadelphia, Saunders, 1996:1137–1174.
18. Rodríguez-Iturbe B, Colic D, Parra G, Gutkowska J. Atrial natriuetic factor in the acute nephritic and nephrotic syndromes. Kidney Int 1990;38:512–517.
19. Geers AB, Koomans HA, Roos JC, Dorhout Mees EJ. Preservation of blood volume during edema removal in nephrotic subjects. Kidney Int 1985;28:652–657.
20. Humphreys MH. Mechanisms and management of nephrotic edema. Kidney Int 1994;45:266–281.
21. Schrier RW, Fassett RG. A critique of the overfill hypothesis of sodium and water retention in the nephrotic syndrome. Kidney Int 1998;53:1111–1117.
22. Warwick GL, Fox JG, Boulton-Jones JM. The relationship between urinary albumin excretion rate and serum cholesterol in primary glomerular disease. Clin Nephrol 1994;41:135–137.
23. Wheeler DC, Bernard DB. Lipid abnormalities in the nephrotic syndrome: Causes, consequences, and treatment. Am J Kidney Dis 1994;23:331–346.
24. Keane WF, St. Peter JV, Kasiske BL. Is the aggressive management of hyperlipidemia in nephrotic syndrome mandatory? Kidney Int 1992;42(suppl 38):S134–S141.
25. Llach F. Hypercoagulability, renal vein thrombosis, and other thrombotic complications of the nephrotic syndrome. Kidney Int 1985;28:429–439.
26. Ginsberg JM, Chang BS, Matarese RA, et al. Use of single voided urine samples to estimate quantitative proteinuria. N Engl J Med 1983;309:1543–1546.
27. Ponticelli C, Passerini P. Treatment of the nephrotic syndrome associated with primary glomerulonephritis. Kidney Int 1994;46:595–604.
28. Klahr S, Levey A, Beck G, et al. The effects of dietary protein restriction and blood pressure control on the progression of chronic renal disease. N Engl J Med 1994;330:877–884.
29. Fliser D, Schroter M, Neubeck M. Coadministration of thiazides increases the efficacy of loop diuretics even in patients with advanced renal failure. Kidney Int 1994;46:482–488.
30. Rudy DW, Voelker JR, Greene PK, et al. Loop diuretics for chronic renal insufficiency: A continuous infusion is more efficacious than bolus therapy. Ann Intern Med 1991;115:360–366.

31. Jacobson HR, Striker GE. Report on a workshop to develop management recommendations for the prevention of progression in chronic renal disease. Am J Kidney Dis 1995;25:103–106.
32. Lewis EJ, Hunsicker LG, Bain RP, et al. The effect of angiotensin-converting-enzyme inhibition on diabetic nephropathy. N Engl J Med 1993;329:977–986.
33. Gansevoot R, Slinter W, Aemmelder M, et al. Antiproteinuric effect of blood pressure lowering agents: A meta analysis of comparative trials. Nephrol Dial Transplant 1995;10:1963–1974.
34. Levey AS, Adler S, Caggiula AW, et al. Effects of dietary protein restriction on the progression of advanced renal disease in the Modification of Diet in Renal Disease Study. Am J Kidney Dis 1996;27:652–663.
35. Praga M, Hernandez E, Montoyo C, et al. Long-term beneficial effects of angiotensin-converting enzyme inhibition in patients with nephrotic proteinuria. Am J Kidney Dis 1992;20:240–248.
36. Gansevoort RT, de Zeeuw D, de Jong PE. Additive antiproteinuric effect of ACE inhibition and a low-protein diet in human renal disease. Nephrol Dial Transplant 1995;10:497–504.
37. Vriesendorp R, Donker AJM, de Zeeuw D, et al. Effects of nonsteroidal anti-inflammatory drugs on proteinuria. Am J Med 1986;81 (suppl 2B):84–94.
38. Heeg JA, de Jong PE, de Zeeuw D. Additive antiproteinuric effect of angiotensin converting enzyme inhibition and non-steroidal anti-inflammatory drug therapy: A clue to the mechanism of action. Clin Sci 1991;81:367–372.
39. Don BR, Kaysen GA, Hutchinson FN, et al. The effect of angiotensin-converting enzyme inhibition and dietary protein restriction in the treatment of proteinuria. Am J Kidney Dis 1991;27:1017.
40. ter Wee PM, Donker AJM. Pharmacologic manipulation of glomerular function. Kidney Int 1994;45:417–424.
41. Velosa JA, Torres VE. Benefits and risks of nonsteroidal antiinflammatory drugs in steroid-resistant nephrotic syndrome. Am J Kidney Dis 1986;8:345–350.
42. Massy ZA, Ma JZ, Louis TA, Kasiske BL. Lipid-lowering therapy in patients with renal disease. Kidney Int 1995;48:188–198.
43. Coleman JE, Watson AR. Hyperlipidemia, diet and simvastatin therapy in steroid-resistant nephrotic syndrome of childhood. Pediatr Nephrol 1996;10:171–174.
44. Thomas ME, Harris KPG, Ramaswamy C, et al. Simvastatin therapy for hypercholesterolemic patients with nephrotic syndrome or significant proteinuria. Kidney Int 1993;44:1124–1129.
45. Keilani T, Schlueter WA, Levin ML, et al. Improvement of lipid abnormalities associated with proteinuria using fosinopril, an angiotensin-converting enzyme inhibitor. Ann Intern Med 1993;118:246–254.
46. Sarasin FP, Schifferli JA. Prophylactic oral anticoagulation in nephrotic patients with idiopathic membranous nephropathy. Kidney Int 1994;45:578–585.
47. Rostoker G, Durand-Zaleski I, Petit-Phar M, et al. Prevention of thrombotic complications of the nephrotic syndrome by the low-molecular-weight heparin enoxaparin. Nephron 1995;69:20–28.
48. Nolasco F, Cameron JS, Heywood EF, et al. Adult-onset minimal change nephrotic syndrome: A long-term follow-up. Kidney Int 1986;29:1215–1223.
49. Jennette JC, Mandal AK. The nephrotic syndrome. In: Mandal AK, Jennette JC, eds. Diagnosis and Management of Renal Disease and Hypertension, 2nd ed. Durham, NC, Carolina Academic Press, 1994: 235–272.
50. A report of the International Study of Kidney Disease in Children: The primary nephrotic syndrome in children. Identification of patients with minimal change nephrotic syndrome for initial response to prednisone. J Pediatr 1981;98:561–564.
51. Brodehl J. The treatment of minimal change nephrotic sundrome: Lessons learned from multicenter co-operative studies. Eur J Pediatr 1991;150:380–387.
52. Tune BM, Mendoza SA. Treatment of the idiopathic nephrotic syndrome: Regimens and outcomes in children and adults. J Am Soc Nephrol 1997;8:824–832.
53. Siegel NJ. Minimal change nephropathy. In: Greenberg A, ed. Primer on Kidney Diseases, 2nd ed. San Diego, Academic Press, 1994: 67–70.
54. Hiraoka M, Takeda N, Tsukahara H, et al. Favorable course of steroid-responsive nephrotic children with mild initial attack. Kidney Int 1995;47:1392–1393.
55. Cade R, Mars D, Privette M, et al. Effect of long-term azathioprine administration in adults with minimal-change glomerulonephritis and nephrotic syndrome resistant to corticosteroids. Arch Intern Med 1986;146:737.
56. A report of the International Study of Kidney Disease in Children: Minimal change nephrotic syndrome in children: Deaths during the first 5 to 15 years' observation. Pediatrics 1984;73:497–501.
57. Niaudel P, Habib R. Cyclosporine in the treatment of idiopathic nephrosis. J Am Soc Nephrol 1994;5:1049–1056.
58. Tejani A, Suthanthiran M, Pomrantz A. A randomized controlled trial of low-dose prednisone and ciclosporin versus high-dose prednisone in nephrotic syndrome of children. Nephron 1991;59:96–99.
59. Meyrier A, Noel H, Auriche P, Gallard P, and the Collaborative Group of the Societe de Nephrologie. Long-term renal tolerance of cyclosporin A treatment in adult idiopathic nephrotic syndrome. Kidney Int 1994;45:1446–1456.
60. Meyrier A, Condamin M-C, Broneer D, and the Collaborative Group of the French Society of Nephrology. Treatment of adult idiopathic nephrotic syndrome with cyclosporin A: Minimal-change disease and focal-segmental glomerulosclerosis. Clin Nephrol 1991; 35(suppl 1):S37–S42.
61. Hulton SA, Neuhans TJ, Dillon MJ, Barratt TM. Long-term cyclosporin A treatment of minimal-change nephrotic syndrome of childhood. Pediatr Nephrol 1994;8:401–403.
62. British Association for Paediatric Nephrology. Levamisole for corticosteroid-dependent nephrotic syndrome in childhood. Lancet 1991; 337:1555–1557.
63. Weiss R. Randomized, double-blind, placebo controlled trial of levamisole for children with frequently relapsing/steroid dependent nephrotic syndrome. J Am Soc Nephrol 1993;4:289.
64. Dayal U, Dayal A, Shastry JCM, Raghupathy P. Use of levamisole in maintaining remission in steroid-sensitive nephrotic syndrome in children. Nephron 1994;66:408–412.
65. Xu J, Qian T, Jiang J, et al. Clinical studies in the use of BCG and levamisole in the treatment of glomerulonephritis. Nephrol Dial Transplant 1991;6:548–553.
66. Black DAK, Rose G, Brewer DB. Controlled trial of prednisone in adult patients with the nephrotic syndrome. Br Med J 1970;3: 421–426.
67. D'Agati V. The many masks of focal segmental glomerulosclerosis. Kidney Int 1994;46:1223–1241.
68. Rennke HG, Klein PS. Pathogenesis and significance of nonprimary focal and segmental glomerulosclerosis. Am J Kidney Dis 1989;13: 443–456.
69. Korbet SM. Primary focal segmental glomerulosclerosis. J Am Soc Nephrol 1998;9:1333–1340.
70. Korbet SM, Schwartz MM, Lewis EJ. Primary focal segmental glomerulosclerosis: Clinical course and response to therapy. Am J Kidney Dis 1994;23:773–783.
71. Banfi G, Moriggi M, Sabadini E, et al. The impact of prolonged immunosuppression on the outcome of idiopathic focal-segmental glomerulosclerosis with nephrotic syndrome in adults. A collaborative retrospective study. Clin Nephrol 1991;36:53–59.
72. Tune BM, Lieberman E, Mendoza SA. Steroid-resistant nephrotic focal segmental glomerulosclerosis: A treatable disease. Pediatr Nephrol 1996;10:772–778.
73. Ponticelli C, Rizzoni G, Edefonti A, et al. A randomized trial of cyclosporine in steroid-resistant idiopathic nephrotic syndrome. Kidney Int 1993;43:1377–1384.
74. Ingulli E, Singh A, Baqi N, et al. Aggressive, long-term cyclosporine therapy for steroid-resistant focal segmental glomerulosclerosis. J Am Soc Nephrol 1995;5:1820–1825.

75. Ingulli E, Tejani A. Severe hypercholesterolemia inhibits cyclosporin A efficacy in a dose-dependent manner in children with nephrotic syndrome. J Am Soc Nephrol 1992;3:254–259.
76. Keane WF, Anderson S, Aurell M, et al. Angiotensin converting enzyme inhibitors and progressive renal insufficiency. Ann Intern Med 1989;11:503–516.
77. Tejani A, Stablein DH. Recurrence of focal segmental glomerulosclerosis posttransplantation: A special report of the North American Pediatric Renal Transplant Cooperative Study. J Am Soc Nephrol 1992;2:S258–S263.
78. Mowry J, Marik J, Cohen A, et al. Treatment of recurrent focal segmental glomerulosclerosis with high dose cyclosporine A and plasmapheresis. Transplant Proc 1993;25:1345–1346.
79. Artero M, Biava C, Amend W, et al. Recurrent focal glomerulosclerosis: Natural history and response to therapy. Am J Med 1992;92: 375–383.
80. Wasserstein AG. Membranous glomerulonephritis. J Am Soc Nephrol 1997;8:664–674.
81. Glassock RJ. The therapy of idiopathic membranous glomerulonephritis. Semin Nephrol 1991;11:138–147.
82. Burstein DM, Korbert SM, Schwartz MM. Membranous glomerulonephritis and malignancy. Am J Kidney Dis 1993;22:5–10.
83. Heidet L, Gagnadoux ME, Beziau A, et al. Recurrence of de novo membranous glomerulonephritis on renal grafts. Clin Nephrol 1994; 41:314–318.
84. Kerjaschi D. Molecular pathogenesis of membranous nephropathy. Kidney Int 1992;41:1090–1105.
85. Bernard DB. Extrarenal complications of the nephrotic syndrome. Kidney Int 1988;33:1184–1202.
86. Winerals CG, Sanderson F. Treatment of aggressive idiopathic membranous glomerulonephritis. Q J Med 1994;87:109–201.
87. Rostoker G, Maadi AB, Remy P, et al. Low-dose angiotensin-converting-enzyme inhibitor captopril to reduce proteinuria in adult idiopathic membranous nephropathy: a prospective study of long-term treatment. Nephrol Dial Transplant 1995;10:25–29.
88. Wheeler DC, Bernard DB. Lipid abnormalities in the nephrotic syndrome: Causes, consequences, and treatment. Am J Kidney Dis 1994;23:331–346.
89. Ponticelli C, Passerini P. The natural history and therapy of idiopathic membranous nephropathy. Nephrol Dial Transplant 1990;5: (suppl 1):37–41.
90. A controlled study of short-term prednisone treatment in adults with membranous nephropathy. Collaborative study of the adult idiopathic nephrotic syndrome. N Engl J Med 1979;301:1301–1306.
91. Cameron JS, Healy MJR, Adu D. The Medical Research Council trial of short-term high-dose alternate day prednisolone in idiopathic membranous nephropathy with nephrotic syndrome in adults. Q J Med 1990;74:133–156.
92. Cattran DC, Delmore T, Roscoe J, et al. A randomized controlled trial of prednisone in patients with idiopathic membranous nephropathy. N Engl J Med 1989;320:210–215.
93. Ponticelli C, Fogazzi GB. Methylprednisolone pulse therapy for primary glomerulonephritis. Am J Nephrol 1989;9(suppl 1):41–46.
94. Hogan S, Muller KE, Jeanette JC, Falk RC. A review of therapeutic studies of idiopathic membranous glomerulopathy. Am J Kidney Dis 1995;25:862–875.
95. Alexopoulos E, Sakellariou G, Memmos D, et al. Cyclophosphamide provides no additional benefit to steroid therapy in the treatment of idiopathic membranous nephropathy. Am J Kidney Dis 1993;21: 497–503.
96. Donadio JV Jr, Holley KE, Anderson CF, et al. Controlled trial of cyclophosphamide in idiopathic membranous nephropathy. Kidney Int 1974;6:431–439.
97. Murphy BF, McDonald I, Fairley KF, et al. Randomized controlled trial of cyclophosphamide, warfarin and dipyridamole in idiopathic membranous glomerulonephritis. Clin Nephrol 1992;37: 229–234.
98. Ponticelli C, Zucchelli P, Passerini P, et al. A randomized trial of methylprednisolone and chlorambucil in idiopathic membranous nephropathy. N Engl J Med 1989;320:8–13.
99. Ponticelli C, Zucchelli P, Passerini P, et al. A 10-year follow-up of a randomized study with methylprednisolone and chlorambucil in membranous nephropathy. Kidney Int 1995;48:1600–1604.
100. Imperiale TF, Goldfarb S, Berns JS. Are cytotoxic agents beneficial in idiopathic membranous nephropathy? A meta-analysis of the controlled trials. J Am Soc Nephrol 1995;5:1553–1558.
101. Glassock RJ. Therapy of idiopathic nephrotic syndrome in adults. A conservative or aggressive approach? Am J Nephrol 1993;13:422–428.
102. Cameron JS. Membranous nephropathy is still a treatment dilemma. N Engl J Med 1992;327:639–640.
103. Hebert LA. Therapy of membranous nephropathy: What to do after (meta) analyses. J Am Soc Nephrol 1995;5:1543–1545.
104. Piccoli A, Pillon L, Passerini P, et al. Therapy for idiopathic membranous nephropathy: Tailoring the choice by decision analysis. Kidney Int 1994;45:1193–1202.
105. Bruns FJ, Adler S, Fraley DS, et al. Sustained remission of membranous glomerulonephritis after cyclophosphamide and prednisone. Ann Intern Med 1991;114:725–730.
106. Jindal K, West M, Bear R, et al. Long-term benefits of therapy with cyclophosphamide and prednisone in patients with membranous glomerulonephritis and impaired renal function. Am J Kidney Dis 1992;19:61–67.
107. Reichert LJM, Huysmans FTM, Assmann K, et al. Preserving renal function in patients with membranous nephropathy: Daily oral chlorambucil compared with intermittent monthly pulses of cyclophosphamide. Ann Intern Med 1994;121:328–333.
108. Warwick GL, Geddes CG, Boulton-Jones JM. Prednisolone and chlorambucil therapy for idiopathic membranous nephropathy with progressive renal failure. Q J Med 1994;87:223–229.
109. Falk RJ, Hogan SL, Muller KE, et al. Treatment of progressive membranous glomerulopathy. A randomized trial comparing cyclophosphamide and corticosteroids with corticosteroids alone. The Glomerular Disease Collaborative Network. Ann Intern Med 1992;116:438–448.
110. Cattran DC, Greenwood C, Ritchie S, et al. A controlled trial of cyclosporine in patients with progressive membranous nephropathy. Kidney Int 1995;47:1130–1135.
111. Lin CY. Treatment of hepatitis B virus-associated membranous nephropathy with recombinant alpha-interferon. Kidney Int 1995;47: 225–230.
112. Lai KN, Tam JS, Lin HJ, et al. The therapeutic dilemma of the usage of corticosteroid in patients with membranous nephropathy and persistent hepatitis B virus surface antigenaemia. Nephron 1990;54: 12–17.
113. Ramos EL, Tisher CC. Recurrent diseases in the kidney transplant. Am J Kidney Dis 1994;24:142–154.
114. Rennke HG. Secondary membranoproliferative glomerulonephritis. Kidney Int 1995;47:643–656.
115. D'Amico G, Ferrario F. Mesangiocapillary glomerulonephritis. J Am Soc Nephrol 1992;2:S159–S166.
116. Donadio JV, Offord KP. Reassessment of treatment results in membranoproliferative glomerulonephritis. Am J Kidney Dis 1989;14: 445–451.
117. Schmitt H, Bole A, Reineke T, et al. Long-term prognosis of membranoproliferative glomerulonephritis type I. Nephron 1990;55: 242–250.
118. Confalonieri P, Schena P, Fellin F, et al. Evoluzione, indici prognostici e terapia in 294 casi di glomerulonefrite idiopatica. Giorn It Nefrologia 1990;7:89–95.
119. Cattran DC. Current status of cyclosporin A in the treatment of membranous, IgA and membranoproliferative glomerulonephritis. Clin Nephrol 1991;35(suppl 1):S43–S47.
120. Galla JH. IgA nephropathy. Kidney Int 1995;47:377–387.
121. D'Amico G. Influence of clinical and histological features on actuarial renal survival in adult patients with idiopathic IgA nephropathy,

membranous nephropathy, and membranoproliferative glomerulonephritis: Survey of the recent literature. Am J Kidney Dis 1992; 20:315–323.

122. Donadio JV, Bergstralh EJ, Offord KP, et al. Clinical and histopathologic associations with impaired renal function in IgA nephropathy. Clin Nephrol 1994;41:65–71.
123. Glassock RJ. Treatment of immunologically mediated glomerular disease. Kidney Int 1992;42(suppl 38):S121–S126.
124. Egido J, Rivera F, Sancho J, Barat A, Hernando L. Phenytoin in IgA nephropathy: a long-term controlled trial. Nephron 1984;38: 30–39.
125. Béné MC, Hurault de Ligny B, Kessler M, et al. Tonsils in IgA nephropathy. Contrib Nephrol 1993;104:153–161.
126. Schena FR, Montenegro M, Scivittaro V. Meta-analysis of randomized controlled trials in patients with IgA nephropathy (Berger's disease). Nephrol Dial Transplant 1990;5(suppl 1):47–52.
127. Donadio JV, Bergstralh EJ, Offord KP, et al. A controlled trial of fish oil in IgA nephropathy. N Engl J Med 1994;331:1194–1199.
128. Dillon JJ. Fish oil therapy for IgA nephropathy: Efficacy and interstudy variability. J Am Soc Nephrol 1997;8:1739–1744.
129. Strihou CY. Fish oil for IgA nephropathy. N Engl J Med 1994; 331:1227–1229.
130. Maschio G, Cagnoli L, Claroni F, et al. ACE inhibition reduces proteinuria in normotensive patients with IgA nephropathy: A multicentre, randomized, placebo-controlled study. Nephrol Dial Transplant 1994;9:265–269.
131. Cattran DC, Greenwood C, Ritchie S. Long-term benefits of angiotensin-converting enzyme inhibitor therapy in patients with severe immunoglobulin A nephropathy: A comparison to patients receiving treatment with other antihypertensive agents and to patients receiving no therapy. Am J Kidney Dis 1994;23:247–254.
132. Hunley T, Julian B, Phillips J. Angiotensin converting enzyme gene polymorphisms: Potential silencer motif and impact on progression in IgA nephropathy. Kidney Int 1996;49:571–577.
133. Rostoker G, Desvaux-Belghiti D, Pilatte Y, et al. High-dose immunoglobulin therapy for severe IgA nephropathy and Henoch–Schönlein purpura. Ann Intern Med 1994;120:476–484.
134. Clarkson AR, Woodroffe AJ, Bannister KM, Odum J. Therapy in IgA nephropathy. Contrib Nephrol 1993;104:189–197.
135. Lai KN, Lai FM, Li PKT, Vallance-Owen J. Cyclosporin treatment of IgA nephropathy. Br Med J 1987;195:1165–1168.
136. Lim EC, Chai D, Gjertson DW, et al. *In vitro* studies to explain high renal allograft survival in IgA nephropathy patients. Transplantation 1993;55:996–999.
137. Mills JA. Systemic lupus erythematosus. N Engl J Med 1994;330: 1871–1879.
138. Kashgarian M. Lupus nephritis: Lessons from the path lab. Kidney Int 1994;45:928–938.
139. Berden JHM. Lupus nephritis. Kidney Int 1997;52:538–558.
140. Schwartz MM, Lan SP, Bernstein J, et al. Role of pathology indices in the management of severe lupus glomerulonephritis. Kidney Int 1992;42:743–748.
141. Gruppo Italiano per lo Studio della Neffrite Lupica (GISNEL). Lupus nephritis: Prognostic factors and probability of maintaining life-supporting renal function 10 years after the diagnosis. Am J Kidney Dis 1992;19:473–479.
142. Donadio JV, Glassock RJ. Immunosuppressive drug therapy in lupus nephritis. Am J Kidney Dis 1993;21:239–250.
143. Austin HA, Klippel JH, Balow JE, et al. Therapy of lupus nephritis: Controlled trial of prednisone and cytotoxic drugs. N Engl J Med 1984;314:614–619.
144. Valleri A, Radhakrishnan J, Estes D, et al. Intravenous pulse cyclophosphamide treatment of severe lupus nephritis: A prospective five-year study. Clin Nephrol 1994;42:71–78.
145. Boumpas D, Austin HA, Vaughn EM, et al. Controlled trial of pulse methylprednisolone versus two regimens of pulse cyclophosphamide in severe lupus nephritis. Lancet 1992;340:741–745.
146. Dooley MA, Hogan S, Jennette C, et al. Cyclosphosphamide therapy for lupus nephritis: Poor renal survival in black Americans. Kidney Int 1997;51:1188–1195.
147. Boumpas DT, Austin HA, Vaughan EM, et al. Risk for sustained amenorrhea in patients with systemic lupus erythematosus receiving intermittent pulse cyclophosphamide therapy. Ann Intern Med 1993; 119:366–369.
148. Hussein MM, Mooij JMV, Roujouleh H. Cyclosporine in the treatment of lupus nephritis including two patients treated during pregnancy. Clin Nephrol 1993;40:160–163.
149. Lewis EJ, Hunsicker LG, Lan SP, et al. A controlled trial of plasmapheresis therapy in severe lupus nephritis. N Engl J Med 1992;326: 1373–1379.
150. Radhakrishnan J, Kunis CL, D'Agati V, et al. Cyclosporine treatment of lupus membranous nephropathy. Clin Nephrol 1994;42: 147–154.
151. Roth D, Milgrom M, Esquenazi V, et al. Renal transplantation in systemic lupus erythematosus: One center's experience. Am J Nephrol 1987;7:367–374.
152. Couser WG. Rapidly progressive glomerulonephritis: Classification, pathogenetic mechanisms, and therapy. Am J Kidney Dis 1988;11: 449–464.
153. Kohler IJ, Gohara AF, Hamilton RW, et al. Crescentic fibrillary glomerulonephritis associated with intermittent rifampin therapy for pulmonary tuberculosis. Clin Nephrol 1994;42:263–265.
154. Jennette JC, Falk RJ. Diagnosis and management of glomerulonephritis and vasculitis presenting as acute renal failure. Med Clin North Am 1990;74:893–908.
155. Kallenberg CGM, Brouwer E, Weening JJ, et al. Anti-neutrophil cytoplasmic antibodies: Current diagnostic and pathophysiological potential. Kidney Int 1994;46:1–15.
156. Levy JB, Winearls CC. Rapidly progressive glomerulonephritis: what should be first-line therapy? Nephron 1994;657:402–407.
157. Bruns FJ, Adler S, Fraley DS, et al. Long-term follow-up of aggressively treated idiopathic rapidly progressive glomerulonephritis. Am J Med 1989;86:400–406.
158. Ponticelli C, Fogazzi GB. Methylprednisolone pulse therapy for primary glomerulonephritis. Am J Nephrol 1989;9(suppl 1):41–46.
159. Bolton W, Couser WG. Intravenous pulse methylprednisolone therapy of acute crescentic rapidly progressive glomerulonephritis. Am J Med 1979;66:495–502.
160. Cole E, Cattran D, Magil A, et al. A prospective trial of plasma exchange as additive therapy in idiopathic crescentic glomerulonephritis. Am J Kidney Dis 1992;20:261–269.
161. Kunis CL, Kiss B, Williams G, et al. Intravenous "pulse" cyclophosphamide therapy of crescentic glomerulonephritis. Clin Nephrol 1992;37:1–7.
162. Falk RJ, Hogan S, Carey TS, et al. Clinical course of anti-neutrophil cytoplasmic autoantibody-associated glomerulonephritis and systemic vasculitis. Ann Intern Med 1990;113:656–663.
163. Pusey CD, Rees AJ, Evans DJ, et al. Plasma exchanges in focal necrotizing glomerulonephritis without anti-GBM antibodies. Kidney Int 1991;40:757–763.
164. Couser WG, Johnson RJ. Postinfective glomerulonephritis. In: Neilson EG, Couser WG, eds. Immunologic Renal Diseases. Philadelphia, Lipponcott–Raven, 1997:915–944.
165. Weinstein L, Le Frock J. Does antimicrobial therapy of streptococcal pharyngitis or pyoderma alter the risk of glomerulonephritis? J Infect Dis 1971;124:229–231.
166. Moudgil A, Bagga A, Fredrich R, et al. Poststreptococcal and other infection-related glomerulonephritides. In: Greenberg A, ed. Primer on Kidney Diseases, 2nd ed. San Diego, Academic Press, 1998:193–199.
167. Baldwin DS. Post-streptococcal glomerulonephritis: a progressive disease? Am J Med 1977;62:1–11.
168. Jennette JC, Falk R. Glomerular clinicopathologic syndromes. In: Greenberg A, ed. Primer on Kidney Disease, 2nd ed. San Diego, Academic Press, 1998;127–141.

47

Drug Therapy Individualization for Patients with Renal Insufficiency

Reginald F. Frye, PharmD, PhD, and Gary R. Matzke, PharmD, FCP, FCCP

Patients with renal insufficiency are commonly encountered in clinical practice. Reductions in renal function can be associated with disease states, drug effects (e.g., drug-induced nephrotoxicity), or the result of the known age-related maturation or diminution of renal function. In children, renal function does not mature to adult values until approximately 1 year of age. In older adults, age-related declines in renal function combined with the increased use of medications make this patient group particularly susceptible to adverse effects secondary to inappropriate pharmacotherapy.[1] The presence of compromised renal function in any patient age group, ranging from pediatric to geriatric, requires that the clinician understand the aspects of drug disposition that are altered in the presence of renal insufficiency and the appropriate methods to individualize drug therapy.[2,3]

Renal insufficiency is accompanied by progressive alterations in several other organ systems and results in the development of anemia, hyperparathyroidism, bleeding abnormalities, hyperlipidemia, hypertension, and changes in gastrointestinal (GI) tract integrity (see Chap. 42). It should not be surprising then that there are now many reports that document changes in the disposition of some drugs in patients with renal insufficiency as the result of changes in bioavailability,[4] protein binding,[5,6] distribution volume,[7] and metabolic activity.[8]

Drug therapy individualization for patients with renal insufficiency may require only a simple dose adjustment based on the fractional reduction in creatinine clearance.[9] However, the use of medications that are extensively metabolized or for which dramatic changes in protein binding and/or distribution volume have been noted may require a more complex adjustment.[7,9] Furthermore, because of the physiologic and biochemical changes associated with progressive renal insufficiency, patients may respond to a given dose or serum concentration of a drug differently than patients with normal renal function.[10]

Knowledge of basic pharmacokinetic principles combined with the drug disposition properties of a particular compound and the degree and type of pathophysiologic alterations associated with renal insufficiency will make it possible for the pharmacotherapist to design an individualized therapeutic regimen. The objectives of this chapter are to describe the influence of renal insufficiency on drug absorption, distribution, metabolism, and elimination and to provide a practical approach for drug dosage individualization for patients with reduced renal function as well as those receiving continuous renal replacement therapy, continuous ambulatory peritoneal dialysis, or hemodialysis.

EFFECT ON DRUG ABSORPTION

There is little quantitative information regarding the influence of impaired renal function on drug absorption and bioavailability. Drug bioavailability in this patient population may be altered by several factors, including changes in GI transit time and gastric pH; edema of the GI tract; vomiting and diarrhea (frequent complications of severe renal insufficiency); and antacid administration. The assessment of bioavailability in this patient population is further complicated, because most patients with severe renal insufficiency receive multiple medications, many of which cannot be discontinued during the course of a bioavailability study.

Some of the drug absorption "bioavailability" studies in patients with renal failure have not provided an assessment of absolute bioavailability (i.e., they have not included intravenous administration of the drug). Rather, they have documented alterations in the peak concentration (C_{max}), time at which the peak concentration was attained (t_{max}), or in the fractional amount of drug recovered in the urine in a finite time period. Unfortunately, this limited information has been extrapolated to suggest that drug absorption is slowed and/or that the extent of absorption is reduced.[4,11,12]

The absolute bioavailability of only a few drug compounds is affected and for several the increase in bioavailability is due to a decrease in metabolism during the first pass through the GI tract and liver. Balant et al.[13] reported an increased bioavailability of three β-blockers, tolamolol, bufuralol, and oxprenolol, in patients with renal failure. These data confirm the observations of increased systemic bioavailability of propranolol,[14] dextropropoxyphene,[15] and dihydrocodeine[16] in patients with renal insufficiency. Although the bioavailability of all these compounds was increased, clinical consequences (development of excessive or unexpected adverse effects) have been demonstrated only with dextropropoxyphene[15] and dihydrocodeine.[17,18] The lack of association between the pharmacokinetic profile and clinical consequences of the β-blockers may be a result of an alteration in the responsiveness of patients with renal disease to these agents, as has been reported with propranolol in the elderly.[19]

EFFECT ON DRUG DISTRIBUTION

Although it is generally assumed that the volume of distribution of drugs is not changed in renal insufficiency, it is

TABLE 47–1. Effect of ESRD on the Volume of Distribution of Selected Drugs[a]

	Normal	ESRD	Change From Normal (%)
Increased			
Amikacin	0.20	0.29	45
Azlocillin	0.21	0.28	33
Bretylium	3.58	4.48	25
Cefazolin	0.13	0.17	31
Cefonicid	0.11	0.14	27
Cefoxitin	0.16	0.26	63
Cefuroxime	0.20	0.26	30
Clofibrate	0.14	0.24	71
Cloxacillin	0.14	0.26	86
Dicloxacillin	0.08	0.18	125
Erythromycin	0.57	1.09	91
Furosemide	0.11	0.18	64
Gentamicin	0.20	0.32	60
Isoniazid	0.6	0.8	33
Minoxidil	2.6	4.9	88
Nalmefene	7.9	14.7	86
Naproxen	0.12	0.17	42
Phenytoin	0.64	1.4	119
Trimethoprim	1.36	1.83	35
Vancomycin	0.64	0.85	33
Decreased			
Chloramphenicol	0.87	0.60	−31
Digoxin	7.3	4.0	−45
Ethambutol	3.7	1.6	−57
Methicillin	0.45	0.30	−33
Pindolol	150 L	80 L	−47
Pipemidic acid	2.0	0.84	−58

[a]All data are in liters per kilogram unless otherwise stated.

clear that the volume of distribution of many drugs may be significantly increased or decreased in patients with renal insufficiency (Table 47–1).[7,20,21] Alterations in distribution volume may result from increased or decreased protein binding; altered tissue binding; or pathophysiologic alterations in body composition, for example, the fractional contribution of total body water to total body weight; or they may be an artifact of the volume term used in the comparison.

Generally, the plasma protein binding of acidic drugs (warfarin, phenytoin) is decreased in uremia[5,6,22,23] (Table 47–2), whereas the binding of basic drugs (quinidine, lidocaine) is usually normal or slightly decreased or increased[5,6,24,25] (Table 47–3). The decrease in binding of acidic drugs in uremic plasma has been attributed to qualitative changes in the binding sites, accumulation of endogenous inhibitors of binding, and decreased concentrations of albumin. The first two of these mechanisms appear to account for most of the observed changes in binding.[26,27] In addition, the high concentrations of metabolites of some compounds that accumulate in patients with renal insufficiency may interfere with the protein binding of the parent compound.

Although the fraction of unbound drug increases in patients with renal insufficiency, a new equilibrium is established as a result of increased drug elimination/distribution such that the free concentrations remain comparable. However, total concentrations are reduced owing to an increase in drug clearance. Thus, the net effect of changes in protein binding is an alteration in the relationship between total drug concentrations and effect. This can be illustrated with the anticonvulsant phenytoin. The protein binding of the acidic drug phenytoin, which binds to albumin, is significantly reduced as a result of endogenous substances that accumulate in renal failure and compete for binding, as well as by conformational changes in albumin in patients with end-stage renal disease.[26] This change in protein binding alters the relationship between total phenytoin concentration and effect or toxicity. The resulting increase in unbound fraction, from the normal of 0.1 to 0.2 or more, results in increased hepatic clearance and decreased total concentrations. Thus, in patients with renal insufficiency, the therapeutic range (normal, 10 to 20 μg/mL) shifts downward as the degree of renal impairment increases. Although the unbound concentration therapeutic range is unchanged in the presence of renal failure, unbound concentrations are often not measured. However, unbound concentration measurements provide the best means for individualizing phenytoin therapy in patients with renal insufficiency. Methods have been presented to equate an observed total concentration in patients with end-stage renal disease receiving hemodialysis treatment to what would be expected in patients with normal renal function.

Predicting the degree of protein binding in individuals improves the ability to interpret total drug concentrations. Liponi et al.[26] have suggested a method by which the total

TABLE 47–2. Change in Percent Unbound of Acidic Drugs in Patients With Normal Renal Function and ESRD

	Normal	ESRD	Change From Normal (%)
Abecarnil	4	15	275
Azlocillin	62.5	75	20
Cefazolin	16	29	81
Cefoxitin	27	59	119
Ceftriaxone	10	20	100
Clofibrate	3	9	200
Cloxacillin	5	20	300
Diazoxide	6	16	167
Dicloxacillin	3	9	200
Diflunisal	12	44	267
Doxycycline	12	28	133
Furosemide	4	6	50
Methotrexate	57.2	63.8	12
Metolazone	5	10	100
Moxalactam	48	64	33
Naproxen	0.2	0.8	300
Pentobarbital	34	41	21
Phenylbutazone	5.5	16	191
Phenytoin	10	21.5	115
Piretanide	6	12	100
Salicylate	8	20	150
Sulfamethoxazole	34	58	71
Valproic acid	8	23	188
Warfarin	1	2	100
Zomepirac	1.3	3.8	192

TABLE 47–3. Change in Percent Unbound of Basic Drugs in Patients With Normal Renal Function and ESRD

	Normal	ESRD	Change From Normal (%)
Decreased			
Bepridil	0.3	0.1	−67
Clonidine	55.6	47.6	−14
Disopyramide	32	28	−13
Propafenone	3.4	2.4	−29
Increased			
Amphotericin B	3.5	4.1	17
Chloramphenicol	45	64	42
Clonazepam	13.9	16	15
Clorazepate	2	5	150
Diazepam	2	8	300
Fluoxetine	5.5	6.5	18
Ketoconazole	1	1.5	50
Morphine	65	71	9
Prazosin	6	10.1	68
Triamterene	19	43	126

phenytoin concentration (C_m^{total}) in patients with creatinine clearance values of 10 to 24 mL/min and less than 10 mL/min can be equated to the concentration that would be observed if plasma protein concentrations and phenytoin-binding characteristics were normal. A patient's "equated" total phenytoin concentration (C_e^{total}) would thus equal:

$$C_e^{total} = \left(\frac{1}{[1] + [(nK_a)(p)]}\right)(C_m^{total})(10)$$

where nK_a is the binding parameter based on the patient's renal function (10 to 24 mL/min = 1.5, and < 10 mL/min = 1.0), and p is the measured serum albumin concentration. This methodology allows one to approximate the equivalent "total" phenytoin concentration in a patient with reduced renal function and can be used to predict dosage requirements via a standard nonlinear approach (see Chap. 3).

The principal binding protein for several basic drug compounds is α_1-acid glycoprotein (AAG), an acute-phase reactant whose plasma concentration is increased in a wide variety of patients, including renal transplant patients and hemodialysis patients.[27,28] The fraction of those drugs principally bound to AAG may be significantly increased in uremic patients.[5,6] Thus, patients with renal insufficiency may experience increased or decreased protein binding depending on the principal binding protein for the drug in question.

Altered tissue binding may also affect the apparent volume of distribution of a drug. The distribution volume of digoxin has been reported to be reduced by 30% to 50% from normal values in patients with renal disease.[29,30] It has been postulated that this reduction in the distribution volume is secondary to a decrease in tissue binding as a result of competitive inhibition by endogenous or exogenous substances. This factor must therefore be taken into consideration in the design of individualized dosage regimens. Multiple methods have been proposed to estimate the degree of reduction in digoxin's distribution volume.[29] Jusko and Szefler[30] have reported that the volume of distribution of digoxin is related to creatinine clearance in the following way:

$$V_{D(liters)} = [226] + \left[\frac{(298)(\text{CrCl})}{29.1 + \text{CrCl}}\right]$$

For a patient weighing 60 kg with a creatinine clearance of approximately 15 mL/min, the volume of distribution for digoxin would be:

$$V_D = [226] + \left[\frac{(298)(15)}{29.1 + 15}\right] = 327 \text{ L or } 5.5 \text{ L/kg TBW}$$

This represents a 30% reduction from the volume of distribution that would have been anticipated in a patient with normal renal function. Acidosis or the presence of digoxin-like immunoreactive substances that bind to and inhibit membrane ATPase may also contribute to this phenomenon.[31,32] In this situation, the absolute amount of digoxin bound to the receptor would be reduced and the resultant serum digoxin concentration from any dose would be greater.

Knowledge of protein and tissue binding changes in patients with renal insufficiency is critically important in the interpretation of serum drug concentrations. Numerous investigations have shown that the unbound concentration of several drugs in plasma correlates more closely with the concentration of drug at the receptor site and, therefore, with the pharmacologic effect, than does the total concentration of drug in plasma.[33] Because an alteration in plasma protein or tissue binding of a drug will likely alter the total drug concentration, the usual expected relationship between total drug concentration and pharmacologic response will be perturbed but the relationship to unbound drug should be unaffected.

Thus, in patients with renal insufficiency, particularly those with end-stage renal disease (ESRD), a "normal" total drug concentration may be associated with either serious adverse reactions secondary to elevated unbound drug concentrations or subtherapeutic responses because of an altered plasma to tissue drug concentration ratio. The monitoring of unbound drug concentrations in this patient population is therefore suggested for those drugs that have a narrow therapeutic range, are highly protein bound (free fraction of < 20%), and for which marked variability in the free fraction has been reported, for example, phenytoin and disopyramide.

Finally, the method used to calculate the volume of distribution may be influenced by renal disease. The three most commonly used volume of distribution terms are volume of the central compartment (V_c), volume of the terminal phase (V_β, V_{area}), and volume of distribution at steady state (V_{ss}). The central compartment volume is calculated as the intravenous bolus dose divided by the initial plasma concentration. V_c for many drugs approximates extracellular fluid volume and thus may be increased or decreased by shifts in this physiologic volume. Renal insufficiency, especially oliguric acute renal failure, is often accompanied by fluid overload and a resultant increased V_c due to reduced renal elimination of water and sodium. V_{area} (V_β) is calculated as the total body clearance divided by the terminal elimination rate constant (k or β). This volume term represents the proportionality constant between plasma concentrations in the terminal elimination phase and the amount of drug remaining in the body. V_β is affected by both distribution characteristics, as well as the elimination rate constant. The third volume term, the steady-state volume of distribution (V_{ss}), is determined by (AUMC × Dose)/AUC^2, where AUMC is the area under the first moment of the concentration–time curve and AUC is the area under the concentration–time curve. V_β and V_{ss} will often be similar in magnitude, with V_β being slightly larger. In situations in which V_β is much larger than V_{ss}, V_β may reflect the elimination rate more than the distribution volume. Because V_{ss} has the advantage of being independent of drug elimination, it may be the most appropriate volume term to use when one desires to compare drug distribution volumes between patients with renal insufficiency and those with normal renal function.[34]

EFFECT ON METABOLISM

Although the role of the kidneys as an excretory organ for drugs and chemicals and their polar metabolites is well described, the fact that the kidney is very metabolically active in the biotransformation of a variety of drugs is not well appreciated.[35,36] The renal cytochrome P450 (CYP) system catalyzes the metabolism of a variety of chemicals and drugs with an activity that may equal that of the liver on an activity per gram of tissue basis. Whole kidney homogenate CYP activity has varied from 14% to 18% of that observed in the liver. Glucuronide, glutathione, and sulfate conjugation activity has also been documented in kidney homogenates. Finally, glucuronyl transferase activity of the kidney in various animal species has been reported to range from 8% to 120% of the liver activity.[37] Prescott and associates[38] demonstrated that *p*-aminohippurate (PAH), a compound frequently used to estimate effective renal plasma flow, is converted to *N*-acetyl-PAH by the human kidney and liver. This metabolism accounts for up to 25% of the total elimination of PAH. These studies clearly suggest that the kidney possesses considerable drug-metabolizing capability; however, the contribution to the total metabolic activity is generally low, because total kidney weight is far less than liver weight.

Investigations of the effect of chronic renal failure on hepatic enzyme activity in animals have demonstrated reductions of 26% to 71% in some, but not all pathways of drug metabolism.[39,40] In each case, the alteration in enzyme activity declined as the extent of renal failure increased.[39] These data suggest that chronic renal impairment may have a detrimental effect not only on drug metabolism in the kidney but also on drug metabolism within the liver. This theory is supported by the observations of reduced nonrenal clearance for several drugs in patients with renal insufficiency.[10] The observed reductions in nonrenal clearance are generally proportional to the reductions in glomerular filtration rate (GFR). The effect(s) of renal failure on nonrenal drug clearance may also depend on whether the renal failure is acute or chronic. Effects observed in acute renal failure do not appear to be as great as those observed in chronic renal failure, potentially due to less accumulation of or exposure to metabolic inhibitors.[10]

Drug metabolism may be increased, decreased, or unaffected by renal failure depending on the drug and the species (animals versus man) investigated[8,35,36,38,41,42] (Table 47–4). These studies should be interpreted cautiously since concurrent drug intake, age, smoking habit, and alcohol intake often were not controlled. Furthermore, the possibility of pharmacogenetic variation must be considered. Prediction of the effect of renal impairment on the metabolism of a particular drug is thus difficult; for example, nifedipine, nitrendipine, and nisoldipine are all apparently metabolized *in vivo* by CYP3A4, yet the metabolism of nifedipine is increased,[43] nitrendipine decreased,[44] and nisoldipine is unaffected by renal failure.[45] The effect of renal insufficiency on other CYP enzymes has not been fully evaluated, but preliminary data suggest a differential effect on the individual isozymes with the activity of some enzymes (CYP2C19) being reduced

TABLE 47–4. Effect of ESRD on Nonrenal Clearance

Decreased		
Acyclovir	Aztreonam	Bufuralol
Captopril	Cefmenoxime	Cefmetazole
Cefonicid	Cefotaxime	Cefotiam
Cefsulodin	Ceftizoxime	Cilastatin
Cimetidine	Ciprofloxacin	Cortisol
Encainide	Erythromycin	Methylprednisolone
Imipenem	Isoniazid	Nicardipine
Metoclopramide	Moxalactam	Procainamide
Nimodipine	Nitrendipine	Zidovudine
Quinapril	Verapamil	
Unchanged		
Acetaminophen	Chloramphenicol	Clonidine
Codeine	Diflunisal	Indomethacin
Insulin[a]	Isradipine	Lidocaine
Morphine	Metoprolol	Nisoldipine
Nortriptyline	Pentobarbital	Propafenone
Quinidine	Theophylline	Tocainide
Tolbutamide		
Increased		
Bumetanide	Cefpiramide	Fosinopril
Nifedipine	Phenytoin	Sulfadimidine

[a]May be unchanged or decreased.

while others (CYP2D6) are not affected.[10] This differential effect on individual enzymes may help to explain some of the conflicting reports of whether drug metabolism is altered in the presence of renal disease. If the metabolism of a drug is known to be increased or decreased in patients with renal failure, then the dose will need to be adjusted appropriately to achieve the desired effect. If the effect of renal failure on metabolism is unknown, then the agent should be used with extreme caution.

Patients with severe renal insufficiency receiving chronic treatment with some agents may experience accumulation of metabolite(s) as well as parent compound. Although metabolites of several drugs have been reported to have significant pharmacologic and/or toxicologic activity in general, the pharmacokinetics and pharmacology of metabolites are not often fully elucidated in humans. In a sense, the patient with severe renal impairment is being exposed to a "new pharmacologic entity" if the serum concentrations of the metabolite exceed those reported in patients with normal renal function.

The metabolite may have pharmacologic activity similar to that of the parent drug and thus contribute significantly to clinical response, for example, oxipurinol and desacetyl cefotaxime.[46] Alternatively, the metabolite may have qualitatively dissimilar pharmacologic action; for example, normeperidine has a CNS-stimulatory activity that has been reported to produce seizures, whereas meperidine has CNS-depressant actions.[47] Because of the multiplicity of potential interactions of compounds that are primarily metabolized, the practical consequences of metabolite accumulation are difficult to predict and are most often identified in those patients at risk by trial and error (Table 47–5).

EFFECT ON RENAL EXCRETION

Net renal excretion (Cl_R) of a drug is the composite of glomerular filtration, tubular secretion, and reabsorption ($Cl_R = (GFR \times f_u) + Cl_{secretion} - Cl_{reabsorption}$), where f_u is the fraction of the drug unbound to plasma proteins. Drug elimination by filtration occurs by a diffusion process, but tubular secretion and reabsorption are bidirectional processes that involve carrier-mediated renal transport systems. The two primary renal transport systems termed the anionic and cationic pathways are responsible for the transport of a number of organic acids and basic drugs, respectively. Other important renal transport systems include the nucleoside and *p*-glycoprotein transporters, which are involved in the renal tubular transport of dideoxynucleosides (e.g., zidovudine, dideoxyinosine) and digoxin, respectively.[48] A reduction in glomerular filtration rate will result in a decrease in renal drug clearance. For drugs that are extensively renally secreted (Cl_R > 300 mL/min), the loss of filtration clearance (up to 120 mL/min) will have less of an impact than for those primarily dependent on GFR. Alterations in one or more of the three renal processes (filtration, secretion, reabsorption) secondary to reductions in functional nephron mass may have a dramatic effect on the pharmacokinetics of a drug.

Although it was once thought that the mechanisms of renal elimination declined in a parallel manner in the presence of renal disease, it is now known that this may not be a valid assumption. Kamiya et al.[49] and Hori et al.[50] demonstrated that the type of renal disease may explain in part the differences in pharmacokinetic parameters observed among patients with similar reductions in glomerular filtration rate. The disposition of antibiotic agents exten-

TABLE 47–5. Pharmacologic Activity of Selected Drug Metabolites

Parent Drug	Metabolite	Pharmacologic Activity of Metabolites
Acetaminophen	*N*-acetyl-*p*-benzo-quinoneimine	Responsible for hepatotoxicity
Allopurinol	Oxipurinol	Metabolite primarily responsible for suppression of xanthine oxidase
Azathioprine	Mercaptopurine	All of the immunosuppressive activity resides in the metabolite
Cefotaxime	Desacetyl cefotaxime	Similiar antimicrobial spectrum, but one-fourth to one-tenth as potent
Chlorpropamide	2-Hydroxychlorpropamide	Similar *in vitro* insulin-releasing activity
Clofibrate	Chlorophenoxyisobutyric acid	Primarily responsible for hypolipidemic effect and direct muscle toxicity
Codeine	Morphine-6-glucuronide	Possibly more active than parent compound; may contribute to prolonged narcotic effect in renal failure patients
Imipramine	Desmethylimipramine	Similar antidepressant activity
Meperidine	Normeperidine	Less analgesic activity than parent, but more CNS-stimulatory effects
Morphine	Morphine-6-glucuronide	Possibly more active than parent compound; may contribute to prolonged narcotic effect in renal failure patients
Procainamide	*N*-acetyl procainamide	Distinct antiarrhythmic activity, the mechanism of which is different from that of the parent compound
Sulfonamides	Acetylated metabolites	Devoid of antibacterial activity, but elevated concentrations are associated with increased toxicity
Theophylline	1,3-Dimethyl uric acid	Cardiotoxicity has been demonstrated
Zidovudine	Zidovudine triphosphate	Primarily responsible for antiretroviral activity

sively secreted by the proximal renal tubules (e.g., ampicillin, cephalexin) was altered to a greater degree in patients with tubulointerstitial disease compared to those with primary glomerular disease. These data suggest that dosage-adjustment methodologies may need to be developed to take into consideration the impact of altered tubular as well as glomerular function.[51] Quantitative investigations of renal handling of new drugs will be required to elucidate the relative contribution of tubular and glomerular function to renal drug clearance. The availability of these data should provide a more rational approach to dosage regimen design for those agents that undergo extensive tubular secretion or reabsorption.

In the absence of data delineating the contribution of tubular function to renal elimination, the clinical measurement or estimation of creatinine clearance remains the guiding factor for drug dosage regimen design.[7,9] The importance of an alteration in renal function on drug elimination thus depends on two factors: the fraction of drug normally eliminated by the kidney unchanged and the degree of renal insufficiency.

Quantitation of the patient's renal function can be accomplished by measurement of creatinine clearance or estimation based on the stable serum creatinine (see Chap. 42). Because of the time delay involved and problems in obtaining complete urine collections, measured creatinine clearance values are infrequently used for initial drug dosage regimen design. Therefore, the calculation of initial drug dosage regimens relies on the estimation of creatinine clearance (CrCl) in adults and children from such routinely available clinical data as age, gender, height, weight, and serum creatinine.[52] We should emphasize that these relationships are most accurate for individuals of average muscle mass for their age, weight, and height. The creatinine clearance of emaciated and obese adult patients is difficult to predict, and incorrect estimates have been obtained with most methods.

Several methods are also available for estimating creatinine clearance in adults with acute renal insufficiency using age, height, weight, serum creatinine, and time data.[52] These methods have not been as rigorously validated as the equations for patients with stable renal function. However, they are one of the few methods we have to approximate renal function in this complex patient situation.

DRUG DOSAGE REGIMEN DESIGNS

PATIENTS WITH RENAL INSUFFICIENCY

Most dosage adjustment guidelines have proposed the use of a fixed dose or interval for patients with broad ranges of renal function.[21,53–55] For example, moderate renal insufficiency may encompass a creatinine clearance range of 10 to 50 mL/min, whereas severe renal insufficiency is often defined as a creatinine clearance of less than 10 mL/min. These categories encompass up to a 10-fold range in renal function and, thus, the drug regimen may not be optimal for all patients whose renal function lies within the range.

The design of the optimal dosage regimen for patients with renal insufficiency requires an individualized assessment and is dependent on the availability of an accurate characterization of the relationship between the pharmacokinetic parameters of the drug and renal function and an accurate assessment of the patient's renal function (creatinine clearance). Secondary references such as the *AHFS Drug Information,*[53] and textbooks[56] are excellent sources of information about a drug's pharmacokinetic characteristics in subjects with normal renal function. However, they often do not provide the explicit relationships of the kinetic parameters of interest (total body clearance, elimination rate constant, and distribution volume) with a continuous index of renal function, such as creatinine clearance. To find this information, you may need to identify the original research study that assessed the drug's disposition or a comprehensive review article on the class of drugs of interest. Ideally, one should be able to identify a relationship between total body clearance (Cl), elimination rate constant (k), or distribution volume (V_D) with CrCl (see Table 47–6). This information along with the patient's CrCl will allow prediction of the patient's kinetic parameters and then formulation of a therapeutic regimen to attain the desired therapeutic outcome.

If specific literature recommendations and/or the relationship of kinetic parameters to CrCl are not available, then one can estimate the kinetic parameters of the patient with the method of Rowland and Tozer,[9] provided you know the fraction of the drug that is eliminated renally unchanged (f_e) in subjects with normal renal function. These approaches assume that the decrease in Cl and k are proportional to CrCl, that renal disease does not alter the drug's metabolism, that the metabolites if formed are inactive and nontoxic, that the drug obeys first-order (linear) kinetic principles, and that it is adequately described by a

TABLE 47–6. Relationship Between Renal Function and Pharmacokinetic Parameters of Selected Drugs

Drug	Total Body Clearance
Acyclovir	Cl = 3.37 (CrCl) + 0.41
Amikacin	Cl = 0.6 (CrCl) + 9.6
Cefmetazole	Cl = 1.18 (CrCl) – 0.29
Ceftazidime	Cl = 1.15 (CrCl) + 10.6
Ciprofloxacin	Cl = 2.83 (CrCl) + 363
Digoxin	Cl = 0.88 (CrCl) + 23
Gentamicin	Cl = 0.983 (CrCl)
Netilmicin	Cl = 0.65 (CrCl) + 3.72
Ofloxacin	Cl = 1.04 (CrCl) + 38.7
Piperacillin	Cl = 1.36 (CrCl) + 1.50
Procainamide	Cl = 3 (CrCl) + 0.23 (ABW)
Teicoplanin	Cl = 7.09 (CrCl) – 16.2
Tobramycin	Cl = 0.801 (CrCl)
Vancomycin	Cl = 0.69 (CrCl) + 3.7

Compiled from Refs. 20, 55, and 56.

one-compartment model. If these assumptions are true then the kinetic parameter/dosage adjustment factor (Q) can be calculated as:

$$Q = 1 - [f_e(1 - KF)]$$

where KF is the ratio of the patient's CrCl to the assumed normal value of 120 mL/min. Thus, for a drug that is 85% eliminated renally unchanged in a patient who has a CrCl of 10 mL/min, the Q factor would be:

$$Q = 1 - [0.85(1 - (10 / 120))]$$
$$= 1 - [0.85(0.92)]$$
$$= 1 - 0.78$$
$$= 0.22$$

The estimated total body clearance for this patient would then be calculated as $Cl_{PT} = Cl_{norm} \cdot Q$, where Cl_{norm} is the mean value in patients with normal renal function as reported in the literature.

Once the kinetic parameters for the patient have been estimated, the best method for dosage regimen adjustment should be selected. Specifically, one must determine if the desired goal is the maintenance of a similar peak, trough, or average steady-state drug concentration. If there is a significant relationship between peak or trough concentration and clinical response[57] (e.g., aminoglycosides and vancomycin) or toxicity[55,58] (e.g., quinidine, phenobarbital, and phenytoin), then attainment of the specific target values is critical. If, however, no specific target values for peak or trough concentrations have been reported (e.g., antihypertensive agents, benzodiazepines, and cephalosporins), then a regimen goal of attaining the same average steady-state concentration may be appropriate.

Although several methods have been proposed to attain the desired average steady-state concentration profile, the principal choices are to decrease the dose or prolong the dosing interval. If the size of the dose is reduced while the dosing interval remains unchanged, the desired average steady-state concentration will be similar; however, the peak will be lower and the trough higher (Fig. 47–1). Alternatively, if the dosing interval is increased and the dose size remains unchanged, the peak and trough concentrations in the patient with reduced renal function will be similar to those in the patient with normal renal function. This dosage adjustment method is generally preferred because it is likely to yield significant cost savings as a result of a reduction in nursing and pharmacy time as well as in the supplies associated with frequent drug administration. Finally, the dose and dosing interval may both need to be changed to attain a desired peak or trough serum concentration time profile.

Regardless of the approach chosen to adjust the dosage regimen, the first step in the process, as previously mentioned, is to estimate the drug disposition parameters in the patient with renal insufficiency. The ratio (Q) of the estimated elimination rate constant or total body clearance of the patient relative to subjects with normal renal function (CrCl = 120 mL/min) may then be calculated. This parameter may be used to determine the dose or dosing interval alterations necessary for the patient.

Scenario	Dose	τ	C_{max}	C_{min}	C_{ave}
A	5	12	26.6	19.8	23.0
B	0.85	12	4.5	3.4	3.9
C	5	70	8.3	1.5	3.9
D	3.4	48	6.7	2.1	3.9

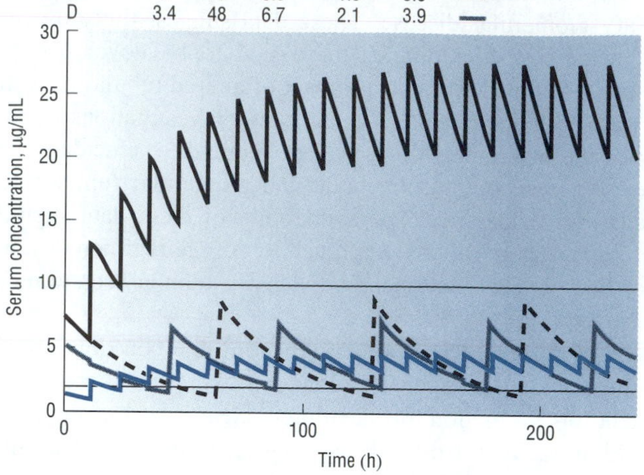

FIGURE 47–1. Without a change in dosage regimen this patient would achieve excessive steady-state serum concentrations (Scenario A). Although the average steady-state concentrations (C_{ave}) are identical, the concentration-time profile will be markedly different if one changes the dose and maintains the dosing interval (τ) constant (Scenario B), versus changing the dosing interval (τ) and maintaining the dose constant (Scenario C) or changing both (Scenario D).

For example, the following relationship between total clearance (Cl) and creatinine clearance has been reported for ganciclovir[59]:

$$Cl(mL/min/1.8\ m^2) = 1.25(CrCl) + 8.57$$

Thus, Cl for a subject with normal renal function (Cl_{norm}) would be calculated as:

$$Cl_{norm} = [1.25(120)] + 8.57$$
$$Cl_{mean} = 158.6\ mL/min/1.8\ m^2$$

Clearance (Cl_{fail}) for a patient with a creatinine clearance of 10 mL/min would be:

$$Cl_{fail} = [1.25\ (10)] + 8.57$$
$$Cl_{fail} = 21.1\ mL/min/1.8\ m^2$$

Neutropenia has been associated with ganciclovir trough concentrations exceeding 10 µmol/L.[60] If this patient received the typical ganciclovir dose for a patient with normal renal function, the predicted trough concentrations would approach 20 µmol/L. Therefore, a dosage modification in this patient is necessary to avoid potential toxicity. The dosing regimen can be modified using the ratio of the predicted clearance values. Therefore, the quotient or Q, for this patient is calculated as:

$$Q = Cl_{fail}/Cl_{norm}$$

$$Q = 21.1/158.6$$

$$Q = 0.133$$

where Cl_{norm} is the clearance in a patient with normal renal function and Cl_{fail} is the clearance of the patient with impaired renal function.

The maintenance dose (D_f) for the patient or the adjusted dosing interval (τ_f) may then be calculated from the following relationships, where D_n is the normal dose and τ_n is the normal dosing interval:

$$D_f = D_n \times Q$$

$$\tau_f = \tau_n/Q$$

For this patient situation, the normal dose of ganciclovir would be 5 mg/kg (D_n) and the τ_n = 12 hours. If we wanted to maintain the dosing interval at 12 hours, then D_f would be calculated as:

$$D_f = (5 \text{ mg/kg}) \times (0.133) = 0.67 \text{ mg/kg}$$

This regimen would result in decreased peak and increased trough concentrations compared to patients with normal renal function (Fig. 47–1, scenario A).

If we want to maintain D_n and extend the dosing interval, τ_f would be calculated as:

$$\tau_f = \tau_n/Q = 12/0.133 = 90.2 \text{ hours}$$

This regimen would yield similar peak and trough concentrations in the renally impaired patient as in the normal renal function patient but there is a risk of missed doses with such an unorthodox interval (Fig. 47–1, scenario B). In addition, the prolonged period below the C_{ss} average concentration may be less than optimal.

Finally, a practical dosing interval may be selected and then a dose based on that interval can be calculated (Fig. 47–1, scenario C). If a dosage interval τ_f of 48 hours were selected, because in many institutions there is an increased risk of missed doses with longer dosing intervals, then the D_f would be calculated as follows:

$$D_f = [D_n \times Q \times \tau_f]/\tau_n$$

$$= [(5 \text{ mg/kg}) \times (0.133) \times (48)]/12$$

$$= 2.66 \text{ mg/kg}$$

This method would likely be most appropriate in this case; prolonged subtherapeutic concentrations are avoided and troughs are reduced from the first method. The selection of which dosage adjustment method to use to calculate an optimal regimen depends on the drug characteristics and the patient care situation. This dosage adjustment method assumes that the protein binding and volume of distribution of the drug are not significantly altered by renal insufficiency. Thus, this approach cannot be used with accuracy for those drugs with demonstrated differences in these pharmacokinetic parameters.

If the volume of distribution (V_D) of a drug is significantly altered in patients with renal insufficiency or in whom one desires to attain a specific maximum or minimum concentration, the estimation of a dosage regimen becomes more complex. If the relationship between V_D and creatinine clearance has been characterized, then V_D may be estimated. If one assumes the drug can be described by a one-compartment linear model, the predicted V_D may then be used with the predicted elimination rate constant (k) of the drug to yield an adjusted dosing interval and intravenous or oral dose.

For orally administered drugs, the τ_f can be calculated as $\tau_f = [(-1/k_f)(\ln[C_{min}/C_{max}])] + t_{peak}$, and the dose can be approximated as:

$$Dose_{PO} = [SFC_p^t V_D(k_a - k)]/[k_a(e^{-kt} / 1 - e^{-k\tau}) - (e^{-kat}/1 - e^{-ka\tau})]$$

where, S equals the sact fraction, F equals bioavailability, C_p^t equals the desired plasma concentration at time t, and k_a is the absorption rate constant. This approach allows for the individualization of a dosage regimen for attainment of specific peak and trough serum concentrations. If the drug is absorbed extremely rapidly, one can approximate the τ_f as: $\tau_f = (-1/k_f)(\ln C_{min}/C_{max})$ and the dose as Dose = $V_D \cdot (C_{max} - C_{min})$.

Digoxin is a frequently used oral medication for which the V_D is decreased in patients with renal insufficiency and for which one usually desires to closely control the plasma concentration time profile. The V_D and Cl_{fail} of digoxin can be estimated for a 70-kg patient with a CrCl of 12 mL/min as follows[29]:

$$V_D = 226 + [(298(\text{CrCl})/(29.1 + \text{CrCl}))]$$

$$= 226 + [(298(12)/(29.1 + 12))]$$

$$= 226 + 87.0$$

$$= 313 \text{ L}$$

$$Cl_{fail} = (0.88\text{CrCl}) + 23 \text{ mL/min}$$

$$= 10.56 + 23$$

$$= 33.6 \text{ mL/min}$$

$$k_f = Cl_{fail}/V_D$$

$$= (33.6 \text{ mL/min} \cdot 1440 \text{ min/day})/313\text{L}$$

$$= 48.3 \text{ L/day}/313 \text{ L}$$

$$= 0.154 \text{ day}^{-1}$$

The t_{peak} is generally at 2 hours and the k_a from the literature is about 0.76 per hour or 18 per day.[56] Thus, one now has all the information needed to calculate the τ_f and dose for this patient:

$$\tau_f = [(-1/k_f)(\ln(C_{min}/C_{max})] + t_{peak}$$

$$= [(-1/0.154)(\ln 0.8/1.4)] + 2 \text{ hours}$$

$$= [(-6.49)(-0.56)]$$

$$= 3.6 \text{ days} + 2 \text{ hours}$$

$$\sim 4 \text{ days}$$

$$\text{Dose}_{PO} = [(1.4)(313)(18 - 0.154)]/[18(e^{-0.154(0.083)}/1 - e^{-0.154(4)}) - (e^{-18(0.083)}/1 - e^{-18(4)})]$$

$$\text{Dose} = 0.226 \text{ mg or } 0.25 \text{ mg oral capsules every 4 days}$$

Alternately, the predicted volume of distribution and elimination rate constant or the total body clearance may be used to calculate a dose regimen that will maintain the desired average steady-state concentration of the drug (C_{ss}).

$$\text{Dose (mg/h)} = C_{ss}\ [(k_f\ V) \text{ or } (\text{Cl}_f)]$$

Depending on how much variance about the average steady state one desires, the dosing interval may range from hourly to as infrequently as every 48 hours or longer. For example, if the calculated dose were 10 mg/h, the desired average steady-state concentration would be maintained with a dosing interval of 60 mg every 6 hours or 480 mg every 48 hours.

PATIENTS RECEIVING CONTINUOUS RENAL REPLACEMENT THERAPY

Continuous renal replacement therapy (CRRT) is used for the management of fluid overload and the removal of uremic toxins in patients with acute renal failure and other conditions.[61] The several forms of CRRT are extensively described in Chapter 41, Acute Renal Failure. Which of these therapies will be optimal for a given patient is dependent on several factors, including bleeding risk, degree of hypercatabolism, acid–base balance, and experience of the health care provider.

Drug therapy individualization for the patient receiving CRRT is complicated by the fact that patients with acute renal failure may have a higher residual nonrenal clearance of some drugs than patients with chronic renal insufficiency who have a similar CrCl.[62,63] For example, the nonrenal clearance of imipenem in patients with acute renal failure (95 mL/min) is between the values observed in chronic renal failure patients (50 mL/min) and normal values (130 mL/min).[63] This may occur because of less exposure to or accumulation of uremic by-products that may alter hepatic function. A nonrenal clearance value in a patient with acute renal failure that is higher than anticipated based on chronic renal failure data would result in lower than expected, possibly subtherapeutic, serum concentrations.

In addition to patient-specific differences, there are marked differences between intermittent hemodialysis and the three primary types of CRRT (continuous arteriovenous or venovenous hemofiltration [CAVH/CVVH]), continuous arteriovenous or venovenous hemodialysis (CAVHD/CVVHD), and continuous arteriovenous or venovenous hemodiafiltration (CAVHDF/CVVHDF)] with regard to drug removal.

During CAVH/CVVH drug removal primarily occurs via convection/ultrafiltration (the passive transport of drug molecules at the concentration at which they exist in plasma water into the plasma ultrafiltrate). The clearance of a drug by either of these methods is thus a function of the membrane permeability for the drug, which is called the sieving coefficient (SC) and the rate of ultrafiltrate formation (UFR). The SC can be calculated as:

$$\text{SC} = (2\text{C}_{\text{UF}})/[(C_a/1-\theta) + (C_v/1-\theta)]$$

where C_a and C_v are the concentration in the plasma going into and returning from the filter, respectively, and θ is 0.0107 times the total protein concentration in plasma. The SC is often approximated by the fraction unbound (f_u) since this information may be more readily available. Thus the clearance by these two modes of CRRT can be calculated as:

$$\text{Cl}_{\text{CVVH}} = \text{UFR} \cdot \text{SC}$$

or

$$\text{Cl}_{\text{CVVH}} = \text{UFR} \cdot f_u$$

Clearance of a drug by CAVHDF/CVVHDF ($\text{Cl}_{\text{CAVHDF}}$/$\text{Cl}_{\text{CVVHDF}}$) is generally greater than by CAVH/CVVH since in addition to the convection/ultrafiltration process, drug is removed by diffusion from the plasma water into the dialysate. The $\text{Cl}_{\text{CVVHDF}}$ can be mathematically approximated as:

$$\text{Cl}_{\text{CVVHDF}} = (\text{UFR} \cdot f_u) + \text{Cl}_{\text{diffusion}}$$

In the clinical setting, it is often not possible to separate these two components of $\text{Cl}_{\text{CVVHDF}}$. In essence the $\text{Cl}_{\text{CVVHDF}}$ is calculated as the product of the combined ultrafiltrate and dialysate volume (V_{df}) and the concentration of the drug in this fluid (C_{df}) divided by the plasma concentration (C_p^{mid}) at the midpoint of the V_{df} collection period:

$$\text{Cl}_{\text{CVVHDF}} = (V_{df} \cdot C_{df})/C_p^{mid}$$

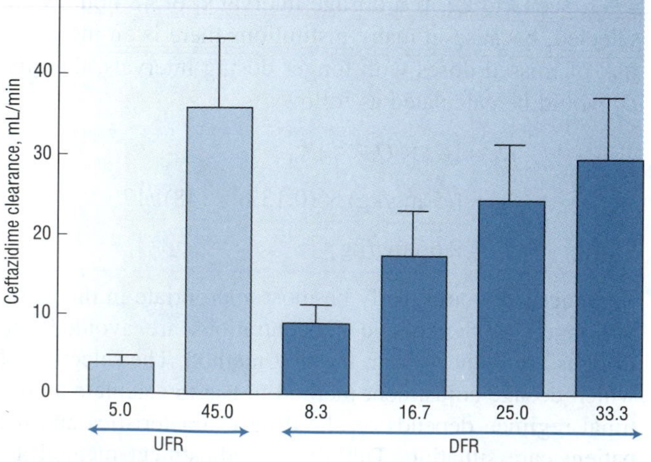

FIGURE 47–2. The effect of increasing ultrafiltration rate (UFR; mL/min) and dialysate flow rate (DFR; mL/min) on the clearance of ceftazidime.

There are differences in the rate of drug removal not only between the three primary modes of CRRT but also within each mode.[61] This is due to differences in the filter membrane composition as the result of variable degrees of drug binding to the membrane and the permeability characteristics of the membrane.[65,66] Important factors to consider that influence drug clearance during CRRT include ultrafiltration rate, blood flow rate, and dialysate flow rate. For example, clearance in CAVH/CVVH is directly proportional to the ultrafiltration rate, whereas clearance in CAVHDF/CVVHDF, which depends on both the ultrafiltration rate and the dialysate flow rate, increases as either flow rate increases. Changes in blood flow rate generally have only a minor effect on drug clearance by any mode of CRRT. These effects are shown for ceftazidime clearance in Figure 47–2, with different ultrafiltration flow rates (5 and 45 mL/min) and increasing dialysate flow rates (8.3 to 33.3 mL/min).

An algorithmic approach for drug dosage adjustment in patients undergoing CRRT has been proposed.[61] Individualization of therapy for a patient receiving CRRT therapy is dependent on the patient's residual renal function and the clearance of the drug by the mode of CRRT they are receiving. The patient's residual drug clearance can be predicted as described in the previous section of this chapter. The CRRT clearance can also be ascertained from published literature reports.[61,67,68] The SCs of frequently used drugs are summarized in Table 47–7, and the clearance of selected drugs by CAVH/CVVH or CAVHD/CVVHD is listed in Table 47–8. These data can be used to design initial dosage regimens for patients receiving CRRT.

For example, WT is a 48-year-old, 60-kg male in acute renal failure with a serum creatinine of 7.2 mg/dL, which has increased from 2.3 mg/dL over 3 days. The residual creatinine clearance value in this patient, calculated using the Jelliffe and Jelliffe equation for changing serum creatinines (see Chap. 40), is 4.8 mL/min. The consulting nephrologist recommends that CVVHDF be initiated using a Fresenius F- 40 filter at a blood and dialysis flow rate of 100 and 33.3 mL/min, respectively. The patient is to receive ceftazidime while on CVVHDF. The patient's residual ceftazidime clearance can be estimated using the regression equation in Table 47–6 relating CrCl and clearance:

$$Cl_{RES}\ (\text{mL/min}) = 1.15\ (\text{CrCl}) + 10.6$$

$$Cl_{RES} = 1.15\ (4.8) + 10.6 = 16.1\ \text{mL/min}$$

TABLE 47–7. Predicted and Measured Sieving Coefficients of Selected Drugs

Drug	Predicted	Measured
Amikacin	0.95	0.88
Amphotericin	0.01	0.32–0.4
Ampicillin	0.80	0.6–0.69
Cefoperazone	0.10	0.27–0.69
Cefotaxime	0.62	0.55–1.1
Cefoxitin	0.30	0.32
Ceftazidime	0.90	0.38–0.78
Ceftriaxone	0.10	0.71–0.82
Clindamycin	0.25	0.49–0.98
Digoxin	0.75	0.96
Erythromycin	0.25	0.37
5-Flurocytosine	0.96	0.98
Gentamicin	0.95	0.81–0.75
Imipenem	0.80	0.78
Metronidazole	0.80	0.80
Mezlocillin	0.68	0.68
Nafcillin	0.20	0.47
N-acetyl procainamide	0.80	0.92
Netilmicin	—	0.85
Oxacillin	0.05	0.02
Phenobarbital	0.60	0.86
Phenytoin	0.10	0.45
Procainamide	0.80	0.86
Theophylline	0.47	0.85
Tobramycin	0.95	0.78–0.86
Vancomycin	0.90	0.5–0.8

Adapted from Ref. 61.

TABLE 47–8. Clearance of Selected Drugs by CAVH/CVVH and/or CAVHD/CVVHD

	CAVH/CVVH		CAVHD/CVVHD		
Drug	*SC*	*Clearance*	*SC*	*Clearance DFR 1 L/h*	*Clearance DFR 2 L/h*
Amikacin	0.93 ± 0.16	10.1			
Amrinone	0.80 – 1.4	2.4–14.4			
Cefuroxime		11.0 ± 5.2	0.90 ± 0.30	14.0 ± 2.2	16.2 ± 3.4
Ceftazidime			0.86 ± 0.07	13.1 ± 1.3	15.2 ± 1.3
Cilastatin	0.77	4.0 ± 2.3	0.68 ± 0.08	10.0 ± 3.0	18.0 ± 4.0
Ciprofloxacin				16.3	19.9
Digoxin				6.4–10.0	11
Gentamicin		3.5 ± 1.9		5.2 ± 1.8	
Imipenem	0.80	13.3	1.05 ± 0.19	16.0 ± 7.0	
Phenytoin	0.37 ± 0.08	1.0		6.5	
Theophylline				14.8	
Tobramycin		3.5 ± 1.9		11.1–29	14.9
Vancomycin	0.80	6.7–13.3	0.66 ± 0.08	12.1 ± 1 5.7	16.6 ± 5.7

Clearance is in mL/min. SC = sieving coefficient; DFR = dialysate flow rate; NR = not reported.
From Ref. 61.

The total clearance while on CVVHDF would be the sum of the patient's residual clearance and the ceftazidime clearance associated with CVVHDF (Cl_{CVVHDF}; Table 47–8) as follows:

$$Cl_T = Cl_{RES} + Cl_{CVVHDF}$$

$$Cl_T = 16.1 \text{ mL/min} + 15.2 \text{ mL/min} = 31.3 \text{ mL/min}$$

This patient clearance value can be used to adjust the ceftazidime dose as described earlier. The ceftazidime clearance in a patient with normal renal function would be calculated as:

$$Cl_{norm} \text{ (mL/min)} = 1.15 \text{ (CrCl)} + 10.6$$

$$Cl_{norm} = 1.15 \text{ (120)} + 10.6 = 148.6 \text{ mL/min}$$

The dosage adjustment factor would then be:

$$Q = Cl_T / Cl_{norm}$$

$$Q = 31.3 / 148.6 = 0.21$$

For this patient situation, the normal regimen of ceftazidime would be 1000 mg (D_n) every 8 hours (τ_n). If we wanted to maintain D_n and extend the dosing interval, then τ_f would be calculated as:

$$\tau_f = \tau_n / Q$$

$$\tau_f = 8 \text{ hours} / 0.21$$

$$\tau_f = 38 \text{ hours or a more practical 36 hours}$$

Therefore, this patient should receive 1000 mg every 36 hours. If the additional clearance associated with CVVHDF (15.2 mL/min) was not considered, the dosing interval would have been considerably longer at approximately 72 hours.

PATIENTS RECEIVING CHRONIC AMBULATORY PERITONEAL DIALYSIS

Although the majority of patients with ESRD receive treatment with hemodialysis, approximately 15% of dialysis patients are maintained with chronic ambulatory peritoneal dialysis (CAPD). A more detailed discussion of CAPD therapeutic principles is provided in Chapter 46. Peritoneal dialysis, like other dialysis modalities, has the potential to affect drug disposition; however, drug therapy individualization is often less complicated in these patients owing to the continuous nature of the CAPD procedure.

Many of the factors that are important in determining drug dialyzability for other treatment modalities pertain to peritoneal dialysis as well.[69] Peritoneal dialysis involves the instillation of 1 to 3 L of dialysis solution into the peritoneal cavity. Waste products and other substances, potentially including drugs, move from the blood and surrounding tissues into the dialysis solution by means of diffusion and ultrafiltration. Factors that influence drug dialyzability in peritoneal dialysis include drug-specific characteristics such as molecular weight, solubility, degree of ionization, protein binding, and volume of distribution. The intrinsic properties of the peritoneal membrane that affect drug removal include blood flow, pore size, and peritoneal membrane surface area, which is approximately equal to the body surface area. There is an inverse relationship between peritoneal drug clearance and molecular weight, protein binding, and volume of distribution. Also, drug compounds that are ionized at physiologic pH will diffuse across the membrane more slowly than un-ionized compounds. In general, hemodialysis is more effective in removing drug substances than peritoneal dialysis such that if a drug is not removed by hemodialysis, it is not likely to be removed by peritoneal dialysis. As shown in Table 47–9, the contribution of peritoneal dialysis to total body clearance is often low and, for most drugs, markedly less than the contribution of hemodialysis. Detailed reviews of the disposition of other drugs in CAPD patients are reported elsewhere.[7,69] Anti-infective agents are the most commonly studied drugs due to concern with therapy during treatment of peritonitis. Most other drugs can generally be dosed according to the residual renal function of the patient because additional clearance by peritoneal dialysis is so small.

TABLE 47–9. Comparison for Selected Drugs of Residual Drug Clearance in ESRD (Cl_{ESRD}) to Clearance by Continuous Ambulatory Peritoneal Dialsysis (Cl_{CAPD}), Intermittent Peritoneal Dialysis (Cl_{IPD}), and Hemodialysis (Cl_{HD})[a]

Drug	Cl_{ESRD}	Cl_{CAPD}	Cl_{IPD}	Cl_{HD}
Aztreonam	1.44	0.13	0.13	2.6
Cefazolin	0.30	0.06		2.1
Cefotaxime	7.13 ± 0.74	0.40 ± 0.08		1.6
Ceftazidime	0.74 ± 0.20	0.10 ± 0.02	0.50	2.3
Gentamicin	0.24	0.17	0.75	2.1
Mezlocillin	6.0		0.44	1.7
Pipericillin	3.90 ± 0.77	0.22		4.4
Ticarcillin	0.96		0.43	2.0
Vancomycin	5.0	0.85 ± 0.22		0.8

[a]All data (mean or mean ± SD) are in liters per hour.
From Refs. 7, 52, and 69.

CHRONIC HEMODIALYSIS PATIENTS

The number of patients with ESRD who receive chronic hemodialysis has steadily increased since the early 1970s and currently over 200,000 patients receive this life-sustaining therapy.[70] Although considerable advances in hemodialysis filter technology have been made in the past 20 years and the efficiency of the hemodialysis procedure has been increased, the effect of hemodialysis on drug disposition is rarely reevaluated after initially reported. Thus, most of the literature probably represents an underestimation of the impact of hemodialysis on drug disposition.

The impact of hemodialysis on a patient's drug therapy is dependent on several factors, including the characteristics of each drug, the dialysis conditions, and the clinical situation for which dialysis is performed. Drug-related factors that affect dialyzability include the molecular weight, protein binding, and distribution volume of each

TABLE 47–10. Drug Disposition During Dialysis Depends on Dialyzer Characteristics

Drug	Hemodialysis Clearance (mL/min)		Half-Life During Dialysis (h)	
	Conventional	*High-Flux*	*Conventional*	*High-Flux*
Ceftazidime	55–60	155[a]	3.30	1.2[a]
Cefuroxime	NR	103[b]	3.75	1.6[b]
Gentamicin	58.2	116[b]	3.0	4.3[b]
Netilmicin	46	87–109	5.0–5.2	2.9–3.4
Vancomycin	9–21	31–60[c]	35–38	12.0[c]
		40–150[b]		4.5–11.8[b]
		72–116[d]		NR[d]

NR, not reported.
[a]Polyamide dialyzer.
[b]Polysulfone dialyzer.
[c]Polyacrylonitrile dialyzer.
[d]Polymethylmethacrylate dialyzer.

drug.[7] The impact of distribution volume (V_D) on drug removal by dialysis is evident in the following example where drug A has a 10-L V_D, whereas drug B has a V_D of 80 L. Both drugs are not bound to plasma proteins, are exclusively eliminated unchanged by the kidney, and have a molecular weight of 300 and a dialyzer clearance of 40 mL/min (2.4 L/h). The half-life in an anuric patient during dialysis [$t_{1/2} = (V_D \times 0.693)/\mathrm{Cl}$] will be markedly different for these two drugs (2.9 hours vs 23 hours) and thus approximately 50% of drug A but only 10% of drug B will be removed during 3 hours of dialysis as a direct result of the larger distribution volume. Prior to the mid-1980s these were the primary factors that needed to be known to assess the degree of dialyzability of a given drug because the vast majority of dialysis filters were composed of cellulose, cellulose acetate, or regenerated cellulose (cuprophane). These "conventional" filter materials were generally impermeable to drugs with a molecular weight over 1000 and the clearance by hemodialysis tended to decline dramatically (by up to 60%) as molecular weight increased from 100 to 500.[71] Drugs that are small but highly protein bound are also not well dialyzed because both of the principal binding proteins, AAG and albumin, have a very high molecular weight. Finally, those drugs that are widely distributed throughout the body are poorly removed by hemodialysis.

The dialysis prescription for the patient can also dramatically affect the degree of drug removal. The primary factors that can vary between patients are the type of hemodialysis they are prescribed, which is primarily reflected in the composition of the dialysis membrane, the filter surface area, blood and dialysate flow rates, and whether or not the dialysis unit reuses the dialysis filter. Dialysis membranes are composed of cellulose-based, semisynthetic or synthetic materials (e.g., polysulfone, polymethylmethacrylate, or acrylonitrile). The synthetic filter materials are now available for low-, medium-, and high-flux modes of dialysis (see Chap. 44), with the principal difference between modes being in the filter pore size, which can range from 25 to 60 angstrom and the degree of water transport. A difference in drug clearance between filters made of the same membrane material but with different pore sizes could be expected, but this has not been studied. The dialysis membranes used in high-flux hemodialysis (HFD) have the greatest pore sizes and more closely mimic the filtration characteristics of the human kidney than the filters used to deliver conventional hemodialysis. This allows the free passage of most solutes, including drugs, that have a molecular weight of 20,000 or less.[71] Thus, high-molecular-weight drugs such as vancomycin are likely to be removed by this mode of dialysis though they are not by conventional dialysis. An increase in removal has also been reported with several other drugs that have lower molecular weights (Table 47–10).[72–78] The clearance of gentamicin in patients receiving dialysis using either a low-clearance or a high-clearance dialyzer is shown in Figure 47–3. When the same doses are given, the gentamicin concentrations will continue to accumulate in the patient receiving dialysis with a low-clearance dialyzer. The net result is that the patients receiving low-flux dialysis will require

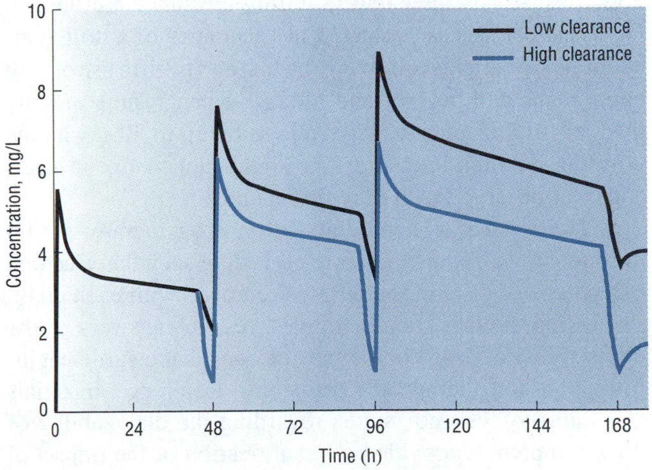

FIGURE 47–3. Clearance of gentamicin by low- and high-clearance dialyzers in patients given the same gentamicin dose. Concentrations in the patient receiving dialysis with a low-clearance dialyzer will continue to accumulate whereas concentrations in the patient receiving dialysis with the high-clearance dialyzer will be maintained at the same peak and predialysis concentrations observed after the third dose.

smaller postdialysis doses relative to the patient receiving high-flux dialysis to maintain similar concentrations.

Two of the primary factors that are increased in newer dialysis modalities compared to conventional dialysis are the blood and dialysate flow rates. These changes have been reported to significantly increase the dialyzer clearance of many endogenous solutes and drugs, especially those with molecular weights of 500 or less. Changes in blood flow rate appear to have the most dramatic impact. Increases in gentamicin clearance of 50% to 100% have been associated with an increase in blood flow rate from 100 to 300 mL/min. Dialysate flow rates are fairly standardized now at 500 mL/min, but in some procedures the dialysate flow rate may be as high as 1000 mL/min. Although no direct comparisons of drug clearances have been reported at these two different dialysate flow rates, urea clearance is increased by only about 11% to 12%.[71] Thus, it is unlikely that changes in this component of the dialysis prescription will significantly alter pharmacokinetic projections.

The final component of the dialysis prescription that may affect drug clearance by dialysis is whether or not the patient has authorized the unit to reuse his or her dialysis filter. Currently more than 75% of all dialysis units in the United States use this procedure to reduce the cost of chronic hemodialysis.[70] The effect of dialysis filter reuse on the clearance of endogenous molecules such as urea, creatinine, and β_2-microglobulin has been evaluated for polysulfone (Fresenius F80B) and cellulose (Terumo T220L) dialysis filters.[81] A progressive decrease (over 20 reuses) in urea and creatinine clearances was observed with the polysulfone but not the cellulose filter. Also, the clearance of the middle-molecular-weight (11,800 daltons) molecule β_2-microglobulin went from negligible (< 5 mL/min) to more than 20 mL/min by the twentieth reuse of the F80B filter; clearance with the cellulose filter remained below 5 mL/min. Unfortunately, reports on the effect of dialysis filter reuse on drug clearance are limited. Only one center has evaluated the clearance of a drug (ceftazidime) in patients following the first and twelfth use of both cuprophane and polysulfone filters.[74] Their results indicate that ceftazidime clearance decreased by up to 30% with the polysulfone filter. In contrast, no significant change in clearance was observed with the cuprophane filter.

The impact of hemodialysis on drug therapy should thus not be viewed as a generic procedure such that a certain percentage of drug in the body is removed with each dialysis session; neither should simple "yes–no" answers on the dialyzability of drug compounds be considered sufficient information for therapeutic decisions. Reference materials that indicate "yes–no" status regarding the dialyzability of drug compounds provide no quantification of the impact of hemodialysis and are thus of little value to the clinician who is attempting to design a rational dosing regimen. Compounds considered nondialyzable with low-flux filters may in fact be significantly removed by high-flux hemodialysis filters. Characteristics of the dialysis prescription such as membrane composition and surface area, and blood and dialysis flow rates, are thus critical data for the design of drug dosing regimens for chronic hemodialysis patients.

The effect of hemodialysis on drug disposition can be estimated in several ways. The determination of drug concentrations at the start and end of dialysis, with the subsequent calculation of the half-life during dialysis ($t_{1/2,\text{onHD}}$), has frequently been used as an index of drug removal by dialysis. Unfortunately, the $t_{1/2,\text{onHD}}$ may not be interpretable because declining plasma drug concentrations during dialysis represent elimination by the body as well as by dialysis. Furthermore, if significant rebound in drug concentrations after dialysis has been reported, the removal of drug by the dialysis procedure may be artificially high depending on when, after dialysis, the concentration is determined (Table 47–11).[73,82–86]

An alternative and more accurate means of assessing the effect of hemodialysis is to calculate the dialyzer clearance of the drug. The dialyzer clearance (Cl_D) can be calculated by several approaches. The C_D^b from blood can be calculated as $Cl_D^b = Q_b\,[(A_b - V_b)/A_b]$, where Q_b is blood flow through the dialyzer, A_b is the concentration of drug in blood going into the dialyzer, and V_b is the blood concentration of drug leaving the dialyzer. This equation is valid only if the drug concentrations are measured in whole blood and if the drug rapidly and completely distributes into red blood cells. Since drug concentrations are generally determined in plasma, the previous equation is usually modified to $Cl_D^p = Q_p\,[A_p - V_p)/A_p]$, where p represents plasma and Q_p is plasma flow, which equals Q_b (1 – hematocrit). This clearance calculation accurately reflects dialysis drug clearance only if the drug does not penetrate red blood cells or bind to formed blood elements.

Because of potential problems in accurately determining Q_b or Q_p, the dialysate recovery method is widely used. In addition, venous plasma concentrations may be concentrated, because plasma water is generally removed from the blood at a faster rate than drug when ultrafiltration is performed simultaneously with diffusion during dialysis. Thus, the recovery clearance approach described as follows has become the benchmark for the determination of dialyzer clearance.[7]

Dialyzer clearance can thus be calculated as:

$$Cl^r_D = R/AUC_{0-t}$$

where R is the total amount of drug recovered unchanged in the dialysate and AUC_{0-t} is the area under the predialyzer

TABLE 47–11. Rebound in Drug Concentrations After the End of Hemodialysis

	t_{max}	% Rebound
Cefmetazole	0.9	17.9
Ceftibuten	0.58	45.9
Gentamicin	1.3	23.3
Netilmicin	1.9	38.3
Tobramycin	1.7	18.3
Vancomycin	6.4	52.4

plasma concentration–time curve during hemodialysis. To determine the AUC_{0-t}, at least two and preferably three to four plasma concentrations should be obtained during dialysis.

The hemodialysis clearance values reported in the literature may vary significantly depending on which of the previous methods was used to calculate Cl_D. The principal reason for this is that for most medications we do not know the degree and rapidity with which the drug crosses the red blood cell (RBC) membrane. Since the Cl^r_D method incorporates no assumption of the degree of RBC permeability, it can be reliably used as the benchmark value. Comparisons of Cl^p_D and Cl^b_D values to the Cl^r_D benchmark thus provide valuable insight to a given drug's dialyzability.[87] Since the Cl^b_D and Cl^r_D clearances of the cephalosporins cefepime, cefmetazole, and ceftibuten were comparable, it can be concluded that these three cephalosporins readily distributed into and out of RBCs. In contrast, since the Cl^p_D and Cl^r_D of netilmicin are approximately the same, one can conclude that netilmicin does not readily penetrate the RBCs. Thus, to evaluate the Cl_D of a new dialysis filter in the clinical setting, the Cl^b_D method would be preferred for these cephalosporins and tobramycin but the Cl^p_D method may be best for netilmicin.

The following principles may be applied to drug dosage regimen design by using a value of Cl_D that is reported in the literature.[7,20,21,55] Because clearance terms are additive, the total clearance during dialysis can be calculated as the sum of the patient's residual clearance during the interdialytic period (Cl_{RES}) and dialyzer clearance (Cl_D):

$$Cl_T = Cl_{RES} + Cl_D$$

The half-life during the period between dialysis treatments and during dialysis can then be calculated from the following relationships using an estimate of the drug's distribution volume (V), which can be obtained from review articles[7,20,21,55]:

$$t_{1/2,\ offHD} = 0.693\ [V/Cl_{RES}]$$

$$t_{1/2,\ onHD} = 0.693\ [V/(Cl_{RES} + Cl_D)]$$

Once the key pharmacokinetic parameters (Cl, Cl_D, and V) have been estimated/calculated, they may be used to simulate the plasma concentration–time profile of the drug for the individual patient and ascertain how much drug to administer and when.

This approach to drug therapy individualization can be accomplished in a stepwise fashion assuming first-order elimination of the drug and a one-compartment model. For example, a 34-year-old male with ESRD was admitted to your institution from the outpatient hemodialysis unit, where he experienced shaking and chills and had a temperature of 40°C. He weighed 70 kg and was 69 inches tall, had a residual creatinine clearance of 3 mL/min, and received conventional dialysis for 4 hours TIW on a CA170 cellulose acetate filter. He received 140 mg of tobramycin at the end of his hemodialysis treatment.

The first step is to estimate this patient's pharmacokinetic parameters of tobramycin on the basis of published population data. The volume of distribution in this patient would be 23.1 L (0.33 L/kg × 70 kg) based on the recent report of Fish and Peter.[88] The patient's residual total body clearance (Cl_{RES}) can be estimated from the relationship between Cl and creatinine clearance, such as the one reported by Matzke et al[89]:

$$Cl_{RES} = CrCl \times 0.801$$

$$Cl_{RES} = 3\ mL/min \times 60\ min/h \times 0.801$$

$$Cl_{RES} = 0.144\ L/h$$

The hemodialysis clearance of tobramycin is dependent on the dialysis filter (Table 47–12), and a value of 69 mL/min can be extrapolated from the report of Fish and St. Peter[88] for the CA170 filter.

Once the patient's kinetic parameters have been approximated, one can predict what the plasma concentrations of tobramycin will be over the next 24 to 48 hours. The concentration at the end of the 30-minute infusion (C_{max}) would be:

$$C_{max} = \frac{(Dose/t')\ 1 - e^{-kt'}}{Cl_{RES}}$$

$$C_{max} = \frac{(140\ mg/0.5\ h)\ 1 - e^{-(Cl_{RES}/V)t'}}{0.144\ L/h}$$

$$C_{max} = \frac{(280\ mg/h)\ 1 - e^{-(0.0062)0.5}}{0.144\ L/h}$$

$$C_{max} = (1944\ mg/L)\ (0.003) = 5.8\ mg/L$$

The plasma concentration prior to the next dialysis session (C_{bD}), which is 44 hours away, and the concentration after dialysis (C_{aD}) can be calculated as:

$$C_{bD} = C_{max} \cdot e^{-(Cl_{RES}/V) \cdot t}$$

$$= 5.8 \cdot e^{-0.0062 \cdot 44}$$

$$= 4.4\ mg/L$$

$$C_{aD} = CbD \cdot e^{-(Cl_{RES} + Cl_D)/V \cdot t}$$

$$= 4.5 \cdot e^{-((0.144 + 4.14)/23.1) \cdot 4}$$

$$= 4.5 \cdot e^{-0.185 \cdot 4}$$

$$= 2.1\ mg/L$$

TABLE 47–12. Variation in CL_D Determinations Are Dependent on the Method of Calculation[a]

	Cl^b_D	Cl^p_D	Cl^r_D
Cefepime	166	116	158
Cefmetazole	83	55	86
Ceftibuten	62	43	77
Netilmicin	78	63	62
Tobramycin	55	44	55

On the basis of these data, one can feel confident that no further therapy is likely be required until after the next dialysis treatment. During this interdialytic interval, however, several blood samples should be collected to characterize this patient's residual tobramycin clearance, distribution volume, and last the clearance of tobramycin during dialysis. Blood samples were therefore collected at the following times after the first dose:

Day 1	7 PM (2 hours after dose)	6.5 mg/L
Day 2	8 AM (39 hours after dose)	4.1 mg/L
Day 3	12 noon (after HD)	2.0 mg/L

The C_{max} can be calculated by back-extrapolation to the end of the infusion. The elimination rate during the interdialytic period (k_{ID}) and during dialysis (k_{DD}), and the V_D can be calculated as:

$$k_{ID} = (\ln C_1 / C_2) / \Delta t$$

$$k_{ID} = (\ln 6.5 / 4.1) / 37 = 0.0125/\text{h}$$

$$k_{DD} = (\ln C_2 / C_3) / \Delta t$$

$$k_{DD} = (\ln 4.1 / 2.0) / 4 = 0.179/\text{h}$$

$$V_D = \frac{\text{Dose} / t'}{k_{ID}} \frac{1 - e^{-k_{ID}t'}}{(C_{max} - C_{min}\, e^{-k_{ID}t'})}$$

$$V_D = \frac{140/0.5}{0.0125} \frac{1 - e^{-(0.0125)0.5}}{(6.7 - 0.0\, e^{-(0.0125)0.5})}$$

$$V_D = \frac{134.4}{6.7} = 20 \text{ L}$$

The patient's residual clearance (Cl_{RES}) and the dialyzer clearance (Cl_D) of tobramycin can then be calculated as:

$$Cl_{RES} = V_d \times k_{ID}$$

$$Cl_{RES} = 20.0 \text{ L} \times 0.0125 = 0.25 \text{ L/h or } 4.2 \text{ mL/min}$$

$$Cl_D = Cl_T - Cl_{RES}$$

$$Cl_D = (k_{DD} \times V_D) - 4.2 \text{ mL/min}$$

$$Cl_D = (0.179/\text{h} \times 20.0 \text{ L}) - 4.2 \text{ mL/min}$$

$$Cl_D = (3.6 \text{ L/h or } 59.6 \text{ mL/min}) - 4.2 \text{ mL/min}$$

$$Cl_D = 55.4 \text{ mL/min}$$

This case illustrates the need for individualizing drug therapy for hemodialysis patients since this patient's V_D was 13% smaller, Cl_{RES} was 75% greater, and Cl_D was 19.7% less than the estimates based on population parameters. The ultimate reason for measuring the plasma concentrations of aminoglycosides and several other agents is to design the patient's dosage regimen. Thus, there remains one important step in our evaluation: the calculation of the dose this patient should receive next. The two factors that enter into this decision are the desired peak and trough concentrations and the degree of rebound in drug concentrations, after the end of dialysis. Since tobramycin concentrations have been noted to increase by about 20% within 1.5 to 2 hours after the end of hemodialysis (Table 47–11), the trough concentration of this patient can be considered to be 2.4 mg/L (2.0 mg/L × 1.2). Although this value is higher than one might like to maintain in an individual with normal renal function, a prolonged period of almost 24 hours would be required just to have the concentration drop below 2.0 mg/L. It is frequently necessary in critically ill individuals to redose the patient even though the postdialysis trough values are between 2 and 3 mg/L. Assuming the desired peak concentration was 7.0 mg/L, the postdialysis dose this patient would need can then be calculated as follows because the elimination half-life is extremely prolonged relative to the infusion time and thus minimal drug is eliminated during the infusion period:

$$\text{Dose} = V_D \times (C_{max} - C_{min})$$
$$= 20.0 \text{ L} \times (7.0 - 2.4) = 92 \text{ mg}$$

Combination antibiotic therapy with aminoglycosides and extended-spectrum penicillins are frequently prescribed for ESRD patients to provide wider antibacterial coverage against gram-negative bacilli through a synergistic effect. It is known, however, that the combined use may result in *in vitro* chemical inactivation of the aminoglycoside, leading to a loss in antibiotic activity. The rate of inactivation is related to the incubation period, temperature, presence of solutes, and β-lactam concentration.[90,91]

The extent of aminoglycoside inactivation *in vivo* may not be clinically significant in human subjects with normal or slightly impaired renal function due to the short contact time. However, in patients with significant renal insufficiency, subtherapeutic aminoglycoside concentrations and a decreased aminoglycoside elimination half-life during combination therapy with broad-spectrum β-lactam penicillins have been reported and will require appropriate dosage modification to maintain the desired serum concentrations. The inactivation of aminoglycosides in patients receiving chronic dialysis therapy has been reported for gentamicin in combination with carbenicillin,[92] ticarcillin,[93] and piperacillin.[92,94] Inactivation of tobramycin given in combination with ticarcillin and piperacillin has also been described,[95,96] though netilmicin disposition is not affected by piperacillin administration.[96]

Tobramycin serum concentrations declined at a faster rate when tobramycin was given with piperacillin, 4 g q 12 hours (half-life alone = 60 ± 25 hours, half-life combined = 25 ± 5 hours), though no significant change was noted in the half-life of netilmicin (41.8 vs 40.0 hours). A similar study recently evaluated the degree of inactivation of isepamicin and gentamicin when they are administered concomitantly with piperacillin.[94] The half-life of gentamicin was reduced significantly from 48 ± 21 hours to 36 ± 11 hours, though no significant difference was noted in the half-life of isepamicin (48 vs 45 hours). No significant changes in V_D were noted for any of the aminoglycosides and thus the inactivation clearances of netilmicin and isepamicin were significantly less than those of tobramycin and gentamicin. From these data tobramycin appears to be affected to the greatest degree followed by gentamicin, netilmicin, and isepamicin in descending order.

Thus, the elimination of aminoglycosides in renal failure patients also receiving antipseudomonal penicillins will be increased; therefore, frequent serum concentration monitoring should be performed. To eliminate any *in vitro* inactivation of aminoglycosides that would complicate assessment of the *in vivo* effects, serum samples should be assayed as soon as possible after collection. If this is not possible, serum samples should be frozen (preferably at –70°C) until they can be assayed.

CONCLUSIONS

Subtherapeutic or supratherapeutic responses to drugs in uremic patients are often misinterpreted and not recognized as such. The adverse outcomes associated with inappropriate drug use and dosing have not been quantified but do warrant future investigations. Sound pharmacokinetic principles as illustrated in this chapter, used in concert with reliable population pharmacokinetic estimates, should ultimately yield the optimal approach to drug dosage regimen design for patients with impaired renal function. Individualization of therapy should be undertaken whenever clinical therapeutic monitoring tools are available.

REFERENCES

1. Vestal RE. Aging and pharmacology. Cancer 1997;80:1302–1310.
2. Sloan RW. Principles of drug therapy in geriatric patients. Am Fam Physician 1992;45:2709–2718.
3. Skaer TL. Drug dosing considerations in the pediatric patient. Clin Ther 1991;13:526–544.
4. Ritschel WA, Denson DD. Influence of disease on bioavailability. In: Pharmacokinetics: Regulatory, Industrial, Academic Perspectives. New York, Marcel Dekker, 1995.
5. Zini R, Riant P, Barre J, et al. Disease-induced variations in plasma protein levels: Implications for drug dosage regimens (Part I). Clin Pharmacokinet 1990;9:147–159.
6. Zini R, Riant P, Barre J, et al. Disease-induced variations in plasma protein levels: Implications for drug dosage regimens (Part II). Clin Pharmacokinet 1990;19:218–229.
7. Matzke GR, Millikin SP. Influence of renal disease and dialysis on pharmacokinetics. In: Evans WE, Schentag JJ, Jusko WJ, eds. Applied Pharmacokinetics: Principles of Therapeutic Drug Monitoring, 3rd ed. Spokane, WA, Applied Therapeutics, 1992.
8. Elston AC, Bayliss MK, Park GR. Effect of renal failure on drug metabolism by the liver. Br J Anaesth 1993;71:282–290.
9. Rowland M, Tozer TN. Clinical Pharmacokinetics: Concepts and Applications, 3rd ed. Philadelphia, Lea & Febiger, 1995.
10. Matzke GR, Frye RF. Drug administration in patients with renal insufficiency: Minimizing renal and extrarenal toxicity. Drug Saf 1997; 16:205–231.
11. Tilstone WJ, Dargie H, Dargie EN, et al. Pharmacokinetics of metolazone in normal subjects and in patients with cardiac or renal failure. Clin Pharmacol Ther 1974;16:322–329.
12. Tilstone WJ, Fine A. Furosemide kinetics in renal failure. Clin Pharmacol Ther 1978;23:644–650.
13. Balant LP, Dayer P, Fabre J. Consequences of renal insufficiency on the hepatic clearance of some drugs. Int J Clin Pharmacol Res. 1983; 3:459–474.
14. Bianchetti G, Graziani G, Brancaccio D, et al. Pharmacokinetics and effects of propranolol in terminal uremic patients and in patients undergoing regular dialysis treatment. Clin Pharmacokinet 1976;1:373–384.
15. Gibson TP, Giancomini KM, Briggs WA, et al. Propoxyphene and norpropoxyphene plasma concentrations in the anephric patient. Clin Pharmacol Ther 1980;27:665–670.
16. Barnes JN, Williams AJ, Tomson MJ, et al. Dihydrocodeine in renal failure: Further evidence for an important role of the kidney in the handling of opioid drugs. Br Med J 1985;290:740–742.
17. Barnes JN, Goodwin FJ. Dihydrocodeine narcosis in renal failure. Br Med J 1983;286:438–439.
18. Redfern N. Dihydrocodeine overdose treated with naloxone infusion. Br Med J 1983;287:751–752.
19. Vestal RE, Wood AJ, Shand DG. Reduced β-receptor sensitivity in the elderly. Clin Pharmacol Ther 1979;26:181–186.
20. St Peter WL, Redickill KA, Halstenson CE. Clinical pharmacokinetics of antibiotics in patients with impaired renal function. Clin Pharmacokinet 1992;22:169–210.
21. St Peter WL, Halstenson CE. Pharmacologic approach in patients with renal failure. In: Chernow B, ed. The Pharmacologic Approach to the Critically Ill Patient. Baltimore, William & Wilkins, 1994:41–79.
22. Vanholder R, Van Landsehoot N, De Smet R, et al. Drug protein binding in chronic renal failure: Evaluation of nine drugs. Kidney Int 1988;33:996–1004.
23. Karara AH, Frye RF, Hayes PE, et al. Pharmacokinetics of abecarnil in patients with renal insufficiency. Clin Pharm Ther 1996;59: 520–528.
24. Chan GL, Axelson JE, Price JD, et al. *In vitro* protein binding of propafenone in normal and uraemic human sera. Eur J Clin Pharmacol 1989;36:495–499.
25. Pritchard JF, Matzke GR, Opsahl JA, et al. Effects of hemodialysis on plasma protein binding of bepridil. J Clin Pharmacol 1995;35: 137–141.
26. Liponi DF, Winter ME, Tozer TN. Renal function and therapeutic concentrations of phenytoin. Neurology 1984;34:395–397.
27. Haughey DB, Kraft CJ, Matzke GR, et al. Protein binding of disopyramide and elevated alpha-1-acid glycoprotein concentrations in serum obtained from dialysis patients and renal transplant recipients. Am J Nephrol 1985;5:35–39.
28. Docci D, Bilancioni R, Pistocchi E, et al. Serum alpha-1-acid glycoprotein in chronic renal failure. Nephron 1985;39:160–163.
29. Job ML. Digoxin. In: Murphy JE, ed. Clinical Pharmacokinetics Pocket Reference, Bethesda, MD, American Society of Hospital Pharmacists, 1993:71–80.
30. Jusko WJ, Szefler SJA. Pharmacokinetic design of digoxin dosage regimens in relation to renal function. J Clin Pharmacol 1974;14:525–535.
31. Malini PL, Strocchi E, Feliciangeli G, Buscaroli A, Bonomini V. Digitalis receptors and digoxin sensitivity in renal failure. Clin Exp Pharmacol Physiol 1985;12:115–120.
32. Rambausek M, Ritz E. Digitalis in chronic renal insufficiency. Blood Purif 1985;3:4–9.
33. Levy RH, Moreland TA. Rationale for monitoring free drug levels. Clin Pharmacokinet 1984;9(suppl 1):1–9.
34. Koup J. Disease states and drug pharmacokinetics. J Clin Pharmacol 1989;29:674–679.
35. Gibson TP. Renal disease and drug metabolism: An overview. Am J Kidney Dis 1986;8:7–17.
36. Milad MA, Ludwig EA, Lew KH, et al. The pharmacokinetics and pharmacodynamics of methylprednisolone in chronic renal failure. Am J Ther 1994;1:49–57.

37. Anders MW. Metabolism of drugs by the kidney. Kidney Int 1980;18:636–647.
38. Prescott LF, Freestone S, McAuslane JA. The concentration-dependent disposition of intravenous *p*-aminohippurate in subjects with normal and impaired renal function. Br J Clin Pharmacol 1993;35:20–29.
39. Patterson SE, Cohn VH. Hepatic drug metabolism in rats with experimental long-term renal failure. Biochem Pharmacol 1984;35:711–716.
40. Terner UK, Wiebe LI, Noujaim AA, et al. The effects of acute and chronic uremia in rats on their hepatic microsomal enzyme activity. Clin Biochem 1978;4:156–158.
41. Touchette MA, Slaughter RL. The effect of renal failure on hepatic drug clearance. Ann Pharmacother 1991;25:1214–1224.
42. Kim YG, Shin JG, Shin SG, et al. Decreased acetylation of isoniazid in chronic renal failure. Clin Pharmacol Ther 1993;54:612.
43. van Bortel L, Bohm R, Mooij J, et al. Total and free steady-state plasma levels and pharmacokinetics of nifedipine in patients with terminal renal failure. Eur J Clin Pharamcol 1989;37:185–189.
44. Aronoff GR. Pharmacokinetics of nitrendipine in patients with renal failure: Comparison to normal subjects. J Cardio Pharmacol 1984;6:S974–S976
45. van Harten J, Burggraaf J, van Brummelen P, et al. Influence of renal function on the pharmacokinetics and cardiovascular effects of nisoldipine after single and multiple dosing. Clin Pharmacokinet 1989;16:55–64.
46. Jones RN, Barry AL. Antimicrobial activity of ceftriaxone, cefotaxime, desacetylcefotaxime, cefotaxime-desacetyl cefotaxime in the presence of human serum. Antimicrob Agents Chemother 1987;31:818–820.
47. Wolfert AI, Sica DA. Narcotic usage in renal failure. Int J Artif Organs 1988;11:411–415.
48. Bendayan R. Renal drug transport—a review. Pharmacotherapy 1996;16:971–985.
49. Kamiya A, Okumura K, Hori R. Quantitative investigation of renal handling of drugs in dogs with renal insufficiency. Pharm Sci 1984;74:892–896.
50. Hori R, Okumura K, Kamiya A, et al. Ampicillin and cephalexin in renal insufficiency. Clin Pharmacol Ther 1983;34:792–798.
51. Hori R, Okumura K, Nihria H, et al. A new dosing regimen in renal insufficiency: Application to cephalexin. Clin Pharmacol Ther 1985;38:290–295.
52. Lam YW, Banerji S, Hatfield C, Talbert RL. Principles of drug administration in renal insufficiency. Clin Pharmacokinet 1997;32:30–57.
53. McEvoy GK, Litvak K, Welsh OH, et al. American Hospital Formulary Service, Drug Information. Bethesda, MD, American Society of Hospital Pharmacists, 1998.
54. Bennett WM, Aronoff GR, Golper TA, et al. Drug Prescribing in Renal Failure: Dosing Guidelines for Adults, 2nd ed. Philadelphia, American College of Physicians, 1991.
55. Murphy JE. Clinical pharmacokinetics pocket reference. Bethesda, MD, American Society of Hospital Pharmacists, 1993.
56. Benet LZ, Williams RL. Design and optimization of dosage regimens: Pharmacokinetic data. In: Goodman GA, Rall TW, Nies AS, Taylor P, eds. The Pharmacological Basis of Therapeutics, 8th ed. Elmsford, NY, Pergamon Press, 1990:1650–1735.
57. Craig WA. Pharmacokinetic/pharmacodynamic parameters: Rationale for antibacterial dosing of mice and men. Clin Infect Dis 1998;26:1–12.
58. Kim SY, Benowitz NL. Poisoning due to class IA antiarrhythmic drugs. Quinidine, procainamide and disopyramide. Drug Saf 1990;5:393–420.
59. Sommadossi JP, Bevan R, Ling T, et al. Clinical pharmacokinetics of ganciclovir in patients with normal and impaired renal function. Rev Infect Dis 1988;10:S507–S514
60. Balfour HH. Management of cytomegalovirus disease with antiviral drugs. Rev Infect Dis 1990;12:S849–S860.
61. Joy MS, Matzke GR, Armstrong DK, Marx MA, Zarowitz BJ. A primer on continuous renal replacement therapy for critically ill patients. Ann Pharmacother 1998;32:362–375.
62. Macias WL, Mueller BA, Scarim SK. Vancomycin pharmacokinetics in acute renal failure: Preservation of non-renal clearance. Clin Pharmacol Ther 1991;50:688–694.
63. Mueller BA, Scarim SK, Macias WL. Comparison of imipenem pharmacokinetics in patients with acute or chronic renal failure treated with continuous hemofiltration. Am J Kidney Dis 1993;21:172–179.
64. Kronfol NO, Lau AH, Barakat MM. Aminoglycoside binding to polyacrylonitrile hemofilter membranes during continuous hemofiltration. ASAIO Trans 1987;33:300–303.
65. Joy MS, Matzke GR, Frye RF, Palevsky PM. Determinants of vancomycin clearance by continuous venovenous hemofiltration and continuous venovenous hemodialysis. Am J Kidney Dis 1998;31:1019–1027.
66. Lau AH, Kronfol NO. Determinants of drug removal by continuous hemofiltration. Int J Artif Organs 1994;17:373–378.
67. Reetze-Bonorden P, Bohler J, Keller E. Drug dosage in patients during continuous renal replacement therapy. Clin Pharmacokinet 1993;24:362–379.
68. Bressolle F, Kinowski JM, de la Coussaye JE, et al. Clinical pharmacokinetics during continuous hemofiltration. Clin Pharmacokinet 1994;26:457–471.
69. Taylor CA, Abdel-Rahman E, Zimmerman SW, Johnson CA. Clinical pharmacokinetics during continuous ambulatory peritoneal dialysis. Clin Pharmacokinet 1996;31:293–308.
70. US Renal Data Systems. USRDS 1998 annual data report. Bethesda, MD, The National Institutes of Health, Institute of Diabetes and Digestive and Kidney Diseases, 1998.
71. Konstantin P. Newer membranes: Cuprophane versus polysulfone versus polyacrylonitrile. In: Bosch JP, ed, Contemporary Issues in Nephrology. Hemodialysis: High Efficiency Treatments, vol 27. New York, Churchill Livingstone, 1993:63–78.
72. Golper TA, Vincent HH, Gleason JR, Vos MC. Drug removal during high efficiency and high-flux hemodialysis. In: Bosch JP, ed. Contemporary Issues in Nephrology. Hemodialysis: High Efficiency Treatments, vol 27. New York, Churchill Livingstone, 1993:175–209.
73. Pollard TA, Lampasona V, Mullins RE, et al. Vancomycin redistribution: Dosing recommendations following high flux hemodialysis. Kidney Int 1994;45:232–237.
74. Toffelmire EB, Reymond JP, Broudar R, et al. Dialysis clearance in high flux hemodialysis with reuse using ceftazidime as the model drug. Clin Pharmacol Ther 1989;45:160.
75. Herrero A, Ruis Alarco F, Garcia-Diez JM, Mahiques E. Pharmacokinetics of netilmicin during hemodialysis: Comparison of four artificial kidneys. Int J Clin Pharmacol Ther Toxicol 1988;26:605–609.
76. Weiss LG, Cars O, Danielson BG, Grahnen A, Wikstrom B. Pharmacokinetics of intravenous cefuroxime during intermittent and continuous arteriovenous hemofiltration. Clin Nephrol 1988;30:282–286.
77. Bastani B, Spyker DA, Minocha A, Cummings R, Westervelt FB. *In vivo* comparison of three different hemodialysis membranes for vancomycin clearance: Cuprophan, cellulose acetate, and polyacrylonitrile. Dial Transplant 1988;17:527–543.
78. Lanese DM, Alfrey PS, Molitoris BA, Gal J. Markedly increased clearance of vancomycin during hemodialysis using polysulfone dialyzers. Kidney Int 1989;35:1409–1413.
79. Minakata T, Fukazawa A, Ikeda Y. Comparison of vancomycin clearance during hemodialysis between high flux and conventional membranes. J Am Soc Nephrol 1991;2:339.
80. Amin NB, Padhi ID, Touchette MA, et al. Gentamicin removal by the F-80 membrane in patients with end-stage renal disease. Pharmacotherapy 1997;17:1129. Abstract.
81. Murthy BVR, Sundaram S, Jaber BL, et al. Effect of formaldehyde/bleach reprocessing on *in vivo* performances of high-efficiency cellulose and high-flux polysulfone dialyzers. J Am Soc Nephrol 1997;9:464–472.
82. Barbhaiya RH, Knupp CA, Forgue ST, et al. Pharmacokinetics of cefepime in subjects with renal insufficiency. Clin Pharmacol Ther 1990;48:268–276.

83. Halstenson CE, Guay DR, Opsahl JA, et al. Disposition of cefmetazole in healthy volunteers and patients with impaired renal function. Antimicrob Agents Chemother 1990;34:519–523.
84. Matzke GR, O'Connell ME, Collins AJ, Keshaviah PR. Disposition of vancomycin during hemofiltration. Clin Pharmacol Ther 1986;40: 425–430.
85. Kelloway JS, Awni WM, Lin CC, et al. Pharmacokinetics of ceftibuten-cis and its trans metabolite in healthy volunteers and in patients with chronic renal insufficiency. Antimicrob Agents Chemother 1991;35:2267–2274.
86. Halstenson CE, Berkseth RO, Mann HJ, Matzke GR. Aminoglycoside redistribution phenomenon after hemodialysis: Netilmicin and tobramycin. Int J Clin Pharmacol Ther Toxicol 1987;25:50–55.
87. Matzke GR, Halstenson CE, Frye RF. Hemodialysis clearance of aminoglycosides and cephalosporins. Pharmacotherapy 1992;1:41. Abstract.
88. Fish JT, St Peter WL. Population pharmacokinetics of vancomycin, netilmicin, amikacin, tobramycin and gentamicin in patients receiving hemodialysis. Pharmacotherapy 1993;13:681. Abstract.
89. Matzke GR, Millikin SP, Kovarik JM. Variability in pharmacokinetic values for gentamicin, tobramycin, and netilmicin in patients with renal insufficiency. Clin Pharm 1989;8:800–806.
90. Flournoy DJ. Factors influencing the inactivation of aminoglycosides by β-lactams. Methods Find Exp Clin Pharmacol 1979;1:233–238.
91. Henderson JL, Polk RE, Kline BJ. *In vitro* inactivation of gentamicin, tobramycin, and netilmicin by carbenicillin, azlocillin, or mezlocillin. Am J Hosp Pharm 1981;38:1167–1170.
92. Thompson MI, Russo ME, Saxon BJ, Atkin-Thor E, Matsen JM. Gentamicin inactivation by piperacillin or carbenicillin in patients with end-stage renal disease. Antimicrob Agents Chemother 1982;21: 268–273.
93. Russo ME, Atkin-Thor E. Gentamicin and ticarcillin in subjects with end-stage renal disease. Clin Nephrol 1981;15:175–180.
94. Halstenson CE, Wong MO, Herman CS, et al. Effect of concomitant administration of piperacillin on the dispositions of isepamicin and gentamicin in patients with end-stage renal disease. Antimicrob Agents Chemother 1992;36:1832–1836.
95. Matzke GR, Luckham DR, Collins AJ, Halstenson CE. Effect of ticarcillin on gentamicin and tobramycin pharmacokinetics in a patient with end-stage renal disease. Pharmacotherapy 1984;4:158–160.
96. Halstenson CE, Hirata CA, Heim-Duthoy KL, Abraham PA, Matzke GR. Effect of concomitant administration of pipericillin on the dispositions of netilmicin and tobramycin in patients with end- stage renal disease. Antimicrob Agents Chemother 1990;34:128–133.

48

ELECTROLYTE HOMEOSTASIS

Nathan J. Schultz, PharmD, BCPS, and Ralph A. Slaker, PharmD

Electrolyte disorders are associated with many disease states and are thus frequently encountered in the acute care setting. A basic understanding of the pathophysiology of these disorders is necessary to determine the etiology of, properly classify, and adequately treat these syndromes. In this chapter, we review the epidemiology, etiology, classification, symptomatology, and therapy of disorders of sodium, potassium, calcium, magnesium, and phosphorus homeostasis.

DISORDERS OF SODIUM AND WATER HOMEOSTASIS

Sodium metabolism and water metabolism are intimately coupled. Sodium is actively excluded from the intracellular milieu, creating an osmotic gradient that maintains water distribution between the intracellular fluid (ICF) and extracellular fluid (ECF). Sodium, accompanied by chloride and bicarbonate, accounts for more than 90% of the osmolality of the extracellular compartment, while potassium is the major osmotic force within the cell.[1]

The kidney has the remarkable ability to maintain body homeostasis over a wide range of dietary sodium intake. A change in effective circulating volume promotes an afferent response from pressure receptors in the renal juxtaglomerular apparatus. This causes an efferent response in which glomerular filtration rate (GFR), aldosterone, oncotic pressure, adrenergic activity, renal hormones, and atrial natriuretic factor contribute to volume expansion through both water and sodium retention.[1] These processes result in the maintenance of adequate ECF volume.

The proper assessment of serum sodium requires recognition that the serum sodium concentration may bear no relationship to total body sodium content. The serum sodium concentration is equal to the amount of total body sodium divided by the amount of ECF water, with normal concentrations ranging from 135 to 145 mEq/L.[2] Hypernatremia and hyponatremia may be associated with conditions of high, low, or normal ECF water and high, low, or normal total body sodium. Because sodium is the major determinant of ECF osmolality, disorders of sodium homeostasis result in disorders of plasma tonicity.

HYPONATREMIA

Hyponatremia (serum sodium < 135 mEq/L) is the most common electrolyte abnormality in hospitalized patients, with a reported incidence of about 2.5%.[3] Brain damage is the cause of the majority of morbidity associated with hyponatremia. Patient age and sex appear to be major determinants of brain damage.[4]

PATHOPHYSIOLOGY

The first step in the proper assessment of hyponatremia is to measure serum osmolality. Hyponatremia associated with normal serum osmolality (isotonic hyponatremia) may be observed in patients with hyperlipidemia or hyperproteinemia. Sodium-free lipid or protein displaces sodium-rich serum water. While the concentration of sodium in serum water remains normal, the laboratory assessment assumes normal plasma solid content, resulting in a falsely decreased serum sodium concentration, termed pseudohyponatremia.[3]

Hyponatremia in the presence of elevated serum osmolality suggests the presence of excess measured or unmeasured osmoles in the serum. This is most frequently encountered in the settings of hyperglycemia or the administration of hyperosmolar glycerin or mannitol solutions. Serum sodium falls by 1.6 mEq/L for each 100 mg/dL increase in blood glucose.[3] These effective osmoles create an osmotic gradient between the isotonic ICF and the hyperosmolar ECF, drawing sodium-free water into the extracellular fluid, diluting the serum sodium, and resulting in hyponatremia.[5] The presence of a milliosmolar gap (measured mOsm/L – calculated mOsm/L > 10) suggests the presence of hyperosmolar compounds not normally measured and provides a clue as to the cause of hyponatremia.

The second step in determining the cause of hyponatremia is the clinical assessment of extracellular fluid volume. Hypotonic hyponatremia may be classified as hypovolemic hyponatremia, hypervolemic hyponatremia, or isovolemic hyponatremia (Fig. 48–1).

Hypovolemic hyponatremia is associated with a deficit of ECF volume and sodium with a proportionally greater deficit of sodium than water. Replacement of sodium-rich fluid losses with sodium-free fluids results in hyponatremia. The ECF volume contraction stimulates the activation of the renin-angiotensin, aldosterone, and antidiuretic hormone (ADH) systems and also changes certain aspects of renal hemodynamics.[5] In patients with extrarenal sodium losses, these changes result in a low urinary sodium concentration (< 20 mEq/L), and patients with renal sodium losses have a high urinary sodium concentration (> 20 mEq/L).[7] In response to volume depletion, the body will attempt to maintain volume even at the expense of tonicity.[8]

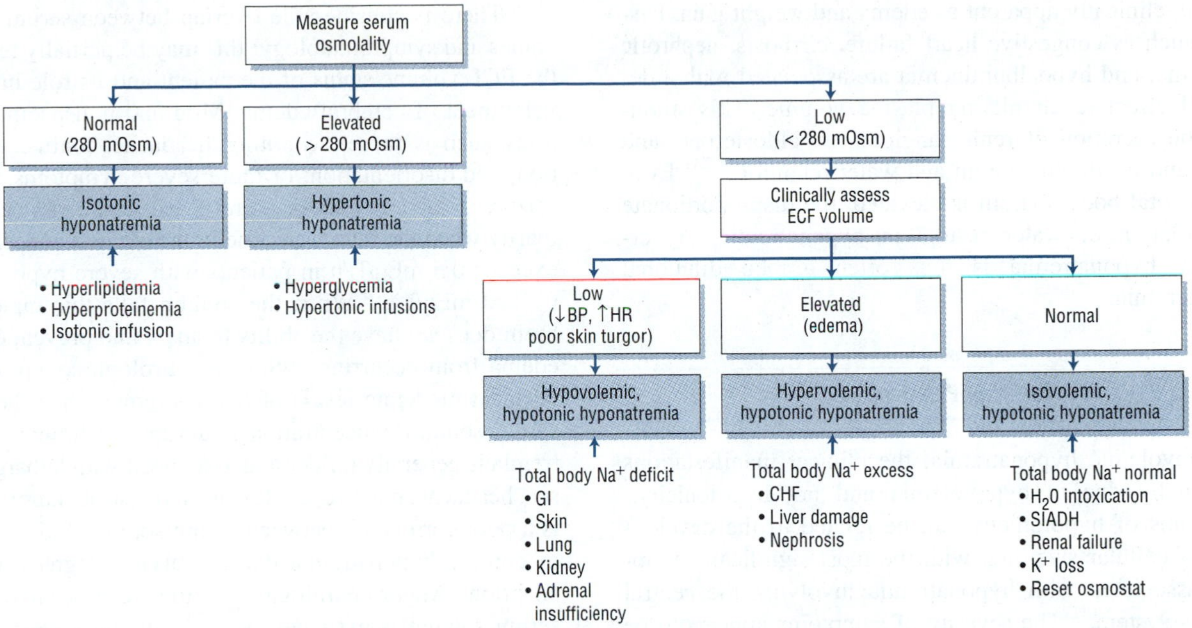

FIGURE 48–1. Diagnostic approach to hyponatremia. *(Adapted from Ref. 6.)*

Diuretic-induced hypovolemic hyponatremia is one of the most common causes of drug-induced hyponatremia. Diuretic action causes a decrease in free water excretion by blocking sodium reabsorption in the thick ascending loop of Henle, thereby decreasing the kidney's ability to dilute urine; causing extracellular fluid volume depletion, which decreases sodium delivery to the proximal tubule and stimulates ADH secretion; causing magnesium and potassium losses in the urine, which decreases renal sensitivity to ADH; and causing urinary sodium excretion.[9] Diuretic-induced hyponatremia may have a quick onset, particularly in elderly females, and may occur as soon as 3 to 15 days after the start of therapy. Diuretic-induced hyponatremia is commonly associated with hypokalemia.

Isovolemic hyponatremia is associated with a normal total body sodium content and small increases in ECF volume. Therefore, the retention of free water present in the setting of isovolemic hyponatremia is always the result of an imbalance of water intake and excretion.[5–8] Isovolemic hyponatremia is thus due to a combination of altered thirst, ADH secretion, and defective renal diluting mechanisms causing water retention and hyponatremia in patients who appear clinically euvolemic. Conditions associated with isovolemic hyponatremia are listed in Table 48–1.

The most common cause of isovolemic hyponatremia is the syndrome of inappropriate antidiuretic hormone secretion (SIADH). SIADH is defined as a sustained or intermittently elevated level of ADH without identifiable osmotic or volume stimuli that normally stimulate ADH secretion.[3–7] SIADH may occur in a wide variety of clinical diseases (Table 48–1). Drugs are an important cause of SIADH and can act by sensitizing the kidney to ADH, stimulating the release of ADH, or both.[3] All diuretics have the propensity to cause hyponatremia by stimulating the release of ADH. The chemotherapeutic agents cyclophosphamide and vincristine have been associated with hyponatremia as well. Hyponatremia occurs in 3% to 4% of patients taking chlorpropamide, which acts by sensitizing the kidney to ADH. Drugs that inhibit prostaglandin synthesis, such as nonsteroidal anti-inflammatory drugs, have demonstrated potentiation of antidiuretic hormone and thus are likely to contribute to hyponatremia, particularly in the elderly or neonates.[10]

Hypervolemic hyponatremia is associated with an elevated total body sodium content and an expanded ECF

TABLE 48–1. Disorders Associated With the Syndrome of Inappropriate Antidiuretic Hormone Secretion

Carcinomas
Lung
Duodenum
Pancreas
Pulmonary Disorders
Viral pneumonia
Bacterial pneumonia
Pulmonary abscess
Tuberculosis
Aspergillosis
Central Nervous System Disorders
Encephalitis, viral or bacterial
Meningitis, viral, bacterial, or tuberculosis
Acute psychosis
Stroke (cerebral thrombosis or hemorrhage)
Acute intermittent porphyria
Brain tumors
Brain abscess
Subdural or subarachnoid hematoma or hemorrhage
Guillain–Barré syndrome
Head trauma

volume, clinically apparent as edema and weight gain. Diseases such as congestive heart failure, cirrhosis, nephrotic syndrome, and hypoalbuminemia are associated with a decreased effective circulating plasma volume. This stimulates the secretion of renin, angiotensin, aldosterone, and ADH, and results in sodium and water retention.[5,7,11] Even though total body sodium is elevated, the disproportionate accumulation of water results in hyponatremia. Hypervolemic hyponatremia is thus often termed dilutional hyponatremia.

Clinical Presentation

In hypovolemic hyponatremia, the clinical manifestations are usually due to hypovolemia and not hypotonicity.[7] Symptoms of hypotonicity can be related to the development of cellular swelling, with the most significant symptoms associated with hyponatremia involving the central nervous system.[11] The severity of symptoms appears to be related to both the degree and the rapidity of development of hyponatremia.[11]

There is considerable overlap between serum sodium values and symptomatology; this may be partially related to the ECF volume status of the patient and its role in the development of cerebral edema. Mild and nonspecific symptoms, such as nausea, vomiting, headache, confusion, agitation, and disorientation; or more severe symptoms, such as seizures, coma, respiratory arrest, and death; can occur primarily when the rate of decline in the sodium concentration exceeds 0.5 mEq/L/h in patients with severe hyponatremia (< 120 mEq/L).[12] When the sodium falls this rapidly, the brain does not have the ability to adapt and prevent cerebral edema from occurring.[12] Severe neurologic symptoms can occur at moderate levels of hyponatremia when the fall in serum sodium concentration is abrupt.[12] Chronic hyponatremia is generally milder and associated with lethargy, nausea, headache, malaise, confusion, and disorientation.[5] There is a poor correlation between serum sodium and symptoms in chronic hyponatremia due to varying degrees of brain adaption.[5] Major neurologic symptoms can occur when the serum sodium is extremely low,[5,12] although patients with serum sodium concentrations of 115 to 120 mEq/L may be free of symptoms in chronic cases of hyponatremia.

▶ TREATMENT: Hyponatremia

DESIRED OUTCOME

The goals of therapy for the treatment of hyponatremia are to treat any life-threatening signs and symptoms that may be present, to raise the serum sodium level back to normal without causing the development of the osmotic demyelination syndrome, and to treat any underlying reversible cause of the hyponatremia. The appropriate treatment of hyponatremia is dependent on the correct classification of hyponatremia, severity of symptoms, concurrent disease states, ECF volume, rate of decline of serum sodium concentration, and degree of hyponatremia. Treatment begins with attention to possible reversible causes of hyponatremia and identification of underlying disorders. Specific therapies are then determined by the type of hyponatremia present in the patient.

PHARMACOLOGIC THERAPY

Because hypovolemic hyponatremia is rarely associated with hypotonic symptoms, therapy is directed at replacing the sodium and volume losses with normal saline.[4] Initially, therapy should begin with normal saline given at a rate of 200 to 300 mL/h or greater depending on the severity of the hemodynamic alterations due to hypovolemia. Once the ECF volume and hemodynamic stability has been restored, the infusion rate can be decreased to a maintenance rate of 75 to 125 mL/h with careful monitoring of the serum sodium level. If the rate of correction of the serum sodium level is greater than 12 mEq/24 h, the solution should be switched to one containing less sodium (1/2NS or $D_5$1/2NS) to prevent the development of the osmotic demyelination syndrome. It is rarely necessary to infuse hypertonic saline (3% or 5% NaCl), because isotonic saline corrects the pathophysiologic factors that lead to impaired free water excretion.[4,5] Ongoing sodium losses must be accounted for by appropriate maintenance fluid adjustments.

Isovolemic hyponatremia associated with a nonacute reduction of serum sodium concentrations to values not less than 115 mEq/L and an absence of symptoms may be treated conservatively by water restriction. Fluids are provided to allow for mandatory urinary solute excretion, allowing insensible water loss to correct the hyponatremia. Because the kidney can concentrate urine up to an osmolality of 1200 mOsm/L, and the average solute load excreted per day is 600 mOsm, a minimum of 500 mL/d is necessary to meet obligatory urine excretion. Initial therapy in this setting is fluid restriction of 500 mL/d or less to correct the hyponatremia.[13] Isovolemic hyponatremia associated with serum sodium concentrations below 115 mEq/L and/or signs and symptoms need rapid correction. Therapy should include an infusion of 3% saline at a rate of 1 to 2 mL/kg/h with close monitoring of the serum sodium concentration.[5] Loop diuretics should also be given to induce a negative water balance and prevent volume overload.[5,13] The goal of therapy with hypertonic saline is to increase the serum sodium concentration by 0.5 to 1.0 mEq/L/h until the signs and symptoms have disappeared. Once the signs and symptoms have been treated, therapy with hypertonic saline and loop diuretics can either be slowed or stopped and a fluid restriction can be instituted. The serum sodium should not be increased by more than 12 mEq/L in the first 24 hours to prevent the osmotic demyelination syndrome from occurring.[5] The serum sodium and potassium should be monitored closely and potassium should be given if the patient develops hypokalemia. Monitoring should also include an assessment of the signs and symptoms, fluid status, and renal function. Isovolemic hyponatremia resulting from chronic SIADH may require pharmacologic intervention in addition to water restriction. Demeclocycline, a tetracycline antibiotic, interferes with the action of ADH at the renal collecting duct, resulting in a nephrogenic diabetes insipidus-like picture. Demeclocycline is effective chronic therapy for isovolemic hyponatremia when SIADH is not self-limiting, when the underlying cause cannot be corrected, and when the patient does not tolerate or is noncompliant with fluid restrictions.[5,12,13] Demeclocycline should be given at doses of 600 to 1200 mg/d, with the onset of action ranging from 3 to 6 days.[12] Because of the delay in onset of action, demeclocycline has no role in the acute treatment of severe hyponatremia. Adverse effects of demeclocycline include nausea, photosensitivity, and nephrotoxicity.[5,12] Acute renal failure and renal tubular toxicity have occurred in patients with cirrhosis or congestive heart failure (CHF).[4] Other agents that have been used in the treatment of SIADH include phenytoin and lithium.[13]

Treatment of hypervolemic hyponatremia is centered on the correction of the underlying disease and the restriction of both water and salt.[8,11] Loop diuretics may be necessary to elicit a loss of free water. Improvement of hemodynamics, renal plasma flow, and glomerular filtration rate may also promote a water and sodium diuresis. Therapy for hypervolemic hyponatremia is often difficult secondary to the severity of the associated illness (CHF, cirrhosis, nephrotic syndrome).

The rapidity of sodium concentration correction has been the subject of some controversy. The term *osmotic demyelinization syndrome* has been used to describe a delayed neurologic deterioration (quadriparesis, mutism, pseudobulbar palsy) that sometimes follows the treatment of symptomatic hyponatremia.[14] Clinical and experimental evidence suggests that this syndrome is most likely to follow a rapid increase in serum sodium concentration in patients with severe hyponatremia of more than 2 days' duration.[14] Patients with acute, rapid development of hyponatremia (acute water intoxication or hypotonic fluid intake in the setting of impaired water excretion) usually tolerate rapid correction (absolute change in serum sodium concentration of 15 mEq/L in 12 hours, 26 mEq/L in 48 hours).[15] However, osmotic demyelination syndrome has occasionally occurred in patients with acute hyponatremia as well.[14] Slow correction of serum sodium concentration (an increase of less than 12 mEq/L/d) is recommended for most cases of nonemergent symptomatic hyponatremia; this treatment approach has been associated with complications even in severe cases of hyponatremia.[14] Rapid correction of hyponatremia should be reserved for true emergencies (seizures or coma in any hyponatremic patient) or in cases of known rapid onset of severe hyponatremia (water intoxication).[14] Treatment of symptomatic hyponatremia may require administration of parenteral hypertonic saline (3% NaCl, which contains 513 mEq/L) in addition to water restriction.

HYPERNATREMIA

Hypernatremia (serum sodium > 150 mEq/L) is always associated with hypertonicity and results from a state of relative water deficit.[11] Because the thirst mechanism is so effective in correcting the hypertonic state, hypernatremia results only when hypotonic fluid loss occurs in combination with a disturbance of water intake.[9] Therefore, patients who cannot express their thirst (infants, unconscious patients) or those who are unable to ambulate (elderly and disabled patients) to obtain fluids are at the highest risk for developing hypernatremia. Hypernatremia occurs in approximately 0.3% to 1.0% of hospitalized patients.[5] Mortality from acute hypernatremia in children ranges from 10% to 70%, while chronic hypernatremia in children has a mortality rate of 10%.[9] In adults, an acute increase in serum sodium to more than 160 mEq/L is associated with a 75% mortality rate, with chronic cases resulting in a 60% mortality rate.[9] Hypernatremia in adults is often associated with serious underlying illness, which may contribute to the high mortality rates.

PATHOPHYSIOLOGY

Hypernatremia may be classified according to the status of the ECF volume (Fig. 48–2). Unlike hyponatremia, which may be associated with low, normal, or even high osmolality, hypernatremia is always associated with hyperosmolality.[8,11]

Hypernatremia that occurs in the setting of ECF volume depletion is termed hypovolemic hypernatremia. It is caused by losses of both sodium and water, with water deficit being of a greater magnitude. Loss of sodium and water from renal and extrarenal sources, when replaced with fluids containing more sodium than present in the fluid lost, will result in the development of hypernatremia (Fig. 48–2). Common extrarenal causes of hypernatremia include profound diarrhea and excessive sweating.[11] Important drug-induced causes include osmotic diuresis with mannitol, diuretics, and laxative-induced diarrhea.

Isovolemic hypernatremia is associated with an isolated pure water loss and is the most common presentation of hypernatremia.[11] Because pure water loss is shared equally across total body water, the ratio of ICF to ECF is not changed; thus, signs of ECF volume depletion are rare unless water losses are massive.[5] Total body sodium content is normal in patients with isovolemic hypernatremia.[8] Mechanisms of pure water loss are listed in Figure 48–2. Iatrogenic causes include failure to replace insensible water loss or the replacement of insensible water losses with relatively hypertonic solutions. Excessive insensible water loss may occur with fever or high ambient temperatures. Insufficient fluid

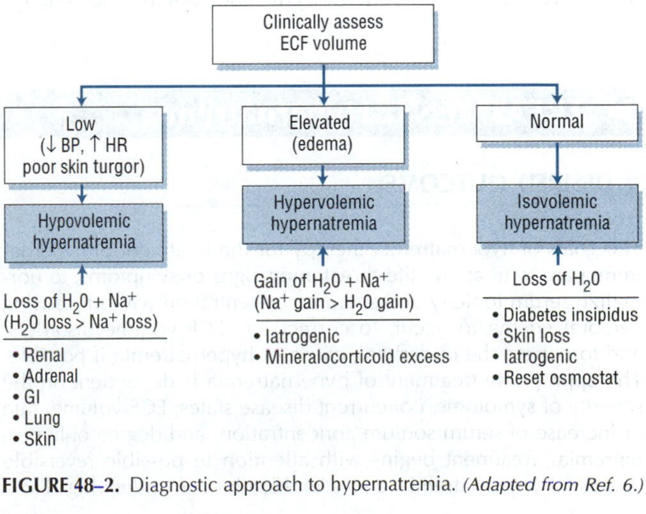

FIGURE 48–2. Diagnostic approach to hypernatremia. *(Adapted from Ref. 6.)*

TABLE 48–2. Causes of Diabetes Insipidus

Central Diabetes Insipidus (CDI)	
Primary	
	Familial (< 1% of cases)
	Idiopathic (50% of cases)
Secondary	
	Trauma (common cause)
	Neoplasms (especially lung and breast; common cause)
	Granulomatous disease (rare cause)
	Eosinophilic granuloma (rare cause)
	Cardiovascular (aneurysm, Sheehan's syndrome)
Nephrogenic Diabetes Insipidus (NDI)	
Primary	
	Congenital
Secondary	
	Electrolyte disorders (sever K^+ depletion
	Renal (ATN, postobstruction, posttransplant)
	Hematologic (sickle cell trail and disease)
	Drugs (lithium, demclocycline)

intake may result from lack of access to water (e.g., elderly patients with decreased levels of consciousness). Isovolemic hypernatremia associated with the production of large amounts of hypotonic urine characterizes diabetes insipidus (DI). Severe, life-threatening hypernatremia may develop if free water intake is not maintained. DI may be categorized as central (characterized by deficient secretion) or nephrogenic (characterized by renal resistance to the antidiuretic effect of ADH).[16] The causes of both central and nephrogenic DI are listed in Table 48–2. Central DI and nephrogenic DI can be distinguished by characteristic responses to water deprivation and exogenous ADH administration.

Central DI is associated with an initial diuretic phase, an antidiuretic phase in which urine output normalizes because of the release of ADH from injured axons, and resumption of the polyuric phase.[9] The degree of polyuria may range from 3 to 15 L/24 h; serum sodium is increased only if water intake is inhibited.[9]

Nephrogenic DI is usually associated with less severe polyuria (3 to 4 L/24 h) than is central DI, especially in the acquired causes of nephrogenic DI (underlying renal disease and drugs).[9] Drugs causing nephrogenic DI include demeclocycline, lithium, methoxyflurane, colchicine, phenytoin, vinblastine, and amphotericin B.[9] Although maximal urine-concentrating ability is impaired in nephrogenic DI, a hypertonic urine may still be produced; thus, the risk of hypernatremia is considerably less than in central DI.

Hypervolemic hypernatremia results from an increase in total body sodium and water, with the gain of sodium exceeding that of water. The increment in sodium results in an expansion of the ECF and the intravascular space, concurrent with a decrease in ICF volume.[11] In patients with renal failure, the inability to diurese the expanded ECF may result in vascular overload and pulmonary edema. Hypervolemic hypernatremia is commonly iatrogenic, because of excessive sodium administration.[8,11] Some examples include sodium bicarbonate therapy, inadvertent intravenous administration of intra-amniotic hypertonic saline for therapeutic abortion, and inadvertent use of salt instead of sugar in preparation of infant formulas. Patients with conditions associated with primary mineralocorticoid excess may also develop hypervolemic hypernatremia, usually of less severity than that caused iatrogenically.

Clinical Presentation

Most of the signs and symptoms of hypernatremia represent central nervous system dysfunction and can be attributed to the effect of hypertonicity on brain cells. Cellular dehydration may lead to symptoms of thirst, restlessness, irritability, tremulousness, spasticity, hyperreflexia, ataxia, seizures, coma, and death.[11] In addition, the shrinking effect of hypernatremia may result in the tearing of cerebral blood vessels, leading to intracranial bleeding.[9] The severity of symptoms is related to both the degree and the rate of rise of serum osmolality; thus, acute hypernatremia is more dangerous than chronic hypernatremia.[5,11] In an attempt to preserve intracellular volume, brain cells form new intracellular solutes, called idiogenic osmoles. Idiogenic osmoles are effective in restoring intracellular brain water to normal during a 7-day period in the presence of chronic hypernatremia.[9] The presence of idiogenic osmoles has important implications with regard to the rate of correction of serum hypertonicity.

▶ TREATMENT: Hypernatremia

DESIRED OUTCOME

The goals of hypernatremia therapy for the treatment of hypernatremia are to treat any life-threatening signs or symptoms, to normalize serum tonicity and sodium concentration without causing cerebral edema to occur, to correct any ECF volume disorders, and to correct the underlying cause of hypernatremia if possible. The appropriate treatment of hypernatremia is dependent on the severity of symptoms, concurrent disease states, ECF volume, rate of increase of serum sodium concentration, and degree of hypernatremia. Treatment begins with attention to possible reversible causes of hypernatremia and identification of underlying disorders. Specific therapies are then determined by the ECF volume status in the patient.

PHARMACOLOGIC THERAPY

In patients with hypovolemic hypernatremia, restoration of intravascular volume with isotonic 0.9% NaCl solution should be accomplished to reverse the hemodynamic alteration.[11] Note that 0.9% NaCl solution will be hypotonic relative to the hypernatremic plasma and thus will aid in correcting hypertonicity as well as intravascular volume. An infusion of 0.9% NaCl can be started at 200 to 300 mL/h or more depending on the severity of

TABLE 48–3. Comparison of Antidiuretic Agents

	Desmopressin	Vasopressin	Lypressin
Pharmacology			
Vasoconstriction/ADH ratio	+	+++	±
ACTH release	—	++++	—
Oxytocicity	+	++++	+
ADH activity	+++ (IV 10 × nasal)	+	+++
Factor VIII	+++	—	?
Pharmacokinetics	(Nasal)	(Parenteral)	(Nasal)
Onset	1 h	?	Minutes
Peak	1–5 h	?	0.5–2 h
Duration	8–20 h	Aqueous SC 2–8 h: oil IM 48–72 h	3–8 h
Route of Administration			
Parenteral	IV/SC	Oil IM/SC Aqueous IM/IV/SC	—
Intranasal	+	—	+
Dose	Nasal: 0.05–0.4 mL (0.01% solution); 5–40 mg in 1–3 doses Parenteral: 2–4 mg/d in 2 doses	Aqueous: 5–10 U SC/IM 2–4 × day prn Oil: 1.5–5 U IM every 2–3 d	1–2 sprays qid

ADH = antidiuretic hormone; IM = intramuscular; IV = intravenous; SC = subcutaneous; ? = unknown.

the hemodynamic alterations. Once intravascular volume is replaced, the infusion rate can be slowed and the water deficit can be replaced. Free water deficit can be estimated by the following formula[8]:

$$\text{water deficit} = \text{normal TBW} - \text{current TBW}$$

where normal TBW = total body water 0.60 × normal body weight in kg, and current TBW = normal TBW × 140/current measured Na concentration.

The free water deficit can be replaced with 5% dextrose or 0.45% NaCl solution, and should be added to the daily fluid requirements of the patients and replaced over 2 to 3 days. Monitoring should include serum electrolytes, fluid status, signs and symptoms of either hypertonicity or hypotonicity, and renal function. Serum sodium concentration must be decreased slowly to avoid the development of cerebral edema, seizures, permanent neurologic damage, or even death.[17] The presence of idiogenic osmoles inside brain cells causes an osmotic gradient to develop between the brain and plasma, and rapid lowering of plasma osmolality may result in the movement of water from plasma into the intracellular space, leading to cerebral edema and increased intracranial pressure. An acceptable rate of decrease in osmolality is 2 mOsm/h (1 mEq/L/h of Na) over a period of 48 to 72 hours.[9,17] Hypernatremia greater than 175 mEq/L should not be corrected by more than 15 mEq/L during the first 24 hours.[17]

Treatment of isovolemic hypernatremia is targeted at replacing water deficit, as outlined earlier, with 5% dextrose or 0.45% NaCl solutions. Initial therapy with 0.9% NaCl is not necessary, because ECF volume is usually not decreased. In addition, potentially reversible or treatable underlying conditions must be addressed. Patients with central DI will respond to administration of natural and synthetic ADH (vasopressin) preparations (Table 48–3).[9] Desmopressin is the most useful agent for chronic therapy.[7] Drugs with antidiuretic properties such as chlorpropamide, carbamazepine, and clofibrate have also been successfully used to manage patients with partial central DI. Thiazide diuretics and nonsteroidal anti-inflammatory drugs may be helpful in some patients with nephrogenic DI.[16]

Hypervolemic hypernatremia should be treated by replacement of water deficit with 5% dextrose or 0.45% NaCl solution in conjunction with diuretics to eliminate sodium excess. Patients with hypervolemic hypernatremia and renal failure may be treated by hemodialysis against a relatively hypotonic dialysate.[9] The rate of correction of hypernatremia should not exceed those previously proposed for hypovolemic and isovolemic hypernatremias.

DISORDERS OF POTASSIUM HOMEOSTASIS

Potassium has two major physiologic functions: (1) cell metabolism, participating in such processes as protein and glycogen synthesis; and (2) determination of the resting potential across cell membranes based on the intracellular to extracellular concentration ratio.[18] Potassium disorders can thus be expected to influence adversely cellular metabolism and neural and muscular function.

Potassium is the primary intracellular cation at a concentration of approximately 150 to 160 mEq/L, while the ECF contains 3.5 to 5 mEq/L. There is approximately 50 to 75 mEq of potassium in ECF (serum), in contrast to 3400 mEq in ICF.[19] Muscle tissue represents the major site of intracellular potassium and varies with age (decreased in elderly), sex (males > females), and muscle mass.[19] Even though the serum potassium represents only a small percentage of total body potassium, it is the ratio of intracellular potassium to serum potassium that is important in maintaining the resting membrane potential, responsible for normal action potential generation in cardiac and noncardiac tissue.[18]

Potassium homeostasis and the maintenance of normal serum potassium concentration (3.5 to 5.0 mEq/L) depend on complex extrarenal and renal factors. Because only 2% of total body potassium resides in the serum (ECF), and the serum potassium level is influenced by shifts between the ICF and ECF as well as potassium balance, estimation of the magnitude of an excess or deficit of total body potassium balance extrapolated from the serum potassium concentration is imprecise.[20] For each 1 mEq/L decrease in serum, the potassium deficit is approximately 150 to 200 mEq. Relatively small incremental increases in total body potassium may result in fatal increases in serum potassium concentration. Thus, the evaluation of serum potassium concentration requires the consideration of factors influencing redistribution of potassium across cell membranes, as well as factors influencing total body potassium balance. The Na^+/K^+-ATPase pump is responsible for maintaining the basal intracellular-to-extracellular gradients of both sodium and potassium. The importance of this homeostatic mechanism is dramatically evident in massive digitalis overdose, which inhibits the Na^+/K^+-ATPase pump, resulting in severe hyperkalemia.

Changes in arterial pH may have important effects on the plasma potassium concentration. In an acidotic state, hydrogen ions enter the cell and obligate sodium and potassium to exit to preserve electrical neutrality. A commonly quoted estimate of the pH effect is that for every decrease of 0.1 unit of pH there is an increase in serum potassium of 0.6 mEq/L.[21,22] The increase in serum potassium is far more variable than the predicted increase of 0.6 mEq/L and ranges from 0.4 to 1.3 mEq/L.[22] Only metabolic acids such as hydrochloric acid cause this increase in serum potassium. Organic acids, such as lactic acid, do not produce a change in potassium concentration, because with H^+ entry into the cell, lactate follows, resulting in minimal hydrogen–potassium exchange and potassium efflux from cells does not occur.[22,23] Respiratory acidosis does not produce large changes in serum potassium concentration.[18]

Metabolic alkalosis causes a shift of potassium into cells; however, this effect is considerably less prominent than the opposite effect produced by metabolic acidosis.[18] The potassium shift associated with alkalosis may not be entirely pH dependent. An increase in the extracellular to intracellular bicarbonate without a change in pH encourages the inward movement of potassium.[23] Respiratory alkalosis has only slight effects on internal and external potassium balance.[24]

Beta-adrenergic agonists stimulate the activity of the Na^+/K^+-ATPase pump via stimulation of cyclic AMP.[23] Alpha-adrenergic stimulation has the opposite effect and inhibits potassium movement into the cell, and may work by inhibiting the activity of the Na^+/K^+-ATPase pump.[20]

Insulin increases potassium uptake of skeletal muscle and hepatic cells by stimulating the Na^+/K^+-ATPase pump.[18,25] Insulin release is stimulated by hyperkalemia and serves as a primary defense against pathologic potassium elevations. Hyperkalemia also causes a concurrent release in glucagon as protection from insulin-associated hypoglycemia. Hypokalemia inhibits insulin release and accounts for the hyperglycemia associated with diuretic use.[25]

Hyperosmolarity produces cellular contraction, increased cellular potassium levels, and potassium movement out of cells.[22] This effect has clinical relevance mainly in the hyperglycemic, insulin-deficient diabetic patient.[22] The glucose-induced hyperkalemia is worse in diabetic patients with hypoaldosteronism.[22]

In addition to the intracellular–extracellular redistribution of potassium, the regulation of serum potassium by renally controlled potassium excretion is paramount in the pathogenesis of potassium disorders. Almost all of the potassium that is filtered in the glomerulus is reabsorbed in the proximal tubule and ascending loop of Henle.[18] Potassium excretion into the urine by secretion from the distal tubule and collecting duct is regulated primarily by aldosterone and plasma potassium concentration.[18] These regulators act to increase tubular intracellular potassium concentration, resulting in increased secretion. Distal tubule urine flow may also influence potassium secretion. Increased distal flow results in a reduced concentration gradient, thus increasing potassium secretion; conversely, decreased tubular flow results in decreasing potassium secretion.[18] The transepithelial potential difference across tubular cell membranes is influenced by sodium reabsorption. Sodium reabsorption makes the tubular lumen relatively electronegative. The enhanced electronegativity favors the movement of positively charged potassium from the cell into the lumen.[18]

HYPOKALEMIA

Hypokalemia is a common disorder that occurs with greater frequency than does hyperkalemia. Hypokalemia may be classified as moderate (serum potassium 2.5 to 3.5 mEq/L) or severe (serum potassium less than 2.5 mEq/L). An approach to evaluation of the hypokalemic patient is shown in Figure 48–3.

PATHOPHYSIOLOGY

The multifactorial causes of hypokalemia can be classified on the basis of body stores—normal body stores (laboratory error, redistribution) or decreased total body stores (gastrointestinal loss, renal loss, other) (Table 48–4). The most frequent causes of hypokalemia are gastrointestinal and diuretic-induced renal losses.[18] Gastrointestinal (GI) losses may be due to direct loss of potassium from GI fluids (vomiting, diarrhea, draining fistulas); metabolic alkalosis from hydrogen ion loss (vomiting, nasogastric suction), resulting in intracellular potassium shift; and plasma volume contrac-

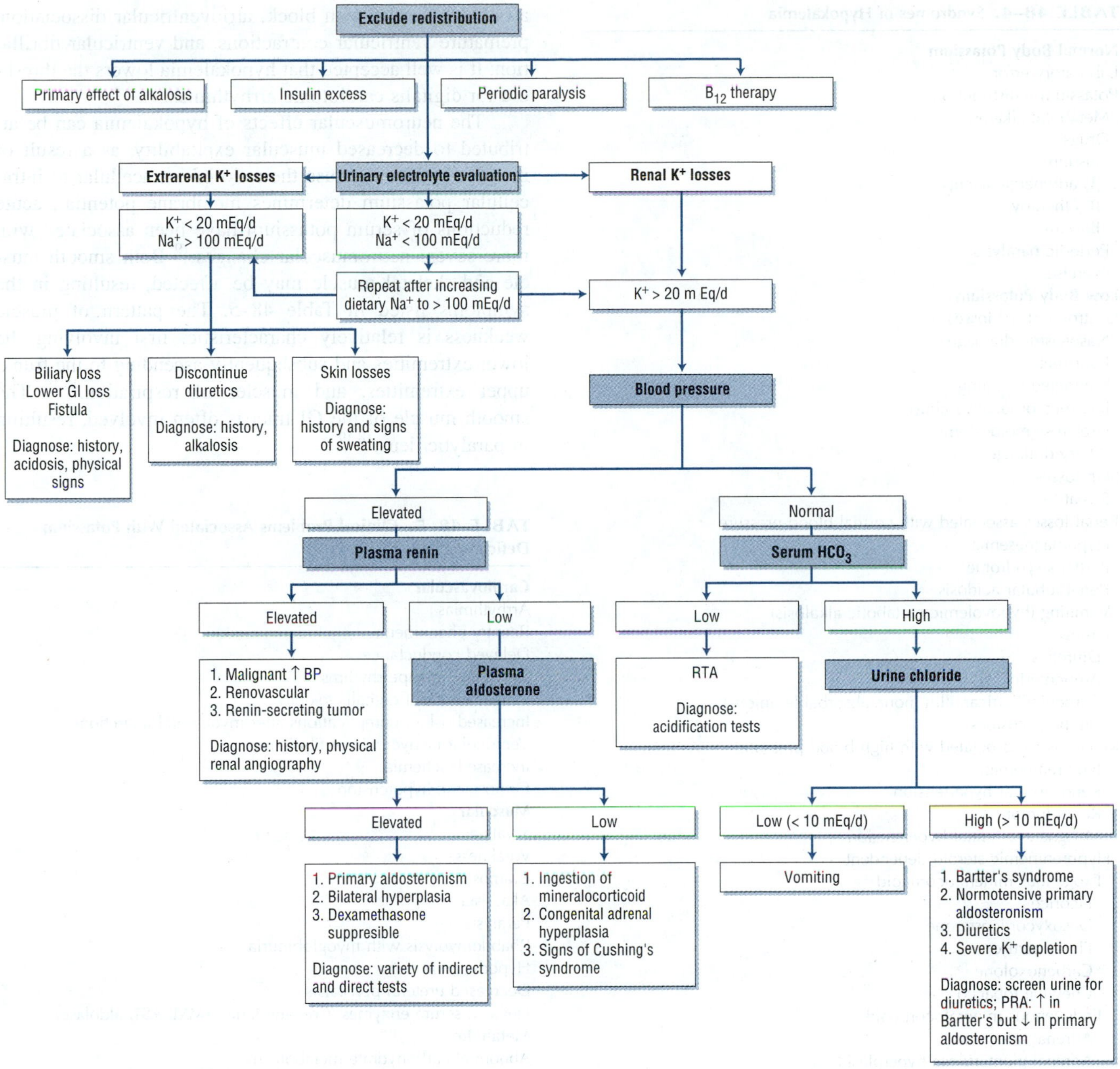

FIGURE 48–3. Diagnostic approach to hypokalemia. (PRA = plasma renin activity; RTA = renal tubular acidosis.) *(From Ref. 6. Reprinted from the American Journal of Medicine.)*

tion, leading to a secondary increase in aldosterone. Diuretics cause hypokalemia by increasing distal tubular flow, resulting in potassium loss down its concentration gradient.[18]

Clinical Presentation

Hypokalemia may cause a wide variety of physiologic abnormalities, resulting in a symptomatology involving several organ systems (Table 48–5). The severity of symptoms is related to the degree and acuteness of hypokalemia, although substantial interindividual variability does exist.[18] Marked symptoms are unusual unless serum potassium concentration is less than 3.0 mEq/L.[18]

The association between serum potassium and arrhythmias can be explained by the effect of potassium on resting membrane potential (RMP) in cardiac tissue. The RMP is proportional to the log of the ratio of extracellular to intracellular potassium; therefore, small changes in serum potassium can have a significant effect on this ratio. Hypokalemia results in an increase in RMP while hypokalemia decreases RMP.[20]

TABLE 48–4. Syndromes of Hypokalemia

Normal Body Potassium
Laboratory error
Potassium redistribution
- Metabolic alkalosis
- Drugs
  - Insulin
  - β_2-adrenergic agents
  - B_{12} therapy
  - Barium
- Periodic paralysis
- Exercise

Low Body Potassium
Gastrointestinal losses
- Nasogastric drainage
- Poor diet
- Protracted vomiting
- Diarrhea or laxative abuse
- Ureterosigmoidostomy
- Biliary drainage

Skin losses
- Sweat

Renal losses associated with normal blood pressure
- Hypomagnesemia
- Bartter's syndrome
- Renal tubular acidosis
- Vomiting (hypovolemic metabolic alkalosis)
- Drugs
  - Diuretics
  - Amphotericin B
  - Carbenicillin/ticarcillin (nonreabsorbable anions)
  - Aminoglycosides

Renal losses associated with high blood pressure
- Hyperreninemic
  - Renovascular hypertension
  - Renin tumor
  - Malignant essential hypertension
- Hyporeninemic steroid dependent
  - Exogenous mineralocorticoid
    - Licorice
    - Desoxycorticosterone
    - Fludrocortisone
    - Carbenoxolone
    - Chewing tobacco
  - Endogenous mineralocorticoid
    - Adrenal adenoma
    - Adrenal glomerulosa hyperplasia
    - Enzyme deficiency (17-hydroxylase, 11-hydroxylase)
  - Exogenous glucocorticoid
  - Endogenous glucocorticoid
    - Cushing's syndrome
    - Excessive ACTH

Adapted from Narins RG, Jones RE, Stom MC, et al. Diagnostic strategies and disorders of fluid, electrolyte and acid base homeostasis. Am J Med 1982;72:502.

The electrocardiographic effects of hypokalemia are characterized by ST segment lowering or flattening, inversion of the T wave, and elevation of the U wave. A widening of the PR interval, widening of the QRS complex, and overall slowing of conduction may also occur, most frequently when serum potassium concentration is less than 2.7 mEq/L.[26] Hypokalemia-associated arrhythmias include bradyarrhythmias, heart block, atrial flutter, paroxysmal atrial tachycardia with block, atrioventricular dissociation, premature ventricular contractions, and ventricular fibrillation. It is well accepted that hypokalemia lowers the threshold for digitalis cardiotoxic arrhythmias.

The neuromuscular effects of hypokalemia can be attributed to decreased muscular excitability, as a result of increased RMP. Because the ratio of extracellular to intracellular potassium determines membrane potential, acute reductions of serum potassium have been associated with more severe neuromuscular changes.[19] Both smooth muscle and skeletal muscle may be affected, resulting in the symptoms listed in Table 48–5. The pattern of muscle weakness is relatively characteristic, first involving the lower extremities and subsequently ascending to the trunk, upper extremities, and muscles of respiration.[18,19] The smooth muscle of the GI tract is often involved, resulting in paralytic ileus.[18,19]

TABLE 48–5. Clinical Problems Associated With Potassium Deficiency

Cardiovascular
Arrhythmias
Reentry phenomena
Delayed conductance
Ventricular escape rhythms
Increased risk of digitalis toxicity
Increased risk of complications after myocardial infarction
Ventricular tachycardia or fibrillation
Increased ischemia
Orthostactic hypotension

Muscular
Myalgia
Weakness
Cramps
Akathisia
Paralysis
Rhabdomyolysis with myoglobinuria
Hypodynamic ileus
Decreased ureteral peristalsis
Elevated serum enzymes (Creatine kinase-MM, AST, aldolase)

Metabolic
Abnormal carbohydrate metabolism
Reduced muscle glycogen content and synthesis
Precipitation of overt diabetes mellitus
Increased glucose intolerance in diabetes mellitus
Reduced normal insulin release during hyperglycemia
Increased risk of complications from electrolyte abnormalities
Hypercalcemia
Hypomagnesemia
Achlorhydria
Hyperlipidemia
Impotence

Renal
Increased production of ammonia by the kidneys
Decreased protein synthesis
Negative nitrogen balance
Growth retardation
Hepatic encephalopathy or coma in susceptible patients with end-stage liver disease
Nephrogenic diabetes insipidus
Increased risk of pyelonephritis

▶ TREATMENT: Hypokalemia

DESIRED OUTCOME

The goals of therapy for the treatment of hypokalemia are to treat or prevent severe life-threatening signs and symptoms, to restore the serum potassium concentration to normal, to correct the underlying cause of hypokalemia if possible, and to prevent hyperkalemia.

Serum potassium levels of less than 3.5 mEq/L in the digitalized patient or when associated with symptoms require treatment. The indications for the treatment of moderate to mild hypokalemia in the asymptomatic, nondigitalized patient have been the subject of much controversy.[24,25] Potassium replacement therapy for these patients has been advocated because diuretic therapy for hypertension has been associated with an increase in sudden death, attributable to ventricular arrhythmias, perhaps mediated by stress-induced intracellular potassium shifts on top of diuretic-induced hypokalemia.[27] A number of trials in patients without heart disease and with diuretic-induced hypokalemia have been done with conflicting results.[25] Using 24-hour ambulatory monitoring, some of these trials have shown an increase in ventricular ectopy, while others have not been able to confirm these results.[24,27] The evidence for implicating hypokalemia in the increased cardiovascular mortality during diuretic therapy remains suggestive but inconclusive.[25] Further controlled clinical trials are necessary to resolve this controversy.

NONPHARMACOLOGIC THERAPY

Alternatives to pharmaceutical dosage forms of potassium chloride include salt substitutes and potassium-rich food sources (bananas, orange juice). Salt substitutes are an effective, inexpensive potassium supplement, which is usually better tolerated than liquid potassium chloride products.[28] Food sources of potassium are generally not recommended for chronic potassium supplementation because they often contain less chloride than other potassium sources and may add unwanted calories to the diets of patients who may benefit from caloric restriction.[28]

PHARMACOLOGIC THERAPY

Potassium replacement therapy is indicated under the following conditions: symptomatic hypokalemia,[20] malnutrition,[20,25] potassium loss associated with vomiting or diarrhea,[29] renal tubular acidosis with hypokalemia,[25] congestive heart failure and digitalis therapy,[24] myocardial infarction with low serum potassium,[24] diabetic ketoacidosis treated with insulin,[20,25] and adrenocortical hyperactivity.[29] Potassium replacement therapy is commonly required for patients on diuretic therapy. Suggested guidelines for potassium administration in nonedematous patients include monitoring serum potassium concentration prior to and at 1- to 2-month intervals during diuretic therapy until a pattern is identified. No treatment is required while serum potassium remains above 3.0 mEq/L unless symptoms develop. If serum potassium falls below 3.0 mEq/L, use 50 to 60 mEq/d KCl oral solution or wax matrix. Caution should be used in patients with renal impairment. For the edematous patient (congestive heart failure, cirrhosis with ascities, severe aldosteronism), potassium replacement should be considered when the risks of treatment with replacement therapy are outweighed by the value of restoring potassium balance. Oral therapy at a dose of 40 to 80 mEq/d should be used to correct mild deficits. With more severe deficits, use up to 100 to 120 mEq/d with careful monitoring. Potassium-sparing diuretics may also be used, but they should be avoided in patients with diabetes, chronic renal failure, advanced age, or those receiving angiotensin-converting enzyme inhibitors.[20]

A variety of potassium salts are available for replacement and prophylactic therapy: chloride, bicarbonate (acetate and citrate are rapidly metabolized to bicarbonate), phosphate, and gluconate. The most frequently used potassium salt is potassium chloride. Metabolic alkalosis is often associated with hypokalemia, and because the causes of metabolic alkalosis (vomiting and diuretics) also cause chloride depletion, the administration of chloride is essential for correction of both the alkalosis and the potassium deficit.[28] Nonchloride salts of potassium are indicated only in treating hypokalemia associated with metabolic acidosis (e.g., renal tubular acidosis).

The route of administration depends on feasibility, severity of hypokalemia, and presence of symptoms. Intravenous potassium is indicated when the oral route is not feasible and/or in the presence of life-threatening hypokalemia (paralysis, arrhythmias). Because of the many factors influencing the internal distribution of potassium, rapid administration of potassium directly into the plasma can potentially result in hyperkalemia. In general, potassium can be intravenously administered safely at a rate of 10 to 20 mEq/h, with careful monitoring. The serum potassium concentration should be measured after each 30 to 40 mEq have been infused to guide further therapy.[28] Potassium administration at rates greater than 10 mEq/h should be accompanied by electrocardiographic monitoring for the signs of hyperkalemia. In rare instances, severe hypokalemia associated with paralysis or life-threatening arrhythmias has been treated by the administration of parenteral potassium at a rate of 40 to 100 mEq/h. This necessitates careful electrocardiographic monitoring and the frequent determination of serum potassium concentration.[20] The generally accepted maximally tolerated potassium concentration for peripheral-vein intravenous administration is 40 to 60 mEq/L.[28,30] Potassium concentrations greater than 50 to 60 mEq/L are often not tolerated by patients because of burning pain and peripheral venous sclerosis. Thus, more centrally located, larger veins are more appropriate sites of administration if large potassium doses are needed. The use of central venous lines for administration of potassium has been discouraged by some authors, because of the potential for adverse cardiac effects as the result of locally high potassium concentrations.[28,30] Data supporting these warnings are scarce, however, and many institutions safely use central line access for the controlled administration of 10 to 20 mEq potassium mixed in 100 mL of dextrose or saline solution given over 1 hour in electrocardiographically monitored ICU patients.[30] Because the rate of intracellular movement and the total body deficit of potassium are unpredictable, caution is advised when parenteral potassium therapy is initiated.

Oral administration, when feasible, is the preferred route for potassium replacement in hypokalemia not associated with life-threatening symptoms and for prophylaxis of diuretic-induced hypokalemia. Liquid potassium preparations are inexpensive, but are often poorly tolerated by patients because of unpleasant taste, aftertaste, nausea, heartburn, and diarrhea.[24,28] Enteric-coated tablets should be avoided, because of the high incidence of small-bowel ulceration and scarring causing obstruction, perforation, or hemorrhage associated with their use.[24,28] Nonetheless, because of poor patient acceptance of liquid potassium preparations and the small-bowel toxicity of enteric-coated potassium products, sustained-release potassium products have enjoyed immense popularity. Potassium crystals embedded in a wax matrix or microencapsulated in polymers result in dosage forms that release potassium in the gut in a sustained, gradual manner, thereby minimizing gastric irritation and ulceration. However, recent studies have shown that even these products may cause endoscopic GI ulceration.[31] Because of their palatability and low side-effect profile, the sustained-release potassium chloride products are excellent dosage forms for oral potassium therapy.

ALTERNATIVE DRUG TREATMENT

Potassium-sparing diuretics are an alternative to exogenous potassium supplementation during diuretic therapy. These agents are widely used in combination with thiazide diuretics. Spironolactone, which antagonizes aldosterone and thereby reduces potassium exchange in the distal tubule, is especially effective as a potassium-sparing agent in conditions associated with primary and secondary hyperaldosteronism. Triamterene and amiloride act by an aldosterone-independent but unknown method to reduce potassium excretion.[24]

Combined use of potassium chloride supplements and potassium-sparing diuretics is unnecessary, except in congestive heart failure, nephrotic syndrome, cirrhosis of the liver, or hypokalemia caused by ectopic ACTH, in which urinary potassium loss can be excessive.[24] The risk of hyperkalemia with combined use is significant, especially in patients with renal dysfunction or diabetes mellitus and in the elderly.[32]

HYPERKALEMIA

Hyperkalemia is defined as a serum potassium concentration greater than 5.5 mEq/L. Hyperkalemia may be classified as mild (serum potassium 5.5 to 6.0 mEq/L), moderate (6.5 to 6.9 mEq/L), or severe (> 7.0 mEq/L).[24] The incidence of hyperkalemia in hospitalized patients is 3% to 8%, with greater prevalence in elderly patients, most likely because of the frequency in this population of diseases and conditions associated with hyperkalemia.[33]

PATHOPHYSIOLOGY

Hyperkalemia may be associated with normal or elevated total body stores of potassium. Hyperkalemia associated with normal total body stores includes redistribution of potassium and "pseudohyperkalemia." Pseudohyperkalemia is an *in vitro* phenomenon in which the measured serum potassium level is falsely elevated compared with the actual *in vivo* level, usually as a result of hemolysis of red blood cells (RBCs).[23] Potassium release from platelets or white blood cells during *in vitro* coagulation can also produce elevations in the serum potassium level in patients with thrombocytosis or extreme leukocytosis.[23,24] Redistribution of potassium from the intracellular to the extracellular space may occur *in vivo*. Acidosis and insulin deficiency may result in ECF movement of potassium, as previously discussed. Release of potassium from ischemic, injured, or lysed cells may occur secondary to crush injury, rhabdomyolysis, burns, and chemotherapy (tumor lysis syndrome).[18] Drugs may cause redistribution of potassium by disruption of the Na^+/K^+-ATPase pump (digitalis intoxication), release of potassium from muscle cells following depolarizing muscle relaxant administration (succinylcholine), β_2 blockade (propranolol), positively charged molecules entering cells to displace potassium (lysine and arginine), inhibition of potassium secretion in a dose-dependent manner (trimethoprim-sulfamethoxazole), and hyporeninemic hypoaldosteronism (NSAIDs and cyclosporine).[23,24]

Hyperkalemia associated with elevated total body potassium stores is due to excessive potassium ingestion, potassium excretion, or both. Although all potassium supplements may cause hyperkalemia, administration by the intravenous route is associated with a higher risk than the oral route. Hyperkalemia resulting from the administration of potassium supplements is rare unless rapid intravenous administration occurs, or there is an underlying

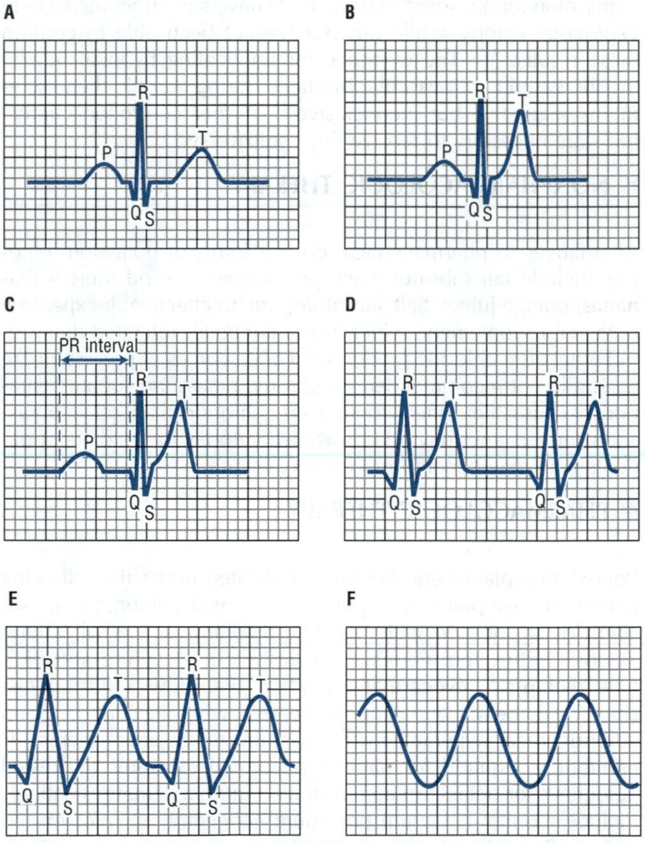

FIGURE 48–4. The earliest ECG manifestation of hyperkalemia is an increase in the rate of ventricular repolarization, which results in a "peaking" of the T wave at serum potassium concentrations of ≈5.5 to 6.0 mEq/L **(B)**, relative to the normal ECG presentation **(A)**. Further increases in the serum potassium concentration above 6 mEq/L result in conduction delays through the His–Purkinje system, the atrial myocardium, and the ventricular myocardium. The ECG manifestations of these conduction delays and the sequence in which they occur are a widening of the PR interval **(C)**, delay through the His–Purkinje system), a loss of the P wave **(D)**, delay through the atrial myocardium), and a widening of the QRS complex **(E)**, delay through the ventricular myocardium). Finally **(F)**, there is a merging of the QRS complex with the T wave, which results in a sine-wave appearance to the tracing.

impairment in its renal or extrarenal disposal.[22] Exogenous administration of potassium to patients receiving concomitant potassium-sparing diuretics or angiotensin-converting enzyme inhibitors should be undertaken with extreme caution and close monitoring. Diabetic patients are especially at risk for development of hyperkalemia because they lack insulin and its vital role in potassium redistribution. Diabetics also have a tendency toward hyporeninemic hypoaldosteronism, which decreases the kidney's ability to excrete potassium. The combination of insulin deficiency and attenuated aldosterone response places the diabetic at greater particular risk for the development of hyperkalemia.[22]

CLINICAL PRESENTATION

The clinical presentation of hyperkalemia is limited primarily to muscle weakness and abnormalities of cardiac conduction, in addition to the symptoms associated with underlying disease. As the resting potential approaches the threshold potential, the cell is unable to sustain an action potential, and weakness or paralysis results.[18] Symptoms often begin in the lower extremities, ascending to the trunk and upper extremities.[18] At serum concentrations of 6.5 mEq/L and above, muscle twitching, weakness, nausea, and cramping can occur.[21]

The cardiac rhythm disturbances associated with hyperkalemia pose the greatest danger to the patient, because they may lead to ventricular fibrillation or cardiac standstill (asystole). The earliest electrocardiogram (ECG) changes are peaked T waves and shortening of the QT interval, reflecting an increased rate of repolarization with occasional ST depression.[21] These changes are seen typically when serum potassium concentrations are 5.5 to 6 mEq/L. With serum concentrations between 6 and 7, the PR interval and QRS duration are prolonged (Fig. 48–4). When the serum concentration exceeds 7 to 8 mEq/L, electrocardiographic manifestations of delayed depolarization occur, resulting in slowed cardiac conduction, and appear as widening of the QRS complex and decreased amplitude, widening, and eventual loss of the P wave.[18] When serum concentrations exceed 9 to 10 mEq/L, the QRS complex merges with the T wave, resulting in a sine-wave pattern, which may deteriorate to ventricular fibrillation or asystole at concentrations from 10 to 12 mEq/L.[21] Depolarization slowing is the result of a reduction in sodium permeability into the cell, caused by a hyperkalemia-induced reduction of resting membrane potential.[18] Note that the serum concentrations at which the characteristic electrocardiographic changes occur are variable, because hypocalcemia, acidosis, hyponatremia, and the rapidity of elevation of serum potassium all may enhance the cardiotoxicity of hyperkalemia.[18] Acute hyperkalemia is generally more dangerous than chronic hyperkalemia, because the protective mechanisms for rapid intracellular movement of potassium may be overwhelmed. Rapid increases in potassium concentration predominately affect conduction and heart rate rather than the T wave or ST segment.[34]

▶ TREATMENT: Hyperkalemia

DESIRED OUTCOME

The goals of therapy for the treatment of hyperkalemia are to antagonize adverse cardiac effects, reverse any symptoms that may be present, and to return the serum and total body stores of potassium to normal. Severe hyperkalemia (> 8 mEq/L) or moderate hyperkalemia (6.5 to 8 mEq/L), when associated with clinical symptoms or electrocardiographic changes, requires immediate treatment. Treatment of hyperkalemia is achieved by antagonism of the membrane actions of hyperkalemia (calcium), decrease in extracellular potassium concentration by promotion of intracellular movement of the cation (glucose, insulin, β_2 agonists, bicarbonate), and removal of potassium from the body (hemodialysis, cation-exchange resins).[19] Exogenous potassium must be withheld, and potentially reversible causes of hyperkalemia must be reversed as well.

PHARMACOLOGIC THERAPY

Initial therapy of severe hyperkalemia or hyperkalemia associated with electrocardiographic changes should be calcium gluconate.[22,23] Calcium chloride would be an appropriate alternative in cardiac arrest with tissue hypoperfusion. (Table 48–6).[23] Calcium administration is an effective rapidly acting but short-lived therapy that dramatically reverses the electrocardiographic manifestations and arrhythmias of hyperkalemia.[19] Calcium changes the relationship between membrane potential and threshold potential, restoring normal conduction in the heart.[18] Calcium administration does not in any way lower serum potassium concentration and, because it is so short acting, must be repeated if symptoms recur, until serum potassium can be lowered. The frequency of repeat administration is dependent on the rate of symptom recurrence.

Once the cardiac effects of potassium have been antagonized with calcium, efforts should be undertaken to lower the extracellular potassium concentration. Promoting intracellular movement of potassium is an effective mechanism for rapidly lowering extracellular potassium concentration. Intravenous glucose and insulin are first-line agents to move potassium intracellularly (Table 48–6). Intravenous glucose enhances endogenous insulin release in nondiabetics, thus promoting cellular uptake of potassium. Insulin is often administered with glucose to facilitate the effect of endogenous insulin. Glucose administration may be omitted and insulin alone administered to the hyperglycemic patient. Albuterol alone or in combination with insulin is an alternative that may substantially decrease serum potassium levels.[23,24] Sodium bicarbonate is another alternative that also promotes the intracellular movement of potassium, by increasing extracellular pH and also by a direct action of the bicarbonate anion itself.[18]

Once rapid reduction of serum potassium is accomplished by moving potassium intracellularly, focus can turn to the reduction of total body stores. Sodium polystyrene sulfonate, a cation-exchange resin, is an effective first-line agent when given orally or rectally (Table 48–6). Each gram of resin may bind as much as

TABLE 48–6. Treatment of Hyperkalemia

Medication	Dose	Route of Administration	Mechanism of Action	Expected Result	Onset/Duration
Albuterol	10–20 mg	Nebulized over 10 min	Stimulates Na^+/K^+-ATPase pump	Redistribution of K+ into the cell	30 min/1–2 h
Calcium chloride	1 g (13.5 mEq)	IV over 5–10 min	Raises threshold potential and reestablishes cardiac excitability	Reverses ECG effects	1–2 min/10–30 min
Dextrose 50%	50 mL (25 g)	IV over 5 min	Increases insulin release	Redistribution of K^+ into the cell	30 min/2–6 h
Dextrose 10%	1000 mL (100 g)	IV over 1–2 h	Increases insulin release	Redistribution of K^+ into the cell	30 min/2–6 h
Sodium bicarbonate	50–100 mEq	IV over 2–5 min	Increases serum pH	Redistribution of K^+ into the cell	30 min/2–6 h
Insulin (regular)	1 unit per 3–5 g dextrose	IV with 10% dextrose SC	Enhances potassium intracellular uptake	Redistribution of K^+ into the cell	30 min/2–6 h
Sodium polystyrene sulfonate	15–60 g	Orally or rectally	Exchanges resin Na^+ for K^+	Increase in K^+ elimination	1 h/variable
Hemodialysis	2–4 h	—	Removal from plasma	Increase in K^+ elimination	Immediate/variable

1 mEq of potassium and release 1 to 2 mEq of sodium.[18] The resin remains in the GI tract and must be removed to be effective. Sodium polystyrene sulfonate should be administered with sorbitol to prevent constipation and retention of the resin. Prepackaged suspensions in sorbitol are commercially available. Sodium polystyrene sulfonate doses of 40 g given orally in four divided doses may decrease serum potassium concentrations by 1.0 mEq/L in 24 hours in patients with renal failure.[19] An effective alternative in pateints without renal failure would be the use of loop diuretics.[22,23]

If hyperkalemia persists, especially if the patient is in renal failure (acute or chronic), hemodialysis is indicated.[21] Peritoneal dialysis is less effective due to the lower efficiency of potassium elimination compared to hemodialysis (see Chap. 41).[23]

DISORDERS OF CALCIUM HOMEOSTASIS

The control and maintenance of calcium concentration in the intracellular and extracellular spaces is vital for the preservation and function of cell membranes, propagation of neuromuscular activity, regulation of endocrine and exocrine secretory functions, blood coagulation cascade, platelet adhesion process, bone metabolism, muscle cell excitation/contraction coupling, and mediation of the electrophysiologic slow channel response in cardiac and smooth muscle tissue. Because of the biologic importance of calcium, the concentration of this cation is closely regulated by a complex system involving parathyroid hormone, vitamin D, and calcitonin. Disruption of these homeostatic mechanisms results in the clinical manifestations of hypercalcemia or hypocalcemia.

The disorders of calcium homeostasis are related to the calcium content of the extracellular fluid, which contains less than 0.52% of the total body stores of calcium. Skeletal bone contains more than 99% of total body stores of calcium.[35] ECF calcium is moderately bound to plasma proteins (46%), with albumin being the primary binding protein.[36] Unbound or ionized calcium is the physiologically active form and is the fraction that is homeostatically regulated.[37] Extracellular calcium is most commonly measured as the total serum calcium level, which includes both bound and unbound calcium.[36] The normal total calcium serum concentration range is 8.5 to 10.5 mg/dL.[37]

Any factor that alters the concentration of albumin or its binding of calcium may be expected to change the fraction of total serum calcium in the ionized form. The most significant cause of changes in calcium binding to albumin is a change in extracellular fluid pH. Metabolic alkalosis and respiratory alkalosis favor an increased binding of calcium to albumin, thus lowering the ionized free calcium fraction while leaving total serum calcium unchanged. This may result in clinically evident, symptomatic hypocalcemia.[35] Conversely, metabolic or respiratory acidosis decreases calcium–protein binding and results in increased ionized calcium. Hypoalbuminemic states are probably the most common cause of low laboratory values of serum calcium. Because of the decreased protein content, however, ionized calcium concentration may be normal. Thus, total serum calcium concentration must be evaluated in light of the serum albumin concentration. A general rule is that for each 1 g/dL that the serum albumin concentration is below 4 g/dL, total serum calcium concentration decreases by 0.8 mg/dL.[35,36]

HYPERCALCEMIA

Hypercalcemia (total serum calcium >10.5 mg/dL) may be due to a multitude of causes (Table 48–7). The most common causes of hypercalcemia are cancer and primary hyperparathyroidism. Hypercalcemia of cancer occurs in approximately 10% to 20% of cancer patients at some time

TABLE 48–7. Causes of Hypercalcemia

Neoplasms	**Drugs**
Bone metastasis	Thiazides
Breast	Lithium
Multiple myeloma	Vitamin A toxicity
Lymphoma	Vitamin D toxicity
Leukemia	Milk–alkali syndrome
Humoral induced	Calcium supplements
Ovary	**Granulomatous Disease**
Kidney	Sarcoidosis
Lung	Tuberculosis
Head and neck	**Berylliosis**
Esophagus	Histoplasmosis
Cervix	Coccidiodomycosis
Lymphoproliferative disease	**Endocrine Disorders**
	Hyperthyroidism
Multiple endocrine neoplasia	Adrenal insufficiency
	Miscellaneous
Pheochromocytoma	Immobilization
Hyperparathyroidism	Paget's disease
Primary	Familial hypocalciuric hypercalcemia
Tertiary (after renal transplant)	

during the course of their disease.[38] The incidence of primary hyperparathyroidism is approximately 270 new cases per million persons per year.[39] Cancer-associated hypercalcemia is most commonly encountered in hospitalized patients, while primary hyperparathyroidism accounts for the vast majority of cases in the outpatient setting.[40,41]

PATHOPHYSIOLOGY

Hypercalcemia of malignancy is most commonly observed in squamous cell carcinomas of the lung, head, and neck, hematologic malignancies such as myeloma and T-cell lymphomas, and carcinomas of ovary, kidney, bladder, and breast.[42] The most frequent types of malignancy associated with hypercalcemia are carcinomas of the lung and breast.[36] The most common example of a hematologic cancer associated with hypercalcemia is multiple myeloma, with 20% to 40% of patients developing hypercalcemia.[41] In most patients with malignancy-associated hypercalcemia, there is evidence for an increase in resorption of calcium from bone.[42] Both metastatic involvement of the skeleton and humoral factors produced by tumors thus contribute to the increase in calcium.[42]

Primary hyperparathyroidism is the most common cause of hypercalcemia in the general population. Increased levels of circulating parathyroid hormone are associated with increased gastrointestinal calcium absorption, renal tubular calcium reabsorption, and calcium resorption from bone. Primary hyperparathyroidism is the result of parathyroid carcinoma in less than 1% of cases.[39,40] Benign parathyroid adenomas account for 80% to 85% of cases of hyperparathyroidism, with parathyroid hyperplasia accounting for the remaining 15%.[40]

CLINICAL PRESENTATION

Mild to moderate hypercalcemia with serum calcium concentrations of less than 13 mg/dL may often be asymptomatic, as is usually the case in drug-induced hypercalcemia and the vast majority of patients with hyperparathyroidism.[43] The signs and symptoms of hypercalcemia may differ depending on the acuteness of onset of elevated serum calcium levels.[36] Symptoms of hypercalcemia associated with malignancy usually have an acute presentation, because the onset of hypercalcemia is often very rapid. The patients may infrequently present in hypercalcemic crisis, manifested by the acute onset of severe hypercalcemia, acute renal failure, and obtundation.[43] If untreated, hypercalcemic crisis may progress to oliguric renal failure, coma, and malignant ventricular arrhythmias, which may result in death.[43] Hypercalcemia more frequently presents with a symptom complex characterized by anorexia, nausea and vomiting, constipation, polyuria, polydipsia, and nocturia.[43] Polyuria and polydipsia secondary to a urinary-concentrating defect constitute some of the most frequent renal effects of hypercalcemia.[43] Disorders associated with long-standing hypercalcemia (hyperparathyroidism) are more likely to present with metastatic calcification, nephrolithiasis, and chronic renal insufficiency caused by deposition of calcium phosphate in soft tissue.[43]

The electrocardiographic changes associated with hypercalcemia include shortening of the QT interval and coving of the ST-T wave.[43] Very high serum calcium concentrations may cause T-wave widening, indicating a repolarization defect that may be associated with spontaneous ventricular tachyarrhythmias.[43] Sensitivity to the pharmacologic and toxic actions of digitalis may be enhanced in the setting of hypercalcemia.[38]

▶ TREATMENT: Hypercalcemia

DESIRED OUTCOME

The indications for treatment of hypercalcemia are dependent on the degree of hypercalcemia, acuteness of development of hypercalcemia, and presence or absence of symptoms. The objectives of treatment of the hypercalcemic patient are reversal of signs and symptoms, restoration of normocalcemia, and treatment of the underlying cause of hypercalcemia. A rational treatment approach for hypercalcemia is outlined in Figure 48–5.

NONPHARMACOLOGIC THERAPY

Patients with hypercalcemic crisis or acute symptomatic severe hypercalcemia should be considered medical emergencies and treated immediately. Such patients require rapid reduction of serum calcium concentration and hemodialysis against a zero or low calcium dialysate solution is considered the treatment of choice, especially in patients with impaired renal function or life-threatening hypercalcemia.[44]

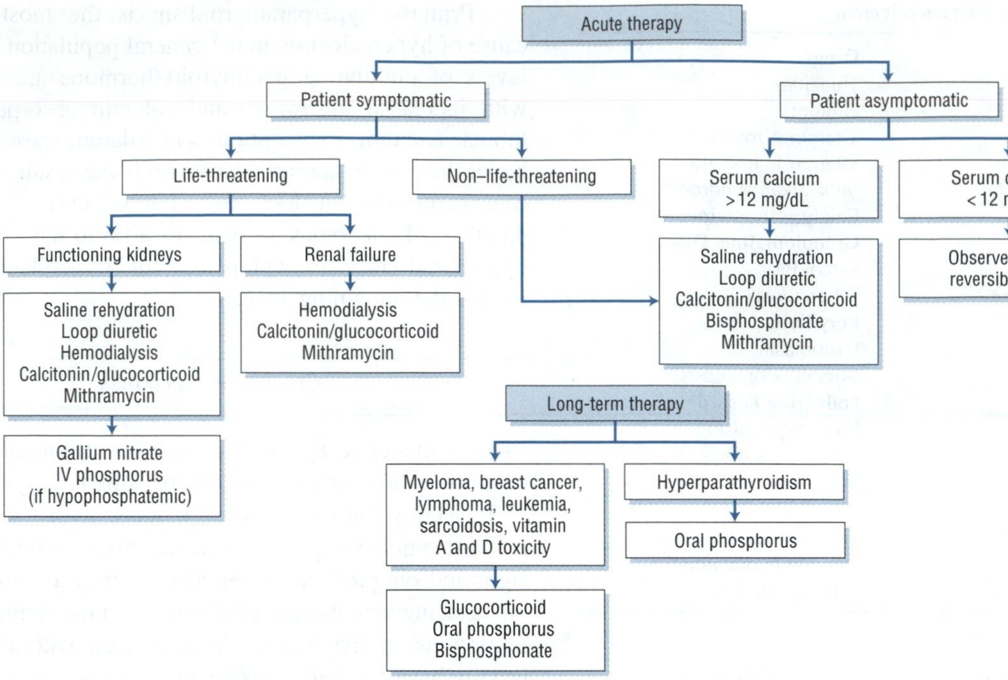

FIGURE 48–5. Pharmacotherapeutic options for the hypercalcemic patient.

PHARMACOLOGIC THERAPY

Intravenous phosphate may rapidly reduce ionized calcium concentrations through the formation of insoluble calcium phosphate salts. However, intravenous phosphate is extremely hazardous because extraskeletal precipitation of calcium phosphate may result in metastatic calcification, hypotension, acute renal failure, or death.[36,46] Therefore, intravenous phosphates should be reserved for the extraordinary patient with severe hypercalcemia and concomitant hypophosphatemia.[36]

Effective treatment of moderate to severe hypercalcemia in the absence of life-threatening symptoms begins with attention to the underlying disorder and correction of associated fluid and electrolyte abnormalities. For example, patients with primary hyperparathyroidism often require surgery, patients with malignancy often require reduction of tumor load, while patients with drug-associated hypercalcemia generally respond to discontinuation of the offending agent. In patients with functioning kidneys, the cornerstone of initial treatment of hypercalcemia is rehydration with normal saline. Patients with symptomatic hypercalcemia are often dehydrated secondary to vomiting and polyuria; thus, rehydration with saline-containing fluids is necessary to interrupt the stimulus for sodium and calcium reabsorption in the kidney tubule.[45] Rehydration can be accomplished by the infusion of normal saline at rates of 200 to 300 mL/h, checking for continued dehydration or fluid overload by monitoring fluid intake and output or by central venous pressure monitoring.[41,44] Once rehydration has been accomplished, loop diuretics such as furosemide (40 to 80 mg intravenously every 1 to 4 hours) may be instituted to inhibit calcium reabsorption by the kidney and to protect against volume overload from the administration of saline.[41] Loop diuretics, such as furosemide, block calcium reabsorption in the thick ascending loop of Henle and augment the calciuric effect of saline alone.[46] Loop diuretics should be employed only after the patient has been fully rehydrated, because the use of a diuretic in a dehydrated patient may lead to increased serum calcium due to enhanced proximal calcium and sodium reabsorption.[36] Potassium chloride should be added to the saline solution after rehydration is accomplished to maintain normokalemia. Serum magnesium levels should also be monitored, and magnesium replacement instituted if diuretic-induced hypomagnesemia occurs. Rehydration with saline and administration of furosemide often leads to decreases of 2 to 3 mg/dL in total serum calcium within 24 to 48 hours.[41]

The pharmacologic therapy of hypercalcemia should be individualized according to the patient's presentation and symptoms. In patients where saline hydration therapy may be contraindicated (e.g., CHF, renal dysfunction) acute, short-term therapy with calcitonin is effective in rapidly reducing serum calcium levels. Calcitonin may be administered subcutaneously or intramuscularly in doses of four Medical Research Council (MRC) units/kg every 12 hours, or intravenously by a constant infusion at rates of 10 to 12 MRC units per hour. Calcitonin side effects are mild and may include nausea, vomiting, and flushing, and rarely an allergic reaction.[46] Calcitonin has a rapid onset of action (within 1 to 2 hours); however, the degree and extent of serum calcium level reduction are often unpredictable.[36] Calcitonin therapy is frequently associated with tachyphylaxis; however, the addition of corticosteroid therapy may prolong calcitonin's actions.[36]

Bisphosphonates (etidronate, pamidronate, alendronate, and risedronate) block bone resorption very efficiently, render the hydroxyapatite crystal of bone mineral resistant to hydrolysis by phosphatases, and also inhibits osteoclast precursors from attaching to the mineralized matrix and therefore blocking their transformation into mature functioning osteoclasts.[41,43,47] Pamidronate is very effective in controlling hypercalcemia associated with malignancy and slightly more effective than etidronate.[42] The usual dose of pamidronate is 60 to 90 mg as an IV infusion given over 4 to 24 hours. Pamidronate also has the advantage of single-day therapy and is currently the bisphosphonate of choice.[41,42] Etidronate, when administered in doses of 7.5 mg/kg/d by slow intravenous infusion over at least 2 hours for 3 days, has also been shown to be effective in the therapy of hypercalcemia of malignancy.[41] Serum calcium concentrations may begin to decline in 2 days and reach a nadir in 7 days;

thus, calcitonin therapy may be necessary if rapid serum level reduction is required.[41,46,48] Duration of normocalcemia varies, but usually does not exceed 2 weeks, depending on the severity and treatment response of the underlying malignancy.[36] Data on the use of these agents for maintenance therapy are limited; however, pamidronate has demonstrated more promise than etidronate.[42]

Gallium nitrate is indicated for the treatment of symptomatic hypercalcemia of malignancy not responsive to hydration therapy. Gallium nitrate inhibits bone resorption, and may be superior to calcitonin in inducing normocalcemia.[42] Gallium nitrate may provide a longer duration of normocalcemia compared to etidronate; however, further studies are needed to clarify the duration of these agents.[42] Gallium nitrate is usually administered as a continuous IV infusion at a dose of 200 $mg/m^2/d$ for 5 consecutive days. Gallium nitrate is potentially nephrotoxic, especially if administered with other nephrotoxic drugs.

Mithramycin (plicamycin), a potent cytotoxic antibiotic, inhibits osteoclast-mediated bone resorption by inhibition of DNA-directed RNA synthesis of proteins.[41] Mithramycin may be administered at a dose of 25 μg/kg via intravenous infusion over 4 to 6 hours in saline or 5% dextrose solution and may be repeated at intervals of 24 to 48 hours.[41,46,49] Serum calcium levels begin to fall within 12 hours of a mithramycin dose with the peak effect generally occurring within 48 to 96 hours.[36,41,42] The most common adverse effects associated with mithramycin are thrombocytopenia, inhibition of platelet function, renal, and hepatotoxicity.[36] Single doses are usually well tolerated.[49] Mithramycin should probably be limited to short-term therapy in patients who have not responded to alternative therapies.[46] Repeated doses may be given every 1 to 2 days as needed, along with frequent determinations of complete blood count, liver function, and renal function. Mithramycin should be avoided in patients with thrombocytopenia, liver disease, or renal disease.[41]

Glucocorticoids are usually effective in the treatment of hypercalcemia resulting from multiple myeloma, leukemia, lymphoma, sarcoidosis, and hypervitaminoses A and D.[36,38,47,49] The mechanisms of glucocorticoid actions include direct tumor lysing and interference in metabolism of vitamin D_2 to calcitriol.[36,46] Daily doses of 40 to 60 mg of prednisone or the equivalent have been effective. The disadvantages of glucocorticoid therapy are a relatively slow onset of hypocalcemic effect and the potential for glucocorticoid side effects.[39,46,47] Treatment of hypercalcemia with inhibitors of prostaglandin synthesis, such as indomethacin, is rarely effective and thus not recommended.[46] The administration of oral phosphorus is minimally effective in the chronic treatment of hypercalcemia associated with hyperparathyroidism and malignancy.[36] Long-term administration of oral phosphorus should be used cautiously because the calcium-phosphate crystals may precipitate in the kidneys or other major organs; thus, serum calcium, phosphorus, and creatinine should be monitored closely. Asymptomatic patients with mild hypercalcemia may be carefully observed, especially if treatment for the underlying condition (malignancy) is initiated.

HYPOCALCEMIA

Hypocalcemia (total serum calcium less than 8.5 mg/dL) occurs when the normal homeostatic mechanisms are disrupted. The incidence of hypocalcemia in ICU patients ranges from 70% to 90% for total to 15% to 50% for ionized calcium.[37]

PATHOPHYSIOLOGY

Hypocalcemia is the result of alterations in the effect of parathyroid hormone and vitamin D on the target end organs (bone, gut, and kidney) (Table 48–8). The majority of cases of hypocalcemia are due to vitamin D deficiency states and hypoparathyroidism.

Vitamin D and its metabolites play an important role in the maintenance of extracellular calcium concentrations and in normal skeletal structure and mineralization. On a worldwide basis, the most common cause of hypocalcemia is nutritional vitamin D deficiency. In malnourished populations, this is manifested by rickets and osteomalacia. Nutritional vitamin D deficiency is uncommon in Western societies because of the supplementation of milk with ergocalciferol.[50] The most common cause of vitamin D deficiency in these societies is GI disease.[43] Gastric surgery, chronic pancreatitis, small-bowel disease, and intestinal resection and bypass surgery have all been associated with decreased levels of vitamin D and metabolites.[43] Decreased production of 1,25-dihydroxyvitamin D_3 may occur as a result of a hereditary defect resulting in vitamin D-dependent

TABLE 48–8. Causes of Hypocalcemia

Hypoalbuminemia
Hypoparathyroidism
Surgical
Infiltrative
Idiopathic
Pseudohypoparathyroidism
Pseudoidiopathic
Hypomagnesemia
Hyperphosphatemia
Pancreatitis
Intestinal malabsorption
Drugs
Oral phosphorus
Furosemide
Calcitonin
Mithramycin
Drugs causing hypomagnesemia
Phenytoin
Barbiturates
Hungry bone syndrome
Recovery from parathyroid surgery
Vitamin D deficiency
Nutritional
Malabsorption
Liver disease
Decreased production of 25-OH-vitamin D_3
Increased metabolism of 25-OH-vitamin D_3
Phenytoin, barbiturates
Accelerated loss of 25-OH-vitamin D_3
Nephrotic syndrome
Decreased production of 1,25-$(OH)_2$-vitamin D_3
Renal disease
Hereditary vitamin D-dependent rickets
Decreased end-organ response of 1,25-$(OH)_2$-vitamin D_3
Hereditary

rickets. It also can occur secondary to chronic renal insufficiency where insufficient 1 α-hydroxylase enzyme is available for the production of the most active metabolite.[51] Treatment of hypocalcemia associated with chronic renal failure is reviewed in Chapter 42.

Symptomatic hypocalcemia most commonly occurs because of parathyroid gland dysfunction secondary to surgical procedures involving the thyroid, parathyroid, and neck.[50] Hypocalcemia in these postsurgical patients is generally transient in nature.[50] Serum calcium concentration should be monitored carefully during the 24 hours following such surgeries.

Proper assessment of total serum calcium levels includes measurement of serum albumin concentrations. Hypoalbuminemia, which may be associated with many disease states, is probably the most common cause of laboratory hypocalcemia. Patients remain asymptomatic because the ionized fraction of serum calcium remains normal. Serum albumin concentration is a vital consideration in the assessment of the cause of hypocalcemia.

Hypomagnesemia of any cause may be associated with severe symptomatic hypocalcemia that is unresponsive to calcium replacement therapy (see the section on hypomagnesemia later in the chapter). The magnesium cation plays an important role in the secretion of and skeletal response to parathyroid hormone. Serum magnesium levels are important in determining the cause of hypocalcemia.

Clinical Presentation

The clinical manifestations of hypocalcemia are characterized by a large degree of individual variability. The acuteness of the development of hypocalcemia plays a large role in whether or not symptoms will occur.[50] The more acute the drop in ionized calcium concentration, the more likely the patient will develop symptoms. Thus, acid–base balance plays a significant role in the likelihood of development of hypocalcemic symptoms, with alkalosis predisposing and acidosis inhibiting symptom development.

Hypocalcemia may manifest as neuromuscular, central nervous system (CNS), dermatologic, and cardiac sequelae.[43] Acute hypocalcemia is more likely to manifest as neuromuscular and cardiovascular symptoms, while chronic hypocalcemia may often present as CNS and dermatologic symptoms associated with an underlying chronic disease (hypoparathyroidism) (Table 48–9). The hallmark sign of acute hypocalcemia is tetany, due to enhanced peripheral neuromuscular irritability.[43] Tetany manifests as paresthesias around the mouth and in the extremities, muscle spasms and cramps, carpopedal spasms, and rarely as laryngospasm and bronchospasm.[43,50]

The cardiovascular manifestations of hypocalcemia result in electrocardiographic changes characterized by a prolonged QT interval and symptoms of decreased myocardial contractility often associated with congestive heart failure.[52] Both acute and chronic hypocalcemia may result in a reversible syndrome characterized by acute myocardial failure. Refractory congestive heart failure may also be precipitated by hypocalcemia.

TABLE 48–9. Signs and Symptoms of Hypocalcemia

Central Nervous System	**Latent Tetany**
Fatigue	Positive Chvostek's sign
Irritability	Positive Trousseau's sign
Memory loss	Weakness
Depression	**Ocular**
Confusion	Cataracts
Delusion	**Cardiovascular**
Hallucinations	Prolonged QT interval
Areflexia	Acute myocardial failure
Seizures	Hypotension
Neuromuscular Tetany	**Skin**
Perioral paresthesias	Hair loss
Carpopedal spasm	Brittle, grooved nails
Muscle spasms	Eczema
Cramps	Psoriasis
	Hyperpigmentation with dermatitis

▶ TREATMENT: Hypocalcemia

DESIRED OUTCOME

Treatment of hypocalcemia is dependent on identification of the pathogenesis of the disorder, acuteness of onset, and presence and severity of symptoms. The goal of therapy is the resolution of signs and symptoms of hypocalcemia, restoration of normocalcemia, management of associated electrolyte abnormalities, and treatment of the underlying cause of hypocalcemia. Asymptomatic hypocalcemia associated with hypoalbuminemia requires no treatment, because ionized plasma calcium concentrations are normal. Acute, symptomatic hypocalcemia requires parenteral administration of soluble calcium salts.

PHARMACOLOGIC THERAPY

The initial therapeutic intervention for patients with acute symptomatic hypocalcemia is to administer 100 to 300 mg of elemental calcium intravenously over 5 to 10 minutes.[53] This may be provided by the administration of 1 g of calcium chloride or 2 to 3 g of calcium gluconate. Calcium gluconate is generally preferred over calcium chloride for peripheral venous administration because calcium gluconate is less irritating to veins.[53] Disadvantages to the use of calcium gluconate are the small amounts of elemental calcium per volume and a less predictable, slightly smaller increase in plasma ionic calcium compared with calcium chloride. Calcium should not be infused at a rate greater than 60 mg of elemental calcium per minute because direct, severe cardiac dysfunction may result.[54] Calcium should not be added to bicarbonate- or phosphate-containing solutions because of the possibility of precipitation.[53] The bolus dose of calcium is only effective for 1 to 2 hours and should be followed by a continuous infusion of elemental calcium at a rate of 0.5 to 2.0 mg/kg/h.[37] The ionized calcium concentration usually normalizes over 2 to 4 hours and the maintenance infusion rate of elemental calcium can be decreased to 0.3 to 0.5 mg/kg/hr.[36] Once the ionized calcium has stabilized, calcium can be administered by the oral route.[37] Intravenous calcium administration should be used with caution in patients receiving digitalis glycosides, because of the possibility of cardiac arrhythmias.[37]

Once acute hypocalcemia is corrected by parenteral administration, further treatment modalities should be individualized according to the cause of hypocalcemia. If hypomagnesemia is present, magnesium supplementation is indicated (see the section on hypomagnesemia later in the chapter). Chronic hypocalcemia associated with hypoparathyroidism and vitamin D-deficient states may be managed by oral calcium and vitamin D supplementation. Therapy is begun with 1 to 3 g/d of elemental calcium.[35] If serum calcium does not normalize, a vitamin D preparation should be added. A comparison of oral calcium and vitamin D preparations is found in Chapter 42.

Treatment of hypocalcemia associated with vitamin D-deficient states should be individualized. In patients with malabsorption, vitamin D requirements vary markedly, and large doses may be required. In contrast, vitamin D deficiency associated with anticonvulsant medication may be corrected with smaller doses of vitamin D.[52] The treatment of vitamin D deficiency associated with chronic renal failure is discussed in Chapter 42. Situations in which 25-hydroxylase activity is reduced (e.g., hepatic disease) may require treatment with calcitriol (1,25-dihydroxyvitamin D_3) or paricalcitol. In selected cases, calcium supplementation may be required if vitamin D replacement alone is ineffective in returning calcium concentrations to normal.

Adverse effects of oral calcium and vitamin D supplementation include hypercalcemia and hypercalciuria, especially in the hypoparathyroid patient, where the renal calcium-sparing effect of parathyroid hormone is absent. Hypercalciuria may increase the risk of calcium stone formation and nephrolithiasis in susceptible patients. The addition of thiazide diuretics for patients at risk for stone formation may result in a reduction of both urinary calcium excretion and vitamin D requirement.[52,54]

DISORDERS OF MAGNESIUM HOMEOSTASIS

Magnesium is ionically bound to the center of chlorophyll molecules; thus, the entire food chain and transfer of energy in biologic systems are dependent on its presence. Magnesium is an important cofactor for hundreds of enzyme systems, including all phosphate transfer reactions involving ATP.[55] Magnesium appears to modulate the neuromuscular activity of the calcium ion; indeed, magnesium has been called "nature's physiologic calcium blocker."[56] Magnesium is the fourth most plentiful cation and the second most abundant intracellular cation. As the clinical significance of magnesium disorders becomes more clearly defined, the need for an understanding of the appropriate therapy for these disorders becomes vital.

Because only about 1% of total body magnesium resides in the ECF space, serum magnesium concentration provides only a rough index of total body magnesium stores. Magnesium is 30% bound to albumin; thus, in contrast to calcium, changes in albumin concentration have much less effect on serum magnesium concentration. Normal serum magnesium concentration is 1.5 to 2.0 mEq/L.[55]

The kidney is the primary regulator of magnesium balance in the body. Magnesium homeostasis is maintained by a balance of glomerular filtration and tubular reabsorption. Renal handling of magnesium seems to follow a tubular maximum mechanism similar to the renal handling of glucose. This tubular maximum is set very close to the filtered load of magnesium that is present at normal serum concentrations. Thus, small increases in serum magnesium concentration are associated with a rise in magnesium excretion.[57] Conversely, decreases in serum magnesium concentration result in the near disappearance of magnesium from the urine.

HYPERMAGNESEMIA

Hypermagnesemia results when magnesium intake exceeds the excretory capacity of the kidneys. Because of the tubular maximum transport threshold is high, hypermagnesemia occurs only in the setting of renal dysfunction or excessive exogenous administration of magnesium. The prevalence of hypermagnesemia (serum magnesium > 2 mEq/L) in hospital patients has been reported to range from 5.7% to 9.3%.[58,59] Fortunately, symptomatic hypermagnesemia is an uncommon clinical problem.[60]

PATHOPHYSIOLOGY

Hypermagnesemia most commonly occurs in the setting of renal insufficiency when glomerular filtration rates are less than 30 mL/min.[56] Use of magnesium-containing laxatives or antacids can lead to hypermagnesemia in renal failure patients.[56] Patients in the intensive care unit with multiple-system organ failure receiving magnesium-containing antacids for stress ulcer prophylaxis or magnesium-containing parenteral fluids (i.e., total parenteral nutrition) constitute a population of patients particularly at risk for developing hypermagnesemia. Parenteral treatment of eclampsia with magnesium sulfate or its use in the therapy of preterm labor can potentially cause hypermagnesemia.[56] Other potential causes of hypermagnesemia are listed in Table 48–10.

TABLE 48–10. Causes of Hypermagnesemia

Decreased Renal Excretion
Acute renal failure
Chronic renal failure with exogenous intake
Excessive Intake
Treatment of toxemia of pregnancy
Ureteral irrigants (hemiacidrin)
Cathartics
Other
Lithium therapy
Hypothyroidism
Milk–alkali syndrome
Addison's disease
Viral hepatitis
Acute diabetic ketoacidosis

Clinical Presentation

Hypermagnesemia manifests as neuromuscular, cardiovascular, and endocrine effects (Fig. 48–6). Signs and symptoms of hypermagnesemia occur when serum magnesium concentration exceeds 4 mEq/L. The neuromuscular manifestations of hypermagnesemia can be ascribed to neuromuscular blockade. Hypermagnesemia may cause diminished or absent deep tendon reflexes, varying degrees of muscle weakness, and respiratory depression or respiratory muscle paralysis and respiratory arrest, depending on the serum concentration of magnesium attained.[55,56,61] Because deep tendon reflexes disappear before the appearance of paralysis of voluntary muscle, monitoring of deep tendon reflexes is a useful tool to evaluate magnesium toxicity. CNS depression may result in varying degrees of lethargy and sedation, which may progress to stupor and coma, especially at high (> 6 mEq/L) serum magnesium concentrations.[61]

Excessively high magnesium concentrations may affect heart rate, cardiac conduction, and blood pressure. Hypotension and cutaneous vasodilation may occur above serum levels of 3 mEq/L.[43,62] A variety of mechanisms have been implicated, including vascular smooth muscle relaxation and sympathetic blockade.[61] Sinus bradycardia, first-degree heart block, nodal rhythms, or bundle branch block may occur at serum magnesium concentrations of 5 to 10 mEq/L or greater.[60] Complete heart block progressing to asystole and cardiac arrest may occur at serum concentrations greater than 14 to 15 mEq/L.[60,62]

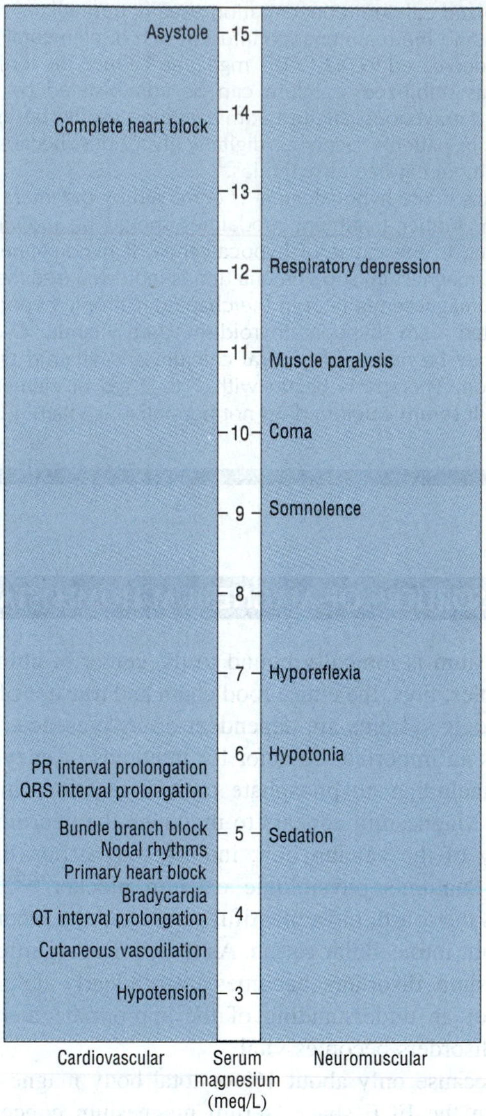

FIGURE 48–6. Clinical findings associated with hypermagnesemia.

▶ TREATMENT: Hypermagnesemia

■ DESIRED OUTCOME

Guidelines for the treatment of hypermagnesemia are based on clinical signs and symptoms and the degree of elevation of serum magnesium. The goals of therapy are to reverse signs and symptoms of hypermagnesemia, restore serum magnesium levels to normal levels, and reverse the underlying cause of hypermagnesemia. Treatment of severe symptomatic hypermagnesemia includes the correction of the cardiovascular and neuromuscular symptoms.[56]

■ PHARMACOLOGIC THERAPY

Because calcium directly antagonizes the neuromuscular and cardiovascular effects of magnesium, intravenous administration of calcium in doses of 100 to 200 mg of elemental calcium is indicated.[55,56] Reversal of symptomatic hypermagnesemia after calcium administration is rapid but transient in nature; thus, repeated doses of calcium may be necessary in life-threatening situations. Hemodialysis is the treatment of choice in patients with end stage renal disease.[55] Supportive care with mechanical ventilation, pressors, and cardiac pacemakers may be necessary until serum magnesium concentrations are lowered.

In patients with adequate renal function and moderate hypermagnesemia, elimination of magnesium intake and promotion of renal magnesium excretion may be accomplished by administering saline and loop diuretics, in a similar fashion as described for hypercalcemia therapy.[56]

HYPOMAGNESEMIA

Hypomagnesemia occurs when magnesium intake is less than renal excretion, or when the renal magnesium-conserving mechanisms fail. Hypomagnesemia (serum magnesium < 1 mEq/L) is a common clinical disorder but is frequently overlooked because of the typically complex clinical setting in which it occurs.[43] Because less than 1% of total body magnesium is extracellular, the serum magnesium concentration may not always reflect the true amount of magnesium in the body.[63] The prevalence of hypomagnesemia among patients admitted to a hospital is approximately 10%, and it may be as high as 65% in intensive care units.[63]

PATHOPHYSIOLOGY

Magnesium depletion is almost always secondary to disturbances of either the intestinal tract or the kidney. Table 48–11 lists many of the potential causes of hypomagnesemia. Magnesium conservation in normal subjects is extremely effective; therefore, dietary magnesium deprivation rarely leads to significant magnesium depletion unless it is prolonged.[43] Generalized malabsorption syndromes associated with hypomagnesemia occur in various intestinal mucosal diseases (e.g., coeliac sprue, Whipple's disease, radiation enteritis), massive intestinal resection, and pancreatic insufficiency.[63,64] Magnesium losses exceeding intake may produce hypomagnesemia. GI disorders may result in hypomagnesemia, secondary to the loss of intestinal fluids. Fluids from the upper intestinal tract contain approximately 1 mEq/L of magnesium and fluids from the lower intestinal tract contain up to 15 mEq/L.[63]

Renal magnesium wasting may be due to intrinsic tubular disorders or drug-, hormone-, ion-, or nutrient-induced renal tubular magnesium losses. Particularly, severe hypomagnesemia may occur during the diuresis

TABLE 48–11. Causes of Hypomagnesemia

Gastrointestinal	**Renal (continued)**
Reduced intake	Pyelonephritis
Protein-calorie malnutrition	Nephrotic syndrome
Total parenteral nutrition without magnesium	Drug-induced renal losses
Prolonged parenteral fluid administration without magnesium	Aminoglycosides
Alcoholism	Amphotericin B
Reduced absorption	Cyclosporine
Primary hypomagnesemia	Diuretics
Malabsorption syndromes (e.g., tropical sprue, celiac disease, radiation enteritis, intestinal lymphectasia)	Digitalis
Short-bowel syndrome (e.g., small-bowel resection, ileal bypass)	Cisplatin
Pancreatic insufficiency	Alcohol
Increased loss	Hormone-induced renal losses
Excessive vomiting	Hyperparathyroidism
Prolonged nasogastric suction	Hyperthyroidism
Excessive laxative use	Aldosteronism
Intestinal and biliary fistulas	Hypoparathyroidism
Prolonged diarrhea (ulcerative colitis, Crohn's disease, cancer of the colon)	"Hungry bone syndrome" after parathyroidectomy
Renal	**Internal Redistribution**
Primary tubular disorders	Diabetic ketoacidosis
Primary renal magnesium wasting	Glucose, amino acid, insulin administration
Bartter's syndrome	Massive blood transfusion (citrate)
Renal tubular acidosis	Pancreatitis with lipidemia (magnesium soap)
Diuretic phase of acute tubular necrosis	**Other**
Postobstructive diuresis	Excessive sweating and lactation
Postrenal transplant diuresis	Hypercalcemia and hypercalciuria
Glomerulonephritis	Phosphate depletion
	Chronic alcoholism
	ECF volume expansion

associated with the recovery or diuretic phase of oliguric acute tubular necrosis, the postobstructive period, and postrenal transplantation.[65]

The most frequent cause of renal magnesium wasting is long-term diuretic therapy.[66] Up to thirty-seven percent of diuretic users develop hypomagnesemia.[67] Other therapeutic agents associated with magnesium wasting include aminoglycosides, amphotericin B, foscarnet, pentamidine, *cis*-platinum, and cyclosporine.[65]

The most common clinical setting for hypomagnesemia is acute and chronic alcoholism. The causes of hypomagnesemia in the alcoholic are multifactorial and include malnutrition, dietary magnesium deficiency, vomiting and diarrhea, increased urinary magnesium excretion, hypophosphatemia, hyperaldosteronism, and pancreatic insufficiency.[65] In addition, upon entry of alcoholic patients into the hospital, acute ethanol withdrawal and IV glucose therapy may lead to further reductions in ECF magnesium levels.[66] It appears likely that magnesium deficiency along with other metabolic disorders associated with alcoholism and alcohol withdrawal contribute to the delirium tremens associated with alcohol withdrawal.[66] Monitoring of serum magnesium concentration is indicated in alcoholic patients, and supplementation is recommended in patients with documented magnesium deficiency, tachyarrhythmias, hypocalcemia, or hypokalemia.[66]

Clinical Presentation

Clinical manifestations of hypomagnesemia are generally not seen until serum magnesium concentrations approach 1 mEq/L (Table 48–12).[17] Magnesium deficiency can result in various nonspecific neuromuscular signs and symptoms. Concomitant hypocalcemia and hypokalemia may contribute as well. Neuromuscular signs and symptoms of hypomagnesemia are the converse of those of hypermagnesemia. Neuromuscular hyperactivity is often the predominant complaint of patients with magnesium deficiency.[63]

Several studies have suggested an association between dietary magnesium deficiency from drinking water with decreased magnesium content ("soft water") and sudden death from coronary artery disease.[66,68] Atrial or ventricular arrhythmias may occur in magnesium deficiency.[57] Magnesium may play an important etiologic role in atypical ventricular tachycardia (torsades de pointes), which is successfully suppressed with magnesium therapy.[65] Hypomagnesemia may also exacerbate digitalis toxicity-induced arrhythmias. The finding of a 19% frequency of hypomagnesemia in hospitalized patients with potential life-threatening manifestations of digitalis toxicity has prompted recommendations for routine monitoring and supplementation of both potassium and magnesium in patients receiving digitalis.[66–68]

The electrocardiograph changes associated with hypomagnesemia are nonspecific and include wide QRS complexes and tall, peaked T waves in moderate magnesium deficiency; and prolonged PR, QRS, and QT intervals, ST segment depression, and flat, broad T waves with prominent U waves in severe magnesium deficiency.[69] These electrocardiographic changes probably reflect alterations in intracellular potassium and calcium in the myocardium.

Magnesium is important in regulating intracellular potassium content.[63] Movement of these intracellular cations appears to be closely linked. Thus, attempts to replace potassium deficits in the presence of magnesium deficiency are difficult. Magnesium deficiency impairs the Na^+/K^+-ATPase pump and allows potassium to escape from the cell.[66] It is estimated that the incidence of hypomagnesemia in hypokalemic patients is 42%.[66]

Hypocalcemia is a prominent manifestation of magnesium deficiency perhaps due to an altered equilibrium between calcium in extracellular fluid and bone, impaired release of parathyroid hormone, impaired formation of parathyroid hormone, and end-organ resistance to parathyroid hormone.[64,66] Serum calcium concentration should be assessed if hypomagnesemia is discovered.

TABLE 48–12. Clinical Manifestations of Hypomagnesemia

Neuromuscular
Muscle twitching and tremor
Muscle weakness
Hyperreflexia
Paresthesias
Positive Chvostek's and Trousseau's signs
Tetany
Seizures
Coma
Nystagmus, ataxia, vertigo
Choreoathetoid movements
Psychiatric
Apathy
Depression
Delirium
Agitation
Confusion
Hallucinations
Cardiac
Premature ventricular beats
Ventricular fibrillation
Ventricular tachycardia
Torsades de pointes
Predisposition to digitalis-mediated arrhythmias
Supraventricular tachycardia
Electrocardiographic changes (PR, QT prolongation, widened QRS)
Coronary artery spasm
Calcium and Potassium
Refractory hypocalcemia
Refractory hypokalemia

▶ TREATMENT: Hypomagnesemia

DESIRED OUTCOME

Treatment goals are the resolution of signs and symptoms of hypomagnesemia, restoration of normal serum magnesium levels, management of concomitant electrolyte abnormalities, and treatment of the underlying etiology.

PHARMACOLOGIC THERAPY

Magnesium supplementation may be administered via the intravenous, intramuscular, or oral route, depending on severity of hypomagnesemia, presence of symptoms, and patient tolerance (Table 48–13). Patients with serum magnesium levels less than 1 mEq/L or who are symptomatic should receive parenteral magnesium therapy. Rapid IV injection of magnesium may be associated with flushing, sweating, and a sensation of warmth; thus, rapid bolus injection of magnesium should be avoided. Direct IV administration of 50% magnesium sulfate may produce pain and venosclerosis; therefore, it should be diluted to 20% before administration. Because intramuscular injections are painful, involve multiple punctures, and have no therapeutic advantage over the IV route, intramuscular therapy should be reserved for situations in which peripheral venous access is not readily available.

Patients with nonsymptomatic hypomagnesemia or with serum magnesium levels greater than 1 mEq/L (1.2 mg/dL) may be treated with oral magnesium supplements. However, diarrhea may be a limiting factor with oral magnesium therapy.

Even if severe magnesium deficiency is present, approximately 50% of an administered dose is excreted in the urine.[66] Magnesium replacement must thus be continued over 3 to 5 days, and subsequent maintenance magnesium administration should continue in patients who are unable to eat or who have continuing magnesium losses. Regardless of route of administration, assessment of renal function is indicated. Patients with renal insufficiency should be treated with lower doses and must be monitored by measuring serum levels frequently.[63]

TABLE 48–13. Guidelines for Treatment of Magnesium Deficiency in Adults

1. Serum Magnesium < 1 mEq/L (1.2 mg/dL) With Life-threatening Symptoms (seizure, arrhythmia)
Day 1
2 g $MgSO_4$ (1 g $MgSO_4$ = 8.1 mEq Mg^{2+}) mixed with 6 mL 0.9% NaCl in 10-mL syringe and administer IV push over 1 min
Follow with 0.5 mEq Mg^{2+}/kg lean body weight IV infusion over 5–6 h, then 0.5 mEq Mg^{2+}/kg lean body weight IV infusion over 17–18 h
Days 2–5
0.5 mEq Mg^{2+}/kg lean body weight per day divided in maintenance IV fluids
2. Serum Magnesium < 1 mEq/L (1.2 mg/dL) Without Life-threatening Symptoms
Day 1
Total of 1 mEq Mg^{2+}/kg lean body weight per day as continuous IV infusion, or divided and given IM every 4 h for five doses
Days 2–5
Total of 0.5 mEq Mg^{2+}/kg lean body weight IV infusion per day as continuous IV infusion or divided and given IM every 6–8 h
3. Serum Magnesium > 1 mEq/L (1.2 mg/dL) and < 1.5 mEq/L (1.8 mg/dL) Without Symptoms
As in no. 2, above, or
Milk of Magnesia 5 mL four times daily as tolerated, or
Magnesium-containing antacid 15 mL three times daily as tolerated, or
Magnesium oxide tablets 300 mg four times daily, increase to two tablets four times daily as tolerated

DISORDERS OF PHOSPHORUS HOMEOSTASIS

Phosphorus is an essential element in phospholipid cell membranes, nucleic acids, and phosphoproteins required for mitochondrial function.[70] Phosphorus regulates the intermediary metabolism of carbohydrates, fats, and proteins. Phosphorus also regulates enzymatic reactions including glycolysis, ammoniogenesis, and the 1-hydroxylation of 25-hydroxyvitamin D.[70] In addition, phosphorus is required for the appropriate generation of 2,3-diphosphoglycerate (2,3-DPG) in red blood cells, which is required for normal modulation of oxygen–hemoglobin dissociation and delivering of oxygen to the tissues.[71] Phosphorus is the source of the high-energy bonds of ATP, thus fueling a wide variety of physiologic processes, including muscle contractibility, electrolyte transport, neurologic function, and other important biochemical reactions.[70] Considering its diverse biologic importance, it is not difficult to appreciate the clinical implications of disorders of phosphorus homeostasis.

Phosphorus is present in living organisms mainly as inorganic phosphate and organic phosphate esters. Potassium is the major intracellular cation, and phosphorus is the major intracellular anion. The majority of intracellular phosphorus exists as organic esters, mainly 2,3-DPG, adenosine and guanosine triphosphate, and fructose 1,6-diphosphate.[72] Only a small fraction of intracellular phosphorus exists as inorganic phosphate; however, this fraction is critical because it is the source from which ATP is resynthesized.[72] The majority of inorganic phosphate is located in the extracellular space. Normal serum phosphorus concentration in the adult is 3.0-4.5 mg/dL.[2] Extracellular inorganic phosphate is the prime determinant of intracellular phosphate; thus, small increments in the organic phosphate pool can profoundly alter both the extracellular and intracellular phosphate pools. Metabolic disturbances, hydrogen ion shifts, and hormones all can cause important syndromes. Because of these phenomena, the serum phosphorus level does not accurately reflect total body stores.[71]

Phosphorus excretion by the kidney is the single most important regulator of steady-state serum phosphorus levels. Renal excretion of phosphorus is regulated by glomerular filtration and active tubular reabsorption. Under normal conditions, 85% to 90% of filtered phosphate is reabsorbed, the majority in the early proximal tubule. Renal tubular reabsorption of phosphorus is inhibited by parathyroid hormone and 1,25-dihydroxyvitamin D_3.[70] Conversely, phosphorus reabsorption is increased by growth hormone and thyroxine.[73] Internal phosphorus balance (transcellular phosphate distribution) is also of importance in the maintenance of normal serum phosphorus, which may vary by as much as 2 mg/dL throughout the day, as the result of acute changes in transcellular distribution of phosphate influenced primarily by carbohydrate intake and insulin secretion.[70]

HYPERPHOSPHATEMIA

Hyperphosphatemia (serum phosphorus concentration greater than 4.5 mg/dL) occurs much less frequently than hypophosphatemia. Serum phosphorus concentration is so closely regulated by the kidneys that it is unusual for hyperphosphatemia to develop in patients with normal renal function. The most frequent causes of hyperphosphatemia are increases in phosphate entrance into the extracellular fluid via either exogenous administration or endogenous intracellular phosphate release, or a decrease in renal excretion of phosphate.

PATHOPHYSIOLOGY

The most common cause of hyperphosphatemia is a decrease in urinary phosphorus excretion secondary to decreased glomerular filtration rate.[74] Patients with excessive exogenous phosphorus administration or endogenous intracellular phosphorus release in the setting of acute renal failure may develop profound hyperphosphatemia. In patients with chronic progressive renal insufficiency, severe hyperphosphatemia is usually encountered in patients with advanced disease, when the glomerular filtration rate is less than 25 mL/min (see Chap. 42). Patients with renal dysfunction thus have the greatest risk for developing hyperphosphatemia of any patient group.

Hypoparathyroidism results in increased renal tubular reabsorption of phosphorus and may result in hyperphosphatemia. Hyperphosphatemia associated with hypoparathyroidism is usually less severe than that associated with severe renal failure or excessive exogenous or endogenous introduction of phosphorus into the ECF space. Hypoparathyroidism is the most important cause of increased tubular phosphorus reabsorption.

Iatrogenic causes of hyperphosphatemia have been widely reported, and awareness of the phosphorus content of intravenous, oral, and rectally administered phosphorus-containing drugs can aid in the prevention of this cause of hyperphosphatemia. Oral and rectal administration of phosphate containing solutions has resulted in severe and life-threatening hyperphosphatemia.[71] Administration and retention of phosphate-containing enemas in patients with moderate and severe renal insufficiency has also been reported to cause hyperphosphatemia with severe symptoms.[74] Large doses of phosphorus administered intravenously to treat patients with hypercalcemia have also been reported to result in severe life-threatening hyperphosphatemia.[74]

Any disorder that causes disruption of skeletal muscle cells can release large amounts of phosphorus into the systemic circulation and cause hyperphosphatemia. Rhabdomyolysis (destruction of skeletal muscle) may result in the release of large amounts of phosphorus from intracellular stores. This condition is frequently associated with acute renal failure as well; thus, hyperphosphatemia of a severe degree may result.

Hyperphosphatemia is not uncommonly observed in patients undergoing treatment for acute leukemia and lymphomas.[74] Chemotherapeutic treatment of acute lymphoblastic leukemia may result in the release of large amounts of phosphorus into the systemic circulation secondary to lysis of lymphoblasts. Initiation of chemotherapy for Burkitt's lymphoma may also result in a rapid lysis of malignant cells, resulting in hyperphosphatemia, hyperuricemia, hyperkalemia, and hypocalcemia (tumor lysis syndrome).[74]

Diabetic ketoacidosis is an unappreciated but common cause of hyperphosphatemia. In one study, hyperphosphatemia was present in 94.7% of patients with diabetic ketoacidosis prior to the initiation of treatment.[75] However, with the institution of treatment, serum phosphorus levels decrease and patients may ultimately develop hypophosphatemia.

CLINICAL PRESENTATION

Some of the signs and symptoms of hyperphosphatemia are due to the low solubility of calcium phosphate. It has been estimated that calcium phosphate crystals are likely to form *in vivo* when the product of the serum calcium and phosphate levels in mg/dL exceeds 70.[74] When the calcium phosphate product is greater than 58 there is a significant risk of calcium phosphate precipitation. Because of this relationship, the major effects of hyperphosphatemia are related to the development of hypocalcemia with its related consequences, as well as damage resulting from the deposition of calcium phosphate crystals. The calcium phosphate solubility relationship may be influenced by the acid–base status of the patient. An alkaline environment would be predicted to decrease the solubility; conversely, an acidic environment would increase the solubility of calcium phosphate.

Hypocalcemia associated with hyperphosphatemia can result in deposition of calcium phosphate in the joints, or soft tissues.[52] Metastatic calcification leading to band keratopathy, "red eye," pruritus, vascular calcification, and periarticular calcification is most common in renal failure patients (see Chap. 42). In addition, soft tissue calcifications in the conjunctiva, skin, heart, cornea, lung, gastric mucosa, and kidney have been observed primarily in chronic renal failure patients.[74] Hyperphosphatemia associated with chronic renal disease may result in renal osteodystrophy (osteitis fibrosis cystica and osteomalacia). This condition is discussed in Chapter 42.

▶ TREATMENT: Hyperphosphatemia

DESIRED OUTCOME

The treatment of hyperphosphatemia should initially be directed at the correction of reversible factors and the treatment of the disease states associated with its development, the management of associated signs and symptoms, management of associated electrolyte abnormalities, and the return of serum phosphate levels to normal.

PHARMACOLOGIC THERAPY

Severe symptomatic hyperphosphatemia manifesting as hypocalcemia and tetany should be treated by the IV administration of calcium salts. In general, the most effective way to treat hyperphosphatemia is to decrease phosphate absorption in the lumen of the GI tract by the use of phosphate binders.[74] Antacids containing divalent cations are the agents most frequently used in the prevention and treatment of hyperphosphatemia. Magnesium salts should be avoided in patients with renal failure, and aluminum hydroxide and aluminum carbonate gels should be used with caution because they are associated with anemia and CNS and bone disease (see Chap. 42). Short-term therapy with these agents is effective, the most frequent adverse effect being constipation. However, long-term treatment with aluminum-containing antacids in patients with chronic renal failure has led to concern over the toxic effects of aluminum accumulation. Thus, calcium salts are now the preferred phosphate binders in this population (see Chap. 42).

HYPOPHOSPHATEMIA

Hypophosphatemia can be differentiated on the basis of severity: Moderate hypophosphatemia is defined as serum phosphorus concentrations from 1 to 2.5 mg/dL, whereas severe hypophosphatemia is considered to be present if the serum phosphorus concentration is less than 1 mg/dL. Hypophosphatemia is found in approximately 2% to 3% of hospital admissions.[73] Hypophosphatemia has been reported to be present in 50% of hospitalized alcoholics.[73] Mild or moderate hypophosphatemia seldom causes recognizable effects.[74]

PATHOPHYSIOLOGY

The causes of hypophosphatemia are many, but can be divided into those associated with phosphate depletion, such as decreased intake or excess renal excretion; those associated with transcellular shifts, resulting in a redistribution of phosphate; or a combination of both[70] (Table 48–14). Patients with moderate hypophosphatemia generally lack significant symptomatology. Although the causes of severe hypophosphatemia are relatively few, these conditions are frequently encountered in patients in the acute care setting and can be associated with life-threatening symptoms.

Phosphate-binding substances such as sucralfate, calcium carbonate, and aluminum/magnesium-containing

TABLE 48–14. Conditions Causing Hypophosphatemia

Inadequate Phosphate Intake
Starvation
Diet deficiency
Malabsorption
Vitamin D deficiency
Vomiting
Gastrectomy
Phosphate-binding drugs
Sucralfate
Antacids
Calcium salts
Intracellular Phosphate Shift
Respiratory alkalosis
Hyperalimentation
Nutritional recovery syndrome
Rapid tumor growth
Exogenous administration of insulin, glucose, epinephrine
Increased Phosphate Excretion
Recovery from severe burns
Glucagon
Diuretics
Volume expansion
Hypomagnesemia
Hyperparathyroidism
Hypothermia
Diabetic ketoacidosis
Acute gout
Renal tubular defects
Aldosteronism
Alcohol withdrawal
May be associated with severe hypophosphatemia

antacids have the potential to bind large amounts of phosphorus in the gut. If phosphate-binding agents are ingested on a chronic basis in conjunction with a dietary phosphorus deficiency, hypophosphatemia may result.[71,74] Patients who are receiving long-term phosphate-binding agents, those with peptic ulcer disease or chronic renal failure, and those who may already possess moderate hypophosphatemia (alcoholics) are at highest risk for the development of severe hypophosphatemia.

The healing process associated with recovery from extensive third-degree burns is associated with a marked diuretic phase. This marked diuresis may be associated with an impressive loss of phosphate through the urine.[71,74] This recovery may also be associated with the development of an anabolic state as stress levels decrease and nutritional therapies take effect. Phosphorus is rapidly taken up by the new cells and this may also result in severe hypophosphatemia.

Rapid refeeding of malnourished patients with high-carbohydrate, high-calorie nutritional diets with inadequate amounts of supplemental phosphorus may result in severe symptomatic hypophosphatemia. This phenomenon is especially significant in patients with other underlying risk factors for the development of hypophosphatemia such as alcoholism.[76] The etiology of severe hypophosphatemia associated with hyperalimentation and nutritional recovery may be separated into two phases: acute, rapid hypophosphatemia secondary to intracellular shifts of phosphorus resulting from glucose-induced insulin secretion; and the gradual decrease in serum phosphorus concentration over 5 to 10 days secondary to tissue repair in the presence of phosphorus deprivation.[72] The development of severe hypophosphatemia secondary to hyperalimentation can be prevented by the administration of 12 to 15 mmol of phosphorus per liter of hyperalimentation solution or 15 mmol per 1000 calories of dextrose administered.[76]

Severe and prolonged respiratory alkalosis may cause profound hypophosphatemia.[71] The mechanism of hypophosphatemia associated with respiratory alkalosis is thought to be secondary to intracellular shifts of phosphorus. Respiratory alkalosis is thought to contribute significantly to the hypophosphatemia observed during alcohol withdrawal.

Patients with diabetic ketoacidosis may present with hyperphosphatemia. With the institution of therapy, however, serum phosphorus levels may rapidly drop as phosphorus shifts back into the intracellular compartment. As the acidosis associated with the diabetic ketoacidotic state causes decomposition of organic compounds inside the cell, inorganic phosphorus is released into the plasma and subsequently excreted into the urine.[72] The combination of intracellular phosphorus breakdown and the shift of phosphorus into cells on initiation of treatment may cause severe hypophosphatemia.

Chronic ethanol abusers are prone to a variety of serum electrolyte disorders including hypocalcemia, hypomagnesemia, hypokalemia, and hypophosphatemia. The etiology of hypophosphatemia in the alcoholic patient is multifactorial. Malnutrition, poor dietary intake, diarrhea, vomiting, and the use of phosphate-binding antacids may contribute to the hypophosphatemia of alcoholism.[72,77] In addition, serum phosphorus levels may decrease after hospitalization in the alcoholic patient with the institution of dextrose-containing IV fluids, as a result of an intracellular shift of phosphorus.[77] Hyperventilation associated with the alcohol withdrawal syndrome may also contribute to the development of hypophosphatemia in the alcoholic patient.[74] Alcoholic patients are particularly susceptible to the complications of hypophosphatemia such as rhabdomyolysis, which is often seen during withdrawal or refeeding.[74,77] Because this complication can be prevented by the administration of phosphorus, serum phosphorus concentrations should routinely be monitored in alcoholic patients.

Clinical Presentation

The clinical manifestations of severe hypophosphatemia are diverse and may affect many major organ systems (Table 48–15). It is likely that two primary biochemical abnormalities are responsible for most of the clinical manifestations of severe hypophosphatemia.[70] First, intracellular energy stores may be decreased secondary to depletion of intracellular ATP, which in itself is dependent on inorganic intracellular phosphate. Second, reduced RBC 2,3-diphosphoglycerate levels are associated with a shift to the left of the oxyhemoglobin saturation curve. This shift to the left is associated with a decrease in the release of oxygen to peripheral tissues and may result in tissue hypoxia.[74] These metabolic disorders can be seen in a wide variety of organ systems.

CNS manifestations of severe hypophosphatemia result in a metabolic encephalopathy syndrome.[72] This progressive syndrome of irritability, apprehension, weakness,

TABLE 48–15. Manifestations of Severe Hypophosphatemia

Central Nervous System	**Gastrointestinal**
Irritability	Anorexia
Apprehension	Nausea
Weakness	Emesis
Numbness	**Skeletal and musclar**
Paresthesias	Weakness
Dysarthria	Myalgia
Confusion	Rhabdomyolysis
Obtundation	Osteomalacia
Seizures	**Hematologic**
Coma	Decreased RBC 2,3-diphosphoglycerate
Pulmonary	Hemolysis
Acute respiratory failure	WBC dysfunction
Slow weaning from ventilator	Platelet dysfunction
Respiratory muscle fatigue	**Renal**
Cardiac	Acute tubular necrosis if myoglobinemia and rhabdomyolysis are present
Congestive cardiomyopathy	Bicarbonate and glucose wasting
Decreased contractility	
Hepatic	
Exacerbation of underlying hepatic insufficiency	
Hepatocellular dysfunction	

numbness, paresthesias, dysarthria, confusion, obtundation, seizures, and coma has been described in patients with severe hypophosphatemia secondary to parenteral nutrition lacking phosphorus.[71,73,74]

Severe hypophosphatemia may result in significant dysfunction of skeletal muscle ranging from myalgia and weakness, with chronic hypophosphatemia, to potentially fatal rhabdomyolysis, with severe, acute hypophosphatemia.[73] Hypophosphatemia has resulted in acute respiratory failure secondary to respiratory muscle weakness and diaphragmatic contractile dysfunction.[53,71] Correction of hypophosphatemia restores diaphragmatic contractility.[71] Close assessment of serum phosphorus concentration is thus indicated in patients at risk for respiratory failure. Treatment of hypophosphatemia in respiratory failure patients may aid in successful weaning from the ventilator.

Cardiac muscle function has also been reported to be impaired in the setting of hypophosphatemia and has resulted in congestive cardiomyopathy.[73] Hypophosphatemia is a potentially reversible cause of heart failure and thus should be considered in patients who experience an acute deterioration in ventricular function.

The hematologic abnormalities of hypophosphatemia constitute a major manifestation of the syndrome.[70] RBC manifestations of hypophosphatemia include decreased levels of 2,3-diphosphoglycerate, decreased RBC ATP, and RBC membrane rigidity.[74] When RBC ATP decreases to below 15% of normal, cells become spherocytic and rigid and are trapped and destroyed in the spleen.[71–73] Therefore, hemolysis may be a manifestation of severe hypophosphatemia.

Reduction in ATP content of white blood cells (WBC) may cause dysfunction of white blood cell mobility, chemotaxis, phagocytosis, and bacteria-killing ability.[73,74] WBC dysfunction may contribute to an increased risk of infection in hypophosphatemic patients.[73] Animal studies have demonstrated thrombocytopenia, shortened platelet survival time, and alteration of clot retraction as manifestations of platelet dysfunction in the setting of hypophosphatemia.[71,73] The implications of hypophosphatemia on human platelet function, however, have not been determined.

▶ TREATMENT: Hypophosphatemia

DESIRED OUTCOME

Treatment is guided by the presence or absence of symptoms and the severity of hypophosphatemia. The goals of therapy are the reversal of signs and symptoms of hypophosphatemia, return to normal serum phosphorus levels, and management of underlying causative conditions. Awareness of the clinical situations in which hypophosphatemia may be anticipated (alcoholism, diabetic ketoacidosis, glucose infusion) is of vital importance in preventing iatrogenic hypophosphatemia. Frequent serum phosphorus determinations should be made in patients at risk. The routine addition of phosphorus in concentrations of 12 to 15 mmol/L of IV hyperalimentation solution is of utmost importance for the prevention of severe hypophosphatemia, which may be associated with the administration of phosphorus-free hyperalimentation solutions.

PHARMACOLOGIC THERAPY

Severe symptomatic hypophosphatemia should be treated with parenteral phosphorus replacement. Similar to potassium, estimation of total body phosphorus deficit is extremely difficult because phosphorus is an intracellular element. Recommendations for parenteral phosphorus replacement are varied and based largely on therapeutic experiences with small groups of patients.[78] Response to IV serum phosphorus supplementation is highly variable. The infusion of 9 to 15 mmol of phosphorus (0.15 to 0.25 mmol/kg) over 4 to 12 hours has been shown to be safe and effective treatment for severe hypophosphatemia.[78] Doses of 15 to 30 mmol of phosphorus given over 1 to 3 hours in patients without hypercalcemia have been shown to be safe and effective.[78]

Parenteral phosphorus supplementation is associated with the risks of hyperphosphatemia, metastatic soft tissue deposition of calcium phosphate, hypocalcemia, and hyperkalemia or hypernatremia, depending on the salt employed. Inappropriate administration of large doses of parenteral phosphorus over relatively short time periods has resulted in symptomatic hypocalcemia and soft-tissue calcification.[74] The rate of infusion and choice of initial dosage should therefore be based on severity of hypophosphatemia and presence of symptoms. Patients should be closely monitored with frequent serum phosphorus determinations. Monitoring should also include assessment of serum potassium, calcium, and magnesium concentrations. Therapy with parenteral phosphorus should be undertaken with great caution and at reduced dosage for patients with baseline hypercalcemia or renal dysfunction.[53,73,74,77] Mild to moderate asymptomatic hypophosphatemia can be treated orally by the administration of oral phosphorus salts (Table 48–16). The dose-limiting adverse effect associated with oral phosphorus replacement is the development of an osmotic diarrhea. Patients with moderate hypophosphatemia and concomitant renal dysfunction should receive reduced daily oral doses (i.e., 1 g or approximately 30 mmol of phosphorus) with careful monitoring of serum phosphorus concentration.

TABLE 48–16. Phosphorus Replacement Therapy

Moderate Hyposphospatemia (serum phosphorus 1.0–2.5 mg/dL)
Oral therapy
1.5–2.0 g (50–60 mmol) phosphorus per day, divided into three or four doses
Parenteral therapy
0.15 mmol/kg lean body weight infused in 250–1000 mL D_5W over 12 h; repeat until serum phosphorus > 2 mg/dL
Severe Hypophosphatemia (serum phosphorus < 1 mg/dL)
Parenteral therapy
0.25 mmol/kg lean body weight infused in 250–500 mL D_5W by infusion pump over 4–6 h; repeat until serum phosphorus > 2 mg/dL

CONCLUSIONS

The pharmacist can play an integral part in the management of electrolyte abnormalities and thus improve the patient's outcome. Most important, the pharmacist is responsible for reviewing the patient's medication history and determining if any of the patient's current drug therapy may have contributed to the existing electrolyte abnormalities. The patient's drug therapy should not be assessed in a vacuum. The acute clinical conditions or chronic diseases the patient has can have a great impact on both existing and future drug therapy. The pharmacist should also assume responsibility for new drug therapy recommendations to reduce the risk of developing new electrolyte problems and to optimize the outcome of the current management plan.

Pharmacists in ambulatory settings may identify existing or potential drug-related electrolyte abnormalities and then suggest dosage adjustments or new drug therapies when appropriate. It is hoped that this proactive interventional approach will facilitate the management of mild disorders in the community and reduce the need for hospitalization. It is critical that the pharmacist be aware of the signs and symptoms of electrolyte problems that patients may have. Pharmacists should attempt to ascertain the presence of mild symptoms due to electrolyte problems in those patients at high risk (e.g., the elderly or the renally impaired).

▶ PRINCIPLES OF PHARMACOTHERAPY

- The rate of correction of hyponatremia should not exceed a change in serum sodium of 12 mEq/L per day to avoid the development of the osmotic demyelination syndrome.
- Idiogenic osmoles are formed in the brain during chronic hypernatremia and can lead to cerebral edema if the hypernatremia is corrected too quickly. The rate should not exceed 15 mEq/L in the first 24 hours.
- When treating electrolyte disorders, patients should be monitored frequently for improvement in signs and symptoms related to the disorder and to ECF volume status.
- Electrolyte concentrations should be monitored frequently to assess therapy and to avoid the development of other electrolyte disorders during treatment.
- Intravenous calcium is a direct antagonist of the adverse cardiac effects of both hyperkalemia and hypermagnesemia.
- In patients with hypokalemia, it is prudent to check a serum magnesium level since concomitant hypomagnesemia is an often overlooked cause of hypokalemia.
- The most common cause of hypercalcemia in hospitalized patients is cancer and in outpatients it is primary hyperparathyroidism.
- Intravenous calcium should be infused at a rate no greater than 60 mg of elemental calcium per minute.
- The development of severe hypophosphatemia secondary to hyperalimentation can be prevented by the addition of 12 to 15 mmol/L TPN.
- Acid-base status can have a profound effect on serum potassium and ionized calcium levels.

REFERENCES

1. Abraham WT, Schrier RW. Renal sodium excretion, edematous disorders and diuretic use. In: Schrier RW, ed. Renal and Electrolyte Disorders, 5th ed. Philadelphia, Lippincott-Raven, 1997:72–129.
2. Systeme international (SI) units conversion table for common laboratory tests. Ann Pharmacother 1996;30:96–103.
3. Mulloy AL, Caruana RJ. Hyponatremic emergencies. Med Clin North Am 1995;79:155–168.
4. Arieff AI. Management of hyponatraemia. Br Med J 1993;307:305–308.
5. Fried LF, Palevsky PM. Hyponatremia and hypernatremia. Med Clin North Am 1997;81:585–609.
6. Narins RG, Jones RE, Stom MC, et al. Diagnostic strategies and disorders of fluid, electrolyte and acid base homeostasis. Am J Med 1982;72:498–504.
7. Oh MS, Carroll HJ. Disorders of sodium metabolism: Hypernatremia and hyponatremia. Crit Care Med 1992;20:94–103.
8. Avner ED. Clinical disorders of water metabolism: Hyponatremia and hypernatremia. Pediatr Ann 1995;24:23–30.
9. Berl T, Schrier RW. Disorders of water metabolism. In: Schier RW, ed. Renal and Electrolyte Disorders, 5th ed. Philadelphia, Lippincott-Raven, 1997:1–71.
10. Rault RM. Case report: Hyponatremia associated with nonsteroidal antiinflammatory drugs. Am J Med Sci 1993;305:318–320.
11. Devita MV, Michelis MF. Perturbations in sodium balance. Hyponatremia and hypernatremia. Clin Lab Med 1993;13:135–148.
12. Soupart A, Decaux G. Therapeutic recommendations for management of severe hyponatremia: Current concepts on pathogenesis and prevention of neurologic complications. Clin Nephrol 1996;46:149–169.
13. Sorensen JB, Andersen MK, Hansen HH. Syndrome of inappropriate secretion of antidiuretic hormone (SIADH) in malignant disease. J Intern Med 1995;238:97–110.
14. Sterns RH. The treatment of hyponatremia: First, do no harm. Am J Med 1990;88:557–560.
15. Cheng JC, Zikos D, Skopicki HA, et al. Long-term neurologic outcome in psychogenic water drinks with severe symptomatic hyponatremia: The effect of rapid correction. Am J Med 1990;88:561–566.
16. Robertson GL. Diabetes insipidus. Endocrinol Metab Clin North Am 1995;24:549–571.
17. Rose BD. Clinical Physiology of Acid–Base and Electrolyte Disorders, 4th ed. New York, McGraw-Hill, 1994:651–694.
18. Rose BD. Clinical Physiology of Acid–Base and Electrolyte Disorders, 4th ed. New York, McGraw-Hill, 1994:346–378.
19. Peterson LN, Moshe L. Disorders of potassium metabolism. In: Schrier RW, ed. Renal and Electrolyte Disorders, 5th ed. Philadelphia, Lippincott-Raven, 1997:192–240.
20. Freedman BI, Burkart JM. Hypokalemia. Crit Care Clin 1991;7:143–153.
21. Innerarity SA. Hyperkalemic emergencies. Crit Care Nurs Q 1992;14:32–39.
22. Williams ME. Hyperkalemia. Crit Care Clin 1991;7:155–174.

23. Clark BA, Brown RS. Potassium homeostasis and hyperkalemic syndromes. Endocrinol Metab Clin North Am 1995;24:573–591.
24. Mandal AK. Hypokalemia and hyperkalemia. Med Clin North Am 1997;81:611–639.
25. Krishna GG. Hypokalemic states: Current clinical issues. Semin Nephrol. 1990;10:515–524.
26. DeAngelis R, Lessig ML. Hypokalemia. Crit Care Nurs 1991;11: 71–75.
27. Isaac G, Holland OB. Drug-induced hypokalemia. Drugs Aging 1992; 2:35–41.
28. Saggar-Malik AK, Cappuccio FP. Potassium supplements and potassium-sparing diuretics: A review and guide to appropriate use. Drugs 1993;46:986–1008.
29. Weiner ID, Wingo CS. Hypokalemia—consequences, causes, and correction. J Am Soc Nephrol 1997;8:1179–1188.
30. Kruse JA, Carlson RW. Rapid correction of hypokalemia. Using concentrated intravenous potassium chloride infusions. Arch Intern Med 1990;150:613–617.
31. Latta K, Hisano S, Chan JCM. Perturbations in potassium balance. Clin Lab Med 1993;13:149–156.
32. Perazella MA, Mahnensmith RL. Hyperkalemia in the elderly drugs exacerbate impaired potassium homeostasis. J Gen Intern Med 1997; 12:646–656.
33. Walmsley RN, White GH, Cain M, et al. Hyperkalemia in the elderly. Clin Chem 1984;30:1409–1412.
34. Wrenn KD, Slovis CM, Slovis BS. The ability of physicians to predict hyperkalemia from the ECG. Ann Emerg Med 1991;20: 1229–1232.
35. Reber PM, Heath H III. Hypocalcemic emergencies. Med Clin North Am 1995;79:93–106.
36. Nussbaum SR. Pathophysiology and management of severe hypercalcemia. Endocrinol Metab Clin North Am 1993;22:343–362.
37. Zaloga GP. Hypocalcemia in critically ill patients. Crit Care Med 1992;20:251–262.
38. Bajorunas DR. Clinical manifestations of cancer-related hypercalcemia. Semin Oncol 1990;17(suppl 5):16–25.
39. Potts JT. Hyperparathyroidism and other hypercalcemic disorders. Adv Intern Med 1996;41:165–212.
40. Rude RK. Hyperparathyroidism. Otolaryngol Clin North Am 1996; 29:663–679.
41. Chisholm MA, Mulloy AL, Taylor AT. Acute management of cancer-related hypercalcemia. Ann Pharmacother 1996;30:507–513.
42. Hall TG, Burns Schaiff RA. Update on the medical treatment of hypercalcemia of malignancy. Clin Pharm 1993;12:117–125.
43. Agus ZS, Wasserstein A, Goldfarb S. Disorders of calcium and magnesium homeostasis. Am J Med 1982;72:473–488.
44. Deftos LJ. Hypercalcemia, mechansims, differential diagnosis, and remedies. Postgrad Med. 1996;100:119–126.
45. Mundy GR, Guise TA. Hypercalcemia of malignancy. Am J Med 1997;103:134–145.
46. Ritch PS. Treatment of cancer-related hypercalcemia. Semin Oncol 1990;17(suppl 5):26–33.
47. Barri YM, Knochel JP. Hypercalcemia and electrolyte disturbances in malignancy. Hemat Oncol Clin North Am 1996;10:775–790.
48. Watters J, Gerrard G, Dodwell D. The management of malignant hypercalcemia. Drugs 1996;52:837–848.
49. Edelson GW, Kleerekoper M. Hypercalcemic crisis. Med Clin North Am 1995;79:79–92.
50. Juan D. Hypocalcemia: Differential diagnosis and mechanisms. Arch Intern Med 1979;139:1166–1171.
51. Fouser L, Disorders of calcium, phosphorus and magnesium. Pediatr Ann. 1995;24:38–46.
52. Lebowitz MR, Moses AM. Hypocalcemia. Semin Nephrol 1992;12: 146–158.
53. Baratta Yucha C, Toto KH. Calcium and phosphorus derangements. Crit Care Nurs Clin North Am 1994;6:747–766.
54. Tohme JF, Bilezikian JP. Hypocalcemic emergencies. Endocrinol Metab Clin North Am 1993;22:363–375.
55. Toto KH, Baratta Yucha C. Magnesium homeostasis, imbalances, and therapeutic uses. Crit Care Nurs Clin North Am 1994;6:767–783.
56. Van Hook JW. Endocrine crises. Hypermagnesemia. Crit Care Clin 1991;7:215–223.
57. Alfrey AC. Normal and abnormal magnesium metabolism. In: Schrier RW, ed. Renal and Electrolyte Disorders, 5th ed. Philadelphia, Lippincott-Raven, 1997:320–348.
58. Whang R, Ryder KW. Frequency of hypomagnesemia and hypermagnesemia. JAMA 1990;263:3063–3064.
59. Wong ET, Rude RK, Singer FR, et al. A high prevalence of hypomagnesemia and hypermagnesemia in hospitalized patients. Am J Clin Pathol 1983;79:348–352.
60. Rude RK, Singer FR. Magnesium deficiency and excess. Annu Rev Med 1981;32:245–259.
61. Clark BA, Brown RS. Unsuspected morbid hypermagnesemia in elderly patients. Am J Nephrol 1992;12:336–343.
62. Mordes JP, Waker WC. Excess magnesium. Pharmacol Rev 1978;29: 273–300.
63. Abbott LG, Rude RK. Clinical manifestations of magnesium deficiency. Miner Electrolyte Metab 1993;19:314–322.
64. Nadler JL, Rude RK. Disorders of magnesium metabolism. Endocrinol Metab Clin North Am 1995;24:623–641.
65. Al-Ghamdi SM, Cameron EC, Sutton RA. Magnesium deficiency: Pathophysiologic and clinical overview. Am J Kidney Dis 1994; 4:737–752.
66. Kobrin SM, Goldfarb S. Magnesium deficiency. Semin Nephrol 1990;10:525–535.
67. Tso EL, Barish RA. Magnesium: Clinical considerations. J Emerg Med 1992;10:735–745.
68. Whang R, Hampton EM, Whang DD. Magnesium homeostasis and clinical disorders of magnesium deficiency. Ann Pharmacother 1994; 28:220–225.
69. Berkelhammer C, Benir RA. A clinical approach to common electrolyte problems. 4. Hypomagnesemia. Can Med Assoc J 1985;1321: 360–368.
70. Stoff JS. Phosphate homeostasis and hypophosphatemia. Am J Med 1982;72:489–495.
71. Peppers MP, Geheb M, Desai T. Hypophosphatemia and hyperphosphatemia. Crit Care Clin 1991;7:201–214.
72. Knochel JP. The pathophysiology and clinical characteristics of severe hypophosphatemia. Arch Intern Med 1977;137:203–220.
73. Rubin MR, Narins RG. Hypophosphatemia: Pathophysiological and practical aspects of its therapy. Semin Nephrol 1990;10:536–545.
74. Bourke E, Yanagawa N. Assessment of hyperphosphatemia and hypophosphatemia. Clin Lab Med 1993;13:183–207.
75. Kebler R, McDonald FD, Cadnapaphornchai P. Dynamic changes in serum phosphorus levels in diabetic ketoacidosis. Am J Med 1985;79:571–576.
76. Silvis SE, DiBartolomeo AG, Aaker HM. Hypophosphatemia and neurological changes secondary to oral caloric intake. Am J Gastroenterol 1980;73:215–222.
77. Hoggson SF, Hurley DL. Acquired hypophosphatemia. Endocrinol Metab Clin North Am 1993;22:397–409.
78. Perreault MM, Ostrop NJ, Tierney MG. Efficacy and safety of intravenous phosphate replacement in critically ill patients. Ann Pharmacother 1997;31:683–688.

49

ACID–BASE DISORDERS

Robert A. Kilroy, PharmD, BCPS, and Gary R. Matzke, PharmD, FCP, FCCP

Acid–base disorders are common and often serious problems that may result in significant morbidity and mortality. This chapter reviews the mechanisms responsible for the maintenance of acid–base balance and the laboratory analyses that aid clinicians in their assessment of acid–base disorders. The pathophysiology of the four most common acid–base disorders is presented, the therapeutic options are critiqued, and guidelines for assessment of the achievement of the desired therapeutic outcomes are presented. Since many drugs affect acid–base homeostasis and many acid–base abnormalities are potentially preventable, pharmacists may have a positive impact on patient outcomes. The pharmacist's responsibility includes anticipation of drug-related problems, avoidance or minimization of clinical consequences, and the design of appropriate treatment regimens. To provide this level of pharmaceutical care, one must have an understanding of the physiology of respiratory and metabolic acid–base regulation.

ACID–BASE DISTURBANCES

Primary alterations in pH may be metabolic or respiratory in origin. Metabolic acid–base disturbances result from processes that alter pH primarily by changing the plasma bicarbonate concentration (HCO_3^-). Respiratory acid–base disturbances result from primary changes in the arterial carbon dioxide tension ($Paco_2$). Changes in pH resulting from these metabolic and respiratory disturbances are dictated by the $HCO_3^-/Paco_2$ ratio.[1]

Nomograms such as the one shown in Figure 49–1 can be used to differentiate between the various acid–base disorders.[2,3] In this nomogram, each pathologic acid–base disorder, together with the appropriate range of *in vivo* physiologic compensation, is represented as a shaded band. Acid–base values—serum bicarbonate, pH, and carbon dioxide tension—falling within a band usually represent a single disturbance; however, a combination of two or more acid–base disorders—a mixed disturbance—may occasionally present in this way. Acid–base values falling outside any band almost certainly represent a mixed acid–base disturbance.[2]

ACID–BASE CHEMISTRY AND PHYSIOLOGY

An acid is a substance that can donate hydrogen ions, H^+. A base is a substance that can accept hydrogen ions, for example,

$$HCl \rightarrow H^+ + Cl^- \text{ (acid)}$$

$$NH_3 + H^+ \rightarrow NH_4^+ \text{ (base)}$$

The acid–base pairs commonly encountered in the body are listed in Table 49–1. A substance capable of accepting and donating hydrogen ions is a buffer. Buffering refers to the ability of a solution containing a weak acid and its anion (a base) to resist a change in pH upon addition of a strong acid or base. The principal extracellular buffer system used by the body is the carbonic acid/bicarbonate (H_2CO_3/HCO_3^-) system. Other buffers include phosphate, hemoglobin, and protein.

The acidity of body fluids is quantified in terms of the hydrogen ion concentration. By convention, the degree of acidity is expressed as pH, or the negative logarithm (base 10) of the hydrogen ion concentration. Hydrogen ion concentration and pH are inversely related. Normally, the pH of blood is maintained at 7.40 (H^+ concentration of 4×10^{-8}) with a range of 7.35 to 7.45. A pH of less than 6.7 (H^+ concentration of 2×10^{-7} represents a fivefold increase) or greater than 7.7 (H^+ concentration of 2×10^{-8} represents a 50% decrease) is considered incompatible with life. Thus, the body tolerates an acidotic state far better than alkalotic.

The hydrogen ion concentration in blood may not be indicative of that in other areas of the body. For example, the pH within cells, within cerebrospinal fluid, and on the surface of bone may all be altered without causing an alteration in blood pH.[1] The blood pH is critically important in determining acid–base status within the body and in diagnosing acid–base disorders. The relationship between pH, pK (the negative logarithm of the dissociation constant for the acid–base buffer pair), and the concentration of the acid [acid] and the base [base] is described by the Henderson–Hasselbach equation:

$$pH = pK + \log(\text{base}/\text{acid})$$

BUFFERS

Because the bicarbonate buffer system is the body's most abundant and measurable buffer, bicarbonate and carbonic acid are most commonly used to assess acid–base status. Because there is abundant carbonic anhydrase in blood, one can assume that equilibrium conditions always apply. The equation describing the dissociation of carbonic acid is thus:

$$H^+ + HCO_3^- \overset{K}{\rightarrow} H_2CO_3 \quad (1)$$

carbonic anhydrase

$$[H^+] = K \times [H_2CO_3]/[HCO_3^-] \quad (2)$$

where K is the dissociation constant for the buffer system.

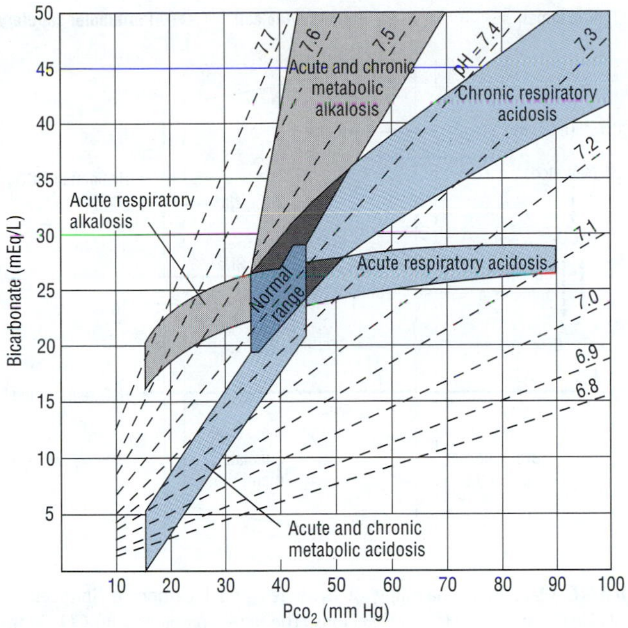

FIGURE 49–1. Acid–base nomogram. *(Reprinted from Ref. 2, with permission.)*

The concentration of carbonic acid (H_2CO_3) is directly proportional to the amount of CO_2 dissolved in blood, which is directly proportional to the partial pressure of CO_2 gas, P_{CO_2}, and the solubility of CO_2 in physiologic fluids. The dissolved CO_2, ($P_{CO_2} \times 0.03$), can be substituted into Eq. (2) because it is more readily measurable than carbonic acid. Taking the negative logarithm of each term along with substitution of the appropriate value for the dissociation constant of the bicarbonate buffer system, the resultant equation is:

$$pH = 6.1 + \log [HCO_3^-/(0.03 \times P_{CO_2})] \quad (3)$$

Thus, hydrogen ion concentration and pH are determined not by the absolute amounts of bicarbonate and P_{CO_2}, but by their ratio.[1] Under normal physiologic conditions, the kidneys maintain the serum bicarbonate at about 24 mEq/L while the lungs control the P_{CO_2} at approximately 40 mm Hg. The normal physiologic pH is, thus, 7.40.

$$HCO_3^- = 24 \text{ mEq/L}$$

$$P_{CO_2} = 40 \text{ mm Hg}$$

$$pH = 6.1 + \log [24/(0.03 \times 40)]$$

$$= 6.1 + 1.3 = 7.4$$

If the P_{CO_2} were acutely increased to 60 as the result of a hypoventilatory state such as pulmonary edema or bronchospasm, the pH would decrease:

$$pH = 6.1 + \log [24/(0.03 \times 60)]$$

$$= 6.1 + 1.12 = 7.22$$

Cellular metabolism of neutral dietary and tissue components results in the production of hydrogen ions and fixed acid anions, both of which need to be excreted to maintain acid–base balance. Small amounts of acid and alkali are presented as such to the body through the diet. On the average, 0.8 mEq/kg/d or 50 to 100 mEq of acid is consumed as part of a normal balanced diet.[4] Digestion of dietary substances and tissue metabolism also result in the production of nonvolatile acids. These acids are derived primarily from the sulfur-containing amino acids, cysteine and methionine, as well as from ingested sulfur. In addition, phosphate is produced from metabolism of proteins and phospholipids. Neutral substances such as glucose are metabolized to intermediates, lactic and pyruvic acids, with the production of hydrogen ion. These intermediates are then metabolized to H_2O and CO_2. Other organic anions, such as citrate and acetoacetate, are also metabolized to CO_2. When respiratory function is normal, the blood CO_2 concentration remains constant, and the amount of CO_2 produced metabolically is equal to the amount lost by respiration. The average adult produces 13,000 to 15,000 mmol of CO_2 each day from the catabolism of carbohydrate, protein, and fat.[5]

Three mechanisms collectively maintain acid–base balance: extracellular buffering, renal regulation of hydrogen ion and bicarbonate excretion, and ventilatory regulation of carbon dioxide elimination. Extracellular buffering is the body's first and fastest defense against an increase in hydrogen ion concentration. The body's buffering system can be broken down into three components: bicarbonate/carbonic acid, proteins, and phosphates. The bicarbonate buffer is the most important of the body's buffers, because (1) there is more bicarbonate present in the extracellular fluid (ECF) than any other buffer component, (2) the supply of carbon dioxide is unlimited, and (3) the acidity of ECF can be regulated by controlling either the bicarbonate concentration or the P_{CO_2}.

EXTRACELLULAR BUFFERING

Carbonic acid represents the respiratory component of the buffer pair because its concentration is directly proportional to the partial pressure of CO_2 (P_{CO_2}), which is determined by ventilation. Bicarbonate represents the metabolic component because the kidney may alter its concentration by reabsorption, generating new bicarbonate, or elimination.[3] The bicarbonate buffer system easily adapts to changes in acid–base status by alterations in ventilatory elimination of acid (P_{CO_2}) and/or renal elimination of base (HCO_3^-).

The phosphate buffer system consists of serum inorganic phosphate (3.5 to 5.0 mg/dL), intracellular organic

TABLE 49–1. Acid–Base Pairs

Carbonic acid/bicarbonate	H_2CO_3 / HCO_3^-
Monobasic/dibasic phosphate	H_2PO_4 / HPO_4^-
Ammonium/ammonia	NH_4^+ / NH_3
Lactic acid/lactate	$H_6C_3O_2$ / $H_5C_3O_2^-$

phosphate, and calcium phosphate in bone. Extracellular phosphate is present only in low concentrations so that its usefulness as a buffer is limited; however, as an intracellular buffer, phosphate is more useful. Calcium phosphate in bone is relatively inaccessible as a buffer, but prolonged metabolic acidosis will result in the release of phosphate from bone.

Intracellular and extracellular proteins also act as buffering systems. The charged side chains of amino acids provide the buffering action. Because the concentration of protein is much greater intracellularly than extracellularly, protein is much more important as an intracellular buffer.

RESPIRATORY REGULATION

The second mechanism of acid–base balance is ventilation. Both the rate and depth of ventilation can be varied to allow for excretion of CO_2 generated by diet and tissue metabolism. Medullary chemoreceptors sense changes in P_{CO_2} or in pH and subsequently alter ventilation. This system rapidly adjusts, within minutes, to changes in acid–base balance so that ventilation can be altered.[5]

RENAL REGULATION

The final and slowest mechanism by which the body maintains acid–base balance is via the renal excretion of acid, reabsorption of filtered HCO_3^-, and generation of new HCO_3^- to replace that which was lost as the result of gastrointestinal disease or secondary to the addition of titratable acid (Fig. 49–2) Essentially all of the approximately 4000 mEq of HCO_3^- filtered daily is reabsorbed, primarily in the proximal tubule. The filtered bicarbonate combines with secreted H^+ to form H_2CO_3, which in the presence of carbonic anhydrase is converted to CO_2 and H_2O. The CO_2 is readily reabsorbed from the renal tubule lumen into the cell, where it can combine with H_2O in the presence of carbonic anhydrase to form H_2CO_3. The H_2CO_3 dissociates in the cell into $H^+ + HCO_3^-$. The H^+ can then cross the cell membrane and enter the tubule lumen. If the H^+ combines with hydrogen monophosphate (HPO_4^{-2}) or ammonia, it will be excreted in the urine as $H_2PO_4^-$ or ammonium (NH_4^+). This process accounts for the kidney's ability to regulate acid excretion.[6]

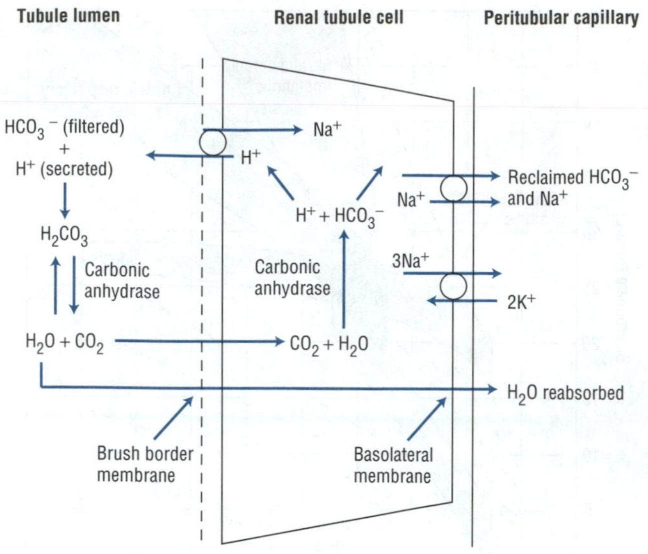

FIGURE 49–2. Renal handling of hydrogen and bicarbonate. Intracellular H_2O dissociates into H^+ and OH^- ions. The latter combines with CO_2 in the presence of carbonic anhydrase to form carbonic acid and then H^+ ion and bicarbonate. The bicarbonate is reabsorbed into the systemic circulation by a Na^+-$3HCO_3^-$ transporter or CL^--HCO_3^- exchanger. Hydrogen ion is secreted into the lumen by the Na^+-H^+ exchanger or H^+-ATPase pump and combines with filtered bicarbonate to form carbonic acid. In the presence of luminal carbonic anhydrase, $CO_2 + H_2O$ are then formed and passively reabsorbed into the tubular cell. Thus, the result of H^+ ion secretion is "reabsorption" of HCO_3^-.

CLINICAL ASSESSMENT OF ACID–BASE STATUS

Arterial blood gases, along with serum electrolytes, physical findings, medical and medication history, and the clinical condition of the patient, are the primary tools to determine the cause of an acid–base disorder and to design a course of therapy.

ARTERIAL BLOOD GASES

Blood gases are measured to determine the patient's oxygenation and acid–base status. Under normal circumstances, there is no clinically significant difference in pH between arterial and mixed venous blood. Arterial samples are designated with the letter "a" (Pa_{O_2} and Pa_{CO_2}), while mixed venous samples are labeled with the letter "v" or not labeled (Pv_{O_2} and Pv_{CO_2}). The normal values for arterial and venous blood gases are shown in Table 49–2. Arterial blood provides the added information of how well the lungs are oxygenating the blood (an accurate measurement of P_{O_2}). Arterial blood rather than venous blood should be used whenever possible because venous blood obtained from an extremity may provide misleading information. If metabolism in the extremity is altered by hypoperfusion, exercise, infection, or some other cause, the differences between arterial and venous blood can be dramatic. Weil and associates[7] reported average mixed venous pH of 7.15 and P_{CO_2} of 74 mm Hg during cardiopulmonary resuscitation, even though the arterial pH was 7.41 and arterial P_{CO_2} was 32 mm Hg. This indicates a severe tissue acidosis from CO_2 accumulation despite adequate arterial blood gases.

TABLE 49–2. Normal Blood Gas Values

	Arterial Blood	Mixed Venous Blood
pH	7.40 (7.35–7.45)	7.38 (7.33–7.43)
P_{O_2}	80–100 mm Hg	35–40 mm Hg
Sa_{O_2}	95%	70%–75%
P_{CO_2}	35–45 mm Hg	45–51 mm Hg
HCO_3^-	22–26 mEq/L	24–28 mEq/L

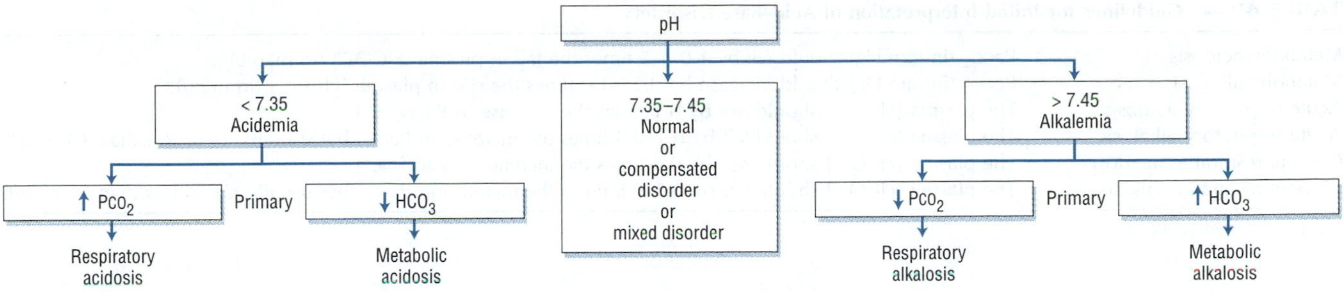

FIGURE 49–3. Analysis of arterial blood gases.

All methods of arterial blood gas analysis are similar and measure pH, PCO_2, and PO_2 of the sample directly. The bicarbonate values and O_2 saturation are calculated. The apparatus for measuring blood gases consists of a pH electrode for measuring the hydrogen ion concentration of the sample, an electrode designed for measuring the partial pressure of carbon dioxide (PCO_2), and an electrode that measures the partial pressure of oxygen (PO_2) in the arterial sample.[8] The temperature of the blood has an effect on pH. For this reason, the analyzer warms the samples to 37°C. Most systems also allow for corrections in temperature when the patient's body temperature differs from 37°C (e.g., during hypothermia for coronary artery bypass).

Clotted samples, samples with air bubbles, and small samples cannot be used to obtain blood gas measurements and should be discarded. Clotted samples may provide misleading information and damage the machinery. Samples that contain air bubbles will also provide distorted blood gas information. Inadequate samples, less than 1 mL, may also provide distorted information because of the concentration of heparin, an acid that is added to anticoagulate the sample.[8]

ANALYSIS OF ARTERIAL BLOOD GAS DATA

Arterial blood gases provide an assessment of the patient's acid–base status. Low pH values (less than 7.35) indicate an acidemia, whereas high pH values (higher than 7.45) indicate an alkalemia (Fig. 49–3). The $PaCO_2$ value helps one to determine if there is a primary respiratory abnormality, whereas the HCO_3^- concentration enables one to ascertain if there is a primary metabolic component.

Acute respiratory acidosis is characterized by an elevated $PaCO_2$, a moderately elevated HCO_3^- concentration (25 to 30 mEq/L), and a decreased pH (see Table 49–3). The renal compensatory response to acute respiratory acidosis is an increase in reabsorption and generation of bicarbonate, leading to a further increase in serum bicarbonate (HCO_3^-) over time. Although buffering occurs almost immediately, the renal response to conserve bicarbonate does not exert a noticeable influence for 12 to 24 hours and requires several days to reach maximal compensation. Acute respiratory alkalosis is characterized by a decreased $PaCO_2$, a decreased HCO_3^- concentration, and an increased pH. The renal compensatory response is increased renal bicarbonate excretion, ultimately leading to an additional decrease in serum bicarbonate (HCO_3^-).

An examination of the bicarbonate concentration helps to determine if there is a primary metabolic abnormality. The two conditions that occur with altered bicarbonate concentration are metabolic acidosis and metabolic alkalosis. Metabolic acidosis is characterized by a decrease in serum bicarbonate concentration (see Fig. 49–2). The body's compensatory response is to increase ventilation, leading to a decrease in $PaCO_2$. Metabolic alkalosis is characterized by an increase in serum bicarbonate concentration; compensatory hypoventilation results in a subsequent increase in $PaCO_2$ (see Table 49–3).

When arterial blood gases differ significantly from those expected on the basis of the patient's clinical condition and previous laboratory determinations, additional venous blood samples should be drawn to assess plasma electrolyte cconcentrations. Then the bicarbonate associated with the patient's $PaCO_2$ and pH can be compared with the bicarbonate value estimated from the total CO_2 content (the amount of CO_2 gas extractable from plasma, consisting of HCO_3^-, H_2CO_3, and $PaCO_2$). Ordinarily, the bicarbonate estimated from the pH and $PaCO_2$ are approximately 1.0 to 2.0 mEq/L less than total CO_2 content.[9] If these values are not

TABLE 49–3. Interpretation of Simple Acid–Base Disorders

Acid–Base Disorder	pH	Primary Disturbances	Compensation
Acidosis			
Respiratory	Decrease	Increase $PaCO_2$	Increase HCO_3^-
Metabolic	Decrease	Decrease HCO_3^-	Decrease $PaCO_2$
Alkalosis			
Respiratory	Increase	Decrease $PaCO_2$	Decrease HCO_3^-
Metabolic	Increase	Increase HCO_3^-	Increase $PaCO_2$

TABLE 49–4. Guidelines for Initial Interpretation of Acid–Base Disorders

Metabolic acidosis	Pa_{CO_2} (in mm Hg) should fall by 1.0–1.5 times the fall in plasma $[HCO_3^-]$ (in mEq/L)
Metabolic alkalosis	Pa_{CO_2} (in mm Hg) should increase by 0.25–1.0 times the rise in plasma $[HCO_3^-]$ (in mEq/L)
Acute respiratory acidosis	The plasma $[HCO_3^-]$ should rise by 0.1 times the increase in $Pa_{CO_2} \pm 3$
Acute respiratory alkalosis	The plasma $[HCO_3^-]$ should fall by 0.1–0.3 times the increase in Pa_{CO_2} but usually not to less than 18 mEq/L
Chronic respiratory acidosis	The plasma $[HCO_3^-]$ should rise by 0.4 times the increase in $Pa_{CO_2} \pm 4$
Chronic respiratory alkalosis	The plasma $[HCO_3^-]$ should fall by 0.2–0.5 times the increase in Pa_{CO_2} but usually not to less than 14 mEq/L

From Ref. 3, with permission.

similar, the results should be interpreted with caution because the difference may reflect an error in the blood collection or storage of the sample, or in the calibration of the blood-gas analyzer.

Several rules of thumb can provide a clinical framework for the interpretation of acid–base disorders (Table 49–4). These guides along with the patient's medical history, physical examination, and other laboratory data provide a means to assess the acuity of respiratory disorders and aid clinicians in their assessment as to the primary cause of the disorder. It is only when the pathologic cause of the disorder is known that one can determine the most appropriate therapeutic plan for the patient. Although occasionally acid–base disorders can be directly addressed, treatment of the underlying cause is usually the most advantageous approach.

METABOLIC ACID–BASE DISORDERS

The two metabolic acid–base disorders, acidosis and alkalosis, are generated by a primary change in bicarbonate concentration. In metabolic acidosis, bicarbonate is lost or a nonvolatile acid is gained, whereas metabolic alkalosis is characterized by a gain in bicarbonate or a loss of nonvolatile acid.

METABOLIC ACIDOSIS

PATHOPHYSIOLOGY

Metabolic acidosis is characterized by a decrease in pH as the result of a primary decrease in serum bicarbonate concentration. This can result from the buffering (consumption of HCO_3^-) of an organic acid that is added to the ECF (e.g., lactic acid, ketoacids) or the progressive accumulation of endogenous acids secondary to impaired renal function (e.g., phosphates, sulfates).[10] The serum HCO_3^- can also be decreased as the result of a loss of bicarbonate-rich body fluids (as with diarrhea) or occur secondary to the rapid administration of nonbicarbonate solutions (dilutional acidosis).

The serum anion gap (AG) as defined below provides an index as to whether an organic acidosis is present. In the serum, the total concentration of cations must equal the total concentration of anions to maintain electroneutrality. The cation concentration is equal to the sodium concentration plus the unmeasured cations (UCs)—magnesium, calcium, and potassium. The anion concentration is equal to the concentration of chloride and bicarbonate and the unmeasured anions (UAs)—proteins, sulfates, phosphates, and organic acids. Therefore,

$$Na^+ + UCs = (Cl^- + HCO_3^-) + UAs$$

$$\text{Anion gap} = Na^+ - (Cl^- + HCO_3^-) = UAs - UCs$$

Normally the serum AG is about 9 mEq/L (range 3 to 11 mEq/L), which is lower than the 12 mEq/L value used in the past. This downward shift of the normal serum AG range occurred in the early 1990s and is primarily owing to the availability of more sensitive Cl^- measurements.[11] In most clinical situations, a major increase in the anion gap can be equated with accumulation of unmeasured anions in ECF.

These unmeasured anions are generated as the result of the consumption of HCO_3^- by endogenous organic acids such as lactic acid, acetoacetic acid, or β-hydroxybutyric acid or from the ingestion of toxic alcohols such as methanol or ethylene glycol. The degree of elevation in the serum AG is dependent on the clearance of the anion, as well as the multiple factors that influence HCO_3^- concentrations. Thus, the serum AG is a relative rather than an absolute indication of the cause of metabolic acidosis.

Normal anion gap metabolic acidosis occurs when bicarbonate losses from the ECF are replaced by chloride or in cases of dilutional acidosis. This decrease in bicarbonate results from losses from the gastrointestinal tract, dilution of bicarbonate in the ECF space by the addition of sodium chloride solutions, or addition of chloride-containing acids to the ECF, which titrates the bicarbonate and replaces it with chloride. Common causes of metabolic acidosis with an increased anion gap or a normal anion gap are listed in Table 49–5.

NORMAL ANION GAP METABOLIC ACIDOSIS

Gastrointestinal disorders such as diarrhea and pancreatic fistula can result in hyperchloremic metabolic acidosis. Diarrhea is by far the most common cause. Severe diarrhea can lead to a daily loss of 5 to 10 L of fluid, which contains 100 to 140 mEq/L of sodium, 20 to 40 mEq/L of potassium, 80 to 100 mEq/L of chloride, and 30 to 50 mEq/L of bicarbonate.[3] Those patients with diseases of the lower urinary tract who require removal of the bladder and urinary diversion into the sigmoid colon or ileal loop may also de-

TABLE 49–5. Common Causes of Metabolic Acidosis

Increased Anion Gap	Normal Anion Gap/ Hyperchloremic States
Alcoholic ketoacidosis	Acid ingestion (hydrochloric acid or ammonium chloride)
Diabetic ketoacidosis	Carbonic anhydrase inhibitors
Lactic acidosis	Cholestyramine
Renal failure (acute or chronic)	Diarrhea
Methanol ingestion	Dilutional acidosis
Ethylene glycol ingestion	Gastrointestinal disorders
Salicylate overdose	Pancreatic fistula
Starvation	Potassium-sparing diuretic
	Renal tubular acidosis
	Ureterosigmoidostomy, ileostomy

velop a hyperchloremic metabolic acidosis. While urine is retained in the colon or bowel loop, water reabsorption, passive chloride reabsorption, and active bicarbonate secretion occur, resulting in a net loss of bicarbonate.

RENAL TUBULAR ACIDOSIS

Renal tubular acidosis (RTA) refers to a group of disorders that result in a metabolic acidosis with a normal anion gap. The primary defect is the kidney's failure to reabsorb sufficient HCO_3^- or to excrete the daily acid load (reduced net acid excretion [NAE]).

The distal RTAs are the most common and are all characterized by impaired NAE, which is in part caused by impaired ammonium (NH_4^+) excretion. These can be subdivided into those that are associated with hypokalemia (type I) and those associated with hyperkalemia (type IV). Type I patients are unable to secrete a sufficient quantity of H^+ to excrete the necessary daily acid load.[3] This disorder of the collecting duct results in hyperchloremic metabolic acidosis as patients are unable to acidify their urine (i.e., attain urine pH of < 5.5) even in the face of an acid challenge. Type I RTA may be the result of a primary tubule defect or the secondary result of hypercalcemia, multiple myeloma, lupus, renal transplant rejection, or following the administration/ingestion of amphotericin B or toluene. The primary form of this disorder usually occurs in children and can result in severe acidosis, growth retardation, nephrocalcinosis, and kidney stones.[12] Hypokalemia is the result of stimulation of the renin–angiotensin–aldosterone axis due to sodium depletion. Thus, renal potassium losses will decrease considerably when bicarbonate therapy is begun.

Type IV, hyperkalemic RTA may be a result of hypoaldosteronism or a generalized distal tubule defect. The most common form of distal RTA is the hyperkalemic, hyporeninemic, hypoaldosteronism associated with diabetic nephropathy. Urine pHs less than 5.5 can be attained, thus indicating that urinary acidification is normal.[3] The cause of this disorder in some patients is impaired NH_4^+ synthesis owing to hyperkalemia. Those patients with pure primary aldosterone deficiency or complete adrenal insufficiency will present with a similar clinical picture. However, the approach to therapy for these patients is directed toward physiologic replacement of the mineralocorticoid. Generalized distal tubule defects are more common than type I RTA, but less so than type IV disorders caused by hypoaldosteronism. Urinary obstruction is the most frequent cause of this disorder followed by chronic cyclosporine nephrotoxicity, renal transplant rejection, and sickle cell nephropathy.

Type II RTA (proximal RTA) is a result of a defect in proximal tubular reabsorption of bicarbonate. Normally, 85% of the filtered load of bicarbonate is reabsorbed in the proximal tubule. With this defect, bicarbonate is delivered to the distal nephron, which has a limited capacity for bicarbonate reabsorption. Thus, ≥ 15% of the filtered bicarbonate load may be lost in the urine when plasma bicarbonate concentration is normal, resulting in a metabolic acidosis. The bicarbonaturia also leads to hypovolemia and hypokalemia secondary to sodium and potassium losses.[3,12] Although uncommon as a primary disorder, it is usually present in infancy or acquired latter in life as the result of other diseases (amyloidosis, multiple myeloma, or nephrotic syndrome) or exposure to toxins (lead, cadmium, mercury, or outdated tetracyclines).

ELEVATED ANION GAP METABOLIC ACIDOSIS

Metabolic acidosis with an increased anion gap commonly results from increased endogenous acid production, such as lactic acidosis or ketoacidosis secondary to diabetes mellitus, starvation, or alcohol ingestion (see Table 49–5). In uremia, accumulation of organic anions (amino acids, proteins) or sulfate and phosphate is responsible for the increased anion gap, which is usually less than 24 mEq/L.[13] The severe metabolic acidosis seen in myoglobinuric acute renal failure due to rhabdomyolysis may be caused by the metabolism of large amounts of sulfur-containing amino acids released from myoglobin.[14]

The presence of an elevated anion gap cannot be automatically attributed to an increase in organic acids. Up to 47% of hospitalized patients have an elevated AG.[15] Furthermore, a mild to moderate increase in AG (10 to 20 mEq/L) is neither sensitive or specific for detection of acidosis, as evidenced by the finding of an increase in AG in some patients who are alkalotic. The usefulness of the serum AG as a marker of acid–base status is dependent on proper interpretation of a patient's clinical status.[16] Despite these limitations, the diagnosis of an organic acidosis has been shown to be highly likely when the anion gap exceeds 26 mEq/L.[17]

The ratio of the change in AG to change in bicarbonate has been proposed as an additional diagnostic parameter, particularly for mixed acid–base disorders. The ratio is usually 1.0 for the common organic acidosis (diabetic ketoacidosis or lactic acidosis). A value greater than 1.2 suggests either coexistent metabolic alkalosis or compensation for a respiratory acidosis.[10] When the ratio is less than 0.8, one must consider the presence of compensation for a respiratory alkalosis or coexistence of hyperchloremic metabolic acidosis. One must remember that as with the anion gap, the predictive ability of a change in this ratio is relative, not absolute.

LACTIC ACIDOSIS

Lactic acidosis is one of the most common causes of metabolic acidosis. Lactic acid is the end product of anaerobic metabolism of glucose (glycolysis). In normal individuals, lactic acid, derived from pyruvate, enters the circulation in small amounts and is promptly removed by the liver. In the liver, lactic acid is reoxidized to pyruvic acid, which is then metabolized to CO_2 and H_2O. The normal plasma lactate concentration in healthy subjects is approximately 1 mEq/L.[10,18]

Normally, the concentration of lactate in blood is 10 times the concentration of pyruvate (L/P ratio). If pyruvate is elevated (e.g., by increased glucose intake), lactate increases, but the L/P ratio remains unchanged. If anaerobic glycolysis increases (e.g., because of tissue hypoxia) and sufficient oxidized nicotinamide adenine dinucleotide (NAD) is not available to reconvert lactate to pyruvate, lactate will increase more than pyruvate and an increase in L/P ratio will result. This increase in L/P ratio is associated with metabolic acidosis. The principle causes of lactic acidosis are (1) an imbalance of production, for example, inadequate oxygen delivery to cells; (2) the inability of the cells to utilize oxygen[3,19]; or (3) altered elimination of lactate, for example, decreased oxidative metabolism or impaired hepatic clearance.[3]

The diagnosis of lactic acidosis should be considered in all forms of metabolic acidosis associated with an increased anion gap. Lactate concentrations of 4.0 to 5.0 mEq/L or greater with a simultaneous decrease in bicarbonate and arterial pH are highly suggestive of lactic acidosis. Each 1 mEq/L increase in plasma lactate will cause an equivalent decrease in serum bicarbonate.[10,19]

Although two types of lactic acidosis have been recognized, those associated with tissue hypoxia (old classification Type A) and those associated primarily with systemic disorders, which alter metabolism (old classification Type B), the distinction between them is blurred (Table 49–6). Cardiovascular collapse with resultant tissue hypoperfusion is the most common cause of lactic acidosis. Poor tissue perfusion and hypoxia influence enzymatic pyruvate and lactate metabolism to stimulate anaerobic glycolysis and decrease lactate utilization. This leads to hyperlactatemia and lactic acidosis. The mortality rate of this type of lactic acidosis may be as great as 80% and appears to be related to blood lactate concentrations.

Lactic acidosis associated with liver disease, drugs (e.g., metformin), toxins, and congenital enzyme deficiency may be due to deranged oxidative metabolism or impaired lactate clearance.[3] The exact role of diabetes mellitus in the induction of lactic acidosis is not clear. It may involve a decrease in pyruvate dehydrogenase activity, the enzyme responsible for pyruvate metabolism. Lactic acidosis in neoplastic disease is uncommon and reported mostly in patients with myeloproliferative disorders. Leukocytes and neoplastic cells in general have high rates of glycolysis. In the case of a large tumor or tightly packed bone marrow, oxygenation can be decreased, favoring the accumulation of lactate. Lactic acidosis has been reported in patients with massive liver tumors, and it has been postulated that the liver uptake of lactate is decreased in these patients. Lactic acidosis associated with seizures is usually transient and occurs because of excessive muscle activity.[10]

TABLE 49–6. Causes of Lactic Acidosis

Primary decrease in tissue oxygenation
Shock
Severe anemia
Congestive heart failure
Asphyxia
Carbon monoxide poisoning
Deranged oxidative metabolism
Diabetes mellitus
Liver failure
Malignancy
Seizures
Medications (iron, isoniazid, metformin, salicylates)
Methanol, ethanol, ethylene glycol
Disorders associated with inborn errors of metabolism

Metabolic acidosis associated with a high AG is also frequently seen in patients with diabetes mellitus (see Chap. 70), alcoholism (see Chaps. 35 and 63), or voluntary or involuntary abstinence from caloric intake (see Chap. 60). Toxic ingestions of methanol, ethylene glycol, and salicylate also have been associated with the development of high-AG metabolic acidosis (see Chap. 7). The mechanisms responsible for the development of acidosis in these settings are diverse and are discussed in the sections of the text identified above.

CLINICAL PRESENTATION

The most common and major consequences of severe acidosis (blood pH < 7.20) are evident on the cardiovascular, respiratory, and central nervous system (Table 49–7). Hyperventilation is often the first sign of metabolic acidosis. At a pH of 7.2, pulmonary ventilation increases about fourfold and an increase of eightfold has been noted at a pH of 7.0.[20] In extremely severe acidosis (pH < 6.8), CNS function is disrupted to such a degree that the respiratory center is depressed. Respiratory compensation may occur as Kussmaul's respirations—the deep, rapid respirations seen commonly in patients with diabetic ketoacidosis.

CNS depression has been found to correlate more closely with spinal fluid pH than with blood pH. For this reason, neurologic symptoms tend to occur more frequently and to a greater degree in patients with respiratory acidosis,

TABLE 49–7. Major Adverse Consequences of Severe Acidemia

Cardiovascular	
	Impairment of cardiac contractility
	Arteriolar dilatation, venoconstriction
	Increased pulmonary vascular resistance
	Reductions in cardiac output, arterial blood pressure, and hepatic and renal blood flow
	Sensitization to reentrant arrhythmias and reduction in threshold of ventricular fibrillation
	Attenuation of cardiovascular responsiveness to catecholamines
Respiratory	
	Hyperventilation
	Decreased strength of respiratory muscles and promotion of muscle fatigue
	Dyspnea
Metabolic	
	Increased metabolic demands
	Insulin resistance
	Inhibition of anaerobic glycolysis
	Reduction in ATP synthesis
	Hyperkalemia
	Increased protein degradation
Cerebral	
	Inhibition of metabolism and cell-volume regulation
	Obtundation and coma

Adapted from Ref. 18.

because the CO_2 accumulated in the respiratory form readily crosses the blood–brain barrier to cause acidosis in the CNS.[1] Because of the slow penetration of administered bicarbonate into the CNS, the CNS pH fails to normalize as rapidly as blood pH. Therefore, patients continue to hyperventilate because of sustained CNS acidity and severe respiratory alkalosis may occur. Sustained lowering of $Paco_2$ within 12 to 36 hours is to be anticipated during the correction of any metabolic acidosis.[1]

Systemic acidosis can cause peripheral arteriolar dilatation characterized by flushing, a rapid heart rate, and wide pulse pressure. Initially, cardiac output may be increased, but as acidosis becomes more severe, it falls as hypotension becomes more pronounced. Experimental work in animals has demonstrated that cardiac contractility decreases as pH declines to values of 7.0 or less by infusion of lactic acid.[21] In contrast, the effects of vagal stimulation were enhanced at pH levels lower than 7.1, probably as a consequence of inhibition of acetylcholinesterase. This increases the danger of vagally mediated bradycardia or arrest during acidosis.

Gastrointestinal symptoms of metabolic acidosis include loss of appetite, nausea, and vomiting. These symptoms occur commonly in patients with renal insufficiency who experience a mild acidosis.[20] Severe acidosis (pH < 7.1) interferes with carbohydrate metabolism and insulin utilization and results in hyperglycemia. The effect of metabolic acidosis on serum potassium depends on the type of acidosis: The effects of mineral acids (e.g., hydrochloric acid) produce a greater pH decrease than organic acids (e.g., lactic acidosis) and, thereby, result in a greater change in potassium levels.

COMPENSATION

The patient's primary means to compensate for metabolic acidosis is to increase carbon dioxide excretion by increasing respiratory rate. This results in a decrease in $Paco_2$. This ventilatory compensation is initiated as the result of stimulation of the respiratory center owing to the changes in cerebral bicarbonate concentration and pH.[1] Arterial blood compensation begins rapidly (within 15 to 30 minutes) but does not reach a steady state for 12 to 24 hours after the onset of metabolic acidosis. For every 1 mEq/L decrease in bicarbonate concentration below the average of 24, the $Paco_2$ decreases by about 1.0 to 1.5 mm Hg from the normal value of 40 (see Table 49–4).

The anticipated $Paco_2$, associated with a given bicarbonate concentration, for patients with uncomplicated metabolic acidosis can be more precisely calculated as[22]:

$$Paco_2 = [(\{HCO_3^-\} \times 1.5) + 8] \pm (2 \times SEM)$$

Where 1.0 is the standard error of the mean (SEM) of the relationship of HCO_3^- to $Paco_2$. For example, 95% of patients with a plasma bicarbonate of 15 mEq/L should have a total plasma Pco_2 of 28.5 to 32.5 mm Hg. An observed plasma Pco_2 in this range is consistent with a diagnosis of primary metabolic acidosis.

▶ TREATMENT: Metabolic Acidosis

CHRONIC METABOLIC ACIDOSIS

Patients with a plasma bicarbonate of 12 to 20 mEq/L and pHs of 7.2 to 7.4 can usually be managed by gradual correction, over a period of days to weeks, with the oral administration of bicarbonate or a substrate that is metabolized to bicarbonate (Table 49–8). A systemic approach to the management of metabolic acidosis in patients with renal failure is described in Chapter 42.

The management of RTAs should be directed at correcting the underlying cause. However, if this is ineffective or if patients have a primary tubular defect, bicarbonate or a suitable substitute should be administered. Once the acute acidosis is corrected, patients with type I (hypokalemic distal) RTA usually require only enough alkali to buffer the amount of acid generated from dietary intake and metabolism. This usually approximates 1 to 3 mEq/kg/d. Potassium supplementation is usually not necessary, because renal potassium losses decrease when appropriate alkali therapy is instituted.

The loading dose of alkali required in addition to the maintenance to correct the acute acidosis can be calculated as follows[23]:

$$\begin{aligned}\text{Loading dose (mEq)} &= (V_D\ HCO_3^- \times BW)\ (\text{desired } HCO_3^- - \text{patient's } HCO_3^-)\\ &= (0.5\ L/kg \times 60\ kg) \times (24\ mEq/L - 15\ mEq/L)\\ &= 30\ L \times 9\ mEq/L\\ &= 270\ mEq\end{aligned}$$

TABLE 49–8. Therapeutic Alternatives for Oral Alkali Replacement

Generic Name	Trade Name(s)	mEq Alkali	Dosage Form(s)	Comment
Shohl's solution Sodium citrate/citric acid	Bicitra (Willen)	1 mEq Na/mL; equivalent to 1 mEq bicarbonate	Solution (500 mg Na citrate, 334 mg citric acid/5 mL)	Citrate preparations increase absorption of aluminum
Sodium bicarbonate	Various (e.g., Rugby)	3.9 mEq bicarbonate/tablet (325 mg) 7.8 mEq bicarbonate/tablet (650 mg)	325 mg tablet 650 mg tablet	Bicarbonate preparations may cause bloating owing to CO_2 production
	Baking soda (various)	60 mEq bicarbonate/tsp (5 g/tsp)	Powder	
Potassium citrate	Urocit-K (Mission)	5 mEq citrate/tablet	5 mEq tablet	See above
Potassium bicarbonate/potassium citrate	K-Lyte (Bristol) K-Lyte DS (Bristol)	25 mEq bicarbonate/tablet 50 mEq bicarbonate/tablet (DS)	25 mEq tablet (effervescent) 50 mEq tablet (effervescent)	See above
Potassium citrate/citric acid	Polycitra-K (Willen)	2 mEq K/mL; equivalent to 2 mEq bicarbonate 30 mEq bicarbonate/UD packet	Solution (1100 mg K citrate, 334 mg citric acid/5 mL) Crystals for reconstitution (3300 mg K citrate, 1002 mg citric acid/UD packet)	See above
Sodium citrate/potassium citrate/citric acid	Polycitra (Willen) Polycitra-LC (Willen)	1 mEq K, 1 mEq Na/mL; equivalent to 2 mEq bicarbonate	Syrup (Polycitra) Solution (Polycitra-LC) (Both contain 550 mg K citrate, 500 mg Na citrate, 334 mg citric acid/5 mL)	See above

The calculated amount of bicarbonate should be administered over a few days to avoid volume overload owing to the increase in sodium intake. For this scenario, a regimen of 60 to 70 mEq tido for 3 to 5 days should result in an increase in HCO_3^- levels toward normal. Once the HCO_3^- reaches 22 to 24 mEq/L, the dosage can be reduced to meet maintenance needs, which can be approximated to be 2 mEq/kg/d (the mean of the range) or 40 mEq tid.

Type II or proximal RTA is a bicarbonate-wasting disorder that requires the administration of large maintenance doses of alkali (10 to 15 mEq/kg/d). Potassium supplementation is almost always necessary, because the potassium losses are increased during alkali therapy owing to the increase in the amount of bicarbonate excreted. The increased amount of HCO_3^- in the urine is the result of the increase in the fractional excretion of bicarbonate. As a result of the increased urinary loses by bicarbonate, the dose of alkali therapy may need to be increased (up to 25 mEq/kg/d), to avoid growth retardation and osteopenia in children. Since the maintenance alkali requirements are much higher in type II than type I patients, there is usually no need to administer a "loading" dose of alkali to acutely correct the acidosis.[25]

The metabolic acidosis associated with hyperkalemic distal RTA owing to hypoaldosteronism often seen in patients with diabetes mellitus may be corrected by the treatment of hyperkalemia alone (see Chap. 48) or in some cases require the administration of pharmacologic amounts of Florinef®.[3] Type IV RTA owing to a generalized tubular defect or hypoaldosteronism often responds to low doses of alkali (1.5 to 2.0 mEq/kg/d).[24] Corrections of the acidosis along with modest dietary potassium restriction (to 80 mEq/d) will often result in the maintenance of serum potassium levels of 5 mEq/L or less.

ACUTE SEVERE METABOLIC ACIDOSIS

The management plan for patients with life-threatening acute metabolic acidosis—plasma bicarbonate of ≤ 8 mEq/L and pH < 7.20—is dependent on the underlying cause and the patient's cardiovascular status. Effective treatment of the underlying cause of some organic acidoses (e.g., ketoacidosis or lactic acidosis) can result in the regeneration of bicarbonate within hours, thus potentially mitigating the need for alkali therapy. Patients with hyperchloremic acidosis (e.g., diarrhea induced) are unable to regenerate bicarbonate, and the generation of new bicarbonate by the kidneys may require several days before one can observe a meaningful change in their status.[18] Thus, intravenous alkali therapy is often required for these patients.

There are several therapeutic alternatives available for the acute correction of severe metabolic acidosis. Sodium acetate, sodium bicarbonate, and sodium lactate are not reliable sources of alkali because their alkalinizing effect is dependent on their oxidative conversion to bicarbonate. This process is often impaired in critically ill patients, especially those with liver disease or circulatory failure. Although sodium bicarbonate is the most widely used intravenous alkalitic agent,[18] several studies have suggested that it is frequently ineffective and may actually be deleterious, especially in patients with lactic acidosis.[27,28] Two of the three remaining alternatives (carbicarb and dichloroacetate) are investigational and, thus, not routinely available in most clinical practice settings. Tromethamine or THAM is a carbon dioxide–consuming, commercially available solution that buffers respiratory as well as metabolic acids.

SODIUM BICARBONATE

Although it has been recommended that sodium bicarbonate be administered to raise the arterial pH to about 7.15 to 7.20, there are no controlled clinical trials demonstrating that sodium bicarbonate administration is significantly better than general supportive care in reducing morbidity and mortality in these patients.[3,18,29] In theory, sodium bicarbonate administration provides fluid and electrolyte replacement and increases arterial pH, thereby improving cardiac function, perfusion and oxygenation of peripheral tissues, intracellular pH, and therefore lactate metabolism. However, sodium bicarbonate administration can actually have an adverse effect on intracellular pH. When bicarbonate is given by IV infusion, the carbon dioxide generated diffuses more readily than bicarbonate across cell membranes and into cerebrospinal fluid. Therefore, the intracellular pH can actually be decreased by administration of bicarbonate.[3]

Excessive sodium bicarbonate administration may result in (1) a shift of the oxyhemoglobin saturation curve to the left and, thereby, impaired oxygen release from hemoglobin to tissues, (2) sodium and water overload with subsequent hypernatremia and hyperosmolality, (3) paradoxical acidosis as a result of the production of CO_2 that freely diffuses into myocardial and cerebral cells,[30] and (4) decreased ionized calcium with resultant decreased myocardial contractility. If there is an endogenous source of bicarbonate, such as can occur in the case of ketoacidosis or lactic acidosis, a bicarbonate "overshoot" may develop because the ketoacids (acetoacetic acid and β-hydroxybutyric acid) or lactic acid are converted in the liver to bicarbonate once the underlying cause of acidosis is corrected.[18,31] Alkalosis may also result if too much is given too fast.[18]

If intravenous sodium bicarbonate is to be used, one must be mindful that the goals are to increase not normalize pH (to approximately 7.20) and plasma bicarbonate (to 8 to 10 mEq/L). There is no calculative method that will assure attainment of these goals with a given dose of sodium bicarbonate because of the multiplicity of competing processes that can affect acid–base status (vomiting, potential increases in endogenous acid production, renal failure) and the marked variability in the distribution volume of biacarbonate (50% of BW in patients with mild acidosis to approximately 100% in those with severe acidosis).[23] Adrogue and Madias[18] have recently recommended that the dose of sodium bicarbonate be calculated using a distribution volume of 50% of BW for all patients to avoid overtreatment. The total dose calculated as described previously in the RTA section should be administered as an infusion over one-half to several hours. Follow-up monitoring of ABGs beginning no sooner than 30 minutes after the end of the infusion should be used to guide further therapeutic decisions.

Bicarbonate therapy is generally not necessary in the routine patient with cardiac arrest, even if the initial arrest was unmonitored. The standards and guidelines from the National Conference on Cardiopulmonary and Emergency Cardiac Care state that sodium bicarbonate is most useful in cardiac life support when combined with ventilation in an attempt to maintain near-normal arterial pH during an arrest.[32] During a cardiac arrest, sodium bicarbonate (initial dose 1 mEq/kg) may be administered by rapid, direct intravenous injection. It should be used only after more proven interventions such as defibrillation, cardiac compression, support of ventilation including intubation, and drug therapies such as epinephrine and antiarrhythmic agents have been employed. Subsequent doses of sodium bicarbonate should be based on measurements of arterial blood pH and $Paco_2$.

TROMETHAMINE

Tromethamine (THAM) available as a 0.3 N solution, is a highly alkaline, sodium-free organic amine that acts as a proton acceptor to prevent or correct acidosis.[33] Tromethamine combines with hydrogen ions from carbonic acid to form bicarbonate and a cationic buffer. THAM also acts as an osmotic diuretic to increase urine flow, urine pH, and the excretion of fixed acids, CO^2, and electrolytes. At pH 7.4, 30% of THAM is not ionized and therefore is capable of reaching equilibrium with total body water. This portion may penetrate into cells and may neutralize acidic anions of the intracellular fluid. Intracellular pH increases have been noted within 1 hour after the infusion of THAM. There is, however, no clinical or physiologic evidence that this action is beneficial or that THAM is more efficacious than sodium bicarbonate.[18,26]

When THAM is used, it must be administered slowly and with careful monitoring to avoid alkalosis. The usual empiric dosage range for tromethamine is 1 to 5 mmol/kg administered intravenously during 1 hour, but doses up to 1.25 mmol/kg may be given over 5 to 15 minutes in acute situations. The dose of THAM can be individualized using the following equation[33]:

$$\text{Dose of 0.3 N THAM (in mL)} = 1.1 \times \text{BW (in kg)} \times (\text{normal } HCO_3^- - \text{patient's } HCO_3^-)$$

The need for additional THAM is determined by serial measurements of the serum bicarbonate concentration and calculation of the base deficit: normal HCO_3^- minus patient's HCO_3^-. Large doses may cause respiratory depression because of a decrease in ventilation secondary to an increase in blood pH and decrease in $Paco_2$ concentration.[26] Tromethamine solution is highly alkaline and may cause severe inflammation, vascular spasm, or tissue damage (necrosis, sloughing, pain, chemical phlebitis, thrombosis) if infiltration occurs. Hyperkalemia, hypoglycemia, hypocalcemia, and impaired coagulation have also been reported.[26,34] This agent should be used with extreme caution in patients with severe liver or kidney failure.

CARBICARB

Carbicarb is an equimolar mixture of sodium carbonate (Na_2CO_3) and sodium bicarbonate ($NaHCO_3$).[35,36] It is no longer commercially available in Canada, and its use in the United States is still investigational. The carbonate ion is a stronger base than is bicarbonate and, thus, preferentially buffers hydrogen ions. The result of this reaction is the formation of bicarbonate rather than CO_2. Thus, carbicarb limits but does not eliminate the generation of CO_2. Unlike bicarbonate, which can result in paradoxical intracellular acidosis and thereby impairment of cardiac function, carbicarb appears to correct intracellular acidosis if present.[37,38] In a prospective, double-blind, randomized, multicenter trial, Leung and colleagues[35] compared carbicarb versus sodium bicarbonate in surgical patients with mild intraoperative metabolic acidosis. Carbicarb proved as effective as sodium bicarbonate in correcting mild metabolic acidosis. Furthermore, cardiac output increased with carbicarb as compared to sodium bicarbonate. Carbicarb also appears to be beneficial in the management of lactic acidosis.[37]

Although the optimal dosage of carbicarb has not been determined, it can be approximated as[35]:

$$\text{Dose (in mEq of Na)} = 0.2 \text{ L/kg} \times \text{BW (in kg)} \times (\text{base deficit})$$

The risk of hypervolemia and hypertonicity after carbicarb administration is similar to that of bicarbonate. The small number of trials reporting the clinical utility of this agent and its continued investigational status in most of the world will obviously limit its use/availability for the foreseeable future.

DICHLOROACETATE

Dichloroacetate (DCA), another investigational agent, has been shown to significantly lower serum lactate levels and increase blood pH in patients with lactic acidosis.[39,40] DCA facilitates aerobic lactate metabolism by stimulating the activity of lactate dehydrogenase, reverses hyperlactatemia, and decreases morbidity in acquired and congenital forms of lactic acidosis. In a randomized, multicenter, placebo-controlled trial, Stacpoole et al.[39] studied the effects of DCA (50 to 100 mg/kg) in 252 patients with lactic acidosis. Serum lactate was significantly lowered and blood pH increased, but there was no improvement in patient outcome compared to conventional management. A subsequent study in patients undergoing liver transplantation demonstrated that DCA attenuated lactate acid accumulation and reduced the need for bicarbonate therapy in this high-risk patient population.[28] The drug also improves cardiac output and left ventricular mechanical efficiency under conditions of myocardial ischemia or failure, probably by facilitating myocardial glucose utilization and inhibiting gluconeogenesis. DCA administration has also been reported to reverse the abnormal glucose metabolism, branch chain amino acid utilization, and muscle catabolism in septic patients.[41] DCA can cause a reversible peripheral neuropathy that may be ameliorated or prevented with thiamine supplementation. Mild drowsiness has been reported in approximately half of the adult recipients, but no other drug-related adverse effects have been reported.[39] The future role of DCA in the management of metabolic acidosis, particularly lactic acidosis, remains to be clarified. For the present, its use is limited by its investigational status.

METABOLIC ALKALOSIS

Metabolic alkalosis is a primary acid–base disorder that is evident as alkalemia (increased arterial pH) and a increase in plasma bicarbonate. It is an extremely common entity that has been observed in 33% to 51% of hospitalized patients with acid–base disturbances.[42,43] The generation of an elevation in plasma HCO_3^- may be the result of renal or extrarenal processes. Extrarenal processes include (1) net loss of hydrogen ion from the extracellular fluid, that is H^+ loss via the gastrointestinal tract that exceeds the daily H^+ generation from diet or metabolism; (2) excessive gain of bicarbonate, which may be the result of oral or parenteral intake of bicarbonate or a bicarbonate presursor such as lactate, acetate, or citrate or the metabolism of other endogenous organic anions to bicarbonate; or (3) the extrarenal loss of chloride-rich, bicarbonate-poor fluids which often leads to volume depletion.[3]

The three factors that often function synergistically within the kidney to increase plasma bicarbonate as the result of an increase in urinary acid excretion are (1) high distal delivery of sodium, (2) mineralcorticoid excess, and (3) potassium deficiency.[44]

PATHOPHYSIOLOGY

INITIATION

Disturbances that initiate metabolic alkalosis can be divided into two categories on the basis of their response to treatment with saline volume expansion. Those categories are sodium chloride–responsive disorders and sodium chloride–resistant disorders (Table 49–9). The most common initiating event for metabolic alkalosis is the loss of chloride-rich, bicarbonate-poor fluid from the body as seen with diuretic use, nasogastric suctioning, or vomiting. Gastric secretory volume is usually less than 50 mL/h in the basal state but may increase fivefold with stimulation. One or more liters of gastric fluid may be lost daily with persistent vomiting. The 24-hour gastric juice output in a 70-kg adult includes 1 to 2 L of fluid that contains 40 to 160 mEq of sodium, 10 mEq of potassium, 200 mEq of chloride, and 25 to 100 mEq of hydrogen ion. Hydrogen ion and bicarbonate are formed from CO_2 and water by gastric parietal cells.[45] The hydrogen ion is secreted into gastric fluid and the bicarbonate is retained in the ECF. Normally, an amount of bicarbonate equal to the bicarbonate generated in the stomach is eliminated in the alkaline pancreatic and small bowel secretions, maintaining hydrogen ion balance. With vomiting and nasogastric suctioning, hydrogen ion is lost externally. Bicarbonate is not eliminated and metabolic alkalosis results.

Diuretic therapy, with agents acting on the cortical and medullary ascending limb of the loop of Henle (e.g., furosemide, bumetamide, and torsemide) and distal convoluted tubule (thiazides), is a common cause of metabolic alkalosis. These agents promote the excretion of sodium and potassium almost exclusively in association with chloride without a proportionate increase in bicarbonate excretion. Net acid excretion is also frequently increased during the diuresis because of both the disproportionate loss of

TABLE 49–9. Courses of Metabolic Alkalosis Differentiated on the Basis of Their Responsiveness to Sodium Chloride

Sodium chloride responsive (urinary chloride concentration < 10 mEq/L)
Gastrointestinal disorders
Vomiting
Gastric drainage
Villous adenoma of the colon
Chloride diarrhea
Diuretic therapy
Correction of chronic hypercapnia
Cystic fibrosis
Excessive bicarbonate therapy of an organic acidosis
Mild/moderate potassium deficiency
Sodium chloride resistant (urinary chloride concentration > 20 mEq/L)
Excess mineralocorticoid activity
Hyperaldosteronism
Cushing's syndrome
Bartter's syndrome
Gitelman's syndrome
Excessive black licorice intake
Profound potassium depletion
Magnesium deficiency
Liddle's syndrome
Unclassified
Alkali administration
Milk–alkali syndrome
Massive blood or plasmanate transfusion
Nonparathyroid hypercalcemia
Carbohydrate refeeding after starvation
Large doses of penicillin

chloride and the loss of hydrogen ion in the urine by increasing tubular flow and sodium delivery to the distal tubule for sodium–hydrogen exchange. Patients at greatest risk from metabolic alkalosis are those with volume depletion, in which the distal tubule and collecting duct exchange sites are stimulated to reabsorb sodium; those on a low-salt diet, which limits the sodium chloride available for reabsorption; and those on diuretics, which continue to deliver sodium to the distal exchange site. Alkalosis caused by diuretic use is usually mild, but the accompanying hypokalemia may be serious. Hypokalemia may also increase net acid excretion by increasing generation of ammonium (NH_4^+).

Metabolic alkalosis resistant to sodium chloride administration is often associated with excess mineralocorticoid activity. Increased mineralocorticoid activity may result from (1) primary adrenal overproduction, as in primary hyperaldosteronism; (2) oversecretion of mineralocorticoid secondary to increased renin activity; or (3) up-regulation of renal mineralocorticoid receptors, secondary to chronic glycyrrhizic acid ingestion, a major component of black licorice.[46] Subjects who ingest about 100 g of licorice per day can develop this reversible syndrome. Mineralocorticoids act on the distal segment of the renal tubule, where they increase sodium reabsorption and enhance secretion of potassium and hydrogen ion into the tubular lumen. For example, in hyperaldosteronism, an increase in aldosterone leads to stimulation of the distal renal tubular secretion of hydrogen by several mechanisms, some of which are linked to sodium reabsorption and potassium secretion. The increased hydrogen ion secreted into the renal tubule causes the generation of new bicarbonate or the reclamation of filtered bicarbonate.[20]

Miscellaneous causes of metabolic alkalosis include large doses of penicillins (e.g., ticarcillin) because they act as a nonreabsorbable anion. High concentrations of the poorly reabsorbable anion in the distal renal tubule result in an increased flow rate and electrical negativity within the tubular lumen. These changes enhance the secretion of potassium and hydrogen ion and result in increased plasma bicarbonate concentration and hypokalemia.

MAINTENANCE

No matter which condition initiated the metabolic alkalosis, the kidney is responsible for its maintenance. Normally, the kidneys are capable of excreting all of the excess bicarbonate presented to them, even during periods of increased bicarbonate loads.[3] The kidney senses changes in the plasma bicarbonate concentration, and if the tubular fluid HCO_3^- concentration exceeds its threshold, proximal reabsorption decreases and the excess HCO_3^- is excreted in the urine. If the kidneys are working properly, excess bicarbonate will rapidly be excreted and metabolic alkalosis will not occur, or will be corrected in a matter of hours.[45]

Several mechanisms tend to increase bicarbonate reabsorption by the kidney, thereby maintaining a metabolic alkalosis.[44] The combination of decreased ECF volume, hypochloremia, and hypokalemia associated with diuretic use or nasogastric suction can maintain a metabolic alkalosis by increasing the tubular HCO_3^- threshold.[3,45] During periods of decreased ECF volume, sodium reabsorption is enhanced in the proximal and distal tubules. Sodium reabsorption from the renal tubule must be associated with a negatively charged ion, such as chloride, or it must be exchanged for an ion in the tubular cell that has a positive charge, such as potassium or hydrogen. In hypochloremia, there is less chloride available for reabsorption and therefore more sodium must be exchanged for potassium or hydrogen. Only a small amount of potassium is available for exchange with sodium, and when the patient becomes hypokalemic, hydrogen is exchanged instead. This loss of hydrogen ions results in hypochloremic metabolic alkalosis.

Metabolic alkalosis may also be maintained by persistent hypokalemia, independent of hypovolemia. Hypokalemic metabolic alkalosis is frequently associated with excess mineralocorticoid activity since mineralocorticoids promote sodium reabsorption and enhance potassium and hydrogen ion excretion in the urine.[45]

Clinical Presentation

There are no unique signs or symptoms associated with mild to moderate metabolic alkalosis, but patients may complain of symptoms related to the underlying cause of the disorder (e.g., muscle weakness with hypokalemia or postural dizziness with volume depletion). They may have a history of vomiting, gastric drainage, or diuretic use, all of which contribute to the development of metabolic alkalosis. Severe alkalemia (blood pH > 7.60) has been associated with cardiac arrhythmias, particularly in those with heart disease, respiratory depression, and hypoventilation.[47] Neuromuscular irritability may be present, with signs of tetany or hyperactive reflexes possibly caused by the decreased ionized calcium concentration that occurs secondary to the increase in pH. This decrease in ionized calcium may be caused by a conformational change in the albumin molecules, to which the calcium is bound, resulting in increased binding, or by decreased competition from hydrogen ions for binding sites on the albumin molecule. Mental confusion, muscle cramping, and paresthesia may also occur.

COMPENSATION

The immediate response to elevated bicarbonate is chemical buffering. This buffering involves the movement of hydrogen ions from within the cells to the ECF in exchange for potassium and sodium. This system is immediate in onset but limited in its capacity to protect the body from sudden life-threatening changes in extracellular pH.

The second phase of the body's response to metabolic alkalosis is respiratory compensation (hypoventilation to raise the Pa_{CO_2}). Using the Henderson–Hasselbach equation, one can see that an increase in the Pa_{CO_2} will return the Pa_{CO_2}/bicarbonate ratio, and therefore the pH, toward normal. Respiratory compensation is initiated when the central and peripheral chemoreceptors sense an increase in pH and occurs within hours. The Pa_{CO_2} increases 6 to 7 mm Hg for each 10 mEq/L increase in bicarbonate, up to a Pa_{CO_2} of about 50 to 60 mm Hg (see Table 49–4) before hypoxia sensors react to prevent further hypoventilation. If the Pa_{CO_2} is normal or less than normal, one should consider the presence of a superimposed respiratory alkalosis, which may be secondary to fever, gram-negative sepsis, or pain.

▶ TREATMENT: Metabolic Alkalosis

Treatment should be aimed at correcting the factor responsible for the maintenance of the alkalosis. If the factors responsible for the generation of the alkalosis are unresolved, interventional efforts should also focus on reducing or correcting them. For example, vomiting should be treated with antiemetics, gastric losses of H^+ may be modulated by giving histamine blockers such as ranitidine, and diuretic therapy may need to be curtailed or dosages reduced.[44,47] Metabolic alkalosis may persist until the renal mechanism responsible for maintaining the disorder is corrected, despite the fact that the original cause of the elevated plasma bicarbonate may have subsided. For example, hypovolemia should be treated with sodium chloride (i.e., diuretic abuse, nasogastric suction) to allow excretion of bicarbonate by the kidney. However, patients with severely compromised cardiovascular function may not be able to tolerate this therapeutic approach. In situations such as this and/or the presence of life-threatening alkalosis, some have advocated reduction in pH by control of ventilation.[3] Although controlled hypoventilation, sometimes using inspired CO_2 and supplemental oxygen to prevent hypoxia, may be lifesaving,[3] this approach is not universally accepted.[44,47] Therapy for metabolic alkalosis can be conceptualized on the basis of the sodium chloride responsiveness of the disorders (Fig. 49–4).

SODIUM CHLORIDE–RESPONSIVE DISORDERS

Sodium chloride–responsive disorders usually result from volume depletion and chloride loss, which may accompany severe vomiting or nasogastric suction. Initially, therapy is directed at expanding intravascular volume and replenishing chloride stores. Sodium chloride and potassium solutions should be administered to patients who can tolerate the administration of fluid and sodium.[44,47] Patients with a metabolic alkalosis who are volume expanded or intolerant to sodium volume loads, as in congestive heart failure, may benefit from the carbonic anhydrase inhibitor acetazolamide. This agent inhibits the action of carbonic anhydrase in the kidney tubule cell, inhibits renal bicarbonate reabsorption, and results in a decreased concentration of bicarbonate in the ECF. Unfortunately, it also increases the renal losses of potassium and phosphate. Administration of acetazolamide (250

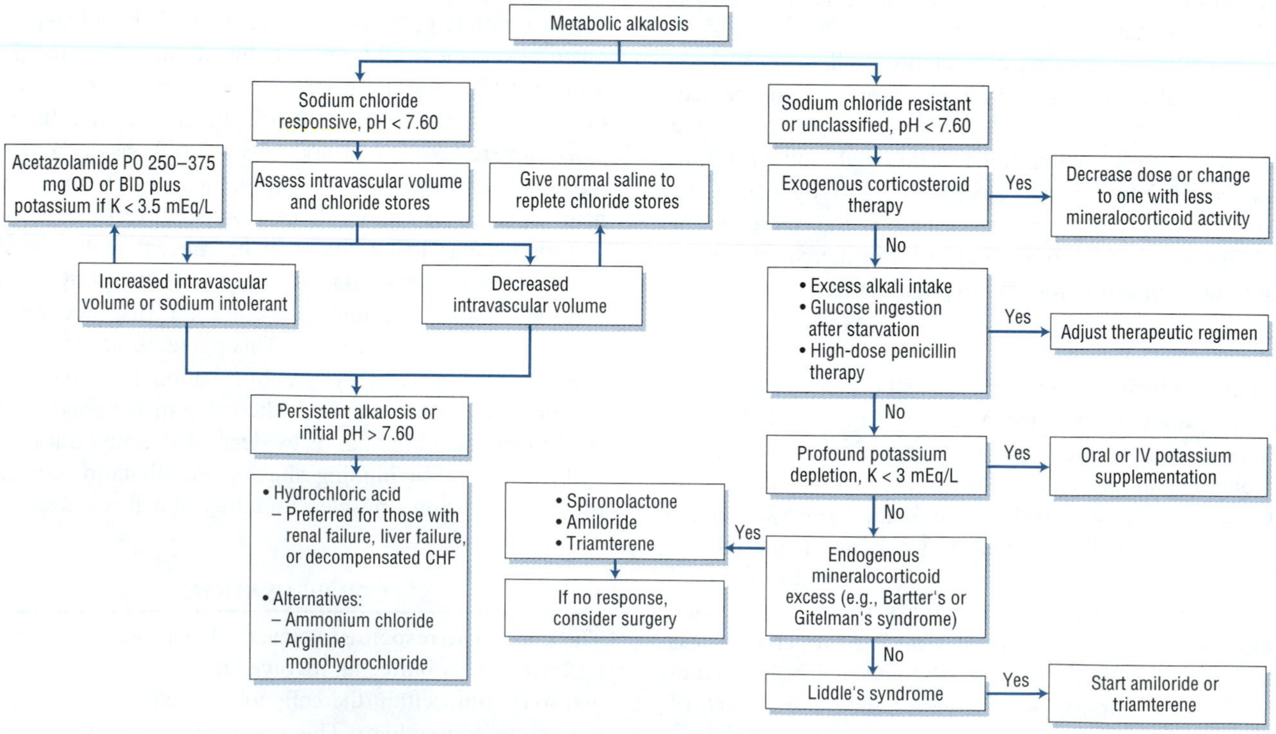

FIGURE 49–4. Treatment algorithm for patients with primary metabolic alkalosis.

to 375 mg once or twice daily) may promote a sufficient bicarbonate diuresis and return the pH toward normal. However, since the clinical effectiveness of the drug declines as the HCO_3^- concentration falls, only rarely will this approach fully correct the alkalosis.[44]

Other agents sometimes used to treat sodium chloride–responsive metabolic alkalosis include hydrochloric acid, ammonium chloride (20 g/L provides 374 mEq hydrogen/L), and arginine monohydrochloride (100 g/L provides 475 mEq hydrogen/L). Indications for the use of hydrochloric acid include severe metabolic alkalosis (pH > 7.60), symptoms of alkali toxicity unresponsive to fluid and electrolyte administration, and the patient's inability to tolerate a large sodium and fluid load (as in decompensated CHF or renal failure with oliguria).[44,47] The dose of hydrochloric acid may be based on an estimate of the chloride deficit[33]:

$$\text{Dose HCl (mEq)} = [0.2 \text{ L/kg} \times \text{BW (kg)}]\,[103 - \text{observed serum chloride}]$$

where the estimated chloride space is 0.2 times the body weight (BW) and the average serum chloride is 103 mEq/L, or base deficit[47]:

$$\text{Dose HCL (mEq)} = [0.5 \text{ L/kg} \times \text{BW (kg)}]\,[(\text{desired } HCO_3^-) - (\text{observed } HCO_3^-)]$$

At present, there are no comparative data that address the relative accuracy of these two formulas to determine the dose of acid. The dose of hydrochloric acid is usually infused intravenously over 12 to 24 hours. Improvement is usually seen within 24 hours of initiating therapy. Arterial blood gases and serum electrolytes should be drawn every 4 to 12 hours to evaluate and adjust therapy. If the Pa_{CO_2} is markedly elevated because of respiratory compensation, the estimated dose of hydrochloric acid should be infused over at least 24 hours.[48] Otherwise, a severe transient respiratory acidosis may occur because of the slower reduction of the elevated bicarbonate concentration in the cerebrospinal fluid than in the extracellular fluid.

Hydrochloric acid is usually infused intravenously via a large central vein as a 0.1 to 0.25 N HCl solution in either 5% dextrose or normal saline, although sterile water has also been used. Extemporaneously prepared solutions can be made by adding 100 to 250 mEq of HCl through a 0.22-mm filter into a glass container of saline or dextrose. Hydrochloric acid may also be added to parenteral nutrient solutions and administered via a central line without serious degradation of proteins.[49] The rate of infusion should be 100 to 125 mL/h (10 to 25 mEq/h), with frequent monitoring of arterial blood gases. The infusion should be stopped when the arterial pH falls to 7.50, to prevent overcorrection.[45]

Ammonium chloride has a limited role in the treatment of metabolic alkalosis. Ammonium chloride is converted by the liver to urea and free hydrochloric acid[33]:

$$2NH_4^+ + 2Cl^- + 2HCO_3^- \rightarrow CO(NH_2)_2 + CO_2 + 3H_2O + 2Cl^-$$

The dose of ammonium chloride can be calculated on the basis of the chloride deficit using the same method as for HCl, but only half of the calculated dose of ammonium chloride should be administered to avoid ammonia toxicity. Ammonium chloride is available as a 26.75% solution containing 100 mEq in 20 mL, which should be further diluted prior to administration. A dilute solution may be prepared by adding 100 mEq of ammonium chloride to 500 mL of normal saline and infusing it at a rate not exceeding 1 mEq/min. Improvement in metabolic status is usually seen within 24 hours of ammonium chloride administration. CNS toxicity, marked by confusion, irritability, seizures, and coma, has been associated with faster rates of administration. It must be administered cautiously to patients with renal or hepatic impairment, because serum ammonia and urea levels may increase. This may lead to encephalopathy in patients with hepatic dysfunction because of impaired conversion of ammonia to urea, and for patients with renal impairment, it may worsen their uremia.[33]

Arginine monohydrochloride at a dose of 10 g/h given intravenously has been used to treat metabolic alkalosis, although it was never FDA-approved for this purpose.[33] Although some have stated that it was taken off the market because of the risk of severe hyperkalemia,[44] it is still commercially available. Like ammonium chloride, arginine must undergo metabolism by the liver to produce hydrogen ions. Unlike ammonium chloride, arginine combines with ammonia in the body to synthesize urea; thus, it may be used in patients with relative hepatic insufficiency. Patients with renal insufficiency should not receive arginine monohydrochloride because it may significantly elevate blood urea nitrogen and has been associated with severe hyperkalemia.[33,34] The increase in potassium is caused by arginine-induced shifts of potassium from the intracellular to the extracellular space.

In patients with metabolic alkalosis caused by nasogastric suction, histamine H_2-receptor antagonists and omeprazole have been used to decrease the volume and hydrogen ion content in gastric fluids. Standard doses of H_2 antagonists produce a marked reduction in volume of gastric aspirate acid production, which has resulted in a significantly decreased H^+ loss during nasogastric suctioning.[50,51]

SODIUM CHLORIDE–RESISTANT DISORDERS

Sodium chloride–resistant disorders are commonly associated with hypermineralocorticoidism and are characterized by plasma volume expansion, hypertension, and a high urinary chloride concentration. Life-threatening alkalemia is a very rare occurrence with these disorders. Their management usually consists of oral regimens, which may be acute or chronic in duration. Chronic therapy is indicated when the underlying cause of the mineralocorticoid excess cannot be corrected. Acute treatment of these disorders involves the removal of the source of excess mineralocorticoid activity. Patients who are taking corticosteroids may require a dosage reduction or may need to be switched to a corticosteroid with less mineralocorticoid activity. Patients with an endogenous source of excess mineralocorticoid activity may require surgery. This can be chronically accomplished for some patients pharmacologically by administering spironalactone, amiloride, or triamterene.[44,47]

Spironolactone limits distal tubule hydrogen secretion and thereby decreases plasma pH as the result of its inhibition of aldosterone-stimulated sodium reabsorption and blockade of aldosterone's direct effect on the hydrogen ion secretory pump. Thus, most patients with mineralocorticoid excess including Bartter's or Gitelman's syndrome respond to this therapy. The sodium channel blockers amiloride and triamterene are effective in these patients, as well as in those with Liddle's syndrome. This disorder is not a result of mineralocorticoid excess but rather is caused by overactivity of the distal tubule sodium channel.[44,52] Although experience is limited, some patients with Bartter's or Gitelman's syndrome may respond to nonsteroidal anti-inflammatory agents or angiotensin-converting enzyme inhibitors.[53,54] Finally, aggressive potassium repletion may correct the alkalosis in those who have not responded to the approaches outlined above.

RESPIRATORY ACID–BASE DISORDERS

There are two types of simple respiratory acid–base disturbances: acidosis and alkalosis. These disorders are generated by a primary alteration in carbon dioxide excretion, which changes the concentration of carbon dioxide and, therefore, the carbonic acid concentration in body fluids. A primary reduction in $Paco_2$ causes a rise in pH (respiratory alkalosis), and a primary increase in $Paco_2$ causes a decrease in pH (respiratory acidosis).

RESPIRATORY ALKALOSIS

Respiratory alkalosis is characterized by a primary decrease in $Paco_2$ that leads to an elevation in pH. The $Paco_2$ falls if the excretion of CO_2 by the lungs exceeds the production of CO_2 by metabolic process. It is the most frequently encountered acid–base disorder, occurring in normal pregnancy and in persons living at high altitudes. Respiratory alkalosis also occurs frequently among hospitalized patients (Table 49–10). In the critically ill patient, this is a bad prognostic sign, since mortality increases in direct proportion to the degree of hypocapnia.[47] Though respiratory alkalosis occurs in a significant number of critically ill patients, treatment of the alkalosis itself has not been shown to produce a change in mortality.

PATHOPHYSIOLOGY

A decrease in $Paco_2$ occurs when ventilatory excretion exceeds metabolic production. Since endogenous production of CO_2 is relatively constant, a negative CO_2 balance is primarily caused by an increase in ventilatory excretion of CO_2 (hyperventilation). The metabolic production of CO_2, however, may be increased during periods of stress or excess carbohydrate administration (e.g., parenteral nutrition). Hyperventilation may develop from an increase in neurochemical stimulation via a central or peripheral mechanism or be the result of physical increase in ventilation either voluntarily or artificially by means of mechanical ventilation.

A decrease in $Paco_2$ may occur in patients with cardiogenic, hypovolemic, or septic shock since oxygen delivery to the carotid and aortic chemoreceptors is reduced. This relative deficit in Pao_2 stimulates an increase in ventilation. Hyperventilation-induced respiratory alkalosis with an elevation in cardiac index and hypotension without peripheral vasoconstriction may therefore be an early sign of sepsis.

TABLE 49–10. Causes of Respiratory Alkalosis

Central stimulation of respiration
Anxiety
Pain
Fever
Brain tumors, vascular accidents
Head trauma
Pregnancy
Progesterone
Catecholamines, theophylline, nicotine
Salicylates
Peripheral stimulation of respiration
Pulmonary emboli
Congestive heart failure
Altitude
Asthma
Pulmonary shunts
Hypotension
Pneumonia
"Stiff lungs" without hypoxemia
Multiple mechanisms
Hepatic cirrhosis
Gram-negative sepsis
Mechanical or voluntary hyperventilation

CLINICAL PRESENTATION

Respiratory alkalosis may cause adverse neuromuscular, cardiovascular, and gastrointestinal effects. During periods of decreased $Paco_2$, there is a decrease in cerebral blood flow, which may be responsible for symptoms of lightheadedness, confusion, decreased intellectual functioning, syncope, and seizures. Nausea and vomiting may occur, probably as a result of cerebral hypoxia. In severe respiratory alkalosis, cardiac arrhythmias may occur, owing to sensitization of the myocardium to the arrhythmogenic effects of circulating catecholamines.[5] Acute respiratory alkalosis has no effect on blood pressure or cardiac output in awake individuals. Anesthetized persons, however, may experience a decrease in both cardiac output and blood pressure, possibly owing to the lack of a tachycardic response.[55]

The concentration of serum electrolytes may also be altered secondary to the development of respiratory alkalosis. The serum chloride concentration is usually slightly increased, and serum potassium concentration may be slightly decreased. Clinically significant hypokalemia can be a consequence of extreme respiratory alkalosis, although the effect is usually very small or negligible.[5,55] Serum phosphorus concentration may decrease by as much as 1.5 to 2.0 mg/dL because of the movement of inorganic phosphate into cells. The amount of ionized calcium is reduced in respiratory alkalosis, which may be partially responsible for symptoms such as muscle cramps and tetany. Approximately 50% of calcium is bound to albumin, and an increase in pH results in an increase in binding secondary to conformational changes in the albumin molecule.[55]

COMPENSATION

BUFFERING

The initial response of the body to acute respiratory alkalosis is to chemically buffer the excess bicarbonate. Hydrogen ions are, therefore, released from the body's buffers—intracellular proteins, phosphates, and hemoglobin—to titrate bicarbonate. Buffering is complete within minutes and the effect persists for at least 2 hours. Acutely, the bicarbonate concentration is decreased by a maximum of no more than 3.0 mEq/L for each 10 mm Hg decrease in $Paco_2$[20] (see Table 49–4).

The second, or compensatory, phase of the body's response to the increase in pH occurs when respiratory alkalosis persists for longer than 6 hours. During this stage, the kidneys attempt to compensate for the decrease in the respiratory acid component, $Paco_2$, by increasing bicarbonate elimination. This compensation consists of a decrease in reabsorption of filtered bicarbonate and/or a reduction in the generation of new HCO_3^-. Renal compensation occurs rapidly (hours) and is probably complete within 1 to 2 days. The kidney's bicarbonaturia and increased sodium losses, as well as decreased NH_4^+ and titrable acid excretion, are direct effects of the $Paco_2$ level on renal reabsorption of HCO_3^- or Cl^-.[5] The acuity of the respiratory alkalosis can be assessed on the basis of the degree of renal compensation (see Table 49–4). The bicarbonate concentration can be reduced in chronic situations by 4 mEq/L below 24 for each 10 mm Hg drop in $Paco_2$. For example, a sustained decrease in $Paco_2$ of 20 mm Hg will lower serum bicarbonate from 24 to 14 mEq/L with a resultant pH of 7.46. Bicarbonate concentrations differing from those anticipated using the preceding guidelines suggest a mixed acid–base disorder (refer to Fig. 49–1).

▶ TREATMENT: Respiratory Alkalosis

Because most patients with respiratory alkalosis, especially chronic cases, have few or no symptoms and pH alterations are usually mild (pH not exceeding 7.50), treatment is often not required.[47] The first consideration in the treatment of acute respiratory alkalosis with pH > 7.50 is the identification and correction of the underlying cause. Relief of pain, correction of hypovolemia with volume, treatment of fever or infection, treatment of salicylate overdose, and other direct measures may prove effective. A rebreathing device, such as a paper bag, may be useful in controlling hyperventilation in some patients, particularly those with the anxiety hyperventilation syndrome. Oxygen therapy should be initiated in patients with severe hypoxemia. Patients with life-threatening alkalosis (pH > 7.60) and complications such as arrhythmia or seizures may require mechanical ventilation with or without sedation and paralysis to control hyperventilation. Simple respiratory alkalosis rarely requires such aggressive therapy, but it may be necessary for patients with mixed respiratory and metabolic alkalosis.

Respiratory alkalosis in patients receiving mechanical ventilation is usually iatrogenic. It may often be corrected by decreasing the minute ventilation (i.e., the number of mechanical breaths per minute, times the volume delivered), although other measures can also be employed. The use of a capnograph and spirometer in the breathing circuit enables a more precise adjustment of the ventilator settings. Another method of treating respiratory alkalosis is to increase the amount of dead space in the ventilator circuit. This involves placing a known length of tubing between the artificial airway and the "Y" piece of the ventilator. This results in "rebreathing" of expired gas and, therefore, an increase in the inspired carbon dioxide concentration. This should increase the carbon dioxide tension of the patient and thereby correct the respiratory alkalosis.

RESPIRATORY ACIDOSIS

PATHOPHYSIOLOGY

Respiratory acidosis, a primary retention of carbon dioxide that lowers the pH, results from a failure of the lungs to excrete carbon dioxide secondary to a disorder that restricts ventilation or is the result of ventilation–perfusion inequality (Table 49–11). Acute respiratory acidosis with hypoxemia, hypercarbia, and acidosis is life threatening. Those disorders that produce an increase in $Paco_2$ and hypoxemia to a degree compatible with life (e.g., chronic obstructive pulmonary disease), with or without oxygen therapy, may result in chronic respiratory acidosis (Table 49–12). These patients can function normally without noticeable neurologic defects with $Paco_2$ concentrations in the range of 90 to 100 mm Hg (normal 40 mm Hg), provided adequate oxygenation is maintained.[55]

CLINICAL PRESENTATION

Neuromuscular symptoms include altered mental status, abnormal behavior, seizures, stupor, and coma. Hypercapnia

TABLE 49–11. Causes of Acute Respiratory Acidosis

Perfusion abnormalities
Massive pulmonary embolism
Cardiac arrest
Airway and pulmonary abnormalities
Severe pulmonary edema
Severe pneumonia
Smoke inhalation
Pneumothorax
Severe bronchospasm
Adult respiratory distress syndrome
Airway obstruction: foreign body, laryngeal edema
Aspiration of vomitus
Neuromuscular abnormalities
Trauma, stroke
Narcotic or sedative overdose
Brainstem or cervical cord injury
Guillain-Barré syndrome
Myasthenia gravis
Status epilepticus
Mechanical ventilator
Ventilator malfunction
Inadequate frequency or tidal volume settings
Large dead space
Total parenteral nutrition (increased CO_2 production)

TABLE 49–12. Causes of Chronic Respiratory Acidosis

Neuromuscular abnormalities
Brainstem infarct
Obesity–hypoventilation (Pickwickian) syndrome
Tumors
Poliomyelitis
Multiple sclerosis
Diaphragmatic paralysis
Pulmonary abnormalities
Chronic obstructive pulmonary disease
Kyphoscoliosis
Interstitial pulmonary disease
Overzealous parenteral feeding

may mimic stroke or central nervous system (CNS) tumor by producing headache, papilledema, focal paresis, and abnormal reflexes. Carbon dioxide acts as a vasodilator in the brain, thus causing an increase in cerebral blood flow.[5] This increase in cerebral blood flow is thought to be partially responsible for the CNS symptoms of respiratory acidosis. The CNS response to hypercapnia is extremely variable between patients and is also influenced by the acuity of presentation. Chronic hypercapnia alters the usual respiratory stimulus of increasing $Paco_2$, and the drive for respiration in these patients is hypoxemia rather than hypercapnia.[55]

The degree to which cardiac contractility and heart rate are altered depends on the severity of acidosis, whether metabolic or respiratory, and the rapidity with which acidosis develops. Modest acute hypercapnia ($Paco_2$ of 50 to 55 mm Hg) stimulates a stress-like response, with elevated catecholamines and corticosteroid hormone levels, and can result in increased cardiac output and pulmonary artery pressure.[56] As the severity increases, cardiac output declines and vascular resistance decreases. Refractory hypotension may be present in some patients.[5]

In respiratory acidosis, serum concentrations of sodium and chloride remain normal or increase slightly. The serum potassium concentration increases modestly secondary to cellular shifts. The increases are less than those seen with inorganic metabolic acidosis and are difficult to predict for individual patients.[55]

COMPENSATION

The body responds to acute respiratory acidosis with chemical buffering. Nonbicarbonate buffers (i.e., proteins, phosphate, hemoglobin) take up the hydrogen ions from the carbonic acid formed as a result of the increase in $Paco_2$. This allows the bicarbonate concentration to increase. Buffering begins almost immediately after an acute increase in $Paco_2$. In general, the bicarbonate concentration will increase by 1 mEq/L above 24 for each 10 mm Hg increase in $Paco_2$ above 40 in acute respiratory acidosis (see Table 49–4).

When respiratory acidosis is prolonged beyond 12 to 24 hours or becomes chronic, renal excretion of hydrogen ions also increases to compensate for acidosis. The kidneys excrete hydrogen ions and generate new bicarbonate, thereby raising the pH toward normal. Renal compensation for chronic hypercapnia generally results in the plasma bicarbonate concentration increasing by 4 mEq/L above 24 for each 10 mm Hg increase in $Paco_2$ above 40 in compensated respiratory acidosis (see Table 49–4). A new steady state in acid–base values generally occurs within 5 days of the onset of hypercapnia in dogs, but the time interval necessary for establishing chronic (i.e., compensated) respiratory acidosis in humans has not been established.

▶ TREATMENT: Respiratory Acidosis

The treatment of respiratory acidosis is dependent on the chronicity of the patient's condition. Respiratory decompensation in patients with chronic elevations in $Paco_2$ are frequently seen in those with acute infections and those recently started on narcotic analgesics or oxygen therapy.[47] Aggressive treatment of these conditions can offer considerable benefit and should be initiated. Furthermore, tranquilizers and sedatives should be avoided and supplemental oxygen, if used, should be minimized. The treatment of chronic respiratory acidosis is discussed in Chapter 25. Acute respiratory acidosis and acute respiratory acidosis superimposed on chronic respiratory acidosis are discussed in detail below.

ACUTE RESPIRATORY ACIDOSIS

When carbon dioxide excretion is severely impaired ($Paco_2 > 80$ mm Hg) and/or life-threatening hypoxia is present ($Po_2 < 40$ mm Hg), the immediate therapeutic goal is to provide adequate oxygenation. Under these circumstances, hypoxia not acidemia is the principle threat to life. A patent airway needs to be established, which may necessitate emergency tracheotomy, bronchoscopy, or intubation. In addition, excessive secretions must be cleared from the airway. Oxygen should be administered to restore adequate oxygenation. Mechanical ventilation may be required in cases of life-threatening hypoxia.

The underlying cause of the acidosis should be treated aggressively (bronchodilators for treatment of severe bronchospasm, discontinuing or reversing the effects of respiratory depressant drugs such as narcotics and benzodiazepines). Bicarbonate administration is rarely necessary in the treatment of respiratory acidosis. Furthermore, rapid correction of acidosis with bicarbonate may eliminate the patient's respiratory drive or precipitate a metabolic alkalosis. Cautious use of alkali (bicarbonate or THAM) can restore the responsiveness of bronchial musculation to β-adrenergic agonists and thus may be exceedingly beneficial for those patients with severe bronchospasm.[57] Arterial blood gases should be monitored closely to ensure that the respiratory acidosis is resolving without creating a metabolic alkalosis as the result of the compensatory elevation in HCO_3^- and decrease in $Paco_2$. Arterial blood gases should be obtained every 2 to 4 hours during the acute phase and less frequently (every 12 to 24 hours) as the acidosis improves.

ACUTE RESPIRATORY ACIDOSIS IN A COMPENSATED CHRONIC RESPIRATORY ACIDOTIC PATIENT

Patients with a history of chronic respiratory acidosis (e.g., those with chronic obstructive pulmonary disease) may experience an acute worsening of their respiratory acidosis. This may result in severe life-threatening hypoxemia. As with acute respiratory acidosis, the goals of therapy are maintenance of a patent airway and adequate oxygenation. Individuals with chronic respiratory acidosis are routinely able to tolerate a low Pa_{O_2} and an elevated Pa_{CO_2} because of compensation (increased number of red blood cells, hemoglobin content, and 2,3-diphosphoglycerate). The drive to breathe in these patients is dependent on hypoxemia rather than hypercarbia. Administration of oxygen to a patient with chronic respiratory acidosis can eliminate this drive to breathe and result in the syndrome of carbon dioxide narcosis. In this case, if the $Pa_{CO_2} \geq 50$ mm Hg, no oxygen treatment is necessary. If the $Pa_{CO_2} < 50$ mm Hg, oxygen therapy should be initiated carefully.[5]

Arterial blood gases should be checked periodically to ensure adequate oxygenation. If the Pa_{CO_2} increases during oxygen therapy, it may be a sign of impending carbon dioxide narcosis and oxygen therapy may need to be discontinued. If the pH remains less than 7.2 and the Pa_{CO_2} remains elevated and/or the patient develops symptoms of acidosis, bicarbonate may be given. The amount of bicarbonate given should increase the pH to no more than 7.25 (for dosage calculation see Metabolic Acidosis section). Arterial blood gases should be monitored to avoid precipitation of metabolic alkalosis.

The underlying cause of the acute exacerbation should be aggressively managed. Pulmonary infections should be treated with the appropriate antibiotics and bronchodilators as necessary. Excess secretions should be cleared from the airway to allow proper gas exchange. This may involve increasing oral fluid intake to decrease secretion viscosity, deep breathing, and postural drainage, suction, or bronchoscopy.

MIXED ACID–BASE DISORDERS

When two or more primary acid–base disturbances occur simultaneously, a mixed acid–base disorder results. A mixed disturbance can be suspected from the clinical setting and medical history, and can be diagnosed with this information together with arterial blood gas and electrolyte data.[5,18,47]

DIAGNOSIS

The diagnosis of a mixed disorder depends on an understanding of the appropriate quantitative response of the compensatory mechanisms for the primary, uncomplicated acid–base disorders. To diagnose mixed disorders, one must know how each of the four simple disorders alters pH, Pa_{CO_2}, and HCO_3^- (see Table 49–4). If a given set of blood gases does not fall within the range of expected responses for a simple acid–base disorder (see Fig. 49–1), a mixed disorder should be suspected. In addition to laboratory information, a clinical evaluation of the patient is important. A thorough history and physical examination will often lead to the diagnosis, even before the laboratory data are available. Examples of common mixed disorders follow.

RESPIRATORY ACIDOSIS AND METABOLIC ACIDOSIS

In mixed respiratory and metabolic acidosis, there is a failure of compensation. The respiratory disorder prevents the compensatory decrease in Pa_{CO_2} expected in the defense against metabolic acidosis. The metabolic disorder prevents the buffering and renal mechanisms from raising the bicarbonate concentration as expected in the defense against respiratory acidosis. In the absence of compensatory mechanisms, the pH decreases markedly.

Mixed respiratory and metabolic acidosis may develop in patients with cardiorespiratory arrest, in those with chronic lung disease who are in shock, and in metabolic acidosis patients who develop respiratory failure. This mixed disorder should be treated by responding to both the respiratory and metabolic acidosis. Improved oxygen delivery must be initiated to improve hypercarbia and hypoxia. Mechanical ventilation may be needed to reduce Pa_{CO_2}. During the initial stage of therapy, appropriate amounts of alkali should be given to reverse the metabolic acidosis (see section on Treatment, under Metabolic Acidosis).

RESPIRATORY ALKALOSIS AND METABOLIC ALKALOSIS

The combination of respiratory and metabolic alkalosis is the most common mixed acid–base disorder. This mixed disorder occurs frequently in critically ill surgical patients with respiratory alkalosis caused by mechanical ventilation, hypoxia, sepsis, hypotension, neurologic damage, pain, or drugs, and with metabolic alkalosis caused by vomiting or nasogastric suctioning and massive blood transfusions. It may also occur in patients with hepatic cirrhosis who hyperventilate, receive diuretics, or vomit, as well as in patients with chronic respiratory acidosis and an elevated plasma bicarbonate concentration who are placed on mechanical ventilation and undergo a rapid fall in Pa_{CO_2}.

The decrease in bicarbonate concentration that usually compensates for respiratory alkalosis is prevented by the complicating metabolic alkalosis. Likewise, the increase in Pa_{CO_2} expected to compensate for metabolic alkalosis is prevented by primary respiratory alkalosis. The failure of compensation that occurs with mixed respiratory and metabolic alkalosis may result in a severe alkalosis.

Correction of the metabolic component by administration of sodium chloride and potassium chloride solutions should be undertaken, and readjustment of the ventilator or treatment of an underlying disorder causing hyperventilation may correct or ameliorate the respiratory component of this mixed disorder.

METABOLIC ACIDOSIS AND RESPIRATORY ALKALOSIS

This mixed disorder is often seen in patients with advanced liver disease, salicylate intoxication, and pulmonary–renal syndromes. The combination of respiratory alkalosis and metabolic acidosis is a disorder of excessive compensation.

The respiratory alkalosis decreases the Pa_{CO_2} beyond the appropriate range of the respiratory compensation for metabolic acidosis. The plasma bicarbonate concentration also falls below the level expected in primary respiratory alkalosis. In a sense, the defense of pH for either disorder alone is enhanced; thus, the pH may be normal or close to normal, with a low Pa_{CO_2} and a low HCO_3^-. Treatment of this disorder should be directed at the underlying cause. Because of the enhanced compensation, the pH is usually closer to normal than in either of the two simple disorders.

METABOLIC ALKALOSIS AND RESPIRATORY ACIDOSIS

This mixed disorder often occurs in patients with chronic obstructive pulmonary disease (COPD) and chronic respiratory acidosis who are treated with salt restriction, diuretics, and possibly glucocorticoids. When diuretics are initiated, the plasma bicarbonate may increase owing to increased renal bicarbonate generation and reabsorption, providing mechanisms for both generating and maintaining metabolic alkalosis. The elevated pH diminishes respiratory drive and may therefore worsen the pulmonary disease.

Although the pH may not deviate significantly from normal, treatment may need to be initiated to maintain Pa_{O_2} and Pa_{CO_2} at acceptable levels. Because it is often difficult to correctly identify this mixed disorder, it is helpful to observe the patient's response to discontinuation of diuretics and administration of sodium and potassium chloride.[5] If the patient has a simple metabolic alkalosis, the Pa_{CO_2} will normalize, but it will only minimally affect the Pa_{CO_2} if it is a mixed disorder. Treatment should be aimed at decreasing plasma bicarbonate with sodium and potassium chloride therapy, allowing the renal excretion of retained bicarbonate from the diuretic-induced metabolic alkalosis. This therapy should be used cautiously to avoid exacerbating the congestive heart failure.

EVALUATION OF THERAPEUTIC OUTCOMES

Because acid–base disorders are such a common and widespread problem, pharmacists may play a key role in identifying, preventing, and properly treating acid–base abnormalities. Acid–base disorders do not occur only in the ICU setting. Patients in ambulatory and extended care settings have many chronic conditions and drug therapies that commonly affect acid–base balance. Thus, pharmacists in all practice settings should use their knowledge to identify patients at high risk for developing drug-related problems and to undertake appropriate prevention and treatment measures to improve the quality of life of the patients they care for.

▶ PRINCIPLES OF PHARMACOTHERAPY

- Primary therapy of most acid–base disorders must include treatment or elimination of the underlying cause, not just correction of the pH and electrolyte disturbances.
- Loss of gastric acid from vomiting or nasogastric suctioning is often responsible for the development of a metabolic alkalosis, characterized by hypochloremia and hyperbicarbonatemia.
- Diarrhea and laxative abuse are common causes of metabolic acidosis, owing to the loss of bicarbonate in the stool.
- Aggressive diuretic therapy may produce a metabolic alkalosis, and the accompanying hypokalemia may be serious.
- Overly aggressive sodium bicarbonate therapy for the treatment of metabolic acidosis can frequently result in "overshoot" alkalosis, paradoxical transient CNS acidosis, hypernatremia, and hyperosmolality.
- The presence of a large anion gap metabolic acidosis may be the result of lactic acidosis, diabetic ketoacidosis, or substance intoxication (methanol, ethylene glycol, aspirin).
- In most cases of acute respiratory acidosis, such as following cardiopulmonary arrest, sodium bicarbonate therapy is not indicated and may be detrimental. Blood gas analysis should guide therapy.
- Significant drug-induced acid–base disorders are usually the result of an overdose; however, some medications can affect acid–base balance when ingested in therapeutic amounts, for example, progesterone derivatives, respiratory stimulants, barbiturates, benzodiazepines, opiates, β-blockers, lithium, metformin, carbonic anhydrase inhibitors, diuretics, and nitroprusside.

REFERENCES

1. Narins RG. Acid–base disorders: Definitions and introductory concepts. In: Narins RG, ed. Maxwell & Kleeman's Clinical Disorders of Fluid and Electrolyte Metabolism, 5th ed. New York, McGraw-Hill, 1994: 765–768.
2. Arbus GS. An in-vivo acid–base nomogram for clinical use. Can Med Assoc J 1973;109:291–293.
3. Shapiro JI, Kaehny WD. Pathogenesis and management of metabolic acidosis and alkalosis. In: Schrier RW, ed. Renal and Electrolyte Disorders, 5th ed. Philadelphia, Lippincott–Raven, 1997: 130–169.
4. Laske ME. Normal regulation of acid–base balance. Med Clin North Am 1983;67:771–780.
5. Kaehny WD. Pathogenesis and management of respiratory and mixed acid–base disorders. In: Schrier RW, ed. Renal and Electrolyte Disorders, 5th ed. Philadelphia, Lippincott–Raven, 1997: 172–191.
6. Halperin ML, Jungas RL, Cheema-Dhadli S, Brosnan JT. Disposal of the daily acid load: An integrated function of the liver, lungs and kidneys. Trends Biochem Sci 1987;12:197–199.
7. Weil MH, Rackow EC, Trenio R, et al. Difference in acid–base state between venous and arterial blood during cardiopulmonary resuscitation. N Engl J Med 1986;315:153–155.
8. Fell WL. Sampling and measurement of blood gases. In: Lane EE, Walker JF, eds. Clinical Arterial Blood Gas Analysis. St. Louis, Mosby, 1987:202–212.
9. Broughton JO. Understanding Blood Gases. Madison, WI, Ohmeda, 1980.

10. Narins RG, Krishna GG, Yee J, et al. The metabolic acidoses. In: Narins RG, ed. Maxwell & Kleeman's Clinical Disorders of Fluid and Electrolyte Metabolism, 5th ed. New York, McGraw-Hill, 1994: 769–826.
11. Winter SD, Pearson JR, Gabow PA, Schultz AL, Lepoff RB. The fall of the serum anion gap. Arch Intern Med 1990;150:311–313.
12. Halperin ML, Carlisle EJ, Donnelly S, et al. Renal tubular acidosis. In: Narins RG, ed. Maxwell & Kleeman's Clinical Disorders of Fluid and Electrolyte Metabolism, 5th ed. New York, McGraw-Hill, 1994: 875–910.
13. Oster JR, Perez GO, Materson BJ. Use of the anion gap in clinical medicine. South Med J 1988;81:229–237.
14. McCarron DA, Elliot WC, Rose JS, et al. Severe mixed metabolic acidosis secondary to rhabdomyolysis. Am J Med 1979;67:905–908.
15. Lolekha PH, Lolekha S. Value of the anion gap in clinical diagnosis and laboratory evaluation. Clin Chem 1983;29:279–283.
16. Salem MM, Mujais SK. Gaps in the anion gap. Arch Intern Med 1992;152:1625–1629.
17. Gabow PA, Kaehny WD, Fennessey PV, et al. Diagnostic importance of an increased serum anion gap. N Engl J Med 1980;303: 854–858.
18. Adrogue HJ, Madias NE. Management of life-threatening acid–base disorders. N Engl J Med 1998;338:26–34.
19. Kraut JA, Madias NE. Lactic acidosis. In: Adrogue HJ, ed. Contemporary Management in Critical Care, Vol 1. Baltimore, Williams & Wilkins, 1995: 449–457.
20. Narins RG, Emmett M. Simple and mixed acid–base disorders: A practical approach. Medicine 1980;59:161–187.
21. Teplinsky K, O'Toole M, Olman M, et al. Effect of lactic acidosis on canine hemodynamics and left ventricular function. Am J Physiol 1990;258:H1193–H1199.
22. Albert MS, Dell RB, Winters RW. Quantitative displacement of acid–base equilibrium in metabolic acidosis. Ann Intern Med 1964; 66:312–322.
23. Kraut JA. The role of metabolic acidosis in the pathogenesis of renal osteodystrophy. Adv Ren Replace Ther 1995;2: 40–51.
24. Morris RC, Ives HE. Inherited disorders of the renal tubule. In: Brenner BM, ed. Brenner and Rector's, The Kidney, Vol II, 5th ed. Philadelphia, W.B. Saunders, 1996:1764–1827.
25. Kamel KS, Briceno LF, Sanchez MI, et al. A new classification for renal defects in net acid excretion. Am J Kidney Dis 1997;29:136–146.
26. Moon PF, Gabor L, Gleed RD, Erb HN. Acid–base, metabolic, and hemodynamic effects of sodium bicarbonate or tromethamine administration in anesthetized dogs with experimentally induced metabolic acidosis. Am J Vet Res 1997;58:771–776.
27. Sing RF, Branas CA, Sing RF. Bicarbonate therapy in the treatment of lactic acidosis: Medicine or toxin? J Am Ostepath Assoc 1995;95: 52–57.
28. Shangraw RE, Winter R, Hromco J, Robinson ST, Gallaher EJ. Amelioration of lactic acidosis with dichloroacetate during liver transplantation in humans. Anesthesiology 1994;81:1127–1138.
29. Cooper DJ, Walley KR, Wiggs BR, Russell JA. Bicarbonate does not improve hemodynamics in critically ill patients who have lactic acidosis: A prospective controlled clinical study. Ann Intern Med 1990; 112:492–498.
30. Adrogue HJ, Rashad MN, Gorin AB, Yacoub J, Madias NE. Assessing acid–base status in circulatory failure: Differences between arterial and central venous blood. N Engl J Med 1989;320:1312–1316.
31. Faber MD, Kupin WL, Heiling CW, Narins RG. Common fluid–electrolyte and acid–base problems in the intensive care unit: Selected issues. Semin Nephrol 1994;14:8–22.
32. Emergency Cardiac Care Committee and Subcomittees, American Heart Association. Guidelines for cardiopulmonary resuscitation and emergency cardiac care. JAMA 1992;268:2171–2302.
33. Drug Information. American Hospital Formulary Service. 1998.
34. Marmarou A, Holdaway R, Ward JD, et al. Traumatic brain tissue acidosis: Experimental and clinical studies. Acta Neurochir 1993;57:160–164.
35. Leung JM, Landow L, Franks M, et al. Safety and efficacy of intravenous carbicarb in patients undergoing surgery: Comparison with sodium bicarbonate in the treatment of mild metabolic acidosis. Crit Care Med 1994;22:1540–1549.
36. Shapiro JI. Functional and metabolic responses of the isolated heart during acidosis: Effects of sodium bicarbonate and carbicarb. Am J Physiol 1990;258:H1835–H1839.
37. Shapiro JI. Pathogenesis of cardiac dysfunction during metabolic acidosis: Therapeutic implications. Kidney Int 1997;51:47–51.
38. Bersin RM, Arieff AI. Improved hemodynamic function during hypoxia with carbicarb, a new agent for the management of acidosis. Circulation 1988;77:227–233.
39. Stacpoole PW, Wright EC, Baumgartner TG, et al. A controlled clinical trial of dichloroacetate for treatment of lactic acidosis. N Engl J Med 1992;327:1564–1569.
40. Stacpoole PW. The pharmacology of dichloroacetate. Metabolism 1989;38:1124–1144.
41. Vary TC, Siegel JH, Zechnich A, et al. Pharmacologic reversal of abnormal glucose regulation, BCAA utilization, and muscle catabolism in sepsis by dichloroacetate. J Trauma 1988;28:1301–1311.
42. Hodgkin JE, Soeprono FF, Chan DM. Incidence of metabolic alkalosis in hospitalized patients. Crit Care Med 1980;8:725–728.
43. Wilson RF, Gibson D, Percinel AK, et al. Severe alkalosis in critically ill patients. Arch Surg 1972;105:197–203.
44. Palmer BF, Alpern RJ. Metabolic alkalosis. J Am Soc Nephrol 1997;8:1462–1469.
45. Sabatini S, Kurtzman NA. Metabolic alkalosis. In: Narins RG, ed. Maxwell & Kleeman's Clinical Disorders of Fluid and Electrolyte Metabolism, 5th ed. New York, McGraw-Hill, 1994: 933–956.
46. Farese RV Jr, Biglieri EG, Shackleton CH, et al. Licorice-induced hypermineralocorticoidism. N Engl J Med 1991;325:1223–1227.
47. Adrogue HJ, Madias NE. Management of life-threatening acid–base disorders II. N Engl J Med 1998;338:107–111.
48. Brimioulle S, Berre J, Dufaye P, et al. Hydrochloric acid infusion for treatment of metabolic alkalosis associated with respiratory acidosis. Crit Care Med 1989;17:232–236.
49. Mirtallo JM, Rogers KR, Johnson JA, et al. Stability of amino acids and the availability of acid in total parenteral nutrition solutions containing hydrochloric acid. Am J Hosp Pharm 1981;38:1729–1731.
50. Rowlands BJ, Tindall SF, Elliot DJ. The use of dilute hydrochloric acid and cimetidine to reverse severe metabolic alkalosis. Postgrad Med J 1978;54:118–123.
51. Barton CH, Vaziri ND, Ness RL, et al. Cimetidine in the management of metabolic alkalosis induced by nasogastric drainage. Arch Surg 1979;1:70–74.
52. Colussi G, Rombola G, De Ferrari ME, Macaluso M, Minetti L. Correction of hypokalemia with antialdosterone therapy in Gitelman's syndrome. Am J Nephrol 1994;14:127–135.
53. Hene RJ, Koomans HA, Dorhout Mees EJ, et al. Correction of hypokalemia in Bartter's syndrome by enalapril. Am J Kidney Dis 1987;9:200–205.
54. Vinci JM, Gill JR Jr, Bowden RE, et al. The kallikrein–kinin system in Bartter's syndrome and its response to prostaglandin synthetase inhibition. J Clin Invest 1987;61:1671–1682.
55. Gennari FJ. Respiratory acidosis and alkalosis. In: Narins RG, ed. Maxwell & Kleeman's Clinical Disorders of Fluid and Electrolyte Metabolism, 5th ed. New York, McGraw-Hill, 1994: 957–990.
56. Giebisch G, Berger L, Pitts RF. The extrarenal responses to acute acid–base disturbances of respiratory origin. J Clin Invest 1955;34: 231–245.
57. Respiratory pump failure: Primary hypercapnia (respiratory acidosis). In: Adrogue HJ, Tobin MJ, eds. Respiratory Failure. Cambridge, MA, Blackwell Science, 1997:125–134.

50
EVALUATION OF NEUROLOGIC ILLNESS

Susan C. Fagan, PharmD, BCPS, FCCP, and K.M.A. Welch, MD

Practitioners and students have long thought of neurology as a specialty primarily concerned with the diagnosis of untreatable diseases. With the notable exception of epilepsy, pharmacists have not played a major role in the care of these patients and have tended to focus their attention on the more pharmacotherapy-intense specialities such as infectious disease and cardiology. In the past decade, however, many novel pharmacologic agents for previously untreatable neurologic diseases have been introduced, making it essential that the pharmacist understands the evaluation tools used to diagnose and manage neurologic disease.[1,2]

The assessment of the neurologic patient follows an orderly progression that may differ from assessment in other specialties. The diagnostic steps of the clinical method are as follows[3]:

1. *Initial assessment.* History and physical examination (including neurologic examination) to determine signs and symptoms.
2. *Syndromic diagnosis.* Identify whether signs and symptoms can be clustered to resemble a known syndrome.
3. *Anatomic localization.* Localize the disease process (localize the lesion) to a part or parts of the nervous system
4. *Pathogenesis.* Determine the etiology of the illness using onset, evolution, course, concommitant diseases, relevant past and family history, and laboratory findings.
5. *Functional assessment.* Assess the degree of disability. Often the most difficult aspect of the neurologic diagnosis is to localize the lesion. This requires an in-depth knowledge of neuroanatomy, neurophysiology, and neuropathology.

The diagnosis of neurologic diseases does not always follow all the steps listed. For example, the diagnosis of disorders such as migraine usually stops at the history and physical examination. Regardless of the steps taken in the assessment of the patient, the accurate identification of signs and symptoms along with an accurate interpretation of the signs elicited (through the neurologic examination) is of paramount importance. Often, repeated examinations are necessary to arrive at a diagnosis with certainty.

SIGNS AND SYMPTOMS FROM HISTORY AND PHYSICAL EXAMINATION

Obtaining an accurate and complete history is of utmost importance in the evaluation of neurologic diseases. In many instances, the diagnosis can be made on the basis of the history, and the remainder of the examination serves to confirm this diagnosis and aid in localizing the problem. The clinician is dependent on the cooperation of the patient in describing symptoms, and special care must be taken to avoid "leading" the patient. In addition to information important for any medical history, the mode of onset, evolution, and course of illness often help to differentiate between different neurologic syndromes. Taking a history may not always be straightforward because many neurologic diseases affect functions such as speech, memory, and orientation.

The physical examination is important in revealing evidence of systemic disease that may have secondarily affected the nervous system (for example, a seizure in a patient with elevated temperature and nuchal rigidity may suggest meningitis). The neurologic examination should be the last component of a complete, general physical examination.

THE NEUROLOGIC EXAMINATION

The neurologic examination consists of six main components: higher cortical function (mental status), cranial nerves, motor function, reflexes, sensory function, and gait. Table 50–1 describes the common approaches to assessing each of the six domains and includes examples of the diseases in which abnormal findings are common. Table 50–2 describes the cranial nerve examination in more detail. The reader is encouraged to consult a patient assessment resource to better understand the intricacies of the neurologic examination.

LABORATORY TESTS AND PROCEDURES FOR DIAGNOSIS

In addition to the neurologic examination, certain imaging techniques and procedures may be essential in the diagnosis of neurologic diorders. Some of the more commonly used procedures are described next.[2]

Lumbar puncture (LP) and cerebrospinal fluid (CSF) evaluation are used in the diagnostic evaluation of a variety

TABLE 50–1. The Neurological Examination

Domain	Tests Performed	Diseases
Mental status	While obtaining the history: general mental and emotional status, speech, memory, alertness, abstract reasoning, ability to follow commands (motor integration), ability to communicate	Dementias, stroke, metabolic encephalopathies
Cranial nerves	Visual acuity, visual fields, eye movements, jaw strength, corneal reflex, facial symmetry, auditory acuity, gag reflex, shoulder and neck strength	Myasthenia gravis, Parkinson's disease, stroke, amyotrophic lateral sclerosis (ALS)
Motor Function	Motor strength with and without resistance, coordination (rapid alternating movements, finger-to-nose), tremors, atrophy, fasiculations	Stroke, myasthenia gravis, Parkinson's disease, ALS
Reflexes	Biceps, triceps, tendon reflexes, plantar response (Babinski sign is an upgoing toe and is abnormal), superficial cutaneous reflexes (abdominal)	Stroke, spinal cord lesions, endocrine diseases (e.g., diabetes, hypothyroidism), peripheral neuropathy
Sensory function	Asymmetry to pin-prick, vibration, temperature	Stroke, peripheral neuropathy, migraine aura, diabetes, spinal cord lesions
Gait	Walking, standing (Romberg test = eyes closed will accentuate disequilibrium)	Stroke, Parkinson's disease, spinal cord lesions

of neurologic disorders including meningitis, subarachnoid hemorrhage, multiple sclerosis, and dementia. The CSF pressure is usually less than 180 mm H_20 if measured appropriately. Low readings may result from excessive removal of CSF prior to measurement, a CSF leak around the needle, spinal block, or herniation of the brain. An LP should be avoided if there is any evidence of increased intracranial pressure, so the optic disks must be checked routinely to exclude papilledema before the procedure. Normal CSF is clear and should not contain any red blood cells (RBCs) or polymorphonuclear cells. The presence of up to 10 mononuclear cells is considered normal. If the white blood cell (WBC) count is high, it should be considered whether blood may have been introduced during the procedure (traumatic tap), leading to a falsely elevated WBC count. A general rule is that 1000 RBCs add 1 WBC to the total count.

CSF glucose should always be compared to a simultaneous blood glucose measurement. The normal CSF glucose concentration is approximately two-thirds that of the blood glucose and is considered abnormal if less than 40 mg/dL. Protein in the CSF is usually 45 mg/dL or less, with IgG making up less than 13% of total protein. Protein may increase with infection, cerebral tumors, stroke, and diabetes. As with WBC, a traumatic tap will add protein to the CSF (allow 1 mg for 1000 RBCs). An increase in IgG is observed in multiple sclerosis and neurosyphilis. Bacteriologic, cytologic, and serologic evaluations are also often performed on the CSF.

TABLE 50–2. Cranial Nerve Function and Examples of Testing

I. Olfactory nerve. Smell: Identify odors (coffee, cinnamon, lemon; test each nostril separately).

II. Optic nerve. Visual acuity: Eye card; Visual fields: Peripheral vision and blind spot; Funduscopic exam; Color vision (rarely done).

III. Oculomotor. (Cranial nerves III, IV, and VI have similar functions and are tested as a unit.) Eye movements: Patient is asked to watch and follow a light as it moved up, down, and on both sides, while eye movements are observed.

IV. Trochlear. See III.

V. Trigeminal nerve. Motor: Tests power of jaw opening and sideways deviation against the resistance of a hand placed against the jaw. Sensory: Test corneal reflex by touching cornea (also nasal mucosa) with a wisp of cotton.

VI. Abducens. See III.

VII. Facial nerve. Observe asymmetry of face at rest or on speaking, baring teeth, raising eyebrows, or wrinkling forehead. Reflex eye closure to a threatening movement. Glabellar tap: Repetitive tapping over bridge of nose—initial blinking should cease after the first few taps.

VIII. Auditory nerve. Vestibular division: Observe for nystagmus, positional testing. Auditory division: Test acuity with light sound; watch, whisper, rubbing of fingers close to ear.

IX. Glossopharyngeal nerve. Test for gag reflex by touching back of throat with tongue depressor; test swallowing and coughing and note any drooling or pooling of saliva. Test symmetry of palate movement on vocalizing "ah."

X. Vagus nerve. Test gag reflex as in IX.

XI. Spinal accessory nerve. Trapezius and sternomastoid muscles: Test power of shrugging shoulders and turning the head to one side against resistance.

XII. Hypoglossal nerve. Motor function of tongue. Look for wasting and abnormal movements.

Electroencephalography (EEG) is used to record the electrical activity of the brain and is used primarily in the assessment of seizure disorders or states of impaired consciousness. Some centers have epilepsy monitoring units, where patients can be monitored around the clock by EEG and video in an attempt to characterize a particular seizure disorder. The EEG recording is evaluated for basic waveform patterns, symmetry of the cerebral activity, transient discharges, and the changes when stimulatory techniques, such as visual activation, are used. The EEG may be used occasionally in localizing cerebral tumors.

Three types of evoked potentials (EPs) are used clinically: visual, auditory (brainstem), and somatosensory. EEG responses to repetitive stimuli (visual patterns, auditory clicks, or electrical skin stimulation) are averaged to produce the evoked potentials. Abnormalities in the latency and amplitude may indicate a lesion in a particular sensory pathway, but give no information regarding the nature of the lesion. Evoked potentials may be useful in the diagnosis of multiple sclerosis, acoustic neuromas, and spinal cord lesions.

Cerebral arteriography is used to visualize the intracranial vasculature by injecting a radioopaque material into the bloodstream, similar to what is done with coronary arteriography. This technique is particularly useful in identifying the location of arterial aneurysms, vascular occlusion, and arteriovenous malformations. Noninvasive assessment of the patency of cerebral arteries can be approximated with the use of transcranial doppler (TCD) ultrasonography, in which cerebral blood flow velocity is measured in the large intracranial vessels (e.g., middle cerebral artery or anterior cerebral artery).

The advent of computed tomography (CT) technology revolutionized the practice of neurology and allowed clinicians a three-dimensional noninvasive view of the brain. X-ray information processed by a computer allows the evaluation of 3- to 12-mm-thick "slices" of brain. Among other things, CT scans are used to differentiate cerebral infarction from cerebral hemorrhage and to identify cerebral tumors and cerebral edema. A second CT using intravenous contrast medium (a contrast-enhanced scan) is often done to enhance the image of blood vessels and areas of blood–brain barrier damage that may be caused by tumors or stroke.

Magnetic resonance imaging (MRI) uses the magnetic properties of the hydrogen atom nucleus and proton to produce computer-processed scans that provide improved anatomic accuracy, compared to CT scans. MRI offers the advantages of differentiating between white and gray matter, delineating lesions close to bone, and no radiation risk; however, it is not as readily available as CT and is more expensive. MRI has a proven advantage over CT in detecting plaques in multiple sclerosis and is also useful in the diagnosis of tumors and very early ischemic stroke.

TABLE 50–3. General Principles Guiding the Evaluation of Neurologic Illness

1. Patients must cooperate with the examiner; therefore, patient reliability and effort must be considered in the interpretation of the findings.
2. The neurologic examination of a patient is often adapted to focus on the patient's specific problem. For example, a patient with Bell's palsy (facial involvement) will have a thorough cranial nerve examination but a less extensive evaluation of hand strength.
3. The importance of symmetry cannot be overemphasized. Rather than comparing a patient's neurologic function to a "normal" standard, asymmetry of strength, sensation, and coordination are often of great importance in detecting neurologic deficits.
4. Although the neurologic examination is important in diagnosing and quantifying neurologic deficits in patients, functional assessment (what the patient can do compared to baseline state—activities of daily living) is also important in making decisions about therapy. For this purpose, functional assessment scales are used with increasing frequency but are usually disease specific, in that they incorporate functions that are most commonly affected by the disease. Often, knowledge of the disease-specific functional scale is necessary to interpret clinical trials of new treatments for neurologic diseases (e.g., Barthel Index for acute ischemic stroke, Expanded Disability Status Scale (EDSS) in multiple sclerosis).

Other imaging techniques such as positron emission tomography (PET) and single-photon emission computed tomography (SPECT) are considered tests of brain function. These tests are being studied extensively in epilepsy as well as in cerebrovascular disorders, cerebral tumors, movement disorders, and dementia. PET scans use a positron-emitting isotope to display chemical activity and the rates of biologic processes within the brain. This method can assess regional metabolic changes in the brain. The expense, technical complexity (a cyclotron is needed), and limited availability of this technique limit its clinical utility.

SPECT scans measure radiotracer uptake by tissues and provide cross-sectional images of the brain. This technique has been used extensively to assess cerebral blood flow. Although the resolution of SPECT is not as good as PET, the availability has led to wide clinical use in disorders such as stroke, dementia, and epilepsy.

General principles guiding the evaluation of neurologic illness are summarized in Table 50–3.

REFERENCES

1. Adams RD, Victor M, Ropper AH. Principles of Neurology, 6th ed. New York, McGraw-Hill, 1996:3–11.
2. Adams RD, Victor M, Ropper AH. Principles of Neurology, 6th ed. New York, McGraw-Hill, 1996:12–40.
3. Longe RL, Calvert JC. Nervous system. In: Young LY, ed. Physical Assessment. A Guide for Evaluating Drug Therapy. Vancouver, WA, Applied Therapeutics, 1994:14-1–14-29.

51

MULTIPLE SCLEROSIS

Barry E. Gidal, PharmD, John O. Fleming, MD, and Christina Dalmady-Israel, PharmD, BCPS

Multiple sclerosis (MS) is an inflammatory disease of the central nervous system that affects between 250,000 and 350,000 persons in the United States.[1] It is one of the major causes of neurologic disability in young and middle-age adults. The term "multiple sclerosis" refers to two characteristics of the disease: the numerous affected areas of the brain and spinal cord producing multiple neurologic symptoms that accrue over time, and the characteristic plaques or sclerosed areas that are the hallmark of the disease.

Although MS was first described almost 130 years ago, the cause remains a mystery, and a cure is still unavailable. Nevertheless, many advances have been made in treating and managing the complications of the disease and improving the quality of life of those individuals affected by MS.

EPIDEMIOLOGY

MS is usually diagnosed in patients between the ages of 20 and 45 years (although cases in children have been reported), with the peak incidence occurring in the fourth decade.[2] Onset can occur as early as age 10 and as late as the eighth decade.[3] Women are afflicted more than men by a ratio of approximately 2 to 1.[3] Men usually develop the first signs of MS at a later age than women, and are also more likely to develop the chronic progressive form of the disease.[3,4] The most important factors in the determination of individuals at risk for developing the disease are geography, age, environmental influences, and genetics.[2,5,6]

Based on rates of prevalence of MS, the world can be divided into three geographic zones.[7] In general, the greater the distance from the equator, the higher the prevalence of the disease.[2,7,8] Within the United States, the prevalence of MS is higher in those states above the 37th parallel. Ethnic differences in prevalence are also observed within the described geographic areas, with MS occurring more frequently in Caucasians of Scandinavian ancestry than in other ethnic groups.[8,9] Asian-Americans, African-Americans, American Hispanics living in California, Australian aborigines, Polynesian Maoris, Lapps, and Hungarian gypsies are among the ethnic groups that have a very low reported incidence of MS, sometimes despite being located in what are considered high-risk areas.[8,9] MS is considered a rare disease in Africa.

It is thought that a crucial environmental agent that may predispose one to developing MS is contracted by susceptible individuals between the ages of 10 and 15 years[4,10] who have usually lived in a high-risk area for at least 2 years.[4] Interestingly, an individual who migrates from a low-risk to a high-risk area prior to the age of 15 years has the same chance of developing MS as those who live in a high-risk area all of their lives.[11] If the move is made in the opposite direction, from a high- to a low-risk area, the individual retains the high risk if the move is made after the age of 15 years, but acquires the lower risk if the move is made prior to this age.[10,11]

The familial recurrence rate of MS is approximately 10%, with siblings being the most commonly reported relationship.[9] Concordance data show a higher prevalence of MS between monozygotic than between dizygotic twins.

Genetic studies also have determined an association between MS and the major histocompatibility complex (MHC) and, in particular, with the human leukocyte antigen (HLA) region on the sixth chromosome that is associated with the genetic control of immune mechanisms.[9,12,13] This association between HLA haplotype and MS susceptibility may vary between ethnic groups. In Caucasians, the strongest association appears to be with the MHC class II allele DR2 haplotype. The relative risk of developing MS is approximately four times as great in $DR2^+$ versus $DR2^-$ individuals.[13] This association is not specific enough to be used for diagnostic purposes, given a 30% to 50% false negative rate, and that the $DR2^+$ haplotype is found in at least 20% of the healthy Caucasian population. Although the significance of the association between MS and the HLA remains unclear, the fact that certain HLA antigens are neither necessary nor sufficient to lead to the development of MS suggests that inheritance is most likely polygenic in nature, and that there may only be a genetic susceptibility to developing this disease following an as-yet unknown etiologic challenge.

ETIOLOGY

AUTOIMMUNE THEORY

In the autoimmune theory (Fig. 51–1), MS results from an autoimmune attack against self-myelin or self-oligodendrocyte antigens. The actual mediator of myelin destruction has not been established, but this activity has been attributed to the action of macrophages, killer T cells, lymphokines, antibodies, or a combination of these elements.[14] T-helper cells ($CD4^+$) appear to be key initiators of myelin destruction in MS. These autoreactive $CD4^+$ cells are activated in the periphery, perhaps following a viral infection, and recognize myelin basic protein (MBP), proteolipid protein, myelin

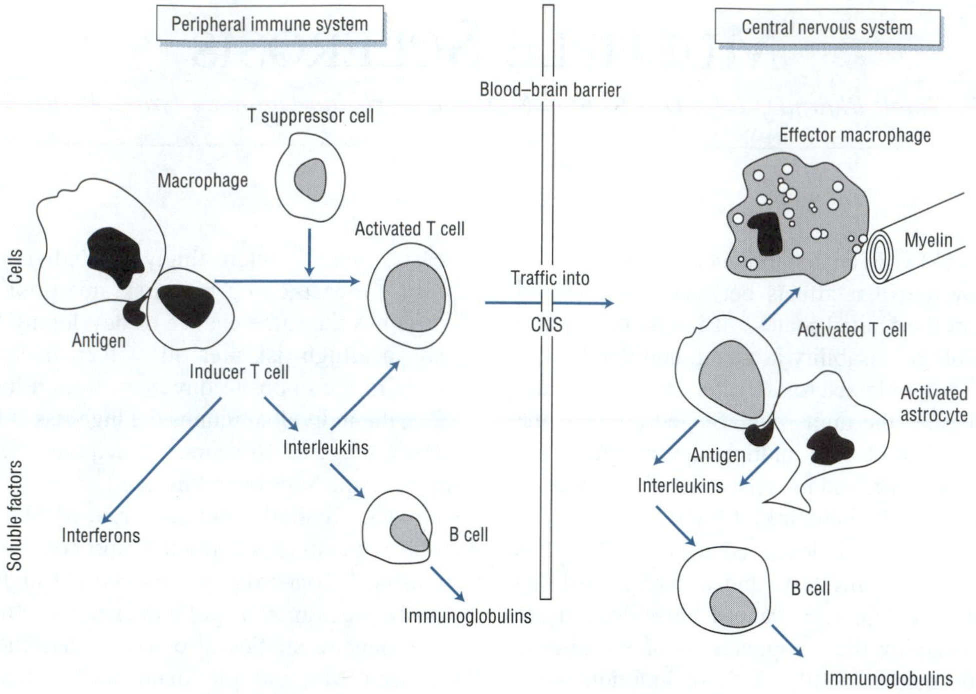

FIGURE 51–1. Autoimmune theory of the pathogenesis of MS. The immune response is initiated in the peripheral immune compartment when antigen is processed and presented to an inducer cell by a macrophage or antigen-presenting cell. The inducer cell becomes activated and releases a number of soluble factors including interleukins and interferons, which act on both B cells and T cells to augment the immune response. T-suppressor cells act to dampen the immune response. Activated T cells traffic into the central nervous system, where they again release factors, presumably after having antigen presented to them. In this regard, astrocytes are capable of presenting antigens to T cells. Other cellular elements also enter the CNS (macrophages, B cells), where the potential for a local immune response occurs. B cells are known to produce immunoglobulin locally within the CNS, and macrophages function within the CNS to phagocytose myelin, in addition to their antigen-presenting properties. *(Reprinted with permission from Ann Neurol, vol 23, p 214, 1988.)*

oligodendrocyte glycoprotein, and myelin-associated glycoprotein in the blood of patients with MS. These antigens are presented by HLA class II molecules on both macrophages and astrocytes. This cellular recognition initiates an inflammatory cascade where $CD4^+$ cells are activated and proliferate. During this process, various cytokines are secreted, and B cells and macrophages are activated. Activated T cells are then able to cross the blood–brain barrier (BBB). Once across the BBB, these cells can interact with specific MHC class II molecules on antigen-presenting cells, and thereby induce an autoimmune response that will eventually lead to the destruction of myelin.[14] Impaired T-suppressor cell function also may play a role in the immunologic process.[15] A reduction in T suppressor cells, or supressor activity, has been reported during active MS and in patients with progressive disease; however, a relative increase in the T helper/suppressor ratio is not consistently found and does not always correlate with disease activity.[16,17]

ROLE OF CYTOKINES

Cytokines are molecules whose physiologic functions are numerous and include modulating inflammatory and anti-inflammatory responses in the immune system. Tumor necrosis factor alpha (TNF-α), interleukin 2 (IL-2), and interferon gamma (INF-γ) have been alleged as contributors to the pathogenesis of MS. TNF-α may contribute to demyelinization by up-regulation of MHC class I expression, direct injury of oligodendrocytes, and/or promotion of BBB breakdown.[18] INF-γ is produced predominantly by $CD4^+$ cells and is involved in antiviral responses. Because of this, INF-γ was at one time evaluated as a potential MS disease-modifying agent. Clinical trials, however, clearly demonstrated that treatment with this compound resulted in an unexpected increase in disease exacerbation.[19] INF-γ up-regulates MHC class II expression on macrophages, microglia, and astrocytes, leading to an inflammatory response. INF-γ also up-regulates adhesion molecules, which are crucial in the early stages of inflammation by facilitating the migration of T cells across the endothelial cells of the BBB.[20]

In contrast, the role of modulating, or down-regulating cytokines has recently been described. In patients with stable or mild disease, increased numbers of cells are found that express mRNA for transforming growth factor beta (TGF-β) and IL-10 as compared to patients with severe disease.[21,22]

VIRAL ETIOLOGY

Although the exact mechanism has not been found, there are several ways in which a virus could play a role in the pathogenesis of MS, including either a direct attack on myelin and/or the oligodendrocyte, or stimulation of an autoimmune response leading to demyelination.[14,23] Evidence to support a viral etiology includes increased IgG synthesis in the CNS, increased antibody titers to certain viruses, and epidemiologic studies indicating a childhood exposure factor and suggesting that "viral" infections may precipitate exacerbations. In addition, viruses have been shown to cause diseases with prolonged incubation periods, myelin destruction, and a relapsing/remitting course in humans and in experimental animal models.[2,24]

The most compelling evidence against a viral etiology is the fact that no single infectious agent has been identified as the causative agent of MS. Many agents have been implicated, including mycoplasma, spirochetes, rabies virus, herpes simplex, canine distemper virus, coronavirus, human T-cell leukemia virus (HTLV)-1, MS-associated retrovirus, and measles. However, studies have been unable to establish a causal relationship.[24]

PATHOPHYSIOLOGY

The basic physiologic derangement in MS is the stripping of the myelin sheath surrounding neurons in the CNS. Demyelination, coupled with an inflammatory response, leads to the formation of the characteristic MS lesions or plaques that are found primarily in the brain, spinal cord, and optic nerves. Neuronal axons, although stripped bare of their myelin sheath, are usually well preserved.[23] It is increasingly appreciated, however, that axons may be lost, especially in the progressive phase of the disease.

Demyelination causes disruption in the transmission of nerve impulses, which leads to neurologic symptoms reflecting the area of the brain affected. Demyelinated nerve fibers have prolonged refractory periods that will impair conduction of electrical impulse volleys. Maximal electrical impulse frequency may be substantially reduced before impulse conduction is interrupted entirely. A single plaque may extend across several nerve pathways producing symptoms involving several nervous system functions. Smaller plaques may cause isolated disturbances; however, typically several plaques develop at the same time, causing multiple but unrelated problems such as disturbed vision and decreased sensation.

The pathology of MS lesions is different in early stages of the disease, during chronic MS, and during acute exacerbations.[25] Active and inactive lesions can be found side by side in the brain. Both types of lesions display some degree of perivascular inflammation, but inflammation is much more pronounced and usually associated with blood–brain barrier damage in active lesions.[25]

Decreased numbers of oligodendrocytes (myelin-producing cells) are observed within the MS plaques, causing speculation as to whether myelin or the oligodendrocyte is the target of an immunologic attack.[16,23,26] Oligodendrocyte destruction appears to occur in a nonspecific manner in early or acute MS, whereas selective destruction of myelin and oligodendrocytes occurs in chronic stages of MS.[25] Although the etiology and pathogenesis of MS remain unclear, it appears that the immune system is crucial in this disease. Many investigators consider MS to be an autoimmune, or immunopathologic disorder, whereby an immune response is directed toward myelin antigens. Although the triggering event for this autoimmune response remains a mystery, an initial viral process is suspected.[14,27]

CLINICAL PRESENTATION

The clinical presentation of MS is extremely variable among patients and may vary over time in a given patient. The transient nature of initial symptoms and the characteristic exacerbations and remissions sometimes make diagnosis difficult.

The signs and symptoms of MS are usually divided into three categories (Table 51–1). Primary symptoms are a direct consequence of conduction disturbances produced by demyelination and reflect the area of the brain or spinal cord that is damaged. Secondary symptoms are complications resulting from primary symptoms. For example, urinary retention, a primary symptom, may lead to frequent urinary tract infections, considered a secondary symptom. Tertiary symptoms relate to the effect of the disease on the patient's everyday life.[28] The most widely used clinical rating scale in MS is the Expanded Disability Status Scale (EDSS), in which a numerical value ranging from 0 (no disability) to 10 (death from MS) is assigned based on the evaluation of several neurologic functions.[29] The limitations to this scale are the relative insensitivity to clinical changes that do not involve impairment of gait

TABLE 51–1. Common Symptomology of Multiple Sclerosis

Primary Symptoms	Secondary Symptoms	Tertiary Symptoms
Visual complaints	Recurrent urinary tract infections	Financial problems
Gait problems	Urinary calculi	Personal/social problems
Paresthesias	Decubiti	Vocational problems
Pain	Muscle contractures	Emotional problems
Spasticity	Respiratory infections	
Weakness	Poor nutrition	
Ataxia		
Speech difficulty		
Psychological changes		
Cognitive changes		
Fatigue		
Bowel/bladder dysfunction		
Sexual dysfunction		
Tremor		

and ambulation, such as changes in cognition, fatigue, and affect. This scale is not linear, and therefore functional changes from 1.0 to 2.0 are not the same as changes from 6.0 to 7.0. This scale is also subject to inter-evaluator inconsistency. Increasingly, magnetic resonance imaging (MRI) is being used as an index of both disease activity and progression.[30,31] Specifically, the appearance of new lesions, or changes in lesional number and volume, are being used as outcome measures. It is important to note, however, that the correlation between MRI lesion load and clinical disability is modest at best.[32]

The unpredictable nature of MS makes it impossible to anticipate when an exacerbation will occur. However, certain factors have been reported to aggravate symptoms or even lead to an acute attack (new episode of demyelination). These implicated factors include infections, hyperventilation, heat (including fever), sleep deprivation, stress, malnutrition, anemia, concurrent organ dysfunction, exertion, and childbirth.[2–4,33] Interestingly, many patients experience a significant reduction in acute relapses during pregnancy, followed by a relative increase postpartum.[33] Physical trauma probably does not play a major role in the onset or exacerbation of MS.[34]

CLINICAL COURSE AND PROGNOSIS

The clinical course of MS is variable, but seems to follow a general pattern of exacerbations and remissions (Fig. 51–2). Based on the course of the disease, MS may be classified into four clinical categories.[35] A benign course—characterized by an abrupt onset, few exacerbations, and no permanent disability—is seen in approximately 20% of patients. Another 20% to 30% of patients develop relapsing/remitting MS, which also begins abruptly, but is subsequently characterized by partial or total remissions, which may last months or years. A large portion of patients (40%) will eventually develop the secondary progressive (or relapsing/progressive) form of the disease, in which a period of initial remissions is followed by progressive disability. The primary progressive (chronic progressive) form of MS, characterized by the slow onset of symptoms, relatively few attacks, and disability that continually worsens over time, is seen in 10% to 20% of patients. In all patients, attack frequency tends to decrease over time, independently of the development of worsening disabilities.[35] Neurologic recovery following an acute exacerbation is usually quite good early in the disease course, but following repeated relapses, recovery tends to be less complete. Typically, relapse rate is usually highest during the first 5 years after the onset of disease. Given these features, interpretation and evaluation of potential therapeutic interventions must be done quite cautiously.

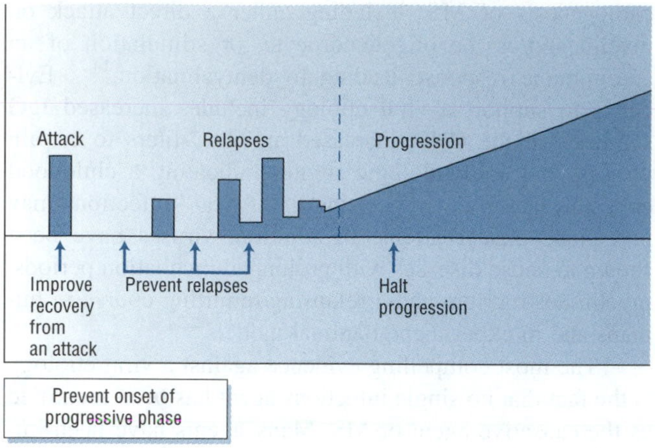

FIGURE 51–2. Clinical course and treatment of multiple sclerosis. The horizontal axis represents time, and the vertical axis represents level of disability. The vertical dotted line represents the onset of the progressive disease phase. The progressive phase may evolve after a number of relapses or, in a subcategory of patients, may be the clinical course of the disease from the onset. *(Reprinted with permission from Ann Neurol, vol 23, p 212, 1988.)*

MS itself usually does not directly diminish life expectancy; however, the development of complications such as pneumonia or septicemia (secondary to decubitus ulcers or urinary tract infections) may lead to a shorter than expected life span. Suicide rates as high as seven times greater than expected in the general population have been reported.[35] Clinical and demographic factors that have been used to predict prognosis of MS are listed in Table 51–2.[35,36] Most likely reflecting improvements in overall care, World Health Organization (WHO) statistics suggest that mortality from MS has decreased up to 25% during the past 30 years.[37]

DIAGNOSIS

MS symptoms can frequently be attributed to other neurologic diseases, just as many syndromes can mimic MS. The unpredictable nature of MS and the lack of laboratory tests and imaging techniques specific for the disease add to the difficulties in making this diagnosis, especially in the early stages of the disease.

TABLE 51–2. Prognostic Indicators In Multiple Sclerosis

Indicator	Favorable Prognosis	Unfavorable Prognosis
Age at onset	< 40 years	> 40 years
Gender	Female	Male
Initial symptoms	Optic neuritis or sensory symptoms	Motor or cerebellar symptoms
Attack frequency in early disease	Low	High
Course of disease	Relapsing/remitting	Progressive

Although MRI techniques have aided in the detection of MS lesions, the diagnosis remains primarily a clinical one that requires the demonstration of "lesions separated in space and time." This statement refers to the occurrence of at least two episodes of neurologic disturbance reflecting distinct sites of damage in the CNS that cannot be explained by another mechanism.[38] MS is currently classified into four major categories based on clinical evidence as well as laboratory studies.[36,39] For purposes of diagnostic classification, an attack is defined as an episode of neurologic dysfunction lasting at least 24 hours. The terms "relapse," "exacerbation," and "bout" also are used synonymously with "attack." The two attacks specified in the criteria must affect different parts of the CNS and must be separated in time by at least 1 month.

LABORATORY STUDIES

To date there are no tests specific for MS. Tests that are frequently used include cerebrospinal fluid (CSF) evaluation, MRI, computed tomography (CT) scans, and evoked potentials. Evidence provided by these studies, used in conjunction with the clinical history, may aid in establishing the diagnosis of MS.

CEREBROSPINAL FLUID EVALUATION

In MS patients, CNS synthesis of IgG is increased, while serum IgG levels are normal. Electrophoretic studies of the CSF show that the IgG separates into a small number of discrete bands called "oligoclonal bands."[36] Although oligoclonal banding of IgG is present in 90% to 95% of patients with clinically definite, established MS, it is significant only if banding is not found in the serum.[36,40] It is important to remember that CSF IgG elevations are not specific for MS and may be seen in a variety of other diseases. Early on (e.g., after initial symptoms), CSF may be positive in only 30% to 50%. Increasingly, CSF analysis is reserved only for atypical cases. Myelin basic protein is detected in the CSF of 90% of patients shortly after an acute attack. Additional CSF abnormalities may include increased CSF protein concentrations in approximately 25% of patients and a mild CSF leukocytosis.[36] The presence of greater than 50×10^6 mononuclear cells in the CSF usually indicates a diagnosis other than MS.[40]

IMAGING STUDIES

MRI, especially with gadolinium enhancement, is much more sensitive than CT scans in the detection of MS lesions and is currently considered the preferred imaging method.[36,41] Lesions that enhance with gadolinium may also indicate new lesions and disruption of the BBB. Lesions are observed on MRI in 70% to 95% of patients with clinically definite MS. More important, they are observed in 65% to 85% of patients with suspected MS.[36]

▶ TREATMENT: Multiple Sclerosis

To date, no therapy has been shown to cure MS, and only recently has any therapy shown the ability to slow the progression of the disease. Symptomatic management of the disease is of utmost importance to maintain the patient's quality of life. A variety of different treatment modalities have been studied; however, many trials had a flawed design.[42] The lack of specific indicators for disease activity and the unpredictable course of the disease make assessment of various therapies difficult. There are no universally accepted treatment protocols, and treatments vary among clinicians and treatment centers. Perhaps more importantly, treatment decisions are frequently based upon the wishes and goals of individual patients. One potential algorithm for the treatment of relapsing-remitting MS is shown in Figure 51–3.

DESIRED OUTCOME

Therapy of MS may be attempted at different stages during the course of the disease as shown in Figure 51–2. The basic goals of therapy are to decrease the severity, intensity, and duration of exacerbations; enhance recovery from exacerbations; prevent relapses and the onset of progressive disease; halt or even reverse progressive disease; and provide symptomatic relief from the complications of MS.

DISEASE-MODIFYING MODALITIES

TREATMENT OF ACUTE EXACERBATIONS

Various immunosuppressive agents have been evaluated for disease-modifying activity in MS.[43–45] Treatment of an acute exacerbation varies depending on the severity of the attack. Mild exacerbations that do not produce functional decline may not require any treatment.[43] When functional ability is affected, treatment is usually started with corticosteroids. In milder cases, oral prednisone is used in a variety of dosing regimens.[43] Intravenous methylprednisolone is the most commonly used agent in the treatment of severe, acute exacerbations.[43,45] Because effects of corticosteroids may be transient and tend to diminish with repeated use, some clinicians stress that steroid therapy should not be used for symptom fluctuations without any functional consequence.

The mechanism of action for corticosteroids in MS is unknown; however, it is speculated that steroids improve recovery by decreasing edema in the area of demyelination.[43] In addition, steroids have been shown to reduce BBB abnormalities observed by CT, reduce CSF IgG synthesis, and decrease concentrations of MBP during acute exacerbations. Unfortunately, the relationship between these parameters and disease activity has not been established.

High-dose methylprednisolone has been shown to shorten the duration of acute exacerbations,[46–48] although it has not been shown to affect the progression of disease.[18,43,49] Comparative trials of adrenocorticoid hormone (ACTH) and high-dose intravenous steroids suggest that steroids produce a quicker and more predictable improvement in acute exacerbations. Although the reasons for this are not entirely clear, differences between agents may be due to the variable adrenal secretion of endogenous glucocorticoids following ACTH stimulation.[50] The use of ACTH, therefore, has been largely supplanted by methylprednisolone.

Methylprednisolone doses may range from 500 to 1000 mg/d, given intraveneously. The duration of therapy is variable and may range from 3 days to 3 weeks depending on clinical response. If improvement occurs it is usually seen in the first 3 to

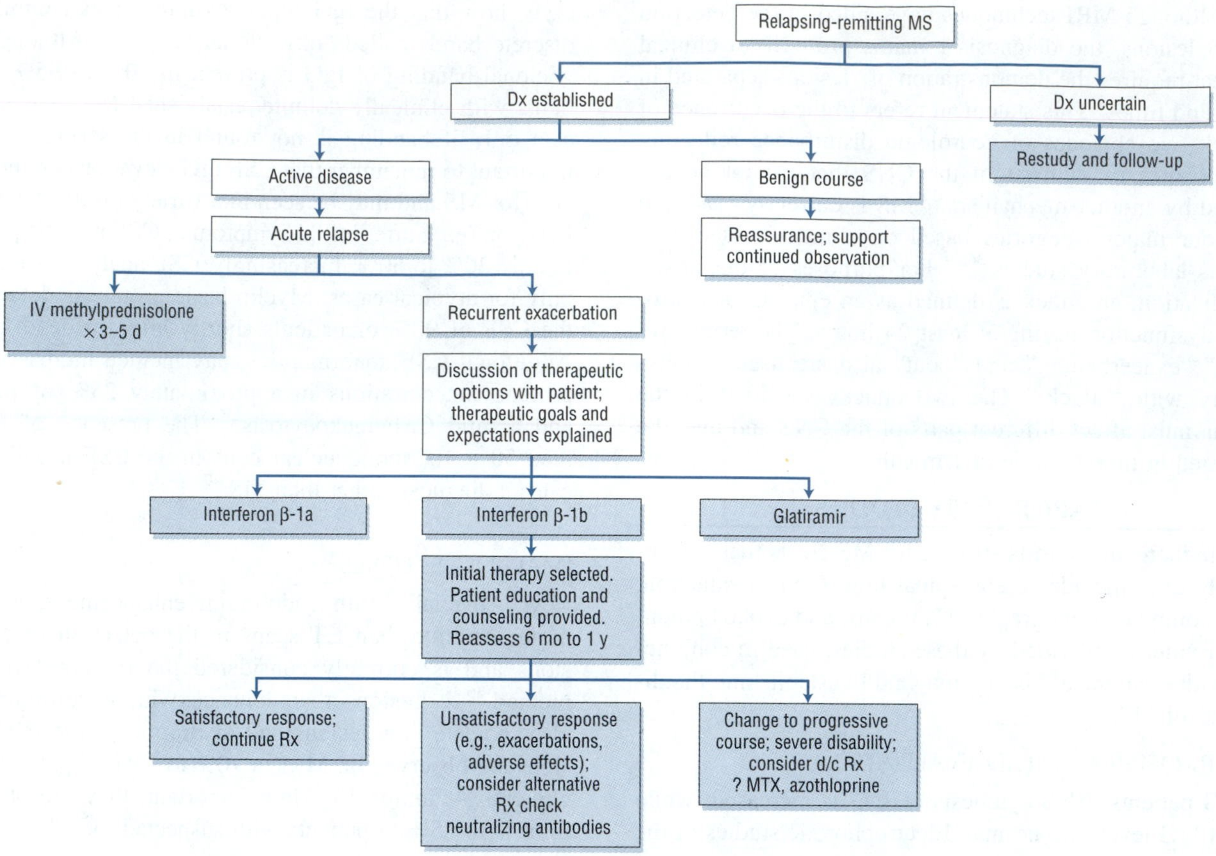

FIGURE 51–3. Algorithm for management of relapsing-remitting MS.

5 days; therefore, parenteral therapy may be continued for up to 5 days, followed by an oral steroid taper. Oral steroid regimens typically begin with 60 to 80 mg of prednisone for 3 to 7 days, and then the dosage is tapered over 7 days or longer depending on the patient's symptoms.[50]

PREVENTION OF RELAPSES AND PROGRESSION

Interferon β-1b and Interferon β-1a

Interferon β-1b (Betaseron), in addition to significantly reducing annual MS exacerbation rates by about one-third, was the first agent to potentially slow the progression of MS.[51] Interferon β-1b is a nonglycosylated synthetic analog of recombinant interferon beta produced in *Escherichia coli*. Although the exact mechanism of action is unknown, its effect in MS may be due to its immunomodulating properties, including the ability to augment suppressor cell function and reduce interferon γ secretion by activated lymphocytes, its macrophage-activating effect and its ability to down-regulate the expression of interferon-γ-induced class II MHC gene products on antigen-presenting glial cells.[42,52,53] Interferon β-1b also suppresses T-cell proliferation and may decrease BBB permeability.[54] The clinical relevance of the interferons, viral inhibiting effects is unclear

Interferon β-1b is administered every other day subcutaneously at a dose of 8 million IU. Clinical trials have demonstrated that at these doses, interferon β-1b can significantly reduce annual relapse rate as compared to placebo. In addition, comparison of serial MRI data showed that at 3 years, placebo-treated patients tended to have an increase in total lesional area of about 20%, while interferon-treated patients had no significant increases. With respect to clinical disability, however, no significant differences were noted between the interferon- and placebo-treated groups.[55] An advisory panel has published guidelines for selection of patients for treatment with interferon β-1b (Table 51–3),[56] which are much broader than the initial treatment guidelines and suggest using interferon β-1b only in ambulatory patients with frequent attacks of relapsing-remitting MS. The patient's motivational level and perceived ability to comply with this therapy are also considered during patient selection.

Baseline hemoglobin, complete blood counts, platelets, and liver function tests should be documented before starting therapy with interferon β-1b. The most common adverse effects include injection site redness and swelling and possibly necrosis, as well as flu-like symptoms (fever, chills, myalgias). These symptoms can be mild or severe and are seen in the majority of patients. Injection site reactions may be lessened by using appropriate injection technique, including site rotation (thighs and buttocks) and hydrocortisone cream. Ice applied before and/or after the injection may also decrease the pain and the redness. Nonsteroidal anti-inflammatory agents or acetominophen taken before and at regular intervals for 24 hours after administration may alleviate the flu-like symptoms. Initiation of one-half the standard dose, then increasing to full dosage over a month may also be beneficial.[57] Some authors suggest that because of the transient immune activation that may occur following the introduction of interferon beta; a short burst of oral prednisone may alleviate some adverse effects.[57] Less commonly reported side effects include shortness of breath, tachycardia, and depression. Clinicians must carefully monitor patients for signs of depression and treat accordingly. Although depression is a common finding in MS patients, recent studies tend to support the notion that interferon β-1b treatment

TABLE 51–3. Patient Selection Criteria for Treatment With Interferon β-1b

A. Class I[a] experimental evidence and expert consensus suggest interferon β-1b may be helpful:
   1. Relapsing-remitting course in patients with clinically definite or laboratory supported MS
   2. Age 18–50 years
   3. Ambulatory with EDSS ≤ 5.5
   4. At least two exacerbations in last 2 years

B. Expert consensus suggests interferon may be helpful:
   1. Relapsing-remitting disease and age > 50 years
   2. Relapsing-remitting disease and EDSS ≥ 6.0
   3. Relapsing-progressive (secondary progressive) disease with clinically definite or laboratory supported MS and at least two exacerbations in last 2 years

C. Neither Class I[a] evidence nor expert consensus support therapy with interferon β:
   1. Primary chronic progressive disease

D. Avoid interferon in patients
   1. At risk for poor compliance
   2. With concurrent illness that will substantially reduce life expectancy

E. Reasons to consider discontinuation of interferon β:
   1. Steady progression of disability for 6 months
   2. Three courses of ACTH or corticosteroids during a 1-year period despite treatment with interferon β-1b
   3. Severe depression or suicidal ideation
   4. Consistent noncompliance
   5. Severe adverse reactions
   6. Planned pregnancy or becoming pregnant

[a]Class I, evidence provided by one or more well-designed clinical trials.
Compiled from Ref. 57.

may be provocative. Patients who develop depressive symptoms should be closely monitored because there may be a risk for suicide. The other side effects are usually transient. Most patients will not feel better when taking this drug, and many will experience side effects; thus compliance may become a major issue. Patients should be reminded that some of the side effects are transient, and they should be counseled to minimize problems associated with local reactions.

Interferon β-1a (Avonex) is a natural-sequence, glycosolated product derived from recombinant Chinese hamster ovary cells. When given 30 μg intramuscularly once weekly for 2 years, patients receiving interferon β-1a demonstrated statistically significant reductions in annual relapse rate (by approximately one-third) as well as disease progression, which was defined as a progression of 1 point on the EDSS. Disease progression was also assessed by MRI studies, where it was found that patients receiving active drug had significantly fewer new lesions as compared to placebo-treated patients.[58] Taken together, these observations suggest that interferon β-1a may possess disease-modifying activity.

Although the adverse effect profile of interferon β-1a resembles interferon β-1b, interferon β-1a may hold several advantages including markedly fewer local tissues reactions and once-weekly administration versus subcutaneous injection every other day. Treatment-emergent depression was no more common with interferon β-1a than placebo. Finally, safety data of interferon-beta in pregnancy and lactation is lacking. Abortifacient activity in primates has been noted, however. Until adequate safety data are available, women should be counselled as to appropriate contraception while using these products.

Despite encouraging results from well-conducted clinical trials, several relevant questions remain. A concern with both products is the development of neutralizing antibodies. In clinical trials, 38% of patients receiving interferon β-1b developed antibodies.[59] In these patients, exacerbation rate was similar to placebo-treated patients. With interferon β-1a, neutralizing antibodies were found in 22% of treated patients. Because assays for these antibodies differ, it is difficult to judge the relative significance of these data. The long-term clinical significance of these findings is still unclear. Whether these antibodies are cross-reactive between products is unknown. The clinical relevance of neutralizing antibodies must be prospectively evaluated. It is also unclear whether the beneficial effects seen with the interferon products in relapsing-remitting MS will be evident in patients with secondary progressive MS. Finally, the optimal dosage and duration of therapy with these agents is unclear, and the lack of comparative trials clouds the question of which agent is superior.

Glatiramir (Copaxone)

Glatiramir (formerly known as copolymer-1) is a synthetic polypeptide consisting of l-alanine, l-glutamic acid, l-lysine, and l-tyrosine. Although the precise mechanism of action of this compound is unknown, glatiramir appears to mimic the antigenic properties of MBP.[60] This agent may also act by directly binding to MHC class II receptors and inhibiting binding of MBP peptides to T-cell receptor complexes.[60] Glatiramir may also suppress T-cell activation. Multicenter trials with glatiramir have demonstrated statistically significant reductions in mean annual relapse rate (~ 25%) that is comparable to the interferons.[61] Currently, it is unclear what effect this agent may have on disease progression.[60] Unfortunately, comparative trials between the interferons and glatiramir have been not been conducted. Intriguingly, *in vitro* data suggest potential synergism between glatiramir and interferon β. Given the cost of these therapies, as well as the potential for additive adverse effects, this therapeutic combination cannot be recommended, however, until clinical evidence demonstrating benefit is available. Glatiramir appears to have a relatively mild adverse effect profile, with mild pain and pruitis at the injection site being the most frequent patient complaints. Approximately 10% of patients will experience a transient reaction consisting of chest tightness, flushing, and dyspnea beginning several minutes after injection, and lasting usually no longer than 20 minutes. If patients have no history or evidence of coronary artery disease, they may be assured that these reactions are almost always self-limiting and appear benign. Several adverse effects that have been associated with the interferons, including flu-like symptoms and depression, do not appear to be provoked by glatiramir. Also unlike the interferons, glatiramir does not seem to induce the formation of *neutralizing* antibodies. The clinical significance of this observation, however, is uncertain.

Other Therapies

Short-term, intensive-pulse doses of corticosteroids, similar to those used in acute exacerbations, may initially decrease disability; however, prolonged steroid therapy has no established effects on the progression of disease.[49] If progression continues, an immunosuppressive agent may be tried.[44,45] Cyclophosphamide has been studied alone and in combination with other treatment modalities in attempts to slow progression of MS.[62] Maintenance therapy with intermittent (monthly) pulse doses of cyclophosphamide may slow the progression of disease in younger patients with secondary progressive disease; however, further study is required to confirm benefit in these patients. Prolonged therapy with cyclophosphamide is usually intolerable; however, it appears that some form of maintenance is necessary.[62] Although cyclophosphamide appears beneficial, toxicities may limit its use to patients with unusually severe disease course.[44]

Conflicting results have been shown when azathioprine is used alone or in combination with other therapies. Reductions in exacerbation rate and slowing of disease progression is only modest.[45] It is usually given in doses of 2 to 3 mg/kg until the white blood cell count drops to less than 4000/mm^3 and is then followed with corticosteroid therapy.[43,45] Although not without serious side effects, azathioprine may be less toxic than cyclophosphamide and may be tolerated for a longer period of time. Methotrexate (MTX) given as 7.5 mg orally each week has also shown modest benefit in slowing disease progression.[43]

Cyclosporine appears to produce only a modest delay in the progression of disability in chronic progressive MS. A significant number of patients may develop severe side effects, in particular nephrotoxicity and hypertension,[63] which may limit the usefulness of this agent.

Other experimental modalities include total lymphoid irradiation (TLI), α-interferon, monoclonal antibodies, mitoxantrone, cladribine, and intraveneous immune globulin (IVIG).[43] IVIG may stimulate remyelinization of neurons in established MS lesions. Further studies are required to confirm the observation of reduced exacerbation and improved neurologic function.

SYMPTOMATIC MANAGEMENT

Many of the symptoms of MS do not require pharmacologic management or do not respond to it. The next section covers those primary symptoms in which pharmacologic management may be of benefit (Table 51–4).

OPTIC NEURITIS

Lesions in the optic nerve will eventually be diagnosed in the majority of MS patients. Patients may complain of variable degrees of visual loss, blurring vision, or hazy vision. The onset of symptoms is typically quite sudden and progressive. High-dose intraveneous steroids are usually given for episodes of severe optic neuritis. In one large clinical trial, methylprednisolone 1 g was given IV for 3 days, followed by oral prednisone 1 mg/kg for 11 days.[64] This regimen was compared to oral prednisone 1 mg/kg alone for 14 days and placebo. Methylprednisolone therapy resulted in a higher rate of symptom recovery. Interestingly, oral prednisone treatment alone was not significantly better than placebo. Improtantly, the subsequent relapse rate was higher in patients treated with oral prednisone alone. At this time, parenteral high-dose steroids would appear preferable to oral treatment for acute attacks of optic neuritis.

GAIT DIFFICULTIES AND SPASTICITY

Problems with gait may be due to spasticity, weakness, ataxia, defective proprioception, or a combination of these factors. Spasticity is amenable to pharmacologic intervention, whereas physical therapy may be required in treating gait disturbances due to any of the other factors. Spasticity is commonly encountered and tends to affect the legs more markedly than the arms. Spasticity may result in falls; however, in the later stages of the disease, the increased muscle tone of a spastic limb often lends strength to patients with underlying weakness. Therefore, when using muscle relaxants, one must be careful not to decrease the tone to an extent where ambulation is actually hindered.[28,65] Baclofen (Lioresal), a γ-aminobutyric acid (GABA) analog, is the preferred agent and is usually started in dosages of 5 mg tid and titrated upward to achieve the desired response. Most patients will achieve a satisfactory response with dosages between 40 and 80 mg/d; however, dosages higher than the recommended daily maximum of 80 mg are required by some patients.[28,65] Continuous intrathecal administration of baclofen may be an option for those patients unable to tolerate, or those who do not respond to oral therapy. Baclofen should not be abruptly discontinued to avoid the possibility of seizures.[65] Small doses of diazepam (for example, 0.5 to 1 mg) are often added to baclofen in patients in whom optimal response has not been achieved. In patients who are unable to tolerate baclofen, diazepam or dantrolene may be considered as alternatives; however they are generally less effective than baclofen. A newer agent, tizanidine (Zanaflex) is a short-acting, centrally acting α-adrenergic agonist that can reduce spasticity by increasing presynaptic inhibition of motor neurons. Tizanidine appears to have efficacy comparable to baclofen.[66] Dosage of this medication must be titrated slowly over 2 to 4 weeks, starting at 4 mg at bedtime, and adjusting based upon clinical response. Effective tolerated dosages have ranged from 2 to 36 mg/d. Sedation, dizziness, and dry mouth are the most commonly reported adverse effects of this agent. Hypotension can also occur, as well as a rare but severe hepatotoxicity. Increased aminotransferase activity was noted in 5% of patients during clinical trials.

TREMOR

Cerebellar symptoms such as tremor can be troubling and difficult to control. Medications that may be helpful include isoniazid, primidone, and propranolol.

BOWEL AND BLADDER SYMPTOMS

Patients commonly complain of incontinence, urgency, frequency, and nocturia, which are indications of a hyperreflexic bladder (i.e., inability to store urine). A number of anticholinergic agents including propantheline bromide (Probanthine 45 to 90 mg/d), oxybutinin chloride (Ditropan 10 to 30 mg/d), and dicyclomine hydrochloride (Bentyl 30 to 80 mg/d) are used to treat this problem, if symptoms are mild.[67] In addition, tricyclic antidepressants, such as imipramine (Tofranil) and amitriptyline (Elavil), also have been used for their anticholinergic properties. As an alternative, the synthetic antidiuretic hormone preparation desmopressin (DDAVP) has been reported effective in the treatment of urgency and incontinence.[67] Intermittent self-catheterization with or without a concomitant anticholinergic agent is recommended in patients with large postvoid urine residual volumes (> 100 mL) or when the urinary problem is hyporeflexic in nature (failure to empty).[65] Patients with large postvoid residual volumes are at risk for developing urinary tract infections and are often prescribed urinary acidifiers such as vitamin C or antiseptics such as methenamine mandelate to prevent infections. For more severe symptoms, urologic referral and urodymanic testing should be considered prior to treatment.

TABLE 51–4. Treatment of Selected Primary MS Symptoms

Spasticity	Bladder Symptoms	Sensory Symptoms	Fatigue
Baclofen	Propantheline	Carbamazepine	Amantadine
Dantrolene	Oxybutinin	Phenytoin	Pemoline
Diazepam	Dicyclomine	Amitriptyline or other TCAs	Antidepressants
Tizanadine	DDAVP		
	Self-catheterization		

Constipation due to either inactivity or medication side effects is the most common bowel complaint. Increases in dietary fiber and hydration may alleviate this problem; however, in some instances laxatives or enemas may be necessary.[28]

MAJOR DEPRESSION

Major depression is common in patients with MS, and the risk of suicide may be markedly increased as compared to healthy subjects.[68,69] Patients should be closely monitored for the development of major depressive symptomatology, and treated accordingly (see Chap. 65).

SENSORY SYMPTOMS

Numbness and paresthesias are frequent sensory complaints, but usually do not require treatment. Some MS patients may develop acute or chronic pain syndromes,[70] such as trigeminal neuralgia and painful dysasthesias, for which treatment is necessary. Carbamazepine is the preferred agent for the treatment of trigeminal neuralgia, and is used in the same doses that are used for the treatment of seizure disorders. Painful dysasthesias are burning sensations that commonly occur in the extremities. These sensory complaints are difficult to treat, but may sometimes respond to treatment with tricyclic antidepressants or carbamazepine. Sexual dysfunction in both men and women is also common in MS, and counseling should be offered to both partners.

Fatigue, one of the most common complaints in MS patients, can be severely disabling. It usually worsens before and during a flare, and with increases in ambient temperature. The cause of fatigue is unclear. Spasticity, weakness, and depression may also contribute to MS-related fatigue. Amantadine hydrocholoride 100 mg bid is sometimes used and may offer modest relief.[65] Studies evaluating this agent are subjective and do not show conclusive evidence for efficacy. Pemoline (Cylert) has also been used in doses starting at 18.75 to 37.5 mg/d.[65] Antidepressants may also be helpful, especially if the patient exhibits symptoms of depression.

The aminopyridines, 4-aminopyridine and 3,4-diaminopyridine,[71] are potassium channel blockers that are currently under investigation in the symptomatic treatment of MS. These agents appear to improve conduction in demyelinated axons and may improve strength and decrease heat sensitivity.[43]

Each symptom should be assessed individually, and therapy with available agents tried and modified when needed. In addition to counseling patients regarding the adverse effects associated with medications, pharmacists should also actively encourage patients to comply with their prescribed regimens.

PHARMACOECONOMIC CONSIDERATIONS

As with many therapeutic decisions, economic cost both to the individual and society must be considered. Currently, the annual cost of the new potentially disease modifying therapies is considerable. The cost to the pharmacist of glatiramir and both currently available interferons is between $10,000 and $11,000 per patient per year. Given this expense, it must be remembered that these therapies are not curative, and that individual patients may experience variable results. Future investigations evaluating these therapeutic modalities will clearly need to address both economic as well as humanistic outcomes.

EVALUATION OF THERAPEUTIC OUTCOMES

Response to treatment of acute exacerbations of MS are commonly seen within days. With respect to disease-modifying treatments, it is important for the clinician to recognize that over the short-term (days to weeks) little or no apparent benefit may be noted by either patient or clinician. Evaluation of therapeutic outcomes, such as decreased MS exacerbations and hospitalizations or perhaps slowed disease progression and disability (as measured using scales such as EDSS), must be conducted over a period of months to years. Patients should be provided with realistic goals and expectations of these treatment options, and encouraged to participate in the evaluation of therapeutic response. Initially, it may be important to reevaluate patients at relatively short time intervals to monitor for adverse effects.

CONCLUSIONS

MS is an inflammatory disease of the CNS that appears to strike young, genetically susceptible individuals living in high-risk geographic areas. Although the exact etiology of MS is unknown, it is likely that MS is an autoimmune disease triggered by a viral infection. There is no cure for MS; however, quality of life can be improved through symptomatic management. Because of the relapsing-remitting nature of MS, it is often difficult to assess whether improvement is due to treatment or due to the course of the disease. The paucity of conclusive evidence for many of the described treatments and the lack of specific guidelines make treatment choices difficult.

▶ PRINCIPLES OF PHARMACOTHERAPY

- The etiology of MS is unknown, and currently there is no cure.
- MS appears to be an immunologic disorder, which is characterized by CNS demyelination.
- Diagnosis of MS is made primarily on the basis of clinical examination and MRI findings.
- Acute exacerbations or relapses are usually treated with high-dose glucocorticoids, such as methylprednisolone.
- In most patients suffering from an acute exacerbation, a clinical response to steroid treatment can be expected within 3 to 5 days.
- Chronic steroid treatment does not appear to alter the course of disease progression.
- Treatment with beta interferon or glatiramir can reduce annual relapse rate, but these drugs are not used for acute exacerbations.
- Disease progression may be altered by chronic beta interferon treatment.

- Patients suffering from MS will frequently have symptoms such as spasticity, bladder dysfunction, fatigue, pain, and depression, which may require treatment. Patients must be counseled that therapies such as interferon and glatiramir will not relieve these symptoms.
- Depression is common in MS and may pose the risk of suicide.

REFERENCES

1. Anderson DW, Ellenberg JH, Leventhal CM, et al. Revised estimate of the prevalence of multiple sclerosis in the United States. Ann Neurol 1992;31:333–336.
2. Wynn DR, Rodriguez M, O'Fallon WM, et al. Update on the epidemiology of multiple sclerosis. Mayo Clin Proc 1989;64:808–817.
3. Sadovnick AD, Ebers GC. Epidemiology of multiple sclerosis: A critical overview. Can J Neurol Sci 1993;20:17–29.
4. Lechtenberg R. Multiple Sclerosis Fact Book. Philadelphia, Davis, 1988.
5. Ebers GC, Bulman D. The geography of MS reflects genetic susceptibility. Neurology 1986;36(suppl 1):108.
6. Compston A. Risk factors for multiple sclerosis: Race or place? J Neurol Neurosurg Psychiatry 1990;53:821–823. Editorial.
7. Kurtzke JF. Epidemiologic contributions to multiple sclerosis: An overview. Neurology (NY) 1980;30(suppl 2):61–79.
8. Ebers GC. Genetics and multiple sclerosis: An overview. Ann Neurol 1994;36:S12–S14.
9. Compston A. The epidemiology of multiple sclerosis: Principles, achievements, and recommendations. Ann Neurol 1994:36; S211–S217.
10. Wolfson C, Wolfson EB, Zielinski JM. On the estimation of the distribution of the latent period of multiple sclerosis. Neuroepidemiology 1989;8:239–248.
11. Detels R, Visscher BR, Haile RW, et al. Multiple sclerosis and age at migration. Am J Epidemiol 1978;108:386–393.
12. Hillert J. Human leukocyte antigen studies in multiple sclerosis. Ann Neurol 1994;36:S15–S17.
13. Genetics and immunology. In: Kesselring J, ed. Multiple Sclerosis. Cambridge, UK, Cambridge, University Press, 1997:30–48.
14. Lucchinetti CF, Rodriguez M. The controversy surrounding the pathogenesis of the multiple sclerosis lesion. Mayo Clin Proc 1997;72: 665–678.
15. De Keyser J. Autoimmunity in multiple sclerosis. Neurology 1988;38:371–374.
16. McDonald WI. The mystery of the origin of multiple sclerosis. J Neurol Neurosurg Psychiatry 1989;49:113–323.
17. Poser CM. Pathogenesis of multiple sclerosis. A critical reappraisal. Acta Neuropathol 1986;71:1–10.
18. Sharief MK, Thompson EJ. *In vivo* relationship of tumor necrosis factor alpha to blood brain barrier damage in patients with active multiple sclerosis. J Neuroimmunol 1992;38:27–33.
19. Panitch HS, Hirsch RL, Schindler J, Johnson KP. Treatment of multiple sclerosis with gamma interferon: Exacerbation associated with activation of the immune system. Neurology 1987;37:1097–1102.
20. Hartung HP, Archelos JJ, Zievasek J, Gold R, et al. Circulating adhesion molecules and inflammatory mediators in demyelination: A review. Neurology 1995;45(suppl 6):22–32.
21. Link J, Soderstrom M, Olsson T. Increased TGFβ, IL-4 and INFα in multiple sclerosis. Ann Neurol 1994;36:379–386.
22. Rieckman P, Albrecht M, Kitze B, et al. Cytokine mRNA levels in mononuclear blood cells from patients with multiple sclerosis. Neurology 1994;44:1523–1526.
23. Sobel RA. The pathology of multiple sclerosis. Neurol Clin 1995;13:1–16
24. Johnson RT. The virology of demyelinating diseases. Ann Neurol 1994;36:S54–S60.
25. Lassman H, Suchanek G, Ozawa K. Histopathology and the blood-cerebrospinal fluid barrier in multiple sclerosis. Ann Neurol 1994; 36:S42–S46.
26. Rodriguez M. Multiple sclerosis. Basic concepts and hypothesis. Mayo Clin Proc 1989;64:570–576.
27. Weiner HL, Hafler DA. Immunotherapy of multiple sclerosis. Ann Neurol 1988;23:211–222.
28. Schapiro RT. Symptom management in multiple sclerosis. Ann Neurol 1994;36:S123–S129.
29. Kurtzke JF. Rating neurologic impairment in multiple sclerosis: An expanded disability status scale (EDSS). Neurology 1983;33:1444–1452.
30. Noseworthy JH. Clinical scoring methods for multiple sclerosis. Ann Neurol 1994;36:S80–S85.
31. Miller DH. Magnetic resonance imaging in monitoring the treatment of multiple sclerosis. Ann Neurol 1994;36:S91–S94.
32. Filippi M, Paty DW, Kappos L, et al. Correlations between changes in disability and T2 weighted brain activity in multiple sclerosis: A follow up study. Neurology 1995;45:255–260.
33. Abramsky O. Pregnancy and multiple sclerosis. Ann Neurol 1994; 36:S38–S41.
34. Kurland LT. Trauma and multiple sclerosis. Ann Neurol 1994;36: S33–S37.
35. Weinshenker BG. Natural history of multiple sclerosis. Ann Neurol 1994;36:S6–S11.
36. Swanson JW. Multiple sclerosis: Update in diagnosis and review of prognostic factors. Mayo Clin Proc 1989;64:577–586.
37. Williams ES, Jones DR, McKeran RO. Mortality rates from multiple sclerosis: Geographical and temporal variations revisited. J Neurol Neurosurg Psychiatry 1991;54:104–109.
38. McDonald WI, Silberberg DH. The diagnosis of multiple sclerosis. In: McDonald WI, Silberberg DH, eds. Multiple Sclerosis. Boston, Butterworth, 1986:1.
39. Lublin F, Reingold S, NMSS Advisory Committee on Clinical Trials of New Agents in Multiple Sclerosis. Defining the clinical course of multiple sclerosis: Results of an international survey. Neurology 1996;46:907–911.
40. Olsson T. Cerebrospinal fluid. Ann Neurol 1994;36:S100–S102.
41. McFarland H, Frank JA, Albert PS, et al. Using gadolinium-enhanced magnetic resonance imaging lesions to monitor disease activity in multiple sclerosis. Ann Neurol 1992;32:758–766.
42. Myers LW, Ellison GW. The peculiar difficulties of therapeutic trials for multiple sclerosis. Neurol Clin 1990;8:119–141.
43. Hunter SF, Weinshenker BG, Carter JL, Noseworthy JH. Rational clinical immunotherapy for multiple sclerosis. Mayo Clin Proc 1997; 72:765–780.
44. Becker C, Gidal BE, Flemming JO. Immunotherapy in multiple sclerosis, part 2 Am J Health Syst Pharm 1995;52:2105–2120.
45. Becker C, Gidal BE, Flemming JO. Immunotherapy in multiple sclerosis, part 1 Am J Health Syst Pharm 1995;52:1985–2000.
46. Rose AS, Kuzma JW, Kurtzke JF, et al. Cooperative study in the evaluation of therapy in multiple sclerosis: ACTH versus placebo, final report. Neurology 1970;20(suppl):1–19.
47. Durelli L, Cocito A, Riccio C, et al. High-dose intravenous methylprednisolone in the treatment of multiple sclerosis: Clinical immunologic correlations. Neurology 1986;36:238–243.
48. Milligan NM, Newcombe R, Compston DAS. A double-blind controlled trial of high-dose methylprednisolone in patients with multiple sclerosis, 1. Clinical effects. J Neurol Neurosurg Psychiatry 1987;50: 511–516.
49. Goodin DS. The use of immunosuppressive agents in the treatment of multiple sclerosis: A critical review. Neurology 1991;41:980–985.
50. Kappos L. Therapy. In: Kesselring J, ed. Multiple Sclerosis. Cambridge, UK, Cambridge University Press, 1997:148–167.

51. The IFNB Multiple Sclerosis Study Group. Interferon beta-1b is effective in relapsing-remitting multiple sclerosis, 1. Clinical results of a multi-center, randomized, double-blind, placebo-controlled trial. Neurology 1993;43:655–661.
52. The IFNB Multiple Sclerosis Study Group. Interferon beta-1b is effective in relapsing-remitting multiple sclerosis, 2. MRI analysis results of a multicenter, randomized, double-blind, placebo-controlled trial. Neurology 1993;43:662–667.
53. Goodkin DE. Interferon β-1b. Lancet 1994;344:1057–1060.
54. Arnason BG, Reder AT. Interferons and multiple sclerosis. Clin Neuropharmacol 1994;17:495–547.
55. The INFB multiple sclerosis study group. The university of British Columbia MS/MRI analysis group. Interferon β-1b in the treatment of multiple sclerosis. Neurology 1995;45:1277–1285.
56. Quality Standards Subcommittee of the American Academy of Neurology. Practice advisory on selection of patients with multiple sclerosis for treatment with betaseron. Neurology 1994;44:1537–1540.
57. Guttman-Weinstock B, Rudick RA. Prescribing recommendations for interferon-beta in multiple sclerosis. CNS Drugs 1997;8:102–112.
58. Jacobs LD, Cookfair DL, Rudick RA, et al. Intramuscular interferon beta-1a for disease progression in relapsing multiple sclerosis. Ann Neurol 1996;39:285-294.
59. The INFB Multiple Sclerosis Study Group and the University of British Columbia MS/MRI Analysis Group. Neutralizing antibodies during treatment of multiple sclerosis with interferon beta 1b: Experience during the first three years. Neurology 1996;47:889–894.
60. Lea AP, Goa KL. Copolymer-1: A review of its pharmacological properties and therapeutic potential in multiple sclerosis. Clin Immunother 1996;6:319–331.
61. Johnson KP, Brooks BR, Cohen JA, et al. Copolymer-1 reduces relapse rate and improves disability in relapsing-remitting multiple sclerosis. Results of a phase III multicenter double-blind placebo controlled trial. Neurology 1995;45:1268–1276.
62. Goodkin DE, Plencner S, Palmer-Saxerud J, et al. Cyclophosphamide in chronic progressive multiple sclerosis. Maintenance versus nonmaintenance therapy. Arch Neurol 1987;44:823–827.
63. The Multiple Sclerosis Study Group. Efficacy and toxicity of cyclosporine in chronic progressive multiple sclerosis: A randomized, double-blinded, placebo-controlled clinical trial. Ann Neurol 1990; 27:591–605.
64. Beck RW, Cleary PA, Anderson MM, et al. A randomized, controlled trial of corticosteroids in the treatment of acute optic neuritis. N Engl J Med 1992;326:581–588.
65. Mitchell G. Update on multiple sclerosis therapy. Med Clin North Am 1993;77:231–249.
66. Wagstaff AJ, Bryson HM. Tizanidine. Drugs 1997;53:435–452.
67. Kinn AC, Larsson PO. Desmopressin: A new principle for symptomatic treatment of urgency and incontinence in patients with multiple sclerosis. Scand J Urol Nephrol 1990;24:109–112.
68. Schubert DS, Foliart RH. Increased depression in multiple sclerosis patients. A meta analysis. Psychosomatics 1993;34:124–130.
69. Stenager EN, Stenager E, Koch Henriksen N, et al. Suicide and multiple sclerosis: An epidemiological investigation. J Neurol Neurosurg Psychiatry 1992;55:542–545.
70. Moulin DE. Pain in multiple sclerosis. Neurol Clin 1989;7:321–331.
71. Beaver CT Jr. The current status of studies of aminopyridine in patients with multiple sclerosis. Ann Neurol 1994;36:S118–S121.

52

EPILEPSY

Nina M. Graves, PharmD, FCCP, and William R. Garnett, PharmD, FCCP

Epilepsy has been recognized for at least 2400 years. It is derived from the Greek "epilepsia," meaning "to come upon, to be grabbed hold of or thrown down, to attack, to seize hold of." Hughlings Jackson, in 1861, first developed the theory that seizures were caused by an excessive discharge of the gray matter of the brain.

Today epilepsy is viewed as a symptom of disturbed electrical activity in the brain caused by a wide variety of disorders. Epilepsy is a general name given to the wide range of symptoms that reflect the many functions of the brain in a pathologically disturbed manner. It is a collection of many different types of seizures that vary widely in severity, appearance, cause, consequence, and management. Epilepsy implies a periodic recurrence of seizures with or without convulsions.[1] Seizures that are prolonged or repetitive can be life threatening (see Chap. 53). The effect epilepsy has on patients' lives can be extremely frustrating. One patient stated:

> While my first seizures were more terrifying than subsequent seizures because I had no idea of what was happening to me, having seizures does not become any easier with familiarity. If anything, each one is a frustrating setback: a reminder that my epilepsy is not under control, an indication that my medication dosage is not sufficient, a signal that I must start over my "countdown" until the day I may drive again, another reason for my family to worry about me.[2]

In the early 1980s, the primary drugs used for epilepsy were phenobarbital, phenytoin, carbamazepine, and valproic acid. Seven new drugs have been approved for use in epilepsy: felbamate, gabapentin, lamotrigine, topiramate, tiagabine, zonisamide, and vigabatrin. Several more are in the latter stages of clinical trials (levetiracetam, losigamone, oxcarbazepine, remacemide, and others). The availability of new drugs for epilepsy offers new opportunities to improve treatment and makes it essential that clinicians review all of their patients to ensure that they are achieving the best outcomes possible.

EPIDEMIOLOGY

Each year 120 per 100,000 people in the United States come to medical attention because of a newly recognized seizure. At least 8% of the general population will have at least one seizure in a lifetime. However, it is possible to have a seizure and not have epilepsy.[3] Recurrence of a first unprovoked seizure within 5 years ranges between 23% and 80%. Children with an idiopathic first seizure and a normal electroencephalogram (EEG) have a particularly favorable prognosis.[4] Some seizures may occur as single events resulting from withdrawal of central nervous system (CNS) depressants (e.g., alcohol, barbiturates, and other drugs) or during acute illnesses (such as meningoencephalitis) or toxic conditions (e.g., uremia or eclampsia). Some patients will have seizures only associated with fever. These febrile seizures do not constitute epilepsy.

Epilepsy is a chronic disorder, indicating recurrent seizures.[1] The age-adjusted incidence of epilepsy is 44 per 100,000 person-years. Each year about 125,000 new epilepsy cases occur; of these, 30% are in people under the age of 18 at the time of diagnosis. There is a bimodal distribution in the occurrence of the first seizure, with one peak occurring in newborn and young children and the second peak occurring in patients older than age 65.[5] The relatively high frequency of epilepsy in the elderly is now being recognized. At least 10% of patients in long-term care facilities are taking at least one antiepileptic drug (AED).[6] At this time, it is unknown if these AEDs are used for seizures or other conditions.[1] The seizure type and the cause of the seizure change with age.[5]

ETIOLOGY

Seizures occur because small numbers of neurons discharge abnormally. Anything that disrupts the normal homeostasis of the neuron and disturbs its stability may trigger abnormal activity and seizures. A hereditary predisposition to seizures has been suggested. Patients with mental retardation and cerebral palsy are at increased risk for seizures. The more profound the degree of mental retardation as measured by IQ, the greater the incidence of epilepsy. However, mental retardation is not synonymous with epilepsy. In the elderly, seizures are primarily (67%) partial in onset. The causes of seizures in the elderly are cerebrovascular disease, tumor, head trauma, metabolic disorders, CNS infections, and multifactorial etiology.[5] In some cases if an etiology can be found, it can be corrected, and the patient will not require chronic AEDs; however, most patients who present with seizures do not have an identifiable cause and thus have idiopathic epilepsy.[5] The incidence of idiopathic epilepsy is higher in children.[7]

Many factors have been shown to precipitate seizures in susceptible individuals.[1] Hyperventilation may precipitate absence seizures. Sleep, sleep deprivation, sensory stimuli, and emotional stress may initiate seizures. Hormonal changes occurring around the time of menses, puberty, or pregnancy have been associated with the onset of, or an increased frequency of, seizures. A history for theophylline, alcohol, phenothiazines, antidepressants (especially maprotiline), and street drug use should be obtained from patients presenting with seizures. Also, AEDs in excessive concentrations may cause seizures. Perinatal factors and subsequent events have been identified as risk factors for the later development of epilepsy. Children who are "small for gestational age" or with neonatal seizures are at increased risk for developing epilepsy. The most clearly established risk factors for epilepsy are severe head trauma, CNS infections, and stroke. Brain surgery increases the risk of developing epilepsy, although the extent of the risk is unknown. Immunizations have not been associated with an increased risk of epilepsy.[5] However, pertussis immunization has been associated with an increase in febrile seizures.

PATHOPHYSIOLOGY

Seizure activity is characterized by paroxysmal discharges occurring synchronously in a large population of cortical neurons. This is characterized on the EEG as a sharp wave or "spike." The basic physiology of a seizure episode is traceable to an unstable cell membrane or its surrounding, supportive cells. The seizure originates from the gray matter of any cortical or perhaps subcortical area. Initially, a small number of neurons fire abnormally. Normal membrane conductances and inhibitory synaptic currents break down and excess excitability spreads, either locally to produce a focal seizure or more widely to produce a generalized seizure.[8] This onset propagates by physiologic pathways to involve adjacent or remote areas. The clinical manifestations depend on the site of the focus, the degree of irritability of the surrounding area of the brain, and the intensity of the impulse.

An abnormality of potassium conductance, a defect in the voltage-sensitive ion channels, or a deficiency in the membrane ATPases linked to ion transport may result in neuronal membrane instability and a seizure. Selected neurotransmitters (e.g., glutamate, aspartate, acetylcholine, norepinephrine, histamine, corticotropin-releasing factor, purines, peptides, cytokines, and steroid hormones) enhance the excitability and propagation of neuronal activity, whereas gamma-aminobutyric acid (GABA) and dopamine inhibit neuronal activity and propagation. A deficiency of inhibitory neurotransmitters such as GABA or an increase in excitatory neurotransmitters would promote abnormal neuronal activity. Normal neuronal activity also depends on an adequate supply of glucose, oxygen, sodium, potassium, chloride, calcium, and amino acids. Systemic pH is also a factor in precipitating seizures. The different kinds of epilepsies probably arise from different physiologic abnormalities.

Control of abnormal neuronal activity with AEDs is accomplished by elevating the threshold of neurons to electrical or chemical stimuli or by limiting the propagation of the seizure discharge from its origin. Raising the threshold most likely involves stabilization of neuronal membranes, whereas limiting the propagation involves depression of synaptic transmission and reduction of nerve conduction.[8]

During a seizure there is a large increase in the demand for blood flow to the brain to carry off CO_2 and to bring substrates for neuronal metabolic activity. The brain has a limited capacity to increase blood flow, and during a seizure the brain may use more energy than it can manufacture. The more prolonged the seizure, the more likely the brain is to suffer ischemia that may result in neuronal destruction and brain damage. The developing brain is especially vulnerable to damage. However, seizure disorders as such do not cause a significant decrease in intelligence.

Seizures beget seizures. There appears to be a positive correlation between the early initiation of appropriate AED therapy and the ability to control seizure activity. The failure to control seizures seems to lead to an increase in seizure activity and also to the occurrence of other seizure types. Therefore, appropriate therapy should be initiated early after the diagnosis of epilepsy.

CLINICAL PRESENTATION

The International League Against Epilepsy (ILAE) has proposed two major schemes for classification of seizures and epilepsies: the International Classification of Epileptic Seizures[9] and the International Classification of the Epilepsies and Epilepsy Syndromes.[10]

The International Classification of Epileptic Seizures (Table 52–1) combines the clinical description with certain electrophysiologic findings, in order to classify epileptic seizures. Seizures are divided into two main pathophysiologic groups, partial seizures and generalized seizures, by EEG recordings and clinical symptomatology.

TABLE 52–1. International Classification of Epileptic Seizures

- I. Partial seizures (seizures begin locally)
  - A. Simple (without impairment of consciousness)
    - 1. With motor symptoms
    - 2. With special sensory or somatosensory symptoms
    - 3. With psychic symptoms
  - B. Complex (with impairment of consciousness)
    - 1. Simple partial onset followed by impairment of consciousness—with or without automatisms
    - 2. Impaired consciousness at onset—with or without automatisms
  - C. Secondarily generalized (partial onset evolving to generalized tonic–clonic seizures)
- II. Generalized seizures (bilaterally symmetrical and without local onset)
  - A. Absence
  - B. Myoclonic
  - C. Clonic
  - D. Tonic
  - E. Tonic–clonic
  - F. Atonic
  - G. Infantile spasms
- III. Unclassified seizures
- IV. Status epilepticus

Compiled from Ref. 9.

Partial (or focal or localization related) seizures begin in one hemisphere of the brain and—unless they become secondarily generalized—result in an asymmetric manifestation. Partial seizures manifest as alterations in motor functions, sensory or somatosensory symptoms, or automatisms. Partial seizures with no loss of consciousness are classified as simple partial. The symptoms (aura) often experienced prior to a generalized tonic clonic seizure may be a simple partial seizure that secondarily generalizes. Partial seizures with a loss or alteration of consciousness are described as complex partial. With complex partial seizures, the patient may have automatisms, periods of memory loss, or aberrations of behavior.[1] Some patients with complex partial epilepsy have been mistakenly diagnosed as having psychotic episodes. Complex partial seizures may progress to a generalized seizure.[1] Partial epilepsy may begin in infancy and may be difficult to recognize in an elderly population.

Generalized seizures have clinical manifestations that indicate involvement of both hemispheres. Motor manifestations are bilateral, and there is a loss of consciousness. Generalized seizures may be further subdivided by EEG and clinical manifestations.[1] A partial seizure that becomes generalized is referred to as a secondarily generalized seizure.

Generalized absence seizures are manifested by a sudden onset, interruption of ongoing activities, a blank stare, and possibly a brief upward rotation of the eyes. They generally occur in young children through adolescence. The EEG during the seizure has a characteristic 2 to 4 cycles/s spike and slow-wave complex.[1] It is important to differentiate absence seizures from complex partial seizures.

Generalized tonic–clonic seizures, formerly known as grand mal, are what many people think of as epilepsy. Although they may be preceded by premonitory symptoms (auras), the majority of patients lose consciousness without warning. The seizure results in a sudden sharp tonic contraction of muscles followed by a period of rigidity and clonic movements. The patient may fall and be injured. During the seizure, the patient may cry or moan, lose sphincter control, bite the tongue, or develop cyanosis. After the seizure, the patient may be unconscious for a variable period of time and frequently goes into a deep sleep. Tonic and clonic seizures may occur separately.[1]

Brief shock-like muscular contractions of the face, trunk, and extremities are known as myoclonic jerks. If they begin in adolescence, they are called juvenile myoclonic epilepsy (JME). They may be isolated events or rapidly repetitive.[1] A sudden loss of muscle tone is known as an atonic seizure. This may be described as a head drop, the dropping of a limb, or a slumping to the ground.[1] These patients often wear protective headware to prevent trauma.

The International Classification of Epilepsies and Epilepsy Syndromes[10] adds components such as age of onset, intellectual development, findings on neurologic examination, and results of neuroimaging studies to more fully define epilepsy syndromes. Syndromes can include one or many different seizure types (e.g., Lennox Gastaut syndrome). The syndromic approach includes seizure type(s) and possible etiologic classifications (idiopathic, symptomatic, or unknown). *Idiopathic* describes syndromes that are presumably genetic but also those in which no underlying etiology is documented or suspected. A family history of seizures is commonly present, and neurologic function is essentially normal except for the occurrence of seizures. *Symptomatic* cases involve evidence of brain damage or a known underlying cause. A cryptogenic syndrome is assumed to be symptomatic of an underlying condition that cannot be documented. *Unknown or undetermined* is used when no cause can be identified. This syndromic classification is more important for prognostic determinations than a classification based simply on seizure type. The syndrome classification scheme requires more information and, in return, provides a more powerful tool for comprehensive clinical management. A patient's epilepsy is classified based on seizure type (generalized versus partial) and syndromic type (idiopathic, symptomatic, cryptogenic).

▶ TREATMENT: Epilepsy

DESIRED OUTCOME

The ultimate goal of treatment for epilepsy is no seizures and no side effects with an optimal quality of life. The best quality of life is associated with a seizure-free state.[11] Often, however, a balance between efficacy and side effects must be reached, because with the older AEDs used as monotherapy, fewer than 50% of patients become seizure free.

Because therapy is extended for many years (often a lifetime), chronic side effects must be considered.[12] If the patient is overly sedated or develops other significant side effects, some seizure control may have to be sacrificed to improve functioning.[13] The patient should be involved in deciding what balance between frequency of seizures and the occurrence of side effects is most appropriate. The newer AEDs offer alternatives for balancing seizure frequency and drug side effects.

Providing optimal quality of life goes beyond balancing seizures and side effects. It involves assessing all the concerns of a patient with epilepsy. For example, patients with epilepsy are concerned about driving, their future, forming relationships, housing, social isolation, social stigma, and so on. Despite public awareness programs, there are still many misconceptions about epilepsy. These misconceptions often liken epilepsy to mental retardation, possession by demons, or punishment by God. Patients may be encouraged to contact or join the Epilepsy Foundation of America (1-800-EFA-1000) or other support groups that encourage patients with epilepsy to lead normal lives. Knowledge about epilepsy has been correlated with an improved quality of life.

GENERAL APPROACH TO TREATMENT

The general approach to treatment involves identification of goals, assessment, development of a care plan, and a follow-up evaluation. During the assessment phase, it is critical to establish an accurate diagnosis of the seizure type and classification. This diagnostic step will help determine the appropriate initial AEDs. Patient-specific treatment goals must be identified, and these may change over time. In patients with new-onset epilepsy, the goal should be "no seizures, no side effects" and an optimal quality of life. Patients with chronic epilepsy ideally have this same goal; however, it may not be possible to achieve it immediately, and thus the goal at a specific point in time must be established (e.g., decrease the number of seizures or alleviate toxicity). Identification of specific goals will help in the development of the short- and long-term treatment plans. Patient characteristics such as age, medical condition, ability to comply with a prescribed regimen, and insurance coverage should also be explored, as these may influence AED choices or help explain lack of response or unexpected side effects.

Once the assessment is complete, the advantages and disadvantages of appropriate AEDs are compared. For patients with new-onset seizures, the choice is whether to use drug therapy and if so, which one. For a patient with long-standing epilepsy, adequacy of the current medication regimen must be evaluated. An AED should not be considered ineffective unless the patient has experienced some concentration-dependent side effects with continued seizures.

If a decision is made to start AED therapy, monotherapy is preferred, and about 70% of all patients with epilepsy can be maintained on one drug.[7] However, not all of these patients are seizure free. The percentage of patients who are seizure free on one drug varies by seizure type. The prognosis for 12-month seizure freedom is best for those who have only generalized tonic clonic seizures (48% to 55%), worst for those who have only complex partial seizures (23% to 26%), and intermediate for those with mixed seizure types (25% to 32%).[14] Drugs may be combined in an attempt to help the patient become seizure free. Combining AEDs with different mechanisms of action may be advantageous, although this approach is as yet unproven. Approximately 65% of patients can be expected to be maintained on one AED and be considered well controlled, though not necessarily seizure free. Of the 35% with unsatisfactory control, 10% will be well controlled with a two-drug treatment. Of the remaining 25%, 20% of these will continue to have unsatisfactory control despite multiple drug treatment. Fifteen percent of these will become surgical candidates.[15]

Once the care plan is established, a prescription is generated for a specific AED. Usually this includes a dose titration schedule. At this point, patient education and assurance of patient understanding of the plan are essential. Detailed directions regarding titration, what to do in the event of a treatment-emergent side effect, and what to do if a seizure occurs must be provided to patients. Documentation of the assessment, care plan, and educational process is essential. Providing the patient with a seizure and side effect diary will assist in the follow-up and evaluation phase. At the follow-up stage of treatment (which can be done in the hospital, clinic, pharmacy, or by phone), the treatment goals must be reviewed. If the goal has been achieved, new goals should be identified. For example, if the generalized tonic–clonic (GTC) seizures are now controlled, the goal may be to control partial seizures. If a patient fails to respond to the first AEDs, trials with other AEDs should be attempted. Completion of the evaluation often requires a reassessment of the patient and development of a new care plan. The assessment at this point should evaluate compliance, efficacy, and safety of the initial treatment.

Noncompliance may be the single most common reason for treatment failure.[16] It is estimated that up to 60% of patients with epilepsy are noncompliant.[17] The rate of noncompliance is increased by the complexity of the drug regimen and by doses taken three and four times a day.[16] Noncompliance is not influenced by age, sex, psychomotor development, seizure type, or seizure frequency.[18]

WHEN TO START AEDs

Drug treatment may not be indicated in patients whose seizures have minimal impact on their lives or those who have had only a single seizure. If a patient presents after a single isolated seizure, one of three treatment decisions can be made: treat, possibly treat, or do not treat. These decisions are based on the probability of the patient having a second seizure (Table 52–2). For patients with no risk factors, the probability of a second seizure is less than 10% in the first year and approximately 24% by the end of 2 years. If risk factors are present, this recurrence rate can increase dramatically and can be as high as 80% after 5 years.[1] Are these rates high enough to warrant AED therapy? That decision often depends on the patient's life-style. Patients who have had two or more seizures should generally be started on AEDs. One study examined whether treatment affected the recurrence rate after a single unprovoked tonic–clonic seizure. The treated group had a 25% risk of seizure recurrence at 24 months, compared to 51% for the untreated group.[19]

WHEN TO STOP AEDs

The AEDs initially used to control seizures may not need to be given for a lifetime. Polypharmacy may be reduced, and some patients can discontinue AEDs altogether. In reducing polypharmacy, the drug considered less appropriate for the seizure type should be discontinued first. In some cases decreasing the number of AEDs a patient is receiving can decrease side effects and increase cognitive abilities.[20] This improvement in cognition may be small, especially if the patient is on a drug that primarily affects psychomotor speed with less effect on higher-order cognitive functioning.

Factors favoring successful withdrawal of AEDs include a seizure-free period of 2 to 4 years, complete seizure control within 1 year of onset, an onset of seizures after age 2 but before age 35 years, and a normal EEG. Factors associated with a poor prognosis in discontinuing AEDs, despite a seizure-free interval, include a history of a high frequency of seizures, repeated episodes of status epilepticus, a combination of seizure types, and development of abnormal mental functioning. Children who have irregular generalized spike and wave activity in EEG recordings prior to discontinuation of treatment may

TABLE 52–2. Recurrence Risk for Patients Experiencing One Unprovoked Seizure

Type of Patient	1st-Yr Risk (%)	5th-Yr Risk (%)
Adults with single unproved seizure		34
No CNS insult	10	29
Influence of family history		
Sibling with seizure	29	46
No sibling with seizures	7	27
EEG patterns		
GSW on EEG	15	58
Normal EEG	9	26
Occurrence of previous seizure	10	39
Due to an illness or childhood febrile seizure		
Remote symptomatic with Todd's paresis	26	48
	41	75
Status epilepticus at onset	37	56
Prior acute seizure	60	80
Idiopathic	10	29

CNS = central nervous system; EEG = electroencephalogram; GSW = generalized spikes and waves.
Compiled from Ref. 138.

TABLE 52–3. American Academy of Neurology Guideline for Discontinuing AEDs in Seizure-Free Patients

After assessing the risks and benefits to both patient and society from a recurrent seizure, the discontinuance of antiepileptic drugs may be considered by the physician and informed patient or parent/guardian if the patient meets the following profile:

- Seizure-free 2 to 5 years on AEDs (mean, 3.5 years)
- Single type of partial seizure (simple partial, complex partial, or secondary generalized tonic–clonic seizure) or single type of primary generalized tonic–clonic seizures
- Normal neurologic examination/normal IQ
- EEG normalized with treatment

have a higher relapse rate (67%) compared to children without epileptiform activity (33%) or children with other types of epileptiform activity (33%) in their last EEG recordings before discontinuation.[21] A 2-year seizure-free period is suggested for absence and rolandic epilepsy, while a 4-year seizure-free period is suggested for simple partial, complex partial, and absence associated with tonic–clonic convulsions. Withdrawal is generally not suggested for patients with juvenile myoclonic epilepsy, absence with clonic–tonic–clonic seizures, or clonic–tonic–clonic seizures.[22] The American Academy of Neurology has issued guidelines for discontinuing AEDs in seizure-free patients (Table 52–3).[23] When the factors likely to be associated with successful withdrawal are present, the relapse rate is expected to be less than 32% for children and 39% for adults.[23] A recent study examined patients who had had a seizure recurrence after randomization to either AED withdrawal or continued AED therapy.[24] The authors suggested that the population that develops epilepsy and then enters a period of remission for 2 or more years may be divided into two groups: (1) patients whose epilepsy has ceased and (2) patients with long interseizure intervals but epilepsy that is still active. Patients are divided about evenly between the two groups.

If the decision is made to attempt AED withdrawal, this should be done gradually. Some patients will have a recurrence of seizures as the AEDs are withdrawn. Sudden withdrawal is associated with the precipitation of status epilepticus. Seizure relapse has been reported to be more common if the AEDs are withdrawn over 1 to 3 months than over 6 months. However, another study found no difference in the rate of seizure recurrence in a 6-week taper versus a 9-month taper.[25]

The risk of seizure relapse has been estimated at 10% to 70%. A meta-analysis determined that the relapse rate was 25% after 1 year and 29% after 2 years.[26] Withdrawal doubles the risk of seizure recurrence for the first 1 to 2 years but does not modify the long-term prognosis of a person's epilepsy. If seizures recur after AED withdrawal, AEDs should be restarted. Ninety percent of patients will regain at least another 2-year remission.[24] In addition to seizure relapse, the withdrawal of AEDs has been associated with the emergence of anxiety and depression.[27]

The patient should agree to the plan to reduce or withdraw AED therapy. Some patients may be reluctant to stop medications because of fear of a seizure. There may be a significant psychosocial benefit to the patient from AED withdrawal.[28] Withdrawal may need to be scheduled at the convenience of the patient (e.g., during a summer vacation). A follow-up of 5 years is suggested for any patient withdrawn from AED therapy.

NONPHARMACOLOGIC THERAPY

Nonpharmacologic therapy for epilepsy includes diet, surgery, and implantation of a vagal nerve stimulator.[29] The vagal nerve stimulator was approved for use in patients in 1997. Recent reports of the effectiveness of sterotactic gamma knife radiosurgery have also been published.[30] Surgery is the most widespread and most useful nonpharmacologic therapy.[31]

The use of surgery for intractable epilepsy that significantly interferes with patients' lives and functioning is increasing. The success rate is reported to be between 80% and 90% in properly selected patients.[31] A National Institutes of Health Consensus Conference identified three absolute requirements for surgery. They are an absolute diagnosis of epilepsy, failure on an adequate trial of drug therapy, and definition of the electroclinical syndrome.[32] A focus in the temporal lobe has the best chance for a positive outcome; however, extratemporal foci may be successfully excised in more than 75% of the patients. The procedure is not without risk. Learning and memory are most susceptible to impairment postoperatively, and general intellectual abilities are also affected in a small number of patients. It may be particularly useful in children with intractable epilepsy.

The ketogenic diet was devised in the 1920s. It is high in fat and low in carbohydrates and protein and thus leads to acidosis and ketosis. Protein and calorie intake are set at levels that will meet requirements for growth. Most of the calories are provided in the form of heavy cream and butter. No sugar is allowed. Vitamins and minerals are supplemented.[33] Medium-chain triglycerides may be substituted for the dietary fats. Fluids are also controlled. It requires strict control and parent compliance. Although some centers find this useful for refractory patients, others have found that it is poorly tolerated by patients. Long-term effects are unknown.

PHARMACOLOGIC THERAPY

DRUG TREATMENTS OF FIRST CHOICE

The drug treatments of first choice depend on the type of epilepsy (Table 52–4) as well as the interface between drug specific adverse effects and patient preferences. Few guidelines or treatment

TABLE 52–4. Drugs of Choice for Specific Seizure Disorders

Seizure Type	Commonly Used Initial Drugs	Alternative Drugs
Partial	Carbamazepine Phenytoin Valproic acid	Felbamate Gabapentin Lamotrigine Phenobarbital Tiagabine Topiramate Vigabatrin
Tonic–clonic	Phenytoin Valproic acid Carbamazepine	Phenobarbital Lamotrigine
Absence	Ethosuximide Valproic acid	Clonazepam Acetazolamide
Bilateral massive epileptic myoclonus, atonic, infantile spasms[a]	Clonazepam ACTH	Phenytoin Phenobarbital Benzodiazepines Acetazolamide Felbamate Topiramate Vigabatrin
Juvenile myoclonic Epilepsy (JME)	Valproic acid	Lamotrigine

[a]Difficult group to treat; combinations are the rule.

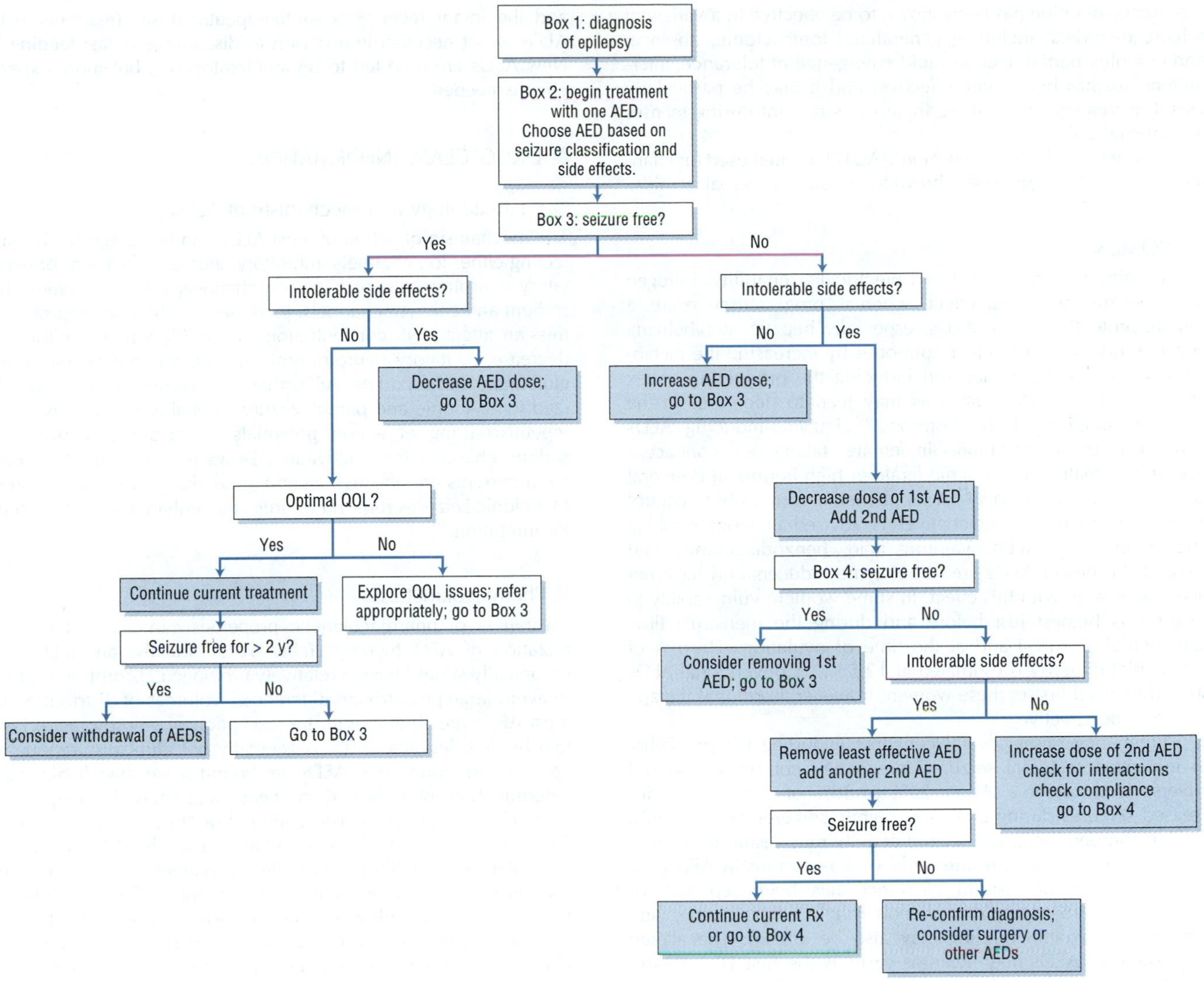

FIGURE 52–1. Algorithm for treatment of epilepsy.

protocols have been published. Figure 52–1 is a suggested algorithm for a general approach to the treatment of epilepsy.

Because the majority of adults have localization-related (partial onset) seizures, the most widely used AEDs are carbamazepine, phenobarbital, phenytoin, and valproic acid. For complex partial seizures, these AEDs have similar efficacy.[34] However, carbamazepine and phenytoin may be preferred, based on two pivotal trials conducted through the Veterans Administration (VA) Epilepsy Cooperative Study Group. In the first of these trials, patients with new-onset partial or generalized epilepsy were randomized to receive either carbamazepine, phenobarbital, phenytoin, or primidone.[35] Doses were titrated upward until seizures were controlled or unacceptable toxicity occurred. At the end of 3 years, patients who received either carbamazepine or phenytoin were equally likely, and patients on phenobarbital or primidone were least likely, to have remained on their originally assigned treatment. Thus, carbamazepine and phenytoin were considered the drugs of first choice in patients with new-onset partial or generalized seizures, though carbamazepine may cause less cognitive and behavioral impairment than phenytoin. A follow-up study, using almost identical methods, compared carbamazepine and valproic acid.[36] Carbamazepine and valproic acid treated groups had equal retention rates for tonic–clonic seizures. Carbamazepine was superior to valproic acid for partial seizures. Valproic acid caused slightly more adverse effects.

These VA cooperative studies directly compared widely used AEDs available at the time the studies were designed, and they are among the very few comparative studies. In clinical trials of newer AEDs, the comparison is between active drug and placebo in patients who continue to have seizures despite current treatment with standard AEDs. Thus, it is difficult to directly compare the efficacy of the newer to the older AEDs. A meta-analysis has recently been published that attempts to compare the newer AEDs.[37]

ALTERNATIVE DRUG TREATMENTS

Some benzodiazepines (e.g., diazepam and lorazepam) are used in the acute treatment of status epilepticus (see Chap. 53). On a chronic basis, other benzodiazepines can be useful, especially in the treatment of seizure types that occur primarily in children, though tolerance may develop. Recently, a rectal formulation of diazepam has been approved for acute repetitive seizures.

Acetazolamide has been shown to be effective in a variety of seizure disorders, including generalized tonic–clonic, absence, and complex partial. Due to rapid emergence of tolerance, intermittent use has been more effective, and it may be particularly useful in treating the increase in seizures present during menses (catamenial epilepsy).[38]

Andrenocorticotropic hormone (ACTH) is often used for infantile spasms.[39] It has not been shown to be superior to oral steroids.

WOMEN

Many hormones influence brain electrical excitability. Estrogen has a seizure-activating effect, whereas progesterone exerts a seizure-protective effect. AEDs, especially hepatic metabolizing enzyme inducers, also affect hormones by increasing the metabolism of steroid hormones and inducing the production of sex hormone binding globulin. This may lead to decreases in the unbound fraction of the hormone.[40] Enzyme-inducing AEDs may cause treatment failures in females taking oral contraceptives; thus, treatment with a moderate or high hormonal dose oral contraceptive is necessary.[41] A supplemental form of birth control in addition to oral contraceptives is advised in women taking enzyme-inducing AEDs. Valproic acid, benzodiazepines, and most of the newer AEDs are not enzyme inducers and have not been associated with this effect. In some women, vulnerability to seizures is highest just before and during the menstrual flow (catamenial seizures) and at the time of ovulation. The risk of catamenial epilepsy is estimated at 12.5%.[42] Conventional AEDs should be tried first in these women; however, hormonal therapy may also be effective.

Pregnancy raises several concerns including the possibility of increased maternal seizures, pregnancy complications, and adverse fetal outcome. About 25% to 30% of women have increased seizures during pregnancy, while seizures decrease in a similar number. Increased seizure activity may result from either a direct effect on seizure threshold or a reduction in AED concentration. An increase in clearance has been reported for phenytoin, carbamazepine, phenobarbital, ethosuximide, and clorazepate. Protein binding may also be altered. The altered disposition of AEDs may begin as early as the first 10 weeks of pregnancy and may take up to 4 weeks postpartum to return to normal. The return to the nonpregnant metabolism and binding requires longer for carbamazepine and phenobarbital than it does for phenytoin.[43] There is a higher incidence of adverse pregnancy outcomes in women with epilepsy. Although the risk of congenital malformations is 4% to 6% (twice as high as in nonepileptic women), more than 90% of pregnancies in epileptic mothers have satisfactory outcomes. Barbiturates and phenytoin are associated with congenital heart malformations, facial clefts, and other malformations. Valproic acid and carbamazepine are associated with spina bifida and hypospadias. Other adverse pregnancy outcomes associated with, but not necessarily caused by, AEDs are growth, psychomotor, and mental retardation. Guidelines have been developed for counseling and managing the pregnant woman with epilepsy.[44] A pregnancy registry (1-888-233-2334) has been established for reporting any pregnancy in women taking AEDs. Many of these teratogenic effects can be prevented by adequate folate intake; therefore, prenatal vitamins with folic acid should be given to any woman of child-bearing potential who is taking AEDs. Higher AED concentrations and polytherapy increase the teratogenic risk, therefore deciding on the most effective single-drug treatment prior to conception is vitally important. AEDs can also lead to neonatal hemorrhagic disorder. Vitamin K given to the mother predelivery can prevent this coagulopathy.[41] Although AEDs pass into the breast milk, the concentrations are very low, and the infant receives a subtherapeutic dose. Treatment with AEDs is not necessarily a reason to discourage breast feeding.[45] New AEDs are reported to be less teratogenic, but more experience is needed.

DRUG CLASS INFORMATION

Pharmacology and Mechanism of Action

The mechanism of action of most AEDs can be categorized as affecting either ion channels, inhibitory neurotransmission, or excitatory neurotransmission. The ion channels affected include the sodium and calcium channels. Increases in inhibitory neurotransmission affect CNS concentrations of GABA, whereas efforts to decrease excitatory neurotransmission are focused primarily on glutatmate and aspartate. AEDs that are effective against generalized tonic–clonic and partial seizures probably reduce sustained repetitive firing of action potentials by delaying recovery of sodium channels from activation. Drugs that reduce T-type calcium currents are effective against generalized absence seizures. Myoclonic seizures respond to drugs that enhance $GABA_A$ receptor inhibition.[46]

Pharmacokinetics

Awareness of pharmacokinetic properties can aid in the optimization of AED therapy (Table 52–5). Ideally, an AED used chronically should have a relatively prolonged absorption profile, to avoid large peak-trough differences. Volumes of distribution of most AEDs are similar, with the exception of valproic acid. Protein binding less than 90% is generally not clinically important. Several commonly used AEDs are bound more than 90%; thus, determination of unbound concentrations may be helpful in some clinical situations. The unbound or "free" concentration is the active drug capable of penetrating the blood–brain barrier and interacting at the receptor site. In patients who are not responding or having side effects at "therapeutic" concentrations of total drug, an unbound concentration may explain the unusual response. For populations known to have conditions that alter plasma protein binding (chronic renal failure, liver disease, hypoalbuminemia, burns, pregnancy, malnutrition, neonates, elderly, and displacing drugs), unbound rather than total drug concentrations should be measured for highly protein-bound drugs.[47] Unbound concentration monitoring is especially useful for phenytoin.

Many AEDs are extensively metabolized through various enzyme systems. The most common is the cytochrome P450 system, though through different subtypes. Many AEDs have active metabolites. Several of the newer AEDs have significant renal elimination.

Neonates may metabolize drugs more slowly but eliminate unchanged drug more rapidly. Infants and children may metabolize drug rapidly.[1] The volume of distribution changes as children grow. The ability to metabolize drugs decreases with age, and lower doses of AEDs are required in the elderly.[1] Although pharmacokinetic differences can be anticipated, pharmacodynamic changes have not been studied in the elderly. However, some elderly have an increased receptor sensitivity to CNS drugs. A change in the pharmacodynamics would mean that the therapeutic range for younger patients would be invalid in the elderly. Because of pharmacokinetic and potential pharmacodynamic changes in the elderly, patient response rather than blood levels is the most important clinical outcome for patients of all ages.

Disease states may alter the pharmacokinetics of AEDs. Liver disease may decrease drug metabolism and protein binding.

TABLE 52–5. Antiepileptic Drug Pharmacokinetic Data

AED	$T_{1/2}$(h)[a]	Time to Steady State (d)	Unchanged (%)	V_D (L/kg)	Clinically Important Metabolite	Removed by Dialysis (%)	Protein Binding (%)
Carbamazepine	12 M; 5–14 Co	21–28 for completion of auto-induction	< 1	1–2	10,11-epoxide	< 20	40–90
Ethosuximide	A 60 C 30	6–12	10–20	0.67	No	~50	0
Felbamate	16–22	5–7	50	0.73–0.82	No	—	~25
Gabapentin[b]	5–40[e]	1–2[b]	100	0.65–1.04	No	Yes	0
Lamotrigine	25.4 M	3–15	0	1.28	No	20	40–50
Phenobarbital	A 46–136 C 37-73	14–21	20–40	0.6	No	30 (H)[c]	50
Phenytoin	A 10–34 C 5-14	7–28	< 5	0.6–8.0	No	4 (H)[c]	90
Primidone	A 3.3–19 C 4.5–11	1–4	40	0.43–1.1	PB[d] PEMA[d]	30 (H)[b]	80
Tiagabine	5–13		Negligible		No	—	95
Topiramate	18–21	4–5	50–70	0.55–0.8 (male) 0.23–0.4 (female)	No	—	15
Valproic acid	A 8–20 C 7–14	1–3	< 5	0.1–0.5	May contribute to toxicity	—	90–95 binding saturates
Vigabatrin	5–14[e]	1–5	50–70	0.8	No		0

[a]A = adult; C = child.; M-monotherapy; Co = combination therapy.
[b]The bioavailability of gabapentin is dose dependent.
[c]H = hemodialysis.
[d]PB = phenobarbital; PEMA = phenylethylmalonamide.
[e]Half-life depends on renal function

Patients with chronic renal failure may have decreased elimination of unchanged drug as well as altered protein binding.

Serum Concentration

Though most AEDs have published therapeutic ranges, the serum concentration should not be the end point. The serum concentration is a target that should be correlated with clinical outcome. Clinicians should treat patients and not numbers.[18] The desired response is the cessation of seizures without side effects. Seizure control may occur before the "minimum" of the published range is achieved, and side effects may appear before the "maximum" of the range is achieved. Some patients may need and tolerate concentrations beyond the "maximum." The therapeutic range for AEDs may be different for different seizure types. Serum concentrations may need to be higher to control complex partial seizures than to control tonic–clonic seizures.[48] Clinicians should define a therapeutic range for an individual patient, above which there are side effects and below which the patient experiences seizures. The response may change as the patient ages.

Efficacy

Classification of seizure types and epilepsy syndromes has improved the ability of clinicians to select drugs of choice for specific seizures (see Table 52–4). Absence seizures are pharmacologically different from other seizure types. Phenytoin, phenobarbital, and carbamazepine, although effective in generalized and partial seizures, are ineffective in treating absence seizures and in some cases may precipitate an increase in seizure activity. Absence seizures are best treated with ethosuximide or valproic acid. If the patient has a combination of absence and other generalized or partial seizures, valproic acid is the preferred first choice because it is the only AED effective against absence and other seizure types. If valproic acid is ineffective in treating a mixed seizure disorder that includes absence, ethosuximide should be used in combination with another AED.[12]

The traditional treatment of tonic–clonic seizures is phenytoin or phenobarbital; however, the use of carbamazepine and valproic acid is increasing because these AEDs have a lower incidence of side effects and equal efficacy. Valproic acid is the drug of first choice for atonic seizures and for juvenile myoclonic epilepsy.[12]

Carbamazepine is recognized as the AED of first choice for partial seizures. Alternatives to carbamazepine are phenytoin, valproic acid, gabapentin, lamotrigine, tiagabine, topiramate, and vigabatrin.[12] The newer antiepileptic drugs were first approved as adjunctive therapy for patients with refractory partial seizures. Monotherapy trials with these drugs are underway. Phenobarbital and primidone are also useful in partial seizures. Felbamate, which has monotherapy approval, is very effective but has been associated with some significant side effects.

TABLE 52–6. Antiepileptic Drug Side Effects

AED	Acute Side Effects: *Concentration Dependent*	Acute Side Effects: *Idiosyncratic*	Chronic Side Effects
Carbamazepine	Diplopia Dizziness Drowsiness Nausea Unsteadiness Lethargy	Blood dyscrasias Rash	Hyponatremia
Ethosuximide	Ataxia Drowsiness GI distress Unsteadiness Hiccoughs	Blood dyscrasias Rash	Behavior changes Headache
Felbamate	Anorexia Nausea Vomiting Insomnia Headache	Aplastic anemia Acute hepatic failure	Not established
Gabapentin	Dizziness Fatigue Somnolence Ataxia	Weight gain	Weight gain
Lamotrigine	Ataxia Diplopia Dizziness Unsteadiness Headache Somnolence Nausea Vomiting Weight gain Nervousness Abnormal thinking	Rash	Not established
Phenobarbital	Ataxia Hyperactivity Headache Unsteadiness Sedation Nausea	Blood dyscrasias Rash	Behavior changes Connective tissue disorders Intellectual blunting Metabolic bone disease Mood change Sedation
Phenytoin	Ataxia Nystagmus Behavior changes Dizziness Headache Incoordination	Blood dyscrasias Rash Immunologic reaction	Behavior changes Cerebellar syndrome Connective tissue changes Skin thickening Folate deficiency Gingival hyperplasia

Adverse Effects

Adverse effects of AEDs can be divided into acute and chronic (Table 52–6). Acute effects can be dose (concentration) related or idiosyncratic. Concentration dependent effects are common and troublesome but not usually life threatening. They are alleviated by decreasing the concentration. Most idiosyncratic reactions due to an allergic reaction are mild, but can be more serious if the hypersensitivity involves one or more organ systems. Other idiosyncratic side effects are rare, but can be serious.

Acute organ failure, if it's going to occur, generally occurs within the first 6 months of AED therapy. No tests are currently available to predict these severe toxic reactions. Screening blood and urine probably does not help detect the early stage of severe reactions and is generally not recommended in asymptomatic patients. Laboratory assessment can be considered if the patient reports an unexplained illness (e.g., lethargy, vomiting, fever, or rash).[49]

Chronic side effects can occur despite serum concentrations within the therapeutic range and multiple organ systems can be affected.[7] The incidence of chronic side effects is greatest with phenytoin (33%), phenobarbital (23%), carbamazepine (15%), and valproic acid (12%). The type and incidence of possible chronic side effects with the newer AEDs is mostly unknown at this time. The incidence of any side effects is lowest in patients on monotherapy and increases with each additional drug.[50]

The comparative effects of AEDs on cognition have been difficult to evaluate because of differences in study design, seizure types, control of drug concentrations, and neuropsychologic tests

TABLE 52–6. (Continued)

AED	Acute Side Effects: *Concentration Dependent*	Acute Side Effects: *Idiosyncratic*	Chronic Side Effects
Phenytoin (cont'd)	Nausea Sedation Lethargy Cognitive impairment Fatigue Visual blurring		Hirsutism Coarsening of facial features Acne Cognitive impairment Metabolic bone disease Sedation
Primidone	Behavior changes Headache Nausea Sedation Unsteadiness	Blood dyscrasias Rash	Behavior change Connective tissue disorders Cognitive Impairment Sedation
Tiagabine	Dizziness Fatigue Difficulties concentrating Nervousness Tremor Blurred vision Depression Speech or language problems Weakness Confusion	Not established	Not established
Topiramate	Difficulties concentrating Psychomotor slowing Speech or language problems Somnolence, fatigue Dizziness Headache Diplopia	Not established	Not established
Valproic acid	Behavior changes GI upset Sedation Unsteadiness Tremor	Acute hepatic failure Acute pancreatitis Thrombocytopenia Blood dyscrasias Rash	Behavior changes Alopecia Sedation Nausea Weight gain Hyperammonemia
Vigabatrin	Sedation Fatigue Unsteadiness	Behavioral disturbances Confusion Psychosis Rash	Behavior changes Confusion Psychosis Sedation Weight gain

used. In general, there are not any large differences between the commonly used AEDs,[51] though some clinicians feel phenobarbital causes more cognitive depression. Some drugs, such as phenytoin, may have a greater effect on motor function, while others, such as carbamazepine, may have a greater effect on speed. For the older AEDs, carbamazepine and valproate may cause less impairment of cognition. Improvement in cognition has been reported in patients switched from phenytoin or phenobarbital to these agents. However, these effects are subtle and may not be pronounced if patients are in the same relative area of the therapeutic range.[52] Patients reduced from polytherapy to monotherapy also demonstrate improvement in cognition.[53] Some of the newer agents are believed to cause fewer neurobehavioral or cognitive effects.

Drug–Drug and Drug–Food Interactions

The AEDs frequently interact with each other via complex mechanisms. Interactions can occur in any of the pharmacokinetic processes: absorption, distribution, or elimination. Caution should be used when AEDs are added to or withdrawn from a drug regimen (Fig. 52–2). Some specific interactions are listed in Tables 52–7 and 52–8. Knowledge of which cytochrome P450 subtype is involved can help predict interactions.

Phenobarbital, phenytoin, primidone, and carbamazepine are potent inducers of cytochrome P450, epoxide hydrolase, and uridine diphosphate glucuronosyltransferase (UDPGT) enzyme systems. Valproic acid can inhibit many hepatic enzyme system activities involved in drug metabolism and significantly displaces some drugs from plasma albumin. Felbamate and topiramate can

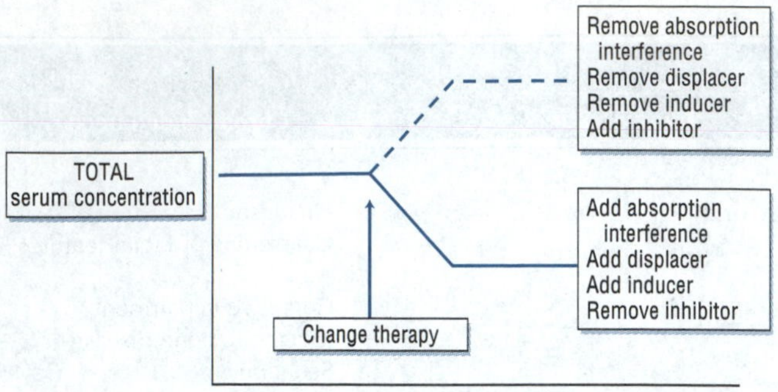

FIGURE 52–2. Effect of drug interactions. If a medication is added to or withdrawn from a patient's AED regimen, serum concentrations of the AED may change. Total serum concentrations will decrease *(bottom line)* if a compound is added that interferes with absorption, displaces from protein binding sites, or induces metabolism. If an inhibitor is removed from the regimen, concentrations will also decrease. Total concentrations will increase *(upper, dashed line)* if a compound is removed that interferes with absorption, displaces from protein binding sites, or induces metabolism, or if an enzyme inhibitor is added.

act as inducers with some isoforms and inhibitors of others. Ethosuximide, gabapentin, lamotrigine, tiagabine, and vigabatrin have little clinically significant effect on hepatic drug metabolism. Other than vigabatrin and gabapentin, which are mainly eliminated unchanged by the renal route, all other AEDs are metabolized wholly or in part by hepatic enzymes, and their disposition may be altered by metabolic changes. Some interactions are clinically unremarkable and some need only careful clinical monitoring, but others require prompt dosage adjustment.[54]

Dosing and Administration

Almost all AEDs (except felbamate) are associated with depressed CNS function (e.g., drowsiness, lethargy, tiredness) early in the course of treatment, but some tolerance usually develops in 7 to 10 days. Therefore, except in life-threatening situations (e.g., status epilepticus), AEDs should be started in low doses and gradually increased until seizure control is achieved or intolerable side effects occur. A general rule is to initiate therapy with one-fourth to one-third of the anticipated maintenance dose and increase the dose to maintenance over 3 to 4 weeks.[18] This allows the clinician to treat the patient and find the therapeutic range for that patient, and not just dose to published values.

Although doses of AEDs are frequently cited in mg/kg (Table 52–9), the individual patient's response is a more definitive therapeutic end point. There is a large interpatient variability in pharmacokinetic parameters, which results in a large variation in the mg/kg dose required to achieve adequate blood concentrations and response.[18] Therefore, the concentration of the drug in the serum or plasma may be a guideline in assessing drug dosing. In compliant patients with low plasma concentrations who are receiving a usual mg/kg dose, the dosage may need to be increased if there are no side effects and seizures are continuing.

SPECIFIC DRUG INFORMATION

Carbamazepine

Pharmacology and Mechanism of Action. Animal studies indicate that carbamazepine depresses transmission in the nucleus ventralis anterior of the thalamus. This area has been associated with the generalization and spread of seizure discharge. The exact mechanism by which carbamazepine suppresses seizure spread is obscure, though it is believed to act primarily through inhibition of voltage-gated sodium channels. There is some depression of posttetanic potentiation (PTP) by carbamazepine, but it is of a lesser magnitude than occurs with phenytoin. It affects ionic conductance only at concentrations far above those normally produced in humans. It may inhibit an increase in cyclic AMP. Other biochemical effects are unknown.[46]

Pharmacokinetics. The absorption of carbamazepine from immediate-release tablets is slow and erratic because of its low water solubility. Because absorption is dissolution rate dependent, dose-dependent absorption may occur, resulting in less bioavailability at higher doses. The variable absorption results in times to peak of 2–24 hours (average, 6 hours). There is also a large variability in the peak-to-trough concentrations of up to 40%. There is no first-pass metabolism. Food may enhance the bioavailability of carbamazepine. The suspension dosage form is absorbed faster than the tablets.[18] Controlled-release (Tegretol XR) and sustained-release (Carbatrol) preparations are also available. These are bioequivalent in twice-daily dosing to dosing four times daily with immediate-release carbamazepine.

TABLE 52–7. Interactions Between Antiepileptic Drugs

AED	Added Drug	Effect[a]
Carbamazepine (CBZ)	Felbamate	Incr. 10,11 epoxide
	Felbamate	Decr. CBZ
	Phenobarbital	Decr. CBZ
	Phenytoin	Decr. CBZ
Felbamate (FBM)	Carbamazepine	Decr. FBM
	Phenytoin	Decr. FBM
	Valproic acid	Incr. FBM
Lamotrigine (LTG)	Carbamazepine	Decr. LTG
	Phenobarbital	Decr. LTG
	Phenytoin	Decr. LTG
	Primidone	Decr. LTG
	Valproic acid	Incr. LTG
Phenobarbital (PB)	Felbamate	Incr. PB
	Phenytoin	Incr. or decr. PB
	Valproic acid	Incr. PB
Phenytoin (PHT)	Carbamazepine	Decr. PHT
	Felbamate	Incr. PHT
	Methsuximide	Incr. PHT
	Phenobarbital	Incr. or decr. PHT
	Valproic acid	Decr. Total PHT
	Vigabatrin	Decr. PHT
Primidone (PRM)	Carbamazepine	Decr. PRM
		Incr. PB
	Phenytoin	Decr. PRM
		Incr. PB
	Valproic acid	Incr. PRM
		Incr. PB
Tiagabine (TGB)	Carbamazepine	Decr. TGB
	Phenytoin	Decr. TGB
Topiramate (TPM)	Carbamazepine	Decr. TPM
	Phenytoin	Decr. TPM
	Valproic acid	Decr. TPM
Valproic acid (VPA)	Carbamazepine	Decr. VPA
	Lamotrigine	Decr. VPA
	Phenobarbital	Decr. VPA
	Primidone	Decr. VPA
	Phenytoin	Decr. VPA

[a]Incr. = increased; Decr. = decreased.

TABLE 52–8. Interactions With Other Medications

AED	Altered By	Result	Alters	Result
Carbamazepine	Cimetidine	Incr. CBZ	Oral contraceptives (OC)	Decr. efficacy of OC
	Erythromycin	Incr. CBZ	Doxycycline	Decr. doxycycline
	Fluoxetine	Incr. CBZ	Theophylline	Decr. theophylline
	Isoniazid	Incr. CBZ	Warfarin	Decr. warfarin
	Propoxyphene	Incr. CBZ		
Phenobarbital	Acetazolamide	Incr. PB	OC	Decr. efficacy of OC
Phenytoin	Antacids	Decr. absorption of PHT	Oral contraceptives	Decr. efficacy of oral contraceptives
	Cimetidine	Incr. PHT	Bishydroxycoumarin	Decr. anticoagulation
	Chloramphenicol	Incr. PHT	Folic acid	Decr. folic Acid
	Disulfiram	Incr. PHT	Quinidine	Decr. quinidine
	Ethanol (acute)	Incr. PHT	Vitamin D	Decr. Vitamin D
	Fluconazole	Incr. PHT		
	Isoniazid	Incr. PHT		
	Propoxyphene	Incr. PHT		
	Warfarin	Incr. PHT		
	Ethanol (chronic)	Decr. PHT		
Primidone	Isoniazid	Decr. metabolism of primidone	Chlorpromazine	Decr. chlorpromazine
	Nicotinamide	Decr. metabolism of primidone	Corticosteroids	Decr. corticosteroids
			Quinidine	Decr. quinidine
			Tricyclics	Decr. tricyclics
			Furosemide	Decr. renal sensitivity to furosemide
Valproic acid	Cimetidine	Incr. VPA		
	Salicylates	Incr. free VPA		

Incr. = increased; decr. = decreased.

Carbamazepine is a neutral and highly lipophilic drug that results in high body tissue binding. Carbamazepine binds to α-1-acid glycoprotein and to albumin to a lesser extent. The percentage bound may decrease at higher concentrations within the therapeutic range. The usefulness of free carbamazepine concentrations remains to be defined.[18]

Most (98% to 99%) of an administered dose of carbamazepine is metabolized by the liver, primarily by CYP3A4.[55] Although 33 metabolites have been identified, the major metabolite is carbamazepine-10,11-epoxide.[18] This metabolite has anticonvulsant activity in animals and humans. In one study, patients switched from carbamazepine to 10,11-epoxide carbamazepine had no loss of seizure control.[56] The formation of the 10,11-epoxide is influenced by other enzyme-inducing or enzyme-inhibiting drugs. The 10,11-epoxide concentration may change with no change in parent carbamazepine concentration.[57]

Carbamazepine has the unique ability to induce its own metabolism (autoinduction).[18] The half-life after a single dose is much longer than the half-life after chronic therapy. The presence of enzyme-inducing drugs reduces the half-life even more. The enzyme induction effect begins within 3 to 5 days after the initiation of therapy and takes 21 to 28 days to complete. Therefore, it is possible to achieve initial concentrations that are within the therapeutic range but have concentrations fall despite continued therapy with good compliance. Some patients who respond well to initial therapy may be labeled refractory or noncompliant if the autoinduction phenomenon is not considered. The autoinduction rapidly reverses if therapy with carbamazepine is temporarily discontinued.[58] This would be very important in epilepsy monitoring units where all drugs are stopped in an attempt to precipitate seizures in patients being evaluated for seizure surgery.

Efficacy. Carbamazepine's relative lack of side effects compared to phenytoin and phenobarbital has resulted in an increased use for a variety of seizure disorders. It may also be useful in selected psychiatric disorders (see Chap. 66) and in trigeminal neuralgia. Carbamazepine is considered the AED of first choice for partial seizures, especially complex partial seizures. It is also useful for generalized seizures other than absence.[1]

Adverse Effects. Side effects (Table 52–6) of carbamazepine may fluctuate daily, paralleling the rise and decline of serum concentrations. The side effect profile may also follow a circadian rhythm.[59] Neurosensory side effects (e.g., diplopia, blurred vision, nystagmus, ataxia, unsteadiness, dizziness, and headache) are the most common, occurring in 35% to 50% of patients. These side effects are more common during initiation of therapy and may dissipate with continued treatment. Patients have variable threshold concentrations for the occurrence of CNS side effects. If the carbamazepine serum concentration is kept below the individual threshold, the CNS side effects can be minimized. Dosage manipulation, including the use of the controlled- or sustained-release preparations, should be tried before the patient is considered to be intolerant of carbamazepine. An analog of carbamazepine, oxcarbazepine, may lead to fewer ADRs.

Carbamazepine may induce a hyponatremic hyposmolar condition that is similar to the syndrome of inappropriate antidiuretic hormone secretion.[60] The incidence may increase with age. Periodic determinations of serum sodium are recommended, especially in the elderly.

The concern over carbamazepine-induced bone marrow suppression has been reinforced by a "black-box" warning in the package insert requiring frequent CBC monitoring. However, only a few cases of aplastic anemia, the most serious complication, have been reported since 1964. In many cases there were confounding factors that precluded a definite cause-and-effect relationship. Thrombocytopenia and anemia have an incidence of less than 5% and usually respond to a cessation of drug

TABLE 52–9. AED Dosing and Target Serum Concentration Ranges

	Trade Name	Manufacturer	Year Introduced	Usual Initial Dose	Usual Maximum Daily Dose	Target Serum Concentration Range
Barbiturates						
Mephobarbital	Mebaral	Sanofi Winthrop	1935	50–100 mg/d	400–600 mg	Not defined
Phenobarbital	Various	Generic	1912	1–3 mg/kg/d (10–20 mg/kg LD)	180–300 mg	10–40 μg/mL
Primidone	Mysoline	Wyeth-Ayerst	1954	100–125 mg/d	750–2000 mg	5–10 μg/mL
Benzodiazepines						
Clonazepam	Klonopin	Roche	1975	1.5 mg/d	20 mg	20–80 ng/ml
Clorazepate	Tranxene	Abbott	1981	7.5–22.5 mg/d	90 mg	Not defined
Diazepam	Valium	Roche/ generic	1968	PO: 4–40 mg IV: 5–10 mg	PO: 4–40 mg IV: 5–30 mg	100–1000 ng/mL
Lorazepam	Ativan	Wyeth-Ayerst generic		PO: 2–6 mg IV: 0.05 mg/kg IM: 0.05 mg/kg	PO: 10 mg IV: 0.044 mg/kg	10–30 ng/mL
Hydantoins						
Ethotoin	Peganone	Abbott	1957	< 1000 mg/d	2000–4000 mg with food	15–50 μL
Mephenytoin	Mesantoin	Sandoz	1947	50–100 mg/d	200–800 mg	25–40 μg/mL
Phenytoin	Dilantin	Parke-Davis	1938	PO: 3–5 mg/kg (200–400 mg) (15–20 mg/kg LD)	PO: 500–600 mg	Total: 10–20 μg/mL Unbound: 0.5–3 μg/mL
Succinimides						
Ethosuximide	Zarontin	Parke-Davis	1960	500 mg/d	500–2000 mg	40–80 μg/mL
Methsuximide	Celontin	Parke-Davis	1957	300 mg/d	300–1200 mg	*N*-desmethyl metabolite 10–40 μg/mL
Other						
Carbamazepine	Tegretol	Novartis, generic	1974	400 mg/d	400–2400 mg	4–14 μg/mL
Felbamate	Felbatol	Carter Wallace	1993	1200 mg/d	3600 mg	Not defined
Gabapentin	Neurontin	Parke-Davis	1993	900 mg/d	4800 mg	Not defined
Lamotrigine	Lamictal	Glaxo-Wellcome	1994	25mg qod if on VPA; 25–50 mg/d if not on VPA	100–150 mg if on VPA; 300–500 mg if not on VPA	Not defined
Tiagabine	Gabitril	Abbott	1997	4–8 mg/d	80 mg	Not defined
Topiramate	Topamax	Ortho McNeil	1997	25–50 mg/d	200–1000 mg	Not defined
Valproic acid	Depakene Depakote Depacon	Abbott	1978	15 mg/kg (500–1000 mg)	60 mg/kg (3000 5000 mg)	50–150 μg/mL
Vigabatrin	Sabril	Hoechst Marion-Roussel	1998?		3000 mg	

LD = loading dose.

therapy. Leukopenia is the most common hematologic side effect. An incidence as high as 10% has been reported. Leukopenia is usually transient even when the drug is continued and may be due to a redistribution of white blood cells (WBCs) rather than a decrease in their production. In about 2% of patients, the leukopenia is persistent, but even patients with WBC counts of $3000/mm^3$ or less do not seem to have an increased incidence of infection. A clinical guide is to continue carbamazepine therapy unless the WBC count drops to less than $2500/mm^3$ and the absolute neutrophil count drops to less than $1000/mm^3$.

Rashes are the most frequent hypersensitivity response. An incidence of 9.9% has been reported.[61] These are usually mildly eczematous but may progress to a Stevens-Johnson syndrome. Other rare side effects reported with carbamazepine include hepatitis, osteomalacia, cardiac conduction defects, and lupus-like reactions. Carbamazepine appears to have minimal effects on cognitive functioning.

Drug–Drug and Drug–Food Interactions. Because of concentration-dependent efficacy and side effects, drug interactions with carbamazepine are often clinically very significant. Valproic acid increases 10,11-epoxide metabolite concentrations without affecting the concentration of carbamazepine. The interaction of erythromycin with carbamazepine is particularly significant. Carbamazepine may interact with other drugs by inducing their metabolism; for example, carbamazepine increases the metabolism of valproic acid, theophylline, warfarin, and ethosuximide (Tables 52–7 and 52–8).[18] The absorption of carbamazepine suspension is slower and diminished when it is given during nasogastric (NG) feeding. This may result from adherence to the NG tube. It is recommended that carbamazepine suspension be mixed with an equal volume of diluent before being administered through NG feeding tubes.[62]

Dosing and Administration. The variable contributions of the 10,11-epoxide metabolite and free carbamazepine concentrations have restricted a precise definition of the therapeutic range. Loading doses of carbamazepine are indicated only for critically ill patients. Carbamazepine suspension has been used to administer a loading dose of 7.4 to 10.4 mg/kg in critically ill patients.[63] Oral loading has also been accomplished with a controlled-release formulation of carbamazepine.[64] There are significant CNS-depressant effects and gastrointestinal complaints (e.g., nausea and vomiting) associated with large initial doses.

During dosage titration, it should be remembered that carbamazepine clearance increases with time. Doses may be started at one-fourth to one-third of the anticipated maintenance dose and increased every 2 to 3 weeks.[18] Because of the auto- and heteroinduction of carbamazepine metabolism, it is necessary to administer the drug two to four times per day. Although some patients, especially those on monotherapy, can be maintained on twice-a-day therapy, others may require more frequent dosage administration. Children are likely to need more frequent administration. Annoying CNS and GI side effects may be minimized by giving larger doses at bedtime.[18] A controlled-released dosage form (Tegretol XR) given twice a day has comparable pharmacokinetics to immediate-release carbamazepine given four times a day.[65] The sustained-release Carbatrol capsules can be opened and used as a sprinkle on food. Carbamazepine tablets should not be stored in places where they would be exposed to high heat and high humidity.[66]

Ethosuximide

Pharmacology and Mechanism of Action. The exact mechanism of action of ethosuximide remains elusive. Ethosuximide inhibits NADPH-linked aldehyde reductase necessary for the formation of gamma-hydroxybutyrate, which has been associated with the induction of absence seizures. It may also inhibit the sodium-potassium ATPase system. Ethosuximide is not believed to have a direct membrane effect or to affect brain metabolism.[67]

Pharmacokinetics and Efficacy. Metabolism occurs in the liver by hydroxylation, and the metabolites are believed to be inactive. There is some evidence of a nonlinear metabolic process at higher concentrations.[18] Ethosuximide has a chiral center, and there may be some stereochemical aspects to its metabolism.[67]

The only indication for the use of ethosuximide is the treatment of absence seizures, for which it is the treatment of choice. It may be used in combination with valproic acid for difficult-to-control absence patients.[67]

Adverse Effects, Drug–Drug Interactions, and Drug–Food Interactions. Ethosuximide is a relatively benign anticonvulsant. The most frequently reported side effects are nausea and vomiting (up to 40%), and these symptoms may be minimized by administration of smaller doses and more frequent dosing. Other common side effects include drowsiness, fatigue, lethargy, dizziness, hiccups, and headaches. Rarely, idiosyncratic reactions such as rashes, lupus, and blood dyscrasias have been reported.[67]

Because ethosuximide is not protein bound, displacement interactions cannot occur. The metabolism of ethosuximide may be induced by carbamazepine. A complex interaction between valproic acid and ethosuximide has been reported. Valproic acid may inhibit the metabolism of ethosuximide, but only if the metabolism of ethosuximide is near saturation.[18]

Dosing and Administration. The therapeutic range of ethosuximide was defined in a relatively small number of patients. Many unresponsive patients became responders when their drug concentrations were raised to equal those of the responsive patients.

A loading dose of ethosuximide is not required. Titration over 1 to 2 weeks to maintenance doses of 20 mg/kg per day usually results in concentrations of approximately 50 μg/mL. Data suggest that patients can be successfully managed on once-a-day therapy; however, GI distress appears to be dose related and the total daily dose is usually divided into two equal doses.[67]

Felbamate

Pharmacology and Mechanism of Action. Felbamate is a structural analogue of meprobamate, but its use does not result in the tolerance or dependence associated with meprobamate. Felbamate appears to act as an antagonist of the glycine receptor site on the *N*-methyl-D-aspartate (NMDA) receptor. This action inhibits the initiation and propagation of seizures.[68] It may also inhibit NMDA/glycine-stimulated increases in intracellular Ca^{2+}.[69]

Pharmacokinetics. Felbamate is rapidly and well absorbed. The absorption is unaffected by food or antacids. About 40% to 50% of a dose of felbamate is metabolized by hydroxylation and conjugation pathways in the liver, with the rest being excreted unchanged in the urine. In patients taking enzyme-inducing drugs, the elimination half-life is shorter. Felbamate displays linear pharmacokinetics, and the concentrations are dose proportional.[70]

Efficacy. Felbamate has been approved for use in adults 14 years and older as monotherapy and adjunctive therapy in partial seizures with and without secondary generalization and for children 2 years and older as adjunctive therapy for the Lennox-Gastaut syndrome.[71] Because of the association of aplastic anemia and acute liver failure with felbamate postmarketing, felbamate is now recommended for patients refractory to other AEDs.[72]

Adverse Effects. The most frequently reported side effects reported with felbamate prior to marketing were anorexia, weight loss, insomnia, nausea, and headache. Less common side effects included diarrhea, rash, diplopia, ataxia, rhinitis, and taste disturbances. The side effects of felbamate are more common with polytherapy than monotherapy.[71] After about 1 year of general use and 100,000 patient care exposures, the use of felbamate was found to be associated with aplastic anemia and acute liver failure. The onset was between 68 and 354 days of therapy. The approximate rate of occurrence of aplastic anemia is 1 in 3000 and of hepatitis is 1 in 10,000.[1] Initially, no relationship with dose and no predictors of who is more likely to develop these life-threatening reactions was apparent. Data are now emerging suggesting an increased risk for aplastic anemia in patients with a history of cytopenia, AED allergy or significant toxicity, viral infection, and/or immunologic problems.

Drug–Drug and Drug–Food Interactions. Significant drug interactions have been reported with felbamate. Felbamate inhibits the clearance, and increases the concentration, of phenytoin and valproic acid.[73] The concentration of carbamazepine decreases in patients on concurrent therapy with felbamate. However, the concentration of the 10,11-epoxide metabolite increases.[74] It is recommended that the dose of phenytoin, carbamazepine, and valproic acid be decreased by about 30% when felbamate is added.[71] These interactions are dose proportional and there is a further change in clearance with each dosage increase of felbamate. Phenytoin and carbamazepine are enzyme inducers and have been shown to increase the clearance of felbamate. Interactions with phenobarbital and warfarin have also been reported.[75]

Dosing and Administration. A therapeutic range for felbamate has not been established. The drug is dosed to clinical response. If felbamate is used as monotherapy, the dose is initiated at 1200 mg/d (15 mg/kg in children) and then is increased by 600 mg every 2 weeks up to a maximum dose of 3600 mg (45 mg/kg in children).

Gabapentin

Pharmacology and Mechanism of Action. Structurally, gabapentin incorporates the inhibitory neurotransmitter GABA into a cyclohexane ring.[76] Gabapentin was designed to be a GABA agonist, but its exact mechanism of action is still undefined. It has been demonstrated that gabapentin does not react at either GABA receptor, alter GABA uptake, or interfere with GABA transaminase. Gabapentin appears to bind to an amino acid carrier protein and act at a unique receptor.[46] It elevates human brain GABA levels.[77]

Pharmacokinetics. Gabapentin is recognized by the *L*-amino acid carrier protein in the gut, as well as in the CNS. This amino acid carrier protein transports the drug across the gut membrane by an active process. The binding of gabapentin to this system saturates, and bioavailability decreases with an increase in dose.[78] The percent of dose excreted unchanged in the urine is 47%, 34%, 33%, and 27% for daily doses of 1200, 2400, 3600, and 4800 mg/d.[79] At doses greater than 1200 mg three times per day, there appears to be a plateauing of the achieved concentration.[80] In one case report of a gabapentin overdose, 49 g of gabapentin led to a concentration of only 62 μg/mL 8.5 hours after ingestion.[81] Concentrations in human cerebrospinal fluid are 5% to 35% of plasma levels, and tissue concentrations are approximately 80% of plasma levels.[76]

Because gabapentin is eliminated exclusively by renal elimination, dosage adjustments will be necessary in patients with significantly impaired renal function. In anuric patients maintained on hemodialysis, the mean elimination half-life on nondialysis days is 132 hours. Approximately 35% of gabapentin is recovered in dialysate. Gabapentin half-life during dialysis is approximately 4 hours.[82]

Efficacy. Gabapentin is approved as adjunctive therapy for partial seizures with or without secondary generalization in adults with epilepsy.[83] It has been used as adjunctive therapy in children with refractory partial seizures.[84] and with benign epilepsy with centrotemporal spikes (BECTS).[85] One case study reported an increase in absence and myoclonic seizures when gabapentin was used in a patient with Lennox-Gastaut syndrome.[86]

Gabapentin has also been used for treatment of pain,[87] amyotrophic lateral sclerosis,[88] and Parkinson's disease.[89] Monotherapy trials have also shown effectiveness.

Adverse Effects, Drug–Drug Interactions, and Drug–Food Interactions. Fatigue, somnolence, dizziness, and ataxia are the most frequently reported side effects. Other side effects reported include nystagmus, tremor, and diplopia. Recently, aggressive behavior has been reported in children.[90] The CNS effects of gabapentin are less than or equal to those of traditional AEDs.[78] Some clinicians have noted that patients may gain weight while on gabapentin.

Gabapentin does not induce or inhibit liver enzymes. Therefore, drug interactions are not likely to occur with gabapentin.[78] There is a 10% reduction in the clearance of gabapentin in patients taking cimetidine and a 20% reduction in the bioavailability if aluminum antacids are taken simultaneously with gabapentin. A high-protein meal increases the maximum concentration achieved by 36% and slightly increases (11%) the area under the curve. Despite these higher maximum concentrations, subjects reported significantly fewer side effects after the high-protein meal.[91]

Dosing and Administration. The manufacturer recommends a gabapentin dose of 300 mg at bedtime on the first day, increasing to 900 mg/d over 3 days. Faster titration rates (e.g., starting at 300 to 900 mg tid) have been well tolerated.[92] The manufacturer recommends maintenance doses of 1800 to 2400 mg/d, but higher doses (5000 to 10,000 mg/d) have been used safely. Most clinicians are using doses of 2400 to 4800 mg/d for epilepsy. It is unclear if higher doses of gabapentin should be given more frequently than three times per day because of saturable absorption. Patients with end-stage renal disease maintained on hemodialysis should receive an initial 300- to 400-mg dose with 200 to 300 mg gabapentin given after every 4 hours of hemodialysis.[82]

Lamotrigine

Pharmacology, Mechanism of Action, and Pharmacokinetics. The most likely mechanism of action of lamotrigine is a use-dependent blocking effect on voltage-sensitive sodium channels, resulting in inhibition of the release of excitatory neurotransmitters, glutamate and aspartate. It does not block the spontaneous release of these neurotransmitters.[93]

Lamotrigine is rapidly and well absorbed. There is no first-pass metabolism, and there is no evidence of saturable pharmacokinetics.[94] One report suggested that there may be some autoinduction in healthy male volunteers.[95] There is no statistically significant difference in the pharmacokinetics of lamotrigine in the elderly versus younger subjects.[96] Children may have a shorter half-life.[93] There is significant intersubject variability in the pharmacokinetic profile of lamotrigine.[94] The half-life is prolonged in patients with renal failure. For patients on dialysis, the half-life is much more prolonged between dialyses (57.4 hours) but shorter during dialysis (13 hours).[93]

Efficacy. Lamotrigine is approved as adjunctive therapy in adult patients with partial epilepsy refractory to other agents.[93] It has been used as monotherapy.[97] In open and small controlled trials, lamotrigine also appears to be effective against many generalized seizure types, and in children.[95] Lamotrigine may lead to improvements in patient's mood.[95]

Adverse Effects. The most frequently reported side effects of lamotrigine include diplopia, drowsiness, ataxia, and headache.[95] It may cause several types of rash, which usually appear in the first 3 to 4 weeks of therapy. A recent "black box" warning has been added to the package insert. The rash is typically generalized, erythematous, and morbilliform and is generally mild to moderate in severity. However, the Stevens-Johnson reaction has also been reported. Some of these rashes, especially a rash that develops early, may necessitate the withdrawal of lamotrigine.[98] The incidence of rash appears to be increased in patients who are also receiving valproic acid and who have a rapid dosage titration. The incidence may be higher in children than in adults.[99]

Drug–Drug and Drug–Food Interactions. Lamotrigine does not inhibit or induce liver enzymes. However, the metabolism of lamotrigine may be altered by concurrent therapy with other drugs. Phenytoin and carbamazepine enhance and valproic acid inhibits the clearance of lamotrigine.[95] A pharmacodynamic interaction may occur with carbamazepine, leading to an increase in CNS side effects. Concomitant valproate markedly increased the half-life of lamotrigine and decreased lamotrigine clearance, without substantial alteration in the linear kinetics of the drug. The addition of lamotrigine was associated with a small but significant (25%) decrease in steady-state valproate plasma concentrations. The formation clearance of the hepatotoxic valproate metabolites, 2-*N*-propyl-4-pentenoic acid (4-ene-valproate) and 2-propyl-2,4-pentadienoic acid, was unaffected by lamotrigine administration.[100]

Dosing and Administration. A therapeutic range for lamotrigine has not been established. In patients who are taking enzyme-inducing drugs, lamotrigine can be started more rapidly than in patients receiving valproic acid. The maintenance doses are also different (Table 52–9). These different doses are critical due to the relationship between rash, concomitant valproic acid, and the dose escalation rate.[97] Removal of inducers from a lamotrigine regimen may necessitate decreases in lamotrigine doses, whereas removal of valproic acid may necessitate an increase in the lamotrigine dose.

Phenobarbital and Primidone

Phenobarbital and primidone may be considered together because primidone is metabolized to phenobarbital. Primidone is an active AED and has a second metabolite that may be active—phenylethylmalonamide (PEMA). In general, because of costs and dosing frequency, phenobarbital should be tried before primidone. In some refractory patients, primidone will be effective where phenobarbital has failed because of additional AED activity.

Mechanism of Action and Pharmacokinetics. Phenobarbital and primidone elevate seizure threshold by decreasing postsynaptic excitation, possibly by stimulating postsynaptic GABA-ergic inhibitor responses.[46] Phenobarbital is rapidly and completely absorbed regardless of whether it is given orally, intramuscularly, or rectally.[18] It has a biphasic distribution. Initially, phenobarbital penetrates highly perfused organs including the brain. It penetrates the brain at a rate comparable to that of phenytoin, and peak concentrations are achieved 3 to 20 minutes after an IV dose. Phenobarbital distributes evenly to all body tissues including fat. Decreasing systemic pH drives phenobarbital into body tissues. Phenobarbital is about 50% bound to plasma proteins, but the free fraction was reported to be 93% in a burn patient with uremia.[18]

Drugs affecting liver enzymes may alter phenobarbital metabolism, but phenobarbital clearance is not affected by liver blood flow. Despite the fact that phenobarbital is a potent enzyme inducer, there is no evidence in humans that it is an autoinducer. The elimination of phenobarbital is linear. Because tubular reabsorption of phenobarbital is pH dependent, the amount excreted renally can be increased by giving diuretics and urinary alkalinizers.[18]

Primidone is metabolized to phenobarbital and PEMA. The primidone to phenobarbital ratio is highly variable. A significant portion of primidone is excreted unchanged. The half-life of primidone may become shorter after chronic therapy because the phenobarbital metabolite may induce the metabolism of primidone.[18]

Efficacy. Phenobarbital is the drug of choice for neonatal seizures. It is also useful in generalized seizures (except absence) and may be useful in patients with partial seizures. Primidone shares the same indications but is less useful in partial seizures.[101] Neither are drugs of first choice because of their adverse effects. The widespread use of phenobarbital in the prophylaxis of febrile seizures has recently been questioned.[102]

Adverse Effects, Drug–Drug Interactions, and Drug–Food Interactions. CNS side effects are the primary factors limiting the use of phenobarbital. Tolerance usually develops to initial complaints of fatigue, drowsiness, sedation, and depression. In children, paradoxically, the primary side effect is hyperactivity. Phenobarbital impairs higher cortical function and depresses cognitive performance.[102] In susceptible patients, phenobarbital may precipitate porphyria. Other rare side effects include rashes, osteomalacia, and hypotension (see Table 52–6).

The side effects of primidone and phenobarbital are similar and may be difficult to separate. The initial side effects of sedation, nystagmus, and ataxia may be minimized by starting at a low dose and gradually increasing the dose.

Phenobarbital is a potent enzyme inducer and may increase the elimination of any drug metabolized by phase I oxidative processes. Valproic acid, phenytoin, cimetidine, and chloramphenicol inhibit phenobarbital metabolism, necessitating a decrease in dose. Ethanol increases the metabolism of phenobarbital. The drug interactions of primidone are similar to those of phenobarbital.[18]

Dosing and Administration. At therapeutic primidone concentrations, most patients have a phenobarbital concentration that is in the therapeutic range. It is rare that a patient on primidone needs supplemental doses of phenobarbital. PEMA concentrations are not routinely monitored.[18]

In nonacute situations, phenobarbital should be started in low doses and titrated upward. The dose–concentration relationship is linear. Because the half-life of phenobarbital is long, doses can be given once daily. Bedtime dosing sometimes minimizes the consequences of CNS depression. Because of its long half-life, phenobarbital takes 3 to 4 weeks to reach steady state. Therefore, rapid dosage adjustments should be avoided in a nonacute situation.

Primidone is not administered as a loading dose. An initial dose of 50 to 125 mg may be increased every 2 to 4 days until the desired concentration is reached. Because of the short half-lives of primidone and PEMA, the drug should be given in divided doses.

Phenytoin

Pharmacology and Mechanism of Action. Phenytoin blocks PTP by influencing synaptic transmission. Proposed mechanisms include altering ion fluxes associated with depolarization, repolarization, and membrane stability; altering calcium uptake in presynaptic terminals; influencing calcium-dependent synaptic protein phosphorylation and transmitter release; altering the sodium-potassium ATP-dependent ionic membrane pump; and preventing cyclic nucleotide buildup and cerebellar stimulation.[46]

Pharmacokinetics. Absorption of phenytoin is primarily from the duodenum, and it may be saturable. Absorption is almost complete, with dissolution being the rate-limiting step. Absorption may be prolonged, and secondary peaks may be seen. Enterohepatic cycling of phenytoin occurs, but there is no first-pass metabolism.[103]

The absorption of orally administered phenytoin is affected by the particle size of the formulation. Therefore, some brands may be absorbed faster than others, and the brand that a patient receives should not be changed without careful monitoring.[18] The intramuscular administration of phenytoin is problematic and best avoided. Fosphenytoin can safely be administered intravenously and intramuscularly (see Chap. 53).

Phenytoin enters the brain quickly, where it is redistributed to other body tissues, including saliva and breast milk. It crosses the placenta to reach an equilibrium between mother and fetus. Phenytoin is bound to serum and tissue proteins. Obesity may increase the volume of distribution.[18]

For most patients, phenytoin binding to albumin is predictable and proportional throughout the therapeutic range. Equations have been developed to normalize the phenytoin concentration in patients with hypoalbuminemia or renal failure. A good correlation has been shown between the free phenytoin concentration and the ratio of total phenytoin to albumin in patients with normal albumin or hyperalbuminemia. The ratio was not predictive for patients with hypoalbuminemia. A recent recalculation[104] of this equation was more reliable in elderly nursing home and trauma patients:

$$C_{calc} = C_{obs}/0.25\ ALB + 0.1$$

where C_{calc} is the calculated serum concentration, C_{obs} is the observed concentration, and ALB is albumin.

Phenytoin is metabolized in the liver primarily by parahydroxylation to 5-(p-hydroxyphenyl)-5-phenylhydantoin (HPPH). The major isoform responsible for phenytoin's metabolism is CYP 2C9 but CYP 2C19 is also involved.[55] HPPH is conjugated and excreted in the urine as a glucuronide. About 80% of an oral dose of phenytoin appears in the urine as HPPH. Abnormally low percentages of HPPH in the urine would indicate a problem with absorption. Phenytoin is a low-extraction drug, and its metabolism is not greatly influenced by changes in liver blood flow; however, because the major route of metabolism is hydroxylation, the clearance may be influenced by drugs that stimulate or inhibit liver microsomal enzymes.[103]

Phenytoin displays Michaelis-Menten elimination (the metabolism changes from first order to zero order) because the enzyme system is saturable. When the enzyme system is saturated, any change in dosage produces significantly disproportional changes in serum concentrations. The process may be described by the equation

$$D = V_{max} \times C_p/K_m + C_p$$

where D is the dose (in mg/d), V_{max} is the maximum rate of metabolism, K_m is the serum concentration at which the rate of metabolism is half-maximal, and C_p is the serum concentration.

Because V_{max} and K_m are both highly and independently variable, the metabolism of phenytoin may saturate at any concentration, and this may occur at doses used clinically. V_{max} has been shown to decline with age, and K_m may be affected by concurrent drug therapy. It is very difficult to predict the resulting outcome of a dosage increase of phenytoin. Also, serum concentrations do not decline by a constant percentage upon discontinuation. Therefore, any dosage change should be followed by careful patient monitoring and serum concentration determinations.[103]

Because of the saturable metabolism, the clinically useful concept of half-life may be inappropriate for phenytoin. Half-life assumes concentration-independent elimination. A more relevant term for phenytoin is the time required to eliminate 50% ($t_{50\%}$) of the serum concentration. The average $t_{50\%}$ for phenytoin is 22 hours, but may range from 7 to 42 hours. Because of saturation, the $t_{50\%}$ increases with increasing serum concentrations and the time to reach steady state may be prolonged.[103]

Less than 5% of a dose of phenytoin is excreted unchanged. Renal impairment does not affect the excretion of HPPH. Although an inhibitory effect of HPPH on phenytoin metabolism has been suggested, it has not been documented in humans. Neither hemodialysis nor peritoneal dialysis affects the clearance of phenytoin. Clinically insignificant amounts of phenytoin are removed by plasmapheresis.[18]

■ *Efficacy and Adverse Effects.* Phenytoin may be used for any generalized seizure type except absence, as it may worsen absence seizures. Partial seizures may also be treated with phenytoin.

When phenytoin is initiated, the CNS depressant effects may result in lethargy, fatigue, incoordination, blurred vision, higher cortical dysfunction, and drowsiness (see Table 52–6). These effects are usually transient and may be minimized by slow dosage titration.

When serum concentrations exceed 20 μg/mL, a significant number of patients exhibit nystagmus at a 45-degree lateral gaze. Ataxia frequently occurs at concentrations greater than 30 μg/mL. At concentrations greater than 40 μg/mL, mental status changes including coma occur. At very high concentrations, phenytoin can exacerbate seizures or precipitate generalized status epilepticus.[49,105]

It is difficult to determine whether the chronic side effects of phenytoin are concentration or duration dependent. One of the more common chronic side effects is gingival hyperplasia, which occurs in up to 50% of the patients. Good oral hygeine should be promoted to possibly minimize the ginginval hyperplasia. Suppression of cognitive abilities is also a concern. Other chronic effects include hirsutism, acne, coarsening of facial features, vitamin D deficiency, osteomalacia, folic acid deficiency, carbohydrate intolerance, immunologic disturbances, hypothyroidism, and peripheral neuropathy. Phenytoin is associated with rare hypersensitivity or idiosyncratic reactions resulting in rashes, Stevens-Johnson syndrome, pseudolymphoma, bone marrow suppression, lupus-like reactions, and hepatitis.[49,105]

■ *Drug–Drug and Drug–Food Interactions.* Phenytoin is prone to many drug interactions (see Tables 52–7 and 52–8), and these have been extensively reviewed. The effects of phenytoin may be enhanced or reduced by drugs that affect its pharmacokinetic parameters. Drug interactions affecting absorption, metabolism, or excretion are potentially more significant because total and free concentrations are affected. The rate of absorption of phenytoin may be decreased if it is given simultaneously with food. The bioavailability of phenytoin suspension may be decreased in patients receiving continuous enteral nutrient tube feedings. A single-dose study of simultaneous administration of enteral feeding found no difference in phenytoin bioavailability, indicating that the mechanism was something other than physical contact.[18] Phenytoin is highly protein bound and may be displaced by other highly protein-bound drugs, resulting in an increase in free phenytoin. The initial increase in free phenytoin is followed by an increase in clearance, a fall in total phenytoin concentrations, and the reestablishment of normal free phenytoin concentrations. Usually no dosage adjustment is necessary. Problems arise when clinicians react to the lower total phenytoin concentration without considering the free concentration. If protein-binding interactions are suspected, free rather than total phenytoin concentrations are a better therapeutic guideline. The metabolism of phenytoin can be inhibited (as by cimetidine) as well as increased (by phenobarbital). Phenytoin may alter the pharmacokinetics of other drugs.

A complex interaction of phenytoin with folic acid has also been described, making vitamin ingestion an important part of the drug history. Phenytoin reportedly decreases folic acid absorption, but folic acid enhances the clearance of phenytoin.[106] Replacement of folic acid can reduce phenytoin concentrations and result in loss of efficacy. It is unknown if the mandatory folic acid supplementation in wheat products (beginning January 1998) will lead to any significant changes in phenytoin concentrations.

TABLE 52–10. Phenytoin Dosage Forms

Dosage Form	Salt or Acid	Extended or Prompt	Amount of Acid Available
Dilantin capsules	Phenytoin sodium	Extended	
100 mg			92 mg
30 mg			27 mg
Dilantin suspension 125 mg/5 mL	Phenytoin acid	Prompt	125 mg/5mL
Dilantin infatabs 50 mg	Phenytoin acid	Prompt	46 mg
Phenytoin injectable 50 mg/mL	Phenytoin sodium	Prompt	46 mg/mL
Fosphenytoin 50 mg PE/mL			50 mg PHT equivalents/mL
Phenytoin capsules (generic)	Phenytoin sodium	Prompt	92 mg

PHT = phenytoin.

Dosing and Administration. Three dosage forms are used for oral administration of phenytoin (Table 52–10). The salt content should be considered in dosage form changes. If given in equal amounts of phenytoin acid, the tablets, capsules, and suspension have the same bioavailability. Changes between dosage forms may lead to changes in phenytoin concentration. Phenytoin capsules are designated as immediate-release or extended-release. Only the extended-release capsules should be used in once-a-day dosing. Particle size rather than formulation may determine the rate of absorption. Phenytoin suspension settles, but resuspension can be accomplished without overzealous agitation.[107]

If oral administration is not feasible, IV administration of phenytoin is preferred over IM administration. Fosphenytoin is a prodrug for phenytoin and is available as a parenteral dosage form (see Chap. 53). It is very water soluble and is rapidly converted to phenytoin systemically. Fosphenytoin can be given rapidly IV and IM with reliable absorption and minimal pain.

Dosing of phenytoin should start at about 5 mg/kg per day for adults. Subsequent dosage adjustments should be done cautiously due to its nonlinearity in elimination. One author has suggested that if the patient's concentration is less than 7 μg/mL, the dose should be increased by 100 mg/d. If the concentration is between 7 and 12 μg/mL, the dose can be increased by 50 mg/d. If the concentration is greater than 12 μg/mL, dose increases of 30 mg/d or less should be made. These increases will result in less than 10% of patients achieving a phenytoin serum concentration greater than 25 μg/mL.[108]

Tiagabine

Pharmacology and Mechanism of Action. Tiagabine (TGB) hydrochloride is a novel AED that is a potent and specific inhibitor of GABA uptake into glial and other neuronal elements. Thus, tiagabine enhances the action of GABA by decreasing its removal from the synaptic space.[109]

Pharmacokinetics. Tiagabine is quickly and nearly completely absorbed after oral administration. There is a linear relationship between daily doses and serum concentrations. Tiagabine is oxidized in the liver by cytochrome P450 3A4 enzymes. Enzyme inducers increase its clearance. Children eliminate tiagabine slightly faster than adults. Subjects with hepatic impairment have higher and more prolonged plasma concentrations of total and unbound drug. Renal dysfunction does not change its pharmacokinetics.[109]

Efficacy. Tiagabine is approved for adjunctive use in patients with partial seizures. Five add-on, placebo-controlled trials and six noncomparative, open-label, long-term multicenter trials have been or are being conducted in Australia, Europe, and the United States. The results of these trials involving 2261 patients indicate that tiagabine is efficacious as add-on therapy in patients with epilepsy difficult to control with existing AEDs. Efficacy of tiagabine is sustained with long-term treatment. These studies included a wide age range of patients, including adolescents and the elderly.[110] In addition, two abstracts have reported success with tiagabine monotherapy.[111]

Adverse Effects. Discontinuation resulting from adverse events in clinical trials was infrequent, occurring in 15% of patients receiving TGB compared to 5% receiving placebo. The most frequently reported adverse event was dizziness, which was usually transient and did not require medical intervention. Adverse events that were significantly more common with TGB than placebo were dizziness, asthenia, nervousness, tremor, diarrhea, and depression (not major depression). Adverse events were usually mild to moderate in severity and transient, and most were associated with dose titration. Serious adverse events were uncommon, and no idiosyncratic events were reported.[112]

Drug–Drug and Drug–Food Interactions. Enzyme inducers, such as carbamazepine and phenytoin, increase tiagabine clearance, reduce area-under-the-curve (AUC), and decrease the half-life. Food decreases the rate, but not the extent, of absorption. Tiagabine is displaced from protein by naproxen, salicylates, and valproate. However, tiagabine does not displace phenytoin, valproic acid, amitryptyline, tolbutamide, and warfarin. The AUC of VPA is reduced 10% to 12% when tiagabine is added. There is approximately a 5% increase in tiagabine AUC when cimetidine is added.[109]

Dosing and Administration. A clear dose response has been demonstrated, and the minimal effective dose level is 30 mg/d.[110] The dosage range studied was 32 to 56 mg daily.[109] Slow dosage titration is essential to decrease adverse CNS effects.

Topiramate

Mechanism of Action and Pharmacokinetics. Topiramate has multiple modes of action involving voltage-dependent sodium channels, GABA receptors, and antagonization of AMPA subtype glutamate receptors.[113]

Mean values for maximal plasma concentration (C_{max}) and AUC increased linearly with dose; however, a greater than proportional increase in both parameters was observed, probably due to saturable binding of the drug to erythrocytes. Approximately 50% of the dose is excreted renally in patients on no other drugs. Renal tubular reabsorption may be prominently involved in the renal handling of topiramate.[114]

Efficacy. Topiramate is approved as adjunctive therapy in adults with partial seizures. Its efficacy as adjunctive treatment in refractory partial epilepsy in adults appears good; over 40% of patients have a 50% or greater reduction in seizure frequency when topiramate is added to their regimen, with up to 7% becoming seizure free.[113] Topiramate may decrease the tonic–clonic seizures associated with Lennox-Gastaut syndrome.[115]

Adverse Effects, Drug–Drug Interactions, and Drug–Food Interactions. The main adverse events of topiramate are ataxia, impaired concentration, confusion, dizziness, fatigue, paresthesia, somnolence, and "thinking abnormally." Most of these occurred during rapid titration and higher doses. During long-term treatment, weight loss also occurred, and nephrolithiasis occurred in 1.5% of patients receiving topiramate.[113]

Food slightly reduces the rate but not the extent of absorption when topiramate was given with food.[114] Topiramate does not change plasma levels of carbamazepine or carbamazepine-epoxide. Oral clearance of digoxin is slightly increased when topiramate is added. *In vitro* studies show an effect of topiramate only on the CYP2C isoform. Carbamazepine increases topiramate clearance; thus, adjustments in topiramate dose may be needed when potent enzyme inducers, such as phenytoin or carbamazepine, are added or discontinued from a topiramate regimen.[116]

Dosing and Administration. Topiramate should be titrated slowly in order to avoid adverse events.[113] Starting doses are 25 to 50 mg/d, increasing by 25 to 50 mg/d every week or every other week. The minimally effective dose of topiramate is approximately 200 mg/d.[117] For patients on other AEDs, doses greater than 600 mg/d do not appear to lead to improved efficacy, and may lead to increased side effects; however, higher doses may prove beneficial to individual patients who tolerate them.[118] Monotherapy doses of 1000 mg/d have been well tolerated and effective.

Valproic Acid /Divalproex Sodium

Mechanism of Action. Initially it was believed that valproic acid increased GABA by inhibiting its degradation or by activating its synthesis. Although this may explain some of valproic acid effects, the time course for the increase in GABA compared with anticonvulsant effects of valproic acid indicates that effects on synthesis and degradation of GABA do not fully explain how valproic acid prevents seizures. It has been proposed that valproic acid may potentiate postsynaptic GABA responses, may have a direct membrane-stabilizing effect, and may affect the potassium channel.[119]

Pharmacokinetics. Valproic acid appears to be completely absorbed from available oral dosage forms when administered on an empty stomach.[119] The rate of absorption differs between preparations. Peak concentrations occur in 0.5 to 1 hour with the syrup, 1 to 3 hours with the capsule, and 2 to 6 hours with the enteric-coated tablet.[119] There is a diurnal decrease in absorption of the enteric-coated preparation following an evening dose. Food delays, but does not decrease, the amount of valproic acid absorbed.[18]

Valproic acid distributes widely throughout the body. The binding sites for valproic acid are saturable, and the free fraction may increase as the total concentration increases. The saturable binding may indicate that the free concentration is a better monitoring parameter than the total valproic acid concentration, especially at higher concentrations.[18] The protein binding of valproic acid is decreased in patients with head trauma.[120]

Valproic acid is metabolized primarily by the liver. There is no first-pass metabolism, and the clearance is independent of hepatic blood flow. As with other highly protein-bound drugs, an increase in free drug results in an increase in clearance. Thus, the clearance of valproic acid changes at higher concentrations.[18]

The primary route of valproic acid metabolism is betaoxidation, although up to 40% of a dose may be excreted as the glucuronide. At least 10 metabolites of valproic acid have been identified. Some of these may have weak anticonvulsant activity, and at least 1 metabolite may be responsible for the hepatotoxicity reported with valproic acid. One of the lesser oxidative metabolites, 4-en-valproic acid, causes significant hepatotoxicity in rats. The formation of this metabolite is increased when valproic acid is given with enzyme-inducing drugs such as phenobarbital.[119]

Efficacy and Adverse Effects. Valproic acid is the drug of first choice for most generalized seizures.[119] and is also useful in the treatment of partial seizures.[121] It is the only AED that is effective against absence and other types of generalized seizures. It may also be useful in neonatal seizures.[119]

The most common side effects are usually mild.[119] The most frequently reported side effects are GI complaints (up to 20%) including nausea, vomiting, anorexia, and weight gain. Pancreatitis is very rare. The GI complaints may be minimized but not totally alleviated with the enteric-coated formulation or by giving the drug with food. Other frequently reported side effects (drowsiness, ataxia, tremor) may respond to a modification of dose (see Table 52–6). Alopecia and hair changes are temporary. Peripheral edema may occur, and weight gain can be significant for many patients. Valproic acid causes minimal cognitive impairment.[119]

The most serious side effect reported with valproic acid is hepatotoxicity. Hyperammonemia is common (50%) but does not necessarily imply liver damage; however, at least 67 fatalities have been attributed to valproic acid hepatotoxicity. Most deaths have occurred in patients who were less than 2 years of age, mentally retarded, and receiving multiple therapy. The hepatotoxicity occurred early in the course of therapy.[122] Patients who complain of nausea, vomiting, lethargy, anorexia, and edema in the first 6 to 12 months of therapy should have liver function tests drawn. Multiple AED therapy may alter the normal metabolism, leading to increased formation of the potentially liver-toxic 4-en-valproic acid. Valproic acid has been shown to alter carnitine metabolism,[123] and it has been postulated that a deficiency of carnitine alters fatty acid oxidation that could lead to liver toxicity. However, valproic acid hepatotoxicity has occurred in a patient taking supplemental carnitine, and a prospective study demonstrated no effect on well-being when carnitine was added. Carnitine is expensive, and there are no data to support routine supplemental carnitine therapy in patients taking valproic acid.[123]

Thrombocytopenia occurs in 6% to 40% of the patients receiving valproic acid, but is responsive to a decrease in dose. Other hematologic toxicities have been reported, including leukopenia with transient neutropenia, transient erythroblastopenia, and bone marrow changes.

Drug–Drug and Drug–Food Interactions. Drugs that affect liver enzymes may alter valproic acid kinetics by increasing or decreasing clearance; for example, phenytoin, phenobarbital, primidone, and carbamazepine all increase valproic acid clearance. Because it is highly protein bound, other highly protein-bound drugs may displace valproic acid. Free fatty acids, aspirin, and phenytoin may alter valproic acid binding.

Valproic acid is an enzyme inhibitor. The most significant reported interaction is with phenobarbital. The addition of valproic acid to patients taking phenobarbital results in a 30% to 50% decrease in the clearance of phenobarbital and toxicity if the dose of phenobarbital is not reduced.[18] Valproic acid may increase concentrations of 10,11-epoxide carbamazepine without affecting concentrations of the parent drug.

Dosing and Administration. The minimal effective concentration of valproic acid is 50 μg/mL; however, there is disagreement on the upper end of the therapeutic range.[119] Although 100 μg/mL is widely quoted as the upper end of the therapeutic range, experience indicates that a significant number of patients have improved seizure control when the concentration is increased. Although some reports have linked tremor, drowsiness, stupor, and decreases in fibrinogen to concentrations greater than 80 to 100 μg/mL, there are very few clearly defined concentration-dependent side effects of valproic acid. In refractory or partially responding patients, the concentration of valproic acid may cautiously be titrated upward, provided the patient is closely monitored. As the concentration is increased, protein binding may become saturated, and concentration monitoring of free drug may be helpful.[18]

Although some patients may have a half-life sufficiently long to permit once-a-day dosing with valproic acid, more frequent dosing is the norm. Based on half-life data, twice-daily dosing is feasible with any valproic acid dosage form; however, children and other patients taking enzyme inducers may require dosing three to four times daily.[18]

The serum concentration–dose relationship is curvilinear (i.e., the concentration–dose ratio decreases with increasing dose), probably because of increasing free concentrations and a resulting increase in clearance.[18]

Valproic acid is available as a soft gelatin capsule, an enteric-coated tablet, a syrup, a "sprinkle," and a recently released IV solution for replacement of oral therapy. The sprinkle is designed to be opened and mixed with food. The soft gelatin capsule is available in several generic forms. The syrup is absorbed more rapidly than either solid. The enteric-coated tablet is not a sustained-release dosage form; it consists of sodium divalproex, which must be metabolized in the gut to valproic acid, and is enteric coated to reduce the incidence of GI distress. The enteric coating does cause delayed absorption, although once the enteric coating dissolves, sodium divalproex has absorption, metabolism, and elimination rates similar to those for other dosage forms. Absorption of the enteric-coated preparation is decreased following an evening dose. The sprinkle formulation has a slower rate of absorption, which results in less fluctuations in the peak-to-trough ratio. Its absorption is unaffected by food.[18]

Vigabatrin

Pharmacology and Mechanism of Action. Vigabatrin acts as an irreversible inhibitor of GABA amino transaminase, thus increasing brain GABA levels.[124]

Pharmacokinetics. Vigabatrin is administered as a racemic [R(−), S(+)] mixture, but the pharmacologic activity of vigabatrin resides in the S(+) enantiomer. The concentration of vigabatrin in saliva was approximately 10% of that in plasma.[125] Though vigabatrin's terminal elimination half-life is only 7 to 14 hours, vigabatrin can be dosed infrequently due to its mechanism of action. Vigabatrin distributes into red blood cells, at concentrations of 30% to 80% of plasma concentrations.[125]

Efficacy. Vigabatrin is used for treatment of partial and secondarily generalized tonic–clonic seizures in both adults and children as well as in infantile spasms.[126] In patients with newly diagnosed epilepsy, as monotherapy, it is similar in efficacy and safety to carbamazepine monotherapy.[127] In routine clinical practice, vigabatrin is beneficial to a significant number of patients with previously uncontrolled seizures.[128]

Adverse Effects. Vigabatrin is generally well tolerated. Sedation and fatigue are the most commonly reported side effects.[126] It has little impact on tests of either cognitive ability or quality of life, even at a high dose.[129] It may cause significant behavioral side effects such as agitation, irritability, depression or psychosis in approximately 2% to 4% of cases. Mild weight gain and possible exacerbation of absence and myoclonic seizures are other reported adverse effects.[130] One study suggested that vigabatrin may interfere with the modulation of the immune system, especially cytotoxic cell populations.[131]

Drug–Drug and Drug–Food Interactions. Addition of vigabatrin leads to increased phenytoin concentrations by approximately 30% by an unknown mechanism.[126] There are no other clinically significant drug interactions known.

Dosing and Administration. Because the effect of vigabatrin is on GABA transaminase, doses necessary to inhibit this enzyme are needed. Doses higher than 4000 mg/d have not shown significant benefit. Due to its prolonged effect on GABA transaminase, doses can be given once or twice daily. With decreased renal function, lower doses can be used.[126]

PHARMACOECONOMIC CONSIDERATIONS

The direct costs of epilepsy include the cost of the drug, treatment for adverse events, emergency room visits, drug levels, laboratory tests, physician visits, rehabilitation, and transportation. Indirect costs include the costs associated with time lost from work, the inability to get a job, decreased productivity, and mortality.

It has been difficult to assess the entire cost of epilepsy to society. Pashko and coworkers[132] used a cohort of Pennsylvania Medicaid patients to estimate that the total direct cost of epilepsy is in excess of $10 billion annually, with the majority of the per-patient cost incurred for inpatient hospitalization (uncontrolled seizures or treatment-related toxicity). Another study suggested that the direct costs of epilepsy made up about 37% of the total costs, with indirect costs accounting for about 63% of the total costs.[133] This study also indicated that the costs were much less for a patient who is well controlled than for a patient who is poorly controlled. Drug costs in the Pashko study accounted for about 10% of the total costs of epilepsy. In another study, the cost-effectiveness of some of the newer drugs (lamotrigine, vigabatrin, and gabapentin) was estimated for the first year of drug therapy. There was little difference in initial costs, but gabapentin, with fewer side effects, resulted in cost savings.[134] The methodology used in this study has been criticized. There have been no pharmacoeconomic studies comparing the older, less expensive AEDs to the newer, more expensive drugs.

Providing the best quality of life possible is a treatment goal for patients with epilepsy. This concept entails more than a balance between side effects and the number of seizures. Quality of life takes into account all of the concerns of patients with epilepsy including their social and economic concerns. This can best be assessed by the patient. Seizure freedom leads to the best quality of life.[11] In one study, driving was listed as the most important concern by 28% of patients, followed by employment (21%), independence (9%), safety (6%), AED side effects (5%), seizure unpredictability (5%), and seizure avoidance (5%).[135] Assessment of quality of life as a therapeutic outcome may ultimately be more meaningful than measuring blood levels of the AEDs. Several quality of life instruments have been used, though primarily as research tools.[136]

It is clear that the cheapest drugs in epilepsy (e.g., phenobarbital) are not the best because of the number of side effects. Further, drug therapy that would control seizures, decrease side effects, improve the quality of life, and reduce the use of other health care resources would be cost effective. Because epilepsy treatment continues to be very patient specific, the drug, or combination of drugs, that controls seizures with the least number of side effects will be the drug of choice for that patient, no matter how expensive the drug acquisition cost.

Because many patients with epilepsy require minimal variation in blood concentrations to prevent seizures and avoid side effects, generic prescribing for epilepsy remains controversial. One study suggested that the money saved by generic prescribing is outweighed by negative health gain for the person with epilepsy, increased work in general practice, and increased social costs.[137]

EVALUATION OF THERAPEUTIC OUTCOMES

MONITORING THE PHARMACEUTICAL CARE PLAN

An individual therapeutic range should be established for a given patient. This range should be the concentrations that result in minimal side effects and optimal seizure control. This therapeutic plasma concentration range should be used to identify the appropriate patient-specific dose. Patients should be chronically monitored for seizure control, social adjustment, drug interactions, compliance, dosage adjustments, and toxicity. The patient's response is more important that the serum drug concentration.

Outcomes can be assessed by prospective clinical monitoring, drug utilization review, and quality of life assessments. Clinical monitoring involves identifying the number and type of seizures. Patients should be given a seizure diary, and the severity as well as the frequency of seizures should be monitored. There should be a decrease in the number or severity of seizures. Patients should be questioned to determine if they are seizure free. If not, they may be candidates for combination therapy. Other clinical monitoring parameters include side effects, dosing, compliance, and drug interactions. Drug utilization reviews can be done for a given drug, or a disease utilization review could be done for all patients with epilepsy. In a utilization review, criteria for acceptable practice are developed, and a given population is measured to determine if these standards are met. Finally, there is a disease-specific quality of life rating scale for epilepsy, and the quality of life of epilepsy patients can be screened or assessed in depth. Uncontrolled seizures can be socially devastating, resulting in impaired progress in school or loss of employment. If the seizures are repetitive and prolonged, there is the possibility of brain injury or death.

CONCLUSIONS

The treatment of epilepsy begins with a careful identification of the seizure type and selection of the most appropriate AED. Therapy should be initiated slowly, except in life-threatening situations, to avoid acute toxicity. Although most patients can be successfully managed on monotherapy, some patients' seizures remain uncontrolled despite use of multiple AEDs. The newer AEDs offer more opportunity for complete seizure control. There is a continuing need for new AEDs and additional research in this area.

▶ PRINCIPLES OF PHARMACOTHERAPY

- Accurate diagnosis and classification of seizure/syndrome type is critical to selection of appropriate pharmacotherapy (see Table 52–4).
- Patient-specific treatment goal(s) should be identified. Often a balance between efficacy and side effects must be reached. Treatment goals may change over time.
- Patient characteristics such as age, medical condition, ability to comply with prescribed regimen, and insurance coverage may also influence choice of AED(s).
- Pharmacotherapy of epilepsy is highly individualized and requires titration of dose to optimize AED therapy (maximal seizure control with minimal or no side effects). About 70% of patients can be maintained on one AED.
- If the therapeutic goal is not achieved, a second drug may be added or a switch to an alternative single AED can be made (see Fig. 52–1).
- When pharmacotherapy is initiated, assurance of patient understanding of the plan is essential to successful treatment. Patient education must be continuously addressed and patient compliance continuously reinforced.
- After assessing risks and benefits, discontinuance of AEDs may be considered if specific criteria are met (see Table 52–3).

REFERENCES

1. Leppik IE. Contemporary Diagnosis and Management of the Patient with Epilepsy, 2nd ed. Newtown, PA, Handbooks in Health Care, 1996.
2. Schachter SC. Brainstorms: Epilepsy in Our Words. New York NY, Raven, 1993:96.
3. Hauser W. The prevalence and incidence of convulsive disorders in children. Epilepsia 1994;35(suppl 2):S1–S6.
4. Shinnar S, Berg A, Moshe S, et al. Risk of seizure recurrence following a first unprovoked seizure in childhood. Pediatrics 1990;85: 1076–1085.
5. Hauser W. Seizure disorders: The changes with age. Epilepsia 1992;33(suppl 4):S6–S14.
6. Cloyd JC, Lackner TE, Leppik IE. Antiepileptics in the elderly. Arch Fam Med 1994;3:589–598.
7. Chadwick D. Epilepsy. J Neurol Neurosurg Psychiatry 1994;57: 264–277.

8. Dichter MA. Emerging insights into mechanisms of epilepsy: Implications for new antiepileptic drug development. Epilepsia 1994;35: S51–S57.
9. Commission on Classification and Terminology of the International League Against Epilepsy. Proposal for revised clinical and electroencephalographic classification of epileptic seizures. Epilepsia 1981; 22:489–501.
10. Commission on Classification and Terminology of the International League Against Epilepsy. Proposal for revised classification of epilepsies and epileptic syndromes. Epilepsia 1989;30:389–399.
11. Vickrey BG, Hays RD, Rausch R, et al. Quality of Life of epilepsy surgery patients as compared with outpatients with hypertension, diabetes,heart disease, and/or depressive symptoms. Epilepsia 1994; 35:597–607.
12. Chadwick D. Standard approach to antiepileptic drug treatment in the United Kingdom. Epilepsia 1994;35:S3–510.
13. Meador KJ. Cognitive side effects of antiepileptic drugs. Can J Neurol Sci 1994;21:S12–S16.
14. Mattson RH, Cramer JA, Collins JF. Prognosis for total control of complex partial and secondarily generalized tonic clonic seizures. Department of Veterans Affairs epilepsy cooperative studies no. 118 and no. 264 group. neurology 1996;47:68–76.
15. Mattson R. Current challenges in the treatment of epilepsy. Neurology 1994;44(suppl 5):S4–S9.
16. French J. The long-term therapeutic management of epilepsy. Ann Intern Med 1994;120:411–422.
17. Cramer JA. Optimizing long-term patient compliance. Neurology 1995;45:S25–S28.
18. Garnett WR. Antiepileptics. In: Schumacher GE, ed. Therapeutic Drug Monitoring. Norwalk, CT, Appleton & Lange, 1995:345–395.
19. First Seizure Trial Group. Randomized clinical trial on the efficacy of antiepileptic drugs in reducing the risk of relapse after a first unprovoked tonic-clonic seizure. Neurology 1993;43:478–483.
20. Duncan JS, Shorvon SD, Trimble MR. Effects of removal of phenytoin, carbamazepine, and valproate on cognitive function. Epilepsia 1990;31:584–591.
21. Andersson T, Braathen G, Persson A, Theorell K. A comparison between one and three years of treatment in uncomplicated childhood epilepsy: a prospective study, 2. The EEG as predictor of outcome after withdrawal of treatment. Epilepsia 1997;38:225–232.
22. Holmes GL. Stopping antiepileptic drugs in children: When and why. Ann Neurol 1994;35:509–510.
23. Quality Standards Subcommittee of AAN. Practice parameter: A guideline for discontinuing antiepileptic drugs in seizure-free patients—Summary statement. Neurology 1996;47:600–602.
24. Chadwick D, Taylor J, Johnson T. Outcomes after seizure recurrence in people with well-controlled epilepsy and the factors that influence it. The MRC antiepileptic drug withdrawal group. Epilepsia 1996; 37:1043–1050.
25. Tennison M, Greenwood R, Lewis D, Thorn M. Discontinuing antiepileptic drugs in children with epilepsy. A comparison of a six-week and a nine-month taper period. N Engl J Med 1994;330: 1407–1410.
26. Berg AT, Shinnar S. Relapse following discontinuation of antiepileptic drugs: A meta-analysis. Neurology 1994;44:601–608.
27. Ketter TA, Malow BA, Flamini R, et al. Anticonvulsant withdrawal—Emergency psychopathology. Neurology 1994;44:55–61.
28. Jacoby A, Johnson A, Chadwick D. Psychosocial outcomes of antiepileptic drug discontinuations. Epilepsia 1992;33:1123–1131.
29. Salinsky MC, Uthman BM, Ristanovic RK, et al. Vagus nerve stimulation for the treatment of medically intractable seizures. Results of a 1-year open-extension trial. Arch Neurol 1996;53:1176–1180.
30. Whang CJ, Kim CJ. Short-term follow-up of stereotactic gamma knife radiosurgery in epilepsy. Stereotact Funct Neurosurg 1995;64: 202–208.
31. Engel J. Surgery for seizures. N Engl J Med 1996;334:647–652.
32. National institutes of Health consensus develoment conference statement. Surgery for epilepsy. Epilepsia 1990;31:806–812.
33. Nordli DRJ, De Vivo DC. The ketogenic diet revisited: Back to the future. Epilepsia 1997;38:743–749.
34. Heller AJ, Chesterman P, Elwes RD, et al. Phenobarbitone, phenytoin, carbamazepine, or sodium valproate for newly diagnosed adult epilepsy: A randomised comparative monotherapy trial. J Neurol Neurosurg Psychiatry 1995;58:44–50.
35. Mattson RH, Cramer JA, Collins JF, et al. Comparison of carbamazepine, phenobarbital, phenytoin, and primidone in partial and secondarily generalized tonic-clonic seizures. N Engl J Med 1985; 313:145–151.
36. Mattson RH, Cramer JA, Collins JF, et al. A comparison of valproate with carbamazepine for the treatment of complex partial seizures and secondarily generalized tonic-clonic seizures in adults. N Engl J Med 1992;327:765–771.
37. Marson AG, Kadir ZA, Chadwick DW. New antiepileptic drugs: a systematic review of their efficacy and tolerability. BMJ 1996;313: 1169–1174. Comments.
38. Resor SR, Resor LD, Woodbury DM, Kemp JW. Sulfonamides and derivatives: Acetazolamide. In: Mattson RH, Meldrum BS, Levy RH, eds. Antiepileptic Drugs. 4th ed. New York, Raven, 1995:969–985.
39. Shields WD, Shewmon DA, Chugani HT, Peacock WJ. Treatment of infantile spasms: Medical or surgical? Epilepsia 1992;33:S26–S31.
40. Morrell MJ. Sexual dysfunction in epilepsy. Epilepsia 1991;32: S38–S45.
41. Morrell MJ. The new antiepileptic drugs and women: Efficacy, reproductive health, pregnancy, and fetal outcome. Epilepsia 1996;37: S34–S44.
42. Duncan S, Read CL, Brodic MJ. How common is catamenial epilepsy? Epilepsia 1993;34:827–831.
43. Lander CM, Eadie MJ. Plasma antiepileptic drug concentrations during pregnancy. Epilepsia 1991;32:257–266.
44. Commission on Genetics, Pregnancy and the Child, International League Against Epilepsy. Guideline for the care of women of childbearing age with epilepsy. Epilepsia 1993;34:588–589.
45. Brodie MJ. Management of epilepsy during pregnancy and lactation. Lancet 1990;336:426–427.
46. Macdonald RL, Kelly KM. Antiepileptic drug mechanisms of action. Epilepsia 1995;36:S2–512.
47. Commission on Antiepileptic Drugs, International League Against Epilepsy. Guidelines for therapeutic monitoring on antiepileptic drugs. Epilepsia 1993;34:585–587.
48. Schmidt D, Einicke I, Haenel F. The influence of seizure type on the efficacy of plasma concentrations of phenytoin, phenobarbital and carbamazepine. Arch Neurol 1986;43:263–265.
49. Camfield P, Camfield C. Acute and chronic toxicity of antiepileptic medications: A selective review. Can J Neurol Sci 1994;21:S7–S11.
50. Collaborative group for epidemiology of epilepsy. Adverse reactions to antiepileptic drugs: A follow-up study of 355 patients with chronic antiepileptic drug treatment. Epilepsia 1988;29:787–793.
51. Vermeulen J, Aldenkamp AP. Cognitive side-effects of chronic antiepileptic drug treatment: A review of 25 years of research. Epilepsy Res 1995;22:65–95.
52. Meador KJ, Loring DW, Huh K, et al. Comparative cognitive effects of anticonvulsants. Neurology 1990;40:391–394.
53. Ludgate J, Keating J, O'Dwyer R, et al. An improvement in cognitive function following polypharmacy reduction in a group of epileptic patients. Acta Neurol Scand 1985;71:448–452.
54. Riva R, Albani F, Contin M, Baruzzi A. Pharmacokinetic interactions between antiepileptic drugs. Clinical considerations. Clin Pharmacokinet 1996;31:470–493.
55. Levy RH. Cytochrome P450 isozymes and antiepileptic drug interactions. Epilepsia 1995;36:S8–S13.
56. Tomson T, Almkvist O, Nilsson BY. Carbamazepine-10,11-epoxide in epilepsy: A pilot study. Arch Neurol 1990;47:888–892.

57. Robbins DK, Wedlund PJ, Buhn R, et al. Inhibition of epoxide hydrolase by valproic acid in epileptic patients receiving carbamazepine. Br J Clin Pharmacol 1990;29:759–762.
58. Schaffler L, Bourgeois BRD, Luders HO. Rapid reversibility of autoinduction of carbamazepine metabolism after temporary discontinuation. Epilepsia 1994;35:195–198.
59. Haefeli WE, Meyer PG, Luscher TF. Circadian carbamazepine toxicity. Epilepsia 1994;35:400–402.
60. VanAmelsvoort TH, Bakshi R, Devaus CB, Schwabe S. Hyponatremia associated with carbamazepine and oxcarbazepine therapy: A review. Epilepsia 1994;35:181–188.
61. Konishi T, Naganuma Y, Hongo K, et al. Carbamazepine-induced skin rash in children with epilepsy. Eur J Pediatr 1993;152:605–608.
62. Clark-Schmidt AL, Garnett WR, Lowe DR, et al. Loss of carbamazepine suspension through nasogastric feeding tubes. Am J Hosp Pharm 1990;47:332–372.
63. Miles MV, Lawless ST, Tennison MB, et al. Rapid loading of critically ill patients with carbamazepine suspension. Pediatrics 1990;86:263–266.
64. Van Der Meyden CH, Kruger AJ, Muller FO, et al. Acute oral loading of carbamazepine-CR and phenytoin in a double-blind randomized study of patients at risk of seizures. Epilepsia 1994;35:189–194.
65. Thakker KM, Mangat S, Garnett WR, et al. Comparative bioavailability and steady state fluctuations of Tegretol commercial and carbamazepine OROS tablets in adult and pediatric epileptic patients. Biopharm Drug Dispos 1992;24:839–841.
66. Wang JT, Shiu GK, Ong-Chen T, et al. Effects of humidity and temperature on *in vivo* dissolution of carbmazepine tablets. J Pharm Sci 1993;83:1002–1005.
67. Wolff D. Ethosuximide. In: Wyllie E, ed. The Treatment of Epilepsy: Principles and Practice, 2nd ed. Baltimore, Williams & Wilkins, 1996:856–864.
68. Macdonald RL, Kelly KM. Mechanisms of action of currently prescribed and newly developed antiepileptic drugs. Epilepsia 1994;35:S41–S50.
69. Taylor LA, McQuade RD, Tice MA. Felbamate, a novel antiepileptic drug, reverses *N*-methyl-D-aspartate/glycine-stimulated increases in intracellular Ca^{2+} concentration. Eur J Pharmacol 1995;289:229–233.
70. Bialer M. Comparative pharmacokinetics of the newer antiepileptic drugs. Clin Pharmacokinet 1993;24:441–452.
71. Graves N. Felbamate. Ann Pharmacother 1993;27:1073–1081.
72. Garnett WR. New opportunities for the treatment of epilepsy. Am J Health Syst Pharm 1995;52:88–91.
73. Graves MN, Holmes GB, Fuerst RH, et al. Effect of felbamate on phenytoin and carbamazepine serum concentrations. Epilepsia 1989;30:225–229.
74. Wagner ML, Remmel RP, Graves NM, Leppik IE. Effect of felbamate on carbamazepine and its major metabolites. Clinl Pharmacol Ther 1993;53:536–543.
75. Tisdel KA, Israel DS, Kilb DW. Warfarin-felbamate interaction: First report. Ann Pharmacother 1994;28.
76. McLean MJ. Gabapentin. Epilepsia 1995;36:S73–86.
77. Petroff OA, Rothman DL, Behar KL, et al. The effect of gabapentin on brain gamma-aminobutyric acid in patients with epilepsy. Ann Neurol 1996;39:95–99.
78. Goa KL, Sorkin EM. Gabapentin. A review of its pharmacological properties and clinical potential in epilepsy. Drugs 1993;46:409–427.
79. Bockbrader HN, Breslin EM, Underwood BA, et al. Multiple-dose, dose-propotionality study of Neurontin (gabapentin) in healthy volunteers. Epilepsia 1996;37:159.
80. McLean MJ. Clinical pharmacokinetics of gabapentin. Neurology 1994;44:S17–S22.
81. Fischer JH, Barr AN, Rogers SL, et al. Lack of serious toxicity following gabapentin overdose. Neurology 1994;44:982–983.
82. Wong MO, Eldon MA, Keane WF, et al. Disposition of gabapentin in anuric subjects on hemodialysis. J Clin Pharmacol 1995;35:622–626.
83. Leiderman DB. Gabapentin as add-on therapy for refractory partial epilepsy: Results of five placebo-controlled trials. Epilepsia 1994;35:S74–S76.
84. Khurana DS, Riviello J, Helmers S, et al. Efficacy of gabapentin therapy in children with refractory partial seizures. J Pediatr 1996;128:829–833.
85. Trudeau VL, Kilgore MB, Poulter CJ, et al. A multicenter, open-label extension study of gabapentin (Neurontin) monotherapy in pediatric patients with benign epilepsy with centrotemporal spikes (BECTS). Epilepsia 1996;37:111.
86. Vossler DG. Exacerbation of seizures in Lennox–Gastaut syndrome by gabapentin. Neurology 1996;46:852–853.
87. Rosner H, Rubin L, Kestenbaum A. Gabapentin adjunctive therapy in neuropathic pain states. Clin J Pain 1996;12:56–58.
88. Romano JG. Reduction of fasciculations in patients with amyotrophic lateral sclerosis with the use of gabapentin. Arch Neurol 1996;53:716.
89. Olson WL, Gruenthal M, Mueller ME, Olson WH. Gabapentin for parkinsonism: A double-blind, placebo-controlled, crossover trial. Am J Med 1997;102:60–66.
90. Lee DO, Steingard RJ, Cesena M, et al. Behavioral side effects of gabapentin in children. Epilepsia 1996;37:87–90.
91. Gidal BE, Maly MM, Budde J, et al. Effect of a high-protein meal on gabapentin pharmacokinetics. Epilepsy Res 1996;23:71–76.
92. Fisher RS, Sachdeo FC, Pellock J, et al. Dose intitiation of gabapentin (CI-945) add-on therapy: A multicenter, randomized, double-blind, comparative study. Epilepsia 1996;37:158.
93. Messenheimer JA. Lamotrigine. Epilepsia 1995;36:S87–S94.
94. Rambeck B, Wolf P. Lamotrigine clinical pharmacokinetics Clin Pharmacokinet. 1993;25:433–443.
95. Gilman JT. Lamotrigine: An antiepileptic agent for the treatment of partial seizures. Ann Pharmacother 1995;29:144–151.
96. Posner J, Holdich CP. Comparison of lamotrigine pharmacokinetics in young and elderly healthy volunteers. J Pharm Med 1991;1:121–128.
97. DeToledo J, Toledo C, Ramsay RE, et al. Conversion to lamotrigine monotherapy: Efficacy and tolerability of previous inducing/non-inducing AEDs on the initiation rates in patients with refractory primary and secondarily generalized seizures. Epilepsia 1996;37:163.
98. French JA, Morris G. Rash associated with lamotrigine use in clinical practice: results of the PADS (postmarketing antepileptic drug survey) study. Epilepsia 1996;37:S203.
99. Richens A. Safety of lamotrigine. Epilepsia 1994;35:S37–S40.
100. Anderson GD, Yau MK, Gidal BE, et al. Bidirectional interaction of valproate and lamotrigine in healthy subjects. Clin Pharmacol Ther 1996;60:145–156.
101. Painter MJ. Benzodiazepines and the barbiturates in the treatment of childhood epilepsy. In: Dodson WE, Pellock JM, eds. Pediatric Epilepsy: Diagnosis and Treatment. New York, Demos, 1993: 281–289.
102. Farwell JR, Lee YJ, Hirtz DG, et al. Phenobarbital for febrile seizures-effects on intelligence and on seizure recurrence. N Engl J Med 1990;322:364–369.
103. Tozer TN, Winter ME. Phenytoin. In: Evans WE, Schentag JJ, Jusko WJ, eds. Applied Pharmacokinetics, 3rd ed. Spokane, Applied Therapeutics, 1992:25-1–25-44.
104. Anderson GD, Pak C, Doane KW, et al. Revised Winter-Tozer equation for normalized phenytoin concentrations in trauma and elderly patients with hypoalbuminemia. Ann Pharmacother 1997;31:279–284.
105. Bourgeois BFD. Pharmacologic intervention and treatment of childhood seizure disorders: Relative efficacy and safety of antiepileptic drugs. Epilepsia 1994;35:S18–S23.
106. Berg MJ, Fincham RW, Ebert BE, et al. Decrease of serum folates in healthy male volunteers taking phenytoin. Epilepsia 1988;29:67–73.
107. Sarkar MA, Garnett WR, Karnes HT. The effects of storage and shaking on the settling properties of phenytoin suspension. Neurology 1989;39:207–209.

108. Privitera MD. Clinical rules for phenytoin dosing. Ann Pharmacother 1993;27:1169–1173. Comments.
109. Schachter SC. Tiagabine: Current status and potential clinical applications. Exp Opin Invest Drugs 1996;5:1377–1387.
110. Ben-Menachem E. International experience with tiagabine add-on therapy. Epilepsia 1995;36:S14–S21.
111. Kalviainen R, Salmenpera T, Aikia M, et al. Tiagaine monotherapy in chronic partial epilepsy. Epilepsia 1996;37:167.
112. Leppik IE. Tiagabine: The safety landscape. Epilepsia 1995;36: S10–S13.
113. Walker MC, Sander JW. Topiramate: A new antiepileptic drug for refractory epilepsy. Seizure 1996;5:199–203.
114. Doose DR, Walker SA, Gisclon LG, Nayak RK. Single-dose pharmacokinetics and effect of food on the bioavailability of topiramate, a novel antiepileptic drug. J Clin Pharmacol 1996;36:884–891.
115. Sachdeo S, Sachdeo RJ, Kugler S. A open label evaluation of topiramate in Lennox–Gastaut syndrome. Epilepsia 1996;37:112.
116. Bourgeois BF. Drug interaction profile of topiramate. Epilepsia 1996;37:S14–S17.
117. Faught E, Wilder BJ, Ramsay RE, et al. Topiramate placebo-controlled dose-ranging trial in refractory partial epilepsy using 200-, 400-, and 600-mg daily dosages. Neurology 1996;46:1684–1690.
118. Privitera M, Fincham R, Penry J, et al. Topiramate placebo-controlled dose-ranging trial in refractory partial epilepsy using 600-, 800-, and 1,000-mg daily dosages. Neurology 1996;46:1678–1683.
119. Davis R, Peters DH, McTavish D. Valproic acid: A reappraisal of its pharmacological properties and clinical efficacy in epilepsy. Drugs 1994;47:332–372.
120. Anderson GD, Gidal BE, Hendryz RJ, et al. Decreased plasma protein binding of valproate in patients with acute head trauma. Br J Clin Pharmacol 1994;37:559–562.
121. Beydoun A, Sackellares JC, Shu V. Safety and efficacy of divalproex sodium monotherapy in partial epilepsy: A double-blind, concentration-response design clinical trial. Depakote monotherapy for partial seizures study group. Neurology 1997;48:182–188.
122. Dreifuss FE, Santilli N. Valproic acid hepatic fatalities: A retrospective review. Neurology 1987;37:379–385.
123. Kelley RI. The role of carnitine supplementation in valproic acid therapy. Pediatrics 1994;93:891–892.
124. Mattson RH, Petroff O, Rothman D, Behar K. Vigabatrin: Effects on human brain GABA levels by nuclear magnetic resonance spectroscopy. Epilepsia 1994;35:S29–S32.
125. Durham SL, Hoke JF, Chen TM. Pharmacokinetics and metabolism of vigabatrin following a single oral dose of [14C]vigabatrin in healthy male volunteers. Drug Metab Dispos 1993;21:480–484.
126. Grant SM, Heel RC. Vigabatrin: A review of its pharmacodynamic and pharmacokinetic properties, and therapeutic potential in epilepsy and disorders of motor control. Drugs 1991;41:889–926.
127. Kalviainen R, Aikia M, Saukkonen AM, et al. Vigabatrin vs carbamazepine monotherapy in patients with newly diagnosed epilepsy. A randomized, controlled study. Arch Neurol 1995;52:989–996.
128. Lhoir A. Vigabatrin in uncontrolled seizures: Belgian clinical experience. Clin Neurol Neurosurg 1994;96:42–46.
129. Dodrill CB, Arnett JL, Sommerville KW, Sussman NM. Effects of differing dosages of vigabatrin (Sabril) on cognitive abilities and quality of life in epilepsy. Epilepsia 1995;36:164–173.
130. Guberman A. Vigabatrin. Can J Neurol Sci 1996;23:S13–S17.
131. Pacifici R, Zuccaro P, Iannetti P, et al. Immunologic aspects of vigabatrin treatment in epileptic children. Epilepsia 1995;36:423–426.
132. Pashko S, McCord A, Sena MM. The cost of epilepsy and seizures in a cohort of Pennsylvania Medicaid patients. Med Interface November 1993:79–84.
133. Begley CE, Annegers JF, Lairson DR, et al. Cost of epilepsy in the United States: A model based on incidence and prognosis. Epilepsia 1994;35:1230–1243.
134. Hughes D, Cockerell OC. A cost minimization study comparing vigabatrin, lamotrigine and gabapentin for the treatment of intractable partial epilepsy. Seizure 1996;5:89–95.
135. Gilliam F, Kuzniecky R, Faught E, et al. Patient-validated content of epilepsy-specific quality-of-life measurement. Epilepsia 1997;38: 233–236.
136. Jacoby A. Assessing quality of life in patients with epilepsy. Pharmaoeconomics 1996;9:399–416.
137. Crawford P, Hall WW, Chappell B, et al. Generic prescribing for epilepsy. Is it safe? Seizure 1996;5:1–5.
138. Hauser WA, Rich SS, Annegers JF, Anderson VE. Seizure recurrence after a first unprovoked seizure: An extended follow-up. Neurology 1990;40:1163–1170.

53

STATUS EPILEPTICUS

Stephanie J. Phelps, PharmD, FCCP, William N. May, MD, Douglas F. Rose, MD

Status epilepticus (SE) is a common neurologic emergency that may be associated with brain damage and death. Convulsive SE accounts for between 1% and 8% of hospital admissions[1] and between 3% and 5% of admissions to neurologic intensive care units.[2] Although there is no consensus on the definition of SE, for practical purposes, SE may be defined as recurrent seizures without an intervening period of consciousness before the next seizure, or any seizure lasting longer than 30 minutes whether or not consciousness is impaired.[3–6]

SE can present in several forms (Table 53–1) and is classified according to the revised International Classification of Epileptic Seizures.[3] The syndrome most commonly associated with the term *status epilepticus* is tonic–clonic or generalized *convulsive* SE (GCSE). This type of SE is characterized by repeated primary or secondary generalized seizures that are associated with a persistent postictal state. *Nonconvulsive* SE (NCSE) is characterized by a fluctuating or continuous "twilight" state that produces altered consciousness (i.e., absence or complex partial) or by repeated simple partial seizures. Simple partial seizures are manifested as focal motor convulsions, focal sensory symptoms, or focal impairment of function not associated with altered consciousness.[7]

EPIDEMIOLOGY

The incidence of SE is difficult to determine, because most studies do not consider the seizure duration or type, etiology, or patient's age. Previous studies using older definitions for SE (seizure lasting longer than 60 minutes) have suggested that between 50,000[1] and 160,000[4] individuals in the United States have an episode of SE yearly. However, a recent community-based study estimated that the incidence of SE in the United States may be as high as 250,000 cases/yr.[8] It is estimated that the global incidence of convulsive SE ranges between 1.2 and 5 million cases/yr.[9] The most common and severe form of SE (GCSE) accounts for approximately 75% of cases, and NCSE accounts for 25%.[10] DeLorenzo and associates[10] reported that more than 70% of adults and 50% of children with GCSE initially presented with partial seizures that became secondarily generalized.[10] The annual incidence of absence SE and complex partial SE is 1 and 35 per million, respectively.[11] It is likely that the incidence of NCSE is higher because of underdiagnosis.[7]

SE may be the initial presentation of epilepsy in 12% to 60% of all patients[12,13] and may be the initial presentation of epilepsy in as high as 48% to 75% of children[14] and in 70% of elderly individuals.[1,10] In children, 21% and 64% of cases are reported by the first and fifth years of age, respectively.[15,16] The incidence of GCSE is higher in nonwhites than whites across all ages.[10]

Although most reports note that the incidence of SE in previously diagnosed epileptics ranges between 0.5%[1] and 6.6%,[17] a recent study noted that the incidence may be as high as 42%.[10] Others have reported that within 5 years of the diagnosis of epilepsy, 20% of patients will have an episode of SE.[5]

ETIOLOGY

Although there has been no change in the pattern of etiologies during the past two decades,[18] precipitating events for SE vary from study to study and generally reflect various populations and referral patterns. Common etiologies and mortality rates for pediatric and adult populations are shown in Table 53–2.[8,10]

Precipitating events for GCSE are divided into two groups. Type I etiologies are not associated with any new structural lesions and include epileptic patients with SE.[19] A variety of prescription, over-the-counter, and recreational medications must also be considered in any patient with new-onset SE. Type II etiologies are associated with structural lesions and have a poor prognosis. These include brain tumor, anoxic encephalopathy, meningitis, stroke, and hemorrhage.

There are major differences in pediatric and adult etiologies. In patients less than 1 year old, the major causes of seizures are acute encephalopathy or metabolic disease (amino acid disturbances).[20] During the neonatal period, it is imperative to consider drug withdrawal-induced seizures (addicted mothers). Although infrequent, a pyridoxine deficiency may exist, and the electroencephalogram (EEG) should normalize within several hours following treatment with an IV dose of pyridoxine (100 mg). In young children the cause is frequently idiopathic but may be associated with fever or a viral illness.[20] Generally, fever-induced SE is not associated with sequelae unless accompanied by an underlying neurologic abnormality.[21] In a study of 44 normal children with fever-induced GCSE, there was no increase in the risk of subsequent febrile or afebrile seizures within 12 months following the episode. However, there was a risk of recurrent seizures in those patients with a prior neurologic abnormality.[22]

In adults, the most frequent precipitating factors are cerebrovascular disease, withdrawal of antiepileptic drugs (AEDs), and low anticonvulsant concentrations. Interest-

TABLE 53–1. International Classification of Status Epilepticus

Convulsive		Nonconvulsive	
International	*Traditional Terminology*	*International*	*Traditional Terminology*
Primary generalized SE • Tonic–clonic[a,b] • Tonic[a,c] • Clonic[c] • Myoclonic[b] • Erratic[d]	Grand mal, epilepticus convulsivus	Absence[c]	Petit mal, spike-and-wave stupor, spike-and-slow-wave or 3/s spike-and-wave, epileptic fugue, epilepsia minora continua, epileptic twilight, minor SE
Secondary generalized SE[a,b] • Tonic • Partial seizures with secondary generalization		Partial SE[a,b]	Focal motor, focal sensory, epilepsia partialis continuans, adversive SE
		Simple partial Somatomotor Dysphasic Other types	Elementary
		Complex partial	Temporal lobe, psychomotor, epileptic fugue state, prolonged epileptic stupor, prolonged epileptic confusional state, continuous epileptic twilight state

[a]Most common in older children.
[b]Most common in adolescents and adults.
[c]Most common in infants and young children.
[d]Most common in neonates.

ingly, infection is not a major cause of SE in adults; however, there have been increasing reports of SE associated with the human immunodeficiency virus (HIV).[6] In elderly patients who have their first seizures after age 60, cerebrovascular disease is the leading cause of SE. The initiating events of NCSE have not been well characterized.[7] Absence SE has been associated with carbamazepine therapy[23] and benzodiazepine withdrawal.[24]

TABLE 53–2. Etiology and Mortality for Pediatric and Adult Cases of Status Epilepticus

Etiology	Pediatric (N = 200) % SE cases (% mortality)	Adult (N = 512) % SE cases (% mortality)
Type I (no structural lesion)		
Infection	55 (5)	6 (35)
CNS infection	11 (0)	2 (20)
Metabolic	20 (5)	12 (36)
Low AED levels	16 (0)	24 (7)
Alcohol	0 (0)	13 (8)
Idiopathic	6 (0)	13 (18)
Type II (structural lesion)		
Anoxia/hypoxia	27 (13)	14 (65)
CNS tumor	3 (50)	5 (22)
CVA	5 (0)	26 (27)
Drug overdose	5 (0)	3 (23)
Hemmorhage	5 (11)	4 (35)
Trauma	13 (0)	3 (23)
Remote causes[a]	33 (5)	7 (13)

Percentages do not add up to 100% because some patients had multiple etiologies. (AED = antiepileptic drug; CVA = cerebrovascular accident)
[a]More than half of remote causes were congential malformations and CVA in pediatric and adult patients, respectively.
Data modified from Refs. 8 and 10.

PATHOGENESIS

Human studies investigating the mechanisms of SE are difficult; hence, scientists have relied largely on experimental animal models. Although the exact mechanisms responsible for GCSE are unknown, it appears there is an activated cascade of changes in excitatory amino acid neurotransmission, γ-aminobutyric acid (GABA) inhibition, and *N*-methyl-D-aspartate (NMDA) receptor-mediated channel events (Fig. 53–1).[25–29] It is unlikely that a single mechanism is responsible for SE, but that multiple interrelated events occur simultaneously at the cellular, brain, and systemic levels.

Neurotransmitters released from the presynaptic terminal may cause either an excitatory or inhibitory effect on neuronal discharge. An increase in excitatory (e.g., glutamate and acetylcholine) or a decrease in inhibitory (e.g., GABA) neurotransmitters can cause sustained seizures with subsequent neuronal death.[30]

The ionic events that occur during SE are associated with opening of ion channels coupled to excitatory amino acid receptors. During GCSE, glutamate activation of the NMDA receptor causes processes that normally suppress the NMDA receptor-coupled channels to be overcome, resulting in opening of the gated calcium channels. This causes cell depolarization and calcium entry, which further depolarizes the cell. Sustained depolarization secondary to NMDA activation may not only sustain GCSE but may eventually cause neuronal death. However, because NMDA receptor antagonists are no more effective than traditional anticonvulsants, it is unlikely that glutamate is the sole

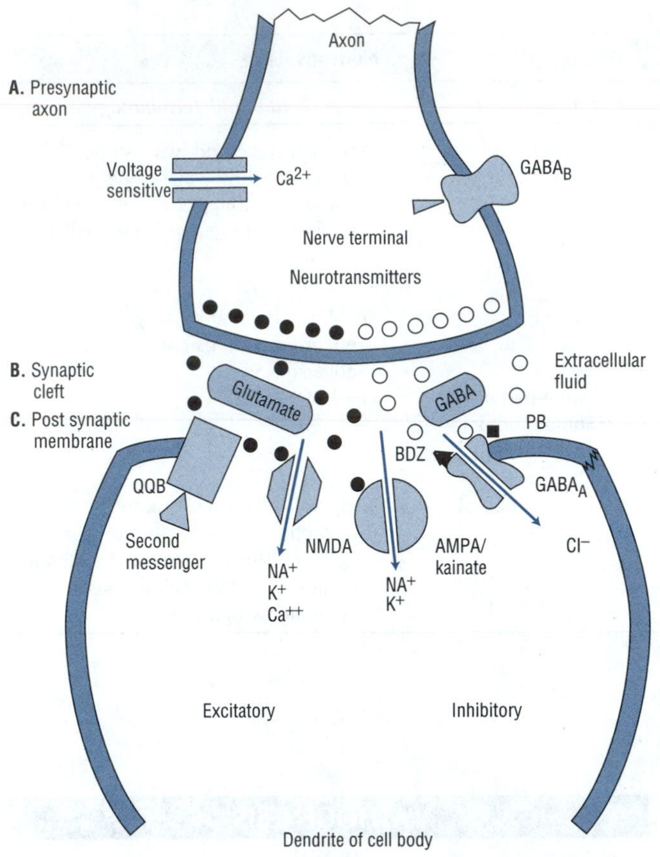

FIGURE 53–1. Neurotransmitters, receptors, and ion channels at nerve synapses. **(A)** Presynaptic axon. When axon action potential arrives at presynaptic nerve terminal, voltage-sensitive calcium (CA^{++}) channels activate and cause release of neurotransmitter into the synaptic cleft. Presynaptic nerve terminals may be excitatory (glutamate) or inhibitory (GABA). $GABA_B$ receptors, activated by presynaptic axo-axonic synapses, decrease Ca^{++} channel influx through a second-messanger pathway and can inhibit presynaptic neurotransmitter release into the synaptic cleft. **(B)** Synaptic cleft. Neurotransmitters (glutamate, GABA) move across the synaptic cleft. **(C)** Postsynaptic membrane of nerve dendrite or cell body. Excitatory neurotransmitters depolarize the postsynaptic membrane. Glutamate receptors are more often on the neuron dendrite than on the neuron cell body. There are four subtypes of receptors: (1) α-amino-3 hydroxy-5 methyl-4 isoxazolepropionate (AMPA), (2) kainate subtypes that are Na^+ and K^+ channels, (3) NMDA subtype permeable to NA^+, K^+, and Ca^{++} and also voltage dependent, and (4) a quisaualate B (QQB) subtype that activates a second-messanger pathway. Inhibitory neurotransmitters: $GABA_A$ receptors are more often on the neuron cell body than on the dendrite and cause Cl^- influx that stabilizes the postsynaptic membrane. The $GABA_A$ receptors have additional binding sites for benzodiazepines (BDZ) and barbiturates (PB) that enhance binding of GABA to the receptor. Glycine, not shown, is an inhibitory neurotransmitter active only in the spinal cord at the postsynaptic membrane.

mechanism for GCSE.[31] Likewise, certain NMDA receptor antagonists may decrease rather than increase the seizure threshold. A second theory suggests that the excitatory amino acid-induced depolarization causes a passive flux of anion, cations, and water into the neuron, producing an osmotic cell lysis. If adenosine triphosphate production also decreases, the sodium pump fails, membrane ion exchange increases, and neurons swell further.

Other non-NMDA receptors (e.g., AMPA, kainate) are activated by quisqualate and kainic acid, producing fast excitatory postsynaptic potentials. Neuronal damage in the hippocampus, similar to that noted after GCSE, has been reported following kainic acid-induced SE. This provides support for the theory that neuron destruction is independent of the systemic metabolic factors discussed in the next section. Antagonists of non-NMDA glutamate transmission can stop or prevent seizures, suggesting that glutamate agonism is important during GCSE.

Although cholinergic drugs can induce SE, they are thought to be secondary neuromodulators that exhibit either presynaptic cholinergic or muscarinic receptor activation. Pilocarpine alone or in combination with lithium activates the acetylcholine receptor to produce SE; however, atropine is an effective anticonvulsant only when used in the first few minutes of SE. Electrically induced SE is not stopped by scopolamine or atropine, suggesting that propagation of SE does not involve the cholinergic system.

The mechanisms that normally terminate seizures are poorly understood. The leading candidate, GABA, binds to postsynaptic receptors to regulate the opening and closing of the GABA channel. GABA binds to two distinct receptor subtypes. $GABA_A$ receptors are postsynaptic receptors that control chloride channels to produce hyperpolarization of the postsynaptic cell membrane. These receptors have binding sites for GABA as well as select anticonvulsants (phenobarbital, benzodiazepines) and enhance $GABA_A$ currents. $GABA_B$ receptors are located pre- and postsynaptically and couple with calcium and potassium to inhibit the presynaptic membrane release of excitatory amino acids.

During SE, the GABA system does not function to inhibit seizures. GABA levels increase during the early phases of GCSE and continue to be elevated during late SE. This may represent increased synthesis or diminished breakdown. Immediately prior to the onset of chemically induced seizures, there is a progressive loss of $GABA_A$ receptor sensitivity to GABA. A diminution of GABAergic inhibition in the hippocampus has been reported in animals after a single, brief seizure.[27] Additionally, many $GABA_A$ antagonists can precipitate SE, and $GABA_A$ agonists (benzodiazepines) can abort SE. Likewise, abrupt withdrawal of a GABA agonist can induce SE. There is growing evidence that $GABA_A$ receptors are modified during SE and that the modification contributes to persistent seizures. Although the role of $GABA_B$ receptor agonists in SE is unknown, inhibition of the presynaptic receptors may inhibit GABA release, causing SE. Although GABA is important, it is unlikely that loss of GABA inhibition is the sole mechanism for SE.

PATHOPHYSIOLOGY

As GCSE progresses, there are systemic alterations, progression of motor phenomena, and specific EEG findings (Fig. 53–2).[32] Two distinct and predictable phases have been identified.[2,20,26,32–36] Phase I occurs during the first 30 minutes of seizure activity, and phase II begins 60 minutes

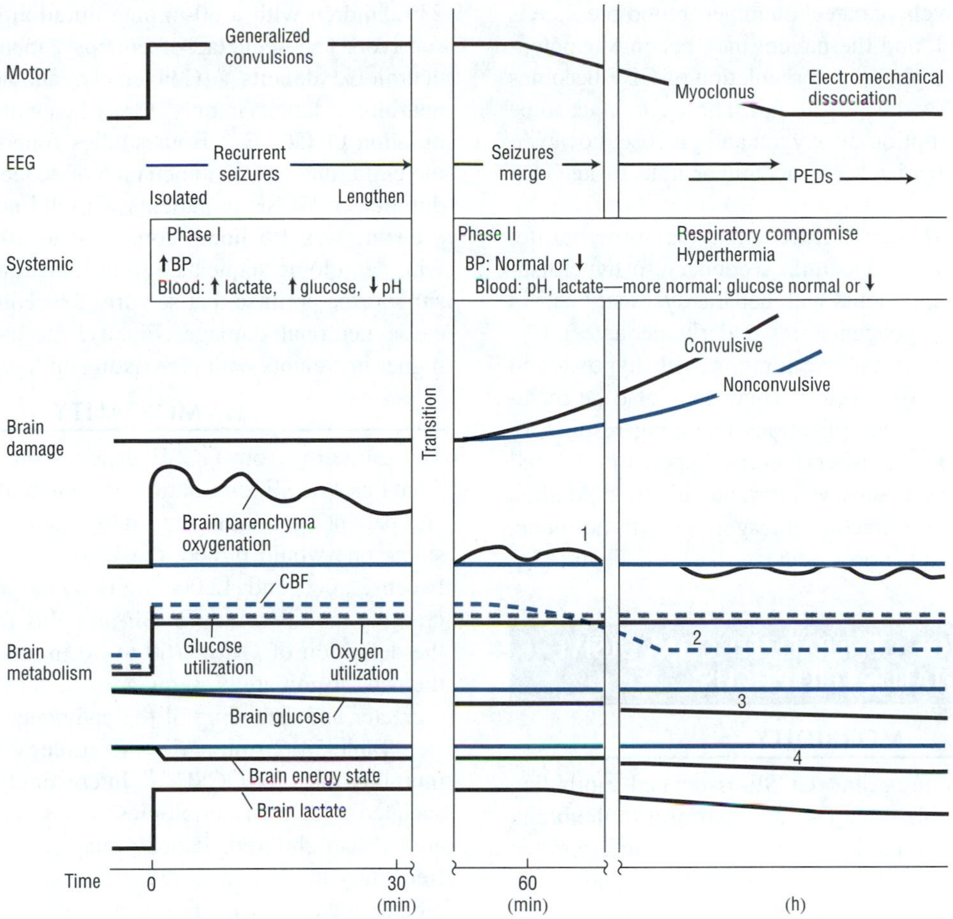

FIGURE 53–2. Systemic alterations, brain physiology, and cerebral metabolic events associated with experimental GCSE. (PEDs = periodic epileptiform discharges.) *(Reproduced from Ref. 1, with permission.)*

later. Although the presence of systemic complications affects the prognosis of SE, one must remember that SE may destroy neurons independent of these systemic events.[37] In fact, the systemic effects of experimentally induced seizures in animals can be blocked, but the damage to the neocortex, cerebellum, and hippocampus persists.

During phase I, each seizure produces marked increases in plasma epinephrine, norepinephrine, and steroid concentrations that may cause hypertension, tachycardia, and cardiac arrhythmias.[35] Within minutes, arterial systolic pressures may rise to values above 200 mm Hg, and heart rate may increase by 83 beats/min. Although blood pressure returns to normal within 60 minutes, mean arterial pressure (MAP) does not fall below 60 mm Hg; hence, cerebral perfusion pressure (CPP) is not compromised. In animals, cerebral blood flow (CBF) is also increased (200% to 600%), thereby protecting neurons.

Seizure-induced increases in sympathetic and parasympathetic stimulation of the heart, in the presence of a hypoxic myocardium, may result in ventricular arrhythmias. Arrhythmias are frequently seen early in GCSE and may prove fatal.[35] Autonomic neuron stimulation can also cause a release of insulin and glucagon. Concurrently, circulating catecholamines cause an elevation of hepatic cyclic adenosine monophosphate (cAMP), producing glycogenolysis. Although the patient may initially be hyperglycemic, serum glucose begins to fall.

Seizure-induced muscular contractions and hypoxia cause lactic acid release that can cause a severe acidosis that may be accompanied by hypotension and shock. Muscle contractions can be so severe that rhabdomyolysis with secondary hyperkalemia, and acute tubular necrosis, may occur. Excessive heat is generated by increased muscle activity, and a correlation has been shown between increased body temperature and severity of brain injury.[38]

The airway may be obstructed, and the patient may become cyanotic or hypoxic at any time. Additionally, an increase in salivation and tracheal and pulmonary secretions may result in aspiration pneumonia. Although transient pleocytosis (WBC up to 20,000/mm^3) may occur, it should not be attributed to SE until infectious causes have been eliminated.

Between seizures, the EEG slows and blood pressure normalizes. Although metabolic demands are increased, the brain is able to adequately compensate for these increased demands. If seizure activity exceeds 60 minutes (phase II), the EEG ictal discharge and clonic motor activity become continuous, and the patient begins to decompensate.

Despite elevated levels of catecholamines, blood pressure is no longer increased, and the patient may become hypotensive. During the late phase, autoregulation of CBF becomes dependent on MAP and begins to fail. There continues to be an excessive consumption of oxygen and glucose; however, compensatory mechanisms are no longer able to keep up with demands.[37]

During phase II, serum glucose may be normal or decreased. Profound hypoglycemia, secondary to hyperinsulinemia, can occur in patients with hepatic dysfunction or in those with reduced glycogen stores (elderly, neonates). Hyperthermia and respiratory deterioration with hypoxia and ventilatory failure may develop. There may also be metabolic and biochemical complications including respiratory and metabolic acidosis, hyperkalemia, hyponatremia, and azotemia. There is increased sweating and salivation. Marked elevations in plasma prolactin, glucagon, growth hormone, and adrenocorticotropic hormone have also been identified.[33]

OUTCOMES OF GENERALIZED CONVULSIVE STATUS EPILEPTICUS

MORBIDITY

Two theories exist regarding GCSE-associated morbidity. Both theories recognize that GCSE is harmful to the brain, but the first theory contends that morbidity occurs from the underlying etiology that caused GCSE.[1] The second theory contends that GCSE itself is responsible for morbidity.[32,39] Although histopathologic changes in animal neurons are evident following 30 minutes of GCSE, it is hard to establish a relationship between long-term outcome and SE because it is difficult to weigh the seizure type, duration, etiology, concurrent physiologic events, and therapy or lack of therapy.

Reports suggest that GCSE may decrease cognitive function in adults and that simple or complex partial SE lasting for days may cause prolonged memory deficits and neuronal death.[6,40,41] Some believe there is an association between GCSE and deterioration in intellectual function,[32] but others have disputed the significance of the association.[39] Animal studies have shown that both single and refractory seizures inhibited brain growth and protein synthesis, causing permanent reduction in brain cell number.[36] Likewise, animal studies have noted that seizures inhibit cell multiplication and reduce the accumulation of myelin and synaptic markers. Importantly, these effects have been observed in the absence of neuronal necrosis. Although extrapolation of these results to humans is difficult, studies have noted that following GCSE, patients may experience a decrease in performance on intelligence quotient and subtle neuropsychometric tests.[39] Development of an epileptic focus (epilepsy) is more likely in patients who have experienced GCSE.[1,32,39] Additionally, these patients are less likely to experience remission of their epilepsy.[1,32,39]

Age,[14] seizure duration,[4] and severe preexisting brain disease[42] are related to SE-induced morbidity. In a study of 239 children with a 60-minute duration of GCSE, 67% of survivors had sequelae of epilepsy, mental retardation, or neurologic deficits.[14] Conversely, another study reported neurologic deficits in only 9.1% of patients with a 30-minute duration of GCSE.[16] Both studies found that the younger the child, the greater the chance of sequelae.[14,16] The mean duration of GCSE in patients who did not have neurologic sequelae was 1.5 hours compared to 10 hours in patients with neurologic sequelae.[4] Both human and animal studies support the premise that seizures exceeding 60 minutes can cause neuronal damage. Finally, morbidity may also be higher in patients with preexisting epilepsy.[16]

MORTALITY

The mortality from GCSE depends on the etiology, time from onset of SE to initiation of treatment, seizure duration, and patient age.[8] Using mortality data from the Richmond study, one would project the U.S. mortality rate to be between 22,000 and 42,000 individuals per year.[10] The decreasing mortality rate for SE probably reflects a change in the definition of GCSE (60 to 30 minutes), recognition of the need to initiate presequenced therapy immediately, and a greater understanding of the pathogenesis.

Table 53–2 summaries the etiology and corresponding mortality rates for GCSE.[8,10] Interestingly, the mortality associated with many etiologies was significantly greater in adults than children. Patients may die from SE, but more frequently they die as a result of the acute illness that precipitated the attack.[5] For example, patients with serious central nervous system (CNS) structural changes (hemorrhage, stroke) have a poor prognosis, while 80% to 90% of patients with no structural lesions generally respond to IV phenytoin.[5] Clearly, the longer the duration of GCSE, the worse the prognosis. GCSE lasting longer than 60 minutes has a higher mortality (32%) than SE lasting less than 60 minutes (2.5%).[8] In one study, the mean duration of GCSE in patients who died was 13 hours.[4]

Recent estimates suggest a 2.5% to 10% mortality rate in children,[10,43] a 14% to 30% rate in adults,[6,10] and a 38% rate in the elderly.[10] Seizures in the neonatal period are associated with higher mortality and neurologic sequelae (mental retardation, cerebral palsy, epilepsy).[44] The best predictors of outcome were a 5-minute Apgar score below 7, the need for resuscitation during the first 5 minutes after birth, early onset of seizures, seizures lasting longer than 30 minutes, and the number of days on which seizures occurred.[44] DeLorenzo and associates reported that race had an effect on mortality, but that gender exerted no influence.[8] Conversely, others have noted no effect of race.[45] There was also no difference in mortality between community hospitals and major medical centers.[8]

CLINICAL PRESENTATION AND DIAGNOSIS

Most generalized tonic–clonic seizures are self-limiting and stop within 5 to 7 minutes. Diagnosis includes observation, physical examination, laboratory assessment, EEG, and neurologic imaging. A careful history of the nature and duration of the seizure should be obtained.[46]

Physical examination should assess language, motor, sensory, and reflex abnormalities. A diagnosis of GCSE should not be made until a trained clinician has observed at least one generalized tonic–clonic seizure in a patient with a history of repeated seizures and impaired consciousness. For NCSE, the diagnosis should not be made until 30 minutes of continuous seizure activity has been observed.[47] For patients without a previous history of NCSE, an EEG is required for diagnosis.

Clinical features of NCSE may vary. Approximately 20% of patients may present mildly obtunded. Marked clouding occurs in two-thirds of patients, and marked lethargy and somnolence with pronounced eyes-open unresponsiveness and waxy rigidity occurs in 15% of patients.[11] Language disturbance (mutism, paucity of speech) and inappropriate behavior (agitation, aggressiveness, hallucinations, emotional liability) can occur.[11] Motor features may include minor eyelid, face, and limb twitching.[11] It should also be remembered that patients with NCSE and patients with GCSE who are comatose or who have been given neuromuscular blockers may not have clinical SE but may continue to have electrical SE.[48]

Laboratory tests are important in the diagnosis of various etiologies. Hypoglycemia, hyponatremia (< 120 mEq/L), hypernatremia, hypomagnesemia, hypocalcemia, and renal failure can all cause seizures. Although hypomagnesemia in alcoholics is often cited as an etiology, its importance is probably overstated. A urine drug screen should be obtained in all patients to rule out the possibility of illicit drug use, drug overdose, or drug withdrawal. It is also necessary to determine serum AED concentration(s) in a patient on chronic anticonvulsants, because loading doses may or may not require adjustment. Likewise, high concentrations of AED can induce seizures, and low or nondetectable levels may reflect noncompliance or rapid withdrawal of anticonvulsants. Assessment of parameters (albumin, renal function, hepatic function) affecting anticonvulsant dosing may also be useful.

A second phase of diagnostic tests is conducted after the seizures have stopped. It is important to determine if the patient is febrile or has a systemic or CNS infection. Many physiologic consequences of SE (e.g., leukocytosis, pleocytosis, and hyperthermia) produce symptoms that may be confused with other conditions such as infections. If a CNS infection is suspected, empiric antibiotics should be started and a spinal tap should be obtained once the patient is stable.

Electroencephalography is a valuable diagnostic tool, but treatment should not be delayed while awaiting results. Patients who do not awaken after clinical control of their seizures should have an EEG performed to rule out NCSE or recurrent subclinical seizures. NCSE patients frequently have abnormalities that begin in one area of the cortex and produce waxing and waning rhythmic activity in one or several brain regions. A trial of benzodiazepines, with concurrent EEG assessment, may be necessary to make a diagnosis of NCSE. Most patients with GCSE have organized discharges that start over the entire cortex simultaneously. Postictal slowing or depressed amplitude may help determine a focal cause of seizures.

In order to rule out vascular, neoplastic, or infectious etiologies, computed tomography (CT) or magnetic resonance imaging (MRI) should be performed in any patient with new-onset seizures. Although MRI is preferred, the use of ancillary technologies (e.g, infusion pumps) may preclude this test. The CT scan is generally adequate and can be done in emergency situations.

If the patient is refractory to treatment, one must consider pseudoseizures. Clinical features of pseudoseizures include resistance to passive eye opening, persistence of a positive conjunctival reflex, downgoing plantar reflexes, and the occurrence of repeated, apparently generalized seizures without cyanosis.[49]

▶ TREATMENT: Status Epilepticus

Although a diagnosis of SE technically cannot be made until seizure activity has persisted for greater than 30 minutes, therapy should not be withheld waiting for this period to pass. Any tonic–clonic seizure that does not automatically stop within 10 minutes should be treated during the diagnostic workup. Anytime doubt exists regarding the diagnosis, the patient should be treated as if they had SE.[5] Additionally, any person experiencing more than three major seizures within 24 hours may be at risk to progress to SE and should be aggressively treated.[40] An algorithm of the choice of anticonvulsants, timing, and dosing for the treatment of GCSE in hospitalized patients is shown in Figure 53–3. Occasionally, patients with a history of frequent prolonged seizures may receive acute treatment at home. For example, rectal diazepam and intramuscular midazolam are easily administered and are rapidly effective.[50,51] However, repeated doses can lead to serious cardiorespiratory complications and are generally discouraged in the home environment.

■ DESIRED OUTCOME

It is imperative that a clear, presequenced management plan be rapidly initiated. There are four immediate goals in the management of SE. The first is patient stabilization and includes adequate oxygenation, preservation of cardiorespiratory function, and management of systemic complications. The second goal is correct diagnosis of the subtype of SE and identification of precipitating factors. Correct diagnosis prevents a delay in initiation of effective therapy and avoids the administration of large doses of unnecessary medications. The third and primary goal is to stop clinical and electrical seizure activity as soon as possible. The final goal is to prevent seizure recurrence.

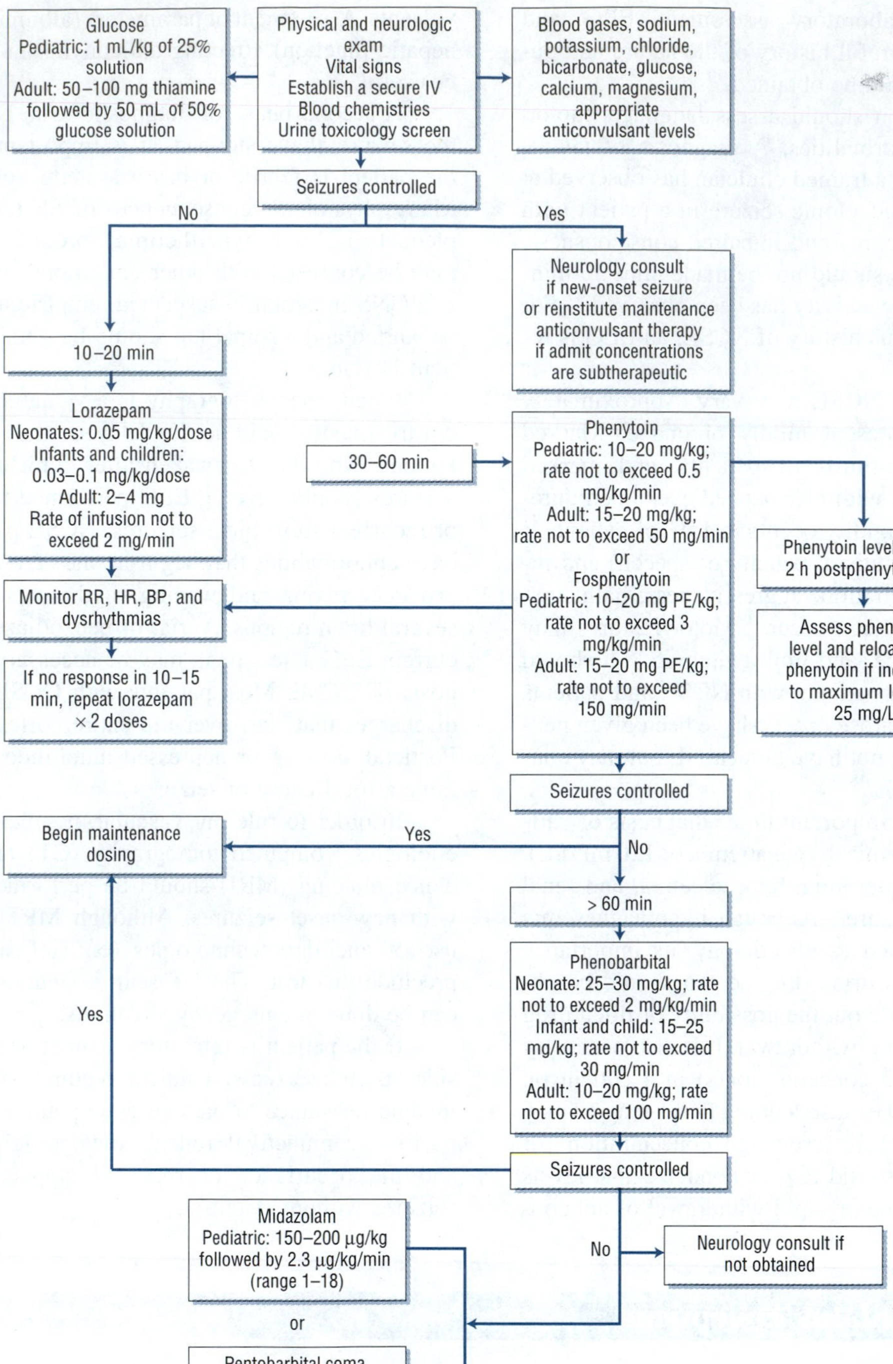

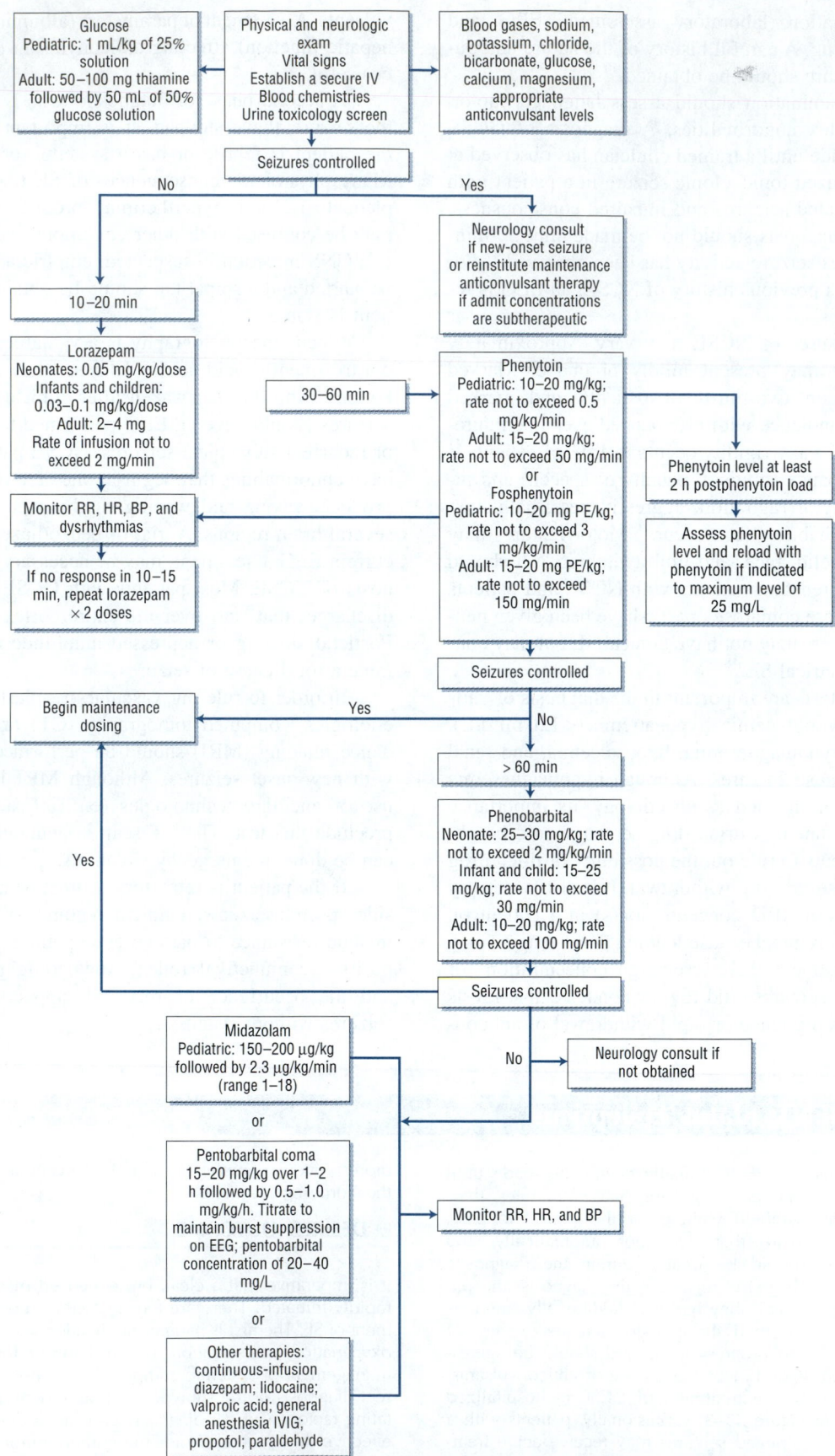

FIGURE 53–3. Algorithm for the management of GCSE.

NONPHARMACOLOGIC THERAPY

Concurrent with initiation of AEDs, vital signs should be assessed, and an adequate airway with ventilation should be established and maintained. The patient should be positioned to protect the airway from aspiration, and oxygen should be administered. If the patient is experiencing poor air exchange, he or she should be intubated and mechanically ventilated and controlled, using arterial blood gas determinations. A short-acting neuromuscular blocker may be required to facilitate intubation; however, it may mask the clinical symptoms of SE but not the electrical activity. EEG monitoring may be necessary in patients on neuromuscular blockers. Because hyperpyrexia can occur following prolonged SE, temperatures should be frequently monitored. If fever occurs, a source of infection should be sought and antipyretics given. Antipyretics are usually not effective in SE-induced hyperthermia, and a cooling blanket may be required.[6]

Several anticonvulsants can cause tissue damage upon extravasation; therefore, a secure IV line should be placed, and an infusion of normal saline should be started. Because all patients have some degree of cerebral edema, overhydration should be avoided.[43] Because cerebral perfusion is dependent on blood pressure, it is imperative that normal to high-normal blood pressure be maintained. Benzodiazepines, phenytoin, fosphenytoin, and phenobarbital can cause hypotension[5]; however, it can generally be controlled by slowing the rate of infusion or by administering dopamine.

Although hypoglycemia is a rare cause of SE, all patients should receive glucose. Wernicke's encephalopathy can develop in alcoholics; hence, thiamine (100 mg) should be given prior to glucose in adults.[43] Initially, adults should receive 50 mL of a 50% solution, and children should be given 2 mL/kg of a 25% solution.[43] Serum glucose should be determined to assess the need for further glucose supplementation.

Most patients who have been seizing for prolonged periods will develop metabolic and/or respiratory acidosis. For this reason, an arterial blood gas should be obtained to determine pH, PaO_2, $PaCO_2$, and HCO_3. Metabolic acidosis quickly resolves following termination of SE; however, if the pH is below 7.2 secondary to a metabolic acidosis, sodium bicarbonate should be given. Persistent metabolic acidosis can be treated with 0.5 to 1 mEq/kg[52] or 50 mEq of sodium bicarbonate to pediatric or adult patients, respectively. If the patient has respiratory acidosis, assisted ventilation should correct the imbalance.

PHARMACOLOGIC THERAPY

The three most commonly used classes of anticonvulsants for the treatment of GCSE are the benzodiazepines, phenytoin/fosphenytoin, and barbiturates. It should be noted that only five prospective, randomized studies have compared therapies for GCSE.[53–57] The first two studies were a blinded comparison of lorazepam versus diazepam in adults[53] and children.[55] The third study was a randomized comparison of phenobarbital to phenytoin plus diazepam.[56] The fourth study compared lorazepam to phenytoin.[54] The fifth study was a multicenter prospective, randomized, double-blind comparison of phenytoin, diazepam followed by phenytoin, lorazepam, or phenobarbital.[57] Therefore, Figure 53–3 is a compilation of the results of limited studies,[53–57] a report of an advisory committee,[43] and clinical observations of the authors.

GENERAL CONVULSIVE STATUS EPILEPTICUS

Benzodiazepines

The benzodiazepines are very effective in the initial treatment of SE and should be administered to patients who are actively seizing as soon as possible. If seizures have stopped, a benzodiazepine is not indicated and a longer-acting anticonvulsant should be given.[43] Generally, one or two doses of an IV benzodiazepine will stop seizures within minutes.[55,58] Treiman reported lasting control of SE with benzodiazepines in 79% of 1455 patients from 47 clinical trials.[59] Diazepam, lorazepam, and midazolam are the only benzodiazepines available in the United States in a parenteral dosage form. Because these are equally effective in GCSE,[53,59,60] the preferred benzodiazepine is determined by differences in the drugs' pharmacokinetic and pharmacoeconomic profiles.

Diazepam is an extremely lipophilic drug with a large volume of distribution (1 to 2 L/kg).[43] Following a single IV dose, 58% of adults had cessation of seizures by a median time of 2 minutes (range, immediate to 10 minutes),[53] and 65% of children had cessation of seizures by a mean time of 26 seconds (range, 20 to 51 seconds).[55] Although its initial distribution phase into the brain is extremely quick (10 seconds), it rapidly redistributes into body fat.[5] This causes its half-life in the brain to be less than 1 hour and results in an extremely short duration of effect (0.25 to 0.5 hours).[43] This rapid fall in concentration may result in seizure recurrence if diazepam is the sole anticonvulsant. For this reason, a longer-acting anticonvulsant (phenytoin, phenobarbital) should be given immediately after diazepam. The recommended initial diazepam dose in neonates, infants and children, and adults is 0.15 to 0.75 mg/kg, 0.1 to 0.5 mg/kg, and 0.15 to 0.25 mg/kg, respectively.[43,61] If the patient does not respond within 5 minutes, the dose should be repeated.[43] The maximum total dosage is 5 mg in children under age 5 years,[62] 10 mg in children 5 years or older,[62] and 40 mg in adults.[2] Although plasma concentrations of 0.2 and 0.8 mg/L have been associated with seizure control,[5] assays are not readily available; hence, therapeutic drug monitoring is impractical.

Although lorazepam is not approved by the Food and Drug Administration (FDA) for SE, it is currently the benzodiazepine of choice.[43,58] In fact, Treiman and associates reported that lorazepam was as effective in overt SE as diazepam plus phenytoin.[57] Lorazepam is less lipid soluble and takes slightly longer to reach peak levels in the brain than diazepam. Following a single IV dose, 78% of adults had cessation of seizures by a median time of 3 minutes (range, immediate to 15 minutes),[53] and in 70% of children by a mean time of 29 seconds (range, 25 to 60 seconds).[55] Redistribution is minimal, leading to a longer duration of action (> 12 to 24 hours). Lorazepam also has a higher-affinity binding to the benzodiazepine receptor than diazepam.[43] For these reasons, significantly fewer patients treated with lorazepam require additional anticonvulsants for seizure termination.[55] Data suggest that a single dose produces serum concentrations above 200 ng/mL and provides seizure protection for 24 hours.[5] The dose of lorazepam is 0.05 to 0.5 mg/kg in pediatric patients and 0.1 mg/kg in adults.[43] If the seizure continues after 5 minutes, a second dose may be given.[43] If there is still no response after 5 minutes, a third (final) dose may be given. The maximum total dosage of lorazepam is 4 and 8 mg in pediatric patients and adults, respectively.[43] It should be remembered that patients chronically on benzodiazepines (such as Klonopin) may have developed tolerance; hence, they may require very large doses before response.

Midazolam is a water-soluble benzodiazepine that diffuses rapidly into the CNS. However, it has an extremely short half-life (0.8 hours), which requires it to be given by continuous infusion. Its cost precludes its use as a first-line benzodiazepine in the hospitalized patient. Although not standard of practice, LeDuc and coworkers recommend intramuscular midazolam as first-line treatment in the out-of-hospital setting by emergency medical technicians.[51]

Diazepam and lorazepam cause vein irritation and should be diluted with an equal volume of compatible diluent before administration. Both diazepam and lorazepam contain propylene glycol, which may cause dysrhythmia and hypotension if administered too rapidly.[43] Therefore, the administration of diazepam and lorazepam should not exceed 5 mg/min and 2 mg/min, respectively.[63] If an IV line cannot be established, lorazepam or midazolam can be given IM, and diazepam can be given rectally.[64] Intramuscular administration of the benzodiazepines may result in delayed or inadequate peak concentrations. This is especially true for diazepam, which has a slow and erratic absorption following IM injection into the gluteal area.[5] For rectal administration, a Foley catheter is inserted rectally, the bulb is inflated, and the catheter is pulled back slightly. Diazepam (0.2 to 0.7 mg/kg) is mixed in an equal volume of saline, injected through the Foley catheter, and flushed with 5 to 10 mL of saline. Peak concentrations occur in 6 to 10 minutes in children and 10 to 20 minutes in adults.[5] Although a rectal diazepam gel (Diastat) has recently been approved by the FDA for a subset of patients with epilepsy, it is expensive.

All benzodiazepines can impair consciousness and interfere with neurologic assessment.[43] A brief period of cardiorespiratory depression (30 to 60 seconds) may occur in 12.5% of patients and can necessitate assisted ventilation or require intubation.[53] This is especially true if benzodiazepines are used concomitantly with barbiturates.[59] Hypotension secondary to a reduction in vasomotor tone may occur following high doses of benzodiazepines.[5]

Phenytoin

The hydantoins are the long-acting anticonvulsants of choice for GCSE.[65] Intravenous phenytoin is effective in terminating GCSE (40% to 91%),[43] has a relatively long half-life (20 to 36 hours),[66] and lacks significant CNS depression[43]; however, it cannot be delivered rapidly enough to be considered a first-line single agent. Treiman and colleagues reported that phenytoin alone was inferior to lorazepam, phenobarbital, or diazepam plus phenytoin at stopping overt SE within 20 minutes of infusion.[57] It takes longer to control seizures than the benzodiazepines, because it is less lipid soluble and enters the brain more slowly.[66] The distribution half-life of phenytoin is 2 to 5 minutes, and complete distribution occurs within 20 to 60 minutes.[66] Phenytoin is also associated with administration-related cardiovascular toxicity and is ineffective in some forms of NCSE.[34]

Although a variety of loading doses have been recommended, doses less than 18 mg/kg do not usually achieve and maintain serum concentrations in the therapeutic range for 24 hours.[34] Provided the patient has not been on phenytoin prior to admission, standard loading doses for adults are 15 to 20 mg/kg and for pediatric patients 20 mg/kg.[43] Reduced doses of 15 mg/kg are recommended for elderly patients.[43] The average volume of distribution of phenytoin in the adult and pediatric patient is 0.75 and 0.6 L/kg, respectively.[34] This means that an 18-mg/kg loading dose in an adult will result in serum concentration immediately after the end of the infusion of approximately 24 mg/L. Very obese patients will require larger loading doses than nonobese patients. In obese patients loading doses should be calculated on adjusted body weight:[67]

$$\text{weight (kg)} = \text{Ideal Body Weight (IBW)} + \frac{1.33\ (\text{weight} - \text{IBW})}{\text{IBW}}$$

If the patient has been on phenytoin prior to admission and the admission phenytoin concentration is known, the following equation can be used to calculate a loading dose:

$$LD_{ADULT} = (\text{Concentration}_{DESIRED} - \text{Concentration}_{ADMISSION}) \times 0.75\ \text{L/kg} \times \text{weight (kg)}$$

As mentioned earlier, phenytoin fully equilibrates into the brain within 20 to 60 minutes.[68] This delayed effect is the reason for waiting 60 minutes for response before administering a second partial loading dose. If seizures continue after the initial loading dose, some have recommended an additional loading dose of 5 mg/kg[40]; however, additional phenytoin may result in toxic serum concentrations and exacerbation of seizures. Additionally, there is no evidence that doses above 20 mg/kg will be of benefit in patients uncontrolled with the initial loading dose.[5] In order to maintain serum concentrations within the therapeutic range, maintenance dosing should be started within 12 to 24 hours of the loading dose. For a review of the distribution and elimination pharmacokinetics of phenytoin, see Chapter 52.

The complications associated with intravenous phenytoin are primarily related to the rate of administration and product pH. The vehicle (propylene glycol) may cause hypotension, especially in older patients with preexisting heart disease and in critically ill patients with marginal blood pressure.[43] Injectable phenytoin must be diluted to 5 mg/mL or less in normal saline. If it is mixed in a glucose-containing solution, microcrystals will precipitate. The maximum rate of infusion is 50 mg/min in adults[66] and 1 mg/kg per minute in children under 50 kg.[43] The rate of infusion should not exceed 25 mg/min in elderly patients or those with a history of atherosclerotic cardiovascular disease.[69] Vital signs and ECG should be obtained during administration and the rate slowed if hypotension develops, the QT interval widens, or arrhythmias develop.[43] In all patients, the rate should be reduced once seizures have stopped.[43] Phenytoin causes less respiratory depression and sedation than the benzodiazepines or phenobarbital.

Because phenytoin has a pH of approximately 13, its intravenous infusion is associated with discomfort. Catheter infiltration during an infusion can cause tissue necrosis. Intramuscular administration is not recommended because it produces extreme pain and may cause tissue necrosis. Crystallized phenytoin has also been found at the injection site for more than 24 hours.[5] Additionally, absorption following IM administration is delayed and erratic. Oral loading has been used in patients not actively seizing; however, 4 to 12 hours may be required before adequate blood concentrations are obtained.[65]

Fosphenytoin

Fosphenytoin is a water-soluble, phosphate ester of phenytoin that has no known pharmacologic activity prior to its conversion to phenytoin.[70] It is rapidly and completely converted to phenytoin after IV and IM dosing.[70] Reported fosphenytoin conversion half-lives following IV administration have ranged from 8 to 15 minutes.[71–73] This inherent delay in conversion to phenytoin was initially a major concern in the use of fosphenytoin for SE. However, protein binding for fosphenytoin is exceedingly high (unbound fraction 0.01 to 0.05) and is nonlinear.[74] Hence, fosphenytoin displaces phenytoin from albumin transiently increasing the unbound phenytoin concentration. This increase in the unbound concentration (the pharmacologically active form of phenytoin) offsets the delay in phenytoin formation from the prodrug, making it bioequivalent to phenytoin at 50 mg/min.[73] Following conversion of fosphenytoin to phenytoin, the fraction unbound and concentrations of unbound phenytoin return to baseline.

Limited studies of fosphenytoin in SE are available. Allen and colleagues reported an open-label study where 54 patients with GCSE received a single IV fosphenytoin loading dose of 18 mg phenytoin equivalents (PE)/kg.[75] Mean rate of administration was 121 mg PE/min (range, 36 to 218 mg PE/min). Benzodiazepine pretreatment was allowed as a standard of care for GCSE. Seizures were aborted in 93% of patients. In another study, 17 adult patients with acute seizures received IV doses of fosphenytoin, while 6 patients received IV phenytoin.[73] Adverse events required adjustment of the infusion rate in 4 of 6 phenytoin patients compared to 2 of 17 fosphenytoin patients. Pain or phlebitis at the injection site occurred in five patients receiving phenytoin compared to no patients receiving fosphenytoin. Complaints of transient, generalized itching and warmth occurred in 9 of 17 fosphenytoin patients. These findings are consistent with other clinical studies that have generally demonstrated that fosphenytoin is safe and significantly better tolerated than phenytoin when administered intravenously.[76,77]

The most frequently observed adverse events reported with parenteral fosphenytoin use are nystagmus, dizziness, and ataxia. These adverse events likely represent effects of the parent drug following conversion. Two side effects that occur more frequently with fosphenytoin than phenytoin are paresthesia and pruritus. These sensations typically have a distribution to the face and groin areas and are associated with dose and infusion rate. Dissipation of symptoms usually occurs within minutes to 1 hour postinfusion. These adverse events do not appear to be allergic reactions (no skin manifestations or vasodilatation) and alone do not warrant cessation of therapy.

In order to minimize dosing errors, all doses and dosing rates are determined using PE, thereby obviating the need for interconversion of doses between phenytoin sodium and fosphenytoin. Pediatric and adult patients with GCSE should receive fosphenytoin loading doses of 15 to 20 mg PE/kg. In adults, the rate of administration should be 100 to 150 mg PE/min. Pediatric patients should receive fosphenytoin at rate between 1 and 3 mg PE/kg per minute. Although efficacy and safety in children under 5 years of age have not been established, trials have been completed and should be available soon.

Patients being treated for GCSE should not be loaded with IM fosphenytoin except when IV access is impossible because of delays in achieving maximum phenytoin concentrations. Fosphenytoin should be diluted prior to IV administration in 5% dextrose or normal saline to a concentration of 1.5 to 25 mg PE/mL. Continuous ECG, blood pressure, and respiratory status monitoring is required for all loading doses of fosphenytoin. Fosphenytoin serum concentrations are not commercially available and are of no value in therapeutic drug monitoring. Serum phenytoin concentrations are the end point for therapeutic drug monitoring, and the desired concentration range in patients receiving fosphenytoin is the same as that for phenytoin (10 to 20 mg/L). Because fosphenytoin cross-reacts with several immunoassays for phenytoin to cause falsely elevated phenytoin concentrations, serum phenytoin concentrations should not be obtained for at least 2 hours or more following fosphenytoin dosing.[78]

Phenobarbital

There are three different opinions regarding the use of phenobarbital in GCSE. The most widely held contention is that because barbiturates cause CNS and respiratory depression, phenobarbital should be the third-line agent when benzodiazepines plus phenytoin have failed.[5] The second group contends that the barbiturates are as safe and effective as other anticonvulsants and argues that phenobarbital should be the initial drug of choice.[56] This belief is especially evident in pediatric institutions with large emergency departments. Clearly, the barbiturates continue to be the anticonvulsant of choice for neonatal seizures.[79] The third emerging opinion is that continuous-infusion midazolam should be the third-line anticonvulsant before the barbiturates.[9]

Two studies have compared the efficacy of phenobarbital to other anticonvulsants. Shaner and colleagues compared phenobarbital alone to diazepam plus phenytoin in adult patients with GCSE.[56] Phenobarbital acted more rapidly and was as safe and effective as the combination of diazepam plus phenytoin.[56] Likewise, Treiman and colleagues reported that phenobarbital was as effective as lorazepam alone, or diazepam plus phenytoin in overt SE and was not associated with serious adverse effects.[57]

Although no one is technically right or wrong, for the present time the Working Group on Status Epilepticus has recommended that phenobarbital be given after benzodiazepines and phenytoin have failed.[43] The results of the multicenter cooperative study should provide definitive support for the selection of an initial anticonvulsant in GCSE.[57] Currently, most would agree that phenobarbital is the long-acting anticonvulsant of choice in patients with a hypersensitivity to the hydantoins or in those with cardiac conduction abnormalities.

Although phenobarbital slowly penetrates into the brain,[66] the highest brain concentrations occur 5 to 15 minutes after an IV infusion.[80] On average, seizures are controlled within 5.5 minutes after initiating the loading dose.[56] Phenobarbital exhibits first-order linear pharmacokinetics, and there is no maximum dose beyond which further doses are likely to be ineffective.

Patients should be given a 20- to 25-mg/kg load of phenobarbital.[43,80] Higher loading doses (30 mg/kg) have been used in neonates without adverse effects.[79] Because the volume of distribution of the barbiturates is 1 L/kg, each mg/kg administered as a loading dose will increase the serum phenobarbital concentration by 1 mg/L.[40] Therefore, a 20-mg/kg loading dose should produce a serum phenobarbital concentration of approximately 20 mg/L. If the initial loading dose does not stop the seizures within 20 to 30 minutes, an additional 10- to 20-mg/kg dose may be given. If the seizures continue, a third 10-mg/kg load may be given.[81] In patients with refractory GCSE, some practitioners have advocated continued escalation of phenobarbital dosing without reference to a predetermined maximum concentration.[81] Once GCSE is controlled, the maintenance dose should be started within 12 to 24 hours.

Although injectable phenobarbital, like injectable phenytoin, contains propylene glycol, it can be given more rapidly than phenytoin. The rate of administration should not exceed 100 mg/min in adults[43] and 2 mg/kg/min[40] or 30 mg/min in pediatric patients.[66] Although phenobarbital can be given IM, its rate of absorption is too slow to be effective in GCSE.[5]

Phenobarbital may cause depression of consciousness and respiration. The risk of apnea and hypopnea may be more profound in patients initially treated with benzodiazepines.[43] Medical personnel should be ready to provide respiratory support whenever the two agents are used together. If significant hypotension develops, the infusion should be slowed or stopped.[43]

REFRACTORY GENERALIZED CONVULSIVE STATUS EPILEPTICUS

Approximately 10% to 15% of patients with overt GCSE will fail therapy with a benzodiazepine, phenytoin, and phenobarbital.[18] Likewise, about 30% of patients with subtle manifestations of GCSE remain in SE after administration of these anticonvulsants.[9] When adequate doses of a benzodiazepine, phenytoin, and phenobarbital have failed, the condition is termed refractory.[9] When a patient develops refractory GCSE, a neurologist with expertise in epilepsy should be consulted, and an intense search should be performed for an acute or progressive cause.[43]

It should be remembered that the longer GCSE lasts, the harder it is treat,[5,43] and that failure to aggressively treat early in the course of SE increases the likelihood of nonresponse.[43] The optimal therapeutic approach for patients with refractory GCSE has not been determined. Approaches used include the benzodiazepines, barbiturate coma, valproate, paraldehyde, propofol, lidocaine, and inhaled anesthetics. Regardless of therapy, the goal is to stop electrical epileptiform activity.

Benzodiazepines

Although refractory GCSE has been treated with a variety of agents, some practitioners have advocated that midazolam should not only be the first-line agent in refractory GCSE, but that it should be the third-line agent in patients unresponsive to lorazepam plus phenytoin.[9] Pediatric patients have been given a midazolam loading dose (0.15 mg/kg) followed by 2.3 μg/kg per minute (range, 1 to 18 μg/kg per minute). The maximum total dose was 1.81 mg (range, 1.78 to 2.02 mg), and seizures were controlled by a mean time of 0.78 hours.[82] Four adult patients were given a midazolam loading dose (0.2 mg/kg) and a continuous infusion of 0.75 to 11 μg/kg per minute for 8 hours to 10 days.[83] Clinical examination and scalp EEG documented termination of seizures in all patients within minutes. Because tachyphylaxis can develop, frequent increases in the infusion rate may be necessary and dosing should be guided by EEG response.[9] Hypotension and poikilothermia can occur and may require supportive therapies.[9] Once seizures are controlled, the midazolam infusion should be gradually discontinued. Bleck recommends that successful discontinuation is enhanced by keeping the patient's phenytoin serum concentration near 20 mg/L and phenobarbital concentration above 40 mg/L.[9]

Labar and colleagues treated nine episodes of refractory GCSE with high-dose intravenous lorazepam.[84] Doses ranged from 0.3 to 9 mg/h with as little as 2 mg/6 h to as much as 9 mg/h. Seizures were terminated in all patients, and lorazepam was slowly discontinued over 24 to 48 hours. Several reports have also noted that continuous-infusion diazepam can successfully control GCSE in patients unresponsive to phenytoin or phenobarbital.[85]

Barbiturate Coma

If there is an inadequate response to high doses of midazolam after 1 hour, anesthetizing the patient to suppress the cerebral ictal discharge is recommended.[9,43] Although it is likely that the patient is already being mechanically ventilated by this time, intubation and respiratory support may be required during barbiturate coma. Likewise, continuous monitoring of vital signs is essential because hypotension is a concern.

Barbiturate coma is usually achieved with either phenobarbital or pentobarbital. Crawford and colleagues reported the use of very high-dose phenobarbital in refractory GCSE.[81] Phenobarbital (10 mg/kg) was given every 30 minutes regardless of serum concentration until seizures stopped or hypotension occurred. Although very high-dose phenobarbital successfully stops refractory GCSE, the long half-life of phenobarbital (90 to 120 hours) produces coma for several days after the anticonvulsant is discontinued. Therefore, a short-acting barbiturate like pentobarbital ($t_{1/2}$ 11 to 23 hours), which allows rapid reversal of coma, is generally preferred.

Although several sources note that the initial loading dose of pentobarbital is 5 mg/kg,[43] this dose is incorrect because it will not produce the concentrations (20 to 40 mg/L) necessary to induce an isoelectric EEG. Pentobarbital should be initiated with a loading dose of at least 15 to 20 mg/kg over 40 to 60 minutes.[5] Should hypotension occur during the loading dose, the rate of administration should be slowed or dopamine should be administered. The loading dose should be immediately followed by an infusion of 0.5 to 3 mg/kg per hour,[43] which should be increased every 5 to 10 minutes until there is evidence of burst suppression on EEG (i.e., flat EEG) or adverse effects occur. Although the duration of barbiturate coma in most studies has been 2 to 3 days, pentobarbital coma has been safely used for 53 days in an 18-year-old.[86] In order to avoid complications (pneumonia, pulmonary edema), the pentobarbital should be discontinued as soon as possible. Twelve hours after a burst suppression pattern is obtained, the rate of pentobarbital infusion should be titrated downward every 2 to 4 hours to enable the clinician to determine if the patient's GCSE is in remission.

Valproate

Limited human data exist regarding the use of valproate in refractory GCSE. Holle and associates reviewed the literature regarding the use of valproic acid in SE.[87] Animal data suggest that even high-dose valproate is not effective because of its delayed access to the site of action.[87] Most of the experience with valproic acid in GCSE has been with the rectal route. Studies have reported that 200 mg every 6 hours or 600 to 4000 mg/d (average dose, 600 mg qid) as a rectal suppository terminated or reduced clinical SE.[87] Snead and Miles described a series of seven pediatric patients who had not responded to benzodiazepines, phenytoin, and phenobarbital.[88] Patients received a loading dose of 10 to 15 mg/kg given as a 1:1 dilution of tap water and valproate syrup enema. Five patients became seizure free within 3 to 12 hours. The Working Group on Status Epilepticus recommends a loading dose of 20 mg/kg.[43]

Although an intravenous dosage form of valproate has recently been approved by the FDA, it is not licensed for SE. Giroud and colleagues evaluated the use of IV valproic acid in 23 adults with SE.[89] Patients received a loading dose of 12 mg/kg followed by a continuous infusion of 0.5 mg/kg per hour; however, serum concentrations were lower than projected, and subsequent patients received a loading dose of 15 mg/kg followed by a continuous infusion of 1 mg/kg per hour. Seizures ceased in 11 of the 12 patients within 20 minutes, and partial status epilepticus ceased in less than 20 minutes in 8 of 11 cases.

Propofol

Propofol is extremely lipid soluble and has a high volume of distribution. It has a very rapid onset of action and an extremely short half-life (2 to 4 minutes), which promotes rapid awakening upon drug discontinuation. Although there are reports of its effectiveness in both GCSE and NCSE, it is not FDA licensed for these indications, and it has not been compared to other anticonvulsants. Patients have been given a 100 mg loading dose followed by continuous infusions ranging from 5 to 11.33 mg/kg per hour.[90,91] Infusion for up to 18 days has been reported.[90] Propofol does not have to be diluted. It may cause respiratory and cerebral depression, bradycardia, and metabolic acidosis. Seizures have also been reported.[92] Additionally, normal adult doses may provide over 1000 calories/d as lipid, and the cost to the patient may exceed $1000/d.

Lidocaine

Although lidocaine has been used in refractory GCSE,[93] its use is not recommended unless other agents have failed. It is administered intravenously and has a rapid onset of action (20 to 30 seconds). The recommended initial dose is 50 to 100 mg (1 to 3 mg/kg) over 2 minutes.[5,93] Because of the short half-life, a lidocaine infusion is initiated at a rate of 1.5 to 3.5 mg/kg per hour in adults or 6 mg/kg per hour in infants.[5,93] Although the therapeutic serum concentration range for the antiarrhythmic effects of lidocaine is 2 to 6 mg/L,[94] the therapeutic range for SE has not been established. Serum lidocaine concentrations should be monitored to avoid drug accumulation and toxicity. CNS toxicity (fasiculations, visual disturbances, tinnitus) may occur at concentrations between 6 and 8 mg/L; seizures and obtundation may develop when concentrations exceed 8 mg/L.[94]

Paraldehyde

Historically, rectal or IV paraldehyde has been used for refractory GCSE.[5,80] Although effective, it is extremely difficult to administer and is associated with serious adverse effects (e.g., hypotension, tachycardia, pulmonary edema, and polyethylene emboli). Intravenous paraldehyde is no longer manufactured in the United States. The only available formulation currently licensed is an enteral product that is difficult to obtain in a timely manner. A dose of 0.3 to 0.5 mL/kg can be given every 20 minutes rectally via a rubber catheter.[43] For rectal administration it should be diluted 1:1 in vegetable oil. Additional references should be consulted before using this product.[5,95,96]

Other Agents

A recent report noted excellent clinical and EEG results following rectal chloral hydrate administration (30 mg/kg) in five adult patients who were refractory to intravenous diazepam, phenytoin, phenobarbital, and valproate.[97]

Halothane, isoflurane, and other inhaled anesthetics have been reported to produce EEG suppression.[5,98] However, these gases are difficult to deliver outside the operating room and require the presence of an anesthesiologist. They have no proven advantages over traditional anticonvulsants (e.g., barbiturate coma or continuous-infusion benzodiazepines) and can raise intracranial pressure.[5] If used, dosing is titrated to obtain EEG burst suppression. Although there are no controlled trials, some have postulated that magnesium has anticonvulsant properties and may be neuroprotective by interacting with the NMDA receptor.[99] Additionally, magnesium deficiency lowers the seizure threshold.

NONCONVULSIVE STATUS EPILEPTICUS

Absence Status Epilepticus

Although absence SE is the most frequent type of nonconvulsive SE, only 3% of all patients with absence seizures develop SE.[7] The clinical manifestations of this disorder include an altered state of consciousness and/or behavior (lethargy, decreased mental function). In one series of 38 patients, the duration of absence SE ranged from 30 minutes to 2 days.[7] The longest reported episode of absence SE is 60 days.[41] The most important diagnostic and management tool in patients with suspected absence SE is an EEG, as absence SE will have a classic 3/s spike-and-slow-wave pattern.[7]

Although the likelihood of morbidity secondary to absence SE is not known, it is not considered life-threatening. Long-acting anticonvulsants (e.g., ethosuximide and clonazepam) are effective, but they are not available in a parenteral dosage form; hence, absence SE is treated with intravenous diazepam/lorazepam or rectal valproic acid. Studies with the intravenous valproic acid product have not been performed. Intravenous acetazolamide (250 to 500 mg) has been used to terminate absence SE; however, it is less effective than the benzodiazepines.[7] Intravenous phenytoin/fosphenytoin or phenobarbital may be tried in patients who do not respond to the other therapies.[7] Currently, general anesthesia or barbiturate coma are not appropriate.[7]

Atypical Absence and Myoclonic Status Epilepticus

Minor motor seizures are difficult to treat. Valproic acid remains the drug of choice for atypical absence. Refractory patients should be tried on a combination of valproic acid plus ethosuximide or clonazepam.[7] Generalized myoclonic SE is rare but may occur during absence or atypical SE. Again, valproic acid is the drug of first choice.[7]

Complex Partial Status Epilepticus

Complex partial SE occurs when a patient experiences clinical and electrical activity that is focal in onset and associated with altered consciousness. Although it is often difficult to differentiate complex partial SE from absence SE, there are some important differences. Unlike absence SE, which is associated with a single prolonged event, complex partial SE is a continuous series of repeated seizures. Additionally, patients with complex partial SE experience phases of total unresponsiveness with stereotypical automatisms, while individuals with absence SE do not. Complex partial SE should be treated aggressively because clinical and experimental data suggest that memory and behavioral alterations may be associated with this type of SE.[7] Management of complex partial SE is similar to that described for GCSE. Although the combination of IV lorazepam or diazepam plus phenytoin is effective, phenytoin alone may be more beneficial because it does not cause sedation.[7] Should the patient continue to experience complex partial SE, administration of phenobarbital is warranted.[7] It is essential that EEG monitoring be performed to evaluate response.

PHARMACOECONOMIC CONSIDERATIONS

Although no pharmacoeconomic studies have been performed in the area of SE, there are a variety of economic issues that may impact formulary considerations. Clearly there are intra- and interclass differences in medication cost and in ancillary tests or technologies associated with select therapies. For example, if one assumes five treatment options[57] and hypothetically initiates anticonvulsant therapy in a patient weighing 70 kg, the following differences in average wholesale prices are noted:

- Lorazepam alone (8 mg), $28.52
- Diazepam (20 mg) plus generic phenytoin (1 g), $13.46
- Phenobarbital (20 mg/kg) alone, $12.50
- Generic phenytoin (1 g) alone, $10
- Diazepam (20 mg) plus fosphenytoin (1 g), $129.46

Although many hospitals have heralded the arrival of fosphenytoin as an important therapeutic advancement, it has created a fiscal and ethical dilemma for many institutions. Fosphenytoin is associated with less infusion pain, IV site complications, and hemodynamic adverse effects than phenytoin; however, the cost of this agent ($126 versus $10/g) has caused many practitioners and administrators to struggle with the practical and ethical importance of the increased safety profile relative to the cost of the product to an institution. When evaluating the difference in cost of these two agents, it is important to remember that phenytoin requires the placement of two intravenous catheters because of its incompatibility with many solutions and medications that are given concurrently. Additionally, some institutions are giving fosphenytoin IM in the ER and avoiding the placement of a catheter and use of an infusion device. Likewise, many institutions do not consider the expense associated with a tissue infiltration of phenytoin. Should an infiltration of phenytoin cause tissue necrosis that necessitates plastic surgery or amputation, the expense of a single million-dollar law suit will likely offset the difference between phenytoin and fosphenytoin cost to several institutions.

If one advocates midazolam as third-line therapy over phenobarbital (20 mg/kg) and administers a loading dose of midazolam (0.15 mg/kg) followed by only a 1-hour continuous infusion (2.3 mg/kg per minute), midazolam will cost $345.78 more than phenobarbital. Conversely, one might argue that should a patient experience phenobarbital-induced respiratory depression and require mechanical ventilation, phenobarbital would be ultimately more expensive. Finally, a 24-hour infusion of propofol to the above patient will cost in excess of $1000.

EVALUATION OF THERAPEUTIC OUTCOMES

Initial success is defined as termination of all clinical and electrical activity, but ultimate success is measured by the patient's quality of life. The morbidity and mortality associated with SE is affected by the underlying etiology; however, these can be minimized by the rapid implementation of a rational therapeutic plan. An EEG is an extremely important tool that may allow the practitioner to not only determine when abnormal electrical activity has been aborted but may assist in determining which AED was effective. Because many of the AEDs affect the cardiorespiratory system, it is imperative that vital signs (e.g., HR, RR, BP) be monitored during drug infusion. It may also be necessary to monitor ECG in some patients. Finally, it is imperative that the infusion site be assessed for any evidence of infiltration before and during administration of phenytoin.

CONCLUSIONS

Our understanding of the cellular basis, physiology, and neuropathology of SE continues to evolve. Over the past decade, research into an activated cascade of pathophysiologic changes in neurotransmission, GABAergic inhibition, and NMDA receptor channel-mediated events has significantly enhanced our understanding of SE. Although anticonvulsants will continue to be the mainstay of therapy in terminating SE, specific agents including antagonists of excitatory amino acid neurotransmitters (glutamate and calcium channel blockers) and agonists of inhibitory neurotransmitters (GABA) may help to block neuronal damage. Likewise, additional trials investigating the role of newer anticonvulsants in SE are warranted.

▶ PRINCIPLES OF PHARMACOTHERAPY

- Status epilepticus is a neurologic emergency that may be associated with brain damage and death.
- For practical purposes, SE is defined as recurrent seizures without an intervening period of consciousness before the next seizure begins or any seizure lasting longer than 30 minutes whether or not consciousness is impaired.
- Although a diagnosis of SE does not officially occur until seizure activity has persisted for greater than 30 minutes, anticonvulsant therapy should not be withheld waiting for this period to pass. Any tonic–clonic seizure that does not automatically stop within 10 minutes should be treated.
- Although the pathophysiology of SE is unknown, experimental models have shown that there is a loss of GABA-mediated inhibitory synaptic transmission and that glutamatergic excitatory synaptic transmission sustains SE.
- The first goal of treatment is patient stabilization and includes adequate oxygenation, preservation of cardiorespiratory function, and management of systemic complications.
- The primary goal of therapy is to stop all clinical and electrical seizure activity as soon as possible.
- Because of its rapid onset and long duration of action, lorazepam is the benzodiazepine of choice in SE.
- Currently, the hydantoins (phenytoin or fosphenytoin) are the long-acting anticonvulsants of choice. One of these should be given concurrently with benzodiazepines.
- The maximum rate of infusion for phenytoin is 50 mg/min in adults and 1 mg/kg per minute in pediatric patients. The maximum rate of infusion should not exceed 25 mg/min in elderly patients or those with a history of atherosclerotic cardiovascular disease. The maximum rate of infusion for fosphenytoin in adults and pediatric patients is 150 mg PE/min and 3 mg PE/kg per minute, respectively.
- Phenobarbital may cause hypotension or respiratory depression and arrest, especially if given in conjunction with the benzodiazepines.

REFERENCES

1. Hauser WA. Status epilepticus: Epidemiologic considerations. Neurology 1990;40:S9–S13.
2. Shorvon S. Tonic clonic status epilepticus. J Neurol Neurosurg Psychiatry 1993;56:125–134.
3. Commission on Classification of Terminology, International League Against Epilepsy. Proposal for revised clinical and electroencephalographic classification of epileptic seizures. Epilepsia 1981;22: 489–501.
4. Delgado-Escueta AV, Wasterlain CG, Trieman DM, Porter RJ. Management of status epilepticus. N Engl J Med 1982;306:1337–1340.
5. Ramsey RE. Treatment of status epilepticus. Epilepsia 1993;34: S71–S81.
6. Treiman DM. Generalized convulsive status epilepticus in the adult. Epilepsia 1993;34:S2–S11.
7. Cascino GD. Nonconvulsive status epilepticus in adults and children. Epilepsia 1993;34:S21–S28.
8. DeLorenzo RJ, Towne AR, Pellock JM, Ko D. Status epilepticus in children, adults, and the elderly. Epilepsia 1992;33:S15–S25.
9. Bleck TP. Advances in the management of refractory status epilepticus. Crit Care Med 1993;21:955–957.
10. DeLorenzo RJ, Pellock JM, Towne AR, Boggs J. Epidemology of status epilepticus. J Clin Neurophysiol 1995;12:316–325.
11. Kaplan PW. Nonconvulsive status epilepticus. Semin Neurol 1996;16: 33–40.
12. Rowan AJ, Scott DF. Major status epilepticus. A series of 42 patients. Acta Neurol Scand 1970;46:573–584.
13. Gross-Tsur V, Shinnar S. Convulsive status epilepticus in children. Epilepsia 1993;34:S12–S20.
14. Aicardi J, Chevrie JJ. Convulsive status epilepticus in infants and children. A study of 239 cases. Epilepsia 1970;11:187–197.
15. Granner MA, Lee SI. Nonconvulsive SE: EEG analysis in a large series. Epilepsia 1994;34:42–47.

16. Maytal J, Shinnar S, Moshe SL,Alvarez LA. Low morbidity and mortality of status epilepticus in children. Pediatrics 1989;83:323–331.
17. Pellock JM. Status epilepticus. In: Dodson WE, Pellock JM, eds. Pediatric Epilepsy: Diagnosis and Therapy. New York, Demos, 1993: 197–206.
18. Lowenstein DH, Alldredge BK. Status epilepticus at an urban public hospital in the 1980s. Neurology 1993;43:483–488.
19. Barry E, Hauser WA. Status epilepticus and antiepileptic levels. Neurology 1994;44:47–50.
20. Brown JK, Hussian IHMI. Status epilepticus. 1. Pathogenesis. Dev Med Child Neurol 1991;33:3–17.
21. Verity CM, Ross EM, Golding J. Outcome of childhood status epilepticus and lengthy febrile convulsions: Findings of national cohort study. Br Med J 1993;307:225–228.
22. Maytal J, Shinnar S. Febrile status epilepticus. Pediatrics 1990;86: 611–616.
23. Callahan DJ, Noetzel MJ. Prolonged absence status epilepticus associated with carbamazepine therapy, increased intracranial pressure, and transient MRI abnormalities. Neurology 1992;42:2198–2201.
24. Thomas P, Lebrun C, Chatel M. De novo absence status epilepticus as a benzodiazepine withdrawal syndrome. Epilepsia 1993;34:355–358.
25. Ditcher MA, Ayala GF. Cellular mechanism of epilepsy: A status report. Science 1987;237:157–164.
26. Fountain NB, Lothman EW. Pathophysiology of status epilepticus. J Clin Neurophysiol 1995;12:326–342.
27. Kapur J, Stringer JL, Lothman EW. Evidence that repetitive seizures in the hipocampus causes a lasting reduction in GABAergic inhibition. J Neurophysiol 1989;61:417–426.
28. Meldrum BS. Anatomy, physiology, and pathology of epilepsy. Lancet 1990;336:231–234.
29. Johnston MV. Neurotransmitters and epilepsy. In: Wyllie E, ed. The Treatment of Epilepsy: Principles and Practice. Philadelphia, Lea & Febiger, 1993:111–125.
30. Lipton SA, Rosenberg PA. Excitatory amino acids as a final common pathway for neurologic disorders. N Engl J Med 1994;330:613–622.
31. Bertram EH, Lothman EW. NMDA receptor antagonists and limbic status epilepticus: a comparison with standard anticonvulsants. Epilepsy Res 1990;5:177–184.
32. Lothman E. The biochemical basis and pathophysiology of status epilepticus. Neurology 1990;40:13–23.
33. Kapur J, MacDonald RL. Status epilepticus: A proposed pathophysiology. In: Shorvon S, Dreifuss F, Fish S, Thomas D, eds. The Treatment of Epilepsy. Cambridge, MA, Blackwell Science, 1996: 258–268.
34. Leppik IE. Status epilepticus. The next decade. Neurology 1990; 40:4–9.
35. Walton NY. Systemic effects of generalized convulsive status epilepticus. Epilepsia 1993;34:S54–S58.
36. Wasterlain CG, Fujikawa DG, Penix L, Sankar R. Pathophysiological mechanisms of brain damage from status epilepticus. Epilepsia 1993; 34:S37–S53.
37. Meldrum BS, Nilsson B. Cerebral blood flow and metabolic rate early and late in prolonged epileptic seizures induced in rats by bicuculline. Brain 1976;99:523–542.
38. Liu Z, Gatt A, Mikati M, Holmes GL. Effect of temperature on kainic acid-induced seizures. Brain Res 1993;63:51–58.
39. Dodill CD, Wilensky AJ. Intellectual impairment as an outcome of status epilepticus. Neurology 1990;40:23–27.
40. Leppik IE. Status epilepticus. In: Wyllie E, ed. The Treatment of Epilepsy: Principles and Practice. Philadelphia, Lea & Febiger, 1993: 678–685.
41. Jagoda A. Nonconvulsive seizures. Emerg Med Clin North Am 1994;12:963–971.
42. Oxbury JM, Whitty CWM. Causes and consequences of status epilepticus in adults. A study of 86 cases. Brain 1971;94:733–744.
43. Working Group on Status Epilepticus. Treatment of convulsive status epilepticus: Recommendations of the Epilepsy Foundation of America's Working Group on Status Epilepticus. JAMA 1993;270: 854–859.
44. Gal P. Anticonvulsant therapy after neonatal seizures: How long should it continue? A case for early discontinuation of anticonvulsants. Pharmacotherapy 1985;5:268–273.
45. Towne AR, Pellock JM, Ko D, DeLorenzo RJ. Determinations of mortality in status epilepticus. Epilepsia 1994;35:27–34.
46. DeLorenzo RJ. Status epilepticus: Concepts in diagnosis and treatment. Semin Neurol 1990;10:396–405.
47. Treiman DM. General principles of treatment: Responsive and intractable status epilepticus in adults. In: Delgado-Escueta AV, Wasterlain CG, Treiman DM, Porter RJ, eds. Status Epilepticus. New York, Raven, 1983:377–384.
48. Munn RI, Farrell K. Failure to recognize status epilepticus in a paralyzed patient. Can J Neurosci 1993;20:234–236.
49. Howell SJL, Owen L, Chadwick DW. Pseudostatus epilepticus. Q J Med 1989;71:507–519.
50. Camfield CS, Camfield PR, Smith E, et al. Home use of rectal diazepam to prevent status epilepticus in children with convulsive disorders. J Child Neurol 1989;4:125–126.
51. LeDuc TJ, Goellner WE, Sanadi NE. Out-of hospital midazolam for status epilepticus. Ann Emerg Med 1996;28:3.
52. Standards and guidelines for cardiopulmonary resuscitation (CPR) and emergency cardiac care (ECC), 6. Pediatric advanced life support. JAMA 1992;268:2262–2275.
53. Leppik IE, Derivan AT, Homan RW, et al. Double-blind study of lorazepam and diazepam in status epilepticus. JAMA 1983;249: 1452–1454.
54. Treiman DM, De Giorgio CM, Ben-Menachem E, et al. Lorazepam versus phenytoin in the treatment of generalized convulsive status epilepticus: Report of an ongoing study. Neurology 1985; 35:284.
55. Appleton R, Sweeney A, Choonara I, et al. Lorazepam versus diazepam in the acute treatment of epileptic seizures and status epilepticus. Dev Med Child Neurol 1995;37:682–688.
56. Shaner DM, McCurdy SA, Herring MO, Gabor AJ. Treatment of status epilepticus: A prospective comparison of diazepam and phenytoin versus phenobarbital and optional phenytoin. Neurology 1988;38: 202–207.
57. Treiman DM, Meyers PD, Walton NY, et al. A comparison of four treatments for generalized convulsive status epilepticus. Veterans Affairs Status Epilepticus Cooperative Study Group. N Engl J Med 1998;339: 792–798.
58. Treiman DM. The role of benzodiazepines in the management of status epilepticus. Neurology 1990;40:32–42.
59. Treiman DM. Pharmacokinetics and clinical use of benzodiazepines in the management of status epilepticus. Epilepsia 1989;30: S4–S10.
60. Giang DW, McBride MC. Lorazepam versus diazepam for the treatment of status epilepticus. Pediatr Neurol 1988;4:358–361.
61. Johnson KB, ed. The Harriet Lane Handbook, 13th ed. Chicago, Year Book, 1993.
62. Diazepam. In: Physicians' Desk Reference, 51st ed. Oradell, NJ, Medical Economics, 1997:2334–2337.
63. Cascino GD. Generalized convulsive status epilepticus. Mayo Clin Proc 1996;71:787–792.
64. Albano A, Reisdorff EJ, Wiegenstein JG. Rectal diazepam in pediatric status epilepticus. Am J Emerg Med 1989;70:168–172.
65. Cloyd JC, Gumnit RJ, McLain W. Status epilepticus. The role of intravenous phenytoin. JAMA 1980;244:1479–1481.
66. Browne TR. The pharmacokinetics of agents used to treat status epilepticus. Neurology 1990;40:28–32.
67. Abernethy DR, Greenblatt DJ. Phenytoin disposition in obesity. Determination of loading dose. Arch Neurol 1985;42:468–471.
68. Wilder BJ, Ramsey E, Willmore J, et al. Efficacy of intravenous phenytoin in the treatment of status epilepticus: Kinetics of central nervous system penetration. Ann Neurol 1977;1:511–518.

69. Donovan PJ. Phenytoin administration by constant intravenous infusion: Selective rates of administration. Ann Emerg Med 1991;20: 139–142.
70. Boucher BA. Fosphenytoin: A novel phenytoin prodrug. Pharmacotherapy 1996;16:777–791.
71. Boucher BA, Bombassaro AM, Rasmussen SN, et al. Phenytoin prodrug 3-phosphoyloxymethyl phenytoin (ACC-9653): Pharmacokinetics following intravenous and intramuscular administration. J Pharm Sci 1989;78:929–932.
72. Eldon MA, Loewen GR, Voightman, et al. Pharmacokinetics and tolerance of fosphenytoin and phenytoin administered intravenously to healthy subjects. Can J Neurol Sci 1993;20:S180.
73. Andrews CO, Turnbull MD, Paloucek FP, et al. Safety and pharmacokinetics of fosphenytoin following intravenous loading dose administration. Pharmacotherapy 1994;14:367.
74. Hussey EK, Dukes GE, Messenheimer JA, et al. Protein binding of phenytoin and a phenytoin prodrug. Pharm Res 1988;5:S214.
75. Allen FH, Runge JW, Legarda S, et al. Safety, tolerance, and pharmacokinetics of intravenous fosphenytoin (Cerebyx) in status epilepticus. Epilepsia 1995;36:S90.
76. Jamerson BD, Dukes GE, Brouwer KLR, et al. Venous irritation related to intravenous administration of phenytoin versus fosphenytoin. Pharmacotherapy 1994;14:47–52.
77. Ramsay RE, Philbrook B, Fischer JH, et al. Safety and pharmacokinetics of fosphenytoin (Cerebyx) compared with dilantin following rapid intravenous administration. Neurology 1996;46:A245.
78. Kugler AR, Olson SC, Webb CL, et al. Cross-reactivity of fosphenytoin (Cerebyx) in two human phenytoin immunoassays. Pharm Res 1994;11:S102.
79. Donn SM, Grasela TH, Goldstein GW. Safety of a higher loading dose of phenobarbital in the term newborn. Pediatrics 1985;75:1061–1064.
80. Ramsey RE. Pharmacokinetics and clinical use of parenteral phenytoin, phenobarbital, and paraldehyde. Epilepsia 1989;30:S1–S3.
81. Crawford TO, Mitchell WG, Fishman LS, Snodgrass SR. Very-high-dose phenobarbital for refractory status epilepticus in children. Neurology 1988;38:1035–1040.
82. Rivera R, Segnini M, Baltodano A, Perez V. Midazolam in the treatment of status epilepticus in children. Crit Care Med 1993;21: 991–994.
83. Parent JM, Lowenstein DH. Treatment of refractory generalized status epilepticus with continuous infusion of midazolam. Neurology 1994;44:1837–1840.
84. Labar DR, Ali A, Root J. High-dose intravenous lorazepam for the treatment of refractory status epilepticus. Neurology 1994;44: 1400–1403.
85. Bell HE, Bertino JS Jr. Constant diazepam infusion in the treatment of continuous seizure activity. Drug Intell Clin Pharm 1984;18:965–970.
86. Mirski MA, Williams MA, Hanlet DF. Prolonged pentobarbital and phenobarbital coma for refractory generalized status epilepticus. Crit Care Med 1995;23:400–404.
87. Holle LM, Gidal BE, Collins DM. Valproate in status epilepticus. Ann Pharmacother 1995;29:1042–1043.
88. Sneed OC, Miles MV. Treatment of status epilepticus in children with rectal sodium valporate. J Pediatr 1985;106:323–325.
89. Giroud M, Gras D, Escousse A, et al. Use of injectable valproic acid in status epilepticus. Drug Invest 1993;5:154–159.
90. Wood PR, Browne GPR, Pugh S. Propofol infusion for the treatment of status epilepticus. Lancet 1988;1:480–481.
91. Pitt-Miller PL, Elcock BJ, Maharaj M. The management of status epilepticus with a continuous propofol infusion. Anesth Analg 1994;78:1193–1194.
92. Makela JP, Iivanainen M, Pieninkeroinen, et al. Seizures associated with propofol anesthesia. Epilepsia 1993;34:832–835.
93. Aggarwal P, Wali JP. Lidocaine in refractory status epilepticus: A forgotten drug in the emergency department. Am J Emerg Med 1993;2: 243–244.
94. Pieper JA, Johnson KE. Lidocaine. In: Evans WE, Schentag JJ, Jusko WJ, eds. Applied Pharmacokinetics, 3rd ed. Spokane, Applied Therapeutics, 1992:21-1-21-37.
95. Curless RG, Holzman BM, Ramsay RE. Paradehyde therapy in childhood status epilepticus. Arch Neurol 1983;40:477–480.
96. Giacoia GP, Gessner PK, Zaleska MM, Boutwell WC. Pharmacokinetics of paraldehyde disposition in the neonate. J Pediatr 1984;104: 291–296.
97. Lampl Y, Eshel Y, Gilad R, Sarova-Ponchas I. Chloral hydrate in intractable status epilepticus. Ann Emerg Med 1990;19:674–676.
98. Meeke RI, Soifer BE, Gelb AW. Isoflurane for the refractory management of status epilepticus. Drug Intell Clin Pharm 1989;23:579–581.
99. Dimple HL. Drugs in status epilepticus. Anaesthesia 1995;50: 824–825.

54

Acute Management of the Head Injury Patient

Bradley A. Boucher, PharmD, BCPS, FCCP, and Stephanie J. Phelps, PharmD, FCCP

An increasing level of interest in neurotrauma has been largely spurred by greater understanding of the pathophysiology of severe head injury and a belief that outcome can be improved through usage of evidence-based management guidelines and administration of neuroprotective agents. This chapter will attempt to capture the level of excitement within this rapidly evolving field by summarizing current understanding of central nervous system (CNS) trauma and highlighting recently developed guidelines for managing the severe head injury patient.

EPIDEMIOLOGY

The 1985 to 1987 National Health Information Survey indicated that nearly 2 million persons sustain a head injury annually in the United States, resulting in 373,000 hospital admissions and 75,000 deaths.[1] Nonetheless, the mortality rate following traumatic brain injury has decreased from nearly 25 to below 20 per 100,000 population per year since 1979.[2] Motor vehicle accidents account for approximately 50% of all adult cases, while falls, assaults, gunshot wounds, sports and recreational accidents, and other miscellaneous causes account for the remaining cases.[3] Most head trauma occurs in early adulthood in persons who are free of medical problems; peak age for acute neurotrauma is 15 to 24 years.[3] Productivity losses secondary to trauma exceed that of heart disease, stroke, and cancer combined.[4] For 1985, it was estimated that the lifetime costs of head trauma in the United States exceeded $64 billion.[4]

PATHOPHYSIOLOGY

PRIMARY HEAD INJURY

The neurologic sequelae of head trauma can occur instantaneously as a consequence of the primary injury or can result from secondary injuries that follow within minutes, hours, or days. Primary injury involves the external transfer of kinetic energy to various structural components of the head (including nerve cells, nerve synapses, supporting cells of the brain such as glial cells, and cerebral blood vessels).[5] The biomechanical forces responsible for primary head injury can be broadly classified as concussive/compressive (blunt object blow, penetrating missile injuries) and acceleration/deceleration (instantaneous head movements following motor vehicle accidents). Primary injuries are further categorized as focal or diffuse.[5] The latter are usually associated with shearing forces, which affect axons within the brain.

SECONDARY BRAIN INJURY

A complex sequence of pathophysiologic events precipitated by primary head injury may seriously disrupt the normal CNS balance between oxygen supply and demand.[6] The end result of this imbalance is cerebral ischemia, the key pathophysiologic event triggering secondary injury. Figure 54–1 is a simplified schematic of the processes that constitute secondary brain injury and their various interrelationships. Readers are referred to a recent review by Luer and associates[7] and the cited reference chapters in the textbook, *Neurotrauma,* for a more detailed discussion of these complex events. The brain is particularly susceptible to ischemia because of its normally high resting energy requirement and its limited capacity to store oxygen, glucose, and high-energy phosphate compounds such as adenosine triphosphate (ATP).[6] Study of ischemia following head injury has documented that it is typically an early event that occurs less than 6 hours after the insult.[8] Patients studied after this 6-hour window frequently have hyperemia ("luxury perfusion"). This latter phenomenon is the result of an uncoupling of oxygen delivery (CDO_2) and consumption ($CMRO_2$) in the brain, a process that is closely autoregulated under normal circumstances.[6] Factors that can diminish cerebral oxygen supply following head injury include cerebral edema, expanding mass lesions (e.g., epidural, subdural, and intracerebral hematomas), cerebral vasospasm, and loss of vasoregulatory control.[6] Hypoxia can further exacerbate local decreases in cerebral oxygen supply following acute respiratory failure and systemic hypotension. Metabolic demand can also increase following neurotrauma secondary to seizures, agitation, and temperature elevation.

Brain tissue affected by focal ischemia has a dense core surrounded by a marginally viable region referred to as the ischemic penumbra.[9] Cells in this area are electrically silent and unable to perform normal neurologic functions. If adequate cerebral blood flow (CBF) is restored, the affected tissue may recover; however, sustained ischemia can result in further loss of cellular integrity and eventual cell death. The loss of ionic homeostasis is postulated to be a key event in fostering secondary brain injury within the ischemic penumbra. Cellular influx of sodium, chloride, and

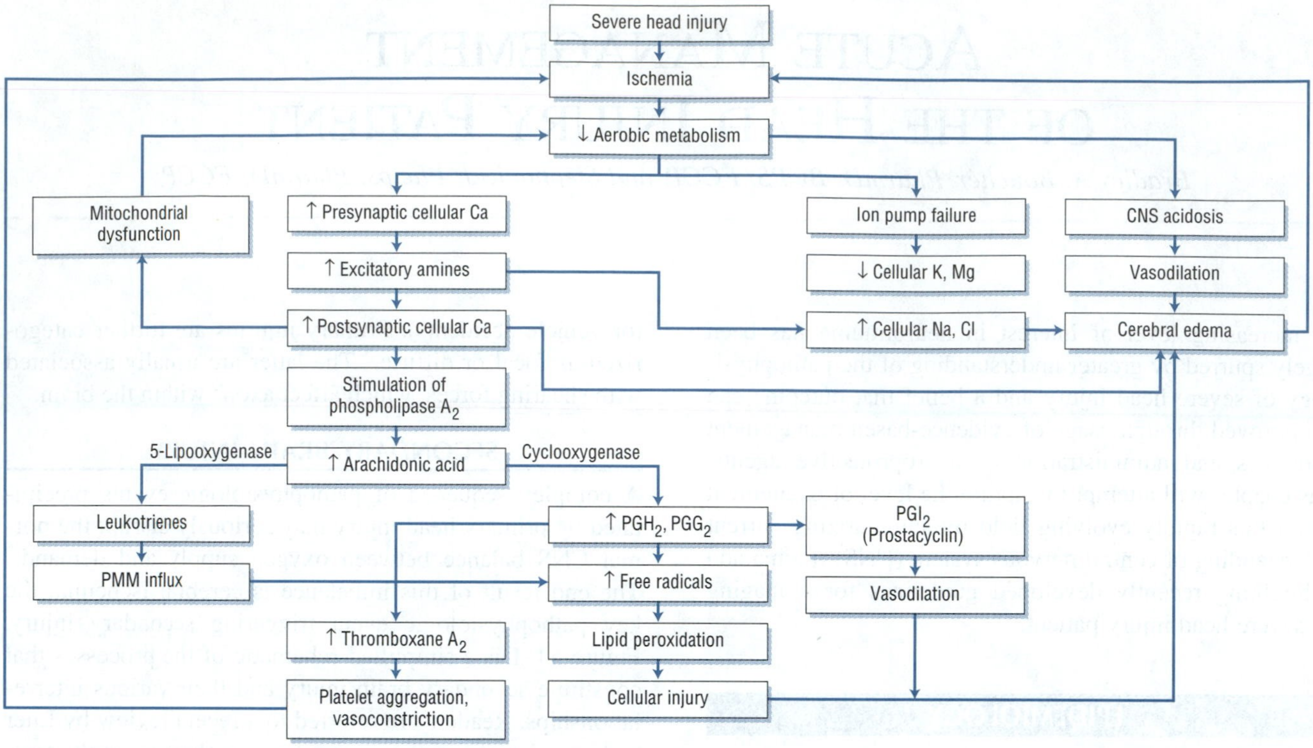

FIGURE 54–1. Schematic illustration of the cascade of events proposed to occur following severe neurotrauma (secondary brain injury).

water with a corresponding efflux of potassium and magnesium begins with Na^+/K^+-ATPase pump dysfunction.[6] An influx of calcium into the presynaptic terminal ends of damaged neurons is mediated by N-type voltage-sensitive calcium channels. This in turn stimulates excessive release of the excitatory amines, glutamate, and aspartate from the affected neurons.[7,10] Influx of calcium and additional sodium is stimulated by activation of the *N*-methyl-D-aspartate (NMDA) receptor.

Calcium influx and its intracellular accumulation initiate a number of events that amplify and perpetuate secondary neuronal injury. High intracellular concentrations of calcium result in mitochondrial dysfunction, which further inhibits cellular respiration, a process already affected by ischemic and/or hypoxic insults.[11] A second major deleterious effect of calcium is to stimulate activation of proteases and phosphatases including calpains, phospholipase A_2, 5-lipooxygenase, and cyclooxygenase.[11,12] The effect of phospholipase A_2 stimulation includes formation of several arachidonic acid metabolites derived from membrane lipids: thromboxane A_2, prostaglandin G_2 (PGG_2), prostaglandin H_2 (PGH_2), prostaglandin I_2 (PGI_2; prostacyclin), and leukotrienes. The subsequent effects of these metabolites include platelet aggregation, vasodilation, vasoconstriction, and lipid peroxidation. A byproduct of lipid peroxidation is the formation of oxygen free radical species.[13] Lipid peroxidation is an especially damaging event, because the formation of oxygen free radicals can propagate itself, resulting in further cellular membrane damage unless quenched by endogenous antioxidants (e.g., vitamin E, ascorbic acid, and superoxide dismutase).[13] Cell-mediated injury involving inflammatory mediators (e.g., cytokines and platelet-activating factor), nitric oxide, and cell adhesion molecules is yet another possible mechanism involved in secondary neuronal injury.[14] Among the cell lines implicated are polymorphonuclear neutrophils, platelets, endothelial cells, and macrophages.

Additionally, vasogenic cerebral edema can develop as a consequence of cerebral capillary endothelial damage.[6] With cytotoxic and vasogenic edema follows the expansion of the intracellular and extracellular fluid spaces, respectively. Elevated intracranial pressure (ICP) is the most detrimental consequence of cerebral edema formation and occurs as the brain tissue volume increases within the nondistensible skull. A significant increase in ICP may further compromise CBF and extend cytotoxic edema. Hence, an increase in ICP can be self-perpetuating unless this cycle is reversed.

CLINICAL PRESENTATION

An initial neurologic examination is essential for assessing the extent of brain injury and establishing a baseline for future comparison. The level of consciousness on admission ranges from awake and alert to completely unresponsive. The Glasgow Coma Scale (GCS) is the most widely used system to grade the arousal and functional capacity of the cerebral cortex.[15] The GCS defines the level of conscious-

TABLE 54–1. Glasgow Coma Scale

	Response	Score
Eyes	Open spontaneously	4
	To verbal command	3
	To pain	2
	No response	1
Best motor response		
To verbal command	Obeys	6
To painful stimulus (pressure to nailbeds)	Localizes pain	5
	Flexion–withdrawal	4
	Flexion–abnormal (decorticate rigidity)	3
	Extension (decerebrate rigidity)	2
	No response	1
Best verbal response (arouse patient with painful stimulus if necessary)	Oriented and converses	5
	Disoriented and converses	4
	Inappropriate words	3
	Incomprehensible sounds	2
	No response	1
TOTAL		3–15

ness according to eye opening, motor response, and verbal response (Table 54–1). A GCS of 15 corresponds to a normal neurologic examination. A GCS of 3 to 8, 9 to 12, and 13 to 14 is consistent with severe, moderate, and minor head injury, respectively.[16] The possibility should always be considered of ethanol or drug intoxication, hypotension, hypoxia, postictal state, or hypothermia altering the neurologic examination. Because narcotics and muscle relaxants affect the neurologic examination, they should not be administered until the initial examination is complete. Significant posttraumatic amnesia (> 1 hour), increasing dizziness, a moderate to severe headache, limb weakness or paresthesia, cerebral spinal fluid otorrhea or rhinorrhea, and seizures indicate more severe injury.[17] A rapid deterioration in mental status strongly suggests the presence of an expanding lesion within the skull. Computed tomography (CT) of the head is an important diagnostic tool for detecting the presence of mass lesions. Poor prognostic signs of survival include advanced age, postresuscitation GCS below 5, uncontrolled ICP elevation, hypotension, and the presence of flaccidity, decerebrate posturing, or fixed dilated pupils.[18,19]

In addition to a profoundly abnormal neurologic examination, patients with severe head injury also may have significant alterations or instability in their vital signs including abnormal breathing patterns (apnea, Cheyne-Stokes respiration, tachypnea), hypotension, or bradycardia. Hypotension and/or hypoxia, although observed in the majority of patients, usually occurs as a result of blood loss, spinal cord injury (e.g., neurogenic shock), impaired cardiac function, or compromised ventilation.[17] After stabilization of vital signs, a thorough physical examination should be performed in order to identify injuries that may contribute to secondary brain injury. For example, airway obstruction and aspiration may compromise pulmonary gas exchange, chest trauma may affect both pulmonary and cardiac function (e.g., rib fractures, tension pneumothorax, cardiac tamponade), and substantial blood loss from intra-abdominal or vascular injuries may decrease the blood's oxygen-carrying capacity. Initial and follow-up laboratory tests should include serum electrolytes, blood glucose, complete blood count (CBC), arterial blood gases (ABG), blood ethanol level (EtOH), and urine drug screen.[17]

▶ TREATMENT: Head Injury

In July 1995, the Brain Trauma Foundation (BTF) published an extensive document entitled *Guidelines for the Management of Severe Head Injury* as a joint initiative with the Guidelines Committee of the American Association of Neurological Surgeons (AANS) and the Joint Section on Neurotrauma and Critical Care of the AANS and the Congress of Neurologic Surgeons.[20] This landmark publication established for the first time a comprehensive series of evidence-based standards, guidelines, and options for the care of the severe head injury patient. Recommendations from this document will be highlighted through the rest of this chapter. Until clinical study results are published that are at variance with the BTF guidelines, their recommendation should serve as the foundation on which all clinical decisions in managing severe head injury are based.

DESIRED OUTCOME

The overall goal in head injury management is not reduction in mortality but rather optimization of long-term, functional outcome for these patients. This requires careful attention to the following short-term therapeutic goals: (1) establishment of an adequate airway, and maintenance of breathing and circulation during the initial period of evaluation; (2) maintenance of balance between CDO_2 and $CMRO_2$; (3) prevention or attenuation of secondary neuronal injury; and (4) prevention and/or treatment of associated medical complications.

INITIAL RESUSCITATION

The first priority in the unconscious patient is the establishment of an airway which ensures adequate oxygenation and prevents aspiration. Thereafter, restoring and maintaining systemic blood pressure to a mean arterial pressure (MAP) of at least 90 mm Hg is of utmost importance. Correcting and preventing early hypotension (systolic BP < 90 mm Hg) and hypoxia (PaO_2 < 60 mm Hg) is essential, because these two factors are among the most powerful predictors of outcome.[21] Isotonic saline (0.9% normal saline [NS]) remains the most commonly used and least expensive resuscitation fluid. Nonetheless, recent attention has focused on the use of hypertonic saline solutions with or without colloids.[22–25] Until a distinct advantage of these latter fluids or agents is demonstrated, it is recommended that the more economical isotonic saline continue to be used. Vasopressors and inotropic agents may be needed to maintain an adequate MAP if hypotension persists after adequate restoration of intravascular volume. Figure 54–2 gives an algorithm summarizing treatment priorities in the initial management of acute head injury.

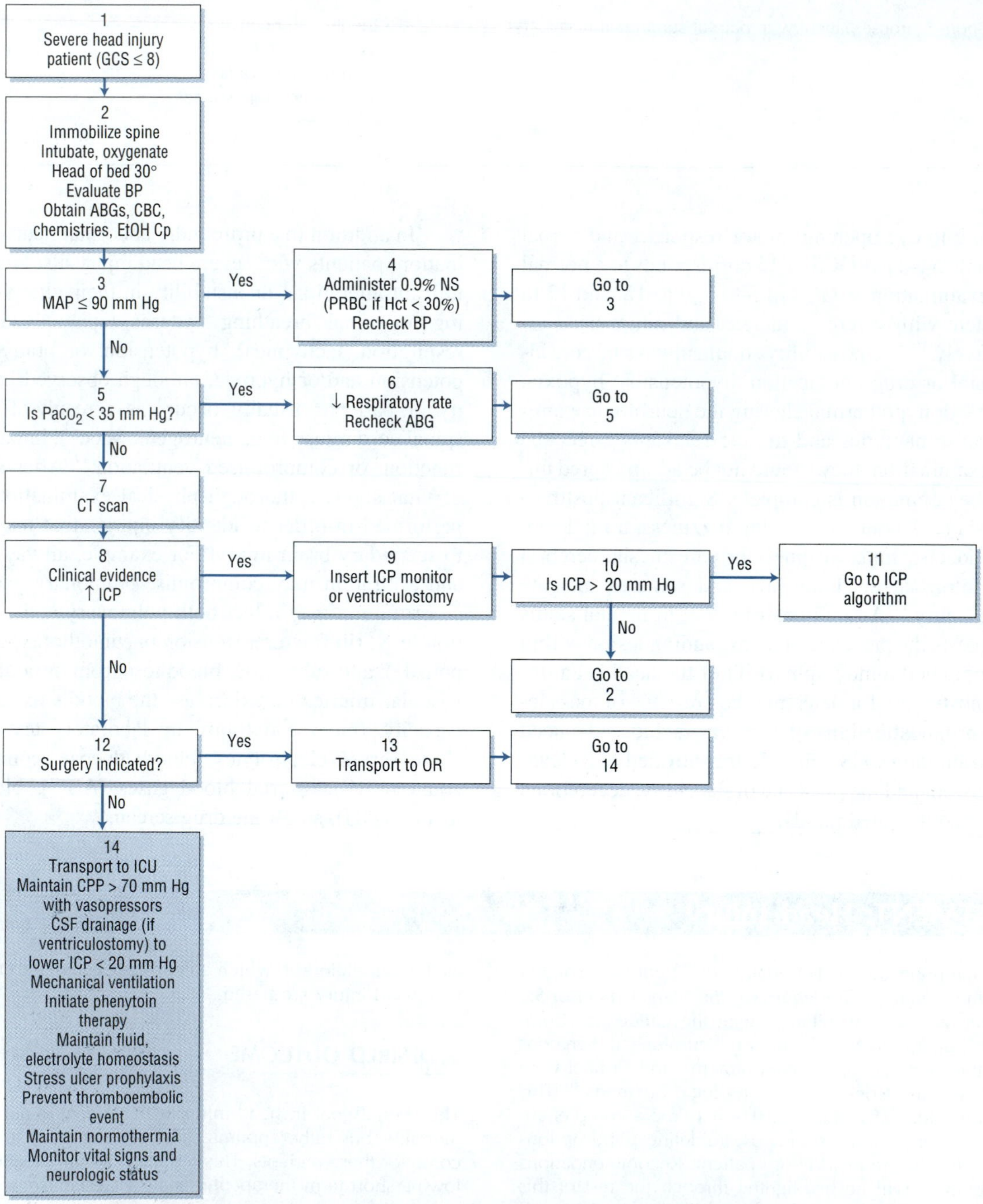

FIGURE 54–2. Algorithm for acute management of the head injury patient. *(Modified from Boucher BA. Neurotrauma. Pharmacotherapy Self-assessment Program, 3rd ed. Module 2 (Critical Care). Kansas City, MO, American College of Clinical Pharmacy, 1995:215–238.)*

POSTRESUSCITATIVE CARE

Following successful resuscitation, priorities shift toward diagnostic evaluation of intracranial and extracranial injuries, and emergent surgical intervention as needed. Approximately 40% of patients with severe head injury have an intracranial mass. Evacuation of intracranial hematomas (i.e., epidural, subdural, and intracerebral hematomas), elevation of depressed skull fractures, and debridement of penetrating wound tracts are essential to control intracranial pressure (ICP) and improve outcome. Continuous ICP monitor placement (ventricular catheter; parenchymal fiber-optic catheter; subarachnoid, subdural, epidural monitors) is indicated in patients with a GCS of 8 or less with an abnormal admission CT scan or in high-risk severe head injury patients with a normal CT scan (age > 40 years, motor posturing, systolic blood pressure < 90 mm Hg).[20] A ventricular catheter has a therapeutic advantage over the other alternatives because cerebrospinal fluid can be drained using this device as a means to lower intracranial pressure. Continuous ICP monitoring is the most important means to objectively evaluate the success of therapies used to decrease ICP. Normal ICP ranges from 0 to 10 mm Hg; once ICP exceeds 20 to 25 mm Hg, therapy should be initiated to decrease ICP below this range.[20]

The principal monitoring parameter for severe head injury patients within the intensive care environment is cerebral perfusion pressure (CPP), which is the difference between MAP and ICP (CPP = MAP − ICP). The CPP is essentially the pressure gradient driving CBF. Therefore, maintenance of an acceptable CPP is critical in reducing cerebral ischemia and secondary injury. Because a number of studies have demonstrated decreased morbidity and mortality in patients when CPP was actively sustained above 70 to 80 mm Hg,[26–30] the BTF guidelines recommend that CPP be maintained above 70 mm Hg.[20] A CPP above 70 mm Hg can be accomplished by increasing MAP to the target level or by lowering elevated ICP.

The MAP can be increased through normalization of the intravascular volume combined with pharmacologically inducing systemic hypertension as needed. The goal of volume expansion should be euvolemia and avoidance of a hypoosmolar state. If the hematocrit is below 30%, transfusion of packed red blood cells is indicated. Volume status should be targeted to a central venous pressure of 5 to 10 mm Hg or a pulmonary artery wedge pressure between 10 and 14 mm Hg.[16] After achievement of euvolemia, the patient's head should be elevated at 30° to promote venous drainage and decrease ICP. If restoration of the intravascular volume is inadequate in elevating MAP to an acceptable level, hypertension should be induced using vasopressors or inotropic support. Although concern has been raised as to the potential for induced hypertension to increase ICP, studies have shown that this does not occur in most patients and that ICP may actually fall.[31,32] The drugs most commonly employed to induce hypertension are the sympathomimetic amines, dopamine, norepinephrine, and phenylephrine. Although none of these agents have shown superiority, norepinephrine is a reasonable selection at a starting dose of 0.02 µg/kg/min.[16] Patients should be monitored for renal dysfunction, lactic acidosis, and signs of peripheral ischemia when these agents are used, especially at high doses.

TREATMENT OF INTRACRANIAL HYPERTENSION

NONPHARMACOLOGIC THERAPY

HYPERVENTILATION

The practice of aggressive hyperventilation (Pa_{CO_2} 25 to 30 mm Hg) to decrease ICP is no longer recommended.[20] Hyperventilation acutely decreases systemic and cerebral P_{CO_2}. The resultant hypocapnia in turn induces cerebral vasoconstriction, thereby decreasing CBF and cerebral blood volume (CBV). For decades, it was a widely held belief that this reduction in CBV and any accompanying decrease in ICP was beneficial. However, recent studies have determined that severe head injury patients with normocapnia versus those receiving aggressive hyperventilation have an improved outcome at 3 and 6 months.[19,20] Therefore, BTF guidelines recommend that Pa_{CO_2} be maintained near 35 mm Hg, especially during the first 24 hours.[20] Thereafter, a Pa_{CO_2} in the range of 30 to 35 mm Hg may be used if ICP control is inadequate.[16]

HYPOTHERMIA

Recent interest in the use of hypothermia as a cerebral protective maneuver has been fueled by the results of several preliminary studies demonstrating trends in improvement in mortality and morbidity rates in severe head injury patients randomized to receive mild to moderate hypothermia.[29,30,33,34] The mechanism underlying this protection is likely multifactorial, although one possibility is that hypothermia reduces CMR_{O_2} in these patients. Although hypothermia can produce shivering that may increase ICP, neuromuscular blockade with controlled ventilation prevents shivering in patients unresponsive to chlorpromazine (5 to 25 mg IM every 8 hours). At present, hypothermia should be considered to be an investigational treatment and reserved for patients refractory to all other forms of therapy.

GENERAL PHARMACOLOGIC THERAPY

Pain, agitation, excessive muscle movement, and resisting mechanical ventilation can cause transient increases in ICP.[33] As such, use of analgesics, sedatives, and paralytics, has an important primary role in the management of intracranial hypertension (Fig. 54–3). Nonetheless, there have been no studies of the effect of sedation on outcome in patients with severe head injury.[20] Morphine sulfate is the most commonly used analgesic and sedative in this setting.[35,36] Alternative sedatives include short-acting benzodiazepines (e.g., midazolam), especially if there is a reasonable suspicion of alcohol withdrawal as the underlying etiology of the agitation; as well as propofol, etomidate, and intermittent low-dose pentobarbital.[35,36] The potential for the latter agents to decrease MAP and CPP must be closely monitored.[37] The use of any sedative agent must also be weighed against their potential to obscure the neurologic examination of the patient. Cautious reversal of the effect of benzodiazepines with flumazenil can be used to allow examination of the patient.[36] Interference with the neurologic examination is also associated with paralytic agents. Prophylactic neuromuscular blockade (unrelated to ICP control) is not recommended based on a study indicating increased complications and length of stay following paralytic use.[38] Hyperthermia should also be avoided, because patients with elevated temperatures have a poorer outcome than normothermic patients.[39] Hence, maintenance of a core temperature below 37.5°C using acetaminophen and cooling blankets is indicated for patients following severe neurotrauma.[16]

SPECIFIC PHARMACOLOGIC THERAPY

DIURETICS

Although a variety of osmotic diuretics (e.g., urea, glycerol) can be used to decrease ICP, mannitol is unquestionably the most widely employed.[40] Despite the common practice of administering mannitol to patients with suspected or actual increase in ICP following head injury, no clinical trial comparing its effects to

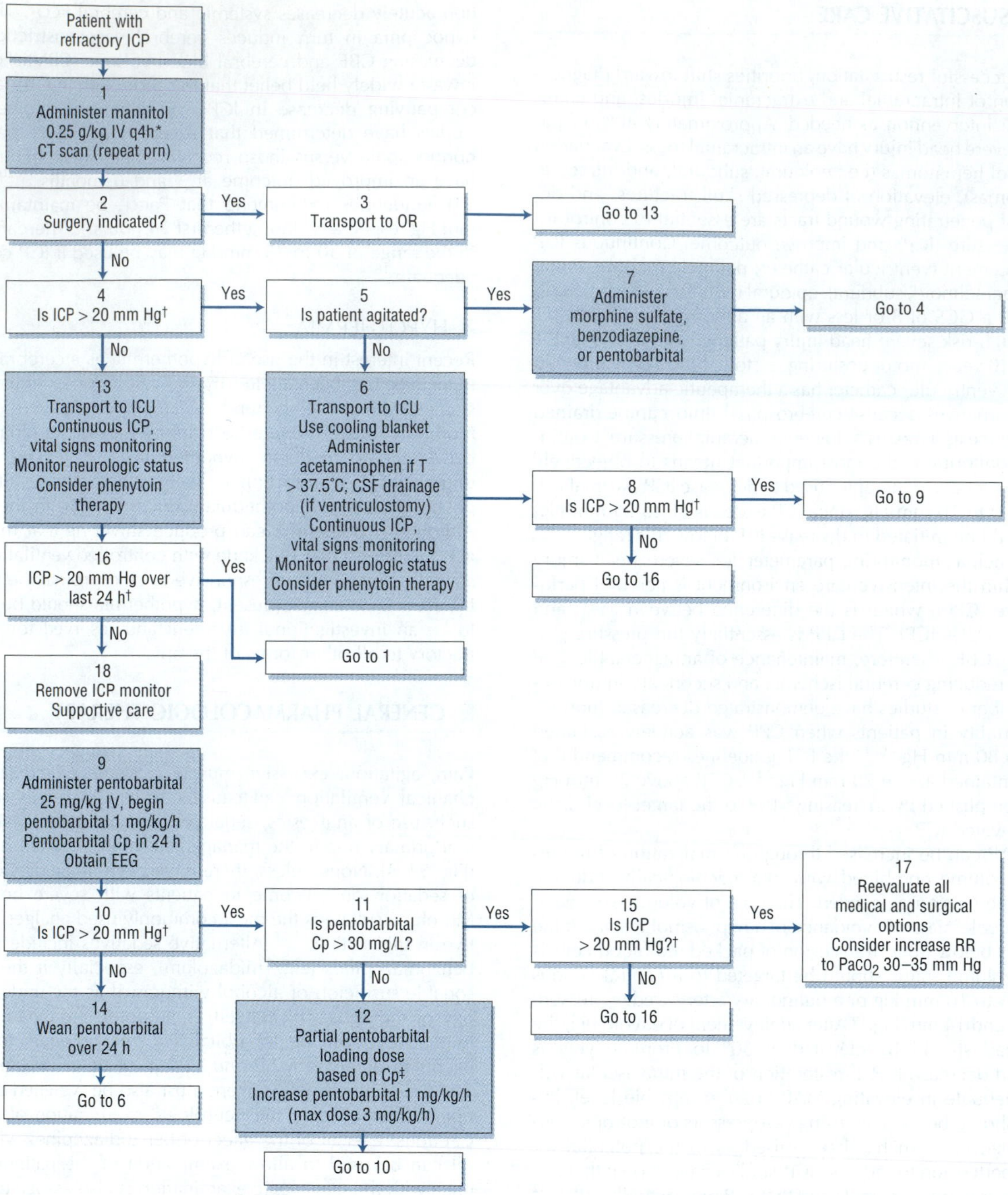

* Hold if serum osmolality > 320 mOsm/kg

† Treatment thresholds: ICP 20–29 mm Hg for > 15 min
ICP 30–39 mm Hg for > 2 min
ICP ≥ 40 mm Hg for > 1 min

Note:
Transient increases may occur following respiratory procedures: (e.g., suctioning, chest physiotherapy, bronchoscopy, intubation).

‡ Partial pentobarbital loading dose (mg) = (30 mg/L – measured Cp) (1 L/kg × wt(kg))

FIGURE 54–3. Algorithm for the management of intracranial pressure (ICP). *(Modified from Boucher BA. Neurotrauma. Pharmacotherapy Self-assessment Program, 3rd ed. Module 2 (Critical Care). Kansas City, MO, American College of Clinical Pharmacy, 1995:215–238.)*

placebo has been conducted.[20] The mechanisms responsible for mannitol's beneficial effects likely relate to (1) an immediate plasma-expanding effect that reduces blood viscosity and increases CBF, and (2) establishing an osmotic concentration gradient across an intact blood–brain barrier; as water diffuses from the brain into the intravascular compartment, ICP decreases.[20,41] If the blood–brain barrier is disrupted as a result of injury or "opened" with prolonged use of the osmotic agent, rebound elevations of ICP may occur as mannitol accumulates in the brain tissue, resulting in an increase in intracellular brain volume.[42]

Effective doses of mannitol range from 0.25 to 1.0 g/kg IV every 4 hours.[20] Increased ICP is reduced within minutes following mannitol administration, while the duration of action ranges from 90 minutes to 6 hours depending on the dose and the clinical conditions that are present.[20] In order to maximize benefit and minimize adverse events, mannitol should not be administered as a continuous infusion in this setting.[20] Monitoring and maintaining serum osmolality below 320 mOsm/kg is important relative to minimizing adverse events.[36] Intravenous furosemide (0.5 to 1 mg/kg) may be used in conjunction with mannitol in refractory cases.

Several adverse effects are associated with mannitol. In addition to hypotension resulting from its diuretic effect, a reversible acute renal dysfunction may occur in adults with previously normal renal function after long-term, high-dose administration, especially if serum osmolality exceeds 320 mOsm/kg.[20] Acute exacerbation of underlying congestive heart failure and pulmonary edema may also occur as a result of rapid intravascular volume expansion. Furosemide is recommended as an alternative diuretic for lowering ICP in these latter patient groups.

CORTICOSTERIODS

Although corticosteroids are effective in preventing or reducing cerebral edema in patients with structural brain damage (e.g., tumors), the majority of studies in patients with severe head injury have not demonstrated that they lower ICP or improve outcome.[20,43,44] In addition, use of corticosteroids following head injury has been associated with increased complications including gastrointestinal (GI) bleeding, glucose intolerance, electrolyte abnormalities, and infection.[16] As such, the BTF guidelines strongly recommend that corticosteroids not be used. This in effect ends the controversy over conventional corticosteroid use in severe head injury patients.

BARBITURATES

High-dose barbiturate therapy ("barbiturate coma") has been used for decades in the management of increased ICP based on the results of several published reports and randomized clinical trials demonstrating improved mortality in responders versus nonresponders.[45–48] This usage is now supported by the BTF guidelines, which recommend high-dose barbiturate therapy be considered in hemodynamically stable severe head injury patients refractory to maximal medical and surgical ICP-lowering therapy.[20] Prophylactic use of barbiturates is not advocated in light of insufficient evidence supporting this practice.[20] Several mechanisms responsible for the cerebral protective effects of barbiturates have been proposed. These include (1) lowering the regional $CMRO_2$ with a coupled reduction in CBF to these areas, (2) inhibition of lipid peroxidation, and (3) altering cerebral vascular tone.[34]

Prior to inducing a barbiturate coma, the severe head injury patient must be mechanically ventilated with continuous monitoring of arterial blood pressure, electrocardiogram, and ICP. Pentobarbital is the most commonly used barbiturate for this indication, although thiopental has also been used over the years. Pentobarbital should be administered as an IV loading infusion totaling 25 mg/kg (10 mg/kg over 30 minutes, then 5 mg/kg/h for 3 hours) followed by a initial maintenance infusion of 1 mg/kg/h.[48] The maintenance infusion can be titrated upward if needed to a maximum of 2 to 3 mg/kg/h.[34] If the systolic blood pressure falls during the loading or maintenance infusions, the rate may need to be slowed temporarily and blood pressure support initiated. The goal of a barbiturate coma is to maintain ICP and CPP at the previously discussed target thresholds in addition to achieving a pentobarbital steady-state concentration between 30 and 40 mg/L and electroencephalogram burst suppression.[20] Initiation of barbiturate therapy withdrawal can occur when ICP has been satisfactorily controlled for 24 to 48 hours.[36] Barbiturates should be tapered over 24 to 72 hours to prevent ICP spikes.

Side effects associated with high-dose barbiturate therapy involve primarily the cardiovascular system. Hypotension, caused by peripheral vasodilation, may occur and necessitate decreasing the barbiturate dose, or the administration of fluids and vasopressors to maintain blood pressure. Gastrointestinal effects of barbiturates include decreased GI muscular tone and decreased amplitude of contraction. On emergence from coma, there may be a period of GI hypermotility. Care should be taken to avoid extravasation of pentobarbital and thiopental solutions because severe tissue damage may occur. Barbiturates should be administered by continuous infusion through a central line dedicated to this purpose.

TREATMENT AND PROPHYLAXIS OF POSTTRAUMATIC SEIZURES

Seizures greatly increase $CMRO_2$. Therefore, it is generally agreed that patients who have experienced one or more seizures following a moderate to severe head injury should receive anticonvulsant therapy to avoid further increases in $CMRO_2$. Initial therapy in these persons should consist of incremental IV doses of diazepam (5 to 40 mg) or lorazepam (2 to 8 mg) to terminate any active seizure activity, followed by IV phenytoin to prevent seizure recurrence. The merits of preventive anticonvulsant therapy in patients who have not had a seizure postinjury has been historically more controversial. Risk factors for early posttraumatic seizures (< 7 days postinjury) include GCS below 10, cortical contusion, depressed skull fracture, subdural hematoma, epidural hematoma, intracerebral hematoma, penetrating head wound, or seizure within the first 24 hours of injury.[20] In a landmark randomized, placebo-controlled study, the incidence of early posttraumatic seizures in patients receiving placebo was 14.2%, compared to 3.6% in patients receiving phenytoin ($P < .05$).[49] Based on these findings and supporting data from other studies, it is recommended that phenytoin (or alternatively, carbamazepine) be used to prevent seizures in head injury patients at high risk within the first 7 days.[20] The benefits of prophylactic anticonvulsants beyond 7 days has not been demonstrated, and thus their use for this indication is not recommended.[20,49,50]

SUPPORTIVE CARE

Although maintaining an adequate CPP and normalizing ICP are the highest priorities in preventing secondary injury following severe neurotrauma, attention must also be given to preventing and/or treating systemic and extracranial complications. This includes careful ongoing fluid and electrolyte management.[51] Specific electrolyte disturbances that should be avoided include hyponatremia, hypomagnesemia, hypokalemia, and hypophosphatemia.[36] Aggressive nutritional support of the head injury patient is another important therapeutic consideration.[52] Infectious complications commonly encountered in severe head injury patients include nosocomial pneumonia, sepsis, urinary tract infections, meningitis, and brain abscesses. Treatment of these potentially devastating infections should be aggressive, with careful attention to antibiotic blood–brain barrier penetration for intracranial infections. Other important therapeutic interventions include correction of any documented coagulopathy, acute gastritis prophylaxis, prevention of thromboembolic events, and temperature control.

PHARMACOLOGIC THERAPY

INVESTIGATIONAL THERAPY

The steady decrease in morbidity and mortality following severe neurotrauma over the last 20 to 30 years can be largely attributed to expeditious and aggressive management of those events resulting in secondary injury (i.e., ischemia, hypoxia, increased ICP). Numerous neuroprotective agents are currently under investigation targeted at specific pathophysiologic processes, which may further enhance the prospects for a meaningful recovery in these patients. For each of these agents, close attention to dose, timing and sequencing of drug administration, duration of therapy relative to the traumatic event, and possibly combination therapy are issues that need to be carefully considered in ultimately maximizing their utility.

MODULATION OF CALCIUM INFLUX

Calcium Antagonists

The calcium antagonists are obvious candidates for attenuating the deleterious effects of calcium influx in acute neurotrauma patients. Nimodipine, a dihydropyridine, has been the most extensively studied among the calcium antagonists that block the postsynaptic L-type calcium channel. Unfortunately, two major trials of nimodipine in head injury patients did not demonstrate a statistically significant improvement in outcome compared to placebo.[53,54] A significant benefit was observed in the subgroup of patients with posttraumatic subarachnoid hemorrhage (SAH) receiving nimodipine, which was corroborated in a follow-up investigation.[55] Systemic hypotension is a relative limitation with the use of other L-type calcium channel antagonists in severe head injury patients.

Another target for calcium modulation is the presynaptic N-type voltage-sensitive calcium channels. Omega conotoxin is one such antagonist currently under clinical investigation for this indication.[56] Systemic hypotension is a significant concern with its use as well.

Glutamate Antagonists

A significant amount of experimental evidence has been accumulated confirming the efficacy of NMDA receptor antagonists in attenuating secondary injury events following model head injury. Based on these results, both competitive and noncompetitive NMDA receptor antagonists have been developed as neuroprotective agents. D-CPP-ene and CGS19755 (Selfotel) are investigational NMDA antagonists competing with glutamate at the receptor site (competitive antagonists). Noncompetitive NMDA antagonists or receptor channel blockers bind to the open NMDA receptor, thereby blocking the ionic current.[7] Compounds within this group include ketamine, phencyclidine, dextromethorphan, dextrorphan, and the investigational agents dizocilpine (MK-801), dexanabinol, and aptiganel (Cerestat).[7] Unfortunately, a phase III trial of aptiganel was recently discontinued based on limited benefit of the active treatment over placebo in the first 340 patients studied.

ANTIOXIDANTS

The potential role of oxygen free radicals in the pathophysiology of head injury has stimulated interest in the use of antioxidants to interrupt the self-perpetuating cycle of membrane destruction in these patients. Tirilazad (Freedox), a 21-aminosteroid, is one such antioxidant that has undergone phase III testing in head injury, stroke, and SAH patients. An attractive feature of this steroid analog is that although a potent inhibitor of lipid peroxidation, it is essentially devoid of glucocorticoid activity. Unfortunately, two major trials of tirilazad in head injury patients were unable to demonstrate efficacy compared to placebo.[7] An enzymatic free radical scavenger that has undergone clinical trials in severe head injury patients is superoxide dismutase conjugated to a polyethylene glycol polymer (PEG-SOD; pegorgotein, Dismutec). Although results of the preliminary phase II trial were promising, no statistically significant improvement in outcome or mortality was observed in the larger phase III trial in severe head injury patients receiving two doses of pegorgotein compared to placebo.[57,58]

OTHER TREATMENT STRATEGIES

Formation of inflammatory mediators including the metabolites of arachidonic acid have been implicated in the latter stages of tertiary injury following neurotrauma. As such, both cyclooxygenase inhibitors (e.g., nonsteroidal anti-inflammatory drugs) and mixed cyclooxygenase–lipooxygenase inhibitors (e.g., BW7544C) have been studied in experimental neurotrauma models with limited success. Inhibitors of inflammatory mediators are also under consideration as neuroprotective agents. These include antagonists to platelet-activating factor, cytokines, and leukotriene LT_4. Last, various growth factors and co-factors such as insulin-like growth factor-1 and GM_1 ganglioside, respectively, may have a future role in the management of head injury by promoting nerve cell regeneration and differentiation.[59,60]

EVALUATION OF THERAPEUTIC OUTCOMES

Achievement of the short-term goals mentioned and eventually returning severe head injury patients to their preinjury neurologic status is the benchmark against which all therapies are measured. One of the most commonly used assessment tools for this purpose in head injury patients is known as the Glasgow Outcome Scale (GOS).[61] This straightforward scale categorizes patient outcome as (1) death, (2) persistent vegetative state, (3) severe disability (conscious but disabled), (4) moderate disability (disabled but independent), and (5) good recovery. The Disability Rating Scale (DRS) is another measurement instrument extensively used in head injury studies that incorporates the GOS in addition to grading activities of daily living (e.g., feeding, toileting, grooming), cognitive functioning, and employability in assessing long-term outcome for these patients.[62] These objective outcome measures, typically measured at 3 and 6 months postinjury, are useful not only to scientists and clinicians, but also to payers in evaluating the relative merits of costly available rehabilitation programs for these patients.[63]

CONCLUSIONS

Publication of the *Guidelines for the Management of Severe Head Injury* published by the BTF in 1995 was a landmark event in establishing evidence-based standards, guidelines, and options for conventional management of the severe head injury patient. Attenuation of secondary neuronal injury through adherence to the recommendations contained in this report offers the greatest likelihood for a meaningful recovery in these patients at present. Combining an ever-increasing understanding of the pathophysiologic processes occurring following a severe head injury with advances in neuroprotective pharmacology offers great promise for further reduction of morbidity and mortality.

▶ PRINCIPLES OF PHARMACOTHERAPY

- Cerebral ischemia is the key pathophysiologic event triggering secondary neuronal injury following severe head injury.
- Intracellular accumulation of calcium is postulated to be a central pathophysiologic process in amplifying and perpetuating secondary neuronal injury via inhibition of cellular respiration and enzyme activation.
- *Guidelines for the Management of Severe Head Injury,* published by the Brain Trauma Foundation, serves as the foundation on which clinical decisions in managing neurotrauma patients are based.
- Correcting and preventing early hypotension (systolic BP < 90 mm Hg) and hypoxia (Pa_{O_2} < 60 mm Hg) are paramount goals during the initial resuscitative and intensive care of severe head injury patients.
- The principal monitoring parameter for severe head injury patients within the intensive care environment is CPP (CPP = MAP − ICP); CPP should be maintained above 70 mm Hg through use of fluids, vasopressors, and/or ICP normalization therapy.
- Nonspecific pharmacologic treatment in the management of intracranial hypertension should include analgesics, sedatives, anxiolytics, antipyretics, and paralytics under selected circumstances.
- Specific pharmacologic treatment in the management of intracranial hypertension includes mannitol, furosemide, and high-dose pentobarbital.
- Neither corticosteroids nor aggressive hyperventilation (maintaining Pa_{CO_2} < 35 mm Hg) should be used in the management of intracranial hypertension.
- Use of phenytoin for the prophylaxis of posttraumatic seizures should be discontinued after 7 days if no seizures are observed.
- Numerous investigational strategies (e.g., calcium antagonists, glutamate antagonists, antioxidants, and free radical scavengers) targeted at interrupting the pathophysiologic cascade of events occurring following severe head injury are being studied.

REFERENCES

1. Collins JG. Types of injuries by selected characteristics: United States, 1985–1987. Vital Health Stat 1990;175:1–68.
2. Sosin DM, Sniezek JE, Waxweiler RJ. Trends in death associated with traumatic brain injury. JAMA 1995;272:1778–1780.
3. Kraus JF, McArthur DL, Silverman TA, Jayaraman M. Epidemiology of brain injury. In: Narayan RK, Wilberger JE Jr, Povlishock JT, eds. Neurotrauma. New York, McGraw-Hill, 1996:13–30.
4. Centers for Disease Control and Prevention (CDC). Cost of injury—U.S.: A report to Congress, 1989. MMWR 1989;743–746.
5. Gennarelli TA. Mechanisms of brain injury. J Emerg Med 1993;11: 5–11.
6. Veremakis C, Lindner DH. Central nervous system injury: Essential physiologic and therapeutic concerns. In: Civetta JM, Taylor RW, Kirby RR, eds. Critical Care, 3rd ed. Philadelphia, Lippincott-Raven, 1997:273–289.
7. Luer MS, Rhoney DH, Hughes M, Hatton J. New pharmacologic strategies for acute neuronal injury. Pharmacotherapy 1996;16: 830–848.
8. Bouma GJ, Muizelaar JP, Choi SC, et al. Cerebral circulation and metabolism after severe traumatic brain injury: The elusive role of ischemia. J Neurosurg 1991;75:685–693.
9. Astrup J, Siesjo J, Symon L. Thresholds in cerebral ischemia—The ischemic penumbra. Stroke 1977;12:723–725.
10. Smith DH, McIntosh TJ. Traumatic brain injury and excitatory amino acids. In: Narayan RK, Wilberger JE Jr, Povlishock JT, eds. Neurotrauma. New York, McGraw-Hill, 1996:1445–1458.
11. Young W. Death by calcium: A way of life. In: Narayan RK, Wilberger JE Jr, Povlishock JT, eds. Neurotrauma. New York, McGraw-Hill, 1996:1421–1431.
12. Pitts LH, McIntosh TK. Dynamic changes after brain trauma. In: Vinken PJ, Bruyn GW, Klawans HL, eds. Handbook of Clinical Neurology, Vol 13. Head Injury. New York, Elsevier, 1990:65–100.
13. Hall ED. Free radicals and lipid peroxidation. In: Narayan RK, Wilberger JE Jr, Povlishock JT, eds. Neurotrauma. New York, McGraw-Hill, 1996:1405–1419.
14. Hsu CY, Hu ZY, Doster SK. Cell-mediated injury. In: Narayan RK, Wilberger JE Jr, Povlishock JT, eds. Neurotrauma. New York, McGraw-Hill, 1996:1433–1444.
15. Teasdale G, Jennett B. Aspects of coma after severe head injury. Lancet 1977;1:878–881.
16. Kelly DF, Doberstein C, Becker DP. General principles of head injury management. In: Narayan RK, Wilberger JE Jr, Povlishock JT, eds. Neurotrauma. New York, McGraw-Hill, 1996:71–101.
17. Valadka AB, Narayan RK. Emergency room management of the head-injured patient. In: Narayan RK, Wilberger JE Jr, Povlishock JT, eds. Neurotrauma. New York, McGraw-Hill, 1996:119–135.
18. Choi SC, Muizelaar JP, Barnes TY. Prediction tree for severely injured patients. J Neurosurg 1991;75:251–255.
19. Muizelaar JP, Marmarou A, Ward JD, et al. Adverse effects of prolonged hyperventilation in patients with severe head injury: A randomized clinical trial. J Neurosurg 1991;75:731–739.

20. Brain Injury Foundation, American Association of Neurological Surgeons, Joint Section on Neurotrauma and Critical Care. Guidelines for the management of severe head injury. J Neurotrauma 1996;13: 641–734.
21. Marmarou A, Anderson RL, Ward JD, et al. Impact of ICP instability and hypotension on outcome in patients with severe head injury. J Neurosurg 1991;75:S59–S66.
22. Feldman JA, Fish S. Resuscitation fluid for a patient with head injury and hypovolemic shock. J Emerg Med 1991;9:465–468.
23 Holcroft JW, Vassar MJ, Turner JE, et al. Three percent NaCl and 7.5% NaCl-dextran in the resuscitation of severely head injured patients. Ann Surg 1987;206:279–288.
24. Freshman SP, Battistella FD, Matteucci M, et al. Hypertonic saline (7.5%) versus mannitol: A comparison for treatment of acute head injuries. J Trauma 1993;35:344–348.
25. Vassar MJ, Fischer RP, O'Brien PE, et al. A multicenter trial for resuscitation of injured patients with 7.5% sodium chloride. The effect of added dextran 70. Arch Surg 1993;128:1003–1011.
26. McGraw CP. A cerebral perfusion pressure greater than 80 mm Hg is more beneficial. In: Hoff JT, Betz AL, eds. Intracranial Pressure, 7th ed. Berlin, Springer-Verlag, 1989:839–841.
27. Fortune JB, Feustel PJ, Weigle CGM, et al. Continuous measurement of jugular venous oxygen saturation in response to transient elevations of blood pressure in head-injured patients. J Neurosurg 1994;80: 461–468.
28. Rosner MJ, Daughton S. Cerebral perfusion pressure management in head injury. J Trauma 1990;30:933–941.
29. Marion DW, Obrist WD, Carlier PM, et al. The use of moderate therapeutic hypothermia for patients with severe head injuries: A preliminary report. J Neurosurg 1993;79:354–362.
30. Clifton GL, Allen S, Barrodale P, et al. A phase II study of moderate hypothermia in severe head injury. J Neurotrauma 1993;10:263–271.
31. Bouma GJ, Muizelaar JP. Relationship between cardiac output and cerebral blood flow in patients with intact and with impaired autoregulation. J Neurosurg 1990;73:368–374.
32. Bouma GJ, Muizelaar JP, Bandoh K, et al. Blood pressure and intracranial pressure–volume dynamics in severe head injury: Relationship with cerebral blood flow. J Neurosurg 1992;77:15–19.
33. Clifton GL, Hayes RL. Hypothermia for the treatment of head injury. In: Narayan RK, Wilberger JE Jr, Povlishock JT, eds. Neurotrauma. New York, McGraw-Hill, 1996:401–412.
34. Shozaki T, Sugimoto H, Taneda M, et al. Effect of mild hypothermia on uncontrollable intracranial hypertension after severe head injury. J Neurosurg 1993;79:363–368.
35. Duhaime AC. Conventional drug therapies for head injury. In: Narayan RK, Wilberger JE Jr, Povlishock JT, eds. Neurotrauma. New York, McGraw-Hill, 1996:365–374.
36. Chesnut RM. Treating raised intracranial pressure in head injury. In: Narayan RK, Wilberger JE Jr, Povlishock JT, eds. Neurotrauma. New York, McGraw-Hill, 1996:445–469.
37. Pinaud M, Lelausque JN, Chetanneu A, et al. Effects of propofol on cerebral hemodynamics and metabolism in patients with brain trauma. Anesthesiology 1990;73:404–409.
38. Hsiang JK, Chesnut RM, Crisp CB, et al. Early, routine paralysis for intracranial pressure control in severe head injury: Is it necessary? Crit Care Med 1994;2:1471–1476.
39. Gopinath SP, Robertson CS, Constant CF, et al. Jugular venous desaturation and outcome after head injury. J Psychiatry Neurosci 1994; 57:717–723.
40. Miller JD, Piper IR, Dearden NM. Management of intracranial hypertension in head injury: Matching results with cause. Acta Neurochir 1993;57(suppl):152–159.
41. Cold GE. Cerebral blood flow in acute head injury. Acta Neurochir 1990;49(suppl):18–21.
42. Kaufman AM, Cardozo E. Aggravation of vasogenic cerebral edema by multiple dose mannitol. J Neurosurg 1992;77:584–589.
43. Braakman R, Schouten HJA, Dishoeck MB, Minerhoud JM. Megadose steroids in severe head injury. Results of a prospective double-blind clinical trial. J Neurosurg 1983;58:326–330.
44. Dearden NM, Gibson JS, McDowell DG, et al. Effect of high dose dexamethasone on outcome from severe head injury. J Neurosurg 1986;64:81–88.
45. Lobato RD, Sarabia R, Cordobes C, et al. Post-traumatic cerebral hemispheric swelling. Analysis of 55 cases studied by CT. J Neurosurg 1988;68:417–423.
46. Marshall LF, Smith RW, Shapiro HM. The outcome with aggressive treatment in severe head injuries, 2. Acute and chronic barbiturate administration in the management of head injury. J Neurosurg 1979;50: 26–30.
47. Nordstrom GH, Messeter K, Sundberg B, et al. Cerebral blood flow, vasoreactivity and oxygen consumption during barbiturate therapy in severe traumatic brain lesions. J Neurosurg 1988;68:424–431.
48. Eisenberg HM, Frankowski RF, Contant CF, et al. High-dose barbiturate control of elevated intracranial pressure in patients with severe head injury. J Neurosurg 1988;69:15–23.
49. Temkin NR, Dikmen SS, Wilensky AJ, et al. A randomized, double-blind study of phenytoin for the prevention of posttraumatic seizures. N Engl J Med 1990;323:497–502.
50. Manaka S. Cooperative prospective study on posttraumatic epilepsy: Risk factors and the effect of prophylactic anticonvulsant. Jpn J Psychiatry Neurol 1992;46:311–315.
51. Andrews BT. Fluid and electrolyte management in the head-injured patient. In: Narayan RK, Wilberger JE Jr, Povlishock JT, eds. Neurotrauma. New York, McGraw-Hill, 1996:331–344.
52. Young B, Ott L. Nutritional and metabolic management of the head-injured patient. In: Narayan RK, Wilberger JE Jr, Povlishock JT, eds. Neurotrauma. New York, McGraw-Hill, 1996:345–363.
53. Teasdale G, Bailey I, Bell A, et al. The effect of nimodipine on outcome after head injury: A prospective randomized clinical trial. The British/Finnish Cooperative Head Injury Trial Group. Acta Neurochir 1990;51:315–316.
54. The European Study Group on Nimodipine in Severe Head Injury. A multicenter trial of the efficacy of nimodipine on outcome after severe head injury. J Neurosurg 1991;80:797–804.
55. Harders A, Kakarieka A, Braakman R. Traumatic subarachnoid hemorrhage and its treatment with nimodipine. German tSAH Study Group. J Neurosurg 1996;85:82–89.
56. Bullock R. Experimental drug therapies for head injury. In: Narayan RK, Wilberger JE Jr, Povlishock JT, eds. Neurotrauma. New York, McGraw-Hill, 1996:375–391.
57. Muizelaar JP, Marmarou A, Young HF, et al. Improving the outcome of severe head injury with the oxygen radical scavenger polyethylene glycol-conjugated superoxide dismutase: A phase II trial. J Neurosurg 1993;78:375–382.
58. Young B, Runge JW, Waxman KS, et al. Effects of pegorgotein on neurologic outcome of patients with severe head injury. A multicenter, randomized controlled trial. JAMA 1996;276:538–543.
59. Hatton J, Rapp RP, Kudsk KA, et al. Intravenous insulin-like growth factor-I (IGF-I) in moderate-to-severe head injury: A phase II safety and efficacy trial. J Neurosurg 1997;86:779–786.
60. Faden AI. Pharmacological treatment approaches for brain and spinal cord trauma. In: Narayan RK, Wilberger JE Jr, Povlishock JT, eds. Neurotrauma. New York, McGraw-Hill, 1996:1479–1490.
61. Jennett B, Bond M. Assessment of outcome after severe brain damage. Lancet 1975;1:480–484.
62. Rappaport M, Hall K, Hopkins K, et al. Disability rating scale for severe head trauma: Coma to community. Arch Phys Med Rehabil 1982; 63:118–123.
63. Hannay HJ, Sherer M. Assessment of outcome from head injury. In: Narayan RK, Wilberger JE Jr, Povlishock JT, eds. Neurotrauma. New York, McGraw-Hill, 1996:723–747.

55

Parkinson's Disease

Merlin V. Nelson, PharmD, MD, Richard C. Berchou, PharmD, and Peter A. LeWitt, MD

While its clinical manifestations had previously escaped attention, *paralysis agitans* had an unmistakable presence following the 1817 publication by an obscure British physician, James Parkinson.[1] Parkinson provided vivid descriptions of features such as an "involuntary tremulous motion" and the tendency to "pass from a walking to a running pace." Later observers added a variety of signs and symptoms, among them rigidity and instability of balance. Idiopathic Parkinson's disease (IPD) is sometimes referred to as Lewy body parkinsonism on the basis of its highly characteristic neuropathologic findings.

EPIDEMIOLOGY

In a series of 100 pathologically proven cases of IPD, the mean age of disease onset was 62.5 years (range, 31 to 83 years).[2] The annual incidence of IPD is about 20 per 100,000 in North America.[3] Extensive research into the epidemiology of the disorder has not clearly identified occupations, regional clusters, or incidence trends implicating specific etiologic environmental factors. Environmental factors continue to be investigated in the search for the etiology of IPD.[4] Interestingly, cigarette smoking has been associated with a slight protection against the illness.[5] The onset of IPD in later life implies that cumulative exposures to putative toxins, factors associated with central nervous system aging, or other as yet uncharacterized cell death mechanisms may be responsible for the onset and progression of the disease. Although IPD appears to be a sporadic disorder in most instances, there may be some role(s) for genetic factors in its etiology. In rare patients with otherwise typical IPD, studies of their families have provided evidence for an inherited disorder. A mutation in a gene coding for a presynaptic protein has recently been identified in a large kindred with early-onset familial Parkinson's disease.[6]

ETIOLOGY

The pathogenesis of IPD is not known. Neurotoxins highly selective to substantia nigra pars compacta (SNc) dopaminergic neurons have been instructive since animal models of parkinsonism can be created with 6-hydroxydopamine and with 1-methyl-4-phenyl-1,2,5,6-tetrahydropyridine (MPTP). The latter compound is converted by monoamine oxidase (MAO) type B to the toxic 1-methyl-4-phenylpyridinium (MPP^+) ion. Inhibition of the oxidase by selegiline eliminates the toxicity of MPTP. MPP^+ is toxic to neurons by interfering with mitochondrial metabolism. Another controversial mechanism of toxicity which has received consideration for the pathogenesis of IPD is cellular damage from oxyradicals.[7,8] Dopamine metabolism generates free radicals from autooxidation and from MAO metabolism (Fig. 55–1). Several antioxidative mechanisms are present within and outside of neurons to limit any damage that might be produced by free radical attack, but it is possible that such protection might be overwhelmed or impaired in IPD.

PATHOPHYSIOLOGY

Dopaminergic projections from the SNc to the striatum (putamen and caudate) synapse on two populations of efferent neurons (Fig. 55–2).[9] The direct pathway involves activation of striatal D_1 dopamine receptors, which stimulate inhibitory γ-aminobutyric acid (GABA)/substance P efferents to the globus pallidus interna (GPi) and substantia nigra pars reticulata (SNr). The indirect pathway involves activation of striatal D_2 dopamine receptors, which inhibit inhibitory GABA/enkephalin efferents to the globus pallidus externa (GPe). The GPe projects inhibitory GABA neurons to the subthalamic nucleus. Here, excitatory glutaminergic neurons project to the GPi. GPi output is inhibitory on the ventroanterior and ventrolateral thalamic projections to the frontal cortex. Thus, loss of nigrostriatal dopamine neurons in IPD results in reduction of cortical activation (Fig. 55–2). Virtually all the motor deficits of IPD are attributable to the marked loss in dopaminergic neurons projecting to the striatum.

The synaptic organization of the basal ganglia involves a variety of neurotransmitters, including acetylcholine, dopamine, GABA, glutamate, substance P, and serotonin. These are all possible targets for interventions in IPD. Drugs enhancing dopaminergic neurotransmission and inhibiting acetylcholine effects have been successful in IPD therapeutics; the role for drug modulation of other neurotransmitters active in the basal ganglia has not been completely explored.

The model of dopaminergic depletion (with reserpine) or blockade in producing parkinsonian features provided much of the impetus for development of therapies to augment stimulation of striatal dopamine receptors. Five classes of human dopamine receptors (D_1 through D_5) have been cloned.[10] Stimulation of D_1 dopamine receptors activates adenylate cyclase. D_2 dopamine receptors are coupled to a guanosine triphosphate (GTP)-binding protein that opens potassium channels to hyperpolarize neurons,

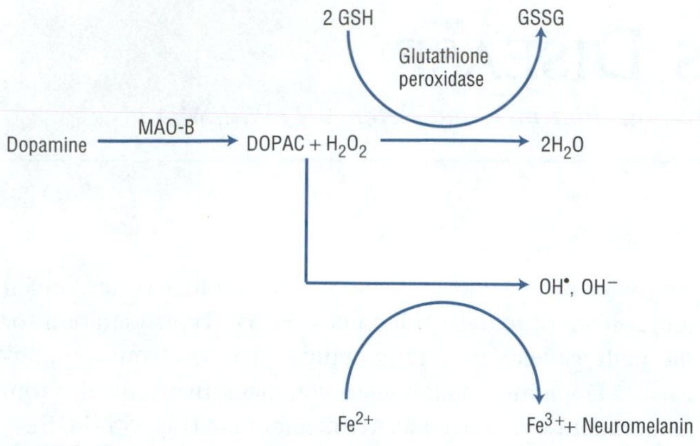

FIGURE 55–1. Dopamine metabolism results in hydrogen peroxide (H_2O_2) formation. If the glutathione system is deficient or excess hydrogen peroxide is present, hydrogen peroxide accepts an electron from ferrous iron (Fe^{2+}) forming ferric iron (Fe^{3+}) and the hydroxyl free radical ($OH^{\bullet}$). The hydroxyl free radical can cause lipid peroxidation, thereby damaging neuronal cell membranes. (MAO-B = monoamine oxidase B; DOPAC = 3,4-dihydroxyphenylacetic acid; H_2O = water; GSH = glutathione; GSSG = glutathione disulfide; and OH^- = the hydroxide ion.)

thereby reducing the excitability of striatal cells.[11] In IPD, activation of the D_2 receptor appears to be of primary importance for mediating both clinical improvements and some adverse effects (such as hallucinations). Dyskinesias are more likely to occur with L-dopa therapy (D_1 and D_2 agonism) than with dopamine agonist therapy (primarily D_2 agonism), suggesting D_1 receptor involvement in producing dyskinesia.

Pathologic findings reveal a markedly decreased number of nigrostriatal dopamine neurons and a positive correlation between the degree of nigrostriatal dopamine loss and the severity of clinical features. The threshold for onset of parkinsonism appears to be the loss of 80% or more of these neurons.[12] Positron emission studies using ^{18}F-fluorodopa clearly demonstrate decreased uptake and use of fluorodopa in IPD.[13] A compensatory increase in striatal dopamine receptors in response to decreased dopamine release has not been supported by positron emission studies, which have shown no difference in dopamine receptor density between sides in hemiparkinsonian subjects.[14] Some *in vivo* imaging studies suggest that chronic dopaminergic stimulation may cause down-regulation of postsynaptic dopamine receptors, leading possibly to a lack of response or fluctuating responses to dopaminergic drugs.[15] Other evidence suggests that fluctuations in stimulation of receptors may predispose to agonist tolerance.[16] Progressive supranuclear palsy and other "Parkinson-plus" disorders are not responsive to dopamine replacement or dopamine agonist therapies, presumably on the basis of decreased dopamine receptors due to damage to postsynaptic elements and other neuropathologic changes beyond those found in IPD.

Dopamine metabolism is shown in Figure 55–3, and the range of therapeutic interventions for IPD are summarized in Table 55–1. Tyrosine, the metabolic precursor of dopamine, is converted by tyrosine hydroxylase (TH) to L-dihydroxyphenylalanine (L-dopa) in a highly regulated synthetic process. Tetrahydrobiopterin is the cofactor required for this process. Attempts to augment dopamine synthesis by supplementing this cofactor have not been effective.[17] L-dopa is decarboxylated to dopamine by the enzyme L-amino acid decarboxylase (L-AAD). L-AAD is present outside of the central nervous system and in some nonaminergic neurons, while TH is found exclusively in aminergic neurons. Peripheral L-AAD can be blocked by administering antagonists such as carbidopa or benserazide, which do not pass the blood–brain barrier. Use of these drugs with L-dopa increases the central nervous system penetration of exogenously administered L-dopa and decreases adverse effects from the peripheral metabolism to dopamine. Dopamine is stored in synaptic vesi-

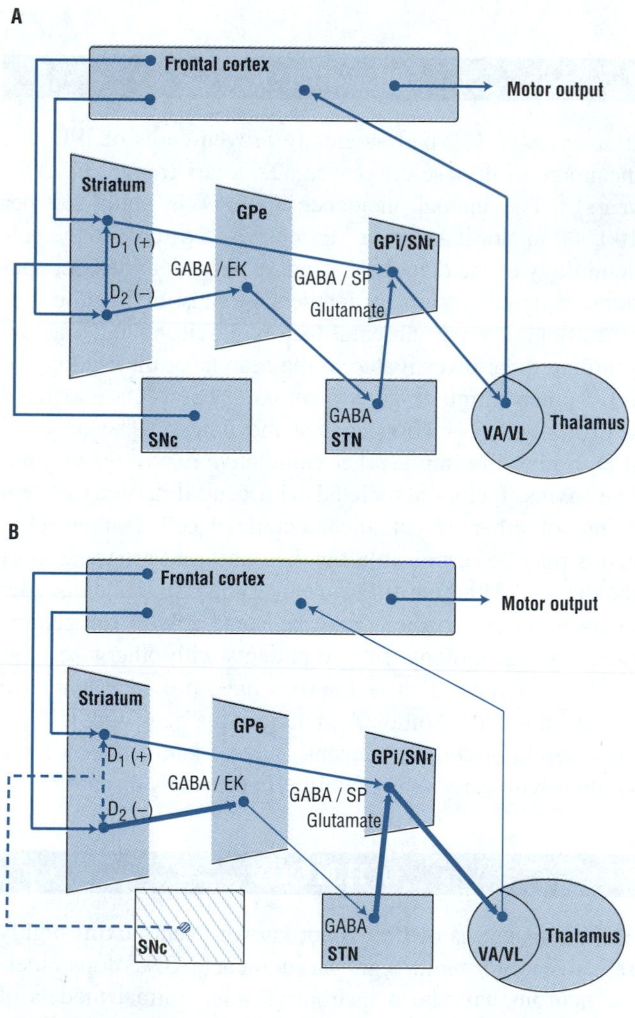

FIGURE 55–2. A. The normal balance of the basal ganglia-thalamo-cortical circuit. (GPe = globus pallidus externa; GPi = globus pallidus interna; SNr = substantia nigra pars reticulata; SNc = substantia nigra pars compacta; VA and VL = ventroanterior and ventrolateral nuclei of the thalamus, respectively; STN = subthalamic nucleus.) **B.** With nigrostriatal degeneration, there is loss of inhibition of the GPi by the direct pathway and activation of the GPi via the indirect pathway resulting in decreased activation of the cortex.

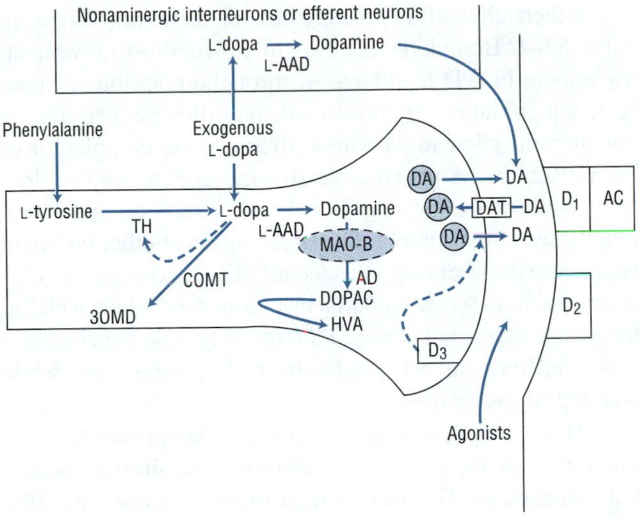

FIGURE 55–3. Dopamine metabolism in presynaptic dopamine neuron. (3OMD = 3-O-methyldopa; AC = adenylate cyclase; AD = aldehyde dehydrogenase; COMT = catechol-O-methyltransferase; D_1 to D_3 = dopamine receptors; DA = dopamine; DAT = dopamine transporter; DOPAC = 3,4-dihydroxyphenylacetic acid; HVA = homovanillic acid; L-AAD = L-aromatic amine decarboxylase; MAO-B = monoamine oxidase B; TH = tyrosine hydroxylase.)

cles until stimulated to be released into the synapse by calcium-dependent mechanisms. Dopamine activity is terminated primarily by reuptake into the presynaptic neuron by means of a specific dopamine transporter. In the presynaptic neurons, sequestration into the storage granules or the actions of catabolic pathways involving MAO or catechol-O-methyltransferase (COMT) lead to inactivation of dopamine.

Because dopamine tonically inhibits acetylcholine neurons in the striatum, the degeneration of nigrostriatal dopamine neurons results in a relative increase of striatal cholinergic interneuron activity. This increased cholinergic activity contributes especially to the tremor of IPD, as evidenced by symptomatic improvement with the use of anticholinergics and worsening with cholinergic agents.

DIAGNOSIS

Although the disorder is unmistakable in its advanced form, distinguishing mild IPD from changes seen with normal aging can be challenging. Diagnostic criteria specify that bradykinesia be present with at least two of the following: limb muscle rigidity, resting tremor (at 4 to 7 Hz and abolished by movement), or postural instability.[18] For the diagnosis of IPD, other conditions must be excluded (Table 55–2). The most common cause of secondary (acquired) parkinsonism is dopamine receptor antagonists (antipsychotics, antiemetics, or metoclopramide). Medication-induced parkinsonism can mimic the idiopathic disorder, so it is important to establish if such medications have been used. A pandemic of encephalitis lethargica in which parkinsonism usually evolved, often with other movement disorders, occurred early in this century. Several neurodegenerative conditions resemble the clinical picture of IPD, including progressive supranuclear palsy, striatonigral degeneration, olivopontocerebellar degeneration, and, rarely, Huntington's or Wilson's diseases. In order to distinguish IPD from secondary parkinsonism, other diagnostic criteria include lack of other neurologic impairments and responsiveness to L-dopa.

IPD has a characteristic neuropathologic picture that permits differentiation from similar clinical syndromes. In the SNc, loss of neurons and the Lewy body (a neuronal inclusion body composed of amyloid neurofilaments) are always found.[18] Lewy bodies appear in degenerating neurons in association with adjacent gliosis. The loss of pars compacta neurons is the basis for loss of dopamine projections to the striatum (caudate nucleus and putamen). Lewy bodies can be found in other neurologic disorders and in normal aging (in from 3.8% to 12.8% of patients from age 60 to 100 years).[18] The occurrence of Lewy bodies in patients

TABLE 55–1. Mechanisms for Potential IPD Treatments

Increase Endogenous Dopamine
- Increase tyrosine hydroxylase
  - Tetrahydrobiopterin
- L-dopa
  - Inhibit peripheral metabolism by dopa decarboxylase
    - Carbidopa
    - Benserazide
  - Sustained-release products
  - Infusions
    - Intravenous
    - Duodenal/jejunal
  - Inhibit catechol-O-methyltransferase
    - Entacapone (peripheral only)
    - Tolcapone (peripheral and central)
  - Inhibit central and peripheral metabolism by MAO-B
    - Selegiline (deprenyl)

Dopamine Agonists
- D_2 specific
  - Bromocriptine
  - Lisuride
- D_2 and D_3 specific
  - Pramipexole
  - Ropinirole
- D_1 and D_2 nonspecific
  - Pergolide
  - Apomorphine
    - Intravenous
    - Subcutaneous infusions
    - Intranasal
    - Sublingual
- Partial agonists
  - Terguride

Anticholinergic
- Benztropine
- Trihexyphenidyl

Surgical Options
- Autologous adrenal tissue or fetal tissue transplantation
- Thalamotomy
- Pallidotomy
- Deep brain stimulation

TABLE 55–2. Differential Diagnosis of Parkinsonism

Idiopathic parkinsonism (Parkinson's disease, Lewy body parkinsonism)
Secondary parkinsonism
- Drug-induced
  - Antipsychotics (phenothiazines, butyrophenones, risperidone, others)
  - Antiemetics (metoclopramide, prochlorperazine)
  - Other drugs (reserpine, α-methyldopa)
- Toxic
  - Carbon monoxide poisoning
  - Hydrogen sulfide
  - Manganese
  - Methanol
  - MPTP (1-methyl-4-phenyl-1,2,5,6-tetrahydropyridine)
  - Petrochemicals
- Neoplasms or strokes in the regions of the nigrostriatal pathways
- Traumatic lesions interrupting substantia nigra projections
- Normal pressure hydrocephalus

Parkinsonism with other neuronal system degenerations
- Wilson's disease (copper deposition in the brain)
- Progressive supranuclear palsy
- Lewy body dementia
- Corticobasalganglionic degeneration
- Alzheimer's disease
- Multiple system atrophy
  - Striatonigral degeneration
  - Shy–Drager syndrome
  - Olivopontocerebellar atrophy

without parkinsonism indicates that the disease can exist as a pathologic entity with less involvement than necessary for causing clinical signs and symptoms (incidental Parkinson's disease). Even cases whose clinical features strongly suggest IPD may lack its characteristic pathology. In a series of 100 autopsied cases of patients diagnosed as IPD during life, 24 had pathologic findings of disorders other than IPD, commonly progressive supranuclear palsy.[18]

CLINICAL PRESENTATION

Idiopathic Parkinson's disease develops insidiously and progresses slowly in most patients, though progression sometimes arrests. Often patients cannot discern exactly when the motor disorder began. Initial complaints may include sensory symptoms, but as the disease progresses, the patient exhibits one or more classic clinical features: resting tremor, rigidity, bradykinesia, or change in posture. Characteristic problems, even in mildly affected patients, include small handwriting (micrographia), decreased facial animation (hypomimia) and blink rate, diminished arm swing while walking, shuffling gait, soft or indistinct speech (hypophonia), and decreased dexterity in everyday activities. Symptoms can progress to severe functional impairment where patients require nursing home placement and are confined to bed or wheelchair. The classification system developed by Hoehn and Yahr[19] is used most frequently to stage disease severity (Table 55–3).

Other clinical characteristics of IPD are listed in Table 55–4. Bradykinesia refers to slowness of movement. Movement in IPD is often slow throughout an intended action, but initiation of movement may display a hesitation out of proportion to slowness affecting the completion of the movement. A progressive slowing and decline in dexterity with repetition may impair tasks such as finger tapping. Intermittent immobility (freezing) is another common characteristic. Freezing is especially likely to occur in situations such as when walking in a crowd or when walking through a narrow doorway. Patients may also experience a slow shuffling gait with difficulty halting their steps while walking, or *festination*.

The pathophysiology of bradykinesia appears to be an impairment in the execution of learned or semireflex sequential motor plans. This has been attributed to a disconnection between basal ganglia structures and the supplementary motor cortex. Many inputs influence the functioning of this system: bradykinesia can on occasion be reversed by sudden changes in emotional state. This type of response, termed *kinesia paradoxica,* suggests that the intrinsic program for movement is intact in IPD.

Tremor occurring at rest is highly typical of IPD and often is the sole presenting feature; however, only two-thirds of parkinsonian patients have tremor on diagnosis, and some will never develop this sign.[20] Tremor in IPD is present most commonly in the hands, sometimes with a characteristic "pill-rolling." It can also involve the jaw or legs. Sometimes, the sensory equivalent is perceived as an "internal" sensation of vibration without outward manifestations. Like other symptoms of IPD, resting tremor often begins unilaterally and may persist in this distribution. Occasionally, maintaining a position of the limbs or volitional movement will elicit tremor. Stressful situations or use of limbs in other activities may increase tremor amplitude in a limb at rest. Usually, resting tremor is abolished by volitional movement, and it is absent during sleep. Rigidity is the increased muscular resistance to passive range of motion and is usually "cogwheel" in nature.

TABLE 55–3. Hoehn and Yahr Staging of Severity of Parkinson's Disease

Stage	Description
0	No clinical signs evident
I	Unilateral involvement
II	Bilateral involvement but no postural abnormalities
III	Bilateral involvement with mild postural imbalance on examination or history of poor balance or falls; patient leads independent life
IV	Bilateral involvement with postural instability; patient requires substantial help
V	Severe, fully developed disease; patient restricted to bed or wheelchair

Compiled from Ref. 19.

TABLE 55–4. Clinical Features of Parkinson's Disease

Primary	**Autonomic Symptoms**
Bradykinesia	Bladder and anal sphincter disturbances
Postural instability	Constipation
Propulsion	Diaphoresis
Retropulsion	Orthostatic blood pressure changes
Resting tremor (may have postural and action components)	Paroxysmal flushing
Rigidity	Sexual disturbances
Motor Symptoms	**Mental Status Changes**
Decreased dexterity	Confusional state
Dysarthria	Dementia
Dysphagia	Psychosis (paranoia, hallucinosis)
Festinating gait	Sleep disturbance
Flexed posture	**Other**
Freezing at initiation of movement	Fatiguability
Hypomimia	Oily skin
Hypophonia	Pedal edema
Micrographia	Seborrhea
Slow turning	Weight loss

Because it can lead to falls, postural instability is one of the most disabling problems of parkinsonism. A disturbance of appropriate responses to the perturbation of balance is common in advanced IPD. Testing for impaired postural responses by means of the "pull test" (in which a patient is unable to recover balance after sudden backward displacement at the shoulders) can help to identify the risk for falling. Many patients with impaired postural responses also have tendencies for propulsive gait (festination) and a forward flexed posture of their axial structures along with partial flexion of the extremities.

IPD is predominantly a disorder of motor capabilities. However, neuropsychologic abnormalities can be detected even in patients with early or mild forms of the disorder with full cognitive abilities. Though intellectual deterioration is not inevitable in IPD, some patients deteriorate in a manner indistinguishable from Alzheimer's disease and other dementing conditions. It is difficult to estimate the number of patients at risk, because medications and concomitant illnesses can confound analysis of the degree of cognitive decline due specifically to IPD. IPD patients are also at increased risk for depression. Although the disabilities of IPD may provoke some instances of depression, the biochemical changes in the brain due to IPD may also predispose for endogenous depression.

▶ TREATMENT: Parkinson's Disease

SURGICAL THERAPY

The transplantation of autologous adrenal medulla tissue or the implantation of dopamine-rich dissociated mesencephalic fetal tissue into the caudate nucleus of patients with Parkinson's disease has been investigated. Autologous tissue transplantation results have been disappointing in view of the risk associated with surgery. Fetal mesencephalic tissue transplantation is fraught with ethical issues and still investigational. Functional neurosurgical techniques are more promising; these include ventrolateral thalamotomy for tremor reduction as well as pallidotomy and deep brain stimulation to decrease the GPi efferent stimulus to the thalamus (as shown in Fig. 55–2B) for reducing akinesia, tremor, dyskinesia, and rigidity.[21–23]

PHARMACOLOGIC THERAPY

A general algorithm for treatment of IPD is shown in Figure 55–4; however, more complete algorithms covering virtually every aspect of IPD management have been published.[24] The optimal management of IPD is best determined by individualized considerations of a patient's disability. The only established pharmacologic therapy for IPD is medication that can transiently reverse signs and symptoms. In patients with mild features of IPD, use of symptomatic medications is often not needed if disabilities have not evolved. Many patients with nothing more than mild slowness and resting tremor can often be managed effectively with only anticholinergics or amantadine.

The most effective drug therapy for IPD involves enhancement of dopaminergic activity. The most efficacious treatment is replacement of the natural neurotransmitter, dopamine, by the use of its immediate precursor, L-dopa. Though L-dopa is more effective than other medications currently available, there has been considerable concern with respect to the possible risks from long-term use. Some clinicians minimize use of L-dopa for this reason. As indicated in the treatment algorithm shown in Figure 55–4, anticholinergic drugs or amantadine can be used for treating resting tremor as an alternative to L-dopa. Although not highly effective against bradykinesia, gait disturbance, or other features of advanced parkinsonism, these medications can be useful for relieving mild disabilities experienced by patients in the first few years after the onset of parkinsonism. The decision to incorporate L-dopa therapy comes from advancing disability and ineffectiveness of these alternative medications to provide adequate symptomatic control. Depending on profession and life-style, the same basic parkinsonian features may result in different degrees of disability, and drug therapy goals may need to

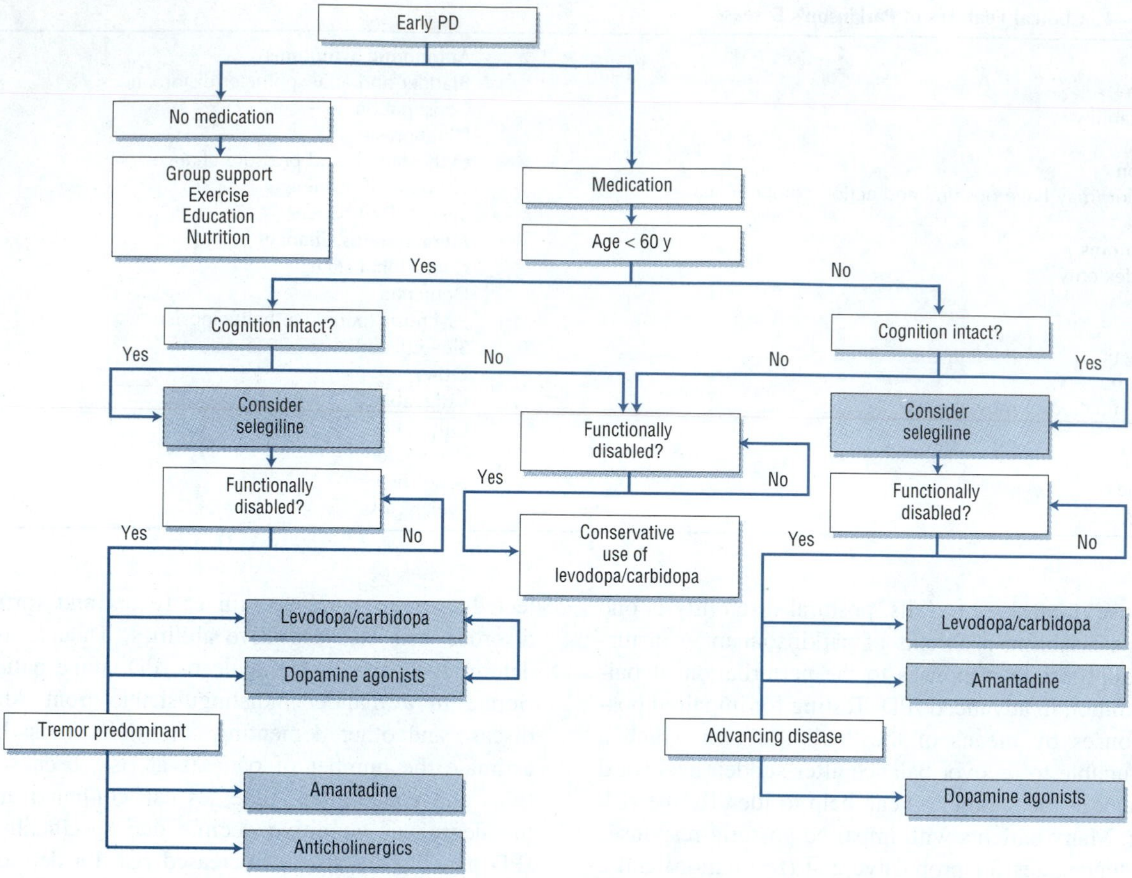

FIGURE 55–4. General algorithm for treating IPD.

be adjusted accordingly. A summary of available antiparkinsonian medications is given in Table 55–5.

SELEGILINE

Selegiline (Eldepryl, Somerset), an MAO-B inhibitor, also known as deprenyl, is marketed for producing extension of L-dopa effects. By blocking the breakdown of dopamine, it has a modest effect on extending the duration of action from each dose of L-dopa. Patients with "wearing-off" of L-dopa actions may experience up to an hour of increased action from each L-dopa dose. The use of selegiline also increases the peak effects of L-dopa, and can thus cause worsening of preexisting dyskinesias or psychiatric symptoms such as delusions and hallucinations. Often, the use of selegiline permits the reduction of L-dopa intake to as little as one-half of its previous optimal dose.

Selegiline has been widely used at a dose of 10 mg/d, although its irreversible inhibition of MAO-B can be achieved at lower doses.[25] In addition, renewal of the enzyme proceeds at a slow rate, so that the effect of the drug lingers for weeks. Selegiline is lipophilic and penetrates the blood–brain barrier rapidly. The metabolic pathway of selegiline leads to end products of L-methamphetamine and L-amphetamine.[26] Adverse effects of selegiline are minimal, and include insomnia and jitteriness. The hypertensive "cheese effect," which occurs from ingesting tyramine with the use of MAO-A inhibitors, does not occur with selegiline.[27] There have been a few case reports of an adverse reaction characterized by hypertension, diaphoresis, and shivering associated with concomitant use of the selective serotonin reuptake blockers.[28] A similar reaction has been reported with meperidine.[29]

In addition to its symptomatic effects at enhancing L-dopa action, selegiline may have neuroprotective properties. It was investigated for an antioxidant effect on the basis of inhibiting the oxidative deamination of dopamine, which generates hydrogen peroxide and ultimately oxyradicals capable of damaging nigrostriatal neurons (see Fig. 55–1). Because MAO-B inhibition diverts dopamine catabolism to an alternate route not generating peroxide, selegiline therapy was proposed as a means for sparing these neurons from oxidative stress. Several studies have investigated this possibility.[30–33] Although initial findings were quite promising, the initial observation of slowing the progression of parkinsonian disability lasted for only 1 year, and afterwards this effect could not be demonstrated as different from the placebo treatment group.[34,35] A report of increased mortality when selegiline was combined with L-dopa as compared to L-dopa alone is of concern,[36] but the study had methodologic flaws.[37]

ANTICHOLINERGIC MEDICATIONS

The anticholinergic drugs can be effective against tremor but rarely show much benefit for bradykinesia or other disabilities of IPD. Not all patients with tremor respond to these medications, but sometimes dystonic features associated with IPD will improve. Adverse effects of these drugs include dry mouth, blurred vision, constipation, and urinary retention. More serious reactions include forgetfulness, sedation, depression, and anxiety. An encephalopathic state can also gradually evolve in some patients. Patients with preexisting cognitive deficits and advanced age are at greater risk for central anticholinergic effects.[38] The anticholinergic drugs differ little in their adverse effects and have essentially the same therapeutic potential. Anticholinergic drugs can be used alone or in conjunction with L-dopa and other antiparkinsonian agents.

AMANTADINE

Amantadine (Symmetrel, DuPont; various generic brands) is often effective for relief of most signs and symptoms of patients with

TABLE 55–5. Drugs Used in Parkinson's Disease

Generic Name	Trade Name	Manufacturer	Dosage Range (mg/d)	Dosage Form (mg)	Cost Index[a]
Amantadine	Symmetrel	DuPont	200–300	100,50/5 mL	8,8
	Generic brands	Various			3,7
Carbidopa/L-dopa	Sinemet	DuPont	[b]	10/100,25/100,25/250	6,7,8
	Generic brands	Various			
Controlled-release carbidopa/L-dopa	Sinemet CR	DuPont	[b]	25/100,50/200	7,14
L-dopa	Larodopa	Roche	[b]	100,250,500	2,3,6
	Dopar	Roberts Pharm			
Selegiline	Eldepryl	Somerset	10	5	21
Tolcapone	Tasmar	Roche	300–600	100,200	16,17
Agonists					
Bromocriptine	Parlodel	Sandoz	[b]	2.5,5	14,22
Pergolide	Permax	Athena	[b]	0.05,0.25,1	2,25,82
Pramipexole	Mirapex	Pharmacia Upjohn	1.5–4.5	0.125,0.25,1,1.5	6,10,21,21
Ropinirole	Requip	SmithKline Beecham	[b]	0.25,1,2,5	9,9,9,19
Anticholinergic Drugs					
Benztropine	Cogentin	Merck	0.5–6	0.5,1,2	2,2,2
	Generic brands	Various			1,1,1
Biperiden	Akineton	Knoll	2–16	2	2
Diphenhydramine	Benadryl	Parke-Davis	25–100	25,50	2,3
	Generic brands	Various			1,1
Procyclidine	Kemadrin	Glaxo-Wellcome	2.5–20	5	4
Trihexyphenidyl	Artane	Lederle	1–15	2,5,2/5 mL,5 LA	1,3,3,4
	Generic brands	Various			1,3

[a]Cost index calculated from June 1994 average wholesale price per 100. Approximate cost per 100 (or per pint for solutions) equivalent to index × $10.00.
[b]Dosage must be individualized.

mild IPD.[39] Like anticholinergics, it can be especially effective against tremor. The drug is used at 200 to 300 mg/d. Adverse effects that may occur at onset of the drug (sedation and vivid dreams) may disappear with time. Dry mouth is a common adverse effect reminiscent of anticholinergic drugs, although amantadine does not block cholinergic receptors. Other adverse central effects seen uncommonly include depression, hallucinations, anxiety, dizziness, psychosis, and confusion. A frequent (and reversible) adverse effect of amantadine is livedo reticularis, a diffuse mottling of the skin.

Amantadine is eliminated renally, and a decreased dose should be administered when renal dysfunction is present (100 mg/d with creatinine clearances from 30 to 50 mL/min, 100 mg every other day for creatinine clearances from 15 to 29 mL/min, and 200 mg every 7 days for creatinine clearances less than 15 mL/min and patients on hemodialysis). Unlike other drugs for IPD, the precise mechanism of action of amantadine is unknown, but it may involve either dopaminergic or nondopaminergic mechanisms such as inhibition of NMDA receptors.[40]

L-DOPA AND CARBIDOPA/L-DOPA

L-Dopa (Larodopa, Roche; various generic brands) was first studied for parkinsonism in the 1960s, and recognition of its unequivocal benefit was reported in 1967.[41] It is still the most effective drug in the management of IPD. L-dopa is the immediate precursor of dopamine. It crosses the blood–brain barrier, whereas dopamine does not. In the striatum and elsewhere, L-dopa is converted by L-amino acid decarboxylase to dopamine. Peripherally formed dopamine is responsible for adverse effects such as nausea, vomiting, cardiac arrhythmias, and postural hypotension. By combining L-dopa with the peripherally acting L-amino acid decarboxylase inhibitors, carbidopa (Sinemet, DuPont; various generic brands) or benserazide (Madopar, not available in the USA), peripheral conversion of L-dopa to dopamine is nearly completely blocked. As a result, increased amounts of L-dopa are transported into the brain.[42]

Today, L-dopa is used almost exclusively as a combination product with decarboxylase inhibitors. Starting L-dopa doses of 200 to 300 mg/d are often adequate for relief of disability. Some patients require larger amounts on a daily basis; however, the usual maximum dose of L-dopa needed by patients even with severe parkinsonism is 800 mg/d. Slow build-up of dose (e.g., increments of 100 mg of L-dopa per week) can help to assess the lowest effective dose, and minimizes the risk for adverse effects, such as postural hypotension, nausea, vomiting, sedation, and vivid dreams.

Several formulations of carbidopa/L-dopa are available. Carbidopa has a maximum effective daily dose of 100 to 125 mg, beyond which there is little increase in L-amino acid decarboxylase inhibitory effect. Some patients may benefit from an increase to as much as 150 mg/d. Carbidopa/L-dopa is most widely used in a 25 mg/100 mg tablet form, although a 25 mg/250 mg and a 10 mg/100 mg form are also available. Controlled-release preparations of carbidopa/L-dopa are available in 50 mg/200 mg and 25 mg/100 mg forms.[43] If peripheral adverse effects are prominent, 25 mg carbidopa (Lodosyn, DuPont) tablets are available from the manufacturer by physician request and can be used to supplement the fixed combination products.

Between 6% and 10% of IPD patients will develop involuntary movements or short-duration responses with each year of L-dopa treatment.[44,45] Movement complications associated with long-term treatment with carbidopa/L-dopa treatment and their suggested treatments are listed in Table 55–6. Debate exists whether these complications are related to treatment or are intrinsic to the disease process itself.

End-of-dose deterioration (the "wearing-off" effect) has been related to increasing loss of neuronal storage capability for dopamine. Initially, exogenous L-dopa is taken up by the remaining presynaptic neurons, converted to dopamine, and stored in synaptic vesicles. With progressive loss of presynaptic neurons, storage capacity declines and patients become more dependent on the rate of L-dopa delivery to the brain for the generation of

TABLE 55–6. Motor Fluctuations and Possible Interventions in IPD

Effect	Possible Treatments
End of dose deterioration ("wearing off")	Increase frequency of doses; controlled-release carbidopa/L-dopa; consider agonists, selegiline, tolcapone, or amantadine; duodenal or intravenous L-dopa infusions; carbidopa/L-dopa oral solution; subcutaneous apomorphine infusions; transdermal dopamine agonists
Delayed onset of response	Give on empty stomach before meals; crush or chew and take with a full glass of water; reduce dietary protein intake; antacids; morning standard release carbidopa/L-dopa if on sustained-release carbidopa/L-dopa; infusions of L-dopa; dopamine agonists
Drug-resistant "off" periods	Increase carbidopa/L-dopa dose and/or frequency; give on empty stomach before meals; crush or chew and take with a full glass of water; infusions of L-dopa or dopamine agonists; apomorphine intranasal spray
"Random" oscillations ("on–off")	Dopamine agonists; selegiline; tolcapone; infusions of L-dopa or dopamine agonists; consider drug holiday
Start hesitation ("freezing")	Increase carbidopa/L-dopa dose; dopamine agonists; gait modifications (tapping, rhythmic commands, stepping over objects, rocking)
Peak-dose dyskinesia ("I-D-I" response[a])	Smaller more frequent doses of carbidopa/L-dopa; controlled-release carbidopa/L-dopa
Diphasic dyskinesias ("D-I-D" response[b])	Reduce anticholinergic medication
Dystonia	Baclofen; nighttime carbidopa/L-dopa; morning standard-release carbidopa/L-dopa if on sustained-release carbidopa/L-dopa; dopamine agonists; anticholinergics
Myoclonus	Decrease nighttime L-dopa doses; clonazepam
Akathisia	Benzodiazepines; propranolol

[a]I-D-I is the "improvement-dyskinesia/dystonia-improvement" pattern of response.
[b]D-I-D is the "dyskinesia-improvement-dyskinesia" pattern of response.

dopamine. Hence, the peripheral pharmacokinetics of L-dopa increasingly become the determinants of dopamine synthesis.

With advancement of IPD and chronic L-dopa therapy, motor response fluctuations emerge. A single carbidopa/L-dopa dose may produce benefits for as little as 1.5 to 2 hours. As a result, carbidopa/L-dopa needs to be given more frequently in order to prevent the wearing-off of its benefits. Alternatively, a controlled-release product is available (Sinemet CR 50/200 and 25/100, DuPont), which can extend the duration of L-dopa effect. A more gradual wearing-off of L-dopa effect and the need for fewer daily doses are associated with this product.[46] Some patients will require an increase of L-dopa intake when switched to the sustained-release form because of its decreased bioavailability. Patients maintained on the sustained-release product may also require a conventional carbidopa/L-dopa dose in the morning for its more rapid absorption and response.[47]

Dopamine agonists also can be added to a carbidopa/L-dopa regimen in an attempt to treat "wearing off." In addition, either intravenous or duodenal L-dopa infusions will produce constant serum L-dopa concentrations (and presumably striatal dopamine concentrations) and thus reduce response fluctuations.[48,49] Although some patients have been maintained on duodenal and IV infusions for long periods of time, these invasive methods of administration require careful planning and are generally not used outside the research setting. Sipping small amounts of carbidopa/L-dopa solution is an easier way to noninvasively titrate drug intake to optimal effect.[50] A solution that is stable for 24 hours can be prepared by adding 10 tablets of carbidopa/L-dopa and 2 g of crystalline ascorbic acid to 1 L of tap water. Finally, MAO-B inhibitors such as selegiline and the COMT inhibitors tolcapone (Tasmar, Roche) and entacapone (currently under development) extend the action of L-dopa.[51] Tolcapone has been shown to significantly decrease "off" time (by about 1.5 hours) and decrease L-dopa requirements with only dopaminergic adverse effects (from the increased dopamine concentrations) and urine discoloration as adverse effects.[52] It remains to be seen whether the use of these adjunctive agents will be more beneficial and cost effective than maximizing therapy with L-dopa/carbidopa alone. Serious liver dysfunction resulting in a few deaths has recently been reported with tolcapone. A boxed warning is being developed which will require every 2-week liver function monitoring for the first year of treatment, then every 4 weeks for the next 6 months, and every 8 weeks thereafter.

Drug-resistant "off" periods or delayed response to carbidopa/L-dopa can be due to delayed stomach emptying or decreased absorption in the upper gastrointestinal tract. Chewing a tablet or crushing it and then drinking a full glass of water may decrease disintegration time and facilitate gastric emptying.

Rapid fluctuations from "on" to "off" motor states (*yo-yoing*) can develop in patients receiving L-dopa chronically. Rapid transitions from normal or dyskinetic "on" motor activity to bradykinetic or "off" states may just be an extension of wearing off. Nonmotor symptoms may also fluctuate.[53] Concentration versus effect data reveal nonlinear (sigmoid E_{max} model) relationships such that small changes in serum L-dopa concentrations may lead to large effect responses, even if the sustained-release product is used.[54] Differences in the pharmacodynamic parameters EC_{50} (concentration at half-maximal effect), K_{eo} (elimination rate constant from the effect compartment), and N (the sigmoidicity constant) have been found between stable and fluctuating IPD patients with no change in pharmacokinetic parameters.[55] These same pharmacodynamic parameters have been found to significantly change in individual patients followed longitudinally over 4 years.[56] With progression of IPD, motor skill performance decreases, so that there will be larger differences between baseline capabilities and maximum therapeutic effect; hence, there will be an even steeper slope at the EC_{50} and more clinically noticeable dose-by-dose effects. These circumstances contribute to rapid fluctuations in motor responses. Simulations of the number of times a patient could alternately tap two levers 25 cm apart using mean pharmacodynamic and kinetic values for stable and fluctuating patients are shown in Figure 55–5 to further illustrate the dramatic differences between these groups. These pharmacodynamic mechanisms have been reviewed in detail by Nutt and Holford.[57]

Infusions of L-dopa or regimens of drugs with long-acting dopaminergic effects tend to alleviate these fluctuations. Dopa-

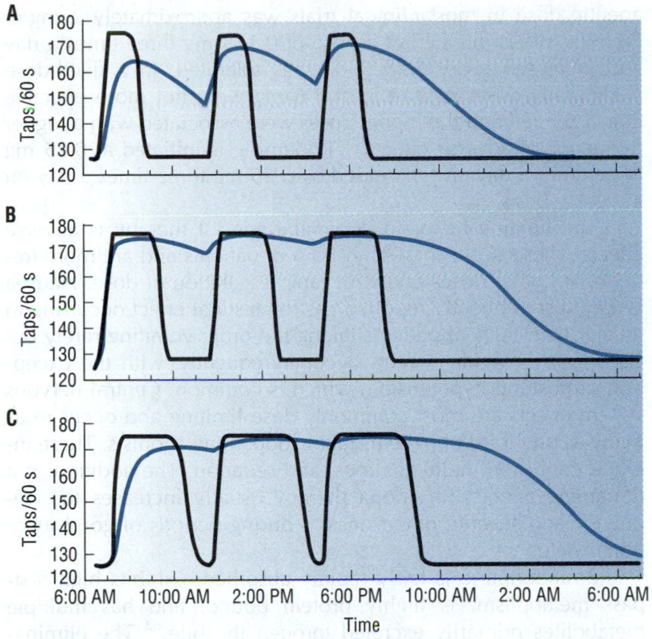

FIGURE 55–5. Effect of change in carbidopa/L-dopa dosage form on tapping effect in stable *(blue line)* and fluctuating *(black line)* patients using pharmacodynamic parameters obtained from Nelson and colleagues.[54] **A.** Carbidopa/L-dopa 25 mg/100 mg (kel of 1.242 hr^{-1}, ka of 3.384 hr^{-1}, and V/f of 35.4 *l*) administered at typical administration times of 7 AM, 12 noon, and 5 PM. **B.** Carbidopa/L-dopa 50 mg/200 mg (same pharmacokinetic parameters as A) administered at the same times. **C.** Carbidopa/L-dopa 50 mg/200 mg with a longer half-life of absorption of 1.4 hr (Ka = 0.5) simulating the controlled-release form.

minergic agonists can also be added to L-dopa to treat "on–off" fluctuations. Other strategies include MAO inhibitors and inhibitors of COMT, which can decrease the clearance of L-dopa. A drug-free period (drug holiday) has been investigated in an attempt to modify postsynaptic dopamine receptors and thus decrease "on–off" fluctuations. Because of the discomforts and risks as well as the limited gains for most patients, drug holiday has not been useful as a therapeutic intervention.

Another complication of L-dopa therapy is dyskinesias (choreiform abnormal involuntary movements involving usually the neck, trunk, and upper extremities) and dystonias (sustained muscle contractions or abnormal postures). These involuntary movements are usually associated with peak antiparkinsonian benefit (peak effect dyskinesia or "improvement-dyskinesia/dystonia-improvement"), although they can also develop during the rise and fall of L-dopa effects (the "dyskinesia-improvement-dyskinesia" or diphasic pattern of response). In the case of peak-effect dyskinesias or dystonias, smaller, more frequent doses of L-dopa or use of the sustained-release preparations can be beneficial. The optimal treatment for the "dyskinesia-improvement-dyskinesia" pattern is unknown, and can actually worsen with strategies useful for extending L-dopa effect. Simplistically, dyskinesias can be thought of as "too much movement" secondary to extension of the pharmacologic effect, or "too much" striatal dopamine receptor stimulation. However, the phenomenology is far more complex, as demonstrated by the occasional patient simultaneously demonstrating parkinsonian features and dyskinesias. An interaction between different classes of dopamine receptors may be involved. Dyskinesias tend to only occur in patients with denervated striatal tissue. A partial dopamine agonist, terguride, has been found to suppress dyskinesias without worsening parkinsonian symptoms, suggesting that some pharmacologic approaches may differentiate the effects of dopaminergic stimulation on different aspects of motor system activation.[58]

Dystonias are especially common in the distal lower extremities. Clenching of the toes or involuntary turning of the foot can precede the development of IPD. Dystonias often occur in the early morning hours or on awakening and improve with the first L-dopa dose of the day. Remedies for this problem include bedtime administration of sustained-release L-dopa, dopaminergic agonists, baclofen, or selective denervation with botulinum toxin. Another problem that can occur during sleep is myoclonus. Lowering nighttime L-dopa doses or use of clonazepam can be beneficial. Akathisia (the sensation of inner restlessness resulting in the need to make movements) can be treated with benzodiazepines or propranolol.

L-Dopa and dopaminergic agonists do not only act in the nigrostriatal system, but also facilitate other dopamine pathways (including the mesolimbic dopaminergic projections). Activation of the latter system may result in occurrence of psychiatric symptoms including delirium, agitation, paranoia, delusions, or hallucinations. These effects occur even more frequently in older patients and in those with underlying confusion or dementia.[59] The atypical antipsychotic clozapine can be quite effective for psychotic symptoms while also improving tremor and other motor symptoms.[60] Other antipsychotics, including olanzapine and risperidone, can also improve psychotic symptoms but worsen parkinsonian features.[61,62]

The decision to start L-dopa early (as soon as the diagnosis of IPD is made) or late (only when symptoms compromise social, occupational, or psychological well-being) has generated controversy.[63,64] Proponents for delaying treatment point to evidence suggesting that long-term L-dopa therapy is associated with increased risk of response fluctuations, increased risk of dementia, and loss of L-dopa efficacy.[65] L-Dopa therapy hypothetically could increase oxidative stress in dopaminergic neurons and thus increase dopaminergic neuronal loss; however, there is no firm evidence that this mechanism actually causes IPD.

The counterargument is that response fluctuations are secondary to disease progression not L-dopa. A multicenter study found that withholding L-dopa therapy for more than 3 years after diagnosis resulted in a doubling of the excess mortality rate compared to early treatment.[66] Despite these conflicting views, there is general consensus that the proper time to initiate L-dopa therapy is at least when the disease interferes with the patient's occupation or activities of daily living, or when the patient wishes to begin therapy after considering all risks and benefits.

L-Dopa pharmacokinetic properties help explain some of the clinical effects seen. There is marked intra- and intersubject variability in the time to peak plasma concentrations after oral L-dopa. Often there may be more than one peak plasma concentration after a single dose, which is attributed to erratic gastric emptying. Meals delay gastric emptying, while antacids (which decrease gastric acidity) promote gastric emptying.[67] Cisapride has been shown to improve "delayed on" and "no on" problems.[68] L-Dopa is primarily absorbed in the proximal duodenum by a saturable LNAA transport system. Competition for this site by dietary or supplemental LNAAs can reduce L-dopa plasma concentrations. The gut wall also contains a saturable decarboxylase, which limits the bioavailability of L-dopa unless it is combined with a peripheral decarboxylase inhibitor such as carbidopa.

L-Dopa is not bound to plasma proteins. It crosses the blood–brain barrier by stereospecific saturable facilitated diffusion and competes with LNAA for transport into the brain. High-dose infusions of phenylalanine and leucine decrease clinical response to L-dopa without altering L-dopa plasma concentrations.[69] This has led to special diets being recommended for these patients, although reduction in protein intake is generally not needed to maintain good L-dopa effect.[70] A metabolite of L-dopa, 3-O-methyldopa (3OMD), also competes for transport, but it is not clear how this affects L-dopa clinical response. Drug holidays may allow the body to clear this longer half-life metabolite, thus restoring L-dopa responsiveness.

L-Dopa elimination is primarily by decarboxylation to dopamine. Additional pathways are by 3-O-methylation and transamination. With adequate decarboxylase inhibition, increased amounts of L-dopa are metabolized by the other pathways. The elimination half-life of L-dopa is about 1 hour, and this is extended to about 1 1/2 hours with the addition of carbidopa; 3OMD has a half-life of about 15 hours and accumulates with chronic dosing. Dose versus area under the curve data suggest a nonlinear relationship for L-dopa, implying a saturable elimination process.[71] There are no peripheral pharmacokinetic differences between patients with stable responses, response fluctuations, and "on–off" fluctuations.[54]

L-Dopa should not be administered with MAO-A inhibitors because of a risk for hypertensive crisis or with antipsychotic agents because of possible antagonism of L-dopa effect.

DOPAMINE AGONISTS

The dopamine agonists pergolide (Permax, Athena), bromocriptine (Parlodel, Sandoz), and the nonergots, pramipexole (Mirapex, Pharmacia Upjohn) and ropinirole (Requip, SmithKline Beecham) are beneficial as adjuncts to L-dopa therapy in prolonging the effective treatment period in patients with deteriorating response to L-dopa, in patients who are experiencing fluctuations in response to L-dopa, and in patients with limited clinical response to L-dopa secondary to inability to tolerate higher doses. The dopamine agonists decrease the frequency of "off" periods and provide an L-dopa–sparing effect. Crossover studies suggest that pergolide with L-dopa is similar or possibly more efficacious with fewer adverse effects than bromocriptine with L-dopa.[72] Pergolide may improve functional status in patients with deteriorating response to bromocriptine,[73] whereas bromocriptine does not appear to improve function in patients with a deteriorating response to pergolide.[74] The dopamine ergot agonists (pergolide and bromocriptine) are not as effective in monotherapy as L-dopa in previously untreated Parkinson's disease patients,[75,76] primarily because of a high incidence of adverse effects and treatment failures necessitating either lowering the dose or the addition of L-dopa. Pramipexole and ropinirole seem to be more effective as monotherapy alternatives to L-dopa.[77] Investigations of the combination of L-dopa with dopamine agonists as initial therapy revealed a decreased risk for the development of response fluctuations.[78,79] This effect is probably secondary to the known symptomatic effect of the agonist.

A recommended initial dose of bromocriptine is 1.25 mg once or twice daily. The dose of bromocriptine should be escalated slowly by 1.25 to 2.5 mg/d every week and maintained at the minimum amount necessary to accomplish the desired therapeutic effect. Average daily dosages less than 30 mg may be effective for several years in many patients; however, some patients may require dosages up to 120 mg/d. Comparison of rapid and slow titration regimens have shown that rapid escalation in dosage produces more adverse effects but has less of a delay in reaching an effective dosage in de novo patients.[80]

A recommended initial dose of pergolide (which is about 13 times more potent than bromocriptine) is 0.05 mg/d for 2 days, gradually increasing the dose by approximately 0.1 to 0.15 mg/d every 3 days over a 12-day period. Should more drug be needed, the dose may then be increased by 0.25 mg every 3 days until symptoms are eliminated or adverse effects occur. The mean therapeutic dose in most clinical trials was approximately 3 mg/d. Pramipexole is initiated at a dose of 0.125 mg three times a day and increased every 5 to 7 days as tolerated. In a fixed-dose study, daily doses of 3, 4.5, and 6 mg were not more effective than 1.5 mg/d and the higher doses were associated with a higher frequency of adverse effects.[81] Ropinirole is initiated at 0.25 mg three times a day and increased by 0.25 mg three times a day on a weekly basis.

The limiting factor in dopamine agonist therapy is adverse effects. These occur in 30% to 50% of patients and are more frequent at higher doses and with rapid escalation of dose. Nausea is the most frequently reported gastrointestinal effect occurring in greater than 50% of patients taking the drug; vomiting rarely occurs. Cardiovascular effects occur infrequently, with the exception of postural hypotension, which is common. Central nervous system effects are most commonly dose limiting and occur in as many as one-third of patients taking dopamine agonists. These include confusion, hallucinations, and sedation. The addition of a dopamine agonist to L-dopa therapy usually increases the frequency and severity of dyskinesias during periods of good functional status.

Bromocriptine is fairly rapidly absorbed, exhibits high first-pass metabolism, is highly protein bound, and has multiple metabolites primarily excreted through the bile.[82] The elimination half-life is about 3 hours. A slow-release bromocriptine product has been investigated but is not clinically available.[83] A significant increase in bromocriptine plasma concentrations has been documented with erythromycin but not with caffeine.[84] Pergolide has approximately the same duration of action as bromocriptine. Pramipexole is primarily renally excreted with an 8- to 12-hour half-life. The initial dosage must be adjusted in renal insufficiency (0.125 mg twice daily for creatinine clearances of 35 to 59 mL/min, 0.125 mg once daily for creatinine clearances of 15 to 34 mL/min). Ropinirole has a 6-hour half-life and is metabolized by CYP1A2.[85] Potent inhibitors (fluroquinolones) and inducers (smoking) of this enzyme will likely lead to alterations in ropinirole clearance.

Apomorphine and lisuride are dopamine agonists being investigated but not available in the United States. Cabergoline is a D_2 agonist with a long half-life as effective as bromocriptine but dosed once a day.[86] N-0923, a D_2 dopamine agonist formulated in a transdermal delivery form, is currently in phase II trials. Apomorphine and lisuride have both been administered as subcutaneous infusions,[87] and a variety of formulations including sublingual and intranasal apomorphine are being investigated.[88,89] Specific D_1 receptor agonists do not appear to have much antiparkinsonian effect.[90] Domperidone is a peripheral dopamine receptor blocker (not available in the United States) that can be used to block some of the adverse effects of the dopamine agonists.[91]

PHARMACOECONOMIC CONSIDERATIONS

No formal pharmacoeconomic assessments have been reported in IPD treatment. Treatment with anticholinergic medications is inexpensive. Carbidopa/L-dopa therapy with the generic products is relatively inexpensive. For cost effectiveness, the lowest dose giving adequate results should be used. In early IPD, a long duration response can be seen, such that a carbidopa/L-dopa dose every 3 days is all that is required.[92] Initial therapy with the more expensive sustained-release product (Sinemet CR) in the absence of response fluctuations is not indicated. As symptoms progress, the addition of dopamine agonists, selegiline or tolcapone, can add considerable expense sometimes with minimal or no benefit.

EVALUATION OF THERAPEUTIC OUTCOMES

A summary of assessment parameters in determining antiparkinsonian drug response is shown in Table 55–7. It is important to educate patients, spouses, or significant others regarding what to expect with treatment. They can participate in treatment by recording medication administration times as well as duration of "on" and "off" times, which can be reviewed upon each office visit. If a bothersome symptom such as dystonia occurs only infrequently, it can be videotaped by the family and reviewed in the office.

The history should always include a detailed medication history because patients may often improvise and adjust their own medication schedule. It is important to determine the times of the day that may be most difficult for them to function. Assessment of general level of functioning including activities of daily living will help determine when L-dopa or dopamine agonists should be added. A history of falls should be investigated further as to the circumstances surrounding the falls to determine whether falls are secondary to IPD or some other etiology. The patient should be assessed for common adverse effects of the antiparkinsonian medications including nausea, hypotension, and psychiatric difficulties.

A focused neurologic examination (Table 55–7) should be undertaken, keeping in mind the timing of the examination in relation to the last dose of medication. Findings should always be considered in view of the patients perception of severity of symptoms.

TABLE 55–7. Assessment of Therapeutic Outcomes

History
Precise medications and frequency
General level of functioning
History of falls
Circumstances of any falls
Problems with activities of daily living
Eating/swallowing
Dressing
Hygiene
Hallucinations
Sleep
Vivid dreams
Depression
Freezing/abnormal involuntary movements/dystonia
Nausea/vomiting
Syncope/presyncope symptoms
Physical Assessment
Appearance
Faces
Salivation
Seborrhea
Speech
Tremor
Rigidity/dyskinesia
Finger tapping
Rapid alternating movements
Foot tapping
Arise from chair with outstretched hands
Standing posture
Stability
Gait
Handwriting
Cognitive assessment

CONCLUSIONS

Although the cause of Parkinson's disease remains unknown, the identification of a neurotoxin and a mechanism to protect against the neurotoxin has advanced the knowledge of this disease. Pharmacologic therapy through manipulation of the dopaminergic system can significantly improve a patient's functional status and prolong meaningful life. Despite problems associated with L-dopa, it remains the standard of therapy for patients with Parkinson's disease. The goal of management remains maintaining acceptable functional control with the minimum amount of antiparkinsonian drug necessary.

▶ PRINCIPLES OF PHARMACOTHERAPY

- Carbidopa/L-dopa is the standard of therapy in IPD.
- Dosages of carbidopa/L-dopa and dopamine agonists must be individualized.
- Most carbidopa/L-dopa–treated patients will eventually develop response fluctuations.
- Response fluctuations may be partially explained by pharmacokinetic and pharmacodynamic properties of L-dopa.
- Medication administration times and dose-by-dose therapeutic and adverse effects must be considered in individualizing therapy to optimize treatment outcome.
- Selegiline, tolcapone, and controlled-release carbidopa/L-dopa decrease response fluctuations through pharmacokinetic mechanisms.
- Anticholinergics should be used with caution in the elderly or those with preexisting cognitive difficulties.
- Amantadine is useful even in the elderly for relieving mild features of IPD.
- The optimal time to start carbidopa/L-dopa is controversial, but in general treatment should be started when the disease interferes with the patient's occupation or activities of daily living.
- Dopamine agonists are L-dopa sparing and decrease response fluctuations, but are more likely than L-dopa alone to cause neuropsychiatric symptoms.

REFERENCES

1. Tyler KL. A history of Parkinson's disease. In: Killer WC, ed. Handbook of Parkinson's Disease, 2nd ed. New York, Marcel Dekker, 1992:1–34.
2. Hughes AJ, Daniel SE, Kilford L, Lees AJ. The accuracy of the clinical diagnosis of Parkinson's disease: A clinicopathological study of 100 cases. J Neurol Neurosurg Psychiatry 1992;55:181–184.

3. Rajput AH, Offord KP, Beard CM, Kurland LT. Epidemiology of parkinsonism: Incidence, classification and mortality. Can J Neurol Sci 1992;19:103–107.
4. Gorell JM, Johnson CC, Rybicki BA, et al. Occupational exposures to metals as risk factors for Parkinson's disease. Neurology 1997; 48:650–658.
5. Morens DM, Grandinetti A, Reed D, et al. Cigarette smoking and protection from Parkinson's disease: False association or etiologic clue? Neurology 1995;45:1041–1051.
6. Polymeropoulos MH, Lavedan C, Leroy E, et al. Mutation in the α-synuclein gene identified in families with Parkinson's disease. Science 1997;276:2045–2047.
7. Calne DB. The free radical hypothesis in idiopathic Parkinsonism: Evidence against it. Ann Neurol 1992;32:799–803.
8. Fahn S, Cohen G. The oxidant stress hypothesis in Parkinson's disease: Evidence supporting it. Ann Neurol 1992;32:804–812.
9. Meara RJ. Review: The pathophysiology of the motor signs in Parkinson's disease. Age Ageing 1994;23:342–346.
10. Jarvie KR, Caron MG. Heterogeneity of dopamine receptors. Adv Neurol 1993;60:325–333.
11. Mercuri NB, Calabresi P, Bernardi G. Physiology and pharmacology of dopamine D_2 receptors: Their implications in dopamine-substitute therapy for Parkinson's disease. Neurology 1989;39:1106–1108.
12. Bernheimer H, Birkmayer W, Hornykiewicz O, et al. Brain dopamine and the syndrome of Parkinson's and Huntington: Clinical, morphological, and neurochemical correlations. J Neurol Sci 1973;20: 415–455.
13. Calne DB, Snow BJ. PET imaging in parkinsonism. Adv Neurol 1993;60:484–487.
14. Rutgers AWF, Lakke JPWF, Paans AMJ, et al. Tracing of dopamine receptors in hemiparkinsonism with positron emission tomography. J Neurol Sci 1987;80:237–248.
15. Pizzolato G, Chierichetti F, Rossato A, et al. Dopamine receptor SPECT imaging in Parkinson's disease: A [^{23}I]-IBZM and [^{99m}Tc]-HM-PAO study. Eur Neurol 1993;33:143–148.
16. Post RM. Intermittent versus continuous stimulation: Effect of time on the development of sensitization or tolerance. Life Sci 1980;26: 1275–1282.
17. LeWitt PA, Miller LP, Newman RP, et al. Tyrosine hydroxylase cofactor (tetrahydrobiopterin) in Parkinsonism. Adv Neurol 1984:40: 459–462.
18. Gibb WRG, Lees AJ. The relevance of the Lewy body to the pathogenesis of idiopathic Parkinson's disease. J Neurol Neurosurg Psychiatry 1988;51:745–752.
19. Hoehn MH, Yahr MD. Parkinsonism: Onset, progression and mortality. Neurology 1967:17:427–442.
20. Martin WE, Loewenson RB, Resch JA, Baker AB. Parkinson's disease. Clinical analysis of 100 patients. Neurology 1973;23:783–790.
21. Goetz CG, DeLong MR, Penn RD, Bakay RAE. Neurosurgical horizons in Parkinson's disease. Neurology 1993;43:1–7.
22. Widner H, Rehncrona S. Transplantation and surgical treatment of parkinsonian syndromes. Curr Opin Neurol 1993;6:344–349.
23. Olanow CW. Gpi pallidotomy—Have we made a dent in Parkinson's disease? Ann Neurol 1996;40:341–343.
24. Koller WC, Silver DE, Lieberman A. An algorithm for the management of Parkinson's disease. Neurology 1994;44(suppl 10)1–52.
25. Hubble JP, Koller WC, Waters C. Effects of selegiline dosing on motor fluctuations in Parkinson's disease. Clin Neuropharmacol 1993;16: 83–87.
26. Heinonen EH, Myllyla V, Sotaniemi K, et al. Pharmacokinetics and metabolism of selegiline. Acta Neurol Scand 1989;80(suppl 126):93–99.
27. Elsworth JD, Glover V, Reynolds GP, et al. Deprenyl administration in man: A selective MAO-B inhibitor without "cheese-effect". Psychopharmacology 1987;57:33–38.
28. Richard IH, Kurlan R, Tanner C, et al. Serotonin syndrome and the combined use of deprenyl and an antidepressant in Parkinson's disease. Neurology 1997;48:1070–1077.
29. Zornberg GL, Bodkin JA, Cohen BM. Severe adverse interaction between pethidine and selegiline. Lancet 1991;337:246.
30. The Parkinson Study Group. Effect of deprenyl on the progression of disability in early Parkinson's disease. N Engl J Med 1989;321: 1364–1371.
31. The Parkinson Study Group. Effects of tocopherol and deprenyl on the progression of disability in Parkinson's disease. N Engl J Med 1993; 328:176–183.
32. Olanow CW, Hauser RA, Gauger L, et al. The effect of deprenyl and levodopa on the progression of Parkinson's disease. Ann Neurol 1995; 38:771–777.
33. Brannan T, Yahr MD. Comparative study of selegiline plus L-dopa-carbidopa versus L-dopa-carbidopa alone in the treatment of Parkinson's disease. Ann Neurol 1995;37:95–98.
34. Landau WM. Clinical neuromythology, 9. Pyramid sale in the bucket shop: DATATOP bottoms out. Neurology 1990;40:1337–1339.
35. Schulzer M, Mak E, Calne DB. The antiparkinsonian efficacy of deprenyl derives from transient improvement that is likely to be symptomatic. Ann Neurol 1992;32:795–798.
36. Lees AJ on behalf of the Parkinson's Disease Research Group of the United Kingdom. Comparison of therapeutic effects and mortality data of levodopa and levodopa combined with selegiline in patients with early mild Parkinson's disease. BMJ 1995;311:1602–1606.
37. Ahlskog JE. Treatment of early Parkinson's disease: Are complicated strategies justified? Mayo Clinic Proc 1996;71:659–670.
38. Van Spaendonick KPM, Berger HJC, Hortink MWI, et al. Impaired cognitive shifting in parksinsonian patients on anticholinergic therapy. Neuropsychologia 1993;31:407–411.
39. Fahn S, Isgreen W. Long-term evaluation of amantadine and levodopa combination in parkinsonism by double-blind crossover analysis. Neurology 1975;25:695–700.
40. Jackisch R, Link T, Neufang B, Koch R. Studies on the mechanism of the antiparkinsonian drugs memantine and amantadine: No evidence for direct dopaminomimetic or antimuscarinic properties. Arch Int Pharmacodyn Ther 1992;320:21–42.
41. Cotzias CG, Van Woert MH, Schiffer LM. Aromatic amino acids and modification of parkinsonism. N Engl J Med 1967;276:374–379.
42. Papavasilou PS, Cotzias GC, Duby SE, et al. Levodopa in parkinsonism: Potentiation of central effects with a peripheral inhibitor. N Engl J Med 1972;285:8–14.
43. Ward CD, Trombley LK, Caine DB, et al. L-dopa decarboxylation in chronically treated patients. Neurology 1984;34:198–201.
44. Poewe WH, Wenning GK. The natural history of Parkinson's disease. Neurology 1996;47(suppl 3):S146–S152.
45. Stocchi F, Nordera G, Marsen CD. Strategies for treating patients with advanced Parkinson's disease with disastrous fluctuations and dyskinesias. Clin Neuropharmacol 1997;20:95–115.
46. LeWitt PA, Nelson MV, Berchou RC, et al. Controlled-release carbidopa/levodopa (Sinemet 50/200 CR4): Clinical and pharmacokinetic studies. Neurology 1989;39(suppl 2):45–53.
47. Stocchi F, Quinn NP, Barbato L, et al. Comparison between a fast and a slow release preparation of levodopa and a combination of the two: A clinical and pharmacokinetic study. Clin Neuropharmacol 1994;17: 38–44.
48. Quinn N, Parkes JD, Marsden CD. Control of on/off phenomenon by continuous intravenous infusion of levodopa. Neurology 1984;34: 1131–1136.
49. Kurth MC, Tetrud JW, Tanner CM, et al. Double-blind, placebo-controlled crossover study of duodenal infusion of levodopa/carbidopa in Parkinson's disease patients with "on-off" fluctuations. Neurology 1993;43:1698–1703.
50. Kurth MC, Tetrud JW, Irwin I, et al. Oral levodopa/carbidopa solution versus tablets in Parkinson's patients with severe fluctuations: A pilot study. Neurology 1993;43:1036–1039.
51. LeWitt PA. Treatment strategies for extension of levodopa effect. Neurol Clin 1992;10:511–526.

52. Kurth MC, Adler CH, St. Hilaire M, et al. Tolcapone improves motor function and reduces levodopa requirement in patients with Parkinson's disease experiencing motor fluctuations: A multicenter, double-blind, randomized, placebo-controlled trial. Neurology 1997;48: 81–87.
53. Hillen ME, Sage JI. Nonmotor fluctuations in patients with Parkinson's disease. Neurology 1996;47:1180–1183.
54. Nelson MV, Berchou RC, LeWitt PA, et al. Pharmacodynamic modeling of concentration-effect relationships after controlled release carbidopa/levodopa (Sinemet CR4) in Parkinson's disease. Neurology 1990;40:70–74.
55. Contin M, Riva R, Martinelli P, et al. Pharmacodynamic modeling of oral levodopa: Clinical application in Parkinson's disease. Neurology 1993;43:367–371.
56. Contin M, Riva R, Martinelli P, et al. Longitudinal monitoring of the levodopa concentration-effect relationship in Parkinson's disease. Neurology 1994;44:1287–1292.
57. Nutt JG, Holford NHG. The response to levodopa in Parkinson's disease: Imposing pharmacological law and order. Ann Neurol 1996;39: 561–573.
58. Baronti F, Mouradian MM, Conant KE, et al. Partial dopamine agonist therapy of levodopa-induced dyskinesias. Neurology 1992;42: 1241–1244.
59. Giorotti F, Soliveri P, Carella F, et al. Dementia and cognitive impairment in Parkinsons's disease. J Neurol Neurosurg Psychiatry 1988;51: 1498–1502.
60. Arevalo GJG, Gershanik OS. Modulatory effect of clozapine on levodopa response in Parkinson's disease: A preliminary study. Mov Disord 1993;8:349–354.
61. Pinter MM, Helscher RJ. Therapeutic effect of clozapine in psychotic decompensation in idiopathic Parkinson's disease. J Neural Transm Park Dis Dement Sect 1993;5:135–146.
62. Wolters EC, Jansen ENH, Tuynman-Qua HG, Bergmans PLM. Onlanzapine in the treatment of dopaminomimetic psychosis in patients with Parkinson's disease. Neurology 1996;47:1085–1087.
63. Fahn S, Bressman SB. Should levodopa therapy for parkinsonism be started early or late? Evidence against early treatment. Can J Neurol Sci 1984;11:200–206.
64. Muenter MD. Should levodopa therapy be started early or late? Can J Neurol Sci 1984;11:195–199.
65. Rajput AH, Stern W, Laverty WH. Chronic low-done levodopa therapy in Parkinson's disease: An argument for delaying levodopa therapy. Neurology 1984;34:991–996.
66. Diamond SG, Markham CH, Hoehn MM, et al. Multi-center study of Parkinson mortality with early versus later dopa treatment. Ann Neurol 1987;22:8–12.
67. Rivera-Calimlim L, Dujovne CA, Morgan JP, et al. L-Dopa treatment failure: Explanation and correction. Br Med J 1970;4:93–94.
68. Djaldetti R, Koren M, Ziv I, et al. Effect of cisapride on response fluctuations in Parkinson's disease. Mov Disord 1995;10:81–84.
69. Nutt JG, Woodward WR, Hammerstad JP, et al. The "on-off" phenomenon in Parkinson's disease: Relation to levodopa absorption and transport. N Engl J Med 1984;310:483–488.
70. Berry EM, Growdon JH, Wurtman JJ, et al. A balanced carbohydrate: protein diet in the management of Parkinson's disease. Neurology 1991;41:1295–1297.
71. Sasahara K, Nitanai T, Habara T, et al. Dosage form design for improvement of bioavailability of levodopa III: Influence of dose on pharmacokinetic behavior of levodopa in dogs and parkinsonian patients. J Pharm Sci 1980;69:1374–1378.
72. Pezzoli G, Martinoni E, Pacchetti C, et al. A crossover, controlled study comparing pergolide with bromocriptine as an adjunct to levodopa for the treatment of Parkinson's disease. Neurology 1995;45 (suppl 3):S22–S27.
73. Lieberman A, Neophytides A, Liebowitz M, et al. Comparative efficacy of pergolide and bromocriptine in patients with advanced Parkinson's disease. Adv Neurol 1983;37:95–108.
74. Olanow CW. Pergolide, parlodel crossover study. Neurology 1988;38: 314–316.
75. Tashiro K, Goto I, Kanazawa I, et al. Eight-year follow-up study of bromocriptine monotherapy for Parkinson's disease. Eur Neurol 1996; 36(suppl 1):32–37.
76. Hely MA, Morris JGL, Reid WGJ, et al. The Sidney multicentre study of Parkinson's disease: A randomised, prospective five year study comparing low dose bromocriptine with low dose levodopa-carbidopa. J Neurol Neurosurg Psychiatry 1994;57:903–910.
77. Watts RL. The role of dopamine agonists in early Parkinson's disease. Neurology 1997;49(suppl 1):S34–S48.
78. Przuntek H, Welzel D, Gerlach M, et al. Early institution of bromocriptine in Parkinson's disease inhibits the emergence of levodopa-associated motor side effects. Long term results of the PRADO study. J Neurol Transm 1996;103;699–715.
79. Montastruc JL, Rascol O, Senard JM, Rascol A. A randomised controlled study comparing bromocriptine to which levodopa was later added, with levodopa alone in previously untreated patients with Parkinson's disease: A five-year follow up. J Neurol Neurosurg Psychiatry 1994;57:1034–1038.
80. UK Bromocriptine Research Group. Bromocriptine in Parkinson's disease: A double blind study comparing "low-slow" and "high-fast" introductory dosage regimens in de novo patients. J Neurol Neurosurg Psychiatry 1989;52:77–82.
81. Parkinson Study Group. Safety and efficacy of pramipexole in early Parkinson disease. A randomized dose-ranging study. JAMA 1997; 278:125–130.
82. Cedarbaum JM. Clinical pharmacokinetics of anti-parkinsonian drugs. Clin Pharmacokinet 1987;13:141–178.
83. Mannen T, Mizuno Y, Iwata M, et al. A multi-center, double-blind study on slow release bromocriptine in the treatment of Parkinson's disease. Neurology 1991;41:1598–1602.
84. Nelson MV, Berchou RC, Kareti D, LeWitt PA. Pharmacokinetic evaluation of erythromycin and caffeine administered with bromocriptine. Clin Pharmacol Ther 1990;47:694–697.
85. Bloomer JC, Clarke SE, Chenery RJ. *In vitro* identification of the P450 enzymes responsible for the metabolism of ropinirole. Drug Metab Dist 1997;25:840–844.
86. Inzelberg R, Nisipeanu P, Rabey JM, et al. Double-blind comparison of cabergoline and bromocriptine in Parkinson's disease patients with motor fluctuations. Neurology 1996;47:785–788.
87. Stocchi F, Bramante L, Monge A, et al. Apomorphine and lisuride infusion: A comparative chronic study. Adv Neurol 1993;60:653–655.
88. Montastruc JL, Rascol O, Senard JM, et al. Sublingual apomorphine in Parkinson's disease: A clinical and pharmacokinetic study. Clin Neuropharmacol 1991;14:432–437.
89. Van Laar T, Jansen ENH, Essink AWG, Neef C. Intranasal apomorphine in parkinsonian on-off fluctuations. Arch Neurol 1992;49:482–484.
90. Tsui JKC, Wolters EC, Peppard RF, Calne DB. A double-blind, placebo controlled, dose ranging study to investigate the safety and efficacy of CY 208-243 in patients with Parkinson's disease. Neurology 1989;39:856–858.
91. Quinn N, Illas A, Lhermitte F, Agid Y. Bromocriptine and domperidone in the treatment of Parkinson's disease. Neurology 1981;31: 662–667.
92. Quattrone A, Zappia M. Oral pulse levodopa therapy in mild Parkinson's disease. Neurology 1993;43:1161–1166.

56

PAIN MANAGEMENT

Terry J. Baumann, PharmD, BCPS

Although the world is full of suffering, it is also full of the overcoming of it.

Helen Keller[1]

Humans have always known and sought relief from pain. The act of relieving pain is probably as old as the medical profession itself. Today, pain's impact on society is still great, and indeed, pain complaints are the number one reason patients seek medical advice.[2]

Regrettably, many health care providers do not receive adequate training in this area, and new information is not widely disseminated and/or understood. Clearly, pain management is enhanced when a multidisciplinary approach is applied. Thus, understanding the pathophysiology of pain therapy, and maintaining a working knowledge of individual pain regimens, are important to clinicians and are key factors in reversing the problem of inadequate pain control.

DEFINITION

An acceptable definition of pain remains an enigma. Once thought to be a punishment from the gods, the word is derived from the Latin *peone* and the Greek *poine,* meaning "penalty" or "punishment."[3] This punishment theory was advanced by Aristotle, who considered pain a feeling and classified it as a passion of the soul. Two thousand years later, Descartes, Galen, and Vaselius postulated that pain was a sensation in which the brain played an important role. In the 19th century, Mueller, Van Frey, and Goldscheider hypothesized the concepts of neuroreceptors, nociceptors, and sensory input.[3] These theories developed into the 20th century's definition of pain: "an unpleasant sensory and emotional experience associated with actual or potential tissue damage or described in terms of such damage."[4] Pain is often so subjective however, that many clinicians define pain as whatever the patient feels it is.

EPIDEMIOLOGY

Most Americans experience three or four different types of pain every year. Over 50 million people are partially or totally disabled because of pain. The annual cost of pain to American society is an estimated $79 billion.[2]

Unfortunately, pain is often undertreated and pain management greatly misunderstood.[5–8] Marks and Sacher[5] studied hospitalized medical patients receiving opiates and found 73% in severe or moderate distress despite their analgesic regimen. Caregivers' misconceptions regarding opiate doses, duration of analgesic effect, and fear of addiction were reportedly responsible for this undertreatment.[5] Cohen demonstrated that despite opiate analgesics, 75% of postsurgical patients were in moderate or marked distress, and 45% "cried out" in pain.[6] Fear of addiction and inadequate knowledge of pharmacologic agents were again considered major factors contributing to pain mismanagement.[6] Similar problems are reported in ambulatory patients.[9]

PATHOPHYSIOLOGY

The pathophysiology of pain involves a complex series of neuronal connections that have not been fully elucidated; however, research over the last 30 years has greatly advanced our understanding of pain transmission.

AFFERENT PAIN TRANSMISSION

PERIPHERAL STIMULATION

The first step leading to the sensation of pain is the stimulation of receptors known as nociceptors. The exact mechanism that underlies the stimulation of nociceptors is not completely understood; however, bradykinins, H^+, K^+, prostaglandins, histamine, leukotrienes, and serotonin sensitize these receptors. Receptor activation leads to action potentials that are transmitted along afferent nerve fibers to the spinal cord.[10,11]

Somatostatin, cholecystokinin, and substance P have been identified as possible neurotransmitters in afferent nociceptive neurons.[11] In addition, substance P may play a role in enhancing the effectiveness of nociceptive neurotransmitters that promote pain.[10] In fact, when substance P is blocked by the neurotoxin capsaicin, pain transmission is significantly reduced, making substance P antagonists a separate class of analgesics.[12] Topical creams containing capsaicin (0.025%, 0.075%, and 0.25%) are available for the treatment of painful neuralgias.[12]

Nociceptive transmission takes place in the A-delta or C afferent nerve fibers.[11] Stimulation of A-delta fibers evokes sharp, acute, well-localized pain, while stimulation of C fibers produces dull, aching, and poorly localized pain.[11]

GATE CONTROL THEORY

Afferent, nociceptive pain fibers synapse in the dorsal horn of the spinal cord along with many other non–pain-transmitting or nonnociceptive neurons. Synapses are made directly onto pain transmission neurons (PTNs) or onto interconnecting neurons (ICNs) that excite PTNs. In addition, large nonnociceptive fibers originating either in the periphery or in neurons descending from the spinal cord may inhibit both PTNs and ICNs in the dorsal horn. When large myelinated fibers are stimulated, they have an inhibitory affect on pain transmission. Therefore, perception of pain is a complex summation of nonnociceptive and nociceptive neuronal stimulation (Fig. 56–1).[13]

Functionally, the importance of the interplay between these different fibers is evident in the analgesic response produced by treatments that stimulate large nonnociceptive neurons, for example, topical irritants, acupuncture, or transcutaneous electrical nerve stimulation. Although modified, this theory was first explained by Melzack and Wall[14] and is referred to as the gate control theory of pain transmission.

SPINAL CORD TRANSMISSION

Pain-initiated processes reach the brain through a complex array of ascending spinal cord pathways. In addition, information other than pain is carried along these pathways. Thus, pain is influenced by many factors supplemental to nociception and precludes simple schematic representation; however, one major ascending pathway, the spinothalamic tract, is known to have a major influence on pain transmission and is classically divided into lateral and ventral pathways. The lateral pathway is associated with sharp localized pain and is responsible for the spatial and temporal discriminative aspects of nociception.[3] The ventral pathway makes possible the perception of aching, dull, nonlocalized pain and the reflexes responsible for aversion motivation.[3] Both pathways eventually merge in the thalamus and connect with the cortex.

PAIN MODULATION

The brain modulates pain through a system that is just beginning to be understood. First evidence of this system was the analgesia produced by selected electrical stimulation of animal brains,[15,16] with subsequent similar results in patients with intractable clinical pain.[17] Almost simultaneously, other investigators discovered opiate receptors within the central nervous system.[18–20] These opiate receptors are found in the ascending and descending pain pathways and in portions of the brain believed to be essential to the pain-modulating system.[10] In 1975, researchers[21,22] identified two pentapeptides (Metenkephalin and Leu-enkephalin) with actions similar to morphine. These enkephalins interact with opiate receptors to form, in part, what is known as the endogenous opiate system.[3] Three classes of opioid peptides are known: the enkephalins, dynorphins, and β-endorphins. Although all three are important in the endogenous opiate system, each class originates from a different precursor and has a distinct anatomic distribution.[10] All are generically referred to as endorphins. As the knowledge of endorphins has expanded, so has the understanding of opiate receptors. Three major classes of such receptors—mu, delta, and kappa—as well as subtypes within each class, have been recognized.[23] These receptors display varying affinities for the endorphins and exhibit varying effects when stimulated (Table 56–1).[23]

The development of opioid antagonists (substances that block endogenous opiate receptors) led to the discovery of a highly integrated network associating pain, opiate receptors, and endorphins. Although the endogenous opioid relationship is still not completely defined, it may moderate pain through a positive and negative feedback system. Thus, a given nociceptive stimulus activates both peripheral pain transmission pathways (causing pain and called *positive feedback*) and the brain's modulatory network (inhibiting pain and called *negative feedback*), making the sensation of pain a partial summation of these two processes.[13] Other neurotransmitter substances known to play a role in pain regulation include norepinephrine and serotonin.[11]

The CNS also contains a highly organized descending system for control of pain transmission. This system influences synaptic transmission of sensory fibers at the dorsal horn level of the spinal cord and is dependent on the biogenic amine neurotransmitters and other networks previously mentioned.[10]

In summary, although progress has occurred in unraveling the pain transmission mystery, understanding of this

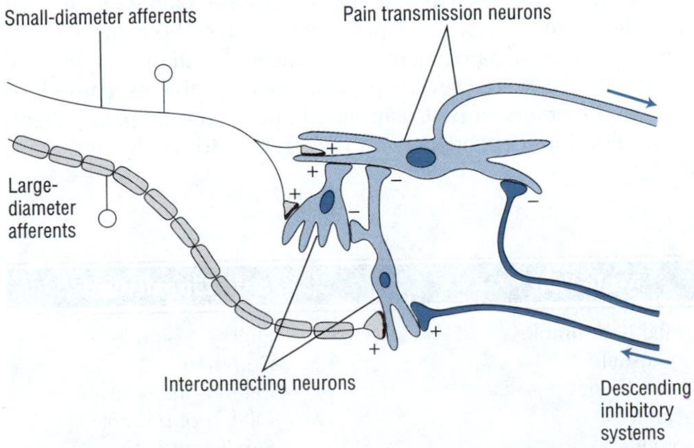

FIGURE 56–1. Schematic representation of dorsal horn nociceptive modulation. (+ = excitatory connection; – = inhibitory connection.) *(Reprinted from Ref. 13, with permission.)*

TABLE 56–1. Opiate Receptor Effects

Opiate Receptor	Function
Mu	Analgesia Respiratory depression Miosis Reduced gastric motility Sedation Euphoria
Kappa	Analgesia Less respiratory depression than mu Less intense miosis than mu Sedation Reduced gastric motility Dysphoria Psychotomimetic effects
Delta	Analgesia

Modified from Ref. 23, with permission.

complex pathway is still limited. Pain without nociception (algodynia), neuropathic pain, sympathetically maintained pain, and phantom limb pain (pain in a limb that has been amputated) are very real phenomena, but defy the nociceptive pathway previously outlined. Future research will augment our present knowledge of neurophysiology and further clarify the roles of neuromodulaters and neurotransmitters.

CLINICAL PRESENTATION

Clinical presentation of pain is best addressed by proper pain assessment. A patient-oriented approach is essential, and evaluation methods should not differ from those used in other medical conditions.[3] Therefore, a comprehensive history and physical examination are imperative to thoroughly evaluate underlying diseases and possible contributing factors.[3] A baseline description of pain can be obtained by assessing PQRST characteristics (Table 56–2).[24] Attention must also be given to mental factors that alter the pain threshold. Anxiety, depression, fatigue, anger, and fear are particularly noted to lower this threshold, whereas rest, mood elevation, sympathy, diversion, and understanding raise the pain threshold.[24]

Clinicians must evaluate all components of the pain experience, including behavioral components (much of our reaction to pain is learned),[25] cognitive components (thinking processes alter pain experiences),[26] social factors (pain expression differs in accordance with social environments),[27] and cultural influences (cultural background may influence pain tolerance).[27] In addition, separating pain with a known organic cause from that with no known cause allows for improved treatment regimens.[3] Pain with a known source is often localized, well described, and relieved with proper analgesic therapy, whereas pain with no obvious origin is often nonlocalized, ill defined, and not easily treated with conventional analgesics.[3] Proper patient assessment must also include an evaluation of pain management. Pain intensity, pain relief, and medication side effects must be assessed and reassessed on a regular basis. The timing and regularity of this assessment will depend on the type of pain and the medications administered. Postoperative pain and acute exacerbation of cancer pain may need to be assessed every hour, while chronic nonmalignant pain may need only daily assessment. Quality of life must also be assessed on a regular basis in all patients.

The clinician must remember, however, that "pain is always subjective. Objective observations of grimacing, limping, and tachycardia may be useful in assessing the patient, but these signs are often absent in patients with chronic pain known to be caused by structural lesions. There is no neurophysiologic or chemical test that can measure pain. The clinician does well in the absence of strong contrary evidence to accept the patient's report of pain."[28]

TABLE 56–2. PQRST Characteristics of Pain

P	Palliative factors	What makes the pain better?
	Provocative factors	What makes the pain worse?
Q	Quality	Describe the pain.
R	Radiation	Where is the pain?
S	Severity	How does this pain compare with other pain you have experienced?
T	Temporal factors	Does the intensity of the pain change with time?

Modified from Ref. 24.

▶ TREATMENT: Acute and Chronic Pain

Acute pain may be a useful physiologic process warning individuals of disease states and potentially harmful situations. Unfortunately, severe, unremitting, undertreated, acute pain, when it outlives its biologic usefulness, can produce many deleterious effects (e.g., psychological problems). When pain is not effectively treated, the stress and concurrent reflex reactions often cause hypoxia, hypercapnia, hypertension, excessive cardiac activity, and emotional difficulties.

Under normal conditions, acute pain quickly subsides as the healing process decreases the pain-producing stimuli; however, in some instances, pain may persist for months to years, leading to a *chronic pain* state with features quite different from those of acute pain (Table 56–3). Chronic pain can be divided into four subtypes: pain that persists beyond the normal healing time for an acute injury, pain related to a chronic disease, pain without identifiable organic cause, and pain that involves both the chronic and acute pain associated with cancer.[29] Patients in chronic pain often develop severe psychological problems caused by fear and memory of past pain. In addition, chronic pain patients may develop dependence and tolerance to analgesics, have

TABLE 56–3. Characteristics of Acute and Chronic Pain

Characteristic	Acute Pain	Chronic Pain
Relief of pain	Highly desirable	Highly desirable
Dependence and tolerance to medication	Unusual	Common
Psychological component	Usually not present	Often a major problem
Organic cause	Common	Often not present
Environmental contributions and family involvement	Small	Significant
Insomnia	Unusual	Common component
Treatment goal	Cure	Rehabilitation, not a cure

Modified from Ref. 3.

trouble sleeping, and more readily react to environmental changes that can intensify the pain response. Distinguishing between chronic and acute pain states is very important because of differing management techniques.[28]

ACUTE PAIN

The obvious way to relieve pain is to eliminate the underlying cause. This is often not possible, however, and symptomatic relief is usually indicated. Therapeutic interventions include pharmacologic treatment, stimulation therapies, and psychological therapies.

NONPHARMACOLOGIC THERAPY

STIMULATION THERAPY

Transcutaneous electrical nerve stimulation (TENS) has shown moderate success in managing postoperative pain.[30] Although opioid-like side effects are certainly prevented, this technique has not gained wide acceptance.

PSYCHOLOGICAL INTERVENTION

Even though the cognitive, behavioral, and social aspects of pain are well established, psychological techniques for the treatment of acute pain are not widely employed. Simple interventions (e.g., introductory information about sensations to expect after certain procedures) reduce patient distress and greatly reduce postprocedure suffering.[30] Other successful psychological techniques include relaxation training, controlled mental imagery, controlled attention or distraction, hypnosis, and biofeedback.

PHARMACOLOGIC THERAPY

NONOPIOID AGENTS

Analgesia should be initiated with the most effective analgesic agent having the fewest side effects. Acetaminophen, acetylsalicylic acid (aspirin), and nonsteroidal anti-inflammatory drugs (NSAIDs) are often preferred over opiates in the treatment of acute, mild to moderate pain (Tables 56–4 and 56–5). These drugs (with the exception of acetaminophen) affect the prostaglandins produced by the arachidonic acid cascade in response to noxious stimuli,[31] thereby decreasing the number of pain impulses received by the CNS. Therapeutic outcomes are also less than desired in those who do not expect "mild" analgesics to relieve pain. Studies comparing the efficacy of these agents have been inconsistent. Therefore, the choice of a particular agent often depends upon availability, cost, and pharmacokinetic and pharmacologic characteristics (Tables 56–4 and 56–5), and the side-effect profile (Table 56–6). It should be noted that all NSAIDs have some analgesic effects, but only those that are FDA approved for the treatment of pain are compared in the tables. There appears to be a great deal of interpatient variability in the therapeutic response to the NSAIDs. After an adequate drug trial of any of these agents, it is considered rational therapy to switch to another member of this drug group for an additional trial period.

OPIOID AGENTS

Most clinicians consider the use of opioids to be the next logical step in the management of acute pain. The classification of these agents, their equianalgesic doses, and dosing guidelines are outlined in Tables 56–7 and 56–8.

The pharmacologic activity of opioids depends on their affinity for opiate receptors.[32] Therapeutic activities and side effects range from those exhibited by the pure opiate agonists (e.g., morphine) to those seen with the pure opiate antagonists (e.g., naloxone). Partial agonists and antagonists (e.g., pentazocine) compete with agonists for opiate receptor sites and, depending on the inherent agonist and antagonist properties, exhibit mixed agonist–antagonist activity. Mixed agonist–antagonist agents with analgesic activity appear to exhibit selectivity for analgesic receptor sites.[32] This may result in analgesia with fewer undesirable side effects.

The effects of the opioid analgesics are relatively selective, and at normal therapeutic concentrations, these agents do not decrease sensitivity to touch, sight, or hearing.[23] As the dosage increases, however, so do the undesirable side effects (Table 56–9). Patients in severe pain may receive very high doses of opioids with no unwanted side effects, but as the pain subsides, will not tolerate even very low doses.[23] Frequently, patients report pain is not eliminated but its unpleasantness is decreased.[23]

TABLE 56–4. Pharmacokinetic and Pharmacodynamic Profiles of FDA-Approved Nonopioid Analgesics

Agent	Time to Peak Concentration (h)	Elimination Half-life (h)	Analgesic Onset (h)	Analgesic Duration (h)
Aspirin	0.25–2	0.25–0.33	0.5	3–6
Choline salicylate	1.5–2	—[a]	—[a]	4
Magnesium salicylate	1.5–2	—[a]	—[a]	4
Sodium salicylate	0.67	—[a]	—[a]	4
Diflunisal	2–3	8–12	1	8–12
Acetaminophen	0.5–2	1–4	0.5–1	3–6
Meclofenamate	0.5–2	2.3–3.3	—[a]	4–6
Mefenamic acid	2–4	2–4	—[a]	6
Etodoloc	1	7	0.5–1	6–8
Diclofenac potassium	1	2	0.5	6–8
Ibuprofen	1–2	1–2.5	0.5	4–6
Fenoprofen	1–2	2–3	0.25–0.5	4–6
Ketoprofen	0.5–2	2–4	1	3–4
Naproxen	2–4	12–15	1	Up to 7
Naproxen sodium	1–2	12–13	1	Up to 7
Ketorolac (parenteral)	0.5–1	4–6	0.17	6
Ketorolac (oral)	0.5–1	4–6	0.5–1	4–6

[a]Data not available.
Compiled from Refs. 35, 36, and 46–50.

TABLE 56–5. FDA-Approved Nonopioid Analgesics

Class and Generic Name	Usual Dosage Range (mg)	Maximum Dose (mg/d)
Salicylates		
Acetylsalicylic acid[a] (aspirin)	325–650 every 4 h	5400
Choline[a]	870 every 3–4 h	5220
Magnesium[a]	500 every 4 h	4800
Sodium[a]	325–650 every 4 h	5400
Diflunisal	250–500 every 8–12 h	1500
Para-aminophenol		
Acetaminophen[a]	325–650 every 4–6 h	4000
Fenamates		
Meclofenamate	50 every 4–6 h	400
Mefenamic acid	250 every 6 h (maximum of 7 days)	1000[b]
Acetic Acid		
Etodoloc	200–400 every 6–8 h	1200
Diclofenac potassium	50 three times a day	150[c]
Propionic Acids		
Ibuprofen[a]	200–400 every 4–6 h	3200
Fenoprofen	200 every 4–6 h	3200
Ketoprofen[a]	25–50 every 6–8 h	300
Naproxen	250 every 6–12 h	1250
Naproxen sodium[a]	220 every 8–12 h	660[d]
Naproxen delayed release[e]	375–500 every 12 h	1250
Naproxen controlled release	750–1000 every 24 h	1000
Ketorolac (parenteral)	15–30 every 6 h (maximum of 5 days)	120
Ketorolac (oral)	10 every 4–6 h (maximum of 5 days)	40

[a]Available both as an over-the-counter preparation and as a prescription drug.
[b]Up to 1250 mg on the first day.
[c]Up to 200 mg on the first day.
[d]Over-the-counter dose.
[e]Not for the initial treatment of acute pain.
Compiled from Refs. 35, 36, and 46.

Opioids share related pharmacologic attributes and exert profound effects on the CNS and gastrointestinal tract.[23] Mood changes, sedation, respiratory depression, nausea, vomiting, decreased gastrointestinal motility, dependence, and tolerance are evident in varying degrees with all agents. Consideration of efficacy and side-effect profile assists in the selection of the most appropriate agent.

The route of administration depends on individual patient needs. Peak analgesic effect usually occurs 1.5 to 2 hours after oral administration and must be considered when immediate relief is needed.[28] The opioids differ greatly in equianalgesic dose. Table 56–7 should be used only as a guide, because the nature of pain makes it necessary to individualize pain regimens. True opioid allergies are rare, but Table 56–7 can also be used when treating a patient hypersensitive to opiates. Although caution is always advised, cross-sensitivity between the morphine-like, meperidine-like, and methadone-like agonists is less likely than among the like agents. When considering cross-sensitivity, the mixed agonist–antagonist class acts much like the morphine-like agonists.[33]

In the initial stages of acute pain, analgesics should be given around the clock. This should commence after administering a typical starting dose and titrating up or down depending on the patient's degree of pain and demonstrated side effects (e.g., sedation).[28] As-needed schedules often produce wide swings in analgesic plasma concentrations that create wide swings in pain and sedation. This may initiate a vicious cycle where increasing amounts of pain medications are needed for relief. As the painful state subsides and the need for medication decreases, however, as-needed schedules can be used. Continuous intravenous and subcutaneous methods of narcotic infusion are effective in some postoperative pain,[28] but the probability of unwanted side effects is

TABLE 56–6. Relative Side Effects of FDA-Approved Nonopioid Analgesics

Agent	GI Irritation	CNS Effects	Hepatic Toxicity	Renal Toxicity
Aspirin	+++++	+	++	++
Choline salicylate	+++	—[a]	—[a]	—[a]
Magnesium salicylate	+++	—[a]	—[a]	—[a]
Sodium salicylate	+++	—[a]	—[a]	—[a]
Diflunisal	++	+	+	+
Acetaminophen	+	+	++	+
Meclofenamate	++	+	+	++
Mefenamic acid	++	+	+	++
Etodolac	++	+	+	++
Diclofenac potassium	++	+	+	++
Ibuprofen	++	+	+	++
Fenoprofen	++	++	+	++
Ketoprofen	++	+	+	++
Ketorolac[b]	++	+	+	+
Naproxen	++	+	+	++

[a]Data not available.
[b]Five-day use only.
Compiled from Refs. 35 and 36.

TABLE 56–7. Opioid Analgesics

Class and Generic Name	Route	Equianalgesic Dose
Morphine-like Agonists		
Morphine	IM, SC	10 mg
	PO	30–60 mg
Hydromorphone	IM, SC	1.3 mg
	PO	7.5 mg
Oxymorphone	IM, SC	1.0 mg
	R	5 mg
Levorphanol	IM, SC	2.0 mg
	PO	4.0 mg
Codeine	IM	130 mg[a]
	PO	200 mg[a]
Hydrocodone	PO	5–10 mg[b]
Oxycodone	PO	5–10 mg[b]
Meperidine-like Agonists		
Meperidine	IM, SC	75 mg
	PO	300 mg[a]
Fentanyl	IM	0.1–0.2 mg
	Transdermal	25 μg/h[c]
	Transmucosal	Not available
Methadone-like Agonists		
Methadone	IM	10 mg
	PO	10–20 mg
Propoxyphene	PO	65 mg[b]
Mixed Agonist–Antagonists		
Pentazocine	IM, SC	30–60 mg
	PO	180 mg[a]
Butorphanol	IM	2.0 mg
	Intranasal	1.0 mg[b] (one spray)
Nalbuphine	IM	10 mg
Buprenorphine	IM	0.4 mg
Dezocine	IM	10 mg
Antagonists		
Naloxone	IV	0.4–1.2 mg[d]
Central Analgesic		
Tramadol	PO	50–100 mg[b]

[a] Starting doses lower (codeine, 15–30 mg; meperidine, 50 mg; pentazocine, 50 mg).
[b] Starting dose only (equianalgesia not shown).
[c] Equivalent IM morphine dose = 8–22 mg/d.
[d] Starting doses to be used in cases of opioid overdose.
Compiled from Refs. 23, 28, 36, 38, 39, and 51–54.

high. An alternative method that has gained prominence is patient-controlled analgesia (PCA). With this technique, patients can self-administer preset amounts of opioids via a syringe pump electronically interfaced with a timing device. Using this procedure, patients balance pain control with sedation.

Administration of opiates directly into the CNS (epidural and intrathecal) has shown considerable promise in the control of acute pain (Table 56–10)[34] and is becoming prominent in both large and small institutions throughout the United States. Because of reports of marked sedation, respiratory depression, pruritus, nausea, vomiting, urinary retention, and hypotension,[11] these methods of analgesia require careful monitoring and are best employed by experienced practitioners. Respiratory depression is of concern and can occur within the first 0.5 hour of opioid administration or manifest as late as 12 hours (especially shown with morphine) after single doses of spinal analgesia.[11] Naloxone is used to antagonize this effect, but continual infusion may be required.[11] Analgesia as well as side effects are evident at lower doses when the opioids are administered intrathecally instead of epidurally. Intrathecally, single morphine doses of 0.25 to 1 mg are common, whereas epidurally 5 to 10-mg doses are the norm. All opioids administered directly into the CNS should be preservative free.

MORPHINE AND CONGENERS

Despite the availability of several newer agents, morphine remains the prototype opiate analgesic. As new opioid and nonopioid compounds are developed, their efficacy and side-effect profiles are compared, with morphine as the standard. Many clinicians consider morphine the first-line agent when treating moderate to severe pain. Morphine can be given parenterally, orally, or rectally.

Morphine's CNS effects are numerous. Through direct stimulation of the chemoreceptor trigger zone, morphine causes nausea and vomiting,[23] which is observed more often in ambulatory patients,[35] and often subsides after the initial dose. Although euphoria and dysphoria have been reported, morphine's unpleasant effects are prominent when administered to those not experiencing pain.[23] As doses of morphine are increased, the respiratory center becomes less responsive to carbon dioxide, resulting in progressive respiratory depression. This effect is less pronounced in those being treated for severe pain. Respiratory depression is most often manifested as a decrease in respiratory rate, and is further compounded because the cough reflex is also depressed. Morphine-induced respiratory depression can be reversed by pure narcotic antagonists.[23] In patients with underlying pulmonary dysfunction, caution must be employed when using morphine or any related opioid. Although these patients may be functioning normally, they are already using compensatory breathing mechanisms and are at risk for further respiratory compromise.[23] Precaution is also urged when using opiate analgesics with alcohol or other CNS depressants. This combination amplifies CNS depression and is potentially quite harmful and possibly lethal.

Therapeutic doses of morphine have minimal effects on blood pressure, cardiac rate, or cardiac rhythm when patients are supine; however, morphine does produce venous and arteriolar vessel dilation, and orthostatic hypotension may result. Hypovolemic patients are more susceptible to morphine-induced cardiovascular changes (e.g., decreases in blood pressure).[23] Because morphine prompts a decrease in myocardial oxygen demand in ischemic cardiac patients, it is often considered the opioid of choice when using opioids to treat pain associated with myocardial infarction.

Morphine decreases the motility of the entire gastrointestinal tract, in turn reducing biliary and pancreatic secretions. The end result, especially when administered over extended time periods, is constipation. Morphine-induced spasms of the sphincter of Oddi have been observed.[23] However, the clinical significance of such an occurrence should be assessed on an individual basis. Although morphine's effect on the urinary bladder varies, urinary retention can become a problem; tolerance develops to this effect over time.[23] Morphine-induced histamine release often manifests as pruritus, and although not seen often, it may exacerbate bronchospasm in patients with a history of asthma.[23] Therapeutic doses of morphine do not directly affect cerebral circulation, but drug-induced respiratory depression can increase intracranial pressure. Thus caution is advised in head trauma patients who are not ventilated because morphine may exaggerate this pressure[23] while clouding the neurologic examination results.

Hydromorphone is more potent, has better oral absorption characteristics, and is more soluble than morphine; however, its overall pharmacologic profile parallels that of morphine. Oxymorphone can be administered rectally and by injection. Although it is more potent than morphine, it offers no real pharmacologic advantages. Although levorphanol has an extended half-life, its overall therapeutic effects are similar to those of morphine.

Codeine is an analgesic that is effective in the treatment of mild to moderate pain. It is often combined with other analgesic

TABLE 56–8. Dosing Guidelines

Agent(s)	Dose (Titrate up or down based on patient response)	Comments
NSAIDs/acetaminophen/ aspirin	Dose to maximum before switching to another agent (see Table 56–5)	Used in mild to moderate pain May use in conjunction with opioid agents to decrease doses of each Regular alcohol use and high doses of acetaminophen may result in liver toxicity Care must be exercised to avoid overdose when combination products containing these agents are used
Morphine	PO 10–30 mg q3–4h[a] IM 5–10 mg q3–4h[a] IV 1–2.5 mg q5min prn[a] SR 15–30 mg q12h (may need to be q8h in some patients) Rectal 10–20 mg q3–4h[a]	Drug of choice in acute severe pain Use immediate-release product with SR product to control breakthrough pain in cancer patients
Hydromorphone	PO 2–4 mg q3–4h[a] IM 0.5–1 mg q3–4h[a] IV 0.1–0.5 mg q5min prn[a] Rectal 2–4 mg q3–4h[a]	Use in severe pain More potent than morphine, otherwise no advantages
Oxymorphone	IM 1–1.5 mg q4–6h[a] IV 0.5 mg initially Rectal 5 mg q3–4h[a]	Use in severe pain No advantages over morphine
Levorphanol	PO 2–4 mg q6–8h IM 2 mg q6–8h IV 2 mg q6–8h	Use in severe pain Extended half-life, useful in cancer patients
Codeine	PO 15–60 mg q3–4h[a] IM 15–60 mg q3–4h[a] IV 15–60 mg q3–4h[a]	Use in moderate pain Weak analgesic, use with NSAIDs, aspirin, or acetaminophen
Hydrocodone	PO 5–10 mg q3–4h[a]	Use in moderate or severe pain Most effective when used with NSAIDs, aspirin, or acetaminophen
Oxycodone	PO 5–10 mg q3–4h[a] Controlled release 10–20 mg q12h	Use in moderate or severe pain Most effective when used with NSAIDs, aspirin, or acetaminophen Use immediate-release product with controlled-release product to control breakthrough pain in cancer patients

products and enjoys a popularity that makes it the standard for other oral opioids. Unfortunately, codeine has the same propensity to produce tolerance, dependence, and constipation as morphine. Hydrocodone, a derivative of codeine, is also most often seen in combination products and has pharmacologic properties similar to those of morphine. Oxycodone is an excellent oral analgesic for moderate to severe pain. This is especially true when the product is used in combination with a peripherally acting nonopioid agent; however, its predilection for causing tolerance and dependence, along with its basic opioid characteristics, likens it to morphine. It should be noted that sustained-release oxycodone is also now available.

MEPERIDINE AND CONGENERS (PHENYLPIPERIDINES)

The prototype phenylpiperidine, meperidine, has a pharmacologic profile comparable to that of morphine; however, it is not as potent and has a shorter analgesic duration. This necessitates larger doses that must be administered more frequently; several studies have shown that this is often not done.[5,6] Although meperidine is effective orally, larger doses must be administered to achieve the same effect as obtained with the parenteral form (see Table 56–7). With high doses or in patients with renal failure, the metabolite normeperidine accumulates, causing CNS excitability manifested as tremor, muscle twitching, and possibly seizures.[35] The combination of monoamine oxidase inhibitors and meperidine should not be used because this mixture can produce an excitation syndrome, hyperpyrexia, and convulsions.[23,35] In most clinical settings meperidine offers no real advantage over morphine.

Fentanyl is a synthetic opioid structurally related to meperidine and is often used in anesthesiology for induction of anesthesia.[35] This agent is more potent and shorter acting than meperidine (see Tables 56–7 and 56–11).[36] Transdermal fentanyl is also available for the treatment of chronic pain in patients requiring opioid analgesics. One patch can provide analgesic support for 72 hours, but because of increasing fentanyl concentrations, the initial evaluation for maximum patch effectiveness cannot be done until 24 hours after it is first applied. In addition, it may take 6 days after increasing a dose before new steady-state levels accumulate. Thus, the patch should not be used in patients with acute pain.[36]

METHADONE AND CONGENERS

Methadone has gained considerable popularity because of its oral efficacy, extended duration of action, and ability to suppress withdrawal symptoms in heroin addicts. With repeated doses, the analgesic duration of action is prolonged, but because of metabolite accumulation excessive sedation may also result. Although methadone is effective in acute pain,[35] it is usually used to treat chronic pain. The pharmacologic profile resembles that of morphine.

Propoxyphene is one-half as potent as codeine, and is more effective than placebo when 65 to 100 mg is ingested.[37] It is usu-

TABLE 56–8. (Continued)

Agent(s)	Dose (Titrate up or down based on patient response)	Comments
Meperidine	PO 50–150 mg q3–4h[a] IM 75–100 mg q3–4h[a] IV 5–10 mg q5min prn[a]	Use in severe pain Oral not recommended Do not use in renal failure May precipitate tremors, myoclonus, and seizures Monoamine oxidase inhibitors can induce hyperpyrexia and/or seizures
Fentanyl	IM 0.05–0.1 mg q1–2h[a] Transdermal 25 μg/h q72h Transmucosal (investigational)	Used in severe pain Do not use transdermal in acute pain
Methadone	PO 5–20 mg q6–8h IM 2.5–10 mg q6–8h	Effective in severe chronic pain Sedation can be major problem Some chronic pain patients can be dosed every 12 hours
Propoxyphene	PO 65–100 mg q3–4h[a]	Use in moderate pain Weak analgesic, most effective when used with NSAIDs, aspirin, or acetaminophen Will cause carbamazepine levels to increase
Pentazocine	PO 50–100 mg q3–4h[b] IM 30 mg q3–4h[b]	3rd-line agent for moderate to severe pain May precipitate withdrawal in opiate-dependent patients
Butorphanol	IM 1–4 mg q3–4h[b] IV 0.5–2 mg q3–4h[b] Intranasal 1 mg (1 spray) q3–4h[b]	2nd-line agent for moderate to severe pain May precipitate withdrawal in opiate-dependent patients
Nalbuphine	IM 10 mg q3–6h[b] IV 10 mg q3–6h[b]	2nd-line agent for moderate to severe pain May precipitate withdrawal in opiate-dependent patients
Buprenorphine	IM 0.3 mg q6h[b] IV 0.3 mg q6h[b]	2nd-line agent for moderate to severe pain May precipitate withdrawal in opiate-dependent patients
Dezocine	IM 5–20 mg q3–6h[b] IV 2.5–10 mg q2–4h[b]	2nd-line agent for moderate to severe pain May precipitate withdrawal in opiate-dependent patients
Naloxone	IV 0.4–1.2 mg	When reversing opiate side effects in patients needing analgesia, dilute and titrate (0.1–0.2 mg q2–3 minutes) so as not to reverse analgesia
Tramadol	PO 50–100 mg q4–6h[a]	Maximum dose is 400 mg/24 h Decrease dose in renal impairment and in the elderly

[a]May start with an around-the-clock regimen and switch to prn if/when the painful signal subsides.
[b]May reach a ceiling analgesic effect.
Compiled from Refs. 30, 35, 36, 39, 55, and 56.

ally used in combination with aspirin or acetaminophen in the treatment of moderate pain. The toxicity profile of propoxyphene is similar to that of codeine.

MIXED NARCOTIC AGONIST–ANTAGONISTS

Analgesic agents that stimulate the analgesic portion of opioid receptors while blocking the toxicity portion would be considered ideal. The mixed agonist–antagonist class was developed with this in mind. The analgesic class produces analgesia and has a ceiling effect on respiratory depression (e.g., after a dose of 30 mg in adults progressively higher doses of nalbuphine do not affect respiratory rate).[32] They have a lower abuse potential than morphine, but psychotomimetic responses (e.g., hallucinations and vivid dreams, seen more often with pentazocine and butorphanol[35]), a ceiling analgesic effect,[32] and a propensity to cause pain and initiate withdrawal in opioid-dependent populations have diminished their widespread clinical use.

TABLE 56–9. Major Adverse Effects of the Opioid Analgesics

Effect	Manifestation
Mood changes	Dysphoria, euphoria
Somnolence	Lethargy, drowsiness, apathy, inability to concentrate
Stimulation of chemoreceptor trigger zone	Nausea, vomiting
Respiratory depression	Decreased respiratory rate
Decreased GI motility	Constipation
Increase in sphincter tone (most evidence with morphine)	Biliary spasm, urinary retention
Histamine release (most evidence with morphine)	Urticaria, pruritus, rarely exacerbation of asthma
Tolerance	Larger doses for same effect
Dependence	Withdrawal symptoms upon abrupt discontinuation

Compiled from Refs. 3 and 23.

TABLE 56–10. Epidural Opioids

Agent	Dose (mg)	Onset of Pain Relief (min)	Duration of Pain Relief (h)
Morphine	5–10	25	12–20
Hydromorphone	1	10–15	12
Fentanyl	0.1	5–10	6

Modified from Ref. 11, with permission.

OPIOID ANTAGONISTS

The pure opioid antagonist, naloxone, binds competitively to opioid receptors but does not produce an analgesic response. Therefore, it is most often used to reverse the toxic effects of agonist and mixed agonist–antagonist narcotics.

CENTRAL ANALGESIC

Tramadol has two basic modes of action: weak opiate receptor binding (predominantly on the mu receptor) and inhibition of norepinephrine and serotonin reuptake. It is indicated for the relief of moderate to moderately severe pain.[38]

Although associated with minimal dependency, tramadol has a side-effect profile similar to that of the previously mentioned opioid analgesics. Tramadol also may enhance the risk of seizures in patients taking MAOIs, neuroleptics, or other drugs that can reduce the seizure threshold, and in patients with seizure disorders.[38]

Tramadol may have a place in treating patients with chronic pain when less dependence and tolerance is desired. However, this agent has little advantage over the previously mentioned opioid analgesics when treating patients for acute pain, and is more expensive.

COMBINATION THERAPY

The combination of opioid and nonopioid oral analgesics often results in analgesia superior to that produced by either agent alone.[30] Attacking pain on two fronts, prostaglandins and opiate receptors, enhances pain relief and facilitates the use of lower doses of each agent. This frequently produces a more favorable side-effect profile and is the reason there are so many aspirin and/or acetaminophen–opioid analgesic combination products marketed. The addition of an injectable NSAID (ketorolac) makes this combination possible also in patients who cannot take oral medications. The clinician should not be limited by the availability of commercially established fixed-ratio combinations. For example, the administration of NSAIDs in combination with scheduled opioid regimens is often very effective in the treatment of pain resulting from bone metastases in advanced cancer.[39]

Agents shown to potentiate the analgesic efficacy of parenteral opioids include hydroxyzine and dextroamphetamine.[39] Promethazine and chlorpromazine, once thought to possess this potentiating property, apparently offer no inherent analgesic or potentiating characteristics when combined with opioids, although unwanted sedation may be increased.[30] Methotrimeprazine, a phenothiazine derivative, does induce some analgesia but also produces sedation and phenothiazine-like side effects (e.g., orthostatic hypotension and extrapyramidal symptoms).[35]

REGIONAL ANALGESIA

Regional analgesia with properly administered local anesthetics can provide complete relief of pain and block pain reflex responses (Table 56–12).[40] They are used epidurally in both acute and chronic pain. Regional analgesics relieve pain by blocking nociceptive transmission, interrupting sympathetic reflexes, and preventing increased skeletal muscle activity.[35] Their lipid solubility, protein-binding characteristics, pK_a, percentage of un-ionized drug, drug concentration, and vasodilator behavior determine the mechanism of action.[40] High plasma concentrations can cause signs of CNS excitation and depression, including dizziness, tinnitus, drowsiness, disorientation, muscle twitching, seizures, and respiratory arrest.[35] Cardiovascular effects include myocardial depression, hypotension, decreased cardiac output, heart block,

TABLE 56–11. Opioid Analgesic Pharmacokinetics[a]

Agent	Time to Peak (h)	Half-life (h)	Analgesic Onset (min)	Analgesic Duration (h)
Morphine	0.5–1	2	15–30,60[b]	4–5
Hydromorphone	0.5–1	2–3	15–30	4–5
Oxymorphone	0.5–1	2–3	5–15	4–6
Levorphanol	0.5–1	12–16	30–90	6–8
Hydrocodone	1.3	4	—[c]	4–5
Codeine	0.5–1	2–4	15–30	4–6
Oxycodone (PO)	0.5–1	—[c]	15–30	4–5
Meperidine	0.5–1	3–4	10–45	3–4
Fentanyl	—[c]	1.5–6	7–8	1–2
Methadone	0.5–1	15–40	30–60	4–5 (acute) > 8 (chronic)
Propoxyphene (PO)	2.0–2.5	6–12	30–60	4–6
Pentazocine	0.25–1	4–5	15–20	4–6
Butorphanol	0.5–1	2.5–3.5	< 10	4–6
Nalbuphine	1	2–3	< 15	4–6
Buprenorphine	1	5	15	4–5
Dezocine	0.17–1.5	0.6–5	15–30	2–4
Naloxone[d]	0.5–2	0.5–1.5	2–5	0.5–1
Tramadol	2–3	6–7	< 60	6

[a]Based on intramuscular data unless otherwise indicated.
[b]Data based intrathecal or epidural administration.
[c]Data not available.
[d]Narcotic antagonist.
Compiled from Refs. 23, 35, 36, 38, 52–54, 57, and 58.

TABLE 56–12. Local Anesthetics

Agent	Onset (min)	Duration (h)
Esters		
Procaine	2–5	0.25–1
Chloroprocaine	6–12	0.50
Tetracaine	15	2–3
Amides		
Mepivacaine	3–5	0.75–1.5
Bupivacaine	5	2–4
Lidocaine	< 2	0.5–1
Prilocaine	< 2	≥ 1
Etidocaine	3–5	5–10

Compiled from Ref. 36.

bradycardia, ventricular arrhythmia, and cardiac arrest.[36] Disadvantages of such methods include the need for skillful technical application, the need of frequent administration, and highly specialized follow-up procedures.

CHRONIC PAIN

CANCER PAIN

Managing the pain of malignant diseases encompasses both acute and chronic management techniques. Thus, pharmacologic treatment and psychological therapies already mentioned are best combined with neurosurgical methods, anesthetic procedures, and supportive care measures in a multidisciplinary approach to pain relief.[41] The goal is to provide patients with enough pain amelioration to tolerate diagnostic and therapeutic manipulation and permit them to function at a level that will allow freedom of movement and choice.[41] Unfortunately, 25% of patients with cancer die without significant relief of severe pain.[41] Assessment techniques described in Table 56–2 apply to these patients. Special attention must be given to continual reassessment of the painful state, and individualization of therapy is always required.[39]

NONPHARMACOLOGIC THERAPY

PSYCHOLOGICAL AND SUPPORTIVE CARE

Previously mentioned psychological techniques, such as relaxation training and controlled mental imagery, are very helpful in relieving pain experienced in malignant disease[39] and prove especially useful in conjunction with pharmacologic therapy.

Supportive care, in and outside the hospital, using programs such as the hospice, is one of the cancer patient's greatest allies not only in coping with pain but in accepting the disease. The positive effect this has on the patient cannot be overstated.

PHARMACOLOGIC THERAPY

Pharmacologic management is the mainstay of therapy, and a typical progression of analgesic use is outlined in Figure 56–2. The objective is to prevent the patient from experiencing constant fluctuation between severe pain and pain relief. This is best accomplished by around-the-clock administration schedules that inhibit serum analgesic concentrations from falling below the point at which a patient experiences the suffering of pain. As-needed (prn) schedules are to be employed in conjunction with around-the-clock regimens and are used only when patients experience breakthrough pain. Again, nonopioid agents are used as first-line agents, with NSAIDs being especially effective in treating bone pain.[39] Bone pain can also be treated with radiopharmaceuticals. Both strontium-89 and samarium SM 153 lexidronam have been shown to provide pain relief.[36] The choice of opiate remains controversial, but should be based on patient acceptance, analgesic effectiveness, and pharmacokinetic, pharmacodynamic, and side-effect profiles. Many clinicians have found morphine both safe and effective when administered by the oral (sustained-release, liquid, and fast-release), subcutaneous, rectal, continual intravenous infusion, patient-controlled intravenous, epidural, or intrathecal routes.[39] Epidural clonidine and/or local anesthetics are effective with epidurally administered opioid analgesics for the treatment of refractory pain.[36] The fentanyl patch may provide a more convenient dosing alternative in patients on stable regimens. Although heroin has shown analgesic and side-effect characteristics equal to those of morphine, it has no proven superiority.[42] Meperidine is usually not recommended for long-term use because of its relatively short duration of action and the CNS hyperirritability of normeperidine, one of its main metabolites.[39] Anticonvulsant drugs, tricyclic antidepressants, antihistamines, amphetamines, and steroids are often used as adjuvant pain medications[39]; however, they have enjoyed only limited success as pain relievers, with anecdotal data or retrospective surveys providing most of the rationale for their use.[41]

Anesthetic and neurosurgical approaches have proven successful in alleviating pain but require special expertise and are usually reserved for patients who are refractory to conventional analgesics. They most commonly involve the sectioning or stimulation of the spinal cord, brain, or peripheral nerves. These techniques block nociceptive pathways and subsequently alleviate pain.[39]

NONMALIGNANT CHRONIC PAIN

The numerous etiologies that produce nonmalignant chronic pain make treatment complex, and its management assumes multidisciplinary aspects. As pain becomes gradually more chronic, it loses many of the autonomic characteristics evident in the acute stage, and additional symptoms such as depression, sleep disturbances, anxiety, irritability, work problems, and family instability tend to dominate.[3] Patients should not be told that the pain they are feeling is "psychosomatic" or in their head. In most cases, etiology is not as important as symptomatic relief. Objectives in evaluation include establishing an accurate diagnosis, identifying iatrogenic factors, obtaining a comprehensive psychiatric and psychosocial assessment, paying special attention to family and social problems, and obtaining a description of factors that alleviate or exacerbate pain.[3]

Pharmacologic approaches to patient care do not differ from those described previously; however, chronic pain patients most often have received a complete pharmacologic regimen. Adding another "pill" to their therapy will promote dependence and not improve pain control.[3] Other noninvasive or psychological techniques may prove more successful. An integrated, systematic approach often provided by pain clinics, with a strong emphasis on patient–clinician relationships, is essential. The goal is to improve or maintain the patient's level of functioning, decrease the rate of physical deterioration, decrease pain perception, improve the patient's sense of well-being, improve family and social relationships, and decrease dependency on drug therapy.[3] Patients and clinicians must realize that maximum effective treatment may take months or even years.

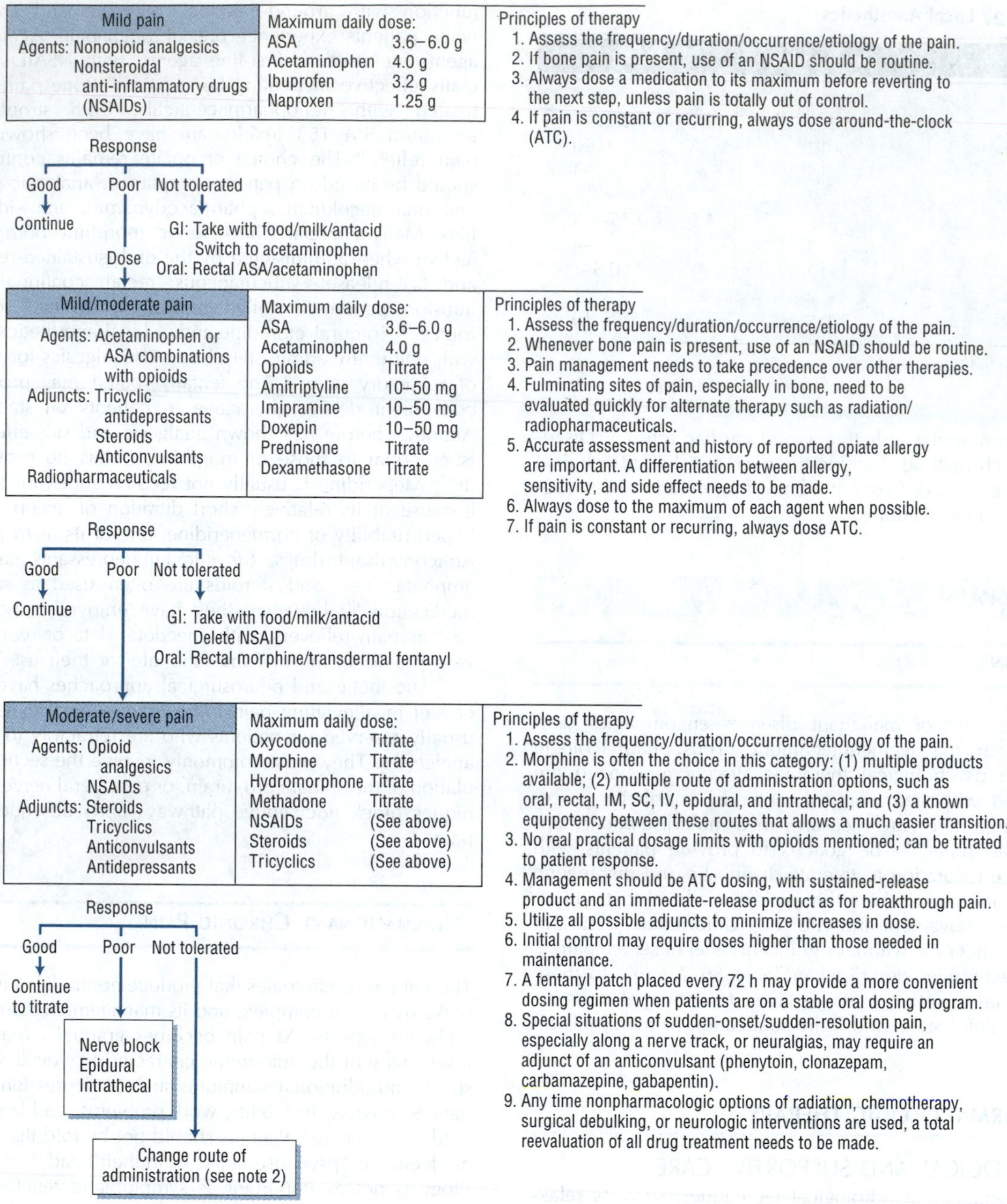

FIGURE 56–2. Algorithm for pain management in oncology patients. *(Modified from Ref. 39.)*

PHARMACOECONOMIC CONSIDERATIONS

One cannot overemphasize the "suffering" component of pain. Most of us know how devastating pain can be to our daily lives. Swift relief from acute and cancer pain and well-planned treatment regimens in chronic pain will allow patients to concentrate on recovery and regaining control of their lives. Although few well-designed pharmacoeconomic studies have been performed,[43,44] most clinicians who treat pain believe that well-planned pain treatment leads to decreased time in the hospital, decreased time away from work, and overall increased quality of life.

EVALUATION OF THERAPEUTIC OUTCOMES

The key to treating pain effectively is to consistently monitor effectiveness (pain relief) versus side effects (e.g., sedation), and titrate treatment accordingly (see Table 56–8). In acute pain, this often needs to be done several times a day (in the early stages, hourly), whereas in chronic pain, this may take place daily or even weekly. The frequency of evaluation also depends on the drug, the administration route, and other therapies being used. When patients, such as those in a coma, cannot be asked about their pain, monitoring agitation and heart rate is appropriate. Given the subjective nature of pain, the most successful therapies will involve not only frequent patient assessment but a large degree of patient control (as with PCA).

All opioids can cause constipation. The best management of constipation is prevention. Patients should be counseled on the proper intake of fluids and fiber. A laxative may be added if needed. As noted earlier, CNS depressants (alcohol, benzodiazepines) amplify CNS depression when used with opioid analgesics, and should be closely monitored and discouraged when possible.

CONCLUSIONS

Pharmacologic agents to treat pain are not always appropriately used. Inadequate dose titration, fear of analgesic side effects, varying analgesic requirements, and failure to appreciate the complications of untreated pain contribute to ineffective and inappropriate pain management. Adherence to the basic principles of pharmacotherapy will promote rational pain-control decisions. Analgesic agents should be given an adequate trial and often require individual dosage titration. Even in acute pain, administering analgesics as needed (prn) may promote anxiety and contribute to future drug dependence. These drugs should be administered on a regular dosing schedule and not on an as-needed schedule. However, as-needed regimens can be used in breakthrough pain (pain despite regular dosing of analgesics) or when acute pain displays great variability or has greatly subsided. Side effects should be well understood and excessive sedation avoided. Finally, placebo therapy should never be used to diagnose psychogenic pain, and the route of administration should always be geared to the analgesic needs of the patient.

It must be remembered that pain is whatever the patient says or feels it is. In acute pain and cancer pain, when patients tell you they are hurting, aggressive drug therapy should be considered. In chronic pain, aggressive assessment and understanding may be more appropriate. If acute pain does not subside within the anticipated duration of the insult (often 1 to 2 weeks), further investigation of the cause is warranted. Cancer pain and chronic pain may need treatment for years.

Clinicians must keep in mind that the risk of dependency is real but often overstated and can often promote inappropriate pain management. In addition, the elderly and the young are at a higher risk for undertreatment because of misunderstandings regarding the pathophysiology of their pain. These populations need special attention to proper titration as outlined earlier.

Poor training of health care practitioners in pain assessment and management, improper patient education, and inadequate communication among health care professionals have been suggested as reasons for inadequate pain relief.[45] The use of an integrated approach, using the expertise of multiple disciplines, as well as individualized pharmacologic and nonpharmacologic strategies may well be the most overlooked principle of pharmacotherapy.[45] Indeed, it is the responsibility of all health care professionals who deal with pain to communicate and ensure proper management in an effort to relieve treatable suffering and pain.

▶ PRINCIPLES OF PHARMACOTHERAPY

- During assessment, always ask the PATIENT if he or she has pain (see Table 56–2).
- Identify the source of pain.
- Use the most effective analgesic with the fewest side effects.
- Properly titrate the dose for each individual and administer for an adequate duration.
- Always consider around-the-clock regimens for acute and chronic pain.
- Use as-needed regimens for breakthrough pain or when acute pain displays great variability and/or has greatly subsided.
- Recognize side effects of analgesics, particularly the constipation seen with the opioids.
- Avoid excessive sedation by carefully titrating the opioids.
- Adjust the route of administration to the needs of the patient; whenever possible, use oral medication.
- Use equianalgesic doses when converting from one agent to another.
- Do not use placebo therapy to diagnose psychogenic pain.
- Use multiple disciplines and nonpharmacologic strategies whenever possible.

REFERENCES

1. Hazelden Foundation. Touchstones. New York, Harper & Row, 1986.
2. Bonica JJ, Procacci P. General considerations of acute pain and general considerations of chronic pain. In: Bonica JJ, Loeser JD, Chapman CR, et al, eds. The Management of Pain. Philadelphia, Lea & Febiger, 1990:159–196.
3. Stimmel B. Pain, Analgesia and Addiction: The Pharmacology of Pain. New York, Raven, 1983.
4. Bonica JJ. Definitions and taxonomy of pain. In: Bonica JJ, Loeser JD, Chapman CR, et al, eds. The Management of Pain. Philadelphia, Lea & Febiger, 1990:18–27.
5. Marks RM, Sacher EJ. Undertreatment of medical inpatient pain with narcotic analgesics. Ann Intern Med 1973;78:173–181.
6. Cohen FL. Postsurgical pain relief: Patients' status and nurses' medication choices. Pain 1980;9:265–274.
7. McCaffery M, Ferrell BR. Opioid analgesics: Nurses' knowledge of doses and psychological dependence. J Nurs Staff 1992;8(2):77–84.
8. Whipple JK, Lewis KS, Quebbeman EJ, et al. Analysis of pain management in critically ill patients. Pharmacotherapy 1995;15:592–599.
9. Lister BJ. Dilemmas in the treatment of chronic pain. Am J Med 1996;101(suppl 1A):2S–5S.
10. Bonica JJ. Biochemistry and modulation of nociception and pain. In: Bonica JJ, Loeser JD, Chapman CR, et al, eds. The Management of Pain. Philadelphia, Lea & Febiger, 1990:95–121.

11. Littrell RA. Epidural analgesia. Am J Hosp Pharm 1991;48: 2460–2474.
12. Cordell GA, Araujo OE. Capsaicin: Identification, nomenclature, and pharmacotherapy. Ann Pharmacother 1993;27:330–336.
13. Field HL, Levins JD. Pain—Mechanisms and management. West J Med 1984;141:347–357.
14. Melzack R, Wall PD. Pain mechanisms: A new theory. Science 1965;150:971–979.
15. Mayer DJ, Leibeskind JC. Pain reduction by focal electrical stimulation of the brain: An anatomical and behavioral analysis. Brain Res 1974;68:73–93.
16. Mayer DJ, Wolfe TL, Akil H, et al. Analgesia from electrical stimulation in the brain stem of the rat. Science 1971;174:1351–1354.
17. Basbaum AL, Fields HL. Endogenous pain control mechanisms: Review and hypothesis. Ann Neurol 1978;4:451–462.
18. Goldstein A, Lowney LL, Pal BK. Stereospecific and nonspecific interactions of morphine narcotic congener levorphanol in subcellular fractions of mouse brain. Proc Natl Acad Sci USA 1971;68: 1742–1747.
19. Pert CB, Pasternak G, Snyder SH. Opiate agonists and antagonists discriminated by receptor binding in brain. Science 1973;182: 1359–1361.
20. Simon EJ, Hiller JM, Edelman I. Stereospecific binding of the potent narcotic analgesic (3-H) etorphine to rat-brain homogenate. Proc Natl Acad Sci USA 1973;38:377–384.
21. Hughes F, Smith TW, Kosterlitz HW, et al. Identification of two related pentapeptides from the brain with potent opiate agonist activity. Nature 1975;258:577–580.
22. Li CH, Chung D. Isolation and structure of an untriakontapeptide with opiate activity from camel pituitary glands. Proc Natl Acad Sci USA 1976;73:1145–1148.
23. Reisine T, Pasternak G. Opioid analgesics and antagonists. In: Hardman JG, Limbird LE, Molinoff PB, et al, eds. The Pharmacological Basis of Therapeutics. New York, McGraw-Hill, 1995:521–555.
24. Twycross RG. Pain and analgesics. Curr Med Res Opin 1978;5: 497–505.
25. Fordyce WE. Learning processes in pain. In: Sternbach RA, ed. The Psychology of Pain. New York, Raven, 1978:49–72.
26. Chapman CR. New directions in the understanding and management of pain. Soc Sci Med 1984;19:1261–1277.
27. Craig KD. Social modelling influences on pain. In: Sternbach RA, ed: The Psychology of Pain. New York, Raven, 1978:73–109.
28. American Pain Society. Principles of analgesic use in the treatment of acute pain and chronic cancer pain. Clin Pharm 1990;9:601–611.
29. Chapman CR, Bonica JJ. Chronic pain. Current concepts. Kalamazoo, MI, Scope, 1985:4.
30. Clinical practice guideline. Acute Pain Management: Operative or Medical Procedures and Trauma. U.S. Department of Health and Human Services, Public Health Service, Agency for Health Care Policy and Research, Rockville, MD, 1992.
31. Cashman J, McAnulty G. Nonsteroidal anti-inflammatory drugs in perisurgical pain management. Drugs 1995;49:51–70.
32. Benedetti C, Butler SH. Systemic analgesics. In: Bonica JJ, Loeser JD, Chapman CR, et al, eds. The Management of Pain. Philadelphia, Lea & Febiger, 1990:1640–1675.
33. Baumann TJ. Analgesic selection when the patient is allergic to codeine. Clin Pharm 1991;10:658.
34. Shafer AL, Donnelly AJ. Management of postoperative pain by continuous epidural infusion of analgesics. Clin Pharm 1991;10: 745–764.
35. American Hospital Formulary Service. McVoy GK, ed. Drug Information. Bethesda, MD, American Society of Hospital Pharmacists, 1987, 1991, 1994, 1997.
36. Drug Facts and Comparisons. Philadelphia, JB Lippincott, 1986, 1991, 1994, 1997.
37. Beaver WT. Mild analgesics: A review of their clinical pharmacology, 4. Am J Med Sci 1966;251:576–599.
38. Package insert, Tramadol. Ortho-McNeil, Raritan, NJ, 1995.
39. Clinical practice guideline no. 9. Management of Cancer Pain. U.S. Department of Health, Public Health Service, Agency for Health Care Policy and Research, Rockville, MD, 1994.
40. Bonica JJ, Buckley PF. Regional analgesia with local anesthetics. In: Bonnica JJ, Loeser JD, Chapman CR, et al, eds. The Management of Pain. Philadelphia, Lea & Febiger, 1990:1883–1966.
41. Foley KM. The treatment of cancer pain. N Engl J Med 1985;313: 84–95.
42. Health and Public Policy Committee, American College of Physicians. Drug therapy for severe chronic pain in terminal illness. Ann Intern Med 1983;99:870–873.
43. Tugwell P. Economic evaluation of the management of pain in osteoarthritis. Drugs 1996;52(suppl 3):48–58.
44. Portenoy RK. Issues in the economic analysis of therapies for cancer pain. Oncology 1995;9(suppl 11):71–78.
45. News. Panel cites need for improved pain management. Clin Pharm 1986;5:777–778.
46. Amadio P. Peripherally acting analgesics. Am J Med 1984;77:17–26.
47. Hopkinson JH, Smith MT, Bare WW, et al. Acetaminophen (500 mg) versus acetaminophen (325 mg) for relief of pain in episiotomy patients. Curr Ther Res 1974;16:194–200.
48. Levy G. Comparative pharmacokinetics of aspirin and acetaminophen. Arch Intern Med 1981;141:279–281.
49. Gaston GW, Mallow RD, Frank JE. Comparison of etodolac, aspirin, and placebo for pain after oral surgery. Pharmacotherapy 1986;6: 199–205.
50. Package insert, Diclofenac potassium. Geigy Pharmaceuticals, Ardsley, NY, 1993–1994.
51. Hare BD. The opioid analgesics: Rational selection of agents for acute and chronic pain. Hosp Formulary 1987;22:64–86.
52. Inturrisi CE. Role of opioid analgesics. Am J Med 1984;77:27–37.
53. Gourlay GK, Cousins MJ. Strong analgesics in severe pain. Drugs 1984;28:79–91.
54. Clotz MA, Nahata MC. Clinical use of fentanyl, sufentanil, and alfentanil. Clin Pharm 1991;10:581–593.
55. Drugs for pain. Med Letter 1993;35:4.
56. Maurer PM, Bartkowski RR. Drug interactions of clinical significance with opioid analgesics. Drug Saf 1993;8:30–48.
57. Schoenle JR, Mullins PM. Dezocine. Pharm Ther November 1990: 1357–1371.
58. Sunshine A. New clinical experience with tramadol. Drugs 1994;47 (suppl 1):8–18.

57

Headache Disorders: Migraine and Cluster

Brian E. Beckett, PharmD, and Katherine C. Herndon, PharmD, BCPS

Headache is one of the most common complaints encountered by health care practitioners.[1,2] Migraine, an episodic headache disorder of moderate to severe intensity, is one of the most common of the primary headache disorders. An estimated 24 million people in the United States have experienced a migraine headache. Approximately one-third of migraineurs report severe disability in association with their headaches.[3] Unfortunately, recent studies indicate that the majority of migraine sufferers have not been diagnosed and take only over-the-counter (OTC) medications for headache relief.[1–3] Thus, it appears that many migraineurs are not receiving adequate treatment of their headaches. A thorough evaluation of the headache history is essential to establish an accurate diagnosis of migraine and identify patients who may benefit from drug therapy.

The International Headache Society (IHS) has developed a classification system that provides precise definitions and standardized nomenclature for primary headache disorders (migraine, tension-type, and cluster headache) as well as secondary organic headache disorders (Table 57–1).[4] Migraine may be classified as migraine without aura (formerly called common migraine) or migraine with aura (formerly called classical migraine) based on the presence of focal neurologic symptoms prior to the onset of headache. Other primary headache disorders also occur frequently. This chapter focuses on the management of migraine and cluster headaches.

MIGRAINE HEADACHE

EPIDEMIOLOGY

Migraine headache accounts for 10% to 20% of all headaches in adults. It is three times more prevalent in women (18%) than men (6%). Gender differences in migraine prevalence have been linked to menstruation; however, these differences persist beyond menopause. The usual age of onset is 15 to 35 years of age, but prevalence is highest between the ages of 35 and 45. An estimated 8.7 million females and 2.6 million males experience moderate to severe migraine-associated disability. Approximately 40% of these patients suffer more than one attack per month. Migraine headaches are more common in lower socioeconomic groups, perhaps the result of diet, stress, increased use of OTC medications, or reduced access to health care. In comparison to other economic groups, lower-income households are also more likely to use emergency care services to treat their migraine attacks. The economic impact of migraine is difficult to ascertain; however, the estimated indirect costs of the illness (e.g., absenteeism, decreased productivity) are between $5.6 and $17.2 billion every year.[5]

PATHOPHYSIOLOGY

The precise etiology and pathophysiologic mechanism of migraine are unknown.[6] The vascular hypothesis of migraine, first proposed by Wolff, theorizes that the aura of migraine is caused by intracerebral vasoconstriction followed by extracranial vasodilation resulting in headache pain.[6] This vascular hypothesis has not been supported by blood flow studies; however, the aura may be related to cerebral blood flow changes. According to recent studies, the aura appears to be a manifestation of spreading depression, a cortical neuronal event characterized by slowly progressing (2 to 5 mm/min) waves of inhibition.[7] Spreading depression may result in a 25% to 35% reduction in regional cerebral blood flow, which falls below critical levels for cortical function and is sufficient to explain the positive (e.g., scintillations) and negative symptoms (e.g., blind spots) as well as the neurologic deficits associated with the aura.

Neuronal dysfunction is now accepted as the primary basis of migraine pathophysiology. Migraine pain is believed to result from activity within the trigeminovascular system, a network of visceral afferent fibers that innervate the cranial vessels and serve to protect the brain from the presence and entry of noxious substances.[8–11] Axons within this system originate from the trigeminal ganglia and upper cervical dorsal root and surround cerebral blood vessels in close proximity to all vessel layers to allow for constant monitoring of the microenvironment of the blood vessel wall. Arteries and venous sinuses have the highest degree of trigeminal innervation. Trigeminal nerves are important initiators and promoters of tissue inflammation. Neuronal activation releases vasoactive neuropeptides—such as substance P, calcitonin gene-related polypeptide, and neurokinin A—from perivascular axons.[6] Released neuropeptides interact with dural blood vessels, promoting vasodilation and plasma protein extravasation, which initiates a sterile, neurogenic inflammatory response. Sterile inflammation

TABLE 57–1. International Headache Society Classification of Migraine Headache

1. Migraine
   - 1.1 Migraine without aura
   - 1.2 Migraine with aura
     - 1.2.1 Migraine with typical aura (aura lasting less than 1 hour)
     - 1.2.2 Migraine with prolonged aura (aura lasting more than 1 hour and less than 1 week)
     - 1.2.3 Familial hemiplegic migraine
     - 1.2.4 Basilar migraine
     - 1.2.5 Migraine aura without headache
     - 1.2.6 Migraine with acute onset aura (aura develops fully in less than 5 minutes)
   - 1.3 Ophthalmoplegic migraine (associated with paresis of one or more ocular cranial nerves)
   - 1.4 Retinal migraine (attacks of monocular scotoma or blindness for less than 1 hour and associated with headache)
   - 1.5 Childhood periodic syndromes that may be precursors to or associated with migraine
     - 1.5.1 Benign paroxysmal vertigo of childhood (brief attacks of vertigo in otherwise healthy children)
     - 1.5.2 Alternating hemiplegia of childhood (attacks of hemiplegia involving each side alternately)
   - 1.6 Complications of migraine
     - 1.6.1 Status migrainosus (headache lasting more than 72 hours despite treatment)
     - 1.6.2 Migrainous infarction (aura symptoms not fully reversible within 7 days and/or associated ischemic infarction)
   - 1.7 Migrainous disorder not fulfilling above criteria

Adapted from Ref. 4.

sensitizes surrounding tissues and produces a hyperalgesic state that prolongs headache pain. In turn, activation of unmyelinated C fibers of the trigeminovascular system stimulates pain-transmitting neurons within the brainstem and upper spinal cord. Activity within the trigeminovascular system is regulated by noradrenergic and, most importantly, serotonergic neurons within the brainstem. Brainstem mechanisms that lead to activation of the nociceptive trigeminovascular system may be stimulated by the cerebral cortex, thalamus, or hypothalamus in response to emotion or stress, excessive afferent stimulation (e.g., glare, noise, smells), or changes in the internal clock or environment.[8] Researchers suggest that all individuals have a predetermined migraine threshold determined by the balance between excitatory and inhibitory pathways within the central nervous system.[6,7] Migraine patients may have a lowered biologic threshold for headache as a result of unstable serotonergic neurotransmission in the dorsal raphe neurons of the brainstem.

Serotonin (5-hydroxytryptamine or 5-HT) is thought to be an important mediator of migraine.[6,7] Of the seven classes of 5-HT receptors (5-HT_1 to 5-HT_7) that have been identified, 5-HT_1 receptors, presynaptic autoreceptors that modulate neurotransmitter release, and the excitatory postsynaptic 5-HT_2 receptors appear to play an important role in migraine pathophysiology as well as in the beneficial effects of antimigraine therapies.[12]

CLINICAL PRESENTATION

Migraines frequently occur in the early morning hours. Approximately 60% of migraineurs experience prodromal symptoms, which may occur for hours or days before the onset of headache.[13] Prodromal features vary widely among migraineurs but are usually consistent within an individual. Symptoms may be psychological (anxiety, depression, euphoria, irritability, fatigue, drowsiness); neurologic (phonophobia, photophobia, hyperosmia); constitutional (polyuria, diarrhea, constipation, stiff neck); or autonomic (yawning, thirst, food cravings).

TABLE 57–2. Diagnostic Criteria for Migraine

Migraine Without Aura

A. At least five attacks fulfilling B through D, below
B. Headache attacks lasting 4 to 72 hours (untreated or unsuccessfully treated)
C. Headache has at least two of the following characteristics:
   1. Unilateral location
   2. Pulsating quality
   3. Moderate or severe intensity (inhibits or prohibits daily activities)
   4. Aggravation by walking stairs or similar routine physical activity
D. During headache, at least one of the following:
   1. Nausea and/or vomiting
   2. Photophobia and phonophobia
E. At least one of the following:
   1. History, physical, and neurologic examinations do not suggest an organic disorder
   2. History and/or physical and/or neurologic examinations do suggest such disorder, but it is ruled out by appropriate investigations
   3. An organic disorder is present, but migraine attacks do not occur for the first time in close temporal relation to the disorder

Migraine With Aura

A. At least two attacks fulfilling B through C, below
B. At least three of the following four characteristics:
   1. One or more fully reversible aura symptoms indicating focal cerebral cortical and/or brainstem dysfunction
   2. At least one aura symptom develops gradually over more than 4 minutes, or two or more symptoms occur in succession
   3. No aura symptom lasts more than 60 minutes (if > 60 minutes, then diagnosis is migraine with prolonged aura). If more than one aura symptom is present, accepted duration is proportionally increased
   4. Headache follows aura with a free interval of less than 60 minutes. (It may also begin before or simultaneously with the aura)
C. At least one of the following:
   1. History, physical, and neurologic examinations do not suggest an organic disorder
   2. History and/or physical and/or neurologic examinations do suggest such disorder, but it is ruled out by approprite investigations
   3. An organic disorder is present, but migraine attacks do not occur for the first time in close temporal relation to the disorder

Adapted from Ref. 4.

Auras are experienced by approximately 10% of migraineurs.[13] The aura typically evolves over 5 to 20 minutes and lasts less than 60 minutes. The headache usually occurs within 60 minutes of the end of the aura. The most common aura is visual and may include both positive (scintillations, teichopsia, photopsia) and negative (visual field defects) features. Hemisensory disturbances (e.g., tingling or numbness in the face or extremities, hemiparesis, or aphasia) may also occur. Migraine without aura occurs in 85% of migraineurs. Five percent of patients experience other types of migraine headache (Table 57–1). A discussion of ophthalmologic and retinal migraines and the complications of migraine headache is beyond the scope of this chapter.

Peak intensity of headache pain typically occurs within 1 hour of onset. Pain is usually unilateral and can occur anywhere on the face or head, but is most often in the temple. Bilateral head pain is also described.[13] Typical headache pain is described as pounding, pulsating, or throbbing. Headaches may be of moderate to severe intensity and may inhibit many activities of daily living. Physical activity may worsen the headache pain. Patients often complain of being incapacitated during the migraine and will seek a dark quiet place for rest or sleep. Patients may complain of a variety of other symptoms such as increased sensitivity to light or sound, anorexia, nausea, vomiting, constipation, or diarrhea. Headache duration can range from 4 to 72 hours. Headache-free periods occur between attacks.[14] Migraineurs may be withdrawn, irritable, or depressed, and may suffer from insomnia, fatigue, and changes in libido. The postheadache syndrome is characterized by exhaustion, scalp tenderness, and recurrence of headache with sudden head movements.

The initial step in establishing an accurate diagnosis of migraine should be a thorough evaluation of the headache history, including the patient's age at onset; the time of day when attacks occur; duration of the attack; precipitating or relieving factors; a description of the aura (if present); the nature, intensity, and location of headache pain; associated symptoms; and the significance of attacks to the patient. Many patients also report a family history of migraine headaches. Diagnostic criteria for migraine without aura and migraine with aura are listed in Table 57–2.[4] Headache may be a manifestation of serious or life-threatening disease processes such as meningitis, cerebral hemorrhage, or brain tumor, but it is rarely caused by organic disease. Physical examination and laboratory tests, including an erythrocyte sedimentation rate, should all be within normal limits to accurately diagnose migraine and rule out organic causes of headache (Table 57–3).[13,14] The use of neuroimaging diagnostic procedures such as CT or MRI is generally not indicated in adult patients with a clear history of migraine with or without aura.[15] These procedures should be considered in patients with an abnormal neurologic examination, new onset of "the worst headache ever," progressive or prolonged headaches, or papilledema.[14] Because migraine headaches usually begin by the second or third decade of life, headaches beginning later in life may suggest an organic etiology such as cerebrovascular disease, cancer, or temporal arteritis.

TABLE 57–3. Evaluation of Patients With Headache

Obtain the headache history
Perform a neurologic examination
Obtain CT of the head if tumor, abscess, or cerebrovascular accident (ischemic or hemorrhagic) is suspected
Perform a lumbar puncture if an infection is suspected
Identify metabolic or electrolyte abnormalities and drug effects or drug withdrawal
Identify emotional disturbances
In elderly patients with new onset of headaches, obtain an erythrocyte sedimentation rate and consider a temporal artery biopsy to rule out temporal arteritis

▶ TREATMENT: Migraines

The management of migraine should begin with the identification and elimination of factors that consistently provoke migraine attacks in susceptible individuals.[16,17] Common migraine triggers are listed in Table 57–4. Many of these factors, including dietary agents and psychological disorders, may provoke migraine by altering neurotransmitter levels within the CNS. A higher incidence of migraines is seen during menstruation, while pregnancy may lower the incidence in 60% to 80% of female migraineurs. Proposed mechanisms for drug-induced migraine include the inhibition (e.g., reserpine) of granular reuptake and storage of 5-HT, blocking neuronal reuptake of 5-HT (e.g., fluoxetine), altered platelet aggregation (e.g., ethinyl estradiol, mestranol), and vasodilation (e.g., nitroglycerin, nifedipine).

Pharmacotherapeutic management of migraine is directed at altering the attack once it is under way (symptomatic or abortive therapy) or preventing the attack altogether (prophylactic therapy).[6,7,18] Abortive therapies must begin at the onset of the attack to achieve their full potential. Although alteration of neurovascular changes that occur early in the headache phase may reduce or eliminate the pain, abortive therapies are less likely to be effective after the attack has fully developed. Only 50% to 80% of patients taking abortive therapies will receive significant relief. Table 57–5 describes medications used for abortive therapy of migraine headaches. In addition to abortive therapy, patients with more frequent or severe headaches may require daily administration of prophylactic agents to reduce the frequency, severity, and duration of attacks.

■ ABORTIVE THERAPY

■ SIMPLE ANALGESICS

Initial therapy for patients with mild and infrequent migraines should be simple analgesics such as aspirin or acetaminophen.[6,7,18–20] Aspirin should be considered the drug of choice, but acetaminophen can be used when aspirin is contraindicated or is not tolerated. Both aspirin and acetaminophen have been combined with the barbiturate butalbital to induce sleep, with narcotics for additional pain relief, and with caffeine to help improve gastrointestinal absorption. Caffeine, however, may interfere with sleep. Butalbital and narcotics have been associated

TABLE 57–4. Precipitating Factors Associated With Migraine

Psychological Factors	**Medications (continued)**
Stress	Ethinyl estradiol
Anxiety	Fluoxetine
Depression	Histamine
Environmental Factors	Hormone replacement therapy
Tobacco smoke	Indomethacin
Glare	Mestranol
Strong odors	Nicotine
Loud noise	Nifedipine
Bright or flickering lights	Nitroglycerin
Weather changes (increase in temperature or humidity)	Oral contraceptives
High altitude	Reserpine
Dietary Factors	**Hormonal Factors**
Alcohol	Menses
Tyramine-containing foods (e.g., red wine, aged cheese)	Pregnancy
Citrus fruit	Menopause
Food additives (e.g., monosodium glutamate, aspartame, sodium nitrite)	**Life-style**
Chocolate	Excessive or inadequate sleep
Caffeine	Fatigue
Medications	Fasting or dieting
Cimetidine	Skipping meals
Cocaine	Strenuous exercise

Compiled from Refs. 16 and 17.

TABLE 57–5. Abortive Migraine Therapies

Medication	Dosage
Simple Analgesics	
Acetaminophen	650 mg at onset; repeat q4h as needed
Aspirin	650 mg at onset; repeat q4h as needed
Aspirin/acetaminophen with butalbital	1 or 2 tablets every 4–6 hours, but not more than 4 tablets/d or usage more than twice per week
Aspirin/acetaminophen with narcotics	Sparingly and infrequently
Nonsteroidal Anti-inflammatory Drugs[a]	
Ibuprofen	400–600 mg at onset; repeat in 1–2 hours
Ketorolac	15–60 mg IM at onset
Naproxen	750 mg at onset; 250 mg prn up to 1375 mg/d
Naproxen sodium	550–750 mg at onset; repeat in 1–2 hours
Ergotamine Preparations	
Ergotamine 1 mg with 100 mg caffeine	2 tablets at onset; then 1 tablet every 30 minutes prn to a maximum of 6 tablets/d or 10 tablets/wk
Ergotamine 2 mg SL tablets	1 tablet every 30 minutes prn to a maximum of 6 tablets/d or 10 tablets/wk. Do not swallow, crush, or chew
Ergotamine 2 mg with 100 mg caffeine suppositories	Insert 1 at onset; repeat in 1 hour prn to a maximum of 2/d or 5/wk
Dihydroergotamine 1 mg/mL injection	0.5–1 mg IV or IM every hour prn to a maximum of 2 mg/d, 6 mg/wk IV, or 3 mg/wk IM
5-HT$_1$ Receptor Agonists	
Sumatriptan 6 mg SC autoinjector	6 mg SC at onset; repeat in 1 hour prn but not more than 12 mg/24 h
Sumatriptan 25 mg tablets	1 tablet at onset; repeat in 2 hours prn to a maximum of 300 mg/d
Sumatriptan intranasal	5, 10, or 20 mg intranasally; repeat in 2 hours to a maximum of 40 mg/d
Zolmitriptan	1.25–2.5 mg initially; repeat in 2 hours to a maximum of 10 mg/d
Naratriptan	1 or 2.5 mg initially; repeat in 4 hours to a maximum of 5 mg/d
Rizatriptan	5–10 mg initially; repeat in 2 hours to a maximum of 30 mg/d
Miscellaneous Agents	
Isometheptene/dichloralphenazone/acetaminophen (Midrin)	2 capsules at onset; repeat 1 capsule every hour to a maximum of 5/d or 12/wk
Metoclopramide	10 mg IV or PO at onset
Prochlorperazine	10 mg IV at onset
Butorphanol nasal spray	1 spray in 1 nostril only; may repeat in 60 minutes if necessary
Chlorpromazine	0.1–1 mg/kg IV at onset

[a]Usage should be limited to three times weekly.
Compiled from Refs. 18, 52, 78–81.

with rebound headaches caused by a pattern of increasing use that induces migraine.[21–23] Increasing use of combination preparations may fail to provide pain relief and worsen headache symptoms when the narcotic wears off, leading to additional medication consumption.

NONSTEROIDAL ANTI-INFLAMMATORY DRUGS (NSAIDs)

Inhibition of prostaglandin synthesis by NSAIDs may prevent neurogenic inflammation in the trigeminovascular system and alleviate migraine pain.[18] NSAIDs have not been associated with rebound headaches; however, NSAIDs are more expensive than simple analgesics and may cause more side effects. Naproxen sodium was superior to placebo and ergotamine in controlled clinical studies.[24,25] Rapidly acting NSAIDs (naproxen, naproxen sodium, ibuprofen) may prove to be superior to agents with a slower onset of action or those used primarily for inflammation. Indomethacin should not be used because of its propensity to cause headaches in a significant number of patients. Migraines that occur before, during, or after menstruation may respond well to NSAIDs. Injectable ketorolac has been used in patients with drug-seeking behavior and in patients with severe nausea and vomiting that prohibit oral therapy.[26]

ERGOTAMINE

As the theories of migraine pathophysiology have changed, so have the proposed mechanisms of action for ergotamine and its derivatives. Recent evidence suggests that their antimigraine action results from the blockade of neurogenic inflammation in the trigeminovascular system through the stimulation of presynaptic 5-HT_1 receptors.[12] They also display activity at α-adrenergic, β-adrenergic, and dopaminergic receptors. Ergotamine and its derivatives are more effective when given early in the migraine attack.[6,7,18,19]

Ergotamine tartrate is available as an oral tablet, a sublingual tablet, and as a suppository.[27] Dihydroergotamine (DHE) is available in an injectable form, and an intranasal spray is in clinical trials.[27–31] Although usually given in emergency rooms, DHE can be safely self-administered at home. Caffeine is added to oral preparations to increase absorption but may interfere with sleep. Other drugs used in combination with ergotamine include antispasmodics, antiemetics, sedatives, analgesics, and CNS stimulants.

Oral ergotamine has poor bioavailability due primarily to extensive first-pass metabolism; sublingual administration may not provide appreciable blood levels.[12,27] Rectal administration has been used for patients suffering from nausea and vomiting, but increased absorption may lead to a worsening of nausea due to stimulation of the vomiting center. Dose and routes of administration should be tailored for individual patients. Intravenous administration is the fastest way to achieve therapeutic drug concentrations and may be preferred by some patients or in more severe attacks.

Ergotamine dosage requirements should be strictly titrated to determine a safe and effective dose for future attacks. Frequent dosing or exceeding the maximum dosage guidelines should be avoided to prevent the development of ergotamine dependency, a self-sustaining cycle of rebound headache and ergotamine usage.[32,33] Withdrawal symptoms—including severe headache, nausea, vomiting, malaise, and prostration—may necessitate hospitalization of patients during detoxification.

Although generally well tolerated, side effects to the ergot products include nausea, vomiting, abdominal pain, weakness, fatigue, vasoconstriction leading to elevation in blood pressure, and severe peripheral ischemia. The syndrome of ergotism is manifested by nausea, diarrhea, thirst, pruritus, vertigo, muscle cramps, paresthesias, cold skin, and decreased pulses in the extremities. Vasoconstrictive complications, including myocardial infarction, hepatic necrosis, and bowel and brain ischemia have been rarely reported.[32] Risk of vasospasm may be increased during concomitant therapy with β-adrenergic blockers or methysergide.[32,33] DHE is rarely associated with side effects.[32] Contraindications to use include coronary, cerebral, or peripheral vascular disease, hypertension, liver or kidney disease, and pregnancy. Ergotamines should be used with caution in patients with prolonged auras (> 60 minutes).

5-HT_1 RECEPTOR AGONISTS

Sumatriptan is a selective 5-HT_1 receptor agonist. It is highly specific for 5-HT_{1D} and to a lesser extent 5-HT_{1A} receptors.[34,35] Stimulation of 5-HT_{1D} receptors produces a direct vasoconstrictive effect. Sumatriptan also appears to inhibit the release of tachykinins and subsequently blocks neurogenic plasma protein extravasation and inflammation.[34,35] Efficacy of oral and subcutaneous sumatriptan is comparable, but patients report a faster onset of headache relief with subcutaneous administration. Efficacy of sumatriptan is consistently superior to placebo in alleviating migraine attacks with significant improvement in approximately 70% of patients in 1 hour and 85% in 2 hours.[36–44] When compared to DHE, subcutaneous sumatriptan provided more rapid headache relief, but both therapies were equally efficacious at 3 hours. Oral sumatriptan provides significant relief in 75% of patients within 4 hours regardless of the size of the dose. Oral sumatriptan was more effective than oral ergotamine[36] or aspirin plus metoclopramide[44] in relieving headaches. Administration of a second dose (oral or subcutaneous) does not improve initial efficacy. Headache recurs within 24 to 48 hours in 40% of patients, probably due to its short half-life. A second dose given at the time of recurrence is usually effective. Higher recurrence rates are reported with sumatriptan than with other abortive therapies.[34,35]

Sumatriptan is generally well tolerated. Adverse effects associated with oral use include bad taste, nausea, vomiting, malaise, fatigue, dizziness, and vertigo, but are usually of short duration. Subcutaneous administration has been associated with minor injection site reactions; chest tightness and pressure have also occurred in 3% to 5% of patients. Isolated cases of coronary vasospasm with ischemia, myocardial infarction, and ventricular dysrhythmias have been reported.

Sumatriptan is contraindicated in patients with a history of ischemic heart disease, angina pectoris, Prinzmetal's angina, previous myocardial infarction, and uncontrolled hypertension. Patients at risk for unrecognized coronary artery disease (e.g., postmenopausal women, men over 40 years of age, and patients with multiple risk factors for coronary artery disease) should receive their initial dose of sumatriptan under medical supervision. Administration of sumatriptan within 2 weeks of therapy with monoamine oxidase inhibitors is not recommended. Sumatriptan should not be given if ergotamine derivatives have been used within the previous 24 hours. An intranasal formulation of sumatriptan is now available.

Three additional agents, zolmitriptan, naratriptan, and rizatriptan, have been approved since 1997.

MISCELLANEOUS AGENTS

Midrin is a combination of isometheptene mucate 65 mg (a sympathomimetic amine), dichloralphenazone 100 mg (a mild sedative), and acetaminophen 325 mg.[19] It can be used in patients who cannot take or do not respond to ergotamine or sumatriptan. Midrin is less effective than ergotamine, but also has fewer side effects. The most frequent side effects are dizziness, insomnia, nausea, vomiting, and transient numbness.

Metoclopramide may be useful in preventing or treating the nausea and vomiting associated with migraines when given with abortive therapies, and it may be beneficial as a single agent for pain relief.[45] Metoclopramide may also help to increase absorption of medications by decreasing gastric stasis.[18] Metoclopramide should be given 15 to 30 minutes before the antimigraine therapy and can be repeated in 4 to 6 hours. Extrapyramidal reactions may occur, but acute dystonic reactions are rare with intermittent use. Anticholinergic agents and narcotics may antagonize the increased gastric emptying seen with metoclopramide.

Chlorpromazine and prochlorperazine have also provided relief of migraine headache when administered parenterally.[46,47] The precise mechanism of action for these agents is unknown. Side effects may include sedation, extrapyramidal effects, and orthostatic hypotension. Tardive dyskinesia can occur after long-term use, but is unusual with lower doses and in younger patients afflicted with migraines.

Corticosteroids may help control prolonged migraines and reduce narcotic requirements.[19] Patients should receive a short course of therapy with rapid dosage reductions to minimize side effects associated with long-term use. Reduced inflammation is the probable mechanism of action, and onset of action is within 8 to 12 hours. Aerobic exercise may also be beneficial for abortive therapy.[48,49]

Parenteral narcotics can be used for pain relief and may allow the patient to sleep through the attack. Use of narcotics should be minimized, however, to prevent abuse. Transnasal butorphanol is an alternative to injectable narcotics.[6,18,19] It has a rapid onset of action and induces sleep in many patients. Use of butorphanol should be monitored closely in patients prone to drug abuse.

Recent studies have investigated the intranasal instillation of 0.4 mL of a 4% lidocaine solution.[50,51] Effective pain relief was provided within 5 minutes for 55% of patients, but the headache recurred in 42% of patients within one hour.

PROPHYLACTIC THERAPY

The daily administration of medications, such as β-adrenergic blockers, tricyclic antidepressants (TCAs), anticonvulsants, NSAIDs, and 5-HT antagonists, may reduce the frequency and severity of migraine attacks and increase responsiveness to symptomatic migraine therapies (Table 57–6).[52] Prophylactic therapy should be considered if attacks occur more than two to three times a month, attacks are severe or prolonged and produce profound impairment, symptomatic therapies have failed or produced serious side effects, the patient is unable to cope with attacks, or headaches occur in a predictable pattern (e.g., menstrual migraine).[18,53] Because most prophylactic drugs have demonstrated similar efficacy in published trials, the selection of an agent should be based on its side effect profile and comorbid conditions of the patient.[53] Drug therapy should be initiated with low doses and advanced slowly until a therapeutic effect is achieved or side effects become intolerable. A therapeutic trial of 2 to 3 months is necessary to judge the efficacy of each medication.[18] Prophylactic treatment is usually continued for 6 or more months after the frequency and severity of headaches has diminished, and then gradually tapered and discontinued. Many migraineurs experience fewer and less severe attacks for lengthy periods following discontinuation of prophylactic medications.[54]

β-ADRENERGIC ANTAGONISTS

β-Adrenergic antagonists are generally regarded as the treatment of choice for the prevention of migraine attacks.[18,53] Propranolol, nadolol, timolol, atenolol, and metoprolol appear to be equally efficacious for the prophylactic management of migraines, reducing the frequency of attacks by 50% or more in 60% to 80% of patients.[18,53,55,56] A β-adrenergic antagonist should be chosen on the basis of such properties as β_1 selectivity, lipid solubility, and convenience of formulation. β-Blockers with intrinsic sympathomimetic activity are ineffective for migraine prophylaxis.[18] Although their precise mechanism of antimigraine action is unknown, they may raise the migraine threshold by modulating serotonergic neurotransmission in cortical or subcortical pathways.[7,10,18] β-Adrenergic antagonists are associated with side effects, including fatigue, sleep disturbances, vivid dreams, memory disturbance, depression, gastrointestinal intolerance, impotence, bradycardia, and hypotension. Use of nonlipophilic β-blockers may lessen CNS side effects.[55] β-Blockers are relatively contraindicated in patients with congestive heart failure, peripheral vascular disease, atrioventricular conduction disturbances, depression, asthma, and diabetes. Bronchoconstrictive and hyperglycemic effects may be minimized with β_1 selective agents.

TABLE 57–6. Prophylactic Migraine Therapies

Medication	Dose
β-Adrenergic antagonists	
Atenolol	25–100 mg/d
Metoprolol[a]	50–300 mg/d in divided doses
Nadolol	40–240 mg/d
Propranolol[a,b]	40–320 mg/d in divided doses
Timolol[b]	10–60 mg/d in divided doses
Methysergide[b]	2–8 mg/d in divided doses
Tricyclic antidepressants	
Amitriptyline	10–200 mg at bedtime
Doxepin	10–200 mg at bedtime
Imipramine	10–200 mg at bedtime
Nortriptyline	10–150 mg at bedtime
Protriptyline	5–30 mg at bedtime
Verapamil[a]	240–360 mg/d in divided doses
Valproic acid/divalproex sodium	750–1500 mg/d in divided doses
Nonsteroidal anti-inflammatory drugs[c]	
Aspirin	1300 mg/d in divided doses
Naproxen sodium[a]	550–1100 mg/d in divided doses
Ketoprofen[a]	150 mg/d in divided doses

[a]Sustained-release formulation available.
[b]FDA approved for prevention of migraine.
[c]Daily or prolonged use limited by potential toxicity.

TRICYCLIC ANTIDEPRESSANTS

Tricyclic antidepressants (TCAs) are effective agents for reducing the frequency and severity of migraine attacks.[55,56] As efficacy has been demonstrated most extensively with amitriptyline, it appears to be the TCA of choice for migraine prophylaxis.[18,55,56] Other TCAs used successfully for migraine prophylaxis include doxepin, nortriptyline, protriptyline, and imipramine.[56] The beneficial effects of TCAs in migraine are independent of their antidepressant activity and may be related to antagonism of $5\text{-}HT_2$ receptors on cerebral vessels or suppression of serotonergic neuronal activity in the brainstem.[7,10] TCAs are generally well-tolerated at the lower doses typically required for migraine prophylaxis. Anticholinergic side effects are common and limit use of these agents in patients with benign prostatic hyperplasia and glaucoma. Evening doses are preferred due to associated sedation. Weight gain, orthostatic hypotension, and cardiac toxicity (slowed AV conduction) are also occasionally reported.

METHYSERGIDE

Methysergide is one of the oldest and most effective agents for migraine prophylaxis.[6] This semisynthetic ergot alkaloid is a potent 5-HT_2 receptor antagonist that appears to stabilize serotonergic neurotransmission in the trigeminovascular system to block the development of neurogenic inflammation.[13] Although methysergide is an effective preventive medication in 60% or more of migraineurs, it is usually reserved for patients with refractory headaches, as rare but potentially serious retroperitoneal, endocardial, and pulmonary fibrotic complications have occurred during long-term, uninterrupted use.[13] Consequently, a medication-free interval of 4 weeks is recommended following each 6-month treatment period.[57] Dosage should be tapered slowly to prevent rebound headaches. Monitoring for fibrotic complications should include periodic auscultation of the heart, chest roentgenography, and urinalysis, as well as monitoring for clinical symptoms (e.g., flank pain, dysuria, chest pain, and shortness of breath).[6] Methysergide is best tolerated when taken with meals. In addition to gastrointestinal intolerance, insomnia, vivid dreams, hallucinations, and muscle cramps are also reported with its use. It is contraindicated in patients with uncontrolled hypertension, coronary or peripheral vascular disease, hepatic or renal dysfunction, and in pregnant women because of its potential vasospastic effects.

VALPROIC ACID AND DIVALPROEX SODIUM

Valproic acid and divalproex sodium (a 1:1 molar combination of valproate sodium and valproic acid) can reduce the frequency, severity, and duration of headaches in up to 86% of migraineurs.[57–59] Efficacy of valproic acid, a facilitator of γ-aminobutyric acid (GABA) neurotransmission, may be due in part to the inhibition of serotonergic neurons of the dorsal raphe nuclei.[10,13] Nausea and vomiting, the most common early side effects, are self-limited and appear to be less common with divalproex sodium and gradual titration of doses. Tremor, weight gain, and hair loss are also common complaints. Hepatotoxicity is the most serious, although rare, side effect of valproate therapy. Clinical guidelines for the use of valproate in migraineurs have recently been published by Silberstein.[60] Clinical monitoring for symptoms suggestive of hepatotoxicity (nausea, vomiting, anorexia, lethargy, abdominal pain, bruising, bleeding, rash, and jaundice) is preferable to routine laboratory screening in patients whose risk of developing valproate hepatotoxicity is negligible (patients over 10 years of age who are receiving monotherapy and have no underlying metabolic or neurologic disorder).[60] However, baseline laboratory studies and patient evaluation every 1 to 2 months during the first 6 to 9 months of therapy is recommended. Valproate levels may be useful for assessing compliance and toxicity; however, rigid adherence to the anticonvulsant therapeutic range of valproate (50 to 100 μg/mL) is not likely to benefit the migraine patient.[60]

NONSTEROIDAL ANTI-INFLAMMATORY DRUGS (NSAIDs)

NSAIDs are effective for reducing the frequency, severity, and duration of migraine attacks; however, potential gastrointestinal and renal toxicity limit the daily or prolonged use of these agents.[18,61,62] Consequently, NSAIDs have been used intermittently to prevent headaches that recur in a predictable pattern, such as menstrual migraine. Administration of NSAIDs in the perimenstrual period may be beneficial in women with true menstrual migraine, which occurs only at the time of menses.[18,55] Their preventive mechanisms are unknown, but are thought to involve the inhibition of prostaglandin synthesis and subsequent neurogenic inflammation in the trigeminovascular system.[18] If long-term NSAID therapy is initiated, monitoring of renal function and occult blood loss is necessary.

VERAPAMIL

Among the calcium channel blockers, verapamil is considered the agent of choice for the prevention of migraines, but it provided only modest benefit in decreasing the frequency of attacks in two placebo-controlled studies.[18,53,62] Verapamil has little effect on the severity of migraine attacks.[18] The therapeutic effect of verapamil, which is thought to be due to the inhibition of 5-HT release, may not be noted for up to 8 weeks after the initiation of therapy.[10,18] It is generally considered a second- or third-line prophylactic agent when other drugs with established clinical benefit are ineffective or contraindicated. Side effects of verapamil may include constipation, hypotension, bradycardia, atrioventricular block, and exacerbation of congestive heart failure.

MISCELLANEOUS AGENTS

Other medications have been suggested as effective alternatives for migraine prophylaxis, including calcitonin, methylergonovine, clonidine, papaverine, cyproheptadine, phenelzine, fluoxetine, and phenytoin.[6,52,55] Although the clinical utility of these agents has not been adequately studied, they may prove useful for patients who are intolerant of standard prophylactic therapies.

PHARMACOECONOMIC CONSIDERATIONS

Although migraine is widely recognized as a disease that exacts an enormous toll on the sufferer, the direct and indirect costs associated with migraine headache impose a substantial burden on society as well. The direct costs associated with migraine diagnosis and treatment are substantial. The volume of health care services used by migraineurs is two to five times that of nonmigraineurs, with 90% of patients reporting visits to a medical clinic and 50% reporting visits to an emergency department.[63,64] However, the indirect costs of the illness related to work absenteeism, decreased productivity, and impairment greatly exceed the direct cost of medical care.[65] The estimated indirect cost of migraine-related disability—the most important determinant of the economic impact of migraine—is between $5.6 and $17.2 billion each year.[5,66]

According to the American Migraine Study, only 41% of women and 29% of men with clear symptoms of migraine had been diagnosed by a physician.[3] Although 95% of severe migraine sufferers take some medication for their headaches, only 40.1% of women and 28.2% of men with moderate to severe headache-related disability take prescription medication.[3] Because many migraineurs not receiving adequate care experience substantial levels of pain and disability, improvement in migraine diagnosis, care, and treatment could potentially result in lower direct and indirect costs of the disease.

Education of headache patients regarding required behavior changes and effective use of acute and prophylactic pharmacotherapy may be time-consuming but is extremely cost effective. Oversights may lead to decreased efficacy of medications resulting in repeat dosing and polypharmacy, decreased compliance, increased emergency department use, increased doctor shopping, and perhaps, increased use of expensive diagnostic procedures and inpatient services.[56] Recent studies have also demonstrated that effective migraine treatment can decrease disability or restore normal function.[65]

SUMMARY

Migraine management should be individualized based on the patient and presentation. Simple analgesics and NSAIDs should be considered the drugs of choice for abortive therapy. Sumatriptan or ergotamine preparations can be used as secondary agents if initial therapies prove ineffective. Abortive therapy should be instituted early in the course of the migraine attack. Prophylactic therapy is indicated for patients with two or more migraines per month, severe or prolonged attacks, migraines refractory to abortive therapy, or migraines occurring in a predictable manner. Therapy should be individualized based on the side effect profiles of available agents and comorbid conditions. Efficacy of a prescribed regimen should be reassessed periodically. Prolonged headache-free intervals could allow for gradual dosage reduction and discontinuation of therapy.

CLUSTER HEADACHE

EPIDEMIOLOGY

Cluster headache, the most severe of the primary headache disorders, is characterized by attacks of severe, unilateral head pain that occur in series lasting for weeks or months (cluster periods) separated by remission periods usually lasting months or years.[4,67,68] Cluster headaches may be episodic or chronic (Table 57–7).[4] It is relatively uncommon among the primary headache disorders, with a prevalence of approximately 1 per 1000.[69] Unlike migraine, more men are afflicted than women. Onset can occur at any age, but it is most common in the late 20s. A family history of migraine or cluster headache is usually not present.

PATHOPHYSIOLOGY

Similar to migraine headache, the basic pathophysiology of cluster headache is thought to involve activation of trigeminovascular neurons with resultant release of vasoactive neuropeptides and the development of sterile, neurogenic inflammation.[67] Triggers of cluster headache attacks may cause periodic discharges of the trigeminovascular system that result in headache pain; however, the mechanisms that activate the trigeminovascular system are not yet understood. The periodicity and regularity of attacks may implicate hypothalamic dysfunction and resulting alterations in circadian rhythms in the pathogenesis of cluster headache.[67,70] Hypothalamus-induced changes in cortisol, prolactin, β-endorphin, and melatonin have been demonstrated during periods of cluster headache attack.[67] Because serotonergic systems modulate activity in both the hypothalamus and trigeminovascular neurons, 5-HT may play a significant role in cluster headache pathophysiology. The association of cluster headache with high-altitude hypoxia, rapid eye movement sleep, and vasodilator therapy, as well as the efficacy of oxygen inhalation therapy in aborting cluster attacks, suggest that hypoxemia may also play a role in the pathogenesis of cluster headache.[67]

TABLE 57–7. Diagnostic Criteria for Episodic and Chronic Cluster Headache

A. At least five attacks fulfilling B through D, below
   Episodic cluster headache: Cluster periods last (untreated) 7 days to 1 year, separated by remissions of at least 14 days
   Chronic cluster headache: Attacks occur for more than 1 year without remission or with remission lasting less than 14 days
B. Severe unilateral orbital, supraorbital, and/or temporal pain lasting 15 to 180 minutes untreated
C. Headache is associated with at least one of the following signs, which have to be present on the painful side:
   1. Conjunctival injection
   2. Lacrimation
   3. Nasal congestion
   4. Rhinorrhea
   5. Forehead and facial sweating
   6. Miosis
   7. Ptosis
   8. Eyelid edema
D. Frequency of attacks: from one every other day to eight per day
E. At least one of the following:
   1. History, physical, and neurologic examinations do not suggest an organic disorder
   2. History and/or physical and/or neurologic examinations do suggest such disorder, but it is ruled out by appropriate investigation
   3. An organic disorder is present, but cluster headache does not occur for the first time in close temporal relation to the disorder

Adapted from Ref. 4.

CLINICAL PRESENTATION

Attacks occur in cluster periods lasting 2 weeks to 3 months in most patients, followed by long pain-free intervals.[4] Periods of remission average 2 years in length, but have been reported from 2 months to 20 years in duration. Cluster headache attacks occur at night in more than 50% of patients and appear to be more common in the spring and fall.[14] Attacks occur suddenly with pain peaking quickly after onset and generally lasting 15 to 180 minutes.[4] Auras are not present with cluster headaches. The pain is excruciating and penetrating, but usually nonthrobbing, and is most often unilateral in orbital, supraorbital, or temporal locations.[4,14] The headache is associated with autonomic features consistent with sympathetic system paresis and parasympathetic overdrive. These features are present on the pain side and include conjunctival injection, lacrimation, and nasal stuffiness or rhinorrhea. Ipsilateral scalp and facial tenderness, ptosis, miosis, and periorbital swelling are also described. Whereas migraine patients retreat to a quiet dark room, cluster headache patients generally move about during an attack and may rub or beat their heads against objects in an attempt to alleviate the pain.[68,70] These patients often have a history of heavy tobacco and/or alcohol use.[67] The IHS diagnostic criteria for cluster headaches are listed in Table 57–7.[4]

▶ TREATMENT: Cluster Headaches

As in migraine, therapy for cluster headaches involves both abortive and prophylactic therapy. Prophylactic therapies are started early in the cluster period and administered daily until the patient is headache free for at least 2 weeks. The medication is then tapered, but may be restarted with the next cluster period. Patients with chronic cluster headache may require prophylactic medications indefinitely.

ABORTIVE THERAPY

OXYGEN

The standard acute treatment of cluster headaches is inhalation of 100% oxygen by facial mask at a rate of 7 L/min for 10 to 15 minutes.[67,68,71] Oxygen inhalation relieves pain almost immediately and is effective in approximately 70% of adult patients. No side effects have been reported.

ERGOTAMINE

The ergot preparations have also provided effective relief of cluster headache attacks when administered orally, sublingually, rectally, or parenterally.[67,68,71] Dosing guidelines are similar to those for migraine headache therapy. Repeated IV administration of DHE for 3 to 7 days can break the cycle of frequent cluster headache attacks with minimal side effects.[32,72] DHE may also be self-administered by IM injection.

SUMATRIPTAN

Subcutaneous sumatriptan is a safe and effective acute treatment for cluster headaches.[73–75] Headache relief is reported within 15 minutes of administration in approximately 75% of patients.[73,74] Adverse events reported in cluster headache patients are similar to those seen in migraineurs. Sumatriptan has been used in the management of cluster headaches for up to 3 months without evidence of tachyphylaxis or increased toxicity.[75] Orally administered sumatriptan has limited use in cluster attacks due to its relatively long onset of action.

PROPHYLACTIC THERAPY

VERAPAMIL

Verapamil, the preferred calcium channel blocker for the prevention of cluster headaches, is effective in approximately 70% of patients.[67,68] The beneficial effects of verapamil often appear after 1 week of therapy. Effective doses usually range from 240 to 360 mg/d for episodic attacks, but higher doses may be necessary to control chronic cluster headaches.

LITHIUM

Lithium carbonate is effective against episodic and chronic cluster headache attacks, with beneficial effects often appearing during the first week of therapy. The usual dose of lithium for cluster headaches is 600 to 900 mg/d administered in divided doses. Tachyphylaxis to lithium has been reported during prolonged therapy.[67] Although therapeutic lithium levels range from 0.6 to 1.2 mEq/L, optimal plasma lithium levels for prevention of cluster headaches have not been established.

Initial side effects are mild and include tremor, lethargy, nausea, diarrhea, and abdominal discomfort. Lithium treatment has been associated with headache symptoms described as episodes of moderately severe, throbbing occipital pain lasting 6 to 12 hours, but these headaches are easily distinguishable from the cluster headaches and disappear when lithium is withdrawn. Lithium should be administered with caution in patients with significant renal or cardiovascular disease, dehydration, pregnancy, or concomitant diuretic use. For a complete review of lithium use, please refer to Chapter 66.

ERGOTAMINE

Ergotamine can be an efficacious agent for prophylactic as well as abortive therapy of cluster headaches.[67,68] A 2 mg bedtime dose is often beneficial for the prevention of nocturnal headache attacks. Daily use of 1 to 2 mg of ergotamine alone or in combination with verapamil or lithium may provide effective headache prophylaxis in patients refractory to other agents with little risk of ergotism.[67,68]

METHYSERGIDE

In patients unresponsive to other therapies, methysergide 4 to 8 mg/d in divided doses is usually effective in shortening the course of cluster headaches.[67,71] Response to treatment usually occurs within 1 week of initiation of the drug. Precautions regarding methysergide use were described earlier in this chapter.

CORTICOSTEROIDS

Corticosteroids are useful for cluster headaches refractory to verapamil, lithium, ergotamine, and methysergide, or combinations of these agents.[67] Therapy is initiated with 40 to 60 mg/d of prednisone and tapered over approximately 3 weeks. Relief appears within 1 to 2 days of initiating therapy. In order to avoid steroid-induced complications, long-term use is not recommended. Headaches may recur when therapy is tapered or discontinued.

MISCELLANEOUS AGENTS

Other therapies that have been used in the management of cluster headaches include valproic acid, transdermal clonidine, intranasal capsaicin, leuprolide, and bright light treatments, but well-designed, controlled studies are lacking.[67,68,76,77] Neurosurgical intervention may be necessary for patients with chronic cluster headaches that are resistant to all medical therapies.[67,68]

EVALUATION OF THERAPEUTIC OUTCOMES

Patients should be monitored for frequency, intensity, and duration of headaches as well as any change in the headache pattern. Careful monitoring is essential to initiate the most appropriate pharmacotherapy, document therapeutic successes and failures, identify medication contraindications, and prevent or minimize adverse events. Patients taking abortive therapy should be monitored for frequency of use of prescription and OTC medications. Patient counseling is necessary to allow for proper medication use (e.g., self-injection with sumatriptan), to encourage early use of medications in the headache cycle, and to enhance patient compliance. Strict adherence to dosing guidelines should be stressed to minimize potential toxicity. Patterns of abortive medication use can be documented to establish the need for prophylactic therapy. Prophylactic therapies should also be monitored closely for adverse reactions, abortive therapy needs, and adequate dosing and compliance. Consultation with other health care practitioners should be encouraged when changes in headache patterns or medication use occur.

CONCLUSIONS

Migraine and cluster headaches appear to occur as a result of neuronal dysfunction, but the precise etiology and nature of the dysfunction are unknown. Serotonergic neurotransmission and the trigeminovascular system appear to play important roles. A careful patient workup, including patient history, physical examination, and appropriate laboratory tests, should identify most headache patients with major disease. A variety of strategies can be helpful for managing both migraines and cluster headaches (Figs. 57–1 and 57–2). Management of primary headache disorders is directed at suppressing an acute attack and preventing recurrences. Continuing research into the problem of headache disorders will better define pathophysiologic mechanisms and aid the search for less toxic and more efficacious pharmacologic agents.

▶ PRINCIPLES OF PHARMACOTHERAPY

- First-line therapy is alteration in life-style and avoidance of risk factors.
- Abortive therapy should be given early in the migraine attack.
- Once an effective abortive agent and dose has been identified, subsequent treatments should begin with that same regimen.
- Strict adherence to maximum daily and weekly doses of antimigraine medications is essential.
- Prophylactic pharmacotherapy for migraine should be considered if attacks occur more than two to three times a month, attacks are severe or prolonged and produce profound impairment, symptomatic therapies have failed or produced serious side effects, the patient is unable to cope with attacks, or headaches occur in a predictable pattern (e.g., menstrual migraine).
- The selection of an agent for migraine prophylaxis should be based on its side-effect profile, convenience of the drug formulation, and comorbid conditions of the patient.
- Each prophylactic medication should be given an adequate therapeutic trial to judge its efficacy, usually 2 to 3 months.

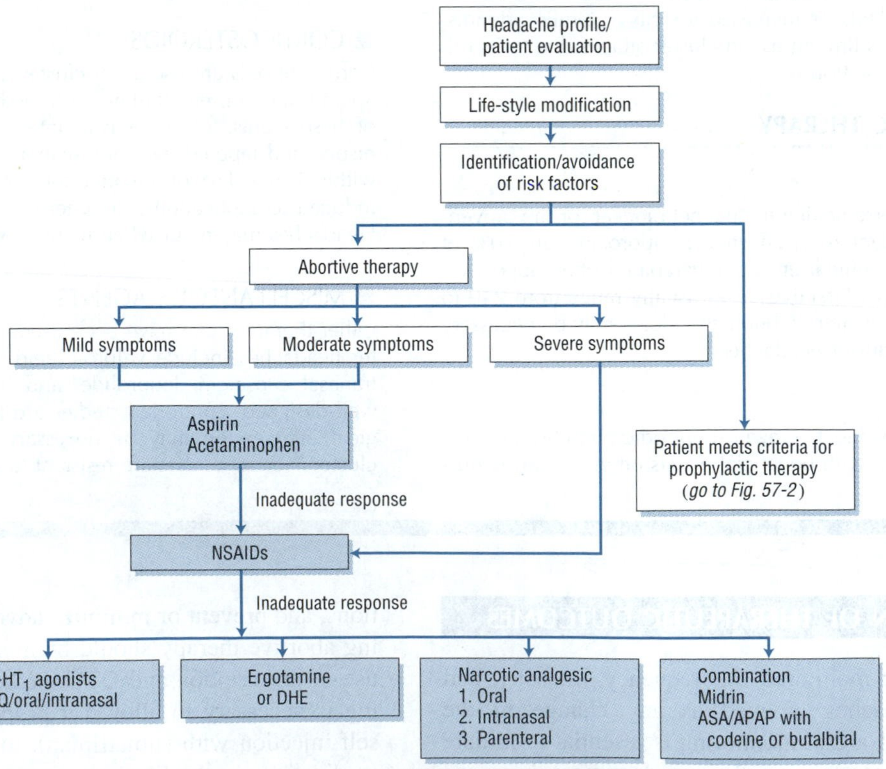

FIGURE 57–1. Treatment algorithm for migraine headaches.

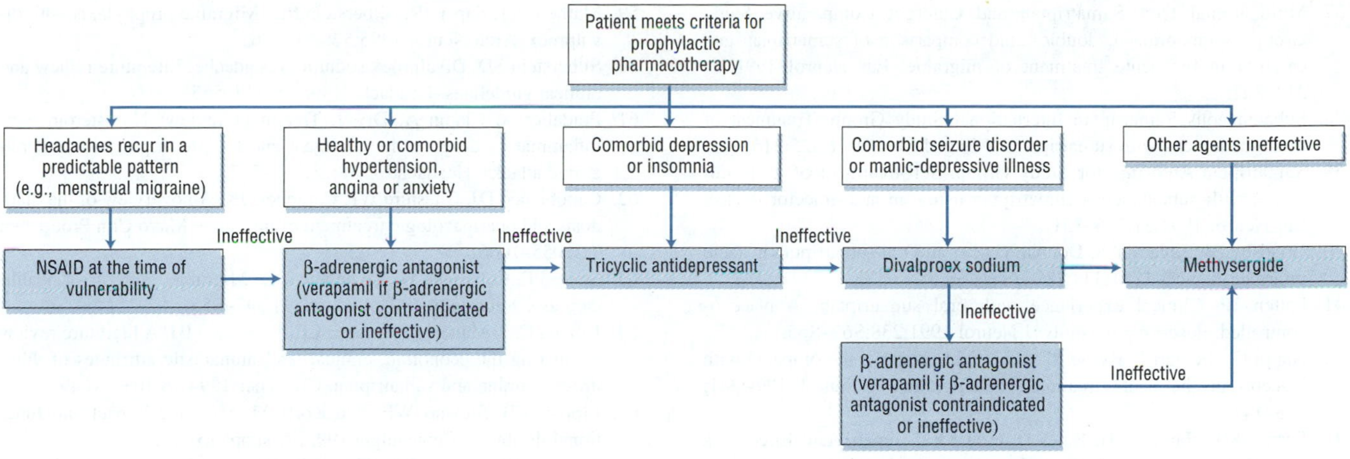

FIGURE 57–2. Treatment algorithm for prophylactic management of migraine headaches.

REFERENCES

1. Stewart WF, Lipton RB, Celentano DD, Reed ML. Prevalance of migraine headache in the United States: Relation to age, income, race, and other sociodemographic factors. JAMA 1992;267:64–69.
2. Linet MS, Stewart WF, Celentano DD, et al. An epidemiologic study of headache among adolescents and young adults. JAMA 1989;261: 2211–2216.
3. Lipton RB, Stewart WF. Migraine in the United States: A review of epidemiology and health care use. Neurology 1993;43(suppl 3): 6–12.
4. Headache Classification Committee of the International Headache Society. Classification and diagnostic criteria for headache disorders, cranial neuralgias, and facial pain. Cephalalgia 1988;8(suppl 7):1–96.
5. De Lissovoy G, Lazarus SS. The economic cost of migraine: Present state of knowledge. Neurology 1994;44:(suppl 4):56–62.
6. Capobianco DJ, Cheshire WP, Campbell JK. An overview of the diagnosis and pharmacologic treatment of migraine. Mayo Clin Proc 1996; 71:1055–1066.
7. Noack H, Rothrock JF. Migraine: Definitions, mechanisms, and treatment. South Med J 1996;89:762–769.
8. Lance JW. Current concepts of migraine pathogenesis. Neurology 1993;43(suppl 3):11–15.
9. Moskowitz MA. Neurogenic inflammation in the pathophysiology and treatment of migraine. Neurology 1993;43(suppl 3):16–19.
10. Silberstein SD. Advances in understanding the pathophysiology of headache. Neurology 1992;42(suppl 2):6–10.
11. Moskowitz MA. The neurobiology of vascular head pain. Ann Neruol 1984;16:157–168.
12. Silberstein SD. The pharmacology of ergotamine and dihydroergotamine. Headache 1997;37(suppl 1)15–25.
13. Silberstein SD, Lipton RB. Overview of diagnosis and treatment of migraine. Neurology 1994;44(suppl 7):S6–S16.
14. Dalessio DJ. Diagnosing the severe headache. Neurology 1994:44 (suppl 3):S6–S12.
15. Frishberg BM. The utility of neuroimaging in the evaluation of headache in patients with normal neurologic examinations. Neurology 1994;33:1191–1197.
16. Solomon S. Migraine diagnosis and clinical symptomatology. Headache 1994;34:S8–S12.
17. Dubose CD, Cutlip AC, Cutlip WD. Migraines and other headaches: An approach to diagnosis and classification. Am Fam Physician 1995; 51:1498–1504.
18. Welch KMA. Drug therapy of migraine. N Engl J Med 1993;329: 1476–1483.
19. Von Seggern RL, Adelman JU. Cost considerations in headache treatment, 2. Acute migraine treatment. Headache 1996;38:493–502.
20. Peters BH, Fraim CJ, Masel BE. Comparison of 650 mg aspirin and 1000 mg acetaminophen with each other, and with placebo in moderately severe headache. Am J Med 1983;75:36–42.
21. Rapoport AM. Analgesic rebound headache. Headache 1988;28: 662–665.
22. Edmeads J. Analgesic-induced headache: An unrecognized epidemic. Headache 1990;30:614–615.
23. Hering R, Steiner TJ. Abrupt outpatient withdrawal of medication in analgesic-abusing migraineurs. Lancet 1991;337:1442–1443.
24. Pfaffenrath V, Scherzer S. Analgesics and NSAIDs in the treatment of the acute migraine attack. Cephalalgia 1995;15(suppl 15):14–20.
25. Treves TA, Streiffler M, Korczyn AD. Naproxen sodium versus ergotamine tartrate in the treatment of acute migraine attacks. Headache 1992;32:280–282.
26. Klapper JA, Stanton JS. Ketorolac versus DHE and metoclopramide in the treatment of migraine headaches. Headache 1991;31: 523–524.
27. Mathew NT. Dosing and administration of ergotamine tartrate and dihydroergotamine. Headache 1997;37(suppl 1):26–32.
28. Raskin NH. Repetitive intravenous dihydroergotamine as therapy for intractable migraine. Neurology 1986;36:995–997.
29. Callaham M, Raskin NH. A controlled study of dihydroergotamine in the treatment of acute migraine headaches. Headache 1986;26:168–171.
30. Gallagher RM for the Dihydroergotamine Working Group. Acute treatment of migraine with dihydroergotamine nasal spray. Arch Neurol 1996;53:1285–1291.
31. Touchon J, Bertin L, Pilgrim AJ, et al. A comparison of subcutaneous sumatriptan and dihydroergotamine nasal spray in the acute treatment of migraine. Neurology 1996;47:361–365.
32. Silberstein SD, Young WB. Safety and efficacy of ergotamine tartrate and dihydroergotamine in the treatment of migraine and status migrainosus. Neurology 1995;45:577–584.
33. Lipton RB. Ergotamine tartrate and dihydroergotamine mesylate: Safety profiles. Headache 1997;37(suppl 1):S33–S41.
34. Hsu VD. Sumatriptan: A new drug for vascular headache. Clin Pharm 1992;11:919–929.
35. Plosker GL, McTavish D. Sumatriptan: A reappraisal of its pharmacology and therapeutic efficacy in the acute treatment of migraine and cluster headache. Drugs 1994;47:622–651.
36. Visser WH, Ferrar MD, Bayliss EM, et al for the subcutaneous sumatriptan international study group. Treatment of migraine attacks with subcutaneous sumatriptan: First placebo controlled study. Cephalalgia 1992;12:308–313.

37. Multinational Oral Sumatriptan and Cafergot Comparative Study Group. A randomized, double-blind comparison of sumatriptan and cafergot in the acute treatment of migraine. Eur Neurol 1991;31: 314–322.
38. Subcutaneous Sumatriptan International Study Group. Treatment of migraine attacks with sumatriptan. N Engl J Med 1991;325:316–321.
39. Sumatriptan Auto-Injector Study Group. Self-treatment of acute migraine with subcutaneous sumatriptan using an auto-injector device. Eur Neurol 1991;31:323–331.
40. Goadsby PJ, Zagami AS, Donnan GA, et al. Oral sumatriptan in acute migraine. Lancet 1991;338:782–783.
41. Patten JP. Clinical experience with oral sumatriptan: A placebo-controlled, dose-ranging study. J Neurol 1991;238:S62–S65.
42. Nappi G, Sicuteri F, Byrne M, et al. Oral sumatriptan compared with placebo in the acute treatment of migraine. J Neurol 1994;241: 138–144.
43. Ferrari MD, James MH, Bates D, et al. Oral sumatriptan: Effect of a second dose, and incidence and treatment of headache recurrences. Cephalalgia 1994;14:330–338.
44. Oral Sumatriptan and Aspirin Plus Metoclopramide Comparative Study Group. A study to compare oral sumatriptan with oral aspirin plus oral metoclopramide in the acute treatment of migraine. Eur Neurol 1992; 32:177–184.
45. Tek DS, McClellan DS, Olshaker JS, et al. A prospective, double-blind study of metoclopramide hydrochloride for the control of migraine in the emergency department. Ann Emerg Med 1990;19: 1083–1087.
46. Lane PL, McLellan BA, Baggoley CJ. Comparative efficacy of chlorpromazine and meperidine with dimenhydrinate in migraine headache. Ann Emerg Med 1989;18:360–365.
47. Jones J, Sklar D, Dougherty J, White W. Randomized double-blind trial of intravenous prochlorperazine for the treatment of acute headache. JAMA 1989;261:1174–1176.
48. Lockett DM, Campbell JF. The effects of aerobic exercise on migraine. Headache 1992;32:50–54.
49. Darling M. The use of exercise as a method of aborting migraine. Headache 1991;31:616–618.
50. Kudrow L, Kudrow DB, Sandweiss JH. Rapid and sustained relief of migraine attacks with intranasal lidocaine: Preliminary findings. Headache 1995;35:79–82.
51. Maizels M, Scott B, Cohen W, Chen W. Intranasal lidocaine for treatment of migraine: A randomized, double blind, controlled trial. JAMA 1996;276:319–321
52. Baumel B. Migraine: A pharmacologic review with newer options and delivery modalities. Neurology 1994:44(suppl 3):S13–S17.
53. Tfelt-Hansen P. Prophylactic treatment of migraine: evaluation of clinical trials and choice among drugs. Cephalalgia 1995;15(suppl 15): 29–32.
54. Raskin NH. Acute and prophylactic treatment of migraine: Practical approaches and pharmacologic rationale. Neurology 1993;43(suppl 3):S39–S42.
55. Walling AD. Drug prophylaxis for migraine headaches. Am Fam Physician 1990;42:425–432.
56. Adelman JU, Von Seggern RL. Cost considerations in headache treatment, 1. Prophylactic migraine treatment. Headache 1995;35:479–487.
57. Hering R, Kuritzky A. Sodium valproate in the prophylactic treatment of migraine: A double-blind study versus placebo. Cephalalgia 1992; 12:81–84.
58. Jensen R, Brinck T, Olesen J. Sodium valproate has a prophylactic effect in migraine without aura: A triple-blind, placebo-controlled crossover study. Neurology 1994;44:647–651.
59. Mathew NT, Saper JR, Silberstein SD. Migraine prophylaxis with divalproex. Arch Neurol 1995;52:281–286.
60. Silberstein SD. Divalproex sodium in headache: Literature review and clinical guidelines. Headache 1996;36:547–555.
61. Pradalier A, Clapin A, Dry J. Treatment review: Non-steroid anti-inflammatory drugs in the treatment and long-term prevention of migraine attacks. Headache 1988;28:550–557.
62. Capobianco DJ, Cheshire WP, Campbell JK. An overview of the diagnosis and pharmacologic treatment of migraine. Mayo Clin Proc 1996; 71:1055–1066.
63. Stang PE, Osterhaus JT, Celentano DD. Migraine: Patterns of health-care use. Neurology 1994;44(suppl 4):S47–S55.
64. Kozma CM, Mauch RP, Reeder CE, Lawrence BJ. A literature review comparing the economic, clinical, and humanistic attributes of dihydroergotamine and sumatriptan. Clin Ther 1994;16:1037–1049.
65. Lipton, RB, Stewart WF, Von Korff M. Migraine impact and functional disability. Cephalalgia 1995;15(suppl 15):4–9.
66. Stewart WF, Lipton RB, Simon D. Work-related disability: Results from the American Migraine Study. Cephalalgia 1996;16:231–238.
67. Mathew N. Cluster headache. Neurology 1992;42(suppl 2):22–31.
68. Lewis TA, Solomon GD. Advances in cluster headache management. Cleve Clin J Med 1996;63:237–244.
69. Mathew NT. Advances in cluster headache. Neurol Clin 1990;8: 867–890.
70. Goadsby PJ. The clinical profile of sumatriptan: Cluster headache. Eur Neurol 1994;34(suppl 2):35–39.
71. Ekbom K. Treatment of cluster headache: Clinical trials, design and results. Cephalalgia 1995;15(suppl 15):33–36.
72. Mather PJ, Silberstein SD, Schulman EA, Hopkins MM. The treatment of cluster headache with repetitive intravenous dihydroergotamine. Headache 1991;31:525–532.
73. Sumatriptan Cluster Headache Study Group. Treatment of acute cluster headache with sumatriptan. N Engl J Med 1991;325:322–326.
74. Ekbom K, Monstad I, Prusinski A, et al. Subcutaneous sumatriptan in the acute treatment of cluster headache: A dose comparison study. Acta Neurol Scand 1993;88:63–69.
75. Ekbom K, Krabbe A, Micelli G, et al. Cluster headache attacks treated for up to three months with subcutaneous sumatriptan. Cephalalgia 1995;15:230–236.
76. Marks DR, Rapoport A, Padla D, et al. A double-blind placebo-controlled trial of intranasal capsaicin for cluster headache. Cephalalgia 1993;13:114–116.
77. Nicolodi M, Sicuteri F, Poggioni M. Hypothalamic modulation of nociception and reproduction in cluster headache, 1. Therapeutic trials of leuprolide. Cephalalgia 1993;13:253–257.
78. Ryan R, Elkind A, Baker CC, et al. Sumatriptan nasal spray for the acute treatment of migraine: Result of two clinical studies. Neurology 1997;49:1225–1230.
79. Reddy P, Lee N. Focus on naratriptan: An oral 5-HT_1 receptor agonist for acute treatment of migraine. Formulary 1998;33:521–533.
80. Rapoport AM, Ramadan NM, Adelman JU, et al. Optimizing the dose of zolmitriptan (Zomig, 311C90) for the acute treatment of migraine. Neurology 1997;49:1210–1218.
81. Teall J, Tuchman M, Cutler N, et al. Rizatriptan (Maxalt) for the acute treatment of migraine and migraine recurrence. A placebo-controlled, outpatient study. Rizatriptan 022 study group. Headache 1998;38(4): 281–287.

58
EVALUATION OF PSYCHIATRIC ILLNESS

Patricia A. Marken, BS Pharm, PharmD, BCPP, and Mark E. Schneiderhan, BS Pharm, PharmD, BCPP

Certain patient assessment skills are common across specialties; however, psychiatry uses additional procedures that are less objective than traditional laboratory tests and physical examination techniques. Mental health clinicians need training in psychiatric assessment in order to participate meaningfully on the treatment team and to provide patient care for the mentally ill. This chapter provides an overview of the assessment of the psychiatric patient in order to facilitate pharmaceutical care planning.

OVERVIEW OF THE *DIAGNOSTIC AND STATISTICAL MANUAL OF MENTAL DISORDERS*

The *Diagnostic and Statistical Manual of Mental Disorders,* fourth edition (DSM-IV), provides a common language for mental health practitioners to describe psychiatric disorders.[1] Common language is essential, because there is considerable overlap of symptoms between many diagnoses. DSM-I was introduced in 1952 and was the first manual on mental disorders to contain a description of diagnostic categories. The most recent edition, DSM-IV, was released in 1994.

The DSM-IV is widely accepted as the most important diagnostic reference for mental illness. It contains many components that provide a comprehensive understanding of the illness and assist clinicians in making an accurate diagnosis. For example, the multiaxial patient evaluation ensures that most factors that could contribute to, or modify, the condition are considered during a patient assessment. The axis I diagnosis lists the principal psychiatric disorder or disorders or provisional diagnoses present. On axis II, developmental and personality disorders are listed. On axis III, existing physical disorders or conditions are listed. On axis IV, the severity of psychosocial stressors that may have contributed to a new or recurrent mental disorder or exacerbation of an existing condition are described. Stressors are rated on a scale of 1 (none) to 6 (catastrophic) and can be acute (lasting less than 6 months) or enduring (lasting longer than 6 months). Examples of stressors include difficulties with interpersonal relationships, parenting, occupation, living circumstances, finances, the legal system, and health. The axis V diagnosis describes the global assessment of functioning (GAF), rated on a scale from 1 (persistent danger to self or others) to 90 (minimal or absent symptoms). A GAF rating should be made for the current level of functioning and the highest level of functioning in the past months to a year prior to the current evaluation. By documenting the baseline level of functioning, the GAF helps in establishing ultimate therapeutic goals.

DSM-IV provides information on all mental disorders recognized by the American Psychiatric Association, including age of onset, clinical course, complications, predisposing factors, prevalence, and differential diagnoses. The specific diagnostic criteria for each mental illness and the number of symptoms required to establish a diagnosis are also listed. The DSM-IV also includes decision trees for differential diagnosis and a glossary of technical terms. *The Clinical Interview Using the DSM-IV* is a companion book that provides extensive information on interviewing techniques to allow the clinician to establish the presence of a DSM-IV diagnosis.[2] Additional information besides the DSM-IV diagnosis is required before a comprehensive treatment plan is developed.[1]

MENTAL STATUS EXAMINATION

The mental status examination (MSE) in psychiatry can be conceptualized as the counterpart to the physical examination in medicine. However, conducting a MSE does not obviate the need for a physical exam in a psychiatric patient. The MSE creates a description of current patient behavior, thoughts, perceptions, and functioning, and provides an objective evaluation used for diagnosis, assessment of course of the illness, and response to treatment. The interview should be completed in a quiet, private, and comfortable area where the patient and the interviewer feel at ease. The interviewer should introduce himself or herself and explain the procedure in order to facilitate establishment of a trusting relationship. Generally, open-ended questions should come first, followed by questions focused on more specific or personal data. Open-ended questions ask the patient to provide descriptions and other information in his or her own words. Even though more specific questions may then be necessary to fill in the gaps, beginning in this manner minimizes the risk of "leading" the patient. Patients may respond to specific questions and "yes" or "no" questions with answers they think the interviewer wants to hear. The interviewer must be nonjudgmental in order to develop trust and rapport with the patient and to ensure completeness and accuracy of the information. A MSE has several components.[2,3]

APPEARANCE AND ATTITUDE TOWARD EXAMINER

The appearance of the patient throughout the interview should be noted, including age, dress, grooming and hygiene, use of cosmetics, and facial expressions. A description of appearance should also include unusual physical characteristics and the general state of physical health. The interviewer should note whether the patient is cooperative, mute, hostile, paranoid, or withdrawn.

ACTIVITY

Changes in motor activity include overactivity, underactivity, and catatonia. Overactivity includes an increase in purposeful movements or agitation, where the movements appear purposeless to the observer. Examples of overactivity include pacing; hand wringing; picking at clothing, skin, or hair; inability to sit still during the interview; and excessive hand gestures. Underactive patients move less than expected. Patients with rigid posture, an absence of movement, and failure to communicate may be catatonic.

SPEECH AND LANGUAGE

The quantity, content, and speed of speech and whether the patient makes eye contact should be noted. Speech should be assessed as to whether it proceeds logically in a goal-directed manner or whether the content is vague and poorly organized. Abnormal speech characteristics include *blocking,* whereby the person suddenly stops speaking without any obvious reason. *Thought blocking* usually occurs when a hallucination or delusion intrudes into the person's thinking or when upsetting issues are discussed. *Circumstantial speech* lacks a clear direction because of excess unnecessary information, but the circumstantial patient will eventually make his or her point. In *tangential speech,* however, the ultimate point is never made. *Perseveration* is repetition of speech despite the patient trying to produce a new answer. *Flight of ideas* is overproductive, rapid speech during which the patient jumps rapidly from one idea to the next. *Mutism* is when the patient does not respond even though she or he is aware of the discussion.

MOOD AND AFFECT

Affect describes the prevailing emotional tone, while mood describes more sustained feelings. To properly evaluate a patient's mood and affect, their appearance and the content of speech must be considered. Change in facial expression and the presence of tears, flushing, sweating, or tremors should be noted. Affect can further be described by its range, appropriateness, intensity, and stability. For example, in schizophrenia or depression, the affect may be flat, whereby no change in expression occurs throughout the interview. In contrast, during a manic episode the affect is very intense and often labile. The range of emotional expression is reduced but not absent with blunted affect. An example of inappropriate affect is when a patient laughs when he is depressed or cries when stating that she is happy. A rapidly shifting affect from one extreme to the other is described as labile.

THOUGHT AND PERCEPTUAL DISTURBANCES

A variety of thought disturbances can occur in mental illness. *Delusions* are fixed, false beliefs that are not based in reality or consistent with the patient's religion or culture. Delusions can be paranoid, somatic, or grandiose in nature, and patients may be deluded that they are controlled by an outside force. Delusions are often unshakable, and one should not attempt to talk a patient out of a delusion. *Obsessions* are unwanted thoughts, ideas, or impulses that intrude into a person's thinking. *Compulsions* are actions often performed in response to the obsessions or to control anxiety associated with the obsession. *Thought broadcasting* is the belief that one's thoughts are audible to others. Hallucinations are false sensory impressions or perceptions that occur in the absence of an external stimulus. *Hallucinations* may be auditory, visual, olfactory, or gustatory and may be continuous or intermittent. In contrast, *illusions* are visual perceptions that are misinterpreted, but have a real sensory stimulus. For example, a patient who perceives a chair sitting in a dark corner to be a threatening figure is experiencing an illusion.

NEUROPSYCHIATRIC EVALUATIONS

A neuropsychiatric evaluation assesses sensorium, attention, concentration, memory, and higher cognitive functions such as orientation, abstraction, and calculation. Prior to initiation of the neuropsychiatric evaluation, it should be documented whether the patient has been prescribed medications with sedative properties, because the outcome of the examination could be altered if central nervous system depressants have been taken.

Sensorium, or level of consciousness, refers to the alertness of the patient and, if he or she is not fully alert, the amount of stimulation needed to awaken the patient. Attention and concentration can be assessed using serial "7s" or "3s," whereby the patient subtracts backward from 100 in increments of 7 or 3, respectively. Another concentration test is to have a patient spell a five-letter word backward. Language skills are initially assessed by having a patient read something aloud and silently. General intelligence can be loosely assessed by asking factual information about current news items, recent presidents, or popular television shows or sporting events. Memory is the ability to recall past experiences and is classified as immediate, recent (past events leading to the patient's current situation), and remote (historical facts). Orientation to time, place, person, and situation assesses immediate and recent memory. Asking a patient to recall three objects 5 minutes after they are learned is another test for recent memory. Remote memory is assessed by asking the patient to recall old facts of their life, such as where they were born or where they went to school. Remote memory usually stays intact the longest in patients with intellectual decline. Abstraction is the ability to interpret information such as a proverb ("people in glass houses shouldn't throw stones") or identify similarities or differences between words (apple and orange). Abstraction ability is influenced by education and linguistic fluency; thus, inability to abstract is not always a sign of a thought disorder.

INSIGHT AND JUDGMENT

Insight refers to patients' awareness that they have a mental illness and the consequences of that illness on their life. Patients typically have a lack of insight when they are psychotic. Patients with poor insight are often noncompliant with prescribed medications. Judgment is the ability to make decisions appropriate to the situation and may be impaired in a variety of mental illnesses.

A MSE is usually completed upon admission to a hospital or intake into a psychiatric facility. The MSE should be used to identify initial target symptoms that are monitored during the course of drug therapy. Table 58–1 provides examples of questions that can be used to gather some information in the MSE. Note that these are additional questions that can be asked for probing and clarification after as much information as possible has been gathered using open-ended (nonleading) questions.

PSYCHIATRIC HISTORY

Both the patient's and the family's history of mental illness provide important information when formulating a diagnosis. Information should be descriptive and include the current and previous psychiatric diagnoses, presentation of each illness, time frame between episodes, level of functioning between episodes, length of each episode, total duration of illness, and treatment given during each episode. Baseline functioning or the highest level of functioning achieved in the past few years is important information because it provides a target or goal for treatment. Information on the history of the current episode and reasons for coming to the clinician should also be gathered. A family history should include a medication history of the immediate relatives, because a family member's response to a given medication may predict an individual patient's response to that same medication.

A social history should include educational and occupational background, religion, marital status, substance use patterns including smoking, and current living situation. By understanding a patient's living environment and social situation, strategies to prevent noncompliance and to reduce stress and increase social support can be developed.

TABLE 58–1. Examples of Interview Questions for Assessing Mental Illnesses

Mania
1. Do your thoughts go faster than you can say them?
2. Have you noticed a change in the amount of sleep that you require?
3. Have you spent a lot of money lately? What did you spend it on?
4. Do you have a lot of extra energy?
(To assess hallucinations and delusions, see Schizophrenia section later in table.)

Depression
1. Do you cry without any reason?
2. Do you still enjoy the same hobbies/activities that you once did?
3. Has your weight changed recently?
4. Have you had changes in your energy level recently?
5. Do you have any guilty feelings?
6. Do you find it difficult to remember phone numbers, names of friends, appointments, and so forth?
(To assess sleep and suicidal potential, see Sleep and Suicide Potential sections later in table.)

Schizophrenia

Delusions
1. Do you feel that people plot against you?
2. Do you feel that you are ever watched or spied on?
3. Do you have any special abilities?
4. Does anyone ever try to mess with you or bother you?
5. Do others read your thoughts?

Hallucinations
1. Does the TV or radio ever tell you things?
2. Do you hear voices that other people don't hear?
3. What do they say? How many voices?
4. How often do they bother you?
5. Do the voices ever tell you to hurt yourself or someone else?
6. Have you ever heard your name called when there is no one there?
7. Have you ever seen anything strange that you can't explain?
8. Do you ever see things that bother you and no one else?
9. Do you want to act on what the voices say?

Thought Broadcasting/Insertion
1. If I stood by you could I hear your thoughts?
2. Does your head ever act like a radio?
3. Do you feel that others can put thoughts in your head?

Insight
1. What reasons did your family give you for coming here?
2. What brought you here?
3. Do you consider yourself in need of help?
4. What does your medication do for you?

Sleep
1. Tell me about your sleep?
2. How many hours do you sleep each night at present?
3. How many hours do you usually sleep at night?
4. Do you sleep all through the night?
5. Is there a reason for your waking up?
6. Do you have trouble falling asleep?
7. How do you feel when you wake up?

Suicide Potential
1. Do you feel your life is worth living?
2. Do you ever think of hurting yourself?
3. Do you see things improving in the future?
4. Do you think you will try to hurt yourself now?
5. How would you do it?
6. Do you have the means to hurt yourself?

MEDICATION HISTORY

A thorough medication history is one of the most important contributions a pharmacist can make to treatment planning. The history should include medication for both psychiatric and medical conditions. The medication history should note not only which medications have been taken, but how they were tolerated and how well the patient responded to them. Because most psychiatric medications have a delay in the onset of effect and many mental illnesses are chronic, it is important to determine whether an adequate trial (adequate duration and adequate dose) was provided before the patient was considered nonresponsive. If a patient has a history of noncompliance, specific causes such as cost, complicated dosing schedules, lack of insight, and adverse effects should be investigated.

MEDICAL ASSESSMENT IN PSYCHIATRY

A careful medical assessment of patients who present with psychiatric symptoms is important for many reasons.[4] Both medical illnesses and medications can cause psychiatric symptoms, making accurate diagnosis very difficult. Patients with psychiatric illnesses, especially depressive and anxiety disorders, may describe only physical complaints. In addition, many patients with chronic psychiatric illnesses receive poor medical care and need a medical referral.

Medical illnesses may be misdiagnosed or undiagnosed in patients with psychiatric illnesses for reasons identified in Table 58–2.[5] An important clue that a physical illness may be causing or contributing to psychiatric symptoms is rapidity of onset of psychiatric symptoms. Most chronic mental illnesses have a prodromal period, whereas medically based psychiatric symptoms often have a more rapid onset of symptoms. Patients over age 40 at first presentation are more likely to have a medical cause for their psychiatric symptoms, because major psychiatric illnesses such as schizophrenia and bipolar affective disorder usually first present at an earlier age. A family history of physical illnesses with a psychiatric component, such as Huntington's chorea and systemic lupus erythematosus, provides an additional clue. Patients with fluctuating levels of consciousness, disorientation, memory impairment, or visual, tactile, or olfactory hallucinations are more likely to have a medical basis for their illness.

Routine laboratory screening in psychiatry is useful for ruling out medical causes of psychiatric illnesses, but extensive testing is usually unnecessary and not cost effective. Laboratory tests should be individualized to the age and physical health of the patient. A complete physical examination along with a detailed medical history and routine blood chemistry (34 panel) are likely to identify possible medical-related causes.[5] Urine drug screens and blood alcohol tests play an important role in identifying the contribution of substances of abuse to the presenting symptoms. In some cases, if available, recent laboratory tests can be used, provided that no change in physical status has occurred. A blood chemistry panel and a complete blood count are usually needed to assess contraindications and complications to drug therapy. Serum concentration monitoring of selected medications is also helpful in increasing probability of response and minimizing the likelihood of adverse effects.

TABLE 58–2. Reasons for Misdiagnosis of Medical Illnesses in the Mentally Ill

Disease Related
Psychiatric symptoms may precede physical signs and symptoms of illness
Impaired memory or perception prevents patients from providing accurate history
Patient Related
Appearance (dirty, strange dress)
Behavior (hostile, threatening, uncooperative)
Physician Related
Incomplete assessments: incomplete medical history, cursory physical examination, failure to interview other informants (old records, friends, family), lack of current physical exam or laboratory tests
Incorrect assumptions: absence of delirium, memory impairment, or disorientation rules out physical disease, psychiatric symptoms imply psychiatric diagnosis, psychosocial stressors explain current symptoms

(Adapted from Ref. 5.)

PSYCHOLOGICAL TESTING

Although pharmacists are not directly involved in psychological testing, they can use the results to evaluate the role of medication in relationship to the diagnosis. Psychological testing alone cannot establish a firm diagnosis, but can be a useful diagnostic tool when coupled with clinical judgment. Types of psychological testing include personality tests, intelligence tests, and neuropsychological tests.[6] Table 58–3 describes common psychological tests.

TABLE 58–3. Common Psychological Tests

Wechsler Intelligence Scales (WAIS-R for adults; WISC-R for children)
Measures abstract thinking, learning from experience, problem solving, adjustment to new situations
Score less than 70 denotes mental retardation
Bender Visual Motor Gestalt Test
Screening test for brain damage, learning problems, emotional difficulties, nonverbal intelligence
Person is asked to reproduce nine geometric designs
Interpretation of Projective Drawings
Patient draws a person, house-tree-person, family, or spontaneously to assess unconscious feeling, conflicts, and strengths
Rorschach
Patient interprets 10 inkblots and explains what they mean
Assesses personality structure
Minnesota Multiphasic Personality Inventory (MMPI-2)
Measures personality traits from 567 true/false questions
Can be affected by intelligence, education, socioeconomic status

PSYCHIATRIC RATING SCALES

Psychiatric rating scales have multiple uses including research, patient care, and education.[7] The purpose of a rating scale is to provide objective data to answer a clinical or research question. A single psychiatric rating scale score provides only a limited picture or snapshot of a complex clinical situation. However, repeated ratings can objectively describe longitudinal change over a defined treatment period. For example, the Hamilton Anxiety Rating Scale (HAM-A) can be used to assess baseline symptoms of anxiety and the change produced by an intervention or time.[8]

Global rating scales, such as the Clinical Global Impression (CGI) scale, assess the overall severity of illness based on a rater's clinical experience.[9] The HAM-A can detect features of somatic and psychic anxiety (e.g., anxious mood, tension, fears, insomnia, somatic, and cardiovascular symptoms). The rating scale will not determine the reason for the symptoms; for example, a patient's anxiety may be secondary to paranoia or a primary anxiety disorder. Second, a patient may have a 15% drop in a rating scale score from one week to the next but remain severely ill. Sensitivity, specificity, reliability, and validity are important considerations when selecting a rating scale. The sensitivity of a test refers to its ability to detect a symptom or illness, given that the symptom or illness is present. Specificity refers to a test's ability to determine that a symptom or illness is absent given that the person does not have the illness.

Reliability is the extent to which the score on the scale reflects the hypothetical "true" score and how much interference occurs from outside influences.[10] Reliability is reported by the correlation coefficient, which represents a chance correlation (zero) or perfect correlation (one). Rating scales with correlation coefficients of less than 0.7 are usually considered unreliable for clinical studies. Interrater reliability—agreement in rating scores among clinicians—is important to achieve when multiple people rate the same patient or population. Interrater reliability is established by having all raters independently rate individual patients at the same time to determine the correlation of their scores. Other types of reliability include test–retest reliability (assesses the stability of the scale in producing the same results with repeated use) and internal consistency (degree to which items in the scale measure different aspects of the same condition without overlap).

Validity, in contrast, is the ability of a scale to measure what it was designed to measure. Content validity measures the extent to which the scale assesses appropriate aspects of the illness. Concurrent validity is a measure of the correlation of the rating scale to an external measure such as diagnosis or clinical change. Construct validity is the extent to which the test appears to measure symptom traits in contrast to measuring a more limited, specific symptom.

TABLE 58–4. Schizophrenia Rating Scales

Rating Scale	Type	Scoring	Comments
Brief Psychiatric Rating Scale (BPRS)	Clinician rated	18 items, 7-point severity scale. Total ≥ 38 indicates moderate severity	The anchored BPRS provides descriptions of each severity rating to increase the interrater reliability The BPRS has four clusters of symptoms: thinking disturbance, anxious depression, withdrawal–retardation, and hostility–suspiciousness
Scale for Assessment of Negative Symptoms (SANS)	Clinician rated	30 items, 6-point severity scale: 0 = normal 5 = severe	Measures degree of affect, alogia, avolition, anhedonia, and attention
Schedule for Affective Disorders and Schizophrenia—Change version (SADS-C)	Clinician rated	29 items, 6-point scale and Global Assessment Scale. Subsets of items can be combinded to score specific affective symptoms	Structured interview to measure change in symptoms and assess anxiety, depression, manic features, and delusions or disorganization
Positive and Negative Syndrome Scale (PANSS)	Clinician rated	30 items, 7-point severity scale	Based on the 18-item Brief Psychiatric Rating Scale
Nurses Observations Scale for Inpatient Evaluation (NOSIE)	Observational	30 items, 4-point severity scale: 0 = never 1 = sometimes 2 = often 3 = usually 4 = always	Patients behavior is rated daily
Clinical Global Impression Scale (CGI)	Observational	Severity of illness, 7-point rating scale Global improvement, 7-point rating scale Efficacy index: 1–4 = marked improvement 5–8 = moderate 9–12 = minimal 13–16 = unchanged/worse	Observational rating scale to compare severity of illness compared to other similar patients and measures improvement from baseline. The efficacy index measures therapeutic effect and side effects to determine the score

TABLE 58–5. Depression Rating Scales

Rating Scale	Type	Scoring	Comments
Hamilton Psychiatric Rating Scale for Depression (HAM-D)	Clinician rated	17-item scale: < 6 = normal mood 17–25 = mild depression > 25 = severe depression	Used to screen patients for drug studies and to determine severity of symptoms and treatment outcome The standard to compare other depression rating scales
Montgomery–Asberg Depression Rating Scale (MADRS)	Clinician rated	10 items, 7-point scale. For each item: 0 = no symptoms 6 = severe symptoms	Differentiates between all the intermediate grades of depression Decreases bias in patients with other medical illness and increased somatization
Beck Depressive Inventory (BDI)	Patient rated	21-item scale: 0–9 = normal 10–15 = mild depression 16–19 = mild to moderate 20–29 = moderate to severe 30–63 = severe depression	The standard for self-rating scales and an objective measure of change in symptoms as a result of treatment
Zung Self-rating Depression Scale (SDS)	Patient rated	20 items, 4-point severity scale: < 50 = normal 50–59 = minimal to mild 60–69 = moderate to marked ≥ 70 = severe depression	Severity rated by frequency of occurrence of symptoms. May not be as sensitive in measuring changes in severity of symptoms
Raskin's Mood Scales and Modified Mood Scales for Depression (RMS)	Patient rated	53-item scale	Measures the presence or absence of symptoms. Sensitive in measuring changes resulting from treatment

Psychiatric rating scales should not be confused with psychological tests such as neuropsychological and intellectual assessments and are best used as only one part of a comprehensive diagnostic plan. Tables 58–4, 58–5, and 58–6 describe commonly used patient-rated and clinician-rated scales for a variety of disease states.[11–16] In clinical research, a combination of clinician- and self-rated rating scales and diagnostic tests provides the most accurate measurement of drug efficacy and treatment outcome.

CONCLUSIONS

Patient assessment is the backbone from which a pharmaceutical care plan evolves. Problem identification and therapeutic monitoring cannot occur unless a thorough assessment is first completed. The initial assessment is also the basis for evaluating response to therapy throughout the course of treatment. Psychiatric assessment requires sensitivity and good listening skills on the part of the clinician

TABLE 58–6. Anxiety Rating Scales

Rating Scale	Type	Scoring	Comments
Hamilton Anxiety Scale (HAM-A, HAM-AS, or HAMRS)	Clinician rated	14 items, 5-point scale. Scores of ≥ 18–20 = moderate anxiety	Consists of subscales to measure somatic and psychic anxiety
Self-rating Anxiety Scale (SAS) (Zung)	Patient rated	20-item scale, 4-point intensity ratings	Correlates with the clinician-rated Anxiety Status Inventory (ASI); however, there is little information on the validity of either test
State–Trait Anxiety Inventory (STAI)	Patient rated	20-item state anxiety (A-state) and 20-item trait anxiety (A-trait) 4-point intensity ratings Total scores range from 20 to 80	A-trait scale reflects the patients general or baseline anxiety. A-state scale reflects the patients most current anxiety and measures changes in anxiety. The A-state score is sensitive to stress-induced testing
Sheehan Panic and Anticipatory Anxiety Scale (SPAAS)	Patient and clinician rated	3-part scale	Measures panic attacks, anticipatory anxiety, and limited symptom attacks. Patient and clinician rated
Yale–Brown Obsessive Compulsive Scale (YBOCS)	Clinician rated	Semistructured interview	Consists of several clusters of obsessions and compulsions. Used to assess change in treatment studies

because it is primarily based on a subjective interview and not objective tests. With careful data collection, pharmacists can make substantial contributions to care that improve patient outcomes.

REFERENCES

1. American Psychiatric Association. Diagnostic and Statistical Manual of Mental Disorders, 4th ed (DSM-IV). Washington, DC, American Psychiatric Press, 1994.
2. Othemer E, Othmer SC. The Clinical Interview Using DSM-IV. Volume 1: Fundamentals. Washington, DC, American Psychiatric Press, 1994.
3. Strauss GD. The psychiatric interview, history and mental status examination. In: Kaplan HI, Sadock BJ, eds. Comprehensive Textbook of Psychiatry/VI, 6th ed. Baltimore, Williams & Wilkins, 1995;1: 521–531.
4. Rosse RB, Deutsch LH, Deutsch SI. Medical assessment and laboratory testing and psychiatry. In: Kaplan HI, Sadock BJ, eds. Comprehensive Textbook of Psychiatry/VI, 6th ed. Baltimore, Williams & Wilkins, 1995;1:601–619.
5. Sternberg DE. Testing for physical illness in psychiatric patients. J Clin Psychiatry 1986;47(suppl 1):3–9.
6. Bulter RW, Satz P. Personality assessment of adults and children. In: Kaplan HI, Sadock BJ, eds. Comprehensive Textbook of Psychiatry/VI, 6th ed. Baltimore, Williams & Wilkins, 1995;1:544–562.
7. Marder SR. Psychiatric rating scales. In: Kaplan HI, Sadock BJ, eds. Comprehensive Textbook of Psychiatry/V, 6th ed. Baltimore, Williams & Wilkins, 1995;1:619–637.
8. Hamilton M. The assessment of anxiety states by rating. Br J Med Psychol 1959;32:50–55.
9. Guy W. ECDEU Assessment Manual for Psychopharmacology, rev ed. DHWE publication (ADM) 76-338. Washington, DC, U.S. Government Printing Office, 1976:158–169.
10. Thompson C. Introduction. In: Thompson C, ed. The Instruments of Psychiatric Research. New York, Wiley, 1989:1–16.
11. Fankhauser MP, German ML. Understanding the use of behavioral rating scales in studies evaluating the efficacy of antianxiety and antidepressant drugs. Am J Hosp Pharm 1987;44:2087–2100.
12. Andreasen NC. The scale for assessment of negative symptoms (SANS): Conceptual and theoretical foundations. Br J Psychiatry 1989;155(suppl 7):49–58.
13. Kay SR, Opler LA, Lindenmayer JP. The positive and negative syndrome scale (PANSS): Rationale and standardization. Br J Psychiatry 1989;155(suppl 7):59–65.
14. Montgomery SA, Asberg M. A new depression scale designed to be sensitive to change. Br J Psychiatry 1979;134:382–389.
15. Sheehan DV. The Anxiety Disease. New York, Bantam, 1983: 114–115.
16. Goodman WK, Price LH, Rasmussen SA, et al. The Yale–Brown Obsessive Compulsive Scale (Y–BOCS): Part II. Validity. Arch Gen Psychiatry 1989;46:1006–1011.

59

CHILDHOOD DISORDERS

Julie A. Dopheide, PharmD, BCPP, and Karen A. Theesen, PharmD, BCPP

Using psychotropic drugs to treat children requires a very different approach than using them for psychiatric disorders in adults. A child's neurologic, physiologic, and psychosocial status are undergoing constant changes throughout the developmental period. Age-related pharmacodynamic and pharmacokinetic differences can alter drug disposition and response. Well-defined diagnostic criteria guide drug selection[1]; however, frequent comorbid disorders present treatment challenges. In addition, children may not be able to verbalize symptom response or adverse effects of a medication. All factors considered, children are generally given psychotropic drugs to control a group of symptoms or behavior in order to facilitate the child's learning and development.

The psychiatric assessment of a child requires obtaining information from the child, parents, caregivers, and teachers. The overall diagnostic impression is formed from psychiatric, social, neuropsychological, and educational evaluations. Before the initiation of psychotropic drugs, the child, family, and caregivers need to be familiar with the risks and benefits of drug therapy and with alternate nondrug therapies. In addition, an explanation of drug monitoring techniques and possible adverse effects, including those of drug withdrawal, should be presented. The risks associated with untreated illness and the possibly related issues of low self-esteem and impaired academic and social functioning should also be discussed.

Pharmacotherapy for children and adolescents is usually administered in conjunction with other therapies (e.g., psychotherapy, family therapy, behavioral therapy). Medication should not be used in place of other therapies or only because other therapies have failed.

ATTENTION DEFICIT HYPERACTIVITY DISORDER

CLINICAL PRESENTATION AND EPIDEMIOLOGY

The three essential features of attention deficit hyperactivity disorder (ADHD) are signs of developmentally inappropriate inattention, impulsivity, and hyperactivity. Inattention typically involves failing to finish tasks, not seeming to listen, being easily distracted, having difficulty concentrating on schoolwork, and having difficulty sticking to a play activity. Impulsivity is often manifested as acting before thinking, shifting excessively from one activity to another, difficulty in organizing work, needing much supervision, frequently calling out in class, and difficulty awaiting a turn in games or group situations. Hyperactivity generally includes excessive running about or climbing on things, difficulty sitting still or staying seated, and excessive movement during sleep. Symptom presence and severity vary with the situation. It is unusual for a child to display signs of the disorder in all settings or even in the same setting at all times.[1] The onset of ADHD is typically by the age of 3 and must be by age 7, although the disorder may not require professional attention until the child enters school. The prevalence in school-age children is estimated to be 3% to 5%, with 4 to 9 boys diagnosed for every girl.[2,3] Girls may be underdiagnosed, as they present with more inattention and less hyperactive and impulsive symptomatology.[2,4] Symptoms may persist across the life cycle for both sexes, but hyperactivity does not usually present beyond middle childhood.[2,5–7]

It is critical to clarify the diagnosis in individuals with these symptoms. Inattention and distractibility can be symptoms of an anxiety disorder, major depression, or bipolar disorder.[7–9] In other cases, these major anxiety or mood disorders can coexist with ADHD, just as learning deficiencies and conduct or oppositional disorders are common comorbid conditions.[2,3,7,9,10] The presence of multiple comorbid conditions, particularly conduct or oppositional disorder, may increase the likelihood of ADHD chronicity.[2,3,9,11]

ETIOLOGY AND PATHOPHYSIOLOGY

Attention deficit hyperactivity disorder is a clinical diagnosis with multiple heterogeneous causes.[2–4,12] Twin studies indicate a genetic component.[2,4,13] One in every four children with ADHD has a biologic parent with a current or prior diagnosis of ADHD. In addition, children with fetal alcohol syndrome, lead poisoning, meningitis, or a genetic resistance to thyroid hormone have a higher incidence of ADHD symptomatology.[2,4] Although not a primary cause, a positive association exists between family environment adversity factors (severe marital discord, low social class, large family size, paternal criminality, maternal mental disorder, foster care) and ADHD.[2,14] Dietary causes are unlikely.[4,15]

Although brain studies show no definitive pathophysiologic markers of ADHD, a dysequilibratory disorder of the frontal–neostriatial dopamine systems with widely varying states of arousal has been proposed. Children with ADHD tend to have phasic outbursts of activity and inactivity, resulting in insufficient alertness during dull and repetitive tasks, and overarousal at other times, resulting in ineffective performance. Stimulant drugs may serve as a homeostat to stabilize arousal and thereby temper the spontaneous fluctuations that are characteristic of ADHD.[2,16] The clinical response associated with stimulants is not paradoxical and is not diagnostic for ADHD, because asymptomatic children also experience increased attention, decreased motor activity, and improvement on learning tasks when given stimulants.[2,4]

▶ TREATMENT: Attention Deficit Hyperactivity Disorder

PHARMACOLOGIC THERAPY

The primary factor in the decision to initiate drug treatment is severity of symptoms. Drug treatment is reserved for moderate to severe symptom intensity; milder cases can often be successfully treated with environmental manipulation alone. Although drug treatment can successfully ameliorate symptoms of ADHD and certain comorbid disorders, multimodal treatment (medication, family therapy, parent training, classroom interventions, behavioral therapy) individualized to the specific needs of the child and family produces better outcomes than drug treatment alone.[2,3] Figure 59–1 provides an algorithm for drug selection in the treatment of ADHD.

Stimulants (dextroamphetamine, methylphenidate, pemoline) are the most effective drug treatment options, with efficacy ranging from 70% to 96% when a trial of each drug is given using wide dosage ranges.[2,7,17] Adderal, a combination of dextroamphetamine and D,l-amphetamine salts, is marketed for use in children with ADHD although there are no published studies demonstrating efficacy.[18] Caffeine has been found to be inferior in efficacy to dextroamphetamine, methylphenidate, and pemoline.[7]

Despite knowledge of the effects of stimulants on neurotransmitter activity, how these drugs affect the primary symptoms of ADHD is unclear. The central nervous system stimulants, in varying degrees, inhibit the reuptake of dopamine and norepinephrine; enhance release of dopamine and norepinephrine from the presynaptic neuron; or inhibit the enzyme monoamine oxidase (MAO). Because stimulants work through slightly different mechanisms, lack of response to one stimulant does not preclude response to another.

Dosing of the stimulants should be titrated for maximum individual efficacy and minimum side effects. Although initiation and dosage titration procedures vary, the following scheme is based on published recommendations of experienced clinicians.[19,20] The initial dose is 2.5 mg of dextroamphetamine or 5.0 mg methylphenidate. Drug response is maximal during the absorption phase, is evident in 15 to 30 minutes, and lasts 2 to 6 hours. Future dosing increments should be 2.5 and 5 mg, respectively. The dosing schedule can be determined by observing when the loss of positive drug effect occurs during the 2 to 6 hours after an oral dose. Most patients require a two or three times daily dosing schedule due to the short half-lives of these drugs (2 to 4 hours for methylphenidate and approximately 6 hours for dextroamphetamine). Controlled studies show substantial symptom reduction from the late afternoon dose with no untoward effects on sleep.[20,21]

Sustained-release products are reported to be either equally or less effective than short-acting products. The convenience of once-daily dosing must be weighed against the potential for difficulty falling asleep with sustained-release products.[22,23] Doses range from 0.3 to 1.0 mg/kg/d for methylphenidate. Maximum daily doses are 40 mg of dextroamphetamine and 60 mg of methylphenidate.[7,20]

The recommended starting dose of pemoline is 37.5 mg, with dosing increments ranging from 18.75 to 37.5 mg/d. Optimal benefit is usually achieved with 56.25 to 75 mg/d, and the maximum dose is 112.5 mg/d. Onset of therapeutic effect is 2 hours postdose.[17] A potential advantage of pemoline is a longer duration of action, allowing once-daily dosing. Pemoline displays wide interindividual variability in metabolism. The plasma half-life varies from 2 to 12 hours acutely and extends to 14 to 34 hours with chronic dosing. Pemoline may accumulate for weeks to months with chronic dosing.[24]

Adults with ADHD are also responsive to methylphenidate using doses up to 1 mg/kg/d.[4,6,25]

Imipramine and desipramine are the most systematically studied tricyclic antidepressants (TCAs) in the treatment of ADHD, although nortriptyline is also effective.[7,26,27] The onset of TCA clinical response occurs within the first 2 weeks, and full response is achieved by week 3. The initial dose of TCA is 10 mg

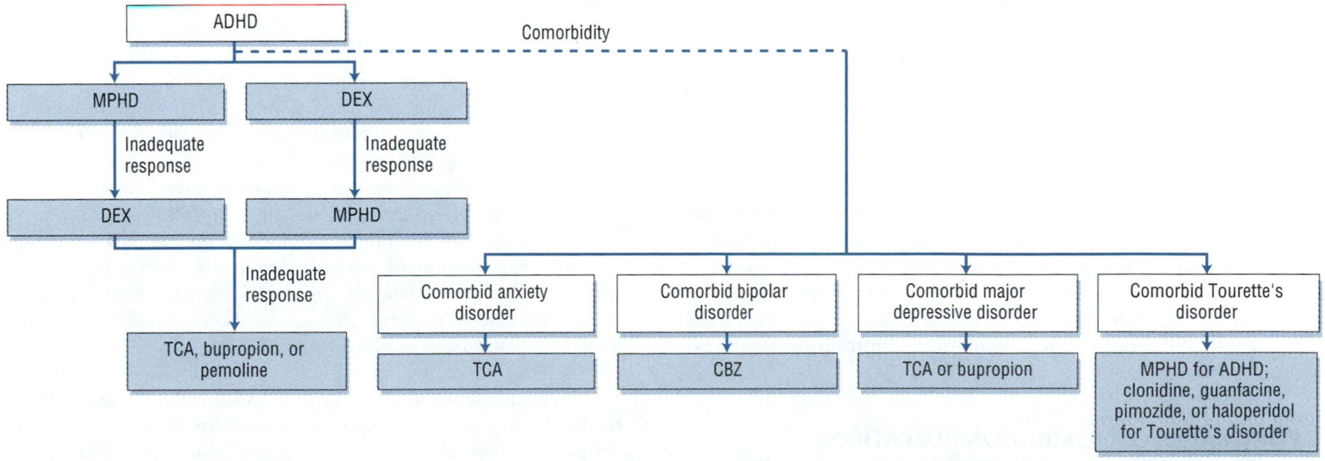

FIGURE 59–1. Algorithm for management of attention deficit hyperactivity disorder. (ADHD = attention deficit hyperactivity disorder; MPHD = methylphenidate; DEX = dextroamphetamine; TCA = tricyclic antidepressant; CBZ = carbamazepine.)

twice daily or 25 mg in the morning. Therapeutic doses of TCA are 1 to 5 mg/kg/d administered in divided doses.[7,26] Variability in dosage requirements may be due to the 10-fold interpatient variability in resultant drug plasma concentration achieved at a given dose. If tolerance seems to develop after months of therapy, a dosage adjustment may be necessary to compensate for age-related changes in distribution and metabolism.

TCAs are second-line alternatives to the stimulants for treatment of ADHD. The potential benefits of TCAs in comparison with stimulants include a longer duration of action, less sleep disturbance, and reduced risk of abuse. Their negative aspects include decreased efficacy, more adverse effects, and the risk of death in overdose.[7,28] TCAs are also effective for adults with ADHD.[6,7,29]

Bupropion, a monocyclic antidepressant, is a weak dopamine uptake inhibitor with no significant direct effect on serotonin or MAO. Its active metabolites augment noradrenergic and dopaminergic function. Preliminary investigations with bupropion at doses of 3 to 6 mg/kg/d titrated over a 2-week period have demonstrated efficacy greater than placebo and in one controlled trial (n = 15 children), comparable efficacy to methylphenidate.[7,30,31] Bupropion may also be effective in adults at antidepressant doses.[32] Further investigations of fluoxetine and venlafaxine are needed to determine their role in ADHD.[7,33,34]

The onset and efficacy of tranylcypromine for ADHD was indistinguishable from that of dextroamphetamine; however, MAOIs are infrequently used largely due to the potential for dangerous drug and dietary interactions.

Clonidine and guanfacine, central α_2-adrenergic agonists, inhibit noradrenergic activity by decreasing the release of norepinephrine from the presynaptic neuron. Both reduce the firing rate within the locus coeruleus and decrease excessive arousal. Two controlled studies suggest that clonidine is more effective than placebo in reducing hyperactivity and impulsivity in children with ADHD at an average dose of 0.2 mg/d after slow upward titration starting at 0.05 mg/d.[7] A retrospective review of clonidine for sleep disturbances associated with ADHD found it was effective in 85% of children for improving sleep at a starting dose of 0.05 mg titrated to an average dose of 0.15 mg/d.[35] An open trial of guanfacine (n = 13) suggests efficacy in decreasing hyperactive behavior and improving attention at doses of 0.5 to 4 mg/d. Guanfacine has a longer elimination half-life (18 hours) compared to clonidine (2.5 hours).[36] Clonidine and guanfacine are alternatives to stimulants and TCAs.

Carbamazepine is an alternative for ADHD. Dosing starts at 100 mg/d or twice daily with gradual titration to response up to 600 mg/d.[37]

Antipsychotics will improve symptoms of hyperactivity and impulsivity, but negative effects on learning and cognitive functioning as well as extrapyramidal side effects (dystonia and tardive dyskinesia) limit their usefulness.[7] For most patients, the disadvantages far outweigh any possible advantage.

Comorbid conditions impact the drug selection process. If a child with ADHD has major depression or an anxiety disorder, an antidepressant may be indicated. Psychostimulants are not effective antidepressants and could make an anxiety disorder worse.[2,3] In children with epilepsy, methylphenidate is effective; however, the child must be stabilized and seizure free on an anticonvulsant prior to the initiation of the stimulant.[38] Bupropion should be avoided in patients with seizure disorders.

PHARMACOECONOMIC CONSIDERATIONS

No cost–benefit studies on the treatment of ADHD have been published. Methylphenidate and dextroamphetamine appear to provide the most effective and economic therapy due to relatively low drug cost and monitoring requirements. The cost of Adderal is approximately twice that of dextroamphetamine. Pemoline's acquisition cost is greater than Adderal, and laboratory monitoring further increases overall costs. Imipramine, desipramine, carbamazepine, and clonidine are relatively inexpensive, but ongoing ECG monitoring increase costs significantly.

EVALUATION OF THERAPEUTIC OUTCOMES

Careful documentation of baseline symptoms and complaints over a 1-month predrug period is essential to the evaluation of therapeutic and adverse outcomes. Baseline symptoms can be measured using videotapes, clinician rating scales, or both. In addition, height, weight, and eating and sleeping patterns should be recorded. After the initiation and titration of any drug treatment, it is necessary that parents, teachers, and clinicians assess the overall functioning of the child to determine if significant therapeutic benefit justifies continuing medication.[39]

Therapeutic effects of the stimulants include decreased motor activity and impulsivity and increased attention span. Improved cognitive performance may result from an overall improvement in attention and concentration, and may not be a direct effect on cognition.[16] This suggests that stimulants are indicated for target behaviors and not for primary learning disorders.

The benefits of drug therapy must outweigh the adverse effects. Anorexia, insomnia, stomach aches, and headaches are frequent but usually mild with stimulant use in children. Anorexia and stomach aches can be minimized by giving the stimulant with or after meals. Insomnia, specifically a delay in onset of sleep, can be minimized by adjusting the dosing schedule and/or the child's bedtime.[39] Occasionally, insomnia persists, and dosage reduction is necessary. Clonidine has been described as an effective treatment for insomnia; however cardiovascular adverse effects and ECG monitoring may limit acceptability.[35,40] Stimulant-induced headache, abdominal pain, and new-onset or exacerbation of tics may require dosage reduction or drug discontinuation. Rare effects include hallucinations (visual or tactile) or delusions, which require dosage reduction or discontinuation. Heart rate and blood pressure are increased with stimulants, but the magnitude is rarely of clinical importance.[7,41]

Pemoline is not a first-line agent due to the risk of hepatotoxicity with long-term use (> 6 months). Twelve cases of hepatotoxicity have been described in the literature with over 20 cases reported to the FDA. Severity of outcomes ranged from full recovery to liver transplantation or death.[42–44] Although not predictive of the onset of liver disease, routine liver function tests are recommended every 3 to 6 months, or as clinical symptoms (fatigue, nausea, vomiting, anorexia) warrant during pemoline therapy. Polypharmacy may increase the risk of hepatotoxicity.

Growth delay is a possibility with stimulant use, but studies in children indicate effects are temporary with normalization in height and weight occurring through midadolescence.[2,45] Proposed mechanisms include alterations in growth hormone secretion and suppression of appetite leading to reduced calorie intake.[41] Heights and weights should be assessed every 3 months for all patients receiving stimulants. Some evidence exists attributing maturational delays to ADHD itself.[45]

A more controversial aspect of stimulant use concerns drug holidays and duration of treatment. Drug holidays are important because they provide time to reassess treatment. All children should be given a drug-free trial every year. Consideration must be given to the risks of negative effects on learning, socialization, and self-image while off of stimulant in determining the frequency and duration of drug holidays. Drug dosage often varies from year to year, largely due to age-related pharmacokinetic changes. As a child develops, hepatic metabolism slows and volume of distribution increases.

The impact of ADHD and its treatment on the development of substance abuse has been investigated in epidemiologic studies. A diagnosis of ADHD confers some risk of adolescent and adult substance abuse, particularly if conduct disorder, antisocial personality, or bipolar disorder coexists.[11,46,47] There is no evidence linking therapy with CNS stimulants for ADHD with substance abuse disorders, and effective treatment may facilitate functioning and participation in substance abuse recovery.[46,48] Nevertheless, practitioners need to pay attention to the presence of an active substance abuse disorder in weighing the risk versus benefit of treatment with stimulants. Alternative therapies may be more appropriate.

TCAs are effective for control of impulsivity and hyperactivity, but they are not as effective as stimulants in increasing attention.[48] Parents should provide doses of TCAs throughout the week and not just during school days. TCA withdrawal effects are common in children and include nausea, vomiting, and diarrhea.

Common adverse effects of TCAs in children are similar to those seen in adults and include sedation, anticholinergic, and cardiovascular effects. Toxic effects include the potential for various arrhythmias and first-degree heart block.[7,49] The effects of TCAs on the ECG should be carefully monitored. Of more concern are reports of sudden death in four children taking desipramine.[49] Children and adolescents given TCAs should have pretreatment and follow-up ECGs to assess the effects of TCA therapy on cardiac rate and rhythm. Possible CNS effects include dizziness, aggressiveness, excitement, nightmares, insomnia, forgetfulness, and irritability. Signs of CNS toxicity are confusion, impaired concentration, hallucinations, and delusions.

Bupropion's adverse effects include nausea, which may resolve over time or with slower dosage titration, and rash, which may require discontinuation of therapy if severe. Bupropion is associated with exacerbation of tics, and therefore should be used with caution in individuals with tics or a family history of tics.[50]

The most common side effect of clonidine is dose-dependent sedation that usually subsides after 2 to 3 weeks of therapy.[7] Of concern are reports of bradycardia, rebound hypertension, heart block, and sudden death.[40,51,52] Concurrent clonidine and stimulant administration, as well as missed doses of clonidine, add to the risk of adverse cardiac events. When clonidine therapy is warranted due to past positive response or comorbid Tourette's disorder, careful ECG, pulse, and blood pressure monitoring is necessary at baseline, after each dosage change, and in response to clinical symptoms of fatigue, shortness of breath, dizziness, anxiety, or mental status changes. Similar adverse effect monitoring is necessary with guanfacine, although its α_{2a} selectivity may result in less sedation and hypotension than clonidine.[53] When discontinuing treatment, clonidine and guanfacine should be withdrawn slowly (0.05 mg q3d) to prevent rebound hypertension or behavioral dyscontrol.[40]

CONCLUSIONS

At this time, the best drug therapy for ADHD is either methylphenidate or dextroamphetamine. The TCAs or bupropion are good options for those unresponsive to or unable to tolerate stimulants. Clonidine, guanfacine, and carbamazepine are alternatives, while other agents require further investigation before their status in the treatment of ADHD can be fully determined.

TOURETTE'S DISORDER

EPIDEMIOLOGY AND CLINICAL PRESENTATION

Once considered rare, Tourette's disorder is present in between 1 and 8 of every 1000 boys and between 0.1 and 4 of every 1000 girls.[54,55] The essential features of this CNS disorder are multiple motor tics and one or more vocalizations. A tic is a sudden, rapid, recurrent, nonrhythmic, stereotyped motor movement or vocalization. Motor tics include eye blinking, facial twitching, lip licking, shoulder shrugging, moving hair out of eyes, and coughing. Vocal tics include throat clearing, hissing, barking, snorting, echolalia, and coprolalia.[1] Tics may be voluntarily suppressed from minutes to hours. The clinical presentation may vary from just noticeable to debilitating, and the type of tic expressed may change over time.[55,56]

Presence of both motor and vocal tics are necessary for more than 1 year before the diagnosis of Tourette's disorder is made. The median age of onset of motor tics is 7 years, with most patients having the onset of symptoms before age 14. Transient tic disorder is diagnosed if motor or vocal tics occur for less than 1 year. If either motor or vocal tics are present for longer than 1 year, chronic motor or vocal tic disorder is diagnosed.[1]

Tics are most prominent during childhood with some plateau and attenuation of symptoms during adolescence. The early 20s frequently bring stabilization of symptoms, although exacerbations occur during adulthood with characteristic "waxing and waning" or fluctuating symptom severity.[55]

ETIOLOGY AND PATHOPHYSIOLOGY

Tourette's disorder is transmitted in a complex polygenic pattern, whereas symptoms and severity of the disorder vary from one generation to another.[55,57] Behavioral disorders commonly occur in children with Tourette's disorder including ADHD (60%) and obsessive-compulsive disorder (50%). Tourette's disorder itself does not cause diminished intellectual functioning; however, the severity of tics and associated attentional and behavioral disorders can result in impaired neuropsychological performance.[55,58] The neurochemical pathophysiology involves an imbalance in the interaction of dopaminergic, serotonergic, and noradrenergic systems in multiple brain regions. The imbalance may cause a lack of regulation of the brain's inhibitory mechanisms, resulting in tics and associated behavior disorders. This multisystem etiology best explains the success of a variety of treatment options.[54,55]

▶ TREATMENT: Tourette's Disorder

PHARMACOLOGIC THERAPY

Whenever symptoms are severe enough to impair the child's ability to function, drug therapy should be initiated. Haloperidol and pimozide (D_2 receptor antagonists) are Food and Drug Administration approved and highly effective with a relatively rapid onset. Clonidine is significantly less effective but has no risk of extrapyramidal side effects. Psychotherapy and behavioral treatment are useful adjuncts.

Therapy with haloperidol or pimozide should be initiated at very low doses of 0.25 to 0.5 mg/d given at bedtime and then increased gradually. Gradual titration over 2 to 3 weeks helps minimize extrapyramidal and sedative effects while permitting careful assessment of response. Symptoms may regress within 48 to 72 hours after dosage initiation. Doses less than 5 mg/d are effective in controlling tics for most patients, but occasionally doses approaching 10 mg/d are required.[54,59]

Pimozide is considered comparable or possibly superior to haloperidol in efficacy when equivalent doses are used. The maximum daily dose is 0.3 mg/kg/d or 20 mg/d. Its elimination half-life in children with Tourette's disorder ranges from 24 to 142 hours, allowing once-daily dosing.[54,59]

Risperidone, a 5-HT_2/D_2 receptor antagonist, was effective in 58% of children and adults in an open trial at an average dose of 2.7 mg/d titrated from a starting dose of 0.5 mg once or twice daily.[60] Clozapine, a 5-HT_2 antagonist with minimal D_1-blocking and no significant D_2-blocking effects, was found to be ineffective with worsening of symptoms in some Tourette's patients.[55]

Clonidine is effective for approximately half of Tourette's disorder patients.[54,55,61] In some patients, the response is limited to attentional and behavioral problems with no changes in the frequency of tics. Clonidine should be initiated with a test dose, usually 0.025 to 0.05 mg given in the morning with gradual titration every 4 to 7 days to the usual therapeutic dose of 0.15 to 0.25 mg/d (maximum 0.5 mg/d).[55] Doses usually need to be divided during maintenance therapy for more continuous symptom control and to minimize adverse effects. The onset of therapeutic effects is slow, ranging from 2 weeks to a few months. Though not well studied, Comings and associates recommend the clonidine patch over oral dosage forms. The starting dose is one-fourth of a 0.1-mg transdermal patch applied every 4 to 7 days, and then gradually increased over weeks to months as needed.[54,62]

COMORBIDITY AND ALTERNATIVES

When Tourette's disorder coexists with other behavioral disorders, the pharmacotherapy can be more challenging, possibly requiring medication combinations. Often the behavioral problems precede and are more disturbing than the involuntary movements, making them a treatment priority. Pharmacotherapy with stimulants increases dopaminergic and noradrenergic activity, which has the potential to aggravate or precipitate tics. One study examined the comparative effects of methylphenidate and dextroamphetamine on tics in children and found the majority experienced improvement in ADHD symptoms with acceptable effects on tics.[63] Methylphenidate was better tolerated than dextroamphetamine. This study confirms previous reports of methylphenidate's efficacy and superior tolerability compared to other stimulants in treating attentional disorders in patients with comorbid Tourette's and ADHD.[64] Patients and caregivers should be aware of the risks of using stimulants in children with Tourette's disorder. Careful monitoring is essential, and worsening of tics is reversible once the stimulant is discontinued.[2,7,55]

Recent reports of TCA therapy for comorbid ADHD and tics show significant improvement in attention without worsening of tics.[7] TCAs may be preferred to clonidine. A controlled trial in children aged 7 to 13 years with Tourette's disorder and ADHD found desipramine 100 mg/d was superior to clonidine 0.2mg/d in improving attention. Neither desipramine nor clonidine demonstrated efficacy for tics or caused worsening of tics.[65]

Clonidine is a less effective alternative to stimulants in the treatment of children with Tourette's disorder and ADHD. However, one chart review of 54 children with ADHD treated over a 4-year period showed that children with a comorbid tic disorder more frequently had a positive response to clonidine than those without tic disorders.[66] In one open trial with 7 patients, the addition of clonazepam at doses of 0.5 to 1.0 mg/d to clonidine therapy decreased tics to an acceptable level.[67]

Guanfacine, a central α_2-noradrenergic receptor agonist, was administered to 10 children with ADHD and Tourette's disorder over a 4- to 20-week open trial at a dose of 1.5 mg/d. Significant decreases in motor and phonic tics as well as improvements in attention were noted, with side effects reported as transient sedation and headache.[68] Due to its similarity to clonidine, guanfacine's cardiovascular effects warrant careful clinical monitoring (mental status, ECG, blood pressure, and pulse).[36,40] Clearly, further investigations are needed to determine the most effective and safest method of treating Tourette's disorder with ADHD.

Therapeutic trials (6 to 8 weeks) of antiobsessional medications such as fluoxetine, fluvoxamine, sertraline, paroxetine, or clomipramine should be tried when obsessional symptoms cause functional impairment in patients with Tourette's disorder.[55] Careful monitoring for behavioral activation, disinhibition, and motor restlessness is essential during therapy, as these symptoms occur in 20% to 40% of children.[69,70] Mania requires drug discontinuation.

Nicotine administration by gum or patch may potentiate the effects of dopamine blocking agents in relieving tics, according to small open trials and case reports.[71] Recently, nicotine has been found beneficial for symptoms of ADHD as well.[72] The adverse effects of nicotine on overall health may limit usefulness. Further investigations are needed.[71–73]

PHARMACOECONOMIC CONSIDERATIONS

No pharmacoeconomic studies have been published on Tourette's disorder. Haloperidol provides the most economic therapy due to high efficacy and low drug cost. Pimozide is more expensive than generic haloperidol. Although generic clonidine is inexpensive, ECG monitoring, delayed onset of effect, and significantly lower efficacy substantially increase total costs of treatment. The clonidine patch (Catapres TTS) is approximately ten times the cost of generic clonidine tablets on a weekly basis. Risperidone is an expensive alternative due to high medication costs.

EVALUATION OF THERAPEUTIC OUTCOMES

Once a drug is selected, Comings' general principles for pharmacologic management of patients with Tourette's disorder are useful.

1. Tourette's disorder patients are very sensitive to medication. Low doses should be started, with gradual (weekly) increases as tolerated.
2. A plateau effect is normal. At first, tics may remit at a very low dose. However, as the body adjusts to this state, tics may slowly return, requiring upward adjustments after 2 to 4 weeks.
3. The treatment goal is not necessarily total elimination of all tics.
4. If tics disappear for a number of weeks, the dose can be decreased.
5. Medication should not be abruptly stopped. Withdrawal effects can be intolerable.[54]

Medication does not impair neuropsychological performance according to one controlled study; however, assessment of individual risk versus benefit is necessary.[74] The use of regular videotaped assessments in conjunction with a standardized rating scale (Yale Global Tic Severity Scale) is helpful in objectively evaluating symptoms and side effects.[75] Adult patients with Tourette's disorder may still be responsive to drug treatments that were effective during childhood, although the dose and schedule may require adjustment.[55]

Typical antipsychotic side effects have been reported with haloperidol doses of 2 mg/d or greater. In one review of 24 patients treated with haloperidol for Tourette's disorder, 66.7% discontinued treatment due to intolerable side effects (e.g., dysphoria, akathisia, nervousness, sedation, dystonia, and cognitive dulling or feeling drugged).[76] Lowering the dose may alleviate side effects. An antiparkinsonian agent such as benztropine (at a starting dose of 0.5 mg orally twice daily) will generally reverse extrapyramidal side effects. Whether a patient with Tourette's disorder is developing a new symptom or is developing tardive dyskinesia can be difficult to determine. Dosage titration of the medication and careful monitoring will assist in this clinical decision-making process.

Pimozide may cause extrapyramidal side effects but at a lower rate than haloperidol. Anticholinergic side effects may occur in addition to drowsiness and occasionally, anxiety. ECG changes, including T- and U-wave abnormalities and prolongation of the QT (corrected) interval, are rarely found in recommended therapeutic doses for Tourette's disorder; however, patients given pimozide should receive baseline and follow-up ECGs.[54,55,59]

Adverse effects reported during clinical studies with risperidone include lightheadedness, sedation, akathisia or agitation, weakness, insomnia, depressed mood, aggressive behavior, weight gain, and extrapyramidal effects including tardive dyskinesia.[77] Two cases of hepatotoxicity have been reported in pediatric patients treated with risperidone for psychosis over 1 to 2 years; therefore, liver function monitoring every 3 months, or when clinical signs and symptoms warrant (weakness, fatigue, nausea, jaundice), is recommended.[78]

For clonidine, the most common adverse effect is sedation. Fortunately, tolerance usually develops to this effect over days to weeks. The most potentially serious side effects are cardiovascular (see the ADHD section earlier in the chapter).[40] Other side effects include dry mouth, headache, mood changes, and even a temporary worsening of tics in 10% of patients. The clonidine patch has the additional adverse effect of skin irritation, which can be minimized by changing the position of the patch every few days or pretreating the skin with beclomethasone dipropionate aerosolized spray.[78]

CONCLUSIONS

Pimozide and haloperidol have the advantage of greatest efficacy and rapid onset in the treatment of Tourette's disorder. Clonidine has the advantage of no extrapyramidal side effects, but it is significantly less effective and requires ongoing cardiovascular monitoring. Drug treatment must be highly individualized, considering comorbid disorders and side-effect sensitivity.

ENURESIS

ETIOLOGY, PATHOPHYSIOLOGY, AND CLINICAL PRESENTATION

The essential feature of enuresis is repeated involuntary or intentional voiding of urine by day or night which is not caused by any physical disorder. Rare physical causes of enuresis (e.g., diabetes mellitus, diabetes insipidus, seizure disorders, or urinary tract infections) should be ruled out. Diagnostic criteria for enuresis include the repeated voiding of urine that is characterized by either a frequency of at least twice per week for at least 3 months or the presence of clinically significant distress, or impairment in social, academic, or other important areas of functioning. The child must be at least 5 years of age.[1] Enuresis may be primary or secondary. Primary enuresis, the most common type, is diagnosed if the child has never established urinary continence. Secondary enuresis follows an established period (3 to 6 months) of urinary continence. At age 5, prevalence is 7% for boys and 3% for girls; at age 10, it is 3% for boys and 2% for girls. Rates decline into adulthood, but 0.3% of individuals continue to experience enuresis even after the age of 20 years.[79]

Factors that predispose a child to either type of enuresis include a positive family history, small bladder capacity, delayed or lax toilet training, and psychosocial stress. The psychiatric disorders most commonly associated with enuresis are depression and developmental delays.[80,81] In addition, some children with nocturnal enuresis lack the normal diurnal nighttime increase in antidiuretic hormone (ADH). Nocturnal enuresis is not associated with a particular sleep stage.[82]

▶ TREATMENT: Enuresis

PHARMACOLOGIC THERAPY

The first step in treating the child with enuresis is to educate the family about the high frequency of the problem, dispel any misconceptions, provide emotional support, and strongly discourage punishment.[83] For younger children who have not been properly toilet trained, the conditioning technique of dry bed training should be tried first. This technique encourages extra fluids during the day and restricts fluids close to bedtime. Children are encouraged to use the toilet before bedtime. If this method is unsuccessful, then a bed-wetting alarm can be used. Teaching continence skills and various behavioral and conditioning methods remain the primary treatment for enuresis, and drug treatment remains a secondary approach.[83,84]

The exact mechanism of action of TCAs in treating enuresis is unknown; proposed mechanisms include an anticholinergic effect, an α-adrenergic agonist effect, and an increase in ADH.[83,85] Imipramine is the most studied TCA, although desipramine, amitriptyline, and nortriptyline are also effective. For children 6 years and older, the initial dose of imipramine should be 25 mg at bedtime, with weekly increases of 25 mg if necessary. A nightly dose greater than 75 mg is rarely necessary, although doses up to 150 mg have been required in teenagers.[86]

Desmopressin acetate, a synthetic analog of the natural human ADH, arginine vasopressin, is currently available in a nasal spray and oral tablet for the treatment of nocturnal enuresis. Desmopressin raises overnight urinary osmotic concentration by increasing water reabsorption and reducing the volume of urine entering the bladder.[82,83,87] For children 6 years of age and older, the initial recommended nasal dose is 20 μg at bedtime, increasing to 40 μg at bedtime after 3 days if there is no response. Some patients may respond to as little as 10 μg. One-half of each dose is administered in each nostril. About 10% of the dose of desmopressin is absorbed from the nasal mucosa, and plasma concentrations reach a maximum about 45 minutes after administration. Less than 1% of oral desmopressin is absorbed, with effective dosages ranging from 200 to 400 μg/d.[87–90] The 400-μg dose provides greater efficacy with comparable tolerability.[88] Biologic half-life is 4 to 6 hours, and the duration of action varies from 6 to 24 hours.[87]

PHARMACOECONOMIC CONSIDERATIONS

No pharmacoeconomic studies on enuresis are available. The use of a bed-wetting alarm provides the highest overall cure rate, and drugs are a secondary approach; however, drug therapy is commonly reimbursed by insurance companies while the alarms are not. The most inexpensive drug therapy is low-dose TCAs. Higher doses require more extensive monitoring of plasma levels and ECGs, which increase overall cost. Therapy with desmopressin is substantially more expensive than with TCAs.

EVALUATION OF THERAPEUTIC OUTCOMES

Before treatment begins, an accurate baseline of bed-wetting frequency must be established. It usually takes 3 to 4 months of using a bed-wetting alarm, but more than 70% of the children are cured using this method. Drug treatment is necessary when nondrug methods fail. Unfortunately, therapeutic efficacy does not extend beyond drug administration.[86] If drug treatment is required for more than several weeks, attempts to discontinue the drug every 3 to 6 months are advisable to assess for spontaneous remission.

TCA efficacy is often immediate and is usually evident within 7 days. Drug plasma concentrations of imipramine plus desipramine correlate with clinical response, and although individual variation exists, a higher percentage of patients responds to higher plasma levels (> 116 ng/mL).[86] In addition, true nonresponders exist at therapeutic doses and plasma levels.[83,86] Imipramine efficacy is about 70% to 85%; one-half of responders experience total elimination of bedwetting, and the other half, a significant decrease in the number of episodes. An initially effective dose often becomes ineffective in 2 to 6 weeks, but increasing the dose usually reestablishes control. One week is needed to evaluate the efficacy of a new dose. Refer to ADHD and the TCAs for monitoring parameters and adverse effects.

Desmopressin is effective in reducing the number of wet nights in 70% of children. In short-term, 2-week studies, 24.5% of children became completely dry.[87] Predictors of best response to desmopressin include older age (> 9 years), fewer initial wet nights, and larger bladder capacity.[89] Patients with colds or allergies that affect the nasal mucosa may have a less-than-optimal response to desmopressin nasal spray.[83,91] Infrequent adverse effects of the spray include nasal irritation, epistaxis, rhinitis, and nasal congestion, while tablet or spray may cause transient headache, chills, dizziness, nausea, and abdominal pain. Rare effects of water intoxication, hyponatremia, and subsequent tonic–clonic seizures have been reported in children with concurrent physical disorders, intentional overdoses, or excessive fluid intake. When desmopressin is administered, evening fluid should be limited to 8 ounces to prevent hyponatremia or water intoxication.[88,91,92]

CONCLUSIONS

Overall, both TCAs and desmopressin are effective in the treatment of nocturnal enuresis as long as the drug is maintained. Drug selection is based on adverse-effect profiles, ease of administration, and cost. Imipramine has a higher incidence of adverse effects than desmopressin, and the risk of accidental overdose is of concern, especially in very disorganized families. In contrast, desmopressin is markedly more expensive than imipramine.

▶ PRINCIPLES OF PHARMACOTHERAPY

- Careful documentation of baseline symptoms and complaints over a 1-month predrug period is essential to the evaluation of therapeutics and adverse outcomes in ADHD.
- Stimulants are the most effective treatment for inattention and impulsivity in ADHD.
- Symptoms of inattention and impulse control can continue in adolescence and adulthood and may require continued treatment.
- Disorders comorbid with ADHD impact drug selection. Bupropion should be avoided in patients with seizure disorder. For a child with ADHD and major depression or an anxiety disorder, an antidepressant may be the drug of first choice.
- Tourette's disorder presents with both motor and vocal tics, which are present during childhood, plateau during adolescence, and may remit during adulthood with a characteristic fluctuating course.
- The decision to medicate for Tourette's disorder is based on the degree of concern perceived by the patient, symptom severity, and comorbid attentional or obsessional symptoms.
- Individuals with Tourette's disorder are particularly sensitive to medication side effects, so medication dosing must be carefully individualized, and close monitoring is essential.
- Nondrug approaches to enuresis management, such as dry bed training and moisture-sensitive alarms, are preferred because of higher cure rates and avoidance of drug side effects.
- Desmopressin is effective orally and intranasally for enuresis, but it is expensive and works better in older than younger children.
- Imipramine is effective in enuresis at wide dosage ranges. It has rapid onset, but side effects may be problematic for some patients.

REFERENCES

1. American Psychiatric Association. Diagnostic and Statistical Manual of Mental Disorders, 4th ed (DSM-IV). Washington, DC, American Psychiatric Press, 1994:37–121.
2. Cantwell DB. Attention deficit disorder: A review of the past ten years. J Am Acad Child Adolesc Psychiatry 1996;35:978–987.
3. Richters JE, Arnold LE, Jensen PS, et al. NIMH collaborative multisite multimodal treatment study of children with ADHD, I. Background and rationale. J Am Acad Child Adolesc Psychiatry 1995; 34:987–1000.
4. Zametkin AJ. Attention-deficit disorder: Born to be hyperactive? Grand rounds at the Clinical Center of the National Institutes of Health. JAMA 1995;273:1871–1874.
5. Faigel HC, Sznajderman S, Tishby O, et al. Attention deficit disorder during adolescence: A review. J Adolesc 1995;16:174–184.
6. Bellak L, Black RB. Attention-deficit hyperactivity disorder in adults. Clin Ther 1992;14:138–147.
7. Spencer T, Biederman J, Wilens T. Pharmacotherapy of attention-deficit hyperactivity disorder across the life cycle. J Am Acad Child Adolesc Psychiatry 1996;35:409–432.
8. Jensen PS, Shervette RE, Xenakis SN, Richters J. Anxiety and depressive disorders in attention deficit disorder with hyperactivity: New findings. Am J Psychiatry 1993;150:1203–1209.
9. Biederman J, Newcorn J, Sprich S. Comorbidity of attention deficit hyperactivity disorder with conduct, depressive, anxiety and other disorders. Am J Psychiatry 1991;148:564–577.
10. Biederman J, Faraone S, Mick E, et al. Attention-deficit hyperactivity disorder and juvenile mania: An overlooked comorbidity? J Am Acad Child Adolesc Psychiatry 1996;35:997–1008.
11. Mannuzza S, Klein RG, Bessler A, et al. Adult outcome of hyperactive boys: Educational achievement, occupational rank and psychiatric status. Arch Gen Psychiatry 1993;50:565–576.
12. Weinberg WA, Harper CR, Schraufnagel CD, et al. Attention deficit hyperactivity disorder: A disease or a symptom complex? J Pediatr 1997;130:6–9.
13. Levy F, Hay DA, McStephen M, et al. Attention-deficit hyperactivity disorder: A category or a continuum? genetic analysis of a large-scale twin study. J Am Acad Child Adolesc Psychiatry 1997;36:737–744.
14. Biederman J. Family–environment risk factors for attention-deficit hyperactivity disorder. Arch Gen Psychiatry 1995;52:464–470.
15. Wolraich ML, Lindgren SD, Stumbo PJ, et al. Effects of diets high in sucrose or aspartame on the behavior and cognitive performance of children. N Engl J Med 1994;330:301–307.
16. Pliszka SR, McCracken JT, Maas JW. Catecholamines in attention-deficit hyperactivity disorder: Current perspectives. J Am Acad Child Adolesc Psychiatry 1996;35:264–272.
17. Pelham WE, Swanson JM, Furman MB, et al. Pemoline effects on children with ADHD: A time–response by dose–response analysis on classroom measures. J Am Acad Child Adolesc Psychiatry 1995;34: 1504–1513.
18. Adderal and other drugs for attention-deficit/hyperactivity disorder. Med Lett Drugs Ther 1994;36:109–110.
19. Barkley RA, DuPaul GJ, Costello A. Stimulants. In: Werry JS, Aman MG, eds. Practitioners Guide to Psychoactive Drugs for Children and Adolescents. New York, Plenum, 1993:224–227.
20. Greenhill LL, Abikoff HB, Arnord E, et al. Medication treatment strategies in the MTA study: Relevance to clinicians and researchers. J Am Acad Child Adolesc Psychiatry 1996;35:1304–1313.
21. Kent JD, Blader JC, Koplewicz HS, et al. Effects of late-afternoon methylphenidate administration on behavior and sleep in attention-deficit hyperactivity disorder. Pediatrics 1995;96:320–325.
22. Pelham WE, Greenslade KE, Vodde-Hamilton M, et al. Relative efficacy of long- acting stimulants on children with ADHD: A comparison of standard methylphenidate, sustained-release methylphenidate, sustained-release dextroamphetamine, and pemoline. Pediatrics 1990;86: 226–237.
23. Fitzpatrick PA, Klorman R, Brumaghim JT, Borgstedt AD. Effects of sustained- release and standard preparations of methylphenidate on attention deficit disorder. J Am Acad Child Adolesc Psychiatry 1992; 31:226–234.
24. Sallee F, Stiller R, Perel J, Bates T. Oral pemoline kinetics in hyperactive children. Clin Pharmacol Ther 1985;37:606–609.
25. Spencer T, Wilens T, Biederman J, et al. A double-blind, crossover comparison of methylphenidate and placebo in adults with childhood-onset attention-deficit hyperactivity disorder. Arch Gen Psychiatry 1995;52:434–443.
26. Biederman J, Baldessarini RJ, Wright V, et al. A double-blind placebo controlled study of desipramine in the treatment of ADD: I. Efficacy. J Am Acad Child Adolesc Psychiatry 1989;28:777–784.
27. Wilens TE, Biederman J, Geist DE, et al. Nortriptyline in the treatment of ADHD: A chart review of 58 cases. J Am Acad Child Adolesc Psychiatry 1993;32:343–349.
28. Spencer T, Biederman J, Wilens T, et al. Nortriptyline treatment of children with attention-deficit hyperactivity disorder and tic disorder

or Tourette's syndrome. J Am Acad Child Adolesc Psychiatry 1993; 32:205–210.
29. Wilens TE, Biederman J, Prince J, et al. Six-week, double-blind, placebo-controlled study of desipramine for adult attention deficit hyperactivity disorder. Am J Psychiatry 1996;153:1147–1153.
30. Conners CK, Casat CD, Gualtieri CT, et al. Bupropion hydrochloride in attention deficit disorder with hyperactivity. J Am Acad Child Adolesc Psychiatry 1996;34:1314–1321.
31. Barrickman LL, Perry PJ, Allen AJ, et al. Bupropion versus methylphenidate in the treatment of attention-deficit hyperactivity disorder. J Am Acad Child Adolesc Psychiatry 1995;34:649–657.
32. Wender PH, Reimherr FW. Bupropion treatment of attention-deficit hyperactivity disorder in adults. Am J Psychiatry 1990;147:1018–1020.
33. Barrickman L, Noyes R, Kuperman S, et al. Treatment of ADHD with fluoxetine: A preliminary trial. J Am Acad Child Adolesc Psychiatry 1991;30:762–767.
34. Findling RL, Schwartz MA, Flannery DJ. Venlafaxine in adults with attention-deficit/hyperactivity disorder: An open clinical trial. J Clin Psychiatry 1996;57:184–189.
35. Prince JB, Wilens TE, Biederman J, et al. Clonidine for sleep disturbances associated with attention-deficit hyperactivity disorder: A systematic chart review of 62 cases. J Am Acad Child Adolesc Psychiatry 1996;35:599–605.
36. Hunt RD, Arnsten AFT, Asbell MD. An open trial of guanfacine in the treatment of attention-deficit hyperactivity disorder. J Am Acad Child Adolesc Psychiatry 1995;34:50–54.
37. Silva R, Munoz D, Alpert M. Carbamazepine use in children and adolescents with features of attention-deficit hyperactivity disorder: A meta-analysis. J Am Acad Child Adolesc Psychiatry 1996;35:352–358.
38. Gross-Tsur V, Manor O, van der Meere J, et al. Epilepsy and attention deficit hyperactivity disorder: Is methylphenidate safe and effective? J Pediatr 1997;130:40–44.
39. Theesen K. The Handbook of Psychiatric Drug Therapy for Children and Adolescents. Binghamton, NY, Haworth, 1995:1–39.
40. Cantwell DP, Swanson J, Connor DF. Case study: Adverse response to clonidine. J Am Acad Child Adolesc Psychiatry 1997;36:539–544.
41. Greenhill LL. Pharmacologic treatment of attention deficit hyperactivity disorder. Psychiatr Clin North Am 1992;15:1–27.
42. Berkovitch M, Pope E, Phillips J, et al. Pemoline-associated fulminant liver failure: Testing the evidence for causation. Clin Pharmacol Ther 1995;57:696–698.
43. Marotta PJ, Roberts E. Pemoline hepatotoxicity in children. J Pediatrics 1998;132:894–897.
44. Rosh JR, Dellert SF, Narkewicz M, et al. Four cases of severe hepatotoxicity associated with pemoline: Possible autoimmune pathogenesis. Pediatrics 1998;101:921–923.
45. Spencer TJ, Biederman J, Harding M, et al. Growth deficits in ADHD children revisited: Evidence for disorder-associated growth delays? J Am Acad Child Adolesc Psychiatry 1996;35:1460–1469.
46. Horner BR, Scheibe KE. Prevalence and implications of attention-deficit hyperactivity disorder among adolescents in treatment for substance abuse. J Am Acad Child Adolesc Psychiatry 1997;36:30–36.
47. Biederman J, Wilens T, Mick E, et al. Is ADHD a risk factor for psychoactive substance use disorders? Findings from a four-year prospective follow-up study. J Am Acad Child Adolesc Psychiatry 1997;36: 21–29.
48. Rapport MD, Carlson GA, Kelly KL, Pataki C. Methylphenidate and desipramine in hospitalized children, I. Separate and combined effects on cognitive function. J Am Acad Child Adolesc Psychiatry 1993;32: 333–342.
49. Biederman J, Thisted R, Greenhill L, et al. Estimation of the association between desipramine and the risk for sudden death in 5-14-year-old children. J Clin Psychiatry 1995;56:87–93.
50. Spencer T, Biederman J, Steingard R, Wilens T. Bupropion exacerbates tics in children with attention-deficit hyperactivity disorder and Tourette's syndrome. J Am Acad Child Adolesc Psychiatry 1993;32: 211–214.
51. Maloney MJ, Schwam JS. Clonidine and sudden death. Pediatrics 1995;96:1176–1177. Letter.
52. Blackman JA, Samson FL, Gutgesell H. Clonidine and electrocardiograms. Pediatrics 1996;98:1223–1224. Letter.
53. Steingard R, Biederman J, Spencer T, et al. Comparison of clonidine response in the treatment of attention-deficit hyperactivity disorder with and without comorbid tic disorders. J Am Acad Child Adolesc Psychiatry 1993;32:350–353.
54. Comings DE. Tourette Syndrome and Human Behavior. Duarte, CA, Hope Press, 1990.
55. Peterson BS. Considerations of natural history and pathophysiology in the psychopharmacology of Tourette's syndrome. J Clin Psychiatry 1996;57:24–34.
56. Cohen DJ, Riddle MA, Leckman JF. Pharmacotherapy of Tourette's syndrome and associated disorders. Psychiatr Clin North Am 1992;15: 109–129.
57. Comings DE. Tourette's syndrome genetics. Child Psychiatry Hum Dev 1997;27:139–150.
58. Randolph C, Hyde TM, Gold JM, et al. Tourette's syndrome in monozygotic twins. Arch Neurol 1993;50:725–728.
59. Sallee FR, Nesbitt L, Jackson C, et al. Relative efficacy of haloperidol and pimozide in children and adolescents with Tourette's disorder. Am J Psychiatry 1997;154:1057–1062.
60. Bruun RD, Budman CL. Risperidone as a treatment for Tourette's syndrome. J Clin Psychiatry 1996;57:29–31.
61. Goetz CG, Tanner CM, Wilson RS, et al. Clonidine and Gilles de la Tourette's syndrome: Double blind study using objective rating methods. Ann Neurol 1987;21:307–310.
62. Comings DE, Comings BG, Tacket T, Li SZ. The clonidine patch and behavior problems. J Am Acad Child Adolesc Psychiatry 1990;29: 667–668. Letter.
63. Castellanos FX, Giedd JN, Elia J, et al. Controlled stimulant treatment of ADHD and comorbid Tourette's syndrome: Effects of stimulant and dose. J Am Acad Child Adolesc Psychiatry 1997;36:589–596.
64. Gadow KD, Sverd J, Sprafkin J. Efficacy of methylphenidate for attention-deficit hyperactivity disorder in children with tic disorder. Arch Gen Psychiatry 1995;52:444–455.
65. Singer HS, Brown J, Quaskey S, et al. The treatment of attention-deficit hyperactivity disorder in Tourette's syndrome: A double-blind placebo-controlled study with clonidine and desipramine. Pediatrics 1995;95:74–81.
66. Steingard R, Biederman J, Spencer T, et al. Comparison of clonidine response in the treatment of ADHD with and without comorbid disorders. J Am Acad Child Adolesc Psychiatry 1993;32:350–353.
67. Steingard RJ, Goldberg M, Lee D, DeMaso DR. Adjunctive clonazepam treatment of tic symptoms in children with comorbid tic disorders and ADHD. J Am Acad Child Adolesc Psychiatry 1994;33: 394–399.
68. Chappell PB, Riddle MA, Scahill L, et al. Guanfacine treatment of comorbid attention-deficit hyperactivity disorder and Tourette's syndrome: Preliminary clinical experience. J Am Acad Child Adolesc Psychiatry 1995;34:1140–1146.
69. Kurlan R, Como PG, Deeley C, et al. A pilot controlled study of fluoxetine for obsessive compulsive symptoms in children with Tourette's syndrome. Clin Neuropharmacol 1993;16:167–172.
70. Leonard HL, March J, Rickler KC, et al. Pharmacology of the selective serotonin reuptake inhibitors in children and adolescents. J Am Acad Child Adolesc Psychiatry 1997;725–736.
71. Silver AA, Shytle D, Philipp MK. Case study: Long-term potentiation of neuroleptics with transdermal nicotine in Tourette's syndrome. J Am Acad Child Adolesc Psychiatry 1996;35:1631–1636.
72. Conners CK, Levin ED, Sparrow E, et al. Nicotine and attention in adult attention deficit hyperactivity disorder (ADHD). Psychopharmacol Bull 1996;32:67–73.
73. McConville BJ, Fogelson MH, Norman AB, et al. Nicotine potentiation of haloperidol in reducing tic frequency in Tourette's disorder. Am J Psychiatry 1991;148:793–794.

74. Bornstein RA, Yang V. Neuropsychological performance in medicated and unmedicated patients with Tourette's disorder. Am J Psychiatry 1991;148:468–471.
75. Leckman JF, Riddle MA, Hardin MT, et al. The Yale global tic severity scale, I. Initial testing of a clinician-rated scale of tic severity. J Am Acad Child Adolesc Psychiatry 1989;28:566–573.
76. Silva RR, Munoz DM, Daniel W, et al. Causes of haloperidol discontinuation in patients with Tourette's disorder: Management and alternatives. J Clin Psychiatry 1996;57:129–135.
77. Feeney DJ, Klykylo W. Risperidone and tardive dyskinesia. J Am Acad of Child Adolesc Psychiatry 1996;35:1421–1422. Letter.
78. Kumra S, Herion D, Jacobsen LK, et al. Case study: Risperidone-induced hepatotoxicity in pediatric patients. J Am Acad Child Adolesc Psychiatry 1997;36:701–705.
79. Gillberg C. Enuresis: Psychological and psychiatric aspects. Scand J Urol Nephrol 1995;173:113–117.
80. Garfinkel BD. The elimination disorders. In: Garfinkel BD, Carlson GA, Weller EB, eds. Psychiatric Disorders in Children and Adolescents. Philadelphia, Saunders, 1990:325–336.
81. Koff SA. Why is desmopressin sometimes ineffective at curing bed-wetting? Scand J Urol Nephrol 1995;173:103–108.
82. Norgaard JP, Rittig S, Djurhuus JC. Nocturnal enuresis: An approach to treatment based on pathogenesis. J Pediatr 1989;114:705–710.
83. Miller K, Atkin B, Moody ML. Drug therapy for nocturnal enuresis. Drugs 1992;44:47–56.
84. Kaplan SL, Breit M, Gauthier B, Busner J. A comparison of three noctural enuresis treatment methods. J Am Acad Child Adolesc Psychiatry 1989;28:282–286.
85. Smellie JM, McGrigor VS, Meadow SR. Nocturnal enuresis: A placebo controlled trial of two antidepressant drugs. Arch Dis Child 1996;75:62–66.
86. Fritz GK, Rockney RM, Yeung AS. Plasma levels and efficacy of imipramine treatment for enuresis. J Am Acad Child Adolesc Psychiatry 1994;33:60–64.
87. Janknegt RA, Zweers HM, Delaere KP, et al. Oral desmopressin as a new treatment modality for primary nocturnal enuresis in adolescents and adults: A double-blind, randomized, multicenter study. Dutch enuresis study group. J Urol 1997;157:513–517.
88. Moffatt ME, Harlos S, Kirshen AJ, Burd L. Desmopressin acetate and nocturnal enuresis: How much do we know? Pediatrics 1993;92:420–425.
89. Rushton HG, Belman AB, Skoog S, et al. Predictors of response to desmopressin in children and adolescents with monosymptomatic nocturnal enuresis. Scan J Urol Nephrol 1995;173:109–111.
90. Stenberg A, Laackgren GL. Desmopressin tablet treatment in nocturnal enuresis. Scand J Urol Nephrol 1995;173:95–99.
91. Miller K, Goldberg S, Atkin B. Nocturnal enuresis: Experience with long-term use of intranasally administered desmopressin. J Pediatr 1989;114:723–726.
92. Robson WL, Norgaard JP, Leung AK. Hyponatremia in patients with nocturnal enuresis treated with DDAVP. Eur J Pediatr 1996;155:959–962.

60
EATING DISORDERS

Patricia A. Marken, BS Pharm, PharmD, BCPP, and Roger W. Sommi, BS Pharm, PharmD, BCPP

The initial descriptions of anorexia nervosa (AN) were published over a century ago[1,2]; however, bulimia nervosa (BN) was described as a distinct disorder in 1979.[3] Extensive research has improved our understanding of these severely disabling and potentially fatal disorders. Eating disorders encompass several biologic, psychological, and developmental etiologies. Pharmacologic management remains only a piece of a comprehensive plan that emphasizes cognitive–behavioral therapy and psychotherapy.

EPIDEMIOLOGY

ANOREXIA NERVOSA

Anorexia nervosa occurs predominantly in females (90%) and usually presents in late adolescence. The median age of onset is 17, with new cases rarely occurring after age 40. The reported prevalence of AN in the United States ranges from 1 in 100 to 1 in 800 for females between the ages of 12 and 18 years.[4] The prevalence of AN may have increased recently, as noted by one epidemiologic study that reported a sixfold increase in the number of documented cases of AN for the period of 1970 to 1976 compared with the period of 1960 to 1969.[5]

BULIMIA NERVOSA

Bulimia nervosa also occurs predominantly in females (90%), and usually presents in adolescence or early adult life.[4] BN has been studied primarily in college students, and therefore knowledge of its prevalence may be limited by the lack of data from other populations. Between 1% and 3% of adolescent and young adult females meet diagnostic criteria for BN, with the prevalence being about one-tenth of that in males.[4]

EATING DISORDER NOT OTHERWISE SPECIFIED/BINGE EATING DISORDER

The American Psychiatric Association's *Diagnostic and Statistical Manual of Mental Disorders,* fourth edition (DSM-IV), includes the diagnosis of eating disorder not otherwise specified (NOS).[4] Individuals with eating disorder NOS manifest symptoms characteristic of eating disorders, but they do not meet the diagnostic criteria for a specific eating disorder. In addition, research diagnostic criteria have been established for further consideration of a binge eating disorder (BED). The diagnostic criteria for BED describe binge eating without the purging behavior requisite for the bulimia diagnosis. The epidemiology of these disorders is unknown, but is likely to be reflective of eating disorders in general.[6]

ETIOLOGY AND PATHOPHYSIOLOGY

The potential etiologic or exacerbating factors for eating disorders represent an array of physiologic, biochemical, developmental, psychological, and psychiatric phenomena. It is difficult to delineate the biologic basis for eating disorders, because it is unclear whether the observed biologic changes are causing the aberrant eating behavior or are a result of the eventual starvation.

Abnormalities of the hypothalamic–pituitary–gonadal (HPG), hypothalamic–pituitary–adrenal (HPA), and hypothalamic–pituitary–thyroid (HPT) axes have been described as potential causes of AN. An extensive review of the psychoendocrinology of AN is provided by the Work Group on Eating Disorders.[6] Although many endocrine abnormalities occur in other forms of starvation, a primary difference with AN is that the dysfunction may not correct despite weight normalization. The finding of amenorrhea in the majority of females with AN supports the role of the HPG axis, and in particular the function of the gonadotropins luteinizing hormone (LH), follicle-stimulating hormone (FSH), and gonadotropin-releasing hormone (GnRH).[7] It should be noted that up to 25% of females had amenorrhea before the onset of AN, and the return of menses lags behind weight normalization.

The role of the neurotransmitter serotonin in eating disorders has been extensively investigated because it plays an important role in feeding. The primary location of serotonin-mediated eating activity is the medial hypothalamus. Serotonin activity in the paraventricular and ventromedial nuclei controls energy balance, while activity in the suprachiasmatic nucleus controls the circadian pattern of feeding. Stimulation of serotonin receptors in these areas decreases carbohydrate intake, enhances satiety, and terminates feeding. In contrast, stimulation of presynaptic serotonin autoreceptors initiates feeding, presumably by inhibiting the release of serotonin. In anorexia, plasma tryptophan (a serotonin precursor), urinary concentration of the major serotonin metabolite 5-hydroxyindoleacetic acid (5-HIAA), platelet serotonin binding, and basal cerebrospinal fluid (CSF) 5-HIAA concentrations are reportedly decreased. These abnormalities all correct with weight normalization.[8]

The role of other neurotransmitters should also be considered. In the presence of decreased food intake, norepinephrine is released in the paraventricular nucleus, which inhibits satiety, while at the same time release of norepinephrine is inhibited at the lateral hypothalamus, which increases the sensation of hunger. Dopamine is associated with self-administration and self-stimulatory behaviors in other disorders, and similarly may be etiologically related to the eating binges observed in BN. Taste and food cues are also regulated by neurotransmitters within the hypothalamus. Hypothalamic dysfunction may account for the food preferences present in BN and the food dislikes exhibited by persons with AN.

A great deal of emphasis is placed on psychological and developmental issues in the pathogenesis of eating disorders, especially regarding the role of the family. Issues surrounding family separations, losses, and dysfunction may trigger abnormal eating behavior.[6,9] Whether family-related issues are truly etiologic for eating disorders remains controversial. It is interesting, however, to note that the prognosis is better in persons with a relatively healthy family environment.[10] Eating disorder patients also commonly have a history of physical and sexual abuse. Finally, athletes are at special risk for eating disorders, especially female gymnasts, figure skaters, distance runners and swimmers, and male wrestlers and body builders.[11] Attention should be given to these variables when diagnostic and treatment decisions are considered.

Eating disorders are very complex and will probably not be explained by any simple physiologic, biochemical, developmental, psychological, or psychiatric model. Instead, a multifaceted view of potential etiologies will best serve the clinician in making decisions about treatment alternatives.

DIAGNOSTIC CRITERIA AND CLINICAL PRESENTATION

Figure 60–1 lists the common clinical signs and symptoms for AN and BN. AN and BN occur together in about 30% to 64% of patients, and may not be distinct diagnostic entities but rather occur along a continuum of symptoms.[12–15] Many patients initially present with either AN or BN and alternate from one eating disorder to the other. The clinician should pay particular attention to these fluctuations and alter therapy accordingly, because patients with AN and BN need different treatment interventions.

Medical consequences of an eating disorder are vast and are related primarily to self-induced starvation and purging. Patients commonly present with vague complaints of lethargy and pain. Metabolic and electrolyte disturbances along with dehydration are common and occur because of poor dietary intake, self-induced vomiting, or chronic laxative and diuretic abuse. Severe electrolyte disturbances can cause cardiac disturbances and even sudden death. Abnormalities of the hypothalamic–pituitary axes are likely the result of starvation. These abnormalities include effects on estradiol, the gonadotropins (e.g., LH, FSH, and GnRH), thyroid function, adrenal function, and growth hormone.[7] Osteoporosis and infertility are potential long-term complications of endocrine changes. Vomiting can cause dental problems, including decalcification, erosion of the enamel and dentin layers, and staining of the surfaces of the teeth.[4] A thorough physical and laboratory evaluation, as described in Table 60–1 is needed to determine the severity of medical complications.[16]

Depression, schizophrenia, obsessive–compulsive disorder, and conversion disorders should be included in the differential diagnosis of AN and BN as eating abnormalities can be a component of these illnesses. The salient difference between these psychiatric disorders and eating disorders is the overriding drive for thinness, a disturbed body image, increased energy level directed toward losing weight, and binge-eating episodes that are relatively specific for the eating disorders. Additionally, many patients

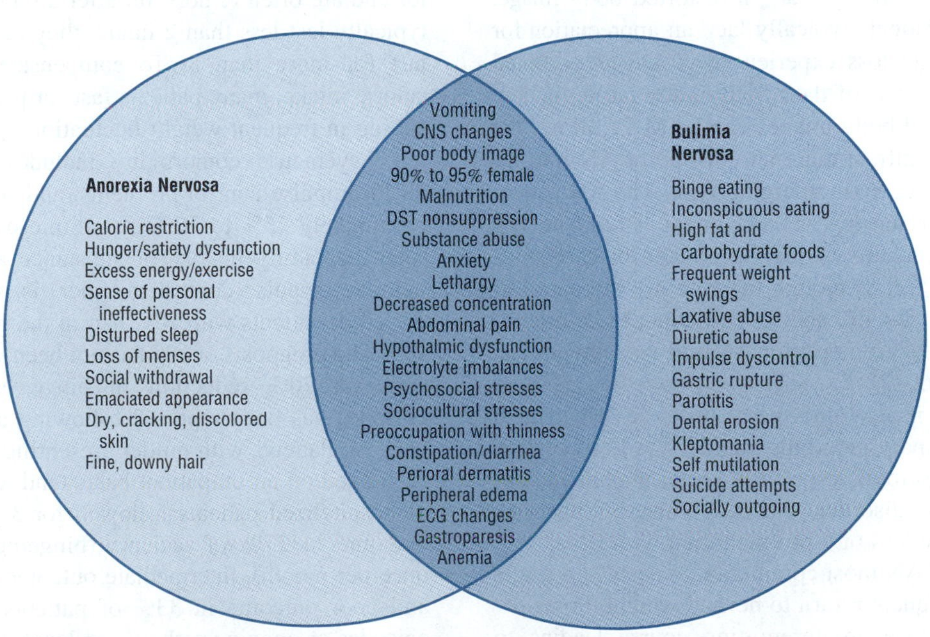

FIGURE 60–1. Signs and symptoms of anorexia nervosa and bulimia nervosa.

TABLE 60–1. Physical and Laboratory Assessment of Eating Disorders

Evaluation	Target Symptoms
Pulse	Bradycardia
Blood pressure	Hypotension, orthostasis
Respiratory rate	Rapid if heart failure occurs during refeeding
Temperature	Hypothermia, cold intolerance
ECG	ST depression, flat T waves, U waves, increased QT, AV block
GI	Hypoactive bowel sounds, gastritis, abdominal distention
Skin	Dry, scaling, lanugo, hair loss, callus on fingers and hands
Menses	Amenorrhea
CBC	Leukopenia, anemias, thrombocytopenia
Electrolytes	Hypokalemia, hypomagnesemia, hypo/hyper-phosphatemia
pH	Metabolic alkalosis (acidosis if laxative abuse)
Amylase	Elevated, pancreatitis rare
Liver	Hypoalbuminemia, gamma-glutamyl transpeptidase if alcohol abuse
Thyroid	Low or low-normal but not true disease
Cortisol	Elevated with lack of dexamethasone suppression test
Bone Density	Osteoporosis

Modified from Ref. 23.

will experience relief of the psychiatric symptoms upon refeeding and not require psychotropics.[6]

ANOREXIA NERVOSA

The essential features of AN include refusal to maintain a minimal normal body weight, intense fear and obsession about weight gain or being "fat," a distorted body image, and amenorrhea. Patients typically lack an appreciation for the degree of weight loss experienced or are preoccupied with the idea that a part of their body is too large, the key feature of a distorted body image. The DSM-IV allows the clinician to further differentiate an episode of AN into restricting type or binge-eating/purging type. The AN patient also has difficulty in sensing when he or she is full (satiety), and commonly complains of feeling bloated or early fullness. Patients also feel as though they are not in control of various aspects of their life and, in particular, of caloric intake. Specific DSM-IV criteria for AN and its subtypes can be found in Table 60–2.

Cormorbidity is also an issue as up to 68% of treated patients have a primary mood disorder.[17–19] A link between AN and anxiety disorders, especially social phobia and obsessive–compulsive disorder, has been noted. Substance abuse appears to be less of a problem than with BN.

The course of AN most commonly consists of a single episode with subsequent return to normal weight. Some patients may experience an unremitting course leading to death, or episodic periods of anorexic behavior.[4] A recent study found that 50% of AN patients had a "good" outcome, 30% had a "medium" outcome, and 20% a "poor" outcome.[20] A poorer prognosis is associated with a longer duration of illness, having a lower initial weight, having a premorbid history of poor family relationships, and the presence of BN or additional symptoms such as vomiting and laxative abuse.[6,21] Varying numbers exist on the mortality of AN, but it is clear that it is among the highest of all psychiatric disorders. Long-term follow-up shows that between 10% and 18% of AN patients eventually died, primarily from cardiac arrest or suicide.[4,21,22]

BULIMIA NERVOSA

The essential feature of BN is binge eating—an excessive intake of calorie-laden food over a short period of time. Persons with BN, as with AN, are overly sensitive about their weight and have a distorted body image. Most have normal weight, although some may be slightly underweight or overweight for body size and age. DSM-IV allows the clinician to further differentiate an episode of BN into purging type or nonpurging type, depending on the patient's recent use of purging methods to offset the effects of binge eating. The DSM-IV diagnostic criteria for BN and its subtypes are listed in Table 60–2.

Patients typically binge one or more times daily and vomit at least once daily. Patients may consume 5000 to 20,000 calories during a single binge, although caloric intake can be smaller. Patients tend to consume foods that are easy to ingest, do not require much chewing or preparation, and are high in carbohydrates or fat (e.g., ice cream, bread, candy, or doughnuts). Binge eating is typically secretive, and episodes are often precipitated by a stressful event. Patients experience a loss of control over their eating behavior and are often remorseful after a binge. Although binges typically last less than 2 hours, they have been reported to last for more than 8. To compensate for the excessive caloric intake, many patients fast for prolonged periods, resulting in frequent weight fluctuations.

Psychiatric comorbidity includes depression (up to 80%), impulse control problems, and substance abuse. Approximately 25% to 30% of bulimic patients report a personal or family history of substance abuse. Kleptomania (another impulse control disorder) is more commonly reported in patients with BN than in the general public.[23]

The prognosis of BN has not been well studied. On average, a 70% reduction in binge eating and purging episodes has been reported following any treatment intervention. Patients with milder presenting symptoms who can be treated on an outpatient basis tend to do better. A study of hospitalized patients followed for 3 years found a good outcome in 27% of patients (bingeing/purging less than once per month), intermediate outcome in 40% of patients, and poor outcome in 33% of patients (daily binge/purge episodes or ongoing cathartic or laxative abuse).[6]

TABLE 60–2. DSM-IV Diagnostic Criteria for Anorexia Nervosa and Bulimia Nervosa

Anorexia Nervosa

1. Refusal to maintain body weight over a minimal normal weight for age and height; or failure to make expected weight gain during period of growth, leading to a body weight 15% lower than expected normal weight for age and height.
2. Intense fear of gaining weight or becoming fat, even though underweight.
3. Disturbance in the way one's body weight, size, or shape is experienced, undue influence of body weight or shape on self-evaluation, or denial of the seriousness of the current low body weight.
4. In postmenarchal females, amenorrhea (absence of at least three consecutive menstrual cycles when otherwise expected to occur [primary or secondary amenorrhea]).

Subtypes are based on findings during the current episode with regard to binge-eating or purging behavior (self-induced vomiting or the misuse of laxatives, diuretics, or enemas):

Restricting type: The person has not regularly engaged in binge-eating or purging behavior.

Binge-eating/purging type: The person has regularly engaged in binge-eating or purging behavior.

Bulimia Nervosa

1. Recurrent episodes of binge eating characterized by both of the following:
   A. Eating, in a discrete period of time, an amount of food that is definitely larger than most people would consume during a similar period of time and under similar circumstances.
   B. A feeling of lack of control over eating behavior during the episode.
2. Recurrent compensatory behavior to prevent weight gain such as self-induced vomiting; misuse of laxatives, diuretics, enemas, or other medications; strict dieting or fasting; or vigorous exercise.
3. Binge-eating episodes and compensatory behaviors occur on average at least twice weekly for 3 months.
4. Self-evaluation is unduly influenced by body shape and weight.
5. Symptoms do not occur exclusively during episodes of AN.

Subtypes are based on findings during the current episode with regard to binge-eating or purging behavior (self-induced vomiting or the misuse of laxatives, diuretics, or enemas).

Purging type: The person has regularly engaged in self-induced vomiting or the misuse of laxatives, diuretics, or enemas.

Nonpurging type: The person has used other inappropriate compensatory behaviors, such as fasting or excessive exercise, but has not engaged in self-induced vomiting or the misuse of laxatives, diuretics, or enemas.

Modified and reprinted from the Diagnostic and Statistical Manual of Mental Disorders, 4th ed. Copyright 1994 American Psychiatric Association.

▶ TREATMENT: Eating Disorders

DESIRED OUTCOME

Various treatment modalities are used to improve the quality of life for patients with AN and BN. Although the approach to individual patients may differ, the basic goals of treatment are to reduce distorted body image, restore and maintain healthy body weight, reestablish normal eating patterns, improve associated psychological and physical problems, resolve contributory family problems, and prevent relapse.

GENERAL APPROACH TO TREATMENT

The initial step in treatment is engaging the patient and important parties into a collaborative treatment plan. Denial is a common problem, and without active patient participation, treatment will not be a success. An individualized treatment plan is based on the specific core and associated features of the eating disorder, and will provide for a team approach to care. Clinicians that provide care to patients with eating disorders include psychiatrists, nutrition specialists, psychologists, specially trained counselors, nurses, and pharmacists. Hospitalization should be based on the criteria outlined in Table 60–3,[6] as most patients can be managed in an outpatient setting. Medications are never indicated as a sole treatment for eating disorders.[11]

ANOREXIA NERVOSA

NONPHARMACOLOGIC THERAPY

Nondrug treatment is the cornerstone of AN treatment. Nondrug treatments include behavioral management, cognitive–behavioral therapy (CBT), individual psychotherapy, and group and family therapy.[24] CBT has emerged as the primary nondrug strategy in

TABLE 60–3. Criteria for Hospitalization of Patients With Eating Disorders

1. Significant weight loss (25% less than normal weight or greater), particularly if weight loss has been recent and rapid, severe starvation symptoms are present or the patient has been ill for more than 2 years
2. Medical complications and metabolic abnormalities from bingeing and purging
3. Suicidal ideation
4. Nonresponsiveness to outpatient treatment (after 3 to 4 months)
5. Demoralization, nonfunctional family
6. Lack of outpatient facilities

Modified from Ref. 6 and 11.

most eating disorder programs and is based on two premises: that AN is a way of coping with negative life experiences and that behaviors leading to food restrictions become entrenched, independent of the initial causative factors. The first stage of treatment is directed towards restoring a healthy weight and treating food phobias. Second, therapy addresses interpersonal problems, and finally skill development for relapse prevention is targeted.[25] Twelve-step programs can also be integrated into a treatment plan, especially for poorly responsive patients.[26]

PHARMACOLOGIC THERAPY

ANTIDEPRESSANTS AND CYPROHEPTADINE

Antidepressants in AN are intended to improve depression, anxiety, and obsessional thought patterns and promote weight gain, although benefit has not been demonstrated in all areas.[27] Cyproheptadine (Periactin), a histamine and serotonin antagonist, is used with variable success to stimulate appetite and decrease depression. Early studies using relatively low doses (12 mg/d) found no difference compared with placebo.[28] A double-blind study compared cyproheptadine in doses up to 32 mg/d to amitriptyline up to 160 mg/d and placebo in 72 subjects. A shorter time to target weight was found for amitriptyline and cyproheptadine patients when compared to placebo. However, cyproheptadine decreased the rate of weight gain in a bulimic subgroup of anorexics.[29] A double-blind comparison of clomipramine 100 mg at bedtime and placebo in 16 subjects found that the clomipramine-treated subjects had significantly more hunger and energy than the placebo subjects. Rate of weight gain was slower in clomipramine-treated subjects, perhaps due to increased activity.[30] Subjects maintained a more stable weight than the placebo patients after discontinuation from the study. Open trials with fluoxetine 20 to 60 mg/d found a reduction in obsessions and depression, maintenance of the target body weight, and restoration of normal eating behavior; however, controlled and long-term trials are needed before fluoxetine can be routinely recommended.[31,32]

As symptom response is generally limited, the overall role of antidepressants in managing AN remains secondary to nondrug treatments.[6] Antidepressants should be initiated only if depression persists after the target weight has been achieved, as many mood symptoms will resolve as weight improves.[6] Selective serotonin reuptake inhibitors (SSRIs) are usually used as first-line antidepressants because they are better tolerated and have greater cardiovascular safety than tricyclic antidepressants (TCAs), especially in low-weight patients.[27] Patients with AN are sensitive to anticholinergic and cardiovascular effects, and if TCAs are used, low starting doses and a slow titration toward an effective dose are needed. The risk of cardiotoxicity in a malnourished population must not be underestimated, especially in chronic purgers who may have hypokalemia. A baseline electrocardiogram (ECG) must be obtained before beginning an antidepressant. Cyproheptadine at higher doses (e.g., 32 mg/d) is an option to promote weight gain and decrease depression in AN.

ANTIPSYCHOTICS

Antipsychotics were the first medications used to treat AN, based on reports of weight gain and reduced eating-related anxiety, agitation, and obsessions.[33] Clinical experience has found little specific improvement from antipsychotic treatment in AN patients. Limited benefit, along with the sensitivity of AN patients to antipsychotic-induced adverse effects, limits their usefulness.

MISCELLANEOUS AGENTS

The effectiveness of lithium has been unimpressive, and the risk of serious adverse effects in patients with AN-associated metabolic and cardiac abnormalities limits its use.[34] Metoclopramide (Reglan) and cisapride (Propulsid) may be helpful in increasing the gastric emptying rate and reducing bloating and abdominal pain common in AN.[35,36] Short-acting benzodiazepines, given before meals, are useful when severe anxiety limits eating.[6] Estrogen replacement (conjugated estrogens 0.3 to 1.25 mg/d) to reduce calcium loss in patients with chronic amenorrhea has also been used.[4,37] Finally, total parenteral nutrition (TPN) is needed during the initial management of severely malnourished patients; however, the decision to administer TPN must be made carefully because of the potentially devastating psychological effect on patients who do not wish to gain weight.

BULIMIA NERVOSA

NONPHARMACOLOGIC THERAPY

Nondrug strategies are similar to those used with AN and play an equally important role in treatment success. Cox and Merkel evaluated 32 studies of individual and group therapy techniques used to manage BN.[38] Most studies had methodologic shortcomings such as failure to use a control group, overreliance on self-reporting as an outcome, and small sample sizes. However, about 40% of patients were totally abstinent from binge eating and purging at follow-up. No intervention was found to be clearly superior to any other. A more recent trial found that interpersonal psychotherapy and CBT were equally effective and superior to behavior therapy alone.[39]

PHARMACOLOGIC THERAPY

ANTIDEPRESSANTS

Antidepressants have been extensively evaluated in BN, although benefit is not universal and design problems are present in several trials. Antidepressants are reported to reduce binge eating, vomiting, and depression, and improve eating habits, although their impact on body dissatisfaction remains unclear. The average number of binge/purge episodes at baseline was 8 to 10 per week, and the mean reduction in episodes about 55%. Placebo-treated patients tended to have a response of about half of that seen with antidepressant-treated patients. Reduction in vomiting episodes tends to mirror reductions in binge episodes. The prevalence of major depression is 15% or less in most studies, suggesting an antibulimic effect independent of an antidepressant effect.[27]

Imipramine, desipramine, and phenelzine demonstrated superiority over placebo in double-blind trials for treating specific symptoms of BN.[40–46] Doses for BN are the same as those used to treat depression, although slow titration is needed to allow time to develop tolerance to adverse effects. Serum concentration monitoring of TCAs is recommended to ensure that absorption is not compromised by purging. The same plasma concentration ranges used in depression are used for patients with AN. Phenelzine should be used only if the patient will reliably follow the dietary and medication restrictions. Trazodone, up to 400 mg/d, has also been beneficial and generally well tolerated.[47]

Fluoxetine is the only antidepressant with Food and Drug Administration approval for treatment of BN. The Fluoxetine Bulimia Nervosa Collaborative Study Group conducted the largest trial evaluating an antidepressant in BN. It should be noted that there was no active control group. Fluoxetine 60 mg/d was found to be superior to both placebo and fluoxetine 20 mg/d for reducing vomiting, bingeing, depression, carbohydrate craving, and pathologic eating habits. The drug was well tolerated, and weight changes were minimal, even at 60 mg/d.[48] Fluvoxamine, mean dose 182 mg a day, has also demonstrated efficacy in a placebo-controlled trial.[49]

Tolerability is the basis for selecting an antidepressant in BN because of heightened sensitivity to adverse effects and lack of a clear difference in efficacy between the classes. For these reasons, SSRIs are usually first-line agents. A careful baseline physical examination and laboratory workup is essential, because underlying ECG changes (U waves, increased Q–T interval, flat T waves) secondary to hypokalemia or bradycardia and arterioventricular block from starvation may be present. All antidepressants can cause seizures; thus, a careful risk–benefit assessment is warranted if the patient has predisposing factors such as a personal or family history of seizures, cerebral vascular disease, or alcohol or sedative–hypnotic withdrawal.[50]

ANTICONVULSANTS

The pharmacotherapy of BN is based on two pathophysiologic models: a relationship to seizure disorders and a relationship to affective disorders. Anticonvulsants were the first medications specifically targeted to treat BN. Green and Rau noted that 38 of 59 patients with binge eating had abnormal electroencephalograms. They subsequently administered phenytoin (Dilantin) to 47 BN patients in an open trial and achieved a 57% improvement in bulimic symptoms.[51] Wermuth and colleagues conducted a double-blind, placebo-controlled trial in 20 subjects and found no significant difference between the placebo and phenytoin-treated groups.[52] Kaplan and colleagues, in a placebo-controlled, double-blind trial of 6 BN patients treated with carbamazepine (Tegretol), found a dramatic response in one patient in both bulimic and affective symptoms.[53] Valproic acid (Depakene) produced a dramatic response in a patient with concurrent bulimia and bipolar affective disorder in a single case report. Subsequent bulimic episodes occurred only after the serum concentration decreased to apparent subtherapeutic values.[54] Anticonvulsants are reserved for the subgroup of BN patients with a comorbid bipolar affective disorder. Doses used and serum concentrations sought are similar to those used for patients with seizure disorders.

MISCELLANEOUS AGENTS

Lithium is reserved for patients with comorbid bipolar affective disorder. It must be used cautiously, as risk of toxicity increases as a result of purging and laxative abuse. Serum concentrations should be maintained between 0.6 and 0.8 mEq/L. The risk of weight gain often makes lithium unacceptable to patients in the long term.[55] Fenfluramine (Pondimin), an indirect serotonin agonist and anorectic agent, appears to be an effective option at 60 mg/d. It was found to be superior to and better tolerated than desipramine in a trial with small sample size.[56] TPN is occasionally needed in metabolically disturbed patients, although the decision to use it must be weighed against the psychological risks of forced refeeding. Low-dose benzodiazepines, such as alprazolam 0.25 mg three times a day administered before meals, may help reduce anxiety associated with refeeding, although long-term use is not warranted for most patients because of the risk of abuse.

COMBINATION THERAPY

A comparison of imipramine and psychotherapy found that the three groups receiving active treatment (imipramine alone, imipramine plus psychotherapy, or placebo plus psychotherapy) showed a better response than did those receiving placebo alone, and that combination treatment was superior to imipramine alone. Imipramine reduced depression and anxiety, but did not improve eating behavior.[57] Angras and associates compared the effectiveness of desipramine (mean dose, 168 mg/d; mean serum concentration, 130.8 μg/mL), cognitive–behavioral therapy, and their combination for 16 or 24 weeks in outpatients with BN. The combination of desipramine and CBT for 24 weeks was found to be superior to any other treatment or duration for reducing bingeing, purging, dietary preoccupation, and hunger.[58] More recently, Walsh and colleagues compared the following treatments: CBT and desipramine (mean dose, 143 mg/d); CBT and placebo; supportive psychotherapy and desipramine (mean dose, 220 mg/d); supportive psychotherapy and placebo; and desipramine alone (mean dose, 198 mg/d). Fluoxetine (mean dose, 55 mg/d) was substituted in the case of inadequate response or poor tolerance to desipramine. Patients receiving CBT and medication had the best response. CBT was the superior psychotherapy intervention, and medication added a modest benefit to nondrug measures. Patients receiving supportive psychotherapy and medication had no better response than medication alone. A significant difference existed in desipramine doses between the CBT and supportive psychotherapy groups, while no difference was found in fluoxetine dose across groups. Finally, two-thirds of patients had to be switched to fluoxetine.[59] In summary, the combination of pharmacologic and nonpharmacologic measures appears to produce the best outcome for patients with BN.

EVALUATION OF THERAPEUTIC OUTCOMES

ANOREXIA NERVOSA

The overall goals of treatment for a patient with AN are to restore healthy weight and eating habits; prevent and resolve physical complications; correct behavioral problems, dysfunctional thoughts, and psychological problems; improve family relationships; and prevent relapse.[6] A diary that records exercise frequency, menses, food intake, patterns of eating, and associated feelings while eating is helpful to monitor progress. Weekly weigh-ins on the same scale, preferably at a clinician's office, help monitor progress early in treatment and reduce the focus on weight and anxiety from variability found between different scales.[25] A patient's use of coping skills and contingencies should also be assessed. Medications (cyproheptadine and antidepressants) are likely to assist in appetite stimulation, alleviation of depression, and perhaps maintenance of target weight. Improvement in mood should occur within approximately 8 weeks. Patients receiving TCAs should be evaluated for anticholinergic effects, especially dry mouth and constipation, hypotension, and sedation. Patients receiving fluoxetine should be monitored for agitation, drug-induced anorexia, nausea, and insomnia. Follow-up laboratory tests and ECGs are not part of routine monitoring, unless signs and symptoms persist necessitating their collection, or the patient continues to lose weight despite treatment. The decision to use long-term medication must be based on specific and sustained improvement in the target symptoms mentioned, balanced with tolerance of adverse effects.

BULIMIA NERVOSA

Treatment can produce a reduction in target behaviors such as bingeing and purging; however, total absence of those behaviors is a less common outcome. The actual definition of recovery

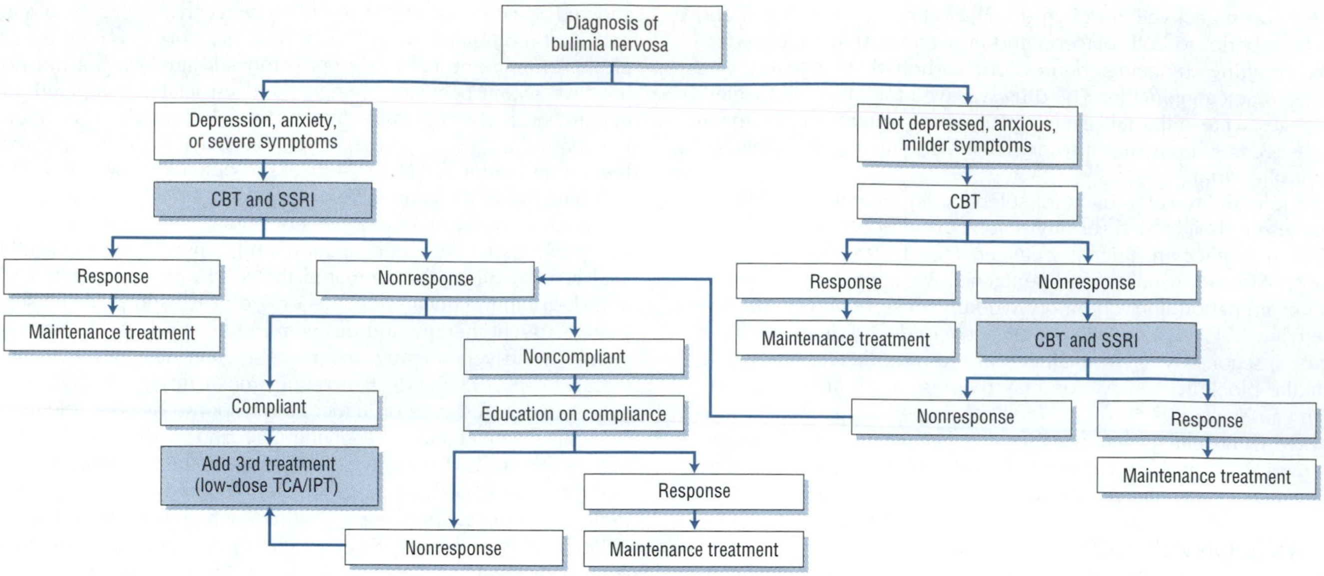

FIGURE 60–2. Proposed treatment algorithm for bulimia nervosa.

varies, as once a month binge/purge episodes is considered by some to be recovery, whereas others consider a patient recovered only when complete absence of these behaviors occurs.[21] Of concern is that ongoing symptoms may predispose patients to relapse.[60] Any individual treatment plan using medication should carefully describe frequency and severity of medication-responsive target symptoms and routinely assess changes from baseline in mood, anxiety, eating behaviors, and laxative abuse.[6] Figure 60–2 describes a proposed treatment algorithm for BN, but it should be noted that no consensus for treatment has been endorsed.[27,60] The time to onset of effect is unclear; however, a 4- to 6-week trial at a therapeutic dose should be tried to fully determine response. Twenty to 40% of subjects are estimated to have a poor or inadequate response to antidepressants, and there are few data on predictors of response or whether switching to another class in an unresponsive patient is effective.[61] Optimal duration of treatment after response is also poorly defined. There is some suggestion that 2 years of continuous treatment is needed in responders to ensure a sustained remission.[41] The impact of antidepressants on the long-term prognosis of BN is also ill defined. Careful evaluation for binge/purge behavior is necessary to ensure that treatment failure is not secondary to vomiting. Evaluation of previously described adverse effects should also be part of the treatment plan. Supportive counseling that encourages compliance may be needed early in treatment while the patient becomes tolerant to adverse effects.

The eating disorder patient presents a challenge to clinicians in ambulatory care. Impulsivity associated with BN may increase the risk for suicide. Prescriptions of the more toxic medications should be limited to small supplies. In addition, the pharmacist should be alert to identify persons who make large or frequent purchases of laxatives or ipecac syrup. If such activity is noted, possible laxative abuse and bulimic behaviors should be considered. Finally, a single case of fluoxetine abuse was reported in a patient with AN, indicating the need for attention to the frequency of refills.[62]

CONCLUSIONS

Our understanding of the pathophysiology and symptomatology of eating disorders has improved significantly over the past several years. Although various models are used to explain the etiology of eating disorders, it is unlikely that any single model will sufficiently explain these complex disorders. Medication serves an adjunctive role to a variety of psychosocial therapies in AN, while it plays a more central role in treatment of BN. By gaining a greater understanding of the underlying physiologic changes and the psychosocial complications associated with eating disorders, treatment plans can be specifically designed for an individual patient with the goal of improving the quality of life.

▶ PRINCIPLES OF PHARMACOTHERAPY

- The cause of eating disorders is multifactorial necessitating interdisciplinary treatment.
- Careful medical and psychiatric assessment is needed at baseline to determine severity of illness and comorbid conditions.
- Outpatient treatment of AN and BN is appropriate for the majority of patients.
- The cornerstone of treatment of AN and BN is nonpharmacologic measures such as cognitive behavioral therapy and psychotherapy.
- Parenteral feeding is a treatment of last resort.

- Antidepressants in AN are generally reserved for patients with mood symptoms that persist after weight has improved.
- Antidepressants can improve both mood and specific target symptoms in BN, but they remain adjunctive to nonpharmacologic treatments.
- SSRIs are usually considered first-line agents when drugs are used because of improved tolerability and safety, but not superior efficacy compared to other antidepressant classes.
- An adequate drug therapy trial is 4 to 6 weeks. Be sure to monitor compliance, especially if patients induce vomiting.
- Long-term course is variable, but there is potential for a fatal outcome.

REFERENCES

1. Gull WW. Anorexia nervosa. Trans Clin Soc (Lond) 1874. In: Kaufman RM, Heifman M, eds. Evolution of Psychosomatic Concepts. Anorexia Nervosa: A Paradigm. New York, International Universities Press, 1964:22–28.
2. Lesegue C. De l'anorexic hysterique. Arch Gen Med 1873. In: Kaufman RM, Heifman M, eds. Evolution of Psychosomatic Concepts. Anorexia Nervosa: A Paradigm. New York, International Universities Press, 1964:385.
3. Russel G. Bulimia nervosa: An ominous variant of anorexia nervosa. Psychol Med 1979;9:429–448.
4. American Psychiatric Association. Diagnostic and Statistical Manual of Mental Disorders, 4th ed (DSM-IV). Washington, DC, American Psychiatric Press, 1994:539–550.
5. Jones DJ, Fox MM, Babigian HM, Hutton HE. Epidemiology of anorexia nervosa in Monroe County, New York, 1960–1976. Psychosom Med 1980;42:551–558.
6. Work Group on Eating Disorders. American Psychiatric Association Practice Guidelines. Practice guidelines for eating disorders. Am J Psychiatry 1993;150:208–228.
7. Weiner H. Psychoendocrinology of anorexia nervosa. Psychiatr Clin North Am 1989;12:187–206.
8. Liebowitz SF. The role of serotonin in eating disorders. Drugs 1990;39(suppl 3):33–48.
9. Garfinkel PE. Eating Disorders. In: Kaplan HI, Sadock BJ, eds. Comprehensive Textbook of Psychiatry, 6th ed. Baltimore, Williams & Wilkins, 1995:1361–1372.
10. Rosenvinge JH, Mouland SO. Outcome and prognosis of anorexia nervosa. Br J Psychiatry 1990;156:92–97.
11. Powers PS. Initial assessment and early treatment options for anorexia nervosa and bulimia nervosa. Psychiatr Clin North Am 1996;19: 639–655.
12. Casper RC, Hedeker D, McClough JF. Personality dimensions in eating disorders and their relevance for subtyping. J Am Acad Child Adolesc Psychiatry 1992;31:830–840.
13. Eckert ED, Halmi KA, Marchi P, et al. Ten-year follow-up of anorexia nervosa: Clinical course and outcome. Psychol Med 1995;25: 143–156.
14. Garner DM, Olmsted MP, Garfinkel PE. Does anorexia nervosa occur on a continuum? Subgroup of weight- preoccupied women and their relationship to anorexia nervosa. Int J Eating Disord 1983;2:11–20.
15. Garner DM, Garfinkel PE, O'Shaughnessy M. Validity of the distinction between bulimia with and without anorexia nervosa. Am J Psychiatry 1985;142:581–587.
16. Carney CP, Anderson AE. Eating disorders: Guide to medical evaluation and complications. Psychiatr Clin North Am 1996;19:657–679.
17. Cantwell DP, Sturzenberger S, Burroughs J. Anorexia nervosa: An affective disorder? Arch Gen Psychiatry 1977;34:1087–1093.
18. Herzog DB. Are anorexic and bulimic patients depressed? Am J Psychiatry 1984;2141:1594–1597.
19. Piran N, Kennedy S, Garfinkel PE, Owens M. Affective disturbance in eating disorders. J Nerv Ment Dis 1985;173:395–400.
20. Steinhaus HC, Rauss-Mason C, Seidel R. Follow-up studies of anorexia nervosa: A review of four decades of research. Psychol Med 1991;21:447–454.
21. Herzog DB, Nussbaum KM, Marmor AK. Comorbidity and outcome in eating disorders. Psychiatr Clin North Am 1996;19:843–859.
22. Theander S. Outcome and prognosis in anorexia nervosa and bulimia: some results of previous investigations compared with those of a Swedish long-term study. J Psychiatr Res 1985;19:493–508.
23. McElroy SL, Keck PE, Pope HG, Hudson JI. Pharmacological treatment of kleptomania and bulimia nervosa. J Clin Psychopharmacol 1989;9:358–360.
24. Bowers WA, Anderson AE. Initial treatment of anorexia nervosa: Review and recommendations. Harvard Rev Psychiatry 1994;2:193–203.
25. Kleifield EI, Wagner S, Halmi KA. Cognitive-behavioral treatment of anorexia nervosa. Psychiatr Clin North Am 1996;19:715–737.
26. Johnson CL, Taylor C. Working with difficult to treat eating disorders using an integration of twelve-step and traditional psychotherapies. Psychiatr Clin North Am 1996;19:829–841.
27. Jimerson DC, Wolfe BE, Brotman AW, Metzger ED. Medication in the treatment of eating disorders. Psychiatr Clin North Am 1996;19: 739–754.
28. Vigersky RA, Loriaux DL. The effect of cyproheptadine in anorexia nervosa: A double-blind trial. In: Vigersky RA, ed. Anorexia Nervosa. New York, Raven, 1977:346–356.
29. Halmi KA, Eckert E, LaDu TJ, Cohen J. Anorexia nervosa. Treatment efficacy of cyproheptadine and amitriptyline. Arch Gen Psychiatry 1986;43:177–181.
30. Lacey JH, Crisp AH. Hunger, food intake and weight: The impact of clomipramine on refeeding an anorexia nervosa population. Postgrad Med J 1980;56:79–85.
31. Gwirtsman HE, Guze BH, Yager J, Gainsley B. Fluoxetine treatment of anorexia nervosa: An open clinical trial. J Clin Psychiatry 1990;51: 378–382.
32. Kaye WH, Weltzin TE, Hsu G, Bulik CM. An open trial of fluoxetine in patients with anorexia nervosa. J Clin Psychiatry 1991;52:464–471.
33. Dally PJ, Sargant W. A new treatment for anorexia nervosa. Br Med J 1960;1:1770–1773.
34. Gross HA, Ebert M, Faden VB, et al. A double-blind controlled trial of lithium carbonate in primary anorexia nervosa. J Clin Psychopharmacol 1981;1:376–381.
35. Saleh JW, Lebwohl SF. Metoclopramide-induced gastric emptying in patients with anorexia nervosa. Am J Gastroenterol 1980;74:127–132.
36. Stacher G, Abatzi-Wentzel TA, Wiesnagrotzki S, et al. Gastric-emptying, body weight and symptoms in promaty anorexia nervosa. Long-term effects of cisapride. Br J Psychiatry 1993;162:398–402.
37. Bachrach LK, Katzman DK, Guido D, Marcus R. Recovery from osteopenia in adolescent girls with anorexia nervosa. J Clin Endocrinol Metab 1991;72:602–606.
38. Cox GL, Merkel WT. A qualitative review of psychosocial treatments for bulimia. J Nerv Ment Dis 1989;177:77–83.
39. Fairburn CG, Jones R, Peveler RC, et al. Psychotherapy and bulimia nervosa. Longer-term effects of interpersonal therapy, behavior therapy and cognitive behavioral therapy. Arch Gen Psychiatry 1993;50:419–428.
40. Pope HG, Hudson JI, Jonas JM, Yurgelun-Todd D. Bulimia treated with imipramine: A placebo-controlled, double-blind study. Am J Psychiatry 1983;140:554–558.
41. Pope HG, Hudson JI, Jonas JM, Yurgelun-Todd D. Antidepressant treatment of bulimia: A two-year follow-up study. J Clin Psychopharmacol 1985;5:320–327.

42. Mitchell JE, Pyle RL, Eckert ED, Hatsakami D, et al. Response to alternative antidepressants in imipramine nonresponders. J Clin Psychopharmacol 1989;9:291–293.
43. Barlow J, Blouin J, Blouin A, Perez E. Treatment of bulimia with desipramine: A double-blind crossover study. Can J Psychiatry 1988;33: 129–133.
44. Hughes PL, Wells LA, Cunningham CJ, Ilstrup DM. Treating bulimia with desipramine. A double-blind, placebo controlled trial. Arch Gen Psychiatry 1986;43:182–186.
45. McCann UD, Angras WS. Successful treatment of nonpurging bulimia nervosa with desipramine: A double-blind, placebo-controlled study. Am J Psychiatry 1990;147:1509–1513.
46. Walsh BT, Gladis M, Roose SP, et al. Phenelzine vs placebo in 50 patients with bulimia. Arch Gen Psychiatry 1988;45:471–475.
47. Pope HG, Keck PE, McElroy SL, Hudson JI. A placebo-controlled study of trazodone in bulimia nervosa. J Clin Psychopharmacol 1989; 9:254–259.
48. Fluoxetine bulimia nervosa collaborative study group. Fluoxetine in the treatment of bulimia nervosa. A multicenter, placebo-controlled, double-blind trial. Arch Gen Psychiatry 1992;49:139–147.
49. Fitcher MM, Kruger R, Rief W, et al. Fluvoxamine in prevention of relapse in bulimia nervosa: Effects on eating-specific psychopathology. J Clin Psychopharmacol 1996;16:9–18.
50. Betts TA, Kabra PL, Cooper R, Jeavons DM. Epileptic fits as a probable side effect of amitriptyline. Lancet 1968;1:390–392.
51. Green RS, Rau JH. Treatment of compulsive eating disorders with anticonvulsant medication. Am J Psychiatry 1974;131:428–432.
52. Wermuth BM, Davis KL, Hollister LE, Stunkard AJ. Phenytoin treatment of binge eating syndrome. Am J Psychiatry 1977;136:1249–1253.
53. Kaplan AS, Garfinkel PE, Darby PL, Garner DM. Carbamazepine in the treatment of bulimia. Am J Psychiatry 1983;140:1225–1226.
54. Herridge PL, Pope HG. Treatment of bulimia and rapid cycling bipolar disorder with sodium valproate: A case report. J Clin Psychopharmacol 1985;5:229–230.
55. Hsu LKG, Clement L, Santhouse R. Treatment of bulimia with lithium: A preliminary study. Psychopharmacol Bull 1987;2:45–48.
56. Blouin AG, Blouin JH, Perez EL, et al. Treatment of bulimia with fenfluramine and desipramine. J Clin Psychopharmacol 1988;8:261–269.
57. Mitchell JE, Pyle RL, Eckert ED, et al. A comparison study of antidepressants, structured interview and group psychotherapy in the treatment of bulimia nervosa. Arch Gen Psychiatry 1990;47:149–157.
58. Angras WS, Rossiter EM, Arnow B, et al. Pharmacological and cognitive-behavioral treatment for bulimia nervosa: A controlled comparison. Am J Psychiatry 1992;149:82–87.
59. Walsh BT, Wilson GT, Loeb KL, et al. Medication and psychotherapy in the treatment of bulimia nervosa. Am J Psychiatry 1997;154: 523–531.
60. Crow SJ, Mitchell JE. Integrating cognitive therapy and medications in bulimia nervosa. Psychiatr Clin North Am 1996;19:755–760.
61. Solyom L, Solyom C, Ledwidge B. The fluoxetine treatment of low-weight chronic bulimia nervosa. J Clin Psychopharmacol 1990;10: 421–425.
62. Wilcox JA. Abuse of fluoxetine by a patient with anorexia nervosa. Am J Psychiatry 1987;144:1100.

61

ALZHEIMER'S DISEASE

M. Lynn Crismon, PharmD, FCCP, BCPP, and Andrea E. Eggert, PharmD, BCPP

"I now begin the journey that will lead me into the sunset of my life."

Ronald Reagan

Alzheimer's disease (AD), first characterized by Alois Alzheimer in 1907, is a gradually progressive dementia affecting both cognition and behavior. The exact pathophysiologic mechanisms underlying AD are not entirely known, and no cure exists.[1] Although drugs may reduce Alzheimer's symptoms for a time, the disease is eventually fatal. This disease profoundly affects the family as well as the patient. A person with AD eventually loses his or her very identity, not just memories, but all associated cognitive, analytical, and physical functioning.[1]

Persons with AD experience something akin to traveling through a time warp, dropped into a foreign universe in which they no longer know how to function. They gradually lose sense of time, date, or year, and become unable to operate simple appliances. Simple day-to-day activities like paying bills, mailing letters, and grocery shopping become beyond their capabilities. Language skills are lost, beginning with the ability to remember less commonly used words and names, and progressing over time to total loss of speech. Calculation of simple figures becomes impossible, such as how much change to expect when paying for a $4 item with a $5 bill. Behavioral problems emerge, and the personality slowly erodes. Men and women with AD slowly become strangers in their own environments, increasingly unable to recognize their homes, neighborhoods, friends, or family members. Personality, memory, and functional ability fade away until the person becomes essentially like a small child, robbed of the ability to dress, feed, bathe, or even use the bathroom without help. The need for supervision and assistance increases until the late stages of the disease, when Alzheimer's sufferers become totally dependent on a family member, spouse, or other caregiver for all of their basic needs. These are all experiences of the over 4 million people in the United States who have AD.[1]

In the *Diagnostic and Statistical Manual for Mental Disorders,* fourth edition (DSM-IV),[2] AD is classified under the heading of Delirium, Dementia and Amnestic and Other Disorders. Dementias are neuropsychiatric disorders defined by widespread symptoms of memory loss and deficits in cognition and reasoning. Dementia is a nonspecific term describing a significant decline in cognitive function, regardless of cause. Dementias, synonymous with the popular lay term "senility," result from underlying disease, and are not part of normal aging. Delirium differs from dementia in that it develops over a short period of time (hours to days), and involves an acute change in the level of consciousness in addition to a decline in cognition. Because the severity, prognosis, and treatment of dementia depends almost entirely on the underlying cause, an accurate diagnosis is essential.

AD is the most common cause of dementia, accounting for over 60% of all cases of late-life cognitive dysfunction.[1] Other subclasses of dementia are based on etiology and listed in Table 61–1. This chapter will focus exclusively on dementia of the Alzheimer's type. However, the reader is encouraged to use the nonspecific treatment portions of this chapter to assist in management of noncognitive behavioral problems associated with other forms of dementia.

EPIDEMIOLOGY

AD is generally thought of as a disease of old age, because most cases present after age 65, but in about 5% of cases onset can be as early as age 40, resulting in the arbitrary age classifications of early-onset (age 40 to 64 years) and late-onset (≥ age 65 years) disease.[3] Studies using standardized diagnostic criteria, gathered by actual patient evaluation, and not limited to institutionalized populations are thought to provide the best estimates of prevalence. One such study found an overall disease prevalence of 10.3% in a large community sample of persons over age 65 years.[4] Both the prevalence and the incidence of AD increase exponentially with age, affecting approximately 3% (incidence, ~1%) of individuals aged 65 to 74, and rising dramatically to 47% (incidence, ~8.4%) of persons age 85 and older.[4–7] AD affects two times as many women as men, and although genetic inheritance is the primary mode of transmission, several environmental factors may also contribute. Factors determining age of onset and rate of progression remain largely undefined.

Although not routinely reported on death certificates, AD is said to be the fourth leading cause of death in U.S. elderly persons.[8] This is somewhat of a misrepresentation, as AD does not cause death directly, but indirectly by predisposing patients to sepsis, pneumonia, choking and aspiration, nutritional deficiencies, and trauma.[9] Severe cognitive impairment and cachexia worsen the prognosis.[10] Approximately 100,000 individuals with AD die every year. Survival following AD onset can be anywhere from 3 to 20 years; however, few people are diagnosed early in the disease course, resulting in an average survival following diagnosis of 4 to 8 years.

TABLE 61–1. Classification of Dementia

- Dementia of the Alzheimer's type
- Vascular dementia (formerly multi-infarct dementia)
- Dementia due to HIV disease
- Dementia due to head trauma
- Dementia due to Lewy body disease
- Dementia due to normal-pressure hydrocephalus
- Dementia due to idiopathic Parkinson's disease
- Dementia due to corticobasal ganglionic degeneration (CBGD)
- Dementia due to progressive supranuclear palsy (PSP)
- Dementia due to Huntington's disease
- Dementia due to Pick's disease
- Dementia due to Creutzfeldt–Jakob disease
- Dementia due to other general medical disorders (indicate disorder, e.g., B_{12} deficiency, hypothyroidism)
- Substance-induced persisting dementia (persistent dementia resulting from exposure to toxins, drugs of abuse, or medications)
- Dementia due to multiple etiologies
- Dementia not otherwise specified (reserved for dementia that cannot be attributed to any other subtype)

Compiled from Refs. 3, 54, and 86.

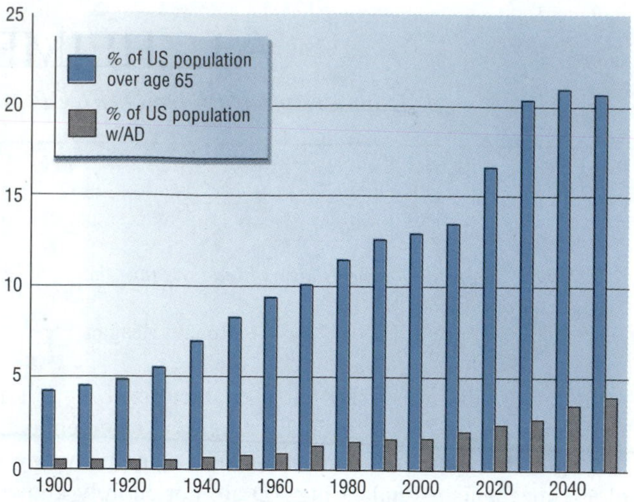

FIGURE 61–1. Our aging population. Increasing percentage of total U.S. population over age 65 and estimated percent with AD from the year 1900 projected to the year 2050. *(Estimates based on data from Refs. 4 and 12.)*

The economic and social costs of AD are staggering. It is the third most expensive illness in the United States after heart disease and cancer. Currently, most insurance plans do not cover AD, and much of the cost of caring for these patients is left to their families. The total national cost of Alzheimer's disease is estimated at $80 to $90 billion annually. To put these numbers in perspective, in 1991 the estimated medical cost of acquired immunodeficiency syndrome (AIDS) was $4.2 billion. Just the Medicaid costs for institutionalized AD patients was estimated at $5.7 billion.[11]

The average life expectancy in 1900 was 47 years. Few people lived long enough to experience the onset of AD. Life expectancy is now 75 years; 4 million people are afflicted with AD, and 250,000 more cases are diagnosed annually.[11,12] By the year 2050, one out of five people will be over age 65, and the number of Alzheimer's patients is projected at 14 million (Fig. 61–1). AD has become a major public health concern, yet in comparison to other major illnesses such as AIDS, heart disease, and cancer, it has received relatively little attention. The potential financial burden of this disease on the health care system could reach crisis proportions unless more effective avenues are developed to provide care for these individuals, prevent the disease from occurring, or slow its progress.

PATHOPHYSIOLOGY

At present, the precise pathophysiologic mechanisms causing AD are a mystery. Each risk factor or cause of AD appears to have the common mechanism of being permissive to neuritic plaque pathogenicity, by allowing increased formation of plaques, enhancing the pathogenicity of plaques, or reducing the reserve of existing brain cells to accommodate the presence of plaques. This section will define the structural changes and lesions present in AD, and attempt to outline how neuritic plaques form and how they destroy neurons.

STRUCTURAL CHANGES

AD is defined by both neuropathologic and clinical criteria. Neuropathologically, AD destroys neurons in the cortex and limbic structures of the brain, particularly the basal forebrain, amygdala, hippocampus, and cerebral cortex. These areas are responsible for higher learning, memory, reasoning, behavior, and emotional control. Anatomically, four major alterations in brain structure are seen: cortical atrophy; degeneration of cholinergic and other neurons; presence of neurofibrillary tangles (NFTs); and the accumulation of neuritic plaques.[13,14] Neurofibrillary tangles and neuritic plaques are considered the signature lesions of AD; without them, AD does not occur. But plaques and tangles may also be present in other diseases and even in normal aging. In order to understand the causes of AD, researchers must discern the circumstances in which these lesions lead to the clinical picture of AD.[15,16]

NEUROFIBRILLARY TANGLES AND NEURITIC PLAQUES

NFTs are comprised of paired helical filaments that aggregate in dense bundles, appearing microscopically like tiny flames filling the neuronal cell body. Paired helical filaments are formed from tau protein. Tau protein provides structural support to microtubules, the cell's transportation and skeletal support system.[17] When tau filaments undergo abnormal phosphorylation at a specific site, they cannot bind effectively to microtubules, and the microtubules collapse. Without an intact system of microtubules, the cell cannot function properly and eventually dies. Overactivity of kinases such as microtubule affinity-regulating kinase (MARK), or underactivity of phosphatases could theoretically produce or prevent breakdown of abnormally phosphorylated tau protein.[18] NFTs are found in other dementing illnesses besides AD, and may represent a common method by which various inciting factors culminate in cell death.[13]

Neuritic plaques (also termed amyloid or senile plaques) are extracellular lesions found in the brain and cerebral vasculature (amyloid angiopathy). Plaques are comprised of beta-amyloid protein (βAP), and an entwined mass of broken neurites (axon and dendrite projections of neurons).[14,19] Many of these broken neurites contain neuropil filaments made up of the abnormally phosphorylated tau protein found in NFTs.[13,14] Two types of glial cells, astrocytes and microglia, are also found in plaques.[19,20] Among other functions, glial cells secrete inflammatory mediators and serve as scavenger cells, which may be important in considering inflammatory mechanisms of AD. Strangely enough, the number of neuritic plaques does not necessarily determine disease severity. Instead, clinical development of AD may correlate inversely with the number of normal neurons and synapses remaining despite plaque presence,[16,21] thus introducing the concept of neurologic reserve. Factors decreasing brain reserve (e.g., stroke, alcohol abuse, small head circumference, decreased synaptic growth [see the section on estrogen later in this chapter], and lower levels of education) all increase the risk of AD.

BETA-AMYLOID PROTEIN

Forming the center of the neuritic plaque are aggregates of a 39 to 43 amino acid protein segment called βAP.[13,19,22] The amyloidoses are a set of diseases marked by amyloid protein deposition in various target organs. The βAP accumulating in the brain and cerebral blood vessels in AD is different from other disease producing amyloid proteins.[20]

Beta-amyloid protein is cleaved from the amyloid precursor protein (APP), a transmembrane protein.[13,14,22] Proteases cleave APP in several different ways (Fig. 61–2) The secretory pathway cleaves APP through the βAP region, using an enzyme called alpha secretase, so βAP is not released intact into the extracellular fluid. The endosomal pathway cleaves on both sides of βAP, using β and γ secretase, allowing intact βAP to be released into the extracellular space, where under the right conditions it can aggregate into fibrils, forming precursors to neuritic plaques.[14,23] Currently, we do not fully understand the conditions that allow βAP to remain in solution and how they differ from those conducive to plaque formation. However, it has been demonstrated that the 42 amino acid form of βAP is more amyloidogenic than other forms of βAP.

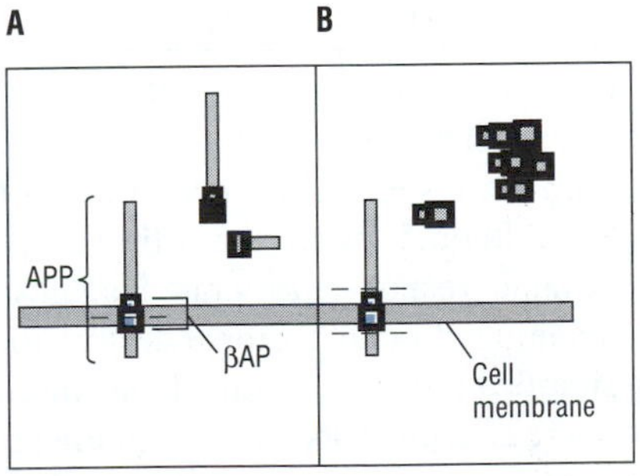

FIGURE 61–2. Representation of two physiologic cleavage sites of APP. APP is pictured as a transmembrane protein, with the βAP subunit anchored within the membrane. In section A, proteases cut APP through the βAP region. In section B, proteases cut βAP on either side of the βAP subunit. βAP is then released intact into the extracellular fluid, where it can aggregate, forming insoluble preamyloid plaques. *(Adapted from Ref. 19.)*

One factor promoting βAP aggregation is the lipophilicity of the carboxy terminal of βAP. The C-terminus of βAP appears to promote plaque formation. Altering this end of the protein could help prevent plaque formation.

Deposits of βAP are assumed to be the initiating cause of AD. Although this theory has not been conclusively proven, it is supported by *in vitro* and animal research. In animal experiments, mice genetically engineered to produce βAP secondarily developed amyloid plaques, dystrophic neurites, loss of synaptic connections, and activated glial cells.[13,24] Injection of beta amyloid into rats' brains causes neuronal breakdown in the exposed areas.[13,14] *In vitro,* hippocampal cells exposed to βAP aggregates develop abnormally phosphorylated tau protein and begin to degenerate.[13,25] Even when not incorporated in plaques, βAP may exert toxic effects. It does this by increasing production of free radicals and disrupting potassium and calcium ion channels across the cell membrane, resulting in depolarization and toxicity from excess calcium influx.[17,26] Taken as a whole, these data suggest βAP deposition occurs early in the disease process, and rather than being simply an end-product of neuronal death, could initiate the process of plaque formation and nerve cell destruction.

APP may play a role in repair of brain injuries. Yet, APP is not limited to the brain, but found in cells throughout the body. It is not known why βAP selectively deposits in the brain in AD as opposed to other anatomic sites.

GENETIC CAUSES

It used to be thought that early-onset cases of AD were genetic, whereas the more common later onset cases were sporadic. Recent genetic research has obliterated the distinctions between familial and sporadic with the discovery of the apolipoprotein E4 allele on chromosome 19, which influences susceptibility to late-onset cases. Almost all early-onset cases of AD can be attributed to alterations on chromosome 1, 14, and 21.

APP is encoded on chromosome 21. Patients with Down's syndrome have three copies of chromosome 21 and show increased amyloid plaque formation at an early age. Although AD has a high incidence in persons with Down's syndrome, some individuals with Down's syndrome do not develop AD, suggesting that increased amyloid deposition is not the sole determinate of disease expression.[14] A small number of early-onset, familial AD cases have also been associated with mutations in the APP, resulting in overproduction of βAP.[13,14,27]

The majority and most aggressive early-onset cases are attributed to mutations of an Alzheimer's gene located on chromosome 14, which produces a protein called presenilin 1.[17] Similar in structure to presenilin 1 is a protein produced by a gene on chromosome 1 called presenilin 2. Presenilin 2 is responsible for early-onset AD in a family of Germans living in Russia's Volga Valley. Both presenilin 1 and presenilin 2 encode for membrane proteins that might be involved in APP processing.

Genetic susceptibility to late-onset AD is influenced by apolipoprotein E genotype.

APOLIPOPROTEIN E

Apolipoprotein E (Apo E) functions as a carrier for cholesterol in the blood and central nervous system. In the brain, Apo E is produced by astrocytes and is important in distributing cholesterol for repair of neuronal membranes and myelin. Thus, its production is increased following injury of neuronal tissue.[21,28] The gene responsible for the production of Apo E is located on chromosome 19 in a region previously associated with late-onset AD. There are three major subtypes or isoforms of Apo E, termed Apo E2, Apo E3, and Apo E4.[29] Humans inherit one copy of the Apo E gene from each parent. Apo E3 is the most common type (90% of individuals have at least one copy), with E2 and E4 occurring less frequently. Inheritance of the Apo E4 isoform increases risk for late-onset AD; however, the degree of risk depends on such factors as number of E4 copies, age, ethnicity, and gender (Fig. 61–3).[30] All individuals homozygous for Apo E4 are at increased risk, such that 90% of persons inheriting two copies of Apo E4 will develop AD by age 80 years. Moreover, onset of symptoms will occur at a relatively younger age compared with patients having no or only one copy of Apo E4 in their genotype.[29,31] In Caucasians, inheriting a single copy of E4 increases AD risk, whereas inheriting the Apo E2 allele protects against AD.[32,33] In African Americans the converse may be true, E4 does not increase risk while E2 may increase it. There are also differences with regard to gender. Inheriting one copy of E4 increases risk in females, but this is less so in males.

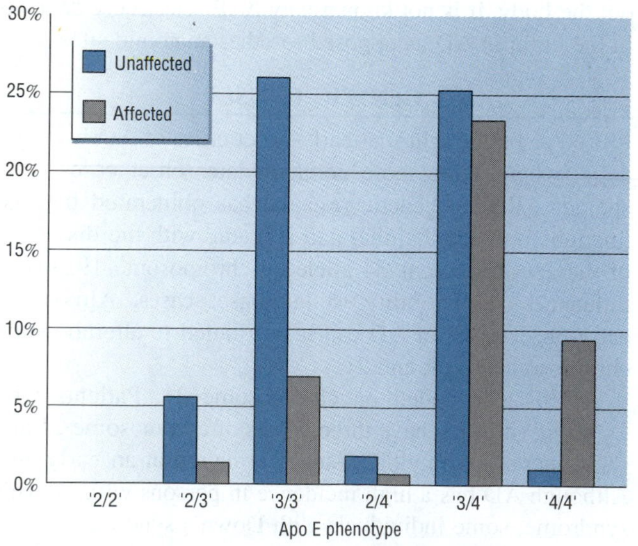

FIGURE 61–3. Ratio of unaffected to affected members by Apo E phenotype in 42 families (total N = 234) with late-onset Alzheimer's disease. Prevalence of Alzheimer's disease increases with number of inherited copies of Apo E4. Phenotype legends indicate Apo E subtypes, (e.g., '2/3' signifies one copy of the Apo E2 allele, and one copy of Apo E3). *(Adapted from Ref. 31.)*

It is important to remember that although inheritance of the Apo E4 subtype might facilitate the development of AD, it is not diagnostic or even essential for disease presence. AD does occur in persons with no copies of Apo E4, and the Apo E4 genotype is also more common in other dementias involving abnormal tau protein such as Pick's disease and progressive supranuclear palsy.[21] Neither is a person with two copies of Apo E4 doomed to get AD. Mitigating factors exist, such that if a person homozygous for E4 does not have AD by age 80, they probably will not develop it.

One of these mitigating factors may be the protein α_1-antichymotrypsin (ACT). ACT binds to βAP and facilitates the formation of amyloid filaments, a possible precursor to plaques. There are two known alleles for ACT: ACT-A and ACT-T. Inheritance of ACT-T appears to protect Apo E4 homozygotes from developing AD.[17] Production of ACT can be increased by interleukin-1, a cytokine involved in the inflammatory response.

Apo E binds to the βAP deposits located in neuritic plaques and cerebral vessels in the brains of patients with AD and is also associated with NFTs. At present, the exact role of Apo E in the genesis of AD is unclear. Links are being discovered, however, like lipoprotein receptor protein (LRP), a receptor for Apo E, which is also responsible for processing released APP. LRP is also found in neuritic plaques.[17]

Tissue plasminogen activator (tPA), an anticoagulant widely known as a treatment for heart attack and stroke, may also play a role in plaque formation. Under certain circumstances, tPA can accelerate neuronal destruction. βAP can bind tPA through LRP, activating tPA and increasing βAP deposition and toxicity.

INFLAMMATORY MEDIATORS

Inflammatory mediators and other immune system constituents are present near areas of plaque formation, suggesting that the immune system plays an active role in the pathogenesis of AD. Although perhaps not the disease-initiating event, an immune response generated against some unknown insult could facilitate neuronal destruction. Evidence supporting significant involvement of the immune system includes the increased presence of acute phase proteins, such as ACT and α-2-macroglobulin, both in the serum and within amyloid plaques of patients with AD.[34] Glial cells (microglial cells and astrocytes), cytokines (e.g., interleukin-1 and interleukin-6), and components of the classic complement cascade are also markedly increased in plaque-infested areas.[34] These inflammatory mediators have been shown to increase βAP toxicity and aggregation. Chronic production of cytotoxic agents and free radicals by activated microglia can result in accelerated neurodegeneration.

Epidemiologic studies suggest that patients who take nonsteroidal antiinflammatory drugs (NSAIDs) have a lower risk of developing AD. In particular, the Boston longitudinal study of aging (BLSA), which attempted to collect data on NSAID use in a more prospective fashion, found a 50% lower risk of developing AD in patients who used NSAIDs regularly (RR, 0.5; 95% CI, 0.3 to 0.85). However, present data are insufficient to determine how long, at what dose, or at what point prior to the development of AD symptoms a person must take NSAIDs to achieve the greatest therapeutic index. Most patents in the BLSA reported using ibuprofen. At this point, it is too early to recommend that all patients with AD take NSAIDs, and more details must be known before NSAIDs can be recommended to prevent AD. We also do not know the most appropriate regimen. Microglial cells located around and within amyloid plaques are thought to release inflammatory mediators, which locally destroy neuronal tissue. Glial cells also function as phagocytes, similar to macrophages and monocytes in the periphery. Another component of the complement cascade, the membrane attack complex (MAC), is found associated with broken neurites and areas containing NFTs, implicating MAC as promoting the vast neuronal destruction characterizing AD.[34] As stated earlier, the acute phase proteins ACT and α-2-macroglobulin also act as protease inhibitors, and could influence proteolytic breakdown of APP into βAP.[20] As is the case in many chronic inflammatory illnesses, specific factors responsible for initiating the immune response are not known. One theory is that breaks in the blood–brain barrier due to trauma, leaky endothelial cells, or other conditions trigger an immune response to brain proteins previously unexposed to the periphery.[34] Another possibility is that the immune system is activated by plaque precursors or byproducts of damaged cells, resulting in further destruction of adjacent neurons.[35]

THE CHOLINERGIC SYSTEM

Multiple neuronal pathways are destroyed in AD. Damage occurs in any nerve cell population located in or traveling through plaque-laden areas.[13,20] Widespread cell destruction results in a variety of neurotransmitter deficits. Most profoundly damaged are the cholinergic pathways, particularly a large system of neurons located at the base of the forebrain in the Nucleus Basalis of Mynert, a brain area believed to be involved in thought integration.[20] Axons of these cholinergic neurons project to the frontal cortex and hippocampus, areas strongly associated with memory and cognition.

The discovery of vast cholinergic cell loss led to the development of a cholinergic hypothesis. The cholinergic hypothesis targeted cholinergic cell loss as the source of memory and cognitive impairment in AD. Therefore, it was presumed that increasing cholinergic function would improve symptoms of memory loss, much the same way that dopamine replacement improves tremor and rigidity in Parkinson's disease. This approach is flawed for two reasons. First, cholinergic cell loss does not appear to be the disease-producing event, but a secondary consequence of Alzheimer's pathology; and second, cholinergic neurons are only one of many neuronal pathways destroyed in AD. Simple addition of acetylcholine cannot compensate for the loss of neurons, receptors, and other neurotransmitters consumed during the course of the illness. Enhancing cholinergic activity no more cures AD than dopamine replacement cures Parkinson's disease.[36] The principle is the same, however: to minimize or improve dementia symptoms through augmentation of cholinergic transmission at remaining synapses.

OTHER NEUROTRANSMITTER ABNORMALITIES

Although the cholinergic system has received a lion's share of attention in AD pharmaceutical research, deficits exist in other neuronal pathways as well. Serotonergic neurons of the raphe nuclei and noradrenergic cells of the locus ceruleus are also lost, while monoamine oxidase type B (MAO-B) activity is increased. MAO-B is found predominately in the brain and in platelets, and is responsible for metabolizing dopamine. The presence of increased MAO-B concentrations may seem counterintuitive considering the vast neuronal loss in AD, unless one considers that MAO-B is also contained in glial cells whose populations are increased. Increased platelet and brain MAO-B concentrations are also seen in Parkinson's disease, but not multi-infarct dementia.[37] Other abnormalities appear in glutamate pathways of the cortex and limbic structures, where a loss of neurons leads to a focus on excitotoxicity models as possible contributing factors to AD pathology.

Glutamate is a major excitatory neurotransmitter in the cortex and hippocampus. Many neuronal pathways essential to learning and memory use glutamate as a neurotransmitter, including the pyramidal neurons (a layer of neurons with long axons carrying information out of the cortex), hippocampus, and entorhinal cortex. Glutamate and other excitatory amino acid neurotransmitters have been implicated as potential neurotoxins in AD.[38,39] If glutamate is allowed to remain in the synapse for extended periods of time, it can act as a toxin, destroying nerve cells. Toxic effects are thought to be mediated through increased intracellular calcium and accumulation of free radicals.[40] The presence of βAP renders cells more susceptible to glutamate-mediated excitotoxicity *in vitro*.[13] Dysregulated glutamate activity is thought to be one of the primary mediators of neuronal injury after stroke or acute brain injury. Although intimately involved in cell injury, the role of excitatory amino acids in AD is as yet unclear.

ESTROGEN

The observation that women appear to be at greater risk for developing AD but not other dementias has fueled interest in estrogen as a possible means of prevention and treatment. In men, circulating testosterone is aromatized to estrogen in the brain. Because men do not undergo drastic changes in testosterone levels with age, they would be relatively protected from loss of estrogen effects on cognition. Estrogen is thought to be involved in promoting neuronal growth and preventing oxidative damage, which would benefit cells exposed to β-amyloid.[26] Estrogen receptors are present in the brain, and are distributed in a pattern consistent with areas destroyed in AD.[41,42] In the hippocampus, cerebral cortex, and basal forebrain, estrogen receptors colocalize with receptors for nerve growth factor on cholinergic nerve terminals.[42,43] The presence of estrogen increases the number of nerve growth factor receptors. The ability of estrogen to interact with nerve growth factor may explain estrogen's ability to promote synaptic growth, stimulating axons and dendrites to sprout new terminals. Estrogen supplementation also prevents decrements in choline uptake and choline acetyltransferase (ChAT) concentrations, occurring in rats following ovarectomy. This suggests estrogen is important in maintaining normal cholinergic neurotransmission.[42] Estrogen may also increase *N*-methyl-D-aspartate (NMDA) receptor numbers in brain areas involved in recording new memory. In addition to promoting growth, estrogen prevents cell damage. Estrogen acts as an antioxidant.[26] In culture, estrogen protects hippocampal neurons exposed to glutamate and β-amyloid from cytotoxic and free radical damage. Progesterone[26] was also effective in preventing cell damage, but less effective than estrogen in specifically preventing damage following exposure to βAP. Estrogen may prevent formation of neuritic plaques by facilitating preferential degradation of APP by α-secretase into soluble products, as opposed to β-secretase, which is potentially amyloidogenic.[41]

The data just reviewed were derived from animal and *in vitro* experiments, so how do we know that these mechanisms will translate into functional benefit in preventing AD? Early epidemiologic studies based on indirectly gathered data gave conflicting results. Recently, however, a longitudinal population study prospectively followed 1124 neurologically healthy women enrolled in a community study of aging.[44] Strengths of this study included face-to-face clinical interviews and diagnosis based on National Institute of Neurological and Communicative Disorders—Alzheimer's Disease and Related Disorders Association (NINCDS—ADRDA) criteria. Age of AD onset in these women was directly related to duration of postmenopausal ERT. The incidence of AD on follow-up was 5.8% in the 156 women taking estrogen at any time after menopause, compared with 16.3% in the 968 nonestrogen users. The relative risk of contracting AD was 0.4 (95% CI, 0.22 to 0.85) for ERT users versus nonusers.

OTHER FACTORS

History of repeated or severe head trauma (dementia pugilistica) is also said to predispose to AD.[45] Increased risk in this population is interesting from the standpoint that glial cells and Apo E are more prevalent in injured brain areas. If inflammatory pathways promote neuronal damage in AD, the increased presence of inflammatory mediators following head injury could explain increased prevalence of dementia in this population. Excitotoxicity has been also implicated as a source of neuronal damage in patient's with head trauma, similar to AD.

The general public still widely believes that aluminum exposure can cause AD. Although ionic aluminum ($Al(OH)^{3+}$) is neurotoxic, it causes a pattern of destruction different from that observed in AD. Patients with AD do not need to avoid aluminum-containing antacids or deodorants. Likewise, there is no evidence to suggest EDTA chelation therapy is an effective treatment of AD.[46]

Another heavy metal ion, zinc, has recently come of interest as a potential facilitator of plaque formation. Following a small study in which Alzheimer's patients treated with zinc showed a rapid deterioration in cognition, Bush and colleagues[47] examined the role of zinc in promoting neuritic plaques using *in vitro* methods. They found zinc accelerated plaque formation from soluble βAP, and hypothesized that abnormalities of zinc homeostasis in the brain could lead to plaque formation. This research is preliminary, and experiments conducted *in vitro* may not represent *in vivo* occurrences. Although the use of zinc supplements should be discouraged in patients with AD, at this time zinc should not be considered a cause of the disease.

Cigarette smoking (nicotine use) may provide some protection from AD. Cigarette smoking upregulates brain nicotine receptors, perhaps partially compensating for generalized loss of these receptors in AD.

One conclusion is that there does not seem to be a single common mechanism for producing disease in all cases. Regardless of the source, however, the features remain the same: degeneration of neurons in higher brain areas; accumulation of NFTs and neuritic plaques; profound destruction of cholinergic pathways; and an insidious dementia, slowly progressive until death.

CLINICAL PRESENTATION

Unlike dementia due to stroke, the onset of AD is almost imperceptible, without abrupt changes in cognition or function. Deficits occur progressively over time and are global, affecting multiple areas of cognition.[1,48,49]

Loss of memory is typically the presenting patient complaint, and is frequently brought to the clinician's attention by a family member. Memory is a nonspecific term representing many diverse areas of cognitive function (e.g., recall, recognition, calculation, and orientation). Crucial to understanding the plight of persons with AD is to understand that "loss of memory" means the inability to extract and use all previously learned information, activity, and experience. Patients' initial complaints of "memory loss" typically refer to disorientation for time or an inability to recall recent events. In early AD, the ability to lay down new memory (learn) and recall recent events is impaired, whereas recall for remote events (childhood/adolescent years) is spared until later in the disease process. Common early problems include forgetting appointments, misplacing items such as keys, getting lost traveling to familiar locations, and difficulties handling money or balancing a checkbook. Patients may notice an increasing need for lists, problems recalling the date or day of the week, and difficulty performing routine tasks at home or work. Anomia is a problem, with difficulty recalling names of familiar objects or people. Speech becomes difficult as details and content words are lost, and patients resort to confabulation or circumlocution (nonspecific, evasive speech) to compensate for their deficits. Problems with speech, recall of events, and comprehension result in decreased socialization and withdrawal from casual conversation.

Persons with AD often conceal their memory problem well at first, and may deny or "forget" that they have a memory problem. Common symptoms of moderate dementia include the inability to use objects properly even though the patient may be able to name the object or even describe how it should be used (apraxia), loss of the ability to draw complex figures or conceptualize their orientation in space (constructional apraxia), inability to work or do routine household chores, forgetting to eat or change clothes, disorientation to place, and difficulty initiating activities. Patients also become unable to determine the appropriate time of day for accomplishing activities and are generally unable to plan or independently follow a daily schedule. As dementia progresses, patients become lost in their own homes, unable to recognize family or spouses, and unable to speak (aphasia). Judgment and reasoning are extremely impaired, and without supervision, patients may burn themselves on appliances, leave water running, wander outside and become lost, or engage in other dangerous activities. Wandering, combativeness, and incontinence are common reasons for placement in a long-term care facility. In the final stages of the disease, patients lose the ability to eat, walk, or communicate. Choking, aspiration, or infection generally result in death within 3 to 20 years of disease onset.

For treatment and assessment purposes, it is helpful to divide Alzheimer's symptoms into two basic categories: cognitive symptoms and noncognitive (behavioral) symptoms (Table 61–2).[49] Cognitive symptoms are present in all patients reaching the final stages of the illness, whereas behavioral symptoms are less predictable.[49]

Noncognitive symptoms such as mood disturbances, disruptive behavior, and psychosis are present at one time or another in most patients and can pose significant management problems for caregivers. Early in the course of the illness, the patient may become depressed, frustrated, or irritable. Anxiety, hostility, misinterpretations, and delusions are common in moderate stages of AD. Personality changes and changes in emotional expression are also frequently reported. Disruptive behavior and psychosis are most often seen in the moderate to severe stages of AD, with severity fluctuating over time. Common disruptive behaviors include wandering, agitation, aggression, uncooperativeness, and purposeless activity. Patients frequently experience "sundowning," or worsening of symptoms at night because of decreased sensory input and fewer orienting stimuli. Suspiciousness, nonsystematized paranoid delusions, and misinterpretation of actual phenomena (illusions) are the most common psychotic symptoms. It is important to recognize that the psychotic symptoms characterizing AD are substantially different from those seen in nondemented patients, such as those with schizophrenia. Delusions in AD more often appear to be an attempt to explain things that have been forgotten. Other delusions may stem from an inability to recognize friends and family members, combined with preferential loss of recent memories. As a consequence of these phenomena, the patient may become agitated, physically or verbally aggressive, or attempt to leave the residence in search of missing persons or to "go home."[50]

TABLE 61–2. Fundamental Symptom Categories in Alzheimer's Disease

Cognitive Deficits[a]	Noncognitive Psychiatric Symptoms and Disruptive Behaviors[b]
• Memory loss Poor recall, agnosia, losing items • Dysphasia Anomia, circumlocution, aphasia • Dyspraxia • Disorientation Impaired perception of time or direction; cannot recognize acquaintances, family, or self • Impaired calculation • Impaired judgment and problem-solving skills	• Depression • Psychotic symptoms Hallucinations, delusions, suspiciousness • Nonpsychotic disruptive behaviors Physical and verbal aggression, motor hyperactivity, uncooperativeness, wandering; repetitive mannerisms/activities, combativeness

[a]Cognitive deficits: Symptoms occurring in all patients as disease progresses.
[b]Noncognitive symptoms: Symptoms that are variably present, consisting mainly of psychiatric and behavioral problems.
Compiled from Ref. 50.

Persons with AD become extraordinarily dependent on those around them. Family and direct caregivers may experience considerable psychological distress through role changes, time commitments, cost, and the hassles of day-to-day care. It is extremely difficult for caregivers to cope with the transformation of someone from an able-bodied companion or parent to a dependent stranger. Any attempts at therapeutic management must take into account the effect of treatment on the caregiver, both with respect to cost and ease of use versus expected therapeutic gain.

DIAGNOSIS

Minor memory loss, sometimes called age-associated memory impairment, is a common complaint associated with normal aging and is not a cause for concern. However, if

TABLE 61–3. NINCDS–ADRDA Criteria and Diagnostic Workup for Probable Alzheimer's Disease

I. History of progressive cognitive decline of insidious onset
 - In-depth interview of patient and caregivers

II. Deficits in at least two or more areas of functioning
 - Confirmation with use of dementia rating scale–Mini-Mental Status Exam MMSE[a] or Blessed Dementia Scale

III. No disturbance of consciousness

IV. Age between 40 and 90 (usually > 65)

V. No other explainable cause of symptoms
 - Normal laboratory tests including hematology, full chemistries, B_{12} and folate, thyroid function tests, VDRL (to rule out syphilis)
 - Normal electrocardiogram and electroencephalogram
 - Normal physical exam, including thorough neurologic exam
 - CT or MRI scanning: No focal lesions signifying other possible causes of dementia present. Abnormalities common, but not diagnostic, for AD include general cerebral wasting, widening of sulci, widening of the ventricles, and lesions of white matter surrounding the ventricle deep in the brain

[a]The Folstein Mini-Mental Status Exam[53] is a commonly used scale measuring orientation, recall, short-term memory, concentration, constructional praxis, and language. The MMSE is scored from 0 to 30, with a score of 10 to ~28 typical of very early to moderate Alzheimer's disease.
Adapted from Ref. 51.

memory loss affects social or occupational functioning, or is noticed by friends and coworkers, patients should be encouraged to visit a neurologist for a formal evaluation. At present, the only way to definitively diagnose AD is through direct examination of brain tissue at autopsy or biopsy. Because no definitive diagnostic laboratory, clinical, or imaging tests are available, AD remains a diagnosis of exclusion. To design criteria that would minimize inaccurate diagnoses, a workgroup was established in 1984 by the NINCDS and the ADRDA. Use of the workgroup's explicit criteria has reduced the percentage of erroneously diagnosed AD cases to under 10%, and the NINCDS-ADRDA criteria (Table 61–3) are the standard.[51] Patient's fulfilling these criteria are given a diagnosis of probable AD. The Agency for Health Care Policy and Research has also published guidelines for the recognition and assessment of AD that are useful tools for the primary care setting.[52] The first step in this diagnostic process is to conduct a thorough history and physical exam. The history should be obtained from the patient and reliable caregivers and confirm a slowly progressive and not precipitous deterioration of functioning. The assessment should include review of prescription drug use, history of alcohol or other substance use, family medical history, and history of trauma, depression, or head injury. It is important to rule out medication use as contributing to dementia symptoms, especially medications with anticholinergic or other central nervous system side effects.

An established dementia screening scale, such as the Folstein Mini-Mental Status Exam (MMSE),[53] can aid in confirming a history of deficits in two or more areas of cognition and establish a baseline to evaluate change in severity.[51,53] Thorough neuropsychological testing is generally not necessary but may be helpful if a diagnosis of dementia is in doubt.[54,55] Other causes of dementia must be excluded, including cerebral vascular disease, subcortical stroke, alcoholism, or vitamin B_{12} deficiency, to name a few (see Table 61–1). Routine laboratory tests and physical and neurologic exams should rule out other disorders. Brain imaging tools help rule out multi-infarct dementia, and although atrophy or other nonspecific abnormalities are often seen on computed tomography (CT) scans or magnetic resonance imaging (MRI), these alone are not sufficient to confer an AD diagnosis. Following diagnosis, AD is staged using a scale such as the Global Deterioration Scale (GDS) (Table 61–4).[56] This seven-point system is widely used, has been validated as correlating to psychometric measures and changes in CT or positron emission tomography scans, and is useful to monitor the global changes in the patient with AD.

TABLE 61–4. Stages of Cognitive Decline: The Global Deterioration Scale (GDS)

Stage 1	Normal	No subjective or objective change in intellectual functioning.
Stage 2	Forgetfulness	Complaints of losing things or forgetting names of acquaintances. Does not interfere with job or social functioning. Generally a component of normal aging.
Stage 3	Early confusion	Cognitive decline causes interference with work and social functioning. Anomia, difficulty remembering right word in conversation, and recall difficulties are present and noticed by family members. Memory loss may cause anxiety for patient.
Stage 4	Late confusion (early AD)	Patient can no longer manage finances or homemaking activities. Difficulty remembering recent events. Begins to withdraw from difficult tasks and give up hobbies. May deny memory problems.
Stage 5	Early dementia (moderate AD)	Patient can no longer survive without assistance. Frequently disoriented with regard to time (date, year, season). Difficulty selecting clothing. Recall for recent events is severely impaired; may forget some details of past life (e.g., school attended or occupation). Functioning may fluctuate from day to day. Patient generally denies problems. May become suspicious or tearful. Loses ability to drive safely.
Stage 6	Middle dementia (moderately severe AD)	Patients need assistance with activities of daily living (e.g., bathing, dressing, toileting). Patients experience difficulty interpreting their surroundings; may forget names of family and caregivers; forget most details of past life; difficulty counting backwards from 10. Agitation, paranoia, and delusions are common.
Stage 7	Late dementia	Patient loses ability to speak (may only grunt or scream), walk, and feed self. Incontinent of urine and feces. Consciousness reduced to stupor or coma.

Adapted from Ref. 56.

Positron emission tomography (PET) and single-photon emission computed tomography (SPECT) have been suggested as potential diagnostic tools for AD, but at present, they remain research probes.[54,55]

Currently, Apo E typing is not recommended on a routine clinical basis. Although Apo E4 is a risk factor for development of Alzheimer's, not all individuals with the E4 allele develop AD. Conversely, some individual have a diagnosis of Alzheimer's without the E4 allele. Better population based estimates of risk are needed in order to provide appropriate genetic counseling.[55] Concern also exists regarding potential discrimination by insurance companies and employers toward individuals who possess one or more copies of Apo E4.

▶ TREATMENT: Alzheimer's Disease

DESIRED OUTCOMES

None of the current treatments for AD are curative or are known to directly reverse or halt the pathophysiologic processes of the disorder. Therefore, the primary goal of treatment in AD is to maintain patient function as long as possible. Secondary goals are aimed toward treating the psychiatric and behavioral sequelae that occur as a result of the disease.

GENERAL APPROACH TO TREATMENT

The primary approach in treating AD is nonpharmacologic. Initial treatment begins with education of the patient, and especially the family or other caregivers, regarding the disease, prognosis, and changes in life-style that are necessary as the disease progresses. Table 61–5 lists basic principles of care for the Alzheimer's patient. While encouraging as much function and self-reliance as possible, the life for the Alzheimer's patients must become progressively more simple and structured in order to compensate for the deficits in cognition. Denial on part of the patient and rationalization on part of the family are common. The caregiver must be prepared to face the changes in life that will occur, and acceptance of this does not come easily. The clinician should encourage the family to address legal and financial matters and designate a durable power of attorney for the point when the patient will not be able to make decisions regarding life matters, including health care decisions. Education and guidance need to be provided regarding the patient's independence in conducting activities of daily living, including use of power tools, household repairs, cooking, and especially driving. The family should be referred to local resources such as the Alzheimer's Association, where detailed information regarding support services can be provided. A list of referral sources and references for caregivers is given in Table 61–6.

TABLE 61–5. Basic Principles of Care for the Alzheimer's Patient

- Keep requests and demands of the patient simple and avoid complex tasks that might lead to frustration.
- Avoid confrontation and defer requests that lead to frustration.
- Remain calm, firm, and supportive if the patient becomes upset.
- Maintain a consistent environment and avoid unnecessary changes.
- Provide frequent reminders, explanations, and orientation cues.
- Recognize declines in capacity and adjust expectations for patient performance.
- Bring sudden declines in function and the emergence of new symptoms to professional attention.

Adapted from Ref. 54.

Latches may need to be installed on doors and cabinets to prevent wandering or rummaging through household items. The patient will need frequent reminders in the beginning, and assistance later, with personal hygiene and other personal activities of daily living. A nightlight and a bedside commode may help prevent confusion and wandering when the patient awakens in the middle of the night for toileting. The caregiver will need to address issues such as respite services to provide time for rest, relaxation, and conduct of personal business. Eventually, the caregiver will need to face critical questions with respect to institutionalization. The two primary reasons for institutionalization are behavioral disturbances and incontinence, problems secondary to Alzheimer's that most caregivers find difficult to manage in the home. This is probably the most difficult decision that the caregiver will have to make, and clinician support and referral to social services is important in assisting the caregiver.

PHARMACOLOGIC THERAPY

Current pharmacotherapeutic interventions for AD are for the most part symptomatic attempts to either improve or maintain cognition. However, there is some evidence that some interventions (e.g., vitamin E, selegiline) may prolong the time to critical functional end points. Secondary pharmacotherapeutic interventions are aimed at treating depression, psychosis, and agitation in the Alzheimer's patient. Figure 61–4 shows pharmacotherapeutic treatment algorithms for AD. These recommendations are made based upon available efficacy, safety, and tolerability data. It is emphasized that nonmedication interventions are the current primary interventions for management of AD, and medications should be used in the context of multimodality interventions.

PHARMACOTHERAPY OF COGNITIVE SYMPTOMS

Research Methodology for Pharmacotherapeutic Studies of Cognition-Enhancing Agents

Early studies with potential cognition-enhancing agents in AD are difficult to interpret. Significant variation existed from study to study with respect to methodology and patient assessments, and in many cases consistency in diagnosis could be questioned. Criticisms of study methodology, including the questionable ability to determine clinically significant effects of a drug in AD, led the Food and Drug Administration (FDA) to recommend minimum, uniform criteria for conducting efficacy studies in Alzheimer's patients.

At a minimum, studies in support of a New Drug Application (NDA) for treatment of AD must be double blind, placebo-controlled, randomized, and of parallel group design. Efficacy must be indicated by statistically significant differences between groups on both the Alzheimer's Disease Assessment Scale–Cognitive Portion (ADAS–Cog) and the Clinical Interview-based Impression of Change (CIBIC).[57] The ADAS–Cog is a structured psychometric assessment measuring patient performance on

TABLE 61–6. Resources for Caregivers of Persons With Alzheimer's Disease

The following organizations provide educational literature, information on diagnosis, treatment, social support, and ongoing research in Alzheimer's disease.

- Administration on Aging
  Department of Health and Human Services
  330 Independence Avenue, SW
  Washington, DC 20201
  202-619-1006
  FAX: 202-619-7586
  Internet address: http://www.aoa.dhhs.gov
- Alzheimer's Disease Education and Referral Center (ADEAR)
  PO Box 8250
  Silver Spring, MD 20907-8250
  1-800-438-4380
  e-mail: adear@alzheimers,org
- Alzheimer's Disease and Related Disorders Association (ADRDA or the Alzheimer's Association)
  919 North Michigan Avenue, Suite 100
  Chicago, IL 60611-1676
  1-800-272-3900 (24-hour line)
  Internet address: http://www.alz.org
- Alzheimer's Disease Society of Canada
  491 Lawrence Ave. West, no. 501
  Toronto, Ontario, Canada M5M1C7
- American Association of Retired Persons (AARP)
  Washington, DC
  1-800-424-3410
- Corporation for National Service
  Office of Public Liaison
  1201 New York Avenue, NW
  Washington, DC 20525
  202-1606-5000
- Elder Care Locator
  1-800-667-1116

Further Reading

- Failure-Free Activities for the Alzheimer's Patient. San Francisco, Cottage Books, 1987.
- Reminiscence: Uncovering a Lifetime of Memories. San Francisco, Elder Press, 1991.
- Living in the Labyrinth. A Personal Journey Through the Maze of Alzheimer's. San Francisco, Elder Press, 1993.
- The 36 Hour Day. Baltimore, Johns Hopkins University Press, 1981.

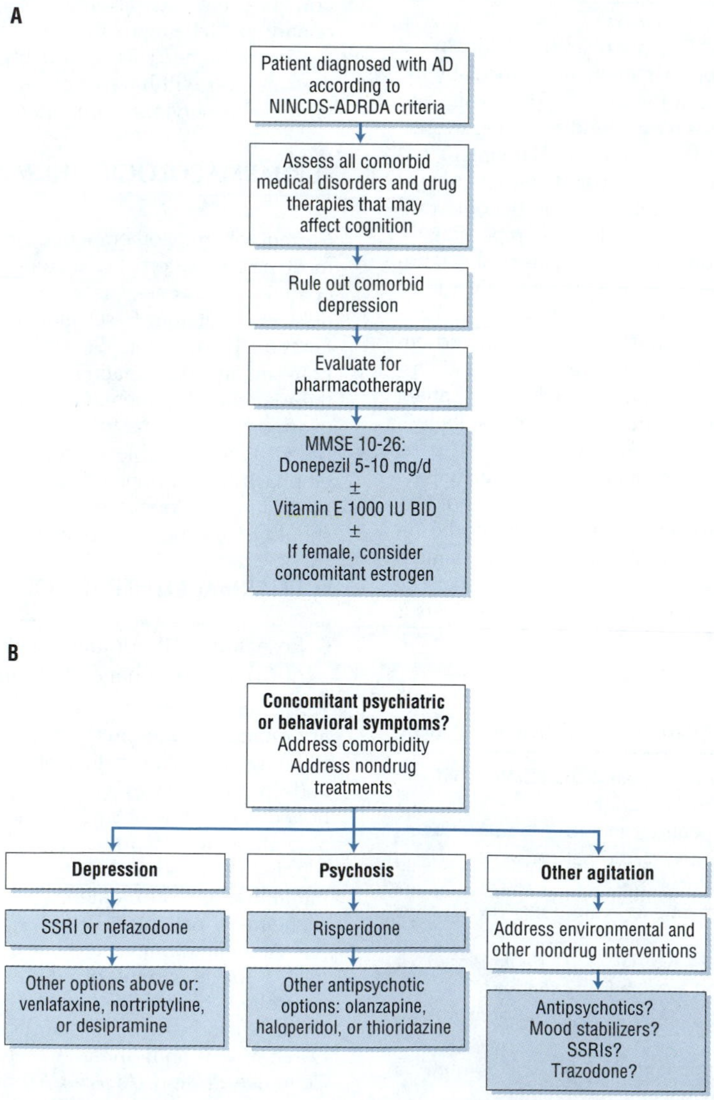

FIGURE 61–4. Proposed treatment algorithm for Alzheimer's disease (AD).

multiple, discrete areas of cognitive function. A decrease in ADAS score indicates improved cognition. In natural disease progression studies, scores on the ADAS-Cog have been shown to worsen (increase) by an average of 4 points over 6 months and 7 points over 1 year. Based upon these findings, the general consensus is that a 4 point change in the ADAS-Cog represents a clinically significant change. Therefore, if a pharmacotherapeutic agent decreases the ADAS-Cog by 4-points, one could think of this as having reversed symptoms of the disease by 6 months. However, the clinical relevancy of the ADAS-Cog is still commonly questioned, as it is difficult to extrapolate how changes in the scale reflect potential changes in a patient's ability to function in life on a daily basis and complete activities of daily living.

The CIBIC is a clinician's assessment based solely on an interview with the patient, and without access to any other patient information.[58] Efficacy based on the CIBIC is deemed important because it is thought to represent a clinically distinguishable change in cognition and to more closely mimic the manner in which a clinician might evaluate a patient in the office setting.[59] More recently, the CIBIC-Plus, a clinical assessment based on an interview with both the patient and the caregiver, has been used in lieu of the CIBIC by many investigators.[59] However, guidelines vary from study to study regarding how the CIBIC is actually conducted. Sometimes the investigator is asked to use a common structured interview and other times the content of the interview is entirely up to individual investigator discretion. Because of the concerns noted regarding the extrapolation of ADAS-Cog results to everyday life, the FDA requires statistical significance on both the ADAS-Cog and the CIBIC (compared with placebo) as requirements for drug approval.

Because of concerns regarding the applicability of psychometric tests to routine clinical practice, some investigators have used critical outcomes (e.g., institutionalization, global severity) as critical end points in Alzheimer's studies.[60] These types of parameters assist in examining the effects of drug therapy on disease progression.

The appropriate duration of Alzheimer's studies remains an important question. Studies with donepezil and tacrine have both established efficacy as compared with placebo over a 6-month period. However, this provides the clinician with limited information regarding the effects of these medications over the duration of the illness. Long-term follow-up studies of medication treatment are important to establish the effects of these agents over the course of the illness.

Cholinesterase Inhibitors

Just as levodopa was developed as replacement therapy for dopaminergic deficiency in Parkinson's disease, in the early 1980s, researchers began to examine means in which to enhance cholinergic activity in patients with AD. Tacrine was the first such drug to be examined in a systematic fashion. However, tacrine is fraught with significant side effects, including hepatotoxicity, that severely limit the ability of patients to adhere to treatment. For all practical purposes, the use of tacrine has been replaced by the advent of safer, more tolerable cholinesterase inhibitors.

Donepezil (Esai 2020, Aricept, Pfizer) is a piperidine, cholinesterase inhibitor with specificity for inhibition of acetylcholinesterase as compared to butyrylcholinesterase. This specificity is claimed to result in fewer peripheral side effects (such as nausea, vomiting, and diarrhea) than with nonspecific cholinesterase inhibitors such as tacrine or physostigmine.[61] Donepezil's overall efficacy in improving cognitive symptoms in AD is probably no greater than that of tacrine. However, due to its more favorable side effect profile, donepezil is much better tolerated, and patients are more likely to continue taking the medication and actually experience a therapeutic benefit. Therefore, donepezil is a significantly more "effective" agent than tacrine.

Although one phase II trial has been published in the literature,[62] neither pivotal trial in support of the donepezil NDA has been published. Therefore, it is difficult to fully assess efficacy. Based upon the summary in the approved product literature,[61] the efficacy appears similar to that of tacrine. Both donepezil 5 and 10 mg daily are effective doses, with no statistically significant difference between the two. However, the data indicate a trend toward superiority with 10 mg daily, and a trial at the higher dosage is reasonable in patients with no side effects. The most common donepezil side effects are nausea, vomiting, and diarrhea—typical cholinergic side effects. However, the medication is well tolerated in most patients. Table 61–7 compares the side effects of donepezil and tacrine.

Donepezil is first-line treatment for cognitive impairment in mild to moderately severe (MMSE 10 to 26) AD. Its efficacy in treatment of patients with severe impairment (MMSE < 10) has not been studied. However, with the severe neuronal degeneration associated with advanced disease, it is doubtful that a cholinesterase inhibitor will produce significant benefit in such patients.

Prior to initiating treatment, a Folstein MMSE or similar cognitive assessment should be performed on the patient to evaluate the severity of cognitive decline and serve as a baseline for change. Donepezil 5 mg daily should be the initial dose. If improvement has not been observed within 4 to 6 weeks and the patient is tolerating the drug, then the dose may be increased to 10 mg daily. In addition to the MMSE, the clinician should evaluate the patient based upon an interview with both the patient and the caregiver. Some caregivers will find it difficult to discuss the patient's symptoms and deficits in front of the loved one, and the clinician should be sensitive to the caregiver's need to talk alone with the clinician. Usually the caregiver is the most reliable source for assessing the patient's progress; however, some caregivers will minimize patient's deficits. Therefore, the clinician must use information from multiple sources in making clinical decisions.

Limited information exists regarding how long to continue donepezil therapy. As long as the patient is not showing rapid decline, it is reasonable to continue treatment. In the face of rapid

TABLE 61–7. Comparative Common Adverse Effects of Donepezil and Tacrine From Clinical Trials Data

Adverse Event	Placebo	Donepezil (n = 747)	Tacrine (n = 634)
Elevated liver function tests	2%	< 1%	29%
Nausea or vomiting	9%	[a]	28%
Nausea	6%	11%	[a]
Diarrhea	5%	10%	16%
Headache	9–15%	10%	11%
Dizziness	6–11%	8%	12%
Muscle cramps	2–5%	6%	9%
Insomnia	6%	9%	6%
Vomiting	3%	5%	[a]
Fatigue	3%	5%	4%
Anorexia	2–3%	4%	9%
Depression	1–4%	3%	4%
Abnormal dreams	0	3%	[b]
Weight decrease	1%	3%	3%
Somnolence	< 1%	2%	4%
Syncope	1%	2%	[b]

[a]The donepezil product literature displays these separately while the tacrine literature lumps nausea and vomiting together.
[b]Not listed.
Compiled from Refs. 62 and 87.

decline, tapering and discontinuation may be tried. However, the clinician should observe the patient carefully for rapid decline upon discontinuation. The decline that occurs after drug discontinuation is thought to be to the point the patient would have been if cholinesterase inhibitor treatment had not been initiated. Because of its adverse effects profile and similar mechanism of action, it is not recommended to use tacrine in patients who do not benefit from or tolerate donepezil.

In the one published donepezil clinical trial, there was a high correlation between both donepezil serum concentrations and percent of acetylcholinesterase inhibition and changes in ADAS-Cog scores.[62] Plateau acetylcholinesterase inhibition of 76% to 84% occurred with donepezil plasma concentrations greater than 50 ng/mL, and donepezil 5 mg daily yielded mean steady-state acetylcholinesterase inhibition, as determined by red blood cell cholinesterase inhibition, of approximately 64%. In this study, donepezil achieved a degree of cholinesterase inhibition significantly greater than usually obtained with clinical doses of tacrine. However, the clinical utility of monitoring either acetylcholinesterase inhibition or donepezil serum concentrations in daily practice is currently unknown.

Potential drug interactions with donepezil have been inadequately evaluated. *In vitro* studies have demonstrated that the CYP 3A3/4 inhibitor ketoconazole and the CYP 2D6 inhibitor quinidine inhibit donepezil metabolism.[61] There have been no reports of this potential interaction in humans; therefore, clinical significance cannot be evaluated. Until the clinical significance of potential drug interactions with these types of enzyme inhibitors is better elucidated, clinicians are urged to use caution when adding CYP 2D6 or 3A3/4 inhibitors to a donepezil regimen. One should monitor the patient for possible increased peripheral cholinergic side effects such as nausea, vomiting, or diarrhea when a medication with potent CYP 2D6 or 3A3/4 inhibition is added to donepezil. The effects of enzyme inducers on donepezil kinetics have not been studied.

In vitro studies have shown donepezil to have a low affinity for CYP 2D6 and 3A4, thus making clinically significant drug interactions through these isoenzymes unlikely.[61] In humans, donepezil is reported by the manufacturer to have no effect on the kinetics of theophylline, warfarin, digoxin, or cimetidine.

Other cholinesterase inhibitors (ENA 713, metrifonate, sustained-release physostigmine) are currently in clinical trials. Preliminary evidence suggests that they all have efficacy similar to donepezil and tacrine. Metrifonate in particular is interesting, as it produces irreversible cholinesterase inhibition and thus has an extremely long duration of action.[63] Whether metrifonate or ENA 713 (Exelon), a pseudoirreversible cholinesterase inhibitor, have any advantages over donepezil remains to be seen. Sustained-release physostigmine is associated with a high incidence of nausea, vomiting, and diarrhea.

Antioxidants

Based upon pathophysiologic theories involving free radicals, there has been significant interest regarding the use of antioxidants in the treatment of AD. A recent study compared the use of vitamin E 1000 IU bid, selegiline 5 mg bid, the combination, and placebo in the treatment of moderately impaired Alzheimer's patients.[60] Instead of using cognition on psychometric assessments as their primary outcomes, time to critical end points (i.e., death, institutionalization, loss of ability to perform activities of daily living, or severe dementia) was used as a measure of efficacy. Both vitamin E and selegiline were superior to placebo, and the combination was actually slightly inferior to either treatment alone. The net result of treatment was a delay of 7 months in reaching one of the specified critical end points. However, the study has been criticized because the placebo and active treatment groups had significantly different baseline MMSE scores, and efficacy could be demonstrated only when the baseline scores were used as a covariate. Although not statistically significant, vitamin E showed slight superiority to either selegiline alone or the combination. Based upon these findings, vitamin E's favorable side effect profile, and low cost, it is considered the preferred treatment, and it can be continued indefinitely. Although potential benefits of vitamin E combined with donepezil have not been evaluated, there are no known complications from their combined use.

Selegiline's use in AD has been evaluated in other studies. In a 15-month double-blind study in mildly demented patients, the only demonstrated effect with selegiline 10 mg daily was a mild decrease in Brief Psychiatric Rating Scale scores. The clinical significance of this effect was questioned by the investigators.[64] Other studies with selegiline alone have shown mixed results. Some studies have shown improvement in cognition, while others have shown improvement in behavior or mood.[64,65] It may be that patients who are more severely demented, particularly those with behavioral symptoms, are more likely to receive benefit than patients with milder disease presentation. Further research is necessary to elucidate its role in AD.

Estrogen

As previously stated, most but not all epidemiologic studies have shown a lower incidence of AD in women who took estrogen replacement therapy (ERT) postmenopausally. One of these studies also showed higher MMSE scores in Alzheimer's patients as compared to matched controls. Schneider and colleagues[66] performed a post hoc analysis of women participating in the 30-week tacrine trial. They found that among women receiving tacrine, the therapeutic benefit occurred almost exclusively in women receiving ERT. Limitations of this study include a small number of women receiving the different treatment conditions and the fact that the report was a post hoc analysis.

Lacking randomized clinical trials evaluating the effects of estrogen in women with AD, the treatment recommendation is a difficult one. The decision should be based upon looking at the benefit to risk profile with respect to using estrogen (see Chap. 78 for discussion of ERT). If the woman is not at risk for either endometrial cancer or breast cancer, a trial of estrogen is reasonable. Doses are the same as for ERT, and it may be used in combination with either donepezil or vitamin E. No data exist regarding its use in men, and it is not recommended at this time.

Anti-inflammatory Agents

A number of epidemiologic studies have shown either a lower incidence of AD or higher MMSE scores in AD if NSAIDs were taken on a regular basis. Indomethacin was studied in a small, double-blind pilot trial with positive results.[67] Although patients treated with indomethacin 100 to 150 mg/d did not appear to show cognitive decline during the 6-month trial, about one-third dropped out due to gastrointestinal (GI) side effects. The outcome measures in this study were poorly defined, and it is difficult to know whether these changes were clinically significant. In a 15-year longitudinal analysis, use of NSAIDs was found to be associated with a lower incidence of AD.[68] Patients with reported use of NSAIDs for greater than 2 years had a relative risk of AD of 0.4 as compared to a relative risk of 0.65 for those taking NSAIDs for less than 2 years.

Although these data are interesting and promising, NSAIDs have a significant incidence of adverse effects, particularly gastritis and the possibility of GI bleeds. Because of the absence of multicenter, controlled trials and the potential side effects, NSAIDs are not recommended for general use in the treatment of AD at the present time.

Ginkgo Biloba

Egb 761, an extract of ginkgo biloba, has been claimed to improve memory. Although it is thought to be an antioxidant and to affect inflammation and neuromodulation, the mechanisms of the multiple compounds in Egb 761 have not been elucidated. Its effects on cognition in uncomplicated dementia were evaluated in 309 patients in a double-blind, placebo-controlled trial of 52 weeks' duration.[69] The study population included patients with multi-infarct and mixed dementia as well as AD (236 patients with Alzheimer's). The dose of Egb 761 was 40 mg tid. Although Egb 761 showed statistically significant superiority over placebo, the differences were small, and only 29% of Egb-treated patients had a 4 point or greater improvement in their ADAS-Cog score. Furthermore, there was little worsening in the ADAS-Cog among the placebo group patients ($\overline{x}$ = 2.1) completing 52 weeks of treatment. The natural decline over 1 year would be an average of 7 points, indicating a significant placebo or nontreatment effect in the study. Egb was not different from placebo on the Clinical Global Impression of Change scale.

The ADAS-Cog differences in this trial are small, and even if the herbal extract is effective, there are significant problems with its use clinically. The content of herbal products is poorly standardized, and significant variation in supposed active ingredient content for some herbals has been shown from lot to lot and among manufacturers. Until these products are better standardized and their manufacturing and stability better assured, it is recommended that they be used with caution. Furthermore, little is known about potential adverse reactions or long-term toxicity with their use.

PHARMACOTHERAPY OF NONCOGNITIVE SYMPTOMS

The majority of patients with AD will manifest noncognitive symptoms at some point in the illness (see the clinical presentation discussion earlier in the chapter).[49,50] These symptoms can be roughly divided into three categories: psychotic symptoms, inappropriate or disruptive behavior, and depression. Effective management of these problems is important because behavioral symptoms are distressing to both the patient and the caregiver, necessitate increased caregiver supervision and patience, and are a leading reason for nursing home placement. In fact, presence of neuropsychiatric symptoms increases caregiver burden more than loss of cognition or self-care. Despite the widespread nature of noncognitive symptoms in AD, there has been surprisingly little formal research on psychotropic drug efficacy in these patients. Most treatment recommendations come from small trials, case reports, and clinical experience. Although information can be extrapolated from studies using psychotropic drugs for similar symptoms in nondemented patients, the widespread neuronal loss seen in AD and different underlying pathology suggest that this approach may not be valid. General guidelines governing therapy can be summarized as follows: Use reduced doses, monitor closely, and document carefully. Periodic attempts to reduce medication are also recommended, as symptoms change with disease progression. Many psychotropic medications have anticholinergic effects that may actually worsen cognition. These anticholinergic effects—as well as sedative effects, medication-induced postural instability, and extrapyramidal side effects—also decrease the clinical utility of many traditional psychotropic agents in this population. An outline of suggested doses of medications is provided in Table 61–8.

Prior to implementing pharmacotherapy for behavioral problems, it should be assured that persons caring for the patient have necessary information on how best to communicate and work with the patient. For example, overly technical or detailed directions may confuse and upset patients. Simple instructions or a demonstration of the desired activity is easier for the patient to understand. Caregivers with good intentions may also try to push patients to continue doing familiar tasks in the hope that this will preserve existing memory as long as possible. As the patient becomes increasingly unable to accomplish a task due to disease progression, he or she may easily become frustrated and upset. A simple change to a less demanding life-style may decrease agitated behaviors substantially. Family members may not realize at first the degree of impairment in the Alzheimer's patient's memory and ability to reason. The patient, for example, may accuse a family member of stealing an item that has been misplaced. The family member becomes upset at this accusation and attempts to rationalize or argue with the patient. This frequently causes agitated behavior to escalate. Although difficult, the caregiver may find that by ignoring accusations or changing the subject, the patient will calm down. Helpful resources for caregivers are provided in Table 61–6.

TABLE 61–8. Medications Used In Treating Noncognitive Symptoms of Dementia

Drugs	Suggested Dosage in Dementia (mg/d)	Indications
Antipsychotics		Psychosis (hallucinations, delusions, suspiciousness), disruptive behaviors (agitation, aggression)
Haloperidol	0.5–5	
Risperidone	0.5–2	
Thioridazine	10–100	
Antidepressants		Depression (poor appetite, insomnia, hopelessness, anhedonia, withdrawal, suicidal thoughts, agitation)
Citalopram	10–30	
Desipramine	50–150[a,b]	
Nortriptyline	25–150[a,b]	
Fluoxetine	5–20	
Sertraline	50–200	
Paroxetine	10–40	
Trazodone	75–400[a]	
Anticonvulsants		Disruptive behaviors, mood instability
Carbamazepine	100–1000[a,b]	
Valproic acid	1000–2500[a,b]	
Other Drugs		
Selegiline	10	Disruptive behaviors, agitation, anxiety, depression
Buspirone	10–45[a]	Disruptive behaviors
Oxazepam	10–60[a]	Disruptive behaviors

[a]Administer in divided doses.
[b]Dosage adjustment should be guided by drug serum concentrations.
Compiled from Refs. 54, 64, 65, 70, and 71.

Depression

Prevalence estimates of depression in AD differ widely, ranging from under 10% to 80%. Actual prevalence rates of major depression in AD are probably about 5% to 15% in community-based patients, and 15% to 20% in institutionalized patients.[70] The inconsistency in these figures is largely attributed to symptom overlap, diagnostic differences, and the patient population sampled. Early in the course of AD, depression presents much the same as in other elderly persons; later in the disease course, diagnosis can be difficult. Apathy, decreased initiative and socialization, decreased concentration, psychomotor retardation, agitation, and changes in appetite and sleep patterns are all symptoms intrinsic to both dementia and depression.[70,71] In determining whether or not a patient with these symptoms is also depressed, it is important to assess particularly the patient's affect and ability to experience pleasure. Affective signs of depression might include crying spells, asking to be killed, moaning, or sorrowful facial expression. An interview with the patient's caregiver can be helpful in obtaining a more accurate record of symptoms. Depression may be more common in the early stages of AD as the patient attempts to adjust to limitations associated with cognitive loss.

The bulk of literature examining antidepressant use in AD is made up of case reports and uncontrolled studies. Most of these report a favorable response to antidepressants.[71] The only available placebo-controlled study, an 8-week trial of imipramine versus placebo, showed significant response in both treatment groups but no advantage of imipramine over placebo.[72] The available literature also suggests that antidepressant response, as measured by reductions in Hamilton Depression Rating scores (HAM-D), is not as dramatic as in depressed nondemented patients. Because depressive target symptoms are difficult to distinguish from dementia, it is unclear whether this modest decrease in HAM-D scores is due to poor drug response or difficulty in assessing symptoms in this population.[71,72] Some clinicians have noted that a longer duration of treatment (e.g., up to 12 weeks) is required before elderly patients experience an antidepressant effect.

Based on the available literature, it would be desirable to document symptoms of depression for several weeks prior to initiating antidepressant therapy in a patient with AD. There appears to be a significant placebo response in this population, and it is possible that simply visiting with a clinician or increasing the patient's activity level may be sufficient to improve symptoms. Should this approach fail, a trial of an antidepressant could be initiated. Pharmacotherapy should be initiated with an antidepressant possessing a favorable side effect profile. Acceptable antidepressants in this population include secondary amine tricyclic antidepressants such as nortriptyline or desipramine, which have a lower incidence of anticholinergic and cardiovascular side effects than the tertiary amines; selective serotonin reuptake inhibitors (SSRIs) such as citalopram, fluoxetine, paroxetine, or sertraline; serotonin/norepinephrine reuptake inhibitors such as venlafaxine; or the triazolopyridines, nefazodone and trazodone.[73] Trazodone, the more sedating of the triazolopyridines, has been reported to decrease insomnia, agitation, and dysphoria in AD patients. Although lacking anticholinergic effects, trazodone tends to cause orthostasis, which may pose disadvantages over other available agents. A placebo-controlled trial of trazodone for agitation in AD is ongoing. Because of their low propensity to cause anticholinergic effects, orthostatic hypotension, and sedation, the SSRIs are often considered to be preferred antidepressants in this population. SSRIs can often be dosed once daily. These medications are not without risk, however. Gastrointestinal adverse effects, confusion, agitation, dizziness, and insomnia have been reported in patients with AD taking fluoxetine, especially at higher doses (> 20 mg of fluoxetine daily).[74] For a more complete discussion of treatment of depression, refer to Chapter 65.

Antipsychotics

Antipsychotic medications have traditionally been used to treat disruptive behaviors and psychosis in AD patients. Rationale for use of these medications is partly derived from their beneficial effects in treating psychosis in schizophrenia, even though the quality of these symptoms is quite different in AD.[50,71] Despite widespread use, available placebo-controlled studies suggest that antipsychotics are only moderately effective at best.[74–77] Symptoms responding include assaultiveness, extreme agitation and hyperexcitability, hallucinations, delusions, suspiciousness, hostility, and uncooperativeness.[74–77] Symptoms not responding include withdrawal, apathy, cognitive deficits, and incontinence.[71] Patients with AD are more sensitive to antipsychotic side effects than other patient groups. Particularly problematic side effects are extrapyramidal side effects, postural instability due to alpha-adrenergic blockade, and anticholinergic effects including increased confusion, urinary retention, constipation, and dry mouth.[71,73] These side effects and worsening cognition seriously limit the usefulness of these medications, especially when behavioral problems are minor. Effective doses of antipsychotic medications are much lower than those typically used to treat schizophrenia (see Table 61–8). For example, the suggested starting dose of haloperidol is 0.5 mg/d.

Increased sensitivity to antipsychotic side effects in the elderly appears to be the result of altered pharmacodynamics rather than altered pharmacokinetics.[71,73] Pharmacotherapy with antipsychotics should be guided by several key concepts. First, if the delusions or behaviors are not particularly disturbing to the patient or caregiver, they may not require treatment. Second, many caregivers have erroneous expectations regarding the effects of these medications, and it should be assured that the anticipated benefits and risks of therapy are understood. Third, disruptive behaviors and delusions wax and wane with disease progression. Attempts to taper and discontinue antipsychotic medication should be undertaken at least every 3 months, because many patients who initially respond to these medications show no change in symptoms and occasionally improve on medication withdrawal.[70]

There is no convincing evidence that one antipsychotic is more efficacious than another. Traditionally, haloperidol and thioridazine have been the most commonly used agents, and they represent opposite ends of the side effect spectrum for typical antipsychotics. More recently, risperidone has begun to be used both in clinical trials and practice.[54] In a double-blind, placebo controlled trial, risperidone 1 and 2 mg was shown to decrease paranoid delusional ideation and aggressiveness on the Behave-AD.[78] However, only risperidone 2 mg daily decreased the total Behave-AD score by more than 30%. It should also be noted that although risperidone demonstrated statistically significant efficacy in this study, there was a high placebo response rate (52%). Side effects, particularly extrapyramidal side effects and somnolence, increased with increased dose, being most prominent with risperidone 2 mg daily. Balancing efficacy with adverse effects, it is recommended to begin with 0.25 mg daily and increase to 1 mg daily if needed, titrating to 2 mg only if the patient is not responding and is tolerating the medication.

Miscellaneous Therapies

Because antipsychotic therapy has shown only modest efficacy and poses a substantial risk of undesirable side effects, medications traditionally used to treat disruptive behaviors and aggression in other psychiatric and neurologic disorders have been suggested as potential alternatives. These include benzodiazepines, buspirone, lithium, carbamazepine, selegiline, valproate, and fluoxetine. Unfortunately, few of these agents have been studied in a controlled fashion in patients with AD. Doses of selected medications are listed in Table 61–8. Benzodiazepines, particularly oxazepam, have been used to treat anxiety, agitation, and aggression, but generally show inferior efficacy when compared to antipsychotics. Because benzodiazepines impair cognition, can result in disinhibition, and may increase the risk of falls in AD patients, their routine use is not advised.[54,71] Conversely, the 5-HT_{1A} partial agonist, buspirone, has shown benefit in treating agitation and aggression in a limited number of patients with minimal adverse effects.[79,80] Selegiline has been shown to decrease anxiety, depression, and agitation in open-label and controlled studies.[64,81,82] Although a longer-term double-blind study using selegiline in mildly demented patients showed no benefit, the more typical patient with AD (greater disease severity) may be more likely to respond.[65] Should antipsychotics fail to manage noncognitive behaviors, a trial of buspirone or selegiline might be reasonable alternatives. Although there is only minimal documentation to support use of the mood stabilizers carbamazepine or valproate, a careful trial is reasonable in patients with treatment-resistant behavioral disturbances. Lithium has shown no benefit and frequent toxicity.[54,71] Clearly, more rigorous placebo-controlled studies would assist in determining the place in therapy, and relative efficacy, of these alternative medications.

PHARMACOECONOMIC CONSIDERATIONS

The cost of caring for an individual with AD is significant, not only from the perspective of dollars expended but also from the viewpoint of uncompensated hours spent in caring for the patient and the effects of the illness on quality of life of both the patient and caregiver. Considering both formal and informal costs, Rice and colleagues estimated that the annual costs for caring for an Alzheimer's patient were $47,000, regardless of whether the person was living at home or in a nursing home.[5]

Few attempts have been made to evaluate the pharmacoeconomics of available medications in Alzheimer's disease. Knopman and associates, in a follow-up of patients completing the 30 week pivotal trial, examined the effects of tacrine on nursing home placement.[83] In their logistic regression analysis, patients receiving greater than 80 mg tacrine daily were less likely to enter a nursing home. However, these data must be interpreted with caution. Due to the high tacrine dropout rate due to adverse effects, the lower institutionalization rate could be secondary to a self-selected healthier patient population that was able to tolerate tacrine. Lubeck and coworkers modeled data from the 30-week trial to predict costs over the course of the illness.[84] They estimated average annual cost savings with tacrine treatment to be $2243 for patients taking 80 to 160 mg daily and $4052 for patients taking 160 mg/d. These formal costs were primarily saved by a projected delay in the time to nursing home placement. A major flaw in this study is an assumption in their model that the patient decline over the course of the illness would be the same as projected from the 30-week study. Unfortunately, the effects of tacrine over the course of the illness are unknown.

The effects of cholinesterase inhibitor therapy on caregiver time was assessed as part of an efficacy trial evaluating the effects of velnacrine (1-hydroxytacrine) in AD.[85] Based upon caregiver report after 24 weeks of treatment, high-dose velnacrine (225 mg/d) reduced unpaid caregiver time by an average of 2.6 hours/d as compared with the placebo group. The primary time savings were reported to be in time spent supervising the patient, and in time bathing the patient. Whether these findings can be extrapolated to other cholinesterase inhibitors is unclear.

As additional treatments for AD are introduced into clinical practice, it is important to perform pharmacoeconomic evaluations of their use. Not only is this important from the perspective of drug efficacy and total formal costs associated with the disease, but also from the perspective of informal, uncompensated costs for the caregiver and quality of life for both the patient and caregiver.

EVALUATION OF THERAPEUTIC OUTCOMES

An evaluation of therapeutic outcomes in the patient with AD begins with a thorough assessment at baseline and a clear definition of therapeutic goals. Cognitive status, physical status, functional performance, mood, thought processes, and behavior all need to be evaluated before initiation of drug therapy. The clinician should interview both the patient and the caregiver to assess the patient's response to the drug. Because caregivers often have difficulty giving honest and frank information about their loved one's condition in his or her presence, it is often necessary to interview family caregivers separately. In evaluating response to cognitive agents, the clinician should ask questions about the patient's ability to perform daily functional tasks and about mood and behavior as well as questions about memory and orientation. Objective assessments, such as the MMSE for cognition and the Functional Activities Questionnaire for activities of daily living, should be used to quantify changes in symptoms and function.[52]

Because target symptoms of psychiatric disorders may respond differently in demented patients, a detailed list of symptoms to be treated should be documented in the pharmaceutical care plan to aid in monitoring. These could include, for example, "striking at spouse because patient believes spouse is an impostor," "verbal threats and refusal to allow clothes to be changed," and so on, as opposed to documenting vague symptoms such as "aggression" or "delusions." To make an accurate assessment of depression, multiple symptoms—including sleep, appetite, and activity and interest levels—need to be assessed in addition to the patient's stated mood.

The patient should be observed carefully for potential side effects of drug therapy. Depending on the therapeutic agent being employed, patients should be assessed for potential side effects such as diarrhea, GI distress, dizziness, sedation, extrapyramidal side effects, or worsening of behavior. The specific side effects to be monitored and the method and frequency of monitoring should be documented. Periodic assessments for drug efficacy, compliance, need for dosage adjustment, or change in treatment should occur at least monthly. However, patients need to be treated for an adequate duration to see a therapeutic effect from a given intervention. Because the effects of cognition-enhancing medications are not great, a treatment period of several months may be necessary before it can be determined whether therapy is beneficial. Cognitive effects of the drug are often noticed only as a plateauing during treatment or a deterioration following drug discontinuation. In general, cognitive agents (e.g., donepezil) should be continued if the patient is demonstrating no change in clinical status. However, if there is doubt, the medication can be tapered and discontinued, and the patient monitored off the drug for 4 to 6 weeks to determine the need for continued therapy.

CONCLUSIONS

Significant advances have been made in our knowledge of the pathophysiology of AD. However, much additional study will be required to allow for development of therapies that will "cure" or arrest progression of the disease. Cholinesterase inhibitors are now available that have modest effects on cognition and a favorable side effect profile. Other medications (e.g., vitamin E and estrogen) that may affect disease progression are also being evaluated. However, the long-term practical benefits of these medications and their effects on function are still unclear. Because these medications are not a panacea, the clinician must carefully screen the patient for appropriateness of treatment, and the family should be active participants in treatment decisions. Families should be educated about AD, appropriate nondrug interventions, available pharmacotherapeutic options, their potential side effects, and the realistic expectations they should have regarding response.

Behavioral and psychiatric manifestations of AD can add significantly to the morbidity of the disease. Carefully chosen psychotropic drugs in combination with consistent behavioral and environmental interventions can often be effective in ameliorating these symptoms.

As new findings become available to unravel the Alzheimer's puzzle, more and more treatments will become available to treat symptoms and hopefully to slow or halt progression of the disease. In future editions, perhaps we will even have the opportunity to discuss genetic treatments that prevent onset of this devastating illness.

▶ PRINCIPLES OF PHARMACOTHERAPY

- A thorough patient evaluation to determine the cause of dementia and rule out other disorders should occur before considering drug therapy.
- The etiology of AD is as yet unknown, and pharmacotherapy neither cures nor arrests the pathophysiology.
- Nondrug therapy and social support for the patient and family are the primary treatment interventions for AD.
- Thorough family and caregiver education should occur regarding the disease prognosis and limitations of treatments. Appropriate referral to social and legal support services should be made.
- Pharmacotherapy is primarily oriented toward treating symptoms and decreasing the rate of cognitive decline.
- A thorough baseline assessment, using rating scales, should be performed before initiating drug therapy for cognitive or behavioral symptoms.
- Slow medication dosage titration with careful monitoring should occur to minimize the incidence of severe adverse drug reactions.
- A thorough behavioral assessment and plan with careful examination of environmental factors should be conducted before initiating drug therapy for behavioral symptoms.
- Pharmacotherapy for behavioral symptoms should be self-limited, and medication tapering and discontinuation attempted in patients with stable symptoms.

REFERENCES

1. Eggert A, Crismon ML. Current concepts in understanding Alzheimer's disease. Clin Pharm Newswatch 1994;1:1–8.
2. Diagnostic and Statistical Manual for Mental Disorders, 4th ed. Washington, DC, American Psychiatric Association, 1994:123–174.
3. Rocca WA, Amaducci LA, Schoenberg BS. Epidemiology of clinically diagnosed Alzheimer's disease. Ann Neurol 1986;19:415–24.
4. Evans DA, Funkenstein HH, Albert MS, et al. Prevalence of Alzheimer's disease in a community population of older persons: Higher than previously reported. JAMA 1989;262: 2551–2552.
5. Rice DP, Fox PJ, Max W, et al. Datawatch: The economic burden of Alzheimer's disease care. Health Affairs 1993;12:164–176.
6. Evans DA. Estimated prevalence of Alzheimer's disease in the United States. The Milbank Q 1990;68:267–289.
7. Hebert LE, Scherr PA, Beckett LA, et al. Age specific incidence of Alzheimer's disease in a community population. JAMA 1995;273: 1354–1359.
8. The Alzheimer's Disease and Related Disorders Association. Statistical Data on Alzheimer's Disease. Chicago, ADRDA, 1992.
9. Chandra V, Bharucha NE, Schoenberg BS. Conditions associated with Alzheimer's disease at death: Case-control study. Neurology 1986;36: 209–211.
10. Evans DA, Smith LA, Scherr PA, et al. Risk of death from Alzheimer's disease in a community population of older persons. Am J Epidemiol 1991;134:403–412.
11. Ernst RL, Hay JW. The US economic and social costs of Alzheimer's disease revisited. Am J Pub Health. 1994;84:1261–1264.
12. U.S. Bureau of the Census. Current Population Reports, Special Studies, P23-190, 65+ in the United States. Washington, DC, U.S. Government Printing Office, 1996.
13. Cordell B. B-amyloid formation as a potential therapeutic target for Alzheimer's disease. Annu Rev Pharmacol Toxicol 1994;34:69–89.
14. Yankner BA, Mesulam MM. β-amyloid and the pathogenesis of Alzheimer's disease. N Engl J Med 1991;325:1849–1857.
15. Travis J. New piece in Alzheimer's puzzle. Science 1993;261:828–829.
16. Mortimer JA. Is Alzheimer's disease a lifelong illness? Risk factors for pathological and clinical disease. In: Heston LL, ed. Progress in Alzheimer's Disease and Similar Conditions. Washington, DC, American Psychiatric Press, 1997:9–20.
17. National Institute on Aging. Progress Report on Alzheimer's Disease. Rockville, MD: U.S. Government Printing Office, 1996. NIH pub. no. 96-4137.
18. Mandelkow EM, Schweers O, Drewes G, et al. Structure, microtubule interactions, and phosphorylation of tau protein. Ann NY Acad Sci 1996;777:96–106.
19. Selkoe D. Amyloid protein and Alzheimer's disease. Sci Am 1991; 265:68.
20. Goldman J, Cote L. Aging of the brain: Dementia of the Alzheimer's type. In: Kandel ER, Scwartz JH, Jessell TM, eds. Principles of Neural Science, 3rd ed. New York, Elsevier, 1991:974–983.
21. Mirra SS. Alzheimer's disease and other dementias: Neuropathological considerations. In: Heston LL, ed. Progress in Alzheimer's Disease and Similar Conditions. Washington, DC, American Psychiatric Press, 1997:21–34.
22. Shoji M, Golde TE, Ghiso J, et al. Production of the Alzheimer amyloid β protein by normal proteolytic processing. Science 1992;258: 126–129.
23. Esch FS, Keim PS, Beattie EC, et al. Cleavage of amyloid β-peptide during constitutive processing of its precursor. Science 1990;248: 1122–1124.
24. Quon D, Wang Y, Catalino R, et al. Formation of β-amyloid deposits in brains of transgenic mice. Nature 1991;357:239–241.
25. Pike CJ, Walencewicz AJ, Glabe CG, Cotman CW. Aggregation-related toxicity of synthetic β-amyloid protein in hippocampal cultures. Eur J Pharmacol 1991;207:367–368.

26. Goodman Y, Bruce AJ, Cheng B, Mattson MP. Estrogens attenuate and corticosterone exacerbates excitotoxicity, oxidative injury, and amyloid B-peptide toxicity in hippocampal neurons. J Neurochem 1996;66:1836–1844.
27. Rosenberg RN. A causal role for amyloid in Alzheimer's disease: The end of the beginning. Neurology 1993;43:851–856.
28. Blass JP, Poirier J. Pathophysiology of the Alzheimer syndrome. In: Gauthier S, ed. Clinical Diagnosis and Management of Alzheimer's Disease. Boston, Butterworth-Heinemann, 1996:17–31.
29. Travis J. New piece in Alzheimer's puzzle. Science 1993;261: 828–829.
30. Tang MX, Maestre G, Tsai WY, et al. Effect of age, ethnicity, and head injury on the association between Apo E genotypes and Alzheimer's disease. Ann NY Acad Sci 1996;802:7–15.
31. Corder EH, Saunders AM, Strittmatter WJ, et al. Gene dose of apolipoprotein type 4 allele and the risk of Alzheimer's disease in late onset families. Science 1993;261:921–923.
32. Talbot C, Lendon C, Craddock N, et al. Protection against Alzheimer's disease with Apo E_2. Lancet 1994;343:1432–1433.
33. Corder EH, Saunders AM, Risch NJ, et al. Protective effect of apolipoprotein E type 2 allele for late-onset Alzheimer's disease. Nat Genet 1994;7:180–184.
34. Aisen PS, Davis KL. Inflammatory mechanisms in Alzheimer's disease: Implications for therapy. Am J Psychiatry 1994;151:1105–1113.
35. Blass JP. Pathophysiology of the Alzheimer's syndrome. Neurology 1993;43(suppl 4):S25–S38.
36. Schneider LS. Clinical pharmacology of aminoacridines in Alzheimer's disease. Neurology 1993;43(suppl 4):S64–S79.
37. Piccini GL, Finali G, Piccirilli M. Neuropsychological effects of L-deprenyl in Alzheimer's type dementia. Clin Neuropharmacol 1990:13:147–163.
38. Francis PT, Sims NR, Procter AW, Bowen DM. Cortical pyramidal neuron loss may cause glutamatergic hypoactivity and cognitive impairment in Alzheimer's disease: Investigative and therapeutic perspectives. J Neurochem 1993;60:1589–1604.
39. Pomara N, Singh R, Deptula D, et al. Glutamate and other CSF amino acids in Alzheimer's disease. Am J Psychiatry 1992;149:251–254.
40. Choi WD. Glutamate neurotoxicity and diseases of the nervous system. Neuron 1988;1:623–634.
41. Jaffe AB, Toran-Allerand CD, Greengard P, Gandy SE. Estrogen regulates metabolism of Alzheimer amyloid B precursor protein. J Biol Chem 1994;269:13065–13068.
42. Simpkins JW, Singh M, Bishop J. The potential role for estrogen replacement therapy in the treatment of the cognitive decline and neurodegeneration associated with Alzheimer's disease. Neurobiol Aging 1994;15:S195–S197.
43. Wickelgren I. Estrogen stakes claim to cognition. Science 1997;276: 675–678.
44. Tang MX, Jacobs D, Stern Y, et al. Effect of estrogen during menopause on risk and age at onset of Alzheimer's disease. Lancet 1996; 348:429–432.
45. Rocca WA, Amaducci LA, Schoenberg BS. Epidemiology of clinically diagnosed Alzheimer's disease. Ann Neurol 1986;19:415–424.
46. Hamdy RC Aluminum toxicity and Alzheimer's disease. Is there a connection? Postgrad Med 1990;88:239–240.
47. Bush AI, Pettingell WH, Multhaup G, et al. Rapid induction of Alzheimer Aβ amyloid formation by zinc. Science 1994;265: 1464–1467.
48. McKhann G, Drachman D, Folstein M, et al. Clinical diagnosis of Alzheimer's disease. Neurology 1984;34:939–944.
49. Mohs RC. Neuropsychological assessment of patients with Alzheimer's disease. In: Bloom FE, Kupfer DJ, eds. Psychopharmacology: The Fourth Generation of Progress. New York, Raven, 1995: 1377–1388.
50. Raskind MA. Geriatric psychopharmacology: Management of late-life depression and the noncognitive behavioral disturbances of Alzheimer's disease. Psychiatry Clin North Am 1993;16:815–827.
51. McKhann G, Drachman D, Folstein M, et al. Clinical diagnosis of Alzheimer's disease: Report of the NINCDS-ADRDA work group under the auspices of the department of health and human services task force on Alzheimer's disease. Neurology 1984;34:939–944.
52. Costa PT Jr., Williams TF, Somerfield M, et al. Recognition and Initial Assessment of Alzheimer's Disease and Related Dementias. Clinical practice guideline no. 19. Rockville, MD, U.S. Department of Health and Human Services, Public Health Service, Agency for Health Care Policy and Research, 1996. AHCPR no. 97-0702.
53. Folstein MF, Folstein SE, McHugh PR. Mini mental state: A practical method for grading the cognitive state of patients for the clinician. J Psychiatr Res 1975;12:189–198.
54. Rabins P, Blacker D, Bland W, and the work group on Alzheimer's disease and related dementias. Practice guideline for the treatment of patients with Alzheimer's disease and other dementias of late life. Am J Psychiatry 1997;154(suppl 5):1–39.
55. Geldmacher DS, Whitehouse PJ. Differential diagnosis of Alzheimer's disease. Neurology 1997;48(suppl 6):S2–S9.
56. Reisberg B, Ferris SH, DeLeon MJ, Crook T. The global deterioration scale for assessment of primary degenerative dementia. Am J Psychiatry 1982;139:1136–1139.
57. Cognex expanded access proposed by FDA as part of "program of further study"; Warner-Lambert will support NDA studies with other data by April 1. FDC Rep, March 25, 1991, 4–9.
58. Knopman DS, Knapp MJ, Gracon SI, Davis CS. The clinical interview-based impression (CIBI): A clinician's global change rating scale in Alzheimer's disease. Neurology 1994;44:2315–2321.
59. Crismon ML. Tacrine: First drug approved for Alzheimer's disease. Ann Pharmacother 1994;28:744–751.
60. Sano M, Ernesto C, Thomas RG, et al. A controlled trial of selegiline, alpha- tocopherol, or both as treatment for Alzheimer's disease. N Engl J Med 1997;336:1216–1222.
61. Roerig Division of Pfizer. Aricept (donepezil hydrochloride tablets) package insert. New York, 1996.
62. Rogers SL, Friedhoff LT, donepezil study group. The efficacy and safety of donepezil in patients with Alzheimer's disease: Results of a U.S. multicentre, randomized, double-blind, placebo-controlled trial. Dementia 1996;7:293–303.
63. Crismon ML. Pharmacokinetics and drug interactions of cholinesterase inhibitors used in Alzheimer's disease. Pharmacotherapy 1998;18(2 Pt 2):475–545.
64. Burke WJ, Roccaforte WH, Wengel SP, et al. L-Deprenyl in the treatment of mild dementia of the Alzheimer type: Results of a 15-month trial. J Am Geriatr Soc 1993;41:1219–1225.
65. Schneider LS, Tariot PN. Emerging drugs for Alzheimer's disease: Mechanisms of action and prospects for cognitive enhancing medications. Med Clin North Am 1994;78:911–934.
66. Schneider LS, Farlow MR, Henderson VW, Pogoda JM. Effects of estrogen replacement therapy on response to tacrine in patients with Alzheimer's disease. Neurology 1996;46:1580–1584.
67. Rogers J, Kirby LC, Hempelman SR, et al. Clinical trial of indomethacin in Alzheimer's disease. Neurology 1993;43:1609–1611.
68. Stewart WF, Kawas C, Corrada M. Risk of Alzheimer's disease and duration of NSAID use. Neurology 1997;48:626–632.
69. Le Bars PL, Katz MM, Berman N, et al. A placebo-controlled, double-blind, randomized trial of an extract of ginkgo bilboa for dementia. JAMA 1997;278:1327–1332.
70. Borson S, Raskind MA. Clinical features and pharmacologic treatment of behavioral symptoms of Alzheimer's disease. Neurology 1997;48:S17–S24.
71. Raskind MA. Alzheimer's disease: Treatment of noncognitive behavioral abnormalities. In: Bloom FE, Kupfer DJ, eds. Psychopharmacology: The Fourth Generation of Progress. New York, Raven, 1995: 1427–1435.
72. Reifler BV, Raskind MA, Veith R, et al. Double-blind trial of imipramine in Alzheimer's disease patients with and without depression. Am J Psychiatry 1989;146:45–249.

73. Crismon ML. Psychotropic drugs in the elderly: Principles of use. Am Pharm 1990;NS30:57–63.
74. Geldmacher DS, Waldman AJ, Doty L, Heilman KM. Fluoxetine in dementia of the Alzheimer's type: Prominent adverse effects and failure to improve cognition. J Clin Psychiatry 1994;55:161.
75. Devanand DP, Sackeim HA, Brown RP, Mayeux R. A pilot study of haloperidol treatment of psychosis and behavioral disturbance in Alzheimer's disease. Arch Neurol 1989;46:854–857.
76. Petrie WM, Ban TA, Berney S, et al. Loxapine in psychogeriatrics: A placebo and standard-controlled clinical investigation. J Clin Psychopharmacol 1982;2:122–126.
77. Schneider LS, Pollock VE, Lyness SA. A meta-analysis of controlled trials of neuroleptic treatment in dementia. J Am Geriatr Soc 1990;38:553–563.
78. Brecher M, Clyde C, risperidone study group. Risperidone in the treatment of psychosis and aggressive behavior in patients with dementia. Eighth congress of the International Psychogeriatric Association, Jerusalem, August, 1997.
79. Sakuye KM, Camp CJ, Ford PA. Effects of buspirone on agitation associated with dementia. Am J Geriatr Psychiatry 1993;1:82–84.
80. Hermann N, Eryavec G. Buspirone in the management of agitation and aggression associated with dementia. Am J Geriatr Psychiatry 1993;1:249–253.
81. Tariot PN, Cohen RM, Sunderland T, et al. L-Deprenyl in Alzheimer's disease. Arch Gen Psychiatry 1987;44:427–433.
82. Schneider LS, Pollock VE, Zemansky MF, et al. A pilot study of low-dose L-deprenyl in Alzheimer's disease. J Geriatr Psychiatry Neurol 1991;4:143–148.
83. Knopman D, Schneider L, Davis K, et al. Long-term tacrine (Cognex) treatment: Effects on nursing home placement and mortality. Neurology 1996;47:166–177.
84. Lubeck DP, Mazonson PD, Bowe T. Potential effect of tacrine on expenditures for Alzheimer's disease. Med Interface 1994;7:130–138.
85. Clipp EC. Moore MJ. Caregiver time use: An outcome measure in clinical trial research on Alzheimer's disease. Clin Pharmacol Ther 1995;58:228–236.
86 Geldmacher DS, Whitehouse PJ. Evaluation of dementia. N Engl J Med 1996;335:330–336.
87. Parke Davis Division of Warner-Lambert. Cognex (tacrine hydrochloride tablets) package insert. Morris Plains, NJ, April 1995.

62

SUBSTANCE-RELATED DISORDERS: OVERVIEW AND DEPRESSANTS, STIMULANTS, AND HALLUCINOGENS

Paul L. Doering, MS

Abuse of alcohol, tobacco, and other drugs (ATOD) is the nation's number one health problem, according to a recent Robert Wood Johnson (RWJ) health care report prepared by the Institute for Health Policy, Brandeis University.[1] Of the \$238 billion the nation spends each year on ATOD abuse, \$34 billion is spent on health care that would otherwise be unnecessary. A heavy smoker will stay 25% longer when hospitalized than a nonsmoker; a problem drinker four times as long as a nondrinker. According to RWJ, "Without a reduction in ATOD abuse, health care costs cannot be curtailed effectively." Each year, there are more deaths and disabilities from ATOD abuse than from any other preventable cause. Of the two million deaths each year in the United States, one in four is attributable to alcohol, illicit drug, or tobacco use: 100,000 people die as a result of alcohol, 19,000 from illicit drug use and related AIDS deaths, and 400,000 from tobacco-related illness.

RWJ also reports a direct link to crime and arrests, with one-half to two-thirds of homicides and serious crimes involving alcohol. Nearly one-half of men arrested for homicide and assault actually test positive for an illegal drug. ATOD abuse contributes to family problems, with one in four Americans reporting that alcohol has been a cause of trouble in the family and alcohol abuse playing a part in one of three failed marriages.[1]

This and the next chapter focus on the problems associated with the abuse of chemical substances and the things clinicians can do to help deal with these problems.

TERMINOLOGY

The lack of a common vocabulary in substance abuse treatment and prevention leads to several problems. There is a large array of terms in common use, many without precise meaning. A variety of professional disciplines are involved in research, treatment, and education regarding alcohol and other drug-related problems, and each discipline tends to use its own terminology. This lack of precise definitions and universal agreement on language hampers effective communication among professionals,[2] and leads to difficulties in formulating public policy and administering third-party reimbursement programs.

To remedy this situation, the American Medical Association's Council on Scientific Affairs, Panels on Alcoholism and Drug Abuse recommended a task force be established to develop standard definitions. Representatives from 23 professional organizations used a four-stage Delphi survey of substance abuse experts to help achieve greater clarity and uniformity in terminology associated with alcohol and other drug-related problems. Their efforts resulted in a list of 50 most important substance abuse terms and their definitions.[3] The following are a few of the terms agreed upon by the panel:

- *Abstinence.* Cessation of use of a psychoactive substance previously abused, or on which the user has developed drug dependence.
- *Abuse potential.* The property of a substance that, by its physiologic or psychological effects, or both, increases the likelihood of an individual's abusing or becoming dependent on the substance.
- *(Drug) addiction.* A chronic disorder characterized by the compulsive use of a substance resulting in physical, psychological, or social harm to the user and continued use despite that harm.
- *Alcohol abuse.* Use of ethyl alcohol in a quantity and with a frequency that causes the individual significant physiologic, psychological, or sociologic distress or impairment.
- *Alcohol dependence.* Chronic loss of control over the consumption of alcoholic beverages, despite obvious psychological or physical harm to the person. Increasing amounts are required over time, and abrupt discontinuance may precipitate a withdrawal syndrome. Following abstinence, relapse is frequent.
- *Alcoholism.* A chronic, progressive, and potentially fatal biogenetic and psychosocial disease characterized by tolerance and physical dependence manifested by a loss of control, as well as diverse personality changes and social consequences.
- *(Drug) dependence.* A generic term that relates to physical or psychological dependence, or both. It is characteristic for each pharmacologic class of psychoactive drugs. Impaired control over drug-taking behavior is implied.

- *Drug abuse.* Any use of drugs that causes physical, psychological, economic, legal, or social harm to the individual user or to others affected by the drug user's behavior.
- *Drug misuse.* Any use of a drug that varies from a socially or medically accepted use.
- *Physical dependence.* A physiologic state of adaptation to a drug or alcohol, usually characterized by the development of tolerance to drug effects and the emergence of a withdrawal syndrome during prolonged abstinence.
- *Psychological dependence.* The emotional state of craving a drug either for its positive effect or to avoid negative effects associated with its absence.
- *Substance abuse.* The use of a psychoactive substance in a manner detrimental to the individual or society but not meeting criteria for substance or drug dependence.
- *Tolerance.* Physiologic adaptation to the effect of drugs, so as to diminish effects with constant dosages or to maintain the intensity and duration of effects through increased dosage.
- *Withdrawal syndrome.* The onset of a predictable constellation of signs and symptoms involving alerted activity of the central nervous system after the abrupt discontinuation of, or rapid decrease in, dosage of a drug.

EPIDEMIOLOGY

NATIONAL HOUSEHOLD SURVEY ON DRUG ABUSE

The National Household Survey on Drug Abuse[4] is the primary source of statistical information on the use of illegal drugs by the United States population. Conducted by the Federal Government since 1971, the survey collects data from a representative sample of the population at their place of residence. Since October 1992 the survey has been supported and directed by the Substance Abuse and Mental Health Services Administration (SAMHSA).

At the time of this writing the most recent data available from the Household Survey are from 1996. These data show that an estimated 13.0 million Americans were current illicit drug users (i.e., they had used an illicit drug in the month prior to interview). This represents 6.1% of the population 12 years old and older. Marijuana is the most commonly used illicit drug, used by 77% of current illicit drug users. About 46% of current illicit drug users in 1996 (an estimated 5.8 million Americans) were current users of illicit drugs other than marijuana and hashish.[4]

The overall use of illicit drugs among Americans of all ages remained unchanged from 1993 to 1996, but illicit drug use among teens 12 to 17 years old declined for the first time since 1992. The number of illicit drug users was at its highest level in 1979 (25.4 million, 14.1%); declined until 1992 (12.0 million, 5.8%); and remained at approximately the same level through 1996.[4]

Half of young adults age 21 to 25 had tried illicit drugs at least once in their lifetime, and 13% were current users. As in prior years, men continued to have a higher rate of current illicit drug use than women (8.1% versus 4.2%) in 1996. Among young adults aged 18 to 34 years in 1996, those who had not completed high school had the highest rate of use (16.8%), while college graduates had the lowest rate of use (6.9%).[4]

THE MONITORING THE FUTURE STUDY

Every year the Institute for Social Research of the University of Michigan conducts its Monitoring the Future Study (MTFS), supported under a series of research grants from the National Institute on Drug Abuse.[5] The project has many purposes. Among them is to study changes in the beliefs, attitudes, and behavior of young people in the United States. This study focuses on youth because of their significant involvement in today's social changes and, most important, because youth in a very literal sense will constitute our future society.[5]

In 1997, approximately 51,000 8th, 10th, and 12th grade students in 429 public and private secondary schools were surveyed. After years of dramatic increases, illicit drug use among 8th graders remained stable for most drugs from 1996 to 1997, and decreased slightly for marijuana, cigarettes, and certain other substances. Daily marijuana use among seniors increased from 4.9% in 1996 to 5.8% in 1997. Marijuana use is still not up to the peak levels reached in the late 1970s (in 1978, nearly 11% were active daily users). Findings regarding other drugs in the 1997 MTFS are summarized as follows:

Cocaine. Rates of cocaine use remained level for 8th and 10th grade students. The percentage of seniors who had used cocaine at least once increased from 7.1% in 1996 to 8.7% in 1997, the highest rates reported since 1990.

Heroin. Past-year use of heroin among 8th graders decreased from 1.6% in 1996 to 1.3% in 1997. In 1997, 2.1% of 8th, 10th, and 12th graders reported having used heroin at least once in their lifetime.

Stimulants. There was no change in the percentage of 8th, 10th, or 12th graders who had tried stimulants at least once. In 1997, 12.3% of 8th graders, 17.0% of 10th graders, and 16.5% of 12th graders used stimulants at least once in their lifetime.

Cigarettes. The percentage of 8th graders reporting heavy cigarette smoking decreased between 1996 and 1997. Daily smoking in the past 30 days decreased from 10.4% to 9.0%, and 8th graders smoking a half pack or more cigarettes per day decreased from 4.3% to 3.5%. Daily cigarette use among seniors increased to 24.6%, its highest level since 1979.

Alcohol. Although rates remained mostly stable, alcohol use remains a problem among adolescents. On the positive side, the percentage of 8th graders reporting having been drunk in the past 30 days decreased from 9.6% in 1996 to 8.2% in 1997. Among 12th graders, past-year use of alcohol increased from 72.5% in 1996 to 74.8% in 1997.

TRENDS IN SUBSTANCE ABUSE EMERGENCIES: THE DAWN PROGRAM

Since the early 1970s, the Drug Abuse Warning Network (DAWN),[6] an ongoing national survey of hospital emergency departments, has collected information on patients seeking hospital emergency department treatment related to their use of an illegal drug or the nonmedical use of a legal drug. The survey provides data that describe the impact of drug use on hospital emergency departments in the United States. More importantly, it serves as an early-warning system to the ever-changing patterns of use of illegal drugs. These data allow health care professionals to be better prepared to react to medical emergencies arising from illegal drug use and to target prevention and education programs to specific drug groups or populations.

Preliminary estimates from the 1996 DAWN survey showed a decline nationally in drug-related emergency room cases from 1995 to 1996 (from 517,800 to 487,600). The number of cases had been steadily increasing from 1990 through 1994, and remained level in 1995.

Cocaine-related episodes remained level between 1994 and 1996 after increasing 78% between 1990 and 1994. Overall, there were 138,000 cocaine episodes reported in 1995 and 144,200 in 1996; this difference was not statistically significant.

Although heroin-related episodes increased steadily since the early 1980s, there was no significant change in the number of heroin-related episodes reported from 1995 (72,200) to 1996 (70,500). However, between 1990 and 1996 there was a 108% increase (from 33,900 to 70,500).

There was a statistically significant *decrease* in methamphetamine-related episodes reported between 1995 (16,200) and 1996 (10,800). However, there was a significant *increase* of 71% between the first half of 1996 and the second half of 1996 (from 4000 to 6800). Reports by local area epidemiologists indicate there was a shortage of methamphetamine in many cities in the western United States in the last half of 1995 and first quarter of 1996.

Marijuana/hashish-related episodes were statistically unchanged in the one-year period between 1995 and 1996, but the trend since 1990 suggests that increases continue. Marijuana/hashish-related episodes rose from 40,200 in 1994 to 50,000 in 1996, a 25% increase. Since 1990, marijuana/hashish-related episodes have increased 219%.

ECONOMIC IMPACT OF SUBSTANCE ABUSE

Substance abuse and addiction have an enormous impact on the economy. In a 1996 study, the Center on Addiction and Substance Abuse (CASA) at Columbia University found that 21 cents out of every tax dollar paid to the City of New York was attributable to substance abuse and addiction.[7] Additionally, in 1994, substance abuse and addiction cost New York City more than $20 billion. Of that $20 billion, less than 4% ($735 million) went toward the actual treatment of substance abuse and addiction and only 0.4% ($80 million) was spent on ways to prevent it. The other $19.2 billion paid for the consequences of the problem.[7]

Another CASA study showed that the total impact of substance abuse on Federal entitlement programs (e.g., Medicare, Medicaid, Veterans Administration, federal employee and other health programs, SSDI, AFDC, food stamps, SSI, and unemployment compensation) can be conservatively estimated to be $77.6 billion. Of that amount, $66.4 billion represents costs directly attributed to substance abuse.[8] The public assistance expenditure for recipients whose substance abuse or addiction must be addressed before they become self-sufficient amounts to $11.2 billion. Although 92% of substance abuse-related health entitlement costs is spent to treat the consequences of tobacco, alcohol, and drug abuse, only 8% is spent to treat alcohol, drug, or tobacco dependence.[8]

CASA has also examined the cost of substance abuse and addiction to our Medicaid[9] and Medicare[10] programs. Nearly 1 out of every 5 dollars ($7.4 billion out of $41 billion) spent by Medicaid in 1994 on inpatient services, and more than 1 out of every 4 dollars ($20 billion out of $87 billion) spent by Medicare during the same period on inpatient hospital care, was attributable to drug, alcohol, and tobacco abuse and addiction. One out of every five Medicaid hospital days is attributable to substance abuse. More than 70 conditions that require hospitalization in the Medicaid population are attributable in whole or part to tobacco, alcohol, and drug abuse.[9,10]

The majority of the substance abuse-related diseases in the Medicaid population are linked to tobacco and illicit drugs, many related to birth complications resulting from cocaine use. More than 60 Medicare ailments are attributable to tobacco, alcohol, and drug abuse. The majority of the substance abuse related diseases in the Medicare population are associated with tobacco, which accounts for 80% of these diseases. If substance abuse and addiction do not decrease, it will cost the Medicare program alone more than one trillion dollars over the next 20 years.[10]

Substance abuse is a major complicating factor in our correctional system today. A study published in 1998 found that 80% of the total population in federal prisons were substance related offenders; that is, they committed a drug offense and/or were substance users whose use of alcohol or drugs was somehow related to their crime. In state prisons, 81% were substance-related offenders. Nearly ten times as many inmates were serving time for drug offenses in 1993 as in 1980. Involvement in criminal activity varied directly with the prevalence, frequency, and seriousness of drug use. Persons testing positive for drugs at the time of arrest have a higher probability of being rearrested. Addicted offenders who receive little or no treatment for their substance abuse problem appear to show an accelerating pattern of criminal activity over time.[11]

ACUTE VERSUS CHRONIC PROBLEMS

Problems brought about by misuse of chemical substances can be categorized into two types: those that occur acutely and those that arise only after continued use of a drug. Acute problems are usually predictable, given the pharmacology of the drug. Acute drug intoxications usually occur at doses in excess of that normally taken. Chronic abuse of chemical substances can cause a wide array of physical, psychological, and psychiatric ailments. The substance-induced disorders to be discussed here mainly include intoxication and withdrawal. Psychiatric problems associated with substance abuse, including dementia, psychosis, mood disorders, and anxiety, are discussed elsewhere. Physical illnesses associated with chronic use of chemicals (e.g., alcoholic liver disease) are likewise covered in other chapters.

The essential feature of substance dependence is the continued use of the substance despite adverse substance-related problems. Repeated use of the drug is often associated with the development of tolerance, withdrawal, and compulsive use, but it is possible to meet criteria for dependence in the absence of physical dependence. The criteria for substance dependence are the same for each of the drugs or drug classes, varying only to fit the unique pharmacologic properties of each drug. To meet criteria for the diagnosis of substance dependence, at least three of the following must be present at any time in a 12-month period:

1. Tolerance.
2. Withdrawal, indicated by the appearance of the characteristic withdrawal syndrome or the use of the same or related drug to relieve or avoid withdrawal symptoms.
3. Substance taken in larger amounts or over a longer period of time than was intended.
4. Persistent desire or unsuccessful efforts to cut down or control substance use.
5. Time spent in activities necessary to obtain the substance, use the substance, or recover from its effects.
6. Social, occupational, or recreational activities given up or reduced because of substance use.
7. Substance use continued despite knowledge of having a persistent or recurrent physical or psychological problem caused or exacerbated by the substance.

The characteristic feature of substance abuse is a maladaptive pattern of substance use indicated by repeated adverse consequences related to the repeated use of substances. Examples include failure to fulfill important obligations at work, school, or home; repeated use in situations in which it is physically dangerous, such as driving under the influence; legal problems; and social or interpersonal problems such as arguments and fights.

Intoxication refers to the development of a substance-specific syndrome after recent ingestion and presence in the body of a substance, and it is associated with maladaptive behavior during the waking state caused by the effect of the substance on the CNS. Examples include belligerence, mood lability, impaired judgment, and impaired social or occupational functioning. Evidence for recent intake of the substance can be obtained from the history, physical examination, or laboratory examination. The most common changes involve disturbances in perception, wakefulness, attention, thinking, judgment, motor behavior, and interpersonal behavior.

Withdrawal, as defined previously, is the development of a substance-specific syndrome after cessation of, or reduction in, intake of a substance that was regularly used by the individual to induce a state of intoxication. Withdrawal causes significant distress to the individual, and is associated with impairment in social, occupational, or other areas of functioning. Withdrawal is usually associated with substance dependence. Withdrawal is generally also associated with a craving to readminister the drug to relieve the symptoms.

As with most illnesses, the course and prognosis of the disorders of substance use and dependence are variable. Untreated physical withdrawal from the CNS depressants is potentially life threatening; however, withdrawal can almost always be successfully managed with proper medical care. Getting patients who are drug dependent to stop using drugs is very difficult, and many patients return to drug use even after treatment. As many as 75% of treated substance-dependent patients relapse at least once. Many patients are, however, able to obtain recovery with treatment and continued care in programs such as Alcoholics Anonymous (AA) or Narcotics Anonymous (NA). Substance dependence or addiction can be viewed as a chronic illness that can be successfully controlled with treatment, but cannot be cured and is associated with a high relapse rate. Without treatment, the course can progress to life-threatening severity, resulting from the effects of the drug, drug contaminants, or medical complications of use.

CENTRAL NERVOUS SYSTEM DEPRESSANTS

BENZODIAZEPINES AND OTHER SEDATIVE–HYPNOTICS

In clinical practice, the benzodiazepines have largely replaced the short-acting barbiturates and other nonbarbiturate sedative–hypnotics. Benzodiazepines with faster onset (e.g., diazepam) tend to be preferred by the recreational drug user because they are reinforcing. Recently, flunitrazepam has burst upon the scene and is rapidly gaining a reputation as a "party drug."[12] It will be discussed in a separate section later. Because all benzodiazepines have abuse and dependence liability, patients cannot be switched from one benzodiazepine to another in hopes of decreasing a pattern of drug abuse or dependence behavior. Zolpidem, a nonbenzodiazepine, nonbarbiturate sedative, has been suggested to have little liability for physical dependence, but tolerance and withdrawal have been reported in association with its use as well.[13]

Unlike the barbiturates, benzodiazepines do not generally cause significant respiratory depression as do the barbiturate-like drugs.[14] Signs and symptoms of withdrawal are similar in many respects to those of alcohol withdrawal, but the time courses may be quite different. While withdrawal from shorter-acting agents (e.g., lorazepam, alprazolam) has an onset within 12 to 24 hours of the last dose, others (e.g., diazepam, chlordiazepoxide, clorazepate, phenobarbital, amobarbital) have elimination half-lives or active metabolites with elimination half-lives of 24 to over 100 hours. As a result, the onset of withdrawal symptoms may be delayed for several days after discontinuation of the drug.[15] Dependence on sedative–hypnotics and benzodiazepines is summarized in Table 62–1.

Long-term use of even therapeutic doses of benzodiazepines may cause physical dependence and withdrawal symptoms after abrupt discontinuation.[15] The likelihood and severity of withdrawal is a function of both dose and duration of exposure. Gradual tapering of dosage is also associated with less withdrawal and rebound anxiety than abrupt discontinuation. Patients who have taken benzodiazepines for the treatment of anxiety often experience a rebound increase in anxiety after discontinuation of the antianxiety drug. The heightened autonomic activity of severe anxiety can be easily mistaken for drug withdrawal. A combination of withdrawal and increased anxiety may also occur, and each may intensify the other. Occurrence of hallucinations or seizures would indicate severe physical withdrawal. For additional information on benzodiazepine withdrawal refer to Chapter 67.

FLUNITRAZEPAM

Anecdotal reports and drug seizures by law enforcement indicate that distribution and abuse of flunitrazepam are increasing domestically, especially in southern and southwestern states. Of particular concern is the drug's low cost, usually below $5 per tablet, and its growing popularity among young people. Flunitrazepam is a benzodiazepine that is used in the short-term treatment of insomnia and as a sedative–hypnotic and preanesthetic medication. It has physiologic effects similar to those of diazepam. A comprehensive review of this drug has been published and will serve as a basis for the discussion below.[12]

Marketed under the trade name Rohypnol, flunitrazepam is manufactured worldwide, including Europe and Latin America, in 1- and 2-mg tablets by Hoffman-La Roche. However, the drug is neither manufactured nor approved for medical use in the United States.

Flunitrazepam has been encountered by U.S. law enforcement agencies in southern states from California to Florida. Authorities in Texas and Florida have observed the most significant activity involving flunitrazepam. Distributors in Texas reportedly travel to Mexico to obtain the drug. In South Florida, the drug is delivered primarily from Columbia via international mail services or commercial airlines. Overnight mail appears to be the preferred method of importation. Several packages seized in Miami over the past 2 years were shipped from Cali, Columbia, and contained up to 11,000 dosage units each.

Flunitrazepam is ingested orally, frequently in conjunction with alcohol or other drugs, including heroin. The

TABLE 62–1. Dependence on Sedative–Hypnotics[a]

Generic Name	Common Trade Names (Manufacturer)	Oral Sedating Dose (mg)	Physical Dependence Dose and Time Needed to Produce Dependence	Time Before Onset of Withdrawal (h)	Peak Withdrawal Symptoms (d)
Benzodiazepines					
Diazepam	Valium (Roche)	5–10	40–120 mg × 42–120 d	12–24	5–8
Chlordiazepoxide	Librium, Libritabs (Roche)	10–25	75–600 mg × 42-120 d	12–24	5–8
Clorazepate	Tranxene (Abbott)	7.5–15	45–180 mg × 42–120 d (est.)	12–24	5–8
Alprazolam	Xanax (Upjohn)	0.25–8	8–16 mg × 42 d (est.)	8–24	2–3
Flunitrazepam	Rohypnol (Roche)	1–2	8–10 mg × 42 d (est.)	24–36	2–3
Barbiturates					
Secobarbital	Seconal, Seco-8 (Lilly)	100	800–2200 mg × 35–37 d	6–12	2–3
Pentobarbital	Nembutal (Abbott)	100	Same	6–12	2–3
Equal parts of secobarbital and amobarbital	Tuinal (Lilly)	100	Same	6–12	2–3
Amobarbital	Amytal (Lilly)	65–100	Same	8–12	2–5
Nonbarbiturate Sedative–Hypnotics					
Ethchlorvynol	Placidyl (Abbott)	200	1–1.5 g × 30 d	6–12	2–3
Chloral hydrate	Noctec (various)	250	Exact dose unknown; 12 g/d chronically has led to delirium upon sudden withdrawal	6–12	2–3
Meprobamate	Equanil, Miltown, Meprotabs (various)	400	1.6-3.2 g × 270 d	8–12	3–8

[a]Withdrawal symptoms are tremor, tachycardia, diaphoresis, nausea, vomiting, blood pressure lability, delirium, seizures, and hallucinations.

drug's effects begin within 30 minutes, peak within 2 hours, and may persist for up to 8 hours or more, depending upon the dosage.[12] Adverse effects associated with the use of flunitrazepam include decreased blood pressure, memory impairment, drowsiness, visual disturbances, dizziness, confusion, gastrointestinal disturbances, and urinary retention.

Flunitrazepam use causes dependence in humans. Once dependence has developed, abstinence induces withdrawal symptoms, including headache, muscle pain, extreme anxiety, tension, restlessness, confusion, and irritability. Numbness, tingling of the extremities, loss of identity, hallucinations, delirium, convulsions, shock, and cardiovascular collapse also may occur. Withdrawal seizures can occur 1 week or more after cessation of use. As with other benzodiazepines, treatment for flunitrazepam dependence includes a gradual tapering of the drug.[12]

Flunitrazepam is often combined with alcohol, marijuana, or cocaine to produce a rapid and very dramatic "high." Even when used by itself, users can appear extremely intoxicated, with slurred speech, poor coordination, swaying, and bloodshot eyes, with no odor of alcohol. The drug has been added to punch and other drinks at fraternity parties and college social gatherings, where it is reportedly given to female party participants in hopes of lowered inhibitions and facilitating potential sexual conquest. Police departments in several parts of the country say that after ingestion of flunitrazepam several young women have reported waking up in strange surroundings with no clothes on, or having actually been sexually assaulted while under the influence of the drug.[16] For this reason, flunitrazepam has come to be called the "date rape drug."

Flunitrazepam is sold under the trade name Rohypnol, from which the street name "Rophy" is derived. In South Florida, street names include "circles," "Mexican valium," "rib," "roach-2," "roofies," "roopies," "rope," "ropies," and "ruffies." In Texas, flunitrazepam is called "R-2," or "roaches."

GAMMA HYDROXY BUTYRATE

Gamma hydroxy butyrate (GHB) is a CNS depressant approved as an anaesthetic in some countries; however, with the exception of investigational research, it is not approved for any use in the United States.[17] Primary groups using GHB include party and nightclub attendees and bodybuilders. In addition, GHB is one of several agents characterized as a "date rape" drug. From August 1995 to September 1996, poison control centers in New York and Texas received reports of 69 acute poisonings and one death attributed to ingestion of GHB.[18]

GHB increases dopamine levels in the brain and has effects through the endogenous opioid system; most GHB is excreted during the first 1 to 2 hours after ingestion.[17] Manifestations of acute GHB toxicity include coma, seizures, respiratory depression, and vomiting. Other documented effects of GHB include amnesia and hypotonia (associated with doses of 10 mg/kg body weight); abnormal sequence of rapid eye movement (REM) and non-REM sleep (doses of 20 to 30 mg/kg); and anesthesia (doses of approximately 50 mg/kg). Doses greater than 50 mg/kg can decrease cardiac output and produce severe respiratory depression, seizure-like activity, and coma[19]; coma and respiratory depression may be potentiated by concomitant use of alcohol.[20] There is no antidote for GHB overdose, and treatment is restricted to nonspecific supportive care.

In the United States, GHB has been produced clandestinely in widely varying degrees of purity. GHB has been marketed as a liquid or powder and has been sold on the street under names such as "grevious bodily harm," "Georgia home boy," "liquid ecstasy," "liquid X," "liquid E," "GHB," "GBH," "soap," "scoop," "easy lay," "salty water," "G-riffick," "cherry menth," and "organic quaalude." Improper preparation of GHB can result in a mixture of GHB and sodium hydroxide that can be severely toxic because of the combined effects of the GHB and the direct caustic effects of sodium hydroxide.[18]

In Dallas, GHB use has been associated with events at which several persons have been found comatose. Some persons who have sustained adverse effects of GHB have reported being given the drug surreptitiously (e.g., having it slipped into their drink), while others have admitted to intentional use. The Drug Enforcement Administration (DEA) is examining the distribution and abuse of GHB in the United States; although distribution has been documented in 27 states, GHB use is highly prevalent in California, Florida, Georgia, and Texas.[18]

In the United States, GHB is being researched for the treatment of narcolepsy. Although it is not a currently controlled substance under federal law, the DEA is considering making it one. In Georgia and Rhode Island, state controlled substances acts have classified GHB into schedule I, and other states are considering similar action.[18]

OPIATES

Incidence and prevalence of opiate use are widely variable depending on the drug. Heroin gained widespread notoriety during the 1960s and 1970s and remains the single most commonly used illicit opiate. The number of heroin-dependent individuals nationally is estimated at around one-half million, a number that pales somewhat in comparison with the approximately 13 million alcohol-dependent individuals.[4]

Collectively, use of opiates other than heroin is far more common. Approximately 6% of adults have tried an opiate or opiate-like analgesic for nonmedical use with around 1% having used an opiate analgesic within 1 month.[4] Hydromorphone has become widely used among the opiate-using population, with single 4-mg tablets selling for as much as $70.[21] Hydromorphone has a pharmaceutical profile very similar to heroin, with the advantage of purity. Drug combinations involving opiates are quite popular. Opiates are commonly combined with stimulant drugs, especially cocaine, a combination known as a "speedball." Opiate users frequently also drink alcohol, especially when their use of opiate drugs declines because of lack of availability or sometimes following treatment.

TABLE 62–2. Signs and Symptoms of Opioid Intoxication and Withdrawal

Intoxication	Withdrawal
Euphoria	Lacrimination
Dysphoria	Rhinorrhea
Apathy	Mydriasis
Motor retardation	Piloerection
Sedation	Diaphoresis
Slurred speech	Diarrhea
Attention impairment	Yawning
Miosis	Fever
	Insomnia
	Muscle aching

Many of the complications of opiate use, especially intravenous use, are related not only to the drug itself but also to varying purity, contaminants, and techniques of administration such as dirty equipment and use of shared needles. Overdoses, anaphylactic reactions to impurities, nephrotic syndrome, septicemia, endocarditis, and acquired immune deficiency syndrome (AIDS) are examples.[22]

Signs and symptoms of opioid intoxication and withdrawal are summarized in Table 62–2[23] Onset of the acute phase of withdrawal varies with the drug consumed, but ranges from a few hours after stopping heroin to 3 to 5 days after stopping methadone. The time course of withdrawal ranges from 3 to 14 days. Opioid withdrawal is significantly different from withdrawal from alcohol or other sedative-hypnotics. Of greatest importance is that opioid withdrawal is not fatal unless there is a concurrent medical problem of major concern. This has significant treatment implications. Although patients in opioid withdrawal may be in great discomfort and incapacitated, they are not delirious. The presence of delirium should raise the question of concurrent withdrawal from another drug, such as alcohol, or another cause of delirium possibly secondary to drug use.

Although the current epidemic of cocaine use has commanded more attention, heroin use remains a serious problem in the United States. In addition, some researchers have noted that snorting and smoking heroin may be growing in popularity as alternatives to injecting the drug.[4] Regardless of how users take the drug, an increase in the purity of heroin could be one reason for the increase in hospital emergency department visits. During 1995, the nationwide average purity for retail heroin from all sources was 39.7%, much higher than the average of 7% reported a decade prior, and considerably higher than the 26.6% recorded in 1991.[24] The significant rise in average purity corresponded directly to the increase in availability of high-purity Southeast Asian and South American heroin.

CENTRAL NERVOUS SYSTEM STIMULANTS

COCAINE

Cocaine is perhaps the most behaviorally reinforcing of all drugs of abuse. Most clinicians estimate that approximately 10% of people who begin to use the drug "recreationally" will go on to serious, heavy use. Once having tried cocaine, an individual cannot predict or control the extent to which he or she will continue to use the drug.

The most characteristic systemic effect of cocaine is stimulation of the CNS.[25] In the CNS, cocaine appears to mediate its effects primarily by blocking reuptake of catecholamine neurotransmitters such as norepinephrine and dopamine. The most common clinical manifestations of cocaine stimulation of the CNS are intense euphoria, decreased fatigue, and increased alertness.

There were an estimated 608,000 (0.3% of the population) frequent cocaine users in 1996. Frequent use, defined as use on 51 or more days during the past year, was not significantly different than in 1995, when there were an estimated 582,000 frequent cocaine users. Since this measure of frequent cocaine use was first estimated in 1985, no significant increases or decreases have been detected.[4]

Cocaine is rapidly absorbed from virtually all sites of application. For many years, cocaine has been administered as the hydrochloride salt form, usually by inhalation, but also by injection. In the last 15 years as the purity of cocaine hydrochloride obtained on the street declined, many users converted the cocaine hydrochloride to cocaine base, also known as "crack" or "rock." Crack cocaine receives its name from the crackling sound that occurs when the rocks are melted into vapors. This form of administration of the drug leads to almost instant absorption and intense euphoria. Peak plasma concentrations of greater than 900 ng/mL have been achieved following inhalation of cocaine base vapors compared with concentrations of only 150 to 200 ng/mL achieved after inhalation of similar amounts of pure cocaine hydrochloride powder.[25]

The high from snorting may last 15 to 30 minutes, while that from smoking may last 5 to 10 minutes. Increased use can reduce the period of stimulation. Some users of cocaine report feelings of restlessness, irritability, and anxiety. An appreciable tolerance to the high may be developed, and many addicts report that they seek but fail to achieve as much pleasure as they did from their first exposure. Scientific evidence suggests that the powerful neuropsychological reinforcing property of cocaine is responsible for an individual's continued use, despite harmful physical and social consequences. In rare instances, sudden death can occur on the first use of cocaine or unexpectedly thereafter. However, there is no way to determine who is prone to sudden death.

High doses of cocaine and/or prolonged use can trigger paranoia. Smoking crack cocaine can produce a particularly aggressive paranoid behavior in users. When addicted individuals stop using cocaine, they often become depressed. This may lead to further cocaine use to alleviate depression. Prolonged cocaine snorting can result in ulceration of the mucous membranes of the nose and can damage the nasal septum enough to cause it to collapse. Cocaine-related deaths are often a result of cardiac arrest or seizures followed by respiratory arrest.

Recent research has helped clarify certain patterns of cocaine use such as combining cocaine and alcohol. Such drug use would seem counterintuitive, because cocaine is a CNS stimulant and alcohol a CNS depressant. In the presence of alcohol, cocaine is metabolized to cocaethylene, a longer-acting but equally potent psychoactive compound as compared to the parent drug.[26] The risk of death from cocaethylene is greater than from cocaine.[27] The cocaine–alcohol combination is one of the most commonly identified among individuals who come to hospital emergency departments with acute substance abuse problems.

Cocaine is rapidly metabolized and eliminated. The elimination half-life of cocaine is approximately 1 hour, and the duration of effect is very short.[25] The short duration of effect provides a powerful incentive for repeated use of the drug. Many users experience intense drug use cycling, sometimes lasting days, characterized by rapidly repeating doses of cocaine until their supply is exhausted. Laboratory monkeys, given a choice between food and cocaine around the clock for 8 days, consistently choose cocaine.[28]

Complications of cocaine use frequently involve cardiovascular events.[29] At higher doses, it increases heart rate because of an overall systemic increase in sympathetic tone. At toxic doses, cocaine causes cardiac failure due to a direct effect on myocardial contractility. Cocaine is also pyrogenic, and hyperthermia is frequently observed in cocaine poisoning. Death is usually related to arrhythmias, shock, or convulsions.

Cocaine is a psychotomimetic drug, sometimes even at systemically nontoxic doses. A kindling phenomenon has been described with cocaine in which neuronal function becomes altered with each dose of the drug. This causes a type of reverse tolerance with increased receptor sensitivity to cocaine, and psychosis may be caused by doses that formerly did not cause psychosis. The toxic psychosis is characterized by auditory, visual, and frequently tactile hallucinations, paranoid thinking, and looseness of associations. The psychosis is qualitatively very similar to a paranoid schizophrenic psychosis.[30]

Recently, research has been conducted to better understand the mechanisms by which cocaine produces its pleasurable effects as they are occurring. Volkow and colleagues[31] have found a significant relationship between the intensity and duration of the "high" induced by cocaine and the degree to which the drug blocks one of the major mechanisms to control the amount of dopamine in the brain. There is a clear relationship between the degree to which cocaine blocks the dopamine transporter and the cocaine abuser's experience of euphoric feelings.

Previously, animal studies[32] have suggested that cocaine works in large part by occupying or blocking dopamine transporter (DAT) sites, thereby preventing reuptake of dopamine by the brain cells that release it. It is this abnormally long presence of dopamine at the synapse that is believed to cause the high and other effects associated with cocaine use.

TABLE 62–3. Signs and Symptoms of Cocaine Intoxication and Withdrawal

Intoxication	Withdrawal
Motor agitation	Fatigue
Elation/euphoria	Sleep disturbance
Grandiosity	Nightmares
Loquacity	Depression
Hypervigilance	Increased appetite
Tachycardia	
Mydriasis	
Elevated or lowered blood pressure	
Sweating or chills	
Nausea and vomiting	

To study the relationship between subjective effects of cocaine and its activity in the brain of humans, Volkow and associates[31] gave injections of cocaine to 17 volunteers who were current cocaine users. Using positron emisson tomography (PET) scans, they produced images of the volunteers' brains showing the concentrations of cocaine occupying DAT sites. They found that doses of cocaine commonly abused by humans blocked about 60% to 77% of the cocaine users' DAT sites. The researchers were able to document a significant relationship between the intensity and duration of the high induced by the cocaine and the concentration of the drug at DAT sites seen in the PET scans. In order for the subjects to perceive cocaine's effects, at least 47% of the DAT sites had to be blocked by cocaine. With a better understanding of the mechanism by which the "high" from cocaine is produced, perhaps specific drugs can be developed that block these subjective effects of the drug, allowing easier detoxification and drug avoidance.

Signs and symptoms of cocaine intoxication are summarized in Table 62–3. Although there is some controversy as to whether cocaine is associated with physical withdrawal upon abrupt discontinuation, most clinicians feel that there is a characteristic syndrome of withdrawal effects although they are not life threatening.[33] Cocaine withdrawal consists primarily of fatigue, sleep disturbance, nightmares, and depression; it begins within hours of discontinuing the drug and lasts up to several days.

AMPHETAMINES AND OTHER STIMULANTS

During World War II, methamphetamine was used by soldiers as an aid to fight fatigue and enhance performance. In Japan, intravenous methamphetamine abuse reached epidemic proportions immediately after World War II, when supplies stored for military use became available to the public.

In the United States in the 1950s, legally manufactured tablets of methamphetamine were used nonmedically by college students, truck drivers, and athletes, who usually did not become severely addicted. This pattern changed drastically in the 1960s with the increased availability of injectable methamphetamine.

According to the DEA,[21] methamphetamine has been the most prevalent clandestinely produced controlled substance in the United States since 1979. The clandestine manufacture of methamphetamine was based primarily in the West and Southwest. Since the 1980s, it has been smuggled from Taiwan and South Korea into Hawaii. However, it was not until the summer of 1988 that its use became relatively widespread in that state. By 1990, distribution of methamphetamine had spread to the U.S. mainland, although distribution remained limited. Today, methamphetamine can be found in cities across the United States.

Street methamphetamine is referred to by many names, such as "speed," "meth," and "crank." Methamphetamine hydrochloride, clear chunky crystals resembling ice, which can be inhaled by smoking, is referred to as "ice," "crystal," and "glass."

The physiologic and psychological effects of amphetamines and other stimulants are qualitatively similar to those of cocaine—they diminish fatigue, increase alertness, and suppress appetite. Pharmacologically, amphetamines increase the activity of catecholamine neurotransmitters (e.g., norepinephrine, dopamine) by blocking reuptake, increasing release of neurotransmitters, and inhibiting the degradative enzyme monoamine oxidase.[34] The primary differences between cocaine and amphetamines are pharmacokinetic.

Methamphetamine is taken orally or intranasally, by intravenous injection, and by smoking. Immediately after inhalation or intravenous injection, the methamphetamine user experiences an intense sensation, called a "rush" or "flash," that lasts only a few minutes and is described as extremely pleasurable.

Because methamphetamine elevates mood, people who experiment with it tend to use it with increasing frequency and in increasing doses, although this was not their original intent. The CNS actions that result from taking even small amounts of methamphetamine include increased wakefulness, increased physical activity, decreased appetite, increased respiration, hyperthermia, and euphoria. Other CNS effects include irritability, insomnia, confusion, tremors, convulsions, anxiety, paranoia, and aggressiveness. Hyperthermia and convulsions can result in death.

Cardiovascular side effects, which include chest pain and hypertension, also can result in cardiovascular collapse and death. In addition, methamphetamine causes increased heart rate and blood pressure and can cause irreversible damage to blood vessels in the brain, producing strokes. Other effects of methamphetamine include respiratory problems, irregular heartbeat, and extreme anorexia.

DESIGNER DRUGS

A designer drug is a chemical compound that is similar in structure and effect to another drug of abuse but differs slightly chemically. Designer drugs are produced in clandestine laboratories to mimic the psychoactive effects of controlled drugs. Theoretically, the number of potential synthetic analogs that can be made and distributed is very large. The most commonly known types of synthetic analog drugs available through the illicit drug market include analogs of fentanyl and meperidine, phencyclidine (PCP), amphetamine, and methamphetamine. The street names of designer drugs vary according to time, place, and manufacturer, and they change frequently.

FENTANYL ANALOGS

Fentanyl was introduced in 1968 as a synthetic narcotic to be used as an analgesic in surgical procedures because of its minimal effect on the heart. In the early 1980s, however, crude clandestine laboratories began manufacturing fentanyl derivatives that were pharmacologically similar to heroin and morphine.[35] These fentanyl analogs create addiction similar to that of the opiate narcotics and present a significant drug abuse problem, including an increased potential for overdose. The most commonly known fentanyl analog is alpha-methylfentanyl, which is known on the streets as China white. Other fentanyl analogs on the street include 3-methylfentanyl (TMF), known on the street as "synthetic heroin," "tango and cash," and "goodfella."

As with other narcotic analgesics, respiratory depression is the most significant acute toxic effect of the fentanyl derivatives. Fentanyl analogs are 80 to 1000 times more potent than morphine, depending on how they are made, and are 200 times more potent than heroin. They are intended to duplicate the euphoric effects of heroin. Fentanyl analogs have a very rapid onset (1 to 4 minutes) and a short duration of action (approximately 30 to 90 minutes), which varies according to the drug.[36] Because of the potency and quick onset, even a very small dose of a fentanyl analog can lead to sudden death.

Alpha-methylfentanyl, which appeared in Orange County, California, in 1979, was the first synthetically produced fentanyl that resulted in overdose deaths. Between 1980 and 1985, China white and several other fentanyl analogs were responsible for 100 unintentional overdose deaths in California.

In 1988, TMF was identified in 16 unintentional overdose deaths in Allegheny County, Pennsylvania.[35] Multiple drug use was common in most of these cases. Because TMF is a powerful opiate, it is possible that it compounded the respiratory suppressant effects of the other drugs ingested, thereby causing death. In 1991, the fentanyl analog tango and cash was implicated in at least 28 deaths, primarily in New York and other northeast areas.[37] In 1992, China white was found to be the cause of death in 21 overdoses during 2 months in Philadelphia. To date, fentanyl analogs are responsible for the drug overdose deaths of more than 150 people in the United States.

The most common route of administration is by injection. Authorities report that a victim can die so suddenly from respiratory paralysis that the needle may still be in the dead user's arm. Recent data indicate that smoking and sniffing are two means of ingestion that are becoming more popular—perhaps because of the attempt on the part of users to avoid the transmission of HIV/AIDS.[21]

MEPERIDINE ANALOGS

Over the past decade, the illicit use of meperidine has increased during periods when heroin was scarce. Two meperidine analogs that have appeared on the streets include MPPP (1-methyl-4-phenyl-4-propionoxypiperidine) and PEPAP (1-[2-phenylethyl]-4-acetyloxypiperdine).[38]

An impurity formed during the clandestine manufacture of MPPP, called MPTP (1-methyl-4-phenyl-1,2,3,6,-tetrahydro-pyridine), has been shown to be a potent neurotoxin and has caused irreversible brain damage in several individuals. The damage is manifested in a syndrome resembling a very severe parkinsonism, which results in increased muscle tone, difficulty in moving and speaking, drooling, and cogwheel rigidity of the upper extremities. Tremor in such patients characteristically involves the proximal muscles and is more pronounced than the typical involuntary resting tremor occurring in idiopathic parkinsonism.[39]

METHAMPHETAMINE ANALOGS

Several dozen analogs of amphetamine and methamphetamine are hallucinogenic. The methamphetamine analogs currently of concern include MDA (3,4-methylenedioxy-amphetamine) and MDMA (3,4-methylenedioxy-methamphetamine).[40]

MDA, known by the street name "Eve" or "love drug," became a drug of abuse in the 1960s. It produces a heightened need for interpersonal relationships, and users report an increased need to talk to and be with other people. Effects of MDA use resemble those of amphetamine intoxication: hyperactivity, hyperthermia, tachycardia, hypertension, and seizures.

MDMA, often known on the streets as "ecstasy" or "Adam," is structurally similar to methamphetamine and mescaline, and stimulates the CNS and produces a mild hallucinogenic effect. It was first synthesized illegally in 1972, but was not widely abused until the 1980s.

Like its chemical first cousin, MDMA can result in a variety of acute psychiatric disturbances, including panic, anxiety, depression, and paranoid thinking.[40] Physical symptoms include muscle tension, nausea, blurred vision, faintness, chills, and sweating. MDMA also increases the heart rate and blood pressure. It has been shown to destroy serotonin-producing neurons in animals.[41] These neurons play a direct role in regulating aggression, mood, sexual activity, sleep, and sensitivity to pain. MDMA also has been reported to cause jaw clenching, tremor, and hallucinations.

In animal studies, the doses of MDA that produce neurotoxicity are only two or three times more than the minimum dose needed to produce a psychotropic response. This suggests that individuals who are self-administering the drug may be getting a neurotoxic dose.[42] The relationship between the neurotoxic dose and the psychotropic dose of MDMA is currently under investigation.

The DEA reports that MDMA is available in at least 21 states and Canada. It is especially popular with college students and young adults.[43] According to the Monitoring the Future survey, 6.1% of high school seniors had used MDMA.[5]

Various claims have been made by a small number of psychiatrists for the usefulness of MDMA in enhancing psychotherapy. No evidence has been presented to document these anecdotal reports.[44]

PHENCYCLIDINE AND KETAMINE

Phencyclidine, commonly referred to as PCP, "angel dust," and "crystal," was popular in the 1970s, but as its adverse effects became better known, use declined. Phencyclidine is most often a substitute for or contaminant of other drugs, and its most common pattern of use may now be unintentional. The actual extent of its use is unclear. It is often misrepresented as lysergic acid diethylamide (LSD) or Δ^9-tetrahydrocannabinol (THC). THC is virtually unavailable on the street because it is highly unstable when isolated from the marijuana plant. When used intentionally, PCP is commonly smoked with marijuana and referred to as a "crystal joint," but may also be taken orally or intravenously.

Phencyclidine has widely varied actions including CNS stimulation, depression, and hallucinogenic properties. Pharmacologically, it is known to block reuptake of serotonin, dopamine, and norepinephrine, but neurotransmitter antagonists do not effectively block its effects. In low doses, phencyclidine causes sedation, ataxia, nystagmus, slurred speech, and paresthesias. At higher doses, users experience an increase in heart rate, blood pressure, temperature, diaphoresis, and muscle rigidity. At acutely toxic doses, coma and seizures may occur.[45]

Behavioral effects of phencyclidine range from sleep to catatonic detachment to paranoid psychosis to violent hostility. Users are sometimes amnestic for events that occur under the influence of the drug. Psychoses sometimes last for weeks. Users with a previous history of schizophrenia are especially susceptible to the psychotomimetic effects of the drug. The only truly characteristic behavioral effect of phencyclidine use is its high unpredictability. The signs and symptoms of phencyclidine intoxication are summarized in Table 62–4.

Ketamine, a compound chemically related to phencyclidine, is used primarily as a veterinary anesthetic but has

TABLE 62–4. Signs and Symptoms of Phencyclidine Intoxication

Nystagmus	Euphoria
Increased blood pressure	Motor agitation
Tachycardia	Anxiety and emotional lability
Paresthesias	Hostility
Ataxia	Delusions
Slurred speech	Hallucinations
Muscle rigidity	

recently gained popularity as a recreational drug.[46] Once used extensively in human medicine, it has fallen out of favor because of "emergence delirium" characterized by hallucinations, delirium, vivid dreams, and other psychiatric effects. This untoward effect as a medicinal agent is precisely the effect that recreational users are seeking. Because it is not currently a controlled substance in the United States, it is often the target of drug diversion schemes or thefts from physicians' or veterinarians' offices.

Known as "special K," "jet," "green," and other names on the street, ketamine is usually injected but can be evaporated to solid crystals, powdered and smoked, snorted, or swallowed. Marijuana cigarettes are sometimes soaked in the ketamine solution, allowed to dry and then smoked. Ketamine has become popular as a "rave" club drug. Side effects include significant transient increases in blood pressure and heart rate, respiratory depression, airway obstruction, apnea, muscular hypertonus, psychomotor, and psychotomimetic and acute dystonic reactions. Following overdosage, seizures, polyneuropathy, increased intracranial pressure, respiratory arrest, and cardiac arrest may occur.[46]

HALLUCINOGENS

The drugs commonly thought of as hallucinogens are LSD, psilocybin, dimethyltryptamine (DMT), mescaline, and other related compounds. LSD is one of the most potent mood-changing chemicals. It is manufactured from lysergic acid, which is found in ergot, a fungus that grows on rye and other grains.[47]

Pharmacologically, LSD and related drugs stimulate both presynaptic (5-HT_{1A}, 5-HT_{1B}) and postsynaptic (5-HT_2) serotonin recognition sites in the brain, which may functionally cause either agonist or antagonist effects on serotonin activity.[48] Precisely how the hallucinogens exert their effects remains unclear. LSD, often referred to as "acid," is an extraordinarily potent compound, producing observable CNS effects at doses as low as 25 μg.[22]

LSD is sold on the street in tablets, capsules, and, occasionally, liquid form. It is odorless, colorless, and tasteless and is usually taken by mouth. Often LSD is added to absorbent paper, such as blotter paper, and divided into small decorated squares, with each square representing one dose.

The DEA[21] reports that the strength of LSD samples obtained currently from illicit sources ranges from 20 to 80 μg of LSD per dose. This is considerably less than the levels reported during the 1960s and early 1970s, when the dosage ranged from 100 to 200 μg, or higher, per unit.

The effects of LSD are unpredictable. They depend on the amount taken; the user's personality, mood, and expectations; and the surroundings in which the drug is used. Usually, the user feels the first effects of the drug 30 to 90 minutes after taking it. The physical effects include dilated pupils, higher body temperature, increased heart rate and blood pressure, sweating, loss of appetite, sleeplessness, dry mouth, and tremors.

Sensations and feelings change much more dramatically than the physical signs. The user may feel several different emotions at once or swing rapidly from one emotion to another. If taken in a large enough dose, the drug produces delusions and visual hallucinations. The user's sense of time and self changes. Sensations may seem to "cross over," giving the user the feeling of hearing colors and seeing sounds. These changes can be frightening and can cause panic.

Many LSD users experience flashbacks, recurrence of certain aspects of a person's experience, without the user having taken the drug again. A flashback occurs suddenly, often without warning, and may occur within a few days or more than a year after LSD use. Flashbacks usually occur in people who use hallucinogens chronically or have an underlying personality problem; however, otherwise healthy people who use LSD occasionally may also have flashbacks.

Most users of LSD voluntarily decrease or stop its use over time. LSD is not considered an addictive drug, because it does not produce compulsive drug-seeking behavior. However, in common with many of the addictive drugs, LSD produces tolerance, so some users who take the drug repeatedly must take progressively higher doses to achieve the state of intoxication that they had previously achieved.

Signs and symptoms of hallucinogen intoxication are summarized in Table 62–5. Psychological symptoms of intoxication include a subjective intensification of perceptions, depersonalization, illusions, hallucinations, and synesthesias, the overflow of one sensory modality to another (colors are heard, sounds are seen). Among the hallucinogenic drugs, LSD is the most potent and long acting; it is hundreds of times more potent than both psilocybin and mescaline. DMT is inactive when ingested orally, but can be smoked, inhaled, or injected. There is cross-tolerance among LSD, psilocybin, and mescaline. There is not an observable physical withdrawal syndrome after abrupt discontinuation of hallucinogenic drugs.[49]

Complications from hallucinogen use are primarily psychologic. Users sometimes experience prolonged episodes of panic, the so-called "bad trip." The flashbacks noted are common, occurring in approximately 15% of users and occurring episodically up to several years after the last

TABLE 62–5. Signs and Symptoms of Hallucinogen Intoxication

Psychologic	Physical
Perceptual intensification	Mydriasis
Depersonalization	Tachycardia
Derealization	Diaphoresis
Illusions	Palpitations
Hallucinations	Blurred vision
Synesthesias	Tremor
	Incoordination
	Dizziness
	Weakness
	Drowsiness
	Paresthesias

exposure to the drug. Flashbacks may occur spontaneously, but are also triggered by other drugs, including marijuana, and by anxiety-provoking stimuli. Physical effects of hallucinogen use are relatively nontoxic. Contrary to a widely held notion in the 1960s and early 1970s, there is no reliable evidence that hallucinogen use causes chromosome damage or genetic defects.[22]

MARIJUANA

Marijuana, referred to as "reefer," "pot," "grass," or "weed," remains the most commonly used illicit drug. In 1995, an estimated 9.8 million Americans had used marijuana or hashish within the last month. This represents 4.7% of the population aged 12 and older.[4] *Cannabis sativa*, the marijuana plant, has been produced with increasingly sophisticated growing techniques to produce a plant of greater potency.[21] The principal psychoactive component of marijuana is THC. Hashish, the dried resin of the top of the plant, is much more potent than the plant itself.

Marijuana has been widely used and is believed by many to be a relatively harmless, nonaddictive intoxicant. Chronic low doses of marijuana are not usually associated with significant physical withdrawal upon abrupt discontinuation, but many chronic users exhibit compulsive drug-seeking and drug-use behavior characteristic of addiction or dependence. As experience with the drug is gained, it is clear that marijuana is far from harmless. Acutely, marijuana has many of the effects of alcohol—sedation, a decrease in reactivity and ability to perform complex tasks, and disinhibition. Marijuana also causes hallucinations with high enough doses. Chronic use is associated with all of the risks of tobacco smoking, although marijuana smokers are commonly also tobacco smokers and thus differentiation of effects is often difficult. Endocrine effects including amenorrhea, decreased testosterone production, and inhibition of spermatogenesis have been demonstrated. Although controversial, marijuana is associated with an amotivational syndrome, characterized by a behavioral pattern of apathy, dullness, impaired judgment, decreased concentration and memory, loss of interest in personal hygiene, and a general reduction of goal-directed behavior.[50]

The signs and symptoms of marijuana intoxication are summarized in Table 62–6. Cardiovascular effects and reddened conjunctivae are the most prominent physical effects with acute use (tachycardia, increased blood pressure with large orthostatic changes). Although the duration of effect of marijuana may be only several hours, THC is detectable upon toxicologic screening for up to 4 to 5 weeks, especially in chronic users.[22]

TABLE 62–6. Signs and Symptoms of Marijuana Intoxication

Tachycardia	Euphoria
Conjunctival congestion	Sensory intensification
Increased appetite	Apathy
Dry mouth	Hallucinations

It has been observed that some people experience a more "pleasurable" effect from marijuana than others, and researchers believe that this is heavily influenced by heredity.[51] A recent study[52] demonstrated that identical male twins were more likely than nonidentical male twins to report similar responses to marijuana use, indicating a genetic basis for their sensations.

Environmental factors such as the availability of marijuana, expectations about how the drug would affect them, the influence of friends and social contacts, and other factors that would be different even for identical twins were also found to have an important effect; however, it was also discovered that the twins' shared or family environment before age 18 had no detectable influence on their response to marijuana.

Taking the environmental and genetic influences together, these results suggest that although exposure to marijuana by factors such as social contacts are important, there are individual differences, perhaps in the brain's reward system, associated with genetic factors that influence whether one will continue using marijuana.

These physiologic differences coupled with the observation that individuals who find pleasure in using marijuana are more likely to use it repeatedly lead to the conclusion that heredity plays a significant role in determining susceptibility to continuing marijuana abuse.

Researchers have found that the daily use of one to three marijuana joints appears to produce approximately the same lung damage and potential cancer risk as smoking five times as many cigarettes.[53] The study results suggest that the way smokers inhale marijuana, in addition to its chemical composition, increases the adverse physical effects. The study findings refute the argument that marijuana is safer than tobacco because users smoke only a few joints a day.

Research findings[54] indicate that smoking marijuana while shooting up cocaine has the potential to cause severe increases in heart rate and blood pressure. In this study, experienced marijuana and cocaine users were given marijuana alone, cocaine alone, and then a combination of both. The heart rate of the subjects in the study increased 29 beats per minute with marijuana alone and 32 beats per minute with cocaine alone. When the drugs were given together, the heart rate increased by 49 beats per minute, and the increased rate persisted for a longer time. In normal circumstances, an individual may smoke marijuana and inject cocaine and then do something physically stressful that may significantly increase risks of overload on the cardiovascular system.

A series of in-depth case studies[55] by a research team at the Center for Psychosocial Studies in New York found that adults who smoked marijuana daily believed it helped them function better, improving self-awareness and relationships with others. However, researchers found that users were more willing to tolerate problems, suggesting that the drug served as a buffer for those who would rather avoid confronting problems than make changes that might increase their satisfaction with life. The study indicated that these subjects used marijuana to avoid dealing with their difficulties, and the avoidance inevitably made their problems worse.

In 1988, it was discovered that the membranes of certain nerve cells contain protein receptors that bind THC. Once securely in place, THC triggers a series of cellular reactions that ultimately lead to the high that users experience when they smoke a marijuana cigarette.[56] It was reasoned that an endogenous THC-like compound must exist and bind to these receptors. In 1992, researchers identified a naturally occurring chemical in the body that binds to these same receptors. Named anandamide, this compound behaves chemically like THC.[57] Studies will continue with anandamide to understand how it interacts with THC receptors to affect memory, movement, hunger, pain, and other functions that are altered by marijuana use.

The issue of whether or not marijuana use is a "gateway" to the use of other drugs has been hotly debated for many years. Very recent research shows that long-term use of marijuana produces changes in the brain that are similar to those seen after long-term use of other major drugs of abuse such as cocaine, heroin, and alcohol. Moreover, these changes may increase a user's vulnerability to addiction to other abusable drugs by "priming" the brain to be more easily changed by drugs in the future.[58]

A substantial number of chronic, high-dose marijuana users become addicted, and previous research with animals has shown that stopping heavy marijuana use suddenly can cause distinct withdrawal symptoms in these individuals.

The purpose of the above referenced study was to discover whether corticotropin-releasing factor (CRF), a brain chemical that increases during emotional times and periods of stress, plays a role in dependence on cannabis. Earlier studies have suggested that CRF plays a role in the neurobiologic and behavioral effects of withdrawal from addiction to cocaine, alcohol, and opiates, and possibly a role in drug dependence in general.[58]

Rats were injected with HU-210, a potent substance that mimics the effects of marijuana. An analysis of the rats' brains showed that one injection of HU-210 reduced the release of CRF in the amygdala, that part of the brain that controls emotions.[58]

After 14 days of HU-210 treatment, the researchers induced drug withdrawal by injecting rats with the antagonist SR 141716A, a substance that blocks many effects of marijuana. The marijuana-treated rats showed many withdrawal symptoms after marijuana antagonist injection. Moreover, these rats showed an increased release of CRF at the same time they demonstrated dramatic behavioral withdrawal symptoms. Importantly, the specific brain areas that were activated during cannabinoid withdrawal are quite active during withdrawal from other drugs of abuse and play a key role in stress responses in general.[58]

Researchers believe that the finding from this and other studies that long-term exposure to cannabinoids can produce changes in the brain that resemble those associated with other major drugs of abuse suggests that addiction to one drug may make a person more vulnerable to abuse and addiction to other drugs. Cannabinoid abuse, by activating CRF mechanisms, may lead to a subtle disruption of brain processes that are then "primed" for further and easier disruption by other drugs of abuse.[58]

INHALANTS

Inhalation of organic solvents including gasoline, glue, aerosols, amyl nitrite, and nitrous oxide has remained fairly constant over the past few years. Approximately 5.7% of persons over age 12 have tried inhalant drugs.[4] According to the Monitoring the Future Study, in 1996 21% of 8th graders reported having used inhalants at least once.[5]

Inhalants are CNS depressants, and symptoms of intoxication are similar to those of alcohol. Intoxication is often accompanied by headache and nausea, and users may experience hallucinations and delusions. The most serious physical risk of acute use is sudden death, usually from cardiac arrhythmias. Some users die from suffocation by plastic bags that contain the solvent. With chronic use, the drugs are toxic to virtually all organ systems. Psychological impairment, impaired pulmonary, renal, and hepatic function; neuropathies; encephalopathy; and brain damage have all been observed.[59]

MECHANISMS OF TOLERANCE, DEPENDENCE, AND WITHDRAWAL

Many factors influence the development of drug dependence. As with any disease, a susceptible host must be combined with favorable conditions. Western society is unquestionably drug oriented. Advertising encourages the reward of good behavior and productivity by the use of alcohol, tobacco, and caffeine.

Drug dependence depends on the reinforcing properties of the drug being used (the drug satisfies a need that demands repetition). Drug dependence most likely evolves in a phasic manner. The euphoriant or other pleasant properties of a drug act initially as reinforcers of drug-seeking behavior; but as tolerance develops, the pleasant effects of the drug are reduced, and higher doses are required to produce the same desirable feelings. Also, the user becomes aware of the need to avoid the pain and discomfort associated with the abstinence syndrome, or drug withdrawal. Many drug-dependent individuals state that their principal motivation for drug use turns relatively quickly from seeking of pleasurable effects to avoidance of unpleasant effects.[60]

Mechanisms of physical dependence involve homeostasis. Drugs disturb biochemical and physiologic systems, which adapt to reduce those effects. Such compensatory adaptation leads to the development of tolerance. Therefore, when the drug is withdrawn, the compensatory changes dominate, and the user experiences withdrawal symptoms. The clinical manifestations of withdrawal syndromes are generally opposite to those effects produced by the drugs. In many cases, the disturbance in homeostatic mechanisms may be long lasting. Withdrawal may consist of an acute, relatively short phase lasting several days, followed by a more subacute, protracted withdrawal syndrome. Protracted withdrawal has been most consistently reported for alcohol and opiates. Opiate dependence, for example, is associated with a "conditioned abstinence syndrome" lasting up to several months or longer after cessation of intake and may be precipitated by environmental stimuli previously associated with drug use.[60] Opiate-dependent individuals have reported the onset of physical withdrawal symptoms after merely coming into contact with their previous environment (e.g., the user's neighborhood, the sight of heroin, or the observation of other individuals using drugs). Conditioned abstinence may be described as a heightened sensitivity to stimuli, abnormal autonomic responses, dysphoria, and intense craving for the effects of the drug.

There are two types of physiologic tolerance to drugs.[22] The first, dispositional tolerance, also called *metabolic* or *pharmacokinetic tolerance,* results from changes in the pharmacokinetics of drugs. Usually, this type of tolerance is related to increased metabolism. Examples of drugs associated with dispositional tolerance are barbiturates and alcohol. The second type of tolerance is pharmacodynamic tolerance, also known as a *cellular* or *functional tolerance.* Pharmacodynamic tolerance results from adaptive changes at the site of action of drugs, such as changes in receptor system binding sensitivity. Examples of drugs that exhibit pharmacodynamic tolerance are alcohol and the opiates.

TOLERANCE TO CNS DEPRESSANTS

The principal mechanism of barbiturate tolerance appears to be dispositional.[22] All barbiturates are potent inducers of liver enzymes and induce their own metabolism. Tolerance to benzodiazepines appears to be primarily pharmacodynamic.[22] The precise cellular mechanism of tolerance to benzodiazepines is not clear, but may be a decrease in the number or sensitivity of benzodiazepine receptors.

Tolerance to opiates appears to be pharmacodynamic.[22] The primary center in the brain for both opiate and noradrenergic-mediated neurons appears to be the locus coeruleus in the midbrain. Neurons from the locus coeruleus project throughout the cerebral cortex. Although there are multiple subtypes of opiate receptors, the opiate receptor appears to be primarily a presynaptic receptor and has an inhibitory effect on the noradrenergic nerve terminal (i.e., stimulation of the presynaptic opiate receptor inhibits neuronal release of norepinephrine). The endogenous ligand for the opiate receptor is enkephalin. Another presynaptic receptor that serves as an inhibitory receptor for noradrenergic activity is the α_2-adrenergic receptor.[61] The presynaptic α_2 receptor is a norepinephrine autoreceptor.

Chronic use of exogenous opiates, such as heroin, hydromorphone, and methadone, causes a decrease in production of the endogenous substance enkephalin, just as administration of exogenous corticosteroids causes a decrease in endogenous production of cortisol. Greater than normal activity at the receptor is associated with a compensatory decrease in the binding sensitivity of the opiate receptor system, also known as down-regulation. Because the opiate receptor is inhibitory to noradrenergic activity, a down-regulation effect would diminish the effect of opiates; thus, larger doses would be required to achieve the same degree of inhibition of noradrenergic activity. Abrupt discontinuation of exogenous opiates produces a down-regulated inhibitory opiate receptor system in the presence of diminished levels of endogenous ligand, enkephalin. Therefore, opiate withdrawal can be conceptualized as a syndrome of noradrenergic hyperactivity.[62]

TOLERANCE TO CNS STIMULANTS

Tolerance to the stimulants, including cocaine, is pharmacodynamic in nature,[22] but the precise cellular mechanism is unclear. Tolerance to different pharmacologic effects of stimulants develops at different rates. Tolerance to appetite suppression, for example, develops within days to weeks, whereas tolerance to the euphoric effects and increased alertness develops more slowly. A type of reverse pharmacodynamic tolerance, kindling, was described earlier and has been observed with both cocaine and amphetamines. The neuropharmacology of cocaine and amphetamine withdrawal is not well understood; however, such withdrawal effects as depression, fatigue, and increased sleep and appetite are the opposite of the usual effects of the drug, as is the case with most drugs. Chronic cocaine use may cause a catecholamine depletion in the brain.

Tolerance develops to phencyclidine and the LSD-type hallucinogens, although the mechanisms are not clearly understood. Phencyclidine may be associated with a dispositional tolerance. Tolerance to marijuana appears to be more pharmacodynamic than dispositional, although marijuana is known to induce microsomal liver enzymes.[63] The mechanism of tolerance to inhalants is not understood.

▶ TREATMENT: Substance-Related Disorders

ACUTE DRUG INTOXICATION

Treatment of drug intoxication, summarized in Table 62–7, is primarily supportive, and vital functions are maintained while waiting for the drug to be eliminated. When absolutely necessary, physical restraint may be required temporarily while a diagnostic evaluation is initiated to rule out other causes for the behavior (e.g., metabolic or fluid and electrolyte disturbances). Whenever possible, drug therapy should be avoided, because psychotropic drug therapy has the potential for worsening a toxic reaction to another psychoactive agent; however, when patients are agitated,

TABLE 62–7. Treatment of Substance Intoxication

Drug Class	Pharmacologic Therapy	Nonpharmacologic Therapy
Benzodiazepines	Flumazenil 0.1–0.2 mg/min IV up to 1 mg	Support vital functions
Alcohol, barbiturates, and sedative–hypnotics (nonbenzodiazepines)	None	Support vital functions
Opiates	Naloxone 0.4–2.0 mg IV every 3 min	Support vital functions
Cocaine and other CNS stimulants	Lorazepam 2–4 mg IM q 30 min to 6 h prn agitation Haloperidol 2–5 mg (or other antipsychotic agent) every 30 min to 6 h prn psychotic behavior	Monitor cardiac function
Hallucinogens, marijuana, and inhalants	Lorazepam and/or haloperidol as above	Reassurance; "talk-down therapy"; support vital functions
Phencyclidine	Lorazepam and/or haloperidol as above	Minimize sensory input

combative, assaultive, hallucinatory, or delusional, drug therapy may be required. Drug therapy may also be indicated in the treatment of an acute, potentially fatal drug overdose. Toxicology screens are useful in the evaluation and treatment process, but knowledge of the metabolism of the suspected drug and its excretion patterns is important for proper interpretation of test results. When toxicology screens are desired, blood or urine should be collected immediately upon the patient's arrival.

For alcohol and barbiturate intoxication, supportive treatment is the rule. For benzodiazepine intoxication, the benzodiazepine antagonist flumazenil (Mazicon, Roche) can be used to reverse toxic effects. It is not indicated in all cases of suspected drug overdosage, however, and is specifically contraindicated in cases in which cyclic antidepressant involvement is known or suspected because of the risk of seizures. In addition, it should be used with caution in patients when benzodiazepine physical dependence is suspected because of the risks of induction of benzodiazepine withdrawal.[64] In the case of opiate intoxication, if the patient is unconscious and respiration is depressed, the opiate antagonist naloxone (Narcan, DuPont) can be used to revive the patient. The usual dosage for naloxone in acute opiate toxicity is 0.4 to 2.0 mg intravenously, given approximately every 3 minutes as necessary.[65] Although naloxone is effective in reversing opiate overdose, it may also precipitate physical withdrawal in physically dependent patients. Patients who fail to respond to a total dosage of 10 mg of naloxone probably have a cause of acute intoxication other than an opiate.

Intoxication with stimulants, including cocaine, is treated pharmacologically only if the patient is overtly psychotic and agitated. Injectable benzodiazepines, usually lorazepam (Ativan, Wyeth) 2 to 4 mg IM every 30 minutes to 6 hours as necessary, can be used for agitation. As a backup to lorazepam, antipsychotic drugs can be used on a short-term basis, primarily in patients with psychotic symptoms, and usually at relatively low doses, such as haloperidol (Haldol, McNeil) 2 to 5 mg IM every 30 minutes to 6 hours as necessary, followed by 5 to 15 mg orally per day in single or divided doses if the patient is still psychotic after initial treatment.[65] Cardiovascular complications are treated symptomatically with antiarrhythmic agents or other interventions as necessary. Seizures are generally treated supportively. Intravenous lorazepam or diazepam can be used if seizures progress to status epilepticus.

Hallucinogen intoxication is treated in a manner similar to stimulant intoxication. Drug therapy can often be avoided, because patients may respond to careful reassurance, or so-called talk-down therapy. When necessary, short-term antianxiety and/or antipsychotic drug therapy can be used as described previously. The same approach applies to marijuana and inhalant intoxication.

Phencyclidine intoxication is more unpredictable and more difficult to treat than other psychosis-producing drugs. Most clinicians suggest that sensory input be minimized to the extent possible; thus, "talk-down therapy" is not recommended and may in fact make the patient worse. If phencyclidine intoxication is suspected, patients should be left alone in a quiet, dimly lit room. If behavior is uncontrollable, antianxiety and/or antipsychotic drug therapy may be necessary.

WITHDRAWAL

Treatment of drug withdrawal is the primary indication for drug therapy in substance-related disorders. Goals of drug therapy include prevention of progression of withdrawal to life-threatening severity, enabling the patient to be sufficiently comfortable and functional in order to participate in a behavioral treatment program, and supportive drug therapy. The clinician should remember that withdrawal is usually part of a substance dependence disorder. Patients with drug dependence generally cope with almost any stress through the use of a drug. In drug therapy for withdrawal, it is important to avoid reinforcing the patient's drug-seeking and drug-use behavior to the extent possible. Drug withdrawal in the best of circumstances is uncomfortable. Patients must be educated to deal with the stress of withdrawal without seeking drugs. The use of drugs as needed for anxiety or insomnia should be avoided. Treatment of drug withdrawal is summarized in Table 62–8.

CNS DEPRESSANT WITHDRAWAL

Benzodiazepines

Treatment of benzodiazepine withdrawal is very similar to the treatment of alcohol withdrawal, and the same drugs and dosages may be used.[15] The major difference in management is the length of treatment. The onset of withdrawal symptoms in patients physically dependent on the long-acting benzodiazepines may be delayed up to 7 days after discontinuation of the drug. A common approach in detoxification of such patients is to initiate treatment at usual dosages (chlordiazepoxide 50 mg three times a day; lorazepam 2 mg three times a day) and to maintain the initial dosage for 5 days, with gradual tapering over an additional 5 days. Detoxification in patients physically dependent on shorter-acting benzodiazepines is similar to treatment of alcohol withdrawal. Among the benzodiazepines, alprazolam has been suggested to be more difficult to taper and discontinue than the other benzodiazepines.[66] Whether the difficulty is related to a different patient population commonly treated with alprazolam (e.g., panic disorder) or to intrinsic differences between alprazolam and other benzodiazepines is not clear. A longer, more gradual taper of the benzodiazepine used for detoxification may be needed. With all benzodiazepines, protracted minor abstinence symptoms—such as anxiety, insomnia, irritability, sensitivity to

TABLE 62–8. Treatment of Withdrawal From Some Common Drugs of Abuse

Drug or Drug Class	Pharmacologic Therapy
Benzodiazepines	
Short to intermediate acting	Chlordiazepoxide 50 mg tid-qid or lorazepam 2 mg tid-qid; taper over 5-7 d
Long acting	Chlordiazepoxide 50 mg tid-qid or lorazepam 2 mg tid-qid; taper over additional 5-7 d
Barbiturates	Pentobarbital tolerance test (see text); initial detoxification at upper limit of tolerance test; decrease dosage by 100 mg every 2–3 d
Opiates	Methadone 20–80 mg PO daily; taper by 5–10 mg daily or clonidine 2 μg/kg tid × 7 d; taper over additional 3 d
Mixed-substance withdrawal	
Drugs are cross-tolerant	Detoxify according to treatment for longer-acting drug used
Drugs are not cross-tolerant	Detoxify from one drug while maintaining second drug (cross-tolerant drugs), then detoxify from second drug
CNS stimulants	Supportive treatment only; pharmacotherapy often not used; bromocriptine 2.5 mg tid or higher may be used for severe craving associated with cocaine withdrawal

light and sound, and muscle spasms—may remain for several weeks in patients with a history of long exposure, even after the acute phase of benzodiazepine withdrawal is complete. Clonidine and CBZ have been used in the treatment of benzodiazepine withdrawal, but are not considered first-line treatments.

Barbiturates and Other Sedative–Hypnotic Drugs

Because of the unpredictability and frequently greater severity of withdrawal from barbiturates and other sedative–hypnotic drugs, it is useful to attempt to determine the patient's level of tolerance before initiating detoxification. Tolerance testing is most often done with pentobarbital (Nembutal, Abbott).[22] The patient is given a single dose of 200 mg of pentobarbital orally and then is observed for 2 to 3 hours for signs of mild intoxication, including sedation, slurred speech, ataxia, and nystagmus. Additional doses are given until one or more signs of intoxication are observed. The total dosage of pentobarbital required to reach the lower levels of the patient's limit of tolerability can be used as an approximate initial daily starting dosage for detoxification. The daily dosage can be reduced in decrements of 100 mg every third day at first, then every other day if the patient tolerates initial dosage reductions without difficulty. The reliability of the test is influenced by the dosage and interval since ingestion of the sedative drug prior to administering the tolerance test. Monitoring parameters for barbiturate detoxification are the same as for alcohol and benzodiazepine detoxification.

Opiates

Opiate withdrawal is not life threatening unless there is a concurrent life-threatening medical condition. Although most patients complain of symptoms of withdrawal, such as cramping or insomnia, these symptoms are tolerable, and initiation of drug therapy may be avoided in many cases. Because opiate withdrawal is not life threatening, observable signs of withdrawal, such as mydriasis, pilomotor erection, diaphoresis, or diarrhea, should be noted before initiation of drug therapy. Unnecessary detoxification with drugs, especially methadone, should be avoided if possible.

The conventional drug therapy for opiate withdrawal has been methadone, a synthetic opiate. Usual starting dosages have been 20 to 80 mg/d orally; but treatment of withdrawal from heroin usually requires no more than 20 mg of methadone, owing to the low purity of street heroin. The dosage of methadone can be tapered in decrements of 5 to 10 mg/d until discontinued. Most patients in withdrawal continue to complain of mild symptoms after detoxification is completed. Some patients who are unable to discontinue methadone completely or habitually return to drug use when methadone is discontinued are placed in methadone-maintenance treatment programs and receive methadone chronically.[22] LAAM (levomethadyl acetate hydrochloride) (Orlaam, Biometric Research Institute) was approved by the Food and Drug Administration (FDA) in 1993 as a potential alternative to methadone maintenance. LAAM forms two long-acting metabolites, which allow three times a week dosing.[67]

Heroin-dependent individuals reduced their use of heroin by nearly 90% after 16 weeks of LAAM treatment.[68] In this first clinical trial comparing different LAAM doses in the treatment of opiate addiction, researchers found that heroin use was reduced for individuals taking a regimen of low, medium, or high doses of LAAM, with effectiveness increasing substantially at the highest dose. This suggests treatment programs need to get patients to the most effective dosage levels as quickly as possible.[68]

Women and men responded equally well to LAAM, and high doses were found to be safe for both male and female heroin addicts. The 17-week study was conducted with 180 heroin-dependent volunteers (70 females, 110 males).[68]

When approved by the FDA, LAAM was the first new drug treatment medication approved in more than two decades.[69] LAAM's main advantage over methadone, widely used in heroin treatment, is that its effects last long enough so that it need be taken only three times per week. Methadone needs to be taken daily, requiring either a daily trip to a clinic or take-home dosages.

An increasingly accepted method of opiate detoxification is the use of clonidine. Use of clonidine can attenuate the noradrenergic hyperactivity of opiate withdrawal without interfering significantly with activity at the opiate receptors. Production of enkephalin and the return of receptors to normal levels of sensitivity can occur as rapidly as possible. Advantages of detoxification with clonidine include a somewhat more rapid detoxification and an absence of the euphoria sometimes observed with methadone.[22,62,70]

Clonidine is often given in an initial dosage of 6 μg/kg/d, in three divided doses. Dosage can be increased if necessary to as high as 17 μg/kg/d. The patient is maintained on the same dosage for 7 days, which is then tapered and discontinued over the next 3 days. A common clonidine side effect is orthostatic hypotension, and the patient's blood pressure should be monitored in the supine and standing positions at least daily. If blood pressure drops to an unacceptably low level (e.g., lying systolic blood pressure less than 90 mm Hg), the dose should be held. If blood pressure has risen in time for the next dose, clonidine can be resumed. Clonidine for treatment of opiate withdrawal has also been administered transdermally, but this method has not been well studied.

Less well established opiate detoxification strategies include the combination of clonidine and naltrexone. Naltrexone, an opiate antagonist, is used to rapidly induce withdrawal that is then attenuated with clonidine. The potential advantage of this method is the shortening of detoxification to as little as 2 days. A similar detoxification regimen using buprenorphine, a partial opiate agonist, and naltrexone has been tried.[70] Buprenorphine has been used as an alternative to methadone maintenance, as well.[71]

WITHDRAWAL FROM OTHER SUBSTANCES

Withdrawal from other drugs, including cocaine and other stimulants, is primarily supportive. Pharmacotherapy has, however, recently assumed a greater role in treating cocaine withdrawal and dependence. Bromocriptine (Parlodel, Sandoz), a dopamine antagonist at low dosages and agonist at high dosages, is usually used in the treatment of parkinsonism and hyperprolactinemia and has been used to treat cocaine withdrawal symptoms and to reduce the craving for cocaine.[72] Use of bromocriptine is based on the hypothesis that chronic use of cocaine causes dopamine depletion; therefore, higher dosages should be used (i.e., 2.5 mg three times daily or higher). Use is generally short term.

MIXED SUBSTANCE ABUSE

Many drug users practice polypharmacy, and it is common for a patient to experience withdrawal from more than one drug. Treatment of withdrawal depends on the individual drug combination. In withdrawal from diazepam and alcohol (cross-tolerant drugs), treatment for withdrawal from diazepam, the longer acting of the two drugs, will also concurrently treat alcohol withdrawal. If the drugs are not cross-tolerant (e.g., alcohol and opiates), withdrawal from each drug must be treated separately. While detoxification for one drug is under way, treatment with the second drug (or a drug that is cross-tolerant to the second drug) must be maintained. When detoxification from the first drug is complete, the second drug can be tapered and discontinued according to usual procedures.

SUBSTANCE DEPENDENCE

The treatment of drug dependence, or addiction, is primarily behavioral. The patient is generally taught that complete abstinence is the only realistic alternative to a life of uncontrollable drug use and despair that will ultimately end in death, and that there is no intermediate, controllable level of drinking or use of another drug. However, complete and permanent abstinence as the sole route to recovery is controversial. There may be an extremely few individuals who can return to controllable levels of drinking alcohol, but it is impossible to predict who these individuals are; thus, most treatment programs continue to advocate complete abstinence. The prospect of life without alcohol or other drugs is incomprehensible to many patients. Entry into treatment is often facilitated by some type of leverage that the drug-dependent person associates with negative consequences, such as potential loss of job, divorce, legal problems, or deteriorating physical health. Early treatment is directed at penetrating the denial of a problem that is always present. The patient must be educated as to the disease of addiction, the effects of drugs, and the permanence of the condition.

In recent years, there has been a trend toward outpatient treatment for drug dependence, due in part to cost-containment efforts. Inpatient treatment programs can cost as much as $20,000 for a 4-week stay. When withdrawal symptoms are mild to moderate and there are no other medical indications for hospitalization, outpatient treatment may be an attractive alternative to inpatient treatment. One critical criterion for outpatient treatment is the patient's compliance with complete abstinence from the dependence producing drug during the treatment experience.

Families must be involved in treatment. The course of the patient's illness often has a devastating effect on other family members. Severely depleted self-esteem, denial of the family member's addiction, feelings of responsibility for the family member's drug use, and other behaviors that parallel the addiction process are often present. Treatment must be a lifelong process. Aftercare, or what is now being called continued care, should include regular and frequent treatment in some form. Most drug-dependence treatment programs embrace a treatment approach based on AA. AA is one of the most successful of all self-help groups. Associated groups include Alanon (a group for family members of alcoholics), NA (self-help groups based on the AA concept for users of other drugs), Overeaters Anonymous (a group for individuals with eating disorders), Gamblers Anonymous, and several other similar programs. Among chemically dependent health care professionals, treatment that incorporates both AA and peer-led self-help groups may be most effective.[73]

COEXISTENT DRUG DEPENDENCE AND PSYCHIATRIC DISORDERS: THE DUAL DIAGNOSIS PATIENT

Although the majority of chemical dependence is primary (no evidence of a preexisting major psychiatric problem prior to the first life problem related to addiction), a significant percentage, up to 50%, coexists with another psychiatric disorder.[74] One way to conceptualize this is that there are two broad categories of persons who receive diagnoses of two or more conditions that occur together. In one type, chemical dependence might be secondary to a complication of a psychiatric disorder. In these individuals, the onset of the psychiatric disorder significantly predated the regular abuse of substances.

A second type has two concurrent primary diagnoses, chemical dependence and a psychiatric disorder. Recognition of this type of patient has been increasing in recent years. Fifty-five percent of male schizophrenics were found to abuse some type of drug, with alcohol, cocaine, and marijuana comprising 88% of the total drug use.[75] In a study of 401 involuntarily hospitalized patients, however, only 8% of the patients with schizophrenia had a positive urine screen.[76] This points out the frequently profound variation among studies that attempt to examine the prevalence of comorbid psychiatric disorders in substance abusers due to the variations in diagnostic methodology, examiner bias, study design, study length, and patient population.[77,78]

When dual problems of a psychiatric disorder and substance use disorder coexist, they are interactive and may be interdependent. This may be particularly true when personality disorder and substance abuse or dependence coexist.[79] Of the personality disorders, antisocial personality disorder (APD) has been subject to the most extensive validity and reliability testing in patients with substance abuse.[77] Even so, there continues to be controversy about the reliability and stability in the APD diagnosis, particularly when substance abuse is involved. The overall prevalence of substance dependence in clinical psychiatric settings is about 50%, but the prevalence of psychiatric disorders in addiction treatment populations is much lower, approximating levels found in the general population.[78]

Treatment of the patient with coexisting substance use and psychiatric disorders involves initial treatment of the substance use disorder, especially when the patient is in physical withdrawal. If symptoms of psychiatric disorder continue after the patient has been drug free for a minimum of 2 weeks, then treatment of the psychiatric disorder must be considered. Psychotropic drug therapy appropriate to the diagnosis may be indicated. Improved relations between psychiatrists and chemical-dependence treatment professionals have led to cooperative efforts to treat all aspects of the patient's illness.

RECOGNIZING ADOLESCENT DRUG ABUSE AND DEPENDENCY

Early recognition of substance abuse problems is a key to successful treatment, especially in young people. Often parents and other family members are unaware that their adolescent may be involved with drugs until it reaches crisis proportions. The checklist in Appendix 62–1 can be used to identify an underlying drug problem, keeping in mind that some of these behaviors can be present even without involvement with drugs.

DRUG ABUSE INFORMATION AND THE INTERNET

With the recent growth of the Internet, information about drug abuse is available with a click of the mouse. Many web sites have been developed to provide factual, reliable information covering a wide array of topics related to abuse of chemical substances. Unfortunately, there are numerous sites where incomplete, misleading, blatantly incorrect or even dangerous information can be found. Browsing just a few newsgroups, web sites, or listserves shows that much of the information is unreliable. It may be useful for the clinician working in the substance area to periodically check the "pro-drug" web sites to see what is being discussed. In this manner, the practitioner can remain up to date on the latest drug fads and can better respond to questions from clients. Appendix 62–1 contains web addresses useful in providing drug abuse prevention and treatment information to professionals and laypersons alike.

CONCLUSIONS

Substance use disorders remain one of the great public health issues of contemporary society. Dependence on drugs is a powerful emotional and political issue. Because we live in a chemically oriented society, everyone is affected in some way by drug abuse and drug dependence. Health care professionals must be particularly vigilant for problems associated with drug use, not only for our patients, but also for ourselves.

REFERENCES

1. Institute for Health Policy, Brandeis University. Substance Abuse: The Nation's Number One Health Problem. Key Indicators for Policy. Princeton, Robert Wood Johnson Foundation, 1993.
2. Brown LS. Federal drug policy and terminolgoy: Foes or allies? J Natl Med Assoc 1980;72:575–581.
3. Rinaldi RC, Steindler EM, Wilford BB, Goodwin D. Clarification and standardization of substance abuse terminology. JAMA 1988;259: 555–557.
4. National Household Survey on Drug Abuse. Rockville, MD, U.S. Department of Health and Human Services, Substance Abuse and Mental Health Services Administration, 1997.
5. Monitoring the Future Study: National High School Senior Drug Abuse Survey. Rockville, MD, US Department of Health and Human Services, National Institute on Drug Abuse, 1997.
6. Substance Abuse and Mental Health Services Administration, Office of Applied Studies, Drug Abuse Warning Network. Advance Report no. 18, 1997.
7. National Center on Addiction and Substance Abuse at Columbia University. Substance Abuse and Urban America: Its Impact on an American City. New York, February 1996.
8. National Center on Addiction and Substance Abuse at Columbia University. Substance Abuse and Federal Entitlement Programs. New York, February 1995.
9. National Center on Addiction and Substance Abuse at Columbia University. The Cost of Substance Abuse to America's Health Care System: Medicaid. New York, July 1993.
10. National Center on Addiction and Substance Abuse at Columbia University. The Cost of Substance Abuse to America's Health Care System: Medicare. New York, May 1994.
11. National Center on Addiction and Substance Abuse at Columbia University. Behind Bars: Substance Abuse and America's Prison Population. New York, January 1998.
12. Woods JH, Winger G. Abuse liability of flunitrazepam. J Clin Psychopharmacol 1997;17(suppl 2):1S–57S.
13. Cavallaro R, Regazzetti MG, Covelli G, Smeraldi E. Tolerance and withdrawal with zolpidem. Lancet 1993;342:868–869.
14. Rall TW. Hypnotics and sedatives; ethanol. In: Gilman AG, Rall TW, Nies AS, Taylor P, eds: The Pharmacological Basis of Therapeutics, 8th ed. New York, Pergamon, 1990:345.
15. Smith DE, Wesson DR. Benzodiazepines and other sedative-hypnotics. In: Galanter M, Kleber HD, eds. Textbook of Substance Abuse Treatment. Washington, DC, American Psychiatric Press, 1994:179.
16. Ledray LE. Date rape drug alert. J Emerg Nurs 1996;22:80.
17. Vayer P, Mandel P, Maitre M. Gamma-hydroxy butyrate, a possible neurotransmitter. Life Sci 1987;41:1547–1557.
18. CDC. Gamma Hydroxy Butyrate Use—New York and Texas, 1995–1996. MMWR 1997;46:281–283.
19. CDC. Multistate outbreak of poisonings associated with illicit use of gamma hydroxy butyrate. MMWR 1990;39:861–863.
20. Mamelak M. Gammahydroxybutyrate: An endogenous regulator of energy metabolism. Neurosci Biobehav Rev 1989;13:187–198.
21. Drugs of Abuse, Drug Enforcement Administration, Department of Justice. Washington DC, U.S. Government Printing Office, 1996.
22. Jaffe JH. Drug addiction and drug abuse. In: Gilman AG, Rall TW, Nies AS, Taylor P, eds. The Pharmacological Basis of Therapeutics, 8th ed. New York, Pergamon, 1990:522.
23. American Psychiatric Association. Diagnostic and Statistical Manual of Mental Disorders, 4th ed (DSM-IV). Washington, DC, American Psychiatric Press, 1994.

24. U.S. Department of Justice, Drug Enforcement Administration. The Supply of Illicit Drugs to the United States. National Narcotics Intelligence, Consumers Committee, August 1996.
25. Gold MS, Miller NS, Jonas JM. Cocaine (and crack): Neurobiology. In: Lowinson JH, Ruiz P, Millman RB, Langrod JG, eds. Substance Abuse: A Comprehensive Textbook, 2nd ed. Baltimore, Williams & Wilkins, 1992:222.
26. Hearn WL, Flynn DD, Hime GW, et al. Cocaethylene: A unique cocaine metabolite displays high affinity for the dopamine transporter. J Neurochem 1991;56:698–701.
27. Hearn WL, Rose W, Wagner J, et al. Cocaethylene is more potent than cocaine in mediating lethality. Pharmacol Biochem Behav 1991;3: 531–533.
28. Aigner TG, Balster RL. Choice behavior in rhesus monkeys: Cocaine versus food. Science 1978;201:534–535.
29. Van Dette JM, Cornish LA. Medical complications of illicit cocaine use. Clin Pharm 1989;8:401–411.
30. Brady DT, Lydiard RB, Malcolm R, Ballenger JC. Cocaine-induced psychosis. J Clin Psychiatry 1991;52:509–512.
31. Volkow ND, Wang GJ, Fischman MW, et al. Relationship between subjective effects of cocaine and dopamine transporter occupancy. Nature 1997;386:827–830.
32. Gatley SJ, Volkow ND, Chen R, et al. Displacement of RTI-55 from the dopamine transporter by cocaine. Eur J Pharmacol 1996;296:145–151.
33. Mendelson JH, Mello NK. Management of cocaine abuse and dependence. N Engl J Med 1996;334:965–972.
34. King GR, Ellinwood EH. Amphetamines and other stimulants. In: Lowinson JH, Ruiz P, Millman RB, Langrod JG, eds. Substance Abuse: A Comprehensive Textbook, 2nd ed. Baltimore, Williams & Wilkins, 1992:247.
35. Hibbs J, Perper J, Winek CL. An outbreak of designer drug—related deaths in Pennsylvania. JAMA 1991;265:1011–1013.
36. Janssen PA. The development of new synthetic narcotics. In: Estafanous FG, ed. Opioids in Anesthesia. Stoneham, MA, Butterworth, 1985:37–44.
37. Henderson GL. Fentanyl-related deaths: Demographics, circumstances, and toxicology of 112 cases. J Forensic Sci 1991;36:422–433.
38. Langston JW, Ballard P, Tetrus JW, Irwin I. Chronic Parkinsonism in humans due to a product of meperidine-analog synthesis. Science 1983;219:979–980.
39. Leads from the MMWR. Street-drug contaminant causing parkinsonism. JAMA 1984;252:331.
40. Miller NS, Gold MS. LSD and ecstasy: Pharmacology, phenomenology, and treatment. Psychiatr Ann 1994;24:131–133.
41. McCann VD, Ridenour A, ShahamY, et al. Evidence for serotonin neurotoxicity in recreational MDMA ("ecstacy") users: A controlled study. Soc Neurosci Abstr 1993;19:1169.
42. Seiden LS, Sabol KE. Methamphetamine and methylenedioxymethamphetamine neurotoxicity: Possible mechanisms of cell destruction. NIDA Res Monogr 1996;163:251–276.
43. Cuomo MJ, Dyment PG, Gammino VM . Increasing use of "ecstasy" (MDMA) and other hallucinogens on a college campus. J Am Coll Health 1994;42:271–274.
44. Barnes DM. Legal limbo for ecstasy. Science 1988;239:865.
45. Zukin SR, Zukin RS. Phencyclidine. In: Lowinson JH, Ruiz P, Millman RB, Langrod JG, eds. Substance Abuse: A Comprehensive Textbook, 2nd ed. Baltimore, Williams & Wilkins, 1992:290.
46. Ghoneim MM, Hinrichs JV, Mewaldt SP, Petersen RC. Ketamine: Behavioral effects of subanesthetic doses. J Clin Psychopharmacol 1985; 5:70–77.
47. Hofmann A. How LSD originated. J Psychedelic Drugs 1979;11: 53–60.
48. Glennon RA. Do classical hallucinogens act as 5-HT_2 agonists or antagonists? Neuropsychopharmacology 1990;3:509–517.
49. Ungerleider JT, Pechnick RN. Hallucinogens. In: Lowinson JH, Ruiz P, Millman RB, Langrod JG, eds. Substance Abuse: A Comprehensive Textbook, 2nd ed. Baltimore, Williams & Wilkins, 1992:280.
50. Grinspoon L, Bakalar JB. Marihuana. In: Lowinson JH, Ruiz P, Millman RB, eds. Substance Abuse: A Comprehensive Textbook, 2nd ed. Baltimore, Williams & Wilkins, 1992;236.
51. Lyons MJ, Toomey R, Meyer JM, et al. How do genes influence marijuana use? The role of subjective effects. Addiction 1997;92: 409–417.
52. Tsuang MT, Lyons MJ, Eisen SA, et al. Genetic influences on DSM-III-R drug abuse and dependence: A study of 3372 twin pairs. Am J Med Genet 1996;67:473–477.
53. Tashkin DP. Pulmonary complications of smoked substance abuse. West J Med 1990;152:525–530.
54. Foltin RW, Fischman MW, Pedroso JJ, Pearlson GD. Marijuana and cocaine interactions in humans: Cardiovascular consequences. Pharmacol Biochem Behav 1987;28:459–464.
55. Hendin H, Haas AP. The adaptive significance of chronic marijuana use for adolescents and adults. Adv Alcohol Subst Abuse 1985;4: 99–115.
56. Devane WA, Dysarz FA, Johnson MR, et al. Determination and characterization of a cannabinoid receptor in rat brain. Mol Pharmacol 1988;34:605–613.
57. Devane WA, Hanus L, Breuer A, et al. Isolation and structure of a brain constituent that binds to the cannabinoid receptor. Science 1992; 258:1946–1949.
58. Rodriguez de Fonseca F, Carrera MRA, Navarro M, et al. Activation of corticotropin-releasing factor in the limbic system during cannabinoid withdrawal. Science 1997;276:2050–2054.
59. Sharp CW, Rosenberg NL. Volatile substances. In: Lowinson JH, Ruiz P, Millman RB, Langrod JG, eds. Substance Abuse: A Comprehensive Textbook, 2nd ed. Baltimore, Williams & Wilkins, 1992:303.
60. Wikler A. Conditioning factors in opiate addiction and release. In: Wilner DI, Kossebaum GG, eds. Narcotics. New York, McGraw-Hill, 1965:85.
61. Lefkowitz RJ, Hoffman BB, Taylor P. Neurohumoral transmission: The autonomic and somatic motor nervous systems. In: Gilman AG, Rall TW, Nies AS, Taylor P, eds. The Pharmacological Basis of Therapeutics, 8th ed. New York, Pergamon, 1990:84.
62. Gold MS, Redmond DE, Kleber HD. Noradrenergic hyperactivity in opiate withdrawal supported by clonidine reversal of opiate withdrawal. Am J Psychiatry 1979;136:100–102.
63. Dewey WL. Cannabinoid pharmacology. Pharmacol Rev 1986;38: 151–178.
64. Hoffman EJ, Warren EW. Flumazenil: A benzodiazepine antagonist. Clin Pharm 1993;12:641–656.
65. Jaffe JH, Martin WR. Opioid analgesics and antagonists. In: Gilman AG, Rall TW, Nies AS, Taylor P, eds. The Pharmacological Basis of Therapeutics, 8th ed. New York, Pergamon, 1990:485.
66. Browne JL, Hauge KJ. A review of alprazolam withdrawal. Drug Intell Clin Pharm 1986;20:837–841.
67. Greenstein RA, Fudala PJ, O'Brien CP. Alternative pharmacotherapies for opiate addiction. In: Lowinson JH, Ruiz P, Millman RB, Langrod JG, eds. Substance Abuse: A Comprehensive Textbook; 2nd ed. Baltimore, Williams & Wilkins, 1992:562.
68. Eissenberg T, Bigelow GE, Strain EC, et al. Dose-related efficacy of levomethadyl acetate for treatment of opioid dependence. A randomized clinical trial. JAMA 1997;277:1945–1951.
69. Anonymous. LAAM—A long-acting methadone for treatment of heroin addiction. Med Lett Drugs Ther 1994;36:52.
70. Kleber HD. Opioids: Detoxification. In: Galanter M, Kleber HD, eds. Textbook of Substance Abuse Treatment. Washington, DC, American Psychiatric Press, 1994:191.
71. Strain EC, Stitzer ML, Liebson IA, Bigelow GE. Comparison of buprenorphine and methadone in the treatment of opioid dependence. Am J Psychiatry 1994;151:1025–1030.
72. Gold MS. Cocaine (and crack): Clinical aspects. In: Lowinson JH, Ruiz P, Millman RB, Langrod JG, eds. Substance Abuse: A Comprehensive Textbook, 2nd ed. Baltimore, Williams & Wilkins, 1992: 205.

73. Galanter M, Talbott D, Gallegos K, Rubenstone E. Combined Alcoholics Anonymous and professional care for addicted physicians. Am J Psychiatry 1990;147:64–68.
74. Schuckit MA. Drug and Alcohol Abuse: A Clinical Guide to Diagnosis and Treatment. 3rd ed. New York, Plenum, 1989:84.
75. Miller FT, Tenebaun JH. Drug abuse in schizophrenia. Hosp Commun Psychiatry 1989;40:847–849.
76. Sanguineti VR, Samuel SE. Comorbid substance abuse and recovery from acute psychiatric relapse. Hosp Commun Psychiatry 1993;44: 1073–1076.
77. Weiss RD, Mirin SM, Griffin ML. Methodological considerations in the diagnosis of coexisting psychiatric disorders in substance abusers. Br J Addict 1992;87:179–187.
78. Raskin VD, Miller NS. The epidemiology of the comorbidity of psychiatric and addictive disorders: A critical review. J Addict Dis 1993; 12:45–57.
79. Walker R. Substance abuse and B-cluster disorders, I. Understanding the dual diagnosis patient. J Psychoactive Drugs 1992;24:223–232.

APPENDIX 62–1

Symptoms of Adolescent Substance Abuse and Useful Drug Abuse Internet Sites

FRIENDS

- ☐ Changing attitude toward straight friends
- ☐ Changing circle of friends
- ☐ Running with new friends unknown to parents
- ☐ Beginning to hang out with an older crowd
- ☐ Receiving strange telephone calls (parties hang up or refuse to identify themselves)
- ☐ Forming superficial relationships based on drug use
- ☐ Suddenly popular

FAMILY

- ☐ Changing attitude towards rules, parents, or siblings
- ☐ Often exhibits negative or defiant behavior; sometimes compliant or agreeable, but failing to follow through on promises
- ☐ Failing to participate in family activities
- ☐ Isolating; frequently staying in room or away from house
- ☐ Breaking curfew or sneaking out of the house
- ☐ Lying and blaming others for irresponsible actions
- ☐ Stealing (money, pills, articles to be sold)
- ☐ Exhibiting mood swings
- ☐ Creating tense family relationships or a sense of "walking on eggshells"
- ☐ Becoming violent and threatening, physically or verbally
- ☐ Showing erratic sleeping patterns, extremes of too much or too little, or frequent naps
- ☐ Acquiring unusual eating habits, possible symptoms of bulimia or anorexia
- ☐ Becoming manipulative

SCHOOL

- ☐ Lacking motivation
- ☐ Sleeping in class
- ☐ Getting poor grades inexplicably
- ☐ Skipping classes or entire days
- ☐ Dropping sports or other activities
- ☐ Disrespectful of teachers, rules, and regulations
- ☐ Frequently disciplined or suspended
- ☐ Expulsion from school entirely

SPIRITUAL

- ☐ Losing interest in church attendance
- ☐ Uncomfortable talking about religion
- ☐ Showing interest in the occult or devil worship (black candles, medallions, pictures or symbols representing the devil)

PHYSICAL/PSYCHOLOGICAL

- ☐ Smelling of alcohol or marijuana
- ☐ Experiencing hangovers (headaches, nausea, flu symptoms, tremors)
- ☐ Frequently using eyedrops (e.g., Visine or Murine)
- ☐ Displaying bloodshot or glassy eyes
- ☐ Chronically suffering a deep, nagging cough or bronchitis
- ☐ Losing or gaining weight
- ☐ Appearing pale and wane
- ☐ Lethargic and apathetic
- ☐ Undisciplined; failure to get things done
- ☐ Sloppy and unkept

- ☐ Sometimes inappropriately happy or inexplicably depressed
- ☐ Experiencing hallucinations or flashbacks
- ☐ Pregnant or has had an abortion
- ☐ Incoherent
- ☐ Smoking cigarettes

LEGAL PROBLEMS

- ☐ Shoplifting
- ☐ Unruly, delinquent, or a runaway
- ☐ Accused of petty or grand theft
- ☐ Breaking and entering
- ☐ Publicly intoxicated
- ☐ Arrested for D.W.I. or D.U.I.
- ☐ In vehicle accidents or near misses
- ☐ Accused of assault
- ☐ Prostituting
- ☐ Vandalizing
- ☐ Selling drugs
- ☐ In possession of drugs and/or paraphernalia

EMOTIONAL

- ☐ Showing impaired judgment; placing self in dangerous situations
- ☐ Mutilating self (tattoos or burn marks)
- ☐ Talking of suicide
- ☐ Attempting suicide
- ☐ Overdosing
- ☐ Violent behavior

INTELLECTUAL

- ☐ Burned out
- ☐ Losing short- and long-term memory
- ☐ Losing IQ points
- ☐ Experiencing blackouts
- ☐ Operating at an inappropriate maturity level

MISCELLANEOUS

- ☐ Managing finances poorly; spending large sums and frequently asking for money
- ☐ Using profanity extensively
- ☐ Displaying “junkie” behavior (slang, T-shirts, acid rock music)
- ☐ Keeping or admiring drug paraphernalia; rolling papers, roach clips, syringes, small mirrors, and razor blades
- ☐ Reading drug-oriented magazines
- ☐ Raiding family liquor supply
- ☐ Promiscuity, acting out sexually
- ☐ Wearing drug jewelry (marijuana leaf motif, tiny cocaine spoons)
- ☐ Carries a beeper or pager device for instant contact with “friends”

USEFUL WEB SITES FOR INFORMATION ON DRUG ABUSE

The following Internet Web sites are useful sources of information about drugs of abuse and the problems they cause. At the time of this writing these sites were funtional. However, Web addresses sometimes change and threrefore it may be necessary to use one of the searching tools to find the updated address.

National Institute on Drug Abuse Capsules

http://www.nida.nih.gov/NIDACapsules/ NCIndex.html

National Institute on Drug Abuse Links

http://www.nida.nih.gov/OtherResources.html

Drug Enforcement Administration Publications

http://www.usdoj.gov/dea/pubs/pblist.htm

Drug Enforcement Administration Home Page

http://www.usdoj.gov/dea/index.htm

Higher Education Center for Alcohol and Other Drug Prevention

http://www.edc.org/hec/

Partnership for a Drug-free America Home Page

http://www.drugfreeamerica.org/legal.html

Partnership for a Drug-free America—Drug-free Resource Net

http://www.drugfreeamerica.org/

National Clearinghouse for Alcohol and Drug Information—Research and Statistics

http://www.health.org/survey.htm

Center for Substance Abuse Prevention (CSAP), Substance Abuse and Mental Health Services Administration (SAMHSA)

http://www.samhsa.gov/csap/CSAP.HTM

National Center on Addiction and Substance Abuse at Columbia University

http://www.casacolumbia.org/

Office of National Drug Control Policy

http://www1.whitehouse.gov/WH/EOP/ondcp/ html/ondcp-plain.html

National Clearinghouse for Alcohol and Drug Information

http://www.health.org/index.htm

63

Substance-Related Disorders: Alcohol, Nicotine, and Caffeine

Paul L. Doering, MS

The use of "socially acceptable" drugs such as alcohol, nicotine, and caffeine causes much more "addiction" than the so-called street drugs, imposing an enormous social and economic cost on our society. More than 430,000 people in the United States die each year as a result of smoking, the leading preventable cause of morbidity and mortality.[1] Smoking is responsible for 85% of all lung cancer deaths, approximately 80% of all chronic obstructive pulmonary disease deaths, and 30% of overall health disease deaths.[2]

Approximately 11 million persons in the United States report current heavy use of alcohol or alcohol abuse, costing almost $100 billion each year.[3,4] Almost one-half of these persons meet DSM-IV criteria for alcohol dependence, and almost 400,000 persons are in treatment for alcoholism at any one time.[3,5,6] The lifetime prevalence of alcohol abuse is 14% and of alcohol dependence is 8%[7,8] It has been estimated that as many as 40% of patients in emergency departments had consumed alcohol recently, and as many as 32% had alcohol levels of at least 80 mg/dL, the legal limit of intoxication in many states.[9]

Caffeine is currently the most widely used psychoactive substance in the world.[10] In the United States more than 80% of adults regularly consume behaviorally active doses of caffeine,[11,12] and the average daily consumption of caffeine is estimated to be 280 mg per adult consumer.[13] Although research has shown that caffeine can cause a compulsive pattern of use, the prevalence of caffeine dependence and its clinical significance is difficult to determine.

The subjects of alcohol, tobacco, and caffeine abuse deserve much more attention than space permits in this chapter. Therefore, the information here should serve as a brief overview of these topics, and the reader desiring more details is urged to consult one or more of the many textbooks and articles devoted to these subjects. Some useful Internet sites are listed in Appendix 63–1

ALCOHOL

EPIDEMIOLOGY OF ALCOHOL USE

In 1996, approximately 109 million persons age 12 and over were current alcohol users, which was about 51 percent of the total population in this age category. About 32 million persons (15.5%) engaged in binge drinking, defined as having five or more drinks on the same occasion at least once in the past month. About 11 million Americans (5.4% of the population) were heavy drinkers, meaning that they drank five or more drinks on the same occasion on at least five different days in the past month.[14]

Among youths age 12 to 17, the rate of current alcohol use was 49.8% in 1979, 32.5% in 1990, 21.1% in 1995, and 18.8% in 1996.[14] Fifty-nine percent of men had used alcohol in the past month, compared with 44% of women. Men were much more likely than women to be binge drinkers (22.8% and 8.7%, respectively) and heavy drinkers (9.3% and 1.9%, respectively).[14] In contrast to the pattern for illicit drugs, the higher the level of educational attainment, the more likely was the current use of alcohol. In 1996, 66% of adults with college degrees were current drinkers, compared with only 39% of those having less than a high school education.

THE DISEASE MODEL OF ADDICTION AS APPLIED TO ALCOHOLISM

Individuals who are drug dependent are frequently regarded as constitutionally weak people who have brought their problems upon themselves and deserve the consequences of their behavior. Even when the lay public and health care professionals acknowledge addiction as a disease process, it is often felt to be self-induced. The disease concept of addiction, using alcoholism as a model, states that addiction is a disease and that individuals who suffer from the disease do not choose to contract the disease any more than someone who suffers from heart disease or diabetes mellitus chooses to contract that illness. A *disease* is defined as "any deviation from or interruption of the normal structure or function of any part, organ, or system (or combination thereof) of the body that is manifested by a characteristic set of symptoms and signs and whose etiology, pathology, and prognosis may be known or unknown."[15] Alcoholism, which is discussed as a prototype, meets all of the definitional criteria. Diagnostic criteria for alcoholism do not specify frequency of drinking or amount of alcohol consumed. The key determinant is whether drinking is compulsive, out of control, and consequential *when one drinks.*

Numerous biologic differences between alcoholics and normals have been demonstrated, but discussions of the disease of alcoholism usually focus on three points. The first point involves interindividual differences in response to alcohol, based on the animal model. When a community of rats is offered two sources of water, one of a solution of glucose, the other of alcohol, approximately 90% of the animals selectively choose glucose–water after testing both supplies. The remainder prefer alcohol. If the alcohol-preferring rats are separated from the remainder of the population, their offspring are significantly more likely to be alcohol preferring.[16]

The experience of the animal studies led researchers to examine family trends in alcoholism and the possibility that alcoholism can be genetically transmitted. Data in human subjects suggest an association between a dopamine D_2-receptor gene and alcoholism,[17] although not all similar studies have replicated these results. More recent data suggest a similar genetic predisposition to polysubstance abuse.[18] A preliminary study in male veterans also showed an association of the D_2-receptor gene with cocaine dependence.[19] Although many researchers think it unlikely that there is a specific gene for addiction, it is possible that interactions among several genes combine in such a way as to be conducive to making a drug an effective reinforcer.[20]

The prevalence of alcoholism among the first-degree relatives of alcoholics (parents, siblings, children) is approximately 25%, versus 8% in the adult population. Concordance for alcoholism among fraternal twins is approximately 31%, but among identical twins concordance is approximately 54%,[21] although data are conflicting. When children of alcoholic parents are separated at birth and placed in nonalcoholic homes, they remain three to five times more likely to become alcoholic than adoptees whose biologic parents are not alcoholic.[21] The opposite is also true—offspring of nonalcoholics adopted by alcoholics do not have elevated rates of alcohol problems.[21]

The difference in concordance between fraternal and identical twins and the greater likelihood of developing alcoholism among adoptees whose biologic parents are alcoholic argue for what some clinicians have called a genetic predisposition, which is the second focus point for the disease model of alcoholism. A genetically predisposed individual will not necessarily manifest alcoholic drinking behavior. As stated previously, a susceptible host and favorable conditions must combine in order for a disease process to occur. Sons of men with early-onset alcoholism appear especially predisposed to developing alcoholism.[21] Research into genetic influences on other forms of drug dependence is limited owing to their being less prevalent, a greater difficulty in recruiting subjects, lack of restriction of use to one class of drugs, and the changes in availability of illicit substances.

A third point regarding the disease of alcoholism regards possible biochemical abnormalities. Research findings are necessarily limited to animal trials and remain controversial. Behavioral genetics studies in drug self-administration in rats across different drugs and genotypes suggest that the drug-seeking behaviors maintained by alcohol, cocaine, and opiates may have some common biologic determinants.[22] Advances in techniques for analysis of brain electrophysiology suggest that alcoholics and their alcohol-naive offspring have similar electroencephalography (EEG) profiles.[21] If these findings are borne out with additional studies, it would support the concept of biologic differences between alcoholics and normals that are innate rather than a consequence of exposure to alcohol. In addition, a family history of alcoholism has been shown to be associated with decreased subjective feelings of acute intoxication, less alcohol-induced anxiety, and fewer alcohol-induced decrements in psychomotor and cognitive test performance. EEGs done on this population of nonalcohol-dependent sons of alcoholics also showed less intense EEG alpha activity in response to alcohol challenge than did matched controls.[21] Other suggested biologic markers for alcoholism include differences in the activity of liver transaminase enzymes and platelet monoamine oxidase activity.

The belief that addiction is a self-induced disease or a constitutional weakness has been dismissed by clinicians in the addiction treatment field. Willpower and self-discipline cannot control genetics and possible biochemical abnormalities. Given that almost all the population will try alcohol and that over half drink alcohol regularly, the determination of who becomes alcoholic is based on more factors than environmental precipitants.

PHARMACOLOGY AND PHARMACOKINETICS OF ALCOHOL

ALCOHOL AS A DRUG

Alcohol is a central nervous system depressant that shares many pharmacologic properties with the nonbenzodiazepine sedative–hypnotic drugs. It affects the CNS in a dose-dependent fashion, producing sedation that progresses to sleep, unconsciousness, coma, surgical anesthesia, and finally, fatal respiratory depression and cardiovascular collapse. Alcohol affects endogenous opiates and several neurotransmitter systems in the brain, including γ-aminobutyric acid (GABA), glutamine, and dopamine. Alcohol intake results in an increase in endogenous opioids,[20] and this may be responsible for the euphoria experienced with alcohol consumption. Currently, there are no clinically useful antagonists that can reverse all of the pharmacologic effects of alcohol.

Alcohol is available in a variety of concentrations, in various alcoholic beverages. There are approximately 14 grams of alcohol in a 12-ounce can of beer, 4 ounces of nonfortified wine, or one shot (1.5 ounce) of 80-proof whiskey. This amount will cause an increase in blood alcohol level of about 25 mg/dL in a healthy 70-kg male.[23] The lethal dose of alcohol in humans is variable, but deaths generally occur when blood alcohol levels are greater than 500 mg/dL.

PHARMACOKINETICS

Absorption of alcohol begins in the stomach within 5 to 10 minutes of oral ingestion. The onset of clinical effects follows fairly rapidly. It is absorbed primarily from the duodenum, but in smaller amounts from the stomach, esophagus, and mucous membranes. Peak serum concentrations of alcohol are usually achieved 30 to 90 minutes after finishing the last drink, although it is quite variable depending on the type of alcoholic beverage consumed, what and when the person last ate, and other factors.[24]

Over 90% of alcohol in the plasma is metabolized in the liver by three enzyme systems that operate within the hepatocyte.[24] The remainder is excreted by the lungs and in urine and sweat. Alcohol is metabolized to acetaldehyde by alcohol dehydrogenase in the cell. In turn, acetaldehyde is metabolized to carbon dioxide and water by the enzyme aldehyde dehydrogenase. A second pathway for oxidation of alcohol uses catalase, an enzyme located in the peroxisome and microsomes. The third enzyme system, the microsomal alcohol oxidase system, has a role in the oxidation of alcohol to acetaldehyde. These last two mechanisms are of lesser importance than the alcohol dehydrogenase–aldehyde dehydrogenase system.[24]

The metabolism of alcohol is generally said to follow zero-order kinetics. This may in fact be an oversimplification, because at very high or very low concentrations of alcohol the metabolism may follow first-order pharmacokinetics.[24] On the average, the blood alcohol concentration is lowered from 15 to 22.2 mg/dL/h in the nontolerant individual, assuming the patient is in the postabsorptive state.[24] Alcohol has a volume of distribution of 0.6 to 0.8 L/kg, representing the total body water.[24]

ACUTE EFFECTS OF ALCOHOL

At lower serum concentrations, euphoria and disinhibition may be noted. Slurred speech, altered perception of the environment, impaired judgment, ataxia, incoordination, nystagmus, and hyperreflexia may occur.[24] As plasma levels increase, or in different individuals, combative and destructive behavior may occur. With higher levels still, somnolence and respiratory depression may ensue.[24] The typical effects on the body of various blood alcohol concentrations (BACs) is shown in Table 63–1, although effects vary from individual to individual.

TABLE 63–1. Specific Effects of Alcohol Related to the Blood Alcohol Concentration (BAC)

BAC (%)[a]	Effect
0.02–0.03	No loss of coordination, slight euphoria and loss of shyness. Depressant effects are not apparent.
0.04–0.06	Feeling of well-being, relaxation, lower inhibitions, sensation of warmth. Euphoria. Some minor impairment of reasoning and memory, lowering of caution.
0.07–0.09	Slight impairment of balance, speech, vision, reaction time, and hearing. Euphoria. Judgement and self-control are reduced, and caution, reason, and memory are impaired.
0.10–0.125	Significant impairment of motor coordination and loss of good judgement. Speech may be slurred; balance, vision, reaction time, and hearing will be impaired. Euphoria. It is illegal to operate a motor vehicle at this level of intoxication.
0.13–0.15	Gross motor impairment and lack of physical control. Blurred vision and major loss of balance. Euphoria is reduced and dysphoria is beginning to appear.
0.16–0.20	Dysphoria (anxiety, restlessness) predominates, nausea may appear. The drinker has the appearance of a "sloppy drunk."
0.25	Needs assistance in walking; total mental confusion. Dysphoria with nausea and some vomiting.
0.30	Loss of consciousness.
≥ 0.40	Onset of coma, possible death due to respiratory arrest.

[a]Grams of ethyl alcohol per 100 mL of whole blood.

ALCOHOL POISONING

If the BAC gets high enough, death becomes a very real possibility, especially with coadministration of other sedative-hypnotics. Acute alcohol poisoning usually occurs with rapid consumption of large quantities of alcoholic beverages, because this type of drinking delivers a large bolus of alcohol to the GI tract. Normally, one passes out before a toxic dose of alcohol can be ingested or the person vomits to rid the stomach of its toxic reservoir. With rapid drinking as described, the person may fall asleep or pass out without vomiting, allowing continued absorption from the GI tract until fatal BACs are achieved.[24]

It is important to differentiate acute alcohol intoxication from certain other medical or surgical illnesses. Mental status changes may result from head trauma, and if the diagnosis is missed, the consequences could be disastrous. Appropriate measures, such as CT, should be performed on any patient with deteriorating mental status, focal neurologic findings, failure to improve over time, new-onset seizures, or mental status out of proportion to the degree of intoxication.[24]

ALCOHOL AND INJURIES

It is estimated that 40% to 50% of traffic fatalities are associated with alcohol intoxication (BAC ≥ 100 mg/dL).[24] By comparison, only 2% to 3% of noninjured drivers have levels this high.[24] One study suggests that persons who consume five or more drinks per occasion are nearly twice as likely to die of injuries (including those from motor vehicle crashes, suicide, homicide, fall, fire, drowning, and poisoning) as persons who drink less than this.[24] It has also been estimated that 25% to 35% of nonfatal motor vehicle injuries, 64% of fires and burns, 48% of hypothermia and frostbite cases, and 20% of suicides are associated with this degree of intoxication.[24]

LABORATORY STUDIES

In the emergency room, a BAC should be ordered in any patient in whom alcohol ingestion is suspected, regardless of the presenting complaint.[24] For clinical purposes most laboratories report BAC in units of milligrams per deciliter. In legal cases results are reported in percent (grams of ethyl alcohol per 100 mL of whole blood). Thus, a blood alcohol level of 150 mg/dL corresponds to 0.15% BAC.

If the diagnosis is unclear, if the intoxication seems atypical, or when there is suspicion of multiple drug ingestions, a complete toxicologic screen to rule out the presence of other substances may be useful.

▶ TREATMENT: Alcohol-Related Disorders

ALCOHOL WITHDRAWAL

The *Diagnostic and Statistical Manual of Mental Disorders,* fourth edition (DSM-IV) definition of alcohol withdrawal includes two main components.[5] The first component is a history of cessation or reduction in heavy and prolonged alcohol use. The second includes the presence of two or more of the symptoms of alcohol withdrawal: autonomic hyperactivity (sweating or tachycardia); increased hand tremor; insomnia; nausea or vomiting; transient tactile, visual, or auditory hallucinations; psychomotor agitation; anxiety; and tonic–clonic seizures. Signs and symptoms of alcohol withdrawal as well as acute alcohol intoxication are given in Table 63–2.

Goals for alcohol-dependent persons decreasing or discontinuing alcohol intake include (1) the prevention and treatment of withdrawal symptoms (including seizures and delirium tremens) and medical or psychiatric complications; (2) long-term abstinence after detoxification; and (3) entry into ongoing medical and alcohol-dependence treatment.

PHARMACOLOGIC THERAPY

Benzodiazepines are the most useful drugs for the management of alcohol withdrawal. The long-acting benzodiazepines are superior for managing the symptoms of alcohol withdrawal and also for preventing seizures and delirium tremens.[25] Chlordiazepoxide (Librium) and diazepam (Valium) are the most effective in preventing the serious complications of seizures and delirium tremens. The shorter-acting benzodiazepines such as alprazolam (Xanax) or oxazepam (Serax) are associated with a higher risk of development of seizures during alcohol withdrawal.[25]

Although phenothiazines, clonidine, and carbamazepine may reduce symptoms of alcohol withdrawal, no evidence supports their ability to prevent seizures or delirium tremens[25]; and in fact the phenothiazines may lower the seizure threshhold. There is a small risk of excessive sedation, particularly in inadequately monitored patients, the elderly, or patients with significant liver disease.[26] Other drugs used to treat symptoms of alcohol withdrawal include the barbiturates, alcohol itself, sympatholytics such as atenolol, neuroleptics such as haloperidol, thiamine, and magnesium.

TABLE 63–2. Signs and Symptoms of Alcohol Intoxication and Withdrawal

Intoxication	Withdrawal
Slurred speech	Tremor
Ataxia	Tachycardia
Nystagmus	Diaphoresis
Sedation	Labile blood pressure
Flushed face	Anxiety
Mood change	Nausea and vomiting
Irritability	Hallucinations
Euphoria	Seizures
Loquacity	Hyperthermia
Impaired attention	Delirium

TREATMENT REGIMENS

Fixed-Schedule Therapy

Benzodiazepines given regularly at a fixed dosing interval are the gold standard therapy for alcohol withdrawal. Chlordiazepoxide 50 to 100 mg orally every 6 hours for 1 day followed by 2 days at 25 to 50 mg every 6 hours is known to prevent delirium tremens and seizures.[25] Patients should be monitored and given additional medication when indicated by symptoms. This type of regimen is useful in patients with a history of seizures, patients with acute medical or surgical illness, or patients with a history of delirium tremens. It also may be preferable for pregnant women.

Front Loading

Front-loading refers to regimens in which frequent, high doses of medication are given to treat the early signs and symptoms of withdrawal.[25] Diazepam is given in 20-mg doses every 2 hours until resolution of withdrawal symptoms. A total of 60 mg is typically required. Because of the long half-life of diazepam and its active metabolites further doses are not required. This regimen has also been shown to decrease rates of seizures. Advantages of front-loading are that medication administration and intensive monitoring are limited to the early symptomatic period of withdrawal.

Symptom-Triggered Therapy

With symptom-triggered therapy, medication is given only when the patient has symptoms.[25] This approach results in treatment that is shorter, potentially avoiding oversedation and allowing the physician to focus on specific therapy for alcohol dependence.

Treatment of Alcohol Withdrawal Seizures. Alcohol withdrawal seizures do not require treatment with an anticonvulsant drug unless they progress to status epilepticus, because seizures usually end before diazepam or another drug can be administered.[25] Phenytoin, which is not cross-tolerant to alcohol, does not prevent or treat withdrawal seizures, and without an intravenous loading dose, therapeutic blood levels of phenytoin are not reached until acute withdrawal is complete. Patients experiencing seizures should be treated supportively. An increase in the dosage and tapering schedule of the benzodiazepine used in detoxification, or a single injection of a benzodiazepine, may be necessary to prevent further seizure activity. Patients with a history of withdrawal seizures can be predicted to experience an especially severe withdrawal syndrome. In such patients, a higher initial dosage of a benzodiazepine drug and a slower tapering period of 7 to 10 days is advisable.

Treatment Settings. Alcohol withdrawal treatment can take place in hospitals, inpatient detoxification units, or outpatient settings. Inpatient treatment may be necessary when there are coexisting acute or chronic medical, surgical, or psychiatric conditions (including pregnancy) that would complicate alcohol withdrawal. Only patients with mild to moderate symptoms should be considered for outpatient treatment, and it is a good idea to have a responsible sober person available to help the patient monitor symptoms and administer medications. Patients with a strong craving for alcohol, those concurrently using other drugs, and those with a history of seizures or delirium tremens are not good candidates for outpatient treatment.

ALCOHOL DEPENDENCE

PHARMACOLOGIC MANAGEMENT

The defining feature of the alcohol dependence syndrome is loss of control over drinking.[27] In the United States, disulfiram and naltrexone are the only two drugs specifically marketed for the treatment of alcohol dependence. Disulfiram acts as a deterrent for the resumption of drinking, and naltrexone is a competitive opioid antagonist that has been shown to reduce craving for alcohol.

DISULFIRAM

Disulfiram deters a patient from drinking by producing an aversive reaction if the patient drinks. In the absence of alcohol, disulfiram has minimal effects. It inhibits the liver enzyme aldehyde-dehydrogenase in the biochemical pathway for alcohol metabolism, allowing acetaldehyde to accumulate. The resulting increase in acetaldehyde causes severe facial flushing, throbbing headache, nausea and vomiting, chest pain, palpitations, tachycardia, weakness, dizziness, blurred vision, confusion, and hypotension. Severe reactions including myocardial infarction, congestive heart failure, cardiac arrhythmia, respiratory depression, convulsions, and death can occur, particularly in vulnerable individuals. A "disulfiram reaction" can occur for up to 2 weeks after therapy has been discontinued, but the time of risk for occurrence of an aversive reaction is usually up to 4 to 7 days. The reaction can occur even from alcohol contained in mouthwashes, certain foodstuffs, and medicinals.[25]

Although disulfiram appeared to be effective in a series of small-scale studies, these were largely uncontrolled.[25] Other studies show conflicting results and generally indicate that factors such as compliance with other aspects of treatment may correlate better with abstinence than use of disulfiram.[28] A well-designed, large scale cooperative study of 605 male veterans treated for 1 year found 250 mg of disulfiram to be no better than placebo or no pill in helping patients remain abstinent.[25]

The disulfiram–alcohol interaction can sometimes be intense, causing serious problems for patients with cerebrovascular, cardiovascular, or severe pulmonary disease, or chronic renal failure. The use of disulfiram in patients who may have occult vascular disease, such as those over 60 years of age and patients with diabetes, should also be avoided.[25] Vomiting during a disulfiram reaction can cause severe bleeding in a patient with esophageal varices, and for this reason disulfiram is contraindicated in cirrhosis with portal hypertension. Disulfiram can lower the seizure threshold and cause peripheral neuropathy and should be avoided in patients with these conditions. It has been linked to birth defects, and therefore should not be used during pregnancy. Because disulfiram can cause drowsiness, it should be first taken on the weekend at bedtime and discontinued if the patient continues to be drowsy on awakening after 2 to 3 days of medication.[29]

A rare but potentially fatal idiosyncratic hepatotoxicity can occur with disulfiram. As a result, baseline liver function tests should be obtained and the patient monitored for hepatotoxicity by symptoms and by repeating the liver function tests at 2 weeks, 3 months, and 6 months, and then twice yearly thereafter.

The prescriber should wait at least 24 hours after the last drink before starting disulfiram, usually at a dose of 250 mg daily. At this dose there are fewer side effects than at 500 mg, although some research suggests that higher doses are needed to reliably produce an aversive reaction if the patient drinks.[25]

NALTREXONE

Naltrexone, an opiate antagonist that has been available in the United States since 1984 for the treatment of opioid dependence, blocks the effects of exogenous opioids. In 1994 it was approved by the Food and Drug Administration (FDA) for use in the treatment of alcohol dependence. Naltrexone is thought to attenuate the reinforcing effects of alcohol,[30] and those who consume alcohol while taking naltrexone report feeling less intoxicated and having less craving for alcohol.[31,32]

The efficacy of naltrexone for use in alcohol dependence has been investigated in two placebo-controlled clinical trials.[33,34] In a combined analysis of the data from the 186 alcohol-dependent patients in these two studies, patients randomized to receive 50 mg of naltrexone daily for 12 weeks were more likely to remain abstinent and to avoid relapse to heavy drinking; 31% of placebo patients remained abstinent compared to 54% of patients on naltrexone; 48% of placebo patients avoided heavy drinking, whereas 75% of naltrexone patient successfully avoided drinking to excess. Craving for alcohol was also significantly lower for patients on naltrexone.[31]

Naltrexone should not be given to patients currently dependent on opiates because it can precipitate a severe withdrawal syndrome. Naltrexone has been shown to have dose-related hepatotoxicity,[35] but this generally occurs at doses higher than those recommended for treatment of alcohol dependence. Nevertheless, it should be considered contraindicated in patients with hepatitis or liver failure, and liver function tests should be monitored monthly for the first 3 months, and then every 3 months thereafter.

Nausea is the most common side effect of naltrexone, occurring in about 10% of patients. Other side effects are headache, dizziness, nervousness, fatigue, insomnia, vomiting, anxiety, and somnolence.

Naltrexone should be given in a dose of 50 mg daily. This dose effectively blocks mu opioid receptors. Documentation is lacking to support routine use of higher doses.

NICOTINE

Cigarette smoking is an enormous national health problem, and we, as health care professionals, are not doing an adequate job in helping people to quit. Only about one-half of the current smokers surveyed in studies conducted in the later 1980s and early 1990s reported that their doctors had ever advised them to quit smoking,[36,37] and only 3.6% of ex-smokers report that their physician helped them quit.[36] Other health care professionals did an even poorer job, with only 22% of dentists, 24% of nurses, and a pitiful 4% of pharmacists helping their patients to quit smoking.[38] The benefits of smoking cessation include a longer life and better health (decreased risk of the health problems that will be cited).[39–41]

EPIDEMIOLOGY OF TOBACCO USE

An estimated 62 million Americans were current smokers in 1996.[14] This represents a smoking rate of 29% for the population age 12 and older. There was no change between 1995 and 1996 in the overall rate of smoking. Current smokers were more likely to be heavy drinkers and illicit drug users. Among smokers, the rate of heavy alcohol use (five or more drinks on five or more days in the past month) was 12.8%, and the rate of current illicit drug use was 14.7%. Among nonsmokers, only 2.5% were heavy drinkers and 2.6% were illicit drug users.

An estimated 6.8 million Americans (3.2% of the population) were current users of smokeless tobacco in 1996.[14] Approximately 4.1 million youths age 12 to 17 were current smokers in 1996, representing 18.3% of this age group. Among adults, men had somewhat higher rates of smoking than women, but rates of smoking were similar for males and females aged 12 to 17. Level of educational attainment was correlated with tobacco usage. Thirty-seven percent of adults who had not completed high school smoked cigarettes, while only 17% of college graduates smoked.[14]

ECONOMIC IMPACT OF SMOKING

In 1993, the estimated direct cost of medical care for smoking-related illnesses in the United States was $50 billion.[42] The annual cost of lost productivity and earnings associated with smoking-related disability is approximately $47 billion.[42] These direct and indirect costs amount to $2.95 for each pack of cigarettes sold, in 1996 dollars.[40]

HEALTH RISKS OF SMOKING

Each year more than 430,000 deaths, or 20% of the total deaths in the United States, are caused by smoking.[39] Cigarette smoking substantially increases the risk of (1) cardiovascular diseases such as stroke, sudden death, and heart attack; (2) nonmalignant respiratory diseases including emphysema, asthma, chronic bronchitis, and chronic obstructive pulmonary disease; (3) lung cancer; and (4) other cancers (e.g., mouth, pharynx, larynx, esophagus, stomach, pancreas, uterus, cervix, kidney, ureter, and bladder).

Exposure to environmental tobacco smoke ("passive exposure") has been cited as the cause of 3000 lung cancer deaths and 35,000 to 40,000 heart disease deaths in the United States every year.[40] When children are exposed to environmental smoke, they have a higher risk of respiratory infection, asthma, and middle-ear infections than those who are not exposed. Sudden infant death syndrome occurs more often in infants whose mothers smoked during pregnancy than in offspring of nonsmoking mothers.[40] The harmful effects of smoking on reproduction and pregnancy include reduced fertility and fetal growth, as well as increased risk of ectopic pregnancy and spontaneous abortion.[41]

PHARMACOLOGY OF NICOTINE

Nicotine is a ganglionic cholinergic receptor agonist whose pharmacologic effects are highly dependent on dose. These effects include central and peripheral nervous system stimulation and depression, respiratory stimulation, skeletal muscle relaxation, catecholamine release by the adrenal medulla, peripheral vasoconstriction, and increased blood pressure, heart rate, cardiac output, and oxygen consumption.[43] Cigarette smoking or low doses of nicotine produces an increased alertness and increased cognitive functioning by stimulating the cerebral cortex. At higher doses, nicotine stimulates the "reward" center in the limbic system of the brain.[43]

Chronic nicotine ingestion may lead to physical and psychological dependence and tolerance to some of its pharmacologic effects. Abrupt smoking cessation in physically dependent smokers results in withdrawal symptoms as shown in Table 63–3. Onset of these symptoms usually occurs within 24 hours and may last for days, weeks, or longer. The craving for tobacco may last for years.

Although some smokers do not develop physical or psychological dependence, most people who smoke 10 to 15 cigarettes daily for several weeks or longer do.[43] Seventy-seven percent to 92% of smokers are addicted to nicotine in cigarettes.[44–46]

FDA's LEGAL AND SCIENTIFIC BASIS FOR CLASSIFYING TOBACCO AS A DRUG

On August 28, 1996, President Clinton announced the final regulations of the FDA restricting the sale and promotion of cigarettes and smokeless tobacco.[47] The FDA's assertion of jurisdiction over tobacco products under the Federal Food, Drug, and Cosmetic Act (the Act) was the culmination of an exhaustive 2.5-year investigation of tobacco products.

The Act defines a "drug" as any article (other than food) "intended to affect the structure or any function of the body."[48] When the FDA last considered this issue, it

TABLE 63–3. Withdrawal Symptoms of Nicotine

Anxiety	Gastrointestinal disturbances
Craving for tobacco	Headache
Decreased blood pressure and heart rate	Hostility
Depression	Increased appetite and weight gain
Difficulty concentrating	Increased skin temperaure
Drowsiness	Insomnia
Frustration, irritability, impatience	Restlessness

declined to assert jurisdiction over cigarettes because it lacked evidence that cigarettes were intended to affect the structure or functions of the body.[47]

As substantial evidence became available to support its argument that cigarettes did, in fact, meet the definition of a drug, the FDA vigorously pursued its classification as such. This evidence included emergence of a scientific consensus that the nicotine in cigarettes and smokeless tobacco causes and sustains addiction. Additionally, there was disclosure of thousands of pages of internal tobacco company documents that the FDA contends prove that the tobacco manufacturers know that nicotine causes significant pharmacologic effects including addiction, and thus design their products to provide pharmacologically active doses of nicotine.[47] As one former senior official at Phillip Morris put it, "a key objective of the cigarette industry over the last 20 to 30 years" was "maintaining an acceptable and pharmacologically active nicotine level" in low-tar cigarettes.[47]

These findings provided the basis for the FDA's determination that cigarettes and smokeless tobacco are subject to FDA jurisdiction as products that contain a "drug" (nicotine) and a "device" (the cigarette itself) for delivering this drug to the body.

According to the agency, nicotine exerts psychoactive effects on the brain that motivate repeated, compulsive use of the substance. These pharmacologic effects create dependence in the user. The pharmacologic processes that cause this addiction to nicotine are similar to those that cause addiction to heroin and cocaine.[47]

The U.S. Surgeon General has also documented that nicotine in cigarettes and smokeless tobacco affects body weight. The FDA concluded that these effects on the structure and function of the body are "significant and quintessentially druglike." They point out that they are the same as the effects of other drugs that FDA has traditionally regulated, including stimulants, tranquilizers, appetite suppressants, and products such as methadone, used in the maintenance of addiction. For these reasons, the agency concluded that cigarettes and smokeless tobacco do "affect the structure or any function of the body" within the meaning of the Food, Drug, and Cosmetic Act.

The FDA contends that manufacturers of cigarettes and smokeless tobacco design their products to provide consumers with a pharmacologically active dose of nicotine.[47] The FDA based this finding in part on industry comments that disclose internal research to determine the dose of nicotine that must be delivered to provide "pharmacological satisfaction for the smoker," as well as estimates by industry scientist of the minimum and optimum doses of nicotine that tobacco products must deliver.[47]

▶ TREATMENT: Nicotine Dependence

AGENCY FOR HEALTH CARE POLICY AND RESEARCH SMOKING CESSATION CLINICAL PRACTICE GUIDELINE

The Agency for Health Care Policy and Research (AHCPR) periodically convenes expert panels to develop clinical guidelines for health care practitioners when the need dictates. Criteria used to determine if a practice guideline is needed include the prevalence of the illness, related morbidity and mortality, the economic burden imposed by the condition, variation in clinical practice related to the condition, the availability of methods for improvement of care, and the availability of data on which to base recommendations for care. Because tobacco addiction in the United States fulfills all of these requirements, AHCPR convened a panel of experts in 1994 to develop guidelines on the treatment of tobacco addiction.[42]

The AHCPR released its guideline for smoking cessation in 1996. In the course of its deliberations, the expert panel reviewed approximately 3000 articles and concluded that smoking cessation interventions are effective. The necessary components of successful programs attack the problem from three directions: (1) skills building, (2) social support for quitting, and (3) nicotine replacement. Some important global recommendations of the guidelines are listed in Table 63–4.

SKILLS BUILDING

Skills building interventions teach the patient how to resist cues to smoke. Patients must be taught to recognize situations that have triggered the urge to smoke in the past and be given the ability to resist the cues, either by avoiding the setting altogether or substituting a behavior for smoking. In the first few weeks of a smoking cessation, planning to avoid alcohol is critical, because so many people find that drinking alcohol triggers the urge to smoke. Making the home, car, and office smoke free is also an effective and legitimate action to take to avoid both cues to smoke and the hazards of environmental tobacco smoke. The full text of the AHCPR guideline should be consulted for further recommendations in this area.[42]

SOCIAL SUPPORT

Social support for quitting is the positive support that the smoker gets from family, friends, coworkers, and health care professionals for taking action toward smoking cessation and for abstaining from tobacco. Encouragement and positive feedback are crucial to the success of a smoking cessation program. It is extremely dif-

TABLE 63–4. Important Information from the Smoking Cessation *Clinical Practice Guideline*

1. Clinicians should ask and record the tobacco use status of every patient.
2. Smoking cessation treatment should be offered to ALL smokers at EVERY office visit.
3. Smoking cessation treatment as brief as 3 minutes is effective.
4. The more intense the treatment, the more effective it is in producing long-term abstinence from tobacco.
5. Nicotine replacement therapy (NRT) combined with social support and skills training delivered by clinicians is the most effective combination of treatments.
6. Health care systems should be modified to identify and intervene routinely with all tobacco users at every visit.

Compiled from Ref. 42.

ficult for one family member to quit smoking if others in the immediate family continue to smoke.

NICOTINE REPLACEMENT

Nicotine replacement therapy (NRT) doubles the probability of a successful quit attempt in most trials. Nicotine replacement can now be obtained through gum, patches, or nasal spray and inhalers. The success of NRT depends in part on the effectiveness of intensive adjuvant treatment.

OTHER FACTORS IMPORTANT TO THE SUCCESS OF A SMOKING CESSATION STATEGY

The AHCPR expert panel emphasized the importance of the type and intensity of the contact with the counselor to the success of the intervention. When interventions last for more than 10 minutes, the increase in cessation rates is much better than when interventions do not involve contact with a professional. Group and individual counseling are more effective than no intervention in increasing abstinence rates, but self-help materials (handouts, pamphlets, brochures) are not. Interventions are more successful when they include social support and training in general problem-solving skills, stress management, and relapse prevention.[42] The number of treatment sessions offered is also important. Providing at least four to seven sessions significantly increased cessation rates, independent of the treatment's intensity.[42]

Comprehensive behavioral interventions are more effective in helping people quit smoking and remain abstinent, but less intensive treatments are beneficial as well. Even minimal contacts lasting less than 3 minutes and simple advice to quit are more successful than intervention involving no contact in increasing cessation rates.[42]

Counseling efficacy is further augmented by the addition of nicotine replacement products. The cessation rates of nicotine patch users are approximately double the cessation rates of smokers who receive placebos, according to a meta-analysis review of the literature.[42] Although absolute quit rates have varied greatly, abstinence rates for the nicotine patch are estimated at 27% (ranging from 14% to 69%) at the end of treatment and 22% (ranging from 13% to 34%) at 6 months posttreatment.[42]

Although comprehensive programs are most effective, few smokers (10% to 15%) seek formal assistance in quitting.[42] A health care professional who merely advises his or her patient to quit smoking is providing at least minimal assistance in the efforts.

NICOTINE REPLACEMENT THERAPY

The ACHPR guidelines (Fig. 63–1) recommend use of NRT in the forms of transdermal nicotine patches or nicotine gum, both of which are now available to consumers without a prescription. At 6 months postcessation, the abstinence rates of persons using nicotine patches are at least two times greater than the rates of patients given placebos (patch, 22% success versus placebo, 9%).[49] Similarly, the use of nicotine gum produced a 40% to 60% increase in abstinence rates at 12-month follow-up when compared with placebo (gum, 16.9% to 18.2% versus placebo, 10.6% to 12.8%).[50–52]

The guideline recommends using the nicotine patch in routine clinical practice because of better compliance and ease of use, although research has shown similar efficacy for both the patch and gum. There is currently little evidence to suggest that combined use of the patch and gum increases abstinence beyond 24 weeks.[53,54]

The use of NRT is relatively safe, but it is not recommended for all smokers. In particular, it may be contraindicated for individuals with cardiovascular disease (e.g., severe arrhythmia, severe or worsening angina pectoris, or a myocardial infarction within the past 4 weeks) or active peptic ulcers.

Although the FDA has approved the use of both patch and gum with pregnant smokers, the agency has stipulated that NRT should be used only when the benefits of its use clearly outweigh the risks incurred by the fetus. Unfortunately, the AHCPR report provided no clear guidelines upon which to make this decision. Pregnant smokers should first be encouraged to quit without pharmacologic intervention. Similar precautions should be exercised for nursing mothers.

Finally, using the nicotine patch may be contraindicated for individuals with skin allergies or dermatologic disease. Similarly, the gum should be used with caution in individuals with jaw problems.

INSTRUCTING PATIENTS IN THE USE OF NRT

Compliance with NRT therapy improves when the patient is presented a clear rationale for its use and a realistic expectation about the response.[55] It should be explained to the patient that nicotine is responsible for addiction and that discontinuation of the nicotine causes craving for cigarettes, tension, irritability, sadness, problems with sleep, and difficulty concentrating. These are partly due to nicotine withdrawal. The patient should be told that using the patch results in less desire to smoke and provides an opportunity for a new nonsmoker to practice all of the new nonsmoking skills without being burdened by craving. The patient should understand that with smoking, there are naturally peaks and valleys in the amount of nicotine in the bloodstream. With the patch there is a steady gradual rise in the blood nicotine concentration that levels off and remains constant for much of the day, then gradually decreases while the person is asleep. Withdrawal symptoms are lessened by maintaining an adequate blood level of nicotine.[55]

A similar rationale can be used if patients are using gum. It should be emphasized that NRT is not a "magic bullet" and that the use of coping skills is essential for abstinence. The patch or the gum only buys time by reducing withdrawal symptoms and giving individuals a chance to figure out alternatives that they can use in place of smoking in many different situations.[55]

SIDE EFFECTS

Both the patch and gum have relatively few side effects. Nausea and light-headedness are possible signs of nicotine overdose that warrant a reduction of the nicotine dose.

The most frequent side effect with the patch is skin irritation related to the adhesive or the medium containing nicotine, and not to the nicotine itself. About 50% of patients report skin irritation during the course of treatment with the patch.[42,43] The patch site can be rotated to diminish this problem. The use of OTC hydrocortisone cream (1%) or triamcinolone cream (0.5%) is recommended as a local treatment for patch-related skin irritations. Switching to a different brand of patch may also alleviate the problem, because different products use a different adhesive or medium. The gum can be used instead of the patch when the skin irritation is severe. Less than 5% of patients were forced to discontinue therapy because of skin reactions.[42]

About 23% of patients using the patch report sleep disturbances,[43] but the insomnia is hard to differentiate from the sleeplessness that often accompanies withdrawal itself, especially during the first few weeks of quitting. If the insomnia is severe and lasts for more than a few weeks, the patient may opt to take off the patch at bedtime and have a new patch ready for the next morning.

DURATION

Those who commit to quitting smoking using the nicotine patch should be told to expect a minimum of 6 to 8 weeks of treatment.

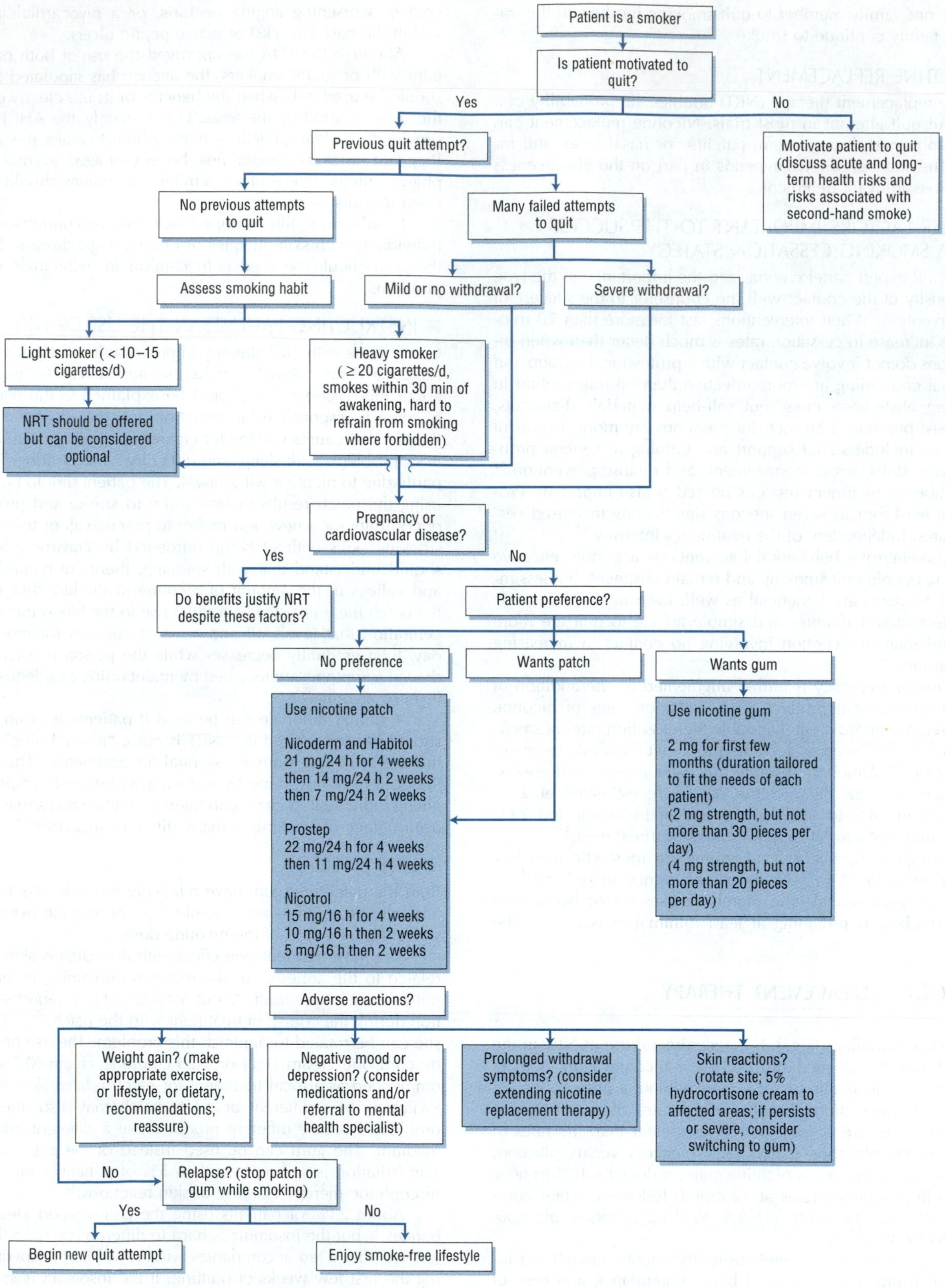

FIGURE 63–1. Algorithm for assessing appropriateness of nicotine replacement therapy (NRT) in patients wishing to quit smoking. *(Adapted from Ref. 42.)*

Using the therapy beyond 8 weeks is not associated with better success rates.[49] However, some patients will experience severe withdrawal even beyond 8 weeks, and these people may need to use the patch longer.

The duration of therapy with the gum should be at least 1 to 3 months on a fixed schedule rather than when one has the urge to smoke.[42] Studies have found, however, that 15% to 20% of abstainers continue to use the gum for longer than 12 months.[56,57] Patients should be encouraged to stick with the patch and/or gum for the minimally acceptable duration of treatment.

DOSAGES AND GRADUAL REDUCTION

Various dosages of the nicotine patch are available. Generally, the maximum dose (21 mg/d for Habitrol and Nicoderm, 22 mg/d for Prostep, and 15 mg/d for the Nicotrol 16-hour patch) is recommended for smokers who smoke 10 to 15 cigarettes or more per day. Traditionally, a gradual fading procedure in which the patch dose is stepped down at 2- to 3-week intervals is used. However, no empirical support exists for using this procedure rather than a single maximum dose for approximately 6 weeks.[49]

Regarding the use of gum, 2 mg should be considered the optimal dose for most patients.[42] Providers may consider using 4-mg gum for those who smoke at least 20 cigarettes a day[42] or those who have failed on the 2-mg gum. No formal empirically based recommendations are available regarding decreasing gum use. Clinical studies found greater efficacy in patients who chewed more than nine pieces per day.[58] Patients tend to cut down gradually or discontinue the gum on their own after using it for some time because of the gum's unpleasant taste or other side effects.

ECONOMIC AND PHARMACOECONOMIC CONSIDERATIONS

Most health insurers provide coverage for the chronic illnesses *caused* by smoking (e.g., chronic obstructive pulmonary disease, cancer, and myocardial infarction) yet few provide coverage for *treating the nicotine addiction* that caused those ailments.[59] For each life saved, smoking cessation programs involving physician counseling costs an estimated $700 to $2000.[60] Even after adding the cost of the nicotine patch to physician counseling, costs from the standpoint of a third-party payer range from $4390 to $10,943 per year of quality-adjusted life saved for males and $4955 to $6983 per year of quality-adjusted life saved for females (based on 15 minutes of physician counseling and 1 to 2 months of NRT).[61] Compared with the cost effectiveness of other preventive treatments, these costs are actually small. For each life saved by treating mild hypertension, the cost ranges from $11,300 to $24,408; and the preventive treatment of hypercholesterolemia is estimated to range from $65,511 to $108,189 per year of life saved.[60] Thus, smoking cessation treatment is clearly more cost effective in comparison.

PHARMACOLOGIC THERAPY FOR SMOKING CESSATION

BUPROPION

In 1997, the antidepressant drug bupropion, available since 1989 under the brand name Wellbutrin, was approved by the FDA in a sustained-release formulation (Zyban) for use as an aid in smoking cessation. Bupropion inhibits neuronal reuptake and potentiates the effects of norepinephrine and dopamine. Although its precise mechanism in smoking cessation is not well understood, dopamine has been associated with the rewarding effects of addictive substances. Withdrawal symptoms may be decreased by virtue of bupropion's inhibition of norepinephrine uptake.

One study compared the effects of 100, 150, or 300 mg/d of sustained-release bupropion, or placebo, for 7 weeks in 615 patients who visited the clinic each week for evaluation and counseling.[62] When the study was concluded, smoking cessation rates were 19% with placebo and 28.8%, 38.6%, and 44.2% with the respective doses of the drug. The differences between the 150- and 300-mg doses and placebo were statistically significant. After 1 year, the respective rates were 12.4%, 19.6%, 22.9%, and 23.1%, indicating a fairly high rate of relapse in all groups.

Bupropion at a dose of 150 mg twice daily of sustained-release tablets was compared to the 21 mg nicotine patch separately, as combined therapy, and placebo in nearly 900 patients studied for 9 weeks. At the 10-week mark, smoking cessation had been accomplished in 20% of the placebo group, 32% using the patch alone, 46% with bupropion alone, and 51% with combined therapy. All three active treatments were significantly better than placebo.[63]

Unlike its use as an antidepressant, no seizures occurred with bupropion in smoking cessation trials. Insomnia and dry mouth were the most frequent adverse effects. Other side effects noted in the trials were tremor, rash, and a few anaphylactoid reactions characterized by pruritus, urticaria, angioedema, and dyspnea. Insomnia was also reported.[63]

For smoking cessation the manufacturer recommends a dosage of 150 mg once daily for 3 days and then twice daily for 7 to 12 weeks or longer, with or without nicotine replacement. Patients are instructed to stop smoking during the second week of treatment and are encouraged to use counseling and support services along with the medication.[64] The clinical utility of this drug will likely be determined only after a few years of its use in typical practice settings. Fluoxetine and other similar agents may have utility in treating depression that occurs when one tries to quit smoking.[65]

CAFFEINE

Caffeinism is the term coined to describe the clinical syndrome produced by acute or chronic overuse of caffeine.[11] The syndrome is usually characterized by CNS and peripheral manifestations, most notably anxiety, psychomotor alterations, sleep disturbances, mood changes, and psychophysiologic complaints. Table 63–5 summarizes typical manifestations of caffeine overuse syndrome.

As many as one in five adults consumes doses of caffeine generally considered large enough to cause clinical symptoms. Controlled double-blind studies demonstrate that caffeine has reinforcement properties in most people with a history of heavy prior use,[66,67] and that this reinforcement is a function of dose and prior exposure.

TABLE 63–5. Signs and Symptoms of Excessive Caffeine Intake

Restlessness	Gastrointestinal disturbances
Nervousness	Muscle twitching
Excitement	Rambling flow of thought or speech
Insomnia	Tachycardia or cardiac arrhythmia
Flushed face	Periods of inexhaustibility
Diuresis	Psychomotor agitation

Pharmacologically, the risk of developing some meaningful clinical manifestations becomes high when intake exceeds 500 mg/d. This places 20% to 30% of North Americans at risk.[68,69] Recognizing that there are individual variations and accepting a conservative approach, these data suggest that perhaps 10% to 20% of the North American adult population probably have meaningful clinical symptoms consistent with diagnosis of caffeinism, a prevalence rate exceeding that of most other substances of abuse.

EPIDEMIOLOGY OF CAFFEINE USE

Caffeine is used by 80% of the population of the United States. In a telephone survey, 17% of 166 respondents fulfilled DSM-III-R criteria for moderate or severe caffeine dependence in the past year. United States caffeine consumption exceeds several billion kilograms annually. Per capita intake for the entire world's population approximated 70 mg/d. In the United States, this figure is considerably larger, at 220 to 240 mg.[68] The majority of caffeine users progress to a pattern of frequent or daily consumption. Approximately one-fourth eventually begin consuming large quantities, exceeding 500 mg/d, and conservatively 10% of all adults then progress to develop the syndrome of caffeinism.[69] Mean daily consumption of caffeine in American children is surprisingly high. Consumption in the age range of 1 to 5 years is 1.20 mg/kg body weight from all sources. This compares with 2.60 mg/kg for people 18 and over.

DIFFERENTIAL DIAGNOSIS

Caffeine intoxication is the only official diagnosis associated with caffeinism in the DSM-IV. Caffeine-induced anxiety may manifest as restlessness, nervousness, excitement, insomnia, diuresis, flushing, gastrointestinal disturbance, muscle twitching, irritability, and jitteriness. If caffeine-induced insomnia requires specific treatment, caffeine-induced sleep disorder (DSM-IV) is an appropriate diagnosis.[11]

Because caffeine consumption is so widespread and at times excessive, a thorough history of caffeine use should be included in the routine assessment of all new patients in primary care medical settings.[69] In this manner, the practitioner can use the information gathered to uncover high levels of caffeine intake and then use the information to pinpoint the cause of clinical signs and symptoms typical of caffeinism. Clinical manifestations of caffeinism will almost always lessen in intensity or disappear completely within 1 to 2 weeks after removing the drug.[11]

PHARMACOLOGY OF CAFFEINE

Caffeine is rapidly and completely absorbed from the gastrointestinal tract,[11] reaching a peak blood level within 30 to 45 minutes of oral ingestion. It easily crosses the blood–brain barrier,[11] and levels achieved in the brain are proportional to the dose administered.

The half-life of caffeine in humans is approximately 3.5 to 5 hours. It is metabolized extensively according to a complex metabolic pathway occurring primarily in the liver.[11] Serious problems rarely result from overdoses of caffeine. In fact, the amount of caffeine needed to cause death in an average adult male is 5 to 10 grams, the equivalent of 50 to 100 cups of regular brewed coffee.[11] Thus, the risk of overdose from dietary sources of caffeine is virtually nonexistent.

Caffeine increases the heart rate and force of contraction.[70] It also has a strong diuretic effect.[70] The key factor promoting caffeine usage and dosage increase may be the drug's reinforcing effect upon pleasure and reward centers of the brain.[70] Caffeine's pharmacologic actions appear comparable (although less potent) in some aspects to those of other stimulants, such as amphetamines and cocaine. After years of uncertainty, it is apparent from both preclinical research and human studies that regular caffeine use does induce tolerance.[11]

CAFFEINE DEPENDENCE

Hughes and colleagues[70,71] and Griffiths and collaborators[72] have demonstrated that abstinence from caffeine induces a distinct withdrawal syndrome. Evidence for the existence of a caffeine dependence syndrome was presented by Strain and associates.[73] In a structured psychiatric interview, subjects self-identified as having problems with caffeine use were evaluated for features of a DSM-IV diagnosis of drug dependence. Those judged as caffeine dependent manifested at least three of four criteria (tolerance, withdrawal, persistent desire, or unsuccessful attempt to reduce consumption and persistent use despite adverse psychological or physical consequences). Of 99 people screened, 27 were evaluated by means of a structured psychiatric interview modified from the diagnosis of caffeine dependence; 16 of those subjects (59%) met the criteria. In a second phase of the study, 11 of the 16 caffeine-dependent individuals participated in a 2-day double-blind cross-over study of caffeine deprivation. Nine showed evidence of caffeine withdrawal during the placebo phase, a finding that validated one of the criteria for the diagnosis of dependence.

CAFFEINE WITHDRAWAL

The frequency of the caffeine withdrawal syndrome is not well known, but it may be common. Withdrawal can occur when individuals who have been previously consuming the drug on a regular basis suddenly discontinue their intake.[11] The syndrome can be characterized by the occurrence of headache, drowsiness, and fatigue. Sometimes the syndrome includes impaired psychomotor performance, difficulty concentrating, nausea, excessive yawning, and craving. These symptoms usually appear within 18 to 24 hours of discontinuation of intake, corresponding to the time required for the drug to leave the body.[11]

The caffeine withdrawal headache is somewhat unique, starting with a sense of fullness in the head and progressing to throbbing and diffuse pain which is made worse by movement. The maximum intensity of the pain occurs 3 to 6 hours after beginning. Symptoms of caffeine withdrawal are summarized in Table 63–6.

When caffeine is reintroduced, relief of withdrawal symptoms tends to occur within 30 to 60 minutes. At present, this appears to be the most effective "treatment" for the caffeine withdrawal syndrome.

EFFECT ON SLEEP

Caffeine interferes with sleep in most nontolerant individuals.[11] Once tolerance has developed, people are much less likely to self-report sleep abnormalities, or they may sense that the insomnia has disappeared altogether. To illustrate, 53% of those consuming less than 250 mg/d agreed that caffeine before bedtime would prevent sleep, compared to 43% of those consuming 250 to 749 mg/d and only 22% of those taking 750 mg/d or more.[11] Even though the higher-level consumers denied that caffeine interferes with their sleep, studies done in the sleep laboratory confirm that caffeine consumers do have greater sleep latency, more frequent awakenings, and altered sleep architecture, and that these effects are dose related.[11]

CAFFEINE-RELATED SOMATIC MANIFESTATIONS

Caffeine can cause other problems in addition to anxiety and nervousness. Users of high doses of caffeine often experience one or more of the following problems: urinary frequency and diuresis, headache, tachycardia, arrhythmias, tremulousness, diarrhea, gastrointestinal pain or discomfort, or light-headedness.[11] Less frequent symptoms include seeing "spots" in front of the eyes, "ringing" in the ears, a feeling of being unable to breathe, "tingling" in fingers and toes, and excessive perspiration. Caffeine may precipitate a true panic attack.

TABLE 63–6. Signs and Symptoms of Caffeine Withdrawal

Headache	Difficulty concentrating
Drowsiness	Nausea
Fatigue	Excessive yawning
Impaired psychomotor performance	Craving

COMORBID SUBSTANCE-RELATED DISORDERS

It is not uncommon for high users of caffeine to also be taking a variety of other psychoactive medications, mostly of the CNS depressant variety. Sedative–hypnotics and antianxiety agents are used significantly more often in those consuming high doses of caffeine than in those consuming low or moderate amounts. Approximately two-thirds of highest caffeine users reported using an antianxiety agent within the past month.[11] Similar effects on the brain reward pathways may help explain why excessive caffeine, alcohol, and tobacco use tend to occur in the same individuals.

▶ TREATMENT: Caffeinism

Caffeinism is treated by reducing or discontinuing the drug. It may be necessary to wean the patient off the drug, as going "cold turkey" may produce such serious symptoms that the drug must be restarted. Decaffeinated beverages may be slowly substituted for the caffeinated type. Relapses are less likely to occur, however, when the drug is discontinued all at once, probably due to the considerable self-discipline required to continue weaning the drug when one knows that an increase in dose will cause the symptoms to abate.

It may be possible for some individuals to simply reduce their dosage of caffeine rather than discontinue it altogether. Others may be particularly sensitive to the drug, and they may not be able to handle even reduced intake of caffeine. Patients with cardiovascular disease, especially arrhythmias, should totally refrain, as should people with prior stroke or transient ischemic attacks. Peptic ulcer patients and those with bipolar mood disorder and schizophrenia should be encouraged to avoid caffeine altogether.

CONCLUSIONS

Use of alcohol, tobacco, and caffeine are so commonly accepted in our society that people take notice only when their use causes serious problems. Yet, when these problems do occur, the human and economic costs are enormous. Health professionals must be committed to helping people free themselves of the addictions that can occur with these common drugs.

REFERENCES

1. Smoking-attributable mortality and years of potential life lost-United States, 1988. MMWR 1991;40:62.
2. Smoking and Health: A National Status Report, 2nd ed. DHHS pub. no. (CDC) 87-8396. Rockville, MD, U.S. Department of Health and Human Services, 1990.
3. Grant BF. Alcohol consumption, alcohol abuse and alcohol dependence: The United States as an example. Addiction 1994;89:1357.
4. Institute for Health Policy, Brandeis University. Substance Abuse: The Nation's Number One Health Problem. Key Indicators for Policy. Princeton, Robert Wood Johnson Foundation, 1993:16.
5. American Psychiatric Association. Diagnostic and Statistical Manual of Mental Disorders, 4th ed (DSM-IV). Washington, DC, APA, 1994.
6. National Institute on Drug Abuse and National Institute on Alcohol Abuse and Alcoholism: National Drug and Alcoholism Treatment Unit Survey (NDATUS) 1989 Main Findings Report. DHHS pub. no. (ADM) 91-1729. Rockville, MD, National Institute of Drug Abuse/National Institute on Alcohol Abuse and Alcoholism, 1990.
7. Fe Caces M, Stinson FS, Dufour MC. Surveillance report 36. Trends in Alcohol-Related Morbidity Among Short-Stay Community Hospital Discharges, United States, 1979–93. Bethesda, MD, Division of Biometry and Epidemiology, National Institute on Alcohol Abuse and Alcoholism, 1995:1.
8. Robins LN, Regier DA, eds. Psychiatric Disorders in America: The Epidemiologic Catchment Area Study. New York, Free Press, 1991:90.

9. Holt S, Stewart IC, Dixon JMJ, et al. Alcohol and the emergency service patient. Br Med J 1983;28:638–640.
10. Gilbert RM. Caffeine consumption. In: Spiller GA, ed. The Methylxanthine Beverages and Foods: Chemistry, Consumption, and Health Effects. New York, Liss, 1984:185–213.
11. Greden JF, Walters A. Caffeine. In: Lowinson JH, Ruiz P, Millman RB, Langrod JG, eds. Substance Abuse—A Comprehensive Textbook. Baltimore, Williams & Wilkins, 1997:294–307.
12. Hughes JR, Oliveto AH, Helzer, et al. Indications of caffeine dependence in a population-based sample. In: Harris L, ed. Problems of Drug Dependence. Proceeding of the 54th annual scientific meeting, College on Problems of Drug Dependence, 1992. Rockville, MD, U.S. Dept of Health and Human Services, National Institute on Drug Abuse, 1993:194. NIDA research monograph no. 132.
13. Barone JJ, Roberts H. Human consumption of caffeine. In: Dews PB, ed. Caffeine: Perspectives From Recent Research. New York, Springer-Verlag, 1984:59–73.
14. National Household Survey on Drug Abuse. Rockville, MD, U.S. Department of Health and Human Services, Substance Abuse and Mental Health Services Administration, 1996.
15. Dorland's Illustrated Medical Dictionary, 28th ed. Philadelphia, Saunders, 1994:478.
16. Li TK, Lumeng L, McBride WJ, Murphy JM. Rodent lines selected for factors affecting alcohol consumption. Alcohol Alcohol 1987; (suppl 1):91–96.
17. Blum K, Noble EP, Sheridan PJ, et al. Allelic association of human dopamine D_2 receptor gene in alcoholism. JAMA 1990;263:2055–2060.
18. Smith SS, O'Hara BF, Persico AM, et al. Genetic vulnerability to drug abuse: The D_2 dopamine receptor Taq IBM restriction fragment length polymorphism appears more frequently in polysubstance abusers. Arch Gen Psychiatry 1992;49:723–727.
19. Noble EP, Blum K, Khalsa ME, et al. Allelic association of the D_2 dopamine receptor gene with cocaine dependence. Drug Alcohol Depend 1993;33:271–285.
20. George FR. Genetic models in the study of alcoholism and substance abuse mechanisms. Prog Neuropsychopharmacol Biol Psychiatry 1993;17:345–361.
21. Anthenelli RM, Schuckit MA. Genetics. In: Lowinson JH, Ruiz P, Millman RB, Langrod JG, eds. Substance Abuse-A Comprehensive Textbook. Baltimore, Williams & Wilkins, 1997:41–51.
22. Gianoulakis C, Angelogianni P, Meany M, et al. Endorphins in individuals with high and low risk for development of alcoholism. In: Reid LD, ed. Opioids, Bulimia, and Alcohol Abuse and Alcoholism. New York, Springer-Verlag, 1990:229.
23. Fisher HR, Simpson RI, Kapur BM. Calculation of blood alcohol concentration (BAC) by sex, weight, number of drinks and time. Can J Public Health 1987;78:300–304.
24. Marco CA, Kelen GD. Acute intoxication. Emerg Med Clin North Am 1990;8:731–748.
25. Saitz R, O'Malley SS. Pharmacotherapies for alcohol abuse. Withdrawal and treatment. Med Clin North Am 1997;81:881–907.
26. Hill A, Williams D. Hazards associated with the use of benzodiazepines in alcohol detoxification. J Subst Abuse Treat 1993;10: 449–451.
27. Morse RM, Flavin DK. The definition of alcoholism. The Joint Committee of the National Council on Alcoholism and Drug Dependence and the Ameriucan Society of Addiction Medicine to Study the Definition and Criteria for the Diagnosis of Alcoholism. JAMA 1992;268: 1012–1014.
28. Gallant D. Alcohol. In: Galanter M, Kleber HD, eds. Textbook of Substance Abuse Treatment. Washington, DC, American Psychiatric Press, 1994:67.
29. Fuller RK. Antidipsotropic medications. In: Hester RK, Miller WR, eds. Handbook of Alcoholism Treatment Approaches: Effective Alternatives. New York, Pergamon, 1989.
30. Swift RM, Whelihan W, Kuznetsov O, et al. Naltrexone-induced alterations in human ethanol intoxication. Am J Psychiatry 1994;151: 1463–1467.
31. O'Malley SS, Croop RS, Wroblewski JM, et al. Naltrexone in the treatment of alcohol dependence: A combined analysis of two trials. Psychiatr Ann 1995;25:681–685.
32. Volpicelli JR, Watson NT, King AC, et al. Effect of naltrexone on alcohol "high" in alcoholics. Am J Psychiatry 1995;152:613–615.
33. O'Malley SS, Jaffe AJ, Chang G, et al. Naltrexone and coping skills therapy for alcohol dependence: A controlled study. Arch Gen Psychiatry 1992;49:881–887.
34. Volpicelli JR, Alterman AL, Hayashida M, et al. Naltrexone in the treatment of alcohol dependence. Arch Gen Psychiatry 1992;49: 876–880.
35. Pfohl DN, Allen JI, Atkinson RL, et al. Naltrexone hydrochloride (Trexan); A review of serum transaminase elevations at high dosage. In: Harris LS, ed. Problems of Drug Dependence, 1985: Proceedings of the 47th annual scientific meeting, the Committee on Problems of Drug Dependence. Rockville, MD, National Institute on Drug Abuse, 1986:213.
36. Frank E, Winkleby M, Altman D, et al. Predictors of physician's smoking cessation advice. JAMA 1991;266:3139–3144.
37. Glynn TJ, Manley MW, Solberg LI, et al. Creating and maintaining an optimal medical practice environment for treatment of nicotine addiction. In: Orleans, C, Slade J, eds. Nicotine Addiction: Principles and Management. New York, Oxford University Press, 1993: 162–181.
38. Marcus E, Emont SL, Corcoran RD, et al. Public attitudes about cigarette smoking: Results from the 1989 smoking activity volunteer executed survey. Public Health Rep 1994;109:124–134.
39. Smoking-attributable mortality and years of potential life lost—United States, 1990. MMWR 1993;42:645–649.
40. American Cancer Society. Cancer Facts and Figures—1996. Atlanta, American Cancer Society, 1996.
41. U.S. Department of Health and Human Services. The Health Benefits of Smoking Cessation: A Report of the Surgeon General. DHHS pub. no. CDC 90-8416. U.S. Department of Health and Human Services, Public Health Services, 1990.
42. Fiore MC, Wetter DW, Bailey WC, et al. Smoking Cessation Clinical Practice Guideline. Rockville, MD, Agency for Health Care Policy and Research, Public Health Service, U.S. Department of Health and Human Services, April 1996. AHCPR pub. 96-0692.
43. McEvoy GK, ed. AHFS Drug Information—96. Bethesda, MD, American Society of Health-System Pharmacists, 1997:1049.
44. Hughes Jr, Gust SW, Pechacek TF. Prevalence of tobacco dependence and withdrawal. Am J Psychiatry 1987;144:205–208.
45. Woody GE, Cottler LB, Cacciola J. Severity of dependence: Data from the DSM-IV field trials. Addiction 1993;88:1573–1579.
46. Cottler LB. Comparing DSM-III-R and ICD-10 substance use disorders. Addiction 1993;88:689–696.
47. Kessler DA, Barnett PS, Witt A, et al. The legal and scientific basis for FDA's assertion of jurisdiction over cigarettes and smokeless tobacco. JAMA 1997;277:405–409.
48. Title 21, United States Code 321(g)(1)(C), 321(h)(3).
49. Fiore MC, Smith SS, Jorenby DE, et al. The effectiveness of the nicotine patch for smoking cessation: A meta-analysis. JAMA 1994;271: 1940–1947.
50. Cepeda-Bernito A. A meta-analytic review of the efficacy of nicotine chewing gum in smoking treatment programs. J Consult Clin Psychol 1993;61:822–830.
51. Silagy C, Mant D, Fowler G, et al. Meta-analysis of efficacy of nicotine replacement therapies in smoking cessation. Lancet 1994;343: 139–142.
52. Tang JL, Law M, Wald N. How effective is nicotine replacement therapy in helping people to stop smoking? BMJ 1994;308:21–26.
53. Kornitzer M, Boiusten M, Dramaix M, et al. Combined use of nicotine patch and gum in smoking cessation: A placebo-controlled clinical trial. Prev Med 1995;24:41–47.
54. Puska P, Korhonen HJ, Vartiainen E, et al. Combined use of nicotine patch and gum compared with gum alone in smoking cessation: A clinical trial in North Karelia. Tobacco Control 1995;4:231–235.

55. Tsoh JY, McClure JB, Skaar, KL, et al. Smoking cessation 2: Components of effective intervention. Behav Med 1997;23:15–27.
56. Hajek P, Jackson P, Belcher M. Long-term use of nicotine chewing gum. JAMA 1988;260:2593–2596.
57. Hughes JR, Wadland WC, Fenwick JW, et al. Effect of cost on self-administration and efficacy of nicotine gum: A preliminary study. Prev Med 1991;20:486–496.
58. Physician's Desk Reference, 50th ed. Montvale, NJ, Medical Economics, 1997:2459.
59. Schauffler HH, Parkinson MD. Health insurance coverage for smoking cessation services. Health Educ Q 1993;20:185–206.
60. Kaplan RM, Orleans, Perkins KA, et al. Marshaling the evidence for greater regulation and control of tobacco products: A call for action. Ann Behav Med 1995;17:3–14.
61. Fiscella K, Franks P. Cost-effectiveness of the transdermal nicotine patch as an adjunct to physicians' smoking cessation counseling. JAMA 1996;275:1247–1251.
62. Hurt RD, Sachs DP, Glover ED, et al. A comparison of sustained-release bupropion and placebo for smoking cessation. N Engl J Med 1997;337:1195–1202.
63. Bupropion (Zyban) for smoking cessation. Med Lett Drugs Ther 1997;39:77–78.
64. Product information, Zyban (bupropion hydrochloride sustained-release tablets). Glaxo Wellcome, May 1997.
65. Dalack GW, Glassman AH, Rivelli S, et al. Mood, major depression, and fluoxetine response in cigarette smokers. Am J Psychiatry 1995; 152:398–403.
66. Griffiths RR, Bigelow GE, Liebson IA. Human coffee drinking: Reinforcing and physical dependence producing effects of caffeine. J Pharmacol Exp Ther 1986;239:416–425.
67. Griffiths RR, Bigelow GE, Liebson IA. Reinforcing effects of caffeine in coffee and capsules. J Exp Anal Behav 1989;52:127–140.
68. Gilbert RM. Caffeine as a drug of abuse. In: Gibben RG, Hiklart YI, Popham RE, et al, eds. Research Addresses in Alcohol and Drug Problems. New York, Wiley; 1976:213.
69. Greden JF. Anxiety and depression associated with caffeinism among psychiatric inpatients. Am J Psychiatry 1978;135:963.
70. Hughes JR, Oliveto AH, Bickel WK, et al. Caffeine self-administration and withdrawal: Incidence, individual differences and interrelationships. Drug Alcohol Depend 1993;32:239–246.
71. Hughes JR, Oliveto AH, Helzer JE, et al. Should caffeine abuse, dependence or withdrawal be added to DSM-IV and ICD-10? Am J Psychiatry 1992;149:33–40.
72. Griffiths RR, Evans SM, Heishman SJ, et al. Low-dose caffeine physical dependence in humans. J Pharmacol Exp Ther 1990;255: 1123–1132.
73. Strain EC, Mumford GK, Silverman K, et al. Caffeine dependence syndrome—Evidence from case histories and experimental evaluations. JAMA 1994;272:1043–1048.

APPENDIX 63–1

Useful Internet Sites on Alcohol, Smoking, and Caffeine

ALCOHOL

National Institute on Alcohol Abuse and Alcoholism (NIAAA)

http://www.niaaa.nih.gov/

National Substance Abuse Web Index

http://nsawi.health.org/cgi-bin/intro.cgi#Indexed_Site

NIAAA Alcohol and Alcohol Problems Science Database (ETOH)

http://etoh.niaaa.nih.gov/

SMOKING

Materials for Physicians and Office Staff—Indiana Tobacco Council Control

http://iumeded.med.iupui.edu/tobacco/ncimatl.htm

American Cancer Society Smokeout Web site

http://www.cancer.org/smokeout/

Agency for Health Care Policy Research Clinical Practice Guideline—Smoking Cessation

http://text.nlm.nih.gov/ftrs/pick?dbName=smkc&ftrsK=52695&cp=1&t=885319560&collect=ahcpr

CAFFEINE

Alcohol and Drug Addiction Research Foundation, Toronto.

http://www.arf.org/isd/pim/caffeine.html

Everything You Need to Know About . . . Caffeine

http://ificinfo.health.org/brochure/caffeine.htm

Caffeine and Women's Health

http://ificinfo.health.org/brochure/caff-wh.htm

64

SCHIZOPHRENIA

M. Lynn Crismon, PharmD, FCCP, BCPP, and Peter G. Dorson, PharmD, BCPP

Schizophrenia is one of the most complex and challenging of psychiatric disorders. It represents a heterogeneous syndrome of disorganized and bizarre thoughts, delusions, hallucinations, inappropriate affect, and impaired psychosocial functioning. From the time that Kraepelin first described dementia praecox in 1896 until publication of the *Diagnostic and Statistical Manual of Mental Disorders,* fourth edition (DSM-IV) in 1994, the description of this illness has continued to evolve.[1] Technological advances that increase our knowledge of central nervous system physiology and pathophysiology will likely improve our understanding of schizophrenia in the future.

EPIDEMIOLOGY

According to the Epidemiologic Catchment Area Study, the U.S. lifetime prevalence of schizophrenia ranges from 0.6% to 1.9%, with an average of approximately 1%.[2] With only a few possible exceptions, the worldwide prevalence of schizophrenia is remarkably similar among all cultures. Schizophrenia most commonly has its onset in late adolescence or early adulthood and rarely occurs before adolescence or after the age of 40. Although the prevalence of schizophrenia is equal in males and females, the onset of illness tends to be earlier in males. Males most frequently have their first episode during their early 20s, whereas with females it is usually during their late 20s to early 30s.[1–3]

PATHOPHYSIOLOGY

Although the etiology of schizophrenia is unknown, research has demonstrated various abnormalities in brain structure and function. However, these changes are not consistent among all individuals with a diagnosis of schizophrenia, and much is yet to be learned about its pathogenesis. The cause of schizophrenia is likely multifactorial, that is, multiple pathophysiologic abnormalities may play a role in producing the similar but varying clinical phenotypes we refer to as schizophrenia.

NEUROTRANSMITTER CHANGES

The most common pathophysiologic theories associated with the etiology of schizophrenia have involved the dopaminergic (DAergic) system. Since the discovery of the role of dopamine (DA) as a neurotransmitter in 1958 and the observations that antipsychotic (AP) drugs are postsynaptic DA receptor antagonists, there has been interest in a DAergic hypothesis for the pathophysiology of schizophrenia. However, these theories may be more appropriately oriented toward the treatment of psychosis with antipsychotics than the etiology of schizophrenia.

There are four DAergic tracts of primary interest (Table 64–1). The nigrostriatal tract originates with cell bodies from the A9 area in the substantia nigra and terminates with synapses in the caudate nucleus and putamen of the basal ganglia. The second tract, the mesolimbic pathway, projects from A10 in the midbrain ventral tegmentum to the cingulate gyrus and to limbic regions such as the amygdala, olfactory tubercle, and septal nuclei. The mesocortical tract extends from A10 to the prefrontal and frontal cortex. The tuberoinfundibular tract projects from the hypothalamus to the pituitary. Each tract is thought to have a primary functional correlate that relates to its anatomic projections (Table 64–1).[4]

Homovanillic acid (HVA, a DA metabolite) concentrations in the cerebrospinal fluid (CSF) are correlated with DAergic turnover in the synapse, and therefore, HVA formation. A hyperactive DA system should result in increased DA release from the presynaptic terminal and increased metabolite formation. However, HVA concentrations are not increased in most chronic schizophrenics, and a subgroup of chronic schizophrenics have decreased CSF HVA. However, even schizophrenic patients with low CSF HVA concentrations during residual phases of the illness have a relative increase in CSF HVA during acute psychotic exacerbations.[5]

Increasing evidence supports the presence of a DA receptor defect in schizophrenia. Numerous positron emission tomography (PET) studies have shown regional brain abnormalities, including increased glucose metabolism in the caudate nucleus and decreased blood flow and glucose metabolism in the frontal lobe and left temporal lobe.[5–7] This may indicate DAergic hyperactivity in the head of the caudate nucleus and DAergic hypofunction in the frontotemporal regions. PET studies using D_2-specific ligands provide data suggesting increased densities of D_2 receptors in the head of the caudate nucleus with decreased densities in the prefrontal cortex.[4] PET studies assessing D_1 function suggest that subpopulations of schizophrenics may have decreased densities of D_1 receptors in the caudate nucleus and the prefrontal cortex. Hypofrontality may be associated with lack of volition, one of the core negative symptoms seen in schizophrenia.[7,8] It is important to emphasize that it is unknown whether these changes represent a primary event or whether they are merely compensatory changes

TABLE 64–1. Dopaminergic Tracts and Effects of Dopamine Antagonists

Dopamine Tract	Origin	Innervation	Function	Dopamine Antagonist Effect
Nigrostriatal	Substantia nigra (A9 area)	Caudate nucleus Putamen	Extrapyramidal system, movement	Movement disorders
Mesolimbic	Midbrain ventral tegmentum (A10 area)	Limbic areas (e.g., amygdala, olfactory tubercle, septal nuclei), Cingulate gyrus	Arousal, memory, stimulus processing, motivational behavior	Relief of psychosis
Mesocortical	Midbrain ventral tegmentum (A10 area)	Frontal and prefrontal lobe cortex	Cognition, communication, social function, response to stress	Relief of psychosis Akathisia?
Tuberoinfundibular	Hypothalamus	Pituitary gland	Regulates prolactin release	Increased prolactin concentrations

secondary to other pathophysiologic abnormalities in schizophrenia. Because of the heterogeneity in the clinical presentation of schizophrenia, it has also been suggested that the DA hypothesis may be more applicable to "neuroleptic-responsive psychosis," with multiple different etiologies possibly being responsible for causing schizophrenia.[5]

Attempts have been made to develop relationships between these abnormal findings and behavioral symptoms present in schizophrenic patients. The positive symptoms are possibly more closely associated with receptor hyperactivity in the mesocaudate, whereas negative symptoms are most closely related to DA receptor hypofunction in the prefrontal cortex.

The potential for phospholipid abnormalities has also been investigated in schizophrenia. Studies have shown a shift from anabolic to catabolic membrane phospholipids in the prefrontal cortex of schizophrenic brains.[7] Phosphoinositide (PI) may serve as a second messenger system for the D_2 receptor, and D_2 stimulation decreases PI turnover. Abnormalities in phospholipid metabolism could therefore result in abnormal DA activity.[5]

Glutamatergic dysfunction has been suggested as being etiologic in schizophrenia. The glutamatergic system is one of the most widespread excitatory neurotransmitter systems in the brain. Alterations in its function, either hypo- or hyperactivity, can result in toxic neuronal reactions.[9] DAergic innervation from the ventral striatum decreases the limbic system's inhibitory activity (perhaps through γ-aminobutyric acid [GABA] interneurons); thus, DAergic stimulation increases arousal. The corticostriatal glutamate pathways have the opposite effect, inhibiting DAergic function from the ventral striatum, therefore allowing the limbic system to have increased inhibitory activity. Descending glutamatergic tracts interact with dopaminergic tracts directly as well as through GABA interneurons. Glutamatergic deficiency produces symptoms similar to those of DAergic hyperactivity and possibly those seen in schizophrenia. Clinical support for this hypothesis comes from the fact that phencyclidine, a potent psychotomimetic, is a noncompetitive antagonist at the *N*-methyl-D-aspartate (NMDA) receptor, a major glutamate receptor. It is proposed that schizophrenia may involve some currently unknown in utero assault that leads to a developmental defect in NMDA receptor function—so-called NMDA hypofunction (NRH). This defect is proposed to have latent clinical expression with neuropsychological pathology from NRH not being seen until late adolescence or early adulthood. According to this theory, if the NRH is accompanied by DAergic hyperactivity, then a DA antagonist responsive psychosis ensues. However, if DA hyperactivity is not present, then the symptoms would likely be poorly responsive to typical antipsychotics.[10,11]

Serotonergic receptors are present on DAergic axons, and it is known that stimulation of these receptors will decrease DA release, at least in the striatum.[4] Although somewhat more diffuse, the distribution of serotonergic neurons is similar to that of DAergic neurons, thus allowing these two neurotransmitter systems to innervate the same areas. In fact, 5-hydroxytryptamine$_2$ (serotonin$_2$; 5-HT$_2$) receptors and D_4 receptors have been found to be colocalized in the cortex.[7] Schizophrenic patients with abnormal brain scans have been shown to have higher whole blood 5-HT concentrations, and these concentrations are correlated with increased ventricular size.[12] Atypical antipsychotics with potent 5-HT$_2$ receptor antagonist effects have been shown to reverse worsening of symptomatology induced by 5-HT agonists in schizophrenic patients.[5]

Increased concentrations of norepinephrine have been observed in limbic structures of patients with chronic paranoid schizophrenia, but not in patients with other subtypes.[5] The relationship of these neurotransmitters to the function of the limbic filtering system is unclear. However, it is possible that they have important functions in modulating the corticostriatal loop, thus modulating limbic input.

A dysregulation hypothesis has been invoked to explain the divergent findings in biochemical and receptor studies.[4,13] The dysregulation hypothesis maintains that aberrant homeostatic control mechanisms cause erratic neurotransmission; that is, the homeostatic mechanisms that control the relationships among neurotransmitter synthesis, release, reuptake, metabolism, activity at receptors, and second messenger systems are defective. This lack of homeostasis can be pictured as resulting in dysfunction among several different processes, including basal neurotransmission, biological rhythm, and return to the basal rate after perturbations on the system. The primary pathophysiologic abnormality in schizophrenia may occur in one of a number of different neurotransmitters (e.g., DAergic, glutamatergic, or serotonergic systems), with changes in other neurotransmitters occurring secondarily. For example, a primary defect resulting in abnormal presynaptic release of DA from the neuron and ineffective feedback mechanisms could lead to postsynaptic DA receptor hypersensitivity. The NRH model is another approach that would lead to dysregulation among neurotransmitter systems.

Schizophrenia is a complex disorder, and multiple etiologies may exist for the clinical syndrome we refer to as schizophrenia. Based on current knowledge, it is naive to think that any currently proposed etiology can adequately explain the genesis of this complex disease. Molecular research involving subtle changes in G-proteins, protein metabolism, and other subcellular processes may more closely identify the biologic disturbances associated with schizophrenia.[13]

STRUCTURAL CHANGES

Computerized axial tomography (CAT) scans and magnetic resonance imaging (MRI) show increased ventricular size, particularly in the third and lateral ventricles, in subtypes of schizophrenics. Recent studies also show a small but definite decrease in brain size as compared with matched controls. These changes appear to be consistent with brain asymmetry, the ventricular enlargement being most pronounced in the left temporal horn, and the decreased cortical size being most obvious in the left temporal lobe.[14] Decreased cortical thickness reflects a decrease in the space between neurons (i.e., increased neuronal density) rather than a decrease in the number of neurons in the prefrontal lobe cortex.[6,7] This may result in a decreased number of axonal and dendritic communications between cells and therefore a loss of connectivity that could be important with respect to neuronal adaptivity and CNS homeostasis.[7] Most studies indicate that patients with enlarged ventricles are more likely to demonstrate abnormal findings on neuropsychologic testing, particularly when mentally stressed. Patients with enlarged ventricles may respond more poorly to AP medications.[14]

GENETICS

Although a specific abnormality has not been discovered, increasing evidence suggests a genetic basis for schizophrenia. Although the risk of developing schizophrenia is 0.5% to 1.5% in the general population, this increases to approximately 10% if a first-degree relative has the illness and 3% for second-degree relatives.[1,15] If both parents have schizophrenia, the risk of producing a schizophrenic offspring increases to approximately 40%. Twin studies in dizygotic twins report that the risk of the second twin developing schizophrenia if one twin has the illness is between 12% and 14%. However, in monozygotic twins the risk increases to 48%.[15] Numerous adoption studies indicate that the risk for schizophrenia lies with the biologic parents, and change in the environment during the child's developmental stages does not alter this. If schizophrenia occurs in siblings, the onset of illness tends to occur at the same age in each, thus lessening the possibility of an environmental precipitant.

A search for a genetic linkage in schizophrenia has been difficult, and any genetic etiology in schizophrenia is multifactorial and follows multiple modes of inheritance. Potential loci have been identified on chromosomes 3, 5, 6, 8, 9, 20, and 22. If confirmed, these may only account for some cases of schizophrenia, and are more likely associated with a predisposition for the illness.[16]

NEURODEVELOPMENTAL CHANGES

A neurodevelopmental model has been evoked as a possible explanation for the etiology of schizophrenia. This model proposes that a genetic predisposition exists for schizophrenia and that an unknown in utero disturbance occurs, probably in the second trimester of pregnancy. Evidence for this is provided by the abnormal neuronal migration demonstrated in most studies of schizophrenic brains. This "schizophrenic lesion" may result in abnormalities in cell shape, position, symmetry, connectivity, and functionally to the development of abnormal brain circuits.[6,7] The resulting secondary "synaptic disorganization" is thought not to produce clinical manifestations until adolescence or early adulthood because this is the corresponding time period of neuronal maturation. Additional support for a developmental model is provided by the fact that although studies have shown decreased cortical thickness and increased ventricular size in many schizophrenics, this typically occurs in the absence of widespread gliosis. Gliosis, or the proliferation of glial cells, is thought to occur as a compensatory change in degenerative diseases of the brain. It is also feasible to integrate neurotransmitter abnormalities, such as the NRH hypothesis, into a developmental model.[10,11] Although this model for the etiology of schizophrenia is far from conclusive, it does provide a useful framework for additional research into the etiology of the disease.

CLINICAL PRESENTATION

Schizophrenia is the most common functional psychosis, and its clinical presentation can be extremely varied. Despite numerous attempts to portray a stereotype in movies and on television, the stereotypic schizophrenic essentially does not exist. Moreover, schizophrenia does not mean "split personality." Schizophrenia is a chronic disorder of thought and affect with the individual having a significant disturbance in interpersonal relationships and ability to function in society on a daily basis.

The first psychotic episode may be sudden in onset with few premorbid symptoms, or commonly may be preceded by withdrawn, suspicious, peculiar behavior (schizoid). During the acute psychotic episodes, the patient loses touch with reality, and, in a sense, the brain creates a false reality to replace it. The patient experiences a variety of acute psychotic symptoms, including hallucinations (especially hearing voices), delusions (fixed false beliefs), ideas of influence (beliefs that one's actions are controlled by external influences), and so on. Thought processes are disconnected (loose associations), the patient may not be able to carry on logical conversation, and may have simultaneous, contradictory thoughts (ambivalence). The patient's affect may be flat (no emotional expression), or it may be inappropriate and labile. The patient is often withdrawn and inwardly directed (autism). Uncooperativeness, hostility, and verbal or physical aggression may be seen because of the patient's misperception of reality. Self-care skills are impaired, and the patient is frequently dirty, unkempt, and in general has poor hygiene. Sleep and appetite are often disturbed.

When the acute psychotic episode remits, the patient typically has residual features. This is an important point in differentiating schizophrenia from other psychotic disorders. Although residual symptoms and their severity vary, patients may have difficulty with anxiety management, suspiciousness, and lack of volition, motivation, insight, and judgment. Therefore, they often have difficulty living independently in the community. Because of poor anxiety management and suspiciousness, they are frequently withdrawn socially, and have difficulty forming close relationships with others. Most do not marry. In addition, impaired volition and motivation contribute to poor self-care skills and make it difficult for the schizophrenic patient to maintain employment. Schizophrenics frequently experience a lack of historicity, or difficulty in learning from their experiences. They may repeatedly make the same mistakes in social conduct and situations requiring judgment. They have difficulty understanding the importance of treatment, including medications, in maintaining their ability to function in society. Therefore, they tend to discontinue medications and other treatments, and this increases the risk of relapse and rehospitalization.

Although the course of the illness is variable, the long-term prognosis for most schizophrenic patients is poor. The disease is marked by intermittent acute psychotic episodes and impaired psychosocial functioning between acute episodes, with most of the deterioration in psychosocial functioning occurring within 5 years after the first psychotic episode.[17] By late life, the patient may appear "burned out," that is, they cease to have acute psychotic episodes but residual symptoms, as previously described, persist. However, functional skills may actually improve as compared with earlier in the patient's life. Although typical AP drugs effectively treat the acute psychotic symptoms and aid in preventing relapse, they do not affect the impairment in psychosocial functioning seen with the disease. In a subpopulation of patients, probably 5% to 15%, psychotic symptoms are nearly continuous, and response to typical antipsychotics poor.[18]

TABLE 64–2. DSM-IV Diagnostic Criteria for Schizophrenia

A. Characteristic symptoms: Two or more of the following, each persisting for a significant portion of at least a 1-month period:
  (1) Delusions
  (2) Hallucinations
  (3) Disorganized speech
  (4) Grossly disorganized or catatonic behavior
  (5) Negative symptoms

  Note: Only one criterion A symptom is required if delusions are bizarre, if hallucinations consist of a voice keeping a running commentary on the person's behavior, or if there are two or more voices conversing with each other.

B. Social/occupational dysfunction: For a significant portion of the time since onset of the disorder, one or more major areas of functioning such as work, interpersonal relations, or self-care are significantly below the level prior to onset.

C. Duration: Continuous signs of the disorder for at least 6 months. This must include at least 1 month of symptoms fulfilling criterion A (unless successfully treated). This 6 months may include prodromal or residual symptoms.

D. Schizoaffective or mood disorder has been excluded.

E. Disorder is not due to a medical disorder or substance use.

F. If a history of a pervasive developmental disorder is present, there must be symptoms of hallucinations or delusions present for at least 1 month.

Adapted from Ref. 1.

DSM-IV places a greater emphasis on the chronicity of schizophrenia and negative symptoms than do previous editions. Schizophrenia is a chronic disorder, and the patient's history must be carefully assessed for dysfunction that has persisted for longer than 6 months. After their first episode, schizophrenics rarely have a level of adaptive functioning as high as before the onset of the disorder. The DSM-IV criteria are summarized in Table 64–2, and this reference should be consulted for a more detailed discussion of the differential diagnosis.[1]

DSM-IV[1] classifies the symptoms of schizophrenia into two categories, positive and negative. Recent research has identified a third separate symptom category, disorganized (Table 64–3).[2] Numerous authors have attempted to construct subtypes of schizophrenia, and it has been suggested that symptom complexes may correlate

TABLE 64–3. Schizophrenia Symptom Clusters

Positive	Negative	Disorganized
Hallucinations	Affective flattening	Disorganized speech
Delusions	Alogia	Disorganized behavior
	Anhedonia	Poor attention
	Avolition	

Adapted from Ref. 2.

with prognosis, cognitive functioning, structural abnormalities in the brain, and response to typical AP drugs.[4] Negative symptoms may be more closely associated with prefrontal lobe dysfunction and positive symptoms with temporolimbic abnormalities. Many patients demonstrate both positive and negative symptoms. Andreasen and associates[19] found that patients with negative symptoms may have more antecedent cognitive dysfunction, poor premorbid adjustment, low level of educational achievement, and a poorer overall prognosis.

▶ TREATMENT: Schizophrenia

DESIRED OUTCOME

Pharmacotherapy is the mainstay of treatment in schizophrenia, and it is essentially impossible in most patients to implement effective psychosocial rehabilitation programs in the absence of antipsychotic treatment. A pharmacotherapeutic treatment plan should be developed that delineates drug-related aspects of therapy. Because most deterioration in psychosocial functioning occurs within the first 5 years of the initial psychotic episode, treatment interventions should be particularly assertive during this period.[17] Explicit end points should be defined, including realistic goals of the target symptoms most likely to respond and the relative time course for response. Other goals include avoiding unwanted side effects, using the minimum effective dose, an emphasis on adequate time as a primary variable in determining response, and the limitation of augmentation medications to severely ill or nonresponsive patients.

NONPHARMACOLOGIC THERAPY

Psychosocial rehabilitation programs oriented toward improving patients' adaptive functioning are the mainstay of nondrug treatment for schizophrenia. These programs may include basic living skills, social skills training, basic education, work programs, and supported housing. In particular, programs aimed at employment and housing have been the more effective interventions and are considered "best practices" for persons with serious and persistent mental disorders. Programs that involve families in the care and lives of the patient have also been shown to decrease rehospitalizations and improve functioning in the community. For particularly low-functioning patients, assertive intervention programs referred to as Active Community Treatment (ACT) have been shown to be effective in improving patients' functional outcomes. ACT teams are available on a 24-hour basis and work in the patient's home and place of employment to provide comprehensive treatment, including medication, crisis intervention, daily living skills, and supported employment and housing.[2,20]

PHARMACOLOGIC THERAPY

ASSESSMENT PRIOR TO TREATMENT

The importance of initial assessment for accurate diagnosis cannot be underestimated in a patient presenting with acute psychosis. A thorough mental status examination, physical and neurologic examination, complete family and social history, and laboratory workup must be performed to exclude medical or substance-induced causes of psychosis, such as acute or chronic drug ingestion. Laboratory tests, biologic markers, and commonly available brain imaging techniques do not assist in diagnosis or selection of medication. A pretreatment patient workup should include the following areas of baseline studies: vital signs, complete blood count, electrolytes, hepatic function, renal function, cardiac function, thyroid function, and urine drug screen.

ANTIPSYCHOTIC MEDICATION CHOICES

Atypical Antipsychotics

Atypical antipsychotics (with the exception of clozapine [CLZ] and sertindole because of side effects) have become the agents of first choice in the treatment of schizophrenia, and practice guidelines and consensus statements support this recommendation.[2,17,21] Controlled trials demonstrate that atypical antipsychotics (AP) such as olanzapine (OLZ), risperidone (RSP), quetiapine, sertindole, and ziprasidone have superior efficacy for the treatment of negative symptoms. Whether this difference in negative symptom response is due to differences in core efficacy or differences in side effect profile is unknown. To date, inadequate maintenance treatment studies have been performed with atypical agents to adequately define the clinical outcomes resulting from their widespread use. However, some experts believe that their use during the first 5 years of onset of the illness could help prevent some of the deterioration associated with the disease.[17,22] Preliminary data on relapse rates and cost effectiveness are presented in the section on pharmacoeconomics later in the chapter.

There is no universally accepted definition for atypical AP. Common to all definitions, however, is the ability of the drug to produce antipsychotic response with few or no acutely occurring extrapyramidal side effects (EPS). Other attributes that have been ascribed to atypical APs include enhanced efficacy, particularly on negative symptoms; absence of tardive dyskinesia (TD); and lack of effect on serum prolactin (PRL). To date, the only approved atypical AP that fulfills all of these criteria is CLZ, the prototypical agent.[23]

RSP fulfills the atypical criterion of having a low incidence of EPS at low to moderate doses. In studies of randomly selected groups of schizophrenic patients in acute exacerbation, RSP has proven efficacy and may be superior to haloperidol in treatment of negative symptoms. The mean optimal dose in parallel, fixed-dose studies was 4 to 6 mg daily. At doses greater than 8 mg daily, RSP's profile is more similar to a typical AP.[22,24] Because RSP appears to lose its atypical profile at higher doses, the lowest possible dose should be used in treatment. This may include dose titration downward if patients do not respond initially, rather than upward titration as has been the traditional approach to dosing APs.[22,23]

OLZ also has superior efficacy in treating negative symptoms, and a very low incidence of extrapyramidal side effects.[25] The optimal dose range is 10 to 20 mg daily. Quetiapine does not appear to have as robust an effect on negative symptoms.[26] Doses above 250 mg are necessary for optimal effects, with mean doses near 350 mg/d. Sertindole also has superior efficacy as compared to traditional antipsychotics, with less EPS when used in doses of 12 to 20 mg daily.[27] Preliminary reports on ziprasidone are similar.[17]

Traditional or Typical Antipsychotics

All typical APs are equal in efficacy when used in equipotent doses. Interindividual variation does occur between individual APs, such that a relatively responsive patient may not respond to each AP. Intraindividual variation has been described but contributing factors, other than progression of disease state, have not been delineated. Selection of medication should be based on the need to avoid certain side effects in concurrent medical or psychiatric disorders. There are no differences in efficacy between low- and high-potency typical APs; and high-potency drugs (e.g., haloperidol [HPD]) are as effective in treating acute agitation as low-potency, highly sedating APs (e.g., chlorpromazine [CPZ]).

Previous patient or family history of response to an AP is helpful in the selection of an agent. Traditional dosage equivalents (expressed in "CPZ equivalent dosages"—the equipotent dosage of any AP compared with 100 mg of CPZ) may assist in determining the range of effective dosage if the need arises to treat a patient with a different typical AP drug. However, because atypical APs differ in mechanism of action, the dose equivalents have little relevance when comparing dosages of atypical APs. APs and their usual dosage ranges are listed in Table 64–4.

Pharmacotherapeutic Algorithm

A suggested pharmacotherapeutic algorithm for schizophrenia is outlined in Figure 64–1.[22] Atypicals are recommended as first-line treatment (i.e., stages 1,2, and 3) because of their superior effect on negative symptoms, a lower incidence of acutely occurring EPS, and growing evidence for a lower incidence of TD. These three atypicals are all considered first-line alternatives as inadequate evidence currently exists to recommend any one of them over the others. Because of safety concerns, it is generally recommended that patients be tried on all three agents as monotherapy before proceeding to a trial of clozapine. As new atypical antipsychotics reach the market, their placement in the algorithm will need to be evaluated. Unless clear evidence of superiority exists, Miller and colleagues[22] recommend that at least 40,000 patient exposures occur before positioning a newly approved medication in the algorithm. This allows minimal clinical experience with the new medication and the opportunity for uncommon, but perhaps severe, adverse reactions to potentially surface before deciding algorithm placement.

If patient noncompliance is primarily because of AP side effects, then two different atypical AP trials are recommended before using a depot antipsychotic. If the patient has never received an adequate trial of a typical AP, then a trial is recommended (stage 3) before proceeding to CLZ at stage 4. The effects of a typical AP in patients who have failed treatment only with atypical APs are unknown, and the risk of agranulocytosis with CLZ is significant enough that it is prudent to try a typical AP in most patients before using CLZ.[22]

Treatment algorithm recommendations after CLZ (stages 4b and 5) are based more on anecdotal experiences and clinical opinions than empirical research data.[22] These combination strategies are aimed at a small percentage of patients who have responded poorly to stages 1 to 4. These interventions should be implemented with careful evaluation of a patient's symptom response and discontinuation of the combination if improvement does not occur. See the later section on the treatment-resistant patient for a discussion of these strategy options.

PREDICTORS OF RESPONSE

Obtaining a thorough medication history is important, and previous AP treatment should help guide the selection of current drug therapy, in that either a good response will favor the use of the same agent or a negative response should influence the selection of a dissimilar drug. Nonprescription and illicit drug use may influence psychiatric presentation and thus diagnosis or AP response. Amphetamine and other CNS stimulants, cocaine, corticosteroids, digitalis glycosides, indomethacin, marijuana, pentazocine, phencyclidine, and other drugs can induce psychosis in susceptible individuals or exacerbate psychosis in patients with preexisting psychiatric illness.[28] Schizophrenic patients who continue to abuse alcohol or drugs usually have poor response to medications. Alcohol, caffeine, and nicotine use potentially result in drug interactions.

Individual differences in patient response have been either proposed or identified, which may be clinically useful predictors of response.[29] Acute onset and short duration of illness, presence of acute stressors or precipitating factors, later age of onset, family history of affective illness, and good premorbid adjustment as reflected in stable interpersonal relationships or employment are all predictors of good response.[29]

TABLE 64–4. Available Antipsychotics: Doses and Dosage Forms

Generic Name	Trade Name	Traditional Equivalent Dose (mg)[a]	Usual Dosage Range (mg/d)	Manufacturer's Maximum Dose (mg/d)	Dosage Forms[b]
Typical (Traditional) Antipsychotics					
Chlorpromazine	Thorazine	100	100–800	2000	T,L,LC,I,C-ER,S
Fluphenazine	Prolixin, Permitil	2	2–20	40	T,L,LC,I
Haloperidol	Haldol	2	2–20	100	T,LC,I
Loxapine	Loxitane	10	10–80	250	C,LC,I
Molindone	Moban	10	10–100	225	T,LC
Mesoridazine	Serentil	50	50–400	500	T,LC,I
Perphenazine	Trilafon	10	10–64	64	T,LC,I
Thioridazine	Mellaril	100	100–800	800	T,LC
Thiothixene	Navane	4	4–40	60	C,LC,I
Trifluoperazine	Stelazine	5	5–40	80	T,LC,I
Atypical Antipsychotics					
Clozapine	Clozaril	NA	50–500	900	T
Olanzapine	Zyprexa	NA	10–20	20	T
Quetiapine	Seroquel	NA	250–500	800	T
Risperidone	Risperdal	NA	2–8	16	T
Sertindole	Serlect	NA	4–20	N	N
Ziprasidone	Zeldox	NA	40–160	N	N

[a]NA, This parameter does not apply to atypical antipsychotics.
[b]T = tablet; C = Capsule; ER or SR = extended or sustained release; I = injection; L = liquid solution, elixir, or suspension; LC = liquid concentrate; R = rectal suppositories; N = not approved by the FDA.

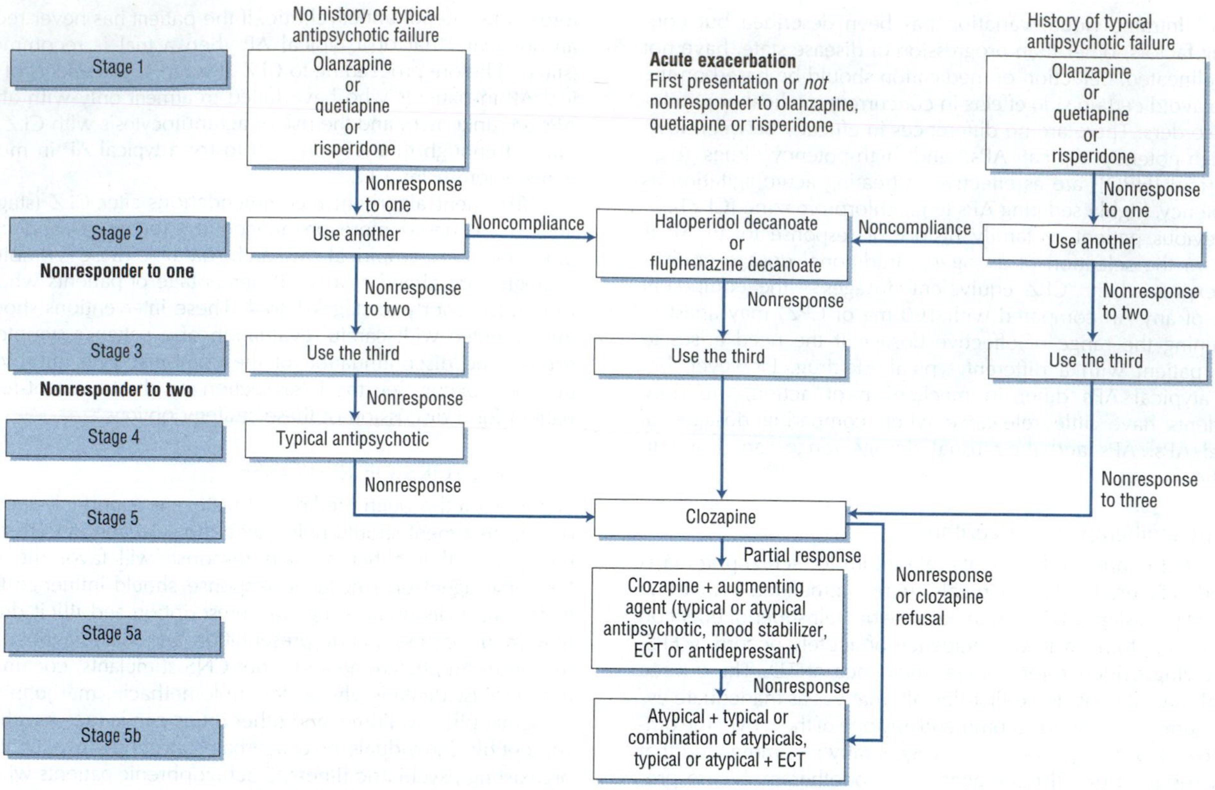

FIGURE 64–1. Suggested pharmacotherapeutic algorithm for schizophrenia. For updates of this algorithm, see the Texas Medication Algorithm Project Website at www.mhmr.state.tx.us.meds/tmap.htm *(From Ref. 22).*

Negative schizophrenic symptoms are less responsive to AP therapy. Although controversial, affective symptoms may correlate with good response. However, other than these caveats, there are few data to support a relationship between drug response and schizophrenic subtypes. Neuropsychologic deficits related to cognition and neurologic soft signs may also correlate with poor AP response.[29]

A patient's subjective response within the first 48 hours after being administered a typical AP may be associated with drug responsiveness.[30] A dysphoric response, demonstrated by stating a dislike of the medication, feeling worse or zombie-like, combined with anxiety or akathisia-like symptoms results in poor drug response, and if continued on the same medication, the patient will likely be noncompliant.

The importance of developing a therapeutic alliance between the patient and the clinician cannot be underestimated. Patients who form good alliances are more likely to be compliant with all aspects of therapy, experience a better outcome at 2 years, and generally require smaller doses of AP medications.[2]

A certain minority of patients fail to benefit from AP therapy, and their psychosocial functioning may actually worsen. Unfortunately, there is no accepted method to identify these people before treatment.[29]

INITIAL TREATMENT

Initial dosing should follow goals described in the pharmacotherapeutic treatment plan. The goals during the first 7 days should be decreased agitation, hostility, combativeness, anxiety, tension, aggression, and normalization of sleep and eating patterns. The usual recommendation is to initiate therapy and titrate over the first few days to an average effective dose unless the patient's physiologic status or history indicates that this dose may result in unacceptable adverse effects.[31] The usual dosage range is listed in Table 64–4, and an average dose is typically midrange. After a week on a stable dose, a modest dosage increase may be considered if the goals have not been achieved (decreased agitation and uncooperativeness). If "cheeking" of medication is suspected, liquid formulations of most APs are available (Table 64–4). If a patient has shown no improvement within 3 to 4 weeks at therapeutic doses, then an alternative AP should be considered, that is, moving to the next treatment stage in the algorithm (Fig. 64–1).[22]

Although some practitioners believe that larger daily doses are necessary in more severely symptomatic patients, fixed-dose studies of low versus high daily doses do not reveal any major differences in degree of symptom improvement, time to response, or length of hospitalization.[32] Some symptoms, such as agitation, tension, aggression, and increased motor activity, may respond more quickly, but side effects, especially EPS, may be more common with higher doses, as well. However, interindividual differences in dosage and patient response do occur. In partial but inadequate responders who are tolerating the chosen AP well, it is reasonable to titrate above usual dose ranges with the exception of thioridazine. However, this tactic should be time limited, and if the patient does not achieve further improvement, the dose should either be decreased or alternative treatment strategies tried.[22]

Rapid neuroleptization is the administration of repeated doses of a high-potency AP (e.g., HPD 5 mg IM) every 30 to 60 minutes in a severely agitated patient to obtain a prompt calming effect. Agitation can be manifested by loud, physically or verbally threatening behavior, motor hyperactivity, or physical aggression. Although this technique may assist in calming an acutely agitated, psychotic patient, it does not improve the extent of or time to remission or the length of hospitalization.

Adjunctive benzodiazepines absorbed rapidly after intramuscular administration (e.g., lorazepam) are equivalent to intramuscular APs in the management of acute agitation or aggression. If the patient is receiving a reasonable daily dose of an AP (as previously described), the use of lorazepam 2 mg IM as needed in combination with the maintenance antipsychotic may actually be more effective in controlling agitation than using additional doses of the antipsychotic. In addition, it may assist in decreasing the injectable antipsychotic dosage requirement, as well as the overall incidence of side effects, especially acute EPS.

STABILIZATION THERAPY

Improvement is usually a slow but steady process over 6 to 8 weeks or longer. During the first 2 weeks, goals should include increased socialization and improvement in self-care habits and mood. Improvement in formal thought disorder should follow and may take an additional 6 to 8 weeks to respond. However, therapeutic onset and time course of AP effects are based mostly on clinicians' impressions and experience, not on placebo-controlled trials.

Historical literature recommends that the average patient requires a dosage of 500 to 800 mg of CPZ equivalents daily, or with atypical antipsychotics, usual labeled dosages, for the acute stabilization phase.[31] An optimum dose of the chosen drug should be estimated in the initial treatment plan. If the patient begins to show adequate response before or at this dosage, then typically the patient should remain at this dosage as long as symptoms continue to improve. If necessary, dose titration may continue every week or two as long as the patient has no side effects. Titration should not continue until the patient can no longer tolerate side effects. During this stage in treatment, most patients can also be switched to once-daily dosing, which can positively affect compliance, cost, and incidence of certain side effects.

An adequate trial to evaluate clinical response is at least 6 weeks of treatment with a typical AP dose of 800 mg CPZ equivalents. If symptom improvement is not satisfactory after 6 to 12 weeks, other considerations are necessary before a change in AP is made. When faced with a poorly responsive patient, the clinician should ask the following questions: Were the initial target symptoms indicative of schizophrenia or did they represent manifestations of a different diagnosis, a long-standing behavioral problem, a substance abuse disorder, or a general medical condition? Is the patient compliant with pharmacotherapy? Are the symptoms unresponsive to AP drugs (e.g., impaired insight or judgment, or fixed delusions)? How does the patient's current status compare with response during previous exacerbations? Would this patient potentially benefit from a change to different treatment stage (see Fig. 64–1)? Does this patient qualify as a treatment-resistant schizophrenic patient?

The conclusion that a partially responding patient has achieved as much symptomatic improvement as possible is one that must be made with great care and after considering all possible treatment alternatives. However, treatment goals must be realistic. Medications are effective at decreasing some of the symptoms of schizophrenia (and are thus referred to as *palliative*), but they are not curative, and all symptoms may not abate.

MAINTENANCE TREATMENT

Maintenance drug therapy prevents relapse, as shown in numerous double-blind studies. The average relapse rate after 1 year is 20% with active drug (including some noncompliant patients) versus 60% to 80% for placebo.[33]

After treatment of the first psychotic episode in a schizophrenic patient, medication should be continued for at least 12 months after remission.[33] Maintenance treatment in patients with multiple acute episodes is more difficult to define. However, it would appear that good medication responders should be treated for at least 5 years; then low-dose strategies or complete drug withdrawal may be attempted to determine the need for continued treatment. When the need for continuous or lifetime pharmacotherapy is established, moderate doses are the most effective.[33]

Targeted medication administration based upon prodromal symptoms has been recommended as an alternative to continuous AP treatment in stabilized patients. However, studies have shown continuous medication to be more effective than targeted medication in preventing decompensation and decreasing need for hospitalization, and improving the extent and quality of employment.[34]

Antipsychotics should be tapered slowly before discontinuation. Abrupt discontinuation of APs, especially low-potency typical APs and CLZ, can result in withdrawal symptoms, felt to be a manifestation of rebound cholinergic outflow. Insomnia, nightmares, headaches, gastrointestinal symptoms (such as abdominal cramps, stomach pain, nausea, vomiting, and diarrhea), restlessness, increased salivation, and sweating are reported. In general, when switching from one AP to another, the first AP should be tapered and discontinued over 1 to 2 weeks after the second AP is initiated. Tapering may need to occur more slowly with CLZ.

Depot Antipsychotic Medications

Depot APs are recommended for patients who are unreliable in taking oral medication on a daily basis. Before a depot AP is initiated it should be determined whether the patient's medication noncompliance is due to side effects. If so, an alternative medication with a more favorable side effect profile should be considered before a depot AP.

The patient's motivation is still a major factor influencing outcome. Conversion from oral therapy to depot therapy is most successful in patients who have been stabilized on oral therapy. The ideal patient for depot therapy is the patient who does not like the daily reminder of oral medication or is unreliable in taking medications. Depot medications should not be used as "forced compliance" in uncooperative patients who refuse to consent to treatment.

Conversion from an oral AP to depot medication should start with stabilization on an oral dosage form of the same agent, or at least a short trial (3 to 7 days) to determine if the patient tolerates the medication without significant side effects. For fluphenazine, the simplest conversion is the Stimmel method, which uses 1.2 times the oral daily dose for stabilized patients, rounding up to the nearest 12.5-mg interval, administered in weekly doses for the first 4 to 6 weeks; or 1.6 times the oral daily dose for more acutely ill patients.[35] Subsequently, fluphenazine decanoate may be administered once every 2 to 3 weeks. Oral fluphenazine may be overlapped for 1 week. For haloperidol, a factor of 10 to 15 times the oral daily dose is commonly recommended, rounding up to the nearest 50-mg interval, administered in a once-monthly dose with an oral haloperidol overlap for the first month. However, this may be inadequate in more acutely psychotic patients. Ereshefsky and associates[36] performed an inpatient conversion study using the standard conversion from European trials (20 times the oral daily dose), but dividing the injection into consecutive doses of 100 to 200 mg every 3 to 7 days until the entire amount was given. With this method, oral medication overlap was not necessary. The depot dose was decreased by 25% at the second and third months. The method was as safe as other methods, and had a lower relapse rate than the most commonly recommended guidelines. Preliminary data suggest that deviation from these conversion protocols may result in poor outcomes and increased adverse effects.[37]

Injection site reactions have been reported with the HPD decanoate 100 mg/mL preparation, consisting of painful pruritic swelling at the injection site.[38] Acute EPS can be seen following injections with FPZ decanoate. Despite the fear of severe or persistent side effects occurring during depot therapy, research indicates that similar depot and oral doses result in a similar incidence of side effects. These issues appear less relevant if patients are stabilized on oral medication before conversion to an appropriate depot dose.

Depot APs should be administered by a deep, "Z-tract" intramuscular method, although there is some evidence that FPZ decanoate can be administered subcutaneously with similar results.

METHODS TO ENHANCE PATIENT ADHERENCE

The chronic mentally ill may be nonadherent with medications based on denial of illness, lack of insight, grandiosity or paranoia, no perceived need for medication, perceived lack of input into choice of medication or dosage, side effects, misperceived "allergies," or the number of medications prescribed or doses received daily.[2] Education geared toward patients becoming more informed about the effectiveness and risks of treatment may help increase compliance. These programs should be staged so that initially patients receive basic information about their disorder and its symptoms and basic information about their medication and self-monitoring. As that patient is capable of dealing with more complex information, more detailed information regarding schizophrenia, psychosocial treatments, and prognosis should be discussed. Patients and families should be taught self-monitoring techniques and when to report symptom exacerbation or medication side effects to the clinician.[2,39] Psychoeducation strategies should involve both individual counseling as well as group activities. Groups facilitated by trained individuals who have the illness may be more effective in enhancing awareness and acceptance of schizophrenia and necessary treatment than groups led only by professionals. Active involvement of family members further increases the likelihood of patient adherence with treatment. In addition to programs provided by community mental health centers, support groups operated by consumer groups such as local chapters of the National Alliance for the Mentally Ill are available in most metropolitan areas. In the hospital, self-medication administration often reinforces the patient's perception of their active role in their own treatment.

When patients miss outpatient appointments, active outreach interventions must be implemented to enhance patient engagement in treatment. These include both phone calls and home visits.[2]

MANAGEMENT OF THE TREATMENT-RESISTANT PATIENT

An official definition of "treatment resistance" does not exist.[18] In general, it reflects a patient who has had inadequate symptom response from antipsychotic treatment. Treatment resistance is usually defined with respect to lack of improvement in positive symptoms, but it can be defined by poor improvement in negative symptoms, or even by medication intolerance. Between 10% and 30% of schizophrenic patients receive minimal symptomatic improvement with typical APs.[18,23,32] An additional group of patients (30% to 60%) has partial but inadequate improvement in symptoms or unacceptable side effects associated with AP use.[2]

Atypical Antipsychotics

Only CLZ has shown superiority in randomized clinical trials for the management of treatment-resistant schizophrenia. Other atypical APs have either not been studied or evaluated in small open trials. For example, one small open trial suggested symptomatic improvement with RSP in patients who had poor symptom response with typical APs.[40] Another report suggests that patients may worsen clinically when switched from CLZ to RSP.[41] In an open label trial, 9 of 25 treatment-resistant patients demonstrated improvement in symptoms of 35% or more on the BPRS with OLZ 15 to 25 mg daily.[42]

In a classic study,[43] CLZ was effective in approximately 32% of refractory schizophrenic patients compared with only 2% treated with a combination of CPZ and benztropine. This study is considered a "classic" because not only did it prove the efficacy of CLZ in this population, but it also provided a definition for treatment-resistant schizophrenia. This definition includes treatment failures on three different APs from at least two different chemical classes and a history of poor social functioning for the past 5 years.[43] It is significant that when using these criteria for treatment-resistant patients, almost no patients improved with trials of HPD and CPZ. These criteria have been subsequently modified to require only two treatment failures. Other treatment candidates for CLZ include those patients who are neuroleptic intolerant and cannot tolerate even conservative doses of other APs.[23]

Symptomatic improvement with CLZ in the treatment-resistant patient often occurs slowly, and as many as 60% of patients may improve if CLZ is used for up to 6 months.[23] This in combination with CLZ's adverse effects profile provides sufficient information to conclude that CLZ is not a panacea for schizophrenia. However, as the only AP with proven efficacy in the treatment-resistant population, a therapeutic trial of CLZ is recommended at algorithm stage 4 for those patients who consent to its use and are willing to have the weekly blood draws for WBCs. Polydipsia and hyponatremia (psychogenic water drinking) is a frequent problem among treatment-resistant patients, and CLZ has been reported to decrease water drinking and increase serum sodium in such patients.[44]

Because of the risk of orthostatic hypotension, CLZ is usually titrated more slowly than other APs. If a 12.5 mg test dose does not produce hypotension, then CLZ 25 mg at bedtime is recommended, increased to 25 mg BID after 3 days, and then increased in 25 to 50 mg/d increments every 3 days until a dose of at least 300 mg/d is reached.[22] Because high doses are associated with significantly increased side effects, including seizures, a CLZ serum concentration is recommended before exceeding 600 mg/d.

Augmentation and Combination Strategies

Little empirical evidence exists to guide treatment decisions for patients who do not respond to CLZ.[22] Numerous suggestions have been made regarding augmentation of CLZ or other atypical APs and using combinations of antipsychotics (see Fig. 64–1).

Augmentation therapy involves the addition of a "non-AP" drug to an AP in a poorly responsive patient, while combination treatment involves using two antipsychotics simultaneously. Theoretically, augmentation is based on the assumption that the mechanism of action of the augmentation agent will interact synergistically with the dopaminolytic to produce efficacy.[45] Several guidelines should be followed regarding augmentation: (1) augmentation should be used only in inadequately responding patients; (2) augmentation agents are rarely effective when used alone; (3) augmentation responders usually improve rapidly; and (4) if augmentation does not improve symptomatology, the augmenting agent should be discontinued.

Mood stabilizers are frequently used as an augmentation strategy. Mood stabilizers do not enhance antipsychotic effect, but may improve labile affect and agitated behavior in selected patients. Therefore, they may improve the overall clinical status in such patients. Lithium augmentation is one of the better evaluated augmentation interventions.[2,32] Valproic acid and carbamazepine have also been used, but no controlled studies exist. Enzyme induction with carbamazepine may cause a decrease in antipsychotic serum concentration and potentially worsen psychotic symptoms in some patients.[32] Dosing of mood stabilizers in treatment-resistant schizophrenia is similar to their use in bipolar disorder.[2]

5-HT reuptake inhibitors (SSRIs) have been used as augmentors with mixed reports. Consistently positive results have been reported when using SSRIs to treat obsessive–compulsive symptoms that worsen or arise during CLZ treatment.

Propranolol reportedly has an antiaggression effect when used in a variety of psychiatric disorders, but particularly in the organic aggressive syndrome. Although its efficacy is probably associated with its pharmacodynamic effects, concomitant use may increase AP plasma concentrations as well.[32] It has been suggested that improvement with propranolol is primarily due to a lessening of akathisia, and whether propranolol is effective as an augmenting agent in patients without symptoms of aggression or akathisia is unclear.[46] Patients should receive a test dose of 20 mg to evaluate tolerance, and if it is acceptable, initial propranolol dosing should be 20 mg three times daily. Dose increases should be in 60 mg/d increments, every 3 days. Patients should be monitored carefully for side effects related to β-adrenergic blockade. Once the patient is β-blocked, the dose may be increased more rapidly as tolerated. Patients may need to be treated with adequate doses for 6 to 8 weeks in order to evaluate an antiaggression response. If appropriate response is not received with a daily dose of 1000 mg, additional response is not usually achieved at higher doses.[47]

Combining a typical antipsychotic with an atypical, and combining different atypicals, have been suggested as intervention strategies for treatment-resistant patients. These treatments are based upon the hypothesis that using antipsychotics with different mechanisms of action will result in greater efficacy than using any medication individually. Critics argue that combining a typical AP with an atypical will negate the advantages of the atypical medications (e.g., fewer EPS). Similarly, it is argued that available data do not exist to suggest that available atypical APs' pharmacodynamic profiles differ sufficiently to obtain added benefit from the combination as compared with monotherapy. Little empirical data exist to either support or refute the use of combination AP strategies. In the absence of information, it is reasonable to cautiously try a combination trial in the treatment-resistant patient (stage 5 of the algorithm in Fig. 64–1).[39] As is evidenced in the treatment algorithm, this is usually indicated only after inadequate response to CLZ. Such combination treatment trials should be time limited (6 to 12 weeks) and the patient carefully evaluated with rating scales for changes in symptomatology. If no apparent improvement is observed, then one of the medications should be tapered and discontinued.

ANTIPSYCHOTIC DRUG MECHANISM OF ACTION

Typical or traditional AP medications are putative DAergic antagonists, with an affinity for D_2 receptors that is greater than for D_1. During chronic treatment with these agents, between 70% and 90% of D_2 receptors in the striatum are usually occupied. In contrast, during CLZ treatment only 38% to 63% of D_2 receptors are occupied.[3] Shortly after beginning treatment with AP drugs, several compensatory processes begin to occur in the brain, particularly in the basal ganglia. These include an increase in DA metabolite formation, increased rate of DA synthesis, and increased rate of cell firing.[48] However, within 21 days of continuous treatment, depolarization block, or decreased DA release or DAergic neuronal inactivation, occurs. With typical APs, depolarization block occurs in both A_9 and A_{10} areas, with the exception of neurons projecting to the prefrontal or cingulate cortex. With at least some atypical APs, depolarization block appears to occur only in the A_{10} region.[4,48,49]

Multiple DA receptor subtypes exist, with D_1 and D_2 being the best studied. Even with these two subtypes, their functioning has not been adequately elucidated. The D_2 receptor is associated with typical AP efficacy; in fact, most studies with typical APs show a high correlation between D_2 blockade and AP efficacy. D_1 receptors may serve as a permissive or modulating receptor for EPS; some D_1 blockade as well as D_2 may be necessary to produce EPS. For example, HPD has high D_2 affinity, but some D_1 binding, and produces a high incidence of extrapyramidal reactions, and CLZ, with greater D_1 and D_4 binding (relative to HPD) and high non-DA affinity, causes almost no EPS.[4,49]

Typical APs have effects on all four DAergic tracts (see Table 64–1). The primary therapeutic effects of typical APs are thought to occur in the limbic system, including the ventral striatum, whereas EPS are thought to be related to DA blockade in the dorsal striatum. Tolerance usually develops to the acutely occurring EPS within a few weeks, but tolerance to the AP effects appear to be less common, if not rare. It is also noteworthy that tolerance develops to an AP drug-induced increase in DA turnover in the striatum and subcortical limbic system, but not in the prefrontal lobe cortex.[4,48] This latter finding is consistent with autoreceptor distribution and with depolarization block not being produced by APs in the prefrontal lobe. It may explain a relative lack of tolerance to the AP effects. In the tuberoinfundibular system, APs block prolactin (PRL) inhibitory factor, which is DA acting at D_2 sites. Tolerance does not appear to develop to this effect, even with long-term treatment.[48]

Typical APs affect other neurotransmitter receptor systems, including blockade of muscarinic, α_1-adrenergic, and histaminic receptors. As a rule, the lower-potency APs, (such as CPZ and thioridazine (TRD), are less specific for DA receptors and block other receptors as well.[4,48] These differences in affinity for non-DAergic receptors are at least partially responsible for the varying side effect profiles among AP agents. This offers a rational explanation for the side effects, such as dry mouth, constipation, sinus tachycardia, and orthostatic hypotension, seen more commonly with the "low-potency" typical APs.

The atypical APs' exact mechanisms of therapeutic action are unknown and likely differ among drugs (Table 64–5). These mechanisms of action may be related to one or more of the following pharmacodynamic effects: relative D_1, D_4, or D_5 specificity; relative selectivity for limbic DAergic receptors; 5-HT_2, 5-HT_6, and 5-HT_7 antagonism; or α_1-adrenergic antagonism.[4,49,50] For example, CLZ has relative D_1 and D_4 selectivity and is an antagonist for 5-HT_2, 5-HT_6, and 5-HT_7 receptors. CLZ and OLZ have also been shown in rodents to block NMDA antagonist neurotoxicity.[11] Blockade of 5-HT_2 receptors on presynaptic neurons in the striatum may lead to increased DA release and therefore less EPS.[12] This has led some investigators to believe that the ratio between 5-HT_2 blockade and D_2 blockade is important in producing an atypical profile. All currently available atypicals APs have potent 5-HT_2 antagonism, and all cause less acute EPS than typical APs. RSP causes EPS less often than typical APs, particularly at low to moderate doses (e.g., 2 to 6 mg/d). However, CLZ and RSP differ clinically, as do all of the atypical APs, indicating potential important differences clinically in their pharmacody-

TABLE 64–5. Receptor Blockade of Atypical Antipsychotics

Agents	Receptors Blocked[a]
Clozapine	D_2, D_1, D_4, 5-HT_{2A}, 5-HT_6, 5-HT_7, α_1, α_2, H_1, M_1
Olanzapine	D_2, D_1, D_3, D_4, 5-HT_{2A}, 5-HT_3, 5-HT_6, α_1, H_1, M_1
Risperidone	D_2, 5-HT_{2A}, α_1, α_1, H_1
Quetiapine	D_2, 5-HT_{2A}, α_1, α_1, H_1
Sertindole	D_2, D_1, 5-HT_{2A}, α_1
Ziprazidone	D_2, 5-HT_{1A}, 5-HT_{2A}, 5-HT_{2C}, 5-HT_{1D}, α_1

[a]Potential mechanisms of action for each respective agent.
Adapted from Refs. 17, 49, and 103.

TABLE 64–6. Cytochrome P450 Isoenzyme Metabolism Profiles of Atypical Antipsychotics

Drug	Major Pathway	Minor Pathway
Clozapine	1A2	2D6, 3A4
Risperidone	2D6	
Olanzapine	1A2, 2D6	
Quetiapine	3A4	
Sertindole	3A4, 2D6	
Ziprasidone	3A4	

Adapted from Ref. 51.

namic profiles. For example, CLZ produces a significantly lower incidence of EPS than RSP, and CLZ does not elevate serum PRL concentrations (through blocking D_2-mediated prolactin inhibitory factor) while RSP does.[23] Although both CLZ and OLZ affect the same common receptor types, they differ in their relative affinities. The clinical utility of these differences requires further investigation.

PHARMACOKINETICS

The APs are highly lipophilic and highly bound to membranes and plasma proteins. They distribute readily into most tissues with a high blood supply and may accumulate in tissues; therefore, they have large volumes of distribution.[51] APs are largely metabolized, primarily through the cytochrome P450 pathways in the liver. The specific hepatic isoenzymes suggested to be responsible for metabolism of selected APs are outlined in Table 64–6. APs have fairly long elimination half-lives, most in the range of 20 to 40 hours. Thus, after dosage stabilization, most APs can be dosed once daily. Exceptions are quetiapine and ziprasidone, which have short half-lives (Table 64–7).[51]

Efforts to develop relationships between AP plasma concentration (Cp) and clinical response have been hampered by several factors, including the variable lag time between beginning AP treatment and symptom change, the subjective and relatively imprecise methods of measuring drug effect or symptom change in schizophrenia, and the presence of multiple metabolites. The most successful research assessing the relationship between AP Cp and response has been performed with HPD, fluphenazine (FPZ), and CLZ.

With HPD, the most well-controlled, fixed-dose studies suggest that the approximate therapeutic Cp range is between 3 and 15 ng/mL. A daily dosage of HPD HCl 10 mg usually results in a HPD Cp in this range in about 50% of patients. HPD may possess a curvilinear Cp response relationship, with less efficacy at Cp values higher than the therapeutic range. It is uncertain whether this truly reflects decreased efficacy or whether patients' clinical presentation is worse at higher Cp values because of increased side effects. Regardless, research indicates that the above proposed range maximizes the therapeutic relationship of efficacy and adverse effects.[32,51]

Although the research with FPZ is not nearly as extensive, preliminary results suggest that the lower end of the FPZ therapeutic range is approximately 0.5 ng/mL.[51] As the Cp increases, efficacy may improve, but adverse effects worsen. The upper end of the suggested therapeutic range is approximately 3 ng/mL.

Early studies indicated that a CLZ plasma concentration greater than approximately 350 ng/mL was associated with a greater probability of efficacy in treatment-resistant patients.[51,52] A recent study investigating the efficacy of three different fixed serum concentration ranges found both the 200 to 300 ng/mL and 350 to 450 ng/mL ranges to be predictive of response.[53] Furthermore, sedation increased with increasing serum concentrations. The authors suggest a 12-hour post dose CLZ serum concentration of at least 250 ng/mL if the patient is receiving divided CLZ doses or 350 ng/mL if the patient is being dosed once daily.

It is not cost effective to monitor AP Cp routinely in all patients, and Cp monitoring should be considered only in patients receiving CLZ, FPZ, or HPD. Cp monitoring should be considered in such patients who do not respond to reasonable doses within a 6-week period, patients who develop unusual or severe adverse experiences, patients who are taking concomitant medications that may cause drug interactions, patients who have age or pathophysiologic changes suggesting a change in pharmacokinetics, or for assessment of patient compliance.

The depot APs, FPZ decanoate (also available in an enanthate salt), and HPD decanoate are esterified APs formulated in sesame seed oil for deep intramuscular injection. Their absorption from the muscle and metabolism to the free base is sufficiently slow to cause absorption to be the rate-limiting step in determining their respective, apparent half-lives. Thus, their pharmacokinetics follow a flip-flop model.[35]

TABLE 64–7. Pharmacokinetic Parameters of Selected Antipsychotics

Drug	Bioavailability (%)	Half-life (h)	Active Metabolites
Typical Antipsychotics			
Chlorpromazine	10–30	8–35	7-hydroxy, others
Fluphenazine	20–50	14–24	?
Fluphenazine decanoate		14.2 + 2.2[a] days	
Haloperidol	40–70	12–36	Reduced haloperidol
Haloperidol decanoate		21 days	
Atypical Antipsychotics			
Clozapine	12–81	11–105	None with significant activity
Olanzapine	80	20–70	N-glucuronide; 2-OH-methyl; 4-N-oxide
Quetiapine	9 ± 4	6.88	7-OH-quetiapine
Risperidone	68	3–24	9-0H-risperidone
Sertindole	74	24–200	None with significant activity
Ziprasidone	59	4–10	None

[a]Based upon multiple-dose data. Single-dose data indicate half-life of 6 to 10 days.
Adapted from Refs. 35 and 51

TABLE 64–8. Relative Side Effect Incidence of Commonly Used Antipsychotics

	Sedation	EPS	Anticholinergic	Orthostasis
Chlorpromazine	++++	+++	+++	++++
Clozapine	+++++	+	+++++	++++
Fluphenazine	++	+++++	++	++
Haloperidol	+	+++++	+	+
Loxapine	+++	++++	++	+++
Molindone	+	+++	++	++
Olanzapine	++	++	+++	++
Perphenazine	++	++++	++	++
Quetiapine	+++	++	–	++
Risperidone	+	++	+	++
Sertindole	++	+	–	++
Thioridazine	++++	++	++++	++++
Trifluoperazine	++	++++	++	++
Thiothixene	++	++++	++	++
Ziprasidone	++	++	+	++

+ = Very low; ++ = low; +++ = moderate; ++++ = high; +++++ = very high.

ADVERSE EFFECTS

Table 64–8 presents the relative incidence of common categories of AP side effects. The precise incidence of many of these side effects has not been systematically evaluated. Side effects will be discussed with respect to organ system affected. Also, many of the side effects can be categorized by the neurotransmitter system affected, as listed in Table 64–9. A general approach to monitoring and assessing side effects requires prospective monitoring by clinicians, preferably using a thorough review of systems approach. Patient-oriented self-rating side-effect scales may also be helpful, because many schizophrenics do not readily complain of side effects, due to lack of volition, lack of perception of having input into their treatment, poor understanding, or because of the actual interference of side effects themselves (e.g., sedation).[54]

With the variety of APs currently available, using an alternative drug should be considered in patients who complain of poorly tolerated side effects. Because medication side effects are one of the primary predictors of patient noncompliance, the clinician should take advantage of the treatment options currently available in attempt to improve patient outcomes.

TABLE 64–9. Adverse Effects by Receptor Blockade

Receptor Type	Adverse Effects
Histamine H_1	Sedation Weight gain Potentiation of CNS-depressant drugs
Muscarinic	Urinary retention Cognition and memory effects Sinus tachycardia Dry mouth Blurred vision Constipation
α_1-adrenergic	Orthostatic hypotension Reflex tachycardia Potentiation of antihypertensives
Dopamine D_2	Extrapyramidal side effects Prolactin elevation
Serotonin 5-HT_2	Orthostatic hypotension Sedation Weight gain

Autonomic Nervous System

Patients receiving APs, or APs in combination with anticholinergics (AChs), may experience ACh side effects (dry mouth, constipation, tachycardia, blurred vision, inhibition or impairment of ejaculation, urinary retention). Lower potency agents are typical offenders, and the elderly are especially sensitive to these effects.[55] Of the atypical antipsychotics, CLZ and OLZ have moderately high rates of anticholinergic effects. System-specific effects are discussed under the appropriate heading.

Dry mouth can be managed with increased intake of fluids, oral lubricants (Xerolube), ice chips, or use of sugarless chewing gum or hard candy. Constipation, caused by slowed peristaltic movement and decreased intestinal fluid content, should be closely monitored and treated, especially in the elderly. Paralytic ileus and necrolyzing colitis may also occur. Constipation can be treated with increases in fluid and dietary fiber intake, and exercise.

Central Nervous System

Extrapyramidal System

DYSTONIA

Dystonia is defined as a state of abnormal tonicity, sometimes described simplistically as a severe "muscle spasm."[56] Dystonias may be dramatic, frightening, and painful. More accurately, they are prolonged tonic contractions, with a rapid onset, usually within 24 to 96 hours of dosage administration or dosage increase. They may be life threatening, as in the case of pharyngeal–laryngeal dystonias, and can contribute to noncompliance. Types of dystonic reactions include trismus, glossospasm, tongue protrusion, pharyngeal–laryngeal dystonia, blepharospasm, oculogyric crisis, torticollis, and retrocollis.

Two pathophysiologic theories for dystonia are proposed[56]: (1) DA release from presynaptic receptors transiently increases (increased synthesis and release) in compensatory response to DA blockade, and (2) heightened sensitivity of postsynaptic DA receptors (as brain AP concentration decreases), such that DA release has an enhanced effect. The actual mechanism may be a combination of these two theories.

Risk factors include younger patients (especially males), the use of high-potency agents, and high dosage. An overall incidence from the 1960s through the mid-1970s ranged from 2.3% to 10%, but as higher-potency agents became more widely used, the rate increased to as high as 64%.

TABLE 64–10. Agents Used To Treat EPS

Generic Name	Equivalent Dose (mg)	Dosage Range (mg)
Antimuscarinics		
Benztropine[a]	1	1–8[b]
Biperiden[a]	2	2–8
Orphenadrine	50	50–250
Procyclidine	2	7.5–20
Trihexyphenidyl	2	2–15
Anithistaminic		
Diphenhydramine[a]	50	50–400
Dopamine Agonist		
Amantadine	N/A	100–400
Benzodiazepines		
Lorazepam[a]	N/A	1–8
Diazepam	N/A	2–20
Clonazepam	N/A	2–8
Beta Blockers		
Propranolol	N/A	20–160

[a]Injectable dosage form can be given intramuscularly for relief of acute dystonia.
[b]Dosage may be titrated to 12 mg with care; nonlinear pharmacokinetics have been demonstrated.

Pharmacotherapeutic treatment options are effective and straightforward, with the choice of intramuscular or intravenous AChs (Table 64–10) or benzodiazepines. Benztropine mesylate 2 mg or diphenhydramine 50 mg may be given intramuscularly or intravenously, with the options of diazepam 5 to 10 mg slow intravenous push or lorazepam 1 to 2 mg intramuscularly. Relief is typically seen within 15 to 20 minutes of an intramuscular injection and within 5 minutes of intravenous administration. This dose should be repeated if no response is seen within 15 minutes of intravenous injection or within 30 minutes of intramuscular injection. AP medication may be continued, with concomitant short-term use of oral ACh agents.

A controversial issue arises regarding the question of prophylaxis of dystonia with ACh medications. Many clinicians prescribe AChs routinely when initiating typical AP therapy, whereas others do so only in patients who may be at greater risk for dystonic reactions or in those patients with a history of dystonic reactions. In general, prophylactic ACh medications are not recommended routinely as prophylaxis with all typical APs. However, prophylaxis is reasonable when using high-potency typical APs (e.g., HPD or FPZ), in young men, and in patients with a history of dystonia.[57] Dystonias may also be minimized by the use of lower initial doses of APs. The AChs are good choices for prophylaxis, whereas amantadine has not been proven effective for this purpose.

Treatment-emergent dystonias are rare with atypical APs, with the exception of reports of dystonia associated with overlapping during a switch from CLZ to RSP.[58]

AKATHISIA

Akathisia is defined as the inability to sit still and as being functionally motor restless. The most accurate diagnosis is made by combining subjective complaints with objective symptoms (pacing, shifting, shuffling, or tapping feet). Subjectively, patients may describe a feeling of inner restlessness or disquiet, a compulsion to move or remain in constant motion. Akathisia occurs in 20% to 40% of patients treated with high-potency agents.[56] Some clinicians believe that the majority of patients experience akathisia, but the reported incidence reflects only patients who can verbalize their feelings or recognize akathisia as being different from psychosis. Akathisia is frequently accompanied by dysphoria. Detection of akathisia requires a high degree of interviewer sensitivity.

The pathophysiology of akathisia is uncertain, but there are two current theories.[56] Theory 1 states that mesocortical postsynaptic DA blockade leads to increased locomotor activity, unlike the cataleptic effect in the striatum. The alternate theory claims that akathisia is caused by DA antagonist-induced dysregulation of noradrenergic tracts that project from the locus ceruleus to the limbic system.[56]

Many treatments for akathisia, although accepted to be effective, are based on anecdotal data. Akathisia research is particularly difficult as the nature of the illness is subjective. Treatment with ACh agents, usually considered the standard treatment for all acute EPS, is disappointing for akathisia, but may be helpful in patients with concomitant pseudoparkinsonism.[56] Traditionally, reduction in AP dosage has been considered the best intervention; however, this may not be a realistic goal in an acutely psychotic patient. A logical alternative is to switch to an atypical antipsychotic or an AP previously used in the patient without adverse effect. However, akathisia also may occur with RSP or OZP. Chronic akathisia that does not respond to multiple interventions including changes in antipsychotic agent may warrant a trial of CLZ therapy.[59]

Benzodiazepines are commonly used for akathisia, probably due to their sedative and anxiolytic properties. Efficacy using diazepam 5 mg three times per day was reported in patients who failed to respond to AChs, whereas other researchers failed to demonstrate efficacy in a series of 25 patients.[56]

Beta-blockers are being used with increasing frequency. Propranolol in doses up to 160 mg daily, nadolol in doses up to 80 mg daily, and metoprolol in β_2-selective doses of 100 mg daily or less were reported as effective doses.[59] The use of clonidine has also been investigated; a mean dose of 0.43 mg/d produced response in 6 patients, with maximum response within 24 to 48 hours of the previous dosage increase. Hypotension and sedation were the only observed side effects.

Preventive measures for akathisia include using the lowest possible typical AP dose or use of atypical APs.

PSEUDOPARKINSONISM

Pseudoparkinsonism, an AP-induced EPS, resembles idiopathic Parkinson's disease. A patient with pseudoparkinsonism may present with any of four cardinal symptoms: (1) akinesia, bradykinesia, or decreased motor activity including difficulty initiating movement as well as extreme slowness, mask-like facial expression, micrographia, slowed speech, and decreased arm swing; (2) tremor, known as pill-rolling type, predominant at rest, decreasing with movement, usually involving the fingers and hands, although it may be seen in the arms, legs, neck, head, and chin (it may often be activated by having the patient perform mechanical movements with one extremity); (3) cogwheel rigidity, seen as the patient's limbs yield in jerky, ratchet-like fashion when passively moved by the examiner (a mild form may present as stiffness); and (4) postural abnormalities and instability manifested as stooped posture, difficulty in maintaining stability when changing body position, and a gait that ranges from slow and shuffling to festinating (a result of dysfunction in autonomic stability combined with a shift in the center of gravity due to the stooped posture).[60] Accessory symptoms include the autonomic manifestations seborrhea, sialorrhea, and hyperhidrosis.[56] Fatigue and weakness may be noted, as well as speech abnormalities including dysphagia and dysarthria, and abnormal palmomental and glabellar reflexes. A variant of pseudoparkinsonism is rabbit syndrome, a perioral tremor.[60]

The overall incidence ranges from 15.4% to 36%, depending on the typical AP used. Akinesia alone can be seen in 59% of patients on high-potency agents. Other risk factors include increasing age and possibly female gender. The onset of symptoms is usually 1 to 2 weeks after initiation of AP therapy or dose increase.

The pathophysiology involves a deficiency of DA. Normal motor function is dependent on a balance between cholinergic and DAergic systems. AP blockade of postsynaptic DA receptors leads to a relative functional DA deficiency and cholinergic excess in the striatum resulting in motor abnormalities approximating those seen in Parkinson's disease.[56,60]

The efficacy of ACh medications in alleviating or attenuating pseudoparkinsonian symptoms is well established.[56,60] Benztropine is advantageous in that its longer half-life allows twice-daily dosing, and in many patients it may be given once daily.[60] Typical dosing is 1 to 2 mg twice a day up to a usual maximum dosage of 8 mg daily, although some patients will continue to respond to doses up to 12 mg. Dosage increases above 6 mg must be slow, as benztropine displays nonlinear pharmacokinetics. Trihexyphenidyl (2 to 5 mg tid), diphenhydramine (25 to 50 mg tid), and biperiden (2 mg tid) usually require three-times daily administration. Diphenhydramine produces more sedation than the other agents. Although it has been suggested that trihexyphenidyl is more likely to be abused, all of the anticholinergics have been abused for their euphorant effects.[61] With all of these agents, symptoms will typically begin to resolve in 3 to 4 days after initiation of treatment, but a minimum of at least 2 weeks of treatment is normally required for full response.

Amantadine is generally as efficacious for pseudoparkinsonism as AChs, with significantly less effect on memory function.[56,60] Amantadine has less potential than other DA agonists (bromocriptine and levodopa) for significant adverse effects. Its mechanism involves enhancement of DAergic tone in the striatum. Excessive doses may produce anxiety, agitation, and restlessness, as well as exacerbation of psychosis. Dosage adjustment is necessary with renal insufficiency.

The need for prophylactic use of these agents against pseudoparkinsonism is less convincing than with dystonias.[56] Trials examining this issue are typically retrospective reviews calculating the incidence of development of pseudoparkinsonism in patients treated with prophylactic agents versus those who were not, or trials examining withdrawal of antiparkinsonian medications in patients on maintenance AP therapy.

The long-term treatment of pseudoparkinsonism with antiparkinsonian medication is controversial.[56] Most investigators believe that it is seldom necessary with maintenance AP therapy, whereas others demonstrate a population of patients who have recurrence or worsening of pseudoparkinsonian symptoms upon discontinuation of ACh medication, even if the medication is withdrawn gradually. An attempt should be made to taper and discontinue these agents 6 weeks to 3 months after symptoms resolve. If symptoms reappear, then either a longer treatment period or switching to an atypical AP should be considered.

RSP, when used in doses of 6 mg/d or less, demonstrates significantly less pseudoparkinsonism than haloperidol.[24] Pseudoparkinsonian symptoms are even less common with other atypical APs. However, in the unusual patient experiencing moderate to severe EPS with all other atypical APs, CLZ is a reasonable alternative.[56,62]

TARDIVE DYSKINESIA

Tardive dyskinesia (TD) is a syndrome characterized by abnormal involuntary movements occurring late in onset in relation to initiation of AP therapy. TD is sometimes irreversible and continues to be a controversial issue, legally and ethically.

The classical description of TD is the bucco-lingual-masticatory (BLM) syndrome, or orofacial movements.[60] The onset of BLM movements is usually insidious. Typically, they are the first detectable signs of TD, and begin with mild forward, backward, or lateral movements of the tongue. As the disorder progresses, more obvious or frank BLM movements appear, including tongue thrusting, rolling, or fly-catching movements, and chewing or lateral jaw movements. TD symptoms may interfere with the patient's ability to chew, speak, or swallow. Further complications include oral ulcerations, inability to wear dentures, and inflammation and loosening of mandibular joints. Eating difficulties and malnutrition may be primary physical complications of TD. Weight loss may be seen in patients with esophageal or respiratory manifestations but not in those with truncal movements.

Facial movements include frequent blinking, brow arching, grimacing, upward deviation of the eyes, and lip smacking. Involvement of the extremities sometimes occurs, with the appearance of restless choreiform (irregular spasmodic) and distal athetosis (slow, writhing movement) of limbs including twisting, spreading, flexion (bending) and extension of fingers, toe tapping, and toe dorsiflexion (upward turning). Unusual posture, hyperextension, pelvic thrusting, axial hyperkinesia (excessive muscular activity of head and trunk), ballismus (jerking or shaking), exaggerated lordosis (bending backward), rocking, and swaying are occasionally observed. Among the more common differential diagnoses are withdrawal dyskinesias occurring after short-term use of APs, spontaneous orofacial dyskinesias in the elderly, orofacial dyskinesias in the edentulous, stereotypic movements in schizophrenics, Huntington's disease, and congenital torsion dystonia.

Orofacial movements are reported more commonly in older patients, whereas the truncal axial movements are classically reported in young adults. Movements may worsen with stress, decrease with sedation, and disappear during sleep. Concentration on motor tasks or attempts to suppress the movements voluntarily may actually increase them.

Early signs of TD may be reversible, but if allowed to persist or if not detected in the early stages, they may be irreversible, even with drug discontinuation. When the AP dose is decreased or tapered and discontinued, there is usually a worsening of abnormal movements and then possibly a slow improvement after months or years if the patient remains on lower doses or discontinues treatment.

There are no standardized criteria for the diagnosis of TD. Abnormal involuntary movements can be detected early through physical assessment and the use of rating scales. Available rating scales include the Abnormal Involuntary Movement Scale (AIMS) and the Dyskinesia Identification System: Condensed User Scale (DISCUS).[63,64] Neither of these scales are diagnostic in themselves.

The pathophysiology of TD is complex and remains to be satisfactorily explained. The traditional theory is that postsynaptic DA receptor blockade in the nigrostriatum leads to disuse hypersensitivity or denervation. This is usually considered in conjunction with a cholinergic dysfunction relative to DAergic activity or the classic DA/acetylcholine imbalance. With DA receptor blockade, there is either an increase in the number of binding sites or an alteration in the sensitivity of the receptor to DA through adenylate cyclase activity. These DA receptors are generally considered to have an inhibitory effect on acetylcholine function in the corpus striatum. DA function may be modulated by a negative feedback system involving two serial sets of GABA-mediated neurons. GABA output to the thalamus and motor cortex is reduced as a result, and this causes the movement disorder. Thus, TD may represent an adaptive change to the loss of gating function usually produced by normal DA activity in extrapyramidal motor circuits. Deficiencies of this theory include the following: (1) It explains withdrawal dyskinesias or a transient movement disorder, but not persistent symptoms; (2) it does not explain concurrent TD and parkinsonism in the same patient; (3) it does not account for the presence of presynaptic DA autoreceptors; (4) postsynaptic receptor hypersensitivity usually develops soon after beginning APs, whereas TD develops after prolonged use; and (5) postmortem studies have found no increase in DA receptors in brains of TD patients.[65] Lack of site specificity and differential effects of APs on D_1 versus D_2 receptors may explain why traditional APs cause TD while some atypical APs do not (see the mechanism of action discussion earlier in the chapter). DA receptor antagonists' effects on decreasing GABA turnover and resulting GABA receptor hypersensitivity have also been theorized as a potential mechanism for TD.[65]

Risk factors include increasing age; diagnoses of organic mental disorder, diabetes mellitus, or mood disorders; and possibly female gender.[65] It is uncertain if a history of significant unresolved acute EPS or lengthy treatment with ACh agents are risk factors.[66] Duration of AP therapy, daily dosage, and possibly total cumulative dosage are probably the most significant risk factors. However, persistent dyskinesias occur with as little as 6 months of therapy. Altered drug metabolism has been suggested, but not proven, to play a role in the development of TD.[67] Overall morbidity and mortality is greater in TD patients, and patients with TD show a greater incidence of respiratory tract infections and cardiovascular illness.

With typical APs, the incidence of TD ranges from 0.5% to 62% (mean, 20% to 30%).[65] Factors causing variation in epidemiologic studies are patient population characteristics, drug dosage, duration of therapy, varieties of methods used in the assessment of TD, inadequacies in differentiating TD from other movement disorders, and bias. In a longitudinal study, Kane and colleagues showed an incidence of 4% per year of drug treatment for the first 4 years.[68] These cases usually were in younger patients (mean age, 29 years) and were mild; follow-up after 2 to 3 years indicates dyskinesia scores did not increase.

AP dosage reduction may have a significant effect on outcome, if the patient can tolerate the reduction without return of psychotic symptoms.[65] Many patients with TD are concerned about the possibility of worsening TD symptoms if they are continued on medication. In one study, the syndrome remained stable over the years, and while a few patients worsened or only modest changes were seen, many improved on lower doses.[65] In another longitudinal study, remissions were seen in 25% of patients with TD after 5 years of continued treatment.[69] However, an increased incidence of pseudoparkinsonism was seen in both of these studies.

Possibly only a small subgroup of patients with TD will develop severe symptoms.[65] Although it is difficult to predict who will develop severe TD, one sample of patients was characterized by a greater number of affective/schizoaffective patients; frequent eye blinking was a prodromal sign in 37%.[70]

Prevention is the single most important aspect of TD, because treatment of the movements is difficult. Because of data suggesting a lower risk of TD with atypical APs, these agents are considered treatments of first choice (see Fig. 64–1). APs should be used only when they are indicated (for psychotic target symptoms), and they should be used at the minimum effective dose. When a patient is treated with APs for more than 3 months for an initial episode of illness, the need for continued treatment should be assessed. Regular neurologic examinations (AIMS or other scales) should be performed at baseline and at least quarterly to assess for early signs of TD. At the first signs of TD, the need for continuing AP treatment should be reassessed. In such situations, if the patient is taking a typical AP and continuing treatment is indicated, the medication should be switched to an atypical AP. In nonpsychotic patients, APs should only be used acutely to abort an aggressive behavior crisis, and always in combination with a behavioral treatment program.

There are no FDA-approved agents for treatment of TD. Numerous drugs have been used, representing various strategies affecting CNS neurotransmission. Older strategies have been aimed at altering the DA, GABA, and cholinergic systems; these are reviewed elsewhere.[65]

Alpha-tocopherol (vitamin E) in doses of 1200 to 1600 IU has been used based on its antioxidant properties. Results from short-term treatment studies have variously shown significant reduction in movements (usually patients with recent onset of TD), and minor benefit in select patients; three studies in patients with longer duration of symptoms have shown no effect.[2,65] Based on its safety and low cost, vitamin E is a reasonable treatment option for mild to moderate TD.[2]

To date, there are no reports of TD with CLZ monotherapy. Although introduced in the United States in 1990, it has been used in some European countries since the early 1970s. In two controlled trials lasting 22 to 52 weeks, it decreased abnormal involuntary movements by 50% or more.[65] Switching AP therapy to CLZ is a favored first-line pharmacotherapeutic strategy, particularly in patients with moderate to severe symptoms.[2] Preliminary information suggests that the atypical antipsychotics RSP and OLZ have rates of emergent dyskinesias significantly lower than with typical APs, and these atypical APs may be considered as alternative treatments in patients with mild to moderate TD.[65]

Sedation. Sedation must be recognized as an AP side effect and not as an indication of therapeutic effect. It occurs more frequently with low-potency APs through their antihistaminic properties. CPZ, TRD, mesoridazine, and CLZ are most frequently implicated. Administration of most or all of the daily dosage at bedtime can decrease daytime sedation and in some patients eliminate the need for hypnotic agents. Sedation occurs early in treatment and may decrease over time. Oversedation plays a large role in cognitive, perceptual, and motor dysfunction.[71] With acute dosing, tasks requiring vigilance, attention, or motor behavior may be affected. However, the positive effects of medication are seen with chronic administration, evidenced by improvements in tasks involving visual-motor skills and attention. Neuropsychologic testing is not affected by chronic drug administration. However, many of these improvements appear to be inversely proportional to dose.

Seizures. APs lower the seizure threshold through GABA depletion, changes in CNS permeability leading to enhanced conduction of a discharge, disruption of DA–acetylcholine balance, or the activation of a latent seizure focus. There is an increased risk of drug-induced seizures in all patients treated with APs. However, this risk is greater if the following predisposing factors are present: preexisting seizure disorder, history of drug-induced seizure, abnormal EEG, and preexisting CNS pathology or head trauma. Seizures are more closely associated with the use of higher doses, rapid dosage increases, and upon initiation of treatment. When an isolated seizure occurs, a dosage decrease is first recommended; anticonvulsant therapy is not recommended. The highest potential seizure risk by an AP drug is with the use of CPZ or CLZ, followed by trifluoperazine and perphenazine. Addition of lithium to a stable CLZ regimen has resulted in seizures in 2 reported cases.[72] If a change in AP therapy is required in the management of AP-induced seizures, atypical antipsychotics (other than CLZ), molindone, TRD, HPD, and FPZ are associated with the lowest potential.[73]

Thermoregulation. Poikilothermia, the body temperature adjusting to the ambient temperature, can be a serious side effect of AP therapy in temperature extremes.[74] Hyperpyrexia can be a danger in hot weather or during exercise. Inhibition of sweating, a result of ACh properties impairing the peripheral mechanisms of heat dissipation, can also contribute to this problem, which in its severest form can lead to heat stroke. Hypothermia is also a risk, particularly in the elderly. All patients receiving APs should be educated about these potential problems. Thermoregulatory problems are reportedly more common with the use of low-potency APs, and may occur with the more anticholinergic atypical antipsychotics (CLZ and OLZ).

■ *Neuroleptic Malignant Syndrome.* Neuroleptic malignant syndrome (NMS) occurs in 0.5% to 1% of patients receiving APs. NMS may occur more frequently in patients receiving high-potency, injectable, or depot APs, and in patients who are dehydrated, with physical exhaustion, or organic mental disorders.[75] NMS has been reported with atypical APs, including CLZ, as well as with typical APs.[23,76] The onset of symptoms varies from early in treatment to months later. It develops rapidly, over the course of 24 to 72 hours. NMS may occur after AP discontinuation, especially when depot agents are used. Possible mechanisms of NMS include disruption of the central thermoregulatory process or excess production of heat secondary to skeletal muscle contractions. The differential diagnosis includes heat stroke, lethal catatonia, anesthetic-associated malignant hyperthermia, ACh toxicity, and monoamine oxidase inhibitor (MAOI) drug interactions.

Cardinal signs and symptoms of NMS are body temperature exceeding 38°C, altered level of consciousness, autonomic dysfunction (tachycardia, labile blood pressure, diaphoresis, tachypnea, urinary or fecal incontinence), and rigidity. Laboratory evaluation, although considered nonspecific, frequently shows leukocytosis with or without left shift, increases in creatine kinase (CK), aspartate aminotransferase (AST), alanine aminotransferase (ALT), lactate dehydrogenase (LDH), and myoglobinuria.

Treatment should always begin with AP discontinuation and supportive care. The DA agonist bromocriptine, used in theory to reverse DA blockade, reduces rigidity, fever, or CK in up to 94% of patients, whereas the use of another DA agonist, amantadine, has been successfully used in up to 63% of patients.[77] Dantrolene has been used as a skeletal muscle relaxant, with effects on temperature, heart, respiratory rate, and CK in up to 81% of patients. AChs and benzodiazepines have been tried but appear to have little effect in most patients, and ACh use can complicate the clinical presentation with possible delirium. Wide recognition and rapid AP discontinuation has drastically reduced mortality from 20% one decade ago to 4% in the mid-1990s.

Many schizophrenics, despite having had NMS, will require future AP pharmacotherapy. Patient selection for rechallenge is important, as only those patients in greatest need of reinstitution of APs (e.g., those who pose risk of harm to society or self) should receive future trials. A review of AP rechallenges suggests that the risk of rechallenge is acceptable in most patients, provided there is careful monitoring, patient selection is appropriate, and the patient is observed for an extended period of time (2 weeks or more is suggested) without APs.[78] Neither patient-specific demographic variables nor AP agent used (neither same or dissimilar, low or high potency) assist in predicting recurrence. Using the lowest effective AP dose is also suggested.

■ *Psychiatric Side Effects.* AP-induced akathisia, akinesia, and dysphoria may have unfortunate sequelae, resulting in what has been termed "behavioral toxicity."[30] Akathisia has resulted in impulsivity and, in extreme cases, violence and suicide. Akinesia, characterized by "diminished spontaneity," results in symptoms of apathy and withdrawal, often mistaken for the negative symptoms of schizophrenia; these patients may actually appear depressed on formal evaluation.

Delirium and psychosis are reported with larger doses of APs or combinations of AChs with APs. Chronic confusion and disorientation can occur in the elderly as a result of AP treatment.[55] Unfortunately, the link is not always made between initiation of AP therapy, and the patient may be misdiagnosed with an organic mental disorder. This clinical presentation, called a "pseudodementia," is easily reversible on discontinuation of the AP.

Exacerbation and new onset of obsessive–compulsive symptoms have been reported with CLZ.[79]

■ Endocrine System

DA blockade in the tuberoinfundibular tract results in increased PRL levels, because DA is the major PRL-inhibiting factor. Galactorrhea may occur in up to 57% of women, and menstrual irregularities or amenorrhea in up to 97%. These effects may be dose related and appear more commonly with the use of high-potency typical APs. Gynecomastia and galactorrhea are reported in men as well. Tolerance does not appear to develop to these effects.[80] Switching to the atypical antipsychotics OLZ, sertindole, or quetiapine, which have no appreciable effect on PRL, is the most reasonable treatment option. Bromocriptine in doses up to 15 mg daily, or amantadine in doses up to 300 mg daily, have also been used.

Weight gain is frequently reported in patients receiving APs.[80] APs can induce weight gain, but dietary factors and activity levels may play a significant role in this population, as does renourishment after a period of poor self-care. Weight gain is seen with most atypical antipsychotics. In particular, significant weight increases have been associated with CLZ and OLZ therapy, and have been shown to be independent of symptomatic improvements.[81] However, the investigational atypical AP ziprasidone is alleged to not cause weight gain.

APs may affect glucose levels and response, a consideration in diabetic patients, although studies in diabetics show little effect in the successful management of their illness. CLZ can exacerbate preexisting diabetes, and has also been linked to a new onset of diabetes; this does not appear to be related to its effect on patient weight.[82]

■ Cardiovascular System

■ *Orthostatic Hypotension.* Postural or othostatic hypotension, defined as a greater than 20 mm Hg drop in systolic pressure, is caused by α-adrenergic blockade, which inhibits reflex vasoconstriction when rising to a sitting or standing position; this appears to be a combination of local vasodilatory effects and central inhibition of the vasomotor center, as well as sympatholysis leading to unopposed β-adrenergic effect.[74] Patients may experience light-headedness or syncope. Associated with lower potency APs (especially on intramuscular or intravenous administration), orthostatic hypotension can occur in any patient, but diabetics, patients with preexisting cardiovascular disease, and the elderly seem particularly predisposed. For the mild case, patient education should address slow changes in posture to allow for adaptation or the use of support hose. For most patients, tolerance to this effect occurs within 2 to 3 months. If this does not occur, lower doses or a change to a higher potency AP can be attempted. Low-potency agents and CLZ should be used with caution in patients with underlying cardiovascular disease.

Severe hypotensive episodes require more vigorous treatment. The patient should be placed in a Trendelenburg position. Volume expansion through intravenous fluids should be attempted before the use of pressor agents. Pure alpha-adrenergic pressor agents, such as phenylephrine (Neo-Synephrine) or metaraminol (Aramine), can be used, as well as norepinephrine (Levophed), which has β_1-adrenergic properties. Epinephrine (Adrenalin), with α- and β-adrenergic effects, should never be used because unopposed β-adrenergic stimulating effects will further lower a patient's blood pressure, potentially leading to cardiovascular collapse.

Isoproterenol (Isuprel), which also has β-adrenergic stimulating effects, should also be avoided.

Electrocardiogram (ECG) Changes. APs have both antiarrhythmic and arrhythmogenic effects. They produce direct myocardial depression and quinidine-like effects on cardiac conduction, and they also antagonize sympathetic nervous system activity in the hypothalamus and stabilize cardiac tissue through local anesthetic properties. Low-potency typical agents, especially piperidine phenothiazines (such as TRD) and CLZ, are more likely to cause these effects. ECG changes include increased heart rate (through sinus tachycardia from Ach effects, or reflex tachycardia from α-adrenergic blockade), flattened T waves, ST segment depression, and prolongation of QT and PR intervals. Torsades de pointes has been reported with TRD, perhaps through its sulfoxide metabolite, which may be a cause of cardiac sudden death. However, most ECG changes are not usually clinically significant at normal therapeutic doses in physically healthy patients.[83] Greater caution is necessary in the elderly and patients with preexisting cardiac disease.[55] In patients older than 40 years, a pretreatment ECG is recommended.

The clinical significance of prolonged QT and QTc intervals associated with use of sertindole is unknown; however, it will probably preclude sertindole from being considered a first-line agent until greater clinical experience is obtained. Baseline and intermittent ECG monitoring will likely be recommended in the product labeling.[26]

Ophthalmologic Effects

Impairment in visual accommodation results from paresis of ciliary muscles, an ACh effect. Although bothersome, the effect is temporary in most cases. Photophobia may also result. Pilocarpine ophthalmic solution may be necessary in severe cases.[84]

Exacerbation of narrow-angle (angle closure) glaucoma can result from increases in intraocular pressure, another ACh effect. APs should be used with great caution in susceptible individuals.[84]

Opaque deposits in the cornea and lens occur with chronic phenothiazine treatment, most frequently with CPZ. Although visual acuity is not usually affected, periodic slit-lamp ophthalmologic examinations are frequently recommended in patients receiving long-term treatment with phenothiazines. Due to cataract development and lenticular changes in animals, baseline and periodic eye exams are also recommended for patients receiving quetiapine.[85]

Retinitis pigmentosis can result from use of TRD doses greater than 800 mg daily. It is caused by melanin deposits, and can result in permanent visual impairment or blindness. There is no evidence that it is a function of dosage accumulation.[84]

Hepatic System

Liver function test (LFT) abnormalities (elevated aminotransferases and alkaline phosphatase) are reported in up to 50% of patients on APs, and may occur without clinical symptoms.[86] This occurs most commonly in patients under 50 years of age and does not appear to be dose related. Mild LFT elevations are typically not significant, although they should be followed closely. If aminotransferases are greater than three times the upper limit of normal, AP therapy should be changed to a chemically unrelated AP.

Cholestatic hepatocanalicular jaundice can occur in up to 2% of patients receiving phenothiazines. It may be a hypersensitivity reaction, or due to either the effects on bile composition or the direct toxic effect of a metabolite on biliary ductile hepatocytes impairing bile flow.[86] The onset is usually within the first 2 weeks of therapy, with prodromal symptoms of malaise, fatigue, fever, chills, arthralgias, myalgias, GI symptoms, and severe pruritis. Symptoms resolve without residual liver damage within 2 to 8 weeks upon discontinuation of the offending AP. Palliative treatment of pruritis with topical or oral antihistamines is frequently necessary. Resumption of AP therapy should be delayed as long as reasonably possible, and it should be done with a nonphenothiazine AP.

Genitourinary System

Urinary hesitancy and retention is commonly reported with low-potency APs. ACh effects cause smooth muscle slowing and paralyze the detrusor muscle of the bladder, requiring greater urine volume to evoke muscle contraction. Men with benign prostatic hypertrophy are especially prone to this effect.[55]

Urinary incontinence is felt by some to be unrelated to urinary retention, as many patients do not complain of problems before it occurs. Instead, it may be mechanistically similar to a dystonic reaction. It is reported more frequently in older patients, especially women.[87]

The AP effects on sexual dysfunction can be frightening or devastating to most schizophrenics and can adversely affect compliance. Erectile dysfunction and impotence, considered an ACh effect, occurs in 25% to 60% of patients, most frequently with TRD. Although this can occur in a large number of untreated psychotic patients, it is most certainly compounded by AP drugs. Anorgasmia and decreased libido in women have also been proposed to be ACh in nature. Alpha-adrenergic blockade is proposed to be the mechanism behind priapism and retarded and retrograde ejaculation. Again, TRD is the most frequently reported AP for these effects and is a potent α-blocker. Decreased libido may also be caused by sedation. In men, another possible, although not fully explored, mechanism of sexual dysfunction is decreased testosterone production secondary to hyperprolactinemia.[88] Changing to an atypical AP, particularly OLZ or quetiapine, is a reasonable intervention. Sertindole causes a significantly reduced ejaculatory volume in 20% of men, but is not associated with any change in sexual functioning.[26]

Hematologic System

Transient leukopenia may occur during initial treatment with APs; however, it typically does not progress to clinically significant parameters.[89] If the WBC count is less than 3000/mm^3 or the absolute neutrophil count (ANC) is < 1000/mm^3, the AP should be discontinued, and the WBC monitored closely until it returns to normal. Agranulocytosis reportedly occurs in 0.01% of patients receiving APs, and with the typical APs may occur most frequently with CPZ and piperazine phenothiazines. The onset is usually within the first 8 weeks of therapy. Agranulocytosis may initially manifest clinically as a local infection, with sore throat, leukoplakia, and erythema and ulcerations of the pharynx. These symptoms in any patient receiving APs should signal the immediate need for a WBC. If either the WBC or ANC falls below these parameters, the drug should be discontinued immediately and the patient monitored closely for the development of secondary infections. There are also isolated, rare case reports of thrombocytopenia and eosinophilia.

Agranulocytosis is the CLZ-related adverse effect receiving the most publicity, from both the medical and political perspectives. Data on the incidence since the release of CLZ in February 1990, following stringent monitoring guidelines, reveal that the 1-year treatment risk of developing agranulocytosis with CLZ appears to be approximately 0.8%, with the 18-month risk at 0.91%.[90] Increasing age and female gender are associated with greater risk. Based on available data, the time period for greatest risk appears to be between months 1 and 6 of treatment.[91] WBC monitoring is mandated in the product labeling. If the total WBC count drops to less than 2000/mm^3, or the ANC is less than

1000/mm^3, CLZ should be discontinued and the patient monitored closely. Some clinicians have used the granulocyte colony stimulating factor, filgrastim, with hopes of improving the outcome by hastening resolution or decreasing morbidity. One case series, using filgrastim (starting dose of 300 μg/d SC, increased by 300 μg/d until 900 μg/d is reached, which is then continued until the agranulocytosis is resolved), demonstrated a decrease in time to resolution and decreased intensive care bed costs when compared with historical controls.[92] In cases of mild to moderate neutropenia (granulocytes between 2000 and 3000/mm^3, or ANC between 1000 and 1500/mm^3), which occurs in up to 2% of patients, CLZ should be discontinued with daily monitoring of complete blood counts until values return to normal. Weekly WBC monitoring after the first 6 months of CLZ therapy is not cost-effective.[93] The FDA recently revised the labeling to allow monitoring every 2 weeks after 6 months of treatment.

Dermatologic System

Allergic reactions are rare and usually occur within 8 weeks of therapy, manifesting as maculopapular, erythematous, pruritic rashes that are evident on the face, neck, trunk, or extremities. Drug discontinuation and topical steroids are recommended.

Contact dermatitis, including the oral mucosa, may occur in patients or medical personnel. For patients, mixing the concentrate in a sufficient quantity of a nonacidic liquid and swallowing it quickly decreases problems in susceptible patients. Care should be taken in the handling and preparation of liquid APs.

Phenothiazine structures can absorb ultraviolet light and energy, resulting in the formation of free radicals, which can have damaging effects on the skin. Erythema and severe sunburns can occur. Exposure to sunlight should be limited, and patients should be educated about the use of a maximally blocking sunscreen, hats, protective clothing, and sunglasses.[74]

Blue-gray or purplish skin coloration in areas exposed to sunlight occurs in patients receiving higher doses of low-potency phenothiazines during long-term administration, especially with CPZ. It commonly occurs with concurrent corneal or lens pigmentation.

Sudden Death Syndromes

Although fewer sudden deaths occurred before AP use, it has been reported in schizophrenics before and after the advent of APs. Most theories emphasize a pharmacologic etiology. The most common theory is that ventricular arrhythmias progress to ventricular fibrillation and death. Another common hypothesis is that an impaired gag reflex from a laryngeal–pharyngeal dystonia leads to aspiration, hypoxia, and death, a syndrome known as "obstructive asphyxia" or "café coronary." Other potentially drug-related theories include hyperpyrexia, NMS, seizures, and toxic megacolon, whereas nondrug-related theories include acute exhaustive mania or Bell's mania, lethal catatonia, coronary artery disease, and the sequelae of alcohol and substance abuse.[94]

Miscellaneous Adverse Effects

A particularly curious and sometimes troubling side effect with CLZ is sialorrhea. Drooling, possibly adrenergic in etiology, occurs in the absence of pseudoparkinsonian symptoms.[91] Some cases respond to the addition of the α-adrenergic blocker clonidine, in doses of 0.1 to 0.2 mg/d.[95] It may also abate with benztropine therapy.

TOXICITY WITH OVERDOSE

Acute overdose with APs rarely results in serious symptomatology. Mild intoxication manifests as sedation, hypotension, and miosis, whereas with severe intoxication, agitation and delirium may typically progress to motor retardation, seizures, cardiac arrhythmias, respiratory arrest, and coma. Dystonias and pseudoparkinsonian symptoms also occur. Supportive measures, gastric lavage, and activated charcoal are recommended. Induction of emesis may be difficult due to effects on the chemoreceptor trigger zone, and dialysis is ineffective due to the degree of drug-protein binding. Phenytoin or sodium bicarbonate are useful in the treatment of quinidine-like cardiac conduction effects on the QRS or QTc intervals. Physostigmine is not generally recommended to reverse anticholinergic toxicity because of deleterious effects on arrhythmias and seizure threshold.[96]

USE IN PREGNANCY AND LACTATION

Currently available data assessing the risk of teratogenesis with AP agents are insufficient. HPD was studied in the treatment of hyperemesis gravidarum without negative effect; it and other high-potency agents appear to be preferred, but unfortunately this is primarily due to a lack of published reports over decades of use. Case reports implicating limb malformations are rare, but should be considered in deciding on the need for first-trimester AP use. The risks of AP use must be weighed against the benefits of pharmacotherapy in patients who may be experiencing disorganized thoughts, delusions about change in body image or pregnancy, or who are unable to provide adequate prenatal care.[97] Other potential but largely unknown risks of APs throughout pregnancy are the incidence of behavioral teratogenicity on the neonate, receptor changes, perinatal effects (e.g., tonicity, strength, sucking), EPS, jaundice, respiratory depression, and intestinal obstruction.

APs appear in breast milk with milk to plasma ratios of 0.5 to 1. Little is known about the effects of these drugs on the neonate. Although not contraindicated, the lowest dosage should be used in the mother, and the infant should be carefully monitored.

DRUG INTERACTIONS

Most AP drug interactions are relatively minor in severity and often involve additive CNS side effects. The most common drug interactions seen in schizophrenia involve anticholinergics and drugs causing sedation. The concurrent use of lithium with APs is generally safe; however, a handful of cases of irreversible encephalopathy (including delirium, ataxia, rigidity, tremors, fever, weakness, and lethargy) have been reported.[98,99] Although anecdotal data report this more commonly with HPD, this is poorly substantiated. Although this interaction can appear similar to NMS, patients recovering from an AP/lithium interaction may more commonly suffer sequelae.

Most antipsychotics are metabolized by the hepatic cytochrome P450 system. CYP 2D6 is the predominant isoenzyme associated with the metabolism of phenothiazines. Atypical antipsychotics are metabolized by multiple different isoenzymes (see Table 64–6). AP pharmacokinetics can be significantly affected by concomitant enzyme inducers or inhibitors. Anticonvulsants, particularly carbamazepine, are the most commonly used enzyme inducers in schizophrenics. However, smoking is a potent inducer of hepatic enzymes and may increase AP clearance by as much as 50%.[21] Potential enzyme inhibition will vary depending on the specific isoenzyme(s) for the substrate antipsychotic as well the isoenzyme(s) affected by the inhibitor. See Table 64–11 for a listing of additional drug interactions.[51]

PHARMACEONOMIC CONSIDERATIONS

It is estimated that approximately 80% of individuals suffering their first schizophrenic break will have recurrent episodes and significant lifetime psychosocial dysfunction. In 1990 prices, the economic cost of schizophrenia in the United States was $38 billion with direct health care treatment costs accounting for 53% of the total.[100] The public mental health care sector provides the

TABLE 64–11. Drug Interactions Involving Antipsychotics

Interacting Medication	Mechanism of Interaction	Clinical Effect or Result Reported
Established, Probable, or Suspected Drug Interactions Regardless of Severity; Possible Interactions of Major Severity		
Anticholinergics	Decreased AP concentrations	Decreased antipsychotic effect
	Additive anticholineric effect	See discussion under autonomic effects
Barbiturates	AP increases neuromuscular excitation with barbiturate anesthesia	Involved only those phenothiazines used as preanesthetic agents
	Phenobarbital induces AP metabolism	Decreased AP Cp
Beta-blockers	Synergistic pharmacologic effect or increases in AP concentrations	Case report of severe hypotension
	AP inhibit metabolism of propranolol, increase plasma concentrations	Increased pharmacologic effects, clinical effect not documented
	Unknown	Potentiated antipsychotic effect
Carbamazepine	Carbamazepine induces AP metabolism	Up to 50% reduction in AP Cp
Charcoal	Reduces GI absorption of AP and adsorbs drug during enterohepatic circulation	May reduce antipsychotic effect or cause toxicity when used during overdose or for GI disturbances
Cigarette smoking	Increase AP clearance if metabolized through CYP 1A2	Decrease AP plasma levels
Epinephrine, norepinephrine	AP antagonizes pressor effect	Hypotension (see discussion of orthostatic hypotension in text)
Ethanol	Additive CNS depression	Impaired psychomotor skills
Fluvoxamine	Inhibits AP metabolism through CYP 1A2	Increased clozapine and perhaps olanzapine Cp
Guanethidine	AP antagonizes guanethidine reuptake	Impaired antihypertensive effect
Lithium	Unknown	Rare reports of neurotoxicity
Meperidine	Additive CNS depression	Hypotension and sedation
Metrizamide	Lowered seizure threshold	Two case reports of seizures
Paroxetine, fluoxetine	Inhibits CYP 2D6 and 2C metabolism	Increased Cp of phenothiazines and sertindole
Quinidine	Inhibits CYP 2D6 metabolism	Increased Cp of phenothiazines and sertindole
Possible Interactions of Minor to Moderate Severity		
Aluminum containing antacids	Forms insoluble complexes in GI tract	Possible reduced antipsychotic effect
Amphetamines, anorexiants	Decreased pharmacologic effect of amphetamine	Diminished weight loss effect
	Drug–disease state interaction	Amphetamines may exacerbate psychosis Amphetamines have been reported to improve psychotic symptoms in treatment-refractory schizophrenics
Angiotensin-converting enzyme inhibitors	Additive hypotensive effects	One case of marked hypotension, postural intolerance
Antidepressants	Decreased metabolism of antidepressants through competitive inhibition	Increased antidepressant concentration, possible increased effect or adverse effect
Benzodiazepines	Increased pharmacologic effect of the benzodiazepine	Case reports of respiratory depression, stupor, hypotension; these effects, along with ataxia and sialorrhea, may be pronounced with clozapine
Bromocriptine	AP antagonize dopamine receptor-stimulating effect; increases prolactin	Should not be coadministered during treatment of prolactin-secreting tumors
Caffeinated beverages	Form precipitates with oral antipsychotic solutions; should not be mixed despite product labelling	Possible diminished antipsychotic effect
Cimetidine	Reduced AP metabolism	Increased AP Cp
Clonidine	AP potentiates alpha-adrenergic hypotensive effect	Hypotension
Disulfiram	Impairs AP metabolism	Increased AP Cp
Erythromycin	Inhibitis CYP 3A metabolism	Increased clozapine Cp and perhaps quetiapine Cp
Fluoxetine	Inhibits CYP 2D6 metabolism	Sudden onset of EPS; also, increase in haloperidol and sertindole Cp
Ketoconazole	Inhibitis CYP 3A metabolism	Increased clozapine Cp and perhaps quetiapine Cp

TABLE 64–11. (Continued)

Interacting Medication	Mechanism of Interaction	Clinical Effect or Result Reported
Possible Interactions of Minor to Moderate Severity (continued)		
Methyldopa	Unknown	Blood pressure elevations
Phenytoin	Induction of AP metabolism Increased phenytoin metabolism	Decreased AP Cp Decreased phenytoin Cp
Valproic acid	AP inhibits valproic acid metabolism	Increases valproic acid half-life and Cp

majority of services for individuals with schizophrenia. Mental health care costs for schizophrenia represent disproportionate expenditures for crisis intervention and hospitalization as compared to outpatient services oriented toward maintaining remission and improving psychosocial functioning. The minimal funding provided for efficient ambulatory mental health services further enhances the demand for hospitalization and detracts additional revenues that might be available for outpatient services. This has created a vicious revolving door cycle with respect to patient care and is one of the major challenges facing public mental health care.

The advent of more expensive atypical APs, accompanied by limited resources, has forced mental health care providers to examine the outcomes and related economics of treating patients with the atypical agents as compared with the traditional, largely generic APs. To date, there are inadequate data to define the true cost effectiveness of using atypical APs. However, some studies have demonstrated potential cost effectiveness of these new interventions, particularly with CLZ. Naturalistic studies have shown that CLZ's use in treatment-resistant patients is associated with a decrease in total patient care costs of nearly $10,000 per patient annually.[23] In a randomized controlled study evaluating CLZ versus HPD in patients with high hospital utilization, CLZ was somewhat more effective in decreasing BPRS scores and better tolerated than HPD while having similar overall costs from a societal perspective.[101] Three different retrospective evaluations using patients' as their own historical controls demonstrated decreased hospitalization days in the year after RSP use with a resulting decrease in direct costs ranging from $4000 to $6100 annually.[102] Although none of these studies adequately address other potential reasons for the decreased costs, they do suggest that total direct costs do not increase with atypical AP use.

EVALUATION OF THERAPEUTIC OUTCOMES

Assessment of response has traditionally been done subjectively or empirically (a relative sense of how the clinician feels the patient is doing). A formal mental status examination (MSE) is used to structure the patient interview and focus on items related to appearance, mood, sensorium, intellectual functioning, and thought processes. However, the MSE is not specific for the measurement of drug response. Realistically, clinicians should be trained to use standardized psychiatric rating scales to assist in objectively rating patients' drug responses.[54] The Brief Psychiatric Rating Scale (BPRS), although not specific for schizophrenia or any other illness, is accepted by the Food and Drug Administration as the primary instrument to determine AP drug efficacy in phase II and III clinical trials. Other scales (e.g., the Comprehensive Psychiatric Rating Scale and the Positive and Negative Syndrome Scale) are also available. Alternatively, the use of symptom subscales (positive or negative symptom clusters) can be used to quantify change in symptoms most often targeted for treatment in schizophrenia.[22] Objectively, the use of a numeric indicator (20% to 30% reduction in BPRS score) can be used to quantify overall symptom reduction. However, individual symptoms considered socially disabling (e.g., delusions or negative symptoms) may become the focus of treatment despite an overall rating scale improvement.

Similarly, the pharmacotherapeutic plan should include specific monitoring parameters for potential side effects. The plan should include the side effects to be monitored (e.g., EPS), how the potential side effect will be monitored (e.g., observation, Simpson Angus Scale, Barnes Akathisia Scale), and the frequency of assessment (e.g., daily, weekly).

Traditionally, clinicians have often accepted partial symptom response in schizophrenia as success, and have not been aggressive in attempting to achieve greater symptomatic remission. In many respects the side effect profile of typical APs encouraged the acceptance of partial response and a tendency to not "rock the boat" in a patient with partial improvement. However, the advent of multiple different atypical APs with favorable side effect profiles should encourage clinicians to be more assertive in attempting to achieve symptom remission. Furthermore, the systematic use and evaluation of augmentation and combination treatment strategies may be of value in more treatment-resistant patients (see Fig. 64–1).

CONCLUSIONS

Schizophrenia is a complex disease with multiple ramifications for patients and their families. Treatment issues remain clouded by the fact that the etiology of the illness is unknown. It is clear, however, that no single treatment modality is adequate to properly manage a patient with schizophrenia. APs are not a panacea and have multiple adverse effects in addition to the limitations of their efficacy. However, the advent of newer medications offers new opportunities for treatment options in schizophrenia. When used within the context of multidisciplinary treatment, APs assist in keeping psychotic symptoms under control so that patients can appropriately participate in psychosocial rehabilitation programs. Technological advances continue to expand our understanding of CNS physiology and abnormalities found in schizophrenia. This, in turn, should greatly enhance the development of safer and more effective treatment interventions.

In practice, it is mandatory that clinicians appropriately use their expanding armamentarium. It is important that clinicians appreciate the pharmacodynamic basis for treatment interventions so that they can effectively design and implement rational pharmacotherapeutic regimens. Finally, it is critical that clinicians more objectively evaluate individual patient response to medication so that treatment can be optimized. With these strategies, the gap between practice and science can be narrowed and patients' lives benefited.

Acknowledgment: The authors thank Richard Wilcox, PhD, for reviewing the basic science sections of the chapter.

▶ PRINCIPLES OF PHARMACOTHERAPY

- A thorough patient evaluation (e.g., history, mental status exam, physical exam, laboratory analysis) should occur to establish a diagnosis of schizophrenia and to determine the possibility of comorbidities, including substance abuse and general medical disorders.
- Patient care must occur in the context of a multidisciplinary mental health care environment that offers medication and comprehensive psychosocial treatment.
- Pharmacotherapy algorithms should emphasize monotherapies with optimal efficacy to side effect ratios and progress to medications with greater side effect risks and to combination regimens in treatment-resistant patients.
- Patients should have input into specific treatment choices for schizophrenia.
- Pharmacotherapy decisions should be guided by systematic monitoring of patient symptoms, preferably with the use of symptom rating scales.
- Adequate time on a given medication at a therapeutic dose is the most important variable in predicting medication response.
- Long-term maintenance antipsychotic treatment is necessary for the vast majority of patients with schizophrenia.
- Depot antipsychotic treatment should, in general, be reserved for patients who are unreliable in taking oral medications on a daily basis.
- Thorough patient and family psychoeducation should occur, including education about the illness, symptoms, prognosis, medication, and psychosocial treatments, and methods to improve adaptive functioning.
- Nondrug treatment should be oriented toward psychosocial rehabilitation programs that improve adaptive functioning, including supported work and housing.

REFERENCES

1. Schizophrenia and other psychotic disorders. In: Diagnostic and Statistical Manual of Mental Disorders, 4th ed (DSM-IV). Washington, DC, American Psychiatric Association, 1994:273–290.
2. Herz MI, work group on schizophrenia, American Psychiatric Association. Practice guideline for the treatment of patients with schizophrenia. Am J Psychiatry 1997;154(suppl 4):1–63.
3. Kane JM. Schizophrenia. N Engl J Med 1996;334:34–41.
4. Ereshefsky L, Tran-Johnson TK, Watanabe MD. Pathophysiologic basis for schizophrenia and the efficacy of antipsychotics. Clin Pharm 1990;9:682–707.
5. Lieberman JA, Koreen AR. Neurochemistry and neuroendocrinology of schizophrenia: A selective review. In: Shore D, ed. Schizophrenia 1993. Rockville, MD, National Institute of Mental Health, 1993: 197–255.
6. Heckers S. Neuropathology of schizophrenia: Cortex, thalamus, basal ganglia, and neurotransmitter-specific projection systems. Schizophr Bull 1997;23:403–421.
7. Goldman-Rakic PS, Selemon LD. Functional and anatomical aspects of prefrontal pathology in schizophrenia. Schizophr Bull 1997;23: 437–458.
8. Gur RF. Functional brain-imaging studies in schizophrenia. In: Bloom FE, Kupfer DJ, eds. Psychopharmacology: The Fourth Generation of Progress. New York, Raven, 1995:1185–1192.
9. Henn FA. The NMDA receptor as a site for psychopathology. Primary or secondary role? Arch Gen Psychiatry 1995;52:1008–1010.
10. Olney JW, Farber NB. Response to commentaries and to the challenge of building a perfect theory to explain schizophrenia. Arch Gen Psychiatry 1995;52:1019–1024.
11. Olney JW, Farber NB. Glutamate receptor dysfunction and schizophrenia. Arch Gen Psychiatry 1995;52:998–1007.
12. Huttunen M. The evolution of the serotonin-dopamine antagonist concept. J Clin Psychopharmacol 1995;15(suppl 1):4S–10S.
13. Heritch AJ. Evidence for reduced and dysregulated turnover of dopamine in schizophrenia. Schizophr Bull 1990;16:605–615.
14. Gur RE, Pearlson GD. Neuroimaging in schizophrenia research. In: Shore D, ed. Schizophrenia 1993. Rockville, MD, National Institute of Mental Health, 1993:163–179.
15. Kendler KS, Diehl SR. The genetics of schizophrenia: A current, genetic, epidemiologic perspective. In: Shore D, ed. Schizophrenia 1993. Rockville, MD, National Institute of Mental Health, 1993: 87–111.
16. Weinberger DR. The biological basis for schizophrenia: New directions. J Clin Psychiatry 1997:58(suppl 10):22–27.
17. Lieberman JA. Atypical antipsychotic drugs as a first-line treatment of schizophrenia: A rationale and hypothesis. J Clin Psychiatry 1996; 57(suppl 11):68–71.
18. Kane JM. Treatment-resistant schizophrenic patients. J Clin Psychiatry 1996;57(suppl 9):35–40.
19. Andreasen NC, Flaum M, Swayze VW, et al. Positive and negative symptoms in schizophrenia. Arch Gen Psychiatry 1990;47:615–621.

20. Keks NA. Impact of newer antipsychotics on outcomes in scizophrenia. Clin Ther 1997;19:148–158.
21. Frances A, Docherty JP, Kahn DA, et al. The expert consensus guideline series: Treatment of schizophrenia. J Clin Psychiatry 1996;57 (suppl 12B):3–58.
22. Miller AL, Chiles JA, Chiles J, Crismon ML. TMAP Procedural Manual: Schizophrenia Module Physician Manual. Texas Medication Algorithm Project, phase 3. Texas Department of Mental Health and Mental Retardation, Austin, August 1998.
23. Meltzer HY. Atypical antipsychotic drugs. In: Bloom FE, Kupfer DJ, eds. Psychopharmacology: The Fourth Generation of Progress. New York, Raven, 1995:1277–1286.
24. Marder SR, Meibach RC, risperidone study group. Risperidone in the treatment of schizophrenia. Am J Psychiatry 1994;151:825–835.
25. Fulton B, Goa KL. Olanzapine. A review of its pharmacological properties and therapeutic efficacy in the management of schizophrenia and related psychoses. Drugs 1997;53:281–298.
26. Small JG, Hirsch SR, Arvanitis LA, et al. Quetiapine in patients with schizophrenia. A high- and low-dose double-blind comparison with placebo. Arch Gen Psychiatry 1997;54:549–557.
27 Zimbroff DL, Kane JM, Tamminga CA, et al. Controlled dose-response study of sertindole and haloperidol in the treatment of schizophrenia. Am J Psychiatry 1997;154:782–791.
28. Drugs that cause psychiatric symptoms. Med Lett Drugs Ther 1993; 35:65–70.
29. Awad AG. Drug therapy in schizophrenia: Variability of outcome and prediction of response. Can J Psychiatry 1989;34:711–720.
30. Van Putten T, Marder SR. Behavioral toxicity of anti-psychotic drugs. J Clin Psychiatry 1987;48(suppl 9):13–19.
31. Mossman D. A decision analysis approach to neuroleptic dosing: Insights from a mathematical model. J Clin Psychiatry 1997;58:66–73.
32. Wirshing WC, Marder SR, Van Putten T, Ames D. Acute treatment of schizophrenia. In: Bloom FE, Kupfer DJ, eds. Psychopharmacology: The Fourth Generation of Progress. New York, Raven, 1995: 1259–1266.
33. Csernansky JG, Newcomer JG. Maintenance drug treatment for schizophrenia. In: Bloom FE, Kupfer DJ, eds. Psychopharmacology: The Fourth Generation of Progress. New York, Raven, 1995: 1267–1275.
34. Herz MI, Glazer WM, Mostert MA, et al. Intermittent vs maintenance medication in schizophrenia: Two year results. Arch Gen Psychiatry 1991;48:333–339.
35. Ereshefsky L, Saklad SR, Jann MW, et al. Future of depot neuroleptic therapy: Pharmacokinetics and pharmacodynamic approaches. J Clin Psychiatry 1984;45:50.
36. Ereshefsky L, Toney G, Saklad SR, Seidel DR. A loading-dose strategy for converting from oral to depot haloperidol. Hosp Comm Psychiatry 1993;44:1155–1161.
37. Pabis DJ, Dorson PG, Crismon ML. Evaluation of inpatient depot antipsychotic prescribing. Ann Pharmacother 1996;30:1381–1386.
38. Hamann GL, Egan TM, Wells BG, et al. Injection site reactions after intramuscular administration of haloperidol decanoate 100 mg/mL. J Clin Psychiatry 1990;51:502–504.
39. Rush AJ, Crismon ML, Biggs M, project management team. Texas Medication Algorithm Project Interim Report. Texas Department of Mental Health and Mental Retardation, Austin, October 20, 1997.
40. Smith RC, Chua JW, Lipetsker B, Bhattacharyya A. Efficacy of risperidone in reducing positive and negative symptoms in medication-refractory schizophrenia: An open prospective study. J Clin Psychiatry 1996;57:460–466.
41. Still DJ, Dorson PG, Crismon ML, Pousson C. Effects of switching inpatients with treatment-resistant schizophrenia from clozapine to risperidone. Psychiatr Serv 1996;47:1382–1384.
42. Martin J, Gomez JC, Garcia-Bernardo E, Cuesta M, et al. Olanzapine in treatment-resistant schizophrenia: Results of an open-label study. J Clin Psychiatry 1997;58:479–483.
43. Kane J, Honigfeld G, Singer J, et al. Clozapine for the treatment-resistant schizophrenic: A double blind comparison with chlorpromazine. Arch Gen Psychiatry 1988;45:789–796.
44. Spears NM, Leadbetter RA, Shutty MS. Clozapine treatment in polydipsia and intermittent hyponatremia. J Clin Psychiatry 1996;57: 123–128.
45. Pickar D, Litman RE, Konicki PE, et al. Neurochemical and neural mechanisms of positive and negative symptoms in schizophrenia. In: Andreason NC, ed. Schizophrenia: Positive and Negative Symptoms and Syndromes. Modern Problems in Pharmacopsychiatry. Basel, Karger, 1990;24:124–151.
46. Lipinski JF, Keck PE, McElroy SL. β-Adrenergic antagonists in psychosis: Is improvement due to treatment of neuroleptic-induced akathisia? J Clin Psychopharmacol 1988;409–416.
47. Yudolfsky SC, Silver JM, Hales RE. Pharmacologic management of aggression in the elderly. J Clin Psychiatry 1990;5(suppl 10): 22–28.
48. Baldessarini RJ. Drugs and the treatment of psychiatric disorders. Psychosis and anxiety. In: Hardman JG, Limbird LE, Molinoff PB, et al, eds. Goodman and GilmanMs The Pharmacological Basis of Therapeutics, 9th ed. New York, Pergamon, 1996:399–430.
49. Richelson E. Preclinical pharmacology of neurolepetics: Focus on new generation compounds. J Clin Psychiatry 1996;57(suppl 11): 4–11.
50. Kahn RS, Davis KL. New developments in dopamine and schizophrenia. In: Bloom FE, Kupfer DJ, eds. Psychopharmacology: The Fourth Generation of Progress. New York, Raven, 1995:1193–1203.
51. Ereshefsky L. Pharmacokinetics and drug interactions: Update for new antipsychotics. J Clin Psychiatry 1996;57(suppl 11):12–25.
52. Perry PJ, Miller DD, Arndt SV, Cadoret RJ. Clozapine and norclozapine plasma concentrations and clinical response of treatment-refractory schizophrenic patients. Am J Psychiatry 1991;148:231–235.
53. VanderZwaag C, Mcgee M, McEvoy JP, et al. Response of patients with treatment-refractory schizophrenia to clozapine within three serum level ranges. Am J Psychiatry 1996;153:1579–1584.
54. Wetzler S. Measuring mental illness: Psychometric assessment for clinicians. Washington DC, American Psychiatric Association Press, 1988.
55. Crismon ML. Psychotropic drugs in the elderly: Principles of use. Am Pharm 1990;NS30:57–63.
56. Holloman LC, Marder SR. Management of acute extrapyramidal effects induced by antipsychotic drugs. Am J Health-Syst Pharm 1997; 54:2461–2477.
57. Arana GW, Goff DC, Baldessarini RJ, Keepers GA. Efficacy of ACh prophylaxis for neuroleptic-induced acute dystonia. Am J Psychiatry 1988;145:993–996.
58. Simpson GM, Meyer JM. Dystonia while changing from clozapine to risperidone. J Clin Psychopharmacol 1996;16:260–261.
59. Fleischhacker WW, Roth SD, Kane JM. The pharmacologic treatment of neuroleptic-induced akathisia. J Clin Psychopharmacol 1990;10:12–21.
60. Crismon ML. Drug induced extrapyramidal syndromes. US Pharmacist 1982;7:33–42.
61. Wells BG, Marken PA, Rickman LA, et al. Characterizing anticholinergic abuse in community mental health. J Clin Psychopharmacol 1989;9:431–435.
62. Spivak B, Mester R, Abesgaus J, et al. Clozapine treatment for neuroleptic-induced tardive dyskinesia, parkinsonism, and chronic akathisia in schizophrenic patients. J Clin Psychiatry 1997;58: 318–322.
63. Anonymous. Tardive dyskinesia scales in current use. In: Fann W, Smith RC, Davis JM, et al, eds. Tardive Dyskinesia Research and Treatment. Jamaica, NY, Spectrum, 1980:243–267.
64. Sprague RL, Kalachnik JE. Reliability, validity, and a total score cutoff for the Dyskinesia Identification System Condensed User Scale (DISCUS) with mentally ill and mentally retarded populations. Psychopharmacol Bull 1991;27:51–58.

65. Egan MF, Apud J, Wyatt RJ. Treatment of tardive dyskinesia. Schizophr Bull 1997;23:583–609.
66. Gardos G, Cole JO. Tardive dyskinesia and anticholinergic drugs. Am J Psychiatry 1983;140:200–202.
67. Yesavage JA, Tanke ED, Sheikh JI. Tardive dyskinesia and steady-state serum levels of thiothixene. Arch Gen Psychiatry 1987;44: 913–915.
68. Kane JM, Woerner M, Borenstein M, et al. Integrating incidence and prevalence of tardive dyskinesia. Psychopharmacol Bull 1986;22: 254–258.
69. Chouinard G, Annable L, Mercier P, Ross-Chouinard A. A five year follow-up study of tardive dyskinesia. Psychopharmacol Bull 1986; 22:259–263.
70. Gardos G, Cole JO, Salomon M, Schniebolk S. Clinical forms of severe tardive dyskinesia. Am J Psychiatry 1987;144:895–902.
71. Cassens G, Inglis AK, Appelbaum PS, Gutheil TG. Neuroleptics: Effects on neuropsychological function in chronic schizophrenic patients. Schizophr Bull 1990;16:477–499.
72. Garcia G, Crismon ML, Dorson PG. Seizures in two patients after the addition of lithium to a clozapine regimen. J Clin Psychopharmacol 1994;14:426–428.
73. Cold JA, Wells BG, Froemming JH. Seizure activity associated with AP therapy. DICP Ann Pharmacother 1990;24:601–606.
74. Simpson GM, Pi EH, Sramek JJ. Adverse effects of AP agents. Drugs 1981;21:138–151.
75. Guze BH, Baxter Jr LR. Neuroleptic malignant syndrome. N Engl J Med 1985;313:163–166.
76. Webster P, Wijeratne C. Risperidone-induced neuroleptic malignant syndrome. Lancet 1994;344:1228–1229.
77. Sakkas P, Davis JM, Hua J, et al. Pharmacotherapy of neuroleptic malignant syndrome. Psychiatr Ann 1991;21:157–164.
78. Wells AJ, Sommi RW, Crismon ML. Neuroleptic rechallenge after neuroleptic malignant syndrome: Case report and literature review. Drug Intell Clin Pharm 1988;22:475–480.
79. Levin Z, Hwang MY, Rotrosen J. The relationship between clozapine and obsessive-compulsive disorder. Comp Psychiatry 1996;37:74.
80. Zito JM, Sofair JB, Jaeger J. Self-reported neuroendocrine effects of APs in women: A pilot study. DICP Ann Pharmacother 1990;24: 176–180.
81. Bustillo JR, Buchanan RW, Irish D, Breier A. Differential effect of clozapine on weight: A controlled study. Am J Psychiatry 1996;153: 817–819.
82. Popli AP, Konicki PE, Jurjus GJ, et al. Clozapine and associated diabetes mellitus. J Clin Psychiatry 1997;58:1089–111.
83. Risch SC, Groom GP, Janowsky DS. The effects of psychotropic drugs on the cardiovascular system. J Clin Psychiatry 1982;43: 16–31.
84. Oshika T. Ocular adverse effects of neuropsychiatric agents: incidence and management. Drug Saf 1995;12:256–263.
85. Zeneca Pharmaceuticals. Quetiapine package insert. Wilmington, DE, July 1997.
86. Regal RE, Billi JE, Glazer HM. Phenothiazine-induced cholestatic jaundice. Clin Pharm 1987;6:787–794.
87. Nurnberg HG, Ambrosini PJ. Urinary incontinence in patients receiving neuroleptics. J Clin Psychiatry 1979;40:271–274.
88. Sullivan G, Lukoff D. Sexual side effects of AP medication: Evaluation and interventions. Hosp Community Psychiatry 1990;41: 1238–1241.
89. Balon R, Berchou R. Hematologic side effects of psychotropic drugs. Psychosomatics 1986;27:119–120, 125–127.
90. Alvir JMJ, Lieberman JA, Safferman AZ, et al. Clozapine-induced agranulocytosis: Incidence and risk factors in the United States. N Engl J Med 1993;329:162–167.
91. Ereshefsky L, Watanabe MD, Tran-Johnson TK. Clozapine: An atypical antipsychotic agent. Clin Pharm 1989;8:691–709
92. Gullion G, Yeh HS. Treatment of clozapine-induced agranulocytosis with recombinant granulocyte colony-stimulating factor. J Clin Psychiatry 1994;55:401–405.
93. Zhang M, Owen RR, Pope SK, Smith GR. Cost-effectiveness of clozapine monitoring after the first 6 months. Arch Gen Psychiatry 1996;53:954–958.
94. Dorson PG, Crismon ML. CPZ accumulation and sudden death in a patient with renal insufficiency. Drug Intell Clin Pharm 1988;22: 776–778.
95. Grabowski J. Clonidine treatment of clozapine-induced hypersalivation. J Clin Psychopharmacol 1992;12:69–70.
96. Perry PJ, Alexander B, Liskow B. Psychotropic Drug Handbook, 6th ed. Cincinnati, Harvey Whitney Books, 1991:3–34, 247–248.
97. Mortola JF. The use of psychotropic drugs in pregnancy and lactation. Psychiatr Clin North Am 1989;12:69–87.
98. Karkji SD, Holden JM. Combined use of HPD and lithium. Psychiatr Ann 1990;20:154–161.
99. Callahan AM, Fava M, Rosenbaum JF. Drug interactions in psychopharmacology. Psychiatr Clin North Am 1993;16:647–671.
100. Knapp M, Kavanaugh S. Economic outcomes and costs in the treatment of schizophrenia. Clin Ther 1997;19:129–137.
101. Rosenheck R, Cramer J, Xu W, et al. A comparison of clozapine and haloperidol in hospitalized patients with refractory schizophrenia. N Engl J Med 1997;337:809–815.
102. Arosnon SM. Cost-effectiveness and quality of life in psychosis: The pharmacoeconomics of risperidone. Clin Ther 1997;19:139–147.
103. Jibson MD, Tandon R. Special report: A summary of research findings on the new antipsychotic drugs. Psychiatry Forum 1996; 16:i–vii.

65

DEPRESSIVE DISORDERS

Judith C. Kando, PharmD, BCPP, Barbara G. Wells, PharmD, FASHP, FCCP, BCPP, and Peggy E. Hayes, PharmD

Mood disorders (affective disorders) are among the most common mental disorders encountered in clinical practice and are divided into bipolar disorders and depressive disorders. The essential feature of these disorders is a major disturbance in mood. Mood is defined as a pervasive and sustained emotion that, in the extreme, markedly affects the person's perception of the world and ability to adequately function in society. A mood disorder occurs when a mood disturbance is combined with certain associated symptoms that impair the person's ability to function for a specific duration of time. Bipolar disorders (discussed in Chap. 66) refer to patients who have episodes of mania and/or hypomania usually alternating with episodes of depression.[1]

Patients with depressive disorders do not have episodes of mania or hypomania. Historically, various names (or classifications) have been used to describe depressive disorders, including reactive, unipolar, psychotic and neurotic, exogenous and endogenous, agitated and retarded, primary and secondary, and involutional melancholia.[2] Currently, the criteria listed in the *Diagnostic and Statistical Manual of Mental Disorders*, fourth edition (DSM-IV), published by the American Psychiatric Association in 1994, are used to diagnose individuals with depressive disorders.[1] The use of these standardized criteria has greatly improved clinicians' ability to correctly diagnose and appropriately treat depressive disorders. Major depressive disorder and dysthymic disorder are two types of depressive disorders listed in the DSM-IV. Dysthymic disorder is a chronic disturbance of mood involving depressed mood combined with at least two other symptoms such as appetite or sleep disturbance, low energy, low self-esteem, hopelessness, poor concentration, and indecisiveness. Also, the patient has experienced a depressed mood more days than not, for at least 2 years.[2] However, these symptoms are not of sufficient severity or duration to meet the specified criteria for major depression. This chapter focuses exclusively on the diagnosis and treatment of major depressive disorder.

Major depressive disorder is a common health problems of patients treated in primary care settings. Depression is associated with a high level of functional disability and increased use of outpatient medical services.[3,4] A 2-year follow-up study concluded that depressed patients have substantial and long-lasting impairments in social and physical functioning that equals or exceeds those of patients with chronic medical conditions.[5]

The most frequent complication of depression is suicide. Approximately 15% of patients with unrecognized or inadequately treated depression commit suicide; this is approximately 30 times the rate of occurrence in nondepressed patients.[2,6] Although adequate treatment reduces the risk of suicide and improves functioning and well-being, studies conducted in primary care settings reported that even when depression is accurately diagnosed, few patients receive an adequate dose and duration of antidepressant treatment. The gap between research findings and clinical practice is especially wide in the management of depression.[3]

The introduction of effective antidepressant drugs with distinctly different adverse event profiles and relatively greater safety in an overdose situation has enabled more patients to be successfully managed.

EPIDEMIOLOGY

The true prevalence of depressive disorders in the United States is unknown. Only 31% of depressed adults actually seek treatment.[7] The National Comorbidity Survey (NCS) reported that 17% of the population studied had a history of major depressive disorder in their lifetime, and more than 10% had an episode within the past 12 months.[8] Evidence supports increasing rates and a decreasing age of onset of depression in persons born after World War II.[9]

Depression is two to three times as frequent in females as males.[1,8,9] Although depression can occur at any age, adults 25 to 44 years of age experience the highest rates of major depression.[8,9] Depressive symptoms occur in about 15% of those 65 years and older living in the community[7,8] and the prevalence of major depression is approximately 10% to 20% among elderly persons in institutions.[6] Depressive disorders are quite common during adolescence. Rates of alcoholism, substance abuse, suicide attempts, and deaths have increased in these young patients.[9] Patients with depressive disorders frequently develop another psychiatric illness (comorbidity), especially anxiety disorders and alcoholism.[2,8]

Depressive disorders and suicide tend to cluster in families, and first-degree relatives of patients with depression are one and a half to three times more likely to develop depression than normal controls.[1,9,10] Approximately 8% to 18% of patients with major depression have at least one first-degree relative (father, mother, brother, or sister) with a history of depression compared to 5.6% of the first-degree relatives of a normal control group.[10,11] Twin studies of major depression estimate the concordance rate for monozygotic (identical) twins to be 54% to 65%, and the rate for dizygotic (fraternal) twins to be 14% to 24%.[11]

ETIOLOGY

The etiology of depressive disorders is too complex to be totally explained by a single social, developmental, or biologic theory. Several factors appear to work together to cause or precipitate depressive disorders. The symptoms reported by patients with major depression consistently reflect changes in brain monoamine neurotransmitters, specifically norepinephrine (NE), serotonin (5-HT), and dopamine (DA).[12]

Although life is filled with unexpected events that cause pain (death of a loved one, loss of a job, major illness), obviously not everyone becomes depressed. Most individuals adjust to life's challenges and suffer only mild, transient dysphoric feelings. However, other individuals exposed to these psychosocial stressors experience a major depressive episode. The initial episodes of depression, in contrast to later episodes, are more likely to be associated with stressful life events.[12] Certain factors (stressful events, medical illness, monoamine-depleting drugs) may place predisposed individuals, especially those with a family or personal history of depression, at high risk for developing a major depressive episode.[12]

PATHOPHYSIOLOGY

BIOGENIC AMINE HYPOTHESIS

Most effective antidepressants increase the availability of certain monoamines at selected brain synapses.[13] Reserpine, an antihypertensive drug known to deplete neuronal storage granules of NE, 5-HT, and DA, produces clinically significant depression in 15% or more of patients.[14] These observations lead to an early hypothesis that depression was caused by inadequate monoamine neurotransmission, most notably NE.[15] However, this early hypothesis failed to explain the actual cause of depression. Although reuptake blockade or monoamine oxidase (MAO) inhibition occurs immediately upon administration of an antidepressant, the clinical effects are generally not observed until after 4 weeks of dosing.[16]

PERMISSIVE HYPOTHESIS

In the early 1970s, Prange and colleagues put forth the "permissive hypothesis of affective illness" regarding the possible role of both NE and 5-HT in causing depression.[17] The theory states that decreased 5-HT levels permit the expression of the affective state, but the type is governed by the level of NE. Decreased NE levels cause depression, and elevated NE levels cause mania. According to this hypothesis, correcting the deficiency in 5-HT activity corrects the affective disease.

THEORIES OF POSTSYNAPTIC CHANGES IN RECEPTOR SENSITIVITY

A more perplexing aspect of the observed effects of antidepressants is the discrepancy between monoamine reuptake blockade (immediate) and any measurable improvement in depressive symptomatology (delayed). Accordingly, theories that focus on adaptive (or chronic) changes in amine receptor systems compared with acute changes have emerged.

In the mid-1970s, it was recognized that chronic, but not acute, administration of antidepressants to animals caused desensitization of NE-stimulated cyclic AMP synthesis. In fact, for most antidepressants, down-regulation of β-adrenergic receptors accompanies this desensitization.[18]

Studies of many antidepressants have demonstrated that either desensitization or down-regulation of NE receptors corresponds to a clinically relevant time course for antidepressant effects.[19] Other studies have revealed down-regulation of 5-HT_2 receptors following chronic administration of antidepressants.[19,20] Thus, a theory based on postsynaptic changes in receptor sensitivity provides a cogent explanation of the delayed onset of activity of antidepressant drugs.[19]

DYSREGULATION HYPOTHESIS

The dysregulation hypothesis incorporates the diversity of antidepressant activity with the adaptive changes occurring in receptor sensitization over several weeks.[21] In this theory, emphasis is placed on a failure of homeostatic regulation of neurotransmitter systems, rather than on absolute increases or decreases in their activities.[21,22] According to this hypothesis, effective antidepressant agents restore efficient regulation to the dysregulated neurotransmitter system.[21,22]

5-HT/NE LINK HYPOTHESIS

It is apparent that no single neurotransmitter theory of depression is adequate. The 5-HT/NE link hypothesis maintains that both the serotonergic and noradrenergic systems need to be functional for an atidepressant effect to be exerted.[23] The 5-HT/NE link hypothesis is also consistent with the rationale of the postsynaptic alteration theory of depression, which emphasizes the importance of β-adrenergic receptor down-regulation for achieving an antidepressant effect.[19] Again, it has been proposed that both NE and 5-HT are necessary for homologous desensitization of central β-adrenergic receptors by antidepressants.[23,24]

ROLE OF DOPAMINE IN DEPRESSION

Traditional explanations of the biologic basis of depressive disorders have focused largely on NE and 5-HT; however, most of the evidence that coalesced into the biogenic amine hypothesis of depression does not clearly distinguish between NE and DA.[25]

Several reviews suggest that elevation of DA neurotransmission in the nucleus accumbens may represent a final common pathway for at least part of the mechanism of action of antidepressant medications.[26,27] The mechanisms by which antidepressant drugs sensitize dopamine transmission remain unclear, but may be indirectly mediated by primary actions at NE or 5-HT terminals.

The evidence supporting a dopaminergic mechanism of antidepressant action is entirely preclinical, and clinical studies evaluating the role of DA mechanisms in the action of classical antidepressants have not been conducted.[25]

The complexity of the interaction between 5-HT, NE, and possibly DA is gaining greater appreciation, but a more in-depth understanding of the precise mechanism is needed.

BIOLOGIC MARKERS

Investigators continue to search for biologic markers to assist in the diagnosis and treatment of depressed patients. Although no biologic marker has been discovered, several interesting biologic abnormalities are present in many depressed patients. Approximately 45% to 60% of patients with major depression have a neuroendocrine abnormality, including hypersecretion of cortisol, lack of cortisol suppression after dexamethasone administration (i.e., a positive dexamethasome suppression test [DST]), or an abnormal or diminished thyroid-stimulating hormone (TSH) response to the administration of thyrotropin-releasing hormone (TRH).[12] The DST is the most specific measure of hypothalamic–pituitary–adrenal (HPA) axis overactivity. Dexamethasone administration suppresses adrenal corticosteroid production in normal subjects for 24 hours. Failure of dexamethasone to suppress plasma cortisol concentrations indicates overactivity or dysregulation of the HPA axis, and in depressed patients this also reflects an increased vulnerability to suicide.[12] The DST is reserved for patients whose diagnosis is in doubt, and then only to confirm clinical impressions. Unfortunately, the high rate of false positives and false negatives limits the usefulness in testing for these markers.

Sleep studies in patients with major depression have identified several abnormalities that become more pronounced with advancing age. The onset of rapid eye movement (REM) sleep occurs sooner in depressed patients (decreased REM latency) than in the normal population. There may also be a decrease in slow-wave sleep, a shift of REM sleep activity to the first half of the night, increased disruption of sleep, and early morning awakening.[28] Sleep abnormalities occur in other psychiatric disorders and are not diagnostic for major depression.

CLINICAL PRESENTATION

When a patient presents with depressive symptoms, it is necessary to investigate the possibility of a medical, psychiatric, and/or drug-induced cause (Table 65–1).[29] Up to 25% of patients with chronic medical conditions (e.g., diabetes, myocardial infarction, carcinomas, stroke) will develop a major depressive episode during the course of their medical condition, and the depression is often not accurately diagnosed, especially in the elderly.[1,6]

All depressed patients, especially the elderly, should have a complete physical examination, mental status examination, and basic laboratory workup, including a complete blood count with differential, thyroid function tests, and electrolyte determinations to identify any potential medical problems. A complete medication review should be performed, because many drugs (e.g., propranolol)[30] may precipitate or worsen a depressive episode (Table 65–1).

Major depressive disorder is characterized by one or more episodes of major depression. A major depressive episode is characterized by five or more of the symptoms described in Table 65–2. At least one of the symptoms is depressed mood (often an irritable mood in children or adolescents) or loss of interest or pleasure in nearly all activities.[1] The five symptoms must have been present nearly every day for at least 2 weeks and must represent a change from previous functioning. The clinician must consider presenting

TABLE 65–1. Common Medical Disorders, Psychiatric Disorders, and Drug Therapy Associated With Depression

Medical Disorders	Metabolic disorders	Anxiety disorders
Endocrine diseases	Electrolyte imbalance	Eating disorders
Hyperthyroidism	Hypokalemia	Schizophrenia
Hypothyroidism	Hyponatremia	**Drug Therapy**
Addison's disease	Hepatic encephalopathy	Alcohol
Cushing's disease	Cardiovascular disease	Antihypertensives
Deficiency states	Cerebral arteriosclerosis	Reserpine
Pernicious anemia	Congestive heart failure	Methyldopa
Wernicke's encephalopathy	Myocardial infarction	Propranolol hydrochloride
Severe anemia	Neurologic disorders	Guanethidine sulfate
Infections	Alzheimer's disease	Hydralazine hydrochloride
Encephalitis	Huntington's disease	Clonidine hydrochloride
Influenza	Multiple sclerosis	Diuretics
Mononucleosis	Parkinson's disease	**Hormonal Therapy**
Tuberculosis	Poststroke	Oral contraceptives
AIDS	Malignant disease	Steroids/ACTH
Collagen disorder	**Psychiatric Disorders**	
Systemic lupus erythematosus	Alcoholism	

Compiled from Ref. 29.

TABLE 65–2. DSM-IV Criteria for Major Depressive Episode

A. Five (or more) of the following symptoms have been present during the same 2-week period and represent a change from previous functioning; at least one of the symptoms is either (1) depressed mood or (2) loss of interest or pleasure.
   1. Depressed mood most of the day, nearly every day.
   2. Markedly diminished interest or pleasure in all, or almost all, activities.
   3. Significant weight loss (not dieting) or weight gain, or decrease or increase in appetite nearly every day.
   4. Insomnia or hypersomnia nearly every day.
   5. Psychomotor agitation or retardation nearly every day (observable).
   6. Fatigue or loss of energy nearly every day.
   7. Feelings of worthlessness or excessive or inappropriate guilt (may be delusional) nearly every day.
   8. Diminished ability to think or concentrate, or indecisiveness.
   9. Recurrent thoughts of death, recurrent suicidal ideation without a specific plan, or a suicide attempt or a specific suicide plan.

B. The symptoms cause clinically significant distress or impairment in social, occupational, or other important areas of functioning.

C. The symptoms are not due to the direct physiologic effects of a substance or a general medical condition (e.g., hypothyroidism).

Modified and reprinted with permission from the Diagnostic and Statistical Manual of Mental Disorders, *4th ed. Washington, DC, American Psychiatric Association, 1994.*

symptoms, their duration, and the patient's current level of social, occupational, or other important areas of functioning. Significant stressors or life events may trigger depression in some individuals, but not others; and there may be an important precipitant at the beginning of the disorder.[1,2]

EMOTIONAL SYMPTOMS

Major depressive episode is characterized by a persistent, diminished ability to experience pleasure. A loss of interest and pleasure in usual activities, hobbies, or work is common. Patients appear sad or depressed, and they are often pessimistic and believe that nothing will help them feel better. Patients often weep or report crying spells. The presence of intense hopelessness and complete or near total loss of interest and pleasure in usual activities may identify patients at risk for suicide.[31] Anxiety symptoms are present in almost 90% of depressed outpatients.

Patients often have guilt feelings that are unrealistic, and these may reach delusional proportions. Patients may feel that they deserve punishment and may view their present illness as a punishment. A depressed patient may hear voices (auditory hallucinations) saying that he or she is a bad person and that he or she should commit suicide. Depression with psychotic features usually requires hospitalization, especially if the patient becomes a danger to self or others.

PHYSICAL SYMPTOMS

Physical symptoms often motivate patients, especially the elderly ones, to seek medical attention. Chronic fatigue is a common complaint, with a decreased ability to perform normal, daily tasks. Fatigue often appears worse in the morning and does not improve with rest. Complaints of pain, especially headache, often accompany fatigue.

Sleep disturbances generally present as frequent early morning awakening (terminal insomnia), with difficulty returning to sleep. This may coexist with difficulty falling asleep (initial insomnia) and frequent nighttime awakening. Less frequently, depressed patients complain of increased sleep (hypersomnia), although they experience daytime exhaustion or fatigue.

Appetite disturbances, including complaints of decreased appetite, often result in substantial weight loss, especially in the elderly.[6] Some patients lose two or more pounds per week without dieting. Other patients, especially in the ambulatory setting, may overeat and gain weight, although they may not actually enjoy eating. They may crave specific foods.

Some patients exhibit gastrointestinal complaints, others cardiovascular complaints, especially heart palpitations. Patients frequently present with a loss of sexual interest or libido.

INTELLECTUAL OR COGNITIVE SYMPTOMS

Intellectual or cognitive symptoms include a decreased ability to concentrate, slowed thinking, and a poor memory for recent events. Patients may appear confused and indecisive. Depression should be considered when cognitive symptoms are present in the elderly.[6]

PSYCHOMOTOR DISTURBANCES

Patients may appear noticeably slowed or retarded in physical movements, thought processes, and speech (psychomotor retardation). Conversely, depression may be accompanied by psychomotor agitation manifesting as purposeless, restless motion (pacing, wringing of hands, outbursts of shouting).

SUICIDE RISK EVALUATION AND MANAGEMENT

Depressed patients should be assessed for suicidal thoughts. Widely held myths regarding suicide include the belief that people are more likely to commit suicide if they are asked about it; that people who attempt or talk about suicide are just looking for attention and are not serious; that suicidal people are crazy; and that most suicides are caused by a sudden traumatic event.

Factors that increase the risk for suicide include increasing age, being widowed, being unmarried, being unemployed, living alone, a history of a previous psychiatric admission, substance abuse, depression, feelings of hopelessness, prior attempts, family history of suicide, anniversary of a loss, presence of a serious medical problem, lack of a social support system, and refusal to seek help.[31] The presence of a very detailed plan with the intention and ability to carry it out indicates strong intent and a high risk of suicide. Although women attempt suicide two to three times more often than men, men succeed about three times more frequently. Completed suicide rates in 80- to 84-year-olds are more than twice the ratio in the general population (26.5 versus 12.4/100,000).[32]

To assess the severity of suicidal thoughts, the clinician must be sensitive to hints of suicidal ideation including a change in personality, a sudden decision to make a will or give away possessions, and any recent purchase of a gun or obtaining (or hoarding) a large supply of medications or other potentially toxic substances. It is not possible to predict accurately whether or when a depressed person will attempt suicide.

When suicidal intent is suspected, it is important to ask, "Are you thinking about harming or killing yourself?" If the risk is significant, the patient must be referred to a health care professional, and a family member must be contacted.

▶ TREATMENT: Depressive Disorders

DESIRED OUTCOME

The goals of treatment of the acute depressive episode are to reduce the symptoms of depression and facilitate the patient's return to a premorbid level (before the onset of the illness) of functioning. Whether or not to hospitalize the patient is the first decision in the treatment plan. This decision is made in consideration of the patient's risk of suicide, physical state of health, social support system, and the presence of a psychotic and/or catatonic depression.

GENERAL APPROACH TO TREATMENT

Studies comparing the efficacy of antidepressants have found that antidepressants are of equivalent efficacy in groups of patients when administered in comparable doses. Because one cannot predict which antidepressant will be the most effective in an individual patient, the initial choice is made empirically. Factors that often influence the choice of an antidepressant include the patient's past history of response, pharmacogenetics (the history of familial antidepressant response), the subtype of depression, the patient's concurrent medical history, the potential for drug–drug interactions, the adverse events profile of the various antidepressants, and drug cost.

Although the pathophysiology of major depression remains elusive, the clinician can now select from multiple drug therapies with different mechanisms of action.[33] Failure to respond to one antidepressant class does not predict a failed response to another drug class.

Approximately 65% to 70% of patients with varying types of depression improve with drug therapy, compared to 30% to 40% who improve with placebo. Melancholic depression appears to respond well to tricyclic antidepressants (TCAs), selective serotonin reuptake inhibitors (SSRIs), and electroconvulsive therapy (ECT).[33] Melancholic depression is characteized by a nearly complete absence of capacity for pleasure, diurnal mood swings (worse in the morning), early morning awakening, psychomotor disturbances, excessive guilt, and weight loss. A preferential response to monoamine oxidase inhibitors (MAOIs) has been reported in patients with atypical depression.[34] In atypical depression, two or more of the following are present: (1) weight gain or increase in appetite, (2) hypersomnia, (3) heavy feelings in arms or legs, and (4) interpersonal rejection sensitivity. Psychotically depressed individuals generally require either ECT or combination therapy with an antidepressant plus an antipsychotic agent.[35]

NONPHARMACOLOGIC THERAPY

In addition to pharmacological interventions, psychotherapy should be employed whenever the patient is able and willing to participate. Psychotherapy alone is not recommended for the acute treatment of patients with severe and/or psychotic major depressive disorder. However, if the depressive episode is mild to moderate in severity, psychotherapy may be the first-line therapy.[36] The effects of psychotherapy and antidepressant medications is considered to be additive. Combined treatment may be advantageous for patients with partial responses to either treatment alone and for those with a chronic course of illness. However, for uncomplicated, nonchronic major depressive disorder, combined treatment may provide no unique advantage.[36] Although not well studied, cognitive therapy, behavioral therapy, and interpersonal psychotherapy appear to be equal in efficacy.[36] Maintenance psychotherapy as the sole treatment to prevent recurrence is generally not recommended unless the patient needs to avoid medication. If there was a full response to combined medication and psychotherapy in the acute or continuation phases of treatment, medication may be all that is necessary in the maintenance phase of treatment to prevent a recurrence.[36]

Other means of treating depression include ECT and light therapy. ECT is a safe and very effective treatment for certain severe mental illnesses. Patients are candidates for ECT when a rapid response is needed, risks of other treatments outweigh potential benefits, there is a history of poor response to drugs and a good response to ECT, and the patient expresses a preference for ECT.[37] ECT is effective for all subtypes of major depressive disorder as well as other selected psychiatric illnesses.

A course of ECT generally consists of 6 to 12 treatments administered either unilaterally or bilaterally two to three times weekly. A rapid therapeutic response (10 to 14 days) has been reported. Although there are no absolute contraindications to the use of ECT, several conditions are associated with increased risk. These include increased intracranial pressure, cerebral lesions, recent myocardial infarction, recent intracerebral hemorrhage, bleeding, or otherwise unstable vascular condition. The use of an anesthetic as well as a nondepolarizing neuromuscular blocking agent decreases the morbidity associated with ECT.[37]

Adverse effects of ECT include cognitive dysfunction, cardiovascular dysfunction, prolonged apnea, treatment-emergent mania, headache, nausea, and muscle aches. Cognitive changes associated with ECT include confusion immediately after the seizure and retrograde and anterograde memory disturbance. Most cognitive disturbances are transient, but some patients may report permanent loss of memory of some events occurring over the months before, after, or during treatment.[37]

Relapse rates during the year immediately following ECT are high unless maintenance antidepressant medication is prescribed. ECT guidelines developed by the American Psychiatric Association include indications and contraindications for the appropriate use of ECT, procedures for obtaining informed consent, and issues in administering ECT.[37]

Some individuals experience depressive episodes during a particular season. This is referred to as seasonal affective disorder (SAD) and most commonly occurs in the winter, with remission in spring or summer.[38] Reduced environmental light may be the main precipitating factor of winter depression.[38] It has been theorized that there is a disturbance of the circadian rhythm caused by desynchronization between the solar clock and the human biologic clock during short photoperiods.[39] Bright light therapy is used to resynchronize the disturbed rhythm.[39] The patient looks into a light box in the morning or evening for approximately 2 hours.[40] Some individuals will require antidepressant therapy in addition to light therapy or antidepressants for nonseasonal episodes of major depression.

The light therapy is generally well tolerated with minor visual complaints being reported most frequently.[41] Consequently, anyone undergoing light therapy should receive baseline and periodic eye examinations.

PHARMACOLOGIC THERAPY

Antidepressants can be classified in several ways. One approach is by chemical structure, and another is by the presumed mechanism of antidepressant activity (Table 65–3). Although the link between the presumed mechanism of drug action and antidepressant response is tenuous, this classification has the advantage of being based on established pharmacology and clearly explains some of the adverse effects of the antidepressants. The knowledgeable clinician can use these facts to tailor treatment to individual patient needs and thereby optimize treatment outcome. Currently available antidepressants, their manufacturers, and initial dosages are shown in Table 65–4.

MIXED SEROTONIN AND NOREPINEPHRINE REUPTAKE INHIBITORS

Among the TCAs, amitriptyline and imipramine are the most extensively studied. Studies comparing the secondary amine TCAs (desipramine and nortriptyline) to the tertiary amine TCAs (amitriptyline and imipramine) found no clinically important difference in efficacy; however, the secondary amines were more potent on a milligram-to-milligram basis.[42]

The TCAs are effective in treating all depressive subtypes, especially the severe melancholic subtype of major depressive disorder. All TCAs potentiate the activity of NE and 5-HT by blocking their reuptake. However, the potency and selectivity of TCAs for the inhibition of NE and 5-HT vary greatly among these agents (Table 65–5). Because TCAs affect other receptor systems, anticholinergic, neurologic, and cardiovascular adverse events are frequently reported during TCA therapy.[21]

Venlafaxine, a structurally novel antidepressant, is a potent inhibitor of 5-HT and NE reuptake and a weak inhibitor of dopamine reuptake. Unlike the TCAs, it has virtually no affinity for muscarinic, histaminergic, and α_1-adrenergic receptors.[43]

TABLE 65–3. Classification of Antidepressant Pharmacotherapy by Presumed Mechanism of Action

Mixed 5-HT/NE reuptake inhibitors	TCAs, venlafaxine
SSRIs	Fluoxetine, paroxetine, sertraline, fluvoxamine, citalopram
Mixed serotonin effects	Trazodone, nefazodone
Mixed NE/DA reuptake inhibitors	Bupropion
Mixed serotonin/ norepinephrine effects	Mirtazapine
MAOIs	Phenelzine, tranylcypromine

Maprotiline and amoxapine are both inhibitors of NE reuptake, with less effect on 5-HT reuptake. Maprotiline is associated with a higher incidence of seizures than is imipramine or amitriptyline.[21] Amoxapine, while less sedating than some antidepressants, blocks cholinergic receptors, causing clinically significant anticholinergic effects.

SELECTIVE SEROTONIN REUPTAKE INHIBITORS

The impetus for the development of the SSRIs was the perceived need for antidepressants with an improved efficacy and adverse effects profile compared with the traditional TCAs. There is a substantial body of knowledge to indicate that the efficacy of SSRIs is superior to placebo and equal to the TCAs in treating patients with major depression.[33] Patients who fail to respond to a TCA often respond to an SSRI, and vice versa.

TRIAZOLOPYRIDINES

Trazodone and nefazodone have dual actions on serotonergic neurons, acting as both a 5-HT_2 antagonist and 5-HT reuptake inhibitor[44]; they also appear to enhance 5-HT_{1A}-mediated neurotransmission. These drugs have negligible affinity for cholinergic and histaminergic receptors. Nefazodone also has low affinity for α_1-adrenergic receptors. Similar to TCAs and SSRIs, the triazolopyridines are effective agents in treating major depression with no substantial evidence to support a unique spectrum of therapeutic activity.

AMINOKETONE

Bupropion, the only marketed aminoketone antidepressant, appears to have a unique mechanism of drug action.[45] It has no appreciable effect on the reuptake of 5-HT, and its most potent neurochemical action is blockade of DA reuptake.

MIXED SEROTONIN/NOREPINEPHRINE EFFECTS

Mirtazapine, a tetracyclic antidepressant agent, enhances central noradrenergic and serotonergic activity through the antagonism of central presynaptic α_2-adrenergic autoreceptors and heteroreceptors.[46]

MONOAMINE OXIDASE INHIBITORS

The MAOIs increase the concentrations of NE, 5-HT, and DA within the neuronal synapse, through inhibition of the MAO enzyme. Studies of several MAOIs have demonstrated that, similar to the TCAs, chronic therapy causes changes in receptor sensitivity (i.e., down-regulation of β-adrenergic, α-adrenergic, and serotonergic receptors).[47,48]

Clinical features that predict preferential response to MAOIs include mood reactivity, irritability, hypersomnia, hyperphagia, psychomotor agitation, and hypersensitivity to rejection,[34] the defining features of atypical depression.

The MAOIs currently marketed in the United States are nonselective inhibitors of MAO A and MAO B. Phenelzine and tranylcypromine inhibit both of these forms (isoenzymes) of MAO. Moclobemide, an antidepressant marketed in Europe, is a selective and reversible inhibitor of MAO A. Clinical trials of moclobemide conducted in Europe have reported efficacy equal to TCAs and superior to placebo.[49]

ADVERSE EFFECTS

Tricyclic Antidepressants and Other Heterocyclics

The most commonly reported adverse effects of antidepressant therapy are summarized in Table 65–5. The TCAs affect several neurotransmitters and produce a wide range of pharmacologic actions, sometimes causing many unwanted adverse effects. The

TABLE 65–4. Adult Dosages for Currently Available Antidepressant Medications[a]

Generic Name	Trade Name	Manufacturer	Suggested Therapeutic Plasma Concentration Range (ng/mL)	Initial Dose (mg/d)	Usual Dosage Range (mg/d)
Tricyclic Antidepressants					
Tertiary amines					
Amitriptyline	Elavil	Stuart	120–250[b]	50–75	100–300
	Endep	Roche			
	Generic	Various			
Clomipramine	Anafranil	Novartis		25	100–250
Doxepin	Adapin	Lotus Biochemical	110–250[b]	50–75	100–300
	Sinequan	Roerig			
	Generic	Various			
Imipramine	Tofranil	Novartis	200–300[b]	50–75	100–300
	Generic	Various			
Trimipramine	Surmontil	Wyeth-Ayerst		50–75	100–300
Secondary amines					
Desipramine	Norpramin	Marion Merrell Dow	125–300	50–75	100–300
	Generic	Various			
Nortriptyline	Pamelor	Novartis	50–150	25–50	50–150
	Generic	Various			
Protriptyline	Vivactil	Merck	70–240	10–20	15–60
Dibenzoxazepine					
Amoxapine	Asendin	Lederle	200–400[c]	50–150	100–400
	Generic	Various			
Tetracyclic					
Maprotiline	Ludiomil	Novartis	200–300[b]	50–75	100–225
	Generic	Various			
Mirtazapine	Remeron	Organon		15	15–45
Triazolopyridines					
Nefazodone	Serzone	Bristol-Myers Squibb		200	300–600
Trazodone	Desyrel	Apothecon		50–150	150–400
	Generic	Various			
Aminoketone					
Bupropion	Wellbutrin	Glaxo Wellcome	50–100	200	300–450
Monoamine Oxidase Inhibitors					
Phenelzine	Nardil	Parke-Davis		15	15–90
Tranlycypromine	Parnate	SmithKline Beecham		20	20–60
Selective Serotonin Reuptake Inhibitors					
Citalopram	Celexa	Forest		20	20–60
Fluoxetine	Prozac	Dista		10–20	10–80
Fluvoxamine	Luvox	Solvay		50	50–300
Paroxetine	Paxil	SmithKline Beecham		20	20–50
Sertraline	Zoloft	Roerig		50	100–200
Serotonin/Norepinephrine Reuptake Inhibitor					
Venlafaxine	Effexor	Wyeth-Ayerst		75	75–375

[a]Doses listed are total daily doses; elderly patients are usually treated with approximately one-half of the dose listed.
[b]Parent drug plus demethylated metabolite.
[c]Parent drug plus hydroxymetabolite.
Compiled from Refs. 16, 21, 47, 54, 56, and 79.

side effects most frequently associated with the TCAs (e.g., dry mouth, constipation, blurred vision, urinary retention, dizziness, tachycardia, memory impairment, and, at higher doses, delirium) may result from blockade of cholinergic receptors.[50] These adverse effects often impact patient tolerance and compliance, particularly in the elderly and those receiving long-term maintenance therapy. In general, anticholinergic effects and sedation are more severe during therapy with tertiary amine TCAs than with secondary amine TCAs.[50]

A common and potentially serious side effect of the TCAs is orthostatic hypotension, which has been attributed to the affinity of the TCAs for adrenergic receptors.[50] Orthostatic hypotension may be symptomatic, resulting in syncope, a particular concern when treating elderly patients due to the increased risk of falls and subsequent fractures.[51] Patients should be advised to rise slowly from a supine position, and prolonged bedrest should be avoided because of the deconditioning and volume-contracting effect. Tilting the head of the bed upward can be helpful for some patients. Adequate fluid intake should be maintained, and blood pressure should be monitored both supine and standing. Antigravity support garments can also be helpful. The risk of symptomatic orthostatic hypotension can be minimized by adequate ambulation and hydration along with proper drug selection, gradual dose increases, and patient education.[52]

TCAs also cause cardiac conduction delays and may even induce heart block in patients with a preexisting conduction

TABLE 65–5. Relative Potencies of Norepinephrine and Serotonin Reuptake Blockade and Side-Effect Profile of Antidepressant Drugs

	Reuptake Antagonism		Anticholinergic Effects	Sedation	Orthostatic Hypotension	Seizures	Conduction Abnormalities
	Norepinephrine	*Serotonin*					
Tricyclic Antidepressants							
Tertiary amines							
Amitriptyline	++	++++	++++	++++	+++	+++	+++
Clomipramine	++	+++	++++	++++	++	++++	+++
Doxepin	++	++	+++	++++	++	+++	++
Imipramine	+++	+++	+++	+++	++++	+++	+++
Trimipramine	++	++	++++	++++	+++	+++	+++
Secondary amine							
Desipramine	++++	+	++	++	++	++	++
Nortriptyline	+++	++	++	++	+	++	++
Protriptyline	+++	++	++	+	++	++	+++
Dibenzoxazepine							
Amoxapine[a]	+++	++	+++	++	++	+++	++
Tetracyclic							
Maprotiline	+++	+	+++	+++	++	++++	++
Mirtazapine	++++	++	+	++	++	++	+
Triazolopyridines							
Nefazodone	0	++	0	+++	+++	++	+
Trazodone	0	++	0	++++	+++	++	+
Aminoketone							
Bupropion	+	+	+	0	0	++++	+
Monoamine Oxidase Inhibitors							
Phenelzine	++	++	+	++	++	+	
Tranylcypromine	++	+	+	+	++	+	+
Selective Serotonin Reuptake Inhibitors							
Citalopram	0	++++	+	+	0	++	0
Fluoxetine	0	+++	0	0	0	++	0
Fluvoxamine	0	++++	0	0	0	++	0
Paroxetine	0	++++	+	+	0	++	0
Sertraline	0	++++	0	0	0	++	0
Serotonin/Norepinephrine Reuptake Inhibitor							
Venlafaxine	++++	++++	+	+	0	++	+

++++ = High; +++ = moderate; ++ = low; + = very low; 0 = none.
[a]Also blocks dopamine receptors.
Compiled from Refs. 16, 21, 47, 54, 55, 59 and 71.

disease. TCA overdose can produce severe arrhythmias.[50] Due to these potential cardiovascular effects, caution should be exercised when prescribing these agents to patients with clinically significant cardiac disease. Other adverse effects that lead to patient noncompliance include weight gain, excessive perspiration, and sexual dysfunction.[50]

Abrupt withdrawal of TCAs is associated with symptoms suggestive of cholinergic rebound (e.g., dizziness, nausea, diarrhea, insomnia, and restlessness), especially if the daily dose exceeds 300 mg.[53]

Clomipramine is a tertiary amine TCA with 5-HT reuptake inhibiting properties. Although it is a commonly used antidepressant in Europe, in the United States it is approved only for the treatment of obsessive–compulsive disorder (Chap. 68).

Amoxapine, the demethylated metabolite of loxapine, has intermediate sedative and anticholinergic potency.[54] Because of its postsynaptic receptor DA-blocking effects, its use may be associated with extrapyramidal side effects including pseudoparkinsonism, dystonia, akathisia, and tardive dyskinesia.[21] Amoxapine offers no advantage over standard TCAs or other antidepressants.

Maprotiline, a tetracyclic drug, blocks reuptake of NE with little effect on 5-HT. It has intermediate sedative and anticholinergic effects and may cause less orthostatic hypotension than imipramine; however, an exanthematous rash occurs in approximately 4% of patients.[21] Maprotiline is also associated with a higher incidence of seizures than standard TCAs and is contraindicated in patients with a history of a seizure disorder.

Venlafaxine

The most commonly reported adverse effects with venlafaxine include nausea, constipation, somnolence, dry mouth, dizziness, nervousness, sweating, asthenia, abnormal ejaculation/orgasm, and anorexia.[43] These side effects are believed to be dose related. Venlafaxine may cause a dose-related increase in diastolic blood pressure, and baseline blood pressure is not a useful predictor of the occurrence of this phenomenon. Blood pressure should be monitored regularly during venlafaxine therapy, and dosage reduction or discontinuation may be necessary if sustained hypertension occurs.[55]

Selective Serotonin Reuptake Inhibitors

The SSRIs include citalopram, sertraline, paroxetine, and fluvoxamine. Fluvoxamine has been approved by the Food and Drug Administration (FDA) for the treatment of OCD (Chap. 68). In general, the SSRIs have a low affinity for histamine, α_1-adrenergic, and muscarinic receptors. They produce fewer anticholinergic and cardiovascular adverse effects than the TCAs, and they are not associated with weight gain.[56] The main adverse effects, which are generally mild and short lived, are gastrointestinal symptoms (nausea, vomiting, diarrhea), sexual dysfunction in both males and females, headache, insomnia, and fatigue.[57]

Although the SSRIs as a group are known to improve the anxiety symptoms associated with depression, a few patients experience an increase in anxiety symptoms or agitation early in treatment. This occurrence may be reported most frequently with fluoxetine.[57]

Triazolopyridines

The adverse effect profile for trazodone and nefazodone is different from the other antidepressants. Trazodone and nefazodone have minimal anticholinergic effects or 5-HT agonist side effects, but can cause orthostatic hypotension. Sedation, cognitive slowing, and dizziness are the most frequent dose-limiting side effects associated with trazodone.[42] Common adverse effects associated with nefazodone use include light-headedness, dizziness, orthostatic hypotension, somnolence, dry mouth, nausea, and asthenia.[44]

A rare but potentially serious adverse effect of trazodone is priapism, which is reported to occur in approximately 1 in 6000 male patients. Some cases have required surgical intervention (1 in 23,000), and permanent impotence may result.[58] There have been no reports of priapism associated with nefazodone use.

Aminoketone

Adverse effects associated with bupropion include nausea, dizziness, tremor, insomnia, vomiting, constipation, dry mouth, and skin reactions. The occurrence of seizures in patients taking bupropion appears to be strongly associated with dose and may be increased by predisposing factors such as history of head trauma and CNS tumor. At daily doses of 450 mg (the ceiling dose) or less, the incidence of seizures is 0.4%.[59]

Mixed Serotonin/Norepinephrine Effects

The most common adverse effects reported in clinical trials in patients taking mirtazapine were somnolence, weight gain, dry mouth, and constipation. Both agranulocytosis and liver function test (LFT) elevations were noted in premarketing clinical trials. Two cases of agranulocytosis and one of neutropenia were reported. The incidence appears to be rare, and therefore, routine monitoring of blood indices is not recommended.[55] Additionally, LFT elevations were observed 1.4 times more frequently than with other antidepressants and 1.6 times higher than with placebo. No specific guidelines for LFT monitoring are recommended, but prescribers should consider obtaining baseline LFTs and monitoring these periodically throughout the course of therapy.

Monoamine Oxidase Inhibitors

The most common adverse effect of MAOIs is postural hypotension; this is more likely to occur with phenelzine than tranylcypromine.[47] Hypotensive reactions may be minimized through divided dosage scheduling. Anticholinergic side effects, especially dry mouth and constipation, are common, but are mild compared with those associated with the TCAs.

Phenelzine, the most frequently prescribed MAOI, has mild to moderate sedating effects. Tranylcypromine may exert a stimulating effect and insomnia may occur, so the last dose of the day should be administered in the early afternoon. Dose-related impotence and anorgasmia in males and orgasmic inhibition in females have been reported.[60,61] In addition, fever, myoclonic jerking, and brisk deep tendon reflexes may occur.[47,62,63]

Phenelzine, a hydrazine, has been associated with hepatocellular damage and weight gain. Tranylcypromine is a nonhydrazine MAOI and should be selected for patients with a history of liver disease if an MAOI is to be used.[47]

Hypertensive crisis, a potentially fatal but rare adverse reaction, occurs when MAOIs are taken concurrently with certain foods, especially those high in tyramine (Table 65–6) or drugs (Table 65–7). Ten milligrams of tyramine can cause a marked pressor effect, and 25 mg can result in serious hypertensive crisis.[64] These incidents may culminate in cerebrovascular accident and death.[47] Symptoms of hypertensive crisis include oc-

TABLE 65–6. Dietary Restrictions for Patients Taking Monoamine Oxidase Inhibitors

Aged cheeses[a]
Sour cream[b]
Yogurt[b]
Cottage cheese[b]
American cheese[b]
Mild Swiss cheese[b]
Wine[c] (especially Chianti and sherry)
Beer
Herring[a] (pickled, salted, dry)
Sardines
Snails
Anchovies
Canned, aged, or processed meats
Monosodium glutamate
Liver (chicken or beef, more than 2 days old)
Fermented foods
Canned figs
Raisins
Pods of broad beans[a] (fava beans)
Yeast extract[a] and other yeast products
Meat extract (Marmite)
Soy sauce
Chocolate[d]
Coffee[d]
Ripe avocado
Sauerkraut
Licorice

[a]Clearly warrants absolute prohibition (e.g., English Stilton, blue, Camembert, cheddar).
[b]Up to 2 oz daily is acceptable.
[c]3 oz white wine or a single cocktail is acceptable.
[d]Up to 2 oz daily is acceptable; larger amounts of decaffeinated coffee are acceptable.

TABLE 65–7. Medication Restrictions for Patients Taking Monoamine Oxidase Inhibitors

Amphetamines	Guanethidine
Appetite suppressants	Levodopa
Asthma inhalants	Local anesthetics containing sympathomimetic vasoconstrictors
Buspirone	Meperidine
Carbamazepine	Methyldopa
Cocaine	Methylphenidate
Cyclobenzaprine	Other antidepressants[a]
Decongestants (topical and systemic)	Other MAOIs
Dextromethorphan	Reserpine
Dopamine	Stimulants
Ephedrine	Sympathomimetics
Epinephrine	Tryptophan

[a]Tricyclic antidepressants may be used with caution by experienced clinicians in treatment-resistant populations.

cipital headache, stiff neck, nausea, vomiting, sweating, and sharply elevated blood pressure. The hypertensive crisis can be treated with 10 to 20 mg of nifedipine sublingually or swallowed or 5 mg of phentolamine IV.[65]

Education of patients taking MAOIs regarding dietary and medication restrictions is extremely important. Printed and verbal patient instructions should be provided. Patients unable to read and those with difficulty understanding or remembering medication instructions should not be given MAOIs unless they have competent caregivers. Patients should be instructed regarding the necessity of consulting a health care professional before taking over-the-counter medications. Patients should also be informed of the symptoms of hypertensive crisis and be advised about what to do should those symptoms occur.

PHARMACOKINETICS

The pharmacokinetics of the antidepressants are summarized in Table 65–8. In general, the TCAs are rapidly absorbed after oral administration. Bioavailability is low (30% to 70% for most TCAs) as a result of the first-pass effect, which shows great interindividual variation.[66]

The TCAs have a large volume of distribution and concentrate in brain and cardiac tissue in laboratory animals. Substantial amounts of TCAs pass into breast milk, and breast feeding is, therefore, inadvisable. They are bound extensively and strongly to plasma albumin, erythrocytes, α_1-acid glycoprotein, and lipoprotein.[66]

The major metabolic pathways are demethylation, aromatic and aliphatic hydroxylation, and glucuronide conjugation. Enterohepatic cycling has been described.[66] Metabolism of TCAs appears to be linear within the usual dosage range. The elimination half-lives of the TCAs vary greatly among individual patients, and this may be genetically determined.[66]

The diversity of the SSRIs is evident not only in their chemical structures but also in their pharmacokinetic profiles. Fluoxetine has an elimination half-life of 2 to 3 days (4 to 5 days with

TABLE 65–8. Pharmacokinetic Properties of Antidepressants

Generic Name	Elimination Half-life (h)[a]	Time of Peak Plasma Concentration (h)	Plasma Protein Binding (%)	% Bioavailable	Clinically Important Metabolites
Tricyclic Antidepressants					
Tertiary amines					
Amitriptyline	9–46	1–5	90–97	30–60	Nortriptyline; 10-Hydroxynortriptyline
Clomipramine	20–24	2–6	97	36–62	
Doxepin	8–36	1–4	68–82	13–45	Desmethyldoxepin
Imipramine	6–34	1.5–3	63–96	22–77	2-Hydroxyimipramine; desipramine; 2-hydroxydesipramine
Trimipramine	7–40	3	94–96	18–63	None
Secondary amines					
Desipramine	11–46	3–6	73–92	33–51	2-Hydroxydesipramine
Nortriptyline	16–88	3–12	87–95	46–70	10-Hydroxynortriptyline
Protriptyline	54–198	6–12	90–94	75–90	None
Dibenzoxazepine					
Amoxapine	8–30[b]	1–2	90	[c]	8-Hydroxyamoxapine
Tetracyclic					
Maprotiline	28–105	4–24	88	79–87	Desmethylmaprotiline
Mirtazapine	20–40	2	85	50	None known
Triazolopyridines					
Nefazodone	2–4	1	99	20	Meta-chlorophenylpiperazine; hydroxynefazodone; triazoledione
Trazodone	6–11	1–2	92	[c]	Meta-chlorophenylpiperazine
Aminoketone					
Bupropion	10–21	3	82–88	[c]	Bupropion threoamino alcohol; bupropion morpholinol
Monoamine Oxidase Inhibitors					
Phenelzine	1.5–4	[c]	[c]	[c]	
Tranylcypromine	1.5–3	[c]	[c]	[c]	
Selective Serotonin Reuptake Inhibitors					
Citalopram	33	2–4	80	≥80	Demethyl- and didemethylcitalopram
Fluoxetine	4–6 days[d]	4–8	94	95	Norfluoxetine
Fluvoxamine	15–26	2–8	77	53	None
Paroxetine	24–31	5–7	95		None
Sertraline	27	6–8	99	36[e]	*N*-Desmethylsertraline
Serotonin/Norepinephrine Reuptake Inhibitor					
Venlafaxine	5	2	27–30		O-Desmethylvenlafaxine

[a]Biologic half-life in slowest phase of elimination.
[b]Amoxapine, 8 hours; 8-hydroxyamoxapine, 30 hours.
[c]No data available.
[d]4–6 days with chronic dosing; norfluoxetine, 4–16 days.
[e]Increases 30% to 40% when taken with food.

multiple dosing). The single-dose half-life of norfluoxetine, the active metabolite, is 7 to 9 days. Paroxetine and sertraline have half-lives of approximately 24 hours. Unlike paroxetine, sertraline has an active metabolite, but the metabolite contributes minimally to the pharmacologic effects. Peak plasma concentrations of citalopram are observed within 2 to 4 hours after dosing, and the elimination half-life is about 30 hours. The SSRIs, with the exception of fluvoxamine and citalopram, are extensively bound to plasma proteins (94% to 99%). The SSRIs are extensively distributed to the tissues, and all, with the possible exception of citalopram, may have a nonlinear pattern of drug accumulation with long-term administration.[67]

Mirtazapine undergoes biotransformation via demethylation and hydroxylation followed by glucuronide conjugation.[46] The IA2 and the IID6 isoenzymes of the cytochrome P450 system may be responsible for the formation of the hydroxymetabolite, while the IIIA4 isoenzyme may be responsible for the formation of the *N*-desmethyl and the *N*-oxide metabolite.[46] Although these metabolites are theoretically active, they are present at such low plasma concentrations as to contribute little to the overall pharmacologic profile of mirtazapine.

Altered Pharmacokinetics

Factors reported to influence TCA plasma concentrations include disease states, genetics, age, cigarette smoking, and concurrent drug administration. Hepatic disease may reduce metabolic clearance of TCAs.[66] Renal failure does not alter nortriptyline metabolism, but the 10-hydroxy metabolite may accumulate, and protein binding may be diminished, with resultant enhanced sensitivity to the drug.[66] Clinicians should be alert to the possibility of higher-than-expected plasma concentrations of some TCAs in the elderly. Because dose-related kinetics cannot be ruled out in the elderly, dosage adjustments based on plasma concentration monitoring may be difficult.

In cirrhotics, the half-lives of fluoxetine and norfluoxetine increased to 7.6 and 12 days, respectively.[68] Patients with hepatic impairment had a twofold increase in plasma concentrations of paroxetine.[69] Similarly, in patients with mild stable cirrhosis, the half-life of sertraline was 2.5 times greater than in patients without liver disease.[70] Patients with renal impairment had a two- to fourfold increase in paroxetine plasma concentrations compared to normal volunteers.[69] Plasma concentrations of SSRIs in the elderly are reported to be greater than in younger patients.[69,70]

The AUC of nefazodone and hydroxynefazodone is 25% greater in cirrhotics than in normal volunteers.[71] Patients with cirrhosis accumulate metabolites of bupropion to concentrations two to three times those in normals.[59]

Plasma Concentration and Clinical Response

Studies in acutely depressed patients have demonstrated a correlation between antidepressant effect and plasma concentrations for some TCAs. The patient's clinical response, not plasma concentration, dictates dosage adjustments. Some patients with plasma concentrations outside the suggested therapeutic plasma concentration range respond, whereas others are nonresponsive regardless of their plasma concentration. See Table 65–4 for a listing of suggested therapeutic plasma concentration ranges.

For four TCAs (nortriptyline, desipramine, imipramine, and amitriptyline) there is more consistent evidence to support a minimal plasma concentration for clinical response. The best established therapeutic range is for nortriptyline.[36] Studies suggest a curvilinear plasma concentration–response relationship for nortriptyline, with a suggested therapeutic range of 50 to 150 ng/mL. Using logistic regression analysis of data from multiple published studies, it was found that within this range, 70% of patients with major depression responded versus only 29% of patients with plasma concentrations outside this range. Interestingly, the response rate was generally higher at the lower end of this range than at the upper limit.[72]

Using the same analysis, the therapeutic window for desipramine was 110 to 160 ng/mL. The remission rate was 50% within this range versus only 20% outside the range.[72] However, in the opinion of many clinicians, the data support a minimal threshold plasma concentration for clinical response, and a more commonly accepted range is 125 to 300 ng/mL.

Unfortunately, data for the tertiary amine TCAs are less convincing. Most investigators conclude that the desired plasma concentration range is defined by a plasma concentration below which patients are less likely to respond clinically and an upper plasma concentration limit that is associated with an increased risk for central nervous system and cardiac toxicity.[32]

Studies suggest that an optimal response in patients taking bupropion is most likely to occur at a plasma concentration of 50 to 100 ng/mL.[32] For the newer antidepressants, a correlation has not been established between plasma concentration and clinical response or adverse effects.

Plasma Concentration Monitoring

Because of interindividual variations in plasma concentrations achieved by a given dose, approximately 40% of patients receiving standard doses of TCAs may not obtain plasma concentrations within the desired therapeutic range.[73] Although plasma level monitoring is not routinely performed, some indications include inadequate response, relapse, serious or persistent adverse effects, use of higher than standard doses, suspected toxicity, elderly patients, pregnant patients, patients of African or Asian descent (because of slower metabolism), cardiac disease, suspected noncompliance, suspected pharmacokinetic drug interactions, and changing brands. Plasma concentration monitoring of TCAs when used appropriately can improve efficacy and minimize drug-related problems. Plasma concentrations should be obtained at steady state, usually after a minimum of 1 week at constant dosage. Sampling should be performed during the drug elimination phase, usually in the morning, 12 hours after the last dose. Samples collected in this manner are comparable for patients on once-daily, twice-daily, or three-times-daily regimens.[66]

DRUG INTERACTIONS

Tricyclic Antidepressants

Because the TCAs are metabolized in the liver through the cytochrome P450 system, they may interact with other drugs that modify hepatic enzyme activity or hepatic blood flow.[21] TCAs are also extensively protein bound, which can cause drug interactions through displacement from protein-binding sites. Many commonly used medications can interact when given concurrently with TCAs. Pharmacokinetic and pharmacodynamic drug interactions involving TCAs are shown in Tables 65–9 and 65–10, respectively.

TCAs may reverse the hypotensive effects of certain sympatholytic antihypertensives (guanethidine, methyldopa, clonidine) because of inhibition of presynaptic uptake of the antihypertensive or desensitization of the α_2-adrenergic receptor.[74] Similarly, because of inhibition of presynaptic uptake, TCAs may increase the vasopressor response to direct-acting sympathomimetics such as phenylephrine, epinephrine, and NE. The vasopressor response to indirect-acting sympathomimetics, such as ephedrine, is decreased.[74] Adverse effects of any TCA would be additive with those of other drugs with similar pharmacologic effects (anticholinergic, sedative, or hypotensive drugs).[74]

TABLE 65–9. Pharmacokinetic Drug Interactions Involving Tricyclic Antidepressants

Elevates Plasma Concentrations of TCAs
Cimetidine
Diltiazem
Ethanol, acute ingestion
SSRIs
Haloperidol
Labetalol
Methylphenidate
Oral contraceptives
Phenothiazines
Propoxyphene
Quinidine
Verapamil
Lowers Plasma Concentrations of TCAs
Barbiturates
Carbamazepine
Ethanol, chronic ingestion
Phenytoin
Elevates Plasma Concentrations of Interacting Drug
Hydantoins
Oral anticoagulants
Lowers Plasma Concentrations of Interacting Drug
Levodopa

Compiled from Ref. 74.

Although MAOIs and TCAs may be safely coadministered in refractory patients with apparent increased efficacy compared with monotherapy, severe reactions and fatalities have occurred. These reactions include hypertensive crises, hyperpyrexia, excitation, and convulsions, and they usually occur when TCAs are added to established MAOI therapy.[75]

Selective Serotonin Reuptake Inhibitors

Table 65–11 summarizes the drug interactions of non-TCA antidepressants. Drug–drug interactions may occur when an SSRI is coadministered with another drug metabolized through the cytochrome P450 system.[74] The long half-lives of fluoxetine (2 to 5 days in young healthy subjects) and of its active metabolite, norfluoxetine (7 to 9 days), ensure that, following discontinuation of the drug, these active compounds will persist in the body for weeks. The very slow elimination of fluoxetine makes it critical to ensure a 5-week washout after fluoxetine discontinuation before starting an MAOI.[76] Serious and potentially fatal reactions may occur when any SSRI is coadministered with an MAOI.[74]

Patients given concurrent fluoxetine and warfarin should be monitored for a possible increased risk of bleeding. Patients prescribed concomitant phenytoin or carbamazepine with fluoxetine may have increased anticonvulsant plasma concentrations and symptoms of toxicity.[74] Markedly increased plasma concentrations of TCAs with resultant symptoms of toxicity have been reported in patients taking fluoxetine.

Although no significant pharmacokinetic changes were present with the coadministration of warfarin, an increased bleeding time was noted.[77] Careful monitoring of prothrombin time is recommended when warfarin and paroxetine are administered concomitantly. No clinically significant drug interactions occurred during coadministration of paroxetine with haloperidol, amobarbital, oxazepam, or alcohol, indicating that paroxetine does not potentiate the CNS-depressant effects of such agents.[56]

Sertraline administration had no clinically significant effects on the pharmacokinetics and protein binding of diazepam or digoxin.[56] Bleeding time was increased with the concurrent administration of sertraline and warfarin, so the prothrombin time should be closely monitored.[56] Sertraline has been reported to increase significantly the plasma concentrations of secondary amine TCAs (e.g., desipramine and nortriptyline) and carbamazepine.

Preliminary studies suggest that citalopram may cause only moderate or no pharmacokinetic interactions when coadministered with TCAs. Coadministration of cimetidine reduced citalopram oral clearance by 29%. Addition of fluvoxamine caused a significant increase in plasma concentrations of citalopram.

Newer Agents

Venlafaxine and its active metabolite, O-desmethylvenlafaxine, are only 30% protein bound, permitting coadministration with other highly protein bound drugs.[55] Venlafaxine did not cause any significant change in the pharmacokinetics of ethanol, diazepam, or lithium.[55] Venlafaxine is metabolized to its active metabolite by the cytochrome P450 IID6 isoenzyme, which is the source of the genetic polymorphism present in the metabolism of many antidepressants. Therefore, the potential exists for interactions between venlafaxine and drugs that inhibit the P450 IID6 system.[55]

Although nefazodone is highly protein bound *in vitro*, nefazodone does not alter the *in vitro* protein binding of chlorpromazine, desipramine, diazepam, phenytoin, lidocaine, prazosin, propranolol, verapamil, or warfarin. However, it is unknown

TABLE 65–10. Pharmacodynamic Drug Interactions Involving Tricyclic Antidepressants

Interacting Drug	Effect
Alcohol	Increased CNS depressant effects
Amphetamines	Increased effect of amphetamines
Androgens	Delusions, hostility
Anticholinergic agents	Excessive anticholinergic effects
Bethanidine	Decreased antihypertensive efficacy
Clonidine	Decreased antihypertensive efficacy
Disulfiram	Acute organic brain syndrome
Estrogens	Increased or decreased antidepressant response; increased toxicity
Guanadrel	Decreased antihypertensive efficacy
Guanethidine	Decreased antihypertensive efficacy
Insulin	Increased hypoglycemic effects
Lithium	Possible additive lowering of seizure threshold
Methyldopa	Decreased antihypertensive efficacy; tachycardia; CNS stimulation
Monoamine oxidase inhibitors	Increased therapeutic and possibly toxic effects of both drugs; hypertensive crisis; delirium; seizures; hyperpyrexia; serotonin syndrome
Oral hypoglycemics	Increased hypoglycemic effects
Phenytoin	Possible lowering of seizure threshold and reduced antidepressant response
Sedatives	Increased CNS depressant effects
Sympathomimetics	Increased pharmacologic effects of direct-acting sympathomimetics; decreased effects of indirect-acting sympathomimetics
Thyroid hormones	Increased therapeutic and possibly toxic effects of both drugs; CNS stimulation; tachycardia

Compiled from Ref. 74.

whether or not displacement of either nefazodone or other drugs occurs *in vivo*.[71] Triazolobenzodiazepines, such as triazolam and alprazolam, interacted significantly with nefazodone. When triazolam is coadministered with nefazodone, a 75% reduction in the dose of triazolam is recommended. If alprazolam is coadministered with nefazodone, a 50% reduction in the initial dose of alprazolam is recommended.[71] Terfenadine and astemizole are both metabolized by the cytochrome P450 IIIA4 isoenzyme. Ketoconazole, erythromycin, and other inhibitors of IIIA4 can block the metabolism of terfenadine and astemizole, resulting in an increased plasma concentration of parent drug. Increased plasma concentrations of terfenadine and astemizole are associated with QT prolongation and with rare cases of serious cardiovascular adverse events, including death. Nefazodone is an *in vitro* inhibitor of IIIA4. Consequently, nefazodone should not be used concomitantly with either terfenadine or astemizole.[71]

The concurrent use of mirtazapine and the MAOIs should be avoided. In addition, 14 days should elapse between the discontinuation of an MAOI and the initiation of mirtazapine and vice versa. Mirtazapine is metabolized by CYP 1A2, IID6, and IIIA4. It is not yet known if medications that induce, inhibit, or serve as substrates for these isoenzymes will lead to significant drug interactions, as they have not yet been systematically studied.

SPECIAL POPULATIONS

Elderly Patients

Depression in the elderly is a major public health problem. Many elderly depressed patients are undiagnosed or inadequately treated. Diagnosis is often missed or mistaken for another disorder, such as dementia. In the elderly depressed patient, depressed mood—the typical signature symptom of depression—may be less prominent than the other depressive symptoms such as loss of appetite, cognitive impairment, sleeplessness, anergia, and loss of interest in and enjoyment of the normal pursuits of life.[79] Somatic complaints are quite frequent in elderly depressed patients.

Before initiating antidepressant treatment, the elderly patient should undergo a complete physical examination including cardiovascular, cerebrovascular, ophthalmologic, gastrointestinal, and urinary systems.

Elderly depressed patients are often over- or undertreated. Overtreatment often occurs when age-related pharmacokinetic and pharmacodynamic factors are overlooked. Undertreatment often results from an overly conservative approach as a result of the patient's advanced age or concurrent medical problems. Plasma concentration monitoring can be a useful tool for managing drug therapy in this patient population. A TCA would not be an appropriate first choice for a depressed patient with cardiac conduction delay. However, in the healthy elderly, cautious use of a secondary amine TCA (desipramine or nortriptyline) are indicated because of their defined therapeutic plasma concentration ranges, well-established efficacy, and well-known adverse effect profiles.[32]

The SSRIs are often selected as first-choice antidepressants, and they may enable the clinician to avoid some of the more problematic adverse effects commonly associated with the TCAs (sedative, anticholinergic, and cardiovascular side effects). Trazodone, nefazodone, and bupropion are also often chosen because of their milder anticholinergic and less frequent cardiovascular side effects.[32]

Although phenelzine has been used safely and effectively in well-selected patients, the MAOIs are usually not recommended for elderly patients because of hypotensive side effects and uncertainty of patient likelihood of adherence to dietary and medication restrictions.[32]

Pediatric Patients

Accumulating evidence indicates that childhood depression occurs quite commonly. Symptoms of depression in children and adults are similar.[80]

Data collected under controlled conditions supporting the efficacy of antidepressants in children and adolescents are sparse. In the double-blind study by Preskorn and associates,[81] imipramine was superior in efficacy to placebo only through the first 3 weeks of treatment.[81] Demonstration of efficacy in this population is confounded by the high placebo response rate. However, the TCAs and the SSRIs remain two viable treatment options. The SSRIs are better tolerated than the TCAs and relatively safer in an overdose. Toxicity in an overdose is important in the adolescent population, where suicide is the second leading cause of death.[32]

Antidepressant compounds are used to treat depressed children and adolescents, because no other definitive therapies are available. Plasma concentration monitoring of TCAs is important to ensure safety. As in the adult population, plasma concentrations above 450 ng/mL are associated with increased risk of serious adverse effects including delirium, seizures, delayed cardiac conduction, and sudden death.[32]

Several cases of sudden death have been reported in children and adolescents taking desipramine. A baseline ECG is recommended before initiating a TCA in children and adolescents, and many clinicians recommend an additional ECG when steady-state plasma concentrations are achieved.[32]

Although three antidepressants are FDA approved for use in children, none are approved for childhood depression. Imipramine is approved only for the treatment of enuresis, clomipramine for obsessive–compulsive disorder in children 12 years and older, and fluvoxamine for obsessive–compulsive disorder in children 8 years and older. Antidepressants should be initiated in this patient population at a dosage somewhat lower than in adults; however, adolescents usually require adult doses of TCAs, and 6 to 8 weeks may be required before an antidepressant response is evident. A typical regimen of imipramine is a starting dose of 1.5 mg/kg/d that is increased by 1.0 to 1.5 mg/kg every third day. The daily dose should not exceed 5 mg/kg.[82]

Pregnant and Lactating Patients

Approximately 10% of pregnant women develop serious depression. No major teratogenic effects have been identified with the TCAs. Although the MAOIs have demonstrated teratogenicity in animals, there are insufficient data in humans to permit firm conclusions. Similarly, there are inadequate data on the use of the newer antidepressants during pregnancy. As a general rule, nondrug approaches to the treatment of depression in the pregnant patient are preferred. The TCAs are usually given first preference, and nortriptyline or desipramine may be the treatment of choice because of the experience gained with these agents in pregnant patients and because therapeutic plasma concentrations have been established. If a TCA is withdrawn during pregnancy, it should be gradually tapered to avoid maternal or fetal withdrawal symptoms. If possible, drug tapering is usually begun 5 to 10 days before the estimated day of confinement.[32]

CLINICAL APPLICATION

A suggested algorithm for the management of depression is shown in Figure 65–1.

Dosing

Recommended initial doses and dosage ranges are shown in Table 65–4. The usual initial adult dose of most TCAs is 50 mg at bedtime, and the dose may be increased by 25 to 50 mg every third day. The recommended initial dose for the SSRIs is fluoxetine, 10 to 20 mg; paroxetine, 20 mg; sertraline, 50 mg; and citalopram, 20 mg.

TABLE 65–11. Drug Interactions of Non-TCA Antidepressants

Non-TCA	Interacting Drug/Drug Class	Effect
Dibenzoxazepine		
Amoxapine	Many of the drugs that interact with the TCAs	Similar response to that seen with TCA interaction
Tetracyclic		
Maprotiline	Many of the drugs that interact with the TCAs	Similar response to that seen with TCA Interaction
Mirtazapine	MAOIs	Theoretically central serotonin syndrome could occur
Triazolopyridines		
Nefazodone	Alprazolam	Increased plasma concentrations of alprazolam
	Astemizole	Theoretically increased plasma concentrations of astemizole with potentially serious cardiovascular adverse effects
	Digoxin	Increased C_{max}, C_{min}, and AUC of digoxin by 29%, 27%, and 15%, respectively
	Haloperidol	Decreased clearance of haloperidol by 35%
	MAOIs	Hypertensive crisis; serotonin syndrome; delirium; coma; seizures; hyperpyrexia
	Propranolol	Decreased C_{max} and AUC of propranolol; increased C_{max}, C_{min}, and AUC of m-CCP metabolite of nefazodone
	Terfenadine	Theoretically increased plasma concentrations of terfenadine with potentially serious cardiovascular adverse effects
	Triazolam	Increased plasma concentrations of triazolam; increased psychomotor impairment
Trazodone	CNS depressants	Increased CNS depression
	Digoxin	Increased serum concentrations of digoxin
	Ethanol	Additive impairment in motor skills
	Fluoxetine	Increased plasma concentrations of trazodone
	MAOIs	Theoretically central serotonin syndrome could occur
	Neuroleptics	Increased hypotension
	Phenytoin	Increased serum concentrations of phenytoin
	Tryptophan	Agitation, restlessness, poor concentration, nausea
	Warfarin	Decreased hypoprothrombinemic response
Aminoketone		
Bupropion	MAOIs	Increased toxicity of bupropion
	Medications that lower seizure threshold	Increased incidence of seizures
	Levodopa	Increased incidence of adverse experiences
Selective Serotonin Reuptake Inhibitors		
Citalopram	Cimetidine	Reduced oral clearance of citalopram
	Fluvoxamine	Increased plasma concentrations of citalopram
	TCAs	Possible increased AUC of TCA
Fluoxetine	Alprazolam	Increased plasma concentrations and half-life of alprazolam; increased psychomotor impairment
	Anticoagulants	Possible increased risk of bleeding
	β-Adrenergic blockers	Increased metoprolol serum concentrations and bradycardia; possible heart block
	Buspirone	Decreased therapeutic response to buspirone
	Carbamazepine	Increased plasma concentrations of carbamazepine with symptoms of carbamazepine toxicity
	Dextromethorphan	Visual hallucinations (one patient only)
	Haloperidol	Increased haloperidol concentrations and increased extrapyramidal side effects
	Lithium	Neurotoxicity—confusion, ataxia, dizziness, tremor, absence seizures
	MAOIs	Severe or fatal reactions—confusion, nausea, double vision, hypomania, hypertension, tremor, serotonin syndrome
	Phenytoin	Increased plasma concentrations of phenytoin and symptoms of phenytoin toxicity

Bupropion is usually initiated at 100 mg twice daily, and this dose may be increased to 100 mg three times daily after 3 days. Most patients will respond at 300 mg/d; however, an increase to 450 mg/d, given as 150 mg three times daily, may be considered in patients with no clinical response after several weeks of treatment at 300 mg/d. Additionally, a sustained-release formulation of bupropion is currently available and may be given as 200 mg twice a day in those individuals requiring higher dosages.

Typically, phenelzine is initiated at 15 mg in the morning and then increased by 15 mg every third day up to 60 mg daily. The dose should be given three times daily to minimize postural hypotension, with the last dose given in the early afternoon to lessen the likelihood of insomnia. Maintenance doses may be as low as 15 mg/d.

The usual starting dose of venlafaxine is 75 mg/d given in two or three divided doses, taken with food. Depending on tolerability,

TABLE 65–11. (Continued)

Non-TCA	Interacting Drug/Drug Class	Effect
	TCAs	Markedly increased TCA plasma concentration with symptoms of TCA toxicity
	Terfenadine	Arrhythmias, shortness of breath, and orthostasis
	Trazodone	Headaches, dizziness, sedation
	Tryptophan	Agitation, restlessness, poor concentration nausea
	Valproate	Increased valproate serum concentrations
Fluvoxamine	Alprazolam	Increased AUC of alprazolam by 96%, increased alprazolam half-life by 71%, and increased psychomotor impairment
	Astemizole	Theoretically increased plasma concentrations of astemizole with potentially serious cardiovascular effects
	β-Adrenergic blockers	Fivefold increase in propranolol serum concentrations; bradycardia and hypotension with combined fluvoxamine and metoprolol
	Carbamazepine	Possible carbamazepine toxicity, although a controlled study did not support this
	Clozapine	Increased clozapine serum concentrations and increased risk for seizures and orthostatic hypotension
	Diazepam	Decreased clearance of diazepam and its active metabolite
	Diltiazem	Bradycardia
	Haloperidol	Increased haloperidol plasma concentrations
	Lithium	Increased serotonergic effects; seizures, nausea, tremor
	MAOIs	Potential for hypertensive crisis, serotonin syndrome, seizures, delirium
	Methodone	Increased methodone plasma concentrations with symptoms of methodone toxicity
	TCAs	Increased TCA plasma concentration
	Terfenadine	Theoretically increased plasma concentrations of terfenadine with potentially serious cardiovascular effects
	Theophylline	Increased serum concentrations of theophylline with symptoms of theophylline toxicity
	Tryptophan	Increased serotonergic effects and severe vomiting
	Warfarin	Increased hypoprothrombinemic response to warfarin
Paroxetine	Cimetidine	Increased paroxetine serum concentrations
	Desipramine	Increased plasma concentrations and half-life of desipramine
	MAOIs	Potential for hypertensive crisis, serotonin syndrome, seizures, delirium
	Warfarin	Possible increased risk for bleeding
Sertraline	Carbamazepine	Increased plasma concentrations of carbamazepine
	Diazepam	Small decrease in clearance of diazepam
	MAOIs	Serotonin syndrome, myoclonus, violent shaking
	TCAs	Increased plasma concentrations of secondary amine TCAs (desipramine, nortriptyline)
	Tolbutamide	Decreased clearance of tolbutamide (16%)
	Warfarin	Increased protime
Serotonin/Norepinephrine Reuptake Inhibitor		
Venlafaxine	Cimetidine	Reduced clearance of venlafaxine by 43%; AUC and peak serum concentration of venlafaxine increased by 60%
	MAOIs	Potential for hypertensive crisis, serotonin syndrome, seizures, delirium

Compiled from Ref. 74.

the dose is then increased to 150 mg/d. If needed, the dose may be further increased to 225 mg/d. Certain patients, including severely depressed patients, may need a dose up to 375 mg/d.

The starting dose of nefazodone is 100 mg given twice daily. Dose increases should occur in increments of 100 mg/d, on a twice-daily schedule, at intervals of no less than 1 week, with the usual effective dose range between 300 and 600 mg/d.

The recommended starting dose of mirtazapine is 15 mg/d administered in a single dose at bedtime. The maximum dose recommended is 45 mg/d. Dosage increases should occur every 1 to 2 weeks as indicated.

Caution is urged when switching from one antidepressant to another. It is important to remember that 3 to 4 weeks is usually required before a mood-elevating response is seen. A 6-week trial at a maximum dosage is considered an adequate trial.[83] It is crucial to explain to the patient about the expected lag time before the onset of clinical response. Patients uneducated in this regard often fail to comply with their prescribed regimens.

In elderly patients, as a general rule, dosing is initiated at half the initial dose administered to younger adults, and the dose is increased at a slower rate. Thus, desipramine or nortriptyline may be initiated at 10 to 25 mg/d or fluoxetine at 10 to 20 mg/d

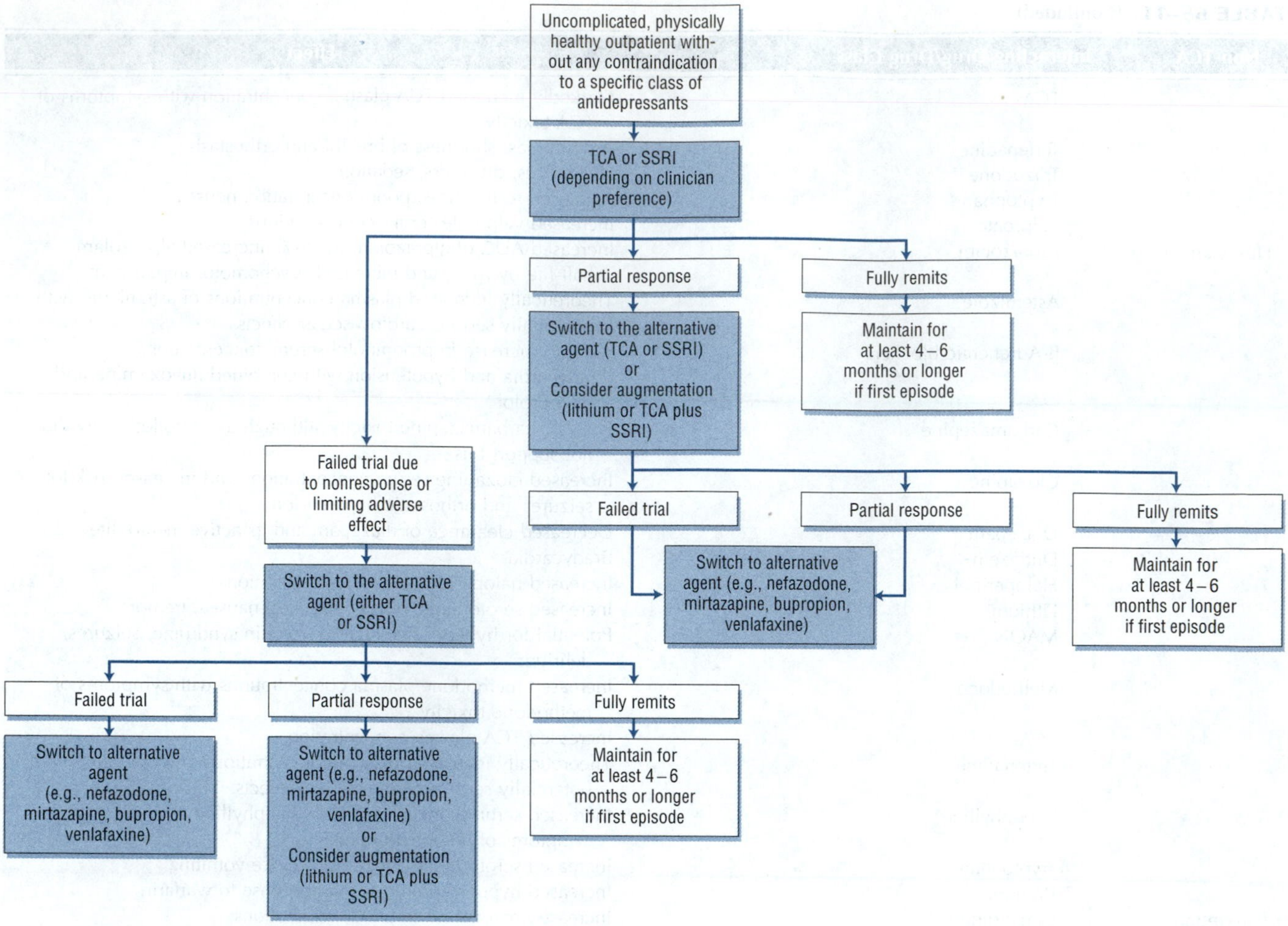

FIGURE 65–1. Algorithum for treatment of uncomplicated major depression.

or alternatively 20 mg every second or third day. Six to 12 weeks of treatment may be required to achieve the desired antidepressant response.[32] A remission is achieved when symptoms of depression are no longer present. A relapse is a return of symptoms within 6 months after remission. To prevent relapse, antidepressants should be continued at full therapeutic doses for 4 to 9 months after remission.[84] This period of treatment is termed *continuation therapy*. A recurrence is a separate episode of depression, which may occur after years of normal functioning. Five years after the first episode of depression, only 25% of patients had recovered and remained well.[85] The risk of recurrence increases as the number of past episodes and age at onset of the first episode increases.[86] The duration of antidepressant therapy depends on the risk of recurrence. Some investigators recommend life-long maintenance therapy for persons at greatest risk for recurrence (persons before 40 years of age and with 2 or more prior episodes and persons of any age with 3 or more prior episodes).[36]

Refractory Patients

The majority of "treatment-resistant" depressed patients are likely the result of inadequate therapy (relative resistance).[32] Issues to be addressed in assessing the patient who has not responded to treatment include the following:

1. Is the diagnosis correct?
2. Does the patient have a psychotic depression?
3. Has the patient received an adequate dose and adequate duration of treatment?
4. Do adverse effects preclude adequate dosing?
5. Has the patient been compliant with the prescribed regimen?
6. Was a stepwise approach to treatment used?
7. Was treatment outcome adequately measured?
8. Is there a coexisting or preexisting medical or psychiatric disorder?
9. Are there other factors that interfere with treatment?[32]

When a patient has failed to respond, nondrug modalities including environmental manipulation, family counseling, cognitive therapy, or interpersonal psychotherapy are often beneficial.[32]

Three primary pharmacologic approaches are used when dealing with treatment nonresponse. The current antidepressant may be stopped and a trial with an unrelated agent initiated. For example, the patient may be switched from a TCA to an SSRI or MAOI. Second, the current antidepressant can be augmented (potentiated) by the addition of lithium, liothyronine, or an anticonvulsant such as carbamazepine or valproic acid. A third approach to the treatment-resistant patient is to use concurrently two different classes of antidepressants (e.g., a TCA plus an MAOI).[32] As previously discussed, the combination of an SSRI and an MAOI should never be used.

There are accumulating data to support that 50% to 60% of previously treatment-resistant depressed patients respond to adequate doses of SSRIs.[32] When separate adequate trials of a heterocyclic antidepressant and an SSRI have failed, many clinicians would switch to an MAOI, especially for the patient with atypical features.[32]

Augmenting strategies, such as the addition of lithium to a TCA regimen, has been found to benefit many previously unresponsive patients, including those with psychotic depression. Lithium augmentation of fluoxetine benefitted five refractory patients. Several trials support that addition of liothyronine to a TCA regimen may induce antidepressant response.[32]

Concurrent use of a TCA and MAOI should be undertaken only by a prescriber experienced in the use of such combinations. When this is undertaken, the MAOI is slowly added to the TCA. Desipramine is not recommended to be used in combination with an MAOI. When the combination is discontinued, the MAOI should be stopped first.[32] Patients with psychotic depression usually require the combination of an antidepressant and an antipsychotic.[32]

The Agency for Health Care Policy and Research offers guidelines in managing patients who fail to respond. They advise that if patients fail to respond to medication after 6 weeks, the diagnosis should be reassessed. Comorbid medical or psychiatric conditions should be identified and treated, because they may complicate treatment. Before changing a patient's treatment, the clinician is advised to evaluate the adequacy of the medication dosage and compliance with the prescribed regimen. A combination of two drugs should not be used when one drug will suffice. Therefore, switching medications is often preferred over augmentation as an initial strategy.[36]

PHARMACOECONOMIC CONSIDERATIONS

Drug costs account for only about 1% to 2% of total costs of the treatment of depression, and about 10% to 12% of direct costs of depression.[87] Other costs associated with depression primarily include the indirect costs associated with lost earnings/productivity and premature death.[87] Therefore, when evaluating the cost of treating depression, more must be considered than the cost of medications. For example, if lack of response to an antidepressant leads to an overdose and subsequent treatment in the intensive care unit, the cost of treating depression will be dramatically increased. Likewise, if the patient suffers intolerable side effects, becomes noncompliant, and relapses requiring hospitalization, the cost of treating the depression becomes very expensive quite rapidly.

When SSRIs were initially introduced, many managed care organizations restricted these medications to those who had failed treatment with the TCAs or been unable to tolerate these agents, with the belief that the SSRIs represented a more expensive approach to the treatment of depression. Subsequent evaluations have shown that in fact the SSRIs represent a more economic approach to the treatment of depression when compared to TCAs when all treatment costs are considered.[88–91] The larger question seems to center around whether one SSRI is more economic than another. Initial findings suggest that fluoxetine may offer an overall cost advantage when compared to other SSRIs, but additional longer-term data are necessary before a final conclusion can be reached.[92]

A recent evaluation examined the cost effectiveness of fluoxetine and nefazodone compared with TCAs in managed care settings.[93] This evaluation found that both nefazodone and fluoxetine were cost effective when compared to imipramine, with nefazodone being slightly more cost effective than fluoxetine.[93] These data further support the notion that a lower cost of drug therapy does not necessarily translate into an overall lesser cost for the treatment of depression

Additional, longer-term studies in more diverse populations are necessary before judgments can be made regarding which of the newer antidepressant agents offers a cost advantage. It would be extremely useful if subpopulations and special populations (the elderly, those with comorbid substance abuse, those with comorbid anxiety disorders, children) were studied and cost-effective agents in these subpopulations were identified.

EVALUATION OF THERAPEUTIC OUTCOMES

Several monitoring parameters, in addition to plasma concentrations, are useful in managing patients. Patients must be monitored for adverse effects, such as sedation, anticholinergic effects, and sexual dysfunction, and for remission of previously documented target symptoms. The presence of side effects does not necessarily indicate adequate dosage. In addition, changes in social and occupational functioning should be assessed. When TCAs are given concurrently with adrenergic neuronal blocking antihypertensives (e.g., guanethidine, methyldopa, clonidine), blood pressure should be regularly monitored. Patients receiving venlafaxine should have their blood pressure monitored at regular intervals. Patients older than 40 should receive a pretreatment ECG before starting TCA therapy, and follow-up ECGs should be performed periodically. Patients should be monitored for the emergence of suicidal ideation after initiation of any antidepressant.

In addition to the clinical interview, psychometric rating instruments (e.g., patient-rated and clinician-rated scales) allow for rapid and reliable measurement of the nature and severity of depressive and associated symptoms (see Chap. 58). Interviewing a family member or friend (with the patient's permission) regarding symptoms and daily functioning can also assist in assessment of progress. It is recommended that patients be monitored closely for relapse or recurrence if the brand of antidepressant is changed. Patients should be monitored at more frequent intervals early in treatment. Monitoring is then continued at regular intervals throughout the continuation and maintenance phases of treatment. Regular monitoring should also be continued for several months after antidepressant therapy is discontinued.

CONCLUSIONS

Major depressive disorder remains one of the most commonly occurring mental illnesses in adults, and it is often undiagnosed and untreated. Pharmacologic intervention remains the cornerstone of antidepressant treatment. Antidepressant medications have a broad spectrum of neurochemical effects and influence a variety of receptors peripherally and centrally. Safe and effective use of antidepressants requires a thorough understanding of the pharmacology of these drugs and of the principles for monitoring efficacy and adverse effects. In addition, clinicians must have a thorough understanding of antidepressant drug interactions and other factors that may influence the pharmacokinetics of antidepressant drugs. Plasma concentration monitoring is unnecessary for most patients, but can improve the outcome in some situations. The search for more effective antidepressants with more favorable adverse effect profiles must continue.

▶ PRINCIPLES OF PHARMACOTHERAPY

- When evaluating a patient for the presence of depression, it is essential to rule out medical causes of depression and drug-induced depression.
- When determining if a patient has been nonresponsive to a particular pharmacotherapeutic intervention, it must be determined whether the patient has received an adequate dose for an adequate duration. If TCAs are being used, a serum level may be useful especially in special populations such as the elderly and those with concurrent medications that may alter the pharmacokinetic profile of the TCAs.
- If the patient exhibits a partial response to a pharmacotherapeutic agent, augmentation therapy should be considered before the trial is abandoned and the patient is treated with an alternative therapeutic agent.
- When counseling patients with depression who are receiving pharmacotherapeutic interventions, the patient should be informed that adverse effects may occur immediately, while a resolution of symptoms may take 2 to 4 weeks.
- The efficacy of the regimen should be based on the resolution of the target signs and symptoms identified before treatment. Rating scales should be used whenever possible to evaluate and document response.
- Family members and friends should be involved in the evaluation and assessment of response if possible, as the patient may not recognize the full extent of the signs and symptoms and their subsequent resolution.
- Whenever other medications are used concurrently with an antidepressant, evaluate the regimen for potential drug interactions, especially those involving the isoenzymes of the cytochrome P450 system.
- When evaluating response to an antidepressant agent, in addition to target signs and symptoms, consider quality of life issues, such as role, social functioning, and occupational functioning. In addition, the tolerability of the agent should be assessed, as the occurrence of side effects may lead to noncompliance.
- An assessment of compliance should be made at every visit. Remember that accurate capsule or tablet counts do not mean the patient has consumed the medication or consumed it in the manner prescribed.

REFERENCES

1. American Psychiatric Association. Diagnostic and Statistical Manual of Mental Disorders, 4th ed (DSM-IV). Washington, DC, American Psychiatric Association, 1994:317–391.
2. Montgomery SA. Efficacy in the long-term treatment of depression. J Clin Psychiatry 1996;57(suppl 2):24–30.
3. Katon W, Von Korff M, Lin E, et al. Collaborative management to achieve treatment guidelines: Impact on depression in primary care. JAMA 1995;273:1026–1031.
4. Wells KB, Stewart A, Hays RD, et al. The functioning and well-being of depressed patients. Results from the medical outcomes study. JAMA 1989;262:914–919.
5. Hays RD, Wells KB, Sherbourne CD, et al. Functioning and well-being outcomes in patients with depression compared with chronic general medical illnesses. Arch Gen Psychiatry 1995;52:11–19.
6. Lebowitz BD, Pearson JL, Schneider LS, et al Diagnosis and treatment of depression in late life. Consensus statement update. JAMA 1997;278:1186–1190.
7. Regier DA, Burke JD, Burke KC. Comorbidity of affective and anxiety disorders in NIMH epidemiologic catchment area program, In: Maser JD, Cloninger CR, eds. Comorbidity of Mood and Anxiety Disorders. Washington, DC, American Psychiatric Press, 1990:113–122.
8. Kessler RC, McGonagle KA, Zhao S, et al. Lifetime and 12-month prevalence of DSM-III-R psychiatric disorders in the United States. Results from the National Comorbidity Survey. Arch Gen Psychiatry 1994;51:8–19.
9. Klerman GL, Weissman MM. Increasing rates of depression. JAMA 1989;261:2229–2235.
10. Weissman MM, Gershon ES, Kidd KK, et al. Psychiatric disorders in the relatives of probands with affective disorder. Arch Gen Psychiatry 1984;41:13–21.
11. McGuffin P, Katz R. The genetics of depression and manic-depressive disorder. Br J Psychiatry 1989;155:294–304.
12. Gold PW, Goodwin FK, Chrousus GP. Clinical and biochemical manifestations of depression in relation to the neurobiology of stress, part I. N Engl J Med 1988;319:348–353.
13. Risch SC. Recent advances in depression research: From stress to molecular biology and brain imaging. J Clin Psychiatry 1997;58 (suppl 5):3–6.
14. Goodwin FK, Bunney WE. Depressions following reserpine: A reevaluation. Semin Psychiatry 1971;3:435–448.
15. Leonard BE. New approaches to the treatment of depression. J Clin Psychiatry 1996;57(suppl 4):26–33.
16. Baldessarini RJ. Drugs and the treatment of psychiatric disorders, II. Drugs used in the treatment of disorders of mood, in Gilman AG, Rall TW, et al, eds. Goodman and Gilman's The Pharmacologic Basis of Therapeutics, 8th ed. New York, Pergamon, 1990:404–435.
17. Prange AJ, Wilson IC, Lynn CW, et al. L-tryptophan in mania. Arch Gen Psychiatry 1974;30:56–62.
18. Vetulani J, Stawarz RJ, Dingell JV, Sulser F. A possible common mechanism of action of antidepressant treatments; reduction in the sensitivity of the noradrenergic cyclic AMP generating system in the rat limbic forebrain. Naunyn Schmiedebergs Arch Pharmacol 1976; 293:109–114.
19. Richelson E. Biological basis of depression and therapeutic relevance. J Clin Psychiatry 1991;52(6 suppl):4–10.

20. Synder SH, Peroutka SJ. A possible role of serotonin receptors in antidepressant drug action. Pharmacopsychiatry 1982;15:131–134.
21. Bryant SG, Brown CS. Current concepts in clinical therapeutics: Major affective disorders, part 1. Clin Pharm 1986;5:304–318.
22. Siever LJ, Davis KL. Overview: Toward a dysregulation hypothesis of depression. Am J Psychiatry 1985;142:1017–1031.
23. Frazer A. Pharmacology of antidepressants. J Clin Psychopharmacol 1997:17(suppl 1):2S–18S.
24. Kalus O, Asnis GM, Van Praag HM. The role of serotonin in depression. Psychiatric Ann 1989;19:348–353.
25. Willner P. Dopaminergic mechanisms in depression and mania. In Bloom FE, Kupfer DJ, eds. Psychopharmacology: The Fourth Generation of Progress. New York, Raven, 1995:921–931.
26. Reddy PL, Khanna S, Subhash MN, et al. CSF amine metabolites in depression. Biol Psychiatry 1992;31:112–118.
27. Willner P. Dopamine and depression: A review of recent evidence. Brain Res Rev 1983;6:211–246.
28. Meltzer HY. Role of serotonin in depression. In Witaker-Azsmitia PM, Peroutka SJ, (eds): The Neuropharmacology of Serotonin. New York, Ann NY Acad Sci 1990:486–499.
29. Katon W, Sullivan MD. Depression and chronic medical illness. J Clin Psychiatry 1990;51(suppl):3–11.
30. Thiessen BQ, Wallace SM, Blackburn JL, et al. Increased prescribing of antidepressants subsequent to beta-blocker therapy. Arch Intern Med 1990;150:2286–2290.
31. Vaillant GE, Blumenthal SJ. Suicide over the life cycle: Risk factors and life span development. In: Blumenthal SJ, Kupfer DJ, eds. Suicide Over the Life Cycle. Washington, DC, American Psychiatric Press, 1990:1–16.
32. Janicak PG, Davis JM, Preskorn SH, Ayd FJ. Principles and practice of psychopharmacotherapy. Baltimore, Williams & Wilkins, 1993: 209–292, 488–489, 506–507.
33. Preskorn SH, Burke MJ. Somatic therapy for major depressive disorder: Selection of an antidepressant. J Clin Psychiatry 1992;53 (suppl 9):5–18.
34. Liebowitz M, Quitkin F, Stewart J, et al. Antidepressant specificity in atypical depression. J Clin Psychiatry 1984;45:19–21.
35. Parker G, Roy K, Hadzi-Pavlovic D, Pedic F. Psychotic (delusional) depression: A meta-analysis of physical treatments. J Affect Disord 1992;24:17–24.
36. Depression guideline panel. Depression in Primary Care, vol 2. Treatment of Major Depression. Rockville, MD, Agency for Health Care Policy and Research, 1993:40–41, 71, 84, 92, 118, 124.
37. APA announces development of guidelines for effective use of electroconvulsive therapy. Hosp Community Psychiatry 1991;41: 208–209.
38. Partonen T, Partinen M. Light treatment for seasonal affective disorder: Theoretical considerations and clinical implications. Acta Psychiatr Scand 1994;377:41S–45S.
39. Chung YS, Daghestani AN. Seasonal affective disorder. Shedding light on a dark subject. Postgrad Med 1989;86:309–314.
40. Lafer B, Sachs GS, Labbate LA, et al. Side effects induced by bright light therapy. Am J Psychiatry 1994;151:1081–1083.
41. Labbate LA, Lafter B, Thibault A, Sachs GS. Phototherapy for seasonal affective disorder: A blind comparison of three different schedules. J Clin Psychiatry 1994;55:189–191.
42. Burke MJ, Preskorn SH. Short term treatment of mood disorders with standard antidepressants. In: Bloom FE, Kupfer DJ, eds. Psychopharmacology: The Fourth Generation of Progress. New York, Raven, 1995:1053–1065.
43. Montgomery SA, Venlafaxine: A new dimension in antidepressant pharmacotherapy. J Clin Psychiatry 1993;54:119–126.
44. Fontaine R. Novel serotonergic mechanisms and clinical experience with nefazodone. Clin Neuropharmacol 1993;16(suppl 3): 45–50.
45. Zung W. Review of placebo controlled trials with bupropion. J Clin Psychiatry 1983;44(suppl 5):104–114.
46. Davis R, Wilde MI. Mirtazapine: A review of its pharmacology and therapeutic potential in the management of major depression. Drugs 1996;5:389–402.
47. Bryant SG, Brown CS. Current concepts in clinical therapeutics: Major affective disorders, part 2. Clin Pharm 1986;5:385–395.
48. Peroutka SJ, Snyder SH. Long term antidepressant treatment decreases spiroperidol-labeled serotonin receptor binding. Science 1980; 210:88–90.
49. Berwish N, Amsterdam J. An overview of investigational antidepressants. Psychosomatics 1989;30:1–17.
50. Cole JO, Bodkin JA. Antidepressant side effects. J Clin Psychiatry 1990;51(suppl):21–26.
51. Ray WA, Griffin MR, Schaffner W, et al. Psychotropic drug use and the risk of hip fracture. N Engl J Med 1987;316:363–369.
52. Jefferson JW. Cardiovascular effects and toxicity of anxiolytics and antidepressants. J Clin Psychiatry 1989;50:368–378.
53. Dilsaver SC, Feinberg M, Greden JF. Antidepressant withdrawal symptoms treated with anticholinergic agents. Am J Psychiatry 1983; 140:249–251.
54. Moller HJ, Volz HP. Drug treatment of depression in the 1990s. An overview of achievements and future possibilities. Drugs 1996;52: 625–638.
55. Venlafaxine prescribing information. Philadelphia, Wyeth-Ayerst Laboratories, 1995.
56. Grimsley SR, Jann MW. Paroxetine, sertraline, and fluvoxamine: New selective serotonin reuptake inhibitors. Clin Pharm 1992;11:930–957.
57. Levinson ML, Lipsy RJ, Fuller DK. Adverse effects and drug interactions associated with fluoxetine therapy. DICP Ann Pharmacother 1991;25:657–661.
58. Aranoff GM. Trazodone associated with priapism. Lancet 1984;1:856.
59. Bupropion prescribing information. Research Triangle Park, NC, Burroughs Wellcome, 1995.
60. Nierenberg AA, Cole JO. Antidepressant adverse drug reactions. J Clin Psychiatry 1991;52(suppl):40–47.
61. Rapp MS. Two cases of ejaculatory impairment related to phenelzine. Am J Psychiatry 1979;136:1200–1201.
62. Barton JL. Orgasmic inhibition by phenelzine. Am J Psychiatry 1979;136:1616–1617.
63. Rabkin JG, Quitkin FM, McGrath P, et al. Adverse reactions to monoamine oxidase inhibitors, II: treatment correlates and clinical management. J Clin Psychopharmacol 1985;5:2–9.
64. Neil JF, Licata SM, May SJ, Himmelhock JM. Dietary noncompliance during treatment with tranylcypromine. J Clin Psychiatry 1979;40: 33–37.
65. Clary C, Schweizer E. Treatment of MAOI hypertensive crisis with sublingual nifedipine. J Clin Psychiatry 1987;48:249–250.
66. Wells BG. Tricyclic antidepressants. In: Taylor WJ, Caviness MHD, eds. A Textbook for the Clinical Application of Therapeutic Drug Monitoring. Irving, TX, Abbott Laboratories, 1986:449–465.
67. DeVane CL. Pharmacokinetics of the selective serotonin reuptake inhibitors. J Clin Psychiatry 1992;53(suppl 2):13–20.
68. Fluoxetine prescribing information. Indianapolis, Dista Products, 1995.
69. Paroxetine prescribing information. Philadelphia, SmithKline Beecham Pharmaceuticals, 1995.
70. Sertraline prescribing information. New York, Roerig Division of Pfizer, 1997.
71. Nefazodone prescribing information. Wallingford, CT, Bristol-Myers Squibb, 1995.
72. Perry PJ, Pfohl BM, Holstad SC. The relationship between antidepressant response and tricyclic antidepressant plasma concentrations. Clin Pharmacokinet 1987;13:381–392.
73. Tricyclic antidepressants—blood level measurements and clinical outcomes: An APA task force report. Am J Psychiatry 1985;142: 155–162.
74. Hansten PD, Horn JR. Drug Interactions and Updates. Vancouver, WA, Applied Therapeutics, 1997:127–842.
75. Hansten PD. Drug Interactions, 6th ed. Philadelphia, Lea & Febiger, 1989.

76. DeVane CL. Pharmacokinetics of the selective serotonin reuptake inhibitors. J Clin Psychiatry 1992;53(suppl):13–20.
77. Bannister SJ, Houser VP, Hulse JD, et al. Evaluation of the potential interactions of paroxetine with diazepam, cimetidine, warfarin, and digoxin. Acta Psychiatr Scand 1989;90(suppl):102–106.
78. Stellamans G. A study to investigate the efficacy, adverse events, safety, and pharmacokinetic effects of coadministration of paroxetine and lithium. Biol Psychiatry 1991;29:628S. Abstract.
79. NIH Consensus Development Panel on Depression in Late Life. Diagnosis and treatment of depression in late life. JAMA 1992;268: 1018–1024.
80. Kelly GL. Childhood depression and suicide. Nursing Clin North Am 1991;26:545–558.
81. Preskorn S, Weller E, Hughes C, et al. Depression in prepubertal children: DST nonsuppression predicts differential response to imipramine versus placebo. Psychopharmacol Bull 1987;23:128–133.
82. Weller EB, Weller RA. Depressive disorders in children and adolescents. In: Garfinkel BD, Carlson GA, Weller EB, eds. Psychiatric Disorders in Children and Adolescents. Philadelphia, Saunders, 1990: 17–19.
83. Hollister LE. Treatment of depression with drugs. Ann Intern Med 1978;89:78.
84. Montgomery SA, Dunbar G. Paroxetine is better than placebo in relapse prevention and the prophylaxis of recurrent depression. Int Clin Psychopharmacol 1993;8:189–195.
85. Keller MB, Lavori PW, Mueller TI. Time to recovery, chronicity, and levels of psychopathology in major depression: A five year prospective follow up of 431 subjects. Arch Gen Psychiatry 1992;49:809–816.
86. Greden JF. Antidepressant maintenance medications: When to discontinue and how to stop. J Clin Psychiatry 1993;54(suppl 8):39–45.
87. Smith W, Sherill A. A pharmacoeconomic study of the management of major depression: Patients in a TennCare HMO. Med Interface 1996.
88. Greenberg PE, Stiglin LE, Finkelstein LM, et al. The economic burden of depression in 1990. J Clin Psychiatry 1993;54:405–418.
89. Sclar DA, Robinson LM, Skaer Tl, et al. Antidepressant Pharmacotherapy: Economic outcomes in a health maintenance organization. Clin Ther 1994;16:715–730.
90. LePen C, Levy E, Ravily V, et al. The cost of treatment dropout in depression. A cost-benefit analysis of fluoxetine vs. Tricyclics. J Affective Disord 1994;31:1–18.
91. Skaer TL, Sclar DA. Robinson LM, et al. Economic evaluation of amitriptyline, desipramine, nortriptyline, and sertraline in the management of patients with depression. Curr Ther Res 1995;56:556–567.
92. Sclar DA, Robinson LM, Skaer TL, et al. Antidepressant Pharmacotherapy: economic evaluation of fluoxetine, paroxetine, and sertraline in a health maintenance organization. J Int Med Res 1995;23: 395–412.
93. Revicki Da, Brown RE, Keller MB, et al. Cost-effectiveness of newer antidepressants compared with tricyclic antidepressants in managed care settings. J Clin Psychiatry 1997;58:47–58.

66
BIPOLAR DISORDER

Martha P. Fankhauser, MS Pharm, FASHP, and William H. Benefield, Jr., PharmD, FASCP, BCPP

Bipolar disorder (previously known as manic–depressive illness) is a cyclical disorder with recurrent fluctuations in mood, energy, and behavior encompassing the extremes of human experiences. This disorder differs from recurrent major depression (or unipolar depression) in the presence of a manic, hypomanic, or mixed episode during the course of the illness. Bipolar disorder is an intriguing psychiatric disorder because it is genetically based, environmentally influenced, and the clinical presentation differs widely from individual to individual.

EPIDEMIOLOGY

Epidemiologic studies report that the lifetime prevalence rate of a manic episode is 1.6% ± 0.3 for men and 1.7% ± 0.3 for women in the United States (approximately 3 million people).[1] The onset of bipolar disorder is rare before puberty, but its prevalence increases during late adolescence and into early adulthood (usually between the ages of 15 and 30). Onset of mania after age 50 is rare and may be related to comorbid neurologic or medical causes instead of a genetic risk for the disorder.[2] Bipolar disorder is not restricted to any educational or social class, race, or nationality.

ETIOLOGY

The exact etiology of bipolar disorder is unknown, but it is believed to be caused from imbalances of certain brain chemicals or abnormalities in secondary messenger systems involved in neuronal transmission.[3]

GENETIC FACTORS

Hereditary risk is an important determinant of who will develop bipolar disorder, but nongenetic factors may be responsible for some cases (perinatal development, head trauma, environmental factors, and stress). Bipolar disorder has a higher genetic risk than major depressive disorders.[3] Approximately 80% to 90% of bipolar patients have a biologic relative, (e.g., parent, sibling, or child) with a mood disorder (bipolar disorder, major depression, cyclothymia, dysthymia). First-degree relatives of bipolar patients have a 15% to 35% risk of developing a mood disorder. Studies show a 78% to 80% concordance rate in monozygotic twins compared with 20% in dizygotic twins. Adoption studies found that 38% of adopted children (if one biologic parent has bipolar disorder) have a mood disorder, whereas only 7% of control, adopted children develop a mood disorder. The exact mechanism of genetic transmission is not known and may involve multifactorial inheritance; linkage studies suggest that loci on the 12, 18, and X chromosome may contribute to genetic susceptibility of bipolar disorder.

SECONDARY MANIA

Several general medical or substance-related causes of mania have been identified (Table 66–1). A complete medical and medication history and physical exam are necessary to rule out any organic causes. Laboratory testing may be warranted if the history or physical examination reveal any abnormalities (e.g., signs or symptoms of hypothyroidism). Medications associated with causing mania, agitation, or insomnia should be discontinued.

PATHOPHYSIOLOGY

Many hypotheses have been proposed regarding the pathophysiology of mood disorders, including neurotransmitter, neuromodulator, neuroanatomic, and physiologic abnormalities.[3–5]

NEUROTRANSMITTER THEORIES

The most prominent and oldest hypotheses regarding mood disorders are those proposing an alteration in monoamine neurotransmitter concentrations in the central nervous system (CNS).[3–5] The monoamine hypothesis suggests a functional deficit of neurotransmitters—primarily norepinephrine (NE), dopamine (DA), and/or serotonin (5-HT)—in depression and an excess of catecholamines (primarily NE and DA) in mania. NE, DA, and 5-HT are highly interdependent and interact or modulate other neurotransmitter and hormone systems.

The "permissive serotonin hypothesis" proposes that there is low central 5-HT activity in both mania and depression. 5-HT plays a critical role in modulating CNS activity (e.g., stabilization of catecholamine system and inhibition of DA). Lithium facilitates the release of 5-HT and increases postsynaptic 5-HT receptor activity. L-Tryptophan (precursor to 5-HT) and fenfluramine (blocks 5-HT reuptake and enhances 5-HT release) have been used with other antimanic agents to enhance efficacy.[5]

Dysregulation between neurotransmitter systems may produce a cyclical rhythm disturbance in the CNS.[3–5] NE and DA dysregulation may play an important role in the development of mania. One hypothesis of the switch phenomenon from depression to mania involves the balance of NE

TABLE 66–1. Medical Conditions, Medications, and Somatic Treatments that Induce Mania

Endocrine or Metabolic Disorders	**Medications (continued)**
Addison's disease	Baclofen—ingestion or withdrawal
Carcinoid tumors	Benzodiazepines—ingestion or withdrawal
Cushing's disease	Bronchodilators: albuterol, isoetharine, isoproterenol, metaproterenol, metaraminol, salmeterol, terbutaline
Hyperthyroidism	Calcium replacement
Vitamin B_{12} deficiency	Cimetidine
Infections	Decongestants/sympathomimetics: ephedrine, epinephrine, methoxamine, midodrine, norepinephrine, phenylephrine, phenylpropanolamine, pseudoephedrine, ritodrine
Acquired immunodeficiency syndrome	Disulfiram
Encephalitis	Dopamine-augmenting agents: amantadine, bromocriptine, levodopa
Neurosyphilis	Hallucinogens: LSD, phencyclidine
Postinfection (viral, encephalitis, influenza)	Isoniazid
Neurologic Disorders	NSAIDs: indomethacin, tolmetin
Epilepsy (temporal lobe)	Procainamide
Huntington's disease	Quinacrine
Multiple sclerosis	Steroids: anabolic, corticosteroids, ACTH
Postcerebrovascular accident	Stimulants: amphetamines, cocaine, methylphenidate, pemoline
Postconcussion	Xanthines: caffeine, theophylline
Right frontotemporal lesions	Yohimbine
Subarachnoid hemorrhage	**Somatic Therapies**
Subcortical lesions	Bright visible spectrum light therapy
Surgical trauma	Electroconvulsive therapy
Medications	Hemodialysis
Alcohol	Sleep deprivation
α_2-Adrenergic agonist—withdrawal	
Anticonvulsants	
Antidepressants: TCAs, MAOIs, SSRIs	

Compiled from Refs. 16, 31, and 32.

to DA. When NE activity is decreased (as in depression), the DA activity predominates, and this may account for the switch to hypomania or mania. Increased dopaminergic activity may play a role in causing hyperactivity and psychosis associated with the severe stages of mania, and reduced DA activity may cause depression. Lithium decreases β-adrenergic receptor number and blocks DA receptor sensitivity.[5] Clonidine, an α_2-noradrenergic agonist, decreases NE release and has been used as an adjunctive agent for agitation and insomnia. Antidopamine medications (e.g., haloperidol, fluphenazine, and risperidone) have antimania properties and are often used during the acute manic phase of the illness.[5] Antidepressants that augment NE, DA, and 5-HT activity have been used to treat bipolar depression; these agents may cause switching to mania.

γ-Aminobutyric acid (GABA), the main inhibitory neurotransmitter in the CNS, is involved in the inhibition of NE and DA activity.[3,5] A GABA deficiency hypothesis has been proposed for mood disorders and is related to the sensitization–kindling theory for mood disorders.[6] Several antimania drugs, including lithium, carbamazepine (CBZ), valproic acid (VPA), clonazepam, and lorazepam, enhance GABAergic activity. Glutamate, an excitatory neurotransmitter, may be involved in mood disorders. Anticonvulsants such as CBZ and lamotrigine decrease glutamate release,[7] and topirimate acts as a glutamate-receptor antagonist.[8]

An acetylcholine (ACh) deficiency hypothesis or a cholinergic–adrenergic imbalance has also been proposed as another explanation of bipolar disorder.[5] Choline interacts with the catecholamine system and is involved in the interaction between phosphatidylinositol and phosphatidylcholine secondary messenger systems. Lithium increases red blood cell levels of choline, and choline supplementation has been used in combination with lithium to treat rapid-cycling bipolar patients.[9]

SENSITIZATION AND KINDLING THEORIES

A supersensitivity and kindling model has been proposed as causing cyclical mood disorders.[4] Recurrences of the illness may result in behavioral sensitivity and electrophysiologic kindling (similar to amygdala-kindling models in animals for seizures). Initially, psychosocial or physical stressors trigger episodes, but later the episodes occur spontaneously due to the increased sensitivity and kindling of the CNS. Anticonvulsants such as CBZ and VPA have antikindling properties and are effective in rapid cyclers and mixed states, whereas lithium does not prevent amygdala kindling and is less effective.[10] Electroconvulsive therapy (ECT) can also inhibit kindling and is used for rapid cyclers and mixed states. Early recognition and successful treatment of initial episodes of bipolar disorder may decrease the likelihood that patients will later develop rapid or continuous cycling.

NEUROENDOCRINE THEORIES

The hypothalamic–pituitary–thyroid axis may be involved in the pathophysiology of mood disorders.[3–5] Excessive thyroid activity may precipitate a manic episode by potentiating β-noradrenergic activity. Thyroid hormones, L-thyroxine (T_4) and triidothyronine (T_3), have been used to speed the response of antidepressant therapy and convert nonresponders to responders. Thyroid supplementation has been used to treat refractory rapid-cycling bipolar disorder including episodes of hypomania and mania. Lithium blocks the release of thyroid hormones and CBZ decreases thyroid indices.[5]

MEMBRANE AND CATION HYPOTHESIS

Abnormal calcium and sodium homeostasis has been proposed as causing mood fluctuations in bipolar disorder.[3–5] Extracellular and intracellular calcium concentrations affect the excitability of neuronal firing and may cause "switches" from depression to mania.[3,4] The calcium secondary messenger system may be involved with neurobiologic abnormalities associated with bipolar disorder.[11] Untreated bipolar patients have higher basal concentrations of intracellular calcium in platelets and lymphocytes compared to unipolar depressed or normal controls.[5,11] Several antimanic drugs have calcium antagonist effects, including lithium, calcium channel blockers, and phenothiazine antipsychotics. Calcium channel blockers, (e.g., nimodipine, verapamil) decrease intracellular calcium; block 5-HT, DA, and endorphin activity; alter sodium–calcium exchange; and act as anticonvulsants.[5] CBZ decreases serum sodium and calcium concentrations and blocks calcium influx through the *N*-methyl-D-aspartate (NMDA) glutamate receptor. Lamotrigine blocks sodium channels, which decreases presynaptic glutamate release and has effects on calcium channels. Lithium decreases calcium transport into cells, inhibits the uptake of calcium into platelets, interferes with the calcium–sodium active transport system, increases renal tubular reabsorption of calcium, and increases serum calcium and parathyroid hormone concentrations.

SECONDARY MESSENGER SYSTEM THEORIES

When neurotransmitters bind to postsynaptic receptors, a series of intracellular events occur that are mediated by chemical systems (or secondary messengers) linked to those receptors. The cyclic adenosine monophosphate (cAMP) and phosphoinositide systems have been the most studied in bipolar disorder.[3] cAMP is involved in the regulation of neuronal excitability and plays an important role in the pathophysiology of bipolar disorder. Both adenylyl cyclase and phospholipase C are involved in G-protein (guanine nucleotide–binding protein) signal transduction systems.[12] G-proteins regulate adenylyl cyclase activity and phosphoinositide responses, modulate sodium/proton exchange and potassium/calcium channels, and activate phospholipases.

Abnormalities in the membrane transport and secondary messenger systems indicate a genetic vulnerability in some bipolar patients.[3–5] A reduction in erythrocyte sodium–potassium–activated adenosine triphosphatase (Na^+/K^+-ATPase) activity has been suggested as a marker for bipolar disorder. ATPase maintains ionic gradients across the cell membranes and responds to neurotransmitter activation. If ATPase activity is reduced, another secondary messenger system involving phosphatidylinositol may become more active, resulting in excessive release of monoamine neurotransmitters. In clinical studies, bipolar manic patients have demonstrated elevated platelet membrane phosphatidylinositol-4,5-biphosphate (PIP2). Cell lines from bipolar patients have shown abnormalities in phosphatidylinositol metabolism.

Lithium exerts major effects on G-protein functioning, which is involved in regulating mood, appetite, and wakefulness.[13] Lithium blocks the enzyme inositol-1-phosphatase (an enzyme that converts inositol-1-phosphatase to inositol), which decreases the neurons' ability to restore normal PIP2 concentrations.[13] By affecting this secondary messenger system, lithium reduces the responsiveness of neurons to muscarinic, dopaminergic, serotonergic, α-adrenergic, and other stimuli. Lithium also interferes with the adenylyl cyclase-catalyzed conversion of ATP to cAMP, which inhibits adenylyl cyclase activity and decreases cellular responses to neurotransmitters. Carbamazepine decreases basal cAMP levels and attenuates stimulated cAMP production. Chronic lithium and VPA therapy down-regulate kinase C isoenzymes, which plays a role in regulating presynaptic and postsynaptic neurotransmission.

BIOLOGIC RHYTHMS HYPOTHESIS

Desynchronization of circadian or seasonal rhythms may cause diurnal variations in mood and sleep and result in seasonal recurrences of episodes.[3,5,14] Abnormalities of circadian rhythms have been reported in bipolar patients, such as alterations in the suppression of the rhythmical hormone melatonin (a metabolite of 5-HT) due to abnormalities in light sensitivity.

Changes in the sleep–wake or light–dark cycle have precipitated episodes of mania or depression.[14] Seasonal peaks of depression are highest in the spring (March to May) and next in the fall (September to November), which parallels the same peaks for suicide.[5] There are less seasonal data for manic episodes, but there appears to be an increased incidence of mania during the summer months when there is more exposure to light and heat.[15] Bright light therapy has been used for the treatment of winter depression and may precipitate hypomanic, manic, or mixed episodes.

Abnormalities in sleep biologic rhythms are implicated in the pathogenesis of bipolar disorder.[14] Switches from depression to mania can happen when a bipolar patient misses a night's sleep.[5] Sleep deprivation has been used to cause a remission in depression, but the clinical response is usually brief.

Environmental, psychosocial, or physical stressors may precipitate mood changes, particularly in vulnerable patients with a genetic predisposition.[4,5] Approximately two-thirds of bipolar patients report a significant stressful life event (especially difficulty at work or interpersonal conflicts) preceding their first manic episode.

CLINICAL PRESENTATION

The essential feature of bipolar disorder is a history of mania or hypomania that is not caused by any other medical condition, substances, or mental disorder.[16] Bipolar disorder is characterized by mood swings (mania and depression) that are outside the range of normal mood states. Bipolar disorder has diverse clinical manifestations that can differ in symptoms, course, severity, and response to treatment among individuals.[17] Patients usually experience periods of mood elevation (mania or hypomania) that alternate with normal mood states (euthymia).

The American Psychiatric Association's *Diagnostic and Statistical Manual of Mental Disorders,* fourth edition (DSM-IV), represents our present understanding of mood (or affective) disorders.[16] DSM-IV divides bipolar disorder into four subtypes based on the identification of specific mood episodes: bipolar I, bipolar II, cyclothymic disorder, and bipolar disorder not otherwise specified (NOS) (Table 66–2).[18] The mood states are further separated into four subcategories to differentiate the current or most recent mood episode: major depressive, manic, hypomanic, or mixed (Table 66–3).

MAJOR DEPRESSIVE EPISODE

The clinical presentation and diagnostic criteria for bipolar depression are the same as those for major depressive episode (Chap. 65). Major depressive episodes are defined by discrete periods of depressed mood or loss of interest or pleasure in life for greater than 2 weeks.[16] In bipolar depression, patients often have changes in sleep patterns, low energy, psychomotor retardation, cognitive impairment, decreased sexual activity, slowed speech, carbohydrate craving, and weight gain (also called atypical depressive features).[19] Approximately 10% to 15% of patients first diagnosed as having major depressive illness will later experience an episode of mania or hypomania. Bipolar women are at increased risk for depressive episodes compared to bipolar men.[20]

MANIC EPISODE

A manic episode is defined by a distinct period when the mood is abnormally and persistently elevated, expansive, or irritable and is accompanied by impairment in judgment and in social and occupational functioning.[16] Acute mania usually begins abruptly, and symptoms escalate over several days. Seasonal changes, stressors, sleep deprivation, antidepressants, bright light, or ECT can precipitate a manic episode.[14,15] Mania is characterized by heightened mood (euphoria), unrealistic grandiosity or optimism, quicker thoughts (flight of ideas), more and faster speech (pressured speech), increased energy, increased physical and mental activities (psychomotor excitement), decreased need for sleep, anger or irritability, heightened perceptual acuity, and impulsivity (e.g., foolish business ventures, illegal activities, increased sexual activity, or buying sprees).[19] A change in the sleep cycle (with a decreased need for sleep) is often the first clue to the beginning of an episode. Attention span is usually very short, resulting in impairment of concentration and "flight of ideas" (thoughts that change rapidly from one topic to another).

The severe stages of a manic episode may resemble paranoid schizophrenia with bizarre behavior, hallucinations, and delusions. Approximately two-thirds of bipolar patients have psychotic symptoms at some point during the depressed or manic episodes, primarily paranoid or grandiose delusions. Psychotic symptoms occur only during severe episodes of

TABLE 66–2. Mood Disorders Defined by Episodes

Disorder	Episode(s)
Major depressive disorder, single episode	Major depressive episode
Major depressive disorder, recurrent	Major depressive episode + major depressive episode
Bipolar disorder, type I	Major depressive episode + manic or mixed episode
Bipolar disorder, type II	Major depressive episode + hypomanic episode
Dysthymic disorder	Chronic subsyndromal depressive episodes
Cyclothymic disorder	Chronic fluctuations between subsyndromal depressive and hypomanic episodes (2 years for adults and 1 year for children and adolescents)
Mood disorder due to a general medical condition	Disturbance in mood that is secondary to a general medical condition: • With depressive features • Major depressive-like episode • With manic features • With mixed features
Substance-induced mood disorder	Disturbance in mood that is due to the effects of a substance (e.g., medication, toxin, drug of abuse, somatic treatments such as ECT or light therapy): • With depressive features • With manic features • With mixed features
Bipolar disorder not otherwise specified	Mood states do not meet criteria for any specific bipolar disorder

Adapted from Ref. 16.

TABLE 66–3. Diagnosis of Mood Episodes

Episode	Impairment of Functioning or Need for Hospitalization[a]	DSM-IV Criteria[b]
Major depressive	Yes	> 2-Week period of either depressed mood or loss of interest or pleasure in normal activities; associated with at least five of the following symptoms: • Depressed, sad mood (adults); may be irritable mood in children • Decreased interest and pleasure in normal activities • Decreased appetite, weight loss • Insomnia or hypersomnia • Psychomotor retardation or agitation • Decreased energy or fatigue • Feelings of guilt or worthlessness • Impaired concentration and decision making • Suicidal thoughts or attempts
Manic	Yes	> 1-Week period of abnormal and persistent elevated mood (expansive or irritable); associated with at least three of the following symptoms (four if the mood is only irritable): • Inflated self-esteem (grandiosity) • Decreased need for sleep • Increased talking (pressure of speech) • Racing thoughts (flight of ideas) • Distractible (poor attention) • Increased activity (either socially, at work, or sexually) or increased motor activity or agitation • Excessive involvement in activities that are pleasurable but have a high risk for serious consequences (buying sprees, sexual indiscretions, poor judgment in business ventures)
Hypomanic	No	At least 4 days of abnormal and persistent elevated mood (expansive or irritable); associated with at least three of the following symptoms (four if the mood is only irritable): • Inflated self-esteem (grandiosity) • Decreased need for sleep • Increased talking (pressure of speech) • Racing thoughts (flight of ideas) • Distractible (poor attention) • Increased activity (either socially, at work, or sexually) or increased motor activity or agitation • Excessive involvement in activities that are pleasurable but have a high risk for serious consequences (buying sprees, sexual indiscretions, poor judgment in business ventures)
Mixed	Yes	Criteria for both a major depressive and manic episode (except for duration) occur nearly every day for at least a 1-week period
Rapid cycling	Yes	> Four major depressive or manic episodes (manic, mixed, or hypomanic) in 12 months

[a]Impairment in social or occupational functioning; need for hospitalization due to potential for self-harm, harm of others, or psychotic symptoms.
[b]The disorder is not due to a medical condition (e.g., hypothyroidism) or substance-induced disorder (e.g., antidepressant treatment, medications, electroconvulsive therapy, light therapy).
Adapted from Ref. 16.

mania or depression and remit when the mood returns to normal. When psychotic symptoms persist into the periods of normal mood, the diagnosis is schizoaffective disorder.

HYPOMANIC EPISODE

Hypomania describes a less severe form of mania in which the patient's mood is elevated, expansive, or irritable and there are associated symptoms such as increased psychomotor activity, decreased need for sleep, pressure of speech, flight of ideas, and distractibility.[16] The hypomanic episode does not have marked impairment in social or occupational functioning to necessitate a hospitalization and no delusions or hallucinations are present. Symptoms found in hypomanic episodes are similar to cocaine- or antidepressant-induced mood disorders; thus the differential diagnosis should rule out any substance-induced or medical conditions that present with elevated mood.

During a hypomanic episode, patients may be more productive and creative.[21] Patients usually find the hypomanic state very desirable because they have a heightened sense of well-being, happiness, exhilaration, feel more powerful and productive, and have increased energy. Hypomanic states are usually associated with euphoria, but some patients have emotional fluctuations with irritability, outburst, rage, and intolerance. Hypomanic states should be closely monitored, because 5% to 15% of patients may rapidly "switch" to a manic episode.

MIXED EPISODE

Bipolar disorder is a dynamic and constantly changing illness, so that manifestations of either phase may occur simultaneously, or patients may cycle or "switch" from one mood state to another. Bipolar "mixed episode" (previously known as mixed state, dysphoric mania, or depressive mania) is defined as the simultaneous occurrence of mania and depressive symptoms for nearly every day for at least a 1-week period.[16] There must be variability and lability in mood that is severe enough to cause impairment in social or occupational functioning or to require hospitalization. Mixed episodes occur in up to 40% of all episodes, are more common in younger and older patients, and may occur more frequently in females.[5,20] Mixed episodes are often difficult to diagnose and treat because of the fluctuating clinical presentation; these patients often have a poorer prognosis and nonresponse to monotherapy with mood stabilizers.[22]

COURSE OF ILLNESS

The average age of onset of a first manic episode is the early 20s, although some episodes may start in adolescence or after age 50.[2] The diagnosis of bipolar disorder does not require a history of depression, but approximately 95% of bipolar patients experience episodes of depression during their lifetime. Unipolar mania (with no depressive episodes) accounts for less than 5% to 9% of bipolar patients. Greater than 80% of patients have more than four episodes during their lifetime.[16] Patients with cyclothymic disorder have a 15% to 50% risk of later developing a bipolar I or II disorder. For bipolar I disorder, 90% of individuals with a manic episode later have multiple recurrent episodes of major depression, mania, hypomania, or mixed episodes alternating with a normal mood state. Usually there is a period of normal functioning between episodes, but approximately 25% to 60% of patients have no period of euthymia due to switching directly to the opposite polarity.

Rapid cyclers have four or more episodes per year (major depressive, manic, mixed, or hypomanic).[16] This subtype of bipolar disorder is seen in approximately 5% to 20% of patients and is more common in women.[5,20] Risk factors associated with rapid cycling include antidepressant or stimulant use, hypothyroidism, and premenstrual mood changes. Rapid-cycling patients may average 50 or more episodes in their lifetime. A rare form of bipolar disorder is characterized by "ultrarapid" cycles (e.g., every 48 hours) or "continuous" cycles with no free interval between episodes. Antidepressant therapy or subclinical hypothyroidism may exacerbate rapid cycling or convert rapid cyclers to a continuous form of the illness.[20]

The length and severity of an episode and the interval between episodes vary from patient to patient.[2] Manic episodes are usually briefer and end more abruptly than major depressive episodes. The average length of untreated manic episodes ranges from 4 to 13 months. Episodes may occur regularly (at the same time or season of the year), and often cluster at 12-month intervals. If a manic episode occurs postpartum, there is an increased risk for recurrences during subsequent postpartum periods. Early postpartum euphoria or mania may be followed by a postpartum depression.[20] Women have more depressive episodes than manic episodes, whereas men have a more even distribution of episodes.[16]

Bipolar disorder usually presents with lability of mood or depression before the onset of bipolar disorder in children and adolescents.[16] Attention deficit/hyperactivity disorder (ADHD) and a manic episode have similar characteristics (hyperactivity, impulsivity, poor judgment), so ADHD should be ruled out if there is an early onset (before age 7 years). Early-onset bipolar disorder has an increased risk of psychotic features, more frequent mood reoccurrences (mixed states and rapid cycling), a more chronic course, and a less favorable response to treatment.

PROGNOSIS

Bipolar disorder can have devastating long-term effects, because recurring episodes may cause deterioration in functioning.[16–19] Between 7% and 32% of bipolar type I patients remain chronically ill throughout their lifetime due to partial or no response to medication, rapid cycling, or mixed episodes. Bipolar type II patients have similar relapse rates compared to type I, and may also have a moderate to poor outcome due to recurrences of mood episodes. Subsyndromal mood episodes may remain in up to 13% to 34% of bipolar patients between major depressive or manic episodes.

Bipolar patients have a 46% lifetime prevalence rate for alcohol abuse or dependence and a 41% rate for drug abuse or dependence.[23] Alcohol or drug abuse can precipitate or modify bipolar episodes (cocaine can lengthen or intensify euphoria, whereas alcohol can cause depression). Substance-induced mania or depression may change the course of the illness and decrease the effectiveness of mood stabilizers. These patients tend to self-medicate during episodes, resulting in impaired judgment, poor impulse control, and a worsening of the clinical course.

Untreated, depressed, or mixed-state bipolar patients have a high risk of suicide (1 in 4 to 5 patients commits suicide and approximately 25% to 50% of patients attempt suicide at least once).[24,25] Inadequately treated bipolar disorder places a significant strain on interpersonal relationships, career, and financial status. Education may be interrupted, and some patients have difficulty keeping a job.

Acutely manic patients may need protection (or hospitalization) because they lack appropriate judgment and insight. Some patients have difficulties accepting that they have a serious, chronic illness and do not receive appropriate treatment until late in the illness or after several hospitalizations. Noncompliance with pharmacologic treatment is a major factor in relapse and hospitalization. Medication discontinuation occurs in up to 50% of patients secondary to intolerance to drug-induced side effects. It is estimated that only one-third of bipolar patients receive treatment due to failure to recognize the disorder, reluctance to acknowledge the disorder, or poor compliance with treatment.

▶ TREATMENT: Bipolar Disorder

DESIRED OUTCOME

The goals of treatment include resolution of bipolar symptoms, prevention of future episodes, minimization of adverse drug effects, compliance with treatment, patient education about the disorder and treatment approaches, and avoidance of stressors that may precipitate an acute episode. The goal for the acute treatment phase is to end the current depression, manic, hypomanic, or mixed episode. Preventive treatment is then given to decrease the risk of relapse after an acute episode has been controlled and to prevent future episodes.[5]

GENERAL APPROACH TO TREATMENT

Treatment of bipolar disorder must be individualized because the clinical presentation, severity, and frequency of episodes vary widely among patients. Treatment approaches include both pharmacologic and nonpharmacologic strategies.[26–33] An algorithm for treatment of bipolar disorder is shown in Figure 66–1.

Three main mood stabilizers are used for the acute and maintenance treatment of bipolar disorder. Lithium is FDA approved for the acute and prophylactic treatment of bipolar depression. VPA is not FDA approved, but divalproex sodium (DVPX) is converted to VPA in the stomach and is FDA approved for the treatment of acute mania. CBZ is not FDA approved for bipolar disorder.

Hypomanic episodes may not require treatment unless the patient has a previous history of manic episodes.[26–28,31] Acute manic episodes can be treated with lithium, CBZ, or VPA along with adjunctive benzodiazepines (BZDs) for anxiety or insomnia. Severe manic episodes associated with psychosis and agitation require antipsychotics alone or with BZDs for sedation along with lithium, CBZ, or VPA until the mania subsides.[31] If the patient has not responded within 2 to 4 weeks, a second mood stabilizer can be added to the regimen for augmentation (e.g., lithium and VPA or CBZ). If patients are nonresponsive to these pharmacologic approaches, the mood stabilizer should be switched to another agent or ECT may be used to rapidly reduce manic symptoms. After the remission of an acute manic episode, patients should be maintained on a 2- to 6-month continuation phase of the mood stabilizer while the adjunctive treatment(s) are tapered and discontinued.[28,31] Bipolar patients who have had only one manic episode and who have responded to treatment should be continued on a mood stabilizer for 12 months, and then the mood stabilizer can be gradually tapered off over several months with close monitoring for recurrence of symptoms.[28] Long-term or lifetime maintenance therapy with a mood stabilizer is recommended for bipolar type I patients after two manic episodes, after one severe manic episode, if there is a strong family bipolar history, with frequent episodes (more than one per year), or with rapid onset of manic episodes.[31] Long-term prophylaxis for bipolar II patients is recommended after three hypomanic episodes or if the patient requires an antidepressant but becomes hypomanic.[31]

Despite adequate maintenance treatment, some patients may have "breakthrough" episodes of hypomania or depression that require short-term adjunctive medication (e.g., BZDs or antipsychotics for mania and antidepressants for depression).[28,31] Depressed patients on lithium should always be evaluated for lithium-induced hypothyroidism, because thyroid supplementation may reverse the depression without the risk of inducing mania. Rapid cyclers may respond to the addition of thyroid supplements to a standard mood stabilizer.

Monotherapy is preferred for long-term maintenance; however, combinations of drugs may be necessary for patients with mixed episodes, rapid cycling, or those with partial or no response to monotherapy. Possible combinations include lithium plus CBZ, lithium plus VPA, and CBZ plus VPA.[31] The concomitant use of multiple drugs may be needed to stabilize refractory patients or continuous cyclers (e.g., lithium plus CBZ and clonazepam; VPA plus an antipsychotic and/or BZD).[31] Rapid discontinuation of effective prophylaxis with lithium therapy has been associated with an increased risk of relapse and possibly a more severe and nonresponsive type of disorder; therefore, gradual tapering down of the dose by 300 mg/mo may reduce the risk of relapse.[28] The risk of relapse after discontinuation of maintenance therapy with CBZ or VPA is not known.

NONPHARMACOLOGIC THERAPY

Several nonpharmacologic treatment strategies (e.g., ECT, high-intensity bright light therapy, phase-advanced sleep schedule, and partial or complete sleep deprivation) have been used for bipolar disorder.[28,30–32] Bilateral ECT is an effective treatment for severe mania, psychotic depression, and mixed states with high suicidal risk (approximately an 80% response rate).[33] ECT may also be used in pregnant women who cannot take lithium, CBZ, or VPA.[28,30]

Acute neurotoxicity and delirium have been reported in patients receiving ECT with lithium (even at reduced doses). Lithium should be withdrawn and discontinued at least 2 days before ECT and should not be resumed until 2 to 3 days after the last ECT.[33] Because CBZ, VPA, and BZDs have anticonvulsant properties, these drugs should also be tapered down and discontinued prior to ECT.

EDUCATION, COUNSELING, THERAPY, AND SUPPORT

Meeting with the patient and family to review the diagnosis and treatment of bipolar disorder, providing verbal education and written materials, and monitoring the patient at regular intervals are important interventions to maximize treatment outcomes.[31] Bipolar disorder is most effectively treated with a combination of medications and adjunctive supportive counseling, insight-oriented psychotherapy (individual or group), couples or family therapy, and cognitive/behavioral therapy. Self-help, support groups, and mental health organizations are found in most communities to provide information, educational materials, and support. For public information, patients may call the National Depressive and Manic–Depressive Association (NDMDA) at 800–826–3632; National Alliance for the Mentally Ill (NAMI) at 800–950–6264; National Foundation for Depressive Illness (NFDI) at 800–248–4344; or National Mental Health Association (NMHA) at 800–969–6642.[31]

Patients (and family members) should be educated or counseled about (1) psychosocial or physical stressors that may precipitate an episode; (2) strategies on coping with stressful life events and using stress-reduction techniques; (3) early recognition of the signs and symptoms of mania and depression and charting mood changes; (4) compliance with treatment recommendations and when to seek treatment; (5) the importance of a stable sleep pattern, good nutrition, and regular exercise; (6) limiting substances and drugs that can trigger mood episodes or affect the course of the illness; and (7) monitoring for adverse effects of medications and avoiding drug–drug interactions.[31]

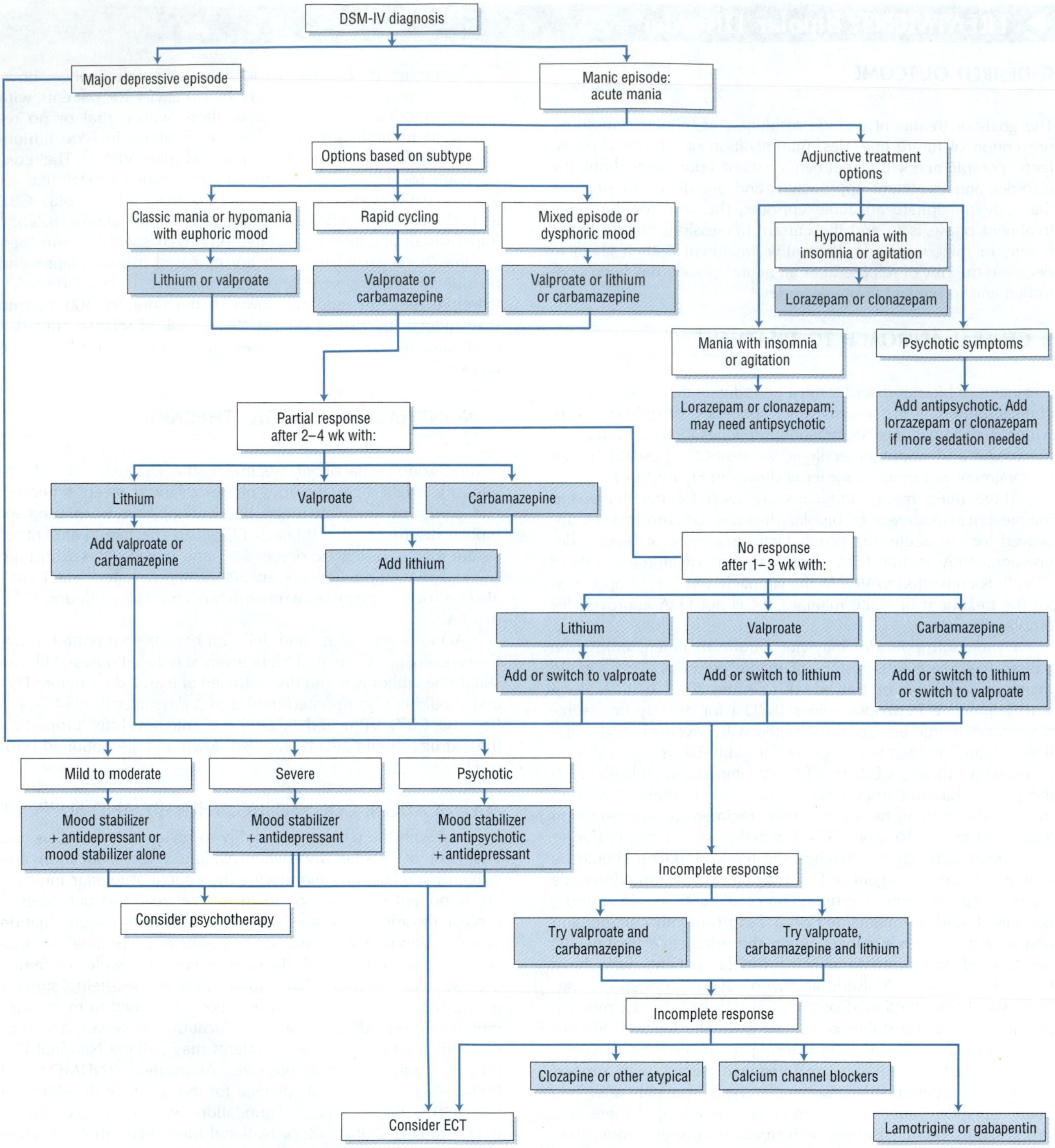

FIGURE 66–1. Algorithm for the treatment of bipolar disorder. *(Adapted from Ref. 31.)*

PHARMACOLOGIC THERAPY

DRUG TREATMENTS OF FIRST CHOICE

Several algorithms have been proposed for selecting mood stabilizers and combinations, but no decision-making tree can accurately reflect the diversity and complexity of bipolar disorder. In 1994, the American Psychiatric Association (APA) published practice guidelines for the treatment of patients with bipolar disorder.[32] These guidelines provide basic information about the diagnosis, clinical course, epidemiology, and treatment strategies for bipolar type I disorder. In 1996, the APA Expert Consensus Guidelines for the Treatment of Bipolar Disorder in adults were published; these are shown in Figure 66–1.[31]

Although lithium has been considered the drug of choice for bipolar disorder, anticonvulsants such as VPA and CBZ are now being used as first-line mood stabilizers.[26–32] Approximately

TABLE 66–4. Names and Formulations of Mood Stabilizers

Generic Name	Brand Name	Formulations
Carbamazepine	Tegretol, Epitol	Tablet: 200 mg
	Tegretol	Chewable tablet: 200 mg Suspension: 100 mg/5 mL
Lithium carbonate	Eskalith	Tablet: 300 mg Capsule: 300 mg
	Lithane	Capsule: 300 mg
	Lithotabs	Tablet: 300 mg
	Lithobid	Extended-release tablet: 300 mg
	Eskalith CR	Extended-release tablet: 450 mg
	Generic, Roxane	Tablet: 300 mg (scored) Capsule: 150, 300, 600 mg
Lithium citrate	Cibalith-S	8 mEq/5 mL
Valproic acid	Depakene	Capsule: 250 mg
Valproate sodium	Depakene	Syrup: 250 mg/5 mL
Divalproex sodium	Depakote	Enteric-coated tablet: 125, 250, 500 mg Sprinkle capsule: 125 mg

20% to 40% of patients cannot tolerate the adverse effects or do not respond to lithium despite therapeutic plasma concentrations.[33] Rapid cycling, mixed episodes, or severe manic stages are often resistant to monotherapy with lithium. VPA and CBZ are now commonly prescribed as first-line treatments for bipolar illness and are more effective than lithium in several mood subtypes.

Newer anticonvulsants (gabapentin, lamotrigine) and calcium channel antagonists (nimodipine, verapamil) are under investigation as mood stabilizers and may be considered alternative agents if a patient cannot tolerate lithium, CBZ, or VPA or is nonresponsive to first-line approaches.[30] BZDs (clonazepam, lorazepam) and antipsychotics (clozapine, haloperidol, olanzapine, risperidone) are often used as adjunctive or augmenting agents with standard mood stabilizers or when patients cannot take mood stabilizers (e.g., during the first trimester of pregnancy).[30] Product information for lithium, CBZ, and VPA is found in Table 66–4, and information about alternative mood stabilizers is listed in Table 66–5. Table 66–6 includes recommendations for baseline and routine laboratory testing for lithium, CBZ, and VPA.

Lithium

In 1970, lithium carbonate was approved for the treatment of mania, and in 1974, it was approved for maintenance therapy of bipolar disorder. Lithium is generally 50% to 70% effective in aborting an acute manic or hypomanic episode within 7 to 14 days after starting therapy.[26,33] Placebo-controlled and naturalistic studies indicate that lithium monotherapy has a response rate against relapse of 70% to 80% at 1 year, 50% at 3 years, and 40% at 5 years.[26] Long-term lithium therapy may be more effective in patients with fewer prior episodes, with a history of euthymia or good functioning between episodes, and with a family history of bipolar illness with a positive response to lithium.[26] Patients maintained on "standard" serum concentrations of lithium (between 0.8 and 1.0 mEq/L) may have fewer relapses than patients maintained on lower serum concentrations (0.4 to 0.6 mEq/L).[34] Lithium has antidepressant effects and is sometimes used to augment other antidepressants in refractory patients. Lithium may be less effective for severe mania with psychotic features, mixed episodes, rapid or continuous cycling, alcohol and drug abuse, and in organic-induced mood states.[26,27]

Divalproex Sodium, Sodium Valproate, or Valproic Acid

Valproic acid (VPA), a branched-chain fatty acid, originally was marketed as an anticonvulsant (as discussed in Chap. 52). In 1995, divalproex sodium (DVPX) was approved by the FDA for the acute treatment of mania. In several controlled studies, DVPX has been shown to be as effective as lithium in patients with pure mania (65% to 70% response rate) and may be more effective than lithium in certain subtypes of bipolar disorder (e.g., secondary bipolar disorder or comorbid substance abuse.)[5,26–29,35–37] Predictors of positive response with VPA include rapid cycling, a high level of dysphoria or depression during the manic episode (mixed episode), concomitant panic attacks, mania associated with organic features (abnormal EEG) or organic mental disorders, history of head trauma, and mental retardation.[26,27,37,38] Antimanic effects may be augmented when VPA is given with lithium, CBZ, antipsychotics, or BZDs.[38] Low-dose VPA (125 to 500 mg/d) has been reported to be effective in reducing mood cycling in bipolar II disorder and cyclothymia.[39] DVPX oral loading of 20 mg/kg/d may produce a rapid reduction in manic and psychotic symptoms (within 3 days) without causing major side effects.[40] VPA also has antianxiety, antipanic, antimigraine, and antiaggressive effects.[35]

Carbamazepine

Carbamazepine (CBZ) is marketed as an anticonvulsant and for paroxysmal pain syndromes, such as trigeminal neuralgia. CBZ

TABLE 66–5. Product Formulations and Daily Dosage Range of Alternative Mood Stabilizers

Generic Name	Brand Name	Formulations	Daily Dose (mg/d)
Benzodiazepines			
Clonazepam	Klonopin	Tablet: 0.5, 1, 2 mg	1.5–20
Lorazepam	Ativan	Tablet: 0.5, 1, 2 mg Oral solution: 2 mg/mL Injection: 2 mg/mL	2–40
Anticonvulsants			
Gabapentin	Neurontin	Capsule: 100, 300, 400 mg	900–3600
Lamotrigine	Lamictal	Tablet: 25, 100, 150, 200 mg	50–500
Calcium Channel Antagonists			
Nimodipine	Nimotop	Capsule: 30 mg	30–120
Verapamil	Verelan	Capsule: 120, 180, 240, 360 mg	80–480
	Calan, Isoptin	Film-coated tablet: 40, 80, 120 mg	
	Calan, Isoptin	Extended-release tablet: 120, 180, 240 mg	

TABLE 66–6. Baseline and Routine Laboratory Testing for Patients Treated With Mood Stabilizers

	Carbamazepine		Lithium		Valproate	
	Baseline	*Follow Up Every 6–12 mo*	*Baseline*	*Follow Up Every 6–12 mo*	*Baseline*	*Follow Up Every 6–12 mo*
Baseline Tests						
Complete physical exam	+	–	+	–	+	–
General chemistry screen	+	–	+	–	+	–
Urine toxicology for substance abuse	+	–	+	–	+	–
Recommended Tests for Mood Stabilizers						
Pregnancy test if needed	+	–	+	–	+	–
Cardiac: ECG	+[a]	–	+[a]	–		
Hematologic						
CBC with differential	+	+[b]	+	+	+	+[b]
Platelet	+	+	–	–	+	+
Hepatic: liver enzymes	+	+[c]	–	–	+	+[c]
Metabolic						
Serum electrolytes	+	+	+	+	–	–
Total T_4, T_4 uptake, and TSH	+	+	+	+	–	–
Renal						
Serum creatinine	–	–	+[d]	+[d]	–	–
Urinalysis/osmolality/specific gravity	–	–	+	+[e]	–	–

[a]If > 40 yr or preexisting cardiac disease.
[b]CBZ and VPA: CBC monthly during first 2 months, then every 3–6 months; discontinue CBZ if platelets are < 100,000/mm^3 or WBC < 3000/mm^3.
[c]CBZ and VPA: LFTs monthly during first 2 months, then every 3–6 months; VPA: < 10 yr should have LFTs every 1–3 months.
[d]24-Hour urine volume and creatinine clearance for impaired renal functioning every 3 months.
[e]If urine volume > 3 L/d.
Compiled from Refs. 5 and 31.

has acute antimanic, antidepressant, and prophylactic effects comparable with lithium in bipolar disorder.[26,28,29,33] Positive predictors for response with CBZ include severe manic episodes, anxiety, dysphoria, schizoaffective or psychotic features, brain damage (abnormal EEG), patients with early-onset manic episodes, and a negative family history for mood disorders.[26,27,38] Preliminary evidence suggests that CBZ may be more effective than lithium in severe mania, rapid or continuous cycling, and in mixed episodes.[5,26,38] Approximately 60% of patients with acute mania respond to CBZ, 33% of bipolar depressed patients show good to moderate response, and effective prophylaxis is provided in approximately 60% of patients. There are some reports that CBZ may lose effectiveness over time; thus, further studies are needed to determine its long-term efficacy compared to lithium and VPA.[41]

ALTERNATE DRUG TREATMENTS

Antipsychotics

An acute manic episode may be treated with a mood stabilizer, an antipsychotic, or a combination of an antipsychotic and mood stabilizer for additive or synergistic effects.[5,28–30,31,42] Low-potency agents (chlorpromazine, thioridazine) are more sedating and cause more orthostatic hypotension, but have the advantage of causing fewer extrapyramidal side effects (EPS). The high-potency agents (haloperidol, fluphenazine) and moderate-potency agents (perphenazine, thiothixene) cause less sedation and fewer blood pressure changes but have increased risk of causing EPS (akathisia may cause agitation). Newer antipsychotic agents that block D_2 and 5-HT_2 receptors (clozapine, olanzapine, quetiapine, risperidone) cause fewer EPS and have been combined with mood stabilizers for treatment-resistant patients.[5,31,43–45] Clozapine appears to be effective in more refractory bipolar disorder, including rapid cyclers, but requires weekly white blood cell tests to monitor for agranulocytosis.[43,44] Risperidone in combination with mood-stabilizing drugs was found to be effective in acute mania with psychotic features.[45] Preliminary studies with olanzapine suggest that it may also have antimanic and antidepressant properties.[42]

Antipsychotics (and possibly CBZ and VPA) may have a more rapid onset of action than lithium (during the first week or two) to control the psychotic symptoms and increased psychomotor activity of acute mania.[30,42] Lower doses of antipsychotics are usually effective, but higher doses (e.g., haloperidol 5 to 10 mg intramuscularly or 10 to 25 mg orally every 4 to 6 hours as needed) may be required for psychotic or agitated patients.[33] Once acute mania is controlled (usually within 7 to 14 days), the antipsychotic should be gradually tapered and discontinued, and the patient maintained on the mood stabilizer alone to avoid neurotoxicity, postmania depression, EPS, supersensitivity psychosis, and tardive dyskinesia (TD). Intermittent use of conventional antipsychotics has been associated with an increased risk of TD in bipolar patients; therefore, antipsychotics should be used only in patients with psychotic symptoms.[30]

Benzodiazepines

An alternative to antipsychotic therapy in acute mania is the use of BZDs that facilitate GABAergic transmission.[5,30] Clonazepam, lorazepam, and other BZDs have been used in conjunction with lithium, CBZ, and VPA during acute mania and added for the treatment of insomnia during maintenance therapy.[28] BZDs cause minimal adverse effects and at higher doses rapidly sedate agitated patients.[33] BZDs have efficacy in the treatment of acute mania or breakthrough mania, but they may not be as effective for prophylactic therapy. Relative contraindications for long-term therapy for BZDs are drug or alcohol abuse or dependency.[5]

The oral dose of lorazepam in acute mania is approximately (0.05 mg/kg) 1 to 4 mg three times daily with the largest dose given at bedtime; gradual dosage increases up to 40 to 80 mg/d can be used to achieve maximum effects.[30] The dose of clonazepam is 0.5 to 2.0 mg three times daily and can be titrated up to 20 mg/d if needed.[30] Lower doses of BZDs should be used if combined with antipsychotics.[33] Lorazepam is available by parenteral injection (2 and 4 mg/mL); lower doses are required if administered IM or IV. Once the patient is stabilized, the dose can be gradually reduced to avoid daytime oversedation or administered at bedtime to promote sleep. BZDs should be gradually tapered over several weeks and discontinued to avoid withdrawal symptoms.

Antidepressants

Bipolar patients with depression may require antidepressants along with mood stabilizers to treat episodes of major depression.[46] Patients with a history of developing mania after a depressive episode or who have frequent cycling should be treated cautiously with antidepressants.[5,28] Bupropion and selective serotonin reuptake inhibitors (SSRIs) are considered first-line antidepressants, and monoamine oxidase inhibitors (MAOIs) and venlafaxine as second-line agents, for the treatment of moderate or severe bipolar depression (Chap. 65).[31] Trazodone, a sedating antidepressant, is sometimes used as an adjunctive medication for insomnia.[31] Bupropion has been recommended as the antidepressant of choice in patients with a high risk of developing mixed states or rapid cycling.[28,31] A psychotic depression can be treated with a mood stabilizer plus an antidepressant and antipsychotic agent or with ECT.[28,31] Lithium may be used as an augmenting agent with standard antidepressants but only has modest antidepressant effects when used alone.[31] Once the depressive episode has resolved, antidepressants should be gradually withdrawn and the patient can be maintained on a mood-stabilizing agent.

Calcium Channel Antagonists

Verapamil, nifedipine, and nimodipine are alternative mood stabilizers if patients cannot be treated with lithium, CBZ, or VPA.[30] Good candidates for calcium channel antagonists are lithium responders who cannot tolerate lithium's adverse effects.[47] Preliminary data suggest that verapamil has acute antimanic effects, although an open trial of verapamil in lithium-resistant mania did not show positive results.[30,33] Nifedipine (in combination with an antipsychotic) was effecting in several treatment-refractory schizoaffective and bipolar manic patients. Nimodipine has anticonvulsant properties; thus, it may be effective in ultra-rapid cycling patients and may have augmenting effects when combined with lithium.[48,49] The most common adverse effects of calcium channel antagonists are bradycardia and hypotension. The agents have low teratogenic effects and may have advantages over standard mood stabilizers for use during pregnancy and with breast feeding.[30]

Alternative Anticonvulsants

Lamotrigine is approved as adjunct therapy for partial seizures and inhibits the release of glutamate, an excitatory amino acid.[49] Lamotrigine has been reported to have antidepressant and mood-stabilizing effects in treatment-resistant bipolar type I and type II patients and may have augmenting effects when combined with VPA.[5,7,30,50,51] Lamotrigine is generally well tolerated and has fewer side effects than other mood stabilizers (e.g., GI upset, headache, dizziness, ataxia, and rash).[30] The incidence of rash appears to be greatest when lamotrigine is combined with VPA. Starting doses are usually 25 mg/d for the first week, with increases to 50 mg/d during the second week. Dosage ranges are 50 to 250 mg/d; some patients may require 500 to 700 mg/d.[30] When patients are on VPA, the starting dose of lamotrigine should be 25 mg every other day for the first 2 weeks due to potential inhibition of VPA's hepatic metabolism and risk of toxicity.

Gabapentin, approved as an adjunct for focal seizures with and without secondary generalization, has a structure similar to GABA, but it does not bind to the GABA receptor.[30] Its mood-stabilizing effects are being investigated, and preliminary case reports show some positive effects.[52,53] Starting dosages are 300 mg tid; titration up to 3600 mg/d may be needed in some patients. Gabapentin is associated with causing GI upset, somnolence, and dizziness, although it is usually well tolerated.

SPECIAL POPULATIONS

Patients with comorbid medical conditions or concomitant substance abuse, those over 65 years of age, and pregnant patients may require different treatment approaches.[31] Recommendations for first-line and second-line mood stabilizers or alternative treatments for special populations are provided in Table 66–7. Approximately 20% to 50% of bipolar women relapse postpartum; therefore, prophylaxis with mood stabilizers is recommended immediately postpartum to decrease the risk of relapse.[20]

DRUG CLASS INFORMATION

Lithium

Pharmacology, Mechanism of Action, and Pharmacokinetics. Despite numerous investigations into the biologic and clinical properties of lithium, there is no unified theory for its mechanism of action.[5,10] Lithium is a monovalent cation and competes with other monovalent and divalent cations (calcium, magnesium, potassium, sodium) in body tissues and at receptor sites. Neuropharmacologic effects of lithium include blockade of dopamine-receptor supersensitivity, decreases of β-adrenoceptor stimulation of adenylate cyclase, and increases of 5-HT, ACh, and GABA function. Lithium stabilizes postsynaptic-receptor sensitivity and has properties similar to calcium channel antagonists. Lithium decreases neurotransmitter activity by acting at the postsynaptic secondary messenger system; for example, it decreases neurotransmitter-coupled adenylate cyclase activity and cyclic AMP formation; decreases receptor–G-protein coupling; and decreases phosphoinositide metabolism. Lithium inhibits the enzyme inositol-1-phosphatase within neurons that are linked to phosphatidylinositol and blocks cAMP stimulation by adrenergic agonists.

Lithium has unique pharmacokinetics because it is a monovalent cation. Lithium is rapidly absorbed, is widely distributed with no protein binding, is not metabolized, and is excreted unchanged in the urine and in other body fluids (see Table 66–8 for pharmacokinetic information).[54,55]

Adverse Effects. Side effects of lithium are divided into those that occur early in therapy but are generally innocuous and transient, those that occur with long-term therapy and are usually not dose related, and toxic effects that occur with high serum concentrations. Common adverse effects of lithium are listed in Table 66–9.[10,31,54–56]

EARLY SIDE EFFECTS

Muscle weakness and lethargy are reported in about 30% of patients, but these symptoms are usually transient, and no intervention is generally needed. Polydipsia with polyuria and nocturia occurs in up to 70% of patients initially; these side effects

TABLE 66–7. Use of Mood Stabilizers in Special Populations

Condition	First Line	Second Line
Aggressive/violent patient	VPA or CBZ or lithium	VPA + lithium CBZ + lithium CBZ + VPA
Cardiac disease/heart failure	VPA	CBZ + lithium may worsen cardiac condition Calcium channel blockers
Drug abuse: alcohol or cocaine	VPA or lithium	CBZ VPA + lithium CBZ + lithium CBZ + VPA
Geriatric patients (in good health)	VPA or lithium	CBZ VPA + lithium CBZ + lithium CBZ + VPA
Liver disease	Lithium	Avoid CBZ + VPA Calcium channel blockers Conventional antipsychotics
Renal disease	VPA or CBZ	VPA + CBZ Calcium channel blockers Conventional antipsychotics
Neurologic disorder	VPA or CBZ	VPA + CBZ; lithium CBZ + lithium VPA + lithium Lamotrigine, gabapentin
Pregnancy[a]	Antipsychotic, benzodiazepine, calcium channel antagonist or ECT; lithium may have fewer teratogenic effects than previously thought and may be considered during first trimester	Lithium or VPA after first trimester Clonazepam or CBZ used as third-line agents after first trimester Lamotrigine

[a]All mood stabilizers (lithium, CBZ, VPA) have teratogenic risk; this risk is greater if the patient is on multiple agents; thus, monotherapy and lower serum levels are recommended.
Compiled from Refs. 7 and 31.

may diminish with time. Patients with polydipsia may experience weight gain, probably because of increased consumption of high-calorie fluids or fluid retention. As many as 40% of patients complain of headache, memory impairment, mental confusion, a decreased ability to concentrate, and impaired fine motor performance. A fine hand tremor may be observed in up to 50% of patients during the first week of lithium therapy, and this usually decreases in intensity with time.[54,56] The tremor is worsened by stress, concomitant use of antidepressants or antipsychotics, caffeine, sympathomimetics, and impending toxicity. Strategies to reduce the tremor include lowering the dose, dividing the dose to decrease peak serum concentrations, switching to an extended-release product, or adding a β-adrenergic antagonist (e.g., propranolol 20 to 120 mg/d, atenolol 50 mg/d, or metoprolol 20 to 80 mg/d).[5]

LONG-TERM SIDE EFFECTS

Lithium reduces the kidney's ability to concentrate urine and in some patients produces a nephrogenic diabetes insipidus (NDI).[54–56] Lithium-induced NDI is associated with normal or elevated serum concentrations of antidiuretic hormone and does not respond to exogenous vasopressin. Lithium-induced NDI is characterized by low urine-specific gravity and low osmolality polyuria (urine volumes of 5 to 6 L/d) and is treated with loop diuretics, thiazide diuretics, or triamterene. Amiloride, a potassium-sparing diuretic, has weaker natriuretic effects than thiazides and appears to be relatively safe with minimal effect on lithium clearance.[57] Fluid restriction is not recommended because dehydration increases the risk of lithium toxicity.

Numerous studies have examined the issue of lithium-induced renal effects (e.g., glomerulosclerosis, tubular atrophy, interstitial nephritis, urinary casts). In general, lithium causes minimal nephrotoxicity if patients are maintained on the lowest effective dose, if adequate hydration is maintained, and if toxicity is avoided.[56] During long-term lithium therapy, there may be a slight decrease in glomerular filtration rate (GFR) that is related to normal aging processes.[58] Because some patients receiving chronic lithium therapy develop rising levels of serum creatinine, renal functioning should be monitored every 6 to 12 months.[59]

Lithium is concentrated in the thyroid gland and interferes with thyroid hormone synthesis.[55,56] It blocks the release of thyroxine (T_4) and triidothyronine (T_3) mediated by thyrotropin, inhibits the organification of iodine, decreases the sensitivity of cell surface receptors to thyroid-stimulating hormone (TSH), inhibits the peripheral conversion of T_4 to T_3, and stimulates the formation of antithyroid antibodies in some patients.[56] Up to 30% of patients on maintenance lithium therapy develop transiently elevated TSH concentrations, and 5% to 15% of patients develop a goiter and/or hypothyroidism. Lithium-induced hypothyroidism is not dose related, is observed 10 times more frequently in women, and usually occurs after at least 18 months of therapy.[5] Subclinical hypothyroidism (normal total and free T_4 with TSH > 6 mIU/mL) is indicative of insufficient thyroid functioning.[56] Hypothyroidism does not require discontinuation of lithium, because exogenous thyroid hormone can be added to the regimen. If the TSH is greater than 5.0 mIU/mL, L-thyroxine 0.05 mg/d can be added (followed by a TSH level in 1 month) and increased up to 0.2 mg/d or higher (to achieve TSH > 0.1 and < 5.0). When

TABLE 66–8. Pharmacokinetics of Mood Stabilizers

	Carbamazepine	Lithium	Valproate
GI tract absorption			
Regular release	Slow and erratic; 85%–90%	Rapid; 95%–100%	Rapid; 100%
Syrup/suspension/solution	Faster rate of absorption	Faster rate of absorption; 100%	Faster rate of absorption
Extended-release/enteric-coated tablets	NA	Delayed absorption	Delayed absorption
Time to reach peak serum concentrations	1–5 h	1–12 h	1–5 h (VPA) 3–5 h (DVPX)
Delay of absorption by food	Yes	Yes	Yes
Volume of distribution	1 L/kg	0.7–1.0 L/kg	11 (total) 92 (free VPA) L/1.73 m^2
Crosses the placenta	Yes	Yes	Yes
Protein binding	70%–80%	No	90%–95%
Renal clearance	Yes	Yes; 10–40 mL/min	Yes
Metabolism	Hepatic microsomal oxidation (P450 2D6/3A4)	No	Hepatic oxidation and conjugation
Metabolites	Yes (active) 10,11-epoxide	No	Yes (inactive)
Kinetics	First order (after initial enzyme induction phase)	First order	First order
Half-life ($t_{1/2}$)			
Adults (normal)	25–60 h (initial)	14–30 h	5–20 h
Adults (epilepsy)	30–40 h (initial)		
After 3 weeks	12–20 h (due to autoinduction)		
During mania		8–20 h	
Geriatric patients		Up to 36 h	
Reduced renal function		40–50 h	
Reduced liver function	↑ $t_{1/2}$		↑ $t_{1/2}$

Compiled from Refs. 5, 54, 55, 65, and 70.

lithium is discontinued, patients should be reassessed for the need of exogenous thyroid hormone, because hypothyroidism is almost always reversible.

Lithium may cause a variety of benign and reversible cardiac effects, particularly T-wave flattening or inversion (in up to 30% of patients) and bradycardia.[55,56] Lithium rarely causes myocarditis, sinus node dysfunction, or sinoatrial block, but may aggravate ventricular arrhythmias and atrial premature contractions.[56] If a patient has significant preexisting cardiac disease, consultation with a cardiologist is recommended before initiation of lithium therapy.

Other long-term lithium side effects include benign reversible leukocytosis, weight gain (20% of patients gain more than 10 kg), and a variety of dermatologic effects (e.g., acne and acneiform eruptions, alopecia, psoriasis, pruritic dermatitis, maculopapular rashes, folliculitis).[56] Decreased libido, sexual dysfunction, dry mouth, alterations in taste, changes in glucose tolerance, hypercalcemia, and hyperparathyroidism have been reported. Severe neurologic disturbances such as myasthenia gravis, EPS, pseudotumor cerebri, and papilledema are occasionally observed.[57]

Toxicity. Lithium is an extremely toxic drug if accidentally or intentionally taken in overdose.[55,56] There are several situations that predispose patients to lithium toxicity: sodium restriction, dehydration, vomiting, diarrhea, and drug interactions that decrease lithium clearance. Heavy exercise, sauna baths, hot weather, and fever may promote sodium loss. Patients should be cautioned to maintain adequate sodium and fluid intake (2.5 to 3 quarts/d of fluids). Excessive use of coffee, tea, cola, and other caffeine-containing beverages and alcohol should be avoided.

Early signs of mild toxicity (1.2 to 1.5 mEq/L) include difficulty with memory and concentration, fine hand tremor, GI upset, muscle weakness, and fatigue. Moderate to severe toxic side effects are usually observed at concentrations greater than 1.5 mEq/L. These include confusion, lethargy, ataxia, dysarthria, nystagmus, emesis, increased deep-tendon reflexes, coarse tremors, and muscle fasciculations. Above 3.0 mEq/L, the syndrome progresses with choreoathetosis, seizures, irreversible brain damage, respiratory complications, coma, and death.

If severe lithium intoxication occurs (concentrations higher than 2.5 mEq/L taken 12 hours after the last dose), lithium should be discontinued and gastric lavage started in cases of overdoses. The patient should be monitored for fluid balance, renal and electrolyte status, and neurologic changes.[5] When lithium concentrations are above 3.5 to 4.0 mEq/L, the serum concentration should be measured every 3 hours until it is below 1.0 mEq/L. If the concentration does not drop greater than 10% every 3 hours or the lithium half-life is greater than 36 hours, intermittent hemodialysis (12 hours on and 12 hours off) should be started and continued until the lithium concentration is below 1.0 mEq/L taken 12 hours after the last dialysis. Hemodialysis can increase lithium clearance by 50 mL/min and peritoneal dialysis by 15 mL/min; rebound increases in serum lithium concentrations may occur 5 to 8 hours after dialysis. Several reports of irreversible neurologic deficits with ataxia, deficits in memory, and kidney damage with reduced GFR have been reported with lithium intoxication.[56]

Teratogenicity. Lithium may have a lower incidence of cardiovascular defects (particularly Epstein's anomaly) if taken during the first trimester than was previously thought.[60] Lithium freely crosses the placenta and is found in equal concentrations in maternal and fetal blood.[61] Neonatal lithium effects include hypotonia, bradycardia, cyanosis, low Apgar scores, hypothyroidism, and goiters.[5] Milk concentrations of lithium range from 30% to 100% of the mother's serum concentration, and serum

TABLE 66–9. Adverse Effects of Mood Stabilizers

System	Carbamazepine	Lithium	Valproate
Cardiac			
Arrhythmias	+		
Atrioventricular block	+		
Sinoatrial block		+	
T-wave flattening/inversion		+	
Widening of QRS		+	
Dermatologic			
Acne		+	
Exfoliative dermatitis (rare)	+	+	
Hair loss/thinning		+	+
Rash (maculopapular)	+	+	+
Erythema multiforme (rare)	+		+
Stevens–Johnson syndrome (rare)	+		+
Psoriasis		+	
Endocrine/Metabolic			
Female abnormalities			
Gynecomastia			+
Dysmenorrhea			+
Galactorrhea			+
Irregular menses			+
Polycystic ovaries			+
Hyperammonemia			+
Hyperandrogenism			+
Hyperparathyroidism		+	
Hyponatremia	+		+
Hypothyroidism		+	
Parotid gland swelling			+
Weight gain		+	
Gastrointestinal			
Abdominal pain	+	+	+
Abdominal bloating		+	
Constipation	+		
Diarrhea	+	+	+
Dyspepsia	+	+	+
Metallic taste		+	
Nausea	+	+	+
Vomiting (high doses)	+	+	+
Hematologic			
Agranulocytosis (rare)	+		
Aplastic anemia (rare)	+		

concentrations in the nursing infant are 10% to 50% of the mother's; for these reasons, breast feeding is discouraged.[5,61]

Drug–Drug Interactions. Several drug–drug interactions and cases of neurotoxicity have been reported with lithium and are summarized in Table 66–10.[55,62] Patients should be instructed to avoid taking diuretics and nonsteroidal anti-inflammatory agents (NSAIAs) unless under close medical supervision. Analgesics such as acetaminophen or aspirin and loop diuretics are less likely to interfere with lithium clearance.

Dosing and Administration. The recommended guidelines for baseline and routine laboratory testing for lithium are listed in Table 66–6. Information about dosing strategies and serum concentrations for the treatment of acute mania and for maintenance therapy are found in Table 66–11. Lithium therapy is usually initiated with moderate doses (600 mg/d) for prophylaxis and higher doses (900 to 1200 mg/d) for acute mania, using a two to three times a day dosing regimen.[63] Lower initial doses should be prescribed in the elderly and in clinical situations of impaired lithium excretion (e.g., concomitant diuretic therapy, low-salt diet, renal disease, dehydration, or decreased cardiac output). Divided dosing regimens and gradual titration of 300 to 600 mg/d every 2 to 3 days to target doses of 900 to 2400 mg/d helps to minimize the early, dose-related side effects of nausea and tremor. Single-daily dosing at bedtime with extended-release products may be used in patients with polyuria, because lower urine volume may occur with the once-per-day schedule than with multiple doses per day.[64] The dose should be adjusted based on the serum steady-state concentration drawn 12 hours ± 30 minutes after the last dose. Approximately 300 mg of lithium carbonate will raise the serum concentration by 0.3 ± 0.1 mEq/L. A therapeutic trial (lithium serum concentrations of 0.8 to 1.2 mEq/L) should last a minimum of 4 to 6 weeks. Acutely manic patients should have a serum concentration of at least 0.8 mEq/L, and some patients may require serum concentrations of 1.2 to 1.5 mEq/L to achieve a therapeutic response. Currently, there is no therapeutic reference range for single-daily dosing with lithium. The 12-hour postdose value may be 12% to 33% higher with extended-release preparations and lower with regular-release tablets compared with divided dosage schedules.

TABLE 66–9. (Continued)

System	Carbamazepine	Lithium	Valproate
Hematologic (continued)			
Anticoagulation			+
Eosinophilia	+		
Hemolytic anemia (rare)	+		
Leukocytosis		+	
Leukopenia	+		
Thrombocytopenia (rare)	+		+
Thrombocytosis		+	
Hepatic			
↑ Liver function tests (mild)	+		+
Hepatotoxicity (rare)			+
Neurologic/Neuromuscular			
Ataxia	+	+	+
Cognitive slowing	+	+	
Diplopia	+		
Dizziness	+		+
Headache	+		
Muscle weakness		+	
Nystagmus (high doses)	+	+	
Sedation	+	+	+
Tremor		+	+
Renal			
Nephrogenic diabetes insipidus (NDI)		+	
Nephrotoxicity (rare)		+	
Polyuria/polydipsia		+	
Syndrome of inappropriate antidiuretic hormone secretion (SIADH)	+		+
Toxicity in Overdoses	+	+	Relatively safe
Teratogenicity	*Class C*	*Class D*	*Class D*
Craniofacial defects	+		
Developmental delays	+		+
Finger hypoplasia	+		+
Neural tube defects	+		+
Cardiac defects		+	+
Cardiac malformations		+	
Hypothyroidism/goiter		+	
Hypotonia/cyanosis		+	

Compiled from Refs. 31, 54, 55, 57, 65, and 70.

Several dose prediction methods have been developed to obtain therapeutic lithium concentrations more rapidly and with fewer blood level determinations.[54] Cooper and associates in 1973 were the first to develop a single-point prediction method (based on a single lithium concentration drawn 24 hours after administering a 600-mg test dose). Other pharmacokinetic methods include a modified Cooper method using a 900- or 1200-mg test dose, a single- and multiple-point method by Perry, a 4-hour urine and a blood sample method by Norman and colleagues, and the Zetin and Pepin method that does not use lithium concentrations.[54] Saliva lithium levels have been used in children, but the exact saliva–serum ratio must be determined (~ 2:1 to 3:1).[54]

Therapeutic Drug Monitoring. When lithium is first started, a non–steady-state serum concentration taken 12 hours after the last dose is recommended every 2 to 3 days in patients prone to toxicity. When the desired serum concentration has been achieved (after dosage adjustments), blood level monitoring should be done every 1 to 2 weeks for 2 months or until lithium concentrations are stabilized.[31] Acutely manic patients may have an increased lithium clearance; once the manic episode abates, the lithium blood levels may increase.[54] Maintenance lithium serum concentrations are usually obtained every 3 to 6 months but can be adjusted to every 6 to 12 months for stabilized patients and every 1 to 2 months for patients with frequent mood episodes. Lithium levels are indicated 5 to 10 days after dosage changes, with the addition or deletion of drugs that affect lithium clearance, or with changes in renal functioning.[54] Lithium clearance increases by 50% to 100% during pregnancy and returns to normal postpartum; thus, monthly lithium levels should be obtained during pregnancy and weekly the month before delivery.[54] Lithium should be discontinued 2 to 3 days before delivery and restarted at prepregnancy doses a few days after delivery.[5]

Valproic Acid

Pharmacology, Mechanism of Action, and Pharmacokinetics. The exact mechanism of action of VPA is not known, but may be related to the inhibition of GABA metabolism, stimulation of GABA synthesis and release, and augmentation of the postsynaptic inhibitory effect of GABA.[10,35]

Valproate sodium is rapidly converted to VPA in the stomach, whereas DVPX sodium delayed-release tablets must pass into the small intestine to be converted to VPA.[65] A summary of the absorption, distribution, metabolism, and elimination data for VPA is found in Table 66–8.

TABLE 66–10. Drug Interactions With Mood Stabilizers

Drugs That Affect Serum Levels of Mood Stabilizers	Carbamazepine	Lithium	Valproate
ACE inhibitors		↑	
Calcium channel blockers	↑	?↓	
Carbamazepine			↓
Cimetidine	↑		↑
Ethosuximide			↓
Danazol	↑		
Diuretics[a]		↑	
Fluoxetine	↑	↑	↑
Fluvoxamine	↑		↑
Isoniazid	↑		
Ketoconazole	↑		
Lamotrigine	↑		↑
Macrolide antibiotics[b]	↑		
Metronidazole	↑		
NSAIAs[c]		↑	
Omeprazole	↑		
Phenobarbital/primidone	↓		↓
Phenytoin	↓		↓
Propoxyphene	↑		
Rifampin			↑
Salicylates			↑
Sodium bicarbonate		↓	
Sodium chloride		↓	
Sodium depletion[d]		↑	
Theophylline		↓	
Valproic acid/valproate	↑		
Carbamazepine (CBZ) Drug Interactions			
CBZ causes ↓ serum levels of the following medications due to induction of cytochrome P450 liver enzymes:			
Anticonvulsants (e.g., carbamazepine, lamotrigine, phenytoin, phenobarbital, primidone, valproic acid)			
Benzodiazepines (e.g., alprazolam, diazepam, midazolam, triazolam)			
Bupropion			
Cyclosporine			
Doxycycline			
Fentanyl			
Glucocorticoids (prednisolone)			
Mebendazole			
Methadone			
Neuroleptics (e.g., clozapine, haloperidol, phenothiazines)			
Neuromuscular blocking agents			

Adverse Effects. Compared with other anticonvulsants, VPA has a lower incidence of adverse effects and is generally well tolerated (Table 66–9).[35,65,66] The most frequent adverse effects reported are GI complaints and sedation. The GI complaints are usually transient and minimized by giving the drug with food, using lower initial doses with gradual increases in doses, or switching to DVPX. Other adverse effects of VPA include ataxia, lethargy, fine hand tremor, alopecia, changes in the texture or color of hair, pruritus, prolonged bleeding due to inhibition of platelet aggregation, transient increases in liver enzymes (transaminase and lactic dehydrogenase), and weight gain.[65,66] Valproate may chelate trace metals such as selenium or zinc, which contributes to hair loss; therefore, supplementation of selenium and zinc may help to manage hair thinning.[31] Thrombocytopenia may occur at higher doses, and patients should be monitored for bleeding and bruising. Rare cases of hepatitis have been reported (1 in 20,000 patients). Fatal hepatotoxicity is a rare, idiosyncratic, and non–dose-related adverse effect that occurs in 1 in 40,000 cases (all fatal cases were in children under the age of 10 with severe seizure disorders that were receiving multiple anticonvulsants).[5,65,66] VPA is not recommended during the first trimester of pregnancy (1% to 2% risk of neural tube birth defects, primarily spina bifida). VPA is excreted into human breast milk in low concentrations (up to 15% of the mother's serum concentrations); so far, no adverse effects in the nursing infant from VPA exposure have been reported.

Drug Interactions. There are several complex drug–drug interactions between VPA and other drugs (see Table 66–10).[62] The antiplatelet effects of VPA may potentiate the anticoagulant effects of warfarin and aspirin.[65,66] VPA also interferes with laboratory tests (e.g., it falsely elevates urine ketones and causes abnormal thyroid function tests). The concomitant administration of VPA with other CNS depressants or anticonvulsants may cause additive CNS-depressant effects. VPA may displace CBZ from serum protein–binding sites and thereby cause CBZ toxicity. CBZ may decrease VPA serum concentrations due to induction of hepatic metabolism.[67] The combination of DVPX and lithium has been used for the maintenance treatment of bipolar I disorder but may result in more adverse effects.[68]

Dosing. The initial starting dose of VPA is 500 to 750 mg/d (5 to 10 mg/kg/d) in divided doses, and the dose is adjusted up by 250 to 500 mg every 2 to 3 days to 1000 to 3000 mg/d (maxi-

TABLE 66–10. (Continued)

CBZ causes ↓ serum concentrations of the following, cont'd:
Oral anticoagulants (warfarin)
Oral contraceptives (estrogens and progestins)
Theophylline
Thyroid supplements (induces metabolism of T_3 and T_4)
Tricyclic antidepressants (e.g., amitriptyline, desipramine, imipramine, nortriptyline)

Adverse Reactions Reported With Combination Therapy

	Neurotoxicity	Impaired Thyroid Function	Cardiotoxicity	Bone Marrow Suppression
Lithium + SSRIs	+			
Lithium + calcium channel blockers	+		+	
Lithium + CBZ[e]	+	+		
Lithium + clonazepam	+			
Lithium + ECT	+			
Lithium + methyldopa	+			
Lithium + neuroleptics[f]	+			
CBZ + calcium channel blockers	+			
CBZ + clozapine[g]				+
CBZ + danazol	+			
CBZ + haloperidol	+			
CBZ + lamotrigine	+			
CBZ + isoniazid	+			
CBZ + macrolide antibiotics	+			
CBZ + monoamine oxidase inhibitors[h]	+			
VPA + clozapine[i]	+			
VPA + lamotrigine[j]	+			
VPA + traditional neuroleptics	+			

[a]Diuretics: Distal tubule (chlorthalidone, metolazone, thiazides); potassium-sparing (spironolactone, triamterene); carbonic anhydrase inhibitors (acetazolamide); loop diuretics (ethacrynic acid, furosemide) are less likely to ↑ lithium levels; amiloride has minimal effect.
[b]Macrolide antibiotics: Clarithromycin, erythromycin, troleandomycin; azithromycin, and dirithromycin are less likely to ↑ CBZ levels.
[c]NSAIAs: Diclofenac, ibuprofen, indomethacin, ketoralac, mefenamic acid, naproxen, phenylbutazone, and piroxicam ↑ lithium levels by 30%–60%; sulindac and aspirin have minimal effects on lithium clearance.
[d]Sodium depletion: diuretics; low-sodium diets; excessive exercise/sweating; protracted diarrhea/vomiting; salt deficiency.
[e]CBZ causes hyponatremia, which may cause lithium toxicity.
[f]Increased risk with higher doses and in elderly patients.
[g]CBZ + clozapine is not recommended due to increased risk of bone marrow suppression.
[h]CBZ may cause a hypertensive crisis with MAOIs (wait 14 days between MAOI and starting CBZ therapy).
[i]Additive side effects (drowsiness, weight gain); VPA may increase levels of clozapine's metabolites.
[j]VPA increases lamotrigine plasma levels; need to lower lamotrigine starting dose and increase more slowly; reports of rash and tremor; possibly synergistic effects.
Compiled from Refs. 5, 55, 62, 65, 70, and 77.

mum of 60 mg/kg/d) (see Table 66–11).[31] Higher initial loading doses of DVPX (20 mg/kg/d or 1200 to 1500 mg/d in divided doses) have been used in acutely agitated manic patients, resulting in therapeutic serum levels within 5 days and a rapid onset of antimanic response.[40,69] Therapeutic serum concentrations have not been established for VPA in bipolar disorder; most clinicians therefore use the anticonvulsant therapeutic range of 50 to 125 μ/mL taken 12 hours after the last dose; some patients may require up to 150 μg/mL during acute mania. Serum VPA levels are usually obtained every 1 to 2 weeks during the first 2 months, and then every 3 to 6 months during maintenance therapy.[31] Recommended baseline and routine laboratory tests for VPA are listed in Table 66–6.

Carbamazepine

Pharmacology, Mechanism of Action, and Pharmacokinetics. CBZ, a dibenzazepine derivative, is structurally related to TCAs. The precise mechanism of action of CBZ in affective disorders remains to be elucidated.[10,49,54] CBZ blocks the reuptake of NE, decreases the release of NE, increases ACh in the striatum, decreases DA and GABA turnover, blocks calcium influx through the NMDA–glutamate receptor, and decreases the activity of adenylate cyclase. In animal models, CBZ is effective in inhibiting amygdala kindling in the temporal lobe stimulated by NE and DA.[10,33] A summary of the absorption, distribution, metabolism, and elimination data for CBZ is found in Table 66–8 and in Chapter 52.

Adverse Effects. The most common adverse effects of CBZ involve CNS toxicity, which occurs in up to 60% of patients.[54,70] Neurologic side effects include drowsiness, dizziness, fatigue, clumsiness, ataxia, vertigo, blurred vision, diplopia, nystagmus, dysarthria, confusion, and headache. These side effects usually occur during the first few weeks of therapy and may be minimized by initiating therapy with low doses, gradually increasing the dose or giving a larger bedtime dose. GI side effects (nausea, vomiting, abdominal pain, diarrhea, constipation, anorexia) occur early in therapy in up to 15% of patients and can be minimized by administering the drug with food or reducing the daily dose.[70]

Serious hematologic dyscrasias are rare, with the exception of leukopenia.[71] Decreased white blood cell counts (WBCs) occur in 25% of patients and return to normal with CBZ discontinuation.[54] Patients with low- or below-normal pretreatment WBC and neutrophil counts should be monitored more closely due to

TABLE 66–11. Dosing Strategies and Serum Concentrations of Mood Stabilizers

	Carbamazepine	Lithium	Valproate
Acute Mania			
Initial dosing	100–200 mg bid with meals	900 mg/d or 15 mg/kg/d in divided doses with meals	500–750 mg/d or 5–10 mg/kg/d in divided doses with meals; oral loading of 20 mg/kg/d with DVPX
Target dose	400–2400 mg/d or 10–15 mg/kg/d; give bid or if ≤ 1200 mg in single hs dose	900–2400 mg/d; give bid or ≤ 1200 mg in single hs dose	1000–3000 mg/d or 20–60 mg/kg/d for mania; lower doses used for hypomania; give bid or single hs dose
Drug serum concentrations			
Adults	4–15 μg/mL[a] (not well established)	0.8–1.5 mEq/L	50–150 μg/mL (not well established)
Elderly/medically ill patients	4–8 μg/mL	0.6–0.8 mEq/L	45–75 μg/mL
Maintenance Therapy[b]			
Dose	400–1800 mg/d	600–1800 mg/d	15–45 mg/kg/d
Drug serum concentrations			
Adults	4–12 μg/mL	0.6–1.2 mEq/L	50–125 μg/mL
Elderly or medically ill patients	4–6 μg/mL	0.4–0.6 mEq/L	40–60 μg/mL

[a]CBZ serum levels decrease during the first 2–4 wk due to autoinduction of metabolism by the cytochrome P450 liver enzymes; higher doses of CBZ may be required to maintain adequate CBZ concentrations.

[b]There is no evidence that dosage reduction should be done for maintenance therapy of bipolar disorder, but lower doses are often tried when the patient is stabilized.

Compiled from Refs. 5, 54, 55, 63, 65, and 70.

increased risks of developing leukopenia (e.g., every 2 weeks for the first 1 to 3 months of treatment).[71] If leukopenia occurs (WBCs < 3000/mm^3 or neutrophil counts < 1000/mm^3), then the dose of CBZ should be decreased or discontinued.[71] CBZ may be restarted at lower doses when WBCs and neutrophils return to normal ranges. Patients should be educated about the signs and symptoms of leukopenia (mouth ulcers, sore throat, easy bruising, fever).

Other side effects include hypersensitivity reactions, dermatologic reactions (e.g., pruritic and erythematous rashes, urticaria, photosensitivity reactions, a lupus erythematosus-like syndrome), hyponatremia, and mild transient elevation of liver enzymes. Acute overdoses of CBZ are potentially lethal and serum levels above 15 μg/mL are associated with ataxia, choreiform movements, seizures, and coma. The safe use of CBZ during pregnancy and lactation has not been established; caution should be used in prescribing CBZ during the first trimester of pregnancy or during breast feeding.[54,70]

Drug–Drug Interactions. CBZ induces the hepatic microsomal P450 enzymes (1A2, 3A4, 2C9/10, and 2D6), which increases the elimination of many commonly coprescribed agents such as anticonvulsants, antidepressants, and antipsychotics. Concomitant drug therapies that inhibit the CYP450 3A4 isoenzyme system may result in CBZ toxicity (e.g., cimetidine, erythromycin, isoniazid, verapamil, diltiazem, propoxyphene, nefazodone, ketoconazole, itraconazole, fluvoxamine, and fluoxetine).[62,70,72,73] For a more complete description of drug interactions with CBZ, see Chapter 52 and Table 66–10.

Dosing and Administration. During an acute manic episode, CBZ should be started at 200 to 400 mg/d in divided doses with meals and increased by 200 mg every 2 to 4 days up to 10 to 15 mg/kg/d.[70] Dose-related side effects are common during the first week of therapy and slower titration may be required for some patients. If there is no response after 2 weeks, then the dose can be gradually increased to obtain serum concentrations between 6 and 12 μg/mL; some treatment-resistant patients may require serum concentrations up to 12 to 14 μg/mL. When patients are symptom free, CBZ can be initiated with lower initial doses (e.g., 100 to 200 mg/d, increased by 100 to 200 mg/d every 3 to 5 days up to 600 to 1200 mg/d). CBZ should be withdrawn slowly to avoid precipitating recurrence of bipolar symptoms or seizures in epileptic patients.

There appears to be no significant correlation between serum concentration and degree of antimanic or antidepressant response.[33] Most clinicians attempt to maintain serum concentrations of CBZ between 6 and 12 μg/mL. During the first month of therapy, serum concentrations of CBZ may decrease (due to autoinduction of hepatic oxidative enzymes that increases CBZ metabolism), and the dose may need to be increased to maintain therapeutic serum concentrations. Autoinduction of CBZ may begin by day 3 and can continue up to 30 days after the last dosage change. CBZ serum levels are usually obtained every 1 to 2 weeks during the first 2 months, and then every 3 to 6 months during maintenance therapy.[31] Recommended baseline and routine laboratory tests for CBZ are listed in Table 66–6.

PHARMACOECONOMIC CONSIDERATIONS

Clinical studies suggest that there are significant differences in the onset of action and the tolerance to adverse effects for lithium, CBZ, and VPA.[31,63] The mood stabilizers may have different efficacies for bipolar subtypes and there are now recognized positive predictors for clinical response to treatment.[26–28,31,37] These factors have a potential impact on drug selection, response rates, noncompliance due to adverse effects, and treatment costs (outpatient and inpatient care).

A recent review of health-economic studies found that DVPX conventional gradual titration or the rapid loading dose method (20 mg/kg/d) was associated with shorter lengths of hospital stays, particularly in patients with rapid cycling or mixed states.[74,75] Other studies have reported cost savings for DVPX sodium and for the combination of CBZ and lithium compared to lithium alone.[75,76] Further studies are needed to compare the different mood stabilizers (monotherapy versus combination therapy), dosing regimens (standard titration versus oral loading), termination of therapy due to adverse effects, and total costs for treatment.

EVALUATION OF THERAPEUTIC OUTCOMES

The evaluation of therapeutic outcomes for bipolar disorder requires frequent laboratory monitoring and regular office visits (every 1 to 2 weeks for acute or frequent episodes or 1 to 3 months for stable patients with infrequent episodes).[31,32] Patients should be actively involved with their treatment and help to monitor target symptoms and adverse effects. Because some patients have a rapid onset or "switching" in episodes, they should be encouraged to call their physician (or mental health professional involved with their care) in order to receive prompt treatment. More frequent office visits, telephone calls, and intensive outpatient programs are first-line strategies to prevent hospitalization during the acute treatment phase of a manic or depressive episode.

CONCLUSIONS

Bipolar disorder has a diversity of manifestations, recurrences of mood states, and clinical subtypes that requires tailoring the pharmacotherapy to the individual patient. Different treatment approaches and a combination of mood stabilizers is often required depending on the clinical state of the patient.[77] Bipolar disorder remains a challenge for clinicians because it is a constantly changing illness that requires close monitoring.

▶ PRINCIPLES OF PHARMACOTHERAPY

- Patients should be educated about their disorder (signs, symptoms, course, causes, outcomes) and treatments (nonpharmacologic and pharmacologic).
- The goal of therapy for bipolar disorder should be to improve the functioning of the patient and to limit adverse effects.
- Baseline and follow-up laboratory tests are required for mood stabilizers; drug level monitoring is required for mood stabilizers and should be obtained 12 hours postdose (preferably before the morning dose) and after steady-state serum concentrations are achieved (four to five times the $t_{1/2}$).
- Different mood episodes and subtypes of bipolar disorder respond differently to mood stabilizers.
- Augmentation strategies may be needed for mood states that do not respond to monotherapy (refractory states).
- Alternative mood stabilizers may be appropriate if the patient cannot tolerate lithium, CBZ, or VPA.
- Lithium, CBZ, and VPA may cause teratogenic effects and may cause adverse effects in the breast-fed infant.
- Maintenance (prophylaxis) therapy is based on the severity of the patient's disorder; the number of episodes; and risk of adverse effects. Patients who have experienced two or more episodes should receive lifelong therapy.

REFERENCES

1. Kessler RC, McGonagle KA, Zhao S, et al. Lifetime and 12-month prevalence of DSM-III-R psychiatric disorders in the United States: Results from the national comorbidity survey. Arch Gen Psychiatry 1994;51:8–19.
2. Goodwin FK, Jamison KR. Course and outcome. In: Goodwin FK, Jamison KR, eds. Manic-Depressive Illness. New York, Oxford University Press, 1990:127–156.
3. Nathan KI, Musselman DL, Schatzberg AF, Nemeroff CB. Biology of mood disorders. In: Schatzberg AF, Nemeroff CB, eds. Textbook of Psychopharmacology. Washington, DC, American Psychiatric Press, 1995:439–477.
4. Goodwin FK, Jamison KR. Biochemical and pharmacological studies. In: Goodwin FK, Jamison KR, eds. Manic-Depressive Illness. New York, Oxford University Press, 1990:416–502.
5. Janicak PG, Davis JM, Preskorn SH, Ayd FJ. Treatment with mood stabilizers. In: Janicak PG, Davis JM, Preskorn SH, Ayd FJ, eds. Principles and Practice of Psychotherapy, 2nd ed. Baltimore, Williams & Wilkins, 1997:403–473.
6. Petty F, Kramer GL, Fulton GK, et al. Low plasma GABA is a trait-like marker for bipolar illness. Neuropsychopharmacology 1993;9: 125–132.
7. Sporn J, Sachs G. The anticonvulsant lamotrigine in treatment-resistant manic-depressive illness. J Clin Psychopharmacol 1997;17: 185–189.
8. Trice SK, Benefield WH. Toprimate. The Habilitative Mental Healthcare Newsletter 1997;16:50–53.
9. Stoll AL, Sach GS, Cohen BM, et al. Choline in the treatment of rapid-cycling bipolar disorder: Clinical and neurochemical findings in lithium-treated patients. Biol Psychiatry 1996;40:382–388.
10. Post RM, Weiss SRB, Chuang D. Mechanisms of action of anticonvulsants in affective disorders: Comparisons with lithium. J Clin Psychopharmacol 1992;12:23S–35S.
11. Dubovsky SL, Murphy J, Christiano J, et al. The calcium second messenger system in bipolar disorders: Data supporting new research directions. J Neuropsychiatr Clin Neurosci 1992;4:3–14.
12. Resenick MM, Chaney KA, Chen J. G protein-mediated signal transduction as a target of antidepressant and antibipolar drug action: Evidence from model systems. J Clin Psychiatry 1996;57(suppl 13): 49–55.

13. Manji HK, Chen G, Hsiao JK, et al. Regulation of signal transduction pathways by mood- stabilizing agents: Implications for the delayed onset of therapeutic efficacy. J Clin Psychiatry 1996;57(suppl 13): 34–46.
14. Goodwin FK, Jamison KR. Sleep and biological rhythms. In: Goodwin FK, Jamison KR, eds. Manic-Depressive Illness. New York, Oxford University Press, 1990:541–574.
15. Faedda GL, Tondo L, Teicher MH, et al. Seasonal mood disorders: Patterns of seasonal recurrence in mania and depression. Arch Gen Psychiatry 1993;50:17–23.
16. Mood disorders. In: Diagnostic and Statistical Manual of Mental Disorders, 4th ed (DSM-IV). Washington, DC, American Psychiatric Press, 1994:317–390.
17. Goodwin FK, Jamison KR. The manic-depressive spectrum. In: Goodwin FK, Jamison KR, eds. Manic-Depressive Illness. New York, Oxford University Press, 1990:74–84.
18. Akiskal HS. The prevalent clinical spectrum of bipolar disorders: Beyond DSM-IV. J Clin Psychopharmacol 1996;16(suppl 1):4S–14S.
19. Goodwin FK, Jamison KR. Clinical description. In: Goodwin FK, Jamison KR, eds. Manic-Depressive Illness. New York, Oxford University Press, 1990:15–55
20. Leibenluft E. Women with bipolar illness: Clinical and research issues. Am J Psychiatry 1996;153:163–173.
21. Goodwin FK, Jamison KR. Manic-depressive illness, creativity, and leadership. In: Goodwin FK, Jamison KR, eds. Manic-Depressive Illness. New York, Oxford University Press, 1990:332–367.
22. Dilsaver SC, Swann AC, Shoaib AM, et al. Depressive mania associated with nonresponse to antimanic agents. Am J Psychiatry 1993; 150:1548–1551.
23. Goodwin FK, Jamison KR. Alcohol and drug abuse in manic-depressive illness. In: Goodwin FK, Jamison KR, eds. Manic-Depressive Illness. New York, Oxford University Press, 1990:210–226.
24. Goodwin FK, Jamison KR. Suicide. In: Goodwin FK, Jamison KR, eds. Manic-Depressive Illness. New York, Oxford University Press, 1990:227–246.
25. Strakowski SM, McElroy SL, Keck PE, West SA. Suicidality among patients with mixed and manic bipolar disorder. Am J Psychiatry 1996;153:674–676.
26. Keck PE, McElroy SL. Outcome in the pharmacologic treatment of bipolar disorder. J Clin Psychopharmacol 1996;16(suppl 1):15S–23S.
27. Calabrese JR, Fatemi SH, Kujawa M, Woyshville MJ. Predictors of response to mood stabilizers. J Clin Psychopharmacol 1996;16(suppl 1): 24S–31S.
28. Sachs GS. Bipolar mood disorder: Practical strategies for acute and maintenance phase treatment. J Clin Psychopharmacol 1996;16(suppl 1): 32S–47S.
29. Bowden CL. Role of newer medications for bipolar disorder. J Clin Psychopharmacol 1996;16(suppl 1):48S–55S.
30. Dubovsky SL, Buzan RD. Novel alternatives and supplements to lithium and anticonvulsants for bipolar affective disorder. J Clin Psychiatry 1997;58:224–242.
31. Frances A, Docherty JP, Kahn DA, et al. The expert consensus guideline series. Treatment of bipolar disorder. J Clin Psychiatry 1996;57 (suppl 12A):1–89.
32. Hirschfeld RMA, Clayton PJ, Cohen I, et al. Practice guideline for the treatment of patients with bipolar disorder. Am J Psychiatry 1994;151 (suppl):1–31.
33. Chou JC. Recent advances in treatment of acute mania. J Clin Psychopharmacol 1991;11:3–21.
34. Gelenberg AJ, Kane JM, Lavori P, et al. Comparison of standard and low serum levels of lithium for maintenance treatment of bipolar disorder. N Engl J Med 1994;331:591–598.
35. Guay DRP. The emerging role of valproate in bipolar disorder and other psychiatric disorders. Pharmacotherapy 1995;15:631–647.
36. Bowden CL, Brugger AM, Swann AC, et al. Efficacy of divalproex vs lithium and placebo in the treatment of mania. The Depakote Mania Study Group. JAMA 1994;271:918–924.
37. Bowden CL. Predictors of response to divalproex and lithium. J Clin Psychiatry 1995;56(suppl 3):25–30.
38. Dilsaver SC. The manic syndrome: Factors which may predict a patient's response to lithium, carbamazepine, and valproate. J Psychiatry Neurosci 1993;18:61–66.
39. Jacobsen FM. Low-dose valproate: A new treatment for cyclothymia, mild rapid cycling disorders, and premenstrual syndrome. J Clin Psychiatry 1993;54:229–234.
40. McElroy SL, Keck PE, Stanton SP, et al. A randomized comparison of divalproex oral loading versus haloperidol in the initial treatment of acute psychotic mania. J Clin Psychiatry 1996;57:142–146.
41. Post RM. Issues in the long-term management of bipolar affective illness. Psychiatr Ann 1993;23:86–93.
42. McElroy SL, Keck PE, Strakowski SM. Mania, psychosis, and antipsychotics. J Clin Psychiatry 1996;57(suppl 3):14–26.
43. Kimmel SE, Calabrese JR, Woyshville MJ, et al. Clozapine in treatment-refractory mood disorders. J Clin Psychiatry 1994;55:91–93.
44. Calabrese JR, Kimmel SE, Woyshville MJ, et al. Clozapine for treatment-refractory mania. Am J Psychiatry 1996;153:759–764.
45. Tohen M, Zarate CA, Centorrino F, et al. Risperidone in the treatment of mania. J Clin Psychiatry 1996;57:249–253.
46. Zornberg GL, Pope HG. Treatment of depression in bipolar disorder: New directions for research. J Clin Psychopharmacol 1993;13: 397–408.
47. Dubovsky SL. Calcium antagonists in manic-depressive illness. Neuropsychobiology 1993;27:184–192.
48. Pazzaglia PJ, Post RM, Keller TA, et al. Preliminary controlled trial of nimodipine in ultra-rapid cycling affective dysregulation. Psychiatry Res 1993;49:257–272.
49. Post RM, Ketter TA, Denicoff K, et al. The place of anticonvulsant therapy in bipolar illness. Psychopharmacology 1996;128:115–129.
50. Calabrese JR, Fatemi SH, Woyshville MJ. Antidepressant effects of lamotrigine in rapid cycling bipolar disorder. Am J Psychiatry 1996; 153:1236. Letter.
51. Walden J, Hesslinger B, van Calker D, Berger M. Addition of lamotrigine to valproate may enhance efficacy in the treatment of bipolar affective disorder. Pharmacopsychiatry 1996;29:193–195.
52. Schaffer CB, Schaffer LC. Gabapentin in the treatment of bipolar disorder. Am J Psychiatry 1997;154:291–292. Letter.
53. Stanton S, Keck PE, McElroy SL. Treatment of acute mania with gabapentin. Am J Psychiatry 1997;154:287. Letter.
54. Perry PJ, Alexander B, Liskow BI. Psychotropic Drug Handbook, 7th ed. Washington, DC, American Psychiatric Press, 1997:221–302.
55. Lithium salts. In: McEvoy GK, Litvak K, Walsh OH, et al, eds. AHFS Drug Information 98. Bethesda, MD, American Society of Health-System Pharmacists, 1998:1987–1995.
56. Kane JM, Lieberman JA, eds. Adverse Effects of Psychotropic Drugs. New York, Guilford Press, 1992.
57. Martin A. Clinical management of lithium-induced polyuria. Hosp Commun Psychiatry 1993;44:427–428.
58. Bendz H, Aurell M, Balldin J, et al. Kidney damage in long-term lithium patients: A cross-sectional study of patients with 15 years or more on lithium. Nephrol Dial Transplant 1994;9:1250–1254.
59. Gitlin MJ. Lithium-induced renal insufficiency. J Clin Psychopharmacol 1993;13:276–279.
60. Cohen LS, Friedman JM, Jefferson JW, et al. A reevaluation of risk of in utero exposure to lithium. JAMA 1994;271:146–150.
61. Schou M. Lithium treatment during pregnancy, delivery, and lactation: An update. J Clin Psychiatry 1990;51:410–413.
62. Hansten and Horn's Drug Interactions Analysis and Management. Vancouver, WA, Applied Therapeutics, 1997.
63. Bowden CL. Dosing strategies and time course or response to antimanic drugs. J Clin Psychiatry 1996;57(suppl 13):4–9.
64. Bowen RC, Grof P, Grof E. Less frequent lithium administration and lower urine volume. Am J Psychiatry 1991;148:189–192.
65. Valproate sodium, valproic acid, and divalproex sodium. In: McEvoy GK, Litvak K, Welsh OH, et al, eds. AHFS Drug Information 98.

Bethesda, MD, American Society of Health System Pharmacists, 1998:1777–1782.

66. Balfour JA, Bryson HM. Valproic acid. A review of its pharmacology and therapeutic potential in indications other than epilepsy. CNS Drugs 1994;2:144–173.
67. Tohen M, Castillo J, Pope HG, Herbstein J. Concomitant use of valproate and carbamazepine in bipolar and schizoaffective disorder. J Clin Psychopharmacol 1994;14:67–70.
68. Solomon DA, Ryan CE, Keitner GI, et al. A pilot study of lithium carbonate plus divalproex sodium for the continuation and maintenance treatment of patients with bipolar I disorder. J Clin Psychiatry 1997; 58:95–99.
69. Keck P Jr, McElroy SL, Tugrul KC, et al. Valproate oral loading in the treatment of acute mania. J Clin Psychiatry 1993;54:305–308.
70. Carbamazepine. In: McEvoy GK, Litvak K, Welsh OH, et al, eds. AHFS Drug Information 98. Bethesda, MD, American Society of Hospital Pharmacists, 1998:1757–1761.
71. Sobotka JL, Alexander B, Cook BL. A review of carbamazepine's hematologic reactions and monitoring recommendations. DICP Ann Pharmacother 1990;24:1214–1219.
72. Ketter TA, Post RM, Worthington K. Principles of clinically important drug interactions with carbamazepine, part I. J Clin Psychopharmacol 1991;11:198–203.
73. Ketter TA, Post RM, Worthington K. Principles of clinical important drug interactions with carbamazepine, part II. J Clin Psychopharmacol 1991;11:306–313.
74. Keck PE, McElroy SL, Bennett JA. Health-economic implications of the onset of action of antimanic agents. J Clin Psychiatry 1996; 57(suppl 13):13–18.
75. Frye MA, Altshuler LL, Szuba MP, et al. The relationship between antimanic agent for treatment of classic or dysphoric mania and length of hospital stay. J Clin Psychiatry 1996;57:17–21.
76. Keck PE Jr, Nabulsi AA, Taylor JL, et al. A pharmacoeconomic model of divalproex vs lithium in the acute and prophylactic treatment of bipolar I disorder. J Clin Psychiatry 1996;57:213–222.
77. Freeman MP, Stoll AL. Mood stabilizer combinations: A review of safety and efficacy. Am J Psychiatry 1998;155:12–21.

67

Anxiety Disorders

Cynthia K. Kirkwood, PharmD

Anxiety is an emotional state commonly caused by the perception of real or potential danger that threatens the security of the individual. Everyone experiences a certain amount of nervousness and apprehension when faced with a stressful situation. Usually the response is reasonable and adaptive, and contains a built-in control mechanism to return to a normal physiologic state.

If anxiety becomes excessive or symptoms are prolonged, it can produce uncomfortable and potentially incapacitating psychological and physical arousal. Some persons experience anxiety symptoms and possess fears that are frequently abnormal, irrational, and severely impair normal daily functioning. These persons often suffer from an anxiety disorder.[1]

Anxiety disorders are among the most frequent mental disorders encountered in clinical practice. One-fourth of the population will experience at least one anxiety disorder in their lifetime. Unfortunately, the majority of patients with anxiety disorder receive no professional treatment.[2]

Failure to diagnose and manage anxiety disorders results in negative outcomes—overuse of health care resources and increased morbidity and mortality.[3] Of the one-third of 6307 primary care clinic outpatients who met initial screening criteria for anxiety, only 44% were diagnosed and treated. These patients had a 52% rate of comorbidity with other psychiatric disorders and showed significant impairment in function and well-being.[4]

To treat anxiety appropriately, the clinician must make a reliable diagnosis. It is essential that the distinction between short-term symptoms of anxiety and anxiety disorders be understood. Common or situational anxiety is a normal response to a stressful situation. Although symptoms may be severe, they are temporary and usually last no more than 2 or 3 weeks. Although short-term, "as-needed" treatment with an anxiolytic agent such as a benzodiazepine (BZ) is common and may provide some symptomatic relief, prolonged drug therapy is unnecessary.[5]

EPIDEMIOLOGY

According to the National Comorbidity Survey of noninstitutionalized persons aged 15 to 54 years, the 12-month prevalence rate for anxiety disorders averaged 17.2%, and the lifetime rate was 24.9%. The lifetime prevalence of generalized anxiety disorder (GAD) was 5.1% and panic disorder was 3.5%.[2] Social phobia was the most common anxiety disorder, with a lifetime prevalence of 13.3% and 12-month rate of 7.9%.[2] Specific phobia has a lifetime prevalence rate of 11.3%; however, patients are not seriously impaired in terms of daily functioning and few persons seek treatment.[1,2]

In general, anxiety disorders are a group of heterogeneous illnesses that develop before age 30 and are more common in women and those with a family history of anxiety and depression. Patients often develop another anxiety disorder, major depression, or substance abuse.[1,2] Anxiety disorders are generally chronic in nature, and although symptoms wax and wane over time, patients are rarely completely symptom free.[1,6] Most patients with anxiety disorders can be treated effectively. However, long-term treatment may be required, and relapse after drug discontinuation is common.[6]

ETIOLOGY

The differential diagnosis of anxiety disorders includes medical and psychiatric illnesses and certain drugs. Evaluation of the anxious patient requires a complete physical and mental status examination, appropriate laboratory tests, toxicologic screen, and a thorough knowledge of the patient's medical, psychiatric, and drug history.[5,7]

MEDICAL DISEASES ASSOCIATED WITH ANXIETY

Anxiety symptoms are an inherent part of the initial clinical presentation in several medical disorders, thus complicating the distinction between anxiety disorders and medical disorders.[7,8] If the anxiety symptoms are secondary to a medical illness, they will usually subside as the medical situation stabilizes.[8] However, the knowledge that one has a physical illness may trigger anxious feelings and further complicate therapy.

Symptoms of anxiety frequently present in medical disorders include palpitations, tachycardia, chest pain or tightness, shortness of breath, and hyperventilation.[5] Medical disorders most closely associated with anxiety are listed in Table 67–1.[8]

Clinically significant anxiety is present as a reaction to postmyocardial infarction (MI), postcardiac surgery, and asthma, and it may influence treatment outcomes. After hospital discharge of MI patients, anxiety and depression may interfere with recovery and subsequent return to work. These patients often require medication for anxiety symptoms.[5]

PSYCHIATRIC DISEASES ASSOCIATED WITH ANXIETY

Anxiety may be a concomitant symptom of several major psychiatric illnesses. Anxiety symptoms are extremely common in patients with mood disorders, schizophrenia, delir-

TABLE 67–1. Common Medical Disorders Associated With Anxiety Symptoms

Cardiovascular	
	Angina, arrhythmias, hypertension, mitral valve prolapse, myocardial infarction
Endocrine and metabolic	
	Anemia, Cushing's disease, hyperthyroidism, hypothyroidism, hypoglycemia, hypokalemia, insulinoma, pheochromocytoma
Gastrointestinal	
	Colitis, irritable bowel syndrome, peptic ulcer
Neurologic	
	Akathisia, essential tremor, seizures, migraine, pain, Parkinson's disease
Respiratory system	
	Asthma, chronic obstructive lung disease, hyperventilation, pneumonia, pulmonary embolus

Compiled from Refs. 7 and 8.

ium, dementia, and substance use disorders.[8] Most psychiatric patients will have two or more concurrent psychiatric disorders (comorbidity) within their lifetime.[2] To appropriately treat patients with anxiety disorders, it is important to adequately assess and diagnose all comorbid psychiatric conditions.

DRUG-INDUCED ANXIETY

The two major drug classes that cause anxiety symptoms are the central nervous system stimulants and depressants (Table 67–2). Anxiety occurs during the use of these drugs in a dose-dependent manner, but ingestion of minimal amounts may result in marked anxiety, including panic attacks, in some individuals.[7,9]

Anxiety occasionally occurs during the use of CNS depressants, especially in children and the elderly; however, anxiety complaints are more common as complications of drug withdrawal after the abrupt discontinuation of these agents.[8]

PATHOPHYSIOLOGY

Data from biochemical and neuroimaging studies indicate that the modulation of normal and pathologic anxiety states is associated with multiple brain structures and abnormal function in several neurotransmitter systems including norepinephrine (NE), γ-aminobutyric acid (GABA), and serotonin (5-HT). Current neuroanatomic models of fear and anxiety include several key brain structures. The amygdala, a temporal lobe structure, plays a critical role in the assessment of fear stimuli and response to danger.[10] The locus ceruleus (LC), located in the brainstem, is the primary NE-containing site in the brain with widespread projections to areas responsible for implementing fear responses (e.g., vagus, lateral and paraventricular hypothalamus). The hippocampus is integral in the consolidation of traumatic memory and, along with the entorhinal cortex, contextual fear conditioning (involved in chronic anxiety). The hypothalamus is the principle site for integrating neuroendocrine and autonomic responses to threat.[10]

NEUROCHEMICAL THEORIES

NORADRENERGIC MODEL

The basic premise of the noradrenergic theory is that the autonomic nervous system of anxious patients is hypersensitive and overreacts to various stimuli. Many anxious patients clearly display symptoms of peripheral autonomic hyperactivity.[10] In response to anxiety or fearful situations, the LC serves as an alarm center, activating NE release and stimulating the sympathetic and parasympathetic nervous systems. Chronic, central noradrenergic overactivity down-regulates α_2-adrenoreceptors in GAD patients. This receptor is hypersensitive in some patients with panic disorder.[10,11]

By administering drugs that have a relatively specific effect on the LC, researchers have further explored the NE theory of anxiety and panic disorder. Drugs with anxiogenic effects (e.g., yohimbine and isoproterenol) stimulate LC firing and increase noradrenergic activity. These agents often produce subjective feelings of anxiety and can precipitate a panic attack in those with panic disorder, but not in normal volunteers or those with other psychiatric illnesses.[11] Drugs with anxiolytic or antipanic effects (e.g., BZs, antidepressants, clonidine) inhibit LC firing, decrease noradrenergic activity, and block the effects of anxiogenic drugs.[12]

BENZODIAZEPINE RECEPTOR MODEL

The BZ receptor is functionally and structurally linked to the GABA type A ($GABA_A$) receptor and a chloride ion channel; this is referred to as the GABA–BZ receptor complex.[13,14] GABA, the major inhibitory neurotransmitter in the CNS, is involved in nerve transmission in nearly one-third of brain impulses. The GABA system also has a strong regulatory or inhibitory effect on the 5-HT and NE systems. When GABA binds to its receptor, the adjacent chloride ion channel opens and permits the influx of negatively charged chloride ions; this results in hyperpolarization of the cell membrane and causes a decrease in nerve cell excitability.

The role of the GABA–BZ receptor complex in anxiety disorders has not been well characterized. Abnormal

TABLE 67–2. Drugs Associated With Anxiety Symptoms

CNS depressant withdrawal	
	Anxiolytics/sedatives, barbiturates, ethanol, narcotic agonists
CNS stimulants	
	Prescription drugs: albuterol, amphetamines, cocaine, diethylpropion, isoproterenol, methylphenidate
	Nonprescription drugs: caffeine, ephedrine, phenylephrine, phenylpropanolamine, pseudoephedrine
Miscellaneous	
	Anticholinergic (toxicity), cycloserine, digitalis (toxicity), dapsone, dopamine, isoniazid, levodopa, lidocaine, antipsychotics, nicotinic acid, selective serotonin reuptake inhibitor antidepressants, steroids, theophylline

sensitivity to the antagonism of the BZ receptor was demonstrated in panic disorder patients. In patients with GAD, down-regulated central BZ receptors and low levels of peripheral lymphocyte and platelet BZ receptors that reverted to normal with treatment were reported.[15]

SEROTONIN MODEL

Although there is increasing evidence that the 5-HT system is altered in patients with anxiety disorders, definitive evidence that shows a clear abnormality in 5-HT function remains to be demonstrated. 5-HT is primarily an inhibitory neurotransmitter that is used by neurons originating in the raphe nuclei of the brainstem and projecting diffusely throughout the brain (e.g., cortex and limbic system).[16] The diverse actions of 5-HT are regulated by approximately 14 different receptor subtypes.[17]

Buspirone is a selective 5-HT_{1A} partial agonist that is effective for GAD but not for panic disorder. Because the selective 5-HT_{1A} partial agonists reduce serotonergic activity, GAD symptoms may reflect excessive 5-HT transmission or overactivity of the stimulatory 5-HT pathways. The role of 5-HT in panic disorder is unclear; however, 5-HT may play a role in the development of anticipatory anxiety.[11] Although buspirone is not an effective antipanic agent, the selective 5-HT reuptake inhibitors (SSRIs) are effective antipanic compounds.[16] Limited data indicate that there is an abnormality in 5-HT function and possibly dopaminergic activity in social phobia.[11]

PEPTIDE THEORY

The role of cholecystokinin (CCK) and other neuropeptides (i.e., neuropeptide Y) in anxiety disorders is a current area of research. CCK is an abundant peptide with receptors located throughout the CNS and high densities in the hypothalamus, limbic system, basal ganglia (BG), cortex, and brainstem. CCK increases the activity of catecholamines in the LC and coexists with GABA-producing neurons. Panic patients may have supersensitive postsynaptic CNS CCK_B receptors.[15]

NEUROIMAGING STUDIES

Functional neuroimaging studies suggest that frontal and occipital brain areas are integral to the anxiety response. There is some evidence that patients with panic disorder have abnormal activation of the parahippocampal region and prefrontal cortex at rest. Panic anxiety is associated with activation of brainstem and BG areas.[11] In GAD patients, there is an abnormal increase in cortical activity and a decrease in BG activity. After BZ treatment, BG activity increases and cortical activity is reduced.[11,15]

CLINICAL PRESENTATION

The *Diagnostic and Statistical Manual of Mental Disorders,* fourth edition (DSM-IV) classifies anxiety disorders into several categories (Table 67–3).[1] The characteristic features of these illnesses are anxiety and avoidance behavior. Obsessive–compulsive disorder is discussed in Chapter 68.

TABLE 67–3. DSM-IV Classification of Anxiety Disorders

A. Generalized anxiety disorder
B. Panic disorder
   With agoraphobia
   Without agoraphobia
C. Agoraphobia without a history of panic disorder
D. Phobic disorders
   Social phobia
   Specific phobia
E. Obsessive–compulsive disorder
F. Posttraumatic stress disorder
G. Acute stress disorder

Compiled and reprinted with permission from the Diagnostic and Statistical Manual of Mental Disorders, 4th ed. Copyright 1994 American Psychiatric Association.

GENERALIZED ANXIETY DISORDER

The diagnostic criteria (Table 67–4) for GAD require persistent symptoms for at least 6 months.[1] The essential feature of GAD is unrealistic or excessive anxiety and worry about a number of events or activities.[1]

GAD has a gradual onset, usually in the early 20s, but may be precipitated in later life by severe psychological stressors. Stressful life events may also play a role in the persistence of symptoms. The course of the illness is

TABLE 67–4. DSM-IV Diagnostic Criteria for Generalized Anxiety Disorder

A. Excessive anxiety and worry (apprehensive expectation), occurring more days than not for at least 6 months, about a number of events or activities (such as work or school performance).
B. The person finds it difficult to control worry.
C. Anxiety and worry, associated with three (or more) of the following six symptoms (with at least some symptoms present more days than not for the past 6 months):
   1. Restlessness or feeling keyed up or on edge
   2. Being easily fatigued
   3. Difficulty concentrating or mind going blank
   4. Irritability
   5. Muscle tension
   6. Sleep disturbance
D. Anxiety and worry, not confined to features of another psychiatric illness (such as having a panic attack, being embarrassed in public).
E. Constant worry causing significant distress, and significant impairment in social, occupational, or other important areas of functioning.
F. Excessive anxiety and worry, not caused by a drug substance (drugs of abuse or medications) or a general medical disorder, and not occurring exclusively as part of another psychiatric disorder (such as a mood disorder).

Adapted and reprinted with permission from the Diagnostic and Statistical Manual of Mental Disorders, 4th ed. Copyright 1994 American Psychiatric Association.

TABLE 67–5. DSM-IV Diagnostic Criteria for Panic Attack

A discrete period of intense fear or discomfort, in which at least four of the following symptoms developed abruptly and reached a peak within 10 minutes:

1. Palpitations or accelerated heart rate
2. Sweating
3. Trembling or shaking
4. Sensations of shortness of breath or smothering
5. Feeling of choking
6. Chest pain or discomfort
7. Nausea or abdominal distress
8. Feeling dizzy, unsteady, lightheaded, or faint
9. Derealization or depersonalization
10. Fear of losing control or going crazy
11. Fear of dying
12. Numbness or tingling sensations (paresthesias)
13. Chills or hot flushes

Adapted and reprinted with permission from the Diagnostic and Statistical Manual of Mental Disorders, 4th ed. Copyright 1994 American Psychiatric Association.

chronic with multiple spontaneous exacerbations and remissions.[1,2,18] Patients report substantial interference with their lives and have a high probability of seeking treatment.[18] The majority of GAD patients will eventually develop another mental disorder.[2,18]

PANIC DISORDER

Panic disorder begins as a series of unexpected (spontaneous) panic attacks, involving an intense, terrifying fear, similar to that caused by life-threatening danger. The unexpected panic attacks are followed by at least 1 month of persistent concern about having another panic attack, worry about the possible consequences of the panic attack, or a significant behavioral change related to the attacks.[1] During an attack, patients often describe an overwhelming sense of doom, a fear of dying or losing control, and numerous physical symptoms (Table 67–5).[1] Panic attacks usually last no more than 20 to 30 minutes, with the peak intensity of symptoms within the first 10 minutes. Often patients seek help at a physician's office or emergency department, only to have their symptoms resolve before or upon arrival. Because panic symptoms mimic those present in several medical conditions, patients are often misdiagnosed, and multiple referrals are common.[1,7]

Secondary to the panic attacks, many patients eventually develop agoraphobia. Agoraphobia is anxiety about being in places or situations where escape might be difficult or where help might not be available in the event of having a panic attack.[1] As a result, patients often avoid specific situations (e.g., crowded places, traveling away from home) where they fear a panic attack might occur.[1]

Panic disorder has an adverse impact on the patient's quality of life, including a significant degree of social and work impairment. Complications include depression (50% to 65% have major depressive disorder), alcohol abuse, and increased use of medications, health services, and emergency rooms.[19] Patients with panic disorder have a high lifetime risk for suicide attempts, compared to the general population.[19] The usual course is chronic but waxing and waning.

SOCIAL PHOBIA

The essential feature of social phobia is a marked and persistent fear of social or performance situations in which embarrassment may occur. Social phobia exists in two distinct forms: (1) generalized, in which anxiety is related to most social situations (e.g., dating or speaking with authority figures); and (2) discrete, in which the anxiety is related to performance and is specific for one or two situations (e.g., public speaking, musical performance).[1,7] Unlike most anxiety disorders, the object of this fearful feeling is clearly recognized. Most often, the social or performance situation is avoided, but it is sometimes endured with dread. The fear and avoidance of the situation must interfere significantly with the person's daily functioning.[1]

SPECIFIC PHOBIA

Specific phobia is marked and persistent fear of a circumscribed object or situation (e.g., animals, water, enclosed places). Apart from contact with the feared object or situation, the patient is usually free of symptoms. Most persons simply avoid the feared object and adjust to certain restrictions on their activities.[1]

▶ TREATMENT: Anxiety Disorders

GENERALIZED ANXIETY DISORDER

DESIRED OUTCOME

The goals of therapy in the acute management of GAD are to reduce the severity, duration, and frequency of the anxiety symptoms and to improve the patient's overall functioning. Long-term goals include prevention of anxiety symptoms and improved quality of life.

Once GAD is diagnosed, a patient-oriented treatment plan, which usually consists of both psychotherapy and drug therapy, is developed. The treatment plan depends on the patient's degree of emotional distress and incapacitation, age, medication history, medical status, personality, and the potential outcomes of pharmacologic treatment. Clinical drug trials in outpatients with GAD indicate a high placebo response rate (50% to 60%), which suggests that some patients have a mild syndrome that may respond to psychotherapy alone.[7] Psychotherapy is the least invasive and safest treatment modality. For those patients experiencing anxiety symptoms severe enough to produce functional disability or discomfort, antianxiety medication is indicated.[7,20]

NONPHARMACOLOGIC THERAPY

Nonpharmacologic treatment modalities in GAD include short-term counseling, stress management, psychotherapy, meditation,

TABLE 67–6. Nonbenzodiazepine Antianxiety Agents

Class/Generic Name	Brand Name	Manufacturer	Usual Dosage Range (mg/d)[a]
Diphenylmethanes			
Diphenhydramine[b]	Benadryl	Parke-Davis	25–200
Hydroxyzine[b,c]	Vistaril	Pfizer	50–400
	Atarax	Roerig	
β-Blockers			
Propranolol[b]	Inderal	Wyeth-Ayerst	80–160
Azapirones			
Buspirone[c]	BuSpar	Bristol-Myers Squibb	15–60[d]

[a]Elderly patients are usually treated with approximately one-half of the dose listed.
[b]Available generically.
[c]FDA approved for anxiety.
[d]The dosage range in elderly patients appears to be the same, but is not established.

or exercise. Anxious patients should be instructed to avoid caffeine, nonprescription stimulants, and diet pills. Most GAD patients require psychological therapy, alone or in combination with antianxiety medication, to overcome fears and learn to improve coping abilities.[7] Consideration of the patient's clinical symptoms, personality, and life problems aids in the choice of psychological therapy. Cognitive therapy is the most effective psychological therapy in GAD patients. Supportive psychotherapy provides explanations and encouragement, and allows formulation of strategies to effectively manage anxiety-provoking situations. Patients with anxiety secondary to impaired interpersonal relations may benefit from group therapy.

PHARMACOLOGIC THERAPY

The BZs are the most effective and safe medications for the amelioration of anxiety symptoms. All BZs are equally effective anxiolytics, and consideration of pharmacokinetic properties and the patient's clinical situation will assist in the selection of the most appropriate agent. Pharmacokinetic differences vary, and the clinician must monitor the patient's response to the initial treatment regimen. Buspirone, autonomic blocking agents, and antidepressants are additional anxiolytic options (Table 67–6). Because of the high risk of adverse effects and toxicity, barbiturates, antipsychotics, antipsychotic/antidepressant combinations, and antihistamines are generally not indicated in the treatment of GAD.[20] Algorithms for the diagnosis, initial treatment with psychotherapy, and pharmacotherapy of GAD were published by Thompson.[21] An algorithm for the pharmacologic management of GAD is shown in Figure 67–1.

BENZODIAZEPINE THERAPY

The BZs are the drugs of choice for treating GAD. Although all BZs possess anxiolytic properties, only 8 of the 15 currently marketed agents have Food and Drug Administration (FDA)-approved labeling for the treatment of GAD (Table 67–7). Estazolam, flurazepam, temazepam, quazepam, and triazolam are marketed as sedative–hypnotic agents. Clonazepam is marketed as an antipanic agent and anticonvulsant,[22] and midazolam is labeled for preoperative sedation. Alprazolam is indicated for the treatment of panic disorder with or without agoraphobia, as well as GAD. Differences in marketed clinical indications often represent the manufacturers' marketing strategy rather than any major inherent differences in pharmacologic properties.

Mechanism of Action

The BZ receptor model of anxiety (described in the Pathophysiology section earlier in the chapter) theorizes that BZs ameliorate anxiety through potentiation of the inhibitory activity of GABA.[14] BZ binding sites are present in high density in the cortical and limbic–forebrain areas of the CNS.[14] The GABA–BZ receptor complex is composed of five protein subunits that form an intrinsic Cl ion channel and BZs bind to the γ_2 subunit.[13] When the BZ receptor is activated in the presence of GABA, the frequency of the Cl ion channels opening and influx of Cl ions into the neuronal cell is increased. The resultant negatively charged, hyperpolarized membrane prevents further depolarization by excitatory neurotransmitters. Other neurotransmitters (e.g., 5-HT, NE, dopamine) may be involved in BZ activity. Animal studies support serotonergic involvement in the anxiolytic effect of BZs downstream from the GABA–BZ receptor complex.[14]

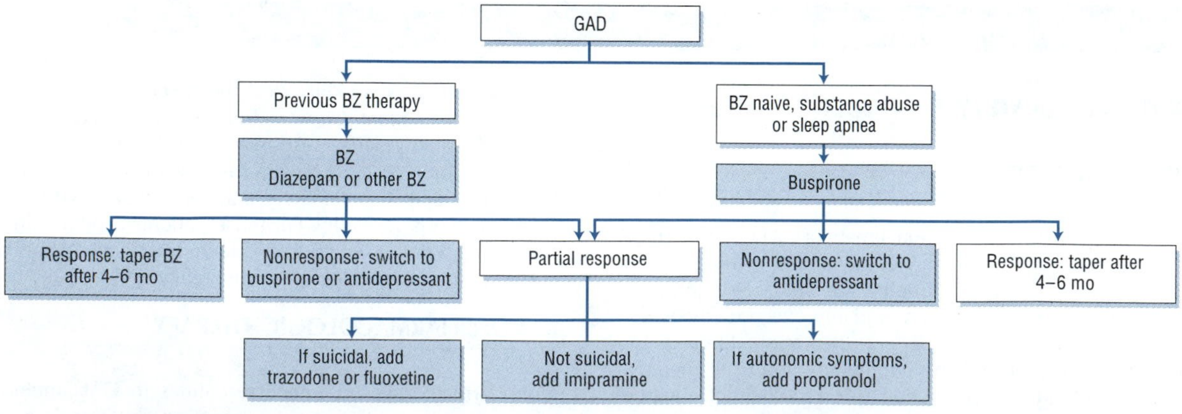

FIGURE 67–1. Algorithm for the management of generalized anxiety disorder. *(Derived from Refs. 7, 21, and 45.)*

TABLE 67–7. Benzodiazepine Antianxiety Agents

Generic Name	Brand Name	Manufacturer	Approved Dosage Range (mg/d)[a]	Approximate Equivalent Dose (mg)
Alprazolam[b]	Xanax	Pharmacia & Upjohn	0.75–4	0.5
Chlordiazepoxide[b]	Librium	Roche	25–100	10
Clorazepate[b]	Tranxene	Abbott	7.5–60	7.5
Diazepam[b]	Valium	Roche	2–40	5
Halazepam	Paxipam	Schering	20–160	20
Lorazepam[b]	Ativan	Wyeth-Ayerst	0.5–10	1
Oxazepam[b]	Serax	Wyeth-Ayerst	30–120	15

[a]Elderly patients are usually treated with approximately one-half of the dose listed. See Table 67–10 for antipanic dosage range.
[b]Available generically.

Pharmacokinetics

A wide difference in milligram potency exists between the BZ compounds; however, when dosage adjustments are made, all agents share similar anxiolytic and sedative–hypnotic activity.[14] Variations in lipid solubility between compounds may influence BZ pharmacokinetic properties. Differences in BZ pharmacokinetic and pharmacodynamic properties may assist the clinician in choosing an appropriate anxiolytic (Table 67–8). After a single dose, the onset, intensity, and duration of pharmacologic effects are important factors to consider when using BZs for the short-term, intermittent, or as-needed treatment of anxiety.

The primary determinant of a drug's onset of effect after a single oral dose is the rate of drug absorption. Because of high lipophilicity, diazepam and clorazepate are rapidly absorbed and quickly distributed into the CNS. Therefore, the onset of anxiolytic effect occurs within 30 to 60 minutes, which results in a rapid and intense relief of anxiety. High lipophilicity increases the extent of drug redistribution into the periphery, particularly adipose tissue, resulting in a shorter duration of effect after a single dose than indicated by single-dose elimination half-life studies.[14] Clinically, patients perceive a rapid onset of action, but some may experience an unpleasant feeling of drowsiness or loss of control. This "rush" may be euphoric and may contribute to an individual BZ's abuse potential. Chlordiazepoxide's onset of action is much slower because of decreased lipophilicity, slower absorption, and delayed passage into the CNS.

Compared with diazepam, lorazepam and oxazepam are relatively less lipophilic and have a slower onset of effect. These BZs have smaller volumes of distribution and a resultant longer duration of action.[14] Oxazepam absorption is slow, and peak levels are not obtained until 2 to 4 hours after a single dose; however, like lorazepam, oxazepam's anxiolytic effects are long lasting because extensive distribution does not occur. BZs with slow absorption rates are not recommended for the acute relief of anxiety symptoms.

Parenteral administration through the intramuscular route should be avoided with diazepam and chlordiazepoxide secondary to variability in the rate and extent of drug absorption. Intramuscular lorazepam provides rapid, reliable, and complete absorption; however, the preparation requires refrigeration.[23]

After multiple dosing, the rate and extent of drug accumulation are functions of the drug's elimination half-life in relation to dosing intervals, clearance, and formation of active metabolites. Differences in clinical effects that occur during and after repeated dosage with the BZs are related in part to variability in metabolism and metabolite accumulation. With dosing intervals less than 24 hours, long-elimination half-life BZs accumulate extensively.[20]

The BZs undergo two primary metabolic processes, hepatic microsomal oxidation (*N*-dealkylation or aliphatic hydroxylation) and glucuronide conjugation. With the exception of lorazepam and oxazepam (which are conjugated only), all BZs are oxidized first, and then conjugated, and excreted renally. Oxidation may be impaired in patients with liver disease, in the elderly, and with the simultaneous use of drugs that inhibit oxidation. Impaired oxidation results in higher levels of the parent drug and/or an active metabolite.

Many BZs are converted (through *N*-demethylation) to *N*-desmethyldiazepam (*N*-DMDZ), an active metabolite with a long-elimination half-life of 36 to 200 hours (Table 67–8).[20]

TABLE 67–8. Pharmacokinetics of Benzodiazepine Antianxiety Agents

Generic Name	Peak Plasma Level (h)	Elimination Half-life, Parent (h)	Metabolic Pathway	Clinically Significant Metabolites	Protein Binding (%)
Alprazolam	1–2	12–15	Oxidation	—	80
Chlordiazepoxide	1–4	5–30	*N*-dealkylation	Desmethylchlordiazepoxide	96
			Oxidation	Demoxepam	—
				N-DMDZ[a]	—
Clorazepate	1–2	Prodrug	Oxidation	*N*-DMDZ	97
Diazepam	0.5–2	20–80	Oxidation	*N*-DMDZ	98
Halazepam	1–3	14	Oxidation	*N*-DMDZ	97
Lorazepam	2–4	10–20	Conjugation	—	85
Oxazepam	2–4	5–20	Conjugation	—	97

[a]*N*-desmethyldiazepam (*N*-DMDZ) half-life 36–200 h.
Compiled from Refs. 20 and 23.

N-DMDZ is further oxidized to oxazepam, then conjugated, and excreted. After multiple dosing, accumulation of *N*-DMDZ is slow and extensive, providing a long-lasting antianxiety effect. If oxidation of *N*-DMDZ is impaired, the half-life is prolonged, and complications of drug accumulation (e.g., drowsiness) may result over time with repeated dosing.[23]

Clorazepate is a prodrug and possesses no anxiolytic effects until metabolism to *N*-DMDZ. Before absorption, clorazepate is rapidly metabolized in the stomach through a pH-dependent process under acidic conditions. Alterations of stomach pH (e.g., administration of antacids) may decrease the rate of *N*-DMDZ formation.

BZs with short half-lives (e.g., alprazolam, lorazepam, oxazepam) reach steady-state plasma concentrations rapidly, and drug accumulation after repeated dosing is minimal. Neither oxazepam nor lorazepam is converted into active metabolites.[23]

BZ protein binding is extensive, especially for the long-elimination half-life drugs. After a single dose of a long-elimination half-life BZ, the expected duration of clinical activity may not parallel the drug's pharmacokinetic half-life because of drug redistribution.[14] After multiple dosing, drugs with long-elimination half-lives and active metabolites may require 1 to 2 weeks to reach steady state.

Special Populations

In the elderly, secondary to a decreased capacity for oxidation and alterations in the volume of distribution, drug accumulation may result. Patients with hepatic disease also are at risk for drug accumulation and subsequent complications. Therefore, intermediate- or short-acting BZs are preferred for chronic use in the elderly and those with liver disorders because of minimal accumulation and achievement of steady state within 1 to 3 days. BZs with long-elimination half-lives may be dosed once a day at bedtime and may provide both hypnotic and daytime anxiolytic activity. Agents with shorter-elimination half-lives should be administered in divided daily doses. Patients with hypoalbuminemia often have increased sensitivity to clinical effects, and BZs with lower protein binding (lorazepam, alprazolam) should be used.

Adverse Events

The most common adverse events associated with BZ therapy involve CNS depression. This is clinically manifested as drowsiness, sedation, psychomotor impairment, and ataxia.[20] A transient mild drowsiness is commonly experienced by patients during the first few days of treatment; however, tolerance often develops. Disorientation, confusion, irritability, aggression, and excitement have been reported.[20]

Impairment of memory and recall may also occur during BZ treatment. The memory loss induced by the BZs is typically limited to events occurring after drug ingestion (or anterograde amnesia).[24] The anterograde amnesia is secondary to disordered consolidation processes that store information and is not an impairment in the perception or retrieval of information.[20,24] BZs with high affinity for binding to the BZ receptor (e.g., lorazepam) appear to possess a higher potential for amnesia. The extent of BZ-induced memory impairment is unknown and may go unrecognized by both clinician and patient.

Abuse, Dependence, Withdrawal, and Tolerance

The widespread use of BZs has generated public concern regarding the potential for abuse. The long-term use of BZs has caused increased interest regarding the development of physical dependence. Most BZ users consume these agents for brief periods, but 15% report daily use that exceeds 1 year.[25] BZ abuse is rare in the general population of users; however, individuals with a history of multiple drug abuse (e.g., alcohol, sedatives) are at the greatest risk for becoming BZ abusers.[20,25] Because of the chronicity of illness, persons with GAD and panic disorder are at high risk of developing BZ dependence.[26]

BZ dependence is a physiologic phenomenon demonstrated by the appearance of a predictable abstinence syndrome (withdrawal symptoms) upon abrupt discontinuation of therapy. Withdrawal symptoms may result because of the sudden dissociation of a BZ from its receptor site. After abrupt BZ discontinuation, an acute decrease in GABA neurotransmission results, producing a less inhibited CNS.[25]

Benzodiazepine Discontinuation

After BZ therapy is suddenly discontinued, several events can occur. Rebound symptoms represent an immediate, but transient return of original symptoms having an increased intensity compared with baseline. Recurrence or relapse is the return of original symptoms with similar intensity as before treatment. In patients treated with BZs for over 1 year, a recurrence of GAD is reported in 50% to 65% of patients.[7] Withdrawal symptoms are the emergence of new symptoms and a worsening of preexisting symptoms after BZ discontinuation. Withdrawal symptoms may persist for days to weeks and be so severe that they interfere with normal functioning.

Common symptoms of BZ withdrawal include anxiety, insomnia, restlessness, agitation, muscle tension, and irritability. Less frequently occurring symptoms are nausea, malaise, coryza, blurred vision, diaphoresis, nightmares, depression, hyperreflexia, and ataxia. Tinnitus, confusion, paranoid delusions, hallucinations, seizures, and psychosis rarely occur.[25] Seizures occur with both therapeutic and high doses of short-elimination half-life BZs, usually within 3 days of drug discontinuation, or approximately 1 week for long-elimination half-life agents. High BZ doses, a long duration of therapy, and concurrent ingestion of drugs that lower the seizure threshold are risk factors for withdrawal seizures.[25]

The onset of withdrawal symptoms in patients ingesting BZs with short-elimination half-lives occurs much earlier (within 24 to 48 hours) than in those taking BZs with long-elimination half-lives (within 3 to 8 days).[26] Other factors associated with an increased incidence or severity of BZ withdrawal include high doses and long-term BZ therapy. Abrupt discontinuation of short-elimination half-life BZs may produce a more severe withdrawal[27] than long-elimination half-life agents. The difference in half-life is less distinct when BZs are gradually tapered.[28]

Factors that increase the likelihood of BZ dependence include high doses for up to 4 to 6 weeks or therapeutic doses for extended periods of time. Rebound symptoms are more intense after the ingestion of short-elimination than long-elimination half-life BZs. In patients who ingest BZs for more than 4 months, withdrawal symptoms are more likely and more severe; patients who experience withdrawal at this time usually do not wish to stop therapy. Therefore, continuous daily usage of BZs for 4 to 8 months may increase the development of dependency.[25]

Several strategies to minimize the severity of BZ withdrawal include a 25% per week reduction in dosage until 50% of the dose is reached, then dosage reduction by one-eighth every 4 to 7 days. The patient should be observed drug free for 3 weeks to monitor for the presence of withdrawal symptoms versus recurrence of original symptoms. If BZ therapy exceeds 6 weeks, a slow dosage taper over several weeks is recommended. Tapering will not entirely eliminate the emergence of withdrawal symptoms, but will prevent severe withdrawal. Slow drug taper is extremely important for the short-elimination half-life drugs because some individuals have greater difficulty with discontinuation.[25,27] Results of studies performed to evaluate the use of adjunctive carbamazepine, clonidine, propranolol, and antidepressants to attenuate BZ withdrawal were inconclusive.[29] If patients experience difficulties, especially with the short-elimination half-life agents, then substitution of a long-elimination half-life BZ should be considered. Diazepam can be initiated as a loading dose (40% of daily consumption), followed by daily tapering of 10%. Clonazepam is an alternative agent. Phenobarbital could be used especially if the patient has mixed BZ and alcohol dependence.[25]

Although tolerance develops to the sedative, muscle relaxant, and anticonvulsant activities, the BZs do not appear to lose anxiolytic or antipanic efficacy.[25] The anxiolytic efficacy of BZs in long-term clinical trials (greater than 4 to 6 months of chronic use) has not been reported; however, some patients derive beneficial anxiolytic effects from chronic BZ ingestion.

Drug Interactions

Drug interactions with the BZs generally fall into two categories—pharmacodynamic and pharmacokinetic (Table 67–9).[20,30–34] Simultaneous use of alcohol and a BZ results in additive CNS depressant effects and lowers the therapeutic index of the BZ. In addition, concurrent use of a BZ and drugs with CNS depressant properties (e.g., antidepressants, narcotic analgesics, antipsychotics, antihistamines) may potentiate the adverse sedative effects. When ingested alone in an overdose attempt, BZs are rarely life-threatening; however, the combination of BZs with alcohol or other CNS depressant agents is potentially fatal. The concomitant use of intravenous lorazepam during clozapine therapy was associated with respiratory suppression and death.[35]

Cimetidine competitively inhibits the metabolism of drugs that require oxidation through the hepatic microsomal P450 enzyme system; thus ranitidine and famotidine are alternatives for patients taking BZs. Nefazodone and fluvoxamine increased alprazolam concentrations; thus the alprazolam dose should be reduced by 50% when these agents are added.[33]

TABLE 67–9. Pharmacokinetic Drug Interactions With the Benzodiazepines

Drug	Effect
Alcohol	Decreased Cl of chlordiazepoxide and diazepam
Antacids	Decreased rate of diazepam and chlordiazepoxide absorption
Cimetidine	Decreased Cl of alprazolam, diazepam, chlordiazepoxide, and clorazepate and increased $t_{1/2}$
Disulfiram	Decreased Cl of chlordiazepoxide and diazepam
Fluoxetine	Decreased Cl of diazepam
Fluvoxamine	Decreased Cl of alprazolam and prolonged $t_{1/2}$
Isoniazid	Decreased metabolism of diazepam
Itraconazole	Potentially decreased Cl of alprazolam
Ketaconazole	Potentially decreased Cl of alprazolam
Nefazodone	Decreased Cl of alprazolam, AUC doubled, and $t_{1/2}$ prolonged
Omeprazole	Decreased Cl of diazepam
Oral contraceptives	Increased free concentration of chlordiazepoxide and slightly decreased Cl; decreased Cl and increased $t_{1/2}$ of diazepam and alprazolam
Rifampin	Increased metabolism of diazepam
Theophylline	Decreased alprazolam concentrations

AUC=area-under-the-plasma-concentration-curve; Cl=clearance; $t_{1/2}$=elimination half-life.
Compiled from Refs. 23 and 30–34.

Dosing and Administration

Benzodiazepine dosage requirements vary widely among patients and must be individualized. Therapy should be initiated using low doses (e.g., diazepam 2 mg tid or its equivalent), and titrated upward to relieve anxiety symptoms and avoid adverse events. After an initial treatment response is achieved, agents with long-elimination half-lives may be dosed at bedtime. Dosage adjustments should be made weekly.

The duration of BZ therapy should be monitored and generally should not exceed 4 to 6 months.[21] Intermittent therapy is indicated in patients with recurring symptoms or anxiety induced by a known cause. Individuals with persistent symptoms may require continuous treatment.[7,36] Drug withdrawal symptoms rarely occur in patients receiving the usual therapeutic doses of BZs for less than 4 months, especially when the BZ is tapered.

The elderly anxious patient requires additional monitoring when a BZ is prescribed. These patients have an enhanced sensitivity to BZs (both to therapeutic and CNS depressant effects) that may possibly be related to pharmacokinetic alterations (e.g., decreased clearance).[23] The elderly may be particularly susceptible to falls, sedation, impaired daytime functioning, and memory problems, which also may be enhanced by other drugs with CNS depressant effects. Thus dosages should be low and short-elimination half-life agents prescribed.[23]

Patient education should include the anticipated length of drug therapy, potential side effects, and consequences of the ingestion of alcohol and other CNS depressants. Patients should understand that medications provide symptomatic relief, but do not solve underlying psychological problems. Patients should be instructed not to decrease or discontinue BZ usage without contacting their physician.

BUSPIRONE THERAPY

Buspirone, an azapirone anxiolytic, is structurally and pharmacologically unlike the BZs; it lacks anticonvulsant, muscle relaxant, hypnotic, motor impairment, and dependence properties. For the treatment of GAD with or without depressive symptoms, clinical trials found buspirone superior to placebo and as efficacious as BZs after 4 weeks.[37]

Mechanism of Action

Buspirone's anxiolytic mechanism of action is unknown; however, it does not interact with the GABA–BZ receptor complex or decrease noradrenergic neuron firing in the LC (it slightly increases firing). Buspirone possesses activity as a 5-HT_{1A} partial agonist, binding presynaptically to the receptors in the dorsal raphe and postsynaptically to receptors in the hippocampus and cortical brain areas.[38] Buspirone also possesses both dopamine agonist and indirect dopamine antagonist properties.[38]

Pharmacokinetics

After an oral dose, buspirone is rapidly and completely absorbed, and undergoes extensive first-pass metabolism. Buspirone is 95% protein bound. The mean elimination half-life is 2.1 to 2.7 hours.[39] Buspirone is eliminated primarily by oxidative metabolism and is converted into both active and inactive metabolites.

Adverse Events

A major advantage of buspirone is its lack of sedative properties. Adverse events include dizziness, nausea, headaches, nervousness, and dysphoria (especially with large single doses of 20 to 40 mg).[7]

Drug Interactions

Buspirone reportedly increases cyclosporine and haloperidol levels and elevates blood pressure in patients taking a MAOI.

Disulfiram caused mania, and clomipramine caused hypertension and anxiety when coprescribed with buspirone.[40]

Dosing and Administration

The recommended initial dose of buspirone is 7.5 mg two times daily with dosage increments of 5 mg/d every 2 to 3 days as needed.[39] The usual therapeutic dose of buspirone is 20 to 30 mg/d, with a maximum dose of 60 mg/d.[39] The onset of anxiolysis is not immediate, requiring a week or more before clinical effects occur; maximum therapeutic benefit may not be evident for 4 to 6 weeks.[41]

Buspirone has minimal sedating properties and is not useful in clinical situations requiring immediate anxiolytic effects or for situations requiring as-needed anxiolytic therapy. Therefore, buspirone is an alternative for GAD patients who are unable to tolerate the sedative effects and psychomotor impairment of BZs, especially the elderly. It may be the agent of choice in the management of chronic, persistent anxiety.[42]

Buspirone is not cross-tolerant with BZs and thus will not prevent or treat symptoms of BZ withdrawal.[41,42] When a patient is switched from a BZ to buspirone, the BZ should be tapered slowly before buspirone is initiated. However, some clinicians advocate pretreatment with buspirone 20 to 40 mg daily for 2 to 4 weeks before initiating the BZ taper.[42]

Previous BZ therapy may lead to certain expectations of anxiolytic drug effects (immediate response and sedation) that buspirone does not demonstrate.[41,42] Therefore, patients who have received BZs should be advised of these differences, particularly at the outset of therapy. Buspirone is an appropriate choice for anxious patients with a history of alcohol or drug abuse because of its low potential for abuse.[42]

ADRENERGIC BLOCKING AGENTS

Propranolol and other β-blocking agents may be useful in patients with prominent cardiovascular symptoms of anxiety (e.g., palpitations or tremors). β-Blocking drugs are less effective anxiolytics than BZs,[43] and their usefulness may be restricted to those anxiety patients whose physical symptoms, especially cardiovascular complaints, have not adequately responded to BZ therapy. Propranolol therapy is usually well tolerated with few adverse effects, provided a complete medical examination is performed and medical contraindications are observed.

Although propranolol has a short-elimination half-life (2 to 6 hours), β-blockade usually lasts for 8 to 12 hours after a single dose.[43] Propranolol 10 mg twice a day should be used initially and gradually titrated to anxiolytic response. Response is usually observed within 1 week of therapy.[7] Emergence of adverse events (e.g., depression, fatigue) may limit the clinical usefulness of propranolol. Upon discontinuation, the dosage should be tapered to avoid rebound anxiety and cardiovascular effects.

ANTIDEPRESSANTS

Because of their adverse events profile, antidepressants are not considered first-line agents in the management of GAD. Recent studies indicated that imipramine, a tricyclic antidepressant (TCA), and trazodone are effective in GAD after 3 to 8 weeks of therapy.[44] The mean daily dosages of imipramine at the end of 1 and 8 weeks were 92 and 143 mg, respectively. The mean daily dosages of trazodone at the end of weeks 1 and 8 were 175 and 235 mg, respectively.[44] Low doses of SSRIs (e.g., fluoxetine 5 mg) have been successful in some GAD patients.[7,45] Antidepressants are alternatives for individuals with contraindications to BZ use or those with concomitant depressive symptoms.[42] They are also useful adjuncts in the treatment of patients with a partial response to BZs or buspirone.[6,45]

PHARMACOECONOMIC CONSIDERATIONS

It is estimated that anxiety disorders account for 31.5% of the total costs of mental illness in the United States.[46] The social costs of anxiety disorders are reflected in increased rates of financial assistance, health care use, and substance abuse.[47] Physical disability was reported by 53% and occupational role disability was reported by 26% of GAD outpatients. The mean number of work days missed secondary to disability in the past month was 4.4 days.[48] These figures increase when GAD is comorbid with one or more other psychiatric disorders. GAD patients tend to use family practitioners and gastroenterologists more frequently than healthy controls.[49] Pharmacoeconomic analyses in the management of GAD have not been conducted.

EVALUATION OF THERAPEUTIC OUTCOMES

The goals of treatment and duration of therapy should be discussed with the patient at the beginning of therapy. Initially, anxious patients should be monitored twice weekly for a reduction in the frequency, duration, and severity of anxiety symptoms and improvement in occupational, social, and interpersonal functioning. The pharmacist should assess the patient for response to treatment by asking about the target symptoms of anxiety and emergence of adverse events. After achieving an optimal drug dosage, the patient can be evaluated monthly until drug discontinuation. Use of an objective measurement of anxiety symptoms (e.g., the Visual Analogue Scale to rate the severity, frequency, and duration of symptoms on scales of 1 to 10, or a standard rating instrument such as the State–Trait Anxiety Inventory or Zung Self-rating Anxiety Scale[50]) may assist in the evaluation of drug response.

PANIC DISORDER

DESIRED OUTCOME

Goals of therapy in panic disorder include a complete resolution of panic attacks, marked reduction in anticipatory anxiety and phobic avoidance, and maintenance of a clinical response that allows the patient to resume normal activities.[51] Despite treatment, only 49% of patients with panic disorder achieve full remission.[52]

Therapeutic options include a single pharmacologic agent, concurrent psychotherapy, or psychotherapy followed by pharmacotherapy. Most patients without agoraphobia will improve with pharmacotherapy alone; however, if agoraphobia is present, cognitive–behavioral therapy (CBT) is typically initiated concurrently. With all effective drug therapies, resolution of phobic avoidance tends to occur slowly, and many patients require concomitant CBT.

NONPHARMACOLOGIC THERAPY

Patients should be educated to avoid substances that may precipitate panic attacks including caffeine, drugs of abuse, and nonprescription stimulants.[10] CBT focuses on the correction of a patient's maladaptive thoughts and behaviors that initiate, perpetuate, or exacerbate panic symptoms.[53] Through CBT, the patient learns to decrease the fear and avoidance of internal and external signals associated with panic attacks. The cognitive restructuring and graded exposure components of CBT target panic

TABLE 67–10. Drugs Used in the Treatment of Panic Disorder

Class/Generic Name	Brand Name	Manufacturer	Starting Dose	Antipanic Dosage Range[a] (mg)
Benzodiazepines				
Alprazolam[b]	Xanax	Pharmacia & Upjohn	0.25–0.5 mg tid	4–10[c]
Clonazepam[b]	Klonopin	Roche	0.25 mg bid	3–4[c]
Diazepam[b]	Valium	Roche	2–5 mg tid	30–40
Lorazepam[b]	Ativan	Wyeth-Ayerst	0.5–1 mg tid	3–4
Tricyclic Antidepressants				
Desipramine[b]	Norpramin	Hoechst Marion Roussel	10–25 mg qd	150–300
Imipramine[b]	Tofranil	Ciba-Geigy	10–25 mg qd	150–300
Monoamine Oxidase Inhibitor				
Phenelzine	Nardil	Parke-Davis	15 mg bid	45–90
Serotonin Reuptake Inhibitors				
Fluoxetine	Prozac	Dista	2.5–5 mg	2.5–20
Fluvoxamine	Luvox	Solvay	25 mg qd	150–300
Paroxetine	Paxil	SmithKline Beecham	10 mg qd	10–60[c]
Sertraline	Zoloft	Roerig	12.5–25 mg qd	25–200[c]

[a]Dosage used in clinical trials but not FDA approved.
[b]Available generically.
[c]Dosage is FDA approved.

attacks and phobic-avoidance behavior.[53] Exposure requires patients to confront phobic situations gradually, starting with the least feared situation.

For patients who cannot or will not take medication, CBT alone is certainly indicated. CBT is associated with short-term improvement in 66% of patients and 6-month improvement in 75% of patients.[54] Combined fluvoxamine and exposure was superior to exposure alone in reducing phobic avoidance.[55]

PHARMACOLOGIC THERAPY

Panic disorder is effectively treated with several drugs including the TCA imipramine, the BZ alprazolam, the MAOI phenelzine, and SSRIs (Table 67–10).[7,45] Alprazolam, clonazepam, sertraline, and paroxetine are approved for this indication. SSRIs are emerging as first-line agents because of their improved tolerability[7,56]; however, these agents are significantly more expensive than TCAs and BZs. In a meta-analysis of the pharmacotherapy of panic disorder, SSRIs and clomipramine had significantly greater effect sizes and improvement ratios than imipramine and alprazolam.[57] An algorithm for the pharmacologic therapy of panic disorder appears in Figure 67–2.

The presence of comorbid psychiatric and/or medical conditions influences the choice of first-line medication.[56] The emergence of depressive symptoms during BZ treatment has been reported. Because most panic disorder patients experience at least one episode of depression, the association with BZ therapy may

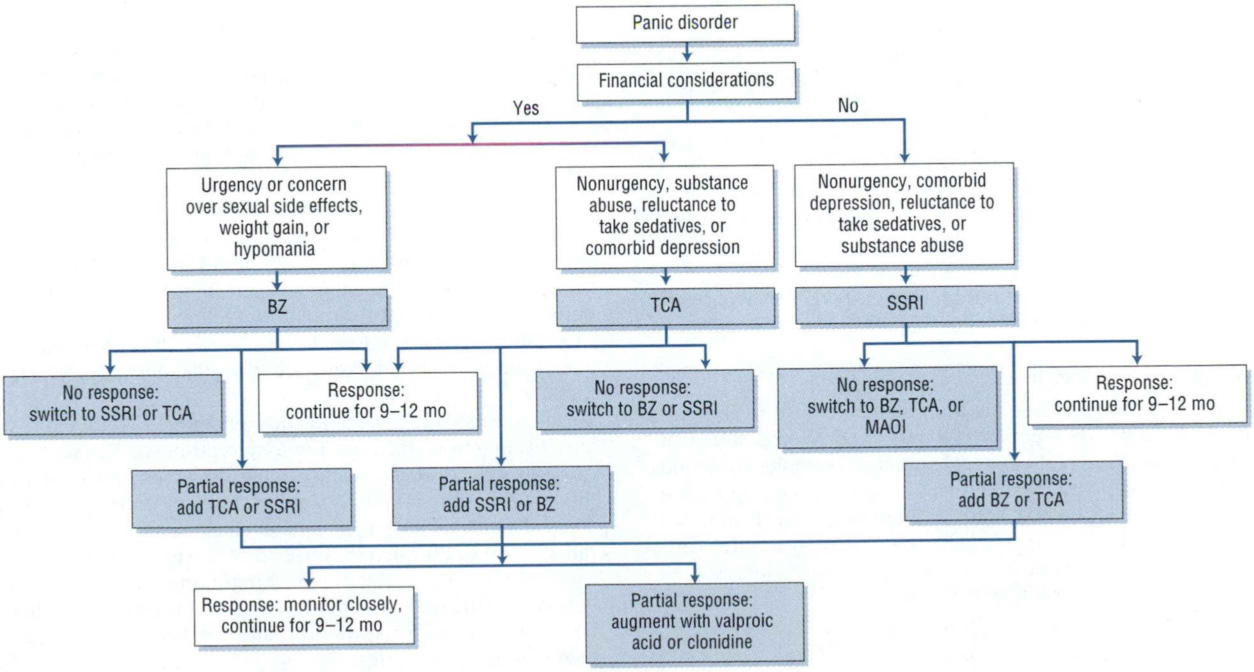

FIGURE 67–2. Algorithm for the management of panic disorder. *(Derived from Refs. 9 and 56.)*

be coincidental.[58] However, because antidepressants are superior to BZs in treating depression, they should be selected first for patients with panic disorder who are clinically depressed or have a history of depression. In patients whose illness is complicated by a history of alcohol or drug abuse, BZs should be cautiously used, and a TCA, SSRI, or MAOI would be more appropriate.[7,59] Initially, concomitant BZ and SSRI therapy for 1 to 3 weeks may be indicated in persons with severe symptoms or anticipatory anxiety.[9]

ANTIDEPRESSANTS

Tricyclic Antidepressants

Double-blind, placebo-controlled studies demonstrated the efficacy of imipramine in blocking panic attacks.[60,61] It is effective in 75% of patients with panic disorder.[7,60,61] Imipramine effectively blocks panic attacks within 3 to 5 weeks; however, maximal improvement (including antiphobic response) does not occur until 6 to 10 weeks. The sequence of patient response is an initial decrease in the number of panic attacks, then diminution of anticipatory anxiety, followed by a reduction in phobic avoidance. Approximately 20% to 30% of patients experience stimulatory (amphetamine-like) side effects including insomnia, jitteriness, irritability, and unusual energy.[51] These side effects often significantly affect patient compliance, prevent medication dosage increases, and interfere with the overall treatment outcome. Reducing the dose may eliminate these unpleasant effects.[61]

Although imipramine and clomipramine are the most studied TCAs for panic disorder, desipramine and nortriptyline may possibly be effective.[62,63] Problems with using TCAs in panic disorder are well documented and include stimulatory side effects, anticholinergic effects, orthostatic hypotension, delayed onset of antipanic effects, and toxicity in an overdose.[10] For patients who cannot tolerate the anticholinergic side effects of TCAs, a switch to an SSRI may be helpful.[7] Approximately 25% to 35% of patients reportedly discontinue treatment because of side effects or nonresponse.[7,51] Weight gain is a problematic side effect associated with long-term therapy.[10]

Selective Serotonin Reuptake Inhibitors

The SSRIs are commonly used in the management of panic disorder. In a 12-week placebo-controlled trial, 82% of combined paroxetine- and CBT-treated patients achieved a 50% or greater reduction in number of panic attacks.[64] Fluvoxamine, fluoxetine, and sertraline have also shown efficacy.[65–67] The antipanic effect of SSRIs is delayed for 3 to 5 weeks.

Typical antidepressant doses of SSRIs can cause side effects of insomnia, jitteriness, restlessness, and agitation, and lead to drug discontinuation in panic patients. Transient gastrointestinal disturbances occur more frequently with SSRIs than with TCAs.[9] Thus, low initial SSRI doses should be prescribed.[9,36] Sexual dysfunction is often problematic.

Monoamine Oxidase Inhibitors

The majority of studies assessing the efficacy of MAOIs in treating panic disorder were poorly designed and lacked sufficient dosage and duration of treatment, sufficient sample size, and valid ratings of panic attacks. The antipanic effect of phenelzine is delayed for 3 to 5 weeks, and the antiphobic effect does not occur for 6 to 10 weeks.[59] Side effects and dietary restrictions adversely affect patient acceptance.[10,59] MAOIs are usually reserved for the most refractory or difficult patient.[7]

Other Agents

Trazodone and maprotiline were effective in some patients, but bupropion was ineffective.[7,45] Limited data suggest that nefazodone reduces panic symptoms in patients with comorbid depression.[68] Venlafaxine may also be effective.[69]

BENZODIAZEPINES

During the past decade, several placebo-controlled studies documented the efficacy of clonazepam and high-dose alprazolam in treating panic disorder.[61,70] Diazepam and lorazepam are possibly effective in treating panic disorder when taken in sufficiently high doses.[7,58,71] Therapeutic response to BZs occurs in 1 to 2 weeks, with further improvement occurring at weeks 4 to 6.[7] It is estimated that 60% to 80% of panic disorder patients respond to BZs.[71] Alprazolam is an ideal agent for patients who need immediate relief. Patient acceptance of alprazolam is not usually a problem and, except for sedation, side effects are rarely reported. Relapse rates of 50% or higher are common, despite slow drug tapering.[53]

TREATMENT RESISTANCE

Common reasons for treatment failures are comorbid psychiatric disorders, rapid dosage increases with resultant intolerable side effects, and underdosage. All standard treatments should be tried before using augmentation strategies. The most common strategy used in patients with a partial response to one agent is to augment with low doses of another antipanic agent (TCA, BZ, or SSRI).[9] Limited data support the use of valproate.[72] Clonidine has shown improvement in a few treatment-resistant patients; however, tolerance developed to its therapeutic effect.[73]

DOSING AND ADMINISTRATION

Acute Phase

The main goal of therapy in the acute phase is reduction of symptoms (e.g., resolution of panic attacks, reduction in anxiety and phobic fears, resumption of the patient's usual activities).[51] The duration of this phase is generally 1 to 3 months depending on the choice of medication. The guiding principle for using medication in panic disorder is to start low, use an adequate dose, and treat for an appropriate period of time.[51] Side effects with the antidepressants, often from too high an initial dose, may prevent achievement of an optimal dosage, compromise treatment response, and contribute to patient noncompliance.[7]

The duration of the acute phase with antidepressants requires a minimum of 8 to 12 weeks. When using imipramine, treatment should be initiated with 10 mg/d at bedtime and slowly increased by 10 mg every 2 to 4 days as tolerated to 100 to 200 mg/d over a 2- to 4-week period.[7,51,62] Although an occasional patient will respond to 50 mg/d or less, most require at least 150 mg/d of imipramine (or a combined imipramine/desipramine plasma concentration of 100 to 150 ng/mL).[51] If this dose is not effective, a higher dose (up to 300 mg/d) should be used. Many patients with panic disorder are extremely sensitive to imipramine and experience an immediate stimulatory feeling or motor restlessness. The starting dose, therefore, is very conservative. Stimulatory side effects are transient and generally dissipate after several weeks of therapy.[51]

Low initial doses of SSRIs are recommended to avoid stimulatory side effects (e.g., insomnia, nervousness). The starting dose of paroxetine is 10 mg with dosage increases of 10 mg weekly; the target dose is 40 mg.[74] Starting doses of fluoxetine are 2.5 to 5 mg/d, with dosage increases every 2 or 3 days to a dosage range of 10 to 20 mg/d by the end of 2 weeks.[7] Fluvoxamine 25 to 50 mg/d was increased to 150 mg/d, in divided doses, over 2 weeks in clinical trials (range, 100 to 300 mg/d).[65] Sertraline, initiated at 12.5 or 25 mg/d and titrated to 100 to 200 mg/d, is effective in panic disorder.[7,67]

The starting dose of phenelzine is 15 mg/d after the evening meal, increased by 15 mg/d every 3 to 4 days until 60 mg/d is reached. A dose of less than 45 mg/d is rarely effective. Dosages may be increased (up to 90 mg/d) if improvement is not achieved after 8 to 12 weeks. If a patient was previously on an antidepressant, it should be discontinued, and 2 weeks should lapse before phenelzine is started to prevent a potential drug interaction. Fluoxetine must be stopped 5 weeks before phenelzine (or another MAOI) can be started. Phenelzine doses taken after meals lessens the risk of orthostatic hypotension. Anticholinergic side effects are less severe with phenelzine than with TCAs, but orthostatic hypotension and insomnia are often more of a problem. After 3 weeks, most unpleasant side effects subside.

Hypertensive crisis following the ingestion of tyramine-containing foods or sympathomimetic drugs is the most serious, potentially life-threatening event encountered with phenelzine.[9,75] Symptoms include a severe headache, usually accompanied by flushing, and a heavy "thumping" of the heart. Patients should be instructed that if symptoms occur, they must go immediately to the nearest emergency department. (See Chap. 65 for food and drug restrictions and side effects.) Patients should observe the food, drink, and drug restrictions for at least 24 hours before starting the first dose of phenelzine, and for 2 weeks after stopping therapy.

The duration of the acute phase with BZs is approximately 1 month because response is rapid and occurs within 1 to 3 weeks. The starting dose of alprazolam is 0.25 or 0.5 mg/d in three divided doses, slowly increased over several weeks. During the initial weeks of therapy, patients may pass through two or three dosage plateaus followed by tolerance to side effects and some loss of benefit before reaching an ideal dose. The duration of action may be as little as 4 to 6 hours, with resultant "breakthrough" symptoms. Although a few patients may respond to doses as low as 2 to 3 mg/d, many patients require 3 to 6 mg/d, and some need doses of 6 to 10 mg/d to obtain a full therapeutic (antipanic and antiphobic) response.[7,51,61] Patients tolerate the initial side effects of alprazolam much better than those of imipramine or phenelzine.[61] Because of its long half-life, clonazepam is an alternative to alprazolam if patients experience breakthrough panic symptoms at the end of a dosing interval.

Continuation Phase

The goals of therapy during the continuation phase are to complete and extend the treatment response obtained in the acute phase, especially with regards to phobic avoidance.[51] During this time the drug dosage necessary to optimally maximize response and minimize adverse drug effects is obtained. Depending on response, this phase lasts for 2 to 4 months.

Maintenance Phase and Discontinuation

The duration of the maintenance phase is 3 to 12 months. In some patients, especially those experiencing adverse events, the drug dosage may be reduced without loss of improvement.[51] The optimal length of therapy is unknown; however, the total duration of therapy appears to be 8 to 12 months before drug discontinuation is attempted.[51] The rate of relapse, measured 6 months after a 3-month imipramine discontinuation, was 83% in panic disorder patients with agoraphobia treated for 6 months and 25% in those treated for 18 months with imipramine.[76] Thus, longer periods of treatment are associated with more sustained response. When medications are discontinued too early, a high rate of relapse occurs.[59] Reinstitution of medication usually results in renewed clinical response.[51] After 3 months, medication taper may be attempted again. Many patients may be successfully tapered off medication during the second year of therapy.[51] Approximately 20% to 40% of patients will require chronic therapy.[59]

Patients taking alprazolam or imipramine for up to 8 months maintained antipanic efficacy without dosage increase. This indicates that tolerance does not develop to the antipanic effects of alprazolam or imipramine.[60]

Some patients receiving high-dose alprazolam (> 4 mg/d) may have an extremely difficult time with drug taper, and the withdrawal schedule for all patients should be individualized. In patients receiving alprazolam doses greater than 3 mg/d, dosage reduction should proceed by 0.5 mg every 2 weeks until 3 mg/d is obtained, then 0.25 mg every 2 weeks until 1 mg is obtained, then 0.125 mg every 2 weeks.[77] The taper phase is most successful when it is accomplished over a 3- to 6-month period.[51] Approximately 30% of the patients receiving high doses, even with slow taper, may experience transient, mild to moderate withdrawal symptoms (as discussed in the earlier section on benzodiazepines) and relapse of panic attacks.[59] Adjunctive CBT reportedly facilitates BZ discontinuation.[36] Also, if a TCA is discontinued abruptly, a substantial number of patients will develop severe cholinergic rebound with upset stomach, nausea, vomiting, and abdominal cramping, thus TCAs should be reduced by 25 mg every 2 to 4 weeks.[59] The dose of phenelzine should be reduced by 15 mg every 2 to 4 weeks.

Patients should be informed regarding the lag time before a therapeutic response will occur and any problematic side effects. Many patients are reluctant to take medications for fear that drugs will worsen their illness or that they will become addicted. Adverse events are often perceived as a worsening of the illness and may contribute to noncompliance and prevent necessary medication increases. Patients receiving alprazolam or another BZ should be told not to decrease or discontinue therapy unless authorized by their physician.

PHARMACOECONOMIC CONSIDERATIONS

Patients with panic disorder have high rates of receipts of welfare and disability benefits and health care use, and have impaired emotional and physical health status. They also experience poor marital and social functioning.[19] Fifty-three percent of patients reported occupational role disability, 34% indicated physical disability, and a mean of 6.7 disability days during the past month.[48] Panic disorder patients had a higher rate of primary care and medical specialist visits (83%) than a healthy control group (36%) for 1 year.[49]

In the year after diagnosis, panic disorder patients reduced the use of general medical services by 94%, increased use of psychiatric services, and demonstrated marked improvement in productivity and well-being.[78] After 6 weeks of clonazepam, work productivity improved (from 71% to 88%) and personal happiness increased.[19]

EVALUATION OF THERAPEUTIC OUTCOMES

During the first 2 weeks of the acute phase of therapy, patients with panic disorder should be seen twice weekly to adjust medication doses based on improvement in panic symptoms and to monitor for adverse events. Once stabilized, the patient can be seen on a weekly basis until antipanic response is achieved. After this, monthly visits should suffice. The patient should be counseled to maintain a diary to record the date, time, frequency, and duration of panic episodes and the severity of panic symptoms, anticipatory anxiety, and phobic avoidance. At scheduled visits, the pharmacist should inquire about the level of disability experienced by the patient. Ratings of functional disability can be achieved by using the Sheehan Disability Scale.[79] During drug discontinuation, the frequency of appointments should be increased to evaluate for emergence of withdrawal symptoms and monitor for relapse.

OTHER ANXIETY DISORDERS

SPECIFIC PHOBIAS

Specific phobia is considered unresponsive to drug therapy, although highly responsive to behavioral therapy. The use of antidepressant medications may be detrimental in patients with specific phobias.

SOCIAL PHOBIA

Although there is no approved treatment for social phobia, patients with generalized social phobia may respond to MAOIs, BZs, or SSRIs. Three double-blind, placebo-controlled trials documented the efficacy of phenelzine in the acute management of social phobia.[80] Approximately 65% of patients treated with phenelzine (doses similar to those used in panic disorder) responded to treatment after 8 to 12 weeks.[80] The BZs, clonazepam 1.5 to 2 mg/d or alprazolam 3 mg/d, were effective after 2 weeks.[7,81] β-Blocking agents are not effective in the management of generalized social phobia; however, evidence supports their use in the management of performance anxiety (discrete phobia). Propranolol 40 mg, 1 hour before the performance may be quite helpful, as physical symptoms of anxiety frequently add to the patient's distress. Results of 12-week, open clinical trials indicate that fluoxetine (range, 10 to 80 mg/d) and paroxetine (range, 20 to 60 mg/d) reduce avoidance and social anxiety and improve social functioning.[7,82] Fluvoxamine 150 mg/d and sertraline (range, 50 to 200 mg/d) evaluated under controlled conditions, significantly improved social and general anxiety compared with placebo.[83,84] Further controlled evaluations of the SSRIs are necessary to define their role in the management of social phobia. In a retrospective review, venlafaxine was effective in patients nonresponsive to SSRIs.[85] Behavioral therapy was useful in controlled studies.[7] Most patients require 6 to 12 months of therapy. Slow medication taper, especially with the BZs, is required to prevent relapse (estimated to be 90% with fast tapers). Patients with social phobia have a significantly lower quality of life, especially for social and role functioning, general health, and work productivity.[86]

CONCLUSIONS

Theories about anxiety disorders have undergone major revisions over the past several years. Anxiety disorders are quite common, occurring in approximately 25% of the population during their lifetime. The proper management of anxiety disorders begins with the correct diagnosis; not all patients should receive antianxiety agents. Nonpharmacologic interventions are often effective alone or when combined with drug therapy.

The current classification for anxiety disorders includes several subtypes. The diagnosis determines the type of drug and nonpharmacologic intervention selected. Although BZs remain the drugs of choice for GAD and situational anxiety, other agents may be preferable for other types of anxiety. The anxiolytic agent buspirone may be useful for patients who need chronic therapy for GAD or who cannot tolerate BZs. Antidepressants, including the SSRIs, and the BZ, alprazolam, are extensively used in patients with panic disorder. The pharmacologic treatment of phobic disorders and posttraumatic stress disorder is not as well studied, and further research is needed to better define appropriate pharmacologic treatment.

▶ PRINCIPLES OF PHARMACOTHERAPY

- GAD is a chronic anxiety disorder that waxes and wanes in intensity over time and causes substantial interference with social and occupational functioning.
- Treatment options for GAD include BZs, buspirone, antidepressants, and psychotherapy; BZs are the drugs of choice for most patients.
- BZs with short-elimination half-lives are recommended for GAD in the elderly, patients with hepatic disorders, and those receiving drugs that impair oxidative metabolism.
- Buspirone is the drug of choice in GAD patients with a history of substance abuse, intolerance to BZs, or for the management of persistent anxiety.
- Buspirone requires 4 to 6 weeks to achieve maximal antianxiety effects for GAD patients and does not have sedative, hypnotic, or muscle relaxant properties.
- The goals of therapy in panic disorder are to eliminate panic attacks and reduce anticipatory anxiety and phobic avoidance, but approximately 50% of patients do not achieve this ideal.
- The sequence of patient response in panic disorder is an initial decrease in the number of panic attacks, then diminution of anticipatory anxiety, followed by a reduction in phobic avoidance.
- Antidepressants should be selected first for patients with panic disorder who are depressed or have a history of depression.
- Many patients with panic disorder are extemely sensitive to TCAs and SSRIs, and experience an immediate stimulatory feeling that may compromise compliance.
- If a TCA is discontinued abruptly, many panic disorder patients will experience severe cholinergic rebound.
- Therapeutic response to BZs for panic disorder occurs in 1 to 2 weeks, with further improvement occurring at weeks 4 to 6.
- Because of its half-life, clonazepam is an alternative to alprazolam for patients having breakthrough panic symptoms at the end of the dosing interval.

- When monitoring the effectiveness of antidepressants in panic disorder, allow an adequate amount of time (10 to 12 weeks) to achieve full therapeutic response.
- The optimal duration of panic therapy is unknown, but at least 12 months is recommended, and some patients require chronic therapy.

REFERENCES

1. American Psychiatric Association. Diagnostic and Statistical Manual of Mental Disorders, 4th ed (DSM-IV). Washington, DC, American Psychiatric Press, 1994:393–444.
2. Kessler RC, McGonagle KA, Zhao S, et al. Lifetime and 12-month prevalence of DSM-III-R psychiatric disorders in the United States. Results from the National Comorbidity Survey. Arch Gen Psychiatry 1994;51:8–19.
3. Zajecka J. Importance of establishing the diagnosis of persistent anxiety. J Clin Psychiatry 1997;58(suppl 3):9–13.
4. Fifer SK, Mathias SD, Patrick DL, et al. Untreated anxiety among adult primary care patients in a health maintenance organization. Arch Gen Psychiatry 1994;51:740–750.
5. Wise MG, Rieck SO. Diagnostic considerations and treatment approaches to underlying anxiety in the medically ill. J Clin Psychiatry 1993;54(suppl 5):22–26.
6. Rickels K, Schweizer E. The clinical course and long-term management of generalized anxiety disorder. J Clin Psychopharmacol 1990; 10:101S–110S.
7. Roy-Burne P, Wingerson D, Cowley D, Dager S. Psychopharmacologic treatment of panic, generalized anxiety disorder, and social phobia. Psychiatr Clin North Am 1993;16:719–735.
8. Wise MG, Griffes WS. A combined treatment approach to anxiety in the medically ill. J Clin Psychiatry 1995;56(suppl 2):14–19.
9. DeVane CL. The place of selective serotonin reuptake inhibitors in panic disorder. Pharmacotherapy 1997;17:282–292.
10. Goddard AW, Charney DS. Toward an integrated neurobiology of panic disorder. J Clin Psychiatry 1997;58(suppl 2):4–11.
11. Johnson MR, Lydiard RB. The neurobiology of anxiety disorders. Psychiatr Clin North Am 1995;18:681–725.
12. Pratt JA. The neuroanatomical basis of anxiety. Pharmacol Ther 1992;55:149–181.
13. Zorumski CF, Isenberg KE. Insights into the structure and function of GABA-benzodiazepine receptors: Ion channels and psychiatry. Am J Psychiatry 1991;148:162–173.
14. Teboul E, Chouinard G. A guide to benzodiazepine selection, part I. Pharmacologic aspects. Can J Psychiatry 1990;35:700–710.
15. Brawman-Mintzer O, Lydiard RB. Biologic basis of generalized anxiety disorder. J Clin Psychiatry 1997;58(suppl 3):16–25.
16. Dubovsky SL, Thomas M. Serotonergic mechanisms and current and future psychiatric practice. J Clin Psychiatry 1995;56(suppl 2):38–48.
17. Lucki I. Serotonin receptor specificity in anxiety disorders. J Clin Psychiatry 1996;57(suppl 6):5–10.
18. Wittchen H, Zhao S, Kessler RC, Eaton WW. DSM-III-R generalized anxiety disorder in the National Comorbidity Survey. Arch Gen Psychiatry 1994;51:355–364.
19. Davidson JRT. Quality of life in panic disorder. J Clin Psychiatry 1997;58:127–129.
20. Shader RI, Greenblatt DJ. Use of benzodiazepines in anxiety disorders. N Engl J Med 1993;328:1398–1405.
21. Thompson PM. Generalized anxiety disorder treatment algorithm. Psychiatr Ann 1996;4:227–232.
22. Klonopin package insert. Nutley, NJ, Roche Laboratories, October 1997.
23. Folks DG, Fuller WC. Anxiety disorders and interactions in geriatric patients. Psychiatr Clin North Am 1997;137:137–165.
24. Barbee JG. Memory, benzodiazepines, and anxiety: Integrations of theoretical and clinical perspectives. J Clin Psychiatry 1993;54(suppl 10):86–97.
25. American Psychiatric Association. Benzodiazepine dependence, toxicity, and abuse: A task force report of the American Psychiatric Association. Washington, DC, American Psychiatric Association, 1990: 1–109.
26. Michelini S, Cassano GB, Frare F, Perugi G. Long-term use of benzodiazepines: Tolerance, dependence and clinical problems in anxiety and mood disorders. Pharmacopsychiatry 1996;29:127–134.
27. Rickels K, Schweizer E, Case G, et al. Long-term therapeutic use of benzodiazepines: Effects of abrupt discontinuation. Arch Gen Psychiatry 1990;47:899–907.
28. Rickels K, Case W, Schweizer E, et al. Benzodiazepine dependence: Management of discontinuation. Psychopharmacol Bull 1990;26: 63–68.
29. Roy-Burne PP, Sullivan MD, Cowley DS, Ries R. Adjunctive treatment of benzodiazepine discontinuation syndromes: A review. J Psychiatr Res 1993;27(suppl 1):143–153.
30. Tuncok Y, Akpinar O, Guven H, Akkaclu A. The effects of theophylline on serum alprazolam levels. Int J Clin Pharmacol Ther 1994; 32:642–645.
31. Massoomi F, Savage J, Destache CJ. Omeprazole: A comprehensive review. Pharmacotherapy 1993;13:46–59.
32. Borcherding SM, Baciewicz AM, Self TH. Update on rifampin drug interactions. Arch Intern Med 1992;152:711–716.
33. Ketter TA, Flockhart DA, Post RA, et al. The emerging role of cytochrome P4503A in psychopharmacology. J Clin Psychopharmacol 1995;15:387–398.
34. Callahan AM, Fava M, Rosenbaum JF. Drug interactions in psychopharmacology. Psychiatr Clin North Am 1993;16:647–671.
35. Klimke A, Klieser E. Sudden death after intravenous application of lorazepam in a patient treated with clozapine. Am J Psychiatry 1994;151:780.
36. Lydiard RB, Brawman-Mintzer O, Ballenger JC. Recent developments in the psychopharmacology of anxiety disorders. J Consult Clin Psychol 1996;64:660–668.
37. Sramek JJ, Transman M, Suri A, et al. Efficacy of buspirone in generalized anxiety disorder with coexisting mild depressive symptoms. J Clin Psychiatry 1996;57:287–291.
38. Yocca FD. Neurochemistry and neurophysiology of buspirone and gepirone: Interactions at presynaptic and postsynaptic $5\text{-}HT_{1A}$ receptors. J Clin Psychopharmacol 1990;10(suppl 10):6–12.
39. BuSpar package insert. Princeton, Bristol-Myers Squibb, April 1996.
40. Watsky EJ, Salzman C. Psychotropic drug interactions. Hosp Comm Psychiatry 1991;42:247–256.
41. Sussman N. The uses of buspirone in psychiatry. J Clin Psychiatry Monograph 1994;12:3–19.
42. Schweizer E, Rickels K. Strategies for treatment of generalized anxiety in the primary care setting. J Clin Psychiatry 1997;58(suppl 3):27–31.
43. Lader M. β-Adrenoreceptor antagonists in neuropsychiatry: An update. J Clin Psychiatry 1988;49:213–223.
44. Rickels K, Downing R, Schweizer E, Hassman H. Antidepressants for the treatment of generalized anxiety disorder. Arch Gen Psychiatry 1993;50:884–895.
45. Hollander E, Cohen LJ. The assessment and treatment of refractory anxiety. J Clin Psychiatry 1994;55(suppl 2):27–31.
46. Rice DP, Miller LS. The economic burden of mental disorders. Adv Health Econ Health Serv Res 1993;14:37–53.
47. Leon AC, Portera L, Weissman MM. The social costs of anxiety disorders. Br J Psychiatry 1995;166(suppl 27):19–22.
48. Ormel J, VonKorff M, Ustun TB, et al. Common mental disorders and disability across cultures: Results from the WHO collaborative study on psychological problems in general health care. JAMA 1994; 272:1741–1748.

49. Kennedy BL, Schwab JJ. Utilization of medical specialists by anxiety disorder patients. Psychosomatics 1997;38:109–112.
50. Hollister LE, Mller-Oerlinghausen B, Rickels K, Shader RI. Clinical uses of benzodiazepines. J Clin Psychopharmacol 1993;13(suppl 1):1S–169S.
51. Ballenger JC. Long-term pharmacologic treatment of panic disorder. J Clin Psychiatry 1991;52(suppl 2):18–23.
52. Keller MB, Yonkers KA, Warshaw MG, et al. Remission and relapse in subjects with panic disorder and panic disorder with agoraphobia: A prospective, short-interval naturalistic follow-up. J Nerv Ment Dis 1994;182:290–296.
53. Spiegel DA, Bruce TJ. Benzodiazepines and exposure-based cognitive behavior therapies for panic disorder: Conclusions from combined treatment trials. Am J Psychiatry 1997;154:773–781.
54. Shear MK, Pilkonis PA, Cloitre M, Leon AC. Cognitive behavioral treatment compared with nonprescriptive treatment of panic disorder. Arch Gen Psychiatry 1994;51:395–401.
55. DeBeurs E, Balkom AJL, Lange A, et al. Treatment of panic disorder with agoraphobia: Comparison of fluvoxamine, placebo, and psychological panic management combined with exposure and exposure *in vivo* alone. Am J Psychiatry 1995;152:683–691.
56. Coplan JD, Pine DS, Papp LA, Gorman JM. An algorithm-oriented treatment approach for panic disorder. Psychiatr Ann 1996;26:192–201.
57. Boyer W. Serotonin uptake inhibitors are superior to imipramine and alprazolam in alleviating panic attacks: A meta-analysis. Int Clin Psychopharmacol 1995;10:45–49.
58. Tesar G, Rosenbaum JF, Pollack MH, et al. Double-blind, placebo-controlled comparison of clonazepam and alprazolam for panic disorder. J Clin Psychiatry 1991;52:69–76.
59. Schatzberg AF, Ballenger JC. Decisions for the clinician in the treatment of panic disorder: When to treat, which treatment to use, and how long to treat. J Clin Psychiatry 1991;52(suppl 2):26–31.
60. Schweizer E, Rickels K, Weiss S, Zavodnick S. Maintenance drug treatment of panic disorder. Arch Gen Psychiatry 1993;50:51–60.
61. Cross-National Collaborative Panic Study, Second Phase Investigators. Drug treatment of panic disorder: Comparative efficacy of alprazolam, imipramine, and placebo. Br J Psychiatry 1992;160:191–202.
62. Jefferson JW. Antidepressants in panic disorder. J Clin Psychiatry 1997;58(suppl 2):20–24.
63. Modigh K, Westberg P, Eriksson E. Superiority of clomipramine over imipramine in the treatment of panic disorder: A placebo-controlled trial. J Clin Psychopharmacol 1992;12:251–261.
64. Oehrberg S, Christiansen PE, Behnke K, et al. Paroxetine in the treatment of panic disorder: A randomized, double-blind, placebo-controlled study. Br J Psychiatry 1995;167:374–379.
65. Hoehn-Saric R, McLeod DR, Hipsley PA. Effect of fluvoxamine on panic disorder. J Clin Psychopharmacol 1993;13:321–326.
66. Schneier FR, Liebowitz MR, Davies SO, et al. Fluoxetine in panic disorder. J Clin Psychopharmacol 1990;10:119–121.
67. Pollack MH, Otto MW, Worthington JJ, et al. Sertraline in the treatment of panic disorder: A flexible-dose multicenter trail. Arch Gen Psych 1998;55:1010–1016.
68. Zajecka JM. The effect of nefazodone on comorbid anxiety symptoms associated with depression: Experience in family practice and psychiatric outpatient settings. J Clin Psychiatry 1996;57(suppl 2):10–14.
69. Garacioti TD. Venlafaxine treatment of panic disorder: A case series. J Clin Psychiatry 1996;56:408–410.
70. Rosenbaum JF, Moroz G, Bowden CL, et al. Clonazepam in the treatment of panic disorder with or without agoraphobia: A dose–response study of efficacy, safety, and discontinuance. J Clin Psychopharmacol 1997;17:390–400.
71. Noyes R, Burrows GD, Reich JH, et al. Diazepam versus alprazolam for the treatment of panic disorder. J Clin Psychiatry 1996;57:349–355.
72. Keck PE, McElroy SL, Tugrul KC, et al. Antiepileptic drugs for the treatment of panic disorder. Neuropsychobiology 1993;27:150–153.
73. Puzantian T, Hart LL. Clonidine in panic disorder. Ann Pharmacother 1993;27:1351–1352.
74. Paxil package insert. Philadelphia, SmithKline Beecham Pharmaceuticals, May 1996.
75. Blackwell B. Monoamine oxidase inhibitor interactions with other drugs. J Clin Psychopharmacol 1991;11:55–59.
76. Mavissakalian M, Perel J. Protective effects of imipramine maintenance in panic disorder with agoraphobia. Am J Psychiatry 1992;149:1053–1057.
77. Noyes R, Garvey MN, Cook B, Suelzer M. Controlled discontinuation of benzodiazepine treatment for patients with panic disorder. Am J Psychiatry 1991;148:517–523.
78. Salvador-Carulla L, Segu J, Fernández-Cano P, Canet J. Costs and offset effect in panic disorder. Br J Psychiatry 1995;166(suppl 27):23–28.
79. Perugi G, Akiskal HS, Musetti L, et al. Social adjustment in panic-agoraphobic patients reconsidered. Br J Psychiatry 1994;164:88–93.
80. Marshall RD, Schneier FR, Fallon BA, et al. Medication therapy for social phobia. J Clin Psychiatry 1994;55(suppl 6):33–37.
81. Davidson JR, Tupler LA, Potts NLS. Treatment of social phobia with benzodiazepines. J Clin Psychiatry 1994;55(suppl 6):28–32.
82. Mancini C, Van Amerigen M. Paroxetine in social phobia. J Clin Psychiatry 1996;57:519–522.
83. Van Vliet IM, den Boer JA, Westenberg HGM. Psychopharmacological treatment of social phobia: A double blind placebo controlled study with fluvoxamine. Psychopharmacology 1994;115:128–134.
84. Katzelnick DJ, Koback KA, Greist JH, et al. Sertraline for social phobia: A double-blind, placebo-controlled crossover study. Am J Psychiatry 1995;152:1368–1371.
85. Kelsey JE. Venlafaxine in social phobia. Psychopharmacol Bull 1995;31:767–771.
86. Wittchen HU, Beloch E. The impact of social phobia on quality of life. Int J Clin Psychopharmacol 1996;11(suppl 3):15–23.

68

Obsessive–Compulsive Disorder

Barbara G. Wells, PharmD, FASHP, FCCP, BCPP, and Peggy E. Hayes, PharmD

Although symptoms of obsessive–compulsive disorder (OCD) have been recognized for centuries and have remained virtually unchanged, OCD has only recently been the focus of extensive research. These investigations have greatly advanced our understanding of the epidemiology, etiology, and pharmacologic treatment of this disorder. Since the mid-1980s, the Food and Drug Administration (FDA) has approved five drugs, as effective for the treatment of OCD: clomipramine (Anafranil), fluoxetine (Prozac), fluvoxamine (Luvox), paroxetine (Paxil), and sertraline (Zoloft). Although OCD is officially classified as an anxiety disorder, it is presented as a separate illness because of its unique clinical presentation and treatment approach. OCD is the most disabling of the anxiety disorders and rarely remits without specific behavioral and pharmacologic interventions. Unfortunately, despite treatment the prognosis often remains poor, and many patients continue to suffer disabling symptoms and a lifelong disability.[1]

EPIDEMIOLOGY

The National Institute of Mental Health, Epidemiologic Catchment Area Study (ECA) provides the most up-to-date, comprehensive data regarding the prevalence of mental illness including OCD. The ECA studies were extensive community surveys conducted from 1980 to 1984 in five areas across the United States. These studies estimated the prevalence of psychiatric illness among community populations and included persons not seeking psychiatric treatment.[2,3]

A most surprising finding was that OCD is approximately 50 times more common than previously reported by surveys conducted using clinical populations (or persons seeking treatment). The ECA studies found a lifetime prevalence of OCD ranging from 1.9% to 3.2% and a 1-year prevalence rate of 1.5% to 2.1%.[1–3] OCD is the fourth most common psychiatric disorder following phobias, substance abuse, and major depression. Unfortunately, many patients do not seek treatment.[2,3]

OCD usually begins in late adolescence or early adulthood, but it may begin in childhood. Childhood-, adolescence-, and adult-onset OCD have a similar clinical presentation. The incidence of OCD is slightly higher in females than males; however, males tend to have an earlier modal age of onset (between ages 6 and 15 years for males versus ages 20 and 29 years for females). The onset is usually gradual with a chronic waxing and waning course.[1,3] OCD may have a familial component to its etiology.[4,5] Approximately 10% of first-degree relatives (mother, father, sibling) of patients with OCD have OCD, and another 8% have a subclinical form of the disorder. In a comparison group of first-degree relatives of normal subjects, there was a prevalence of only 2% for OCD and another 2% for the subclinical form.[4] When one twin has OCD, the concordance rate is higher for monozygotic twins than for dizygotic twins.[3,5]

PATHOPHYSIOLOGY

Although OCD occasionally begins following a brain injury, especially involving the basal ganglion (e.g., encephalitis or trauma), there is usually no neurologic precipitant. The most compelling evidence suggesting a biologic basis for OCD is the consistent successful treatment using selective and potent serotonin (5-HT) reuptake-blocking drugs. Treatment trials with drugs having other mechanisms of action have not been effective. The neurotransmitter 5-HT appears to play an important role in the pathogenesis of OCD.[6,7] Although studies of 5-HT function dominate research into the pathophysiology of OCD, a clear model of serotonergic dysfunction to explain the pathophysiology of OCD is lacking. (For example, is there a decrease or increase in serotonergic function, and what specific subtypes of 5-HT receptors are involved?)

SEROTONERGIC PROBES

Important evidence for an abnormality in 5-HT functioning comes from pharmacologic challenge studies that assess serotonergic responsiveness in OCD patients.[8,9] The most frequently used probe in studies of OCD has been *m*-chlorophenylpiperazine (*m*-CPP). A nonspecific postsynaptic 5-HT agonist and metabolite of the antidepressant trazodone, *m*-CPP produced very limited behavioral effects in normal volunteers. In untreated OCD patients, *m*-CPP produced a marked, but transient, increase in obsessions, depression, and anxiety symptoms.[3,5,8] These findings indicate an increased sensitivity to *m*-CPP in some untreated OCD patients. Treatment with clomipramine[3,5] and fluoxetine[8] abolished the pretreatment *m*-CPP-induced exacerbation of obsessive–compulsive symptoms. Several other 5-HT probes have been studied in OCD patients (metergoline, ipsapirone, L-tryptophan, fenfluramine). However, the serotonergic probes have been disappointing in their failure to identify a consistent 5-HT defect in OCD.[9]

BRAIN-IMAGING STUDIES

Structural brain-imaging studies with computed tomography (CT) and magnetic resonance imaging (MRI) have not identified the presence of a clear lesion (structural pathology) in patients with OCD.[10,11] However, brain-imaging studies to assess the biochemical and physiologic function of the brain using single-photon emission computed tomography (SPECT) and positron emission tomography (PET) have produced consistent findings that identify three areas of increased/abnormal metabolic activity—the orbitofrontal cortex, cingulate cortex, and head of the caudate nucleus.[10,11] These areas may be involved in the pathophysiologic origin of OCD symptoms and may form a circuit that is "hyperactive" in OCD. However, these areas of increased metabolic activity may be merely compensating for areas of decreased brain activity. Successful pharmacologic treatment of OCD patients with increased metabolic activity in the caudate nucleus and the orbitofrontal cortex was associated with a return to normal metabolic functioning.

DOPAMINE MODEL

Because neurologic symptoms (tics) are part of the clinical presentation in some OCD patients, and because some patients have a family history of Tourette's syndrome, a disorder of dopamine (DA) dysfunction, DA dysregulation may contribute to some forms of OCD. The neurotransmitter DA is found in high concentrations in the caudate nucleus, an area believed to be "hyperactive" in OCD. OCD patients with tics often benefit from the addition of an antipsychotic to their treatment regimen.[3,12]

CLINICAL PRESENTATION

The *Diagnostic and Statistical Manual of Mental Disorders,* fourth edition (DSM-IV) requires the presence of either obsessions and/or compulsions (although most patients have both) that are severe enough to cause marked distress, to be time consuming (occupy more than 1 hour a day), and to cause significant impairment in social or occupational functioning (Table 68–1).[1] These individuals often recognize that their obsessions or compulsions are excessive or unreasonable. An obsession is a recurrent, persistent idea, thought, impulse, or image that is experienced as intrusive and inappropriate and produces marked anxiety. Common obsessions involve thoughts about contamination (such as a concern with germs, dirt, or toxic chemicals), repeated doubts (e.g., whether a door was left unlocked), and needing to have things in a particular order.[1,5] Individuals recognize obsessions as products of their own mind and attempt to ignore or suppress them. "No matter how hard I try, I cannot get this crazy thought out of my mind." An obsession produces a marked feeling of anxiety and is not simply excessive worry about a real life situation.[1,5]

A compulsion is a repetitive, purposeful, intentional behavior or mental act usually performed in response to an obsession. The most common compulsions involve washing and cleaning, counting, checking, and requesting or demanding assurances. Compulsive behavior is not pleasurable and is designed to prevent discomfort or the occurrence of a dreaded event that is often unknown. For example, many patients are obsessed with feelings of doubt (e.g., whether a door was left unlocked), causing them marked distress, and leading to repetitive checking (or compulsive behaviors). These behaviors are usually performed according to certain rules or in a stereotyped fashion.[1,5]

TABLE 68–1. DSM-IV Diagnostic Criteria for Obsessive–Compulsive Disorder

A. Either obsessions or compulsions:
Obsessions as defined by (1), (2), (3), and (4):
(1) Recurrent and persistent thoughts, impulses, or images that are experienced, *at some time during the disturbance,* as intrusive and *inappropriate and that cause marked anxiety or distress.*
(2) The thoughts, impulses, or images are not simply excessive worries about real-life problems.
(3) Attempts are made to ignore or suppress the thoughts, impulses, or images or to eliminate them.
(4) It is recognized that the obsessional thoughts, impulses, or images are a product of the person's own mind (not imposed from without).
Compulsions as defined by (1) and (2):
(1) Repetitive behaviors (e.g., hand washing, ordering, checking) or mental acts (e.g., praying, counting, repeating words silently) that the person feels driven to perform in response to an obsession, or according to certain rules.
(2) The behaviors or mental acts are aimed at preventing or reducing distress or preventing some dreaded event or situation; however, these behaviors or mental acts either are not connected in a realistic way with what they are designed to eliminate or they are clearly excessive.

B. The person has recognized that the obsessions or compulsions are excessive or unreasonable.

C. The obsessions or compulsions cause marked distress, are time consuming (take more than 1 hour a day), or significantly interfere with the person's normal routine, occupational (or academic) functioning, or usual social activities or relationships.

Modified and reprinted with permission from the Diagnostic and Statistical Manual of Mental Disorders, 4th ed. Copyright 1994, American Psychiatric Association.

Compulsions are also recognized by the individual as senseless. Because patients recognize their behavior as silly, they become extremely adept at denying symptoms, disguising their rituals, and concealing their illness from friends and family members.[1,5]

In addition to primary symptoms, about 20% to 40% of patients have involuntary motor movements (e.g., facial tics and grimaces).[3,5] The overlap between Tourette's syndrome and OCD is well documented. Tourette's syndrome, a neurologic disorder that begins in childhood, is characterized by repetitive, involuntary, multiple motor and vocal tics.[13] Some OCD patients meet criteria for Tourette's syndrome, and some Tourette's patients have symptoms of OCD.[3,5]

Many patients experience disabling symptoms for several years before seeking treatment.[2,3] Typically, almost 7.5 years elapse between the onset of clinical symptoms and the first psychiatric visit.[2,3] Although the consequences of untreated OCD have not been systematically studied, OCD produces significant work and social disability. Depression and anxiety symptoms are also present in many patients with OCD, and depression often prompts patients to seek treatment.[1,3] The ECA study reported that approximately 50% of patients with OCD had another major psychiatric disorder (e.g., major depression, alcohol abuse or dependence, panic disorder, or schizophrenia). In most patients, OCD occurred first.[2,5] This means that certain illnesses (e.g., major depression, alcohol abuse, and panic disorder) might be consequences of untreated OCD or part of the natural course of OCD. Therefore, OCD patients seeking treatment commonly require treatment for a comorbid psychiatric disorder. OCD is a chronic disorder that for most patients continues throughout adult life.[1,5]

DIFFERENTIAL DIAGNOSIS

Patient with OCD are aware of the irrationality of their symptoms, are often ashamed to admit their symptoms, and are skilled at hiding them.[1–3,5] Therefore, most cases of OCD are not recognized by the primary care physician. Certain disorders have symptoms resembling OCD (known as OCD spectrum disorders), including trichotillomania (an urge to pull out one's hair), Tourette's syndrome, complex motor or vocal tics, eating disorders (15% of adult women with OCD had anorexia in adolescence), compulsive gambling, and compulsive sexual behaviors.[1,3] Patients with OCD often initially seek treatment from primary care physicians or dermatologists because of severe dermatitis from excessive washing.[3,5]

A distinction should be made between OCD and obsessive–compulsive personality disorder. Obsessions and compulsions are not present in obsessive–compulsive personality disorder. These individuals are preoccupied with orderliness, perfectionism, and control beginning early in childhood. Unlike individuals with OCD, those with obsessive–compulsive personality disorder do not view their behavior as irrational and do not wish to change, as they consider these personality features to be beneficial.[1,3,5]

▶ TREATMENT: Obsessive–Compulsive Disorder

DESIRED OUTCOME

A goal of treatment for OCD is to achieve as great a level of symptom reduction as possible while recognizing that a complete cure or elimination of all symptoms is unlikely.[14] An additional goal is to minimize adverse consequences on quality of life and to restore the patient to an optimal level of psychosocial and occupational functioning. However, most patients generally have symptom reduction far short of total symptom relief. Although several nondrug and drug therapies are superior to placebo, many patients continue to demonstrate significant symptomatology.

GENERAL APPROACH TO TREATMENT

In adolescents with OCD, cognitive–behavioral therapy (CBT) is generally selected first for milder OCD, but CBT plus a selective serotonin reuptake inhibitor (SSRI), such as fluoxetine, fluvoxamine, sertraline, or paroxetine, are selected for more severe OCD. In adults, CBT is selected first for milder OCD; CBT plus an SSRI or an SSRI alone is selected first for more severe OCD.[15] An algorithm for the treatment of OCD is presented in Figure 68–1.

NONPHARMACOLOGIC THERAPY

For OCD, CBT involves exposure plus response prevention combined with cognitive therapy. When available, CBT should be offered to every OCD patient.[15] Two-thirds to three-fourths of patients who continue in therapy often respond,[16] but patients who agree to CBT must tolerate high levels of anxiety that often eventually causes them to discontinue therapy.[17] CBT should be added to the regimen when a patient has been a nonresponder or partial responder to a serotonin reuptake inhibitor (SRI) alone. SRIs include the SSRIs and clomipramine. CBT should be used alone if the patient is intolerant to side effects of medication, is pregnant, or has a medical condition that contraindicates medication.[15]

Exposure with response prevention is particularly helpful for contamination or other fears, symmetry rituals, counting/repeating, hoarding, and aggressive urges. Cognitive therapy is especially helpful for scrupulosity, moral guilt, and pathologic doubt. Thirteen to 20 sessions are typically required to treat uncomplicated OCD,[15] and an adequate trial is considered to be at least 20 hours.[18]

OCD patients with concomitant depression, psychosis, or mania are unlikely to respond to behavior therapy until these symptoms are well controlled with pharmacotherapy.[19] Eighty percent of patients will experience at least moderate improvement with combined treatment. Behavior therapy has little to offer the patient with severe obsessions who does not have compulsions (approximately 20% of OCD patients). In OCD patients who suffer from obsessive thoughts only (without compulsions), a trial of antiobsessional medication is a reasonable first choice.[19]

PHARMACOLOGIC THERAPY

MECHANISMS OF ACTION

Current evidence strongly indicates that 5-HT is important for the antiobsessional effects of medication. The SRIs inhibit 5-HT reuptake into the presynaptic neuron. Reuptake is the first and most important step in reducing 5-HT neurotransmission. Inhibiting reuptake of 5-HT makes more 5-HT available to postsynaptic receptors and reduces formation of the 5-HT metabolite, 5-hydroxyindoleacetic acid (5-HIAA). Although other antidepressants, such as imipramine and amitriptyline, inhibit 5-HT reuptake, they are less potent and selective than the SRIs. Prolonged exposure to increased amounts of 5-HT following chronic antidepressant treatment (2 to 3 weeks) leads to altered responsiveness of postsynaptic 5-HT receptors or presynaptic autoregulatory receptors that may govern 5-HT release in specific brain regions.[14]

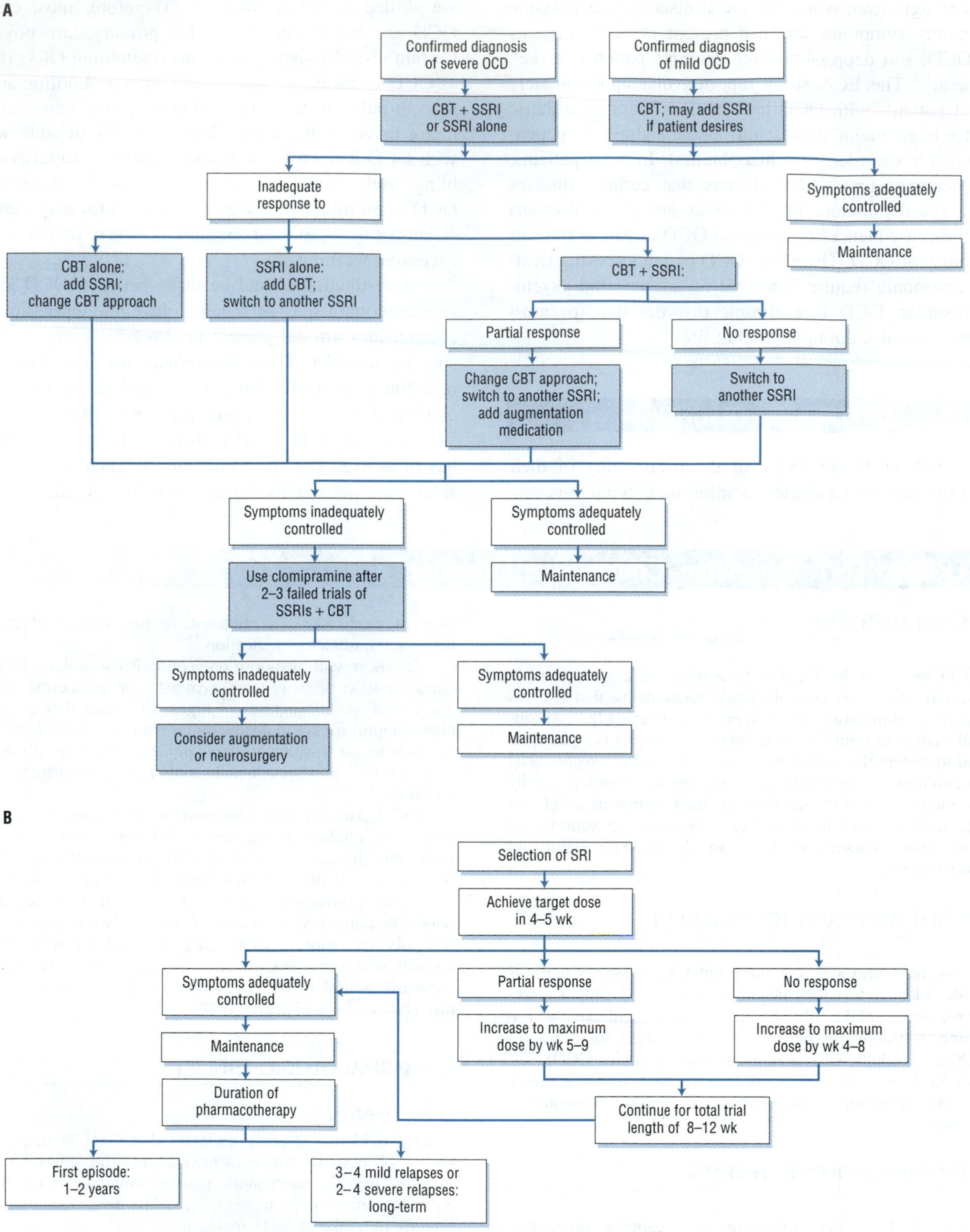

FIGURE 68–1. Algorithm for management of OCD in adults. **A.** Overall approach to treatment. **B.** Pharmacotherapeutic approach to treatment. (CBT = cognitive–behavioral therapy; SRI = serotonin reuptake inhibitor; SSRI = selective serotonin reuptake inhibitor.) *(Derived from Refs. 15 and 76.)*

The most impressive and consistent evidence to support a role for 5-HT in treating OCD is that only potent 5-HT reuptake inhibitors appear to be consistently effective. Further, an improvement in obsessional symptoms may correlate with plasma concentrations of clomipramine but not desmethylclomipramine, the metabolite of clomipramine with less selectivity for 5-HT reuptake inhibition. With clomipramine treatment, the decrease in obsessional symptoms correlates with a decrease in the concentration of 5-HIAA in cerebrospinal fluid, and a decrease in platelet 5-HT content.[14] The effectiveness of serotonergic agents in treating OCD lends support to the role of 5-HT in the etiology of OCD. However, because many patients fail to respond to these agents, the role of other neurotransmitter systems in the pathophysiology of OCD must continue to be explored.

GENERAL PRINCIPLES

SRIs may be combined with CBT or used alone in adults with moderate to severe symptoms. An SSRI should be added when there has been no response or partial response to CBT alone. Generally, an SSRI is selected before clomipramine and whenever anticholinergic, cardiovascular, sexual, sedative, or weight gain side effects are a major concern. If one SSRI is ineffective, then another SSRI should be tried. Treatment resistance can be defined as failure to achieve at least a 25% reduction in baseline score on the Yale Brown Obsessive Compulsive Scale (Y-BOCS). Clomipramine may be selected after 2 to 3 failed SSRI trials. Clomipramine may also be used to augment an SSRI in partially responsive or nonresponsive patients.[15]

When OCD is complicated by comorbid illness, treatment strategies are individualized to the comorbid illness and to patient needs. In general, OCD in the pregnant patient is treated with CBT alone. OCD in a patient with cardiac or renal disease may be treated with CBT alone or CBT plus an SSRI. OCD in patients with Tourette's disorder may be treated with CBT plus a conventional antipsychotic and an SRI. OCD in the presence of attention-deficit hyperactivity disorder may be treated with CBT plus an SSRI and psychostimulant. OCD with panic disorder or social phobia may be treated with CBT and an SSRI. In a patient with OCD and major depression, CBT plus an SRI can be used, and the SRI should be started first for severe symptoms. CBT plus a mood stabilizer with or without an SRI may be used in patients with bipolar disorder. OCD may be treated with an SRI and antipsychotic in patients with comorbid schizophrenia.[15]

The only medications consistently demonstrating efficacy in controlled clinical trials are the SRIs.[6,7,17,20–28] These studies confirm the gradual improvement of obsessive and compulsive symptoms over a 4- to 10-week treatment period. It is unlikely that clinical trials will be able to demonstrate significant differences in efficacy between the SRIs, because 600 to 700 patients would probably be required to show a statistically significant difference.[17] A meta-analysis suggested that the efficacy of clomipramine was slightly superior to fluvoxamine, which was slightly superior to sertraline.[23] However, these data must be viewed with caution, because of varying methodologies between studies and differences in numbers of treatment-resistant patients and placebo responders. An additional meta-analysis supported the superiority of clomipramine over fluoxetine, fluvoxamine, and sertraline, but head-to-head double-blind comparisons would be the best evaluation of comparative efficacy.[7]

Responders often experience only a 50% reduction in symptom severity. A patient showing partial response after 4 to 5 weeks of treatment may improve considerably if treatment is continued for several additional weeks. Approximately 60% to 70% of patients experience at least a moderate response to the SRIs compared to 5% to 10% who respond to placebo.[6,17] Therefore, most patients continue to have symptoms severe enough to limit their functioning. Although this degree of improvement seems modest, patients usually find this improvement clearly preferable to their pretreatment condition and are often willing to tolerate substantial adverse effects to maintain partial symptom remission.

Approximately 89% of 18 OCD patients chronically treated with clomipramine had a substantial recurrence of symptoms after a 7-week placebo period.[29] However, in a study of 35 OCD patients who discontinued fluoxetine after a good response, only 23% relapsed without medication during the first year.[30] Behavior therapy that accompanies pharmacotherapy may not only increase the extent of symptom reduction, but may also enhance the persistence of improvement after drug therapy is discontinued.

No predictors of response to pharmacotherapy have been firmly identified. Most investigators agree that factors failing to predict response include severity of illness, presence of depression, duration of illness, type of symptoms (obsessions versus compulsions), dexamethasone resistance, reduced rapid-eye movement (REM) sleep latency, and platelet 5-HT measures.[14] However, Alarcon and associates[31] found that higher initial scores on the Y-BOCS were associated with poorer response to clomipramine. Further, this group reported that the presence of cleaning rituals, such as washing or cleaning sinks, bathtubs, walls, and ovens, was a predictor of poor or modest response to clomipramine. An additional report found that the presence of panic or phobia with OCD is a positive predictor of response to clomipramine.[32] The SRIs may be more likely to be effective for pathologic doubt, mental rituals, and aggressive obsessions and urges than for slowness, hoarding, and tic-like symptoms.[15]

Table 68–2 summarizes dosing guidelines. If there is inadequate response to an average SRI dose, then the dose should be pushed to the maximum dose within 4 to 9 weeks from the start of treatment. If there is an inadequate response after 4 to 6 weeks at the maximum dose, then another SRI should be tried. Eight to 13 weeks is considered an adequate trial before changing to another medication or augmenting with another agent.

Once patients have responded to the acute phase of treatment, treatment gains are maintained with maintenance-phase strategies. Monthly follow-up visits are recommended for at least 3 to 6 months, and a medication taper can be considered after 1 to 2 years of treatment. Medication should not be rapidly discontinued, and booster CBT sessions may reduce the risk of relapse when medication is withdrawn. Medication doses can be decreased by 25%, and then 2 months should lapse before again decreasing the dose, depending on response. Long-term or lifelong prophylactic maintenance medication is recommended after two to four severe relapses or three to four mild to moderate relapses.[15] Although the appropriate maintenance dose of the SRIs is unknown, it is notable that one investigator was successful in reducing the dose of clomipramine from a mean of 270 mg/d to 165 mg/d in the maintenance phase. Mundo and colleagues[33] studied patients successfully treated with clomipramine or fluvoxamine and reduced their doses by 33% to 66% for maintenance therapy. They found that maintenance therapy was successful with reduced dosages of the antiobsessional drug, with clear advantages for tolerability and compliance. However, study duration was only 102 days.[33]

Most experts agree that the SSRIs are better tolerated than clomipramine. The SSRIs are less likely than clomipramine to cause cardiovascular, sedative, anticholinergic, and weight gain side effects. Clomipramine is less likely than the SSRIs to cause insomnia, akathisia, nausea, and diarrhea. Side effects may be more severe when larger doses are used and with faster dose escalation. Tolerance to adverse effects often develops over 6 to 8 weeks of treatment, and tolerance may be more likely to develop to nausea, diarrhea, sedation, diminished libido and/or orgasm, anxiety, restlessness, insomnia, and anticholinergic side effects than to akathisia.[15]

TABLE 68–2. Dosing of SRIs in Treatment of OCD

Generic Name	Usual Initial Daily Dose (mg)	Usual Daily Dosage Range (mg)	Average Target Daily Dose (mg)
Clomipramine	10	100–250	150–200
Fluoxetine	20	20–80	40–60
Fluvoxamine	50	100–300	200
Paroxetine	20	20–60	50
Sertraline	50	75–225	150

Modified from Ref. 15.

SSRIs must not be given concurrently with monoamine oxidase inhibitors (MAOIs). It is usually recommended that 2 weeks elapse between administering an SSRI and an MAOI in either direction. However, 5 weeks should elapse after stopping fluoxetine before starting an MAOI, because of fluoxetine's long half-life of elimination. SSRIs variably inhibit multiple components of the cytochrome P450 system that is responsible for metabolism of many psychotropic and other medications. Refer to Chapter 65 for a more complete discussion of drug interactions involving the SRIs.

ALTERNATIVE PHARMACOLOGIC THERAPIES

Jenike and colleagues[34] conducted a 10-week, placebo-controlled trial in 64 patients with OCD, and found that only a subgroup of patients with symmetry or other atypical obsessions responded to therapy with phenelzine. Fluoxetine-treated patients (80 mg/d) improved significantly more than phenelzine-treated patients (60 mg/d) or placebo-treated patients. There was no efficacy of phenelzine overall or in a subgroup of patients with high levels of anxiety.[34] Based on limited data, the efficacy of MAOIs in OCD appears limited.

Benzodiazepines are rarely useful despite occasional case reports of response.[35] Limited evidence suggests that buspirone, a 5-HT_{1A} partial agonist, may occasionally be beneficial in the treatment of OCD.[36,37] These finding are preliminary, and further controlled studies with larger sample sizes are needed to assess whether buspirone is an effective agent in the treatment of OCD.

SPECIAL POPULATIONS

Hepatic and Renal Disease

Clomipramine, fluoxetine, paroxetine, and fluvoxamine are extensively metabolized in the liver, and patients with significant liver disease should be prescribed these drugs cautiously and in lower doses than those used in healthy subjects. The pharmacokinetics of fluoxetine and fluvoxamine were similar in patients with renal failure and in healthy subjects; however, the manufacturer recommends starting with a lower dose in patients with renal impairment. The pharmacokinetics of sertraline in patients with significant renal dysfunction have not been determined. Increased plasma concentrations of paroxetine occur in subjects with renal impairment. The initial dose of paroxetine should be reduced in patients with severe renal impairment, and upward titration should occur more slowly.

Elderly Patients

There is little available information on treating OCD in the elderly. Case reports and anecdotal information suggests that the antiobsessional medications are likely to be equally effective in the elderly and in younger adults.[38,39] Selection of medication for an elderly person with OCD, however, should be based on history of response and adverse side-effect profile. Treatment should be initiated with low doses in elderly patients, and doses should be increased slowly, with vigilance for emergence of side effects. Some elderly patients may ultimately require doses similar to those used in younger adults, but doses must be individualized according to response and tolerance of side effects.

In elderly patients refractory to SSRIs, an augmentation strategy with minimal risk is to add buspirone to SSRI therapy. Buspirone has few side effects and appears to be a good choice for augmentation. On the other hand, clonazepam causes excessive sedation and may accumulate over time. It should not be prescribed as augmentation for the frail elderly or those with gait disturbances.[40]

Approximately 150 elderly patients received clomipramine in U.S. clinical trials. Although no unusual age-related adverse effects were identified, age-related differences in efficacy or safety cannot be ruled out. This is especially true for elderly patients with coexisting diseases and those receiving concurrent drugs. Elderly patients receiving clomipramine may experience more sedation and anticholinergic adverse effects than younger adults.[6,41] Because of clomipramine's sedative and anticholinergic side effects, it is not usually chosen as first-line therapy for elderly OCD patients.

Plasma concentrations of fluoxetine are 127% higher in the elderly than in younger individuals receiving the same dose.[42] The overall cardiovascular profile of fluoxetine appears quite favorable; however, Buff and associates[43] reported that atrial fibrillation and bradycardia developed in an 87-year-old woman shortly after fluoxetine was initiated. On fluoxetine rechallenge, these dysrhythmias recurred.

The multiple-dose elimination half-life of fluvoxamine was 17.4 and 25.9 hours in the elderly compared to 13.6 and 15.6 hours in younger subjects at steady state for 50- and 100-mg doses, respectively.[44] The safety of fluvoxamine has not been adequately studied in the elderly and patients with cardiovascular disease. Dosage should be titrated slowly during initiation of fluvoxamine therapy in elderly patients.

Sertraline plasma clearance in elderly patients was approximately 40% lower than in a group of younger individuals. Clearance of desmethylsertraline was also decreased in elderly males, but not in elderly females. To date, the pattern of adverse reactions in the elderly appears to be similar to that in younger adults.

In a multiple-dose study in the elderly, paroxetine C_{min} concentrations were 70% to 80% greater than in nonelderly subjects. The manufacturer recommends that the initial dose be reduced in the elderly. In worldwide premarketing trials, the adverse event profile was similar in elderly and nonelderly patients, but the patients in these studies were healthy.[45]

Children and Adolescents

Childhood and adult OCD appear to respond similarly to drug therapy. Data suggest that at least 50% of patients with childhood-onset OCD remain symptomatic as adults and have a chronic and debilitating course.[46]

Flament and colleagues[47] treated 19 children and adolescents with clomipramine in a 10-week, double-blind, placebo-controlled, crossover trial. Clomipramine was significantly superior to placebo, and 75% of patients had a moderate to marked improvement. In a double-blind, crossover study comparing clomipramine with desipramine, 48 children and adolescents completed the 10-week trial. Clomipramine was more effective than desipramine; however, desipramine was no more effective than placebo.[48] In both studies clomipramine was well tolerated at doses of 3 mg/kg/d.

Pregnant and Lactating Patients

In general, CBT alone should be used for pregnant patients except in cases where the risks of untreated OCD outweigh the risks of medication use in pregnancy (for example, a pregnant mother who will not eat because of contamination fears).[15] Women with a history of OCD should be informed that OCD may worsen during pregnancy and the postpartum period. OCD symptoms may exacerbate during the first trimester, especially if pharmacotherapy is discontinued just before conception or early in pregnancy. Symptoms often improve during the second trimester and worsen during the third.[49]

Data suggest that exposure to fluoxetine in the first trimester does not increase the risk of congenital malformations.[50,51] Transient withdrawal syndromes have been reported in infants exposed to imipramine and nortriptyline.[49] Prenatal clomipramine exposure has resulted in cases of infant hypothermia, respiratory acidosis, and seizures.[52,53]

If drug therapy during pregnancy is required, fluoxetine appears to be the safest choice. However, the neurobehavioral effects of prenatal exposure on the neonate and the child have not been fully elucidated. Clomipramine should probably be avoided during pregnancy.[49] Clonazepam may be considered for OCD symptoms in pregnant women with disabling anxiety, but with higher doses (2.0 to 5.0 mg) hypotonia, apnea, and failure to feed have been observed.[49]

In general, prescribing SSRIs during nursing is considered inadvisable. All SRIs are excreted into breast milk, and therefore, a decision must be made whether to discontinue nursing or discontinue drug therapy, weighing benefits against risks. With fluoxetine, one case of colic symptoms and unexplained high serum levels was reported in a breast-fed 5-week-old,[54] but several infants have been safely breast fed during maternal fluoxetine use.[55,56] Sertraline was undetectable in the plasma of a breast-fed infant whose mother was taking a dosage of 100 mg/d.[57] Paroxetine and fluvoxamine appear in milk in amounts similar to or less than fluoxetine,[58,59] but there is less clinical experience with their use during nursing.

SPECIFIC AGENTS

Clomipramine

The adverse effect profile of clomipramine is similar to the other tricyclic antidepressants (TCAs; refer to Chap. 65). The most frequently reported adverse effects are dry mouth, dizziness, tremor, fatigue, somnolence, constipation, and nausea. Other side effects include weight gain and sexual dysfunction, such as ejaculation failure, libido change, and impotence.

Because of the risk of seizures, the maximum daily dose should not exceed 250 mg, and caution should be used in prescribing clomipramine to patients with a history of seizures, alcoholism, or brain damage.[6,41] Similarly, caution should be used when prescribing clomipramine concomitantly with other drugs known to lower the seizure threshold.[41] Caution is also advised when prescribing clomipramine for patients with a history of liver disease, as rare reports of severe liver injury, some fatal, have been reported.[41]

Protein binding is approximately 97%, and the elimination half-life ranges from 31 to 37 hours. However, given reports of non-first-order elimination kinetics, these estimates should be viewed with caution.[60] Studies have reported that plasma clomipramine concentrations positively correlated with improvement in compulsions[61] and obsessions,[62] whereas plasma desmethylclomipramine levels were related to improvement in depression.[61] Mavissakalian and others[63] reported that plasma concentrations of clomipramine, but not desmethylclomipramine, correlated significantly with clinical response. Plasma concentrations of neither compound predicted response in children and adolescents. Clomipramine's drug–drug interactions are similar to those of the other TCAs. Refer to Chapter 65 for a review of these.

Clomipramine should be initiated at a dose of 25 mg/d (usually at bedtime) and gradually increased during the first 2 weeks to approximately 100 mg/d. Over the next several weeks, the dose may be increased gradually to a maximum of 250 mg/d. Initially clomipramine should be administered in divided doses with meals to reduce gastrointestinal side effects, but after titration, the total daily dose may be given once daily at bedtime.[6,41] For maintenance therapy, many patients may have their dose reduced by 25% to 50%.

Fluoxetine

The most commonly reported fluoxetine-related side effects in OCD patients include nausea, headache, anxiety, sedation, insomnia, diarrhea, sexual dysfunction, and tremor.[64]

Absorption of fluoxetine is delayed when it is administered with food. It is approximately 95% bound to plasma proteins. With multiple daily dosing, the half-life of elimination of fluoxetine is 5.7 days, and that of norfluoxetine has been reported to be 7 to 15 days.[65] No relationship has been established between plasma concentrations of fluoxetine or norfluoxetine and clinical response in treatment of OCD.[66]

Several fatal reactions have occurred with coadministration of MAOIs and fluoxetine. Therefore, MAOIs should not be administered until at least 5 weeks after discontinuation of fluoxetine. Fluoxetine is a potent inhibitor of CYP2D6 and CPY2C9, a moderate inhibitor of CYP3A3/4 and CYP2C19, and a weak inhibitor of CYP1A2.[67] The metabolism of both methylated and demethylated TCAs is impaired by fluoxetine. Therefore, the dose of a TCA should be reduced by 75% when fluoxetine is added, and 3 months should be allowed for a new steady-state TCA plasma concentration to be attained.[65] Multiple other drug–drug interactions have been associated with fluoxetine. Refer to Chapter 65 and the drug interaction literature for a more complete discussion.

The effective dose of fluoxetine in treating OCD is 20 to 80 mg/d. The manufacturer recommends an initial dose of fluoxetine of 20 mg/d given in the morning. An average target dose of 40 to 60 mg/d is recommended, and 80 mg/d is considered the maximum.[15] Doses greater than 20 mg/d may be administered once daily in the morning or on a twice-daily schedule (morning and noon).[64] Fixed-dose studies revealed no significant difference in efficacy between the 20-, 40-, and 60-mg doses, but individual patients may have a better response at the higher doses.

Fluvoxamine

The most commonly observed fluvoxamine-related adverse effects are insomnia, nausea, somnolence, fatigue, abnormal ejaculation, nervousness, dry mouth, tremor, anorexia, anorgasmia, sweating, and decreased libido.[44]

The half-life of elimination of the parent compound is 15 hours, and there are no known active metabolites. It is 77% plasma protein bound. The pharmacokinetics of fluvoxamine are not affected by food intake.[68]

Fluvoxamine is a weak inhibitor of CYP2D6, and a potent inhibitor of CYP3A3/4, CYP1A2, CYP2C9, and CYP2C19.[67] Drug–drug interactions are reported between fluvoxamine and warfarin, theophylline, MAOIs, carbamazepine, alprazolam, propranolol, clozapine, phenytoin, TCAs, and selected other drugs. Coadministration of fluvoxamine with terfenadine, astemizole, and MAOIs should be avoided.[69] Refer to Chapter 65 and the drug interaction literature for a more complete discussion.

The recommended initial dose of fluvoxamine is 50 mg at bedtime. This dose should be increased in 50-mg increments every 4 to 7 days to an average target dose of 200 mg/d. The maximal dose is 300 mg/d. The manufacturer recommends that total daily doses of more than 100 mg be given in two divided doses. In many cases, a larger dose is given at bedtime.[44]

Paroxetine

The most commonly observed side effects from paroxetine are nausea, somnolence, dry mouth, headache, dizziness, insomnia, weakness, and sexual dysfunction.[45] It is more likely to cause sedation than insomnia. The half-life of elimination of paroxetine is 24 hours, and it is metabolized to inactive metabolites. It is approximately 95% bound to plasma proteins.[45]

Paroxetine is a potent inhibitor of CYP2D6 and a weak inhibitor of CYP3A3/4 and CYP1A2.[67] Drug interactions may occur between paroxetine and tryptophan, MAOIs, warfarin, cimetidine, phenobarbital, phenytoin, TCAs, phenothiazines, type 1C antiarrhythmics, quinidine, and theophylline.[45] For a more complete discussion of paroxetine interactions, refer to Chapter 65.

The recommended initial dose of paroxetine is 20 mg/d, and the dose can be increased in 10-mg increments at intervals of at least 1 week. Once-daily administration is usually preferred (in the morning). The average target dose is 40 to 50 mg/d, and the maximal dose is 60 mg/d. Patients should be placed on the lowest effective dose for maintenance therapy.[45]

Sertraline

The adverse effects of sertraline are similar to the other SSRIs and include nausea, headache, diarrhea, insomnia, dry mouth, sexual dysfunction, and dizziness.[70]

The mean terminal elimination half-life of sertraline is about 26 hours. When administered with food, the area under the plasma concentration time curve is slightly increased, the C_{max} was 25% greater, and the T_{max} decreased from 8 hours to 5.5 hours. *N*-desmethyl sertraline has an elimination half-life of 62 to 104 hours, but it is substantially less active than sertraline. Sertraline is 98% bound to plasma proteins.[70]

Sertraline is considered to have moderate potency as an inhibitor of CYP2D6, and to have low potency as an inhibitor of CYP3A3/4 and CYP1A2.[67] Sertraline was reported to cause a mean increase in prothrombin time of 8%. Cimetidine increased the sertraline area under the curve by 50%, the C_{max} by 24%, and the half-life by 26%. Sertraline caused a 32% decrease in diazepam clearance. Like other SSRIs, sertraline increases the plasma concentrations of TCAs, and should not be administered concurrently with the MAOIs. Sertraline also caused a 16% decrease in the clearance of tolbutamide.[70] For a more complete discussion of drug interactions associated with sertraline, refer to Chapter 65.

Dosage of sertraline is usually initiated at 50 mg/d. If the initial dose is not effective, the dose may be increased at intervals of not less than 1 week up to a maximum of 200 mg/d. Sertraline may be administered as a once-daily dose in the morning or evening.[70] The dose–response curve for sertraline appears flat across doses of 50, 100, and 200 mg/d.

REFRACTORY PATIENTS

For most patients who respond to SRIs, the improvement is incomplete, and approximately 50% of patients are clinically unchanged after an adequate trial of SRIs.[71] If there is no response or partial response to CBT alone, an SRI should be added, and more intensive CBT can be undertaken. If there is no response or partial response to an SRI alone, CBT should be added, or another SRI can be tried. If there is no response to combined CBT and an SRI, then another SRI should be tried. If there is a partial response to combined CBT and SRI therapy, a switch to another SRI, more intensive CBT, or augmentation therapy can be initiated. After failing separate trials of two or three SSRIs and CBT, clomipramine should be tried. If there is no response or partial response to combined CBT and three SRI trials (one of which was clomipramine), then augmentation with another medication can be undertaken, and more intensive CBT can be tried.[15]

Although case reports of lithium have reported encouraging findings, in controlled studies of lithium augmentation of clomipramine and fluvoxamine, no clinically meaningful improvement was noted.[71]

Two open-label studies reported that addition of buspirone to ongoing fluoxetine treatment led to a greater reduction of obsessive and compulsive symptoms than did fluoxetine alone. Three separate controlled studies of the addition of buspirone to clomipramine, fluvoxamine, and fluoxetine failed to corroborate these initial reports.[71] When buspirone is used as augmentation therapy, the initial dose is 5 mg three times daily, and the target dose should be 60 to 90 mg/d.[15]

The DA system may play a role in the pathobiology of Tourette's disorder. Furthermore, some forms of OCD, especially those comorbid with chronic tic disorders, may be associated with abnormal DA function.[72] Some investigators have studied SRI/DA receptor antagonist combination treatments in subgroups of OCD patients with SRI-resistant symptoms. However, DA receptor antagonists alone are not effective in the treatment of the core symptoms of OCD.

In an open-case series of 17 fluvoxamine nonresponders, 88% of patients with comorbid tic disorder diagnoses responded after pimozide was added, whereas only 22% of patients without these comorbid diagnoses responded.[12] The recommended initial dose of pimozide is 0.5 mg, and the target dose is 1 to 6 mg/d. Pimozide may cause cardiovascular problems and probably should not be used with clomipramine.[15] In a double-blind, placebo-controlled study, haloperidol or placebo was added to fluvoxamine in patients who had failed to respond to fluvoxamine monotherapy. Haloperidol was significantly more effective than placebo in reducing obsessive–compulsive symptoms. Furthermore, those with a concurrent chronic tic disorder demonstrated a preferential response to the fluvoxamine–haloperidol combination.[12] The recommended initial dose of haloperidol is 0.5 mg, and the target dose is 0.25 to 6 mg/d.[15]

Preliminary results from a 6-week, double-blind, placebo-controlled trial of low-dose risperidone (0.5 to 2.0 mg/d) added to an SRI in SRI-refractory OCD patients are encouraging. The authors report that treatment response was rapid and well-maintained.[71] An additional 8-week, open-label study reported that 50% of patients previously unresponsive to clomipramine responded after risperidone 3 mg/d was added.[73] The recommended initial dose of risperidone is 0.25 mg, and the target dose is 0.5 to 5 mg/d.[15]

PHARMACOECONOMIC CONSIDERATIONS

In 1990, the total cost to the U.S. economy for OCD was $8 billion. This figure includes expenditures for direct costs ($2.1 billion) and indirect costs ($5.9 billion). Direct costs include costs of hospitalization, outpatient professional services, and medications. Indirect costs include costs associated with lost productivity, work loss, early retirement, and absenteeism. As OCD frequently has its onset in childhood or adolescence, loss of income over a lifetime is substantial. An estimated 2% of completed suicides in 1990 were attributable to OCD.[74] It is estimated that $2.2 billion is spent annually for inappropriate outpatient treatment, with 25% of survey respondents requiring hospitalization with average total hospital costs of $12,500. On average, a person with OCD loses 3 full years of wages over a lifetime.[75]

EVALUATION OF THERAPEUTIC OUTCOMES

OCD patients receiving pharmacotherapy should be monitored for target symptom response, adverse effects (including the emergence of suicidal ideas), and drug interactions. Symptom severity can be effectively monitored through periodic assessment using the Y-BOCS. In addition, changes in social and occupational functioning should be assessed. Regular monitoring should be assured for several months after OCD treatment is discontinued.

Patients older than 40 years should receive a pretreatment electrocardiogram (ECG) before starting clomipramine. In patients with a history of liver disease, baseline and periodic liver function tests are recommended when clomipramine is used. If clomipramine is given concurrently with sympatholytic antihypertensives, blood pressure should be regularly monitored. Although controversial, patients failing to respond to clomipramine may benefit once the dose is adjusted to bring the plasma concentration of clomipramine between 100 and 250 ng/mL. Patients taking clomipramine who develop fever and sore throat should have leukocyte and differential white blood counts assessed to evaluate for agranulocytosis.

CONCLUSIONS

OCD is a chronic and often profoundly disabling anxiety disorder with a lifetime prevalence rate of 2.5% in adults and 1% in children. Traditional psychotherapies have failed to offer significant benefit to OCD patients, but the effectiveness of both CBT and the SRIs is well established. These complementary treatments effect a substantial reduction in symptomatology in most patients. Although currently approved medications are far superior in efficacy compared with placebo, many responders continue to demonstrate disabling symptoms. Further, the SRIs are associated with an adverse effect profile that is often problematic for a significant percentage of patients. A high rate of relapse is reported after medication discontinuation. Marked progress has been made in the treatment of this disorder over the last 10 years, and with continued research, the future holds still greater promise.

▶ PRINCIPLES OF PHARMACOTHERAPY

- When evaluating a person for OCD, remember that patients are often ashamed to admit their symptoms and are skilled at hiding them.
- In adults, CBT is selected first for milder OCD; CBT plus an SSRI or an SSRI alone is selected first for more severe OCD; when available, CBT should be offered to every OCD patient.
- Placebo-controlled trials confirm the efficacy of clomipramine, fluoxetine, fluvoxamine, sertraline, and paroxetine over a 4- to 10-week period.
- If one SSRI is ineffective, then another should be tried; clomipramine may be selected after two or three failed SSRI trials.
- Most successfully treated patients continue to have residual symptoms severe enough to limit functioning.
- Tolerance to SSRI adverse effects often develops over 6 to 8 weeks of treatment, and tolerance is more likely to develop to nausea, diarrhea, sedation, diminished libido and/or orgasm, anxiety, restlessness, insomnia, and anticholinergic side effects than to akathisia.
- Pharmacotherapy in elderly patients should be initiated with low doses, and doses should be increased slowly, with vigilance for emergence of side effects; some elderly patients will require doses similar to those used in younger adults.
- If there is no response or partial response to combined CBT and three separate SRI trials (one of which was clomipramine), then augmentation with another medication can be undertaken, and more intensive CBT can be tried.
- After successful treatment, a medication taper can be considered after 1 to 2 years of treatment. Long-term or lifelong prophylactic maintenance medication is recommended after two to four severe relapses or three to four mild to moderate relapses.

REFERENCES

1. American Psychiatric Association. Diagnostic and Statistical Manual of Mental Disorders, 4th ed (DSM-IV). Washington, DC, American Psychiatric Press, 1994, pp 417–423.
2. Karno M, Golding J, Sorenson S, Burnam A. The epidemiology of obsessive-compulsive disorder in five U.S. communities. Arch Gen Psychiatry 1988;45:1094–1099.
3. Robertson MM, Yakeley J. Gilles de la Tourette syndrome and obsessive compulsive disorder. In: Fogel BS, Schiffer RB, eds. Neuropsychiatry. Baltimore, Williams & Wilkins, 1996:827–870.
4. Pauls DL, Alsobrook JP, Goodman W, et al. A family history of obsessive-compulsive disorder. Am J Psychiatry 1995;152:76–84.
5. Pato MT, Pato CN. Obsessive-compulsive disorder in adult life. In: Pato MT, Steketee G, eds. OCD Across the Life Cycle. Section III of Review of Psychiatry, vol 16. Washington, DC, American Psychiatric Press, 1997: 30–55.
6. Clomipramine collaborative study group. Clomipramine in the treatment of patients with obsessive-compulsive disorder. Arch Gen Psychiatry 1991;48:730–738.
7. Greist JH, Jefferson JW, Kobah KA, et al. Efficacy and tolerability of serotonin transport inhibitors in obsessive-compulsive disorder. Arch Gen Psychiatry 1995;52:53–60.
8. Hollander E, DeCaria CM, Nitescu, A, et al. Serotonergic function in obsessive-compulsive disorder: Behavioral and neuroendocrine responses to oral m-chlorophenylpiperazine and fenfluramine in patients and healthy volunteers. Arch Gen Psychiatry 1992;49:21–28.
9. Barr LC, Goodman WK, Price LH, et al. The serotonin hypothesis of obsessive compulsive disorder: Implications of pharmacologic challenge studies. J Clin Psychiatry 1992;53(suppl 4):17–28.
10. Insel TR. Toward a neuroanatomy of obsessive-compulsive disorder. Arch Gen Psychiatry 1992;49:739–744.
11. Baxter LR. Neuroimaging studies of human anxiety disorders: Cutting paths of knowledge through the field of neurotic phenomena. In: Bloom FE, Kupfer DJ, eds. Psychopharmacology: Fourth Generation of Progress. New York, Raven, 1995:1287–1300.
12. McDougle CJ, Goodman WK, Price LH. Dopamine antagonists in tic-related and psychotic spectrum obsessive compulsive disorder. J Clin Psychiatry 1994;55(suppl 3):24–31.
13. Hyde TM, Weinberger DR. Tourette's syndrome: A model neuropsychiatric disorder. JAMA 1995;273:489–501.
14. Insel TR. New pharmacologic approaches to obsessive compulsive disorder. J Clin Psychiatry 1990;51(suppl 10):47–51.
15. Expert Consensus Panel for Obsessive-Compulsive Disorder. Obsessive compulsive disorder executive summary: Recommendations for first line treatments by clinical situation. J Clin Psychiatry 1997; 58(suppl 4):11–12.

16. Baer L. Behavior therapy for obsessive compulsive disorder in the office-based practice. J Clin Psychiatry 1993;54(suppl 6):10–15.
17. Rasmussen SA, Eisen JL, Pato MT. Current issues in the pharmacologic management of obsessive compulsive disorder. J Clin Psychiatry 1993;54(suppl 6):4–9.
18. Jenike MA, Rauch SL. Managing the patient with treatment-resistant obsessive compulsive disorder: Current strategies. J Clin Psychiatry 1994;55(suppl 3):11–17.
19. Jenike MA. Approaches to the patient with treatment-refractory obsessive compulsive disorder. J Clin Psychiatry 1990;51(suppl 2):15–21.
20. Mundo E, Bianchi L, Bellodi L. Efficacy of fluvoxamine, paroxetine, and citalopram in the treatment of obsessive-compulsive disorder: A single-blind study. J Clin Psychopharmacol 1997;17:267–271.
21. Greist J, Chouinard G, DuBoff E, et al. Double-blind comparison of three doses of sertraline and placebo in the treatment of outpatients with obsessive-compulsive disorder. Arch Gen Psychiatry 1995;52: 289–295.
22. Flament MF, Bisserbe JC. Pharmacologic treatment of obsessive-compulsive disorder: Comparative studies. J Clin Psychiatry 1997;58(suppl 12):18–22.
23. Jenike MA, Hyman S, Baer L, et al. A controlled trial of fluvoxamine in obsessive compulsive disorder: Implications for a serotonergic theory. Am J Psychiatry 1990;147:1209–1215.
24. Goodman WK, Price LH, Delgado PL, et al. Specificity of serotonin reuptake inhibitors in the treatment of obsessive-compulsive disorder: Comparison of fluvoxamine and desipramine. Arch Gen Psychiatry 1990;47:577–585.
25. Dominguez RA. Serotonergic antidepressants and their efficacy in obsessive compulsive disorder. J Clin Psychiatry 1992;53(suppl 10): 56–59.
26. Jenike MA, Baer L, Summergrad P, et al. Sertraline in obsessive compulsive disorder: A double-blind comparison with placebo. Am J Psychiatry 1990;147:923–928.
27. Pigott TA, Pato MT, Bernstein SE, et al. Controlled comparisons of clomipramine and fluoxetine in the treatment of obsessive-compulsive disorder: Behavioral and biological results. Arch Gen Psychiatry 1990;47:926–932.
28. Tamimi RR, Mavissakalian MR, Jones B, Olson S. Clomipramine versus fluvoxamine in obsessive-compulsive disorder. Ann Clin Psychiatry 1991;3:275–279.
29. Pato MT, Zohar-Kadouch R, Zohar J, Murphy DL. Return of symptoms after discontinuation of clomipramine in patients with obsessive compulsive disorder. Am J Psychiatry 1988;145:1521–1525.
30. Fontaine R, Chouinard G. Fluoxetine in the long-term maintenance treatment of obsessive compulsive disorder. Psychiatr Ann 1989;19: 88–91.
31. Alarcon RD, Libb JW, Spitler D. A predictive study of obsessive compulsive disorder response to clomipramine. J Clin Psychopharmacol 1993;13:210–213.
32. Austin LS, Lydiard B, Fossey MD. Panic and phobic disorders in patients with obsessive compulsive disorder. J Clin Psychiatry 1990;51: 45–48.
33. Mundo E, Bareggi SR, Pirola R, et al. Long-term pharmacotherapy of obsessive-compulsive disorder: A double-blind controlled study. J Clin Psychopharmacol 1997;17:4–10.
34. Jenike MA, Baer L, Minichiello WE, et al. Placebo-controlled trial of fluoxetine and phenelzine for obsessive-compulsive disorder. Am J Psychiatry 1997;154:1261–1264.
35. Hewlett WA, Vinogradov S, Agras WS. Clonazepam treatment of obsessions and compulsions. J Clin Psychiatry 1990;51:158–161.
36. Pato MT, Pigott TA, Hill JL, et al. Controlled comparison of buspirone and clompramine in obsessive compulsive disorder. Am J Psychiatry 1991;148:127–129.
37. Jenike MA, Baer L. An open trial of buspirone in obsessive compulsive disorder. Am J Psychiatry 1988;145:1285–1286.
38. Sheikh JL, Salzman C. Anxiety in the elderly. Psychiatr Clin North Am 1995;18:871–883.
39. Stoudemire A, Moran MG. Psychopharmacologic treatment of anxiety in the medically ill elderly patient: Special considerations. J Clin Psychiatry 1993;54(suppl):27–33.
40. Pollard CA, Carmin CN, Ownby R. Obsessive-compulsive disorder in later life. In: Pato MT, Stekette G, eds. OCD Across the Life Cycle. Section III of Review of Psychiatry, vol 16. Washington, DC, American Psychiatric Press, 1997:63.
41. Ciba-Geigy. Anafranil package insert. Summit, NJ, 1998
42. Preskorn SH. Recent pharmacologic advances in antidepressant therapy for the elderly. Am J Med 1993;94(suppl SA):2S–12S.
43. Buff DD, Brenner R, Kirtane SS, Gilboa R. Dysrhythmia associated with fluoxetine treatment in an elderly patient with cardiac disease. J Clin Psychiatry 1991;52:174–176.
44. Solvay Pharmaceuticals. Luvox package insert. Marietta, GA, 1998.
45. SmithKline Beecham Pharmaceuticals. Paxil package insert. Philadelphia, 1998.
46. Hollingsworth C, Tanguay P, Grossman L, et al. Long-term outcome of obsessive compulsive disorder in childhood. J Am Acad Child Psychiatry 1980;19:134–144.
47. Flament MF, Rapoport JL, Berg CJ, et al. Clomipramine treatment of childhood compulsive disorder. Arch Gen Psychiatry 1985;42: 977–983.
48. Leonard HL, Swedo S, Rapoport JL, et al. Treatment of obsessive compulsive disorder with clomipramine and desipramine in children and adolescents. Arch Gen Psychiatry 1989;46:1088–1092.
49. Diaz SF, Grush LR, Sichel DA, Cohen LS. Obsessive-compulsive disorder in pregnancy and the puerperium. In: Pato MT, Steketee G, eds. OCD Across the Life Cycle. Section III of Review of Psychiatry, vol 16. Washington, DC, American Psychiatric Press. 1997:97–112.
50. Goldstein DJ. Effects of third trimester fluoxetine exposure on the newborn. J Clin Psychopharmacol 1995;15:417–420.
51. Pastuszak A, Schick-Poschetto B, Zuber C, et al. Pregnancy outcome following first trimester exposure to fluoxetine (Prozac). JAMA 1993; 269:2246–2248.
52. Ben Musa A, Smith CS. Neonatal effects of maternal clomipramine therapy (case report). Arch Dis Child 1979;54:405.
53. Schimmell MS, Katz EZ, Shaag Y, et al. Toxic neonatal effects following maternal clomipramine therapy. Clin Toxicol 1991;29:479–484.
54. Lester BM. Possible association between fluoxetine hydrochloride and colic in an infant. J Am Acad Child Adolesc Psychiatry 1993;32: 1253–1255.
55. Burch KJ, Wells, BG. Fluoxetine/norfluoxetine concentrations in human milk. Pediatrics 1992;89:676–677.
56. Taddio A. Excretion of fluoxetine and its metabolite, norfluoxetine, in human breast milk. J Clin Pharmacol 1996;36:42–27.
57. Altshuler LL. Breastfeeding and sertraline: A 24-hour analysis. J Clin Psychiatry 1995;56:243–245.
58. Spigset O. Paroxetine levels in breast milk. J Clin Psychiatry 1996; 57:29.
59. Wright S. Excretion of fluvoxamine in breast milk. Br J Clin Pharmacol 1991;31:209.
60. Jermain DM, Crismon LC. Pharmacotherapy of obsessive compulsive disorder. Pharmacotherapy 1990;10:175–198.
61. Stern RS, Marks IM, Mawson D, Luscombe DK. Clomipramine and exposure for compulsive rituals, I. Plasma levels, side effects, and outcome. Br J Psychiatry 1980;136:161–166.
62. Insel TR, Murphy DL, Cohen RM, et al. Obsessive compulsive disorder. Arch Gen Psychiatry 1983;40:605–612.
63. Mavissakalian MR, Jones B, Olson S, Perel JM. Clomipramine in obsessive compulsive disorder: Clinical response and plasma levels. J Clin Psychopharmacol 1990;10:261–268.
64. Dista Products. Prozac package insert. Indianapolis, 1998.
65. Van Harten J. Clinical pharmacokinetics of selective serotonin reuptake inhibitors. Clin Pharmacokinet 1993;24:203–220.
66. Koran LM, Cain JW, Dominguez RA, et al. Are fluoxetine plasma levels related to outcome in obsessive-compulsive disorder? Am J Psychiatry 1996;153:1450–1454.

67. Ereshefsky L, Riesenman C, Lam YWF. Serotonin selective reuptake inhibitor drug interactions and the cytochrome P450 system. J Clin Psychiatry 1996; 57(suppl 8):17–25.
68. Finley PR. Selective serotonin reuptake inhibitors: Pharmacologic profiles and potential therapeutic distinctions. Ann Pharmacother 1994;28:1359–1369.
69. Goodman WK, Ward H, Kablinger A, Murphy T. Fluvoxamine in the treatment of obsessive-compulsive disorder and related conditions. J Clin Psychiatry 1997;58(suppl 5):32–49.
70. Pfizer. Zoloft package insert. New York, 1998.
71. McDougle CJ. Update on pharmacologic management of OCD: Agents and augmentation. J Clin Psychiatry 1997;58(suppl 12):11–17.
72. Goodman WK, McDougle CJ, Price LH, et al. Beyond the serotonin hypothesis: A role for dopamine in some forms of obsessive compulsive disorder? J Clin Psychiatry 1990;51:36–43.
73. Ravizza L. Therapeutic effect and safety of adjunctive risperidone in refractory obsessive-compulsive disorder (OCD). Psychopharmacol Bull 1996;32:677–682.
74. Dupont R, Rice D, Shiraki S, et al. Economic costs of obsessive-compulsive disorder. Pharmacoeconomics April:1995;2:102–109.
75. Hollander E, Kwon JH, Stein MB, et al. Obsessive-compulsive and spectrum disorders: Overview and quality of life issues. J Clin Psychiatry 1996;57(suppl 8):3–6.
76. American Pharmaceutical Association. Management of obsessive-compulsive disorder. In: APhA Guide to Drug Treatment Protocols: A Resource for Creating and Using Disease-specific Pathways. Washington, DC, American Pharmaceutical Association, 1997:OCDi–ii.

69

SLEEP DISORDERS

Donna M. Jermain, PharmD, BCPP

Sleep is essential to human life, providing both emotional and physical restoration in ways not completely understood. Approximately one-third of our lives is spent sleeping with a wide interindividual variability in the amount of sleep required per night (3 to 10 hours).[1] Abnormalities in the normal physiology of sleep often cause three types of sleep problems: insomnia, excessive daytime sleepiness, and abnormal sleep behaviors.[2]

SLEEP PHYSIOLOGY

A circadian rhythm of sleep and waking is established shortly after birth and changes over the life cycle. Two oscillators with different period lengths control the circadian rhythm of sleep. One oscillator is located in the suprachiasmic nucleus (biologic clock) and the other occurs through neurobiologic mechanisms. Two peptides, delta-sleep-inducing peptide and factor S, also appear to be involved in the biochemical regulation. Synchronization of the sleep–wake cycle, which naturally lasts 25 hours, with the 24-hour cycle imposed by the earth's rotation, requires routinely occurring zeitgebers or cues (clock, light, shower, breakfast time) to set the internal clock.[3]

NEUROCHEMISTRY

Sleep is a complex psychophysiologic phenomenon that ensues as wakefulness abates. Neuronal complexes involved in regulating the cyclic alteration of sleep and wakefulness are located in the brainstem, basal forebrain, and hypothalamus, with projections into the cortex and thalamus. The reticular activating system (RAS) is responsible for maintaining wakefulness. Norepinephrine (NE) and acetylcholine in the cortex and histamine and neuropeptides (e.g., substance P and corticotropin-releasing factor) in the hypothalamus modulate neuronal activity during wakefulness.[4] Neuron systems in the brainstem raphe nuclei, solitary tract, ventricular thalamus, anterior hypothalamus, and basal forebrain are involved in sleep promotion. As the RAS decelerates, information transfer to the cortex ceases, and serotonin (5-HT) neurotransmission in the raphe nuclei reduces sensory input to inhibit motor activity.[4] NE is involved in dreaming, while 5-HT is active during nondreaming sleep.

SLEEP CYCLE

Wakefulness is characterized by an electroencephalogram (EEG) of low voltage, fast activity, random eye movements and blinks, and a high muscle tone. The two types of sleep are non-rapid eye movement (non-REM or NREM; stages 1 to 4) and REM. During NREM sleep, skeletal muscle tone and eye movements are low in comparison to wakefulness, and respiratory activity occurs at a slow, regular pace. Stage 1 sleep represents a transition between wakefulness and sleep that lasts between 0.5 and 7 minutes; the EEG reveals low-voltage (3- to 7-Hz), desynchronized activity. Stage 2 sleep is a low-voltage EEG, and frequent "sleep spindles" (10- to 16-Hz spindle-shaped waves) and "K-complexes" (high-voltage spikes). Stages 3 and 4 are called delta sleep, and consist of high-amplitude, slow waves.[5] Stages 1 to 4 occur within 45 minutes of falling asleep. Most delta sleep occurs during the first half of the night.

REM sleep is characterized by the onset of low-voltage, mixed frequency EEG and bursts of bilaterally conjugate REMs.[5] During REM sleep, muscle tone is low, but autonomic fluctuations (heart rate, perspiration, penile erection) are active.[6] Within 90 minutes of falling asleep, the first REM period commences and lasts only 5 to 7 minutes. The cycle lasts approximately 70 to 120 minutes and is repeated 4 to 6 times during the night.[5] REM periods progressively lengthen throughout the night.[7] A typical young adult spends approximately 75% of the night in NREM sleep and the remainder in REM sleep.[5] Dream reports occur in 80% to 90% of subjects if awakened during or at the end of a REM period.

In elderly individuals the sleep pattern is altered, with a considerable decrease in delta sleep, REM sleep, and total sleep time.[5] Correspondingly, there is an increase in the number of awakenings and total time spent awake at night.[8] The contribution of daytime napping and specific sleep pathology (including sleep apnea and periodic leg movements) to this apparent decrease in sleep is unclear.

CLASSIFICATION

The Association of Sleep Disorders Center's International Classification of Sleep Disorders (ICSD) organizes more than 80 sleep disorders (based on pathophysiology) under the major headings of dyssomnias, parasomnias, medical/psychiatric sleep disorders, and proposed sleep disorders.[9] Similar to the ICSD, the *Diagnostic and Statistical Manual of Mental Disorders,* fourth edition (DSM-IV), classifies sleep disorders based on presumed etiology into three major categories (Table 69–1) and requires a period of duration of 1 month before a sleep disorder is diagnosed.[10] Pri-

TABLE 69–1. DSM-IV Classification of Sleep Disorders

Primary Sleep Disorders
Dyssomnias
Primary insomnia
Primary hypersomnia
Breathing-related sleep disorder
Narcolepsy
Circadian rhythm sleep disorder
Delayed sleep phase type
Jet lag type
Unspecified type
Dyssomnias not otherwise specified
Parasomnias
Nightmare disorder
Sleep terror disorder
Sleepwalking disorder
Parasomnias not otherwise specified
Sleep Disorders Related to Another Mental Disorder
Insomnia related to another mental disorder
Hypersomnia related to another mental disorder
Other Sleep Disorders
Sleep disorder due to a general medical condition
Substance-induced sleep disorder

Adapted from Ref. 10.

mary sleep disorders result from endogenous abnormalities in the sleep–wake timing or generating processes and are further classified as dyssomnias (abnormalities in the amount, timing, or quality of sleep) or parasomnias (abnormal behaviors associated with sleep). Sleep disorders secondary to another mental disorder, medical condition, or substance (concurrent use or discontinuation of a substance or a drug) are classified separately.

Polysomnography (PSG) measures multiple electrophysiologic parameters simultaneously during sleep and typically includes an electroencephalogram (EEG), electrooculogram (EOG), and electromyogram (EMG).[2] Two EOGs, one EEG, and one EMG are the minimal recordings used in scoring sleep stages.[11] Commonly measured objective parameters of sleep include sleep onset latency (amount of time to fall asleep), number of awakenings, number of stage shifts during the night, and first REM latency period. Other polysomnographic measures (oral and nasal airflow, respiratory effort, oxygen desaturation, periodic leg movements [PLM], gross motor activity, and nocturnal penile tumescence) may also be used to diagnose sleep disorders.[2,5]

INSOMNIA

Insomnia is a subjective complaint of difficulty falling asleep, maintaining sleep, or of not feeling rested despite a sufficient opportunity to sleep.[3,10] A concurrent disturbance of daytime functioning (decreased concentration, fatigue, myalgia) usually accompanies the sleep complaint.[12] Younger individuals usually complain of delays in sleep onset, while older patients complain of nocturnal awakening and shorter time periods of sleep.[10] The most important aspect in evaluating a sleep complaint is its duration. Transient (2 to 3 nights) and short-term (less than 3 weeks) insomnia are typical of individuals without a history of sleep problems; however, long-term or chronic insomnia has a duration exceeding 3 weeks and may be related to medical or psychiatric disorders, or may be psychophysiologic in nature.[3] Psychophysiologic insomnia is caused by arousal or anxiety at bedtime, usually surrounding a negative expectation about sleep. Patients may have tension and maladaptive, conditioned behavior typified by a marked overconcern about their inability to fall asleep.[2,3,8]

EPIDEMIOLOGY

Insomnia is the most prevalent sleep complaint in the general population.[2] A 1-year prevalence study of insomnia in the United States reported that one-third of individuals surveyed complained of insomnia, and 17% reported the symptoms to be serious.[3] Data from the National Institute of Mental Health Epidemiologic Catchment Area (ECA) study indicated that the 6-month prevalence of insomnia, defined as symptoms for 2 weeks, was 10.2%. Females; individuals who are unemployed, elderly, separated, or widowed; and those in the lower socioeconomic sector reported significantly higher rates of insomnia. Forty percent of those with insomnia had a concurrent psychiatric disorder (e.g., anxiety, depression, alcohol or substance abuse).[13]

Despite the widespread prevalence of insomnia, only 5% of individuals seek medical assistance for management.[12] Approximately 10% to 20% of insomniacs use

TABLE 69–2. Common Etiologies of Insomnia

Situational
Work or financial stress
Interpersonal conflicts
Major life events
Jet lag, shift work
Medical
Cardiovascular (angina, arrhythmias, heart failure)
Respiratory (asthma, sleep apnea)
Chronic pain
Endocrine disorders (diabetes, hyperthyroidism)
Gastrointestinal (gastroesophageal reflux, ulcers)
Neurologic (delirium, epilepsy, Parkinson's disease)
Pregnancy
Psychiatric
Mood disorders (depression, mania)
Anxiety disorders (generalized anxiety disorder, obsessive–compulsive disorder, panic disorder)
Substance abuse (alcohol or sedative/hypnotic withdrawal)
Pharmacologically Induced
Anticonvulsants
Central adrenergic blockers
Diuretics
Selective serotonin reuptake inhibitors
Steroids
Stimulants

Compiled from Refs. 2 and 4.

nonprescription drugs or alcohol to alleviate symptoms. Of the 3% of the population who ingest hypnotics for insomnia, 11% report a duration of use exceeding 1 year.[14]

DIFFERENTIAL DIAGNOSIS

The causes of insomnia may be multidimensional and related to underlying situational stressors, medical or psychiatric illnesses, or medication use. Common identifiable causes of insomnia are listed in Table 69–2. Evaluation of transient insomnia should focus on possible acute stress, environmental disruptions (change in job, recent surgery, examinations), and drug-related causes. In patients with chronic sleep disturbances, a complete diagnostic evaluation should include physical and mental status examinations and routine laboratory tests, as well as medication and substance abuse histories to rule out medical and psychiatric etiologies.

▶ TREATMENT: Insomnia

Assessment of insomnia should include a history of the specific symptomatology, time course of onset, duration, frequency, daytime symptoms, sleep hygiene habits, and history of previous treatments. The therapeutic management of insomnia is determined by the duration of insomnia and may consist of a combination of general measures to improve sleep, psychotherapy, and pharmacotherapy. A treatment plan should be individualized based on the type of insomnia, severity of daytime impairment in functioning, patient age, and concurrent medical conditions. All unnecessary or high dosages of medications should be discontinued.[3,12] The expected duration of therapy and desired pharmacologic profile must be considered when choosing a hypnotic.

NONPHARMACOLOGIC THERAPY

General measures to improve insomnia are useful adjuncts to the specific treatment of identifiable etiologies. Cognitive, behavioral, and educational interventions include cognitive therapy, relaxation therapy (e.g., progressive muscle relaxation), stimulus control therapy, light therapy, sleep deprivation, and sleep hygiene education.[15,16] Results of a meta-analysis of nonpharmacologic treatments for chronic insomnia indicate that stimulus control and sleep restriction were the most effective treatment modalities compared to placebo or no treatment, and improvements were sustained for 6 months.[15]

Changes in sleep hygiene habits can improve the patient's sleep–wake routine and augment recovery from transient or short-term insomnia (Table 69–3).[3] Alcohol, stimulants, and nicotine use should be avoided by patients with insomnia. Although alcohol enhances sleep onset, the subsequent sleep is disturbed and fragmented. Alcoholics frequently have insomnia for months to years after recovery.[4] Individuals with insomnia are sensitive to the arousal effects of mild stimulants and should avoid all caffeine-containing products and chocolate for at least 8 hours before bedtime. Nicotine withdrawal often arouses smokers from quiescence.[1]

PHARMACOLOGIC THERAPY

NONBENZODIAZEPINE HYPNOTIC AGENTS

The benzodiazepines (BZs) have largely replaced barbiturates (butalbital, pentobarbital, secobarbital) because of the latter's propensity for the rapid development of tolerance, fatalities by overdose, development of physical and psychological dependence, withdrawal syndromes, and significant drug interactions.[5] Because of safety considerations, the barbiturates have few indications for use as hypnotics.[3,4]

Chloral hydrate therapy, which also offers no clinical advantage, may be complicated by gastrointestinal irritation, drug interactions, and fatalities in overdosage. Chloral hydrate interacts with other sedatives, and the combination of chloral hydrate and alcohol has been termed a "Mickey Finn" or "knockout drops."[3]

The antidepressants (including amitriptyline, doxepin, and trazodone) are alternatives for patients with nonrestorative sleep who should not receive BZs.[3,17] Prescriptions for antidepressants as hypnotics doubled from 11.6% in 1987 to 26.4% of all hypnotic prescriptions in 1991.[14] Trazodone 50 to 100 mg is an effective hypnotic in patients with antidepressant-induced insomnia.[17]

Antihistamines are less effective than the BZs, and their use may be complicated by anticholinergic side effects.[3] Nonprescription sleep aids commonly contain antihistamines and analgesics. The amino acid L-tryptophan is no longer recommended for use as a hypnotic because of reports of eosinophilia–myalgia syndrome.[18]

Zolpidem, an imidazolpyridine chemically unrelated to BZs or barbiturates, acts selectively at the BZ_1 receptor and has minimal anxiolytic and no muscle relaxant or anticonvulsant effects. It is comparable in effectiveness to BZ hypnotics, reducing latency to sleep, and increasing total sleep time and efficiency.[19] Zolpidem has little effect on sleep stages.[20] Zolpidem is metabolized by methyloxidation and hydroxylation to inactive metabo-

TABLE 69–3. Nonpharmacologic Recommendations for Insomnia

Stimulus Control Procedures

1. Establish a regular time to wake up and to go to sleep (including weekends).
2. Sleep only as much as necessary to feel rested.
3. Go to bed only when sleepy. Avoid long periods of wakefulness in bed. Use the bed only for sleep or intimacy; do not read or watch television in bed.
4. Avoid trying to force sleep. If you do not fall asleep within 20–30 minutes, leave the bed and perform a relaxing activity (read, listen to music, watch television) until drowsy. Repeat this as often as necessary.
5. Avoid daytime naps.
6. Schedule worry time during the day. Do not take your troubles to bed.

Sleep Hygiene Recommendations

1. Exercise routinely (three to four times weekly), but not close to bedtime because this may cause arousal.
2. Create a comfortable sleep environment by avoiding temperature extremes, loud noises, and illuminated clocks.
3. Discontinue or reduce the use of alcohol, caffeine, and nicotine.
4. Avoid excessive fullness or hunger at bedtime.
5. Avoid drinking large quantities of liquids in the evening to prevent nighttime trips to the restroom.
6. Do something relaxing and enjoyable before bedtime.

Adapted from Ref. 30.

lites. Its half-life is approximately 2.5 hours, and duration of effect is 6 to 8 hours.

The most common adverse effects of zolpidem are drowsiness, amnesia, dizziness, headache, and gastrointestinal complaints.[19] Several cases of brief psychotic reactions have been reported in women.[21–23] Compared with BZs, zolpidem use is not associated with the development of tolerance or rebound insomnia after 35 days of continuous use.[24] Zolpidem may also have no significant effects on next-day psychomotor performance.[25] However, it is more expensive. The recommended daily dosage is 10 mg, and 5 mg in elderly patients and those with hepatic impairment. The dosage can be increased up to 20 mg nightly, but the incidence of adverse events is dose related.[20]

Melatonin, a hormone released by the pineal gland at night, is available over the counter and is promoted as a sleep aid. It may be promising in neurologically devastated children and the elderly, and in individuals experiencing jet lag.[26,27] Marketed as a dietary supplement, no Food and Drug Administration controls are imposed. Thus, manufacturing and purity concerns should not be ignored.

BENZODIAZEPINE HYPNOTICS

In the United States, five BZs are marketed with a therapeutic indication for insomnia (Table 69–4); however, other BZs also are effective. BZs relieve insomnia by reducing the latency to sleep onset and number of awakenings and by increasing the total sleep time. BZs decrease the duration of stages 1 and 4 sleep and increase stage 2 sleep. Unlike the barbiturates, BZs do not decrease REM sleep to cause a severe REM withdrawal syndrome.[28]

Pharmacokinetics

BZ onset and duration of activity are the most important characteristics to be considered when choosing an agent.[6,29] As a single dose, the extent of distribution and elimination half-life are important in predicting BZ duration of action. However, after multiple dosing the elimination half-life and formation of active metabolites will determine the extent of drug accumulation and resultant clinical effects.[29]

BZ pharmacokinetic properties are summarized in Table 69–4. The onset of action is dependent on the rate of absorption. Flurazepam and triazolam are rapidly absorbed. Temazepam is less lipophilic and has a slower onset of effect. Sedation after flurazepam, estazolam, and quazepam occurs within 1 to 2 hours after ingestion.[30]

Triazolam is redistributed quickly because of its high lipophilicity and thus has a short duration of effect.[29] Estazolam and temazepam are intermediate in their duration of action. The therapeutic effects of flurazepam and quazepam are long in comparison because of the active metabolites.

With the exception of temazepam, which is eliminated via conjugation, all BZ hypnotics are metabolized by hepatic microsomal oxidation and then undergo glucuronide conjugation. Oxidation may be inhibited in patients with impaired liver function, advanced age, or concurrent use of drugs that inhibit oxidation. Drugs that inhibit the cytochrome P-450 IIIA4 enzyme (e.g., erythromycin, nefazodone, fluvoxamine, ketoconazole) reduce the clearance of triazolam and increase its plasma concentrations.[31,32]

Triazolam (a short-elimination half-life BZ), estazolam, and temazepam (intermediate-elimination half-life BZs) lack clinically significant metabolites. Flurazepam and quazepam have long elimination half-lives. Flurazepam is rapidly metabolized to two short-acting metabolites, hydroxyethylflurazepam and flurazepam aldehyde. These metabolites contribute to sleep induction on the first night of therapy but are eliminated within 12 hours. *N*-Desalkylflurazepam (*N*-DAF) is an active metabolite that peaks 10 hours after a single dose and accumulates extensively during multiple dosing.[3] *N*-DAF accounts for most of flurazepam's pharmacologic effects. Quazepam and one of its metabolites, 2-oxo-quazepam, have elimination half-lives of 39 hours. Quazepam's oxo-quazepam metabolite is metabolized to *N*-DAF.[33] If oxidation of *N*-DAF is impaired, its half-life becomes prolonged, and complications of drug accumulation may result with repeated dosing; however, tolerance may develop to these effects.[29] *N*-DAF is beneficial when daytime anxiety or early morning awakening are complaints, but daytime sedation and impaired psychomotor performance may complicate therapy.[3]

Adverse Effects

High dosages of BZs with long- or intermediate-elimination half-lives have a greater potential for producing daytime sedation and performance decrements. These effects include excessive drowsiness, psychomotor incoordination, decreased concentration, and cognitive deficits.[3] Tolerance to the CNS carryover effects may develop with time. Rapidly eliminated BZs have less potential for producing daytime sedation.

Tolerance to BZ hypnotic effect develops sooner with triazolam (after 2 weeks of continuous use) than with other BZ hypnotics.[6] Laboratory studies indicate that the hypnotic efficacy of flurazepam, quazepam, and temazepam is maintained for 1 month of continuous nightly use.[34] Estazolam reportedly maintains the duration and quality of sleep at the maximum dosage (2 mg nightly) for up to 12 weeks.[35] Long-term use (greater than 6 months) of BZs was associated with a low risk of abuse, side

TABLE 69–4. Pharmacokinetics of Benzodiazepine Hypnotic Agents

Generic Name	t_{max} (h)[a]	Parent $t_{1/2}$ (h)	Daily Dose Range (mg)	Metabolic Pathway	Clinically Significant Metabolites
Estazolam	2	12–15	1–2	Oxidation	—
Flurazepam	1	8	15–30	Oxidation	Hydroxyethylflurazepam Flurazepam aldehyde
				N-dealkylation	*N*-DAF[b]
Quazepam	2	39	7.5–15	Oxidation *N*-dealkylation	2-Oxo-quazepam *N*-DAF[b]
Temazepam	1.5	10–15	15–30	Conjugation	—
Triazolam	1	2	0.125–0.25	Oxidation	—

[a]Time to peak plasma concentration.
[b]*N*-desalkylflurazepam, mean half-life 47 to 100 hours.

effects, and tolerance in patients with severe, chronic sleep disorders; however, efficacy has not been established.[36]

Anterograde amnesia is an impairment of memory and recall after drug ingestion reported to occur during BZ therapy. Anterograde amnesia occurs more frequently with triazolam than with temazepam[37]; however, anterograde amnesia has been reported with most BZs.[3,30] The lowest effective dosage should be used to avoid adverse effects on memory. When compared with temazepam, triazolam usage was associated with a higher reported rate of confusion, bizarre behavior, agitation, and hallucinations. These central nervous system effects occurred with higher doses (68% of patients ingested 0.5 to 1.5 mg) and in older patients (mean of 63 years).[37] Because of the high incidence of CNS adverse effects, the United Kingdom suspended sales of triazolam in October 1991.[38] Controversy surrounding triazolam led the FDA to review the agent in 1990 and 1992. Triazolam was considered safe and effective, but caution was noted about possible memory problems.

Daytime anxiety and rebound insomnia are associated with use of triazolam.[3] Rebound insomnia is characterized by increased wakefulness beyond baseline amounts that usually lasts for 1 to 2 nights after abrupt discontinuation of BZ hypnotics with short- or intermediate-elimination half-lives. Rebound insomnia occurs more frequently after high doses of triazolam, even when intermittently ingested.[39] The occurrence of rebound insomnia can be minimized by using the lowest effective dose and tapering the dose upon discontinuation.[40]

The incidence of CNS side effects increases with age secondary to increased sensitivity to pharmacologic effects and prolonged BZ half-lives, which may increase the potential for drug accumulation. Impaired judgment, excessive daytime sedation, and confusional states may result.[41] Short- and intermediate-elimination half-life drugs are associated with fewer performance deficits; however, they may increase the chance of daytime anxiety in elderly patients. There is an association between falls and hip fractures and the use of long-elimination half-life BZs; thus flurazepam and quazepam should be avoided in elderly patients.[3]

GUIDELINES

Hypnotic therapy is indicated in individuals with transient or short-term insomnia.[2] Patients should be counseled that sleep will return to normal when the precipitating stressor is eliminated, and also be educated on strategies for stimulus control and good sleep hygiene (Table 69–3). If the stressor is expected to last more than 1 week, intermittent hypnotic use (three or four nights per week) should be prescribed for no more than 3 weeks. For patients with chronic insomnia, medical, psychiatric, and pharmacologic causes should be identified and managed.[3] If treatment of an underlying disorder fails to result in improvement, intermittent pharmacotherapy may be indicated. If the insomnia is psychophysiologic, several months of supervised hypnotic therapy may help alleviate anxiety and reestablish a regular sleep pattern upon drug discontinuation; however, these patients require nonpharmacologic therapy as well.[15]

Tolerance and dependence can be avoided by using hypnotics at the lowest possible dose, intermittently, and for the shortest duration possible. Patients should receive instruction on frequency of drug use and the expected duration of therapy to prevent development of dependence. Withdrawal symptoms can be diminished by gradually tapering the dosage. Patients should be counseled on rebound insomnia when BZ therapy is terminated.

Patients with difficulty initiating sleep and those who require daytime alertness should receive the short-acting BZ hypnotics. Those with difficulty maintaining sleep or early morning awakening may benefit from intermediate-elimination half-life agents if daytime performance is required. Long-elimination half-life BZs should be considered if management of daytime anxiety is required. There is no rationale for the concurrent use of two BZs to treat anxiety and insomnia.

BZ hypnotics should not be prescribed for individuals with sleep apnea, a history of substance abuse, or during pregnancy. Patients should be instructed to avoid alcohol; even alcohol on the day after ingestion of a long-elimination half-life BZ can result in additive CNS impairment. Prescriptions for BZ hypnotics should be accompanied by printed information and verbal counseling on precautions.

SLEEP APNEA

Sleep-related respiratory abnormalities are commonly diagnosed in sleep labs using PSG. Apnea is defined as the cessation of airflow at the nose and mouth lasting at least 10 seconds. It is classified into two major categories, obstructive and central. Patients with sleep apnea have a high risk of morbidity and mortality.[42]

OBSTRUCTIVE SLEEP APNEA

Obstructive sleep apnea (OSA) is a potentially life-threatening condition characterized by repeated episodes of nocturnal breathing cessation with loud snoring and gasping, often reported by the bed partner.[43] OSA is estimated to occur in 1% to 9% of the population, predominantly in males.[2] OSA is caused by an occlusion of the upper airway (causes include obesity, polyps, enlarged tonsils, adenoids, or tongue) that occurs only during sleep.[43]

In OSA patients, airflow ceases while respiratory effort continues. The apneic episode is terminated by a reflex action to the fall in O_2 saturation that causes a brief "mini-arousal" during which breathing resumes. Patients may be unaware of the "mini-arousals," however, the EEG clearly indicates activity that may cause fragmented sleep. Thus, patients usually present with excessive daytime sleepiness. In severe cases, excessive somnolence may cause sleep attacks that can result in decrements in performance (leading, for example, to motor vehicle accidents). Additional daytime symptoms include morning headache, poor memory, and irritability.[43] Most individuals with OSA are overweight. Complications include arrhythmias, hypertension, cor pulmonale, and sudden death during somnolence.[43]

Treatment of OSA must be individualized and depends on the severity of the disordered breathing and the amount of sleep disruption.[44] Patients with severe apnea (greater than 20 apneas/h on PSG and excessive daytime somnolence), and those with moderate apneas (5 to 20 apneas/h on PSG and excessive daytime sleepiness or other daytime symptoms) have shown significant improvement and reduction in mortality with treatment.[43] Nonpharmacologic measures are the treatments of choice. Weight loss may eliminate the apnea and reduce daytime hypersomnia[44]; however, improvement is only limited. Treatment of underlying causes of obstruction (tonsillectomy, nasal septal repair, nonsedating antihistamines for allergic rhinitis) may eliminate apneas during sleep. In patients with mild apnea and snoring with no daytime symptomatology, management may include avoidance of a supine sleep position.[44]

Nasal continuous positive airway pressure (CPAP) during sleep is the standard treatment for most patients with OSA.[42] CPAP elevates the pressure in the oropharyngeal space to maintain positive airway pressure during the respiratory cycle. Patient tolerance and compliance are the major limitations of CPAP. Although tracheostomy is an effective surgical procedure, it is reserved for use in treatment-resistant patients. Uvulopalatopharyngoplasty is a surgical procedure to enlarge the pharyngeal airspace that successfully reduces apnea in 50% of patients and snoring in 90%.[42,44] Upper airway resection can also be performed with new laser surgical techniques.[42]

The single most important pharmacologic intervention is the avoidance of all CNS depressants (alcohol, anxiolytics, hypnotics, narcotics, zolpidem).[42] CNS depressant use is potentially lethal because it interferes with the brain's ability to produce the resumption of breathing. Drug therapy should be reserved for patients with mild forms of OSA and those who have failed other treatments. Protriptyline, in doses of 10 to 30 mg daily, reduces the frequency of apneas and increases O_2 saturation.[42] Protriptyline may be used for mild OSA without hypercapnia. The mechanism of action may be related to a decrease in REM sleep or an increase in the tonus of the musculature of the oropharynx. Anticholinergic side effects often complicate therapy.[44] Fluoxetine 20 mg/d was effective in reducing apneas in some patients.[45] Respiratory stimulants, such as theophylline[46] and clonidine (in males),[47] also have been tried; however, efficacy is limited, and research has not documented long-term effectiveness. Medroxyprogesterone 60 mg has improved persons with sleep apnea and obesity-hypoventilation syndrome; however, controlled studies show no beneficial effects.[44]

CENTRAL SLEEP APNEA

Central sleep apnea (CSA) is characterized by repeated episodes of apnea caused by temporary loss of respiratory effort during somnolence. It accounts for less than 10% of all apneas. Hypercapnic patients usually present with morning headache and daytime somnolence, while nonhypercapnic patients complain of insomnia and nocturnal awakenings with shortness of breath or gasping. Although the majority of CSA cases are idiopathic, identifiable causes are nasal obstruction, autonomic system lesions (e.g., cervical cordotomy), neurologic diseases (poliomyelitis, encephalitis, myasthenia gravis), and congestive heart failure.[48] The primary treatment approach for the hypercapnic CSA patient is ventilatory support with O_2 and CPAP; acetazolamide, theophylline, and medroxyprogesterone have shown mixed results.[48] In refractory cases, diaphragmatic pacing, tracheostomy, or positive pressure ventilation are helpful. In nonhypercapnic CSA patients, treatment may consist of BZs (triazolam or temazepam) to reduce arousals, and acetazolamide, CPAP, and O_2 to stabilize breathing patterns.[48]

NARCOLEPSY

Narcolepsy is a chronic disease that typically begins before the age of 25 years. About 0.5% of the adult population has narcolepsy, with men and women being equally affected. There appears to be a genetic predetermination for narcolepsy, as 3% of patients have a first-degree relative with the disorder.[49] An association between narcolepsy and the human leukocyte antigens (HLA) HLA-DR2 and HLA-DQ1 (HLA-DR15 and HLA-DQ6 under new nomenclature) has been identified.[50] Recently, across all ethnic groups, a closer association is with a DQB1 allele, DQBI*0602, than HLA-DR2.[51] DQBI*0602 is found in 98% of persons with narcolepsy; however it is also found in 25% of the general population.

The essential feature of narcolepsy is excessive daytime sleepiness with sleep attacks that may last up to 30 minutes. Individuals often complain of hypersomnia, fatigue, impaired performance, and disturbed nighttime sleep. Excessive daytime sleepiness occurs before the second decade of life, and the auxiliary symptoms (cataplexy, hypnagogic hallucinations, sleep paralysis) appear several years later.[49]

Cataplexy, often precipitated by emotionally charged stimuli (laughter, anger, excitement), occurs in 70% to 80% of narcoleptics and is characterized by brief episodes (seconds to several minutes) of muscle weakness and/or paralysis that may cause the individual to collapse while remaining conscious. Sleep paralysis is a loss of muscle tone while the patient is still awake. Hypnagogic (at the threshold of sleep) and hypnopompic (upon awakening) hallucinations are brief dreamlike experiences with more fragmentation and bizarre features than a typical dream.[49]

Sleep laboratory evaluation of the narcoleptic confirms the existence of excessive daytime sleepiness, disturbed nighttime sleep, and sleep-onset REM periods. The occurrence of sleep paralysis, cataplexy, and sleep-onset REM indicates that narcolepsy represents an abnormality in the regulatory mechanisms of REM sleep (possibly in the cholinergic system).[49]

▶ TREATMENT: Narcolepsy

Symptomatic management is both nonpharmacologic and pharmacologic. Counseling the patient and significant others is essential, because family members often think that narcolepsy is voluntary and the patient is lazy and nonproductive. Good sleep habits should be encouraged. If the patient's daily schedule allows, two or more brief daytime naps can be beneficial. Following a 15-minute nap, the patient may be refreshed for several hours. Support groups exist locally and nationally for narcoleptics.[52]

Pharmacologic treatment consists of the use of psychostimulants for excessive daytime sleepiness and antidepressants for cataplexy (Table 69–5).[49] Stimulants exert their effects by enhancing norepinephrine release from presynaptic neurons.[49] Only methylphenidate and dextroamphetamine are FDA-approved for use in narcolepsy. Amphetamines and methylphenidate have a fast onset of effect and durations of 3 to 4 hours and 6 to 10 hours, respectively. The dose may range from 5 to 60 mg/d and divided daily doses are recommended; however, more expensive sustained-release formulations are available. Pemoline has a delayed onset of effect, but its duration is 8 to 10 hours; maximal effect may take several weeks. Pemoline's dose range is 18.75 to 112.5 mg/d. Liver function tests must be monitored (at 1 month and yearly) during pemoline therapy. Amphetamine use is associated with more likelihood of abuse and tolerance, especially when prescribed in high doses.[53]

The tricyclic antidepressants (TCAs), through blockade of NE and 5-HT reuptake, are effective in reducing cataplexy and sleep paralysis. Imipramine, protriptyline, and nortriptyline are effective in approximately 80% of patients.[53] Selegiline improves hypersomnolence and cataplexy, presumably through REM suppression and increase in REM latency.[54,55] Tranylcypromine and codeine may improve cataplexy and increase daytime alertness.[56,57] Gamma-hydroxybutyrate is a therapeutic option without anticholinergic side effects.[58]

GUIDELINES

General principles of drug therapy for narcolepsy include using the lowest effective dose possible, employing gradual titration, and carefully monitoring for therapeutic and adverse events. The goal of therapy is to maximize alertness during normal waking hours or at selected times of the day. Scheduled naps can help to maintain wakefulness.[50] Naps should be encouraged instead of taking drugs. In addition, cataplexy may be treated on an as-needed basis in some patients. If the patient can predict the occurrence of cataplexy (associated with an anticipated specific stimulus), then a TCA can be ingested for only the day or two before and during the expected occurrence.

TABLE 69–5. Drugs Used to Treat Narcolepsy

Generic Name	Trade Name (Manufacturer)	Daily Dosage Range (mg)
Excessive Daytime Somnolence		
Dextroamphetamine	Dexedrine (SmithKline Beecham), generics (various)	5–60
Dextroamphetamine/amphetamine salts[a]	Adderall (Richwood)	5–60
Methamphetamine[b]	Desoxyn (Abbott)	5–15
Methylphenidate	Ritalin (Ciba), generics (various)	30–80
Pemoline	Cylert (Abbott)	37.5–112.5
Adjunct Agents for Cataplexy		
Imipramine	Tofranil (Geigy), generics (various)	50–250
Protriptyline	Vivactil (Merck), generics (various)	5–30
Nortriptyline	Aventyl (Lilly), Pamelor (Sandoz), generics (various)	50–200
Selegiline	Eldepryl (Somerset)	20–40
Gamma-hydroxybutyrate	(Orphan Medical)	60 mg/kg/night

[a]Dextroamphetamine sulfate, dextroamphetamine saccharate, amphetamine aspartate, amphetamine sulfate.
[b]Not available in some states.
Compiled from Refs. 50 and 53.

CIRCADIAN RHYTHM DISORDERS

The etiology of circadian rhythm disorders is a mismatch between an individual's biologic clock and the external time cues of the environment. Two commonly occurring circadian rhythm sleep disorders are jet lag and shift work sleep problems.

JET LAG

Jet lag follows rapid travel over multiple time zones and results in varying degrees and durations of sleep onset or maintenance insomnia complaints and daytime sleepiness. Insomnia usually occurs every other night. Sleep disturbances last for 2 to 3 days, but may prevail for 7 to 10 days if time zone changes are 8 to 12 hours. Compared with westward travel, eastward travel is associated with a longer duration of jet lag. Affected individuals also may suffer from decreased performance and alertness and gastrointestinal disturbances.[59]

Treatment of jet lag includes preventive measures and pharmacologic management. Jet lag can be avoided during coast-to-coast travel in the United States for durations of stay less than 7 days in a new time zone by adhering to the normal sleep–wake schedule from home. For longer lengths of stay, adjustment to a westbound time zone can be made by staying up and arising 1 to 2 hours later several days before the trip. Eastbound travelers also can adjust their schedule by retiring and arising earlier for several days before the trip.[59]

Pharmacologic treatment of jet lag includes the use of short-acting BZs. Melatonin has been used investigationally to rapidly entrain the circadian rhythm.[4,59] Patients should also be instructed to avoid ingestion of alcohol.

SHIFT WORK SLEEP PROBLEMS

Shift workers comprise approximately 20% of the workforce.[59] Working at night causes a misalignment in the sleep–wake cycle and circadian rhythms associated with a decrease in alertness, performance, and quality of daytime sleep. On nonworking nights many night-shift workers experience insomnia.[59] Treatment may consist of recommending a daytime job, extending daytime sleep by sleeping in the afternoon, or scheduling a 2- to 3-hour afternoon nap on days off from work. Hypnotics may be useful.[60] Scheduled exposure to bright lights at night and darkness during the daytime improves psychologic and behavioral adaptation to night work and daytime sleep.[61]

DYSSOMNIAS NOT OTHERWISE SPECIFIED

A dyssomnia that is not primary, due to a general medical condition, or substance induced is categorized as not otherwise specified. Idiopathic restless legs syndrome and idiopathic periodic limb movements are examples.

RESTLESS LEGS SYNDROME

Restless legs syndrome (RLS), also known as Ekbom's syndrome, is a discomfort, not pain, verbalized as pins and needles, a crawling sensation, or cramping mainly in the calves but sometimes noted in the thighs or arms.[62] Males and females are equally affected, and RLS occurs most commonly in the elderly. Iron deficiency, pregnancy, and renal failure are associated with RLS. Caffeine, stress, or fatigue may worsen the symptoms. The diagnosis is generally made based on the clinical presentation.

The sensation is generally bilateral and occurs only during rest and inactivity and is quickly relieved by walking or moving the legs.[63] When the person tries to resume sleep, the discomfort returns, thus resulting in insomnia. Mild or intermittent symptoms generally require no treatment, but patients should be reassured that this is benign and chronic. Depression and suicidal ideation may occur in more severe cases.

BZs may be the first-line agents for less severe cases and younger patients. Clonazepam, lorazepam, triazolam, and temazepam have been effective. Clonazepam 0.5 to 2.0 mg is the most studied.[30] Opiates, such as methadone 5 to 20 mg, codeine 30 to 120 mg, and oxycodone 2.5 mg, are very effective, but tolerance develops and abuse potential is a concern because the condition is chronic. Other agents used include bromocriptine, clonidine, and carbamazepine. Tolerance may develop with any agent used; thus one approach is to alternate chemically unrelated agents weekly or biweekly.[63] Patients should take the agent early enough prior to bedtime to allow time for drug absorption.

In the most severe cases, levodopa is considered the drug of choice.[62,63] Generally, the initial dose of levodopa is 50 mg 30 minutes before bedtime. This dose may be titrated, and most patients achieve benefit from levodopa 200 mg with carbidopa 50 mg.[64] However, rebound symptoms during the night and possibly during the day are noted. Dosing during the day or using the sustained-release product may alleviate rebound symptoms.

NOCTURNAL MYOCLONUS (PERIODIC LIMB MOVEMENTS)

Most patients with RLS also have periodic limb movements (PLMs), and approximately one-third of patients with PLM have RLS.[62,63] However, the two disorders are distinct. Unlike RLS, PLM is diagnosed in the sleep laboratory. A burst of muscle activity lasting 0.5 to 5 seconds is noted in the anterior tibialis EMG recording. Confirmation of diagnosis is at least 40 bursts in an 8-hour period of sleep.

The PLM is described as stereotypic, repetitive, periodic movements of the legs that occurs every 20 to 40 seconds and lasts 10 minutes to several hours.[62,63] The movement generally involves the big toe, but the ankle, knee, and hip may also flex. PLM occurs during sleep. It may be terminated by a violent kick or other bodily movement. The person does not recognize the problem and notes only the daytime consequence of excessive daytime somnolence. Often the bed partner describes the person as a restless sleeper and notes that the bedcovers are in disarray. Renal failure is likely a predisposing condition to PLM. BZ withdrawal and TCAs may precipitate the condition.

The treatment approach is similar to RLS. Milder cases do not require treatment. Clonazepam 0.5 to 2 mg is frequently used, as is baclofen 20 to 40 mg and opiates. TCAs generally worsen the problem; however, in one series, imipramine 25 mg improved symptoms in five patients.[30] Lamotrigine 100 mg has also improved symptoms.[65] The most severe cases are begun on levodopa. Alternating medications and allowing drug holidays may be helpful. Patients should take their medications early enough before bedtime to allow for drug absorption.

PARASOMNIAS

Parasomnias refer to a group of acute, episodic, physical phenomena that occur either exclusively during sleep or are exaggerated by sleep. Sleep walking (somnambulism) and sleep terrors are seen in children and may be considered normal to some degree at a certain age.[66] Somnambulism treatment consists primarily of protection from injury (e.g., putting safety latches on doors and windows, removing hazardous objects from bedrooms, and covering glass doors with heavy curtains). Theoretically, sleepwalking may be prevented by suppressing delta sleep. Although BZs suppress delta sleep, the risks of long-term, continuous exposure of a developing child to delta sleep suppressants is unknown. BZs, selective serotonin reuptake inhibitors

(SSRIs), or TCAs may be beneficial in adults.[66] Sleep terrors treatment consists of counseling the parents to wait until the disorder is outgrown. As with somnambulism, sleep terrors occur during delta sleep; BZs may be useful in adults secondary to delta sleep suppression.[66]

Nightmares are a REM phenomenon associated with frequent, elaborate recall of frightening dream content (e.g., dreams of physical attacks and death). Treatment usually consists of psychological intervention. This may be as simple as a parent providing comfort and reassurance to a child with an occasional nightmare, or as complex as intensive psychotherapy and use of cyproheptadine for an adult with frequent, highly disturbing nightmares.[67]

PHARMACOECONOMIC CONSIDERATIONS

Insomnia affects all three domains of quality of life: the ability to perform activities of daily living, emotional concerns, and interpersonal life.[68,69] Scores of patients with dyssomnias were compared to the general United States population norms from a health-related quality of life questionnaire. Results reflected significantly worse quality of life in persons with dyssomnias.[70] The estimated cost from absenteeism and sleep-related accidents is $92.5 to $107.5 billion per year. Direct and indirect costs include medications and treatment, absenteeism, decreased productivity, accidents, hospitalizations, and increased morbidity (both psychiatric and nonpsychiatric) and mortality. Treatment of the sleep disorder is beneficial. For example, treatment with nasal CPAP for obstructive sleep apnea improved the number of years of expected good health by 5.5 quality-adjusted life years.[68]

Quality of life was severely impaired in shift workers, but hypnotic therapy markedly improved the disorder and quality of life.[60] Persons were once again able to enjoy their free time, and alertness was not affected by sedative use. Quality of life can be improved by smoking cessation, reductions in caffeine and alcohol intake, and reduction in intake of over-the-counter sleep aids. If the sleep disturbance is related to a side effect of an antidepressant, quality of life, compliance, and overall outcome can be improved by managing the side effect.[71]

EVALUATION OF THERAPEUTIC OUTCOMES

A decision analysis for dyssomnias is shown in Figure 69–1. Patients with short-term or chronic insomnia should be evaluated after 1 week of therapy to assess for drug effectiveness, adverse events, and adherence to nonpharmacologic recommendations. Patients should be instructed to maintain a daily sleep diary. The diary requires daily recording of bedtime, arising time, sleep onset latency,

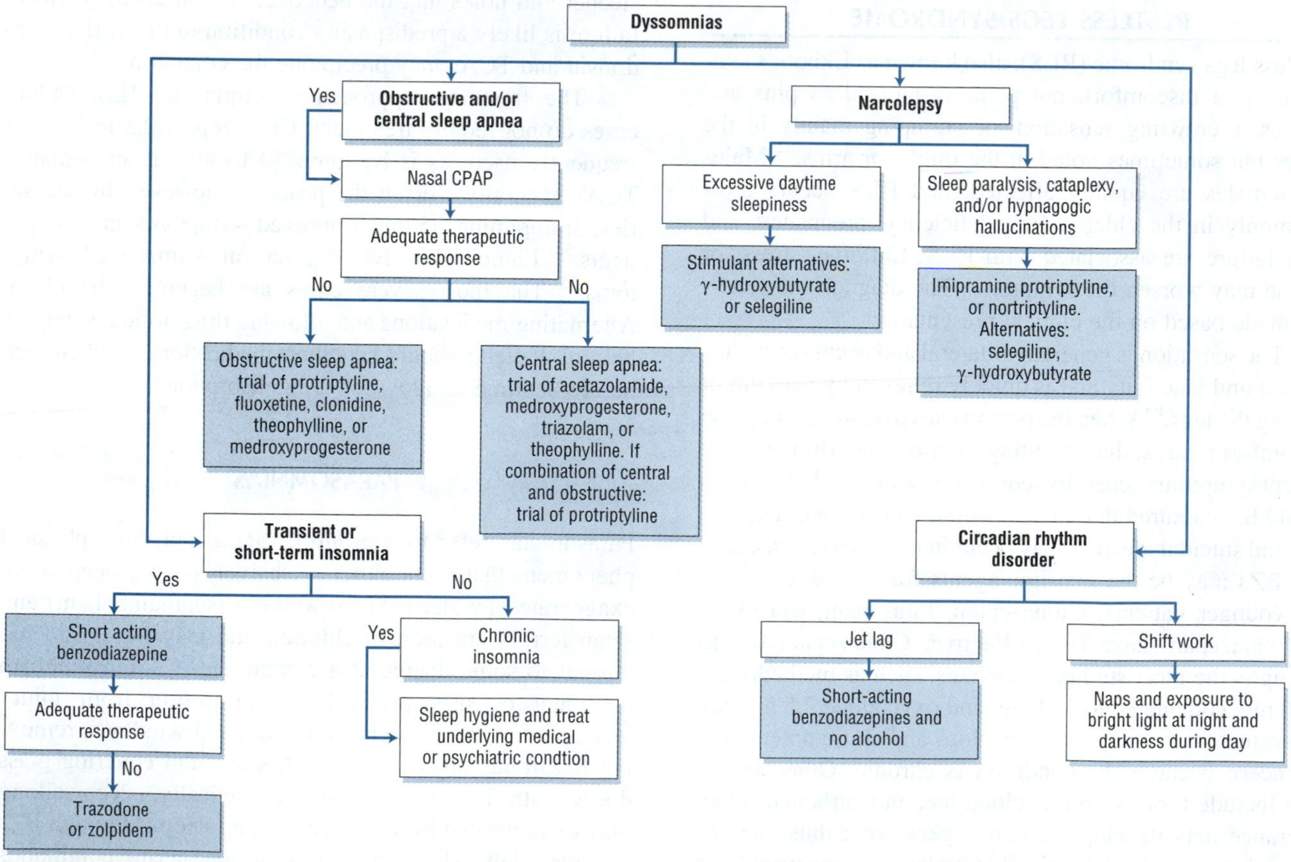

FIGURE 69–1. Algorithm for treatment of dyssomnias. *(Adapted and reprinted with permission from Jermain DM. Sleep disorders. In Jann M, ed.: Pharmacotherapy Self-assessment Program, 2nd ed. Kansas City, MO, American College of Clinical Pharmacy, 1995:139–154.)*

number and durations of awakenings, medication ingestion, naps, and an index of sleep quality.[72]

Individuals with sleep apnea treated with weight reduction and CPAP or drug therapy should be evaluated after 2 to 4 weeks of treatment for improvement in alertness and daytime symptoms (reduction in headache frequency and severity, improvement in memory, decreased irritability), and weight reduction. The bed partner can be consulted regarding reduced snoring and gasping episodes. A repeat PSG is indicated if the patient has not shown clinical improvement. Overall, the goals of therapy are to reduce the number of apneic episodes and improve O_2 saturation.

Reduction in daytime sleepiness, cataplexy, hypnogogic and hypnopompic hallucinations, and sleep paralysis is monitored in narcoleptics. Patients should be evaluated monthly until an optimal dose is achieved, and then every 6 to 12 months to assess for the development of adverse drug events (mood changes, sleep disturbances, cardiovascular abnormalities). If symptoms increase during therapy, PSG should be performed.

Patients with RLS and/or PLM should be evaluated monthly to monitor excessive daytime somnolence, tolerance, efficacy, and adverse effects of the medications. Because the conditions are chronic, assessment should occur every 6 to 12 months, and should include monitoring for depression, as it is a frequent complication that should be treated.

CONCLUSIONS

Disturbances of sleep affect approximately one-third of the population. Effective management of sleep disturbances is dependent on a proper diagnosis. Treatment of sleep disorders includes both pharmacologic and nonpharmacologic modalities.

Identifiable causes of insomnia should be managed before pharmacologic therapy is considered. BZs are the preferable agents for the short-term treatment of insomnia; however, their use is contraindicated in sleep apnea. Antidepressants are an alternative for insomnia, and they effectively manage sleep apnea and symptoms of narcolepsy. The psychostimulants and TCAs are effective treatments for patients with narcolepsy. Parasomnias and circadian rhythm disorders are usually managed nonpharmacologically. Mild cases of RLS and PLM are often managed nonpharmacologically, but the more severe cases are treated with clonazepam, levodopa, or opiates.

▶ PRINCIPLES OF PHARMACOTHERAPY

- Insomnia for greater than 3 weeks should be viewed as a symptom of a medical or psychiatric disorder.
- Common causes of insomnia include jet lag, significant psychosocial stress, excessive alcohol use, caffeine intake, and nicotine use.
- Sleep hygiene principles, such as relaxing before bedtime, exercising regularly, establishing a regular bedtime and wake up time, and discontinuing or reducing alcohol, caffeine, and nicotine, should be taught to patients with insomnia.
- Benzodiazepine tolerance and dependence is avoided by using low-dose, intermittent therapy for the shortest possible duration.
- Long-acting benzodiazepines should be avoided in the elderly.
- Bedtime doses of antidepressants such as trazodone may be considered as an alternative for patients experiencing insomnia.
- Monitoring mood symptoms of a patient experiencing a sleep disturbance after a significant loss or during a difficult time is important to prevent a long-term problem with insomnia and provide appropriate therapy if a mood disorder occurs.
- Obstructive and obstructive/central sleep apnea patients should avoid benzodiazepines, zolpidem, and alcohol.
- Nonpharmacologic interventions such as weight loss, removing an obstruction in the airway, and/or nasal continuous positive airway pressure should be considered first-line therapy for patients with obstructive sleep apnea.
- Therapeutic naps should be used rather than stimulants if possible for excessive daytime sleepiness associated with narcolepsy.

REFERENCES

1. Doghramji K. Causes, pathogenesis, and management of sleep disorders. Compr Ther 1990;16:49–59.
2. Farney RJ, Walker JM. Office management of common sleep–wake disorders. Med Clin North Am 1995;79:391–414.
3. Gillin JC, Byerley WF. The diagnosis and management of insomnia. N Engl J Med 1990;322:239–248.
4. Culebras A. Update on disorders of sleep and the sleep–wake cycle. Psychiatr Clin North Am 1992;15:467–489.
5. Neylan TC, Reynolds CF, Kupfer DJ. Sleep disorders. In: Hales RE, Yudofsky SC, Talbott JT, eds. American Psychiatric Press Textbook of Psychiatry, 2nd ed. Washington, DC, American Psychiatric Press, 1994:833.
6. Lader MH. Management of insomnia. Br J Clin Pract 1990;44: 125–130.
7. Morin CM. Insomnia: Psychological Assessment and Management. New York, Guilford Press, 1993:16.
8. Prinz PN, Vitiello MV, Raskind MA, et al. Geriatrics: Sleep disorders and aging. N Engl J Med 1990;323:520–526.
9. American Sleep Disorders Association Diagnostic Classification Steering Committee. International Classification of Sleep Disorders: Diagnostic and Coding Manual. Rochester, American Sleep Disorders Association, 1990:1.
10. American Psychiatric Association. Sleep disorders. In: Diagnostic and Statistical Manual of Mental Disorders, 4th ed. Washington, DC, American Psychiatric Press, 1994:551.
11. Rechtschaffen A, Kales A. A manual of standardized terminology, techniques and scoring system for sleep stages of human subjects. Washington, DC, U.S. Government Printing Office, 1968:1. Publication 204, Public Health Service Publications.

12. Dement WC. The proper use of sleeping pills in the primary care setting. J Clin Psychiatry 1992;53(suppl 12):50–56.
13. Ford DE, Kamerow DB. Epidemiologic study of sleep disturbances and psychiatric disorders. JAMA 1989;262:1479–1484.
14. Walsh JK, Engelhardt CL. Trends in the pharmacologic treatment of insomnia. J Clin Psychiatry 1992;53(suppl 12):10–17.
15. Morin CM, Culbert JP, Schwartz SM. Nonpharmacological interventions for insomnia: A meta-analysis of treatment efficacy. Am J Psychiatry 1994;151:1172–1180.
16. Bootzin RR, Perlis ML. Nonpharmacologic treatments of insomnia. J Clin Psychiatry 1992;53(suppl 6):37–41.
17. Nierenberg AA, Alder LA, Peselow E, et al. Trazodone for antidepressant-associated insomnia. Am J Psychiatry 1994;151:1069–1072.
18. Hertzman PA, Blevins WL, Mayer J. Association of eosinophilia–myalgia syndrome with the ingestion of tryptophan. N Engl J Med 1990;322:869–873.
19. Hoehns JD, Perry PJ. Zolpidem: A nonbenzodiazepine hypnotic for treatment of insomnia. Clin Pharm 1993;12:814–828.
20. Zolpidem for insomnia. Med Lett Drugs Ther 1993;35:35–36.
21. Ansseau M, Pichot W, Hansenne M, Gonzales-Moreno A. Psychotic reactions to zolpidem. Lancet 1992;339:809.
22. Markowitz JS, Brewerton TD. Zolpidem-induced psychosis. Ann Clin Psychiatry 1996;8:89–91.
23. Hoyler CL, Tekell JL, Silva JA. Zolpidem-induced agitation and disorganization. Gen Hosp Psychiatry 1996;18:452–453.
24. Scharf MB, Roth T, Vogel GW, Walsh JK. A multi-center, placebo-controlled study evaluating zolpidem in the treatment of chronic insomnia. J Clin Psychiatry 1994;55:192–199.
25. Roth T, Roehrs T, Vogel G. Zolpidem in the treatment of transient insomnia: A double-blind, randomized comparison with placebo. Sleep 1995;18:246–251.
26. Jan JE, O'Donnell ME. Use of melatonin in the treatment of paediatric sleep disorders. J Pineal Res 1996;21:193–199.
27. Turow V. Melatonin for insomnia and jet lag. Pediatrics 1996;97:439.
28. Ashton H. Guidelines for the rational use of benzodiazepines: When and what to use. Drugs 1994;48:25–40.
29. Greenblatt DJ. Benzodiazepine hypnotics: Sorting the pharmacokinetic facts. J Clin Psychiatry 1991;52(suppl 9):4–10.
30. Jermain DM. Sleep disorders. In: Pharmacotherapy Self-Assessment Program, 2nd ed. Kansas City, MO, American College of Clinical Pharmacy, 1995:139–154.
31. Nefazodone for depression. Med Lett Drugs Ther 1995;37:33–35.
32. Greenblatt DJ, von Moltke LL, Harmatz JS, et al. Interaction of triazolam and ketaconazole. Lancet 1995;345:191.
33. Maczaj M. Pharmacological treatment of insomnia. Drugs 1993;45:44–55.
34. Mendelson WB. Hypnotics in the treatment of chronic insomnia. In: Thorpy MJ, ed. Handbook of Sleep Disorders. New York, Dekker, 1990, 737.
35. ProSom package insert. Chicago, Abbott Labs, October 1991.
36. Schenck CH, Mahowald MW. Long-term, nightly benzodiazepine treatment of injurious parasomnias and other disorders of disrupted nocturnal sleep in 170 adults. Am J Med 1996;100:333–337.
37. Wysowski DK, Barash D. Adverse behavioral reactions attributed to triazolam in the Food and Drug Administration's spontaneous reporting system. Arch Intern Med 1991;151:2003–2008.
38. Ghaeli P, Dufresne RL, Stoukides CA. Triazolam treatment controversy. Ann Pharmacother 1994;28:1038–1040.
39. Kales A, Manfredi RL, Vgontzas AN, et al. Rebound insomnia after only brief and intermittent use of rapidly eliminated benzodiazepines. Clin Pharmacol Ther 1991;49:468–476.
40. Roehrs T, Vogel G, Roth T. Rebound insomnia: Its determinants and significance. Am J Med 1990;88(suppl 3A):39–42.
41. Monane M. Insomnia in the elderly. J Clin Psychiatry 1992;53(suppl 6):23–28.
42. Rapoport DM. Treatment of sleep apnea syndromes. Mt Sinai J Med 1994;61:123–130.
43. Brown LK. Sleep apnea syndromes: Overview and diagnostic approaches. Mt Sinai J Med 1994;61:99–112.
44. Kaplan J, Staats BA. Obstructive sleep apnea syndrome. Mayo Clin Proc 1990;65:1087–1094.
45. Hanzeol DA, Proia NG, Hudgel DW. Response of obstructive sleep apnea to fluoxetine and protriptyline. Chest 1991;100:416–421.
46. Mulloy E, McNicholas WT. Theophylline in obstructive sleep apnea: A double-blind evaluation. Chest 1992;101:753–757.
47. Issa FG. Effect of clonidine in obstructive sleep apnea. Am Rev Respir Dis 1992;145:435–439.
48. Hanly PJ. Mechanisms and management of central sleep apnea. Lung 1992;170:1–17.
49. Aldrich MS. Narcolepsy. Neurology 1992;42(suppl 6):34–43.
50. Mitler MM, Aldrich MS, Koob GF, Zarcone VP. ASDA standards of practice: Narcolepsy and its treatment with stimulants. Sleep 1994;17:352–371.
51. Lamberg L. Narcolepsy researchers barking up the right tree. JAMA 1996;276:765–766.
52. Garma L, Murchand F. Non-pharmacological approaches to the treatment of narcolepsy. Sleep 1994;17:S97–S102.
53. Standard of Practice Committee of the American Sleep Disorders Association. Practice parameters for the use of stimulants in the treatment of narcolepsy. Sleep 1994;17:348–351.
54. Mayer G, Meier KW, Hephata K. Selegiline hydrochloride treatment in narcolepsy. A double-blind, placebo-controlled study. Clin Neuropharmacol 1995;18:306–319.
55. Reinish LW, MacFarlane JG, Sandor P, Shapiro CM. REM changes in narcolepsy with selegiline. Sleep 1995;18:362–367.
56. Gernaat HBPE, Haffmans PMJ, Knegtering H, Birkenhager TK. Tranylcypromine in narcolepsy. Pharmacopsychiatry 1995;28:98–100.
57. Benbadis SR. Effective treatment of narcolepsy with codeine in a patient receiving hemodialysis. Pharmacotherapy 1996;16:463–465.
58. Lammers GJ, Arends J, Declerck AC, et al. Gammahydroxybutyrate and narcolepsy: A double-blind placebo-controlled study. Sleep 1993;16:216–220.
59. Wagner DR. Circadian rhythm sleep disorders. In: Thorpy MJ, ed. Handbook of Sleep Disorders. New York, Dekker, 1990:493.
60. Puca FM, Perrucci S, Prudenzano MP, et al. Quality of life in shift work syndrome. Funct Neurol 1996;11:261–268.
61. Czeisler CA, Johnson MP, Duffy JF, et al. Exposure to bright light and darkness to treat physiologic maladaptation to night work. N Engl J Med 1990;322:1253–1259.
62. Ambrogetti A, Olson LG, Saunders NA. Disorders of movement and behaviour during sleep. Med J Aust 1991;155:336–340.
63. Krueger BR. Restless legs syndrome and periodic movements of sleep. Mayo Clin Proc 1990;65:999–1006.
64. Becker PM, Jamieson AO, Brown WD. Dopaminergic agents in restless legs syndrome and periodic limb movements of sleep: Response and complications of extended treatment in 49 cases. Sleep 1993;16:713–716.
65. Staedt J, Stoppe G, Riemann H, et al. Lamotrigine in the treatment of nocturnal myoclonus syndrome (NMS): Two case reports. J Neural Transm 1996;103:355–361.
66. Mahowald MW, Schenck CH. NREM sleep parasomnias. Neurol Clin 1996;14:675–696.
67. Schenck CH, Mahowald MW. REM sleep parasomnias. Neurol Clin 1996;14:697–720.
68. Idzikowski C. Impact of insomnia on health-related quality of life. Pharmacoeconomics 1996;10:15–24.
69. Stoller MK. Economic effects of insomnia. Clin Ther 1994;16:873–897.
70. Wagner AK. Health related quality of life of people with dyssomnias. American Society of Health System Pharmacists (ASHP) annual meeting Philadelphia, PA, 1995;52:FGF-3.
71. McElroy SL, Keck PE, Friedman LM. Minimizing and managing antidepressant side effects. J Clin Psychiatry 1995;56:49–55.
72. Morin CM. Insomnia: Psychological Assessment and Management. New York, Guilford Press, 1993:61.

70
DIABETES MELLITUS

Condit F. Steil, PharmD, CDE

Diabetes mellitus is a term that describes a series of complex and chronic metabolic disorders characterized by symptomatic glucose intolerance. Since diabetes appears to be a heterogeneous group of disorders, there is no commonality in regard to the age of onset, genetic predisposition or development of complications. It is known that all diabetes patients eventually show abnormalities of insulin secretion and complications of the disease, such as vascular and neurologic abnormalities, and most manifest some degree of cellular resistance to insulin in type 2 diabetes. Recent data show some dramatic trends in the incidence of diabetes. Approximately 15.7 million people (5.9% of the population) in the United States have diabetes, though about one third of these individuals have not been diagnosed. It is more prevalent in minority populations, including Hispanics, African-Americans, American Indians, and Asian-Americans, in whom there is a two to five times higher rate of diabetes and a subsequently greater burden from its complications. As detection and screening methods become more common, the identification of patients will increase. The annual costs of diabetes care during 1992 was estimated at $91.8 billion for both direct and indirect costs, with $46.7 billion of this total representing direct costs of care. Diabetes is the leading cause of blindness in adults ages 20 to 74, is the leading cause by category of end-stage renal disease, and accounts for approximately 67,000 lower extremity amputations annually.[1,2]

PATHOGENESIS AND CLASSIFICATION

Diabetes has usually been classified primarily by age of onset and ease of control. Such terms as *juvenile onset, adult onset, insulin* or *noninsulin dependent, brittle, chemical, overt,* and *latent* often made the understanding of diabetes difficult. In 1997 the American Diabetes Association Expert Committee on the Diagnosis and Classification of Diabetes Mellitus recommended the use of the terms type 1 and type 2 to simplify the labels for the primary forms of diabetes.[3] Type 2 diabetes can range from a predominantly insulin resistance defect with relative insulin deficiency to a predominantly insulin secretory defect. The levels for diagnosis were altered, and a new category of risk, impaired fasting glucose, was described. The new system provides a method of differentiating insulin sensitive and insulin resistant type 2 disease. Smaller etiologic categories include secondary diabetes, impaired glucose tolerance (IGT), impaired fasting glucose (IFG), and gestational diabetes mellitus (GDM) (see Table 70–1 for a more complete classification).

TYPE 1

This type of diabetes usually develops in childhood or early adulthood and accounts for up to 10% of all diabetes patients. They are often thin, have an absolute lack of insulin, and are prone to develop diabetic ketoacidosis (DKA) if insulin is withheld. Type 1 diabetes results from a cellular-mediated autoimmune destruction of the β cells of the pancreas and islet cell, and tyrosine phosphatases autoantibodies are seen in 85% to 90% of patients.[3] There are strong genetic linkages to the DQA and B genes and certain human leukocyte antigens (HLA) may be predisposing (DR3 and DR4) or protective (DRB1*04008-DQB1*0302 and DRB1*0411-DQB1*0302) on chromosome 6. Other candidate gene regions have been identified on several other chromosomes as well. Because twin studies do not show 100% concordance, environmental factors such as infectious agents, chemical agents, and dietary agents are likely contributing factors in the expression of the disease.

TYPE 2

Type 2 diabetes usually manifests in adulthood around age 40 or later. About 90% of patients with diabetes develop type 2 diabetes. Type 2 diabetes genetics are complex and manifest tremendous variability across populations. Numerous candidate gene studies have been conducted: genes such as the insulin and insulin receptor gene, glucose transporter genes, the HLA region of chromosome 6 (including DR3 and DR4), and genes controlling fatty acid, glycogen, and apo- and lipoprotein metabolism. Though there is evidence that type 2 diabetes has a strong genetic predisposition, no single gene defect explains the protean manifestations of this syndrome.[3] About 90% of patients are obese and may not display the classic symptoms of diabetes. Plasma insulin levels in type 2 diabetes may be high, normal, or low, and the metabolic defects include (1) impaired basal and stimulated insulin secretion, (2) an increased rate of endogenous hepatic glucose production, and (3) inefficient peripheral tissue glucose use. Inactive receptors, densensitized receptors, or inadequate insulin action may contribute to these defects. Thus, type 2 diabetics may exhibit a range of problems from insulin hypersecretion to exhaustion of islet cell activity

TABLE 70–1. Classification of Diabetes Mellitus, Impaired Fasting Glucose, and Impaired Glucose Tolerance

Diabetes mellitus
- Type 1—insulin mediated, idiopathic
- Type 2—may range from predominantly insulin resistance with relative insulin deficiency to predominantly secretory defect with insulin resistance

Other specific causes/types of diabetes mellitus
- Pancreatic disease and endocrinopathies
- Chronic pancreatitis, cystic fibrosis, pancreatectomy, hemochromatosis
- Acromegaly, Cushing's disease, glucagonoma, pheochromocytoma, primary aldosteronism, somatostatinoma, hyperthyroidism
- Drugs: catecholamines, glucocorticoids, oral contraceptives, thiazide and loop diuretics, niacin (induced hyperglycemia), vacor, pentamidine, phenytoin, α-interferon
- Genetic syndromes: Huntington's chorea, hyperlipidemia, muscular dystropy, leprechaunism, Rabson–Mendenhall syndrome, Turner's syndrome, Friedreich's ataxia, Down's syndrome, porphyria, myotonic dystrophy, Prader Willi syndrome

Causes of impaired glucose tolerance
- Pre-diabetes mellitus
- Secondary to pancreatic disease, drugs, and genetic syndromes (see secondary causes of diabetes mellitus above)

accompanied by resistance of insulin action on various tissues. Type 2 patients do not usually progress to ketoacidosis except during periods of stress; therefore, insulin replacement is not an absolute necessity for initial therapy, but may ultimately be needed by many patients as their insulin production declines. This classification is under current study (see Table 70–2 for a more thorough differentiation between type 1 and 2 diabetes).

OTHER TYPES

Genetic defects of the β cell or in insulin action (insulin receptor mutations or postreceptor defects) as well as disease of the exocrine pancreas (e.g., pancreatitis, cystic fibrosis) are less common causes of diabetes. Endocrinopathies may antagonize the effect of insulin or produce hormone excesses (e.g., Cushing's syndrome—ACTH and cortisol; acromegaly—growth hormone) resulting in diabetes. Diabetes may also result from the use of certain medications or chemicals (e.g., corticosteroids, thiazide diuretics, pentamidine, niacin, α-interferon).

Gestational diabetes mellitus (GDM) refers to the onset of glucose intolerance during pregnancy, usually in the second or third trimester, and occurs in ~ 4% of pregnancies. GDM patients who require drug therapy in addition to diet must use insulin, but usually return to normal glucose tolerance immediately postdelivery. Most pregnant women should have a general screening by week 24 to 28 of the pregnancy, though new recommendations state that low-risk patients (< 25 years of age, normal body weight, no family history of diabetes, and not a member of an ethnic group with high incidence of diabetes) do not require screening. Screening for GDM is based on a glucose load of 50 g and is positive if the 1-hour glucose is > 140 mg/dL. The diagnostic challenge is with 100 g of glucose and plasma glucose sampling at fasting, 1, 2, and 3 hours; two or more glucose concentrations exceeding 105 mg/dL, 190 mg/dL, 165 mg/dL, and 145 mg/dL, respectively, are considered to be diagnostic of GDM.[3] Subsequent follow-up is needed because up to 40% of persons with GDM will develop diabetes within the next 10 years.[4,5]

IMPAIRED GLUCOSE TOLERANCE AND IMPAIRED FASTING GLUCOSE

Impaired glucose tolerance (IGT) and impaired fasting glucose (IFG) are terms to describe patients whose plasma glucose levels are higher than normal (fasting glucose ≥ 110 mg/dL but < 126 mg/dL nor random glucose > 140 mg/dL

TABLE 70–2. General Characteristics of Type 1 and Type 2 Diabetes

Characteristic	Type 1 Diabetes	Type 2 Diabetes
Age of onset	Usually during childhood or adolescence	Usually age 40 or older
Rapidness of onset	Usually abrupt	Usually gradual
Family studies	Increased prevalence of type 1	Increased prevalence of type 2
Etiology	Unknown; postulated causes include heredity, autoimmune diseases, and viral infections	Unknown, but heredity is highly associated with occurrence
Twin studies	< 50% concordance in monozygotic twins	Close to 100% concordance in monozygotic twins
Islet cell antibodies and pancreatic cell-mediated immunity	Yes	No
Body weight	Usually thin and undernourished	Obesity is common
Insulin	Secretion is markedly diminished early in the disease and may be totally absent later in the disease; insulin therapy is mandatory	Levels may be low (indicating deficiency), normal, or high (indicating insulin resistance); insulin therapy may not be required decreasing as the disease progresses indicating the pancreas loses its insulin production capability
Ketosis	Common, especially with proper insulin control	Uncommon; if present, usually associated with severe stress or infection
Symptoms	Polyuria, polydipsia, polyphagia, weight loss	May be asymptomatic; polyuria and/or polydipsia may be present

TABLE 70–3. Drugs Causing Significant Elevations in Plasma Glucose Concentration

Drug	Mechanism of Action	Clinical Significance
Alcohol	Chronic ingestion increases tolbutamide metabolism	+
Asparaginase	Related to inhibition of insulin synthesis	++
β-Adrenergic antagonists	Inhibit insulin secretion	++
Calcium channel blockers	Inhibit insulin secretion	+/–
Combination oral contraceptives	Unknown	++
Diazoxide	Inhibits insulin secretion	+++
Diuretics	May be related to hypokalemia	++
Glucocorticoids	Increase gluconeogenesis, depress insulin action	+++
Glycerol	Unknown	++
Lithium salts	May decrease insulin secretion	+
Niacin	Unknown	++
Pentamidine isethionate	Promotes pancreatic toxicity	+++
Phenytoin sodium	Inhibits insulin secretion	++
Rifampin	Enhances metabolism of tolbutamide	+
Sympathomimetics	Increase glycogenolysis and gluconeogenesis	++

From: White J, Hartman J, Campbell RK. Drug interactions in diabetic patients. Postgrad Med 1993;93:137.

but < 200 mg/DL), but are not diagnostic for diabetes. IGT and IFG are risk factors for diabetes and cardiovascular disease and are associated with insulin-resistance syndrome (insulin resistance, hyperinsulinemia, dyslipidemia, and hypertension). Although about 25% of thesc patients will develop diabetes mellitus, it is important not to label these patients with diabetes until a definite diagnosis has been made because there are often social, insurance, and job limitations for persons with diabetes. Medications may be identified as the cause of IǴT (Table 70–3). Current studies are investigating the value of aggressive early therapy of IGT and IFG.

METABOLISM AND UTILIZATION OF CARBOHYDRATES, PROTEINS, AND FATS

INSULIN: DIABETES-RELATED CHANGES

Before understanding the etiology, manifestations, or complications of diabetes, one must first be familiar with normal carbohydrate, protein, and fat metabolism. Carbohydrates are metabolized in the body to glucose, the body's main source of energy. The glucose is absorbed from the gastrointestinal tract into the bloodstream, where it is oxidized in skeletal muscle to produce energy. Glucose is also stored in the liver in the form of glycogen and utilized in adipose tissue to build fats and triglycerides. Insulin is produced, stored, and released from the β cells of the pancreas and facilitates glucose use by increasing uptake of glucose by the tissues, increasing liver glycogen levels, decreasing glycogen breakdown (glycogenolysis) by the liver, increasing synthesis of fatty acids and inhibiting the breakdown of fatty acids into ketone bodies, and promoting incorporation of amino acids into proteins.[6]

Insulin is released from a functioning pancreas at a rate of 0.5 to 1 U/h and also in response to blood sugar in excess of 100 mg/dL. A normal adult pancreas secretes 25 to 50 U of insulin per day. Insulin is cleared by the liver, peripheral tissues, and kidneys. It is not unusual for patients with renal disease to require less insulin simply owing to reduced clearance by the kidneys.

Glucose can diffuse into the brain without the aid of insulin, but muscle and fat require the presence of insulin to receive glucose. If glucose is not available or cannot enter muscle and adipose tissue, these tissues will convert amino acids and fatty acids to carbohydrate (gluconeogenesis). As this tissue deprivation continues, the tissue eventually metabolizes stored fats, resulting in the production of free fatty acids that are eventually oxidized to ketone bodies.[6]

The body normally maintains plasma glucose concentrations between 40 and 160 mg/dL. A plasma glucose concentration of at least 40 mg/dL is necessary for brain function. Symptoms of hypoglycemia will usually be present at these concentrations or earlier. A high plasma concentration implies that glucose is not being transported into cells for energy production. Plasma concentrations in excess of 180 mg/dL usually exceed the renal tubular maximal reabsorption rate or "threshold" for reabsorption; consequently, glucose spills into the urine with significant interpatient variation

Insulin secretion is under the control of counterregulatory hormones and insulin secretagogues (Table 70–4). The balance of these systems determines blood glucose.

CLINICAL PRESENTATION

The classic symptoms of diabetes include polyuria (excessive urination), polydipsia (increased thirst), and polyphagia (increased appetite with increased calorie intake). As plasma glucose levels increase to about 180 mg/dL, the reabsorptive capacity of the kidneys for glucose is exceeded, causing spillage of glucose into the urine. The ensuring osmotic diuresis produces polyuria and a risk of dehydration. Because glucose cannot be properly transported into cells, the

TABLE 70–4. Counterregulatory Hormones and Insulin Secretagogues

	Origin	Action
Counterregulatory Hormones		
Glucagon	α cells of the endocrine pancreas	Stimulated during fasting to prevent blood glucose values from dropping too low. Glucagon increases blood glucose by increasing glycogenolysis and gluconeogenesis in the liver.
Growth hormone	Anterior pituitary	Opposes the action of insulin by interfering with the body's ability to utilize glucose. One stimulus for growth-hormone secretion is hypoglycemia.
Somatostatin	γ cells of the pancreas	Inhibits both insulin and glucagon secretion and suppresses growth hormone. This results in a fall in blood glucose levels because of the suppression of glucagon. In addition, somatostatin inhibits absorption of glucose from the gastrointestinal tract.
Epinephrine	Secreted by the adrenal medulla	Stimulates the conversion of glycogen to glucose in the liver. Similarly, drugs such as ephedrine and phenylpropanolamine, which stimulate the release of epinephrine and other catecholamines, can also produce an elevation in plasma glucose levels via the same mechanism.
Glucocorticoids	Secreted by the zona reticularis of the adrenal cortex	Stimulate gluconeogenesis, causing a marked increase in liver glycogen. They do not increase glycogen in any other body cells. In fact, glucocorticoids decrease glycogen stores in all other cells because they decrease glucose uptake and utilization by these cells.
Thyroid hormone	Secreted by the thryoid gland	Elevates blood glucose by increasing the rate of absorption of glucose from the gastrointestinal tract. Moreover, thyroid hormone increases liver gluconeogenesis and glycogenolysis.
Insulin Secretgogues		
Glucose	Diet, gluconeogensis, glycogenolysis	Hyperglycemia stimulates insulin release
Amino acids	Diet, muscle catabolism	Less potent than carbohydrates in stimulating insulin release and also stimulate glucagon release
Fats	Diet, adipose tissue catabolism	No direct effect
Gastrointestinal hormones		
Gastric insulinotropic polypeptide	Duodenum and jejunum	GI hormones are responsible for extra insulin release with oral feeding compared with intravenous glucose
Cholecystokinin	Duodenum and proximal jejunum	
GLP-1	L cells—distal small intestine	
Vasoactive intestinal polypeptide	GI tract	
Neuropeptide tyrosine	GI tract	
Acetylcholine	Parasympathetic nerves innervating the pancreas	Stimulates insulin release through activation of a muscarinic receptor
Norepinephrine	Sympathetic neurons innervating the pancreas	Net effect of inhibiting glucose-mediated insulin secretion

"hunger sensation" is triggered, inducing polyphagia. These symptoms are common in type 1 patients along with weight loss, weakness, and dry skin. The onset of these symptoms is rapid, and secondary ketoacidosis is common.[6]

In contrast, the onset of type 2 diabetes is insidious, and patients may be asymptomatic for years. Because the type 2 patient is usually obese, weight changes and/or polyphagia may be absent or go unnoticed. Polyuria and/or fatigue may be presenting complaints, but most type 2 patients are discovered because of an abnormal blood or urine glucose on routine physical examination or screening.[7]

SCREENING TESTS

Current recommendations call for routine glucose determination for all people over age 45 years, with subsequent screening every 3 years.[3,8] This practice was advocated by the ADA Task Force previously mentioned to build the sense

TABLE 70–5. Criteria for Testing for Diabetes in Asymptomatic, Undiagnosed Individuals

1. Testing for diabetes should be considered in all individuals at age 45 years and above and, if normal, it should be repeated at 3-year intervals.
2. Testing should be considered at a younger age or be carried out more frequently in individuals who:
   - are obese (≥ 120% desirable body weight or a BMI ≥ 27 kg/m^2)
   - have a first-degree relative with diabetes
   - are members of a high-risk ethnic population (e.g., African-American, Hispanic, Native American)
   - have delivered a baby weighing > 9 lb or have been diagnosed with GDM
   - are hypertensive (≥ 140/90)
   - have an HDL cholesterol ≤ 35 mg/dL and/or a triglyceride level ≥ 250 mg/dL
   - on previous testing, had IGT or IFG

From Ref. 3 with permission.

in the practice community and the public that diabetes must be identified by monitoring actively rather than passively. Testing should be considered earlier if the high-risk features are present (Table 70–5). The oral glucose tolerance test (OGTT) may be used to diagnose diabetes; however, the fasting plasma glucose (FPG) may be preferred by patients owing to cost convenience and availability.

DIAGNOSTIC TESTS

Three methods of diagnosing diabetes are currently recommended. Each of the three methods must be confirmed on a subsequent day by any of the three techniques. The criteria include:

1. Symptoms of diabetes plus casual plasma glucose concentration of ≥ 200 mg/dL. Casual is defined as any time of day for the test without regard to time since the last meal. The classic symptoms of diabetes include polyuria, polydipsia, and unexplained weight loss.

   OR

2. FPG ≥ 126 mg/dL. Fasting is defined as no caloric intake for at least 8 hours.

   OR

3. Two-hour postprandial plasma glucose ≥ 200 mg/dL during an OGTT. The test should be performed using a glucose load containing the equivalent of 75 g of anhydrous glucose dissolved in water.

For a meaningful glucose tolerance test, the patient should have fasted for the past 8 hours and should have discontinued glucose-altering medications 3 days before the test day. The patient must not be carbohydrate depleted and should have an adequate carbohydrate intake 3 days prior to testing. He or she should be instructed not to smoke or drink coffee just before and during the test, because misleading elevations in plasma glucose may occur. A fasting plasma glucose is then drawn. The patient is administered a standard glucose-containing solution (75 g for nonpregnant adults, 100 g for pregnant women, and 1.75 g/kg ideal body weight up to 75 g for children). In nonpregnant adults and children, blood samples are drawn every 30 minutes for 2 hours. In pregnant women, blood samples are drawn every hour for 3 hours. Plasma glucose values should peak in about 1 hour, remain under 200 mg/dL throughout the test, and return to fasting values by the 2-hour interval.[3,6] Those patients who have abnormal test results and cannot be diagnosed with diabetes are classified as having impaired glucose tolerance (IGT). IGT exists when the random glucose (e.g., 2 hours postprandial) level is ≥ 140 mg/dL but < 200 mg/dL. Impaired fasting glucose is defined as FPG > 110 mg/dL but < 126 m/dL.

Once the diagnosis of diabetes has been made, it is important to classify the patient as having either type 1 or type 2 diabetes. Usually the classification can be made on the basis of age, suddenness of onset, and physical characteristics of the patient. C-peptides have also been used to distinguish between type 1 and 2 diabetics. Proinsulin is cleaved in the pancreas to form insulin and C-peptide molecules. Therefore, patients with no insulin production have little, if any, production of C-peptides.[9] Regardless of the criteria used for classification, it is important to remember that the type 1 patient has an absolute lack of insulin and must be given exogenous insulin to sustain life and prevent ketoacidosis. Therapy for type 2 diabetes, on the other hand, can often be started with diet and no medication.

▶ TREATMENT: Diabetes Mellitus

GOALS AND INTENSIVE THERAPY

The basic goals of diabetes therapy have largely remained unchanged for several years. Many clinicians assumed that tighter management of glucose was beneficial to the patient's welfare, though few clinical data supported this belief. The results of several long-term studies that reviewed the importance of tight glycemic control have been reported. One study was the Diabetes Control and Complications Trial (DCCT) involving 1441 patients treated for over seven thousand patient-years. The two hypotheses for the study were: "Does tight management prevent the initiation of complications"—primary prevention; and "Does tight management prevent or limit the progression of diabetes complications?—(secondary intervention). Retinopathy was the complication used for assigning patients to the prevention or intervention cohort. The study was limited to patients with type 1 diabetes and they were divided into intensive and conventional treatment groups. A similar approach was taken with type 2 patients in a study based in Japan. The studies' results on complications are listed in Table 70–6. The primary adverse event of intensive treatment appears to be an increase in severe hypoglycemia.[10,11] An epidemiologic review in an 11-county area of Wisconsin demonstrates similar trends to these studies with regard to retinopathy progression.[12] Any improvement in glycemic control decreased the risk for complications, and thus metabolic control matters.

These studies' findings have changed the therapy goals for diabetes patients, though some limitations to applying the same intensive principles to all patients exist. Persons who have significant hypoglycemia unawareness or significant cardiovascular

TABLE 70–6. Results—Diabetes Control and Complications Trial: Risk Reductions from Conventional to Intensive Cohorts Both Primary and Secondary Interventions and the Risk Reductions From the Type 2 Study at Kumamoto University

Complication	DCCT Reduction (%)	Kumamoto Reduction (%)
>3 step sustained retinopathy	63	65
Macular edema	26	
Severe nonproliferative or proliferative retinopathy	47	40
Laser treatment	51	
Urinary albumin excretion (mg/24 h)		
> 40	39	
> 300	54	57
Clinical neuropathy at 5 yr	60	52

TABLE 70–7. Goals of Therapy

Parameter	Normal	Acceptable	Fair	Poor
Fasting plasma glucose (mg/dL)	< 110	< 140	< 200	> 200
Postprandial plasma glucose (mg/dL)	< 140	< 175	< 235	> 235
Glycosylated hemoglobina[a] (%)	< 6	< 8	8–9.5	> 10

[a]Increase limits 10% for elderly patients.

disease may be poor candidates for tight control owing to the potential for hypoglycemia. Although clinicians desire good control, young patients must receive adequate nutrition for growth and development. However, the important point of these studies is that any improvement in glucose and the glycosylated hemoglobin resulted in a decreased incidence of complications.

The treatment of diabetes varies considerably between type 1 and type 2 diabetes. Type 1 patients have an absolute lack of insulin, so diet, exercise, self-monitoring of blood glucose, and insulin are necessary for proper management. Type 2 therapy also consists of nutrition and physical activity; however, oral medications or insulin may or may not be required. The nutritional goals for the two types of diabetes also differ. The overall goal of therapy, however, is consistent: to maintain the plasma glucose in an acceptable range throughout the day so that the patient remains asymptomatic. Desirable plasma glucose concentrations are listed in Table 70–7.

PATIENT EDUCATION

Successful treatment of diabetes involves life-style changes for the patient (e.g.,nutrition, physical activity, self-monitoring of blood and possibly urine, and/or taking medication). Standards of diabetes self-management have been established through field testing and include 14 specific content areas listed in Table 70–8. The patient must be involved in the decision-making process. He or she must learn as much as possible about diabetes. The long-term complications of diabetes and other issues must be explained to the patient, stressing that newer evidence indicates that many of these complications can be curtailed or prevented with a well-controlled blood glucose concentration. Recognition of this need for proper patient involvement in care has spawned a new specialty practice of diabetes education, including a certification process whose requirements are noted in Table 70–9. Most educators follow a two-phase education structure, with survival skills taught initially and then self-care management, which mandates behavior change and patient motivation.[13–15]

TABLE 70–8. Content Areas of Instruction From the National Standards for Diabetes Self-Management Training

Diabetes overview
Stress and psychosocial adjustment
Family involvement and social support
Nutrition
Exercise and activity
Medications
Monitoring and use of results
Relationships among nutrition, exercise, medication, and blood glucose monitoring
Prevention, detection, and treatment of acute complications
Prevention, detection, and treatment of chronic complications
Foot, skin, and dental care
Behavior change strategies, goal setting, risk factor reduction, and problem solving
Preconception, pregnancy, and postpartum management
Use of health care systems and community resources

TABLE 70–9. Certified Diabetes Educator Requirements

1. Professional education: Currently hold a U.S. license as an RN, RD, RPh, MD, licensed PA, Podiatrist, Reg. PT
   OR
   Hold at least a master's level education in the chosen health profession.
2. Experience: At least 1000 h of direct diabetes patient education in the U.S. in an organized education program in at least 2 yr and within the past 5 yr.
3. Successfully pass the certification examination.[a]

[a]Recertification by examination every 5 yr.

DIET AND NUTRITION

Recent changes in the American Diabetes Association's nutrition guidelines have altered the approach of dietary management of diabetes. Effective self-management requires an individualized approach for building a diet plan, usually involving the input of a dietitian. The goal of the diet plan for type 1 patients is to build a healthy daily nutrition intake into a regimen that allows flexibility in insulin therapy and home monitoring. The emphasis for type 2 patients should be placed on achieving blood glucose, lipid, and blood pressure goals. Weight loss has been the mainstay of previous therapy goals and usually improves short-term glucose levels, but most patients have not achieved long-term weight loss. Therefore, the emphasis shifts to glucose and lipid goals. Healthy food choices may be the first step used for the type 2 patient, to obtain the calories with less saturated fat and protein.

Limited data are available to establish firm protein nutritional recommendations for diabetes patients. The recommendation is the same as for the general population, about 10% to 20% of total calories. This is reduced for patients with renal failure. Less than 10% of the total daily intake should come from saturated fats, and up to 10% from polyunsaturated fats, leaving 60% to 70% of the total calories between carbohydrates and monounsaturated fats. The distribution of calories between these two remaining categories varies from patient to patient depending on the assessment and treatment goals. For individuals with near-normal body weight and lipid levels, the recommendations of 30% or less of the calories from total fat could be implemented, leaving 50% to 60% of the calories as carbohydrates. If obesity and weight loss are major issues, a reduction in dietary fat can be effective in achieving positive change. One may also want to consider the Step 2 diet guidelines of the National Cholesterol Education Program, which calls for < 7% of the total calories from saturated fat, with < 200 mg cholesterol.

The percentage of calories from carbohydrates will vary and should be individualized with the patient's eating habits and therapy goals. For many years, patients with diabetes were taught to avoid simple sugars. There is little evidence that the assumed rapid absorption and increase in glucose actually occurs when the sugar is part of the basic meal plan. Rather than a concern for the type of carbohydrate source (starch, bread) one should be concerned with the total amount consumed.

The patient should understand the need for attention to the amount of other nutritive sweeteners (fructose, sorbitol) consumed and their being "hidden" in several foods. The polyols of course carry the potential for a laxative effect. Sodium intake should receive attention with the risk link for hypertension. Similar precautions for alcohol consumption apply to persons with diabetes as to the public at large. The risk for hypoglycemia acutely can be enhanced when alcohol is consumed on an empty stomach. Though it has no nutritional value, its calories must be accounted for, and moderation is the key, avoiding binges. One should consider the potential for combinations of concurrent pancreatitis, neuropathy, and alcohol consumption as well as individual occurrences[16,17]

EXERCISE AND PHYSICAL ACTIVITY

Unless contraindicated, appropriate physical activity should be recommended to improve insulin sensitivity and possibly improve glucose tolerance. Exercise can also help promote weight loss and maintain ideal body weight when combined with restricted caloric intake.[18] Prior to embarking on a moderate-to-high intensity exercise program, evaluation of cardiovascular and peripheral vascular disease as well as the presence of retinopathy, nephropathy, and peripheral and autonomic neuropathy should be performed. In type 2 diabetes, the desired level of exercise is 50% to 80% of maximal uptake of oxygen (approximately 60% to 80% of maximal heart rate) three or four times per week. In type 1 diabetes care must taken to have adequate metabolic control (FPG > 250 mg/dL, ketones present or glucose > 300 mg/dL if no ketones present) prior to exercise and to monitor blood glucose before and after exercise. Exercise is not recommended if the patient has poorly controlled, labile blood glucose levels or is at increased risk from diabetic complications. Strenuous exercise is not wise in the patient prone to developing hypoglycemia unless the patient is well educated about the symptoms and consequences of hypoglycemia and takes proper measures to anticipate and treat this condition. Patients with progressive complications involving the eyes or feet should avoid strenuous activity that may cause further damage.[18]

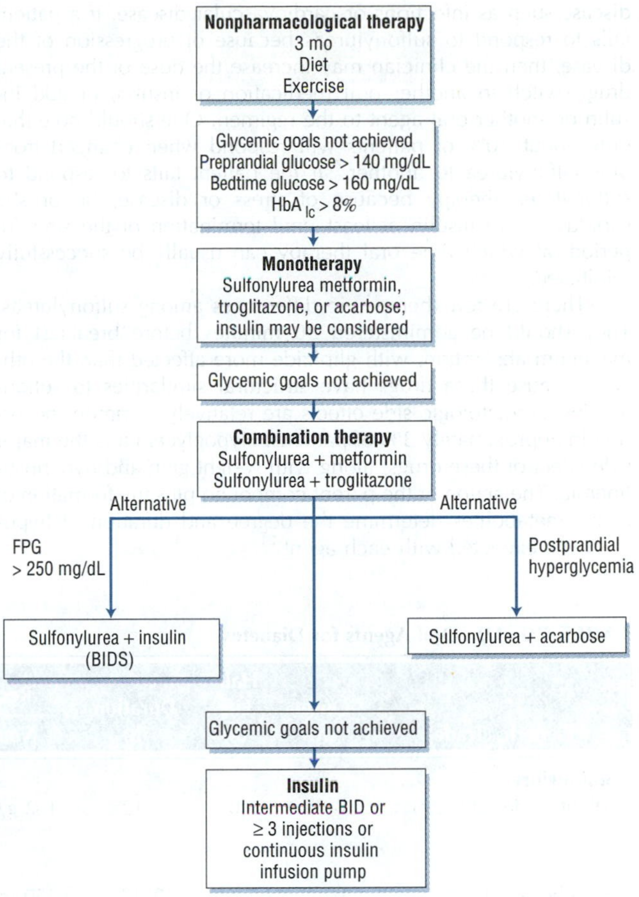

FIG. 70–1. Treatment algorithm for type 2 diabetes mellitus.

PHARMACOLOGIC THERAPY

ORAL AGENTS FOR DIABETES CONTROL

Pharmacologic intervention for type 2 diabetes is necessary if an appropriate diet and exercise program does not improve glycemic control adequately (Fig. 70–1).[19] The dilemma of which agent to prescribe, an oral agent or insulin, reaches back to 1960s and the University Group Diabetes Program (UGDP) study, which examined diet alone versus diet plus oral hypoglycemic (tolbutamide) versus diet plus insulin.[20] The doses of each of the medications were fixed and no home blood glucose monitoring was available at that time. The study concluded that prolonged use of an oral sulfonylureas greatly increased cardiovascular mortality. However, numerous flaws in the design and conduct of the study were discovered, and patients on sulfonylureas are no longer believed to be at greater risk owing to sulfonylurea therapy. Although controversy regarding the overall safety and long-term efficacy of oral sulfonylureas still exists, this form of therapy is preferred by many clinicians and type 2 patients as initial therapy.

The sulfonylureas have been the only class of oral hypoglycemics marketed in the United States from 1978 to 1995. Metformin (Glucophage, Bristol-Myers Squibb), a biguanide, was approved for use by FDA in April 1995. Although structurally in the same class as a product called phenformin, its ability to induce the life-threatening lactic acidosis is much lower. Another category of oral agents for diabetes control, α-glucosidase inhibitors, was introduced to the U.S. market in 1996. Acarbose (Precose, Bayer) was the first of these agents, which work by inhibiting or slowing the breakdown of carbohydrates in the gastrointestinal tract for absorption. Another group of products, the thiazolidinediones, were first approved in 1997. Troglitazone (Rezulin, Parke Davis) is the first of these agents, which primarily sensitize peripheral tissue (primarily skeletal muscle) to the effects of insulin. Finally, another product class, meglitinide, which is the nonsulfonylurea moiety of glyburide, is available in the United States as the drug repaglinide (Prandin, Novo Nordisk). Repaglinide closes or prevents activation of ATP-sensitive K^+ channels and increases intracellular Ca^{2+}, resulting in an increase in insulin secretion (insulinotropic action). This is a short-duration hypoglycemic agent, which must be taken immediately before eating. The starting dose is 0.5 mg prior each meal with a maximum dose of 4 mg prior to each meal.

Sulfonylureas

Sulfonylureas are classified into two groups or generations based on their potency, duration of action, and drug interaction–side-effect profiles and exert their initial effect by increasing β-cell insulin secretion. After several months, insulin levels return to pretreatment values but glucose levels remain improved. This suggests that sulfonylureas exert extrapancreatic as well as pancreatic effects on glucose metabolism. The extrapancreatic mechanisms of action may include reducing the rate of hepatic glucose production, increasing insulin receptor sensitivity and/or number, and potentiation of postreceptor insulin effects; enhancing insulin release remains their major action.[20,21]

Approximately 75% to 90% of all patients with type 2 diabetes have an initial response to sulfonylurea therapy. Primary failure with a sulfonylurea occurs when a patient does not respond initially to the drug, perhaps owing to weight gain or inability of sulfonylureas to potentiate insulin action or release; however, when initial glycemic control has been achieved with an oral agent and then is lost, the patient is considered to be a secondary drug failure. About 5% to 20% of patients experience secondary failure annually because of the patient's failure to follow a dietary plan, because of the development of unrecognized type 1 diabetes, or because of the occurrence of intercurrent disease such as infections or cardiovascular disease. if a patient fails to respond to sulfonylureas because of progression of the disease, then the clinician may increase the dose of the present drug, switch to another oral medication or insulin, or add insulin or another oral agent to the regimen. One should note that only about 10% of patients will respond when changed from one sulfonylurea to another.[7] If the patient fails to respond to sulfonylurea therapy because of stress or disease, he or she should receive insulin at least until termination of the stressful period, at which time oral therapy can usually be successfully reinitiated.

There are few therapeutic differences among sulfonylureas. They should be administered 30 minutes before breakfast for maximum absorption, with glipizide more affected than the others. Because these drugs have structural similarities to sulfonamides, dermatologic side effects are relatively common, occurring in approximately 3% of patients. Hypoglycemia is the major side effect of these drugs, along with weight gain and hyperinsulinemia. The action of the parent compound plus the formation of active metabolites determine the degree and duration of hypoglycemia expected with each agent.[21]

The first-generation oral hypoglycemics include tolbutamide, chlorpropamide, tolazamide, and acetohexamide, (Table 70–10). Tolbutamide is the shortest acting sulfonylurea (6 to 12 hours) and is metabolized in the liver to inactive metabolites and excreted in the urine. On a weight basis, tolbutamide is the least potent of the first-generation hypoglycemics, but the net hypoglycemic effect from the maximum dose is usually equivalent. Tolbutamide is usually administered two or three times a day to control plasma glucose. Many clinicians consider this drug safer than other agents in patients with renal impairment or in the elderly.[20,21]

Tolazamide and acetohexamide are intermediate-acting sulfonylureas that are metabolized by the liver. Exhibiting a duration of action of 12 to 24 hours, tolazamide is usually administered once or twice a day.[20,21] Because its three active metabolites are eliminated renally, hypoglycemia may result in the patient with renal failure. Acetohexamide's primary metabolite is 2 to 2.5 times more potent than the parent compound. Acetohexamide and its metabolite exhibit diuretic and potent uricosuric activity. Chlorpropamide has the longest duration of action of any of the sulfonylureas (60 to 72 hours) and is usually prescribed once per day. The drug is more than 80% metabolized in the liver to active compounds; the other

TABLE 70–10. Oral Agents for Diabetes

Generic (Trade)	Onset (h)	Half-Life (h)	Duration (h)	Recommended Starting Dose: *Nonelderly*	*Elderly*	Maximum Dose per Day	Metabolism/ Elimination
Sulfonylureas							
Tolbutamide (Orinase)	1	5.6	6–12	1–2 g/d	500 mg/d to 500 mg twice daily	2–3 g	Metabolized in liver to inactive metabolites that are excreted renally
Acetohexamide (Dymelor)	1	5	10–14	250 mg–1.5 g/d	125–250 mg/d	1.5 g	Metabolized in liver; metabolite's potency is equal to or greater than that of parent compound; renally eliminated
Tolazamide (Tolinase)	4–6	7	10–14	100–250 mg/d	100 mg/d	750 mg–1 g	Metabolized in liver; metabolite less active than parent compound; renally eliminated
Chlorpropamide (Diabinese)	1	35	72	250 mg/d	100 mg/d	500 mg	Metabolized in liver; also excreted unchanged in the urine
Glyburide (DiaBeta, Micronase)	1.5	2–4	18–24	2.5 mg/d	1.25–2.5 mg/d	20 mg	Metabolized in liver; 50% of metabolites eliminated in urine, 50% in feces
Glyburide, micronized (Glynase)	1.5	2–4	18–24	1.5 mg	1.5–3 mg	12 mg	Metabolized in liver; 50% metabolites eliminated urine, 50% in feces
Glipizide (Glucotrol, Glucotrol XL)	1	3–7	10–24	5 mg/d	2.5–5 mg/d	40 mg	Metabolized in liver to inactive metabolites; renally eliminated
Glimepiride (Amaryl)	2	4–6	18–28	1–2 mg/d	0.5–1 mg/d	8 mg	Metabolized in liver to inactive metabolities
Biguanides Metformin (Glucophage)	1.5	1.5–4.9	16–20	500 mg	500–1000 mg	2550 mg	Urinary excretion
α-Glucosidase Inhibitors Acarbose (Precose)	0.5	1–2	4	25 mg/d	25 mg/d	300 mg/d	Nonabsorbed, excreted in feces
Thiazolidinediones Troglitazone (Rezulin)	1–2	4–6	16–24	200 mg w/food	200 mg w/food	600 mg	

20% is excreted unchanged in the urine. In elderly or renally impaired patients, chlorpropamide has been associated with more side effects than sulfonylureas. It can also cause significant water retention and hyponatremia, primarily by promoting the release of antidiuretic hormone. A disulfiram-like reaction is experienced in 30% of patients who ingest alcohol while using this medication. Because of chlorpropamide's long half-life, accumulation of metabolites in the elderly and in patients with renal failure, and its side-effect profile, there is no pharmacologic advantage in using this drug as a first-line agent in the treatment of type 2 diabetes.

Three second-generation agents are marketed in the United States: glyburide and a micronized form, glipizide and a longer acting form, and glimepiride. These agents are at least 100 times more potent on a weight basis than first-generation drugs and have a duration of action of up to 24 hours. Their effect on FPG and HbA_{1c} is similar to first-generation sulfonylureas. Moreover, except for hypoglycemia, the second-generation oral hypoglycemics appear to produce fewer side effects than do the older drugs.

Glyburide has an onset of action of approximately 1.5 hours and is more effective when administered at least 30 minutes before breakfast.[22] The pharmacokinetic half-life has been reported as 2 to 10 hours (more specific assays show the half-life to be closer to 2 to 4 hours), whereas the biologic half-life is much longer. The micronized preparation provides a higher plasma level and perhaps more predictable absorption, and thus the recommended dose is 60% of the regular glyburide. The duration of activity is approximately 24 hours, and many patients require only one dose per day.

Glyburide is metabolized completely by the liver, with 50% of the metabolites excreted renally and the other 50% eliminated via the biliary–gastrointestinal tract. Elderly patients are usually started on 1.25 mg a day, and younger patients are usually started on a daily dose of 2.5 mg. Because of the long duration of activity of glyburide, several case reports of glyburide-induced hypoglycemia (some of which have been fatal) have been reported.[23,24] Other side effects of glyburide include a mild diuresis with an increase in free-water clearance.

Glipizide has a half-life similar to that of glyburide but a duration of action of only 10 to 24 hours, whereas glimepiride's duration is thought to be 18 to 28 hours with once-daily dosing possible. The absorption of glipizide is impaired by meals, so it should be administered 30 minutes before meals. The drug is hydroxylated in the liver to inactive compounds that are renally excreted. Once-daily dosing can be achieved with doses of 15 mg or less; however, larger doses should be divided and administered twice a day.

Glyburide was approved by the FDA as twice as potent as glipizide on a weight basis;[21] therefore, the maximum daily dose of glyburide is 20 mg and that of glipizide is 40 mg. More recent studies have shown that adequate glycemic control can be produced by equal doses.[22] Further controversy surrounds long-term control with these agents.[22]

Side Effects. Hypoglycemia is the major complication of all sulfonylurea drugs. It is particularly troublesome with chlorpropamide because of the drug's long duration of action. Elderly patients are more susceptible to the hypoglycemia, especially when they skip meals or when there is some degree of renal or liver dysfunction. Other side effects of sulfonylureas include hematologic reactions such as leukopenia, thrombocytopenia, and hemolytic anemia; skin reactions, particularly rashes, purpura, and pruritus; antithyroid activity; and diffuse pulmonary reactions. Renal side effects of these drugs include mild diuresis, seen especially with tolazamide and acetohexamide, as well as significant fluid retention and hyponatremia occurring with chlorpropamide.[7,21] Gastrointestinal side effects include nausea, vomiting, and cholestasis (with or without jaundice). Cholestatic jaundice has been identified more often with chlorpropamide than with any other oral agent.

Those patients who are at least 40 years of age at the onset of diabetes, have been diabetic for less than 5 years prior to the initiation of sulfonylurea therapy, and have a fasting plasma glucose concentration of less than 300 mg/dL appear to be the best candidates for sulfonylurea therapy.[7,25] The dosage of these agents should be increased every 1 to 2 weeks until satisfactory control has been achieved or until the maximum dose has been reached.

Biguanides

Metformin has a twofold mechanism to enhance peripheral muscle glucose uptake and inhibit glucose release (hepatic glucose production) from the liver (principle effect). Metformin is also observed to induce some increased insulin sensitivity more consistently in obese versus lean type 2 patients. This may explain the modest weight loss in some patients. The most frequent side effects of metformin are gastrointestinal, with diarrhea incidence as high as 30% and up to 4% of patients stopping the therapy owing to this action. A drug with a similar structure, phenformin, was removed from the U.S. market in the 1970s secondary to the production of lactic acidosis. Metformin does not interfere with glucose oxidation and undergoes little mitochondrial binding, unlike phenformin. Worldwide incidence of lactic acidosis over the past four decades is about 3 cases per 100,000 patient-years of use. Metformin has some prescribing restrictions/warnings in patients with renal disease ($S_{cr} > 1.5$ for males, > 1.4 for females), or elderly patients with abnormal creatinine clearance, renal impairment, liver disease, history of alcohol abuse, acute or chronic metabolic acidosis, and patients with conditions that predispose them to renal insufficiency or hypoxia. Patients who are undergoing radiographic dye studies are advised to stop the metformin for 2 days prior to the study since hyperosmolar contrast dyes cause dehydration and predispose patients to metformin accumulation secondary to renal insufficiency. This agent is best classified an "antihyperglycemic agent" because it does not induce significant hypoglycemia when used alone.[26]

α-Glucosidase Inhibitors

The α-glucosidase family[27] of enzymes, which include glucoamylase, sucrase, maltase, isomaltase, and lactase, hydrolzye complex starches into oligo- and monosaccharides and glucose, which are readily absorbed. Acarbose inhibits the action of intestinal amylase and α-glucosidase action and causes a delay in the breakdown of complex carbohydrates into glucose. This results in a reduced peak effect of postprandial plasma glucose. Acarbose was the first of these agents approved for use and is indicated for monotherapy or in combination with insulin, sulfonylurea, or metformin. Acarbose is not absorbed from the gastrointestinal tract and will not induce hypoglycemia if used as monotherapy. A second agent, miglitol, has recently been approved for use but is not yet marketed. Miglitol is absorbed orally to some extent, but its clinical significance is not understood.

α-Glucosidase inhibitors, by delaying the absorption of carbohydrate, cause the production of abdominal gas as a result of gut bacterial action on carbohydrate. This results in a high incidence of flatulence, diarrhea, and abdominal cramps. Patients with a history of inflammatory bowel diseases are not good candidates for the products. These products can also alter liver function, usually only at high doses. Patients should be counseled to start the dosage at a low level and gradually increase it. They need to adjust their diets (complex carbohydrates, limit ethanol) to limit the production of the gas and refrain from sitting for long periods of time.[28]

Thiazolidinediones

A new class of drugs that reduce insulin resistance is the thiazolidinediones. Troglitazone was approved for marketing in the United States in January 1997. Initially the use was limited to type 2 patients currently using insulin (at least 30 units with a

HbA_{1c} > 8.5%), but was later expanded to include monotherapy or use combined with a sulfonylurea. These agents reduce insulin resistance in peripheral tissue by their effects on enzyme systems including the P-Par γ system, and thus require several weeks of use to determine the clinical effect in a patient. Thiazolidinediones enhance insulin action in muscle, liver, and fat tissue and require several weeks to assess the effectiveness. They also reduce hepatic glucose output and have lipid-lowering and mild antihypertensive effects.

Thiazolidinediones do not induce hypoglycemia when used alone and should be taken with a meal. However, during the fall of 1997, several case reports of liver dysfunction were noted. At the time of this writing, approximately 150 reports of altered liver function, including four deaths, had been received from use in approximately 800,000 patients in the United States, Japan, and Europe. The reaction appears to be an idiosyncratic reaction of hepatocellular damage. If the medication is discontinued when liver function tests (LFT) rise to three times normal, the liver function returns to normal. The important factor appears to be the inclusion of monitoring (LFT) routinely and withholding therapy if LFT results rise above three times the upper limit of normal. New monitoring guidelines were implemented in early December 1997 requiring baseline and monthly LFT in the first 6 months of therapy, then every 2 months for 6 months, and periodically thereafter. The reaction appears to be more common in the early months of therapy. Troglitazone can enhance clearance of estrogens such as ethinyl estradiol or norethindrone, potentially rendering oral contraceptives ineffective. Troglitazone can also enhance the clearance of cimetidine. Although troglitazone does have P450 activity, most data demonstrates that it is not clinically significant.[29,30]

ORAL HYPOGLYCEMIC COMBINATIONS

Combination therapy should be considered when FPG and HbA_{1c} are not adequately controlled (see Table 70–7). If initial therapy was a sulfonylurea, then adding metformin, troglitazone, or acarbose is the most rational next step. Individual patient characteristics such as obesity (e.g., metformin to induce weight loss), renal function (e.g., troglitazone is hepatically eliminated), and time of day for lack of glycemic control (acarbose for postprandial hyperglycemia) are important in the selection of the second agent. A common mistake is to discontinue the initial drug and substitute another class of drug (e.g., sulfonylurea → metformin); because different classes have different and complementary mechanisms of action, it is more rational to add a second drug. Combination therapy has demonstrated the capability of lowering blood glucose a greater amount than one of the agents alone.[28] Several investigators have studied insulin versus the combination of insulin plus an oral agent to control plasma glucose or the combination of two oral drugs. Most of these studies have found a statistically significant improvement in fasting glucose concentrations using combination therapy.[31,32] When sulfonylurea is combined with insulin, the insulin is initially given at bedtime and the sulfonylurea in the morning (BIDS—bedtime insulin, day-

TABLE 70–11. Insulins

Brand Name	Manufacturer	Origin	Concentration
Short-Acting Insulins			
Regular Iletin I	Lilly	Beef–pork	U-100
Pork Regular Iletin II	Lilly	Pork	U-100, U-500
Regular purified pork insulin	Novo-Nordisk	Pork	U-100
Humulin R	Lilly	Human (recombinant DNA)	U-100
Humulin R cartridge	Lilly	Human (recombinant DNA)	U-100
Humalog	Lilly	Human (recombinant DNA)	U-100
Velosulin	Novo-Nordisk	Human (recombinant DNA)	U-100
Novolin R	Novo-Nordisk	Human (recombinant DNA)	U-100
Novolin R PenFill	Novo-Nordisk	Human (recombinant DNA) (for use with NovoPen)	U-100
Intermediate-Acting Insulins			
NPH			
NPH Iletin I	Lilly	Beef–pork	U-40, U-100
Pork NPH Iletin II	Lilly	Pork	U-100
NPH purified pork	Novo-Nordisk	Pork	U-100
Humulin N	Lilly	Human (recombinant DNA)	U-100
Humulin N cartridge	Lilly	Human (recombinant DNA)	U-100
Novolin N	Novo-Nordisk	Human (recombinant DNA)	U-100
Novolin N PenFill	Novo-Nordisk	Human (recombinant DNA) (for use with NovoPen)	U-100
Lente			
Lente Iletin I	Lilly	Beef–prok	U-40, U-100
Lente Iletin II	Lilly	Pork	U-100
Lente purified pork	Novo-Nordisk	Pork	U-100
Novolin L	Novo-Nordisk	Human (recombinant DNA)	U-100
Humulin L	Lilly	Human (recombinant DNA)	U-100
NPH–Regular Combinations			
Human	Novolin 70/30	Novo-Nordisk Human (recombinant DNA)	U-100
Novolin 70/30 PenFill	Novo-Nordisk	Human (recombinant DNA) (for use with NovoPen)	U-100
Humulin 70/30	Lilly	Human (recombinant DNA)	U-100
Humulin 70/30 cartridge	Lilly	Human (recombinant DNA)	U-100
Humulin 50/50	Lilly	Human (recombinant DNA)	Long-acting insulins
Ultralente			
Ultralente Humulin U	Lilly	Human (recombinant DNA)	U-100

time sulfonylurea). This regimen takes advantage of increased insulin secretion secondary to the sulfonylurea while the bedtime insulin suppresses hepatic glucose production. Patients poorly controlled on this regimen may eventually require multiple injections of insulin throughout the day.

INSULIN

Characteristics

Insulins are categorized according to their strength, onset and duration of action, species source, and purity. Each of these factors plays a role in determining the insulin type and dose best suited to an individual patient.

Strengths. Most patients in the United States use U-100 insulin, although U-500 is also available. (The numeral following the "U" indicates the number of units of insulin per milliliter.) U-500 is available for patients who require greater than 100 units of insulin as a single injection. For those patients who require other strengths of insulin (e.g., U-10), special diluents and empty sterile vials are available from the manufacturer to prepare appropriate dilutions.

Species Source. All insulins currently on the market are of three types: pork, beef–pork mixture, or "biosynthetic" human. Beef insulin differs from human insulin by three amino acids, whereas pork insulin differs from human insulin by one amino acid. It has been cited that beef insulin is more antigenic than pork insulin, although rarely has this proven to be clinically significant.[33,34] Biosynthetic insulins are also known as "human" insulins because their amino acid structure is identical in composition to human insulin and they are less antigenic than either beef or pork insulins. The biosynthetic insulins are produced by recombinant-DNA technology using yeast or bacteria. There may be slight differences in pharmacokinetics between pork and human insulins or between human insulins from different manufacturers. If these differences are significant, they would be more noticeable in the type 1 patient.[34] The ability to use recombinant-DNA technology to produce human insulin has stimulated research for other products, so-called insulin analogues. Altering the insulin molecule (inversion of lysine and proline at B-28 and B-29) to keep more insulin in the monomeric state rather than the hexamers while retaining the physiologic action on blood glucose has resulted in a product called lispro (Humalog, Lilly). Lispro (marketed in 1996) has more rapid absorption and can be administered immediately before a meal, thus allowing more flexibility in dosing.[35] Lispro may also cause fewer severe hypoglycemic episodes than unmodified regular insulin and be associated with improved quality of life. A more detailed listing of the current insulins is given in Table 70–11.

Purity. Purity refers to the amount of proinsulin and other impurities present in a given insulin product. Prior to 1980, most insulins contained enough impurities (300 to 10,000 ppm) to cause local reactions upon injection as well as systemic adverse effects from antibody induction. This led to production of a "purified" insulin, containing fewer than 10 parts per million (ppm) of proinsulin. Because of the expense of this purification technique, these insulins were initially more expensive than "standard" insulin. Modern technology, however, has made the purification process less expensive; consequently, all "purified" insulins produced in the United States contain 10 or less ppm of proinsulin, and none is considered to be antigenic.[36] Only purified insulins are now marketed in the United States.

Pharmacokinetics

Table 70–12 compares the onset, peak, and duration of various insulin preparations. Regular insulin and insulin lispro are clear, colorless solutions. Until the advent of the insulin infusion pump,

TABLE 70–12. Onset, Peak, and Duration of Various Insulin Preparations by Species

Type of Insulin	Onset (h)	Peak (h)	Effective Duration (h)
Animal			
Short acting			
Regular	0.5–2	3–4	6–8
Intermediate acting			
NPH	4–6	8–14	16–20
Lente	4–6	8–14	16–20
Long acting			
Ultralente	8–14	Minimal	24–36
Human			
Rapid acting			
Lispro	0.25	0.5–1.5	2–4
Short acting			
Regular	0.5–1	2–3	4–6
Intermediate acting			
NPH	2–4	4–10	10–16
Lente	3–4	4–12	12–18
Long acting			
Ultralente	6–10	Minimal	20–24

regular insulin was rarely used by itself for maintenance therapy because of its short duration of action. Lispro is also useful for pump therapy. Regular insulin with added buffers (Velosulin) is recommended for the pump to avoid crystal formation and possible plugging in the microbore tubing. It was found that the addition of acetate buffers, protamine, and/or zinc to regular insulin could greatly prolong its effect. Consequently, the addition of protamine and zinc led to protamine zinc insulin (PZI; Iletin II), with a predetermined amount of protamine and zinc in a neutral fluid, producing NPH. The addition of acetate buffers and zinc led to the Lente series to avoid allergic reactions to protamine. Because regular insulin is a solution, it can be administered by the intravenous, intramuscular, or subcutaneous route. All other types of insulin, however, are suspensions and can be administered subcutaneously *only*.[36]

NPH and Lente insulins are considered "intermediate-acting" insulins because their duration of action ranges from 18 and 24 hours. Single injections of either NPH or Lente were usually the first step in chronic maintenance of the type 1 diabetes patient. NPH (neutral, protamine, Hagedorn) is produced by combining zinc, protamine, and regular insulins. Protamine is a foreign protein and can produce high antibody titers and symptoms of allergy in a small number of patients. Lente insulin is produced by adding acetate buffers and zinc to regular insulin. The resultant product may produce local allergic manifestations in patients with metal allergies.[36]

Although NPH and Lente are similar in their onset, peak, duration of action, and cost, they differ in their ability to be mixed with other types of insulin. NPH and regular insulins can be combined in the same syringe and refrigerated for up to 21 days without changes in potency.[37] If larger quantities of NPH and regular insulins are mixed in a vial, the preparation is stable for 1 month if unrefrigerated or for 3 months under refrigeration. Opened vials of insulin should be used within 1 month.[38]

A well-documented and clinically significant interaction between regular and Lente insulins exists.[38] Lente insulin is formed by adding zinc to regular insulin, with an excess of zinc in the mixture. The addition of regular insulin in the same syringe produces an interaction within 15 minutes, which proceeds for 24 hours. The zinc binds with the regular insulin and delays insulin action, by producing more Lente insulin. Patients should be instructed either to inject the mixture immediately or to wait 24 hours before administration consistently. Patients who use syringes that have been prefilled and stored in the refrigerator should be instructed to use only those that have been prepared at least 24 hours in advance.[39] Prefilled syringes should be stored with the needle tips facing upward to prevent insulin suspensions from settling and plugging the needle.

Phosphate-buffered insulins (e.g., NPH) should not be combined with insulins in the Lente series. Zinc is precipitated by the phosphate buffer, thus forming a product that acts similar to regular insulin. Similar interactions also occur with the human insulins. It appears that human NPH and human regular preparations can be mixed with no adverse consequences.

Dosing

Insulin doses can range anywhere from 0.1 U/kg to more than 2.5 U/kg of actual body weight (Table 70–13). Because the type 2 patient is usually not prone to ketoacidosis, there is less urgency to initiate aggressive therapy.[40] He or she can be started on a single injection of 15 to 20 U/d of an intermediate-acting insulin, and dosage adjustments can be made according to plasma glucose levels. Although this is a typical starting dose, most type 2 patients will eventually require ≥1 U/kg whereas type 1 patients are often well controlled on 0.5 to 0.7 U/kg. Either NPH or Lente insulin can be selected as the intermediate-acting insulin; however, many patients will eventually require regular insulin to be added to the regimen. To avoid the problems associated with the regular–Lente interaction, NPH may be a better initial choice, with premixed NPH and regular (70:30) being available. Patients receiving insulin for the first time should receive human insulin, whereas those who have used a pork or a beef–pork combination can remain on that product unless resistance or other complications arise.

Many specialists discourage single daily injections of intermediate-acting insulin, citing evidence that the majority of their patients do not exhibit 24-hour control on this regimen. A common regimen instead calls for two thirds of the dose in the morning and one third in the evening with the first injection consisting of an intermediate-to-regular ratio of 2:1, given 30 minutes before breakfast. The second injection is given 30 minutes before the evening meal; the ratio of intermediate-acting to regular insulin is 1:1. These regimens are known as "intensive-dose" regimens.[25,41,42] These regimens mimic the activity of a functioning pancreas. Figure 70–2 illustrates the effects of a nondiabetic glucose–insulin release pattern around meals and throughout the day with considerations of age and complications. The goal of the therapy is to fit the schedule to the patient's needs. The regimen for a college scholarship athlete with variable practice times will differ from a schoolteacher with a very predictable schedule.

TABLE 70–13. Average Daily Insulin Requirements

Diabetes Type	Dosage in U/kg Actual Body Weight
Type 1	
Initial dose	0.5–0.6
Honeymoon phase	0.1–0.4
Split-dose therapy	0.5–1.2
With ketosis or during acute illness	0.5–1.0
Type 2	
Initial dose	0.2–0.6
Split-dose therapy	0.5–1.2
With insulin resistance	0.7–2.5

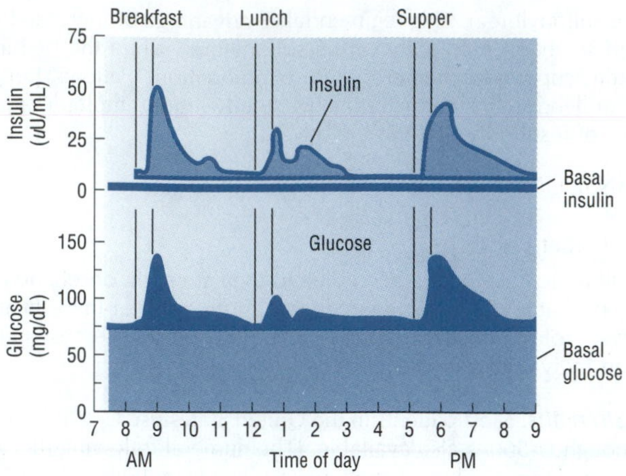

Intensive insulin therapy regimens

	7A	11A	4–5P	HS
1. 2 doses, intermediate	X		X	
2. 2 doses, regular or intermediate	Regular and intermediate		Regular and intermediate	
3. 3 doses, regular or regular and intermediate	Regular and intermediate	Regular	Regular and intermediate	
4. 4 doses, regular and long acting	Regular	Regular	Regular	Long-acting

FIG. 70–2. Relationship between insulin and glucose over the course of a day and how various insulin regimens could be given. *(Adapted from Ref. 41, p 24.)*

Another intensive dose regimen uses regular insulin only. The patient's total daily insulin requirement is divided into four equal doses, each given 30 minutes before meals and at bedtime. This regimen attempts to mimic insulin release that occurs in nondiabetics with ingestion of meals. The bedtime dose is given with a snack and is used to suppress glycogen and fat catabolism, which occur at night during the fasting state. Obviously, it requires an intelligent patient with a great deal of motivation to optimally use this regimen.

A different method uses regular insulin via an insulin pump, termed a continuous subcutaneous insulin infusion (CSII). Regular insulin is administered continuously and as bolus doses before meals. A high incidence of complications, including hypoglycemia, ketoacidosis, dermatologic problems, and mechanical pump problems occur with this regimen. As a result, the American Diabetes Association recommends restricting insulin pump use to those patients who are knowledgeable, stable, and well motivated and who are receiving care from a physician properly trained in the use of these pumps. Figure 70–2 lists several dosing regimens options.[43]

For the hospitalized patient, some clinicians prefer a "sliding scale" approach to start insulin. Blood glucose levels are obtained several times a day (e.g., every 4 or 6 hours, or at specified times), so that fasting premeal values are obtained. Subcutaneously administered regular insulin is then ordered in an amount that increases with the increase in blood glucose. When the patient's insulin requirement has stabilized over 2 to 3 days, the number of units required during the previous 24 hours is totaled to determine the patient's dose. Although sliding scale regimens have long been used, this approach should be discouraged and therapy should be based on the patient's previous dose or his or her estimated requirements, and the therapy adjusted from that starting point.

New technology is leading to the development of novel insulin delivery systems, including sustained-release injections and nasal insulin administration. Amylin is a substance produced by the pancreas that apparently facilitates insulin's action. Perhaps amylin should be used along with insulin; current studies are assessing the usefulness of this concept.[44]

Dosing Insulin During the "Honeymoon" Phase

It is important to note that type 1 diabetes patients may experience a "honeymoon" phase after the initial diagnosis of diabetes. During this period, insulin requirements diminish so that the patient is taking a very low dose of insulin. Regardless of how low the dose may become, patients should be encouraged to still use insulin during this period to decrease the production to antibodies to the insulin and to lessen the probability of becoming insulin resistant.[44] Patients should be taught proper storage, dosage preparation, and administration techniques for their insulin. These guidelines are presented in Table 70–14.

MONITORING THERAPY

Regardless of whether the patient's therapy consists of diet and exercise, diet and exercise plus an oral agent(s), or diet and exercise plus insulin, the success of the therapy must be closely monitored by such methods as home blood or plasma glucose testing or urine testing. Glycosylated hemoglobins, C-peptides, and blood glucose levels are more suited for clinic-based assessments. The choice of method depends on the severity of the diabetes, the progression of the disease, economic factors, and the patient's willingness and ability to monitor therapy. More health plans are including home blood glucose monitoring in diabetes care, following suit with the Balanced Budget Act of 1997 coverage for Medicare patients.[45]

In the home setting, urine glucose concentrations were the mainstay of assessing glycemic control until recent years, when most patients have begun using whole-blood glucose determinations as a means of monitoring. Urine testing uses a less

TABLE 70–14. Patient Information on the Storage and Administration of Insulin

1. Unopened vials of insulin should be stored in the refrigerator but should not be frozen; storage on the refrigerator door is preferred usually. Freezing may alter the desired effect of the insulin. An opened vial of insulin that is being used daily should be stored at room temperature (59–85°F), away from windows, lamps, or any other places in which temperature could be altered. Insulin injected at room temperature causes less pain and fewer local reactions than does refrigerated insulin. Insulin that is refrigerated is usable until the expiration date stamped on the vial. Insulin stored at room temperature loses 1.5% of its activity each month; many clinicians recommend use within 1 month.
2. All supplies for administering an insulin dosage should be close at hand. These include insulin syringes, cotton balls, and 70% isopropyl alcohol or alcohol swabs, and the insulin. The alcohol should be clear in appearance and should not contain any soaps or perfumes that might cause a local irritation resembling an insulin allergy. U-100 syringes are available as standard or Lo-Dose. The Lo-Dose (25-U, 30-U, 50-U) syringes can accurately measure single units of insulin, and the numbers on the barrel of the syringe are easy to read; these syringes are useful for patients who are administered lower doses of insulin per injection. Syringes can be capped after use, stored in the refrigerator, and reused until the needle starts to dull.
3. All insulins except Regular and Lispro are cloudy—like skim milk—in appearance and need to be gently agitated before a dosage is drawn. If the insulin appear different—color change, particles sticking to the vial, clumps in the vial—or the suspension settles after agitation momentarily), the insulin should be replaced. The vial should not be shaken vigorously but should be gently agitated or rolled between the palms of the hands.
4. The plunger on the syringe should be pulled back to the appropriate number of units desired.
5. The insulin vial should be inverted and the needle should be inserted into the rubber stopper in the vial. The plunger should be pressed all the way into the barrel of the syringe; the plunger should then be pulled back, allowing the correct number of units of insulin to enter the barrel of the syringe.
6. Air bubbles should be tapped toward the needle and gently expelled from the syringes. Injecting an air bubble subcutaneously is not harmful; however, air in the syringe indicates that the full dose of insulin has not been properly drawn up. Therefore, every attempt should be made to ensure that air bubbles have been expelled from the syringe, leaving the correct number of units of insulin in the syringe for injection.
7. A subcutaneous injection is made into fat (not merely "under the skin" as many people think). The most popular places for injecting insulin are the backs of the arms (triceps area), the abdomen, and the inner thigh areas. Patients who administer their own injections usually prefer the abdomen or thighs. Absorption is usually fastest from the abdomen, slowest from the thigh, inducing some changes in injection-site-use recommendations. Many centers advocate use of one site with rotation before switching (e.g., several injections in the left leg, then to the right leg). Also, some centers now have patients rotate around the abdomen only. Not alternating sites with each injection may lead to a "calloused" area, affecting the actual subcutaneous tissue and altering insulin's absorption from that area.
8. After the site for injection is chosen, the area should be cleaned with alcohol. This should be done in a circular fashion, beginning in the center of the circle working outward about 2 in. Allow a few seconds for the alcohol to evaporate.
9. If you are right-handed, pinch up the fat at the site of injection with your left hand, being careful not to touch the area where the needle will enter the skin. Hold the syringe in your right hand as you would a pencil. The needle should be aimed perpendicular (90 deg) to the skin unless the patient is very thin and has too little subcutaneous tissue (in which case the needle should be inserted at a 45 deg angle). Using a slight wrist action, quickly insert the needle through the skin into the subcutaneous tissue. The entire length of the needle should be below the skin surface.
10. While the needle is still in the subcutaneous tissue, gently pull back on the plunger about 2 units—this is called aspirating. (If you are right-handed, this can be done by using the thumb of your right hand or by letting go of the pinched-up area with your left hand and using your left hand to aspirate.) If any blood comes back into the syringe, you may have inserted the needle into a vein. DO NOT INJECT! If no blood appears in the syringe after aspirating, you can assume it is okay to inject. Note: Many health professionals are no longer teaching the technique of aspiration, because they claim it is rare for the needle to be inserted into a large vein. Check with providers in your practice setting.
11. Slowly push the plunger in all the way until it stops. Gently pull out the needle. You may use a cotton ball to GENTLY wipe the injected area after pulling out the needle, but do NOT massage the area of injection because this will alter the rate of insulin absorption.

TABLE 70–15. Tests for Urine Glucose Determination

Product	Detection Method	Range Detected (%)
Chemstrip G	Glucose oxidase	0, , , 1, 2, 3, 5
Clinitest (5-drop)	Copper reduction	0, , , , 1, __2
Clinitest (2-drop)	Copper reduction	0, __, , 1, 2, 3, 5
Diastix	Glucose oxidase	0, , , , 1, __2

TABLE 70–16. Drugs That Cause False-Positive Results With Copper Reduction Tests for Glucosuria

para-Aminosalicyclic acid	Methyldopa
Ascorbic acid	Nalidixic acid
Cephalosporins	Penicillins (large doses)
Chloral hydrate	Probenecid
Isoniazid	Salicylates
Levodopa	Streptomycin
Metaxalone	

expensive monitoring device, but the results are not always easily interpretable. The tests, listed in Table 70–15, use either the glucose-oxidase or the copper-reduction method to detect glucose in the urine. The glucose-oxidase method is a qualitative test, which is specific for glucose and yields few false-positive results. The copper-reduction method is a better quantitative test but will react with any reducing substance, producing false-positive results (Table 70–16). With either test, the presence of glucose results in a color change, which is correlated with a relative urine glucose concentration.

Urine glucose tests, although inexpensive and relatively easy to perform, have some limitations. First, a randomly collected urine specimen may correspond to a blood glucose concentration several hours previously. Using a "double-voided" specimen, whereby the patient urinates, drinks a full glass of water, and in approximately 30 minutes recollects and tests a second urine specimen, can alleviate this concern. Urine-testing results may lack correlation to blood glucose values. The tests are time and technique dependent.

Although it is commonly stated that the average person begins to spill glucose into the urine when the serum glucose approaches 180 mg/dL, the level fluctuates greatly among patients. In addition, there can even be intrapatient variation depending on progression of the disease and day-to-day stress factors. A negative urine glucose cannot distinguish among normoglycemia, hypoglycemic, or hyperglycemia. Though urine glucose is now used less frequently for patient monitoring, urine ketone determination is commonly recommended to patients with type 1 or who are ketosis prone (Ketostix, etc.). These home-based tests that can indicate general trends in control should be used as the sole monitoring parameter.[46]

Blood glucose determination is the standard for diabetes home monitoring. In the laboratory, serum or plasma is used for glucose determinations. These concentrations may be slightly higher than those obtained on whole blood, although in almost all cases, the differences have no clinical significance. More-recent advances in blood glucose monitoring have allowed patients and health professionals to monitor glucose levels using chemically impregnated strips or hand-held electronic glucose monitoring machines that use these strips. These systems are designed to be able to monitor whole-blood glucose from a drop of blood obtained by a fingerstick.[47]

Differences in the various commercially available strips exist. The strip itself cannot monitor a true blood glucose level but measures a range for the patient's value. Many of these strips, are used with a machine that can then measure and display an accurate blood glucose value. When used without the machine, the patient's blood interacts with the chemicals on the strip to produce a color change that corresponds to a range of blood glucose values. Some strips maintain this color for several hours or days, whereas other strips begin to fade after a few minutes. A drawback to the use of blood glucose monitoring is the relative expense, especially if the patient has to monitor blood values several times a day.[41] The monitors have become increasingly user friendly, in large part from two conferences reviewing their use.[48] These monitors have allowed patient to become involved in the day-to-day management of their disease.[49,50] Keep in mind the need to maintain a good quality-assurance program for the use of the monitors as noted in a user error study.[50] The strips or machines are not useful in detecting ketones.

The glycosylated hemoglobin (hemoglobin A_{1c} or HbA_{1c}) is useful for monitoring long-term control of diabetes. Glucose can react in a concentration-dependent manner with amino groups of amino acids to produce glycosylated products.[51] Chronic elevation of blood glucose results in an increase in the presence of glycosylated hemoglobins, of which HbA_{1c} is a major component. HbA_{1c} usually constitutes 4% to 6% of the total hemoglobin, but may constitute up to 15% of the total with chronic hyperglycemia. Because the life span of an average red blood cell is 120 days, bringing the blood glucose under control for 4 to 6 weeks will result in a fall in the percentage of HbA_{1c}. On the other hand, a patient must have experienced hyperglycemia for 1 to 4 weeks before the HbA_{1c} concentration rises substantially.[51,52] Methods for measuring glycosylated hemoglobins have become more standardized, with two home-based kits available for mailing to labs. Some tests that measure other glycosylated derivatives may be affected by short periods of hyperglycemia. Other conditions, such as sickle cell anemia, bleeding, or hemolysis, that affect the average life span of the red blood cell, can also yield misleading results. Fructosamine is another protein that binds glucose in the blood and can be measured to determine glucose control for the previous 1 to 3 weeks.[53]

Most patients show an interest in monitoring their urine or blood glucose initially but seem to lose interest after a short time. Factors contributing to this loss of interest include expense and lack of knowledge of how to use the results of these tests. Patients must be educated as to the short- and long-term benefits of day-to-day monitoring of glucose. Daily monitoring of glucose allows the patient to fine-tune dietary intake and medications. Follow-up visits to review the patient's monitoring technique are recommended.[50] Patients should become more involved in their own therapy.

Exercise also affects daily blood glucose concentrations throughout the day. Monitoring daily urine or blood glucose values allows the patient to define the appropriate exercise habits. For the type 1 patient, the amount and type of exercise may dictate which parts of the body to use for insulin injections. Running may increase the absorption of insulin that has been injected into the thighs, resulting in hypoglycemia or shorter duration of action of the insulin.[34]

Certain prescription and nonprescription drugs can alter blood glucose concentrations (listed in Table 70–3). Daily monitoring of glucose allows the patient to determine the effect on glycemic control of taking these drugs. Other short-term factors affect daily insulin requirements, including those that increase insulin needs such as infection, trauma, stress, and the second and third trimesters of pregnancy.[1] Exercise and early pregnancy decrease insulin requirements in most individuals. Consequently, daily monitoring of blood glucose not only can detect the aforementioned factors but can also help to define to what extent they affect an individual patient.

Self-monitoring of blood glucose, therefore, is essential in helping the patient and caregiver detect acute and chronic factors that affect the patient's control of diabetes. Moreover, daily monitoring actively involves the patient in his or her own therapy, and involvement is essential to the success of any regimen. Without monitoring, the patient really is not an active participant in his or her care. Home glucose monitoring can allow the patient to adjust his or her insulin on a daily basis to achieve "tight" glucose control.

ADJUSTING THERAPY

RECOGNIZING, TREATING, AND PREVENTING HYPOGLYCEMIA

Hypoglycemia is the most common side effect from sulfonylurea or insulin therapy. During the waking hours, the usual symptoms of hypoglycemia include sweating, tachycardia, palpitations, and tremor as driven by adrenergic innervation. When the blood glucose level falls below 40 mg/dL, central nervous system (neuroglycopenia) signs such as headache, confusion, visual disturbances, irritability or other personality changes, seizures, or unconsciousness may occur. Hypoglycemia may occur during the night or early morning hours while the patient is asleep, producing such symptoms as nightmares, night sweats, and headache. All of these symptoms result from a release of epinephrine, which is triggered by low plasma-glucose concentrations. Patients who have had diabetes for 5 years or more often lose this response and remain asymptomatic with a fall in plasma-glucose concentrations.

In some diabetes patients (especially the elderly) and nondiabetic individuals, a mildly depressed blood glucose level (50 to 70 mg/dL) can produce epinephrine release with resulting symptoms. It is often hard in these cases to document the hypoglycemia; thus, the patient may experience such episodes for months or years before making a definitive diagnosis. Unexplained hypoglycemia in previously well-controlled patients may also result from microinfarcts of the pituitary gland with loss of growth-hormone secretion.

Although there are several causes of hypoglycemia, by far the most frequent cause in type 1 diabetes is not eating at the proper times. Other possible causes of hypoglycemia in type 1 or 2 diabetes include a high level of exercise or too much insulin or sulfonylurea (type 2). Many patients let their life-style dictate their eating habits, like other people in society. It is not uncommon for someone to skip breakfast because he or she is late for work. Working through lunch or making a late dinner engagement are other causes. Intensive insulin management and blood glucose self-monitoring allow patients to achieve some flexibility in life's activities. Other causes of hypoglycemia, especially in type 1 diabetes, include a defect in glucagon secretion and renal insufficiency leading to prolonged insulin action.[54] Other counterregulatory mechanisms may also be adversely affected, such as the impairment of epinephrine's action resulting from the administration of a β-adrenergic blocking drug or from hypopituitarism.

Hypoglycemia occurring in the early morning hours can produce a rebound hyperglycemia because of the release of counterregulatory hormones (glucagon, cortisol, or growth hormone). This rebound hyperglycemia, often accompanied by glucosuria and possibly ketonuria, is known as the Somogyi phenomenon.[56,57] Although often hard to diagnose, this phenomenon must be distinguished from the "dawn phenomenon," which is a relative resistance to insulin's effect during the early morning hours, or just too much insulin. The dawn phenomenon also results in hyperglycemia and is thought to result from excessive action of growth hormone and cortisol.[56]

The immediate treatment of hypoglycemia in a conscious patient involves the administration of food, preferably sugar. Eight Lifesavers, 4 to 6 ounces of a sugar-containing soft drink, a piece of fruit (equivalent to 1/4 to 1/3 cup raisins), 1/2 cup fruit juice, 2 or 3 glucose tablets (5 g each), a tube of glucose gel, or 1 cup skim milk usually reverses the symptoms in 10 to 20 minutes. In the unconscious patient, 1 mg of glucagon injected subcutaneously should provide relief within 10 to 15 minutes. Patients who weigh less than 20 kg should receive 0.5 mg. A common side effect is nausea and vomiting. Once the patient regains consciousness, oral liquids containing sugar should then be administered. In the hospitalized hypoglycemic patient, 50 mL of $D_{50}W$ provides rapid reversal of symptoms.

The long-term prevention of hypoglycemia involves altering the patient's dietary habits, exercise plan, or medication. If insulin is implicated as the cause of hypoglycemia, the dosage regimen may have to be altered to deliver the proper effect when needed. Hypoglycemia (ultimately leading to hyperglycemia) resulting from the Somogyi phenomenon can be corrected by decreasing the insulin dose by 10% in the type 1 patient and by 30% to 40% in the type 2 patient.[56,57]

CORRECTING HYPERGLYCEMIA WITH ORAL AGENTS FOR DIABETES

Many patients taking sulfonylureas mistakenly assume that the drug by itself will adequately control their diabetes. Any patient taking an oral agent who has been controlled but who is now hyperglycemic should be asked the following questions:

1. Tell me how you have been taking your medication.
2. Have you run out of your medication during the past several days?
3. Tell me about your diet and exercise plan and how you have followed it since you were last here.
4. Have you experienced any recent "stresses" (infection, trauma—physical or emotional, altered life-style, increased pressures)?
5. Are you self-monitoring your blood sugar? Show me how you do this. Is this hyperglycemia a new reaction or has it evolved over the past few weeks?
6. Have you experienced any symptoms of low blood sugar (i.e., increased heart rate, irritability, night sweats, nightmares) recently?
7. Have you experienced any symptoms of high blood sugar (i.e., increased urination, increased thirst) recently?
8. Have you taken any new medicine—prescription or nonprescription—during the past month?

Correctable factors should first be determined. If the patient has deviated from the prescribed diet and exercise plans, every attempt should be made to reinstitute the previous plan, or determine if the plan should be changed. If increased work or family pressures have triggered the hyperglycemia, the duration of these pressures must be ascertained. If there is evidence of infection or other "stress," then many times the patient will not respond to an oral agent. In such cases, the patient must be started on short-term insulin therapy (preferably "human" insulin to minimize production of antibodies)[36] until the problem subsides, at which time the patient can be restarted on an oral agent. Blood glucose determinations performed three or four times per day will be beneficial in deciding the need for regimen change. Usually if the patient's blood glucose is not adequately controlled with near maximum doses of one oral agent, addition of another category of drug may be indicated.

CORRECTING HYPERGLYCEMIA WITH INSULIN

It is not uncommon for patients who have begun insulin therapy, whether they have type 1 or type 2 diabetes, to reject the course of treatment—insulin injections, finger glucose sticks, diet adherence, exercise plans, and so on. This nonadherence results from a set of reactions to the diagnosis including fear, anger, denial, and guilt. Sometimes a patient becomes overwhelmed with the demands of working to control the diabetes. Therefore, in the patient who is not properly controlled on his or her current insulin regimen, one should try to find answers to the following questions:

1. Is the patient administering the correct number of units of the correct insulin(s) at the correct time(s) per day and visually inspected the insulin vial(s) to assure its quality?
2. How does the patient store the insulin?
3. If the patient is using an insulin suspension, have him or her show you how he swirls it for resuspending.
4. Have the patient show you how he or she draws up a dose.
5. What site(s) does the patient use? How does the patient alternate the sites?
6. Is the patient injecting the insulin correctly? Check the technique.
7. Has the patient experienced any itching, redness at the site of injection, or any other evidence of insulin allergy?
8. Have there been any recent dietary modifications (time of meals, type of food consumed, amount of food consumed)?
9. Has the patient continued to follow the same exercise plan during the past month?
10. Has the patient gained or lost any weight during the past month?
11. Has the patient experienced any daytime or nocturnal symptoms of hypoglycemia recently?
12. Has the patient experienced any recent "stresses" (infection, trauma, altered life-style, increased pressures, etc.)?
13. Has the patient tested urine or blood consistently during the past month? Is the hyperglycemia new or has it evolved over several weeks?
14. Has the patient experienced any recent symptoms of hyperglycemia?
15. Has the patient taken any new medications—prescription or nonprescription—during the past month?

WEIGHT

A weight gain may indicate that the patient's insulin dosage is too large. Excess insulin promotes fat storage and hypoglycemia, with a rebound hyperglycemia, seeming to require extra insulin to reduce the high blood glucose.[24,55] This can be a caveat to intensive therapy, ultimately resulting in the patient remaining hyperglycemic while simultaneously gaining weight. Symptoms of hypoglycemia and hyperglycemia can verify this suspicion. In this case, the insulin dosage must actually be adjusted downward.

SOMOGYI EFFECT

Hyperglycemia occurring during the early morning hours may be caused by a shorter-than-anticipated duration of action of the insulin with a pronounced dawn effect to raise glucose or by nocturnal hypoglycemia resulting from rebound hyperglycemia (Somogyi effect). Measuring blood glucose levels several times during the early morning hours (3 AM) will determine the cause of the morning hyperglycemia. Assessing the patient's symptoms of nocturnal hypoglycemia (nightmares, night sweats) may help determine the cause of the problem. If a Somogyi reaction is confirmed, the insulin dose should be reduced.

TIMES OF HYPERGLYCEMIA

This is the most important factor in determining adjustments to insulin therapy. Blood glucose levels collected at various times throughout the day can pinpoint the times the patient consistently loses control. The simplest way of starting to determine insulin dose issues is to examine blood glucose patterns and to "fall back" from the abnormal glucose to the quadrant of the day from abnormal glucose levels, that is, fall back to the most recent insulin peak action. If a patient experiences hyperglycemia during the night and/or has a high fasting value using one dose daily, splitting the dose of intermediate-acting insulin such that the patient received two thirds of the total dose before breakfast and one third before supper will help achieve tighter control. A patient who exhibits hyperglycemia during the evening hours may benefit from a dose of regular insulin just before supper. Examples of the "fall back" principle for multiple daily injections are included in Table 70–17.

COMPLICATIONS

Much of the concern for optimal treatment of diabetes is focused around the long-term complications of the disease. Diabetes, especially if untreated or poorly treated, induces complications involving numerous organ systems through changes in neurologic and macro- and microvascular function. Most diabetes-related deaths result from the long-term complications of the disease, with only 10% resulting from direct causes such as ketoacidosis and hypoglycemia.[1,58] Study results confirm that good diabetes management is perhaps the best current method for preventing the progression of the complications.[10–12] Knowledge that some large macromolecules are altered in diabetes patients and undergo glycation during high blood glucose episodes may play a large role in setting treatment options for the future. These macromolecule–glucose complexes undergo further change to form advanced glycation end products (AGE products), which deposit in tissue and induce many of the complications and organ damage.[59,60] Some medications, notably aminoguanidine, have been noted to prevent the formation of AGE product and are currently in clinical research.[60]

MACROVASCULAR EFFECTS

Diabetes complications are generally categorized as either neurologic, macrovascular, or microvascular. Macrovascular complications involve large blood vessels such as coronary, cerebral, or peripheral vessels. With diabetes, blood vessels are more prone to occlusion, leading to coronary heart disease, stroke, or peripheral vascular disease. Although uncontrolled chronic hyperglycemia may be causal, most clinicians believe macrovascular complications are secondary to alterations in lipid metabolism and hypertension.[61,62]

HYPERLIPIDEMIA

Obesity, hyperlipidemia, hypertension, insulin resistance or hyperinsulinemia, and diabetes cluster together creating syndrome X and this syndrome accelerates the rate of development of the long-term complications of diabetes. Specifically, people with diabetes develop a unique dyslipidemia, including a high VLDL, small dense LDL, and low HDL. Hypertension is also about two times

TABLE 70–17. Adjusting Insulin Dosages Based on Clinical Response

Problem	Time Problem Experienced	Possible Solutions
Hyperglycemia	Fasting	If the patient is receiving a single dose of an intermediate-acting insulin, split into 2 doses: 2/3 of total dose before breakfast, 1/3 of dose before supper. If the patient is receiving split-dose intermediate insulin, increase presupper dose or move present dose to a later time in the evening.
	Midmorning	Add regular to morning dose.
	Midafternoon	Increase morning NPH or Lente dose, **OR** add regular at lunch time.
	Bedtime	Add regular with presupper dose if not currently receiving, **OR** increase regular at presupper dose.
	Early morning (2:00–3:00 AM)	Consider pronounced dawn effect. Give the presupper dose later in the evening.
Hypoglycemia	Fasting	Decrease evening insulin dose, but first check timing of AM test and dose.
	Midmorning	Decrease or omit prebreakfast dose of regular insulin.
	Midafternoon	Decrease morning NPH or Lente dose. Be sure patient is withdrawing correct dosage into syringe in the correct order if he or she is receiving more than one type of insulin.
	Bedtime	Instruct patient to eat a bedtime snack and/or check dose of afternoon NPH/Lente dose (again, "fall back"). Decrease presupper dose of regular insulin.
	Early morning (2:00–3:00 AM)	Decrease presupper dose of intermediate-acting insulin if it is being administered earlier in the afternoon. Consider Somogyi effect. Decrease the evening dose of intermediate-acting insulin.

If more than one monitoring time throughout the day is abnormal, try to adjust only one insulin dose at a time. Adequately titrating more than one dose adjustment and gauging the effects is quite difficult and often creates more adjustment problems.

more common in diabetes. Data suggest that these metabolic changes may be related to increased abdominal fat. The glycation or modification of proteins and lipoproteins enhances the atherogenicity of low-density lipoprotein (LDL) cholesterol and delays egress of LDL from the artery wall. Free fatty acids also seem to inhibit liver metabolism of insulin, which inhibition may, in turn, predispose patients to hypertension and contribute to peripheral insulin resistance, causing glucose derangements.[63,64]

Obesity is more often associated with type 2 diabetes, and abdominal obesity induces insulin resistance and hyperinsulinemia. Hyperinsulinemia, hypertension, and diabetic dyslipidemia all contribute to macrovascular complications. In fact, 60% of deaths in type 2 diabetes results from macrovascular complications, whereas there is only a 30% mortality rate in type 1 diabetes. Evidence now shows that increases in glucose correlate with coronary heart disease (CHD) and that HbA_{1c} may be a predictor of myocardial infarction.[64] There is a recognized association between blood glucose control and cholesterol levels. Controllable risk factors (smoking, hypertension, dyslipidemia) should be addressed along with weight reduction. Reduced intake of saturated fats and cholesterol will decrease atherogenic proteins, especially LDL. The National Cholesterol Education Program has set the goal for LDL-cholesterol in patients with multiple risk factors, including diabetes, at < 130 mg/dL. Some experts believe that the LDL target in diabetes should be < 100 mg/dL even in the absence of CHD. If a diabetic patient also has CHD, the goal is < 100 mg/dL.)[63] The use of lipid-lowering agents in diabetes patients may prove beneficial in decreasing the risk of coronary heart disease (see Chap. 19). Because the typical diabetic dyslipemic patient has low HDL, high triglycerides, and normal or modestly elevated total and LDL cholesterol, the most commonly used drugs are either HMG CoA reductase inhibitors (statins) or fibric acid derivatives such as gemfibrozil or fenofibrate. Nicotinic acid use is limited in diabetes owing to its ability to increase blood glucose. The statins are often used as initial agents when the LDL cholesterol is elevated with the additional changes described in HDL and triglycerides. Gemfibrozil or fenofibrate can also be useful in diabetics because these drugs increase HDL and lower triglycerides. Bile acid sequestrants should generally be avoided because they increase triglycerides in patients with baseline elevation in triglycerides. In addition, estrogen replacement therapy can be considered for postmenopausal women. The clinician should realize the potential for these agents to aggravate other complications (Table 70–18).[63,65]

HYPERTENSION

Treating coexistent hypertension and diabetes represents a challenge for choosing appropriate antihypertensive therapy (see Chap. 10). Many available agents can induce adverse effects that potentiate the risk of long-term complications. β-Blockers and diuretics can increase serum glucose and lipid levels and increase the incidence of sexual dysfunction. β-Blockers also exacerbate claudication and block the normal physiologic response

TABLE 70–18. Possible Complications Associated With Antilipidemics

Drug	Possible Complication	Notes
Bile acid–binding resins	Hypertriglyceridemia	Increased triglycerides is a major risk factor for diabetic vascular disease
	Constipation, abdominal pain	Diabetics are predisposed to GI disease
Nicotinic acid	Hyperuricemia	Diabetics are predisposed to hyperuricemia and gout
	Glucose intolerance	May increase blood glucose; can be significant
	Constipation, abdominal pain	Diabetics are predisposed to GI disease
Fibric acid derivatives	Gallstone formation	Diabetics are predisposed to cholelithiasis

to hypoglycemia, making them potentially dangerous additions to the diabetic drug regimen. Orthostasis is worsened by many of the antiadrenergic agents. Other antihypertensive medications that can aggravate diabetic-induced complications include guanethidine, guanadrel, methyldopa, and reserpine. Many of the newer agents, such as angiotensin-converting enzyme (ACE) inhibitors, calcium channel blockers, and β_1-blockers (e.g., prazosin, terazosin), do not potentiate the adverse complications of diabetes. Recent data have demonstrated that ACE inhibitors are also beneficial in slowing the progression of nephropathy.[66,67] Additional possible influences leading to the development of atheromatous macrovascular complications include genetic predisposition, racial characteristics, stressful personality types, obesity, and smoking.[68] Important aspects that should be addressed to help prevent macrovascular complications include cholesterol control, treatment of hypertension, diet and weight control, stress management, and smoking cessation.

MICROVASCULAR EFFECTS

Aberrations of arterioles and capillaries result in microvascular complications. Data from the DCCT demonstrate that microvascular complications arise related to the degree and duration of hyperglycemia and that good metabolic control minimizes complications (see Table 70–6). Although microvascular complications occur in both types of diabetes, their prevalence increases with the progression and duration of the disease and eventually can lead to diabetic nephropathy, retinopathy, and neuropathy. The mechanism for the development of these complications is unclear, but hyperglycemia induces metabolic aberrations that lead to structural tissue damage and long-term complications. Recent studies have implicated alterations in the polyol (sorbitol) pathway and the aforementioned AGE products as major mechanisms for inducing metabolic complications. This results in damaged, leaky capillary-wall vessels, causing capillary membrane thickening and functional impairment. The capillary abnormality primarily affects the eyes and kidneys as well as autonomic nerves, leading to painful neuropathies.[69]

NEUROPATHY

Up to 50% of diabetics patients will experience painful neuropathies after several years of diabetes. The DCCT demonstrated the value to intensive diabetes care in preventing and limiting or reversing the neuropathy with early detection.[10,70] Neuropathy is categorized as motor–sensory or autonomic neuropathies. Symptoms may begin as tingling or burning sensations, particularly in the distal tissues, with a definite loss in vibratory sensation.[71] As these neuropathic problems progress, the patient may lose all sensation in a particular area, thus not being able to detect hot, cold, or pain. The combination of neuropathic changes and peripheral vascular disease leads to injury and infection and all too often amputation. Diabetes is the leading cause of nontraumatic amputations in the United States.[1]

Treatment for painful neuropathy remains symptomatic and unsatisfactory. Many drugs have been tried for the treatment of diabetic peripheral neuropathy, but none has proven very effective. The wide variety of analgesic and anti-inflammatory agents can provide some relief for this painful complication. These include narcotics, nonsteroidal anti-inflammatory agents, anticonvulsants, and psychotropic agents. Of the anticonvulsants used, phenytoin and carbamazepine have been effective at doses ranging from 100 to 200 mg three or four times daily. Because of the incidence of side effects, such as dizziness, drowsiness, gastrointestinal (GI) disturbances, and ataxia, and because of inconsistent therapeutic benefits, these agents should not be used routinely for the treatment of diabetic peripheral neuropathy.[72,73] A short trial may be warranted only in severe cases that have been resistant to other treatments.[70,74] Psychotropic drugs, such as tricyclic antidepressants, trazodone, fluoxetine, and phenothiazines, have mixed favorable responses but seem to provide greater pain relief than do anticonvulsant agents. Doses for the treatment of painful neuropathies should be initially low and titrated to effect.[74,75] Antiarrhythmics such as mexiletine have been beneficial in resistant cases of neuropathy. Capsaicin is an over-the-counter preparation indicated for painful neuropathies. Capsaicin, obtained from red chili peppers, is an approved FDA, category 1 counterirritant, for external use. Few data support benefit from this product; however, subjective response from patients appears promising.[76]

Because impairment of nerve conduction is thought to be owing, in part, to abnormalities in the polyol pathway, newer therapy has focused on the pathway's rate-limiting enzyme, aldose reductase.[69] One should keep in mind that this enzymatic path is only one of several that play a role in development of neuropathy, and thus inhibiting aldose reductase does not alter neuropathic changes. Alteration to the polyol pathway results in sorbitol accumulation in peripheral nerves with fluid accumulation, capillary membrane thickening, and functional impairment leading to axonal degeneration, myelin damage, and decreased nerve conduction with painful neuropathies. Aldose reductase inhibitors prevent the conversion of glucose to sorbitol, thus minimizing these changes. The initial studies with these investigational agents indicated promising improvements in motor and sensory nerve conduction and reduction in pain and weakness, but their place in therapy is not well defined. The incidence of side effects is low with these agents. Hypersensitivity reactions, such as skin rash and fever, are the most common and can occur in up to 10% of patients.

Autonomic neuropathies are the other form of nerve changes in diabetes. These complications may induce changes in function of organ systems controlled by the autonomic nervous system.[77,78] Neurogenic bladder, with loss of autonomic-mediated urinary continence, may require bethanechol and/or anticholinergics. As many as 50% of men with diabetes for longer than 25 years may become impotent.[70] The symptoms of hypoglycemia may not be sensed by many patients, especially the elderly. This so-called hypoglycemia unawareness is a significant danger in attempting an aggressive, intensive control program. Vision changes affecting eye focus are reported. Orthostasis can be a significant problem in patients who develop significant autonomic neuropathy. In its final states, drops in pressure of more than 30 mm Hg upon standing are not uncommon.

Gastroparesis is a complication that affects approximately 20% to 30% of patients with diabetes, but is often overlooked. It is most common in type 1 diabetes and is believed to be a result of autonomic dysfunction. Symptoms include nausea, vomiting, and abdominal distension and perhaps a rapid satiety from delayed gastric emptying. Variation in gastric emptying time can lead to fluctuation of blood glucose levels, and improved glycemic control is linked to limiting the effects of gastroparesis. The goals of therapy are to provide good glycemic control and relief of symptoms. Although antiemetics have been used with some success, most clinical attention has centered on use of agents to stimulate or regulate gastric emptying. Two agents currently in use in the United States are metoclopramide, an antidopaminergic agent, and cisapride, a cholinergic stimulant with apparently more potency. Because cisapride has fewer adverse effects (e.g., extrapyramidal) and works at least as well as metoclopramide, it is usually the drug of choice.[79,80] Other agents such as clonidine and erythromycin have shown limited success.[81]

Diabetic diarrhea occurs in about 20% of patients and may also be a neuropathic disorder. It is characterized as episodic, voluminous, and watery brown stools alternating with normal bowel function. This is most common in middle-age people with long-standing diabetes. Treatment has included anticholinergic agents, dietary change, antibiotics, bulk and bile salt resins, kaolin–pectin, and diphenoxylate–atropine. Ocetreotide has shown some promise in this disorder.[82,83]

RETINOPATHY

Diabetic retinopathy is the leading cause of new blindness in the United States. Good glycemic control significantly slows the progression of retinopathy (see Table 70–6). Diabetes-related retinopathy may be either nonproliferative or proliferative. Nonproliferative retinopathy develops with little vision impairment, whereas proliferative retinopathy can greatly diminish vision or cause sudden blindness.[84] It is estimated that after 15 years' duration of type 1 diabetes, 75% of patients will develop some degree of retinopathy. All persons with diabetes should be encouraged to have an annual dilated eye examination. The majority will have little significant visual impairment, however, because the retinopathy is minimal. Only 5% or fewer of type 1 diabetics in the United States are totally blind from diabetic-induced retinopathy.[2,58] The prevalence of significant retinopathy in patients with type 2 diabetes is much less than it is in type 1 diabetes. Nonproliferative retinopathy presents with microaneurysms progressing to hard yellow exudates, retinal edema, and hemorrhage. Nonproliferative retinopathy is treated with laser photocoagulation therapy that may help to arrest progression and decrease the loss of vision associated with macular edema. Because hypertension and smoking lead to more rapid progression of ocular damage, it is very important to halt or to eliminate these risk factors.[85]

Aldose reductase inhibitors may prove beneficial in progressive retinopathy by preventing sorbitol-induced osmotic swelling and halting lenticular cataract development.[69] Because platelet aggregation may play a role in occluding retinal capillaries, there is some evidence that aspirin therapy may help to prevent the development of diabetic retinopathy. There is debate in the diabetes clinical community regarding the positive value of low-dose aspirin for the vascular changes.[86] Once retinopathy has developed, aspirin is contraindicated owing to the increased risk of retinal hemorrhage. The patient should be cautioned to avoid strenuous physical activity that might increase venous pressure and cause hemorrhage from the weakened ocular vessels.[58]

NEPHROPATHY

Diabetic nephropathy syndrome, defined as persistent proteinuria, decreased glomerular filtration, and increased arterial blood pressure, is the primary cause of increased morbidity and mortality in the type 1 patient. The DCCT and Kumamoto studies demonstrated the positive benefits of glycemic control in limiting progression of nephropathy.[10,11] Again, one must weigh the relative risks of increased incidence of hypoglycemia and the patients' skill and motivation against their limitations for participating in their control. Roughly 35% of diabetic patients will develop nephropathy, and the cumulative death rate is 50% to 75% 10 years after the diagnosis of diabetic nephropathy. This means that about 14,000 patients develop end-stage diabetic renal disease annually. Factors such as hypertension, hyperlipidemia, poor diet control, and smoking all contribute to the development of progressive renal insufficiency.[1,58]

Microalbuminuria (albumin excretion of 30 to 300 mg/d or 20 to 200 μg/min) is a harbinger of diabetic nephropathy. Aggressive management of hypertension and microalbumuria delays the worsening of microalbumuria and diabetic nephropathy in type 1 and 2 diabetes. The current standard of care is to screen all new diabetics at first visit and yearly thereafter if diabetes has been present for 5 years for the presence of microalbumuria and, if present, to begin an ACE inhibitor such as captopril or linsinopril to stabilize and prevent worsening of renal microalbumuria.[86] ACE inhibitors should be given to all type 1 diabetics with microalbumuria even if normotensive; in normotensive type 2 diabetics there is less evidence substantiating a positive effect, but many clinicians would use ACE inhibitors in this setting as well. If cough or hyperkalemia occurs with ACE inhibitors angiotensin-receptor antagonists could be substituted for ACE inhibitors, according to preliminary studies.

The renin–angiotensin system regulates glomerular and tubular function and systemic blood pressure. As diabetes-related changes evolve in the kidney, hyperfiltration will be the initial alteration in glomerular filtration. With progression of diabetes the filtration rate shifts to normal and then to loss of renal function. Hypertension results in greater glomerular capillary pressure, which, in turn, leads to progressive glomerular damage, proteinuria, and azotemia, a common risk link with diabetes. ACE inhibitors normalize systemic and glomerular capillary pressures, and reduce proteinuria and glomerulosclerosis. When the ACE inhibitors are started, the patient may have a transient rise in serum creatinine, which usually returns to baseline within a few days. Caution must be advised, however, when using these agents in severe renal disease, because ACE inhibitors can worsen or cause renal impairment. ACE inhibitors, therefore, seem to be most useful during the early stages of diabetic nephropathy.[66]

The American Diabetes Association estimates that more than 10 million persons with diabetes have experienced long-term complications. Once these conditions develop, they are irreversible. Strong support to achieve optimal glycemic control and identifying therapies to prevent the progression of the complications must be a priority. Foot care and lower extremity complications are a particular worry. At least half of amputations from diabetes-related disease can be prevented with good self-care and -monitoring. This combined neurologic–vascular complication requires very close monitoring. Finally, a recent ADA position statement reviewed the use of aspirin therapy in diabetes patients.[87] Citing its effects on thromboxane and cyclo-oxygenase, the statement recommends aspirin use for diabetes patients with a history of myocardial infarct, vascular bypass, stroke or transient ischemic attack, peripheral vascular disease, claudication, and/or angina in a dose of 81–325 daily. Aspirin can also be used for prevention; however, the following may be exclusions for aspirin therapy: patients under 30 years of age without cardiovascular risk factors and individuals with aspirin allergy or bleeding abnormalities.[87]

SPECIAL PROBLEMS ASSOCIATED WITH THERAPY

DIABETIC KETOACIDOSIS AND HYPERGLYCEMIC HYPEROSMOLAR NONKETOTIC SYNDROME

Hyperglycemia from uncontrolled diabetes can lead to two types of metabolic crises that may result in a medical emergency. Diabetic ketoacidosis (DKA) is more common in type 1 diabetics, from complications from inadequate glycemic control, stress (such as infection, myocardial infarction, stroke), failure to take insulin, or an acute presentation of previously undiagnosed diabetes mellitus. Another condition is termed hyperglycemic hyperosmolar nonketotic syndrome (HHNS). This is a life-threatening emergency usually seen in the elderly. HHNS is characterized by severe hyperglycemia (> 800 mg/dL), absence of ketoacidosis, profound dehydration, and neurologic signs of depressed sensorium to coma. Plasma insulin concentrations are usually higher in HHNS than in DKA. Because the mortality associated with these conditions averages 5% to 10%,[88] they should be regarded as a medical emergency that requires immediate diagnosis and prompt treatment.

Pathophysiology of DKA

For DKA to develop, a relative insulin deficit must be present with increased levels of stress hormones (glucagon, cortisol, catecholamines, or growth hormone) and a precipitating factor.[89] Insulin deficiency results in postmeal hyperglycemia with impaired protein synthesis and increased protein degradation. Usually some internal or external stress causes increases in counterregulatory factors, creating either direct hyperglycemia or insulin resistance. Examples of precipitating events are listed in Table 70–19.

The counterregulatory hormones cause increased glucose production by the liver, and glycerol is an important gluconeogenic precursor (see Fig. 70–3). These two events in tandem produce moderate to severe hyperglycemia. Insulin deficiency also causes glycogen catabolism to glucose in the liver, and glycogen is depleted within several hours with subsequent mobilization of fatty acids from peripheral tissues that undergo hepatic lipolysis. Insulin deficiency also reduces peripheral clearance of glucose, causing increased hyperglycemia. Moreover, protein from muscles is metabolized in the liver to amino acids. Increased levels of glucagon can also increase glucose and ketone production by altering hepatic metabolism.[89] This series of events results in ketosis and metabolic acidosis. Hyperglycemia, ketonuria and ketonemia, and acidosis comprise the triad producing diabetic ketoacidosis.[90]

TABLE 70–19. Factors Precipitating Diabetic Ketoacidosis

Relative insulin deficiency: ~50% of cases
Insulin withdrawal or noncompliance
Insulin resistance/inappropriate dose
β Cell dysfunction, undiagnosed patient
Triggers diabetes diagnosis: ~25% of cases
Production of excess counterregulatory hormones
Dehydration
Infection–illness: ~25% of cases
Surgery
Psychologic stress
Sustained strenuous exertion
Pregnancy
Trauma
Pancreatitis
Hyperthyroidism
Hyperthermia
Acute myocardial infarction

Diabetic ketoacidosis profoundly affects the body's fluid and electrolyte status, renal function, and central nervous system. Renal tubular glucose levels surpass the reabsorption threshold to "spill" into the urine, producing an osmotic diuresis and dehydration. Because the plasma glucose cannot be transported into cells, an osmotic gradient between intracellular and extracellular compartments is established. Movement of fluid from the intracellular to extracellular space ensues, reducing hemodynamic signs of dehydration.[89] Many patients with DKA experience vomiting, which worsens the dehydration and preventing patients from taking enough fluids to improve their fluid status. Osmotic diuresis and dehydration lead to a decrease in glomerular filtration rate, further impairing glucose, free fatty acid, and ketone elimination and lead to serum hyperosmolality. Kussmaul respiration pattern (rapid, deep breathing) may occur in response to metabolic acidosis.

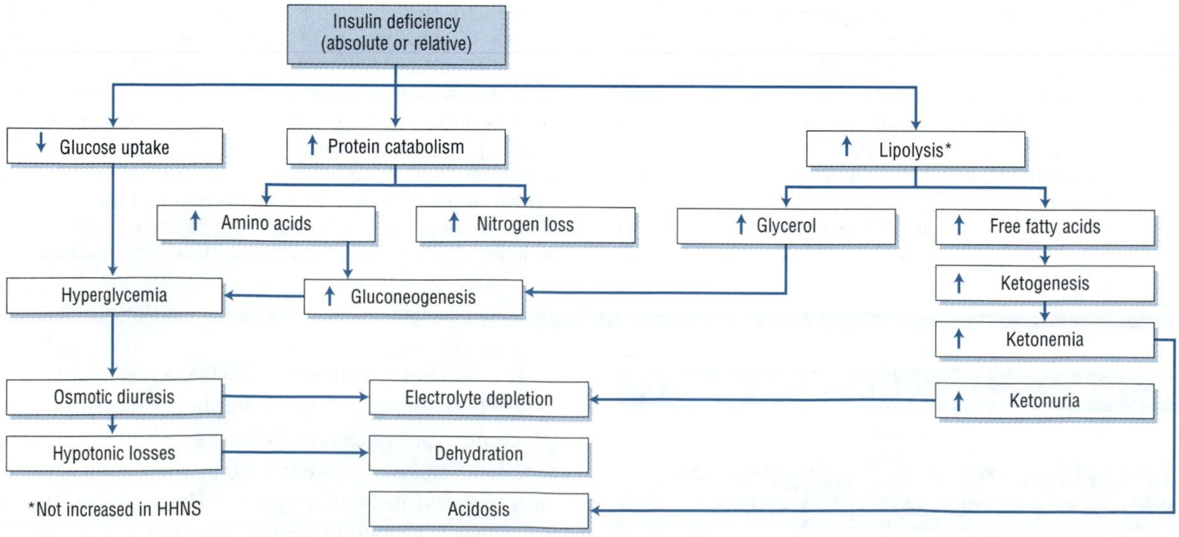

FIG. 70–3. DKA–HHNS pathways.

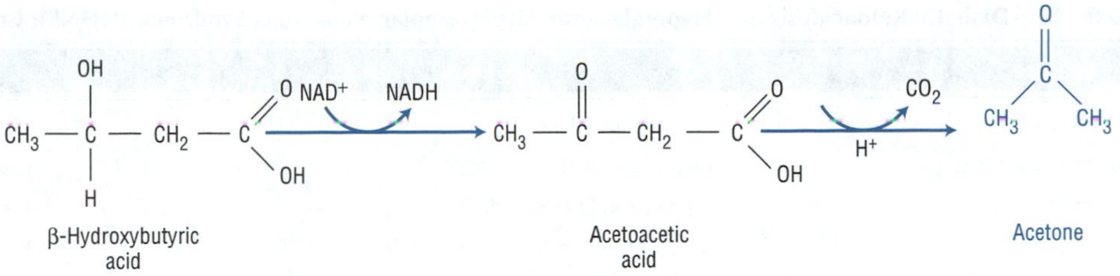

FIG. 70–4. Precursors of acetone.

Kussmaul respiration results in hyperventilation, reducing P_{CO_2} and producing a secondary respiratory alkalosis.

Hypovolemia decreases tissue perfusion, leading to lactic acidosis. Up to 25% of the acidemia seen in DKA may be a result of lactic acid accumulation.[90] Decreased GFR impairs the excretion of organic acids and ketones. β-Hydroxybutyric acid (BOHB) and acetoacetate (AcAc) are precursors of acetone, as depicted by Fig. 70–4.

BOHB is converted to AcAc by oxidation; AcAc is further decarboxylated to acetone. Normally the ratio of BOHB to AcAc in the serum is 3:1, but the ratio in DKA increases from 6:1 to 12:1; acetone concentration is much lower. Because the common method of measuring serum or urinary ketones (nitroprusside method) detects only AcAc, the quantification of ketones will most likely be low prior to therapy and not reflect the true contribution of BOHB to the acidosis. Ketone concentrations may increase during therapy as oxidative metabolism improves and converts BOHB to AcAc.[90] The osmotic diuresis causes losses of electrolytes, primarily sodium, potassium, phosphate, and bicarbonate. Typical losses of fluid and electrolytes are quantitated in Table 70–20. Serum sodium may appear normal or low in patients in DKA, even though dehydration may be severe. This is owing partially to fluid shifts from the intravascular to extravascular compartments caused by the increased osmotic pressure exerted by hyperglycemia. Each 100 mg/dL elevation of plasma glucose lowers the serum sodium by 1.6 mEq/L.[91] The following equation is often used for "correcting" the serum sodium concentration; $Na^+ = Na^+$ (measured) + 1.6 × (Glucose − 100)100.

Potassium is shifted to the extracellular compartment during acidosis and is lost through osmotic diuresis. Stimulation of aldosterone secretion by dehydration may also lead to hypokalemia. Whereas the serum potassium concentration appears normal or elevated in the early stages of DKA owing to the extracellular shift of potassium and the decreased GFR. Rehydration and insulin therapy improve the GFR and correct the acidosis, thereby producing evidence of hypokalemia. If serum potassium prior to therapy is low, one should expect a precipitous drop in potassium during therapy with fluids and insulin. In such instances, potassium-containing intravenous fluids should be administered *prior to insulin*. The patient should have a cardiac monitor at all times to detect the effects of hyper- or hypokalemia. Phosphate is depleted owing to acidosis and diuresis, although serum phosphate concentrations in patients with DKA may be normal or somewhat decreased. The clinical significance of phosphate depletion in patients with DKA is unclear; however, most clinicians begin repleting phosphate if the plasma concentration falls below 1.5 mg/dL.

TABLE 70–20. Fluid and Electrolyte Losses in Diabetic Ketoacidosis

Bicarbonate	0.1–2 mmol/kg body weight
Free water	50–150 mL/kg body weight
Sodium	4–11 mEq/kg body weight
Potassium	3–10 mEq/kg body weight
Phosphate	0.1–2 mmol/kg body weight
Bicarbonate	3–6 mEq/kg body weight

Serum bicarbonate concentrations in patients with DKA are low because the bicarbonate buffer system is one of the body's defenses against metabolic acidosis. Though the serum bicarbonate concentration appears low, ketoacids and lactic acid are eventually metabolized via the Corey cycle to regenerate bicarbonate so that serum bicarbonate is restored to a near-normal level.[91]

Clinical Manifestations

Patients in diabetic ketoacidosis often present with lethargy (from hyperglycemia, hyperosmolality, ketonemia, and acidosis), hyperventilation with possible Kussmaul respirations (from compensatory respiratory alkalosis), fruity odor to the breath (from acetonemia), changes in mental status (from hyperosmolality), nausea and vomiting (from metabolic acidosis), abdominal pain (from gastric distention), thirst and polyuria (from osmotic diuresis) or decreased urine output (from progressive DKA causing hypovolemia and decreased GFR), dry mucous membranes and poor skin turgor (from dehydration), and tachycardia. Diagnosis is established by testing for one or a combination of the following: presence of urine ketones, serum ketones, lowered serum bicarbonate level, and or a lowered arterial pH. Initial laboratory data are included in Table 70–21. Patients usually have an increased anion gap ($AG = [Na^+ + K^+] - [HCO_3^- + Cl^-]$) owing to accumulation of BOHB and AcAc as unmeasured anions. Acid–base status is usually determined by calculating the anion gap as a marker for acidemia and may be used in place of pH determined by arterial blood gas (ABG) once therapy is started. Over three fourths of DKA patients will exhibit an increased serum amylase, although the cause and significance of this finding is unclear.[92]

TABLE 70–21. Diabetic Ketoacidosis and Hyperglycemic Hyperosmolar Nonketotis Syndrome (HHNS): Comparison

Feature	DKA	HHNS
Age of patients	Usually < 40 yr	Usually > 60 yr
Duration of symptoms	Usually < 2 d	Usually > 5 d
Glucose level	Usually < 600 mg/dL	Usually > 800 mg/dL
Sodium concentration	More likely to be normal or low	More likely to be normal or high
Potassium concentration	High, normal, or low	High, normal, or low
Bicarbonate concentration	Low	Normal
Ketone bodies	At least 4+ in 1:1 dilution	< 2+ in 1:1 dilution
pH	Low	Normal
Serum osmolality	Usually < 350 mOsm/kg	Usually > 350 mOsm/kg
Cerebral edema	Often subclinical	Subclinical has not been evaluated
Prognosis	3–10% mortality	1–20% mortality
Subsequent course	Insulin therapy required in virtually all cases	Insulin not needed in many cases

▶ TREATMENT: Diabetic Ketoacidosis

If DKA is diagnosed, it is imperative for the physician to initiate immediate treatment and to search for and correct the precipitating event. Treatment of DKA should be targeted toward correcting dehydration, reducing the plasma glucose concentration to normal, reversing the acidosis and ketosis, replenishing electrolyte and volume losses, and identifying the underlying cause. Patients in DKA have fluid deficits of 4 to 10 L (with an average deficit of 5 L).[90] Administration of the proper type and amount of intravenous fluids will correct the dehydration and hyperglycemia associated with DKA. Plasma glucose concentrations greater than 600 mg/dL denote dehydration greater than 10%. Plasma glucose concentrations of this magnitude can be reduced to 300 mg/dL by administering fluids alone without insulin.[91] Volume replacement lowers the plasma glucose concentration by increasing urine flow and glucose excretion, through a dilutional effect, and by decreasing circulating levels of counterregulatory hormones. There is some consensus regarding fluid replacement in these patients, with such factors as the patient's hemodynamic status, age, concurrent medical problems, and suspected precipitating event influencing the decision. Most clinicians believe that 0.9% sodium chloride should be administered initially, at a rate of 1 L/h for 2 to 3 hours.[89,92] After the patient's vascular status has been stabilized, with heart rhythm and blood pressure normalized, intravenous fluids can be changed to 0.45% sodium chloride. When the patient's plasma glucose concentration approaches 250 mg/dL, the IV fluid should be changed to 5% dextrose in 0.45% sodium chloride. This is to prevent hypoglycemia and to avoid hyperchloremic acidosis.

Insulin lowers plasma glucose and ketone levels. Inhibition of lipolysis and ketogenesis is much more sensitive than glucose-lowering effects. Investigators have discovered that a relatively low dose of insulin is just as effective without producing postrecovery hypoglycemia.[89,93] Counterregulatory hormone activity diminishes at similar rates with high-dose versus low-dose regimens. Consequently, most clinicians now use low-dose IV regular insulin to treat DKA.

Because the half-life of insulin is approximately 5 to 6 minutes,[93] giving a loading dose is probably not needed. To avoid time delays encountered in preparing intravenous fluids containing insulin, some practitioners prefer administering a bolus of 0.1 U/kg before starting a continuous infusion. The maintenance infusion may be prepared by adding 100 units of regular to 100 mL of 0.9% sodium chloride piggybacked and infusing the drug at an initial rate of 0.1 U/kg/h.[89] Plasma glucose determinations should be made hourly. If there has been less than a 10% drop in 2 hours, then the insulin drip rate should be doubled.[89,93] The need for increased levels of insulin in some patients may indicate insulin resistance, which will improve with continued therapy.

When the patient's plasma glucose concentration approaches 250 mg/dL, the primary intravenous fluid should be changed from 0.45% sodium chloride to 5% dextrose in 0.45% sodium chloride, and the infusion rate of the insulin drip should be cut in half.[89] It is important to emphasize that the end point of insulin therapy is not euglycemia but correction of acidosis (AG) and ketonemia. The insulin infusion should be continued until the acidosis has been corrected (arterial pH, > 7.30; plasma glucose concentration, < 250 mg/dL, anion gap 13 to 17; serum bicarbonate > 15 mEq/L, no ketonemia).[89]

Electrolytes depleted from osmotic diuresis and acidosis should be replaced as quickly as possible to prevent development of cardiovascular problems. Sodium and potassium are the primary electrolytes that need to be replaced, although some clinicians also replace phosphate, magnesium, and bicarbonate. Sodium is replaced by administering 2 to 4 L of normal saline during the initial management of DKA. Sodium balance is maintained by changing the patient's IV fluids to 0.45% sodium chloride and later to 5% dextrose in 0.45% sodium chloride.

Osmotic diuresis produces a total body deficit of potassium ranging from 300 to 600 mEq. The serum potassium concentration falls to its lowest point approximately 1 to 4 hours after treatment of ketoacidosis is initiated. Potassium levels should be monitored closely every hour initially, then every 2 to 4 hours because hypokalemia can induce cardiac arrhythmias. Potassium can be replaced by adding 40 to 60 mEq to each liter of IV fluid and administering it at a rate of 10 to 20 mEq/h.[89,93] Electrocardiogram (ECG) monitoring is necessary to monitor the patient's status. Oral potassium replacement is possible provided the patient is not experiencing nausea or vomiting or is comatose.[93]

There is no agreement on the routine administration of phosphate, bicarbonate, or magnesium in DKA. Phosphate is necessary to maintain adequate levels of 2,3-dephosphoglycerate in red blood cells and to improve tissue oxygenation by shifting the oxygen–hemoglobin dissociation curve to the right. Phosphate is also necessary to produce ATP and enhance proper function of cardiac and respiratory tissues. Serum phosphate concentrations may drop during treatment of ketoacidosis. Therefore, phosphate replacement should be instituted when the serum level approaches the lower end of the normal range.[92] If phosphate is replaced as the potassium salt, it should be kept in mind that each milliliter of potassium phosphate contains 3 mM phosphate and

4.4 mEq potassium and that hyperkalemia is possible with this product. High doses of phosphate can induce hypocalcemia.

Significant amounts of bicarbonate are lost in ketoacidosis. However, most clinicians agree that replacement of this electrolyte has the potential of causing hypokalemia, acidification of cerebrospinal fluid, systemic alkalosis, impaired oxygen delivery to tissues, increased carbon dioxide production, and ketoacid overproduction.[91,92] During therapy to correct DKA, ketoacids and lactic acid are metabolized by the liver to bicarbonate. Generally, bicarbonate is administered only to patients whose arterial pH is below 7.0 and/or when serum bicarbonate is very low (< 5 mEq/L). When indicated, bicarbonate should be administered via infusion of 50 mEq (or 1 mEq/kg) over 1 hour. The goal of therapy is to raise the arterial pH to 7.10 to 7.15.[93]

MONITORING

Plasma or whole-blood glucose concentrations should be monitored hourly until they have stabilized below 250 mg/dL. Electrolytes, especially potassium, should be monitored every hour until stabilized within the normal range, then every 2 to 4 hours until the acidosis has been corrected. Heart rhythm should be monitored, especially in comatose patients. Patients with HHNS are managed in a similar manner to DKA, with fluid and electrolyte replacement the cornerstone of treatment rather than insulin. Usually lower doses of insulin are needed for treating HHNS because of higher circulating insulin levels. The troubling component of HHNS is that many times the diagnosis is missed owing to the patient's history.

INSULIN REQUIREMENTS OF THE SURGICAL PATIENT

Diabetics patients scheduled for surgery usually do not receive breakfast on the day of surgery, and administration of insulin might lead to profound hypoglycemia; however, the "stress" of surgery has a tremendous hyperglycemic effect such that withholding insulin can lead to dehydration, an impaired inflammatory response, and possible ketoacidosis (in the type 1 patient). Plasma glucose values should ideally be between 150 and 200 mg/dL. In an insulin-dependent patient, the dose the day of surgery is 50% of the normal dose. Postoperatively, insulin requirements may remain elevated for a day or so but should return to typical requirements once the surge of counterregulatory hormones ceases.

Patients whose diabetes is controlled by diet only usually need no exogenous insulin but should at least be covered by a sliding scale order should the need for insulin arise. Human insulin should be used to minimize the formation of insulin antibodies. The patient controlled with oral agents should have the medication held on the day of surgery and needs a sliding scale order. The insulin-requiring patients should receive half of the usual dose of an intermediate-acting insulin and should likewise have an order for sliding scale insulin after surgery.[94]

"SICK-DAY" GUIDELINES FOR INSULIN-DEPENDENT PATIENTS

When a patient with type 1 diabetes feels too ill to eat, the question often arises as to how much (if any) insulin is needed. Insulin needs vary, but the stress of the causative event can increase blood glucose. Extra clear fluids (up to 12 glasses) should be consumed, especially if the patient has a fever. Patients should record the amount of fluid they consume along with the number of times they urinate, vomit, or have loose stools. Blood glucose concentrations should be measured several times during the day up to hourly, and urine should be tested for ketones with each urination. Most patients are instructed to contact their health care provider when a "sick day" starts for specific guidelines; the provider should also consider the patient's mentation in the monitoring. If the blood glucose concentration is greater than 300 mg/dL and urine ketones are present, the patient needs to be formally evaluated. Similarly, any patient having difficulty breathing or breathing over 24 times per minute (symptoms of respiratory compensation for metabolic acidosis) should seek medical attention. Although it is normal to feel tired or sleepy when sick, any patient who is very sleepy or cannot pay attention should have someone seek medical help immediately.[95]

▶ PRINCIPLES OF PHARMACOTHERAPY

- Diabetes mellitus is classified as type 1 (~10% to 15% of diabetes) and type 2 (~85% to 90% of diabetes); diagnostic criteria for diabetes are set at a level consistent with promptly limiting complication progression.
- The pathophysiology of diabetes is directly linked to a relative or absolute lack of insulin with resultant abnormalities in utilization of energy sources such as fat, carbohydrate, and protein.
- Intensive diabetes screening and detection are important processes to limit progression of chronic complications of diabetes.
- Type 1 diabetes patients are managed pharmacologically with insulin, and the regimen may range from a single daily injection to multiple injections of different types of insulin to constant infusions using pump devices.
- Type 2 diabetes patients are managed pharmacologically initially with oral agents including sulfonylureas, metformin, troglitazone, and acarbose.
- The initial oral drug for type 2 diabetes is often a sulfonylurea, although metformin or troglitazone may be used initially as well in diet-failed patients; sulfonylureas and metformin have similar effects on lowering FPG and HbA_{1c}, whereas troglitazone is slightly less potent.
- Patients failing monotherapy (after maximizing the dose) for diabetes should be given combination therapy rather than switching because improved control of FPG and HbA_{1c} is seen with combination therapy compared with any single agent.
- Acarbose is useful primarily for reduction in postprandial blood glucose and has little effect on FPG or HbA_{1c}.
- Many type 2 diabetes patients will eventually require insulin (BIDS therapy) to achieve FPG and HbA_{1c} goals set by the American Diabetes Association.
- Metabolic control of diabetes is directly related to evolution and occurrence of long-term complications.

REFERENCES

1. American Diabetes Association. Direct and indirect costs of diabetes in the United States in 1992. Alexandria, VA, American Diabetes Association, 1993.
2. Harris MI. Third National Health and Nutrition Examination Survey (NHANES III), 1988–1994.
3. Report of the Expert Committee on the Diagnosis and Classification of Diabetes Mellitus of the American Diabetes Association. Diabetes Care 1997;20:1183–1197.
4. Rifkin H, Porte D Jr, eds. Ellenberg and Rifkin's Diabetes Mellitus: Theory and Practice, 4th ed. New York, Elsvier Science, 1990.
5. Metzger BE, Organizing Committee. Summary and Recommendations of the Third International Workshop-Conference on Gestational Diabetes Mellitus. Diabetes 1991;40(suppl 2):197–201.
6. Shulman GI, Barrett EJ, Sherwin RS. Integrated fuel metabolism. In: Porte D Jr, Sherwin RS, eds. Ellenberg & Rifkin's Diabetes Mellitus, 5th ed. Stamford, CT, Appleton & Lange, 1997:1–17.
7. Raskin P, ed. Medical Management of Non-Insulin-Dependent (Type 2) Diabetes, 3rd ed. Alexandria, VA, American Diabetes Association Clinical Education Series, 1994.
8. American Diabetes Association. Clinical Practice Recommendations 1997. Diabetes Care 1997;20(suppl 1):S1–S70.
9. Hoekstra JBL, van Rijn HJM, Erkelens DW, et al. Review: C-peptide. Diabetes Care 1982;5:438–446.
10. The Diabetes Control and Complications Trial Research Group. The effect of intensive treatment of diabetes on the progression of long-term complications in insulin-dependent diabetes mellitus. N Engl J Med 1993;319:977–986.
11. Ohkubo Y, Kishikawa H, Araki E, et al. Intensive insulin therapy prevents the progression of diabetic microvascular complications in Japanese patients with non-insulin-dependent diabetes mellitus: A randomized prospective 6-year study. Diabetes Res Clin Pract 1995;28:103–117.
12. Klein R, Klein BEK, Moss SE, Cruikshanks KJ. Relationship of hyperglycemia to the long-term incidence of diabetic retinopathy. Arch Intern Med 1994;154:2169–2178.
13. American Diabetes Association Clinical Practice Guidelines, 1996. The pharmacological treatment of hyperglycemia in NIDDM. Diabetes Care 1996;19(suppl 1):S54–S61.
14. Funnell MM, Anderson RM, Arnold MS, et al. Empowerment: An idea whose time has come in diabetes education. Diabetes Educ 1991; 17:37–41.
15. National Diabetes Data Group. Diabetes in America, 2nd ed. Washington, DC, National Institutes of Health Publication 95-1468, 1995.
16. Franz MJ, Horton ES, Bantle JP, et al. Technical review: Nutrition principles for the management of diabetes and related complications. Diabetes Care 1994;17:490–518.
17. American Diabetes Association Position Statement. Nutrition recommendations and principles for people with diabetes mellitus. Diabetes Care 1998;21(suppl 1) S32–S35.
18. American Diabetes Association Position Statement. Diabetes and exercise. Diabetes Care 1998;21(suppl 1):S40–S44.
19. Lebovitz HE. The oral hypoglycemic agents. In Porte D Jr, Sherwin RS, eds. Ellenberg & Rifkin's: Diabetes Mellitus, 5th ed. Stamford CT, Appleton & Lange, 1997:761–788.
20. The University Group Diabetes Program. A study of the effects of hypoglycemic agents on vascular complications in patients with adult onset diabetes. Diabetes 1970;19(suppl 2):1–26.
21. Lebovitz HE. Sulfonylurea drugs. In: Lebovitz HE, ed. Therapy for Diabetes Mellitus and Related Disorders. Alexandria, VA, American Diabetes Association, 1991:114–122.
22. Antidiabetic agents. In: American Hospital Formulary Service Drug Information 95. Bethesda, American Society of Hospital Pharmacists, 1997:1782–1837.
23. Gavin JR. Dual actions of sulfonylureas and glyburide: Receptor and post-receptor effects. Am J Med 1985;79(suppl 3B):34–43.
24. Lebovitz HE. Oral antidiabetic agents. In: Kahn CR, Weir GC, eds. Joslin's Diabetes Mellitus, 13 ed. Malvern, PA, Lea & Febiger, 1994: 508–529.
25. Davis SN, Granner DK. Insulin, oral hypoglycemic agents, and the pharmacology of the endocrine pancreas. In: Hardman JG, Limbird LE, Molinoff PB, Goodman & Gilman's The Pharmacologic Basis of Therapeutics, 9th ed. New York, McGraw-Hill, 1996;1486–1517.
26. Bailey CJ. Biguanides and NIDDM. Diabetes Care 1992;15:755–772.
27. Chiasson J-L, Josse RG, Hunt JA. The efficacy of acarbose in the treatment of patients with non-insulin-dependent diabetes mellitus: A multicenter controlled clinical trial. Ann Intern Med 1994;121: 928–935.
28. White JR. Combination oral agent/insulin therapy in patients with type 2 diabetes mellitus. Clin Diabetes 1997;15:8–28.
29. Suter SL, Nolan JJ, Wallace P, Gumbiner B, Olefsky JM. Metabolic effects of new oral hypoglycemic agents CS-045 in NIDDM subjects. Diabetes Care 1992;15:193–203.
30. Saltiel AR, Horikoshi J. Thiazolidinediones are novel insulin-sensitizing agents. Curr Opin Endocrinol Diabetes 1995;2:341–347.
31. Lewitt MS, Yu VKF, Rennie GC, et al. Effects of combined insulin-sulfonylurea in type 2 patients. Diabetes Care 1989;12:379–383.
32. Reaven GM, Johnston P, Hollenbeck CB, et al. Combined metformin-sulfonylurea treatment of patients with non-insulin-dependent diabetes in fair to poor glycemic control. J Clin Endocrinol Metab 1992;74: 1020–1026.
33. Deckert T. The immunogenicity of new insulins. Diabetes 1985;34 (suppl 2):94–96.
34. Galloway JA, Spradlin CT, Nelson RL, et al. Factors influencing the absorption, serum insulin concentration, and blood glucose responses after injections of regular insulin and various mixtures. Diabetes Care 1981;4:366–376.
35. Holleman F, Hoekstra JBL. Drug therapy: Insulin lispro. N Engl J Med 1997;337:176–183.
36. Brange J, Owens DR, Kang S, Valund A. Monomeric insulins and their experimental and clinical implications. Diabetes Care 1990;13: 923–954.
37. Kotsanos JG, Vignati L, Huster W, et al. Health-related quality-of-life results from multinational clinical trials of insulin lispro. Diabetes Care 1997;20:948–958.
38. Peters AL, Davidson MB. Effect of storage on action of NPH and regular insulin mixtures. Diabetes Care 1986;14:180–183.
39. White J, Campbell RK. Guide to mixing insulins. Hosp Pharm 1991; 26:1046–1048.
40. Genuth S. Insulin use in NIDDM. Diabetes Care 1990;13:1240–1264.
41. Schade D, Santiago J, Skyler J, Rizza R. Intensive Insulin Therapy. Geneva, Excerpta Medica, 1983.
42. Cahill GF, McDevitt HO. Insulin-dependent diabetes mellitus: The initial lesion. N Engl J Med 1981;304:1454–1465.
43. Strowig SM. Initiation and management of insulin pump therapy. Diabetes Educ 1993;19:50–59.
44. Rink TJ, Beaumont K, Koda J, Young A. Structure and biology of amylin. Trends Pharmacol Sci 1993;14:113–118.
45. Peters AL, Legorreta AP, Ossorio RC, Davidson MB. Quality of outpatient care provided to diabetic patients: A health maintenance organization experience. Diabetes Care 1996;19:601–606.
46. Guthrie D, Guthrie R, Hinnen D. Urine tests: Still useful after all these years. Diabetes Forecast 1985;38:43–45.
47. American Diabetes Association. Tests of glycemia in diabetes. Diabetes Care 1998;21(suppl 1):S69–S71.
48. American Diabetes Association. Consensus statement. Self-monitoring of blood glucose. Diabetes Care 1994;17:76–87.
49. Farkas-Hirsch R, ed. Monitoring in intensive diabetes management. American Diabetes Association Clinical Education Series, Alexandria, VA, 1994:80–87.
50. National Steering Committee for Quality Assurance in Capillary Blood Glucose Monitoring. Proposed strategies for reducing user error in capillary blood glucose monitoring. Diabetes Care 1993;16:493–498.

51. Gebhart SSP, Wheaton RN, Mullins RE, Austin GE. A comparison of home glucose monitoring with determinations of hemoglobin A_{1c}, total glycated hemoglobin, fructosamine, and random serum glucose in diabetic patients. Arch Intern Med 1991;151:1133–1137.
52. The relationship of glycemic exposure to the risk of development and progression of retinopathy in the Diabetes Control and Complications Trial. Diabetes 1995;44:968–983.
53. Steen G, Weber RF. Clinical usefulness of serum fructosamine and HbA_1 as markers for metabolic control in patients with changing insulin regiments. Diabetes Res 1990;13:177–182.
54. Lefebvre PJ. Biosynthesis, secretion and action of glucagon. In: Alberti KGMM, DeFronzo RA, Keen H, Zimmet P, eds. International Textbook of Diabetes Mellitus. Chichester, UK, Wiley, 1992:333–339.
55. Galloway JA. The complications of insulin therapy. In: Bressler R, Johnson DG, eds. Management of Diabetes Mellitus. Boston, John Wright—PSG, 1982:91–114.
56. Stephenson JM, Schernthaner G. Dawn phenomenon and Somogyi effect in IDDM. Diabetes Care 1989;12:245–251.
57. Bolli GB, Gerich JE. The dawn phenomenon—a common occurrence in both non-insulin-dependent and insulin-dependent diabetes mellitus. N Engl J Med 1984;310:746–750.
58. Nathan DM. Long-term complications of diabetes mellitus. N Engl J Med 1993;328:1676–1685.
59. Brownlee M. Glycation of macromolecules. In Alberti KGM, DeFronzo RA, Keen H, Zimmet P, eds. International Textbook of Diabetes Mellitus. West Sussex, UK, Wiley, 1993:669–684.
60. Brownlee M. Glycation products and the pathogenesis of diabetic complications. Diabetes Care 1992;15:1835–1843.
61. Kaplan NM. The deadly quartet: Upper-body obesity, glucose intolerance, hypertriglyceridemia, and hypertension. Arch Intern Med 1989; 149:1514–1519.
62. Klein R. Hyperglycemia and microvascular and macrovascular disease in diabetes. Diabetes Care 1995;18:258–268.
63. Lyons T. Lipoprotein glycation and its metabolic consequences. Diabetes 1992;41(suppl 2):67–76.
64. Stanlee J. Glycosylated hemoglobin and predictive data (MRFIT Study Analysis). Diabetes Care 1993;16:434–445.
65. The Scandinavian Simvastatin Survival Study Group. Randomized trial of cholesterol lowering in 4444 patients with coronary heart disease: The Scandinavian Simvastatin Survival Study. Lancet 1994;344: 1383–1389.
66. Lewis EJ, Hunsicker LG, Bain RP, et al. The effect of angiotensin-converting-enzyme inhibition on diabetic nephropathy. N Engl J Med 1993;328:1456–1462.
67. Greenfield S, Rogers W, Mangotich M, Carney MF. Outcomes of patients with hypertension and non-insulin dependent diabetes mellitus treated by different systems and specialties: Results from the medical outcomes study. JAMA. 1995;274:1436–1444.
68. Mitchell BD, Hawthorne VM, Vinik AI. Cigarette smoking and neuropathy in diabetic patients. Diabetes Care 1990;13:434–437.
69. Zenon GJ, Abobo CV, Carter BL, et al. Potential use of aldose reductase inhibitors to prevent diabetic complications. Clin Pharm 1990;9: 446–457.
70. Daniels JS. Abnormal nerve conduction in impotent patients with diabetes mellitus. Diabetes Care 1989;12:449–454.
71. Greene DA, Sima AAF, Albers JW, Pfeifer MA. Diabetic neuropathy. In: Rifkin H, Porte D, eds. Diabetes Mellitus, 4th ed. New York, Elsevier, 1990:710–755.
72 Vinik AI, Holland MT, LeBeau JM, et al. Diabetic neuropathies. Diabetes Care 1992;15:1926–1975.
73. Moss SE, Klein R, Klein BE, et al. The association of glycemia and cause-specific mortality in a diabetic population. Arch Intern Med. 1994;154:2473–2479.
74. Theesan KA, Marsh WR. Relief of diabetic neuropathy with fluoxetine. DICP Ann Pharmacother 1989;23:572–574.
75. Mendel CM, Klein RF, Chappell DA, et al. A trial of amitriptyline and fluphenazine in the treatment of painful diabetic neuropathy. JAMA 1986;255:637–639.
76. Capsaicin Study Group. Effect of treatment with capsaicin on daily activities of patients with painful diabetic neuropathy. Diabetes Care 1992;15:159–165.
77. Cahill GF, Arky RA, Perlman AJ. Diabetes mellitus. In: Rubenstein E, Federman DD, eds. Scientific American Medicine. New York, Scientific American, 1987;9(VJ):1–19.
78. Cyrus J, Broadstone VL, Pfeifer MA, Greene DA. Diabetic peripheral neuropathy. Part II. Autonomic neuropathies. Diabetes Educ 1987;13: 111–114.
79. Singh PJ, Santella RN, Zawada ET. Gastrointestinal prokinetic agents for enhancing drug response in gastroparesis. Am J Health Syst Pharm 1997;54:2609–2612.
80. Kendall BJ, Kendall ET, Soykan I, McCallum RW. Cisapride in the long-term treatment of chronic gastroparesis: A 2-year open-label study. J Intl Med Res 1997;25:182–189.
81. Jassens J, Peeters TL, Vantrappen J, et al. Improvement of gastric emptying in diabetic gastroparesis by erythromycin. N Engl J Med 1990;322:1028–1031.
82. Ogbonnaya KI, Arem R. Diabetic diarrhea pathophysiology, diagnosis, and management. Arch Intern Med 1990;150:262–267.
83. Rosenberg JM. Ocetreotide: A synthetic analog of somatostatin. DICP 1988;22:748–754.
84. Merimee TJ. Diabetic retinopathy: A synthesis of perspectives. N Engl J Med 1990;322:978–983.
85. The Prevention and Treatment of Complications of Diabetes: A Guide for Primary Care Practitioners. Atlanta, GA, Department of Health and Human Services, Centers for Disease Control and Prevention, 1991.
86. American Diabetes Association. Current practice standards. Diabetic nephropathy. Diabetes Care 1998;21(suppl 1):S50–S53.
87. Aspirin Therapy in Diabetes. American Diabetes Association Position Statement. Diabetes Care 1997;20:1772–1773.
88. Genuth SM. Diabetic ketoacidosis and hyperglycemic hyperosmolar coma. Curr Ther Endocrinol Metab 1997;6:438–447.
89. Davidson MB. Diabetic ketoacidosis and hyperosmolar non-ketotic coma. In: Davidson MB, ed. Diabetes Mellitus: Diagnosis and Treatment, 3rd ed. New York, Churchill Livingstone, 1991:175–212.
90. Lebovitz HE. Diabetic ketoacidosis. Lancet. 1995;345:767–772.
91. Green SM, Rothrock SG, Ho JD, et al. Failure of adjunctive bicarbonate to improve outcome in severe pediatric diabetic ketoacidosis. Ann Emerg Med 1998;31:41–48.
92. Kitabchi AE, Wall BM. Diabetic ketoacidosis. Med Clin North Am 1995;79:9–37.
93. Peragallo-Dittko V, Godley K, Meyer J, eds. A Core Curriculum for Diabetes Education, 2nd ed. Chicago, American Association of Diabetes Educators, 1993.
94. Gill GV, Alberti KGMM. The care of the diabetic patient during surgery. In: Alberti KGMM, DeFronzo RA, Keen H, Zimmet P, eds. International Textbook of Diabetes Mellitus. West Sussex, UK, Wiley, 1993.
95. Ley B, Goldman D. Sick-day management: Preparing for the unexpected. Diabetes Spectrum 1991;4:173–176.

71

THYROID DISORDERS

Charles A. Reasner, II, MD, FACE, and Robert L. Talbert, PharmD, FCCP, BCPS

Thyroid hormones affect the function of virtually every organ system. In the child, thyroid hormone is critical for normal growth and development. In the adult, the major role of thyroid hormone is to maintain metabolic stability. Substantial reservoirs of thyroid hormone in the thyroid gland and blood provide constant thyroid hormone availability. In addition, the hypothalamic–pituitary–thyroid axis is exquisitely sensitive to small changes in circulating thyroid hormone concentrations, and alterations in thyroid hormone secretion maintain peripheral free thyroid hormone levels within a narrow range. Patients seek medical attention for evaluation of symptoms owing to abnormal thyroid hormone levels or because of diffuse or nodular thyroid enlargement.

THYROID HORMONE PHYSIOLOGY

THYROID HORMONE SYNTHESIS

The thyroid hormones thyroxine (T_4) and triiodothyronine (T_3) are formed on thyroglobulin, a large glycoprotein synthesized within the thyroid cell (Fig. 71–1). Because of the unique tertiary structure of this glycoprotein, iodinated tyrosine residues present in thyroglobulin are able to bind together to form active thyroid hormones.[1,2]

IODIDE TRANSPORT AND ORGANIFICATION

Iodide is actively transported from the extracellular space into the thyroid follicular cell against both electrical and biochemical gradients. Structurally related anions such as SCN^- (thiocyanate), ClO_4^- (perchlorate), and TcO_4^- (pertechnetate) are competitive inhibitors of iodine transport.[3] In addition, bromine, fluorine, and lithium block iodide transport into the thyroid (Table 71–1). Inorganic iodide that enters the thyroid follicular cell is oxidized by thyroid peroxidase and is covalently bound (organified) to tyrosine residues of thyroglobulin (Fig. 71–2). It is interesting that although salivary glands and the gastric mucosa are able to actively transport iodide, they are unable to effectively incorporate iodide into proteins. Similarly, when tyrosine molecules are iodinated on proteins other than thyroglobulin, they lack the proper tertiary structure needed to allow the formation of active thyroid hormones.

IODOTYROSINE COUPLING

The iodinated tyrosine residues monoiodotyrosine (MIT) and diiodotyrosine (DIT) combine to form iodothyronines (Fig. 71–3). Thus, DIT and DIT combine to form T_4, whereas MIT and DIT constitute T_3. In addition to its role in iodine organification, the hemoprotein thyroid peroxidase also catalyses the formation of iodothyronines (coupling).

Iodine deficiency causes an increase in the ratio of MIT to DIT in thyroglobulin and leads to a relative increase in the production of T_3. Because T_3 is more potent than T_4, the increase in T_3 production in iodine-depleted areas may be beneficial. The thionamide drugs used to treat hyperthyroidism inhibit thyroid peroxidase and thus block thyroid hormone synthesis.

THYROID HORMONE SECRETION

Thyroglobulin is stored in the follicular lumen and must reenter the cell, where the process of proteolysis liberates thyroid hormone into the bloodstream. Thyroid follicles active in hormone synthesis are identified histologically by columnar epithelial cells lining follicular lumens, which are depleted of colloid. Inactive follicles are lined by cuboidal epithelial cells and are replete with colloid. Both iodide and lithium block the release of preformed thyroid hormone, through poorly understood mechanisms.

CHARACTERISTICS OF CIRCULATING THYROID HORMONES[4]

T_4 and T_3 are transported in the bloodstream by three proteins: thyroid-binding globulin (TBG), thyroid-binding prealbumin (TBPA), and albumin. It is estimated that 99.96% of T_4 and 99.5% of T_3 are bound to these proteins. Only the unbound (free) thyroid hormone is able to diffuse into the cell, elicit a biologic effect, and regulate thyroid-stimulating hormone (TSH) secretion from the pituitary.

Whereas T_4 is secreted solely from the thyroid gland, less than 20% of T_3 is produced in the thyroid. The majority of T_3 is formed from the breakdown of T_4 catalyzed by the enzyme 5′-monodeiodinase found in peripheral tissues. Because T_3 may be five times more active than T_4, the deiodinase enzymes play a pivotal role in determining overall metabolic activity. Three different 5′-monodeiodinase enzymes are present in the body.[5] Type I enzymes are present in peripheral tissues, whereas type II enzymes are found in the central nervous system, pituitary, and thyroid. Type III enzymes, found in the placenta, skin, and developing brain, inactivate T_4 and T_3.[4] The principal characteristics of these enzymes are listed in Table 71–2. T_4 may also be acted on by the enzyme 5′-monodeiodinase to form reverse T_3. Reverse T_3 has no known significant biologic activity. T_3 is removed from the body by deiodinative degradation and through the action of sulfotransferase enzyme systems to T_3 sulfate and 3,3-diiodothyronine sulfate.[6]

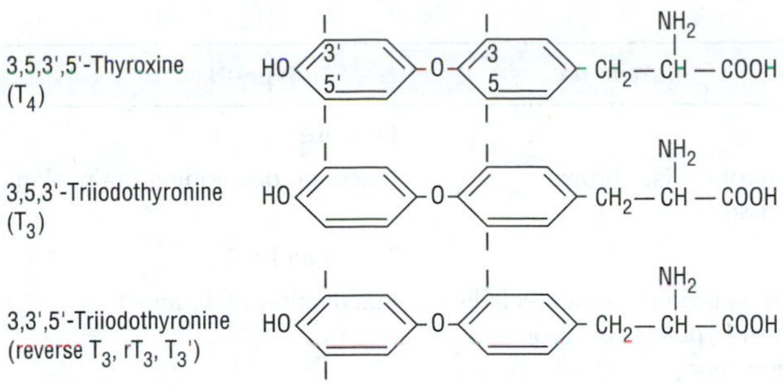

FIGURE 71–1. Structure of thyroid hormones.

TABLE 71–1. Thyroid Hormone Synthesis and Secretion Inhibitors

Mechanism of Action	Substance
Blocks iodide transport into thyroid	Bromine Fluorine Lithium
Impairs organification and coupling of thyroid hormones	Thionamides Sulfonylureas Sulfonamide (?) Salicylamide (?) Antipyrine (?)
Inhibits thyroid hormone secretion	Iodide (large doses) Lithium

THYROTROPIN RECEPTORS[7]

The growth and function of the thyroid are stimulated by activation of the thyrotropin receptor by thyroid-stimulating hormone. This receptor belongs to the family of G-protein-coupled receptors. The thyrotropin receptor is coupled to the α subunit of the stimulatory guanine-nucleotide-binding protein ($G_s\alpha$) activating adenylate cyclase and increasing the accumulation of cyclic AMP. This regulates the expression of thyroglobulin and thyroid peroxidase genes. A mutation in the receptor that results in chronic stimulation causes diffuse thyroid enlargement and hyperthyroidism (germ-line mutations) or autonomously functioning thyroid nodules (somatic mutation in an epithelial cell).[8] Conversely, thyrotropin resistance would result from point mutations, leading to abnormalities in the thyrotropin receptor–adenylate cyclase system.[7] Individuals with this abnormality have high levels of TSH but decreased thyroglobulin levels and a normal or small gland.

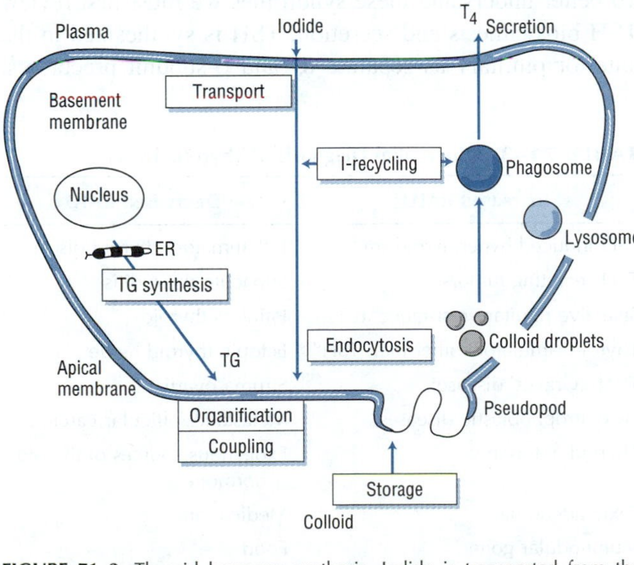

FIGURE 71–2. Thyroid hormone synthesis. Iodide is transported from the plasma, through the cell, to the apical membrane, where it is organified and coupled to thyroglobulin (TG) synthesized within the thyroid cell. Hormone stored as colloid reenters the cell through endocytosis and moves back toward the basal membrane, where T_4 is secreted. Nonhormonal iodide is recycled.

THYROID HORMONE RECEPTORS

Thyroid hormone receptors[9,10] regulate the transcription of target genes in the presence of physiologic concentrations of T_3. Thyroid receptors translocate from the cytoplasm to the nucleus and interact in the nucleus with T_3, target genes, and other proteins required for basal and T_3-dependent gene transcription. Thyroid receptors exist in multiple isoforms such as TRb2, TRb1, TRa1, and others in man and animals.

REGULATION OF THYROID HORMONE PRODUCTION

The production of thyroid hormone is regulated in two main ways. First, thyroid hormone is regulated by TSH secreted by the anterior pituitary. The secretion of TSH is itself under negative feedback control by the circulating level of free thyroid hormone and the positive influence of hypothalamic thyrotropin-releasing hormone (TRH). Second, extrathyroidal deiodination of T_4 to T_3 is regulated by a variety of factors including nutrition, nonthyroidal hormones, drugs, and illness.

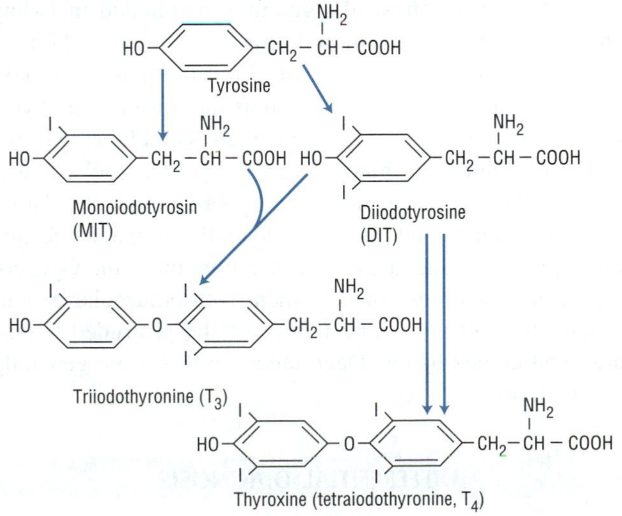

FIGURE 71–3. Scheme of coupling reactions. After tyrosine is iodinated to form MIT or DIT (organification of the iodine), MIT and DIT combine to form T_3, or two molecules of DIT form T_4.

TABLE 71–2. Properties of Iodothyronine 5′-Deiodinase Isoforms

Property	Type I	Type II	Type III
Effect of propylthiouracil	Increase	Decrease	Increase
Tissue localization	Thyroid, liver, kidney	Pituitary, thyroid, CNS, brown adipose tissue	Placenta, developing brain, skin
Preferred substrate	$rT_3 > T_4 > T_3$	$T_4 > T_3$	T_3 (sulfate) $> T_4$
Physiologic role	Extracellular T_3 production for peripheral tissue	Intracellular T_3 production, especially for brain in hypothyrodism or iodine deficiency	Inactivation of T_4 and T_3
Developmental expression	Expressed latest in development, predominant deiodinase in adult	Expressed second, especially high in brain and brown adipose tissue	Expressed first, high in developing brain, may be important for fetal thyroid hormone metabolism

T_4 = thyroxine; T_3 = triiodothyronine; rT_3 = reverse T_3; PTU = propylthiouracil.

THYROTOXICOSIS

Thyrotoxicosis[11] results when tissues are exposed to excessive levels of T_4, T_3, or both. Like many endocrine disorders, thyrotoxicosis occurs more frequently in women, with an estimated annual incidence of 3 per 1000.

CLINICAL PRESENTATION

The clinical manifestations of thyrotoxicosis include nervousness, emotional lability, easy fatigability, and heat intolerance. A cardinal sign is loss of weight concurrent with an increased appetite. In the elderly patient and in the patient with very severe disease, anorexia may be present as well. The frequency of bowel movements may increase but frank diarrhea is unusual. Palpitations are a prominent and distressing symptom, particularly in the patient with preexisting heart disease. Proximal muscle weakness is common and is noted on climbing stairs or in getting up from a sitting position. Women may note their menses are becoming scanty and irregular.

A variety of physical signs may be elicited including warm, smooth, moist skin and unusually fine hair. Separation of the end of the fingernails from the nail beds (onycholysis) may be noted. Ocular signs that result from thyrotoxicosis include retraction of the eyelids and lagging of the upper lid behind the globe when the patient looks downward (lid lag). Physical signs of a hyperdynamic circulatory state are common and include tachycardia at rest, a widened pulse pressure, and a systolic ejection murmur. Gynecomastia is sometimes noted in men. Neuromuscular examination often reveals a fine tremor of the protruded tongue and outstretched hands. Deep tendon reflexes are generally hyperactive.

DIFFERENTIAL DIAGNOSIS

Measurement of the radioactive iodine uptake (RAIU) is critical in the evaluation of the clinically thyrotoxic patient (Table 71–3). The normal 24-hour RAIU ranges from 10% to 30% with some regional variation owing to differences in iodine intake. An elevated RAIU indicates *true hyperthyroidism,* that is, the patient's thyroid gland is actively overproducing T_4, T_3, or both. Conversely, a low RAIU indicates the excess thyroid hormone is not a consequence of thyroid gland hyperfunction. The importance of differentiating true hyperthyroidism from other causes of thyrotoxicosis lies in the widely different prognosis and treatment of the diseases in these two categories. Therapy of thyrotoxicosis associated with thyroid hyperfunction is mainly directed at decreasing the rate of thyroid hormone synthesis, secretion, or both. Such measures are ineffective in treating thyrotoxicosis that is not the result of true hyperthyroidism, because hormone synthesis and regulated hormone secretion are already at a minimum.

CAUSES OF THYROTOXICOSIS ASSOCIATED WITH ELEVATED RAIU

TSH-INDUCED HYPERTHYROIDISM

To better understand these syndromes we must first review TSH biosynthesis and secretion. TSH is synthesized in the anterior pituitary as separate α- and β-subunit precursors.

TABLE 71–3. Differential Diagnosis of Thyrotoxicosis

Increased RAIU	Decreased RAIU
TSH-induced hyperthyroidism	Inflammatory thyroid disease
TSH-secreting tumors	Subacute thyroiditis
Selective pituitary resistance to T_4	Painless thyroid
Thyroid simulators other than TSH[a]	Ectopic thyroid tissue
TSAb (Graves' disease)	Struma ovarii
HCG (trophoblastic diseases)	Metastatic follicular carcinoma
Thyroid autonomy	Exogenous sources of thyroid hormone
Toxic adenoma	Medication
Multinodular goiter	Food

RAIU = radioactive iodine uptake; TSH = thyroid-stimulating hormone; TSAb = thyroid-stimulating antibodies; HCG = human chorionic gonadotropin.

[a]The RAIU may be decreased if the patient has been recently exposed to excess iodine.

Adapted from Ingbar SH, Braverman LE, Werner SC. The Thyroid, 5th ed. Philadelphia, JB Lippincott, 1986, with permission.

The α subunits from luteinizing hormone (LH), follicle-stimulating hormone (FSH), human chorionic gonadotropin (HCG), and TSH are similar whereas the β subunits are unique and confer immunologic and biologic specificity. Free β subunits are devoid of receptor binding and biologic activity and require combination with an α subunit to express their activity. Criteria for the diagnosis of TSH-induced hyperthyroidism include (1) evidence of peripheral hypermetabolism, (2) diffuse thyroid gland enlargement, (3) elevated free thyroid hormone levels, and (4) elevated serum immunoreactive TSH concentrations. Because the pituitary gland is extremely sensitive to even minimal elevations of free T_4, a detectable TSH level in any thyrotoxic patient indicates the inappropriate production of TSH.

TSH-SECRETING PITUITARY ADENOMAS

TSH-secreting pituitary tumors[12,13] occur sporadically and release biologically active hormone that is unresponsive to normal feedback control. The mean age at diagnosis is around 40 years with women being diagnosed more commonly than men (8:7). These tumors may cosecrete prolactin or growth hormone; therefore, the patients may present with amenorrhea/galactorrhea or signs of acromegaly. Most patients present with classic symptoms and signs of thyrotoxicosis. Visual-field defects may be present owing to impingement of the optic chiasm by the tumor. Tumor growth and worsening visual-field defects have been reported following treatment of thyrotoxicosis.

Diagnosis of a TSH-secreting adenoma should be made by demonstrating lack of TSH response to TRH stimulation, elevated α-subunit levels, and radiologic imaging. Note that some small tumors are not identified by MRI. Moreover, 10% of "normal" individuals may have pituitary tumors noted on pituitary imaging.[14]

Transphenoidal pituitary surgery is the treatment of choice for TSH-secreting adenomas. Pituitary gland irradiation is often given following surgery to prevent tumor recurrence. Bromocriptine has been used to treat tumors that cosecrete prolactin.

PITUITARY RESISTANCE TO THYROID HORMONE[15,16]

Pituitary resistance to thyroid hormone (PRTH) refers to selective resistance of the pituitary thyrotrophs to thyroid hormone. About twice as many women as men have been reported with this rare, probably familial syndrome. Multiple abnormalities have been reported in the initial 50 reported cases including schizophrenia (3 patients), mental retardation (2 patients), short fourth metacarpals (1 patient), and Marfanoid habitus (1 patient). About 90% of patients studied have an appropriate increase in TSH in response to TRH; conversely, the TSH will be suppressed by T_3 administration.

Patients with PRTH require treatment to reduce their elevated thyroid hormone levels. Determining the appropriate serum T_4 level is difficult because TSH cannot be used to evaluate adequacy of therapy. Any reduction in thyroid hormone carries the risk of inducing thyrotroph hyperplasia. Ideally, agents that suppress TSH secretion could be used to treat these individuals. Glucocorticoid, dopaminergic drugs, somatostatin and its analog, and thyroid hormone analogs with reduced metabolic activity have all been tried. None is ideal.

THYROID STIMULATORS OTHER THAN TSH[11]

GRAVES' DISEASE

Graves' disease[17,18] is an autoimmune syndrome that may include hyperthyroidism, diffuse thyroid enlargement, exophthalmus, pretibial myxedema, and thyroid acropachy (Figs. 71–4 and 71–5). The prevalence of Graves' disease is estimated to be 3 per 1000 population in the United States. Hyperthyroidism results from the action of thyroid-stimulating antibodies (TSAb), which are directed against the thyrotropin receptor on the surface of the thyroid cell. When these immunoglobulin G (IgG) antibodies bind to the receptor, they activate the enzyme adenylate cyclase in the same manner as TSH. Autoantibodies that react with orbital muscle and fibroblast tissue in the skin are responsible for the extrathyroidal manifestations of Graves' disease, and these autoantibodies are encoded by the same germ-line genes that encode for other autoantibodies for striated muscle and thyroid peroxidase. The defect leading to abnormal antibody production may be a genomic point mutation in the extracellular domain of the thyrotropin receptor.[7] Clinically, the extrathyroidal disorders may not appear at the same time that hyperthyroidism develops.

There is now compelling evidence that heredity and gender both play a role in the development of clinically overt

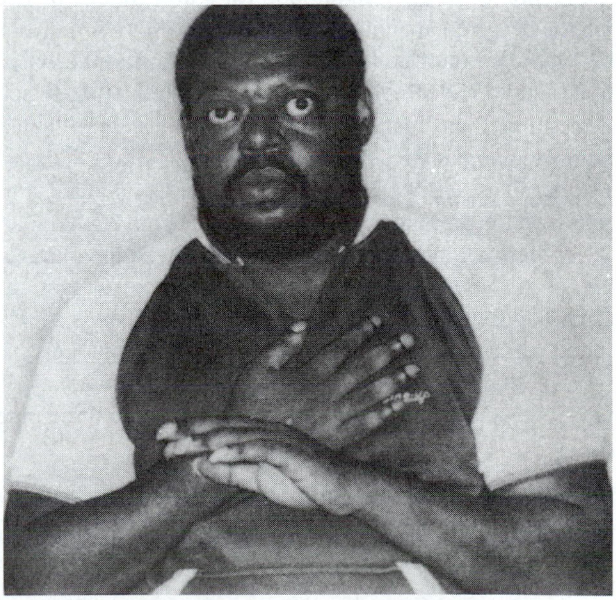

FIGURE 71–4. A 33-year-old man with Graves' disease manifested by bilateral exophthalmos, achropachy (clubbing), and extensive pretibial myxedema. When this photograph was taken, he already had been treated with radioactive ^{131}I, had become hypothyroid, and was receiving replacement therapy with exogenous L-thyroxine. *(From Becker KL, ed. Principles and Practice of Endocrinology and Metabolism. Philadelphia, Lippincott, 1990, with permission.)*

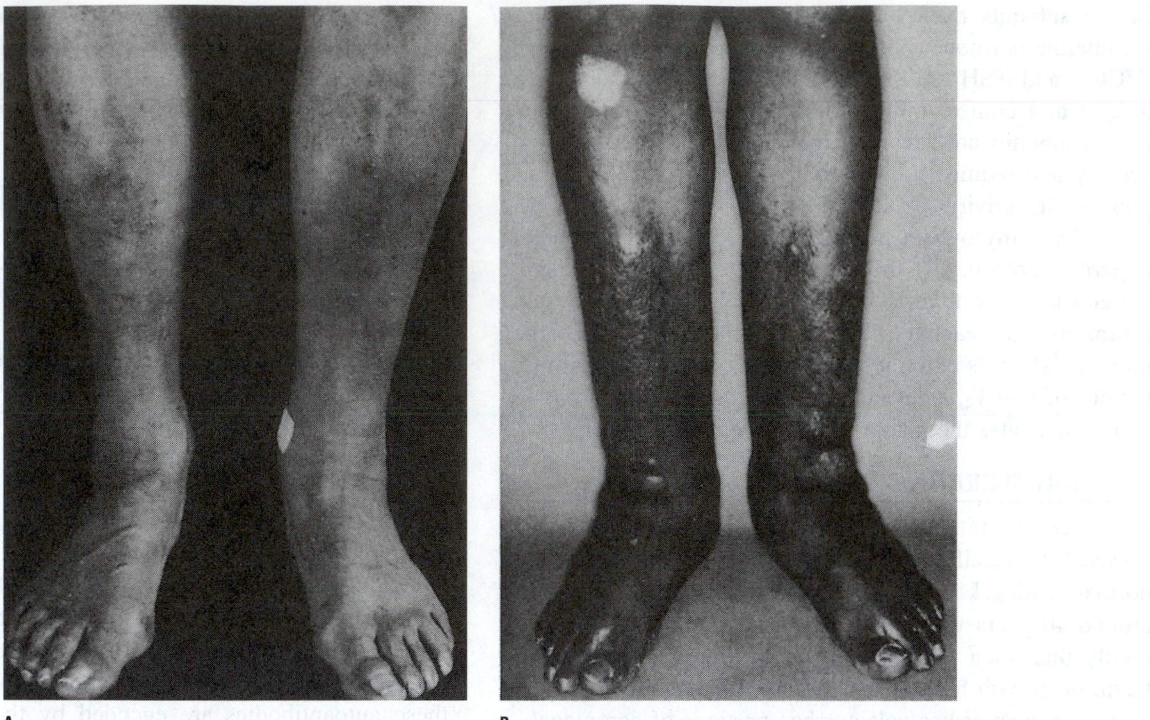

A B

FIGURE 71–5. (A and B): Different degrees of involvement of tissues with pretibial myxedema. *(From Becker KL ed. Principles and Practice of Endocrinology and Metabolism. Philadelphia, Lippincott, 1990, with permission.)*

thyroid disease. Several lines of evidence support a role for heredity. First, there is a well-recognized clustering of Graves' disease within some families. Twin studies in patients with Graves' disease have revealed that a monozygotic twin has a 50% likelihood of ultimately developing the disease compared to a 9% likelihood for a dizygotic twin. Second, the occurrence of other autoimmune diseases, including Hashimoto's thyroiditis, is also increased in families of patients with Graves' disease. Third, several studies have demonstrated an increased frequency of certain human leukocyte antigens (HLAs) in patients with Graves' disease. In Caucasians, HLA-D3 is present in at least one-half of patients, and the presence in an individual of both HLA-B8 and -D3 confers a fourfold greater risk for developing Graves' disease. A role for gender in the emergence of Graves' disease is suggested by the fact that hyperthyroidism is approximately eight times more common in women than men.

The thyroid gland is diffusely enlarged in the majority of patients and is commonly 40 to 60 g (two to three times the normal size). The surface of the gland is smooth and the consistency varies from soft to firm. In patients with severe disease, a thrill may be felt and a systolic bruit may be heard over the gland. The presence of any of the extrathyroidal manifestations of this syndrome including exophthalmus, thyroid acropachy, or pretibial myxedema in a thyrotoxic patient is pathognomonic of Graves' disease (see Fig. 71–4). An important clinical feature of Graves' disease is the occurrence of spontaneous remissions. The abnormalities in thyroid-stimulating antibody production may decrease or disappear over time in many patients.

The results of laboratory tests in thyrotoxic Graves' disease include an increase in the overall hormone production rate with a disproportionate increase in T_3 relative to T_4 (Table 71–4). In an occasional patient, the disproportionate overproduction of T_3 is exaggerated with the result that only the serum T_3 concentration is increased (T_3 toxicosis). The saturation of thyroid-binding globulin (TBG) is increased owing to the elevated levels of serum T_4 and T_3. This is re-

TABLE 71–4. Thyroid Function Test Results in Different Thyroid Conditions

	Total T_4	Free T_4	Total T_3	T_3 Resin Uptake	Free Thyroxine Index	TSH
Normal	4.5–12.5 μg/dL	0.8–1.5 ng/dL	80–220 ng/dL	22%–34%	1.0–4.3 U	0.2–4.8 mIU/mL
Hyperthyroid	↑↑	↑↑	↑↑↑	↑	↑↑↑	↓↓
Hypothyroid	↓↓	↓↓	↓	↓↓	↓↓↓	↑↑
Increased TBG	↑	Normal	↑	↓	Normal	Normal

TSH = thyroid-stimulating hormone; TBG = thyroid-binding globulin.

flected in elevated values for the T_3 resin uptake. As a result, the concentration of free T_4, free T_3, and the free T_4 and T_3 indices are increased to an even greater extent than are the measured serum total T_4 and T_3 concentrations. The TSH level will be undetectable owing to negative feedback by elevated levels of thyroid hormone at the pituitary.

In the patient with manifest disease, measurement of the serum T_4 concentration, T_3 resin uptake (or free T_4), and the TSH value will confirm the diagnosis of thyrotoxicosis. If the patient is not pregnant, a 24-hour RAIU should be obtained. An increased RAIU documents that the thyroid gland is inappropriately utilizing the iodine to produce more thyroid hormone at a time when the patient is thyrotoxic.

Hypokalemic periodic paralysis is a rare complication of hyperthyroidism commonly observed in Asian and Hispanic populations. It presents as recurrent proximal muscle flaccidity ranging from mild weakness to total paralysis. The paralysis may be asymmetric and usually involves muscle groups that are strenuously exercised before the attack. Cognition and sensory perception are spared whereas deep tendon reflexes are commonly markedly diminished. Hypokalemia results from a shift of potassium from extracellular to intracellular sites. High carbohydrate loads and exercise provoke the attacks. Treatment includes correcting the hyperthyroid state, potassium administration, spironolactone to conserve potassium, and propranolol to minimize intracellular shifts.[9]

TROPHOBLASTIC DISEASES

In the past decade several lines of evidence have shown that HCG is a thyroid stimulator and may cause hyperthyroidism.[11,20] The basis for the thyrotropic effect of HCG is the structural similarity of HCG to TSH (similar α subunits and unique β subunits). In hyperthyroid patients with very high HCG levels, serum TSH may be inappropriately detectable owing to the weak cross-reactivity of HCG in the radioimmunoassay for TSH. In patients with hyperthyroidism caused by trophoblastic tumors, serum HCG levels usually exceed 300 U/mL and always exceed 100 U/mL. The mean peak HCG level in normal pregnancy is 50 U/mL. On a molar basis, HCG has only 1/10,000 the activity of pituitary TSH in mouse bioassays. Nevertheless, this thyrotropic activity may be very substantial in patients with trophoblastic tumors, whose serum HCG concentrations may reach 2000 U/mL.

THYROID AUTONOMY

TOXIC ADENOMA[21,22]

An autonomous thyroid nodule is a discrete thyroid mass whose function is independent of pituitary control. The prevalence of toxic adenoma ranges from about 2% to 9% of thyrotoxic patients and depends on iodine availability and geographic location. Toxic adenomas arise from gain-of-function somatic or germ-line mutations of the $G_s\alpha$ protein or the TSH receptor; more that a dozen TSH receptor mutations have been described.[21] These nodules may be referred to as a toxic adenoma or a "hot" nodule because of their appearance on a radioiodine thyroid scan (Fig. 71–6). The amount of thyroid hormone produced by an autonomous nodule is mass related. Therefore, hyperthyroidism usually

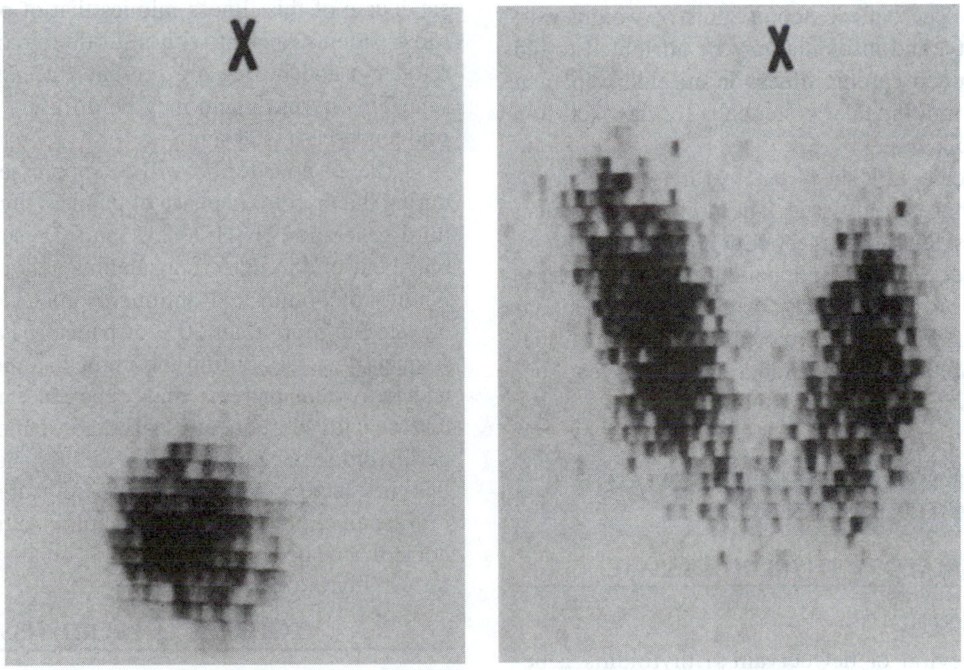

FIGURE 71–6. Left, autonomously functioning nodule is suppressing the remainder of thyroid gland. Right, previously suppressed lobes of thyroid gland are visualized 3 months after radioiodine treatment of hyperfunctioning nodule. The "X" is a marker for thyroid cartilage. *(From Becker KL, ed. Principles and Practice of Endocrinology and Metabolism. Philadelphia, Lippincott, 1990, with permission.)*

occurs with larger nodules, that is, those more than 4 cm in diameter. Older patients (~ 60 years) are more likely (up to 60%) to be thyrotoxic from autonomous nodules than are younger patients (~ 12%). There are many reports of isolated elevation of serum T_3 in patients with autonomously functioning nodules. Therefore, if the T_4 level is normal, a T_3 level must be measured to rule out T_3 toxicosis. Once a radioiodine scan has demonstrated that the toxic thyroid adenoma would collect more radioiodine than the surrounding tissue, independent function may be documented by a failure of the autonomous nodule to decrease its iodine uptake during exogenous T_3 administration. RAI ablation, subtotal thyroidectomy, thionamides, and percutaneous ethanol injection are treatment options but since thionamides do not halt the proliferative process in the nodule, definitive therapies are recommended. Because thyroid carcinoma is not a major consideration in an autonomously functioning thyroid nodule, observation is usually recommended for patients with autonomously functioning nodules who are euthyroid.

MULTINODULAR GOITERS

In multinodular goiters (MNGs; Plummer's disease),[21] follicles with a very high degree of autonomous function coexist with normal or even nonfunctioning follicles. Thyrotoxicosis in a multinodular goiter occurs when the follicles with a high degree of autonomy generate enough thyroid hormone to exceed the needs of the patient. The pathogenesis of multinodular goiter is thought to be similar to toxic adenoma.[23] It is not surprising that this type of hyperthyroidism develops insidiously over a period of several years and predominantly affects older individuals with longstanding goiters. Often, elderly women present with subtle signs of hyperthyroidism that are superimposed on underlying heart disease. The patient's complaints of weight loss, depression, anxiety, and insomnia may be attributed to old age. Any unexplained chronic illness in an elderly patient presenting with a multinodular goiter calls for the exclusion of hidden thyrotoxicosis.

A thyroid scan will show patchy areas of autonomously functioning thyroid tissue. The preferred treatment for toxic MNG is RAI or surgery. Surgery is usually selected for younger patients and patients in whom large goiters impinge on vital organs. Alternatively, percutaneous injection of 95% ethanol has also been used to destroy single or multinodular adenomas with a 5-year success rate approaching 80%.[24]

CAUSES OF THYROTOXICOSIS ASSOCIATED WITH SUPPRESSED RAIU

INFLAMMATORY THYROID DISEASE

SUBACUTE THYROIDITIS

Painful subacute (viral or deQuervain's) thyroiditis is believed to be caused by viral invasion of thyroid parenchyma. Typically, patients complain of severe pain in the thyroid region, which often extends to the ear on the affected side. With time, the pain may migrate from one side of the gland to the other. Low-grade fever is common. Systemic symptoms owing to thyrotoxicosis are present. On physical examination, the thyroid gland is firm and exquisitely tender. Signs of thyrotoxicosis are present.

Thyroid function tests typically run a triphasic course. Initially, serum thyroxine levels are elevated owing to release of preformed thyroid hormone from disrupted follicles. The 24-hour RAIU during this time is less than 2% owing to thyroid inflammation and TSH suppression by the elevated thyroxine level. As the disease progresses, intrathyroidal hormone stores are depleted and the patient may become mildly hypothyroid with an appropriately elevated TSH level. During the recovery phase thyroid hormone stores are replenished and serum TSH elevation gradually returns to normal. Recovery is generally complete within 2 to 6 months. Most patients remain euthyroid and recurrences of painful thyroiditis are extremely rare. The patient with painful thyroiditis should be reassured that the disease is self-limited and is unlikely to recur. Thyrotoxic symptoms may be relieved with β-blockers. Aspirin (650 mg orally every 6 hours) will usually relieve the pain. Occasionally, prednisone (20 mg orally three times a day) must be used to suppress the inflammatory process. Antithyroid drugs are not indicated because they do not decrease the release of preformed thyroid hormone.

PAINLESS THYROIDITIS

Since its description in 1975, painless (silent, lymphocytic, postpartum) thyroiditis has been recognized as a common cause of thyrotoxicosis and may represent up to 15% of cases of thyrotoxicosis in North America. The etiology is not fully understood and may be heterogeneous. The triphasic course of this illness mimics that of painful thyroiditis. Most patients present with mild thyrotoxic symptoms. Lid retraction and lid lag are present but exophthalmos is absent. The thyroid gland may be diffusely enlarged but thyroid tenderness is absent.

The 24-hour RAIU will be suppressed to less than 2% during the thyrotoxic phase of painless thyroiditis; however, third-generation TSH assays and T_3 suppression testing may be useful in detecting subclinical hyperthyroidism.[25,26] Antithyroglobulin and antimicrosomal antibody levels are elevated in more than 50% of patients. Painless thyroiditis frequently occurs during the immediate postpartum period, and individual patients may experience recurrence of the disease with subsequent pregnancies. Patients with mild hyperthyroidism and painless thyroiditis should be reassured that they have a self-limited disease. Adrenergic symptoms may be ameliorated with propranolol. Antithyroid drugs are not indicated because they do not decrease the release of preformed thyroid hormone.

ECTOPIC THYROID TISSUE

STRUMA OVARII

Struma ovarii is a teratoid tumor of the ovary that is capable of making thyroid hormone. This extremely rare cause of thyrotoxicosis is suggested by the absence of thyroid enlargement in a thyrotoxic patient with a suppressed RAIU. The diagnosis is established by localizing functioning thyroid tissue in the ovary with whole-body radioactive iodine (^{131}I) scanning. Interestingly, struma ovarii without associated hyperthyroidism is much more common than struma ovarii associated with hyperthyroidism. Because the tissue is neoplastic and potentially malignant, combined surgical and radioiodine treatment of malignant struma ovarii for both monitoring and therapy of relapse is the recommended treatment.[27]

FOLLICULAR CANCER

In widely metastatic follicular carcinomas with relatively well-preserved function, sufficient thyroid hormone can be synthesized and secreted to produce thyrotoxicosis. In most instances, a previous diagnosis of thyroid malignancy has been made. The diagnosis can be confirmed by whole-body ^{131}I scanning. Treatment with ^{131}I is generally effective at ablating functioning thyroid metastases.

EXOGENOUS SOURCES OF THYROID HORMONE

MEDICATION

The term *thyrotoxicosis factitia* denotes hyperthyroidism produced by the ingestion of exogenous thyroid hormone. Obesity is the most common nonthyroidal disorder for which thyroid hormone is used, but thyroid hormone has been used for almost every conceivable problem from menstrual irregularities and infertility to baldness. Because these patients do not benefit from treatment with thyroid hormone, the physician or patient may gradually increase the dose of hormone employed in an attempt to gain the desired effect. Obviously, thyrotoxicosis factitia can also occur when too large a dose of thyroid hormone is employed for conditions in which it is likely to be beneficial, such as hypothyroidism or nontoxic goiter. Rarely, thyrotoxicosis factitia is caused by the purposeful and secretive ingestion of thyroid hormone by disturbed patients (usually with a medical background) who wish to obtain attention or lose weight.

Thyrotoxicosis factitia should be suspected in a thyrotoxic patient without infiltrative ophthalmopathy or thyroid enlargement. The RAIU uptake is at low levels because the patient's thyroid gland function is suppressed by the exogenous thyroid hormone. Measurement of plasma thyroglobulin (TG) is a valuable laboratory aid in the diagnosis of thyrotoxicosis factitia. TG is normally secreted in small amounts by the thyroid gland; however, when thyroid hormone is taken orally, very low amounts of thyroglobulin are detectable in the plasma. In other entities characterized by a low RAIU, such as silent thyroiditis, leakage of preformed thyroid hormone results in elevated thyroglobulin levels. If a history of thyroid hormone ingestion is elicited or deduced, exogenous thyroid hormone should be withheld for between 4 and 6 weeks and thyroid function tests repeated to document that the euthyroid state has been restored.

Amiodarone may induce thyrotoxicosis (2% to 3% of patients) or hypothyroidism. Amiodarone contains 37.2% iodine by weight and approximately 6 mg/d of iodine is released for each 200 mg of amiodarone.[3,28] The recommended daily amount of iodine is 200 μg/d. Amiodarone interferes with type I 5′-deiodinase, leading to reduced conversion of T_4 to T_3, and iodide released from the drug owing to deiodination contributes to iodine excess, especially in iodine-deficient areas. Amiodarone also causes a destructive thyroiditis with loss of thyroglobulin and thyroid hormones. Iodine-induced thyroid dysfunction occurs primarily in patients with preexisting thyroid disease (Graves' disease, nodular goiter, Hashimoto's thyroiditis) known as type I or in patients who have apparently normal thyroid glands (type II). The two types may be differentiated using color flow Doppler ultrasonography.[29] Type I amiodarone-induced hyperthyroidism responds well to thionamides whereas type II may require glucocorticoids. An inflammatory process induced by amiodarone or iodine, which also leads to follicular cell damage and subacute thyroiditis with leakage of thyroid hormones into the circulation, is associated with elevated interleukin-6 (IL-6) levels. The manifestations may be untypical symptoms such as ventricular tachycardia and exacerbation of underlying chronic obstructive pulmonary disease. Prednisone has been reported to normalize IL-6 and thyroid hormone values.[30]

Iodinated glycerol improves some symptoms of chronic obstructive pulmonary disease but no objective measures of pulmonary function. This compound contains 15 mg of organic iodine per tablet or 25 mg/mL of solution. Thyroid dysfunction has been reported with this preparation, and patients with underlying thyroid disease need to be monitored carefully if iodinated glycerol is used.[31]

▶ TREATMENT: Hyperthyroidism

Three common treatment modalities are used in the management of hyperthyroidism: surgery, antithyroid medications, and radioactive iodine (RAI) (Table 71–5). The overall therapeutic objectives are to eliminate the excess thyroid hormone and minimize the symptoms and long-term consequences of hyperthyroidism. Therapy must be individualized based on the type and severity of hyperthyroidism, patient age and gender, existence of nonthyroidal conditions, and response to previous therapy.[11,32,33] Minimum clinical guidelines for the treatment of hyperthyroidism have been published by the American Thyroid Association.[34]

SURGERY

Surgical removal of the thyroid gland became feasible in 1923 when Plummer discovered that iodine reduced the gland's vascularity, making this definitive procedure possible. Traditional

TABLE 71–5. Management of Hyperthyroidism

Modality	Maintenance Dose (mg/d)	Maximum Dose (mg/d)	Actions	Indications
Thiourea drugs			Inhibit thyroid hormone synthesis (PTU also inhibits peripheral conversion of T_4 to T_3); may exert immunosuppressive actions	First-line therapy for Graves' hyperthyroidism, short-term therapy before ^{131}I or surgery
Propylthiouracil (PTU), 50-mg tablets	200–600	1200		
Methimazole (Tapazole), 5- and 10-mg tablets	10–60	120		
β-Adrenergic antagonists[a]			Ameliorate action of thyroid hormone in tissues	Adjunctive therapy; often therapy required for thyroiditis
Propranolol	80–160	480		
Nadolol	80–160	320		
Iodine-containing compounds			Inhibit T_4 and T_3 release	Preparation for surgery; thyrotoxic crisis
Lugol's solution	750	750		
Potassium iodide (SSKI)	10–300	400		
Miscellaneous				
Potassium perchlorate	NA	NA	Inhibits iodine transport	No routine indications
Lithium carbonate	NA	NA	Inhibits thyroid hormone synthesis and release	No routine indications
Glucocorticoids			Ameliorates actions of thyroid hormones in tissues; exerts hyperthyroidism, short-term immunosuppressive action (Graves' disease)	Severe subacute thyroiditis; thyrotoxic crisis
Radioactive iodine (RAI, ^{131}I)	NA	5–29 mCi	Ablation of thyroid gland	First-line therapy for Graves' hyperthyroidism, treatment of choice for recurrent thyrotoxicosis; young adults to elderly; contraindicated in pregnancy, children, and active ophthalmopathy
Surgery	NA	NA	Removal of thyroid gland	Patients should be euthyroid prior to surgery; caution in elderly; cold iodine given prior to surgery

SSKI = saturated solution of potassium iodide; NA = not applicable.
[a]Not approved in the United States by the FDA for the treatment of thyrotoxicosis.

preparation of the patient for thyroidectomy includes propylthiouracil (PTU) or methimazole (MMI) until the patient is biochemically euthyroid (usually 6 to 8 weeks), followed by the addition of iodides (500 mg/d) for 10 to 14 days before surgery to decrease the vascularity of the gland. Levothyroxine may be added to maintain the euthyroid state while the thionamides are continued. Propranolol for several weeks preoperatively and 7 to 10 days after surgery has also been used to maintain a pulse rate of less than 90 beats/min. Combined pretreatment with propranolol and 10 to 14 days of potassium iodide also has been advocated.

The overall morbidity rate with surgery is 2.7%. Hyperthyroidism persists or recurs in 0.6% to 17.9% of patients after thyroidectomy for Graves' disease and is more common in children. The most common complications of surgery include hypothyroidism (up to about 49%), hypoparathyroidism (up to 3.9%), and vocal cord abnormalities (up to 5.4%). The frequent occurrence of hypothyroidism following surgery requires periodic follow-up for identification and treatment of these patients.[35]

PHARMACOLOGIC THERAPY

ANTITHYROID MEDICATIONS[36]

THIOUREA DRUGS

Two drugs within this category, PTU and MMI, are approved for the treatment of hyperthyroidism in the United States. They are classified as thioureylenes (thionamides), which incorporate a N—C—S=N group into their ring structures.

Mechanism of Action

PTU and MMI share several mechanisms to inhibit the biosynthesis of thyroid hormone.[33] These drugs serve as preferential substrates for the iodinating intermediate of thyroid peroxidase and divert iodine away from potential iodination sites in thyroglobulin.[36] This prevents subsequent incorporation of iodine into iodotyrosines and ultimately iodothyronine ("organification"). Second, they inhibit coupling of monoiodotyrosine and diiodotyrosine to form T_4 and T_3. The coupling reaction may be more sensitive to these drugs than the iodination reaction. Experimentally, these drugs exhibit immunosuppressive effects, although the clinical relevance of this finding is unclear. In patients with Graves' disease, antithyroid drug treatment has been associated with lower TSAb titers and restoration of normal suppressor T-cell function. However, perchlorate, which has a different mechanism of action, also decreases thyroid-stimulating antibodies, suggesting that normalization of the thyroid hormone level may itself improve the abnormal immune function. PTU inhibits the peripheral conversion of T_4 to T_3. This effect is acutely dose related and occurs within hours of PTU administration. MMI does not have this effect. Over time, depletion of stored hormone and lack of continuing synthesis of thyroid hormone results in the clinical effects of these drugs.

Pharmacokinetics

Both antithyroid drugs are well absorbed (80% to 95%) from the gastrointestinal tract, with peak serum concentrations about 1 hour after ingestion. The plasma half-life ranges of PTU and MMI are 1 to 2.5 hours and 6 to 9 hours, respectively, and are not appreciably affected by thyroid status. Urinary excretion is about 35% for PTU and less than 10% for MMI. These drugs are actively concentrated in the thyroid gland, which may account for the disparity between their relatively short plasma half-lives and the effectiveness of once-daily dosing regimens even with PTU. Approximately 60% to 80% of PTU is bound to plasma albumin whereas MMI is not protein bound. Methimazole readily crosses the placenta and appears in breast milk. Older studies suggested that PTU crosses the placental membranes only one-tenth as well as MMI; however, these studies were done in the course of therapeutic abortion early in pregnancy. Newer studies show little difference between fetal concentrations of PTU and MMI and both are associated with elevated TSH in about 20% and low T_4 in about 7% of the fetuses.[37]

Dosing and Monitoring

PTU is available as 50-mg tablets and MMI as 5- and 10-mg tablets. MMI is approximately 10 times more potent than PTU. Initial therapy with PTU ranges from 300 to 600 mg daily, usually in 3 or 4 divided doses. MMI is given in three divided doses totaling 30 to 60 mg/d. Although the traditional recommendation is for divided doses, evidence exists that both drugs can be given as single daily doses.[38] Patients with severe hyperthyroidism may require larger initial doses, and some may respond better at these larger doses if the dose is divided. The maximal blocking doses of PTU and MMI are 1200 and 120 mg daily, respectively. Once the intrathyroidial pool of thyroid hormone is reduced and new hormone synthesis is sufficiently blocked, clinical improvement should ensue. Usually within 4 to 8 weeks of initiating therapy, symptoms are diminished and circulating thyroid hormone levels are returning to normal. At this time the tapering regimen can be started. Changes in dose for each drug should be made on a monthly basis, because the endogenously produced T_4 will reach a new "steady-state" concentration in this interval. Typical ranges of daily maintenance doses for PTU and MMI are 50 to 300 mg and 5 to 30 mg, respectively.

If the objective of therapy is to induce a long-term remission, the patient should remain on continuous antithyroid drug therapy for 12 to 24 months. Antithyroid drug therapy induces permanent remission rates of 10% to 98% with an overall average of about 40% to 50%. This is much higher than the remission rate seen with propranolol alone, which is reported to range from 22% to 36%. Patient characteristics for a favorable outcome include older patients (> 40 years), low ratio of T_4 to T_3 (< 20), a small goiter (less than 50 g), short duration of disease (less than 6 months), no previous history of relapse with antithyroid drugs, duration of therapy 1 to 2 years or longer, and low TSAb titers at baseline or a reduction with treatment.[36] It is important that patients be followed every 6 to 12 months after remission occurs. If a relapse occurs, alternate therapy with RAI is preferred to a second course of antithyroid drugs. Relapses seem to plateau after about 5 years and eventually 5% to 20% of patients will develop spontaneous hypothyroidism.

Concurrent administration of thyroxine with thionamide therapy for thyrotoxicosis and subclinical hyperthyroidism may reduce autoantibodies directed toward the thyroid gland and improve the remission rate; however, these effects have not been consistently observed in all studies.[36] In a Japanese study, adjunctive treatment with thyroxine was associated with a 20-fold reduction in the recurrence rate of Graves' disease compared to the recurrence rate seen in patients treated with antithyroid drugs alone. Attempts to reproduce these results in American and European patients with Graves' disease have failed to show any delay or reduction in the recurrence of Graves' disease with thyroxine administration.[39]

Adverse Effects

Minor adverse reactions to PTU and MMI have an overall incidence of 5% to 16% depending on the dose and the drug, whereas major adverse effects occur in 1.5% to 4.6% of patients receiving these drugs.[40] Pruritic maculopapular rashes (sometimes associated with vasculitis based on skin biopsy), arthralgias, and fevers occur in up to 5% of patients and may occur at greater frequency with higher doses and in children. Rashes often disappear spontaneously, but if persistent, may be managed with antihistamines.

Perhaps one of the most common side effects is a benign transient leukopenia characterized by a white blood cell (WBC) count of less than 4000/mm. This condition occurs in up to 12% of adults and 25% of children and sometimes can be confused with mild leukopenia seen in Graves' disease. This mild leukopenia is not a harbinger of the more serious adverse effect of agranulocytosis, so therapy can usually be continued. If a *minor* adverse reaction occurs with one antithyroid drug, the alternate thiourea may be tried, but cross-sensitivity occurs in about 50% of patients.[36]

Agranulocytosis is the most serious adverse effect of thiourea drug therapy and is characterized by fever, malaise, gingivitis, oropharyngeal infection, and a granulocyte count less than $250/mm^3$.[36] These drugs are concentrated in granulocytes and this reaction may represent a direct toxic effect rather than hypersensitivity. This toxic reaction has occurred with both thioureas, and the incidence varies from 0.5% to 6%. It is higher in patients over age 40 receiving a methimazole dose greater than 40 mg/d or the equivalent dose of PTU and is linked to HLA class II genes containing the DRB1*08032 allele.[41] Agranulocytosis almost always develops in the first 3 months of therapy. Because the onset is sudden, routine monitoring is not recommended. Colony-stimulating factors have been used with some success to restore cell counts to normal. Peripheral lymphocytes obtained from patients with PTU-induced agranulocytosis undergo transformation in the presence of other thioamides, suggesting that these severe reactions are immunologically mediated and patients should not receive other thionamides. Aplastic anemia has been reported with MMI and may be associated with an inhibitor to colony-forming units. Once antithyroid drugs are discontinued, clinical improvement is seen over several days to weeks. Patients should be counseled to discontinue therapy and contact their physician when flu-like symptoms such as fever, malaise, or sore throat develop.

Arthralgias and a lupus-like syndrome (sometimes in the absence of antinuclear antibodies) has been reported in 4% to 5% of patients. This generally occurs after 6 months of therapy. Uncommonly, polymyositis, presenting as proximal muscle weakness and elevated creatine phosphokinase, has been reported with PTU administration. Gastrointestinal intolerance is also reported to occur in 4% to 5% of patients. Hepatotoxicity, which usually occurs within the first 3 months of therapy, may be seen with both methimazole and PTU with a prevalence of about 1.3%.[42,43] At moderate doses, some authors have found that initial enzyme elevations eventually normalize in most patients with continued therapy. High doses of PTU are more likely to produce severe hepatitis and even death. Discontinuation of therapy usually results in complete resolution of hepatitis. Patients receiving interferon products for hepatitis C or other disorders may develop hyper- or hypothyroidism along with liver enzyme abnormalities.[44] Although older reports suggested that congenital skin defects (aplasia cutis) may be caused by methimazole and carbimazole, a recent registry review from the Netherlands could not find an association between maternal use of these drugs and skin defects.[45] Hypoprothrombinemia is a rare complication of thionamide therapy. Patients who have experienced a *major* adverse reaction to one thiourea drug should not be converted to the alternate drug because of cross-sensitivity.

IODIDES

Iodide was the first form of drug therapy for Graves' disease. Its mechanism of action is to acutely block thyroid hormone release, inhibit thyroid hormone biosynthesis by interfering with intrathyroidal iodide utilization (the Wolff–Chaikoff effect), and decrease the size and vascularity of the gland. This early inhibitory effect provides symptom improvement within 2 to 7 days of initiating therapy, and serum T_4 and T_3 concentrations may be reduced for a few weeks. Despite the reduced release of T_4 and T_3, thyroid hormone synthesis continues at an accelerated rate, resulting in a gland rich in stored hormones. The normal and hyperfunctioning thyroid soon escapes from this inhibitory effect within 1 to 2 weeks by decreasing the active transfer of iodide into the gland. Iodides are often used as adjunctive therapy to prepare a patient with Graves' disease for surgery, to acutely inhibit thyroid hormone release and quickly attain the euthyroid state in severely thyrotoxic patients with cardiac decompensation,[36] or to inhibit thyroid hormone release following radioactive iodine therapy. However, large doses of iodine may exacerbate hyperthyroidism or indeed precipitate hyperthyroidism in some previously euthyroid individuals (Jod–Basedow disease). This Jod–Basedow phenomenon is most common in iodine-deficient areas, particularly in patients with preexisting nontoxic goiter. Iodide is contraindicated in toxic multinodular goiter.

Potassium iodide is available either as a saturated solution (SSKI), which contains 38 mg of iodide per drop, or as Lugol's solution, which contains 6.3 mg of iodide per drop. The typical starting dose of SSKI is 3 to 10 drops daily (120 to 400 mg) in water or juice. There is no documented advantage to using doses in excess of 6 to 8 mg/d. When used to prepare a patient for surgery, it should be administered 7 to 14 days preoperatively. As an adjunct to RAI, SSKI should not be used before, but rather 3 to 7 days after RAI treatment so that the radioactive iodide can concentrate in the thyroid. The most frequent toxic effect with iodide therapy is hypersensitivity reactions (skin rashes, drug fever, rhinitis, conjunctivitis); salivary gland swelling; "iodism" (metallic taste, burning mouth and throat, sore teeth and gums, symptoms of a head cold, and sometimes stomach upset and diarrhea); and gynecomastia.

Other compounds containing organic iodide have also been used therapeutically for hyperthyroidism. These include various radiologic contrast media that share a triiodo- and monoaminobenzene ring with a propionic acid chain (e.g., iopanoic acid and sodium ipodate). The effect of these compounds is a result of the iodine content inhibiting thyroid hormone release as well as competitive inhibition of 5′-monodeiodinase conversion related to their structures, which resemble thyroid analogs.[3]

ADRENERGIC BLOCKERS

Because many of the manifestations of hyperthyroidism are mediated by β-adrenergic receptors, β-blockers (especially propranolol) have been used widely to ameliorate thyrotoxic symptoms such as palpitations, anxiety, tremor, and heat intolerance. Although β-blockers are quite effective for symptom control, they have no effect on the urinary excretion of calcium, phosphorus, hydroxyproline, creatinine, or various amino acids, suggesting a lack of effect on peripheral thyrotoxicosis and protein metabolism. Furthermore, β-blockers do not reduce TSAb nor prevent thyroid storm. Propranolol and nadolol partially block the conversion of T_4 to T_3 but this contribution to the overall therapeutic effect is small in magnitude. Inhibition of conversion of T_4 to T_3 is mediated by D-propranolol, which is devoid of β-blocking activity, and L-propranolol, which is responsible for the antiadrenergic effects, has little effect on the conversion.

β-Blockers are usually used as adjunctive therapy with antithyroid drugs, RAI, or iodides when treating Graves' disease or toxic nodules; in preparation for surgery; or in thyroid storm. The only conditions for which β-blockers are primary therapy for thyrotoxicosis are thyroiditis and iodine-induced hyperthyroidism. The dose of propranolol required to relieve adrenergic symptoms is variable, but an initial dose of 20 to 40 mg four times daily is effective (heart rate less than 90 beats/min) for most patients. Younger or more severely toxic patients may require as much as 240 to 480 mg/d because there seems to be an increased clearance rate in these patients. β-Blockers are contraindicated in patients with congestive heart failure unless it is caused solely by tachycardia (high output) and in patients who have developed cardiomyopathy and heart failure. Nonselective agents and those lacking intrinsic sympathomimetic activity (ISA) should be used with caution in patients with asthma, chronic obstructive lung disease, and diabetes mellitus (particularly insulin-dependent diabetes). Cardioselective and ISA β-blockers may have a slight margin of safety in these situations. Other patients in whom contraindications exist are those with sinus bradycardia, those receiving monoamine oxidase inhibitors or tricyclic antidepressants, and those with spontaneous hypoglycemia. β-Blockers may also prolong gestation and labor during pregnancy. Other side effects include nausea, vomiting, anxiety, insomnia, light-headedness, bradycardia, and hematologic disturbances.

Antiadrenergic agents such as centrally acting sympatholytics and calcium channel antagonists may have some role in the symptomatic treatment of hyperthyroidism. These drugs might be useful when contraindications to β-blockade exist. When compared to nadolol 40 mg twice daily, clonidine 150 μg twice daily reduced plasma catecholamines, whereas nadolol increased both epinephrine and norepinephrine after 1 week of treatment. Diltiazem 120 mg given every 8 hours reduced heart rate by 17%; fewer ventricular extrasystoles were noted after 10 days of therapy, and diltiazem has been shown to be comparable to propranolol in lowering heart rate and blood pressure.

RADIOACTIVE IODINE[17,46]

Although other radioisotopes have been used to ablate thyroid tissue, sodium iodide 131 (^{131}I) is considered to be the agent of choice for Graves' disease, toxic autonomous nodules, and toxic multinodular goiters. RAI is administered as a colorless and tasteless liquid that is well absorbed and concentrates in the thyroid. Sodium iodide 131 is a β-emitter with a tissue penetration of 2 mm and a half-life of 8 days. Other organs take up ^{131}I but the thyroid gland is the only organ in which organification of the absorbed iodine takes place. Initially, RAI disrupts hormone synthesis by incorporating into thyroid hormones and thyroglobulin. Over a period of weeks, follicles that have taken up RAI and surrounding follicles develop evidence of cellular necrosis, breakdown of follicles, development of bizarre cell forms, nuclear pyknosis, and destruction of small vessels within the gland, leading to edema and fibrosis of the interstitial tissue. Pregnancy is an absolute contraindication to the use of RAI.

β-Blockers may be given anytime without compromising RAI therapy, accounting for their role as a mainstay of adjunctive therapy to RAI treatment. If iodides are administered, they should be given 3 to 7 days *after* RAI to prevent interference with the uptake of RAI in the thyroid gland. Because thyroid hormone levels will transiently increase following RAI treatment owing to release of preformed thyroid hormone, patients with cardiac disease and elderly patients are often treated with thionamides prior to RAI ablation. Occasionally, in patients with underlying cardiac disease, it may be necessary to reinstitute antithyroid drug therapy following radioactive iodine abalation.

The standard practice is to withdraw the thionamide 4 days prior to RAI treatment and to reinstitute it 4 days after therapy is concluded. Administering antithyroid drug therapy following RAI treatment may result in a higher rate of posttreatment recurrence or persistent hyperthyroidism.[46]

Corticosteroid administration will blunt and delay the rise in antibodies to the TSH receptor, thyroglobulin, and thyroid peroxidase while reducing T_3 and T_4 concentrations following RAI. Bartalena et al. found no progression in ophthalmopathy in patients receiving prednisone after RAI compared with methimazole (2% to 3% worsened) or no other treatment (5% with persistent worsening).[47] Theoretically, if shared thyroidal and orbital antigen is involved in the pathogenesis of Graves' ophthalmopathy, antigen released with RAI treatment could aggravate preexisting eye disease. Note also that thyroid ablation may decrease eye disease in the long term by removing the source of antigen, but it is unclear if RAI differs from surgery or thionamide for the risk of worsening eye disease.[48]

Destruction of the gland attenuates the hyperthyroid state, and hypothyroidism commonly occurs months to years following RAI. The goal of therapy is to destroy overactive thyroid cells, and a single dose of 4000 to 8000 rads results in a euthyroid state in 60% of patients at 6 months or less. The remaining 40% become euthyroid within 1 year, requiring two or more doses. It is advisable that a second dose of RAI be given 6 months after the first RAI treatment if the patient remains hyperthyroid. Variables that influence the outcome of RAI include gender (men are less likely to develop hypothyroidism), race (blacks are more resistant to ^{131}I), the size of the thyroid, severity of disease, and perhaps the level of TSAb. The acute, short-term side effects of ^{131}I therapy are minimal and include mild thyroidal tenderness and dysphagia. Concern over the development of thyroid carcinoma and leukemia and increased risk of mutations and congenital defects now appears to be unfounded because long-term follow-up studies have not revealed increased risk for these complications.[36] Although RAI is very effective in the treatment of hyperthyroidism, long-term follow-up from Great Britain suggests that among patients with hyperthyroidism treated with RAI, mortality from all causes and mortality resulting from cardiovascular and cerebrovascular disease and fracture are increased.[49]

A common approach to Graves' hyperthyroidism is to administer a single dose of 5 to 15 mCi (80 to 120 μCi/g of tissue).[36,46] Thyroid glands estimated to > 80 g may require larger doses of RAI. Larger doses are likely to induce hypothyroidism and are seldom given outside the United States owing to the imposition of stringent safety restrictions. For example, in the United Kingdom, a nursery school teacher is advised to stay out of school for 3 weeks following a 15-mCi dose of ^{131}I.[33]

EVALUATION OF THERAPEUTIC OUTCOMES: HYPERTHYROIDISM

After therapy (surgery, thionamides, or RAI) for hyperthyroidism has been initiated, patients should be evaluated on a monthly basis until they reach a euthyroid condition. Clinical signs of continuing thyrotoxicosis (tachycardia, weight loss, heat intolerance, etc.) or the development of hypothyroidism (bradycardia, weight gain, lethargy, etc.) should be noted. β-Blockers may be used to control symptoms of thyrotoxicosis until the definitive treatment has returned the patient to a euthyroid state. Once thyroxine replacement is initiated, the goal is to maintain both the free thyroxine level and the TSH concentration in the "normal range." Once a stable dose of thyroxine is identified, the patient may be followed up every 6 to 12 months.

Finally, a common, potentially confusing clinical situation should be mentioned. Why are the TSH concentrations suppressed in some patients who are clinically hypothyroid and who have a low free T_4 level? In patients with long-standing hyperthyroidism, the pituitary thyrotrophs responsible for making TSH become atrophic. The average amount of time required for these cells to resume normal functioning is 6 to 8 weeks.[50] Therefore, if a thyrotoxic patient has his/her free T_4 concentration lowered rapidly, before the thyrotrophs resume normal function, a period of "transient central hypothyroidism" will be observed.

SPECIAL CONDITIONS

GRAVES' DISEASE AND PREGNANCY[51–53]

Inappropriate production of human chronionic gonadotropin (hCG) is the leading cause of abnormal thyroid function tests during the first half of pregnancy, and hCG can cause either subclinical (normal T_4, suppressed TSH) or overt hyperthyroidism. This is owing to the homology of hCG and TSH as well as their receptors. Hyperthyroidism during pregnancy is almost solely caused by Graves' disease, with approximately 0.1% to 0.4% of pregnancies affected. Although the increased metabolic rate is usually well tolerated in pregnant women, two symptoms suggestive of hyperthyroidism during pregnancy are failure to gain weight despite good appetite and persistent tachycardia. There is no increase in maternal mortality or morbidity in well-controlled patients; however, postpartum thyroid storm has been reported in about 20% of untreated individuals. Fetal loss is also more common, owing to spontaneous abortion and premature delivery in untreated pregnant women. Transplacental passage of thyroid-stimulating antibodies may occur, causing fetal as well as neonatal hyperthyroidism.[54]

Because RAI is contraindicated in pregnancy and surgery is usually not recommended (especially during the first trimester), antithyroid drug therapy is usually the treatment of choice. Methimazole readily crosses the placenta and appears in breast milk.

PTU is considered to be the drug of choice in pregnancy with the lowest possible doses used to maintain the maternal T_4 level in the high-normal range, but as described previously, there appears to be little difference between PTU and methimazole.[37] To prevent fetal goiter and suppression of fetal thyroid function, PTU is usually prescribed in daily doses of 300 mg or less and tapered to 50 to 150 mg daily after 4 to 6 weeks. PTU doses of less than 200 mg daily are unlikely to produce fetal goiter. During the last trimester, TSAbs fall spontaneously, and some patients will go into remission so that antithyroid drug doses may be reduced. A rebound in maternal hyperthyroidism occurs in about 10% of women and may require more intensive treatment postpartum than in the last trimester of pregnancy.[55]

NEONATAL AND PEDIATRIC HYPERTHYROIDISM[56]

Following delivery, some babies will be hyperthyroid owing to placental transfer of TSAbs, which stimulates thyroid hormone production in utero and postpartum. This is likely if the maternal TSAb titers were quite high. The disease is usually expressed 7 to 10 days postpartum and treatment with antithyroid drugs (PTU 5 to 10 mg/kg/d or methimazole 0.5 to 1 mg/kg/d) may be needed for as long as 8 to 12 weeks until the antibody is cleared (IgG half-life is about 2 weeks). Iodide (potassium iodide 1 drop/d or Lugol's solution 1 to 3 drops/d) and sodium ipodate may be used for the first few days to acutely inhibit hormone release.

Childhood hyperthyroidism is usually managed with either PTU or methimazole. Long-term follow-up studies suggest that this form of therapy is quite acceptable, with 25% of a cohort experiencing remission every 2 years.[57]

THYROID STORM[58,59]

Thyroid storm is a life-threatening medical emergency characterized by severe thyrotoxicosis, high fever (often greater than 103°F), tachycardia, tachypnea, dehydration, delirium, coma, nausea, vomiting, and diarrhea. Precipitating factors for thyroid storm include infection, trauma, surgery, RAI treatment, and withdrawal from antithyroid drugs. It may occur at any age and has an average duration of 72 hours, although symptoms may persist up to 8 days if treatment is not aggressive. With aggressive treatment, the mortality rate has been lowered to 20%. The following therapeutic measures should be instituted promptly: (1) suppression of thyroid hormone formation and secretion, (2) antiadrenergic therapy, (3) administration of corticosteroids, and (4) treatment of associated complications or coexisting factors that may have precipitated the storm. Specific agents used in thyroid storm are outlined in Table 71–6. PTU in large doses is the preferred thionamide because it interferes with the production of thyroid hormones and blocks the peripheral conversion of T_4 to T_3. If patients are unable to take medications orally, the tablets can be crushed into suspension and instilled by gastric tube. Iodides, which rapidly block the release of preformed thyroid hormone, should be administrated *after* PTU is initiated to inhibit iodide utilization by the overactive gland. If iodide is administered first, it may provide the substrate permitting the synthesis and storage of a large amount of thyroid hormone in the thyroid gland, which would prolong the duration of hyperthyroidism thereafter.

Antiadrenergic therapy with the short-acting agent esmolol may be used in the patient with pulmonary disease or at risk for cardiac failure because its effects may be rapidly reversed.[60] Corticosteroids are generally recommended, although there is no convincing evidence of adrenocortical insufficiency in thyroid storm, and the benefits derived from steroids may be owing to their antipyretic action and

TABLE 71–6. Drug Dosages Used in the Management of Thyroid Storm

Drug	Regimen
Propylthiouracil	900–1200 mg/d PO in four or six divided doses
Methimazole	90–120 mg/d PO in four or six divided doses
Sodium iodide	Up to 2 g/d IV in single or divided doses
Lugol's solution	5–10 drops tid in water or juice
Saturated solution of potassium iodide	1–2 drops tid in water or juice
Propranolol	40–80 mg every 6 h
Esmolol	50–150 mg/kg/min IV
Dexamethasone	5–20 mg/d PO or IV in divided doses
Prednisone	25–100 mg/d PO in divided doses
Methylprednisolone	20–80 mg/d IV in divided doses
Hydrocortisone	100–400 mg/d IV in divided doses

their effect of stabilizing blood pressure.[61] General supportive measures, including acetaminophen as an antipyretic (do not use aspirin or other nonsteroidal anti-inflammatory agents because they may displace bound thyroid hormone), fluid and electrolyte replacement, sedatives, digitalis, antiarrhythmics, insulin, and antibiotics should be given as indicated. Plasmapheresis and peritoneal dialysis have been used to remove excess hormone when the patient has not responded to more conservative measures, although these measures do not always work.[62]

HYPOTHYROIDISM[63]

Hypothyroidism is defined as the clinical and biochemical syndrome resulting from decreased thyroid hormone production. Overt hypothyroidism occurs in 1.5% to 2% of women and 0.2% of men, and its incidence increases with age.[64–66] The vast majority of hypothyroid patients have thyroid gland failure (primary hypothyroidism). Pituitary failure is an uncommon cause of hypothyroidism but should be suspected in a patient with decreased levels of thyroxine and inappropriately normal or low TSH levels. Most patients with secondary hypothyroidism will have clinical signs of more generalized pituitary insufficiency such as abnormal menses and decreased libido, or evidence of a pituitary adenoma such as visual-field defects, galactorrhea, or acromegaloid features. Generalized (peripheral and central) resistance to thyroid hormone is extremely rare.

Thyroid hormone is essential for normal growth and development during embryonic life. Thyroid hormone deficiency during fetal and neonatal development results in mental retardation. In the child, thyroid hormone deficiency may manifest as growth retardation. In the adult, manifestations of hypothyroidism are varied and nonspecific. There is slowing of physical and mental activity as well as of cardiovascular, gastrointestinal, and neuromuscular function.

Common symptoms of hypothyroidism include dry skin, cold intolerance, weight gain, constipation, and weakness. Complaints of lethargy and fatigue or loss of ambition and energy are also common but are less specific. Depression may result from untreated hypothyroidism.

The most common signs of decreased levels of thyroid hormone include coarse skin and hair, cold skin, periorbital puffiness, and bradycardia. Speech is often slow as well as hoarse. Reversible neurologic syndromes such as carpal tunnel syndrome, polyneuropathy, and cerebellar dysfunction may also occur. Muscle cramps, myalgia, and stiffness are frequent complaints of hypothyroid patients. Objective weakness is common, with proximal muscles being affected more than distal muscles. Slow relaxation of deep tendon reflexes is common.

A rise in the TSH level is the first evidence of primary hypothyroidism. Many patients will have a T_4 level within the normal range (compensated hypothyroidism) and few, if any, symptoms of hypothyroidism. As the disease progresses the T_4 concentration will drop below the normal level. Interestingly, the T_3 concentration will often be maintained in the normal range in spite of a low T_4. The RAIU is not a useful test in the evaluation of a hypothyroid patient.

CAUSES OF HYPOTHYROIDISM (TABLE 71–7)

CHRONIC AUTOIMMUNE THYROIDITIS

Autoimmune thyroiditis (Hashimoto's disease) is the most common cause of spontaneous hypothyroidism in the adult. Patients may present with either goitrous thyroid gland enlargement and mild hypothyroidism or thyroid gland atrophy and more severe thyroid hormone deficiency. Both forms of autoimmune thyroiditis probably result from cell- and antibody-mediated thyroid injury. The bulk of evidence suggests that the presence of specific defects in suppressor T-lymphocyte function leads to the survival of a randomly mutating clone of helper T lymphocytes, which are directed against normally occurring antigens on the thyroid membrane. Once these T lymphocytes interact with thyroid membrane antigen, B lymphocytes are stimulated to produce thyroid antibodies.[67,68]

TABLE 71–7. Causes of Hypothyroidism

Primary hypothyroidism
Hashimoto's disease
Iatrogenic hypothyroidism
Others
Iodine deficiency
Enzyme defects
Thyroid hypoplasia
Goitrogens
Secondary hypothyroidism
Pituitary disease
Hypothalamic disease

Antimicrosomal antibodies are present in virtually all patients with Hashimoto's thyroiditis and appear to be directed against the enzyme thyroid peroxidase, thyroglobulin, and other thyroid cell-membrane antigens. These antibodies are capable of fixing complement and inducing cytotoxic changes in thyroid cells. Antibodies that are capable of stimulating thyroid growth are also present in the goitrous variety of Hashimoto's disease; conversely, antibodies that inhibit the trophic effects of TSH are present in the atrophic type.[69]

IATROGENIC HYPOTHYROIDISM

Iatrogenic hypothyroidism follows exposure to radiation (radioiodine or external radiation) or surgery. Hypothyroidism occurs within a year after ^{131}I therapy in most patients treated for Graves' disease. Thereafter, it occurs at a rate of approximately 2.5% each year. External radiation therapy to the region of the thyroid using doses of greater than 2500 rads for therapy of neck carcinoma also causes hypothyroidism. This effect is dose dependent, with more than 50% of patients developing hypothyroidism who have received more than 4000 rads to the thyroid bed. Total thyroidectomy causes hypothyroidism within 1 month.

OTHER CAUSES OF PRIMARY HYPOTHYROIDISM

Iodine deficiency, enzymatic defects within the thyroid gland, thyroid hypoplasia, and maternal ingestion of goitrogens during fetal development may cause cretinism. Early recognition and treatment of the resultant thyroid hormone deficiency is essential for optimal mental development. Large-scale screening programs in North America, Europe, Japan, and Australia are now in place. The frequency of congenital hypothyroidism in North America and Europe is 1 per 3500 to 4000 live births. In the United States, there are racial differences in the incidence of congenital hypothyroidism, with whites being affected seven times as frequently as blacks.[70]

In the adult, hypothyroidism may rarely be caused by iodine deficiency and goitrogens. Rarely, iodine ingestion in the form of expectorants can lead to hypothyroidism. In sensitive persons, the iodide blocks the synthesis of thyroid hormone, leading to an increased secretion of TSH, which causes thyroid enlargement.[3] Thus, both iodine excess and iodine deficiency can cause decreased secretion of thyroid hormone.

CAUSES OF SECONDARY HYPOTHYROIDISM

PITUITARY DISEASE

TSH is required for normal thyroid secretion. Thyroid atrophy and decreased thyroid secretion follow pituitary failure. Pituitary insufficiency may be caused by destruction of thyrotrophs by either functioning or nonfunctioning pituitary tumors, surgical therapy, external pituitary radiation, postpartum pituitary necrosis (Sheehan's syndrome), infiltrative processes of the pituitary such as metastatic tumors, tuberculosis, histiocytosis, and autoimmune mechanisms. In all these situations, TSH deficiency most often occurs in association with other pituitary hormone deficiencies.

In most hypothyroid patients with pituitary disease, serum TSH concentrations are low or normal. A serum TSH concentration in the normal range is clearly inappropriate if the patient's T_4 is low.

Note that pituitary enlargement in hypothyroidism does not invariably indicate the presence of a primary pituitary tumor. Pituitary enlargement is seen in patients with severe primary hypothyroidism owing to compensatory hyperplasia and hypertrophy of the thyrotrophs. Serum TSH concentrations and pituitary enlargement decline during thyroid hormone replacement therapy, indicating that the TSH secretion is not autonomous. These patients are easily separated from patients with primary pituitary failure by measuring a TSH.

HYPOTHALAMIC HYPOTHYROIDISM

TRH deficiency also causes hypothyroidism. In both adults and children it may occur as a result of cranial irradiation, trauma, infiltrative diseases, or neoplastic diseases. Hypothalamic hypothyroidism is rare.

▶ TREATMENT: Hypothyroidism

PHARMACOLOGIC THERAPY

The goals of therapy are to restore normal thyroid hormone concentrations in tissue, provide symptomatic relief, prevent neurologic deficits in newborns and children, and reverse the biochemical abnormalities of hypothyroidism. Any of the commercially available thyroid preparations accomplish this goal (Table 71–8); however, levothyroxine (L-thyroxine) is considered to be drug of choice. The thyroid preparations are either natural (i.e., desiccated thyroid, thyroglobulin) or synthetic (levothyroxine, liothyronine, liotrix) in origin. The availability of sensitive and specific assays for total and free hormone levels as well as TSH now allow more definitive dose titration to allow adequate replacement without inadvertent overdose. The response of TSH to TRH had been advocated by some for "fine-tuning" thyroid replacement, but this is not necessary if the sensitive immunoradiometric assays (IRMA) for TSH are used. Minimum clinical guidelines for the treatment of hypothyroidism have been published by the American Thyroid Association.[34]

NATURAL THYROID HORMONES

Desiccated thyroid is derived from hog, beef, or sheep thyroid gland. The *United States Pharmacopeia,* 23th edition, requires Thyroid USP to contain 38 µg (±15%) of levothyroxine and 9 µg (±10%) of liothyronine for each 65 mg (1 grain) of the labeled content of thyroglobulin. Thyroglobulin USP should contain 36 µg (±15%) of levothyroxine and 12 µg (±10%) of liothyronine for each 65 mg (1 grain) of the labeled content of thyroglobulin. Not all generic brands may be bioequivalent, and switching among brands in patients stabilized on one product should be discouraged. Thyroid USP, as an animal protein–derived product, may be antigenic in allergic or sensitive patients. Even though desiccated thyroid is inexpensive, its limitations preclude it from being considered as a drug of choice for hypothyroid patients. Thyroglobulin is a purified hog-gland extract but it has no clinical advantages and is not widely used.

SYNTHETIC THYROID HORMONES[71]

Levothyroxine (T_4, L-thyroxine) is the drug of choice for thyroid replacement and suppressive therapy because it is chemically

TABLE 71–8. Thyroid Preparations Used in the Treatment of Hypothyroidism

Drug/Dosage Form	Content	Relative	Comments/Equivalency
Thyroid, USP Armour Thyroid, USV ¼-, ½-, 1½-, 2-, 3-, 4-, and 5-grain tablets	Desiccated hog, beef, or sheep thyroid gland	1 grain (equivalent to 60 µg of T_4)	Unpredictable hormonal stability; inexpensive generic brands may not be bioequivalent
Thyroglobulin, 32 mg (½ grain), 65 mg (1 grain), 100 mg (1½ grains), 130 mg (2 grains), and 200 mg (3 grains)	Partially purified hog thyroglobulin	1 grain	Standardized biologically to give T_4:T_3 ratio of 2.5:1; more expensive than thyroid extract; no clinical advantage
L-Thyroxine Synthroid, Flint; Levothyroid, USV 25-, 50-, 75-, 100-, 125-, 150-, 175-, 200-, and 300-µg tablets; 100 µg/mL, 5 mL	Synthetic T_4	100 µg	Stable; predictable potency; generics may be bioequivalent; when switching from natural thyroid to L-thyroxine, lower dose by ½ grain; variable absorption between products; $t_{1/2}$ = 7 d, so daily dosing
Liothyroine Cytomel, Smith Kline and French, 5-, 25-, and 50-g tablets	Synthetic T_3	25 µg	Uniform absorption; rapid onset; $t_{1/2}$ = 1.5 d, multiple daily dosing; monitor response with TSH assays
Liotrix Euthyroid, Parke-Davis; Thyrolar, USV ¼-, ½-, 1-, 2-, and 3-strength tablets	Synthetic T_4:T_3 in 4:1 ratio		Stable, predictable, expensive; lacks therapeutic rational because T_4 is converted to T_3 peripherally

stable, relatively inexpensive, and free of antigenicity and has uniform potency. Whereas T_3 and not T_4 is the biologically more active form of thyroid hormone, levothyroxine administration results in a pool of thyroid hormone that is readily and consistently converted to T_3; in this regard levothyroxine may be thought of as a prohormone. The half-life of levothyroxine is approximately 7 days. This long half-life is responsible for a stable pool of prohormone and the need for only once-daily dosing with levothyroxine. Older studies with levothyroxine suggested that bioavailability was low and erratic; however, this product has been reformulated and the average bioavailability is now approximately 80%.[72] The bioavailability of Synthroid, Levoxine, and generic levothyroxine preparations were compared in a blinded, randomized, four-way cross-over trial.[73] The study was sponsored by the manufacturers of Synthroid, who have challenged the author's conclusions that the levothyroxine preparations are bioequivalent and should be interchangeable for the majority of patients. The time to maximal absorption is 2 hours, and this should be considered when T_4 and TSH concentrations are determined.[74] Mucosal diseases such as sprue, diabetic diarrhea and ileal bypass surgery may also reduce absorption. Cholestyramine, sucralfate, aluminum hydroxide,[75] ferrous sulfate,[76] soybean formula,[77] and dietary fiber supplements[78] may also impair the absorption of levothyroxine from the gastrointestinal tract. Drugs that increase nondeiodinative T_4 clearance include rifampin, carbamazepine, and possibly phenytoin. Selenium deficiency and amiodarone may block the conversion of T_4 to T_3.

Liothyronine (T_3) is chemically pure with known potency and has a shorter half-life of 1.5 days. Although it is widely used diagnostically in the T_3-suppression test, T_3 has some clinical disadvantages including a higher incidence of cardiac adverse effects, higher cost, and difficulty in monitoring with conventional laboratory tests. Liotrix is a combination of synthetic T_4 and T_3 in 4:1 ratio that attempts to mimic the natural hormonal secretion. It is chemically stable and pure and has a predictable potency. The major limitations to this product are high cost and lack of therapeutic rationale, because about 35% of T_4 is peripherally converted T_3.

DOSING AND MONITORING

During the mid-1980s the average dose of levothyroxine was about 160 µg/d. With the advent of more sensitive assay methods for TSH and the reformulation of levothyroxine, it is now apparent that many patients have been treated with excessive amounts of levothyroxine. More recent studies suggest that the average maintenance dose for most adults should be closer to about 110 to 120 µg/d. Indeed, as many as one-third of patients receiving levothyroxine 150 µg daily will be overreplaced.[71] There is, however, a wide range of replacement doses, necessitating individualized therapy and appropriate monitoring to determine an adequate but not excessive dose.

The initial dose of levothyroxine is dependent on the patient's age, the presence of associated disorders, as well as the severity and duration of hypothyroidism.[79] In young patients with long-standing disease and patients over age 45 without known cardiac disease, therapy should be initiated with 50 µg daily of levothyroxine and increased to 100 µg daily after 1 month. The recommended initial daily dose for older patients or those with known cardiac disease is 25 µg/d titrated upward in increments of 25 µg at monthly intervals to prevent stress on the cardiovascular system. Some patients may experience an exacerbation of angina with higher doses of thyroid hormone. Although the TSH is very sensitive for under- or overreplacement, clinicians often fail to alter the dose of T_4 based on TSH clearly outside of the normal range.[80]

Patients with subclinical hypothyroidism (seen more commonly in the elderly and particularly in women) have no or few signs or symptoms, normal serum T_3 and T_4 concentrations, and an elevated basal TSH concentration. The prevalence of this disorder is thought to be about 8%, but the reported range is quite wide.[26,65] Although the treatment of subclinical hypothyroidism is controversial, patients presenting with marked elevations in TSH (>10 mU/L) and high titers of TSAb or prior treatment with ^{131}I may be most likely to benefit from treatment.[81] Other patients who may improve with replacement include those with mild symptoms of hypothyroidism and depression. It should be noted that some studies find that only one of four treated patients experienced improvement.[82] Conservative treatment goals in this situation would be to maintain serum T_4 and T_3 levels in the normal range and reduce TSH to a value of 1.0 mU/L.

Once euthyroidism is attained, the daily maintenance dose of levothyroxine does not fluctuate greatly. As patients age, the dosing requirement may need to be reduced.[63] The ability to measure serum TSH concentrations has improved the accuracy with which thyroid hormone replacement can be monitored. Many clinicians now consider serum TSH concentration to be the most sensitive and specific monitoring parameter for adjustment of levothyroxine dose, and using TSH with ankle reflex and cholesterol measurements may be useful in some patients.[83] Plasma TSH concentrations begin to fall within hours and are usually normalized within 2 weeks, but may take up to 6 weeks in some patients, depending on the baseline value. TSH and T_4 concentrations are both used to monitor therapy, and they should be checked every 6 weeks until a euthyroid state is achieved. Serum T_4 concentrations can be useful in detecting noncompliance, malabsorption, or changes in levothyroxine product bioequivalence. An elevated TSH concentration indicates insufficient replacement. The appropriate dose maintains the TSH concentration in the normal range.

In patients with hypothyroidism caused by hypothalamic or pituitary failure, alleviation of the clinical syndrome and restoration of serum T_4 to the normal range are the only criteria available for estimating the appropriate replacement dose of levothyroxine. Concurrent use of dopamine, dopaminergic agents (bromocriptine), somatostatin or somatostatin analogs (octreotide), and corticosteroids suppresses TSH concentrations and may confound the interpretation of this monitoring parameter.[84]

Thyroid-stimulating hormone suppressive levothyroxine therapy may also be given to patients with nodular thyroid disease and diffuse goiter, to patients with a history of thyroid irradiation, and to patients with thyroid cancer. The rationale for suppression therapy is to reduce TSH secretion, which promotes growth and function in abnormal thyroid tissue. In patients with soliditary nodules who have not received radiation, TSH should be suppressed to 0.05 to 0.1 mU/L in premenopausal women and in men <60 years old. A dose of levothyroxine of 100 to 150 µg/d is usually sufficient. In men over 60 years of age and postmenopausal women, TSH levels should be reduced to 0.1 to 0.3 mU/L owing to the risk of more serious adverse effects in this population and reduced clearance of levothyroxine with advanced age. Levothyroxine may be given in nontoxic multinodular goiter to suppress the TSH to low-normal levels of 0.5 to 1.0 mU/L if the baseline TSH is >1.0 mU/L. Goiter size and thyroid volume may be reduced with suppression therapy. Diffuse goiter associated with autoimmune thyroiditis may also be treated with levothyroxine to reduce goiter size and thyroid volume. In patients with follicular or papillary thyroid cancer, current recommendations are to suppress the TSH to < 0.02 mU/L. Doses of levothyroxine of up to 2.2 to 2.5 µg/kg may be needed to provide TSH levels of < 0.02 mU/L in this population, and free T_4 levels are useful in detecting hyperthyroidism.[85,86]

ADVERSE EFFECTS

Serious untoward effects are unusual if dosing is appropriate and the patient is carefully monitored during initial treatment. Levothyroxine replacement in athyreotic hypothyroid patients restores systolic and diastolic left ventricular performance within 2 weeks, and the use of levothyroxine may increase the frequency of atrial premature beats but not necessarily ventricular premature beats. Excessive doses of thyroid hormone may lead to heart failure, angina pectoris, and myocardial infarction; rarely, the latter may be caused by coronary artery spasm.[87] Allergic or idiosyncratic reactions can occur with the natural animal-derived products such as desiccated thyroid and thyroglobulin, but these are extremely rare with the synthetic products used today. The 0.05-mg Synthroid tablet is the least allergenic (owing to lack of dye and few excipients) and should be tried in the patient suspected to be allergic to thyroid hormone.

Hyperremodeling of cortical and trabecular bone due to hyperthyroidism leads to reduced bone density and may increase the risk of fracture. Compared with normal controls, excess exogenous thyroid hormone results in histomorphometric and biochemical changes similar to those observed in osteoporosis and untreated hyperthyroidism; however, at routinely used replacement doses, bone mineral density loss is less than with untreated hyperthyroidism and only slightly greater than in controls.[88–91] The risk for this complication of therapy seems to be related to the dose of levothyroxine, patient age, and gender. Markers for bone turnover include urinary cross-linked *N*-telopeptides pyridinoline of type I collagen, osteocalcin, and bone-specific alkaline phosphatase. When doses of levothyroxine are used to suppress TSH concentrations to below normal values (less than 0.3 mU/L) in postmenopausal women, this adverse effect is more likely to be seen. Cortical bone is affected to a greater degree than trabecular bone at suppressive doses of L-thyroxine.[92] In contrast, it appears to be much less likely in men and in premenopausal women. Maintaining the TSH between 0.7 and 1.5 mU/L with approximately 150 μg/d of levothyroxine does not alter bone mineral density in premenopausal women.[93]

SPECIAL CONDITIONS

MYXEDEMA COMA[94,95]

Myxedema coma is the end stage of long-standing, uncorrected hypothyroidism. Clinical features include hypothermia, advanced stages of hypothyroid symptoms, and altered sensorium ranging from delirium to coma. Mortality rates of 60% to 70% necessitate immediate and aggressive therapy with intravenous bolus thyroxine 300 to 500 μg. Glucocorticoid therapy with intravenous hydrocortisone 100 mg every 8 hours should be given until coexisting adrenal suppression is ruled out. Consciousness, lowered TSH concentrations, and normal vital signs are expected within 24 hours. Maintenance doses are typically 75 to 100 μg given intravenously until the patient stabilizes and oral therapy is begun. Supportive therapy must be instituted to maintain adequate ventilation, euglycemia, blood pressure, and body temperature. Any underlying disorder, such as sepsis, myocardial infarction, and the like obviously must be diagnosed and treated.

CONGENITAL HYPOTHYROIDISM[96,97]

In congenital hypothyroidism, full maintenance therapy should be instituted early to improve the prognosis for mental and physical development. The average maintenance dose in infants and children depends on the age and weight of the child. Several studies demonstrate that aggressive therapy with levothyroxine is important for normal development and current recommendations are for initiation of therapy within 45 days of birth at a dose of 10 to 15 μg/kg/d.[96] This dose is used to keep T_4 concentrations at about 10 μg/dL within 30 days of starting therapy and is associated with improved IQs in treated infants. The dose is progressively decreased to a typical adult dose as the child ages, the adult dose being given in the age range of 11 to 20 years. In utero treatment of fetal goiter and hypothyroidism has been accomplished with the injection of thyroxine into the amniotic fluid.[98]

HYPOTHYROIDISM IN PREGNANCY[52,99,100]

Hypothyroidism during pregnancy leads to an increased rate of stillbirths and possibly lower psychological scores in infants born of women who received inadequate replacement during pregnancy.[101] Thyroid hormone is necessary for fetal growth and must come from the maternal side during the first 2 months of gestation. Although liothyronine may cross the placental membrane slightly better than levothyroxine, the latter is considered to be the drug of choice. The objective of treatment is to decrease TSH to 1 U/mL and maintain T_4 concentrations in the normal range. Based on elevated TSH levels during pregnancy, Mandel et al.[102] found that the mean dose of levothyroxine had to be increased by 36 μg/d to suppress TSH into the normal range. Increased need for thyroid hormone during pregnancy may be a result of pharmacokinetic alterations, although this has not been studied. Increase in thyroxine metabolism by the fetal–placental unit also contributes to increased thyroid hormone demand, and the need for increased doses decreases after delivery. Consequently, after delivery the levothyroxine may need to be reduced based on T_3 concentrations and measurement of TSH.

EFFECTS OF HYPOTHYROIDISM ON SELECTED MEDICATIONS

Hypothyroidism may affect the metabolism and clinical efficacy of several medications. Digitalis preparations have a decreased volume of distribution in the hypothyroid state, resulting in increased sensitivity to the digitalis effect.

Therefore, many hypothyroid patients achieve a therapeutic effect at lower digitalis doses. Insulin degradation may be delayed in hypothyroidism, thereby requiring a lower insulin dose.[103] Hypothyroidism delays the catabolism of clotting factors, and if a patient stabilized on warfarin is made euthyroid with levothyroxine, the patient may become excessively anticoagulated. Respiratory depressants such as barbiturates, phenothiazines, and opioid analgesics should be avoided, because increased sensitivity may increase carbon dioxide retention and precipitate myxedema coma.

NONTHYROIDAL ILLNESS

A wide variety of abnormalities of pituitary–thyroid function, serum thyroid hormone binding, and extrathyroidal thyroid hormone metabolism occur in patients with nonthyroidal illness. These abnormalities frequently result in decreased serum T_3 concentrations and less often lead to a decreased serum T_4 concentration. Serum TSH concentrations are usually within the normal range. The presence of coexisting primary hypothyroidism can be recognized in patients who have other illnesses by an elevation in the TSH concentration.

The degree and extent of the abnormality in thyroid function generally correlates with the severity of the nonthyroidal illness. These conditions are frequently referred to as the "euthyroid sick syndrome." It is likely that these changes represent adaptive forms of hypothyroidism that serve to reduce the availability of thyroid hormones to lessen the impact of the nonthyroidal illness.[104]

Decreased serum T_3 concentrations occur in patients with both acute and chronic illnesses. The fundamental cause of decreased serum T_3 concentrations in these situations is decreased extrathyroidal conversion of T_4 to T_3. This reaction is normally mediated by T_4-5′-deiodinase. A circulating inhibitor of this enzyme, perhaps interleukin-6, is present in patients with nonthyroidal illness.[105] Serum total and free T_4 concentrations are usually normal. The serum reverse T_3 concentration is characteristically high because the same enzyme, 5′-deiodinase, that is necessary to convert T_4 to T_3 is necessary to convert reverse T_3 to its breakdown products. Acute respiratory infections and surgery acutely elevate interleukin-6, and T_3 concentration is inversely correlated.[106]

Low serum T_4 is seen in most critically ill patients. This change is caused by diminished serum T_4 binding resulting either from decrease serum concentrations of TBG, TBPA, albumin, or from inhibitors of T_4 binding. The free T_4 concentration is generally normal. This more severe degree of hypothyroidism, which occurs in severely ill patients, produces a greater reduction in thyroid hormone availability. The low serum T_4 concentrations in patients with nonthyroidal illness indicates a grave prognosis. In two studies, more than 60% of hospitalized patients with a low serum free-T_4 index died. T_4 or T_3 supplementation has been of no benefit in this situation and in fact has increased morbidity.

To confuse matters, some patients with nonthyroidal illness have elevation of their serum T_4 concentration. Most commonly, this is seen in patients with psychiatric disorders during acute psychotic breaks. Thyroid hormone levels return to normal within 2 weeks after successful treatment of the underlying psychiatric disease. The occurrence of these abnormalities requires that care be taken in diagnosing hypothyroidism or hyperthyroidism in patients who have nonthyroidal illnesses.

GOITROUS THYROID DISEASE

Endemic goiter is the major thyroid disease throughout the world, affecting more than 200 million people. Many goitrous glands contain one or more nodules. The introduction of iodide supplementation has eliminated goiter as a major medical problem in developed countries, though it continues to be a problem in developing countries whose geographic position makes them more susceptible to iodide deficiency. In 1924, Marine postulated that periods of iodide deficiency resulted in cyclic hyperplasia and involution of thyroid follicular cells with eventual development of nodular hyperplasia.[107] This hypothesis is still used to explain goiter formation today. Whatever the specific cause, the final common pathway appears to result from an inadequate thyroid hormone secretion with compensatory TSH secretion and eventual thyroid gland enlargement. The essential factor for the conversion of a hyperplastic iodine-deficiency goiter into a colloid goiter appears to be an acute reduction of TSH stimulation; therefore, any situation that would result in a cyclical increase and decrease in TSH secretion might eventually result in the production of a nodular goiter.

There has been an interest in the possibility that growth factors other than TSH play a role in the development of a goiter. Immunoglobulin fractions capable of stimulating thyroid growth have been found in patients with nontoxic goiter and Graves' disease. In these patients, thyroid growth promoting immunoglobulin titers correlates with goiter size rather than with the thyroid hormone concentration.

Sporadic goiter is defined as a goiter occurring in a nonendemic goiter region. Although a number of known goitrogens and errors in thyroid hormone biosynthesis may cause goiter, the majority of cases of sporadic goiter have no known etiology.

Treatment of all goiters is a trial of thyroid hormone suppression in an effort to eliminate TSH as a possible stimulus for continued thyroid growth. Large, long-standing goiters seldom undergo significant reduction in size. If the patient is symptomatic (with dysphagia or dyspnea) or there is a question of malignant thyroid involvement, surgery is recommended.

▶ PRINCIPLES OF PHARMACOTHERAPY

- The molecular biology of the thyroid hormones and their receptors has provided an in-depth understanding of the various mutations that give rise to hyper- and hypothyroidism.
- Thyrotoxicosis is most commonly caused by Graves' disease, which is an autoimmune disorder in which TSAb directed against the thyrotropin receptor elicits the same biologic response as TSH.
- Hyperthyroidism may be treated with antithyroid drugs such as propylthiouracil (PTU) or methimazole (MMI), radioactive iodine, or surgical removal of the thyroid gland; selection of the initial treatment approach is based on patient characteristics such as age, concurrent physiology (e.g., pregnancy) or comorbidities (e.g., chronic obstructive lung disease), and convenience.
- PTU and MMI reduce the synthesis of thyroid hormones and are similar in efficacy and adverse effects but their dosing range differs by 10-fold.
- Response to PTU and MMI is seen in 4 to 6 weeks with a maximal response in 4 to 6 months; treatment usually continues for 1 to 2 years and therapy is monitored by clinical signs and symptoms and by measuring the serum concentrations of TSH and free T_4.
- Many patients choose to have ablative therapy with ^{131}I rather than undergo repeated courses of PTU or MMI; most receiving RAI eventually become hypothyroid and require thyroid hormone supplementation.
- Surgery is typically performed in patients with large goiters that compress surrounding structures. Surgery should be done in high-volume centers to minimize complications.
- Adjunctive therapy with β-blockers controls the adrenergic symptoms of thyrotoxicosis but does not correct the underlying disorder; iodine may also be used adjunctively in preparation for surgery and acutely for thyroid storm.
- Hypothyroidism is most often to an autoimmune disorder known as Hashimoto's thyroiditis, and the drug of choice for replacement therapy is thyroxine (T_4).
- Monitoring of thyroxine replacement therapy is done by clinical signs and symptoms and by measuring the TSH (elevated for underreplacement) and free T_4 (below normal for underreplacement).

REFERENCES

1. Cavalieri RR. Iodine metabolism and thyroid physiology: Current concepts. Thyroid 1997;7:177–181.
2. Arvan P, Kim PS, Kuliawat R, et al. Intracellular protein transport to the thyrocyte plasma membrane: Potential implications for thyroid physiology. Thyroid 1997;7:89–105.
3. Wolff J. Perchlorate and the thyroid gland. Pharmacol Rev 1998; 50:89–105.
4. Motomura K, Brent GA. Mechanisms of thyroid hormone action. Endocrinol Metab Clin North Am 1998;27:1–23.
5. Salvatore D, Tu H, Harney JW, Larsen PR. Type 2 iodothyronine deiodinase is highly expressed in human thyroid. J Clin Invest 1996;98:962–968.
6. LoPresti JS, Nicoloff JT. 3,5,3′-Triiodothyronine (T_3) sulfate: A major metabolite in T_3 metabolism in man. J Clin Endocrinol Metab 1994;78:688–692.
7. Paschke R, Ludgate M. The thyrotropin receptor in thyroid diseases. N Engl J Med 1997;337:1675–1681.
8. Leclere J, Bene MC, Aubert V, et al. Clinical consequences of activating germline mutations of TSH receptor, the concept of toxic hyperplasia. Horm Res 1997;47:158–162.
9. Brent GA. The molecular basis of thyroid hormone action. N Engl J Med 1994;331:847–853.
10. Lazar M. Thyroid hormone receptors: Multiple forms, multiple possibilities. Endocrinol Rev 1993;14:184–193.
11. Kannan CR, Seshadri KG. Thyrotoxicosis. Dis Mon 1997;43: 601–677.
12. Russo D, Arturi F, Wicker R, et al. Genetic alterations in thyroid hyperfunctioning adenomas. J Clin Endocrinol Metab 1995;80: 1347–1351.
13. Beck-Peccoz P, Brucker-Davis F, Persani L, Smallridge RC, Weintraub BD. Thyrotropin-secreting pituitary tumors. Endocr Rev 1996; 17:610–638.
14. Hall W, Luciano M, Doppman J. Pituitary magnetic resonance imaging in normal human volunteers. Occult adenomas in the general populations. Ann Intern Med 1994;120:817–820.
15. Refetoff S, Weiss R, Usala S. The syndromes of resistance to thyroid hormone. Endocr Rev 1993;14:348–399.
16. Clifton-Bligh RJ, Gregory JW, Ludgate M, et al. Two novel mutations in the thyrotropin (TSH) receptor gene in a child with resistance to TSH. J Clin Endocrinol Metab 1997;82:1094–1100.
17. Wartofsky L. Radioiodine therapy for Graves' disease: Case selection and restrictions recommended to patients in North America. Thyroid 1997;7:213–216.
18. Prummel MF, Wiersinga WM. Medical management of Graves' ophthalmopathy. Thyroid 1995;5:231–234.
19. Ober K. Thyrotoxic periodic paralysis in the United States. Report of 7 cases and review of the literature. Medicine 1992;71:109–120.
20. Yamazaki K, Sato K, Shizume K, et al. Potent thyrotropic activity of human chorionic gonadotropin variants in terms of ^{125}I incorporation and de novo synthesized thyroid hormone release in human thyroid follicles. J Clin Endocrinol Metab 1995;80:473–479.
21. Siegel RD, Lee SL. Toxic nodular goiter. Toxic adenoma and toxic multinodular goiter. Endocrinol Metab Clin North Am 1998;27: 151–168.
22. Mazzaferri EL. Management of a solitary thyroid nodule. N Engl J Med 1993;328:553–559.
23. Tonacchera M, Chiovato L, Pinchera A, et al. Hyperfunctioning thyroid nodules in toxic multinodular goiter share activating thyrotropin receptor mutations with solitary toxic adenoma. J Clin Endocrinol Metab 1998;83:492–498.
24. Monzani F, Caraccio N, Goletti O, et al. Five-year follow-up of percutaneous ethanol injection for the treatment of hyperfunctioning thyroid nodules: A study of 117 patients. Clin Endocrinol 1997;46:9–15.
25. Ito M, Takamatsu J, Yoshida S, et al. Incomplete thyrotroph suppression determined by third generation thyrotropin assay in subacute thyroiditis compared to silent thyroiditis or hyperthyroid Graves' disease. J Clin Endocrinol Metab 1997;82:616–619.
26. Charkes ND. The many causes of subclinical hyperthyroidism. Thyroid 1996;6:391–396.
27. Brenner W, Bohuslavizki KH, Wolf H, Sippel C, Clausen M, Henze E. Radiotherapy with iodine-131 in recurrent malignant struma ovarii. Eur J Nucl Med 1996;23:91–94.

28. Ross DS. Syndromes of thyrotoxicosis with low radioactive iodine uptake. Endocrinol Metab Clin North Am 1998;27:169–185.
29. Bogazzi F, Bartalena L, Brogioni S, et al. Color flow Doppler sonography rapidly differentiates type I and type II amiodarone-induced thyrotoxicosis. Thyroid 1997;7:541–545.
30. Ajjan RA, Watson PF, Weetman AP. Cytokines and thyroid function. Adv Neuroimmunol 1996;6:359–386.
31. Gittoes NJ, Franklyn JA. Drug-induced thyroid disorders. Drug Saf 1995;13:46–55.
32. Lazarus JH. Hyperthyroidism. Lancet 1997;349: 339–343.
33. Franklyn JA. The management of hyperthyroidism [published erratum appears in N Engl J Med 1994 Aug 25;331(8):559]. N Engl J Med 1994;330:1731–1738.
34. Singer PA, Cooper DS, Levy EG, et al. Treatment guidelines for patients with hyperthyroidism and hypothyroidism. Standards of Care Committee, American Thyroid Association. JAMA 1995;273: 808–812.
35. Razack MS, Lore JM Jr, Lippes HA, Schaefer DP, Rassael H. Total thyroidectomy for Graves' disease. Head Neck 1997;19:378–383.
36. Cooper DS. Antithyroid drugs for the treatment of hyperthyroidism caused by Graves' disease. Endocrinol Metab Clin North Am 1998; 27:225–247.
37. Momotani N, Noh JY, Ishikawa N, Ito K. Effects of propylthiouracil and methimazole on fetal thyroid status in mothers with Graves' hyperthyroidism. J Clin Endocrinol Metab 1997;82:3633–3636.
38. Roti E, Gardini E, Minelli R. Methimazole and serum thyroid hormone concentrations in hyperthyroid patients: Effects of single and multiple daily doses. Ann Intern Med 1989;111:181–182.
39. McIver B, Rae P, Becke H. Lack of effect of thyroxine in patients with Graves' hyperthyroidism who are treated with an antithyroid drug. N Engl J Med 1996;334:220–224.
40. Werner M, Romaldini J, Bromberg N. Adverse effects related to thionamide drugs and their dose regimen. Am J Med Sci 1989;297: 216–219.
41. Tamai H, Sudo T, Kimura A, et al. Association between the DRB1*08032 histocompatibility antigen and methimazole-induced agranulocytosis in Japanese patients with Graves' disease. Ann Intern Med 1996;124:490–494.
42. Williams KV, Nayak S, Becker D, Reyes J, Burmeister LA. Fifty years of experience with propylthiouracil-associated hepatotoxicity: What have we learned? J Clin Endocrinol Metab 1997;82: 1727–1733.
43. Hardee JT, Barnett AL, Thannoun A, Eghtesad B, Wheeler D, Jamal MM. Propylthiouracil-induced hepatotoxicity. West J Med 1996; 165:144–147.
44. Benelhadj S, Marcellin P, Castelnau C, et al. Incidence of dysthyroidism during interferon therapy in chronic hepatitis C. Horm Res 1997;48:209–214.
45. Van Dijke C, Heydendael R, De Kleine M. Methimazole, carbimazole, and congenital skin defects. Ann Intern Med 1987;106:60–61.
46. Kaplan MM, Meier DA, Dworkin HJ. Treatment of hyperthyroidism with radioactive iodine. Endocrinol Metab Clin North Am 1998;27: 205–223.
47. Bartalena L, Marcocci C, Bogazzi F, et al. Relation between therapy for hyperthyroidism and the course of Graves' ophthalmopathy. N Engl J Med 1998;338:73–78.
48. Tallstedt L, Lundell G. Radioiodine treatment, ablation, and ophthalmopathy: A balanced perspective. Thyroid 1997;7:241–245.
49. Franklyn JA, Maisonneuve P, Sheppard MC, Betteridge J, Boyle P. Mortality after the treatment of hyperthyroidism with radioactive iodine. N Engl J Med 1998;338:712–718.
50. Uy HL, Reasner CA, Samuels MH. Pattern of recovery of the hypothalamic–pituitary–thyroid axis following radioactive iodine therapy in patients with Graves' disease. Am J Med 1995;99:173–179.
51. Mestman JH. Hyperthyroidism in pregnancy. Endocrinol Metab Clin North Am 1998;27:127–149.
52. Thyoid disease in pregnancy. ACOG Technical Bulletin Number 181—June 1993. Int J Gynaecol Obst 1993;43:82–88.
53. Glinoer D. The regulation of thyroid function in pregnancy: Pathways of endocrine adaptation from physiology to pathology. Endocr Rev 1997;18:404–433.
54. Burrow GN, Fisher DA, Larsen PR. Maternal and fetal thyroid function. N Engl J Med 1994;331:1072–1078.
55. Momotani N, Noh J, Ishikawa N, Ito K. Relationship between silent thyroiditis and recurrent Graves' disease in the postpartum period. J Clin Endocrinol Metab 1994;79:285–289.
56. Zimmerman D, Lteif AN. Thyrotoxicosis in children. Endocrinol Metab Clin North Am 1998;27:109–126.
57. Sills IN. Hyperthyroidism. Pediatr Rev 1994;15:417–421.
58. Rennie D. Thyroid storm. JAMA 1997;277:1238–1243.
59. Dillmann WH. Thyroid storm. Curr Ther Endocrinol Metab 1997; 6:81–85.
60. Reasner C, Isley W. Thyrotoxicosis in the critically ill. Crit Care Clin 1991;7:57–94.
61. Kidess Al, Caplan RH, Reynertson RH, Wickus G. Recurrence of ^{131}I-induced thyroid storm after discontinuing glucocorticoid therapy. Wis Med J 1991;90:463–465.
62. Samaras K, Marel GM. Failure of plasmapheresis, corticosteroids and thionamides to ameliorate a case of protracted amiodarone-induced thyroiditis. Clin Endocrinol 1996;45:365–368.
63. Lindsay RS, Toft AD. Hypothyroidism. Lancet 1997;349:413–417.
64. Wang C, Crapo LM. The epidemiology of thyroid disease and implications for screening. Endocrinol Metab Clin North Am 1997;26: 189–218.
65. Arem R, Escalante D. Subclinical hypothyroidism: Epidemiology, diagnosis, and significance. Adv Inter Med 1996;41:213–250.
66. Massoudi MS, Meilahn EN, Orchard TJ, et al. Prevalence of thyroid antibodies among healthy middle-aged women. Findings from the thyroid study in healthy women. Ann Epidemiol 1995;5:229–233.
67. Mukuta T, Yoshikawa N, Arreaza G, et al. Activation of T lymphocyte subsets by synthetic TSH receptor peptides and recombinant glutamate decarboxylase in autoimmune thyroid disease and insulin-dependent diabetes. J Clin Endocrinol Metab 1995;80:1264–1272.
68. Roura-Mir C, Catalfamo M, Sospedra M, Alcalde L, Pujol-Borrell R, Jaraquemada D. Single-cell analysis of intrathyroidal lymphocytes shows differential cytokine expression in Hashimoto's and Graves' disease. Eur J Immunol 1997;27:3290–3302.
69. Kasagi K, Kousaka T, Higuchi K, et al. Clinical significance of measurements of antithyroid antibodies in the diagnosis of Hashimoto's thyroiditis: Comparison with histological findings. Thyroid 1996;6: 445–450.
70. Grant DB. Congenital hypothyroidism: Optimal management in the light of 15 years' experience of screening. Arch Dis Child 1995;72: 85–89.
71. Nuovo J, Ellsworth A, Christensen DB, Reynolds R. Excessive thyroid hormone replacement therapy. J Am Board Fam Pract 1995;8: 435–439.
72. Fish L, Schwartz H, Cavanaugh J. Replacement dose, metabolism, and bioavailability of levothyroxine in the treatment of hypothyroidism. Role of triiodothyronine in pituitary feedback in humans. N Engl J Med 1987;316:764–770.
73. Dong BJ, Hauck WW, Gambertoglio JG, et al. Bioequivalence of generic and brand-name levothyroxine products in the treatment of hypothyroidism. JAMA 1997;277:1205–1213.
74. Wennlund A. Variation in serum levels of T_3, T_4, FT_4 and TSH during thyroxine replacement therapy. Acta Endocrinol 1986;113:47–49.
75. Sperber A, Liel L. Evidence of interference with the intestinal absorption of levothyroxine sodium by aluminum hydroxide. Arch Intern Med 1992;152:183–184.
76. Shakir KM, Chute JP, Aprill BS, Lazarus AA. Ferrous sulfate–induced increase in requirement for thyroxine in a patient with primary hypothyroidism. South Med J 1997;90:637–639.

77. Jabbar MA, Larrea J, Shaw RA. Abnormal thyroid function tests in infants with congenital hypothyroidism: The influence of soy-based formula. J Am Coll Nutr 1997;16:280–282.
78. Liel Y, Harman-Boehin I, Shavy S. Evidence for a clinically important adverse effect of fiber-enriched diet on the bioavailability of levothyroxine in adult hypothyroid patients. J Clin Endocrinol Metab 1996;81:857–859.
79. Kabadi UM. Influence of age on optimal daily levothyroxine dosage in patients with primary hypothyroidism grouped according to etiology. South Med J 1997;90:920–924.
80. De Whalley P. Do abnormal thyroid stimulating hormone level values result in treatment changes? A study of patients on thyroxine in one general practice. Br J Gen Pract 1995;45:93–95.
81. Kabadi UM, Cech R. Normal thyroxine and elevated thyrotropin concentrations: Evolving hypothyroidism or persistent euthyroidism with reset thyrostat. J Endocrinol Invest 1997;20:319–326.
82. Jaeschke R, Guyatt G, Gerstein H, et al. Does treatment with L-thyroxine influence health status in middle-aged and older adults with subclinical hypothyroidism? J Gen Intern Med 1996;11:744–749.
83. Zulewski H, Muller B, Exer P, Miserez AR, Staub JJ. Estimation of tissue hypothyroidism by a new clinical score: Evaluation of patients with various grades of hypothyroidism and controls. J Clin Endocrinol Metab 1997;82:771–776.
84. Surks M, Chopra I, Mariash C. American Thyroid Association guidelines for use of laboratory tests in thyroid disorders. JAMA 1990;263:1529–1532.
85. Burmesiter L, Goumaz M, Mariash C, Oppenheimer J. Levothyroxine dose requirements for thyrotropin suppression in the treatment of differentiated thyroid cancer. J Clin Endocrinol Metab 1992;75:344–350.
86. Taimela E, Koskinen P, Nuutila P, et al. Free thyroid hormones and a third-generation TSH assay in the detection of hyperthyroidism during long-term thyroxine treatment in thyroid carcinoma patients. Scand J Clin Lab Invest 1995;55:181–186.
87. Aronow WS. The heart and thyroid disease. Clin Geriatr Med 1995;11:219–229.
88. Hanna FW, Pettit RJ, Ammari F, Evans WD, Sandeman D, Lazarus JH. Effect of replacement doses of thyroxine on bone mineral density. Clin Endocrinol 1998;48:229–234.
89. Guo CY, Weetman AP, Eastell R. Longitudinal changes of bone mineral density and bone turnover in postmenopausal women on thyroxine. Clin Endocrinol 1997;46:301–307.
90. Fowler PB, McIvor J, Sykes L, Macrae KD. The effect of long-term thyroxine on bone mineral density and serum cholesterol. J R Coll Physicians Lond 1996;30:527–532.
91. Langdahl BL, Loft AG, Eriksen EF, Mosekilde L, Charles P. Bone mass, bone turnover and body composition in former hypothyroid patients receiving replacement therapy. Eur J Endocrinol 1996;134:702–709.
92. McDermott M, Perloff J, Kidd G. A longitudinal assessment of bone loss in women with levothyroxine-suppressed benign thyroid disease and thyroid cancer. Calcif Tissue Int 1995;56:521–525.
93. Marcocci C, Golia F, Bruno-Bossi G. Carefully monitored levothyroxine suppressive therapy is not associated with bone loss in premenopausal women. J Clin Endocrinol Metab 1994;78:818–823.
94. Pittman CS, Zayed AA. Myxedema coma. Curr Ther Endocrinol Metab 1997;6:98–101.
95. Jordan RM. Myxedema coma. Pathophysiology, therapy, and factors affecting prognosis. Med Clin North Am 1995;79:185–194.
96. American Academy of Pediatrics AAP Section on Endocrinology and Committee on Genetics, and American Thyroid Association Committee on Public Health. Newborn screening for congenital hypothyroidism: Recommended guidelines. Pediatrics 1993;91:1203–1209.
97. Kannan CR, Seshadri KG, Gruters A, et al. Guidelines for neonatal screening programmes for congenital hypothyroidism. Working group on congenital hypothyroidism of the European Society for Paediatric Endocrinology. Dis Mon 1997;43:601–677.
98. Bruner JP, Dellinger EH. Antenatal diagnosis and treatment of fetal hypothyroidism. A report of two cases. Fetal Diagn Ther 1997;12:200–204.
99. Roti E, Minelli R, Salvi M. Clinical review 80: Management of hyperthyroidism and hypothyroidism in the pregnant woman. J Clin Endocrinol Metab 1996;81:1679–1682.
100. Montoro MN. Managemnt of hypothyroidism during pregnancy. Clin Obstet Gynecol 1997;40:65–80.
101. Delange F. Neonatal screening for congenital hypothyroidism: Results and perspectives. Horm Res 1997;48:51–61.
102. McDougall IR, Maclin N. Hypothyroid women need more thyroxine when pregnant. J Fam Pract 1995;41:238–240.
103. Reasner C. Autoimmune thyroid disease and type 1 diabetes. Diabetes Rev 1993;1:343–351.
104. Chopra IJ. Clinical review 86: Euthyroid sick syndrome: Is it a misnomer? J Clin Endocrinol Metab 1997;82:329–334.
105. Yamazaki K, Yamada E, Kanaji Y, et al. Interleukin-6 (IL-6) inhibits thyroid function in the presence of soluble IL-6 receptor in cultured human thyroid follicles. Endocrinology 1996;137:4857–4863.
106. Murai H, Murakami S, Ishida K, Sugawara M. Elevated serum interleukin-6 and decreased thyroid hormone levels in postoperative patients and effects of IL-6 on thyroid cell function *in vitro*. Thyroid 1996;6:601–606.
107. Delange F. The disorders induced by iodine deficiency. Thyroid 1994;4:107–128.

72

ADRENAL GLAND DISORDERS

John G. Gums, PharmD, and Jerry D. Smith, PharmD

The adrenal glands were first characterized by Eustachius in 1563 (Table 72–1). After Addison identified a case of adrenal insufficiency in man, adrenal anatomy and physiology flourished. Most of the work done in the early and mid-1900s centered on the glucocorticoid cortisol. With the discovery of aldosterone by Simpson and Tait in 1952, adrenal pharmacology turned toward the mineralocorticoid. Conn[1] followed with his classical description of primary aldosteronism in 1955, and numerous clinicians and investigators have continued the discovery of the variety of disease processes promoted through the adrenal gland.

PHYSIOLOGY, ANATOMY, AND BIOCHEMISTRY

There are two adrenal glands located extraperitoneally to the upper poles of each kidney (Fig. 72–1). On average, each adrenal gland weighs 4 g and is 2 to 3 cm in width and 4 to 6 cm in length. The gland is fed by small arteries from the abdominal aorta and renal and phrenic arteries. Drainage of the adrenal gland occurs via the renal vein on the left and the inferior vena cava on the right.

The adrenal cortex occupies 10% of the total gland and is responsible for the secretion of catecholamines. The adrenal cortex accounts for the remaining 90% and is responsible for the secretion of three types of hormones (Fig. 72–2) from three separate zones.[2]

The zona glomerulosa, 15% of the total adrenal cortex, is responsible for mineralocorticoid production, of which aldosterone is the principle end product. Aldosterone maintains electrolyte and volume homeostasis by altering potassium and magnesium secretion and renal tubular sodium reabsorption. The zona reticularis, the innermost zone, makes up 60% of the cortex and is responsible for basal and stimulated glucocorticoid production. Glucocorticoids, mainly cortisol, are responsible for the regulation of fat, carbohydrate, and protein metabolism. The zona fasiculata occupies 25% of the adrenal cortex, is high in cholesterol, and is responsible for all androgen production. The androgens, testosterone and estradiol, are the major end products and have influence within the reproductive system as well as affecting primary and secondary sex characteristics.

HORMONE PRODUCTION AND METABOLISM

Cortisol production is accomplished via two successive hydroxylations: the first at the 21-position by 21-hydroxylase (yielding 11-deoxycortisol) and the second at the 11-position by 11-hydroxylase, yielding cortisol or hydrocortisone.

Aldosterone is a by-product of the 21-hydroxylation of pregnenolone to form deoxycorticosterone. The oxidation of 18-hydroxycorticosterone to aldosterone is a unique feature of the zona glomerulosa, explaining why aldosterone is not affected during disease processes limited to the fasiculata and/or reticularis.

Androgens have a 19-carbon nucleus and serve as precursors to more potent analogs produced in the periphery. The adrenal gland can synthesize estradiol and estrone from testosterone and androstenedione, respectively; however, the quantities are extremely small. The rates of production for the various steroids produced by the adrenal gland are listed in Table 72–2.

Metabolism of glucocorticoids is responsible for converting inactive steroids to active metabolites as well as deactivating the active steroids to less active or inactive metabolites. Most steroid products administered are active; however, in the case of prednisone and cortisone, metabolism is necessary for the conversion to the active prednisolone and cortisol, respectively. Following metabolic conversion, glucocorticoids are excreted renally as less active or inactive metabolites.

After metabolism, glomerular filtration is primarily responsible for the elimination of endogenously produced glucocorticoids. The half-life of cortisol is 70 to 120 minutes; with aldosterone, the half-life is only 15 minutes because of an extremely high first-pass effect.

Metabolism and conversion of the various steroids can be altered by a variety of disease states and medicinal compounds. Drugs and diseases known to result in enhanced clearance of steroids include phenytoin, phenobarbital, rifampin, mitotane, aminoglutethimide, hyperthyroidism, and renal disease (dexamethasone only). Drugs and diseases known to result in reduced clearance of steroids include estrogens and estrogen-containing oral contraceptives, liver disease, age, pregnancy, hypothyroidism, anorexia nervosa, protein–calorie malnutrition, and renal disease (prednisolone only). Plasma glucocorticoids are bound to one of three plasma proteins in varying degrees. Corticosteroid-binding globulin (CBG), albumin, and α_1-glycoprotein are capable of binding glucocorticoids, with CBG being the principle binding protein.

The function of steroid binding is to serve as a reservoir of steroids in their inactive state. This binding may change the availability of glucocorticoids to receptor-activating sites. Therefore, a final but important variable in altered plasma concentration of free (active) steroids is concentration of plasma proteins.

TABLE 72–1. Landmarks in Adrenal Cortical History

Date	Discovery	Investigator
1563	Adrenal described	Eustachius
1855	Adrenal insufficiency in man	Addison
1856	Adrenalectomy fatal in dog	Brown
1895–1904	Discovery of epinephrine	Oliver
1910	Hypoglycemia of Addison's disease	Porges
1927	First active adrenal cortical extract	Hartman
1932	Life of patient with Addison's disease prolonged with salt	Loeb
1936	The "alarm reaction"	Selye
1938	Synthesis of deoxycorticosterone	Reichstein
1948	Partial synthesis of cortisone	Sarrett
1949	First anti-inflammatory use of cortisone	Hench/Kendall
1952	Discovery of aldosterone	Simpson/Tait
1955	Discovery of primary aldosteronism	Conn

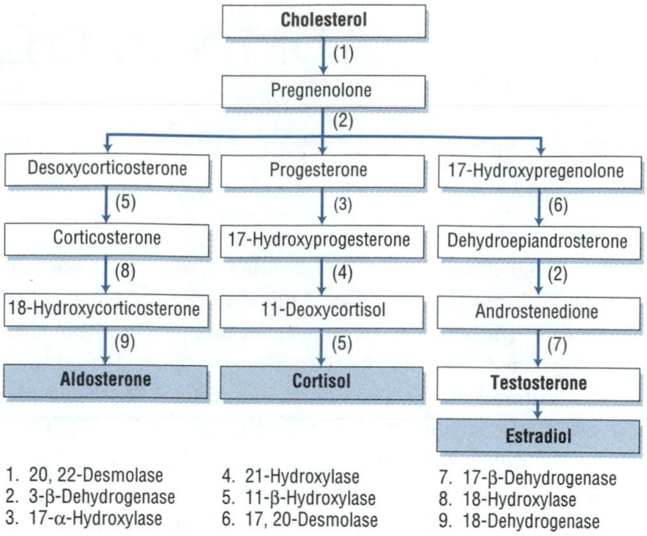

FIG. 72–2. The cholesterol pathway with the major enzymes and end points. *(From Ref. 1, with permission.)*

REGULATION OF HORMONE SECRETION

The regulation of glucocorticoid secretion is accomplished by the pituitary hormone, adrenocorticotropic hormone (ACTH). Under normal conditions, ACTH is released from the anterior pituitary in response to corticotropin-releasing factor (CRF), which is secreted by the median eminence of the hypothalamus (Fig. 72–3).

Additionally, histochemical studies have demonstrated that certain neurotransmitters have unique ability to stimulate production of CRF or ACTH directly. 5-Hydroxytryptamine (5-HT) and norepinephrine (NE) have both been shown to increase levels of ACTH. 5-HT causes a release of CRF through excitation of a cholinergic intervention. NE can cause direct stimulation of ACTH release, although this effect is still controversial. After release ACTH stimulates the adrenal gland to release cortisol and to a lesser extent aldosterone and androgens. The rising cortisol concentration inhibits the secretion of CRF and ACTH through a negative-feedback mechanism.

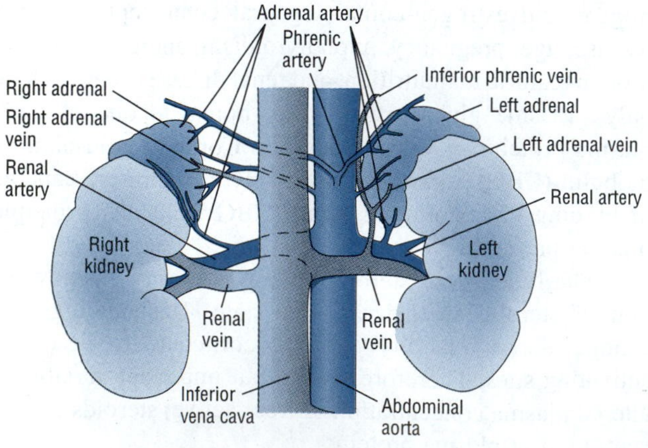

FIG. 72–1. Anatomy of the adrenal gland.

Regulation of adrenal androgens is accomplished in a manner similar to cortisol regulation. Therefore, when plasma androgen reaches sufficient concentrations, production is terminated via a negative-feedback loop. Androgen release is increased during puberty and in women with hirsutism. Adrenal androgen release is decreased in fasting, anorexia nervosa, and aging.

Regulation of aldosterone secretion is considerably more complex. The renin–angiotensin system has the ability to respond to electrolyte and volume changes to increase or decrease aldosterone secretion. Renin production and subsequent aldosterone secretion is stimulated by blood pressure lowering, erect posture, salt depletion, β-adrenergic stimulation, and central nervous system excitation. Renin production is inhibited by salt loading, angiotensin

TABLE 72–2. Rates of Production of Plasma Concentrations of Various Steroids

Steroid	24-Hour Secretion (mg)	Plasma Concentration (ng/mL)
Aldosterone	0.15	0.15–0.17
Androstenedone	2.50 (female)	1.80 Å 0.21 (female)
	2.20 (male)	1.14 Å 0.21 (male)
Corticosterone	1–4	2.4 Å 1.5 (female)
		4.2 Å 2.2 (male)
Cortisol	8.00–25.00	85.00 (female)
		116.00 (male)
11-Deoxycorticosterone	0.60	0.15–0.17
11-Deoxycortisol	0.40	0.95–2.50
Progesterone	0.0	0.20 Å 0.09 (female)[a]
		11.80 Å 7.00 (female)[b]
		0.18 Å 0.10 (male)
Testosterone	0.23	0.48 Å 0.14 (female)
		5.59 Å 1.51 (male)

[a]Follicular phase of menstrual cycle.
[b]Luteal phase of menstrual cycle.

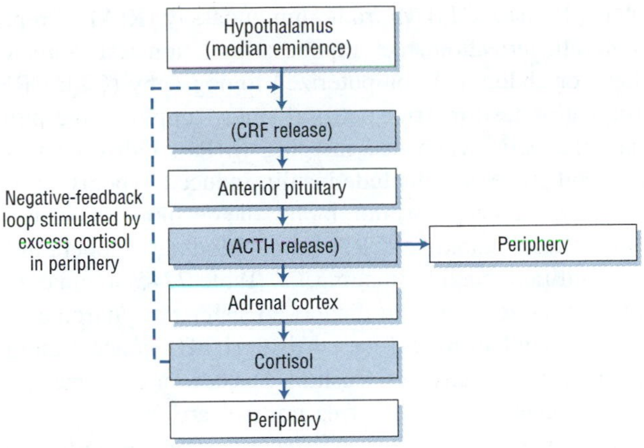

FIG. 72–3. Regulation of cortisol secretion under normal conditions. CRF = corticotropin-releasing factor; ACTH = adrenocorticotropic hormone.

II, vasopressin, potassium, calcium, blood pressure increases, and a variety of drugs. The conversion of renin substrate angiotensinogen to angiotensin I and subsequently to angiotensin II is the initial stimulus for aldosterone synthesis. Angiotensin II is acted on by aminopeptidase and converted to angiotensin III. Angiotensin II and III are both capable of stimulating the zona glomerulosa to secrete aldosterone. Following aldosterone secretion, increases in renal sodium and water retention as well as blood pressure are seen, thereby turning off the stimulus for renin release.

HYPERFUNCTION OF THE ADRENAL GLAND

CUSHING'S SYNDROME

In 1932, Cushing first described a syndrome of pituitary basophilism that attracted national attention. It was not until this time that patients with unexplained central obesity, cutaneous striae, osteoporosis, weakness, hypertension, diabetes mellitus, and congestion had a definite diagnosis. Cushing emphasized that the disease was of pituitary origin. Ten years later, Albright[3] focused his attention on the sugar hormone, which he believed originated from the adrenal cortex.

After the development of the method for measuring urinary steroids, Daughaday discovered elevated steroids in the urine of Cushing's disease patients. Finally, the end product was identified and Cushing's disease was correctly explained as an excess of cortisol in the plasma (hypercortisolism).

ETIOLOGY

Cushing's syndrome results from the effects of supraphysiologic levels of glucocorticoids originating either from exogenous administration or from endogenous overproduction by the adrenal glands (ACTH-dependent) or by abnormal adrenocortical tissues (ACTH-independent). Corticotropin-dependent Cushing's syndrome is usually (~ 70% of Cushing's cases) caused by overproduction of ACTH by the pituitary gland, causing adrenal hyperplasia (Cushing's disease). Pituitary adenomas account for approximately 85% of these cases. Ectopic ACTH-secreting tumors (12%) and nonneoplastic corticotrophin hypersecretion possibly secondary to excess corticotropin releasing hormone (CRH) production are felt to be responsible for the remainder of ACTH-dependent causes. The remaining 18% of Cushing's syndrome cases are ACTH-independent and are almost equally divided between adrenal adenomas and adrenal carcinomas, with rare cases caused by micronodular or macronodular hyperplasia.[4,5]

The majority of adrenal cortex tumors are benign adenomas. Adrenal carcinoma is found more often in children than in adults with Cushing's syndrome. Ectopic ACTH syndrome refers to excessive ACTH production resulting from a nonendocrine tumor, usually of the pancreas, thyroid, or lung. Small cell carcinoma of the lung will lead to ectopic ACTH secretion in 0.5% to 2% of cases. To distinguish between the various etiologies, a careful history and some pertinent laboratory work are required (Table 72–3).

CLINICAL PRESENTATION

The clinical symptoms most commonly seen with Cushing's syndrome are listed in Table 72–4.[5] The most common of these findings include central obesity and facial

TABLE 72–3. Various Etiologies of Cushing's Syndrome and Their Respective Differences

	Pituitary Dependent	Ectopic ACTH Syndrome	Adrenal Adenoma	Adrenal Carcinoma
Course	Slow	Rapid	Slow	Rapid
Symptoms	Mild to moderate	Atypical	Mild to moderate	Severe
Dominant sex/age	Female/male	Male	None noted	Children
Virilization	+	+	+	+++
Abdominal mass	0	0	0	++
Plasma ACTH concentration	Slightly elevated	0	0	0
Dexamethasone suppression test	≥ 50% suppression	No suppression	No suppression	No suppression
Iodocholesterol scan	Bilateral uptake	Unilateral uptake	Unilateral uptake	No uptake

TABLE 72–4. Clinical Features in Patients With Hypercortisolism

Feature	% Patients
Obesity	90
Hypertension	85
Facial plethora	84
Glucose intolerance	80
Menstrual dysfunction	76
Hirsutism	72
Striae	67
Myopathy	65
Muscular weakness	58
Osteoporosis	55
Psychiatric changes	55

rounding. About 50% of patients will exhibit some peripheral obesity and fat accumulation. Facial plethora is caused by an underlying atrophy of the skin and connective tissue. Patients often are described as having moon fascies with a buffalo hump. Fat accumulation in the dorsocervical area (buffalo hump) can be associated with any major weight gain, whereas increased supraclavicular fat pads are more specific for Cushing's syndrome.[5] Striae are usually present along the lower abdomen and take on a red to purple color.

Hypertension is seen in 75% to 85% of patients with Cushing's syndrome. Diastolic blood pressures greater than 119 mm Hg have been noted in over 20% of patients with Cushing's syndrome.[6] Hypertensive complications have traditionally been major contributors to the mortality and morbidity of Cushing's syndrome.

Gonadal dysfunction is common in patients with hypercortisolism. The abnormalities are principally a result of elevated levels of androgens in the females and cortisol in the males. Most common in females is amenorrhea, which is seen in up to 75% of females with the diagnosis. Excess androgen secretion is also responsible for the 80% of female patients who present with hirsutism.

Approximately 50% to 60% of patients will develop Cushing's-induced osteoporosis. Of these patients 40% will present with back pain and about 20% of these will progress to compression fractures of the spine.

DIAGNOSIS

Diagnosis of Cushing's syndrome is relatively easy, but the differentiation between etiologies can be difficult[4,5] (Fig. 72–4). The diagnostic evaluation involves two steps. First, the presence of hypercortisolism must be established via the following tests: 24-hour urine free cortisol, midnight cotrisol of > 7.5 μg/dL, and/or the low-dose dexamethasone-suppression test (DST) (using 1 mg for the overnight test or 0.5 mg/6 h for the "classic" 2-day study). Second, because these tests cannot determine the etiology of Cushing's syndrome, other tests and procedures will be employed and may include any of the following: high-dose DST; plasma ACTH via radioimmunoassay (RIA); adrenal vein catheterization; metyrapone stimulation test; adrenal, chest, or abdominal computerized tomography (CT); CRH stimulation test; inferior petrosal sinus sampling; and pituitary magnetic resonance imaging (MRI). Other possible tests and procedures include insulin-induced hypoglycemia; somatostatin receptor scintigraphy; the desmopression stimulation test; naloxone CRH stimulation test; loperamide test; and radionuclide imaging.[4–16] Table 72–5 summarizes some of the tests used to diagnose Cushing's syndrome.

Elevated urinary free cortisol (UFC) concentrations are highly suggestive of Cushing's syndrome. Normal reference values for urinary free cortisol are 20 to 90 g per 24-hour period. It is not unusual to detect a twofold or threefold increase in urine cortisol in the patient with hyperfunction of the adrenal gland. Starvation, topical steroid application, hydration from water loading, and acute stress all are capable of elevating the urine cortisol concentrations. Because other pathologic conditions can increase the amount of free cortisol, additional tests should be performed to confirm the diagnosis, or the diagnostic evaluation should be repeated when the acute stress has resolved. Of all urinary measures, UFC is the most useful for assessment of any patient with suspected Cushing's syndrome.[7]

In the overnight DST, 1 mg of dexamethasone is administered at 11:00 PM. The following morning at 8:00 AM plasma cortisol is obtained for analysis. The Cushing's patient will not exhibit a suppressed cortisol concentration via the negative-feedback loop, and the morning cortisol concentration will be elevated (greater than 5 g/100 mL).[5] The overnight DST is useful only as a screening tool for Cushing's syndrome because of a high sensitivity, but a rather low specificity. Phenytoin, rifampin, phenobarbital, and

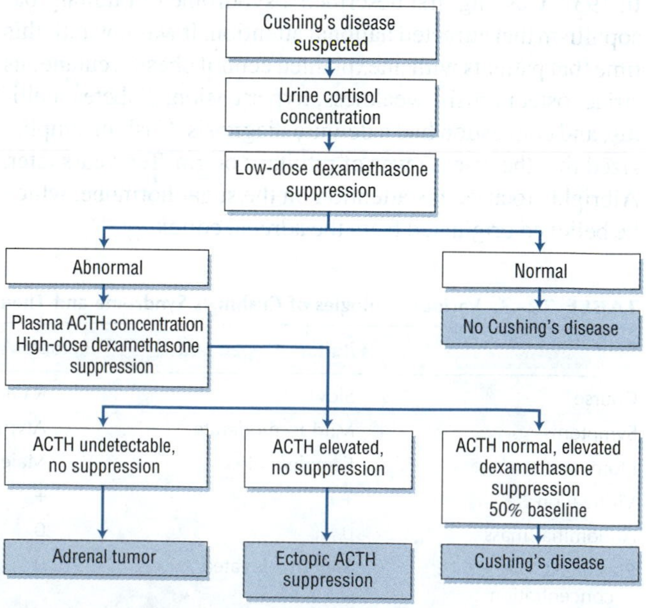

FIG. 72–4. Algorithm for diagnosing Cushing's disease. ACTH = adrenocorticotropic hormone.

TABLE 72–5. Summary of Tests Used to Diagnose Cushing's Syndrome[a]

Test	Normal	Hyperplasia	Adenoma	Carcinoma
Plasma				
Cortisol (μg/100 mL, AM/PM)	17/8	↑/↑	↑↑/↑↑	↑↑↑/↑↑↑
ACTH (pg/mL)	10–80	↑↑↑	↑	↑
Urine 17-Hydroxycorticosteroid (mg/d)				
Basal	2–10	15	30	50
After ACTH[b]	2–5 × ↑	3–5 × ↑	↔	↔
Dexamethasone 2 mg/d[b]	↓/↔	↓	↔	↔
Dexamethasone 8 mg/d[b]	↓/↔	↓	↔	↔
Nuclear				
Iodocholesterol uptake pattern	Bilateral	Bilateral	Unilateral	No uptake

[a]↑ = increase; ↓ = decrease; ↔ = no change.
[b]Compared to basal.

other drugs that induce liver enzymes may cause an increase in the clearance rate of the dexamethasone, causing decreased levels leading to a falsely positive suppression test.[7] Plasma dexamethasone measured at the conclusion of this test can clarify results clouded by differences in metabolism from these drug interactions, individual variability, or patient noncompliance.

Urinary examination of steroids can be used in the diagnosis of Cushing's disease. The normal circadian rhythm of cortisol will demonstrate a 60% to 80% decline between 8:00 AM and 11:00 PM. This rhythm is lost in the Cushing's syndrome patient. Critics of the use of urinary steroids in the diagnosis of Cushing's syndrome point out that urinary 17-OHCS levels may be decreased in the presence of starvation, renal failure, liver disease, pregnancy, and hypothyroidism. Additionally, drugs that induce hepatic microenzymes such as phenytoin, phenobarbital, carbamazepine, and mitotane may indirectly reduce levels of urinary 17-OHCS. Drugs that have direct assay interference with urinary 17-OHCS include spironolactone, hydroxyzine, chlordiazepoxide, phenothiazines, and troleandomycin.[17] The false-negative and false-positive rates from clinical studies of 11% and 27%, respectively, exclude urinary 17-OHCS from being a screening test.[7]

Additionally, plasma ACTH concentrations can be measured via RIA.[16] In the ACTH-dependent Cushing's syndromes, ACTH may be normal or elevated. Very high levels of ACTH favor the ectopic production. ACTH values are low in ACTH-independent (adrenal) Cushing's syndrome. ACTH levels may appear artificially low in some ectopic ACTH-producing tumors because ACTH can be secreted as an active prohormone that is not detected by the assay.

The high-dose DST operates under the same principle as the low-dose test.[5] The main difference is in total dose (16 mg) and the time to test the patient (48 hours). The high-dose test has its main application in differentiating the adrenal hyperplasia patient from the patient with another form of hypercortisolism. The adrenal hyperplasia patient will generally demonstrate a 50% reduction in urinary steroids over baseline, whereas the others will generally not suppress. The high-dose test is based on the principle that patients with Cushing's syndrome not caused by adrenal tumors or ectopic ACTH production will suppress their hypothalamic–pituitary axis in the presence of glucocorticoids, but it takes higher than normal doses. An overnight high-dose DST has been developed, whereby the patient has a baseline serum cortisol drawn at 8:00 AM and dexamethasone 8 mg is taken at 11:00 PM. The next morning, at 8:00 AM, another serum cortisol is drawn.[16] The high-dose test is most useful when the low-dose test and other diagnostic studies have confirmed the diagnosis of Cushing's syndrome. The high-dose DST has been studied in combination with ACTH and metapyrone testing and results in better specificity than either test alone.

Abnormal adrenal anatomy is effectively identified using high-resolution CT scanning and perhaps MRI. Nodules as small as 1 to 1.5 cm on the adrenal cortex are easily identified by CT. With the use of thin-section scanning, nodules as small as 3 to 5 mm can be visualized.[18,19]

Differential Diagnosis

Although the diagnosis of Cushing's disease is not a difficult one, at times the clinician will need to differentiate it from syndromes that mimic Cushing's. Pseudo-Cushing's syndrome refers to a group of diseases that can mimic Cushing's disease. Patients with obesity, chronic alcoholism, depression, and acute illness of any type can cloud the diagnosis of Cushing's disease. Depressed patients, though mimicking the urinary steroid abnormalities of Cushing's disease, will not resemble a Cushinoid patient in appearance. The chronic alcoholic will have his laboratory panel returned to baseline after he or she stops drinking. The obese patient often will have normal cortisol concentrations of both serum and urinary screening. Iatrogenic Cushing's syndrome, induced by glucocorticoid administration, often can be indistinguishable from Cushing's disease. A careful history and serum determination in a basal state can aid the clinician in making the diagnosis. If exogenous glucocorticoids are being taken, plasma cortisol levels may increase while corticosterone levels remain low.[20]

▶ TREATMENT: Cushing's Syndrome

If left untreated, Cushing's syndrome is associated with a high percentage of morbidity and mortality owing to associated disorders such as diabetes mellitus, cardiovascular disease, and electrolyte abnormalities. These disorders limit the survival of the Cushing's disease patient to 4 to 5 years following initial diagnosis. The desired outcomes of treatment are to limit the morbidity and mortality and return the patient to a normal functional state by removing the source of hypercortisolism without causing any pituitary or adrenal deficiencies.

Once the etiology of the disease is identified, the treatment of choice for both ACTH-dependent and -independent Cushing's syndrome is surgical resection of any offending tumors.[21] However, many secondary treatment plans are available depending on the etiology of the disease (Table 72–6)[4,5] The next section will discuss the different pharmacologic agents, followed by differential treatment.

PHARMACOLOGIC THERAPY

Pharmacotherapy of Cushing's syndrome (dosing can be found in Table 72–6)[22,23] can be divided into four categories based upon the anatomic site of action of the agent: (1) steroidogenic inhibitors; (2) adrenolytic agents; (3) neuromodulators of ACTH release; and (4) glucocorticoid-receptor blocking agents.[24–26]

Steriodogenic inhibition may be accomplished with the following agents: metyrapone, aminoglutethimide, and ketoconazole. Either metyrapone or aminoglutethamide used alone has limited efficacy, with relapse occurring after discontinuation of therapy. Neither agent should be used after successful surgery. Their use should be restricted to the refractory patient who is not a surgical candidate. Combination therapy with these agents appears more effective than single-agent therapy and may cause fewer side effects.

Metyrapone (Metopirone, Novartis) inhibits 11-hydroxylase activity, resulting in cortisol-synthesis inhibition. Initially, patients may demonstrate an increase in plasma ACTH concentrations because of a sudden drop in cortisol. Metyrapone is biologically active following oral administration. Nausea, vomiting, vertigo, headache, dizziness, abdominal discomfort, and allergic rash have been reported following administration.[22,27]

Initially, aminoglutethimide (Cytadren, Novartis) was used to treat refractory forms of epilepsy, but it was later discovered to be a potent inhibitor of cortisol synthesis. Aminoglutethimide inhibits the conversion of cholesterol to pregnenolone early in the cortisol pathway.[27,28] Plasma cortisol concentrations are reduced by up to 50% following aminoglutethimide therapy. Side effects include severe sedation, nausea, ataxia, and skin rashes.[22,26,28] Most of these reactions are dose-dependent and limit the use of aminoglutethimide in most patients. Aminoglutethimide may decrease the anticoagulant effect of warfarin. Caution is advised if aminoglutethimide is given to patients already receiving corticosteroids. Alone, aminoglutethimide is indicated for short-term use in inoperable Cushing's disease with ectopic-ACTH syndrome as the suspected underlying etiology.

Aminoglutethimide may be used in combination with metyrapone. Smaller doses of both drugs can be used, therefore minimizing the toxicity associated with either agent. The combination therapy appears effective for various etiologies of Cushing's disease and is useful in the inoperable patient.

The imidazole derivative antifungal ketoconazole[22,24–27] (Nizoral, Janssen) is highly effective in lowering cortisol in Cushing's disease, resulting in normal corticosteroid values in 84% of patients with an additional 11% of patients reporting improvement. In addition to lowering serum cortisol levels, ketoconazole can cause gynecomastia and lower plasma testosterone values. All of these effects are attributed to its inhibition of a variety of cytochrome P450 enzymes including 11-hydroxylase and 17-hydroxylase. The most

TABLE 72–6. Possible Treatment Plans in Cushing's Disease Based on Etiology

	Treatment				
			Dosing		
Etiology	*Nondrug*	*Drug*	*Initial*	*Usual*	*Md*
Adrenal carcinoma	Surgery	Mitotane (Lysodren) 500-mg tabs	1–6 g/d, increased by 1–2 g/d q3–7d	9–10 g/d, divided tid–qid	16g/d
Ectopic ACTH syndrome	Surgery Chemotherapy Irradiation	Metyrapone (Metopirone) 250-mg tabs	1–1.5 g/d divided q4–6h	1–6 g/d divided q4–6h	6g/d
		Aminoglutethimide, (Cytadren) 250-mg tabs	0.5–1 g/d divided bid–qid × 2 wk	1 g/d divided q6h	2g/d
Pituitary dependent	Surgery Irradiation	Cyproheptadine (Periactin) 2 mg/5 mL syrup and 4-mg tabs	8 mg/d divided bid	24–32 mg/d divided qid	32 mg/d
		Metyrapone Mitotane	See above	See above	See above
Adrenal adenoma	Surgery plus postoperative replacement therapy	Ketoconazole (Nizoral) 200-mg tabs	200 mg qd–bid	600–800 mg/d divided bid	1200 mg/d

common adverse effects are reversible elevation of hepatic transaminases, gynecomastia, and gastrointestinal upset.

The adrenolytic agent mitotane (*ortho-, para*-dichlorodiphenyldichloroethane, Lysodren, Bristol-Myers Squibb) is a cytotoxic drug that structurally resembles the insecticide chlorophenothane (DDT). Mitotane inhibits the 11-hydroxylation of 11-desoxycortisol and 11-desoxycorticosterone in the cortext. The net result is a reduced synthesis of cortisol and corticosterone. It decreases cortisol secretion rate, plasma cortisol concentrations, urinary free cortisol, and plasma concentrations of the 17-substituted steroids.[22] This drug appears to selectively inhibit adrenocortical function without causing cellular destruction. Degeneration of cells within the zona fasiculata and reticularis occurs with resultant atrophy of the adrenal cortex. The zona glomerulosa is minimally affected during acute therapy but can become damaged following long-term treatment.

Because mitotane can severely reduce urinary excretion of 17-OHCS, before initiating therapy the patient should be hospitalized. Mitotane should be continued as long as clinical benefits occur. Cortisol secretion rate, plasma cortisol concentration, urinary free cortisol, and urinary steroid production should be monitored to assess response to mitotane. If necessary, steriod replacement therapy can be given. Approximately 80% of mitotane-treated patients develop lethargy and somnolence, and other central nervous system adverse drug reactions occur in approximately 40% of patients.

Neuromodulatory agents include cyproheptadine, bromocriptine, valproic acid, and octreotide. None of the neuromodulatory agents has demonstrated consistent clinical efficacy in the treatment of Cushing's disease. The existence of a bromocriptine-responsive subset of patients remains controversial.[26]

Cyproheptadine (Periactin, Merck) can decrease ACTH secretion in the Cushing's disease patient. Morning plasma cortisol concentrations, as well as 24-hour urinary cortisol (free) concentrations should be monitored. Side effects are minor and include sedation and hyperphagia. Cyproheptadine should be reserved for nonsurgical candidates who fail more conventional therapy. Because response rate is no more than 30%, patients should be followed closely for relapses.

Glucocorticoid receptor antagonism may be accomplished via RU-486 (mifepristone). RU-486 is a progesterone and glucocorticoid receptor antagonist that inhibits dexamethasone suppression and raises endogenous cortisol and ACTH values in normal subjects.[26,27,29,30] Limited clinical experience in Cushing's suggests that RU-486 is highly effective in reversing the manifestation of hypercortisolism. Because of its novel site of action as a receptor antagonist leading to higher cortisol and ACTH levels, the diagnosis of treatment-induced glucocorticoid insufficiency must rest on clinical signs only. The efficacy and long-term effects of RU-486 remain to be determined.

Spironolactone has been used for its competitive antagonism of aldosterone in the treatment of Cushing's syndrome. Spironolactone can provide symptomatic relief of the hypertension and hypokalemia often seen in Cushing's syndrome.

Daily monitoring of 24-hour urinary free-cortisol levels and serum cortisol levels are essential to monitor for adrenal insufficiency. Steroid secretion should be monitored with all of these drugs and steroid replacement given as needed. Whatever the choice, pharmacologic therapy in pituitary-dependent disease is mainly centered around patient stabilization prior to surgery or in patients waiting for potential response to other therapies.

PITUITARY-DEPENDENT CUSHING'S DISEASE

The etiology of Cushing's disease of pituitary origin is unknown. A solitary corticotrophic adenoma is almost always the cause.[4] The tumor is usually a microadenoma (< 1 cm in diameter) with macroadenomas being rare and corticotrophic hyperplasia and carcinomas being extremely rare.[5] A minority of cases may be caused by excessive ACTH secretion by nonneoplastic corticotrophin cells.[27] Currently the optimal form of therapy uses the hypothalamic, pituitary, and adrenal glands as avenues for intervention.

▶ TREATMENT: Pituitary-Dependent Cushing's Disease

NONPHARMACOLOGIC THERAPY

SURGERY

During the last decade, the treatment of choice for Cushing's disease has been transsphenoidal resection of the pituitary microadenoma.[4,5,30] The advantages to this procedure include preservation of pituitary function, low complication rate, and high clinical improvement rate. The overall cure rate of histologically proven tumors approaches 90%.

Bilateral adrenalectomy surgery had been the mainstay of therapy for years. It is used now only in patients for whom transsphenoidal surgery and pituitary irradiation have failed or cannot be used.[5,27] Bilateral adrenalectomy rapidly reverses hypercortisolism. However, patients may develop Nelson's syndrome, which involves sella turcica enlargement and hyperpigmentation, caused by postoperative hypothalamic stimulation. Therefore, if bilateral adrenalectomy is used, it should be accompanied by some form of hypothalamic inhibition.

IRRADIATION

Irradiation (4000 to 5000 rads) of the pituitary has provided clinical improvement in approximately 50% of patients.[27] Improvement is usually not seen until 6 to 12 months after therapy and can create pituitary-dependent hormone deficiencies. Most clinicians will reserve pituitary irradiation for the patient with a mild case of Cushing's disease or as an adjunct to another therapy.

TABLE 72–7. Alternative Steroid Replacement Regimens in the Adrenal Adenoma Patient

Time	Hydrocortisone Dose (mg) IV	IM	PO
Operation day	300	50 before surgery/ 50 after surgery	
Postoperative day 1	200	50 q12h	
2	150	50 q12h	
3	100	50 q12h	
4		50 q12h	25 q6h
5		25 q12h	25 q6h[a]
7			25 q6h
8–10			25 q8h
11–20			25 q12h
21+			20 at 8 AM 10 at 4 PM

[a]Add fludrocortisone 0.05–0.2 mg PO daily starting on postop day 5 and adjust dose based on blood pressure, body weight, and serum electrolytes.

ETIOLOGY-BASED THERAPY

ADRENAL ADENOMA

Surgical resection of benign adrenal adenoma is associated with relatively few side effects and a high cure rate (95%). The contralateral gland in the patient with adrenal adenoma is usually atrophic. Therefore, steroid replacement is needed both perioperatively and postoperatively. Table 72–7 outlines an approach to steroid replacement for three separate routes of hydrocortisone. Therapy should be continued for 6 to 12 months following surgery. Before replacement therapy is discontinued, recovery of the adrenal axis may be assessed by administering (ACTH) and measuring cortisol response at 30 and 60 minutes. Cortisol levels should exceed 18 g/dL before discontinuance of the exogenous steroids.[4]

ADRENAL CARCINOMA

Unlike the benign adenoma patient, patients with adrenal carcinoma have an unpredictable and unfavorable outcome with surgical resection.[5] Often, the complete tumor cannot be excised, leaving the patients with some degree of symptomatology and extra-adrenal involvement. Irradiation can be used if metastases are discovered. In the patient with adrenal carcinoma who is not a surgical candidate, the focus of treatment is on palliative pharmacologic intervention (e.g., mitotane).

Mitotane appears to be the drug of choice in inoperable functional and nonfunctional adrenal carcinoma. Tumor regression is seen in approximately 35% to 50% of the patients, with most regression occurring between the second and fourth month of therapy. Seventy-five percent of patients will exhibit a 30% fall in urinary steroids, with 50% of patients showing an improved clinical response after 5 months of treatment. Patient survival appears prolonged, although no adequate clinical trials are available to support this assumption.

Metyrapone, aminoglutethimide, and ketoconazole may be given to attempt control of steroid hypersecretion. 5-Fluorouracil has also been used in combination therapy.[30]

ECTOPIC ACTH SYNDROME

In the ectopic ACTH syndrome multiple sites of tumors exist, and location of the ectopic site is essential but often difficult. Therefore, only approximately 10% of patients are cured following surgery and the remaining 90% receive postoperative medication.

Pharmacologic management with metyrapone was shown to be effective and remains the agent of choice in the ectopic ACTH syndrome.[30] Aminoglutethimide and are alternative agents.[4,27] Mitotane has been tried in patients with ectopic ACTH syndrome; however, its side-effect profile generally limits its use.

Ketoconazole, RU-486 (mifepristone), and the somatostatin analog (octreotide) have been reported to reduce the clinical signs of the ectopic ACTH syndrome.[25,30,31] Further evaluation of these agents is needed.

HYPERALDOSTERONISM

Excess aldosterone is categorized as either primary or secondary forms of hyperaldosterone (Table 72–8).[32-40]

Primary Aldosteronism

Etiology. Primary aldosteronism implies that the physiologic abnormality is within the adrenal cortex. The most common causes include a solitary adrenal adenoma (60%) or idiopathic adrenocortical hyperplasia (35% bilateral and 5% unilateral). Other rare causes include adrenal cortex carcinoma, glucocorticoid-suppressible hyperaldosteronism, renin-responsive adrenocortical adenoma, and primary adrenocortical hyperplasia.[35,41]

Clinical Presentation. The incidence of primary aldosteronism is relatively uncommon, occurring in approximately 0.05% to 2% of all hypertensive patients. The disease is more common in women aged 30 to 50 years. Signs and symptoms include arterial hypertension, muscle weakness, fatigue, tetany, parasthesia, paralysis, nocturnal polyuria, polydipsia, reduced glucose tolerance (25%), metabolic alkalosis, and headache. Hypokalemia (80% to 90%), suppressed renin activity, elevated plasma aldosterone concentrations, hypernatremia (> 142 mEq/L), hypomagnesemia, and an elevated bicarbonate concentration (> 31 mEq/L) all the characteristic laboratory findings in primary aldosteronism.[42]

TABLE 72–8. Syndromes of Mineralocorticoid Excess

Primary Aldosteronism	Secondary Aldosteronism: Hypertensive	Secondary Aldosteronism: Nonhypertensive
Aldosterone-producing adenoma (APA)	Accelerated and renal vascular hypertension	Sodium depletion Hemorrhage
Bilateral adrenal hyperplasia (BAH)—idiopathic	Renin-secreting tumors Necrotizing vasculitis	Pregnancy Edema
Adrenal carcinoma Glucocorticoid-remediable hyperaldosteronism	Estrogen therapy	Bartter's syndrome Diuretic therapy

TABLE 72–9. Differential Diagnosis of Primary Aldosteronism

Disease	Plasma Renin Concentration	Plasma Aldosterone Concentration	Blood Pressure
Primary aldosteronism	Low	High	High
Edematous disorders	High	High	Normal
Malignant hypertension	High	High	High
Congenital adrenal hyperplasia	Low	Low	High
Cushing's syndrome	Low to normal	Low to normal	High
Liddle's syndrome	Low	Low	High
Bartter's syndrome	High	High	Low to normal
Licorice ingestion	Low	Low	High
Low-renin essential hypertension	Low	Low to normal	High

Diagnosis. The absolute diagnosis is relatively easy based on clinical findings and pertinent laboratory findings.[43] However, as in Cushing's disease, the discovery of the underlying etiology is mandatory to ensure proper treatment. Table 72–9 lists the various abnormalities that must be ruled out when suspicion of hyperaldosteronism is high.

A serum potassium concentration of less than 3.5 mEq/L with a concurrent urinary potassium content greater than 30 mEq per 24 hours is suggestive of primary aldosteronism.[44] Normokalemia does not exclude the diagnosis of primary aldosteronism. Between 7% and 38% of patients with primary aldosteronism will have serum potassium concentrations greater than 3.6 mEq/L.[45] The diagnosis of primary aldosteronism can be made with a plasma-aldosterone-to-plasma-renin-activity ratio (PA:PRA). A PA:PRA of > 30 with a PA value of > 20 ng/dL has been shown to be 90% sensitive and 91% specific.[40]

Differentiating between an aldosterone-producing adenoma (APA) and bilateral adrenal hyperplasia (BAH) is imperative to formulate a proper treatment plan. A majority of the adenomas are singular and small, less than 1 cm. The left adrenal gland is affected at a higher rate than the right. Patients with APA generally have more severe hypertension, more profound hypokalemia, and higher plasma and urinary aldosterone levels compared to patients with BAH.[42]

The underlying abnormality in BAH remains a mystery, but some investigators believe that a hormone factor stimulates the zona glomerulosa, resulting in increased sensitivity to angiotensin II.[41] In contrast to APA patients, patients with BAH are able to maintain control of the renin–angiotensin system, with little effect following doses of ACTH. The use of 50 mg of captopril given orally with subsequent determination of plasma renin and plasma aldosterone can be a useful method of screening for primary aldosternism.[44] The false-negative rate was 6.3% and the false-positive rate was 0.6%.

Therapeutic Management: BAH-Dependent Hyperaldosteronism. Spironolactone (Aldactone, Searle), a competitive inhibitor of aldosterone, is the drug of choice in BAH-dependent hyperaldosteronism.[36,42] Spironolactone inhibits aldosterone biosynthesis within the adrenal gland, making it extremely useful in overstimulated BAH patients. Spironolactone is available in oral form, with most patients responding to doses in the 200 to 400 mg/d range. The clinician should wait 4 to 8 weeks before reassessing the patient for urinary electrolytes and blood pressure control. Adverse effects of spironolactone include gastrointestional discomfort, impotence, gynecomastia, and menstrual irregularities. Additionally, because salicylates increase the renal secretion of canrenone, the active metabolite, patients should be advised to avoid concomitant therapy with salicylates. Because spironolactone blocks testosterone biosynthesis, it often is not used in men. The drug of choice in men and patients intolerant of spironolactone is amiloride (Midamor, Merck).[42,45] The usual dose is 5 mg twice a day up to 30 mg/d if necessary.

Second-line therapy is often required to control the blood pressure of patients with BAH. Agents useful as second-line choices include the calcium channel blockers, ACE inhibitors, and low-dose diuretics such as HCTZ.[42,45]

Therapeutic Management: APA-Dependent Hyperaldosteronism. The treatment of choice for APA-dependent aldosteronism remains surgical resection of the adenoma. If no primary lesion is found, resection of one and a half of the adrenal glands can be attempted, followed by supplemental spironolactone therapy.

Summary. The diagnosis of primary aldosteronism is made through the observation of elevated blood pressure, low serum potassium, high urinary potassium, elevated serum and urinary aldosterone, and an elevated PA:PRA (Fig. 72–5).

Differentiating between the various etiologies is mandatory. Patients with adrenal adenomas can be distinguished from patients

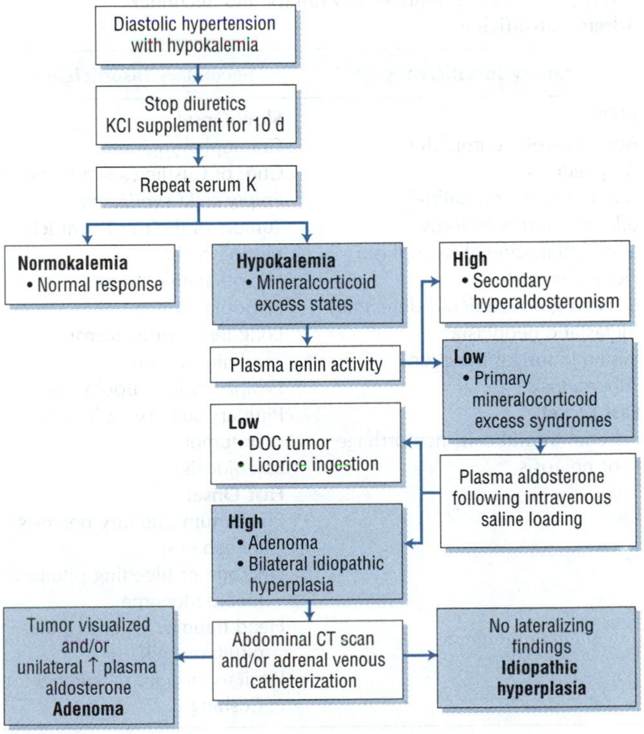

FIG. 72–5. Flow chart in the diagnosis of primary aldosteronism.

with hyperplasia by CT scan. Treatment depends on the etiology with surgical resection, well accepted as the treatment of choice in adenomas, and spironolactone or amiloride plus second-line agents in patients with hyperplasia.

Secondary Aldosteronism

Secondary hyperaldosteronism results from stimulation of the zona glomerulosa by an extra-adrenal factor, usually the renin–angiotensin system. Excessive potassium intake can create a physiologic increase in aldosterone, as can oral contraceptive use, pregnancy (10 times normal by third trimester), and menses. Congestive heart failure, cirrhosis, renal artery stenosis, and Bartter's syndrome also can lead to elevated aldosterone concentrations.

Treatment of secondary aldosteronism is dictated by etiology. Removal of the extra-adrenal source of the excess aldosterone should resolve the disorder. Medical therapy with spironolactone is the mainstay of treatment until an exact etiology can be located.

HYPOFUNCTION OF THE ADRENAL GLAND

Primary adrenal insufficiency, or Addison's disease, involves the destruction of all regions of the adrenal cortex. Deficiencies arise in cortisol, aldosterone, and the various androgens.[46] Approximately 40% to 53% of patients with idiopathic primary adrenal insufficiency present with one or more clinical disorders involving multiple endocrine organs. The organs involved can include ovary, thyroid, pancreas, and parathyroid gland. This polyglandular failure syndrome is associated with the idiopathic etiology only and has not been seen with adrenal insufficiency associated with tuberculosis or other invasive diseases.

Secondary insufficiency most commonly results from exogenous steroid use, leading to suppression of the hypothalamic–pituitary axis, resulting in a deficiency of ACTH, producing low concentrations of androgen and cortisol. Secondary disease classically presents with normal concentrations of mineralocorticoids.

Approximately 90% of the adrenal cortex must be destroyed before adrenal insufficiency symptoms will occur.[47] Specific etiologies for both primary and secondary insufficiency are listed in Table 72–10.

Symptoms common in patients with adrenal insufficiency include weakness (100%), weight loss (100%), increased pigmentation (95%), hypotension (90%), gastrointestinal symptoms (55%), postural dizziness (10%), and vitiligo (20%).[48]

Adrenal hemorrhage can result from multiple etiologies, traumatic shock, coagulopathies, ischemic disorders, and other situations of severe stress, but septicemia is the most common.[48] Symptoms include truncal pain, fever, shaking, chills, hypotension preceding shock, anorexia, headache, vertigo, vomiting, rash, psychiatric symptoms, abdominal rigidity or rebound, and death in 6 to 48 hours if not treated. The most common organisms found on autopsy are *Streptococcus pneumoniae, Staphylococcus, and Haemophilus influenzae.*

TABLE 72–10. Etiologies of Primary and Secondary Adrenal Insufficiency

Primary Insufficiency	Secondary Insufficiency
AIDS	**Slow Onset**
Adrenomyeloneuropathy	Craniopharyngioma
Amyloidosis	Cure of Cushing's syndrome
Autoimmune adrenalitis[a]	Empty-sella syndrome
Bilateral adrenalectomy	Tumors of the third ventricle
Congenital adrenal hypoplasia	Histiocytosis
Hemochromatosis	Hypothalamic tumors
Isolated glucocorticoid deficiency	Hypopituitarism
Metastatic neoplasia	Long-term corticosteroid administration
Systemic fungal infection	Lymphocytic hypophysitis
Tuberculosis[b]	Pituitary surgery, radiation, or tumor
Fast Onset	Sarcoidosis
Adrenal thrombosis, hemorrhage, or necrosis	**Fast Onset**
	Postpartum pituitary necrosis (Sheehan's)
	Necrotic or bleeding pituitary macroadenoma
	Head trauma, lesions of the pituitary stalk
	Pituitary or adrenal surgery for Cushing's

[a]Accounts for approximately 70% of total cases.
[b]Accounts for approximately 20% of total cases.

ADDISON'S DISEASE

Distinguishing Addison's disease from secondary insufficiency is difficult; however, the following guidelines may be helpful:

1. Hyperpigmentation usually is not seen in secondary adrenal insufficiency because of low amounts of melanocyte-stimulating hormone (MSH). Low amounts of MSH are present owing to a deficient pituitary secretion of ACTH and β-lipotropin.
2. Aldosterone secretion usually is preserved in secondary insufficiency.
3. Weight loss, dehydration, hyponatremia, hyperkalemia, and elevated blood urea nitrogen are common in Addison's disease.
4. Addison's disease will have an abnormal response to the rapid ACTH-stimulation test. Plasma ACTH levels are usually 400 to 2000 pg/mL in primary insufficiency versus 0 to 50 pg/mL in secondary insufficiency. A normal ACTH-stimulation test does not rule out secondary adrenal insufficiency.

The short cosyntropin-stimulation test can be used to assess patients suspected of hypocortisolism. Patients are given 250 μg of synthetic ACTH IV or IM, with serum cortisol levels drawn at baseline and 30 to 60 minutes after the injection. An increase to a cortisol level ≥ 18 μg/dL at 30 minutes or an absolute cortisol level above 20 μg/dL rules out adrenal insufficiency. In some patients with secondary adrenal insufficiency, this test will be normal. This result may be owing to the high dose of corticotropin given. Studies have demonstrated that the same results can be seen using 1 to 5 g of cosyntropin. The normal response is 18 g/dL at baseline or 20 to 60 minutes after the injection. Other tests include the insulin tolerance test, the prolonged ACTH stimulation test, the metyrapone test, and the corticotropin-releasing hormone stimulation test.[46,48]

Treatment of Addison's disease must include adequate patient education, so that the patient is aware of treatment complications, expected outcome, missed doses, and drug side effects. The agents of choice are prednisone, hydrocortisone, and cortisone, with the treatment objective being the establishment of the lowest effective dose while mimicking the normal diurnal adrenal rhythm[47,49] (Table 72–11). Usually, a twice-daily dosing schedule is adequate, with the dose used dependent on the steroid chosen. A morning dose of cortisone (25 mg), hydrocortisone (20 mg), or prednisone (5 mg) followed by an evening dose of the same agent at 50% of the morning dose is usually sufficient to duplicate the normal circadian rhythm of cortisol production. To replace the mineralocorticoid loss, 9-fluohydrocortisone can be used. A dose of 0.05 to 0.2 mg by mouth once a day is adequate. If parenteral therapy is needed, 2 to 5 mg of deoxycorticosterone trimethylacetate in oil intramuscularly every 3 to 4 weeks can be used. The main reason for adding the mineralocorticoid is to minimize the development of hyperkalemia. Adverse effects must be monitored closely. Symptoms include gastric upset, edema, hypertension, hypokalemia, insomnia, excitability, and diabetes mellitus. In addition, patient weight, blood pressure, and electrocardiogram should be monitored regularly.[46,48]

The end point of therapy is difficult to assess in most patients, but a reduction in excess pigmentation is a good clinical marker. The development of features of Cushing's syndrome indicates excessive replacement. Treatment of secondary adrenal insufficiency is identical to primary disease treatment with the exception that mineralocorticoid replacement usually is not necessary. Patient education still should be stressed with emphasis placed on establishing an alternate-day regimen.

ACUTE ADRENAL INSUFFICIENCY

Adrenal crisis, or Addisonian crisis, is characterized by an acute adrenocortical insufficiency. Adrenal crisis represents a true endocrine emergency. Anything that increases adrenal requirements dramatically can precipitate an adrenal crisis. Stressful situations, surgery, infection, and trauma all are potential triggering events, especially in the patient with some underlying adrenal or pituitary insufficiency. The most common cause of adrenal crisis is adrenal insufficiency brought on by chronic use of glucocorticoids.

TABLE 72–11. Congenital Adrenal Hyperplasia (CAH)

Enzyme Deficiency (Disorder)	Symptoms	Lab Tests	Comments
20-Hydroxylase (nonvirilizing CAH)	Enlarged adrenal gland (owing to cholesterol) and female genitalia	All steroids are low in blood and urine	Poor prognosis for infants
17-Hydroxylase (nonvirilizing CAH)	Hypertension usually present	Low concentrations of cortisol and estrogens	Mineralocorticoid replacement not necessary
21-Hydroxylase (virilizing CAH)	Pubertal irregularities (acne, early pubic hair, voice lowering, increased muscularity) Mature normally w/replacement	High progesterone, renin, 17-hydroxyprogesterone and ACTH Low cortisol, sodium, and aldosterone	Most common form of CAH (90% of total), incidence of 1/10,000 Monitor growth velocity, bone age renin, and 17-hydroxyprogesterone
11-Hydroxylase (virilizing CAH)	Hypertension, secondary aldosterone excess, and virilism from androgen excess Mistaken for Cushing's, but no glucose intolerance	Low plasma cortisol and aldosterone High ACTH and MSH concentrations	Second most common cause of CAH (9%); incidence of 1/100,000 (final step in biosynthesis of corticosterone and cortisol; found only in adrenal cortex)
3-Hydroxysteroid dehydrogenase (mixed CAH)	Both cortisol and aldosterone deficiencies	Decreased aldosterone, cortisol, estrogens, and androgens Increased pregnenolone and cholesterol	Defect involves the adrenals and gonads
18-Hydroxysteroid dehydrogenase (corticosterone methyloxidase deficiency)	Hypotension	Restricted to zona glomerulosa—sole aldosterone defect: hyponatremia, hyperkalemia, increased renin activity	Treatment is identical to Addison's disease—mineralocorticoid replacement without glucocorticoid replacement

Early symptoms of acute adrenal insufficiency include myalgias, malaise, anorexia, weakness, and weight loss. As the situation continues, vomiting, fever, hypotension, and shock will develop. Hyponatremia, hypoglycemia, and hypercalcemia also may be present.

Treatment of adrenal crisis involves the administration of parenteral glucocorticoids. Hydrocortisone (Solu-cortef, Upjohn) is the agent of choice owing to its mineralocorticoid activity plus glucocorticoid effects. Hydrocortisone is started at 100 mg intravenously through rapid infusion and followed by a continuous infusion of 100 mg every 6 to 8 hours. Intravenous administration is continued for 24 to 48 hours, at which time, if the patient is stable, oral hydrocortisone may be started at a dose of 50 mg every 8 hours for another 48 hours. Following oral maintenance therapy, a hydrocortisone taper is initiated until the dosage is 30 to 50 mg/d in divided doses. Fluid replacement often is required and may be accomplished with 5% dextrose and isotonic saline (D_5NS) at a rate to support blood pressure. If hyperkalemia is present after the hydrocortisone maintenance phase, additional mineralocorticoid usually is required. Fludrocortisone acetate (Florinef, Apothecon) in a dose of 0.1 mg by mouth daily is the agent of choice.

Patients with adrenal insufficiency should be instructed to carry a card or wear a bracelet or necklace, such as Medic Alert, that contains information about their condition. Patients should also have easy access to injectable hydrocortisone or glucocorticoid suppositories in case of an emergency or during times of physical stress, such as febrile illness or injury.[48]

HYPOALDOSTERONISM

Hypoaldosteronism is rare and usually is associated with low renin status, diabetes, complete heart block, or severe postural hypotension, or it may occur postoperatively following tumor removal.[2]

Hypoaldosteronism may be part of a larger adrenal insufficiency or be the only defect the patient has. In nonselective hypoaldosteronism, the etiology of the low aldosterone is most likely generalized adrenocortical insufficiency (see Addison's disease). In selective hypoaldosteronism, the etiology is usually a specific defect in the stimulation of adrenal aldosterone secretion (21-hydroxylase deficiency most common) or a defect in peripheral aldosterone action (decreased aldosterone receptors).

Laboratory analysis reveals low serum sodium and high serum potassium concentrations. Patients often will present with hyperchloremic metabolic acidosis. Because the deficiency is in the mineralocorticoid, replacement with fludrocortisone in a dose of 0.1 to 0.3 mg is usually effective. Patients should be followed for blood pressure response as well as electrolyte status.

CONGENITAL ADRENAL HYPERPLASIA

ADRENAL VIRILISM

Virilism, excessive secretion of androgens from the adrenal gland, is more commonly seen in females, with hirsutism being the dominant feature. Women who present with hirsutism also may have voice deepening, increased muscle mass, menstrual abnormalities, clitoral enlargement, redistribution of body fat and loss of female body contour, breast atrophy, and hair recession and crown balding.[50] Though virilism may be easy to diagnose based on clinical symptoms, making the diagnosis on a biochemical basis is difficult. The most common etiology of virilism involves one of many possible congenital enzyme defects. Depending on the enzyme deficiency, accumulation of a variety of androgens, notably testosterone, can develop.

Treatment of virilism centers around suppression of the pituitary–adrenal axis with exogenous glucocorticoids. Choice of steroids is variable, with the focus of treatment being the establishment of an alternate-day therapy. In adults, the usual steroid used is dexamethasone (0.23 mg/m^2 per 24 hours) or hydrocortisone (18 mg/m^2 per 24 hours).

HIRSUTISM

Hirsutism (hypertrichosis) is defined as more hair than is cosmetically acceptable. The majority of cases occur in women with no underlying endocrine abnormality. Some cases of hypertrichosis are related to a wide variation in hairiness as well as hereditary factors. In general, people who are dark-haired, pigmented Caucasians of either sex from the Mediterranean and southern European stock are more prone to genetic hypertrichosis. If virilism and/or defeminization are concurrently present, the chances of the hirsutism arising from an endocrine abnormality increase.[50–53]

Endocrinopathies without masculinization can predispose to hirsutism in patients with documented pituitary tumors, Cushing's disease, or excessive use of steroids/androgens. Certain drug-related hirsutisms have been documented, namely with phenytoin, oral contraceptives, methyldopa, danazol, metoclopramide, phenothiazines, reserpine, and diazoxide. In the patient with hirsutism, congenital adrenal hyperplasia, adrenal tumors, and ovarian tumors should be ruled out.[50–53]

Only when cosmetic surgery is ineffective should suppressive therapy be used. Glucocorticoids, such as dexamethasone, can be used, but may induce cushingnoid symptoms even in doses of 0.5 mg/d. Oral contraceptives can be used in patients who require contraception concurrently. If oral contraceptives are used, a progestin with low androgen activity (norethynodrel or ethynodiol diacetate) should be employed.

Because many enzyme systems are needed to complete the complex cholesterol-to-cortisol pathway, enzyme deficiencies may lead to disruptions of the normal cascade of events (see Fig. 72–2). This group of enzyme disorders is known as congenital adrenal hyperplasia, mainly because of the resultant chronic adrenal gland stimulation that occurs following enzyme deficiency.[51,54] Any enzyme deficiency is capable of affecting any one or all three of the steroid pathways.[55] Therefore, treatment should be focused on replacement of the deficient hormone as well as cessation of chronic stimulation causing the hyperplasia. In Table 72–11, six of the most common enzyme deficiencies are briefly outlined. Antiandrogens are often added to the more specific therapies or for the treatment of idiopathic hirsutism. The most common include spironolactone, flutamide (Eulexin, Schering), and finasteride (Proscar, Merck), although none of these is FDA approved for the treatment of hirsutism. It can take 4 months for the antiandrogens to alleviate the hirsutism, and duration of therapy is unclear.[50]

PRINCIPLES OF GLUCOCORTICOID ADMINISTRATION

Originally, the term *glucocorticoid* was given to these agents to describe their glucose-regulating properties. However, carbohydrate metabolism is only one of a multitude of effects that steroids can exhibit. The activity produced is a function of the receptor activated (glucocorticoid vs mineralocorticoid) as well as the agent and dose prescribed.

The mechanism of steroids is complex and not fully known. The steroid enters the cell through passive diffusion and binds to the steroid receptor. There are between 5000 and 100,000 receptors per cell. Steroids exhibit various binding affinities to the vast number of receptors in almost every tissue and therefore elicit a wide variety of biologic effects.

After binding to the receptor, there is a structural change that occurs in the receptor, known as activation. After activation, the receptor–steroid complex binds to DNA sites in the cell called glucocorticoid regulatory elements (GREs). This binding to the GREs affects stimulates or inhibits transcription of nearby genes.

The pharmacokinetics of the glucocorticoids varies with the agent given and the route of administration. In general, most steroids given by the oral route are well absorbed. Water-soluble agents are more rapidly absorbed following intramuscular injection than are lipid-soluble agents. Intravenous administration is recommended when a quick onset of action is needed. A summary of the steroids is provided in Table 72–12.

In addition to systemic steroids causing iatrogenic Cushing's syndrome, they also can lead to increased susceptibility to infection, osteoporosis,[56] sodium retention with resultant edema, hypokalemia, hypomagnesemia, cataracts, peptic ulcer disease, seizures, and generalized suppression of the hypothalamic–pituitary–adrenal (HPA) axis. Long-term complications tend to be insidious and less likely to respond to steroid withdrawal.

Suppression of the HPA axis is a major concern whenever systemic steroids are tapered or withdrawn. Single doses of glucocorticoids can prevent the axis from responding to major stressors for several hours. In general, the longer the steroid is administered and the higher the dose used, the more suppression of the axis that occurs. The possibility of suppression occurs anytime the patient is exposed to supraphysiologic doses of a steroid. Symptoms of steroid withdrawal resemble those seen in a patient with adrenocortical deficiency.

A variety of recommendations for steroid tapering are available.[57] In general, patients who have been on long-term steroid therapy will need to be gradually withdrawn toward physiologic doses over months. On average, the normal adult produces approximately 20 to 30 mg of cortisol per day with the peak concentration occurring around 8:00 AM. As the steroid or steroid-equivalent dose approaches the 20- to 30-mg level, the taper should be slowed and the patient checked for axis function. The primary mode to test HPA integrity is the rapid ACTH test. A normal ACTH test would indicate that daily steroid maintenance therapy is not needed. More recently, the use of exogenous human corticotropin-releasing hormone (CRH) was found to be nearly as useful in the assessment of pituitary–adrenal function.[58] Caution should be used to prevent disease exacerbation during the steroid taper to prevent the need for rebolusing the patient with another course of high-dose steroids. The dilemma of prolonged steroid administration is sometimes lessened by the use of an alternate-day

TABLE 72–12. Relative Potencies of Glucocorticoids

Glucocorticoid	Anti-inflammatory Potency	Equivalent Potency (mg)	Approximate Half-Life (min)	Sodium-Retaining Potency
Cortisone	0.8	25.0	30	2.0
Hydrocortisone	1.0	20.0	90	2.0
Prednisone	3.5	5.0	60	1.0
Prednisolone	4.0	5.0	200	1.0
Triamcinolone	5.0	4.0	300	0.0
Methylprednisolone	5.0	4.0	180	0.0
Betamethasone	25.0	0.60	100–300	0.0
Dexamethasone	30.0	0.75	100–300	0.0

TABLE 72–13. Factors in Successful Glucocorticoid Therapy[60,61]

Monitoring	Glucose concentrations (serum and urine) Electrolytes (serum and urine) Ophthalmologic exams Stool tests for occult blood loss Growth and development (children and adolescents)
Counseling	Take with food to minimize gastrointestinal upset. Never discontinue medication on your own; check with physician. Gradual dosage reduction is usually necessary. Carry or wear medical identification indicating that you are on long-term glucocorticoid therapy. Dosage increases may be necessary at times of increased stress (surgery or emergency treatments). Be aware of potential side effects (i.e., visual disturbances, bruising, delayed wound healing. What to do if you miss a dose. If dosing schedule is: Every other day: Take as soon as possible if remembered that morning; if not remembered until later, skip that day; take the next morning, then skip a day. Every day: Take as soon as possible but skip if almost time for the next dose; never double doses.
Recognizing complications	Early in therapy and essentially unavoidable: insomnia, enhanced appetite and/or weight gain. Common in patients with underlying risk factors: hypertension, diabetes mellitus, peptic ulcer disease. Long-term intense treatment: cushingoid habitus, hypothalamic–pituitary–adrenal suppression, impaired wound healing. Delayed and insidious: osteoporosis, cataracts, atherosclerosis. Rare and unpredictable: psychosis, glaucoma, pancreatitis.

From Refs. 60 and 61.

therapy (ADT) regimen.[57,59] ADT minimizes the hypothalamic–pituitary suppression as well as some of the adverse effects seen with once-daily therapy. This can be especially important in the treatment of the child and young adult, in whom growth suppression is a major concern. ADT is not recommended for initial management, but rather in the management of the stabilized patient who needs long-term therapy. The patient will be exposed to "on" and "off" days, with the "on" day dose gradually increased with concurrent reduction in the "off" day dose over a period of 14 days. By the 14th day, the patient will be consuming medication only on the "on" day.

EVALUATION OF THERAPEUTIC OUTCOMES

Successful glucocorticoid therapy involves counseling the patient, monitoring the patient, and recognizing complications of therapy (Table 72–13). The risk–benefit ratio of glucocorticoid administration should always be considered, especially with concurrent disease states such as hypertension, diabetes mellitus, peptic ulcer disease, and uncontrolled systemic infections.

▶ PRINCIPLES OF PHARMACOTHERAPY

- Corticotropin-releasing factor (CRF) is secreted from the hypothalamus and stimulates the release of corticotropin (adrenocorticotropic hormone or ACTH) from the anterior pituitary, which in turn stimulates glucocorticoid secretion from the adrenal cortex.
- Cushing's syndrome results from hypercortisolism originating either from exogenous administration or from endogenous overproduction by the adrenal glands or abnormal adrenocortical tissues.
- Surgery is the treatment of choice for both ACTH-dependent and -independent Cushing's syndrome, and pharmacologic treatment is reserved for use as adjunctive therapy or in refractory or inoperable disease.
- Pharmacologic agents for Cushing's syndrome can be divided into three categories: (a) steroidogenic inhibitors (mitotane, metyrapone, aminoglutethimide, ketoconazole); (b) neuromodulators of ACTH release (cyproheptadine, bromocriptine, valproic acid, octreotide); and (c) glucocorticoid-receptor blocking agents (mifepristone).
- Hyperaldosteronism is classified as excess aldosterone production from adrenal cortex (primary) or from stimulation of the zona glomerulosa by an extra-adrenal factor, usually the renin–angiotensin system.
- Primary aldosteronism is usually caused by aldosterone-producing adenoma (APA), treated with surgery; or bilateral adrenal hyperplasia, treatable with spironolactone or amiloride.
- Addison's disease (primary adrenal insufficiency) involves the loss of function of all regions of the adrenal cortex and a resulting deficiency in cortisol, aldosterone, and various androgens.
- Secondary adrenal insufficiency usually results from exogenous steroid use, leading to suppression of the hypothalamic–pituitary axis and decreased release of ACTH, resulting in low levels of androgens and cortisol.
- Virilism, the excessive secretion of androgens from the adrenal gland, is usually seen as hirsutism in fe-

males and is usually treated with glucocorticoid suppression of the pituitary–adrenal axis.

- Glucocorticoid suppression of the HPA axis occurs whenever a patient is exposed to supraphysiologic doses of a steroid and becomes a concern whenever the steroids are tapered or withdrawn.

REFERENCES

1. Conn JW. Primary aldosteronism, a new clinical syndrome. J Lab Clin Med 1955;45:6–17.
2. Orth DN, Kovacs WJ. The adrenal cortex. In: Wilson JD, Foster DW, Kronenberg HM, Larsen PR, eds. Williams' Textbook of Endocrinology. Philadelphia, Saunders, 1998:517–664.
3. Albright F. Cushing syndrome. Harvey Lect 1942–1943;38:123–186.
4. Neiman L, Cutler GB. Cushing's syndrome. In: Degroot LJ, ed. Endocrinology, 3rd ed. Philadelphia, Saunders, 1995:1741–1769.
5. Orth DN. Cushing's syndrome. N Engl J Med 1995;332:791–803.
6. Danese RD, Aron DC. Cushing's syndrome and hypertension. Endocrinol Metab Clin North Am 1994;23:299–324.
7. Trainer PT, Grossman A. The diagnosis and differential diagnosis of Cushing's syndrome. Clin Endocrinol 1991;34:317–330.
8. Fiad TM, Kirby JM, Cunningham SK, McKenna TJ. The overnight single-dose metyrapone test is a simple and reliable index of the hypothalamic–pituitary–adrenal axis. Clin Endocrinol 1994;40:603–609.
9. de Herder WW, Krenning EP, Malchoff CD, et al. Somatostain receptor scintigraphy: Its value in tumor localization in patients with Cushing's syndrome caused by ectopic corticotropin or corticotropin-releasing hormone secretion. Am J Med 1994;96:305–312.
10. Malerbi DA, Liberman B, Corradini MC, et al. The desmopressin stimulation test in the differential diagnosis of Cushing's syndrome. Clin Endocrinol 1993;38:463–472.
11. Jackson RV, Hockings GI, Torpy DJ, et al. New diagnostic tests for Cushing's syndrome: Uses of naloxone, vasopressin and alprazolam. Clin Exp Pharmacol Physiol 1996;23:579–581.
12. Ambrosi B, Bochicchio D, Colombo P, Fadin C, Faglia G. Loperamide to diagnose Cushing's syndrome. JAMA 1993;270:2301–2302.
13. de Herder WW, Uitterlinden P, Pieterman H, et al. Pituitary tumour localization in patients with Cushing's disease by magnetic resonance imaging: Is there a place for petrosal sinus sampling? Clin Endocrinol 1994;40:87–92.
14. Snow K, Nai-Siang J, Kao P, Scheithauer BW. Biochemical evaluation of adrenal dysfunction: The laboratory perspective. Mayo Clin Proc 1992;67:1055–1065.
15. Avgerinos PC, Yanovski JA, Oldfield EW, Nieman LK, Cutler GB. The metyrapone and dexamethasone suppression tests for the differential diagnosis of the adrenocorticotropin-dependent Cushing's syndrome: A comparison. Ann Intern Med 1994;121:318–327.
16. Kaye TB, Crapo L. The Cushing's syndrome: An update on diagnostic tests. Ann Intern Med 1990;112:434–444.
17. Boruskek S, Gold JJ. Commonly used medications that interfere with routine endocrine laboratory procedures. Clin Chem 1964;10:41.
18. Dunnick NR, Leight GS Jr, Roubidoux MA, et al. CT in the diagnosis of primary aldosteronism: Sensitivity in 29 patients. AJR Am J Roentgenol 1993;160:321–324.
19. Shamma FN, Abrahams JJ. Imaging in endocrine disorders. J Reprod Med 1992;37:39–45.
20. Tsigos C, Crousus GP. Differential diagnosis and management of Cushing's syndrome. Annu Rev Med 1996;47:443–461.
21. Gumowski J, Loughran M. Diseases of the adrenal gland. Nurs Clin North Am 1996;31:747–768.
22. McEvoy GK, ed. American Hospital Formulary Service (AHFS) Drug Information. American Society of Hospital Pharmacists, Inc., 1997: 19–20, 96–101, 837–839, 1909–1910.
23. United States Pharmacopeial Convention Inc. USPDI: Drug information for the health care professional, Vol. I, 13th ed. Taunton, MA: Rand-McNally, 1997:65–68, 2898–2900.
24. Engelhardt D. Steroid biosynthesis inhibitors in Cushing's syndrome. Clin Invest 1994;72:481–488.
25. Engelhardt D, Weber MM. Therapy of Cushing's syndrome with steroid biosynthesis inhibitors. J Steroid Biochem Molec Biol 1994; 49:261–267.
26. Miller JW, Crapo L. The medical treatment of Cushing's syndrome. Endocr Rev 1993;14:443–458.
27. Schteingart DE. Cushing's syndrome. Endocrinol Metab Clin North Am 1989;18:311–338.
28. Cocconi G. First generation aromatase inhibitors—aminoglutethimide and testololactone. Breast Cancer Res Treat 1994;30:57–80.
29. Agarwal MK. The antiglucocorticoid action of mifepristone. Pharmacol Ther 1996;70:183–213.
30. Atkinson AB. The treatment of Cushing's syndrome. Clin Endocrinol 1991;34:507–513.
31. Winquist EW, Laskey J, Crump M, Khamsi F, Shepherd FA. Ketoconazole in the management of paraneoplastic Cushing's syndrome secondary to ectopic adrenocorticotropin production. J Clin Oncol 1995;13:157–164.
32. Bravo EL. Primary aldosteronism: Issues in diagnosis and management. Endocrinol Metab Clin North Am 1994;23:271–283.
33. Corry DB, Tuck ML. Secondary aldosteronism. Endocrinol Metab Clin North Am 1995;24:511–529.
34. Gordon RD. Mineralcorticoid hypertension. Lancet 1994;344:240–243.
35. Grondal S, Hamberger B. Primary aldosteronism. Br J Surg 1992;79: 484–485.
36. Holland OB. Primary aldosteronism. Semin Nephrol 1995;15:116–125.
37. Opocher G, Rocco S, Carpene G, Mantero F. Differential diagnosis in primary aldosteronism. J Steroid Biochem Molec Biol 1993;45: 49–55.
38. Vallotton MB. Primary aldosteronism: Part I. Diagnosis of primary aldosteronism. Clin Endocrinol 1996;45:47–52.
39. Vallotton MB. Primary aldosteronism: Part II. Differential diagnosis of primary hyperaldosteronism and pseudoaldosteronism. Clin Endocrinol 1996;45:53–60.
40. Weinberger MH, Fineberg NS. The diagnosis of primary aldosteronism and separation of two major subtypes. Arch Intern Med 1993; 153:2125–2129.
41. White PC. Disorders of aldosterone biosynthesis and action. N Engl J Med 1994;331:250–258.
42. Young WF, Hogan MJ, Klee GG, et al. Primary aldosteronism: Diagnosis and treatment. Mayo Clinic Proc 1990;65:96–110.
43. Ganguly A. Glucocorticoid-suppressible hyperaldosteronism: An update. Am J Med 1990;88:321–324.
44. Iwaoka T, Umeda T, Naomi S, et al. The usefulness of the captopril test as a simultaneous screening for primary aldosteronism and renovascular hypertension. Am J Hypertens 1993;6:899–906.
45. Blumenfield JD, Sealey JE, Schlussel Y, et al. Diagnosis and treatment of primary hyperaldosteronism. Ann Intern Med 1994;121:877–885.
46. Oelkers W. Adrenal insufficiency. N Engl J Med 1996;335:1206–1212.
47. Stoffer SS. Addison's disease: How to improve patients' quality of life. Postgrad Med 1993;93:265–278.
48. Werbel SS, Ober KP. Acute adrenal insufficiency. Endocrinol Metab Clin North Am 1993;22:303–328.
49. Davenport J, Kellerman C, Reiss D, Harrison L. Addison's disease. Am Fam Physician 1991;43:1338–1342.
50. Gilchrist VJ, Hecht BR. A practical approach to hirsutism. Am Fam Physician 1995:52:1837–1844.

51. Kalve E, Klein JF. Evaluation of women with hirsutism. Am Fam Physician 1996;54:117–124.
52. Watson RE, Bouknight R, Alguire PC. Hirsutism: Evaluation and management. Gen Intern Med 1995;10:283–292.
53. Rittmaster RS. Hirsutism. Lancet 1997;349:191–195.
54. Thorn GW. The adrenal cortex. Johns Hopkins Med J 1968;123: 49–77.
55. Kuttenn F, Couillin P, Girard F, et al. Late-onset adrenal hyperplasia in hirsutism. N Engl J Med 1985;313:224–231.
56. Zelissen PM, Croughs RJ, van Rijk PP, et al. Effects of glucocorticoid replacement therapy on bone mineral density in patients with Addison's disease. Ann Intern Med 1994;120:207–210.
57. Kountz DS, Clark CL. Safely withdrawing patients from chronic glucocorticoid therapy. Am Fam Physician 1997;55:521–552.
58. Schlaghecke R, Kornely E, Santen RT, et al. The effect of long-term glucocorticoid therapy on pituitary–adrenal responses to exogenous corticotropin-releasing hormone. N Engl J Med 1992;326:226–230.
59. Holland EG, Taylor AT. Glucocorticoids in clinical practice. J Fam Pract 1991;32:512–519.
60. United States Pharmacopeial Convention Inc. USPDI: Advice for the patient: Drug information in lay language, Vol. II, 13th ed. Taunton, MA: Rand-McNally 1997: 583–588.
61. Barlow JE. Complications of therapy. In: Boumpas DT, moderator. Glucocorticoid therapy for immune mediated diseases: Basic and clinical correlates. Ann Intern Med 1993;119:1198–1208.

73

Pituitary Gland Disorders

Amy M. Heck, PharmD, Karim A. Calis, PharmD, MPH, BCPS, BCNSP, FASHP, and Jack A. Yanovski, MD, PhD

In the 1950s Geoffrey Harris and his colleagues uncovered the physiologic importance of pituitary hormones and proposed the theory of neurohormonal regulation of the pituitary by the hypothalamus.[1] Today the pituitary gland is recognized for its essential role in body homeostasis, and for this reason, it is often referred to as the "master gland." The hypothalamus and the pituitary gland are closely connected, and together they provide a means of communication between the brain and endocrine organs of the body. The hypothalamus uses nervous input and metabolic signals from the body to control the secretion of pituitary hormones that regulate growth, thyroid function, adrenal activity, reproduction, lactation, and fluid balance.

ANATOMY AND PHYSIOLOGY

The hypothalamus (Fig. 73–1) is a small region at the base of the brain that receives autonomic nervous input from different areas of the body to regulate limbic functions such as motivation, emotion, sexual behavior, food and water intake, body temperature, cardiovascular function, respiratory function, and diurnal rhythms. In addition, the hypothalamus controls the release of hormones from the anterior and posterior regions of the pituitary gland. Neurons in the hypothalamus produce the vasopressin and oxytocin that are secreted by the posterior pituitary and make many hormone-releasing factors that stimulate or inhibit the release of trophic hormones from the anterior pituitary. At the base of the hypothalamus, a projection known as the median eminence is connected to the pituitary stalk. The median eminence is rich with nerve axons and blood vessels that provide both chemical and physical connections between the hypothalamus and the pituitary gland.

The pituitary gland, also referred as the hypophysis, is located at the base of the brain in a cavity of the sphenoid bone known as the *sella turcica.* The pituitary is separated from the brain by an extension of the dura mater known as the *diaphragma sella* and is not in direct contact with cerebrospinal fluid. The pituitary is a very small gland, weighing between 0.4 and 1 g in adults. It is divided into two distinct regions, the anterior lobe, or adenohypophysis, and the posterior lobe or the neurohypophysis (see Fig. 73–1).

The posterior pituitary gland secretes two major hormones, oxytocin and vasopressin (antidiuretic hormone) (Table 73–1). Oxytocin release from the posterior pituitary causes contraction of the smooth muscles in the breast during lactation and also plays a role in uterine contraction during parturition. Vasopressin is essential for proper fluid balance and acts on the renal collecting ducts to conserve water. Oxytocin and vasopressin are synthesized in the paraventricular and supraoptic nuclei of the hypothalamus. The posterior pituitary gland contains the terminal nerve endings of these two nuclei as well as specialized secretory granules that release hormones in response to appropriate signals. Osmoreceptors located in the hypothalamus stimulate the supraoptic nuclei to release vasopressin in response to hyperosmotic extracellular fluid, and a negative-feedback control system exists to regulate fluid osmolarity. Suckling stimuli to the breast nipple cause nervous stimulation of the hypothalamus and release of oxytocin, which is responsible for milk ejection. It is important to note that loss of anterior pituitary function does not necessarily affect the release of vasopressin or oxytocin, because these hormones are actually synthesized in the hypothalamus.

Unlike the posterior pituitary, the release of anterior pituitary hormones is not regulated by direct nervous stimulation, but rather is controlled by specific hypothalamic releasing and inhibitory hormones. The median eminence of the hypothalamus contains a large number of capillaries that converge to form a network of veins known as the hypothalamic–hypophysial portal circulation. Inhibiting and releasing hormones synthesized in the neurons of the hypothalamus reach the anterior pituitary via the hypothalamic–hypophysial portal vessels to control release of anterior pituitary hormones. Although there is a direct arterial blood supply to the anterior pituitary lobe, the hypothalamic–hypophysial portal vessels provide the primary blood supply (see Fig. 73–1). In contrast to the posterior pituitary, the anterior pituitary lobe is extremely vascular and has the highest rate of blood flow of all body organs.

The specialized secretory cells of the anterior pituitary lobe secrete six major polypeptide hormones (Table 73–1). These include growth hormone (GH) or somatotropin, adrenocorticotropic hormone (ACTH) or corticotropin, thyroid-stimulating hormone (TSH) or thyrotropin, prolactin (PRL), follicle-stimulating hormone (FSH), and luteinizing hormone (LH). The release of these hormones is regulated primarily by hypothalamic releasing and inhibiting hormones. Thyrotropin-releasing hormone (TRH) stimulates anterior pituitary release of TSH and prolactin, corticotropin-releasing hormone (CRH) stimulates anterior pituitary release of ACTH, growth-hormone releasing hormone (GHRH) stimulates anterior pituitary release of GH, and gonadotropin-releasing hormone (GnRH) stimulates anterior pituitary release of LH and FSH. Hypothalamic release of dopamine

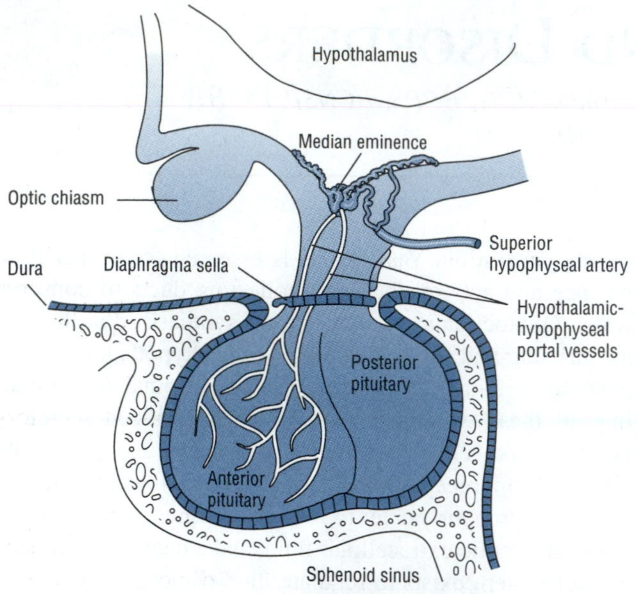

FIG. 73–1. Illustration showing anatomic relationships of the pituitary gland to surrounding structures. *(From Kohler PO. Clinical Endocrinology. John Wiley and Sons, 1986, p 12, Fig 2-1 with permission.)*

(prolactin inhibitory hormone) inhibits the release of prolactin. Prolactin differs from the other anterior lobe hormones in that an inhibiting factor, rather than a stimulating factor, from the hypothalamus is primarily responsible for controlling its release. Therefore, in the absence of hypothalamic input, an excess of prolactin is produced, whereas a deficiency state of other anterior pituitary hormones results.

Somatotropes comprise approximately one-third to one-half of the anterior pituitary lobe and secrete growth hormone. Growth hormone is essential for growth and development of all body cells and has important effects on carbohydrate and lipid metabolism. GH increases protein synthesis, hepatic glucose output, and lipolysis, while decreasing glucose utilization. The secretion of growth hormone is stimulated primarily by GHRH from the hypothalamus. The release of growth hormone is enhanced by ACTH, vasopressin (ADH), sleep, exercise, physical or psychological stress, fasting, and a number of pharmacologic agents such as α-adrenergic agonists, β-adrenergic antagonists, dopamine agonists, and GABA agonists.[2] The hypothalamic hormone somatostatin is the most substantial inhibitor of growth-hormone secretion. Other factors that inhibit growth-hormone secretion include postprandial hyperglycemia, elevated free fatty acids, elevated insulin-like growth factor-I (IGF-I, also known as somatomedin C), progesterone, and a number of pharmacologic agents including α-adrenergic antagonists, β-adrenergic agonists, serotonergic antagonists, dopamine antagonists, and chronic administration of glucocorticoids.[2]

Corticotropes, the second most abundant type of secretory cells found in the anterior pituitary, secrete ACTH. ACTH stimulates the adrenal cortex to release glucocorticoids, mineralocorticoids, and androgenic steroid hormones. Secretion of ACTH from the anterior pituitary is stimulated by CRH and is ultimately controlled by an internal diurnal rhythm, nervous input secondary to physical or psychological stress, and a negative-feedback mechanism based on concentrations of circulating cortisol.

Thyrotropes secrete TSH, which stimulates the thyroid gland to synthesize thyroglobulin, thyroxine (T_4), and triiodothyronine (T_3). The secretion of TSH is stimulated by hypothalamic TRH and is regulated by negative feedback of elevated concentrations of circulating thryroxine and triiodothyronine. Thyrotropin secretion is inhibited by somatostatin and dopamine and can be stimulated by norepinephrine and serotonin.

Gonadotropes secrete both LH and FSH, which control the development and function of both male and female reproductive organs. FSH stimulates the growth of ovarian follicles and promotes testicular spermatogenesis. LH promotes sex-steroid production, produces ovulation in females, and maintains the function of testicular Leydig cells in males. Secretion of LH and FSH is regulated by hypothalamic release of GnRH. The release of LH and FSH is inhibited by negative feedback of sex steroids and inhibin.

Lactotropes comprise approximately 15% to 20% of the normal pituitary and secrete prolactin. During pregnancy, the number of lactotropes can increase significantly because prolactin is needed for the formation of mammary tissue, production of milk, and lactation. The regulation of prolactin secretion by the nervous and endocrine systems is mainly inhibitory, and dopamine has been identified as the strongest inhibitor of prolactin secretion. Prolactin secretion is stimulated by TRH, vasoactive intestinal polypeptide (VIP), pregnancy, nursing, exercise, sleep, stress, and many pharmacologic agents including dopamine antagonists, GABA agonists, histamine H_2-receptor antagonists, estrogens, and opioids.[3]

Destruction of the pituitary gland may result in secondary hypothyroidism, hypogonadism, adrenal insufficiency, growth hormone deficiency, and hypoprolactinemia. The formation of certain types of pituitary tumors may result in pituitary hormone excess. Pituitary tumors may also physically compress the pituitary and prevent the release of the trophic hypothalamic factors that regulate pituitary hormones. In this chapter, the pathophysiology and role of pharmacotherapy in the treatment of acromegaly, short stature, hyperprolactinemia, and panhypopituitarism will be discussed.

ADRENOCORTICOTROPIC HORMONE

See Chapter 72.

THYROID-STIMULATING HORMONE

See Chapter 71.

LUTEINIZING HORMONE AND FOLLICLE-STIMULATING HORMONE

See Chapters 71 to 78.

TABLE 73–1. Regulation and Action of Pituitary Hormones

Hormone	Stimulation	Inhibition	Physiologic Effects
Anterior Pituitary Hormones			
Growth hormone (GH)	*Physiologic* GH-releasing hormone ACTH ADH GABA Norepinephrine Dopamine Serotonin Estrogen Sleep Stress Exercise *Pharmacologic* α-Adrenergic agonists (e.g., clonidine) β-Adrenergic antagonists (e.g., propanolol) Dopamine agonists (e.g., bromocriptine) GABA agonists (e.g., muscimol)	*Physiologic* Somatostatin Elevated IGF-I Growth hormone Progesterone Glucocorticoids Postprandial hyperglycemia Elevated free fatty acids *Pharmacologic* Dopamine antagonists (e.g., phenothiazines) α-Adrenergic antagonists (e.g., phentolamine) β-Adrenergic agonists (e.g., isoproterenol) Serotonin antagonists (e.g., methysergide)	Stimulates IGF-I production IGF-I and GH promote growth in all body tissues
Prolactin (PRL)	*Physiologic* TRH VIP Estrogen Serotonin Histamine Endogenous opioids Pregnancy and nursing *Pharmacologic* Dopamine antagonists (e.g., phenothiazines, haloperidol, methyldopa) Opiates Estrogens H_2-blockers (cimetidine) MAO inhibitors	*Physiologic* Dopamine GABA *Pharmacologic* Dopamine agonists (e.g., levodopa, bromocriptine, pergolide, cabergoline)	Lactation
Adrenocorticotropic hormone (ACTH)	CRH	Elevated cortisol	Gluccocorticoid effects pigmentation
Thyroid stimulating hormone (TSH)	TRH Estrogens Norepinephrine Serotonin	Thyroxine Triiodothyronine Somatostatin Glucocorticoids Dopamine	Iodine uptake and thyroid hormone synthesis
Luteinizing hormone (LH)	*Physiologic* GnRH *Pharmacologic* Clomiphene	Estradiol Testosterone Fasting	Ovulation Corpus luteum progesterone Sex-hormone-binding globulin
Follicle-stimulating hormone (FSH)	*Physiologic* GNRH Menopause Ovarian disorders *Pharmacologic* Clomiphene	Estradiol Inhibin Fasting	Ovarian follicle and stimulation of estradiol and progesterone Sex-hormone-binding globulin
Posterior Pituitary Hormones			
Vasopressin (ADH)	Hyperosmolality Volume depletion	Hypervolemia Hypoosmolality	Acts on renal collecting ducts to prevent diuresis
Oxytocin (OT)	Parturition Suckling		Uterine contraction Milk ejection

TRH = thyrotropin-releasing hormone; ADH = antidiuretic hormone; GABA = γ-aminobutyric acid; IGF-I = insulin-like growth factor; VIP = vasoactive intestinal peptide; CRH = corticotropin-releasing hormone.

VASOPRESSIN

See Chapter 48.

OXYTOCIN

See Chapter 74.

GROWTH HORMONE

PHYSIOLOGIC EFFECTS

Growth hormone has direct "anti-insulin" effects on lipid and carbohydrate metabolism. GH decreases utilization of glucose by peripheral tissues, increases lipolysis, and increases muscle mass. GH also stimulates gluconeogenesis in hepatocytes, impairs tissue glucose uptake, decreases insulin-receptor sensitivity, and impairs postreceptor insulin action. The growth-promoting effects of GH are largely mediated by insulin-like growth factors, also known as somatomedins. GH stimulates the formation of IGF-I primarily in the liver, as well as in other peripheral tissues. This anabolic peptide acts as a direct stimulator of cell proliferation and growth. There are two types of insulin-like growth factors, IGF-I and IGF-II. IGF-I regulates growth to some extent before, and largely after, birth. In contrast, IGF-II is thought to primarily regulate growth in utero.[4] Growth hormone is secreted by the anterior pituitary in a pulsatile fashion with several short bursts that occur mostly at night. Because of the short half-life of growth hormone in the plasma (approximately 30 minutes), measurements of circulating GH concentrations throughout the waking hours are usually very low or undetectable. Daytime GH pulses are most likely to occur after meals, following exercise, or during periods of stress. The greatest amount of GH secretion occurs during the night within the first 1 to 2 hours of slow-wave sleep (stages III or IV). Secretion of growth hormone is lowest during infancy, increases slightly during childhood, reaches its peak during adolescence, and then begins to gradually decline during the middle-age years.[2]

GROWTH HORMONE EXCESS

Acromegaly is a pathologic condition characterized by excessive production of growth hormone. This is a rare disorder that affects approximately 50 to 70 adults per million.[5] Gigantism, which is even more rare than acromegaly, is the excess secretion of growth hormone prior to epiphysial closure in children.[6] Patients diagnosed with acromegaly are reported to have a two- to threefold increase in mortality.[5,7,8] The cause of mortality is usually related to cardiovascular, respiratory, or neoplastic disease.[7–10] Most patients are middle-aged at the time of diagnosis, and this disorder does not appear to affect one gender to a greater extent than the other. The most common cause of excess GH secretion in acromegaly, accounting for approximately 98% of all cases, is a growth hormone–secreting pituitary adenoma.[7–9] Rarely, acromegaly may be caused by ectopic GH-secreting adenomas, GH cell hyperplasia, excess growth hormone–releasing hormone secretion, or as one of the manifestations of McCune–Albright syndrome or Carney complex, very rare hypersecretory endocrinopathies.[8]

The clinical signs and symptoms of acromegaly develop gradually over an extended period of time. In fact, because of the subtle and slowly developing changes in physical appearance that GH excess causes, most patients are not definitively diagnosed with acromegaly until 10 to 15 years after the presumed onset of excessive growth-hormone secretion.[5,7] Excessive secretion of growth hormone affects several organ systems. Almost all acromegalic patients have physical signs of soft-tissue overgrowth, manifested as coarsening of facial features, increased hand volume, increased ring size, increased shoe size, and an enlarged tongue. Other common symptoms include headache, fatigue, visual disturbances, excessive sweating, neuropathies, parasthesias, and dermatologic abnormalities.[5,7,9–11] At presentation, approximately 90% of acromegalic patients have symptomatic osteoarthritis and joint damage secondary to soft-tissue overgrowth.[7,10,11] Because of GH effects on glucose utilization, 50% of acromegalic patients experience glucose intolerance, and up to 25% have overt diabetes.[7,10] Cardiovascular diseases such as hypertension, coronary heart disease, cardiomyopathy, and increased left-ventricular mass have also been noted in acromegalic patients.[5,7,9–11] Upper airway obstruction caused by soft-tissue overgrowth contributes to respiratory disorders in this population, and sleep apnea occurs in 60% of patients.[7,9,10] In addition, epidemiologic studies have reported that patients with acromegaly have an increased risk for the development of esophageal, colon, and stomach malignancies.[7,9,10] Some patients with acromegaly may present with few of these classic signs and symptoms, making recognition of this disease extremely difficult.

The diagnosis of acromegaly is based on a combination of diagnostic tests and clinical signs and symptoms. Random measures of plasma GH levels are not dependable because of the pulsatile pattern of release. The oral glucose tolerance test (OGTT) is commonly used as an important diagnostic tool. Postprandial hyperglycemia inhibits the secretion of growth hormone for at least 1 to 2 hours. Therefore, an oral glucose load would be expected to suppress growth-hormone concentrations (below 2 μg/L). However, patients with acromegaly continue to secrete growth hormone during the OGTT, and GH concentrations remain elevated (> 2 μg/L) after oral glucose loads of 50 to 100 g in 80% of acromegalics.[5,9,11] Since GH stimulates the production of IGF-I, serum IGF-I concentrations can also be measured to aid in the diagnosis of acromegaly. Circulating IGF-I is cleared from the body at a much slower rate than is GH, and measurements can be collected at any time of the day to identify patients with GH excess.[5,9,11] In addition, IGF-I-binding-protein-3 (IGFBP-3) can be measured because it is positively regulated by GH and binds to circulating IGF-I with high affinity.[9] These laboratory tests are also useful in monitoring response to therapy. Computed tomography (CT) and magnetic resonance imaging (MRI) of the pituitary are also important diagnostic tests to confirm the presence of a pituitary adenoma.[5,9,11]

▶ TREATMENT: Growth Hormone Excess

The goal of treatment for patients diagnosed with acromegaly is to reduce GH secretion and improve the clinical signs and symptoms of the disease. Many clinicians define cure of acromegaly as suppression of GH concentrations to lower than 2 μg/L after a standard OGTT.[5,9,11] The treatment of choice for acromegaly is transsphenoidal surgical resection of the growth-hormone secreting adenoma.[5,9,11] Postsurgical cure rates have been reported to range from 50% to 90% depending on the type of adenoma that is removed.[9,11,12] Complications of transsphenoidal surgery are relatively infrequent and include cerebrospinal fluid leak, meningitis, arachnoiditis, diabetes insipidus, and pituitary failure.[5,9,12] For patients who are poor surgical candidates, those who have failed surgical interventions, or others who refuse surgical treatment, radiation therapy may be considered. Radiation, however, may take several years to relieve the symptoms of acromegaly. Because neither radiation therapy nor surgery will cure all patients with acromegaly, adjuvant drug therapy is often needed to control symptoms.[5,9,11]

PHARMACOLOGIC THERAPY

Drug therapy should be considered for patients in whom surgery and irradiation are contraindicated, when rapid control of symptoms is indicated, or when other treatments have failed to normalize GH concentrations. Dopamine agonists such as bromocriptine, pergolide, or cabergoline may be effective in a small subset of patients. Recently, the somatostatin analog octreotide has become the most commonly used pharmacologic agent for the management of acromegaly.

DOPAMINE AGONISTS

In normal healthy adults, dopamine agonists cause an increase in growth hormone production. However, when these agents are given to patients with acromegaly, there is a paradoxical decrease in GH production.[13,14] Most clinical experience with the use of dopamine agonists in acromegaly is with bromocriptine. Other agents such as pergolide, cabergoline, and lisuride have also been used. Bromocriptine is a semisynthetic ergot alkaloid that acts as a dopamine-receptor agonist. Most clinical trials assessing the efficacy of bromocriptine in the treatment of acromegaly were conducted in the 1970s and early 1980s. It was determined from these studies that certain subsets of acromegalic patients have a favorable response to drug therapy with bromocriptine. These patients include individuals with high circulating concentrations of prolactin and patients who experience GH suppression following a single dose of 2.5 mg of bromocriptine, known as a bromocriptine challenge.[13,14] A recent review evaluating 34 studies concluded that therapy with bromocriptine was effective in suppressing mean serum GH levels to less than 5 mg/L in approximately 20% of patients.[15] Only 10% of patients experience normalization of IGF-I concentrations with bromocriptine therapy, but over 50% of patients treated with bromocriptine experience improvement in acromegalic symptoms.[9,13,15]

Bromocriptine (Parlodel) is commercially available in the United States as 2.5-mg oral tablets and 5-mg oral capsules. Bromocriptine is well absorbed from the gastrointestinal tract, with oral bioavailability ranging from 60% to 100% and peak serum concentrations occurring within 1 to 3 hours of administration. Concurrent ingestion of food with bromocriptine can increase the time to peak serum concentrations, but the overall extent of absorption is not affected. Bromocriptine is extensively metabolized by the liver with very high hepatic first-pass metabolism, and it is primarily eliminated through the bile. For the treatment of acromegaly, bromocriptine is initiated at a dose of 1.25 mg at bedtime and is increased by 1.25-mg increments every 3 to 4 days as needed.[5,9,11,13,15] Doses as high as 60 mg per day have been used for the treatment of acromegaly, but clinical studies have shown that dosages greater than 20 or 30 mg daily do not offer additional benefits in the suppression of GH.[9,13,15] When used for the treatment of acromegaly, the duration of action of bromocriptine is shorter than for the treatment of hyperprolactinemia. Therefore, the total daily dose of bromocriptine should be separated in three to four divided doses.[13,14]

The most common adverse effects of bromocriptine therapy include central nervous system symptoms such as headache, lightheadedness, dizziness, nervousness, and fatigue. Gastrointestinal effects such as nausea, abdominal pain, or diarrhea are also very common. Some patients may need to take bromocriptine with food to decrease the incidence of adverse gastrointestinal effects. Most adverse effects are seen early in the course of therapy and tend to decrease with continued treatment.[3,13] Bromocriptine may cause thickening of bronchial secretions and nasal congestion. There have been rare cases of psychiatric disturbances, pleural diseases, and an erythromelalgic syndrome reported with the use of bromocriptine. These conditions appear to be associated with higher doses and prolonged duration of therapy.[13,15]

According to the product labeling, bromocriptine is contraindicated in pregnancy, and the medication should be discontinued immediately if a woman becomes pregnant while taking the drug. However, case reports of women who took the medication throughout pregnancy do not suggest that bromocriptine is associated with an increased risk of birth defects.[3,13] If a woman becomes pregnant while taking bromocriptine, the risks and benefits of therapy should be fully considered. In most cases the benefits of successful therapy outweigh the risks, and bromocriptine therapy should be continued if it is effective in improving symptoms and reducing the elevated GH concentrations.

Other dopamine agonists that have been used to treat acromegaly include pergolide, cabergoline, lisuride, and quinagolide. Recently, quinagolide, a dopamine agonist available in Europe, has been shown to be more effective than both bromocriptine and cabergoline in normalizing GH and IGF-I values in acromegalic patients.[16] Dopamine agonists should be considered for all patients with acromegaly, prior to initiating therapy with a somatostatin analog, because of the potential cost advantages and convenience of oral administration.

SOMATOSTATIN ANALOGS

Octreotide

The pharmacotherapy of acromegaly has improved significantly with the development of synthetic somatostatin analogs. Octreotide is a long-acting somatostatin analog that is approximately 40 times more potent in inhibiting GH secretion than endogenous somatostatin.[9,17,18] It also suppresses the LH response to GnRH; decreases splanchnic blood flow; and inhibits the secretion of vasoactive intestinal peptide (VIP), gastrin, secretin, motilin, serotonin, and pancreatic polypeptide. Octreotide (Sandostatin) injection is commercially available in the United States for subcutaneous or intravenous administration. In addition to the treatment of acromegaly, octreotide has many other therapeutic uses including the treatment of carcinoid tumors, vasoactive intestinal peptide tumors (VIPomas), gastrointestinal fistulas, variceal bleeding, diarrheal states, and irritable bowel syndrome.

The efficacy of octreotide for the treatment of acromegaly has been determined by two major multicenter trials.[19,20] These studies determined that drug therapy with octreotide suppresses mean serum GH concentrations to less than 5 μg/L and normalizes serum IGF-I concentrations in 50% to 60% of acromegalic patients. Octreotide is also beneficial in reducing the clinical signs and symptoms of acromegaly. In a 6-month, multicenter trial, 70% of patients experienced significant relief of headaches.[20] In some patients, relief of headache symptoms occurred within minutes of octreotide administration. In addition, middle-finger circumference was reduced significantly, and 50% to 75% of the patients experienced improvement in symptoms of excessive perspiration, fatigue, joint pain, and cystic acne. A 2-year follow-up of 103 patients treated with octreotide showed that octreotide therapy is safe and effective for long-term use in acromegalic patients.[21] Several small studies have shown that octreotide improves the cardiovascular manifestations of acromegaly, resulting in decreased left-ventricular mass, decreased heart rate, and increased exercise capacity.[22–24] Octreotide also improves oxygen desaturation, sleep quality, and subjective symptoms of sleepiness in acromegalic patients suffering from sleep apnea.[25] Data from two major multicenter trials indicate that pituitary-tumor growth is halted during octreotide treatment, and a small number of patients actually experience tumor regression.[19,20] A recent study determined that the growth of pituitary tumors during octreotide therapy is suppressed by approximately 83%.[26]

Response to long-term therapy with octreotide is related to the presence and quantity of somatostatin receptors located in the pituitary adenoma.[17,18] Identification of patients who will most likely respond to octreotide, prior to the initiation of therapy, is important when considering the high cost of this medication and the inconvenience of subcutaneous drug administration. Suppression of serum GH concentrations after a single 50-μg dose of octreotide has been used to predict a favorable long-term response to octreotide therapy.[17] Somatostatin-receptor imaging and serum GH concentrations after short-term (1 month) administration of octreotide appear to be even more accurate in predicting which patients will respond to long-term octreotide therapy than acute suppression of GH by a single dose of octreotide.[27]

The initial dose of octreotide for the treatment of acromegaly is 100 μg administered every 8 hours.[5,15,18] Some clinicians recommend a starting dose of 50 μg every 8 hours, then increasing the dose to 100 μg every 8 hours after 1 week, to improve the patient's tolerance of the adverse gastrointestinal effects.[11,17] The dose may be increased by increments of 50 μg every 1 to 2 weeks based on mean serum GH and IGF-I concentrations. Patients who experience a significant rise in GH prior to the end of the 8-hour dosing interval may benefit from decreasing the dosing interval to every 4 to 6 hours. Although doses as high as 1500 μg per day have been used, doses above 600 μg daily generally do not offer additional benefits, and most patients are adequately managed with 100 to 200 μg three times daily.[17,19–21] In an effort to provide continuous suppression of GH throughout a 24-hour period, several small studies have evaluated the use of continuous subcutaneous infusions or pulsatile subcutaneous infusions of octreotide via portable battery-powered pumps. Octreotide delivery in this manner results in improved suppression of serum GH and IGF-I concentrations with fewer adverse effects than intermittent subcutaneous injections.[28]

Following subcutaneous injection, octreotide is rapidly absorbed, with peak serum concentrations occurring within 15 to 30 minutes. GH suppression lasts from 4 to 8 hours.[9,17] The elimination half-life of octreotide is approximately 90 minutes, and this is substantially longer than that of physiologic somatostatin, which has a half-life of only 3 minutes in the plasma.[14,17] Octreotide is extensively metabolized by the liver, and 32% of the drug is eliminated unchanged in the urine. Elderly patients may require lower doses of octreotide owing to decreased clearance of the drug and a prolonged elimination half-life.

The most common adverse effects of octreotide therapy are gastrointestinal disturbances such as diarrhea, nausea, abdominal cramps, malabsorption of fat, and flatulence.[5,11,14,15,17,18] These effects are dose dependent and can be seen within a few hours of the first octreotide injection. Gastrointestinal adverse effects occur in approximately 75% of patients, but usually subside within 10 to14 days of continued treatment.[5,11,14,15,17,18] Octreotide has also been reported to cause injection-site pain (8%), clinically insignificant sinus bradycardia (15% to 20%), conduction abnormalities and arrhythmias (9%), and biochemical hypothyroidism (12%).[5,14,17] Because octreotide slows gastric emptying, long-term therapy may predispose patients to the development of gastritis and *Helicobacter pylori* infection.[29]

Octreotide also inhibits cholecystokinin release and gallbladder motility, predisposing patients to the development of cholelithiasis.[30–32] The development of gallstones is a long-term adverse effect of octreotide use and is largely dependent on geographic factors, dietary habits, and length of therapy.[5,11,14,15,17,18] Octreotide-induced gallstones are three times more common in China than in the United States and may be more prevalent in patients who ingest low-fat diets.[5,14] The incidence of gallstones in acromegalic patients receiving octreotide increases with length of therapy and has been reported to range from 20% to 50%.[5,11,18–21] Most patients, however, are asymptomatic, and the diagnosis of cholelithiasis is usually made following an ultrasonographic study that is not prompted by patient symptoms. It has been estimated that only 1% of patients will develop symptomatic gallstones during 1 year of octreotide treatment.[5,11,18] Because octreotide-induced gallstones are usually present without clinical symptoms, the 1994 U.S. Acromegaly Therapy Consensus Development Panel recommended that treatment of octreotide-induced gallstones be the same as that for gallstones in the general population.[5] Prophylactic cholecystectomy or medical therapy with ursodeoxycholic acid for acromegalic patients with asymptomatic gallstones is usually not considered. Ursodeoxycholic acid has not been evaluated in acromegalic patients receiving octreotide.

The effect of octreotide on glucose metabolism in patients with acromegaly is multifactorial. Decreases in serum GH concentrations induced by octreotide should result in decreased hepatic gluconeogenesis and increased insulin-receptor sensitivity. However, octreotide also decreases insulin secretion and increases IGFBP-1, which is known to inhibit the insulin-like effects of IGF-I. In addition, octreotide delays the gastrointestinal absorption of glucose, which may further alter glucose metabolism in acromegalic patients. Small studies conducted in acromegalic patients with glucose intolerance have reported improvement in insulin sensitivity associated with octreotide therapy.[33,34] However, one study of 90 acromegalics reported that 11 (12%) patients developed impaired glucose tolerance and 16 (18%) patients developed frank diabetes mellitus while receiving octreotide.[35] In the same study, 27% of subjects who were diabetic at the beginning of the trial experienced an improvement in their glycemic control by the end of the 6-month study period.[35] Risk factors associated with worsening glucose tolerance included female gender and elevated baseline insulin values. Although octreotide appears to have a beneficial effect on glucose tolerance in most patients, glucose determinations should be obtained frequently in the early stages of octreotide therapy in all acromegalic patients.

Octreotide has very few significant drug–drug interactions. However, it can alter the absorption of some orally administered medications. Octreotide may substantially reduce serum concentrations of cyclosporine by decreasing its intestinal absorption, and the dosage of cyclosporine may need to be increased when these two medications are given concomitantly. Since octreotide has variable effects on glucose metabolism in patients with acromegaly, adjustments in the dose of insulin or oral antihyperglycemic agents may be needed. When bromocriptine and octreotide are administered concomitantly, the bioavailability of bromocriptine is increased by 40%.[36]

Bromocriptine and Octreotide Combination Therapy

Based on previous trials, octreotide is generally considered to be more effective than bromocriptine in reducing mean serum GH concentrations and normalizing IGF-I.[13,15,19,20] Several small studies have suggested that combination therapy with octreotide and bromocriptine may be more beneficial than either drug alone.[14,36] Because of the potential for additive adverse effects while using both medications, combination therapy should be considered as a therapeutic option only for refractory patients who have not fully responded to either octreotide or bromocriptine therapy alone.

Long-Acting Octreotide

A long-acting intramuscular (Sandostatin LAR) formulation of octreotide is currently in phase III clinical trials in the United States, with FDA-approval anticipated during 1999. This once-monthly intramuscular injection was developed by incorporating octreotide into the microspheres of a biodegradable polymer.[37] The pharmacodynamic effects of this formulation are similar to those of subcutaneously administered octreotide. Single monthly doses of long-acting octreotide have been shown to be at least as effective as 300 or 600 μg of subcutaneous octreotide in maintaining suppression of mean serum GH concentrations and normalizing IGF-I levels.[37] The tolerability of long-acting octreotide is similar to that of the intermittent subcutaneous injections. In patients who are adequately controlled with subcutaneous octreotide doses of 300 to 600 μg per day, the initial dose of long-acting intramuscular octreotide is 20 mg every 4 weeks. After 3 months of therapy, the dose may be increased or decreased based on clinical response.[37] Long-acting octreotide offers a more convenient method of octreotide administration for acromegalic patients. It can result in improved patient compliance, quality of life, and overall disease management. Lanreotide, another promising new agent, is a slow-release somatostatin analog that is administered intramuscularly twice monthly and is currently in phase III clinical trials.[14]

PHARMACOECONOMIC CONSIDERATIONS

Cost-effectiveness comparisons of the various treatment options for patients with acromegaly have not been performed. Considering that approximately 40% of patients are not completely cured after transsphenoidal surgery, pharmacologic treatment may become necessary. Bromocriptine is considerably less expensive than octreotide. However, it is not effective in the majority of patients, and octreotide is often the only viable therapeutic option. The drug therapy of choice in specific acromegalic patients should be determined by an individual's clinical response, suppression of serum GH concentrations, and normalization of IGF-I.[38]

CONCLUSIONS

Acromegaly is a chronic debilitating disease characterized by excess growth-hormone secretion most commonly caused by a GH-secreting pituitary adenoma. Transsphenoidal surgical resection of the adenoma is the treatment of choice for patients with acromegaly. Patients who are poor surgical candidates may receive radiation therapy or long-term pharmacologic therapy. Drug therapy options for acromegaly are limited to dopamine agonists and the somatostatin analog octreotide. Dopamine agonists are generally not as effective as octreotide in suppressing GH concentrations or normalizing IGF-I values. However, a small subset of patients may respond to dopamine agonists, and these agents should be considered for all patients because of the potential cost advantages and convenience of oral administration. Octreotide has proved to be the most effective pharmacologic agent for the treatment of acromegaly and is typically administered by intermittent subcutaneous injections. Improved somatostatin analog delivery formulations, such as long-acting octreotide and lanreotide, should improve patient compliance, quality of life, and therapeutic outcomes.

GROWTH HORMONE DEFICIENCY

Short stature is a condition that is commonly defined by a physical height that is more than two standard deviations below the population mean and lower than the third percentile for height in a specific age group.[39–41] It has been estimated that greater than 1.8 million children in the United States can be characterized as having short stature.[41] Short stature is a very broad term describing a condition that may be the result of many different causes. A true lack of GH is among the least common causes and is known as growth-hormone-deficient (GHD) short stature. Absolute GH deficiency is a congenital disorder that can result from various genetic abnormalities such as GHRH deficiency, GH gene deletion, or developmental disorders including pituitary aplasia or hypoplasia.[39,42] GH insufficiency is an acquired condition that can result secondary to hypothalamic or pituitary tumors, cranial irradiation, head trauma, pituitary infarction, and various types of CNS infections. In addition, psychosocial deprivation; hypothyroidism; poorly controlled diabetes mellitus; treatment of precocious puberty with LHRH agonists; and pharmacologic agents such as glucocorticoids, methylphenidate, and dextroamphetamine may induce transient GH insufficiency.[39,42]

Short stature also occurs with several conditions that are not associated with a true GH deficiency or insufficiency. These conditions include intrauterine growth retardation; constitutional growth delay; malnutrition; malabsorption of nutrients associated with inflammatory bowel disease, celiac disease, and cystic fibrosis; chronic renal failure; skeletal and cartilage dysplasia; and genetic syndromes such as Turner's syndrome.[39,42] In addition, many children are diagnosed with idiopathic or normal variant short stature. These patients have heights that are significantly lower than the third percentile, but present with normal GH serum concentrations and no specific underlying explanation for short stature.[41,42]

Children with GHD short stature are usually born with an average birth weight. Decreases in growth velocity generally become evident between the age of 6 months and 3 years.[39,42] In contrast, GH insufficiency may arise at any age during growth and development. GH-deficient or -insufficient children appear to be short and centrally obese with a prominent forehead and an immature face.[39] Because

GH deficiency may be accompanied by the loss of other pituitary hormones, characteristics such as small genitalia, hypoglycemia, and hypothyroidism may also be noted.

Several factors must be considered in the diagnosis of GH deficiency or insufficiency. Standard epidemiologic growth charts developed by the National Center for Health Statistics (NCHS) are typically used to determine the percentile of anthropometric measurements such as height, weight, and head circumference. Pubertal stage is typically determined using the Tanner method. The bone age is determined according to published standards, and growth velocity is calculated to determine the patient's height velocity percentile using standard growth-velocity charts.[39,42] Growth-hormone deficiency is rarely seen in the absence of delayed bone age and decreased growth velocity. In addition, several different provocative stimuli that induce GH secretion are used diagnostically to determine GH status. Common provocative pharmacologic GH stimuli include insulin-induced hypoglycemia, clonidine, L-dopa, arginine, glucagon, and growth hormone-releasing hormone.[40] A subnormal GH response is arbitrarily defined as a maximum GH serum concentration of < 7 μg/L for 2 hours after administration of one of these agents.[40,43] Some centers use 10 μg/L as the maximum GH serum concentration to determine a subnormal GH response. The three generally accepted criteria for the definitive diagnosis of GH deficiency are a subnormal growth velocity, a delayed bone age, and a subnormal GH response to at least two provocative stimuli.[43] For prepubertal patients, priming with sex hormones is needed to improve specificity.[44] Some patients may exhibit clinical signs of GH deficiency, subnormal growth velocity, and delayed bone age, despite GH levels that are within normal limits after provocative testing. This makes diagnosis in this group of patients very difficult. Diagnosis based on GH stimulation tests becomes further complicated because of the paucity of data reporting the normal range of GH concentrations after provocative testing in healthy children and the fact that commercial GH assays currently available may not be equivalent.[40,43] One study comparing several different GH assays found a significant variation between measured GH serum concentrations.[43] Because of these limitations, careful consideration of multiple factors by a pediatric endocrinology specialist is required to diagnose growth-hormone deficiency correctly.

▶ TREATMENT: Growth Hormone Deficiency

PHARMACOLOGIC THERAPY

The treatment of growth-hormone deficiency with pituitary-derived human growth hormone was first reported in 1958.[45] The National Pituitary Agency was founded by the National Institutes of Health in 1963 to coordinate the collection of human pituitary glands and purification of GH for administration to children with GHD. In 1985, three deaths linked to Creutzfeldt–Jakob disease (CJD) were identified in young individuals who were previously treated with human pituitary growth hormone.[46] In the United States, a total of seven cases of CJD were reported in patients who had received human pituitary growth hormone prior to 1970.[46] Human pituitary growth hormone was withdrawn from the U.S. market because of the strong likelihood that the agent of CJD was transmitted through contaminated human pituitary-derived growth hormone. Shortly after the withdrawal of human pituitary growth hormone, the U.S. Food and Drug Administration approved the first recombinant DNA–derived growth hormone for the treatment of GH insufficiency.[45] Prior to the introduction of recombinant growth hormone, the number of individuals who received treatment for GH insufficiency was relatively small owing to the limited availability of human pituitary tissue for GH extraction. Currently, with the widespread availability of recombinant growth-hormone products, a large number of children can receive growth-hormone-replacement therapy at higher doses (Table 73–2). Unfortunately, human pituitary-derived growth hormone continues to be used today in some underdeveloped countries.

GH replacement therapy in children with documented GHD short stature produces a significant improvement in growth velocity within the first year of therapy.[43] This initial increase in growth velocity is often referred to as catch-up growth. Most of the initial studies evaluating the efficacy of GH therapy in GHD children were conducted for short periods of time in small numbers of patients, and, until recently, information about the long-term outcome of GH therapy was limited. Although growth velocity improves initially following GH therapy, the available data from patients receiving long-term growth hormone therapy suggest that final adult height is not substantially improved. The average final adult height typically reported in the literature has been two standard deviations below the population mean.[47–49] Analysis of data compiled by the French National Register from 3233 children with short stature, who received growth hormone replacement therapy between 1973 and 1993, also reported a mean final height that was two standard deviations below the population mean after an average of 4 years of GH therapy.[50] Although these results are disappointing, it is important to note that a substantial percentage of patients included in these studies had initially received human pituitary growth hormone in relatively low doses because of its limited availability. In addition, current growth-hormone dosing regimens have changed with regard to frequency of administration, making these data difficult to apply to patients who are receiving GH-replacement therapy today. More recently, a study evaluating the adult height of children who received only recombinant-GH therapy with currently recommended dosing regimens suggests that current recombinant-GH therapy may have a greater impact on final adult height than previously reported.[51] Additionally, several studies have suggested that initiation of GH therapy at an early chronologic age, prior to the onset of puberty, may be associated with a more favorable increase in final height.[49–51] Therefore, prompt diagnosis of growth hormone deficiency and initiation of replacement therapy with recombinant GH may be a crucial factor in optimizing the final adult height of children with GHD. Recombinant GH is currently considered the mainstay of therapy for the treatment of GHD short stature. However, additional well-controlled studies are needed to define the optimal use of GH therapy in patients with this disorder. A number of studies evaluating the effect of GH therapy on final adult height are ongoing.

Recombinant growth hormone has also been shown to increase short-term growth rate in patients with chronic renal fail-

TABLE 73–2. Recombinant-Growth-Hormone Products

Product	Formulation	Recommended Dosing Regimen	FDA-Approved Indications
Protropin	Somatrem lyophilized powder for injection	Doses up to 0.1 mg/kg SQ 3 times weekly	Growth failure associated with chronic renal failure Growth hormone–deficient growth failure
Genotropin	Somatropin lyophilized powder for injection	0.16–0.24 mg/kg/wk SQ 6–7 times per week iin divided doses	Growth failure associated with chronic renal failure Growth hormone–deficient growth failure
Norditropin	Somatropin lyophilized powder for injection	0.024–0.034 mg/kg SQ 6–7 times weekly	Growth failure associated with chronic renal failure Growth hormone–deficient growth failure
Nutropin	Somatropin lyophilized powder for injection	0.3 mg/kg/wk SQ or IM	Growth failure associated with chronic renal failure Growth hormone–deficient growth failure Short stature associated with Turner's syndrome
Nutropin AQ	Somatropin injection	0.3 mg/kg/wk SQ or IM	Growth failure associated with chronic renal failure Growth hormone–deficient growth failure Short stature associated with Turner's syndrome
Humatrope	Somatropin lyophilized powder for injection	0.18–0.3 mg/kg/wk SQ or IM administered on 3 alternate days or 6 times per week in divided doses	Growth failure associated with chronic renal failure Growth hormone–deficient growth failure Adult-onset somatropin deficiency syndrome
Serostim	Somatropin lyophilized powder for injection	0.1 mg/kg SQ daily	Growth failure associated with chronic renal failure AIDS wasting or cachexia
Saizen	Somatropin lyophilized powder for injection	0.06 mg/kg SQ or IM 3 times weekly	Growth failure associated with chronic renal failure Growth hormone–deficient growth failure

ure and Turner's syndrome and is FDA approved for the treatment of growth failure associated with these conditions.[43,45] GH is also FDA approved for the treatment of adult growth-hormone deficiency. Long-term GH therapy in growth-hormone deficient adults significantly decreases body fat, increases muscle mass, and improves exercise capacity.[52] In small studies GH therapy in adults has been shown to improve cardiac and renal function as well as psychological well-being.[53–55] In addition, the use of GH is currently being studied in a variety of different disorders including infertility, obesity, AIDS, and natural aging and for use as an anabolic agent in trauma and other catabolic states.[45]

The majority of short children in the United States do not have an identifiable medical cause for their condition, but with widespread availability of several recombinant-growth-hormone formulations, many children have received GH therapy regardless of the underlying etiology of their short stature. The use of recombinant-growth-hormone therapy in children with non-growth-hormone-deficient, or normal variant, short stature has been studied by several investigators.[56–59] Most of these studies indicate that these patients experience an improvement in short-term growth velocity, but improvements in final height have not been proven.[56–59] A subset of patients may maintain better growth with continued GH therapy, but the specific characteristics of this patient population remain to be determined.[56–58] The use of GH therapy in patients with non-growth-hormone-deficient short stature is controversial. For example, although guidelines established for the use of growth hormone by the Lawson Wilkins Pediatric Endocrine Society do not consider GH to be a safe and effective treatment for non-GHD short stature,[43] a national survey of physicians revealed that a majority of pediatric endocrinologists regard GH therapy to be an appropriate treatment in certain patients with non-GHD short stature.[60] Additional long-term studies evaluating the efficacy and safety of GH therapy are needed to determine the role of GH therapy in non-GHD children.

Eight different recombinant-growth-hormone products are currently available for use in the United States. Somatrem (Protropin) was the first recombinant-GH product developed and used for the treatment of GH deficiency. This formulation contains the same 191 amino-acid sequence as human pituitary growth hormone with the exception of the terminal addition of a methionine amino-acid group. The remaining GH formulations (Genotropin, Norditropin, Nutropin, Nutropin AQ, Humatrope, Serostim, and Saizen) contain somatropin. Somatropin is composed of the same amino-acid sequence as human pituitary GH. Recombinant-GH formulations must be administered by intramuscular or subcutaneous injection. Nutropin AQ is the only GH product that is available as a liquid formulation. The remaining products are formulated as lyophilized powders for injection, and patients must to be instructed regarding proper reconstitution, storage, and administration. The potency of GH products is expressed as International Units per milligram (IU/mg) with 1 mg containing approximately 2.6 IU of growth hormone.[61] Direct comparisons between the different recombinant-growth-hormone products have not been published. Although some differences exist in recommended dosages, all GH products are generally considered to be equally efficacious. Usual recommended doses range from 0.15 to 0.3 mg/kg/wk.[43] Recombinant GH is usually administered subcutaneously in equal doses 3 to 7 times per week depending on the specific GH product used.[42,43] Dosing regimens with greater frequency of administration have been shown to provide more favorable short-term growth responses.[43] Growth-hormone-replacement therapy should be initiated as early as possible after diagnosis of GH insufficiency and continued until a desirable height is reached or growth velocity has decreased to less than 2.5 cm/yr after the pubertal growth spurt.

The bioavailability of recombinant GH is approximately 75% after subcutaneous administration and 60% after intramuscular administration. Following systemic administration, recombinant GH localizes to highly perfused organs, such as the kidney and liver, where it is metabolized to amino acids that then return to the systemic circulation. The elimination half-life of exogenous GH is approximately 3 to 5 hours.

Glucocorticoids may inhibit the growth-promoting effects of recombinant GH, and concomitant administration of androgens, estrogens, thyroid hormones, or anabolic steroids may accelerate epiphyseal closure and compromise final height.

Three large databases, the National Cooperative Growth Study (NCGS), the Kabi International Growth Study (KIGS), and the Australian OZGROW, have been developed to collect post-marketing adverse-effect data or reports associated with recombinant growth hormone. Development of these databases was prompted by the unexpected and tragic cases of CJD reported in patients treated with human pituitary growth hormone. These databases are maintained by pharmaceutical companies that manufacture GH products.[62] Recombinant GH is generally well tolerated in children, and adverse effects are relatively uncommon.[63,64] A small number of patients may complain of injection-site pain or arthralgias. Idiopathic intracranial hypertension (IIH), also known as pseudotumor cerebri, has been reported in a very small number of children receiving GH therapy. This condition usually develops within the first 8 to 12 of weeks treatment and presents with symptoms such as headache, blurred vision, diplopia, nausea, and vomiting.[62] The symptoms of IIH usually resolve after discontinuation of GH therapy, and long-term complications are rare. Cases of slipped capital femoral epiphysis (SCFE) have been reported in children with growth-hormone deficiency who are receiving GH therapy.[62] This condition is thought to occur as a result of the increased width of the femoral plate during GH treatment, but it has also been reported in GH-deficient children who are not receiving GH replacement. Patients with this condition typically complain of hip or knee pain. SCFE can be managed by an orthopedic surgeon, and GH therapy does not need to be withdrawn. Because growth hormone is known to cause decreased insulin sensitivity, hyperglycemia and diabetes mellitus may develop. A very small number of patients have developed frank diabetes mellitus during GH treatment, and all of these patients had specific predisposing risk factors for diabetes mellitus.[62–64] GH may promote the growth of various types of neoplasms and increase tumor recurrence rates in patients with a history of malignancy.[63,64] For this reason, GH should not be administered to patients with an active malignant tumor or a history of recurrent tumor growth. In 1988, a Japanese report indicated that children receiving GH therapy were twice as likely to develop leukemia as children who were not receiving the hormone.[65] A more recent analysis of all collected reports of leukemia associated with GH therapy determined that these children had other leukemia risk factors (Fanconi anemia, Bloom's syndrome, or a prior history of cancer).[66] GH therapy in children without these risk factors does not appear to predispose children to develop leukemia.[62–64] Finally, some patients may develop antibodies to recombinant GH. The development of antibodies during replacement therapy with recombinant-GH products has been reported to be relatively low, affecting approximately 15% to 20% of patients.[67,68] More importantly, the presence of GH antibodies has not been shown to adversely affect growth response and appears to be clinically insignificant except in patients with GH gene deletions.

Appropriate monitoring of GH therapy includes regular assessments of height, weight, growth velocity, serum alkaline phosphatase, and bone age every 6 to 12 months. Additional laboratory tests to monitor for potential adverse effects include serum glucose and thyroid function. The dose of GH will periodically need to be increased as weight increases in growing children.

GROWTH HORMONE-RELEASING HORMONE

The U.S. Food and Drug Administration has recently approved a synthetic growth hormone–releasing hormone (GH-RH) product, known as sermorelin (Geref), for the treatment of idiopathic growth-hormone deficiency in children. Sermorelin (GH-RH (1-29)-NH_2) is composed of 29 amino-acid residues that are identical to the amino-terminal segment of human GH-RH. Although not as effective as recombinant-GH therapy, sermorelin has been shown to increase short-term growth velocity in children with idiopathic growth-hormone deficiency.[69,70] This product has also been shown to increase growth velocity in children who have GH deficiency secondary to hypothalamic damage rather than pituitary abnormalities, as is observed with radiation-induced GH deficiency.[71] In most cases of radiation-induced GH deficiency, pituitary somatotropes are capable of secreting endogenous GH, and stimulation of these cells by exogenously administered GH-RH may restore the natural pulsatile secretion of GH and result in increased growth rate.

The recommended dose of sermorelin is 0.03 mg/kg administered daily by subcutaneous injection. No serious adverse events have been identified. The most common adverse effect reported by patients receiving sermorelin therapy is pain at the site of injection. Because normal pituitary function is needed for sermorelin to stimulate GH secretion, children should not receive GH-RH therapy with sermorelin unless adequate capacity to secrete GH is documented by provocative GH-stimulation testing. Sermorelin may prove to be a beneficial therapeutic option in the treatment of various types of non-GHD short stature. However, owing to its mechanism of action, sermorelin does not have a role in the treatment of true GHD short stature.

FUTURE THERAPIES

A number of biosynthetic growth hormone–releasing peptides (GHRPs), including examorelin (Hexarelin), are currently under investigation for use in the treatment of various types of short stature.[72] Like synthetic GHRH, GHRP stimulates the secretion of GH. However, GHRPs act through different receptor mechanisms and can potentially be used synergistically with synthetic GH-RH formulations. A significant advantage of GHRPs is that they are biologically active when administered intravenously, subcutaneously, nasally, and orally.[72–74] Small studies have shown that GHRPs are generally well tolerated, and short-term use in children with growth-hormone deficiency, normal-variant short stature, and idiopathic short stature results in increased growth velocity.[73,74] This new class of medications may offer significant therapeutic benefits in specific patient populations with short stature.

The use of insulin-like growth factor-I (IGF-I) for the treatment of growth disorders associated with GH insensitivity is also currently under investigation. Because the growth-promoting effects of GH are primarily mediated by IGF-I, patients who are resistant to GH may benefit from IGF-I therapy. Growth-hormone resistance may result from hereditary abnormalities characterized by defective GH receptors, such as Laron-type dwarfism, or antibody formation to recombinant-growth-hormone products. Several studies in a limited number of patients have documented increased growth in children with GH insensitivity receiving IGF-I.[45] The safety and efficacy of IGF-I is currently being studied in phase III clinical trials.

PHARMACOECONOMIC CONSIDERATIONS

The treatment of short stature with recombinant GH is very expensive. Despite the prohibitive cost, recombinant GH remains the mainstay of therapy for children with GHD short stature. However, treatment of non-GHD short stature with recombinant GH is not widely accepted. Though the benefits in final adult height reported in the literature are equivocal for those with non-GHD short stature, and clearly less than ideal for those with GHD short stature, the increases in growth velocity, particularly in children with true GH deficiency, are associated with significant psychosocial benefits. Many clinicians believe that GH therapy can improve quality of life and should be made available to all children with short stature, regardless of whether or not they are GH deficient.[75] Until studies using recombinant GH more definitively demonstrate improvements in both final adult height and quality of life, the cost-effectiveness of GH, particularly for non-GHD short stature, remains uncertain.

CONCLUSIONS

Growth-hormone deficiency during childhood results in short stature. Replacement with recombinant GH is considered the mainstay of therapy for patients with GHD short stature, but its use for the treatment of non-GHD short stature remains controversial. Recombinant GH has proven to be safe for use in children and is associated with very few adverse effects. Although GH improves initial growth velocity, the long-term benefits with respect to final adult height remain to be determined. New therapeutic agents such as the synthetic growth hormone–releasing hormone sermorelin and other growth hormone–releasing peptides may provide benefits for patients with non-GHD short stature. Because growth-hormone regimens can be particularly demanding and inconvenient for patients, knowledge of the long-term benefits is critical to the development of rational, cost-effective treatments for patients with short stature.

PROLACTIN

PHYSIOLOGIC EFFECTS

Prolactin is secreted in a pulsatile fashion by the lactotroph cells of the anterior pituitary, with the highest peak concentrations observed during sleep.[3] The secretion of prolactin is regulated primarily by tonic hypothalamic inhibitory effects of dopamine. As described earlier in this chapter and listed in Table 73–1, many factors can affect prolactin secretion. During pregnancy, prolactin serum concentrations rise substantially above the normal. All other conditions characterized by excess prolactin serum concentrations, known as hyperprolactinemia, are considered pathologic.

HYPERPROLACTINEMIA

Hyperprolactinemia is a state of persistent serum prolactin elevation. Prolactin concentrations greater than 20 μg/L observed on multiple occasions are generally considered indicative of hyperprolactinemia.[76,77] Hyperprolactinemia usually affects women of reproductive age and has been noted in 25% of women with secondary amenorrhea.[76,77] The incidence of hyperprolactinemia in the general population is reported to be less than 1%.[76]

Hyperprolactinemia has several etiologies. The most common causes are benign prolactin-secreting pituitary tumors, known as prolactinomas, and various medications. Prolactinomas are classified according to size. Prolactin-secreting microadenomas are less than 10 mm in diameter and often do not increase in size.[3,78,79] In contrast, macroadenomas are tumors with a diameter greater than 10 mm that continue to grow and can cause invasion of surrounding tissues.[3,78,79] In the presence of a prolactinoma, prolactin serum concentrations may remain normal or may be markedly elevated to thousands of micrograms per liter.

Any pharmacologic agent that antagonizes dopamine or increases the release of prolactin can induce hyperprolactinemia (Table 73–3). Serotonin is a strong stimulator of prolactin secretion, and serotonin-reuptake inhibitors (SSRIs) such as fluoxetine (Prozac), paroxetine (Paxil), sertraline (Zoloft), and fluvoxamine (Luvox) are the medications most frequently associated with hyperprolactinemia.[80] Prior to the increased use of SSRIs, antipsychotic medications with potent dopamine-receptor blockade, such as the phenothiazine derivatives and haloperidol (Haldol), were most often identified as the cause of drug-induced hyperprolactinemia.[3,81] Metoclopramide (Reglan) and domperidone, an antiemetic available in Europe, are potent dopamine-receptor antagonists reported to induce hyperprolactinemia.[80] Hormones such as estrogen and progesterone, commonly prescribed as oral contraceptives, can stimulate lactotroph growth to promote prolactin secretion and have been implicated in drug-induced hyperprolactinemia.[80] Although the exact mechanism of action remains to be determined, the calcium-channel-blocking agent verapamil (Calan, Isoptin, etc.) has been associated with cases of hyperprolactinemia.[3,80] Methyldopa (Aldomet) and reserpine, although not used frequently in clinical practice today, are antihypertensive agents that can stimulate

TABLE 73–3. Drug-Induced Hyperprolactinemia

Dopamine antagonists	Gonadotropin-releasing-hormone analogs
Phenothiazines	Benzodiazepines
Haloperidol	Tricyclic antidepressants (clomipramine and nortriptyline)
Metoclopramide	Monoamine oxidase inhibitors
Domperidone	H_2-Receptor antagonists (cimetidine)
Prolactin Stimulators	Opioids
Methyldopa	**Other**
Reserpine	Verapamil
Serotonin reuptake inhibitors (SSRIs)	
Dexfenfluramine	
Estrogens	
Progestins	

prolactin secretion.[80] Prolactin concentrations may increase with the administration of gonadotropin-releasing hormone analogs like leuprolide (Lupron) or goserelin (Zoladex).[80] Other medications rarely reported to cause hyperprolactinemia include H_2-receptor blocking agents, benzodiazepines, tricyclic antidepressants, dexfenfluramine, opioids, and monoamine oxidase inhibitors.[3,76,78,80] Prolactin levels do not typically rise to greater than 150 μg/L in cases of drug-induced hyperprolactinemia. Measurement of serum prolactin concentrations prior to the initiation of therapy with medications known to cause prolactin elevation may obviate the need for extensive examination of pituitary function and aid with the appropriate diagnosis of drug-induced hyperprolactinemia.

Less common etiologies include CNS lesions that physically compress the pituitary stalk and interrupt tonic hypothalamic dopamine secretion resulting in hyperprolactinemia.[76,78] Increased thyroid-releasing hormone (TRH) concentrations in hypothyroidism can stimulate prolactin secretion and cause hyperprolactinemia.[76,78] During conditions of renal or liver compromise, the clearance of prolactin is decreased, resulting in elevated prolactin concentrations.[76] Despite vigorous diagnostic effort, the cause of hyperprolactinemia cannot always be determined. This is known as idiopathic hyperprolactinemia and is most likely a result of the presence of very small tumors that are not detected by standard imaging techniques.[79] It should be noted that many physiologic factors, such as stress (including the stress of phlebotomy), sleep, exercise, coitus, and eating can also induce transiently elevated prolactin levels.[3,77] This emphasizes the importance of obtaining multiple prolactin measurements to confirm the diagnosis. Ideally, after an intravenous line is placed in the patient's arm, the patient should rest in a supine position or in a chair for 2 hours before prolactin samples are collected.

Elevated prolactin serum concentrations inhibit gonadotropin secretion and sex-steroid synthesis.[77] Because prolactin concentrations higher than 60 μg/L are associated with anovulation, women with hyperprolactinemia typically present with menstrual irregularities such as oligomenorrhea or amenorrhea and infertility.[76–78] In addition, approximately 40% to 70% of women with hyperprolactinemia will have galactorrhea.[77,78] Hyperprolactinemia in men, although rare, may cause decreased libido, erectile dysfunction, infertility, galactorrhea, or gynecomastia.[77,78] In the presence of a prolactin-secreting pituitary tumor, many patients with hyperprolactinemia may first present with headaches and visual-field disturbances that result from tumor compression of the optic chiasm.[78] The prolonged suppression of estrogen in premenopausal women with hyperprolactinemia leads to a decrease in bone mineral density and significant risk for the development of osteoporosis.[76,78] In addition, untreated hyperprolactinemia in women may increase the risk of ischemic heart disease.[78]

The diagnosis of hyperprolactinemia, as defined by multiple prolactin serum concentrations above 20 μg/L, is relatively simple. However, identifying the underlying cause of this abnormality may be more challenging. Patients with modest prolactin elevations should have multiple prolactin serum determinations to minimize the potential for detecting only transient increases in prolactin. A careful medication history is essential, and the presence of hypothyroidism, renal failure, or hepatic dysfunction should be evaluated. If the cause of hyperprolactinemia remains ambiguous, a CT scan or MRI study should be performed to determine the presence of a pituitary tumor.[76–78] If an underlying cause of elevated prolactin serum concentration is not determined, the hyperprolactinemia is considered to be idiopathic.

▶ TREATMENT: Hyperprolactinemia

The treatment of hyperprolactinemia depends on the underlying cause of the abnormality. In cases of drug-induced hyperprolactinemia, discontinuation of the offending medication and initiation of an appropriate therapeutic alternative usually normalizes serum prolactin concentrations.[80] In cases for which an appropriate therapeutic alternative does not exist, medical therapy with dopamine agonists is warranted. Sex-steroid replacement should also be considered.[80] Treatment options for the management of prolactinomas include clinical observation, medical therapy with dopamine agonists, radiation therapy, and transsphenoidal surgical removal of the tumor.[76–78,82] Because prolactin-secreting microadenomas are very small and typically do not increase in size, treatment of these tumors is primarily directed toward alleviating symptoms.[78,79,82] The goal of therapy is to normalize prolactin serum concentrations and reestablish gonadotropin secretion to restore fertility and reduce the risk of osteoporosis. In patients with asymptomatic elevations in serum prolactin, observation and close follow-up are appropiate.[76,77,79] Treatment goals are more aggressive in patients with prolactin-secreting macroadenomas because these tumors are larger and can cause invasion of local tissues with significant visual defects.[82] Therefore, in addition to normalizing prolactin concentrations, tumor shrinkage and correction of visual defects are primary goals of treatment.

Medical therapy with dopamine agonists is usually more effective than transsphenoidal surgery for both types of pituitary prolactinomas.[77–79,82] Postsurgical cure rates differ depending on tumor type and are reported to be approximately 70% for microprolactinomas and only 30% for macroprolactinomas.[3] In addition, long-term follow-up of patients with prior transsphenoidal surgical removal of prolactinomas has indicated a relatively high recurrence rate (approximately 40%) within 5 years.[78] A more recent, 10-year follow-up of patients with microprolactinomas found a recurrence rate of only 27%.[83] This marked improvement in outcome has been largely attributed to advancements in neurosurgical techniques. Transsphenoidal surgery for the removal of prolactinomas is usually reserved for patients who are refractory to or cannot tolerate therapy with dopamine agonists and for patients with very large tumors that cause severe compression of adjacent tissues.[77,82] Radiation therapy may require several years for effective tumor shrinkage and reduction in serum prolactin concentrations and is usually used only in conjunction with surgery.[82]

PHARMACOLOGIC THREAPY

Medical therapy with dopamine agonists has proven to be very effective in normalizing prolactin serum concentrations, restoring menstruation, and reducing tumor size in approximately 70% to 100% of patients within 3 to 6 months of therapy.[84,85] Bromocriptine (Parlodel) has been the mainstay of therapy since the 1970s, and pergolide (Permax) has been used as an effective alternative in patients who are intolerant of the adverse effects associated with bromocriptine. Cabergoline (Dostinex) is a new long-acting dopamine agonist that offers the advantage of less-frequent dosing and may eventually replace bromocriptine as the agent of choice for the medical management of prolactinomas.

BROMOCRIPTINE

Bromocriptine was the first D_2-receptor agonist to be used in the treatment of hyperprolactinemia and has been the mainstay of therapy for over 20 years. Medical therapy with bromocriptine normalizes prolactin serum concentrations, restores gonadotropin production, and shrinks tumor size in approximately 90% of patients with prolactinomas.[82]

For the management of hyperprolactinemia, bromocriptine therapy is typically initiated at 1.25 to 2.5 mg once daily at bedtime to minimize adverse effects.[76,77,82] The dose can be gradually increased by 1.25-mg increments every week to obtain desirable serum prolactin concentrations. Usual therapeutic doses of bromocriptine range from 2.5 to 15 mg per day, although some patients may require doses as high as 40 mg per day.[76,77,86] Bromocriptine is usually administered in two or three divided doses, but once-daily dosing has also been shown to be effective.[86]

The most common adverse effects associated with bromocriptine therapy include central nervous system symptoms such as headache, lightheadedness, dizziness, nervousness, and fatigue. Gastrointestinal effects such as nausea, abdominal pain, and diarrhea are also common. Bromocriptine should be administered with food to decrease the incidence of adverse gastrointestinal effects. Although most of these adverse effects diminish with continued treatment, about 12% of patients will not tolerate the adverse effects associated with bromocriptine therapy.[86] New extended-release dosage forms of bromocriptine are currently being investigated to improve tolerability and compliance. These include a long-acting injectable form of bromocriptine (Parlodel LAR), which can be administered as monthly intramuscular injections in doses of 50 to 75 mg monthly, and a slow-release oral formulation (Parlodel SRO) that is given as a single daily dose of 5 to 15 mg. These formulations have been shown to be as effective as immediate-release bromocriptine and may improve compliance.[87–89] Vaginal preparations of bromocriptine have also been studied in an effort to decrease the incidence of adverse effects associated with oral dosage forms.[90]

Because most patients with hyperprolactinemia are women with a principal complaint of infertility, the safety of bromocriptine in pregnancy must be considered. One report of over 2000 pregnancies in women who received bromocriptine during part or all of their gestation did not detect an increase in the risk for spontaneous abortion or incidence of congenital abnormalites.[86] Although bromocriptine does not appear to be teratogenic, some clinicians discontinue therapy as soon as pregnancy is detected because the effects of in utero exposure to bromocriptine on gonadal function and fertility of the offspring remains to be determined.[79,82] In some patients with macroprolactinomas undergoing rapid tumor expansion, bromocriptine therapy must be continued throughout pregnancy.

PERGOLIDE

Pergolide (Permax) is a dopamine-receptor agonist with affinity for both D_1- and D_2-receptors. In the United States, pergolide is not FDA approved for the treatment of hyperprolactinemia and is most commonly prescribed for the treatment of parkinsonism. However, pergolide has been used for many years as a safe and effective alternative to bromocriptine in the management of patients with hyperprolactinemia and offers the advantage of one-daily dosing.[91,92]

For the treatment of hyperprolactinemia, pergolide therapy is initiated at a dose of 25 μg given once daily at bedtime. The average dose that achieves optimal suppression of prolactin serum concentrations is 50 μg per day given as a single dose.[91] Adverse effects of pergolide are similar to those of bromocriptine and include nausea, headache, vomiting, and dizziness in about 30% of patients.[91] The use of pergolide during pregnancy has not been evaluated as extensively as has bromocriptine and should be avoided until additional data become available.

CABERGOLINE

Cabergoline (Dostinex) is a new long-acting dopamine agonist with high selectivity and affinity for dopamine D_2-receptors. This agent was approved by the U.S. FDA in 1996 for the treatment of hyperprolactinemia and has been shown to effectively reduce serum prolactin concentrations in 80% to 90% of hyperprolactinemic patients.[93–95] Cabergoline also effectively reduces tumor size in patients with both micro- and macroprolactinomas.[93,96] In a multicenter randomized trial comparing the efficacy of cabergoline and bromocriptine, serum prolactin levels were normalized in 83% of patients receiving cabergoline and 58% of patients receiving bromocriptine after 6 months of therapy.[97] Cabergoline may also be effective in patients who are intolerant of or resistant to bromocriptine.[98]

Cabergoline is commercially available as 0.5-mg oral tablets. The initial dose of cabergoline for the treatment of hyperprolactinemia is 0.5 mg once weekly or in divided doses twice weekly. This dose may be increased by increments of 0.5 mg at 4-week intervals based on serum prolactin concentrations. The usual dose is 1 to 2 mg weekly; however, doses as high as 4.5 mg weekly have been used.[99] Recent studies have also evaluated the efficacy of a vaginal dosage form of cabergoline to reduce the adverse effects associated with oral therapy.[100]

Following oral administration, peak serum concentrations are obtained within 2 hours, and food does not affect absorption. Data from animal studies indicate that cabergoline is widely distributed to well-perfused organs, including the pituitary gland.[99] The elimination of cabergoline from the pituitary appears to be very slow; this rate may explain the long duration of action. Cabergoline is extensively metabolized in the liver by hydrolysis, and the dose should be reduced in patients with severe hepatic failure.[99] This drug is eliminated primarily in the feces, and the elimination half-life ranges from 79 to 155 hours in hyperprolactinemic patients.[99]

The most common adverse effects reported with the use of cabergoline are nausea, vomiting, headache, and dizziness.[93–96,99] These are similar to the adverse effects reported with bromocriptine and pergolide. However, in a large comparative study evaluating bromocriptine and cabergoline, fewer patients receiving cabergoline reported adverse effects than patients receiving bromocriptine, and only 3% of the patients in the cabergoline group withdrew from the study because of adverse effects versus 12% of patients taking bromocriptine.[97] Other adverse events associated with the use of cabergoline include gastrointestinal complaints, drowsiness, fatigue, paresthesias, dyspnea, suffocation sensation, and epistaxis.[97,99] As with other dopamine agonists, adverse events usually occur early in therapy and subside with continued treatment. However, in one study 15% to 20% of patients receiving cabergoline experienced a recurrence of early symptoms or an onset of new symptoms after several weeks of treatment.[97] Mild to moderate decreases in blood pressure have been observed in up to 50% of patients taking cabergoline;

however, the incidence of symptomatic orthostatic hypotension has not been significant.[93,94,97] Several patients have experienced clinically insignificant decreases in hemoglobin.[94,95] This was attributed to the restoration of menses in previously amenorrheic patients. Transient increases in serum alkaline phosphatase, bilirubin, and aminotransferases have been reported in small numbers of patients receiving cabergoline.[94,97] Pleuropulmonary disease has been reported with cabergoline, but only with larger doses used in the treatment of Parkinson's disease.[99]

The use of cabergoline in pregnancy has not been extensively studied. However, several case reports of women who received cabergoline therapy during the first and second trimesters of pregnancy have not documented an increased risk of spontaneous abortion, congenital abnormalities, or tubal pregnancy.[99] However, prospective data in large numbers of pregnancies is lacking. Owing to the long half-life and limited data on cabergoline use in pregnancy, most clinicians recommend that women receiving cabergoline therapy who plan to become pregnant should discontinue the medication 1 month before planned conception.

Other dopamine agonists that have been used in the treatment of hyperprolactinemia but are not commercially available in the United States include lisuride, terguride, metergoline, dihydroergocristine, and quinagolide.[86] Quinagolide is a D_2-receptor agonist, used frequently in Europe, that is dosed once daily. Quinagolide has been shown to be as effective as bromocriptine for the management of hyperprolactinemia and may also be effective in the treatment of patients who are resistant to or intolerant of bromocriptine.[86]

MONITORING

Prolactin serum concentrations should be monitored every 3 to 4 weeks after the initiation of any dopamine-agonist therapy to assess efficacy and appropriately titrate medication dosage.[77] In addition, symptoms such as headache, visual disturbances, menstrual cycles in women, and sexual function in men should be evaluated to assess clinical response to therapy. Once prolactin concentrations have normalized and clinical symptoms of hyperprolactinemia have resolved with dopamine-agonist therapy, prolactin serum concentrations should be monitored every 6 to 12 months. In patients receiving long-term treatment, the medication can be discontinued every 5 years to determine if remission has occurred.

PHARMACOECONOMIC CONSIDERATIONS

Medical therapy with dopamine agonists is more effective than transsphenoidal surgery or radiation for the management of hyperprolactinemia, and bromocriptine has been the mainstay of therapy. Because most patients receive therapy for long periods of time, the medical management of hyperprolactinemia may result in considerable costs. Although bromocriptine is most frequently used to manage hyperprolactinemia, therapy with pergolide, which has been shown to be equally effective, costs considerably less and offers the advantage of single-daily dosing. With the more recent approval of cabergoline, further cost comparisons must be made. The cost of cabergoline therapy is approximately two times greater than that of bromocriptine, and the costs associated with monitoring the response to therapy should be similar. However, cabergoline has been shown to be more effective than bromocriptine in at least one study and may offer additional advantages such as a decreased incidence of adverse effects and improved patient compliance. Pharmacoeconomic studies are needed to assess whether the higher cost of cabergoline therapy is balanced by the potential added benefits.

CONCLUSIONS

Hyperprolactinemia is a common disorder that can have a significant impact on fertility. Hyperprolactinemia is most commonly caused by the presence of prolactin-secreting pituitary tumors and various medications that antagonize dopamine or increase the secretion of prolactin. Available treatment options for this disorder include medical therapy with dopamine agonists, radiation therapy, and transsphenoidal surgery. In most cases, medical therapy with dopamine agonists is considered the most effective treatment, and bromocriptine has been the mainstay of therapy. Cabergoline, a new dopamine agonist, appears to be better tolerated than bromocriptine and is at least as effective as if not more effective than bromocriptine. Although additional studies are needed to confirm its benefits, cabergoline may soon replace bromocriptine as the mainstay of medical therapy.

PANHYPOPITUITARISM

Panhypopituitarism is a condition of complete or partial loss of anterior and posterior pituitary function resulting in a complex disorder characterized by multiple pituitary-hormone deficiencies. Patients with panhypopituitarism may have ACTH deficiency, gonadotropin deficiency, growth-hormone deficiency, hypothyroidism, and hyperprolactinemia. Panhypopituitarism can be classified as either primary or secondary depending on the etiology. Primary panhypopituitarism involves an abnormality within the secretory cells of the pituitary, whereas secondary panhypopituitarism is caused by a lack of proper external stimulation needed for normal release of pituitary hormones. Some of the most common causes of panhypopituitarism include primary pituitary tumors, ischemic necrosis of the pituitary, surgical trauma, irradiation, and various types of CNS infections. Pharmacologic treatment of panhypopituitarism is essential and consists of replacement of specific pituitary hormone after careful assessment of individual deficiencies. This is accomplished by administration of glucocorticoids, thyroid-hormone preparations, and sex steroids. The administration of recombinant growth hormone may be also considered in growing children and, more recently, for GH-deficient adults. Patients with panhypopituitarism will need life-long replacement therapy and constant monitoring of multiple homeostatic functions.

▶ PRINCIPLES OF PHARMACOTHERAPY

- Drug therapy should be considered for acromegalic patients in whom surgery and irradiation are contraindicated, when rapid control of symptoms is indicated, or when other treatments have failed to normalize GH concentrations. Dopamine agonists, such as bromocriptine, should be considered for all patients with acromegaly, prior to initiating therapy with a somatostatin analog, because of the potential cost advantages and convenience of oral administration.

- Octreotide (Sandostatin) suppresses mean serum GH concentrations to less than 5 μg/L and normalizes serum IGF-I concentrations in 50% to 60% of acromegalic patients. It halts tumor growth and is also effective in reducing the clinical signs and symptoms of acromegaly. The most common adverse effects of octreotide therapy include gastrointestinal disturbances such as diarrhea, nausea, abdominal cramps, malabsorption of fat, and flatulence, which occur in approximately 75% of patients and usually subside within 10 to 14 days of continued treatment.
- Octreotide inhibits cholecystokinin release and gallbladder motility, predisposing acromegalic patients to the development of cholelithiasis. The incidence of gallstones in acromegalic patients receiving octreotide increases with length of therapy and has been reported to range from 20% to 50%. However, most patients are asymptomatic, and the diagnosis of cholelithiasis is usually made following routine ultrasonographic evaluation that is not prompted by patient symptoms. The treatment of octreotide-induced gallstones is the same as that for gallstones in the general population, and prophylactic cholecystectomy or medical therapy with ursodeoxycholic acid is usually not warranted.
- Recombinant GH is currently considered the mainstay of therapy for the treatment of children with GHD short stature. Prompt diagnosis of GHD and initiation of replacement therapy with recombinant GH is crucial in optimizing the final adult heights of children with GHD. The use of GH therapy in patients with non-GHD short stature is controversial.
- Eight different recombinant growth hormone products are currently available in the United States. The potency of GH products is expressed as International Units per milligram (IU/mg) with 1 mg containing approximately 2.6 U of growth hormone. Although recommended dosages may vary, all GH products are generally considered to be equally efficacious.
- Sermorelin (Geref), a synthetic growth hormone–releasing hormone (GH-RH), was recently approved by the FDA for the treatment of idiopathic growth-hormone deficiency in children and has been shown to increase short-term growth velocity in children with idiopathic growth-hormone deficiency. Because normal pituitary function is needed for sermorelin to stimulate GH secretion, children should not receive GH-RH therapy with sermorelin unless the capacity to secrete GH is documented by provocative GH-stimulation testing.
- Pharmacologic agents that antagonize dopamine or increase the release of prolactin can induce hyperprolactinemia. Medications commonly reported to induce hyperprolactinemia include selective serotonin-reuptake inhibitors (SSRIs), phenothiazine derivatives, haloperidol (Haldol), metoclopramide (Reglan), domperidone, estrogens, progestins, verapamil (Calan, Isoptin, etc), methyldopa (Aldomet), reserpine, gonadotropin-releasing hormone analogs, H_2-receptor antagonists, benzodiazepines, tricyclic antidepressants, dexfenfluramine, opioids, and monoamine oxidase inhibitors. Discontinuation of the offending medication and initiation of an appropriate therapeutic alternative usually normalizes serum prolactin concentrations. In cases for which an appropriate therapeutic alternative does not exist, medical therapy with dopamine agonists may be warranted. Sex-steroid replacement may also be considered.
- Medical therapy with dopamine agonists is usually more effective than transsphenoidal surgery for the treatment of pituitary prolactinomas. Bromocriptine (Parlodel) has been the mainstay of medical therapy since the 1970s. However, up to 12% of patients do not tolerate the adverse effects associated with this medication. Pergolide (Permax), although not FDA approved for the treatment of hyperprolactinemia, has been used as a cost-effective alternative in patients who are intolerant of the adverse effects associated with bromocriptine.
- Cabergoline (Dostinex), a new long-acting dopamine agonist, may be more effective than bromocriptine for the medical management of prolactinomas and offers the advantage of once-weekly dosing. Cabergoline may also be effective in patients who are intolerant of or resistant to bromocriptine.
- Pharmacologic treatment of panhypopituitarism consists of replacement of specific pituitary hormones such as glucocorticoids, thyroid-hormone preparations, sex steroids, and recombinant growth hormone where appropriate. Patients with panhypopituitarism will need life-long replacement therapy and constant monitoring of multiple homeostatic functions.

REFERENCES

1. Raisman G. An urge to explain the imcomprehensible: Geoffrey Harris and the discovery of the neural control of the pituitary gland. Ann. Rev Neurosci 1997;20:533–566.
2. Cuttler L. The regulation of growth hormone secretion. Endocrinol Metab Clin North Am 1996;25:541–571.
3. Molitch ME. Pathologic hyperprolactinemia. Endocrinol Metab Clin North Am 1992;21:877–901.
4. D'Ercole AJ. Insulin-like growth factors and their receptors in growth. Endocrinol Metab Clin North Am 1996;25:573–590.
5. Acromegaly Therapy Consensus Development Panel. Consensus Statement: Benefits versus risks of medical therapy for acromegaly. Am J Med 1994;97:468–473.
6. Daughaday WH. Pituitary giantism. Endocrinol Metab Clin North Am 1992;21:633–647.
7. Molitch ME. Clinical manifestations of acromegaly. Endocrinol Metab Clin North Am 1992;21:597–614.
8. Melmed S. Etiology of pituitary acromegaly. Endocrinol Metab Clin North Am 1992;21:539–551.
9. Melmed S, Ho K, Klibanski A, et al. Recent advances in pathogenesis, diagnosis, and management of acromegaly. J Clin Endocrinol Metab 1995;80:3395–3402.

10. Melmed S. Unwanted effects of growth hormone excess in the adult. J Pediatr Endocrinol Metab 1996;9(suppl 3):369–374.
11. Ezzat S, Wilkins GE, Patel Y, et al. The diagnosis and management of acromegaly: A Canadian consensus report. Clin Invest Med 1996; 19:259–270.
12. Fahlbusch R, Honegger J, Buchfelder M. Acromegaly—The place of the neurosurgeon. Metabolism 1996;45:65–66.
13. Jaffe CA, Barkan AL. Treatment of acromegaly with dopamine agonists. Endocrinol Metab Clin North Am 1992;21:713–735.
14. Giustina A, Zaltieri G, Negrini F, Wehrenberg WB. The pharmacological aspects of the treatment of acromegaly. Pharmacol Res 1996; 34:247–268.
15. Jaffe CA, Barkan AL. Acromegaly recognition and treatment. Drugs 1994;47:425–445.
16. Colao A, Ferone D, Marzullo P, et al. Effect of different dopaminergic agents in the treatment of acromegaly. J Clin Endocrinol Metab 1997;82:518–523.
17. Lamberts S, Reubi JC, Krenning EP. Somatostatin analogs in the treatment of acromegaly. Endocrinol Metab Clin North Am 1992;21: 737–752.
18. Lamberts SE, Van der Lely A, de Herder WW, Hofland LJ. Drug therapy; octreotide. N Engl J Med 1996;334:246–254.
19. Vance ML, Harris AG. Long-term treatment of 189 acromegalic patients with the somatostatin analog octreotide. Results of the international mulicenter acromegaly study group. Arch Intern Med 1991; 151:1573–1578.
20. Ezzat S, Snyder PJ, Young WF, et al. Octreotide treatment of acromegaly: A randomized, multicenter study. Ann Intern Med 1992; 117:211–218.
21. Newman CB, Melmed S, Snyder PJ, et al. Safety and efficacy of long term octreotide therapy of acromegaly: Results of a multicenter trial in 103 patients—A clinical research center study. J Clin Endocrinol Metab 1995;80:2768–2775.
22. Merola B, Cittadini A, Colao A, et al. Chronic treatment with the somatostatin analog octreotide improves cardiac abnormalities in acromegaly. J Clin Endocrinol Metab 1993;77:790–793.
23. Padayatty SJ, Perrins EJ, Belchetz PE. Octreotide treatment increases exercise capacity in patients with acromegaly. Eur J Endocrinol 1996;134:554–559.
24. Giustina A, Boni E, Romanelli G. Cardiopulmonary performance during exercise in acromegaly, and the effects of acute suppression of growth hormone hypersecretion with octreotide. Am J Cardiol 1995;75:1042–1047.
25. Grunstein RR, Ho KKY, Sullivan CE. Effect of octreotide, a somatostatin analog, on sleep apnea in patients with acromegaly. Ann Intern Med 1994;121:478–483.
26. Thapar K, Kovacs KT, Stefaneanu L, et al. Antiproliferative effect of the somatostatin analogue octreotide on growth hormone-producing pituitary tumors: Results of a multicenter randomized trial. Mayo Clin Proc 1997;72:893–900.
27. Coloa A, Ferone D, Lastoria S, et al. Prediction of efficacy of octreotide therapy in patients with acromegaly. J Clin Endocrinol Metab 1996;81:2356–2362.
28. Harris AG, Kokoris SP, Ezzat S. Continuous versus intermittent subcutaneous infusion of octreotide in the treatment of acromegaly. J Clin Pharmacol 1995;35:59–71.
29. Anderson JV, Catnach S, Lowe DG, et al. Prevalence of gastritis in patients with acromegaly: Untreated and during treatment with octreotide. Clin Endocrinol 1992;37:227–232.
30. Eastman RC, Arakaki RF, Shawker T, et al. A prospective examination of octreotide-induced gall-bladder changes in acromegaly. Clin Endocrinol 1992;36:265–269.
31. Ewins DL, Javaid A, Coskeran PB, et al. Assessment of gall bladder dynamics, cholecystokinin release and the development of gallstones during octreotide therapy for acromegaly. Q J Med 1992;300:295–306.
32. Stolk MFJ, van Erpecum KJ, Koppeschaar HPF, et al. Effect of octreotide on fasting gall bladder emptying, antroduodenal motility, and motilin release in acromegaly. Gut 1995;36:755–760.
33. Ho KK, Jenkins AB, Furier SM, et al. Impact of octreotide, a long-acting somatostatin analogue, on glucose tolerance and insulin sensitivity in acromegaly. Clin Endocrinol 1992;36:271–279.
34. Sato K, Takamatsu K, Hashimoto K. Short-term effects of octreotide on glucose tolerance in patients with acromegaly. Endocr J 1995;42: 739–745.
35. Koop BL, Harris AG, Ezzat S. Effect of octreotide on glucose tolerance in acromegaly. Eur J Endocrinol 1994;130:581–586.
36. Flogstad AK, Halse J, Grass P, et al. A comparison of octreotide, bromocriptine, or a combination of both drugs in acromegaly. J Clin Endocrinol Metab 1994;79:461–465.
37. Gillis JC, Noble S, Goa KL. Octreotide long-acting release (LAR): A review of its pharmacological properties and therapeutic use in the management of acromegaly. Drugs 1997;53:681–699.
38. Weekes LM, Ho KK, Seale JP. Treatment options in acromegaly: Benefits and costs. Pharmacoeconomics 1996;10:453–459.
39. Hindmarsh PC, Brook CGD. Short stature and growth hormone deficiency. Clin Endocrinol 1995;43:133–142.
40. Audi L, Granada ML, Carrascosa A. Growth hormone secretion assessment in the diagnosis of short stature. J Pediatr Endocrinol Metab 1996;9:313–324.
41. Hintz R. Growth hormone treatment of idiopathic short stature. Horm Res 1996;46:208–214.
42. Grunt JA, Schwartz ID. Growth, short stature, and the use of growth hormone: Considerations for the practicing pediatrician. Curr Prob Pediatr 1992;22:390–412.
43. Lawson Wilkins Pediatric Endocrine Society Executive Committee. Guidelines for the use of growth hormone in children with short stature. A report by the drug and therapeutics committee of the Lawson Wilkins Pediatric Endocrine Society. J Pediatr 1995;127:857–867.
44. Marin G, Domene HM, Barnes KM, et al. The effects of estrogen priming and puberty on the growth hormone response to standardized treadmill exercise and arginine-insulin in normal girls and boys. J Clin Endocrinol Metab 1994;79:537–541.
45. Hintz R. Current and potential therapeutic uses of growth hormone and insulin-like growth factor-I. Endocrinol Metab Clin North Am 1996;25:759–773.
46. Fradkin JE, Schonberger LB, Mills JL, et al. Creutzfeldt–Jakob disease in pituitary growth hormone recipients in the United States. JAMA 1991;265:880–884.
47. Rikken B, Massa GG, Wit JM and the Dutch Growth Hormone Working Group. Final height in a large cohort of Dutch patients with growth hormone deficiency treated with growth hormone. Horm Res 1995;43:136–137.
48. Chipman JJ, Hicks JR, Holcombe JH, Draper MW. Approaching final height in children treated for growth hormone deficiency. Horm Res 1995;43:129–131.
49. Serveri F. Final height in children with growth hormone deficiency. Horm Res 1995;43:138–140.
50. Coste J, Letrait M, Carel JC, et al. Long term results of growth hormone treatment in France in children of short stature: Population, register based study. BMJ 1997;315:708–713.
51. Blethen SL, Bapitista J, Kuntze J, et al. Adult height in growth hormone (GH)-deficient children treated with biosynthetic GH. J Clin Endocrinol Metab 1997;82:418–420.
52. Jorgensen JO, Thuesen L, Muller J, et al. Three years of growth hormone treatment in growth hormone-deficient adults: Near normalization of body composition and physical performance. Eur J Endocrinol 1994;130:224–228.
53. Jorgensen JL, Pedersen SA, Thusen L, et al. Beneficial effects of growth hormone treatment in GH-deficient adults. Lancet 1989;1: 1221–1225.
54. Cuneo RC, Saloman F, Wilmshurst P, et al. Cardiovascular effects of growth hormone treatment in growth-hormone-deficient adults: Stimulation of the renin–aldosterone system. Clin Sci 1991;81:587–592.
55. McGauley GA, Cuneo RC, Salomon F. Psycho-social well-being before and after growth hormone treatment in adults with growth hormone deficiency. Horm Res 1990;33(suppl 4):52–54.

56. Moore WV, Moore KC, Gifford R, et al. Long-term treatment with growth hormone of children with short stature and normal growth hormone secretion. J Pediatr 1992;120:702–708.
57. Loche S, Cambiaso P, Setzu S, et al. Final height after growth hormone therapy in non-growth-hormone-deficient children with short stature. J Pediatr 1994;125:196–200.
58. Wit J, Boersma B, DeMuinch Keizer-Schrama SM, et al. Long-term results of growth hormone therapy in children with short stature, subnormal growth rate and normal growth hormone response to secretagogues. Clin Endocrinol 1995;42:365–372.
59. Schmitt K, Blumel P, Walkhor T, et al. Short- and long-term (final height) data in children with normal variant short stature treated with growth hormone. Eur J Pediatr 1997;156:680–683.
60. Cuttler L, Silvers JB, Singh J, et al. Short stature and growth hormone therapy; A national study of physician recommendation patterns. JAMA 1996;276:531–537.
61. Recombinant human growth hormone. Med Lett Drugs Ther 1992; 32:77–78.
62. Blethen SL, MacGillivray MH. A risk-benefit assessment of growth hormone use in children. Drug Saf 1997;17:303–316.
63. Cowell CT, Dietsch S. Adverse events during growth hormone therapy. J Pediatr Endocrinol Metab 1995;8:243–252.
64. Blethen SL, Allen DB, Graves D, et al. Safety of recombinant deoxyribonucleic acid-derived growth hormone; the National Cooperative Growth Study experience. J Clin Endocrinol Metab 1996;81: 1704–1710.
65. Wantanabe S, Tsunematsu Y, Fujimoto J, et al. Leukaemia in patients treated with growth hormone. Lancet 1988;1:1159–1160.
66. Stahnke N. Leukemia in growth-hormone-treated patients: An update. Horm Res 1992;38(suppl 1):56–62.
67. Rougeot C, Marchand P, Dray F, et al. Comparative study of biosynthetic human growth hormone immunogenicity in growth hormone deficient children. Horm Res 1991;35:76–81.
68. Pirazzoli P, Cacciari E, Mandini M, et al. Follow-up of antibodies to growth hormone in 210 growth hormone-deficient children treated with different commercial preparations. Acta Paediatr 1995;84: 1233–1236.
69. Grunt JA, Schwartz ID, Buchanan C, et al. Effects of long-term growth hormone releasing hormone 1-29 in significantly short children. Acta Paediatr 1995;85:631–633.
70. Thorner M, Rochiccioli P, Colle M, et al. Once daily subcutaneous growth hormone-releasing hormone accelerates growth in growth-hormone deficient children during the first year of therapy. J Clin Endocrinol Metab 1996;81:1189–1196.
71. Ogilvy-Stuart AL, Stirling HF, Kelnart CJH, et al. Treatment of radiation-induced growth hormone deficiency with growth hormone-releasing hormone. Clin Endocrinol 1997;46:571–578.
72. Deghenghi R. Examorelin. Drugs Future 1996;21:366–368.
73. Pihoker C, Badger TM, Reynolds GH, et al. Treatment effects of intranasal growth hormone releasing peptide-2 in children with short stature. J Endocrinol 1997;155:79–86.
74. Bellone J, Ghizzoni L, Aimaretti G. Growth hormone-releasing effect of oral growth hormone-releasing peptide 6 (GHRP-6) administration in children with short stature. Eur J Endocrinol 1995;133: 425–429.
75. American Academy of Pediatrics Committee on Drugs and Committee on Bioethics. Considerations related to the use of recombinant human growth hormone in children. Pediatrics 1997;99:122–129.
76. Kaye TB. Hyperprolactinemia. Causes, consequences, and treatment options. Postgrad Med 1996;99:265–268.
77. Yuen BH. Etiology and treatment of hyperprolactinemia. Semin Reprod Endocrinol 1992;10:228–235.
78. Jones TH. The management of hyperprolactinaemia. Br J Hosp Med 1995;53:374–378.
79. Sarapura V, Schlaff WD. Recent advances in the understanding of the pathophysiology and treatment of hyperprolactinemia. Curr Opin Obstet Gynecol 1993;5:360–367.
80. Davies PH. Drug-related hyperprolactinaemia. Adverse Drug React Toxicol Rev 1997;16:83–94.
81. Marken PA, Haykal RF, Fisher JN. Management of pychotropic-induced hyperprolactinemia. Clin Pharm 1992;11:851–856.
82. Cunnah D, Besser M. Management of prolactinomas. Clin Endocrinol 1991;34:231–235.
83. Thompson JA, Davies DL, McLaren EH, et al. Ten-year follow-up of microprolactinomas treated by transsphenoidal surgery. BMJ 1994; 309:1409–1410.
84. Dalkin AC, Marshal JC. Medical therapy of hyperprolactinemia. Endocrinol Metab Clin North Am 1989;18:259–276.
85. Bevan JS, Bebster J, Burke CW, et al. Dopamine agonists and pituitary tumor shrinkage. Endocr Rev 1992;13:220–220.
86. Webster J. A comparative review of the tolerability profiles of dopamine agonists in the treatment of hyperprolactinaemia and inhibition of lactation. Drug Saf 1996;14:228–238.
87. Weingrill CO, Portes E, Mussio W, et al. Long-acting oral bromocriptine (Parlodel SRO) in the treatment of hyperprolactinemia. Fertil Steril 1992;57:331–335.
88. Merola B, Colao A, Caruso E, et al. Oral and injectable long-lasting bromocriptine preparations in hyperprolactinemia: Comparison of their prolactin lowering activity, tolerability, and safety. Gynecol Endocrinol 1991;5:267–276.
89. Ciccarelli E, Grottoli S, Miola C, et al. Double blind randomized study using oral or injectable bromocriptine in patients with hyperprolactinaemia. Clin Endocrinol 1994;40:193–198.
90. Dash RJ, Ajmani AK, Sialy R. Prolactin (PRL) response to oral or vaginal bromoergocriptine in hyperprolactinemic women. Horm Metab Res 1994;26:164.
91. Lamberts SWJ, Quik RFP. A comparison of the efficacy and safety of pergolide and bromocriptine in the treatment of hyperprolactinemia. J Clin Endocrinol Metab 1991;72:635–641.
92. Berezin M, Avidan D, Baron E. Long-term pergolide treatment of hyperprolactinemic patients previously unsuccessfully treated with dopaminergic drugs. Isr J Med Sci 1991;27:375–379.
93. Ferrari C, Paracchi A, Mattei AM, et al. Cabergoline in the long-term therapy of hyperprolactinemic disorders. Acta Endocrinol 1992;126: 489–494.
94. Webster J, Piscitelli G, Polli A, et al. Dose-dependent suppression of serum prolactin by cabergoline in hyperprolactinaemia: A placebo controlled, double blind, multicentre study. Clin Endocrinol 1992;73: 534–541.
95. Webster J, Piscitelli G, Polli A, et al. The efficacy and tolerability of long-term cabergoline therapy in hyperprolactinaemic disorders: An open, uncontrolled multicentre study. Clin Endocrinol 1993;39: 323–329.
96. Ferrari CI, Abs R, Bevan JS, et al. Treatment of macroprolactinoma with cabergoline: A study of 85 patients. Clin Endocrinol 1997;46: 409–413.
97. Webster J, Piscitelli G, Polli A, et al. A comparison of cabergoline and bromocriptine in the treatment of hyperprolactinemic amenorrhea. N Engl J Med 1994;331:904–909.
98. Delgrange E, Maiater D, Donckier J. Effects of the dopamine agonist cabergoline in patients with prolactinoma intolerant or resistant to bromocriptine. Eur J Endocrinol 1996;134:454–456.
99. Rains CP, Bryson HM, Fitton A. Cabergoline: A review of its pharmacological properties and therapeutic potential in the treatment of hyperprolactinaemia and inhibition of lactation. Drugs 1995;49:255–279.
100. Motta T, Colombo N, DeVincentiis S, et al. Vaginal cabergoline in the treatment of hyperprolactinemic patients intolerant to oral dopaminergics. Fertil Steril 1996;65:440–442.

74

PREGNANCY AND LACTATION: THERAPEUTIC CONSIDERATIONS

Janet McCombs, PharmD, and Margaret K. Cramer, MD, FACOG

Pregnancy is a normal, natural life event through which most women progress with minimal problems. Although modern medicine and advanced technology have reduced obstetric risks and decreased complications, new problems such as the teratogenicity of medications have emerged. Since the thalidomide tragedy in 1956 and, more recently, the problems associated with diethylstilbestrol use, medical practitioners are more cautious about recommending medications for pregnant patients.

Although very little information is available about drug effects on the fetus, many women ingest both prescription and nonprescription medications during pregnancy. Although it would be ideal to avoid all drugs, the health and well-being of the mother must also be considered. The patient may have an acute or chronic medical problem that requires medication. A mother who is uncomfortable and ill for the duration of her pregnancy is less likely to approach delivery and the newborn with a positive attitude. Some pregnant patients may take medication before realizing that they are pregnant or before consulting a physician. Some patients erroneously assume that because nonprescription medications are widely available, they are safe to take during pregnancy.

DIAGNOSIS

Amenorrhea is usually the first sign of pregnancy; however, some women may experience other symptoms of pregnancy before they miss their first menstrual period. These symptoms include morning nausea and vomiting (morning sickness), frequent urination, and tender breasts with enlargement and increased pigmentation of the nipple and areola. Pregnancy may be confirmed by the presence of human chorionic gonadotropin (HCG) in serum or urine. Some assays used in professional laboratories are sensitive enough to detect the presence of HCG within 7 to 9 days after fertilization. HCG is produced by the placenta very early in pregnancy and the concentration doubles approximately every 2 to 3 days and peaks between 8 and 12 weeks in a normal pregnancy. HCG is comprised of α and β subunits; the α subunit is identical to the α subunit of luteinizing hormone (LH), thyroid-stimulating hormone (TSH), and follicle-stimulating hormone (FSH). In some of the earlier diagnostic tests, cross-reactivity with these hormones occasionally produced a false-positive result. The β subunit is unique to HCG, and the newer pregnancy tests specifically detect the β subunit. Serum tests such as radioimmunoassay (RIA) and enzyme-linked immunosorbent assay (ELISA) can detect concentrations of HCG as low as 5 mIU/mL (present about 6 to 10 days after implantation).[1] This is especially useful when a pregnancy loss is suspected, because HCG levels will begin to fall, rather than increase. Urine tests using monoclonal antibodies can usually detect concentrations of HCG in the 20 to 40 mIU/mL range (1 to 2 weeks after fertilization). Ectopic pregnancies (those in which the embryo implants outside the endometrial cavity) may not produce enough HCG to be detected by urine tests, and a negative urine test should not eliminate the possibility of pregnancy. Quantitative serum assays for HCG should be used in the diagnosis of ectopic pregnancies or suspected pregnancy loss. The current home pregnancy tests using monoclonal antibodies are sensitive and specific and are 97% accurate when used correctly.[2] False negatives occur about 25% of the time with the home testing products, usually due to errors in performing the test, but false positives occur less than 3% of the time.[2] The home tests fail to detect 50% of ectopic pregnancies, and women who get a negative result should be counseled about this possibility and the fact that many ectopic pregnancies rupture and require emergency surgery. A patient who has a negative result and still believes she is pregnant should be encouraged to see a physician; otherwise, she should repeat the test in 7 days if menses have not begun. A second negative result should prompt the patient to make an appointment with her physician for further evaluation.

NORMAL PREGNANCY

The normal duration of human gestation is 267 days from conception or 280 days from the first day of the last menstrual period, usually spanning 40 weeks. There are charts and "wheels" available to aid the practitioner in determining the expected date of confinement (EDC) or "due date," but Nagele's rule, a mathematical method, also provides a reasonable estimate of the delivery date. To apply Nagele's rule, take the date of the first day of the last menstrual period, subtract 3 months, and add 7 days.[2] (Example: June 20 − 3 months = March 20 + 7 days = March 27.) These methods are usually correct to within 2 weeks of delivery and work best in patients who have regular 28-day cycles. Most EDCs are now confirmed by ultrasound.

Gestational age is the number of completed weeks of pregnancy since the first day of the last menstrual period. The conceptus is referred to as an embryo for the first 8 weeks and thereafter as a *fetus.* The *gravidity* of a female patient is the total number of pregnancies including ectopic, premature, spontaneous or induced terminations, and normal pregnancies. A *gravid* patient is pregnant; a *primigravida* is pregnant for the first time, and a *nulligravida* has never been pregnant. The *parity* of a patient refers to the number of deliveries after the twentieth week of gestation. *Parity* may be further defined for an individual patient by a series of four numbers. In order, these numbers indicate the number of term deliveries, number of premature deliveries, number of aborted and/or ectopic pregnancies, and the number of living children. Deliveries involving multiple births add only one parous experience to the mother's obstetric history. For example, G_3P_{1112}, is a woman who has had three pregnancies—one full-term baby, one preterm delivery, one miscarriage or abortion—and has two living children. A woman who has had one full-term delivery, one preterm delivery of twins, no miscarriages or abortions, and has three living children is a G_2P_{1103}.

During pregnancy, it is common to give a multivitamin supplement, although this may not be necessary in a patient consuming a well-balanced diet. Many pregnant patients may require supplemental iron, and most prescription prenatal vitamins contain at least 60 mg of elemental iron. Adequate calcium intake is necessary for normal growth of fetal bones and teeth; therefore, pregnant women should consume at least 1.2 g of elemental calcium daily, either from their diet or through supplementation.

The Committee on Genetics of the American Academy of Pediatrics currently recommends that all women of childbearing age who are capable of becoming pregnant take at least 0.4 mg of folic acid daily to reduce the incidence of neural tube defects.[3] Studies indicate that maximal benefit is received when women receive supplemental folic acid at least 1 month prior to conception and through the first trimester. Most multivitamin products that are available over the counter contain 0.4 mg of folic acid; nonprescription prenatal vitamins usually contain 0.8 mg of folic acid; and prescription prenatal vitamins contain 1 mg of folic acid. No patient, whether pregnant or not, should take more than 0.8 mg of folic acid daily without physician supervision. Women who have had an infant with a neural tube defect are at higher risk and should receive prenatal counseling and testing in addition to larger doses of folic acid; sometimes a dose as high as 4 mg/d is recommended.[4] Folic acid in large doses may also be prescribed for women whose mother or sister delivered a child with a neural tube defect.

DRUG EFFECTS ON THE FETUS

Any medication administered to a pregnant patient may affect the fetus directly or indirectly. Drugs and environmental agents that have the potential to cause abnormal fetal growth and development are called teratogens. Teratogenicity is the capability to produce congenital abnormalities. These may be major or minor malformations or functional abnormalities.[5] Major structural abnormalities (defects incompatible with life or requiring major surgery for correction) occur in about 2% to 4% of births in the United States. If minor malformations, such as ear tags or extra digits, are included, the incidence increases to as much as 10%. Approximately 10% of children have abnormal physical or mental development. About 25% of abnormalities are caused by genetic predisposition, 2% to 3% are drug induced, and the cause is unknown in the remainder of cases. Although the number of infants with defects due to drug exposure is relatively small, it is important to avoid as many defects as possible. The use of any drug, prescription or nonprescription, should be avoided during pregnancy unless its use is absolutely necessary.

Ethically, studies to ascertain outcomes of drug exposure cannot be performed in pregnant women, and unfortunately, outcomes in animal studies do not always correlate with human fetal risk. A prime example is thalidomide, a sedative marketed in Europe that was very close to being approved in the United States when its teratogenic potential was recognized. Thalidomide is extremely teratogenic in humans; up to one-third of all infants exposed in utero to thalidomide developed abnormalities. Standard animal studies had failed to demonstrate this risk. There is no good method of predicting or determining the safety of a particular drug given during pregnancy. Most reports of teratogenicity are case reports following the birth of a child exposed to a particular medication.

Factors that influence the teratogenicity of a drug include the genotypes of the mother and fetus, the embryonic stage at exposure, the dose, the specificity of the agent, and the simultaneous exposure to other drugs or environmental agents that may increase or decrease potential abnormalities.[5] Teratogens may cause spontaneous abortion, congenital abnormalities, intrauterine growth retardation (IUGR), mental retardation, carcinogenesis, and mutations.

Timing of exposure to medication is of the utmost importance when considering the teratogenic risk. Exposure around the time of conception and implantation may kill the embryo, and the patient may never realize that she was pregnant. If the exposure occurs in the first 12 to 15 days after conception when the cells are still totipotential, meaning that if one cell is damaged or killed, another can assume its function, the embryo may not be damaged.[5] It has long been known that the first 3 months of pregnancy are the most critical in terms of physical malformations.[6] More recently, functional and behavioral defects have been associated with exposure to drugs or other environmental factors later in gestation. This may be explained by the fact that the central nervous system including the brain continues developing and growing throughout pregnancy.[7] Functional defects are more difficult to recognize and diagnose, and it is more difficult to establish cause and effect. It should also be remembered that long-term effects of medication may not be recognized for many years. For example, the carcinogenic potential of diethylstilbestrol (DES) in exposed daughters did not become evident until after puberty.

PLACENTAL TRANSPORT

The amount of drug reaching the fetus depends on many factors, which may vary among patients and which depend on the stage of gestation. In the past, the placenta was mistakenly considered a barrier; however, the placenta does not protect the fetus from the effects of all drugs. Drugs with molecular weights less than 400 daltons cross the placenta more readily than do highly un-ionized and lipophilic drugs. Since most drugs have molecular weights between 250 and 400 daltons, they have potential to cross the placenta and enter the fetal circulation. Other factors that influence the placental transfer of drugs include the degree of protein binding, maternal and fetal blood flow, the area available for exchange, and the metabolic activity of the placenta. Most drugs cross the placenta by simple diffusion. Because simple diffusion depends on the concentration gradient, fetal serum concentrations usually equal maternal levels. However, the extent to which drugs cross the placenta varies, and many drugs reach concentrations in the fetus at 50% to over 100% of maternal blood levels. The total concentration of blood proteins is lower in the fetus than in the mother, often resulting in an increased free drug concentration, especially for drugs that are highly bound in maternal blood. Excretion of medications by the fetus occurs primarily via the fetal liver and the placenta. Clearance may be much slower in the fetus than in healthy adults.

Late in pregnancy, effects of medications on labor and delivery should also be considered. For example, salicylate use late in gestation can cause increased bleeding at delivery or even delay the onset of labor by decreasing prostaglandins. Very near delivery, the effect of a medication on the neonate must be considered because any medication present in the infant at delivery must be metabolized and excreted by the newborn. Because these functions are generally slower in neonates, prolonged exposure and toxicity may result.

Drugs are placed in categories that describe the potential risk in pregnancy based on available animal and human studies. The Food and Drug Administration (FDA) published definitions for pregnancy risk categories in 1979[8] (Table 74–1). Unfortunately, only drugs marketed after December 1983 are required to have an assigned pregnancy risk category; thus, most drugs currently available do not have risk categories assigned by the manufacturer. Practitioners who need to assess teratogenic risk for particular medications are referred to the primary literature and selected reference texts.[2,6,9]

TABLE 74–1. FDA Categories for Drug Use in Pregnancy

Category A—Controlled studies in women fail to demonstrate a risk to the fetus in the first trimester, and the possibility of fetal harm appears remote.

Category B—Either animal studies do not indicate a risk to the fetus and there are no controlled studies in pregnant women, or animal studies have indicated fetal risk, but controlled studies in pregnant women failed to demonstrate a risk.

Category C—Either animal studies indicate a fetal risk and there are no controlled studies in women, or there are no available studies in women or animals.

Category D—There is positive evidence of fetal risk, but there may be certain situations where the benefit might outweigh the risk (life-threatening or serious diseases where other drugs are ineffective or carry a greater risk).

Category X—There is definite fetal risk based on studies in animals or humans or based on human experience, and the risk clearly outweighs any benefit in pregnant women.

From Ref. 8.

Although there is a great deal of concern about the risks associated with medication use during pregnancy, drugs are a welcome addition to managing the obstetric patient with chronic medical disorders. An example is the use of insulin in diabetic patients. In the past, many diabetic patients had virtually no chance of a successful pregnancy without complications, but today with close monitoring and control of blood glucose levels and appropriate use of insulin, these patients have a much improved pregnancy outcome.

Pregnancy is a time for nurturing the developing fetus, but it is also a time of great physical change for the mother. These changes may cause symptoms in the pregnant patient that lead to use of more medications than prior to pregnancy. All patients who are considering pregnancy or have a confirmed pregnancy should be advised about the risks associated with use of any medication during pregnancy. Often a patient has already taken a medication before she seeks professional advice about the teratogenic risk. In this situation, it is important to accurately determine the drug, dose, route of administration, exact gestational age at the time of exposure, length of exposure, and any other drugs taken concurrently. Information about the patient's general health, previous obstetric history, and family history may be useful in assessing the possible risk. The physician can be helpful in providing information and offering an opinion as to the possible risk. If the risk of severe deformity is extremely high, it may be appropriate to offer the option of termination; but, ultimately, the decision to terminate or to continue the pregnancy should be made by the patient.

Before any drug is prescribed during pregnancy, several factors should be considered. First, the risk to benefit ratio must be evaluated. The practitioner must be confident that the selected drug is indicated and is the most effective with the least risk of teratogenicity. To make this determination, appropriate references should be consulted to ascertain whether or not there are any reports of abnormalities and the nature of possible problems. Once the decision has been made to use medication, the lowest effective dose should be prescribed for the shortest possible duration.

Every parent desires and expects a normal, healthy baby with normal physical and mental development. The birth of a child with an abnormality is a personal tragedy for the parents and the medical professionals caring for the family. In searching for a reason, the mother often tries to recall any medication taken during pregnancy. As discussed previously, medications are probably implicated in a very few cases, but for legal reasons, all medications prescribed or recommended for a pregnant patient should be carefully documented in the patient's medical record.

SPECIFIC AGENTS

Several classes of drugs and their effects on the fetus will be discussed in other sections of this chapter. This section will discuss other potentially teratogenic medications. Because this is not an all inclusive list, the reader is referred to the primary literature and other reference resources about drug use in pregnancy.

BENZODIAZEPINES

These drugs cross the placenta and are associated with congenital malformations. The incidence of malformations is greater when exposure occurs during the first trimester. The benzodiazepine most often implicated is diazepam, which has been associated with facial clefts. Large studies both refute and confirm the teratogenicity of benzodiazepines.[2] The floppy infant syndrome, neonatal central nervous system (CNS) depression, and withdrawal symptoms may occur following chronic benzodiazepine use during the last trimester and when large doses are administered shortly before delivery.[9]

LITHIUM

Infants exposed to lithium during the first trimester of pregnancy have an increased risk of developing abnormalities, 75% of which are cardiovascular. Ebstein's anomaly, a rare heart defect, is the most common.[5] When lithium is administered late in pregnancy, manifestations of neonatal toxicity include cyanosis, hypotonia, bradycardia, and electrocardiographic abnormalities. These toxic effects usually reverse as the lithium is excreted by the newborn.[5]

SEX HORMONES

Estrogens, progestogens, and androgens are associated with congenital abnormalities. Progestogens and androgens, including danazol, are associated with masculinization of the female fetus. Other abnormalities found in female infants exposed in utero to progestogens or androgenic agents include ambiguous genitalia, clitoral hypertrophy, and labial fusion.[2] Progestogens, primarily those present in oral contraceptives, may produce the VACTERL syndrome: vertebral, anal, cardiovascular, tracheal, esophageal, renal, and limb defects. Recent studies indicate only a 0.07% risk of the VACTERL syndrome in a fetus exposed to these agents.[6] It is more likely that these agents would cause abnormal reproductive organ development. DES causes a number of reproductive tract abnormalities in both female and male infants exposed in utero.[5] Vaginal clear cell adenocarcinoma is the most common problem seen in offspring of mothers who took DES while pregnant. Estrogens and progestogens are contraindicated in pregnancy owing to reports of congenital abnormalities.

ISOTRETINOIN

Isotretinoin, a vitamin A isomer, is a potent human teratogen. Indicated only for the treatment of severe cystic acne, the drug should never be used during pregnancy. Recognized as a teratogen before marketing, the manufacturer issued warnings about its use in pregnant women or in women who might become pregnant while taking isotretinoin. Women of childbearing age should have a negative pregnancy test before initiating treatment and must use at least two reliable methods of contraception during the course of therapy and for 1 month after the last dose. Major malformations reported with isotretinoin include craniofacial, CNS, and cardiac defects.

ANTINEOPLASTIC AGENTS

All the drugs in this class, except cyclosporin A,[10] have teratogenic potential in animals. Fortunately, the occurrence of anomalies in exposed infants is less than that reported in animals. The highest rate of malformations occurs with first-trimester exposure. Since most treatment regimens for neoplasms include several drugs, it is difficult to ascertain cause and effect for individual agents. Reports of teratogenicity from neoplastic medications are limited, probably owing to a high rate of elective and spontaneous abortions during treatment. Because these drugs are designed to kill rapidly proliferating malignant cells, it is logical to assume that the rapidly growing fetus might be subject to the same effect.

Handling of chemotherapeutic agents by those health care professionals in the reproductive age group should be done with caution to minimize direct contact with these drugs.

ANTIBIOTICS

Teratogenicity of the tetracyclines first became recognized in the early 1960s.[6] All members of the class—tetracycline HCl, demeclocycline, minocycline, doxycycline—have been reported to cause congenital abnormalities, particularly, staining of the teeth and retardation of the developing skeletal system. Other miscellaneous congenital malformations have also been reported, and some cases of maternal liver toxicity have been mentioned.

Fluoroquinolones were tested in animals prior to marketing and were shown to cause erosion of the cartilage and other arthropathies in fetuses and immature offspring exposed to the medication. Thus, fluoroquinolones should not be used during pregnancy.

TABLE 74–2. Medications Known to be Teratogens

Alcohol	Isotretinoin
Androgens	Lithium
Anticonvulsants	Live vaccines
Antineoplastics	Methimazole
Cocaine	Penicillamine
Diethylstilbestrol	Tetracyclines
Etretinate	Warfarin
Iodides (including radioactive iodine)	

TABLE 74–3. Medications Suspected to be Teratogens

ACE inhibitors	Estrogens	Progestogens
Benzodiazepines	Oral hypoglycemic agents	Quinolones

TABLE 74–4. Medications With No Known Teratogenic Effects[a]

Acetaminophen	Erythromycin	Phenothiazines
Cephalosporins	Multiple vitamins	Thyroid hormones
Corticosteroids	Narcotic analgesics	Tricyclic antidepressants
Docusate sodium	Penicillins	

[a]No drug is absolutely without risk during pregnancy. These drugs appear to have a minimal risk when used judiciously in usual doses under clinical supervision.

TABLE 74–5. Medications With Nonteratogenic Adverse Effects in Pregnancy

Antithyroid drugs	Diuretics
Aminoglycosides	Isoniazid
Aspirin	Narcotic analgesics (chronic use)
Barbiturates (chronic use)	Nicotine
Benzodiazepines	Nonsteroidal anti-inflammtory agents
β-Blockers	Oral hypoglycemic agents
Caffeine	Prophylthiouracil
Chloramphenicol	Sulfonamides
Cocaine	

SUMMARY

Selecting medications for use during pregnancy and understanding their effects on the fetus is at best an inexact science. No drug is absolutely safe and no drug produces abnormalities in all exposed infants. Drugs with known, suspected, and no known teratogenic effect are listed in Tables 74–2, 74–3, 74–4, and 74–5. Every patient must be treated individually. Possible risks and benefits should be carefully weighed before the patient and her physician make a decision to use medication during pregnancy.

▶ TREATMENT: Conditions Caused or Exacerbated by Pregnancy

Physiologic and functional changes during pregnancy may cause exacerbation or development of medical problems commonly diagnosed in the general population. Pregnancy and concern for the fetus may dictate management of these disorders in a manner different from that used in the nonpregnant patient.

NAUSEA AND VOMITING

The nausea and vomiting associated with pregnancy are usually mild and are commonly referred to as *morning sickness.* About half of all pregnant patients experience some degree of nausea and vomiting during the first trimester of pregnancy. The symptoms usually begin within a few weeks after conception and continue through weeks 12 to 14 of gestation. Nausea usually occurs upon arising and diminishes as the day progresses. Some women, however, experience nausea throughout the day, and in some patients it persists until delivery.

Hyperemesis gravidarum is severe nausea and vomiting that cannot be controlled and may result in dehydration and malnutrition. It can progress to a life-threatening problem requiring immediate therapy. Left untreated, maternal neurologic, renal, retinal, and hepatic damage may occur and are similar to changes observed in starvation. These patients should be hospitalized and treated with intravenous fluids, electrolytes, antiemetics, and sedatives. In severe cases, peripheral or central parenteral nutrition may be useful. Total parenteral nutrition has been shown to be effective in providing the mother and fetus with adequate nutrition, as evidenced by normal birth weight and lack of adverse effects.[11] Enteral feeding has been used successfully by some investigators; however, possible complications include risk of aspiration, less absorptive capacity of the gut, nausea, and vomiting.[12]

The cause of nausea and vomiting in pregnancy is unknown. Proposed etiologies include increased levels of hormones during pregnancy and emotional or psychological factors. Because the etiology has not been found, treatment is directed at symptoms. A patient who experiences only early morning nausea may be advised to eat two or three soda crackers upon awakening, then to wait 15 to 20 minutes before arising. Often, keeping the stomach from becoming completely empty will also help alleviate the nausea. Dietary suggestions include small, dry meals high in carbohydrates, with avoidance of spicy foods and foods with noxious odors.

Medication must be considered for patients whose vomiting persists despite dietary alterations. Although teratogenic risk cannot be ruled out for any drug, the risk involved with the antiemetic agents currently used for nausea and vomiting in pregnancy seems to be minimal.[13] Medications used most often include the phenothiazines, meclizine, cyclizine, dimenhydrinate, doxylamine, and pyridoxine. Bendectin® (Merrell-Dow; doxylamine 10 mg, pyridoxine 10 mg) was the most widely used agent for morning sickness until its withdrawal from the market by the manufacturer in 1983. Despite lack of evidence associating Bendectin® with birth defects, damaging publicity and decreasing patient confidence prompted the decision to stop manufacture of the medication. This tablet had a special coating that delayed activity, making a bedtime dose effective during the morning hours.

Antihistamines and phenothiazines have been used often to treat nausea and vomiting during pregnancy without any evidence of association with teratogenic effects.[14] When considering the use of medications for nausea and vomiting during pregnancy, the possible effects of malnutrition, dehydration, and electrolyte status of the mother as well as her general health must be considered. Ondansetron, a medication used to treat nausea and vomiting associated with cancer chemotherapy, has recently been given to women who are experiencing nausea and vomiting of pregnancy. It is a manufacturer's assigned category B drug, it is effective clinically, and it does not seem to have any harmful effects on the mother or the fetus.[15]

HEARTBURN

Many patients experience heartburn during the latter half of pregnancy. This probably results from relaxation of the esophageal sphincter and increased pressure on the stomach caused by the enlarging uterus, allowing regurgitation of the stomach contents into the lower esophagus. Relaxation of the lower esophageal sphincter is probably caused by a combination of mechanical and intrinsic factors. Dietary management of heartburn should be attempted before medication. Smaller, more frequent meals often help to alleviate the symptoms. Some women find that avoiding food and liquids other than water for at least 3 hours before bedtime and elevating the head of the bed with blocks helps to relieve discomfort that is exacerbated by reclining.

Antacids may be used judiciously in patients who do not respond to dietary alterations. Magnesium and/or aluminum hydroxides are usually effective for relieving the pain, and their duration of action is several hours. Calcium carbonate may be used, but as with sodium bicarbonate, the duration of action is very short. Other problems with sodium bicarbonate include rebound symptoms and metabolic alkalosis with chronic use.

Sucralfate is poorly absorbed by the gastrointestinal tract and has been suggested as a reasonable alternative for heartburn in pregnancy. Although it is an aluminum salt and aluminum has been associated with neurobehavioral and skeletal toxicity in animals, there is no evidence that aluminum is absorbed from the gastrointestinal tract, and there have been no reports of associated congenital defects.[6,14]

CONSTIPATION

Constipation is a common problem in pregnancy and is most likely a result of decreased peristalsis. Patients experiencing constipation should be encouraged to add bulky, high-fiber foods to their diet and increase their fluid intake to at least eight 8-oz glasses of water daily. Moderate exercise, such as walking, is also helpful for most patients.

Surfactants and bulk laxatives are the agents of choice in the pregnant patient. Bulk laxatives are not absorbed and thus pose the least threat to the fetus. Adequate fluid intake (at least 16 oz) with each dose should be emphasized to prevent possible bowel obstruction with the fiber laxatives. Mineral oil in any dosage form should be avoided because there is a possibility of impairment of vitamin K absorption, which could decrease vitamin K availability to the fetus and result in hypoprothrombinemia.

HEMORRHOIDS

Hemorrhoids often develop or worsen during pregnancy because of constipation and increased venous pressure below the uterus. Correction of constipation, use of stool softeners, and taking sitz baths are usually helpful in reducing the discomfort from hemorrhoids. External medications are preferred over those inserted into the rectum because many drugs are well absorbed from the rectal mucosa. Products containing topical anesthetics and steroids should be avoided during pregnancy except under the supervision of a physician (with a prescription). These medications can be systemically absorbed with consequent effects on the fetus.

COAGULATION DISORDERS

Thromboembolic phenomena are uncommon during pregnancy, but anticoagulation is necessary when a patient has a history of deep vein thrombosis, a prosthetic heart valve, deficiencies of certain clotting factors, or antiphospholipid antibodies. Warfarin should be avoided in pregnancy because about 30% of pregnancies exposed to warfarin result in fetal malformations, developmental deficiencies, stillbirths, or hemorrhage.[2] Another danger of use of oral anticoagulants during pregnancy is the risk of bleeding in the mother or fetus if delivery occurs while the mother is taking the medications.

Subcutaneous heparin and low-molecular-weight heparin (LMWH) are the anticoagulants of choice for chronic use during pregnancy because the large molecular weight of heparin prevents it from crossing the placenta.[16,17] They are also preferred because the effect of anticoagulation produced by heparin and LMWH can be reversed by protamine sulfate. This is especially important because the onset of labor and the necessity for an operative delivery are not always predictable There are no reports of congenital malformations associated with heparin or LMWH.[2] Most of the fetal risks associated with heparin and LMWH are indirect, such as maternal hemorrhage, or from the underlying disease requiring anticoagulation. Although heparin appears to be a safe anticoagulant for the mother and fetus, the risk of osteoporosis in the mother must be considered. Osteoporosis occurs as a result of interference with vitamin D metabolism and is dose related.[18] It may or may not be reversible. Heparin-induced thrombocytopenia is another complication sometimes encountered in pregnancy.

Reproductive-age females requiring long-term anticoagulation with oral agents should be counseled about the risks of pregnancy and provided with effective contraception. Conversion from oral anticoagulants to subcutaneous heparin or LMWH should be considered for those patients planning pregnancy. LMWH has several advantages over heparin. It causes less thrombocytopenia, requires only once-daily dosing, has a decreased risk of osteoporosis, and does not require any monitoring. It is, however, more expensive. Ambulatory patients should be capable of self-administering either medication subcutaneously and compliant with appointments for follow-up monitoring.

▶ TREATMENT: Pregnancy-Specific Conditions

PREGNANCY-INDUCED HYPERTENSION

Pregnancy-induced hypertension can be a serious and life-threatening obstetric complication. Gestational hypertension is diagnosed when the blood pressure exceeds 140/90 mm Hg in the absence of proteinuria or pathologic edema. Preeclampsia is divided into mild and severe forms. Mild preeclampsia is hypertension accompanied by proteinuria (≥ 300 mg/24 h or 100 mg/dL in two random samples 6 hours apart) and/or pathologic edema. Preeclampsia is considered severe when proteinuria exceeds 4 g/24 h or persistent dipstick values of 2+, blood pressure is 160/110 mm Hg, or severe headache, visual disturbances, or epigastric pain is noted. Eclampsia is the development of generalized tonic–clonic seizures in a patient with pregnancy-induced hypertension. Pregnancy-aggravated hypertension is diagnosed in a patient with preexisting essential hypertension who experiences a 15 mm Hg increase in her diastolic or 30 mm Hg increase in systolic blood pressure after week 24 of gestation. If pathologic edema or proteinuria develop, the patient has superimposed preeclampsia.

The incidence of preeclampsia in the United States is 5% to 8%.[2] Hypertensive disorders induced by pregnancy are diagnosed after week 20 of gestation but can also occur postpartum and in the presence of trophoblastic disease. Of patients diagnosed with the disorder, 85% are primiparas, particularly those who are very young or at the upper end of the reproductive age group.[19] Other risk factors include essential hypertension, diabetes, family history of preeclampsia, multiple fetuses, and molar pregnancies.

Although the specific causes of preeclampsia are still unknown, three mechanisms seem to be involved in the development of this disorder. First, increased vasospasm with increased vascular resistance and increased sensitivity to angiotensin II is noted in preeclamptic patients. Second, preeclampsia occurs after 20 weeks of pregnancy, suggesting possible immunologic reaction to pregnancy. Third, the five-fold increase in prostacyclin production seen in normal pregnancies is decreased in preeclamptic patients, thus producing a relative increase in the thromboxane A_2 to prostacyclin ratio and explaining the vasoconstriction, increased platelet aggregation, and decreased uteroplacental blood flow seen in preeclamptic patients. The only cure for preeclampsia/eclampsia is termination of the pregnancy.

Prevention of preeclampsia with low-dose aspirin has been suggested for patients at high risk for development of this disorder. If an imbalance of prostaglandins is a causative factor in this condition, then perhaps prophylactic aspirin would be useful in some women. Low-dose aspirin has been shown to decrease thromboxane A_2 synthesis to a greater degree than the decrease in prostacyclin synthesis,[20,21] theoretically normalizing the ratio of prostacyclin and thromboxane A_2. The dose of aspirin used in most studies is 60 mg/d beginning in week 24 to 28 of gestation and continued until the onset of labor.[21,22] The usefulness of low-dose aspirin in preventing preeclampsia has now been verified in several studies,[21–23] but further investigation is needed to determine which patients are at the highest risk for preeclampsia and might benefit from the prophylaxis. Although there have been no adverse effects noted in infants or mothers exposed to low-dose aspirin during pregnancy,[23] pregnancies at low risk for development of preeclampsia should not be exposed unnecessarily. Low-dose aspirin has not been shown to be useful in the treatment of existing preeclampsia/eclampsia.

Treatment for preeclampsia consists of delivery if the pregnancy is at term. If not at term, the treatment is bedrest with frequent monitoring of blood pressure, urine protein, serum chemistries, and platelets. This may be accomplished at home or in the hospital depending on the severity of the disease, patient compliance, and response to treatment. Antihypertensive medications have not been shown to be useful in prolonging gestation in pregnancies complicated by pregnancy-induced hypertensive conditions.[2]

Severely preeclamptic women must be hospitalized, begun on a regimen of parenteral magnesium sulfate to prevent seizures, and delivered. Several different methods for the administration of magnesium sulfate in preeclamptic patients have been described.[2,19] Both IM and IV routes of administration are effective in achieving adequate serum concentrations, and both have advantages and disadvantages in the treatment of the preeclamptic/eclamptic patient. IV administration may be preferred because magnesium carries risk of toxicity, and an IV infusion may be quickly discontinued and the magnesium more quickly excreted if toxicity does occur. IV administration is initiated with a loading dose of 4 g and followed with an infusion of 1 to 3 g/h. The infusion must be delivered via a reliable controlled-infusion pump. Another regimen begins with a 4-g IV loading dose with simultaneous intramuscular injection of 10 g (5 g in each buttock) followed by 5 g IM every 4 hours. The disadvantages of IM administration are the large volume of solution required to administer the dose and the pain associated with the injection. Lidocaine may be used to minimize the discomfort of the injection. Seizures not controlled by adequate serum concentrations of magnesium may respond to IV diazepam or phenytoin.

Monitoring for signs of toxicity in a patient receiving magnesium sulfate is essential. The optimal serum concentration is 4 to 7 mEq/L.[2] At 9 to 10 mEq/L, the patellar reflexes become hypoactive and may disappear; reflexes should be checked every hour. Urine output should be greater than 25 mL/h because magnesium is excreted only in the urine, and impaired excretion can result in toxicity. Respirations should be greater than 10/min. Respiratory depression and cardiac conduction abnormalities may occur if the magnesium serum concentration reaches 13 to 15 mEq/L. The IV administration of 1 g of calcium gluconate (10 mL of 10% solution) usually reverses mild magnesium toxicity. An ampule of calcium gluconate should be kept at the bedside of any patient receiving magnesium therapy for preeclampsia/eclampsia. Reversal of respiratory depression occurs rapidly in the mother, but calcium gluconate adminstration to the mother may not be effective for hypermagnesemia in the fetus. Magnesium levels should be determined in "floppy" neonates exposed to magnesium prior to delivery.

Magnesium sulfate is not an antihypertensive, and blood pressure should continue to be monitored frequently. A systolic reading of 160 to 180 mm Hg or greater or a diastolic reading of 110 mm Hg or greater should be treated with an intravenous antihypertensive medication to prevent cerebral hemorrhage. Intravenous hydralazine in a dose of 5 to 10 mg should be given initially, followed by 10 mg every 20 minutes as needed to decrease diastolic blood pressure to below 100 mg Hg. An IV infusion may also be used if necessary. To prevent shock, it is important not to decrease blood pressure too quickly. Parenteral hydralazine often produces tachycardia, palpitations, flushing, and headache; propranolol may be useful in opposing the cardiac side effects of hydralazine but should not be used alone to control blood pressure. Intravenous labetalol, an α- and β-adrenergic blocking agent, may be an alternative choice to hydralazine in the acute treatment of hypertension in preeclampsia/eclampsia.[24] The drug is given IV at a dose of 10 to 20 mg, doubling the dose every 10 minutes until the blood pressure is controlled or a cumulative dose of 300 mg is reached. An infusion of labetalol may be given at a rate of 1 to 2 mg/min until blood pressure is controlled, then decreased to 0.5 mg/min to maintain control. It seems to have a faster onset than IV hydralazine with less reflex tachycardia; however, IV hydralazine tends to be more effective overall. If IV hydralazine is unavailable, labetalol is a good alternative.[24] Calcium channel blockers, especially nifedipine, are being used in some centers.

Diazoxide is not recommended for control of blood pressure in the preeclamptic/eclamptic patient because of multiple, serious adverse effects. These include sodium and water retention, serious hyperglycemia in the mother and neonate, and irreversible hypotension when given with other antihypertensive agents. The drug has a relaxant effect on the uterus and is likely to inhibit labor; thus, the use of diazoxide to control blood pressure in the obstetric patient is best reserved for postpartum hypertension. Diuretics are not recommended for use in preeclampsia/eclampsia because of the possibility of decreasing placental perfusion following intravascular fluid depletion. Nitroprusside is not used in obstetrics owing to the lack of experience with the drug in pregnancy and concern about fetal thiocyanate toxicity.[25] It is used only when all other medications fail or when left ventricular failure is present.

The goal of therapy in preeclampsia/eclampsia is to decrease blood pressure, prevent or control seizures and deliver a viable infant. In most cases, the response to any therapy is temporary; the only cure for preeclampsia/eclampsia is delivery. Labor often begins spontaneously in these patients but, if not, plans for induction of labor or cesarean section should be made.

PRETERM LABOR

Uterine contractions with cervical changes beginning before week 37 of gestation are considered preterm labor. There is controversy about the earliest gestational age at which preterm labor should be treated. Labor occurring before week 20 of amenorrhea usually results in expulsion of an nonviable fetus; inhibition of labor is not usually attempted before week 20.

Many patients with preterm contractions respond to bedrest, hydration, and sedation. Pharmacologic intervention is most successful when the cervix is dilated less than 4 cm and membranes are intact. If there is significant cervical change, pharmacologic treatment should not be delayed because it may be unsuccessful later. Certain maternal and fetal conditions preclude the use of tocolytic agents (medications that inhibit uterine contractions). Although premature rupture of membranes is usually considered a contraindication to tocolysis, it may be advantageous to administer pharmacologic agents to delay delivery 24 to 48 hours to provide an opportunity to administer glucocorticoids to enhance fetal lung maturity.

Recently, several investigators have questioned the efficacy of tocolytic agents, β-agonists specifically, to prolong gestation, decrease perinatal mortality, and increase birth weight.[26] Most clinicians, however, choose to treat preterm labor to give the fetus the greatest chance of survival.

β-AGONISTS

The most widely used tocolytic agents are the β-agonists. Ritodrine is the only β-adrenergic agonist approved in the United States for the treatment of preterm labor, but terbutaline is used often. No data are available to suggest that one agent is more efficacious or has fewer side effects than the other. Isoxsuprine was used in the past but is associated with significant tachycardia and hypotension.

Before ritodrine was released in 1980, terbutaline was the drug used most often for the inhibition of preterm labor. Terbutaline is effective and much less expensive than ritodrine. Ritodrine is available only for intravenous infusion, but terbutaline is used intravenously, subcutaneously, and orally.[27]

Terbutaline and ritodrine have similar side effects, including hypotension and tachycardia. In many patients, hypokalemia occurs secondary to an intracellular shift of potassium, but resolves after discontinuation of the drug. This intracellular shift occurs only with parenteral therapy, and unless hypokalemia is detrimental to the patient for other medical reason, no treatment is required. Other side effects include palpitations, tremor, nervousness, angina, and headache.

Hyperglycemia is a common side effect of the β-agonist drugs, but it is not usually important unless the patient is diabetic. Diabetic patients should be closely monitored, and the use of an insulin pump may be advantageous. Some women receiving terbutaline maintenance dosing develop hyperglycemia or unmasking of gestational diabetes; evaluating glucose tolerance after a week of therapy is suggested. Hyperglycemia caused by β-agonist drugs is treated as if it were gestational diabetes.

Pulmonary edema has occurred with the β-agonists.[28] The incidence is greater when the infusion solution is isotonic saline.[29] Therefore, the fluid of choice is 5% dextrose in water injection. Limiting the fluid intake to 2500 mL per 24 hours may also decrease the likelihood of pulmonary edema. A concentrated solution of ritodrine (300 mg in 500 mL D_5W) will help minimize fluid intake.

The intravenous infusion of ritodrine or terbutaline is usually continued for 12 hours after the contractions cease. Oral medication is initiated 30 minutes before the infusion is stopped to allow for absorption. Some investigators have used terbutaline via subcutaneous pump for maintenance with no reported serious side effects and acceptable efficacy.[30,31] However, several women have experienced serious side effects and even death while using the pump.[2] It has been suggested that some β-agonist failures are caused by β-receptor down-regulation (tachyphylaxis) and that using very small doses of terbutaline continuously with a subcutaneous pump may prevent this occurrence. The effectiveness of using terbutaline prophylactically has not been investigated for use in single or twin gestations.

MAGNESIUM SULFATE

Magnesium sulfate is also effective in inhibiting preterm labor, although it is more often[32] used as an anticonvulsant in preeclampsia/eclampsia. Magnesium sulfate probably antagonizes calcium to prevent the actin–myosin interaction, thus reducing uterine activity. Serum magnesium levels of 6 to 8 mEq/L are effective in suppressing uterine contractions.

The patient should be closely observed for signs of hypermagnesemia. In addition to monitoring the patellar reflex, urine output, and respirations, some protocols require serial magnesium levels every 6 hours as an added precaution (see Pregnancy-induced Hypertension). Magnesium sulfate does not alter carbohydrate metabolism and may be the agent of choice in the diabetic patient.

Magnesium sulfate crosses the placenta and can produce fetal serum levels comparable to maternal levels.[6] Serious neonatal effects are uncommon unless the treatment fails and the delivery occurs during the infusion. Respiratory depression in the mother can be reversed by administration of 10 mL of 10% calcium gluconate.

PROSTAGLANDIN SYNTHETASE INHIBITORS

Prostaglandins are present in amniotic fluid during labor and delivery but are absent during pregnancy. The production and release of prostaglandins is postulated as a key factor in the initiation of labor. Therefore, the prostaglandin synthetase inhibitors (nonsteroidal anti-inflammatory agents) may be useful in stopping labor. Indomethacin (oral or rectal) is effective in the treatment of preterm labor;[33] however, its usefulness is limited by serious potential side effects in the fetus. The possibility of premature closure of the ductus arteriosus and poor cardiopulmonary adaptation after delivery are of great concern. Other reported problems in premature neonates exposed to indomethacin include necrotizing enterocolitis, intracranial hemorrhage, and renal dysfunction. Oligohydramnios has also been reported in pregnancies exposed to these medications. Because of these concerns,[33,34] use of these drugs is limited to 72 hours. Maternal side effects are the same as those in the nonpregnant patient.

CALCIUM CHANNEL BLOCKERS

Because calcium is necessary for muscle contraction, calcium channel blocking agents should be useful in the treatment of preterm labor. Two agents, verapamil and nifedipine, relax the myometrium *in vitro.*[35]Clinically, nifedipine has been shown to be effective in decreasing uterine contractions in severe dysmenorrhea[36] and following prostaglandin-induced abortions.[37] Nifedipine is currently used as a tocolytic agent; but the large doses of verapamil required to stop contractions are not tolerated by the mother.

OXYTOCIN ANTAGONISTS

Oxytocin antagonists, a new class of medications, are being studied for tocolysis in the United States. Atosiban®, the first of this class to reach human testing, is currently undergoing trials to demonstrate its effectiveness in inhibiting premature labor.[27,29,38] Atosiban appears to lack cardiovascular, pulmonary, and CNS effects, and side effects such as nausea and vomiting are minimal. It seems to have great promise for the management of preterm labor.

INDUCTION OF LABOR

Labor is not generally induced in normal pregnancies because the uterus is the preferred environment for the fetus until labor occurs. Induction is most successful when the cervix is soft, effaced, and partially dilated. Induction should not be attempted unless an operative delivery would be indicated if the induction fails. Appropriate indications include severe maternal infection, uterine bleeding (usually caused by partial placenta previa or abruptio placentae), preeclampsia/eclampsia or chronic hypertension, diabetes mellitus, macrosomia, maternal renal insufficiency, premature rupture of membranes after week 36, polyhydramnios, oligohydramnios, evidence of placental insufficiency such as intrauterine growth retardation, isoimmunization, and postdate pregnancy.

Three classes of drugs are effective for stimulating uterine contractions: oxytocin, ergot alkaloids, and prostaglandins. The ergot alkaloids are not used to induce labor at term or in late pregnancy because of the possibility of violent, sustained uterine contractions that could compromise the fetus or rupture the uterus. They are used to terminate early pregnancies and to stimulate contractions to decrease postpartum or postabortion bleeding. They are administered orally and parenterally.

The prostaglandin dinoprostone is available in a gel that comes in a prefilled applicator and in an extended release vaginal insert; both are approved for labor induction. The vaginal suppository that has been available for quite some time is approved only for termination in early pregnancy. The gel or insert is applied to the cervix in the labor and delivery suite with electronic fetal and uterine monitoring because of the possibility of uterine hyperstimulation. These agents are usually used in one or more applications for ripening of the cervix, which includes softening, effacement, and some dilatation; oxytocin is usually administered several hours later. Recently, misoprostol has been used for labor induction by both vaginal and oral routes of administration.[39] This is not an approved indication but many investigators have reported excellent efficacy. Most of these reports of induction at term have used vaginal administration.[39] Using tablets, 25 to 50 μg is placed in the posterior vaginal fornix. Misoprostol has several advantages over dinoprostone. It costs significantly less and can be stored at room temperature. It is so effective in many patients that oxytocin is not needed. Because it is not yet approved for labor induction, many clinicians are awaiting the results of larger studies and determination of optimal protocols prior to using it. Hyperstimulation with any of the above agents can be reversed with β-adrenergic tocolytic agents.

Oxytocin is the drug used most often to induce labor and to augment inadequate labor, as well as to decrease postpartum bleeding. Oxytocin is administered by an intravenous infusion, usually a solution of 10 U of oxytocin to 1 L of fluid. Various dosing protocols are used; some of these begin with 1 mU/min increasing by 1 mU every 20 to 30 minutes; others call for as much as 6 mU/min increasing by 6 mU every 20 to 30 minutes. The maximum dose of 20 mU/min should generally not be exceeded, unless internal monitoring of the magnitude of uterine contractions is being used. The goal of therapy is contractions that last 45 to 60 seconds at intervals of 2 to 3 minutes. An IV infusion is recommended because it results in more predictable absorption, distribution, and drug response. IM administration is not recommended because the absorption is not consistent, and the medication cannot be discontinued if complications or side effects arise.

The patient should be attended continually by experienced obstetric nurses. Electronic fetal monitoring including monitoring of frequency and duration of uterine contractions is essential for the early recognition and treatment of side effects. If higher doses of oxytocin are necessary, it is important to internally monitor the intensity of uterine contractions and resting pressure, because a resting pressure greater than 15 to 20 mm Hg increases the incidence of complications such as uterine rupture, uteroplacental hypoperfusion, and fetal distress from hypoxia.[40] If the resting pressure exceeds this level, oxytocin should be discontinued. Maternal blood pressure and pulse rate should be checked frequently.

Side effects of oxytocin are limited if appropriate monitoring is performed. Oxytocin does not cross the placenta;[40] any effects on the fetus are indirect secondary to the drug effects on the uterus. The most notable side effect, however infrequent, is uterine rupture. Oxytocin can also reduce uteroplacental blood flow, resulting in deceleration of fetal heart rate and possible fetal hypoxia. Other side effects are maternal hypotension, hypoglycemia, and fluid retention. Oxytocin is structurally very similar to antidiuretic hormone, and some fluid retention is unavoidable. Water intoxication is a rare but serious complication.

Contraindications include abnormal fetal positions or presentations, cephalopelvic disproportion, previous classical cesarean section, some other previous uterine surgeries, and a firm, closed, uneffaced, posterior cervix. Patients with functional class III or IV heart disease are not good candidates for oxytocin use. Grand multiparas (greater than 7 previous deliveries) have a significantly increased risk of uterine rupture when oxytocin is used.

▶ TREATMENT: Chronic Medical Disorders in Pregnancy

DIABETES

The management of the pregnant diabetic patient differs from that in the nonpregnant state because of the significant metabolic changes during pregnancy. The White classification of diabetes in pregnancy[41] (Table 74–6) is used for determining the prognosis and management of the pregnant diabetic. This classification is based on the duration and severity of disease and remains in use for describing the pathologic complications of the disease.

Preconception planning of pregnancy in the diabetic patient is important, because prevention of complications provides the best management. The patient should be assessed for other risk factors, undergo ophthalmic evaluation and electrocardiography, and have a 24-hour urine collection for creatinine and protein values. The incidence of congenital abnormalities in diabetics is 4% to 11% depending on the degree of glycemic control,[42] compared with 2% to 4% in the normal population. It is especially important that the patient be normoglycemic before conception

TABLE 74–6. White Classification of Diabetes in Pregnancy

Class A: Chemical diabetes
Class B: Maturity onset (age over 20 years), duration under 10 years, no vascular lesions
Class C^1: Age 10 to 19 years at onset
Class C^2: 10 to 19 years duration
Class D^1: Under 10 years at onset
Class D^2: Over 20 years' duration
Class D^3: Benign retinopathy
Class D^4: Calcified vessels of legs
Class D^5: Hypertension
Class F: Nephropathy
Class H: Cardiomyopathy (heart disease)
Class R: Proliferating retinopathy
Class T: Renal transplant

Adapted from Ref. 41.

and during the first trimester, because the congenital malformations associated with diabetes seem to be related to poor glucose control during the first 8 weeks of gestation.[42] Determination of glycosylated hemoglobin (A_{1c}) before conception helps to assess the degree of glucose control.

Patients with the highest risk of complications include those with vasculopathy, poor glucose control, a previous stillbirth, and noncompliance. The complications of diabetic pregnancies include fetal macrosomia, polyhydramnios, malformations, and respiratory distress syndrome. Patients with vascular disease are more likely to have a fetus with intrauterine growth retardation. With careful prenatal management, diabetic patients now have a 96% chance of delivering a healthy child.[43]

During pregnancy, diabetic patients have an increased risk of hypoglycemia and ketoacidosis. Thus, the goal of therapy is the avoidance of fasting and postprandial hyperglycemia and hypoglycemia. The quality of maternal glucose control is the best indicator of perinatal risk, and the use of glucose reflectance monitors has significantly improved control. Tests using whole blood are preferred over urine tests for glucose monitoring during pregnancy because the renal threshold for glucose is decreased in pregnancy, giving an inaccurate estimate of blood sugar. Glucose should be monitored fasting, before meals, and at bedtime daily. Some physicians also ask their patients to monitor glucose 1 hour after meals 1 day each week. Evaluation of glycosylated hemoglobin once each trimester helps assess control.

Pregnant patients usually require a diabetic diet of 35 kcal/kg ideal body weight daily, or about 2200 to 2400 calories. Only intermediate- and fast-acting insulins should be used. Long-acting insulins should not be used because of the variable rates of onset and prolonged duration of activity. NPH or Lente insulin combined with regular insulin should be given SQ, usually in two divided doses daily, although some women require more doses. The dose and frequency of administration should be adjusted to maintain glucose levels between 60 and 120 mg/dL.[44] About 70% of pregnant patients have increased insulin requirements after week 24, and requirements will usually double by the end of pregnancy. Insulin has a large molecular weight and very little, if any at all, crosses the placenta; thus, the effects on the fetus are indirect. Close prenatal monitoring by the patient's obstetrician, internist, or perinatologist is essential for promoting compliance and for early recognition of problems.

Oral hypoglycemic agents are contraindicated during pregnancy because they cross the placenta and stimulate the fetal pancreas, which can produce fetal and neonatal hypoglycemia. They may also cause some teratogenic effects[6] and do not appear to have any advantage over insulin in the control of blood sugar in the pregnant patient. These agents should be discontinued before conception if at all possible. If pregnancy occurs in a patient who is taking one of these agents, the drug should be stopped when pregnancy is confirmed, and insulin therapy initiated.

Gestational diabetes (glucose intolerance of pregnancy) develops during the second half of pregnancy in about 2% to 3% of patients.[45] Initially, the patient is placed on a diabetic diet and home glucose monitoring. If this does not control the glucose, insulin therapy should be started and the patient managed as a pregnant diabetic.

Tight control should be maintained during labor and delivery to reduce the risk of neonatal hypoglycemia. This may be accomplished by an IV infusion of 1 L of 5% dextrose solution with 10 units of regular insulin given at a rate of 100 mL/h. Additional glucose or insulin is given to maintain glucose at approximately 100 mg/dL. Another regimen includes IV administration of 50 g of glucose every 6 hours, with regular insulin given SQ to maintain glucose. In either case, blood glucose should be checked every 1 to 2 hours with a portable glucose monitor.

Immediately after delivery of the placenta, insulin requirements drop and remain lower for 24 to 72 hours. During this period, hypoglycemic shock is common, and the patient must be monitored very closely and insulin dosage lowered accordingly. Breast-feeding is encouraged in diabetic patients, and lower insulin requirements during lactation should be expected owing to the increased caloric consumption during lactation. Patients also may be allowed to keep their glucose levels slightly elevated to prevent the possibility of hypoglycemia while caring for the baby.

THYROID DISEASE

The incidence of hyperthyroidism in pregnancy is about 0.2%.[46] It is important that these patients be treated to minimize maternal and fetal morbidity and mortality. Preeclampsia, maternal heart failure, and stillbirths are more common in hyperthyroid pregnancies than normal pregnancies or those adequately treated. Two thioamides, methimazole and prophylthiouracil (PTU), have both been used with equal efficacy in pregnancy. Both medications cross the placenta and have the potential for causing fetal hypothyroidism and goiter. However, PTU is used most often because of its dual mechanism of action and some belief that it crosses the placenta to a lesser degree than methimazole.[47] There are also reports of aplasia cutis in infants exposed in utero to methimazole.[6] The dose is empirical and may need to be adjusted in pregnancy to maintain the total serum T_4 level in the upper range of normal, the TSH within normal limits, and the patient clinically euthyroid.

Hypothyroidism in pregnancy should be treated with l-thyroxine replacement sufficient to maintain the patient in the euthyroid state. Patients with uncorrected hypothyroidism have a greater incidence of preeclampsia, placental abruption, low-birthweight and stillborn infants, and heart failure. Infants born to mothers with corrected hypothyroidism are usually healthy. Infants born in the United States are screened for congenital hypothyroidism at birth.[2]

CHRONIC HYPERTENSION

Chronic hypertension in pregnancy is described as hypertension present at conception or developing before 20 weeks' gestation. Obstetric patients with chronic hypertension are considered high risk and require close observation during pregnancy, with prenatal visits scheduled every 1 to 2 weeks. Hypertensive patients have a greater incidence of fetal growth retardation because of decreased placental function. At delivery, the placenta may be small, and multiple infarcts may be present. Up to 25% of hypertensive patients have superimposed preeclampsia,[2] which occurs earlier and progresses more rapidly than in otherwise normal pregnancies. These patients have higher maternal and fetal mortality rates and are less responsive to treatment. Abruptio placentae (premature separation of the placenta) occurs more often in patients with vascular disease. Cerebral hemorrhage is a more common cause of maternal mortality than preeclampsia in these patients. To minimize complications, blood pressure should be controlled during pregnancy. It is common for blood pressure to decrease in the second trimester, and it may be possible to discontinue therapy and reinstate it later if necessary.

Given the relatively young age of many pregnant patients, most chronic hypertension is usually mild with minimal sequelae. Mild hypertension should first be treated with bedrest and home blood pressure monitoring. The patient should have complete bedrest for at least 1 hour at lunchtime and 1 hour in the afternoon in addition to 10 hours of rest each night.

Blood pressure not responding satisfactorily to bedrest may be treated with methyldopa. Methyldopa has been used for many years and continues to be the most commonly used antihypertensive medication in pregnancy. It is effective, with no significant fetal or neonatal problems reported.[48] Using methyldopa reportedly increases fetal survival rates and decreases midtrimester fetal loss.[49]

Propranolol, labetalol, and hydralazine are the second-line drugs of choice. There are reports of intrauterine growth retardation, bradycardia, neonatal respiratory distress syndrome, and hypoglycemia with the use of propranolol. The true incidence of these effects is not known and may be more likely when used immediately prior to delivery. If it becomes necessary to use propranolol during pregnancy, it should be discontinued 1 to 2 weeks before delivery and the neonate observed closely for adverse effects. Trials using other β-blockers, including atenolol, labetalol, and metoprolol, are ongoing and may give more definitive information about the efficacy and safety of these drugs in pregnancy.[49] Oral hydralazine may be less effective than propranolol, but it may be useful in controlling blood pressure if the patient is near delivery.

Cardiac output and intravascular volume are often reduced in hypertensive pregnancies; therefore, diuretics should not be used during pregnancy because these drugs cause a 5% to 10% decrease in plasma volume that may be detrimental to the fetus if uteroplacental blood flow is decreased. Diuretics also cause fluid depletion, electrolyte imbalance, and carbohydrate imbalance in the mother.

Reserpine is also avoided in pregnancy because of the possibility of fetal and neonatal bradycardia, congenital abnormalities, and alteration of thermal equilibrium at birth.

Calcium channel blockers are being used extensively in the treatment of chronic hypertension in the nonpregnant population, but there are no published reports of large, controlled studies using these agents in pregnancy. Until these data are available, calcium channel blockers should be avoided in pregnancy.

Angiotensin-converting enzyme (ACE) inhibitors are contraindicated during pregnancy owing to reports of fetal and neonatal renal impairment, oligohydramnios, congenital malformations, and neonatal death.[48–50]

Although fetal loss is about 16% in mild hypertension and may reach 40% in severe hypertension,[51] the primary goal of blood pressure management is to prevent maternal complications while ensuring adequate uterine perfusion for optimal fetal growth.

EPILEPSY

There are about 1.1 million women with epilepsy in the United States who could become pregnant by choice or accident.[52] As with diabetes, the patient and her fetus benefit from preconception planning and careful management during pregnancy. The primary goal in managing these patients is prevention of seizures with the fewest possible effects on the fetus. Pregnancy has unpredictable effects on the frequency and severity of seizures. About 25% of patients experience an exacerbation of the disease, about 25% have fewer seizures, and the remaining 50% do not have any change in seizure frequency.[53] Patients with epilepsy, whether they are taking medications or not, have a greater chance of delivering an infant with congenital abnormalities and mental retardation.[53] Though it is difficult to separate the effects of medication from the effects of the disease, most evidence supports the role of anticonvulsants in causing congenital problems.[2] The most common abnormalities seen in babies exposed to anticonvulsants during pregnancy include orofacial clefts, skeletal anomalies, CNS malformations, cardiac abnormalities, as well as mental retardation. Although teratogenicity does occur with the anticonvulsants, the risk of a seizure is considered more harmful to the fetus.

The American Academy of Pediatrics Select Committee on Anticonvulsants in Pregnancy recommends that for the patient who has been seizure-free for several years, an attempt should be made to discontinue her medication for several months. If she remains seizure-free, she may attempt to become pregnant without medication; however, if the seizures return, she must take the medication during pregnancy. A patient with recurrent epilepsy on medication should be advised that she has a 90% chance of having a normal child, but that the risk of congenital abnormalities and mental retardation is twice that of the normal population.[53]

Treatment with one medication is preferred when possible to decrease fetal exposure, thus minimizing teratogenic risk. When monotherapy fails, an assessment of compliance and evaluation of serum concentrations should be considered. If necessary, the dose should be adjusted. If the first drug does not successfully control seizures, a second drug should be initiated and the first drug gradually withdrawn over 7 days. A trial using a third drug may be tried. If monotherapy with the third medication fails, a trial of two medications simultaneously should be given.

Serum concentrations of most anticonvulsants are lower during pregnancy despite maintenance of prepregnancy dosage.[52,54] Although serum concentrations may be decreased, seizure frequency may not increase because free concentrations of the drug do not decline proportionally with the total concentration. Reasons for decreased serum concentrations include noncompliance due to fears of teratogenic potential of the medication, inadequate dosage, incomplete absorption secondary to nausea and vomiting, increased hepatic clearance, abnormally rapid excretion, and an increased volume of distribution resulting from passage into fetal tissues. The increased extracellular fluid volume occurring in pregnancy may cause dilutional lowering of serum concentrations. Anticonvulsant serum concentrations should be evaluated at least every other month during pregnancy and the dose adjusted according to the concentration, frequency of seizures, and adverse effects.

In a large percentage of neonates exposed to anticonvulsants, a severe coagulopathy occurs during the first 24 hours after delivery.[52,54] This is because of a deficiency of the vitamin K–dependent clotting factors. All babies exposed to anticonvulsants should be treated with 2 mg of vitamin K at birth. Cord blood should be sent for clotting studies and, if necessary, additional vitamin K administered. Some physicians give their pregnant patients receiving anticonvulsants prophylactic oral vitamin K, 20 mg daily, during the last 1 to 3 weeks before delivery is expected.[52,54] Prophylaxis is suggested because treatment may not be successful once there is clinical evidence of bleeding. Folate deficiency also occurs in patients taking anticonvulsants, and folate supplementation is suggested to prevent megaloblastic anemia.

Phenobarbital has been recommended as the anticonvulsant of choice during pregnancy by the American Academy of Obstetrics and Gynecology.[55] The choice of phenobarbital most likely reflects the vast experience with this medication; however, it can be teratogenic, with some infants displaying some hydantoin features, and some studies have associated its use with behavioral abnormalities and impaired intellect.[48,52] Others have suggested that carbamazepine is the best choice.[48] During pregnancy, higher dosages are usually required to maintain serum levels, and the dose should be adjusted to maintain therapeutic concentrations. Neonates exposed to phenobarbital may experience CNS depression at delivery and may experience withdrawal symptoms. Because of the long half-life in neonates, withdrawal symptoms do not usually begin for 4 to 7 days after delivery; therefore, it is likely that the symptoms will begin after hospital discharge. Parents should be advised to report neuromuscular excitability, hyperactivity, sleep disturbances, excessive crying, tremulousness, and persistent vomiting or diarrhea, because these may indicate barbiturate withdrawal. The withdrawal may last 2 to 6 weeks and may be treated by avoiding excessive stimulation of the infant and by inducing sedation with phenobarbital if necessary. Primidone is metabolized to phenobarbital and, thus, would be expected to cause the same problems.

Phenytoin causes the fetal hydantoin syndrome. The teratogenic potential of phenytoin may be more closely related to the metabolites than to the parent drug. The fetal hydantoin syndrome includes craniofacial abnormalities, growth retardation, limb defects, cardiac lesions, hernias, and distal digital and nail hypoplasias. Many congenital malformations are surgically correctable. About 10% of infants exposed to phenytoin will manifest the full syndrome, and about 30% have some features. Genetic variations would help explain why some infants exposed to phenytoin are affected and others are not. Phenytoin dosages may need to be increased during pregnancy, and serum concentrations should be monitored because of individual variation.[56] Phenytoin is probably more teratogenic than phenobarbital, suggesting that phenobarbital should be used in reproductive-age women when possible.

Carbamazepine was thought to be less teratogenic than other anticonvulsants and was often considered the drug of choice for pregnant patients with seizure disorders. Recent reports, however, suggest that carbamazepine causes a greatly increased risk of neural tube defects.[48,57] Other defects reported include craniofacial defects, nail hypoplasia, and developmental delays.

Valproic acid has been noted as the anticonvulsant that causes the highest incidence of malformations.[55] It is associated with cleft palate, renal defects, and neural tube defects, which are often not surgically correctable. It should be avoided in women of childbearing age.

Trimethadione is the most potent teratogen in the anticonvulsant class of drugs. There is an approximate 87% incidence of major malformations, including developmental delays, low-set ears, palatal abnormalities, V-shaped eyebrows, and speech impediments.[55] It should never be used in pregnancy.

Felbamate and gabapentin, the most recently approved anticonvulsants for partial seizures, have not been studied in pregnancy and have been assigned a pregnancy risk category of C. Lamotrigine has also been assigned a pregnancy risk category of C.

ASTHMA

Approximately 1% to 4% of pregnant patients have asthma.[58] The effect of pregnancy on asthma is not predictable; one-third of patients experience improvement of their disease, one-third worsen, and one-third have no change. Mild and well-controlled asthma does not increase complications in pregnancy, and treatment is usually the same as in the nonpregnant state. Impairment of respiratory function causing decreased oxygen delivery to the fetus can cause pregnancy complications including intrauterine growth retardation, fetal asphyxia, and intrauterine fetal death. Therefore, the benefit to the fetus from control of asthma far outweighs the risks from exposure to the drugs currently used.

Of the drugs that have been used to treat asthma in nonpregnant patients, only the iodides are absolutely contraindicated in pregnancy. Iodides cross the placenta and may cause congenital thyroid problems. Iodides are not routinely used as expectorants in asthma but are often "hidden" in other products used to treat asthma.

Inhaled steroids, cromolyn sodium, inhaled and oral β-agonists, and oral theophylline appear to be without significant fetal harm. When oral steroids are required, prednisone and prednisolone are suggested because fetal serum concentrations of these are lower than other steroids. Severe attacks and status asthmatics are managed as in the nonpregnant patient.

Prostaglandins for cervical ripening or induction of labor should be avoided in asthmatic patients as they can precipitate severe acute attacks. For postpartum hemorrhage, prostaglandin E_2 is preferred over prostaglandin $F_{2\alpha}$ because it is less likely to cause significant bronchospasm.[3]

HIV

It is well known that a mother who is infected with HIV can transmit this disease to her fetus. Zidovudine given during pregnancy can significantly decrease the perinatal transmission of HIV-1. All seropositive pregnant women should be offered zidovudine; it is not teratogenic and the only effect on the infant appears to be a small transient anemia that resolves after the neonate finishes the therapy at 6 weeks postpartum. According to the AIDS Clinical Trials Group Protocol 076,[59] the drug is given orally to the mother as early as 14 weeks' or as late as 34 weeks' gestation. It is given IV during labor and orally to the infant for 6 weeks after delivery. ACTG Protocol 076 demonstrated safety, tolerance, and efficacy with zidovudine and showed a 67.5% relative reduction in perinatal HIV transmission. It is suggested that all pregnant women who are HIV positive be counseled about taking the medication and reminded that they should not breast-feed their infants, to further reduce the transmission of HIV.

LACTATION

The renewed interest and participation in breast-feeding in recent years is very positive. Breast-feeding accelerates uterine involution and promotes bonding between mother and baby. Breast milk is the ideal food for neonates. It contains immunologic factors, is not allergenic, is inexpensive, and is readily available on a supply and demand basis.

The increase in breast-feeding has presented clinicians with a new challenge: the need to know what medications are transferred into breast milk, the extent of transfer, and the effect on the infant. As with using medications during pregnancy, the possible risks and benefits of drug therapy should be assessed. There are few controlled studies documenting drug levels in breast milk and their subsequent effects on the infant. Most available information is from case reports or small studies.

When using medications in lactating women, the effect on both quality and quantity of milk produced must be considered. Drugs that decrease milk production include sympathomimetics, nicotine, levodopa, bromocriptine, ergot alkaloids, pyridoxine, monoamine oxidase inhibitors, and androgens. Drugs that decrease prolactin inhibition factor may increase milk production and often have galactorrhea as a side effect. Examples are the antipsychotics, cimetidine, metoclopramide, reserpine, amoxapine, and methyldopa.

Some women choose not to nurse because of personal preference, working conditions, or their babies' inability to nurse (e.g., babies who require intensive care or have palate abnormalities). These mothers can pump their breasts to establish lactation in the event that the baby can later breast-feed. Mothers who have inverted nipples that cannot be successfully corrected are unable to breast-feed. Breast-feeding is contraindicated in some women with medical conditions requiring medication that could harm the infant. A patient with a chronic medical condition requiring medication should consult her physician before delivery to determine if she may consider nursing. A woman who requires short-term drug therapy with a medication that is contraindicated may pump her breasts and discard the milk until the therapy is completed. Her pharmacist, pediatrician, obstetrician, or lactation counselor should consider the half-life of the drug and other characteristics to determine when she may resume breast-feeding.

To minimize the effects of drugs during breast-feeding, sustained-release products or drugs with long half-lives should be avoided. Scheduling a dose immediately after a feeding or before a long sleep period would help decrease the dose reaching the infant, depending on the drug's half-life. If several drugs are equally useful, the drug that is excreted in breast milk in the lowest concentration, with the least effect on the infant, should be selected. As a general guide, the practitioner could consider whether or not the medication is typically given to neonates. The infant should be closely observed for problems after a nursing mother has taken any medication. Drugs contraindicated by the American Academy of Pediatrics include amphetamines, bromocriptine, cocaine, ergotamine, lithium, nicotine, most antineoplastic medications, and drugs of abuse.[60]

In the past, estrogens and bromocriptine were given to women postpartum to suppress lactation. Estrogens suppress lactation by a local effect on breast tissue; bromocriptine acts centrally to inhibit prolactin secretion. Both were associated with serious side effects and are no longer used. Estrogens were associated with thromboembolic disorders originating from the hypercoagulable state that exists in the later stages of pregnancy and during parturition. The most significant concern reported with bromocriptine was the risk of stroke, seizure, and myocardial infarction after its use postpartum.

Breast engorgement is usually self-limiting, begins about the third to fourth day postpartum, and resolves within 48 to 72 hours. During this time, the breasts are swollen, firm, and tender. Some patients report severe pain, whereas others have only mild discomfort. Nondrug treatment includes application of ice packs and binding of the breasts with wide elastic bandages. The patient should be reminded not to express the milk as this will only result in further production. Depending on the severity of pain, nonprescription and prescription analgesics may be provided.

USE OF SELECTED AGENTS DURING LACTATION

ALCOHOL

There is no evidence that occasional, moderate intake of alcohol during lactation is harmful to the infant.[6] However, ingestion of large quantities or chronic use may cause sedation, CNS depression, weakness, and abnormal growth.[60,61]

CAFFEINE

Caffeine is excreted in breast milk at low levels. Mothers who are breast-feeding should be cautioned about ingestion of large amounts of beverages containing caffeine. Moderate use (1 to 2 cups a day) of caffeine-containing beverages is considered acceptable if tolerated by the infant. Caffeine can cause irritability and sleeplessness in breast-fed infants.[6,60]

NICOTINE

Nicotine causes a decrease in milk production and is excreted in breast milk. Nausea, vomiting, diarrhea, tachycardia, and restlessness may occur in nursing infants exposed to nicotine.[60,61] Smoking is harmful to the newborn, both via nicotine in breast milk and from secondhand smoke. It is recommended that nicotine replacement products used as smoking deterrents not be used during nursing unless the risk from continued maternal cigarette smoking is considered greater than the risk of nicotine replacement in the mother.[62]

ANALGESICS

Most analgesics, both narcotic and nonnarcotic, are excreted in breast milk in low concentrations and should not be harmful to the baby if the mother takes only regular therapeutic doses. However, large doses or chronic use should be considered with more caution. For example, a mother taking antiarthritic doses of aspirin may excrete enough drug to alter a baby's prothrombin time.[61]

ANTIBIOTICS

Antibiotics are perhaps the drugs most often required by nursing mothers. All cross into breast milk but at less than pharmacologic doses; however, there remains the potential to cause candidiasis, diarrhea, and thrush in the infant. Penicillins, cephalosporins, and erythromycins are usually considered to be permissible for nursing mothers. Sulfonamides are permitted if the infant is healthy and full-term. Chloramphenicol, tetracyclines, and isoniazid should be avoided. If metronidazole is required, a single 2-g dose should be used, and the breasts pumped for 24 to 48 hours to allow for excretion of the drug before nursing is resumed.[61]

ANTICONVULSANTS

Anticonvulsants are generally considered safe during breast-feeding, although the drugs appear in breast milk at low concentrations. Infants should be observed for sedation and poor feeding.[60]

LAXATIVES

All laxatives, with the exception of bulk-forming products, potentially cross into breast milk. Infants should be observed for diarrhea; however, occasional use is not likely to be harmful.[14,60,61]

HYPOGLYCEMIC AGENTS/INSULIN

There is little information available about oral hypoglycemic agents and breast-feeding. Diabetic mothers using insulin may breast-feed because the large molecular weight of insulin prevents its excretion into breast milk. The diabetic mother may have an increased incidence of nipple candidiasis with accompanying thrush in the baby. This is usually treated with topical nystatin applied to the nipple and concurrent suspension given to the nursing infant. Keeping the nipples clean and dry will decrease the potential for fungal infections.

CONCLUSIONS

All medication use in pregnancy, during labor and delivery, and during breast-feeding should include patient education, informed consent, and careful documentation. The risks and benefits of any drug's use must be carefully considered from the viewpoint of both patients—mother and fetus. What is in the best interest of one may not be in the best interest of the other, and difficult therapeutic decisions must sometimes be made by clinicians and patients. Medication use in pregnancy and lactation is a complex issue. Physicians and pharmacists must work together to provide the patient with the most effective and least potentially harmful medication when treatment is indicated.

REFERENCES

1. Jacobs DS, Kasten BL Jr, Demott WR, Wolfson, WL. Laboratory Test Handbook, 2nd ed. Baltimore, Williams & Wilkins, 1990:222–224, 305–307.
2. Cunningham FG, MacDonald PC, Gant NF, et al. Williams Obstetrics, 20th ed. Stamford, CT: Appleton & Lange, 1997.
3. Committee on Genetics of the American Academy of Pediatrics. Folic acid for the prevention of neural tube defects. Pediatrics 1993:92 493–494.
4. Centers for Disease Control. Recommendations for use of folic acid to reduce number of spina bifida cases and other neural tube defects. JAMA 1993;269:1233–1238.
5. Dicke JM. Teratology: Principles and practice. Med Clin North Am 1989;73:567–582.
6. Briggs GG, Freeman R, Yaffe SJ. Drugs in Pregnancy and Lactation. 4th ed. Baltimore, Williams & Wilkins, 1994.
7. Blake DA, Niebyl JR. Requirements and limitations in reproductive and teratogenic risk assessment. In: Niebyl JR, ed. Drug Use in Pregnancy, 2nd ed. Philadelphia, Lea & Febiger, 1988:1–9.
8. Content and format for labeling of human prescription drugs. Fed Reg 1979;44:37434–37467.
9. Scialli AR. Anticonvulsants and pregnancy. In: Nieby JR, ed. Drugs in Pregnancy, 2nd ed. Philadelphia, Lea & Febiger, 1988:44–54.
10. Buscema J, Stern JL, Johnson TRB. Antineoplastic drugs and pregnancy. In: Niebyl JR, ed. Drug Use in Pregnancy, 2nd ed. Philadelphia, Lea & Febiger, 1988:101.
11. Watson LA, Bammarito AA, Marshall JF. Total peripheral parenteral nutrition in pregnancy. JPEN 1990;14:485–489.
12. Hsu JJ, Clark-Glena R, Nelson DK, Kim CH. Nasogastric enteral feeding in the management of hyperemesis gravidarum. Obstet Gynecol 1996;88:343–346.
13. Kousen M. Treatment of nausea and vomiting in pregnancy. Am Fam Physician 1993;48:1279–1283.
14. Baron TH, Ramirez B, Richter JE. Gastrointestinal motility disorders during pregnancy. Ann Intern Med 1993;118:366–375.
15. Tincello DG, Johnstone MJ. Treatment of hyperemesis gravidarum with the 5-HT_3 antagonist ondansetron (Zofran). Postgrad Med J 1996;72:688–689.
16. Greaves M. Anticoagulants in pregnancy. Pharmacol Ther 1993;59: 311–327.
17. Ginsberg JS, Hirsh J. Use of antithrombotic agents during pregnancy. Chest 1995;108:305S–311S.
18. Barbour LA, Kick SD, Steiner JL, et al. A prospective study of heparin-induced osteoporosis in pregnancy using bone densitometry. Am J Obstet Gynecol 1994;170:862–869.
19. Zuspan FP, Zuspan KJ. Antihypertensive therapy during pregnancy. In: Rayburn WF, Zuspan FP, eds. Drug Therapy in Obstetrics and Gynecology, 3rd ed. St. Louis, Mosby–Year Book, 1992:105–126.
20. Sibai BM, Mirro R, Chesney CM, Leffler C. Low-dose aspirin in pregnancy. Obstet Gynecol 1989;74:551–557.
21. Sibai BM, Caritis SN, Thom E, et al. Prevention of preeclampsia with low-dose aspirin in healthy, nulliparous pregnant women. N Engl J Med 1993;329:1213–1218.
22. Hauth JC, Goldenberg RL, Parker CR Jr, et al. Low-dose aspirin therapy to prevent preeclampsia. Am J Obstet Gynecol 1993;168:1083–1093.
23. Imperiale TF, Pertrulis AS. A meta-analysis of low-dose aspirin for the prevention of pregnancy-induced hypertensive disease. JAMA 1991; 266:261–265.
24. Kyle PM, Redman CWG. Comparative risk-benefit assessment of drugs used in the management of hypertension in pregnancy. Drug Saf 1992;7:223–234.
25. Shoemaker CT, Meyers M. Sodium nitroprusside for control of severe hypertensive disease of pregnancy: A case report and discussion of possible toxicity. Am J Obstet Gynecol 1984;149:171–173.
26. The Canadian Preterm Labor Investigators Group. Treatment of preterm labor with the β-adrenergic agonist ritodrine. N Engl J Med 1992;327:308–312.
27. Sullivan CA, Morrison JC. Emergent management of the patient in preterm labor. Obstet Gynecol Clin North Am 1995;22:197–214.
28. Phelan JP. Pulmonary edema in obstetrics. Obstet Gynecol Clin North Am 1991;18:319–331.
29. Keirse MJNC. New perspectives for the effective treatment of preterm labor. Am J Obstet Gynecol 1995;173:618–628.
30. Fischer JR, Kaatz BL. Continuous subcutaneous infusion of terbutaline for suppression of preterm labor. Clin Pharm 1991;10:29
31. Allbert JR, Johnson C, Roberts WE, et al. Tocolysis for recurrent preterm labor using a continuous subcutaneous infusion pump. J Reprod Med 1994;39:614–618.
32. Gonik B, Creasy RK. Preterm labor: Its diagnosis and management. Am J Obstet Gynecol 1986;154:3–8.
33. Norton ME, Merrill J, Cooper BAB, et al. Neonatal complications after the administration of indomethacin for preterm labor. N Engl J Med 1993;329:1602–1607.
34. Schoenfeld A, Bar Y, Merlob P, Ovadia Y. NSAIDs: Maternal and fetal considerations. Am J Reprod Immunol 1992;28:141–147.
35. Saade GR, Taskin O, Belfort MA, et al. *In vitro* comparison of four tocolytic agents alone and in combination. Obstet Gynecol 1994;84: 374–378.
36. Andersson KE, Ulmsten U. Effects of nifedipine on myometrial activity and lower abdominal pain in women with primary dysmenorrhoea. Br J Obstet Gynecol 1978;85:142–148.

37. Andersson KE, Ingemarsson I, Ulmsten U, Wingerup L. Inhibition of prostaglandin-induced uterine activity by nifedipine. Br J Obstet Gynecol 1979;86: 175–179.
38. Goodwin TM, Valenzuela G, Silver H, et al. Treatment of preterm labor with the oxytocin antagonist atosiban. Am J Perinatol 1996;13: 143–146.
39. Bauer TA, Brown DL, Chai LK. Vaginal misoprostol for term labor induction. Ann Pharmacother 1997;31:1391–1393.
40. Thurman GR, Rayburn WF. Cervical ripening agents and uterine stimulants. In: Rayburn WF, Zuspan FP, eds. Drug Therapy in Obstetrics and Gynecology, 3rd ed. St. Louis, Mosby–Year Book, 1992:229–246.
41. White P. Classification of obstetric diabetes. Am J Obstet Gynecol 1978;130:228–230.
42. Steel JM, Johnstone FD. Guidelines for the management of insulin-dependent diabetes mellitus in pregnancy. Drugs 1996;52:60–70.
43 Schneider JM. Pregnancy complicated by diabetes mellitus. In: Pernoll ML, ed. Current Obstetric and Gynecologic Diagnosis and Treatment. 7th ed. Stamford, CT: Appleton & Lange, 1991: 364–372.
44, Landon MB, Gabbe SG. Diabetes mellitus and pregnancy. Obstet Gynecol Clin North Am 1992;19:633–654.
45. Barss VA. Diabetes and pregnancy. Med Clin North Am 1989;153: 824–828.
46. Mestman JH, Goodwin TM, Montoro MM. Thyroid disorders of pregnancy. Endocrinol Metab Clin North Am 1995;24:41–71.
47. Sipes SL, Malee MP. Endocrine disorders in pregnancy. Obstet Gynecol Clin North Am 1992;19:655–677.
48. Rayburn WF. Chronic medical disorders during pregnancy. J Reprod Med 1997;42:1–24.
49. Remuzzi G, Ruggenenti P. Prevention and treatment of pregnancy-associated hypertension: What have we learned in the last 10 years? Am J Kidney Dis 1991;18:285–305.
50. Shotan A, Widerhorn J, Hurst A, Elkayan U. Risks of angiotensin-converting enzyme inhibition during pregnancy: Experimental and clinical evidence, potential mechanisms, and recommendations for use. Am J Med 1994;96:451–456.
51. Zuspan FP, Zuspan KJ. Antihypertensive therapy during pregnancy. In: Rayburn WF, Zuspan FP, eds. Drug Therapy in Obstetrics and Gynecology, 3rd ed. St. Louis, Mosby–Year Book, 1992:105–126.
52. Yearby MS, Devinsky O. Epilepsy and pregnancy. Adv Neurol 1994; 64:45–63.
53. Patterson RM. Seizure disorders in pregnancy. Med Clin North Am 1989;73:661–665.
54. Brodie MJ, Dichter MA. Antiepileptic drugs. N Engl J Med 1996; 334:168–175.
55. Yerby MS. Pregnancy, teratogenesis, and epilepsy. Neurol Clin 1994; 12:749–771.
56. Buehler BA, Stempel LE. Anticonvulsant therapy during pregnancy. In: Rayburn WF, Zuspan FP. eds. Drug Therapy in Obstetrics and Gynecology, 3rd ed. St. Louis, Mosby–Year Book, 1992:147–163.
57. So EL. Update on epilepsy. Med Clin North Am 1993;77:203–214.
58. Clark SL, National Asthma Education Program Working Group on Asthma and Pregnancy, National Institutes of Health, National Heart, Lung and Blood Institute. Asthma in pregnancy. Obstet Gynecol 1993; 82:1036–1040.
59. Mofenson LM. The role of antiretroviral therapy in the management of HIV infection in women. Clin Obstet Gynecol 1996;39:361–385.
60. Committee on Drugs of the American Academy of Pediatrics. Transfer of drugs and other chemicals into human milk. Pediatrics 1994;93: 137–150.
61. Gardner DK. Drugs in breast milk. In: Rayburn WF, Zuspan FP, eds. Drug Therapy in Obstetrics and Gynecology, 3rd ed. St. Louis, Mosby–Year Book, 1992: 312–352.
62. Hebel SK, Rivard R, Threlkeld DS, et al. Facts and Comparisons, 52nd ed. St. Louis, Facts and Comparisons, Inc., 1998:3679.

75

INFERTILITY

Deborah Stier Carson, PharmD, BCPS, and Kathryn K. Bucci, PharmD, BCPS

Infertility is defined as 1 year of unprotected coitus without conception. Conception rates of 20% to 25% per month are expected in normal couples trying to achieve pregnancy. If couples had been using oral contraceptives (OCs) previously, this period may be extended to 15 months.[1] A series of complex and interrelated events must occur for successful conception, implantation, and maintenance of a pregnancy (Table 75–1). Dysfunction in one or more of these events can result in infertility. Although new assisted reproduction techniques (ART), including *in vitro* fertilization (IVF), gamete intrafallopian transfer (GIFT), zygote intrafallopian transfer (ZIFT), intracytoplasmic sperm injection (ICSI), and surgical correction of abnormalities, contribute greatly to successful pregnancies in previously infertile couples, drug therapy directed toward induction of ovulation still plays an important role in treating infertility.

EPIDEMIOLOGY

Impaired ability to have children occurs in an estimated 8.4% of women 15 to 44 years of age in the United States, with about 25% of women having an episode of infertility at some point in their reproductive lives.[2] The prevalence of infertility has increased in the past 15 years. Contributing factors are a delay in childbearing, contraceptive practices, sexual practices, and an increase in therapeutic abortions.

Male factors are wholly or partially responsible for 40% to 50% of infertility problems. Although assessment and treatment of the male factors are beyond the scope of this chapter, they should be investigated before an extensive workup and hormonal manipulation begins in the woman.

Uterine and tubal disease (including endometriosis) are present in 20% to 50% of female infertility patients. Cervical and immunologic factors and various infectious diseases cause infertility in approximately 5% to 10% of infertility cases, and failure to ovulate occurs in 30% to 40%.

PHYSIOLOGY OF THE NORMAL MENSTRUAL CYCLE

Comprehension of the mechanisms of hormonal regulation of the normal menstrual cycle is essential to understanding infertility in women.[3] Undeveloped follicles in the ovaries are present during early fetal development. Each follicle consists of an oocyte (undeveloped ovum) that remains in a resting phase until puberty, when the stimulus for further development occurs. At puberty, hypothalamic and pituitary activation cause cyclic changes in the ovaries that in turn affect the endometrium and cervix. Infertility can result from quantitative or chronologic alterations in the normal hormonal cycle.

Until their numbers are exhausted, follicles begin to grow, and then degenerate under a variety of physiologic circumstances, including ovulatory and anovulatory cycles. The stimulus for successful follicular development and the normal menstrual cycle depends on pulsatile secretion of gonadotropin-releasing hormone (GnRH) from the hypothalamus in a changing but critical range, frequency, and concentration. GnRH is responsible for stimulating the synthesis, storage, and secretion of the specific hormones (gonadotropins) from the anterior pituitary. These gonadotropins, follicle-stimulating hormone (FSH) and luteinizing hormone (LH), direct events in the ovarian follicles that result in the production of a fertile ovum. Prolactin is also secreted from the anterior pituitary. Whereas a low concentration of prolactin is expected in the normal menstrual cycle, elevated prolactin concentrations can alter the menstrual cycle, leading to ovulation failure. Although follicles begin to grow independent of gonadotropin control, FSH and LH are necessary for full follicular development and production of estrogen (specifically estradiol) and progesterone. Each month of a normal female menstrual cycle, gonadotropins and ovarian hormones cyclically increase and decrease (Fig. 75–1). The ovarian hormones cause sequential changes in the endometrium that sustain a suitable environment for growth of a fertilized ovum within the uterus if conception occurs. With relation to events in the ovary, the cycle can be divided into three phases: the follicular phase, ovulation, and the luteal phase. Events in the uterus can be divided into the menstrual, proliferative, and secretory phases, with the first two corresponding temporally to the follicular phase and the latter coinciding with the luteal phase.

FOLLICULAR (MENSTRUAL AND PROLIFERATIVE) PHASE

Follicular development begins during the menstrual flow when FSH concentrations are high. The follicular or proliferative phase ends with ovulation of usually only one follicle, called the dominant follicle. As the concentration of FSH rises at the end of the previous cycle, a series of hormonal events over 10 to 14 days matures the dominant follicle and causes the degeneration or atresia of the remaining follicles recruited during the cycle.

Once a follicle has received FSH stimulation, it must continue to be stimulated by FSH or die. As

TABLE 75–1. Complex and Interrelated Events That Must Occur for Normal Fertilization, Implantation, and Maintenance of Pregnancy

1. The male must produce an adequate number of viable spermatozoa and must be able to deposit them in the upper vagina at the time when a mature oocyte has been released from the ovary.
2. The female's ovulatory cycle must be normal, including sufficient estrogen in the proliferative phase to stimulate the endometrial lining and produce the quantity and quality of cervical mucus necessary to allow passage of spermatozoa and enough progesterone in the secretory phase to support implantation and maintenance of pregnancy.
3. The oviducts must be patent and sufficiently mobile to allow fertilization as well as transport of the ovum from the ovary to the uterus.
4. The uterus must be capable of supporting implantation and fetal growth throughout pregnancy.

Adapted from Ref. 1.

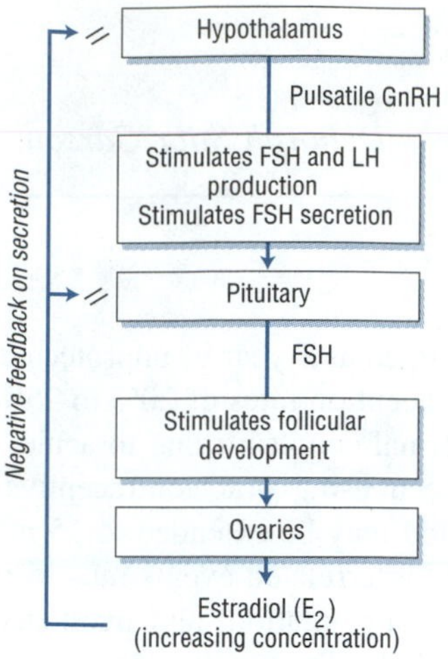

FIGURE 75–2. Hypothalamic–pituitary–ovarian (HPO) feedback loop during the follicular phase of the normal menstrual cycle.

gonadotropin-dependent growth is initiated in the follicle, the follicle enlarges and develops other layers of cells capable of further developing receptors for FSH and LH, as well as synthesizing estradiol (E_2), progesterone, and androgen. Estradiol increases its own follicular receptors, stimulates cell growth (independent of FSH), and amplifies the effect of FSH action in the follicle. The developing follicles cause a rise in the E_2 level that serves to stop the menstrual flow from the previous cycle, thicken the endometrial lining of the uterus, increase the uterine gland size, and thin the cervical mucus. Follicles receiving the most FSH stimulation will have the greatest rate of cell proliferation and produce the highest E_2 concentrations. FSH also regulates an aromatase enzyme system that converts androgens to estrogens in the follicles. Follicles that become androgenic do not survive. Therefore, follicles with the most FSH stimulation have the lowest androgen to estrogen ratios.

Although estrogen positively influences FSH action within the maturing follicle, a rising serum E_2 concentration has a negative feedback for FSH release at the hypothalamic–pituitary level, leading to diminished FSH support for the other less developed follicles (Fig. 75–2). Follicular atresia of the nondominant follicles parallels the rise in plasma estrogen concentration. The dominant follicle can be observed as early as cycle days 5 to 7, corresponding to the gradual fall of FSH levels observed at midfollicular phase.

FSH, with estrogen as a coordinator, is also responsible for the production of LH receptors on the dominant follicle. The dominant follicle produces increasing amounts of E_2, reaching a peak approximately 24 to 36 hours before ovulation. As the estrogen concentration slowly increases, gonadotropin secretion diminishes, but accumulation continues within the pituitary. At a critical E_2 concentration (greater than 200 pg for at least 50 hours), GnRH is triggered, leading to a midcycle LH and FSH surge (Fig. 75–3). While providing the ovulatory stimulus to the dominant follicle, the LH surge ensures atresia of the remaining follicles with their lower estrogen and FSH content. LH also promotes production of a small amount of preovulatory progesterone, specifically 17-OH progesterone, from the dominant follicle which enhances the LH surge at the level of the pituitary. A growing body of knowledge also indicates that a host of ovarian peptides—such as inhibin, activin, follistatin, and insulin-like growth factor—are important to regulation of follicular development.[4]

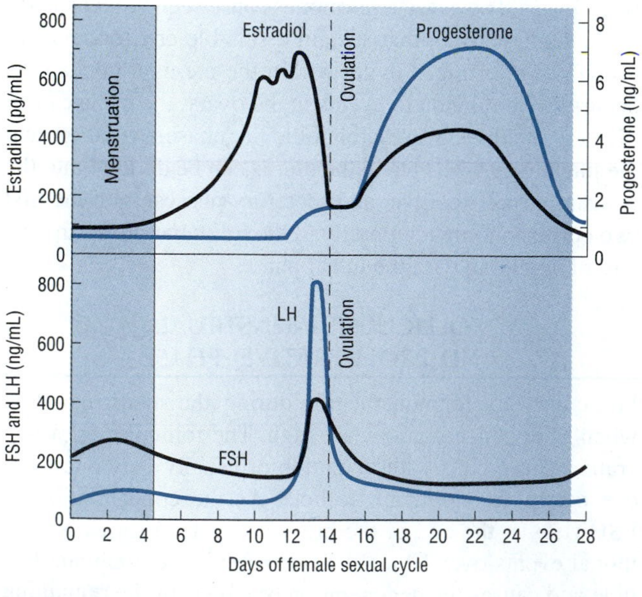

FIGURE 75–1. Approximate plasma concentrations of the gonadotropins and ovarian hormones during the normal female menstrual cycle. *(From Guyton AC, ed. Textbook of Medical Physiology, 8th ed. Philadelphia, Saunders, 1991: p 900.)*

OVULATION

Ovulation is dependent on both adequate gonadotropin levels and a follicle being sufficiently mature to respond to an appropriate stimulus. Although considerable variation exists from cycle to cycle, ovulation is estimated to occur approximately 10 to 12 hours after the LH peak and 24 to 36

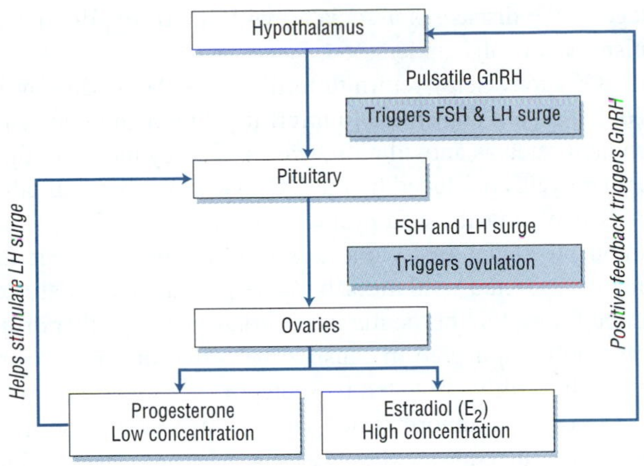

FIGURE 75–3. HPO feedback loop just prior to ovulation in a normal menstrual cycle.

hours after peak E_2 concentrations. The LH surge, occurring 28 to 32 hours before follicle rupture, is the most clinically useful indicator of approaching ovulation.

Progesterone may increase the distensibility of the follicle wall, allowing it to accommodate accumulating fluid. Proteolytic enzymes and prostaglandins appear necessary for induction of follicular rupture from the ovary. After ovulation, the plasma E_2 concentration dramatically decreases, possibly related to LH-induced down-regulation of its own receptors on the follicle or to an inhibitory action of midcycle progesterone on further cell proliferation. The actual mechanism for LH withdrawal is not known.

LUTEAL (SECRETORY) PHASE

The remaining luteinized follicular cells in the ovary, known as the corpus luteum, synthesize androgen, estrogen, and progesterone. Concentrations of progesterone and E_2 from the corpus luteum peak by day 8 or 9 after ovulation. Progesterone, the most abundant ovarian hormone during the luteal phase, antagonizes estrogen action through depletion of estrogen receptors as well as inhibiting gonadotropin release at the hypothalamic level. Negative feedback actions of both estrogen and progesterone on gonadotropins inhibit new follicular growth during the luteal phase. Progesterone also stimulates glands in the endometrium to release a glycogen-rich secretion that prepares the uterus to receive a fertilized ovum and causes cervical mucus to become more viscous. Because estrogen is necessary for synthesis of progesterone receptors, luteal phase estrogen may be necessary to prepare the endometrium for progesterone stimulation after ovulation. Without adequate estrogen priming, progesterone receptor content may be inadequate and cause infertility or early abortion.

The life span and hormone-producing capacity of the corpus luteum are dependent on the continuous presence of small amounts of LH. If conception does not occur, the corpus luteum function rapidly declines over 9 to 11 days. As progesterone concentration decreases, the endometrial lining cannot be maintained and partially sloughs, thus beginning another menstrual cycle. With pregnancy, the corpus luteum is maintained by the emergence of human chorionic gonadotropin (HCG), which first appears 9 to 13 days after ovulation, thus preventing luteal regression. HCG maintains the vital hormonal production from the corpus luteum until placental progesterone production is well established by weeks 6 to 8 of gestation.

PATHOGENESIS OF FEMALE INFERTILITY

Numerous causes of infertility exist, and the more common ones are listed in Table 75–2. More than one cause can be found in 10% to 30% of infertile couples.[2] Failure to ovulate or anovulation secondary to chronic hypothalamic dysfunction is probably the most frequent cause of menstrual disorders in women with normal prolactin and androgen

TABLE 75–2. Common Causes of Infertility, Estimated Pregnancy Rates, and Conventional Treatments

	Pregnancy Rate in a Couple With a Single Infertility Factor		
Cause of Infertility	Actual[a] (%)	Life Table Expected With Indefinite Follow-up[a] (%)	Conventional Treatment
Endometriosis	31	52	Ablation of ectopic endometrial tissue, danazol; sex steroids; GnRH analogs; assisted reproduction
Male factor	38	74	Assisted reproduction or donor insemination
Anovulation	44	79	Clomiphene, gonadotropins, GnRH
Tubal factor	26	48	Tubal surgery
Luteal phase abnormalities	46	58	Correction of cause, progesterone, clomiphene citrate, gonadotropins
Cervical factor	26	45	Estrogen; guiafenesin, intrauterine insemination
Uterine factor (congenital anomalies, adhesions, polyps, hyperplasia)	33	38	Surgical correction of congenital abnormalities; cerclage; dilation and curettage; appropriate antibiotic therapy

[a]Pregnancy rate is a function of time. Actual rates are based on conventional measures (number of patients achieving pregnancy compared to number of patients treated in a defined period of time) while life-tables are calculated based on the assumption that patients are followed indefinitely.

Compiled from Refs. 1 and 2.

levels. Stress, trauma, alterations in body weight, or excessive athletic activity often contribute. Patients with hypothalamic dysfunction exhibit a variety of patterns ranging from luteal phase defects to amenorrhea.

Another common cause of chronic anovulation results from hyperandrogenicity, and is often diagnosed as polycystic ovary syndrome (PCOS) or Stein–Leventhal syndrome. Since puberty, many patients with PCOS have chronically increased LH secretion, which continuously stimulates follicles to produce excess androgen. Elevated androgen levels may lead to prolonged periods of anovulation by enhancing follicular atresia and estrogen overproduction from peripheral conversion of the androgens to estrogens. Ovarian cysts, amenorrhea, or oligomenorrhea, acne, obesity, and hirsutism in association with normal or elevated testosterone concentrations and an inappropriately high LH to FSH ratio (often greater than 3 to 1) are classically associated with this disease. Insulin resistance and hyperinsulinemia are also present with this syndrome. In obese women with hyperandrogenic chronic anovulation, weight loss can significantly reduce circulating levels of androgens.[5]

Age-related changes in the reproductive system eventually result in loss of ovulatory function. During the perimenopausal period, a woman may still have follicular growth, but does not consistently ovulate because of potential refractoriness to FSH and LH. Although changes in fertility rates related to age are difficult to quantify, fertility rates decline after age 30; however, the rate does not fall dramatically until a woman enters her 40s. Approximately one-third of the women who defer pregnancy to their mid to late 30s have infertility problems.

Luteal phase deficiency or inadequacy is linked to inappropriate or inadequate LH support. The inability of the corpus luteum to maintain the luteal phase causes recurrent miscarriages. A deficient luteal phase is (1) the production of adequate progesterone concentrations, but not for an appropriate length of time (less than 11 days); or, more commonly, (2) progesterone produced in suboptimum quantities for the full luteal phase. Whether luteal deficiency causes infertility is controversial, because sporadic luteal deficiency occurs in fertile women, and treatment is not always beneficial.[2] Premature luteinization, another defect related to the luteal phase, is an untimely LH surge in response to rising estrogen when the follicle is still immature and unable to ovulate. This defect may represent an exaggerated sensitivity of the pituitary to rising levels of estrogen, resulting in a premature LH surge.

Infectious processes, particularly pelvic inflammatory disease, that result in scarring of the reproductive system are increasingly identified as a cause of infertility and ectopic pregnancy in young women. Tubal damage contributing to later infertility problems may occur in women who have had a septic abortion or a ruptured appendix, used an intrauterine device, or had tubal surgery.

Endometriosis is a disease indicating the presence of ectopic endometrial tissue. Although endometriosis at any stage of the disease is associated with infertility, the mechanism is not fully understood.

OCs may delay return to fertility after being discontinued, but do not contribute to infertility. Often an underlying problem, such as anovulation, was masked by the seemingly regular cycles produced by the OCs. However, several other drugs may contribute to problems with fertility. Drugs that inhibit prostaglandin synthesis should be avoided near the time of expected ovulation, because prostaglandins are required for rupture of the mature ovarian follicle. Other drugs commonly implicated in causing menstrual disturbances or female infertility are listed in Table 75–3.

Endocrine abnormalities such as thyroid disease, prolactinoma, diabetes, excessive adrenal androgen production, and hepatic disease can alter the metabolism or feedback of hormones in the hypothalamus or pituitary, thus preventing follicular development, ovulation, or the survival of the corpus luteum. Diseases that cause increased prolactin concentrations can cause luteal phase inadequacy, progressing to anovulation and amenorrhea with complete GnRH suppression. Prolactin may work both centrally and in the ovaries to prevent ovulation. The presence of galactorrhea, with or without elevated serum prolactin levels, tends to indicate the presence of excessive prolactin stimulation. Prolactin levels are normally elevated during lactation but can also be increased in response to prolactin-producing tumors, stress, and drugs (antipsychotics, opiates, and reserpine derivatives).

Although sperm are very antigenic, only a small percentage of infertility cases can be explained by an immunologic reaction to sperm. The treatment options are controversial, and include sperm washing, high-dose corticosteroids, vitamin C, and ART.

DIAGNOSIS OF INFERTILITY

An estimated 43% of infertile couples seek help for infertility problems.[6] The history and physical examination are important, and close attention should be paid to details that provide clues to ovulation, previous infections or surgery, androgenicity, or other factors that could contribute to infertility.[7] In addition to history and physical exam of both partners, the current workup of the infertile couple consists of (1) semen analysis after 2 to 3 days of abstinence; (2) evaluation of pelvic anatomy and tubal patency via laparoscopy, fluoroscopically controlled hysterosalpingography, and/or hysteroscopy; (3) postcoital testing; and (4) evaluation of ovulatory function. Other tests such as sperm penetration assay, immune screen, karyotype, and human leukocyte antigen screening may be employed in certain cases.

If an approximate time of ovulation can be determined, coitus can be scheduled 3 to 4 days prior to and 2 to 3 days after expected ovulation. The human egg is fertilizable for 12 to 24 hours after ovulation and sperm may retain ability to fertilize for 24 to 48 hours. Although serial ultrasound examination by an experienced operator is an

TABLE 75–3. Drugs Associated With Female Infertility or Menstrual Irregularities

Agent	Type of Problem
Androgens (including danazol and leuprolide)	Inhibition of follicular development, menstrual derangement
Atenolol	Hyperprolactinemia
Nonsteroidal anti-inflammatory agents	Block release of mature follicle through inhibition of prostaglandin
Opiates	Hyperprolactinemia, suppresses LH secretion
Cimetidine	Mild androgenic properties (dose related)
Corticosteroids	Amenorrhea with high doses; inhibition of ovulation if given early in cycle
Coumarin derivatives	Follicular (corpus luteum) bleeding, ovarian hemorrhage
Cyproterone acetate	Inhibition of ovulation
Domperidone	Hyperprolactinemia
Reserpine	Hyperprolactinemia
Metoclopramide	Hyperprolactinemia
Oral contraceptives	Inhibition of ovulation
Progestogens	Alter FSH:LH ratio
Spironolactone	Menorrhagia, metrorrhagia, amenorrhea
Cannabis	Increase in HCG when used in testicular cancer. Concerns are mostly related to male fertility
Serotonin reuptake inhibitors	Serotonin pathways are involved with regulation of prolactin secretion
Cytostatic/cytotoxic agents	Amenorrhea, early menopause, dyspareunia, decreased libido
Neuroleptics	Hyperprolactinemia, galactorrhea, hirsutism, amenorrhea
Licorice (glycyrrihiza glabra)	Amenorrhea and hyperprolactinemia
Diethylstilbestrol (history of exposure in utero)	Cervical, uterine and vaginal changes resulting in infertility, spontaneous abortion and premature labor

Adapted from Dukes MNG, ed. Meyler's Side Effects of Drugs. Amsterdam, Elsevier, 1996.

accurate noninvasive method of determining follicular growth and ovulation, ovulatory function can be evaluated with home test kits for detection of increase in urinary LH, measurement of serum progesterone concentration, endometrial biopsy, or measurement of basal body temperature (BBT). BBT, the body temperature after a night's rest, is often lower than 98.6°F and varies throughout the menstrual cycle. Although not completely reliable, charting BBT allows indirect confirmation that ovulation has taken place. BBT can be taken orally or rectally with a regular thermometer or with special thermometers that show a range of only a few degrees, making it easier to read small differences. It is very important that women take the reading upon awakening and before any activity. In women who have an ovulatory menstrual cycle, BBT will reach a nadir at about the time of the LH surge and rise about 0.5°F at the time of ovulation when progesterone is secreted from the corpus luteum.

▶ TREATMENT: Infertility

PRINCIPLES OF OVULATION INDUCTION

When infertility is related to anovulation or luteal phase defects, hormonal manipulation is often successful. Some therapeutic agents augment the patient's natural endocrine process, while other agents will take control of, and in some cases replace, the natural cycle (Table 75–4). To induce ovulation, FSH is necessary in the early phase of the cycle to recruit and select follicles. For follicular growth and maturation, both FSH and LH are necessary. Adequate estrogen is necessary in the follicular phase to stimulate the endometrial lining and alter the cervical mucus, making it favorable for sperm penetration. If the aim is to develop one or two mature follicles, then gonadotropin stimulation should be delayed until the dominant follicle has been selected. Once ovulation has occurred, progesterone is required in the luteal phase to maintain and transform the endometrial lining into one suitable for implantation by a fertilized ovum. In cases of IVF where the aim is to obtain many oocytes, increased gonadotropin stimulation is commenced before or during the early follicular recruitment phase.

Determination of the likely cause of infertility will direct the management (Figs. 75–4 and 75–5). Pregnancy rates achieved in patients with single infertility factors are listed in Table 75–2. Case reports of ovarian cancer occurring in women taking fertility drugs has caused concern that ovulation induction increases the risk. However, infertility and low parity are known risk factors for ovarian cancer, making causal relationship between the fertility drugs and ovarian cancer difficult to establish.[8–11]

PHARMACOLOGIC THERAPY

SPECIFIC AGENTS

Clomiphene Citrate

Clomiphene citrate (CC) is a nonsteroidal estrogen agonist–antagonist that causes the hypothalamus to release GnRH as if estrogen concentrations were low. The FSH and LH pulse frequency (but not amplitude) rise, increasing the peripheral serum concentrations of FSH and LH (Fig. 75–6). Enhancement of the natural hypothalamic–pituitary–ovarian (HPO) axis is recognized as the primary mechanism of action, although pituitary and ovarian effects may occur. The predominant indication for CC is for anovulatory or oligo-ovulatory infertility, including PCOS. Suitable patients are likely to have a chronic anovulatory disorder often

TABLE 75–4. Drugs Used To Induce Ovulation

Category	Trade Name (Manufacturer)	Content	How Supplied	Indications/Adjunct Therapy	Contraindications & Precautions	Common Adverse Effects
Estrogen agonist/ antagonist	Clomid (Marion Merrell Dow) Milophene (Milex) Serophene (Serono)	Clomiphene citrate	50-mg tablets	Anovulation or oligo-ovulation with intact pituitary/ovarian response and endogenous estrogen	Contraindications: liver disease, ovarian cysts, undiagnosed, abnormal uterine bleeding, pregnancy Precautions: PCOS[a]	Multiple pregnancy, hot flushes, ovarian enlargement, visual disturbances Possible association with ovarian cancer after ≥ 12 cycles
Human chorionic gonadotropin (HCG)	Various	HCG from human placenta and urine of pregnant women (activity is essentially identical to activity of LH)	Reconstituted products available in following strengths: 200, 500, 1000, & 2000 IU/mL	Used after pretreatment with clomiphene, human menotropins, and other agents in women with secondary ovarian failure	Contraindications: PCOS,[b] previous episode of OHSS, prior allergic reaction Precautions: Large or numerous ovarian follicles, high serum estrogen levels	OHSS, fluid retention, headache, irritability, fatigue, depression, edema, breast tenderness
Menotropin (hMG)	Pergonal (Serono) Humegon (Organon)	FSH & LH	75 IU FSH, 75 IU LH activity /2-mL ampule 150 IU FSH, 150 IU LH activity /2-mL ampule	Hypothalamic–pituitary failure: Ovaries must be responsive (secondary ovarian failure); stimulates follicular growth and maturation: HCG needed for ovulation	Contraindications: Primary ovarian failure, overt thyroid or adrenal dysfunction, undevelopment, ovarian enlargement or abnormal uterine bleeding, pituitary tumor Precautions: Thrombotic tendency	OHSS, multiple pregnancy, breast tenderness, nausea and vomiting, hypercoagulability
Urofollitropin (FSH via urinary extraction)	Metrodin (Serono)	FSH (IM)	0.83 mg (75 IU FSH activity)/2-mL ampule	Ovulation induction. Especially useful in women with PCOS where LH:FSH is elevated. Used sequentially with HCG	Contraindications: Primary ovarian failure, overt thyroid or adrenal dysfunction, undiagnosed ovarian enlargement or abnormal uterine bleeding, pituitary tumor. Precautions: thrombotic tendency	OHSS, multiple pregnancy, breast tenderness, nausea and vomiting, hypercoagulability
	Fertinex (Serono)	Highly purified FSH (SQ)	75 IU or 150 IU FSH (powder for reconstitution)			
Follitropin (recombinant FSH)	Gonal-F (Serono) *Follitropin Alpha*	FSH (SQ)	75 IU or 150 IU FSH (powder for reconstitution)			
	Follistim (Organon) *Follitropin Beta*	FSH (SQ or IM)	75 IU FSH (powder for reconstitution)			

Synthetic GnRH	Factrel (Wyeth Ayerst)	Gonadorelin HCl (IV or SQ)	100 μg (as HCl)/vial 500 μg (as HCl)/vial	Anovulation due to primary hypothalamic failure or dysfunction: Must be given in a pulsatile fashion	Contraindications: Pregnancy Precautions: Low risk of ovarian enlargement	Moderate risk of multiple pregnancies
	Lutrepulse (Ferring)	Gonadorelin acetate (IV)	0.8 or 3.2 mg as powder for reconstitution[c]			
GnRH agonists	Synarel (Syntex)	Nafarelin acetate	2 mg/mL nasal spray	Endometriosis; adjunct to hMG/HCG for ovulation induction	Contraindications: Pituitary tumor, primary ovarian failure Precautions: PCOS,[d] thyroid or adrenal dysfunction	Multiple pregnancy, nausea, headache, abdominal pain
	Lupron (TAP)	Leuprolide acetate	5 mg/mL for SC injection (depot formulation should NOT be used for ovulation induction)			
	Superfact (Hoechst)	Buserilin	Nasal spray, subcutaneous injection	Adjunct to HMG/HCG for ovulation induction (not available in U.S.)		
	Triptorelin pamoate (Organon)	Decapeptyl	Injection	Orphan drug; palliative treatment for ovarian carcinoma of epithelial origin; may be more prone to ovarian hyperstimulation than other GnRHa		
	Zoladex (ICI Pharma)	Goserelin acetate	3.6-mg implant	Not used for ovulation induction because of duration to effect		
GnRH antagonists	Ganirelex Cetrorelix		Nasal spray SQ	Investigational		

PCOS = polycyctic ovarian syndrome; OHSS = ovarian hyperstimulation syndrome.
[a]May be an exaggerated response.
[b]Risk of OHSS.
[c]FDA currently requires that product must be marketed with components for administration via pump. Because the pump components became unavailable in 1997, product may be unavailable unless labeling changes.
[d]Ineffective.
Compiled from Refs. 12, 18, and 22.

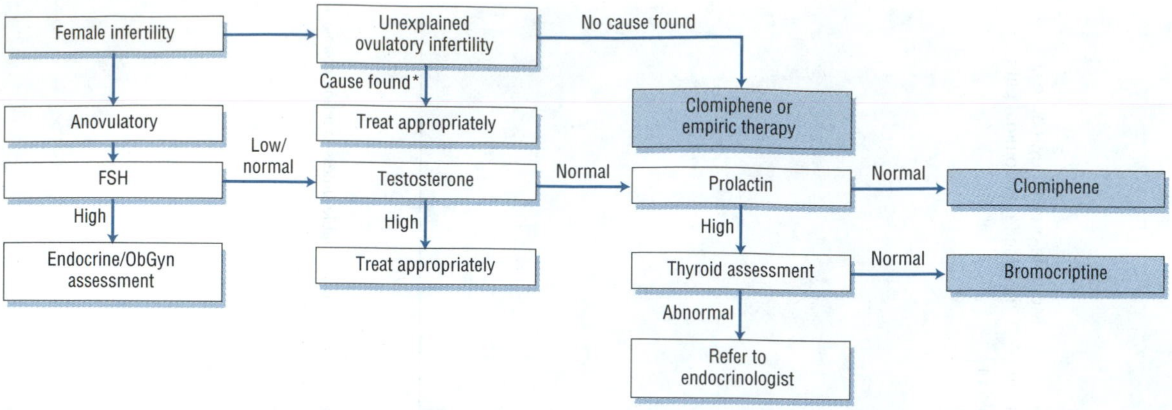

FIGURE 75–4. Flow diagram for treatment of female-factor infertility. *Hostile cervical mucus; luteal phase defects; obstructed tubes; congenital abnormalities; endometriosis; infection; immunologic abnormalities. *(Adapted from Ref. 18.)*

dating back to puberty. Appropriate candidates for CC therapy have endogenous estrogen activity and an intact HPO axis. Although generally less successful in inducing ovulation in women with reduced estrogen levels, a trial of CC therapy may be warranted unless galactorrhea or hyperprolactinemia suggest other therapy (see the section later in the chapter on dopamine agonists). Patients with an FSH level of 40 mIU/mL or more have absent or resistant follicles and are not likely to respond to ovulation induction.

Because there is a possible association between CC dosage and multiple birth, a low dose of CC should be used initially and then increased, if necessary, with each cycle. The recommended starting dosage is 50 mg/d for 5 days. Because women with PCOS may be ultra-sensitive, the starting dose may be lowered to 25 mg. Treatment is most commonly started on or about the 5th day of the cycle after the start of progestin-induced bleeding or spontaneous uterine bleeding. An earlier starting date (day 3 or 4) is sometimes used, but waiting until day 9 may be too late to induce ovulation. Ovulation is expected 5 to 10 days after the last dose and is determined by BBT charts, urinary LH monitoring, plasma progesterone assay, or endometrial histology.

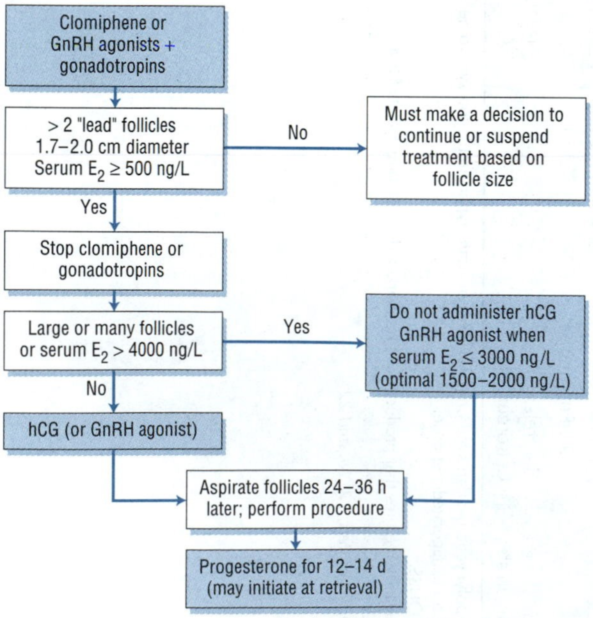

FIGURE 75–5. Flow diagram for follicular development for assisted reproductive techniques. *(Adapted from Ref. 22.)*

If the initial CC dosage is ineffective, the dosage is usually increased by 50 mg/d for the next cycle. No benefit is obtained by increasing the dose in subsequent cycles, once an ovulatory dose is found. Greater than 70% of pregnancies occur at daily dosages of 100 mg/d or less.[12] Doses of above 150 mg/d are not generally recommended. If there is a lack of ovulatory response to 150 mg daily for 5 days, or if pregnancy fails to occur after 4 to 6 ovulatory cycles, further evaluation and other treatment measures are needed. Adjuncts to CC, such as corticosteroids, estrogen, or HCG (adjunct therapy is discussed later in the chapter), or an increased duration of CC therapy, may improve chances of ovulation in some women who are unresponsive to standard therapy.[12–15] To ensure optimal timing for conception after ovulation, intercourse can be timed according to results of ultrasound or urinary LH monitoring kits, or should occur every other day for 1 week beginning 4 to 5 days after the last day of CC administration.

Precautions and contraindications are listed in Table 75–4. A uterine ultrasound can be performed prior to initiation of therapy to rule out the presence of ovarian cysts. Rates of multiple births have ranged from 5% to 12.3%, with the vast majority being twins. The antiestrogenic properties of CC cause reversible hot flushes in 11% of patients. Visual disturbances occur at an estimated rate of less than 2%. Blurring and spots or flashes (scintillating scotomata) are dose related and are an indication to discontinue therapy. Although midcycle pain (mittelschmerz) may be accentuated, abnormal ovarian enlargement is infrequently associated with normal doses of CC. However, CC is capable of causing ovarian enlargement and cyst formation with high or prolonged doses. Abdominal symptoms (discomfort, distention, bloating, and abnormal uterine bleeding) occur in 5% to 6% of patients. Miscellaneous symptoms including nausea, vomiting, breast tenderness, headache, and dizziness occur in 1% to 2.5% of patients. Until more data are available regarding a possible association between drugs used for ovulation induction and cancer, CC use should be limited to 6 or less cycles if pregnancy does not occur.[16,17]

The use of CC generally does not require intense monitoring. BBT charting as an adjunctive measure is recommended. Some experts employ pelvic ultrasound with dosage increases or serum progesterone concentration determination in an attempt to verify an adequate luteal phase.[7] Up to 85% of well-selected patients treated with CC are expected to ovulate with a conception rate of approximately 40%.[7,18] When no other causes of infertility are identified, reported conception rates range from 50% to 70%.[18]

Human Chorionic Gonadotropin

In some cases, CC and other agents cause follicular maturation with an adequate rise in the follicular phase E_2 concentration, but

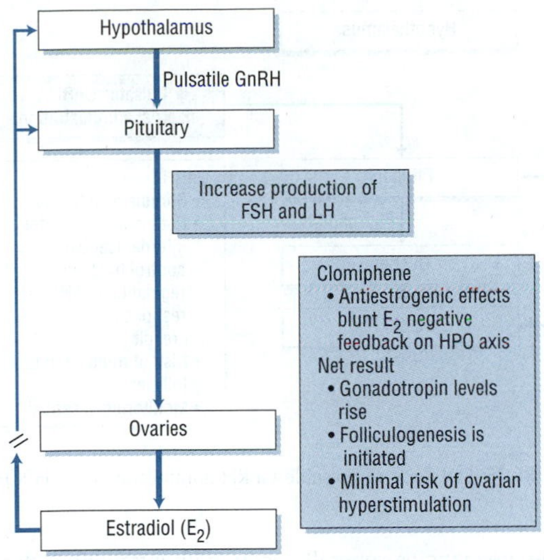

FIGURE 75–6. Effects of clomiphene on HPO axis.

ovulation fails to occur. If a lack of a midcycle gonadotropin surge is causing ovulation failure, that can be bypassed by exogenous administration of HCG (5000 to 10,000 IU intramuscularly) 3 or 4 days after the last dose of CC or when follicular diameter is 20 mm or greater by ultrasound.[7] The activity of HCG is essentially identical to that of LH, but with a longer half-life (> 24 hours versus 60 minutes). Hormonal monitoring and follicle ultrasound measurements help determine the appropriate timing of HCG administration.

Gonadotropin Therapy (hMG, FSH, and LH)

Gonadotropin replacement therapy is indicated in amenorrheic women with anovulation due to hypothalamic–pituitary insufficiency or failure. It also is used for follicular recruitment for IVF. The ovaries must be able to respond normally to FSH and LH stimulation. Gonadotropins are relatively safe when administered as ovulation-inducing drugs to properly selected patients, in correct dosages, and with appropriate monitoring. Gonadotropins are expensive, must be administered parenterally on a daily basis, and require more extensive monitoring than other methods. They are indicated only after a thorough infertility workup and careful counseling of the couple. *These agents should only be prescribed and monitored by individuals who are expert in their use.* Once exogenously administered gonadotropins are employed, the menstrual cycle, including the follicle selection process (ovarian stimulation) and ovulation, is controlled by external manipulation. Without proper monitoring, women may be at risk for severe consequences.

Human menopausal gonadotropin (hMG), obtained from the urine of postmenopausal women, contains both FSH and LH. Each vial of hMG (Pergonal) for intramuscular administration should contain equal amounts of FSH and LH activity; however, radioimmunoassay suggests a dominance of FSH. Purified FSH may be of particular benefit for women with PCOS with an increased LH to FSH ratio who have failed CC therapy, or those in ART programs. A highly purified form of extracted FSH (Fertinex) is preferred, because it can be administered subcutaneously, has better batch-to-batch consistency than earlier FHS preparations, and can be manufactured in large quantities. Recombinant technique for production of both FHS and LH is likely to represent an important step for the future of reproductive medicine.[19,20] The first recombinant FSH preparations became available in the United States in 1997.

Administration of hMG or FSH overrides the normal mechanism of ovarian follicular selection and can produce more than one mature follicle (Fig. 75–7). The earlier exogenous gonadotropin stimulation occurs during the cycle, the more follicles can reach maturity. Gonadotropins are administered daily until at least one follicle is ready to ovulate; then HCG is delivered to induce ovulation. The effective gonadotropin dose, the length of time required for follicular maturation, and the appropriate time to trigger ovulation with HCG are determined by close monitoring of follicular growth and ovarian hormone production. In some cases, CC is used in combination with gonadotropins, but it is questionable whether the pregnancy rate is enhanced.[21]

A suggested initial dose (based on FSH) is 75 to 150 IU/d beginning the third or fourth day of the cycle. The dose may need to be increased based on response. Once the serum estrogen concentration has risen steadily and is not excessive (< 1500 pg/mL), the same dosage is continued until the serum concentration is between 500 and 2000 pg/mL and one or two follicles have reached a diameter of 17 to 20 mm via ultrasound monitoring (exact criteria vary). The injections should be given at a consistent time each day (at times twice daily), and can be administered by the patient or her partner, if properly trained. Generally, gonadotropin administration should not exceed 12 days, although a longer time may be required in poor responders. Ovulation is triggered by the intramuscular administration of HCG 5000 to 10,000 IU 1 day after the last dose of gonadotropin. Intercourse is advised the day after HCG administration and for the next 2 days. Subsequent lower doses of HCG may be needed to support the luteal phase in women with low levels of estrogen and gonadotropins.

Most treatment protocols aim to induce multifollicular development; therefore, the main complications are ovarian hyperstimulation syndrome (OHSS) and obstetric and postnatal complications due to multiple gestation. When many large follicles (for example, three or more follicles larger than 15 mm in diameter) are present, or when serum E_2 concentrations are excessive (>2000 pg/mL) (exact criteria may vary), HCG administration is generally withheld and the treatment cycle terminated in order to prevent complications. In centers that perform assisted reproductive procedures, multiple follicles pose less risk of OHSS because excess follicles are punctured during the surgical procedure, thus reducing the estrogen stimulation.

However, the risk of OHSS remains even with carefully controlled ovulation because HCG has a sustained half-life compared to LH, thus allowing multiple corpus lutea to produce supraphysiologic concentrations of E_2 and progesterone throughout the luteal phase.

Although mild to moderate in most cases, OHSS occurs in 8% to 23% of artificially induced ovulatory cycles.[22] The incidence of severe hyperstimulation has declined and with proper

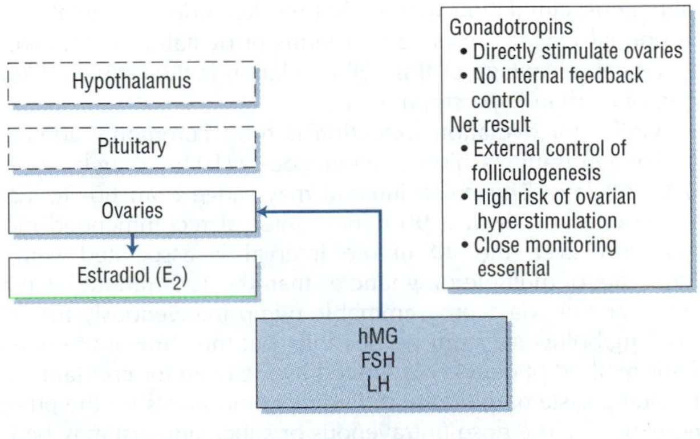

FIGURE 75–7. Effects of exogenous gonadotropins on HPO axis.

monitoring is rare. Hyperstimulation can develop rapidly over 3 to 4 days and generally within 2 weeks after HCG administration. If OHSS results in rupture of ovarian cysts, serious complications may arise from the subsequent hemoperitoneum, ascites, hypovolemia, and electrolyte imbalance. Patients should be advised to seek medical attention if they experience an increase in abdominal girth or weight gain, nausea or dizziness, pelvic pain, decrease in urine output, or shortness of breath.[22] If moderate or severe hyperstimulation is detected, discontinue treatment, begin supportive fluid and electrolyte therapy if needed, and strongly consider hospitalization for severe cases.[12,23] The ovaries slowly return to normal within 2 to 3 weeks in nonpregnant women, but will take longer in pregnant women because of endogenous HCG stimulation. A baseline ultrasound in patients who have experienced hyperstimulation in previous cycles should be performed before a new cycle of hMG stimulation is started.

Monitoring is not only necessary for adjusting therapy, but helps early recognition or prevention of OHSS. Monitoring includes ultrasonography, serum estrogen concentrations, and cervical mucus changes. In addition, the patient is usually examined clinically at least every other day during the administration of hMG and for at least 2 weeks posttreatment for signs of hyperstimulation.

The pregnancy rate with hMG–HCG therapy in amenorrheic patients with hypothalamic–pituitary insufficiency or failure may be as high as 80%, but the success rate is lower in patients with PCOS.[7] The cumulative pregnancy rate is significantly affected by age, with 90% of patients younger than 35 years of age conceiving after six treatment cycles but only 60% of patients older than 35 conceiving.[12] More than 25% of births are multiple, and of these, 74% are twins. Overall, women older than 35 years of age have a relatively poor chance of becoming pregnant. Evidence suggests that production of antibodies to FSH and LH (older, not highly purified products) may be partially responsible in women who have a poor response to exogenous gonadotropin therapy.[23]

Clinical evidence does not indicate that hMG–HCG ovulation induction places fetuses at any greater risk of malformation than the normal population. However, fetal loss due to spontaneous abortion or premature delivery of multiple gestations is of concern.[12] Hypersensitivity and febrile reactions are also reported with hMG–HCG.

Gonadotropin-Releasing Hormone for Ovulation Induction

GnRH is also commonly known as luteinizing hormone-releasing hormone (LH-RH) or luteinizing hormone-releasing factor (LRF). When given in a pulsatile fashion that mimics its release from the hypothalamus, GnRH is effective in inducing ovulation in women with hypothalamic dysfunction. GnRH therapy is also effective in women with hyperprolactinemia who are resistant to traditional therapy and to a lesser degree in women with PCOS. Continuous stimulation with GnRH results in down-regulation of the normal FSH/LH response. In terms of ovulation induction, a theoretical advantage of this self-regulation is the reduced likelihood of ovarian hyperstimulation.

GnRH for ovulation induction is most commonly administered in a pulsatile fashion subcutaneously (10 to 20 μg/bolus) for 10 to 20 days. The pulse interval may range from 60- to 120-minute intervals, with a 90-minute interval recommended most often. However, the 90-minute interval is associated with a higher rate of multiple pregnancies than the 120-minute interval. Administration via a programmable pump intravenously (usually 3 to 5 μg/bolus) may still be possible, but the clinical usefulness of this method of delivery is limited by the need for constant care of a pump system, difficulty in finding components for the pump, and expense. The dose (intravenous or subcutaneous) may be increased by 3- to 5-μg increments if the patient fails to ovulate.

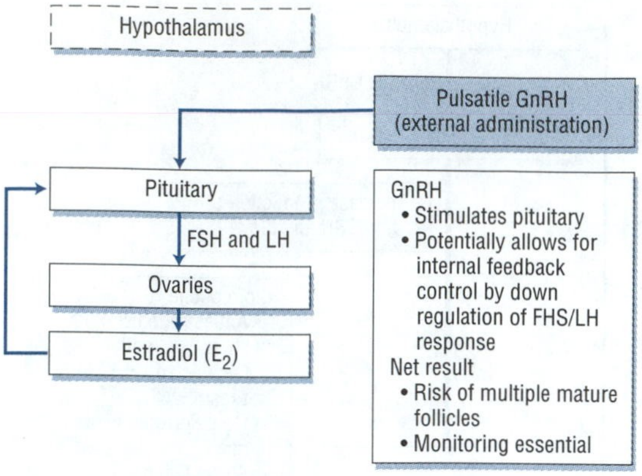

FIGURE 75–8. Effects of pulsatile GnRH administration on HPO axis.

Multiple pregnancies generally occur with intravenous dosages of 5 μg and greater. Hyperphysiologic responses occur at intravenous dosages of 4 to 5 μg (75 ng/kg).[24]

Although the subcutaneous route is better tolerated and is effective in most women with hypothalamic dysfunction, higher doses are necessary and this route does not appear to be as successful in inducing ovulation in patients with PCOS[25] or obesity.[26] Heparin (1000 IU/mL diluent) should be added if GnRH is to be administered via the intravenous route. After reconstitution, GnRH can remain biologically potent for more than 1 month.[27] Regardless of the route of administration, GnRH given at a fixed interval can produce normal gonadotropin stimulation resulting in follicular development, adequate LH surge, ovulation, and development of a healthy corpus luteum (Fig. 75–8).

The administration of a combined OC or medroxyprogesterone acetate (5 to 10 mg) for 7 to 10 days to induce withdrawal bleeding serves as a useful reference point to begin treatment. GnRH is begun 7 days after the first day of flow. Ovulation should occur within 10 to 20 days of treatment.[12] Low-dose HCG (1500 to 2500 IU IM), beginning the day after ovulation and administered every third day thereafter for three doses, is often used following pulsatile GnRH to support the luteal phase. However, continuous treatment with pulsatile GnRH alone is effective for maintaining the corpus luteum.[3] Progesterone is commonly given intramuscularly or intravaginally during the luteal phase.[28] A slow-release intravaginal progesterone gel (Crinone) appears to be as effective as larger doses of oral micronized progesterone in maintaining pregnancies brought about by ART,[29] and is the only progesterone product approved for use in assisted reproduction in the United States.

Ultrasound monitoring is recommended to decrease the risk of unrecognized ovarian hyperstimulation and multiple pregnancy even though the risk is small with this therapy (5%). Ultrasound monitoring may be used to adjust the GnRH dosage in hyporesponders. Ovulation rates of more than 90% are observed in hypothalamic insufficiency, and most patients become pregnant within 6 months of subcutaneous GnRH therapy. In women with PCOS, the ovulation rates are about 50% per treatment cycle. The addition of CC, glucocorticoids, or low-dose hMG may increase GnRH responsiveness in otherwise resistant patients.

GnRH Analogs

Analogs of GnRH are more potent, with a longer half-life than GnRH. Antagonists rapidly produce gonadotropin suppression through direct receptor blockade. GnRH agonists (GnRHa) initially cause gonadotropin stimulation during the first week followed by suppression that results from hypothalamic desensitization (Fig. 75–9).[30] Suppression of endogenous gonadotropin

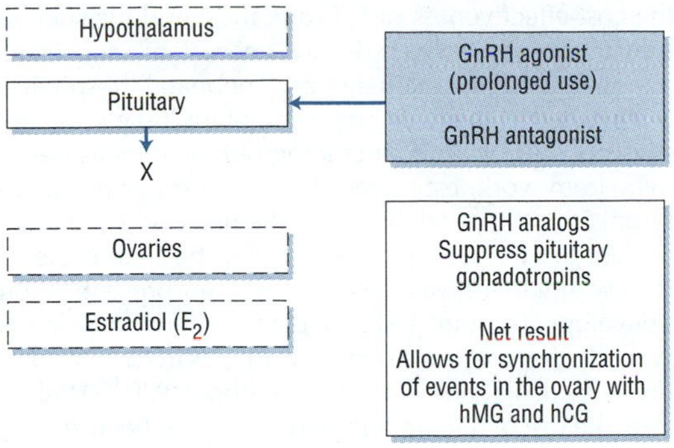

FIGURE 75–9. Effects of GnRH analogs on HPO axis.

secretion allows better follicular synchronization with exogenous gonadotropins. The use of GnRH analogs improves the predictability of ovarian response, especially in CC-resistant patients with PCOS and in superovulation regimens used with IVF.[31] Although not FDA approved for ovulation induction, GnRHa therapy is commonly used in the United States. Introduction of GnRH antagonists has been delayed because of low biologic potency and allergic reactions in the first-generation agents. Newer agents appear to have fewer problems with histamine release and are effective when administered intranasally.[32]

GnRHa is administered via nasal spray or by subcutaneous injection for up to 3 weeks starting in the luteal phase of the previous cycle or, more commonly, early in the follicular phase of a new cycle. Administration beginning in the luteal phase effectively blocks endogenous gonadotropin secretion, especially the LH surge, which could prove detrimental if premature. When a hypogonadotropic hypogonadal state is achieved, ovulation can be induced with gonadotropins. However, when given during the luteal phase, GnRHa may "rescue" the corpus luteum from the previous cycle, thus introducing unwanted progesterone into the follicular phase of the new cycle. Waiting to begin GnRHa therapy in the follicular phase takes advantage of the initial gonadotropin stimulating effects ("flare" effect) and reduces the amount of exogenous gonadotropin that is necessary to induce ovulation.[31]

The effect of GnRH analogs on pituitary and ovarian function is temporary and persists only as long as administration of the analog is continued. HPO function returns to baseline within 1 to 2 months after discontinuation of the GnRH analog. Monitoring with ultrasound and measuring E_2 response to screening tests with a GnRH agonist may help individualize ovarian stimulation and possibly reduce the risk of ovarian hyperstimulation or multiple pregnancy.[33,34]

Hormonal changes caused by the gonadotropins, particularly the GnRH analogs, can produce symptoms of estrogen deficiency, including hot flushes, vaginal dryness, and decreased libido. GnRH and its analogs also can cause allergic reactions with production of antibodies.[35] The development of anti-GnRH antibodies may reduce treatment effectiveness and contribute to the higher than expected miscarriage rate (about 20%) that occurs in GnRH-induced pregnancies. Other adverse effects are determined by route of administration (local irritation at the site of injection, or nasal irritation and bad taste in the mouth after nasal sprays). Most adverse risks involve pump function or local reactions to the needle placement and to the concurrent use of hMG. Women with myocardial valvular disease that is prone to microbial seeding of the valve should be evaluated prior to pump use. Multiple pregnancy occurs in 5% of patients. Ovarian hyperstimulation, although rare, may occur with GnRH doses greater than 10 μg/pulse intravenously or 20 μg/pulse subcutaneously. Allergic reactions may occur in patients receiving long-term treatment.

Dopamine Agonists (Bromocriptine, Cabergoline)

Dopamine agonists are clearly indicated for women whose infertility is related to hyperprolactinemia with or without galactorrhea (80% fertility rate after therapy). Bromocriptine, a semisynthetic ergotamine derivative, acts as a dopamine agonist to directly inhibit pituitary prolactin secretion. Cabergoline is a long-acting dopamine agonist with a high affinity for the D_2 receptors. Normalizing prolactin concentration restores central gonadotropin function. The use of dopamine agonists may reduce the size of prolactin-producing pituitary tumors and return serum prolactin concentrations to normal. Hyperprolactinemia also occurs in up to 20% to 40% of patients with PCOS. Dopamine agonists may help correct the inappropriate release of LH in these patients by normalizing prolactin.[36] Bromocriptine has been sometimes used with variable success in combination with CC in patients who appear to have normal prolactin levels with or without galactorrhea.

Bromocriptine treatment is usually initiated with a bedtime dose of 1.25 mg for 1 week, and then titrated up based on prolactin concentrations. Doses greater than 15 mg/d are rare.[12] Once ovulation begins to occur, bromocriptine should be taken during the follicular phase. If pregnancy does not occur in a cycle as determined by a sensitive pregnancy test, the drug can be stopped during the luteal phase and begun again after the next menses starts. Cabergoline is initiated at a dose of 0.25 mg twice weekly and titrated to a dose of 1 mg twice weekly based on serum prolactin concentrations.

Ovulatory menses and pregnancy occur in 80% of individuals with galactorrhea or hyperprolactinemia. If there is no objective indication that ovulation is occurring within 3 months despite normal prolactin, then CC and/or gonadotropins may be added.

Nausea, headache, and dizziness are common side effects of dopamine agonists. Psychiatric symptoms may occur in less than 1% of patients. Other complaints include orthostatic hypotension, nasal congestion, vomiting, constipation, and abdominal cramps. Side effects from oral administration can be minimized by slow dosage titration and by taking the dose at bedtime and with food. Intravaginal and intramuscular administration of bromocriptine may also prove to be beneficial and reduce the incidence of side effects.[37] There is no evidence of increased teratogenicity with use of dopamine agonists, but barrier contraception is recommended until normal menstrual cycles are established.[12]

ADJUNCTIVE THERAPY

Corticosteroid supplementation may act synergistically with CC to promote folliculogenesis and ovulation.[14,38] The primary mechanism is thought to be lowering the circulating levels of adrenal androgens that might otherwise inhibit folliculogenesis or aromatase activity, but other mechanisms may exist. Dexamethasone (0.5 to 1 mg/d) or prednisone (5 to 10 mg/d) should be taken at bedtime until pregnancy occurs. The dose of CC usually remains unchanged from the previous cycle.

Clomiphene citrate has associated antiestrogen effects causing thick, tenacious cervical mucus that can hinder sperm migration. Although the increased amount of estrogen being produced by multiple maturing follicles usually overrides this effect, exogenous estrogen (ethinyl estradiol, 10 to 20 μg/d, or conjugated equine estrogens 0.3 to 2.5 mg/d on cycle days 10 to 16) in combination with CC may improve the quality of the cervical mucus. The lower doses (conjugated equine estrogens 0.3 mg) may be begun as early as cycle day 4. The addition of estrogen to progesterone during the luteal phase after CC stimulation for IVF may also improve pregnancy rates.[39] Other therapeutic attempts to improve the cervical mucus quality include guaifenesin and potassium iodide. If sperm penetration through the cervical mucus remains a problem, artificial intrauterine insemination with the partner's sperm may be attempted.

Tamoxifen, a nonsteroidal antiestrogen primarily indicated for adjuvant treatment of breast cancer, has successfully treated infertility in anovulatory women who have failed CC. The usual dose is 20 to 40 mg/d for 4 to 5 days commencing after menstruation, or at any time in amenorrheal women.[40] A proposed mechanism is lowering prolactin levels by reducing estrogen stimulation.[25]

Growth hormone (GH) may be involved with the regulation of ovarian activity, but the exact role is unknown. The addition of GH to poor responders to gonadotropin therapy has been tried with variable success.[41–44]

PHARMACOECONOMIC CONSIDERATIONS

Third party health insurance coverage for infertility treatments varies considerably with respect to the type and amount of treatments covered.[45,46] Generally, payers do not recognize infertility as a disease, and some view it as a condition to be addressed on an individual basis.[46] Many couples have limited or no health care coverage, and the high cost of infertility treatments places a burden on their life savings. Despite the significant cost implications, very few analyses of the relative cost-effectiveness of infertility treatments in the United States have been conducted.[45] The cost of a treatment cycle of IVF ranges from $7000 to 11,000. However, when considering the cost-effectiveness of IVF, one must add the success rates measured in women delivered and the cost of "successful" IVF pregnancies including antenatal and neonatal hospitalizations, usually attributed to the high incidence of multiple pregnancies.[47] An analysis of these factors, including outcome measures such as time away from work, estimated that the cost per delivery of IVF ranges from $50,000 per delivery for the first cycle in women with tubal disease to $800,000 per delivery for the sixth cycle in older women in whom there was also a male factor present.[47] Some advocate developing a managed care plan for infertility, claiming the cost savings to the insurance company ranges from 10% to 20% for infertility-related diagnoses, with or without IVF.[48] Within managed care, the use of a financial model has also been suggested as a way to identify treatment algorithms that can be used to calculate how capitation rates will affect practice revenue and profit, while educating physicians on the cost of their medical decisions.[49]

One study compared the cost-effectiveness of infertility treatments at an academic institution. Intrauterine insemination (IUI), CC-IUI, and hMG-IUI were found similar in terms of cost per delivery, and all were more cost-effective procedures than ART. These procedures are preferred in infertile couples with open fallopian tubes. For women with blocked fallopian tubes, IVF appears to be cost effective when compared to surgery (e.g., neosalpingostomy performed by laparotomy).[45]

EVALUATION OF THERAPEUTIC OUTCOMES

Few pharmacists are directly involved with therapeutic management of infertility because most of the treatment and close monitoring occurs within the setting of the infertility center. With the exception of CC and bromocriptine, which are relatively safe, the drugs needing to be monitored require high technology and expert supervision. Similarly, the treatment regimens, including drug and dose, are often based on a complex combination of the underlying disorder and the individual patient's response to follicular development and ovulation as indicated by ultrasound or laboratory parameters. Patients who have received any ovulation-stimulating agent should receive close clinical surveillance for ovarian cancer, even after therapy.[18] However, pharmacists need to understand and respect the psychological component of the patient and/or couple receiving treatment for infertility. The process of diagnosing and treating infertility has a dramatic impact on the lives of the couple. The emotional pain and impact of infertility, combined with the time-consuming and expensive therapeutic manipulations and monitoring procedures, can take a toll on relationships, self-esteem, health, and security. Couples seeking treatment often experience severe anxiety, grief, and depression as a result of the process. In addition to being understanding and supportive, pharmacists may help relieve some of the fears and frustration by explaining the purpose of drugs being used, side effects to expect, and the importance of adhering to the prescribed monitoring regimen. Pharmacists should advise patients to notify their physician if they experience an increase in abdominal girth, nausea, pelvic pain, decreased urine output, weight gain greater than 2.25 kg, dizziness, or shortness of breath. If properly trained, pharmacists could assist in the administration of or education regarding intramuscular or subcutaneous gonadotropin therapy. Pharmacists can also educate patients on the proper method for obtaining and interpreting basal body temperature and using home kits for detecting LH surge. Pharmacists should also be alert to serious psychological disturbances that may manifest in the infertile couple, encourage them to discuss these issues with each other and their infertility therapist, or refer patients for appropriate psychological consultation.

► PRINCIPLES OF PHARMACOTHERAPY

- Customarily, treatment for infertility should not be sought until after 1 year of unprotected coitus without conception.
- Approach to treatment is based on the likely cause of infertility. More than one factor in one or both of the partners may contribute to the infertility.
- Investigation of the male partner should be completed before beginning treatment of the female partner.
- Some therapeutic agents used for induction of ovulation augment the patient's natural endocrine process (e.g., clomiphene citrate), while other agents take control of, and in some cases replace, the natural cycle (e.g., menotropins, gonadotropins).
- Clomiphene should be used at the lowest effective dose, because multiple births and adverse effects are dose dependent.

- Clomiphene should not be used for more than 6 cycles because of the potential risk of ovarian cancer.
- Menotropins/gonadotropins are second-line therapeutic options because of cost, the high risk of multiple pregnancies, and ovarian hyperstimulation syndrome (OHSS).
- Close daily monitoring by trained experts is *essential* when menotropins or gonadotropins are used.
- OHSS is a possible side effect of fertility drugs and is rare with proper monitoring. Patients taking fertility drugs should be advised to notify their physician if they experience an increase in abdominal girth, nausea, pelvic pain, decreased urine output, weight gain of more than 2.25 kg, dizziness, or shortness of breath.
- For unknown reasons, the rate of fetal loss is higher in pregnancies derived through assisted reproductive technology.

REFERENCES

1. Talbert LM. Overview of the diagnostic evaluation, In: Hammond MG, Talbert LM, eds. Infertility: A Practical Guide for Physicians, 3rd ed. Boston, Blackwell, 1993:1–10.
2. Jones HW, Toner JP. The infertile couple. N Engl J Med 1993;329: 1710–1712.
3. Speroff L, Glass RH, Kase NG. Clinical Gynecologic Endocrinology and Infertility, 5th ed. Baltimore, William & Wilkins, 1994:183–230, 897–930.
4. Taymor ML. The regulation of follicle growth: Some clinical implications in reproductive endocrinology. Fertil Steril 1996;65:235–247.
5. American College of Obstetrics and Gynecologists (ACOG). Hyperandrogenic chronic anovulation. ACOG Technical Bulletin 202. Washington, DC, ACOG, 1995.
6. Wilcox L, Mosher W. The use of infertility services in the United States. In: Proceedings and Abstracts of the 48th Annual Meeting of the American Fertility Society, New Orleans, October–November 1992. Birmingham, American Fertility Society, 1993:S138. Abstract.
7. American College of Obstetrics and Gynecologists (ACOG). Infertility. ACOG Technical Bulletin 125. Washington, DC, ACOG 1989.
8. Bristow RE, Karlan BY. Ovulation induction, infertility, and ovarian cancer risk. Fertil Steril 1996;66:499–507.
9. Shushan A, Paltiel O, Iscovich J, et al. Human menopausal gonadotropin and the risk of epithelian ovarian cancer. Fertil Steril 1996; 65:13–18.
10. Mosgaard BJ, Lidegaard Ø, Kjaer SK, et al. Infertilty, fertility drugs, and invasive ovarian cancer: A case control study. Fertil Steril 1997; 67:1005–1012.
11. Rossing MA, Daling JR, Weiss NS, et al. Ovarian tumors in a cohort of infertile women. N Engl J Med 1994;331:771–776.
12. American College of Obstetrics and Gynecologists (ACOG). Managing the anovulatory state: Medical induction of ovulaton. ACOG Technical Bulletin 197. Washington, DC, ACOG, 1994.
13. Fluker MR, Wang IY, Rowe TC. An extended 10-day course of climiphene citrate (CC) in women with CC-resistant ovulatory disorders. Fertil Steril 1996;66:761–764.
14. Isaacs JD Jr, Lincoln SR, Cowan BD. Extended clomiphene citrate (CC) and prednisone for the treatment of chronic anovulation resistant to CC alone. Fertil Steril 1997;67:641–643.
15. Kelly AC, Jewelewicz R. Alternate regimens for ovulation induction in polycystic ovarian disease. Fertil Steril 1990;54:195–202.
16. King TM. Ovarian cancer and fertility drugs. Cancer Bull 1994;46: 181–184.
17. Rossing MA, Dailing JR, Weiss NS, et al. Ovarian tumors in a cohort of infertile women. N Engl J Med. 1994;331:771–776.
18. Investigation of anovulatory infertility guides treatment. Drugs Ther Perspect 1997;9:6–9.
19. Shoman Z, Insler V. Recombinant technique and gonadotropin production: New era in reproductive medicine. Fertil Steril 1996;66: 187–201.
20. Lunenfeld B, Lunenfeld E. Gonadotropic preparations—Lessons learned. Fertil Steril 1997;67:812–814. Editorial.
21. Ransom MX, Doughman NC, Garcia AJ. Menotropins alone are superior to a clomiphene citrate and menotropin combination for superovulation induction among clomiphene citrate failures. Fertil Steril 1996;65:1169–1174.
22. Safety factors important with drug use in assisted reproduction. Drugs Ther Perspect 1997;10:1–5.
23. Borenstein R, Elhalah U, Lunenfeld B, Schwartz ZS. Severe ovarian hyperstimulation syndrome: A reevaluated therapeutic approach. Fertil Steril 1989;51:791–795.
24. Santoro N, Wierman ME, Filicori M, et al. Intravenous administration of pulsatile gonadotropin-releasing hormone in hypothalamic amenorrhea: Effects of dosage. J Clin Endocrinol Metab 1986;62:109–116.
25. Sakamoto H, Den K, Kondo Y, et al. Evidence that estrogen may be a key factor in hyperprolactinemic anovulation: A case report. Am J Obstet Gynecol 1987;157:318–319.
26. Lyles R, Elkind-Hirsch K, Goldzieher, Besch PK. Plasma gonadotropin releasing hormone profiles after intravenous and subcutaneous bolus injection in thin and obese women. Obstet Gynecol 1988;71:44–48.
27. Hahn PM, Van Vugt DA, Reid RL. The stability of synthetic gonadotropin-releasing hormone in solution. Fertil Steril 1987;48:155–158.
28. Hammond MG. Management of ovulatory dysfunction. In: Hammond MG, Talbert LM, eds. Infertility: A Practical Guide for Physicians, 3rd ed. Boston, Blackwell, 1993:151–181.
29. Pouly JL, Bassil S, Frydman R, et al. Luteal support after in-vitro fertilization: Crinone 8%, a sustained release vaginal progesterone gel, versus Utrogestan, an oral micronized progesterone. Human Reprod 1996;11:2085–2089.
30. Hall JE. Gonadotropin-releasing hormone antagonists: Effects on the ovarian follicle and corpus luteum. Clin Obstet Gynecol 1993;36: 744–752.
31. Grosskinsky CM, Hammond MG. Ovulation induction in the anovulatory woman with GnRH agonists. Semin Reprod Endocrinol 1993;11: 136–141.
32. Fujimoto VY, Monroe SE, Nelson LR, et al. Dose-related suppression of serum luteinizing hormone in women by a potent new gonadotropin-releasing hormone antagonist (Ganirelix) administered by intranasal spray. Fertil Steril 1997;67:469–473.
33. Itskovitz-Eldor J, Levron J, Kol S. Use of gonadotropin-releasing hormone agonist to cause ovulation and prevent ovarian hyperstimulation syndrome. Clin Obstet Gynecol 1993;36:701–710.
34. Garcia JE. Gonadotropin-releasing hormone and its analogs: Applications in gynecology. Clin Obstet Gynecol 1993;36:719–723.
35. Meyer WR, Lavy G, DeCherney AH, et al. Evidence of gonadal and gonadotropin antibodies in women with a suboptimal ovarian response to exogenous gonadotropin. Obstet Gynecol 1990;75:795–799.
36. Paoletti AM, Cagnacci A, Depau GF, et al. The chronic administration of cabergoline normalizes androgen secretion and improves menstrual cyclicity in women with polycyctic ovary syndrome. Fertil Steril 1996:66;527–532.
37. Katz E, Adashi EY. Treatment of infertility using bromocriptine mesylate, In: Seibel MM, ed. Infertility: A Comprehensive Text. Norwalk, CT, Appleton & Lange, 1990:351–362.
38. Trott EA, Plouffe Jr L, Hansen K, et al. Ovulation induction in clomiphene-resistant anovulatory women with normal dehydroepiandrosterone sulfate levels: Beneficial effects of the addition of dexamethasone during the follicular phase. Fertil Steril 1996;66:484–486.

39. Hurd WW, Randolph JF, Christman GM, et al. Luteal support with both estradiol and progesterone after clomiphene citrate stimulation for *in vitro* ferilization. Fertil Steril 1996;66:587–592.
40. Buckley MMT, Goa KL. Tamoxifen, a reappraisal of its pharmacodynamic and pharmacokinetic properties and therapeutic use. Drugs 1989;37:451–490.
41. Schoolcraft W, Schlender T, Gee M, et al. Improved controlled ovarian hyperstimulation in poor responders *in vitro* fertilization patients with a microdose follicle-stimulating hormone flare, growth hormone protocol. Fertil Steril 1997;67:93–97.
42. Homburg R, West C, Torresani T, Jacobs HS. Cotreatment with human growth hormone and gonadotropins for induction of ovulation: A controlled clinical trial. Fertil Steril 1990;53:254–260.
43. Ibrahim ZHZ, Lieberman BA, Matson PL, et al. The use of biosynthetic growth hormone to augment ovulation induction with buserelin acetate/human menopausal gonadotropin in women with a poor ovarin response. Fertil Steril 1991;55:202–204.
44. Hughes SM, Huang ZH, Morris ID, et al. A double-blind cross-over controlled study to evaluate the effect of human biosynthetic growth hormone on ovarian stimulation in previous poor responders to in-vitro fertilization. Hum Reprod 1994;9:13–18.
45. VanVoorhis BJ, Sparks AE, Allen BD, et al. Cost effectiveness of infertility treatments: A cohort study. Fertil Steril 1997; 67:830–836.
46. Soules MR. Now that we have painted ourselves in a corner. Fertil Steril 1996; 66:693–696.
47. Goldfarb JM, Austin C, Lisbona H, et al. Cost-effectiveness of in-vitro fertilization. Obstet Gynecol 1996;87:18–21.
48. Bates GW. The economics of infertility: Developing an infertility managed-care plan. Am J Obstet Gynecol 1996;174:1200–1207.
49. Rabin DS, Qadeer U, Steir VE. A cost and outcome model of fertility treatment in a managed care enviroment. Fertil Steril 1996;66: 896–903.

76

CONTRACEPTION

Kathryn K. Bucci, PharmD, BCPS, and Deborah Stier Carson, PharmD, BCPS

Comprehension of mechanisms involved in the hormonal regulation of the normal menstrual cycle is essential to understanding contraception and infertility in women. Please refer to Chapter 75 for a review of the menstrual cycle. Contraception generally implies the prevention of pregnancy following sexual intercourse by inhibiting viable sperm from coming into contact with a mature ovum (methods act as barriers or prevent ovulation) or by preventing a fertilized ovum from successfully implanting in the endometrium (mechanisms that create an unfavorable uterine environment).

COMPARATIVE EFFECTIVENESS OF VARIOUS METHODS OF CONTRACEPTION

Commonly used methods of reversible contraception include oral contraceptives, long-acting injectable or implantable progestins, condoms, spermicides, withdrawal, the diaphragm, periodic abstinence, and the intrauterine device. These methods differ in their relative effectiveness, safety, and patient acceptability.[1–4]

The actual effectiveness of any contraceptive method is difficult to determine because many factors affect contraceptive failure. Failure inherent in the proper use of the contraceptive alone is considered a "method failure" or "perfect use failure." "User failure" or "typical use failure" takes into account the user's ability to follow directions correctly and consistently (Table 76–1).

ORAL CONTRACEPTIVES

Oral contraceptives (OCs), the most popular method of reversible contraception in the United States, are highly effective for birth control (Table 76–1).[2] When used correctly, their effectiveness approaches that of surgical sterilization.

COMPOSITION AND FORMULATIONS

The currently available OCs contain either a combination of a synthetic estrogen and synthetic progestin, or a progestin alone. Estrogens suppress follicle-stimulating hormone (FSH) and thus prevent the development of a dominant follicle. Estrogens also potentiate the action of the progestin component, which suppresses the luteinizing hormone (LH) surge. Thus, even if follicular growth is not adequately blunted by the estrogenic component, ovulation is blocked by action of the progestin. Estrogen also serves to stabilize the endometrial lining (bleeding cycle control), while the progestin contributes to other contraceptive effects on cervical mucus (thickened/impermeable) and the endometrium (involution/atrophy).[4,6,7]

The currently available low-dose combination OCs (21 days of active hormones/cycle) are modifications of the original products introduced in 1960 and contain approximately three- to fourfold less estrogen and one-tenth the progestin dose found in earlier pills.[7] Over the past decade, combination multiphasic (biphasic and triphasic) formulations have further lowered the total monthly hormonal dose without clearly demonstrating a significant clinical advantage.[1,4,7] Also introduced in 1960, the progestin-only "minipills" (28 days of active hormone/cycle) are still available. Containing even lower doses of progestin than found in combination OCs and lacking the contribution of estrogen, minipills tend to be less effective that combination OCs with typical use and are generally reserved for women who must avoid estrogen.

COMPONENTS

Two synthetic estrogens commonly used in OCs in the United States, ethinyl estradiol (EE) and mestranol, differ only by the presence of a methyl group attached to mestranol at the C-3 site. Mestranol, which must be converted by the liver to EE before it is pharmacologically active, is estimated to be 50% less potent than EE.[3,8] Progestins currently used in OCs include ethynodiol diacetate, desogestrel, gestodene (not available in the United States), norgestimate, norethindrone, norethindrone acetate, norethynodrel, norgestrel, and its active isomer levonorgestrel. Progestins vary in their progestational activity and differ with respect to inherent estrogenic, antiestrogenic, and androgenic effects.[2,3,8] Estrogenic and antiestrogenic properties are secondary to the extent of progestin's metabolism to estrogenic substances, whereas androgenic activity is determined by structural similarity of the progestin to testosterone (receptor binding and activity) and the ability to affect free testosterone concentrations through impact on sex hormone binding globulin, a major carrier protein for testosterone.[9]

Third-generation OCs contain newer progestins (e.g., norgestimate, desogestrel, and gestodene). These progestins are potent progestational agents that appear to have no estrogenic effects and are less androgenic when compared to levonorgestrel on a weight basis. Unfortunately, clinical trials comparing the differences between OCs are few and sample size is small, so determining actual relevance of these purported improvements in progestational selectivity and lower androgenic activity remains

TABLE 76–1. Comparison of Reversible Methods of Contraception

Method	Absolute Contraindications	Advantages	Disadvantages	Percent of Women With Pregnancy[a]	
				Lowest Expected	*Typical Use*
Episodic Contraceptive Methods					
Spermicides alone	Allergy to spermicide	Inexpensive No office visit required Some protection against STDs	High user failure rate Must be reapplied before each act of intercourse May cause local irritation in either partner May enhance HIV transmission (?)	3.0	21.0
Condoms, male	Allergy to latex or rubber	Inexpensive Readily available No office visit required STD protection, including HIV (latex only)	Poor acceptance Possibility of breakage Efficacy decreased by oil-based lubricants Latex can cause allergic reactions in either partner	2.0	12.0
Condoms, female (Reality)	Allergy to polyurethane History of toxic shock syndrome	Can be inserted just before intercourse or ahead of time; provides protection for 48 hours STD protection, including HIV	Dislike ring hanging outside vagina Cumbersome	5	21
Diaphragm with spermicide	Allergy to latex, rubber, or spermicide Recurrent UTIs History of toxic shock syndrome Abnormal gynecologic anatomy	Low cost Decreased incidence of cervical neoplasia STD protection, including HIV Can be inserted for up to 6 hours before intercourse	Office visit required Decreased efficacy with increased frequency of intercourse Must be refitted after significant change in weight (± 10 pounds) Increased incidence of vaginal yeast and UTI infections Increased incidence of toxic shock syndrome Efficacy affected by oil-based lubricants Cervical irritation	6.0	18.0
Cervical cap (Prentif)	Allergy to rubber or spermicide History of toxic shock syndrome Abnormal gynecologic anatomy Abnormal Pap smear	Low cost STD protection, including HIV Can be inserted just before or ahead of time; provides protection for 48 hours.	Office visit required May be difficult for patient to use correctly Decreased efficacy with parity Not possible to fit all patients	6.0	18.0
Hormonal Methods					
OCs	Hepatic adenomas Thromboembolic disorders or history thereof Cerebrovascular or coronary artery disease Known or suspected breast cancer Undiagnosed abnormal gynecologic bleeding Cardiovascular risk factors (relative contraindication) Jaundice with pregnancy or previous pill use	Decreased risk of pelvic inflammatory disease, ovarian and endometrial cancer Improvement in endometriosis (probably) Fewer functional ovarian cysts (possibly) Less salpingitis; ectopic pregnancy Prevention of benign breast disease (fibroadenoma and fibrocyctic changes) Less rheumatoid arthritis (possibly) Increased bone density (possibly) Improvement in acne/hirsutism *Significant improvement in menstrually related problems:* Fewer cramps; less flow for fewer days; less iron-deficiency anemia; more predictable menses; elimination of mittelschmerz; less dysmenorrhea/premenstrual tension syndrome	Increased risk of benign hepatocellular adenomas Mild increased risk of thromboembolism and stroke May elevate blood pressure No protection against most STDs Estrogenic side effects (nausea, breast tenderness, fluid retention) Progestogen side effects (acne, increased appetite, depression) Increased risk of myocardial infarction in older smokers, nausea, headache	0.1	3.0
Progestin-only OCs	Undiagnosed abnormal gynecologic bleeding	May be used by lactating women and women with cardiovascular risk Allows avoidance of estrogen-related side effects Protection against PID, iron deficiency anemia, and dysmenorrhea	Frequent spotting/amenorrhea Increased risk of ectopic pregnancy Must take every day at the same time	0.5	3.0

Progestin Implants Norplant and Norplant II (levonorgestrel) Capronor (levonorgestrel) Implanon (3-ketodesogestrel) Uniplant (nomegestrol acetate)	Undiagnosed abnormal gynecologic bleeding Acute liver disease Benign or malignant liver tumors Known or suspected breast cancer Active thrombophlebitis or thromboembolic disease	Passive contraception Duration of efficacy varies; effective up to 5 years with Norplant in women < 154 pounds Effects are quickly reversible Less menstrual cramping/mittelschmerz pain No suppression of lactation No metabolic disturbances Can be considered for use in women who have diabetes, hypertension, gall bladder disease, history of cardiovascular or thromboembolic disease, SLE, or sickle-cell disease; in women who are smokers or lactating.	Requires outpatient surgical procedure Irregular menstrual bleeding, headaches, weight gain (?), acne Progestin side effects Local infection or bruising on insertion; removal may be difficult Expensive initially High discontinuation rate Unacceptable in patients using some anti-convulsants	0.2	0.2
Depo-Provera	Pregnancy Undiagnosed abnormal gynecologic bleeding Known or suspected breast cancer Liver disease (relative contraindication) Severe depression (relative contraindication) Severe cardiovascular disease (relative contraindication)	No suppression of lactation No increased risk of thromboembolism Passive contraception No drug interactions May decrease seizures Effective for 3 months Can be considered for use in women who have seizure disorders, diabetes, hypertension, gall bladder disease, history of cardiovascular or thromboembolic disease, SLE, or sickle-cell disease; in women who are smokers or lactating.	Irregular menstrual bleeding, headache, weight gain, acne Delayed return of fertility Possible increased risk of breast cancer in younger users Decreased HDL Progestin side effects Decreased bone density in long-term users Office visit required	0.3	0.3
Intrauterine Devices (Hormonal and Nonhormonal)					
Copper-T 380A (Paragard)	Multiple sexual partners/partner with multiple partners (high risk for STDs) History of PID or ectopic pregnancy, acute pelvic infection Abnormal uterine cavity/pelvic surgery/undiagnosed vaginal bleeding Uterine or cervical cancer	Passive contraception Long-term contraception (can remain in place up to 10 years) Less expensive per year and easier for some patients No delay in return of fertility after removal	Increased heavy bleeding Spotting between periods increased cramping and dysmenorrhea Increased risk of ectopic pregnancy Office visit required Rarely uterine perforation	0.8	<1.0
Progesterone T (Progestasert)	Postpartum endometritis or infected abortion in previous 3 months Acute cervicitis or vaginitis (including BV) until infection controlled	Remains in place for 1 year Decreased cramping and dysmenorrhea Decrease in menstrual blood loss No delay in return of fertility after removal	Office visit required Must be changed each year Increased risks of ectopic pregnancy Rarely uterine perforation	2.0	<2.0
Levonorgestrel IUD	Conditions associated with increased susceptibility to infections, including leukemia, AIDS, IV drug abuse, and corticosteroid use Valvular heart disease (±) Nulliparity (±) Genital actinomyces Wilson's disease[b] Allergy to copper[b]	Constant rate of hormone release for 5 years Possibly the single most effective reversible contraceptive method over 5-year period Decreased cramping and dysmenorrhea Reduced incidence of ID and menorrhagia Combines benefits of Norplant and Copper-T	Office visit required Irregular menstrual bleeding (?) Rarely uterine perforation	Not available	Not available

STD = sexually transmitted disease; UTI = urinary tract infection; PID = pelvic inflammatory disease; SLE = systemic lupus erythematosus; HDL = high density lipoprotein cholesterol; BV = bacterial vaginosis.
[a]Failure rates during first year of use, United States.
[b]Contraindication for copper IUD only.

TABLE 76–2. Composition of Commonly Prescribed Oral Contraceptives[a]

Product	Composition				Spotting & BTB[b] (%)
	Estrogen	*μg*	*Progestin*	*mg*	
50-μg Estrogen					
Ovral	E. estradiol	50	norgestrel	0.5	4.5
Norlestrin 2.5/50	E. estradiol	50	nor. acetate	2.5	5.1
Genora/Norethin/Norinyl/Ortho-Novum 1/50	Mestranol	50	norethindrone	1.0	10.6
Ovcon 50	E. estradiol	50	norethindrone	1.0	11.9
Demulen 50	E. estradiol	50	ethy. diacetate	1.0	13.9
Norlestrin 1/50	E. estradiol	50	nor. acetate	1.0	13.6
Sub-50-μg Estrogen Monophasic					
Lo-Ovral	E. estradiol	30	norgestrel	0.3	9.6
Desogen/Ortho-Cept	E. estradiol	30	desogestrel	0.15	9.9
Ovcon 35	E. estradiol	35	norethindrone	0.4	11.0
Levlen/Nordette/Min-Ovral[c]	E. estradiol	30	levonorgestrel	0.15	14.0
Ortho-Cyclen	E. estradiol	35	norgestimate	0.25	14.3
Brevicon/Modicon/Nelova 0.5/35 Brevicon/Ortho 0.5/35[c]	E. estradiol	35	norethindrone	0.5	14.6
Genora/Nelova/Norethin/Norinyl/Ortho-Novum 1/35 Ortho 1/35[c]	E. estradiol	35	norethindrone	1.0	14.7
Loestrin 1.5/30	E. estradiol	30	nor. acetate	1.5	25.2
Loestrin/Minestrin[c] 1/20	E. estradiol	20	nor. acetate	1.0	29.7
Alesse/Levlite	E. estradiol	20	levonorgestrel	0.1	
Demulen 1/35	E. estradiol	35	ethy. diacetate	1.0	37.4
Sub-50-μg Estrogen Multiphasic[d]					
Ortho Novum 7/7/7	E. estradiol E. estradiol E. estradiol	35(7) 35(7) 35(7)	norethindrone norethindrone norethindrone	0.5(7) 0.75(7) 1.0(7)	12.2
Jenest	E. estradiol E. estradiol	35(7) 35(14)	norethindrone norethindrone	0.5(7) 1.0(14)	14.1
Tri-Levlen/TriPhasil Triquilar[c]	E. estradiol E. estradiol E. estradiol	30(6) 40(5) 30(10)	levonorgestrel levonorgestrel levonorgestrel	0.05(6) 0.075(5) 0.125(10)	15.1
Tri-Norinyl/Synphasic[c]	E. estradiol E. estradiol E. estradiol	35(7) 35(7) 35(7)	norethindrone norethindrone norethindrone	0.5(7) 1.0(9) 0.5(5)	14.7
Estrostep 21/Estrostep FE	E. estradiol E. estradiol E. estradiol	20 (5)▲ 30 (7)■ 35 (9)●	nor. acetate	1.0	18 (first cycle)
Tri-Cyclen	E. estradiol E. estradiol E. estradiol	35(7) 35(7) 35(7)	norgestimate norgestimate norgestimate	0.180(7) 0.215(7) 0.250(7)	17.5
Ortho Novum 10-11	E. estradiol E. estradiol	35(10) 35(11)	norethindrone norethindrone	0.5(10) 1.0(11)	19.6
Progestin Only					
Ovrette	None	—	norgestrel	0.075	34.9
Micronor/Nor Q.D.	None	—	norethindrone	0.35	42.3

E. = estradiol-ethinyl estradiol; Ethy. diacetate = ethynodiol diacetate; Nor. acetate = norethindrone acetate; BTB = breakthrough bleeding.

▲, ■, ● = tablet shapes.

[a]Oral contraceptives containing greater than 50 μg of estrogen are not included in this chart. These products are generally not necessary to prevent conception and are associated with an increase in serious complications. Women who may need to use the higher strength estrogen include women who have had a contraceptive failure while *properly* taking a product containing 50 μg of estrogen, women who are concomitantly taking a medication that decreases the efficacy of the estrogen, or women who have severe acne. The higher-dose estrogen products are also used to treat other conditions such as ovarian cysts, endometriosis, and dysfunctional uterine bleeding.

[b]Reported prevalence of BTB and spotting in the third cycle of use. Information was submitted to the FDA by the manufacturer. These rates are derived from individual studies conducted by various investigators, and therefore information should not be precisely compared.

[c]Canadian trade name.

[d]Number in parentheses indicates number of tablets (days) in each phase.

Adapted from Ref. 8

unknown.[7,10] Table 76–2 lists available OC products by brand name and specifies hormonal composition.

CONSIDERATIONS WITH ORAL CONTRACEPTIVE USE

Oral contraceptives are highly effective and, when used properly, extremely safe.[7,11] However, a complete medical history and physical examination should be obtained before a patient is started on an OC, and the risks and contraindications to OC use must be carefully considered (Tables 76–3 to 76–5).[3,4,7,8,11]

Generally, OCs are an acceptable form of birth control for nonsmoking women up to the age of menopause, with women over 40 using the lowest-dose estrogen products.[2–4,12] An exsmoker for at least 1 year can be regarded as a nonsmoker.[4] Oral contraceptives containing estrogen are absolutely contraindicated in smokers over the age of 35, and relatively contraindicated in younger women who are heavy smokers (15 or more cigarettes per day). One possible exception may be a 20-μg estrogen formulation. This extremely low dose OC does not appear to have an impact on clotting factors and platelet activation, even in smokers.[13] Progestin-only pills are generally acceptable for women in whom an estrogen is contraindicated.[7,14] Numerous noncontraceptive benefits, including relief from menstrually related problems and prevention of several diseases, have been attributed to OC use (Table 76–1). However, certain patient-specific characteristics and concomitant disease states increase the patient's risk for adverse effects relating to OC use (Table 76–4).[4,7,15]

Combination OCs, even those containing less than 35 μg of estrogen, can cause small increases in blood pressure, although clinically significant increases are rare with low dose OCs.[16] If an OC-related increase in blood pressure occurs, discontinuing the OC usually results in a return to pretreatment blood pressure values within 3 to 6 months.[4]

OCs appear to affect carbohydrate and lipid metabolism, possibly through the progestin component.[17–24] With the exception of some levonorgestrel-containing products, formulations containing low dose of progestins do not significantly alter insulin, glucose, or glucagon release after a glucose load in healthy women or in those with a history of gestational diabetes.[19–21] The new progestins

TABLE 76–3. Absolute and Relative Contraindications to the Use of Oral Contraception

Absolute Contraindications

1. Thrombophlebitis, thromboembolic disorders, cerebral vascular disease, coronary occlusion, or a past history of these conditions, or conditions predisposing to these problems.
2. Markedly impaired liver function. Steroid hormones are contraindicated in patients with hepatitis until liver function tests return to normal.
3. Known or suspected breast cancer.
4. Undiagnosed abnormal vaginal bleeding.
5. Known or suspected pregnancy.
6. Smokers over the age of 35.

Relative Contraindications Requiring Clinical Judgment and Informed Consent

1. **Migraine headaches.** In retrospective studies of high-dose formulations, migraine headaches have been associated with an increased risk of stroke; however, some women report an improvement in their headaches.
2. **Hypertension.** A woman under 35 who is otherwise healthy and whose blood pressure is controlled by medication can elect to use OCs. If an OC-related increase in blood pressure occurs, discontinuing the OC usually results in a return to pretreatment blood pressure values within 3 to 6 months.
3. **Uterine leiomyoma.** This is no longer a contraindication with the low-dose formulations. There is evidence that the risk of leiomyomas is decreased by 31% in women who used higher-dose oral contraception for 10 years. However, a case-control study with lower-dose OCs found neither a decrease nor an increase in risk. The administration of low-dose oral contraceptives to women with leiomyomata does not stimulate fibroid growth and is associated with a reduction in menstrual bleeding.
4. **Gestational diabetes.** Low-dose formulations do not produce a diabetic glucose tolerance response in women with previous gestational diabetes, and there is no evidence that oral contraception increases the incidence of overt diabetes mellitus. Women with previous gestational diabetes can use oral contraception with annual assessment of the fasting glucose level.
5. **Elective surgery.** The recommendation that oral contraception should be discontinued 4 weeks before elective surgery to avoid an increased risk of postoperative thrombosis is based on data derived from high-dose products. If possible, it is safer to follow this recommendation, but it is probably less critical with low-dose OCs. It is more prudent to maintain contraception right up to the performance of a sterilization procedure, and this short, outpatient operation probably carries very minimal risk.
6. **Epilepsy.** Oral contraceptives do not exacerbate epilepsy, and in some women, improvement in seizure control has occurred. Antiepileptic drugs, however, may decrease the effectiveness of oral contraception.
7. **Obstructive jaundice in pregnancy.** Not all patients with this history will develop jaundice on OCs, especially with the low-dose formulations.
8. **Sickle-cell disease or sickle-C disease.** Patients with sickle-cell trait can use oral contraception. The risk of thrombosis in women with sickle-cell disease or sickle-C diseases is theoretical (and medicolegal). Effective protection against pregnancy in these patients warrants the use of low-dose oral contraception.
9. **Diabetes mellitus.** Effective prevention of pregnancy outweighs the small risk of complicating vascular disease in diabetic women who are under age 35 and otherwise healthy.
10. **Gallbladder disease.** Oral contraceptives do not cause gallstones, but may accelerate the emergence of symptoms when gallstones are already present.

From Ref. 4, with permission.

TABLE 76–4. OC Use and Medical Problems

- **Coagulation disorders.** Estrogens increase the risk of thrombotic events, including MI, in a dose related manner. The use of estrogen-containing OCs in women who are predisposed to coagulation disorders is contraindicated. However, the use of OCs in women with coagulation disorders *who have been properly anticoagulated* may be considered, because OCs lower the risk of fetal exposure to warfarin, bleeding corpus luteum cysts, and excessive blood loss during menses.
- **Gestational diabetes.** There is no contraindication to OC use following gestational diabetes.
- **Diabetes mellitus.** Oral contraception can be used by diabetic women less than 35 years old, who do not smoke and are otherwise healthy (especially in an absence of diabetic vascular complications).
- **Hypertension.** Low-dose oral contraception can be used in women less than 35 years old with hypertension controlled by medication, who are otherwise healthy and do not smoke.
- **Pregnancy-induced hypertension.** Women with pregnancy-induced hypertension can use OCs as soon as the blood pressure is normal in the postpartum period.
- **Hemorrhagic disorders.** Women with hemorrhagic disorder and women taking anticoagulants can use OCs. Inhibition of ovulation can avoid the problem of hemorrhagic corpus luteum in these patients. A reduction in menstrual blood loss is another important benefit.
- **Gallbladder disease.** Oral contraceptive use may precipitate a symptomatic attack in women known to have stones or a positive history for gallbladder disease, and therefore should either be used very cautiously or not at all.
- **Obesity.** An obese woman who is otherwise healthy can use low-dose OCs.
- **Hepatic disease.** Oral contraception can be used when liver function tests return to normal. Follow-up liver function tests should be obtained after 2 to 3 months of use.
- **Seizure disorders.** There is no impact of OCs on pattern or frequency of seizures; anticonvulsant drugs can decrease efficacy of OCs and Norplant, increasing the risk of contraceptive failure. Some clinicians advocate the use of higher-dose (50 mg estrogen) products or Depo-Provera.
- **Mitral valve prolapse.** Oral contraception use is limited to nonsmoking patients who are asymptomatic (no evidence of regurgitation). Patients with atrial fibrillation, migraine headaches, or clotting factor abnormalities should consider progestin-only methods or the IUD (prophylactic antibiotics should cover IUD insertion in mitral regurgitation if present).
- **Systemic lupus erythematosus.** Oral contraceptive use can exacerbate systemic lupus erythematosus, and the vascular disease associated with lupus represents a contraindication to estrogen-containing OCs. The progestin-only methods can be considered.
- **Migraine headaches.** Low-dose OCs (the lowest estrogen formulations) can be tried with careful surveillance in women with common migraine headaches. Daily administration can prevent menstrual migraine headaches. Oral contraception is best avoided in women with classic migraine headaches associated with neurologic symptoms.
- **Sickle-cell disease.** Patients with sickle-cell trait can use OCs. The risk of thrombosis in women with sickle-cell disease or sickle C is theoretical (and medicolegal). Effective protection against pregnancy in these patients warrants the use of low-dose OCs.
- **Benign breast disease.** Benign breast disease is not a contraindication for oral contraception; with 2 years of use, the condition may improve.
- **Congenital heart disease or valvular heart disease.** Oral contraception is contraindicated only if there is marginal cardiac reserve or a condition that predisposes to thrombosis.
- **Hyperlipidemia.** Because low-dose OCs have negligible impact on the lipoprotein profile, hyperlipidemia is not an absolute contraindication, with the exception of very high levels of triglycerides (which can be made worse by estrogen). If vascular disease is already present, OCs should be avoided. If other risk factors are present, especially smoking , OCs are not recommended. Dyslipidemic patients who begin OCs should have their lipoportein profiles monitored monthly for a few visits to ensure no adverse impact. If the lipid abnormality cannot be held in control, an alternative method of contraception should be used. OCs containing desogestrel, norgestimate, or gestodene can increase HDL levels, but it is not known if this change is clinically significant.
- **Depression.** Low-dose oral contraceptives have minimal, if any, impact on mood.
- **Smoking.** Oral contraception is absolutely contraindicated in smokers over the age of 35. In patients 35 years old and less, heavy smoking (15 or more cigarettes per day) is a relative contraindication. The relative risk of cardiovascular events is increased for women of all ages who smoke and use OCs; however, because the actual incidence of cardiovascular events is so low at a young age, the real risk is very low for young women, although it increases with age. An exsmoker (for at least 1 year) should be regarded as a nonsmoker. Risk is only linked to active smoking.
- **Pituitary prolactin-secreting adenomas.** Low-dose OCs can be used in the presence of microadenomas.
- **Infectious mononucleosis.** Oral contraception can be used as long as liver function tests are normal.
- **Ulcerative colitis.** There is no association between oral contraception and ulcerative colitis; women with this problem can use OCs. Oral contraceptives are absorbed mainly in the small bowel.

Compiled from Refs. 4, 7, and 15.

(e.g., desogestrel and norgestimate) are believed to have little if any effect on carbohydrate metabolism.[6,10] Use of an OC is not absolutely contraindicated in a woman with diabetes, and poses much less risk than pregnancy.

Generally, synthetic progestins adversely affect lipid metabolism by decreasing high-density lipoprotein (HDL) and increasing low-density lipoprotein (LDL). Estrogens tend to have more beneficial effects by increasing removal of LDL from the circulation and increasing HDL as increases in $ApoA_1$. Estrogens may also alter the composition of very-low-density lipoprotein (VLDL) and increase triglycerides.[15] Most low-dose combination OCs, with the possible exception of monophasic levonorgestrel (0.150 mg), do not significantly impact HDL, LDL, triglycerides, or total cholesterol.[4,22–25] Although the lipid effects of OCs can theoretically influence cardiovascular risk, the mechanism of the increased incidence of both venous and arterial cardiovascular disease in OC users, including myocardial

TABLE 76–5. Symptoms of a Serious or Potentially Serious Nature

Symptom	Possible Cause
Serious: OCs Should Be Stopped Immediately	
Loss of vision, proptosis, diplopia, papilledema	Retinal artery thrombosis
Unilateral numbness, weakness, or tingling	Hemorrhagic or thrombotic stroke
Severe pains in chest, left arm, or neck	Myocardial infarction
Hemoptysis	Pulmonary embolism
Severe pains, tenderness or swelling, warmth, or palpable cord in legs	Thrombophlebitis
Slurring of speech	Hemorrhagic or thrombotic stroke
Hepatic mass or tenderness	Liver neoplasm
Potentially Serious: OCs May Be Continued With Caution While Patient Is Being Evaluated	
Absence of menses	Pregnancy
Spotting or breakthrough bleeding	Cervical, endometrial, or vaginal cancer
Breast mass, pain, or swelling	Breast cancer
Right upper-quadrant pain	Cholecystitis, cholelithiasis, or liver neoplasm
Midepigastric pain	Thrombosis of abdominal artery or vein, myocardial infarction, or pulmonary embolism
Migraine (vascular or throbbing) headache	Vascular spasm which may precede thrombosis
Severe nonvascular headache	Hypertension, vascular spasm
Galactorrhea	Pituitary adenoma
Jaundice, pruritus	Cholestatic jaundice
Depression	Vitamin B_6 deficiency
Uterine size increase	Leiomyomata, adenomyosis, pregnancy

From Ref. 8, with permission.

infarction, is believed to be secondary to thromboembolic and thrombotic changes, not atherosclerosis.[2]

Estrogens play a dose-related role in development of venous thrombosis and consequent pulmonary embolism (PE), especially in women who smoke or have other underlying inherited (deficiencies in antithrombin III, protein C, protein S; factor V Leiden mutation) or acquired (immobility, trauma, surgery, and certain malignancies) conditions that predispose them to coagulation abnormalities.[4] Early observational studies reported the incidence of venous thromboembolism (VTE) to be as high as 12 times greater in OC users than in nonusers.[26,27] Recent reevaluation of these data suggest that although the association between non-third-generation OC use and VTE is valid, the risk is much less (less than threefold increase in the relative risk) than originally thought.[28] In addition, the absolute risk is low (15 cases/100,000 woman-years). Increased risk of VTE and PE appears to be limited to current users, with disappearance of the risk within 3 months after stopping the OC.[4,29] The 20-μg EE formulations do not appear to have an effect on clotting parameters, even in smokers, but whether or not these products lower the risk of thrombotic events has not been studied.[13,30]

European literature recently reported that some progestins also appear to have a role in the procoagulant effects of OCs. Users of third-generation OCs containing gestodene or desogestrel had a twofold greater risk of nonfatal venous thromboembolism than women using the older *low-dose* combination OCs.[31–34] Some clinicians argue this difference reflects "preferential prescribing" of the newer, and perceived safer, progestin products for women at greater risk for venous thrombosis.[35]

OCs are currently contraindicated in any woman at risk for VTE or with a history of deep venous thrombosis (see Table 76–3). Women who develop thrombotic complications while taking a low-dose OC should be evaluated for underlying coagulation disorder.[4] This having been said, some experts support the use of OCs in women with coagulation disorders *who have been properly anticoagulated,* citing the potential advantages of lowering the risk of fetal exposure to warfarin, bleeding corpus luteum cysts, and excessive blood loss during menses.[4,15]

Both thrombotic and hemorrhagic stroke have been associated with OC use. However, early studies used higher-dose products and did not take into account independent risk factors for vascular disease (e.g., smoking, hypertension and advancing age). Two recent studies evaluating low-dose OCs found the risk for stroke to be extremely low in healthy young women.[36,37] These results suggest that the effect of smoking in women less than 35 years old is minimal in the absence of hypertension and that hypertension appears to be the major risk factor for stroke.[38] Cerebrovascular accidents (CVAs) are often preceded by persistent headaches (for weeks or months) and/or by temporary hemiparesis. Patients should be carefully screened and counseled to recognize warning signs of CVAs in order to decrease risk.

Myocardial infarction (MI) occurs primarily in OC users over 35 years of age who have additional risk factors for cardiovascular disease (smoking, diabetes, hypertension, obesity).[4,7] These risk factors, in particular smoking, appear to act synergistically with OCs to increase the risk of cardiovascular disease.[7,39] A large British study found a 21-fold increase in MI among women who smoke more than 15 cigarettes daily with no apparent increased risk in healthy nonsmoking women, regardless of age.[40] Since the Food and Drug Administration (FDA) lifted its restrictions on OC use in healthy nonsmoking women over 40 in 1989, OCs containing 30 μg estrogen or less are being used more frequently in healthy, nonsmoking women up to the age of menopause without evidence of significantly increased risk of cardiovascular events.[4,12]

The risk for ovarian and endometrial cancer decreases by 40% to 50% with OC use, and the beneficial effect is believed to persist for at least 15 years after OC use ceases.[2,4,7] The relationship between OCs and other cancers is controversial. Worldwide epidemiologic data from 54 studies in 25 countries (many of which studied high-dose OCs) were recently reanalyzed to assess the relationship between OC use and the risk of breast cancer.[41,42] Researchers concluded that women who began OC use before age 20 had a higher relative risk compared with recent users who began at later ages. They also found that women currently taking OC and those within 10 years of stopping OCs have a small increase in the risk of breast cancer, but these cancers were less clinically advanced than in women who had never used OCs.[41,42] Prospective U.S. data from the Nurses' Health Study cohort found no overall relationship between duration of OC use and breast cancer, even in long-term users (≥ 10 years), and researchers concluded that long-term past use, either overall or prior to a full-term pregnancy, does not result in an increased risk of breast cancer in women over 40 years of age.[43] It will take many years to discover what, if any, impact the low-dose OCs will have on breast cancer risk. OCs increase cervical ectopy, but the association with cervical cancer is unclear.

CHOICE OF AN ORAL CONTRACEPTIVE

Before prescribing an OC, several questions must be answered. Are there any contraindications to the use of OCs (Tables 76–3 to 76–5)? Does this form of contraception fit the patient's life-style, and will the patient be compliant? The advantages and disadvantages of all available forms of contraception should be discussed with the patient to ensure that an informed choice can be made (see Table 76–1).

Minipills tend to be less effective than combination OCs with typical use and are associated with irregular and unpredictable menstrual bleeding and an increased frequency of functional ovarian cysts.[3,4,44] Irregular menstrual cycles indicate that ovulation has been inhibited; however, this is one of the most frequent reasons for discontinuation of this method.[1,3] Unlike combination OCs, minipills are always begun on the first day of menses and must be taken every day at approximately the same time to maintain contraceptive efficacy.[7] In that ovulation is often not blocked with minipills (nearly 40% of women continue to ovulate normally), the risk of ectopic pregnancy increases when compared to other hormonal contraceptives.[3,4]

Most clinicians routinely prescribe a combination OC that contain less than 50 μg of EE (Table 76–2). This strategy is based on evidence that the most serious side effects of combination OCs (thromboembolic stroke, MI) result from excessive estrogen content.[2–4,8]

Many symptoms occurring in the first cycle of OC use (e.g., breakthrough bleeding and side effects related to estrogen excess) improve spontaneously by the second or third cycle of use as the body adjusts to the altered hormonal level.[4,8] Therefore, initial OC use should be reevaluated during the first 3 to 6 months of therapy to determine if the patient is experiencing any adverse effects and if the patient wishes to continue medication.[3,4]

If the patient complains of symptoms related to OC use, it should be determined if the symptom indicates the presence or potential development of a serious illness (see Table 76–7).[8] Nearly all OC-induced side effects parallel the symptoms and physiologic changes of pregnancy (hormone excess) or perimenopausal period (hormone deficiency).[8] In some cases, symptoms relating to the hormonal imbalance may benefit from adjustments in the specific combination of estrogen and progestin, because progestins can contribute to estrogenic and antiestrogenic activity.[8] However, the clinically significant differences between the low-dose OCs used today are hard to distinguish.[4] Several useful handbooks and articles are available to the practitioner in managing side effects associated with OCs.[1–4,7,8]

DRUG INTERACTIONS

The effectiveness of OCs is sometimes limited by drug interactions resulting in interference with gastrointestinal absorption; increased intestinal motility by alteration of gut bacteriologic flora; and alterations in the metabolism, excretion, or binding of the OC (Table 76–6).[8,45,46]

PATIENT INSTRUCTIONS

Many women who take OCs are poorly informed about the proper use of these medications. The patient should first be given the patient package insert required for all estrogen products, and be instructed to read it carefully. The written information in the package insert should be supplemented with verbal information describing how the medication works (primarily by stopping the release of the egg from the ovary) and recognition of both common and serious side effects and their management. Although there are often several transient self-limiting side effects (breast tenderness, bloating, breakthrough bleeding, spotting, nausea), the patient should be aware of the danger signals (Table 76–7) that require immediate medical attention (Table 76–5).[3] Also, benefits and risks should be discussed in terms the patient can understand, including the fact that OCs provide no physical barrier to the transmission of STDs (including HIV). Detailed instructions for when to start taking the medication should be provided (either Sunday start or on the first day of the next menses). Patients should be told the importance of routine daily administration to ensure consistent plasma concentrations and improve compliance, and specific instructions should be given regarding what to do if a pill is missed. Important drug interactions should be dis-

TABLE 76–6. OC Interactions with Other Drugs

Interacting Drugs	Adverse Effects (Probable Mechanism)	Comments and Recommendation
Acetaminophen (Tylenol and others)	Possible decreased pain-relieving effect (increased metabolism)	Monitor pain-relieving response
Alcohol	Possible increased effect of alcohol	Use with caution
Ampicillin	Decreased contraceptive effect	Low but unpredictable incidence; use backup method of contraception
Anticoagulants (oral)	Decreased anticoagulant effect	Use with caution, monitor INR
Antidepressants (Elavil, Norpramin, Tofranil, and others)	Possible increased antidepressant pharmacologic effect	Monitor for adverse effects
Barbiturates (phenobarbital and others)	Decreased contraceptive effect	Avoid simultaneous use; use alternative contraceptive for patients with epilepsy (DMPA)
Benzodiazepine tranquilizers (Ativan, Librium, Serax, Tranxene, Valium, Xanax, and others)	Possible increased or decreased tranquilizer effects including psychomotor impairment	Use with caution; greatest impairment during drug-free week in oral contraceptive dosage
β-Blockers (Corgard, Inderal, Lopressor, Tenormin)	Possible increased β-blocker pharmacologic effect	Monitor cardiovascular status
Carbamazepine (Tegretol)	Possible decreased contraceptive effect	Avoid simultaneous use; use alternative contraceptive for patients with epilepsy (DMPA)
Corticosteroids (cortisone)	Possible increased corticosteroid toxicity	Clinical significance not established
Griseofulvin (Fulvicin, Grifulvin V, and others)	Decreased contraceptive effect	Use backup method of contraception
Hypoglycemics (Tolbutamide, Diabinese, Orinase, Tolinase)	Possible decreased hypoglycemic effect	Monitor blood glucose
Methyldopa (Aldoclor, Aldomet, and others)	Possible decreased antihypertensive effect, especially with high-dose OCs	Monitor blood pressure
Phenytoin (Dilantin)	Decreased contraceptive effect, possible increased phenytoin effect	Use alternative contraceptive (DMPA); monitor phenytoin concentration
Primidone (Mysoline)	Decreased contraceptive effect	Use alternative contraceptive (DMPA)
Rifampin	Decreased contraceptive effect	Use backup method of contraception; use alternate method if planned concomitant use is long term
Tetacycline	Decreased contraceptive effect	Use backup contraception
Theophylline (Bronkotabs, Marax, Primatene, Quibron, Tedral, TheoDur, and others)	Decreased contraceptive effect, increased theophylline effect	Monitor theophylline concentration
Troglitazone (Rezulin)	Decreased contraceptive effect	Use alternative contraceptive
Troleandomycin (TAO)	Jaundice (additive)	Avoid simulanteous use
Vitamin C	Increased serum concentration and possible increased adverse effects of estrogens with 1 g or more per day of vitamin C	Avoid high dose of vitamin C

INR = International Normalized Ratio; DMPA = depomedroxyprogesterone acetate.
Compiled from Refs. 3, 8, 45, and 46.

cussed. Some prescription drugs, including certain antibiotics and anticonvulsants, may decrease OC effectiveness.

The patient taking combination OCs should expect her menses to start within 1 to 3 days after taking the last active pill. She should start another pack of pills immediately after finishing a 28-day pack (no days between) or 1 week after finishing the previous 21-day pack, whether or not her menses is completed.[3] An additional contraceptive method should be recommended during the first pack of pills (especially if begun 5 days or more after start of menses), if the patient misses more than one pill per cycle, or if she experiences severe diarrhea or vomiting for several days.[13] Patients taking minipills should be advised to use a backup method for 48 hours if they are 3 or more hours late in taking their daily progestin dose.[4]

STOPPING THE OC, RETURN OF FERTILITY, AND BREAST FEEDING

Women who have previously used OCs may take longer to return to their baseline fertility than women who have used

TABLE 76–7. Which Symptoms May Be Warnings of Serious Trouble?[a]

Five Signals	Possible Problem
Abdominal pain (severe)	Gallbladder disease, hepatic adenoma, blood clot, pancreatitis
Chest pain (severe), shortness of breath, or coughing up blood	Blood clot in lungs or myocardial infarction (heart attack)
Headaches (severe)	Stroke, hypertension, or migraine headache
Eye problems: blurred vision, flashing lights, or blindness	Stroke, hypertension, or temporary vascular problem of many possible sites
Severe leg pain (calf or thigh)	Blood clot in legs

[a]See your clinician if you have any of these problems, or if you develop depression, yellow jaundice, or a breast lump.
From Ref. 3, with permission.

barrier contraception methods.[2] Eventually, the percentage of women who conceive after stopping OCs becomes the same as for barrier-method users.[47]

Traditionally, women are counseled to allow for two to three normal menstrual periods before becoming pregnant to permit the reestablishment of menses and ovulation.[3] However, in several large cohort and case-controlled studies, the infants conceived in the first month after an OC was discontinued had no greater chance of being born with a birth defect than those born in the general population.[2,48–50]

Any method of hormonal contraception is acceptable to begin immediately after first- or second-trimester termination of pregnancy (spontaneous or induced). Following third-trimester childbirth, ovulation does not usually begin again for 3 weeks, even in a non-breast-feeding woman,[51] and the risk of maternal thromboembolic disease is increased for approximately the same time period.[52] Ideally, estrogen-containing contraceptives are withheld until the third week after delivery, but progestin-only methods can be initiated immediately. However, it is because the hormones in OCs are excreted into breast milk that breast feeding is generally regarded as a relative contraindication to OC use. This contraindication was based on earlier formulations containing higher doses of hormones, and probably does not apply to current formulations. Another concern is that estrogens inhibit the action of prolactin in breast tissue receptors resulting in decreased milk production and protein content.[2] Although this is not a particular problem when used in well-nourished breast-feeding women, many practitioners recommend progestin-only contraceptives because progestins do not diminish the amount of breast milk and provide highly effective contraception in breast-feeding women.[2,4]

POSTCOITAL "MORNING AFTER" PILLS OR EMERGENCY CONTRACEPTION

High doses of estrogens can cause almost immediate shedding of the endometrium and prevent implantation of the fertilized ovum.[1,53] Recently the FDA declared OCs in one-time high-doses as safe and effective as "emergency contraception" to prevent pregnancy after unprotected intercourse (e.g., condom breakage, diaphragm dislodging, sexual assault).[54] Specifically, a dose of one of the following 6 brands can be taken within 72 hours of unprotected intercourse with a follow-up dose 12 hours after the first: Ovral (2 tablets/dose); Nordette, Lo/Ovral, Triphasil, Levlen, or Tri-Levlin (4 tablets/dose).[54] Begun more than 72 hours after intercourse, the efficacy of this regimen declines, and treatment is totally ineffective by 7 days, when implantation usually occurs.[54] Patients may experience nausea, vomiting, and breast tenderness with this regimen. Although some clinicians will prescribe antiemetics prophylactically, others will recommend simply repeating the dose if the patient vomits within an hour of taking the pills.[53]

LONG-ACTING INJECTABLE AND IMPLANTABLE PROGESTINS

Steroids are useful for long-term contraception when injected or implanted into the skin. The most commonly used steroids for contraception are progestins. Sustained progestin exposure blocks the LH surge, thus preventing ovulation. Should ovulation occur, progestins reduce ovum motility in the fallopian tubes, and even if fertilization occurs, progestins thin the endometrium, reducing the chance of implantation. Progestins also thicken the cervical mucus, producing a barrier for sperm penetration. However, FSH is not intensely suppressed by progestin-only contraception; therefore, follicular growth and estrogen concentrations, although lower than normal at times, are maintained. Women who particularly benefit from progestin-only methods, including minipills, are those who are breast feeding; those who have contraindications or intolerance to estrogens (those with systemic lupus erythematosus, sickle-cell hemoglobinopathies, a history of estrogen-related headache, or hypertension); or those who smoke and are older than 35 years of age.[1,3,4,7] Women who report premenstrual weight gain, nausea, or acne may also benefit from these methods.[3,5] Pregnancy failure rates with long-acting progestin contraception are comparable to female sterilization.[1] However, if pregnancy does occur while using one of the progestin-only methods, the risk of it being ectopic is increased.[4] These methods of contraception do not offer protection from STDs, but the thickened cervical mucus may help prohibit entry of bacteria into the upper pelvic region, thus preventing pelvic inflammatory disease.

MEDROXYPROGESTERONE ACETATE

Medroxyprogesterone is a C21-17 acetoxy-progestogen that is similar in structure to naturally occurring progesterone. Depomedroxyprogesterone acetate (DMPA), 150 mg administered by deep intramuscular (IM) injection in the gluteal or deltoid muscle within 5 days after the onset of menstrual bleeding, inhibits ovulation for over 3 months.

The half-life of DMPA is approximately 50 days after IM injection.[55] Although DMPA 150 mg IM may inhibit ovulation for up to 14 weeks, the dose should be repeated every 3 months (12 weeks) to ensure continuous contraception.[56] The manufacturer recommends excluding pregnancy in women more than *1 week* late for repeat injection. No apparent weight restrictions apply in women using DMPA.[55] Although two strengths of DMPA are available (Depo-Provera 100 and 400-mg/mL suspensions), the 400-mg/mL concentrated form has inconsistent bioavailability, may be less effective, and is more painful than the less concentrated formulation. It is not approved for contraception.[3,4,56]

DMPA can be used in lactating women, and it may increase the length of time a woman can breast-feed.[3] Although DMPA is safe postpartum and no adverse effects have occurred in infants exposed to DMPA through breast milk, the manufacturer recommends initiating DMPA at 6 weeks postpartum in women who are breast feeding.[55,56] DMPA is also safe in women with sickle-cell disease and may reduce the propensity of red blood cell sickling.[57] DMPA does not alter blood pressure or increase the risk of thromboembolic disorders. It may be used in women with SLE or seizure disorders, and it may decrease the frequency of seizures.[58] Noncontraceptive benefits observed in women using DMPA include reducing the risk of anemia due to less menstrual blood loss and decreasing the incidence of menstrual cramps and pain at ovulation. The incidence of candida vulvovaginitis, ectopic pregnancy, and pelvic inflammatory disease (PID), and endometrial and ovarian cancer are decreased in women using DMPA for contraception compared with women using no contraception.

Return of fertility may be delayed after discontinuation of DMPA. The median time to conception from the first omitted dose is 6 months.[3] Sixty-eight percent of women will be able to conceive within 12 months, 83% within 15 months, and 93% within 18 months of the last injection.[56]

Menstrual irregularities, including irregular unpredictable spotting or, more rarely, continuous heavy bleeding, are the most frequent adverse effects from DMPA. In some cases, bleeding may be severe enough to cause a significant drop in hemoglobin. Women who cannot tolerate prolonged bleeding may benefit from a short course of oral estrogen (e.g., 7 days of 2 mg estradiol or 1.25 mg conjugated estrogen).[4] The incidence of irregular bleeding decreases from 30% in the first year to 10% thereafter (such that most women are amenorrheic after the first year).[1] After 12 months of therapy, 57% of women report amenorrhea, with the incidence increasing to 68% after 2 years.

Because estrogen concentrations may be lower than normal in women using DMPA, women can lose bone density.[59,60] The clinical significance of this bone loss is unknown. Breast tenderness, weight gain, and depression are reported less commonly (< 5%). Weight gain averages 1 kg annually and may not resolve until 6 to 8 months after the last injection.[4,61,62] Whether or not weight gain can be directly attributed to DMPA is debatable.[63]

Minor elevations in serum total triglycerides and decreases in serum HDL cholesterol, particularly HDL-2, have been noted after DMPA exposure.[59] LDL cholesterol and total cholesterol concentrations have been increased in some studies with no change reported in others.[59,64] Carbohydrate metabolism and coagulation factors are not affected.[64,65] The clinical significance of these minor alterations in metabolism is unknown.

Although used in developing countries for decades, DMPA was not approved as a contraceptive in the U.S. market until 1992 because of a concern about a possible increased incidence of breast cancer.[1] Overall, the risk of breast cancer in women who have used DMPA is not increased. However, two studies suggest that the risk may be increased in some groups. One study from the World Health Organization found a very slight increased risk in the first 4 years of use, but the risk did not increase with longer duration of use.[66,67] Another study found a possible increased risk in women initiating use at an early age.[68] These studies suggest that if any effect exists at all, medroxyprogesterone may enhance the growth of already existing tumors. DMPA was approved for use in the United States as a contraceptive because worldwide data in millions of women showed benefit on maternal mortality and demonstrated other noncontraceptive benefits, outweighing any possible increased risk of breast cancer. Other side effects are similar to those seen with progestogen-only oral contraceptives. Common side effects (> 5%) include abdominal pain or discomfort, asthenia, dizziness, headache, and nervousness.

PROGESTIN SUBDERMAL IMPLANTS

Norplant, developed by the Population Council, was the first progestin subdermal implant approved for use in the United States in 1990. The Norplant contraceptive system is a set of six implantable, nonbiodegradable, soft, silicone rubber capsules, each filled with 36 mg of crystalline levonorgestrel. These capsules are inserted just under the skin to provide continuous contraception for up to 5 years. In early clinical trials, both hard and soft Norplant capsules were used, with the soft capsules allowing more levonorgestrel to be released into the blood. Not surprisingly, cumulative failure rates were higher among women who used the hard capsules (9.3% with hard capsules versus 2.4% with soft capsules), particularly women over 70 kg (154 pounds).[69] Because the cumulative pregnancy rate in all groups of women significantly increases during the sixth year, Norplant should be replaced after 5 years. Even with the softer capsules currently available in the United States, failure rates may be unacceptable during the fourth and fifth years of use in women weighing over 154 pounds. Replacement after 3 years in heavier women helps ensure effectiveness.[1]

A new system can be inserted immediately after removal of the old system. Removal of a Norplant system often becomes complicated as a result of poor insertion technique, broken capsules, or impedance by fibrous tissue. A "U" technique of Norplant removal using a 4-mm incision located parallel to the third and fourth implant appears to be an improvement over the manufacturer-recommended technique, especially for personnel who are not highly experienced in this procedure.[70] Norplant II, a levonorgestrel two-rod, 150-mg implant system providing 3 years of contraception, may prove to be easier to insert and remove than the older system.[71,72] Other progestin implants, some of which are biodegradable, are under development.[72]

Similar to other progestin-only methods, the most common side effect of subdermal progestin implants is irregular menstrual bleeding. Irregular bleeding occurs in approximately 60% to 70% of women using Norplant during the first year after insertion. Prolonged bleeding can be treated with a short course of estrogen (e.g., 2 mg estradiol or 1.25 mg conjugated estrogen for 7 to 10 days).[4] Spotting and bleeding decrease in amount and duration with time. However, by the fifth year of use, regular bleeding cycles may resume in over 60% of users. Regular cyclic bleeding while using Norplant indicates return of ovulation and a higher risk of method failure.[73]

Unlike Depo-Provera, fertility returns quickly after removal of Norplant. Most women return to baseline ovulatory patterns within the first month after removal of the system. Other progesterone-related adverse effects that usually occur in the first year include headache (common), depression, nervousness, breast discharge, mastalgia, dizziness, acne, hirsutism, hair loss, changes in appetite, and weight gain. Because of the extremely low concentrations of levonorgestrel released from the Norplant system, drugs that significantly increase hepatic enzymes, including most antiseizure medications and rifampin, lower the efficacy of the contraceptive. Ovarian cysts may occur, but usually regress spontaneously within 1 month of detection.[4]

Noncontraceptive benefits are similar to those of Depo-Provera, and no clinically significant adverse effects have been observed on carbohydrate metabolism in nondiabetic women, blood coagulation, liver function, lipid metabolism, serum cortisol, renal function, or electrolytes.

PERIODIC ABSTINENCE

The avoidance of sexual intercourse during the days of the menstrual cycle when conception is likely to occur may be used by highly motivated couples. Using the abstinence (rhythm) method, women rely on physiologic changes, such as basal body temperature and cervical mucus, during each cycle, to determine the fertile period. The major reasons for lack of acceptance are the relatively high pregnancy rates among users and the need to avoid intercourse for several days during each menstrual cycle. To overcome these drawbacks, many women use barrier methods or spermicides during the fertile period.[2,74]

BARRIER TECHNIQUES AND SPERMICIDES

The effectiveness of barrier methods and spermicides depends almost exclusively on a couple's motivation to use them consistently and correctly. These methods include the diaphragm, cervical cap, sponge (no longer available in the United States), condom, and spermicide. Besides contraception, an advantage to using these methods is that they can reduce the rate of transmission of STDs.[2]

The diaphragm, a reusable dome-shaped rubber cap with a flexible rim, is inserted vaginally and fits over the cervix in order to decrease access of sperm to the ovum. The diaphragm is available in 11 sizes and requires a prescription from a physician who has fitted the patient for the correct size.[4,75] The effectiveness of the diaphragm depends on its function as a barrier and on the spermicidal cream or jelly placed in the diaphragm before insertion.[2] The diaphragm may be inserted as long as 6 hours before intercourse and must be left in place for at least 6 hours after intercourse.[4] If intercourse occurs more than once within 6 hours, the patient must not remove the diaphragm, but rather insert more spermicide and wear the diaphragm for 6 hours after subsequent acts of intercourse or use a condom.[3] Contraindications to the diaphragm are listed in Table 76–1. Users of diaphragms appear to have a lower incidence of cervical neoplasia, which may be attributed to the adjunctive spermicide and the diaphragm's barrier effect against the human papillomavirus.[5] Diaphragm use has also been associated with an increased incidence of urinary tract and yeast infections.[5]

The Prentif cervical cap is a soft, deep, rubber cup with a firm round rim smaller than a diaphragm that fits over the cervix like a thimble.[1,3] Spermicide, used to fill the cap one-third full prior to insertion, is held in place against the cervix until removed.[3] The cap remains effective for more than one episode (up to 48 hours) of intercourse without adding more spermicide and is less messy to use than a diaphragm. However, because of the limited number of sizes, it may not be possible to fit some women with this device.[1,3] It is recommended that women not wear the cap for longer than 48 hours, to reduce the risk of toxic shock syndrome.[3]

Condoms are devices that create a mechanical barrier, preventing direct contact with semen, genital lesions and discharges, and infectious secretions.[1,3] Most condoms made in the United States are made of latex rubber, which is impermeable to viruses; a small proportion (5%), however, is made from young lamb intestine, which is not.[1,3] Condoms are used worldwide as protection from STDs. When used in conjunction with any other barrier methods, their effectiveness theoretically approaches 95%.[3] Spillage of semen or perforation and tearing of the condom can occur, but is minimized by proper use.[4,76,77] Mineral-oil-based vaginal drug forumations (Cleocin vaginal cream, Premarin vaginal cream, Vagistat 1, Femstat, Monistat Vaginal suppositories), lotions, or lubricants can decrease the barrier strength of latex by 90% in just 60 seconds; thus making water-soluble lubricants preferable if they are to come in contact with latex condoms.[1] A condom for women (Reality) was approved in April 1993 by the FDA and appears to be as effective as the diaphragm in preventing pregnancy.[77] The female condom is a prelubricated, soft, loose-fitting polyurethane sheath, closed at one end, with flexible rings at both ends. Properly positioned, the ring at the closed end covers the cervix, and the sheath lines the walls of the vagina. The outer ring remains outside the vagina, covering the labia; this may make it more effective than the male condom in preventing transmission of diseases such as herpes because it protects the labia from coming in contact with the base of the penis.[77] The manufacturer reports a use-effective pregnancy rate of 26% per year, based on a 6-month follow-up study of 200 women.[5]

Spermicides, most of which contain nonoxynol-9, are chemical surfactants that destroy sperm cell walls and offer some protection against STDs and cervical cancer.[1] Spermicides are available as foams, creams, suppositories, jellies, and film.[2] Spermicidal tablets or suppositories require 10 to 30 minutes to dissolve.[1] Spermicides can cause local irritation in both men and women. Additional spermicide must be used each time intercourse is repeated.[1]

INTRAUTERINE DEVICES

Intrauterine devices (IUDs) cause low-grade intrauterine inflammation and increased prostaglandin formation. These effects appear to be primarily spermicidal with interference of implantation being a backup mechanism.[4,9,78,79] The IUD has several contraindications (Table 76–1). The risk of PID among IUD users ranges from 1% to 2.5%.[5] The increase in risk appears to be related to the introduction of bacteria into the genital tract during IUD insertion. Therefore, the risk of infection is highest during the first 20 days after the procedure.[1] Ideal patients for IUD use include parous, monogamous women, who are not at risk for STDs or PID.[5] Two IUDs are currently marketed in the United States; both are shaped like a "T" and are medicated, one with copper (ParaGard) and the other with progesterone (Progestasert). ParaGard provides better contraceptive effectiveness than previous copper devices and can be left in place for 10 years.[1,5] A disadvantage of Progestasert is that it must be replaced annually, but it has been associated with less blood loss during menstruation and less dysmenorrhea.[1]

ECONOMIC AND PHARMACOECONOMIC CONSIDERATIONS

More than half of all pregnancies in the United States are unintended.[80] That is not to say that all unintended pregnancies are unwanted; many are just "mis-timed." Nevertheless, the United States has a higher rate of induced abortions than most other industrialized Western nations. Regardless of the method used, preventing unintended pregnancy is highly cost effective.[81] When considering the acquisition cost of reversible contraception, spermicides alone are the least expensive method, followed by their use with condoms. Depo-Provera is slightly less expensive than Norplant and IUDs. Implantable and injectable methods carry a higher initial cost that can be prohibitive for some women, and the annual cost will be greater if they are removed prior to their expiration. The diaphragm and cervical cap (with spermicide) are midrange in cost, with the female condom being slightly more expensive that the other female barrier methods. Oral contraceptives are the most expensive form of reversible contraception. These cost estimates are based on the assumption of 100 acts of intercourse annually.[3] However, when considering direct medical costs (method use, side effects, and unintended pregnancies) over 5 years, the copper IUD, vasectomy, Norplant, and Depo-Provera are the most cost effective. OCs are more cost effective than methods with high failure rates (barrier methods, spermicides, withdrawal, and periodic abstinence), but even these methods are more cost effective than no method.[81]

EVALUATION OF THERAPEUTIC OUTCOMES

Both verbal and written instructions concerning the chosen method should be given to the patient, and follow-up appointments can increase compliance, allow time for the patient to ask questions, and provide opportunities to address other health maintenance issues (self-breast exam, Pap smears, STD risk).[5] At least annual blood pressure monitoring is recommended in all users of OCs. When an OC is started or stopped in a patient with a history of glucose intolerance or overt type 1 diabetes mellitus, glucose should be more closely monitored for deterioration of the condition. OC users should receive at least annual (more frequent if they are at risk for a sexually transmitted disease) cytology screening.[2,4] Finally, the OC users should be evaluated for clinical problems possibly relating to the OC (breakthrough bleeding, amenorrhea, weight gain, acne).[4] Women using Norplant should be monitored for menstrual cycle disturbances, weight gain, local inflammation or infection at the implant site, acne, breast tenderness, headaches, and hair loss.[3] Women using DMPA should be asked at 3-month follow-up visits about weight gain, any problems or concerns they may have, menstrual cycle disturbances, and STD risks. Patients on DMPA should also be weighed and have their blood pressure checked and receive annual exams (e.g., complete physical exam, Pap smear, mamogram) as indicated based on the patient's age.[3]

CONCLUSIONS

Choosing a contraceptive method most suited to the patient's needs will significantly reduce the chance of unintended pregnancy. Typical use failure rates for some of the commonly used methods of reversible contraception are listed in Table 76–1. Information from a medical and sexual history and a thorough physical exam are essential when evaluating the various available methods. Understanding the risks and contraindications of the available methods is essential for both the patient and prescriber (Table 76–1)

▶ PRINCIPLES OF PHARMACOTHERAPY

- The attitude of both the patient and sexual partner toward various contraceptive methods, the effectiveness of the method, reliability of the patient to use it correctly, and the patient's ability to pay must be carefully considered when selecting a contraceptive method.

- Patient specific factors (such as frequency of intercourse, age, smoking status, and concomitant diseases or conditions) that may prove to be a consideration or absolute or relative contraindication for use of a specific method must be evaluated when selecting a contraceptive method.
- Side effects or difficulties using the chosen method should be carefully monitored and managed in consideration of patient-specific factors.
- The utility and satisfaction of the patient and partner(s) with a contraceptive method must be periodically reevaluated.
- Many practitioners recommend progestin-only contraceptives for breast-feeding women because progestins do not diminish the amount of breast milk and provide highly effective contraception.
- Accurate and timely counseling on the optimal use of the contraceptive method and strategies to minimize STD transmission must be provided to all patients when contraceptive pharmacotherapy is initiated and on an ongoing basis.
- Certain OCs in high doses can be used as "emergency contraception" to prevent pregnancy after unprotected intercourse. Administration must occur within 72 hours of unprotected intercourse with a follow-up dose 12 hours after the first.

REFERENCES

1. Choice of contraceptives. Med Lett Drug Ther 1995;37:9–12.
2. Mishell DR. Contraception. N Engl J Med 1989;320:777–785.
3. Hatcher RA, Trussell J, Stewart F, et al. Contraceptive Technology, 16th ed. New York, Irvington, 1994:145–171, 223–272, 285–318.
4. Speroff L, Darney P. A Clinical Guide for Contraception, 2nd ed. Baltimore, Williams & Wilkins, 1996:25–117, 129–174, 175–189, 229–262.
5. Heath CB. Helping patients choose appropriate contraception. Am Fam Physician 1993;48:1115–1124.
6. Baird DT, Glasier AF. Hormonal contraception. N Engl J Med 1993;328:1543–1548.
7. Hormonal contraception. ACOG Technical Bull 1994;198:1–11.
8. Dickey RP. Managing Contraceptive Pill Patients, 7th ed. Durant, OK, Essential Medical Information Systems, 1993:18–34, 58–65.
9. Van der Vange N, Blankenstein MA, Kloosterboer HJ, et al. Effects of seven low-dose combined oral contraceptives on sex hormone binding globulin, corticosteroid binding globulin, total and free testosterone. Contraception 1990;41:345–352.
10. Kaplan B. Desogestrel, norgestimate, and gestodene: The newer progestins. Ann Pharmacother 1995;29:736–742.
11. Colditz GA. Oral contraceptive use and mortality during 12 years of follow-up: the Nurses' Health Study. Ann Int Med 1994;120:821–826.
12. FDA Drug Bull 1990;20:5.
13. Fruzzetti F, Ricci C, Fioretti P. Haemostasis profile in smoking and nonsmoking women taking low-dose oral contraceptives.Contraception 1994;49:579–592.
14. Speroff L. Contraception for older women. OB/GYN Clin Alert, September 1994; 38–39.
15. Corson SL. Contraception for women with health problems. Int J Fertil 1996;41:77–84.
16. Chasan-Taber L, Willett WC, Manson JE, et al. Prospective study of oral contraceptives and hypertension among women in the United States. Circulation 1996;94:483–489.
17. Kalkhoff RK. Relative sensitivity of postpartum gestational diabetic women to oral contraceptive agents and other metabolic stress. Diabetes Care 1980;3:421–424.
18. Perlman JA, Russell-Briefel R, Ezzati T, Lieberknecht G. Oral glucose tolerance and the potency of contraceptive progestins. J Chronic Dis 1985;38:857–864.
19. Van der Vange N, Kloosterboer HJ, Haspels AA. Effect of seven low-dose combined oral contraceptive preparations on carbohydrate metabolism. Am J Obstet Gynecol 1987;156:918–922.
20. Kung AW, Ma JT, Wong VC, et al. Glucose and lipid metabolism with triphasic oral contraceptives in women with a history of gestational diabetes. Contraception 1987;35:257–269.
21. Godsland IF, Crook D. Update on the metabolic effects of steroidal contraceptives and their relationship to cardiovascular disease. Am J Obstet Gynecol 1994;170:1528–1536.
22. Skouby SO, Kuhl C, Molsted-Pedersen K, Christensen MS. Triphasic oral contraception: Metabolic effects in normal women and those with previous gestational diabetes. Am J Obstet Gynecol 1985;153: 495–500.
23. Kloosterboer HJ, van Wayjen RG, van den Ende A. Comparative effects of monophasic desogestrel plus ethinyl estradiol and triphasic levonorgestrel plus ethinyl estradiol on lipid metabolism. Contraception 1986;34:135–144.
24. Percival-Smith RK, Morrison BJ, Sizto R, Abercrombie E. The effect of triphasic and biphasic oral contraceptive preparations on HDL-cholesterol and LDL-cholesterol in young women. Contraception 1987; 35:179–187.
25. Kloosterboer HJ, Rekers H. Effects of three combined oral contraceptive preparations containing desogestrel plus ethinyl estradiol on lipid metabolism in comparison with two levonorgestrel preparations. Am J Obstet Gynecol 1990;163:370–373.
26. Helmrich SP, Rosenberg L, Kaufamn DW, et al. Venous thromboembolism in relation to oral contraceptive use. Obstet Gynecol 1987;69: 91–95.
27. Meade TW. Risks and mechanism of cardiovascular events in users of oral contraceptives. Am J Obstet Gynecol 1988;158:1646–1652.
28. Douketis JD, Ginsberg JS, Holbrook A, et al. A reevaluation of risk for venous thromboembolism with use of oral contraception and hormone replacement. Arch Int Med 1997;157:1522–1530.
29. Grodstein F, Stampfer MJ, Goldhaber SZ, et al. Prospective study of exogenous hormone and risk of pulmonary embolism in women. Lancet 1996;348:983–987.
30. Basdevant A, Conrad J, Pelissier C, et al. Hemostatic and metabolic effects of lowering the ethinyl estradiol dose from 30 mcg to 20 mcg in oral contraceptives containing desogestrel. Contraception 1993;48: 193–204.
31. Hume AL, Barbour MM, Lapane KL. Correlates of oral contraceptive use in two New England communities:1981–1993.Pharmacotherapy 1996;16:1173–1178.
32. Spitzer WO, Lewis MA, Heinemann LAJ, et al. Third generation oral contraceptives and risk of venous thromboembolic disorders: An international case-control study. Br Med J 1996;312:83–88.
33. World Health Organization. WHO Collaborative Study of Cardiovascular Disease and Steroid Hormone Contraception. Venous thromboembolic disease and combined oral contraceptives: Results of international multicentre case-control study. Lancet 1995;346:1589–1593.
34. Jick H, Jick SS, Gurewick V, et al. Risk of idiopathic cardiovascular death and nonfatal venous thromboembolism in women using oral contraceptives with differing progrestin components. Lancet 1995; 346:1589–1593.

35. Speroff L. Third-generation oral contraceptives and venous thrombosis.OB/GYN Clin Alert, June 1997; 11–12.
36. Petitti DB, Sidney S,Bernstien A, et al. Stroke in users of low-dose oral contraceptives. N Engl J Med 1996;335:8–15.
37. Poulter NR, Chang CL, Farley TMM, et al. Haemorrhagic stroke, overall stroke risk, and combined oral contraceptives: Results of an international, multicentre, case-control study. Lancet 1996;348: 498–510.
38. Speroff L. Low-dose oral contracpetives and stroke.OB/GYN Clin Alert 1996;13:49–51.
39. Slone D, Shapiro S, Kaufman DW, et al. Risk of myocardial infarction in relation to current and discontinued use of oral contraceptives. N Engl J Med 1981;305:420–424.
40. Croft P, Hannaford PC. Risk factors for acute myocardial infarction in women: Evidence from the Royal College of General Practitioners' oral contraception study. Br Med J 1989;298:165–168.
41. Collaborative group on hormonal factors in breast cancer. Breast cancer and hormonal contraceptives: Collaborative reanalysis of individual data on 53,297 women with breast cancer and 100,239 women without breast cancer from 54 epidemiological studies. Lancet 1996;347:1713–1727.
42. Collaborative group on hormonal factors in breast cancer. Breast cancer and hormonal contraceptives: Further results.Contraception 1996; 54(suppl 3):1S–106S.
43. Hankinson SE. Colditz GA, Manson JE, et al. A prospective study of oral contraceptive use and risk of breast cancer (Nurses' health study, United States). Cancer Causes and Control 1997;8:65–72.
44. Tayob Y, Adams J, Jacobs HS, Guillebaud J. Ultrasound demonstration of increased frequency of functional ovarian cysts in women using progestogen-only oral contraception. Br J Obstet Gynecol 1985;92:1003–1009.
45. D'Arcy PF. Drug interactions with oral contraceptives. Drug Intell Clin Pharm 1986;20:353–362.
46. Stoehr GP, White J. Managing drug interactions with oral contraceptives. J Obstet Gynecol Nurs 1983;12:327–332.
47. Vessey MP, Lawless M, McPherson K, Yeates D. Fertility after stopping use of intrauterine contraceptive device. Br Med J 1983;286:106.
48. Rothman KJ, Louik C. Oral contraceptives and birth defects. N Engl J Med 1978;299:522–524.
49. Janerich DT, Piper JM, Glebatis DM. Oral contraceptives and birth defects. Am J Epidemiol 1980;112:73–79.
50. Harlap S, Shiono PH, Ramcharan S. Congenital abnormalities in the offspring of women who use oral and other contraceptives around the time of conception. Int J Fertil 1985;30:39–47.
51. Gray RH, Campbell OM, Zacur HA, et al. Postpartum return of ovarian activity in nonbreastfeeding women monitored by urinary assays. J Clin Endocrinol Metab 1987;64:645–651.
52. American Academy of Pediatrics Committee on Drugs. Transfer of drugs and other chemicals into human milk. Pediatrics 1989;84: 924–936.
53. Ovral as a "morning-after" contraceptive. Med Lett Drug Ther 1989; 31:93–94.
54. "Morning after" pill declared safe and effective for emergency contraception. RXtra Facts 1997;2:3.
55. Depo-Provera Contraception Injection package information. Kalamazoo, MI, Upjohn, December 1992.
56. American Health Consultants. Depo-Provera update: Not FDA-approved, but experts recommend Depo-Provera. Contracept Tech Update 1992;13:1–20.
57. Kaunitz AM. Injectable contraception. Clin Obstet Gynecol 1989; 32:356–368.
58. Mattson RH, Rebar RN. Contraceptive methods for women with neurologic disorders. Am J Obstet Gynecol 1993;168:2027–2032.
59. Olin BR, ed. Drug Facts and Comparions. St. Louis, Lippincott, 1994:108n–108p.
60. Cundy T, Evans M, Roberts H, et al. Bone density in women receiving depot medroxyprogesterone acetate for contraception. Br Med J 1991;303:13–16.
61. Nash HA. Depo Provera: A review. Contraception 1975;12:377–393.
62. Garza-flores J, De la Cruz DL, Valles de Bouges V, et al. Long-term effects of depo-medroxyprogesterone acetate on lipoprotein metabolism. Contraception 1991;44:61–71.
63. Moore LL, Valuck R, McDougall C, Fink W. A comparative study of one-year weight gain among users of medroxyprogesterone acetate, levonorgestrel implants, and oral contraceptives. Contraception 1995; 52:215–219.
64. Fahmy K, Khairy M, Allam G, et al. Effects of depo-medroxyprogesterone acetate on coagulation factors and serum lipids in Egyptian women. Contraception 1991;44:431.
65. Fahmy K, Abdel-Razik M, Shaaraway M, et al. Effects of long acting progestagen-only injectable contraceptives on carbohydrate metabolism and hormonal profile. Contraception 1991;44:419–430.
66. World Health Organization Collaborative Study of Neoplasia and Steroid Contraceptives. Breast-cancer and depot-medroxyprogesterone acetate: A multinational study. Lancet 1991;338:833–838.
67. Bonhomme MG, Potts DM, Fortnry JA, Allen MY. Safety of depot medroxyprogesterone acetate. Lancet 1991;338:942. Letter.
68. Paul C, Skegg DCG, Spears GFS. Depo-medroxyprogesterone (Depo-Provera) and risk of breast cancer. Br Med J 1989;299: 759–762.
69. Sivin I. International experience with Norplant and Norplant II. Contraception 1988;19:81–94.
70. Rosenberg MJ, Alverez F, Barone MA, et al. A comparison of "U" and standard techniques for Norplant removal. Obstet Gynecol 1997; 89:168–173.
71. Levonorgestrel approved. RXtra Facts 1997;2:4.
72. Newton JR. New hormonal methods of contraception. Balliere's Clin Obstet Gynaecol 1996;10;87–101.
73. Shoupe D, Mishell DR, Jr, Bopp BL, Fielding M. The significance of bleeding patterns in Norplant implant users.Obstet Gynecol 1991; 77:256–260.
74. Zinaman MJ. Why you should know about natural family planning. Contemp Ob/Gyn 1988;32:69–86.
75. Heaton CJ, Smith MA. The diaphragm. Am Fam Physician 1989;39: 231–236.
76. Can you rely on condoms? Consumer Reports, March 1989.
77. The female condom. Med Lett 1993;35:123–124.
78. The intrauterine device. ACOG Technical Bull May 1987.
79. Ortiz ME, Croxatto HB. The mode of action of IUDs. Contraception 1987;36:37–53.
80. Harlap S, Kost K, Forrest JD. Preventing Pregnancy, Protecting Health: A New Look at Birth Control Choices in the United States. New York, Alan Guttmacher Institute, 1991.
81. Trussel J, Leveque J, Koenig J, et al. The economic value of contraception: A comparison of 15 methods. Am J Public Health 1995; 85:494–503.

77

MENSTRUAL-RELATED DISORDERS

Martha P. Fankhauser, MS Pharm, FASHP

Premenstrual, postpartum, and premenopausal mood and physical changes are commonly experienced by women during their reproductive years.[1–5] *Dysmenorrhea* is associated with painful cramps and backache at the onset of menses. *Premenstrual molimina* describes the mild physical symptoms of breast tenderness and bloating that occur premenstrually. *Premenstrual tension* or *premenstrual syndrome* (PMS) is the cyclic recurrence during the luteal phase of a combination of psychological, behavioral, and physical symptoms. A more severe subtype of PMS, called *late luteal phase dysphoric disorder* (LLPDD) and later renamed *premenstrual dysphoric disorder* (PMDD), is associated with significant mood changes (comparable to a major depressive episode) with impairment of functioning.[6] *Maternity blues* is characterized by postpartum tearfulness, emotional lability, anxiety, and sleep disturbance.[5] Severe postpartum mood syndromes are called *postpartum depression* and *postpartum psychosis.* The *perimenopausal phase* (or premenopause) is associated with irregular menstrual cycles, a worsening of premenstrual symptoms (sleep disturbances, irritability, anxiety, depression, cognitive changes), and vasomotor complaints (hot flashes, night sweats).[3–4,7]

EPIDEMIOLOGY

Over 75% of women experience one or more physical or behavioral symptoms just before or during menses.[2,3] The prevalence of dysmenorrhea increases from early to late adolescence and decreases after age 30 to 35; 40% to 50% of women have painful menstrual cramps, and up to 10% have impaired functioning for 1 to 3 days per month such as missing work or school due to pain. Approximately 5% of women have severe PMS symptoms (meeting the diagnostic criteria for PMDD) such that their functioning is significantly affected.[6] PMDD may worsen with age secondary to the decline in ovarian production of estrogen starting 10 years before menopause.[7] Women with a history of major depressive disorder, bipolar disorder, postpartum depression, mood changes induced by oral contraceptives, and a family history of mood disorders or premenstrual depression have an increased risk for premenstrual depression.[6]

Maturity blues occurs in 50% to 80% of women 3 to 14 days after delivery, 10% to 15% have postpartum depression, and 0.1% experience postpartum psychosis.[5] Women with PMDD and premenstrual irritability have an increased risk of experiencing depression during pregnancy and the postpartum period.[8] Risk factors for postpartum mood disorders include current stressful life events; depressive symptoms during pregnancy; a past history of depression, bipolar disorder, postpartum depression, or premenstrual irritability; and a family history of mood disorders.

ETIOLOGY

Several biologic, psychological, cognitive, and social theories have been proposed for premenstrual and postpartum mood disorders, but there are no definite conclusions regarding the etiology.[2–5,7–16] Changes in mood, behavior, eating habits, and sexual activity occur in other mammalian species that have cyclical fluctuations in hormone levels. The occurrence of physical and psychological symptoms associated with the premenstrual or postpartum period or with pregnancy is closely linked to the rise and fall of gonadotropins, ovarian hormones, serotonin (5-hydroxytryptamine or 5-HT), endorphins, and prostaglandins.[14,15] During pregnancy and the postpartum period, there are more extreme and sustained hormonal changes compared to the normal menstrual cycle.[8] There is a genetic risk in the development of premenstrual depression (concordance rates of 93% in monozygotic twins, 44% in dizygotic twins, and 31% in nontwin controls).[9] Premenstrual and postpartum depression may be genetically linked.[5]

Several medical conditions, emotional/behavioral symptoms, and physiologic indices change during the menstrual cycle and worsen premenstrually (Table 77–1).[2,15,16] Dysmenorrhea may be "primary," which occurs during ovulatory cycles, or "secondary" to pelvic pathology (intrauterine devices, endometriosis, pelvic inflammatory disease, ovarian cyst, endometrial cancer, adhesions, benign uterine tumors).

PATHOPHYSIOLOGY

The menstrual cycle is a rapidly changing biologic process that involves the hypothalamic–pituitary–ovarian axis with input from gonadotropin-releasing hormones (GnRHs), gonadotropins, ovarian hormones, neurotransmitters, and neuropeptides.[3,4,11,14,17,18] The hormonal feedback system that controls neuroendocrine balance is extremely complex and vulnerable to psychosocial and environmental stresses and circadian rhythms.[3]

TABLE 77–1. Symptoms and Conditions That Change or Worsen Premenstrually

Medical Conditions	Emotional/Behavioral Changes
Acute porphyria	Aggression/anger/irritability/hostility
Arthritis	Altered libido/sex drive
Asthma	Amotivation
Chronic fatigue syndrome	Anxiety/nervousness
Dysmenorrhea	Depression/feeling blue/crying
Endometriosis	Food cravings (sugar, carbohydrates, salty foods)
Fibrocystic breast disease	Impulse control problems
Genital herpes	Mood lability/mood swings
Irritable bowel syndrome	Obsessive–compulsive behaviors
Migraine headaches	Panic attacks
Seizures	Poor concentration/memory impairment
Systemic lupus erythematosus	Psychosis/paranoia/hallucinations
Thyroid disorders	Sleep changes (insomnia, hypersomnia)
Physical Changes	Suicidal ideation/tendencies
Abdominal bloating	**Physiologic Changes**
Acne	Weight
Breast swelling/tenderness	Body temperature
Cold sores	Blood pressure and pulse
Constipation	Respiration
Dizziness	Arteriolar responses to hormones and catecholamines
Fatigue	GI transit time
Fluid retention/edema	Hepatic metabolism
Headaches	Mucus cytology
Hot flashes	Renal clearance/elimination
Muscle aches/pains	Sodium retention
Palpitations	Urinary excretion
Weight gain	

Compiled from Refs. 2, 4, 15, and 16.

HYPOTHALAMUS AND ANTERIOR PITUITARY HORMONES

The hypothalamus produces GnRH, a neurohormone that regulates the release of luteinizing hormone (LH) and follicle-stimulating hormone (FSH) from the anterior pituitary. GnRH must be released in the correct amounts and at the right pulse rate to stimulate gonadotropin secretion and to cause ovulation.[4] Release of GnRH is regulated by positive and negative feedback effects from neurotransmitters (including 5-HT, norepinephrine [NE], epinephrine [Epi], dopamine [DA], and endorphins) and by LH, FSH, and ovarian hormones.[17,18] 5-HT, NE, and Epi promote GnRH secretion, whereas endogenous opiates decrease FSH and LH by inhibiting GnRH release from the hypothalamus. Continuous activation of GnRH pituitary receptors by GnRH agonists (GnRH-As) causes a desensitization of receptors, which stops gonadotropin secretion and shuts down the reproductive cycle.[18] GnRH-As have been used to inhibit ovulation (described as a medical ovariectomy or pseudomenopausal state).

Prolactin is primarily secreted from the anterior pituitary during sleep in a pulsatile manner. Several physiologic factors influence the secretion of prolactin (e.g., stress, hypoglycemia, exercise, sleep). Prolactin peaks at midcycle and during the luteal phase if ovulation occurs. Prolactin causes proliferation and differentiation of mammary tissues during pregnancy and milk production postpartum. Estrogens, 5-HT agonists (e.g., fenfluramine), and DA antagonists (e.g., antipsychotics) stimulate prolactin release, whereas 5-HT antagonists (e.g., cyproheptadine), DA agonists (e.g., bromocriptine), and antiestrogenic agents suppress prolactin release.[3,19] Changes in DA and prolactin activity may cause mania and psychotic symptoms prior to menses and during the postpartum period.[18]

OVARIAN HORMONES

FSH stimulates follicle development in the ovaries and is the main hormone controlling estrogen secretion. LH stimulates ovulation at midcycle and is the main hormone-controlling progesterone secretion from the corpus luteum. Both estrogen and progesterone have negative feedback effects on hormonal secretion from the hypothalamus and anterior pituitary.

The rate of decline in ovarian hormones during the late luteal phase has been proposed as being more important in causing premenstrual symptoms than absolute basal values.[3,18] Rapid decline in hormone and neurotransmitter levels, and an increase in prolactin levels, immediately after delivery contribute to postpartum mood changes.[5] The premenstrual decline in ovarian function and hypoestrogenic state may play a role in the pathogenesis of PMDD and a worsening of symptoms during the perimenopausal phase.[7,20]

Estrogens are mainly synthesized by the ovary and placenta and in small amounts by the adrenal cortex.[21] Estradiol is the principal estrogen secreted by the ovary. Estrogen receptors occur primarily in the reproductive system (vagina, uterus, and mammary glands), but are also found in the pituitary, hypothalamus, bone, liver, and other tissues. Estrogen is involved in the modulation of neurotransmitter activity (for example, it increases 5-HT receptor density and augments cholinergic neurotransmission).[3] Estrogens are involved in endometrial proliferation, bone growth, metabolic action (glucose and insulin), lipid metabolism (serum lipoprotein and triglycerides), and coagulability of blood.[21] Estrogen causes sodium and water retention by increasing aldosterone levels.

Hypoestrogenic states are associated with causing hot flashes, night sweats, insomnia, vaginal dryness and atrophy, irritability, depression, anxiety, panic, and memory/cognitive impairment.[7,22,23] Menopause estrogen replacement therapy is used to decrease the risk of osteoporosis, vasomotor symptoms, cardiovascular disease, and dementia.[20–23] Continuous estrogen therapy has been effective in treating PMDD and has mood-elevating effects in perimenopausal women.[14]

Progestational agents, called *progestins,* are secreted by the corpus luteum, placenta, and in small amounts by the adrenal cortex.[24] Progesterone receptors are found in the female reproductive tract, mammary gland, hypothalamus, and pituitary. Progestins bind to $GABA_A$/benzodiazepine receptors and are involved in LH secretion.[3] Progesterone levels increase during the luteal phase and induce the formation of a secretory endometrium (which decreases the estrogen-induced endometrial proliferation) and prepare the uterus for implantation of the fertilized egg. The abrupt decline in the release of progesterone from the corpus luteum at the end of the cycle is the main determinant of the onset of menstruation. Progestins suppress menstruation and uterine contractility and are important for the maintenance of pregnancy. Physiologic effects of progesterone include reduction of arterial and alveolar P_{CO_2} in the luteal phase and during pregnancy; stimulation of lipoprotein lipase activity; enhancement of fat storage; and changes in aldosterone, sodium reabsorption, and mineralocorticoid secretion.[24] Early PMS research focused on a progesterone-deficiency theory, but several studies have found no difference in progesterone levels during the menstrual cycle in women with or without PMS.[3,10,18] Progestins may cause breakthrough bleeding, amenorrhea, edema, nausea, cholestatic jaundice, rashes, thromboembolic disorders, drowsiness, sleep disturbances, and mental depression.

NEUROTRANSMITTERS AND NEUROPEPTIDES

The activity of neurotransmitters, neurohormones, and peptides (e.g., endogenous opiates, 5-HT, DA, and GABA) parallels gonadal and ovarian hormonal fluctuations and is involved in the feedback regulation of the ovulatory cycle.[18,19] Endogenous opiates are naturally occurring neuropeptides and play a role in gonadal and neurotransmitter activity (estrogen decreases β-endorphins levels; progesterone increases β-endorphin levels; and GnRH stimulates β-endorphin release).[3] Levels of β-endorphin drop premenstrually (similar to an opiate-like withdrawal syndrome) and decrease at menopause. β-endorphins facilitate prolactin release and inhibit oxytocin, vasopressin, and LH release. Opiate antagonists increase LH release and decrease sexual drive and activity in humans.[3]

Serotonin has a reciprocal relationship with the gonadal hormones and inhibits DA activity. A 5-HT deficiency theory has been proposed as a cause for depression, premenstrual dysphoria, postpartum depression, and binge-eating behavior.[3,19,25,26] Compared to normal controls, women with PMDD have a blunted prolactin response to fenfluramine (a 5-HT releasing agent).[27] Platelet uptake of 5-HT (a model for measuring serotonergic activity) has been reported to be decreased in patients with depression and during the week before menstruation among women with PMS. Lower platelet content of 5-HT, lower whole-blood 5-HT concentrations, and lower levels of melatonin (MLT) during the luteal phase have been reported in women with PMS compared to normal controls.[25,26] Lower levels of plasma-free tryptophan (a precursor of 5-HT) have been associated with postpartum depression and PMDD.[3] Dietary tryptophan depletion can aggravate depression, PMS, and postpartum depression.[28] MLT, a metabolite of 5-HT, is secreted by the pineal gland under the influence of darkness. MLT is a neurohormone and its secretion is controlled by circadian rhythms that are synchronized by the light–dark cycle.[29] Bright light increases 5-HT levels during the day, whereas darkness promotes the synthesis of melatonin. Worsening of PMS in the winter may be caused by a reduction in daytime sunlight, which increases melatonin secretion; this type of seasonal PMS may respond to phototherapy.

Monoamine oxidase (MAO) and catechol-o-methyltransferase (COMT) metabolize monoamines, and in animal models the activity of MAO and COMT is decreased by estradiol and increased by progesterone.[18] MAO inhibitors (MAOIs) inhibit the MAO enzyme and prolong the activity of 5-HT, NE, and DA.[4] Tricyclic antidepressants (TCAs) block the reuptake of 5-HT and NE; and selective serotonin reuptake inhibitors (SSRIs) block the reuptake of 5-HT into the presynaptic neuron, which increases the amount available for neurotransmission. 5-HT augmenting antidepressants are effective in treating depression (e.g., PMDD, postpartum depression, seasonal affective disorder); anxiety (e.g., panic disorder, social phobia, obsessive–compulsive disorder); and bulimia.[26] Buspirone, a 5-HT_{1A} agonist, is used to decrease anxiety symptoms. The strong relationship between premenstrual and postpartum depression, eating disorders, and anxiety disorders suggests that 5-HT plays an important role in menstrual-related disorders.[3,25,26]

GABA, a major inhibitory neurotransmitter, is linked with steroid activity (e.g., the GABA receptor binds with progesterone; $GABA_B$ receptors inhibit LH secretion; and $GABA_A$ receptors enhance LH secretion).[3] High doses of synthetic progestins have sedative properties similar to benzodiazepines and barbiturates. Low GABA plasma levels have been reported in patients with depression and during the luteal phase in women with PMDD.[30] Benzodiazepines (agonists at the $GABA_A$/benzodiazepine receptor) have been used in the treatment of anxiety disorders and insomnia.

PROSTAGLANDINS

At menstruation, the shedding of the uterine lining releases arachidonate and stimulates prostaglandin synthesis. Prostaglandins are found in the menstrual fluid and cause uterine and gastrointestinal (GI) smooth muscle contraction.[17] Prostaglandin inhibitors (e.g., nonsteroidal anti-inflammatory agents, or NSAIAs) are effective in treating dysmenorrhea, headaches, and other pain syndromes. A deficiency of prostaglandin E_1 (PGE_1) has been proposed as causing breast pain (e.g., low levels of PGE_1 may increase prolactin's effect on breast tissue and cause mastodynia).[31] *Cis*-linolenic acid, an essential fatty acid contained in vegetable oils, is converted to γ-linolenic acid, the precursor to PGE_1. *Cis*-linolenic acid, magnesium, pyridoxine, zinc, and vitamin C are involved in the synthesis of PGE_1. Products that promote the synthesis of

PGE_1 (e.g., evening primrose oil contains γ-linolenic acid) have been used for breast pain.

VITAMIN AND MINERAL DEFICIENCY

Pyridoxine (vitamin B_6) is a cofactor in the synthesis of DA and 5-HT; a coenzyme in the metabolism of protein, carbohydrate, and fat; and involved in the production of prostaglandins from essential fatty acids. A deficiency of pyridoxine decreases the synthesis of DA and 5-HT and may be involved in causing depression.[31] Although pyridoxine is commonly used as a vitamin treatment, there is no evidence of pyridoxine deficiency in women with PMS.[2] Low blood levels of calcium and low intracellular magnesium levels have been reported in women with PMS compared to controls.[31] Low magnesium levels may cause a depletion of DA, resulting in increased prolactin concentrations. Dairy products and calcium can interfere with GI absorption of magnesium, but the significance of this is not known.

CLINICAL PRESENTATION

Before a diagnosis of a menstrual-related disorder is made, other medical or psychiatric causes should be excluded (Table 77–2). Approximately 50% of women with PMS complaints have an underlying mood disorder that requires long-term treatment. Premenstrual and postpartum exacerbation of an underlying disorder (anxiety, panic, depression, mania, bulimia, migraine headaches, seizures) has been reported.

Although some women experience positive premenstrual changes such as increased energy and productivity, the majority of women experience negative changes in mood, appetite, sleep, and energy. Physical changes (back pain, breast tenderness, headaches, water retention, and bloating sensations) may be better tolerated than the mood or behavioral changes. The most distressing PMS symptoms include depression, anxiety, mood swings, irritability, anger attacks, oversensitivity, crying episodes, difficulty concentrating, and clumsiness.[1,2] Severe PMDD may include episodes of psychosis, mania, and suicidal ideation and has resulted in marital discord, physical and verbal abuse of others, difficulties in parenting, criminal behavior, poor work or school performance, work absenteeism, social isolation, accidents, hospitalizations, suicide, and homicide.[1–3]

Postpartum psychiatric disorders often require hospitalization and are associated with marital conflict, impaired functioning, poor bonding with the infant, suicide, and infanticide.[5] In the climacteric phase preceding menopause (ages 35 to 50 years), women report more sleep disturbances, hot flashes, anxiety attacks, depression, irritability, and decreased short-term memory.[7]

TABLE 77–2. Evaluation of Menstrual-Related Disorders

Type of Evaluation	Tests/Procedures/Assessments
Psychiatric evaluation	Past psychiatric history (particularly mood disorders and alcohol/substance abuse) History of symptoms: onset, duration, course, precipitating factors, previous treatments, and response Family history for PMS and mood disorders; treatment of other family members
Medical evaluation	Past and current history for endocrine and gynecologic disorders (dysmenorrhea, endometriosis, fibrocystic breast disease, thyroid abnormalities, abnormal PAP, irritable bowel syndrome) Physical and pelvic exam
Laboratory tests	Chemistry panel, complete blood count with differential, and thyroid function tests—to rule out anemia, hypothyroidism, or other disease states Other tests: FSH and estradiol, to rule out estrogen deficiency if perimenopausal or symptoms of irregular bleeding or hot flashes Prolactin, to rule out cause of irregular menses or amenorrhea Vitamin B_6, B_{12}, folate, magnesium, and calcium, to rule out deficiencies
Medication use	History of OTC and prescription medications (psychoactive agents, those that can induce psychiatric conditions); caffeine; alcohol; and substances/illicit drugs; oral or injectable hormonal contraceptives
Nutritional evaluation	Assessment of diet (protein, complex carbohydrates, phytoestrogens, salt, minerals, calcium, trace elements, vitamins) Well-balanced, regular meals
Exercise and sleep evaluation	Assessment of adequate and regular exercise and good sleep habits
Self-rating for PMS	Two months of prospective daily rating of symptoms using a PMS rating scale.[a] Compare average ratings of luteal phase to follicular phase (5–7 days postmenses and 5–7 days premenses); > 30–50% change in severity ratings required for PMS plus a symptom-free week postmenses
Other evaluations	Daily basal body temperatures to determine ovulation Morning and evening weights to monitor fluid retention

[a]Menstrual Distress Questionnaire (MDQ), PMS Diary (PMSD) Daily Rating Form (DRF).
Compiled from Refs. 9,12 and 92.

▶ TREATMENT: Menstrual-Related Disorders

The goals of treating menstrual-related disorders are to minimize symptoms and improve functioning and well-being without causing adverse effects. A stepwise approach is recommended so that the least toxic agent is used first before resorting to experimental treatments. The weighing of risk versus benefit of pharmacologic interventions is important, because some medications cause significant adverse effects.[32]

For PMS, a treatment trial of three menstrual cycles is recommended to adjust dosages based on adverse effects and efficacy. For women with premenstrual exacerbation of an underlying depression, PMDD, or postpartum depression, a 6- to 12-month duration of antidepressant therapy is recommended.[32] Some women benefit from continuous antidepressant dosing with an intermittent increase in dose prior to the onset of symptoms

TABLE 77–3. Pharmacologic Treatments for Menstrual-Related Disorders

Agent/Drug	Dose	Clinical Reason for Use
Vitamins and Minerals		
Pyridoxine	50–100 mg/d	A cofactor in the synthesis of DA and 5-HT; reduces irritability, depression, fatigue, edema, and headache
Calcium (Ca)	1 g/d before menopause; 1.5 g/d after menopause	Intracellular Ca plays a role in cellular function; bone loss of Ca results in osteoporosis (↑ risk as estrogen levels decline)
Magnesium (Mg)	50–100 mg bid up to 360 mg/d	Intracellular Mg plays an essential role in neuromuscular function and protein and carbohydrate enzyme systems
Vitamin E (α-tocopherol)	200–600 IU/d	A fat-soluble vitamin that is involved in the functioning of many organs and systems: reproductive, muscular, cardiovascular, hematopoietic, and central nervous system; antioxidant effects
Other OTC Products		
Diphenhydramine	25–50 mg hs	Antihistamine: used for sedative-hypnotic effects to induce sleep
Evening primrose oil	0.5–2 g bid during cycle or luteal phase	Contains γ-linolenic acid (a precursor to prostaglandin E_1) and reported to reduce breast pain
Kava-kava	100 mg tid	Used for anxiety, stress, restlessness, and premenstrual cramps
Melatonin	0.1–2 mg hs	Metabolite of 5-HT, OTC sleep inducing agent used for jet lag, sleep–wake cycle disorder, insomnia
Passion flower	4–8 gm of herb qid prn	Used for anxiety and restlessness
St. John's wort (hypericin)	300 mg tid	Folk remedy for depression, anxiety, and insomnia
Valerian	1/2–1 teaspoon tincture or 2–3 gm extract	Sedative–hypnotic effects; used for insomnia and restlessness
Diuretics		
Spironolactone	25–50 mg qd, bid on days 14–28	Synthetic steroid aldosterone antagonist with K^+-sparing effects
Hydrochlorothiazide	25–50 mg qd, bid on days 14–28	Diuretic that enhances the excretion of Na, Cl, K, and H_2O
Triamterene	50–100 mg qd, bid on days 14–28	K^+-sparing diuretic; structurally related to folic acid
NSAIAs		
Ibuprofen	200–400 mg q4–6h; or 600 mg bid	Prostaglandin inhibitors: reduces pain, swelling, headache, and cramping; start regular dosing 7–10 d prior to menses
Mefenamic acid	250–500 mg tid	See ibuprofen; not to exceed 7 d
Naproxen	500 mg, then 250–500 mg bid	See Ibuprofen
Naproxen sodium	550 mg, then 275–550 mg bid	See Ibuprofen
Hormones		
Estradiol		
Oral	0.5–2 mg/d	Used for perimenopause to decrease emotional and physical symptoms; use concomitant natural progesterone if uterus is present to ↓ risk of endometriosis; intermittent therapy for estrogen withdrawal headache
Transdermal	100-μg patch: 1 or 2 every 3 d during cycle	See oral, above
Progesterone		
Oral	100 mg/d and 200 mg/d on days 17–28	Not recommended for monotherapy for PMS; combined with estrogen to reduce risk of endometriosis
Suppository	200–400 mg bid on days 17–28	See oral form, above
Oral contraceptives	1 pill/d estrogen + progesterone; use monophasic or biphasic with low progesterone	Suppresses the hypothalamic-pituitary system and prevents ovulation; regulates the menstrual cycle; used for the treatment of endometriosis or dysfunctional uterine bleeding

and a reduction in dose at the onset of menses.[4] Varying the antidepressant dosage and adding supplemental medications based on menstrual-related symptoms has empirically been shown to be helpful. It may be necessary to try several different treatments before an acceptable therapy is identified.

GENERAL APPROACH

A wide variety of nonpharmacologic and pharmacologic treatments are available for menstrual-related disorders.[1,2,9,12,13,33–38] Treatment approaches should be tailored to the primary symptom complaints (or target symptoms). In general, five different treatment strategies are used for PMS: (1) life-style changes to minimize precipitants, (2) physical and behavioral symptom relief, (3) modification of neurotransmitter/hormonal imbalances, (4) suppression of ovulation, and (5) removal of ovaries.[9,33]

NONPHARMACOLOGIC THERAPY

Nonpharmacologic treatments for menstrual-related disorders include (1) education about the symptoms, treatment approaches, and strategies to reduce target behaviors; (2) daily charting for

TABLE 77–3. (Continued)

Agent/Drug	Dose	Clinical Reason for Use
Hormones (Continued)		
Antiestrogen		
Danazol	200–400 mg/d: onset of breast pain until first day of menses	Synthetic androgen with antiestrogenic effects; used for mastalgia and to suppress ovarian function prior to ovariectomy
Gonadotropin-releasing hormone agonists		
Leuprolide	3.75 mg IM q4wk	Causes anovulation and drops estrogen levels to menopausal levels; add-back estrogen ± progestin
Buserelin	Intranasal spray/d	See Leuprolide
Dopamine Agonist		
Bromocriptine	2.5 mg bid on days 10–26	DA agonist: ↓ prolactin and reduce breast swelling and pain; use only for severe mastodynia
Antidepressants		
Selective serotonin reuptake inhibitors (SSRIs)		
Citalopram	10–40 mg/d	5-HT augmenting agent with antidepressant and antianxiety effects; use for PMDD and postpartum depression; continuous or intermittent dosing
Fluvoxamine	50–200 mg/d	
Fluoxetine	20–40 mg/d	
Paroxetine	10–30 mg/d	
Sertraline	50–100 mg/d	
Serotonin–norepinephrine reuptake inhibitors		
Venlafaxine	75–375 mg/d in divided doses	5-HT and NE-augmenting agent with antidepressant effects
Norepinephrine–dopamine reuptake inhibitor		
Bupropion	75 mg tid; 100–150 mg SR bid	NE- and DA-augmenting agent with antidepressant effects; avoid in eating disorder patients due to potential ↑ seizure risk at > 450 mg/d
Tricyclic antidepressants (TCAs)		
Amitriptyline	25–50 mg hs, prn sleep	Sedating TCA with high anticholinergic and antihistamine effects; used for insomnia and migraine prophylaxis
Clomipramine	25–125 mg/d	5-HT > NE-augmenting agent with antianxiety and antidepressant effects
Doxepin	25–50 mg hs	See Amitriptyline; primarily used for insomnia
Nortriptyline	50–125 mg/d	5-HT- and NE-augmenting agent with antianxiety and antidepressant effects
Serotonin antagonists		
Nefazodone	100–400 mg/d	5-HT antagonist with antidepressant and antianxiety effects
Trazodone	150–400 mg/d in divided doses; 25–150 mg hs	5-HT antagonist with antidepressant effects; primarily used for insomnia
Antianxiety Agents		
Alprazolam	0.25–4 mg/d in divided doses continuous or days 16–28	BZD that augments $GABA_A$ receptor; antianxiety effects; do not use in patients with a history of substance abuse; taper down by 25%/d
Buspirone	15–60 mg/d in divided doses continuous or days 16–28	$5\text{-}HT_{1A}$ agonist with antianxiety effects
Hypnotic Agents		
Temazepam	7.5–30 mg hs	BZD that augments $GABA_A$ receptor; marketed as a hypnotic agent
Triazolam	0.125–0.25 mg hs	See temazepam
Zolpidem	5–10 mg hs	Non-BZD that binds to same BZD-chloride channel as BZDs; rapid hypnotic effects with no significant antianxiety effect

Compiled from Refs. 1, 2, 12, 13, 33, and 34.

two menstrual cycles to identify target symptoms; (3) reduction or discontinuation of alcohol, caffeine, nicotine, and drugs of abuse; (4) regular conditioning or aerobic exercise with an increase in the daily workout routine by 30 minutes during the premenstrual week; (4) bright white morning and evening light for 1 week premenstrually for seasonal worsening of PMS; (5) regular, well-balanced, scheduled meals with adequate fiber, protein, carbohydrates, vitamins, calcium, and minerals; (6) reduction of salt, caffeine, fat, and simple sugars; (7) increase in phytoestrogen-rich foods (soybean products) and tryptophan-containing foods (fish, poultry, and dairy products); (8) adequate rest and regular sleep patterns or partial sleep deprivation for premenstrual depression; (9) stress reduction, relaxation training, yoga, massages, biofeedback, and self-hypnosis; and (10) individual, group, or family therapy, cognitive–behavioral therapy, support groups, and assertiveness training.[1–2,31–36]

PHARMACOLOGIC THERAPY

There are no FDA-approved medications or published guidelines for the treatment of premenstrual or postpartum mood disorders. NSAIAs are the treatment of choice for dysmenorrhea, whereas perimenopausal symptoms usually respond to estrogen replacement therapy. PMDD and postpartum depression are generally treated with 5-HT augmenting antidepressants. A list of pharmacologic treatments used for menstrual-related symptoms is found in Table 77–3. An example of first-line and second-line treatment approaches for PMS is shown in Table 77–4, and an algorithm for the treatment of PMDD is shown in Fig. 77–1.

VITAMIN, MINERAL, HERBAL, NUTRITIONAL, AND HORMONAL THERAPIES

Daily supplementation of vitamins, minerals, and calcium along with a well-balanced diet is recommended as a first-line therapy for all menstrual-related disorders. Adequate postpartum replacement of vitamins and minerals is important to reduce deficiency states, particularly in women who breast-feed their infants. OTC products containing megadoses of vitamins along with minerals and trace elements have been marketed for PMS without scientific testing.

Vitamin B_6 is recommended for women taking oral contraceptives and estrogen therapy because estrogenic substances increase the demand for pyridoxine. Although pyridoxine has been reported to reduce premenstrual depression, fatigue, irritability, headache, and edema,[31] a review of 12 controlled studies revealed little support for its efficacy in PMS.[39] A few studies have investigated single-mineral therapy (calcium, magnesium, zinc, copper) in the treatment of PMS. Elemental calcium reduced premenstrual mood changes, fluid retention, and pain,[40] and magnesium improved mood symptoms in PMS studies.[41]

Herbal products and nutritional supplements are promoted for PMS but they cannot be recommended, as little is known about their dosing, efficacy, or safety.[38] *St. John's wort* extract is used for the treatment of depression in doses of 300 mg (standarized to contain 0.3% hypericin) taken three times daily. The exact mechanism of action for hypericin (hypericum extract) is

TABLE 77–4. First-Line and Second-Line Treatment Approaches for Premenstrual Syndrome

PMS Symptoms	First-Line	Second-Line
Standard approaches	Counseling/education; charting for PMS; good nutrition/diet; aerobic exercise; good sleep hygiene	Eliminate caffeine, nicotine, alcohol, drugs of abuse
General mild symptoms (low energy, poor diet)	Multiple vitamins + minerals	Add pyridoxine, calcium, magnesium, vitamin E, zinc, herbal therapies
Dysmenorrhea	Aspirin, ibuprofen, ketoprofen, naproxen	Meclofenamic acid, mefenamic acid
Migraine headaches	Aspirin, ibuprofen, ketoprofen, naproxen	Prophylaxis with atenolol, propranolol; amitriptyline; verapamil; valproic acid; estradiol; or combination therapy
Bloating/edema	Spironolactone	Amiloride, metolazone, hydrochorothiazide, triamterene ± HCTZ
Breast pain/mastalgia	Mild: Stop caffeine; vitamin E Moderate: Bromocriptine Severe: Leuprolide	Evening primrose oil Danazol Other GnRH-As
Insomnia	Mild: Melatonin; herbal sleep aids Moderate: Trazodone Severe: Lorazepam, temazepam, triazolam	Diphenhydramine, doxylamine Amitriptyline, doxepin, imipramine Zolpidem
Anxiety	Buspirone; nefazodone	Alprazolam, lorazepam
Binge-eating/craving foods/weight gain	Fluoxetine, fluvoxamine, paroxetine, sertraline	Bupropion, amphetamines; fenfluramine and D-fenfluramine taken off the market
Depression/irritability PMDD	Citalopram, fluoxetine, fluvoxamine, paroxetine, sertraline	Clomipramine, nortriptyline, venlafaxine, nefazodone
Seasonal PMS/PMDD	Bright-light,	Citalopram, fluoxetine, fluvoxamine, paroxetine, sertraline
Mood swings (severe)	Valproic acid, carbamazepine	Lithium, verapamil, investigational; gabapentin, lamotrigine
Perimenopausal symptoms	Estradiol: Oral, transdermal, implants	± Progestins ± testosterone
Moderate PMS/PMDD	Oral contraceptives: monophasic or biphasic	Leuprolide + estrogen add-back ± progestin; other GnRH-As
Severe PMS/PMDD	Combine SSRIs with other therapies: OCs, estradiol, GnRH-As	Bilateral ovariectory + estrogen add-back ± progestin

Adapted from Refs. 1, 2, 12, 13, 33, 34, 36, and 38.

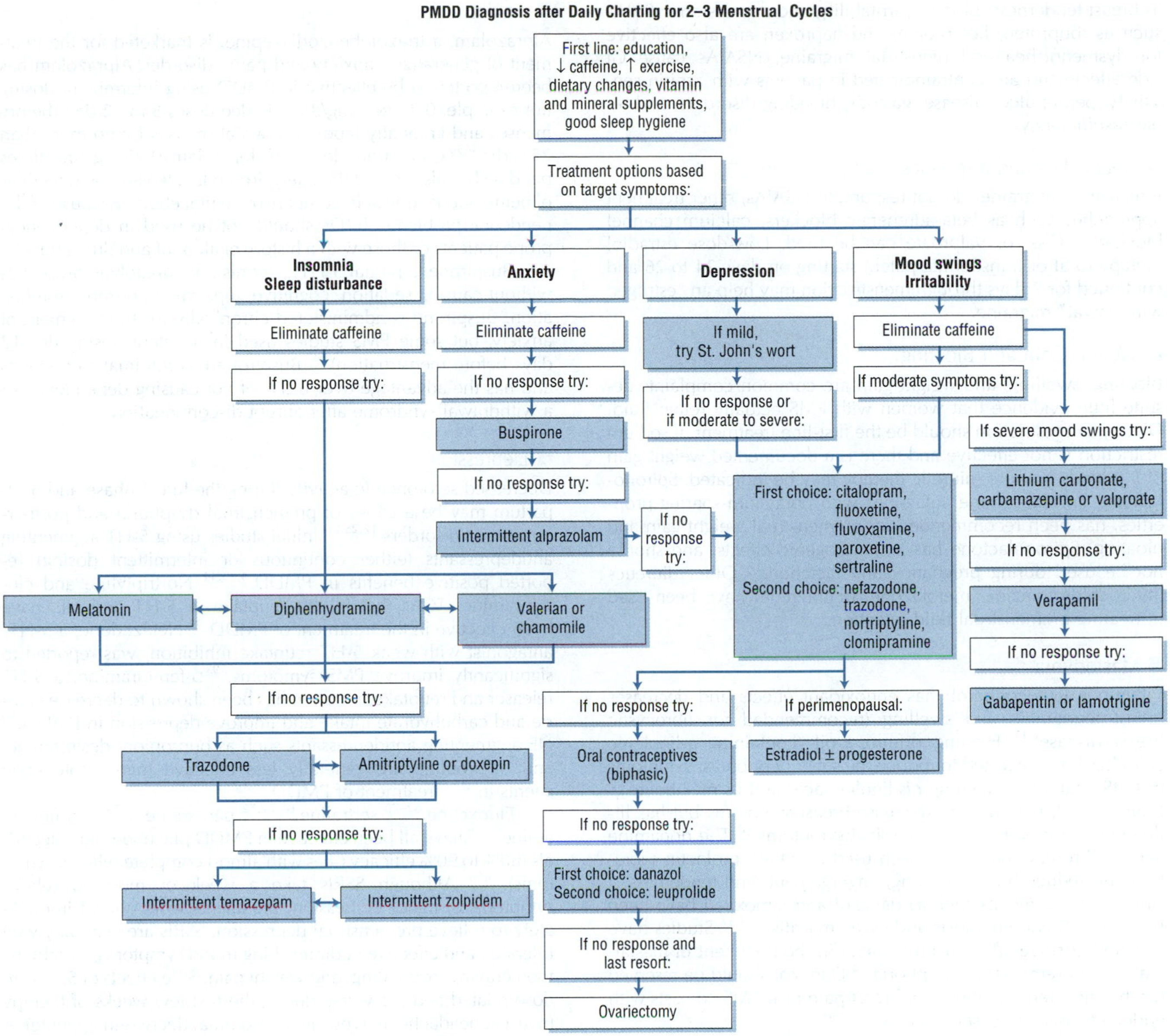

FIGURE 77–1. Algorithm for the treatment of premenstrual dysphoric disorder.

not known, and no information is available about its use in PMS or in postpartum depression. *Dong quai,* which contains coumarin derivatives, is widely used in China for menstrual cramps and irregular menses.[42] *Black cohosh* has been used for the treatment of dysmenorrhea and menopausal hot flashes,[43] and *blue cohosh* has been used for menstrual cramps and stimulation of menstrual flow.[44] Valerian is an herbal sleep aid,[45] and *chamomile* is a sedative, antispasmodic, antipyretic, and anti-inflammatory agent.[46]

Tryptophan (the amino acid precursor to 5-HT) was used for insomnia until it was withdrawn from the market in 1989 because of several deaths associated with an eosinophilia myalgia syndrome (EMS). EMS was probably caused by a contaminant in the manufacturing process of trytophan by one Japanese company.[47] Tryptophan is found in high concentrations in dairy products, beef, chicken, and fish. Dietary tryptophan or exogenous tryptophan increases the production of 5-HT and MLT. MLT regulates the sleep–wake cycle and has been used for the treatment of premenstrual and menopausal insomnia. MLT is not recommended during pregnancy and breast feeding due to lack of information about its safety. Lower doses of MLT (e.g., 0.1 to 1 mg hs) are effective in initiating sleep; higher doses may not improve the hypnotic effect.[48]

Products promoted for perimenopausal symptoms without scientific testing include *dehydroepiandrosterone* (a steroid hormone produced by the adrenal glands and ovaries that is a precursor hormone for testosterone and estrogen); passion flower (for insomnia, pain, and climacteric complaints); wild yam root (contains diosgenin, a precursor to progesterone); and phytoestrogens (plant-based hormones found in soybean food such as tofu and flax seeds that promote estrogenic effects).[49]

SYMPTOM-BASED APPROACHES

Dysmenorrhea and Cramps

NSAIAs inhibit prostaglandin synthesis and exhibit anti-inflammatory, analgesic, and antipyretic activity.[17] Mefenamic acid has been reported to be effective in reducing menstrual pain, as well as breast tenderness, bloating, irritability, and depression. NSAIAs such as ibuprofen, ketoprofen, and naproxen are also effective for dysmenorrhea and menstrual migraine. NSAIAs cause GI side effects and are contraindicated in patients with aspirin sensitivity, peptic ulcer disease, gastritis, bleeding disorders, and renal insufficiency.

Headaches and Migraines

If menstrual migraines do not respond to NSAIAs, other treatment approaches such as beta-adrenergic blockers, calcium channel blockers, TCAs, or valproate can be tried. Low-dose estradiol therapy (oral or transdermal patch) starting on days 24 to 26 and continued for 7 days through menstruation may help an "estrogen withdrawal" migraine.

Weight Gain and Bloating

Bloating, swelling, and weight gain are common complaints despite little evidence that women with PMS actually retain fluid. Dietary salt restriction should be the first-line treatment. If sodium restriction is not effective and there is a documented weight gain of 5 pounds or more, diuretic therapy may be indicated. Spironolactone, an aldosterone antagonist with potassium-sparing properties, has been recommended for premenstrual weight gain and bloating. Spironolactone has antiandrogenic effects, and should not be used during pregnancy and lactation.[17] Other diuretics (hydrochlorothiazide, metolazone, triamterene) have been used in treating premenstrual fluid retention.

Mastodynia

Vitamin E (α-tocopherol) has antioxidant effects and decreases breast tenderness and swelling (recommended for fibrocystic breast disease).[17] Evening primrose oil (containing γ-linolenic acid) has been reported to reduce the severity of breast symptoms in PMS. Efamol (containing *cis*-linoleic acid and its metabolite γ-linoleic acid) may help to decrease breast symptoms but has little effect on mood or other physical symptoms.[50] The dopamine agonist, bromocriptine, has been used to inhibit prolactin secretion and reduce breast swelling, engorgement, and tenderness.[17] Antiestrogenic agents such as danazol and tamoxifen have been used to treat endometriosis and cystic mastitis.[2,14,17] Studies have reported positive effects with danazol in the treatment of mastalgia [51] and premenstrual dysphoria.[52] Danazol should be reserved for the short-term treatment of breast pain or if PMS coexists with endometriosis and cystic mastitis.

Insomnia

Histamine$_1$ antagonists (e.g., diphenhydramine) can be tried for acute sleep disturbances but may cause anticholinergic side effects and daytime sedation. Antidepressants with high histamine$_1$ blockade (doxepin, amitriptyline) have been used for insomnia but may not be tolerated due to significant anticholinergic and α-adrenergic antagonist effects. Trazodone (a 5-HT$_2$ and α-adrenergic antagonist) has sedative properties at lower doses and may be used to promote sleep; higher doses may cause dizziness and daytime sedation. Trazodone has been used in combination with SSRIs, MAOIs, and bupropion as a hypnotic to reverse antidepressant-induced insomnia.[53]

Chronic use of benzodiazepines (BZDs) is not recommended for insomnia because tolerance and physical dependence may result. If BZDs are used for the acute treatment of insomnia, agents with shorter ($t_{1/2}$) half-lives should be used (e.g., lorazepam or temazepam). Ultra-short-acting hypnotic BZDs (triazolam) are less likely to cause daytime sedation but have an increased risk of causing anterograde amnesia, early-morning insomnia, delirium, and withdrawal reactions. Zolpidem, a nonbenzodiazepine, is an alternative treatment for premenstrual insomnia but should be used only for short-term or intermittent therapy.

Anxiety

Alprazolam, a triazolobenzodiazepine, is marketed for the treatment of generalized anxiety and panic disorder. Alprazolam has been reported to be effective in PMDD using intermittent dosing (for example, 0.25 to 4 mg/d in divided doses 8 to 12 days before menses and gradually tapered down at menses by no more than 25%/d).[54–56] Continuous dosing of alprazolam (0.25 mg three times per day) has also reduced anxiety, irritability, tension, and feelings of being out of control in comparison to placebo.[57] Because of dependency problems, BZDs should not be used in dependency-prone patients or those with a history of alcohol and drug abuse.

Buspirone, a partial 5-HT$_{1A}$ agonist, has anxiolytic properties without causing sedation, cognitive impairment, or muscle relaxation. Buspirone is administered chronically for the treatment of anxiety, but some PMS studies used intermittent dosing (for 12 days before menstruation).[58] Buspirone has minimal side effects and has the advantage over BZDs of not causing dependence or a withdrawal syndrome after abrupt discontinuation.

Depression

Decreased serotonergic activity during the luteal phase and postpartum may be a cause of premenstrual dysphoria and postpartum mood disorders.[17,25,26] Initial studies using 5-HT augmenting antidepressants (either continuous or intermittent dosing) reported positive benefits in PMDD.[4,33,34] Nortriptyline and clomipramine, TCAs that inhibit reuptake of 5-HT and NE, have been effective in the treatment of PMDD.[34] Nefazodone, a 5-HT$_2$ antagonist with weak 5-HT reuptake inhibition, was reported to significantly improve PMS symptoms.[59] D-fenfluramine, a 5-HT releaser and reuptake inhibitor, has been shown to decrease calorie and carbohydrate intake and improve depression in PMDD.[60] NE augmenting antidepressants such as bupropion, desipramine, and maprotiline are generally less effective than serotonergic agents in the treatment of PMDD.[61,62]

Fluoxetine,[62–70] sertraline,[61,71,72] paroxetine,[73,74] and fluvoxamine[75,76] have all been effective in PMDD placebo-controlled trials (60% to 90% efficacy rates with almost complete relief of symptoms).[33,34] Although SSRIs take a week or more to relieve symptoms of major depression, the agents work almost immediately to relieve premenstrual depression. SSRIs are generally well tolerated and effective in diminishing mood symptoms, irritability, food craving, overeating, and weight gain. Side effects of SSRIs are dose related and are worse during the first few weeks of therapy (nausea, headache, nervousness, insomnia, decreased appetite). A common long-term adverse effect of SSRIs is sexual dysfunction (decreased libido and delayed orgasm).[68] SSRIs have the advantage of not causing significant weight gain, drowsiness, cardiovascular changes, and anticholinergic side effects compared to TCAs.[32]

Mood Swings

Lithium carbonate, carbamazepine, and valproate are used as mood stabilizers and may be appropriate for women with predominant mood swings or those with a history of recurrent mood disorders. Mood stabilizers should be used with caution during pregnancy because of potential teratogenic effects. Lithium has numerous adverse effects (such as hypothyroidism) and requires routine blood level monitoring. Low dose valproate (range, 125 to 500 mg/d with mean serum levels of 32.5 μg/mL) was reported to decrease PMS symptoms and migraine headaches in a small study.[77] Other investigational mood stabilizers such as verapamil, lamotrigine, and gabapentin have not been evaluated for PMS.

HORMONAL THERAPIES

Progesterone

For many years, administration of progesterone by vaginal suppositories during the luteal phase was a common hormonal treatment for PMS.[78] After several double-blind, placebo-controlled studies, it is now thought that progesterone is no better than placebo for treating PMS.[14,17,78] However, controversy still surrounds the form (natural versus synthetic), length of treatment (luteal phase versus chronic therapy), and route of administration (oral, buccal/sublingual, vaginal, rectal, or implants). If progesterone is used, an oral micronized form of natural progesterone is better absorbed and has advantages over synthetic progestins.[79] Progesterone may make some PMS symptoms worse (fatigue, depression, fluid retention, irritability, acne, increase in appetite), and it should be used with caution in certain medical conditions (including migraine, seizure disorders, asthma, and cardiac or renal disease). Progestins are contraindicated in patients with thrombophlebitis and thromboembolic disorders. Because of its questionable efficacy and risk of adverse effects, progesterone-only therapy is not recommended as a treatment in PMS.

Estrogen

Estradiol, the active estrogen produced by the ovaries, is effective for menstrual migraines and for estrogen replacement therapy to control menopausal symptomatology. Estradiol implants and transdermal estradiol patches have been beneficial in reducing premenstrual symptoms.[14] Chronic estradiol therapy suppresses ovulation and is more effective than oral conjugated estrogens. Available products include a micronized and an ethinyl estradiol tablet; a cypionate and a valerate estradiol parenteral oil injection; a transdermal estradiol topical system; and a vaginal estradiol cream. The transdermal estradiol patches may cause skin irritation and should be replaced at a new application site every 3 to 4 days. Estradiol with intermittent progestin therapy (e.g., norethisterone 5 mg/d for 7 days each month to induce regular menses) may cause PMS-like side effects.[78] Estrogen–progestin combinations have an increased risk of causing thrombophlebitis, pulmonary embolism, and cerebral thrombosis due to the progestin effects. Chronic estrogen-only therapy has certain risks (e.g., increasing endometrial, ovarian, and breast cancer and gallbladder disease) and should not be administered during pregnancy. Oral or transdermal estradiol (combined with cyclical or continuous progesterone if the uterus is present) should be tried in perimenopausal women with significant premenstrual mood and physical symptoms.

Estrogen–Progestin Combinations

Oral contraceptives (OCs) cause anovulation and may reduce dysmenorrhea, depression, and irritability.[14,78] OCs can worsen PMS symptoms in approximately 30% of women, but some women may derive benefit.[16] Biphasic or triphasic products have been used in PMS, but triphasic products are associated with causing more mood changes.[3,80] OCs high in progestin may produce breakthrough bleeding and/or spotting, amenorrhea, acne, hirsutism, fatigue, and depression. Pyridoxine replacement therapy, 50 mg/d, is recommended for women who become depressed while taking OCs. OCs should be used with caution in women who smoke because of an increased risk of thromboembolism.

GnRH-As

Initial administration of GnRH-As stimulate the release of FSH and LH from the pituitary, and then a down-regulation of the pituitary decreases ovarian stimulation to release estrogen and progesterone.[14] GnRH-As (administered subcutaneously, intranasally, by implants, or by intramuscular depot injections) are used to inhibit ovulation and suppress estradiol and progesterone levels.[81] Initially, some women report a "flare" in PMS symptoms during the first few weeks of GnRH-A treatment, which is followed by a reduction in the physical and behavioral symptoms of PMS. The use of a combination of GnRH-A plus an "add-back" of estrogen/progestin may help to reverse antiestrogenic and antiprogesterone effects without decreasing the effectiveness of GnRH-As.

Depot leuprolide (3.75 mg/mo) was found to reduce physical and behavioral symptoms in women without premenstrual depression but was not effective in women with severe premenstrual depression.[82,83] Long-term treatment with depot leuprolide along with estrogen and progestin add-back therapy was reported to be effective in PMS over a 12-month period; however, 4 out of 10 subjects exhibited bone loss during the study.[84] Nafarelin acetate is approved as a nasal spray for the management of endometriosis, but little is known about its effectiveness in PMS. A double-blind study comparing depot goserelin (3.6 mg/mo) with a placebo reported that it significantly improved physical symptoms of PMS (e.g., breast discomfort) but did not reduce the psychological symptoms (depression, anxiety, irritability).[85] Buserelin was shown to have beneficial effects in PMS when administered intranasally in two PMS studies[86,87] and no improvement in one placebo-controlled study.[88] Histrelin was administered by daily subcutaneous injections in 8 women with severe PMS, resulting in a 75% improvement in luteal phase symptoms.[89]

GnRH-As may improve cyclical mood changes during short-term therapy, but the chronic effects of suppressing ovarian hormone secretion could result in significant antiestrogen effects (osteoporosis and cardiovascular disease) and worsening of mood without low-dose hormone replacement therapy. Until the long-term safety is established, GnRH-As should be used only for the most severe cases of PMS.[81]

SURGICAL THERAPY

OVARIECTOMY

Surgical ablation of the ovaries should be reserved as the last-resort treatment for severe PMDD.[90,91] A 3- to 6-month trial of a GnRH-A or danazol is recommended before radical surgery to determine if anovulation is effective, because the ovariectomy is not reversible. A hysterectomy without a ovariectomy is not effective for PMS. If an ovariectomy is done without a hysterectomy, women need both estrogen and progestin replacement therapy. Unopposed estrogen increases the risk for endometrial hyperplasia; therefore, intermittent (for 7 or more days of a cycle) or continuous progestin therapy is recommended. Women who have both the ovariectomy and hysterectomy can receive continuous estradiol without intermittent progestin therapy because there is no risk for endometrial cancer.[91]

EVALUATION OF THERAPEUTIC OUTCOMES

Self-rating of PMS symptoms using a severity rating scale (PMS Diary, Menstrual Distress Questionnaire, the Daily Rating Form) helps to monitor the efficacy of different treatment approaches.[92] Reduction of baseline premenstrual ratings (the average score for 5 to 7 days prior to menses) by 50% should be the minimum goal of therapy. Ideally, complete relief would show that premenstrual ratings are similar to postmenstrual ratings 5 to 7 days after the cessation of menses for several menstrual cycles. A trial of at least three menstrual cycles is needed to determine treatment efficacy and to adjust dosing before resorting to another therapy.

CONCLUSIONS

Menstrual-related disorders are very common and cause significant disability and impairment in functioning if not properly treated. Therapeutic strategies should be individualized and targeted to the most distressing symptoms. If possible, medications should not be prescribed unless nonpharmacologic approaches have failed or unless symptoms cause disruption in functioning. The regular assessment and monitoring of menstrual-related disorders is necessary throughout the woman's reproductive years.

▶ PRINCIPLES OF PHARMACOTHERAPY

- A correct diagnosis of dysmenorrhea, PMS, PMDD, postpartum psychiatric disorders, and perimenopause is essential. An evaluation and careful workup should rule out other possible causes and identify target symptoms.
- A stepwise treatment approach using safer agents first and reserving more toxic agents or combination therapies for refractory or severe symptoms is recommended for PMS and PMDD.
- Combination therapies (hormonal agents plus antidepressants; NSAIAs plus antianxiety agents) may be needed if monotherapy is ineffective or if multiple symptoms are present for PMS and PMDD.
- Education, supportive therapy, regular exercise, dietary changes (limiting caffeine, salt, and alcohol), and good sleep hygiene are first-line approaches for all menstrual-related disorders.
- NSAIAs are the treatment of choice for dysmenorrhea and menstrual headaches.
- Serotonin-augmenting agents (SSRIs) are the most effective treatment for PMDD. Some women may require an increase in dose during the luteal phase if symptomatic.
- Postpartum depression should be treated with antidepressants (and antipsychotics if needed for psychosis). Electroconvulsive therapy should be considered for severe cases that involve psychosis or suicidality. Prophylaxis at the time of delivery is recommended for women with at least one previous postpartum depression.
- Perimenopausal women should be evaluated for hormone replacement therapy, because estrogen deficiency causes numerous health-related problems.
- After a 3-month trial of a pharmacologic agent, the risks versus benefits of treatment should be evaluated based on severity of adverse effects and efficacy for treating the menstrual disorder.

REFERENCES

1. Fankhauser MP. Treatment of dysmenorrhea and premenstrual syndrome. J Am Pharm Assoc 1996;NS36:503–513.
2. Parker PD. Premenstrual syndrome. Am Family Physician 1994;50: 1309–1317.
3. Janowsky DS, Halbreich U, Rausch J. Association among ovarian hormones, other hormones, emotional disorders, and neurotransmitters. In: Jensvold MF, Halbreich U, Hamilton JA, eds. Psychopharmacology and Women: Sex, Gender, and Hormones. Washington, DC, American Psychiatric Press, 1996:85–106.
4. Jensvold MF. Nonpregnant reproductive-age women, part I. The menstrual cycle and psychopharmacology. In: Jensvold MF, Halbreich U, Hamilton JA, eds. Psychopharmacology and Women: Sex, Gender, and Hormones. Washington, DC, American Psychiatric Press, 1996: 139–169.
5. Suri R, Burt VK. The assessment and treatment of postpartum psychiatric disorders. J Pract Psychiatr Behav Health 1997;3:67–77.
6. American Psychiatric Association. Diagnostic and Statistical Manual of Mental Disorders, 4th ed. Washington, DC, American Psychiatric Press, 1994:715-718.
7. Arpels JC. The female brain hypoestrogenic continuum from the premenstrual syndrome to menopause. A hypothesis and review of supporting data. J Reprod Med 1996;41:633–639.
8. Sugawara M, Toda MA, Shima S, et al. Premenstrual mood changes and maternal mental health in pregnancy and the postpartum period. J Clin Psychol 1997;53:225–232.
9. Severino SK, Moline ML. Premenstrual syndrome: Identification and management. Drugs 1995;49:71–82.
10. Rubinow DR, Schmidt PJ. The neuroendocrinology of menstrual cycle mood disorders. Ann NY Acad Sci 1995;771:648–659.
11. Parry BL. Biological correlates of premenstrual complaints. In: Gold JH, Severino SK, eds. Premenstrual Dysphorias: Myths and Realities. Washington, DC, American Psychiatric Press, 1994:47–66.
12. Burt VK, Hendrick VC. Premenstrual dysphoric disorder. In: Concise Guide to Women's Mental Health. Washington, DC, American Psychiatric Press, 1997:11–24.
13. Altshuler LL, Hendrick V, Parry B. Pharmacologic management of premenstrual disorder. Harvard Rev Psychiatry 1995;2:223–245.
14. Roca CA, Schmidt PJ, Bloch M, Rubinow DR. Implications of endocrine studies of premenstrual syndrome. Psychiatr Ann 1996;26: 576–580.
15. Leibenluft E, Fiero P, Rubinow DR. Effects of the menstrual cycle on dependent variables in mood disorder research. Arch Gen Psychiatry 1994;51:761–781.
16. Henrick V, Altshuler LL, Burt VK. Course of psychiatric disorders across the menstrual cycle. Harvard Rev Psychiatry 1996;4:200–207.
17. Severino SK, Moline ML. Premenstrual Syndrome: A Clinician's Guide. New York, Guilford Press, 1989.
18. Backstrom T. Neuroendocrinology of premenstrual syndrome. Clin Obstet Gynecol 1992;35:612–628.
19. Steiner M. Female-specific mood disorders. Clin Obstet Gynecol 1992;35:599-611.
20. Gilbaldi M. Hormone replacement therapy: Estrogen after menopause. Pharmacotherapy 1996;16:366–375.
21. Hardman JG, Limbaird LE, eds. Goodman & Gilman's The Pharmacological Basis of Therapeutics. 9th ed. New York, McGraw-Hill, 1996:1412–1426.
22. Fink G, Sumner BE, Rosie R, et al. Estrogen control of central neurotransmission: Effect on mood, mental state, and memory. Cell Molec Neurobiol 1996;16:325–344.
23. Sherwin BB. Estrogen, the brain, and memory. Menopause 1996;3: 97–105.
24. Hardman JG, Limbaird LE, eds. Goodman & Gilman's The Pharmacological Basis of Therapeutics, 9th ed. New York, McGraw-Hill, 1996:1426–1430.

25. Rapkin AJ. The role of serotonin in premenstrual syndrome. Clin Obstet Gynecol 1992;35:629–636.
26. Severino SK. A focus on 5-hydroxytryptamine (serotonin) and psychopathology. In: Gold JH, Severino SK, eds. Premenstrual Dysphorias: Myths and Realities. Washington, DC, American Psychiatric Press, 1994:67–98.
27. FitzGerald M, Malone KM, Li S, et al. Blunted serotonin response to fenfluramine challenge in premenstrual dysphoric disorder. Am J Psychiatry 1997;154:556–558.
28. Menkes DB, Coates DC, Fawcett JP. Acute tryptophan depletion aggravates premenstrual syndrome. J Affective Disord 1994;32:37–44.
29. Cavallo A. The pineal gland in human beings; relevance to pediatrics. Pediatriacs 1993;123:843–851.
30. Halbreich U, Petty F, Yonkers K, et al. Low plasma γ-aminobutyric acid levels during the late luteal phase of women with premenstrual dysphoric disorder. Am J Psychiatry 1996;153:718–720.
31. Chuong CJ, Dawson EB. Critical evaluation of nutritional factors in the pathophysiology and treatment of premenstrual syndrome. Clin Obstet Gynecol 1992;35:679–692.
32. Mortola JF. A risk–benefit appraisal of drugs used in the management of premenstrual syndrome. Drug Saf 1994;10:160–169.
33. Rivera-Tovar A, Rhodes R, Pearlstein TB, Frank E. Treatment efficacy. In: Gold JH, Severino SK, eds. Premenstrual Dysphorias: Myths and Realities. Washington, DC, American Psychiatric Press, 1994: 99–148.
34. Yonkers KA, Brown WA. Pharmacologic treatments for premenstrual dysphoric disorder. Psychiatr Ann 1996;26:586–589.
35. Pearlstein T. Nonpharmacologic treatment of premenstrual syndrome. Psychiatr Ann 1996;26:590–594.
36. Parry BL, Mahan AM, Mostofi N, et al. Light therapy of late luteal phase dysphoric disorder: An extended study. Am J Psychiatry 1993; 150:1417–1419.
37. Parry BL, Cover H, Mostofi N, et al. Early versus late partial sleep deprivation in patients with premenstrual dysphoric disorder and normal comparison subjects. Am J Psychiatry 1995;152:404–412.
38. Carter J, Verhoef MJ. Efficacy of self-help and alternative treatments of premenstrual syndrome. WHI 1994;4:130–135.
39. Kleignen J, Ter Riet G, Knipschild P. Vitamin B_6 in the treatment of the premenstrual syndrome: A review. Br J Obstet Gynaecol 1990;97: 847–852.
40. Alvir JMJ, Thys-Jacobs S. Premenstrual and menstrual symptoms clusters and response to calcium treatment. Psychopharmacol Bull 1991;27:145–148.
41. Facchinetti F, Borela P, Sances G, et al. Oral magnesium successfully relieves premenstrual mood changes. Obstet Gynecol 1991;78: 177–181.
42. Dong quai. The Lawrence Review of Natural Products. St. Louis, Facts and Comparisons, April 1990.
43. Black cohosh. The Lawrence Review of Natural Products. St. Louis, Facts and Comparisons, September 1992.
44. Blue cohosh. The Lawrence Review of Natural Products. St. Louis, Facts and Comparisons, October 1992.
45. Valerian. The Lawrence Review of Natural Products. St. Louis, Facts and Comparisons, October 1991.
46. Chamomile. The Lawrence Review of Natural Products. St. Louis, Facts and Comparisons, March 1991.
47. Kaufman LD, Philen RM. Tryptophan: Current status and future trends for oral administration. Drug Saf 1993:8:89–98.
48. Zhdanova IV, Wurtman RJ, Lynch HJ, et al. Sleep-inducing effects of low doses of melatonin ingested in the evening. Clin Pharmacol Ther 1995;57:552–558.
49. Brzezinski A, Adlercreutz H, Shaoul R, et al. Short-term effects of phytoestrogen-rich diet on postmenopausal women. Menopause 1997; 4:89–94.
50. Collins A, Cerin A, Coleman G, Landgren BM. Essential fatty acids in the treatment of premenstrual syndrome. Obstet Gynecol 1993;81: 93–98.
51. Derzko CM. Role of danazol in relieving the premenstrual syndrome. J Reprod Med 1990;35:97–102.
52. Halbreich U, Rojansky N, Palter S. Elimination of ovulation and menstrual cyclicity (with danazol) improves dysphoric premenstrual syndromes. Fertil Steril 1991;56:1066–1069.
53. Nierenberg AA, Adler LA, Peselow E, et al. Trazodone for antidepressant-associated insomnia. Am J Psychiatry 1994:151:1069–1072.
54. Harrison WM, Endicott J, Nee J. Treatment of premenstrual dysphoria with alprazolam. Arch Gen Psychiatry 1990;47:270–275.
55. Smith S, Rinehart JS, Ruddock VE, Schiff I. Treatment of premenstrual syndrome with alprazolam: Results of a double-blind, placebo-controlled, randomized crossover clinical trial. Obstet Gynecol 1987; 70:37–43.
56. Freeman EW, Rickels K, Sondheimer SJ, Polansky M. A double-blind trial of oral progesterone, alprazolam, and placebo in treatment of severe premenstrual syndrome. JAMA 1995;274:51–57.
57. Berger CP, Presser B. Alprazolam in the treatment of two subsamples of patients with late luteal phase dysphoric disorder: A double-blind placebo-controlled crossover study. Obstet Gynecol 1994;84:379–385.
58. Rickels K, Freeman E, Sondheimer S. Buspirone in the treatment of premenstrual syndrome. Lancet 1989;4:777.
59. Freeman EW, Rickels K, Sondheimer SJ, et al. Nefazodone in the treatment of premenstrual syndrome: a preliminary study. J Clin Psychopharmacol 1994;14:180–186.
60. Brzezinski AA, Wurtman JJ, Wurtman RJ, et al. D-Fenfluramine suppresses the increased calorie and carbohydrate intakes and improves the mood of women with premenstrual depression. Obstet Gynecol 1990;76:296–300.
61. Freeman EW, Rickels K, Sondheimer SJ, Wittmaack FM. Sertraline versus desipramine in the treatment of premenstrual syndrome: An open-label trial. J Clin Psychiatry 1996;57:7–11.
62. Pearlstein TB, Stone AB, Lund SA, et al. Comparison of fluoxetine, bupropion, and placebo in the treatment of premenstrual dysphoric disorder. J Clin Psychopharmacol 1997;17:261–266.
63. Rickels K, Freeman EW, Sondheimer S, Albert J. Fluoxetine in the treatment of premenstrual syndrome. Curr Therapeutic Res 1990;48: 161–166.
64. Stone AB, Pearlstein TB, Brown WA. Fluoxetine in the treatment of late luteal phase dysphoric disorder. J Clin Psychiatry 1991;52: 290–293.
65. Menkes DB, Taghavi, Mason PA, et al. Fluoxetine treatment of severe premenstrual syndrome. Br Med J 1992;305:346–347.
66. Menkes DB, Taghavi, Mason PA, Howard RC. Fluoxetine's spectrum of action in premenstrual syndrome. Int Clin Psychopharmacol 1993; 8:95–102.
67. Wood SH, Mortola JF, Chan YF, et al. Treatment of premenstrual syndrome with fluoxetine: A double-blind, placebo-controlled, crossover study. Obstet Gynecol 1992;80:339–344.
68. Pearlstein TB, Stone AB. Long-term fluoxetine treatment of late luteal phase dysphoric disorder. J Clin Psychiatry 1994;5:332–335.
69. Steiner M, Steinberg S, Stewart D, et al. Fluoxetine in the treatment of premenstrual dysphoria. N Engl J Med 1995;332:1529–1534.
70. Su TP, Schmidt PJ, Danaceau MA, et al. Fluoxetine in the treatment of premenstrual dysphoria. Neuropsychopharmacology 1997;16:346–356.
71. Yonkers KA, Halbreich U, Freeman E, et al. Sertraline in the treatment of premenstrual dysphoric disorder. Psychopharmacol Bull 1996;32:41–46.
72. Yonkers KA, Halbreich U, Freeman E, et al. Symptomatic improvement of premenstrual dysphoric disorder with sertraline treatment: A randomized controlled trial. JAMA 1997;278:983–988.
73. Eriksson E, Hedberg MA, Andersch B, et al. The serotonin reuptake inhibitor paroxetine is superior to the noradrenaline reuptake inhibitor maprotiline in the treatment of premenstrual syndrome: A placebo-controlled trial. Neuropsychopharmacology 1995;12:167–176.
74. Yonkers KA, Gullion C, Williams A, et al. Paroxetine as a treatment for premenstrual dysphoric disorder. J Clin Psychopharmacol 1996; 16:3–8.

75. Veeninga AT, Westenberg HGM, Weusten JTN. Fluvoxamine in the treatment of menstrually related mood disorders. Psychopharmacology 1990;102:414–416.
76. Freeman EW, Rickels K, Sondheimer SJ. Fluvoxamine for premenstrual dysphoric disorder: A pilot study. J Clin Psychiatry 1996;57 (suppl 8):56–59.
77. Jacobsen FM. Low-dose valproate: A new treatment for cyclothymia, mild rapid cycling disorders, and premenstrual syndrome. J Clin Psychiatry 1993;54:229–234.
78. Muse K. Hormonal manipulation in the treatment of premenstrual syndrome. Clin Obstet Gynecol 1992;35:658–666.
79. McAuley JW, Kroboth FJ, Kroboth PD. Oral administration of micronized progesterone: A review and more experience. Pharmacotherapy 1996;16:453–457.
80. Graham CA, Sherwin BB. A prospective treatment study of premenstrual symptoms using a triphasic oral contraceptive. J Psychosom Res 1992;36:257–266.
81. Mortola JF. Applications of gonadotropin-releasing hormone analogues in the treatment of premenstrual syndrome. Clin Obstet Gynecol 1993;36:753–763.
82. Brown CS, Ling FW, Andersen RN, et al. Efficacy of depot leuprolide in premenstrual syndrome: Effect of symptom severity and type in a controlled trial. Obstet Gynecol 1994;84:779–786.
83. Freeman EW, Sondheimer SJ, Rickels K, Albert J. Gonadotropin-releasing hormone agonist in treatment of premenstrual symptoms, with and without comorbidity of depression: A pilot study. J Clin Psychiatry 1993;54:192–195.
84. Mezrow G, Lobo R, Shoupe, et al. Depot leuprolide acetate with estrogen and progestin add-back for long-term treatment of premenstrual syndrome. Fertil and Steril 1994;62:932–937.
85. West CP, Hillier H. Ovarian suppression with the gonadotropin-releasing hormone agonist goserelin (Zoladex) in management of the premenstrual tension syndrome. Hum Reprod 1994;9:1058–1063.
86. Hammarback S, Backstrom T. Induced anovulation as treatment of premenstrual tension syndrome: A double-blind cross-over study with GnRH-agonist versus placebo. Acta Obstet Gynecol Scand 1988;67: 159–166.
87. Hussain SY, Massil JH, Matta WH, et al. Buserelin in premenstrual syndrome. Gynecol Endocrinol 1992;6:57–64.
88. Bancroft J, Boyle H, Warner P, Fraser HM. The use of an LHRH agonist, buserelin, in the long-term management of premenstrual syndromes. Clin Endocrinol 1987;27:171–182.
89. Mortola JF, Girton L, Fischer U. Successful treatment of severe premenstrual syndrome by combined use of gonadotropin-releasing hormone agonist and estrogen/progestin. J Clin Endocrinol Metab 1991; 72:252A–252F.
90. Casson P, Hahn PM, Van Vugt DA, Reid RL. Lasting response to ovariectomy in severe intractable premenstrual syndrome. Am J Obstet Gynecol 1990;162:99–105.
91. Casper RH, Hearn MT. The effect of hysterectomy and bilateral oophorectomy in women with severe premenstrual syndrome. Am J Obstet Gynecol 1990;162:105–109.
92. Thys-Jacobs S, Alvir JAJ, Fratarcangelo P. Comparative analysis of three PMS assessment instruments: The identification of premenstrual syndrome with core symptoms. Psychopharmacol Bull 1995;31: 389–396.

78

Hormone Replacement Therapy

Mark C. Pugh, PharmD, and Patricia Moynahan Mullins, PharmD

Menopause is simply defined as the loss of ovarian function leading to a state of permanent amenorrhea.[1,2] It is but one event in a series of physiologic, endocrinologic, and psychologic changes that signify the transition from reproductive to nonreproductive life, which are termed the *climacteric.*

The terms *menopause* and *climacteric* are not synonymous.[1] The main distinction between these two terms is that menopause is a discrete event while events of the climacteric span several years. The term *perimenopausal* is often used to refer to an arbitrarily defined time period of the climacteric, including the first few years before and after menopause.[1,3]

Although menopause is usually thought of as a discrete event, in reality the change from regular menstruation to permanent amenorrhea is marked by a series of irregular cycles. Mean menstrual-cycle length is increased, and the intermenstrual interval may vary widely. These irregular cycles continue until no more ovarian follicles capable of responding to gonadotropin stimulation exist. A period of amenorrhea lasting at least 1 year is used clinically to define the onset of menopause.[3]

EPIDEMIOLOGY

Based on both historical writings and modern data, the average age of onset of natural menopause has remained remarkably constant, and is estimated to be 51.4 years.[1,4] Premature menopause, defined as a loss of ovarian function before the age of 35 years, is secondary to a variety of causes including ovarian surgery (surgical castration), endocrinologic, and autoimmune disorders (Table 78–1).[4] Age of onset appears to be unaffected by race, socioeconomic status, alcohol consumption, age of menarche, or age of last pregnancy. However, women who are cigarette smokers may undergo menopause up to 2 years earlier than nonsmokers, possibly because of the gametotoxic effects of cigarette smoke constituents or effects on steroid hormone metabolism by the liver.[1,4]

Although the age of onset of natural menopause is constant, the proportion of women living a significant number of years beyond the age is increasing. Projections estimate that 50 million will be over the age of 50 years in the United States by the end of the 20th century.[5] Given the current life expectancies in the United States, by the end of the century women can expect to live one-third of their life span after the onset of menopause.[1]

PHYSIOLOGY

The underlying cause of the climacteric is an age-related loss of ovarian function that results in a decline in estrogen secretion by the ovarian follicular unit. Most follicles are lost due to follicular atresia, a normal physiologic process of degeneration of the oocyte and its surrounding stroma.[1] Although some follicles remain in postmenopausal women, they are less sensitive to gonadotropin stimulation, implying that the more hormonally sensitive or functionally normal follicles are depleted earlier in life.[1]

The gradual but complete loss of functional follicles as a woman ages results in alterations of endocrine function involving the gonadotropins and estrogens (Fig. 78–1).

ESTROGENS

The major circulating estrogen during the reproductive years is 17 β-estradiol (E_2). Estradiol, in the premenopausal woman, is produced primarily by the ovary with additional amounts being synthesized in the peripheral tissue by conversion from testosterone or estrone (BE_1). Once the functional follicles are exhausted after menopause, estradiol secretion from the ovary ceases, and the primary circulating estrogen is estrone. Estrone concentrations exceed estradiol by about fourfold after menopause, but estrone has approximately one-third the estrogenic potency of estradiol. In postmenopausal women, the majority of estrone is derived by the peripheral conversion of androstenedione by an extraglandular aromatase found primarily in adipose tissue. Virtually all circulating estradiol in the postmenopausal period is derived from conversion of estrone. Unlike the cyclic fluctuations of estrogen in the reproductive years, the levels of estrone and estradiol remain relatively constant after menopause.[1]

GONADOTROPINS

Postmenopausal decline in ovarian estradiol production causes diminished negative-feedback effects on the anterior pituitary gland, which results in a compensatory increase in secretion of the gonadotropins, follicle-stimulating hormone (FSH), and luteinizing hormone (LH).[2] Therefore, for the first time since puberty, the level of FSH exceeds LH (Fig. 78–1) and is the inverse of the ratio found in the premenopausal period. The peak levels of FSH and LH are reached 2 to 3 years after menopause and remain stable or decline slightly over the remaining years of life.[1]

TABLE 78–1. Potential Causes of Premature Menopause

Idiopathic	Iatrogenic
Identifiable karyotypic abnormalities	Ovarian surgery (surgical castration)
Exposure to gametotoxic environmental agents	Radiation therapy
	Cytotoxic chemotherapy
Viral oophoritis	Defective gonadotropin action
Autoimmune oophoritis	Congenital absence of the thymus
Isolated ovarian failure	17-Hydroxylase deficiency
Associated with other autoimmune disease	Galactosemia

Compiled from Ref. 4.

Even though postmenopausal FSH and LH levels are substantially elevated compared to those during the premenopausal period, the remaining follicles generally do not respond to gonadotropin stimulation because of their relative gonadotropin insensitivity. However, occasionally a follicle will mature and release a burst of estradiol. Corpus luteum formation may follow, but progesterone secretion is limited. The result is unopposed estrogen stimulation without cyclic progesterone secretion. These events may be responsible for the occurrence of dysfunctional uterine bleeding during the perimenopausal period.[3]

DIAGNOSIS

The diagnosis of menopause should be approached with the idea of excluding physical or laboratory changes unrelated to decreasing estrogen. Many signs and symptoms observed during menopause can be attributed to aging. Body systems affected by aging include the cardiovascular system, respiratory system, nervous system, immune system, skin, and musculoskeletal system. With the exception of the gonads, the endocrine system undergoes very little change during aging. Specifically, the diagnosis of menopause should involve a comprehensive medical history and thorough physical exam with complete blood count and with measurement of serum FSH. Altered thyroid function, which may mimic menopausal symptoms, and pregnancy must be excluded. A breast exam and mammography should be performed. In the absence of other disease processes, an elevated FSH concentration of 30 pg/mL or greater indicates that the woman is menopausal.[1,6] In symptomatic patients with either elevated or borderline (15 to 30 pg/mL) FSH concentrations, hormone replacement therapy (HRT) may be considered. Until recently, HRT was not usually recommended for asymptomatic women in the absence of other medical risk factors even though FSH is elevated.[6] A growing body of clinical data now supports the use of HRT for prevention or treatment of osteoporosis and for its cardioprotective benefits.

CLINICAL PRESENTATION

Symptom complexes specifically related to estrogen deprivation include genitourinary atrophy and vasomotor instability. Insomnia and psychosexual symptoms may also occur. Osteoporosis and cardiovascular disease in women, while related to estrogen deficiency, are more appropriately considered as long-term sequelae.

GENITOURINARY ATROPHY

Large numbers of estrogen receptors are located in the vagina, vulva, urethra, and trigone of the bladder. Atrophy of these tissues begins with diminished estrogen concentrations and continues, at different rates for the specific tissues, over many years. The vulva undergoes atrophy, and there is thinning of hair of the mons and shrinkage of the labia minora. A decrease in subcutaneous fat and elasticity of the tissue causes the labia majora to flatten. Atrophic changes of the vulva (Kraurosis vulvae) lead to pruritus and pain.[1,7] Vaginal epithelium becomes pale and thin, leading to diminished distensibility and reduced secretion; the tissue is easily traumatized and may bleed. The vaginal pH

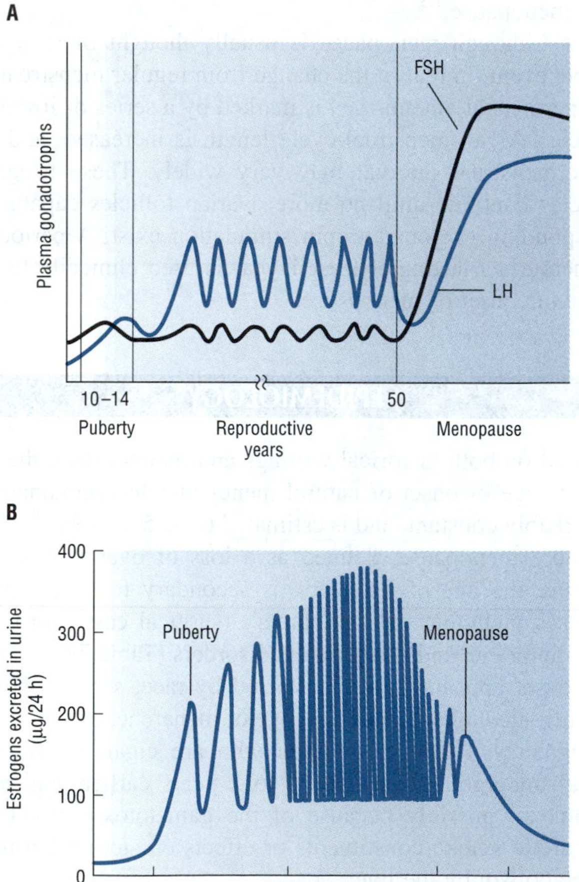

FIGURE 78–1. A. Comparison of gonadotropin production at various ages. **B.** Comparison of estrogen production at various ages in sexual life. *(**A** reproduced from Carr BR, Wilson JD. Disorders of the ovary and female reproductive tract. In: Petersdorf RG, Adams RD, Braunwald E, et al, eds. Harrison's Principles of Internal Medicine, 10th ed. New York, McGraw-Hill, 1983: 700–720, with permission of the publisher. **B** reproduced from Guyton AC. Female physiology before pregnancy, and the female hormones. In: Textbook of Medical Physiology, 7th ed. Philadelphia, Saunders, 1986:968–982, with permission.)*

rises to an alkaline range (6 to 8; usual premenopausal vaginal pH is 4.5 to 5), creating a favorable environment for bacterial colonization by various pathogens. The incidence of atrophic vaginitis increases during postmenopausal years, producing symptoms of itching, bleeding, or dyspareunia. Decreased estrogen is probably not the direct cause of uterine prolapse; hernias in the anterior (cystocele) and posterior (rectocele) vaginal wall, coupled with a decrease in tissue elasticity, could account for the higher incidence of these conditions in the climacteric.[1,7]

The urethra may become rigid and inelastic and undergo epithelial thinning. The urethral syndrome, a recurrent nonbacterial urethritis, is more common in postmenopausal women. Despite changes in the urethra and supporting pelvic tissue, there does not appear to be any increase in stress urinary incontinence in postmenopausal women compared with premenopausal women. Bacteriuria is found in 7% to 10% of postmenopausal women versus 4% of premenopausal women. Postmenopausal women may be more prone to bacteriuria due to mucosal atrophy and increased vaginal contamination caused by vaginal foreshortening.[1,7] Treatment with local (intravaginal) or systemic estrogen reverses the thinning of the vaginal mucosa through epithelial proliferation and decreases vaginal pH to its more normal acidic state. Estrogen therapy often relieves symptoms of vaginitis and frictional dyspareunia and improves urinary frequency, dysuria, nocturia, urgency, postvoiding dribbling, and, to some extent, stress urinary incontinence.[1,7]

VASOMOTOR INSTABILITY

Vasomotor symptoms or hot flushes most often prompt the postmenopausal woman to seek medical care. The cause of these symptoms is estrogen deficiency, possibly leading to aberrant surges of LH or gonadotropin-releasing hormone (GnRH), which affect the hypothalamic neurons that control central thermoregulation centers. The rate of decrease in estrogen concentrations is directly related to the severity of vasomotor responses. Hot flushes (or flashes) are experienced by 75% to 85% of women following natural menopause and by 37% to 50% of premenopausal women who undergo bilateral oophorectomy, but only 30% of women describe them as severe and seek medical treatment.[8] They are most common within 12 to 24 months after the last menstrual period, gradually subsiding thereafter. The hot flush is an acute, episodic event that initially occurs several times a day, often during sleep. Peripheral blood flow increases, causing increased skin temperature. Perspiration occurs as a homeostatic response designed to dissipate heat; an increase in heart rate probably reflects a sympathetic response to change in skin temperature.[9] Hot flushes are frequently associated with nausea, dizziness, headache, palpitations, diaphoresis, and night sweats that interrupt sleep.[1,7] Estrogen has traditionally been the drug of choice for relieving hot flushes, but medroxyprogesterone in relatively high doses, some ergot alkaloids, or α-adrenergic agonists such as clonidine are also effective.[9] When prescribed to control vasomotor symptoms, estrogen should be started at the lowest dose that controls the hot flushes, and continued for 3 to 5 years, when it can be tapered and discontinued by most women, in the absence of other justification for HRT.[10]

OSTEOPOROSIS

Osteoporosis is a universal, gradual loss of bone mass that eventually compromises the skeleton and results in fractures after minimal trauma (see Chap. 82 for a more detailed discussion of osteoporosis). Rather than a single pathologic condition, osteoporosis is a heterogeneous disease process involving multiple etiologies and affecting both men and women.

The medical and socioeconomic considerations of managing postmenopausal osteoporosis is a major concern. About 1.2 million fractures annually are related to osteoporosis. Vertebral crush fractures are most common (500,000/y), but hip fractures have the most serious sequelae. Annually, about 300,000 hip fractures occur, and 12% to 20% of patients who suffer a hip fracture die from complications within 6 months. At least one-half of the survivors will require assistance with daily living and 15% to 25% will enter a long-term care facility.[11] By age 70, 15% of women will experience a wrist fracture, 25% will experience a vertebral fracture, and 15% will experience a hip fracture.[12] The greatest risk of postmenopausal osteoporosis occurs in slender, sedentary females of Caucasian or Asian descent. Social history (smoking, alcohol use), diet (low intake of calcium and vitamin D), family/medical history (illness such as malignancy, rheumatoid arthritis, or endocrine disorders), and chronic use of specific drugs (corticosteroids) are also risk factors. Prophylaxis against osteoporosis should be considered when two or more of these risk factors are present.[8]

CARDIOVASCULAR DISEASE

Cardiovascular disease (CVD) includes a group of disorders of the heart and circulatory system such as atherosclerosis, hypertension, angina, and stroke. Although death rates for CVD in women lag approximately 10 years behind those in men, CVD is the leading cause of death in both men and women. As the number one killer of American women, CVD is responsible for slightly more than one-half of all deaths in women over age 50.[11]

Coronary artery disease is a multifactoral problem associated with identifiable risk factors including hypertension, hyperlipidemia, diabetes, and cigarette smoking. After menopause, the incidence of coronary artery disease rapidly increases; after surgical menopause the risk is more than 2.2-fold greater. Each year coronary artery disease is responsible for the deaths of approximately 500,000 women in the United States.[13] The years after menopause, which now account for more than one-third of a woman's total life, are the period when a woman is at greatest risk for CVD.[11]

OTHER SYMPTOMS

Insomnia and fatigue, which affect 30% to 40% of postmenopausal women, may be related to estrogen deficiency. Some estrogen-deficient women suffer from chronic sleep deprivation, which can be verified by sleep polygraphs documenting a close temporal relationship between hot flushes and waking episodes.[1] Mood changes—such as irritability, depression, insomnia, impaired memory, and crying spells—are usually regarded as "hormone-related" symptoms that precede and postdate menopause. Although many of these changes are estrogen dependent, depression and anxiety may be caused by numerous nonhormonal conditions.[10]

Estrogens may modify the metabolism of several central nervous system neurotransmitters, thus accounting for their behavioral effects.[1] Response of some psychological symptoms to estrogen have been attributed to a placebo response.[1] However, some prescribers use an estrogen trial for symptomatic patients with no other clinical evidence of a CNS problem.[10]

Most women experience some change in sexual function in the years immediately before and after menopause. Sexual function is influenced by the interaction between complex hormonal factors and nonbiologic factors, including psychological and sociocultural factors and interpersonal relationships. That estrogen deficiency may be a possible cause for a change in libido and sexual response rests on the hypothesis that sexual disinterest is a consequence of dyspareunia, resulting from atrophic changes of the genitourinary tract. However, dyspareunia occurs in less than 8% of postmenopausal patients, and oophorectomy before menopause does not affect libido unless the uterus is also removed.[1] In 1966, Masters and Johnson characterized the physiologic changes in menopause that are related to sexual function. These changes are classified into five disorder categories: desire phase; excitement phase (touch sensations impairment, clitoral sensation impairment, vaginal dryness, urinary incontinence); orgasmic phase (primary or secondary nonorgasmic responses); dyspareunia (including vaginismus, a conditioned response to painful penetration); and a dysfunctional male partner. The effects of decreased estrogen on the CNS, the peripheral nervous system, and the cardiovascular system, as well as on specific tissues, may account for most changes and may explain why estrogen therapy can markedly improve sexual function in some women. Counseling and referral to a specialist is not required in the majority of cases of sexual dysfunction associated with menopause.[14]

▶ TREATMENT: Menopause

DESIRED OUTCOME

Treatment goals for postmenopausal women receiving HRT include reduction of the symptom complexes specifically related to estrogen deprivation including genitourinary atrophy and vasomotor instability. Relief of these symptoms is often accompanied by increased psychosocial or sexual well-being. The greatest impact of HRT on women's health is the long-term benefits. These include prevention of osteoporosis and its risk of bone fractures and associated morbidity and mortality. Reduction of mortality associated with cardiovascular disease is also a long-term goal of HRT.

NONHORMONAL TREATMENT OF MENOPAUSE

Most clinical symptoms present in the menopausal period are associated directly with estrogen deficiency, thus nonpharmacologic measures are not generally helpful. Some of the problems in menopausal women—including CVD, obesity, muscle weakness, and osteoporosis—are also related to life-style and aging. These symptoms may respond to dietary modification, aerobic exercise, and resistance training. Behavioral symptoms may respond to counseling.[5,15,16] Alternative medicine and natural remedies (nonvalidated) include vitamins (B complex, C, and E), zinc, ginseng tea, and bee pollen.[16] The safety and efficacy of these treatments has not been established.

Response of vasomotor symptoms to various nonhormonal agents including clonidine, β-blockers, veralapride, naloxone, methyldopa, clomifene, and androgens has been studied, but these investigations have generally not been well designed. In noncontrolled trials, clonidine increased LH and had peripheral vascular effects; both effects may improve hot flushes. Placebo-controlled studies have not demonstrated a significant reduction in hot flushes with clonidine. Veralapride, an investigational dopaminergic agent similar to metoclopramide, eliminated hot flushes in 60% to 80% of women in several clinical studies. Patients remained free of symptoms for up to 3 months after discontinuing veralapride. Adverse effects included galactorrhea and breast tenderness. Clomifene, a weak estrogenic/antiestrogenic compound, may be beneficial in the treatment of some symptoms of menopause, but it is not effective in relieving hot flushes.[5]

Adequate dietary calcium or supplementation and weight-bearing exercise are primary nonhormonal preventions and treatments for osteoporosis. Clomifene, which decreases urinary calcium loss and may block parathyroid hormone-induced bone resorption, may be particularly useful in the prevention of osteoporosis. Other agents, including calcitonin and alendronate or etidronate, may also be beneficial for treating and preventing osteoporosis.[5,17]

Atrophic vaginitis can be minimized by continued sexual activity.[16] Pelvic exercises called Kegel exercises (alternately tensing and relaxing the muscles of the urethra, vagina, and anus) may help reduce urinary incontinence.[16] For the treatment of vaginal dryness and dyspareunia, a mucoadherent compound, polycarbophil, is available on a nonprescription basis. This long-acting lubricant lowers vaginal pH, and may be preferable to water-soluble lubricants.[5] Exercise and diet along with other life-style practices such as smoking abstinence, moderation in alcohol consumption, and stress reduction form the primary approach to prevention of CVD.[13,18]

ESTROGEN REPLACEMENT THERAPY

Indications for estrogen replacement therapy include relief from vasomotor symptoms, genitourinary dysfunction, and certain psychological changes and prevention or treatment of osteoporosis. Estrogen replacement therapy (ERT) is also effective in reducing cardiovascular morbidity and mortality.[10]

PHARMACOLOGY

Estrogens attach to tissue-specific receptor proteins in the cytoplasm of target organs including the ovaries, uterus, fallopian tubes, vagina, bladder, urethra, and breast. Other target organs include the skin, adrenals, cardiovascular system, gastrointestinal tract (colon, pancreas, and liver), and the CNS (pituitary, hypothalamus, and spinal cord).[1,2,19] This estrogen–protein complex diffuses through the nuclear membrane and ultimately binds to materials in the cell nucleus. Synthesis of DNA, RNA, and other proteins increases, resulting in characteristic changes in the responsive tissues. Any estrogen capable of binding to the estrogen receptors in target organs should alleviate menopausal symptoms. Exogenous estrogens administered orally, transdermally, or vaginally are the major useful forms of therapy (Table 78–2). Injectable estrogens are not generally used for treating menopausal symptoms because of poor patient acceptance and because of fluctuating plasma concentrations, with initial peaks and subsequent low estrogen levels.[19,20] The precise mechanism by which estrogen prevents bone loss is unknown. Exogenous estrogen administration reverses biochemical changes (decreases in serum calcium, phosphorus, alkaline phosphatase, and osteocalcin) and urinary output of calcium and hydroxyproline associated with estrogen withdrawal. Conflicting changes are seen in the regulatory hormones that control calcium homeostasis, particularly parathyroid hormone. Overall, the response of bone to estrogen therapy is a reduced rate of resorption with normal mineralization of the remodeling unit.[12]

Several oral estrogen products are commercially available. Conjugated equine estrogens are purified from the urine of pregnant mares. The product obtained from horse urine is a mixture of estrogen compounds, mostly sulfates and glucuronides, some of which are not found in humans. The pharmacokinetics of orally administered equine estrogens is complex because of the many different estrogen compounds in the products.[19]

Absorption of oral estradiol tablets has become more reliable with micronized formulations, but estradiol is metabolized significantly on first pass through the liver to other less active metabolites. Oral estrone tablets also provide relief of symptoms at appropriate doses.[19,20]

Estrogen, in vaginal creams, is readily absorbed through the vaginal epithelium and is a feasible treatment not only for urogenital symptoms but for other menopausal symptoms as well. Estradiol is metabolized very little as it is absorbed from the vagina, and this route of administration results primarily in increased estradiol serum concentrations. Unfortunately, these concentrations return to baseline in approximately 6 hours. Because of the short duration of increased serum concentrations and because vaginal creams are messy and dosage is difficult to control, they are not widely used.[19]

A transdermal patch containing estradiol is the newest commercially available dosage form. One patch is applied to the skin, usually on the lower trunk. This dosage form offers parenteral therapy with little metabolism of estradiol, convenient administration, and precise dosing.[19]

TABLE 78–2. Estrogen Products

Agent	Dosage Form	Dose	Indications
Estrone aqueous suspension	Injection	0.1–5 mg IM 2 or 3 times/week	A,B
Estrogenic substance or estrogen aqueous suspension (primarily estrone) injection	Injection	0.1–1.0 mg IM 2 or 3 times/week	A,B
Estradiol cypionate (in oil)	Injection	1–5 mg IM weekly for 3 to 4 weeks	C
Estradiol valerate (in oil)	Injection	10–20 mg every 4 weeks	A,B,C
Conjugated estrogens	Oral	0.03–1.25 mg/d[a]	A,B,C,D
Conjugated estrogens/medroxyprogesterone acetate	Oral	0.625 mg/d for 14 days,[b] then 0.625 mg/5 mg/d for 14 days[b]	C,D
Estradiol, micronized	Oral	0.5–2 mg/d[a]	A,B,C,D
Esterified estrogens (75% to 85% estrone sulfate and 6% to 15% sodium equilin)	Oral	0.3–1.25 mg/d[a]	A,B,C,D
Estropipate (piperazine estrone sulfate)	Oral	0.75–6 mg/d[a]	A,B,C
Ethinyl estradiol	Oral	0.02–1.5 mg/d[a]	A,C
Quinestrol	Oral	0.1 mg/d for 7 days, then 0.1 mg once weekly	A,B,C
Chlorotrianisene	Oral	12–25 mg/d for 21 days	A,B,C
Estropipate vaginal cream	Topical	3–6 mg daily for 3 weeks	B
Estradiol micronized vaginal cream	Topical	Daily[c]	B
Conjugated estrogens vaginal cream	Topical	1.25–2.5 mg daily for 3 weeks	B
Dienestrol vaginal cream	Topical	Once or twice daily[c]	B
Estrone vaginal cream	Topical	2–4 mg daily	B
Estradiol transdermal	Transdermal	0.05–0.1 mg system twice weekly	A,B,C,D

A = replacement therapy of estrogen deficiency-associated conditions (e.g., female hypogonadism); B = senile vaginitis and Kraurosis vulvae; C = moderate to severe vasomotor symptoms associated with menopause; D = osteoporosis.

[a]May administer continuously or cyclically with 3 weeks of daily estrogen followed by 1 week off.

[b]Blister pack dosage cards used for single prescription convenience in continuous or cyclic combination regimens.

[c]Typical regimen: Initial therapy one dose daily for 2 weeks, followed by 2 additional weeks of daily therapy at one-half dose, followed by maintenance therapy of one dose 1–3 times/week for 3 weeks.

Check drug information references for specific regimens.

Compiled from Ref. 19.

A complicating pharmacokinetic feature of exogenous estrogen replacement is the relatively high first-pass metabolism of orally administered estrogens. Approximately 60% to 90% of an orally administered dose of estrogen is converted to estrone or inactive metabolites. Consequently, high doses of exogenous estrogens need to be administered to compensate for this effect.[21] Transdermal administration of estrogens, such as 17 β-estradiol, results in estradiol levels equivalent to those in the early to midfollicular phase and an estrone-to-estradiol ratio of approximately 1 to 1, which closely resembles the premenopausal state.[22] Oral administration can also achieve similar estradiol levels, but only at the expense of a higher estrone-to-estradiol ratio.[23] Unlike oral estrogen replacement, transdermal estrogen delivery has no significant effect on production of certain hepatic proteins, renin substrate, sex-hormone-binding globulin, thyroxine-binding globulin, and cortisol-binding globulin. Elevations in these proteins may be associated with some of the adverse effects of oral estrogen therapy including hypertension, gallbladder disease, and thrombosis, although the clinical significance of this effect is not yet established.[20,24]

The effects of transdermal estrogen administration on the lipid profile appear to be less favorable than with orally administered estrogens, presumably because of the lack of a first-pass effect on the liver. Short-term and some longer term (6 months or more) studies report no alteration in lipid profiles with transdermal administrations.[22] However, other long-term studies report increased HDL[25] and decreased LDL.[26]

The typical transdermal estrogen regimen involves the application of one patch twice weekly. Administration may be either continuous, or in 3-week cycles with 1 week estrogen free. As with oral estrogen therapy, the addition of a progestin is recommended for the last 10 to 13 days of the cycle in women receiving cyclic therapy who have an intact uterus.[27]

CLINICAL USE

By the year 2005, it is estimated that 25.3 million women in the United States will be candidates for ERT.[28] However, it is greatly underused, with only 30% of eligible women receiving prescriptions for estrogens. Compounding this problem is the fact that many women either do not fill these prescriptions or discontinue therapy after the first year.[29] In light of these findings, it is clear that the decision to take estrogen is one of the most difficult that a woman and her physician face. Recent decision analysis models that factor in the major benefits and risks of ERT may aid clinicians and women in their decision.[30] Figure 78–2 provides a set of guidelines based on achievement of therapeutic benefit by women with various degrees of risk for developing coronary heart disease (CHD), breast cancer, or hip fracture. The authors of this study estimate that 99% of healthy postmenopausal women would benefit from HRT. Only those women with the greatest risk of breast cancer and the least risk for CHD would not benefit.[30]

Vasomotor Instability

The symptoms of vasomotor instability respond to exogenous estrogen therapy.[31,32] In most women, the period of bothersome vasomotor symptoms lasts from 3 to 5 years, and therapy for these symptoms can be limited to that time span.[10] A variety of estrogens, including dosage forms and schemes for administration, exist (Table 78–2). A popular regimen is oral therapy with conjugated equine estrogens starting at doses of 0.3 to 0.625 mg/d given in 25-day cycles, with 5 estrogen-free days. The addition of a progestin is standard therapy in women with an intact uterus because of the adverse consequences of unopposed estrogen therapy, specifically the increased risk of endometrial cancer. One common regimen is the addition of medroxyprogesterone acetate 5 to 10 mg daily during the last 10 to 12 days of the cycle.[33] Other progestins used in cyclic therapy include norethindrone 2.5 mg, norgestrel 150 μg, or micronized oral progesterone 300 mg.[34] This cyclic regimen results in the return of regular menstrual periods, which some women find objectionable.

For women in whom cyclical bleeding is unacceptable, an alternative regimen involves the continuous administration of estrogens, with the addition of a progestin for 10 to 12 days during the calendar month. Advantages include a less complicated schedule and less likelihood of return of symptoms during the estrogen-free period.[34] Continuous combined estrogen–progestin therapy may be associated with a 40% incidence of breakthrough bleeding, especially during the first 6 months.[35] Some clinicians have advocated the continuous administration of estrogens and lower-dose progestins (2.5 to 5 mg daily medroxyprogesterone acetate) as an effective alternative to cyclic therapy, with the benefit of avoidance of withdrawal bleeding.[36–38] See Table 78–2 for combination product availability. The long-term effects of these treatments are unknown, especially their effects on cardiovascular morbidity and mortality, although using surrogate markers of

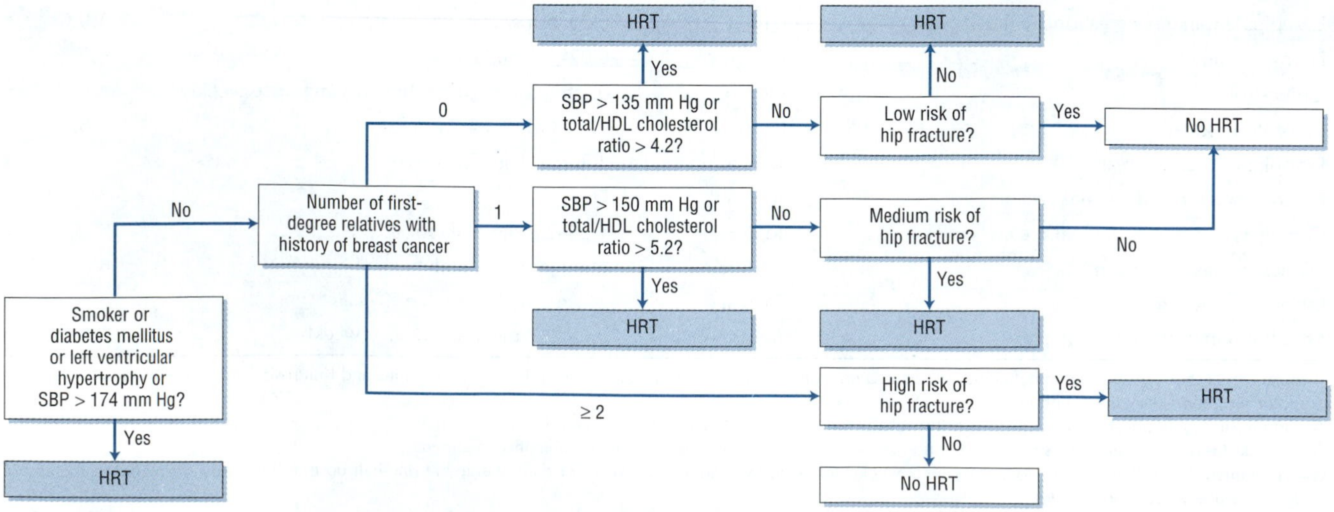

FIGURE 78–2. Decision analysis model to determine patients who would achieve at least 6 months of additional life expectancy from HRT. (HDL = high density lipoprotein; SBP = systolic blood pressure.) *(Adapted from Ref. 30.)*

cardiovascular disease and a follow-up period of 3 years showed effects comparable to estrogen alone.[39]

Urogenital Atrophy

Various vaginal preparations of estrogen are effective in the treatment of vaginal itching, dryness, burning, and other symptoms associated with changes in the vaginal epithelium caused by menopause. The goal of therapy is to restore the epithelium to its premenopausal state and thereby reduce these symptoms. Therapy is generally initiated with the smallest dose to restore the vaginal epithelium, usually 2 to 4 g of estradiol cream (0.1 mg estradiol/g) given once daily for 1 to 2 weeks initially. Therapy is tapered to half-doses for an additional 2 weeks. Maintenance therapy can be continued with 1 g given one to three times weekly in the usual cyclic manner.[40] Alternatives to estradiol cream include dienestrol (0.01 mg/g) 5 to 6 g/d, conjugated estrogens (0.625 mg/g) 2 to 4 g/d, or estropipate (1.5 mg/g) 2 to 4 g/d given in the same cyclic manner as estradiol. Oral or transdermal administration of estrogens may also be used to treat the symptoms of urogenital atrophy in the same doses and regimens discussed for use in the earlier section on vasomotor instability.

Osteoporosis

Studies show a correlation between gains in bone density and the serum levels of estrogen achieved with HRT. For maximal benefit, estrogen replacement should begin as soon as possible after menopause, preferably within 3 years. After 6 to 24 months of therapy, bone resorption and formation return to a state of equilibrium, and bone mass stabilizes. If HRT therapy is discontinued, bone loss begins immediately at approximately the pretreatment rate. The question of optimal duration of HRT for osteoporosis benefits remains unresolved. Traditionally, HRT was initiated at or shortly after menopause and continued for a fixed number of years, such as 10 to 15 years. At least 7 years of HRT is necessary to achieve persistent bone density; this benefit extends to women of age 75 years, but not thereafter. Protective effects against hip fracture also wane, but are not eliminated, with age. Thus some investigators recognize the need to start HRT treatment at menopause and never stop, while others recommend starting HRT many years after menopause, for example, at age 65 or 70, and treating for life as the most cost-effective regimen.[8] Despite their preventive effect, estrogens alone do not restore bone that has been lost. Fractures may still occur despite estrogen replacement if bone demineralization was severe before replacement therapy. Progestins, in combination with estrogen, do not impair estrogen's bone-preserving actions.[41] Some progestins used as single-agent therapy will protect against bone loss, but clarification of the overall role of progestins in osteoporosis awaits further study.[12]

The dose of estrogen required to prevent bone loss is 0.625 mg daily. Lower doses of conjugated estrogen (e.g., 0.312 mg/d) may prevent bone loss if used in conjunction with high daily doses of elemental calcium (at least 1500 mg/d).[34] Esterified estrogens at doses of 0.625 mg/d, oral ethinyl estradiol 0.02 mg/d, micronized 17 β-estradiol 1 mg/d, and transdermal estrogen patches (delivering estradiol at 0.05 to 0.10 mg/d, administered as one patch twice weekly) are alternative regimens. Adequate intake of calcium and regular weight-bearing exercise are also important adjunctive treatments to be used in conjunction with HRT.

Cardiovascular Disease

Most studies investigating the use of estrogens in protecting the cardiovascular system have used oral estrogen in doses similar to those used for prevention of osteoporosis. The most effective regimen has not been established.[13,18]

In most studies, estrogen replacement produces a potentially beneficial effect on cardiovascular risk by favorably altering the serum lipid profile. Prospective studies suggest that high-density lipoprotein (HDL) cholesterol is the best predictor of coronary heart disease risk in women. Estrogens lower low-density lipoprotein (LDL) cholesterol and increase HDL cholesterol, the latter accounting for up to one-half of the apparent benefit.[39] Other mechanisms, such as platelet effects and direct effects on vessel wall physiology, may also be cardioprotective. Although triglycerides may be higher in estrogen users, blood pressure and fasting blood glucose levels are unchanged or lower.[18,42] Certain estrogens increase insulin secretion and decrease insulin resistance; central obesity may be reversed.[43] In most studies, estrogen therapy has shown a 50% or greater reduction in cardiovascular disease and related mortality.[42,44] Recent evidence suggests that the beneficial cardiovascular effects of estrogen replacement after menopause are most pronounced in the presence of angiographically defined coronary artery disease and in women with at least one major cardiovascular risk factor (smoking, high cholesterol, hypertension, diabetes, previous myocardial infarction, or body mass index greater than 29).[18,44]

In contrast, experimental data show that progestins, unlike natural progesterone, may attenuate or eliminate the benefits on HDL cholesterol.[42] A 3-year placebo-controlled trial (postmenopausal estrogen/progestin interventions, or PEPI) compared estrogen alone with three estrogen/progestin combinations and observational data from the nurses health study. This study confirmed the cardiovascular benefits of combined treatment on HDL cholesterol.[39,44–46]

PROGESTIN THERAPY

Progesterone, a secretory product of the corpus luteum, is the primary natural progestational substance. Progestins act on the endometrium to change proliferative endometrial tissue into secretory tissue. Progestins alone are as effective as estrogens for relief of vasomotor symptoms. These agents also are useful in the treatment and prevention of osteoporosis, by increasing the formation of new bone. Synthetic progestins appear to stimulate bone formation via androgenic or anabolic effects.[5]

The administration of a progestin for 12 days each month with estrogen replacement therapy serves three major purposes: to decrease the risk of estrogen-induced irregular bleeding, endometrial hyperplasia, and carcinoma; to protect against breast carcinoma; and to enhance estrogen prophylaxis of osteoporosis.[34]

Natural progesterone is poorly absorbed when administered orally, and thus synthetic forms of 17-hydroxy progesterone and 19-nortestosterone are used clinically. The 19-nortestosterone derivatives must be converted to norethisterone in order to be biologically active. Because the 19-nortestosterone derivatives possess androgenic activity, they tend to cause acne and increase oil production on the skin and scalp. These products are used primarily in oral contraceptives.[19,34] The 17-hydroxyprogesterone derivatives, used primarily in hormone replacement therapy, are less androgenic but are associated with depression and anxiety symptoms.[20,34] Micronized natural progesterone is used clinically; however, large doses are required due to significant first-pass metabolism. Medroxyprogesterone acetate is the progestin generally used in treating menopausal symptoms because it is relatively well absorbed orally and has a more acceptable side-effect profile.

CLINICAL USE

In addition to using a progestin in cyclic ERT to prevent endometrial hyperplasia, progestins alone are used successfully to treat vasomotor instability. Medroxyprogesterone acetate 20 mg/d orally has been employed.[47] Depot medroxyprogesterone acetate 50 to 100 mg intramuscularly given every 2 to 3 months is as effective as conjugated estrogens in relieving vasomotor symptoms.[48] In women for whom estrogen therapy is contraindicated, progesterone may be a suitable alternative for treatment of osteoporosis. Recommended dosages are oral medroxyprogesterone acetate 5 to 10 mg/d or the depot injection form 100 to 200 mg every 2 to 3 months.[5]

ADVERSE EFFECTS

Progestins may cause certain dose-related physical, psychological, and metabolic side effects. When used alone or during the progestin phase of a combination regimen, an iatrogenic premenstrual tension-like syndrome may occur. Breast tenderness or mastalgia, bloating, edema, and abdominal cramping, as well as anxiety, irritability, and depression, are frequent complaints. Weight gain, headache, and drowsiness may occur. Approximately 5% of patients are intolerant to all types of progestins, but others may benefit from a dosage reduction or change to another type of progestin. There are no convincing data to support the premise that continuous-combined HRT reduces progesterone-induced adverse effects relative to sequential HRT.[34]

Progestins alone or with estrogen cause monthly bleeding in 80% to 90% of women; unopposed estrogen causes monthly withdrawal bleeding in 25% of patients. For women with moderate to severe postmenopausal symptoms, the inconvenience of bleeding may be offset by symptom relief. However, for the asymptomatic woman receiving estrogen for its cardiovascular or bone effects, or for the woman who has been postmenopausal for a number of years, regular withdrawal bleeding may be unacceptable. Some women choose not to begin or to continue HRT because of bleeding.[34] Continuous therapy with an estrogen–progestin combination is an option for women who wish to avoid monthly bleeding.

Progestins, both the C-19 nortestosterone derivatives and the C-21 derivatives, cause a dose-related decrease in HDL cholesterol and an increase in LDL cholesterol levels. To minimize the possibility of negating the cardioprotective effects of estrogens, progestins should be used in the minimum dosage required for endometrial protection when prescribed with estrogen.[34] Some data exist that suggest this adverse effect of progestins on HDL cholesterol may be a short-term effect. Women using combined therapy and those using unopposed estrogens for more than 3 years had HDL levels 11% higher and LDL levels 10 to 14% lower than women not receiving hormonal therapy. Much research is currently being done to find a synthetic progestin without this adverse effect on lipids.[49] Although not yet available for clinical use as progestin replacement agents, three 19-nortestosterone derivatives or gonanes—gestodene, norgestimate, and desogestrel—with relatively fewer androgenic effects than the estranes (norethindrone and norethindrone acetate) are of interest.[35]

PHARMACOECONOMIC CONSIDERATIONS

Because the benefits and risks of HRT can span as many as 30 years, pharmacoeconomic analysis based on clinical databases can be problematic. Consequently economic studies of HRT rely mostly on disease modeling and decision analysis. Most models incorporate reduction in mortality from hip fracture and cardiovascular and cerebrovascular events, relief of menopausal symptoms, and increase in risk for breast cancer as the possible outcomes. Costs include cost of therapy (drugs, monitoring, physician visits), and cost of adverse events (breast cancer). Costs avoided include nursing home costs and treatment costs for CHD and hip fracture. Some studies adjust life expectancy based on quality factors such as morbidity of hip fracture, relief of menopausal symptoms, and adverse effects of HRT.[29]

Tosteston and colleagues have published one of the most comprehensive models of HRT, which includes most of the relevant outcomes and costs.[28] Their analysis is based on a Markov state transition model of women aged 50 years who were treated for 10 or 15 years with either cyclic combination therapy (estrogen and medroxyprogesterone) or estrogen alone in women with previous hysterectomy. The model encompassed breast cancer risk, adverse effects of HRT, bothersome menopausal symptoms, avoidance of hip fracture, nursing home placement, and CHD. Costs varied greatly depending on the combination of risk factors and outcomes. In general, cost per quality-adjusted life-year (QALY) ranged from $5600 in symptomatic women with no increased breast cancer risk and no HRT side effects treated for 10 years, to $139,000 in women with increased risk of breast cancer, who had no menopausal symptoms but did suffer HRT adverse effects. Cost per QALY saved for women with menopausal symptoms, no HRT adverse effects but increased risk for breast cancer was $13,000.

EVALUATION OF THERAPEUTIC OUTCOMES

Before initiating HRT, menopause should be verified. Because periods of amenorrhea are not sufficiently reliable to signal the beginning of menopause, other diagnostic means are necessary. An FSH level of 30 pg/mL or greater indicates the beginning of menopause. If FSH levels are unavailable, the progestin challenge test can be used for diagnosis. This method, whereby a progestin is given for 10 days, is relatively inexpensive and easy to administer. Absence of withdrawal bleeding indicates lack of significant estrogen secretion and endometrial stimulation. If withdrawal bleeding occurs, the progestin can be repeated in monthly cycles until withdrawal bleeding fails to occur.[20]

The presence of any estrogen-dependent cancer should be ruled out before the initiation of HRT. Mammography should be performed if the woman has not recently undergone this procedure. A complete physical exam including breast exam and lipid profile should be performed to establish a baseline. Screening endometrial biopsy is not necessary before HRT is initiated in asymptomatic perimenopausal women in the absence of nulliparity or obesity. Periodic endometrial biopsy to screen for endometrial hyperplasia should be performed in women receiving unopposed estrogen.[50] Routine follow-up visits with breast and pelvic examinations are recommended at yearly intervals.[20]

The most immediate benefits of HRT are relief of vasomotor symptoms and genitourinary atrophy. The frequency and severity of hot flushes is a good measure of the therapeutic benefits of HRT. The patient should be asked how frequently hot flushes disrupt her normal activities of daily living and her sleep. Relief of genitourinary atrophy can be measured by reduction in the symptoms of atrophic vaginits (itching, bleeding, dyspareunia) and the frequency of nonbacterial urethritis and bacteriuria. Long-term benefits of HRT are more difficult to monitor because they result from prevention of CVD and osteoporosis. Postmenopausal women should receive regular medical examinations with emphasis on the health of the cardiovascular system (blood pressure, lipid profile, symptoms), and skeleton.

RISKS AND BENEFITS

Only about 15% to 30% of women who are eligible for HRT are now receiving it; that leaves 70% to 85% who do not want, need, or know about HRT.[8] Many of those for whom HRT is prescribed will not fill the prescription; for those who do, only one-third will continue treatment for more than 3 months.[8] Patients who do not understand the purpose, risks, and side effects of HRT may refuse treatment, exhibit poor compliance, or discontinue therapy. Although acceptance of HRT is ultimately a decision for the patient and her physician, family and friends may offer opinions about what constitutes appropriate use, providing anecdotal details to support these opinions. HRT has also captured the attention of the media, and much of the patient's education, sometimes reflecting misinformation or misinterpretation of facts presented in an abbreviated format, may arise from lay publications or programs.[51]

Among the risks of therapy that may figure prominently in the patient's decisions about HRT are concerns about endometrial and breast cancer, coagulation and thrombosis, cardiovascular events, and neurologic effects.[10,51] Concerns about endometrial (uterine) and breast cancer are primary therapy considerations for many women. Although estrogen is not a carcinogen, it may act as an accelerative growth factor when cancer is present. Breast cancer is a contraindication to ERT,[10,51] except in patients where powerful overriding indications exist and where careful follow-up can be assured.[52] Studies examining the risk of breast cancer in women receiving estrogen replacement at menopause have not shown a consistent pattern of increased risk, possibly due to methodologic differences and deficiencies and flaws in study design. Recently, three large observational studies have addressed the risk of breast cancer associated with HRT.[44,53,54] Overall, HRT use was associated with a 37% decrease in mortality from any cause, but the apparent benefit declined after 10 or more years to a 20% decrease in overall mortality due to increase in incidence of breast cancer.[44] Because there does appear to be an increased risk of breast cancer with long-term HRT, all women receiving estrogen replacement should practice regular breast self-examination along with annual physician breast examinations and routine mammography.[52]

In contrast to the more questionable association of HRT and breast cancer, the association between endometrial cancer and estrogen use has been recognized since 1975. Increased frequency of uterine cancer is related to endometrial hyperplasia, a predictable result of unopposed estrogen therapy (estrogen therapy without progestional agents).[52] Studies have shown that 3% to 75% of women will develop endometrial cancer subsequent to the diagnosis of hyperplasia, depending on the length of follow up and the baseline severity of hyperplasia at the time of diagnosis.[55] Overall, estrogen users have a fourfold to eightfold increase (range, 1.7 to 20-fold) in risk of developing endometrial cancer relative to the risk in the normal population of 1 case per 1000. Risk, which persists after discontinuation of estrogens, is related to various factors including duration of use, dosage, method of administration, drug-free interval, and concomitant progestin use.[12,52] The addition of progestin to estrogen therapy confers protection against hyperplasia and is generally recommended, either cyclically for at least 10 days per month or continuously in patients with an intact uterus.[10,52,55]

Because estrogens and progestins produce a complex variety of effects on coagulation, a history of thromboembolism is a relative contraindication to estrogen therapy.[52] Progestins may increase or reduce prostacyclin production, while synthetic estrogens specifically or preferentially increase prostacyclin activity. Platelet aggregation is generally unchanged by estrogens, although there are limited data to the contrary. Virtually all clotting factors—particularly factors II, VIII, IX, X, XII, and fibrinogen—are elevated by synthetic estrogens such as ethinyl estradiol and diethylstilbestrol. The effects on clotting factors are primarily related to estrogen potency. Elevations are relatively marked with ethinyl estradiol, but are either not observed or are not clinically significant after use of estrogen patches and ointment or natural estrogens.[10,52] In general, total estrogen potency in HRT is less than that received by most women taking oral contraceptives.

Despite producing increased amounts of clotting factors, estrogens do not produce a hypercoagulable state because the clotting proenzymes remain inactive until exposed to injured vascular endothelium. Also, antithrombin III is not reduced to a clinically significant degree by either oral or transdermal estrogens. Plasminogen, a major factor in the fibrinolytic pathway, and plasminogen activity are elevated by estrogens. These effects are enhanced by estrogen–progestin combination therapy. Plasminogen effects, along with normal antithrombin III activity, ensure against inappropriate venous thrombosis. Clinical trials have shown no increase in risk of thromboembolism in postmenopausal women receiving estrogen replacement.[10,52]

Recent studies have demonstrated significant benefit of HRT on the risk of cardiovascular disease, including stroke and CHD, and cardiovascular death. Among HRT users the largest reduction in mortality risk (49%) was seen in women with high cardiovascular risk versus women at low risk (11%).[44] The benefits of estrogen in cardiovascular disease are generally attributed to their favorable effects on lipids and lipoproteins. Enhanced prostacyclin production, resulting in vasodilation, is also beneficial. LDL cholesterol is reduced and HDL cholesterol is increased. These changes are seen with both oral and nonoral ethinyl estradiol and with oral, but not vaginal, conjugated estrogens. Transdermal estrogen patches do not appear to produce favorable effects on lipids and lipoproteins.

In contrast, synthetic progestins have an effect on prostacyclin and on lipoproteins that is opposite that of estrogens, at least in the short term. At conventional doses of progestin, HDL cholesterol is decreased, an effect that may ameliorate or abolish estrogen's beneficial effects. In balancing the effects of unopposed estrogens on the intact uterus in the patient at high cardiovascular risk, some authorities recommend relatively high-dose estrogen (e.g., conjugated estrogens 1.25 mg) with cyclic progestin (e.g., medroxyprogesterone acetate 5 mg) for the first 2 weeks of the cycle, a regimen associated with a favorable lipid profile.[10] Most women do not need added progestins after a hysterectomy.[10]

The concern that hypertension may be caused or exacerbated by estrogens has contributed to the belief that hypertension is a contraindication to estrogen therapy.[10] Most clinical evidence shows no causal relationship between ERT and hypertension. Oral estrogen therapy, particularly potent synthetic products, but not transdermal estrogen, causes increased renin substrate and may increase angiotensin II and aldosterone, although the clinical significance of these changes is unknown.[52] Progestins, however, produce a dose-related elevation in blood pressure by causing sodium and water retention.[9]

Estrogen therapy may potentiate headaches, including migraine headache. Therefore, a history of migraine headache is a relative contraindication to ERT. In some patients, the frequency of headache may be reduced over a period of about 4 weeks by a reduction in estrogen dosage. Parenteral testosterone has also been used to alleviate estrogen-induced headache.[1]

Some epidemiologic data and observational studies suggest that HRT may decrease the risk of colon and colorectal cancer.[56] HRT has been associated with nearly 30% decrease in mortality risk from all cancers.[44] Preliminary findings also suggest benefit in prevention of Alzheimers disease.

CONCLUSIONS

Menopause is caused by an age-related loss of ovarian function and the resultant decline in estrogen secretion by the ovarian follicles. Symptoms related to estrogen deprivation include genitourinary atrophy and vasomotor instability; long-term sequelae include osteoporosis and cardiovascular disease. Other symptoms experienced during menopause may be insomnia and fatigue, behavioral changes, and changes in libido. HRT with a combination of estrogen and progestin is the most effective treatment modality. Benefits of ERT include relief of hot flushes and genitourinary symptoms, as well as long-term positive effects on bone and lipids. Observational data indicate decreased mortality from all causes in women receiving HRT; those with high cardiovascular risk benefited most. Therapy for 10 years or more significantly increased breast cancer mortality despite lower overall death rates.

Risks of HRT include concerns about breast and endometrial cancer, coagulation disturbances, and thrombosis. The return of regular monthly bleeding, in response to cyclic HRT regimens, is unacceptable to many women; continuous therapy should be considered. Further investigation is needed in several areas, particularly in clarifying the relative role of HRT in breast cancer, in defining the optimal HRT treatment regimen for women with specific treatment goals and risk factors, and in identifying synthetic progestins with no negative effects on lipids. HRT plays an important role in the preventive medical care of postmenopausal women, and most postmenopausal women without an absolute contraindication should receive HRT.

▶ PRINCIPLES OF PHARMACOTHERAPY

- Estrogen deficiency following natural or surgical menopause may lead to symptoms of genitourinary atrophy, vasomotor instability, and morbidity and mortality associated with the long-term sequelae of osteoporosis and cardiovascular disease.
- Administration of estrogen alone or in combination with progestin effectively treats or prevents symptoms and sequelae of estrogen deficiency and is associated with a 37% decrease in mortality from all causes.
- Despite clear benefits, HRT may be associated with troublesome adverse effects, including monthly menstrual bleeding, that greatly compromise patient acceptance and compliance, and significant risks of endometrial cancer and breast cancer.
- The choice of specific estrogen product, the need for a progestin, when to initiate therapy, dose, treatment regimen, route of administration, and duration of treatment should be based on indication(s) for use and medical history, with specific attention to risk factors that define potential benefit as well as contraindications.
- Because HRT is prescribed for less than one-third of eligible women and the percent who fill their prescriptions or continue therapy for more than 6 months is much less, there appears to be much need for a better-informed professional community and female population.
- Although the growing body of scientific data suggest that the benefits of HRT outweigh the known risks for most women, the decision to receive HRT is highly personal and must be based on informed collaboration between patient and prescriber; the clinician may play a pivotal role in patient compliance and acceptance of therapy.

REFERENCES

1. London SN, Hammond CB. The climacteric. In: Danforth DN, Scott JR, eds. Obstetrics and Gynecology, 5th ed. Philadelphia, Lippincott, 1986:905.
2. Utian WH. Biosynthesis and physiologic effects of estrogen and pathophysiologic effects of estrogen deficiency: A review. Am J Obstet Gynecol 1989;161:828–831.
3. Korenman SG. Menopausal endocrinology and management. Arch Intern Med 1982;142:1131–1136.
4. Haney AF. The physiology of the climacterium. Clin Obstet Gynecol 1986;20:397–406.
5. Young RL, Kumar NS, Goldzieher JW. Management of menopause when estrogen cannot be used. Drugs 1990;40:220–230.

6. Wells RG. Hormone replacement before menopause. Is it a good idea? Postgraduate Med 1989;86:61–71.
7. Mishell DR. Estrogen replacement therapy: An overview. Am J Obstet Gynecol 1989;161:1825–1827.
8. Gibaldi M. Hormone replacement therapy: Estrogen after menopause. Pharmacotherapy 1996;16:366–375.
9. Ravnikar V. Physiology and treatment of hot flushes. Obstet Gynecol 1990;75:3S–8S.
10. Notelovitz M. Estrogen replacement therapy: Indications, contraindications, and agent selection. Am J Obstet Gynecol 1989;161:1832–1841.
11. Menopause. National Institutes of Health, National Institute on Aging, NIH pub. no. 94-3886. U.S. Government Printing Office, 1995.
12. Genant HK, Baylink DJ, Gallagher JC. Estrogens in the prevention of osteoporosis in postmenopausal women. Am J Obstet Gynecol 1989; 161:1842–1846.
13. Hammond CB. Estrogen replacement therapy: What the future holds. Am J Obstet Gynecol 1989;161:1864–1868.
14. Sarrel PM. Sexuality and menopause. Obstet Gynecol 1990;75: 26S–30S
15. Shangold MM. Exercise in the menopausal woman. Obstet Gynecol 1990;75:53S–58S.
16. Wildasin EM. Menopause: Important points to include in the pharmacist and patient interaction. Am Druggist 1997;214:49–54.
17. Watts NB, Harris ST, Genant HK, et al. Intermittent cyclical etidronate treatment of postmenopausal osteoporosis. N Engl J Med 1990;323:73–79.
18. Sullivan JM, Zwaag RV, Hughes JP, et al. Estrogen replacement and coronary artery disease. Arch Intern Med 1990;150:2557–2562.
19. Estrogens (systemic and vaginal). In: Johnson KW, ed. USPDI. Rockville, MD, U.S. Pharmacopoeial Convention, 1994:1304.
20. Sitruk-Ware R. Estrogen therapy during menopause: Practical treatment recommendations. Drugs 1990;39:203–217.
21. Lievertz RW. Pharmacology and pharmacokinetics of estrogens. Am J Obstet Gynecol 1987;156:1289–1293.
22. Chetkowski RJ, Meldrum DR, Steingold KA, et al. Biologic effects of transdermal estradiol. N Engl J Med 1986;314:1615–1620.
23. Powers MS, Schenkel L, Darley PE, et al. Pharmacokinetics and pharmacodynamics of transdermal dosage forms of 17-estradiol: Comparison with conventional oral estrogens used for hormone replacement. Am J Obstet Gynecol 1985;152:1099–1106.
24. Mashchak CA, Lobo RA, Dozono-Takano R, et al. Comparison of pharmacodynamic properties of various estrogen formulations. Am J Obstet Gynecol 1982;144:511–518.
25. Stanczyk FZ, Shoupe D, Nunez V, et al. A randomized comparison of nonoral estradiol delivery in postmenopausal women. Am J Obstet Gynecol 1988;159:1540–1546.
26. Jensen J, Riis BJ, Strom V, et al. Long-term effects of percutaneous estrogens and oral progesterone on serum lipoproteins in postmenopausal women. Am J Obstet Gynecol 1987;156:66–71.
27. Balfour JA, Heel RC. Transdermal estradiol: A review of its pharmacodynamic and pharmacokinetic properties, and therapeutic efficacy in the treatment of menopausal complaints. Drugs 1990;40:561–582.
28. Tosteson ANA, Weinstein MC, Shiff I. Cost-effectiveness analysis of hormone replacement therapy. In: Lobo RA, ed. Treatment of the Postmenopausal Woman: Basic and Clinical Aspects. New York, Raven, 1994:405–413.
29. Armstrong EP. Pharmacoeconomic analysis of hormone replacement therapy—Implications for managed care. J Managed Care Pharm 1997; 3:200–209.
30. Col NF, Eckman MH, Karas RH, et al. Patient-specific decisions about hormone replacement therapy in postmenopausal women, JAMA 1997;277:1140–1147.
31. Jensen J, Christiansen C. Dose response and withdrawal effects on climacteric symptoms after hormonal replacement therapy: A placebo-controlled therapeutic trial. Maturitas 1983;5:125–133.
32. Lauritzen CH. The female climacteric syndrome: Significance, problems and treatment. Acta Obstet Gynecol 1976;53(suppl):47–61.
33. Lufkin EG, Carpenter PC, Ory SJ, et al. Estrogen replacement therapy: Current recommendations. Mayo Clin Proc 1988;63:453–460.
34. Whitehead MI, Hillard TC, Crook D. The role and use of progestogens. Obstet Gynecol 1990;74(suppl):59S–76S.
35. Belchetz PE. Hormonal treatment of postmenopausal women. N Engl J Med 1994;330:1062–1071.
36. Staland B. Continuous treatment with natural oestrogens and progestogens: A method to avoid endometrial stimulation. Maturitas 1981; 3:145–156.
37. Jensen J, Riis BJ, Strom V, Christiansen C. Continuous estrogen-progestogen treatment and serum lipoproteins in postmenopausal women. Br J Obstet Gynaecol 1987;94:130–135.
38. Sporrong T, Hellgren M, Samsioe G, Mattsson LA. Comparison of four continuously administered progestogen plus oestradiol combinations for climacteric complaints. Br J Obstet Gynaecol 1988;95: 1042–1048.
39. PEPI Trial Group. Effects of estrogen or estrogen/progestin regimens on heart disease risk factors in postmenopausal women. JAMA 1995; 273:199–208.
40. McEvoy GK, ed. AHFS Drug Information 95. Bethesda, MD, American Society of Health-System Pharmacists, 1995:2150.
41. Speroff L, Rowan J, Symons J, et al. The comparative effect on bone density, endothelium, and lipids of continuous hormones as replacement therapy (CHART study). JAMA 1996;275:1397–1403.
42. Lobo RA. Cardiovascular implications of estrogen replacement therapy. Obstet Gynecol 1990;75:18S–25S.
43. Stevenson JC, Crook D, Godsland IF, et al. Hormone replacement therapy and the cardiovascular system. Drugs 1994;47(suppl 2):35–41.
44. Grodstein F, Stampfer MJ, Colditz GA, et al. Postmenopausal hormone therapy and mortality. N Engl J Med 1997;336:1769–1775.
45. Grodstein F, Stampfer MJ, Manson J, et al. Postmenopausal estrogen and progestin use and the cardiovascular risk of cardiovascular disease. N Engl J Med 1996;335:453–461.
46. Whitcroft SI, Crook D, Marsh S, et al. Long-term effects of oral and transdermal hormone replacement therapies on serum lipid and lipoprotein concentrations. Obstet Gynecol 1994;84:222–226.
47. Schiff I, Tulchinsky D, Cramer D, Ryan KJ. Oral medroxyprogesterone in the treatment of postmenopausal symptoms. JAMA 1980; 244:1443–1445.
48. Lobo RA, McCormick W, Singer F, Roy S. Depo-medroxyprogesterone acetate compared with conjugated estrogens for the treatment of postmenopausal women. J Am Coll Obstet Gynecol 1984;63:105.
49. Nachtigall LE. Enhancing patient compliance with hormone replacement therapy at menopause. Obstet Gynecol 1990;75:77S–80S.
50. Korbonen MO. Histologic classification and pathologic findings for endometrial biopsy specimens obtained from 2964 perimenopausal and postmenopausal women undergoing screening for continuous hormones as replacement therapy (CHART 2 study): Am J Obstet Gynecol 1997;176:377–380.
51. Barrett-Connor E, Winhard DL, Criqui MH. Postmenopausal estrogen use and heart disease risk factors in the 1980s. JAMA 1989;261: 2095–2100.
52. Lufkin EG, Carpenter PC, Ory SJ, et al. Estrogen replacement therapy: Current recommendations. Mayo Clin Proc 1988;63:453–460.
53. Stanford JL, Weiss NS, Voigt LF, et al. Combined estrogen and progestin hormone replacement therapy in relation to risk of breast cancer in middle-aged women. JAMA 1995;274:137–142.
54. Colditz GA, Hankinson SE, Hunter DJ, et al. The use of estrogens and progestins and the risk of breast cancer in postmenopausal women. N Engl J Med 1995;332:1589–1593.
55. Writing group for the PEPI trial. Effects of hormone replacement therapy on endometrial histology in postmenopausal women. The postmenopausal estrogen/progestin interventions (PEPI) trial. JAMA 1996;275:370–375.
56. Calle EE, Miracle-McMahil HL, Then MJ, Heath CW. Estrogen replacement therapy and risk of fatal colon cancer in a prospective cohort of postmenopausal women. J Natl Cancer Inst 1995;87:517–523.

79
FUNCTION AND EVALUATION OF THE IMMUNE SYSTEM

Philip D. Hall, PharmD, BCPS, and Janet L. Karlix, PharmD

Knowledge of the immune system has rapidly expanded over the past few years, enabling an understanding of normal immune system function as well as identification of the role of immune system dysfunction in a multitude of disease states. To adequately analyze the immune system in disease processes, it is vital to comprehend normal immune function and to recognize immune dysfunction. This chapter presents first an overview of the immune system and then a discussion of the evaluation of immune function in the clinical setting. The term "immune system" encompasses a wide range of components including mechanical immunodefenses and soluble mediators as well as cellular and humoral immune responses. Cells involved in the immune response (e.g., neutrophils, lymphocytes, etc.) develop from a common pluripotent stem cell. Please refer to Chap. 90 for a review of the hematopoiesis. The section illustrating immune function will also focus on those laboratory examinations commonly available in clinical settings or likely to be available in the near future.

The immune system primarily serves to protect the body against infectious pathogens. To accomplish this task, the immune system exhibits specificity, memory, mobility, and replicability. Specificity indicates that the immune system can distinguish between non-cross-reacting antigens. Memory allows a quicker and more vigorous response to pathogenic invasion. Because elements of the immune system are mobile, local reactions may provide systemic protection. All cellular components of the immune system can replicate, allowing the immune response to be amplified.[1] In addition, the immune response normally distinguishes "self" from "nonself," preventing damage to the host. This discrimination between "self" and "nonself" is done by the adaptive or specific arm of the immune response. The immune system is commonly separated into two functional divisions: innate (nonspecific) and adaptive (specific) (Table 79–1).[2] Despite this simple separation, both divisions heavily interact.

The innate arm provides the first line of defense against pathogens. One of the most frequently overlooked methods of host defense is the body's ability to provide a physical and chemical defense against invading pathogens. The skin, the largest organ of the body, has the primary role of providing this physical defense. Alterations in the skin, such as burns or abrasions, allow an easier route of entry for pathogens. The gastrointestinal tract also plays an important role in providing a physical defense against pathogenic invasion. The low pH of the stomach (pH 1 to 2) kills many organisms. The constant sloughing of intestinal cells also limits systemic infection because infected cells are frequently replaced. Drugs, such as cell-cycle specific antineoplastics, which disrupt the sloughing process, leave the patient at an increased risk of infection. Likewise, the respiratory tract has its forms of physical defense, namely the cilia lining the epithelium of the lungs, which have the ability to remove organisms in that area. Mucus that coats the epithelial cells serves in part to prevent microorganisms from adhering to cell surfaces. The combination of cilia, mucus, and coughing provides a natural barrier to invasion via the respiratory tract. Other examples of mechanical or nonspecific defenses include lysozymes in tears and saliva, the normal flora of the lower gastrointestinal tract, and normal urine flow. It is these physical and chemical defenses that often play the first line of defense against antimicrobial infections. It is well known that conditions or devices that allow microorganisms to transgress these normal barriers predispose patients to infections. As such, patients with a substantial loss of the skin from a burn or requiring mechanical ventilation, bladder catheterization, or central venous access are at increased risk of infection.

THE IMMUNE RESPONSE

When an infectious pathogen eludes the physical defenses of the body, an immune response involving both soluble mediators and leukocytes is generated against the pathogen.

INNATE RESPONSE

Innate immunity is present from birth and involves the stimulation of cells that nonspecifically recognize foreign invaders and destroy them. The innate leukocytes are monocytes, macrophages, neutrophils, basophils, mast cells, and eosinophils. Monocytes, macrophages, neutrophils, and eosinophils act as phagocytes whereas mast cells and basophils secrete inflammatory mediators when stimulated. The phagocytes recognize, internalize, and destroy invading pathogens. These cells use nonspecific recognition systems

TABLE 79–1. Functional Divisions of the Immune System

	Innate	Adaptive
Physical barriers	Skin & mucous membranes	None
Specificity	None	Yes
Memory	No	Yes
Soluble factors	Lysozymes, complement, acute phase proteins	Antibodies, lymphokines
Cells	Neutrophils, monocytes, macrophages, NK[a] cells, eosinophils	B lymphocytes, T lymphocytes

[a]NK = natural killer.
From Ref. 37, with permission.

to identify the pathogen. On the surface of phagocytic cells exist receptors for complement (complement receptors [CR] 1, 2, 3, 4) and antibody (Fc receptors). Complement or antibodies coat infectious pathogens in a process termed "opsonization," and then the antibody or complement binds to the receptors on the innate leukocyte (Fig. 79–1), thereby activating the phagocytic process.

The granulocytic cells of the body include neutrophils, eosinophils, and basophils. The cytoplasmic granules of these cells often contain inflammatory mediators or digestive enzymes. Neutrophils are polymorphonuclear cells (often denoted as PMNs for this reason), which constitute the primary human defense against pathogenic bacteria and make up the majority of leukocytes in the bloodstream. Neutrophils respond to chemotactic factors, such as interleukin-8 and C3a and C5a, breakdown products of complement, that are released from infected or inflamed tissue. Neutrophils migrate to sites of infection in a process termed "chemotaxis," whereupon they recognize, adhere to, and phagocytose pathogens. Neutrophils can recognize only pathogens coated with either complement or IgG (antibody) via the complement and antibody receptors located on the surface of the neutrophil. Once bound, the neutrophil then releases its granular contents into vacuoles and generates the release of oxidative metabolites, thereby killing engulfed pathogens.[3]

Eosinophils are also granulocytic cells but have a minor role in combatting bacterial infections. Patients with drug-induced neutropenia or other neutrophil deficiency states are not protected against microbial pathogens by

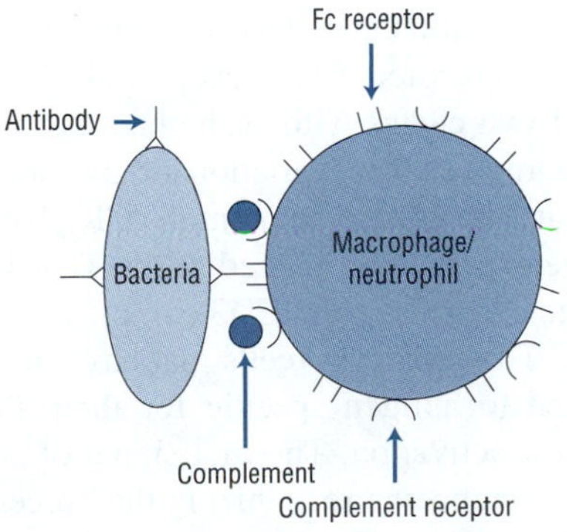

FIGURE 79–1. Phagocytosis of bacteria by macrophages and neutrophils. Macrophages and neutrophils recognize bacteria opsonized (coated) with antibody or complement. On the surface of the macrophages and neutrophils reside receptors for the antibody (Fc receptor) and complement (CR1, CR2, CR4).

eosinophils. However, eosinophils play a major role against nonphagocytable multicellular pathogens, such as parasites. With their cytoplasmic granules and ability to generate oxidative substances, the eosinophils are capable of destroying multicellular parasites even when the eosinophil is unable to phagocytose the parasite. Eosinophils recognize pathogens coated by complement or IgE (antibody). Because of their ability to bind IgE, eosinophils contribute to the pathogenesis of allergic disorders (e.g., asthma).[4]

Macrophages and monocytes are mononuclear cells capable of phagocytosis. These cells also have the ability to release soluble factors with inflammatory properties. Monocytes are found within the bloodstream whereas macrophages are found in the tissues. Tissue macrophages are believed to arise from the migration of monocytes. Macrophages differ from monocytes by possessing an increased number of Fc and complement receptors. Macrophages are found within specific tissues such as the liver, spleen, gastrointestinal tract, lymph nodes, brain, and others. These specific types of macrophages are often called histiocytes or are referred to by a specialized name depending on the site where they are found (Kupffer cells in the liver, Langerhans' cells in the skin, osteoclasts in the bone, microglial cells in the central nervous system, etc.). The term "reticuloendothelial system" (RES) was commonly used to refer to macrophages found in reticular connective tissue, but the term "mononuclear phagocyte system" is now the preferred nomenclature.

In addition to phagocytosing pathogens, monocytes/macrophages act as antigen-presenting cells (APCs) to stimulate the adaptive (specific) system. Macrophages internalize the organism, digest it into small peptide fragments, and then place these antigenic fragments together with major histocompatibility complex (MHC) proteins. Once the APC has formed the antigen/MHC complex, it places the complex on the surface of the APC. This complex is recognized by the T-cell receptor on the surface of T lymphocytes, which will activate the T lymphocyte (Fig. 79–2). Other cells, B lymphocytes and dendritic cells, can act as APCs.[2,5,6]

Mast cells and basophils act primarily by releasing inflammatory mediators. Mast cells are tissue cells predominantly associated with IgE-mediated inflammation. They are especially abundant in the skin, lungs, and nasal mucosa. Granules within the mast cells contain large amounts of preformed mediators, including histamine, heparin, serotonin, and others. Mast cells can phagocytize, destroy, and present bacteria to other immune cells. Basophils are similar to mast

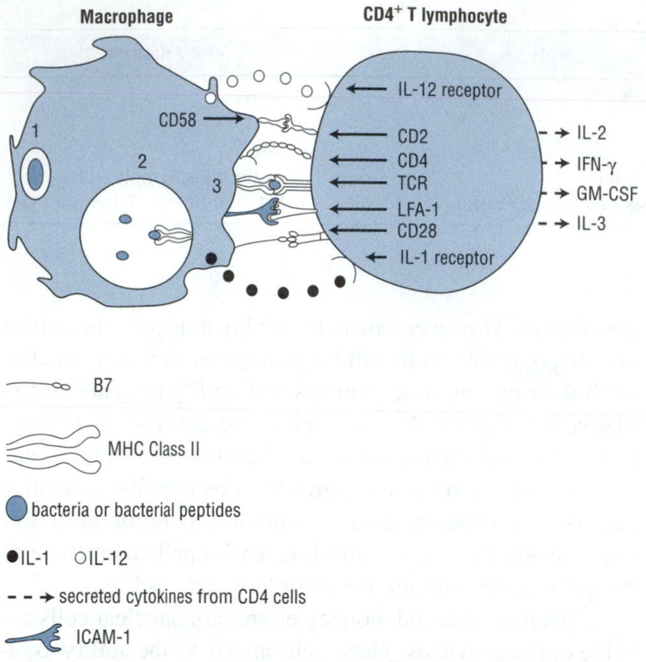

FIGURE 79–2. Macrophage presentation to CD4$^+$ T lymphocytes. After phagocytosis of the bacteria by the macrophage (1), the bacteria is digested into small peptides and becomes associated with MHC class II within the endosome (2). Finally the MHC class II plus antigen is expressed on the surface of the macrophage (3). CD4$^+$ T lymphocyte activation requires the T-lymphocyte receptor (TCR) to recognize the antigenic peptide plus MHC class II as well as the B7-CD28 interaction. IL-1 and IL-12 secreted by macrophage also activates the T lymphocyte. The CD2-CD58 and LFA-1-ICAM-1 (adhesion molecules) interaction allows for adherence between the T lymphocyte and macrophage. Upon activation, CD4$^+$ lymphocytes secrete numerous cytokines to up-regulate the immune response (IL-2, γ-IFN) and growth factors (IL-3, GM-CSF).

cells because they contain granules filled with histamine; however, they are typically found circulating in the blood and are not found in connective tissue. Like mast cells and eosinophils, basophils also express high-affinity IgE Fc receptors. IgE-mediated anaphylaxis (type I hypersensitivity, Chap. 81) is caused by the stimulation of mast cell and/or basophil degranulation (release of preformed mediators) by allergen binding to IgE bound on the surface of mast cells or basophils.[7]

Soluble mediators of innate immunity include complement and C-reactive protein (CRP). The complement system consists of 20 plasma proteins and five regulatory membrane proteins that play a key role in immune defense. The three major functions of the complement system include (1) the ability to lyse certain microorganisms and cells, (2) the ability to stimulate the chemotaxis of phagocytic cells, and (3) the ability to coat or opsonize foreign pathogens, thus allowing phagocytosis of the pathogen by leukocytes expressing complement receptors. Complement factors (C3a, C5a) act as chemotaxis factors for phagocytic cells.

Two different pathways are used in stimulating the complement cascade. In the classic pathway, antibody binding to its target antigen or CRP binding to bacteria or fungi activates the first component of complement (C1), thereby initiating the complement cascade. The alternative complement pathway does not require the presence of a specific complement-fixing antibody but is stimulated directly by microorganisms. Mannose-binding protein, an acute-phase reactant, binds to mannose-rich glycoconjugates on microorganisms and can activate both the classic and alternative pathways. Patients with hereditary deficiencies of complement have recurrent bacterial infections.[2,8]

ADAPTIVE RESPONSE

To amplify the immune response, activation of the adaptive immune system is required. The adaptive immune response differs from the innate immune response in two critical areas: specificity and memory. Lymphocytes (T and B) comprise the cells of the adaptive response. These cells have surface receptors specific for the invading organism. In a manner that uses genetic rearrangement of their DNA, it is estimated that lymphocytes have the ability to recognize more than 10^{16} different types of antigens. Generally, the body will use both the innate and adaptive immune responses to kill foreign pathogens.

The adaptive immune response can be divided into two major arms: humoral or cellular-mediated. The B lymphocytes and activated B lymphocytes (plasma cells) that secrete antibody compose the humoral arm of adaptive immune response. The humoral response is so denoted because it was found that the factors that provided the immune protection could be found in the humor or serum. The cell-mediated arm is controlled primarily by T lymphocytes. The immune protection provided by these cells could not be transferred by serum alone. Rather, it is essential to actually have T lymphocytes present, thus the term cell-mediated immunity. T lymphocytes are specially tailored to defend against infections that are intracellular, such as virally infected cells, whereas B lymphocytes secrete antibodies that can neutralize pathogens prior to their entry into host cells.

T lymphocytes do not recognize intact antigen. T lymphocytes recognize processed antigen in association with MHC. APCs (macrophages, dendritic cells, Kupffer cells) phagocytose the pathogen and then break down the pathogen and express peptide fragments (processed antigen) in association with MHC on their surface. T lymphocytes express a specific antigen receptor, T-cell receptor (TCR). The TCR is comprised of two chains with each chain having a variable and constant region. The variation of the amino acid sequence within the variable domain of TCR gives the cell its unique antigen specificity. Linked to the TCR is a complex of single chains known as the CD3 complex.

"Naive" T lymphocyte (cells that have not been previously exposed to antigen specific for their TCR) require two signals for activation. The first signal of activation involves the T lymphocyte recognizing the processed antigen in the MHC molecule. The second signal involves the interaction of the B7-1 (CD80) or B7-2 (CD86) molecule on the APC with the CD28 molecule on the surface of T lymphocyte (Fig. 79–2). Without the second signal, the T lymphocyte becomes anergic or inactive. Memory T lymphocytes are less dependent on the second signal than naive T lymphocytes. CD28 is expressed on both resting and activated T lymphocytes whereas CTLA-4 (a second ligand for B7 on T lymphocytes) is expressed only on activated T lymphocytes. CTLA-4 binding B7 transduces a negative signal, so its function may be to terminate T-lymphocyte activation.[9] After the two activation signals, a message is sent through the TCR to the CD3 complex into the cell. Then a calcium influx occurs with subsequent activation of the T-lymphocyte. Activated $CD4^+$ T lymphocytes release various soluble factors (IL-2, γ-interferon, etc.) to stimulate other cells of the immune system (Fig. 79–2). T-lymphocyte populations can be classified by cell surface markers or functional activity. Typically, T lymphocytes are divided into helper cells ($CD4^+$), suppressor cells ($CD8^+$), and cytotoxic cells ($CD8^+$). Each of the subclasses appears to play a distinct role in the cell-mediated immune response.

The primary role of $CD4^+$ cells is to stimulate other cells in the immune response. Based on surface markers, two subgroups of $CD4^+$ T lymphocytes have been identified: helper/inducer ($CD4^+$, $CD29^+$) and helper/suppressor ($CD4^+$, $CD45RA^+$). The helper/inducer subtype amplifies the immune response and $CD8^+$ cytotoxic cells.[10] The helper/suppressor induces $CD8^+$ suppressor cells.[11] Functionally, $CD4^+$ cells can be divided into TH_1 and TH_2. This functional system was first described in mice. TH_1 cells secrete interleukin-2 (IL-2) and γ-interferon and stimulate $CD8^+$ cytotoxic cells whereas TH_2 cells secrete IL-4, IL-5, and IL-10 and stimulate B-lymphocyte production of antibody.[12] This functional classification of $CD4^+$ T lymphocytes is not as distinct in humans as in mice, but has been well described in several disease states. For example, HIV patients exhibit a shift from normally predominant TH_1 subclass to the TH_2 subclass.[13]

$CD8^+$ suppressor cells down-regulate the immune response once the pathogen has been destroyed. Obviously, continued activation of the immune response may not be beneficial to the host. Down-regulation of autoreactive cells may also occur to prevent autoimmune disease. $CD8^+$ cytotoxic cells are instrumental in killing cells recognized as foreign, such as those that have become infected by a virus. These cells also play an important beneficial role in the eradication of tumor cells, but also are responsible for rejection of transplanted organs. $CD8^+$ T lymphocytes recognize antigen in association with MHC class I.

B lymphocytes recognize antigen via its associated antibody or immunoglobulin located on the surface of the cell. The antibody on the surface can recognize an intact pathogen, such as a bacteria, and present antigen to T lymphocytes (acting as APC). However, the major function of B lymphocytes is to produce antibody to bind to the invading pathogen, a process that first entails activation of the lymphocyte. The activation of B lymphocyte also requires two steps: (1) recognition of antigen by the surface immunoglobulin, and (2) the presence of B-lymphocyte growth factors (IL-4, -5, -6) secreted by activated $CD4^+$ T lymphocytes. Once activated, the B lymphocyte becomes a plasma cell, a differentiated cell capable of producing and secreting large quantities of antibody. A fraction of activated B lymphocytes do not differentiate into plasma cells, but rather form a pool of memory cells. The memory cells will respond to subsequent encounters with the pathogen and allow for a quicker and more vigorous response to the pathogen. Some B lymphocytes can become activated without help from T lymphocytes, but these responses are generally weak and do not invoke memory.

When binding of a specific antigen to the surface immunoglobulin receptor of B lymphocytes occurs, the B lymphocyte matures into a plasma cell and produces large quantities of antibody that have the ability to bind to the inciting antigen. The secreted antibodies may be of five different isotypes. On primary exposure to the pathogen, the plasma cell will secrete IgM, but there is a switch to predominantly IgG during the first exposure. On second exposure the memory B lymphocytes will predominantly produce IgG. Isotype switching from IgM to IgG, IgA, or IgE is controlled by T lymphocytes. Table 79–2 illustrates normal serum concentrations for the five different isotypes.[14]

An antibody or immunoglobulin is a glycoprotein comprised of two different chains, heavy and light (Fig. 79–3). The basic structure of every immunoglobulin consists of four peptide chains: two identical heavy chains and two identical light chains held together by disulfide bonds. The basic structure of the antibody is a Y-shaped figure.

TABLE 79–2. Five Immunoglobulin Classes in Man and Their Characteristics

	IgG	IgA	IgM	IgD	IgE[a]
Serum conc. (mg/dL)	600–1200	140–260	70–120	0.3–30	0.002–0.2
Serum half-life (d)	23	6	5	3	2
Antibacterial lysis	+	+	+++	?	?
Antiviral activity	+	+++	+	?	?
Complement fixation	+	0	++++	0	0
Placental transfer	Yes	No	No	No	No
Location	Serum, amniotic fluid	Serum, colostrum, GI and respiratory tracts, saliva, tears	Serum	Serum, membrane receptor on B lymphocytes	Serum

[a]IgE is involved in allergic response and parasitic infections; also measured in IU/mL with a normal concentration range of 1–150 IU/mL.

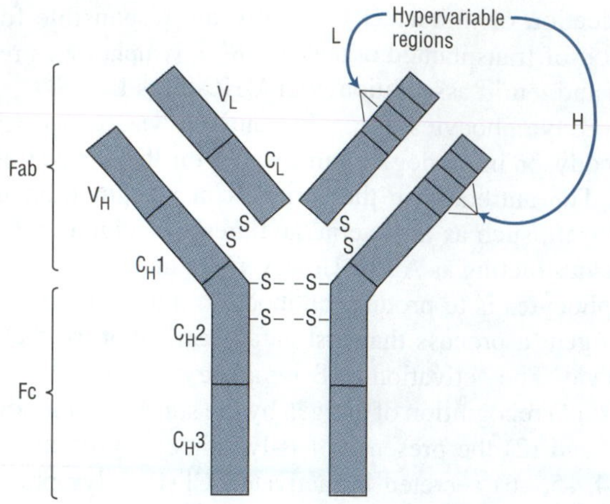

FIGURE 79–3. IgG molecule. Prototype of immunoglobulin molecule showing heavy (H) and light (L) chains, each with common (C) and variable (V) regions, each of which has hypervariable regions. Antigen combines with antibody in the cavity formed by hypervariable ends of H and L chains. These two chains are joined by disulfide bonds (S–S). Light chains consist of one variable (V_L) and one constant (C_L) region whereas heavy chains consist of one variable (V_H) and three or four constant (C_H1 through C_H3) regions, but IgE has an additional C_H4 region. Light chains and V_H and C_H1 make up the Fab region. The COOH ends of the molecules are in the constant regions, and the NH_2 ends of the molecules are in the variable regions. *(Reprinted from Ref. 1, with permission. Copyright 1992 American Medical Association).*

Each arm of the Y is formed by the linkage of the end of the light chain to its heavy-chain partner. These arms contain the portions described as the Fab fragments (fragments of antigen binding). The stem of the Y contains the heavy chains that comprise the Fc (crystallizable fragment) portion of the antibody. It is within the Fc portion that complement is activated once the antibody has bound its target. Likewise, it is the Fc portion of the antibody that is recognized by Fc receptors on the surface of phagocytes (see Fig. 79–1). The amino acid composition of the same isotype is homogeneous except in the variable regions of the light (V_L) and heavy chains (V_H). The variation in amino acid composition of the variable region gives the antibody its unique specificity (see Fig. 79–3).

IgG, the most prevalent of the antibody classes, comprises approximately 80% of serum antibody. IgG is usually the second isotype of antibody to be produced in an initial humoral immune response. IgG is the only isotype of antibody that can cross the placenta. Therefore, maternal humoral protection of neonates is primarily owing to maternal IgG that has crossed the placenta in utero.

Four different subclasses of IgG have been described: IgG_1, IgG_2, IgG_3, and IgG_4. These subclasses differ slightly in their constant amino acid sequences. IgG_1 constitutes the majority (60%) of the subclasses. It appears that different subclasses recognize different types of antigen. IgG_1 and IgG_3 are principally responsible for recognition of protein antigens whereas IgG_2 and IgG_4 commonly bind to carbohydrate antigens.[15] Other differences in the subclasses are the ability to activate complement, with IgG_3 and IgG_1 being the most efficient and IgG_4 unable to activate complement.

IgM can be found on the surface of B lymphocytes as a monomeric Y-shaped structure. IgM, secreted from plasma cells, is a pentamer in which five of the monomers are joined by a joining chain (J chain). IgM is the first class of antibody to be produced on initial exposure to an antigen. Because the pentameric form of IgM has no Fc portions exposed, phagocytic cells cannot bind pathogens opsonized by IgM. However, IgM is an excellent activator of the complement cascade (classic pathway).

IgA is found primarily in the fluid secretions of the body–tears, saliva, nasal fluids–and also in the gastrointestinal and respiratory tract. IgA functions by preventing pathogens from adhering to and infecting the epithelial cells at these sites. IgA is also secreted in a nursing mother's breast milk as well as are IgG and IgM in lower concentrations. In bodily secretions, IgA is in a dimeric form in which two monomers are held together by a J chain and secretory chain.

IgD is the least understood isotype. IgD is found on the surface of B lymphocytes at different stages of maturation and may be involved in the differentiation of these cells. The main function of IgD has not yet been determined.

IgE is the least common of the serum antibody isotypes. Most of the IgE in the body is bound to the IgE Fc receptors on mast cells. When antigen is bound by the IgE on the surface of mast cells, it causes the release of various inflammatory substances from the mast cell. The overall effect is the stimulation of inflammation. Asthma and hay fever are a few examples of allergic reactions primarily caused by antigen binding to IgE.[16]

Natural killer (NK) cells, often referred to as large granular lymphocytes, are the third type of lymphocyte. NK cells do not express on their surface specific receptors like the TCR on T lymphocytes and are not restricted by MHC, but they do express Fc receptors for IgG. NK cells were originally described and named because of their ability to lyse tumor cells without prior sensitization. Upon exposure to IL-2, NK cells exhibit greater cytotoxic activity against a wide variety of tumors. The majority of lymphokine-activated killer (LAK) cells used to treat melanoma and renal cell carcinoma are NK cells. NK cells play important roles in surveillance against tumors and virally infected host cells, and in the regulation of hematopoiesis.[17]

MAJOR HISTOCOMPATIBILITY COMPLEX

The MHC, an association of genes found on chromosome 6 in humans, is also known as the HLA complex. The genes from this complex encode for molecules that play a pivotal role in immune recognition and response. The MHC is divided into three different classes: I, II, and III. The molecules encoded by class I HLA genes include HLA-A, HLA-B, and HLA-C antigens. These molecules can be found on all nucleated cells within the body as well as on platelets. Class I antigens are not found on mature red blood cells. Molecules encoded by class II HLA genes include HLA-DP, HLA-DQ, and HLA-DR molecules. The expression of these molecules is more restricted and can be found primarily on antigen-presenting cells such as macrophages and B lymphocytes. The class III HLA antigens encode for soluble factors, complement, and tumor necrosis factors.

For a $CD4^+$ T lymphocyte to become activated, the $CD4^+$ T lymphocyte must recognize the antigenic peptide in association with MHC class II (see Fig. 79–2). $CD8^+$ T lymphocytes recognize antigenic peptide in association with class I molecules. Class I molecules generally contain endogenous peptides from within the cell such as viruses, whereas class II molecules contain exogenous peptides from antigen that has been phagocytosized, such as bacteria (see Fig. 79–2). For it to destroy a virally infected cell, a $CD8^+$ cytotoxic T lymphocyte requires two steps. First, its TCR must recognize the antigenic fragment such as a viral protein in association with MHC class I. The second step involves the costimulatory step of B7-CD28 binding. Because any cell can become infected, it is advantageous that

TABLE 79–3. Cytokines

Cytokines	Sources	Principal Effects
Regulatory		
IL-1	Macrophages	Activation of T and B lymphocytes, hematopoietic growth factor
IL-2	$CD4^+$ T lymphs	Activation of T lymphs, B lymphs, and NK cells
IL-4	$CD4^+$ T lymphs, mast cells	Induce TH_2 cells, B and T lymph growth factor, activation of macrophages, promotes IgE production, proliferation of bone marrow precursors
IL-5	$CD4^+$ T lymphs, mast cells	Activation of B lymphs and eosinophils, promotes IgE production
IL-6	$CD4^+$ T lymphs, macrophages, mast cells, fibroblasts	T and B lymph growth factor, hematopoietic growth factor, augments inflammation
IL-8	T lymphs, monocytes, endothelial cells, fibroblasts	Neutrophil and T lymph chemotaxis
IL-10	T and B lymphs, macrophages	Cytokine synthesis inhibitory factor, growth of mast cells
IL-12	Macrophages, neutrophils dendritic and Langerhans' cells	Induce TH_1 cells, ⇑ NK cell activity, ⇑ generation of cytotoxic T lymphs
IL-13	Activated T lymphs	Proliferation of B lymphs, suppression of proinflammatory cytokines, directs IgE isotype switching
IL-14	T lymphs	Induces B-lymph proliferation, inhibits secretion of Igs
IL-15	Macrophages, fibroblasts, epithelial cells	T-lymph proliferation
IL-16	$CD8^+$ T lymphs, epithelial cells	Chemoattractant for $CD4^+$ T lymphs and eosinophils; stimulation of secondary cytokine secretion from and proliferation of $CD4^+$ T lymphs
TNF-α	Macrophages, T lymphs	Activation of neutrophils, endothelial cells, lymphs, and liver cells to produce acute phase proteins
TNF-β	T lymphs	Tumoricidal
IFN-α	Monocytes, other cells	Antiviral, activation of NK cells and macrophages, up-regulation of MHC class I
IFN-γ	T lymphs, NK cells	Activation of macrophages, NK cells; up-regulation of MHC classes I and II
Hematopoietic Growth Factors		
IL-3	T lymphs	Maturation and differentiation of hematopoietic and mast cells
IL-7	BM stromal cells	Lymphopoietin
IL-9	T lymphs	Maturation and proliferation of T lymphs and mast cells
IL-11	BM stromal cells	Maturation of B lymphs and megakaryocytes
G-CSF	Macrophages, endothelial cells, fibroblasts	Maturation and activation of neutrophils
GM-CSF	T lymphs, macrophages, endothelial cells, fibroblasts	Maturation and activation of granulocytes and monocytes/macrophages and eosinophils
M-CSF	Macrophages, endothelial cells, fibroblasts	Maturation and activation of monocytes/macrophages
Erythropoietin	Kidney, liver	Maturation of RBCs
Stem cell factor	BM stromal cells, hepatocytes	Activation of mast cells, early acting growth factor for myeloid and lymphoid precursors
c-MPL ligand	BM stromal cells, liver, kidney	Lineage-specific growth factor for megakaryocytes (platelets)
FLT3 ligand	BM stromal cells	Early-acting growth factor, dendritic cells

Lymphs = lymphocytes; BM = bone marrow.

the $CD8^+$ cytotoxic T lymphocyte recognize the MHC class I molecule, which is expressed on all cells except red blood cells. The ability of the MHC class I to present endogenous peptides allows the $CD8^+$ cytotoxic T lymphocytes to constantly screen cells for infections.[6]

CYTOKINES

Research has shown that many of these cytokines have a broad spectrum of effects dependent on their concentration, the presence of other factors, and the target cell. Cytokines orchestrate the complex homeostasis of cells and tissues by acting in both an autocrine and paracrine fashion. For example, activated $CD4^+$ T lymphocytes secrete IL-2 to activate itself as well as $CD8^+$ T lymphocytes and NK cells. Cytokines, soluble factors released or secreted by cells, affect the activity of other cells or the secreting cell itself. Cytokines can also be membrane bound (e.g., IL-1α) and require direct cell-to-cell contact. It is also important to remember that *in vivo* cytokines do not act alone but in combination with other cytokines. For example, activated $CD4^+$ T lymphocytes secrete both IL-2 and interferon-γ, which are synergistic in activating NK cells. As shown in Table 79–3, cytokines are broadly classified as regulatory or hematopoietic growth factors.[18–23] It should be remembered that this classification does not describe all their activities. Granulocyte-macrophage colony stimulating factor (GM-CSF) released by activated T lymphocytes acts as a hematopoietic growth factor, but also activates granulocytes and macrophages to phagocytize foreign pathogens.

The division of the immune system into the two functional groups does not imply that the divisions do not interact. To generate a vigorous immune response, both soluble mediators (complement, antibody, and cytokines) and cells (neutrophils, macrophages, T lymphocytes, and B lymphocytes) are needed. Generally, the innate system will respond first. Macrophages and neutrophils in the tissues will recognize the opsonized pathogen (see Fig. 79–1). To amplify the immune response, the macrophages will present antigen to $CD4^+$ T lymphocytes (see Fig. 79–2). The activated $CD4^+$ T lymphocytes will then secrete cytokines to activate B lymphocytes, $CD8^+$ T lymphocytes, NK cells, macrophages, and neutrophils. The next section of the chapter will look at evaluating the immune system.

EVALUATION OF COMPONENTS OF THE IMMUNE SYSTEM

Assessment of a patient's immune function requires consideration of multiple components, including mechanical defenses, cell phenotypes and numbers, and soluble components. Recent developments in biotechnology have allowed extraordinary progress in characterization of immune function. Despite technological advances, careful patient evaluations are required to properly identify patients with compromised immune systems. Specific methods for assessment of patient immune status are discussed below.

TABLE 79–4. Examples of Alteration in Mechanical Immunodefenses That Result in Impaired Immune Status

Reduced gastric pH
Achlorhydria
Use of histamine$_2$ blockers and proton pump inhibitors
Patients with acquired immunodeficiency syndrome (AIDS)
Break in skin barrier
Burns
Surgical incision
Penetrating trauma
Vascular access devices
Impaired mucociliary function of the lungs
Smoking
Impaired esophageal or epiglottal function
Endotracheal intubation
Stroke
Recumbent position
Altered urine flow
Urinary stones
Anatomic deformities obstructing flow
Bladder catheter
Anatomic alterations of the heart resulting in turbulent blood flow and endocarditis

MECHANICAL AND NONSPECIFIC IMMUNODEFENSES

As discussed earlier, the mechanical aspects of host defense are extremely important in protection from infection; therefore, assessment of mechanical defenses is critical. Much of the assessment of mechanical immunodefense is accomplished by recognition of situations in which it is compromised. Careful patient examination usually reveals the extent of compromise, and laboratory tests are generally not necessary for evaluation of this component. To evaluate the extent of compromise in mechanical immunodefenses, the clinician should carefully examine the patient and identify the specific types of risks present. Specific examples of altered mechanical defenses are listed in Table 79–4.

CELLULAR ASPECTS OF IMMUNE FUNCTION

A major aspect of the assessment of immune function relates to the cells of the immune system. Assessment of cells in the clinical setting includes determination of cell number, cell type, and/or function. Generally, quantification of the cell types and numbers is performed first because of its rapid turnaround and correlation with clinical picture.

QUANTIFICATION

To quickly screen cell numbers, a white blood count (WBC) with differential is performed. Normal cell counts are shown in Table 79–5.[24,25] This test often steers the differential diagnosis. In interpreting a WBC with differential, several factors must be considered. A normal cell count does not mean that a leukocyte disorder does not exist. For example, in

TABLE 79–5. Leukocytes in Adults

Cell	Absolute count[a] (range)	Percent (range)
White blood cell	7.5 (4.5–11.0)	100
Neutrophils	4.5 (2.3–7.7)	60 (50–70)
Eosinophils	0.2 (0.0–0.45)	3 (0–5)
Basophils	0.04 (0.0–0.2)	1 (0–2)
Monocytes	0.3 (0.0–0.8)	4 (0–10)
Lymphocytes	2.1 (1.6–2.4)	32 (28–39)
T lymphocytes	1.4 (1.1–1.7)	72 (67–76)[b]
$CD4^+$ cells	0.8 (0.7–1.1)	42 (38–46)[b]
$CD8^+$ cells	0.7 (0.5–0.9)	35 (31–40)[b]
B lymphocytes	0.3 (0.2–0.4)	13 (11–16)[b]
NK cells[c]	0.3 (0.2–0.4)	14 (10–19)[b]
CD4:CD8 ratio	1.2 (1.0–1.5)	

[a]$\times 10^3$ cells/mm^3.
[b]Percent of lymphocyte subpopulations expressed as percentage of total lymphocyte population.
[c]NK = natural killer.

chronic granulomatous disease, a child has a normal neutrophil count, but the neutrophils are unable to destroy the bacteria. Second, a differential comes back as percentage of the WBC; therefore, one must assess the absolute number as well as the percentage of white cell subtypes. For example, a patient admitted to the hospital with pneumonia has an elevated WBC (15.0×10^3 cells/mm^3), which is predominantly neutrophils (segs + bands = 80%). The percentage of lymphocytes appears low at 15%, but the absolute number of lymphocytes is actually normal (2250 cells/mm^3). A third factor to consider is that the majority of lymphocytes are in secondary lymphoid organs (e.g., lymph nodes, spleen), and changes in peripheral blood lymphocytes do not mirror changes in the secondary lymphoid organs.[26] Additionally, the majority of granulocytes, macrophages, and mast cells are in the tissues, not the bloodstream.

Generally, the numbers of granulocytes (neutrophils, basophils, eosinophils) and monocytes are assessed by a WBC with differential. It long has been recognized that the lower the absolute neutrophil count, the greater the risk of infection. Drugs (e.g., chemotherapy) and diseases (e.g., collagen vascular disorders) may lower the neutrophil count and make the patient more susceptible to infections. Patients with a neutrophil count below 1500 cells/mm^3 are considered to have neutropenia. Functional analysis of these cell types is rarely done in routine clinical practice. Patients with functional deficits in these cell types are generally referred to tertiary medical centers for evaluation and treatment.

A count of lymphocytes may be performed for overall number by a routine WBC with differential. Total lymphocyte count has been used as a measure of nutritional status, because this rapidly changes with nutrient loss or repletion. This is a relatively gross measure of a patient's immune status, although it has been correlated to patient outcome and risk of infection. Quantification of specific lymphocyte subsets is also important in some situations.

The availability of monoclonal antibodies against lymphocyte cell surface markers (CDs) and the invention of flow cytometry have allowed specific quantification of lymphocyte subsets. These evaluations are valuable for assessment of patients with immune deficiency states such as AIDS or leukemias, and for patients who have received organ transplants. They allow the detection of specific lymphocyte subsets such as $CD4^+$ and $CD8^+$ T lymphocytes. Quantification of $CD3^+$ and $CD4^+$ cells is used to monitor OKT3 immunosuppression and in the clinical management of AIDS patients, respectively.

The principle underlying the determination of lymphocyte subsets is a characteristic cell surface marker (cluster designation or CD) that distinguishes one subset from another. The CD is usually a protein or glycoprotein on the surface of the cell. Cells can be detected by monoclonal antibodies that bind to the specific CDs such as CD4 or CD8. The monoclonal antibodies have been bound to substances such as fluorescein or phycoerythrin dyes, which fluoresce green or red, respectively, when exposed to light of a certain wavelength. This fluorescence then allows detection and enumeration of the lymphocyte subsets by a flow cytometer. The flow cytometer analyzes individual cells to determine their fluorescence (presence or absence of surface-bound antibody) as well as light scatter (to determine cell size). Flow cytometry can be used for leukocyte phenotyping and tumor cell phenotyping, as well as for some types of DNA analysis. Some of the most common CD antigens and their respective cellular distribution are listed in Table 79–6.[27]

FUNCTIONAL EVALUATION OF THE IMMUNE RESPONSE

IN VIVO

The most common *in vivo* assay of lymphocyte function is the delayed hypersensitivity skin test. This test specifically

TABLE 79–6. Cluster of Differentiation (CD) Guide: Characterization of Human Leukocyte Antigens

CD	Predominant Cellular Distribution
CD1	Thymocytes, Langerhans' cells
CD3	T lymphocytes
CD4	Helper T lymphocytes, monocytes, macrophages
CD5	T lymphocytes, B-lymphocyte subset
CD8	Cytotoxic/suppressor T lymphocytes, NK cells
CD14	Monocytes, neutrophils
CD19	B lymphocytes
CD25	Activated T lymphocytes, B lymphocytes; IL-2 receptor α chain (Tac)
CD29	$CD4^+$ T-lymphocyte subset (helper/inducer)
CD34	Lymphoid and myeloid precursors (stem cell)
CD45RA	$CD4^+$ T-lymphocyte subset (helper/suppressor), B lymphocytes, NK cells
CD56	NK cells

NK = natural killer.

evaluates the presence of delayed-type hypersensitivity or memory T lymphocytes. By injecting a small amount of test material (antigen to which the patient has previously been exposed) into the patient's skin, one can make a visual assessment of the patient's ability to react to the antigen.

When an antigen to which a normal patient has previously been exposed is injected into the skin, the area of the injection becomes infiltrated with lymphocytes within a few hours. In the next stage, additional lymphocytes and phagocytes (macrophages, neutrophils) infiltrate. The maximal intensity of the inflammatory reaction is 24 to 72 hours. This reaction is often referred to as type IV hypersensitivity (cell mediated; Chap. 81). In type I hypersensitivity, a positive skin reaction is evident usually within 15 minutes and always within 24 hours. Type I hypersensitivity involves the release of histamine from basophils and mast cells when antigen binds to the IgE on the surface of these cells.

There are a number of reasons that a patient will not react to an antigen injected intradermally. Most commonly, the patient may not have had a previous exposure to the antigen. Nonresponsiveness may occur from anergy (dysfunction of cell-mediated immunity) owing to immunosuppression from drugs (corticosteroids, cyclosporine) or disease (AIDS, cancer). A small subset of patients may be genetically unresponsive to the antigen.

A delayed hypersensitivity skin test can be performed by two methods. In one method, the patient can be administered a dose of antigen at a time sufficiently preceding the skin test so that the immune response can develop. Then the skin test with the same antigen is applied and the extent of reactivity measured. The most common method is to administer a panel of five or six recall antigens. The most common antigens are Candida, coccidiodin, mumps, Trichophyton, and purified protein derivative of tuberculin (PPD). More than 90% of the population will show a positive reaction to two or more of these antigens. After injection of the recall antigens, the patient should be carefully observed for the occurrence of immediate reactions. Measurements in millimeters of induration and erythema at the site of injection should be taken 24, 48, and 72 hours after injection. A reaction is considered positive if the diameter of induration and erythema is 5 mm or greater. Reaction to even a single antigen indicates a functioning cell-mediated immunity. The degree of sensitivity relates to the area of induration.[27]

The accepted indications for delayed hypersensitivity skin testing include evaluation of immune disorders and chronic diseases that cause cellular immune dysfunction (e.g., uremia, cancer, AIDS), exposure to infectious pathogens (e.g., *Mycobacterium tuberculosis*), evaluation of nutritional status because malnutrition can result in cellular immune deficit, and, in some cases, assessment of immune senescence.

In vivo assessment of B-lymphocyte function involves immunizing the patient with a protein (e.g., tetanus toxoid) and a polysaccharide (e.g., Pneumovax) antigen to quantitate antibody response after immunization. After 2 to 3 weeks, the patient's serum is tested for antibodies specific for the immunized antigen. This test measures B-lymphocyte responsiveness to the inoculated antigens. It is used to evaluate responsiveness to a vaccine but is reserved for patients who are suspected to have impaired B-lymphocyte function.[27]

IN VITRO

There are a number of specific lymphocyte functional assays, but most of these assays are used in the research setting. Many of these assays are performed at most tertiary-care medical centers. One of these tests is the lymphocyte proliferation assay. In this assay, lymphocytes are obtained from a patient's peripheral blood and cultured *in vitro*. The cells are exposed to nonspecific mitogen such as pokeweed mitogen, phytohemagglutin, or concanavalin A. Then the cells are incubated in growth media containing tritium-labeled (^{3}H) thymidine (a DNA precursor). In the presence of the mitogens, normal lymphocytes will be stimulated to proliferate. Proliferation results in incorporation of ^{3}H thymidine, which can be measured on a β-scintillation counter. The patient sample would be compared to normal, healthy controls. Patients with immune deficiencies (AIDS, cancer) have fewer active or less-active lymphocytes, as detected by this test.

A modification of the lymphocyte proliferation assay is used in allogeneic bone marrow transplantation to evaluate how closely a donor and host are matched, to predict a patient's risk for graft-versus-host disease. A mixed lymphocyte culture (MLC) assesses the potential of the donor cells to attack the host cells: graft-versus-host disease (Chap. 125). In this test, donor cells and host cells are incubated *in vitro*. The host lymphocytes are irradiated prior to the incubation so that they cannot proliferate. *In vitro,* ^{3}H thymidine is provided to the cells and uptake is measured. The degree of uptake is related to proliferation of donor lymphocytes. If the cells are well matched, proliferation is minimal. If the cells are mismatched, proliferation will be noted with the level of proliferation predictive of the potential extent of graft-versus-host disease.

In addition to the test described above, a number of other tests have been devised to evaluate the function of $CD8^+$ T lymphocytes, natural killer cells, and monocytes/macrophages. Although these evaluations are not commonly performed, they may be helpful in some specific diseases. A thorough discussion of these tests is available.[28]

HUMORAL ASPECTS OF IMMUNE FUNCTION

The humoral components of the immune system (immunoglobulins, complement, cytokines) are often assessed. Assays of humoral components may be either quantitative to determine the absolute concentration of the factor or qualitative to determine the function of the component.

IMMUNOGLOBULINS

The most common evaluation of immunoglobulins is the estimation of total immunoglobulin concentration. This is obtained by subtracting the albumin concentration from the total protein concentration. This difference gives a gross estimation of the total immunoglobulin concentration. Actual determination of the total immunoglobulin concentration is done by serum protein electrophoresis (SPEP). Five separate zones are detected by this method, albumin, α_1-globulin, α_2-globulin, β-globulin, and γ-globulin. The γ-globulin fraction contains the five isotypes of immunoglobulin (IgG, IgA, IgM, IgE, IgD). A normal total immunoglobulin or γ-globulin concentration ranges from 0.8 to 1.6 g/dL. This test is used to determine if patients have hypogammaglobulinemia (primary and secondary immunodeficiencies), a monoclonal peak (multiple myeloma, Waldenstrom's macroglobulinemia), or a polyclonal hypergammaglobulinemia (chronic inflammatory conditions such as systemic lupus erythematosus and chronic active hepatitis). Total immunoglobulin or γ-globulin concentrations cannot measure antigen-specific antibodies or specific isotypes.

In a patient suspected of having humoral immune deficiency or B-lymphocyte failure (primary and secondary immunodeficiency), specific immunoglobulin isotypes in the plasma should be measured. These are usually determined by radial immunodiffusion or byrate nephelometry. Refer to Table 79–2 for the normal concentrations of different isotypes.

There are many indications for the measurement of antigen-specific antibody. Some common indications are listed in Table 79–7. The most common methods to perform these measurements include enzyme-linked immunosorbent assay (ELISA), radioimmunoassay (RIA), Western blot, and radioallergosorbent test (RAST). The most common reason to measure antigen-specific antibody is to determine whether a patient has been exposed to an infectious agent. Generally, IgM antibodies directed against the pathogen indicates an active infection whereas IgG antibodies directed against the pathogen indicates prior exposure. For example, in hepatitis A and cytomegalovirus infections, the presence of the IgM antibody against the virus supports the diagnosis of an active infection whereas the presence of the IgG antibody signifies immunity to the virus. Initially, plasma cells produce IgM in response to an infection, but memory B lymphocytes produce IgG. Therefore, IgG concentrations will go up in a second exposure, but IgM antibodies will be present during an active infection and shortly after recovery from the infection. Other uses of antigen-specific antibody include determining if a patient has had exposure and is likely to be protected from further infection (e.g., rubella virus) or indicating adequate response to vaccination (e.g., hepatitis B).

Antigen-specific IgE is commonly measured in patients with allergies. Because the presence of antigen-specific IgE is related to clinical allergy, measurement of these antibodies can be helpful in diagnosing allergies and determining offending substances. A standard method for determination of allergen-specific IgE is the RAST. The basic technique involves adding the antigen of interest, which is bound to beads or disks, to the patient's serum *in vitro*. After precipitation and several washings, the antibody bound to the bead or disk is isolated. Finally, a radiolabeled antibody that binds to IgE is added. After further washings, the radiolabeled antibody bound to IgE that is bound to the antigen on the bead or disk is counted on a γ counter.

TABLE 79–7. Potential Indications for Measurement of Antigen-Specific Antibody

Environmental or drug allergy
Exposure to or infection with bacteria
Streptococci (ASO titer)
Staphylococcus aureus (teichoic acid antibody)
Neisseria gonorrhoeae
Legionella pneumophila
Exposure to or infection with viruses
Human immunodeficiency virus
Cytomegalovirus
Epstein-Barr virus
Hepatitis A, B, or C
Rubella
Exposure to or infection with other pathogens
Syphilis
Lyme disease
Typhoid
Chlamydia
Immune disorders
Rheumatoid factor antibody—rheumatoid arthritis
Anti-nuclear antibodies—systemic lupus erythematosus
Platelet-associated IgG—idiopathic thrombocytopenia
Blood typing and cross-matching
Transplantation
HLA antibodies

Antigen skin testing is the preferred method to determine the presence of allergen-specific IgE. When it is produced, IgE binds to high-affinity IgE Fc receptors on basophils or mast cells. Contact of an allergen with the specific IgE on the basophil or mast cell surface causes activation of these cells and the release of inflammatory mediators (e.g., histamine). When this occurs systemically, it can cause anaphylaxis. When it occurs in a confined area such as the skin, erythema and induration are observed within a few minutes of allergen injection. This is the principle used for detection of penicillin allergy as well as for environmental or food allergies. A positive skin reaction (5 mm or greater of induration) within 15 to 20 minutes is indicative of the presence of allergen-specific IgE.

IgG SUBCLASSES

There are four subclasses of IgG: IgG_1, IgG_2, IgG_3, and IgG_4. They make up 65%, 20%, 10%, and 5% of total plasma IgG, respectively. Concentrations of the subclasses are often measured in patients with primary and secondary immunodeficiencies. IgG_2 and IgG_4 deficiencies are associated with chronic infections. IgG_4 deficiencies are also associated with autoimmune disorders. Measurement of the subclasses can be performed by ELISA.

COMPLEMENT SYSTEM

The complement system consists of a group of over 20 different plasma proteins involved in lysing and opsonizing invading pathogens as well as serving as chemotactic factors. The various proteins of the complement system are named by numbers following the letter C (C1, C2, etc.). A global assessment of the complement system is the CH_{50}. The CH_{50} (total hemolytic complement test) measures the ability of the patient's entire classic complement system to lyse sheep red blood cells opsonized with antibody. This test does not provide an indication of the function of any specific complement component but is used as a screening test for any complement system defects. If a defect is found, individual complement proteins can then be evaluated by functional or immunochemical methods. Assessment of the complement system is important in patients suspected of having humoral immune deficiencies (i.e., recurrent infections).

Several disease states can alter complement concentrations. Systemic lupus erythematosus, rheumatoid arthritis with vasculitis, poststreptococcal glomerulonephritis, gram-negative infections, and subacute bacterial endocarditis are associated with a decrease in CH_{50} assay and various components of the complement system. The liver is the primary source of several components of the complement system (C2, C3, C4, factors B and D); therefore in liver failure, a decrease in complement levels is observed. Inherited complement deficiencies have been described in patients with systemic lupus erythematosus, recurrent gonococcal and meningococcal infections, Raynaud's phenomenon, and hereditary angioedema.[27]

CYTOKINES

Scientists have identified and cloned many of the various natural cytokines within the body that are responsible for altering immune function. Methods to detect levels of these cytokines within the blood have been developed. For nearly all the currently identified cytokines, commercial kits are available to measure endogenous and exogenously administered cytokines. Most of the commercial cytokine measurements are done by ELISA or RIA. ELISAs and RIAs are easy to run but measure immunoactivity, not biologic activity. Bioassays measure biologic activity, but are cumbersome and extremely variable. Therefore, most researchers prefer ELISAs and RIAs.[29,30]

We are still at the very early stages of interpreting the clinical relevance of endogenous cytokine concentrations. Not only is the immune system affected by cytokines such as IL-1, IL-6, and TNF-α, but other systems (skeletal, endocrine, central nervous system) also are affected. Measurement of cytokine concentrations may be important in the evaluation of the immune system as well as of other systems.

When we administer cytokines in therapeutic trials, we may change not only the concentration of that particular cytokine, but also the concentration of other cytokines. Several studies have demonstrated that the systemic administration of GM-CSF to patients increases concentrations not only of GM-CSF but also of TNF-α, IL-6, macrophage colony-stimulating factor, and erythropoietin.[31,32] Secondary endogenous cytokine release should be taken into account when monitoring cytokine concentrations.

In the future, tissue concentrations as well as blood concentrations may be measured. For example, although many centers currently measure cyclosporine concentrations to estimate the potential for immunosuppressive effects, it may be more advantageous to monitor IL-2 concentrations. One of the primary actions of cyclosporine is the inhibition of IL-2 production. Furthermore, perhaps it would be beneficial to measure tissue concentrations of IL-2 in the transplanted organ to get a better estimate of the state of immunologic suppression.

SOLUBLE RECEPTORS AND RECEPTOR ANTAGONISTS

Two types of cytokine inhibitors have been described: (1) receptor-binding antagonists and (2) cytokine-binding inhibitors. The best characterized receptor-binding antagonist is the interleukin-1 receptor antagonist (IL-1RA), which inhibits binding of IL-1 to its receptor by competing for the same binding site.[33,34]

Cytokine-binding inhibitors bind the cytokine before it is able to reach its target receptor. The cytokine-binding proteins may act to inhibit the cytokine's activity by preventing the cytokine from binding to its receptor, or the cytokine-binding protein may also serve as binding proteins that protect the cytokine from degradation.[33] The best characterized cytokine-binding inhibitors are soluble cytokine receptors. Several soluble cytokine receptors have been described both *in vitro* and *in vivo:* soluble IL-2 receptor (sIL-2R), sIL-4R, sIL-6R, sIL-7R, sIFN-γR, and sTNFR. The best characterized soluble cytokine receptor is the sIL-2R. Although patients with normal immune systems have relatively low concentrations of sIL-2R, it has been demonstrated that patients with a wide variety of diseases exhibit an increase in sIL-2R concentrations. This may reflect an increase in the activity of the immune system. Because sIL-2R has the ability to bind free IL-2, it has been postulated that IL-2R is shed from the surface of cells to down-regulate the immune response. In hairy cell leukemia, the neoplastic cells secrete sIL-2R, and sIL-2R concentrations correlate with tumor burden. A reduction in sIL-2R closely parallels the clinical response of leukemia to α-interferon therapy. Relapse is preceded by a rise in the sIL-2R concentrations.[35] sIL-2R concentrations have also been correlated with rejection of transplanted organs.[36] Our better understanding of soluble receptors and receptor antagonists may allow us to mimic natural mechanisms for minimizing the toxicity of administering cytokines (e.g., IL-1, IL-2,

TNF-α) as well as immunomodulation of various diseases (solid organ transplant rejection, collagen vascular disorders, sepsis, etc).

CONCLUSION

Our understanding of the immune system has dramatically increased over the past decade. An immune response encompasses dynamic events involving both immunologic cells (phagocytes, lymphocytes, etc.) and soluble mediators (complement, cytokines, antibodies, etc.). A better understanding of the normal immune response allows us to investigate the pathophysiology of diseases for which the immune response is inappropriate. All clinicians need a basic understanding of the immune system and familiarity with parameters to monitor immune system function to refine the development of immunologic treatments for diseases ranging from diabetes mellitus to collagen vascular disorders to cancer.

REFERENCES

1. Claman HN. The biology of the immune response. JAMA 1992;268: 2790–2796.
2. Male D, Roitt I. Introduction to the immune system. In: Roitt I, Brostoff, Male D, eds. Immunology. London, Mosby, 1998:1–12.
3. Lehrer RI, Ganz T, Selsted ME, Babior BM, Curnutte JT. Neutrophils and host defense. Ann Intern Med 1988;109:127–142.
4. Weller PF. The immunobiology of eosinophils. N Engl J Med 1991; 324:1110–1118.
5. Selijelid R, Eskeland T. The biology of macrophages. Eur J Haematol 1993;51:267–275.
6. Restifo NP. Antigen processing and presentation: An update. In: DeVita VT, Hellman S, Rosenberg SA, eds. Biologic Therapy of Cancer Updates, Vol 2. Philadelphia, Lippincott, 1992:1–10.
7. Galli SJ. New concepts about the mast cell. N Engl J Med 1993;328: 257–265.
8. Johnston RB. The complement system in host defense and inflammation: The cutting edges of a double edged sword. Pediatr Infect Dis J 1993;12:933–941.
9. Reiser H, Stadecker MJ. Costimulatory B7 molecules in the pathogenesis of infectious and autoimmune diseases. N Engl J Med 1996; 335:1369–1377.
10. Morimoto C, Letvin NL, Boyd W, et al. The isolation and characterization of human helper inducer T cell subset. J Immunol 1985;134: 3762–3769.
11. Morimoto C, Letvin NL, Distaso JA, Aldrich WR, Schlosssman SF. The isolation and characterization of human suppressor inducer T cell subset. J Immunol 1985;134:1508–1515.
12. Romagnani S. Human TH_1 and TH_2 subsets: Regulation of differentiation and role in protection and immunopathology. Int Arch Allergy Immunol 1992;98:279–285.
13. Clerici M, Hakim F, Venzon DJ, et al. Changes in interleukin-2 and interleukin-4 production in asymptomatic, human immunodeficiency virus-seropositive individuals. J Clin Invest 1993;91:759–765.
14. Feldmann M. Cell cooperation in the antibody response. In: Roitt I, Brostoff, Male D, eds. Immunology. London, Mosby, 1998:139–150.
15. Heiner DC. IgG subclass composition of intravenous immunoglobulin preparations: Clinical relevance. Rev Infect Dis 1986;8(suppl 4): S391–S395.
16. Goodman JW. Immunoglobulin structure & function. In: Stites DP, Terr AI, eds. Basic and Clinical Immunology. East Norwalk, CT, Appleton & Lange, 1991:109–121.
17. Robertson MJ, Ritz J. Biology and clinical relevance of human natural killer cells. Blood 1990;76:2421–2438.
18. Basic components. In: Chapel H, Haeney M, eds. Essentials of Clinical Immunology. London, Blackwell Scientific, 1993:1–32.
19. Oppenheim JJ, Ruscetti FW, Faltynek C. Cytokines. In: Stites DP, Terr A, eds. Basic and Clinical Immunology. Norwalk, CT, Appleton & Lange, 1991:78–100.
20. Du XX, Williams DA. Interleukin-11: A multifunctional growth factor derived from the hematopoietic microenvironment. Blood 1994;83: 2023–2030.
21. Zurawski G, de Vries JE. Interleukin 13, an interleukin 4-like cytokine that acts on monocytes and B cells, but not on T-cells. Immunol Today 1994;15:19–26.
22. Trinchieri G. Function and clinical use of interleukin-12. Curr Opinion Hematol 1997;4:59–66.
23. Kennedy MK, Park LS. Characterization of interleukin-15 (IL-15) and the IL-15 receptor complex. J Clin Immunol 1996;16:134–143.
24. Hannet I, Erkeller-Yuksel F, Lydyard P, Deneys V, DeBruyere M. Developmental and maturational changes in human blood lymphocyte subpopulations. Immunol Today 1992;13:215–218.
25. Bakerman S. White blood count and differential. In: Bakerman S, ed. ABC's of Interpretive Laboratory Data. Greenville, NC, Interpretive Laboratory Data, 1984:444–447.
26. Westermann J, Pabst R. Lymphocyte subsets in the blood: A diagnostic window on the lymphoid system? Immunol Today 1990;11: 406–410
27. Lopez M, Gleisher T, deShazo RD. Use and interpretation of diagnostic immunologic laboratory tests. JAMA 1992;268:2970–2990.
28. Rose NR, Friedman H, Fahey JL, eds. Manual of Clinical Laboratory Immunology, 3rd ed. Washington, DC, American Society of Microbiology, 1986:43–46.
29. Van Brunt J. Assaying cytokines. Biotechnology 1991;9:439–441.
30. Rabinowitz J, Petros WP, Peters WP. Cytokine kinetics: Clinical pharmacology studies complementing recombinant growth factor trials. Cancer Bull 1994;46:40–47.
31. Rabinowitz J, Petros WP, Stuart A, Peters WP. Characterization of endogenous cytokine concentrations after high-dose chemotherapy with autologous bone marrow support. Blood 1993;81:2452–2459.
32. Stehle B, Weiss C, Ho A, Hunstein W. Serum levels of tumor necrosis factor alpha in patients treated with granulocyte-macrophage colony stimulating factor. Blood 1990;75:1895–1896.
33. Heaney ML, Golde DW. Soluble cytokine receptors. Blood 1996;87: 847–857.
34. Larrick JW, Wright SC. Native cytokine antagonists. Baillieres Clin Haematol 1992;5:681–702.
35. Ho AD, Grossman M, Knauf W, et al. Plasma levels of soluble CD8 antigen and interleukin-2 receptor antigen in patients with hairy cell leukemia, relationship with splenectomy and with clinical response to therapy. Leukemia 1989;3:718–723.
36. Lawrence EC, Holland VA, Young JB, et al. Dynamic changes in soluble interleukin-2 receptor levels after lung and heart-lung transplantation. Am Rev Respir Dis 1989;140:789-796.
37. Hall PD. Immunomodulation with intravenous immunoglobulin. Pharmacotherapy 1993;13:564–573.

80

Systemic Lupus Erythematosus and Other Collagen Vascular Diseases

Mark B. Burlingame, PharmD, BCPS, and Jeffrey C. Delafuente, MS, FCCP

The collagen vascular diseases are a heterogeneous group of diseases that can involve the musculoskeletal system, integument, and blood vessels. Each collagen vascular disease has its own set of diagnostic criteria, although diagnosis can be difficult because of overlapping and nonspecific clinical presentations. The etiology of the various collagen vascular diseases is often unknown, although the immune system is usually involved in mediation of disease. Therefore, pharmacotherapy usually includes anti-inflammatory or immunosuppressive drugs.

Although the prevalence of other collagen vascular diseases may be greater than that of systemic lupus erythematosus (e.g., polymyalgia rheumatica), SLE is discussed most extensively in this chapter because it is a major collagen vascular disease with numerous clinical manifestations; its pharmacotherapy can be complex; and a plethora of data is available on the therapy of SLE. Since all the diseases discussed in this chapter have an immune-mediated pathogenesis, the therapeutic principles of lupus can be applied to other autoimmune collagen vascular diseases. The collagen vascular diseases discussed include systemic sclerosis, polymyositis/dermatomyositis, polymyalgia rheumatica, and systemic vasculitis; these were chosen because they are seen in general practice.

SYSTEMIC LUPUS ERYTHEMATOSUS

Systemic lupus erythematosus (SLE) is a fluctuating, multisystem disease with a diversity of clinical presentations. Abnormal immunologic function and formation of antibodies against "self" antigens underlie the pathogenesis of SLE.

Lupus is the Latin word for wolf and was first used in the tenth century to describe erosive skin lesions that looked as though a wolf had eaten away the flesh. The term *lupus erythemateux* was first used in 1851 by Cazenave, a Frenchman who described an illness in a patient with manifestations occurring in the skin. It is not surprising that SLE was first recognized as a skin disorder, because cutaneous manifestations constitute one of the most common clinical features of the disease. Further descriptions by Kaposi in 1872 and Osler in 1895 led to the concept of a multisystem disease, as it became recognized that patients developed complications in other organ systems.[1,2]

Autoantibodies in this disease became apparent with the development of the lupus erythematosus (LE) cell test in 1948 and the fluorescent antinuclear antibody test in 1957.[1] Recognition of SLE as an autoimmune disease of multisystemic nature led the American Rheumatism Association (ARA) to develop criteria for identifying lupus patients (Table 80–1). These criteria were originally developed in 1971 and revised in 1982. The criteria do not include all the clinical manifestations of the disease and are used primarily for distinguishing SLE from other collagen vascular diseases and determining patients for clinical studies.[3] To classify a patient as having SLE, 4 or more of the 11 criteria must be present. Although these criteria may be helpful, diagnosis requires additional serologic, immunopathologic, and clinical evaluations.

EPIDEMIOLOGY

The incidence of SLE has been reported as 1.0 to 7.6 per 100,000 population per year[4–6] with a prevalence of 14.6 to 51 per 100,000 population.[5,6] International studies report similar ranges with an incidence of 3.0 to 4.8 per 100,000 per year[4–6] and a prevalence of 12.5 to 52 per 100,000 population.[5,6] The disease occurs predominantly in women, with a reported female-to-male ratio approaching 10:1. This predominance is most in the 15- to 64-year age group.[4–6] The reported incidence in blacks in the United States is higher than in whites, including an earlier peak incidence in black females compared to white females.[4] Although the most typical SLE patient is a young adult woman, the disease can occur in people of any age or race and either gender.

ETIOLOGY

The etiology of abnormal autoantibody production and development of SLE is still unknown. Genetic, environmental, and hormonal factors all may have a role in loss of self-tolerance and expression of disease. A popular theory is that autoimmune disease, such as SLE, develops in genetically susceptible individuals after exposure to a "triggering" agent, possibly something in the environment.[7]

Family and twin studies suggest a genetic predisposition for the development of SLE. For example, one study in twins shows a monozygotic concordance rate of 24%, similar to other autoimmune diseases.[8] However, the risk in dizygotic twins is the same as that in first-degree relatives. Genetic analysis suggests that at least three or four genes are required in the expression of lupus in humans.[9] Evi-

TABLE 80–1. The 1982 Revised Criteria for Classification of Systemic Lupus Erythematosus[a]

Criterion	Definition
Malar rash	Fixed erythema, flat or raised, over the malar eminences, tending to spare the nasolabial folds
Discoid rash	Erythematous raised patches with adherent keratotic scaling and follicular plugging; atrophic scarring may occur in older lesions
Photosensitivity	Skin rash as a result of unusual reaction to sunlight, by patient history or physician observations
Oral ulcers	Oral or nasopharyngeal ulceration, usually painless, observed by a physician
Arthritis	Nonerosive arthritis involving two or more peripheral joints, characterized by tenderness, swelling, or effusion
Serositis	Pleuritis—convincing history of pleuritic pain or rub heard by a physician or evidence of pleural effusion or Pericarditis—documented by ECG or rub or evidence of pericardial effusion
Renal disorder	Persistent proteinuria greater than 0.5 g/d or greater than 3+ if quantitation not performed or Cellular casts—may be red cell, hemoglobin, granular, tubular, or mixed
Neurologic	Seizures—in the absence of offending drugs or known metabolic derangements, e.g., uremia, ketoacidosis, or electrolyte imbalance or Psychosis—in the absence of offending drugs or known metabolic derangements, e.g., uremia, ketoacidosis, or electrolyte imbalance
Hematologic disorder	Hemolytic anemia—with reticulocytosis or Leukopenia—fewer than 4000/mm^3 total on two or more occasions or Lymphopenia—fewer than 1500/mm^3 on two or more occasions or Thrombocytopenia—fewer than 100,000/mm^3 in the absence of offending drugs
Immunologic disorder	Positive LE cell preparation or Anti-DNA; antibody to native DNA in abnormal titer or Anti-Sm; presence of antibody to Sm nuclear antigen or False-positive serologic test for syphilis known to be positive for at least 6 months and confirmed by *Treponema pallidum* immobilization or fluorescent treponemal antibody absorption test
Antinuclear antibody	An abnormal titer of antinuclear antibody by immunofluorescence or an antibody equivalent assay at any point in time and in the absence of drugs known to be associated with "drug-induced lupus" syndrome

[a]The proposed classification is based on 11 criteria. For the purpose of identifying patients in clinical studies, a person shall be said to have systemic lupus erythematosus if any 4 or more of the 11 criteria are present, serially or simultaneously, during any interval of observation.
From Ref. 3, with permission.

dence indicates that major histocompatibility complex (MHC) genes, such as the human leukocyte antigen (HLA) genes in humans, may be important in lupus. However, non-MHC-linked genes, such as complement receptor genes and immunoglobulin receptor genes, may also contribute to disease susceptibility.[10] Environmental agents that may have a role in induction or activation of SLE include sunlight (i.e., ultraviolet light), drugs, chemicals such as hydrazine and aromatic amines (found in hair dyes), foods, and infection with viruses or bacteria.[7,11] Additionally, androgen may inhibit, and estrogen enhance, the expression of autoimmunity, and elevated circulating prolactin levels have been associated with lupus in males and females.[12,13]

PATHOPHYSIOLOGY

A major event in the development of SLE is excessive and abnormal autoantibody production and the formation of immune complexes. Patients may develop autoantibodies against multiple nuclear, cytoplasmic, and surface components of multiple types of cells in multiple organ systems; this fact underlines the multisystemic nature of the disease.

Excessive autoantibody production results from hyperactive B lymphocytes and helper T lymphocytes. Multiple mechanisms may be involved in the development of hyperactive lymphocytes, including impairment of immune regulatory processes involving T lymphocytes (suppressor T cells), cytokines (e.g., interleukins, interferon γ, tumor necrosis factor α, transforming growth factor β), and natural killer cells. Many autoantibodies are directed against nuclear constituents of the cell and are called collectively *antinuclear antibodies*. Several antinuclear antibodies are important because their presence or absence may aid in the diagnostic and clinical evaluation of the patient with SLE. The SLE patient usually has more than one antigen-specific antinuclear antibody in his or her serum and tissues.[14]

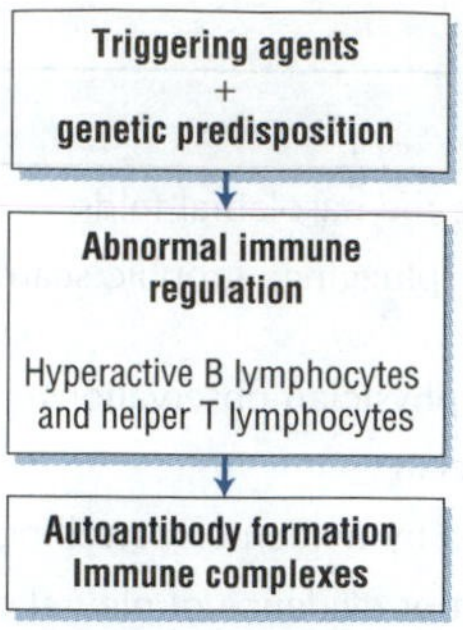

FIGURE 80–1. Pathogenesis of systemic lupus erythematosus. Environmental factors, such as infectious organisms, drugs, and chemicals, serve as triggering agents in genetically susceptible individuals to induce a state of immune dysregulation. These abnormal immune responses lead to hyperactive T helper lymphocyte and B lymphocyte function. Suppressor T lymphocyte function, cytokine production, and other immune regulatory mechanisms also are abnormal and fail to down-regulate autoantibody formation from hyperactive B lymphocytes. The autoantibodies formed from this immune dysregulation become pathogenic and form immune complexes that lead to damage of host tissue.

These are antibodies against such nuclear constituents as double-stranded or native DNA (dsDNA), single-stranded or denatured DNA (ssDNA), and RNA. Four RNA-associated antigens frequently occurring in SLE are the Sm antigen, ribonuclear protein (RNP), Ro (SS-A) antigen, and La (SS-B) antigen. Histone, a basic component of chromatin and nucleosomes, is another important nuclear component against which antinuclear antibodies are formed in lupus patients.[2,15]

Antibodies may also be directed against the phospholipid moiety of the prothrombin activator complex (lupus anticoagulant) and against cardiolipin. The lupus anticoagulant and anticardiolipin antibody are cross-reactive and constitute the two main types in a group of autoantibodies called antiphospholipid antibodies.[16]

The mechanism of tissue injury in SLE is thought to be related to immune complex formation and deposition in the kidney and other tissues, resulting in cell damage, complement fixation, and inflammation.[17] An overview of the pathogenesis[18] of SLE is illustrated in Figure 80–1.

CLINICAL PRESENTATION

As previously mentioned, SLE is a multisystem disease. Table 80–2 lists many of the signs and symptoms and incidences[19,20] in patients with SLE. Though certain of these may be more common than others, each patient presents differently and the course of the disease is highly unpredictable. Furthermore, SLE is not static, and most patients have fluctuations or "flare-ups" during the course of the disease.

Nonspecific signs and symptoms such as fatigue, fever, anorexia, and weight loss are frequently seen in patients with active disease. Musculoskeletal involvement (e.g., arthralgia, myalgia, arthritis) is very common in SLE,[19,20] with arthritis and arthralgia frequently the chief complaint upon initial presentation of the disease.[20] Joint involvement tends to be symmetric and may affect multiple sites. Objective evidence of musculoskeletal disease is often missing, although a few patients may present with deforming arthritis or subcutaneous nodules.

Manifestations in the skin and mucous membranes are nearly as common as those involving the musculoskeletal system.[19,20] The most well known of these is the butterfly rash, which occurs over the bridge of the nose and the malar eminences. The classic butterfly rash is seen in approximately one-half of patients and is often observed after sun exposure. In fact, photosensitivity is common to many SLE patients who present with cutaneous manifestations. Skin lesions characteristic of discoid lupus occur in up to 25% of patients with SLE and may occur without other clinical or serologic evidence of lupus.[19] Some individuals are said to develop *subacute cutaneous lupus erythemato-*

TABLE 80–2. Clinical Signs and Symptoms of SLE and Incidence[19,20]

Sign/Symptom	Incidence (%)
Musculoskeletal	
Arthritis and arthralgia	53–95
Myalgia	42–79
Constitutional	
Fatigue	80–100
Fever	41–86
Weight loss	31–71
Mucocutaneous	55–85
Butterfly rash	10–61
Photosensitivity	11–58
Raynaud's phenomenon	10–34
Discoid lesions	9–29
Central nervous system	12–75
Psychosis	5–52
Seizures	6–26
Pulmonary	
Pleuritis	31–57
Pleural effusion	12–40
Cardiovascular	
Pericarditis	2–48
Myocarditis	8–40
Heart murmur	12–44
ECG changes	34–70
Renal	31–65
Gastrointestinal	
Nausea	7–53
Abdominal pain	8–34
Bowel hemorrhage (vasculitis)	1–6
Hepatomegaly	25
Splenomegaly	10–20
Hematologic	
Anemia	30–78
Leukopenia	35–66
Thrombocytopenia	7–30
Lymphadenopathy	10–59

From Refs. 19 and 20, with permission.

sus, the nature of whose lesions falls between discoid (one type of *chronic cutaneous lupus erythematosus*) and the butterfly rash (an example of *acute cutaneous lupus erythematosus*).[21] Other cutaneous manifestations include vasculitis (which may be ulcerative), levido reticularis, periungual erythema, Raynaud's phenomenon, and alopecia.

Another common source of symptomatology in SLE is the pulmonary system, with manifestations such as pleurisy, coughing, or dyspnea. Pleurisy may present as pleuritic pain, a pleural rub, or a pleural effusion that is usually exudative in nature. Lupus pneumonitis may present acutely with fever, dyspnea, tachypnea, cough, rales, and patchy infiltrates or chronically with interstitial fibrosis. Lupus pneumonitis is an uncommon manifestation of SLE and has a poor prognosis.[19,21]

Cardiac manifestations of SLE often present as pericarditis, myocarditis, ECG changes, or valvular heart disease, including the classic cardiac lesion of Libman–Sacks endocarditis (nonbacterial verrucous endocarditis).[19,22] Coronary artery disease is occurring with increasing frequency, as the life expectancy of lupus patients increases.[23,24] It is thought that the development of heart disease in these patients is multifactorial. Hypertension, obesity, and hyperlipidemia are common in patients with SLE. Corticosteroid therapy and underlying renal disease may be contributing factors in the development of these cardiac risk factors.[22]

Neuropsychiatric manifestations of SLE may present in a diversity of ways, including psychosis, depression, seizure, stroke, peripheral neuropathy, organic brain syndrome, and others. This aspect of lupus may be an important factor contributing to morbidity and mortality.[21,25]

Symptoms associated with gastrointestinal manifestations are often nonspecific for lupus and include dyspepsia, abdominal pain, nausea, and difficulty swallowing. Mesenteric vasculitis may be problematic, particularly if arterial perforations occur. Hepatomegaly may present in some patients, although liver dysfunction is not characteristic of lupus. Pancreatitis may also be present in an occasional patient.[19]

HEMATOLOGIC MANIFESTATIONS

Anemia is found in many cases of SLE. It is usually an anemia of chronic inflammation, with a mild normochromic, normocytic smear, and low serum iron but adequate iron stores. Some patients may develop a hemolytic anemia with a positive Coombs test. Leukopenia, usually mild, is present in approximately half of SLE patients. Both granulocytes and lymphocytes may be affected but there is usually a larger decrease in the amount of circulating granulocytes. The absolute number of both T lymphocytes and B lymphocytes decreases. Thrombocytopenia may occur in SLE and is usually caused by antiplatelet antibodies resulting in phagocytosis by macrophages in the spleen, liver, lymph nodes, and bone marrow.[19,22]

Another significant finding associated with SLE is the presence of antiphospholipid antibodies such as the lupus anticoagulant (LA) and anticardiolipin antibodies. Although the LA is directed against the prothrombin activator complex and implies potential bleeding complications, this is not the case. In fact, the presence of LA and other antiphospholipid antibodies may be associated with thrombosis, neurologic disease, thrombocytopenia, and fetal loss, and is termed the *antiphospholipid syndrome*.[16,26] Not all patients with antiphospholipid syndrome have lupus. If a patient has no concomitant autoimmune disease, the syndrome is "primary." If a patient has accompanying SLE, the syndrome is "secondary."[27]

LUPUS NEPHRITIS

Clinical evidence of renal involvement, such as a rising serum creatinine or proteinuria, is generally associated with a poorer outcome compared with patients without renal involvement. Progression to end-stage renal disease is a major cause of morbidity and mortality in SLE. However, the extent and course of renal disease are quite variable and many lupus nephritis patients do very well. The World Health Organization (WHO) has classified lupus nephritis on the basis of histologic characteristics observed following renal biopsy. This system identifies lupus nephritis as normal (class I), mesangial, (class IIA and IIB), focal proliferative (class III), diffuse proliferative (class IV), or membranous (class V) glomerulonephritis.[2] Many patients progress from one form of nephritis to another during the course of the disease. Renal biopsy findings such as diffuse proliferative glomerulonephritis and high activity and/or chronicity indices may be associated with a poor outcome.[28–30]

DIAGNOSIS

As mentioned earlier, the diagnostic criteria listed in Table 80–1 should not be the primary means for diagnosing SLE, although many of the criteria may be valuable in the diagnostic process. Epidemiologic characteristics, clinical signs and symptoms, and common laboratory abnormalities are all used in diagnosing SLE.

TABLE 80–3. Antinuclear Antibody Test: Patterns, Antigens, and Specificities

Pattern	Antigen	Disease
Peripheral	Double-stranded DNA	SLE
Speckled	Acidic nuclear protein Ribonucleoprotein Extractable nuclear antigen	Rheumatoid arthritis SLE Scleroderma Mixed connective tissue disease
Homogeneous	Deoxyribonucleoprotein Histone	Rheumatoid arthritis SLE, drug-induced lupus
Nucleolar	Nucleolar RNA	Progressive systemic sclerosis

Once the disease is suspected, serologic tests may be helpful in making the diagnosis. A serologic test extensively used to aid in the diagnosis of SLE is the fluorescent antinuclear antibody (ANA) test. Nearly all SLE patients are ANA positive, but other disease states can also be associated with a positive test (Table 80–3); however, in other diseases many of the positive ANA tests are of a lower titer. The pattern of immunofluorescence of the ANA test may also be of diagnostic value (Table 80–3), with a peripheral (also called rim) pattern being specific for SLE. Detecting antibodies to specific nuclear constituents may also be diagnostically useful. Antibodies to native (dsDNA) and to Sm antigen are quite specific for and are considered diagnostic of SLE.[31,32]

PROGNOSIS

In earlier years, SLE was associated with a poor prognosis. For example, the classic report of cases diagnosed between 1949 and 1953 showed a 4-year survival rate of 51%.[33] Today, probably as a result of improved treatment and improved diagnostic techniques that allow earlier diagnosis, the 10- and 20-year survival rates approaches 90% and 70%, respectively.[13,34]

Historically, an important prognostic sign has been that of lupus nephritis. In 1981, a10-year survival rate of 87% in patients without evidence of nephritis compared with 65% in patients with nephritis was reported.[35] However, with the ability to better manage patients with kidney disease (e.g., dialysis), infection has replaced renal disease as the most common cause of death from SLE.[13] Lupus involving the central nervous system (CNS) also contributes to mortality, although to a lesser extent in recent years.[34,36] Cardiovascular disease, especially that resulting from atherosclerosis such as coronary artery disease, has emerged as a prominent cause of death as lupus patients live longer.[21]

▶ TREATMENT: Systemic Lupus Erythematosus

Desired treatment outcomes for the patient with SLE are twofold: (1) management of symptoms and induction of remission during times of disease flare; and (2) maintenance of remission for as long as possible between disease flares. An approach to the management of the patient with SLE is outlined in Figure 80–2. Because of the variability in clinical presentation of disease, treatment will vary accordingly and should be highly individualized. Optimal care of the patient with SLE will offer education and support services in addition to nonpharmacologic and pharmacologic treatments discussed below. Numerous lupus organizations

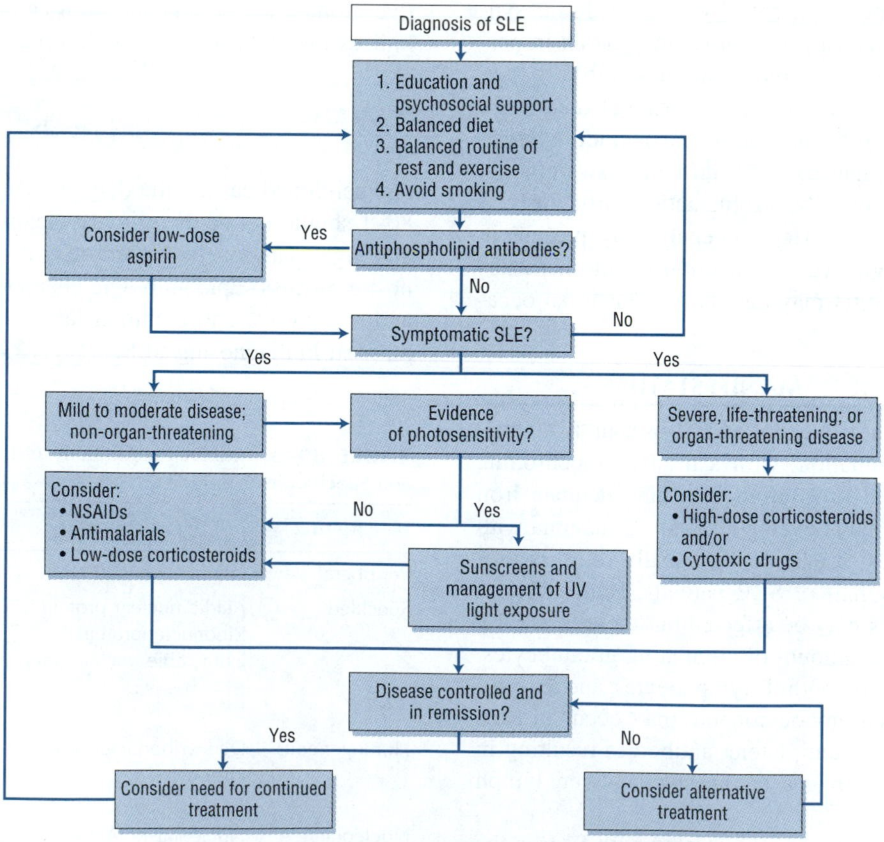

FIGURE 80–2. General approach to the management of SLE.

exist throughout the world and can be located by contacting the Lupus Foundation of America, Inc.[37] (http://www.lupus.org/lupus.index.html).

NONPHARMACOLOGIC THERAPY

Several nonpharmacologic measures can be employed to manage symptoms and help maintain remission. Fatigue is a common symptom in patients with lupus.[38,39] A balanced routine of rest and exercise, while avoiding overexertion, is essential in managing fatigue.[40] Avoidance of smoking may be particularly important because hydrazines in tobacco smoke may be an environmental trigger of lupus.[7,40] No specific dietary measures are known to definitively affect the clinical course of lupus. However, fish oil derivatives might prevent miscarriages in pregnant women with antiphospholipid antibodies,[40] but alfalfa sprouts should be avoided because they contain the amino acid L-canavanine, which is thought to alter T- and B-cell responses and may exacerbate lupus.[7,40] Many patients with SLE will need to limit exposure to sunlight and use sunscreens to block the possible exacerbating effects of ultraviolet light. The amount of sunlight exposure limitation should be individualized.

PHARMACOLOGIC THERAPY

In general, drug therapy for SLE is designed to suppress the immune response and inflammation. Table 80–4 lists common agents and doses used to control SLE. In general, the choice of drug therapy depends on the extent and severity of disease.

NONSTEROIDAL ANTI-INFLAMMATORY DRUGS

As discussed earlier, signs and symptoms such as fever, arthritis, and serositis are among the most common in patients with active disease. Therefore, in many patients with mild disease, initial treatment with a nonsteroidal anti-inflammatory drug (NSAID) is a logical choice. The choice of NSAIDs in SLE is empiric. The dose used should be adequate to provide anti-inflammatory effects, although low-dose aspirin may be useful in the management of patients with antiphospholipid syndrome.[41]

Patients with SLE taking NSAIDs may experience a decline in renal function because of drug effects and not the underlying disease. Prostaglandins may be important mediators of renal hemodynamics in patients with SLE, possibly increasing susceptibility to the renal sequelae from prostaglandin inhibition.[42] Awareness of this effect is important, because declining renal function might be mistakenly attributed to progression of lupus nephritis. There also exist reports of an association between aseptic meningitis in SLE patients and the use of ibuprofen, sulindac, diclofenac, tolmetin, and naproxen.[25,43]

ANTIMALARIAL DRUGS

Antimalarial agents such as chloroquine and hydroxychloroquine have been used successfully in the management of discoid lupus and SLE. A few controlled trials provide evidence for the role of antimalarial therapy in controlling disease exacerbations and as steroid-sparing agents.[44–46] In general, the manifestations of SLE that can be managed with antimalarials are cutaneous manifestations, arthralgia, pleuritis, mild pericardial inflammation, fatigue, cognitive dysfunction, and mild anemia, and leukopenia.[47] Because these drugs are not effective immediately, they are best used in long-term management. Response to chloroquine occurs in 1 month, whereas the maximal effect of hydroxychloroquine may not occur for 3 to 6 months.[25] Hydroxychloroquine is probably safer than chloroquine and is considered the antimalarial of first choice.

The mechanism of action of the antimalarial drugs is uncertain. It has been proposed that antimalarials interfere with antigen processing in macrophages and other cells.[48] Other effects of antimalarials that may benefit patients with SLE include inhibition of cytokines, decreased sensitivity to ultraviolet light, anti-inflammatory activity, antiplatelet effects, and antihyperlipidemic activity.[47]

Dosage and duration of therapy depend on patient response, tolerance of side effects, and development of retinal toxicity, which is a potentially irreversible adverse reaction associated with long-term therapy, especially with chloroquine. Current recommended doses of antimalarials in SLE are hydroxychloroquine 200 to 400 mg daily and chloroquine 250 to 500 mg daily. After 1 or 2 years of treatment, gradual tapering of dosage can be attempted. Some patients may require only one or two tablets per week to suppress cutaneous manifestations.[49]

Side effects of these drugs include CNS effects (e.g., headache, nervousness, insomnia, and others), dermatitis, pigmentary changes of the skin and hair, gastrointestinal disturbance (e.g., nausea), flu-like symptoms, and reversible cycloplegia resulting from deposition of the drug in the cornea. Retinal toxicity is uncommon when the currently recommended doses are used and is least common with hydroxychloroquine;[25] however, because of the possibility of permanent damage associated with the retinopathy, an ophthalmologic evaluation should be done at baseline and every 3 months with chloroquine and every 6 to 12 months with hydroxychloroquine.[25] If retinal abnormalities are noted, antimalarial therapy should be discontinued.

TABLE 80–4. Drug Treatment of Systemic Lupus Erythematosus

Drug Class	Drug and Dose	Indication
NSAID	Various agents Anti-inflammatory dose	Mild disease: fever, arthritis, skin rash, serositis
Antimalarial	Hydroxychloroquine, 200–400 mg PO daily Chloroquine, 250–500 mg PO daily	Mild disease: arthritis, skin rash, serositis
Corticosteroid	Prednisone 1–2 mg/kg/d PO (or equivalent) <1 mg/kg/d (or equivalent)	Initial control of severe disease Control of mild disease or maintenance after disease suppression with higher doses
	Methylprednisolone, 500–1000 mg IV daily × 3–5 d	Life-threatening disease
Cytotoxic	Cyclophosphamide, 0.5–1.0 g/m^2 IV monthly for 6 mo; then, every 3 mo for 2–3 yr Azathioprine, up to 4 mg/kg/d PO Cyclophosphamide, up to 4 mg/kg/d PO	Most commonly used in severe lupus nephritis; may be necessary for other severe disease manifestations

CORTICOSTEROIDS

Corticosteroid therapy is commonplace in therapeutic regimens for SLE. Although evidence for improved survival with corticosteroid therapy is inadequate, these agents are known to be effective for suppressing the clinical expression of disease and are considered by many to be a major factor in the improved prognosis of recent years. Although most controlled trials of corticosteroid therapy have been conducted in patients with severe lupus nephritis, evidence suggests that corticosteroids are also effective in the management of severe cases of CNS disease, pneumonitis, polyserositis, vasculitis, thrombocytopenia, and others.[50]

A patient with the diagnosis of SLE does not automatically require corticosteroid therapy. Mild disease with such manifestations as fever, arthralgia, pleuritis, or skin manifestations may respond adequately to NSAIDs or antimalarials, but patients with clinical manifestations that are more serious or unresponsive to other drugs may require corticosteroids. Some patients with chronic or subacute cutaneous lupus erythematosus may benefit from topical or intralesional administration of corticosteroids.[51]

The goal of treatment when using corticosteroids in SLE is to suppress and maintain suppression of active disease with the lowest dose possible. In patients with mild disease, low-dose therapy (prednisone 15 to 20 mg daily) is adequate, but in patients with more severe disease (severe hemolytic anemia or cardiac involvement) higher doses, such as prednisone 1 to 2 mg/kg daily, may be required. Once adequate suppression of disease is achieved, the dose should be tapered to the minimum amount required for continued disease suppression. When analyzing the need to treat with corticosteroids, the clinician should consider other conditions that may increase the risk of corticosteroid therapy such as infection, hypertension, diabetes, obesity, osteoporosis, and psychiatric disease.[50]

Steroid pulse therapy is the administration of short-term, high-dose, intravenous corticosteroids with the goal of inducing remission in SLE patients with serious, life-threatening disease, such as diffuse proliferative glomerulonephritis, CNS involvement, or hemolytic disease. A standard pulse regimen consists of intravenous methylprednisolone 500 to 1000 mg for 3 to 5 consecutive days. Pulse therapy is usually followed by high-dose oral therapy that is rapidly tapered to low-dose maintenance therapy.[50] Potential advantages of pulse therapy over high-dose oral steroids include a quicker response and avoidance of side effects associated with the longer duration of therapy required with oral steroids. Although generally well tolerated, methylprednisolone pulse therapy may result in significant adverse effects, including infection, gastrointestinal disturbances, rapid increases in blood pressure, arrhythmias, seizures, and sudden death.[50–52] Furthermore, there is insufficient data from controlled clinical trials to clearly define the role of pulse steroids in the management of SLE. One controlled trial indicated that pulse methylprednisolone was less effective than pulse cyclophosphamide in severe lupus nephritis.[53] Thus, pulse therapy represents an alternative mode of treatment for patients with life-threatening disease or disease unresponsive to other pharmacotherapy.

CYTOTOXIC DRUGS

A considerable amount of literature exists describing the use of cytotoxic and immunosuppressive drugs in SLE, although few of these are reports of controlled clinical trials. Included in this category are the alkylating agent cyclophosphamide and the antimetabolite azathioprine. These agents, usually used in combination with corticosteroids, have been the mainstays of immunosuppressive therapy. Although both are known to suppress and stabilize extrarenal disease activity, much of the evaluation of these agents has focused on lupus nephritis, a major factor associated with morbidity and mortality in SLE.

Both cyclophosphamide and azathioprine have been shown to delay the onset of nephritis and prolong survival in the New Zealand mouse, the animal model of SLE.[28] Results in human trials, however, have been inconclusive and contradictory, probably because of a paucity of adequately controlled trials, because of the variable presentation and course of disease, because trials were short and included few patients, and because subjects are usually studied late in the course of severe renal disease (e.g., diffuse proliferative glomerulonephritis).[28] However, a recent meta-analysis concluded that cytotoxic drugs combined with prednisone are more effective than prednisone alone for both total mortality and progression to end-stage renal disease.[54]

Azathioprine has not been studied as extensively as cyclophosphamide for lupus nephritis. Additionally, azathioprine has not been shown to be clearly more effective than prednisone alone. Although some studies have shown azathioprine to be associated with improved survival and a steroid-sparing effect, other studies indicate no significant advantage.[28] Azathioprine is given orally in doses up to 4 mg/kg/d. Azathioprine is generally less toxic than cyclophosphamide, but adverse reactions may be serious and include suppression of hematopoiesis, opportunistic infection, cancer, hepatotoxicity, pulmonary fibrosis, pancreatitis, and teratogenesis.[28]

The case for cyclophosphamide is only slightly more convincing. Although controlled studies indicate a benefit in controlling renal disease, a reduced risk for death in lupus nephritis patients receiving cyclophosphamide has not been shown.[22] Controlled studies that indicate a possible advantage of cyclophosphamide are usually of longer duration, such as the series of clinical trials examining the role of various cytotoxic drug regimens in lupus nephritis reported from the National Institutes of Health (NIH).[28,55–57] The longer NIH trials have used a chronicity index based on renal biopsy information as a predictor of renal functional outcome. The most significant benefit was observed in high-risk patients who were identified as having chronic histologic change based on the chronicity index. The duration of treatment was variable, from about 2 to 4 years, and differences in outcome were not observed until more than 5 years of follow-up. The probability of progression to end-stage renal disease was less in groups treated with intravenous cyclophosphamide, or oral cyclophosphamide, or combined oral cyclophosphamide and azathioprine compared to prednisone alone.

Other reports of more recent investigations have indicated variable rates of success using intravenous cyclophosphamide for lupus nephritis.[53,58,59] Cyclophosphamide is often administered intravenously in intermittent pulse doses to minimize toxicity. Mesna may be used to prevent hemorrhagic cystitis. Additionally, following the initial induction of remission over the first several months, follow-up treatment may be necessary to maintain disease control. Therefore, a typical pulse regimen would be intravenous cyclophosphamide (0.5 to 1.0 g/m^2 of body surface area) every month followed by intermittent pulse doses every 3 months for 2 to 3 years.

Of course, cyclophosphamide therapy is not without risk. Serious toxic effects include suppression of hematopoiesis, opportunistic infection, bladder complications (hemorrhagic cystitis and cancer), sterility, and teratogenesis.[28]

Cyclophosphamide may be of benefit to some patients with other serious, refractory manifestations of lupus, including neuropsychiatric manifestations.[60,61] Reports of other cytotoxic drugs for lupus in recent years include methotrexate[62,63] and mechlorethamine (nitrogen mustard).[64]

The evidence supporting the usefulness of cytotoxic drugs for patients with SLE is questionable; however, many clinicians consider these drugs to be important therapeutic agents in the management of patients with serious disease such as severe lupus nephritis.

TABLE 80–5. Alternative and Experimental Treatments for SLE

Treatment	Symptom	Reference
Plasmapheresis	Multiple severe symptoms—nephritis, CNS, thrombocytopenia, anemia, leukopenia	65
Cyclosporine	Nephritis	66
	Multiple symptoms—anemia, leukopenia, thrombocytopenia, nephritis	67
Immune globulin	Multiple symptoms—anemia, thrombocytopenia, nephritis	68, 69
Thromboxane A_2 synthetase inhibitor	Nephritis	70, 71
Prostaglandin E_1	Nephritis	72
	Cutaneous vasculitis, peripheral neuropathy	73
Ultraviolet-A1 irradiation	Multiple symptoms—rash	74
Monoclonal antibodies	Nephritis	75, 76
Dihydroepiandrosterone (DHEA)	Multiple symptoms	77
Bromocriptine	Multiple symptoms—fatigue, rash, Raynaud's, arthritis/arthralgia	78
Danazol	Thrombocytopenia, hemolytic anemia	79

ALTERNATIVE AND EXPERIMENTAL TREATMENTS

As the pathogenesis of SLE continues to be elucidated, new and promising treatments are being developed. Several alternative treatments reportedly successful in managing various manifestations of SLE are listed in Table 80–5. However, the pharmacotherapist should be aware that many of these are reports of uncontrolled trials. Furthermore, in addition to reports of success, the literature contains reports of unsuccessful treatment for many of these therapies (e.g., plasmaphersis[80] or immune globulin[81] for lupus nephritis).

SPECIAL POPULATIONS

PREGNANCY AND SLE

Pregnancy in SLE patients has been associated with exacerbation of disease during pregnancy, exacerbation during early postpartum, a greater incidence of spontaneous abortion, and a greater chance of developing preeclampsia or pregnancy-induced hypertension (particularly those patients with nephritis).

Exacerbation of lupus during pregnancy seems to be less likely if the disease is in remission at conception.[82] Disease exacerbations can be aggressively managed with corticosteroids, if needed, with little concern about harm to the fetus.[83] The decision to use other classes of drug therapy to control disease exacerbation should be highly individualized, although hydroxychloroquine or NSAIDs can probably be used safely, if needed.[83] In fact, it may be safer to continue hydroxychloroquine during pregnancy than to discontinue the drug.[84] The decision to use cytotoxic drugs during pregnancy should be made with extreme caution because of potential harmful effects (e.g., teratogenesis, fetal loss) to the fetus, particularly during the first trimester. Azathioprine may be the safest of the cytotoxic drugs if needed during pregnancy.[83,85]

Antiphospholipid antibodies may be associated with a greater likelihood of spontaneous abortion. Corticosteroids, aspirin, and heparin, alone and in various combinations, have been used to try to improve fetal outcome.[86] The optimal treatment regimen for pregnant patients with antiphospholipid antibodies is yet to be determined, although it has been recommended that women with prior fetal loss after the first trimester receive low-dose aspirin.[87] Additionally, women with a history of preeclampsia or nephritis with or without a history of hypertension should be considered for low-dose aspirin.[87]

Women with SLE are as capable as other women of becoming pregnant and having children, although there is an increased chance of a high-risk pregnancy.[88] However, appropriate planning and management will result in a high likelihood of a successful pregnancy and a healthy child.

ANTIPHOSPHOLIPID SYNDROME AND THROMBOSIS

As mentioned earlier, the presence of antiphospholipid antibodies may result in several clinical manifestations including thrombosis. If desired, patients positive for antiphospholipid antibodies but without a history of thromboembolism may be treated prophylactically with low-dose aspirin, although no treatment is also acceptable.[41] Patients with an acute thrombotic event should receive standard treatment with anticoagulants (e.g., heparin). Follow-up treatment with warfarin to prevent recurrence may require an INR of 3 or greater in patients with antiphospholipid syndrome.[89] However, currently, there is no consensus on the intensity of anticoagulation or duration of secondary prophylaxis.[27]

DRUG-INDUCED LUPUS

One of the earliest descriptions of a drug-induced SLE-like syndrome was reported in 1945 and was associated with the use of sulfadiazine.[90] Today, procainamide and hydralazine are most commonly associated with drug-induced lupus (DIL), although numerous other drugs have been implicated (Table 80–6).[91] A consensus on diagnostic criteria for DIL does not exist and many reported cases do not satisfy the 1982 revised ARA criteria for identification of SLE patients.[91] It has been suggested that DIL be suspected in patients with no history of idiopathic lupus, who develop antinuclear antibodies and at least one clinical feature of SLE, and whose symptoms resolve following drug discontinuation.[91]

The epidemiologic characteristics of DIL are different from those of idiopathic SLE. In general, patients with procainamide- or hydralazine-induced lupus develop the disease much later in life compared to idiopathic SLE, probably because the majority of people who use these drugs are older. Other observations include a greater percentage of white patients and an absence of female predominance when compared with idiopathic SLE.[90,91]

Patients of the slow acetylator phenotype may have a greater risk for developing DIL, particularly with procainamide and

TABLE 80–6. Medications Implicated in Drug-Induced Lupus

Acebutolol	Leuprolide	Phenylbutazone
Aminoglutethimide	Levodopa	Phenytoin
Atenolol	Lithium	Prazosin
Captopril	Lovastatin	Primidone
Carbamazepine	Mephenytoin	**Procainamide**
Chlorpromazine[a]	Methimazole	Promethazine
Chlorprothixene	**Methyldopa**	Propylthiouracil
Clonidine	Methysergide	Psoralen
Danazol	Metrizamide	**Quinidine**
Diclofenac	Minoxidil	Spironolactone
Disopyramide	Nalidixic acid	Streptomycin
Ethosuximide	Nitrofurantoin	Sulindac
Gold salts	Nomifensine	Sulfasalazine
Griseofulvin	Oral contraceptives	Tetracycline
Hydralazine	Para-aminosalicylate	Thioridazine
Ibuprofen	**Penicillamine**	Timolol
Interferon (α,γ)	Penicillin	Tolazamide
Isoniazid	Perphenazine	Tolmetin
Labetalol	Phenelzine	Trimethadione

[a]Drugs in boldface represent those with best evidence of association.
Adapted from Ref. 91, with permission.

hydralazine.[90,91] In DIL, the development of a positive ANA test occurs more rapidly and symptoms present more often with a slow acetylator phenotype.[90] Procainamide-induced lupus can present as early as 1 month or as late as 12 years after starting therapy. Hydralazine-induced lupus is related to dose and appears in patients receiving 100 mg/d or more.[91]

Musculoskeletal symptoms are the most common clinical manifestations, whereas renal and CNS involvement is much less common compared to idiopathic SLE.[90] Pleuropulmonary manifestations are also common, particularly in procainamide-induced disease. Fever is also common in DIL.[90,91]

A positive ANA test is found in nearly all procainamide- or hydralazine-induced cases.[90,91] The immunofluorescence pattern is usually homogeneous and antibodies are primarily against ssDNA and not dsDNA as in idiopathic SLE. Antibodies to Sm antigen are absent in DIL.[90] Antihistone antibodies are associated with DIL but are not specific for DIL and are found in idiopathic SLE and other diseases (e.g., rheumatoid arthritis).[91]

If signs and symptoms of SLE appear in a patient and are thought to be drug related, the drug should be discontinued. If the lupus is drug induced, the clinical manifestations should disappear in days to weeks, although it may take up to 1 year or longer for symptoms and serologic abnormalities to resolve completely.[90,91] An NSAID might be useful in treating musculoskeletal manifestations. Other, more aggressive drug therapy should not be necessary unless manifestations are deemed more serious.

PHARMACOECONOMIC CONSIDERATIONS

Patients with SLE have been shown to have higher rates of hospitalization and greater need for ambulatory care medical services.[92] Therefore, it is particularly important in the management of a potentially debilitating chronic disease such as SLE to achieve desired treatment outcomes in an optimal manner to minimize the impact on use of health care resources. Furthermore, because the cost of treating lupus patients is greater in the United States than in other countries,[93] SLE may have a greater impact on health care resources in the United States than elsewhere.

Lupus patients with physical impairment, lupus nephritis, CNS involvement, and poor psychological functioning have been shown to incur higher direct medical costs, whereas patients with CNS involvement, psychological impairment, and pain incur higher indirect costs (costs associated with loss of productivity such as days of work missed).[94,95] This implies that a targeted, multidisciplinary approach incorporating treatment for physical and psychological manifestations of SLE might reduce use of health care resources.[94]

One study targeting a cohort of patients with severe lupus nephritis found that, compared to prednisone alone, combined treatment with IV cyclophosphamide and prednisone resulted in slightly higher costs early in therapy (0 to 4 years) but substantial savings later (5 to 10 years) as a result of less need for dialysis and transplantation and increased productivity of patients.[96] Another study examined antiemetic therapy in patients with lupus nephritis receiving pulse cyclophosphamide and found that a regimen of combined oral ondansetron plus dexamethasone was completely effective in preventing emesis and was less expensive than a conventional intravenous regimen in patients who had previously failed conventional antiemetic therapy.[97]

As the field of pharmacoeconomics grows and as clinicians and researchers attempt to define the optimal management of patients in our cost conscious environment, the pharmacotherapist can expect additional examination of the economics of treating patients with lupus.

SYSTEMIC SCLEROSIS

CLINICAL MANIFESTATIONS

Systemic sclerosis is characterized by alteration of the microvasculature and by massive deposition of collagen. This disease can present as a spectrum of differing manifestations depending on affected areas and the extent of disease. Sclerosis of the skin is a hallmark for this disease. There can be a proximal diffuse (truncal) sclerosis, with skin tightness and marked skin thickening involving most of the body. There can also be internal organ involvement, such as the gastrointestinal tract, lung, kidney, or heart, which can result in death. Scleroderma refers to patients with only skin involvement. Disease that affects only the fingers and toes is referred to as sclerodactyly.

Most patients with systemic sclerosis have Raynaud's phenomenon, where the digits turn white, followed by a bluish color, which is then followed by reddening in response to an appropriate stimulus. Usually the precipitating event is cold temperature or emotion. The pallor is due to vasospasm; the bluish color is from ischemia; and the reddish color is caused by a reactive hyperemia. Raynaud's phenomenon is a common manifestation of other syndromes, and most patients with Raynaud's phenomenon do not have systemic sclerosis. Approximately 70% of patients with systemic sclerosis have symptoms of gastroesophageal reflux.[98]

In patients who have only sclerodactyly there is about an 80% incidence of survival at 5 years following diagnosis.[99] Patients with diffuse sclerosis have a 5-year survival rate of about 50%.[99] Elderly individuals and patients with poor renal function, anemia, or pulmonary involvement have a poorer prognosis.

ETIOLOGY AND PREVALENCE

The cause of systemic sclerosis is unknown. Ninety-five percent of patients have identifiable autoantibodies. Patients with limited cutaneous involvement often have the CREST syndrome (*C*alcinosis, *R*aynaud's, *E*sophageal dysmotility, *S*clerodactyly, *T*elangiectasias). Most of these patients have anticentromere antibodies.[98] The prevalence of the disease is estimated between 4 and 290 cases per million population.[99] These are the high and low values published. The large range may be due to differences in diagnostic criteria, regional variation, or sample sizes used to estimate the prevalence.

▶ TREATMENT: Systemic Sclerosis

There are no well-controlled trials evaluating and comparing various forms of therapy. The available data are difficult to interpret because of the heterogeneity of the disease and spontaneous remissions that can occur. There is also a lack of objective measures to assess changes in clinical status. D-Penicillamine is most often used for skin involvement. This drug does seem to improve the skin manifestations and prolong survival.[99] The initial dose of D-penicillamine is 250 mg daily, with gradual increases in dose every 2 to 3 months, to an optimal dose of 750 to 1000 mg/d. Response occurs over many months and the drug is not always effective.[98] The high incidence of severe adverse events and dropout rates from D-penicillamine limits its usefulness. Anti-inflammatory agents and corticosteroids have not been effective in systemic sclerosis.

Angiotensin-converting enzyme (ACE) inhibitors have dramatically improved survival in patients with renal involvement. Patients with sclerosis of the kidneys develop hypertension leading to a renal crisis. In these patients plasma renin activity and angiotensin concentrations can be more than twice normal. Renal involvement should be anticipated in all systemic sclerosis patients who develop hypertension. Patients with systemic sclerosis and hypertension should be treated and maintained with an ACE inhibitor regardless of renal involvement. ACE inhibitors have allowed some dialysis-dependent systemic sclerosis patients to discontinue dialysis.[100] Prior to the use of ACE inhibitors in systemic sclerosis, renal disease was the major cause of death.[101]

Treatment of Raynaud's phenomenon requires patient education and sometimes drug therapy. Patients must maintain their peripheral extremity and core body temperatures. Wearing appropriate clothing in cold environments is essential. Reaching into a freezer with unprotected hands should be avoided. Smoking causes cutaneous vasoconstriction and should be eliminated, including passive smoke. When preventive measures are not sufficient, calcium channel blocking agents have become the agents of choice for Raynaud's phenomenon. Nifedipine, 10 to 20 mg tid or qid, decreases the frequency and duration of attacks.[100] Diltiazem, 60 mg tid or qid, can also be used. The sustained-release formulations of these agents may enhance patient compliance.

POLYMYOSITIS AND DERMATOMYOSITIS

CLINICAL MANIFESTATIONS

Polymyositis and dermatomyositis (PM and DM) are chronic inflammatory diseases of skeletal muscle and skin of unknown etiology. Dermatomyositis is distinguished from polymyositis by a typical rash, which is red, scaly, and plaque-like over the knuckles, wrists, elbows, and knees. A blue-purple discoloration on the upper eyelids with edema can also occur in dermatomyositis. In PM and DM there is proximal muscle weakness in the shoulder and hip girdles and trunk. The onset is insidious and patients usually notice lower extremity weakness and may complain of difficulty in rising from a chair or climbing stairs. There is an increase in serum creatine kinase concentration and electromyography abnormalities. The creatine kinase concentration may be as much as 50 times normal.[102] Other serum enzymes, such as the ALT, AST, and LDH may also be increased.[103] Muscle biopsies show a necrotizing inflammatory process. The skin lesions of dermatomyositis show an immune complex–mediated necrosis of the microvasculature. Polymyositis appears to be related to cytotoxic T-cell activity, and up to 20% of patients with inflammatory myopathies have ANA and cytoplasmic antibodies.[103] Patients may develop features associated with other connective tissue diseases, such as arthritis, Raynaud's phenomenon, or overlap syndromes in which the patient has SLE, rheumatoid arthritis, Sjögren's syndrome, or scleroderma, in addition to the myositis.[104]

▶ TREATMENT: Polymyositis and Dermatomyositis

Large controlled trials of drug therapy have not been conducted. The goal of therapy is to increase muscle strength so as to improve function in activities of daily living (bathing, dressing, feeding, toileting). Treatment consists of physical therapy during periods of remission and rest during periods of disease activity. Corticosteroids are the first line of drug therapy for PM/DM. There is no consensus as to the optimal dose of corticosteroid to use. Most clinicians use prednisone at a starting dose of 40 to 100 mg/d or approximately 1 mg/kg/d as a single morning dose.[102–104] Patients who do not have an initial response may benefit from higher prednisone doses of 1.5 mg/kg/d.[104] The initial dose of prednisone is continued for 1 to 2 months or until maximum benefit is achieved or a remission is induced. The full effect of prednisone may not be evident for several months. Approximately 90% of patients treated with prednisone will have some improvement.[105] The prednisone dose is tapered when muscle strength improves and serum creatine kinase concentrations decrease. If the prednisone is working and there are no serious side effects, then the drug is slowly tapered. Again, there is no consensus on how to accomplish this. One author advocates tapering the dose over 10 weeks to 80 to 100 mg every other day, with alternate day doses decreased by 5 to 10 mg/wk every 3 to 4 weeks.[103] The dose that maintains a good clinical response can be used as maintenance. Tapering too quickly can cause an exacerbation of disease activity. Monitoring serum creatine kinase concentrations is useful because they tend to increase several weeks before clinical symptoms become apparent. Although some have advocated tapering to an every-other-day regimen,[102,103] others have found qod dosing not to be as good as daily dosing.[104] Patients with milder disease tend to have better results with every other day dosing than those patients with more severe disease. Some clinicians will treat patients with daily prednisone for 1 or more years, while others may use qod therapy for many years.

One complication from corticosteroid use is the development of a myopathy. Based on symptoms it is difficult to know if increased muscle weakness is due to the corticosteroid or to worsening disease status. Lowering the prednisone dose may be useful. If patients get better on a lower dose of prednisone, then most likely the muscle weakness was due to the drug. It may take 2 to 8 weeks for this to become clinically evident. Use of serum creatine kinase concentration may also be useful because this does not increase with steroid myopathy. It is possible that a steroid myopathy and worsening disease can coexist.

Although most patients with PM/DM improve with prednisone, some will not and some will develop corticosteroid resistance. In these patients azathioprine has been used at a dose of 1.5 to 3 mg/kg/d.[102] Clinical response may take 3 to 6 months. Another alternative is methotrexate at a dose of 7.5 to 20 mg once weekly. With patients resistant to these therapies, cyclophosphamide, cyclosporine, or chlorambucil can be tried. Intravenous γ-globulin at a dose of 2 g/kg/month for 3 months may be effective in patients with refractory disease.[106] There are no large series of data available on clinical outcomes in patients on alternative therapies for PM/DM. These alternative therapies may also be beneficial in patients who cannot take corticosteroids because of serious adverse effects.

POLYMYALGIA RHEUMATICA

CLINICAL MANIFESTATIONS

Polymyalgia rheumatica (PMR) is characterized by aching and morning stiffness of the neck, shoulder, and pelvic girdle musculature and torso. Stiffness is greatest following periods of inactivity, such as sleeping. Pain and morning stiffness may last from 1 to 6 hours. Fatigue, anorexia, and low-grade fever are common signs and symptoms. The erythrocyte sedimentation rate (ESR) is generally more than 40 mm/h, and often is more than 100 mm/h. Some patients go from exhibiting no symptoms to overt clinical manifestations overnight, whereas others have a gradual onset of symptoms over a number of weeks. The etiology is unknown. There is a close association between PMR and temporal arteritis or giant cell arteritis. Some researchers suggest that these disease entities are variants of the same disorder. PMR occurs primarily in individuals older than 50 years of age, with a mean age onset of approximately 70 years.[107]

▶ TREATMENT: Polymyalgia Rheumatica

The treatment of choice for PMR is prednisone at a dose of 10 to 20 mg/d. This therapy is so effective that if improvement does not occur within a week, another diagnosis should be considered. The ESR should decrease by 2 weeks and be normal after 4 weeks of therapy. The prednisone should be tapered beginning several weeks following control of symptoms. The rate of tapering is based on clinical response. A taper of 2.5 mg/d at 2- to 4-week intervals to 10 mg/d followed by a slower tapering of 1 mg/d at monthly intervals has been suggested.[108,109] The lowest dose of prednisone that controls symptoms should be used for maintenance, which is usually between 7 and 15 mg/d.[108] Maintaining the ESR in the normal range is a good monitoring parameter. For elderly patients the normal ESR may be slightly higher than that usually given as a reference value by the clinical laboratory. PMR is a self-limited disease, and patients usually continue maintenance therapy for 2 to 5 years.[107,108] Patients may experience a relapse when the prednisone is discontinued and may require prednisone therapy for up to 15 years.[110] Every-other-day prednisone has not been as successful as daily therapy. Methotrexate has been tried in patients refractory to prednisone, but it does not improve the disease activity or allow for a prednisone dose reduction.[111]

PMR-associated temporal arteritis and giant cell arteritis require aggressive therapy with high-dose corticosteroids, such as prednisone at a dose of 40 to 60 mg/d or higher. These forms of arteritis can cause permanent loss of vision if not treated promptly. Patients should be educated to seek immediate medical care for possibly related symptoms such as jaw pain on chewing, temporal headache, visual changes, or mental status changes.

SYSTEMIC VASCULITIS

CLINICAL MANIFESTATIONS

Clinical manifestations of vasculitis are heterogeneous and are due to inflammation and damage to blood vessels. Vasculitis can be primary, as in Wegener's granulomatosis and polyarteritis nodosa, or secondary from other disease states, such as rheumatoid arthritis or SLE. Immune complexes can develop at the site of the vessel damage, or circulating immune complexes can be deposited in the vessel wall. The immune complexes can then activate the humoral immune system, leading to inflammation and damage. Cellular-mediated immunity may also be involved in some vasculitides.[112] There are numerous forms of vasculitis, and there is currently no universally accepted scheme to classify them. Table 80–7 lists some systemic vasculitis syndromes.

TABLE 80–7. Classification of Systemic Vasculitis Syndromes

Hypersensitivity Vasculitis
Due to exogenous agents
Drugs
Infection
Henoch–Schönlein purpura
Serum sickness-like reactions
Due to endogenous agents
Autoimmune disease
Malignancy
Systemic connective tissue diseases
Cryoglobulinemia
Systemic Necrotizing Vasculitis
Polyarteritis nodosa
Polyangiitis overlap syndrome
Allergic granulomatosis
Wegener's Granulomatosis
Giant Cell Arteritis
Temporal arteritis
Takayasu's arteritis
Thromboangiitis Obliterans (Buerger's Disease)

▶ TREATMENT: Systemic Vasculitis

There are few controlled trials of pharmacologic treatments for the various forms of vasculitis. Treatment is guided by the severity, prognosis, and response of the vasculitis. For example, a drug-induced hypersensitivity vasculitis resulting in a rash may require only that the drug be discontinued. At the other end of the spectrum, Wegener's granulomatosis is a fatal vasculitis if not aggressively treated with corticosteroids, often in combination with cyclophosphamide. Each type of vasculitis has its recommended therapeutic protocol, which usually includes the use of anti-inflammatory agents and immunosuppressive agents, either alone or in combination.

EVALUATION OF THERAPEUTIC OUTCOMES

The diversity of clinical features and disease severity associated with the collagen vascular diseases leads to a number of possible clinical outcomes with a broad range of desired therapeutic outcomes. Achieving desired therapeutic outcomes for most of the collagen vascular diseases is highly variable. Currently, it is not possible to predict which patients will have a satisfactory therapeutic response and which patients will have unrelenting progressive disease. These diseases often have fluctuating courses, necessitating frequent changes in drug therapy and drug doses.

Evaluation of drug therapy of several of the collagen vascular diseases often only requires monitoring for resolution of symptoms such as rash or muscle pain. However, patients with life-threatening disease receiving aggressive pharmacotherapy may require intensive monitoring and evaluation of therapy. For example, the patient receiving cytotoxic drug therapy for severe lupus nephritis requires close monitoring of laboratory indices of renal function as well as monitoring symptomatology and laboratory indices for possible bone marrow suppression, infection, cystitis, or other possible undesired therapeutic outcomes.

Evaluation of therapeutic outcomes should also include an awareness of the possibility of drug therapy mimicking signs and symptoms of disease such as the lupus patient receiving NSAID therapy and presenting with renal insufficiency or the patient with polymyositis receiving prednisone presenting with an exacerbation of muscle weakness.

TABLE 80–8. Instruments Used for Assessing Outcome Measures in Patients with SLE

Outcome Domain	Instrument
Disease activity	Systemic Lupus Activity Measure (SLAM) Systemic Lupus Erythematosus Activity Index (SLEDAI) British Isles Lupus Activity Group (BILAG)
Accumulated damage	Systemic Lupus International Collaborating Clinics/American College of Rheumatology (SLICC/ACR) damage index
Quality of life	Health Assessment Questionaire (HAO) functional ability index Medical Outcome Survey short form (MOS SF-20 and MOS SF-36)

As patients live longer, as is the case with SLE, outcome measures other than mortality will be needed to assess the effect of treatment. Clinicians and researchers working with lupus patients have developed and continue to refine some of these alternative outcome measures. Three important domains for assessing lupus patients include disease activity, accumulated damage, and quality of life.[113] Several instruments useful for assessing patients with SLE are listed in Table 80–8.[113] Pharmacotherapists can expect to see increased use of these and similar instruments for assessment of treatment outcomes in patients with SLE.

CONCLUSION

SLE is a disease that affects multiple organ systems and consists of abnormal immunologic function and the development of autoantibodies. The disease is quite variable in clinical presentation and progression. The cause of lupus is unknown, although several factors (e.g., genetics, environment, hormones) may predispose an individual to the development of the disease. Although SLE was once thought to be rapidly fatal, today nearly 90% of patients survive 10 years.

Drug therapy is nonspecific and is aimed at suppressing the inflammation and abnormal immune response associated with active disease. Clinical trials with various agents have often been inadequate and contradictory, and the therapeutic management of lupus is not optimal. Nevertheless, drug therapy of recent years probably has contributed significantly to the improved survival of these patients. As the understanding of SLE progresses, we can expect to see the development of more specific and optimal treatment and further improvement in survival.

Each of the collagen vascular diseases has its own recommended form of therapy. For most of these diseases, there are few well-controlled clinical trials evaluating pharmacotherapy. Treatment of most of these diseases requires anti-inflammatory or immunosuppressive drugs. Monitoring therapeutic outcomes is essential because drugs and drug doses may need to be modified frequently.

▶ PRINCIPLES OF PHARMACOTHERAPY

- SLE can have a tremendous psychological impact on patients in addition to its physiologic effects. Therefore, education and support services are essential for optimal management upon diagnosis of lupus.
- Nonspecific symptoms, especially fatigue, present frequently in SLE patients and are often debilitating. Therefore, a balanced routine of rest, exercise, and diet is an essential component of treatment.
- Because of the fluctuating, diverse presentation of SLE and other collagen vascular diseases, pharmacologic and nonpharmacologic treatment should be highly individualized.
- Drug therapy options for patients with mild to moderate manifestations of SLE should include NSAIDs, antimalarials, and low-dose corticosteroids.
- Drug therapy options for patients with severe manifestations of SLE should include high-dose corticosteroids and cytotoxic drugs (usually cyclophosphamide).
- Monitoring therapeutic outcomes is critical because the drugs used to treat collagen vascular diseases frequently cause severe adverse events and the disease process can fluctuate between spontaneous remissions and disease exacerbations.

REFERENCES

1. Benedek TG. Historical background of discoid and systemic lupus erythematosus. In: Wallace DJ. Hahn BH, eds. Dubois' Lupus Erythematosus, 5th ed. Baltimore, Williams & Wilkins, 1997:3–16.
2. Kotzin BL, O'Dell JR. Systemic lupus erythematosus. In: Frank MM, Austen KF, Claman HN, Unanue ER, eds. Samter's Immunologic Diseases, 5th ed. Boston, Little, Brown, 1995:667–697.
3. Tan EM, Cohen AS, Fries JF, et al. The 1982 revised criteria for the classification of systemic lupus erythematosus. Arthritis Rheum 1982;25:1271–1277.
4. McCarty DJ, Manzi S, Medsger TA. Incidence of systemic lupus erythematosus. Arthritis Rheum 1995;38:1260–1270.
5. Hopkinson N. Epidemiology of systemic lupus erythematosus. Ann Rheum Dis 1992;51:1292–1294.
6. Hochberg MC. The epidemiology of systemic lupus erythematosus. In: Wallace DJ, Hahn BH, eds. Dubois' Lupus Erythematosus, 5th ed. Baltimore, Williams & Wilkins, 1997:49–65.
7. Mongey AB, Hess EV. The role of environment in systemic lupus erythematosus and associated disorders. In: Wallace DJ, Hahn BH, eds. Dubois' Lupus Erythematosus, 5th ed. Baltimore, Williams & Wilkins, 1997:31–47.
8. Deapen D, Escalante A, Weinrib L, et al. A revised estimate of twin concordance in systemic lupus etythematosus. Arthritis Rheum 1992; 35:311–318.
9. Winchester RJ. Systemic lupus erythematosus: Pathogenesis. In: Koopman WJ, ed. Arthritis and Allied Conditions: A Textbook of Rheumatology, 13th ed. Baltimore, Williams & Wilkins, 1997: 1361–1391.
10. Vyse TJ, Kotzin BL. Genetic basis of systemic lupus erythematosus. Curr Opin Immunol 1996;8:843–851.
11. Hess EV. Environmental lupus syndromes. Br J Rheum 1995;34: 597–599.
12. Lahita RG. Sex hormones as immunomodulators of disease. Ann N Y Acad Sci 1993;685:278–287.
13. Mills JA. Systemic lupus erythematosus. N Engl J Med 1994;330: 1871–1879.
14. Olhoffer IH, Peng SL, Craft J. Revisiting autoantibody profiles in systemic lupus erythematosus. J Rheumatol 1997;24:297–302.
15. Harley JB. Autoantibodies in systemic lupus erythematosus. In: Koopman WJ, ed. Arthritis and Allied Conditions: A Textbook of Rheumatology, 13th ed. Baltimore, Williams & Wilkins, 1997:1347–1360.
16. Tomer Y, Buskila D, Shoenfeld Y. Pathogenic significance and diagnostic value of lupus autoantibodies. Int Arch Allergy Immunol 1993;100:293–306.
17. Condemi JJ. The autoimmune diseases. JAMA 1992;268:2882–2892.
18. Hahn BH. An overview of the pathogenesis of systemic lupus erythematosus. In: Wallace DJ, Hahn BH, eds. Dubois' Lupus Erythematosus, 5th ed. Baltimore, Williams & Wilkins, 1997:69–75.

19. Schur PH. Clinical features of SLE. In: Kelley WM, Harris ED, Ruddy S, Sledge CB, eds. Textbook of Rheumatology, 4th ed. Philadelphia, Saunders, 1993:1017–1042.
20. Wallace DJ. The clinical presentation of systemic lupus erythematosus. In: Wallace DJ, Hahn BH, eds. Dubois' Lupus Erythematosus, 5th ed. Baltimore, Williams & Wilkins, 1997:627–633.
21. Boumpas DT, Fessler BJ, Austin HA III, et al. Systemic lupus erythematosus: Emerging concepts. Part 2: Dermatologic and joint disease, the antiphospholipid antibody syndrome, pregnancy and hormonal therapy, morbidity and mortality, and pathogenesis. Ann Intern Med 1995;123:42–53.
22. Boumpas DT, Austin HA III, Fessler BJ, et al. Systemic lupus erythematosus: Emerging concepts. Part 1: Renal, neuropsychiatric, cardiovascular, pulmonary, and hematologic disease. Ann Intern Med 1995;122:940–950.
23. Manzi S, Meilahn EN, Rairie JE, et al. Age-specific incidence rates of myocardial infarction and angina in women with systemic lupus erythematosus: Comparison with the Framingham Study. Am J Epidemiol 1997;145:408–415.
24. Petri M, Spence D, Bone LR, Hochberg MC. Coronary artery disease risk factors in the Johns Hopkins lupus cohort: Prevalence, recognition by patients, and preventive practices. Medicine 1992;71: 291–302.
25. Barr WG, Merchut MP. Systemic lupus erythematosus with central nervous system involvement. Psychiatr Clin North Am 1992;15: 439–454.
26. Love PE, Santoro SA, Antiphospholipid antibodies: Anticardiolipin and the lupus anticoagulant in systemic lupus erythematosus (SLE) and in non-SLE disorders. Ann Intern Med 1990;112:682–698.
27. Lockshin MD. Answers to the antiphospholipid-antibody syndrome? N Engl J Med 1995;332:1025–1027.
28. Donadio JV, Glassock RJ. Immunosuppressive drug therapy in lupus nephritis. Am J Kidney Dis 1993;21:239–250.
29. McLaughlin J, Gladman DD, Urowitz MB, et al. Kidney biopsy in systemic lupus erythematosus. II. Survival analyses according to biopsy results. Arthritis Rheum 1991;34:1268–1273.
30. McLaughlin JR, Bombardier C, Farewell VT, et al. Kidney biopsy in systemic lupus erythematosus. III. Survival analysis controlling for clinical and laboratory variables. Arthritis Rheum 1994;37:559–567.
31. Craft J, Hardin JA. Antinuclear antibodies. In: Kelley WM, Harris ED, Ruddy S, Sledge CB, eds. Textbook of Rheumatology, 4th ed. Philadelphia, Saunders, 1993:164–187.
32. Pisetsky DS, Gilkeson G, St. Clair EW. Systemic lupus erythematosus. Diagnosis and treatment. Med Clin North Am 1997;81:113–129.
33. Merrell M, Shulman LE. Determination of prognosis in chronic disease, illustrated by systemic lupus erythematosus. J Chron Dis 1955; 1:12–32.
34. Abu-Shakra M, Urowitz MB, Gladman DD, Gough J. Mortality studies in systemic lupus erythematosus. Results from a single center. 1. Causes of death. J Rheumatol 1995;22:1259–1264.
35. Wallace DJ, Podell T, Weiner J, et al. Systemic lupus erythematosus—survival patterns. Experience with 609 patients. JAMA 1981; 245:934–938.
36. Rosner S, Ginzler EM, Diamond HS, et al. A multicenter study of outcome in systemic lupus erythematosus. II. Causes of death. Arthritis Rheum 1982;25:612–617.
37. Lupus Foundation of America, Inc., 1300 Picard Drive, Suite 200, Rockville, MD, 301–670–9292 or 1–800–558–0121.
38. Krupp LB, LaRocca NG, Muir J, Steinberg AD. A study of fatigue in systemic lupus erythematosus. J Rheumatol 1990;17:1450–1452.
39. Wysenbeek AJ, Leibovici L, Weinberger A, Guedj D. Fatigue in systemic lupus erythematosus. Prevalence and relation to disease expression. Br J Rheumatol 1993;32:633–635.
40. Wallace DJ. Principles of therapy and local measures. In: Wallace DJ, Hahn BH, eds. Dubois' Lupus Erythematosus, 5th ed. Baltimore, Williams & Wilkins, 1997:1099–1108.
41. Lockshin MD. Which patients with antiphospholipid antibody should be treated and how? Rheum Dis Clin North Am 1993;19:235–247.
42. ter Borg EJ, de Jong PE, Meijer S, Kallenberg CGM. Renal effects of indomethacin in patients with systemic lupus erythematosus. Nephron 1989;53:238–243.
43. Weksler BB, Lehany AM. Naproxen-induced recurrent aseptic meningitis. Ann Pharmacother 1991;25:1183–1184.
44. The Canadian Hydroxychloroquine Study Group. A randomized study of the effect of withdrawing hydroxychloroquine sulfate in systemic lupus erythematosus. N Engl J Med 1991;324:150–154.
45. Williams HJ. Egger MJ, Singer JZ, et al. Comparison of hydroxychloroquine and placebo in the treatment of the athropathy of mild systemic lupus erythematosus. J Rheumatol 1994;21:1457–1462.
46. Meinao IM, Andrade LEC, Ferraz MB, et al. A controlled trial with diphosphate chloroquine (DPC) in systemic lupus erythematosus (SLE). Arthritis Rheum 1994;37(suppl):S406. Abstract.
47. Wallace DJ. Antimalarial agents and lupus. Rheum Dis Clin North Am 1994;20:243–263.
48. Fox RI. Mechanism of action of hydroxychloroquine as an antirheumatic drug. Semin Arthritis Rheum 1993;23(2 suppl 1):82–91.
49. Wallace DJ. Antimalarial therapies. In: Wallace DJ, Hahn BH, eds. Dubois' Lupus Erythematosus, 5th ed. Baltimore, Williams & Wilkins, 1997:1117–1139.
50. Hahn BH. Management of systemic lupus erythematosus. In: Kelley WM, Harris ED, Ruddy S, Sledge CB, eds. Textbook of Rheumatology, 4th ed. Philadelphia, Saunders, 1993:1043–1056.
51. Redford TW, Small RE. Update on pharmacotherapy of systemic lupus erythematosus. Am J Health Syst Pharm 1995;52:2686–2695.
52. Baethge BA, Lidsky MD, Goldberg JW. A study of adverse effects of high-dose intravenous (pulse) methylprednisolone therapy in patients with rheumatic disease. Ann Pharmacother 1992;26:316–320.
53. Boumpas DT, Austin HA III, Vaughn EM. Controlled trial of pulse methylprednisolone versus two regimens of pulse cyclophosphamide in severe lupus nephritis. Lancet 1992;340:741–745.
54. Bansal VK, Beto JA. Treatment of lupus nephritis: A meta-analysis of clinical trials. Am J Kidney Dis 1997;29:193–199.
55. Carette S, Klippel JH, Decker JL, et al. Controlled studies of oral immunosuppressive drugs in lupus nephritis. A long-term follow-up. Ann Intern Med 1983;99:1–8.
56. Austin HA, Klippel JH, Balow JE, et al. Therapy of lupus nephritis. Controlled trial of prednisone and cytotoxic drugs. N Engl J Med 1986;314;614–619.
57. Steinberg AD, Steinberg SC. Long-term preservation of renal function in patients with lupus nephritis receiving treatment that includes cyclophosphamide versus those treated with prednisone only. Arthritis Rheum 1991;34:945–950.
58. Valeri A, Radhakrishnan J, Estes D, et al. Intravenous pulse cyclophosphamide treatment of severe lupus nephritis: A prospective five-year study. Clin Nephrol 1994;42:71–78.
59. Martinelli R, Pereira LJC, Santos ES, Rocha H. Clinical effects of intermittent, intravenous cyclophosphamide in severe systemic lupus erythematosus. Nephron 1996;74:313–317.
60. Neuwelt CM, Lacks S, Kaye BR, et al. Role of intravenous cyclophosphamide in the treatment of severe neuropsychiatric systemic lupus erythematosus. Am J Med 1995;98:32–41.
61. Ramos PC, Mendez MJ, Ames PRJ, et al. Pulse cyclophosphamide in the treatment of neuropsychiatric systemic lupus erythematosus. Clin Exp Rheumatol 1996;14:295–299.
62. Walz LeBlanc BAE, Dagenasis P, Urowitz MB, Gladman DD. Methotrexate in systemic lupus erythematosus. J Rheumatol 1994; 21:836–838.
63. Wise CM, Vuyyuru S, Roberts WN. Methotrexate in nonrenal lupus and undifferentiated connective tissue disease—a review of 36 patients. J Rheumatol 1996;23:1005–1010.
64. Wallace DJ, Metzger AL. Successful use of nitrogen mustard for cyclophosphamide resistant diffuse proliferative lupus glomerulonephritis: Report of 2 cases. J Rheumatol 1995;22; 801–802. Letter.
65. Euler HH, Schroeder JO, Harten P, et al. Treatment-free remission in severe systemic lupus erythematosus following synchronization of

plasmapheresis with subsequent pulse cyclophosphamide. Arthritis Rheum 1994;37:1784–1794.

66. Radhakrishnan J, Kunis CL, D'Agati V, Appel GB. Cyclosporine treatment of lupus membranous nephropathy. Clin Nephrol 1994; 42:147–154.
67. Caccavo D, Lagana B, Mitterhofer AP. Long-term treatment of systemic lupus erythematosus with cyclosporin A. Arthritis Rheum 1997;40:27–35.
68. Francioni C, Galeazzi M, Fioravanti A, et al. Long term I.V. Ig treatment in systemic lupus eyrthematosus. Clin Exp Rheumatol 1994; 12:163–168.
69. Schroeder JO, Zeuner RA, Euler HH, Loffler H. High dose intravenous immunoglobulins in systemic lupus erythematosus: Clinical and serological results of a pilot study. J Rheumatol 1996;23:71–75.
70. Yoshida T, Kameda H, Ichikawa Y, et al. Improvement of renal function with a selective thromboxane A_2 synthetase inhibitor, DP-1904, in lupus nephritis. J Rheumatol 1996;23:1719–1724.
71. Pierucci A, Simonetti BM, Pecci G, et al. Improvement of renal function with selective thromboxane antagonism in lupus nephritis. N Engl J Med 1989;320:421–425.
72. Lin CY. Improvement in steroid and immunosuppressive drug resistant lupus nephritis by intraveous prostaglandin E_1 therapy. Nephron 1990;55:258–264.
73. Yoshikawa Y, Mizutani H, Shimizu M. Systemic lupus erythematosus with ischemic peripheral neuropathy and lupus anticoagulant: Response to intravenous prostaglandin E_1. Cutis 1996;58:393–396.
74. McGrath H. Ultraviolet-A1 irradiation decreases clinical disease activity and autoantibodies in patients with systemic lupus erythematosus. Clin Exp Rheumatol 1994;12:129–135.
75. Stafford FJ, Fleisher TA, Lee G, et al. A pilot study of anti-CD5 ricin A chain immunoconjugate in systemic lupus erythematosus. J Rheumatol 1994;21:2068–2070.
76. Wacholtz MC, Lipsky PE. Treatment of lupus nephritis with CD5 Plus, an immunoconjugate of an anti-CD5 monoclonal antibody and ricin A chain. Arthritis Rheum 1992;35:837–839.
77. Van Vollenhoven RF, Engleman EG, McGuire JL. Dehydroepiandrosterone in systemic lupus erythematosus. Results of double-blind, placebo-controlled, randomized clinical trial. Arthritis Rheum 1995;38:1826–1831.
78. McMurray RW, Weidensaul D, Allen SH, Walker SE. Efficacy of bromocriptine in an open label therapeutic trial for systemic lupus erythematosus. J Rheumatol 1995;22:2084–2091.
79. Cervera H, Jara LJ, Pizarro S, et al. Danazol for systemic lupus erythematosus with refractory autoimmune thrombocytopenia or Evans' syndrome. J Rheumatol 1995;22:1867–1871.
80. Lewis EJ, Hunsicker LG, Lan SP, et al. A controlled trial of plasmapheresis therapy in severe lupus nephritis. N Engl J Med 1992; 326:1373–1379.
81. Barron KS, Sher MR, Silverman ED. Intravenous immunoglobulin therapy: Magic or black magic. J Rheumatol 1992;19(suppl 3): 94–97.
82. Hayslett JP. The effect of systemic lupus erythematosus on pregnancy and pregnancy outcome. Am J Reprod Immunol 1992;28: 199–204.
83. Khamashta MA, Ruiz-Irastorza G, Hughes GRV. Systemic lupus erythematosus flares during pregnancy. Rheum Dis Clin North Am 1997;23:15–30.
84. Parke A, West B. Hydroxychloroquine in pregnant patients with systemic lupus erythematosus. J Rheumatol 1996;23:1715–1718.
85. Ramsey-Goldman R, Schilling E. Immunosuppressive drug use during pregnancy. Rheum Dis Clin North Am 1997;23:149–167.
86. Petri M. Systemic lupus erythematosus and pregnancy. Rheum Dis Clin North Am 1994;20:87–118.
87. Brennecke SP, Brown MA, Crowther CA, et al. Aspirin and prevention of preeclampsia. Aust N Z J Obstet Gynaecol 1995;35:38–41.
88. Mintz G, Niz J, Gutierrez G, et al. Prospective study of pregnancy in systemic lupus erythematosus. J Rheumatol 1986;13:732–739.
89. Khamashta MA, Cuadrado MJ, Mujic F, et al. The management of thrombosis in the antiphospholipid-antibody syndrome. N Engl J Med 1995;332:993–997.
90. Price EJ, Venables PJW. Drug-induced lupus. Drug Saf 1995;12: 283–290.
91. Yung RL, Richardson BC. Drug-induced lupus. Rheum Dis Clin North Am 1994;20:61–86.
92. Clarke AE, Esdaile JM, Bloch DA, et al. A Canadian study of total medical costs for patients with systemic lupus erythematosus and the predictors of costs. Arthritis Rheum 1993;36:1548–1559.
93. Gironimi G, Clarke AE, Hamilton VH, et al. Why health care costs more in the US. Comparing health care expenditures between systemic lupus erythematosus patients in Stanford and Montreal. Arthritis Rheum 1996;39:979–987.
94. Clarke AE, Bloch DA, Danoff DS, Esdaile JM. Decreasing costs and improving outcomes in systemic lupus erythematosus: Using regression trees to develop health policy. J Rheumatol 1994;21:2246–2253.
95. Lacaille D, Clarke AE, Bloch DA, et al. The impact of disease activity, treatment and disease severity on short term costs of systemic lupus erythematosus. J Rheumatol 1994;21:448–453.
96. McInnes PM, Schuttinga J, Sanslone WR, et al. The economic impact of treatment of severe lupus nephritis with prednisone and intravenous cyclophosphamide. Arthritis Rheum 1994;37:1000–1006.
97. Yarboro CH, Wesley R, Amantea MA, et al. Modified oral ondansetron regimen for cyclophosphamide-induced emesis in lupus nephritis. Ann Pharmacother 1996;30:752–755.
98. Miller M. Scleroderma. Aust Fam Physician 1993;22:2112–2119.
99. Perez MI, Kohn SR. Systemic sclerosis. J Am Acad Dermatol 1993;28:525–547.
100. Yost JH, Spencer-Green G. Diagnosis and management of vascular disease in systemic sclerosis. Compr Ther 1993;19:53–59.
101. Black CM. Scleroderma—clinical aspects. J Intern Med 1993;234: 115–118.
102. Dalakas MC. Clinical, immunopathologic, and therapeutic considerations of inflammatory myopathies. Clin Neuropharmacol 1992;15: 327–351.
103. Dalakas MC. Immunopathogenesis of inflammatory myopathies. Ann Neurol 1995;37(suppl 1):S74–86.
104. Targoff IN. Diagnosis and treatment of polymyositis and dermatomyositis. Compr Ther 1990;16:16–24.
105. Cronin ME. Treatment, pp 153–155, in Plotz PH (moderator): Current concepts in the idiopathic inflammatory myopathies: Polymyositis, dermatomyositis, and related disorders. Ann Intern Med 1989; 111:143–157.
106. Dalakas MC. Update on the use of intravenous immune globulin in the treatment of patients with inflammatory muscle disease. J Clin Immunol 1995;15(suppl 6):70S–75S.
107. Stander PE. Polymyalgia rheumatica. Clinical features and management. Postgrad Med 1989;86:131–138.
108. Goodwin JS. Progress in gerontology: Polymyalgia rheumatica and temporal arteritis. J Am Geriatr Soc 1992;40:515–525.
109. Lestico MR, Boh LE, Schuna AA. Polymyalgia rheumatica. Clin Pharm 1993;12:571–580.
110. Brooks RC, McGee SR. Diagnostic dilemmas in polymyalgia rheumatica. Arch Intern Med 1997;157:162–168.
111. Feinberg HL. Sherman JD, Schrepferman CG, et al. The use of methotrexate in polymyalgia rheumatica. J Rheumatol 1996;23: 1550–1552.
112. Fauci AS, Leavitt RY. Vasculitis. In: McCarty DJ, Koopman WJ, eds: Arthritis and Allied Conditions, 12th ed. Philadelphia, Lea & Febiger, 1993:1301–1322.
113. Gladman DD, Urowitz MB, Fortin P, et al. Systemic lupus international collaborating clinics conference on assessment of lupus flare and quality of life measures in SLE. J Rheumatol 1996;23: 1953–1955.

81

Allergic and Pseudoallergic Drug Reactions

Joseph T. DiPiro, PharmD, FCCP, Chester T. Stafford, MD, and Lauren S. Schlesselman, PharmD

"Allergic drug reactions" are adverse medication effects that involve immunologic mechanisms. Adverse drug effects not proven to be immune mediated, but resembling allergic reactions in their clinical presentation, are referred to as "allergic-like" or "pseudoallergic" reactions.[1]

Allergic reactions are responsible for up to 5% of reactions to medications among hospitalized patients.[2–5] The true frequency of allergic drug reactions is difficult to determine, because many reactions may not be reported and others may be difficult to distinguish from nonallergic adverse events. Dermatologic reactions represent the most common form of allergic drug reactions.

MECHANISMS OF ALLERGIC DRUG REACTIONS

Drugs can cause allergic reactions by a variety of immunologic mechanisms. Although some reactions are relatively well defined, the majority are due to mechanisms that are either unknown or poorly understood.

The following criteria suggest that a drug reaction may be immunologically mediated:[6] (1) The reaction occurs in a small percentage of patients receiving the drug, (2) the observed reaction does not resemble the drug's pharmacologic effect, (3) the type of manifestation is similar to that seen with other allergic reactions (e.g., anaphylaxis, urticaria, serum sickness), (4) there is a lag time between first exposure of the drug and reaction, (5) the reaction is reproduced even by minute doses of the drug, (6) the reaction is reproduced by agents with similar chemical structures, (7) eosinophilia is present, and (8) the reaction resolves after the drug has been discontinued. Exceptions to each of these criteria are commonly observed.

Many allergic reactions can be classified into one of four immunopathologic categories, types I, II, III, and IV (Table 81–1 and Figure 81–1).[7] Some drug reactions suspected of being immunologically mediated are considered possibly allergic. Examples include drug-associated skin eruptions, drug fever, drug-induced hepatitis, and interstitial nephritis. Other drug reactions can be classified as "pseudoallergic" or idiosyncratic. Examples include anaphylactoid (anaphylaxis-like) reactions to radiocontrast media, sulfite sensitivity, and reactions to local anesthetics.

EFFECTORS OF ALLERGIC DRUG REACTIONS

Allergic drug reactions can involve most of the major components of the immune system including the cellular elements, immunoglobulins, complement, and cytokines. Most immunoglobulin isotypes have been implicated in immunologically mediated drug reactions. Immunoglobulin E (IgE) bound to basophils or mast cells mediates immediate (anaphylactic-type) reactions. IgG or IgM antibodies may also be involved in allergic reactions, resulting in destruction of cells and tissues.

CELLULAR ELEMENTS

A variety of cells may be involved in immunologic drug reactions. Basophils, mast cells, eosinophils, and lymphocytes are most frequently involved. Platelets and vascular endothelial cells are also important because they can also release a number of inflammatory mediators. Most cells of the body, including nerve cells, can become directly or indirectly involved in allergic drug reactions.

Basophils and mast cells play prominent functional roles in immediate allergic reactions. They each have approximately 10^5 high-affinity cell surface receptors for IgE. Cross-linking of at least two cell surface IgE molecules by multivalent antigen is necessary to trigger mediator release. Bridging of cell surface IgE molecules and the resultant effect on histamine release for a type I hypersensitivity reaction is illustrated in Figure 81–1.

Basophils account for 0.5% to 2% of all circulating leukocytes. Mast cells are morphologically and biochemically distinct cells that reside in a variety of tissues of the skin and the respiratory and digestive tracts.[8] Both cells are believed to originate from a common hematopoietic stem cell.

MEDIATORS OF ALLERGIC REACTIONS[9]

The release of a number of preformed, pharmacologically active chemical mediators (histamine, serotonin, eosinophil chemotactic factor [ECF-A], neutrophil chemotactic factor [NCF-A], and bradykinin-generating factor, also known as basophil kalikrein of anaphylaxis [BK-A]) is triggered by antigen cross-linking IgE molecules on the surface of circulating basophils and tissue mast cells. Newly generated mediators include platelet-activating factor and arachidonic acid metabolites (prostaglandins, thromboxanes, leukotrienes). Each of these mediators is discussed in the following sections.

Histamine

Histamine is a low-molecular-weight amine compound formed by decarboxylation of histidine and stored in basophil and mast cell granules. The release of histamine

TABLE 81–1. Classification of Allergic Drug Reactions

Type	Descriptor	Characteristics	Typical Onset	Drug Causes
I	Anaphylactic (IgE mediated)	Allergen binds to IgE on basophils or mast cells resulting in release of inflammatory mediators	Within 30 min	Penicillin immediate reaction Blood products Polypeptide hormones Vaccines Dextran
II	Cytotoxic	Cell destruction occurs because of cell-associated antigen that initiates cytolysis by antigen-specific antibody (IgG or IgM). Most often involves blood elements.	Typically 5–12 h	Penicillin, quinidine, phenylbutazone, thiouracils, sulfonamides, methyldopa
III	Immune complex	Antigen–antibody complexes form and deposit on blood vessel walls and activate complement. Result is a serum-sickness-like syndrome.	3–8 h	May be caused by penicillins, sulfonamides, radiocontrast agents, hydantoins
IV	Cell mediated (delayed)	Antigens cause activation of lymphocytes, which release inflammatory mediators.	24–48 h	Tuberculin reaction

from these cells is triggered by antigen cross-linking with IgE on surface membranes of mast cells and basophils. One function of histamine is believed to be as a host defense against invasion by parasites. The tissue effects of histamine are evident within 1 to 2 minutes, but it is rapidly metabolized within 10 to 15 minutes. The major effects of histamine on target tissues include increased capillary permeability, contraction of bronchial and vascular smooth muscle, and hypersecretion of mucous glands.

Serotonin

Serotonin is also a low-molecular-weight amine stored in and released from platelets and mast cells. Its effects are similar to those of histamine. It may cause vasoconstriction or vasodilatation in some animal species but has no proven role in human anaphylaxis.

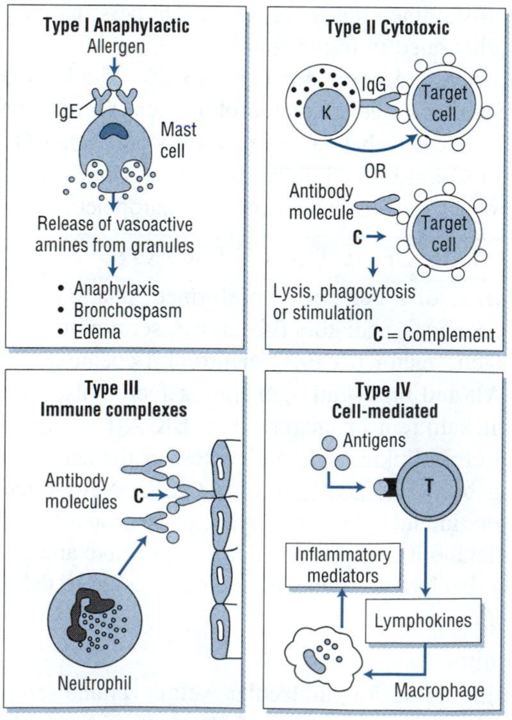

FIGURE 81–1. Types of hypersensitivity reactions.

Eosinophil Chemotactic Factor(s)

This group of preformed cellular tetrapeptides and dodecapeptides is released by stimulated mast cells. They attract eosinophils to inflammatory sites and participate in phagocytosis.

Neutrophil Chemotactic Factor

Neutrophil chemotactic factor is a high-molecular-weight protein that enhances neutrophil migration to areas of mast-cell activation.

Bradykinin Generating Factor

Bradykinin generating factor is a series of proteases that activate Hageman factor, resulting in the production of kinins, including bradykinin, which is more potent than histamine on a molar basis in causing vascular permeability and contraction of smooth muscle.

Platelet-activating Factor

Platelet-activating factor (PAF) is a glyceride-derived substance that is released by mast cells, alveolar macrophages, neutrophils, platelets, and other cells but not by basophils. It has potent bronchoconstrictor effects and also causes platelet aggregation and lysis. It attracts neutrophils and causes their activation. Also, PAF enhances vascular permeability and can cause pain, pruritus, and erythema.

Leukotrienes

The leukotrienes (LT) are metabolites of arachidonic acid produced through the 5-lipoxygenase pathway. They have potent effects on bronchial and vascular smooth muscle. Three important leukotrienes, LTC_4, LTD_4, and LTE_4, are produced by mast cells; however, LTC_4 is the major leukotriene produced by basophils and eosinophils. The leukotrienes have more potent bronchoconstrictor effects than histamine and can also increase vascular permeability and cause arteriolar vasoconstriction followed by vasodilatation. Their effects are slower in onset but longer lasting than those of histamine. They have previously been called the "slow-reacting substance of anaphylaxis" (SRS-A). Another product, leukotriene B_4 (LTB_4), is a potent chemoattractant, particularly for neutrophils. It is also produced by neutrophils, macrophages, and monocytes.

Prostaglandins and Thromboxanes

These are metabolites of arachidonic acid produced through the cyclooxygenase pathway. The actions of prostaglandins (PGs) vary considerably. Some have vasoconstrictive and/or bronchodilatory properties, whereas others are vasodilatory (e.g., PGD_2) and/or bronchoconstrictive (e.g., $PGF_{2\alpha}$). PGD_2 is the major prostaglandin product of mast cells. It is a potent inhibitor of platelet aggregation. Thromboxanes cause platelet aggregation and are important regulators of coagulation.

Complement

The complement system consists of approximately 20 plasma proteins. They are involved in a variety of immunologic responses, including enhancement of phagocytosis through opsonization of target cells, cell lysis, and generation of anaphylatoxins (C3a, C4a, and C5a), which can cause non–IgE-mediated activation of mast cells and release of inflammatory mediators.

CLASSIFICATION OF IMMUNOPATHOLOGIC DRUG REACTIONS

Immunologic mechanisms have been identified for some drug reactions. Many can be classified into one of four immunopathologic reactions, as follows.

TYPE I

Type I reactions require the presence of IgE specific for the drug antigen or other allergen. It is assumed that on initial exposure to the antigen, predisposed individuals produce IgE specific for the drug allergen. IgE binds to basophils and mast cells. On repeat exposure to the antigen, two or more IgE molecules on the basophil or mast cell surface may be bound by one multivalent antigen molecule (referred to as cross-linking) (Figure 81–1). This binding initiates a signal to the cell and the cell becomes activated. Activation causes the extracellular release of granules with preformed inflammatory mediators including histamine, serotonin, heparin, proteases (tryptase in the mast cell), bradykinin-generating factor, eosinophil chemotactic factors, and neutrophil chemotactic factor, as well as generation of newly formed mediators as previously discussed. Substances in the latter category are mostly lipid metabolites from arachidonic acid, which is a major component of cell walls. Arachidonic acid metabolites include leukotrienes, prostaglandins, thromboxanes, and PAF among others. Most of these substances are produced by the activated mast cell; however, only one leukotriene (LTC_4) is produced by the basophil.

Generation of a type I reaction can be evident as an immediate hypersensitivity reaction, or anaphylaxis. Anaphylaxis can occur on a local basis, typically in the nasal mucosa (rhinitis), respiratory tract (acute asthma), skin, or GI tract; or anaphylaxis may be generalized.

A prototype of a type I reaction is the immediate anaphylactic reaction after benzylpenicillin exposure in sensitized individuals. It is assumed that a person has had an initial exposure to benzylpenicillin and then produces IgE specific for the benzylpenicilloate or other penicillin metabolites. On subsequent exposure the benzylpenicillin or metabolite bound to a macromolecule (e.g., albumin) cross-links IgE that is on the surface of basophils and mast cells. The result is an immediate hypersensitivity or anaphylactic reaction.

TYPE II

Type II immunopathologic reactions involve destruction of host cells (usually blood cells) through cytotoxic antibodies by one of two mechanisms (Figure 81– 1). First, the drug as antigen binds to the cell (e.g., the platelet or red blood cell). Antibodies (IgG or IgM) specific for the bound drug, or to a component of the cell surface that has been altered by the drug, then bind, initiating a cytolytic reaction. The cell destruction may be mediated by complement or by phagocytic cells that have Fc receptors on their surface. Activation of complement near the cell surface can result in loss of cell membrane integrity and cell death. Alternatively, neutrophils, monocytes, or macrophages may bind to the cell coated with antibody bound by IgG Fc receptors on the attacking cell surface. The result is phagocytosis of the target cell. The process of enhancement of phagocytosis by antibody-covered cell surface is referred to as opsonization. In addition, cell-bound IgG may direct the nonphagocytic action of T cells or natural killer cells, which results in cell destruction by a process called antibody-dependent cellular cytotoxicity (ADCC). This process can proceed in a nonspecific fashion, as T cells bind to the target cell through IgG Fc receptors on the T-cell surface. Contact is necessary between the target and effector cell.

Cells commonly affected by these types of reactions include erythrocytes, leukocytes, and platelets, resulting in hemolytic anemia, agranulocytosis, or thrombocytopenia, respectively. This process may be initiated by drugs such as penicillin, quinidine, quinine, phenacetin, cephalosporins, and sulfonamides, among others. For a complete discussion of this topic see Chapter 94.

Another type of reaction that may affect the formed elements in blood is the "innocent bystander" reaction. With this type of reaction, antigen–antibody complexes formed in blood bind nonspecifically to cells. Complement is then activated, resulting in cell lysis.

TYPE III

Type III immunologic reactions are caused by antigen–antibody complexes that are formed in blood. The complexes form with drug allergen and antibody in varying ratios, and may deposit in tissues, resulting in local or disseminated inflammatory reactions. Antigen–antibody complex formation can result in platelet aggregation, complement activation, or macrophage activation. When complement is activated, C3a, C4a, and C5a (anaphylatoxins) may be formed and can cause vascular permeability changes and mast-cell activation. The latter leads to release and production of inflammatory mediators as discussed previously. Chemotactic substances such as C4b are also produced, and they cause the influx of neutrophils and result in the release of a number of toxic substances from the neutrophil (e.g., proteinases, collagenases, kinin-generating enzymes, and reactive oxygen and nitrogen substances), which can cause local tissue destruction.

Platelet aggregation may also occur as a result of immune complex formation. Activation of platelets may result in the formation of microthrombi and the release of vasoactive mediators. Also, insoluble complexes may be phagocytized by macrophages and activate these cells.

The formation of antigen–antibody complexes can lead to a number of clinical syndromes. The Arthus reaction is an example. In this model, a high level of preformed specific IgG antibody combines with antigen to produce a localized edematous, erythematous reaction within 5 to 8 hours. The reaction involves local formation of insoluble antigen–antibody complexes, complement activation with anaphylatoxin release, mast cell degranulation, and influx of polymorphonuclear cells.

TYPE IV

Type IV immunopathologic reactions are mediated by T cells and involve delayed hypersensitivity. Type IV reactions require memory T cells specific for the antigen in question. On exposure to the antigen the T cells become activated and produce an inflammatory response. Although these reactions may be associated with adverse effects (e.g., contact dermatitis), they may also be useful for diagnostic purposes. Examples of the latter include the use of the purified protein derivative (PPD) antigen from *Mycobacterium tuberculosis* used in the tuberculin skin test and other recall skin test antigens, such as mumps. After intradermal injection, these antigens produce a local reaction (erythema and induration) within 48 to 72 hours. Delayed contact hypersensitivity can also be caused by a wide variety of chemicals and drugs.

OTHER ALLERGIC REACTIONS

The mechanism of many allergic reactions is not known, although they are believed to be immune mediated. Perhaps most common are the delayed dermatologic reactions that occur with a variety of drugs (especially penicillins and sulfonamides). These reactions may be evident as macropapular, morbilliform, or erythematous rashes; exfoliative dermatitis; photosensitivity reactions; or eczema. These reactions often cause pruritus, urticaria, and angioedema.

Other serious dermatologic syndromes may be the result of immunologic reactions. These include Stevens–Johnson syndrome, characterized by rash, erythema multiforme with mucous membrane involvement, and toxic epidermal necrolysis (widespread blister formation in the epidermis), which are referred to as febrile mucocutaneous syndromes. Drugs commonly associated with these syndromes include the penicillin and sulfonamide antibiotics as well as a number of other agents. Drug-induced fever may also involve immunologic mechanisms. Other general types of reactions believed to be immune mediated include hepatic drug reactions (cholestatic or hepatocellular) and pulmonary reactions, for example, interstitial pneumonitis, which has been associated with nitrofurantoin.

ANAPHYLACTOID REACTIONS

A number of substances can produce an anaphylactoid (anaphylaxis-like) reaction that is similar to anaphylaxis in clinical signs and symptoms. The substances causing these reactions can produce the direct release of inflammatory mediators from cells, possibly by a pharmacologic effect, but this is not believed to occur through cell-bound IgE. These reactions are sometimes referred to as "pseudoallergic." Drugs that can produce anaphylactoid reactions include opiates, iodinated radiocontrast agents, vancomycin, amphotericin, and D-tubocurarine. A number of other agents may produce anaphylactoid reactions by altering the metabolism of inflammatory mediators such as prostaglandins or kinins.

CLINICAL MANIFESTATIONS OF ALLERGIC AND ALLERGIC-LIKE REACTIONS

ANAPHYLAXIS

Anaphylaxis is an acute, life-threatening allergic reaction involving multiple organ systems.[10,11] Although many drugs have been reported to cause anaphylaxis those most commonly reported are aspirin and other nonsteroidal anti-inflammatory drugs, penicillins, and insulins.[12] The manifestations of anaphylaxis may include signs and symptoms referable to the skin, gastrointestinal (GI) tract, respiratory tract, and cardiovascular system. Patients may experience adverse effects involving any combination of these systems. Common dermatologic manifestations include urticaria, angioedema, and pruritus.[12] GI manifestations include nausea, abdominal pain, vomiting, and diarrhea. With respiratory tract involvement the patient may experience dyspnea or wheezing. The major cardiovascular manifestations include hypotension, tachycardia, and arrhythmias.

Anaphylactic reactions generally begin within 30 minutes, but almost always within 2 hours after exposure to the inciting allergen. The risk of fatal anaphylaxis is greatest within the first few hours. After apparent recovery, anaphylaxis may recur 6 to 8 hours after antigen exposure. Because of the possibility of these "late-phase" reactions, patients should be observed for at least 12 hours after an anaphylactic reaction. Fatal anaphylaxis most often results from asphyxia due to laryngeal edema or from cardiovascular collapse.

SERUM SICKNESS

Serum sickness is a clinical syndrome resulting from the effects of soluble circulating immune complexes that form under conditions of antigen excess. The reaction commonly results from the use of heterologous antisera containing foreign (donor) antigens such as equine serum in the form of antitoxins or antivenins. The onset of serum sickness usually occurs 7 to 14 days after antigen administration. Fever, malaise, and lymphadenopathy are the most common clinical manifestations. Arthralgias, urticaria, and morbilliform skin eruption may also be present. Although often associated with administration of heterologous antisera, serum sickness may also be caused by drugs, including sulfonamides, hydantoins, penicillins, and cephalosporins (especially cefaclor). In addition, immune complex–mediated systemic lupus erythematosus–like syndrome has been attributed to reactions from drugs such as hydralazine, procainamide, isoniazid, and phenytoin.

DRUG FEVER

Fever may occur in response to an inflammatory process, or develop as a manifestation of a drug reaction. Drug fever occurs in as many as 10% of hospital inpatients.[13] A large number of drugs have been reported to cause fever, including methyldopa, procainamide, phenytoin, barbiturates, quinidine, and a variety of antibiotics. These drugs may directly affect the central nervous system to alter temperature regulation, or stimulate the release of endogenous pyrogens (e.g., interleukin-1 and tumor necrosis factor) from white blood cells. Drugs may also cause fever as a result of their pharmacologic effects on tissues, for example, fever resulting from massive tumor cell destruction caused by chemotherapy. However, the mechanism of drug fever remains unknown for agents such as amphotericin B and radiographic contrast agents.

The temperature pattern of drug-induced fever is quite variable. It may be low grade and continuous or spiking and intermittent. A temporal relationship between drug administration and occurrence of fever has been noted for some medications. Generally, withdrawal of the causative agent results in prompt defervescence as soon as the drug is completely metabolized. Fever usually recurs on readministration of the causative agent.

DRUG-INDUCED AUTOIMMUNITY

Autoimmune diseases have been associated with drugs and may involve a variety of tissues and organs. A commonly recognized drug-related autoimmune disorder is systemic lupus erythematosus (SLE) induced by procainamide, hydralazine, or isoniazid (see Chap. 80). Other drugs associated with SLE include methyldopa, β-adrenergic blockers, penicillamine, quinidine, interferon-α, and sulfasalazine.[14] The most common clinical manifestations include arthralgias, myalgias, and polyarthritis. Facial rash, ulcers, and alopecia occur less frequently. Renal or pulmonary involvement may also occur. These reactions typically develop several months after beginning the drug and generally resolve soon after it is discontinued.[15]

Other syndromes believed to involve autoimmune mechanisms include drug-induced hemolytic anemia due to methyldopa, renal interstitial nephritis produced by methicillin, and hepatitis caused by phenytoin and halothane. Interstitial nephritis is characterized by fever, rash, and eosinophilia associated with proteinuria and hematuria. Hepatic damage due to drugs is generally manifested as either hepatocellular necrosis or cholestatic hepatitis. Drug-induced hepatitis has been associated with phenothiazines, sulfonamides, halothane, phenytoin, and isoniazid (see Chap. 36). Hepatocellular destruction is evidenced by elevations in serum transaminases. Hepatomegaly and jaundice may sometimes be evident. Cholestasis may be manifested by jaundice and elevations in serum alkaline phosphatase, and sometimes by rash, fever, and eosinophilia.

VASCULITIS

Vasculitis is a clinicopathologic process characterized by inflammation and necrosis of blood vessels. The vasculitic process may be limited to the skin or may involve multiple organs, including the liver or kidney, joints, or central nervous system. Characteristically, cutaneous vasculitis is manifested by purpuric lesions that vary in size and number. Vasculitis may also be manifested as papules, nodules, ulcerations, or vesiculobullous lesions, generally occurring on the lower extremities, but the upper extremities, including the hands, may also be involved. Drugs associated with vasculitis include allopurinol, β-lactam antibiotics, sulfonamides, thiazide diuretics, and phenytoin.

DERMATOLOGIC REACTIONS

A wide variety of dermatologic drug reactions have been reported to have an immunologic basis.[16] As previously noted, cutaneous reactions are the most common manifestations of allergic drug reactions. Although most dermatologic reactions are mild and resolve promptly after discontinuing the drug, some may progress to serious or even life-threatening reactions (e.g., toxic epidermal necrolysis or Stevens–Johnson syndrome). Serious dermatologic drug reactions are estimated to occur in 1.9 cases per one million people per year and can have a mortality rate as high as 40%.[17,18] Table 81–2 lists drugs and agents most commonly associated with cutaneous reactions.[19] Antimicrobials are implicated most frequently. The clinical presentation of dermatologic drug reactions is discussed in more detail in Chapter 89.

TABLE 81–2. Top 10 Drugs or Agents Reported to Cause Skin Reactions

	Reactions per 1000 Recipients
Amoxicillin	51.4
Trimethoprim-sulfamethoxazole	33.8
Ampicillin	33.2
Iopodate	27.8
Blood	21.6
Cephalosporins	21.1
Erythromycin	20.4
Dihydralazine hydrochloride	19.1
Penicillin G	18.5
Cyanocobalamin	17.9

Adapted from Ref. 19.

RESPIRATORY REACTIONS

Drugs may also produce upper or lower respiratory tract reactions, including rhinitis and asthma. Respiratory tract manifestations may result from direct injury to the airway or may occur as a component of a systemic reaction (e.g., anaphylaxis). Asthma may be induced by aspirin and other nonsteroidal anti-inflammatory agents as discussed in the following paragraphs, or by sulfites used as preservatives in foods and medications. Other pulmonary drug reactions believed to be immunologic include acute infiltrative and chronic fibrotic pulmonary reactions. The latter is often caused by antineoplastics such as bleomycin. For a more detailed discussion of drug-induced pulmonary disease see Chapter 94.

HEMATOLOGIC REACTIONS

Most formed elements and soluble components of the hematopoietic system may be affected by immunologic drug reactions. Eosinophilia is a common manifestation of drug hypersensitivity and may be the only presenting sign. Hemolytic anemia may result from hypersensitivity to drugs. Other hematologic reactions include thrombocytopenia, granulocytopenia, and agranulocytosis. For a detailed discussion of hematologic drug reactions see Chapter 94.

FACTORS RELATED TO OCCURRENCE OR SEVERITY OF ALLERGIC DRUG REACTIONS

A number of factors influence the likelihood of allergic drug reactions. Among these are the dose of the allergen, the route of exposure, and the sensitivity of the individual as determined by age, genetics, or environmental factors. For many drugs, the severity of a reaction is determined by the dose and the duration of exposure. A relatively larger dose or longer duration of treatment encourages development of drug sensitivity. The route of administration also influences drug sensitivity. The topical route of drug administration appears to be the most likely to sensitize and predispose to drug reactions. The oral route is the safest and the parenteral route is the most hazardous for administration of drugs in sensitive individuals. There are relatively few reported cases of immediate hypersensitivity-associated deaths with oral β-lactam antimicrobials. Although intravenous administration is more likely to result in severe immediate reactions in a sensitized individual, it may be the least likely route for initially inducing sensitivity. One possible explanation is that intravenous administration results in systemic drug exposure for the shortest period of time.

Individual host factors are also important in determining drug sensitivity. There may be a genetic predisposition for some types of allergic reactions. Slow acetylators of procainamide and hydralazine are at increased risk for lupus erythematosus.

In general, the risk of drug allergy appears to be increased in patients who are atopic (history of allergic rhinitis, asthma, and/or atopic dermatitis). In addition, patients with a history of drug allergy appear to be at increased risk of adverse reactions to other pharmacologic agents. Age seems to be related to the risk of allergic reactions since they occur less frequently in children. This may be related to immaturity of the immune system or decreased exposure. The presence of concurrent diseases predisposes to drug reactions. Examples include the morbilliform rash, which occurs after ampicillin administration to patients with infectious mononucleosis, the reactions that occur with trimethoprim-sulfamethoxazole in AIDS patients, and allergic reactions with blood products, which occur in patients with IgA deficiency.

DRUGS COMMONLY CAUSING ALLERGIC OR ALLERGIC-LIKE DRUG REACTIONS

In general, small-molecular-weight (MW) compounds (less than 10,000 MW) are not immunogenic. Most drugs are less than 1000 MW. To become immunogenic, these small compounds must first combine with carrier proteins in plasma or tissue. Penicillin G (356 MW) is an example of a drug that binds covalently to serum proteins through amide or disulfide linkages. For drugs like sulfonamides, the parent compound must first be converted to a metabolite before it can combine with the macromolecule. The species that combines with the carrier macromolecule is referred to as a hapten or an incomplete antigen. Some macromolecular drugs such as insulin are referred to as complete antigens because they do not require binding with another molecule to evoke an immune response.

In some cases the inciting allergen may not actually be the drug itself but contaminants of the drug product. For example, frequent reactions to early penicillin preparations were attributed to impurities. In addition, drug additives may also cause allergic reactions. Dyes, preservatives, and a variety of excipients have been implicated.

β-LACTAM ANTIMICROBIALS

Allergic reactions to penicillin occur in 0.7% to 8% of treatment courses.[20] The most common reactions to penicillin include urticaria, pruritus, and angioedema. One in 10 allergic reactions is life-threatening and about 10% of these are fatal. All four of the major types of hypersensitivity reactions have been reported with penicillin, as well as some reactions that do not fit into these categories. A wide variety of idiopathic reactions occur, for example, maculopapular eruptions, eosinophilia, Stevens–Johnson syndrome, and exfoliative dermatitis. Maculopapular rash occurs in about 2% of treatment courses of penicillin and in 5.2% to 9.5% with ampicillin. The incidence of ampicillin rash increases to 69% to 100% in patients with Epstein–Barr virus infection, cytomegalovirus infection, or acute lymphocytic leukemia.

Some aspects of the mechanism of penicillin immunogenicity have been determined. Because benzylpenicillin is a relatively small molecule (MW 356), it must combine with macromolecules (usually proteins) to elicit an immune response. Penicillin may covalently bind to the lysine residues of proteins such as albumin through an amide linkage involving the β-lactam ring (Figure 81–2). This is the penicilloyl–protein conjugate and is referred to as the "major antigenic determinant." In addition, a number of other penicillin metabolites may covalently bind to proteins. These are referred to as "minor antigenic determinants." The terms major and minor refer to the relative proportions of these conjugates that are formed and not to the clinical severity of the reactions generated. In fact, the minor antigenic determinants are more likely to cause anaphylactic reactions. The humoral immune response to penicillin has been well studied. From one report of 60 patients that received 3 or more grams per day of penicillin for at least 10 days, 38% had detectable IgG response to benzylpenicilloyl groups and 18% had detectable IgE response.[21] Immediate hypersensitivity reactions may be mediated by IgE for minor as well as major determinants.

Patients who are allergic to penicillins may also be sensitive to other β-lactams. The exact incidence of cross-reactivity between cephalosporins and penicillins is not known, although it is believed to be low.

Some allergists would administer cephalosporins to patients who had history of hives from penicillin.[22] Results of skin testing with cephalosporins may not be reliable because the mechanism of cephalosporin sensitivity has not been clearly defined. The incidence of cephalosporin reactions is minimally if at all increased in patients with histories of penicillin allergy.[23] At present, patients with positive penicillin skin tests are advised not to receive cephalosporins if they can be avoided. Patients who have experienced only mild, cutaneous reactions, such as maculopapular rashes, may receive cephalosporins with caution.

Other new β-lactam derivatives (monobactams and carbapenems) have been studied for potential cross-reactivity with penicillins. *In vitro* and *in vivo* studies have demonstrated that the monobactam aztreonam only weakly cross-reacts with penicillin and that it may be safely administered to most patients who are penicillin allergic.[24,25] In contrast, there appears to be considerable cross-reactivity between imipenem (a carbapenem), and penicillin. Therefore, imipenem (and other carbapenems) should not be administered to patients who have positive penicillin skin tests.

RADIOCONTRAST MEDIA

Radiocontrast agents frequently cause allergic-like reactions because these agents are commonly used in medical practice. Five percent to 10% of patients receiving radiocontrast agents experience some type of adverse reaction. Of the variety of reactions reported, approximately 1% are urticarial, 0.25% dyspnea, and severe reactions occur as frequently as 0.01%. In addition, radiocontrast agents may cause dose-dependent toxic reactions that can cause cardiovascular effects, arrhythmias, changes in renal blood flow, diuresis, or proteinuria.[26,27]

The mechanism of reactions to radiocontrast agents is not clearly understood. Allergic-like reactions are not IgE mediated. Potential mechanisms of reactivity include the

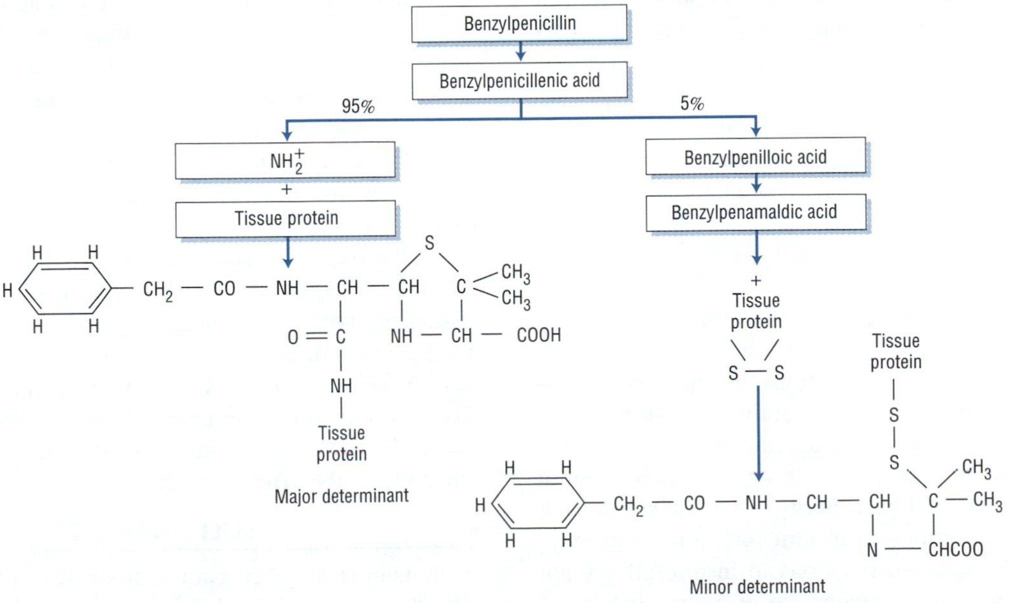

FIGURE 81–2. Formation of the benzyl penicilloyl hapten–protein complex.

activation of complement directly by the radiocontrast agents.[28] Also, the older radiocontrast agents have a high osmolarity, and it is possible that they can directly activate mast cells and basophils (IgE-independent mechanism), resulting in the release of inflammatory mediators.[29] Relatively new, low-osmolar contrast agents appear to result in fewer anaphylactoid reactions. In a report of 800 intravascular procedures, the frequency of immediate generalized reactions to high-osmolar radiocontrast agents was 9.1%. This contrasted with a frequency of 0.5% of 181 intravascular procedures, using low-osmolar agents in patients who had previously experienced an immediate generalized reaction with high-osmolar agents.[30] The relative risk of having a reaction to a lower osmolarity, nonionic agent is estimated to be at least five times lower than with conventional agents.[26]

Patients at risk of reactions from radiocontrast agents are difficult to identify. History is helpful, because a patient who has experienced previous reactions is more likely to experience subsequent reactions. The risk of allergic reactions to radiocontrast media is greater in patients with a history of atopy or asthma.[26] Despite a common misconception, a seafood allergy does not appear to predispose to radiocontrast media reactions. Skin testing or oral testing is not useful with these agents. Some regimens have been recommended to prevent reactions in patients who have previously experienced them. One pretreatment regimen includes the administration of prednisone 50 mg orally 13, 7, and 1 hours before the procedure, diphenhydramine 50 mg orally or intramuscularly 1 hour before the procedure, and 25 mg ephedrine orally 1 hour before.[31] The ephedrine should be omitted if the patient has angina, arrhythmia, or hypertension. Guidelines have been published for treatment of acute reactions to contrast media.[26,32]

INSULIN

Insulin is capable of producing a variety of allergic reactions. A protein molecule, insulin is a complete antigen. It may be of beef, pork, or human (recombinant) origin. Allergic reactions to insulin have been reported from all three sources. Reactions to insulin may involve the insulin molecule itself or other substances that have been added to insulin (e.g., protamine). Insulin may cause reactions through a variety of immunologic mechanisms. The majority of patients have anti-insulin antibodies after a few months of therapy.

Insulin reactions may be limited to the site of injection or they may produce systemic reactions. Local reactions most often present as a wheal and flare at the injection site and may occur immediately after injection or up to 8 to 12 hours later. Generally, these reactions are mild, do not require treatment, and resolve with continued insulin administration. If a patient does not tolerate the local reaction well, antihistamines may be given or a different insulin source (or product of higher purity) may be substituted. Rarely, systemic reactions to insulin (urticaria or anaphylaxis) occur. IgE-mediated reactions to insulin allergy appear to be declining with greater use of human insulins.[33] Skin testing with various products can aid in selecting the type of insulin least likely to cause a systemic reaction. Human insulin appears to be least allergenic but may occasionally cause reactions. In some patients, insulin desensitization may be indicated.

ASPIRIN AND NSAIDs

Aspirin and other nonsteroidal anti-inflammatory drugs (NSAIDs) produce characteristic reactions in susceptible patients.[34,35] The two general types of reactions to aspirin are urticaria/angioedema and rhinosinusitis/asthma. Approximately 1% of the population exposed to NSAIDs experiences urticaria or angioedema whereas about 0.5% experiences rhinosinusitis/asthma.[36,37]

The rhinosinusitis/asthma syndrome typically develops in middle-aged patients who are nonatopic and have no history of aspirin intolerance. Generally, it progresses from rhinitis to sinusitis with nasal polyps and steroid-dependent asthma. It is uncommon in children and young adults. However, children with asthma may be aspirin sensitive. In retrospective studies 1.9% to 5.6% of asthmatics are aspirin sensitive,[38] whereas up to 40% of steroid-dependent asthmatics may be aspirin sensitive.[39] In aspirin-sensitive asthmatics, administration of aspirin and NSAIDs may provoke an asthmatic attack. Ketorolac can cause severe, life-threatening bronchospasm in aspirin-sensitive asthmatics.[40] The mechanism of aspirin sensitivity is not completely understood. One suspected mechanism of aspirin and NSAID sensitivity is cyclooxygenase blockade, which may facilitate production of alternative arachidonic acid metabolites (e.g., leukotrienes). This is supported by the observation that the reaction occurs with other NSAIDs but infrequently with acetaminophen or salicylates. It is possible that aspirin and NSAIDs may directly stimulate mast cells to release inflammatory mediators. Also, subjects with aspirin-induced asthma have a marked increase in airway responsiveness to leukotrienes.[41]

In patients with asthma or those suspected of being sensitive to aspirin, an oral or inhalation challenge can be performed. This should be performed with great caution, in a hospital setting, with resuscitation equipment at hand. For patients known to be aspirin sensitive the major preventive measure is avoidance. Other agents reported to be cross-reactive with aspirin include tartrazine dye, indomethacin, and phenylbutazone.

NSAIDs have also been associated with pulmonary infiltrates and eosinophilia (PIE) syndrome. This syndrome is associated with fever, cough, dyspnea, infiltrates on chest roentgenogram, and a peripheral eosinophilia that develop 2 to 6 weeks after initiating treatment. PIE syndrome has been reported more frequently for naproxen compared with other NSAIDs and is noted to resolve rapidly after discontinuation of the offending agent.[42]

SULFONAMIDES

Sulfonamide drugs are a common cause of allergic reactions. These agents are included in a number of drug classes including antimicrobials, diuretics, oral hypoglycemics, and carbonic anhydrase inhibitors. Although immediate reactions can occur, sulfonamides typically cause delayed cutaneous reactions, often beginning with fever then followed by a rash (morbilliform eruptions, erythema multiforme, or, less frequently, toxic epidermal necrolysis).[43] Other reactions to sulfonamides may include mucocutaneous, GI, hepatic, renal, or hematologic complications, which may be fatal. It is believed that sulfonamide reactions are immune mediated and involve the production of reactive metabolites (hydroxylamines).[44]

Trimethoprim-sulfamethoxazole (TMP-SMZ) is frequently used for preventive or active treatment of *Pneumocystis carinii* pneumonia in patients with the acquired immunodeficiency syndrome (AIDS). Adverse reactions to TMP-SMZ have been observed to occur much more frequently in these patients compared to those without AIDS. Adverse effects to TMP-SMZ occur in 50% to 80% of AIDS patients compared with 10% in other immunocompromised patients.[45] TMP-SMZ was associated with an adverse event rate of 26.3 per 100 person-years and hypersensitivity events at 22 per 100 person-years. Adverse event rate was related to lower $CD4^+$ cell count. When $CD4^+$ cell count was < 100, the adverse drug event rate was 31 per 100 person-years.[46]

EXCIPIENTS

Pharmaceutical products contain a number of "inert" additives (e.g., dyes, fillers, buffers, stabilizers) in addition to the therapeutic ingredient. These ingredients are not always inert and may cause adverse effects, including allergic reactions.

TARTRAZINE

The azo dye tartrazine (FD&C Yellow 5) is associated with anaphylactoid reactions, acute bronchospasm, urticaria, rhinitis, and contact dermatitis. Although the immunologic mechanisms are unclear, approximately 10% of aspirin-sensitive asthmatics are also intolerant to tartrazine,[47–49] suggesting a role of tartrazine as a cyclooxygenase inhibitor. As little as 0.85 μg or as much as 25 mg of tartrazine have provoked positive responses.[47]

SULFITES

Sulfites (including sulfur dioxide, sodium sulfite, sodium and potassium bisulfite, and sodium and potassium metabisulfite) are commonly used as antioxidants in pharmaceutical products and some foods. Over 250 cases of adverse reactions associated with ingestion of sulfites (usually in foods) have been reported to the FDA,[50] including wheezing, dyspnea, chest tightness, urticaria, angioedema, flushing, weakness, nausea, anaphylaxis, and death. Although the FDA has banned the use of sulfites in fresh fruits and vegetables, they were not banned in drug products because of the lack of a suitable substitute.

IgE-mediated and nonimmunologic sulfite hypersensitivity has been demonstrated in children with a history of chronic asthma. Adverse reactions to sulfite-preserved injectables, such as gentamicin, metoclopramide, and doxycycline, have been reported. In contrast to reactions caused by foods, these reactions do not occur more frequently in steroid-dependent asthmatics and do not always coincide with a positive oral sulfite challenge.[51] Blunted bronchodilation may be observed in asthmatics following inhalation of sulfite-containing nebulizer solutions. Although many nebulizer solutions contain sulfites, metered-dose inhalers do not. Many aqueous epinephrine products also contain sulfites. The FDA labeling states that, in emergency situations when sulfite-free preparations are not available, sulfite-containing epinephrine should not be withheld from a sulfite-intolerant individual because small subcutaneous doses of sulfites are usually well-tolerated. However, an increased risk of anaphylaxis exists after subcutaneous injection in those rare patients with a positive oral challenge to 5 to 10 mg of sulfite.

PARABENS

Parabens (including methyl, ethyl, propyl, and butylparaben) are widely used in pharmaceutical products as a biocidal agent. The majority of allergic reactions to parabens are observed after topical exposure. Delayed hypersensitivity contact dermatitis occurs more often in individuals with preexisting dermatitis.[47] Immediate hypersensitivity after parenteral administration is rare. Although chemically related to benzoic acid and *p*-aminobenzoic acid, the evidence for cross-sensitivity is lacking.[47]

LATEX AS AN ALLERGEN

The recognition of latex sensitivity has increased dramatically over the past decade. Several hundred reports of immediate and delayed hypersensitivity reactions to latex have been reported to the FDA, including more than a dozen deaths.[52] Adverse reactions include dyspnea, bronchospasm, anxiety, urticaria, flushing, and anaphylaxis.

Reactions due to dry rubber latex products (e.g., vial stoppers, syringe plungers, and injection ports) are less frequent than to natural rubber products (e.g., medical gloves, condoms, and catheters).[53] Several latex proteins (e.g., rubber elongation factor, prenyltransferase, and hevein) have been implicated in the IgE-mediated reactions.[52] Cross-sensitivity has been documented in individuals allergic to various foods, including bananas, kiwi, chestnut, papaya, plums, avocados, and peaches.

Although the prevalence of latex allergy among the general population remains less than 5%, high-risk individuals have been identified, including spina bifida patients, patients having undergone recurrent surgical procedures, and health care professionals. An increased exposure to latex may account for the increased incidence of latex-specific IgE found among these individuals. Atopic individuals within these groups may be at an even greater risk.

The frequency of latex allergy among patients with neural tube defects ranges from 12% to 65%.[54] These patients undergo frequent catheterization, enemas, and bowel disempactions, allowing for increased exposure to latex-containing medical supplies.

Because of the ubiquity of latex-containing supplies within the medical setting, patients undergoing recurrent surgical procedures experience increased exposure to latex. Latex is readily absorbed through internal tissue during invasive procedures. Patients undergoing urologic procedures involving instumentation of the bladder appear to have a greater risk of developing latex sensitivity.

With the institution of universal precautions as a means to avoid occupational hazards of blood-borne pathogens, the use of protective gloves became standard practice. The appearance of latex allergy as a serious medical problem has been associated with this regulation. An estimated 250,000 health care professionals are allergic to latex.[54]

Patient and health care provider education is crucial to decrease latex exposure through environment modification. Health care providers should be alerted to high-risk groups. Lists of latex-containing medications and devices, along with reasonable substitutes, are necessary in high-risk environments, including pharmacies, nursing homes, and surgical suites.

▶ TREATMENT: Allergic Reactions

The basic principles for management of allergic reactions to drugs or biologic agents includes (1) discontinuation of the medication or agent when possible, (2) treatment of the adverse clinical signs and symptoms, and (3) substitution, if necessary, of another agent.[1]

Identification of patients at high risk for allergic drug reactions requires a careful history and, where appropriate, performance of specific tests to evaluate sensitivity. One of the most helpful tests to evaluate risk is the allergen skin test. For some drugs, skin testing can demonstrate the presence of drug-specific IgE and predict a relatively high risk of immediate hypersensitivity reactions. Note that skin testing does not predict the risk of delayed or most dermatologic reactions.

A higher proportion of patients report an "allergic reaction" to penicillin than actually experience a reaction. However, patients with a history of penicillin allergy are recognized to have a fourfold to sixfold greater risk of subsequent reactions.[20] In addition, a negative history of penicillin allergy does not eliminate the risk of immediate reactions, because many serious and even fatal allergic reactions to β-lactam antibiotics occur in patients who have no history of penicillin allergy.[20]

Skin testing can reduce the uncertainty of β-lactam sensitivity and should be performed in all patients who have a history of β-lactam allergy and require treatment with these agents. Testing for the major penicillin determinant is accomplished with penicilloyl-polylysine (PPL; Pre-Pen, Kremers-Urban). If this agent alone is used, patients reacting only to minor determinants will be missed. At present, there is no commercially available product that can be used to test for most of the minor determinants. Benzylpenicillin (at a concentration of 10,000 U/mL) has been used; however, some reactive patients will still be missed. Penicillin skin testing can facilitate the safe use of penicillin in 90% of patients with a history of penicillin allergy.[55] The procedure for performing penicillin skin testing is presented in Table 81–3.

The National Institute of Allergy and Infectious Diseases reported a collaborative trial to test the predictive value of skin testing with major and minor penicillin derivatives.[56] The frequency of IgE-mediated reactions was 1.2% and 0% (568 patients) with positive and negative history of penicillin allergy, respectively, who were all skin test negative. Of skin-test-positive patients who received penicillin, 22% experienced immediate or accelerated penicillin allergy. Of skin-test-positive patients, 84% had dermal reactions to skin testing with the major determinant (benzyl penicilloyl-octalysine) whereas 16% reacted only to an experimental minor determinant mixture of benzylpenicillin, benzylpenicilloate, and benzylpenicilloyl-*N*-propylamine.

Immediate hypersensitivity reactions to penicillin are rare after a properly performed negative skin test. Dermatologic reactions occur in 1% of skin-test-negative patients.[20] A negative penicillin skin test indicates that the risk of life-threatening reactions is extremely low with administration of penicillin or other β-lactams.

Occasionally, patients may experience systemic reactions after skin testing. Also, certain types of patients (e.g., those with dermatographism or taking antihistamines) may be unsuitable for skin testing because a false-positive or false-negative test may result. No reliable skin testing protocol or *in vitro* assay is presently available to predict a reaction to sulfonamides.

TREATMENT OF ANAPHYLAXIS

Anaphylaxis requires prompt treatment to minimize the risk of death or serious morbidity. On presentation, attention should first

TABLE 81–3. Procedure for Performing Penicillin Skin Testing

A. Percutaneous (prick) skin testing

Materials	Volume
Pre-Pen 6 × 10^6M	1 drop
Penicillin G 10,000 U/mL	1 drop
β-Lactam drug 3 mg/mL	1 drop
0.03% albumin-saline control	1 drop
Histamine control (1 mg/mL)	1 drop

1. Place a drop of each test material on the volar surface of the forearm.
2. Prick the skin with a sharp needle inserted through the drop at a 45° angle gently tenting the skin in an upward motion.
3. Interpret skin responses after 15 minutes.
4. A wheal at least 2 × 2 mm with erythema is considered positive.
5. If the prick test is nonreactive, proceed to the intradermal test.
6. If the histamine control is nonreactive, the test is considered uninterpretable.

B. Intradermal skin testing

Materials	Volume
Pre-Pen 6 × 10^6M	0.02 mL
Penicillin G 10,000 U/mL	0.02 mL
β-Lactam drug 3 mg/mL	0.02 mL
0.03% albumin-saline control	0.02 mL
Histamine control (0.1 mg/mL)	0.02 mL

1. Inject 0.02–0.03 mL of each test material intradermally (amount sufficient to produce a small bleb).
2. Interpret skin responses after 15 minutes.
3. A wheal at least 6 × 6 mm with erythema and at least 3 mm greater than the negative control is considered positive.
4. If the histamine control is nonreactive, the test is considered uninterpretable.

Antihistamines may blunt the response and cause false-negative reactions.

From Sullivan TJ. Current Therapy in Allergy. St Louis, Mosby, 1985:57–61.

TABLE 81–4. Treatment of Anaphylaxis

1. Place patient in recumbent position and elevate extremities.
2. Monitor vital signs often (or continuously if possible).
3. Apply tourniquet proximal to site of antigen injection; remove every 10–15 min.
4. Administer epinephrine 1:1000 into nonoccluded site: 0.3–0.5 mL subcutaneously or intramuscularly in adults and 0.01 mL/kg subcutaneously or intramuscularly in children.
5. Administer aqueous epinephrine 1:1000 into site of antigen injection; 0.15–0.25 mL subcutaneously in adults and 0.005 mL/kg subcutaneously in children.
6. Establish and maintain airway with oropharyngeal airway device, endotracheal intubation, transtracheal catheterization, or cricothyrotomy.
7. Administer oxygen at 6–10 L/min.
8. Institute rapid fluid replacement with 0.9% sodium chloride, lactated Ringer's, or colloid solution (e.g., 5% albumin or 4% hetastarch).
9. For hypotension in adults, administer norepinephrine, 32 μg/min (use 8 mg in 500 mL dextrose 5%) with the rate adjusted to maintain low-normal blood pressure. Alternatively, administer dopamine at 2–10 μg/kg/min intravenously.
10. If refractory hypotension is present, administer cimetidine 300 mg or ranitidine 50 mg, intravenously over 3–5 min.
11. If bronchospasm is present, administer aminophylline 6 mg/kg intravenously over 20 min.
12. Administer hydrocortisone sodium succinate 100 mg intravenously (push) and 100 mg intravenously in saline every 2–4 h to block the late-phase reaction.
13. Administer diphenhydramine 1–2 mg/kg intravenously (up to 50 mg) over 3 min to block histamine-1 receptors.
14. For adults taking a β-adrenergic blocker, administer atropine (0.5 mg intravenously) every 5 min until heart rate is greater than 60 beats/min, or isoproterenol 2–20 μg/min intravenously titrated to heart rate of 60 beats/min, or glucagon 0.5 mg/kg intravenously (push) followed by 0.07 mg/kg/h continuously intravenously.

From Weiss ME, Adkinson NF. Clin Allergy 1988;18:515–540.

be given to restoration of respiratory and cardiovascular function. A protocol for the treatment of anaphylaxis is presented in Table 81–4. Epinephrine is administered as primary treatment to counteract bronchoconstriction and vasodilatation. Epinephrine should be administered subcutaneously or intramuscularly and at the site of antigen injection to delay absorption of the antigen. Crystalloids should be administered intravenously to restore intravascular volume. Typically, 1 L of 0.9% sodium chloride or lactated Ringer's solution will be administered over 10 to 15 minutes. This may be repeated if the patient is still believed to be volume depleted. Intravenous fluids should be given early in the course in an attempt to prevent shock. A maintenance intravenous fluid will then be initiated. An immediate priority is establishment and maintenance of an airway. This should be achieved by the use of endotracheal intubation if necessary. When a patient with anaphylaxis is hypotensive, vasopressors will also be needed in addition to crystalloids. Norepinephrine is the vasoconstrictor agent of choice for treatment of anaphylactic shock, although dopamine may also be useful.

A number of other agents may be required for treatment of anaphylactic reactions. Corticosteroids (hydrocortisone sodium succinate intravenously) are recommended to prevent the late-phase reaction. Aminophylline may be used as adjunctive therapy for bronchospasm. Histamine (H_1)-receptor blockers (such as diphenhydramine) may be administered to reduce some of the symptoms associated with anaphylaxis; however, these agents are not effective as primary therapy. H_2-receptor blockers such as cimetidine have been used for treatment of refractory hypotension,[57] although routine use is controversial.

TABLE 81–5. Protocol for Oral Desensitization

	Phenoxymethyl Penicillin			
Step[a]	*Concentration (U/mL)*	*Volume (mL)*	*Dose (U)*	*Cumulative Dose (U)*
1	1000	0.1	100	100
2	1000	0.2	200	300
3	1000	0.4	400	700
4	1000	0.8	800	1500
5	1000	1.6	1600	3100
6	1000	3.2	3200	6300
7	1000	6.4	6400	12,700
8	10,000	1.2	12,000	24,700
9	10,000	2.4	24,000	48,700
10	10,000	4.8	48,000	96,700
11	80,000	1.0	80,000	176,700
12	80,000	2.0	160,000	336,700
13	80,000	4.0	320,000	656,700
14	80,000	8.0	640,000	1,296,700
Observe for 30 min				
15	500,000	0.25	125,000	
16	500,000	0.5	250,000	
17	500,000	1.0	500,000	
18	500,000	2.25	1,125,000	

[a]The interval between steps is 15 min.
From Ref. 58.

TABLE 81–6. Parenteral Desensitization Protocol

Injection No.	Benzylpenicillin Concentration (U)	Volume (mL)	Route
1[a,b]	100	0.1	ID
2	100	0.2	SC
3	100	0.4	SC
4	100	0.8	SC
5[b]	1000	0.1	ID
6	1000	0.3	SC
7	1000	0.6	SC
8	10,000	0.1	ID
9	10,000	0.2	SC
10	10,000	0.4	SC
11	10,000	0.8	SC
12[b]	100,000	0.1	ID
13	100,000	0.3	SC
14	100,000	0.6	SC
15[b]	1,000,000	0.1	ID
16	1,000,000	0.2	SC
17	1,000,000	0.2	IM
18	1,000,000	0.4	IM
19	Continuous IV infusion at 1,000,000 U/h		

[a]Administer doses at intervals of not less than 20 min.
[b]Observe and record skin wheal-and-flare response.
From Ref. 59.

DESENSITIZATION

For some patients allergic to penicillin, no reasonable alternatives exist and penicillin therapy may be necessary for treatment of severe, life-threatening infection. In this situation, penicillin desensitization should be considered. Desensitization can reduce the risk of anaphylaxis, but does not influence the likelihood of other types of reactions such as exfoliative dermatitis or Stevens–Johnson syndrome.

Penicillin desensitization should be performed in a hospital setting where resuscitation equipment is readily available. Prior to initiating the protocol, the patient should be stabilized and fluid, pulmonary, and cardiovascular function optimized. The use of premedicants (antihistamines or corticosteroids) is controversial because these agents may mask the early signs of acute reactions and do not reliably reduce the severity of acute reactions. About one-third of patients who have undergone desensitization experience mild, transient allergic reaction either during the desensitization procedure or during penicillin therapy.[20] Patients who can take oral medication should undergo desensitization with oral penicillin. Protocols for oral and intravenous penicillin desensitization[58,59] are presented in Tables 81–5 and 81–6. It is important that once the desensitization protocol is begun it not be interrupted except for severe reactions. Antihistamines may be administered to treat reactions. Also, if the patient completes the desensitization regimen and then undergoes penicillin treatment, a lapse between doses of as little as 8 hours can allow for reemergence of sensitivity.

Desensitization of TMP-SMZ can be achieved within 2 days in most HIV patients.[60] This can be accompanied by using the following schedule of doses (mg of sulfamethoxazole/trimethoprim): Day 1: 9 AM 4/0.8, 11 AM 8/1.6, 1 PM 20/4, 5 PM 40/8; Day 2: 9 AM 80/16, 3 PM 160/32, 9 PM 200/40; Day 3: 9 AM 400/80 and 400/80; daily thereafter.

Skin tests often become negative during and shortly after desensitization. The mechanism by which desensitization is protective is unclear. It does not seem to be that penicillin-specific IgE is neutralized or that IgG as "blocking antibody" is produced. One possible explanation is that basophils and mast cells attain some degree of tolerance on exposure to the antigen.

▶ PRINCIPLES OF PHARMACOTHERAPY

- Allergic reactions are responsible for up to 5% of reactions to medications among hospitalized patients.
- The following criteria suggest that a drug reaction may be immunologically mediated: (a) The reaction occurs in a small percentage of patients receiving the drug, (b) the observed reaction does not resemble the drug's pharmacologic effect, (c) the type of manifestation is similar to that seen with other allergic reactions (anaphylaxis, urticaria, serum sickness), (d) there is a lag time between first exposure of the drug and reaction, (e) the reaction is reproduced even by minute doses of the drug, (f) the reaction is reproduced by agents with similar chemical structures, (g) eosinophilia is present, and (h) the reaction resolves after the drug has been discontinued. Exceptions to each of these criteria are commonly observed.
- Factors that influence the likelihood of allergic drug reactions are the dose of the allergen, the route of exposure, and the sensitivity of the individual as determined by age, genetics, or environmental factors. For many drugs, the severity of a reaction is determined by the dose and the duration of exposure.
- Anaphylaxis is an acute, life-threatening allergic reaction involving multiple organ systems that generally begins within 30 minutes, but almost always within 2 hours after exposure to the inciting allergen. Anaphylaxis requires prompt treatment to restore respiratory and cardiovascular function. Epinephrine is administered as primary treatment to counteract bronchoconstriction and vasodilatation. Intravenous fluids should be administered to restore intravascular volume.
- Patients with positive penicillin skin tests are advised not to receive cephalosporins if they can be avoided. Patients who have experienced only mild, cutaneous reactions, such as maculopapular rashes, may receive cephalosporins with caution.
- Five percent to 10% of patients receiving radiocontrast agents experience some type of adverse reaction. Low-osmolar contrast agents appear to result in fewer anaphylactoid reactions. A regimen recommended to prevent reactions in patients who have previously experienced them includes prednisone 50 mg orally 13, 7, and 1 hours before the procedure, diphenhydramine 50 mg orally or intramuscularly 1 hour before the procedure, and 25 mg ephedrine orally 1 hour before. The ephedrine should be omitted if the patient has angina, arrhythmia, or hypertension.
- The two general types of reactions to aspirin are urticaria/angioedema (1% of the population) and rhinosinusitis/asthma (0.5%). Aspirin-sensitive patients may also be sensitive to NSAIDs.
- Adverse reactions to TMP-SMZ have been observed to occur much more frequently in AIDS patients compared to those without AIDS (50% to 80% of AIDS patients compared with 10% in other immunocompromised patients).
- The basic principles for management of allergic reactions to drugs or biologic agents includes (a) discontinuation of the medication or agent when possible, (b) treatment of the adverse clinical signs and symptoms, and (c) substitution, if necessary, of another agent.
- One of the most helpful tests to evaluate risk is the allergen skin test. For some drugs, skin testing can demonstrate the presence of drug-specific IgE and predict a relatively high risk of immediate hypersensitivity reactions. Skin testing does not predict the risk of delayed or most dermatologic reactions.

REFERENCES

1. Anderson JA. Allergic reactions to drugs and biologic agents. JAMA 1992;268:2845–2857.

2. Parker CW. Drug allergy (a review in three parts). N Engl J Med 1975;292:511, 732, 957.
3. Jick H. Adverse drug reactions: The magnitude of the problem. J Allergy Clin Immunol 1984;74:555.
4. DeWeck AI. Drugs as allergens. J Allergy Clin Immunol 1986;78:1047.
5. Stafford CT. Adverse drug reactions. Med Times 1988;116:31–42.
6. DeSwarte RD. Drug allergy. In: Patterson R, ed. Allergic Diseases, 4th ed. Philadelphia, Lippincott, 1993.
7. Roitt I, Brastoff J, Male D. Immunology, 4th ed. London, Mosby, 1996.
8. Schwartz LB, Austen KF. The mast cell and mediators of immediate hypersensitivity: In: Samter M, Talmage DW, Frank MM, et al, eds. Immunologic Diseases, 5th ed. Boston, Little, Brown, 1995.
9. Serafin WF, Austen KF. Mediators of immediate hypersensitivity reactions. N Engl J Med 1987;317:30–34.
10. Stafford CT. Life-threatening allergic reactions. Postgrad Med 1989; 86:235–241.
11. Bochner BS, Lichtenstein LM. Anaphylaxis. N Engl J Med 1991;324: 1785–1790.
12. Kemp SF, Lockey RF, Wolf BL, Lieberman P. Anaphylaxis: A review of 266 cases. Arch Intern Med 1995;155:1749–1754.
13. Johnson DH, Cuhna BA. Drug fever. Infect Dis Clin North Am 1996; 10:85–91.
14. Prince EJ, Venables PJ. Drug-induced lupus. Drug Safety 1995;12: 283–290.
15. Rich MW. Drug-induced lupus. The list of culprits grows. Postgrad Med 1996;100:299–302.
16. Roujeau JC, Stern RS. Severe adverse cutaneous reactions to drugs. N Engl J Med 331;1994:1272–1285.
17. Mockenhaupt M, Schopf E. Epidemiology of drug-induced severe skin reactions. Semin Cutaneous Med Surg 1996;15:236–243.
18. Stern RS, Steinberg LA. Epidemiology of adverse cutaneous reactions to drugs. Dermatoepidemiology 1995;13:681–688.
19. Bigby M, Jick S, Jick H, et al. Drug-induced cutaneous reactions. A report from the Boston Collaborative Drug Surveillance Program on 15,438 consecutive inpatients, 1975 to 1982. JAMA 1986;256: 3359–3363.
20. Weiss ME, Adkinson NF. Immediate hypersensitivity reactions to penicillin and related antibiotics. Clin Allergy 1988;18:515–540.
21. Adkinson NF. Risk factors for drug allergy. J Allergy Clin Immunol 1984;74:567–572.
22. Wickern GM, Nish WA, Bitner AS, Freeman TM. Allergy to β-lactams: A survey of current practices. J Allerg Clin Immunol 1994;94: 725–731.
23. Anne S, Reisman RE. Risk of administering cephalosporin antibiotics to patients with histories of penicillin allergy. Ann Allergy Asthma Immunol 1995;74:167–170.
24. Saxon A, Beall GN, Rohr AS, et al. Immediate hypersensitivity reactions to β-lactam antibiotics. Ann Intern Med 1987;107:204–215.
25. Kishiyama JL, Adelman DC. The cross-reactivity of beta-lactam antibiotics. Drug Safety 1994;10:318–327.
26. Bush WH, Swanson DP. Acute reactions to intravascular contrast media: Types, risk factors, recognition, and specific treatment. Am J Radiol 1991;157:1153–1161.
27. Murphy KJ, Brunberg JA, Cohan RH. Adverse reactions to gadolinium contrast media. Am J Roentgenol 1996;167:847–849.
28. Lieberman. Radiocontrast reactions. Clin Rev Allergy 1986;4:229–245.
29. Lasser EC, Walter AJ, Lang JH. An experimental basis for histamine release in contrast material reactions. Radiology 1974;110:49–59.
30. Greenberger PA, Patterson R. The prevention of immediate generalized reactions to radiocontrast media in high-risk patients. J Allergy Clin Immunol 1991;87:867–872.
31. Greenberger PA. Contrast media reaction. J Allergy Clin Immunol 1984;74:600.
32. Cohan RH, Leder RA, Ellis JH. Treatment of adverse reactions to radiographic contrast media in adults. Radiol Clin North Am 1996;34: 1055–1076.
33. Patterson R, Roberts M, Grammer LC. Insulin allergy: Re-evaluation after two decades. Ann Allergy 1990;64:459–462.
34. Samter M, Stevenson DD. Reactions to aspirin and aspirin-like drugs. In: Samter M, Talmage DW, Frank MM, et al, eds. Immunologic Diseases, 5th ed. Boston, Little, Brown, 1995.
35. Stevenson DD. Diagnosis, prevention and treatment of adverse reactions to aspirin and non-steroidal antiinflammatory drugs. J Allergy Clin Immunol 1984;74:617.
36. Chafee FH, Settipane GA. Aspirin intolerance: I. Frequency in an allergic population. J Allergy Clin Immunol 1974;53:193.
37. MacDonald JR, Mathison DA, Stevenson DD. Aspirin intolerance in asthma, detection by oral challenge. J Allergy Clin Immunol 1972;50: 198.
38. Falliers CJ. Aspirin and subtypes of asthma risk factor analysis. J Allergy Clin Immunol 1973;52:141.
39. Kowalski M. Aspirin sensitive rhinosinusitis and asthma. Allergy Proc 1995;16:77–80.
40. Vicks SD, Dean JR, Tenholder MF. Ketorolac induced respiratory failure in an aspirin-sensitive asthmatic. Immunol Allergy Pract 1991; 13:23–25.
41. Lee TH. Mechanisms of aspirin sensitivity. Am Rev Respir Dis 1992; 145:S34–S36.
42. Goodwin SD, Glenny RW. Nonsteroidal anti-inflammatory drug-associated pulmonary infiltrates with eosinophilia. Arch Intern Med 1992; 152:1521–1524.
43. Anonymous. Serious adverse reactions with sulfonamides. FDA Drug Bull 1984;14:5–6. Bulletin.
44. Reider MJ, Uetrecht J, Shear NH, et al. Diagnosis of sulfonamide hypersensitivity reactions by *in vitro* "rechallenge" with hydroxylamine metabolites. Ann Intern Med 1989;110:286–289.
45. Santomauro JT, Stover DE. *Pneumocystis carinii* pneumonia. Med Clin North Am 1997;81:299–318.
46. Moore RD, Fortgang I, Keruly J, Chaisson RE. Adverse events from drug therapy for human immunodeficiency virus disease. Am J Med 1996;101:34–40.
47. Weiner M, Bernstein IL. Adverse Reactions to Drug Formulation Agents: A Handbook of Excipients. New York, Marcel Dekker, 1989.
48. American Academy of Pediatrics Committee on Drugs. "Inactive" ingredients in pharmaceutical products. Pediatrics 1985;76:635–642.
49. Lockey SD. Hypersensitivity to tartrazine (FD&C Yellow No. 5) and other dyes and additives present in foods and pharmaceutical products. Ann Allergy 1977; 38:206–210.
50. Stevenson DD, Simon RA. Sensitivity to ingested metabisulfites in asthmatic subjects. J Allergy Clin Immunol 1981;68:26–32.
51. Smolinski SC. Review of parenteral sulfide reactions. J Toxicol Clin Toxicol 1992;30:597–606.
52. Landwehr LP, Boguniewicz M. Current perspectives on latex allergy. J Pediatrics 1996;128:305–312.
53. Senst BL, Johnson RA. Latex allergy. Am J Health Syst Pharm 1997; 54:1071–1075.
54. Steelman WM. Latex allergy precautions: A research-based protocol. Nursing Clin North Am 1995;30:475–493.
55. Gadde J, Spence M, Wheeler B, Adkinson NF. Clinical experience with penicillin skin testing in a large inner-city STD clinic. JAMA 1993;270:2456 –2463.
56. Sogn DD, Evans R, Shepherd GM, et al. Results of the National Institute of Allergy and Infectious Diseases collaborative clinical trial to test the predictive value of skin testing with major and minor penicillin derivatives in hospitalized patients. Arch Intern Med 1992;152: 1025–1032.
57. Yarbrough JA, Moffitt JE, Brown DA, et al. Cimetidine in the treatment of refractory anaphylaxis. Ann Allergy 1989;63:235–238.
58. Sullivan TJ. Current Therapy in Allergy. St. Louis, Mosby, 1985: 57–61
59. Weiss ME, Adkinson NF. Immediate hypersensitivity reaction to penicillin and related antibiotics. Clin Allergy 1988;18:515–540.
60. Caumes E, Guermonprez G, Lecomte C, et al. Efficacy and safety of desensitization with sulfamethoxazole and trimethoprim in 48 previously hypersensitive patients infected with human immunodeficiency virus. Arch Dermatol 1997;133:465–469.

82
OSTEOPOROSIS AND OSTEOMALACIA

Mary Beth O'Connell, PharmD, BCPS, FASHP, FCCP

Osteopenia, osteoporosis, and osteomalacia, disorders of bone metabolism, constitute a major cause of disability in women and older men. Disability results from kyphosis, fractures, and pain. Osteopenia and osteoporosis are conditions associated with low bone mass density. Severe osteoporosis is osteoporosis with fractures. Osteomalacia is deficient bone mineralization, leading to unmineralized osteoid and decreased bone strength. This chapter examines the physiology of normal bone and the pathophysiology of osteopenia, osteoporosis, and osteomalacia; describes different methods for assessing bone mass and remodeling; and explores nonpharmacologic and pharmacologic treatment options to prevent or treat osteoporosis and osteomalacia.

NORMAL FUNCTION OF BONE

Bone has two basic functions in humans: (1) structural support, which allows movement and vital organ protection; and (2) a depot for calcium, phosphorus, magnesium, sodium, and carbonate. The maintenance of normal ion and buffer concentrations takes precedence over the supportive role. Bone will be destroyed to maintain homeostasis.

TYPES AND COMPOSITION OF BONE

About 80% of adult bone is cortical bone and 20% is trabecular bone. Cortical bone is found in the midshafts and on the surfaces of long and flat bones. Trabecular bone is found in the inner aspects of the long bones and between the cortical surfaces of the vertebrae, ribs, and pelvic bones. The composition of each type of bone varies (Table 82–1). Because of a larger surface area and more abundant cell population, trabecular bone is more metabolically active than cortical bone, and responds more quickly to hormonal stimuli.

The three primary components of bone are the protein matrix, mineralized bone, and bone cells. The matrix provides tensile strength and the mineralized bone provides compressional strength. The bone matrix is composed of type I collagen fibers and proteoglycans. Mineralized bone consists primarily of hydroxyapatite ($Ca_{10}(PO_4)_6(OH)_2$). The hydroxyapatite crystals also contain substantial amounts of sodium, potassium, magnesium, and carbonate. Cortical bone consists of 70% mineralized bone and 30% protein matrix.[1] Bone cells—osteoblasts, osteocytes, and osteoclasts—occupy only about 3% of the total bone volume.

BONE REMODELING AND HORMONAL CONTROL

Normally, 25% of trabecular bone and 3% of cortical bone is remodeled each year.[2] At any given time, about 4% of bone is undergoing osteoblastic activity and 1% is undergoing osteoclastic activity.[1] The control and feedback mechanisms of bone remodeling are still being unraveled (Figs. 82–1 and 82–2 and Table 82–2).[1–7] Osteoblastic and osteoclastic activity are coupled to each other, influencing the activity of the other. Theoretically, coupling keeps bone resorption and formation equalized, which maintains the skeletal bone mass. The balance usually exists until the third decade, when an age-related imbalance begins favoring resorption over formation, creating a loss in bone mass. Some conditions such as hormonal deficiencies and certain medications (Table 82–3) can also cause a disproportionate shift in bone formation or resorption, resulting in bone mass loss and later osteoporosis.

The remodeling process can take 3 to 4 months (Fig. 82–1). Osteoclasts produce projections that attach to bone via integrin molecules. With the help of H^+-ATPase and carbonic anhydrase II, acids such as citric and lactic acid are formed, which work with proteolytic enzymes to dissolve the bone mineral salts and create a bone cavity. Osteoblasts then secrete alkaline phosphatase and collagen monomers to fill in the cavity. These monomers are polymerized to collagen fibers. Possibly under the control of osteonectin, osteocalcin, and phosphoproteins, calcium precipitates in the osteoid, first as amorphous salts and then as hydroxyapatite. Osteoblasts also secrete hormonal compounds that prevent osteoclasts from creating a larger or new cavity.

This remodeling process is under the control of various hormones, cytokines, and feedback systems (Fig. 82–1 and Table 82–2).[1–7] Bone remodeling begins with the maturation of colony forming units (CFU) from the mesenchymal lineage of marrow stroma. Stromal cells can also develop into fibroblasts, chondrocytes, adipocytes, or muscle cells. Estrogen, interleukin-1 (IL-1), tumor necrosis factor (TNF), parathyroid hormone (PTH), and 1,25-dihydroxyvitamin D may control the differentiation of stromal cells to os-

TABLE 82–1. Bone Composition

Bone	Cortical Bone (%)	Trabecular Bone (%)
Total body	80	20
Midradius	95	5
Distal radius	30–50	30–50
Femur neck	75	25
Trochanter	50	50
Lumbar spine	40	60

teoblasts. IL-1 and TNF-α from monocytes potentially also activate osteoblasts. The osteoblast has receptors for estrogen, androgens, 1,25-hydroxyvitamin D, growth hormone (GH), and PTH. Osteoblasts may produce osteoclast-activating factors (OAFs) such as peptides, prostaglandins, colony-stimulating factors (CSFs), transforming growth factors (TGFs), insulin-like growth factor-1 and 2 (IGF-1 and IGF-2), TNF, IL-1, IL-3, IL-6, IL-11, and other cytokines. These compounds either promote the proliferation of CFU-GM cells from the hematopoietic stem cell to osteoclast precursors or initiate the differentiation of precursors to osteoclasts. The hormonal compounds predominantly controlling the differentiation are PTH, 1,25-hydroxyvitamin D, and IL-1. Osteoclasts have receptors for estrogen and calcitonin but no receptors for PTH and 1,25-hydroxyvitamin D. The precise processes and influencing factors that control resorption and formation are still being discovered and explored including the relationship between vitamin K and carboxylation of bone proteins such as osteocalcin.[8] Genetics may also play a role via the genes for the vitamin D receptor, TGF-β, procollagen, and the estrogen receptor.[9]

VITAMIN D METABOLISM AND REGULATION OF SERUM CALCIUM AND PHOSPHATE

Vitamin D_2 (ergocalciferol) and vitamin D_3 (cholecalciferol) enter the body from the diet; vitamin D_3 is also created by the action of ultraviolet rays on skin 7-dehydrocholesterol (Fig. 82–2).[1,10,11] Vitamin D_2 and vitamin D_3 act similarly in the human body; thus they are referred to as "vitamin D." In the liver, 25-hydroxylase produces 25-hydroxyvitamin D, which is then metabolized in the kidney to the active moiety, 1-25-dihydroxyvitamin D (calcitriol), by 1-α-hydroxylase. If too much active metabolite exists, the kidneys can produce inactive compounds such as 24,25-dihydroxyvitamin D.

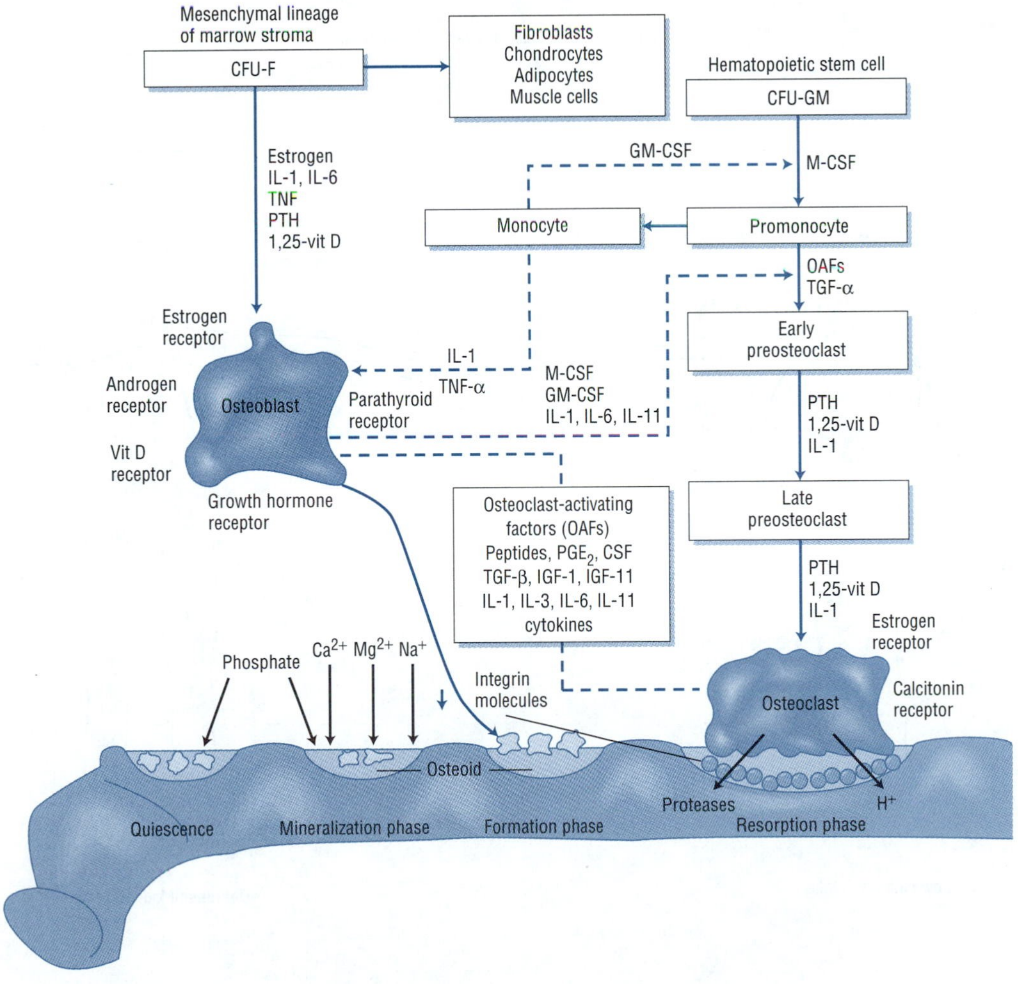

FIGURE 82–1. Tentative feedback and control systems for bone remodeling.

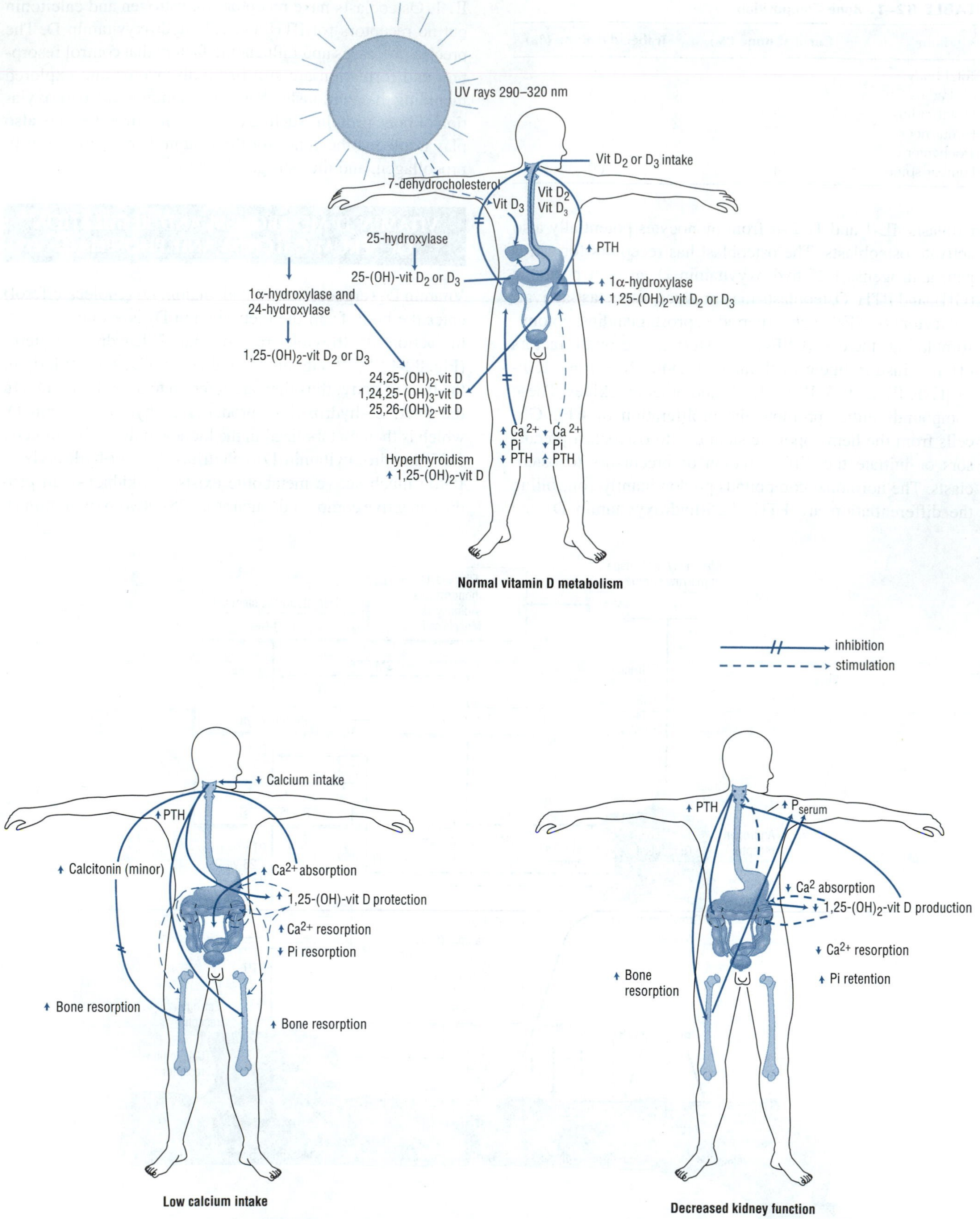
UV rays 290–320 nm
Vit D_2 or D_3 intake
7-dehydrocholesterol
Vit D_3
Vit D_2
Vit D_3
25-hydroxylase
↑ PTH
25-(OH)-vit D_2 or D_3
↑ 1α-hydroxylase
↑ 1,25-$(OH)_2$-vit D_2 or D_3
1α-hydroxylase and
24-hydroxylase
1,25-$(OH)_2$-vit D_2 or D_3
24,25-$(OH)_2$-vit D
1,24,25-$(OH)_3$-vit D
25,26-$(OH)_2$-vit D
↑ Ca^{2+} ↓ Ca^{2+}
↑ Pi ↓ Pi
↓ PTH ↑ PTH
Hyperthyroidism
↑ 1,25-$(OH)_2$-vit D
Normal vitamin D metabolism
inhibition
stimulation
↓ Calcium intake
↑ PTH
↑ Calcitonin (minor)
↑ Ca^{2+} absorption
↑ 1,25-(OH)-vit D protection
↑ Ca^{2+} resorption
↓ Pi resorption
↑ Bone resorption
↑ Bone resorption
Low calcium intake
↑ PTH
↑ P_{serum}
↓ Ca^2 absorption
↓ 1,25-$(OH)_2$-vit D production
↓ Ca^{2+} resorption
↑ Pi retention
↑ Bone
resorption
Decreased kidney function

FIGURE 82–2. Feedback systems for vitamin D, calcium, and phosphate.

TABLE 82–2. Hormones and Local Factors Involved in Bone Remodeling and Their Effect on Bone Cell Function

	Action	
	Resorption	*Formation*
Hormones		
Steroid		
$1,25(OH)_2D_3$	↑	↓[a]
Sex steroids (estrogen, progesterone, androgen)	↓	—
Glucocorticoids	—	↓
Polypeptide		
PTH	↑	↓↑[b]
Calcitonin	↑	—
Growth hormone	—	↑
Thyroid hormone	↑	—
Local factors		
Produced by bone cells or bone tissue		
IGF-I, IGF-II	?	↑
TGF-β	↓	↑
FGFs	—	↑
PDGF	↑	↑
Granulocyte colony-stimulating factor (G-CSF)	↑	?
GM-CSF	↑	?
Bone morphogenetic protein (BMP)	?	↑
Osteoinductive factor (OIF)	↓	↑
Synthesized by bone-related tissue		
Cartilage-derived IGF-1, basic FGF, TGF-β	↓	↑
Blood-cell-derived		
IL-1	↑	?
TNF	↑	↓
Gamma interferon (γ-IFN)	↓	—
Other factors		
Prostaglandins	↑	↑↓
Binding proteins	?	?

↑ = increase; ↓ = decrease; — = no effect; ? = effect unknown.
[a]Decreases proliferation of osteoblast-like cells at high concentrations and stimulates proliferation at low concentrations; decreases collagen synthesis.
[b]Decreases collagen synthesis; intermittent administration promotes increased collagen synthesis and increased osteoblast number and activity. (From Ref. 5.)

The movement of calcium and phosphorus in and out of bone is primarily under the control of PTH and 1,25-dihydroxyvitamin D.[1,10,11] Figure 82–2 shows the interrelationships of these hormones on mineral metabolism in cases of low calcium ingestion, low or high phosphate ingestion, and decreased kidney function with concomitant hyperphosphatemia. When the serum calcium is low, PTH increases, resulting in increased bone resorption and 1,25-dihydroxyvitamin D production. The 1,25-dihydroxyvitamin D metabolite increases calcium absorption from the gut, tubular reabsorption from the kidneys, and bone resorption. When the serum calcium concentration returns to normal, PTH production decreases, and so does bone resorption and 1,25-dihydroxyvitamin D production. The feedback system for phosphorus is less complicated and basically controlled directly by the kidneys with minor PTH influences.

OSTEOPOROSIS

Osteoporosis is a very heterogeneous disease involving numerous processes (Fig. 82–1) and contributing etiologic factors (Table 82–3).[7,12–15] The precursor condition, osteopenia, is defined by the World Health Organization (WHO) as bone density of 1 to less than 2.5 standard deviations (SDs) below the average young adult peak bone mass. The osteoporosis WHO definition is bone density of 2.5 or more SDs below the average young adult peak bone mass. Severe osteoporosis includes fractures.

Three categories of osteoporosis have been described: postmenopausal, age-related, and secondary. Postmenopausal osteoporosis affects primarily trabecular bone in women within the first 5 to 15 years after menopause. Consequently, fractures of the vertebrae and distal forearm are more common. Age-related osteoporosis affects women and men (2:1 ratio) older than age 70. Cortical and trabecular bone density both decrease. The clinical manifestations are multiple wedge, hip, and radius fractures. Secondary osteoporosis is caused by other diseases or medications. It occurs in either sex at any age and affects both bone types. All types of fractures are possible.

EPIDEMIOLOGY

Based on NHANES III data and WHO definitions for total femur bone density, the respective prevalences of osteopenia and osteoporosis are as follows[16]:

- White women, 42% and 17%
- African-American women, 28% and 8%
- Hispanic women, 37% and 12%
- Men of all races, 16% and 2%, using women's bone-density cutoff points
- Men of all races, 33% and 4%, using men's bone-density cutoff points.

Based on age and the WHO definitions, the percent of women with osteoporosis is 15% for ages 50 to 59, 22% for ages 60 to 69, 39% for ages 70 to 80, and 70% for those 80 years and older.[17]

About 1.5 million fractures are reported each year in the United States: 47% vertebral, 16.5% wrist, 16.5% hip, and 20% other limb sites.[18] The lifetime risks of a 50-year-old woman experiencing fractures are 16% for the spine, 16% for the wrist, 18% for the hip and 40% for any fracture.[17,18] The lifetime risks of a 50-year-old man experiencing fractures are 5% for the spine, 2.5% for the wrist, 6% for the hip, and 13% for any fracture. The relative risk of a hip fracture increases for women with low bone density from 5.7 for women 65 to 79 years old to 16.8 for women at least 80 years old.[19]

RISK FACTORS

Multiple genetic, environmental, medical, social, and fall-related conditions can influence both a woman's[7,12–14] and a

TABLE 82–3. Risk Factors Associated with Osteoporosis and Hip Fractures

Genetic	Cushing's syndrome
White or Asian ethnicity	Diabetes
Family history of osteoporosis or fractures	Altered GI or hepatobiliary function
Small body frame (tall, thin, low body mass index)	Occult osteogenesis imperfecta
Lifestyle	Mastocytosis
Minimal exercise	Arthritis
Sedentary	Prolactinoma
Smoking	Hemolytic anemia, hemochromatosis, thalassemia
Excessive alcohol	Ankylosing spondylitis
Minimal sun exposure	Gastric surgery
Location with minimal seasonal sunlight exposure	Poor self-rated health
Diet	Stroke
Low calcium intake any time in life	**Medications**
Lactose intolerance	Excessive thyroid replacement
High caffeine intake	Glucocorticoids
High phosphorus intake	Long-term heparin
High animal protein intake	Chronic lithium therapy
Weight loss greater than 10% after age 50	Chemotherapy
Anorexia nervosa	Gonadotropin-releasing hormone agonist or antagonists
Long-term parenteral nutrition	Anticonvulsants
Obstetric/Gynecology History	Drugs altering calcium absorption: tetracycline, some diuretics, phenothiazine derivatives, cyclosporine, aluminum-containing antacids
Late menarche	**Fall-related Conditions**
Early natural menopause	Medications: anxiolytics, long-acting benzodiazepines
Surgical menopause	Physical disability
Oophorectomy without replacement therapy	Slow gait, difficult tandem walk
Nulliparity	Decreased visual acuity
Amenorrhea associated with anorexia nervosa, medications, or excessive exercise	Poor depth perception
Chronic Illnesses	Decreased quadriceps and grip strength
Low bone mineral density	Inability to rise from a chair
Hyperthyroidism	Use of walking aids

man's[15] likelihood of developing osteoporosis with or without fractures (Table 82–3). The magnitude and significance of all these risk factors vary for the elderly,[12,14] African-American women,[13] and men.[15] Women, predominantly because of the combination of lower peak bone mass, estrogen deficiency, and longevity, generally have lower bone density and more fractures than men. Caucasian and Asian heritage is associated with osteoporosis more so than African heritage, although osteoporosis does occur in those of African descent at a much lower incidence.[13] With an elderly cohort, additional risk factors are associated with conditions causing falls.

Considerable overlap exists between the bone density measured in normal subjects and patients with osteoporosis with or without previous fractures. However, bone densities 1 SD below peak bone mass have been associated with a 1.7 to 2.4-fold increased likelihood of vertebral fractures, 1.6 to 2.6-fold increased likelihood of forearm fractures, and a 1.5 to 9-fold increased likelihood of hip fractures.[20–22] Low bone density at one site does not always predict fractures at another site.

PATHOPHYSIOLOGY

POSTMENOPAUSAL OSTEOPOROSIS

Estrogen deficiency is associated with an increase in bone resorption without an increase in bone formation. The secretion of cytokines and other compounds by the osteoblasts most likely is influenced by estrogens. Human and animal studies indicate that estrogen deficiency increases the release of IL-1, TNF, and granulocyte–macrophage colony-stimulating factor (GM–CSF) from peripheral blood monocytes, and IL-6 and colony-stimulating factors from stromal cells and osteoblasts.[4] Interleukin-1 is a potent inducer of resorption. TNF-α induces osteoclast differentiation and maturation and bone resorption. Estrogen replacement therapy (ERT) decreased cytokine production, thus decreasing resorption, increasing calcitonin concentrations, decreasing prostaglandin E_2 (a stimulator of osteoblast collagen production and bone resorption), decreasing IGF-I secretion, and increasing calcium absorption.[4,11]

AGE-RELATED OSTEOPOROSIS

Peak bone mineral density occurs in women and men sometime in the second to fourth decade of life, followed by a plateau and then a slow decline. Women have less bone mass at skeletal maturity, thus requiring less bone to be lost before the threshold for fractures is reached. In women, bone loss proceeds at a rate of 3% per decade until menopause, at which time it accelerates to about 9% per decade.[23] The rate returns to age-related rates 10 to 20 years after menopause. Men lose bone at a rate of 3% to 4% per decade throughout life. Over a lifetime, women lose about 35% of their cortical bone, men about 23%. The rate of bone loss increases in the older old. The following rates of bone loss have been reported, respectively, for women 67 to 70 years old and greater than 85 years old: calcaneous, 1.2% and 2.8% per year; femur, 0.4% and 1.1% per year; and trochanter, 0.4% and 1.7% per year.[19]

Age-related bone loss results from decreased osteoblast function, calcium and vitamin D intake and absorption, sex hormone concentrations, and mechanical bone stress. Secondary causes—such as concomitant diseases and medications—may also contribute. After age 40, bone formation is less than bone resorption. Calcium absorption and intake decreases with age in both sexes, especially after the age of 70. Decreased sun exposure (and thus decreased skin conversion) and impaired liver or kidney vitamin D metabolism can lead to decreased, 1,25-dihydroxyvitamin D concentrations. PTH concentrations are increased secondary to the decreased serum calcium and potentially secondary to aging, leading to increased bone loss. In some studies, aging has been associated with decreased calcitonin concentrations. Androgen and estrogen deficiencies are documented with aging. With less physical activity, less mechanical stress is experienced by the bones, thereby decreasing bone remodeling. Other changes increase the likelihood for falls—and thus fractures.[24]

OSTEOPOROSIS IN MEN

Although often thought of as a disorder of women, osteoporosis also occurs in men. Hip and vertebral fractures are common in men but occur at half the rate as in women; forearm fractures are uncommon.[15,25] The lower osteoporosis incidence in men may result from higher peak bone mass at skeletal maturity, shorter life expectancy, lower bone loss rate during aging, fewer falls, and/or a gradual (versus a distinct) cessation of hormone production. The pathogenesis, risk factors, and clinical features of male osteoporosis are similar to those of postmenopausal women with osteoporosis (Table 82–3). Decreased testosterone, calcium, vitamin D, GH, and IGF concentrations and increased PTH concentrations are also seen in aging men.[15,25] Overt male hypogonadism is associated with fractures. Secondary causes of osteoporosis exist for 50% to 60% men with osteoporosis versus 5% to 10% for women.[15]

DRUG-INDUCED OSTEOPOROSIS

Glucocorticoids, heparin, excessive thyroid replacement, and anticonvulsants have been associated with low bone density and fractures.[26] Glucocorticoids produce the greatest amount of drug-induced disease and will be discussed later in further depth.[27,28] Generally, prednisone doses of 7.5 mg or greater and high-dose inhaled glucocorticoids decrease bone formation and increase bone resorption. Transplant patients can develop osteoporosis as a function of glucocorticoid therapy, decreased renal function, increased PTH, or possibly cyclosporine therapy.

Heparin therapy in excess of 15,000 to 30,000 units per day for greater than 3 to 6 months has been associated with decreased bone density and vertebral fractures. The mechanism is unknown.

Thyroid hormones can increase osteoclasts, decrease calcitonin concentrations, and increase bone resorption. Doses greater than 200 μg/d (or 1.6 μg/kg/d) or those producing excessive thyroid concentrations decrease bone mass.[26,29] Sensitive TSH assays should be used to detect clinical and subclinical hyperthyroidism. Women using thyroid with concomitant ERT had less bone loss.[29]

Anticonvulsants increase vitamin D metabolism to inactive compounds, thus producing osteomalacia, and may directly increase bone loss.[26,30] Monitoring 25-hydroxyvitamin D levels may help identify patients at risk. Replacement therapy with vitamin D or its metabolites may be required.

CLINICAL PRESENTATION AND FRACTURE OUTCOMES

The usual presentation of osteoporosis is shortened stature; kyphosis; lordosis; vertebra, hip, or forearm fracture; and/or bone pain. Fractures can occur after minor trauma, such as bending, lifting, or falling. Vertebral fractures are the most common. Recurrent fractures—especially vertebral—are common. Multiple vertebral fractures may lead to dorsal kyphosis and exaggerated cervical lordosis, frequently referred to as Dowager's or widow's hump. Subsequent chest wall changes can lead to pulmonary and cardiovascular complications. Collapsed vertebra rarely lead to spinal cord compression.

The consequences of fractures can be devastating. One half of hip fracture patients are unable to walk independently after the fracture heals.[18] About 25% of them will reside in a nursing home within 1 year of the fracture. Hip fractures are associated with a 5% to 20% mortality rate in the first year. Acute fracture pain usually resolves in 2 to 3 months. Chronic fracture pain can occur, manifested as a nagging, deep, dull pain localized to the general area of the fracture.

PATIENT ASSESSMENT

A comprehensive patient history should be obtained in the following areas: family history, medical diseases, surgeries, medications (current and past), diet, smoking, alcohol use, exercise, menstruation, pregnancies, menopause, and in the elderly, falls. Accurate measurements of height and weight should be included. On physical examination, additional attention should be directed to the spine and sites of pain. The onset, duration, severity, and quality of life impact of bone pain and fractures should be explored. For the elderly, gait, sway, and muscle strength should be evaluated and sometimes an assessment for assistive walking devices should be performed.

RADIOLOGIC QUANTIFICATION OF BONE LOSS

Regular chest radiographs are not helpful for diagnosis of osteoporosis, because 30% to 40% of bone loss is required before visualization; but radiographs are helpful in diagnosing acute fracture. Various bone densitometry techniques exist.[31] Single-photon absorptiometry (SPA) is recommended for measurement of the forearm and dual-energy X-ray absorptiometry (DEXA) for the spine and hip. Computed tomography provides a three-dimensional picture and directly measures both trabecular and cortical bone densities, but it is expensive and has the highest radiation exposure. Ultrasound evaluations of the heel, a procedure that is feasible for community pharmacies and clinics, involves no radiation, is inexpensive, is portable, and can predict hip[21] and vertebral fracture risk.[22]

An international panel developed consensus statements on bone densitometry.[32] They concluded that bone densitometry can predict fracture risk, diagnose osteoporosis, and provide useful information for patient and health care providers for treatment decisions and effectiveness. For every 1 SD below average young adult peak bone mass, the fracture risk increases 1.5 to 2.5 times.[20,32] Because bone mass changes slowly, measurements are repeated every 1 to 4 years to determine rate of bone loss or response to therapy. Bone densitometry is not always reimbursed by insurance providers.

BIOCHEMICAL AND BIOPSY EVALUATION

The initial routine screen for osteoporosis includes a complete blood count, chemistry panel, and urinalysis.[31] Depending on these findings, other tests are required to evaluate secondary causes of bone disorders.[31] A bone biopsy can provide information on bone quality, quantity, and turnover rate, and thus can differentiate osteoporosis from osteomalacia. This test is also used when treatment is ineffective or no identifiable reasons exist for disease.[31]

Various serum and urinary markers of bone resorption, formation, and turnover exist, and are sometimes used to identify bone-remodeling problems or responses to therapy.[33] These tests do not quantify bone mass. Markers for bone resorption are hydroxyproline; total, free, or peptide-bound deoxypyridinoline; and C-terminal (Crosslaps) or N-terminal telopeptides (NTX). Markers for bone formation include total and bone-specific alkaline phosphatase and C-terminal (PICP) and N-terminal (PINP) procollagen extension peptides. A marker of bone turnover is intact, fragmented, carboxylated, or undercarboxylated osteocalcin. These tests vary by specificity, assay variability, sensitivity to monitor response to therapy, predictability of future disease, cost, and availability. They are also influenced differently by body composition, diet, and diurnal factors.

▶ PREVENTION AND TREATMENT: Osteoporosis

A general guideline for osteopenia and osteoporosis prevention and treatment is given in Table 82–4. Osteoporosis prevention begins with increasing peak bone mass in children, adolescents, and young adults. In women and men under the age of 35 to 40 years, maintenance of bone mass is critical. Finally, prevention focuses on eliminating or decreasing bone loss in postmenopausal women and preventing bone loss, falls, and fractures in older women and men. Pain control may be important for patients with new fractures or severe osteoporosis.

NONPHARMACOLOGIC PREVENTION AND THERAPY

DIET CHANGES

American diets, especially in the elderly, are usually deficient in calcium and may be deficient in vitamin D. Children, adolescents, and adults should ingest an adequate amount of daily calcium and vitamin D (Table 82–5).[34,35] The maximum upper calcium intake limit is 2500 mg/d.[35] Diet changes precede supplementation (see Table 82–6 for calcium-containing foods).[34,35] Dairy products are the best source, because the calcium contained in fruits, vegetables, and grains may be less absorbable due to binding with oxalates (from spinach and rhubarb) and phytates (from bran and whole cereals).[34] Vitamin D-containing foods include oily fishes, liver, butter, and fortified milk. Direct sunlight exposure without sunscreen of 5- to 20-minute duration two or three times a week may fulfill a person's vitamin D needs.

Caffeine increases urinary calcium excretion, and adaptation does not occur with long-term usage. Older women are more prone to caffeine-induced calcium excretion. Restricting caffeine ingestion to less than 2 cups of caffeine beverages per day is recommended.[36]

A potential concern is the increased phosphates and phosphorus in American diets from cola beverages and food preservatives.[37] In some studies, phosphates—especially with low calcium intakes—have been associated with secondary hyperparathyroidism,[37] lower calcitriol concentrations,[37] or increased bone resorption. In the gut, calcium and phosphates can bind to each other and become nonabsorbable salts.[36] However, an effect on calcium is not seen in all studies.[36,37] Thus, dietary phosphorus should be decreased to prevent decreased calcium absorption.[37]

The National Research Council recommends the calcium/phosphorus ratio for intake should be greater than or equal to 1:1; however, the average American diet is less than 1:1 due to both low calcium intake and high phosphorus intake.[37] The adequate intakes for phosphorus are 100 mg for ages 0 to 6 months and 275 mg for ages 6 to 12 months.[35] The recommended daily phosphorus allowances are 460 mg for ages 1 to 3 years, 500 mg for ages 4 to 8 years, 1250 mg for 9 to 18 years, and 700 mg for those 19 years or older.[35]

SOCIAL HABIT CHANGES

Tobacco smoking has been associated with lower bone mass[38,39] and increased fracture rates.[39] Based on a study of twins, every 10 pack–year increase in smoking decreased spine bone density by 2% and femoral bone density by 1%.[39] Smoking can cause earlier menopause and can increase endogenous and exogenous sex hormone metabolism. Smoking cessation is beneficial, yielding higher bone mass than continued smoking.[38]

TABLE 82–4. Osteoporosis Prevention and Treatment Guidelines for Children, Women, and Men

Age (years)	0–18	19–45	45[a]–65			≥ 65		
Goal	Increase bone mass	Maintain bone mass	Prevent bone loss			Prevent bone loss and falls		
Exercise	Yes	Yes	Yes			Yes, may need physical assessment		
Lifestyle changes[b]	Yes	Yes	Yes			Yes		
Calcium[c]	Adequate intake	Adequate intake	Adequate intake			Adequate intake		
Vitamin D[d]	Adequate intake	Adequate intake	Adequate intake			Adequate intake		
Bone density[e]			< 1 (P)	1–2.5 (P/T)	>2.5 (T)	<1 (P)	1–2.5 (P/T)	>2.5 (T)
ERT/HRT[f]		OC[h] if amenorrheic	Yes, especially if risks[i]	Yes	Yes	Yes, especially if risks[i]	Yes	Yes
Alendronate (A)			OK	OK, especially if no ERT	Yes[j]	OK, especially if no ERT	Yes[j]	Yes[j]
Nasal calcitonin[g]				Bone pain	Bone pain or if no ERT & A		Bone pain	Bone pain, if no ERT & A

[a]Beginning age for women is postmenopausal age.
[b]Lifestyle changes—stop smoking, increase calcium and vitamin D in diet, decrease caffeine and phosphates in diet, minimize alcohol use.
[c]See National Institute of Health and Institute of Medicine Recommendations in Table 82–5.
[d]Daily adequate intakes for vitamin D (cholecalciferol): birth to 50 years is 200 IU, 51 to 70 years is 400 IU, older than 70 years is 600 IU.
[e]Standard deviation below young adult peak bone mass, <1 = prevention (P), 1-2.5 = prevention or treatment (P/T), > 2.5 = treatment (T).
[f]ERT = estrogen replacement therapy, HRT = hormonal (estrogen and progestin) replacement therapy, for women as long as no absolute contraindications exist; if intact uterus, need concomitant progestin or annual endometrial biopsy.
[g]May consider sooner for treatment of acute fracture or chronic bone pain.
[h]Oral contraceptives.
[i]Risks include cardiovascular disease, family history of Alzheimer's (investigational), urogenital disorders.
[j]Combination therapy with ERT or HRT under investigation, use in patients with ongoing bone loss or fracture while on ERT/HRT (non–FDA-approved indications).

TABLE 82–5. Daily Calcium and Vitamin D Requirements

	NIH Ca^{2+} Consensus[33] Recommendations (mg)	Institute of Medicine[34] Adequate Ca^{2+} Intake (mg)	Institute of Medicine[34] Adequate Vitamin D Intake (IU)
Infant			
Birth–6 mo	400	210	200
6 mo–1 yr	600	270	200
Children			
1–3 yr		500	200
1–5 yr	800		
4–8 yr		800	200
6–10 yr	800–1200		
9–13 yr		1300	200
Adolescents			
11–18 yr	1200–1500		
14–18 yr		1300	200
Women			
19–24 yr	1200–1500	1000	200
Pregnant or nursing	1200–1500	1000	200
Premenopause (25–50 yr)	1000	1000	200
51–70 yr		1200	400
Postmenopause without estrogens	1500		400
Postmenopause with estrogens	1000		400
Women well beyond menopause	1500		400
>70 yr		1200	600
Men			
19–24 yr	1200–1500	1000	200
25–50 yr	1000	1000	200
51–65 yr	1000	1200	400
65–69 yr	1500	1200	400
≥70 yr	1500	1200	600
Maximum dose (upper limit)		≤2500	≤2000

TABLE 82–6. Dietary Sources of Calcium

Food	Serving Size	Calcium Content
Whole milk	1 cup	291
Skim milk	1 cup	302
Ice cream	1 cup	200
Yogurt (low-fat)	1 cup	345–415
American cheese	1 oz	150
Cheddar cheese	1 oz	211
Swiss cheese	1 oz	250
Cottage cheese (low-fat)	1 cup	154
Sardines	3 oz	372
Salmon with bones	3 oz	167
Bokchoy	1/2 cup	126
Broccoli	1 cup	100–136
Collards, raw	1/2 cup	179
Soybeans	1 cup	131
Spinach	1/2 cup	113
Tofu	4 oz	106
Turnip greens	1/2 cup	126
Figs, dried	5 medium	126
Cheese pizza	1 slice	150
Macaroni and cheese	1 cup	362

An association between alcohol use and low bone density and fractures has been found in some but not in all studies, especially when more significant variables were also analyzed.[40] Potentially, alcohol directly decreases calcium absorption and affects bone remodeling through prostaglandins, granulocyte–macrophage progenitor cells, and mineralization rate. Alcohol may induce nutritional deficiencies in calcium, vitamin D, and magnesium; decrease vitamin D liver metabolism to its active metabolite; alter PTH concentrations; and increase falls. Although possibly only a minor factor in osteoporosis, reduced alcohol intake will improve a patient's overall health.

EXERCISE

Increased weight-bearing aerobic and strengthening exercises may prevent bone loss and may decrease falls and fractures.[41–43] Exercise early in life will increase peak bone mass. The type, duration, and style of exercise produce variable results on bone mass and fractures. Generally, bones most directly stressed by exercise have the greatest bone density effect. Running is better than walking; swimming and cycling may offer no benefit. The primary benefit of exercise may be improved balance, muscle strength, range of motion, endurance, and posture, along with decreased falls and pain. Elderly persons and those with severe osteoporosis should have a medical examination and potentially a physical therapist's prescription for an exercise program. Calcium and estrogen therapy are enhanced with concomitant exercise.[41–43] Of note, very vigorous exercise programs, such as for elite athletes, can produce amenorrhea, which leads to low bone density and fractures in women.[44]

ANTIRESORPTIVE PREVENTION AND THERAPY

CALCIUM

Most of the body's calcium content is stored in bone. A feedback system between serum calcium concentration, PTH, and vitamin D controls the destruction of bone to meet the body's calcium needs (Fig. 82–2). To prevent bone destruction, adequate calcium should be ingested (Table 82–5).[34,35] Because the American diet is generally insufficient in calcium,[37] patients should either increase dietary calcium intake (Table 82–6) and/or use supplements (Table 82–7).

Clinical Effectiveness

Supplemental calcium can significantly slow the rate of bone loss and may decrease fractures. Calcium works better to prevent bone loss in cortical bones, in women with the lowest dietary or life history of calcium intake, and in women before or after the first 5 years of menopause. Its effect is enhanced when combined with other osteoporosis medications or exercise.[41,45] The combination of calcium and vitamin D slows bone loss and decreases nonvertebral,[46,47] hip,[47] and vertebral[47] fractures. Thus, calcium alone is insufficient to prevent osteoporosis and should be combined with other therapies.

Calcium Administration

Pharmacists should assist patients in designing the appropriate calcium regimen to fulfill NIH[34,35] daily calcium requirements (see Table 82–5). Oral calcium supplements are convenient and may be needed for patients with certain characteristics or conditions: lactose intolerance, nondairy vegetarians, malnutrition, insufficient calcium intake, glucocorticoid therapy, and low-fat diets. The various calcium salt preparations provide different amounts of calcium (Table 82–7). Calcium carbonate contains the most elemental calcium by weight (40%) and is the least expensive. Pharmacists should suggest calcium carbonate products with good disintegration and dissolution rates, because these can vary significantly between products and lots.[48]

Calcium carbonate tablets should be ingested with meals to enhance absorption from meal-stimulated acid secretion. Calcium citrate is acid-independent and thus does not need to be taken with meals. Some elderly patients may have decreased acid secretion and therefore should take their calcium carbonate with meals or use calcium citrate, a more expensive product. The calcium absorption fraction decreases as tablet size increases; divided doses (500 to 600 mg or less) should be ingested to enhance the amount absorbed.

Because the goal of supplementation is to provide the amount of calcium the body needs, few side effects are experienced. However, caution and/or monitoring should be conducted for patients with a history of kidney stones. The most common side effect is constipation, which can have a higher incidence in the elderly. Calcium should not be administered with fiber laxatives. Calcium can decrease absorption of iron, tetracycline, quinolones, alendronate, etidronate, phenytoin, and fluoride when given concomitantly.

DIURETICS

Thiazide diuretics promote a decrease in renal calcium excretion, while loop diuretics increase renal calcium excretion. A recent meta-analysis of 13 thiazide diuretic observational studies yielded a relative risk of 0.8 (95% confidence interval, 0.73 to 0.91) for hip fracture, with the benefit greater with longer use; past users showed no continued benefit.[49] Concurrent thiazides and estrogens resulted in greater bone mineral density than did thiazides alone.[50]

VITAMIN D AND METABOLITES

Vitamin D deficiency can result from insufficient dietary intake, decreased skin conversion (decreased sun exposure, use of sunscreens), decreased conversion to 1,25-dihydroxyvitamin D (liver or renal dysfunction), or receptor resistance (aging, possibly genotypes). Vitamin D deficiency or decreased responsiveness occurs in some elderly and patients with osteoporosis.

TABLE 82–7. Calcium Product Selection[a]

Product	Calcium Content	Calcium (mg)	Tablets for 1 g[b]
Calcium Carbonate	40		
Generic		200–600	2–6
Generic + Vit D (125 IU)		600	2
Generic suspension		500/5 mL	10mL
Calcilyte + Vit D (200 IU)		500	2[c]
Calel-D + Vit D (200 IU)		500	2
Caltrate		600	2
Caltrate + Vit D (125 IU)		600	2
OsCal		500	2
OsCal + Vit D (125 IU)		500	2
Titralac Chewable		168	5
Extra Strength		300	4
Liquid		400/5 mL	12.5 mL
Tums		200	5
E-X		300	4
Ultra		500	2
Calcium Citrate	24		
Citracal 950		200	5
Citracal Liquitab		500	2
Citracal + Vit D (200 IU)		316	4
Calcium Lactate	18		
Generic		42–84	12–24

[a]Not all calcium products listed, only those with 500–600 mg per tablet or with an alternative dosage form (i.e., chewable, liquid, dissolvable tablet).
[b]When using a combination product, determine if total vitamin D ingestion is appropriate for the age of the person.
[c]Tablet for solution.

Clinical Effectiveness

Although agreement may exist on ensuring adequate vitamin D intake (see Table 82–5),[35] the pharmacologic use and appropriate dose of vitamin D_3 or calcitriol to prevent fractures are controversial.[41] Vitamin D_3 700[45] or 800 IU[46] with 500 to 1200 mg calcium resulted in significantly increased femur bone density and decreased hip and nonvertebral fractures in ambulatory[45] and nursing home elderly,[47] while 400 IU with 800 to 1000 mg of calcium in ambulatory women did not decrease hip or peripheral fractures.[51] when compared with placebo. Calcitriol 0.25 mg twice daily for 3 years decreased new vertebral fractures in women with fewer than five vertebral fractures at baseline and also decreased peripheral fractures.[41]

Vitamin D Administration

Vitamin D supplementation should be given to patients with inadequate sun exposure or ingestions less than the newly established adequate vitamin D intakes (see Table 82–5).[35] Seasonal variations due to sun exposure may require periodic adjustments in vitamin D supplementation. In patients with kidney failure, calcitriol or dihydrotachysterol administration may be needed. In those with liver disease, calcifediol or calcitriol may be needed. A 25- or 1,25-dihydroxyvitamin D metabolite concentration may be required for dosage determination, especially in patients with advanced osteoporosis or liver or renal dysfunction.

Hypercalcemia and hypercalciuria can develop with high vitamin D doses or calcitriol. With calcitriol therapy, lower supplemental or dietary calcium intake may be required, especially at initiation. Serum calcium and sometimes urinary calcium concentrations should be monitored for patients receiving calcitriol; adequate vitamin D supplementation generally requires no monitoring. Vitamin D-induced high serum calcium concentrations could aggravate verapamil and digoxin activity. Concomitant use of thiazide diuretics may increase the serum calcium concentrations, while cholestyramine, mineral oil, phenytoin, and barbiturates can decrease vitamin D concentrations.

HORMONAL THERAPY

Estrogen

The osteoporosis consensus development conference in 1993 stated estrogen replacement therapy (ERT) was the treatment of choice for preventing osteoporosis.[52] The Food and Drug Administration (FDA) has approved conjugated equinine estrogens (CEEs) for osteoporosis prevention and treatment and other estrogen products for prevention. Based on a recent Markov model including coronary artery disease, hip fracture, and breast and endometrial cancer, women with at least 1 coronary heart disease risk factor should receive ERT/HRT (ERT plus progestin) regardless of relatives with breast cancer.[53] Women with at least one risk factor for hip fracture should receive ERT/HRT, but in this case the number of risk factors required for treatment increases with the number of relatives with breast cancer.

Estrogen receptors exist on osteoblasts, osteoclasts, macrophage cells, intestinal cells, and many other tissue sites. Estrogens decrease osteoclast recruitment and activity, decrease bone resorption, inhibit PTH peripherally, increase calcitriol concentrations (oral therapy), increase intestinal calcium absorption, and decrease renal calcium excretion.[4,6,43] Estrogens decrease cytokines and other bone-influencing compounds, leading to decreased bone resorption.

Clinical Effectiveness

BONE DENSITY AND FRACTURES

ERT consistently increases both cortical (1% to 3%) and trabecular (2% to 5%) bone density.[43] The initial increase over the first

1 to 2 years of therapy results from the uncoupling of bone remodeling, slowing resorption and allowing formation to continue until a new equilibrium is established.

Some clinical trials suggest the greatest effect is seen when ERT is administered during accelerated bone loss, which occurs for 3 to 6 years after menopause. However, women who were 55 to 64 years old with low initial bone density or no previous ERT use had a greater response to CEE than women 45 to 54 years old.[54] Significant effects are also seen with ERT use in elderly women. Serum estradiol concentrations above 60 pg/mL are associated with increased bone density.[43] About 10% to 15% of women will still lose bone mass with ERT.[43] Immediately after ERT discontinuation, bone loss is accelerated at rates similar to those after menopause.

A dose of CEE of 0.625 mg or equivalent generally produces the best balance between increase in bone density and adverse reactions; however, esterified estrogens of 0.3 mg or equivalent may at least maintain or slightly increase bone density when combined with calcium,[55] progestins, or other osteoporosis treatments. Oral and transdermal estrogens at equivalent doses have similar bone density effects. ERT implants and intrauterine impregnated devices have also shown positive effects. Similar effects are seen with continuous or cyclic ERT/HRT administration. Initially, at least 10 years of ERT was advocated starting as soon as possible after menopause; however, based on the following study and future research, duration for preventing bone loss may be changed to either life-long use or initial use beginning later in life. In an elderly cohort, current continuous ERT (mean, 20 years) started around menopause was associated with the highest bone densities at four different body sites.[56] However, the bone densities in women with current continuous use for about 9 years starting after age 60 were slightly less but not significantly different than values in current continuous users of 20 years. Both of these groups produced greater responses than the other groups of women (early past users for 10 years, current late users for short duration, and women who had never used ERT).

ERT/HRT decreases osteoporotic fracture risk, but the effect varies by bone type, age, onset of therapy, and duration of ERT.[43,57] Pooled results from epidemiology hip fracture studies conducted from 1979 to 1991 yielded a relative risk of 0.75 (95% confidence interval, 0.68 to 0.84) for HRT use.[57] Not all studies report a decrease in hip fractures.[57,58] Wrist and nonspinal fractures were significantly decreased in elderly women with ERT use.[58] Only women older than 75 with current ERT use had significantly fewer hip fractures compared to women 65 to 75.[58] In contrast, ERT use produced fewer hip fractures in black women younger than 75.[13] Longer duration had a greater fracture-protective effect.[57,58] The risk of hip and lower forearm fracture returned to near baseline after HRT had been discontinued for at least 6 years.[57] More definitive answers about ERT/HRT will come from the Women's Health Initiative (WHI) clinical trial begun in 1993, which enrolled 10,000 women of ages 50 to 79 for a 10-year study. The study goals are to evaluate the effect of ERT/HRT, low-fat diets, calcium and vitamin D supplementation, and counseling programs on cardiovascular disease, cancer, and osteoporotic fracture incidences.

CARDIOVASCULAR DISEASE AND LIPIDS

The decision to use ERT/HRT to prevent osteoporosis must include ERT/HRT's other potential benefits, most notably the cardiovascular benefit.[53] This benefit is currently based on outcome epidemiology studies and clinical trials exploring possible cardiovascular mechanisms.[57–60] In the most recent cohort studies, the relative risk for cardiovascular morbidity was 0.39 (95% confidence interval, 0.19 to 0.78),[59] and the relative risk for all-cause mortality in current users was 0.63 (95% confidence interval, 0.56 to 0.7).[60] The greatest mortality effect was for patients with greater cardiovascular risk. More definitive answers will be provided by the WHI study.

The mechanisms for ERT/HRT prevention of cardiovascular disease include favorable lipid alterations; decreased vascular tone; preserved endothelial function; decreased fibrinogen, antithrombin III, and thromboxane A_2 formation; increased factor VII and protein C; decreased fasting glucose and insulin; increased prostacyclin I_2, blood flow, stroke volume, and antioxidant activity; and decreased plasminogen activator inhibitor.[61,62] ERT decreases or maintains total cholesterol; decreases LDL, apolipoprotein B, and lipoprotein (a); and increases HDL, HDL-2, HDL-3, apolipoprotein A-1, and triglycerides.[62–65] ERT's positive lipid effect is maintained while on therapy. Because transdermal ERT bypasses the liver, less positive lipid effects occur, which are achieved later than with oral ERT.[64] Progestins and androgens can minimize or eliminate the positive ERT lipid effect.[62,63] CEE combined with pravastatin produced a greater decrease in LDL, a similar effect on HDL, and reversal of the triglyceride rise seen with CEE alone.[65]

OTHER BENEFITS

Other potential benefits of ERT have been validated to various degrees.[57,58,66] ERT can decrease urge and stress incontinence, vaginal atrophy, dyspareunia, urinary tract infections, and tooth loss and slow the aging of skin. Many women experienced more energy and a positive mood, but the contrary can also be experienced, especially when progestins are added. Although cerebral blood flow may be increased, the effect on stroke is less remarkable.[57,58] In some cohort studies, ERT/HRT users had less dementia.[66] Effects on patients with Alzheimer's disease and cognitive function is variable. More research needs to be conducted in the areas of stroke, cognitive function, and Alzheimer's disease.

ERT/HRT Administration. Absolute contraindications to ERT/HRT therapy include active or suspected estrogen-dependent cancer, abnormal vaginal bleeding, severe liver disease, and active vascular thrombosis. Relative contraindications include migraine headaches, history of thromboembolic disease especially with pregnancy or past oral contraceptive use, migraines, hypertriglyceridemia, uterine fibroids, endometriosis, gallbladder disease, strong family history of breast cancer, and chronic hepatic dysfunction.

The suggested ERT doses for osteoporosis prevention and treatment are CEE 0.625 mg, ethinyl estradiol 0.02 mg, estropipate 0.625 mg, esterified estrogens 0.625 mg, micronized estradiol 1 mg, 17-β estradiol 2 mg, estrone sulfate 1.5 mg, and transdermal estradiol 0.05 mg/d.[43,67] Vaginal administration from creams or rings results in significant systemic absorption. ERT products are not considered interchangeable. Each product produces different estradiol and estrone concentrations. Estradiol is the predominant estrogen before menopause, while estrone is the predominant estrogen after menopause. Oral estradiol is converted via the first-pass effect to estrone, while transdermal estradiol bypasses liver metabolism and is associated with the highest estradiol concentrations. The major and minor components of CEE and other combination estrogen products may have some bone, cardiovascular, and breast protective effects.

ERT is usually administered continuously with continuous or cyclic progestin. Continuous HRT therapy is usually initiated because 60% to 80% of women will be amenorrheic 6 to 12 months after starting therapy and fewer women will have hyperplasia.[68] However, until then, random spotting and bleeding will occur. If amenorrhea does not develop after 1 year, predictable bleeding patterns with cyclic therapy may be preferred. Continuous ERT alone is used for women with a hysterectomy. If used for women with an intact uterus, 85% of the women will be amenorrheic, but all should have annual endometrial biopsies.

For continuous therapy, CEE 0.625 mg or equivalent is administered daily and medroxyprogesterone (MPA) 5 to 10 mg is administered for 12 to 14 days at the beginning of the month or 2.5 to 5.0 mg is administered daily. A combination tablet of CEE 0.625 mg with MPA 2.5 or 5 mg exists. For the cyclic regimen, CEE 0.625 mg or equivalent is administered for 3 or 4 weeks, with MPA 5 to 10 mg administered for the last 12 to 14 days of ERT. A blister packet is marketed of 28 CEE 0.625-mg tablets with the last 14 containing MPA 5 mg. Duration of therapy is for at least 10 years and potentially for life. Response, tolerance, and other ERT benefits such as cardiovascular protection will influence duration of therapy.

ERT Side Effects. The risks of ERT/HRT must be discussed with all women. Use of unopposed ERT is associated with up to a 12-fold increase in endometrial cancer, with the risk rising with longer duration.[57,69] Concomitant progestin therapy for at least 12 to 14 days a month usually eliminates this risk and may even be protective.[57,69] Numerous case-control, cohort, and meta-analysis studies have been done on the relationship between ERT and breast cancer.[57,70] Generally, the relative risk values for breast cancer are between 1 and 1.5, with the risk increasing slightly with longer duration (≥ 15 to 20 years). Small studies have reported beneficial effects of ERT in women with breast cancer remission, most of whom have had no recurrence.[70] Data from the WHI study will assist in elucidating this relationship. ERT/HRT can cause benign increased breast density on mammography. Of note, women who develop endometrial or breast cancer while on ERT/HRT generally have longer survival. Proposed theories include better access to health care, more preventive health behaviors, earlier detection with better survival rates, and less cardiovascular disease/mortality.

Common adverse reactions for ERT/HRT include vaginal spotting and bleeding, breast tenderness and enlargement (especially in older women), pedal edema, and weight gain. These effects may decrease over time. During cyclic therapy, vaginal bleeding should be evaluated if bleeding occurs on days 1 to 9 or 16 to 31 if progestin is given for the first 10 days.[71] For the continuous regimen, vaginal bleeding needs to be evaluated if bleeding is heavier than premenopause periods, lasts for more than 10 days, occurs more than once a month, or persists after 10 months of therapy.[71] Use of an exercise or more supportive bra and/or wearing the bra to bed may decrease breast tenderness. Lower estrogen dose, estrogen break, different progestin, decreased caffeine, or a short course of hydrochlorothiazide can also decrease breast tenderness.[67]

Less common adverse reactions are facial hair growth, bloating, nausea, vomiting, leg pain, headache/migraines, increase or decrease in sexual desire, dizziness, and mood changes. If migraines occur, a transdermal estrogen product may eliminate the side effect.[67] HRT taken at bedtime or with food can avoid problems with nausea.[67] If bloating occurs, a different progestin or low-dose hydrochlorothiazide may help.[67] In patients experiencing mood changes, the clinician may switch to a different progestin, decrease the intermittent dose, or use a continuous low dose.[67] Rare adverse events with ERT include skin darkening, acne, rash, loss of pubic hair, stomach pain, jaundice, and venous thromboembolism (VTE). A 2.5-fold increase in cholelithiasis exists. Although the rate of VTE is two to three times that of nonusers, it is very rare, with only 2 to 3 cases per 10,000 women.[72] The highest incidence of VTE was within 1 year of ERT/HRT initiation.

ERT/HRT may decrease the metabolism of corticosteroids, oral anticoagulants, and tricyclic antidepressants, resulting in increased effect and/or toxicity. Enzyme inducers and smoking may increase estrogen metabolism.

ERT/HRT Usage and Compliance. In 1992, 1 out of every 4 to 6 American women used ERT.[73] Users are generally better educated, have a higher socioeconomic status, have better insurance coverage, have more access to health care, and/or practice preventive health. The majority of ERT/HRT prescriptions were written by gynecologists (50% to 60%), while 20% came from family medicine or general practitioners. Between 1990 and 1992, only 17% of an elderly cohort were using ERT/HRT.[74] The most common reasons for current ERT/HRT use included hysterectomy, postmenopausal symptoms, physician prescription, and prevention or treatment of osteoporosis. The primary reasons for never using hormones were that they were perceived harmful or of no benefit. Past users quit ERT/HRT predominantly because they saw no perceived benefit; however, 16% quit because of side effects.[73] The two adverse reactions causing women to discontinue use are vaginal bleeding and breast tenderness. Bone density measurements can influence a woman's decision to use HRT.[43,75]

Low usage and compliance with ERT/HRT are important issues for pharmacists to address. Pharmacists' access to healthy and/or ambulatory clients creates an opportunity for them to educate and help adolescents and women practice preventive health and resolve medication-related problems. Women need to be educated about adverse reactions. Dosage manipulation can decrease or eliminate adverse events. The long-term benefits versus the adverse reactions must be continually reemphasized. The lifetime probabilities for a 50-year old woman without ERT/HRT are coronary artery disease, 46%; stroke, 20%; hip fracture, 15%; breast cancer, 10%; and endometrial cancer, 3%.[57] Without risk factors, HRT would increase life by 1 year; for those with risk factors, it would increase life by 0.6 to 2.2 years.[56]

Progestins

Progestins are used only in women with an intact uterus to prevent and potentially protect them from endometrial cancer.[69] They may affect ERT's beneficial and adverse effects.

Clinical Effectiveness. The addition of progestins to ERT (termed hormone-replacement therapy, or HRT) results in no change or a slight increase in bone density.[54,76,77] Compared with ERT alone, when a progestin was added to ERT, a smaller rise in HDL[62] but similar LDL, triglyceride, and apoliproprotein A-1 and B effects occurred.[78] MPA and CEE increased 2-hour glucose concentration and produced similar blood pressure, insulin, and fibrinogen responses to CEE alone.[62] Based on the Nurses' Health Study, both HRT and ERT were associated with decreased risk for major coronary disease.[59]

Progestin Administration. Daily doses of MPA 2.5 to 5 mg or cyclic 5 to 10 mg for 12 to 14 days every month can be used. Daily administration improves compliance and increases amenorrhea. Progestin implants and intrauterine devices, micronized progesterone, and quarterly progestin administration are under investigation. With the continuous MPA regimen, the percentage of women with amenorrhea is 55% to 92% at 6 months and 75% to 100% at 1 year.[68] Investigational MPA 10 mg for 14 days every 3 months produced a longer and sometimes heavier and/or unscheduled menses, but less frequently and was preferred over the monthly cyclical regimen.[79] Micronized progesterone is under review by the FDA for HRT. The combination patch with estradiol 0.05 mg and norethindrone either 0.14 or 0.25 mg has been approved for treatment of vasomotor symptoms of menopause, valvular atrophy, and hypoestrogenic conditions. It is under investigation for osteoporosis prevention and treatment. The Nurses' Health Study and other investigations have revealed no significant increase in breast cancer with HRT versus ERT.[70] Progestins, more likely responsible for breast changes and discomfort, acne, fluid retention, and psychological side effects, should be altered before ERT to resolve these problematic adverse effects.

Selective Estrogen Receptor Modulators

Tamoxifen, the first selective estrogen receptor modulator (SERM), is both an estrogen antagonist in breast tissue and an agonist in bone and uterine tissue. Small (0.6% to 2%) but significant increases in bone density occur with standard breast cancer prevention doses (20 mg/d).[76,80] Tamoxifen decreased total cholesterol, LDL, apolipoprotein B, fibrinogen, and antithrombin III; increased apolipoprotein A-1; and had no effect on HDL.[80,81] Women who received continuous tamoxifen had a lower incidence of fatal myocardial infarction.[76] However, tamoxifen has been associated with endometrial cancer, requiring women to have routine follow-up and sometimes endometrial biopsies.

Raloxifene and droloxifene (investigational) are also SERMs, but unlike tamoxifen, they are antagonists in uterine tissue.[76,83,84,85] Short term raloxifene 200 mg daily produced similar biochemical bone marker and LDL-C changes to CEE 0.625 mg but no HDL-C increase.[84] Raloxifene 60 mg daily increased bone mineral density (BMD) by about 2% and decreased LDL and total cholesterol.[85] No endometrial changes were seen.[84,85] The only major raloxifene adverse reaction was hot flashes. Women with current or past thromboembolic events should not use raloxifene. Raloxifene may be preferred for women with current, past, or strong family history for breast cancer (investigational).

Testosterone and Anabolic Steroids

Methyltestosterone 1.25 or 2.5 mg and testosterone patches and implants (investigational) are being coadministered with ERT/HRT in women with depression or decreased libido, sexual function, or energy level.[82] Concomitant methyltestosterone or testosterone therapy has either no effect, or an additive effect, on bone density[43,63]; reverses the increased HDL[63,82]; and increases virilizing side effects such as hirsutism, acne, and hoarseness.[82]

Although anabolic steroids enhance osteoblast activity, in clinical trials their effect is predominantly decreased resorption. Their effect may be more related to increased muscle mass and strength. Nandrolone decanoate 50 mg IM every 3 to 4 weeks minimally increased bone density, with a plateau after 1 year.[83] Most women develop adverse reactions such as liver function alterations, negative lipid effects, hirsutism, hoarseness, acne, and other virilizing adverse effects, thus limiting androgen use.

Oral Contraceptives

Past or current use of oral contraceptives by pre-, peri-, or postmenopausal women has been associated with an increase in bone density in some but not all epidemiologic studies.[86] Use of oral contraceptives showed no protective effect on fracture rate in an older cohort.[87] Oral contraceptives given to women with anorexia nervosa and primary or secondary amenorrhea showed increased bone densities in some but not all types of bone.[88] In perimenopausal women with oligomenorrhea, oral contraceptive use was associated with higher lumbar spine[89,90] but not femoral neck bone[89] densities. Because estrogen deficiency is associated with an accelerated rate of bone loss, in the future oral contraceptive use during the perimenopausal time frame may eliminate any period of estrogen deficiency. However, the safety of oral contraceptives in older women needs further study.

Tibolone

Tibolone is a synthetic hormone with weak estrogenic, progestogenic, and androgenic activity. After 2 years of treatment, metacarpal, lumbar spine, and femoral neck bone densities increased or were maintained versus bone loss with placebo.[76,91] Vaginal bleeding occurs less frequently (20% of patients) than with ERT/HRT therapy.[91] Tibolone decreased HDL and lipoprotein(a) and had no effect on LDL or triglycerides.[92] Long-term effects on fracture rate, cardiovascular disease, and breast and uterine cancer are unknown.

Bisphosphonates

Bisphosphonates adsorb to bone hydroxyapatite, later becoming a permanent part of bone structure. They are resistant to enzymatic hydrolysis; thus, their estimated half-lives are similar to that of bone (1 to 10 years). When osteoclasts bind to the bisphosphonate-covered or bisphosphonate-contained bone surface, their structure and function are altered, preventing adherence and resorption. Etidronate—but not alendronate—also inhibits bone mineralization, which can cause osteomalacia. Alendronate is FDA approved for prevention and treatment.

Clinical Effectiveness. Alendronate at prevention doses[93] produced similar or lower BMD effects than HRT, while treatment doses[94–96] produced greater BMD effects. From the EPIC (Early Postmenopausal Intervention Cohort) study, alendronate 5 mg (prevention dose) increased lumbar (3.5%), femoral neck (1.3%), and trochanter (3%) BMD.[93,94] Alendronate 10 mg (treatment dose) significantly increased lumbar (5% to 10%), femoral neck (1% to 5%), trochanter (7%), and distal forearm (0.3% to 2%) bone densities in women with bone densities greater than 2 to 2.5 SDs of young adult peak bone mass.[94] The 5-mg dose was effective treatment in elderly women, but less effective than the 10-mg dose.[95] The bone effect is greatest in the first year but continues in subsequent years.[93] After discontinuation, the rate of bone loss will eventually return to average age-related losses but the BMD will be higher than for nonusers. Vertebral[92] and nonvertebral[96] (relative risk, 0.71; 95% confidence interval, 0.5 to 0.997; P = 0.048) fractures were decreased. Alendronate produced greater BMD effects than a low dose of nasal calcitonin (100 IU).[94]

Intermittent administration of etidronate has been evaluated. Five years of intermittent cyclical etidronate (400 mg/d for 2 weeks, then calcium and vitamin D for 13 weeks) continually increased vertebral bone density and decreased vertebral fracture rate.[97] Intermittent cyclical etidronate evaluated for up to 4 years had an additive effect with HRT on vertebral and hip bone densities, with no reported osteomalacia; while 33% of those on etidronate alone had osteomalacia.[98]

Bisphosphonate Administration. Currently, alendronate is the preferred bisphosphonate because it does not inhibit mineralization. Bisphosphonates are poorly absorbed (1% to 5%), with food and calcium significantly decreasing absorption. Alendronate should be taken 30 to 120 minutes before breakfast with a full glass of water (not coffee, juice, or milk). The patient should remain in an upright position for at least 30 minutes. Calcium and, when needed, vitamin D should also be used but administered at different times. Nausea and diarrhea are the most common side effects of the drug. Esophageal irritation and ulceration can result when alendronate directions are not followed or when prescribed for patients with contraindications. Investigational bisphosphonates for osteoporosis include clodronate, pamidronate, and residronate.

Calcitonin

Calcitonin is FDA approved for postmenopausal osteoporosis treatment. Calcitonin opposes the action of PTH; thus, when calcium is high, calcitonin is released, decreasing osteoclastic activity and resorption. Stimulation of calcitonin osteoclastic receptors results in a decreased osteoclast bone attachment, motility, life span, and numbers; altered osteoclastic cellular structure; and decreased tubular reabsorption of sodium and calcium. In some elderly, calcitonin concentrations are decreased.

Clinical Effectiveness. Calcitonin increases lumbar spine bone density (1% to 3%), with less effect on cortical bone.[98,99] Nasal calcitonin decreases vertebral fractures.[100] Patients with high bone turnover or late-onset menopause respond better than those with normal or low bone turnover rates or early-onset menopause. However, elderly women, those assumed to have low bone turnover rate, have been shown to have decreased bone resorption with calcitonin.[99] Neutralizing antibodies, which develop in 40% to 70% of patients treated with subcutaneous calcitonin, can sometimes minimize calcitonin's effect and may be partly responsible for the tolerance sometimes observed with continuous long-term treatment. To overcome the plateau effect, various intermittent dosing regimens have been investigated and are usually less effective than daily administration. The rate of bone loss reverts to age-related losses after discontinuation.

Calcitonin provides pain relief within days to weeks for many patients with osteoporotic, Paget's disease, or metastatic bone pain.[99,101] Potential mechanisms of action include decreased prostaglandins, altered intracellular calcium concentrations, increased β endorphins, cholinergic or serotonergic effects, direct effect on receptors, or neuromodulator effect.

Calcitonin Administration. Because it is not as effective as other osteoporosis medications, calcitonin is generally reserved for treating patients with acute fractures or chronic osteoporotic pain and for those in whom hormonal or bisphosphonate therapy is contraindicated, not tolerated, or refused. The intranasal dose is 200 IU daily, alternating nares. Calcitonin nasal absorption is 0.3% to 30.6%. The subcutaneous dose is 100 IU daily. If the primary reason for use is pain control, attempts at decreasing the weekly dose can be tried after pain is controlled. Concomitant calcium and, when needed, vitamin D should be used.

Nasal administration produces fewer side effects; rhinitis, epistaxis, and nasal irritation. Subcutaneous side effects are nausea, anorexia, diarrhea, stomach discomfort, abdominal pain, salty taste, injection site pain, and flushing; these decrease with nighttime administration and duration of use.

INVESTIGATIONAL ANTIRESORPTIVE AGENTS

PHYTOESTROGENS

Phytoestrogens such as isoflavones (genistein, daidzein) and lignans (enterodiol, enterolactone) may have weak estrogenic or antiestrogenic activity.[102] Isoflavones are metabolized from soybeans, soyflour, textured vegetable protein, tempeh, and tofu. Lignans are metabolized from flaxseed and some cereals, vegetables, legumes, and fruits. Ipriflavone, a synthetic isoflavone partially metabolized to diadzein, is void of estrogenic activity but may increase the effect of estrogens.[76,83,102] It can decrease bone resorption by inhibiting osteoclast production or differentiation, decreasing PTH responsiveness, and potentially increasing osteoblast maturation.

MISCELLANEOUS AGENTS

In animal studies, low doses of strontium uncouple resorption and formation, while high doses interfere with mineralization.[83] Short-term therapy decreases osteoclastic activity; long-term therapy increases formation. Other trace minerals such as boron, manganese, copper, and zinc are under investigation. Because prostaglandins may have a role in bone remodeling, aspirin and nonsteroidal anti-inflammatory drugs (NSAIDs) could influence bone by decreasing prostaglandin production, as has been suggested with diclofenac.[83] By changing osteoclast ability to attach to bone, compounds such as echistatin, amylin, proton pump inhibitors, and potassium bicarbonate may also minimize bone loss.[76] Vitamin K has a role in bone metabolism, with ongoing research to determine if supplementation is beneficial, especially in vitamin K deficiency.[8]

INVESTIGATIONAL BONE FORMATION THERAPY

FLUORIDE

Sodium fluoride and monofluorophosphate are under investigation for treatment of osteoporosis. Fluoride ions serve as hydroxy radicals in the hydroxyapatite crystals, forming fluorapatite. Fluorapatite alters the size and structure of crystals, resulting in increased bone crystallinity and a decrease in solubility. Adequate calcium concentrations are required. Fluoride also produces an uncoupling of the remodeling process and a prolongation of the remodeling cycle, which favors formation over resorption. With lower doses, bone density increases; however, with larger doses the increased bone density has altered structure, leading to decreased strength and more microfractures. This new bone forms on existing bone but does not build new bridges between segments of old bone.

Clinical Effectiveness

Fluoride's therapeutic window is 95 to 190 ng/mL, which can be maintained with the lower-dose, sustained-release products but not with older higher-dose, rapid-release products.[103] Sustained-release sodium fluoride doses of 25 mg twice a day administered with 312 to 400 mg of calcium citrate daily increased lumbar (4% to 5%) and femoral bone density (2% to 4%), but it produced no effect on radial bone density and vertebral fracture rate.[103] Lumbar bone density increased for at least 4 years, although the femoral bone density leveled off after 2 years. Patients with mild to moderate osteoporosis had a greater response than patients with severe osteoporosis. To enhance efficacy and safety, intermittent regimens are under investigation. Results with monofluorophosphate and enteric-coated sodium fluoride are not as favorable as with the sustained-release products.

Fluoride Administration

In the future, sustained-release fluoride 25 mg twice a day with calcium therapy administered at a different time may be advocated for patients with severe osteoporosis. Fluoride, a renally eliminated drug, will require dosage adjustments in patients with decreased renal function. Antacids and calcium decrease fluoride absorption. Adverse effects with the sustained-release product are gastrointestinal (8%) and musculoskeletal (6%). So far the sustained-release product has not yielded microfractures and nonvertebral fractures, which had been seen with the higher dose rapid-release fluoride products.

GROWTH HORMONES AND FACTORS

Growth hormone (GH) and insulin-like growth factor (IGF) stimulated bone formation and bone resorption; but transforming growth factor (TGF), only increased bone formation.[76,83] GH's effect may be due to increasing IGF levels. Aging decreases both GH and IFG-I. Within the few human studies, results of GH, IGF, and TGF reveal little or no effect on bone density. Side effects include glucose intolerance, hyperinsulinemia, hypertension, edema, and aggravated carpel tunnel syndrome. These products may have a future role as components of combination therapy.

PARATHYROID HORMONE

Parathyroid hormone (PTH) controls calcium and phosphorus concentrations and bone turnover through its effect on bone, kidney, and calcitriol production and activity in the gut. Subcutaneous injections of hPTH (1-34 fragment) 400 to 800 IU given daily or for short intervals have increased lumbar bone density without femoral neck bone density changes.[76,83] Various combinations with other medications have been investigated with mixed results.

COHERENCE THERAPY

Coherence therapy, a theoretical model now referred to as the activation-depression-free-repeat (ADFR) regimen, tries to mimic the normal remodeling sequence. The first phase requires an agent to increase the activation of new bone modeling, and the second phase uses an agent to shift the bone balance, inhibiting osteoclasts but not osteoblasts. The net result would increase bone mass. In practice, these regimens have not produced better results or fewer side effects.

SPECIAL POPULATIONS

WOMEN WITH AMENORRHEA

Women with amenorrhea secondary to excessive exercise, anorexia nervosa, or certain medications are at risk for bone loss due to estrogen deficiency and may respond to hormone replacement. Generally, oral contraceptives[88] are the preferred estrogen product, but HRT has been used.[44]

MEN

Adequate intakes of calcium and vitamin D (see Table 82–5) should be achieved through diet or diet and supplementation.[35] Smoking cessation; decreased alcohol, caffeine, and phosphate intake; and increased exercise should be advocated. Fall prevention should be employed for older men. Current thiazide use had minimal effect on bone density for men.[50]

Testosterone replacement therapy has been used in hypogonadal men,[104] but its use for prevention of bone loss—especially in older men—has been minimally studied. Transdermal patches were as effective as intramuscular testosterone in these men. Testosterone is contraindicated in men with prostatic cancer and should be used cautiously in men with prostatic hypertrophy. Adverse reactions include liver toxicity, gynecomastia, and painful erections. Alendronate increased femoral neck and vertebral bone density in a small sample of men.[105] Calcitonin decreased bone loss in castrated men.[25] Many studies are currently underway to develop better treatment regimens for men.

ELDERLY

In elderly patients, prevention of falls gains greater importance.[24] Because decreased muscle strength is associated with falls, exercise should be conducted to increase muscle strength. Home environments should be redesigned, eliminating opportunities for falls. Slip rugs and extension cords should be removed, handrails should be placed on the bathtub, and nonslip tape should be placed inside tubs. A patient's medication profile should be reviewed for psychotropic, sedative/hypnotic, antidepressant, antihypertensive, NSAIDs, and diuretic medications, all of which are associated with falls. Sedatives should be discontinued or switched to short-acting agents. Other central nervous system medications should also be eliminated or changed if altered balance or confusion result. Diuretics should be given during the day to prevent nocturnal voiding. Orthostatic blood pressure changes should be evaluated, and problems should be resolved through slow arousal from lying and sitting positions or medication changes. The use of hip protectors may decrease fractures after falls,[83] but most patients do not like wearing them.

Through diet or supplements, adequate amounts of calcium and vitamin D should be ingested daily (see Table 82–6). Due to age-associated decreases in renal and liver function, a serum 25- or 1,25-hydroxyvitamin D level may be appropriate to determine the ability of the patient to convert vitamin D to the active metabolite. Smoking cessation and exercise begun late in life still have a positive effect on bones.

Estrogens can decrease bone loss in the elderly. In fact, future recommendations may be to delay the onset of ERT/HRT until later in life, and then to continue it for 10 years or for life.[56] Elderly patients have a greater incidence of ERT/HRT breast enlargement and tenderness, which decreases over time. A very small body of literature has identified a lower estrogen dose (0.3 mg esterified estrogens or equivalent) to be effective in the elderly. Starting at a lower dose and increasing it later to 0.625 mg may decrease side effects, increase acceptance and adherence, and prevent bone loss.

For elderly with significant bone loss or fracture history and no cardiovascular or Alzheimer's disease or family history of these diseases, alendronate may be preferred over estrogens. If estrogens are contraindicated, then alendronate would be the drug of choice. However, the elderly must not have significant gastrointestinal problems, especially of the esophagus; must be able to follow the complicated administration directions; and must have judgment capabilities to respond to GI problems.

Nasal calcitonin may decrease osteoporotic bone pain, decreasing the need for the more toxic narcotics and NSAIDs.

PHARMACOECONOMIC CONSIDERATIONS

The annual cost for osteoporotic fractures is about $5 to $10 billion, not including long-term care expenses.[18] Health expenses related to osteoporosis fractures in 1986 resulted in 492,000 hospitalizations for a total of 4,290,000 hospital days, 83,000 long-term care stays with an average 1-year duration, and 2.3 million physician visits.[18]

Based on eight cost-effectiveness studies, controversy still exists over universal preventive treatment of all women with ERT/HRT versus select women with low bone density measurements or certain risk factors.[106] If the pharmacoeconomic models include changes in cardiovascular mortality and/or treatment of menopausal symptoms, universal treatment is preferred.

The other controversial issue is when to begin therapy—at age 50 or age 70 years.[20,56] Women who start HRT at age 50 most likely need to use this therapy for life to maintain or increase the fracture protection. Among 10,000 50-year-old women using ERT for 5 years, 54 lives would be saved, 79 nonfatal events would be prevented, and 969 quality-adjusted life years (5% discount) would be gained.[107] Among 10,000 50-year-old women using ERT for 25 years, 574 lives would be saved, 859 nonfatal events would be prevented, and 2968 quality-adjusted life years (5% discount) would be gained. If a 50-year-old woman used HRT for 15 years, her life expectancy would increase by 0.8 years if she had no risks, and by 1.8 years if she had a history of coronary disease.[17] Even when at risk for breast cancer, she would gain 0.4 years of life. In terms of elderly women (70 years or older), screening and treating is cost effective and will prevent some hip fractures.[19]

Further research using new models is still needed for ERT/HRT and other osteoporosis medications.

EVALUATION OF THERAPEUTIC OUTCOMES

Precise monitoring plans for patients at risk for osteoporosis are difficult to define. Minimally, a person receiving prevention or treatment with ERT/HRT, alendronate, or calcitonin should be examined annually. For women on ERT/HRT, this visit includes an annual breast and pelvic examination, mammography, and Papanicolaou smear.[31] Excessive bleeding should be evaluated with an endometrial biopsy, transvaginal ultrasonography, or a dilation and curettage if needed.[31] Medication adherence and tolerance should be evaluated at each visit.

The use of bone mineral density (BMD) measurements is increasing, especially with the availability of portable heel ultrasonography. The American Association of Clinical Endocrinologists' guidelines recommend BMD every 2 to 3 years if baseline BMD T-score was more than −1.5.[31] For prevention programs, BMD should be assessed every 1 to 2 years until BMD is stabilized and then every 2 to 3 years thereafter. For treatment programs, BMD should be measured every year for 3 years. If stable, BMD measurement can be done every 2 years; otherwise, annual BMD determinations should be continued until stable. The role of biochemical markers of bone remodeling for routine patient monitoring and routine evaluation of medications is still being defined.

GLUCOCORTICOID-INDUCED OSTEOPOROSIS

Although the incidence of glucocorticoid-induced osteoporosis is unknown, the incidence of fractures is estimated to be 30% to 50%.[27] Osteonecrosis, also called aseptic necrosis, is associated with glucocorticoid therapy. It usually involves the femoral and humeral heads, causing intense pain and decreased mobility. Bone is lost throughout the duration of steroids; however, the greatest loss is experienced during the first 6 to 12 months of therapy.[27,28] Trabecular bone is affected more than cortical bone. Men and women are both prone to steroid-induced osteoporosis. Younger patients may lose more bone than older patients. Oral doses greater than 7.5 mg of prednisone or equivalent are generally required for significant bone loss, but bone loss has been reported with lower doses and high-dose inhaled steroids. Some of the inhaler studies may have been confounded by patients' previous oral steroid use and short-course oral burst therapies.

PATHOPHYSIOLOGY

Glucocorticoids decrease bone formation and increase bone resorption as a result of steroid effects on calcium balance, osteoblasts, osteoclasts, and muscle strength.[27,28] The decrease in calcium gastrointestinal absorption and increase in renal excretion leads to a negative calcium balance and secondary hyperparathyroidism. Steroids do not affect vitamin D concentrations. A decrease occurs in the replication, differentiation, life span, and osteoid production of osteoblasts and osteoblast sensitivity to prostaglandins, growth factors, and 1,25-dihydroxyvitamin D. Decreases in gonadal hormone secretion (ovarian, testicular, and adrenal) lead to decreased production of estrogen, testosterone, and androstenedione. Effects on prostaglandins, IGF, and TGF also influence bone density. Muscle weakness, resulting from myopathy, may cause immobility or decreased mobility, thus contributing to bone loss by removing the normal forces on bone produced by strong muscle contraction.

DIAGNOSIS

Measurement of 24-hour urinary calcium excretion may be helpful in assessing calcium balance, need for calcium therapy, and need for medication adjustment. Because vitamin D levels are not altered by glucocorticoids, they only need to be monitored for assessing malnutrition or other metabolism problems. Markers of bone formation and resorption can be used, but generally calcium excretion and bone density measurements will be better and less expensive.

X-ray examination can indicate steroid-induced osteoporosis. Vertical and horizontal trabeculae tend to be equally thin and translucent. Pseudocallus formations occur in large numbers around stress fractures. These are hallmark findings because they are not seen with postmenopausal or senile osteoporosis.

The American College of Rheumatology (ACR) Task Force on Osteoporosis Guidelines recommends hip bone density measurements for all patients beginning or on glucocorticoids and spine bone density measurements for patients 60 years or older.[28] Their treatment decisions are based on these measurements. All abnormal laboratory values should be worked up for other causes of osteoporosis.

▶ PREVENTION AND TREATMENT: Glucocorticoid-Induced Osteoporosis

The best recommendation for preventing steroid-induced osteoporosis is to discontinue the agent when possible. If this is not possible, steroid exposure should be minimized by using the lowest possible dose for the shortest duration. Alternate-day therapy does not eliminate this adverse effect. Inhaled steroids have less effect on bone than does oral therapy, with lower doses potentially having no effect. Although not yet available in the United States, deflazacort may produce less bone loss than other steroids.

All patients should adopt life-style changes promoting good bone density and decreased fracture likelihood: stop smoking; increase exercise; decrease caffeine, phosphate, and alcohol intake; and prevent falls. All secondary causes of osteoporosis should be treated appropriately. Antiresorptive and formation medications have been evaluated for prevention and treatment.[27,28]

According to the ACR calcium guidelines,[28] children between 1 and 5 years should take 800 mg, and between 6 and

10 years should take 1200 mg. Everyone else should ingest 1500 mg daily from diet and supplements. Thiazide diuretics can be used for patients with greater than 300 mg of calcium excreted in the urine over 24 hours. All children should receive 400 IU per day of vitamin D, and all adults should take 800 IU per day or 50,000 IU ergocalciferol three times a week.

HRT should be given to all women on steroids if they agree, regardless of their bone density measurements. Oral contraceptives with an equivalent of 50 μg of estradiol should be given to premenopausal or perimenopausal women with menstrual irregularities or amenorrhea. Testosterone should be given to men if their measured testosterone concentrations are low.

Older patients who already have had a fracture or have low bone density at the onset of glucocorticoid therapy could use a bisphosphonate or calcitonin. Intermittent etidronate has been shown effective for primary and secondary prevention in men and women.[28] Of note, etidronate produced osteomalacia in 33% of women users (no steroid use).[98] Daily pamidronate also decreased lumbar bone loss.[28] Studies with alendronate are being conducted. The ACR does not recommend bisphosphonates for younger patients until the long-term effects of these medications are known.

All patients should receive follow-up bone density measurements after 6 to 12 months of starting glucocorticoids or osteoporosis preventive/treatment therapy.

OSTEOMALACIA

Osteomalacia results from abnormal mineralization of new bone matrix. In children and adolescents, osteomalacia is called rickets, and it affects growth due to defective calcification of the epiphyseal cartilage. Because bone remodeling occurs in all bones throughout life, unmineralized matrix can produce abnormal and weak bone structure at any age.

EPIDEMIOLOGY

The incidence of osteomalacia is not known but is probably low in the United States due to vitamin D supplemented foods and sun exposure. However, low vitamin D concentrations are frequently seen in the elderly and in patients of all ages during the winter months in cold climates. Osteomalacia occurs in countries with vitamin D-deficient diets or decreased dermal exposure to sun (such as women fully clad due to religious or cultural beliefs). Asian diets are high in phytates, which decrease calcium absorption, and lignins, which decrease vitamin D absorption. Due to a lack of detection or misdiagnosis, some women with osteoporosis may have osteomalacia (or both diseases concomitantly).

PATHOPHYSIOLOGY

Numerous causes of osteomalacia exist, each with its own special characteristics.[10,11,30,108] The main pathologic categories are vitamin D, calcium, and phosphate dietary deficiencies or absorption problems; vitamin D metabolism abnormalities; acquired or hereditary kidney diseases; tumor-related osteomalacia; or medications. Defective matrix mineralization results from lack of calcium and phosphate substrate and/or osteoblast or cellular dysfunction. The amount of calcium and phosphate in the body is controlled by a feedback system among serum calcium and phosphate concentrations, PTH, 1,25-dihydroxyvitamin D, and calcitonin (see Fig. 82–2). Cortical and trabecular bone are both affected. Faulty or deficient bone mineralization results in weak bones with irregular structure. Aging can result in osteomalacia due to decreased calcium and vitamin D concentrations from less intake and sun exposure and decreased kidney or liver function.

DRUG-INDUCED OSTEOMALACIA

Osteomalacia can result when drugs induce the hepatic microsomal oxidase enzymes, thereby accelerating the conversion of vitamin D and its metabolites to inactive compounds. Potentially any hepatic oxidase-inducing drug could reduce levels of vitamin D metabolites, but phenytoin and phenobarbital are most commonly implicated. Etidronate and fluoride can also alter bone mineralization. Excessive aluminum-containing antacids and high-dose calcium supplementation ingestion can create a phosphate deficiency due to binding. Aluminum can also be absorbed and accumulate in patients with severe renal impairment or in patients undergoing hemodialysis. Potential mechanisms for aluminum-induced osteomalacia include suppression of PTH secretion, inhibition of osteoblasts, or interference with hydroxyapatite crystal formation.

CLINICAL PRESENTATION

Patients with osteomalacia complain of fatigue, malaise, bone pain and tenderness, muscle weakness and wasting, and altered gait. The pain is diffuse, dull, aching, and poorly localized. Hypophosphatemia may explain some of the muscle weakness. Skeletal deformities are caused by softening of the bone and include bowing, gibbosity, pigeon chest, scoliosis, kyphosis, and shortening of the spine. Growth retardation, abnormal teeth, and changes in the skull bones occur in children with untreated rickets. The various etiologies produce a different biochemical picture. Evaluating plasma calcium, phosphate, alkaline phosphatase, urea, creatinine, 25- and 1,25-hydroxyvitamin D, and PTH and urinary calcium and creatinine excretion may help in identifying the underlying cause, determining treatment, and monitoring treatment efficacy and safety.[10,108]

▶ TREATMENT: Osteomalacia

The goals of therapy are to correct hypocalcemia, decrease skeletal deformities, prevent hypercalcemia and hypercalcuria, and promote normal growth. First, the underlying disease state needs to be eliminated or treated. The needed viamin D product, dose, and duration differ markedly according to the specific osteomalacia etiology, patient, and time of year. Vitamin D-containing foods include oily fishes, fortified milk, liver, butter, and eggs. When sun exposure is minimum, such as in the winter, more vitamin D may be needed. The clinical, biochemical, and radiologic effects may take weeks to resolve. Patients debilitated by the disease can become asymptomatic within 2 to 3 months. If osteoporosis exists concurrently, appropriate therapy should also be instituted.

Various vitamin D compounds and metabolites are available. Vitamin D_2 (ergocalciferol, a plant product) and vitamin D_3 (cholecalciferol) undergo the same metabolic conversion; 25-hydroxylation in the liver and then 1-hydroxylation in the kidney to the active moiety 1,25-hydroxyvitamin D_2 or D_3. Both metabolites are equally effective. Steady-state equilibrium is reached in 4 to 6 weeks. Calcifediol, 25-hydroxyvitamin D, does not require liver metabolism and may be a preferred agent in patients with severe liver disease. The half-life is 2 to 3 weeks.

Calcitriol, 1,25-hydroxyvitamin D, requires no metabolism, has a 6-hour half-life, and has a rapid onset of action. Steady state will be achieved within a week. Dihydrotachysterol is a synthetic compound that undergoes liver but not kidney conversion to the active compound. Calcitriol and dihydrotachysterol could be used in renal failure patients. Patients with renal dysfunction should also decrease oral phosphate ingestion, use a phosphate binder, and avoid aluminum-containing products such as certain antacids.

Initially, a lower vitamin D dose than recommended is initiated and adjusted according to patient needs. The dose of vitamin D can be monitored using serum alkaline phosphatase, calcium, phosphate, and/or 25-hydroxyvitamin D levels in patients without renal disease. When the serum alkaline phosphatase concentration starts to fall, the dose of vitamin D should be reduced until the lowest possible dose is found. In most circumstances, the final maintenance dose is slightly lower than the dose needed to produce healing. Calcium and phosphorus may need to be supplemented.

CONCLUSIONS

Osteoporosis is a disease that can be prevented with positive life-style changes throughout life. Postmenopausal estrogen deficiency, age-associated bone loss, and various diseases and medications can lead to osteoporosis. Bone resorption can be decreased, but new strong bone cannot be created. Thus, prevention is the key to controlling this disease. Prevention of osteoporosis includes smoking cessation, exercise, adequate calcium and vitamin D intake, hormone therapy, and alendronate.

Treatment of established osteoporosis relies on preventing further bone loss, preventing falls, and controlling pain, which can include calcium and vitamin D supplementation, hormone therapy, alendronate, and nasal calcitonin. Many medications are under investigation to build bone or prevent its loss.

Pharmacists can have a major role in preventing and treating osteoporosis, resolving medication-related problems, and ensuring compliance.

Osteomalacia is a disease of decreased bone mineralization with multiple etiologies all of which have some impairment of calcium, phosphorus, or vitamin D homeostasis. After treating or eliminating the underlying cause, vitamin D is the predominant therapy, with the dose, duration, and product variable according to the underlying etiology and liver and kidney function.

ADDENDUM

Since the writing of this chapter, the first results from an estrogen controlled trial evaluating cardiovascular protection has been published. The Heart and Estrogen/progestin Replacement Study (HERS) randomized 2763 postmenopausal women under 80 years and with coronary disease to either 0.625 mg conjugated equine estrogens plus 2.5 mg medroxyprogesterone daily or placebo for an average follow-up period of 4.1 years. HRT did not provide secondary prevention in terms of nonfatal myocardial *infarction or coronary* heart disease. However, a trend existed for HRT women to have less cardiovascular events than the placebo group after 4 or 5 years of therapy. HRT did lower LDL, increase HDL, but also increased venous thromboembolic events and gallbladder disease.[109]

▶ PRINCIPLES OF PHARMACOTHERAPY

- Osteoporosis prevention begins at birth, by ensuring that everyone has adequate calcium and vitamin D in the diet and exercises regularly.
- Life-style changes such as stopping smoking, decreasing dietary phosphate and caffeine, minimizing alcohol intake, and decreasing falls will help prevent bone loss and fractures.
- To ensure adequate calcium intake, most Americans will need calcium supplementation with doses of 500 mg calcium once or twice a day.
- Estrogen-replacement therapy (ERT), with medroxyprogesterone (HRT) for women with an intact uterus, should begin at menopause and potentially be continued for life.
- ERT/HRT will also prevent bone loss in elderly women.

- ERT/HRT improves lipid profiles, decreases cardiovascular disease and mortality, and decreases urogenital symptoms.
- Alendronate can be used for prevention in postmenopausal women if ERT/HRT is contraindicated or adverse reactions occur.
- Alendronate can be used to treat osteoporosis, with bone mass increasing for at least 3 years.
- Nasal calcitonin can be used to treat acute and chronic bone pain and in some cases to treat osteoporosis.
- Pharmacists need to educate patients on osteoporosis prevention and the use of their medications, especially alendronate; help ensure adherence; and identify and resolve medication-related problems.

REFERENCES

1. Guyton AC, Hall JE. Parathyroid hormone, calcitonin, calcium and phosphate metabolism, vitamin D, bone and teeth. In: Guyton AC, Hall JE, eds. Textbook of Medical Physiology. Philadelphia, W.B. Saunders Co., 1996;985–1002.
2. Manolagas SC, Jilka RL. Bone marrow, cytokines, and bone remodeling. Emerging insights into the pathophysiology of osteoporosis. N Engl J Med 1995;332:305–311.
3. Zerwekh J. Bone metabolism. Semin Nephrol 1992;12:79–90.
4. Horowitz M. Cytokines and estrogen in bone: Anti-osteoporotic effects. Science 1993;260:625–626.
5. Murray TM. Mechanisms of bone loss. J Rheumatol 1996;23(suppl 45):6–10.
6. Duursma SA, Raymakers JA, Boereboom FTJ, Scheven BAA. Estrogen and bone metabolism. Obstet Gynecol Surv 1991;47:38–44.
7. Dempster D, Lindsay R. Pathogenesis of osteoporosis. Lancet 1993; 341:797–801.
8. Vermeer C, Gijsbers BLMG, Craciun AM, et al. Effects of vitamin K on bone mass and bone metabolism. J Nutr 1996;126:1187S–1191S.
9. Kelly PJ. Is osteoporosis a genetically determined disease? J Obstet Gynaecol 1996;103:20–27.
10. Mankin HJ. Rickets, osteomalacia, and renal osteodystrophy: An update. Orthop Clin North Am 1990;21:81–96.
11. Doppelt SH. Vitamin D, rickets, and osteomalacia. Orthop Clin North Am 1984;15:671–686.
12. Cummings SR, Nevitt MC, Browner WS, et al. Risk factors for hip fracture in white women. N Engl J Med 1995;332:767–773.
13. Grisso JA, Kelsey JL, Strom BL, et al. Risk factors for hip fracture in black women. N Engl J Med 1994;330:1555–1559.
14. Dargent-Molina P, Favier F, Grandjean H, et al. Fall-related factors and risk of hip fracture: The EPIDOS prospective study. Lancet 1996;348:145–149.
15. Ringe JD. Hip fractures in men. Osteoporosis Int 1996;3:S48–S51.
16. Looker AC, Orwoll ES, Johnston CC, et al. Prevalence of low femoral bone density in older U.S. adults from NHANES III. J Bone Miner Res 1997;12:1761–1768.
17. Kanis JA, WHO group. Assessment of fracture risk and its application to screening for postmenopausal osteoporosis: Synopsis of a WHO report. Osteoporosis Int 1994;4:368–381.
18. Riggs BL, Melton LJ. The worldwide problem of osteoporosis: Insights afforded by epideminology. Bone 1995;17(suppl 5): 505S–511S.
19. Black DM. Why elderly women should be screened and treated to prevent osteoporosis. Am J Med 1995;98:(suppl 2A):67S–75S.
20. Marshall D, Johnell O, Wedel H. Meta-analysis of how well measures of bone mineral density predict occurrence of osteoporotic fractures. Br Med J 1996;312:1254–1259.
21. Bauer DC, Gluer CC, Cauley JA, et al. Broadband ultrasound attenuation predicts fractures stongly and independently of densitometry in older women. Arch Intern Med 1997;157:629–634.
22. Bauer DC, Gluer CC, Genant HK, Stone K. Quantitative ultrasound and vertebral fracture in postmenopausal women. Fracture intervention trial research group. J Bone Miner Res 1995;10:353–358.
23. Mazess RB. On aging bone loss. Clin Orthop 1982;165:239–252.
24. Rubenstein LZ, Josephson KR, Robbins AS. Falls in the nursing home. Ann Intern Med 1994;121:442–451.
25. Wolinsky-Friedland M. Drug-induced metabolic bone disease. Endocrinol Metab Clin North Am 1995;24:395–420.
26. Seeman E. The dilemma of osteoporosis in men. Am J Med 1995; 98(suppl 2A):S76–S88.
27. Adachi JD. Corticosteroid-induced osteoporosis. Am J Med Sci 1997;313:41–49.
28. American College of Rheumatology Task Force on Osteoporosis Guidelines. Recommendations for the prevention and treatment of glucocorticoid-induced osteoporosis. Arthritis Rheum 1996;39: 1791–1801.
29. Schneider DL, Barrett-Connor EL, Morton DJ. Thyroid hormone use and bone mineral density in elderly women. JAMA1994;271: 1245–1249.
30. Hutchinson FN, Bell NH. Osteomalacia and rickets. Semin Nephrol 1992;12:127–145.
31. Osteoporosis task force. AACE Clinical practice guidelines for the prevention and treatment of postmenopausal osteoporosis. J Fla Med Assoc 1996;83:552–566.
32. Miller PD, Bonnick SL, Rosen CJ, et al. Clinical utility of bone mass measurement in adults: Consensus of an international panel. Semin Arthritis Rheum 1996;25:361–372.
33. Kleerekoper M. Biochemical markers of bone remodeling. Am J Med Sci 1996;312:270–277.
34. NIH Consensus Development Panel on Optimal Calcium Intake. Optimal calcium intake. JAMA 1994;272:1942–1948.
35. Institute of Medicine, National Research Council. Summary statement on calcium and related nutrients. 1997;S1–S14. Available at: www.nas.edu/new.
36. Hasling C, Sondergaard K, Charles P, Mosekilde L. Calcium metabolism in postmenopausal osteoporotic women is determined by dietary calcium and coffee intake. J Nutr 1992;122:1119–1126.
37. Calvo MS, Park YK. Changing phosphorus content of the U.S. diet: Potential for adverse effects on bone. J Nutr 1996;126: 1168S–1180S.
38. Hollenbach KA, Barrett-Connor E, Edelstein SL, Holbrook T. Cigarette smoking and bone mineral density in older men and women. Am J Public Health 1993;83:1265–1270.
39. Hopper JL, Seeman E. The bone density of female twins discordant for tobacco use. N Engl J Med 1994;330:387–392.
40. Moniz C. Alcohol and bone. Br Med Bull 1994;50:67–75.
41. Reid IR. Therapy of osteoporosis: Calcium, vitamin D, and exercise. Am J Med Sci 1996;312:278–286.
42. ACSM position stand on osteoporosis and exercise. Med Sci Sports Exer 1995;27:1–7.
43. Notelovitz M. Estrogen therapy and osteoporosis: Principles and practice. Am J Med Sci 1997;313:2–12.
44. Cumming DC. Exercise-associated amenorrhea, low bone density, and estrogen replacement therapy. Arch Intern Med 1996;156: 2193–2195.
45. Cumming RG, Nevitt MC. Calcium for prevention of osteoporotic fractures in postmenopausal women. J Bone Miner Res 1997;12: 1321–1329.
46. Dawson-Hughes B, Harris SS, Krall EA, Dallal GE. Effect of calcium and vitamin D supplementation on bone density in men and women 65 years of age or older. N Engl J Med 1997;337: 670–676.

47. Chapuy MC, Arlot ME, Duboeuf F, et al. Vitamin D_3 and calcium to prevent hip fractures in elderly women. N Engl J Med 1992;327: 1637–1642.
48. Carr CJ, Shangraw RF. Nutritional and pharmaceutical aspects of calcium supplementation. Am Pharm 1987;27–57.
49. Jones G, Nguyen T, Sambrook PN, Eisman JA. Thiazide diuretics and fractures: Can meta-analysis help? J Bone Miner Res 1995;10: 106–111.
50. Morton DJ, Barrett-Connor EL, Edelstein SL. Thiazides and bone mineral density in elderly men and women. Am J Epidemiol 1994; 139:1107–1115.
51. Lips P, Graafmans WC, Ooms ME, et al. Vitamin D supplementation and fracture incidence in elderly persons: A randomized, placebo-controlled clinical trial. Ann Intern Med 1996;124:400–406.
52. Consensus development conference: Diagnosis, prophylaxis, and treatment of osteoporosis. Am J Med 1993;94:646–650.
53. Col NF, Eckman MH, Karas RH, et al. Patient-specific decisions about hormone replacement therapy in postmenopausal women. JAMA 1997;277:1140–1147.
54. Writing group for the PEPI Trial. Effects of hormone therapy on bone mineral density: Results from the postmenopausal estrogen/ progestin interventions (PEPI) trial. JAMA 1996;276:1389–1396.
55. Genant HK, Lucas J, Weiss S, et al. Low-dose esterified estrogen therapy: Effects on bone, plasma estradiol concentrations, endometrium, and lipid levels. Arch Int Med 1997;157:2609–2615.
56. Schneider DL, Barrett-Connor EL, Morton DJ. Timing of post-menopausal estrogen for optimal bone mineral density: The Rancho Bernardo study. JAMA 1997;277:543–547.
57. Grady D, Rubin SM, Petitti DB, et al. Hormone therapy to prevent disease and prolong life in postmenopausal women. Ann Intern Med 1992;117:1016–1037.
58. Miller KL. Hormone replacement therapy in the elderly. Clin Obstet Gynecol 1996;29:912–932.
59. Grodstein F, Stampfer MJ, Manson JE, et al. Postmenopausal estrogen and progestin use and the risk of cardiovascular disease. N Engl J Med 1996;335:453–461.
60. Grodstein F, Stampfer MJ, Colditz GA, et al. Postmenopausal hormone therapy and mortality. N Engl J Med 1997;336:1769–1775.
61. Wild RA. Estrogen: Effects on the cardiovascular tree. Obstet Gynecol 1996;87:27–35S.
62. Writing Group for the PEPI Trial. Effects of estrogen or estrogen/ progestin regimens on heart disease risk factors in postmenopausal women: The postmenopausal estrogen/progestin interventions (PEPI) trial. JAMA 1995;273:199–208.
63. Watts NB, Notelovitz M, Timmons MC, et al. Comparison of oral estrogens and estrogens plus androgen on bone mineral density, menopausal symptoms, and lipid–lipoprotein profiles in surgical menopause. Obstet Gynecol 1995;85:529–537.
64. Taskinen MR, Puolakka J, Pyorala T, et al. Hormone replacement therapy lowers plasma Lp(a) concentrations: Comparison of cyclic transdermal and continuous estrogen-progestin regimens. Arterioscler Thromb Vasc Biol 1996;16:1215–1221.
65. Davidson MH, Testolin LM, Maki, KC, et al. A comparison of estrogen replacement, pravastatin, and combined treatment for the management of hypercholesterolemia in postmenopausal women. Arch Intern Med 1997;157:1186–1192.
66. McBee WL, Dailey ME, Dugan E, Shumaker SA. Hormone replacement therapy and other potential treaments for dementias. Endocrinol Metab Clin North Am 1997;26:329–345.
67. Evans MP, Fleming KC, Evans JM. Hormone replacement therapy: Management of common problems. Mayo Clin Proc 1995;70: 800–805.
68. Udoff L, Langenberg P, Adashi EY. Combined continuous hormone replacement therapy: A critical review. Obstet Gynecol 1995;86: 306–316.
69. Grady D, Gebretsadik T, Kerlikowske K, et al. Hormone replacement therapy and endometrial cancer risk: A meta-analysis. Obstet Gynecol 1995;85:304–313.
70. Speroff L. Postmenopausal hormone therapy and breast cancer. Obstet Gynecol 1996;87:44–54S.
71. American College of Physicians. Guidelines for counseling postmenopausal women about preventive hormone therapy. Ann Int Med 1992;117:1038–1041.
72. Gutthann SP, Rodriguez LAG, Castellsague J, Oliart AD. Hormone replacement therapy and risk of venous thromboembolism: Population based case-control study. Br Med J 1997;314:796–800.
73. Wysowski DK, Golden L, Burke L. Use of menopausal estrogens and medroxyprogesterone in the United States, 1982–1992. Obstet Gynecol 1995;85:6–10.
74. Salamone LM, Pressman AR, Seeley DG, Cauley JA. Estrogen replacement therapy: A survey of older women's attitudes. Arch Intern Med 1996;156:1293–1297.
75. Silverman SL, Greenwald M, Klein RA, Drinkwater BL. Effect of bone density information on decisions about hormone replacement therapy: A randomized trial. Obstet Gynecol 1997;89: 321–325.
76. Patel S. Current and potential future drug treatments for osteoporosis. Ann Rheum Dis 1996;55:700–714.
77. Yun S, Hart LL. Medroxyprogesterone in osteoporosis. Ann Pharmacother 1993;27:448–449.
78. Folsom AR, McGovern PG, Nabulsi AA, et al. Changes in plasma lipids and lipoproteins associated with starting or stopping postmenopausal hormone replacement therapy. Am Heart J 1996;132: 952–958.
79. Ettinger B, Selby J, Citron JT, et al. Cyclic hormone replacement therapy using quarterly progestin. Obstet Gynecol 1994;103(suppl 13):693–700.
80. Chang J, Powles TJ, Ashley SE, et al. The effect of tamoxifen and hormone replacement therapy on serum cholesterol, bone mineral density and coagulation factors in healthy postmenopausal women participating in a randomised, controlled tamoxifen prevention study. Ann Oncol 1996;7:671–675.
81. Love RR, Wiebe DA, Newcomb PA, et al. Effects of tamoxifen on cardiovascular risk factors in postmenopausal women. Ann Intern Med 1991;115:860–864.
82. Kaunitz AM. The role of androgens in menopausal hormonal replacement. Endocinol Clin North Am 1997;26:391–397.
83. Reginster JY. Miscellaneous and experimental agents. Am J Med Sci 1997;313:33–40.
84. Draper MW, Flowers DE, Huster WJ, et al. A controlled trial of raloxifene (LY139481) HCL: Impact on bone turnover and serum lipid profile in healthy postmenopausal women. J Bone Miner Res 1996;11:835–842.
85. Delmas PD, Bjarnson NH, Mitlak BH, et al. Effects of raloxifene on bone mineral density, serum cholesterol concentrations and uterine endometrium in postmenopausal women. N Engl J Med 1997;337: 1641–1647.
86. DeCherney A. Bone-sparing properties of oral contraceptives. Am J Obstet Gynecol 1996;174:15–20.
87. Cooper C, Hannaford P, Croft P, Kay CR. Oral contraceptive pill use and fractures in women: A prospective study. Bone 1993;14: 41–45.
88. Haenggi W, Casez JP, Birkhaeuser H, et al. Bone mineral density in young women with long-standing amenorrhea: Limited effect of hormone replacement therapy with ethinylestradiol and desogestrel. Osteoporosis Int 1994;4:99–103.
89. Seeman E, Szmukler GI, Formica C, et al. Osteoporosis in anorexia nervosa: The influence of peak bone density, bone loss, oral contraceptive use, and exercise. J Bone Miner Res 1992;7:1467–1474.
90. Gambacciani M, Spinetti A, Taponeco F, et al. Longitudinal evaluation of premenopausal vertebral bone loss: Effects of a low-dose oral contraceptive preparation on bone mineral density and metabolism. Obstet Gynecol 1994;83:392–396.

91. Bjarnason NH, Bjarnason K, Haarbo J, et al. Tibolone: Prevention of bone loss in late postmenopausal women. J Clin Endocrinol Metab 1996;81:2419–2422.
92. Hanggi W, Lippuner K, Riesen W, et al. Long term influence of different postmenopausal hormone replacement regimens on serum lipids and lipoprotein(a): a randomized study. Br J Obstet Gynaecol 1997;104:708–717.
93. Hosking D, Chilvers CED, Christiansen C, et al. Prevention of bone loss with alendronate in postmenopausal women under 60 years of age. N Engl J Med 1998;338:485–492.
94. Jeal W, Barradell LB, McTavish D. Alendronate: A review of its pharmacological properties and therapeutic efficacy in postmenopausal osteoporosis. Drugs 1997;53:415–434.
95. Bone HG, Downs RW, Tucci JR, et al. Dose-response relationships for alendronate treatment in osteoporotic elderly women. J Clin Endocrinol Metab 1997;82:265–274.
96. Karpf DB, Shapiro DR, Seeman E, et al. Prevention of nonvertebral fractures by alendronate: A meta-analysis. JAMA 1997;277: 1159–1164.
97. Storm T, Kollerup G, Thamsborg G, et al. Five years of clinical experience with intermittent cyclical etidronate for postmenopausal osteoporosis. J Rheumatol 1996;23:1560–1564.
98. Wimalawansa SJ. Combined therapy with estrogen and etidronate has an additive effect on bone mineral density in the hip and vertebrae: Four-year randomized study. Am J Med 1995;99:36–42.
99. Silverman SL. Calcitonin. Am J Med Sci 1997;313:13–16.
100. Stock JL, Avioli LV, Baylink DJ, et al. Calcitonin-salmon nasal spray reduces the incidence of new vertebral fractures in postmenopausal women: Three year interim results of the PROFF study. J Bone Miner Res 1997;12:S149. Abstract.
101. Braga PC. Calcitonin and its antinociceptive activity: Animal and human investigations 1975–1992. Agents Actions 1994;41:121–131.
102. Knight DC, Eden JA. A review of the clinical effects of phytoestrogens. Obstet Gynecol 1996;87:897–904.
103. Pak CYC, Sakhaee K, Rubin CD, et al. Sustained-release sodium fluoride in the management of established postmenopausal osteoporosis. Am J Med Sci 1997;313:23–32.
104. Behre HM, Kliesch S, Leifke E, et al. Long-term effect of testosterone therapy on bone mineral density in hypogonadal men. J Clin Endocrinol Metab 1997;82:2386–2390.
105. Sisson de Castro JA. Alendronate treatment of osteoporosis in men: Short term bone mass response. J Bone Miner Res 1996;11(suppl 1):S341. Abstract.
106. Taylor TN, Chrischilles EA. Economic evaluation of interventions in endocrinology. Endocrinol Metab Clin North Am 1997;26: 67–87.
107. Gorsky RD, Koplan JP, Petersen HB, Thacker SB. Relative risks and benefits of long-term estrogen replacement therapy: A decision analysis. Obstet Gynecol 1994;83:161–166.
108. Stamp TCB. Rickets and osteomalacia. In: Klippel JH, Dieppe PA, eds. Rheumatology. 1994;7:35.1–35.12.
109. Hulley S, Grady D, Bush T, et al. Randomized trial of estrogen plus progestin for secondary prevention of coronary heart disease in postmenopausal women JAMA 1998;280:605–613.

83

RHEUMATOID ARTHRITIS

Arthur A. Schuna, MS, FASHP, Michael J. Schmidt, PharmD, and Denise Walbrandt Pigarelli, PharmD

Rheumatoid arthritis is the most common systemic inflammatory disease characterized by symmetrical joint involvement. Extra-articular involvement including rheumatoid nodules, vasculitis, eye inflammation, neurologic dysfunction, cardiopulmonary disease, lymphadenopathy, and splenomegaly are manifestations of the disease. Although the usual disease course is chronic, some patients will spontaneously enter a remission.

EPIDEMIOLOGY

Rheumatoid arthritis is estimated to have a prevalence of 1% to 2% and does not have any racial predilections. It can occur at any age with increasing prevalence up to the seventh decade of life. The disease is three times more common in women. In people age 15 to 45 years, women predominate by a ratio of 6 to 1; the sex ratio is approximately equal among patients in the first decade of life and in those more than 60 years old.

Epidemiologic data suggest that a genetic predisposition and exposure to unknown environmental factors may be necessary for expression of the disease. The major histocompatibility complex (MHC) molecules, located on T lymphocytes, appear to have an important role in most patients with rheumatoid arthritis. These molecules can be characterized using human lymphocyte antigen (HLA) typing. A majority of patients with rheumatoid arthritis have HLA-DR4, HLA-DR1, or both antigens found in the MHC region. Although the MHC region is important, it is not the sole determinant, as patients can have the disease without these HLA types. Rheumatoid arthritis is six times more common among dizygotic twins and nontwin children of parents with rheumatoid factor-positive, erosive rheumatoid arthritis when compared with children whose parents do not have the disease. If one of a pair of monozygotic twins is affected, the other twin has a 30 times greater risk of developing the disease.[1,2]

PATHOPHYSIOLOGY

Chronic inflammation of the synovial tissue lining the joint capsule results in the proliferation of this tissue. The inflamed, proliferating synovium characteristic of rheumatoid arthritis is called *pannus* (Fig. 83–1). This pannus invades the cartilage and eventually the bone surface, producing erosions of bone and cartilage, leading to destruction of the joint.

The factors that initiate the inflammatory process are unknown. Infectious agents have been postulated as a cause of rheumatoid arthritis. The evidence supporting this possibility includes the similarity between rheumatoid arthritis and acute inflammatory arthritides associated with known infectious agents (e.g., rheumatic fever following streptococcal infection, Lyme arthritis, postviral arthritis). Also, synovitis resembling rheumatoid arthritis can be produced experimentally in animals by injection of bacterial cell wall fragments. No specific infectious agent has been isolated from the joints of patients suffering from rheumatoid arthritis.

The immune system is a complex network of checks and balances designed to discriminate self from nonself (foreign) tissues. It helps rid the body of infectious agents, tumor cells, and products associated with the breakdown of cells. In rheumatoid arthritis this system no longer can differentiate self from nonself tissues, and attacks the synovial tissue and other connective tissues.

The immune system has both humoral and cell-mediated functions. The humoral component is necessary for the formation of antibodies. These antibodies are produced by plasma cells. Most patients with rheumatoid arthritis form antibodies called rheumatoid factors. Rheumatoid factors have not been identified as pathogenic nor does the quantity of these circulating antibodies always correlate with disease activity. Seropositive patients tend to have a more aggressive course of their illness than do seronegative patients. Immunoglobulins can activate the complement system. The complement system amplifies the immune response by encouraging chemotaxis, phagocytosis, and the release of lymphokines by mononuclear cells.

The cellular component of the inflammatory process consists of polymorphonuclear cells, macrophages, and lymphocytes (Fig. 83–2). Antigen-presenting cells (including macrophages) engulf and process antigens, which are then presented to T lymphocytes. The processed antigen is recognized by MHC proteins on the lymphocyte, which activates it to stimulate the production of T and B cells. Lymphocytes may be either B cells (derived from bone marrow) or T cells (derived from thymus tissue). T cells may be either T-helper (which promote inflammation) or T-suppressor cells (which attenuate the inflammatory response). Activated T cells produce cytotoxins, which are directly toxic to tissues, and cytokines, which stimulate further activation of inflammatory processes and attract cells to areas of inflammation. Macrophages are stimulated to release prostaglandins and cytotoxins. Activated

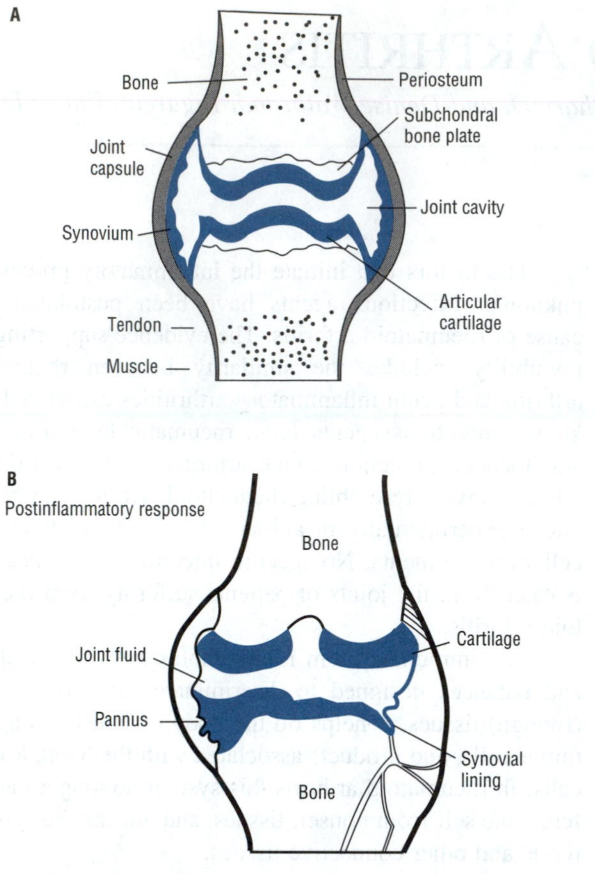

FIG. 83–1. A. Schematic diagram of a normal diarthrodial joint. **B.** Schematic diagram of a knee joint with active rheumatoid arthritis showing pannus invading and destroying the cartilage and bone. *(Reproduced from the Arthritis Foundation Allied Health Professions Teaching Slide Collection, Copyright © 1980, with permission.)*

B cells produce plasma cells, which form antibodies. These antibodies in combination with complement result in the accumulation of polymorphonuclear leukocytes (PMNs). These PMNs release cytotoxins, free oxygen radicals, and hydroxyl radicals, which promote cellular damage to synovium and bone. Patients with rheumatoid arthritis appear to have an excessive amount of T-helper cell activity in synovial tissues.

Vasoactive substances also play a role in the inflammatory process. Histamine, kinins, and prostaglandins are released at the site of inflammation. These substances increase both blood flow to the site of inflammation and the permeability of blood vessels. These substances cause the edema, warmth, erythema, and pain associated with inflamed joints and also make it easier for granulocytes to pass from blood vessels to the site of inflammation.

The end results of the chronic inflammatory changes are variable. Loss of cartilage may result in a loss of the joint space. The formation of chronic granulation or scar tissue can lead to loss of joint motion or bony fusion (called ankylosis). Laxity of tendon structures can result in a loss of support to the affected joint, leading to instability or subluxation. Tendon contractures may also occur, leading to chronic deformity.[3–9]

CLINICAL PRESENTATION

The symptoms of rheumatoid arthritis usually develop insidiously over the course of several weeks to months. Prodromal symptoms include fatigue, weakness, low-grade fever, loss of appetite, and joint pain. Stiffness and muscle

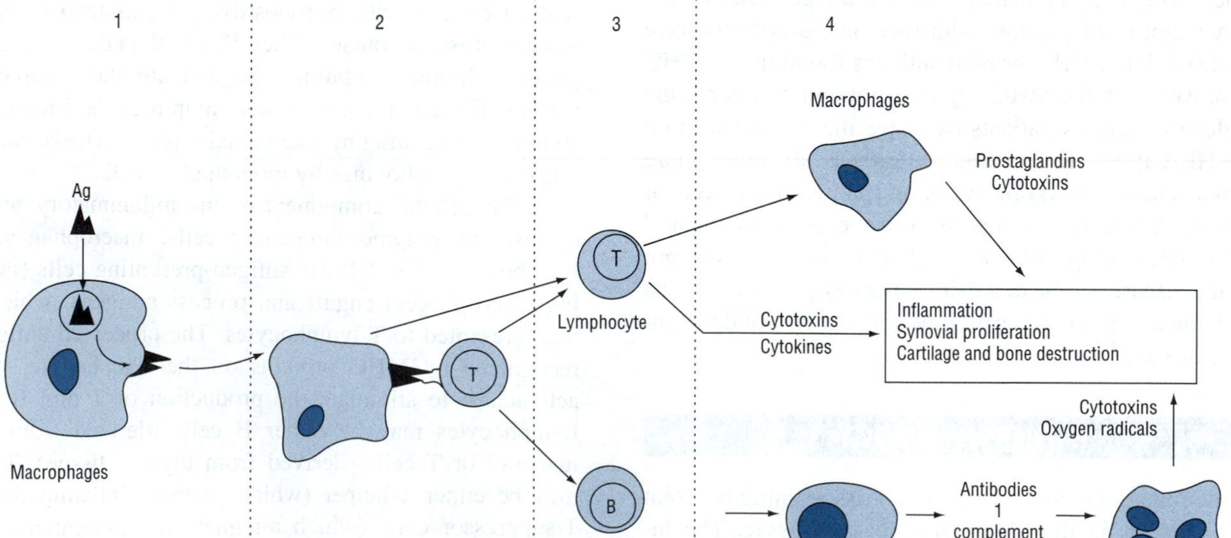

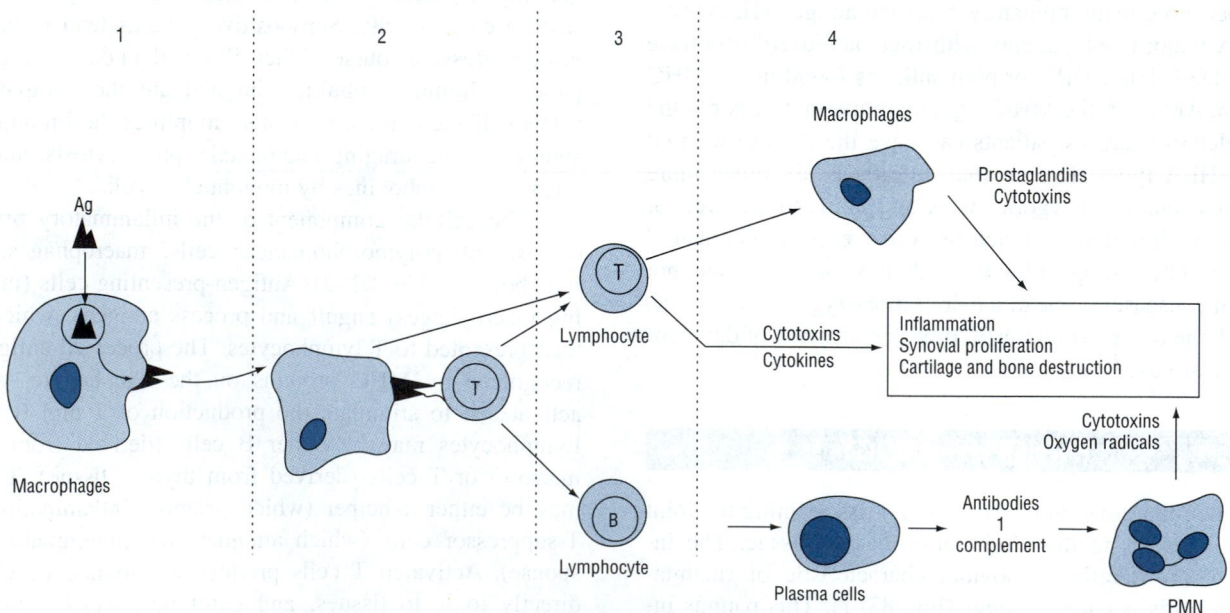

FIGURE 83–2. Pathogenesis of the inflammatory response. Phase 1: Antigen-presenting cells phagocytizes antigen. Phase 2: Antigen is presented to T lymphocyte. T lymphocyte attaches to antigen at MHC portion of cell wall, causing activation. Phase 3: Activated T cell stimulates T- and B-lymphocyte production, promoting inflammation. Phase 4: Activated T cells and macrophages release factors that promote tissue destruction, increase blood flow, and result in cellular invasion of synovial tissue and joint fluid. *(Ag = antigen; PMN = polymorphonuclear leukocyte.)*

TABLE 83–1. American Rheumatism Association Criteria for Classification of Rheumatoid Arthritis—1987 Revision

Criteria[a]	Definition
1. Morning stiffness	Morning stiffness in and around the joints lasting at least 1 hour before maximal improvement.
2. Arthritis of three or more joint areas simultaneously	At least three joint areas have had soft tissue swelling or fluid (not bony overgrowth alone) observed by a physician. The 14 possible joint areas are (right or left): PIP, MCP, wrist, elbow, knee, ankle, and MTP joints[b]
3. Arthritis of hand joints	At least one joint area swollen as above in wrist, MCP, or PIP joint.
4. Symmetric arthritis	Simultaneous involvement of the same joint areas (as in 2) on both sides of the body (bilateral involvement of PIP, MCP, or MTP joints is acceptable without absolute symmetry).
5. Rheumatoid nodules	Subcutaneous nodules, over bony prominences, or extensor surfaces, or in juxtaarticular regions, observed by a physician.
6. Serum rheumatoid factor	Demonstration of abnormal amounts of serum "rheumatoid factor" by any method that has been positive in less than 5% of normal control subjects.
7. Radiographic changes	Radiographic changes typical of RA on posterior–anterior hand and wrist x-rays, which must include erosions or unequivocal bony decalcification localized to or most marked adjacent to the involved joints (osteoarthritis changes alone do not qualify).

[a]For classification purposes, a patient is said to have rheumatoid arthritis (RA) if he or she has satisfied at least four of the above seven criteria. Criteria 1 through 4 must be present for at least 6 weeks. Patients with two clinical diagnoses are not excluded. Designation as classic, definite, or probable rheumatoid arthritis is not to be made.

[b]PIP = proximal interphalangeal; MCP = metacarpophalangeal; MTP = metatarsophalangeal.

aches (myalgias) may precede the development of joint swelling (synovitis). Fatigue may be more of a problem in the afternoon. During disease flares, the onset of fatigue begins earlier in the day and subsides as disease activity lessens. Most commonly, joint involvement tends to be symmetric; however, early in the disease some patients present with an asymmetric pattern involving one or a few joints, which eventually develops into the more classic presentation. About 20% of patients develop an abrupt onset of their illness with fevers, polyarthritis, and constitutional symptoms (e.g., depression, anxiety, fatigue, anorexia, weight loss).[1,2] No single test or physical finding can be used to make the diagnosis of rheumatoid arthritis, but criteria have been developed to aid in its diagnosis (Table 83–1).

JOINT INVOLVEMENT

The joints most frequently affected by rheumatoid arthritis are the small joints of the hands, wrists, and feet (Fig. 83–3). In addition, elbows, shoulders, hips, knees, and

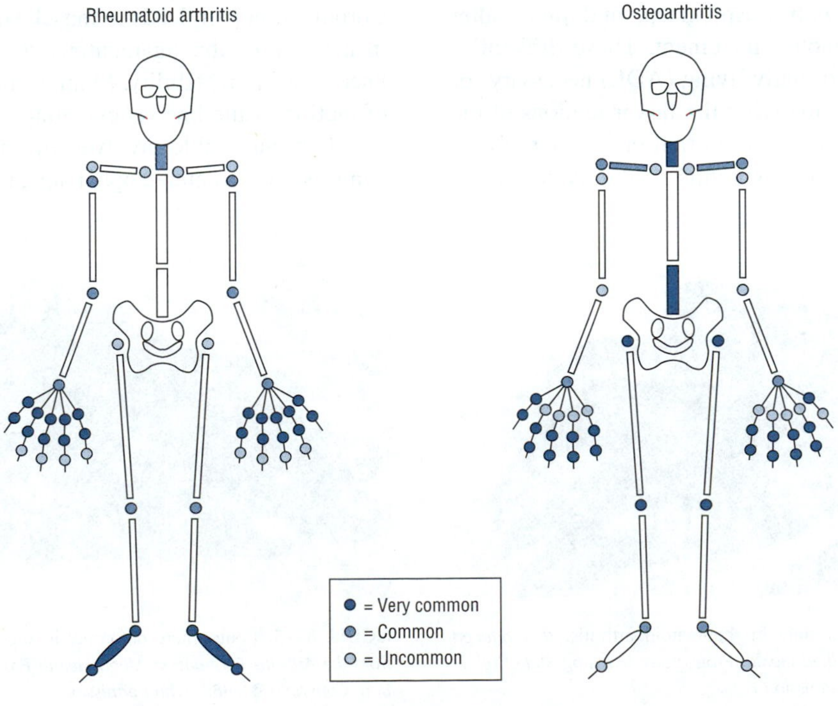

FIGURE 83–3. Patterns of joint involvement in rheumatoid arthritis and osteoarthritis.

TABLE 83–2. Functional Classifications of Rheumatoid Arthritis

Class I	Capable of all activities without handicap
Class II	Able to conduct normal activities despite handicap of discomfort or limited mobility of one or more joints
Class III	Functional capacity only adequate to perform a few of the normal duties of usual occupation
Class IV	Confined to bed or wheelchair, capable of little or no self-care

ankles may be involved. Patients usually experience joint stiffness that is typically worse in the morning. The duration of stiffness tends to be directly correlated with disease activity, usually exceeds 30 minutes, and may persist all day. Chronic inflammation with lack of an adequate exercise program results in loss of range of motion, atrophy of muscles, weakness, and deformity. A functional classification scale to indicate a patient's degree of impairment is frequently used (Table 83–2).

On examination, the swelling of the joints may be visible or may be apparent only by palpation. The swelling feels soft and spongy, because it is caused by proliferation of soft tissues or fluid accumulation within the joint capsule. The swollen joint may appear erythematous and feel warmer than nearby skin surfaces, especially early in the course of the disease. In contrast, the swelling associated with osteoarthritis is usually bony (caused by osteophytes) and is infrequently associated with signs of inflammation.

Involvement of the hands and wrists is common in rheumatoid arthritis. Hand involvement is manifested by pain, swelling, tenderness, and grip weakness during the acute phase and by subluxation, instability, ulnar deviation, and muscle atrophy in the chronic phase of the disease. Functional difficulties with clasp, grasp, and pinch alter both strength and fine motor movement. These difficulties can affect the activities of daily living (ADL) necessary for self-care. Tenosynovitis involving the flexor tendons of the hands can result in restriction of motion or locking of digits in a flexed position. Tenosynovitis of the extensor tendons of the hand may result in pain, swelling, and spontaneous rupture with loss of function.

Deformity of the hand may be seen with chronic inflammation. Subluxations of the wrists and metacarpophalangeal (MCP) joints may be seen. The thumbs may develop flexion at the MCP joint and hyperextension of the interphalangeal (IP) joint, which may make pinch grip difficult. Involvement of tendons in the hands can result in either hyperextension at the proximal interphalangeal (PIP) joint and flexion of the distal interphalangeal (DIP) joint (called a swan-neck deformity; see Fig. 83–4) or flexion at PIP with hyperextension of the DIP (called a boutonniere deformity; see Fig. 83–5). Ulnar deviation of the fingers may also occur as a result of tendon abnormalities associated with rheumatoid arthritis (Fig. 83–6).

Wrist involvement can result in joint space narrowing, collapse, and subluxation leading to grip weakness. Destruction of the cartilage at the radioulnar joint results in pain with rotational movement of the forearm. Carpal tunnel syndrome is caused by entrapment of the median nerve by inflamed synovium. This results in pain and tingling in the fingers and grip weakness.

Swelling at the elbow is most evident at the radial-humeral joint. Shoulder pain may result from involvement of the joint itself or from tendon inflammation (tendinitis) or inflammation of the bursa (bursitis) near the deltoid muscle.

The knee can also be involved, with loss of cartilage, instability, and joint pain. Synovitis of the knee may cause the formation of a cyst behind the knee called a popliteal or Baker's cyst. These cysts may become painful as they get tense or they may rupture, producing a clinical picture similar to thrombophlebitis secondary to the release of inflammatory components into the area of the calf muscle. Chronic joint pain leads to muscle atrophy, which can result in a laxity of the ligamentous structures that support the knee, causing instability. Maintenance of an adequate range of motion of the knee is essential to normal gait.

Foot and ankle involvement in rheumatoid arthritis is common. The metatarsophalangeal (MTP) joints are com-

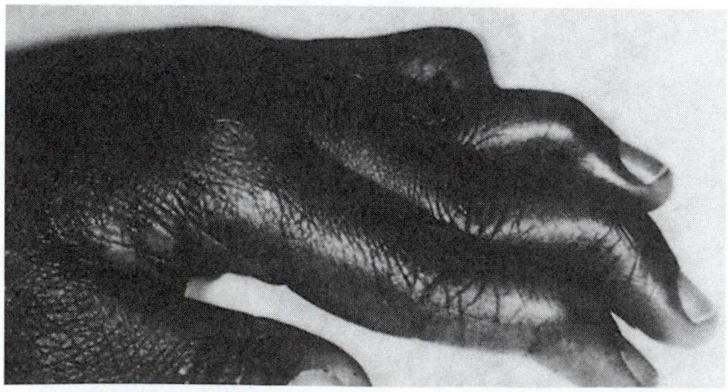

FIGURE 83–4. Swan-neck deformity in rheumatoid arthritis. *(Reproduced from the Arthritis Foundation Allied Health Professions Teaching Slide Collection, Copyright © 1980, with permission.)*

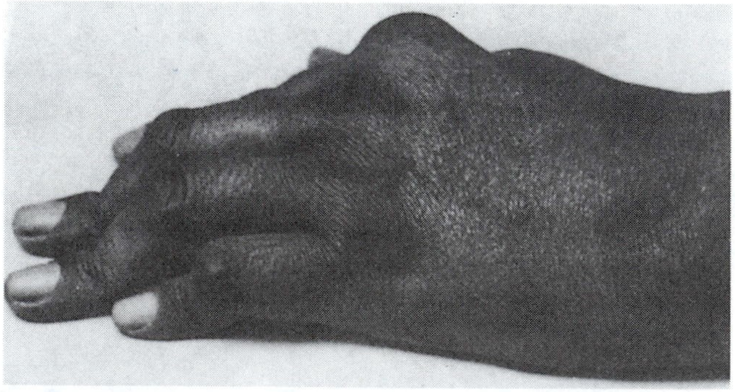

FIGURE 83–5. Boutonniere deformity in rheumatoid arthritis. *(Reproduced from the Arthritis Foundation Allied Health Professions Teaching Slide Collection, Copyright © 1980, with permission.)*

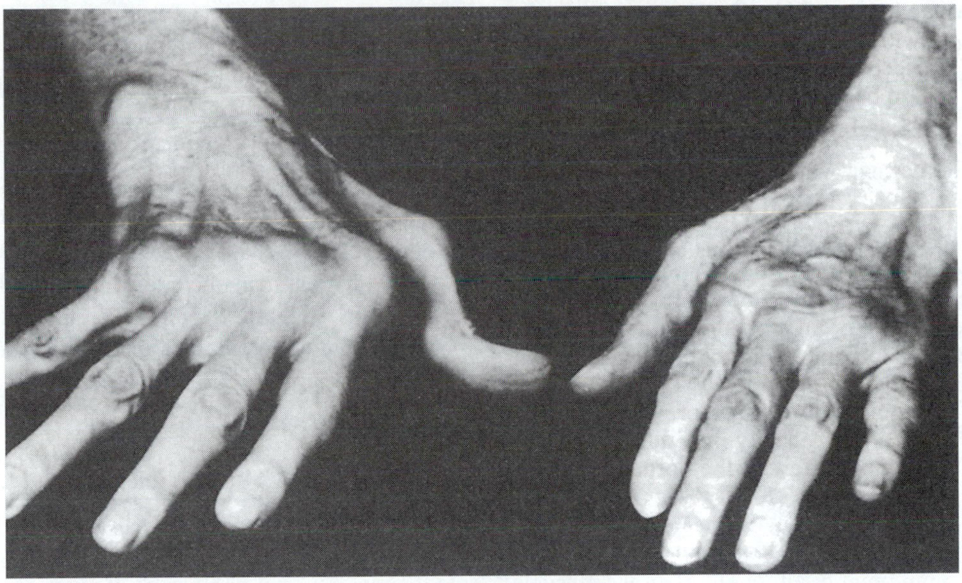

FIGURE 83–6. Ulnar deviation of the fingers of the right hand. *(Reproduced from the Arthritis Foundation Allied Health Professions Teaching Slide Collection, Copyright © 1980, with permission.)*

monly involved in rheumatoid arthritis, making walking difficult. Subluxation of the metatarsal heads leads to "cock-up" toe deformities. Subluxation may also cause a flexion deformity at the PIP joint of the toe, leading to pressure necrosis of the skin over the joint secondary to irritation caused by shoes. Hallux valgus (lateral deviation of the digit) and bunion or callus formation may occur at the great toe (Fig. 83–7). A widening of the foot commonly occurs with long-standing disease.

Involvement of the spine usually occurs in the cervical vertebrae; lumbar vertebral involvement is rare. Involvement of the first and second cervical vertebrae (C1 to C2) can lead to instability of this joint. Patients with this problem are at a greater risk for spinal cord compression, although this complication is rare.

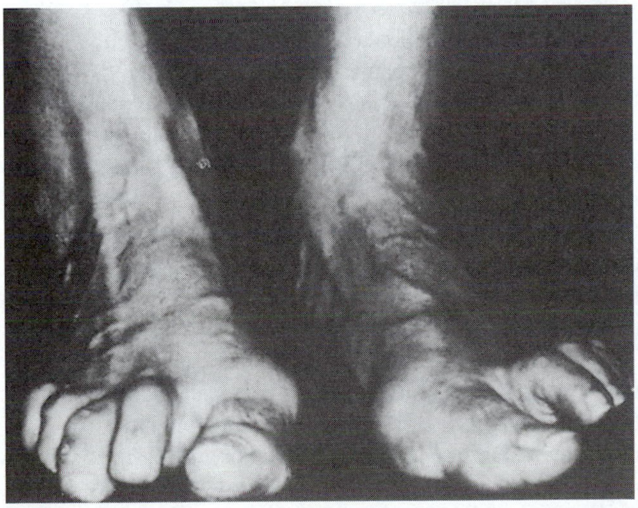

FIGURE 83–7. Foot involvement of rheumatoid arthritis with hallux valgus deformity of the first digit and hammer toe deformity of second through fifth digits bilaterally. *(Reproduced from the Arthritis Foundation Allied Health Professions Teaching Slide Collection, Copyright © 1980, with permission.)*

The temporomandibular joint (jaw) can be affected, resulting in malocclusion and difficulty in chewing food. Inflammation of cartilage in the chest can lead to chest wall pain. Hip pain may occur as a result of destructive changes in the hip joint, soft-tissue inflammation (e.g., bursitis), or referred pain from nerve entrapment at the lumbar vertebrae.

EXTRA-ARTICULAR INVOLVEMENT

RHEUMATOID NODULES

Rheumatoid nodules occur in 20% of patients with rheumatoid arthritis. These nodules are most commonly seen on the extensor surfaces of the elbows, forearms, and hands but may also be seen on the feet and at other pressure points. They may also develop in the lung or pleural lining of the lung and rarely, in the meninges. Rheumatoid nodules are usually asymptomatic and do not require any special intervention. Nodules are more commonly observed in patients with erosive disease.[8]

VASCULITIS

Vasculitis is usually seen in those patients with long-standing rheumatoid arthritis. Vasculitis may result in a wide variety of clinical presentations. Invasion of blood vessel walls by inflammatory cells results in an obliteration of the vessel, producing infarction of tissue distal to the area of involvement. Most commonly, small-vessel vasculitis produces infarcts near the ends of the fingers or toes, especially around the nail beds. These infarcts are usually of little consequence.

Vasculitis may also cause the breakdown of skin, especially in the lower extremities, producing ulcers that may be indistinguishable in appearance from stasis ulcers. However, these ulcers do not heal with the usual modes of treatment used for stasis ulcers. Involvement of larger vessels with vasculitis can result in life-threatening complications. Infarction of vessels supplying blood to nerves can cause irreversible motor deficits. Involvement of vessels supplying other organ systems can lead to visceral involvement and a polyarteritis nodosa-like illness. Aggressive treatment of the inflammatory process is necessary in these patients. Fortunately, the more serious vasculitic picture is rarely seen.

PULMONARY COMPLICATIONS

Rheumatoid arthritis may involve the pleura of the lung, which is often asymptomatic although pleural effusions may result. Pulmonary fibrosis may also develop as a result of rheumatoid involvement; smoking appears to increase the risk of this complication. Rheumatoid nodules may develop in lung tissue and appear similar to neoplasms on chest x-ray films. Interstitial pneumonitis and arteritis are rare, potentially life-threatening complications of rheumatoid arthritis.

OCULAR MANIFESTATIONS

Ocular manifestations include keratoconjunctivitis sicca and inflammation of the sclera, episclera, and cornea. Atrophy of the lacrimal duct may result in a decrease in tear formation, causing dry and itchy eyes, termed keratoconjunctivitis sicca. When this is observed in association with rheumatoid arthritis, it is referred to as Sjögren's syndrome. Artificial tears may be used to relieve symptoms. Inflammation of the superficial layers of the sclera (episcleritis) is generally self-limiting. Involvement of deeper tissues (scleritis) usually results in a more serious, painful, and chronic inflammation. Rheumatoid nodules may develop on the sclera.

CARDIAC INVOLVEMENT

Cardiac involvement occurs in rheumatoid arthritis but is rarely symptomatic. Pericarditis may occur, resulting in the accumulation of fluid. Although many patients show evidence of previous pericarditis at autopsy, the development of clinically evident pericarditis with tamponade is a rare complication. Cardiac conduction abnormalities and aortic valve incompetence, caused by aortic root dilatation, may occur. Myocarditis is a rare complication of rheumatoid arthritis.

FELTY'S SYNDROME

Rheumatoid arthritis in association with splenomegaly and neutropenia is known as Felty's syndrome. Thrombocytopenia may also be a manifestation of the syndrome. Patients with Felty's syndrome and severe leukopenia are more susceptible to infection. The decrease in granulocytes appears to be mediated by the immune system, because splenectomy does not result in improvement of the patient.[10]

OTHER COMPLICATIONS

Lymphadenopathy may occur in patients with rheumatoid arthritis, particularly in nodes proximal to more actively involved joints. Renal involvement is rare but can be associated with treatment including nonsteroidal anti-inflammatory drugs (NSAIDs), gold salts, and penicillamine. Amyloidosis is a rare complication of long-standing rheumatoid arthritis. It appears to be more common in Europe than in the United States.

LABORATORY FINDINGS

Hematologic tests often reveal a mild to moderate anemia with normocytic, normochromic indices. The hematocrit may fall as low as 30%. The anemia is usually inversely related to inflammatory disease activity and is referred to as an anemia of chronic disease. This type of anemia does not respond to iron therapy and can present a diagnostic dilemma, because NSAIDs may induce gastritis and chronic blood loss leading to iron-deficiency anemia. Laboratory tests useful in differentiating these anemias include stool guaiac (or other stool tests for occult blood), serum iron/iron binding capacity ratio (decreased in iron deficiency), and mean corpuscular volume (more likely to be decreased in iron deficiency). Other causes of anemia must also be considered in the differential diagnosis (see Chap. 93).

Thrombocytosis is another common hematologic finding with active rheumatoid arthritis. Platelet counts rise and fall in direct correlation with disease activity in many patients. Thrombocytopenia may result from toxicity of gold salts, penicillamine, or immunosuppressive therapy. Thrombocytopenia may also be observed in Felty's syndrome or vasculitis.

Although leukopenia is associated with Felty's syndrome, it may also result from toxicity of gold, penicillamine, and immunosuppressive drugs. Leukocytosis is commonly seen as a result of corticosteroid treatment.

The erythrocyte sedimentation rate (ESR) is usually elevated in patients with rheumatoid arthritis and other inflammatory diseases. This test is very nonspecific, and although the ESR usually falls as patients respond to therapy, there is a large variability among patients in response to treatment.

Rheumatoid factor is present in 60% to 70% of patients with rheumatoid arthritis. The usual laboratory test for rheumatoid factor is an antibody specific for IgM rheumatoid factor. Patients with rheumatoid arthritis and a negative test for rheumatoid factor may have IgG or IgA rheumatoid factors, but tests for these are not routinely available. Rheumatoid factor tests are usually reported positive at a specific serum dilution. Serum is diluted to a standard series of dilutions; the greatest dilution that yields a positive test result will be reported (e.g., rheumatoid factor positive at 1:640). Higher dilutional titers of rheumatoid factors usually indicate a more severe disease, but like the ESR, the large interpatient variability makes this test difficult to use as a means of assessing patient progress. Rheumatoid factor may be positive in patients without rheumatoid arthritis (Table 83–3).

Antinuclear antibodies (ANA) are detected in 25% of patients with rheumatoid arthritis. These antibodies usually have a diffuse pattern of immunofluorescence. Tests for antibodies to double-stranded DNA (usually positive in systemic lupus erythematosus, SLE) are negative. Serum complement is usually normal, although complement concentrations of joint fluid are often depressed from consumption secondary to the inflammatory process. In patients with vasculitis, serum complement concentrations may be low.

Synovial fluid usually is turbid because of the large number of leukocytes in inflammatory fluid. White cell counts of 5000 to 50,000/mm^3 are not uncommon in inflamed joints. The fluid is usually less viscous than that in normal joints or in fluid associated with osteoarthritis. Glucose concentrations of joint fluid are normal or low compared with those in serum drawn at the same time as synovial aspirates. The decrease is not as profound as the decrease associated with joint infection or SLE.

Radiologic manifestations of rheumatoid arthritis include soft-tissue swelling and osteoporosis near the joint (periarticular osteoporosis). Erosions tend to occur later in the course of the disease and are usually seen first in the MCP and PIP joints of the hands and the MTP joints of the feet. Erosions are usually first seen at the margin of the joint near the interface of the head of the bone with the synovial tissue (Fig. 83–8).

TABLE 83–3. Diseases Associated with a Positive Rheumatoid Factor

Rheumatic Diseases	Syphilis
Rheumatoid arthritis	Infectious mononucleosis
Sjögren's syndrome (with or without arthritis)	Infectious hepatitis
Systemic lupus erythematosus	Leprosy
Progressive systemic sclerosis	**Other Causes**
Polymyositis/dermatomyositis	Aging
Infectious Diseases	Interstitial pulmonary fibrosis
Bacterial endocarditis	Cirrhosis of the liver
Tuberculosis	Chronic active hepatitis
	Sarcoidosis

SERONEGATIVE INFLAMMATORY ARTHRITIS

Although rheumatoid arthritis may have a negative rheumatoid factor titer, a number of other systemic inflammatory arthritic conditions exist including psoriatic arthritis, ankylosing spondylitis, and arthritis associated with inflammatory bowel disease. These conditions often tend to be less aggressive than those typical seen with rheumatoid arthritis. Detailed discussion about these conditions is beyond the scope of this chapter, but further information may be found elsewhere.[2] Management principles are similar to those for rheumatoid arthritis.

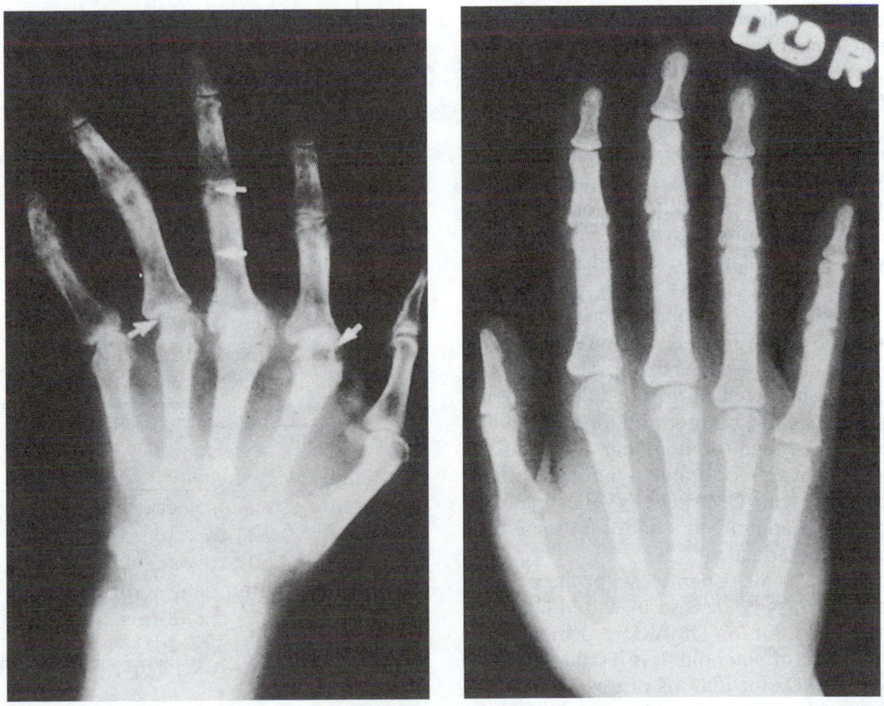

FIGURE 83–8. Radiograph of normal hand *(right)* and rheumatoid arthritis *(left)* with joint space narrowing, periarticular osteoporosis, and erosions *(arrows)*. *(Reproduced from the Arthritis Foundation Allied Health Professions Teaching Slide Collection, Copyright © 1980, with permission.)*

▶ TREATMENT: Rheumatoid Arthritis

The primary objective is to improve or maintain functional status, thereby improving quality of life. Treatment of rheumatoid arthritis is a multifaceted approach that includes pharmacologic and nonpharmacologic therapies. Recent emphasis has been placed on aggressive treatment early in the disease course. The ultimate goal is to achieve complete disease remission, though this goal is seldom achieved. Additional goals of treatment include control of disease activity, joint pain, maintaining ability to function in daily activities or work, improve quality of life, and slow destructive joint changes.

NON-PHARMACOLOGIC THERAPY

Nondrug therapy consists of rest, occupational therapy, physical therapy, use of assistive devices, weight reduction, and surgery. Rest is an essential component of a nonpharmacologic treatment plan. It relieves stress on inflamed joints and prevents further joint destruction. Rest also aids in alleviation of pain. Too much rest and immobility, however, may lead to decreased range of motion and, ultimately, muscle atrophy and contractures.

Occupational and physical therapy can provide the patient with skills and exercises necessary to increase or maintain mobility. These disciplines may also provide patients with supportive and adaptive devices such as canes, walkers, and splints.

Other nondrug therapeutic options include weight loss and surgery. Weight reduction helps to alleviate inflamed joint stress. This should be instituted and monitored with close supervision of a health care professional. Tenosynovectomy, tendon repair, and joint replacements are surgical options for patients with rheumatoid arthritis. Such management is usually reserved for patients with severe disease.[11]

PHARMACOLOGIC THERAPY

Figure 83–9 presents a treatment algorithm for RA. This figure reflects a more aggressive treatment approach than has been previously suggested. Prevention of destructive disease is the basis for this treatment strategy. Many rheumatologists believe early introduction of disease-modifying antirheumatic drugs (DMARDs) results in a more favorable outcome. DMARDs include methotrexate, gold, hydroxychloroquine, sulfasalazine, penicillamine, and azathioprine. Some factors identified as predictors for poor outcome include early age of disease onset, high titer rheumatoid factor, elevated erythrocyte sedimentation rate, and swelling of more than 20 joints.

NSAIDs alone do not prevent the debilitating complications seen in RA, possibly because of the limited role prostaglandins play in the inflammatory cascade (see Fig. 83–2). Used as primary therapy, NSAIDs should be given on a scheduled basis in anti-inflammatory doses. This should be used only in those with milder disease and should not be tried for more than 3 months as monotherapy unless the patient demonstrates a satisfactory response. When in combination with DMARDs, NSAIDs may be used as adjunctive therapy for symptomatic control. In some patients, as-needed dosing may be adequate.

DMARDs should be used in all patients except those with limited disease or those with class IV disease in whom little reversibility of disease is expected. Of the DMARDs, methotrexate appears to have the best long-term outcome. It is less likely to be discontinued than other DMARDs for reasons of toxicity or lack of efficacy. Gold or hydroxychloroquine should be considered in patients who have contraindications or are refractory to methotrexate. The other agents in Fig. 83–9 should be considered second- or third-line drugs in the treatment of RA. Combination therapy with two or more DMARDs may be effective when single DMARD treatment is unsuccessful.[11a,12–14a]

Corticosteroids can be used in various ways. They are valuable in controlling symptoms before the onset of action of DMARDs. A burst of corticosteroids can be used in acute flares. Continuous low doses may be adjuncts when DMARDs do not provide adequate disease control. Corticosteroids may be injected into joints and soft tissues to control local inflammation. Steroids should seldom be used as monotherapy because of their high risk of toxicity. NSAIDs and DMARDs have steroid-sparing properties that permit reductions of steroid doses.

For monitoring parameters and dosing guidelines for DMARDs and NSAIDs used in rheumatoid arthritis, see Tables 83–4 and 83–5.[14–18]

NONSTEROIDAL ANTI-INFLAMMATORY DRUGS

NSAIDs are generally accepted as first-line therapy for the symptomatic treatment of mild RA (Table 83–6). NSAIDs possess both analgesic and anti-inflammatory properties and reduce stiffness

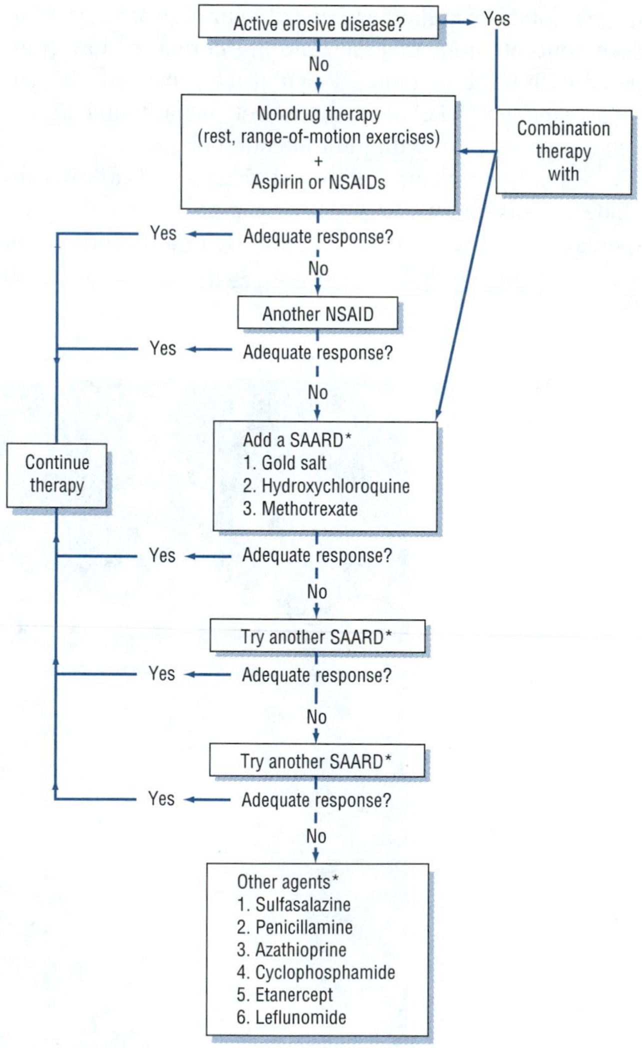

FIGURE 83–9. Algorithm for treatment of rheumatoid arthritis. *Corticosteroids may be necessary for patients with severe inflammatory disease in any of these phases to enable the patient to be more functional while awaiting the beneficial effects of therapy or in patients with partial responses to therapy.

TABLE 83–4. Usual Doses and Laboratory Monitoring Parameters for Antirheumatic Drugs

Drug	Usual Dose	Initial	Maintenance
NSAIDs	Table 83–6	Scr or BUN, CBC q 2–4 wk p starting therapy × 1–2 mo salicylates: serum salicylate levels if therapeutic dose and no response	Same as initial plus stool guaiac q 6–12 mo
Methotrexate	Oral or IM: 7.5–15 mg q wk	Baseline: AST, ALT, alk phos, alb, t. bili, hep B & C studies, CBC w/plt, Scr	CBC w/plt, AST, alb q 1–2 mo
Auranofin (gold)	Oral: 3 mg daily to bid	Baseline: UA, CBC w/plt	Same as initial q 1–2 mo
Gold sodium thiomalate or aurothioglucose	IM: 10 mg test dose, then weekly dosing 25–50 mg, after response may ↑ dosing interval	Baseline and until stable: UA, CBC w/plt preinjection	Same as initial every other dose
Hydroxychloroquine	Oral: 200–300 mg bid, after 1–2 months may ↓ to 200 mg bid or daily	Baseline: color fundus photography and automated central perimetric analysis	Ophthalmoscopy q 9–12 mo and Amsler grid at home q 2 wk
Sulfasalazine	Oral: 500 mg bid, then ↑ to 1 g bid max	Baseline: CBC w/plt, then q wk × 1 mo	Same as initial q 1–2 mo
Azathioprine	Oral: 50–150 mg daily	CBC w/plt, AST q 2 wks × 1–2 mo	Same as initial q 1–2 mo
D-penicillamine	Oral: 125–250 mg daily, may ↑ by 125–250 mg q 1–2 mo, max 750 mg/d	Baseline: UA, CBC w/plt, then q wk × 1 mo	Same as initial q 1–2 mo, but q 2 wk if dose change
Cyclophosphamide	Oral: 1–2 mg/kg/d	UA, CBC w/plt q wk × 1 mo	Same as initial q 2–4 wk
Cyclosporine	Oral: 2.5 mg/kg/d	Scr, blood pressure q mo	Same as initial
Corticosteroids	Oral, IV, IM, IA, and soft-tissue injections; variable	Glucose, blood pressure q 3–6 mo	Same as initial
Leflunomide	100 mg daily × 3 d, then 20 mg daily	AST or ALT q mo	AST or ALT periodically
Etanercept	25 mg 2 × weekly	None	None

Alb = albumin; alk phos = alkaline phosphatase; ALT = alanine aminotransferase; AST = aspartate aminotransferase; BUN = blood urea nitrogen; CBC = complete blood count; hep = hepatitis; IA = intraarticular; IM = intramuscular; IV = intravenous; p = after; plt = platelet; q = every; Scr = serum creatinine; t. bili = total bilirubin; UA = urinalysis.

TABLE 83–5. Clinical Monitoring of Drug Therapy in Rheumatoid Arthritis

Drug	Toxicities Requiring Monitoring	Symptoms to Inquire About[a]
NSAIDs and salicylates	GI ulceration and bleeding, renal damage	Blood in stool, black stool, dyspepsia, nausea/vomiting, weakness, dizziness, abdominal pain, edema, weight gain, shortness of breath
Corticosteroids	Hypertension, hyperglycemia, osteoporosis[b]	Blood pressure if available, polyuria, polydipsia, edema, SOB, visual changes, weight gain, headaches, broken bones or bone pain
Azathioprine	Myelosuppression, hepatotoxicity, lymphoproliferative disorders	Symptoms of myelosuppression (extreme fatigue, easy bleeding or bruising, infection), jaundice
Gold (intramuscular or oral)	Myelosuppression, proteinuria, rash, stomatitis	Symptoms of myelosuppression, edema, rash, oral ulcers, diarrhea
Hydroxychloroquine	Macular damage, rash, diarrhea	Visual changes including a decrease in night or peripheral vision, rash, diarrhea
Methotrexate	Myelosuppression, hepatic fibrosis, cirrhosis, pulmonary infiltrates or fibrosis, stomatitis, rash	Symptoms of myelosuppression, SOB, nausea/vomiting, lymph node swelling, coughing, mouth sores, diarrhea, jaundice
Penicillamine	Myelosuppression, proteinuria, stomatitis, rash, dysgeusia	Symptoms of myelosuppression, edema, rash, diarrhea, altered taste perception, oral ulcers
Sulfasalazine	Myelosuppression, rash	Symptoms of myelosuppression, photosensitivity, rash, nausea/vomiting
Leflunomide	Hepatotoxicity	Jaundice
Etanercept	Sepsis	Chills, fevers, infection

[a]Altered immune function increases infection, which should be considered particularly in those patients taking azathioprine, methotrexate, and corticosteroids or other drugs as a symptom of myelosuppression.
[b]Osteoporosis is not likely to manifest itself early in treatment but all patients should be taking appropriate steps to prevent bone loss.
From American College of Rheumatology Ad Hoc Committee on Clinical Guidelines. Guidelines for monitoring drug therapy in rheumatoid arthritis. Arthritis Rheum 1996;39:723–731.

associated with RA. NSAIDs mainly inhibit prostaglandin synthesis, which is only a small portion of the inflammatory cascade (see Fig. 83–2). NSAIDs alone will not prevent joint erosions, and most rheumatologists advocate early combination therapy with DMARDs except in very minimal disease. For discussion of the mechanism of action, adverse effects, and drug interactions, see the anti-inflammatory drugs section of (Chap. 84).[19–21]

METHOTREXATE

Methotrexate (MTX) was first used to treat psoriatic arthritis and was approved by the FDA for RA in 1988. MTX is now the DMARD of choice by many rheumatologists. MTX is contraindicated in pregnant and nursing women. It is also contraindicated in patients with chronic liver disease, immunodeficiency, pleural or peritoneal effusions, leukopenia, thrombocytopenia, preexisting blood disorders, and creatinine clearance of less than 40 mL/min.

Absorption of MTX is variable and averages about 70% of an oral dose. MTX is 35% to 50% bound to albumin; it may be displaced by highly protein-bound drugs such as NSAIDs, but the clinical importance of this interaction is not known. MTX is extensively metabolized intracellularly to polyglutamated derivatives. It is excreted renally, 80% unchanged, by glomerular filtration and active transport. Some MTX may be reabsorbed, but this transport process may be saturated even with low doses, resulting in increased renal clearance.

MTX has a fairly rapid onset of action; results may be seen as early as 2 to 3 weeks after starting therapy. Some 45% to 67% of patients remain on MTX therapy in studies ranging from 5 to 7 years.[22,23] Sustained efficacy is also reported in patients receiving MTX for up to 15 years.[24] MTX may be given intramuscularly or orally. Doses greater than 15 mg/wk are generally given parenterally because of decreased oral bioavailability of larger doses.

The toxicities of MTX therapy are mainly gastrointestinal, hematologic, pulmonary, and hepatic. Stomatitis occurs in 3% to 10% of patients and may be painful or painless. Diarrhea, nausea, and vomiting may occur in up to 10% of patients. The most common hematologic toxicity is thrombocytopenia in 1 to 3% of patients. Leukopenia may also occur, but in a smaller number of patients. Although pulmonary fibrosis and pneumonitis are severe adverse effects, they are rare. Elevated liver enzymes may occur in up to 15% of patients; cirrhosis is rare. Guidelines for monitoring hepatotoxicity in patients taking MTX for rheumatoid arthritis have been established. Liver biopsy is now recommended before beginning MTX therapy only for patients with a history of excessive alcohol use, ongoing hepatitis B or C infection, or recurring elevation of aspartate aminotransferase. Biopsies during MTX therapy are recommended only for patients who develop consistently abnormal liver function tests.[25] Since the drug is teratogenic, patients should use contraception to avoid pregnancy and discontinue the drug if conception is planned.

Because it is a folic acid antagonist, MTX can induce a folic acid deficiency. This deficiency is thought partly responsible for MTX toxicity, and supplementation with folic acid has been shown to alleviate some adverse effects. Addition of folic acid to an MTX regimen for rheumatoid arthritis does not compromise drug efficacy.[24,26–28]

GOLD

Gold is available as oral (auranofin) or intramuscular (aurothioglucose or gold sodium thiomalate) dosage forms. The antirheumatic effects of oral or injectable gold may be delayed 3 to 6 months. Auranofin is poorly absorbed from the gastrointestinal tract, and the extent of distribution to various body compartments is unknown. Urinary excretion accounts for ap-

TABLE 83–6. Dosage Regimens and Durations of Antiplatelet Effect for Nonsteroidal Anti-inflammatory Drugs

Drug	Recommended Anti-inflammatory Total Daily Dosage		Dosing Schedule	Approximate Duration of Anti-platelet Effect
	Adult	*Children*		
Aspirin	2.6–5.2 g	60–100 mg/kg	qid	14 d
Diclofenac	150–200 mg	—	tid to qid Extended release, bid	5–10 h
Diflunisal	0.5–1.5 g	—	bid	2–7 d
Etodolac	0.2–1.2 g (max 20 mg/kg)	—	tid to qid	36 h
Fenoprofen	0.9–3.0 g	—	qid	15–24 h
Flurbiprofen	200–300 mg	—	bid to qid	24—48 h
Ibuprofen	1.2–3.2 g	20–40 mg/kg	tid to qid	5–10 h
Indomethacin	50–200 mg	2–4 mg/kg (max 200 mg)	bid to qid Extended release, daily	24–48 h
Ketoprofen	150–300 mg	—	tid to qid Extended release, daily	5–10 h
Meclofenamate	200–400 mg	—	tid to qid	24–48 h
Nabumetone	1–2 g	—	daily to bid	4–7 d
Naproxen	0.5–1.0 g	10 mg/kg	bid Extended release, daily	4 d
Naproxen sodium	0.55–1.1 g	—	bid	4 d
Nonacetylated salicylates	1.2–4.8 g	—	bid to 6/d	None
Oxaprozin	0.6–1.8 g (max 26 mg/kg)	—	daily to tid	8–10 d
Piroxicam	10–20 mg	—	daily	7–20 d
Sulindac	300–400 mg	—	bid	4 d
Tolmetin	0.6–1.8 g	15–30 mg/kg	tid to qid	8–16 h

proximately 60% of the drug absorbed, fecal elimination the other 40%. Aurothioglucose and gold sodium thiomalate are rapidly absorbed after intramuscular injection, although aurothioglucose may be absorbed more slowly because it is an oil suspension. Injectable gold is 85% to 95% protein bound. Metabolism of parenteral gold is unknown, but the compounds are probably not degraded to elemental gold. Urinary elimination averages 70%. After cumulative dosing of 1 g of these drugs, they may be detected in the urine 12 to 15 months after drug discontinuation.

Toxicities of gold compounds are similar, whether taken orally or parenterally. Metallic taste can be a harbinger of other adverse effects. Dermatologic effects such as skin rash and stomatitis require discontinuation of gold therapy; patients may be rechallenged with gold after resolution of these side effects if they are not severe. Renal toxicity manifests as proteinuria or hematuria; hematologic toxicity presents as anemia, leukopenia, or thrombocytopenia. These toxicities are reversible if the drug is discontinued. Gastrointestinal events such as nausea, vomiting, and diarrhea resolve with time or dosage decrease and are more common with auranofin. Injectable gold preparations, particularly gold sodium thiomalate, may cause nitritoid reactions that may involve flushing, palpitations, hypotension, tachycardia, headache, or blurred vision. Such reactions are self-limiting and usually respond to change of gold salt.

Patients may experience increased joint symptoms for 1 to 2 days after an injection. This is referred to as a postinjection disease flare. If the flare is severe, therapy must be changed.[29]

HYDROXYCHLOROQUINE

The pharmacokinetics of hydroxychloroquine (HCQ) are poorly understood but are probably similar to chloroquine. It is well absorbed orally and widely distributed to body tissues. HCQ is partially metabolized in the liver and is excreted renally. The onset of action of HCQ may be delayed up to 6 weeks, but the drug is considered a therapeutic failure only when 6 months of therapy without a response has elapsed.

The main advantage of HCQ is the lack of myelosuppressive, hepatic, and renal toxicities that may be seen with other slow-acting agents. Monitoring of HCQ toxicity is, therefore, simplified in comparison with other DMARDs. Short-term toxicities of HCQ include gastrointestinal effects such as nausea, vomiting, and diarrhea, which can be managed by taking doses with food. Ocular toxicity includes accommodation defects, benign corneal deposits, blurred vision, scotomas (small areas of decreased or absent vision in the visual field), and night blindness. Although the risk of true retinopathy with HCQ approaches zero, pre-retinopathy may occur in 2.7% of patients. All patients must understand the importance of adhering to HCQ monitoring guidelines. Any visual change must be reported immediately. Dermatologic toxicities include rash, alopecia, and increased skin pigmentation; neurologic adverse effects such as headache, vertigo, and insomnia are usually mild.[29,30]

SULFASALAZINE

Sulfasalazine, a prodrug, is cleaved by bacteria in the colon into sulfapyridine and 5-aminosalicylic acid (5-ASA). It is believed that the sulfapyridine moiety is responsible for the agent's antirheumatic properties, although the exact mechanism of action is not known. Once the colonic bacteria have cleaved sulfasalazine, sulfapyridine and 5-ASA are rapidly absorbed from the gastrointestinal tract. Sulfapyridine rapidly distributes throughout the body, but higher concentrations are found in certain tissues such as serous fluid, liver, and intestines. Both sulfasalazine and its metabolites are excreted in the urine. Antirheumatic effects should be seen in 1 to 2 months.

Use of sulfasalazine is often limited by its adverse effects. Gastrointestinal adverse effects such as nausea, vomiting, diarrhea, and anorexia are the most common. These can be minimized by initiating therapy with low doses and gradually titrating to higher doses, dividing the dose more evenly throughout the day, or using enteric-coated preparations. Rash, urticaria, and serum sickness-like reactions can be managed with antihistamines and, if indicated, corticosteroids. If a hypersensitivity reaction occurs, therapy should be stopped immediately and another DMARD substituted. Sulfasalazine has been associated with leukopenia, alopecia, stomatitis, and elevated hepatic enzymes. It may also cause the patient's urine and skin to turn a yellow-orange color.

Sulfasalazine's absorption can be decreased when antibiotics are used that destroy the colonic bacteria. Sulfasalazine also binds iron supplements in the gastrointestinal tract that can lead to a decreased absorption of sulfasalazine. The administration of these two agents should be temporally separated to avoid this interaction. Sulfasalazine can potentiate warfarin's effects by displacing it from protein-binding sites. Close monitoring of the patient's international normalized ratio (INR) is indicated.[29,31]

AZATHIOPRINE

Azathioprine is an antimetabolite that is generally considered safer but slower acting than cyclophosphamide. Azathioprine is a purine analog that is biologically converted to 6-mercaptopurine and is believed to interfere with DNA and RNA synthesis.

Azathioprine is rapidly absorbed after oral dosing and is approximately 30% bound to plasma proteins. The major route of elimination is renal, and doses should be reduced by 25% for patients with creatinine clearance (CrCl) of 10 to 50 mL/min and by 50% for CrCl below < 10 mL/min.

Antirheumatic effects can be seen within 3 to 4 weeks. If no response is seen after 12 weeks at maximal dosages, azathioprine should be discontinued.

The major adverse effect associated with azathioprine use is reversible bone-marrow suppression (e.g., leukopenia, macrocytic anemia, pancytopenia, thrombocytopenia) that appears to be dose related. When this occurs, it is common practice to stop the drug temporarily until the marrow recovers. Therapy may be reinstituted at a 25% dose reduction. Other adverse effects include gastrointestinal intolerance, oncogenic potential, stomatitis, infections, drug fever, and hepatotoxicity. Allopurinol inhibits xanthine oxidase, which decreases the metabolism of 6-mercaptopurine and increases the likelihood of myelosuppression. If the two agents must be used together, azathioprine should be reduced to approximately 30% of the usual dose.[32,33]

D-Penicillamine

The pharmacokinetics of D-penicillamine (DP), a heavy metal chelating agent, are not well known. The drug is quickly absorbed from the gastrointestinal tract, but food, antacids, and iron will decrease the amount absorbed. The extent of distribution to body tissues is unknown. DP is metabolized in the liver and excreted mainly as inactive disulfide metabolites in the urine and feces.

Therapeutic effects may be delayed 1 to 3 months after starting therapy. Most clinical responses are seen within 6 months. Early adverse effects of DP include a pruritic, erythematous skin rash, metallic taste, and hypogeusia (decreased taste sensation). Hypogeusia may last 2 to 3 months and resolves without intervention. A rash or metallic taste occurring after 6 months of therapy with DP requires the drug to be decreased or withheld. It may be reinstituted at a lower dose. Stomatitis, which may be painful or painless, usually improves with a decrease in DP dose. Nausea, vomiting, anorexia, and dyspepsia may occur and are managed by dosage reduction. DP may induce glomerular nephritis, which manifests as proteinuria and hematuria. Other autoimmune diseases include polymyositis, Goodpasture's syndrome, myasthenia gravis, systemic lupus erythematosus, and pemphigus. If any of these develop, DP must be discontinued. Although autoimmune diseases are rare, they are the primary reason most clinicians reserve DP for patients with RA resistant to other therapies.[34]

CYCLOSPORINE

Cyclosporine (CSA) may be considered for treating rheumatoid arthritis in patients who fail more conventional therapies. It is a potent modulator of the immune system reducing the production of cytokines involved in T-cell activation as well as direct effects on B cells, macrophages, bone, and cartilage cells. Its absorption is variable and incomplete, and the drug has a large volume of distribution (about 13 L/kg). CSA undergoes hepatic metabolism and has many metabolites; one or more of these may have pharmacologic action. The principal route of elimination is biliary; less than 10% is excreted in the urine.

The onset of action of CSA appears to be 1 to 3 months. Clinically important toxicities of CSA 1 to 10 mg/kg/d include hypertension, hyperglycemia, nephrotoxicity, tremor, gastrointestinal intolerance, hirsutism, and gingival hyperplasia. Hypertension and nephrotoxicity appear to be reversible after CSA is discontinued.

Because drug therapy for rheumatoid arthritis is long term (perhaps lifelong) and is commonly administered to older adults, the current recommendation is to reserve CSA for patients refractory to or intolerant of other disease-modifying antirheumatic drugs. The drug should be avoided in patients with current or past malignancy, uncontrolled hypertension, renal dysfunction, immunodeficiency, low white blood cell or platelet count (unless secondary to Felty's syndrome), or liver function test results greater than twice the upper limits of normal. It should be used cautiously in patients 65 years or older or with controlled hypertension, premalignant conditions, active infection pregnancy, or lactation. Also patients taking antiepileptic drugs, ketoconazole, fluconazole, trimethoprim, erythromycin, verapamil, diltiazem, or nonsteroidal anti-inflammatory drugs, or with concurrent or previous use of alkylating agents such as cyclophosphamide, should use CSA with caution.[35–38]

NEWER AGENTS

Leflunomide

Leflunomide is a DMARD that acts by inhibiting pyrimidine synthesis. It was approved for the treatment of RA by the FDA in 1998. It is given as a loading dose of 100 mg daily for 3 days followed by 20 mg daily. A 10-mg tablet is also available for patients who may experience dose-related side effects from the usual dose. The loading dose is necessary due to the long (14–16 days) half-life, which would result in a delayed time to onset of activity if only the maintenance dose is prescribed. With use of the loading dose, patient response is usually seen in 1 month.

Leflunomide has been demonstrated to reduce the progression of erosions in RA. The drug may cause liver function abnormalities, and ALT should be monitored monthly initially and periodically thereafter. Leflunomide has no bone marrow toxicity, so blood cell monitoring is not needed. The drug is teratogenic, so it should be avoided in pregnancy, and contraceptives should be used to prevent pregnancy. Both men and women seeking to conceive should discontinue leflunomide and not attempt conception until plasma levels of the drug's metabolites drop below 0.02 μg/mL. Cholestyramine administration is recommended to help clear the drug from plasma more rapidly.[44,45]

Etanercept

Etanercept is a human tumor necrosis factor receptor (TNF) p75-fusion protein. It competitively binds to the cytokine TNF, preventing its binding to inflammatory cell surface receptors. By doing this, it neutralizes the pro-inflammatory activity of TNF and reduces RA activity. No dose-limiting toxicities have been identified and the drug requires no laboratory monitoring. It must be administered by subcutaneous injection, 25 mg twice weekly. Local inflammation at the injection site has been reported. Patients with life-threatening infections or who are at high risk for sepsis should discontinue etanercept as blocking TNF activity may increase risk of mortality in patients who develop sepsis.[45,46]

Both etanercept and leflunomide are too new at this point to know how they fit into the approach for treating RA, but the drugs probably should be reserved for patients who fail more conventional treatments. This recommendation is based on the lack of long-term outcome studies and use in a large population of patients.

CORTICOSTEROIDS

Corticosteroids are used in RA for their anti-inflammatory and immunosuppressive properties. Given early in the course of the disease, they appear to reduce the progression of erosive joint changes.[38,42a] They interfere with antigen presentation to T lymphocytes, inhibit prostaglandin and leukotriene synthesis, and inhibit neutrophil and monocyte superoxide radical generation. Corticosteroids also impair migration and cause redistribution of monocytes, lymphocytes, and neutrophils, thus blunting the inflammatory and autoimmune responses.

Oral corticosteroids are rapidly and completely absorbed from the gastrointestinal tract. They are primarily metabolized and inactivated by the liver and excreted in the urine. The elimination half-life of most corticosteroids is sufficiently long that once-daily dosing is possible.

Oral corticosteroids can be used in several ways. They can be used in "bridging" therapy, continuous low-dose therapy, and short-term high-dose bursts to control flares of RA. Oral steroids (e.g., prednisone, methylprednisolone) can be used to control pain and synovitis while DMARDs are taking effect. This is termed "bridging" therapy, and is often used in patients with debilitating symptoms when DMARD therapy is initiated. Patients with difficult-to-control disease may be placed on low-dose, long-term corticosteroid therapy to control their symptoms. Prednisone doses below 7.5 mg daily are well tolerated but are not devoid of the long-term adverse effects associated with corticosteroids. The lowest dose of corticosteroid that controls symptoms should be used to reduce adverse effects. Alternate-day dosing of low-dose oral corticosteroids is usually ineffective in RA; symptoms usually flare on days without medication. High-dose corticosteroid bursts are often used to suppress flares of the disease. High doses are sustained for several days until symptoms are controlled, followed by a taper to the lowest effective dose.

Corticosteroids may also be delivered by injection. The intramuscular route is preferable in patients with compliance problems, since a depot effect is achieved. Depot forms of corticosteroids include triamcinolone acetonide, triamcinolone hexacetonide, and methylprednisolone acetate. This provides the patient with 2 to 8 weeks of symptomatic control. The depot effect provides a physiologic taper, avoiding hypothalamic–pituitary axis (HPA) suppression. It should be noted that the onset of effect via this route may be delayed by several days. Intravenous corticosteroids may be used to provide the patient with large amounts of drug during a steroid burst to control severe symptoms of RA. Intra-articular injections of depot forms of corticosteroids can be useful in treating synovitis and pain when a small number of joints are affected. The onset and duration of symptomatic relief is similar to those of intramuscular injection. The intra-articular route is often preferred because it is associated with the fewest number of systemic adverse effects. If efficacious, intra-articular injections may be repeated every 3 months. No one joint should be injected more than two or three times per year, because of the risk of accelerated joint destruction and atrophy of tendons. Soft tissues such as tendons and bursa may also be injected. This may help control the pain and inflammation associated with these structures. The onset and duration of symptomatic relief is similar to those of intramuscular and intra-articular injections.

Adverse effects are the major limitations to the long-term use of corticosteroids. They include HPA suppression, Cushing's syndrome, osteoporosis, myopathies, glaucoma, cataracts, gastritis, hypertension, hirsutism, electrolyte imbalances, glucose intolerance, skin atrophy, and increased susceptibility to infections. To minimize these effects, use the lowest effective corticosteroid dose and limit the duration of use. Patients on long-term therapy should be given calcium and vitamin D (and estrogen supplements for postmenopausal women) to minimize bone loss. Alendronate, etidronate, or calcitonin may be necessary in patients with evidence of clinically important bone loss. There is no evidence that corticosteroids alone increase the risk of gastrointestinal ulcerations, even though they have been often implicated. Therefore, gastrointestinal protective measures are not usually indicated.[39,40]

MISCELLANEOUS THERAPIES

Minocycline has been shown to have antirheumatic activity and may be of benefit in some patients. The mechanism of action is not known. When to use this antimicrobial agent in the management of RA remains to be determined.[41]

Although cyclophosphamide has been used in the past for severe rheumatoid arthritis when vasculitis is present, the benefit in most cases is outweighed by potential risks. Of primary concern is the oncogenic potential, but also hematologic complications as well as risks associated with immunosupression have limited its usefulness.

Investigational inhibitors of tumor necrosis factor are currently under investigation and appear to be promising for treating rheumatoid arthtitis. Monoclonal antibodies directed against the T-cell receptor may help to turn off the inflammatory process. T-cell "vaccination," which down-regulates the immune response, has been successful in treating experimental arthritis in mice. Monoclonal antibodies against adhesion molecules, which prevent the migration of immune cells to the synovium, have been tried with some success in humans.[42] Finally, type II collagen, and omega III fatty acids have been reported to be of some benefit in treating RA.

PHARMACOECONOMIC CONSIDERATIONS

The total cost of treating a patient with RA is estimated to be between $5000 and $7300 annually (1991 dollars). Of this, drugs account for roughly 10% of the total, excluding monitoring costs. These costs are approximately three times the cost of medical care for patients of similar age and gender without RA. The costs must be balanced against the high cost of disability on earning potential in these patients. Men with RA have average annual wages 50% of those of similar age without RA. Women with the disease have average annual wages only 25% of those without. The costs of disability make treatment worth the price if disability can be prevented or delayed and patients can continue to function as productive members of society.[43]

EVALUATION OF THERAPEUTIC OUTCOMES

The evaluation of therapeutic outcome is based primarily on improvements of clinical signs and symptoms of rheumatoid arthritis. Clinical signs of improvement include a reduction in joint swelling, decreased warmth over actively involved joints, and decreased tenderness to joint palpation. Improvement in RA symptoms includes reduction in perceived joint pain and morning stiffness, longer time to onset of afternoon fatigue, and improvement in ability to perform ADL. Joint radiographs may be of some benefit in assessing the progression of the disease, but have limitations.[43a] Laboratory monitoring is of little value in monitoring individual patient response to therapy. Monitoring of toxicity of drugs is shown in Tables 83–4 and 83–5. Routine monitoring of patients is essential to the safe use of these drugs. In addition, patients should be questioned about symptoms of the adverse effects outlined in the drug monograph section of this chapter.

CONCLUSIONS

Rheumatoid arthritis is the most common inflammatory arthritis, affecting approximately 1% of the population. The disease is characterized by symmetric swelling and stiffness of the involved joints. The stiffness is usually more prominent in the morning. Extra-articular features of rheumatoid arthritis include rheumatoid nodules, vasculitis, and ocular, cardiac, and pulmonary complications. The course of the disease is highly variable. Treatment is aimed at relieving pain and inflammation and maintaining and preserving joint function. The initial drug treatment in patients with mild disease is either aspirin or NSAIDs. Nondrug therapy, including exercise and adequate rest periods, should be used early in the course of treatment. One of the DMARDs such as methotrexate, gold, or hydroxychloroquine may be added to NSAID therapy in patients with inadequate response to initial treatment or those with more active disease. Sulfasalazine, penicillamine, and azathioprine may be effective in patients failing to respond to or having serious toxicity to other DMARDs. Combination DMARDs may be considered in those who fail adequate trials of single agent therapy. Corticosteroids are a useful adjunct for treatment, but because of adverse effects should be used in the lowest possible dose for the shortest possible treatment interval.

▶ PRINCIPLES OF PHARMACOTHERAPY

- Consider multiple drug regimens, including NSAIDs and DMARDs with or without corticosteroids, in all but the mildest forms of rheumatoid arthritis.
- NSAIDs as monotherapy should be given a trial of no greater than 3 months before considering adding a DMARD in patients who do not achieve adequate response to NSAID alone. If adequate response is achieved with a DMARD, NSAID use can be as needed in many patients.
- Corticosteroids can be used in these three situations: early in treatment to provide symptomatic relief while waiting for a DMARD to work, in low doses chronically for patients who fail to get adequate response from a DMARD, and in bursts to treat acute flairs of disease.

- When DMARDs used singly are ineffective, combination therapy induce a response.
- Pharmacotherapy is only part of the therapeutic regimen that should include physical therapy, exercise, and rest. Assistive devices and orthopedic surgery may also be necessary in some patients.
- Patients require careful monitoring for toxicity and therapeutic benefit for the duration of treatment.

REFERENCES

1. Harris ED. The clinical features of rheumatoid arthritis. In: Kelly WN, Harris ED, Ruddy S, Sledge CB, eds. Textbook of Rheumatology, 5th ed. Philadelphia, Saunders, 1997:898–932.
2. Schumacher HR, Klippel JH, Koopman WJ, eds. Primer of the Rheumatic Diseases, 10th ed. Atlanta, Arthritis Foundation, 1993.
3. Claman HN. The biology of the immune response. JAMA 1992;268: 2790–2796.
4. Condemi JJ. The autoimmune diseases. JAMA 1992;268:2882–2892.
5. Firestein GS. Etiology and pathogenesis of rheumatoid arthritis. In: Kelley WN, Harris ED, Ruddy S, Sledge CB, eds. Textbook of Rheumatology, 5th ed. Philadelphia, Saunders, 1997.
6. Harris ED. Rheumatoid arthritis: Pathophysiology and implications for therapy. N Engl J Med 1990;322:1277–1289.
7. Sewell KL, Trentham DE. Pathogenesis of rheumatoid arthritis. Lancet 1993;341:283–290.
8. Snyderman R. Mechanisms of inflammation and leukocyte chemotaxis in the rheumatic diseases. Med Clin North Am 1986;70: 217–235.
9. Weyand CM, Goronzy JJ. Pathogenesis of rheumatoid arthritis. Med Clin North Am 1997;81:29–55.
10. Hard ER. Extraarticular manifestations of rheumatoid arthritis. Semin Arthritis Rheum 1979;8:151–176.
11. Harris ED. The treatment of rheumatoid arthritis. In : Kelley WN, Harris ED, Ruddy S, Sledge CB, eds. Textbook of Rheumatology, 5th ed. Philadelphia, Saunders, 1997:933–950.

11a. American College of Rheumatology Ad Hoc Committee on Clinical Guidelines. Guidelines for the management of rheumatoid arthritis. Arthritis Rheum 1996;39:713–722.

12. O'Dell JR, Haire CE, Erickson N, et al. Treatment of rheumatoid arthritis with methotrexate alone, sulfasalazine and hydroxychloroquine, or a combination of all three medications. N Engl J Med 1996; 334:1287–1291.
13. Cash JM, Wilder RL. Refractory rheumatoid arthritis: Therapeutic options. Rheum Dis Clin North Am 1995;21:1–18.
14. Luqmani R, Gordon C, Bacon C. Clinical pharmacology and modification of autoimmunity and inflammation in rheumatoid disease. Drugs 1994;47:259–285.

14a. Pincus T, Callahan LF. Remodeling the pyramid or remodeling the paradigms concerning rheumatoid arthritis: Lessons from Hodgkin's disease and coronary artery disease. J Rheumatol. 1990;17:1582– 1585.

15. Jain R, Lipsky PE. Treatment of rheumatoid arthritis. Med Clin North Am 1997;81:57–83.
16. American College of Rheumatology Ad Hoc Committee on Clinical Guidelines. Guidelines for monitoring drug therapy in rheumatoid arthritis. Arthritis Rheum 1996;39:723–731.
17. Cash JM, Klippel JH. Second-line therapy for rheumatoid arthritis. N Engl J Med 1994;330:1368–1375.
18. Conaghan PG, Brooks P. Disease-modifying antirheumatic drugs including methotrexate, gold, antimalarials, and penicillamine. Curr Opin Rheumatol 1995;7:167–173.
19. Green JM, Winickoff RN. Cost-conscious prescribing of non-steroidal anti-inflammatory drugs for adults with arthritis. Arch Intern Med 1992;152:1995–2002.
20. Brooks PM, Day RO. Nonsteroidal antiinflammatory drugs—differences and similarities. N Engl J Med 1991;324:1716–1725.
21. Paulus HE. Current medicinal approaches to the treatment of rheumatoid arthritis. Clin Orthop 1991;265:96–102.
22. Pincus T, Marcum SB, Callahan LF. Long-term drug therapy for rheumatoid arthritis in seven rheumatology private practices: II. Second line drugs and prednisone. J Rheumatol 1992;19:1885–1894.
23. Wolfe F, Hawley DJ, Cathey MA. Termination of slow acting antirheumatic therapy in rheumatoid arthritis: A 14-year prospective evaluation of 1017 consecutive starts. J Rheumatol 1990;17:994–1002.
24. Weinblatt ME, Maier AL. Long-term experience with low dose weekly methotrexate in rheumatoid arthritis. J Rheumatol 1990; 17(suppl 22):33–38.
25. Kremer JM, Alarcon GS, Lightfoot RW Jr, et al. Methotrexate for rheumatoid arthritis. Suggested guidelines for monitoring liver toxicity. Arthritis Rheum 1994;37:316–328.
26. Morgan SL, Baggott JE, Vaughn WH, et al. The effect of folic acid supplementation on the toxicity of low-dose methotrexate in patients with rheumatoid arthritis. Arthritis Rheum 1990;33:9–18.
27. Schnabel A, Gross WL. Low-dose methotrexate in rheumatic diseases: Efficacy, side effects and risk factors for sided effects. Semin Arthritis Rheum 1996;39:310–327.
28. Barnworth B, Labat L, Moride Y, Schaeverbeke T. Methotrexate in rheumatoid arthritis: An update. Drugs 1994;47:25–50.
29. McConkey B. Disease-modifying antirheumatic drugs: Gold, penicillamine, antimalarials, and sulfasalazine. Curr Opin Rheumatol 1991;3: 348–354.
30. Ruiz RS, Saatci OA. Chloroquine and hydroxychloroquine retinopathy: How to follow affected patients. Ann Ophthalmol 1991;23: 290–291.
31. Rains CP, Noble S, Faulds D. Sulfasalazine:A review of its pharmacological properties and therapeutic efficacy in the treatment of rheumatoid arthritis. Drugs 1995;50:137–156.
32. Luqmani RA, Palmer RG, Bacon PA. Azathioprine, cyclophosphamide and chlorambucil. Baillieres Clin Rheumatol 1990;4:595–619.
33. Brooks PM. Clinical management of rheumatoid arthritis. Lancet 1993;341:286–290.
34. Munro R, Capell HA. Penicillamine. Br J Rheumatol 1997;36:104– 109.
35. Horton S, Resman-Targoff BH, Thompson DF. Use of cyclosporinee in rheumatoid arthritis. Ann Pharmacother 1993;27:44–46.
36. Tugwell P. Cyclosporinee in rheumatoid arthritis: Documented efficacy and safety. Semin Arthritis Rheum 1992;21(suppl 3):30–38.
37. Richardson C, Emery P. Clinical use of cyclosporine in rheumatoid arthritis. Drugs 1995;50(suppl 1):26–36.
38. Tugwell P. International consensus recommendations on cyclosporine use in rheumatoid arthritis. Drugs 1995;50(suppl 1):48–56.
39. Moeser PJ. Corticosteroid therapy for rheumatoid arthritis: Benefits and limitations. Postgrad Med 1991;90:175–182.
40. Caldwell JR, Furst DE. The efficacy and safety of low-dose corticosteroids for rheumatoid arthritis. Semin Arthritis Rheum 1991;21: 1–11.
41. Trentham DE, Dynesius-Trentham RA. Antibiotic therapy for rheumatoid arthritis: Scientific and anecdotal appraisals. Rheum Dis Clin North Am 1995;21:817–834.
42. Moreland LW, Heck LW Jr, Koopman WJ. Biologic agents for treating rheumatoid arthritis. Arthritis Rheum 1997;40:397–409.

42a. Kirwan JR, Arthritis and Rheumatism Council Low-Dose Glucocorticoid Study Group. The effect of glucocorticoids on joint destruction in rheumatoid arthritis. N Engl J Med 1995;333:142–146.

43. Pincus T. Underestimated long term medical and economic consequences of rheumatoid arthritis. Drugs 1995;50(suppl 1)1:1–14.

43a. Brower AC. Use of the radiograph to measure the course of rheumatoid arthritis: The gold standard of fool's gold. Arthritis Rheum 1990;33:316–324

44. Arava (package insert). Kansas City, Mo, Hoescht Marion Roussel, 1998.
45. Schuna AA. Update on treatment of rheumatoid arthritis. J Am Pharm Assoc 1998;38:728–737.
46. Enbrel (package insert). Seattle, Wa, Immunex, 1998.

84

OSTEOARTHRITIS

Larry E. Boh, MS

Osteoarthritis (OA), the most common form of joint disease, affects nearly 50% of the population older than the age of 65 and virtually everyone over the age of 75.[1] It remains an important public health problem. It ranks second only to cardiovascular diseases in producing severe chronic disability.[1-3] Because of the costs associated with the care of individuals and the progress in understanding of this disease, we have seen a renewed interest in its etiology and treatment.

OA affects primarily the weight-bearing joints of the peripheral and axial skeleton, causing pain, limitation of motion, deformity, and progressive disability. Throughout the literature, terms such as osteoarthrosis, degenerative joint disease (DJD), or hypertrophic arthritis are widely used to describe this disease, although none of these terms is truly adequate. Osteoarthrosis, a term used primarily in Europe, implies a general lack of inflammation and excess materials in the joint. DJD suggests a wearing out, deterioration, or breakdown of the joint. Hypertrophic arthritis, the earliest historic designation, describes only one aspect of the disease, the overgrowth of bone and cartilage.

In general, the term osteoarthritis is preferred as it best reflects the changes that occur in this highly anabolic, synthetic, and reparative tissue. With this term, it remains important to remember that osteoarthritis is not a single disorder but a sequence of events or a pattern of reactions that lead to joint injury. It is often best viewed as a disorder of both mechanical and biologic events that alter the normal synthesis and degradation of the articular cartilage. These events which affect the underlying bone, ultimately lead to clinical features of pain in the affected joint, tenderness, decreased or altered motion, crepitus, and varying degrees of local inflammation.[4–9]

Unlike rheumatoid arthritis or other inflammatory musculoskeletal disease, if inflammation is present, it is often mild or localized. Therefore, the major goals of therapy are to control the pain and other symptoms, minimize disability, and educate the patient.[8,9] Nonpharmacologic therapy serves as the foundation of treatment strategies, involving patient education, strengthening and range of motion exercises, use of assistive devices, joint protection, and as necessary, weight loss. The pharmacologic therapy is anchored by the use of nonopioid analgesics such as acetaminophen, followed by nonsteroidal anti-inflammatory drugs (NSAIDs), often in lower doses, and the topical analgesics such as capsaicin or methylsalicylate creams. Intra-articular steroid therapy and the use of opioid analgesics are reserved for individuals with specific clinical features or when patients have failed to respond to the other therapies. New therapy approaches, which are best described as in their infancy, focus on the attempting to account for the pathophysiology of the articular cartilage by providing compounds that stimulate chondrocyte metabolism or alter the degrading enzymes in the joint.

EPIDEMIOLOGY

Osteoarthritis remains the most prevalent of the rheumatic diseases and a common cause of decreased worker productivity and disability.[1,11–16] The overall disease prevalence increases with age. Radiographic data confirm the presence of OA at some site in the body in the majority of individuals older than 65 years of age and in most individuals ages 75 and older.[1,10,11] Although numerous epidemiologic studies have reported on the prevalence of OA, estimates of the true prevalence remain imprecise because of a lack of a clear diagnostic definition and variations in the reporting mechanisms (autopsy data, self-report).[10,13] Further, many patients with radiographic evidence of OA do not have symptoms or disabilities for which they seek health care, thus making estimates of disease extent and severity difficult without large-scale controlled population data.

PREVALENCE BY AGE, SEX, AND RACE

In the United States, the most frequently cited series of prevalence data is reported by the National Centers for Health Statistics (NCHS).[14] These data, referred to as the National Health Interview Survey (NHIS) and the National Health and Nutrition Examination Survey (NHANES), are based on probability samples of the U.S. civilian, noninstitutionalized population more than 20 years ago. Using this information, an estimated 15.8 million adults, or 12% of those between 25 and 74 years of age, have signs and symptoms of OA. As anticipated, the proportion of moderate to severe cases also increases with age. In the less than 45-year-old group, 19.3% of hands and 23.9% of feet were categorized as mild to severe. By comparison, in the 75- to 79-year-old group, 85% and 51% have this degree of changes in the hands and feet, respectively. OA of the knee also increased from less than 0.1% in people between the ages of 25 and 34 to 10% to 20% for those 65 to 74 years old. Likewise, the proportion of individuals with OA classified as moderate to severe increased with age, reaching 33% of knees and about 50% of hips for individuals between 65 and 74 years of age.

In the United States, both sexes tend to be equally affected by OA. However, older women are about twice as likely as men to be affected with OA of the knee and hands.[1,11,12] Women are also more likely to have the inflammatory form of OA, which involves the distal and proximal joints of the hands, giving rise to the formation of Heberden's and Bouchard's nodes.[1] In Europe, a report of a Dutch village of 6585 randomly selected individuals also confirms the increased prevalence and severity of OA by sex.[14] In women ages 65 to 70 years, 75% had OA of their distal interphalangeal joint (DIP), in contrast to less than 60% of men in that same age group (Fig. 84-1). Changes in articular cartilage from older individuals without OA differs from that observed in individuals with OA. The normal joint use throughout life has not been shown to cause degeneration in all individuals.[2] Although these data identify age as a risk factor for developing OA, age alone is not the sole cause.

Racial, ethnic, and urban–rural differences in the prevalence of OA are often difficult to establish because of the variations in sampling procedures and diagnostic criteria. OA of the knee has been reported to be twice as prevalent in black than white women.[14] Chinese, East Indian, and Native American people have a lower prevalence of hip OA than do Caucasians.[10] These differences, whether related to life-style, occupation, or genetic differences, further underscore the importance of a variety of factors that must be considered when evaluating the prevalence data.

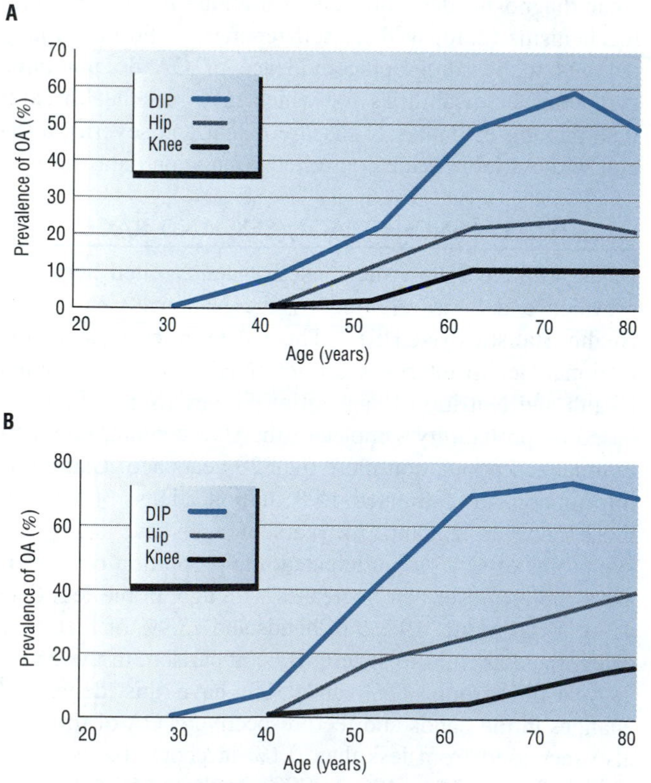

FIGURE 84–1. Prevalence of radiographic osteoarthritis of the hip, knee, and distal interphalangeal (DIP) joints. **A.** Men. **B.** Women. *(Adapted from Van Saase JL, Van Romunde LK, Cats A, et al. Epidemiology of osteoarthritis: Zoetermeer survey. Comparison of radiological osteoarthritis in a Dutch population with that in 10 other populations. Ann Rheum Dis 1989;48:271–280.)*

INCIDENCE

The overall incidence of newly diagnosed OA of the hip or knee was about 200 per 100,000 person-years in a population-based study in 1985 of 98 individuals.[16] The incidence of hip OA was greater in women than in men, while the rate for knee disease was similar in both sexes. Rates at both the knee and hip increase with age in men but plateau after menopause in women. With this population-based data, it is estimated that approximately 500,000 new symptomatic cases of idiopathic OA occur annually in the United States Caucasian population.

RISK FACTORS

OBESITY

Increased body mass has been closely associated with OA at the knee and less strongly with hip OA.[1,3,13,17,18] Historically, until the Framingham data, it was difficult to establish whether obesity preceded or even caused OA, or whether the obesity occurred as a result of the sedentary life-style in patients with OA. From this report, individuals who were in the highest quintile for body mass, at the beginning of this 36-year follow-up study, demonstrated a relative risk for developing knee OA of 1.5 for men and 2.1 for women. The relative risk for developing severe knee OA increased further to 1.9 for men and 3.2 for women. A subsequent report demonstrated that, in obese individuals, a weight loss of as little as 5 kg could further reduce the risk by up to 50% of developing symptomatic knee OA.[17]

OCCUPATION, SPORTS, AND TRAUMA

The role of repetitive use either through work or leisure activities has been implicated as a risk factor for developing OA. In certain workers who perform repetitive activities, such as dock workers, basket weavers, cotton mill workers, or jackhammer operators, a higher incidence of OA of the hand has been observed.[3,5,18,19] Likewise, a similar finding is observed in individuals engaged in activties that involve lower limbs such as road workers. In professional sports such as football, there appears to be a higher incidence in the development of lower extremity OA. However, in those individuals engaged in long-distance running the development of OA does not occur with increased frequency.[20,21] This increased occurrence of developing OA in certain types of occupations or activities is believed to be related to the repeated exposures throughout the day. Thus duration and intensity of the activity appear to play a major role. Further, trauma to the joint, loss of ligament integrity, or damage of the meniscus can lead to the development of knee OA.[5] Individuals who injure knee ligaments at a later age appear to be more likely to develop OA of the knee sooner than those at an earlier age.[3] This model of joint instability, used to study the development of OA in dogs, may also account for the higher incidence of OA in football players who have trauma-associated knee injuries.

GENETIC FACTORS

Heredity is a determinant with certain types of osteoarthritis.[3,10,18] Heberden's nodes are 10 times more prevalent in women than men, and their occurrence is about twice as likely if a woman's mother has these findings. Other types of osteoarthritis associated with genetic links include involvement of the first metatarsophalangeal joints, generalized osteoarthritis, and the recently described genetic defect in type II procollagen.[1,22,23] This discovery—of a genetic link that alters the cartilage matrix and leads to premature development of osteoarthritis—enhances understanding of the disease and may ultimately lead to screening at-risk patients and the targeting of therapeutic modalities in selected patients.

OSTEOPOROSIS

In individuals with osteoporosis, several reports have descibed an inverse relationship associated with osteoarthritis of either the knee or hip, although this remains a controversial issue.[5,18,24,25] Less dense bone in osteoporosis may be better able to distribute the load across the joint, thus slowing the development of OA. However, a confounding variable is that obesity—common in OA—is often associated with increased bone mass in almost all skeletal sites.[10,18,24,25]

PATHOPHYSIOLOGY

The major changes associated with osteoarthritis involve cartilage and the associated joint. Over the past several years, considerable interest has led to advances in the understanding of articular cartilage function and physiology. This knowledge has dispelled the wear-and-tear theory and focused attention on the dynamic changes occurring within the joint as normal functioning is sought to be maintained.[1,4,5,26–31] Thus the pathogenesis of OA involves not only the biomechanical forces but inflammatory, biochemical, and immunologic factors.

Before discussing these factors, it is useful to clinically classify OA. Generally, OA can be classified into two major categories. The categories are based on the etiology of the disease. *Primary* (idiopathic) OA occurs without any previous triggering event or known cause; this reflects the majority of cases. It can be further subclassified into localized OA, which often involves a single site such as a hip or knee, and generalized OA, which involves three or more sites. Erosive, a third category, reflects changes to the underlying bone. The *secondary* classification is based on occurrence attributed to other known abnormalities or trauma (Table 84–1).[26,32,33] This includes factors such as trauma, metabolic or endocrine disorders, and congenital factors. To assist in uniform reporting of rheumatic diseases, a classification scheme and criteria for OA of the hip, knee, and hand have been reported by the American College of Rheumatology (ACR).[34] These criteria include both subjective and objective factors such as pain, bony changes on examination, sedimentation rate, and radiographic features consistent with OA.

TABLE 84–1. Classification of Osteoarthritis

Primary (Idiopathic)	Secondary
Localized	Trauma—acute/chronic
Generalized	Underlying joint disorder
	Local (fracture/infection)
	Diffuse (rheumatoid arthritis)
Erosive	Systemic metabolic or endocrine disorders
	Wilson's disease
	Acromegaly
	Hyperparathyroidism
	Hemochromatosis
	Paget's disease
	Diabetes mellitus
	Obesity
	Crystal deposition disease
	Basic calcium phosphate crystal disease
	Calcium pyrophosphate dihydrate
	Hydroxyapatite
	Other calcium-containing crystals
	Monosodium urate monohydrate
	Neuropathic disorders
	Intra-articular corticosteroid overuse
	Avascular necrosis
	Bone dysplasia

Compiled from Refs. 26, 32, and 33.

To assist the reader in understanding the relationships and changes associated with osteoarthritis, normal cartilage function, biochemistry, and mechanics of a diarthroidal joint are reviewed. Several excellent and more detailed discussions of cartilage and bone biochemistry and function can be found elsewhere.[4,5,26,30,31]

NORMAL CARTILAGE

FUNCTION

In the free-moving diarthrodial joint (Fig. 84–2), cartilage provides a low-friction surface covering the concave and convex ends of the bone. Its major features are to (1) provide for movement within the required range of motion; (2) distribute load across the joint tissues, thereby preventing damage; and (3) promote stability during use. It is avascular, aneural, and alymphatic with a calcified base covering a thin layer of cortical bone known as the subchondral plate. Because of its frictionless surface, cartilage provides a smooth gliding surface during movement of the joint and serves as a shock absorber or load support. Upon compression from weight loading, it is easily deformed; up to 40% of its height can be compressed. As a result, when a load is applied, cartilage can provide a large contact area and disperse this force more uniformly to the underlying

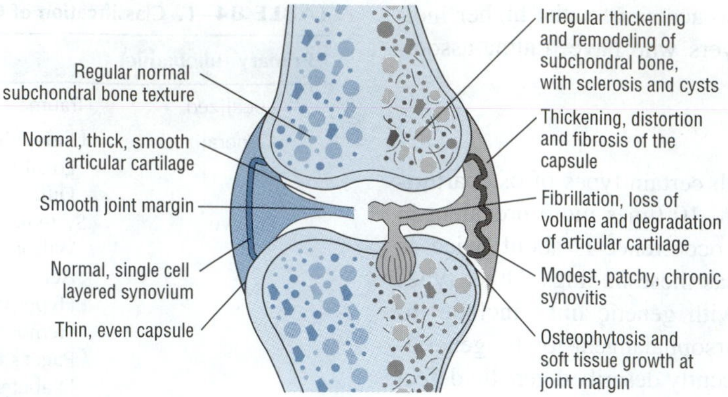

FIGURE 84–2. Characteristics of osteoarthritis in the diarthrodial joint (right).

bone. Despite these characteristics, cartilage is relatively thin (2 to 5 mm thick), so that loading energy is not taken up there but actually transmitted directly to the bone. Therefore, the greatest share of loading energy is taken up within the tendons, ligaments, and surrounding muscles of that joint.

STRUCTURE AND BIOCHEMICAL COMPOSITION OF CARTILAGE

Histologically, articular cartilage is a hydrated (75% to 80% water by weight) extensive extracellular matrix (ECM) comprising a small number of chondrocytes (<5%). The remainder (20% to 25%) of the cartilage matrix consists of three classes of molecules: collagens, large aggregates of proteoglycans or aggrecans, and noncollagenous proteins. Cartilage can be divided into four zones: a superficial or tangential zone, an intermediate or transitional zone, the deep or radial zone, and the calcified cartilage zone located below the tidemark and above the subchondral bone. These zones typically reflect the changes between composition of chondrocytes, distribution of collagen, and heterogeneity of

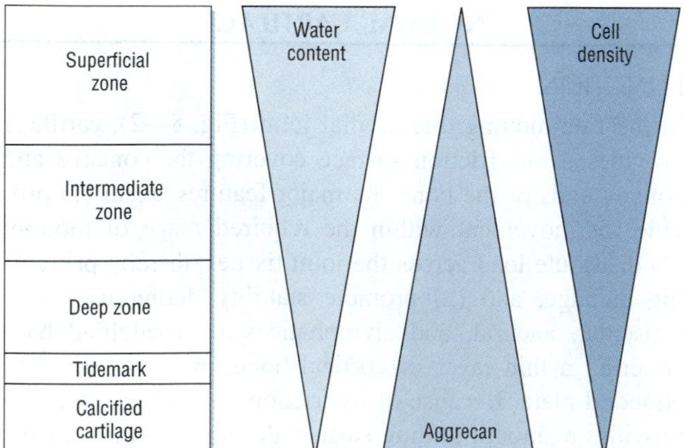

FIGURE 84–3. Structure and composition of articular cartilage by zone. *(Adapted from Ref. 4, 5.)*

proteoglycan components in the cartilage matrix (Fig. 84–3). At the basal zone, the type II collagen fibers are perpendicular and serve to anchor cartilage to the subchondral bone. At the superficial zone, these collagen fibers are densely packed and are parallel to the the surface.

Chondrocytes

Cartilage is not the simple inert tissue that it appears. Instead it is metabolically active tissue that undergoes a continual internal remodeling of the ECM. The control of this process rests with the chondrocytes, which control the synthesis and degradation of this matrix by affecting the production of collagen and proteoglycans. Because adult articular cartilage is avascular, the chondrocytes must receive their nutrition from the synovial fluid. With the cyclic movement and loading of joints, nutrients flow into the cartilage, while immobilization reduces nutrient supply.

Considerable interest has developed in the role peptide growth factors play in regulating chondrocyte function.[4,5,29] Some of these growth factors—such as low concentrations of insulin-like growth factor, epidermal growth factor, or fibroblast growth factor—cause an enhanced proliferation of chondrocytes and synthesis of proteoglycans. At the same time, the cytokines such as interleukin-1 (IL-1) and tumor necrosis factor (TNF-α) have been shown to induce chondrocytes to release major matrix metalloproteinases (MMP) such as collagenase (MMP-1) and stromelysin (MMP-2), which have the ability to degrade most if not all of the matrix proteins. These cytokines also have the ability to suppress the synthesis of proteoglycans and collagen within the ECM.[4,5,29]

This role of growth factors has raised considerable interest in how these factors may ultimately interact to regulate chondrocyte function and enhance articular cartilage repair. Despite enthusiasm in reviewing these effects, it is important to use caution in applying findings from one type of tissue to another, extrapolating *in vitro* to *in vivo* data, and developing therapeutic agents that may affect a particular factor. Because the actions of growth factors and cytokines have multiple complex roles in the regulation of articular cartilage, they should be viewed more as messengers, effectors, or signaling agents.[5,26,29]

The role of biomechanical factors such as defined loads and strains also appears to affect how chondrocytes alter the production of proteoglycans. In some studies, joint loading has markedly improved the production of proteoglycans.[5] Therefore, this area of biochemical and biomechanical study appears to hold considerable promise for improving our understanding about osteoarthritis.

Collagen

Of the approximately 14 distinct types of collagen, five types (II, IX, X, XI, and VI) are primarily located in cartilage. The most predominant type (about 90% to 95%) of collagen found in articular cartilage is type II.[4,5,26] The other types of collagen are found in reduced amounts. Type VI appears to form a link between the chondrocytes and their attachment to the matrix. It does appear that type IX may play a role in linking to other matrix molecules; interestingly, this molecule is also a proteoglycan. The network of type II collagen fibrils and their cross-linking among collagen molecules and other ECM proteins provides the tensile strength and maintenance of the tissue's volume and shape. This is accomplished by the ordering of the collagen fibers. Near the surface, the fibers remain in a direction parallel to the surface, thereby providing the ability to dissipate forces. In contrast, collagen fibers located near the basal layer are perpendicular to the surface. This allows the collagen fibers to assume a role in anchoring of the uncalcified cartilage to the calcified zone or subchondral bony endplate.

Proteoglycans

The large aggregates of proteoglycans (PGs) provide the "stuffing material" for the matrix. The proteoglycans consist of a protein core and at least one or more glycosaminoglycan chains. The glycosaminoglycans (GAGs) include chondroitin sulfate, keratan sulfate, and dermatan sulfate. By covalently binding to the protein core, these molecules form a proteoglycan subunit. The subunits then combine with long hyaluronate molecules to form aggregates. The aggregates retain and maintain the water content of the cartilage because of their highly hydrophilic and anionic properties. These characteristics give cartilage its resilience and load-bearing properties.

Under pressure, these compounds release water and enhance solute flux and chondrocyte nutrition; then, on removal of pressure, the compounds regain their water content. It is also this property that renders the PG molecular structure vulnerable to degradation by the matrix metalloproteases; cleavage of only one or two peptide bonds can totally alter the properties of this molecule. Thus PG turnover occurs at a faster rate than does collagen turnover. When protease degradation of proteoglycans has been experimentally induced, cartilage has maintained its shape but lost its elastic properties.[4,5]

With the degradation of the ECM there is a release of collagen and proteoglycan fragments into the synovial fluid. This liberation of contents eventually reaches the blood and urine. Various experimental assays have been created to identify and measure these compounds to assist with diagnosis or as monitoring tools. Although experimental, these tools provide additional approaches to aid understanding of the metabolic changes within the joint.

OSTEOARTHRITIC CARTILAGE

BIOCHEMICAL CHANGES

Several changes have been reported in the composition of osteoarthritic cartilage (Table 84–2). An initial biochemical change in cartilage appears to be an increase in water content of the cartilage matrix despite a reduction in the hydrophilic proteoglycans. This initial change results in a thickened articular cartilage but one less able to withstand mechanical forces. Although the reason for this change is not clearly understood, it may relate to damage of the collagen fiber network, which is no longer able to restrain the PGs. This allows the molecules to increase hydration and expand.[4,5,26] The decrease in proteoglycan content appears to correlate with the severity of the disease and may relate to the release of the many matrix metalloproteases.

Soon after these changes in water content occur, the GAG composition changes, reflecting changes in keratan sulfate and the ratio of chondroitin 4-sulfate to chondroitin 6-sulfate. These changes may result in decreased PG–collagen interaction in the cartilage. The collagen content does not appear to change until severe disease is present. Increases in collagen synthesis and in the distribution and diameter of the fibers have been noted.[4,5,26]

Originally, researchers believed that cartilage passively eroded away. However, cellular activity actually increases, suggesting that the articular cartilage is responding with a reparative process.[4,5,25] This increase in activity appears to continue only until the disease is advanced and may suggest a possible failure of the chondrocytes.

Despite the increase in matrix synthesis controlled by the chondrocytes, there continues to be a loss of proteoglycan and an increase in water content. This implies that degradation is proceeding faster than synthesis. Further, an

TABLE 84–2. Changes in Osteoarthritic Cartilage

Increase in water content
Increase in chondroitin sulfate-4 to chondroitin sulfate-6 ratio
Increase in proteases, especially neutral metalloproteinases
Decrease in glycosaminoglycans—chondroitin sulfate and keratan sulfate
Decrease in proteoglycan aggregation
Decrease in proteoglycan monomer size
Minimal change in collagen content

Compiled from Refs. 4, 5, and 26.

increase in enzymes such as matrix metalloproteinases and collagenolytic enzymes directed toward collagen appears in the osteoarthritic cartilage. The action of the MMPs are normally inhibited by tissue inhibitors of the metalloproteinases (TIMPs). When the concentration or effectiveness of these inhibitors occur, the imbalance causes the proteolysis of the ECM, promoting osteoarthritic changes.

In summary, the slow progressive changes in osteoarthritis consist of an increase in water content, loss of PG, and reduction of PG aggregates of cartilage. The net result is the failure of the cartilage to repair itself. An overview of the evolution of osteoarthritis and the interactions of the multiple complex factors or mechanisms is shown in Fig. 84–4. The series of pathologic changes results in loss of cartilage, eburnation of bone, and, ultimately, severe pain.

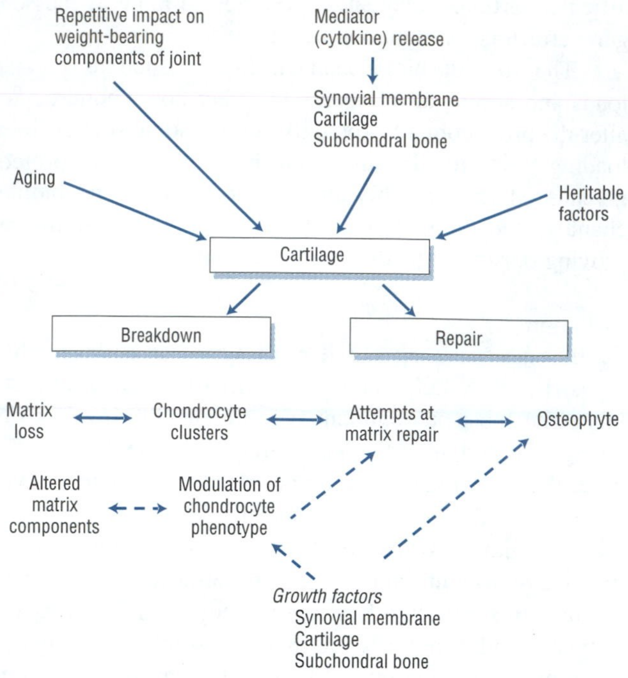

FIGURE 84–4. Factors contributing to the evolution of osteoarthritis. *(From Hamerman D. The biology of osteoarthritis. N Engl J Med 1989;320: 1322–1330, with permission.)*

PATHOLOGIC CHANGES

Coexistent with the biochemical changes are a series of pathologic changes in the cartilage and bone. Although the early pathologic changes are not well defined in humans, the intermediate- and late-stage changes in osteoarthritis are well characterized. To address the early changes, two animal models, the canine cruciate-deficient and the rabbit meniscectomy models, have provided useful information. Further, changes are similar for weight-bearing and non-weight-bearing joints and for idiopathic OA and secondary osteoarthritis. Specifically, the following changes are observed in cartilage:

1. An initial thickening of the articular cartilage. This reflects the damage to the ECM at the molecular level and an increase of water content.
2. Proliferation of chondrocytes in response to tissue damage or alterations in ECM structure. An increase in the anabolic and catabolic activity occurs within the ECM.
3. Decline in response of chrondrocytes to stabilize or restore tissue. This results in progressive loss of articular cartilage.
4. Joint synovial lining may show moderate degrees of inflammation.
5. Fibrillation, a splitting of the noncalcified cartilage, believed to be related to the biochemical changes described earlier. This exposes the underlying bone, which may ultimately lead to microfractures of the subchondral bone.[4,5,26,30,31]

As destruction of the cartilage progresses, pathologic changes in subchondral bone occur. The appearance varies considerably depending on the site of cartilage loss; areas lacking the protective layer of cartilage demonstrate the most change. The superficial portion of subchondral bone contains necrotic osteocytes. Increased osteoblastic and osteoclastic activity with osteolytic foci or cysts is observed below the superficial layer. The exposed area of bone may contain fibrous or chondroid tissue, presumably reflecting reactive bone resorption and vascular changes. With continued progression, the cartilaginous layer is completely eroded, leaving denuded subchondral bone that becomes dense, smooth, and glistening (eburnation). This alters the physical properties of the bone and results in a brittle, stiffer bone less able to resist the stress of bearing weight.[4,5,26,30,31] The subchondral bone then develops sclerosis and microfractures. Microfractures result in the production of callus and increased amounts of osteoid. New bone formation at the joint margins, away from the area of cartilage destruction, is referred to as *osteophytes.* An interesting observation is that osteophytes can occur in the absence of cartilage destruction and, conversely, cartilage destruction can occur in the absence of osteophytes. Osteophytes may be an attempt to stabilize the joints and may not be part of the destructive aspects of osteoarthritis.

The joint capsule and synovium also show a variety of pathologic changes secondary to OA. Inflammation, such as synovitis, is seen and may result from the release of inflammatory mediators such as prostaglandins secreted by the chondrocytes.[4,5,26,29] Again, the inflammation is localized to the affected joint in contrast to rheumatoid or other inflammatory arthridities.

SIGNS AND SYMPTOMS

The clinical presentation (Table 84–3) depends on the duration of disease, joints affected, and severity of joint in-

TABLE 84–3. Clinical Presentation of Osteoarthritis

Age	
Usually elderly	
Sex	
Age <45 more common in men	
Age >45 more common in women (hands)	
Symptoms	
Pain	
Deep, aching	
Pain on motion	
Early in disease—pain with use	
Late in disease—pain at rest	
Stiffness	
Rarely exceeds 15 min; related to weather	
Localized to involved joints	
Limited joint motion	
Instability of weight-bearing joints	
Crepitus, crackling	
Signs/Physical Examination	
Monoarticular or oligoarticular; asymmetrical involvement	
Joints frequently involved	
Hands—DIP, PIP, first carpometacarpal joint	
Foot—first metatarsophalangeal joint	
Hips, knees, cervical spine, lumbar spine	
Observations on Joint Examination	
Bony proliferation or occasional synovitis	
Local tenderness	
Crepitus	
Muscle atrophy	
Limited motion with passive/active movement	
Effusions	
Characteristics of Synovial Fluid	
High viscocity	
Mild leukocytosis (<2000 WBC/mm^3)	
Laboratory Values	
No specific test	
ESR, hematologic survey, chemistry survey are normal	
No systemic manifestations	

DIP = distal interphalangeal; PIP = proximal interphalangeal; ESR = erythrocyte sedimentation rate.
Compiled from Refs. 6, 18, 29, and 32.

volvement. The predominant symptom is a localized deep, aching pain associated with the affected joint. If more than one joint is involved or if systemic symptoms are present, another form of arthritis or connective tissue disease should be considered. However, many patients with documented OA (either pathologically or radiographically) remain asymptomatic.

Early in the course of the disease, pain occurs when the joint is first used and becomes relieved by rest or removal of weight from the affected joint. Later, the pain occurs with minimal motion or activity and may be present even during rest. The pain is not related to the destruction of cartilage, because cartilage is aneural. Rather, the pain arises from the activation of nociceptive nerve endings by the mechanical and chemical irritants related to joint pathology.[35] Pain caused by a bursitis, tendinitis, or muscular pain may also confuse the patient's presentation and require an accurate diagnosis. Weather or changes in the barometric pressure also seem to aggravate the pain associated with OA.

The joints most commonly affected in primary OA are the distal and proximal interphalangeal (DIP and PIP) joints of the hand, the first carpometacarpal (CMC) joint, knees, hips, cervical and lumbar spine, and the first metatarsophalangeal (MTP) joint of the toe. In addition to pain in the affected joint, limitation of motion, stiffness, crepitus, and deformities may be present. The limitation of motion that develops as the disease progresses is related to the loss of articular surfaces, muscle spasms, capsular contracture, and mechanical blockage secondary to osteophytosis. Patients may also notice a decreased range of motion (ROM) of an affected joint by describing limitations in performing normal activities of daily living (ADLs). A sense of weakness or instability (described by patients as the joint "gives way") is yet another feature observed in patients with lower extremity involvement.

Joint stiffness is often another complaint expressed by patients with OA. The joint stiffness is of a relatively short duration, unlike that described by patients with rheumatoid arthritis. Most important, the stiffness lasts less than 30 minutes and often occurs after sitting or resting for some time. However, after movement it seems to resolve, leading some to describe this as a "gelling phenomenon." Crepitation, or the crackling-grating sound heard as the joint moves, is related to irregularity of the joint surface and loss of cartilage. Joint enlargement is typically related to bony proliferation or in some cases thickening of the synovium and joint capsule. The presence of a warm, red, tender joint may suggest an inflammatory type of synovitis.

Joint deformity may be present in the later stages of OA and is the result of subluxation, collapse of subchondral bone, formation of bone cysts, or bony overgrowths. Patient descriptions of joint swelling require close clinical inspection to separate synovial thickening (inflammation) from the bony proliferation observed in OA.

PHYSICAL EXAMINATION

Physical examination of the affected joint or joints reveals pain, tenderness, crepitus, and possible joint enlargement.[18,32,34] The specific findings reported on physical examination of the commonly affected joints in OA in contrast to RA are shown in Fig. 83–3.

HANDS

Hand involvement in OA primarily involves the DIP, PIP, and first carpometacarpal joints. Heberden's and Bouchard's nodes are bony enlargements (osteophytes) of the DIP and PIP joints, respectively. Heberden's nodes usually develop slowly, are nonpainful, occur on both lateral and medial aspects of the joint, and are approximately 10 times more common in women than men.[18,32,34] Occasionally, these nodes become red, warm, swollen, and painful, usually as a result of trauma or use. As discussed earlier on the genetic association, a strong female hereditary predominance is demonstrated on questioning of the patient concerning whether they recall their mother having bony-appearing digits.

In patients with first carpometacarpal joint involvement, pain and tenderness are common. The increase in osteophytosis gives the radial aspect of the hand the characteristic square appearance termed the *shelf sign.* Difficulty pinching and opening the tops of bottles or jars is a frequent complaint.

KNEES

The knee is one of the most commonly affected joints. It is important to localize the symptoms because the joint has three separate articulations: the patellofemoral, medial, and lateral compartments. Pain related to climbing stairs is typically associated with patellofemoral joint involvement. Presentation with a bowlegged deformity (genu varum or varus deformity) is caused by medial compartment involvement; knock-knee deformity (genu valgum or valgus deformity) results from lateral compartment involvement. The symptoms include pain, tenderness, crepitation, limited extension with passive or active motion, and joint instability. These symptoms may cause the patient to limit the use of this joint, thereby causing muscle atrophy. Transient joint effusions may also occur. The synovial fluid is typically noninflammatory (white blood cell [WBC] count <2000/mm^3 with normal protein).

HIPS

The symptoms of OA of the hip frequently appear in older individuals and can be described by the three patterns of hip joint involvement: superolateral, medial pole, and concentric. Hip osteoarthritis is associated with buttock or groin pain exacerbated when the patient is bearing weight, standing up, or walking. Pain located on the outside of the hip is typically bursitis and should not be confused with hip disease. Stiffness is common, especially after inactivity, and joint motion may be limited.

SPINE

Degenerative changes result from involvement of the intervertebral disks, vertebral bodies, or posterior apophyseal articulations. In the lumbar spine area, L3-4 involvement is most common. The resulting nerve root compression can cause pain, paresthesias, loss of reflexes, and muscle weakness in the distribution of the affected nerve root.

FEET AND OTHER JOINTS

The involvement in the feet is limited primarily to the first metatarsophalangeal joint. Pain, tenderness, and stiffness are the predominant symptoms.

Other joints not commonly involved include the shoulder, elbow, acromioclavicular, sternoclavicular, and temporomandibular joint.

LABORATORY FINDINGS

No specific clinical laboratory abnormalities occur in *primary* OA.[18,32,34] Erythrocyte sedimentation rate (ESR), routine chemistry studies, complete hematologic surveys, and urinalysis are generally normal. However, the ESR may be slightly elevated in patients with generalized or erosive inflammatory OA. The rheumatoid factor test is negative. Analysis of the synovial fluid reveals fluid with high viscosity. This fluid demonstrates a mild leukocytosis (<2000 WBC/mm^3) with predominantly mononuclear cells. In the case of secondary osteoarthritis associated with an underlying metabolic disorder or endocrinopathy, specific laboratory tests are indicated to identify the cause.

RADIOLOGIC EVALUATION

Radiologic evaluation is an absolute necessity in the diagnosis of OA.[18,32,34] In early, mild OA, radiographic changes may be normal. With the progression of degenerative changes in cartilage, the joint space may begin to narrow, subchondral bony sclerosis occurs, and marginal osteophyte and cyst formation may develop. Late in the disease process, subluxation and deformity sometimes occur. In general, osteoporosis and joint erosions are not seen, but they do occur in a subset of patients with erosive OA. A variety of published radiographic grading scale criteria are available for use in the clinical outcome assessment of various clinical trials; however, there is considerable need to standardize the evaluative process to ensure repoducibility of the measurements.[34,35]

Technetium-99m bone imaging has also been used to demonstrate the appearance of OA and may actually precede the development seen on plain radiographs of the affected joint. Specifically, weight-bearing radiographs at the knee provide better definition of the joint space. Newer imaging techniques such as computed tomography (CT) scans and magnetic resonance imaging (MRI) or ultrasonographic techniques are also used, but often provide limited useful information during the routine examination of OA joints.[18,26,29,32,34,35] Joint arthroscopic examination can also confirm the diagnosis or extent of OA present in a particular joint; however, few clinical situations require this procedure to establish a diagnosis of OA.

DIAGNOSIS

The diagnosis of osteoarthritis is strongly dependent on an evaluation of the patient's history, clinical examination of the affected joint(s), and radiologic findings. The major diagnostic goals are to (1) distinguish patients with OA from other connective tissue diseases that may exhibit DIP joint involvement, such as psoriatic arthritis or Reiter's syndrome (see Chap. 83); and (2) identify patients with the secondary form of OA. Although the diagnosis is relatively straightforward, a complete examination of all clinical information is required, and not until all clinical data are evaluated can an accurate diagnosis be made. The American College of Rheumatology (ACR) has published algorithms for the classification of patients with OA of the hands, knees, and hips.[34] These criteria serve as useful guidelines for evaluating patients in clinical practice and assessing outcomes in those involved in clinical trials.

PROGNOSIS

The prognosis for patients with primary OA is variable and depends on the joint involved. If a weight-bearing joint or the spine is involved, considerable morbidity and disability are possible. In the case of secondary OA, the prognosis depends on the underlying cause of osteoarthritis. Presently, treatment of the cause may prevent further progression but does not reverse joint changes already present.

▶ TREATMENT: Osteoarthritis

DESIRED OUTCOME

Successful therapeutic management of the patient with OA depends on accurate diagnosis of the degree and extent of joint involvement. Because many patients are commonly asymptomatic, radiologic diagnosis and clinical examination and history are paramount. Further, the optimal treatment approach must be individualized to include, as appropriate, physical therapy, occupational therapy, dietary considerations, drug therapy, surgery, and patient education. The major goals are to (1) educate the patient, caregivers, and relatives; (2) relieve symptoms such as pain and stiffness; (3) preserve the joint motion and function by limiting disease progression; and (4) minimize the disability.

GENERAL APPROACH TO TREATMENT

The major treatment strategies are highly patient specific (Fig. 84–5). They are based on the distribution and severity of joint involvement as well as the presence or absence of other comorbid disease states, concomitant medications, or allergies. In general, the foundation of all treatment approaches consists of nonpharmacologic approaches, which include patient education, physical and occupational therapy, weight loss, and assistive devices. At the same time, pharmacologic approaches aimed at pain relief, as opposed to treating inflammation as in rheumatoid arthritis, are instituted. At present, no drugs are approved to reverse the structural or biochemical abnormalities of OA. The medications used to provide pain relief should begin with trials of a simple analgesic, acetaminophen (up to 4 g/d), followed by low-dose NSAIDs, unless significant joint inflammation is present. Opioid analgesics are usually avoided for long-term use; however, short-term intermittent use may be considered for those patients when treating acute exacerbations of joint pain. For localized joints, symptomatic pain relief may be supplemented with the use of topical analgesic creams such as capsaicin cream. For knee effusions, aspiration of the joint and injection with steroids may provide some relief. In general this approach must be used cautiously because of the risk for infection and possibility of progressive cartilage destruction when repeated injections (3 or 4 times per year) are given.[9] Recently approved intra-articular (IA) injections of hyaluronate may provide limited and temporary relief for some patients, and may serve as approach to consider prior to surgery. However, when patients have inadequate symptom control despite the measures outlined here, or they have functional joint impairment, referral for an orthopedic surgical procedure is indicated. Lastly, for patients interested in participating in clinical trials, investigational strategies involving oral doxycycline, major metal metalloprotease inhibitors (MMPIs), intramuscular injection of pentosan polysulfate and polysulfated glycosaminoglycans, or cartilage transplants may be considered as options.

NONPHARMACOLOGIC THERAPY

An effective management plan requires more than drug therapy. The first step is to educate the patient about the extent, degree of involvement, prognosis, and management approach. OA is often thought of by both the public and some within the medical community as a "wear-and-tear" disease. Patients often will accept that belief, and attribute symptoms to just "one of those things" associated with getting older and therefore not seek medical care.

To relieve their symptoms, patients may resort to the use of various alternative medications or arthritis-quackery schemes. Patients should be warned about these and encouraged to access several excellent sources of patient information on osteoarthritis available from the local or national units of the Arthritis Foundation (Atlanta, Georgia) or via the Internet at http://www.arthritis.org. Specifically, the Arthritis Foundation provides literature about the disease and information about clinics and other local agencies offering physical and economic assistance and information about the various medications. The Arthritis Foundation also sponsors various support groups and public education programs.

In addition, contact between OA patients and trained lay personnel to review self-care status has demonstrated a beneficial effect in reducing pain and improving physical function in individuals at high risk of morbidity.[36–38] This approach again highlights the importance of personal contact and interventions as a way to positively influence patient outcomes.

DIET

For the overweight patient, dietary counseling is an important recommendation. The excess weight can contribute not only to the progression of the disease but also to the contraction of the muscles that span and stabilize the joint. Further, obese patients scheduled to undergo total joint replacement of the hips or knees generally have a poorer surgical outcome and postoperative prognosis than patients of normal weight. Weight reduction requires a motivated patient and participation in a supervised program.

Recently, there has been considerable interest in dietary supplements that contain glucosamine, a basic constituent of cartilage glycosaminoglycans.[39,40] With publication in the lay press and discussions on television shows, patients have sought this therapy. Glucosamine stimulates cartilage cells to synthesize, at least *in vitro,* glycosaminoglycans and proteoglycans. Several short-term trials in humans have demonstrated benefits

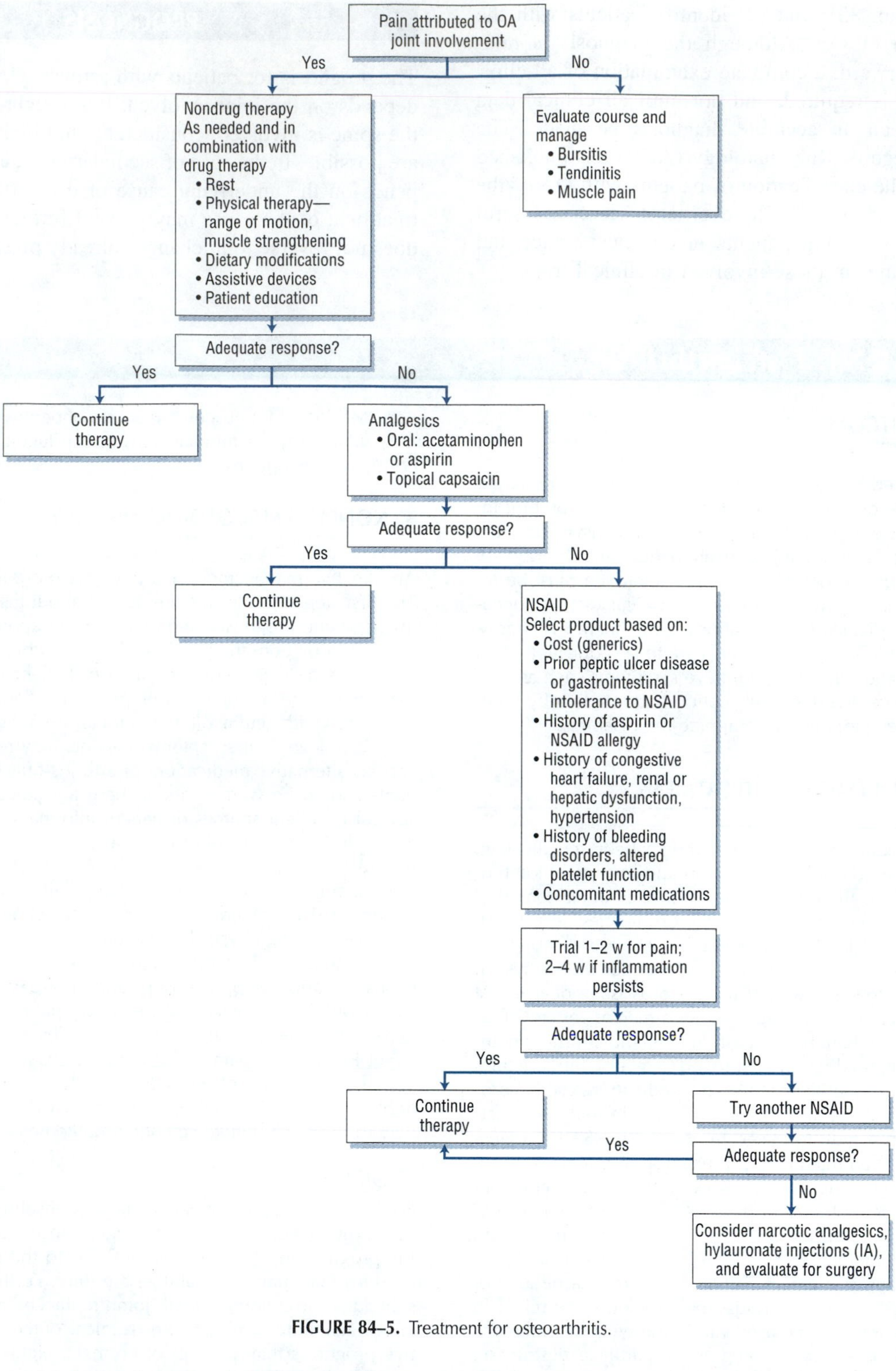

FIGURE 84–5. Treatment for osteoarthritis.

in relieving symptoms when administered as 500 mg tid PO therapy in comparison to NSAIDs in low doses. However, most of these trials have been of a limited nature and lack long-term outcome clinical or radiologic assessment. In general, commercial products may be combined with chondroitin sulfate, another cartilage constituent that plays a role in cartilage repair and prevention of further breakdown. The products appear well tolerated, but as a "dietary supplement" neither the products nor their purity are approved by the FDA. The use of these compounds in patients is of questionable value. However, if they are effective, a benefit should be observed within 4 to 8 weeks.

PHYSICAL AND OCCUPATIONAL THERAPY

Physical therapy—with heat or cold treatments and an exercise program—helps to maintain and regain joint range of motion, relieve pain, and reduce muscle spasms. Such simple measures as a warm bath or warm water soaks may be effective in reducing pain and diminishing stiffness. With heat application, patients should be cautioned to avoid lying on the heat source for longer than 30 minutes to minimize the risk of burns. Other heat-application techniques consist of diathermy or ultrasound to the affected joints (but not in patients with artificial metal joints because the potential for deep thermal burns exists). These techniques are reserved primarily for deep-seated joints (hips/spine) and are more costly than simpler forms of heat application. Transcutaneous electrical nerve stimulation (TENS), the transmission of an electrical current from the skin to a peripheral nerve, may provide some pain relief primarily for acute pain; however, it is cumbersome and expensive.[34,36]

Exercise programs using isometric techniques are designed to strengthen the muscles and improve joint function and motion.[41] The program should favor isometric over isotonic exercises because the latter can aggravate the affected joint. Typical exercises for knee involvement consist of quadriceps-setting exercises and straight leg raises designed to strengthen knee and leg muscles. Each exercise should be taught and then observed before the patient is allowed to exercise at home. The exercises should be performed three to four times daily. If severe pain develops during exercise, the patient should be instructed to decrease the number of exercises.

Supervised fitness walking has also been shown to improve a patient's functional status and should be encouraged in selected patients.[38] To assist with walking, various assistive devices—including splints, canes, walkers, and braces—can be used during exercise or daily activities. These devices should be carefully selected to meet each patient's functional abilities and limitations. Patients should then be carefully instructed and their understanding evaluated on the use of the various devices. Other orthotic devices such as heel cups or insoles may also be tried to help relieve pain and improve a patient's ability to walk.

SURGERY

Surgical procedures are indicated for patients with severe disease or with substantial pain or marked functional disabilities and in whom conservative therapy has not been effective.[41,42] Often the main indication for surgery in OA is pain of the degree and extent that it hinders a patient's life-style. For patients with mild disease of the knee, an osteotomy will correct the malalignment seen with genu varum or genu valgum. Joint debridement may also be indicated to remove free cartilage fragments, eliminate locking, and reduce pain. If osteophytes are large, removal may be attempted to increase joint range of motion. For severe, advanced disease a partial or total arthroplasty is performed primarily to relieve pain, although improvement of motion is also possible. The increased motion occurs more commonly with hip than with knee joint replacements. An arthrodesis or joint fusion can also be performed to reduce the pain associated with degenerative changes, but it will restrict motion of that joint. Restorative approaches to articular cartilage involve soft-tissue grafts, penetration of subchondral bone, cell transplantation, and use of growth factors or use of artificial matrices.[5,29,43,44] The cartilage that is formed does not appear to duplicate normal articular cartilage in its composition, structure, or mechanical properties. These approaches are all investigational and have shown varying degrees of success at decreasing symptoms and improving joint function.

PHARMACOLOGIC THERAPY

Drug therapy in OA is directed at the symptomatic relief of pain and inflammation when present. Because OA is a disease often occurring in an older individual who may also have other preexisting medical conditions, a conservative approach to the use of medications is warranted (Fig. 84–5). This does not imply that patients should not use medications for pain relief, but that the regimen of choice requires a very individualistic approach. Some patients with mild symptoms may require simple topical or oral analgesics; those receiving no relief from the analgesics or those with signs of active inflammation may benefit from the use of an anti-inflammatory medication.

ANALGESICS

The pain in OA is not related to the degenerating cartilage because cartilage is aneural. Rather, pain occurs primarily at three local sites: synovium, soft tissue around the joint, and bone.[32,36] The major oral analgesic of choice is acetaminophen in doses of 325 to 650 mg four times daily; maximum dose of 4 g/d. Aspirin may also be considered, but its use has largely been replaced by the nonaspirin-containing NSAIDs. However, the discussion here is aimed at providing some fundamental concepts relating to the broad use of aspirin in inflammatory arthritis. If aspirin is used, a dose of greater than 3.6 g/d is needed to achieve anti-inflammatory activity. The zero-order kinetics of anti-inflammatory doses of aspirin may warrant the monitoring of serum salicylate concentrations for efficacy or toxicity, especially when anti-inflammatory doses are being administered or if toxicity is suspected. The use of serum salicylate levels is not routine in the treatment of OA. The serum half-life of salicylates ranges from 2 hours for analgesic doses to more than 20 hours for anti-imflammatory doses. Serum concentrations should be measured after five half-lives. Therapeutic salicylate concentrations are between 15 and 25 mg/dL, while plasma levels greater than 30 mg/dL generally correlate with the onset of tinnitus, except in children or in the elderly patient with preexisting hearing loss.

Aspirin is also highly protein bound; increasing doses result in an increase in the apparent volume of distribution as protein-binding site saturation occurs. Low albumin concentrations, increasing age, and highly protein-bound drugs can increase the toxic effects from salicylates. Urinary pH changes can affect the excretion of salicylates several-fold, because an alkaline urine increases the excretion of salicylates. In the choice of a particular aspirin product, several factors related to toxicity should be considered; a large variety of acetylated and nonacetylated salicylate products exist (Table 84–4).

First, salicylates can cause adverse gastrointestinal effects ranging from mild discomfort to gastric ulcers.[45,46] To minimize these effects, the salicylates should be taken with food or milk. Also, enteric-coated products cause less gastric mucosal injury compared with buffered or plain aspirin.[46] However, caution should be used if the enteric products are taken with antacids or milk because the coating can be altered, resulting in an increase in abdominal symptoms in susceptible individuals. The nonacetylated salicylate products also produce less gastrointestinal irritation and bleeding than plain aspirin.[47,48]

Second, the decreased platelet aggregation observed with aspirin is not seen with the nonacetylated salicylate products.[47,48] These nonacetylated salicylates are a safer alternative in the patient with a bleeding disorder or in those patients scheduled to undergo a surgical procedure. Third, a clinically important syndrome of aspirin intolerance exists in some patients.[49] Administration of aspirin can result in two kinds of reactions: type A, with bronchoconstriction, vasomotor rhinitis, and nasal polyps or laryngeal edema; and type B, with urticaria and angioedema. Type A occurs in 2% to 4% of asthmatics with cross-sensitivity to other nonsteroidal anti-inflammatory drugs (although a nonacetylated salicylate may be tolerated).

Type B reactions generally occur with other salicylates.[49] Other toxic responses to aspirin products include impaired renal function and increases in serum transaminases. Another factor to consider in selection of a product is cost. Nonacetylated products are considerably more expensive than plain aspirin.

TABLE 84–4. Medications Commonly Used in Treatment of Osteoarthritis

Medication	Dosage and Frequency	Maximum Dosage (mg/d)
Oral Analgesics		
Acetaminophen	325–650 mg every 4–6 h or 1 g 3 or 4 times per day	4000
Tramadol	50–100 mg every 4–6 h	400
Topical Analgesic		
Capsaicin 0.025% or 0.075%	Apply to affected joint 3 or 4 times per day	—
Nonsteroidal Anti-inflammatory Drugs (NSAIDs)		
Carboxylic acids		
Acetylated salicylates		
Aspirin, plain, buffered, or enteric coated	325–650 mg every 4–6 h pain. Anti-inflammatory doses start at 3600 mg/d in divided doses	3600[a]
Nonacetylated salicylates		
Salsalate	500–1000 mg 2 or 3 times per day	3000[a]
Diflunisal	500–1000 mg 2 times per day	2000
Choline salicylate[b]	500–1000 mg 2 or 3 times per day	3000[a]
Choline magnesium salicylate	500–1000 mg 2 or 3 times per day	3000[a]
Acetic acids		
Etodolac	800–1200 mg/d in divided doses	1200
Diclofenac	100–150 mg/d in divided doses	200
Indomethacin	25 mg 2–3 times a day; 75 mg SR once daily	200; 150
Ketorolac[c]	10 mg every 4–6 h	40
Nabumetone[d]	500–1000 mg 1 or 2 times a day	2000
Propionic acids		
Fenoprofen	300–600 mg 3 or 4 times per day	3200
Flurbiprofen	200–300 mg/d in 2–4 divided doses	300
Ibuprofen	1200–3200 mg/d in 3 or 4 divided doses	3200
Ketoprofen	150–300 mg/d in 3 or 4 divided doses	300
Naproxen	250–500 mg twice per day	1500
Naproxen sodium	275–550 mg twice per day	1375
Oxaprozin	1200 mg/d	1800
Fenamates		
Meclofenamate	200–400 mg/d in 3 or 4 divided doses	400
Mefenamic acid[e]	250 mg every 6 h	1000
Pyrazoles		
Phenylbutazone[f]	100–200 mg twice per day	400
Oxicams		
Piroxicam	20 mg/d	20

[a]Monitor serum salicylate levels over 3–3.6 g/d.
[b]Only available as a liquid; 870 mg salicylate/5 mL.
[c]Not approved for treatment of OA for more than 5 days.
[d]Nonorganic acid but metabolite is an acetic acid.
[e]Not approved for treatment of OA.
[f]Not to exceed 1 week in patients greater than 60 years old.

For patients who need only analgesic therapy, acetaminophen 650 mg four times daily provides analgesia comparable with that provided by aspirin 650 mg four times daily without the associated gastrointestinal toxicity of aspirin. The lack of anti-inflammatory properties of acetaminophen limits its usefulness in patients with evidence of inflammation. However, several recent reports have demonstrated the comparable efficacy of acetaminophen (2.6 to 4 g/d) to either ibuprofen at doses of 1200 or 2400 mg/d or naproxen 750 mg/d in relieving the pain symptoms associated with OA of the knee.[50–52] This has lead some clinicians as well as practice guidelines by the ACR, to recommend the use of acetaminophen in doses less than 4 g/d as first-line therapy for the short-term symptomatic relief of OA pain.[4,8,9,33,52]

Generally, acetaminophen is well tolerated by patients, but when taken in excess, for prolonged periods of time, or by at-risk populations, hepatic and renal toxicity has been reported.[53–55] The National Kidney Foundation has issued guidelines on the use of analgesics based on concerns related to the renal toxicity of simple analgesics like aspirin or acetaminophen and the nonsteroidal anti-inflammatory drugs. In their recommendations, acetaminophen was recommended as the analgesic of choice for episodic use in patients with underlying renal disease. The habitual consumption of acetaminophen should be discouraged and only used under the supervision of a physician. The guidelines also strongly discouraged the use of combination analgesic over-the-counter (OTC) products because of their increased prevalence of kidney injury and chronic renal failure. Finally, it is important to remember the potential toxicity that exists when nonprescription acetaminophen products (especially extra-strength ones) are used concurrently with prescription acetaminophen-containing products.

To avoid the systemic effects associated with various medications, the use of topical products may also be tried either alone or as an adjunct to oral analgesics or NSAIDs. Topical administration of capsaicin, an extract of red peppers that produces release of and ultimately depletion of substance P, has been beneficial in providing pain relief in OA. The depletion of substance P, a principal transmitter of nociceptive impulses from the periphery to central nervous system, was first used for temporary relief of neuralgia associated with herpes zoster infections or in patients with diabetic neuropathy.[56–58] This product is administered either two to four times a day by gently rubbing the cream around the affected joint. Pain relief often takes several weeks of *consistent* application before maximal pain relief is noted. It is generally well tolerated by most patients, though some will report a burning or stinging sensation when it is first applied. Patients need to be warned of the irritant effect that may occur if they inadvertently touch their mouth or eyes after administration. To avoid this problem, patients should be instructed to wash their hands after application.

Other analgesics include tramadol, a centrally acting analgesic, or propoxyphene or stronger narcotics such as codeine. These agents are often reserved for patients who have failed single- or multiple-agent therapy with simple analgesics, topical agents, or NSAIDs. Patients should be instructed to use these products primarily for severe pain and for the shortest duration possible. Ideally, prescriptions should be written for a limited quantity with only one or two refills, to minimize the abuse potential associated with these agents and to assist with assessing the degree of patient discomfort experienced. If the pain becomes unbearable and limits a patient's activities of daily living, then surgery is indicated rather than using more or stronger narcotics.

NONSTEROIDAL ANTI-INFLAMMATORY DRUGS

NSAIDs provide analgesic effects at lower doses and anti-inflammatory activity at higher doses. Several NSAIDs from a variety of chemical classes are available (Table 84–4); more products are in various phases of clinical testing in Europe and the United States.[59–61]

As a class of compounds, the NSAIDs are all comparably effective in reducing pain and modifying or diminishing the inflammatory process. Although the exact mechanism of action is unknown, a major component of the activity of all NSAIDs is believed to be related to a reduction of prostaglandin biosynthesis by inhibition of cyclooxygenase (COX-1 and COX-2) (Fig. 84–6).[3,47,48,60–62] COX-1 concentrations within the body are relatively constant, being present in vascular endothelial cells, platelets, and kidney collecting tubules. COX-2 concentrations are relatively low but increase during the inflammatory response. Considerable attention has focused on which isoenzyme is inhibited by the various NSAIDs, because selective inhibition of COX-2 appears to result in less toxicity (gastrointestinal, antiplatelet, renal) while still maintaining anti-inflammatory effects.

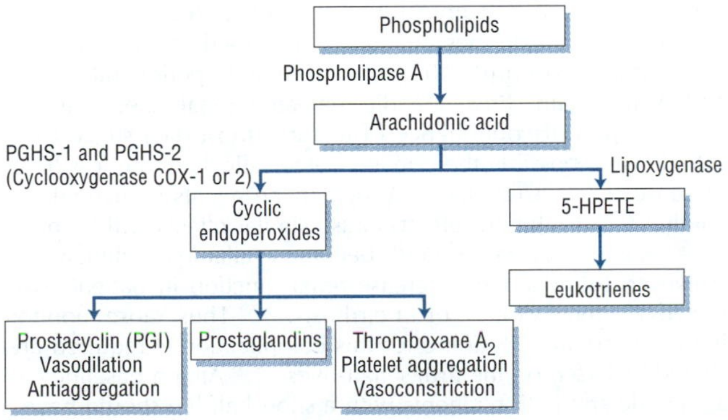

FIGURE 84–6. Pathway of synthesis of prostaglandins and leukotreine. COX-1 and COX-2 are cyclooxygenase 1 and 2 enzymes.

Several COX-2 inhibitor products, including celecoxib (Celebra) and rofecoxib (Vioxx), were reaching the U.S. market as this book was going to press. Of interest will be how effective these products are in not only preventing or minimizing the gastrointestinal and other toxicities related to COX-1 inhibition, but the extent of their therapeutic efficacy in providing pain relief and anti-inflammatory effects.

Other actions of the NSAIDs at various dose ranges include inhibiting a variety of enzymes, proteoglycan synthesis, transmembrane ion fluxes, cell–cell binding, and the immune system.[47,48,60–63]

The choice of a particular NSAID is frequently a matter of prescriber preference based on past treatment, cost, patient preference, toxic effects, and compliance. In general, the NSAIDs are indicated after simple analgesics have failed to relieve pain, toxic effects have developed, or inflammation is present. All NSAIDs are as effective as aspirin in terms of analgesia or anti-inflammatory properties and cause fewer gastrointestinal complaints than aspirin.[47,48,60–62] These characteristics have encouraged many clinicians to select the NSAIDs before aspirin; however, often the NSAIDs are considerably more expensive, unless generic products are available (e.g., ibuprofen, naproxen).

The pharmacokinetics of the individual NSAIDs are generally similar except for serum half-lives.[47,48] All are well absorbed after oral administration, are highly protein bound (greater than 90%), and have a low volume of distribution (< 0.2 L/kg). Elimination is via hepatic biotransformation to inactive metabolites (except sulindac or nabumetone, which are metabolized to an active form), with renal excretion of less than 5% of unchanged drug. Total body clearance is low (for most NSAIDs, less than 200 mL/min). They readily penetrate the joint fluid in concentrations approximately 60% of the mean plasma concentration, regardless of the elimination half-life of the drug. This may account for a portion of the relatively prolonged biologic effects of NSAIDs with a short half-life.[47,48] Therapeutic monitoring of serum and synovial drug concentrations has not been successfully applied.[47,48] The anti-inflammatory effect generally peaks after 2 to 3 weeks, irrespective of the half-life. Analgesic effectiveness usually occurs 1 to 2 hours after taking the NSAID and lasts up to 24 hours. The most variable property appears to be the serum half-life, which ranges from 1 hour for tolmetin to 60 to 90 hours for phenylbutazone.

Patient response to the NSAIDs is typically variable and highly individual.[47,48] A patient may respond well to one drug in a particular chemical class but experience little or no benefit from another NSAID in the same class. NSAIDs are then selected, often based on prior experience of the prescriber. The NSAID selected is given an adequate trial (2 to 3 weeks) and at an adequate dose (either anti-inflammatory or analgesic). If therapy fails, another NSAID either in the same chemical class or another class is selected and the process is repeated until an effective agent is found or toxicity develops. Patients should always be instructed that a trial with more than one product may be necessary and compliance with the scheduled regimen is important in evaluating effectiveness. Combination of NSAIDs with other NSAIDs or aspirin increases adverse gastrointestinal effects while providing no added benefit.[45–48]

Gastrointestinal complaints are the most common adverse effects observed with NSAIDs and account for many treatment failures.[45,46,60,64] Minor gastrointestinal complaints include nausea, dyspepsia, anorexia, abdominal pain, flatulence, and diarrhea, and affect between 10% and 60% of patients.[64,65] To minimize adverse effects, administration with food or milk should be encouraged, except for the enteric-coated products (milk or antacids may destroy the enteric coating and cause increased gastrointestinal symptoms in selected patients). Diarrhea can occur but is more commonly observed with meclofenamate than the other NSAIDs.

All NSAIDs have the potential to cause gastrointestinal bleeding through a variety of mechanisms related to direct topical or systemic effects of the NSAIDs.[45,46,60,64] As organic acids, most NSAIDs are weak acids (except nabumetone), which results in compounds being nonionized at a pH below 3.5 in the stomach. This results in the transport across the cell membrane and "ion trapping" within the cell, thereby causing cell death and releasing by back diffusion hydrogen ion. The systemic manifestations of the NSAIDs are related to inhibition of prostaglandins responsible for providing gastric mucosal protection.

No patient or subgroup of patients is completely free from the risk of NSAID-associated complications or ulcers. Some NSAIDs are more likely than others to cause gastrointestinal toxicity. However, attempts to define a true incidence are often difficult because of the considerable variability in defining the problem.[62] This variability is related to definition of gastrointestinal symptoms or ulcers, time course to develop toxicity, prevalence of NSAID use by the population, age of the population being studied, disease state being treated, and concomitant medications. Most importantly, patient symptoms correlate poorly with the endoscopic appearance and severity of mucosal injury. Up to 50% of patients with dyspepsia have mucosa with normal appearance, while approximately 40% of asymptomatic patients have endoscopic evidence of erosive gastritis.[45] However, several factors have been shown to increase the risk of ulcers and complications related to NSAIDs. These include age above 65 years; prior ulcer disease or complications; therapy with high-dose or multiple NSAIDs; concomitant corticosteroid therapy; and NSAID therapy duration less than 3 months; and cardiovascular disease.[46,60,64,65] These risk factors also appear to be additive, and an increased risk occurs when several factors occur in the same patient.[65] Although testing for fecal occult blood has been recommended as a way to predict NSAID-induced ulcers, it has not been proven reliable. Instead, other pathologic processes that may cause gastrointestinal bleeding may be present and require further investigation.[46,47]

The location of the mucosal injury secondary to NSAIDs is important when reviewing trials of therapies designed to prevent this injury. The most common site of mucosal injury is to the gastric mucosa, which occurs with an 11% to 13% incidence of gastric ulcers (GU), followed by duodenal damage with an incidence of 7% to 10% of duodenal ulcers (DU).[64–73] The incidence of these lesions is highly dependent on the classification system used to define the lesions based on size (3-mm versus 5-mm ulcers).[46,64] The NSAIDs can also cause injury throughout the entire gastrointestinal tract involving the small intestine and colon.[64,66] Ulcer complications consisting of gastrointestinal bleeding, perforation, and gastric outlet obstruction occur in 1.5% to 4% of patients per year.[64–66] Patients with an increased age, history of peptic ulcer or bleeding, and cardiovascular disease have a 9% risk of a major complication.[65] H_2-receptor antagonists (H_2RAs) appear effective in preventing NSAID-induced *duodenal* ulcer lesions but not *gastric* ulcers.[46,64] Recent data have questioned whether higher doses may have protective effects on gastric ulcers as well.[67,68] However, caution should be exercised in interpreting these data, as the incidence of ulcers in the placebo group has exceeded the usual expected incidence, in part because of the smaller size (3 mm) used to define ulcer occurrence. Together with this and other study concerns relating to concurrent use of other medications and a lack of information relating to ulcer complication rates, the value of H_2RAs still appears to be limited to preventing NSAID-induced duodenal ulcers. A further concern has been reported, that the use of H_2RAs and antacids may actually increase the risk of serious gastrointestinal complications by masking the symptoms.[68]

Presently, only misoprostol has demonstrated the ability to protect against both NSAID-induced gastric and duodenal ulcers and their associated complications.[64,65,70,71] Furthermore, misoprostol did not interfere with the anti-inflammatory effects of the NSAIDs. The major drawbacks to this therapy have been the occurrence of diarrhea, abdominal cramps associated with its administration, and a lack of gastrointestinal pain relief. This product also is not indicated in women of child-bearing age because of its abortifacient properties. Dispensing of the product is intended to be in the original container, which carries this warning on the prescription bottle.

Other agents have been evaluated in an attempt to prevent NSAID-induced gastrointestinal toxicity. Sucralfate appears less effective than misoprostol in preventing gastric ulcers in patients on NSAIDs. Data on duodenal ulcer prevention are limited, and no data on reduction of complication rate are available.[70] Only recently, has an international multicenter clinical trial been published comparing the effects of omeprazole with misoprostol, and omeprazole with rantidine, in promoting healing of NSAID-induced ulcers (gastric and duodenal) as well as preventing further GU or DU formation. In both of the trials, omeprazole was more effective than either misoprostol or ranitidine in promoting healing and preventing a recurrence of both duodenal and gastric ulcers.[72,73] This therapy also was more effective at improving patient's quality of life and promoting symptom relief, especially when compared with misoprostol. Limitations of the study appear to be similar to those previously described with high-dose H_2RAs. The incidence of gastric and duodenal ulcers was higher than expected, even when using the definition of greater than 5 mm for ulcer size. The incidence of *Helicobacter pylori* appears to be lower than expected for the study population, and though its influence appears to be an indicator of a higher probability of continued remission, concerns relating to not treating duodenal ulcers in patients who are positive for *H. pylori* remains a confounding variable in the interpretation of the data. Concomitant medications such as prednisone, a known risk factor, were allowed to be continued. Lastly, the study did not examine issues relating to a reduction in complications, as has been done with misoprostol.[65] Instead, the authors expect a similar incidence to misoprostol data, by inference, though not proven in the study. Despite these concerns, it is positive that data on this therapeutic option have finally been reported in the medical literature and are available for critique.

NSAIDs cause a variety of renal complications, including peripheral edema, transient acute renal insufficiency, tubulointerstitial nephropathy, hyperkalemia, and renal papillary necrosis.[74–76] Many of these complications may be mediated by inhibition of prostaglandins, which have an important role in the regulation of intrarenal blood flow in vasoconstricted states. Highly prone to developing renal insufficiency are patients with congestive heart failure, cirrhosis/ascites, volume contraction (from any cause), and advanced age. Clinical findings associated with NSAID-induced renal syndromes include an increased serum creatinine, blood urea nitrogen (BUN), serum potassium, peripheral edema, and weight gain. Prostaglandin-mediated renal effects are reversible upon discontinuance of therapy. Most data suggest that sulindac and possibly the nonacetylated salicylates are less likely to cause renal insufficiency. Whether the agents with predominantly COX-2 inhibitor effects cause similar effects will be of interest as these new compounds become available for clinical use. However, sulindac can decrease renal function in patients with underlying renal disease or in cirrhosis.[74–76] Thus, close monitoring of the serum creatinine for this complication is required and should be based on the drugs' half-lives.[74–76] After a baseline creatinine determination, agents with a short half-life should have a follow-up creatinine determination within several days, while those with longer half-lives may require a follow-up creatinine level after 5 to 7 days.

All NSAIDs can cause drug-induced hepatitis. Fortunately, this adverse effect is relatively uncommon. The NSAIDs used in the treatment of OA most frequently implicated include diclofenac and sulindac.[77–79] Patient monitoring should include baseline liver studies consisting of the transaminases, AST, and ALT, with therapy stopped if these values exceed two to three times the upper limit of normal.

Other toxic effects include hypersensitivity reactions, rash, or central nervous system complaints such as drowsiness, dizziness, headaches, depression, confusion, and tinnitus.[47,48,60,61] Additionally, all the agents that inhibit COX-1 affect platelet function to some extent. Aspirin inhibition is irreversible, and platelet function returns to normal only after 5 to 7 days, whereas the other NSAIDs cause a reversible inhibition that allows platelet function to return to normal sooner (1 to 3 days) after discontinuance. In either case, the nonacetylated salicylate products and nabumetone (which appear to affect only COX-2 synthetase) may be preferable for the patient with a bleeding disorder or as a temporary treatment before elective surgical procedures.[47,48,60,61] Finally, NSAIDs should be used cautiously during pregnancy because of risk to the fetus.[80]

Important drug interactions with the NSAIDs are frequently related to either pharmacokinetic or pharmacologic interactions. These interactions have been described in several excellent reviews.[47,48,81–83] The most potentially serious interactions include the concomitant use of NSAIDs with lithium, warfarin, oral hypoglycemics, methotrexate, lithium, antihypertensives, angiotensin-converting enzyme (ACE) inhibitors, β-blockers, and diuretics. Although these effects are variable and often only have been reported with certain NSAIDs, anticipation and careful monitoring can prevent serious adverse effects. Patient monitoring should also include the use of over-the-counter (OTC) NSAIDs and the H_2-receptor antagonists famotidine, ranitidine, cimetidine, or nizatidine, because a combination of NSAIDs may increase the risk of gastrointestinal toxicity leading to self-medication with an OTC H_2 antagonist product.

A continuing controversy in the treatment of OA with NSAIDs is whether these agents actually help or hinder the progression of osteoarthritis.[47,60,84] The data for this issue are primarily based on animal studies, with limited information in humans. Experimental data in animals have demonstrated the ability of salicylates and some NSAIDs to suppress proteoglycan biosynthesis in articular cartilage, while tiaprofenic acid, diclofenac, and piroxicam have been shown to stimulate proteoglycan synthesis. Limited human data seem to suggest a twofold risk for further progression of knee osteoarthritis if indomethacin therapy is continued.[84] Although the study had limitations, and further clinical trial data are needed in humans, the findings clearly raise some interesting issues concerning selection of NSAIDs and duration of therapy. This appears to be another reason to consider starting therapy with simple analgesics like acetaminophen.

CORTICOSTEROIDS

Systemic corticosteroid therapy is not recommended in the treatment of osteoarthritis.[6,8,9] The side effects associated with prolonged use outweigh any potential benefits of therapy. The use of intra-articular corticosteroids (IACs) may temporarily be helpful in patients with knee effusions, but their long-term benefit remains controversial.[6,8,9] If used, IACs should be administered infrequently at intervals of 4 to 6 months for any given joint and not to exceed 3 to 4 injections per year. If no improvement occurs from one or two injections, then further treatment is not likely to succeed. After injection, the patient should be instructed to minimize joint activity and the joint stress load for several days. The use of injection of corticosteroids into the ligaments or pericapsular areas can be beneficial and is associated with reduced risks relative to IAC administration.

HYALURONATE INJECTIONS

Recently new intra-articular injection agents that contain hyaluronic acid (e.g., sodium hyaluronate, Hyalgan, Synvisc) have become commercially available for the treatment of pain associated with OA of the knee.[85–88] These products are intended to assist in the reconstitution of the synovial fluid, thereby improving joint function. Hyaluronic acid also plays an important role in cartilage matrix formation through its role in aggregation with proteoglycanen. Several of the published studies have indicated benefit with this therapy.[85,86] However, most of the studies used symptom relief as outcome assessments. Additionally, most of the studies have been of relatively short duration and longer-term study is clearly warranted. These products require once weekly administration for either 3 or 5 consecutive weeks. Currently, the side effects profile indicates that the products are relatively well tolerated. There are reports of pain on injection and local skin reactions, including rash, ecchymosis, and purititis. With repeated knee injections, the risk of infection is possible, and sterile preparation of the area is important. Based on the information to date, these products may have value in patients who have failed to respond to conventional therapy or are interested in delaying surgery. However, further long-term trial and clinical use in patients will determine the ultimate value of these modestly expensive therapies, which include not only the medication costs but therapeutic procedure expenses.

DISEASE-MODIFYING DRUGS

Disease-modifying drugs used in the treatment of OA are not principally analgesic. These agents are aimed at preventing, retarding, or reversing the changes to the articular cartilage matrix.[89] Most of the products have been tested in animal models with limited data in humans. For example, heparinoid compounds that contain glycosaminoglycans such as Rumalon (glycosaminoglycan peptide complex from bovine trachea or bronchial cartilage) or Arteparon (chondroitin-4-sulfate and chondroitin-6-sulfate, which are extracts of calf cartilage and bone marrow) have been used in some experiments. These compounds appear to stimulate the synthesis of cartilage but may also play a role in inhibiting the degradative enzyme reactions of articular cartilage. However, a concern has been reports of bleeding attributed to the heparinoid structure of the glycosaminoglycans and anaphylaxis associated with the presence of the antigenic proteins in the compounds.[89] Other approaches have involved the use of tetracycline or doxycycline, which appear to inhibit the degradative MMPs.[29,89,90] Still other approaches have centered on affecting the chondrocytes controlling the articular cartilage through the use of various inhibitors of cytokines, such as IL-1 and TNF, which may produce cartilage degradation.

Despite the interest and excitement in these various regimens, the majority of approaches have undergone limited controlled trials in humans and should be considered experimental. Ongoing clinical trials have begun with some of these therapies. To provide the most accurate interpretation of the data, in a disease that progresses very slowly, it will be important to identify outcome measures and assessment tools for evaluation of disease-modifying drugs carefully. Patient selection for these trials needs to be focused on those who have a high risk of osteoarthritis.[89]

PHARMACOECONOMIC CONSIDERATIONS

Over the past 15 years, considerable interest has been shown in economic evaluations in the field of rheumatology.[91–93] At least 36 full economic evaluations were published over a 10-year period: 1984 to 1990 (31%) and 1991 to 1995 (61%).[91] Of these, the majority of evaluations focused on prevention, treatment, or a combination. Diagnostic economic evaluations were the least-studied area. The disease state that was evaluated most frequently was OA (36%) followed by osteoporosis (22%) and rheumatoid arthritis (14%). Within OA, more than 38% of the studies evaluated misoprostol use in patients receiving NSAIDs.

Recently, data on the cost-effectiveness of misoprostol in preventing NSAID-associated ulcers has been reported.[93] In this study, the authors examined the original data from the (MUCOSA) trial reported by Silverstein and associates.[65] The important observation from this work concluded that the cost of prophylactic therapy with misoprostol would be greatly reduced if only patients with a higher risk of developing serious gastrointestinal complications were selected to receive misoprostol. The cost reduction would be reduced from $94,766 if all patients received the misoprostol to $4101 for those with higher and several risk factors. This work is consistent with the belief that only selected high-risk patients should receive prophylactic therapy.

Other pharmacoeconomic considerations involve the selection of therapy for the initial treatment of patients with OA. The initial recommendation of a simple OTC analgesic (acetaminophen) as the initial therapy has greatly reduced the prescription medication cost associated with the use of NSAIDs. This cost ranges from $20 to $100 per month depending on the medication, daily dose, and regimen selected. Though this may appear within some budgets as a reduction in the cost of prescription medications, much of this cost shifting to "out of pocket" expense still greatly affects patients on fixed incomes. Many elderly patients, who are likely to use the medications, often receive limited if any prescription reimbursement from their insurance or governmental plans. Careful attention to this cost shifting to OTC products—acetaminophen or NSAIDs—needs to be given for all patients receiving therapy for OA.

NSAIDs as a chemical category of analgesics and anti-inflammatory agents are considered therapeutically equivalent. This does not imply that the agents are therapeutically interchangeable. Patient response to these agents is highly individualized. When starting therapy, it is often useful to consider the cost of the product and its generic availability among factors for product selection. Both of these factors are of importance to patients on fixed incomes and those on limited budgets, as well as for the health care system costs.

EVALUATION OF THERAPEUTIC OUTCOMES

Pharmacotherapy monitoring is patient specific, focusing on the degree and extent of joint involvement, patient age, concomitant medications and disease states, and the nondrug and drug therapy selected. Generally, the monitoring plan for assessing therapeutic efficacy consists of establishing the patient's baseline pain through the use of a pain visual analog scale (VAS) and identifying the range of motion for the affected joint (flexion, extension, abduction, or adduction). Depending on the joint affected, measurement of grip strength and 50-foot walking time may aid in the assessment of hand or hip/knee OA, respectively. Baseline radiographs of the respective joint are often performed to assist with establishing the degree and/or extent of joint involvement, and may be repeated when the clinical course indicates a worsening of patient symptoms. Other measures include the clinician's global assessment based on the patient's history of activities and limitations caused by the OA as well as documentation of analgesic or NSAID use. Lastly, disease-specific quality of life (QOL) questionnaires for arthritis provide yet another valuable tool in assessing a patient's clinical response to various therapeutic interventions.[94–96]

Establishment of monitoring parameters for adverse effects depends on the therapeutic regimen chosen. Often, the most effective approach is through direct patient questioning. Patients should be questioned directly to establish if they are having any "problems" with their medications rather than first just listing a series of adverse effects. This approach is quite useful and can be followed up with more direct questions relating to the most common adverse effects associated with the respective medication. With most NSAIDs, symptoms of abdominal pain, heartburn, nausea, or change in stool color are often valuable questions to identify gastrointestinal complaints. Patients should also be monitored for any signs of skin rash, headaches, drowsiness, weight gain, or alterations in blood pressure. Baseline serum creatinine determinations, hematology profiles, and serum transaminases with repeat levels as needed are useful in identifying specific toxicities to the kidney, liver, gastrointestinal tract, or bone marrow.

CONCLUSIONS

Osteoarthritis is a very common, slowly progressive disorder that affects diarthrodial joints. It is characterized by a progressive deterioration of articular cartilage resulting in loss of articular cartilage and osteophyte formation. Clinically, the manifestations occur later in life and consist of gradual onset of joint pain, stiffness, and limitation of motion. The primary treatment goal is to reduce pain, maintain function, and prevent further destruction. An individualized approach consisting of nondrug therapy such as rest/exercise regimens and drug therapy can be successful in attaining these goals. Currently, the mainstay of therapy consists of starting therapy with acetaminophen below 4 g/d and when necessary use of topical analgesics and NSAIDs. Experimental therapy aimed at preventing the progression of OA requires further clinical investigation before becoming widely accepted.

▶ PRINCIPLES OF PHARMACOTHERAPY

- The most common form of arthritis is osteoarthritis (OA). It affects individuals in the mid to later years of life, with women more commonly affected than males after age 45.

- Osteoarthritis is primarily a disease of cartilage that reflects a failure of the chondrocyte to maintain the balance between cartilage production and destruction.
- The most common symptom associated with OA is pain, which leads to decreased function and motion.
- Patients have bony proliferation of their affected joints that can be confused with the swelling associated with rheumatoid or inflammatory arthritis.
- OA is not a systemic disease like rheumatoid arthritis. The joint distribution often involves primarily the knees, hips, and hands (DIPs and PIPs), though other joints are also affected.
- Nonpharmacologic therapy is the foundation of any pharmaceutical care plan in treating patients. It should be started at the same time as simple analgesics like acetaminophen (< 4 g/d) are instituted.
- Failure with simple analagesics warrants the trial with a NSAID in low doses unless inflammation is present.
- NSAIDs are associated with gastrointestinal, renal, liver, or central nervous system toxicity. The appropriate monitoring with CBC, Scr, AST, or ALT laboratory tests is valuable to detect potential toxicity.
- Prevention of NSAID-induced gastrointestinal toxicity includes using enteric-coated products, nonacetylated salicylates, or compounds that inhibit the COX-2 enzyme. The use of misoprostol has shown to be effective in both reducing gastric and duodenal ulcers and the associated complications. H_2RAs are effective in preventing DU but not GU; sucralfate appears equal to placebo; and omeprazole may have comparable effects to misoprostol, though reduction in complications has not been studied.
- OA is a chronic disease that has a wide spectrum of disease progression. New therapies are being studied that may prevent further joint progression, thereby limiting or delaying the need for surgery.

REFERENCES

1. Fife RS. Epidemiology, pathology and pathogenesis. In: Klippel JH, ed. Primer on the Rheumatic Diseases, 11th ed. Atlanta, Arthritis Foundation, 1997:216–217.
2. Yelin E, Callahan LF. The economic cost and social and psychological impact of muscloskeletal conditions. Arthritis Rheum 1995;38: 1351–1362.
3. Oddis CV. New perspectives on osteoarthritis. Am J Med 1996; 100(suppl 2A):2S–10S.
4. Buckwalter JA, Mankin HJ. Articular cartilage. Part I: Tissue design and chondrocyte–matrix interactions. J Bone Joint Surg 1997;79A: 600–611.
5. Buckwalter JA, Mankin HJ. Articular cartilage. Part II: Degeneration and osteoarthrosis, repair, regeneration, and transplantation. J Bone Joint Surg 1997;79A:612–632.
6. Hochberg MC. Clinical features and treatment. In: Klippel JH, ed. Primer on the Rheumatic Diseases, 11th ed. Atlanta, Arthritis Foundation, 1997:218–221.
7. Dieppe P. Osteoarthritis: Introduction. In: Klippel JH, Dieppe PA, eds. Rheumatology. London, Mosby-Year Book, 1994:1–2.
8. Hochberg MC, Altman RD, Brandt KD, et al. Guidelines for the medical management of osteoarthritis: Part I. Osteoarthritis of the hip. Arthritis Rheum 1995;38:1535–1540.
9. Hochberg MC, Altman RD, Brandt KD, et al. Guidelines for the medical management of osteoarthritis: Part II. Osteoarthritis of the knee. Arthritis Rheum 1995;38:1541–1546.
10. Lawrence RC, Hochberg MC, Kelsey JL, et al. Estimates of the prevalence of selected arthritic and musculoskeletal diseases in the United States. J Rheumatol 1989;16:427–441.
11. Felson DT, Anderson JJ, Naimark A, et al. The prevalence of chondrocalcinosis in the elderly and its association with knee osteoarthritis: The Framingham study. J Rheumatol 1989;16:1241–1245.
12. Spector TD, Hochberg MC. Methodological problems in the epidemiological study of osteoarthritis. Ann Rheum Dis 1994;53:143–146.
13. Davis MA, Ettinger WH, Neuhaus JM, et al. Knee osteoarthritis and physical functioning: Evidence from the NHANEWSI epidemiologic follow-up study. J Rheumatol 1991;18:591–598.
14. Van Saase JL, Van Romunde LK, Cats A, et al. Epidemiology of osteoarthritis: Zoetermeer survey. Comparison of radiological osteoarthritis in a Dutch population with that in 10 other populations. Ann Rheum Dis 1989;48:271–280.
15. Wilson MG, Michet CJ, Strup DM, Melton IJ. Idiopathic symptomatic osteoarthritis of the hip and knee: A population-based incidence study. Mayo Clin Proc 1990;60:1214–1221.
16. Cooper C. Osteoarthritis: Epidemiology. In: Klippel JH, Dieppe PA, eds. Rheumatology. London, Mosby-Year Book, 1994:3.1–3.4.
17. Felson DT, Zhang Y, Anthony JM, et al. Weight loss reduces the risk for symptomatic knee osteoarthritis in women. Ann Intern Med 1992;117:535–539.
18. Solomon L. Clinical features of osteoarthritis. In: Kelly WN, Harris ED, Ruddy S, Sledge CB, eds. Textbook of Rheumatology, 5th ed. Philadelphia, Saunders, 1997:1383–1393.
19. Bergenudd H, Lindgarde F, Nilsson B. Prevalence and co-incidence of degenerative changes of the hands and feet in middle age and their relationship to occupational workload, intelligence and social background. Clin Orthop 1989;239:306–310.
20. Lane NE, Bloch DA, Hubert HB, et al. Running, osteoarthritis, and bone density: Initial 2-year longitudinal study. Am J Med 1990;88: 453–459.
21. Panush RS, Schmidt C, Caldwell JR, et al. Is running associated with degenerative joint disease? JAMA 1986;255:1152–1154.
22. Eye DR, Weis MA, Moskowitz RW. Cartilage expression of a type II collagen mutation in an inherited form of osteoarthritis associated with a mild chondrodysplasia. J Clin Invest 1991;87:357–361.
23. Vikkula M, Palotie A, Ritvaniemi P. Early onset osteoarthritis linked to the type II procollagen gene. Arthritis Rheum 1993;36:401–409.
24. Knight SM, Ring EFJ, Bhalla AK. Bone mineral density and osteoarthritis. Ann Rheum Dis 1992;51:1025.
25. Hannan MT, Anderson JJ, Zhang Y, et al. Bone mineral density and knee osteoarthritis in elderly men and women: The Framingham study. Arthritis Rheum 1993;12:1671–1680.
26. Mankin HJ, Brandt KD, Pathogenesis of osteoarthritis. In: Kelly WN, Harris ED, Ruddy S, Sledge CB, eds. Textbook of Rheumatology, 5th ed. Philadelphia, Saunders, 1997:1369–1382.
27. Sipe JD. Acute-phase proteins in osteoarthritis. Semin Arthritis Rheum 1995;25:75–86.
28. Westacott CI, Sharif M. Cytokines in osteoarthritis: Mediators or markers of joint destruction. Semin Arthritis Rheum 1996;25:254–272.
29. Kraus VB. Pathogenesis and treatment of osteoarthritis. Med Clin North Am 1997;81:85–112.
30. Buckwalter JA, Glimcher MJ, Cooper RR, Recker R. Bone Biology. Part I: Structure, blood supply, cells, matrix, and mineralization. J Bone J Surg Am 1995;77A:1256–1275.
31. Buckwalter JA, Glimcher MJ, Cooper RR, Recker R. Bone Biology. Part II: Formation, form, modeling, remodeling, and regulation of cell function. J Bone J Surg Am 1995;77A:1276–1288.

32. Dieppe P. Osteoarthritis: Clinical features and diagnostic problems. In: Klippel JH, Dieppe PA, eds. Rheumatology. London, Mosby-Year Book, 1994:1–16.
33. Mankin HJ, Brandt KD, Shulman LE. Workshop on the etiopathogenesis of osteoarthritis. J Rheumatol 1986;13:1130–1134.
34. Mazzuca S. Plain radiography in the evaluation of knee osteoarthritis. Curr Opin Rheumatol 1997;9:263–267.
35. Ravaud P, Dougados M. Radiographic assessment in osteoarthritis. J Rheumatol 1997;24:786–791.
36. Altman RD, ed. Pain in osteoarthritis. Semin Arthritis Rheum 1989;18:(suppl 2):1–104.
37. Rene J, Weinberger M, Mazzuca SA, et al. Reduction of joint pain in patients with knee osteoarthritis who have received monthly telephone calls from lay personnel and whose medical treatment regimens have remained stable. Arthritis Rheum 1992;35:511–515.
38. Kovar PA, Allegrante JP, MacKenzie CR, et al. Supervised fitness walking in patients with osteoarthritis of the knee. Ann Intern Med 1992;116:529–534.
39. McCarty MF. Glucosamine may retard atherogenesis by promoting endothelial production of heparan sulfate proteoglycans. Med Hypotheses 1997;48:245–251.
40. Glucosamine for osteoarthritis. Med Lett Drugs Ther 1997;39:91–92.
41. Puett DW, Griffin MR. Published trials of nonmedicinal and noninvasive therapies for hip and knee osteoarthritis. Ann Intern Med 1994; 121;133–140.
42. Harris WH, Sledge CB. Total hip and total knee replacement (part I). N Engl J Med 1990;323:725–731.
43. Harris WH, Sledge CB. Total hip and total knee replacement (part II). N Engl J Med 1990;323:801–807.
44. Wirth CJ. Techniques of cartilage growth enhancement: A review of the literature. Arthroscopy 1996;12:300–308.
45. Hollander D. Gastrointestinal complications of nonsteroidal anti-inflammatory drugs: Prophylactic and therapeutic strategies. Am J Med 1994;96:274–281.
46. Lichtenstein DR, Syngal S, Wolfe MM. Nonsteroidal anti-inflammatory drugs and the gastrointestinal tract. Arthritis Rheum 1995;1:5–18.
47. Furst DE. Are there differences among nonsteroidal anti-inflammatory drugs? Arthritis Rheum 1994;1:1–9.
48. Brooks PM, Day RO. Nonsteroidal anti-inflammatory drugs—differences and similarities. N Engl J Med 1991;324:1716–1725.
49. Morassut P, Yang W, Karsh J. Aspirin intolerance. Semin Arthritis Rheum 1989;19:22–30.
50. Bradley JD, Brandt KD, Katz BP, et al. Comparison of an anti-inflammatory dose of ibuprofen, an analgesic dose of ibuprofen, and acetaminophen in the treatment of patients with osteoarthritis of the knee. N Engl J Med 1991;325:87–91.
51. Williams HJ, Ward JR, Egger MJ, et al. Comparison of naproxen and acetaminophen in a two-year study of treatment of osteoarthritis of the knee. Arthritis Rheum 1993;36:1196–1206.
52. Brandt KD. NSAIDs in the treatment of osteoarthritis. Friends or foes? Bull Rheum Dis 1993;42:1–3.
53. Henrich WL, Agodoa LE, Barrett B, et al. Analgesics and the kidney: Summary recommendations to the scientific advisory Board of the National Kidney Foundation from an ad hoc committee of the National Kidney Foundation. Am J Kidney Dis 1996;27:162–165.
54. Whitcomb DC, Block GD. Association of acetaminophen hepatotoxicity with fasting and ethanol use. JAMA 1994;272:1845–1850.
55. Perneger TU, Whelton PK, Klag MJ. Risk of kidney failure associated with the use of acetaminophen, aspirin and nonsteroidal anti-inflammatory drugs. N Engl J Med 1994;331:1675–1679.
56. Rumsfield JA, West DP. Topical capsaicin in dermatologic and peripheral pain disorders. DICP Ann Pharmacother 1991;25:381–387.
57. Mapp P, Kidd B. The role of substance P in rheumatic disease. Semin Arthritis Rheum 1994;23(suppl 3):3–9.
58. Altman RD, Aven A, Holmburg CE, et al. Capsaicin cream 0.025% as monotherapy for osteoarthritis: A double-blind study. Semin Arthritis Rheum 1994;23(suppl 3):25–39.
59. Mossinghoff GJ. In: Development of New Medicines for Arthritis. Washington, Pharmaceutical Manufacturers Association, 1991.
60. Simon LS. Biologic effects of nonsteroidal anti-inflammatory drugs. Curr Opin Rheumatol 1997;9:178–182.
61. DeWitt DL, Meade EA, Smith WL. PGH synthase isoenzyme selectivity: The potential for safer nonsteroidal anti-inflammatory drugs. Am J Med 1993;95(suppl 2A):40S.
62. Miwa LJ, Jones JK, Pathiyal A, Hatoum H. Value of epidemiologic studies in determining the true incidence of adverse events. The nonsteroidal anti-inflammatory drug story. Arch Intern Med 1997;157: 2129–2136.
63. Abramson SB. Treatment of gout and crystal arthropathies and uses and mechanism of action of nonsteroidal anti-inflammatory drugs. Curr Opin Rheumatol 1992;4:295–300.
64. Wallace JL. Nonsteroidal anti-inflammatory drugs and gastroenteropathy: The second hundred years. Gastroenterology 1997;112:1000–1016.
65. Silverstein FE, Graham DY, Senior JR, et al. Misoprostol reduces serious gastrointestinal complications in patients with rheumatoid arthritis receiving nonsteroidal anti-inflammatory drugs. Ann Intern Med 1995;123:241–249.
66. Allison MC, Howatson AG, Torrance CJ, et al. Gastrointestinal damage associated with the use of nonsteroidal anti-inflammatory drugs. N Engl J Med 1992;327:749–754.
67. Taha AS, Hudson N, Trye P, et al. Prevention of NSAID related gastric and duodenal ulcers by famotidine: A placebo controlled double blind study. N Engl J Med 1996;334:1435–1439.
68. Hudson N, Taha AS, Russell RI, et al. Famotidine for healing and maintenance in nonsteroidal anti-inflammatory drug-associated gastroduodenal ulceration. Gastroenterology 1997;112:1817–1822.
69. Singh G, Ramey DR, Morfeld D, et al. Gastrointestinal tract complications of nonsteroidal anti-inflammatory drug treatment in rheumatoid arthritis. Arch Intern Med 1996;156:1530–1536.
70. Agrawal NM, Roth S, Graham DY, et al. Misoprostol compared with sucralfate in the prevention of nonsteroidal anti-inflammatory drug-induced gastric ulcer: A randomized, controlled trial. Ann Intern Med 1991;115:195–200.
71. Graham DY, White RH, Moreland LW, et al. Duodenal and gastric ulcer prevention with misoprostol in arthritis patients taking NSAIDs. Ann Intern Med 1993;119:257–262.
72. Yeomans ND, Tulassay Z, Juhasz L, et al. A comparison of omeprazole with ranitidine for ulcers associated with nonsteroidal anti-inflammatory drugs. N Engl J Med 1998;338:719–726.
73. Hawkey CJ, Karrasch JA, Szczepanski L, et al. Omeprazole compared with misoprostol for ulcer associated with nonsteroidal anti-inflammatory drugs. N Engl J Med 1998;338:727–734.
74. Bennett WM, Henrich WL, Stoff JS. The renal effects of nonsteroidal anti-inflammatory drugs: Summary and recommendations. Am J Kid Dis 1996;28(suppl 1):S56–S62.
75. Murray MD, Brater DC. Adverse effects of nonsteroidal anti-inflammatory drugs on renal function. Ann Intern Med 1990;112: 559–560.
76. Murray KM, Keane WR. Review of drug-induced acute interstitial nephritis. Pharmacotherapy 1992;12:462–467.
77. Rodriguez LA, Williams R, Derby LE, et al. Acute liver injury associated with nonsteroidal anti-inflammatory drugs and the role of risk factors. Arch Intern Med 1994;154:311–316.
78. Rabinovitz M, Van Thiel DH. Hepatotoxicity of nonsteroidal anti-inflammatory drugs. Am J Gastroenterol 1992;87:1696–1704.
79. Furst DE, Anderson W. Differential effects of diclofenac and aspirin on serum glutamic oxaloacetic transaminase elevations in patients with rheumatoid arthritis and osteoarthritis. Arthritis Rheum 1993;36: 804–810.
80. Roubenoff R, Hoyt J, Petri M, et al. Effects of anti-inflammatory and immunosuppressive drugs on pregnancy and fertility. Semin Arthritis Rheum 1988;18:88–110.
81. Furst DE. Clinically important interactions of nonsteroidal anti-inflammatory drugs with other medications. J Rheumatol 1988;15 (suppl 17):58–62.

82. Hansen P, Horn JR, eds. All NSAID are not alike with regard to drug interactions. Drug Int Newsl 1987;7:7–11.
83. Johnson AG, Nguyen TV, Day RO. Do nonsteroidal anti-inflammatory drugs affect blood pressure. Ann Intern Med 1994;121:289–300.
84. Brandt KD. Should nonsteroidal anti-inflammatory drugs be used to treat osteoarthritis? Rheum Dis Clin North Am 1993;19:29–45.
85. Lohmander LS, Dalen N, Englund G, et al. Intra-articular hyaluronan injections in the treatment of osteoarthritis of the knee: A randomized, double blind, placebo controlled multicentre trial. Ann Rheum Dis 1996;55:424–431.
86. Puhl W, Bernau A, Greiling H, et al. Intra-articular sodium hyaluronate in osteoarthritis of the knee: A multi center, double-blind study. Osteoarthritis Cartilage 1993;1:233–241.
87. Creamer P, Dieppe PA. Novel drug treatment strategies for osteoarthritis. J Rheumatol 1993;20:1461–1463.
88. Ghosh P. Osteoarthritis and hyaluronan. Palliative or disease-modifying treatment? Semin Arthritis Rheum 1993;22(suppl 1):1–3.
89. Brandt KD. Toward pharmacologic modification of joint damage in osteoarthritis. Ann Intern Med 1995;122:874–875.
90. Yu LP, Smnith GN, Brandt KD, et al. Reduction of the severity of canine osteoarthritis by prophylactic treatment with oral doxycycline. Arthritis Rheum 1992;35:1150–1159.
91. Ferraz MB, Maetzel A, Bombardier C. A summary of economic evaluations published in the field of rheumatology and related disciplines. Arthritis Rheum 1997;40:1587–1593.
92. Gabriel SE, Crowson CS, Campion ME, O'Fallon WM. Indirect and nonmedical costs among people with rheumatoid arthritis and osteoarthritis compared with nonarthritic controls. J Rheumatol 1997;24:43–48.
93. Maetzel A, Ferraz MB, Bombardier C. The cost-effectiveness of misoprostol in preventing serious gastrointestinal events associated with the use of nonsteroidal anti-inflammatory drugs. Arthritis Rheum 1998;41:16–25.
94. Dougados M. Clinical assessment of osteoarthritis in clinical trials. Curr Opin Rheumatol 1995;7:87–91.
95. Gill TM, Geinstein AR. A critical appraisal of the quality of quality-of-life measurements. JAMA 1994;272:619–626.
96. Wilson IB, Cleary PD. Linking clinical variables with health-related quality of life: A conceptual model of patient outcomes. JAMA 1995;273:59–65.

85

GOUT AND HYPERURICEMIA

David W. Hawkins, PharmD, and Daniel W. Rahn, MD

The term *gout* describes a disease spectrum including hyperuricemia, recurrent attacks of acute arthritis associated with monosodium urate crystals in leukocytes found in synovial fluid, deposits of monosodium urate crystals in tissues (tophi), interstitial renal disease, and uric acid nephrolithiasis.[1]

Hyperuricemia may be an asymptomatic condition, with an increased serum uric acid as the only apparent abnormality. Statistically, hyperuricemia is defined as a serum urate concentration greater than two standard deviations above the population mean. But for determination of the risk for gout, hyperuricemia is defined as a supersaturated urate concentration.[2] By this definition, a urate concentration greater than 7.0 mg/dL is abnormal and is associated with an increased risk for gout. This corresponds to a measured value greater than 7.5 mg/dL by most autoanalyzers.

EPIDEMIOLOGY

Population studies have shown that serum urate concentration (and consequently the risk of gout) correlates with age, serum creatinine, blood urea nitrogen, male gender, blood pressure, body weight, and alcohol intake. Serum urate concentration are normally distributed with slight skewing toward higher values. Mean values are 6.8 mg/dL for men and 6.0 mg/dL for women.

There is a direct correlation between the serum uric acid concentrations and both the incidence and prevalence of gout. The incidence of gout varies from 20 to 35 per 100,000 persons with an overall prevalence of 1.6 to 13.6 per thousand. Prevalence increases with age, especially in men.[1] Men are affected by gout approximately 10 times more often than women. Although no genetic marker has been isolated for gout, the familial nature of gout strongly suggests an interaction between genetic and environmental factors.

ETIOLOGY AND PATHOPHYSIOLOGY

In humans, uric acid is the end product of the degradation of purines. It serves no known physiologic purpose and therefore is regarded as a waste product. In lower animals, the enzyme uricase breaks down uric acid to the more soluble allantoin, and thus uric acid does not accumulate. Gout occurs exclusively in humans in whom a miscible pool of uric acid exists. Under normal conditions, the amount of cumulated uric acid is about 1200 mg in men and about 600 mg in women. The size of the urate pool is increased severalfold in individuals with gout. This excess accumulation may result from either overproduction or underexcretion.

OVERPRODUCTION OF URIC ACID

The purines from which uric acid is produced originate from three sources: dietary purine, conversion of tissue nucleic acid to purine nucleotides, and de novo synthesis of purine bases. The purines derived from these three sources enter a common metabolic pathway, leading to the production of either nucleic acid or uric acid. Under normal circumstances, uric acid may accumulate excessively if production exceeds excretion. The average human produces about 600 to 800 mg of uric acid each day.

Several enzyme systems regulate purine metabolism. Abnormalities in these regulatory systems can result in overproduction of uric acid. Uric acid may also be overproduced as a consequence of increased breakdown of tissue nucleic acids, as with myeloproliferative and lymphoproliferative disorders. Dietary purines play an unimportant role in the generation of hyperuricemia in the absence of some derangement in purine metabolism or elimination.

Two enzyme abnormalities resulting in an overproduction of uric acid have been well described (Fig. 85–1). The first is an increase in the activity of phosphoribosyl pyrophosphate (PRPP) synthetase, which leads to an increased concentration of PRPP. PRPP is a key determinant of purine synthesis and thus uric acid production. The second is a deficiency of hypoxanthine-guanine phosphoribosyl transferase (HGPRT).

HGPRT is responsible for the conversion of guanine to guanylic acid and hypoxanthine to inosinic acid. These two conversions require PRPP as the cosubstrate and are important reutilization reactions involved in the synthesis of nucleic acids. A deficiency in the HGPRT enzyme leads to increased metabolism of guanine and hypoxanthine to uric acid and more PRPP to interact with glutamine in the first step of the purine pathway.[3] Complete absence of HGPRT results in the childhood Lesch–Nyhan syndrome, characterized by choreoathetosis, spasticity, mental retardation, and markedly excessive production of uric acid. A partial deficiency of the enzyme may be responsible for marked hyperuricemia in otherwise normal, healthy individuals.

UNDEREXCRETION OF URIC ACID

Uric acid does not accumulate as long as uric acid production is balanced with elimination. Uric acid is eliminated in two ways. About two-thirds of the uric acid produced each

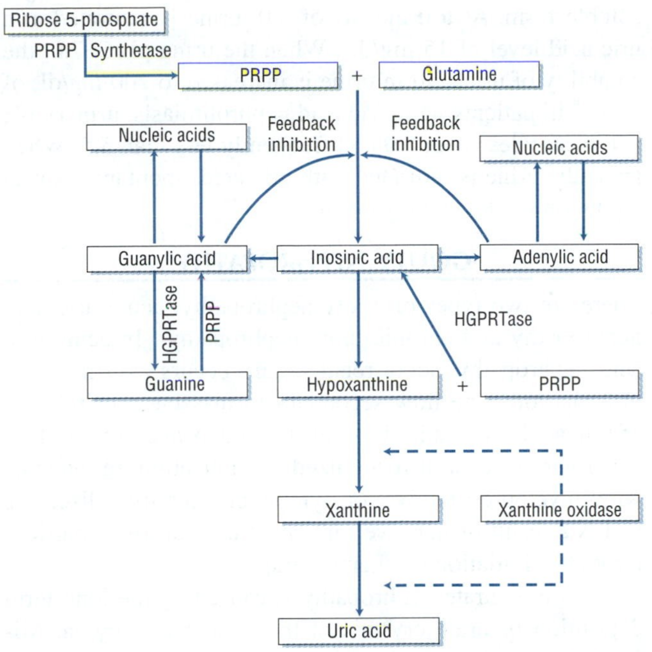

FIGURE 85–1. Purine metabolism.

day is excreted in the urine. The rest is eliminated through the gastrointestinal tract, after enzymatic degradation by colonic bacteria.

A decline in the urinary excretion of uric acid to a level below the rate of production leads to hyperuricemia and an increased miscible pool of sodium urate. Almost all the urate in plasma is freely filtered across the glomerulus. The concentration of uric acid appearing in the urine is determined by multiple renal tubular transport processes in addition to the filtered load. Evidence favors a four-component model including glomerular filtration, tubular reabsorption, tubular secretion, and postsecretory reabsorption.[2]

Approximately 90% of filtered uric acid is reabsorbed in the proximal tubule, probably by both active and passive transport mechanisms. There is a close linkage between proximal tubular sodium reabsorption and uric acid reabsorption; so states that enhance sodium reabsorption (e.g., dehydration) also lead to increased uric acid reabsorption. The exact site of tubular secretion of uric acid has not been

TABLE 85–1. Conditions Associated with Hyperuricemia

Primary gout	Obesity
Diabetic ketoacidosis	Sarcoidosis
Myeloproliferative disorders	Congestive heart failure
Lactic acidosis	Renal dysfunction
Lymphoproliferative disorders	Down's syndrome
Starvation	Lead toxicity
Chronic hemolytic anemia	Hyperparathyroidism
Toxemia of pregnancy	Acute alcoholism
Pernicious anemia	Hypoparathyroidism
Glycogen storage disease type 1	Acromegaly
Psoriasis	Hypothyroidism

TABLE 85–2. Drugs Capable of Inducing Hyperuricemia and Gout

Diuretics	Ethanol	Ethambutol
Nicotinic acid	Pyrazinamide	Cytotoxic drugs
Salicylates (< 2 g/d)	Levodopa	Cyclosporine

determined; this too appears to involve an active transport process. Postsecretory reabsorption occurs somewhere distal to the secretory site.

Factors that decrease uric acid clearance or increase its production will result in an increase in serum urate concentration. Some of these factors are listed in Table 85–1. Drugs that decrease renal clearance of uric acid through modification of filtered load or one of the tubular transport processes are listed in Table 85–2.

The pathophysiologic approach to the evaluation of hyperuricemia requires determining whether the patient is overproducing or underexcreting uric acid. This can be accomplished by placing the patient on a purine-free diet for 3 to 5 days and then measuring the amount of uric acid excreted in the urine in 24 hours. Normal individuals produce 600 to 800 mg of uric acid daily and excrete less than 600 mg in urine. Individuals who excrete more than 600 mg on a purine-free diet may be considered overproducers. Hyperuricemic individuals who excrete less than 600 mg of uric acid per 24 hours on a purine-free diet may be classified as underexcretors of uric acid. It is very difficult in clinical practice, however, to maintain someone on a purine-free diet for several days. On a regular diet, excretion of greater than 1000 mg per 24 hours reflects overproduction; less than this is probably normal.

CLINICAL PRESENTATION

Gout is a disease manifested by acute attacks of arthritis, nephrolithiasis, gouty nephropathy, and aggregated deposits of sodium urate (tophi) in cartilage, tendons, synovial membranes, and elsewhere.

ACUTE GOUTY ARTHRITIS

Acute attacks of gouty arthritis are characterized by rapid onset of excruciating pain, swelling, and inflammation. The attack is typically monoarticular at first, most often affecting the first metatarsophalangeal (MTP) joint (great toe) and then, in order of frequency, the insteps, ankles, heels, knees, wrists, fingers, and elbows. In one-half of initial attacks, the first MTP joint is affected. Of gouty patients, 90% experience attacks in the great toe at some point in their disease.

The predilection of acute gout for peripheral joints of the lower extremity is probably related to the low temperature of these joints combined with high intra-articular urate concentration. Synovial effusions are postulated to occur transiently in weight-bearing joints in the course of a day with routine activity. At night, water is reabsorbed from the joint space, leaving behind a supersaturated solution of monosodium urate, which can precipitate attacks of acute arthritis. Attacks generally begin at night with the patient awakening from sleep with excruciating pain.

The development of crystal-induced inflammation involves a number of chemical mediators causing vasodilation, increased vascular permeability, and chemotactic activity for polymorphonuclear leukocytes.[4] Phagocytosis of urate crystals by the leukocytes results in rapid lysis of cells and a discharge of proteolytic enzymes into the cytoplasm. The ensuing inflammatory reaction is associated with intense joint pain, erythema, warmth, and swelling. Fever is common, as is leukocytosis. Untreated attacks may last from 3 to 14 days before spontaneous recovery.

Although acute attacks of gouty arthritis may occur without apparent provocation, a number of conditions may precipitate an attack. These include stress, trauma, alcohol ingestion, infection, surgery, rapid lowering of serum uric acid by ingestion of uric acid–lowering agents, and ingestion of certain drugs known to elevate serum uric acid concentrations. The diagnosis is best accomplished by aspiration of synovial fluid from the affected joint and identification of intracellular crystals of monosodium urate monohydrate in synovial fluid leukocytes. Other crystal-induced arthropathies that may resemble gout on clinical presentation are caused by calcium pyrophosphate dihydrate crystals (pseudogout) and calcium hydroxyapatite crystals, which are associated with calcific periarthritis, tendinitis, and arthritis.[5,6]

URIC ACID NEPHROLITHIASIS

Nephrolithiasis occurs in 10% to 25% of patients with gout.[7] Factors that predispose individuals to uric acid nephrolithiasis include excessive urinary excretion of uric acid, an acidic urine, and a highly concentrated urine. The risk of renal calculi approaches 50% in individuals whose renal excretion of uric acid exceeds 1100 mg/d. In addition to pure uric acid stones, hyperuricosuric individuals are at increased risk for mixed uric acid–calcium oxalate stones, and pure calcium oxalate stones. Uric acid stones are usually small, round, and radiolucent. Uric acid stones containing calcium are radiopaque.[7]

Uric acid has a pK_a of 5.5. Therefore, when the urine is acidic, uric acid exists primarily in the un-ionized, less soluble form. At a urine pH of 5.0, urine is saturated at a uric acid level of 15 mg/dL. When the urine pH is 7.0, the solubility of uric acid in urine is increased to 200 mg/dL of urine.[8] In patients with uric acid nephrolithiasis, urinary pH is typically less than 6.0 and frequently less than 5.5. When an acidic urine is saturated with uric acid, spontaneous precipitation of stones may occur.

GOUTY NEPHROPATHY

There are two types of gouty nephropathy: acute uric acid nephropathy and chronic urate nephropathy.[9] In acute uric acid nephropathy, acute renal failure occurs as a result of blockage of urine flow secondary to massive precipitation of uric acid crystals in the collecting ducts and ureters. This syndrome is a well-recognized complication in patients with myeloproliferative or lymphoproliferative disorders and is a result of massive malignant cell turnover, particularly after initiation of chemotherapy.

Chronic urate nephropathy is caused by the long-term deposition of urate crystals in the renal parenchyma. Microtophi may form, with a surrounding giant cell inflammatory reaction. A decrease in the kidney's ability to concentrate urine and the presence of proteinuria may be the earliest pathophysiologic disturbances. Hypertension and nephrosclerosis are common associated findings. Although renal failure occurs in a higher percentage of gouty patients than expected, it is not clear that hyperuricemia per se has a harmful effect on the kidney. The chronic renal impairment seen in individuals with gout may result largely from the co-occurrence of hypertension, diabetes mellitus, and atherosclerosis.

TOPHACEOUS GOUT

Tophi (urate deposits) are uncommon in the general population of gouty subjects and are a late complication of hyperuricemia. The most common sites of tophaceous deposits in patients with recurrent acute gouty arthritis are the base of the great toe, helix of the ear, olecranon bursae, Achilles tendon, knees, wrists, and hands.[2] Eventually even the hips, shoulders, and spine may be affected. In addition to causing obvious deformities, tophi may damage surrounding soft tissue, cause joint destruction and pain, and even lead to nerve compression syndromes including carpal tunnel syndrome.

▶ TREATMENT: Gout and Hyperuricemia

The goals in the treatment of gout are to terminate the acute attack, prevent recurrent attacks of gouty arthritis, and prevent complications associated with chronic deposition of urate crystals in tissues.[10] Distinction must be made between the goals of therapy for the acute attack and the chronic management of hyperuricemia.

ACUTE GOUTY ARTHRITIS

Acute attacks of gouty arthritis may be treated successfully with colchicine or any of a variety of nonsteroidal anti-inflammatory drugs (NSAIDs; Fig. 85–2).

Colchicine can be given orally or parenterally. Unless contraindications exist or the patient has renal insufficiency, the usual oral dose is 1 mg initially, followed by 0.5 mg every 2 hours until the joint symptoms subside, until the patient develops abdominal discomfort or diarrhea, or until a total dose of 8 mg has been administered.[11] About 75% to 95% of patients with acute gouty arthritis respond favorably to colchicine when ingestion of the drug is begun within 24 to 48 hours of the onset of joint symptoms.[12] If the initiation of colchicine is delayed longer than 48 hours after the onset of acute symptoms, the probability of success with the drug diminishes substantially.

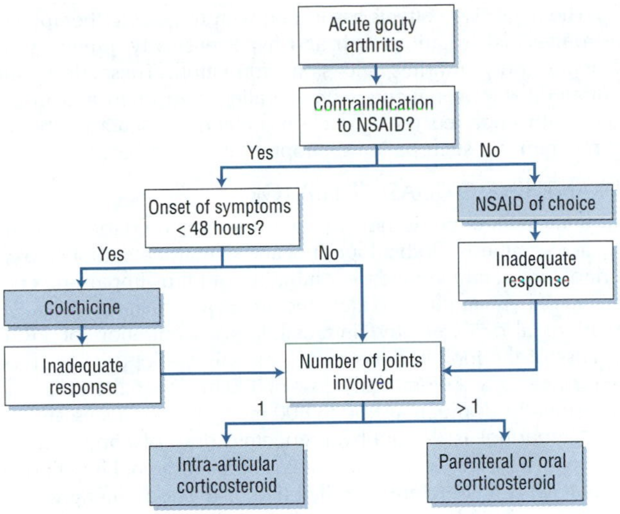

FIGURE 85–2. Treatment algorithm for acute gouty arthritis.

The major problem associated with the use of oral colchicine is that it causes gastrointestinal side effects in 50% to 80% of patients before the relief of the attack.

This high incidence of GI side effects may be circumvented by administering colchicine intravenously. Except in patients with renal insufficiency, the initial intravenous dose of colchicine is 2 mg. If relief is not obtained, an additional 1-mg dose may be given at 6 and 12 hours to a total dose of 4 mg for a specific attack. The colchicine should be diluted with 20 mL of normal saline before administration to minimize sclerosis of the vein. The intravenous administration of colchicine eliminates most of the gastrointestinal symptoms associated with the oral dose but subjects the patient to the risk of local extravasation, which can cause inflammation in and necrosis of the surrounding tissue. Very small difficult-to-inject veins and renal impairment represent relative contraindications to intravenous colchicine therapy.

Because of the risk of bone marrow toxicity, colchicine should be discontinued for 7 days following initial therapy with either oral or IV administration. Colchicine should not be used intravenously in individuals who are neutropenic, have severe renal impairment (creatinine clearance less than 10 mL/min), or have combined renal and hepatic insufficiency. The dose should be decreased by 50% in individuals with renal insufficiency (creatine clearance 10 to 50 mL/min) and limited to a total dose of 2 mg in patients receiving oral maintenance colchicine.[13]

Indomethacin is as effective as colchicine in the treatment of acute gouty arthritis. Because acute gastrointestinal toxicity occurs far less frequently with indomethacin than with colchicine, it is preferred. Side effects unique to indomethacin include headache and dizziness. All NSAIDs have been implicated in the cause of gastric ulceration and bleeding, but with short-term therapy this is not likely.

For treatment of acute gouty arthritis, indomethacin may be begun with a relatively large dose for the first 24 to 48 hours and then tapered over 3 to 4 days to minimize the risk of recurrent attacks. For example, 75 mg of indomethacin should be given initially, followed by 50 mg every 6 hours for 2 days, then 50 mg every 8 hours for 1 or 2 days.

A number of other NSAIDs (e.g., naproxen, fenoprofen, ibuprofen, piroxicam) are also effective in relieving the inflammation of acute gout. There is no evidence that any given NSAID is superior to all the others in the management of acute gout.[14] All NSAIDs should be used with caution in individuals with a history of acid peptic disease, heart failure, chronic renal failure, or coronary artery disease.

Corticosteroids may be used to treat acute attacks of gouty arthritis, but they are reserved primarily for resistant cases or for patients with a contraindication to colchicine and NSAID therapy.[14] Doses of 40 to 80 USP units of adrenocorticotropic hormone gel are given intramuscularly every 6 to 8 hours for 2 to 3 days and then the doses are reduced in stepwise fashion and discontinued. Intra-articular administration of triamcinolone hexacetonide in a dose of 20 to 40 mg may be useful in treating acute gout limited to a single joint. Prednisone may be administered orally in doses of 30 to 60 mg for 3 to 5 days in patients with multiple-joint involvement. Because rebound attacks may occur upon steroid withdrawal, the dose should be gradually tapered by 5-mg decreases over 10 to 14 days and discontinued.

NEPHROLITHIASIS

The medical management of uric acid nephrolithiasis includes hydration sufficient to maintain a urine volume of 2 to 3 L/d, alkalinization of urine, avoidance of purine-rich foods, moderation of protein intake, and reduction of urinary uric acid excretion.

Maintenance of a 24-hour urine volume of 2 to 3 L with an adequate intake of fluids is desirable for all gouty patients, but especially for those with excessive (> 1.0 g/d) uric acid excretion. Alkalinizing agents should be used with the objective of making the urine less acidic. Urine pH should be maintained at 6.0 to 6.5. In this pH range, up to 85% of uric acid will be in the form of the soluble urate ion.

Reduction of urine acidity can be accomplished by the administration of sodium bicarbonate or Shohl's solution (40 g citric acid and 98 g sodium citrate per liter). With the former, 2 to 6 g/d is given in equally divided doses at 6- to 8-hour intervals. A dose of 20 to 60 mL of Shohl's solution per day, given in three or four divided doses, provides an equivalent amount of alkali. If use of a sodium salt is contraindicated, potassium citrate may be used instead.

One must keep in mind that the older patient with uric acid kidney stones may also have hypertension, congestive heart failure, or renal insufficiency and obviously should not be exposed to overload with alkalinizing sodium salts or unlimited fluid intake. Acetazolamide, a carbonic anhydrase inhibitor, produces rapid and effective urinary alkalinization and is sometimes used in conjunction with alkali therapy. When a 250-mg dose of acetazolamide is given at bedtime, the excretion of an acidic urine in the early morning hours is avoided. The usual tachyphylaxis (rapid tolerance) to this drug is obviated by a daily repletion dose of bicarbonate.

Since the advent of allopurinol, a low-purine, low-protein diet in the patient with uric acid lithiasis is no longer as critical as it once was; however, it is still advisable to instruct the patient to avoid foods rich in purine and to limit the protein to no more than 90 g/d. Such a diet is still palatable and reduces appreciably the amount of uric acid in the urine.

The mainstay of drug therapy for recurrent uric acid lithiasis is allopurinol. It is effective in reducing both serum and urinary uric acid levels, thus preventing the formation of calculi. Allopurinol is also recommended as prophylactic treatment in the patient who will receive cytotoxic agents for the treatment of lymphoma or leukemia. The marked increase in uric acid production associated with cytolysis of a neoplasm predisposes a patient to the development of uric acid nephrolithiasis.

PROPHYLACTIC THERAPY

After the first attack of acute gouty arthritis or after the passage of the first renal stone, a decision to institute prophylactic therapy must be entertained. If the first episode was mild and responded promptly to treatment, the patient's serum urate concentration was only minimally elevated, and the 24-hour urinary uric acid excretion was not excessive (< 1000 mg/24 hours on a regular diet), then prophylactic treatment can be withheld. Some patients never have a second attack or a second stone. Others may not experience a second gouty episode for 5 to 10 years. A wait-and-see attitude, therefore, seems justified in patients who meet these conditions.[5]

On the other hand, if the patient had a severe attack of gouty arthritis, a complicated course of uric acid lithiasis, a substantially elevated serum uric acid (> 10.0 mg/dL), or a 24-hour urinary excretion of uric acid of more than 1000 mg, then prophylactic treatment should be instituted immediately after resolution of the acute episode. Prophylactic therapy is also appropriate for patients with frequent (more than two or three per year) attacks of gouty arthritis even if the serum uric acid concentration is normal or only minimally elevated.

Recurrences of acute gouty arthritis may be prevented with continuous low-dose daily oral colchicine or by uric acid–lowering therapy with either uricosuric agent or inhibition of xanthine oxidase with allopurinol. Combination therapy consisting of colchicine plus a uricosuric agent or allopurinol may be employed in resistant cases. The choice of treatment depends on the serum urate concentration, the amount of uric acid excreted in a 24-hour period, and the renal function status of the patient.

Prophylactic therapy with low-dose oral colchicine, 0.5 to 0.6 mg twice daily, may be effective in preventing recurrent arthritis in patients with no evidence of visible tophi and a normal or slightly elevated serum urate concentration.[11] Patients do not become resistant to or tolerant of daily colchicine, and, if they sense the beginning of an acute attack, they should increase the dose to 1 mg every 2 hours; in most instances the attack will abort after 1 or 2 mg of colchicine. If the serum urate concentration is within the normal range, and the patient has been symptom-free for 1 year, maintenance colchicine may be discontinued. The patient should be advised, however, that discontinuation of the treatment program may be followed by an exacerbation of acute gouty arthritis.

Patients with a history of recurrent acute gouty arthritis and a significantly elevated serum uric acid concentration are probably best managed with uric acid–lowering therapy. Colchicine at a dose of 0.5 mg twice daily should be administered during the first 6 to 12 months of antihyperuricemic therapy to minimize the risk of acute attacks that may occur during initiation of uric acid–lowering therapy. The therapeutic objective of antihyperuricemic therapy is to reduce the serum urate concentration below 6 mg/dL, well below the saturation point.

Reduction of the serum urate concentration can be accomplished pharmacologically by increasing the renal excretion of uric acid or by decreasing its synthesis. The drugs most widely used to increase uric acid excretion are probenecid and sulfinpyrazone. Several other uricosuric drugs are available in Europe, but they have not been approved for use in the United States.

URICOSURIC DRUGS

Uricosuric drugs increase the renal clearance of uric acid by inhibiting the renal tubular reabsorption of uric acid. Therapy with uricosuric drugs should be started at a low dose to avoid marked uricosuria and possible stone formation. The maintenance of adequate urine flow and alkalinization of the urine with sodium bicarbonate or Shohl's solution during the first several days of uricosuric therapy further diminish the possibility of uric acid stone formation. Probenecid is given initially at a dose of 250 mg twice a day for 1 to 2 weeks, then 500 mg twice a day for 2 weeks. Thereafter, the daily dose is increased by 500-mg increments every 1 to 2 weeks until satisfactory control is achieved or a maximum dose of 2.0 g is reached. The initial dose of sulfinpyrazone is 50 mg twice a day for 3 to 4 days, then 100 mg twice a day, increasing the daily dose by 100-mg increments each week up to 800 mg/day.

The major side effects associated with uricosuric therapy are gastrointestinal irritation, rash and hypersensitivity, precipitation of acute gouty arthritis, and stone formation. These drugs are contraindicated in patients who are allergic to them and in patients with impaired renal function (creatinine clearance below 50 mL/min); for such patients, allopurinol should be used.

XANTHINE OXIDASE INHIBITOR

Currently, allopurinol is the only approved drug used for inhibiting uric acid synthesis. Both allopurinol and its major metabolite, oxypurinol, are xanthine oxidase inhibitors, and thus impair the conversion of hypoxanthine to xanthine and xanthine to uric acid. Allopurinol also lowers the intracellular concentration of PRPP. Because of the long half-life of its metabolite, allopurinol can be given once daily. An oral daily dose of 300 mg is usually sufficient. Occasionally, as much as 600 to 800 mg/d may be necessary.

Allopurinol is the antihyperuricemic drug of choice in patients with a history of urinary stones or impaired renal function, in patients who have lymphoproliferative or myeloproliferative disorders and need pretreatment with a xanthine oxidase inhibitor before initiation of cytotoxic therapy to protect against acute uric acid nephropathy, and in patients with gout who are overproducers of uric acid. The major side effects of allopurinol are skin rash, leukopenia, occasional gastrointestinal toxicity, and increased frequency of acute gouty attacks with the initiation of therapy.

ASYMPTOMATIC HYPERURICEMIA

Questions are often raised regarding the indications for drug therapy for asymptomatic hyperuricemia. The purported benefits from treatment include prevention of acute gouty arthritis, tophi formation, nephrolithiasis, and chronic urate nephropathy. The first three complications are easily controlled should they develop; therefore, antihyperuricemic therapy is not warranted to prevent these conditions. The prevention of urate nephropathy might be a stronger indication because it is irreversible even with proper treatment. Available data indicate, however, that gouty nephropathy is extremely rare in the absence of clinical gout, and evidence that elevation of uric acid by itself may cause renal disease is weak and inconclusive.[15] As previously discussed, renal impairment is very rare in the absence of concurrent hypertension and atherosclerosis. In addition, it is unclear whether uric acid–lowering therapy protects renal function in such individuals. Available data thus do not justify therapy for most patients with asymptomatic hyperuricemia.

PHARMACOECONOMIC CONSIDERATIONS

Assuming no treatment of asymptomatic hyperuricemia, pharmacoeconomic considerations apply only to the management of the acute and chronic clinical manifestations of gout.

In a cost-effectiveness analysis in patients with nontophaceous recurrent gouty arthritis, urate-lowering therapy was found to reduce costs if patients experienced two or more recurrent attacks per year.[16] Generic allopurinol was associated with a lower incremental cost-effectiveness ratio than were either probenecid or sulfinpyrazone.

In the case of chronic tophaceous gout, a need to continue long-term therapy with a urate-lowering drug clearly exists. Allopurinol is generally less expensive than uricosuric therapy and may be more effective. Comparative trials are lacking. For severe cases, combination therapy may be indicated. Many clinicians will add colchicine to the regimen to reduce the likelihood of precipitating acute gouty arthritis, but this does not appear to be a cost-effective measure.

CONCLUSION

Hyperuricemia may lead to acute arthritis, chronic gout, or kidney stones or remain asymptomatic. Asymptomatic hyperuricemia need not be treated, especially if the serum urate concentration remains below 10 mg/dL.

Acute gouty arthritis requires either colchicine or an NSAID to treat the underlying inflammatory condition. The management of uric acid kidney stones includes hydration and alkalinization of the urine. Prevention of recurrent gouty arthritis or recurrent nephrolithiasis and treatment of chronic gout require hypouricemic therapy with either a uricosuric drug or allopurinol. Allopurinol is the hypouricemic drug of choice in patients with a history of uric acid stones or renal insufficiency and in patients known to be overproducers of uric acid.

▶ PRINCIPLES OF PHARMACOTHERAPY

- Asymptomatic hyperuricemia discovered incidentally requires no therapy.
- Acute gouty arthritis may be treated effectively with short courses of high-dose nonacetylated NSAID or colchicine.
- Individuals with contraindications to NSAID (active peptic ulcer disease, renal impairment, heart failure, or history of hypersensitivity) or individuals who cannot ingest medications orally may be treated with intravenous corticosteroids or intra-articular corticosteroids.
- Intravenous colchicine is rapidly effective but cannot be administered to individuals with renal impairment or extrahepatic biliary obstruction. A single intravenous dose should not exceed 2 to 3 mg, with a cumulative total dose not exceeding 4 to 5 mg per episode.
- Recurrent attacks of gouty arthritis can be prevented effectively through administration of uric acid–lowering therapy.
- Treatment with urate-lowering drugs is considered cost-effective for acute gouty arthritis in patients having two or more attacks of gout per year.
- When allopurinol is used, start with a low dose (100 mg/d) after the acute attack has settled, and adjust the dose every 4 weeks until the goal is reached (serum urate of < 6 mg/dL). Give colchicine (0.5 mg twice daily) during the first 3 months of therapy, and stop allopurinol if rash develops or liver function tests become abnormal.
- Uricosuric agents should be avoided in patients with renal impairment (creatinine clearance below 50 mL/min), a history of renal calculi, and overproduction of uric acid.
- Uric acid nephrolithiasis should be treated with adequate hydration (2 to 3 L/d), a daytime urinary-alkalinizing agent, and a 250-mg bedtime dose of acetazolamide.
- Individuals with tophaceous deposits have a large uric acid pool and benefit from allopurinol adminstration.

REFERENCES

1. Kelley WN, Worthman RL. Gout and Hyperuricemia. In: Kelley WN, Harris EP, Ruddy S, Sledge CB, eds. Textbook of Rheumatology. Philadelphia, Saunders, 1997:1313–1351.
2. Levinson DJ, Becker MA. Clinical gout and the pathogenesis of hyperuricemia. In: Koopman WJ, ed. Arthritis and Allied Conditions, 13th ed. Baltimore, Williams & Wilkins, 1997:2041–2071.
3. Wilson JM, Young AB, Kelley WN. Hypoxanthine-guanine phosphoribosyltransferase deficiency. N Engl J Med 1983;309:900–910.
4. Beutler A, Schumacher HR. Gout and "pseudogout": When are arthritis symptoms caused by crystal deposition? Postgrad Med 1994;95: 103–116.
5. McGill NW. Gout and other crystal arthropathies. Med J Aust 1997; 166:33–38.
6. Schumacher HR. Crystal-reduced arthritis: An overview. Am J Med 1996;100(suppl2A):46S–52S.
7. Yu T. Nephrolithiasis in patients with gout. Postgrad Med 1978;63: 164–170.
8. Worthman RL. Management of hyperuricemia. In Koopman WJ, ed. Arthritis and Allied Conditions, 13th edition. Baltimore, Williams & Wilkins, 1997:2073–2083.
9. Klineberg JR. Role of the kidneys in the pathogenesis of gout. Postgrad Med 1978;63:145–150.
10. Star VL, Hochberg MC. Prevention and management of gout. Drugs 1993;45:212–222.
11. Emmerson BT. The management of gout. N Engl J Med 1996;334: 445–451.
12. Tan N, Lertratanalcul, Barr WG. Acute gouty arthritis. Postgrad Med 1993;94:73–87.
13. Evans TI, Wheeler MT, Small RE, et al. A comprehensive investigation of inpatient intravenous colchicine use shows more education is needed. J Rheumatol 1996;23:143–148.
14. Conaghan PG, Day RO. Management and prevention of gout—risks and benefits of drugs used. Curr Therap 1995;(Apr):75–80.
15. Dykman D, Simon EE, Avioli W. Hyperuricemia and uric acid nephropathy. Arch Intern Med 1987;147:1341–1345.
16. Ferrgz MB, O'Brien B. A cost effectiveness analysis of urate lowering drugs in nontophaceous recurrent gouty arthritis. J Rheumatol 1995; 22:908–914.

86
GLAUCOMA

Timothy S. Lesar, PharmD

The glaucomas are a group of ocular disorders involving optic neuropathy characterized by changes in the optic nerve head (optic disk) and loss of visual sensitivity and field. Increased intraocular pressure (IOP), a traditional diagnostic criterion for glaucoma, plays an important role in the pathogenesis of glaucoma but is no longer a diagnostic criterion for glaucoma. Two major types of glaucoma have been identified: open angle and closed angle. Open-angle glaucoma accounts for the great majority of cases. Either type may be a primary, inherited disorder; secondary to disease, trauma, or drugs; or congenital. Both primary and secondary glaucomas may be caused by a combination of open-angle and closed-angle mechanisms (Table 86–1). Glaucoma affects up to 15 million Americans, resulting in 12,000 new cases of blindness annually. The prevalence rate varies with age, race, diagnostic criteria, and other factors. In the United States, open-angle glaucoma occurs in 1% to 2% of the population over the age of 40, the incidence increasing with age. The incidence of glaucoma varies by ethnic group, with blacks having a higher incidence (over 11% in those over the age of 80 years) than whites.[1,2] In this chapter, the pathophysiology, clinical findings, and drug therapy of glaucoma are reviewed.

PATHOPHYSIOLOGY

The specific cause of glaucomatous optic neuropathy is presently unknown. Previously, increased IOP was considered to be the sole cause of the visual damage; however, it is now recognized that IOP is only one of many factors associated with the development and progression of glaucoma. Increased susceptibility of the optic nerve due to neuropathy factors such as retinal ischemia, a reduced or dysregulated blood flow, or physiologic processes of the extracellular matrix of the optic nerve head are likely additional contributory factors. Indeed, open-angle glaucoma may represent a number of distinct diseases or conditions that simply manifest the same symptoms. Susceptibility to visual loss at a given IOP varies considerably; some patients do not demonstrate damage at high IOPs, whereas other patients have progressive visual field loss despite an IOP in the "normal" range (normal-tension glaucoma). Although IOP poorly predicts which patients will have visual field loss, the risk of visual field loss clearly increases with increasing IOP within any range. Reduction of IOP, no matter what the level of pretreatment IOP, slows or prevents progression of visual field and optic disk changes in most patients. The mechanism by which an IOP too great for the susceptibility of a given eye produces optic nerve damage remains controversial. Pressure-sensitive astrocytes and other cells in the optic disk supportive structure matrix may produce changes and remodeling of the disk, resulting in axonal death. Vasogenic theories suggest that optic nerve damage results from insufficient blood flow to the retina secondary to the perfusion pressure required in the eye, dysregulated perfusion, or vessel wall abnormalities, and results in degeneration of axonal (axoplasmal) fibers of the retina. Another theory suggests that the IOP may disrupt axoplasmal flow at the optic disk. These mechanisms, as well as others, could be operative alone or in a spectrum of combinations to produce the optic nerve damage observed in glaucoma.[1–10]

AQUEOUS HUMOR DYNAMICS AND IOP

Presently, the drug therapy of glaucoma is designed to reduce IOP, even if in the normal range, thereby reducing the risk for progression of visual loss. An understanding of IOP and aqueous humor dynamics will assist the reader in understanding the drug therapy of glaucoma.

Aqueous humor is formed in the ciliary body (Fig. 86–1) through both filtration and secretion. Because ultrafiltration depends on pressure gradients, blood pressure and IOP changes influence aqueous humor formation. Osmotic gradients produced by active secretion of sodium and bicarbonate and possibly other solutes such as ascorbate from the ciliary body epithelial cells into the aqueous humor result in movement of water from the pool of stromal ultrafiltrate into the posterior chamber, forming the aqueous humor. Carbonic anhydrase appears to be involved in this secretion of the solutes sodium and bicarbonate, and may explain the IOP-lowering effects of carbonic anhydrase inhibitors.

Receptor systems controlling aqueous inflow have not been fully elucidated. Pharmacologic studies suggest that beta-adrenergic agents increase inflow; while α_2-adrenergic, α-adrenergic blocking, β-adrenergic blocking, dopamine blocking, and adenylate cyclase-stimulating agents

TABLE 86–1. General Classification of Glaucoma

I. Primary glaucoma
   A. Open angle
   B. Angle closure
      1. With pupillary block
      2. Without pupillary block
II. Secondary glaucoma
   A. Open angle
      1. Pretrabecular
      2. Trabecular
      3. Posttrabecular
   B. Angle closure
      1. With pupillary block
      2. Without pupillary block
III. Congenital glaucoma

decrease aqueous inflow. Aqueous humor produced by the ciliary body is secreted into the posterior chamber at a rate of approximately 2 to 3 μL/min. The pressure in the posterior chamber produced by the constant inflow pushes the aqueous humor between the iris and lens and through the pupil into the anterior chamber of the eye.[1,2,11]

Aqueous humor in the anterior chamber leaves the eye by two routes: (1) filtration through the trabecular meshwork to Schlemm's canal (85% to 90%) and (2) traversal of the anterior face of the iris and absorption into iris blood vessels (uveoscleral outflow). Cholinergic agents such as pilocarpine increase outflow by physically pulling open the meshwork pores through ciliary muscle contraction. Cholinergic agents such as pilocarpine may decrease uveoscleral outflow; however, the net effect of cholinergic agents is a decrease in IOP. The uveoscleral outflow of aqueous is also increased by prostaglandin $F_{2\alpha}$ analog, and β and α_2-adrenergic agonists. Constant inflow of aqueous humor from the ciliary body and resistance to outflow result in an IOP great enough to produce an outflow rate equal to the inflow rate (Fig. 86–2).

The average IOP measured in large populations is 15.5 ± 2.5 mm Hg; however, the distribution of pressures around the mean is skewed to the right (toward higher readings). Intraocular pressure is not constant and changes with pulse, blood pressure, forced expiration or coughing, neck compression, and posture. The IOP is measured by tonometry—indentation tonometry, applanation tonometry, or a noncontact method using an air pulse. These methods may result in slightly different pressure readings. Intraocular pressures consistently greater than 21 mm Hg are found in 5% to 8% of the general population. The incidence increases with age such that abnormal IOP is found in 15% of those 70 to 75 years old. Intermittently very high IOP (>40 mm Hg) is found in patients with angle-closure glaucoma.

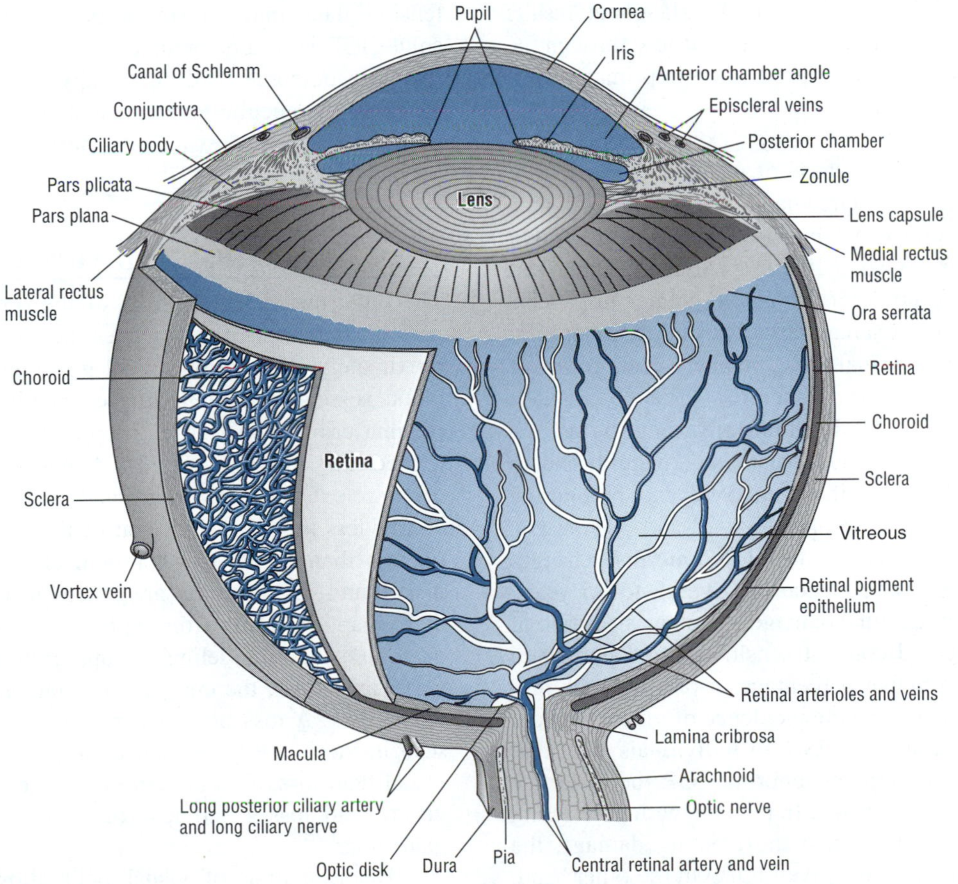

FIGURE 86–1. Anatomy of the eye. *(Redrawn from an original by Paul Beck and reproduced with permission from Anatomy of the Eye. Courtesy of Lederle Laboratories. In Vaughn D, Asbury T, Riordan-Eva P. General Ophthalmology, 14th ed. Stamford, CT, Appleton & Lange, 1995, with permission.)*

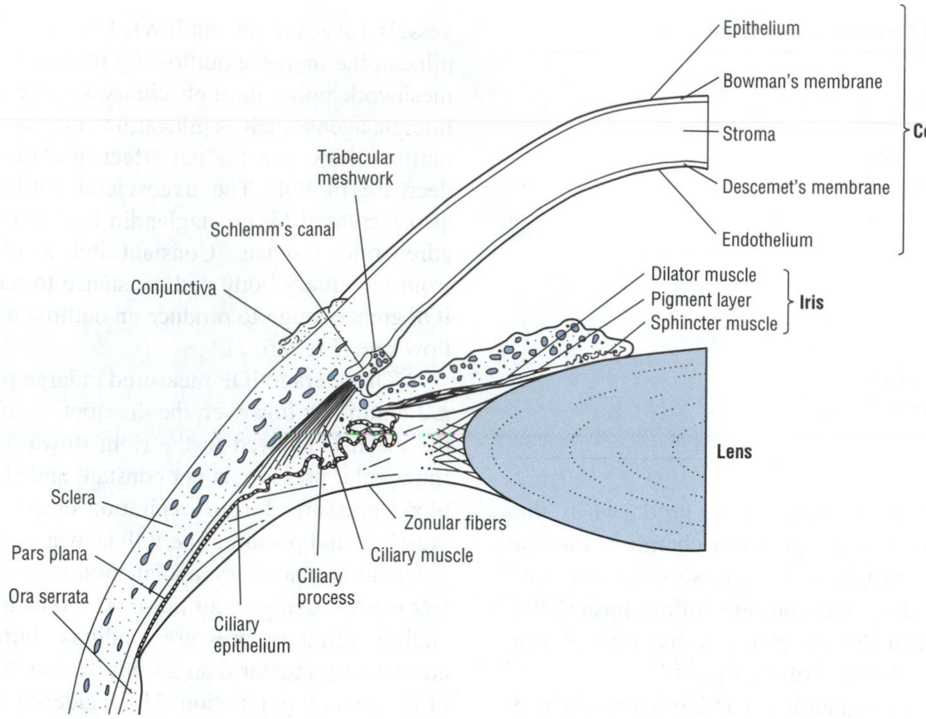

FIGURE 86–2. The anterior chamber of the eye. *(From Vaughn D, Asbury T, Riordan-Eva P. General Ophthalmology, 14th ed. Stamford, CT, Appleton & Lange, 1995, with permission.)*

The increased IOP in open-angle glaucoma results from the decreased facility for aqueous outflow through the trabecular meshwork. Aqueous production in primary open-angle glaucoma is normal.[1,2]

Intraocular pressure demonstrates considerable circadian variation, primarily because of changes in the rate of aqueous formation. This circadian variation results in a minimum IOP at approximately 6 PM and a maximum IOP at awakening. The circadian IOP variation is usually less than 3 to 4 mm Hg; however, it may be greater in patients with glaucoma. This circadian variation, and the poor relationship of IOP with visual loss, makes measurement of IOP a poor screening test for glaucoma.

Although increased IOP within any range is associated with a higher risk of glaucomatous damage, it is both an insensitive and nonspecific diagnostic and monitoring tool. Of individuals with IOP between 21 and 30 mm Hg, only 0.5% to 1% per year will develop optic disk changes and visual field loss (i.e., glaucoma) over 5 to 15 years. However, more subtle retinal damage—such as alteration of color vision, decreased contrast sensitivity, and peripheral acuity—occurs in a higher percentage of patients with IOP greater than 21 mm Hg, and the incidence of visual field defects increases to as high as 28% in individuals with IOP above 30 mm Hg. For a given abnormal IOP, the incidence of glaucoma increases with age. In patients with preexisting optic nerve damage, the worse the existing damage, the more sensitive the eye is to a given IOP. On the other hand, about 35% to 50% of patients with glaucomatous visual field loss have an IOP of less than 21 mm Hg (called normal-tension glaucoma, referring to normal IOP). Thus, the absolute IOP is a poor predictor of optic nerve damage and therefore outcome of drug therapy. More direct measurements of therapeutic outcome such as optic disk examination and visual field evaluation must also be used as monitors of drug therapy.[1,2,11–15]

OPTIC DISK AND VISUAL FIELDS

The optic disk is the portion of the optic nerve ophthalmoscopically visible as it leaves the eye. It consists of approximately one million retinal ganglion nerve cell axons, blood vessels, and supporting connective tissue structures (lamina cribosa). The small depression within the disk is termed the cup (Fig. 86–3). A normal physiologic cup does not extend below the retinal surface and has a diameter of less than one-third that of the disk (cup to disk ratio less than 0.33). The common alterations of the optic disk found in glaucoma are listed in Table 86–2. These disk changes result from optic nerve degeneration and death and the remodeling of supporting structures. As the nerve axons die, the cup becomes larger in relation to the whole disk. A loss of retinal nerve fiber layer visibility is seen in the majority of glaucoma patients with detectable visual field loss. This pattern of changes is consistent with visual field losses and loss of visual sensitivity seen in glaucoma.[1,2,14]

Determination of visual field allows assessment of optic nerve damage and is a primary monitoring parameter in treatment. However, visual field changes lag behind op-

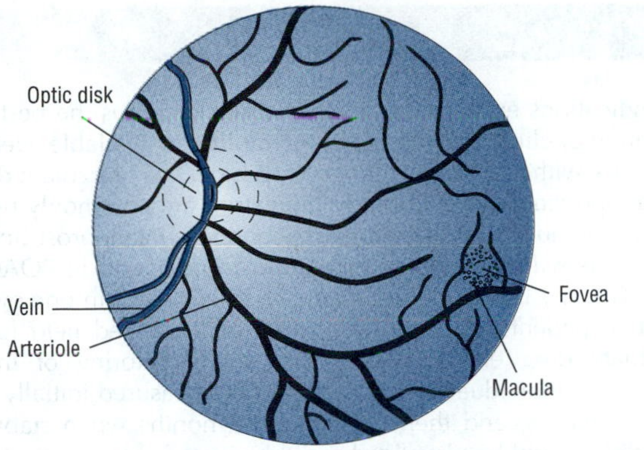

FIGURE 86–3. The normal disk fundus. *(From Vaughn D, Asbury T, Riordan-Eva P. General Ophthalmology, 14th ed. Stamford, CT, Appleton & Lange, 1995, with permission.)*

tic disk changes and a loss of 20% of axons is usually required before detectable visual field defects are noted. The peripheral visual field is measured using an automated visual field instrument called a *perimeter.* Characteristic visual field loss occurs in glaucoma (Fig. 86–4 and Table 86–2), but loss of central visual acuity does not occur until late in the disease. Other indicators such as color vision changes and contrast sensitivity may allow earlier and more sensitive detection of glaucomatous changes.[1,2]

OPEN-ANGLE GLAUCOMA

SYMPTOMS AND DIAGNOSIS

Primary open-angle glaucoma (POAG) is a bilateral, genetically determined disorder constituting 60% to 70% of all glaucomas and 90% to 95% of primary glaucomas. POAG manifests as optic nerve degeneration characterized by disk changes and visual field loss (Table 86–2). An increased IOP is not required for diagnosis of POAG. POAG is a chronic, slowly progressive disease found primarily in individuals older than 50 years, although it may occur earlier. Symptoms do not present until substantial visual field constriction occurs. Central visual acuity is typically maintained, even in the late stages of the disease. POAG is a bilateral disease; however, one eye may have greater progression of disease than the other. Detection and diagnosis involve evaluation of the optic disk and retinal nerve fiber layer, assessment of the visual fields, and measurement of IOP. The presence of characteristic disk changes and visual field loss with or without increased IOP confirms the diagnosis of glaucoma. Typical disk changes and field loss occurring at an IOP of less than 21 mm Hg account for 35% to 50% of patients, and are referred to as normal-tension glaucoma. Elevated IOP (greater than 21 mm Hg) without disk changes or visual field loss is observed in 5% to 7% of individuals (known as "glaucoma suspects"), and is referred to as ocular hypertension.[1,2,11]

TABLE 86–2. Optic and Visual Field Findings in Glaucoma

Optic Disk Findings
Cup to disk ratio greater than 0.5
Progressive increase in cup size
Cup to disk ratio asymmetry greater than 0.2
Vertical elongation of the cup
Excavation of the cup
Deepening of the cup
Increased exposure of lamina cribrosa
Pallor of the cup
Splinter hemorrhages
Cupping to edge of disk
Notching of the cup (usually superior or inferior)
Visual Field Defects in Glaucoma
General peripheral visual field constriction
Isolated scotomas (blind spots)
Nasal visual field depression (nasal step)
Enlargement of the blind spot
Large arclike scotomas
Reduced contrast sensitivity

Secondary open-angle glaucoma has many causes, including systemic diseases, trauma, surgery, rubeosis, lens changes, ocular inflammatory diseases, and medications. A system for classifying secondary glaucomas into pretrabecular, trabecular, and posttrabecular forms has been proposed. This classification allows drug therapy to be chosen on the basis of the pathogenic mechanism involved. In pretrabecular forms, a normal meshwork is covered that does not permit aqueous outflow. Trabecular forms of secondary glaucoma result from either an alteration of meshwork or an accumulation of material in the intertrabecular spaces. The posttrabecular forms result primarily from disorders causing increased visceral venous blood pressure.[1,2]

PROGNOSIS

In most cases of POAG the overall prognosis is excellent. Progression to severe visual loss is rare when POAG is discovered early and adequately treated. Patients with advanced visual field loss rarely have continued field loss if the IOP is maintained at less than 15 to 18 mm Hg; however, of patients with IOP greater than 22 mm Hg, 30% have visual loss. Thus, the keys to medical treatment of POAG are an effective, well-tolerated drug regimen, close monitoring of therapy, and compliance. Medications will successfully control IOP in 60% to 80% of patients over a 5-year period. Availability of newer highly effective, well-tolerated agents may improve the prognosis further.[1,2,14,15]

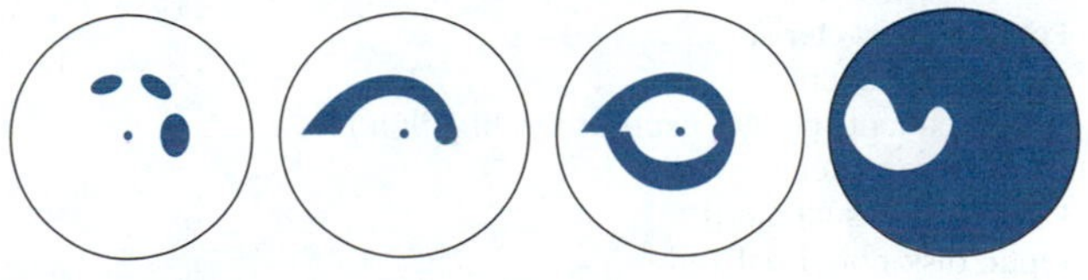

FIGURE 86–4. Schematic representation of the progression of visual field loss.

TREATMENT: Open-Angle Glaucoma

Treatment of the patient with possible glaucoma (ocular hypertension, patients with IOP > 22 mm Hg) remains controversial, because only 0.5% to 1% per year develop visual field loss. Based on the presence or absence of risk factors known to increase the chance of developing visual field loss and on the presence of certain individual traits, therapy is initiated in selected patients with elevated IOPs (Table 86–3). Patients with significant risk factors usually will be treated with a well-tolerated topical agent such as a β-blocking agent, dipivefrin, or dorzolamide, depending on individual patient characteristics. Optimally, therapy is initiated in one eye to assess efficacy and tolerance. The cost, inconvenience, and frequent side effects of combination therapies, anticholinesterase inhibitors, and oral carbonic anhydrase inhibitors result in an unfavorable risk to benefit ratio in the patient with possible glaucoma, and they are thus indicated only in high-risk patients. The goal of therapy is to lower the IOP to a level associated with a decreased risk of optic nerve damage—usually a 25% to 30% decrease, but greater decreases may be required in high-risk patients or those with higher initial IOP. Drug therapy should be monitored by measurement of IOP, examination of the optic disk, assessment of the visual fields, and evaluation of the patient for drug side effects and compliance with therapy. Patients who are unresponsive to, or intolerant of, a drug should be switched to an alternative agent rather than given an additional drug. Many clinicians prefer to discontinue all medications in patients failing to respond adequately to simple topical therapy, closely monitor for development of disk changes or visual field loss, and treat when such changes occur.[1,2,14]

All patients with characteristic optic disk changes and/or visual field defects not due to other factors (i.e., glaucoma by definition) should be treated. Some controversy exists as to whether the initial therapy of glaucoma should be surgical trabeculectomy (filtering procedure), argon laser trabeculectomy, or medical therapy.[1,2,15,16] Presently, drug therapy remains the most common initial treatment modality. Drug therapy of patients with documented glaucomatous change is initiated in a stepwise manner (Fig. 86–5), starting with lower concentrations of a single well-tolerated topical agent. Usually a β-blocker is used if no contraindications exist, as this class of drugs provides the best combination of clinical efficacy and tolerability of available agents. In patients with contraindications to β-blockers, dorzolamide, pilocarpine, and epinephrine (or dipivefrin) are commonly used as initial therapy. With additional experience, latanoprost and brimonidine will likely be considered first-line agents in POAG.

Therapy is optimally started as a single agent in one eye (except in patients with very high IOP or advanced field loss) to evaluate drug efficacy and tolerance. Monitoring of therapy should be individualized: IOP should be measured initially every 1 to 2 weeks, and then every 1 to 3 months when stabilized; the disk should be visualized and the visual field measured every 6 to 12 months (more frequently after any change in drug therapy). Patients should always be questioned regarding compliance with prescribed therapy. Initial IOP response does not predict long-term IOP control, requiring continuous regular monitoring of IOP. In patients who fail therapy, the drug concentration and/or frequency (depending on the agent being used) should be increased. Using more than one drop per dose does not improve response, but it increases the likelihood of side effects and cost of therapy. When using more than one medication, apply drops at least 5 to 10 minutes apart to provide optimal ocular contact for each agent.

The value of an agent to which the patient has shown a loss of IOP control following an initial response can be measured by discontinuing the medication completely and determining if an increase in IOP occurs. Patients responding to, but intolerant of, initial therapy may be switched to another drug or an alternative dosage form of the same medication. For patients failing to respond to the highest tolerated concentrations of an initial drug, a switch to an alternative agent after 1 day of concurrent therapy—or, if only a partial response occurs, addition of another topical drug to be used in combination—should be considered. A number of drugs or drug combinations may need to be tried before an effective and well-tolerated regimen is identified. Because of the frequency of side effects, topical cholinesterase inhibitors and oral carbonic anhydrase inhibitors are considered last-line agents to be used in patients who fail less toxic combination topical therapy.

TABLE 86–3. Considerations in Treating the "Glaucoma Suspect"

Risk Factors
IOP over 30 mm Hg
Suspicious optic disk findings
Family history of glaucoma
Systemic vascular disease
Increased age (over 65 to 70 years)
Asymmetric cups
High myopia
Optic disk hemorrhages
Increasing IOP over time
Retinal nerve fiber defects
Diabetes mellitus
Black patients
Patient Characteristics
One-eyed patients
Young patients (longer exposure to high IOP)
Unreliable patients
Unreliable visual fields
Optic disk not visualized
Patient desires treatment
Patient with retinal vascular occlusion

NONPHARMACOLOGIC THERAPY

SURGERY

When drug therapy fails, is not tolerated, or is excessively complicated, surgical procedures such as argon-laser trabeculoplasty (ALT) or a surgical trabeculectomy (filtering procedure) to produce aqueous drainage paths may be performed to improve aqueous outflow. Laser trabeculeculoplasty is usually an intermediate step between drug therapy and trabeculectomy. Procedures with higher complication rates, such as those involving placement of draining tubes or destruction of the ciliary body (cyclodestructive), may be required when other methods fail (see Fig. 86–3).[1-3,12–19]

PATIENT EDUCATION

An important consideration in patients failing to respond to drug therapy is compliance. Poor compliance or noncompliance occurs in 25% to 60% of glaucoma patients. A large percentage of patients also fail to use topical ophthalmic drugs correctly. The patient should be taught the following procedure:

- Wash and dry the hands; shake bottle if it contains a suspension.

- With a forefinger, pull down the outer portion of the lower eyelid to form a "pocket" to receive the drop.
- Grasp the dropper bottle between the thumb and fingers with the hand braced against the cheek or nose with the head upward.
- Place the dropper over the eye while looking at the tip of the bottle; then, look up and place a single drop in the eye.
- The lids should be closed (but not squeezed or rubbed) for 1 to 3 minutes after instillation. This increases the ocular availability of the drug.
- Recap bottle and store as instructed.
- Note that many patients are physically unable to administer their own eyedrops without assistance.

Nasolacrimal occlusion (NLO) should also be used to improve ocular bioavailability and reduce systemic absorption.[1,2,20] The patient induces NLO for 1 to 3 minutes by closing the eyes and placing the index finger over the nasolacrimal drainage system in the inner corner of the eye. This maneuver as well as eyelid closure itself decreases punctal drainage of drug, thereby decreasing the amount of drug available for systemic absorption from the nasopharyngeal mucosa. The use of NLO may significantly improve drug response, reduce side effects, and allow less frequent dose intervals and the use of lower drug concentrations.

Use of more than one drop per dose does not significantly improve response but may increase side effects. When two drugs are to be administered, instillations should be separated by at least 3 to 5 minutes (preferably 10 minutes) to prevent the drug administered first from being washed out. The patient should be taught not to touch the dropper bottle tip with eye, hands, or any surface.

Compliance with glaucoma therapy is commonly inadequate, and it should always be considered as a possible cause of drug therapy failure. Assessment of compliance by health care providers is generally poor, so that all patients should be continually encouraged to diligently administer prescribed therapy as instructed. To improve compliance, the patient, family, and care providers should be fully informed of the expectations of therapy and the need to continue therapy despite a lack of symptoms. Possible side effects of the medication and ways of reducing them should be discussed. Compliance will be improved by good communication, close monitoring, and use of well-tolerated and convenient drug regimens.[1–3,14]

PHARMACOLOGIC THERAPY

β-BLOCKING DRUGS

The topical β-blocking agents are the most commonly used antiglaucoma medications. β-blockers lower intraocular pressure by 20% to 30% with a minimum of local ocular side effects. These are commonly the agents of choice in treating POAG if no contraindications exist. The β-blocking agents produce ocular hypotensive effects by decreasing the production of aqueous by the ciliary body, without producing substantial effects on aqueous outflow facility. The mechanism by which blockers decrease aqueous inflow remains controversial, but it is most frequently attributed to β_2-adrenergic receptor blockade in the ciliary body.

Five ophthalmic β-blockers are presently available: timolol, levobunolol, metipranolol, carteolol, and betaxolol. Timolol, levobunolol, and metipranolol are nonspecific β-blocking agents, whereas betaxolol is a β_1-adrenergic-selective agent. Carteolol is a nonspecific blocker with intrinsic sympathomimetic activity (ISA). Despite differences in potency, selectivity, lipophilicity, and ISA, the five agents reduce IOP to a similar degree, though betaxolol has been reported to produce somewhat less lowering of IOP than timolol and levobunolol. Levobunolol may be more effective than timolol and betaxolol in reducing postcataract surgery IOP increases. Levobunolol solution is more effective in controlling IOP than other agents when given as aqueous solutions on a once-daily schedule. Timolol in the form of a gel-forming solution (Timolol XE, Merck, West Point, PA) provides equivalent IOP control with once-daily administration when compared with an equal concentration of the aqueous solution administered twice daily. The choice of a specific β-blocking agent is generally based on differences in side-effect potential and individual patient response.[1–3,12–14,18,19]

Local side effects with blockers are usually minimal, though stinging upon application occurs commonly, particularly with

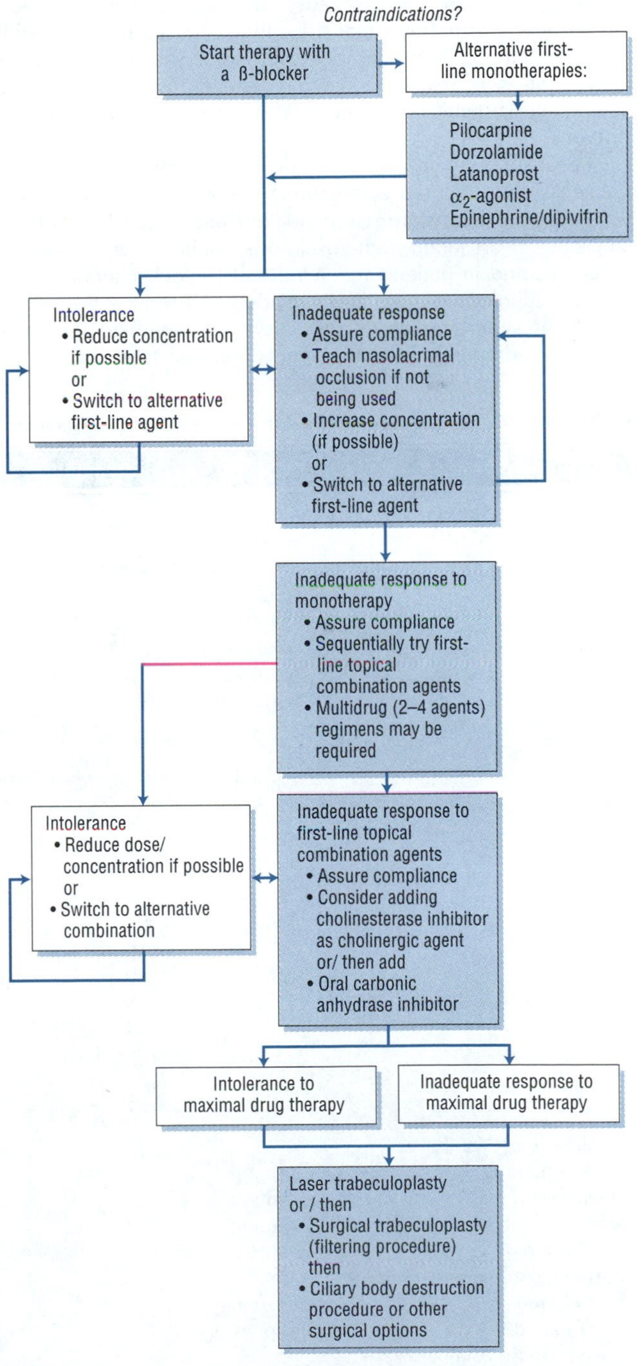

FIGURE 86–5. Algorithm for the pharmacotherapy of open-angle glaucoma.

betaxolol solution (less with betaxolol suspension) and metipranolol. Other local effects include dry eyes, corneal anesthesia, blepharitis, blurred vision, and, rarely, conjunctivitis, uveitis, and keratitis. Some local reactions may be a result of preservatives used in the commercially available products. Switching from one agent to another, or switching the type of formulation, may improve local tolerance in patients experiencing local side effects.

Systemic effects are the most important adverse effects of blockers. Drug absorbed systematically may produce decreased heart rate, reduced blood pressure, negative inotropic effects, conduction defects, bronchospasm, block symptoms of hypoglycemia, central nervous system effects, and alteration of serum lipids. The β_1-specific agents betaxolol and possibly carteolol (due to ISA) are less likely to produce the systemic side effects caused by β-adrenergic blockade, such as the cardiac effects and bronchospasm; but a real risk still exists. The use of timolol as a gel-forming liquid, or betaxolol as a suspension, allows administration of less drug per day, and therefore reduces the chance for systemic side effects compared with the aqueous solutions.

Because of their systemic side effects, all ophthalmic β-blockers should be used with caution in patients with pulmonary diseases, sinus bradycardia, second- or third-degree heart block, congestive heart failure, atherosclerosis, diabetes, and myasthenia gravis, and in patients receiving oral β-blocker therapy. Use of NLO technique during administration will reduce the risk or severity of systemic side effects as well as optimize response. Overall, β-adrenergic blocking agents are well tolerated by patients and most potential problems can be avoided by appropriate patient evaluation, drug choice, and monitoring of drug therapy. In patients failing or having an inadequate response to single drug therapy with a β-blocking agent, the addition of carbonic anhydrase inhibitor, parasympathomimetic agent, latanoprost, or an α_2-adrenergic receptor agonist will usually result in additional IOP reduction. Epinephrine or dipivefrin added to a β-blocking agent (particularly nonspecific β blockers) usually results in only minimal additional IOP reduction.[1–3]

PARASYMPATHOMIMETIC AGENTS

The parasympathomimetic (cholinergic) agents reduce IOP by increasing aqueous humor trabecular outflow. The increase in outflow is a result of physically pulling open the trabecular meshwork secondary to ciliary muscle contraction, thereby reducing resistance to outflow. These agents reduce uveoscleral outflow.

Pilocarpine, the parasympathomimetic agent of choice in POAG, is available as an ophthalmic solution, an ocular insert, and a hydrophilic polymer gel (Table 86–4). Pilocarpine produces similar (20% to 30%) reductions in IOP as seen with β-blocking agents, but limited data suggest effects on visual outcome may be poorer.[21] Pilocarpine in POAG or "glaucoma suspects" is initiated as 0.5% to 1% solution, one drop three to four times daily. The use of NLO improves response and reduces the need for an every-6-hour dosing frequency. Use of one drop of 2% pilocarpine every 6 to 12 hours and NLO provides optimal response in many patients. Both drug concentration and frequency may be increased if IOP reduction is inadequate. Patients

TABLE 86–4. Topical Agents Used in the Treatment of Glaucoma

Drug	Form	Strength (%)	Brand Name	Dose Frequency[a]	Mechanism of IOP Reduction
β-adrenergic Blockers					Decreased aqueous flow
Betaxolol	Solution	0.5	Betoptic	q 12 h	
	Suspension	0.25	Betoptic S	q 12 h	
Carteolol	Solution	1	Ocupress	q 12 h	
Levobunolol	Solution	0.25, 0.5	Betagan	q 12–24 h	
Metipranolol	Solution	0.3	OptiPranolol	q 12 h	
Timolol	Solution	0.25, 0.5	Timoptic, other	q12–24 h	
	Gelling soln.	0.25	Timoptic XE	q 24 h	
Adrenergic Agents					
α/β-agonists					Increased aqueous outflow
Epinephrine HCl	Solution	0.25, 0.5, 1, 2	Epifrin, Glaucon	q 12 h	
Epinephrine bitartrate	Solution	2		q 12 h	
Epinephryl borate	Solution	0.5, 1, 2	Epinal	q 12 h	
Dipivefrin	Solution	0.1	Propine	q 12 h	
α_2-agonists					Decreased aqueous inflow
Apraclonidine	Solution	1	Iopidine	Pre- and postop	
	Solution	0.5	Iopidine	q 8–12 h	
Brimonidine	Solution	0.2	Alphagan	q 8–12 h	
Parasympathomimetics					
Direct acting					Increased aqueous outflow
Pilocarpine	Solution	0.25–10	Numerous	q 4–12 h	
Pilocarpine	Gel	4	Pilopine HS	q 24 h	
Carbachol	Solution	0.75, 1.5, 2.25	IsoptoCarbachol	q 8–12 h	
Cholinesterase inhibitors					Increased aqueous outflow
Physostigmine	Solution	0.25, 0.5	Isopto Eserine	q 8–12 h	
Demecarium	Solution	0.125	Humorsol	q 8–72 h	
Echothiophate	Solution	0.03–0.25	Phospholine Iodide	q 12–24 h	
Isoflurophate	Ointment	0.25	Floropryl	q 8–72 h	
Carbonic Anhydrase Inhibitors					Decreased aqueous inflow
Dorzolamide	Solution	2	Trusopt	q 8–12 h	
Brinzolamide	Suspension	1	Azopt	q 8–12 h	
Prostaglandin Analog					Increased uveoscular outflow
Latanoprost	Solution	0.005	Xalatan	q 24 h	

[a]Use of nasolacrimal occlusion (NLO) may allow use of lower concentrations at longer intervals.

with darkly pigmented eyes frequently require higher concentrations of pilocarpine than patients with lightly pigmented eyes. Concentrations of pilocarpine above 4% rarely improve IOP control in patients other than those with darkly pigmented eyes.

Pilocarpine 4% gel (Pilocarpine HS) once daily is equivalent to treatment with pilocarpine solution 4% four times daily or timolol 0.5% twice daily. When using every-24-hour dosing of pilocarpine gel, the adequacy of IOP control late in the dosing interval should be confirmed.

The pilocarpine Ocusert is a solid, elliptical, sustained-release device designed for placement in the conjunctival sac and delivery of pilocarpine over a 7-day period. The Ocusert should be placed in the eye at bedtime so early side effects occur during sleep. The advantages of the Ocusert are convenience of weekly placement, possibly improved control of diurnal IOP increases, and decreased frequency of side effects. The disadvantages include a "burst" release of drug upon insertion, increased cost, discomfort, undetected loss of the device, and increased dexterity required for unit placement.

Ocular side effects of pilocarpine include miosis, which decreases night vision and vision in patients with central cataracts. Constriction of the visual field occurs secondary to miosis and should be considered when evaluating visual field changes in a glaucoma patient. Pilocarpine ciliary muscle contraction produces accommodative spasm, particularly in young patients still able to accommodate (prepresbyopic). Pilocarpine also may produce frontal headache, browache, periorbital pain, eyelid twitching, and conjunctival irritation or injection early in therapy, which tends to decrease in severity over 3 to 5 weeks of continued therapy. Cholinergics produce a breakdown of the blood–aqueous barrier and may result in a worsening of an ocular inflammatory reaction or condition. Systemic cholinergic side effects of pilocarpine—such as diaphoresis, nausea, vomiting, diarrhea, cramping, urinary frequency, bronchospasm, and heart block—are rare, but may be seen in patients using high concentrations (6% to 8%) or with overzealous use in treatment of acute angle closure. Other side effects associated with direct-acting miotics include retinal tears or detachment, allergic reaction, permanent miosis, cataracts, precipitation of angle-closure glaucoma, and rarely, miotic cysts of the pupillary margin.

Carbachol is a potent, direct-acting miotic agent; its duration of action is longer than that of pilocarpine (8 to 10 hours) because of resistance to hydrolysis by cholinesterases. This drug may also act as a weak inhibitor of cholinesterase. Patients with an inadequate response to, or intolerance of, pilocarpine as a result of ocular irritation or allergy frequently do well on carbachol. The ocular and systemic side effects of carbachol are similar but more frequent, constant, and severe than those of pilocarpine.[1–3]

The cholinesterase inhibitors most commonly used in the treatment of POAG are the long-acting, relatively irreversible agents demecarium, echothiophate, and isoflurophate (Table 86–4). These agents are potent inhibitors of pseudocholinesterase, but they also inhibit true cholinesterase. Because of the serious ocular and systemic toxic effects of these agents, the cholinesterase inhibitors are reserved primarily for patients not responding to or intolerant of other therapy. Because of their cataractogenic properties, many ophthalmologists will use these agents only in patients without lenses (aphakia) or those with artificial lenses (pseudophakia). The ocular and periocular parasympathomimetic side effects are more common and more severe than with pilocarpine or carbachol. In addition to the parasympathomimetic effects, the cholinesterase inhibitors may produce severe fibrinous iritis (particularly with the irreversible inhibitors), synechiae, iritic cysts, conjunctival thickening, and occlusion of the nasolacrimal ducts. Cataracts occur at high frequency with the use of cholinesterase inhibitors, particularly echothiophate, after about 10 to 18 months of therapy. The incidence of cataracts appears to increase with increasing concentration, with up to 60% of patients developing cataracts at higher concentrations. The inhibition of systemic pseudocholinesterase by these agents decreases the rate of succinylcholine hydrolysis, resulting in prolonged muscle paralysis. Cholinesterase inhibitors should be discontinued at least 2 weeks before procedures in which succinylcholine is to be used.

The role of cholinesterase inhibitors in glaucoma is limited by the frequency and potential toxicity of these agents. In phakic patients, cholinesterase inhibitors should be administered only if intolerance or failure results with other antiglaucoma medications. Cholinesterase inhibitors have been shown to provide additional IOP lowering effects when used with β-blockers, carbonic anhydrase inhibitors, and sympathomimetic (adrenergic) agents. Like all agents for glaucoma, therapy should be initiated with lower concentrations of these agents. A once-daily administration frequency should be used in most patients unless very high IOP is present. Use of NLO will likely improve response and reduce systemic side effects and should be done by all patients administering cholinesterase inhibitors. The cholinesterase inhibitors should be used with caution in patients with asthma, retinal detachments, narrow angles, bradycardia, hypotension, heart failure, Down's syndrome, epilepsy, parkinsonism, peptic ulcer, and ocular inflammation, and in those receiving cholinesterase inhibitor therapy for myasthenia gravis or exposure to carbamate or organophosphate insecticides and pesticides.[1–3,14]

EPINEPHRINE AND DIPIVEFRIN

The mechanism of action by which epinephrine lowers IOP has not been fully elucidated; however, a β_2-receptor mediated increase in outflow facility through the trabecular meshwork and uveoscleral route appears to be the primary mechanism. Compared with β-blockers or miotics, epinephrine and dipivefrin reduce IOP less. For this reason, epinephrine is generally used as initial therapy in patients with mild to moderate increases in IOP or in combination with other agents when only modest IOP decrease is needed. Epinephrine used in combination with parasympathetic agents, latanoprost, or carbonic anhydrase inhibitors (CAIs) result in additional IOP lowering. Epinephrine plus betaxolol may result in greater IOP reduction than when it is used in combination with nonspecific β-blockers.

Epinephrine is available as epinephrine hydrochloride, epinephrine bitartrate, and epinephryl borate solutions. Epinephryl borate and epinephrine hydrochloride are labeled as the concentration of epinephrine base; however, epinephrine bitartrate 2% is equivalent to epinephrine base 1.1%. The various salts of epinephrine produce equivalent IOP-lowering effects and adverse reactions. Patients with minor ocular irritation from one salt of epinephrine may occasionally benefit from use of another salt because of differences in pH of the commercial solutions. Use of the prodrug dipivefrin allows use of lower concentrations secondary to improved intraocular absorption (10- to 15-fold). The 0.1% dipivefrin produces equivalent IOP reduction to 1% to 2% epinephrine. Dipivefrin may therefore be tolerated by patients unable to tolerate epinephrine solutions, and it is often chosen over other epinephrine products when this class of drugs is indicated.

A factor limiting the usefulness of epinephrine is the high frequency of local ocular side effects. Tearing, burning, ocular discomfort, browache, conjunctival hyperemia, punctate keratopathy, allergic blepharoconjunctivitis, rare loss of eyelashes, stenosis of the nasolacrimal duct, and blurred vision may occur. Prolonged use (over 1 year) may result in deposition of pigment (adrenochrome) in the conjunctiva and cornea. Pigment may also deposit in soft contact lenses, turning them black. These side effects occur less frequently with dipivefrin. Epinephrine may produce mydriasis (particularly when combined with a β-blocker) and may precipitate acute angle-closure glaucoma in patients with narrow anterior chambers. A transient increase in IOP may occur with initial therapy, particularly in patients not using other antiglaucoma medications. A relative contraindication to the use of epinephrine (and dipivefrin) is aphakia (i.e., after cataract removal) or lens dislocation because of the development of degeneration of the macular portion of the retina. The edema is dose dependent and disappears with drug discontinuation.

Systemic side effects of epinephrine include headache, faintness, increased blood pressure, tachycardia, arrhythmias, tremor, pallor, anxiety, and increased perspiration. Epinephrine should be used with caution in patients with cardiovascular diseases, cerebrovascular diseases, aphakia, angle-closure glaucoma, hyperthyroidism, and diabetes mellitus, and in patients undergoing anesthesia with halogenated hydrocarbon anesthetics. Using NLO with epinephrine and dipivefrin will improve therapeutic response and reduce risk of systemic side effects.[1–3,12,13]

α_2-ADRENERGIC AGONISTS

Apraclonidine and the more lipid-soluble brimonidine are relatively selective α_2-adrenergic agonists structurally similar to clonidine. Apraclonidine is indicated (brimonidine is also effective) for prevention or control of postsurgical increases in IOP, and both are indicated as adjunctive agents in the treatment of open-angle glaucoma. Preliminary data suggest these agents may be useful in acute angle-closure glaucoma. α_2-Agonists reduce IOP by decreasing the rate of aqueous humor production (some increase in uveoscleral outflow may also occur). The drugs reduce IOP by 18% to 27% at peak (2 to 5 hours) and by 10% at 8 to 12 hours. Comparative trials demonstrate a reduction of IOP similar to that obtained with 0.5% timolol. Use of apraclonidine 0.5% or brimonidine 0.2% every 8 to 12 hours appears to provide the maximum IOP lowering effects in long-term use. Use of NLO may improve response and allow the longer dosing frequency (i.e., every 12 hours). Some patients have demonstrated a loss of IOP control with use of apraclonidine agonists for periods greater than 1 to 2 months; however, many patients demonstrate long-term IOP control. A similar loss of IOP control has not been found with brimonidine. Confirmation of continuing IOP-lowering effects with α_2-agonists is required for all patients using the class for prolonged periods. Combinations of α_2-agonists with β-blockers, latanoprost, or CAIs produces additional IOP reduction.

Local adverse effects occur frequently with apraclonidine and brimonidine. An allergic-type reaction characterized by lid edema, eye discomfort, foreign object sensation, itching, and hyperemia occurs in approximately 10% to 30% of patients and commonly necessitates drug discontinuation. Systemic side effects may be greater with brimonidine than apraclonidine and include dizziness and somnolence, dry mouth, and a reduction in blood pressure and pulse. α_2-Agonists should be used with caution in patients with cardiovascular diseases, renal compromise, cerebrovascular disease, and diabetes, and in those taking antihypertensives and other cardiovascular drugs, monoamine oxidase inhibitors, and tricyclic antidepressants.

Presently, the role of α_2-adrenergic agonists in the treatment of POAG is primarily as an alternative for patients not tolerating, with contraindications, or not responding to initial-step agents such as β-blockers, an adjunctive therapy in patients not responding adequately to other drug therapy, and for postlaser or postsurgical IOP elevation.[1–3,22,23]

CARBONIC ANHYDRASE INHIBITORS

Carbonic anhydrase inhibitors (CAI) reduce IOP by decreasing ciliary body aqueous humor secretion by up to 40% to 60%. CAIs appear to inhibit aqueous production by blocking active secretion of sodium and bicarbonate ions from the ciliary body to the aqueous humor.[1–3,24] Topical CAIs such as dorzolamide and brinzolamide are well tolerated and indicated for monotherapy or adjunctive therapy of open-angle glaucoma and ocular suspects. Relatively specific inhibitors of carbonic anhydrase enzyme II, dorzolamide, and brinzolamide reduce IOP by 15% to 26%. Administration every 8 hours provides maximal IOP reduction; however, they are not as effective as oral CAIs. Topical CAIs commonly provide additional IOP reductions when combined with other classes of antiglaucoma agents such as β-blockers, epinephrine, latanoprost, and cholinergic agents. The drug may provide additional IOP lowering in patients on maximal medical therapy for glaucoma.

CAIs are generally well tolerated. Local side effects encountered with dorzolamide include transient burning and stinging, ocular discomfort and transient blurred vision, tearing, and rare conjunctivitis, lid reactions, and photophobia. A superficial punctate keratitis occurs in 10% to 15% of patients. Systemic side effects are unusual despite the accumulation of dorzolamide in red blood cells (RBCs). Because of their favorable side-effect profile, topical CAIs provide a useful alternative agent for monotherapy, or adjunctive therapy in patients with inadequate response to, or those unable to use, a β-blocking agent. The drugs may add additional IOP reduction in patients using other single or multiple topical agents. The usual dose of dorzolamide is one drop every 8 to 12 hours. Administration every 12 hours produces less IOP reduction than administration every 8 hours. Use of NLO should optimize response to CAI given at any interval.[1,2]

Systemic CAIs are indicated in patients failing to respond to or tolerate maximum topical therapy. Systemic and topical CAIs should not be used in combination because no data exist concerning improved IOP reduction, and the risk for systemic side effects is increased. Oral CAIs reduce aqueous inflow by 40% to 60% and IOP by 25% to 40%. The available systemic CAIs (Table 86–5) produce equivalent IOP reduction but differ in potency, side effects, dosage forms, and duration of action. Despite their excellent effects on elevated IOP of any etiology, the systemic CAIs frequently produce intolerable side effects. As a result, CAIs are considered second- or third-line agents in the treatment of POAG.

TABLE 86–5. Carbonic Anhydrase Inhibitors

Drug	Strength Form	(mg)	Brand Name	Dose	IOP Reduction (h) Onset	Peak	Duration
Acetazolamide	Injection	500	Diamox	500 mg IV or IM	2 min	0.25–0.5	2–5
	Tablets	125, 250	Diamox	125–250 mg bid-qid	1–1.5	2–4	8–12
	Capsules	500	Diamox Sequels[a]	500 mg bid	2	8–12	12–24
Dichlorphenamide	Tablets	50	Daranide	25–50 mg bid-qid	0.5–1	2–4	6–12
Methazolamide	Tablets	50	Neptazane	25–100 mg bid-tid	2–4	6–8	10–12

[a]Sustained-release capsule.

On average, only 30% to 60% of patients are able to tolerate CAI therapy for prolonged periods. Intolerance to CAI therapy most commonly results from a symptom complex thought to result from systemic acidosis that includes malaise, fatigue, anorexia, nausea, weight loss, altered taste, depression, and decreased libido. Other side effects include renal calculi, increased uric acid, blood dyscrasias, diuresis, and myopia. Elderly patients do not tolerate CAIs as well as younger patients. The three available CAIs produce the same spectrum of side effects; however, the drugs differ in the frequency and severity of the side effects listed. Acetazolamide (standard or sustained-release capsules) and methazolamide are commonly considered the best-tolerated CAIs.

CAIs should be used with caution in patients with sulfa allergies, sickle-cell disease, respiratory acidosis, pulmonary disorders, renal calculi, electrolyte imbalance, hepatic disease, renal disease, diabetes mellitus, or Addison's disease. Concurrentuse of a CAI and a diuretic may rapidly produce hypokalemia. High-dose salicylate therapy may increase the acidosis produced by CAIs, while the acidosis produced by CAIs may increase the toxicity of salicylates.[1–3,12,13]

PROSTAGLANDIN $F_{2\alpha}$ ANALOGS

Analogs of prostaglandin $F_{2\alpha}$ such as latanoprost reduce IOP by increasing the uveoscleral outflow of aqueous humor. Reduction in IOP with one drop of 0.005% latanoprost is similar to or greater than that seen with timolol 0.5% twice daily. In addition, nocturnal control of IOP is improved compared to timolol. Interestingly, administration of latanoprost twice daily may reduce the IOP control compared to single daily dosing. Latanoprost is well tolerated, and produces fewer systemic side effects than timolol, but an increase in the frequency of ocular reactions such as punctate corneal erosions and conjunctival hyperemia occurs. Altered iris pigmentation occurs in 7% to 22% of patients, particularly those with mixed-color irisis (blue-brown, green-brown, blue-gray-brown, or yellow-brown eyes), which become more brown in color over 3 to 12 months. The frequency of iris pigmentation changes increases with corresponding increases in the duration of treatment. The long-term consequences of this pigment change are unknown. Latanoprost can be used in combination with other antiglaucoma agents for additional IOP control due to its unique mechanism of action. Given its excellent efficacy and side-effect profile, latanoprost provides an alternative monotherapy or adjunctive therapy in patients not responding to or tolerating other agents. Studies of long-term tolerance, efficacy, and the implications of iris pigmentation changes are needed to clearly define the place of latanoprost in glaucoma therapy.[1–3,25,26]

FUTURE DRUG THERAPIES

New agents, improved formulations, and novel approaches to the reduction of IOP and other methods of prevention of glaucomatous visual field loss will hopefully provide more effective and better-tolerated therapies. A number of drug classes have been shown to reduce IOP including cannabinoids, dopamine-blocking agents, angiotensin-converting enzyme (ACE) inhibitors, and calcium channel blockers.[1,2,4–9] Ethacrynic acid improves aqueous outflow through the trabecular meshwork by making it more permeable. Other agents such as steroid receptor antagonists, which act to improve trabecular meshwork aqueous outflow, are being investigated.

Agents that act through mechanisms other than IOP reduction are likely to be part glaucoma therapy in the future. Such agents may act as either "retinal nerve protectants" or through regulation of retinal blood flow. Examples of this approach include oral calcium channel blockers and nitrates, which may improve or maintain visual fields in patients with glaucoma by regulating retinal blood flow.

ANTIPROLIFERATIVES USED IN GLAUCOMA SURGERY

Surgical methods for reduction of IOP involve the creation of a channel through which aqueous humor can flow from the anterior chamber to the subconjunctival space ("filtering bleb"), where it is reabsorbed by the vasculature. A major reason for failure of the procedure is healing and scarring of the sight. Modification of the healing process to maintain patency is possible with the use of antiproliferative agents. The antiproliferative agents 5-fluorouracil (5-FU) and mitomycin are used in patients undergoing glaucoma filtering surgery to improve success rates by reducing the inflammatory response and fibroblast proliferation. Although most commonly used in patients with increased risk for suboptimal surgical outcome (postcataract and previous failed filtering procedure), use of these agents also improves success in low-risk patients.[27]

EVALUATION OF THERAPEUTIC OUTCOMES

The ultimate goal of drug therapy in the glaucoma patient is to preserve visual function through the reduction of the IOP to a level at which no further optic nerve damage occurs. Because of the poor relationship between IOP and optic nerve damage, no specific target IOP exists. Indeed, drugs used to treat glaucoma agents may partially act to halt visual loss through mechanisms separate from, or in addition to, IOP reduction such as improvements in retinal or choroidal blood flow. Often a 25% to 30% reduction is desired, but greater reductions (40% to 50%) may be desired in patients with initially high IOP. For patients with glaucoma, an IOP less than 21 mm Hg is generally desired, with progressively lower target pressures desired for greater levels of glaucomatous damage. Even lower IOP (possibly even below 10 mm Hg) is required in patients with very advanced disease, those showing continued damage at higher IOP, and those patients with normal-tension glaucoma and pretreatment pressures in the low to mid-teens. The IOP considered acceptable for a patient is often a balance of desired IOP and acceptable treatment related toxicity.

ANGLE-CLOSURE GLAUCOMA

Primary angle-closure glaucoma accounts for 5% or less of primary glaucomas; however, when acute angle-closure occurs, it must be treated as an emergency to avoid visual loss. Angle-closure glaucoma results from mechanical blockage of the (usually normal) trabecular meshwork by the peripheral iris. Partial or complete blockage of the meshwork occurs intermittently, resulting in extreme fluctuations between normal IOP with no symptoms and very high IOP with symptoms of acute angle-closure glaucoma. Between attacks of angle-closure glaucoma, the IOP is usually normal unless the patient has concomitant POAG. Primary angle-closure glaucoma occurs in patients with inherited shallow anterior chambers, which produce a narrow angle between the cornea and iris or tight contact between the iris and lens ("pupillary block"). Secondary angle-closure glaucoma results from any cause (synechiae) of trabecular meshwork blockade by the iris. The presence of a narrow angle is determined by visualization of the angle by gonioscopy. Other tests for angle-closure glaucoma involve provocation of an angle-closure-induced IOP increase. These tests attempt to produce angle closure through mydriasis (dark room test, mydriasis test) or by gravity (prone test) and measure any increase in IOP resulting from the provocative test.

Two major types of primary angle-closure glaucoma have been described: angle closure with pupillary block and angle closure without pupillary block. Angle closure with pupillary block results when the iris is in firm contact with the lens. This produces a relative block of aqueous flow through the pupil to the anterior chamber, resulting in a bowing forward of the iris, which blocks the trabecular meshwork. Angle closure with pupillary block most commonly occurs when the pupil is in mid-dilation. In this position the combination of pupillary block and relaxed iris allows the greatest bowing of the iris; however, angle closure may occur during miosis or mydriasis.

Angle-closure glaucoma without pupillary block occurs in patients with an abnormality called a plateau iris. The iris root of these patients is inserted anteriorly, very close to the trabecular meshwork. Mydriasis causes the peripheral iris to bunch up and block the meshwork. The mydriasis produced by anticholinergic drugs or any other drug results in precipitation of both types of angle-closure glaucoma, whereas drug-induced miosis may produce pupillary block.

Patients with untreated angle-closure glaucoma typically experience intermittent prodromal symptoms brought on by precipitating events. The symptoms include blurred or hazy vision with halos around lights, caused by a hazy, edematous cornea, and occasionally headache.

Increased IOP during such prodromal episodes is not great enough or long enough to produce the other symptoms of a full-blown attack. Such prodromal attacks last 1 to 2 hours, at which time pupillary block is broken by further mydriasis or miosis, or miosis occurs in patients with plateau iris. Acute angle closure produces the symptoms associated with a cloudy, edematous cornea, ocular pain or discomfort, nausea, vomiting, abdominal pain, and diaphoresis. On examination, the patient is found to have a closed angle, narrow anterior chamber, hyperemic conjunctiva, and an edematous and hyperemic optic disk. The rate at which IOP increases may be a determinant of when full-blown symptoms occur. Visual fields demonstrate generalized constriction. In prolonged attacks, total loss of vision may occur if the IOP is high enough. Tonometry reveals IOPs as high as 40 to 90 mm Hg.

The goal of initial therapy for angle-closure glaucoma is rapid reduction of the IOP to preserve vision and to avoid surgical or laser iridectomy on a hypertensive, congested eye. Iridectomy is the definitive treatment of angle-closure glaucoma; it produces a hole in the iris that permits an aqueous flow to move directly from the posterior chamber to the anterior chamber. Drug therapy of an acute attack typically involves administration of pilocarpine, hyperosmotic agents, and a secretory inhibitor (β-blocker, α_2-agonist, topical or systemic CAI). With miosis produced by pilocarpine, the peripheral iris is pulled away from the meshwork. Though traditionally the drug of choice, the use of pilocarpine as initial therapy is controversial. Miotics may worsen angle closure by increasing pupillary block and producing anterior movement of the lens because of drug-induced accommodation.

At IOPs greater than 60 mm Hg, the iris may be ischemic and unresponsive to miotics; as the pressure drops and the iris responds, miosis occurs. During this time, the tendency to use excessive amounts of pilocarpine must be avoided. The dose of pilocarpine commonly used is a 1% to 2% solution instilled every 5 minutes for 2 or 3 doses, then every 4 to 6 hours. However, many practitioners withold application of pilocarpine until IOP has been reduced by other agents, and then apply a single drop of 1% to 2% pilocarpine to produce miosis. In either case, the unaffected contralateral eye should be treated with the miotic every 6 hours to prevent development of angle closure. An osmotic agent is also commonly administered because these drugs produce the most rapid decrease in IOP (Table 86–6). Oral glycerin or isosorbide can be used if an oral agent is tolerated; if not,

TABLE 86–6. Osmotic Agents Used in Glaucoma

Drug	Molecular Weight	Strength (%)	Dose (g/kg)	Route	Ocular Distribution[a]	Penetration[b]	IOP Reduction (h)		
							Onset	Peak	Duration
Mannitol	182	5, 10, 15, 20, 25	1–2	IV	Extracellular	Poor	025	0.5–1	6–9
Urea	60	30	1–1.5	IV	Total	Good	0.25	1–2	5–6
Glycerin	92	50, 75	1–2	PO	Extracellular	Moderate	0.25	0.5–1.5	4–6
Isosorbide	146	45	1–2	PO	Total	Good	0.25	0.5–1.5	4–6

[a]Distribution in body water.
[b]Prefer poor intraocular penetration for greater blood–eye osmotic gradient and IOP reduction.

intravenous mannitol should be used. Osmotic agents reduce IOP by withdrawing water from the eye secondary to the osmotic gradient between the blood and the eyes. These drugs are among the first-line agents in the treatment of angle-closure glaucoma or other forms of acute IOP elevations. Topical corticosteroids are often used to reduce the ocular inflammation in angle-closure eyes. Once the IOP is controlled, pilocarpine should be given every 6 hours until iridectomy is performed. Patients failing therapy altogether will require an emergency iridectomy. Because peripheral iridectomy essentially "cures" primary angle-closure glaucoma, long-term drug therapy is not used.[1,2]

DRUG-INDUCED GLAUCOMA

A number of medications have been associated with increased IOP or carry labeling that cautions against use of the medication in glaucoma patients. The potential for a medication to produce or worsen glaucoma depends on the type of glaucoma and whether or not the patient is adequately treated.

Patients with treated, controlled POAG are at minimal risk of induction of an increase in IOP by systemic medications with anticholinergic properties or vasodilators; however, in the patient with untreated glaucoma or uncontrolled POAG, the potential of these medications to increase IOP should be considered. Topical anticholinergic agents used to produce mydriasis may result in an increase in IOP. Potent anticholinergic agents such as atropine or homatropine are most likely to increase the IOP. Weaker anticholinergics such as tropicamide that produce less cycloplegia are less likely to increase the IOP and are favored, along with phenylephrine, when mydriasis is desired in the POAG patient. Inhaled, nasal, topical, or systemic glucocorticoids may produce increased IOP in both normal individuals and patients with POAG.

Patients with POAG appear to be particularly susceptible to glucocorticoid-induced increases in IOP. Glucocorticoids reduce the facility of aqueous outflow through the trabecular meshwork. The decreased facility of outflow appears to result from the accumulation of extracellular material blocking the trabecular channels. The potential of a glucocorticoid to increase IOP is related to its anti-inflammatory potency and intraocular penetration. Thus, patients should be treated with the lowest potency and dose and for the shortest time possible when steroids are indicated.

In patients predisposed to angle-closure glaucoma (i.e., narrow anterior chambers), angle closure may be produced by any drug that produces mydriasis or swelling of the lens (such as sulfa compounds). The topical use of anticholinergics or sympathomimetic agents is most likely to result in angle closure. Systemic anticholinergic and sympathomimetic agents must also be used with caution in such patients. As previously discussed, potent miotic agents such as echothiophate may produce angle closure by increasing pupillary block. Drugs associated with potentiation of glaucoma are listed in Table 86–7.[1,2]

TABLE 86–7. Drugs That May Induce or Potentiate Glaucoma

Open-angle Glaucoma
Ophthalmic corticosteroids (high risk)
Systemic corticosteroids
Nasal/inhaled corticosteroids
Fenoldapam
Ophthalmic anticholinergics
Vasodilators (low risk)
Cimetidine (low risk)
Angle-closure Glaucoma
Topical anticholinergics (high risk)
Topical sympathomimetics (high risk)
Antihistamines
Systemic anticholinergics
Heterocyclic antidepressants
Phenothiazines
Ipratropium
Benzodiazepines
Theophylline (low risk)
Vasodilators (low risk)
Systemic sympathomimetics (low risk)
CNS stimulants (low risk)
Tetracyclines (low risk)
Carbonic anhydrase inhibitors (low risk)
Monoamine oxidase inhibitors (low risk)
Topical cholinergics (low risk)

CONCLUSIONS

Glaucoma is a group of primary and secondary diseases, management of which presents a considerable challenge to the pharmacotherapist. Successful therapy requires rational use of antiglaucoma medications by the clinician and patient compliance with the selected regimen, combined with conscientious monitoring for side effects and disease progression. The reward for successful therapy is considerable: the maintenance of vision. The overview of the clinical findings, pathology, and drug therapy presented in this chapter provides the clinician with the fundamentals necessary to understand and treat glaucoma.

▶ PRINCIPLES OF PHARMACOTHERAPY

- The objective of treating primary open-angle glaucoma is to reduce intraocular pressure.
- Effective glaucoma therapy stops progression of visual field loss.
- Each patient needs an effective, well-tolerated, and convenient drug regimen for treating glaucoma.
- Topical glaucoma medications have the potential to produce systemic adverse effects.
- Patient and family education is necessary to assure compliance and successful outcomes for treating glaucoma.

REFERENCES

1. Ritch R, Shields MB, Krupin T. The Glaucomas, 2nd ed. St. Louis, Mosby, 1996.
2. Epstein DL, ed. Chandler and Grant's Glaucoma. 4th ed. Baltimore, Williams & Wilkins, 1997.
3. Fiscella RG, Winarko T. Glaucoma. New therapeutic options. US Pharmacist 1996;21:55–64.
4. Schumer RA, Podos SM. The nerve of glaucoma. Arch Ophthalmol 1994;112:37–44.
5. Nernandez MR, Pena JDO. The optic nerve head in glaucomatous optic neuropathy. Arch Ophthalmol 1997;115:389–395.
6. Fechtner RD, Weinreb RN. Mechanisms of optic nerve damage in primary open angle glaucoma. Surv Ophthalmol 1994;39:23.
7. Drance SM. Glaucoma: A look beyond intraocular pressure. Am J Ophthalmol 1997;123:817–819.
8. Mao LK, Stewart WC, Shields MB. Correlation between intraocular pressure control and progressive damage in primary open angle glaucoma. Am J Ophthalmol 1991;111:51–55.
9. Grunwald R, DuPont J, Dreyer EB. Effect of chronic nitrate treatment on retinal vessel caliber in open-angle glaucoma. Am J Ophthalmol 1997;123:753–758
10. Bose S, Piltz JR, Breton ME. Nimodipine, a centrally active calcium antagonist, exerts a beneficial effect on contrast sensitivity in patients with normal-tension glaucoma and in control patients. Ophthalmology 1995;102:1236–1241.
11. Caprioli J. The aqueous. In: Hart WM, ed. Adler's Physiology of the Eye: Clinical Applications, 9th ed. St. Louis, Mosby, 1992.
12. Serle JB. Pharmacologic advances in the treatment of glaucoma. Drugs Aging 1994;5:156–170.
13. Novack GD, Robin AL, Derick RJ. New medical treatments for glaucoma. Int Ophthalmol Clin 1993:33:183–202.
14. Taniguchi T, Kitazawa Y. A risk-benefit assessment of drugs used in the management of glaucoma. Drug Saf 1994;11:68–74.
15. Sherwood MB, Migdal CS, Hitchings RA, et al. Initial treatment of glaucoma: Surgery or medications. Surv Ophthalmol 1993:37:293–305.
16. Stewart WC, Sine CS, LoPresto C. Surgical vs medical management of chronic open-angle glaucoma. Am J Ophthalmol 1996;122:767–774.
17. Sorenson SJ, Abel SR. Comparison of the ocular beta blockers. Ann Pharmacother 1996;30:43–54.
18. Brooks AMV, Gilies WE. Ocular beta-blockers in glaucoma management. Drugs Aging 1992;2:208–221.
19. Kaiser H, Flammer J, Stumpfig D, Hendrickson P. Long term visual field follow up of glaucoma patients treated with beta-blockers. Surv Ophthalmol 1994;38(suppl):S156–S160.
20. Zimmerman TJ, Sharir M, Nardin GF, Fuqua M. Therapeutic index of pilocarpine, carbachol, and timolol with nasolacrimal occlusion. Am J Opthalmol 1992;114:1–7.
21. Vogel R, Crick RP, Mills KB, et al. Effect of timolol versus pilocarpine on visual field progression in patients with primary open angle glaucoma. Ophthalmology 1992;99:1505–1511.
22. Stewart WC, Ritch R, Shin DH, et al. The efficacy of apraclonidine as an adjunct as timolol therapy. Arch Opthalmol 1995;113:287–292.
23. Schuman JS, Horwitz B, Choplin NT, et al. A 1-year study of brimonidine twice daily in glaucoma and ocular hypertension. Arch Ophthalmol 1997;115:847–852.
24. Wikerson M, Cyrlin M, Lippa EA, et al. Four-week safety and efficacy study of dorzolamide, a novel, active topical carbonic anhydrase inhibitor. Arch Ophthalmol 1993;111:1343–1350.
25. Camras CB. Comparison of latanoprost and timolol in patients with ocular hypertension and glaucoma. Ophthalmology 1996;103:138–147.
26. Watson P, Stjernschantz J. A six-month, randomized, double masked study comparing latanoprost with timolol in open angle glaucoma and ocular hypertension. Opthalmology 1996;103:126–137.
27. Skuta GL. Antifibrotic agents in glaucoma filtering surgery. Int Ophthalmol Clin 1993;33:165–182.

87

ALLERGIC RHINITIS

J. Russell May, PharmD

Rhinitis is inflammation of the nasal mucous membrane. Allergic rhinitis is caused by mucous membrane exposure to inhaled allergenic materials that elicit a specific immunologic response. It is characterized by sneezing, nasal itching, and watery rhinorrhea, often associated with nasal congestion. Itching of the throat, eyes, and ears frequently accompanies allergic rhinitis. There are two types of allergic rhinitis. Seasonal allergic rhinitis, commonly known as hay fever, occurs in response to specific allergens present seasonally—in the spring or fall. Seasonal allergens include pollen from trees, grasses, and weeds and typically cause more acute symptoms. Perennial allergic rhinitis is a year-round disease caused by nonseasonal allergens such as house dust mites, animal dander, and molds, typically resulting in subtle, chronic symptoms. Unfortunately, some patients have a combination of these two types of allergic rhinitis, suffering all year with seasonal exacerbations.

EPIDEMIOLOGY AND ETIOLOGY

Allergic rhinitis is one of the most common medical disorders found in humans. It affects 20% of the American population and ranks as the sixth most prevalent chronic illness in the United States.[1] Patients are limited in their ability to do normal daily functions, concentration is impaired, sleep is disturbed, social interaction is limited, and emotional well-being is affected.[2] The impact of allergic rhinitis goes well beyond these minor inconveniences. Potentially serious complications may occur, such as those related to the paranasal sinuses, eustachian tube, olfaction, and possibly lower airways. Patients with allergic rhinitis have a threefold increase in risk of asthma.[3]

PREDISPOSING FACTORS

There is a strong genetic predisposition to allergic rhinitis. A family history of allergic rhinitis, atopic dermatitis, or asthma suggests that rhinitis is allergic. Likewise, a personal history of other atopic diseases (e.g., atopic dermatitis as an infant) predisposes a person to the development of allergic rhinitis later in life.[4,5] The risk of developing allergic rhinitis is approximately 30% for children with one atopic parent and approaches 50% for those with two allergic parents.[1] Peak incidence occurs in childhood and adolescence, with approximately 70% of patients developing symptoms by the age of 30 years.[6]

Allergen exposure is another predisposing factor. For allergic rhinitis to occur, an individual must be exposed to a protein that elicits the allergic response in that individual. Many potential sufferers never develop symptoms because they never come into contact with the appropriate allergen.

For reasons that are unclear, positive skin tests indicating allergen sensitization have been observed more frequently in people in higher socioeconomic classes and in people who live in suburban areas compared with those living in more crowded and polluted inner city areas.[7,8] Further epidemiologic studies are needed to confirm and explain these findings. Once symptoms have started, they can be exacerbated by various nonspecific irritants, such as cigarette smoke, strong odors, air pollution, and climatic changes.

ALLERGENS

Allergens that produce seasonal rhinitis are the protein components of airborne pollen grains from a variety of trees, grasses, and weeds. Ragweed and grass pollen are the most common offenders in the United States; however, this changes with the geographic region. In general, tree pollens cause symptoms in the spring, grass pollens cause symptoms in the late spring to summer, and weed pollens are the culprits in the late summer to early fall. Patients who are hypersensitive to all three may have overlapping problem periods that can lead to a misdiagnosis of perennial rhinitis. Flowering plants that depend on insect pollination do not usually cause allergic rhinitis.

To complicate matters further, the antigenic components of many grasses are similar, resulting in cross-allergenicity. These include fescue, Kentucky bluegrass, orchard, redtop, and timothy. Fortunately, the trees that produce many of the offending airborne pollens produce pollens that are antigenically distinct. These trees include ash, beech, birch, cedar, hickory, maple, oak, poplar, and sycamore.

Mold spores are also significant allergens. Spores are present year-round; however, there are seasonal increases because of mold growth on decaying vegetation. Thus mold spores can be responsible for both perennial and seasonal allergies.

Indoor allergens are usually present perennially; most important among these are house dust mites, animal dander, cockroaches, and certain mold species.

PHYSIOLOGY AND PATHOPHYSIOLOGY

NASAL PHYSIOLOGY

Knowledge of nasal physiology aids in the understanding of allergic rhinitis. The nose performs three air-conditioning

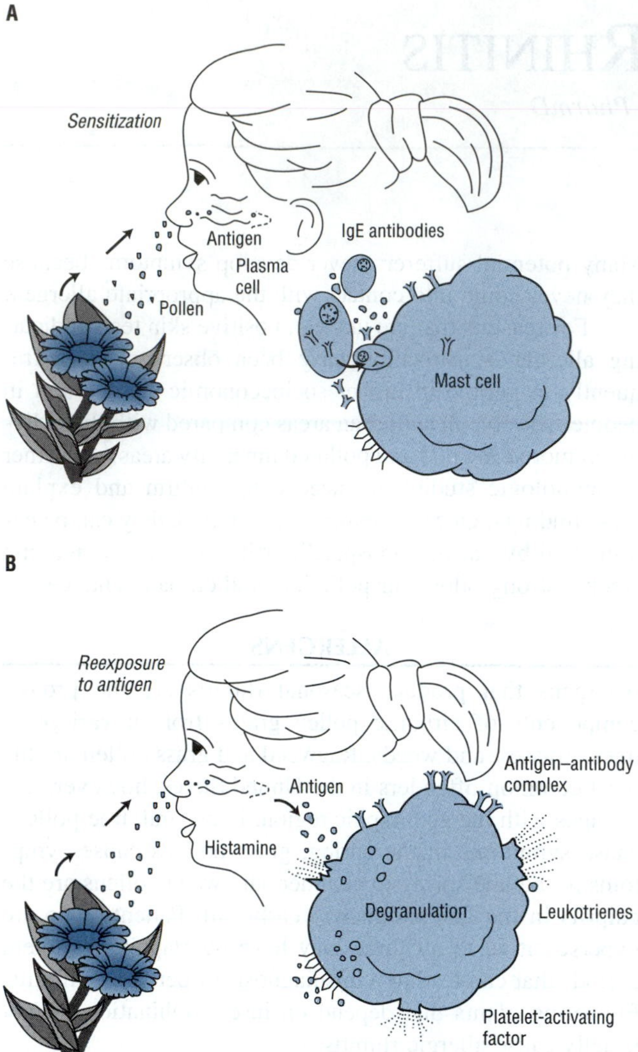

FIGURE 87–1. Allergen sensitization and the allergic response. **A.** Exposure to antigen stimulates IgE production and sensitization of mast cells with antigen-specific IgE antibodies. **B.** Subsequent exposure to the same antigen produces an allergic reaction when mast cell mediators are released.

functions to prepare the air for the lungs. During the fraction of a second that air is in the nose, it is heated, humidified, and cleaned. The cleaning process plays a role in the development of allergic rhinitis. As the air passes through the nose, the turbulence throws particulate matter against a mucous blanket. The rhythmic movements of the nasal cilia cause the mucous blanket to move posteriorly at approximately 9 mm/min, where it is eventually swallowed; therefore, foreign particles are removed via the gastrointestinal tract and do not reach the lungs.

The vascular tissue in the nose is erectile. Stimulation of sympathetic fibers causes vasoconstriction, reduction in erectile tissue size, and airway widening. Parasympathetic stimulation causes vasodilatation, increase in erectile tissue size, and airway narrowing.[9]

Located in the nasal mucosa are the mast cells, which participate in the regulation of nasal patency by releasing mediators such as histamine and others as described below.

IMMUNE RESPONSE

Allergic reactions in the nose are mediated by antigen–antibody responses involving allergens interacting with specific IgE molecules bound to nasal mast cells and basophils. In allergic subjects these cells are increased in both number and reactivity. During inhalation, airborne allergens enter the nose and are processed by lymphocytes, which produce antigen-specific IgE, thereby sensitizing genetically predisposed hosts. Upon nasal reexposure, IgE bound to mast cells interacts with the airborne allergen, triggering release of inflammatory mediators (Fig. 87–1).[10]

Both immediate and late-phase reactions are observed after allergen exposure. The immediate reaction occurs within minutes, resulting in the rapid release of preformed mediators and newly generated mediators from the arachidonic acid cascade as the mast cell membrane is disturbed (Table 87–1).[11] These mediators of immediate hypersensitivity include histamine, leukotrienes C4, LTD4, LTE4, prostaglandin D_2, tryptase, and kinins.[9,12] In addition the mast cell has been found to be a source of several cytokines that are probably relevant to the chronicity of the mucosal inflammation that characterizes allergic rhinitis.[13] The physiologic responses to these inflammatory mediators include vasodilatation, increased vascular permeability, and

TABLE 87–1. Mast Cell Mediators

Mediator	Effect
Performed and Rapidly Released	
Histamine	Stimulates irritant receptors Pruritis Vascular permeability Mucosal permeability Smooth muscle contraction
Neutrophil chemotactic factor	Influx of inflammatory cells
Eosinophil chemotactic factor	Influx of inflammatory cells
Kinins	Vascular permeability
N-α-tosyl L-arginine methyl esterase	Vascular permeability
Newly Generated	
Leukotrienes	Smooth muscle contraction Vascular permeability Mucus secretion Chemotaxis Mucus secretion Neutrophil chemotaxis
Thromboxanes	Smooth muscle spasm
Platelet-activating factor	Mucus secretion Airway permeability Chemotaxis Vascular permeability
Granule Matrix Contents	
Heparin	Anti-inflammatory
Tryptase	Protein hydrolysis
Kallekrein	Protein hydrolysis

the production of nasal secretions.[9,14] Histamine, probably the most important mediator,[11] causes vascular engorgement leading to nasal congestion, directly stimulates secretion of mucus, and increases glandular secretion.

Several hours after the initial exposure to an allergen, a late-phase reaction may occur. This reaction involves an influx of inflammatory cells (e.g., eosinophils, monocytes, macrophages, basophils) and activation of the rich lymphocyte population.[15,16] The patient experiences renewed allergic symptoms without additional allergen exposure. With repeated allergen exposure this late-phase reaction may become virtually continuous, resulting in persistent nasal inflammation.[17] The inflamed mucosa becomes hyperresponsive, characterized by exacerbation of nasal symptoms when the patient is exposed to nonspecific or irritant triggers. Subsequent exposure to lower doses of the same allergen produces repeated or persistent nasal symptoms in the "primed" host.

CLINICAL PRESENTATION

The patient with allergic rhinitis typically complains of clear rhinorrhea, paroxysms of sneezing, nasal congestion, postnasal drip, and pruritic eyes, ears, nose, or palate. Symptoms of allergic conjunctivitis are more frequently associated with seasonal than perennial allergic rhinitis. A majority of the perennial allergens, such as dust mites and molds, are indoors where air velocity is too low for substantial deposition of allergenic particles on the conjunctiva.

Symptoms secondary to the late-phase reaction, predominantly nasal congestion, begin 3 to 5 hours after antigen exposure and peak at 12 to 24 hours. Subsequent symptoms, both allergic and irritant, are more easily elicited because of the "priming effect." For instance, a ragweed-sensitive patient, when exposed to ragweed pollen out of season, responds with modest symptoms and may be very tolerant of irritants such as air pollution or tobacco smoke. During the ragweed season, however, when the nasal mucosa is already inflamed, exposure to small doses of pollen or to irritants to which the patient is usually tolerant elicits a more severe response.

DIAGNOSIS

Allergic rhinitis is differentiated from other causes of rhinitis by a thorough history, physical examination, and certain diagnostic tests. The medical history consists of a careful description of symptoms, environmental factors and exposures, results of previous therapy, use of other medications, previous nasal injuries, previous nasal or sinus surgery, family history, and the presence of other medical problems. Identification of specific causative allergens may be difficult. For example, a reaction induced by mowing the yard may not be caused by grass pollens, but by the disturbance of various weeds, molds, or other plants in the lawn. With perennial allergic rhinitis the cause-and-effect relationship is less clear, making the diagnosis more difficult.[18] This is especially true with such covert allergens as house dust mites and molds.

Physical examination may reveal allergic shiners, a transverse nasal crease caused by repeated rubbing of the nose, and adenoidal breathing. Pale, bluish, edematous nasal turbinates coated with thin, clear secretions are characteristic. Tearing, conjunctival injection and edema, and periorbital swelling may be present.

Nasal scrapings will provide a representative sample of cells infiltrating the nasal mucosa and can be helpful in supporting the diagnosis.[19] Microscopic examination of the nasal smear from an allergic individual will typically show numerous eosinophils. The peripheral eosinophil count may be elevated in allergic rhinitis, but it is nonspecific and has limited usefulness.[20]

The diagnostic evaluation is supported by determination of the presence or absence of specific IgE by allergen skin testing or *in vitro* assays (e.g., the radioallergosorbent test, or RAST). Two different methods of skin testing are available. The epicutaneous test, also known as the scratch or prick test, is performed by making a superficial wound in the outermost layer of skin. A drop of antigen is placed in the wound and allowed to diffuse into the underlying skin. The intradermal test is performed by injecting 0.01 to 0.05 mL of diluted allergen between the layers of skin. With both procedures, a positive test produces a wheal and flare reaction within 15 to 30 minutes. The epictaneous-prick test is the fastest and least expensive screening tool; intradermal tests should be reserved for patients who give negative prick tests but in whom there is a high degree of suspicion of an allergic etiology.[21]

The variability in potency and stability of skin testing extracts has led to a movement for the development of standardized extracts, which have a defined potency and are labeled with a common unit, the bioequivalent allergy unit (BAU).[22] This provides the allergist with guidance in selecting common safe and effective doses for diagnosis and treatment. Skin test results may vary depending on the anatomic site, method of skin testing, or even time of day at which the test is performed.[21] Also, the concurrent use of antihistamines or sympathomimetics may alter the test response. The allergens available for testing are numerous and include extracts of tree, grass, and weed pollens, and molds, foods, and other miscellaneous inhalants. Selection should be based on patient history.

RAST is an *in vitro* assay for measurement of specific IgE that is rarely justified in clinical practice because it is more expensive and less sensitive than skin tests.[23] Such *in vitro* testing may be useful when appropriate specific skin test extracts are not available, when negative controls produce a wheal reaction, when antihistamine therapy cannot be discontinued, or in the presence of dermatographia.[8] Total IgE levels are elevated in only 30% to 40% of allergic rhinitis patients, and it is also elevated in some nonallergic conditions, thus limiting its diagnostic usefulness.[8,20]

COMPLICATIONS

Not only is allergic rhinitis aggravating, it frequently leads to further complications, particularly if the patient does not receive adequate treatment. Untreated rhinitis symptoms may lead to inability to sleep, chronic malaise, fatigue, and poor work or school efficiency. Patients are often plagued by loss of smell or taste, with sinusitis or polyps underlying many cases of allergy-related hyposmia.[24,25] Postnasal drip with cough can also be bothersome.

The role of allergic rhinitis in the development of acute otitis media or chronic middle ear effusion remains controversial. Children with allergic rhinitis appear to be at greater risk due to nasal obstruction, insufflation of nasal secretions into the middle ear via the eustachian tube, and eustachian tube obstruction and negative middle ear pressure.[26] Hearing problems in children related to middle ear effusion may lead to delayed development of language in young children or school problems in older children.[27]

Structural facial and dental problems can result from chronic allergic rhinitis.[28,29] The chronic edema and venous stasis may contribute to the development of a high-arched, V-shaped palate. Mouth breathing caused by nasal obstruction can be responsible for dental malocclusion and orthodontic problems.[28,29] Constant upward rubbing of the nose *(allergic salute)* can cause a permanent transverse crease across the lower nose; nasal congestion leads to venous pooling and dark circles under the eyes known as *allergic shiners.*

Allergic rhinitis is clearly a risk factor for asthma, with approximately 90% of asthmatics younger than 16 years having allergies.[20] Asthma is more common in those with perennial than seasonal allergic rhinitis, and it is less likely to be "outgrown" when associated with allergic rhinitis.[30–32]

Recurrent and chronic sinusitis are relatively common complications of allergic rhinitis.[33] Nasal polyps are less common but nonetheless bothersome; they require specific therapy but may improve with management of the underlying allergic state. Epistaxis can also be a problem; it is related to mucosal hyperemia and inflammation.

▶ TREATMENT: Allergic Rhinitis

DESIRED OUTCOME

The therapeutic goal for patients with allergic rhinitis is to minimize or prevent symptoms. This goal should be accomplished with no drug side effects or at least minimal and tolerable side effects with minimal medication expense. The patient should be able to maintain a normal life-style including participating in outdoor activities, yard work, and playing with pets as desired.

GENERAL APPROACH TO TREATMENT

Once the causative allergens and the specific symptoms are identified, management consists of three possible approaches: (1) allergen avoidance, (2) pharmacotherapy for prevention or treatment of symptoms, and (3) specific immunotherapy. The pharmacotherapy for preventing or treating symptoms includes several options that are based on patient-specific information (Table 87–2).

AVOIDANCE

Avoidance of offending allergens is the most direct method of preventing allergic rhinitis, but it is often the most difficult to accomplish, especially with perennial allergens. Mold growth can be reduced by maintaining household humidity below 50% and removing obvious growth with bleach or disinfectant. Patients

TABLE 87–2. Pharmacotherapeutic Options

Medication Class	Symptoms Controlled	Comments
Antihistamines		
Systemic	Sneezing, rhinorrhea, itching, conjunctivitis	For seasonal allergic rhinitis, begin treatment before allergen exposure. Older, less expensive agents should be tried first. If sedation is a problem, move to nonsedating choices. For perennial allergic rhinitis, use as an alternative to or in combination with an intranasal steroid.
Ophthalmic	Conjunctivitis	Logical addition to nasal steroids if ocular symptoms are present.
Intranasal	Sneezing, rhinorrhea, nasal pruitis	Option for seasonal allergic rhinitis. Warn patients of potential drowsiness.
Decongestants		
Systemic	Nasal congestion	Only needed when nasal congestion is present.
Topical	Nasal congestion	Only needed when nasal congestion is present. Do not exceed 3 to 5 days.
Intranasal corticosteroids	Sneezing, rhinorrhea, itching, nasal congestion	For seasonal allergic rhinitis, an option when congestion is present. Must begin therapy before allergen exposure. Excellent choice for perennial rhinitis.
Mast cell stabilizers	(See Comments)	Prevents symptoms therefore, for seasonal allergic rhinitis, use before offending allergen's season. For perennial rhinitis, improvement may not be seen for up to a month.
Intranasal anticholinergics	Rhinorrhea	Reserve for use when above therapies fail or cannot be tolerated.

sensitive to animals will benefit most by removing pets from the home; however, most animal lovers are reluctant to comply. Cats may be more of a problem than dogs. Cat allergen is so prevalent that 25 percent of cat-free houses surveyed contained detectable cat allergen.[34] Species differences may exist with dogs; therefore a person may be allergic to one dog but not another.

Efforts to eliminate dust mites should be rigorous, particularly in the bedroom. Exposure to dust mites can be reduced by encasing mattresses and pillows with impermeable covers and washing bed linens in hot water.[35] Washable area rugs are preferable to wall-to-wall carpeting. Acaricide treatment of carpets has been shown to denature the dust mite allergen. Atopic infants who are exposed to high levels of dust mites are at increased risk for developing asthma.[36] Environmental control of these allergens may be helpful in forestalling further rhinitis and preventing later asthma.

Older central air-filtration systems for houses were expensive and minimally effective. High-efficiency particulate air (HEPA) filters have minimal effect on the heavy mite allergens, but are effective in removing lightweight particulates including pollens, mold spores, and cat allergen, thus reducing allergic respiratory symptoms.[37]

Patients with seasonal allergic rhinitis should keep windows closed and minimize time spent outdoors during pollen seasons. Using fans that direct outside air into the house should be avoided. Filter masks can be worn while gardening or mowing the lawn.

When avoidance is impractical, unacceptable to the patient, or produces only a partial response, pharmacotherapeutic approaches can be used to prevent and treat allergic rhinitis.

PHARMACOLOGIC THERAPY

First-line therapeutic modalities for treating allergic rhinitis are directed at relief of symptoms. This group includes antihistamines and decongestants (both oral and topical). Knowledge of pathophysiology and the inflammatory state has led to prophylactic therapy for more severe disease with cromolyn and topical steroids. One may have difficulty interpreting the medical literature for a variety of reasons, including lack of uniformity in the research methodologies, inappropriate drug controls, and failure to identify types of rhinitis (perennial versus seasonal and allergic versus nonallergic).

ANTIHISTAMINES

Histamine H_1-receptor antagonists are competitive antagonists to histamine. They bind to H_1 receptors without activating them, preventing histamine binding and activity.[38] Newer antihistamines may also inhibit mediator release; however, the exact mechanism is not understood. Antihistamines are now available in oral, ophthalmic, and intranasal dosage forms.

Antihistamines are more effective in preventing the actions of histamine than in reversing these actions once they have taken place. Reversal of symptoms is, at least in part, caused by the anticholinergic properties of these drugs. This activity is responsible for the drying effect of antihistamines, which reduces the problem of nasal, salivary, and lacrimal gland hypersecretion. Antihistamines antagonize capillary permeability, wheal-and-flare formation, and itching.

Histamine H_2-receptor antagonists, such as cimetidine and ranitidine, may have some effect on histamine-induced nasal blockage.[8] Combining one of these agents with an H_1 antagonist may result in decreased nasal congestion.[39] At the present time, the H_2 antagonists have no established role in treating allergic rhinitis.

In general, the antihistamines are well absorbed, have a large volume of distribution, and are metabolized by the liver. There appears to be considerable interpatient variation in mean serum half-life.[38] Also, the therapeutic effects of these agents are more prolonged than might be predicted by their half-lives.

Drowsiness is usually the chief complaint of patients who take antihistamines. Drowsiness can interfere with a patient's ability to drive a car or operate machinery and may interfere with a patient's ability to function adequately at the workplace. The sedative effects of antihistamines vary from class to class. Table 87–3 lists common antihistamines and their relative potential for causing sedation. The table also gives the agents' relative anticholinergic effects.

The sedative effects of antihistamines can be useful in patients who suffer from sleeplessness caused by the symptoms of allergic rhinitis. In these patients, a bedtime dose may prove beneficial. The mechanism for sedation is not well understood, but its central effect depends on the drug's ability to cross the blood–brain barrier.[40] Most older antihistamines are lipid soluble and cross this barrier easily.

Most of the newer "second generation" agents are highly selective peripheral histamine H_1-receptor antagonists with little or no central or autonomic nervous system effects. The term "nonsedating" antihistamines has been used to describe these agents. This group includes: astemizole, fexofenadine, and loratadine. Cetirizine is also peripherally acting, but the sedation rate is greater than with the other agents.

Another important differentiation between second generation agents is the potential for drug interactions. Astemazole may cause arrhythmias (QT prolongation syndrome and torsade de pointes), especially in patients with hepatic impairment or when combined with drugs that inhibit their metabolism (e.g., azole antifungals and macrolide antibiotics). Fexofenadine, an active metabolite of terfenadine (recently removed from the market), is renally eliminated unchanged, and therefore the drug interactions are not a problem.

The second-generation agents should not be automatically substituted for older agents. Many patients respond to and tolerate the older agents quite well. Because many of the older agents are generically available, they are much less expensive. Average wholesale price of many of the generically available agents is less than \$5 for a 30-day supply, compared with more than \$50 for some of the nonsedating agents.

Anticholinergic (drying) effects lend to the agents' therapeutic efficacy. Dry mouth, difficulty in voiding urine, constipation, and potential cardiovascular effects may be troublesome. Table 87–3 lists several antihistamines and their relative anticholinergic effects. Keep in mind that the differences may be small. Patients with a predisposition to urinary retention (e.g., elderly men, those on concurrent anticholinergic therapy) should use antihistamines with caution. Caution should also be used in patients with increased intraocular pressure, hyperthyroidism, and cardiovascular disease.

Other side effects of antihistamines include loss of appetite, nausea, vomiting, and epigastric distress.

Antihistamines are more effective when taken approximately 1 to 2 hours before the anticipated exposure to the offending allergen. If tolerance develops to the therapeutic effect, change to an agent in a different chemical class may be effective.

Patients should be counseled about the proper use of antihistamines. Side effects, especially drowsiness, should be emphasized. Patients should be warned against taking other central nervous system depressants, including alcohol. Patients should be told not to take a double dose when a dose is missed. Taking the antihistamine with meals or at least a full glass of water will help prevent the gastrointestinal side effects (e.g., nausea, vomiting, epigastric distress). Patients should check with their pharmacists and read labels before taking nonprescription medications. Many cold products and sleep aids contain antihistamines. Patients

TABLE 87–3. Relative Side-Effect Profile of Antihistamines

Agent	Relative Sedative Effect	Relative Anticholinergic Effect
Alkylamine Class		
Brompheniramine maleate	Low	Moderate
Chlorpheniramine maleate	Low	Moderate
Dexchlorpheniramine maleate	Low	Moderate
Ethanolamine Class		
Carbinoxamine maleate	High	High
Clemastine fumarate	Moderate	High
Diphenhydramine hydrochloride	Low	High
Ethylenediamine Class		
Pyrilamine maleate	Low	Low to none
Tripelennamine hydrochloride	Moderate	Low to none
Phenothiazine Class		
Methdilazine hydrochloride	Low	High
Promethazine hydrochloride	High	High
Trimeprazine	Moderate	High
Poperadine Class		
Azatadine maleate	Moderate	Moderate
Cyproheptadine hydrochloride	Low	Moderate
Diphenylpyraline hydrochloride	Low	Moderate
Phenindamine tartrate	Low to none	Moderate
"Second-generation" Peripherally Selective Class		
Astemizole	Low to none	Low to none
Cetirizine	Low to moderate	Low to none
Fexofenadine	Low to none	Low to none
Loratadine	Low to none	Low to none

should be instructed not to use more than one antihistamine at a time. Table 87–4 lists the recommended dosages of the commonly prescribed agents.

For seasonal allergic rhinitis, an intranasal antihistamine, azelastine is available. Intranasal azelastine has been shown to be comparable to oral chlorpheniramine and cetirizine.[41,42] Patient satisfaction seems to be high due to the rapid relief of symptoms. Patients should be warned of the potential for drowsiness. The systemic availability of this product is approximately 40%.[43]

Allergic conjunctivitis, often associated with allergic rhinitis, can be treated with an ophthalmic antihistamine such as levocabastine or olopatadine. Systemic antihistamines usually are effective for allergic conjunctivitis making the ocular product unnecessary. However, these agents are a logical addition to nasal steroids when ocular symptoms occur.

TABLE 87–4. Oral Dosages or Commonly Prescribed Antihistamines and Decongestants

Drug	Dosage and Interval	
	Adults	*Children*
Antihistamines		
Chlorpheniramine maleate, plain	4 mg every 6 h	6–12 yr: 2 mg every 6 h 2–6 yr: 1 mg every 6 h
Chlorpheniramine maleate, sustained release	8–12 mg at HS or 8–12 mg every 8 h	6–12 yr: 8 mg at bedtime < 6 yr: not recommended
Diphenhydramine HCl	25–50 mg every 8 h	5 mg/kg/d divided every 8 h (up to 25 mg per dose)
Clemastine fumerate	1.34 mg twice daily to 2.68 mg three times daily	Not recommended
Astemizole	10 mg once daily	< 6 yr: 0.2 mg/kg daily
Loratadine	10 mg once daily	10 mg once daily
Fexofenadine	60 mg twice daily	Not recommended
Cetirizine	5 to 10 mg once daily	> 6 yr: 5 mg once daily
Decongestants		
Pseudoephedrine	60 mg every 4–6 h 120 mg every 12 h for sustained release	6–12 yr: 30 mg every 4–6 h 2–5 yr: 15 mg every 4–6 h
Ephedrine sulfate	25–50 mg every 4 h	2–3 mg/kg/d divided every 4 h (up to 25 mg every 4 h)
Phenylpropanolamine	25 mg every 4 h or 50 mg every 8 h for sustained release	6–12 yr: 12.5 mg every 4 h 2–5 yr: 6.25 mg every 4 h

DECONGESTANTS

Topical and systemic decongestants are sympathomimetic agents that act on adrenergic receptors in the nasal mucosa, producing vasoconstriction. Decongestants shrink swollen mucosa and improve ventilation. When nasal congestion is part of the clinical picture, decongestants work well in combination with antihistamines.

Topical Decongestants

Topical decongestants are applied directly to swollen nasal mucosa via drips or sprays. Table 87–5 lists some of the common topical decongestants and their duration of action. The use of these agents results in little or no systemic absorption.

Because these agents are extremely effective and available to patients over the counter (OTC), they are widely used. Prolonged use of these agents (more than 3 to 5 days) can result in a condition known as rhinitis medicamentosa or rebound vasodilation with associated congestion. Patients who develop this condition use more spray more often with less response. Although the methods used to treat this "addiction" have not been formally studied, several are commonly used. Abrupt cessation works, but it is difficult because of rebound congestion that may leave the patient congested for several days or weeks. Sleeping may become difficult. Nasal steroids have been used successfully, but they take several days to work. Weaning the patient off topical decongestants can be accomplished by decreasing the dosing interval or the concentration over several weeks. Combining the weaning process with nasal steroids may prove useful.

Other side effects of topical decongestants include burning, stinging, sneezing, and dryness of the nasal mucosa.

Patients should be counseled on the use of topical decongestants to prevent rhinitis medicamentosa. Patients should be instructed to use as small a dose as possible as infrequently as possible and only when absolutely necessary (e.g., at bedtime to aid in falling asleep). Duration of therapy should always be limited to 3 to 5 days.

Systemic Decongestants

Oral decongestants are not as effective on an immediate basis as the topical agents but they may last longer and cause less local irritation. Also, rhinitis medicamentosa is not a problem. The most commonly used agents are pseudoephedrine, phenylpropanolamine, and ephedrine.

The pharmacokinetic variables for pseudoephedrine, phenylpropanolamine, and ephedrine are summarized in Table 87–6.

The therapeutic index for phenylpropanolamine is very low. It can produce severe or life-threatening hypertension at less than three times the usual OTC dose of 37.5 mg.[44,45] The therapeutic index for ephedrine is also low; doses exceeding two to three times the therapeutic dose can cause clinically important hypertension.[44]

TABLE 87–5. Duration of Action of Topical Decongestants

Drug	Duration (h)
Short acting	
Phenylephrine hydrochloride	Up to 4
Intermediate acting	
Naphazoline hydrochloride	4–6
Tetrahydralazine hydrochloride	
Long acting	
Oxymetazoline hydrochloride	Up to 12
Xylometazoline hydrochloride	

TABLE 87–6. Pharmacokinetic Variables of Systemic Decongestants

Drug	Half-life (h)	Mechanism of Metabolism or Elimination
Pseudoephedrine	3–8	Partially metabolized; majority excreted unchanged in urine
Ephedrine	3–6	Majority excreted unchanged in urine
Phenylpropanolamine	3–4	Majority excreted unchanged in urine

Pseudoephedrine appears to be the safest of the three. Doses of 180 mg have been shown to produce no measurable change in blood pressure or heart rate.[46] In higher doses (210 to 240 mg), pseudoephedrine has raised both blood pressure and heart rate.[47] All three systemic decongestants can cause mild central nervous system stimulation, even at therapeutic doses.

Table 87–4 lists the usual doses for pseudoephedrine, phenylpropanolamine, and ephedrine. Because most of the studies on the effect of decongestants on blood pressure were performed in normotensive patients, hypertensive patients should, unless absolutely necessary, avoid these drugs, especially phenylpropanolamine and ephedrine. Severe antihypertensive reactions can occur with any of these agents when given with monoamine oxidase inhibitors.[48]

As with antihistamines, patients should be encouraged to read product labels to avoid therapeutic duplications. Because most OTC appetite suppressants contain phenylpropanolamine, they should not be taken in combination with decongestants.

COMBINATION PRODUCTS

Numerous products combining an antihistamine with a decongestant are available. The combination seems rational because of the different mechanisms of action. Two well-controlled studies have documented the efficacy of pseudoephedrine in combination with triprolidine.[49,50] On the basis of these two studies, the Food and Drug Administration upgraded this product's designation to "effective." Some of the second-generation antihistamines are available in combination with a decongestant. As previously mentioned, patients should read labels to avoid therapeutic duplication. The therapeutic benefit of products containing more than one antihistamine has not been demonstrated.

NASAL STEROIDS

Nasal steroids are an excellent choice for treating perennial rhinitis and can be useful in seasonal rhinitis especially if dosed in advance of symptoms. Nasal steroids appear to be effective with minimal side effects. In one consensus report, nasal steroids are recommended as initial therapy with avoidance of allergens in seasonal allergic rhinitis and perennial rhinitis.[51]

Multiple mechanisms are involved with the effects of nasal steroids on the nasal mucosa, including reducing inflammation by blocking mediator release, suppressing neutrophil chemotaxis, reducing intracellular edema, causing mild vasoconstriction, and inhibiting mast cell-mediated late-phase reactions.[52] Table 87–7 lists the available nasal steroids and their usual doses.

Topical steroids produce only minor side effects, the most common being sneezing, stinging, headache, and epistaxis. Suppression of the hypothalamic–pituitary–adrenal axis has not been a problem with therapeutic doses.[53] Local infections with *Candida albicans* have occurred rarely.

TABLE 87–7. Dosages of Topical Steroids

Drug	Dosage and Interval
Beclomethasone dipproprionate	> 12 yr: 1 inhalation (42 μg) per nostril 2–4 times a day (maximum, 336 μg/d) 6–12 yr: 1 inhalation per nostril 3 times per day
Budesonide	> 6 yr: 2 sprays (64 μg) per nostril in AM and PM, or 4 sprays per nostril in AM (maximum, 256 μg)
Flunisolide	Adults: 2 sprays (50 μg) per nostril twice daily (maximum, 400 μg) Children: 1 spray per nostril 3 times a day
Fluticasone	Adults: 2 sprays (100 μg) per nostril once daily; after a few days decrease to 1 spray per nostril Adolescents: (> 12 yr): 1 spray per nostril once daily (maximum, 200 μg/d)
Triamcinolone acetonide	> 12 yr: 2 sprays (110 μg) per nostril once daily (maximum, 440 μg/d)

The therapeutic benefits of topical steroids are not immediate. Patients need to understand this to ensure cooperation and continuation of therapy. Some patients notice improvement in a few days, but peak responses may not be observed for 2 to 3 weeks. Once a response is achieved the dosage may be reduced. Blocked nasal passages should be cleared with a decongestant before administration to ensure adequate penetration of the spray. Patients should be advised to try to not sneeze or blow their nose for at least 10 minutes after administration. Topical steroids should not be used in patients with nasal septum ulcers or recent nasal surgery or trauma.

OTHER INHALANT MEDICATIONS

Cromolyn sodium and ipratropium bromide offer two additional approaches to treating allergic rhinitis. Cromolyn sodium is a mast cell stabilizer. Increased interest in this product has resulted from it becoming available over-the-counter. Ipratropium bromide is an anticholinergic agent useful in perennial allergic rhinitis.

Cromolyn sodium nasal solution spray is used for the symptomatic prevention and treatment of allergic rhinitis. It has the unique property of preventing antigen-triggered mast cell degranulation and release of the mediators of allergic reactions, including histamine. Cromolyn sodium has no direct antihistaminic, anticholinergic, or anti-inflammatory properties. Similar to topical steroids, the most common side effects result from local irritation—sneezing and nasal stinging. The dose in adults and children older than 6 years is one spray in each nostril three to four times per day at regular intervals. Cromolyn sodium must come into contact with the entire nasal lining; therefore, patients should be instructed to clear nasal passages before administration. Inhaling through the nose during administration aids in this process.

For seasonal rhinitis, treatment with cromolyn sodium should be initiated just before the usual start of the offending allergen's season. Treatment should continue throughout this season. In perennial rhinitis, the effects may not be seen for 2 to 4 weeks; therefore, antihistamines or decongestants may be needed during this initial phase of therapy. As the cromolyn sodium begins to work, the need for these medications should decrease.

Ipratropium nasal spray is an anticholinergic agent that exhibits antisecretory properties when applied locally. It provides symptomatic relief of rhinnorhea associated with allergic rhinitis. The 0.03% solution is given as two sprays (42 μg) two to three times daily. The optimal dose should be determined based on the specific patient's symptoms and response. Side effects are mild, with the most common being headache, nose bleeds, and nasal dryness.

IMMUNOTHERAPY

The first report of the successful use of grass pollen extract injections to treat allergic rhinitis was published in 1911 by Noon.[54] The therapy was first called desensitization; however, this did not seem appropriate because skin reactivity remained. The name was changed to hyposensitization. Although the term *hyposensitization* is still used today, immunotherapy has become the most accepted term.

Immunotherapy is the slow, gradual process of injecting increasing doses of antigens responsible for eliciting allergic symptoms in a patient with the hope of increasing tolerance to the allergen when natural exposure occurs. Several immunologic changes have been documented resulting from immunotherapy that likely result in its effectiveness.[55] The changes include: diminished IgE production, increased IgG production, changes in T lymphocytes, reduced inflammatory mediator release from sensitized cells, and diminished tissue responsiveness.

Immunotherapy is expensive, has significant potential risks, and requires a major time commitment from the patient. For these reasons it should only be considered in a select group of patients. These patients should have a strong history of severe symptoms unsuccessfully controlled by avoidance and drug therapy. Patients who have been unable to tolerate the side effects of drug therapy should also be considered as candidates. Patients must be committed to the regular office visits required to complete this long course of therapy.

The selection of antigens should be based on patient history and skin test results. Numerous regimens for administration of selected allergens have been suggested. In general, very dilute solutions (1:100,000 to 1:1,000,000,000 wt/vol) are given one or two times per week. The concentration is increased until the maximum tolerated dose is achieved. This maintenance dose is continued every 2 to 6 weeks, depending on clinical response. Best results are usually obtained when injections are given year-round rather than seasonally.

Adverse reactions can occur with immunotherapy and range from mild to life threatening. Among the most common are mild local reactions consisting of induration and swelling at the site of the injection. Other more serious reactions (e.g., generalized urticaria, bronchospasm, laryngospasm, vascular collapse) occur rarely, including deaths from anaphylactic reactions. Severe reactions are treated with epinephrine, antihistamines, and systemic corticosteroids.

Several patient types have been identified as poor candidates for immunotherapy, including patients with any medical condition that would compromise the ability to tolerate an anaphylactic type reaction, patients with impaired immune systems, and patients with a history of noncompliance.[55]

PHARMACOECONOMIC CONSIDERATIONS

The economic impact of allergic rhinitis is enormous. When looking at both prescription and nonprescription drug expenditures, the estimated medication cost in the United States was $2.3 billion ($56 for prescription drugs and $56 for over-the-counter drugs per patient per year).[56] Because the majority of these patients visited a physician, an additional $1.1 billion must be added to account for physician billing. Indirect costs related to missed school or work days and loss of productivity may approach the amount for the direct costs.[57]

The most cost-effective choice will be a individualized decision. Seasonal allergic rhinitis patients who see improvement and can tolerate over-the counter, generic antihistamines will have the least impact on their pocketbook. From there, the economic picture becomes complicated. Choices should follow the logical path based on symptoms, tolerance, and efficacy as described earlier in this chapter.

EVALUATION OF THERAPEUTIC OUTCOMES

With allergic rhinitis, the major outcome issues include the effect of the disease on a patient's life, the efficacy and tolerability of treatment, and patient satisfaction. How the condition affects the patient's job or school performance, family and social interactions, and other aspects of their quality of life is vital. The drug therapy should prevent or minimize symptoms with minimal or no side effects. The patient should not have difficulty obtaining medication for financial or any other reasons. Patients should be questioned about their satisfaction with the management of their allergic rhinitis. The management should result in minimal disruption to their life.

Both the Medical Outcomes Study 36-item short-form Health Survey (SF-36) and the Rhinoconjunctivitis Quality of Life Questionnaire have been used to evaluate outcomes of treatment for seasonal and perennial allergic rhinitis.[58–60] These tools go beyond measuring improvement in symptoms and include such items as sleep quality, nonallergic symptoms (e.g., fatigue, poor concentration), emotions, and participation in a variety of activities. How well each of the current treatment modalities perform and how they compare in improving patient outcomes remains to be determined.

Currently, the therapeutic goal for patients with allergic rhinitis is to minimize or prevent symptoms. Evaluation of success is primarily accomplished through discussions with the patient where both relief of symptoms and tolerance of drug therapy must be discussed.

▶ PRINCIPLES OF PHARMACOTHERAPY

- Many pharmacotherapeutic options are used to prevent symptoms. Patients must be thoroughly knowledgeable about the proper timing and administration of prophylactic regimens. If the patient cannot tolerate or is unable to remain compliant with the chosen drug regimen, alternatives should be discussed and mutually selected. The least expensive regimen that controls symptoms with minimal side effects should be selected.
- Allergic rhinitis is one of the most common human diseases. Treatment is justified in most cases because of the potential for complications. Therapeutic modalities include avoidance of allergens and pharmacologic management with antihistamines, topical and systemic decongestants, topical steroids, cromolyn sodium, and immunotherapy.
- Patient counseling regarding the proper selection and use of available drug therapy is crucial to successful management of allergic rhinitis.

REFERENCES

1. Naclerio R. Allergic rhinitis. N Engl J Med 1991;325:860–869.
2. Juniper E, Guyatt G, Andersson B, Ferrie P. Comparison of powder and aerosolized budesonide in perennial rhinitis: Validation of rhinitis quality of life questionaire. Ann Allergy 1993;70:225–230.
3. Meltzer EO. Introduction. J Allergy Clin Immunol 1997;99:S807.
4. Weeke E. Epidemiology of allergic diseases in children. Rhinology 1992;13(suppl):5–12.
5. Sibbald B, Rink E. Epidemiology of seasonal and perennial rhinitis: Clinical presentation and medical history. Thorax 1991;46: 895–901.
6. Evans R. Epidemiology and natural history of asthma, allergic rhinitis, and atopic dermatitis. In: Middleton E Jr, Reed CE, Ellis EF, et al, eds. Allergy: Principles and Practice, 4th ed. St. Louis, Mosby-Year Book, 1993:1109–1136.
7. Sibbald B. Epidemiology of allergic rhinitis, In: Burr ML, ed. Epidemiology of Clinical Allergy. Monographs in Allergy. Basel, Karger, 1993:61–79.
8. International rhinitis management working group. International consensus report on the diagnosis and management of rhinitis. Allergy 1994;49:1–34.
9. Raphael G, Baraniuk J, Kaliner M. How and why the nose runs. J Allergy Clin Immunol 1991;87:457–467.
10. Gomez E, Corrado O, Baldwin D, et al. Direct *in vivo* evidence for mast cell degranulation during allergen-induced reactions in man. J Allergy Clin Immunol 1986;78:637–645.
11. Naclerio R, Togias A. The nasal allergic reaction: Observations on the role of histamine. Clin Exp Allergy 1991;21(suppl 2):13–19.
12. White M, Kaliner M. Mediators of allergic rhinitis. J Allergy Clin Immunol 1992;90:699–704.
13. Bradding P, Iain H, Wilson S, et al. Immunolocalization of cytokines in the nasal mucosa of normal and perennial rhinitic subjects. J Immunol 1993;151:3853–3865.
14. Mygind N. Glucocorticosteroids and rhinitis. Allergy 1993;48: 476–490.
15. Naclerio R. Inflammation in allergic rhinitis. Res Clin Forums 1992; 14:49–55.
16. Lozewicz S, Davies R. Inflammatory cells in allergic rhinitis. Respir Med 1991;85:259–261.
17. Bentley A. Immunohistology of the nasal mucosa in seasonal allergic rhinitis: Increases in activated eosinophils and epithelial mast cells. J Allergy Clin Immunol 1992;89:877–883.
18. Sibbald B, Rink E. Labeling of rhinitis and hayfever by doctors. Thorax 1991;46:378–381.
19. Romero J, Scadding G. Eosinophilia in nasal secretions compared to skin prick and nasal challenge in the diagnosis of nasal allergy. Rhinology 1992;30:169–175.

20. Kalliner M, Lemanske R. Rhinitis and asthma. JAMA 1992;268: 2807–2829.
21. Turkeltaub P. Skin testing. In: Creticos PS, ed. Immunotherapy: A Practical Guide to Current Procedures. Milwaukee, American Academy of Allergy and Immunology, 1994;2:2–11.
22. Turkeltaub P. Standardized extracts in practice. In: Creticos PS, ed. Immunotherapy: A Practical Guide to Current Procedures. Milwaukee, American Academy of Allergy and Immunology, 1994;4:4.
23. Badhwar A, Druce H. Allergic rhinitis. Med Clin North Am 1992;76: 789–803.
24. Cowart B, Flynn-Rodden K, McGeady S, Lowry L. Hyposmia in allergic rhinitis. J Allergy Clin Immunol 1993;91:747–751.
25. Apter A, Mott A, Cain W, et al. Olfactory loss and allergic rhinitis (clinical conference). J Allergy Clin Immunol 1992;90:670–680.
26. Ziering RW, Klein Gl. Allergic rhinitis: Measures to control the misery. Postgrad Med 1992;91:225–232.
27. Nuss R, Berman S. Medical management of persistent middle ear effusion. Am J Asthma Allergy Pediatr 1990;4:17–22.
28. Trask G, Shapiro G, Shapiro P. The effects of perennial allergic rhinitis on dental and skeletal development: A comparison of sibling pairs. Am J Orthodont Dentofac Orthoped 1987;92:286–293.
29. Shapiro G, Shapiro P. Nasal airway obstruction and facial development. Clin Rev Allergy 1984;2:225–236.
30. Linna O, Kokkonen J, Lukin M. A 10-year prognosis for childhood allergic rhinitis. Acta Paediatr 1992;81:100–102.
31. Aberg N, Engstrom I. Natural history of allergic diseases in children. Acta Paediatr Scand 1990;79:206–211.
32. Verdiani P, Di CS, Baronti A. Different prevalence and degree of nonspecific bronchial hyperreactivity between seasonal and perennial rhinitis. J Allergy Clin Immunol 1990;86:576–582.
33. Guarderas JC. Rhinitis and sinusitis: Office management. Mayo Clin Proc 1996;71:882–888.
34. Ferguson BJ. Allergic rhinitis: Recognizing signs, symptoms and triggering allergens. Postgrad Med 1997;101:110–116.
35. Colloff M, Ayres J, Carswell F, et al. The control of allergens of dust mites and domestic pets: A position paper. Clin Exp Allergy 1992; 22(suppl 2):1–28.
36. Sporik S, Holgate S, Platts-Mills T. Exposure to house dust mite allergen and the development of asthma in childhood: A prospective study. N Engl J Med 1990;323:502.
37. Reisman R, Mauriello P, Davis G, et al. A double-blind study of the effectiveness of a high efficiency particulate air (HEPA) filter in the treatment of patients with perennial allergic rhinitis and asthma. J Allergy Clin Immunol 1990;85:1050–1057.
38. Simons FE, Simons KJ. The pharmacology and use of H1-receptor antagonist drugs. N Engl J Med 1994;330:1663–1670.
39. Wang D, Clement P, Smitz J. Effect of H1 and H2 antagonists on nasal symptoms and mediator release in atopic patients after nasal allergen challenge during the pollen season. Acta Otolaryngol 1996;116: 91–96.
40. Garrison JC. Histamine, bradykinin, 5-hydroxytryptamine and their antagonists. In: Gilman AG, Rall TW, Nies AS, et al, eds. The Pharmacological Basis of Therapeutics, 8th ed. New York, Macmillan, 1990:575–599.
41. LaForce C, Dockhorn RJ, Prenner BM, et al. Safety and efficacy of azelastine nasal spray for seasonal allergic rhinitis: A 4 week comparative multicenter trial. Ann Allergy Asthma Immunol 1996;76: 181–188.
42. Charpin D, Godard P, Baehre M, et al. A multicenter clinical study of the efficacy and tolerability of azelastine nasal spray in the treatment of seasonal allergic rhinitis: A comparison with oral cetirizine. Eur Arch Otorhinolaryngol 1995;252:455–458.
43. Astelin product information. Wallace Laboratories, 1997.
44. Pentel P. Toxicity of over-the-counter stimulants. JAMA 1984;252: 1898–1903.
45. Horowitz JD, Lang WJ, Howes LG, et al. Hypertensive response induced by phenylpropanolamine in anorectic and decongestant preparations. Lancet 1980;1:60–61.
46. Empey DE, Young GA, Letley E, et al. Dose response study of the nasal decongestant and cardiovascular effects of pseudoephedrine. Br J Clin Pharmacol 1980;9:351–358.
47. Drew CDM, Knight GT, Hughes DTD, et al. Comparison of the effects of D-(−)ephedrine and L-(+)-pseudoephedrine on the cardiovascular and respiratory systems in man. Br J Clin Pharmacol 1978;6: 221–225.
48. Drug interaction facts. Tatro DS, ed. Facts and Comparisons. St. Louis, 1997:680.
49. Diamond L, Gerson K, Cato A, et al. An evaluation of triprolidine and pseudoephedrine in the treatment of allergic rhinitis. Ann Allergy 1981;47:87–91.
50. Connell JT, Williams BO, Allen S, et al. A double-blind controlled evaluation of Actifed and its individual constituents in allergic rhinitis. J Intern Med Res 1982;10:341–347.
51. International rhinitis management working group. International consensus report on the diagnosis and management of rhinitis. Allergy 1994;49(suppl 19):1–34.
52. Quintiliani R. Hypersensitivity and adverse reactions associated with the use of newer intranasal corticosteroids for allergic rhinitis. Curr Ther Res 1996;57:478–488.
53. Small P, Black M, Frenkiel S, et al. Beclomethasone dipropionate in the management of rhinitis—a review. Ann Allergy 1982;49:127–130.
54. Noon L. Prophylactic inoculation against hayfever. Lancet 1911;1: 1572–1573.
55. Schoenwetter WF. Safe allergen immunotherapy. Postgrad Med 1996; 100:123–135
56. Storms W Meltzer EO, Nathan RA, Selner JC. The economic impact of allergic rhinitis. J Allergy Clin Immunol 1997;99:S820–S824.
57. Rossoff LJ, Stempel DA, Alam R, et al. The health and economic impact of allergic rhinitis. Am J Man Care 1997;3:S8–S18.
58. Bousquet J, Duchateau J, Pignat JC, et al. Improvement of quality of life by treatment with cetirizine in patients with perennial allergic rhinitis as determined by a French version of the SF-36 questionnaire. J Allergy Clin Immunol 1996;98:309–316.
59. Meltzer EO, Nathan RA, Selner JC, Storms W. Quality of life and rhinitc symptoms: Results of a nationwide survey with the SF-36 and RQLQ questionnaires. J Allergy Clin Immunol 1997;99:S815–S819.
60. Harvey RP, Comer C, Sanders B, et al. Model for outcomes assessment of antihistamine use for seasonal allergic rhinitis. J Allergy Clin Immunol 1996:97:1233–1241.

88
ACNE AND PSORIASIS

Nina H. Han, PharmD, Phillip A. Nowakowski, PharmD, and Dennis P. West, PhD, FCCP

Nearly 2000 different skin disorders are readily visible and brought to the attention of health care practitioners daily. Patients may be screened to identify dermatologic disorders, identify drug-induced causes of dermatoses, initiate drug therapy (considering vehicle and active ingredients), and monitor for therapeutic effect, adverse reactions, and patient compliance. A practical reference for nondermatologists is *Primary Care Dermatology.*[1]

The clinical approach to solving dermatologic problems involves analysis, assessment, establishment, and initiation of a treatment plan followed by careful drug monitoring (Table 88–1). This algorithm is similar to problem-solving approaches in other specialties, but major differences include the development of an objective database by physical examination of lesions on the integument and mucous membrances as well as description of the dermatoses in specific, brief, concise, and uniform terminology. Important aspects of the physical examination of skin and definitions of lesion types are presented. This is designed to assist in identification of common dermatologic disorders and appropriate treatment regimens. Examination of the skin should include observations on color and consistency of lesions, anatomic localization and distribution, configuration, size, border, and other superficial characteristics.

LESION CHARACTERISTICS

COLOR

Lesion color, attributed to a variety of causes, is of major diagnostic importance. The consistency of color should also be noted. Some lesions have consistent color throughout, while others may vary in color from the border to an area of central clearing or may demonstrate multiple colors and hues (Table 88–2).

DISTRIBUTION

Distribution of lesions may be helpful in determining a diagnosis (Figs. 88–1 and 88–2). Lesions may be localized to an anatomic area or generalized over the body surface. Lesions limited to specific anatomic regions such as photo-exposed areas or body-fold areas (intertriginous) should be differentiated.

CONFIGURATION

Configuration is also essential to diagnosis and may be defined as the relationship of one lesion to another or how lesions are grouped (Table 88–3). Lesion size can be approximated in centimeters or using familiar objects (e.g., 5 cm or the size of a dime); borders should be categorized as demarcated (sharply circumscribed) or diffuse (ill defined). Superficial characteristics such as elevations or depressions in skin, changes in texture, presence of moisture or dried exudate, and firmness should also be noted. Usually, the characteristics of a lesion are communicated in a few singular terms describing the morphologic type of lesion. Description of lesion type, along with color, distribution, size, and configuration, is the most accepted method of communicating what is noted by physical assessment. Use of uniform terminology aids in diagnosis and allows others to visualize the lesions.

TABLE 88–1. An Approach to Solving the Dermatologic Problems of Patients

Knowledge Base	Action	Patient Database
Dermatologic manifestations	Analyze the problem	Subjective data Objective data
Therapeutic end points Risk versus benefit Pharmaceutic and pharmacokinetic considerations Drug/disease/lab interactions Monitoring parameters	Assess the problem Establish optimal treatment plan for the patient	
	Monitor the patient Therapeutic effect Adverse effects Compliance	

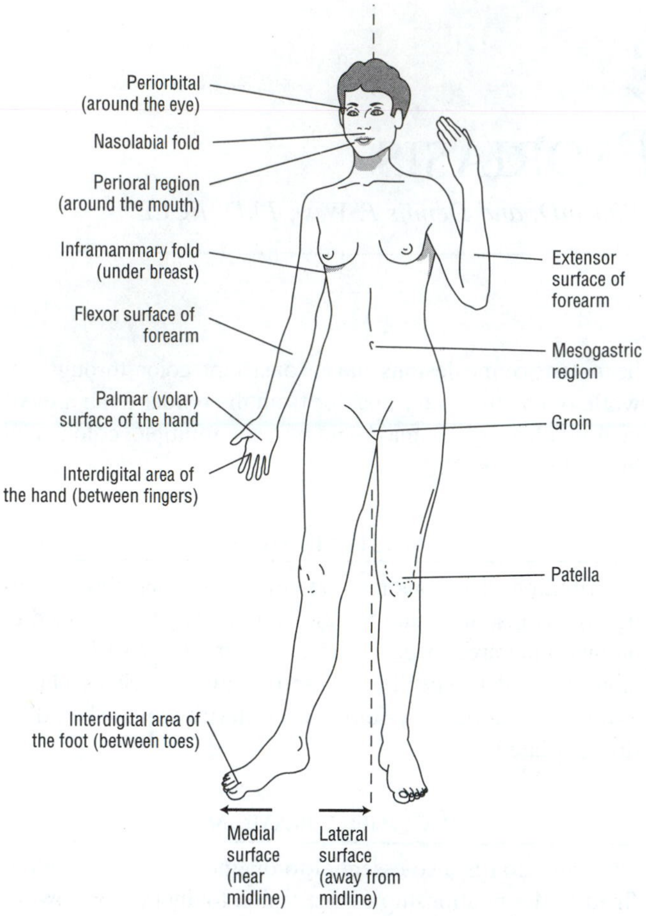

FIGURE 88–1. Anterior (ventral) surfaces of the body.

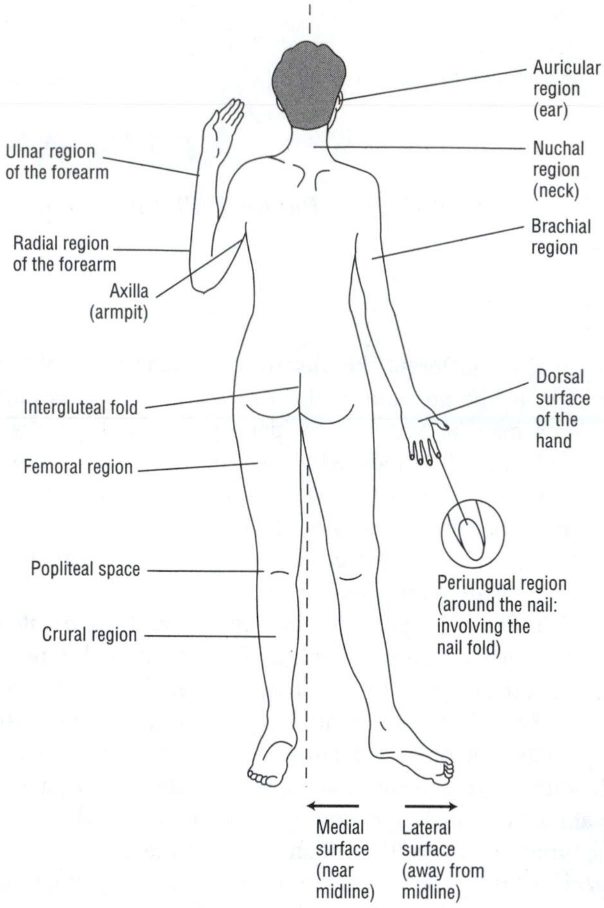

FIGURE 88–2. Posterior (dorsal) surfaces of the body.

ACNE

Acne vulgaris, the most common skin disease, affects 80% of the population between the ages of 12 and 25.[2] Although acne is generally self-limiting, it can persist for years and can result in disfigurement and scarring and have profound psychological effects on patients.[2–5] It is important for the health care professional to play a major role in educating patients on causes of acne, recommending treatment regimens, and counseling on proper medication use.

DIAGNOSIS

Generally, the diagnosis of acne vulgaris consists of a finding that includes a mixture of lesions of acne (comedones, pustules, papules, nodules, cysts) on the face, back, or chest. Although there is no precise definition for acne, most consider the presence of 5 to 10 comedones to be diagnostic. Other dermatologic conditions, such as folliculitis, acne rosacea, and other various acneform disorders, may sometimes be confused with acne vulgaris.[6]

TABLE 88–2. Examples of Lesional Color Variation

Lesion Description	Color	Pathophysiologic Mechanism	Precipitating Factor(s)
Hyperpigmented	Darkened areas	Melanin deposition	Pregnancy, sunlight, oral contraceptives
Hypopigmented	Lightened	Lack of melanin	Autoimmune phenomena
Jaundiced	Yellowish	Increased bilirubin or carotene	Hepatitis
Cyanotic	Bluish	Excess reduced hemoglobin	Hypoxia
	Reddish blue	Capillary stasis	Increased red blood cells
Erythematous	Red	Dilation of blood vessels	Inflammation, sunburn
Violaceous	Purple	Aging lesion, formerly erythematous	Bruising trauma

TABLE 88–3. Examples of Lesional Configuration

Type	Description
Clustered	Grouped lesions
Linear	Straight line
Annular	Circular
Polycyclic	Two or more adjacent, circular lesions
Serpiginous	Snake like with wavy borders
Geographic	Irregular map-like borders

CLINICAL MANIFESTATIONS

Acne is primarily found on the face, and to a lesser degree, the upper back, chest, and shoulders. Lesions can vary morphologically and are primarily classified as either inflammatory or noninflammatory. The clinical presentation of acne can range from a mild comedonal form to severe inflammatory necrotic acne of the face, chest, and back. Formation of the primary lesion, the comedo, may be simplistically thought of as plugging of the pilosebaceous follicle. In acne, the follicular canal widens and an increase in cell production is seen.[2] Sebum mixes with excess loose cells in the follicular canal to form a keratinous plug. The resulting lesion appears as a "blackhead" or open comedo. The brown or black color is not a result of dirt accumulation but that of melanin.[2] Inflammation or trauma to the follicle may lead to formation of a whitehead," or closed comedo. If the follicular wall is damaged or ruptured, the contents of the follicle may extrude into dermis and present clinically as a pustule. Closed comedones are of clinical importance as these may presage larger, inflammatory lesions.[2]

Acne lesions may take months to heal completely and fibrosis associated with healing may lead to permanent scarring. Most forms of adolescent acne are self-limiting, but more severe forms may be persistent and require aggressive treatment.

PATHOPHYSIOLOGY

Although an exact cause of acne is unknown, the pathogenesis of acne is multifactorial, and thus treatment is directed at these factors (Table 88–4). Pathogenic theories of acne development include the roles of androgens, sebum production, *Propionibacterium acnes,* and follicle growth.[2,4,5] Sebaceous glands, normally found on the face, chest, back, and shoulders, develop at puberty in response to androgen stimulation. Sebum produced in these glands is transported through ducts to the canal and onto the surface of the skin. The follicular canal also contains fine vellus hair, keratinous material, and bacteria (primarily *P. acnes*). Acne formation is believed to be caused by a derangement in the structure or function of normal sebaceous follicles (Fig. 88–3).

ANDROGENS

Increased androgen activity at puberty triggers growth of sebaceous glands and enhanced production of sebum. Although testosterone is the most potent androgen, its metabolites and weaker androgens (androstenedione, dehydroepiandrosteone, dehydroepiandrosterone sulfate) are increased in acne patients and may also stimulate sebaceous gland activity.[2] Skin, hair follicles, and sebaceous glands metabolize

TABLE 88–4. Major Pathophysiologic Features of Acne and Responsive Pharmacotherapeutic Agents

Feature	Systemic Drug	Topical Drug
Sebum production/secretion	Estrogens Antiandrogens Spironolactone Isotretinoin	None established
Abnormal desquamation of follicular epithelium	Isotretinoin Antibiotics	Tretinoin Salicylic acid Adapalene Tazarotene
Propionibacterium acnes proliferation	Tetracycline Minocycline Doxycycline Erythromycin Clindamycin Cotrimoxazole Isotretinoin	Erythromycin Clindamycin Benzoyl peroxide Azelaic acid
Inflammation	Corticosteroids Isotretinoin Nonsteroidal anti-inflammatory agents	Metronidazole Intralesional corticosteroids Sulfur Adapalene Azelaic acid

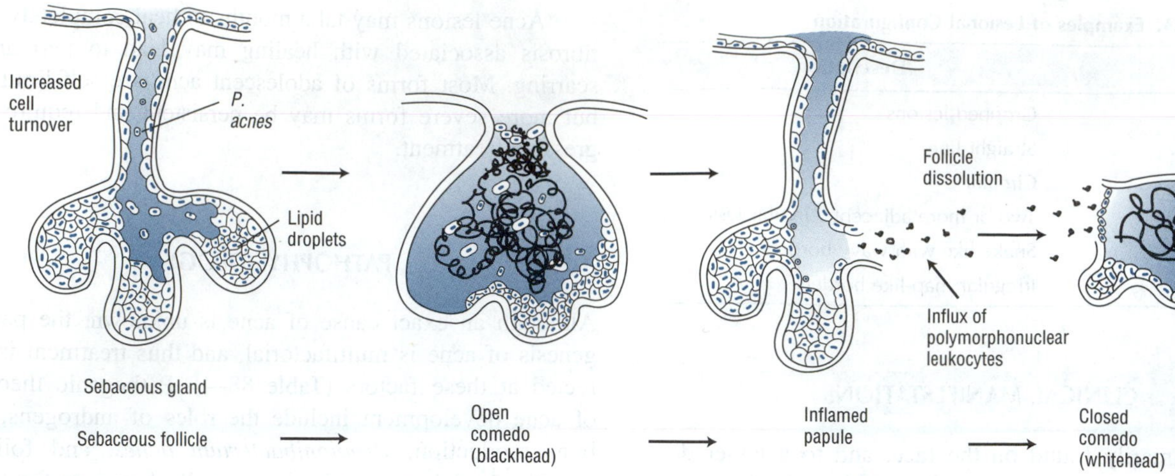

FIGURE 88–3. Cross-sectional view of the sebaceous follicle.

androgens to active dihydrostestosterone, and acne-prone areas of skin demonstrate increased metabolic activity.[2]

SEBUM PRODUCTION

Sebum is produced in the sebaceous glands and consists of glycerides, wax esters, squalene, and cholesterol. The glyceride component of sebum is converted to free fatty acids and glycerol by lipases, products of *P. acnes.*[2] Free fatty acids may irritate the follicular wall and cause increased cell turnover and inflammation. Recently glycerol has been identified as a substrate for *P. acnes,* while free fatty acids may function as a measure of *P. acnes* activity and viability.[2] Though patients with acne have been shown to have increased sebum production, there is variation among patients with acne, indicating that this disease is not solely related to sebaceous gland activity.[2]

FOLLICLE ACTIVITY

The primary change in acne is an alteration in the pattern of keratinization within the follicle. Abnormal alterations in the follicle wall and its cell growth have been noted histologically in association with acne.[2] Increased production of loosely adherent keratin cells has been correlated with obstruction of the follicles seen in comedo formation. It is unknown whether this abnormality is inherent or secondary to irritation and other factors.

BACTERIA

Propionibacterium acnes, a resident anaerobic organism, proliferates in the environment created by the mixture of excessive sebum and follicular cells and may lead to inflammation.[2] Although *P. acnes* counts are typically higher in patients with acne, the pathogenic role of this organism is not that of a simple infection. *P. acnes* may be considered antigenic and capable of causing increased antibody formation (IgG, IgM), leading to an inflammatory response.[2] Immune complex–mediated complement activation as a result of *P. acnes* may lead to vascular leakage, mast cell degranulation, and leukocyte chemotaxis.[7] Levels of antibodies to *P. acnes* are higher in patients with severe forms of acne than in normal controls. *P. acnes* may activate the complement cascade via both classic and alternate pathways and produce direct tissue damage.[2] Also, chemotactic factors may be secreted by *P. acnes,* diffuse through the follicle wall, and activate neutrophil chemotaxis and complement. Hydrolytic enzymes released by complement activation may damage the follicle wall and lead to more severe, inflammatory acne. Neutrophils are an important factor in severe inflammatory acne and patients may demonstrate neutrophil defects of either very high or low chemotaxis as well as impaired phagocytosis. *P. acnes* may also evoke a cell-medicated immune response.[2] Although the exact cause of acne is unclear, its pathogenesis involves various factors that are apparently interrelated (Fig. 88–4).

PATIENT ASSESSMENT

In assessing a patient with acne, an in-depth drug and medical history should be obtained to determine if there are any exacerbating factors that can be eliminated (Table 88–5).

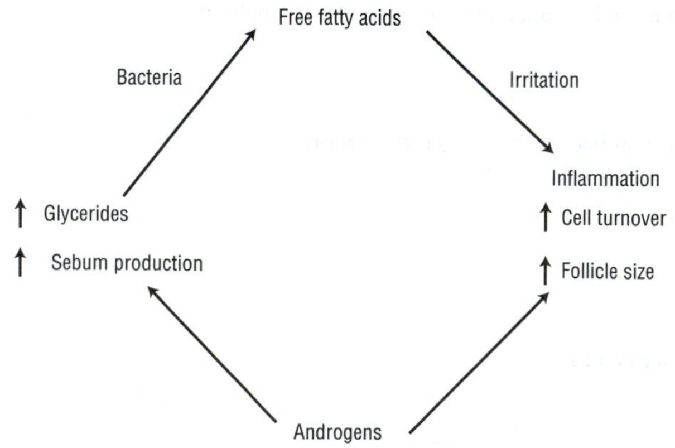

FIGURE 88–4. Acne pathogenesis.

TABLE 88–5. Examples of Components to Patient History for Acne

Onset and duration of acne	All current and recent topical and systemic medications
Family history	All topical products such as soaps, moisturizers, astringents, and cosmetics
Exacerbating factors	Environmental and occupational exposures to chemicals and toxins
Previous history of antiacne agents with efficacy and adverse effect data	Allergies (food, drug, environmental)

▶ TREATMENT: Acne Vulgaris

TOPICAL PHARMACOLOGIC THERAPY

Aggressive therapy may be required to modify or inhibit inflammatory acne. An important goal of therapy is to prevent or minimize scarring, and the treatment of choice depends on severity and individual patient tolerance. Because acne is a multifactorial process, multiple treatment approaches may be required for control. Tables 88–6 and 88–7 summarize treatment guidelines for acne vulgaris.

BENZOYL PEROXIDE

Benzoyl peroxide is an effective treatment for mild and moderately severe acne. However, the Food and Drug Administration (FDA) currently does not categorize it as generally recognized as safe; studies are ongoing and being analyzed to assess the tumorigenic potential of benzoyl peroxide in humans. The mechanism of action is uncertain, although it is known that benzoyl peroxide is decomposed on the skin by cysteine, liberating free oxygen radicals that oxidize bacterial proteins.[7] Daily application of 10% benzoyl peroxide for 2 weeks can reduce free fatty acid levels by 50% and *P. acnes* levels by 98%.[7] Benzoyl peroxide increases the sloughing rate of epithelial cells, loosens the follicular plug structure, and thus possesses some degree of comedolytic activity.[8]

Dryness and irritation from a primary irritant such as benzoyl peroxide may limit therapy in some patients; allergic contact dermatitis may occur in 1% to 3% of patients.[9] To limit irritation and increase patient tolerance to benzoyl peroxide, one may initiate therapy with a low-potency formulation (2.5%) and increase either strength (5% to 10%) or application frequency (every other day, each day, then twice a day).

Benzoyl peroxide is available in soaps, lotions, creams, and gels. Gel formulations are usually most potent, while the lotions and soaps are weaker. Gels are usually alcohol, propylene glycol, or water based; the alcohol-based preparations generally cause more dryness and irritation. Fair or moist skin is usually more sensitive to irritation from benzoyl peroxide; thus, patients should be advised to apply medication to dry skin (at least 30 minutes after washing) to decrease irritation. The oxidizing capability of benzoyl peroxide may bleach colored fabrics (washcloths, pillowcases).

SULFUR, RESORCINOL, AND SALICYLIC ACID

Sulfur, resorcinol, and salicylic acid are keratolytic and mildly antibacterial. The term *keratolytic* refers to the effect of solubilization of intracellular cement of keratin cells in the stratum corneum. Although evidence for efficacy in treatment of acne is conflicting, each agent has been classified as safe and effective by an advisory review panel of the FDA. Combinations of these agents are often considered synergistic (e.g., sulfur and resorcinol, salicylic acid and benzoyl peroxide). Keratolytic products, in

TABLE 88–6. Topical Acne Treatment Guidelines

Active Ingredient	Formulation	Strength (%)	Regimen	Potential Side Effects
Benzoyl peroxide	Soaps, lotions creams, gels	2.5–10	Initially every other day, or daily, then twice daily	Irritation based on form/strength Bleaching/staining of clothing
Tretinoin	Creams, gels, solution, microsphere gel, liquid polymer	0.025–0.05	Initially every other day or daily	Moderate erythema, burning, stinging, pruritus Concomitant use of other irritants increases likelihood of undue irritation
Sulfur/resorcinol/ salicylic acid	Creams, lotions, gels, soaps	0.5–10 in various combinations	Daily	
Clindamycin	Solution, gel, lotion	1	Twice daily	Drying, gastrointestinal effects (Pseudomembranous colitis)
Tetracycline	Solution	2.2	Twice daily	Burning and stinging following application, skin discoloration
Erythromycin	Solution, powder, gel	1.5–2	Twice daily	Drying, erythema
Adapalene	Gel, lotion	0.03–0.1	Daily	Moderate erythema, drying, stinging, burning, pruritus
Azelaic acid	Cream	20	Twice daily	Mild, transient, local erythema, burning, pruritus
Tazarotene	Gel	0.1	Daily or twice daily	Moderate erythema, burning, stinging, pruritus

TABLE 88–7. Oral Acne Treatment Guidelines

Active Ingredient	Formulation	Strength (mg)	Regimen	Potential Side Effects
Tetracycline	Tablets, capsules	250–500	1 g/d initially; if no response in 2–3 weeks or severe acne, 2–3 g/d Maintenance 125–500 mg/d	Gastrointestinal upset, photoreactivity, drug and food interactions
Minocycline	Tablets, capsules, suspension	50–100	100 mg twice daily	CNS effects (dizziness, drowsiness) Discoloration of skin
Doxycycline	Tablets, capsules, suspension, syrup	50–100	50–100 mg twice daily	Discoloration, gastrointestinal upset (esophagitis), photoreactivity
Erythromycin	Tablets as various salts	250–500	1 g/d as base; if no response in 2–3 weeks or severe acne, 2–3 g/d. Maintenance 250–500 mg/d	Gastrointestinal upset, cutaneous reactions, drug interactions
Clindamycin	Capsules	75, 150, 300	300–450 mg/d	Diarrhea, pseudomembranous colitis
Isotretinoin	Capsules	10, 20, 40	0.5–1 mg/kg/d in two divided doses Maximum of 2 mg/kg/d	Cheilitis, erythema, dryness, gastrointestinal effects, teratogenicity

the concentration allowed, may be less irritating than benzoyl peroxide and tretinoin; however, they are not considered effective comedolytic agents as are benzoyl peroxide and tretinoin. Disadvantages of these agents include the odor created by hydrogen sulfide upon reaction of sulfur with the skin, the brown scale from use of resorcinol, and the remote possibility of salicylism from repeated use of sufficient concentrations of salicylic acid on highly permeable (inflamed and/or abraded) skin.

TOPICAL ANTIBACTERIAL PRODUCTS

Topical antibacterials other than benzoyl peroxide and salicylic acid (e.g., clindamycin, erythromycin, tetracycline) have been used effectively to treat acne by concentrating local antimicrobial activity in the skin and subsequently decreasing risk of systemic toxicity. Many clinical trials that compare efficacy of topical versus systemic antibacterials are difficult to evaluate because formulations may have been prepared extemporaneously or different vehicles were used.[10,11]

Although it does not necessarily correlate with clinical response, inhibition of *P. acnes* is most effectively accomplished by clindamycin. In one study, *in vivo* topical clindamycin significantly reduced the numbers of *P. acnes,* while topical erythromycin and tetracycline did not.[12] Reduction of the percentage of free fatty acids in sebum has been noted with the use of topical tetracycline and erythromycin.[12]

A topical preparation of erythromycin plus zinc has been reported to be significantly better than 500 mg/d oral tetracycline in reducing overall acne severity and papule lesion counts.[13] In a randomized, double-blind study of 122 patients with acne vulgaris, a 4% erythromycin and zinc combination lotion was more effective than 2% erythromycin lotion. The higher concentration of erythromycin may have been more effective, or the zinc acetate complex may enhance the penetration of erythromycin into the pilosebaceous unit.[14]

Disadvantages of topical antibiotic dosage forms include occasional irritation and stinging upon application. Although tetracycline is the most frequently prescribed oral antibiotic for acne, it is one of the least frequently prescribed topical antibiotics. On the skin, tetracycline photooxidizes to produce a visible yellow tinting.[12] Diarrhea and pseudomembranous colitis may occur from the use of topical clindamycin.[15,16] Antimicrobial resistance from widespread use of topical antibiotics for acne has been postulated but not substantiated as a serious clinical problem.[12]

AZELAIC ACID

Azelaic acid is a naturally occuring substance that interferes with DNA synthesis in some of the bacteria associated with acne vulgaris.[17] Inhibition of thioredoxin reductase by azelaic acid provides a rationale for this property.[18] Azelaic acid also demonstrates a potential anti-inflammatory role. In a series of investigations using 20% azelaic acid cream as a therapy for acne, it was found that the treatment, compared with vehicle, significantly reduced inflammatory lesions at 1 month and noninflammatory lesions at 2 months.[19] In an open study of 100 unselected patients of either gender, the attained rates of improvement indicate that topical 20% azelaic acid cream can be considered an effective therapy.[20] Although uncommon, mild transient erythema, burning, and pruritus are the most frequently reported side effects. Azelaic acid is not a primary irritant and is generally well-tolerated by acne patients. It is distinct, in that it is antibacterial, has comedolytic activity, and is not a primary irritant. Because of its combined activity, topical azelaic acid offers a twice-daily, cost-effective, single product option for the treatment of mild to moderate acne.

TRETINOIN

Tretinoin, a topical vitamin A analog, is a comedolytic agent that increases cell turnover in the follicular wall and decreases cohesiveness of cells, leading to extrusion of existing comedones and inhibition of the formation of new comedones.[21] Tretinoin also decreases the number of cell layers in the stratum corneum from 14 to 5.[7] A "flare" of acne may suddenly appear after initiation of treatment followed by clinical clearing in about 8 to 12 weeks.[7] Irritation, erythema, and peeling often limit successful therapy, and allergic contact dermatitis has been reported in a few cases, although not as frequently as with benzoyl peroxide.[21] Tolerance to irritation may be managed by titrating strength and frequency of application. Tretinoin is currently available in 0.05% solution (most irritating); 0.01% and 0.025% gel; and 0.025%, 0.05%, and 0.1% cream (least irritating). Treatment initiation with 0.025% cream is usually recommended for mild acne in people with easily irritated and nonoily skin, 0.01% gel for moderate acne in easily irritated skin with oily complexion, and 0.025% gel for moderate acne with nonsensitive and oily skin. Two newer reformulations of tretinoin, Retin-A Micro® and Avita®, have been introduced. Although Retin-A Micro® contains a microsphere vehicle consisting of porous beads, Avita® contains a liquid polymer vehicle. These newer reformulations are less irritating than standard vehicles for tretinoin.

Once control is established, therapy should be continued at the lowest effective concentration and at the maximum effective interval sufficient to minimize acne exacerbations.[22] Concomitant use of an antibacterial agent with tretinoin can decrease keratinization, inhibit *P. acnes,* and decrease inflammation. In addition, both benzoyl peroxide and tretinoin have shown additive or synergistic effects in the treatment of inflammatory acne.[22,23] A combination of benzoyl peroxide each morning and tretinoin at bedtime may enhance efficacy and be less irritating than either agent used alone.[23] When using tretinoin, patients should be advised to apply the medication to dry skin approximately 30 minutes after washing to minimize erythema and irritation. Slowly increasing application frequency from every other day, to daily, then twice daily, may increase tolerance to tretinoin. Increased sensitivity to sun exposure, wind, cold, and other irritants has also been evident in patients using tretinoin.

ADAPALENE

Adapalene, available as 0.1% aqueous gel or as an alcoholic solution, is a retinoid-mimetic compound used for treatment of mild to moderate acne.[4,24] Adapalene has been shown to have selective affinity for retinoic acid receptor (RAR) subtypes RAR-γ and RAR-β , found in the epidermis.[4,24] It also has comedolytic and anti-inflammatory effects.[24] Vehicle-controlled and comparative studies have demonstrated the utility of adapalene in the treatment of acne.[24–26] Adapalene 0.1% gel produced a greater reduction in total lesion counts than tretinoin 0.025% gel at week 12, and it was significantly better tolerated, resulting in less erythema, pruritus, burning, stinging, and peeling.[25] Thus, adapalene 0.1% gel can be used as an alternative to tretinoin 0.025% gel in patients with mild to moderate acne, with better patient tolerability.[24,25]

TAZAROTENE

Tazarotene, a prodrug, is a synthetic acetylenic retinoid that is converted to an active metabolite, tazarotenic acid, following topical application. This new-generation retinoid also selectively binds to retinoic acid receptors and can alter expression of genes involved in cell proliferation, cell differentiation, and inflammation.[4] Tazarotene 0.1% and 0.05% gel have been shown to be more effective than vehicle in the treatment of acne vulgaris.[26] The 0.1% gel was slightly more effective than the 0.05% gel in decreasing lesion counts. Dose-related adverse effects included erythema, pruritus, stinging, and burning.[26] Although effective for the treatment of acne, as currently formulated and used, this product is similar to tretinoin gel for its primary irritant effects on the face in the treatment of acne.

SYSTEMIC PHARMACOLOGIC THERAPY

ORAL ANTIBACTERIAL AGENTS

Few well-controlled, double-blind studies have been conducted on the efficacy of oral antibiotics in acne. Nevertheless, oral antibiotics are considered effective and relatively safe for inflammatory acne.[12,27] Tetracycline (and derivatives), erythromycin, clindamycin, and cotrimoxazole can significantly decrease the percentage of free fatty acids in skin surface lipids and also decrease numbers of *P. acnes.*[12] Tetracycline exhibits additional activity by reducing the amount of keratin in sebaceous follicles and by inhibiting chemotaxis, phagocytosis, complement activation (by the alternate pathway), and cell-mediated immunity.[12] Tetracycline also appears to have an affinity for inflammatory cells and bacteria, resulting in higher drug concentrations in areas of inflamed skin.[12] Drawbacks to the use of tetracycline include a drug–food interaction with dairy products, photosensitivity, gastrointestinal disturbances, hepatoxicity, and predisposition to superinfections (vaginal candidiasis). In refractory cases, minocycline or doxycycline may be effective because of greater lipid solubility and enhanced penetration into tissue and sebaceous follicles.[28] Minocycline has been used as long-term therapy for acne vulgaris. Disadvantages of minocycline include vestibular toxicity, discoloration of skin and visceral tissues, and drug-induced lupus erythematosus.[28,29]

Clindamycin use for acne is limited by diarrhea and risk of pseudomembranous colitis. Erythromycin has a somewhat safer adverse effect profile when compared with tetracycline; however, efficacy profiles are similar.[12,30]

Although cotrimoxazole may be effective in tetracycline-resistant acne, it should perhaps be reserved for refractory cases to minimize risk of resistance.[12,31] Another consideration in the use of oral antibiotics for acne is a potential interaction with oral contraceptives. Ampicillin and tetracycline decrease intestinal flora necessary for hydrolysis of conjugated ethinyl estradiol excreted into bile; thus, enterohepatic recirculation is interrupted and active estrogen is reduced.[32] The clinical importance of this interaction is not well established, but several pregnancies have been reported with concurrent use of ampicillin or tetracycline and oral contraceptives.[32] Women taking oral contraceptives (especially agents containing less than 50 μg estrogen) should be informed of the potential for this interaction, especially before initiation of long-term oral antibiotics.[33]

ORAL CONTRACEPTIVES

Androgen levels correlate with sebum production and may affect the development of acne.[34] Based on this evidence, alteration of androgen levels represents a potential hormonal treatment for acne in women.[34] The combination of norgestimate and ethinyl estradiol has been shown to increase sex hormone–binding globulin (SHBG), causing a decrease in unbound, biologically active androgens such as free testosterone.[34,36] In January 1997, the FDA approved Ortho Tri-Cyclen for use as antiacne therapy.[6] This triphasic combination oral contraceptive, containing a fixed dose of ethinyl estradiol 0.035 mg and increasing doses of norgestimate 0.180 mg, 0.215 mg, and 0.250 mg, was studied in 2 multicenter, randomized, double-blind, placebo-controlled trials, which concluded that oral contraceptives containing 0.035 mg of ethinyl estradiol along with a triphasic dose of norgestimate can be an effective treatment alternative for moderate acne in women.[34,36]

ANTIANDROGENS AND OTHER HORMONAL THERAPIES

Androgen receptor blockers, such as spironolactone, flutamide, and cyproterone acetate, have been studied.[35] The most widely used agent in this group is cyproterone acetate (not available in the United States). Other drugs that can reduce androgen levels include gonadotropin-releasing hormone agonists, 5-α-reductase inhibitors, and corticosteroids.[35]

ISOTRETINOIN

Isotretinoin is a compound that affects most of the etiologic factors involved in inflammatory acne including (1) decreased sebum production and change in sebum composition, (2) inhibition of *P. acnes* growth within follicles, (3) inhibition of inflammation, and (4) altered patterns of keratinization within follicles (decreased size and increased differentiation).[37,38] Oral isotretinoin is indicated for patients with severe recalcitrant nodular or inflammatory acne unresponsive to conventional therapies. In a recent survey of dermatologists, it was concluded that, for patients with moderate or mild acne who respond with less than 50% improvement after 6 months of conventional therapies, oral isotretinoin should be considered for therapeutic use.[39] After a 16-week course, isotretinoin produces a greater than 70% success rate followed by a prolonged remission of more than 20 months.[40]

Isotretinoin dosing guidelines range from 0.5 to 1.0 mg/kg/d, while the cumulative dose taken by patients during a treatment course may be the major factor influencing long-term outcome.[41] Optimal results have generally occurred when *cumulative* doses have attained a range of 120 to 150 mg/kg.[41] Although the costs of therapy with isotretinoin are greater in the first year, it has been demonstrated that isotretinoin can be more cost effective than long-term antibiotic treatment.[42]

Adverse effects from isotretinoin are numerous, frequent, and often dose related.[43,44] About 90% of patients receiving isotretinoin therapy suffer from mucocutaneous effects. Drying of the mucosae of the mouth, nose, and eyes is the most common problem, with relatively rare involvement of the genitoanal mucosae. Chelitis and skin desquamation occurs in over 80% of patients receiving therapy. Less frequently, the conjunctiva and nasal mucosa are affected. Systemic side effects mostly involve arthralgias and muscle stiffness, occurring in 15% of patients. These muscle and joint pains, including complaints of backache, may be attributed to catabolic effects on mesenchymal tissues of cartilage, connective tissue, and bone. Disturbances in lipid metabolism may also occur, resulting in hypertriglyceridemia in more than 25% of patients.[41,43,44]

An increase in creatinine phosphokinase and blood glucose, as well as photosensitivity, pseudotumor cerebri, and excess granulation tissue, has occurred during use of isotretinoin.[40] The incidence of teratogenicity after maternal exposure to isotretinoin is high and well documented.[45] Of 16 case reports of adverse pregnancy outcomes in women exposed to isotretinoin, 9 were spontaneous abortions and 7 were babies with major birth defects (i.e., hydrocephalus, small or partially occluded external auditory canals, and cardiac abnormalities). Though five normal pregnancies were reported, the timing of exposure to isotretinoin was uncertain.

EVALUATION OF THERAPEUTIC OUTCOMES

Contrary to popular belief, environmental factors such as diet, lack of appropriate hygiene, certain hairstyles, and early cosmetic use do not necessarily play a role in acne formation.[6] Though various etiologic theories exist, acne is primarily due to an alteration in the pattern of keratinization within the follicle.[2,6] In most patients, therapy should be directed at correcting abnormal follicular keratinization and inhibition of *P. acnes* to control inflammatory acne. Systemic therapy should be reserved for those patients who do not respond to topical therapy or who are at risk for scarring. Mild inflammatory acne, which consists of scattered small papules or pustules, tends to develop in teenage and young adult women. Treatment with once or twice daily application of a topical antibacterial in combination with a comedolytic agent is recommended.[2] Agents that combine both activities include azelaic acid and benzoyl peroxide.

In patients with moderate severity (inflammatory lesions on the face and trunk), the combination of a topical comedolytic agent applied once or twice daily with either a topical or a systemic antibiotic is appropriate. A possible alternative for women unresponsive to typical therapies is hormonal therapy with estrogen or an antiandrogen.[2] Patients with nodular lesions and significant scarring potential are candidates for systemic isotretinoin therapy if conventional treatments have failed.

Concepts of therapy should be conveyed to the patient and the importance of compliance and prevention of new acne activity should be emphasized. Achievement of clinical response by any given therapeutic regimen may require 6 to 8 weeks. Patients may also notice an "exacerbation" of acne after initiation of topical comedolytic therapy. Follicular plugging may take approximately 4 weeks to evolve into an inflammatory lesion; therefore, new follicular plugging should be significantly less likely to occur by 2 months of effective therapy. For topical agents, all acne-prone areas should be treated, because the purpose of therapy is to prevent or minimize the formation of new lesions[8] and to minimize the risk of scarring, a permanent end point for moderate to severe disease.

PSORIASIS

Psoriasis is a common chronic disease characterized by recurrent exacerbations and remissions of thickened, erythematous, and scaling plaques. It is universal in occurrence and affects approximately 2% of the U.S. population.[46] This debilitating disease occurs in all racial groups but more frequently in Caucasians. It is equally common in males and females.[47] The mean age of onset is 27 years, with approximately 50% of cases occurring in the most productive years between ages 20 and 60; however, the age of onset is widely variable from infancy to old age.[48] About 80% of patients are affected by the most common form, stable plaque psoriasis, which covers up to 20% of the body surface (mean body surface area of involvement is about 7%).

PATHOPHYSIOLOGY

The exact cause of psoriasis is unknown. A validated, adequate animal model using human skin implants has only recently been developed. In immunodeficient mice, it was established that psoriasis may be primarily caused by immunocytes inducing secondary activation and disordered growth of keratinocytes and vascular endothelium.[49] There are several hypotheses regarding the pathophysiology of psoriasis (Table 88–8).

DEFECTS IN EPIDERMAL CELL CYCLE

The search for an inherent skin defect as a pathogenic mechanism for psoriasis has provided numerous hypotheses. Psoriatic epidermal cells proliferate at a rate sevenfold faster than normal epidermal cells.[2,50,51] The germinative cell pop-

TABLE 88–8. Pathophysiologic Aspects of Psoriasis

Defects in epidermal cell cycle
Disruption in arachidonic acid metabolism
Genetics
Exogenous trigger factors
Climate
Stress
Infection
Trauma
Drugs
Immunologic mechanisms

ulation increases in psoriatic skin, and duration of the cell cycle is calculated at 37.5 hours (versus 300 hours in normal skin).[51] Lesion-free skin in psoriatic patients is generally considered to be involved because epidermal proliferation is elevated in apparently normal skin of psoriatic patients.[52]

DISRUPTION IN ARACHIDONIC ACID METABOLISM

Other abnormalities found in psoriatic skin include evidence of increased metabolic activity and increased cGMP, DNA, RNA, IgG, and C3.[51,52] In psoriatic lesions, arachidonic acid levels are 30 times normal, 12-L-hydroxy-5,8,10,14-eicosatetraenoic acid (HETE) levels are 80 times normal, and prostaglandin E_2 levels are 50% higher than normal. Glucocorticoids normalize levels of arachidonic acid and HETE by inhibition of phospholipase A, and these activities may be partly responsible for regression of psoriatic lesions.[51]

GENETICS

There is a significant genetic component in psoriasis, but the exact mode of inheritance is uncertain.[53] Approximately 36% of patients with psoriasis have at least one immediate relative with the disorder.[48] Monozygotic twins have a higher concordance for psoriasis than do dizygotic twins.[48] Studies of histocompatibility antigens in psoriatic patients indicate statistically significant associations on the B, C, and D loci, more specifically, HLA-B13, HLA-B17, and HLA-B37.[52,54] The most significant association is with HLA-CW6, where the relative likelihood for developing psoriasis is 9 to 15 times normal. In addition, the B13 and B17 loci appear to be linked with the gene that expresses CW6.[52]

EXOGENOUS TRIGGER FACTORS

Factors such as climate, stress, infection, trauma, and drugs may aggravate psoriasis. Warm seasons and sunlight reportedly improve psoriasis in 80% of patients, while 90% report worsening in cold weather. Also, stress worsens psoriasis in 30% to 40% of patients; however, the exact role stress plays in exacerbation of psoriasis is uncertain.

Infection has been identified retrospectively as a common precipitating factor in psoriasis. A review of 245 cases of psoriatic children indicates that 25% had initial onset of the disease after clinically documented infections, while 54% had exacerbation during a 2- to 3-week interval after an upper respiratory infection.[55] Another study indicates that exacerbation of psoriasis is common 1 to 2 weeks after acute streptococcal infection.[56]

Lesions may occur at the site of injury to normal-appearing skin (Koebner response). The incidence is variable, ranging up to 76% of patients in retrospective studies and 51% in prospective studies.[52] The Koebner response may be induced by a variety of traumatic causes including rubbing, venipuncture, bites, surgery, and pressure. The mechanism for development of the Koebner response is unknown and is not unique to psoriasis. The length of time between injury and lesion development, although variable, is usually a few days to weeks. Lithium carbonate and β-adrenergic–blocking agents are among the most commonly noted drugs to exacerbate psoriasis.[57,58]

CLINICAL PRESENTATION

The clinical appearance of psoriasis, although not scarring, may be cosmetically disfiguring, especially for patients with severe disease. In general, psoriatic lesions are characterized by sharply demarcated, erythematous papules and plaques often covered with silver-white fine scales. Initial lesions are usually small papules that enlarge over time and coalesce into plaques, sometimes as serpiginous or geographic forms. If the fine scale is removed, a salmon-pink lesion is exposed, perhaps with punctate bleeding from prominent dermal capillaries (Auspitz sign).

The appearance of psoriatic lesions also varies depending on the area of the body affected and the variant type of psoriasis. Scalp psoriasis ranges from diffuse scaling on an erythematous scalp to thickened plaques with exudation, microabscesses, and fissures. Trunk, back, arm, and leg lesions may be generalized, scattered, discrete, guttate (drop-like) lesions, or large plaques. Palms, soles, face, and genitalia may be involved as well. Affected nails are often pitted and associated with subungual keratotic material. Yellow spots under the nail plate may also be seen.

Psoriatic arthritis is a distinct clinical entity in which both psoriatic lesions and inflammatory "arthritis" occur. Classically, distal interphalangeal joints and adjacent nails are involved, but knees, elbows, wrists, and ankles may also be involved. Skin lesions usually precede joint involvement, although the reverse may occur, or skin lesions and joint disease may occur simultaneously. The clinical appearance of psoriasis may sometimes be confused with numerous other dermatologic diseases; thus, the differential diagnosis is important and histopathology is often useful.

PATIENT ASSESSMENT

Evaluation and education of the psoriatic patient is of great importance because of the myriad drug therapy options available as nonprescription and prescription products (Table 88–9).

TABLE 88–9. Psoriatic Patient Assessment

Onset and duration of psoriasis
Family history
Exacerbating factors
Previous history of antipsoriasis agents with efficacy and side-effect data
All current and recent topical and systemic medications
Environmental and occupational exposure to chemicals and toxins
Allergies (food, drug, environmental)

▶ TREATMENT: Psoriasis

Although the exact cause of psoriasis is unknown, in a majority of patients, treatment approaches are usually reliable and offer good clinical control. Psoriasis is often a lifelong relapsing and remitting disease, so modes of therapy should be selected with long-term consequences in mind. Major factors for consideration include the extent and site of disease involvement and the age of the patient. The goal of therapy is to achieve resolution of lesions, but partial clearing is acceptable at times, using regimens with decreased toxicity and increased patient acceptability. Drug treatments for psoriasis are listed in Table 88–10. Treatment guidelines are listed in Tables 88–11 and 88–12.

TOPICAL PHARMACOLOGIC THERAPY

EMOLLIENTS AND KERATOLYTICS

Moisturizers or emollients hydrate the stratum corneum (after application of an occlusive oily film) and minimize evaporation of water from the stratum corneum.[59] Hydration causes the stratum corneum to swell and flatten the surface contour. Moisturizers may decrease the binding forces within the horny layer, enhance desquamation, and eliminate scaling.[59] Moisturizers may also increase pliability of the skin, have antipruritic activity, and possess mild vasoconstrictor activity. Moisturizers often need to be applied several times a day to achieve a beneficial response. Adverse effects include folliculitis and allergic or irritant contact dermatitis.

Keratolytics are used to remove scale, smooth the skin, and decrease hyperkeratosis.[59] Salicylic acid, the most frequently used keratolytic agent, is generally applied in concentrations of 2% to 10%. A possible mechanism of salicylic acid keratolysis is that it causes a decrease in corneocyte-to-corneocyte cohesion in the abnormal horny layer of psoriatic skin. Lower concentrations of salicylic acid exhibit a keratin-dispersing effect, while concentrations of 5% or higher have a corneolytic (exfoliative) action.[60] Although salicylic acid may enhance percutaneous penetration of some drugs, it also produces local irritation.[59] Application of salicylic acid to large, inflamed areas of skin is capable of inducing salicylism with symptoms of nausea, vomiting, tinnitus, or hyperventilation.[61]

COAL TAR

Although tar derivatives have been used to treat skin diseases for two millennia, relatively little is known about their composition or mechanism of action.[62] Tars are derived from wood such as pine or juniper, shale (ichthammol), and bituminous coal (coal tar). In recent years, wood and shale tars have fallen out of use because they possess relatively less efficacy than coal tar.[62] Coal tar contains numerous hydrocarbon compounds formed from distillation of bituminous coal.[62] When applied to normal skin, coal tar causes predominantly transient epidermal hyperplasia during the first 2 weeks of therapy followed by a cytostatic effect with epidermal thinning.[63] There is additional evidence that UVB light-activated coal tar photoadducts with epidermal DNA, and inhibits DNA synthesis. This normalized epidermal replication rate leads to reduction in plaque elevation.[64,65]

Coal tar is an effective treatment for psoriasis; however, it is a burdensome, time-consuming treatment with disadvantages that include unpleasant odor, ability to stain skin and clothing, ability to reversibly darken or alter light hair colors, and ability to tarnish silver in jewelry. Coal tar is usually applied topically to lesions (often at bedtime), but may also be used in bath water and as a shampoo. Short-contact treatment allows for application of tar just 2 hours before light treatment and avoids overnight applications that may interfere with sleep.

Risk of carcinogenicity is a concern with the long-term use of topical coal tar. Crude coal tar contains numerous polynuclear aromatic hydrocarbons that are known carcinogens. Retrospective studies of psoriatic patients treated with crude coal tar have not indicated any increase in cancer cases compared with controls[62]; however, there are cases indicating a higher rate of cutaneous carcinoma in patients exposed to tar and UVB light. Controlled studies are lacking to assess the carcinogenicity risk associated with clinical use of crude and refined coal tars.

TABLE 88–10. Examples of Drug Treatments for Psoriasis

Topical	Systemic
Emollients and keratolytics	Ultraviolet A and oral psoralens (systemic PUVA)
Coal tar	Methotrexate
Anthralin	Retinoids
Calcipotriene	Sulfasalazine
Acitretin	Cyclosporine
Tazarotene	Tacrolimus
Mycophenolate mofetil	
Methotrexate	
Ultraviolet A and topical psoralens (topical PUVA)	

TOPICAL CORTICOSTERIODS

Topical corticosteroids play an important *adjunctive* role in the treatment of psoriasis by decreasing erythema, pruritus, and scaling. The mechanism of action for topical corticosteroid efficacy in psoriasis is uncertain. Steroid receptors have been identified in the skin, and synthesis and mitosis of DNA in epidermal cells have been halted by topical corticosteroids in hairless mice.[66,67] However, humans mount a tachyphylactic response to topical corticosteroid antimitotic effect after only 72 hours of treatment. Topical corticosteroids appear to inhibit phospholipase A, lowering amounts of arachidonic acid, prostaglandins, and leukotrienes in the skin.[68] Coupled with local vasoconstriction, these agents are useful to reduce erythema and pruritus, but as antipsoriatic agents they are best used adjunctively with a product that specifically functions to normalize epidermal hyperproliferation.

A wide variety of topical corticosteroids are available in various potencies and vehicles as described in USP-DI.[69]

1. Products with a *low-potency* ranking have a modest anti-inflammatory effect and are safest for long-term application. These products are also the safest products for use on the face and intertriginous areas, in infants and young children, and with occlusion.

2. Products with a *medium-potency* ranking are used in moderate inflammatory dermatoses. Examples of conditions for which these products are frequently used include chronic eczematous dermatoses such as hand eczema and atopic eczema. Medium-potency preparations may be used on the face and intertriginous areas for limited periods of time.

3. *High-potency* preparations are used in severe inflammatory dermatoses. Examples of conditions for which these products are frequently used include more severe eczematous dermatoses, lichen simplex chronicus, and psoriasis. They are used for

TABLE 88–11. Topical Psoriasis Treatment Guidelines

Active Ingredient	Formulation	Strength (%)	Regimen	Potential Side Effects
Emollients	Lotions, creams, ointments	N/A	Three to four times daily	Folliculitis, contact dermatitis
Salicylic acid (keratolytic)	Gels, lotions	2–10	Two to three times daily	Can be irritating Has resulted in salicylism
Coal tar	Creams, gels, lotions, ointments, solutions	1–48.5	Apply in evening, allowing to remain through the night	Messy and burdensome Can be irritating Photoreactions
Anthralin	Creams, ointments	0.1–1	Usually in the evening, allowing to remain through the night. Short contact regimens have also been used	Stains skin and clothing Can be irritating
Calcipotriene	Ointment, solution, cream	0.005	Apply twice daily, no more than 100 g/wk, for up to 8 days	Burning and stinging in 10% of patients
Corticosteroids	Creams, lotions, ointments, solutions	Variable potency	Two to four times daily for maintenance; may use occlusion at night	Local tissue atrophy, striae, epidermal thinning, glucocorticoid systemic effects
Methoxsalen	Lotion	1	Apply to area prior to UVA therapy	Photoreaction, exaggerated burning

intermediate duration of treatment, or for longer periods in areas with thickened skin secondary to chronic conditions. High-potency preparations may also be used on the face and intertriginous areas but only for short periods of time.

4. *Very-high-potency* products are used primarily as an alternative to systemic adrenocorticoid therapy when local areas are involved. Examples of conditions for which very-high-potency products are frequently used include thick, chronic lesions caused by psoriasis, lichen simplex chronicus, and discoid lupus erythematosus. There is a high likelihood of skin atrophy with the use of very-high-potency preparations. They are used for only short periods of time and on relatively small surface areas. Occlusive dressings should not be used with these products.

The choice of corticosteroid and vehicle depends on severity and extent of involvement, the anatomic region of the body to be treated, and the anticipated duration of treatment. Topical corticosteroids are available in ointments, creams, lotions, gels, sprays, shampoos, mousses, and impregnated adhesive tapes.

An ointment is considered the most clinically effective dosage form in psoriasis treatment because it consists of an oily phase that is occlusive and conveys a hydrating effect as well as enhancement of penetration of the corticosteroid into the dermis by its lipophilicity.[70] Ointments are not suited for use in areas such as the axilla, groin, or other intertriginous areas where maceration and folliculitis may develop secondary to the occlusive effect. Creams typically are emulsified products with an aqueous phase and are occasionally preferred by patients as more cosmetically desirable. They may be used in intertriginous areas even though their lower oil content makes them more drying than ointments.

In severe, acute forms of psoriasis, and other inflammatory dermatoses, a patient may be instructed to apply a high-potency topical steroid every 2 hours for 24 to 48 hours, followed by gradual tapering down of applications to the rate of three or four times a day. For maintenance, application one to two times a day conveys cost-effective and nearly maximal vasoconstriction. Adverse reactions are not uncommon. Local tissue atrophy,

TABLE 88–12. Oral Psoriasis Treatment Guidelines

Active Ingredient	Formulation	Strength	Regimen	Potential Side Effects
Sulfasalazine	Suspension, tablets	250 mg/5mL; 500 mg	3–4 g/d	Gastrointestinal upset
Methoxsalen	Capsules	10 mg	Dosed on a mg/kg 2 hours before UVA exposure	Burns, erythema, gastrointestinal upset, CNS effects, ocular damage
Methotrexate	Tablets, injection	2.5 mg; 20–25 mg/mL	2.5–5 mg every 12 hours for three doses every week	Anemia, leukopenia, thrombocytopenia, gastrointestinal upset
Acitretin	Capsules	10 mg, 25 mg	25–50 mg daily	Dry mouth and lips, eye irritation, arthralgia, monitor liver function tests
Cyclosporine	Capsules, solution	25 mg, 100 mg; 100 mg/mL	3–4 mg/kg/d in two divided doses; may increase to 5 mg/kg/d in one month if no response	Nephrotoxicity, gastrointestinal upset, hypertension, tremor, monitor liver function tests
Tacrolimus	Capsules	1 mg, 5 mg	0.15 mg/kg twice daily; titrate based on side effects	Nephrotoxicity, gastrointestinal upset

degeneration, and striae are manifestations of corticosteroid effect on collagen synthesis and fibroblast growth. If detected early, atrophy and striae may be reversible upon drug discontinuation, but in numerous cases of prolonged therapy with high-potency agents, these changes may be long-lasting. Thinning of the epidermis may result in visible distended capillaries (telangiectasias) and purpura. Acneform eruptions and masking of symptoms of bacterial or fungal skin infections have also been reported with topical corticosteriod use.

Systemic consequences of topical corticosteroid use include risk of suppression of the hypothalamic–pituitary–adrenal axis, hyperglycemia, and development of cushingoid features. Avoidance of prolonged therapy with high-potency agents minimizes the risk of these side effects. Tachyphylaxis and rebound flare of psoriasis after abrupt cessation of topical corticosteroid therapy can also occur. With proper monitoring, topical corticosteroids are a safe and effective adjunctive approach to psoriasis treatment.

ANTHRALIN

Anthralin, an anthrone derivative of chrysarobin (from the South American araroba tree), is used topically to treat psoriasis.[71] Although anthralin (under the name dithranol) has been used for 70 years in Great Britain, it has only recently been extensively used in the United States. Anthralin appears to inhibit DNA synthesis by intercalation between DNA strands.[72] Another possible mechanism is that anthralin may decrease epidermal proliferation by mitochondrial inhibition. Irritation and inflammation are common with anthralin therapy and, to some degree, may correlate with clinical efficacy.[71,73] Other hypotheses support the role of anthralin-generated free radicals in producing both antipsoriatic effects and irritation.[74]

Inflammation, irritation, and staining of skin and clothing (via oxidation and binding to keratins) are often therapy-limiting effects. Fortunately, anthralin exerts its clinical effects at low cellular concentrations; therefore, short-contact therapy regimens (application for 20 minutes) have been found effective with decreased side effects.[75] Titrating the strength of anthralin gradually from a low concentration (0.1% to 0.25%) to a higher concentration (0.5% to 1%) may minimize irritation.

Anthralin was traditionally formulated in stiff paste bases to provide adherence to plaques. More recently, cream formulations have been developed that are more cosmetically appealing and appear to be as clinically effective. The patient must apply anthralin products only to affected areas of skin, because contact with uninvolved skin may result in excessive and unwanted irritation and staining, which usually disappears within 1 to 2 weeks of discontinuation. Staining of affected plaques is a sign of resolution as cell turnover has been slowed enough to take up the stain.[72] Despite the demonstrated efficacy of anthralin, some patients will not tolerate local irritation and staining.

CALCIPOTRIENE

Calcipotriene, a synthetic 1,25-dihydroxyvitamin D_3 analog, is used in the treatment of mild to moderate plaque psoriasis.[76] Calciprotriene binds to receptors in epidermal keratinocytes, resulting in the inhibition of cell proliferation and induction of cell differentiation.[77] Calcium metabolism may be altered by the application of calcipotriene, even with restricted use according to FDA labeling. Hypercalcemia has been reported with application of calcipotriene.[76,78,79] The long-term effects of altered calcium homeostasis are unknown. Calcipotriene has been evaluated in several open label or randomized, double-blind controlled studies and has been shown to be effective in improving or clearing psoriatic plaques.[78,80–82] On average, improvement was seen within 2 weeks of treatment, with approximately 70% of the patients demonstrating marked improvement after 8 weeks of therapy. Adverse effects include lesional and perilesional irritation, occurring in approximately 10% of treated patients and consisting of mild burning and stinging. Irritant dermatitis occurs more commonly on the face.[76,83] Dry skin, peeling, rash, and worsening of psoriasis have also been reported.

ACITRETIN

Acitretin, a retinoic acid analog, is the active metabolite of etretinate and has demonstrated clinical effects similar to etretrinate. Acitretin is indicated for the treatment of severe psoriasis, including erythrodermic and generalized pustular types, and is expected to replace etretinate, though some cases of patients responding to etretrinate and not acitretin exist.[84] Though the mechanism for treatment in patients with severe psoriasis is not clearly defined, it has shown significant clearing when administered. The initial recommended dose is 25 or 50 mg, with therapy being continued until lesions have resolved.

As with other retinoids, acitretin is associated with side effects such as hypervitaminosis A (i.e., dry lips/cheilitis, dry mouth, dry nose, dry eyes/conjuncitivitis, dry skin, pruritus, scaling, and hair loss). Other systemic side effects include hepatotoxicity, skeletal changes, hypercholesterolemia, and hypertriglyceridemia. To counteract hyperlipidemic effects, gemfibrozil has been studied for concomitant use with acitretin.[85] In addition, acitretin is a known teratogen and thus is contraindicated in females who are pregnant or who plan pregnancy within the 3 years following drug discontinuation. Acitretin is eliminated more rapidly and thus only a short period of contraception following treatment has been suggested as compared with etretinate.[86] A major drawback is that acitretin metabolizes to some degree to etretinate, which in turn poses the original hazard identified with etretinate use (prolonged retention in the host).

TAZAROTENE

Tazarotene, a synthenic retinoid, is a prodrug that exerts its pharmacologic activity when hydrolyzed to its active metabolite, tazarotenic acid. Though this metabolite has similar pharmacologic actions to other retinoids, it has been shown to have specific affinity for the retinoic acid receptors, RAR-γ and RAR-β, which enhance gene expression.[87] Tazarotene appears to affect the primary pathogenic factors involved in psoriasis: abnormal differentiation, hyperproliferation of the keratinocyte, and inflammation.[87,88] It has been evaluated for use in large, multicenter, vehicle-controlled trials. Treatment with 0.1% gel resulted in substantial reduction in the severity of erythema, scaling, and plaque elevation with 12-week therapies. In these studies, the 0.1% gel was somewhat more efficacious, but the 0.05% formulation was associated with less irritation.[88,89] Predominant treatment-related adverse effects were mild to moderate pruritus, burning/stinging, or erythema. These local reactions have been shown to be dose and frequency related.[89–91] Application of the gel to eczematous skin or to more than 20% of body surface area is not recommended, as this may lead to extensive systemic absorption.[90] Based on the results of these clinical trials, tazarotene 0.05% and 0.1% gels, applied once daily, are effective for the treatment of mild to moderate plaque psoriasis.[87,89,90]

SYSTEMIC PHARMACOLOGIC THERAPY

CYCLOSPORINE

Systemically administered cyclosporine demonstrates immunosuppressive activity by inhibiting an early step of T-cell activation, and also has anti-inflammatory activity by inhibiting the release of inflammatory mediators from mast cells, basophils, and polymorphonuclear cells.[92] Given these mechanisms, cyclosporine has been evaluated for use in the treatment of both cutaneous and articular manifestations of psoriasis.[92–94] An oral microemulsion formulation of cyclosporine (Neoral) has shown a better pharmacokinetic profile, resulting in a more consistent and predictable rate of absorption.[95]

Adverse effects of cyclosporine include hypertension, paresthesia, hypertrichosis, gingival hyperplasia, and renal dysfunction.[92,96] Recent evaluation of 30 psoriatic patients receiving long-term cyclosporine therapy indicated a need for renal biopsies or change of treatment after 2 years as all biopsies demonstrated features consistent with cyclosporine-related nephropathy.[96] A 1-year multicenter trial investigated the efficacy and safety of intermittent use of the immunosuppressant in the microemulsion form. Patients received three courses of therapy, with a maximum 12-week duration per course, but significant increases in serum creatinine were still found.[97] Lower maintenance doses of cyclosporine have also been studied to alleviate or prolong progression to cyclosporine-induced nephropathy.[98]

TACROLIMUS

Tacrolimus, an immunosuppressant indicated for organ allograft rejection, has been found to be efficacious in the treatment of recalcitrant psoriasis, on the basis of psoriasis as a T-cell mediated disease.[99–101] In a double-blind, placebo-controlled trial, patients receiving tacrolimus at oral doses of 0.05 mg/kg/d (increased up to 0.15 mg/kg/d as needed) resulted in efficacious treatment of recalcitrant plaque-type psoriasis.[101] Frequently reported adverse effects included diarrhea, paresthesia, and insomnia. Other toxicities, including renal insufficiency, have also been reported. As a topical agent, tacrolimus is advancing in clinical trials for eventual approval in the treatment of atopic dermatitis; however, trials establishing efficacy of topical tacrolimus in psoriasis are lacking to date.

MYCOPHENOLATE MOFETIL

Therapy with oral mycophenolic acid, a weak organic acid, was investigated in the 1970s for the treatment of moderate to severe psoriasis. Its ability to inhibit purine biosynthesis and show immunosuppressive activity was demonstrated by several multicenter, double-blind, placebo-controlled studies. Recent introduction of mycophenolate mofetil, a morpholinoester of mycophenolic acid, has recreated interest in its antipsoriatic properties. Commonly reported side effects include genitourinary symptoms (such as urgency, frequency, and dysuria), hematologic effects (including anemia, neutropenia, and thrombocytopenia), and an increased incidence of viral and bacterial infections. Oral mycophenolate mofetil, as well as topical mycophenolic acid, may undergo further clinical studies to determine usefulness in the treatment of patients with severe psoriasis.[102]

SULFASALAZINE

Oral sulfasalazine (3 to 4 g/d for 8 weeks) has been reported to be an effective therapy for plaque-type psoriasis in some patients.[103] When used as a single agent in the treatment of psoriasis, it is not as effective as is therapy with methotrexate, psoralens plus ultraviolet A light (PUVA), or etretinate. One possible advantage of sulfasalazine therapy compared with other systemic treatments is its lower incidence of severe side effects.[103]

COMBINATION THERAPY

SYSTEMIC THERAPY–PHOTOCHEMOTHERAPY: ORAL AND TOPICAL PSORALEN AND LONG-WAVE ULTRAVIOLET A LIGHT

The use of psoralens with UVA (PUVA) has been studied since the early 1970s and was approved by the FDA in 1982. Efficacy studies indicated that control of psoriasis occurred in nearly 90% of patients.[104]

Psoralens react with nucleic acids and intercalate between base pairs. When DNA is irradiated with long-wave ultraviolet light (320 to 400 nm, UVA), the psoralens covalently bind to pyrimidine bases, forming a cross-link.[105] PUVA may also affect immune responses in the skin and circulating lymphocytes, as demonstrated by a decreased ability to mount delayed hypersensitivity responses to contact sensitizers and increased risk of cutaneous cancer in treated patients.[106,107]

Candidates for PUVA therapy usually have severe incapacitating psoriasis unresponsive to topical therapies and are without history of photosensitivity, skin cancers, cataracts, or x-ray therapy of the skin. Methoxsalen (8-methoxypsoralen or 8-MOP) is usually dosed at 0.6 to 0.8 mg/kg and is given 2 hours before exposure to UVA. Serum methoxsalen concentrations usually peak within 0.5 to 2 hours of ingestion; however, a large interindividual and intraindividual variation in absorption may complicate titration of effective therapy.[108] Dosing of UVA is determined by patient skin type and history of previous response to ultraviolet radiation.

TOPICAL PSORALENS

The use of PUVA has been proven to be beneficial for psoriasis.[109–112] Several studies involving plaque psoriasis, comparing oral and bath-water delivery of 8-MOP, have found that the bath-water form was as effective, required reduced amounts of UVA, and was associated with fewer side effects.[113,114] Recently, local bath-PUVA therapy has also been studied in the management of chronic palmoplantar eczema.[115]

EVALUATION OF THERAPEUTIC OUTCOMES

Psoriasis is a relatively common hyperproliferative epidermal disorder for which several effective therapeutic modalities control rather than cure the condition. Recognition of the pathogenic factors associated with psoriasis, selection of an appropriate treatment regimen, and monitoring for adverse effects as well as disease progression often lead to a satisfactory outcome. Concepts of therapy should be adequately conveyed to the patient and the importance of compliance should be emphasized.

Achievement of clinical efficacy by any given therapeutic regimen requires days to weeks. Initial dramatic response may be achieved with some agents such as tazarotene and/or corticosteroids; however, sustained benefit with pharmacologically specific antipsoriatic therapy usually requires a range of about 2 to 8 weeks for noticeable response with most other therapies. Positive response to therapy is noted as normalization of involved areas of skin as measured by reduced erythema and scaling as well as reduction of plaque elevation.

As with most pharmacotherapy choices, risk–benefit issues are of great importance in treating an epidermal-based disorder that may be seriously debilitating to the patient. The purpose of pharmacotherapy in this disorder is often to keep or establish the patient functional in his or her social and job environments as well as to preserve emotional and physical health.

Rational dermatologic therapy must be principled in the pathogenesis of the disorder. Major advances in recent years have allowed a better understanding of disease mechanisms and have produced a high level of interest in the development of pharmacotherapeutic approaches to treatment. Common skin disorders such as acne and psoriasis are excellent clinical models for demonstrating broad areas of pharmacologic intervention and therapeutic benefit. For many other common dermatologic disorders, these same principles apply.

▶ PRINCIPLES OF PHARMACOTHERAPY

- The pathogenesis of acne is multifactorial, including androgen-stimulated sebum production, follicular abnormalities, and bacterial *(Propionibacterium acnes)* action on sebum to create breakdown products that produce inflammation.
- Contrary to popular belief, diet, hygiene, cosmetic use, and certain hairstyles do not necessarily play a role in the development of acne.
- In mild inflammatory acne, topical treatment with once to twice daily application of an antibacterial agent as well as a comedolytic agent is recommended.
- Acne patients with scarring potential and those not responding to topical therapy may use the combination of a topical comedolytic agent with a systemic antibiotic.
- Acne patients with nodular lesions and scarring potential are candidates for systemic isotretinoin therapy.
- The clinical response in acne is delayed and is not fairly assessed, regardless of therapeutic regimen, until 6 to 8 weeks of therapy.
- Since topical agents are disease preventive, all acne-prone areas should be treated to prevent or minimize the formation of new lesions and to minimize the risk of scarring.
- Exogenous factors such as climate, stress, infection, trauma, and drugs may aggravate or trigger psoriasis in an individual who is otherwise genetically predisposed to expression of the disease.
- Warm seasons and sunlight improve psoriasis in 80% of patients, whereas a majority report worsening with cold or hot temperature extremes.
- Adjunctive topical therapies include psoriasis emollients, keratolytics, and corticosteroids.
- A positive response to psoriasis therapy is noted as "normalization" of involved areas measured by reduced erythema and scaling as well as reduction of plaque elevation.
- The risk–benefit ratio is an important consideration in the treatment of psoriasis, and the goal is to maintain a functional status for the patient.
- Disease-modifying therapies for psoriasis include topical calcipotriene and tazarotene, light-source treatments such as coal tar plus UVB and PUVA, and systemic treatments such as methotrexate, hydroxyurea, cyclosporine, and acitretin.

REFERENCES

1. Arndt KA, Wintroub BU, Robinson JK, et al, eds. Primary Care Dermatology, Philadelphia, Saunders, 1997.
2. Leyden JJ. Therapy for acne vulgaris. N Engl J Med 1997;336: 1156–1162.
3. Morgan M, McCreedy R, Simpson J, et al. Dermatology quality of life scales—A measure of the impact of skin diseases. Br J Dermatol 1997;136:202–206.
4. Thiboutot DM. Acne: An overview of clinical research findings. Dermatol Clin 1997;15:97–109.
5. Layton AM, Seukeran D, Cunliffe WJ. Scarred for life? Dermatology 1997;195(suppl 1):15–21.
6. Landow K. Dispelling myths about acne. Postgrad Med 1997; 102:94–112.
7. Arndt KA, ed. Acne. In: Manual of Dermatologic Therapeutics, 5th ed. Boston, Little, Brown, 1995:3–15.
8. Melski JW, Arndt KA. Topical therapy for acne. N Engl J Med 1980;302:503–506.
9. Eaglstein WH. Allergic contact dermatitis to benzoyl peroxide. Arch Dermatol 1968;97:527.
10. Franz TJ. On the bioavailability of topical formulations of clindamycin hydrochloride. J Am Acad Dermatol 1983;9:66–73.
11. Eady EA, Holland KT, Cunliffe NJ. Should topical antibiotics be used for the treatment of acne vulgaris? Br J Dermatol 1982;107: 235–246.
12. Eady EA, Holland KT, Cunliffe WJ. The use of antibiotics in acne therapy: Oral or topical administration? J Antimicrob Chemother 1982;10:89–115.
13. Schachner L, Eaglstein W, Kittles C, Mertz P. Topical erythromycin and zinc therapy for acne. J Am Acad Dermatol 1990;22:253–260.
14. Habbema L, Koopmans B, Menke HE, et al. A 4% erythromycin and zinc combination (Zineryt) versus 2% erythromycin (Eryderm) in acne vulgaris: A randomized double-blind comparative study. Br J Dermatol 1989;121:497–502.
15. Becker LE, Bergstresser PR, Whiting DA, et al. Topical clindamycin therapy for acne vulgaris. Arch Dermatol 1981;117:482–485.
16. Parry MF, Rha CK. Pseudomembranous colitis caused by topical clindamycin phosphate. Arch Dermatol 1986;122:583–594.
17. Mackrides PS, Shaughnessy AF. Azelaic acid therapy for acne. Am Fam Physician 1996; 54:2457–2459.
18. Schallreuter KU, Wood JW. A possible mechanism of action for azelaic acid in the human epidermis. Arch Dermatol Res 1989;202: 168–171.
19. Cunliffe WJ, Holland KT. Clinical and laboratory studies on treatment with 20% azelaic acid cream for acne. Acta Derm Venereol (Stockh) 1989;143(suppl):31–34.
20. Cavicchini S, Caputo R. Long-term treatment of acne with 20% azelaic acid cream. Acta Derm Venereol (Stockh) 1989;143(suppl): 40–44.
21. Thomas JR III, Doya JA. The therapeutic uses of topical vitamin A acid. J Am Acad Dermatol 1981;4:505–513.
22. Berson DS, Shalita AR. The treatment of acne: The role of combination therapies. J Am Acad Dermatol 1995;32:S31–S41.
23. Hurwitz S. The combined effect of vitamin A acid and benzoyl peroxide in the treatment of acne. Cutis 1976;17:585–590.
24. Brogden RN, Goa KL. Adapalene: A review of its pharmacological properties and clinical potential in the management of mild to moderate acne. Drugs 1997;53:511–519.
25. Shalita A, Weiss J, Chalker D, et al. A comparison of the efficacy and safety of adapalene gel 0.01% and tretinoin gel 0.025% in the treatment of acne vulgaris: A multicenter trial. J Am Acad Dermatol 1996;34:482–485.
26. Shalita A, Chalker D, Griffith R, et al. Double-blind study of AGN 190168, a new retinoid gel, in the topical treatment of acne vulgaris. J Invest Dermatol 1993;100:542.
27. Ad Hoc Committee on the Use of Antibiotics in Dermatology. Systemic antibiotics for treatment of acne vulgaris, efficacy and safety. Arch Dermatol 1975;111:1630–1636.
28. Jonas M, Cunha BA. Minocycline. Ther Drug Monit 1982;4:137–145.
29. Shapiro LE, Knowles SR, Shear NH. Comparative safety of tetracycline, minocycline, and doxycycline. Arch Dermatol 1997;133: 1224–1230.

30. Gammon WR, Meyer C, Lantis S, et al. Comparative efficacy of oral erythromycin versus oral tetracycline in the treatment of acne vulgaris. J Am Acad Dermatol 1986;14:183–186.
31. Nordin K, Hallander H, Fredriksson T, Rylander C. A clinical and bacteriological evaluation of the effect of sulphamethoxazole–trimethoprim in acne vulgaris, resistant to prior therapy with tetracyclines. Dermatologica 1978;157:245–253.
32. Hansten PD, Horn JR. Inhibition of oral contraceptive efficacy. Drug Interactions Newslett 1985;5:7–10.
33. Miller DM, Helms SE, Brodell RT. A practical approach to antibiotic treatment in women taking oral contraceptives. J Am Acad Dermatol 1994;30:1008–1011.
34. Lucky AW, Henderson TA, Olson WH, et al. Effectiveness of norgestimate and ethinyl estradiol in treating moderate acne vulgaris. J Am Acad Dermatol 1997;37:746–754.
35. Shaw JC. Antiandrogen and hormonal treatment of acne. Dermatol Clin 1996;14:803–811.
36. Redmond GP, Olson WH, Lippman JS, et al. Norgestimate and ethinyl estradiol in the treatment of acne vulgaris: A randomized, placebo-controlled trial. Obstet Gynecol 1997;89:615–622.
37. Rumsfield JA, West DP, Tse CST, et al. Isotretinoin in severe, recalcitrant cystic acne: A review. Drug Intell Clin Pharm 1983;17: 329–333.
38. Saurat JH. Oral isotretinoin: Where now, where next? Dermatology 1997;195(suppl 1):1–3.
39. Ortonne JP. Oral isotretinoin treatment policy: Do we all agree? Dermatology 1997;195(suppl 1):34–37.
40. Shalita AR, Cunningham WJ, Leyden JJ, et al. Isotretinoin treatment of acne and related disorders: An update. J Am Acad Dermatol 1983;9:629–638.
41. Meigel WN. How safe is oral isotretinoin? Dermatology 1997; 195(suppl 1):22–28.
42. Newton JN. How cost-effective is oral isotretinoin? Dermatology 1997;195(suppl 1):10–14.
43. Gilchrest BA. Retinoid pharmacology and skin. In: Mukhtar H, ed. Pharmacology of the Skin. Boca Raton, CRC, 1995:167–181.
44. Goulden V, Cunliffe WJ. The long-term experience with isotretinoin treatment of acne. In: Dahl MV, Lynch PJ, eds. Current Opinion in Dermatology. Philadelphia, Current Science, 1995:231–234.
45. Adverse effects with isotretinoin. FDA Drug Bull 1983;13:21–23.
46. Krueger GG, Bergstresser PR, Lowe NJ, et al. Psoriasis. J Am Acad Dermatol 1984;11:937–947.
47. Watson W. Psoriasis: Epidemiology and genetics. Dermatol Clin 1984;2:363–371.
48. Farber EM, Nail ML. The natural history of psoriasis in 5,600 patients. Dermatologica 1974;148:1–18.
49. Wrone-Smith T, Nickoloff BJ. Dermal injection of immunocytes induces psoriasis. J Clin Invest 1996;98:1878–1887.
50. Weinstein GD, McCullough JL, Ross PA. Cell kinetic basis for pathophysiology of psoriasis. J Invest Dermatol 1985;85:579–583.
51. Baden HP. Biology of the epidermis and pathophysiology of psoriasis and certain ichthyosiform dermatoses. In: Soter NA, Baden HP, eds. Pathophysiology of Dermatologic Diseases. New York, McGraw-Hill, 1984:101–126.
52. Krueger GG. Psoriasis: Current concepts of its etiology and pathogenesis. In: Dobson RL, Thiers BH, eds. Yearbook of Dermatology. Chicago, Year Book, 1981.
53. Elder JT. Cytokine and genetic regulation of psoriasis. In: Callen JP, ed. Advances in Dermatology, vol 10. St. Louis, Mosby-Year Book, 1995:99–134.
54. Russell TJ, Schultes LM, Kuban DJ. Histocompatibility (HLA) antigens associated with psoriasis. N Engl J Med 1972;287: 738–740.
55. Nyfors A, Lemholt K. Psoriasis in children: A short review and a survey of 245 cases. Br J Dermatol 1975;92:437–442.
56. Whyte HJ, Baughman RD. Acute guttate psoriasis and streptococcal infection. Arch Dermatol 1964;89:350–356.
57. Skoven I, Thormann J. Lithium compound treatment and psoriasis. Arch Dermatol 1979;115:1185–1187.
58. Neumann HAM, van Joost T. Adverse reactions of the skin to metoprolol and other beta-adrenoreceptor-blocking agents. Dermatologica 1981;162:330–335.
59. Marks R. Topical therapy for psoriasis: General principles. Dermatol Clin 1984;2:383–388.
60. Weirich EG. Dermatopharmacology of salicylic acid. I: Range of dermatotherapeutic effects of salicylic acid. Br Med J 1979;1:661.
61. Davies MG, Briffa DV, Greaves MW. Systemic toxicity from topically applied salicylic acid. Br Med J 1979;1:661.
62. Lin AN, Moses K. Tar revisited. Int J Dermatol 1985;24:216–218.
63. Polano MK. Topical Skin Therapeutics. London, Churchill Livingstone, 1984:95.
64. Lavker RM, Grove GL, Kligman AM. The atrophogenic effect of crude coal tar on human epidermis. Br J Dermatol 1981;105: 77–82.
65. Lowe NJ, Breeding J, Wortzman MS. The pharmacological variability of crude coal tar. Br J Dermatol 1982;107:475–479.
66. Cornell RC, Stoughton RB. The use of topical steroids in psoriasis. Dermatol Clin 1984;2:397–409.
67. Cornell RC. Topical glucocorticoids in dermatology. In: Dahl MV, Lynch PJ, eds. Current Opinion in Dermatology, 2nd ed. Philadelphia, Current Science, 1995:193–197.
68. Hammarstrom S, Hamberg M, Duell EA, et al. Glucocorticoid in inflammatory proliferative skin disease reduces arachidonic and hydroxyeicosatetraenoic acids. Science 1977;197:994–996.
69. Corticosteroids (topical). In: United States Pharmacopeia Drug Information (USP-DI), 18th ed, vol 1. Taunton, MA, 1998:931–950.
70. Burdick KH, Haleblian JK, Poulsen BJ, Cobner SE. Corticosteroid ointments: Comparison by two human bioassays. Curr Ther Res 1973;15:233–242.
71. Ashton RE, Andre P, Lowe NJ, Whitefield M. Anthralin: Historical and current perspectives. J Am Acad Dermatol 1983;9:173–192.
72. Swanbeck G, Thyresson N. Interaction between dithranol and nucleic acids. Acta Derm Venereol (Stockh) 1965;45:344–348.
73. Barr RM, Misch KJ, Hensby CN, et al. Arachidonic acid and prostaglandin levels in dithranol erythema: Time course study. Br J Clin Pharmacol 1983;16:715–717.
74. Finnen MJ, Lawrence CM, Shuster S. Inhibition of dithranol inflammation by free-radical scavengers. Lancet 1984;2:1129–1130.
75. Gorsulowsky DC, Voorhees JJ, Ellis CN. Anthralin therapy for psoriasis: A new look at an old compound. Arch Dermatol 1985;121: 1509–1511.
76. Kirsner RS, Federman D. Treatment of psoriasis: Role of calcipotriene. Am Fam Physician 1995;52:137–239.
77. Berth-Jones J, Fletcher A, Hutchinson PE. Epidermal cytokeratin and immunocyte responses during treatment of psoriasis with calcipotriol. In: Norma AW, Bouillon R, Thomasset M, eds. Vitamin D: Gene Regulation, Structure-Function Analysis and Clinical Application. Berlin, de Gruyter, 1991:424.
78. Cunliffe WJ, Claudy A, Faiross G, et al. A multicenter comparative study of calcipotriol and betamethasone 17-valerate in patients with psoriasis vulgaris. J Am Acad Dermatol 1992;26:736–743.
79. De Jong EM, van de Kerkhof PM. Simultaneous assessment of inflammation and epidermal proliferation in psoriatic plaques during long-term treatment with the vitamin D analogue MC 903: Modulations and interrelations. Br J Dermatol 1991;124:221–229.
80. Kragballe K, Fogh K. Treatment of psoriasis by the topical application of the novel cholecalciferol analogue calcipotriol (MC 903). Arch Dermatol 1989;125:1647–1652.
81. Kragballe K, Gjertsen BT, DeHoope D, et al. Double-blind, right/left comparison of calcipotriol and betamethasone valerate in treatment of psoriasis vulgaris. Lancet 1991;337:193–196.
82. Berth-Jones J, Chu AC, Dodd WAH, et al. A multicenter parallel-group comparison of calcipotriol ointment and short contact dithranol therapy in chronic plaque psoriasis. Br J Dermatol 1992;127:266–271.

83. Fisher DA. Allergic contact dermatitis to propylene glycol in calcipotriene ointment. Cutis 1997;60:43–44.
84. Bleiker TO, Bourke JF, Graham-Brown RAC, et al. Etretrinate may work where acitretin fails. Br J Dermatol 1997;136:368–370.
85. Vahlquist C, Olsson AG, Lindholm A, et al. Effects of gemfibrozil on hyperlipidemia in acitretin-treated patients. Results of a double-blind cross-over study. Acta Derm Venereol 1995;75:377–380.
86. Lambert WE, Meyer E, DeLeenheer AP, et al. Pharmacokinetics of acitretin. Acta Derm Venereol 1994;186:122–123.
87. Duvic M, Nagpal S, Asano AT, et al. Molecular mechanisms of tazarotene action in psoriasis. J Am Acad Dermatol 1997;37:S18–S24.
88. Chandraratna RAS. Tazarotene: The first receptor-selective topical retinoid for the treatment of psoriasis. J Am Acad Dermatol 1997; 37:S12–S17.
89. Weinstein GD, Krueger GG, Lowe NJ, et al. Tazarotene gel, a new retinoid, for topical therapy of psoriasis: Vehicle-controlled study of safety, efficacy, and duration of therapeutic effect. J Am Acad Dermatol 1997;37:85–92.
90. Weinstein GD. Tazarotene gel: Efficacy and safety in plaque psoriasis. J Am Acad Dermatol 1997;37:S33–S38.
91. Marks R. Clinical safety of tazarotene in the treatment of plaque psoriasis. J Am Acad Dermatol 1997;37:S25–S32.
92. Olivieri I, Salvarani C, Cantini F, et al. Therapy with cyclosporine in psoriatic arthritis. Semin Arthritis Rheum 1997;27:36–43.
93. Tourne L, Durez P, Van Vooren JP, et al. Alleviation of HIV-associated psoriasis and psoriatic arthritis with cyclosporine. J Am Acad Dermatol 1997;37:501–502.
94. Jones G, Crotty M, Brooks P, Psoriatic Arthritis Meta-analysis Study Group. Psoriatic arthritis: A qualitative overview of therapeutic options. Br J Rheumatol 1997;36:95–99.
95. Erkko P, Granlund H, Nuutinen M, et al. Comparison of cyclosporin A pharmacokinetics of a new microemulsion formulation and standard oral preparation in patients with psoriasis. Br J Dermatol 1997;136:82–88.
96. Zachariae H, Kragballe K, Hansen HE, et al. Renal biopsy findings in long-term cyclosporin treatment of psoriasis. Br J Dermatol 1997;136:531–535.
97. Berth-Jones J, Henderson CA, Munro CS, et al. Treatment of psoriasis with intermittent short course cyclosporin (Neoral). A multicentre study. Br J Dermatol 1997;136:527–530.
98. Shupack J, Abel E, Bauer E, et al. Cyclosporine as maintenance therapy in patients with severe psoriasis. J Am Acad Dermatol 1997;36: 423–432.
99. Thompson AW, Carroll PB, McCauley J, et al. FK506: A novel immunosuppressant for treatment of autoimmune disease. Springer Semin Immunopathol 1993;14:323–344.
100. Jegasothy BV, Ackerman CD, Todo S, et al. Tacrolimus (FK 506)—A new therapeutic agent for severe recalcitrant psoriasis. Arch Dermatol 1992;128:781–785.
101. European FK 506 Multicentre Psoriasis Study Group. Systemic tacrolimus (FK 506) is effective for the treatment of psoriasis in a double-blind, placebo-controlled study. Arch Dermatol 1996;132: 419–423.
102. Kitchin JE, Pomeranz MK, Pak G, et al. Rediscovering mycophenolic acid: A review of its mechanism, side effects and potential uses. J Am Acad Dermatol 1997;37:445–449.
103. Gupta AK, Ellis CN, Siegel MT, et al. Sulfasalazine improves psoriasis. Arch Dermatol 1990;126:487–493.
104. Bickers DR. Position paper—PUVA therapy. J Am Acad Dermatol 1983;8:265–270.
105. Cole RS. Light-induced crosslinking of DNA in the presence of a furocoumarin (psoralen). Biochem Biophys Acta 1970;217:30–39.
106. Thorvaldsen J, Volden G. PUVA-induced diminution of contact allergic and irritant skin reactions. Clin Exp Dermatol 1980;5:43–46.
107. Elmets CA, Bergstresser PR. Ultraviolet radiation effects on immune processes. Photochem Photobiol 1982;36:715–719.
108. Goldstein DP, Carter DM, Ljunggren B, Burkholder J. Minimal phototoxic doses and 8-MOP plasma levels in PUVA patients. J Invest Dermatol 1982;78:429–433.
109. Fischer T, Alsins J. Treatment of psoriasis with trioxsalen baths and dysprosium lamps. Acta Derm Venereol (Stockh) 1976;56:383–390.
110. Salo OP, Lassus A, Taskinen J. Trioxsalen bath plus UVA treatment of psoriasis. Acta Derm Venereol (Stockh) 1981;61:551–554.
111 Berne B, Fischer T, Michealsson G, Noren P. An 8-year follow-up of 149 psoriasis patients. Photodermatol 1984;1:18–22.
112. Turjanma K, Salo H, Reunala T. Comparison of trioxsalen bath and oral methoxsalen PUVA in psoriasis. Acta Derm Venereol (Stockh) 1985;86–88.
113. Lowe NJ, Weingarten D, Bourget T, et al. PUVA therapy for psoriasis: Comparison of oral and bath-water delivery of 8-methoxypsoralen. J Am Acad Dermatol 1986;14:754–760.
114. David M, Lowe NJ, Halder RM, Borok M. Serum 8-methoxypsoralen (8-MOP) concentrations after bath water delivery of 8-MOP plus UVA. J Am Acad Dermatol 1990;23:931–932.
115. Schempp CM, Muller H, Czech W, et al. Treatment of chronic palmoplantar eczema with local bath-PUVA therapy. J Am Acad Dermatol 1997;36:733–737.

89

DRUG-INDUCED SKIN REACTIONS

Nina H. Han, PharmD, Phillip A. Nowakowski, PharmD, and Dennis P. West, PhD, FCCP

Cutaneous drug reactions occur in approximately 2% to 3% of medical inpatients, and skin rash is a frequent reason for patient visits to physicians.[1,2] Establishment of a relationship between medication use and subsequent development of cutaneous reactions, however, is often difficult. Unfortunately, mechanisms underlying adverse drug reactions are poorly understood and few diagnostic tests are available to properly establish cause and effect. Patients with drug-induced reactions are often taking more than one drug, making detection of the causative agent difficult. The picture is further complicated because small doses of a drug may evoke severe reactions even if that agent was previously well tolerated.[3]

DRUG HISTORY

A thorough and organized approach is essential to proper diagnosis of a drug-induced skin reaction. Patient evaluation should include (1) a comprehensive drug history, (2) awareness of various clinical manifestations of drug allergy and cutaneous reactions, (3) awareness of factors that favor development of allergic reactions to drugs, and (4) awareness of the immunologic and nonimmunologic mechanisms involved in cutaneous reactions to drugs.[4–6]

A patient may experience a skin reaction while on multiple drugs. Most authorities advise that the first drug(s) to consider is that initiated within the week preceding the reaction. This short temporal relationship does not hold for all drugs (e.g., onset perhaps 2 weeks after discontinuation of semisynthetic penicillins, onset perhaps 6 months for β-blocker–induced psoriasiform eruptions, onset of 2 months to perhaps 5 years for some forms of drug-induced systemic lupus erythematosus [SLE]).[7] Each drug should be individually considered as a potential cause. Adverse drug reactions can be classified into two categories: types A and B (Table 89–1).[8] Type A reactions, accounting for 80% of reported adverse drug reactions, are produced by known pharmacologic drug actions and are usually dose dependent and predictable to some extent. Reactions classified as type B are generally uncommon and unpredictable.

A Guide to Drug Eruptions[9] is updated at 4- to 5-year intervals and is a useful source of confirmed and tabulated information on drug-induced skin reactions. Other resources include an online reference, the Dartmouth Database (gopher://gopher.Dartmouth.edu/1/Research/BioSci/CDRD), and *Cutaneous Drug Reactions,*[10] which cites over 6500 references and is categorized by drug name and skin disorder. With an increased number of drugs undergoing shorter premarketing phases, a greater number and variety of skin reactions are expected to occur during postmarketing surveillance. The pharmacist plays an important role in identifying and reporting possible drug-induced skin reactions and in monitoring or preventing recurrence.

DIAGNOSIS

Although several *in vitro* and *in vivo* tests have been used to diagnose drug allergy, the availability and reliability of these tests are limited.[11–13] The *in vitro* radioallergosorbent test (RAST) may be used to detect IgE or IgG antibodies and has produced reasonably reliable results in detecting penicillin allergy. The modified Coombs test and bacteriophage inhibition test have even higher sensitivity for detecting IgG and IgE antibodies, although more elaborate laboratory resources are required. The lymphocyte transformation test is an *in vitro* test for diagnosis of both immediate and delayed drug reactions, but results depend on the drug and type of skin eruption.[9]

Patch testing, useful in assessing allergic and irritant contact dermatitis, has limited to no utility for other types of skin reactions such as delayed hypersensitivity reactions and fixed-drug eruptions.[9] Scratch or prick testing with drugs and/or metabolites may be useful in immediate-type reactions, but there are practical limitations to this method. Dechallenge/rechallenge continues to be regarded as the most definitive method for ascertaining drug-induced reactions. However, it is often not an option if a patient has experienced a potentially life-threatening reaction or if the suspected agent cannot be discontinued. In some cases, rechallenge may not result in the same reaction, which further clouds the picture. Symptoms of an allergic drug reaction usually have an acute onset, may last several minutes to months, or may occur periodically throughout an exposure period. An accurate description of the characteristics of a cutaneous drug reaction should be obtained. Although drug hypersensitivity is impossible to predict, certain drug and host factors increase the likelihood of a reaction.

CLINICAL PRESENTATION

Drug allergy is more frequent in older individuals[14] and may be related to immune response capability and to increased exposure to drugs. Individual genetic factors may also predispose an individual to drug allergy: variability in

TABLE 89–1. Classification of Adverse Drug Reactions

Type A: Common and Predictable Adverse Reactions
I. Effects of overdosage
II. Immediate or delayed adverse effects
III. Secondary or indirect effects
  A. Related to drug alone
  B. Related to both disease and drug
IV. Interactions between/among drugs
Type B: Uncommon and Unpredictable Reactions
I. Intolerance
II. Idiosyncratic reaction
III. Hypersensitivity reactions

Compiled from Ref. 8.

drug metabolism, immune response, tissue receptor sites, and elaboration of immunologic mediators may all play a role.[15] In addition, a previous history of allergic drug reactions may increase the likelihood of developing a new allergic reaction. Hepatic and renal disorders may alter drug biotransformation and increase the likelihood of an allergic response.[16]

To induce an immune response (i.e., hypersensitivity reaction), the drug or its metabolite must act as, or form, a complete antigen. For example, proteins contained in sera, vaccines, biologicals, and allergens may act as complete antigens; however, many drugs are small molecules and must bind with larger molecules to create a complete antigen. Haptens are often drugs capable of such binding. Once a complete antigen is formed, the immune system reacts to neutralize, destroy, or eliminate it from the host.

The route of administration may influence drug allergy. For example, topical application of drugs has the greatest propensity to induce allergy, followed by the intravenous route and the oral route. Although not strictly dose related, such factors as the number of drugs, the dose of drug, and the duration of therapy may influence the likelihood of developing a hypersensitivity reaction.

The host's ability to react to antigenic material is the basis for specific immune reactions. The ultimate physiologic role of the immune system is to differentiate "self" from "nonself" and eliminate foreign materials from the body. The type of immunologic mediation of hypersensitivity may determine the category of reaction and thus the clinical presentation of drug-induced skin disorders.

For a discussion of allergic drug reaction mechanisms, see Chapter 81.

Because any drug may induce cutaneous reactivity, a complete review of drug-induced skin reactions is not practical; however, for common cutaneous drug reactions, their clinical course, possible mechanisms, etiologies, and management are described in the next sections. Maculopapular reactions and urticaria occur most often. The clinical type and frequency of cutaneous reactions to drugs for a series of 225 patients are listed in Table 89–2.[16]

TABLE 89–2. Type and Frequency of Cutaneous Drug Reactions

Eruption Type	Total no. (%)	Verified by Provocation no. (%)
Fixed-drug eruption	77 (34.2)	51 (66.2)
Exanthematous eruption	71 (31.6)	47 (66.2)
Urticaria/angioedema	45 (20.0)	26 (57.8)
Gold dermatitis	15 (6.7)	0 (0)
Purpuric eruption	5 (2.2)	0 (0)
Erythema multiforme	4 (1.8)	2 (50.0)
Toxic epidermal necrolysis	3 (1.3)	0 (0)
Stevens–Johnson syndrome	2 (0.9)	1 (50.0)
Exfoliative dermatitis	2 (0.9)	1 (50.0)
Systemic lupus erythematosus–like eruption	1 (0.4)	0 (0)
TOTAL	225 (100.0)	128 (56.9)

Compiled from Ref. 16.

MACULOPAPULAR ERUPTIONS

CLINICAL PRESENTATION

Maculopapular eruptions are the most common drug-induced skin reactions. Lesions are somewhat nonspecific, but may be "measles-like" in their clinical manifestations in that they resemble viral exanthems and may be called morbilliform, scarlatiniform, or rubelliform eruptions. These reactions often start on the trunk or in areas of pressure or trauma and are frequently symmetrical. Individual lesions may be flat or raised and vary in size from a few millimeters to large, confluent areas. In some cases, vesicles may also be present. Mild fever and involvement of mucous membranes or palms and soles, though less frequent, may also occur.[17,18]

The course of a maculopapular eruption is classified as an "early" or "late" reaction. Individual patient responses may vary, with reactions occuring between the first day of exposure to 2 or more weeks after therapy. In the early reaction, the eruption usually appears within hours or up to 3 days after drug administration to previously sensitized patients. The late reaction appears most commonly at about 9 days but with wide variability after drug exposure.[17,18] Maculopapular rashes generally do not persist for prolonged periods, although recurrence may present as more serious and extensive exfoliative skin reactions.[12] Occasionally, eruptions decrease or disappear even with continued medication use and may not always recur with drug rechallenge.[17] Although the penicillins have been well documented as a cause of drug-induced maculopapular eruption, many other drugs have been associated with maculopapular eruptions (Table 89–3).[9,19,20]

TABLE 89–3. Selected Drugs Associated With Maculopapular Eruptions

Allopurinol	Nitrofurantoin
Barbiturates	Ofloxacin
Benzodiazepines	Penicillamine
Captopril	Penicillins
Carbamazepine	Phenothiazines
Chloramphenicol	Phenylbutazone
Ciprofloxacin	Phenytoin
Enalapril	Piroxicam
Erythromycin	Pyrazolon derivatives
Ethionamide	Rifampin
Etoposide	Streptomycin
Gold salts	Sulfonamides (includes sulfonylureas and thiazides)
Hydantoin derivatives	
Ibuprofen	Sulindac
Indomethacin	Tetracyclines
Isoniazid	Tolmentin

Compiled from Refs. 8, 9, 19, and 20.

PATHOGENESIS

Although the variable and unpredictable course of these eruptions make classification of the reaction difficult, some maculopapular reactions are possibly due to cell-mediated immune response. This has been suggested by skin testing, lymphocyte transformation, and macrophage migration inhibition tests.[12,18] Humoral immune complex mechanisms have also been suggested.[12]

▶ TREATMENT: Maculopapular Eruptions

Generally, maculopapular reactions fade within a few days after discontinuation of the offending agent, and thus patient history and temporal relation to drug exposure may often be major diagnostic clues. Patients usually receive palliative treatment with tepid or cool water baths or compresses. Systemic antihistamines may be added for pruritus. Severe reactions may be treated with a short-term course of a systemic corticosteroid.[6]

URTICARIA, ANGIOEDEMA, AND ANAPHYLAXIS

CLINICAL PRESENTATION

Urticarial reactions are the second most common cutaneous manifestation of drug allergy. Lesions consist of raised, well-defined, pruritic, erythematous wheals (hives) that are highly variable in size and number. Urticarial lesions may manifest as a single focus at the site of an injection or may appear as a large, generalized eruption with numerous lesions extending over the chest or trunk. These lesions are unique in that they are evanescent or transient, disappearing within a matter of hours; however, new ones may continue to appear until the offending agent is eliminated from the system. Urticaria can also occasionally be accompanied by vesicle formation.

Typically the course of drug-induced urticaria is acute, occuring within 12 to 36 hours and resolving within 1 to 3 days of exposure. Chronic urticaria usually has been present at least 6 weeks and has a more prolonged, sometimes relatively indefinite, course. Other symptoms that may accompany urticaria in late reactions include fever, lymphadenopathy, joint swelling, and arthralgias. In some cases urticaria may be the first manifestation of anaphylaxis, thus indicating close monitoring for any swelling around the lips or tongue or for tightness of breath. Anaphylactic syndrome is characterized by the acute onset of skin and mucosal lesions and progression to GI symptoms, peripheral vascular collapse, and shock. Urticarial reactions can be caused by food, allergens, infection, temperature changes, and drugs (Table 89–4).[9,19–21]

PATHOGENESIS

Immunologically, urticarial lesions are caused by IgE-dependent circulating immune complexes. Mast cells and basophils play a central role in the pathogenesis of these immediate reactions by their affinity for IgE. Various drugs or foreign substances do not require an allergic mechanism to liberbate histamine and can produce urticaria. Certain amines may displace histamine from intracellular storage sites, while other drugs directly degranulate mast cells through complement or arachidonic acid–dependent pathways.[9,17,22] Examples of nonimmunologic drug–induced histamine release include acetylsalicylic acid, atropine, opiates, quinine, thiamine, pilocarpine, iodinated radiocontrast dyes, and nonsteroidal anti-inflammatory drugs. Because immunologic and nonimmunologic reactions are clinically indistinguishable, differential diagnosis can be made by immunologic investigations.[9,12,18]

TABLE 89–4. Selected Drugs Associated With Urticaria, Angioedema, and Anaphylaxis

Acetylsalicylic acid	Indomethacin	Nizatidine
Amitriptyline	Insulin	Omeprazole
Bisacodyl	Interleukin-2	Opiates
Cyclophosphamide	Iodinated radiocontrast media	Penicillins
Gold		Ranitidine
Granulocyte colony–stimulating factor	Mannitol	Senna
	Mesna	Sulfonamides
Heparin	Metoclopramide	Sulindac
Ibuprofen	Naproxen	Tolmentin

Compiled from Refs. 9 and 19–21.

▶ TREATMENT: Urticaria, Angioedema, and Anaphylaxis

The primary treatment of urticaria involves identification of the offending agent and subsequent discontinuation. Because urticaria is mediated by histamine, various antihistamines such as diphenhydramine, chlorpheniramine, hydroxyzine, as well as newer less sedating agents, have been used. Doxepin exhibits affinity for both H_1 and H_2 receptors, and has been shown to be effective in those unresponsive to conventional antihistamines.[22,23] Topical doxepin 5% cream has also been evaluated but does not appear to be as effective and has potential for systemic absorption and sensitization.[23] Other topical agents other than mild antipruritic agents are not very useful, and classical topical antihistamines (such as diphenhydramine) are best avoided because of their high incidence of contact sensitization.[22,24]

FIXED-DRUG ERUPTIONS

CLINICAL PRESENTATION

A typical fixed-drug reaction, presenting as an erythematous or hyperpigmented round or oval lesion, is distinctive in behavior and appearance. Lesions may range in size from a few millimeters to nearly 20 cm in diameter.[9] These lesions usually change color from a pale red to a dusky-red or violaceous hue over a brief period of time. A gray-brown hyperpigmented spot persists and deepens in color with each exposure to the medication. Although lesions can occur on any part of the skin or mucosal membranes, there seems to be a preference for the oral mucosa and gentalia.[18,25] Often patients complain of pruritus and a painful burning sensation. An important characteristic of this disease is recurrence of the eruption (within 30 minutes to 8 hours) in the exact location as the previous reaction upon reexposure, hence the term "fixed-drug eruption."[25]

PATHOGENESIS

The pathogenesis of this cutaneous reaction is still not well understood. Typically, a single drug is responsible for the reaction, though some patients react to chemically related compounds.[25] The sole cause of fixed-drug reactions is thought to be due to drugs or chemicals (Table 89–5).[9,20,21] Diagnosis is typically confirmed by histology.[9,25] Histopathologic examinations suggest that there is a lymphocyte-mediated attack on epidermal cells, which leads to the lichenoid tissue injury.[26]

TABLE 89–5. Selected Drugs Associated With Fixed-drug Eruptions

Barbiturates	Gold	Phenothiazines
Carbamazepine	Griseofulvin	Phenylbutazone
Dapsone	Hydralazine	Quinidine
Digoxin	Hydroxyurea	Sulfasalazine
Diphenhydramine	Ibuprofen	Sulfonamides
Disulfiram	Ipecac	Sulindac
Epinephrine	Metronidazole	Tetracyclines
Erythromycin	Phenolphthalien	Trimethoprim

Compiled from Refs. 9, 20 and 21.

▶ TREATMENT: Fixed-drug Reactions

Systemic corticosteroids and antihistamines are often used, but they typically have minimal or no apparent effect on the course of fixed-drug eruptions.[25] The offending drug should be removed and not readministered as the reaction may extend to additional areas of skin and mucous membranes and may also progress to formation of bullous lesions in some patients.[9] Conservative measures are occasionally useful, including cool water compresses during the short acute phase and perhaps bleaching creams for hyperpigmentation in the chronic phase.[18,25,26]

PHOTOSENSITIVITY

CLINICAL PRESENTATION

Photosensitivity is a broad term used to describe adverse reactions to light energy. Sun and drug-induced photoreactions are more common due to increased use of tanning booths and increased number of photosensitizing chemicals in cosmetics and drugs (Table 89–6).[9,12,18,19,21,27] Clinically, these reactions appear very similar to a sunburn and can include erythema, edema, papules, and plaque-like perhaps urticarial lesions, sometimes with vesicle formation. The

TABLE 89–6. Selected Drugs Associated With Photosensitivity Reactions

Amiodarone	Phenylbutazone
Barbiturates	Piroxicam
Benzodiazepines	Promethazine
Carbamazepine	Protryptyline
Chlorothiazide	Psoralens
Chlorpromazine	Quinidine
Dacarbazine	Simvastatin
5-Fluorouracil	Sulfonamides
Furosemide	Sulfonylureas
Ketoprofen	Sulindac
Mitomycin C	Tetracyclines
Naproxen	Thiazides
Oral contraceptives	

Compiled from Refs. 9, 12, 18, 19, 21, 27, and 33.

hallmark of photosensitivity eruptions is appearance on areas of skin that receive the greatest exposure to sunlight (the tops of the ears, nose, cheeks, lateral and lower posterior surfaces of the neck, extensor surfaces of the forearms, and dorsa of the hands).[9] In some cases, the eruption can occur on non–sun-exposed areas and become generalized over the body.[28] Chronically, reactions may become hyperpigmented or hypopigmented, perhaps atrophic, and with yellowish papules as well as telangiectasias.

PATHOGENESIS

Photosensitivity is a phenomenon that can be further subgrouped into phototoxic reactions and photoallergic reactions. Phototoxicity, a nonimmunologic reaction, resembles a sunburn and appears to be dose dependent.[21] It occurs secondary to ingestion or topical application of an agent that potentiates solar energy. The drug acts as a chromophore and absorbs ultraviolet light (potentially UVA and/or UVB), causing damage to adjacent tissue. Clinically, patients respond with erythema, pain, and possibly frank blistering within 30 minutes to several hours after exposure. Most of the damage is present on exposed skin only. Histologically, dermal edema, dyskeratosis, and necrosis of keratinocytes can be seen.[27]

A photoallergic reaction is less common and involves an immunologic mechanism; thus, there is a delay between exposure to the drug and the onset of eruption.[19,21] The presumed mechanism is that of a type IV cell–mediated hypersensitivity response. It is postulated that ultraviolet light (UVA and UVB are both capable of having active spectra, depending on the drug) reacts with the drug or metabolite in the skin to produce a hapten. This hapten combines with a tissue antigen to form a complete antigen, eliciting an allergic response upon subsequent exposure.[9] Once sensitization is achieved, minimal amounts of drug are usually needed to produce a reaction.[9] The initial eruption, a papulovesicular eczematous dermatitis, occurs from 1 to 14 days after exposure. Histopathologic findings are similar to that of contact dermatitis.[9,27]

▶ TREATMENT: Photosensitivity

Appropriate treatment of photosensitivity depends on the type of reaction. Managing patients with phototoxic reactions parallels that of routine burn care and avoidance of agents that may cause phototoxicity. Systemic and topical antihistamines and corticosteroids have been shown to be ineffective.[27] For patients with acute photoallergic reactions, topical corticosteroids and antihistamines can be used for symptomatic relief. Prednisone, starting at 1 mg/kg/d, and tapered over 3 weeks, can be effective for highly symptomatic individuals. In both scenarios, avoidance of sunlight and appropriate use of sunscreens that block UVA and UVB are indicated.[18,27,29,30]

ALOPECIA

CLINICAL PRESENTATION

Alopecia, most commonly affecting the scalp, is characterized by localized or generalized hair loss. Drug-induced hair loss usually presents as a diffuse, nonscarring alopecia that is reversible after drug discontinuation. Because of other causes of alopecia—such as infections, thyroid disease, anemia, and trauma—diagnosis of drug-induced hair loss may be difficult.[21] Selected offending agents are included in Table 89–7.[19,21,31,32]

PATHOGENESIS

Drug-induced alopecia results from damage to proliferating cells in the anagen (actively growing) hair follicle. This results in a thin, fragile hair shaft that breaks even with minor trauma.[31] Certain agents, such as thioamides, used to treat hyperthyroidism, cause a dose-dependent hair loss and also change the texture of hair to dry, brittle, and lusterless.[9] In women on oral contraceptive therapy, sufficient progesterone stimulation via androgenic effects may cause reversible alopecia.[34]

▶ TREATMENT: Alopecia

Management of drug-induced alopecia may be dependent on the etiology of the hair loss. Most cases are reversible upon discontinuation of the drug. To best determine a particular drug cause, hair regrowth with drug discontinuation and reexacerbation of the problem upon reexposure should be observed. In some patients receiving chemotherapy, a scalp-cooling method has been evaluated to induce vasoconstriction of blood vessels, thus resulting in decreased drug levels to hair follicles. The efficacy of this treatment has been highly variable.[31] Other methods of treatment include topical minoxidil and oral finasteride.[19]

TABLE 89–7. Selected Drugs Associated With Alopecia

Anticonvulsants	Hydantoin derivatives
Busulfan	Hydroxyurea
Carbamazepine	Interferon-α
Clofibrate	Isotretinoin
Colchicine	Methotrexate
Cyclophosphamide	Mitoxantrone
Doxorubicin	Oral contraceptives
Ethionamide	Propranolol
Etretinate	Tricyclic antidepressants
Granulocyte colony–stimulating factor	Valproate sodium
Heparin	Vitamin A, high dose
	Warfarin

Compiled from Refs. 19, 21, 31, and 32.

VASCULITIS

CLINICAL PRESENTATION

Vasculitis is characterized by inflammation and damage of blood vessels that may affect various organ systems. It commonly appears on the lower extremities or pressure-dependent areas of the skin as erythematous or violaceous lesions. Lesions, ranging in size from a pinpoint to several centimeters, are often macular, but may be palpable with variable morphology.[35] Urticarial lesions may coexist with purpura, and in severe cases, development of vesicular, bullous, hemorrhagic, ulcerating, or necrotic lesions may be seen. Lesions may persist for weeks and in some cases become yellow to brown during resolution.[35] Systemic symptoms such as burning, stinging, malaise, arthralgias, and fever may also be present. Other manifestations, such as involvement of the liver, kidney, brain, and joints, may also be present. Some drug causes of vasculitis are listed in Table 89–8.[9,12,17]

PATHOGENESIS

Though difficult to pinpoint the etiology of most vasculitides, it is possible that free antigen is present in circulating blood. Complexation with IgE antibodies and resultant release of histamine leads to increased vascular permeability and allows immune complexes from the circulation to migrate to target tissue, fix complement, and lyse cells.

▶ TREATMENT: Vasculitis

Palliative treatment with bedrest and compression of lesions may promote healing. Oral corticosteroids, cyclophosphamide, plasmapheresis, indomethacin, dapsone, colchicine, and aspirin have also been used in treatment.[35]

TABLE 89–8. Selected Drugs Associated With Vasculitis

Allopurinol	Ibuprofen	Piroxicam
Anticoagulants	Indomethacin	Propylthiouracil
Cimetidine	Penicillins	Quinine
Fluoxetine	Phenylbutazone	Sulfonamides
Hydralazine	Phenytoin	Thiazides

Compiled from Refs. 9, 12, and 17.

HYPERPIGMENTATION

DRUGS THAT MAY CAUSE PIGMENTARY CHANGES

Changes in skin color may be caused by the drug itself, disturbances in melanin formation, or both.[28] Drugs known to induce pigmentary changes include hydantoins, metals (Table 89–9),[9,30] antimalarials, phenothiazines, oral contraceptives, tetracyclines, chemotherapeutic agents (Table 89–10), and amiodarone.[36,37]

ANTICONVULSANTS

Anticonvulsants, such as phenytoin, phenobarbital, and carbamazepine, have reported a brown patchy hyperpigmentation on light-exposed areas.[9] Those individuals who take these anticonvulsants for longer than 1 year are at a 10% risk of developing this change. Although the hyperpigmentation deepens with light exposure, it usually does not disappear during winter months.[38] Hydantoin derivatives appear to cause an increase in melanin of the basal layer and induce dispersion of melanin granules in an animal model.[37] Women appear to be affected more than men, suggesting a hormonal origin with light as a triggering factor.[38]

ANTIMALARIALS

Approximately 25% of patients taking antimalarials for more than 3 or 4 months develop pigmentation changes.[36] The pigmentation patterns vary and may commonly manifest as patchy, irregular blue-black or gray lesions on pretibial areas or diffuse facial hyperpigmentation. Transverse bands in nails have also been reported.[36] The onset of pigmentation changes has ranged from 4 to 20 months, with discontinuation of therapy resulting in some lightening but commonly a persistence of lesions.[36] Quinacrine causes a diffuse lemon-yellow skin discoloration that gives the patient a jaundiced appearance. Scleral coloration is slight and pigmentation usually returns to normal 1 to 4 months after therapy.[36]

PHENOTHIAZINES

Pigmentation changes induced by phenothiazines (e.g., chlorpromazine, thioridazine) range from a bronze color in sun-exposed areas to a violet, purplish gray with long-term exposure.[36] Forehead, cheeks, nose, hands, and upper extremities are most commonly affected. An increased deposition of melanin occurs in the dermis, and phenothiazine–melanin complexes are believed responsible for color changes. Pigmentation is not usually totally reversible but may fade slowly in winter months or upon discontinuation of therapy.[36]

TABLE 89–9. Heavy Metal–induced Hyperpigmentation

Agent	Color	Region Involved	Special Features
Mercury	Gray-brown, Slate green	Skin folds (topical), gingival pigmentation (systemic)	Caused by deposition of metallic granules and increased melanin production; formerly used in bleaching agents.
Silver	Slate gray, Blue-gray	Sun-exposed areas, mucosa, sclerae, nails	Silver granule deposition that activates melanin production; occurs months to years after ingestion.
Bismuth	Blue-gray	Skin, conjunctiva, oral and vaginal mucosa, black line along gingival margin	Deposition of metallic granules or interaction with bacteria in mouth; more common with parenteral use.
Arsenic	Brown, bronze	Trunk, "raindrop"-shaped hyperkeratotic papulonodular lesions; palms, soles	Activates enzymes that form melanin and deposit in skin; used systemically for psoriasis and as a health tonic; pigmentation appears 1–20 years after exposure.
Gold	Blue-gray	Periorbital, generalized chrysiasis, sun-exposed areas	Caused by deposition of metallic particles in epidermis; occurs months to years after exposure and is permanent.

Compiled from Refs. 9 and 36.

ORAL CONTRACEPTIVES

Melasma, characterized by irregular brown macules on the cheeks, forehead, or upper lip, is a frequent cutaneous reaction to oral contraceptives.[34] Estrogen, progesterone, or sun exposure may be responsible for the increased melanin deposition in the dermis and epidermis.[36] Onset usually occurs within 1 to 20 months, but hyperpigmentation may persist after discontinuation.[34] Sunscreens may be helpful in minimizing the extent of hyperpigmentation.

TETRACYCLINES

Bluish pigmentation of previously inflamed skin may result from tetracycline deposition after prolonged high-dose therapy.[9,36] Several types of pigmentation changes have been reported with the use of minocycline. Blue-black coloration in areas of active scarring, generalized blue-gray pigmentation on sun-exposed areas, generalized muddy hue, and discoloration of teeth have been noted.[36] Black pigmentation of the thyroid gland has been reported in patients receiving long-term minocycline. The dimethylamino group at the 7 position, which is specific to minocycline and not the other tetracyclines, may cause an oxidation reaction resulting in this pigmentation.[37,39] Coloration commonly fades after cessation of therapy but may persist for months to years in some individuals.[39,40]

CLOFAZIMINE

Clofazimine has been used extensively to treat lepromatous leprosy.[41] It has also been used in the treatment of mycobacterial infections in patients with AIDS,[42] discoid lupus erythematosus,[43] and pyoderma gangrenosum.[44] This phenazine compound crystalizes in tissues and can result in a frequent side effect of deep brown pigmentation, which may concentrate at sites of leprosy lesions.[41]

AMIODARONE

A gray-blue coloration in sun-exposed areas has been reported in up to 10% of patients receiving amiodarone.[45] The discoloration may be caused by the incorporation of amiodarone into lysosomes, causing an accumulation of polar lipids.[46] Symptom onset has ranged from 6 to 39 months after initiation of therapy, and discontinuation may cause slow fading of the lesion.[40]

CYTOTOXIC AGENTS

Patients receiving bleomycin have reported a reticulated patchy hyperpigmented area with some cases being associated with erythematous plaques. Symptomatic treatment

TABLE 89–10. Chemotherapeutic Agents Associated With Hyperpigmentation

Agent	Color	Region Involved	Special Features
Busulfan	Brown	Face, forearms, chest, trunk, hands	Accelerates melanin formation by enzymes; incidence more frequent in dark-skinned patients; resolves on discontinuation.
Bleomycin	Brown	Linear bands on chest, back	Incidence 8%–20%; reversible on discontinuation.
Doxorubicin	Black-brown	Tongue, palms, soles, nails	Increased incidence in dark-skinned patients; reversible on discontinuation.
Mechlorethamine (topical)	Brown	Areas of contact	Toxic effect on keratinocytes; increased melanocytes; some aggregation.

Compiled from Refs. 36 and 37.

with antihistamines for pruritis is recommended, and resolution of hyperpigmentation is seen over time.[19] Patients treated with mitomycin C and thiotepa have also shown areas of hyperpigmentation.[19]

ACUTE GENERALIZED EXANTHEMATOUS PUSTULOSIS

CLINICAL PRESENTATION

Acute generalized exanthematous pustulosis (AGEP) is characterized by an acute onset of pustular eruption and a burning, pruritic, edematous erythema associated with fever greater than 38°C. The eruption can begin on the face or intertriginous areas and within a few hours move to the trunk and lower limbs. AGEP typically involves the mucous membranes, particularly on the mouth and tongue. Diagnosis can sometimes be difficult, as this disease can be confused with pustular psoriasis. In an analysis of 63 cases, the major distinction between AGEP and pustular psoriasis was the acute onset and shorter duration (8 versus 16 days) for those patients with AGEP.[47,48]

PATHOGENESIS

Acute generalized exanthematous pustulosis generally occurs shortly after onset of a respiratory infection. Because the physiologic mechanisms are hypothetical, AGEP is classified as a syndrome. Leukocytosis, hypocalcemia, and an increase in aminotransferases can also been seen. The most common cause of AGEP is drug related, especially antibiotics, typically presenting with a very short interval between drug exposure and onset of eruption.[47,49,50] Selected drugs suspected of being responsible are listed in Table 89–11.[47–51]

TABLE 89–11. Selected Drugs Associated With AGEP

Acetaminophen	Diltiazem	Methoxalen (plus PUVA)
Acetazolamide	Doxycycline	Metronidazole
Allopurinol	Enalapril	Nifedipine
Amoxacillin	Erythromycin	Phenytoin
Amphotericin	Furosemide	Pyrimethamine
Ampicillin	Gentamicin	Quinidine
β-lactam penicillins	Griseofulvin	Quinolones
Carbamazepine	Hydroxychloroquine	Streptomycin
Cephalosporins	Imipenem	Sulfonamides
Chloramphenicol	Isoniazid	Terbinafine
Chloroquine	Itraconazole	Tetracycline
Clindamycin	Macrolides	Vancomycin
Clobazam	Mercury	
Cotrimazole		

Compiled from Refs. 47–51.

▶ TREATMENT: Acute Generalized Exanthematous Pustulosis

Although patients present with fever and impressive skin eruptions, AGEP is often simply treated by discontinuation of the offending drug, which allows for self-healing.[48]

DRUG HYPERSENSITIVITY SYNDROME

CLINICAL PRESENTATION

Drug hypersensitivity syndrome, or drug rash with eosinophilia and systemic symptoms (DRESS), includes a severe skin eruption, fever, lymphadenopathy, hepatitis, hematologic abnormalities with eosinophilia, and may involve internal organs. Cutaneous reactions usually begin as a morbilliform eruption on the face and upper trunk. Eventually, the lower extremities are affected and erythroderma may occur. Sterile follicle-centered pustules and nonfollicular small pustules may also present. Other patients can present with exfoliative dermatitis and edema of the face and periorbital areas. Mortality is approximately 10% in this syndrome; thus, prompt diagnosis and treatment are necessary. Overall prognosis is poor, as the median survival rate is 24 to 30 months.[52] Commonly implicated drugs are listed in Table 89–12.[53]

PATHOGENESIS

The skin contains active isozymes of cytochrome P450, making it metabolically active. A defect in the enzymes can lead to an accumulation of toxic metabolites, thus initiating immune responses. Langerhans cells and dendritic cells present in the skin contribute to the pathogenesis of cutaneous reactions.[49,52] Although this is the proposed pathogensis for some anticonvulsants, hypersensivity syndrome secondary to sulfonamides is considered to be due to another mechanism. Slow acetylation and an increased susceptibility of lymphocytes to toxic metabolites are associated with an increased risk of developing this type of sulfonamide hypersensitivity.

▶ TREATMENT: Drug Hypersensitivity Syndrome

Symptoms after drug withdrawal may persist for weeks. Skin manifestations are often treated with high-potency topical corticosteroids, and in some cases systemic use is indicated. Because of the immunodeficiency that results from chemotherapy or the disease itself, death is usually secondary to infection. Development of lymphoma has also been observed in 30% of patients.[49,52]

TABLE 89–12. Selected Drugs Associated With DRESS

Allopurinol	Diltiazem	Phenytoin
Atenolol	Isoniazid	Ranitidine
Captopril	Mexiletine	Sulfasalazine
Carbamazepine	Minocycline	Sulfonamides
Chlorpropramide	Phenobarbital	Thalidomide
Dapsone	Phenylbutazone	Zalcitabine

Compiled from Refs. 39, 52, and 53.

DRUG-INDUCED SYSTEMIC LUPUS ERYTHEMATOSUS

CLINICAL PRESENTATION

As many as 10% of reported cases of systemic erythematosus lupus (SLE) are induced by medications. Although epidemiologic characteristics of the two types of SLE are quite different (Table 89–13),[54] the presenting features—arthralgias, myalgias, and pulmonary involvement—are somewhat similar. The clinical course of drug-induced lupus is much more benign, as idiopathic SLE commonly involves the renal, central nervous, and lymphatic systems.[54] Drug-induced SLE can be subdivided into four types[10]:

1. Induction of SLE in patients who have never had SLE.
2. Aggravation of SLE, usually systemic.
3. Induction of cutaneous discoid or subacute lupus erythematosus.
4. Induction of serologic changes only: antinuclear antibodies are of a different type, lupus erythematosus cells.

Selected drugs implicated for inducing lupus are listed in Table 89–14.[10,18,20,37,39,55,56]

PATHOGENESIS

Autoantibody responses in idiopathic and drug-induced lupus are similar in that both are characterized by antinuclear antibodies. However, titers of anti-double stranded DNA can be seen in idiopathic lupus, while it is rarely (< 1%) found in drug-induced lupus. In addition, antihistone antibody occurs in a higher percentage of patients with drug-induced lupus.[56]

TABLE 89–13. Epidemiologic Characteristics of Two Types of SLE

Characteristic	Idiopathic SLE	Drug-induced SLE
Age at onset	20–50 years	50–70 years
Sex	Females > males	Equal between males and females
Race	Blacks > whites	Whites > blacks
Acetylator status	Equal between slow and fast acetylators	Slow > fast

Compiled from Ref. 54.

TABLE 89–14. Selected Drugs Associated With Drug-induced SLE

Most Common	Good Evidence	
Hydralazine	Atenolol	Minocycline
Procainamide	Carbamazepine	Penicillamine
Quinidine	Chlorpromazine	Phenytoin
	Isoniazid	Sulfasalazine
	Methyldopa	Thiazides

Compiled from Refs. 10, 18, 20, 37, 39, 55, and 56.

▶ TREATMENT: Drug-Induced SLE

Withdrawal of the offending medication is the mainstay of treatment for drug-induced lupus. Symptomatic treatment, such as nonsteroidal anti-inflammatory agents for arthralgias, may also be helpful. In cases with cutaneous or systemic manifestations, corticosteroids and/or immunosuppressants may be administered.[54]

ANTICOAGULANT-INDUCED SKIN NECROSIS AND "PURPLE TOE SYNDROME"

Although anticoagulants such as heparin and warfarin are commonly used medicines, an estimated 0.01% to 0.1% of patients receiving anticoagulant therapy develop skin necrosis.[57]

WARFARIN

Clinical Presentation

Of patients with reported warfarin-induced skin necrosis, 85% are female, while the purple toe syndrome predominately occurs in males. Skin necrosis generally occurs between the third and tenth day of treatment. Patients typically complain of a sudden onset of cold or painful sensation, followed by well-demarcated erythematous lesions that usually progress to purpuric and hemorrhagic areas. These lesions occur in areas of subcutaneous fatty tissue and commonly involve the breasts, thighs, buttocks, and penis. Histologically, skin necrosis due to warfarin presents very specifically with hemorrhage and breakdown of precapillary arterioles.[58]

The "purple toe syndrome" is a rare complication of warfarin therapy. Most lesions typically develop 3 to 8 weeks after initiation of anticoagulation and are characterized by the sudden appearance of bilateral violaceous discoloration on toes and sides of feet. The affected area is cold and tender to touch, although some have reported a burning sensation. Most patients who develop warfarin-induced skin necrosis have been receiving anticoagulation for venous thrombosis, while those who develop purple toe syndrome have typically been patients receiving anticoagulation in association with atrial fibrillation or chronic heart failure.[57,59]

Pathogenesis

Patients receiving excessive initial doses of warfarin, thus causing a severe and rapid depression of factor VII and protein C, have been associated with skin necrosis attributed to a hypercoagulable state.[57,58] Other mechanisms including cytokines such as tumor necrosis factor (TNF) and direct toxicity to epithelial cells by warfarin have been proposed. Finally, immunologically mediated hypersensitivity has also been considered.[60]

▶ TREATMENT: Warfarin-induced Skin Necrosis

Rapid reversal with vitamin K can be initiated if skin necrosis is discovered early in anticoagulant therapy. Intravenous anticoagulation with heparin should be initiated while warfarin is discontinued. As most indications for warfarin require long-term treatment, reinitiation of warfarin at lower doses has been well-documented. Interestingly, a majority of patients previously affected with skin necrosis are not likely to redevelop lesions upon reinitiation of anticoagulant therapy.[57–59] Approximately 50% of cases require surgical intervention, such as debridement, skin grafting, and amputation.[59] Other immediate treatments such as vasodilation, steroids, vitamin C, and sympathetic nerve blocks have been evaluated without documented success.[58]

HEPARIN

Clinical Presentation

The frequency of heparin-induced skin necrosis is extremely low and clinically indistinguishable from warfarin-induced skin necrosis. Lesions typically involve the abdominal wall, upper and lower extremities, and hands. Generally occuring within the 5th to 10th day of therapy, heparin-induced skin necrosis can occur regardless of the route administered.[57] Case reports of low-molecular-weight heparins inducing skin necrosis have also been documented.[61]

Pathogenesis

Contrary to warfarin-induced skin necrosis, patients who have developed heparin-induced necrosis did not have deficiencies in the coagulation pathways. Heparin-induced thrombocytopenia has been postulated as a possible etiologic factor. In addition, although the significance of the association is unknown, greater than 80% of these reported cases had comorbid conditions such as hypertension, diabetes mellitus, malignancy, and connective tissue disorder.[57]

▶ TREATMENT: Heparin-induced Skin Necrosis

Immediate cessation of the offending agent is required as heparin-induced skin necrosis is associated with high mortality. The risk of redevelopment of skin necrosis due to reinstitution of heparin therapy has not been evaluated; thus, the risk is unknown.[57]

NEUTROPHILIC ECCRINE HIDRADENITIS

CLINICAL PRESENTATION

Neutrophilic eccrine hidradenitis (NEH) is an inflammatory dermatosis that primarily affects eccrine glands and is most commonly seen in patients undergoing chemotherapy. Erythematous macules, papules, plaques, and nodules are clinical manifestations, while the neutrophilic infiltrate of eccrine glands and degeneration of these cells are seen histologically.[62] In some cases, fever has been the presenting symptom; thus, infection must be ruled out.

PATHOGENESIS

There are three described mechanisms of NEH: (1) a cutaneous manifestation of acute myelogenous leukemia, (2) a toxic effect of cytarabine, and (3) a neutrophilic dermatosis within a spectrum.[62] Chemotherapeutic agents capable of concentrating in the eccrine sweat glands are dependent on the partitition coefficient and dissociation constant of the drug. The drug concentrates in sweat and causes local cutaneous reactions secondary to inflammation and destruction of sweat glands. Some drugs associated with NEH are listed in Table 89–15.[62,63]

TABLE 89–15. Selected Drugs Associated With Neutrophilic Eccrine Hidradenitis

Acetaminophen	Cytarabine
Bleomycin	Mitoxantrone
Chlorambucil	Zidovudine

Compiled from Refs. 62 and 63.

▶ TREATMENT: Neutrophilic Eccrine Hidradenitis

Typically, clinical manifestations of neutrophilic eccrine hidradenitis resolve within 1 to 4 weeks without treatment. Systemic corticosteroids may be useful in patients with fever and symptomatic lesions (SJS), but preferably with no evidence of infection.[63]

SEVERE SKIN REACTIONS

For several decades, the nomenclature and classification of severe, sometimes life-threatening, skin reactions have been much debated. There is disagreement whether erythema multiforme (EM), Stevens–Johnson syndrome (SJS), and toxic epidermal necrolysis (TEN) are distinctive diseases or are all within a single "erythema multiforme spectrum."[64–66] A consensus classification was proposed by an international group of dermatologists that is based on the patterns of skin lesions and on the extent of epidermal detachment (Table 89–16).[64]

TABLE 89–16. Classification of Severe Skin Reactions

Type	Lesions	Epidermal Detachment
Bullous erythema multiforme	Localized typical lesions, or raised atypical targets, primarily on extremites	< 10% of body surface area
Stevens–Johnson syndrome (SJS)	Purpuric macules or flat atypical targets on trunk	< 10% of body surface area
SJS/Toxic epidermal necrolysis (TEN) overlap	Widespread purpuric macules or flat atypical targets	10%–30% of body surface area
TEN with maculae	Purpuric macules or flat atypical targets	> 30% of body surface area
TEN on large erythema	Large epidermal sheets without purpuric macules or target lesions	> 10% of body surface area

Compiled from Ref. 64.

ERYTHEMA MULTIFORME AND STEVENS–JOHNSON SYNDROME

Clinical Presentation

Erythema multiforme is an acute, cutaneous reaction of variable morphology that evolves and changes over time. Typically, the hands, feet, face, limbs, and mucous membranes are the sites affected, with possible nonspecific prodromal symptoms such as an upper respiratory infection. Initially, a round 1- to 10-cm erythematous macule may appear, which becomes edematous and papular over time.[67] These lesions may enlarge into plaques or form an erythematous periphery, while the center clears, becoming cyanotic or purpuric and forming an "iris" or "target" lesion.[68] Lesions begin to resolve in 4 to 5 days, with complete healing in 2 to 4 weeks, although new lesions can continue to appear during this period.[67] In addition, postinflammatory hyperpigmentation can occur without healing.

SJS is considered a severe variant of erythema multiforme with extensive mucosal and conjunctival edema, erosions, high fever, myalgias, vomiting, diarrhea, and arthralgias. Skin lesions may be severe with large bullae and areas of denudation. The onset of these lesions is variable, but healing usually occurs within 6 weeks. Complications include keratitis, conjunctival scarring, blindness, pneumonia, dehydration, and esophagitis.[67]

Pathogenesis

Although various etiologic factors have been identified, the exact pathogenesis remains unknown. There is evidence that indicates that both an immune complex mechanism and cell-mediated immune reactivity may be involved.[65] Another theory suggests cytotoxic T cells release tumor necrosis factor (TNF-α), causing keratinocyte degeneration.[65] Further, it has also been proposed that patients with EM/SJS are phenotypically slow acetylators of drugs.[65,68] Identification of the etiologic factor is also difficult, because erythema multiforme may be precipitated by a wide variety of factors. Although various medications (Table 89–17) and herpes simplex virus (HSV) are the most frequent causes of erythema multiforme, there are other precipitating causes such as bacteria, fungi, vaccines, and other diseases.[66–69]

Diagnosis of erythema multiforme is based primarily on history, clinical appearance, and histology. Histopathologically, it has been shown that eosinophils were present more commonly in EM/SJS than other severe diseases, such as toxic epidermal necrolysis.[70] Often, prodromal symptoms are treated with antibiotics; thus, etiology (virus, bacteria, or drug) is difficult to clarify.

TABLE 89–17. Selected Drugs Associated With Erythema Multiforme/Stevens–Johnson Syndrome

Acetaminophen	Macrolides	Propranolol
Allopurinol	Methazolamide	Quinolones
Carbamazepine	Penicillins	Sulfadiazine
Cephalosporins	Phenobarbital	Sulfonamides
Cotrimoxazole	Phenylbutazone	Thiazides
Ibuprofen	Phenytoin	Valproic acid

Compiled from Refs. 65, 73, 74, 78, and 79.

▶ TREATMENT: Erythema Multiforme and Stevens–Johnson Syndrome

Because mild forms of erythema multiforme are self-limiting, symptomatic therapy such as antihistamines for pruritus, tap water compresses for blisters and necrosis, and half-strength hydrogen peroxide gargles for oral lesions may be instituted. Careful monitoring for progression to more severe forms or development of complications is essential. The efficacy of using systemic corticosteroids for severe erythema multiforme and SJS is not clearly defined.[71–73] Typically erythema multiforme resolves within 2 to 3 weeks but recurrences are common, especially if the EM is due to recurrent herpes simplex virus infections.[69]

TOXIC EPIDERMAL NECROLYSIS

Clinical Presentation

Toxic epidermal necrolysis (TEN) is a severe reaction of the skin, characterized by erythema and extensive detachment of the epidermis (necrolysis). Though it is a rare disease, TEN is associated with a relatively high mortality rate.[65,74] Typically, there is a prodromal state with nonspecific symptoms such as fever, cough, sore throat, pyrexia, and myalgia, followed by an acute onset of cutaneous manifestations occuring within 1 to 3 days. The eruption may present in various forms, often as a macular lesion with a burning sensation that becomes widespread over the body. The lesions may form large flaccid bullae within the erythema or directly progress to massive detachment of the epidermis. At this point, the epidermis is easily sloughed by light mechanical pressure, with outer coverings of ruptured bullae clinging to underlying tissue. This appearance of a sheet-like loss of epidermis is most characteristic of toxic epidermal necrolysis. Because lesions may appear on any area of skin (palms, soles, mouth, throat, nose, trachea, eyelids, conjunctiva, cornea, vagina), the picture may be similar to a second-degree burn or scald. Though virtually the entire skin surface may be involved with close to 100% of the epidermis, the hairy areas of the scalp seem not to be affected.[74]

Complications are numerous and include fluid and electrolyte imbalance from the loss of epidermis, septicemia, corneal ulcerations, and conjunctivitis. Systemic involvement is also common and may be due to the same process that destroys the epidermis.[74] Internal manifestations include dysphagia, gastrointestinal ulceration, hepatocellular damage, pneumonia, nephritis, and myocardial damage. Normocytic anemia, leukopenia, granulocytopenia, and neutropenia are also commonly present.[74–76]

Pathogenesis

Pathogenic mechanisms responsible for TEN remain unknown. The onset of TEN after drug exposure suggests an immunologic-mediated reaction.[74,75] A TEN-like eruption has occurred in patients with a graft-versus-host reaction after bone marrow transplant or blood transfusion.[68,76] Although there is no reliable test to prove correlations, drugs are the main cause of toxic epidermal necroysis (Table 89–18). Other reported causes include bacterial, viral, and fungal infections; chemicals; immunizations; and malignancies.[77–79]

The prognosis for TEN depends on the patient's age, extent of skin involvement, concurrent diseases, and complications.[12] Mortality is estimated at about 3% within the first 3 to 4 days of the acute episode.[12,74] After the acute episode, the epidermis may regenerate within 2 to 3 weeks, with complete healing usually in less than 6 weeks.

▶ TREATMENT: Toxic Epidermal Necrolysis

Management of TEN must include immediate identification and withdrawal of the precipitating factor. The principles of symptomatic treatments are essentially the same as for burn patients.[74] Therapy includes fluid and electrolyte maintenance, treatment or prevention of infections, prevention of ocular complications, and aggressive nutritional support.

Although the empiric use of systemic corticosteroid therapy is well documented, it is controversial because of a lack of well-controlled studies.[71,72] Some clinicians advocate corticosteroid use only within the first 48 to 72 hours of onset to prevent progression of complications[78]; others attribute delayed morbidity to systemic steroid use.[75] Other treament modalities include plasmapheresis, cyclosporine, and cyclophosphamide.[74]

TABLE 89–18. Selected Drugs Associated With Toxic Epidermal Necrolysis

Allopurinol	Lamotrigine	Quinolones
Barbiturates	Macrolides	Sulfonamides
Carbamazepine	Penicillins	Sulindac
Chloramphenicol	Phenylbutazone	Tolmentin
Ibuprofen	Phenytoin	Valproic acid
Indomethacin	Quinine	

Compiled from Refs. 74, 77, and 78.

REFERENCES

1. Shapiro S, Slone D, Siskind V, et al. Drug rash with ampicillin and other penicillins. Lancet 1969;2:969–972.
2. Johnson M, Johnson KG, Engel A. Prevalence, morbidity, and cost of dermatologic diseases. J Am Acad Dermatol 1984;11:930–936.
3. Baer RL, Witten VM, eds. Drug eruptions. In: Yearbook of Dermatology 1960–1961 Series. Chicago, Year Book, 1961:9–37.
4. Witte K, West DP. Immunology of adverse reactions to drugs. Pharmacotherapy 1982;2:54–65.
5. Witte KW, West DP. Immunology of adverse reactions to antimicrobial agents. In: Jeljaszewicz J, Pulverer G, eds. Antimicrobial Agents and Immunity. London, Academic Press, 1986:217–249.
6. Arndt KA. Drug eruptions, allergic. In: Arndt KA, ed. Manual of Dermatologic Therapeutics, 5th ed. Boston, Little, Brown, 1995: 60–63.
7. Bruinsma W. Drug monitoring in dermatology. Int J Dermatol 1986;25:166–168.
8. DeShazo RD, Kemp SF. Allergic reactions to drugs and biologic agents. JAMA 1997;278:1895–1906.
9. Bruinsma W. A Guide to Drug Eruptions, 6th ed. Oosthuizen, Netherlands, De Zwaluw, 1995.
10. Zurcher K, Krebs A, eds. Cutaneous drug reactions: An integral synopsis of today's systemic drugs. Switzerland, Karger, 1992.
11. Merk HF, Mukhtar H, Hertl M. Drug-induced skin disorders. In: Mukhtar H, ed. Pharmacology of the Skin. Boca Raton, CRC, 1992: 151–166.
12. Schulz KH. Cutaneous manifestations of drug allergy. In: De Weck AL, Bundgaard H, eds. Allergic Reactions to Drugs. Berlin, Springer-Verlag, 1983:135–162.
13. Roujeau JC, Stern RS. Severe adverse cutaneous reactions to drugs. N Engl J Med 1994;331:1272–1285.
14. Nelson HS. Allergic reactions to drugs. Adv Asthma Allergy 1976; 3:18–35.
15. Sullivan TJ. Drug allergy. In: Middleton E Jr, Reed CE, Ellis EF, et al, eds. Allergy Principles and Practice. St. Louis, Mosby-Year Book, 1993: 1726–1746.
16. Alanko K, Stubb S, Kauppinen K. Cutaneous drug reactions: Clinical types and causative agents. Acta Derm Venereol (Stockh) 1989;69: 223–226.
17. Wintroub BU, Stern R. Cutaneous drug reactions: Pathogenesis and clinical classification. J Am Acad Dermatol 1985;13:167–179.
18. Merk HF, Hertl M. Immunologic mechanisms of cutaneous drug reactions. Semin Cut Med Surg 1996;15:228–235.
19. Prussick R. Adverse cutaneous reactions to chemotherapeutic agents and cytokine therapy. Semin Cut Med Surg 1996;15:267–276.
20. Gruppo Italiano Studi Epidemiologici in Dermatologica. Cutaneous reactions to alimentary tract medications: Results of a seven-year surveillance program and review of the literature. Dermatology 1996;193:11–16.
21. Garnis-Jones S. Dermatologic side effects of psychopharmacologic agents. Dermatol Clin 1996;14:503–507.
22. Greene SL, Reed CE, Schroeter AL. Double-blind crossover study comparing doxepin with diphenhydramine for the treatment of chronic urticaria. J Am Acad Dermatol 1985;12:669–675.
23. Smith PF, Corelli RL. Doxepin in the management of pruritus assocaited with allergic cutaneous reactions. Ann Pharmacother 1997;31:633–634.
24. Yaffe SJ, Bierman CW, Cann HM, et al. Antihistamines in topical preparations. Pediatrics 1973;51:299–301.
25. Korkij W, Soltani K. Fixed drug eruption. Arch Dermatol 1984;120: 520–524.
26. Shiohara T, Nickoloff BJ, Sagawa Y, et al. Fixed drug eruption: Expression of epidermal keratinocyte intercellular adhesion molecule-1. Arch Dermatol 1989;125:1371–1376.
27. Wolverton SE. Update on cutaneous reactions. In: James WD, Cockerell CJ, eds. St. Louis, Mosby-Year Book, 1997:65–83.
28. Epstein JH, Wintroub BU. Photosensitivity due to drugs. Drugs 1985;30:42–57.
29. Mammen L, Schmidt CP. Photosensitivity reactions: A case report involving NSAIDs. Am Fam Physician 1995;52:575–578.
30. Robison HN, Morison WL, Hood AF. Thiazide diuretic therapy and chronic photosensitivity. Arch Dermatol 1985;121:522–524.
31. Dawber RBR, Ebling FJG, Wojnarowska FT. Disorders of hair, alopecia of chemical origin. In: Champion RH, Burton JL, Ebling FJG, eds. Textbook of Dermatology, 5th ed. Oxford, Blackwell, 1992: 2582–2584.
32. Brodin MB. Drug-related alopecia. Dermatol Clin 1987;5:571–579.
33. Drugs that cause photosensitivity. Med Lett 1986;28:51–52.
34. Jelinek JE. Cutaneous side effects of oral contraceptives. Arch Dermatol 1970;101:181–186.
35. Mackel SE. Treatment of vasculitis. Med Clin North Am 1982; 6:941–954.
36. Granstein RD, Sober AJ. Drug and heavy metal-induced hyperpigmentation. J Am Acad Dermatol 1981;5:1–18.
37. Shapiro LE, Knowles SR, Shear NH. Comparative safety of tetracycline, minocycline, and doxycycline. Arch Dermatol 1997;133:1224–1230.
38. Moller H. Pigmentary disturbances due to drugs. Acta Derm Venereol (Stockh) 1966;46:423–431.
39. Knowles SR, Shapiro L, Shear NH. Serious adverse reactions induced by minocycline: Report of 13 patients and review of the literature. Arch Dermatol 1996;132:934–939.
40. Basler RSW. Minocycline-related hyperpigmentation. Arch Dermatol 1985;121:606–608.
41. Job CK, Yoder L, Jacobson RR, Hastings RC. Skin pigmentation from clofazimine therapy in leprosy patients: A reappraisal. J Am Acad Dermatol 1990;23:236–241.
42. Masur H, Tuazon C, Gill V, et al. Effect of combined clofazimine and ansamycin therapy on *Mycobacterium avium–Mycobacterium intracellulare* bacteremia in patients with AIDS. J Infect Dis 1987;155:127–129.
43. Crovato F, Levi L. Clofazimine in the treatment of annular lupus erythematosus. Arch Dermatol 1981;117:249–250.
44. Michaelson G, Molin L, Ohman S, et al. Clofazimine, a new agent for the treatment of pyoderma gangrenosum. Arch Dermatol 1976;112:344–349.
45. Trimble JW, Mendelson DS, Fetter BF, et al. Cutaneous pigmentation secondary to amiodarone therapy. Arch Dermatol 1983;119:914–918.
46. Huff JC, Weston WL, Tonnesen MG. Erythema multiforme: A critical review of characteristics, diagnostic criteria, and causes. J Am Acad Dermatol 1983;8:763–775.
47. Roujeau JC, Bioulac-Sage P, Bourseau C, et al. Acute generalized exanthematous pustulosis. Arch Dermatol 1991;127:1333–1338.
48. Lazarov A, Livni E, Halevy S. Generalized pustular drug eruptions: confirmation by *in vitro* tests. J Eur Acad Dermatol Venereol 1998; 10:36–41.
49. Shapiro LE, Shear NH. Mechanisms of drug reactions: The metabolic track. Semin Cut Med Surg 1996;15:217–227.
50. Beylot C, Doutre MS, Beylot-Barry M. Acute generalized exanthematous pustulosis. Semin Cut Med Surg 1996;15:244–249.

51. Knowles S, Gupta AK, Shear NH. The spectrum of cutaneous reactions associated with diltiazem: Three cases and a review of the literature. J Am Acad Dermatol 1998;38:201–206.
52. Bocquet H, Bagot M, Roujeau JC. Drug-induced pseudolymphoma and drug hypersensitivity syndrome (drug rash with eosinophilia and systemic symptoms: DRESS). Semin Cut Med Surg 1996;15:250–257.
53. Callot V, Roujeau JC, Bagot M, et al. Drug-induced pseudolymphoma and hypersensitivity syndrome. Arch Dermatol 1996;132:1315–1321.
54. Rich MW. Drug-induced lupus: The list of culprits grows. Postgrad Med 1996;100:299–307.
55. McGuiness M, Frye RA, Deng JS. Atenolol-induced lupus erythematosus. J Am Acad Dermatol 1997;37:298–299.
56. Yung RL, Johnson KJ, Richardson BC. New concepts in the pathogenesis of drug-induced lupus. Lab Invest 1996;73:746–759.
57. Sallah S, Thomas DP, Roberts HR. Warfarin and heparin-induced skin necrosis and the purple toe syndrome: Infrequent complications of anticoagulant treatment. Thromb Haemost 1997;78:785–790.
58. DeFranzo AJ, Marasco P, Argenta LC. Warfarin-induced necrosis of the skin. Ann Plast Surg 1995;34:203–208.
59. Jillella AP, Lutcher CL. Reinstituting warfarin in patients who develop warfarin skin necrosis. Am J Hematol 1996;52:117–119.
60. Hermes B, Haas N, Henz BM. Immunopathological events of adverse cutaneous reactions to coumarin and heparin. Acta Derm Venereol 1997;77:35–38.
61. Tonn ME, Schaiff RA, Kollef MH. Enoxaparin-associated dermal necrosis: A consequence of cross-reactivity with heparin-mediated antibodies. Ann Pharmacother 1997;31:323–326.
62. Beutner KR, Packman CH, Markowitch W. Neutrophilic eccrine hidradenitis associated with Hodgkin's disease and chemotherapy. Arch Dermatol 1986;122:809–811.
63. Bernstein EF, Spielvogel RL, Topolsky DL. Recurrent neutrophilic eccrine hidradenitis. Br J Dermatol 1992;127:529–533.
64. Bastuji-Garin S, Rzany B, Stern RS, et al. Clinical classification of cases of toxic epidermal necrolysis, Stevens–Johnson syndrome, and erythema multiforme. Arch Dermatol 1993;129:92–96.
65. Mockenhaupt M, Schopf E. Epidemiology of drug-induced severe skin reactions. Semin Cut Med Surg 1996;15:236–243.
66. Assier H, Bastuji-Garin S, Revuz J, et al. Erythema multiforme with mucous membrane involvement and Stevens–Johnson syndrome are clinically different disorders with distinct causes. Arch Dermatol 1995;131:539–543.
67. Huff JC, Weston WL, Tonnesen MG. Erythema multiforme: A critical review of characteristics, diagnostic criteria, and causes. J Am Acad Dermatol 1983;763–775.
68. Fitzpatrick TB, Elsen AZ, Wolff K, et al. Erythema multiforme. In: Fitzpatrick TB, et al, eds. Dermatology in General Medicine, 3rd ed. New York, McGraw-Hill, 1987:555–563.
69. Choy AC, Yarnold PR, Brown JE, et al. Virus induced erythema multiforme and Stevens–Johnson syndrome. Allergy Proc 1995;16:157–161.
70. Rzany B, Hering O, Mockenhaupt M, et al. Histopathological and epidemiological characteristics of patients with erythema exudativum multiforme major, Stevens–Johnson syndrome and toxic epidermal necrolysis. Br J Dermatol 1996;135:6–11.
71. Barton P, Flowers F. Controversies in the management of erythema multiforme and toxic epidermal necrolysis. In: Dahl MV, Lynch PJ, eds. Current Opinion in Dermatology, 2nd ed. Philadelphia, Current Science, 1995.
72. Duarte AM, Pruksachatkunakorn C, Schachner LA. Life-threatening dermatoses in pediatric dermatology. In: Callen JP, ed. Advances in Dermatology, vol 10. St. Louis, Mosby-Year Book, 1995:329–371.
73. Cheriyan S, Patterson R, Greenberger PA, et al. The outcome of Stevens–Johnson syndrome treated with corticosteroids. Allergy Proc 1995;16:151–155.
74. Revuz JE, Roujeau JC. Advances in toxic epidermal necrolysis. Semin Cut Med Surg 1996;15:258–266.
75. Westly ED, Wechsler HL. Toxic epidermal necrolysis. Arch Dermatol 1984;120:721–726.
76. Goeens J, Song M, Fondu P. Haematological disturbances and immune mechanisms in toxic epidermal necrolysis. Br J Dermatol 1986; 114:255–259.
77. Chaffin JJ, Davis SM. Suspected lamotrigine-induced toxic epidermal necrolysis. Ann Pharmacother 1997;31:720–723.
78. Roujeau JC, Kelly JP, Naldi L, et al. Medication use and the risk of Stevens–Johnson syndrome or toxic epidermal necrolysis. N Engl J Med 1995;333:1600–1607.
79. Shirato S, Kagaya F, Suzuki Y, et al. Stevens–Johnson syndrome induced by methazolamide treatment. Arch Ophthalmol 1997;115: 550–553.

90
HEMATOPOIESIS

William P. Petros, PharmD, FCCP, and Gwynn D. Long, MD

Hematopoiesis is defined as the formation and maturation of blood cells and their derivatives. There is a tremendous daily turnover rate of cells in this system, with more than 6 billion cells produced per kilogram of body weight every 24 hours.[1] These accelerated processes result in vastly exaggerated and rapid responses to the slightest perturbation.

In humans, hematopoiesis takes place primarily in the bone marrow. Hematopoietic cells were among the first to be evaluated for their biologic functions and pattern of maturation and recent identification of the protein molecules (cytokines) that seem to regulate this system has yielded an extraordinary amount of new information regarding its control. The process of continual hematopoietic cell production is complicated, involving interactions between immature cells, the surrounding microenvironment, and cytokines.

This chapter discusses the regulation, proliferation, and some functions of hematopoietic cells. This information is essential to understanding the pathophysiologic and therapy-related hematopoietic effects covered elsewhere in the text. Directly related chapters include Chapter 79, Immune System; Chapter 91, Anemias; Chapter 92, Coagulation Disorders; Chapter 94, Drug-Induced Hematologic Disorders; Chapter 115, Cancer Treatment and Chemotherapy; and Chapter 125, Bone Marrow Transplantation.

HEMATOPOIETIC SYSTEM

The hematopoietic system consists of three primary cell components: erythrocytes, platelets, and leukocytes. The last term encompasses a functionally diverse group of cells that includes neutrophils, lymphocytes, monocytes/macrophages, eosinophils, plasma cells, and basophils. Typical concentrations of mature hematopoietic cells found in the peripheral blood of adults are shown in Table 90–1.

LEUKOCYTES

NEUTROPHILS (SEGS AND BANDS)

The major functions of neutrophils (also known as polymorphonuclear leukocytes) are to prevent pathogenic microorganism invasion and to localize and kill these microorganisms. These effects are mediated by a series of events, including migration to the site (chemotaxis), recognition/attachment to the invader, phagocytosis, lysosomal fusion, degranulation, and local generation of oxidants (respiratory burst) and degrading enzymes (Fig. 90–1).[2] A neutrophil is attracted to the site of infection by chemotactic factors. Once migration to the site has occurred, the neutrophil ingests the opsonized microorganism (opsonization is the process whereby antibody and complement coat the microorganism, allowing for increased neutrophil recognition). Following ingestion or phagocytosis, the cytoplasmic granules within the neutrophil fuse with the phagosome or phagocytosed microorganism, thereby initiating degranulation and release of enzymes. These degrading enzymes kill the microorganism through oxygen reduction. Secretion of these enzymes may also result in localized host-tissue injury. Neutrophil activity may be intensified by the actions of cytokines such as granulocyte colony-stimulating factor (G-CSF) and granulocyte–macrophage colony-stimulating factor (GM-CSF).[3]

EOSINOPHILS

Effector functions similar to those of neutrophils are elicited by eosinophils, although they are done with less efficiency. Eosinophil activity is primarily directed against large invaders such as helminths and other parasites that cannot be phagocytized. During an allergic reaction, activated mast cells secrete chemicals that attract and stimulate eosinophils, which in turn produce substances that neutralize or degrade the reaction products of mast cells. Unfortunately, the eosinophil constituents may also damage normal tissue and cause secondary histamine release. High concentrations of eosinophils for prolonged periods may result in damage to the cardiac and central nervous systems, with possible pulmonary and dermatologic involvement.[4]

BASOPHILS AND MAST CELLS

These cells function as mediators of inflammatory processes via massive release of their granule contents upon stimulation. The released chemicals include heparin, histamine, and other substances. The mediator may be vasoactive, bronchoconstrictive, and/or chemotactic (attractive) for eosinophils.[5,6]

MONOCYTES/MACROPHAGES

Monocytes are derived from the granulocyte–monocyte colony-forming unit. They are peripheral cells in transit

TABLE 90–1. Average (Normal Range) Adult Blood Cell Concentrations

White cell count (× 10^9/L)		7.8 (4.4–11.3)
Red cell count (× 10^{12}/L)	Male	5.21 (4.52–5.90)
	Female	4.60 (4.10–5.10)
Hemoglobin[a] (mg/dL)	Male	15.7 (14.0–17.5)
	Female	13.8 (12.3–15.3)
Hematocrit	Male	0.46 (0.42–0.50)
	Female	0.40 (0.36–0.45)
Mean corpuscular volume (fL/red cell)		88.0 (80.0–96.1)
Platelet count (× 10^9/L)		311 (172–450)

[a]May be 0.5–1.0 mg/dL lower in black patients.

from the bone marrow to tissues. Once in the tissues, under the influence of local factors, monocytes are transformed to macrophages.

Macrophages exist in the liver (Kupffer's cells), spleen, lymph nodes, microglial (CNS) cells, skin (Langerhans cells), and bone. A variety of functions are performed by monocytes and macrophages, including initiation of immune responses for recognition by lymphocytes, regulation of immune response intensity, phagocytosis of foreign invaders, tumor cytotoxicity, degradation of cellular debris, and secretion of peptide molecules called monokines (a subclassification of cytokines).[7] Examples of monokines include interferons, tumor necrosis factor, and interleukin-1. Monokines and other cytokines regulate the activity of these cells.

LYMPHOCYTES

The primary functions of lymphocytes are to control and be the effector cells for the immune system. Many of these cells also are important synthetic sites for various cytokines. Lymphocytes can be functionally divided into cells that display cell-mediated immunity (T cells) and those that are responsible for humoral immunity (B cells) (Table 90–2). B lymphocytes ultimately become plasma cells, which produce immunoglobulin specific for an antigen attached to the cell's surface. Several different T-cell subtypes are found in peripheral blood. These include the cytotoxic suppressor T cells (CD8), which attack intracellular pathogens and regulate the size and duration of the immune response, as well as helper T cells (CD4). The latter cells are responsible for delayed hypersensitivity, stimulation of B-cell differentiation (maturation), and antibody production, in addition to regulation of inflammatory reactions. Null cells are a separate subset of lym-

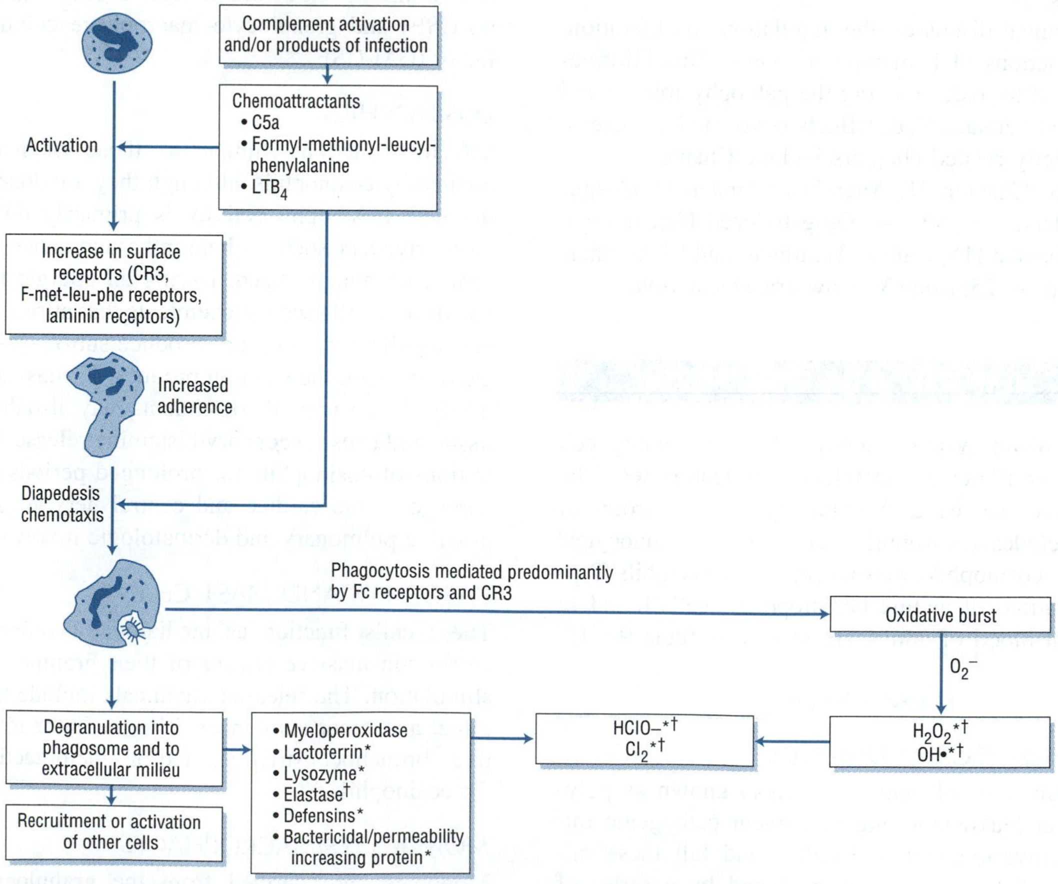

FIGURE 90–1. Neutrophil responses to infection or inflammation (*Microbicidal; †Damage to host tissues).

TABLE 90–2. Lymphocyte-Mediated Immune Function

Cellular Immunity (T Cells)	
1.	Provides resistance against intracellular pathogens such as viruses, protozoa, fungi, and bacteria
2.	Mediates allogeneic transplant rejection
3.	Responsible for contact dermatitis
4.	Provides autologous reaction to tumor cells
Humoral Immunity (B Cells)	
1.	Major component of allergic reactions and other autoimmune diseases
2.	Aids in eradication of encapsulated bacteria
3.	Inactivates circulating toxins
4.	May play role in antitumor reactions

phocytes that lack surface markers of B or T origin. These cells, also referred to as LGL or large granular lymphocytes, are thought to perform functions such as direct cytotoxicity to foreign entities, and they act either alone (natural killer cells) or in concert with immunoglobulin (antibody-dependent cellular cytotoxicity).[8,9] Further details regarding lymphocytes are found in Chapter 79, Immune System.

PLATELETS

Platelets (thrombocytes) interact to facilitate blood coagulation by several mechanisms. These include localization of the thrombus; providing a specific receptor site for clotting factors as well as the necessary phospholipid surface for the conversion of prothrombin to thrombin; and protection of thrombin from antithrombin. The process is initiated with a vascular injury that causes platelets to adhere to the exposed collagen fibers of the damaged wall as blood flows out. These events require the presence of other plasma proteins, namely, von Willebrand factor. Platelets then aggregate through a process that is calcium dependent. Following aggregation, various platelet mediators are released (thromboxane, serotonin, platelet factor V), resulting in the formation of an irreversible platelet aggregate with subsequent formation of a stable fibrin cross-linked clot.[10,11]

ERYTHROCYTES

The primary function of the erythrocyte is to carry oxygen from the lungs to the peripheral tissues. Its optimal design enables efficient oxygen transport via the hemoglobin molecule. Oxygen release is controlled by the general metabolic state of the patient and local factors.

HEMATOPOIETIC STRUCTURE AND COMPARTMENTS

Embryonic development of hematopoietic tissue occurs in the yolk sac mesenchyme, with fetal transition occurring in the liver and spleen. Very immature hematopoietic cells can also be found in umbilical cord blood, but not many are evident in the peripheral blood of adults.[12] The ultimate location of immature hematopoietic cells is in the bone marrow. The average adult has approximately 1.7 L of bone marrow, which provides an optimal environment for the development and proliferation of hematopoietic cells. The hematopoietic bone marrow is primarily located in the central portion of the pelvis, ribs, vertebrae, skull, and femora/ humeri epiphyses. The anatomic structure of the bone marrow is characterized by the central venous marrow sinus, which is linked by coarse vascular sinusoids that intertwine a reticulin mesh where the cells are suspended. Thus, hematopoiesis occurs in the extravascular marrow spaces, which also contain endothelial cells, fibroblasts, macrophages, and adipocytes, collectively termed *bone marrow stroma.*[13] Stromal cells are thought to be important hematopoietic components, providing growth factors, collagen, and cell-adhesion proteins.[14] When these cells are combined with accessory cells (lymphocytes/monocytes) and cytokines, the mixture is referred to as the *hematopoietic microenvironment.* Egress of more mature cells from the bone marrow occurs through the endothelial cell barrier. Release of cells such as neutrophils may be stimulated by complement, steroids, or endotoxin. Immature (progenitor) cells that may ultimately become any one of the blood cellular components can be transiently mobilized from the bone marrow into peripheral blood by administration of a cytotoxic chemotherapy drug (e.g., cyclophosphamide)[15] or a colony-stimulating factor (G-CSF or GM-CSF).[16] This process is commonly referred to as "priming" the bone marrow for peripheral blood progenitor or stem cells (see Chap. 125).

The least mature hematopoietic cell, accounting for only a fraction of a percent of bone marrow cells, is referred to as the *stem cell.* These cells have the unique potential to ultimately become any of the mature hematopoietic cells, and thus they are termed *pluripotent* and, importantly, have self-renewal capacity (Fig. 90–2).[17] Extensive research has been conducted describing the morphologic and immunologic characteristics indicative of the earliest stem cell, but investigators have yet to arrive at a consensus model. Only a small percentage of these cells is likely to be dividing at any one time, and thus most are dormant in the cell cycle. Stem cell renewal and differentiation occur within the bone marrow under the influence of the marrow microenvironment. Stromal endothelial cells, fibroblasts, and fat cells (adipocytes) are necessary to support stem cell proliferation and division by providing anchorage for adhesion and secreting various hematopoietic growth factors necessary for differentiation. It is the characteristics of the local microenvironment (cellular matrix and growth-factor concentrations) that influence the differentiation of a particular hematopoietic lineage, favoring it over another.

The next step in hematopoietic cell differentiation is thought to be represented by committed pluripotent stem cells that can still differentiate into any cell line (red blood cells [RBCs], white blood cells [WBCs], platelets); however, they have a limited capacity for self-renewal (see Fig. 90–2).

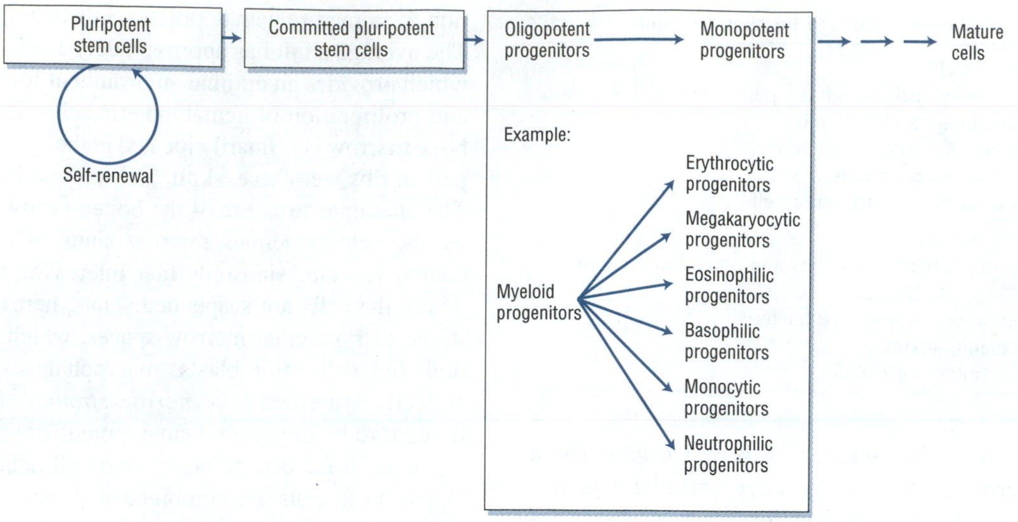

FIGURE 90–2. This rudimentary model of hematopoiesis displays the basic steps a cell may take from its inception as a stem cell in the bone marrow, through stages in which it can become multiple (oligopotent) or only one specific (monopotent) type of mature blood cell.

Cells that choose to differentiate can proceed to either myeloid or lymphoid cell precursors (oligopotent progenitors). These cells may ultimately become B or T lymphocytes in the case of lymphoid cells. Myeloid progenitors may become granulocytes, erythrocytes, macrophages, or megakaryocytes as outlined in the following and displayed in Fig. 90–2. Nomenclature for immature hematopoietic cells often uses terms developed during *in vitro* experiments of cell proliferation. Thus, the term burst-forming unit (BFU) or colony-forming unit (CFU) is added to the suffix of the cell lines ultimately produced by the specific cell.

Leukocytes found in the peripheral blood can generally be classified into neutrophils (most frequently occurring blood leukocyte subdivided into the more mature segs and less mature bands), lymphocytes, monocytes, eosinophils, basophils, and the tissue derivative of basophils, the mast cell. Immature neutrophils such as metamyelocytes are rarely seen in peripheral blood. Strictly speaking, the group of cells referred to as granulocytes includes neutrophils, eosinophils, and basophils, although common use tends to include only the first cell type. The terminally differentiated leukocytes, which are usually not seen in blood, include the macrophage or histiocyte (derived from monocytes) and plasma cells (derived from B lymphocytes).

Most of the body's neutrophils and neutrophilic precursors reside in the bone marrow (approximately 9 billion cells) in contrast to the circulation (approximately 700 million). Similarly, only 1% of the eosinophils in the body are found in peripheral blood, whereas the skin, lungs, and gastrointestinal tract are the preferred sites of residence.[4] There is no marrow reserve pool of monocytes. Neutrophil development in the bone marrow initiates with the stem cell and proceeds through intermediate precursors such as the myeloblast, promyelocyte, myelocyte, and metamyelocyte.

Only a small fraction of the total body pool of lymphocytes resides in the blood. Mature B lymphocytes express surface immunoglobulin, which functions as an antigen receptor. Most of these cells migrate from the bone marrow to areas such as the lymph nodes (dense collections of lymphocytes, plasma cells, and macrophages that are supplied by postcapillary venules and drained by a system of efferent lymphatics) and spleen, where antigenic stimulation results in specific immunoglobulin production.[13] Immature T cells are found in the circulation on their way to full maturation in the thymus. Approximately 75% of blood lymphocytes are T cells, 15% null cells, and 10% B cells. Various antigens expressed on the lymphocyte surface, depending on the degree of cell maturity and function, are termed *clusters of differentiation* (CD).

Progenitor cells that give rise to platelets are referred to as *colony-forming unit megakaryocyte* (CFU-MK). Megakaryocytes account for only 0.05% to 0.02% of marrow cells. Maturation of megakaryocytes is accompanied by morphologic changes in both the cytoplasm and nucleus. At differing stages of maturation, one can therefore see granules, organelles, and increasing segmentation of the nucleus. Cells in this lineage progress through three stages of development: commitment, proliferation, and differentiation, similar to that of leukocytes.[18,19]

The term *erythron* has been used to describe collectively the erythropoietic cellular structure, composed of all cells that lie along this pathway starting with the earliest committed erythroid progenitor and ending with the mature circulating RBC. The earliest cell committed to the erythroid lineage is known as a BFU-E (erythroid). One BFU-E can proliferate into several hundred progeny using *in vitro* culture systems. These cells are followed in differentiation by the CFU-E cell and subsequently to the nucleated normoblast and the immediate RBC precursor, the circulating anuclear reticulocyte as

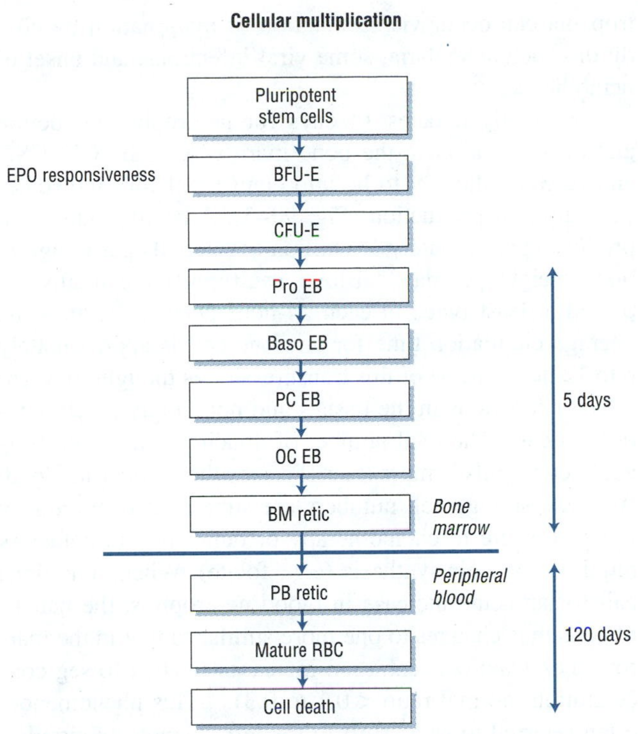

FIGURE 90–3. The proposed differentiation pattern of cells into mature erythrocytes is shown, including the various immature cell types that have been identified. In addition, the cells that may be stimulated by the cytokine erythropoietin are identified. BFU = burst-forming unit; E = erythroid; CFU = colony-forming unit; EB = erythroblast; PC = polychromatophilic; OC = orthochromatophilic; BM = bone marrow; retic = reticulocyte; EPO = erythropoietin.

outlined in Figure 90–3. The remaining RNA is typically lost from the RBC within 2 days of its appearance in the peripheral blood; thus, the mature cell does not synthesize new proteins such as enzymes.[20]

The erythrocyte precursor cell types display a continuum of changes in shape, hemoglobin concentration, Rh antigen, and erythropoietin (EPO) receptor expression with maturity. However, mature erythrocytes express significantly lower EPO receptor density than do proerythroblasts.[21]

Neonatal RBCs primarily contain fetal hemoglobin (HbF), which is replaced within a few months by adult hemoglobin (HbA), 85% of which is synthesized in the erythropoietic marrow. Heme-synthesizing cells must have a mitochondria; therefore, its synthesis cannot occur in the mature erythrocyte. Genetic alterations in hemoglobin structure may dramatically alter the stability or solubility of the hemoglobin and also cell confirmation. The characteristic biconcave-disk shape of the normal RBC is approximately 8 × 2 μm. Pathologic alterations in plasma lipids may affect the outer phospholipid membrane of the RBC, thus changing the cell's shape and survival. Blood types are characterized by the antigenic structure of the external surface of the cell membrane. Membrane function, integrity, and phagocytosis of the cells are affected by interactions of antibodies with RBC surface antigens.

NATURAL REGULATION OF CELL PROLIFERATION AND DIFFERENTIATION

A generic model of cell maturation is presented in Figure 90–2. The model includes a population of stem cells, thought to be capable of self-renewal, that provides the initial cell (committed progenitor) for subsequent maturation, differentiation (i.e., commitment to a cell line), and expansion into all blood cell types. This is followed by an initial differentiation step when a cell is produced (oligopotent progenitor) that will ultimately become one of only several mature blood cell types. Finally monopotent progenitors are noted in which differentiation is restricted to one cell type. The latter cells then undergo a series of maturation steps, ultimately resulting in a mature cell.

STEM CELL

The decision of a stem cell to self-renew versus differentiate and the selection of lineage by a multipotential progenitor cell during the differentiation process are thought to be stochastic (random) events. Conversely, survival and proliferation of the subsequent progenitor cells is thought to be regulated by the group of cytokines referred to as colony-stimulating factors (also known as CSFs, hematopoietins, hematopoietic cytokines, or hematopoietic growth factors).[22] Receptors for a variety of CSFs are present on the surface of stem cells, which agrees with *in vitro* studies demonstrating stimulatory activity for cytokines such as stem cell factor (SCF), IL-6, G-CSF, IL-11, IL-12, and leukemia inhibitory factor when present in combinations. Whether or not therapeutic use of a CSF that is thought to act primarily on more mature cells will result in exhaustion (depletion) of the stem cell pool over the course of multiple cycles of therapy is under active debate and study.[23] Proposed "cascades" of hematopoiesis are represented in Figures 90–3 through 90–6. Inserted within some figures are

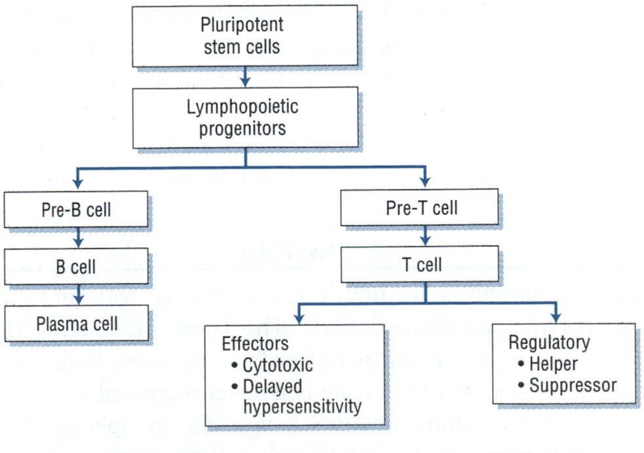

FIGURE 90–4. The pattern of lymphocyte maturation and differentiation into T and B cells is displayed. The plasma cell is a factory for antibodies whereas the T cells have both effector and regulatory functions on the immune system.

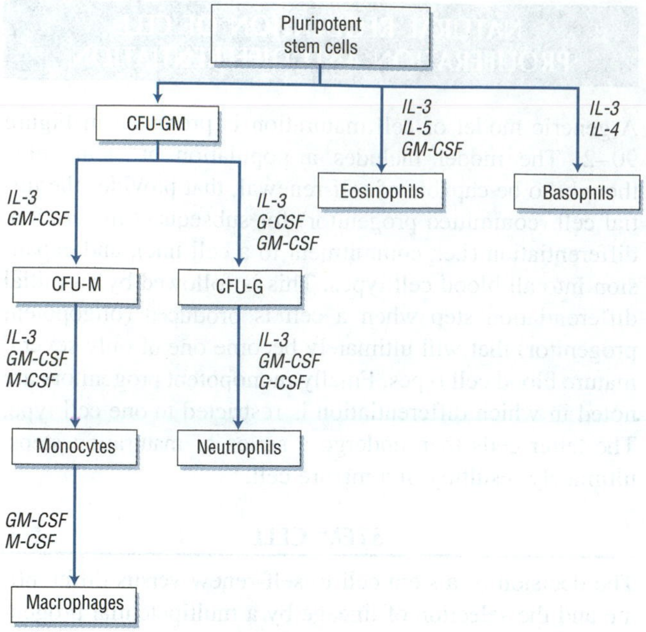

FIGURE 90–5. Maturation of precursor cells into granulocytes and macrophages, including some intermediate precursor cells (CFU-GM, G, and M) is depicted. The CSFs that affect the more terminal (mature) pathways are also shown. (CSFs that regulate immature cell types are not displayed.) CFU = colony-forming unit; G = granulocyte; M = monocyte.

the suspected sites in the process where CSFs are thought to interact by promoting the production, proliferation, and survival of hematopoietic cells. These schema are simple representations of a system of complex interactions between stimulatory and inhibitory cytokines that may not be adequately described by the *in vitro* models used thus far to define them. Details regarding the clinical pharmacology of individual CSFs are presented in Chapter 115.

Immature bone marrow precursor cells such as the myeloblast (first recognizable cell of granulocytic differentiation), promyelocyte, myelocyte, and erythroblast are thought to be capable of replication. This is in contrast to most mature hematopoietic cells, which are incapable of division. Exceptions to the latter statement include monocytes, macrophages, and tissue mast cells. Evaluation of reasons for a change in hematopoietic cellular concentration over time must be conducted with a thorough knowledge of the mechanisms of both cellular production and destruction.

NEUTROPHILS

Blood neutrophils are in constant exchange with an equal number of "marginated" cells. The latter are stuck to the walls of vessels in the peripheral blood, liver, lungs, and spleen. Demargination or the converse, increased adhesion, can therefore dramatically change the peripheral neutrophil concentration even though cell production remains constant. A variety of stimuli can result in demargination including infection, exercise, epinephrine, corticosteroids, and sickle-cell anemia.[24] Conversely, transient neutropenia can occur via stimulation of margination by conditions such as malaria, some viral infections, and onset of hemodialysis.[25]

Normally it takes 14 days for neutrophil production and differentiation in the bone marrow. G-CSF, GM-CSF, and IL-3 are thought to be important regulatory molecules of neutrophil production (Fig. 90–5). A healthy adult will produce approximately 1.6 billion neutrophils per kilogram body weight per day.[26] Blood neutrophils are totally replaced at least twice in each 24-hour period, and thus the average circulation time for any one cell is approximately 6 to 12 hours. Most of this transgression is thought to be for effector functions in the tissues and not simply an elimination process. The total number of noncirculating (i.e., storage) neutrophils is more than 15 times the number in blood. Absolute storage cell numbers are subject to alteration by prior exposure to chemotherapy or deficiency in cofactors required for their synthesis (e.g., folate). When conditions call for an acute increase in blood neutrophils, the pattern of cells thus changes to one more similar to that in the marrow (i.e., band concentration increases relative to seg concentration; normal ratio < 0.1 to 0.3).[27] This phenomenon, often referred to as a "shift to the left," denotes a circulating neutrophil population made of less-mature cells. Infectious processes are often accompanied by such a shift as well as increased outflow of cells from storage forms in the bone marrow, but extreme cases may require so many granulocytes at the infection site that marrow pools are depleted, resulting in neutropenia. Cytokine expression, and thus hematopoiesis, may be impaired in the elderly, resulting in a reduced ability to tolerate myelosuppressive chemotherapy.[28]

EOSINOPHILS

The typical blood circulation time for an eosinophil is approximately 6 hours but it may survive weeks within tissues. Cytokines thought important in eosinophil production or function include IL-1, IL-3, GM-CSF, G-CSF, and, per-

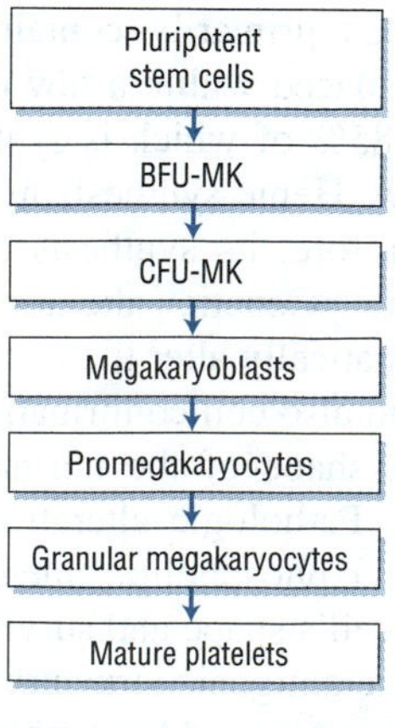

FIGURE 90–6. Megakaryocyte precursors undergo several maturation steps prior to becoming mature platelets as outlined in this figure. BFU = burst-forming unit; MK = megakaryocyte; CFU = colony-forming unit.

haps most important, IL-5. Corticosteroids cause a transient margination of eosinophils and inhibit release of mature cells from the bone marrow.[4]

MONOCYTES AND MACROPHAGES

Both macrophages and T lymphocytes secrete cytokines that stimulate monocytopoiesis.[29] Examples of cytokines that act on relatively mature monocytes include M-CSF and GM-CSF. Blood monocytes have a shorter marrow transit time than neutrophils (6 vs 13 days, respectively) and there is no monocyte reserve in the marrow.[27] The peripheral blood turnover of these cells is much slower (circulation half-life 3 days) than for neutrophils; similarly, tissue macrophages are thought to be very long lived. Macrophages may be able to produce their own progeny as well as attract additional monocytes for differentiation in the local environment.

LYMPHOCYTES

Immature T cells produced in the bone marrow ultimately migrate to the thymus, where they both expand and mature into immunologically competent cells (see Fig. 90–4). Lymphopoiesis is facilitated by a variety of cytokines including IL-2, IL-4, and IL-7, whereas others such as transforming growth factor-β may decelerate this process.[30] T lymphocytes are probably the longest lived hematopoietic cell because experimental evidence exists for the life span of some to be greater than 10 years. The term *lymphokine* is used to describe cytokines secreted by T cells. Lymphokines such as interleukin-2 are important in both activation and proliferation of the immune response while monokines are also important regulators of lymphocyte development. T and B lymphocytes have important interactions with each other in both lymphocyte development and activation, which seem necessary for immunocompetence. There is some evidence for age-associated reductions in circulating helper and suppressor T cells and B cells.[31]

PLATELETS

Thrombopoiesis is the term used to describe the process of platelet production. The bone marrow manufactures 40,000 platelets/μL of blood each day. Proliferation and differentiation of platelet precursors are thought to be primarily influenced by cytokines such as IL-6, IL-11, leukemia inhibitory factor, and perhaps most specifically by thrombopoietin (megakaryocyte growth and development factor; see Fig. 90–6).[32,33] Other hematopoietins that may act in concert, producing synergistic effects include IL-3, IL-1, GM-CSF, EPO, and SCF.[34] The platelet survival time is a clinical test that can estimate the rate of platelet turnover.[35] In normal individuals, this time is 9.5 ± 0.6 days.[36]

ERYTHROCYTES

The normal life span of an RBC is approximately 100 to 120 days, with a circulating cell turnover rate of 1% per day. This translates into a typical adult producing approximately 200 billion reticulocytes every day. Conditions such as anemia or hypoxemia primarily stimulate the renal peritubular interstitial cells to produce EPO by interaction with the renal oxygen sensor. The degree of elevation in blood EPO concentrations is dependent on the severity of anemia or hypoxemia. This in turn recruits RBC precursors and shortens the normal time for differentiation if adequate cofactors such as iron, folate, and vitamin B_{12} are present. Although the overall time for differentiation is shortened (as is the duration of time a reticulocyte spends in the marrow), the blood maturation time is lengthened. The increase in EPO concentrations are relatively quick (within hours), but the effects on marrow transpire over several days. The ultimate increase in RBC mass occurs at an even slower pace, generally over weeks to months (see Fig. 90–3). Multiple other endogenous cytokines are also thought to play a role in either stimulating or inhibiting erythropoiesis by acting on the early progenitors. These include GM-CSF, G-CSF, IL-1, IL-3, IL-6, IL-9, SCF, and some stromal proteins.[21]

Adequate production of RBCs for a degree of anemia is best assessed by evaluation of the number of circulating reticulocytes. Although the normal range is approximately 0.4% to 1.7% of the RBCs, this would obviously be higher in anemic patients with adequate productive capacity. A corrected reticulocyte count is calculated by multiplying this value by the hemoglobin and dividing by the normal hemoglobin expected for a healthy patient with similar characteristics. Additional correction accounts for the increased life span of reticulocytes in the peripheral blood of patients depending directly on their degree of anemia. Figure 90–7 displays correction factors that can be used to accommodate for these changes.[37] Direct assessment of

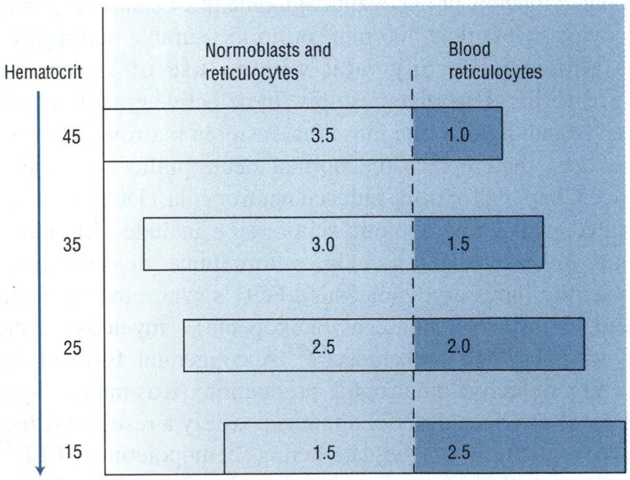

FIGURE 90–7. Correction of hematocrit with the marrow and blood reticulocyte maturation times. With a hematocrit of 45 the blood reticulocytes circulate for 1 day, whereas reduction in hematocrit to 15 results in a 2.5-day circulation time. The numbers found under the blood reticulocyte column can be used as a correction factor in evaluation of reticulocyte concentrations as described in the text. *(From Hillman RS, Finch CA. Red Cell Manual. Philadelphia, FA Davis, 1992, p 59. Reprinted with permission.)*

erythropoiesis in the bone marrow can be performed by estimating the myeloid to erythroid (M/E) cell ratio from a marrow aspirate. The normal adult ratio is 3:1 to 5:1 but can obviously be influenced by changes in erythroid or myeloid production. RBCs lose flexibility with age and eventually undergo lysis or are phagocytized and removed by the monocyte–macrophage system (primarily via the spleen). Accelerated red cell destruction can be grossly quantitated by increases in plasma concentrations of bilirubin and lactate dehydrogenase (LDH).[37]

Although clinical laboratories measure RBC concentrations with excellent accuracy, the most useful tool for assessment of the blood's oxygen-carrying capacity is the hemoglobin because of the variability in RBC size. The average RBC and hemoglobin concentrations in healthy adult male and female patients are approximately 5.21 and 4.60 × 10^6/mm^3, respectively, and 15.7 and 13.8 g/dL, respectively. Variations in normal concentrations will also be evident depending on age, menstruation status, race, environmental factors, and pregnancy.[38]

DISEASE-ASSOCIATED HEMATOPOIETIC CHANGES

NEUTROPHILS

The usual definition of neutropenia is an absolute neutrophil count below 1800/mm^3 in white patients, 1400/mm^3 in black patients, and 1500/mm^3 for children 1 month to 10 years old. Clinical manifestations of neutropenia (i.e., infection) are not typically evident without other cofactors until the concentration drops below 1000/mm^3.[39] Accompanying factors that may influence the risk of infection for a particular patient include skin and mucous membrane integrity; vascular tissue supply; nutritional status; and lymphocytopenia, monocytopenia, or hypogammaglobinemia. Persistent agranulocytosis (less than 500/mm^3 or no measurable neutrophils) is almost uniformly fatal without use of supportive antibiotics. Disorders resulting in defective granulopoiesis can be subdivided into those that result in marrow aplasia or diseases that replace the normal neutrophilic component. (See Chap. 94 for drug-induced neutropenia.) Diseases associated with granulopoietic suppression include viral infection, tuberculosis, anorexia, autoimmune diseases (e.g., systemic lupus erythematosus), Felty's syndrome (rheumatoid arthritis/splenomegaly/leukopenia), myelodysplastic syndromes, and leukemias.[39,40] A congenital form of severely defective neutrophil production (Kostmann's syndrome) has been described that is possibly a result of defective regulation of the late-acting hemopoietin G-CSF.[41] Patients with the rare disorder of cyclic neutropenia display periodic wide fluctuations in the WBCs at approximately 3-week intervals that last for 3 to 6 days. Other forms of chronic neutropenias may occur with adequate marrow stores and can be relatively benign in symptomatology.

Neutrophilia is typically defined as an absolute neutrophil count greater than 7.5 × 10^9 cells/L blood and is sometimes referred to as a leukemoid reaction, if extreme.[24] Acute neutrophilia may be a result of emotional or physical stimuli (e.g., exercise, seizures, labor, pain, temperature changes), infections, inflammation or tissue necrosis, or drugs or toxins (e.g., CSFs, epinephrine, corticosteroids, lithium, vaccines, endotoxin). Chronic causes of increased neutrophils include persistent infections, inflammation, malignancies, drugs, metabolic or endocrine disorders, cigarette smoking, hereditary or congenital abnormalities, and myeloproliferative diseases such as polycythemia vera.[24]

EOSINOPHILS

Eosinophilia (absolute count greater than 700/mm^3) may result from neoplastic processes, parasitic or fungal infections, gastrointestinal disorders, malignancies, dermatitis, granulomatous disorders (e.g., sarcoidosis, Wegener's disease), or collagen–vascular diseases in addition to the more typical cause, allergic reactions.[42] One mechanism that may be common to several of these etiologic factors has been postulated to be antigenic stimulation of T cells, which produce a cytokine (IL-5) that mediates eosinophil proliferation.[43] Infections may cause eosinopenia; however, its significance is not thought to be of concern in that setting.

BASOPHILS

Basophilia may be seen frequently in patients with myeloproliferative disorders and in association with inflammatory reactions and diseases. Viral infections, iron deficiency, or lung cancer can sometimes increase basophil counts. Mastocytosis is usually evident only on analysis of tissue or bone marrow mast cells. Causes include hypersensitivity reactions, malignancy, osteoporosis, and chronic liver or renal disease.

MONOCYTES

Monocytosis (> 0.8 × 10^9 cells/L) occurs with some infections (e.g., tuberculosis, histoplasmosis, toxoplasmosis, bacterial endocarditis, salmonellosis), collagen–vascular diseases (rheumatoid arthritis, systemic lupus erythematosus), gastrointestinal disorders (ulcerative colitis, alcoholic liver disease), leukemias, and up to 60% of nonhematologic malignancies, whereas abnormally low monocyte concentrations occur in patients with hairy cell leukemia or aplastic anemia.[44]

LYMPHOCYTES

Significant reductions in lymphocyte concentration (< 1 × 10^9 cells/L) can be evident without apparent cause or in a variety of diseases, including acute inflammatory disorders, severe uremia, immune deficiency diseases such as systemic lupus erythematosus, chronic infections such as tuberculosis or human immunodeficiency virus infection, malignancies, and connective tissue diseases.[45] Lymphocytosis (> 4 × 10^9 cells/L) may occur with mononucleosis, pertussis, measles, or chickenpox, and in lymphoid malignancies. A progressive increase in mature lymphocytes may be indicative of chronic lymphocytic leukemia. Increased atypical lymphocytes may be demonstrated in patients with infections (mononucleosis, hepatitis, cytomegalovirus, etc), allergic reactions, or lymphomas.[46]

PLATELETS

Both qualitative and quantitative platelet disorders have important pathophysiologic consequences. Thrombocytopenia, defined as a platelet count < 150,000 cells/mm^3, may result from a defect in production, increased sequestration, or accelerated destruction.[47]

Certain stimuli may cause injury to the marrow by reducing the number of megakaryocytes available. Drugs, chemicals, radiation, and infection are among the potential causes of marrow injury. Diseases producing general bone marrow failure or those that invade the bone marrow may result in thrombocytopenia. Examples of the latter include cancers such as leukemia, lymphoma, myelofibrosis, myelodysplasia, and metastatic solid tumors (breast and prostate cancer) and infections such as those caused by mycobacterium. Suboptimal platelet production may also result from defects in maturation seen with vitamin B_{12} and/or folate deficiency or in congenital syndromes.[48]

Alteration in platelet distribution may also result in thrombocytopenia. Splenomegaly is the most frequent cause of increased platelet sequestration.

Idiopathic thrombocytopenic purpura (ITP) is a common cause of thrombocytopenia owing to accelerated destruction of platelets. Antiplatelet antibodies combine with platelets in ITP, thus sensitizing them to removal by the immune system. Accelerated platelet destruction can also be seen in patients with connective tissue disorders. Approximately 14% of patients with systemic lupus erythematosus experience thrombocytopenia similar to ITP.

ERYTHROCYTES

Suboptimal erythropoiesis can be classified by changes in the size of RBCs noted on exam of the peripheral blood. The excretory and endocrine functions of the kidney usually mirror each other, and thus renal dysfunction can result in anemia by reduction in EPO production, resulting in a normochromic, normocytic pattern. Other causes of insufficient erythropoiesis include replacement of bone marrow by fibrosis, solid tumors, or leukemia, as well as defects in erythroid maturation. Relative deficiencies in the cofactors required for heme–RBC synthesis such as iron, folate, and vitamin B_{12} may also be important contributors. Structurally, RBC macrocytosis denotes defects in the maturation of the nucleus, whereas microcytosis is indicative of cytoplasmic defects (reduced hemoglobin synthesis). A detailed description regarding the pathogenesis and treatment of anemic disorders is found in Chap. 91.

Exaggerated erythropoiesis with increased RBC mass (polycythemia) can be mistaken for a reduction in plasma volume. Symptoms are not always immediately evident but may progress to reduced tissue oxygenation, thrombosis, and congestive heart failure. The most common etiology is hypoxia; alternative causes can be subdivided based on their ability to stimulate EPO production. EPO (or a similar cytokine) may be produced in response to genetic alterations or a variety of malignancies including angioblastoma, hepatomas, and hypernephroma.[49] Polycythemia vera, a malignancy of the bone marrow stem cells, results in an increased sensitivity of RBC precursors to stimulation by EPO and is accompanied in many patients by thrombocytosis and leukocytosis.

CLINICAL USES OF HEMATOPOIETIC CELLS

BONE MARROW TRANSPLANTATION

High-dose chemotherapy with or without irradiation is beneficial in the treatment of a number of malignant diseases (see Chap. 125). The dose of chemotherapy that can be administered, however, is limited by hematopoietic toxicity, resulting in prolonged periods of pancytopenia with the attendant risks of serious infection and bleeding. This hematopoietic toxicity can be overcome by the infusion (transplantation) of bone marrow, following the high-dose therapy with subsequent repopulation of the bone marrow and recovery of hematopoiesis. Bone marrow transplantation (BMT) involves the removal of bone marrow from the donor, administration of intensive doses of chemotherapy (with or without irradiation) to the recipient, and infusion of the donor bone marrow to the recipient. If the donor and recipient are the same individual (i.e., the patient serves as his or her own donor), the procedure is termed *autologous bone marrow transplantation.* If the marrow comes from another individual, the procedure is termed *allogeneic bone marrow transplantation.* Most allogeneic donors are HLA-matched siblings, but the use of alternative donors such as matched related volunteer donors or umbilical cord blood cells (see below) is increasing.

Allogeneic transplantation is complicated by the immune recognition of host tissues by donor T lymphocytes, resulting in a syndrome called graft-versus-host disease. Immune recognition of tumor cells also occurs (graft-versus-tumor effect), resulting in lower relapse rates compared to autologous transplants for similar disease stages. Allogeneic transplantation is used more commonly for diseases primarily involving the bone marrow, such as acute and chronic leukemias, aplastic anemia, thalassemia, and severe combined immunodeficiency. Autologous transplantation is more commonly used in lymphoma and Hodgkin's disease and selected solid tumors such as breast cancer, ovarian cancer, and germ cell tumors.

A number of laboratory techniques are evolving to allow the harvested bone marrow to expand in the laboratory prior to infusion and to cleanse the marrow of potential malignant cell contamination in the autologous transplant setting.

PERIPHERAL BLOOD PROGENITOR CELL TRANSPLANTATION

Small numbers of hematopoietic progenitor cells capable of reconstituting hematopoiesis circulate in the peripheral blood under normal circumstances.[50] The number of circulating progenitor cells is increased during recovery from myelosuppressive chemotherapy or after treatment with cytokines such as G-CSF or GM-CSF.[51,52] These cells can be collected by a process called leukopheresis and stored for reinfusion following high-dose therapy. Hematopoietic recovery is generally more rapid following rescue with peripheral blood progenitor cells (PBPC) as compared with bone marrow. Potential tumor cell contamination may also be less with PBPC transplants. The use of PBPC has essentially replaced the use of bone marrow in the autologous setting and is increasing in allogeneic transplants.

UNRELATED-DONOR BONE MARROW TRANSPLANTATION

Only approximately one-third of patients who would otherwise be eligible for allogeneic bone marrow transplantation have HLA-matched related donors. One alternative is the use of closely HLA-matched, unrelated-donor marrow. The National Marrow Donor Program (NMDP) is a registry of volunteer marrow donors now containing over 2 million members. The NMDP facilitates the identification of potential donors and the procurement of marrow and coordinates the activities of a network of donor, collection, and transplant centers. Unrelated-donor marrow transplants are associated with an increased incidence of graft-versus-host disease compared to related-donor transplants; however, recent advances in tissue typing and donor matching and graft-versus-host disease prophylaxis have resulted in comparable overall survival rates for many diseases.

CORD BLOOD TRANSPLANTATION

Many patients, however, do not have matched family members or unrelated donors in the marrow registries. Another alternative is the use of human umbilical cord blood, which contains hematopoietic stem cells capable of reconstituting bone marrow function following high-dose therapy.[53] An almost unlimited number of cord blood donors is potentially available because the cord and its associated blood are commonly discarded following delivery. Cord-blood banks have been established in which cord blood cells are HLA typed and cryopreserved and are available for transplantation for appropriate recipients. The majority of cord-blood progenitor cell transplants performed to date have been in children because of the relatively small number of cells available from a cord blood unit, although the number of cord blood transplants in adults is increasing. Laboratory methods to expand the number of progenitor cells in cord blood units are under investigation. Cord blood transplants are thought to be associated with less graft-versus-host disease than transplants from matched unrelated bone marrow donors with similar degrees of matching and may prove to be an important source of progenitor cells for transplantation in the near future.

GENE THERAPY

Hematopoietic progenitor cells are the focus of intense research in gene therapy. The self-renewal capacity of these cells makes them an obvious target for delivering corrective genetic information for a variety of both hematologic and metabolic inherited disorders such as sickle cell anemia, thalassemia, immunodeficiency syndromes, and glycogen storage diseases.

TRANSFUSION AND BLOOD PRODUCT SUPPORT

Advances in blood banking and transfusion support have been critical to the improved outcome of therapy for patients with hematologic and malignant diseases. Platelet transfusions are indicated for the prevention and treatment of bleeding. In general, prophylactic platelet transfusions are not indicated for platelet counts above 10,000/μL unless the patient is febrile or actively bleeding. Platelets are available as pooled random donor concentrates obtained from red blood cell donations (six to eight donors per transfusion) or single-donor platelets collected by apheresis. The use of ABO-compatible platelets and leukocyte filters has been shown to decrease the development of alloimmunization and refractoriness to platelet transfusions and is cost effective. Leukocyte filters also decrease the risk of transmission of cytomegalovirus and febrile transfusion reactions. Packed red blood cell transfusions are indicated to keep hemoglobin levels greater than 7 to 8 g/dL to maintain adequate-oxygen carrying capacity. Each unit of packed red blood cells should increase the hemoglobin level by approximately 1 g/dL unless active blood loss is evident. Red blood cells should also be filtered to reduce the risk of nonhemolytic, febrile transfusion reactions. Patients who are candidates for bone marrow transplantation should also receive blood products that have been irradiated with 2500 cGy to prevent transfusion-associated graft-versus-host disease.

Fresh frozen plasma (FFP) contains the components of the coagulation system and is indicated for the replacement of deficient coagulation factors II, V, VII, X, XI, and XIII. Factors VIII and IX deficiencies are treated with specific factor concentrates. FFP is also used for the rapid reversal of warfarin anticoagulation and in the treatment of disseminated intravascular coagulation. Thrombotic thrombocytopenic purpura is treated with therapeutic plasma exchange using FFP as the replacement fluid. Cryoprecipitate contains factor VIII, von Willebrand's factor, and fibrinogen and is indicated for the treatment of von Willebrand's disease that does not respond to desmopressin acetate (DDAVP) and for fibrinogen replacement.

Intravenous immunoglobin (IVIg) has been used in a variety of hematologic disorders, but for most of these situations it is still considered experimental or indicated only when other therapeutic options have been exhausted. Patients with deficient immunoglobin production (e.g., agammaglobinemia, hypogammaglobulinemia) or function (e.g., chronic lymphocytic leukemia, multiple myeloma, children with human immunodeficiency virus [HIV]) may benefit from this therapy with the goal of raising the IgG level such that there is less chance for bacterial infection (< 500 mg/dL). IVIg also has other pharmacologic properties which include Fc-receptor blockade, modification of complement activation, and modulation of the immune response by anti-idiotypic antibodies.[54] Additional clinical indications include patients with ITP who are at high bleeding risk or need higher platelet counts prior to surgery.[55] Posttransplant prophylaxis (approximately 3 months) with IVIg is also sometimes used in patients receiving allogeneic BMT for prevention of bacterial sepsis and acute graft-versus-host disease. Treatment with IVIg may benefit patients whose platelet counts do not increase substantially despite transfusions owing to the formation of alloantibodies.

REFERENCES

1. Erslev AJ, Lichtman MA. Structure and function of the marrow. In: Williams WJ, Beutler E, Erslev AJ, Lichtman MA, eds. Hematology, 4th ed. New York, McGraw-Hill, 1990:37.
2. Lehrer RI, Ganz T, Selsted ME, et al. Neutrophils in human diseases. N Engl J Med 1987;317:687–694.
3. Lieschke GJ, Burgess AW. Granulocyte colony-stimulating factor and granulocyte–macrophage colony-stimulating factor. N Engl J Med 1992;327:28–35.
4. Weller PF. The immunobiology of eosinophils. N Engl J Med 1991;324:1110–1118.
5. Kitamura Y, Kasugai T, Arizono N, Matsuda H. Development of mast cells and basophils: Processes and regulation mechanisms. Am J Med Sci 1993;306:185–191.
6. Galli SJ, Dvorak AM, Dvorak HF. Morphology, biochemistry, and function of basophils and mast cells. In: Williams WJ, Beutler E, Erslev AJ, Lichtman MA, eds. Hematology, 4th ed. New York, McGraw-Hill, 1990:840.
7. Johnston RB. Monocytes and macrophages. N Engl J Med 1988; 318:747–752.
8. Kipps TJ, Carson DA. Functions of B lymphocytes and plasma cells in immunoglobulin production. In: Williams WJ, Beutler E, Erslev AJ, Lichtman MA, eds. Hematology, 4th ed. New York, McGraw-Hill, 1990:932.
9. Kipps TJ, Carson DA. Functions of T lymphocytes: T-cell receptors for antigen. In: Williams WJ, Beutler E, Erslev AJ, Lichtman MA, eds. Hematology, 4th ed. New York, McGraw-Hill, 1990:939.
10. Thompson AR, Harker LA. Manual of Hemostasis and Thrombosis, 3rd ed. Philadelphia, Davis, 1983:47.
11. Mustard JF, Packham MA, Kinlough-Rathbone RL. Platelets, blood flow, and the vessel wall. Circulation 1990;81(suppl 1):I40–I41.
12. Gordon MY. Physiological mechanisms in BMT and haematopoiesis-revisited. Bone Marrow Transplant 1993;11:193–197.
13. Weiss LP. Functional organization of the hematopoietic tissues. In: Hoffman R, Benz EJ, Shattil SJ, et al, eds. Hematology—Basic Principles and Practice. New York, Churchill Livingstone, 1991:82.
14. Greenberger J. The hematopoietic microenvironment. Crit Rev Oncol Hematol 1991;11:65–84.
15. To LB, Shepperd KM, Haylock DN, et al. Single high doses of cyclophosphamide enable the collection of high numbers of hematopoietic stem cells from the peripheral blood. Exp Hematol 1990;18: 442–447.
16. Peters WP, Rosner G, Ross M, et al. Comparative effects of granulocyte–macrophage colony-stimulating factor and granulocyte colony-stimulating factor on priming peripheral blood progenitor cells for use with autologous bone marrow after high-dose chemotherapy. Blood 1993;81:1709–1719.
17. Spangrude GJ, Heimfeld S, Wessman IL. Purification and characterization of mouse hematopoietic stem cells. Science 1988;241:58–62.
18. Williams N, Levine RF. The origin, development and regulation of megakaryocytes. Br J Hematol 1982;52:173–180.
19. Hoffman R. Regulation of megakaryocytopoiesis. Blood 1989;74: 1196–1212.
20. Papayannopoulou T, Abkowitz J. Biology of erythropoiesis, erythroid differentiation, and maturation. In: Hoffman R, Benz EJ, Shattil SJ, et al, eds. Hematology—Basic Principles and Practice. New York, Churchill Livingstone, 1991:252.
21. McGuire MJ, Spivak JL. Erythropoiesis. In: Anderson KC, Ness PM, eds. Scientific Basis of Transfusion Medicine—Implications for Clinical Practice. Philadelphia, Saunders, 1994:1.
22. Ogawa M. Differentiation and proliferation of hematopoietic stem cells. Blood 1993;81:2844–2853.
23. Moore MAS. Does stem cell exhaustion result from combining hematopoietic growth factors with chemotherapy? If so, how do we prevent it? Blood 1992;80:3–7.
24. Dale DC. Neutrophilia. In: Williams WJ, Beutler E, Erslev AJ, Lichtman MA, eds. Hematology, 4th ed. New York, McGraw-Hill, 1990:816.
25. Coates T, Baehner R. Leukocytosis and leukopenia. In: Hoffman R, Benz EJ, Shattil SJ, et al, eds. Hematology—Basic Principles and Practice. New York, Churchill Livingstone, 1991:552.
26. Gabrilove J. Granulopoiesis. In: Anderson KC, Ness PM, eds. Scientific Basis of Transfusion Medicine—Implications for Clinical Practice. Philadelphia, Saunders, 1994:17.
27. Boggs DR, Winkelstein A. White Cell Manual. Philadelphia, Davis, 1983:29.
28. Rothstein G. Hematopoiesis in the aged: A model of hematopoietic dysregulation? Blood 1993;82:2601–2604.
29. Bagby GC, Segal GM. Growth factors and the control of hematopoiesis. In: Hoffman R, Benz EJ, Shattil SJ, et al, eds. Hematology—Basic Principles and Practice. New York, Churchill Livingstone, 1991:97.
30. Jordan SC. Cytokines and lymphocytes. In: Kunkel SL, Remick DG, eds. Cytokines in Health and Disease. New York, Marcel Dekker, 1992:309.
31. Yamashiki M, Nishimura A, Kosaka Y, James SP. Two-color analysis of peripheral lymphocyte surface antigens in inherently healthy adults. J Clin Lab Anal 1994;8:22–26.
32. Du XX, Williams DA. Interleukin-11: A multifunctional growth factor derived from the hematopoietic microenvironment. Blood 1994; 83:2023–2030.
33. Metcalf D. Thrombopoietin—at last. Nature 1994;369:519–520.
34. Gordon MS, Hoffman R. Growth factors affecting human thrombocytopoiesis: Potential agents for the treatment of thrombocytopenia. Blood 1992;80:302–307.
35. Shulman NR, Jordan JV Jr. Platelet kinetics. In: Colman RW, Hirsh J, Marder VJ, Saltzman EW, eds. Hemostasis and Thrombosis. Basic Principles and Clinical Practice, 2nd ed. Philadelphia, Lippincott, 1987:341–351.
36. Harker LA, Finch CA. Thrombokinetics in man. J Clin Invest 1969; 48:963–974.
37. Hillman RS, Finch CA. Red Cell Manual. Philadelphia, Davis, 1992:59.
38. Glassman AB. Anemia: Diagnosis and clinical considerations. In: Harmening DM, ed. Clinical Hematology and Fundamentals of Hemostasis, 2nd ed. Philadelphia, Davis, 1992:54.
39. Lichtman MA. Classification and clinical manifestations of neutrophil disorders. In: Williams WJ, Beutler E, Erslev AJ, Lichtman MA, eds. Hematology, 4th ed. New York, McGraw-Hill, 1990:802.

40. Malech HL, Gallin JI. Neutrophils in human disease. N Engl J Med 1987;317:687–694.
41. Dong F, Hoefsloot LH, Schelen AM, et al. Identification of a nonsense mutation in the G-CSF receptor in severe congenital neutropenia. Proc Natl Acad Sci 1994;91:4480–4484.
42. Boggs DR, Winkelstein A. White Cell Manual, 4th ed. Philadelphia, Davis, 1983:54.
43. Sanderson CJ. Interleukin-5, eosinophils and disease. Blood 1992; 79:3101–3109.
44. Lichtman MA. Classification and clinical manifestations of disorders of monocytes and macrophages. In: Williams WJ, Beutler E, Erslev AJ, Lichtman MA, eds. Hematology, 4th ed. New York, McGraw-Hill, 1990:879.
45. Williams WJ. Lymphocytopenia. In: Williams WJ, Beutler E, Erslev AJ, Lichtman MA, eds. Hematology, 4th ed. New York, McGraw-Hill, 1990:964.
46. Williams WJ. Lymphocytosis. In: Williams WJ, Beutler E, Erslev AJ, Lichtman MA, eds. Hematology, 4th ed. New York, McGraw-Hill, 1990:963.
47. Rutherford CJ, Frenkel EP. Thrombocytopenia. Issues in diagnosis and therapy. Med Clin North Am 1994;78:555–575.
48. Williams WJ. Classification and clinical manifestations of disorders of hemostasis. In: Williams WJ, Beutler E, Erslev AJ, Lichtman MA, eds. Hematology, 4th ed. New York, McGraw-Hill, 1990:1338.
49. Tabbara IA. Erythropoietin biology and clinical applications. Arch Intern Med 1993;153:298–304.
50. Kessinger A, Armitage JO, Landmark JD, et al. Autologous peripheral hematopoietic stem cell transplantation restores hematopoietic function following marrow ablative therapy. Blood 1988;71:723–727.
51. Peters WP, Rosner G, Ross M, et al. Comparative effects of granulocyte–macrophage colony-stimulating factor (GM-CSF) and granulocyte colony-stimulating factor (G-CSF) on priming peripheral blood progenitor cells for use with autologous bone marrow after high-dose chemotherapy. Blood 1993;81:1709–1719.
52. To LB, Shepperd KM, Haylock DN, et al. Single high doses of cyclophosphamide enable the collection of high numbers of hematopoietic cells from the peripheral blood. Exp Hematol 1990;18:442–447.
53. Auerbach AD, Liu Q, Ghosh R, et al. Prenatal identification of potential donors for umbilical cord blood transplantation for Fanconi anemia. Transfusion 1990;30:682–687.
54. Otten A, Bossuyt PMM, Vermeulen M, Brand A. Intravenous immunoglobulin treatment in hematological diseases. Eur J Haematol 1998;60:73–85.
55. George JN, Woolf SH, Gary E, et al. Idiopathic thrombocytopenic purpura: A practice guideline developed by explicit methods for the American Society of Hematology. Blood 1996;88:3–40.

91

ANEMIAS

Thomas T. Sproat, PharmD, BCPS, PA-C

Anemias are a group of diseases characterized by a decrease in either hemoglobin (Hgb) or red blood cells (RBCs); this decrease results in decreased oxygen-carrying capacity of blood. Anemias represent problems with RBC production, an accelerated loss of RBC mass, or a manifestation of a host of systemic disorders such as infection, chronic renal disease, or malignancy. Anemias are often a sign of underlying pathology; a rapid diagnosis of the etiology of the anemia is essential. The goals of this chapter are to review the maturation, development, and destruction cycle of RBCs; classification systems; definitions; pathophysiology; and laboratory tests and procedures used in the diagnosis and treatment of anemias.

Anemias can be classified on the basis of morphology of the RBCs, etiology, or pathophysiology. Table 91–1 gives some examples of anemias in these classifications. Iron deficiency anemia (IDA), anemia of chronic disease (ACD), and anemias associated with acute bleeding account for roughly 75% of all anemias.[1] The remaining anemias result from such conditions as bone marrow damage, decreased erythropoiesis, and hemolysis.

MATURATION AND DEVELOPMENT OF RBCs

In adults, RBCs are formed in the marrow of the vertebrae, ribs, sternum, clavicle, pelvic (iliac) crest, and the proximal epiphyses of the long bones. In children, most bone marrow space is hematopoietically active to meet increased RBC requirements.

In normal RBC formation, an undifferentiated progenitor cell, a pluripotent stem cell, yields an erythroid burst–forming unit. This cell is stimulated by erythropoietin (EPO) and cytokines such as interleukin-3 (IL-3) and granulocyte-macrophage colony-stimulating factor (GM-CSF) to form an erythroid colony–forming unit [CFU-E] in the marrow. The CFU-E is very sensitive to EPO and produces proerythroblasts. Subsequent divisions yield basophilic erythroblasts, polychromatic erythroblasts, pyknotic erythroblasts, reticulocytes, and finally an erythrocyte. During this evolution, the nucleus becomes smaller with each division, finally disappearing in the normal erythrocyte (Fig. 91–1). This process is accompanied by incorporation of hemoglobin and iron into the gradually maturing RBC, which is released from the marrow into the circulating blood as a reticulocyte. The maturation process takes about 1 week; several days are then required for the reticulocyte to lose its nucleus and become an erythrocyte.

STIMULATION OF ERYTHROPOIESIS

Production of RBCs is initiated by the hormone EPO, 90% of which is produced by the kidneys in response to a decrease in tissue oxygen concentration. Decreased tissue oxygen signals the kidneys to increase production and release EPO into the plasma, which (1) stimulates stem cells to differentiate into proerythroblasts, (2) increases the rate of mitosis, (3) increases the release of reticulocytes from the marrow, and (4) induces hemoglobin formation. When hemoglobin synthesis is accelerated, the critical hemoglobin concentration necessary for maturity is reached more rapidly and a feedback mechanism stops further RBC nucleic acid synthesis such that the last mitotic division is skipped, causing an earlier release of reticulocytes. Early appearance of reticulocytes, in larger quantities, in the peripheral circulation (reticulocytosis) is another indication that RBC production is being stimulated.

SYNTHESIS OF HEMOGLOBIN

Hemoglobin consists of a protein component comprised of two α- and two β-chains; each chain is linked to a heme group consisting of a porphyrin ring structure with an iron atom chelated at its center, which is capable of binding oxygen. The hemoglobin formed in an adult is composed of 96% hemoglobin A (two α- and two β-chains), 3% hemoglobin A_2 (two α- and two δ-chains), and 1% fetal hemoglobin (two α- and two χ-chains). These polypeptide chains are attached to and folded around each heme structure, giving hemoglobin its unique tetrahedron shape.

The initial step in the synthesis of heme from the substrate succinyl CoA and glycine requires the presence of pyridoxine phosphate (vitamin B_6) as a catalyst. Following synthesis of heme in the cytoplasmic mitochondria of the RBC, it diffuses into the extramitochondrial space to combine with the completed α- and β-chains forming hemoglobin.

Under normal conditions, the body produces approximately 6.25 g of hemoglobin daily. Maximal output of hemoglobin in the event of a hemolytic disease has been estimated at about 40 g daily. Consequently, the normal RBC survival time of 120 days can be decreased to 18 to 20 days before occurrence of an anemia if the bone marrow functions at maximal capacity. When hemolytic destruction of RBCs exceeds marrow production capacity, anemia will develop, causing the hemoglobin value to decrease to a steady-state level at which production is equal to destruction. Hemoglobin values in these hemolytic anemias, such as sickle cell anemia, will remain stable unless other factors further shorten RBC life span.

TABLE 91–1. Classification Systems for Anemias

- I. Morphology. Classifies anemias based on the red blood cell's size (microcytic, normocytic, macrocytic) and hemoglobin content (hypochromic, normochromic, hyperchromic)
  - Macrocytic
    - Megaloblastic anemias
      - Vitamin B_{12} deficiency
      - Folic acid deficiency anemia
  - Hypochromic, microcytic
    - Iron deficiency anemia
    - Genetic anomaly
      - Sickle cell anemia
      - Thalassemia
      - Other hemoglobinopathies (abnormal hemoglobins)
  - Normocytic anemias
    - Recent blood loss
    - Hemolysis
    - Bone marrow failure
    - Anemias of chronic disease
    - Renal failure
    - Endocrine disorders
    - Myeloplastic anemias
- II. Etiology. Classifies anemias on the basis of three fundamental mechanisms
  - Deficiency
    - Iron
    - Vitamin B_{12}
    - Folic acid
    - Pyridoxine
  - Central—caused by impaired bone marrow function
    - Anemia of chronic disease
    - Anemia of the elderly
    - Malignant bone marrow disorders
  - Peripheral
    - Bleeding (hemorrhage)
    - Hemolysis (hemolytic anemias)
- III. Pathophysiology. Classifies anemias based on an evaluation of the pathophysiologic etiology
  - Excessive blood loss
    - Recent hemorrhage
      - Trauma
      - Peptic ulcer
      - Gastritis
      - Hemorrhoids
    - Chronic hemorrhage
      - Vaginal bleeding
      - Peptic ulcer
      - Intestinal parasites
      - Aspirin and other nonsteroidal anti-inflammatory agents
  - Excessive red cell destruction
    - Extracorpuscular (outside the cell) factors
      - RBC antibodies
      - Drugs
      - Physical trauma to RBC (artificial valves)
      - Excessive sequestration in the spleen
    - Intracorpuscular factors
      - Heredity
      - Disorders of hemoglobin synthesis
    - Inadequate production of mature RBCs
      - Deficiency of nutrients (B_{12}, folic acid, iron, protein)
      - Deficiency of erythroblasts
        - Aplastic anemia
        - Isolated (often transient) erythroblastopenia
        - Folic acid antagonists
        - Antibodies
      - Conditions with infiltration of bone marrow
        - Lymphoma
        - Leukemia
        - Myelofibrosis
        - Carcinoma
      - Endocrine abnormalities
        - Hypothyroid
        - Adrenal insufficiency
        - Pituitary insufficiency
      - Chronic renal disease
      - Chronic inflammatory disease
        - Granulomatous diseases
        - Collagen–vascular diseases
      - Hepatic disease

The affinity of hemoglobin for oxygen is influenced by three intracellular components. Increasing hydrogen ion concentration (decreasing pH), carbon dioxide, and 2,3-bisphosphoglycerate (2,3-BPG), as well as increased temperature, all facilitate the ability of hemoglobin to release oxygen into tissue by decreasing oxygen affinity.

TOTAL BODY IRON

The average adult body contains about 4 g of iron, approximately two-thirds of which exists in the form of hemoglobin. Another 13% exists as myoglobin, while the same percentage exists as a combination of ferritin and hemosiderin. Because inorganic iron is quite toxic, the body has an intricate system for iron absorption, transport, storage, assimilation, and elimination.

ABSORPTION OF IRON

The normal daily Western diet contains approximately 12 to 15 mg of iron, mainly in the ferric (Fe^{3+}) nonabsorbed form. This is first ionized by stomach acid and then reduced to the ferrous state (Fe^{2+}) and absorbed primarily in the duodenum and, to a smaller extent, in the jejunum via intestinal mucosal cell uptake and subsequent transfer across the cell into the plasma.[2] The average intake of iron from this diet is about 6 mg per 1000 calories (about 10 to 30 mg of iron per day).[3]

Daily losses, and thus requirements for iron, are 1 mg in adult males and postmenopausal females, and 1.5 to 3 mg in menstruating females. Children and pregnant women have increased iron demands. Children require more iron because of growth-related increases in blood volume, whereas pregnant women have an increased iron demand from fetal development. Iron overload is prevented because only the amount of iron lost per day is absorbed. This represents about 5% to 10% (1 mg) of daily dietary intake. However, up to 8 to 12 mg daily can be absorbed if iron requirements increase.

Absorption of nonheme iron is increased by gastric acid and by other dietary components such as most meats and ascorbic acid. Absorption is decreased by dietary com-

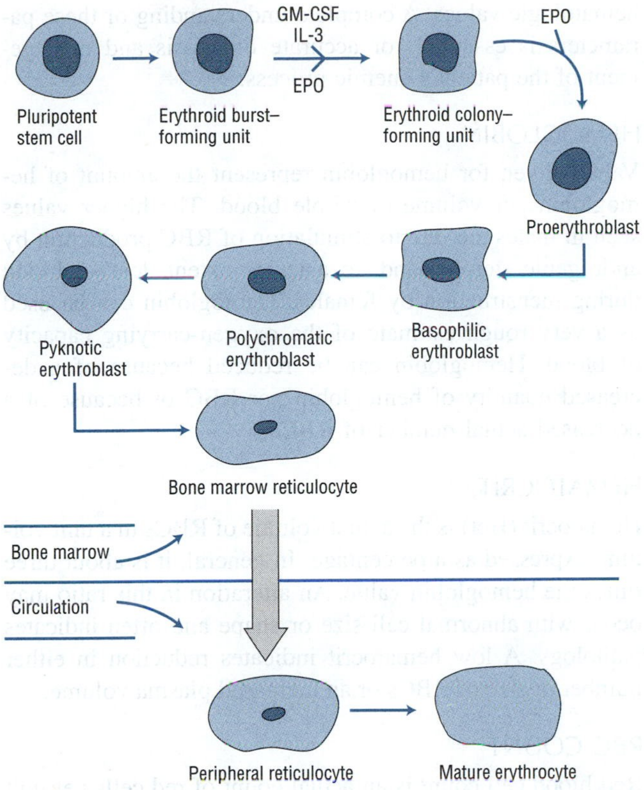

FIGURE 91–1. Erythrocyte maturation sequence.

ponents that form insoluble complexes or chelates with iron (phytates, tannates, and phosphates).[4] Phytates, a natural component of grains, brans, and some other vegetables, form stable, poorly absorbed complexes and partially explain the increased prevalence of iron deficiency anemia in poorer countries, where grains and vegetables compose a disproportionate part of the normal diet, while the more readily absorbed heme iron is lacking in their diet. Last, because gastric acid improves iron absorption, patients who have undergone a gastrectomy or have achlorhydria will have decreased iron absorption.

INCORPORATION OF IRON INTO HEME

The delivery of iron to the bone marrow for incorporation into the RBC hemoglobin molecule is carried out by a specific plasma transport protein called *transferrin.* Transferrin enters cells by binding to transferrin receptors; these circulate and then attach to cells needing iron. Likewise, there is a reduction in transferrin receptors on the surface of cells not currently needing iron, thus preventing iron-replete cells from receiving excess iron.[5]

Circulating transferrin is normally about 30% saturated with iron. Transferrin delivers extra iron to other body storage sites such as the liver, marrow, and spleen for later use. This iron is stored within macrophages of the reticuloendothelial system as ferritin or hemosiderin. Ferritin consists of a ferric hydroxyphosphate core surrounded by a protein shell called *apoferritin.* Hemosiderin can be described as compacted ferritin molecules with an even greater iron–protein shell ratio; physiologically, it is a more stable but less available form of storage iron.

NORMAL DESTRUCTION OF RBCs

Older blood cells are destroyed primarily in the spleen and also in the marrow by phagocytic breakdown (Fig. 91–2). Amino acids from the globin chains return to an amino acid pool; the porphyrin heme structure splits, forming biliverdin and releasing its iron. Iron returns to the iron pool for reuse while biliverdin is further enzymatically reduced to bilirubin. This bilirubin is released into the plasma, where it binds to albumin and is transported to the liver for glucuronide conjugation and excretion via bile. If the liver is unable to perform this conjugation, as seen with intrinsic liver disease or oversaturation of conjugation enzymes by excessive cell hemolysis, the result would be an elevated indirect (unconjugated) bilirubin laboratory value. Should

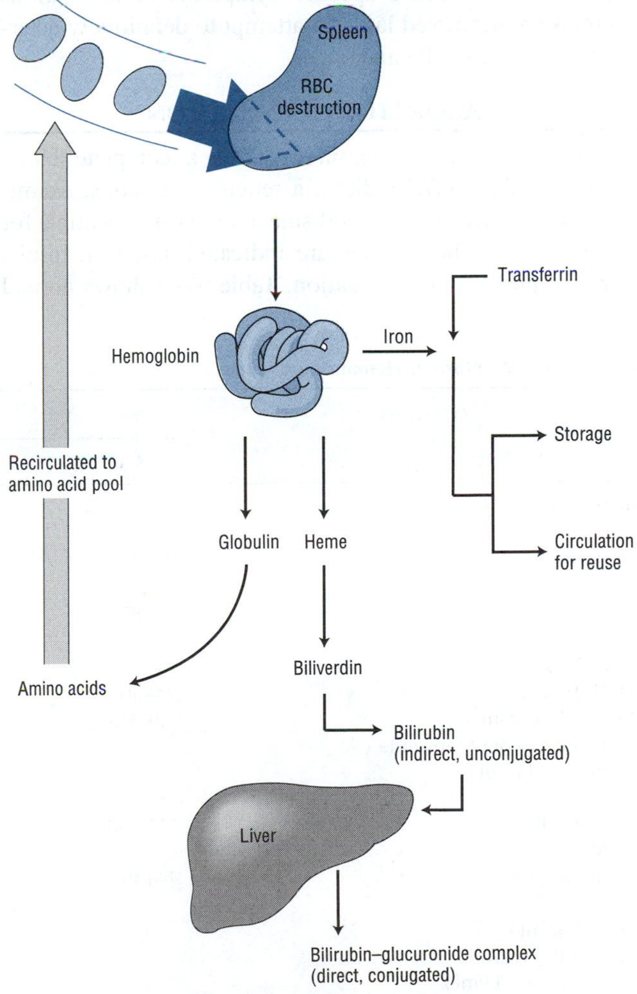

FIGURE 91–2. Destruction of red blood cells (RBCs).

there be an obstruction in the biliary excretion pathway for the already conjugated bilirubin, an elevated direct bilirubin would result. Comparison of direct and indirect bilirubin values helps determine if the defect in bilirubin clearance occurs before or after bilirubin enters the liver.

The hemoglobin in RBCs, which is destroyed by intravascular hemolysis, becomes attached to haptoglobin and is carried back to the marrow for processing in the normal manner.

DIAGNOSIS OF ANEMIA

GENERAL PRESENTATION

Presenting signs and symptoms of anemias depend on the rate of development of the anemia, age, and cardiovascular status of the patient. Anemia of recent onset is most likely to present with cardiorespiratory symptoms such as tachycardia, lightheadedness, and breathlessness, whereas if onset is more chronic in nature, the presenting symptoms may include fatigue, weakness, headache, vertigo, faintness, sensitivity to cold, pallor, and loss of skin tone. These symptoms represent the manifestation of an illness, not a specific disease. More specific symptoms of the various anemias are discussed later, to attempt to definitively determine the cause of the anemia.

LABORATORY EVALUATION

Initial evaluation of anemia involves a complete blood count including RBC indices, a reticulocyte index, examination of the peripheral blood smear, and a stool sample for occult blood. Other studies are indicated based on results from the preliminary evaluation. Table 91–2 shows normal hematologic values. A complete understanding of these parameters is essential for accurate diagnosis and management of the patient's anemic process.

HEMOGLOBIN

Values given for hemoglobin represent the amount of hemoglobin per volume of whole blood. The higher values seen in males are due to stimulation of RBC production by androgenic steroids and, to a lesser extent, loss of blood during menstruation by females. Hemoglobin can be used as a very rough estimate of the oxygen-carrying capacity of blood. Hemoglobin can be reduced because of a decreased quantity of hemoglobin per RBC or because of a decreased actual number of RBCs.

HEMATOCRIT

Hematocrit (Hct) is the actual volume of RBCs in a unit volume expressed as a percentage. In general, it is about three times the hemoglobin value. An alteration in this ratio may occur with abnormal cell size or shape and often indicates pathology. A low hematocrit indicates reduction in either number or size of RBCs or an increased plasma volume.

RBC COUNT

Red blood cell count is an actual count of red cells per unit of blood; it is an indirect estimate of the hemoglobin content of the blood.

RBC INDICES

Wintrobe indices were introduced in 1934 by Maxwell Wintrobe to describe the size and hemoglobin content of the RBCs; these parameters are calculated from the hemoglobin, hematocrit, and RBC count.

TABLE 91–2. Normal Hematologic Values

Test	Reference Range (yr)			
	2–6	6–12	12–18	18–49
Hemoglobin (g/dL)	11.5–15.5	11.5–15.5	M 13.0–16.0 F 12.0–16.0	M 13.5–17.5 F 12.0–16.0
Hematocrit (%)	34–40	35–45	M 37–49 F 36–46	M 41–53 F 36–46
MCV (fL)	75–87	77–95	M 78–98 F 78–102	80–100
MCHC (%)	—	31–37	31–37	31–37
MCH (pg/cell)	24–30	25–33	25–35	26–34
RBC (million/mm^3)	3.9–5.3	4.0–5.2	M 4.5–5.3	M 4.5–5.9
Reticulocyte count, absolute (%)				0.5–1.5
Serum iron (μg/dL)		50–120	50–120	M 50–160 F 40–150
TIBC (μg/dL)	250–400	250–400	250–400	250–400
RDW (%)				11–16
Ferritin (ng/mL)	7–140	7–140	7–140	M 15–200 F 12–150
Folate (ng/mL)				1.8–16.0[a]
Vitamin B_{12} (pg/mL)				100–900[a]
Erythropoietin (U/mL)				0.01–0.03

[a]Varies by assay method.

MEAN CORPUSCULAR VOLUME (HCT/RBC COUNT)

Mean corpuscular volume (MCV) represents the average volume of RBCs. Cells are said to be macrocytic if they are larger than normal, microcytic if they are smaller than normal, and normocytic if their size falls within normal limits. Folic acid and vitamin B_{12} deficiency anemias yield macrocytic morphology, whereas iron deficiency and thalassemias are examples of microcytic anemias. A falsely elevated MCV is seen with reticulocytosis due to the fact that reticulocytes are larger than erythrocytes. A falsely elevated MCV is also seen in the presence of cold agglutinins and hyperglycemia.

MEAN CORPUSCULAR HEMOGLOBIN (HGB/RBC COUNT)

Mean corpuscular hemoglobin (MCH) is the percent volume of hemoglobin in an RBC. Two morphologic changes, microcytosis or hypochromia, can reduce MCH. A microcytic cell contains less hemoglobin because it is a smaller cell, whereas a hypochromic cell has a low MCH because of the decreased amount of hemoglobin present in a normocytic cell. Cells commonly are both microcytic and hypochromic, as seen with iron deficiency anemia. MCH alone cannot distinguish between microcytosis and hypochromia. The most common cause of an elevated MCH is macrocytosis (e.g., folate deficiency). A falsely elevated MCH is seen in patients with hyperlipidemia.

MEAN CORPUSCULAR HEMOGLOBIN CONCENTRATION (HGB/HCT)

Mean corpuscular hemoglobin concentration (MCHC) is the weight of hemoglobin per volume of cells. MCHC is independent of cell size and, therefore, is more useful than the MCH in distinguishing between microcytosis and hypochromia. A low MCHC always indicates hypochromia; a microcyte with a normal hemoglobin concentration will have a low MCH but a normal MCHC. A falsely elevated MCHC is seen in patients with hyperlipidemia. It is routinely low in iron deficiency anemia, but it can also be decreased in other hemoglobin-synthesis disorders.

TOTAL RETICULOCYTE COUNT

The total reticulocyte count is an indirect assessment of the new RBC production. In a normal situation, 1% of RBCs are replaced daily; this would represent a reticulocyte count of 1%. The reticulocyte count in normocytic anemia can be used to differentiate hypoproliferative marrow from a compensatory marrow response to an anemia. Occasionally, a patient's hematocrit decreases while the absolute number of reticulocytes remains the same, resulting in a falsely elevated reticulocyte percentage. For example, if a patient's hematocrit decreases by 50% (from 50% to 25%), the corresponding reticulocyte percentage doubles. This problem is corrected by expressing the reticulocyte count as an absolute number; to do this, the percentage of reticulocytes (expressed as a decimal) is multiplied by the total RBC count. A corrected percentage of reticulocytes can also be calculated by multiplying the reticulocyte percentage by the patient's hematocrit and then dividing the product by an average normal hematocrit (for men or women).

RED BLOOD CELL DISTRIBUTION WIDTH

The red blood cell distribution width (RDW) measures variation in RBC volume; the higher the RDW, the more variable the size of the RBCs. The RDW increases in early iron deficiency anemia (often prior to changes in other parameters); however, this is not specific for this disease state. The RDW is also helpful in the diagnosis of a mixed anemia. A patient could have a normal MCV yet have a wide RDW. This would indicate presence of microcytes and macrocytes, which would yield a "normal" average RBC size.

SERUM IRON

Serum iron is the concentration of iron bound to transferrin. Normally transferrin is about one-third bound (saturated) to iron. Unfortunately, the serum iron level of many patients with IDA remains within the lower limits of normal, giving a false-negative test. There is also a 20% to 30% diurnal variation in serum iron levels (it is best to draw blood levels in the morning) and a 20% to 25% day-to-day variation among individuals.[6] Consequently, as a diagnostic tool, serum iron levels are best interpreted in conjunction with the total iron-binding capacity (TIBC). Serum iron is decreased with IDA and ACD and is increased with hemolytic anemias and iron overload.

TOTAL IRON-BINDING CAPACITY

Total iron-binding capacity is an indirect measurement of the iron-binding capacity of serum transferrin, performed by adding an excess of iron to plasma to saturate all transferrin with iron. The excess (unbound) iron is then removed and the serum iron concentration is determined. Unlike the serum iron level, the TIBC is remarkably constant. The finding of a low serum iron and a high TIBC indicates IDA. In patients with infection, malignancy, and uremia, a decreased TIBC and a decreased serum iron level may be observed; this is consistent with ACD.

PERCENTAGE TRANSFERRIN SATURATION

Transferrin saturation is the ratio of the serum iron to the TIBC expressed as a percentage, that is, transferrin saturation = (serum iron/TIBC) $\times$ 100. In IDA, the serum iron decreases and the TIBC increases, making the percent saturation of the iron-binding capacity less than 13% to 15%. This is a common measure of IDA.

SERUM FERRITIN

The concentration of ferritin (storage iron) in the serum is proportional to total iron stores and, consequently, is a reliable indicator of body iron stores. Low serum ferritin levels are virtually diagnostic of IDA as they are decreased only in IDA. In contrast, serum iron may be decreased in IDA and in ACD.

FOLIC ACID LEVEL

Folic acid values may vary depending on assay method used. Decreased levels indicate a folate deficiency megaloblastic anemia that may coexist with a vitamin B_{12} deficiency anemia. An erythrocyte folic acid level is less volatile; it is slow to decrease in an acute process such as drug-induced folic acid deficiency and slow to increase in patients receiving oral folic acid replacement. However, the clinical utility of the erythrocyte folic acid level is questionable; it should be reserved for cases in which folic acid depletion is suspected in which the serum folic acid may be falsely elevated or depleted as described above.

VITAMIN B_{12} LEVEL

Vitamin B_{12} (cyanocobolamine) levels may vary depending on assay method used. Low levels indicate vitamin B_{12} deficiency anemia.

SCHILLING TEST

This test is used to diagnose vitamin B_{12} deficiency anemia caused by a B_{12} absorption defect resulting from lack of intrinsic factor (pernicious anemia). An oral dose of cobalt-labeled vitamin B_{12} is administered. If sufficient gastrointestinal (GI) intrinsic factor is being produced gastrointestinally, the B_{12} will be absorbed. Concomitantly, a large intramuscular dose of nonlabeled vitamin B_{12} is given to saturate tissue-binding sites and flush the radiolabeled B_{12} into the urine. Normally, approximately 33% of the absorbed radiolabeled B_{12} appears in the urine over 24 hours. Patients with pernicious anemia excrete less than 8% of the original oral radiolabeled dose. If impaired oral absorption is demonstrated, this test is repeated, except that the oral radiolabeled B_{12} is administered along with a sufficient amount of intrinsic factor. Results within the normal range indicate that the defect is in intrinsic factor production as opposed to other causes of vitamin B_{12} deficiency such as dietary deficiency or small bowel pathology.

COOMBS TEST

Antiglobulin tests are used to indicate hemolytic anemia caused by an immune response. A direct antiglobulin test detects antibodies bound to erythrocytes, whereas an indirect antiglobulin test measures antibodies present in the serum. A positive direct antiglobulin test is usually indicative of immune hemolysis.

ERYTHROPOIETIN

In healthy individuals, 10 to 30 mU/mL (IU/L) of EPO are required to maintain normal hemoglobin and hematocrit concentrations. Endogenous EPO levels can increase up to 100- to 1000-fold during hypoxia or anemia. This marked increase is not seen in patients with end-stage renal disease, patients receiving chemotherapy, and AIDS patients, especially those taking azidothymidine (AZT). These patients will have an erythropoietin response that is insufficient to correct their anemia.

Figure 91–3 provides a broad, general algorithm for the diagnosis of anemias based on laboratory data. Keep in mind that many exceptions and additions exist with respect to this algorithm, many of which are addressed in the text. It is meant to be a guide to the typical presentation of the most common types and causes of anemia.

PATHOPHYSIOLOGY AND TREATMENT

ANEMIAS CAUSED BY ABNORMAL HEMOGLOBIN SYNTHESIS

A defect in hemoglobin synthesis as well as acquired defects in EPO precursor cell metabolism may cause changes in iron incorporation, producing a cell with an excess of nonheme iron within the cytoplasm. These cells, called sideroblasts, cause sideroblastic anemia, which is usually microcytic. Sideroblastic anemia can be congenital (hereditary-sex linked in males) or acquired. The acquired forms can be either primary or secondary to drugs, toxins (lead, alcohol), or other disease states. Hypocupremia has long been associated with sideroblastosis. Excess zinc intake will also cause sideroblastic anemia by binding preferentially to copper, causing impaired copper absorption and hypocupremia.[7] Primary acquired sideroblastic anemia is usually classified as a myelodysplastic syndrome and may eventually transform into acute myeloblastic leukemia in some patients.

Other hereditary defects in heme synthesis can lead to an overproduction of heme precursors, resulting in porphyria. The most common form, acute intermittent porphyria (AIP), results from a hereditary (autosomal dominant) partial deficiency in the enzyme uroporphyrinogen I synthetase, responsible for converting porphobilinogen to uroporphyrinogen. This causes an inhibition of the normal feedback mechanism of porphyrin synthesis, leading to an excess production of heme intermediate pigments uroporphyrin I and coproporphyrin I. These products can be detected in abnormal amounts in urine and feces to confirm the diagnosis of AIP.

AIP is characterized by neuropsychiatric, neuromuscular, and autonomic dysfunction and intense abdominal pain. In the liver, this enzyme deficiency results in increased inducibility of abnormal heme intermediates by certain drugs. Drugs and agents known to induce hepatic cytochrome P450 or to increase hepatic heme turnover are theoretically capable of precipitating porphyria. Barbiturates,[8] estrogens,[9] alcohol,[10] and heavy metals such as lead have been documented to induce porphyria in genetically susceptible people.

Genetic expression of an abnormal amino acid substitution in either the α- or β-globin chains can lead to a vari-

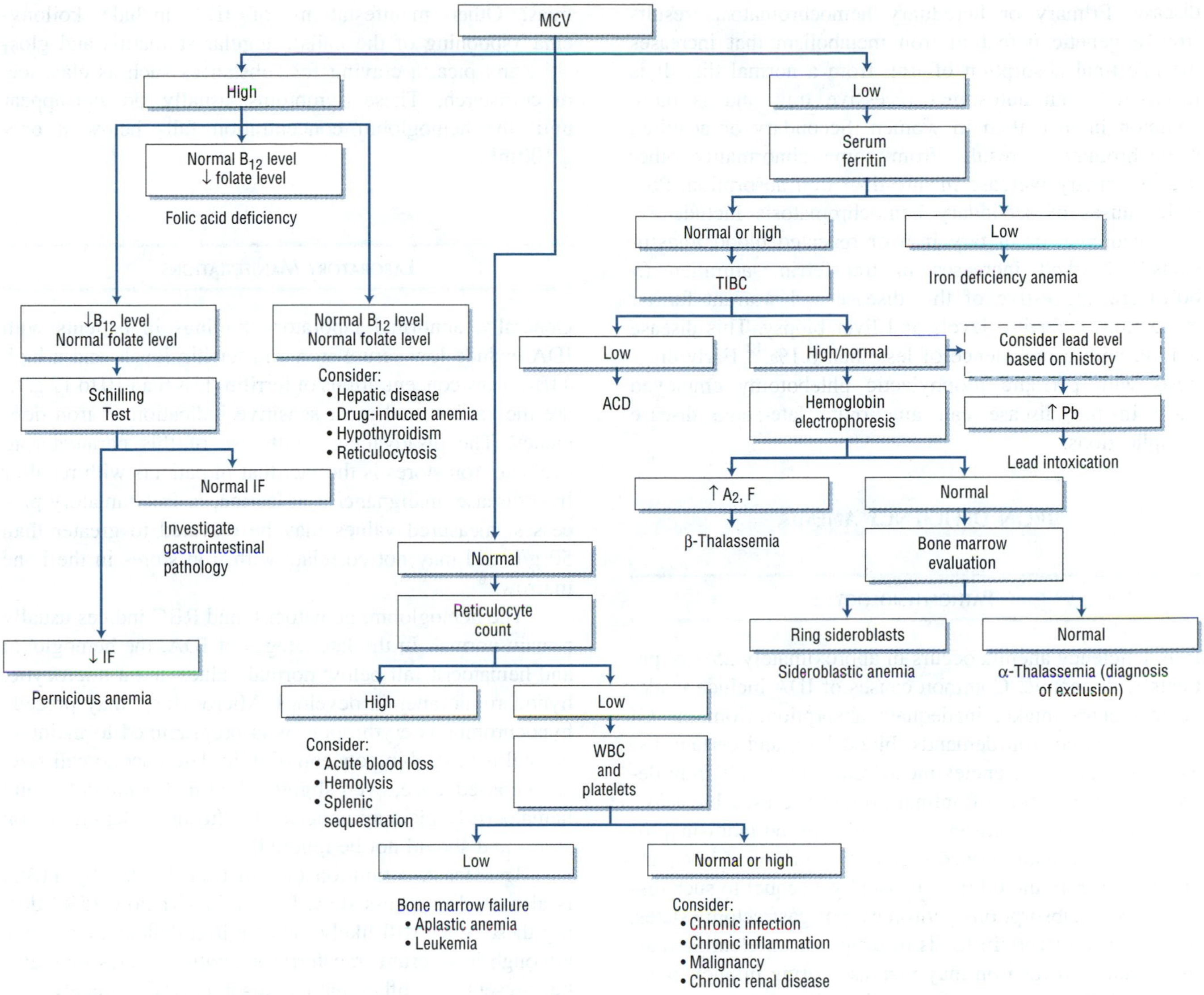

FIGURE 91–3. General algorithm for the diagnosis of anemias. ↑ = increased; ↓ = decreased; MCV = mean corpuscular volume; IF = intrinsic factor; TIBC = total iron-binding capacity; ACD = anemia of chronic disease; Pb = lead; A_2 = hemoglobin A_2; F = hemoglobin F.

ety of hemoglobinopathies causing hemolytic diseases such as sickle cell anemia and thalassemia (see Chap. 93, Sickle Cell Anemia). Four genes control α-chain production and two genes regulate β-chain production. Thalassemias result when these genes are defective. If three or four α-genes or both β-genes are not functioning properly, a major thalassemia, which is often incompatible with life, develops. Fortunately, thalassemia minor (trait) is more common. This results from deficiencies in one or two α-genes or one β-gene. For example, if α-genes are affected, normal β-chains would accumulate in the cell and result in membrane damage. This cell would then be prematurely cleared from the circulation, exacerbating the anemia. Surviving cells have inadequate hemoglobin and are microcytic and hypochromic. Thalassemia is most commonly seen in patients of Asian, Mediterranean, or African descent and are frequently asymptomatic, requiring no treatment. It is important to distinguish thalassemia from IDA to avoid inappropriate iron therapy. Although both are microcytic, the MCV tends to be much lower with thalassemia than with IDA. Also, target cells may be seen on the peripheral smear in patients with thalassemia. Finally, in contrast to IDA, ferritin levels are normal or increased in patients with thalassemia. Hundreds of these abnormal hemoglobin diseases exist and are best diagnosed by hemoglobin electrophoresis.

HEMOCHROMATOSIS (IRON OVERLOAD)

A hereditary GI disease, hemochromatosis, results from a loss of regulation of iron absorption. As a result, iron deposition in various tissues causes multiple organ system failure including cirrhosis and various forms of heart disease. Primary or hereditary hemochromatosis results from a genetic defect in iron metabolism that increases the intestinal absorption of iron from a normal diet. It is inherited as an autosomal recessive trait and is more common in men than in women. Secondary or acquired hemochromatosis results from some abnormality other than a primary increase in intestinal iron absorption. Possible causes of secondary hemochromatosis include excess medicinal or dietary iron or repeated blood transfusions.[11] Marked increases in transferrin saturation (> 60%) are suggestive of this disease and warrant further evaluation of ferritin levels and liver biopsy. This disease is rare, with a prevalence of less than 0.1%.[12] Early diagnosis with periodic prophylactic phlebotomy employed early in the disease can ameliorate late-stage disease complications.

IRON DEFICIENCY ANEMIA

PATHOPHYSIOLOGY

Iron deficiency anemia occurs in approximately 25% of patients with anemia. Common causes of IDA include inadequate dietary intake, inadequate absorption from the GI tract, increased iron demands, blood loss, and certain diseases. Dietary deficiencies most frequently result from decreased consumption of animal protein and ascorbic acid[13] as a consequence of chronic alcoholism, food faddism, prolonged illness with anorexia, or poor nutrition. Inadequate absorption from the GI tract is usually a sequel to such disorders as malabsorption syndromes, postgastrectomy states, the presence of certain foods or drugs, or unrelenting diarrhea. Demands for iron may increase during infancy, pregnancy, adolescence, or old age. Blood loss may occur as a result of many disorders, including trauma, angiodysplasia, hemorrhoids, peptic ulcers, gastritis, GI malignancies, diverticular disease, copious menstrual flow, nose bleeds, or postpartum bleeding.[14] Occult blood loss from a single GI lesion has been shown to be a frequent cause of "idiopathic" IDA.[15]

Diseases contributing to the development of IDA include rheumatoid arthritis (with chronic aspirin ingestion), various malignancies, and renal disease. With IDA, the possibility of multifactorial etiology must always be considered. Other causes of hypochromic, microcytic anemia that must be considered include thalassemia (especially thalassemia minor) and heavy metal (mostly lead) poisoning (see Fig. 91–3).

SIGNS AND SYMPTOMS

Patients with IDA may be asymptomatic or have vague, general signs and symptoms associated with most anemias. Other manifestations of IDA include koilonychia (spooning of the nails), angular stomatitis and glossitis, and pica, a craving for substances such as clay, ice, or cornstarch. These symptoms usually do not appear until the hemoglobin concentration falls below 8 or 9 g/100 mL.

LABORATORY MANIFESTATIONS

Generally, abnormal laboratory findings in patients with IDA include low serum iron and ferritin levels and a high TIBC. Low concentrations of ferritin (less than 10 to 12 g/L) are the earliest and most sensitive indication of iron deficiency. The disadvantage with use of this parameter to evaluate iron stores is the fact that in patients with renal or liver disease, malignancies, infection, or inflammatory processes, measured values may be elevated to greater than 50 g/L and may not correlate with iron stores in the bone marrow.[16]

The hemoglobin, hematocrit, and RBC indices usually remain normal. In the later stages of IDA, the hemoglobin and hematocrit fall below normal values and a microcytic, hypochromic anemia develops. Microcytosis may precede hypochromia as erythropoiesis is programmed to maintain normal hemoglobin concentration in deference to cell size. As a consequence, even slightly abnormal hemoglobin and hematocrit levels may indicate significant depletion of iron stores and should not be ignored.

Transferrin saturation (serum iron divided by TIBC) is also used to assess IDA. Low values (below 15%) during these times will likely indicate iron deficiency anemia, although low serum transferrin saturation values may also be present in inflammatory disorders. Fortunately, the TIBC usually helps to differentiate the diagnosis in these patients; a TIBC greater than 400 g% suggests IDA, whereas values below 200 g% usually represent inflammatory disease.

Free erythrocyte protoporphyrin can also be used in the diagnosis of IDA. Iron normally binds with protoporphyrin to form heme. When iron levels are low, the serum concentration of protoporphyrin not bound to iron is elevated. This test is very helpful in distinguishing between iron deficiency and thalassemia minor, because values are normal in patients with thalassemia and elevated in patients with IDA. Unfortunately, free erythrocyte protoporphyrin is also elevated in inflammatory disorders and lead poisoning and, thus, is less effective in distinguishing IDA in patients in whom these other two conditions may be present.

Finally, in rare cases, a bone marrow examination can be performed to assess bone marrow iron stores. Documentation of decreased hemosiderin will confirm the diagnosis of IDA.

▶ TREATMENT: Iron Deficiency Anemia

DIETARY SUPPLEMENTATION AND THERAPEUTIC IRON PREPARATIONS

Treatment of IDA usually consists of dietary supplementation and administration of therapeutic iron preparations. Iron absorption varies greatly with different foods. Iron is poorly absorbed from vegetables, grain products, dairy products, and eggs and is best absorbed from meat, fish, and poultry. Substitution of meat for eggs, milk, or cheese in a mixed meal has been shown to quadruple the absorption of iron from the entire meal.[17] Beverages have also been shown to affect iron absorption. For example, orange juice doubles the absorption of iron from an entire meal, whereas tea or milk will reduce absorption to less than one-half.[18,19] It is recommended that meat, orange juice, and other ascorbic acid–rich foods be included in meals and that if milk and tea are used, they be consumed in moderation between meals.

In most cases of IDA, oral iron therapy with soluble ferrous iron salts is appropriate therapy. Iron is best absorbed in the reduced ferrous form with maximal absorption occurring in the duodenum, primarily because the iron is maintained in a soluble form by the acid medium of the stomach and by mucopolysaccharide chelator substances that prevent the iron from precipitating. In the alkaline environment of the small intestines, iron tends to form insoluble complexes that are unavailable for absorption. Based on these considerations, the preferred iron preparation is nonenteric-coated ferrous salts. Slow-release or sustained-release iron preparations do not undergo sufficient dissolution until reaching the small intestines, and consequently, iron absorption is significantly reduced,[20,21] which can cause an attenuation in the hematinic effects. The dose of iron to be administered depends on the patient's ability to tolerate the administered iron. In patients with IDA, it is generally recommended that approximately 200 mg elemental iron be administered daily, usually in two or three divided doses to maximize tolerability.[22] Table 91–3 shows the percent elemental iron of commonly available iron salts. Note that ferrous sulfate is also available as an exsiccated form that contains approximately 30% elemental iron as opposed to the nonexsiccated form that is only 20% elemental iron. The percentage of iron absorbed progressively decreases as the dose increases, but the absolute amount absorbed increases. Since food interferes with the absorption of iron, it should preferably be administered one or more hours before meals. Many patients must take their iron with food because they experience nausea and diarrhea when iron is administered on an empty stomach. However, these effects may be offset by giving smaller amounts of iron with each administration. Although some forms of iron are combined with ascorbic acid or antacids, previous studies have shown that addition of ascorbic acid or other ingredients does not enhance absorption from oral iron preparations when given on an empty stomach.

TABLE 91–3. Iron Products

Salt	Elemental Iron (%)	Amount of Iron Provided
Ferrous sulfate	20	60–65 mg/300–325-mg tablet
Ferrous sulfate, exsiccated	30	65 mg/200-mg tablet
Ferrous gluconate	12	37–39 mg/300–325-mg tablet
Ferrous fumarate	33	33 mg/100-mg tablet
Ferric pyrophosphate	12	
Ferrous carbonate	48	

EVALUATION OF THERAPEUTIC OUTCOMES

Therapeutic doses of iron should increase hemoglobin values by 1 g% to 2 g% weekly. As the hemoglobin level approaches normal, the rate of increase slows progressively. A hemoglobin response of less than 2 g% over a 3-week period is unacceptable and should be further evaluated. Reticulocytosis occurs within 7 to 10 days after initiation of iron therapy. If the patient does not develop reticulocytosis, the diagnosis or therapy needs to be reevaluated.

Iron therapy should continue for a period sufficient for complete restoration of iron stores. The time interval required to accomplish this goal varies, although at least 3 to 6 months of therapy is usually necessary.[23] Patients with negative iron balances caused by bleeding may require iron replacement therapy for only a month after correction of the underlying lesion, whereas patients with recurrent negative balances may require long-term treatment. This latter group may require as little as 30 to 60 mg of elemental iron daily.

Adverse reactions to therapeutic doses of iron are primarily gastrointestinal in nature and consist of discoloration of feces (dark), constipation or diarrhea, nausea, and vomiting. Failure to develop at least some of these symptoms, even mildly, may indicate noncompliance. If these side effects become intolerable, the dose may be taken with meals or the total daily dose may be decreased to 110 to 120 mg elemental iron. Administration of iron with meals, however, reduces the amount of iron absorbed by more than one-half.

Failure to respond to appropriate treatment regimens necessitates reevaluation of the patient. Common causes of treatment failure include noncompliance with therapy, misdiagnosis, presence of a concomitant anemia-inducing disease state, malabsorption, and blood loss equal to the rate of production. Malabsorption can be ruled out by the iron test in which plasma iron levels are determined at half-hour intervals for 2 hours following the administration of 50 mg of elemental iron as liquid ferrous sulfate. If plasma iron levels increase by more than 50 ng% during this time, absorption is satisfactory.

PARENTERAL IRON THERAPY

Parenteral iron therapy may be necessary when there is evidence of iron malabsorption or intolerance of orally administered iron or when long-term noncompliance is a problem. Another condition that may warrant parenteral iron therapy includes patients with significant blood loss who refuse transfusions and in whom oral iron therapy is not possible. Parenteral iron is commonly given with EPO to patients receiving chronic hemodialysis and chronic ambulatory peritoneal dialysis.

Iron dextran, a complex of ferric hydroxide and dextran containing 50 mg of iron/mL, may be given IM or intravenously (IV). Methods of IV administration include multiple slow injections of undiluted iron dextran solution or an infusion of a diluted preparation. This latter method is often referred to as total dose infusion. IM iron dextran is given via Z-tract administration in order to minimize staining of the skin. Because each IM dose is limited to 2 mL (100 mg of iron), multiple injections are often required.

TABLE 91–4. Equations for Calculating Doses of Iron Dextran

In patients with iron deficiency anemia:

mg of iron = $W \times (100 - \%Hgb) \times 0.3$

where *W* is the patient's weight in pounds and %Hgb is the patient's observed hemoglobin expressed as a percentage of the normal hemoglobin concentration (assuming 14.8 g of hemoglobin per 100 mL is equivalent to 100% concentration).

If the patient weighs 13.6 kg (30 lb) or less, the dose is 80% of the calculated amount.

In patients with anemia secondary to blood loss (hemorrhagic diathesis or long-term dialysis):

mg of iron = blood loss × hematocrit

where blood loss is in milliliters and hematocrit is expressed as a decimal fraction.

Problems with IM administration include patient discomfort, sterile abscesses, tissue necrosis, or atrophy. In addition, up to 30% of an administered dose remains physiologically unavailable. For these reasons, the IV route is the preferred route of administration.

Equations for calculating the dose in patients with IDA and patients with anemia secondary to blood loss can be found in Table 91–4. When given by IV administration, the dose should not exceed 50 mg iron per minute (1 mL/min). The manufacturer suggests no more than 100 mg of iron dextran be administered daily. However, numerous reports have been made in which the total dose of iron dextran needed was administered as a single dose by IV infusion.[24,25] Although not FDA approved, this method is efficacious and convenient. If the total dose required to correct the anemia is given in a single dose, there is an increased possibility of adverse reactions such as arthralgias, myalgias, flushing, malaise, and fever. Other adverse reactions include staining of the skin, pain at the injection site, allergic reactions, and rarely anaphylaxis. Patients most likely to experience adverse effects with iron dextran include individuals with a history of allergies, asthma, or an inflammatory disease. Patients with preexisting immune-mediated diseases such as active rheumatoid arthritis or systemic lupus erythematosus are considered high risk because of their hyperreactive immune response capabilities. It is suggested that all patients receiving an iron dextran injection receive a test dose of 25 mg IM or IV, or a 5- to 10-minute infusion of the diluted solution. Patients should then be observed for more than 1 hour for untoward reactions. Patients receiving total dose infusions can have the remaining solution infused during the next 2 to 6 hours if no adverse effects are noted.

EVALUATION OF THERAPEUTIC OUTCOMES

Iron dextran must be processed by macrophages for the iron to be biologically available. The absorption and metabolism characteristics vary with the route and amount of drug given. Absorption of an IM dose of iron dextran occurs in two phases. During the first 72 hours, iron dextran is absorbed primarily through the lymphatics into the left superior vena cava. A smaller amount is absorbed directly through the intramuscular capillary network into the blood.[23] A second, slower phase involves uptake of the iron dextran complex by macrophages, with subsequent transport through the lymphatics into the blood. About 60% of an IM dose of iron dextran is absorbed after 3 days and up to 90% is absorbed within 3 weeks.[26] The remainder is absorbed slowly over several months or longer.

IV doses of iron dextran are taken up immediately by the reticuloendothelial system.[27] Small to intermediate IV doses (50 to 500 mg of elemental iron) can be cleared from the plasma within 3 days of administration. In contrast, larger IV doses of iron dextran (> 500 mg of elemental iron) are processed by the reticuloendothelial system at a constant rate of 10 to 20 mg/h.[28] Doses this large are associated with increased plasma concentrations of iron dextran for as long as 3 weeks.

Once iron is absorbed into the blood, cells of the reticuloendothelial system (such as macrophages) phagocytize the iron dextran complex and cleave the dextran moiety, making free iron available to the body as circulating iron, transferrin-bound iron, or storage iron (ferritin and hemosiderin). Iron dextran can remain within these cells for many months.

When large amounts of parenteral iron are administered, either by total dose infusion or by multiple IM or IV doses, iron status should be closely monitored. Hemoglobin and hematocrit should be measured weekly and serum iron and ferritin levels should be measured at least every month.

TRANSFUSIONS

Another form of treatment of IDA is blood transfusions. However, this form of therapy should be used with extreme caution when cardiovascular compromise exists. Once the hematocrit value falls below 30, oxygen-carrying capacity in older patients drops precipitously, predisposing them to ischemia. Tachycardia, angina, ischemic patterns on ECG, cerebrovascular insufficiency, postural hypotension, and prerenal azotemia are strong indications for transfusions to maintain the hematocrit above 30. An exception to this treatment option is the patient who has developed low hematocrit values over extended time periods. These patients often demonstrate cardiac compromise after transfusion despite hematocrits in the 20s. Therapy in these patients should consist of iron therapy, followed by transfusion only if necessary.

MEGALOBLASTIC ANEMIAS

Megaloblastosis results from interference in folic acid– and vitamin B_{12}–interdependent nucleic acid synthesis in the immature erythrocyte. Because DNA and RNA synthesis is slowed, one or more mitotic cell divisions are skipped, resulting in an abnormally large cell. Synthesis of the RNA and DNA necessary for cell division depends on a series of reactions catalyzed by vitamin B_{12} and folic acid (Fig. 91–4). As shown in the figure, in this process, dietary folates are absorbed and converted (A) to 5-methyl tetrahydrofolate (5-MTHF), which is then converted via a B_{12}-dependent (B) reaction to tetrahydrofolate (THF) (C). After gaining a carbon, THF is converted to a folate cofactor (D), 5,10-methylene tetrahydrofolate (5,10-METHF), used by thymidylate synthetase enzyme (E) in the biosynthesis of nucleic acids. The 5,10-METHF cofactor is converted to dihydrofolate (DHF) (F) during biosynthesis. Normally, dihydrofolate reductase enzyme reduces DHF back to tetrahydrofolate (C), which can again pick up a carbon and be recycled to produce more 5,10-METHF (D).

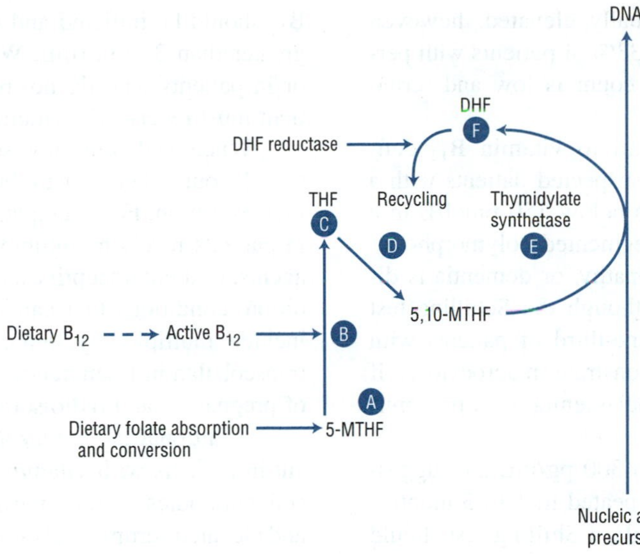

FIGURE 91–4. Drug-induced megaloblastosis. DHF = dihydrofolate; THF = tetrahydrofolate; 5-MTHF = 5 methyl THF; 5,10-METHF = 5,10-methylene THF.

VITAMIN B_{12} DEFICIENCY ANEMIA

Etiology and Pathophysiology

Adult-onset pernicious anemia has an estimated annual incidence of 100 per one million population, and it is slightly more common in women. There is a sharp increase in incidence with increasing age, suggesting that it is a consequence of gastric epithelial aging.

The three major causes of vitamin B_{12} deficiency are inadequate intake, decreased absorption, and inadequate utilization. Vitamin B_{12} is a water-soluble vitamin obtained by ingestion of primarily meat and dairy products. Body stores of vitamin B_{12} range from 2 to 5 mg, with daily requirements being approximately 1 to 5 μg. The average daily diet contains more than 20 μg of B_{12}; it would take 1360 days (3 to 4 years) to become B_{12} deficient in a person deprived of vitamin B_{12}. Vitamin B_{12} is necessary for DNA synthesis, is important in metabolic reactions involving folic acid, and is essential in maintaining the integrity of the neurologic system.

Inadequate dietary consumption of vitamin B_{12} is rare. It is usually only seen in patients who are strict vegetarians, because body stores are large and meats and vegetables are readily available sources of this nutrient.

Decreased absorption of vitamin B_{12} occurs in patients with a deficiency of intrinsic factor and can be diagnosed with the Schilling test. A decrease in the production of intrinsic factor results in acquired pernicious anemia, while dysfunction of the intrinsic factor causes congenital pernicious anemia. Vitamin B_{12} deficiency may also result from overgrowth of bacteria in the bowel that utilize B_{12} or from injury or removal of ileal receptor sites where vitamin B_{12} and the intrinsic factor complex are absorbed. Blind-loop syndrome, fish tapeworm infestations, intestinal resections, tropical sprue, regional enteritis, and Crohn's disease may all contribute to development of vitamin B_{12} deficiency.[29]

In portal blood, vitamin B_{12} is bound to the transport protein, transcobolamin II, which rapidly delivers the vitamin to sites of utilization and storage. In persons with a transcobolamin II deficiency, B_{12} cannot be transported from the blood to utilization and storage sites. Consequently, the patient has a normal B_{12} level but clinical evidence of frank B_{12} deficiency.

Signs and Symptoms

As in most forms of anemia, symptoms result when the body can no longer tolerate the increased cardiac output stimulated by the anemia. Clinically, vitamin B_{12} deficiency can present with gastric mucosal atrophy, followed by neuropsychiatric abnormalities as a result of combined degeneration of the spinal cord and brain. The most frequently reported neurologic symptoms are paresthesias and ataxia. Other reported symptoms include glossitis, diminished vibratory sensation in the lower extremities, muscle weakness, dysphagia, anorexia, irritability, dementia, and psychosis.[30]

Laboratory Findings

In macrocytic anemias, MCV is usually elevated above 100 fL. Mild leukopenia and thrombocytopenia may be present. A peripheral blood smear demonstrates macrocytosis accompanied by hypersegmented polymorphonuclear leukocytes (one of the earliest and most specific indications of this disease) and oval macrocytes. Serum lactate dehydrogenase (LDH) and bilirubin levels may be elevated as a result of hemolysis or ineffective erythropoiesis. Serum iron and transferrin saturation are usually elevated; however, iron levels may be low in 21% to 33% of patients with pernicious anemia. The reticulocyte count is low and serum B_{12} levels are usually low.[31]

Recommendations with regard to vitamin B_{12} deficiency include a screening of all suspected patients with a low B_{12} level. Vitamin B_{12} values below 150 pmol/L in a patient with macrocytosis, hypersegmented polymorphonuclear leukocytes, peripheral neuropathy, or dementia is diagnostic of B_{12} deficiency, even though the Schilling test may be normal. Approximately one-third of patients with pernicious anemia will not demonstrate macrocytosis if complicated by iron deficiency, thalassemia, or a predominant neurologic involvement.

Vitamin B_{12} values of 200 to 300 pg/mL are suggestive of depletion and should be repeated in 1 to 3 months. If this value is less than 200 pg/mL, a Shilling test should be performed. In patients with a normal Schilling test, oral B_{12} should be initiated and continued until the B_{12} level is greater than 300 pg/mL. With an abnormal Schilling test, or in patients who do not respond to oral therapy, the patient must receive IM vitamin B_{12}.[32]

When evaluating low serum B_{12} levels, it is important to rule out other causes besides dietary deprivation and malabsorption. For example, falsely low levels may be seen in patients receiving antibiotics, anticonvulsants, cytotoxic agents, oral contraceptives, and high-dose vitamin C. In addition, conditions that can result in falsely low B_{12} levels include multiple myeloma, malignancy, aplastic anemia, transcobalamin I deficiency, gastrectomy, the third trimester of pregnancy, and radioisotope diagnostic studies.

Additional laboratory abnormalities that may be present in patients with vitamin B_{12} deficiency include parietal cell antibodies, serum intrinsic factor–blocking antibody, and elevated serum levels of both homocysteine and methylmalonic acid.

▶ TREATMENT: Vitamin B_{12} Deficiency Anemia

ORAL VITAMIN B_{12} THERAPY

In the rare cases of nutritional deficiency, oral administration of vitamin B_{12} may be given. Oral vitamin B_{12} (cobalamin) can also be used effectively to treat pernicious anemia but in much larger doses than those used to treat B_{12} deficiency. Cobalamin can be absorbed by both an intrinsic factor–dependent and –independent route. The independent route is less effective and requires large B_{12} doses to provide adequate absorption.[33] Observed clinical response to oral doses of 1000 mg/d has been confirmed by cyanocobalamin absorption rate studies. The mean absorption rate in patients with pernicious anemia is 1.2% across a wide range of doses.[34]

PARENTERAL VITAMIN B_{12} THERAPY

A commonly used parenteral vitamin B_{12} regimen consists of initiation with daily injections of 800 to 1000 μg of cyanocobalamin or hydroxycobalamin for 1 to 2 weeks. This initial 2-week therapy should saturate B_{12} stores in the body and resolve clinical manifestations of the deficiency. At that time, the dose can be decreased to 100 to 1000 μg once weekly until normalization of the hemoglobin and hematocrit occurs. Thereafter, monthly injections of 100 to 1000 μg for life should be administered.[29]

EVALUATION OF THERAPEUTIC OUTCOMES

A rapid response to vitamin B_{12} therapy is observed in most patients. Bone marrow becomes normoblastic after 24 hours, reticulocytosis is noted within 2 to 3 days, the hemoglobin begins to rise after the first week, and the leukocyte and platelet counts normalize after about 7 days. Failure to observe these findings usually indicates an incorrect diagnosis or other factors contributing to the anemia, such as iron deficiency or thalassemia trait. Demands for iron may be greater during initiation of therapy as a result of increased erythropoiesis.[35]

Potential adverse effects that may be associated with B_{12}-induced reticulocytosis include hyperuricemia and hypokalemia. Rebound thrombocytosis may precipitate thrombotic events. Another side effect of vitamin B_{12} therapy is sodium retention. This effect is more likely to occur in the patient with compromised cardiovascular status because of an expansion of the intravascular volume secondary to the sudden increase in production of RBCs.

FOLIC ACID DEFICIENCY ANEMIA

ETIOLOGY AND PATHOPHYSIOLOGY

Folic acid is a heat-labile vitamin necessary for production of nucleic acids, proteins, amino acids, purines, and thymine and hence DNA and RNA. Because humans are unable to synthesize total daily folate requirements, they depend on a dietary source of this vitamin. Major dietary sources of folate include fresh vegetables and fruits, yeast, mushrooms, and such animal organs as liver and kidney. Even though body demands for folate are high owing to high RBC synthesis and turnover, the minimum daily requirement is 50 to 100 μg. The body stores approximately 10 to 20 mg folate; therefore, cessation of dietary folate intake would result in depletion of all body stores within a few months. Folic acid deficiency results in the development of large functionally immature erythrocytes termed megaloblasts.

Major causes of folic acid deficiency include inadequate intake, decreased absorption, hyperutilization, and inadequate utilization. Folic acid deficiency is associated with poor eating habits seen in elderly patients, alcoholics, food faddists, the poverty stricken, and those who are chronically ill or in demented states. Decreased absorption of folic acid may occur in patients with malabsorption syndromes such as nontropical and tropical sprue, or after administration of certain drugs. Celiac disease is a common cause of malabsorption of folate, but other conditions such as Crohn's disease and extensive small bowel resection can also reduce absorption.[36] Alcoholism often results in a diet deficient in folic acid; alcohol also interferes with folic acid absoprtion, interferes with folic acid utilization at the cellular level, and decreases hepatic stores of folic acid.

Hyperutilization of folic acid may occur in states in which the rate of cellular division is increased. Examples include pregnancy, hemolytic anemia, myelofibrosis, malignancy, chronic inflammatory disorders such as Crohn's disease, rheumatoid arthritis or psoriasis, long-term dialysis, and growth spurts seen in adolescence and infancy. This is primarily of importance when the daily intake of folate is borderline, resulting in inadequate replacement of folate stores.

Several drugs have been reported to cause a folic acid deficiency megaloblastic anemia by either interfering with folate absorption or inhibiting the dihydrofolate reductase enzyme necessary for conversion of DHF to its active tetrahydrofolate form (see Chap. 94).

Although phenytoin may induce a megaloblastic anemia, folic acid supplementation in these patients may decrease phenytoin's anticonvulsant activity by increasing the metabolism of phenytoin.[37] Although routine supplementation is therefore not recommended, close monitoring for this potential interaction is advised.

SIGNS AND SYMPTOMS

Symptoms associated with folate deficiency are similar to those seen in patients with B_{12} deficiency. The major difference between these two disease entities is the relative absence of neurologic manifestations in folate deficiency megaloblastic anemia. Symptoms have an insidious onset that often precludes early identification of the etiology.

LABORATORY FINDINGS

Laboratory changes associated with folate deficiency megaloblastic anemia are similar to those seen in vitamin B_{12} deficiency anemia. A decreased serum and RBC folate level are also seen. Because serum folate levels are quite sensitive to short-term changes in folate balance, the erythrocyte folate level is a better predictor of true tissue folate stores. Erythrocyte folate levels are established during erythrocyte formation and persist throughout the life span of the cell, making this test less sensitive to daily folate variations.

▶ TREATMENT: Folic Acid Deficiency Anemia

Folic acid deficiency is treated by administration of exogenous folic acid. For replenishment of folate stores, it is generally recommended that therapy be initiated orally with 1 to 5 mg daily, even in patients with documented absorption problems; 1 mg daily is usually sufficient in most patients. Therapy should be continued for approximately 4 months, which is a sufficient amount of time for all folate-deficient RBCs to be cleared from the circulation. Once the cause of the deficiency is corrected, therapy can usually be discontinued. Long-term folate administration may be necessary in chronic hemolytic states, refractory malabsorption, and myelofibrosis. It is also recommended that patients with a folic acid deficiency be placed on diets containing foods high in folates. For patients with cardiovascular problems, the approach is the same as that for B_{12} deficiency anemia. Low-dose folate therapy (500 μg daily) may be administered when anticonvulsant drugs produce a megaloblastic anemia. Such therapy may obviate the need to remove the anticonvulsant.

Although megaloblastic anemia during pregnancy is rare, the most common cause is folate deficiency. This usually manifests itself as underweight, premature infants and suboptimal health for the mother. Prophylactic folate therapy during pregnancy in women with poor diets, multiple pregnancies, and thalassemia minor may be a useful preventive measure. The recommended dose is 200 to 300 μg daily. Folic acid supplementation (800 to 1000 μg daily) prior to conception and during pregnancy reduces the incidence of neural tube defects in the general population.[38] Higher doses (4 mg daily) have been demonstrated to reduce the incidence of neural tube defects in the children of patients who have given birth to previous offspring with these disorders.[39] Finally, it has been suggested that supplementation with 10 mg of folic acid daily may reduce the incidence of cleft lip.[40] It is clearly essential that women in their childbearing years maintain adequate folic acid intake.

EVALUATION OF THERAPEUTIC OUTCOMES

Symptomatic improvement as evidenced by increased alertness, appetite, and cooperation are often noted early during a course of treatment. Reticulocytosis occurs within 2 to 3 days and peaks within 5 to 8 days after beginning therapy. Hematocrit begins to rise within 2 weeks of beginning therapy and should reach normal levels within 2 months. MCV will initially increase due to an increase in reticulocytes, but will then gradually decrease to normal.

ANEMIA OF CHRONIC DISEASE

Pathophysiology

Anemia of chronic disease is a hypoproliferative anemia that has traditionally been associated with infectious, inflammatory, or neoplastic diseases lasting more than 1 or 2 months.[41,42] Pathologically, the RBC life span is shortened and the bone marrow's capacity to respond to erythropoietin is inadequate to maintain normal hemoglobin concentration. The cause of this defect is still not certain but appears to involve a block in the release of iron from the reticuloendothelial cells of the marrow. It is thought that various cytokines released during these illnesses inhibit the production or action of erythropoietin or inhibit RBC production.[43]

Laboratory Findings

Examination of the bone marrow reveals an abundance of iron, so it appears that the release mechanism for this iron is the central defect. Serum iron is usually decreased, but, unlike IDA, serum ferritin is normal or increased and iron-binding capacity is decreased. ACD is usually normocytic; hematocrits as low as 25% have been reported in 20% of patients.[44] The diagnosis is usually one of exclusion, with particular emphasis on evaluation of possible IDA as the primary anemia or coexistent with ACD due to chronic disease-associated conditions such as GI blood loss from aspirin, other nonsteroidal anti-inflammatory agents, or steroids, or malignancy-associated bleeding. Although usually referred to as anemia of chronic disease, it can occur in conditions with fairly rapid onset of several weeks, such as a pneumonia. It can also often coexist with anemia of renal disease and IDA. Table 91–5 lists common diseases associated with ACD.

TABLE 91–5. Diseases Causing Anemia of Chronic Disease

Common Causes
Chronic infections
Tuberculosis
Other chronic lung infections
Subacute bacterial endocarditis
Osteomyelitis
Chronic urinary tract infections
Chronic inflammation
Rheumatoid arthritis
Systemic lupus erythematosus
Rheumatoid (collagen–vascular) diseases
Inflammatory osteoarthritis
Gout
Chronic inflammatory liver diseases
Malignancies
Carcinoma
Hodgkin's disease
Leukemia
Multiple myeloma
Less Common Causes
Alcoholic liver disease
Congestive heart failure
Thrombophlebitis
Chronic obstructive lung disease
Ischemic heart disease

► TREATMENT: Anemia of Chronic Disease

The treatment of ACD is somewhat less specific than treatment of other anemias. Usually, recovery from the anemia occurs with resolution of the underlying process. During inflammation, iron therapy is ineffective by either the oral or parenteral route. Red cell transfusions are effective but should be limited to situations where oxygen transport is inadequate due to concomitant medical problems.

Exogenous EPO has been used to stimulate erythropoiesis in patients with chronic diseases. These patients have a relative erythropoietin deficiency; EPO levels are not as elevated as they should be for the degree of anemia they have. They also have a relatively impaired response to erythropoietin. Treatment with human recombinant erythropoietin is controversial. ACD has been successfully treated with recombinant human erythropoietin in several studies using rheumatoid arthritis patients,[45] but other studies have found no role for erythropoietin in treatment of ACD.[46]

ANEMIA OF CHRONIC RENAL FAILURE

Pathophysiology

Patients with chronic renal failure (CRF) have several reasons to be anemic. Decreased EPO production by the kidneys is the primary mechanism of severe anemia associated with end-stage renal disease.[47] The uremic environment of CRF decreases RBC life span, requiring an increased demand for RBCs that often cannot be supplied with decreased serum erythropoietin levels.[48] An increased demand for folic acid for new RBC production coupled with the body's limited folic acid stores can cause a folic acid deficiency anemia. Finally, many CRF patients become iron deficient due to blood and iron loss from hemodialysis[49] (see Chapter 41, Acute Renal Failure).

▶ TREATMENT: Anemia of Chronic Renal Failure

Patients with CRF are unable to produce appropriate levels of EPO, and many of these patients are transfusion dependent. Due to inherent risks associated with repeated transfusions (febrile reactions, iron overload, hepatitis, AIDS, rejection of future transplants), recombinant human EPO, or epoetin alfa, is often used to reverse the anemia of CRF. Epoetin has become the mainstay in the management of anemia associated with renal failure.

The goal of epoetin therapy is to raise the hematocrit to a target range of up to 36%. Starting doses of epoetin are 50 to 100 U/kg, administered three times weekly. Doses should be reduced as the hematocrit approaches 36%. The dose of epoetin should then be individualized to maintain the hematocrit within 30% to 36%. It is important to remember that considerable interpatient half-life variations exist for this product and administration may require individual regimens for optimum therapeutic value.

Epoetin may be administered IV or subcutaneously (SC). The SC route provides more sustained epoetin concentrations, which are more advantageous than the peak and trough levels achieved with IV bolus administration. This suggests that the amount of time the levels remain above baseline EPO concentrations may be most important in determining hematopoietic response.[50]

The major side effect encountered with epoetin therapy is an elevation of diastolic blood pressure. Approximately 30% to 47% of patients receiving this product experience this effect, which is thought to occur as a consequence of an increase in peripheral vascular resistance. It is estimated that 25% of these patients will experience an increase of greater than 10 mm Hg, thus producing or aggravating existing hypertension, which often requires adjustments in blood pressure medications.[51] No evidence exists that this blood pressure change is related to a direct pressor effect of epoetin. It appears that the major risk factor for the development of hypertension is severe anemia and not the rate of rise of hematocrit with therapy.

One major reason for failure to respond with epoetin therapy is the development of iron depletion. Iron deficiency arises during epoetin therapy primarily because raising hematocrit levels requires a massive transfer of iron from storage areas to RBCs for manufacturing new hemoglobin. Other causes of iron deficiency include blood loss secondary to bleeding, retention of blood in dialyzer and tubing, or laboratory test phlebotomy. Chronic renal failure patients with transferrin saturations of at least 20% and serum ferritin levels below 100 ng/mL are probably candidates for concurrent iron therapy.[52] The agent of choice for prevention of iron storage deficiency is ferrous sulfate, 325 mg at bedtime. As with any IDA, if a patient does not respond to oral iron supplementation, parenteral iron therapy is indicated. Fortunately, most patients respond appropriately to oral iron.

ANEMIA IN THE ELDERLY AND PEDIATRIC POPULATIONS

One of the most common clinical problems observed in the elderly is anemia.[53] Although it is often assumed that anemia is an inevitable part of the aging process, studies in normal healthy elderly populations demonstrate that this is not necessarily true.[54] What is observed in these patients is a progressive decrease in bone marrow reserve with age and a decrease in hormonal response to hematologic stress.[51] Although hemoglobin levels usually remain normal, the diminished marrow reserve leaves the elderly patient more susceptible to other causes of anemia. Such causes may include the presence of multiple minor and often unrecognized diseases that negatively affect erythropoiesis.[55] One major factor often overlooked that may contribute to the presence of anemia in the older population is nutritional status. Anemia is rarely encountered in affluent and healthy elderly communities.[56] On the other hand, cross-sectional studies demonstrate a higher prevalence of anemia in low socioeconomic populations, which also have been shown to have a high prevalence of other nutritional deficiencies. Thus, nutritional deficiencies not usually severe enough to affect the hematopoietic system in the younger population may account for anemia in the aged.

Clinically, anemias in the pediatric population are more often due to a primary hematologic abnormality such as a hypoplastic or hemolytic anemia compared with adults, in which anemias tend to be manifestations of some broader underlying pathology.[57] The age of the child can yield some clues to the etiology of the anemia. In neonates, blood loss and hemolysis are common causes of anemia. Owing to the increased survival of premature infants, more children are born with decreased iron stores. Dietary deficiency of iron in the first 6 to 12 months of life is less common today, however, due to increased use of iron supplementation during breast feeding and use of iron-fortified formulas. Iron deficiency becomes more prominent when children change to regular diets. Adolescents are also prone to iron deficiency anemia, especially those who participate in faddish diets. Many more children are attending daycare centers at an earlier age. This is resulting in an increased incidence of anemia due to frequent infections and acute inflammation. Also, as more children in the United States are born to parents of Asian and African backgrounds, an increased incidence of hemoglobin-related disorders has been realized. A full assessment of pediatric anemias is beyond the scope of this chapter; this topic has been reviewed in detail elsewhere.[57,58]

HEMOLYTIC ANEMIA

PATHOPHYSIOLOGY

Hemolytic anemia results from decreased survival time of RBCs secondary to destruction in the spleen or circulation.

The severity of hemolytic anemia varies with the mechanism. Hemolysis may be mild, chronic, compensated, and lifelong or acute, severe, and life threatening.

The normal 120-day life span of an RBC comes from its inherent flexibility in passage through the microvasculature and spleen without disruption of the cell membrane or sequestration and phagocytosis by reticuloendothelial cells. Hemolysis, as defined by an RBC life span of less than 120 days, results from one of three primary defects: (1) membrane defects, (2) alterations in hemoglobin solubility or stability, and (3) changes in intracellular metabolic processes. These changes in membrane integrity, hemoglobin stability, and cell metabolism can be from intrinsic or extrinsic origin. Intrinsic defects are intracorpuscular changes and are often genetically determined; extrinsic defects, or extracorpuscular changes, are usually the cause of acquired hemolytic anemia. Acquired disorders result mainly from a direct effect on the membrane and less often from alterations in hemoglobin or metabolism. Table 91–6 lists examples of the different classes of hemolytic anemias.

Causes of hemolytic anemia differ in the younger patient compared to the elderly patient. Most younger patients exhibit congenital disease, whereas older patients most often experience autoimmune hemolytic anemia. A positive Coombs test is diagnostic in the latter group.

Hereditary spherocytosis is the most common inherited disorder of the RBC membrane. In this disorder, RBCs lose their flexible biconcave characteristics and become tight spheres. These altered cells can still deliver oxygen to body cells, but when these rigid cells enter the splenic microcirculation, they cannot pass through the pores lining the sinusoids of the spleen and consequently become trapped in the splenic pulp, where they are eventually destroyed by the reticuloendothelial cells. These patients are at risk of developing cholelithiasis or cholecystitis, pigment bile stones, mild jaundice, and splenomegaly. The treatment of choice for hereditary spherocytosis is splenectomy. Although the spherocytosis persists, the hemolysis is no longer a problem once the spleen has been removed.

Alterations in hemoglobin's solubility or stability, as seen with sickle cell anemia and the thalassemias, cause cell deformations leading to hemolysis (see Chap. 93).

Finally, alterations in cell metabolism (enzymopathies) lead to hemolytic disease by causing an alteration in cell dimensions and hemoglobin solubility. The two major metabolic pathways necessary for normal RBC metabolism are the hexose monophosphate shunt, with its associated enzyme systems, and the Embden–Myerhof pathway of anaerobic glycolysis. The former is responsible primarily for maintaining hemoglobin in the reduced state and thus preventing the formation of methemoglobin, while the latter metabolizes glucose to lactic acid, which leads to adenosine triphosphate formation.

The most common metabolic abnormality resulting in a hemolytic syndrome is glucose-6-phosphate dehydrogenase (G6PD) deficiency in the hexose monophosphate shunt pathway. Hemoglobin is oxidized to methemoglobin and then to sulfhemoglobin. Heinz bodies of denatured hemoglobin form, resulting in damage to the RBC membrane. Hemolysis results from the action of the spleen and reticuloendothelial system on these damaged cells. The disease more typically presents in whites of Mediterranean descent on exposure to oxidant drugs (sulfamethoxazole, dapsone) and chemicals or with infection.

TABLE 91–6. Common Classes of Hemolytic Anemias

Intrinsic (intracorpuscular; are usually genetically inherited)
Membrane defect
Spherocytosis and elliptocytosis
Hemoglobin defect
Sickle cell anemia
Thalassemia syndrome
Metabolic defect
Glucose-6-phosphate dehydrogenase (G6PD) deficiency
Many other enzyme deficiencies
Extrinsic
Membrane defect
Autoimmune hemolytic anemias
Oxidants, may cause unstable hemoglobin to clump

LABORATORY FINDINGS

Hemolytic anemias tend to be normocytic and normochromic (see Fig. 91–3). An increased reticulocyte count is seen in an attempt to maintain RBC mass. Peripheral smear may reveal sickle cells, target cells, spherocytes, elliptocytes, and fragmented RBCs. Decreased haptoglobin is seen, caused by increased hemoglobin–haptoglobin complex formation. LDH increases secondary to release from RBCs; however, this is a very nonspecific enzyme. Hemoglobinuria may result, and an increase in indirect bilirubin is often seen.

▶ TREATMENT: Hemolytic Anemia

Therapy of this condition consists of managing the underlying cause of the anemia. Clearly, avoidance of precipitating oxidant medications and chemicals in patients with G6PD deficiency is essential. Currently, there is no specific therapy that compensates for this enzyme deficiency. Steroids and other immunosuppressive agents have been used for management of autoimmune hemolytic anemias. In some instances, a splenectomy is indicated in an attempt to reduce RBC destruction.

▶ PRINCIPLES OF PHARMACOTHERAPY

- Anemias are a group of diseases characterized by a decrease in either hemoglobin or red blood cells, which results in decreased oxygen-carrying capacity of blood.
- Anemias are often a sign of underlying pathology; a rapid diagnosis of the etiology of the anemia is essential.
- Patients with acute-onset anemias are most likely to present with tachycardia, lightheadedness, and dyspnea; those with chronic anemia often present with weakness, fatigue, headache, vertigo, faintness, sensitivity to cold, pallor, and loss of skin tone.
- Defects in hemoglobin synthesis can result in a wide variety of disorders, including sideroblastic anemia (excessive nonheme iron in RBCs), acute intermittent porphyria (enzyme deficiency leading to neuromuscular symptoms), and thalassemia (dysfunction of genes controlling globulin-chain production).
- Iron deficiency anemia is characterized by decreased ferritin (most sensitive marker), serum iron, and transferritin saturation; the hemoglobin and hematocrit fall late in the disease. TIBC is increased. RBC morphology includes anisocytosis, hypochromia, and microcytosis. Most patients are adequately treated with oral ferrous sulfate, although parenteral iron is necessary in selected patient populations.
- Vitamin B_{12} deficiency can be due to inadequate intake, decreased absorption, and inadequate utilization. Anemia owing to lack of intrinsic factor resulting in decreased vitamin B_{12} absorption is called pernicious anemia. Vitamin B_{12} deficiency is manifested as a macrocytic anemia with hypersegmented polymorphonuclear leukocytes and oval macrocytes. Vitamin B_{12} levels and the reticulocyte count are usually low. Neurologic symptoms may also be present. Oral replacement is appropriate for dietary deficiency, but most patients with intrinsic factor deficiency or other absorption problems require parenteral replenishment.
- Folic acid deficiency is also manifested as a macrocytic anemia. It occurs due to inadequate intake, decreased absorption, hyperutilization, and inadequate utilization. Treatment consists of oral folic acid, even in patients with absorption problems. Adequate folic acid intake is essential in women of childbearing years to decrease the incidence of neural tube defects in their children.
- Anemia of chronic disease is a diagnosis of exclusion. This anemia results from chronic inflammation, infection, or malignancy; however, it can occur as soon as 1 to 2 months after the onset of these processes. Serum iron is usually decreased; however, in contrast to IDA, serum ferritin is normal or increased and TIBC is usually decreased. Treatment is aimed at correcting the underlying pathology.
- Patients with chronic renal failure have several reasons to be anemic. The primary mechanism is decreased EPO production. Epoietin alfa is now the standard of care for management of anemia associated with chronic renal failure. Iron supplementation may also be necessary in some patients.
- Hemolytic anemia results in decreased survival time of RBCs secondary to destruction in the spleen or in the circulation. There are many etiologies of hemolytic anemia. Hemolytic anemias are normocytic and normochromic. An increased reticulocyte count, LDH, and indirect bilirubin are seen. Peripheral smear may reveal sickle cells, target cells, spherocytes, elliptocytes, and fragmented RBCs. Haptoglobin is decreased. As with ACD, treatment is directed toward correcting or controlling the underlying pathology.

REFERENCES

1. Bergin JJ. Evaluation of anemia. Postgrad Med J 1985;77:253–269.
2. Charlton RW, Bothwell TH. Iron absorption. Ann Rev Med 1983; 34:55–68.
3. Committee on Iron Deficiency of the AMA Council on Foods and Nutrition. Iron deficiency in the United States. JAMA 1968;203:407.
4. Hallberg L, Rossander L, Skanberg A-B. Phytates and the inhibitory effort of bran on iron absorption in man. Am J Clin Nutr 1987;45:965–988.
5. Cook JD, Skikne BS, Baynes RD. Serum transferrin receptor. Ann Rev Med 1993;44:63–74.
6. Long R. Diurnal variation of serum iron in normal individuals. Clin Chem 1978;24:842–847.
7. Ramadurai J, Shapiro C, Kozloff M, Telfer M. Zinc abuse and sideroblastic anemia. Am J Hematol 1993;42:227–228.
8. Hryhorczuk DO, Hogan MM. Variegate porphyria and heavy metal poisoning from ingestion of moonshine. South Med J 1983;76: 1027–1031.
9. McKenzie AW, Acharya U. Oestrogen-induced familial porphyria. Br J Dermatol 1975;92:707–709.
10. Doss M, Baumann H, Sixel F. Alcohol in acute porphyria. Lancet 1982;1:1307. Letter.
11. Kirking MH. Treatment of chronic iron overload. Clin Pharm 1991;10:775–783.
12. Edwards CQ, Griffen LM, Goldgar D, et al. Prevalence of hemochromatosis among 11,065 presumably healthy blood donors. N Engl J Med 1988;318:1355–1362.
13. English EC, Finch CA. Iron deficiency: A systematic approach. Drug Therapy 1984(April);19–20, 25–27.
14. Stucky WJ. Common anemias: A practical guide to diagnosis and management. Geriatrics 1983;38:42–48.
15. Rockey DC, Cello JP. Evaluation of the gastrointestinal tract in patients with iron-deficiency anemia. N Engl J Med 1993;329: 1691–1695.
16. Beissner RS, Trowbridge AA. Clinical assessment of anemia. Postgrad Med 1986;80:83–95.
17. Cok JD. Food iron absorption in human subjects—III. Comparison of the effect of animal proteins on non-heme iron absorption. Am J Clin Nutr 1976;29:859–867.
18. Dallman PR, Siimes MA, Stekel A. Iron deficiency in infancy and childhood. Am J Clin Nutr 1980;6:86–118.
19. Monsen ER, Hallberg L, Layrisse M. Estimation of available dietary iron. Am J Clin Nutr 1978;31:134–141.

20. McGrath K. Treatment of anaemia caused by iron, vitamin B_{12} or folate deficiency. Med J Aust 1989;151:693–697.
21. Beutler E. The common anemias. JAMA 1988;259:2433–2437.
22. Dallman PR. Iron deficiency: Diagnosis and treatment. West J Med 1981;134:496–505.
23. Beresford CR, Goldberg L, Smith JP. Local effects and mechanism of absorption of iron preparations administered intramuscularly. Br J Pharmacol 1957;12:107–114.
24. Auerbach M, Witt D, Toler W, et al. Clinical use of the total dose intravenous infusion of iron dextran. J Lab Clin Med 1988;111: 566–570.
25. Halpin TC, Bertino JS, Rothstein FC. Iron-deficiency anemia in childhood inflammatory bowel disease: Treatment with intravenous iron-dextran. JPEN 1982;6:9–11.
26. Will G. The absorption, distribution and utilization of intramuscularly administered iron-dextran: A radioisotopy study. Br J Haematol 1968;14:395–406.
27. Grime AJ, Hutt MSR. Metabolism of ^{59}Fe-dextran complex in human subjects. Br J Med 1957;2:1074–1077.
28. Henderson PA, Hillman RS. Characteristics of iron dextran utilization in man. Blood 1969;34:357–375.
29. Clementz GL, Schade SG. The spectrum of vitamin B_{12} deficiency. Am Fam Physician 1990;41:150–162.
30. Healton EB, Savage DG, Brust JC. Neurologic aspects of cobalamin deficiency. Medicine 1991;70:229–245.
31. Christensen DJ. Diagnosis of anemia: Clues to greater precision. Postgrad Med J 1983;73:293–297, 300.
32. McRae TD, Freedman ML. Why vitamin B_{12} deficiency should be managed aggressively. Geriatrics 1989;44:70–79.
33. Doscherholmer A, Hager PS, Liu M. A dual mechanism of vitamin B_{12} plasma absorption. J Clin Invest 1957;36:1551–1557.
34. Berlin H, Berlin R, Brante G. Oral treatment of pernicious anemia with high doses of vitamin B_{12} without intrinsic factor. Acta Med Scand 1968;184:247–258.
35. Carmel R, Weiner JM, Johnson CS. Iron deficiency occurs frequently in patients with pernicious anemia. JAMA 1987;257:1081–1083.
36. McGrath K. Treatment of anaemia caused by iron, vitamin B_{12} or folate deficiency. Med J Aust 1989;151:693–697.
37. MacCosbe PE, Toomey K. Interaction of phenytoin and folic acid. Clin Pharm 1983;2:362–369.
38. Cziezel AE, Dudas I. Prevention of the first occurrence of neural tube defects by periconceptual vitamin supplementation. N Engl J Med 1992;327:1832.
39. MRC Vitamin Study Research Group. Prevention of neural tube defects. Results of the Medical Research Council Vitamin Study. Lancet 1991;338:131.
40. Tobarova M. Periconceptual supplementation with vitamins and folic acid to prevent recurrence of cleft lip. Lancet 1982;2:217.
41. Lee GR. The anemia of chronic disease. Semin Hematol 1983;20: 465–479.
42. Samson D. The anaemia of chronic disorders. Postgrad Med J 1983; 59:543–550.
43. Means RT, Krantz SB. Progress in understanding the pathogenesis of the anemia of chronic disease. Blood 1992;80;1639–1647.
44. Cash JM, Sears DA. The anemia of chronic disease: Spectrum of associated diseases in a series of unselected hospitalized patients. Am J Med 1989;87:638–644.
45. Pincus T, Olsen NJ, Russell IJ. Multicenter study of recombinant human erythropoietin in correction of anemia in rheumatoid arthritis. Am J Med 1990;89:161–166.
46. Nielsen OJ, Anderson LS, Ludwigsen E. Anaemia of rheumatoid arthritis: Erythropoietin concentrations and red cell distribution width in relation to iron status. Ann Rheum Dis 1990;49:349–353.
47. Paganini EP. Overview of anemia associated with chronic renal disease: Primary and secondary mechanisms. Semin Nephrol 1989;9:3–8.
48. Shaw AB. Haemolysis in chronic renal failure. Br Med J 1967;2: 213–216.
49. Van Wyck DB. Iron deficiency in patients with dialysis-associated anemia during erythropoietin replacement therapy: Strategies for assessment and management. Semin Nephrol 1989;9:21–24.
50. Eschbach JW, Adamson JW. Recombinant human erythropoietin: Implications for nephrology. Am J Kidney Dis 1988;11:203–209.
51. Lipschitz DA, Udupa KB, Milton KY, Thompson CO. Effect of age on hematopoiesis in man. Blood 1984;63:502–509.
52. Adamson JW, Eschback JW. Treatment of the anemia of chronic renal failure with recombinant human erythropoietin. Ann Rev Med 1990; 41:349–360.
53. Guyatt GH, Patterson C, Ali M. Diagnosis of iron deficiency anemia in the elderly. Am J Med 1990;88:205–209.
54. Baldwin JG, Lichtenstein LS. Longitudinal study of hemoglobin and hematocrit in the elderly. Blood 1986;68(5, suppl 1):52a.
55. Mansouri A, Lipschitz DA. Anemia in the elderly patient. Med Clin North Am 1992;76:619–630.
56. Gary PJ, Goodwin JS, Hunt WE. Iron status and anemia in the elderly: New findings and a review of previous studies. J Am Geriatr Soc 1983;31:389–399.
57. Berliner N, Duffy TP, Abelson HT. Approach to the adult and child with anemia. In: Hoffman R, Benz EJ, Shattil SJ, et al, eds. Hematology: Basic Principles and Practice, 2nd ed. New York, Churchill Livingstone, 1995:468–483.
58. Graham EA. The changing face of anemia in infancy. Pediatr Rev 1994;15:175–183.

92

COAGULATION DISORDERS

Mariela Diaz-Linares, PharmD, and Keith A. Rodvold, PharmD, FCCP, BCPS

This chapter describes a pathophysiologic approach to diagnosis and management of patients with common coagulation disorders. The chapter is divided into two sections: fundamental concepts of hemostasis and thrombosis, and clinical application of these fundamentals with regard to hemostatic disorders and thrombotic disorders. The general categories of disorders contrast congenital bleeding illnesses with acquired disorders of coagulation. Treatment of each coagulation disorder is discussed.

REGULATION OF HEMOSTASIS

Hemostasis is the spontaneous arrest of bleeding from damaged blood vessels. Hemostasis and thrombosis are regulated by a series of complex actions and reactions of procoagulant and anticoagulant events.[1,2] The exact mechanisms that precisely regulate the balance between clot formation and lysis are not completely understood. The following is a brief description of the physiologic interaction and regulation of four major components of the normal hemostatic system: (1) the vessel wall, (2) platelets, (3) the coagulation system, and (4) the fibrinolytic system.

VESSEL WALL AND PLATELETS

The blood vessel and circulating platelets play central roles in primary hemostasis. The involvement of vessel wall includes vasoconstriction, formation of platelet plugs, and regulation of coagulation and fibrinolysis (Fig. 92–1). Platelet function in response to vascular injury includes four phases: (1) adhesion, (2) aggregation, (3) secretion, and (4) elaboration of procoagulant activity. Formation of a platelet plug proceeds through the sequence of platelet adhesion to exposed subendothelial connective tissue structures; platelet aggregation by adenosine diphosphate, thromboxane A_2, and thrombin recruitment; contribution of platelet coagulant activity to the coagulation process, which stabilizes the plug with a fibrin mesh; and retraction of the platelet mass to provide a dense thrombus.

The endothelial cell, and especially its surface, is intimately involved in the balance between clotting and bleeding. Procoagulant molecules, such as von Willebrand's factor, and anticoagulant proteins, such as tissue plasminogen activator, are secreted by these cells. Prostaglandins, such as prostacyclin, inhibit platelet aggregation, whereas thromboxane A_2, released by platelets, promotes aggregation. Thrombomodulin on the surface of the cell reacts with thrombin to activate proteins C and S, which inhibit the plasma cascade of coagulation factors. There is a dynamic balance of fibrinolysis and fibrin formation, both of which interact with platelets at the cell surface to keep the blood in fluid phase and prevent bleeding at the same time.[2,3]

COAGULATION SYSTEM

The coagulation and fibrinolytic systems serve two interrelated and opposing functions. The formation of a fibrin clot occurs as a result of the coagulation system, whereas the fibrinolytic system dissolves the polymerized clot and restores blood flow. To generate fibrin for the formation of the clot, fibrinogen is cleaved by thrombin. Thrombin, generated by the intrinsic or extrinsic pathways, plays a key role in the hemostatic system (see Fig. 92–1); it is involved in platelet aggregation, fibrin formation, and the modulation of fibrinolysis.

Twelve plasma proteins are considered coagulation factors (Table 92–1). It is convenient to divide the coagulation factors into three groups on the basis of biochemical properties. These groups include vitamin K–dependent factors (II, VII, IX, and X), contact activation factors (XI and XII, prekallikrein, high-molecular-weight kininogen), and thrombin-sensitive factors (V, VIII, XIII, and fibrinogen).

Coagulation factors and enzymes of the fibrinolytic system circulate as inactive precursors (zymogens). Coagulation of blood entails a cascading series of proteolytic reactions. At each step a clotting factor undergoes limited proteolysis and becomes an active protease (designated by a lowercase "a," as in Xa). This clotting factor enzyme activates the next clotting factor until ultimately an insoluble fibrin clot is formed.

Clotting is initiated by either an intrinsic or an extrinsic pathway, with subsequent factor interactions converging at the common pathway (see Fig. 92–1). Both pathways can be activated when normal components of the vascular endothelium come into contact with blood. Tissue factor catalyzes factor VII. Tissue factor is found in many organs (brain, lungs, kidneys, and liver) extrinsic to blood; therefore, it initiates the extrinsic clotting pathway by catalyzing factor VII. In the extrinsic system, factor VII undergoes proteolytic activation by tissue factor. Factor VIIa, calcium, tissue thromboplastin, and factor X form a lipoprotein complex that results in activation of factor X. After this step, the extrinsic system is identical to the intrinsic system.

In the intrinsic pathway, all the protein factors necessary for coagulation are present in the circulating blood. Contact by circulating factor XII with subendothelial membrane initiates the intrinsic pathway. This activation phase

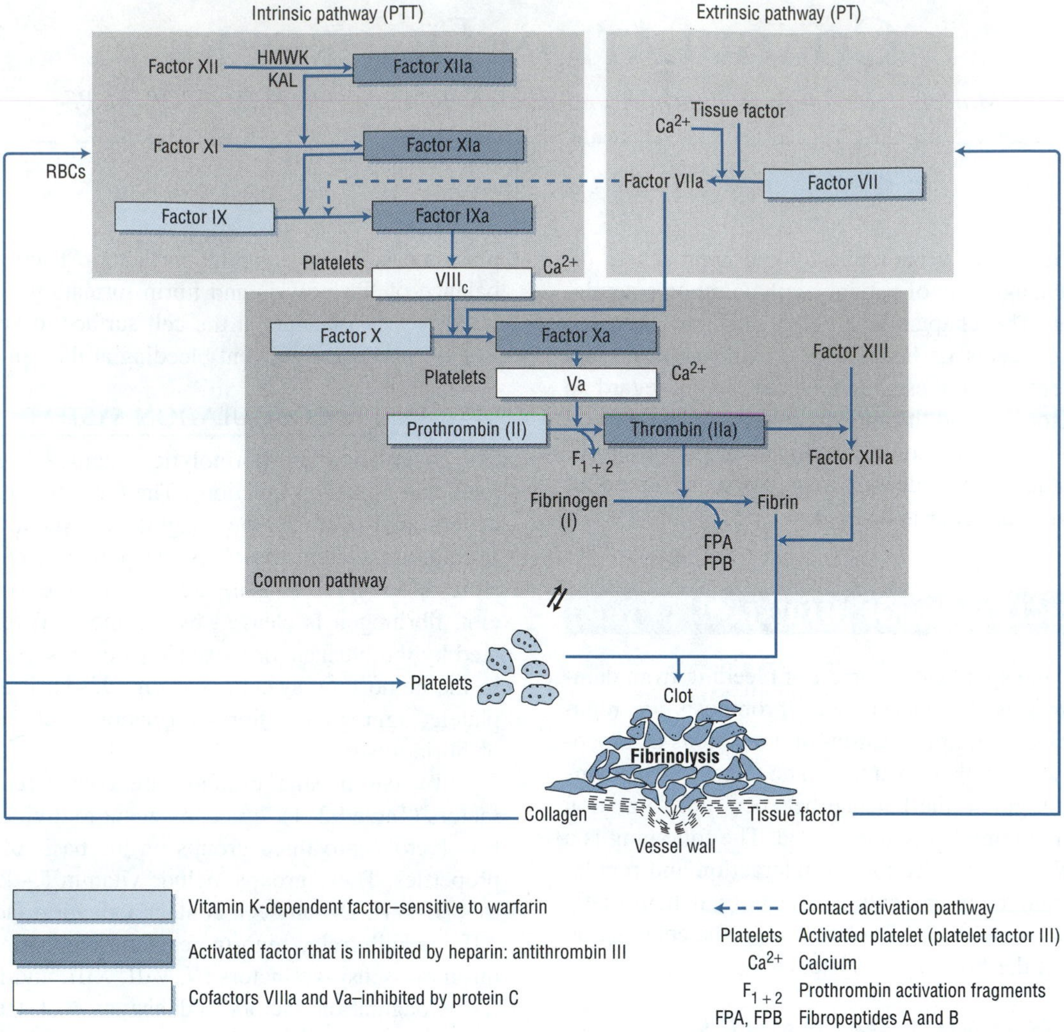

FIGURE 92–1. Scheme of the hemostatic system, showing interaction of vessel wall, platelets, coagulation pathways, and fibrinolytic system. Important features of the coagulation pathways include the contact activation phase, vitamin K–dependent factors (affected by warfarin), the activated serine proteases that are inhibited by heparin: antithrombin III, and the role of platelets and calcium. Factors VIIIc and Va are nonenzymatic cofactors that are inactivated by protein C. The protime (PT) measures the function of the extrinsic and common pathways; the partial thromboplastin time (PTT or APTT) measures the function of the intrinsic and common pathways. HMWK, high-molecular-weight kininogen; KAL, kallikrein. *(Adapted from Ref. 91.)*

includes several other factors including high-molecular-weight kininogen and prekallikrein. Factor XIIa, with cofactor high-molecular-weight kininogen, activates factor IX to factor IXa. Factor VIII, factor IXa, calcium, and platelet phospholipid form a lipoprotein complex with prothrombin and activate it to thrombin. A fibrin clot is formed after thrombin converts fibrinogen to fibrin.

Because thrombin has a central role in coagulation, its generation is the focus of two important regulatory systems. Antithrombin III complexes to thrombin and inactivates thrombin as well as several other serine proteases (IXa, Xa, XIa, XIIa). Patients with a hereditary or acquired deficiency of antithrombin III have a high incidence of recurrent thromboembolic disease. Heparin enhances the inhibitory capacity of antithrombin III and is present on the surface of endothelial cells. The second system involves thrombin exerting an inhibitory influence on clot formation by activating protein C.[2–4] Protein C and its cofactor, protein S, are vitamin K–dependent proteins that inactivate factors V and VIII of the coagulation cascade (see Fig. 92–1).

FIBRINOLYSIS

The fibrinolytic system is part of the localized repair of damaged endothelium as a regulatory mechanism in clot formation. Plasminogen is incorporated into the clot formation by binding to fibrin. Plasminogen activators (tissue-type plasminogen activator and urokinase-like plasminogen activator) are released in response to thrombin or venous stasis. Plasmin, converted from zymogen plasminogen, enzymatically digests fibrin, dissolves the clot, and releases a number of fibrin degradation products (fibrin split products). The interaction between plasminogen activators, plasminogen, and fibrin restricts the fibrinolytic activity to the site of the clot.

TABLE 92–1. Blood Coagulation Factors

Factors[a]	Synonym	Pathway	Role
I	Fibrinogen	Common	Terminal substrate of the coagulation system, polymerizes into fibrin fibers upon proteolysis by thrombin
II	Prothrombin	Common	Vitamin K–dependent zymogen of the serine protease thrombin
V	Proaccelerin, labile factor	Common	Nonenzymatic procofactor for factor Xa in the prothrombinase complex
VII	Proconvertin	Extrinsic	Vitamin K–dependent zymogen of factor VIIa that activates factor X via the extrinsic pathway and factor IX via the alternate pathway
VIII	Antihemophilic factor A	Intrinsic	Nonenzymatic procofactor of factor IXa in the factor X activation complex
IX	Antihemophilic factor B, Christmas factor	Intrinsic	Vitamin K–dependent zymogen of factor IXa that activates factor X
X	Stuart–Power factor	Common	Vitamin K–dependent zymogen of factor Xa, the protease of the prothrombinase complex
XI	Plasma thromboplastin antecedent	Intrinsic	Zymogen of protease factor XIa that converts factor IX to factor IXa
XII	Hageman factor	Intrinsic	Zymogen of factor XIIa that activates factor XI and prekallikrein
XIII	Fibrin-stabilizing factor		Zymogen of a transglutaminase that covalently cross-links fibrin monomers with each other
Prekallikrein	Fletcher factor	Intrinsic	Zymogen of kallikrein that activates factor XII and cleaves high-molecular-weight kininogen to liberate bradykinin
High-molecular-weight kininogen	Flaujeac's, Fitzgerald's, or Williams' factor	Intrinsic	Nonenzymatic contact activation cofactor of factor XIIa and kininogen

[a]Coagulation factors are numbered with roman numerals in order of their discovery. The most frequent synonyms are listed. Factor III (tissue factor) and factor IV (calcium ions) have been omitted from the table.
Adapted from Refs. 3 and 92.

Plasminogen-activator inhibitor and α_2-plasmin inhibitor inactivate plasmin to prevent systemic fibrinolysis.

SIMPLE LABORATORY TESTS

The initial diagnosis of coagulation disorders can be established from a detailed clinical history, a physical examination, and the results of a few laboratory tests.[3–8] The most common screening tests include bleeding time, prothrombin time, activated partial thromboplastin time, thrombin time, and platelet count. The results of these standard laboratory procedures can distinguish bleeding disorders caused by defects in the intrinsic, extrinsic, and common coagulation pathways (see Fig. 92–1) or from alterations in the number of functioning platelets. Specific assays of individual coagulation factors and platelet function tests can be determined after abnormalities are identified by initial screening tests. The following is a brief review of simple tests that are available in most hospital or clinical settings. These tests are summarized in Table 92–2.

BLEEDING TIME

In conjunction with the platelet count, determination of the bleeding time[5] allows the examiner to make fundamental decisions regarding abnormalities of primary hemostasis. Patients with an abnormal bleeding time but a normal platelet count are arbitrarily designated as having qualitative abnormalities of platelet function (thrombocytopathy). Such patients include those with von Willebrand's disease, those who have recently ingested various antiplatelet drugs (i.e., aspirin), and those with uremia or dysproteinemia.

PROTHROMBIN TIME

The prothrombin time (PT)[6] assesses the function of the extrinsic system and common pathway of the coagulation system. In particular, the test measures the activity of the vitamin K–dependent factor, factor VII. PT reflects the time required for fibrin strands to appear after the addition of tissue thromboplastin and calcium to a patient's plasma. Thus, the PT yields evidence about the current synthetic capacity of the liver, the adequacy of vitamin K absorption, and the inhibition of clotting factor synthesis by warfarin.

ACTIVATED PARTIAL THROMBOPLASTIN TIME

The activated partial thromboplastin time (APTT)[7] measures the activity of the intrinsic system and common pathway. APTT reflects the time required for a fibrin clot to form after calcium and an activating agent are added to the patient's plasma. APTT is widely used for monitoring heparin therapy.

THROMBIN TIME

The thrombin time (TT)[8] assesses the clotting of plasma by thrombin and is affected by quantitative and qualitative abnormalities of fibrinogen. The TT measures the time required for the formation and the appearance of the fibrin clot. The test bypasses all earlier steps of the coagulation pathway. It is commonly used to monitor the effect of systemic fibrinolytic therapy and can be modified for monitoring heparin therapy.

TABLE 92–2. Laboratory Procedures

Procedure (Normal Range)	Identifies	Test Result	Pathogenesis	Clinical Manifestations
Bleeding time (3–8 min)	Platelet functions: adhesion, aggregation, and release	8–15 min	Moderately low levels of vWF Antiplatelet drugs Circulating anticoagulants Factor V deficiency Factor XI deficiency	Bleeding from the gums Easy bruising Bleeding following surgery and teeth extraction Nose bleeds
		> 15 min	Very low levels of vWF Inherited qualitative platelet defects Thrombocytopenia Afibrinogenemia Antiplatelet drugs	Spontaneous hemorrhage, especially CNS
Prothrombin time [PT] (10.3–12.7 s)	Identifies factors I, II, V, VII, X Selective to plasma level changes: factor I, V, VII	< 1% deficiency Factor V: 48–50 s Factor VII: 28–30 s Factor X: 50–52 s Fibrinogen: 6 mg/L, 32–35 s	Newborn Inherited factor deficiencies Aged plasma Warfarin Liver disease Lupus anticoagulant Polycythemia Afibrinogenemia	Bleeding: umbilical cord, uterine, surgery, childbirth, trauma, etc
Activated partial thromboplastin time [APTT] (21.5–30.5 s)	Identifies: factors of the contact phase: prekallikrein, HMW-K, XII	< 1% deficiency HMW-K: 142–158 s Prekallikrein: 80–90 s Factor XII: 280–300 s	Inherited deficiencies	Decreased fibrinolytic activity Increased incidence of thrombotic disease
	Factors of the intrinsic pathway: XI, IX, VIII	Factor XI: 68–82 s Factor IX: 78–82 s Factor VIII: 77–80 s	Inherited deficiencies	Hemarthrosis and muscle bleeding Pseudo-tumors
	Factors of the common pathway: I, II, V, X Selective for: Factors of the contact phase and intrinsic pathway	Factor X: 144–150 s Factor V: 135–140 s	Inherited deficiencies	Joint and muscle bleeding
	Sensitivity conferred by activating agent Kaolin and silica recommended Ellagic acid and soy extract unreliable	High degree of variability with heparin therapy	Lupus anticoagulant Heparin therapy Liver disease Polycythemia Afibrinogenemia	
Thrombin time [TT]	Fibrinogen Inhibitors of the thrombin–fibrinogen interaction, such as acquired or inherited abnormal fibrinogens and heparin Inhibitors of fibrin aggregation, such as paraproteins and specifically abnormal immunoglobulins associated with multiple myeloma	1 unit thrombin activity clots 200 μL plasma fibrinogen in 15 min	Inherited afibrinogenemia and dysfibrinogenemia	Life-long hemorrhagic disease

Adapted from Ref. 3, with permission.

CONGENITAL DISORDERS

HEMOPHILIA

Inherited plasma coagulation disorders result from rare defects in single coagulation proteins. The two X-linked disorders, hemophilia A (factor VIII deficiency) and hemophilia B (factor IX deficiency), account for almost all known congenital coagulation defects.

Hemophilia A is also called classic hemophilia and is the oldest known congenital coagulopathy.[9–12] In general, only males are affected by the disease, but females are carriers. The incidence of hemophilia A in the overall population is approximately 1 or 2 per 10,000 males.[11,12] The National Heart and Lung Institute estimates the frequency to be 25 per 100,000 males in the United States. Approximately 85% of those affected have hemophilia A (factor VIII deficiency); the remaining have hemophilia B (factor IX deficiency). Both hemophilia A and hemophilia B are recessive sex-linked diseases; the defective gene is located on the X chromosome. Affected males have the abnormal allele on their X chromosome and no matching allele on their Y chromosome; thus, their sons would be normal (assuming the mother is not a carrier), and their daughters would be obligatory carriers. Female carriers have one normal allele and, therefore, do not have a hemorrhagic tendency. Sons of a female carrier and a normal male have a 50% chance of being hemophiliacs, whereas daughters have a 50% chance of being carriers. This mode of inheritance with a "skipped generation"—the female carriers who are children of the hemophiliacs do not express the disease but pass it on to the next male generation—was first described accurately early in the 19th century.

Hemophilia has been observed in few females.[10–13] This can occur if a hemophiliac marries a female carrier or if the normal X chromosome in the carrier female undergoes extreme lyonization. Lyonization is the process by which one of the X chromosomes in a female degenerates and does not produce effective gene products. There have been extremely rare cases where patients have had either one X chromosome or an autosomal dominant mode of transmission. In the older literature, many of these cases of female hemophilia are now thought to have been von Willebrand's disease.[14–17]

Before 1947, it was thought that all patients with sex-linked, hereditary bleeding disorders had classic hemophilia resulting from factor VIII (antihemophilic factor) deficiency.[16] In 1947, blood from one patient with presumed classic hemophilia was found to correct the clotting abnormality in another patient. Subsequent investigators showed that both of these disorders were inherited as sex-linked recessive disorders with identical means of inheritance, but one resulted from a deficiency of factor IX (plasma thromboplastin component, or Christmas factor).

Modern techniques of molecular biology have been successful in cloning the gene for factor VIII production.[9] The gene is 186,000 bases long. The coagulant material encoded by the gene originates from liver cells, although other tissues such as the kidney, spleen, and lymph glands have also been found to be sources of the coagulant material (factor VIII). This protein cofactor is missing in hemophilia A. The entire factor VIII molecule consists of this factor VIII coagulant material, along with a larger molecule, von Willebrand's factor, which is the protein that mediates adhesion of platelets to the subendothelium.[16] The larger part of the molecule is absent, decreased, or defective in von Willebrand's disease. Von Willebrand's factor circulates as a complex with factor VIII in normal plasma and appears to stabilize the latter. Antibodies have been produced to both the factor VIII coagulant material and the von Willebrand's factor and are called factor VIII antigen and von Willebrand's factor antigen, respectively.

At least 500 hemophiliac factor genes have been examined and many different mutations have been pinpointed. The kind of mutations that can affect the factor VIII gene include deletions and missense and nonsense mutations. Deletions and nonsense mutations are associated with the more severe forms of hemophilia A. A wider range of clinical conditions has been associated with more than 80 missense mutations.[10,16] Classic hemophilia A is caused by a deficiency of factor VIII coagulant material, with the degree of deficiency depending on the degree of genetic defect. In patients with classic hemophilia, there is a deficiency of factor VIII coagulant material but not of von Willebrand's factor, which appears to be synthesized in endothelial cells.

All patients with hemophilia B have decreased factor IX clotting activity.[18] The molecular basis for this decrease varies; some patients have decreased synthesis of a normal molecule, whereas others appear to have normal amounts of factor IX antigen with markedly decreased coagulant activity and thus are thought to have an abnormal protein with retained antigenic characteristics. There are several variants of factor IX deficiency, one of which is hemophilia B_m.[13,18] This disorder is characterized by a prolonged PT, whereas in most patients with hemophilia B this test is normal. The subscript "m" refers to the family name of the original patient. These patients have been shown to have the factor IX molecule by the presence of cross-reactive material, but the protein does not have normal coagulant activity. The specific protein abnormality has been identified in several different types of these variants. It is this abnormal protein that is believed to interfere with a factor VII–tissue factor activation of factor X, thereby prolonging the PT. The mechanism of this interference is unknown. About 5% of hemophilia B patients are hemophilia B_m variants. There are several other variants of hemophilia B, but they all have similar clinical manifestations.

The complete amino acid sequence for the circulating factor IX molecule has been delineated, and the gene for factor IX has been cloned. The entire gene is 35,000 nucleotides long.[13,18]

Molecular biologists use various techniques to detect carriers of either hemophilia A or B. In addition, prenatal diagnosis can be carried out if sufficient fetal DNA is obtained by cell culture of amniotic fluid or by biopsy of the chorionic villi.[9,10,18]

Hemophilia has been cured following liver transplantation.[10,11] Three patients who underwent liver transplant secondary to end-stage liver disease normalized their factor VIII levels. However, the need for lifelong immunosuppression and the risks associated with the surgical procedure preclude this option for most patients. It should be possible to cure hemophiliacs by introducing the appropriate gene into their cells.[10,19] Gene therapy for hemophilia is currently in the developmental stages and holds promise of a cure for this disease.[20,21]

Clinical Presentation

HEMOPHILIA A

Clinical bleeding is usually correlated with the degree of deficiency of factor VIII. Patients with less than 1% factor VIII are classified as severe hemophiliacs; those with 1% to 5% are moderate hemophiliacs, and those with greater than 5% are mild hemophiliacs (Table 92–3).[10,11] Most bleeding episodes are characterized by joint and muscle hemorrhage, with prolonged bleeding after trauma or surgery. Minor trauma and abrasions, which are frequently controlled with platelet plugs, do not pose clinical problems in patients with hemophilia.

Joint hemorrhages frequently involve the large joints, especially the weight-bearing ones. These episodes are frequently spontaneous, begin in childhood, and can lead to disabling arthropathies.

Muscle hematomas, especially psoas hematomas, can lead to false diagnoses, including appendicitis, and can also compress nerves, leading to weakness or paralysis. Bleeding into vital organs can cause significant dysfunction. Retroperitoneal bleeding can obstruct one or both kidneys or bleeding into the oral cavity can obstruct the airway. Occasionally, bleeding into the subperiosteum after trauma can cause pseudotumors with bone necrosis.

Although mucous membrane bleeding is more common in disorders affecting platelet function, genitourinary, gastrointestinal, and intracranial bleeding may occur.

HEMOPHILIA B

Hemophilia B (factor IX deficiency) is similar in all of its clinical manifestations to hemophilia A, with the severity of the disorder paralleling the degree of factor deficiency.[16]

Diagnosis

Patients who have spontaneous bleeding or bleeding out of proportion to what is expected clinically from an injury or surgical procedure may have a coagulopathy. Screening tests to detect coagulopathies include platelet count, bleeding time, PT, and APTT (Table 92–4).[3,4,22] TT can provide rapid information on the later stages of the coagulation mechanism and may also be useful. Depending on the results of these tests, additional tests including specific factor assays may be utilized to establish the specific diagnosis.

The APTT is an excellent test for screening deficiencies in the pathways of coagulation and has been reported to detect 99% to 100% of hemophilia A patients.[3,4,7] The

TABLE 92–3. Laboratory and Clinical Manifestations of Hemophilia

	Severe (< 0.01 U/mL)	Moderate (0.01–0.05 U/mL)	Mild (> 0.05 U/mL)
Factor VIII/IX activity level[a]			
% of all hemophilia A	70%	15%	15%
% of all hemophilia B	50%	30%	20%
Bleeding manifestations			
Age of onset	≤ 1 y	1–2 y	2 y–adult
Neonatal symptoms	PCB: usually ICH: occasionally	PCB: usually ICH: uncommonly	None Rare
Muscle/joint hemorrhage	"Spontaneous"; requires no trauma	Requires minor trauma	Requires minor trauma
CNS hemorrhage	High risk (2%–8%)	Moderate risk	Rare
Postsurgical hemorrhage (without prophylaxis)	Frank bleeding, severe	Wound bleeding, common	Wound bleeding, with factor < 0.3 U/mL
Oral hemorrhage following trauma, tooth extraction	Usual	Common	Often

[a]Normal range of factor VIII/IX activity level is 0.5–1.5 U/mL (50%–150%). 1 U/mL corresponds to 100% of the factor found in 1 mL of normal plasma.
PCB = postcircumcisional bleeding; ICH = intracranial hemorrhage; CNS = central nervous system.
From Ref. 10, with permission.

TABLE 92–4. Typical Laboratory Findings in von Willebrand's Disease Variants

	Hemophilia[a]		von Willebrand's Disease					
	A	*B*	*1*	*2A*	*2B*	*2M*	*2N*	*3*
Factor VIII	↓↓	N	↓	↓	↓ or N	↓ or N	↓↓	↓↓
vWF:Ag	N	N	↓	↓	N or ↓	↓	N or ↓	ND
vWF:RCof	N	N	↓	↓↓	↓↓	↓↓	N or ↓	ND
RIPA	N	N	↓ or N	↓	↑	↓ or N	N or ↓	↓↓
vWF multimers in plasma	N	N	N	Largest and ↑ intermediate absent	Largest absent	N	N	All absent

[a]N = normal; Ag = antigen; RCof = ristocetin cofactor activity; RIPA = ristocetin-induced agglutination; ND = not detected; vWF = von Willebrand factor.
Adapted from Ref. 17, with permission.

sensitivity of the test is therefore excellent. If clinically normal patients are screened, there is an approximately 2% false-positive rate; this rate is approximately 11% for patients being evaluated for abnormal bleeding. Normal APTT and PT essentially rule out a significant plasma coagulation defect. Preoperative screening for coagulation disorders with the APTT shows that the incidence of clinically inapparent coagulopathies is so low that false-positive results greatly outnumber true-positive results and make screening pointless. The most critical piece of information is an adequate clinical assessment, including a medical history related to any prior history of bleeding problems. In patients for whom a clinical assessment is not possible, patients who have clinical evidence to suggest a bleeding disorder, such as liver disease and malabsorption, or patients undergoing procedures that may interrupt normal coagulation, such as extracorporeal circulation, screening tests are recommended.

Ideally, the APTT is sensitive to factor deficiency states of less than 30% activity. Patients with a normal PT but an abnormal APTT typically have deficiencies of factors that are unique to the intrinsic system (factors VIII, IX, XII, and XI). The specific factor assay for factor VIII or IX will reveal the appropriate defect. The exception to this is the deficiency of factor IX in hemophilia B_m in which case the PT and APTT are prolonged.

In addition, any patient with factor VIII deficiency should undergo the laboratory tests necessary to define von Willebrand's disease to be sure that the patient does not have this disorder or a variant thereof (see Table 92–4).

▶ TREATMENT: Hemophilia

Comprehensive care of hemophilia requires a multitude of medical and paramedical personnel.[10–12] In the United States and the United Kingdom, the treatment of hemophilia has become centralized because of federally funded regional comprehensive hemophilia programs. In addition to centralizing the treatment, the federal government has supported the high cost of hemophilia treatment, thus decreasing the difficulty of providing care to both the institution and the patient. These patients frequently require primary care physicians, hematologists, orthopedic surgeons, nurses, physical medicine specialists, dentists, genetic counselors, psychologists, social workers, and vocational counselors along with pharmaceutical services and inpatient and outpatient treatment facilities associated with adequate coagulation testing.

In addition to some of the previously mentioned preventive medicine aspects necessary from birth, children need to be educated about physical protection during usual play. Passenger restraints in automobiles are especially important to children with hemophilia. Physical exercise is encouraged along with a daily program to improve muscle and joint function.

Newborn male infants who may be hemophiliacs should not be circumcised until the diagnosis is excluded. Blood should be obtained from a peripheral vein and not from a femoral or jugular vein puncture because of the danger of hematoma formation. Babies with hemophilia should receive routine immunizations, including immunization against hepatitis B. These small-gauge needles do not usually cause hematomas.

Genetic counseling with a neutral attitude should be offered and female relatives who may be carriers should be tested. Female relatives who are carriers may have a mild to moderate bleeding diathesis and can be forewarned of any difficulty with either trauma or surgery.

As children grow they may be taught to administer their own factor concentrate so that they may achieve independence. Concurrent illnesses can complicate hemophilia. Minor infections are frequently associated with bleeding into the site of inflammation and need to be followed closely.

HEMOPHILIA A

The degree of severity determines the choice of treatment among these patients. Those with severe or moderate disease are treated with either cryoprecipitate or factor VIII concentrate.[10–12] Lyophilized factor VIII concentrate is easy to store, reconstitute, and administer. In addition, these products are subject to various purification processes, decreasing the chances of transmitting blood-borne viruses.[23] Recombinant-DNA technology has made it possible to have two products with structural and functional characteristics similar to plasma-derived factor VIII. The safety and efficacy of these products have been demonstrated in large-scale trials.[24,25]

Opinions of which factor concentrate to use vary widely among physicians. These physician opinions can be grouped into four general categories: (1) those who use plasma-derived products on all their patients because they are satisfied with viral-inactivation methods and do not think that plasma-derived products would have any degree of immunosuppression; (2) those who are concerned for the previously mentioned reasons and advocate only recombinant products; (3) those who are worried about the potential immunosuppressant effects of plasma-derived products and choose recombinant products for patients who have the human immunodeficiency virus (HIV positive) and plasma-derived products for patients without the human immunodeficiency virus (HIV negative); and (4) those who choose recombinant products for patients previously untreated and plasma-derived products for the rest of their patients.

Table 92–5 summarizes the factor VIII products currently available in the United States. All products are equally effective with similar rates of antibody development. However, plasma-derived products carry the potential for transmission of blood-borne viruses other than HIV and hepatitis, although the implications of this small chance are unknown at this time. The main factors that influence choice are cost and the preferences of the physician and/or patient; however, there is no solid evidence to support the preference for one product.

The factor is quantitated in units, where 1 unit of factor VIII is the amount found in 1 mL of pooled plasma. By definition, 1 unit of factor VIII per milliliter is 100% of normal. Dosing factor VIII will depend on several factors including the severity of the bleeding episode, desired plasma level, half-life of the infused factor, body weight, and plasma volume.[10–12,16,26] The usual half-life of factor VIII is 8 to 12 hours; thus, to maintain a specific factor level, it is necessary to infuse the factor at least twice daily or as a continuous infusion.

One way of calculating the appropriate initial dose is based on the observation that each unit of factor VIII infused per kilogram of body weight yields a 2% rise in plasma factor VIII levels. The following equation may also be used to calculate an initial dose of factor VIII:

$$\text{Factor VIII (units)} = (\text{Desired level} - \text{Actual level}) \times 0.5\ (\text{Weight})$$

This equation assumes a plasma volume of 5% of the patient's body weight in kilograms. It is usually necessary to administer half the loading dose every 12 hours to sustain a desired level of factor VIII. As previously mentioned, dosing factor VIII depends on several variables and the approach to replacement therapy is generally empiric. Each case must be considered individually.

Table 92–6 is designed to provide general guidelines for dosing factor VIII based on the site and severity of the bleeding episode.[10,14] Mild bleeding episodes are not included in the table because they should be managed without the use of blood products. The general goal is to achieve a factor VIII level of 30% to 50% to maintain hemostasis. To achieve this in 8 to 12 hours, it is necessary to have twice this level immediately after the infusion to allow for the decay with time. This level of factor is satisfactory for joint or muscle hemorrhage, but with severe bleeding or major surgical procedures the level should be raised to and maintained at 75% to 100% for up to a week.

Administration via continuous infusion has been shown to be safe and effective and may be more convenient than bolus therapy for inpatients.[27,28] Advantages of using continuous infusion include steady-state plasma concentrations of factor VIII and the use of coagulation factor when the infusion rate is adjusted to maintain a certain level.[29] A decrease in clearance of the factor concentrate is observed after 5 to 6 days of continuous infusion. Adjustments on the infusion rate with the following equation have been proposed to account this decrease in clearance:

$$\text{Dose (IU/kg/h)} = \text{Clearance (mL/kg/h)} \times \text{Measured plasma level (IU/mL)}$$

The adjusted infusion rate can decrease dose requirements by up to 50% to 90%.[29] The savings gained by the decreased dose of concentrate should be weighed against its limitations, such as limited data on the stability of the formulations (current FDA la-

TABLE 92–5. Factor VIII and IX Preparations

Manufacturer	Brand Name	Viral Inactivation or Exclusion Method	Annual Costs ($)[a]
Plasma derived, factor VIII			
Alpha	Alphanine	Solvent-detergent	60,000
American Red Cross	AHF, Method M	Monoclonal antibody	66,400
Baxter	Hemophil-M	Solvent-detergent	72,000
Centeon	Humate-P	Heat-treated, pasteurized	104,000
Bayer	Koate-HP	Solvent-detergent	72,000
Bayer	Monoclate-P	Heat-treated, pasteurized monoclonal antibody	72,000
Recombinant, factor VIII			
Centeon	Bioclate, Helixate		94,000
Bayer	KoGENate		94,000
Hyland/Genetics Institute	Recombinate		94,000
APCC			
Hyland	Autoplex-T	Heat-treated	104,000
Immuno-US	Feiba VH Immuno	Heat-treated	104,000
Plasma derived, factor IX			
Alpha	Alphanine SD	Solvent-detergent	84,000
Centeon	Mononine	Monoclonal antibody	88,000
Plasma derived, factor IX complex (PCC)			
Immuno	Bebulin VH Immuno Konyne 80	Heat-treated	44,000
Recombinant, factor IX			
Genetics Institute	BeneFIX		94,000
Porcine, factor VIII: C			
Seywood	Hyate: C	Freeze-dried	139,200

[a]Based on 1997 average wholesale price *(Red Book)*, and consumption of 80,000 units/year.

TABLE 92–6. Guidelines for Factor-Replacement Therapy for Hemorrhage in Hemophilia A and B

Site of Hemorrhage	Hemostatic Factor Level (% of normal)	Factor Dosing		Comment
		Hemophilia A	*Hemophilia B*	
Joint	30%–50%, minimum	20–40 U/kg qd PRN	30–40 U/kg qod PRN	Rest/immobilization/physical therapy rehabilitation following bleed. Several doses may be necessary to prevent or treat target joint.
Muscle	40%–50%, minimum	20–40 U/kg qd PRN	40–60 U/kg qod PRN	Calf/forearm bleed is limb threatening, significant blood loss with femoral/retroperitoneal bleed.
Oral mucosa	Initially 50%; then antifibrinolytic coverage usually suffices	25 U/kg	50 U/kg	Antifibrinolytic therapy is critical. Do not use with PCCs or APCCs.
Epistaxis	Initially 80%–100%; then 30% until healing occurs	40–50 U/kg; then 30–40 U/kg qd	80–100 U/kg; then 70–80 U/kg qod	Local measures: pressure/packing/cautery useful for severe or recurrent bleed.
Gastrointestinal	Initially 100%; then 30% until healing occurs	40–50 U/kg; then 30–40 U/kg qd	80–100 U/kg; then 70–80 U/kg qod	Lesion is usually found; endoscopy highly recommended. Antifibrinolytic therapy may be useful.
Genitourinary	Initially 100%; then 30% until healing occurs	40–50 U/kg; then 30–40 U/kg qd	80–100 U/kg; then 70–80 U/kg qod	Evaluate for stones or urinary tract infection. Lesion usually not found. Prednisone 1–2 mg/kg/d × 5–7 d may be useful.
Central nervous system	Initially 100%; then 50%–100% for 10–14 d	50 U/kg; then 25 U/kg q12h *or* CI	100 U/kg; then 50 U/kg q24h CI of HPPs may be possible	Anticonvulsants frequently used preventatively, neuro follow-up. Lumbar puncture requires prophylactic factor coverage.
Trauma or surgery	Initially 100%; then 50% until wound healing begins; then 30% until wound healing complete	50 U/kg; then dose q12h *or* by CI	100 U/kg; then dose q24h *or* as above	Perioperative and postoperative management plan must be in place preop; evaluation for inhibitors crucial prior to elective surgery.

CI = continuous infusion; HPP = high-purity product.
From Ref. 10, with permission.

beling and recommendations are for immediate injection of factor VIII), the use of infusion pumps, and complications associated with venous access.

Cryoprecipitate is rich in factor VIII, fibrinogen, and von Willebrand's factor, and still in use in some hemophiliac centers, although it has been replaced, for the most part, by factor VIII concentrates. In general, each bag of cryoprecipitate contains approximately 70 to 100 units of factor VIII activity per 10- to 20-mL bag. The potency of cryoprecipitate will vary from bag to bag; therefore, the dose can only be estimated. The number of bags necessary to achieve a desired level of factor VIII may be estimated by calculating the amount of factor VIII in units required as previously discussed.[16]

Mild factor VIII deficiency may be treated with 1-desamino-8-D-arginine vasopressin (desmopressin acetate, DDAVP), which transiently increases factor VIII and von Willebrand's factor levels and shortens prolonged bleeding time.[30] DDAVP is a synthetic analog of the antidiuretic hormone vasopressin. If the patient has a mild bleeding episode, such as a hemarthrosis, DDAVP 0.3 to 0.4 μg/kg IV infused over 15 to 30 minutes may be given. Factor levels should be measured to ensure that an adequate response has been achieved.[31] DDAVP can result in a fourfold to sixfold rise in factor VIII levels, with maximum levels occurring at about 90 to 120 minutes postinfusion with persistent activity for greater than 6 hours. The injection can be repeated within 12 to 24 hours depending on the severity of the bleeding episode and the clinical response. It is important to realize that the factor increments become attenuated with frequent dosages.

A concentrated DDAVP formulation is available for subcutaneous administration.[31] When administered at the same dose as the IV formulation, it has been shown to be as effective. This formulation offers the advantage of self-adminstration at home.[32]

Intranasal administration of DDAVP via a concentrated nasal spray (Stimulate) has become available in the United States.[33] It effectively increases factor VIII levels but to a lesser extent than that of parenteral DDAVP.[10,31,34] The nasal spray may serve as an alternative to the parenteral formulation, especially in patients with mild bleeding episodes who need to self-administer DDAVP. Before starting intranasal DDAVP, a test dose should be performed to assure adequate response to this particular formulation.

Very few adverse effects are associated with DDAVP. Most side effects are probably secondary to mild vasodilation.[31] The most commonly observed side effect is facial flushing. Side effects less frequently reported include mild headaches, increased heart rate, and decreased blood pressure. DDAVP has the potential to cause water retention, which may lead to severe hyponatremia secondary to its potent antidiuretic effects. Since DDAVP can also increase plasminogen activator, some experts suggest the concomitant use of ε-aminocaproic acid (EACA) to inhibit the potential fibrinolysis that may occur. Use of DDAVP reduces exposure to blood-borne viruses. Caution should be exercised when administering DDAVP to patients with a history of recurrent thrombosis.

Traditional therapy for hemophilia has been given on demand, as the bleeding episode occurs. Recurrent joint bleeding in severe cases of hemophilia can lead to the development of chronic arthropathies. This can further lead to severe physical disability, loss of time from normal activities, and in most instances surgical interventions. Prophylactic use of factor VIII concentrates in severe hemophilia has been explored.[35–37] The rational comes from observations where patients with moderate disease rarely develop arthropathy. The goal of prophylactic replacement is to maintain a level of factor VIII of a least 1% in these patients. Infusion of the factors at least three time a week in a dose range between 24 and 40 IU factor VIII/kg can maintain this goal. Patients who have received this approach since age 1 year have almost no bleeding episodes and have had completely normal joints during follow-up.[35–37] When compared to on-demand administration, patients receiving prophylaxis had better orthopedic outcomes.[37,38]

Prophylactic regimens can increase the use of factor VIII concentrates by more that fourfold.[10] Despite the widespread use of these regimens in many European countries, the increase in direct cost has resulted in low acceptance of this modality by many centers in the United States. Other issues to consider besides cost are the need for permanent venous access and compliance with the weekly infusions. Prospective studies are currently ongoing to address these issues and to determine the optimal time for initiation of prophylaxis.

HEMOPHILIA B

High-purity factor IX plasma concentrate is currently considered the treatment of choice for hemophilia B.[39] These products have rapidly replaced the older products, known as prothrombin complex concentrate (PCC). PCC, in addition to factor IX, contains vitamin K–dependent factors responsible for the thromboembolic complications observed with their administration.[23] Available high-purity factors include Alphanine and Alphanine-SD (Alpha Therapeutic) and Mononine (Centeon). The first two products contain 50 units of factor IX activity per milligram of protein and Mononine contains at least 150 units per milligram of protein. No thromboembolic complications have been reported with either product, and excellent hemostasis during bleeding episodes is observed.[40]

The half-life of factor IX is approximately 24 hours, with normal hemostasis being achieved when plasma levels are approximately 10% to 25%. Each unit of factor IX infused per kilogram body weight yields a 1% rise in the level of factor IX. As with factor VIII, the success of infusion depends on achievement of appropriate factor IX levels, which requires monitoring with factor IX assays.

Table 92–5 provides general guidelines for dosing factor IX based on the site and severity of the bleed episode. In addition, concomitant antifibrinolytic agents and factor IX concentrates have been used without thrombotic complications.[41] This has been proposed as a cost-effective way of controlling bleeding episodes because of a reduction in the requirements for factor IX concentrate. Finally, a recombinant human factor IX (BeneFix, Genetics Institute) has recently been licensed.[42]

TREATMENT OF INHIBITORS IN HEMOPHILIA

Antibodies to factor VIII and IX, also known as inhibitors, develop in a group of patients with hemophilia, challenging the management of these patients. The development of antibodies is probably the most common serious complication of factor replacement therapy, because transmission of blood-borne pathogens is now a rare occurrence. The incidence of inhibitors was thought to be around 15%; however, prospective studies with more intensive screening surveillance reports the incidence to be as high as 52%.[43–46] The two most important factors that influence the development of inhibitors seem to be host-related and product-related (plasma-derived versus recombinant).[47]

These inhibitors are usually IgG immunoglobulin. They do not precipitate human factor VIII or IX and do not fix complement. They are directed against the factor coagulant portion of the complex. Advances in the characterization of these antibodies have allowed differentiation between alloantibodies and autoantibodies.[48,49] These antibodies may be recognized when a calculated dose of factor does not produce the expected plasma level. In such cases, inhibitor levels should be determined to guide therapy in these patients. Inhibitor titers are reported in Bethesda units (BU) in the United States. Patients with inhibitors to factor VIII/IX are divided into two groups: low responders, who have low levels of inhibitors (2 to 5 BU/mL) with little or no rise in antibody titers after exposure to the factor; and high responders, who have an anamnestic response after exposure to factor VIII/IX and usually have higher inhibitor levels (> 10 BU/mL). Approximately 20% of this population are low responders and 50% to 60% are high responders.

The treatment of patients with factor inhibitors will depend on the titer of the inhibitor and can be approached in two ways.[46,47] First, one may attempt to reduce inhibitor levels prophylactically with immunosuppressive agents (i.e., cyclophosphamide), γ-globulin infusions, plasmapheresis, or by-production of immune tolerance using high-dose or frequent regular infusions of the factor.[50] This approach can have up to 80% success rate and different institutions have developed various protocols to achieve immune tolerance.[51,52] The second method is used to achieve hemostasis in acute bleeding episodes or for surgery. If the patient has low inhibitor titers (< 5 BU/mL) an anamnestic response is unlikely, and hemostasis may be achieved with a high dose of factor (usually twice the dose ordinarily indicated). These patients should have an inhibitor level taken 7 to 10 days after therapy to assure that inhibitor titers do not rise. Patients with high inhibitor titers (> 10 BU/mL), however, usually have an anamnestic response to the factor. Hemostasis can usually be achieved in these patients with PCC, activated prothrombin complex concentrate (APCC), or porcine factor VIII.[50,53,54] The dose of PCC required is usually at least twice the dose of factor VIII/IX used in noninhibitor patients. Initial doses are usually in the range of 50 to 75 units/kg every 12 hours depending on the severity of the bleeding episode.

The patients must be clinically monitored since there are no laboratory tests to measure effectiveness of therapy. If the patient does not appear to be responding to PCC infusions, then APCC should be used in similarly high doses. Porcine factor VIII concentrate is intended primarily for use in patients who have developed inhibitors against factor VIII. The neutralizing activity of these inhibitors is usually absent or weaker against nonhuman as opposed to human factor VIII. The dose of porcine factor VIII may be estimated using the same criteria that are used for human factor VIII. Response to therapy may be monitored with factor VIII levels. Tolerance may be induced by the use of porcine factor VIII, and the inhibitor may not recur.[55]

Recombinant factor VIIa (rFVIIa) seems to offer an alternative treatment for patients with inhibitors.[47,53] In a series of 57 patients, none developed antibodies to factor VII. Hemostasis was achieved for hemophilia A and B using doses of 70 to 100 μg/kg every 2 to 3 hours and prolonging the interval of administration as clinical improvement occurred. An optional approach is to use a dose of 90 to 120 μg/kg or higher every 5 to 6 hours.[56] Prothrombin time has been suggested as a monitoring parameter for rFVIIa response.[57]

Figure 92–2 summarizes the therapeutic options in the management of hemophilia A patients with inhibitors.[50] The same algorithm can be applied to the management of hemophilia B patients, except that factor IX should be substituted for factor VIII. The use of porcine factor VIII is not indicated for the inhibitors in hemophilia B.

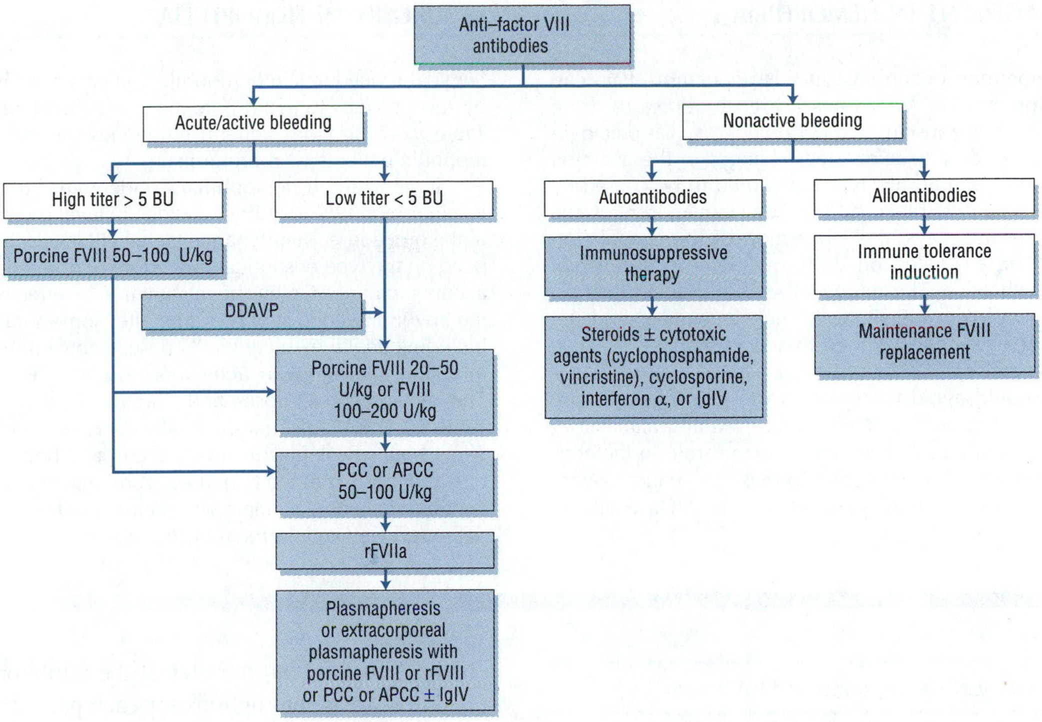

FIGURE 92–2. Treatment algorithm for the management of patients with hemophilia and factor VIII antibodies. *(Adapted from Ref. 50.)*

TABLE 92–7. Guidelines for Managing Hemophilic Patients Who Require Surgery

Before surgical procedure
1. Complete coagulation workup
2. Incubate test for inhibitors
3. Calculate needs and stockpile therapeutic material in hospital
4. Perform survival study for recovery and half-life of therapeutic material
5. Determine red cell type, crossmatch
Minor surgical procedures
1. Give dose calculated to bring patient's plasma level to 100% 1 h before procedure (50 IU/kg)
2. Maintain plasma level above 60% for 4 d
3. Maintain plasma level above 20% for the subsequent 4 d
4. Assay daily prior to dose
Major surgical procedures
1. Give dose calculated to bring patient's plasma level to 100% 1 h before procedure (50 IU/kg)
2. Maintain plasma level above 60% for 4 d
3. Maintain plasma level above 20% for the subsequent 4 d or until all drains and sutures are removed
4. Assay daily prior to dose
Orthopedic surgical procedures
1. Give dose calculated to bring patient's plasma level to 100% 1 h before procedure (50 IU/kg)
2. Maintain plasma level above 80% for 4 d
3. Assay daily prior to dose
4. Maintain plasma level above 40% for the subsequent 4 d
5. If patient is casted, discontinue replacement until rehabilitation program is begun
6. If not casted, maintain above 20% for ambulation
7. For rehabilitation program, maintain above 10% for 3 wk
Dental procedures
1. Give EACA 100 mg/kg IV 4 h before surgery or tenexamic acid to 10 mg/kg
2. Give factor replacement dose calculated to bring patient's plasma level to 100% 1 h before procedure
3. Continue EACA 100 mg/kg orally q6h for 7 d or tenexamic acid for 7 d (adults, 2 g 3 times a day for 7 d)
4. Repeat one dose of replacement therapy in 3 d if procedure is extensive

From Ref. 58, with permission.

PAIN MANAGEMENT IN HEMOPHILIA

Pain can be a common occurrence in this population. Pain can be either acute or chronic. Acute pain is a result of pressure from hemorrhage into joints, muscle, or other tissues.[10,11] Chronic pain usually occurs secondary to permanent changes in the anatomy of joints. Acute pain should always be assumed to be caused by bleeding. Control of the bleeding episode should control the pain. Pain that persists days after correction of the coagulation problem should be evaluated on the basis of the possibility of permanent joint changes. The relief of the chronic pain may require nonpharmacologic interventions such as surgery and the use of narcotic analgesics in addition to acetaminophen.[12]

Hemophilic patients, as well as other patients with coagulation disorders, should avoid the use of drugs that affect platelet aggregation such as aspirin and nonsteroidal anti-inflammatory agents (NSAIDs). Pharmacists have an important role in the education of these patients. It is important to make the patient aware of the various aspirin-containing drugs and NSAIDs available over the counter.

SURGERY IN HEMOPHILIA

Surgical procedures in hemophilic patients must be accompanied by several steps to avoid potentially life-threatening hemorrhage. Table 92–7 provides general guidelines for management of hemophilic patients who require surgery.[58]

In general, all hemophiliacs undergoing surgery—whether it is minor or major—require a factor VIII level of 100% 1 hour prior to the procedure. Maintenance factor VIII levels, however, will depend on the type of surgical procedure performed. Antifibrinolytic agents such as EACA has been shown to be effective as adjunctive therapy in the control of bleeding after some surgical procedures, including dental extractions.[10] These agents inhibit fibrinolysis by inhibiting plasminogen activators resulting in clot preservation. The recommended doses and duration of therapy are listed in Table 92–7. EACA is mainly renally excreted and has a half-life of 1 to 2 hours. Peak plasma levels occurr at 2 hours. Side effects are rare and mostly limited to nausea, vomiting, and diarrhea. EACA is contraindicated in patients with hematuria because of the potential for ureteral or intrarenal obstruction by blood clots.

EVALUATION OF THERAPEUTIC OUTCOMES

Pharmacists can assume an active role in the management of patients with hemophilia as members of the multidisciplinary team taking care of these patients. In view of the fact that the main goal in the treatment of hemophilia is to control and prevent bleeding episodes and their long-term sequelae, like arthropathies, pharmacologic and nonpharmacologic interventions should be aimed at achieving this goal. Appropriate selection of product according to the type and site of bleeding (e.g., factor concentrates vs DDAVP), an adequate dose corresponding to the desired level and patient weight, and the optimal duration of therapy are required for each particular episode. The institution of home therapy for the administration of factor concentrates is frequent in these patients, especially because this can lead to the early establishment of therapy and more independence to the patient. Assuring compliance with the regimen instituted as soon as the onset of bleeding symptoms, along with adequate education regarding proper storage, handling, and administration of these products, is integral to a successful home program. In addition, the patient should become familiar with common side effects and how to react to them. Fear of acquiring viral infections, in particular HIV, through plasma-derived products can lead to poor compliance with therapy or to delayed medical attention during a bleeding episode. Patient counseling can serve as a tool to overcome these fears.

Surveillance for the development of inhibitors, especially in patients with severe disease and high usage of factor concentrates, should be part of the pharmaceutical intervention, so that the discovery of the presence of inhibitors when the patient fails to respond to therapy is avoided. Development of inhibitors challenges the management and control of bleeding episodes. A full understanding of the clinical situation and the titer of the inhibitor is mandatory to address treatment options for each patient. Dose and frequency of administration for the product selected (e.g., porcine factor VIII or rFVIIa) vary from patient to patient. Because there is no laboratory test to measure effectiveness of therapy in this scenario, close clinical monitoring for worsening or resolution of the symptoms is required to optimize the outcome.

Preparation for any surgical intervention and assurance of the required levels of factor VIII or IX depending on the type of procedure are maintained through surgery and afterward are vital for a successful surgery with minimal or no complications. The above-mentioned scenarios are examples of different areas where management interventions can have a positive impact on the overall quality of the care and outcome of hemophiliacs.

VON WILLEBRAND'S DISEASE

Von Willebrand's disease is probably the most common inheritable coagulopathy.[14,15,17] The first clinical description of the disease was made by von Willebrand in 1926. Von Willebrand's disease is caused by an abnormality, quantitative or qualitative, of von Willebrand's factor and results in both abnormal platelet function and defective plasma clotting. Von Willebrand's factor (vWF) is a glycoprotein that can be found in classic hemophiliac plasma and normal plasma. At first, it was called factor VIII-related antigen or protein, because antibodies had been raised against protein fractions containing factor VIII coagulant activity. It is now known that factor VIII is distinct from vWF, but forms a dissociable complex with it.[59] Von Willebrand's factor can normally be detected in plasma, vessel walls, and platelets. Almost all of the vWF in platelets is located in the α granules. Within endothelial cells, vWF has been located on the plasma membrane and in the endoplasmic reticulum of the cytoplasm, as well as in cell-specific organelles.

Von Willebrand's factor has a dual role in hemostasis, facilitating platelet adhesion to injured vessel walls and binding the antihemophilic factor (factor VIII) in a complex, thus serving as a carrier of factor VIII in plasma.

The basic subunit of vWF is a protein chain with a molecular weight of approximately 230,000. The subunits are held together in a very complex way by disulfide bonds, forming proteins that vary widely in molecular weight. Von Willebrand's factor consists of a series of multimers ranging from 800,000 to 14,000,000 in molecular weight. The large multimers are thought to be the most hemostatically efficient with a greater potential for interaction with platelets and binding to the subendothelium. Von Willebrand's factor must join the platelets with the subendothelium to cause effective platelet function.

The antibiotic ristocetin causes platelet aggregation dependent on vWF.[14,17] Platelet aggregation with ristocetin became a model system in the study of platelet–vWF interactions. Von Willebrand's factor activity was measured on the basis of platelet aggregation and expressed as ristocetin cofactor activity. Because ristocetin and vWF agglutinate platelets fixed with paraformaldehyde or formalin, formalin-fixed platelets are now used to measure this activity.

High-molecular-weight forms of vWF seem to have the highest ristocetin cofactor activity and appear to be the most efficient in promoting adhesion in these systems. Some commercial factor VIII concentrates contain only low-molecular-weight multimers of vWF and are less efficient in promoting platelet adhesion.

Von Willebrand's factor appears to be the carrier protein for factor VIII as it circulates in normal blood. Although the site of factor VIII has not been established, factor VIII antigen has been demonstrated in the endothelial cells lining liver sinusoid, but not in other types of endothelium. Von Willebrand's factor also seems to be a stimulator of factor VIII production, because when vWF is given to a patient who lacks the complete complex, the factor VIII activity in the patient's blood increases more than can be explained by the factor VIII activity in the infused material.

Clinical Presentation

Von Willebrand's disease is usually inherited in the heterozygous form as an autosomal dominant disorder.[15,17] Genetic variants are defined according to the qualitative and quantitative abnormalities of vWF, which run true in affected kindreds. One affected person may be markedly different from another within a kindred with respect to the amount of factor deficiency but not the type of deficiency.

Patients with von Willebrand's disease frequently present with mucosal bleeding such as epistaxis, gingival bleeding, easy bruising, menorrhagia, and postsurgical bleeding, especially after operations on mucosal surfaces such as tonsillectomy, vaginal surgery, and dental surgery. In the most severe forms of the disease the bleeding starts in early childhood and tends to decrease with age or with pregnancy. In milder forms the disease may not be discovered until an episode of trauma or surgery when the patient is an adult. The bleeding into joints and muscles characteristic of hemophilia is rare in von Willebrand's disease.

Diagnosis

Von Willebrand's disease and its variants are defined by the type of abnormality in vWF: quantitative, qualitative, or both.[15,17] Von Willebrand's factor activity is measured as the bleeding time and by the ristocetin cofactor test. The bleeding time has been shown to be reasonably reproducible and accurate when obtained by the template technique. The ristocetin cofactor test measures the ability of the patient's plasma to agglutinate normal washed, fresh, or formalin-fixed platelets in the presence of ristocetin. Ristocetin-induced platelet aggregation (RIPA) is measured on platelet-rich plasma with an aggregometer.

Von Willebrand's factor is also measured by quantitation of von Willebrand's antigen, usually by electrophoresis with precipitating antibody to von Willebrand's factor or by radioimmunoassay.

The multimeric structure of von Willebrand's factor is demonstrated by electrophoresis in sodium dodecyl sulfate agarose or acrylamide gels. The multimers are then identified with radiolabeled antibody to vWF and autoradiography. The bands separate on the basis of their molecular size, and the relative proportions of large and small multimers can be demonstrated. Genetic variants are defined by the results of these tests. Factor VIII coagulant activity is usually low and commensurate with the degree of vWF deficiency. In some patients, however, factor VIII levels may approach normal.

Recent advances in the genetic analysis of patients with von Willebrand's disease have improved the understanding of the genetic and biochemical differences among this heterogeneous group of patients. An increasing number of subtypes have been described, and this pattern is expected to continue as genetic analysis becomes of widespread use in clinical practice.[59,60] In addition, a new and revised classification (Table 92–8) for vWD has replaced the old classification system.[61] As the complexity of vWD subtypes increased the nomenclature and classification of vWD grew confusing and hard to follow. The new classification categorizes subtypes of vWD by the mechanism of bleeding.

ACQUIRED VON WILLEBRAND'S DISEASE

Patients with altered immune status or polycythemioa rubra vera have been reported to develop a disorder resembling von Willebrand's disease, with prolonged bleeding times

TABLE 92–8. Revised Classification of von Willebrand's disease

Revised Type	Defect	Previous Type
1	Partial quantitative	I, I platelet normal, I platelet low, IA, I-1, I-2, I-3
2A	Qualitative; decreased platelet-dependent function associated with the absence of high-molecular-weight vWF multimers	IIA, IIA-1, IIA-2, IIA-3, IB, I platelet discordant, IIC, IID, IIE, IIF, IIG, IIH, II-I
2B	Qualitative; increased affinity for platelet glycoprotein 1b	IIB, I New York, Malmö
2M	Qualitative; decreased platelet-dependent function not caused by the absence of high-molecular-weight vWF multimers	B, Vicenza, IC, ID
2N	Decreased affinity of factor VIII	Normandy, defective binding factor VIII
3	Quantitative; complete deficiency of vWF	III

Adapted from Ref. 17, with permission.

and reduced levels of factor VIII–related activities.[60] Patients with systemic lupus erythematosus and other connective tissue diseases, monoclonal gammopathies, lymphoproliferative disease, and Wilms' tumor have been reported to have this disease. In some cases, inhibitors (antibodies) have been detected in the plasma that are capable of binding to factor VIII–von Willebrand's factor complex, removing it at an accelerated rate.

▶ TREATMENT: von Willebrand's Disease

The goals of therapy are to improve factor VIII level and to improve the bleeding time. Diagnosis of von Willebrand's disease and the type is important to guide therapy. However, during serious trauma or other acute situations presenting with severe bleeding, this information may not be available. In this scenario, replacement therapy should be the treatment of choice (Table 92–9). The use of cryoprecipitate carries the risk of transmitting bllod-borne viruses; different strategies have been attempted to reduce the size of the donor pool. Repetitive plasmapheresis of a single donor to extract cryoprecipitate or pretreatment with DDAVP to augment the donor's preexisting factor VIII and vWF levels are examples of these strategies.[15,17,62,63]

The majority of the commercial concentrates used for the treatment of hemophilia A are not suitable because they lack high-molecular-weight multimers and, therefore, fail to correct the bleeding time.[23,64] Humate-P is a commercial concentrate that contains sufficient large vWF multimers to provide adequate hemostasis. Many physicians have advocated the use of Humate-P for replacement therapy instead of cryoprecipitate.[15,17,65] Koate-HS and Koate-HP have been reported to achieve clinical hemostasis prior to surgery.[66] A vWF concentrate has been developed in Europe.[67] *In vitro* characterization of this concentrate has shown a multimer pattern and composition similar to that of plasma.[53]

In mild von Willebrand's disease, DDAVP should be used because any plasma product carries the risk of transmitting hepatitis.[15,17,30,63,68] Intravenous DDAVP, at 0.3 to 0.4 μg/kg over 15 to 30 minutes, usually induces a dose-dependent increase in all factor VIII–related activities, with both factor VIII and vWF increasing fourfold to sixfold. This usually lasts 4 to 8 hours and is effective in mild or moderate type 1 disease and in type 2A disease. The dose may be repeated in 8 to 12 hours, but the response diminishes with repeated treatment. Laboratory monitoring should be initiated if treatment is extended. Intranasal DDAVP also can be considered. The side effects of DDAVP were described under the treatment of hemophilia A.

Patients with mild hemophilia A may also be treated with DDAVP, but patients with either severe type 1 von Willebrand's disease or severe hemophilia do not respond well. In type 2A, DDAVP increases plasma vWF, but the qualitative abnormality is not corrected and the bleeding time may be shortened but not normalized.[63] DDAVP should not be used before the type of von Willebrand's disease is defined by multimeric analysis, because in type 2B, *in vivo* platelet aggregation and severe thrombocytopenia may occur.[66]

Menorrhagia is a frequent problem in women with von Willebrand's disease. Oral contraceptives may be very effective in controlling this symptom. Inhibitors of the fibrinolytic system may be of special value in those tissues rich in fibrinolytic activity such as the ear, nose, and throat region and especially with tooth extractions. Patients with von Willebrand's disease should be encouraged to avoid aspirin and NSAIDs because of their effects on platelet function.

Inhibitors can develop in severe type 3 von Willebrand's disease. In severe bleeding situations, PCC has been used with favorable results. Plasmapheresis is another approach used in these situations.[62]

TABLE 92–9. Replacement Therapy in von Willebrand's Disease[a]

Condition	Therapy
Major surgery	Maintain factor VIII level ≥ 50% for 1 wk Prolonged treatment in type 3 patients (up to 10 d)
Minor surgery	Maintain factor VIII level ≥ 50% for 1–3 d Maintain factor VIII level > 20%–30% for additional 4–7 d
Dental extraction	Single infusion to reach factor VIII level > 50%
Spontaneous or posttraumatic bleeding	Usually single infusion (20–40 U/kg)

[a]The yield of factor VIII after first infusion is similar to that observed in hemophilia A (about 2% increment over basal level for 1 U/kg of factor VIII infused).
Adapted from Ref. 93, with permission.

Evaluation of Therapeutic Outcomes

Hemorrhagic manifestations will depend on the type and severity of the disease; thus, to provide optimal management, it is instrumental to know the subtype of von Willebrand's disease and the patient's prior response to therapy if available. Currently, the goal in the treatment of von Willebrand's disease is to improve factor VIII and bleeding time (Fig. 92–3). The choice of cryoprecipitate, Humate-P, or DDAVP will depend on the von Willebrand's disease subtype and the severity of the bleeding episode. Awareness of common side effects and how to respond to them must be part of the treatment plan. Patient education is needed regarding self-management of superficial bleeding with pressure maneuvers or topical hemostatic agents. If DDAVP is indicated, proper storage and adequate subcutaneous administration techniques must also be covered. Good oral hygiene can prevent mucosal bleeding. Patients should avoid activities that can predispose them to bleeding. Risks of complications during surgery will depend on the type of procedure and the subtype of von Willebrand's disease; these factors will also determine the replacement product to use and duration of therapy. Awareness of aspirin-containing products and over-the-counter NSAIDs would ensure patient avoidance of these products and prevention of bleeding episodes.

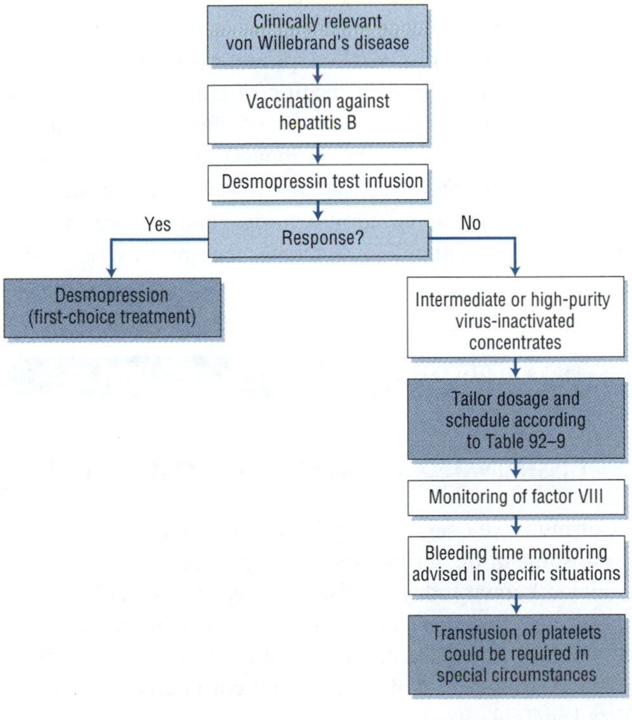

FIGURE 92–3. Guidelines to the treatment of von Willebrand's disease. In the setting of gastrointestinal bleeding, the use of concentrates able to completely or partially correct bleeding times, such as "Haemate P" or "8Y," is recommended; desmopressin could be used after concentrate infusion. *(Adapted from Ref. 93, with permission.)*

Other Congenital Factor Deficiencies

In addition to deficiencies in factors VIII and IX, congenital deficiencies in fibrinogen, in factors II, V, VII, X, XI, XII, XIII, contact factors, and combinations of factor deficiencies have been reported to form multiple defects.[69] Contact factor abnormalities, including deficiencies in factor XII (the Hageman factor) and prekallikrein (Fletchers factor), prolong the APTT but do not lead to any bleeding diathesis. The only contact factor deficiency that causes bleeding diathesis is factor XI deficiency. Most other deficiencies are inherited as autosomal recessive disorders and are rare. Some patients with abnormal molecules, such as fibrinogen, may have an increased tendency to develop thromboembolic disease. The usual treatment for these deficiencies is fresh-frozen plasma, although there may be instances in which PCC is necessary to treat factor II, VII, or X deficiencies. Cryoprecipitate may be used to treat a fibrinogen deficiency (Table 92–10).[31,65]

Complications of Replacement Therapy

Transmission of blood-borne viruses is always a concern when blood and blood-derived products are used. The infection of a large number of hemophiliac patients with hepatitis viruses and HIV during the 1980s prompted the development of virucidal methods to inactivate infectious agents.[23] All currently available factor concentrates undergo donor screening and viral inactivation methods in an effort to minimize donor exposure in patients who do require large amounts of factor. The most common method of inactivation is heat treatment, which includes dry and wet heat. Wet heat is applied while the concentrate is in suspension or in solution (pasteurization) and appears to be more effective than dry heat. Other methods of viral inactivation include chemical (solvent/detergent) and affinity chromatography with monoclonal antibodies. These methods effectively eliminate lipid-coated viruses such as HIV and hepatitis B; however, there is still some risk of acquiring blood-borne viruses.[70] Hepatitis A virus has been transmitted in Europe. Protein-coated viruses such as B19 parvovirus are not inactivated by current methods.[23] This last one can be a concern for the HIV-positive hemophiliac, because of the potential for chronic anemia in patients with immune deficiency.

Other complications associated with factor administration include allergic reactions, fever, chills, urticaria, and nausea. Factor concentrates also contain blood group isoagglutinins (anti-A or anti-B) and, when administered in large amounts to patients with blood group A or B, hemolysis can occur.

In addition to the complications listed previously, PCC also has the potential for causing thromboembolic phenomenon (deep vein thrombosis, pulmonary embolism, myocardial infarction, disseminated intravascular coagulation)

TABLE 92–10. Replacement Therapy for Coagulation Factor Deficiency

Factor	Desired Hemostatic Level in Bleeding Surgical Patients	*In Vivo* Recovery	Biologic Half-Life	Therapeutic Dose	Component or Derivative
Fibrinogen	50–100 mg/dL	50%–70%	72–144 h	1 unit cryoprecipitate per 5 kg body weight	Cryoprecipitate (100–250 mg fibrinogen/bag)
Prothrombin	10%–25%	50%	48–120 h	10–20 mL plasma per kg weight	Plasma or PCC
Factor V	10%–30%	~80%	4.5–36 h (avg: 12 h)	20 mL fresh-frozen plasma per kg body weight, then 2–6 mL fresh-frozen plasma per kg body weight every 12 h × 5–10 d	Fresh-frozen plasma
Factor VII	> 10%	100%	2–5 h	10–20 mL plasma per kg body weight every 12 h	Plasma or PCC
Factor X	10%–40%	50%–95%	20–42 h	10–20 mL plasma per kg body weight, then 3–6 mL plasma per kg body weight every 12 h	Plasma or PCC
Factor XI	20%–30%	90%	40–80 h	10–20 mL plasma per kg body weight, then 5 mL/kg body weight daily	Plasma
Factor XIII	< 5%	50%–100%	12 d	4–6 bags cryoprecipitate or 500 mL plasma every 3 wk	Cryoprecipitate or plasma

Modified from Ref. 31, with permission.

thought to be secondary to the presence of activated vitamin K–dependent factors. Antifibrinolytics should be avoided in patients receiving PCC to avoid thrombotic complications.[71]

Porcine factor VIII, used in patients with inhibitors to factor VIII, is not known to transmit hepatitis or HIV. However, allergic-type reactions including fever, chills, skin rashes, nausea, and headaches have been reported. Patients who experience these reactions may be treated with hydrocortisone and/or diphenhydramine.[72]

Recombinant factor VIII lacks the risk of transfusion-transmitted diseases associated with human factor VIII. Newly diagnosed hemophiliacs or those who are HIV seronegative would benefit most from this product. Adverse effects with these products include metallic taste, mild dizziness, mild rash, burning at the infusion site, and a small drop in blood pressure.[25,26]

PHARMACOECONOMIC CONSIDERATIONS

The lack of prospective comparative trials for the treatment of hemophilia makes it difficult to objectively evaluate the optimal approach for this disease. The selection of factor concentrate remains a matter of clinician preference. Prevention of hermathroses and subsequent joint injury has been achieved through prophylactic regimens. This has the potential to positively impact patient lifestyle and integration into society. These benefits should be weighed against the increased use of factor concentrate and subsequently increased cost, the need for permanent venous access, and patient compliance with weekly infusions. A prospective study evaluating the impact of this modality is ongoing and will aid in answering these issues.

No pharmacoeconomic information is available to guide the treatment of vWD. Optimal management of vWD starts with adequate identification of patient's disease type. DDAVP should be the treatment of choice for all patients responsive to the test dose. Intranasal or subcutaneous formulations are preferred to the intravenous formulation. These allow for home administration and a more independent lifestyle without significantly compromising clinical efficacy.

ACQUIRED COAGULATION DISORDERS

DISSEMINATED INTRAVASCULAR COAGULATION

"Consumptive coagulopathy" and "defibrination syndrome" were some of the terms used in the past to describe the phenomena known today as disseminated intravascular coagulation (DIC).[73] This is a serious complication of several clinical disorders and can be acute or chronic. Some known clinical settings in which acute and chronic DIC occurs are listed in Table 92–11.

Although the causes for DIC can be diverse, once the triggering event is provided the pathophysiology leading to DIC is the same. An overwhelming insult will lead to the

TABLE 92–11. Conditions Associated With Disseminated Intravascular Coagulation

Infectious	Obstetrics	Pulmonary
Bacterial	Amniotic fluid embolism	Adult respiratory distress syndrome
Gram-negative	Placental abruption	Pulmonary embolism
Gram-positive	Missed abortion	Pulmonary infarction
Mycoplasmal	Eclampsia	Hyaline membrane disease
Rickettsial	Malignancy	Miscellaneous
Rocky Mountain spotted fever	Leukemia	Snake bite
Viral	Most carcinomas	Heat stroke
Cytomegalovirus	Other	Hypothermia/hyperthermia
Hepatitis	Pheochromocytoma	Organic solvent poisoning
Varicella	Myeloma	Aspirin poisoning
Chlamydial	Sarcomas	Fat embolism
Psittacosis	Neuroblastoma	Severe anoxia
Fungal	Histiocytosis X	Liver disease
Aspergillosis	Polycythemia vera	Hematologic
Candidiasis	Intravascular hemolysis	Sickle cell crisis
Histoplasmosis	Hemolytic transfusion reaction	Paroxysmal nocturnal hemoglobinuria
Mycobacterial	Minor hemolysis	Collagen vascular disease
Protozoal	Massive transfusion	Immune complex
Malaria (falciparum)	Cardiovascular	Anaphylaxis
Tissue injury	Postcardiac arrest	Systemic lupus
Burns	Aortic aneurysm	
Extensive surgery	Prosthetic device (aortic balloon)	
Crush injuries	Giant hemangiomas	
Multiple trauma	Acute myocardial infarction	
Head trauma	Peripheral vascular disease	

From Ref. 75, with permission.

formation of thrombin and plasmin beyond the control of the regulatory systems. This process is summarized in Figure 92–4. Once thrombin is formed, it leads to the cleavage of fibrinopeptide A and B from fibrinogen, leaving a fibrin monomer. The monomer polymerizes into a clot, leading to microvascular and macrovascular thrombosis. Thrombosis will ultimately decrease blood flow to multiple organs, leading to organ damage. Plasmin, also circulating systemically, cleaves fibrinogen into fibrinogen degradation products (FDPs). FDPs can combine with the fibrin monomer before polymerization and the monomer becomes solubilized (also known as soluble fibrin monomer), impairing hemostasis and leading to hemorrhage. Also, some of the FDP may adhere to platelets, causing platelet dysfunction that may contribute to clinically significant hemorrhage. In addition, plasmin is a proteolytic enzyme that can degrade factors V, VIII, IX, XI, and other plasma proteins. Circulation of plasmin can activate the complement system, leading to red cell and platelet lysis. The activated complement system also increases vascular permeability that can cause hypotension and shock.[73,74]

Acute DIC is characterized by a rapid and extensive depletion of coagulation factors and inhibitors as well as evidence of excessive fibrinolysis, which presumably is an attempt to compensate for microvascular clotting. Normally, a constant, balanced dynamic process of clotting and fibrinolysis operates to prevent organ dysfunction, bleeding, or clotting. In acute DIC, this process is disrupted by some sort of injury that causes excessive intravascular coagulation, overcoming normal inhibitory processes. In subacute or chronic DIC, the balance between depletion and synthesis of coagulation factors in the circulation may make diagnosis difficult.

In summary, bleeding problems observed during DIC can be the product of consumption of coagulation factors during clotting, depletion or dysfunction of platelets, interference in fibrin formation by FDP, and lysis of clots by plasmin. It is important to remember that in parallel with the bleeding process, thrombosis is occurring, and the extent of microvascular obstruction will determine the degree of organ damage.

Clinical Presentation

Acute DIC occurs secondary to many clinical conditions as listed Table 92–11.[73,75] Sepsis is one of the more common causes, and although more frequently linked to gram-negative bacteria, it may occur with gram-positive organisms, fungi, and viruses. Acute DIC may be seen in late pregnancy associated with either abruptio placentae and placenta previa or with a dead fetus or amniotic fluid embolism. Patients who have severe hypotension, who require prolonged surgery, or who suffer tissue injury such as burns or heat stroke may experience DIC.

Subacute and chronic DIC is more commonly associated with malignancies, especially solid tumors. Mucin-producing adenocarcinomas, especially those originating in the gastrointestinal tract or the prostate and sometimes in other organs such as the lung or breast, may be associated

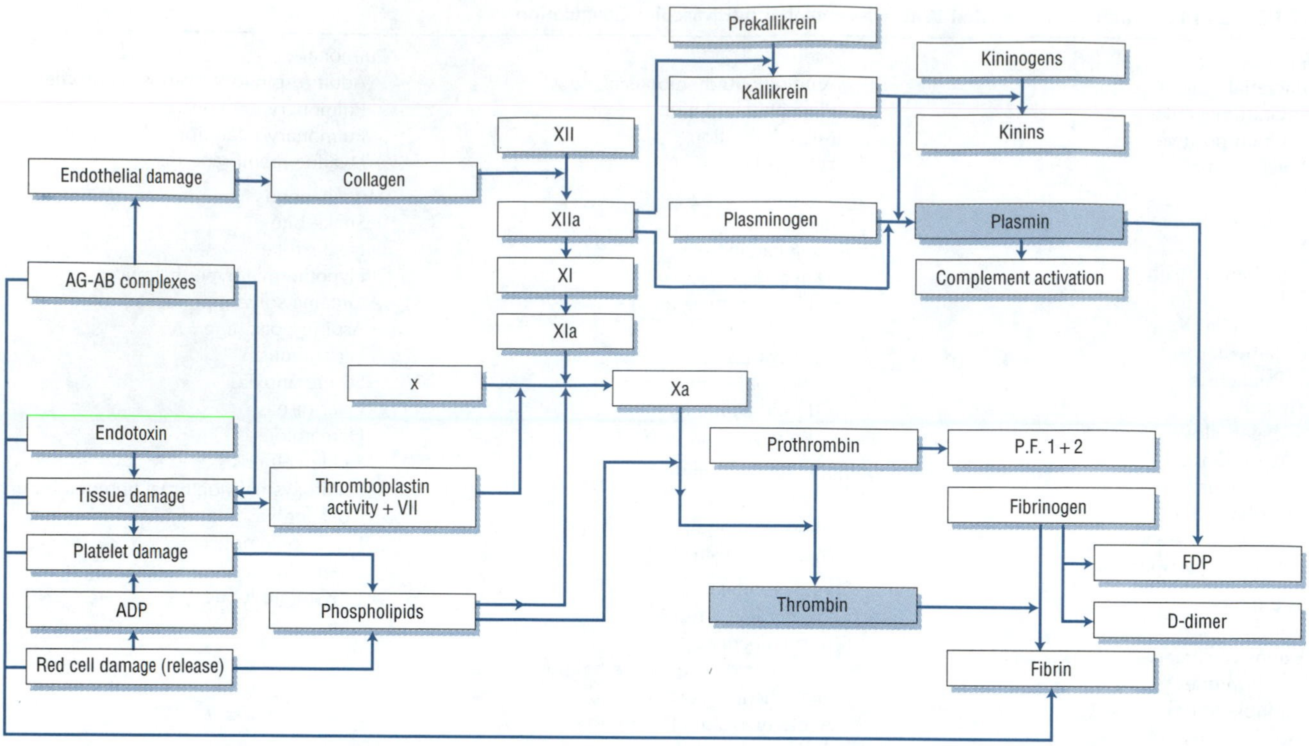

FIGURE 92–4. Triggering mechanisms of disseminated intravascular coagulation. *(From Ref. 73, with permission.)*

with smoldering DIC. Promyelocytic leukemia is almost always associated with DIC to the point that prophylactic treatment has been recommended. In addition, vascular disorders (such as giant hemangiomas) and chronic liver disease have been associated with smoldering DIC.

DIAGNOSIS

Disseminated intravascular coagulation should be suspected on clinical grounds in any of the previously mentioned clinical situations. It should also be considered if the patient develops bleeding from many sites, including oozing from intravenous lines or from invasive procedures. DIC should be suspected with multiple-organ-system failure. Massive bleeding from the gastrointestinal tract or genitourinary system, peripheral cyanosis of the extremities, renal and/or cardiopulmonary failure, or purpura fulminans may dominate the clinical picture.

The laboratory diagnosis of DIC is based on a complete battery of laboratory tests.[73–75] A single laboratory abnormality is insufficient for a diagnosis of DIC. The relative importance of any particular laboratory test is controversial. Routine tests of blood coagulation including PT, APTT, and TT should be done. The PT is usually prolonged, whereas the APTT is more variable and frequently normal. Occasionally, both tests may be decreased rather than increased. The TT is usually prolonged, because of the absolute decrease in fibrinogen as well as the presence of fibrin split products, which inhibit the conversion of fibrinogen to fibrin. D-dimer is a neoantigen formed as a result of plasmin digestion of cross-linked fibrin; thus, D-dimer is a more specific measure of fibrin degradation products. Because liver disease frequently causes abnormalities in these tests, it can be difficult to separate patients who have decreased synthesis of coagulation factors secondary to liver disease from those with DIC.

Fibrinogen levels below 150 mg/dL and platelet counts below 150,000/mm^3 are seen in 95% of DIC patients. In addition, 75% of patients have schistocytes (red blood cell fragments). Unfortunately, these findings may also be observed in severe liver disease and hypersplenism. Depressed antithrombin III, protein C, and protein S levels are seen in most patients. Severe initial decreases in antithrombin III levels is a constant finding in septic DIC, and the degree of suppression correlates with mortality in this group. Fibrin split products are not usually greater than 100 μg/dL in chronic liver disease but are quite elevated in patients with DIC; thus, this finding is more specific. Mild elevations in fibrin split products may be seen in many other inflammatory diseases and in association with hematomas and deep vein thrombosis, but these are usually less than 40 μg/dL.

Paracoagulation tests, such as the ethanol gelation or the protamine sulfate precipitation test, measure fibrin monomers and should be specific for DIC but are of low specificity in most series. Factor VIII and V levels should be decreased in DIC; however, these tests may be quite variable. The most specific findings are a low platelet count associated with elevated fibrin split products and depressed antithrombin III and fibrinogen levels. Because the generation of thrombin is the sine qua non of DIC, it would be useful to measure thrombin in plasma. Thrombin cleaves fibrinopeptides A and B from fibrinogen; thus, fibrinopeptides A and B should be elevated in patients with DIC. Initial studies of fibrinopeptide A in patients suspected of having DIC have shown a good correlation, but other inflammatory conditions such as systemic lupus erythematosus, infections, and thrombosis may also result in elevated levels, thus decreasing the specificity of this test.

▶ TREATMENT: Disseminated Intravascular Coagulation

The diagnosis of DIC is very difficult, and if left unrecognized it may lead to death as a result of hemorrhage and/or thrombosis. Because of the different mechanisms and clinical manifestations that can occur with DIC, controversy regarding optimal treatment exists. However, there is a consensus that the most important step in the treatment of DIC is treatment of the underlying disease (Table 92–12).[73–75] In a pregnant woman with abruptio placentae or retained placenta in whom the disease is self-limited, delivery of the fetus with the products of conception usually returns hemostasis to normal. In those patients who have overwhelming sepsis or shock, antibiotics and treatment of hypotension are the mainstays of therapy. In patients who are receiving maximum treatment for the underlying condition, but in whom the process is worsening or in whom bleeding develops, either replacement of deficient factors or the use of anticoagulants has been tried. Fresh-frozen plasma provides volume to expand intravascular space and replaces clotting factors including fibrinogen. If hypofibrinogenemia is severe, cryoprecipitate may be useful, because in addition to the factor VIII in each unit there is a significant amount of fibrinogen. Although it has been argued that replacement of coagulation factors "adds fuel to the fire," in practice this does not appear to make the situation worse, and frequently hemostasis is improved. Antithrombin III (which should remove thrombin from the circulation) is present in fresh-frozen plasma and may be beneficial.

The use of purified antithrombin III has been evaluated in septic shock with DIC.[76] Administration of antithrombin III did not have a significant impact on mortality, although a trend toward improved mortality was observed. Doses used in this trial were higher than doses recommended for replacement: 90 to 120 IU/kg was the loading dose followed by a continuous infusion of 100 IU/kg. When antithrombin III was administered to critically ill patients with low-level DIC, it did not have any impact on hemostasis or clinical outcomes.[77] Based on these trials and anecdotal experiences, the routine use of antithrombin III for all patients with DIC is not recommended at this time.

TABLE 92–12. Sequential Therapy for Disseminated Intravascular Coagulation

Individualize therapy Site(s) and severity of hemorrhage Site(s) and severity of thrombosis Hemodynamic status Age	Stop intravascular clotting problem Subcutaneous or intravenous heparin Antithrombin concentrate Antiplatelet agents ?
Treat or remove triggering process	Inhibit residual fibrino(geno)lysis EACA
Component therapy as indicated Fresh-frozen plasma Antithrombin concentrate Platelet concentrates Packed red cells Cryoprecipitate	

Adapted from Ref. 73.

Anticoagulation is controversial in patients with DIC, and specific guidelines are not available.[73,74,78] The main pathogenic factor of DIC is considered to be the generation of intravascular thrombin. Interference of thrombin activity with an agent such as heparin appears to be a logical therapeutic step. The main advantage of heparin is to prevent further consumption of hemostatic factors, since it has no influence on already established microthrombus within the vasculature. Because the major complication of heparin therapy is bleeding, some experts argue against the anticoagulation of patients with an already existing bleeding disorder. There are numerous anecdotal reports of improvement in individual patients, but controlled clinical studies are lacking. Heparin has not been shown to reduce morbidity or mortality in uncontrolled series. Heparin rarely restores the coagulopathy to normal, although both the deficiency of coagulation factors and the thrombocytopenia may improve. If the patient does not respond to the replacement of coagulation factors, heparin followed by factor replacement may improve the coagulopathy. If the patient has an underlying condition that can be brought under control, improvement of the coagulopathy may provide sufficient time for the DIC to abate.

Heparin may be given either as an intravenous bolus (every 4 hours) or as a continuous intravenous infusion via pump. The dose of heparin in DIC is controversial, ranging anywhere from full-dose to low-dose heparin.[73] Full-dose heparin requires that 5000 units as intravenous bolus be administered followed by a continuous infusion at 1000 U/h or weight-based heparin dosing. Some experts advocate the use of low-dose heparin such as 500 U/h and adjusting the dose based on clinical and laboratory data. Low-dose subcutaneous heparin of 80 to 100 U/kg every 4 to 6 hours has been used with success.[73] It is difficult to monitor the APTT, because it is often elevated before initiation of heparin therapy. Therefore, it is best to follow fibrin degradation products and fibrinogen levels.

Clinical situations in which heparin may be useful have been identified. These include patients who have progressive organ dysfunction, evidence of dermal necrosis or ischemia, retained dead fetus syndrome, aortic aneurysms, or hemangiomas and patients who require replacement of hemostatic factors. Anticoagulation is contraindicated in patients who have evidence of bleeding into a closed space (intracranial, intraperitoneal, pericardial).[78]

Heparin with replacement of coagulation factors, including fresh-frozen plasma, cryoprecipitate, and platelets, has been recommended routinely for patients with acute promyelocytic leukemia. In those patients with metastatic carcinoma of the prostate, in whom hormonal therapy may be very efficacious, prophylactic anticoagulation prior to hormonal therapy may be life-saving if the patient has DIC.[78]

Antifibrinolytics, such as EACA, have been used in patients in whom the dominant clinical picture is one of excessive fibrinolysis.[73,75] It is important that an accurate distinction between defibrination and fibrinolysis be made prior to institution of antifibrinolytic agents. Because EACA can increase fibrin deposition, many experts believe that it is contraindicated more often than not. Most clinicians prefer to use EACA only in conjunction with heparin, unless the patient has recently had cardiopulmonary bypass surgery or has carcinoma of the prostate, the two clinical conditions in which isolated fibrinolysis without generation of thrombin has been well documented. In patients with chronic liver disease, who manifest dominant fibrinolysis, inhibition of the fibrinolytic system has been attempted but is generally unsuccessful.

The procoagulant role of tumor necrosis factor-α (TNF-α) has been proposed as a cause of DIC in sepsis.[79] Treatment against TNF-α such as monoclonal antibodies may prove to be helpful against DIC in the future. Other treatment modalities may include infusion of protein C, the use of protease inhibitors like gabexate mesylate (FOY), or the use of thrombin inhibitors like dermatan sulphate.[80–82]

EVALUATION OF THERAPEUTIC OUTCOMES

The management of DIC is surrounded with controversy and the optimal approach to these patients is still to be determined. Diagnosis and treatment of the underlying disease should be the goal in all cases. Determination, if possible, of the dominant process between hemorrhage and thrombosis can help focus the treatment approach toward the dominant process. This is often impossible, however, leading to the institution of replacement therapy of the deficient clotting factors and an attempt to control the clotting problems with agents such as heparin. Table 92–12 delineates a sequential approach for DIC, although it is important to remember that treatment for each patient must be individualized.

Risk versus benefit should be considered at the start of any given therapy along with contraindications of the therapy for each patient. Monitoring therapy with laboratory tests can be difficult because the underlying process can cause a variety of laboratory abnormalities. For example, monitoring heparin using APTT can be a complex task, especially when the patient has an abnormal baseline APTT; in this case, monitoring fibrinogen and D-dimer to adjust therapy may be more useful. In addition, it is important to combine laboratory parameters with clinical assessment to make rational treatment adjustments. Aggressive hemodynamic stabilization and other supportive measures to prevent development of organ failure are also important in the overall management and outcome of these patients, especially since the development of organ failure carries a poor prognosis.

VITAMIN K DEFICIENCY

Vitamin K_1 is necessary for carboxylation of factors II, VII, IX, and X to make complete γ-carboxyglutamic acid molecules from glutamic acid residues.[83] When vitamin K deficiency occurs, the inactive precursors of these coagulation factors, which do not bind calcium, accumulate in the plasma and act as vitamin K antagonists. These have been called protein-induced vitamin K antagonists. Vitamin K is also necessary for the active form of protein C, which inhibits the activated factor V and VIII molecules. In most clinical situations, vitamin K deficiency causes a bleeding diathesis as a result of the marked deficiency of factors II, VII, IX, and X.

Vitamin K is found in green vegetables and is synthesized by bacteria in the large intestine. Naturally occurring vitamin K_1 is fat soluble, but the synthetic analogs are water soluble so that they may be administered parenterally.

ETIOLOGY

HEMORRHAGIC DISEASE OF THE NEWBORN

Infants may become deficient in vitamin K because of the absence of this vitamin in human milk and because their gut has not had sufficient time to be colonized by bacteria. In addition, some infants may be too immature to have the ability to synthesize vitamin K–dependent clotting factors from the liver. These infants may bleed from the umbilical cord, from the gastrointestinal tract, or occasionally into the brain after birth.

The risk for bleeding originally was thought to be during the first week of life, but it can occur up to the 12th week of life. Risk factors identified for late hemorrhagic diseases of the newborn include exclusive breast-feeding and failure to give vitamin K. The use of oral vitamin K_1 in Japan and Europe is associated with a higher incidence of late hemorrhagic diseases of the newborn. It has been hypothesized that intramuscular vitamin K_1 acts as a depot preparation and may explain the low rate of late-onset hemorrhagic diseases.[84] This remains a speculation that needs to be confirmed in a prospective study. The committee on Fetus and Newborn of the American Academy of Pediatrics recommends that all infants receive prophylactic vitamin K_1 at birth, preferably using parenteral formulations.[85]

Although the normal neonate has a mild deficiency of coagulation factors, if vitamin K deficiency exists, the vitamin K–dependent factors are usually less than 25% of normal. In this situation the PT and APTT are prolonged, but TT, fibrinogen, and platelet count are normal. Levels of vitamin K–dependent factors will substantiate the diagnosis.

Infants usually respond to 1 mg of vitamin K_1 parenterally on the first day, which can be repeated every 8 hours until the clotting tests have returned to normal. If there is life-threatening hemorrhage, fresh-frozen plasma should correct the defect immediately. In the United States, it is a common practice to use prophylactic parenteral vitamin K_1 on obstetric units.

MALABSORPTION

Patients may become vitamin K deficient because of poor nutrition or malabsorption.[86] A careful dietary history is important in this regard. Patients with a poor diet may have other manifestations of malabsorption, such as vitamin deficiencies and anemia. Broad-spectrum antibiotics may sterilize the large intestine postoperatively, and if vitamin K_1 is not administered, the patient may become vitamin K deficient even more quickly.

Malabsorption resulting from diseases of the small intestine such as celiac disease, amyloidosis, Whipple's disease, and short-bowel syndrome may cause abnormal development in children, weight loss, muscle wasting, and steatorrhea, as well as other manifestations of malnutrition such as vitamin deficiencies and anemia. Significant malabsorption can occur even without symptoms of diarrhea or steatorrhea, requiring quantitation of fat excretion to confirm the presence of malabsorption.

Severe vitamin K deficiency is also seen in obstructive jaundice, in which bile salts do not reach the small intestine and therefore vitamin K cannot be absorbed. Patients with malabsorption from small-bowel disease or obstructive jaundice require parenteral administration of vitamin K. Vitamin K_1 10 mg weekly is usually sufficient.

▶ TREATMENT: Vitamin K Deficiency

The treatment of vitamin K deficiency is vitamin K_1. The dose, frequency, and duration of vitamin K_1 depend on the severity of the deficiency and the patient's response.[86] The dose of vitamin K_1 ranges from 2 to 25 mg and may be administered orally, intramuscularly, subcutaneously, or intravenously. After an oral dose of vitamin K_1 one can expect an increase in blood coagulation factors 6 to 12 hours later. Even when administered parenterally, the PT will take 24 to 48 hours to normalize. Close monitoring of PT in these patients can help to guide therapy. Failure to correct PT after 48 hours should raise suspicion about the etiology of the coagulation abnormality (e.g., liver disease).

The route of administration is dependent on the severity as well as the etiology of prothrombin deficiency. For instance, in patients with severe hypoprothrombinemia, it is best to avoid the intramuscular route owing to the risk of forming a hematoma. Because of the rare anaphylactic reaction associated with the intravenous route of administration, this route is often restricted to patients who are thrombocytopenic and unable to absorb the drug via the gastrointestinal tract. Vitamin K_1 can be administered subcutaneously to those patients without an intravenous site or postoperatively. In cases of severe hemorrhage, patients should receive fresh-frozen plasma as a source of vitamin K–dependent factors to assure immediate correction. Because patients on long-term total parenteral nutrition (TPN) can become vitamin K deficient, it is good practice to prophylactically add 10 mg of vitamin K_1 to the TPN solution weekly.

Identification of patients at risk for vitamin K deficiency and institution of treatment are key components in pharmaceutical care. Selection of the best route of administration and dose is decisive for an optimal outcome.

LIVER DISEASE

CLINICAL PRESENTATION

Liver disease can be associated with bleeding disorders.[87] The degree of coagulopathy correlates with the degree of hepatocellular disease. The liver synthesizes the majority of blood coagulation factors including fibrinogen (factor I) and factors II, VII, IX, X, XII, XIII, and V. In addition, clotting inhibitors of the fibrinolytic system like plasminogen, α_2-antiplasmin, and α_2-macroglobulin are regulated by the hepatic cells. Furthermore, the clearance of activated clotting or fibrinolytic factors and of end products of the fibrinogen–fibrin conversion can be impaired, leading to a fibrinolytic state. Decreased platelet count and function are fairly common findings in liver disease. In addition to the defect in synthesis of these coagulation factors, DIC may occur. The development of DIC can potentially have an additive effect to the coagulopathy observed. Patients have a poor prognosis if hepatocellular disease is so severe that a coagulopathy occurs.[88]

PT, APTT, and TT are useful in screening for a deficiency of liver-dependent factors. The PT is sensitive to deficiencies in the vitamin K–dependent factors (factors II, VII, IX, and X). The APTT helps to determine deficiencies in factor IX as well as some other factors. The TT is helpful in detecting hypofibrinogenemia and dysfibrinogenemia as well as the presence of fibrin degradation products that interfere with fibrin polymerization. Another test that is sometimes useful in hepatic disease is the measurement of clotting time using snake venom, which is not affected by heparin. This test indicates the degree of dysfibrinogenemia. Because defects in polymerization may occur before severe hypofibrinogemia, this may be an indication of the degree of liver dysfunction.

Factor V is synthesized by hepatic cells but is not dependent on vitamin K. Therefore, it may be useful in distinguishing vitamin K deficiency from liver disease. The deficiency of antithrombin III occurs with severe hepatocellular disease and may contribute to the development of DIC. Tests of the lytic system, such as an euglobulin clot lysis time, may show increased activity, either because of decreased clearance of fibrinolytic factors or because of DIC. In acute hepatic failure, plasminogen may be low, reflecting both decreased synthesis and increased catabolism associated with DIC.

▶ TREATMENT: Liver Disease

Treatment of the coagulopathy may occur under two different scenarios: overt bleeding or the correction of the coagulation parameters (e.g., PT, APTT) prior to an invasive procedure. In addition, treatment for other conditions (e.g., encephalopathy) may be necessary.

Patients with liver disease should be evaluated with a PT, APTT, TT, and platelet count.[88,89] Although patients can have severe abnormalities in these tests, bleeding may not occur. Patients who are not bleeding should not be treated. Conversely, major bleeding may occur with normal tests secondary to esophageal varices or peptic ulcer disease. To be sure that a vitamin K deficiency is not contributing to the abnormalities, most clinicians administer 10 to 25 mg of vitamin K_1 for one or several days to be sure that the liver is synthesizing to its capacity.

When a patient bleeds in association with a coagulopathy, replacement therapy may decrease bleeding tendency. Overt bleeding requires aggressive management with blood products. Fresh-frozen plasma supplies all the missing coagulation factors, but fluid overload may be a serious problem. Intensive monitoring to determine frequency of administration is needed for each patient and to evaluate signs and symptoms of fluid overload. Usually 1 to 2 units (250 to 500 mL) of fresh-frozen plasma is necessary every 6 hours in a seriously ill patient. Repeated PT or APTT after completion of infusion can be used to determine if extra units are needed. Additional fresh-frozen plasma may be required if the PT or APTT is greater than 1.5 times the upper limits of the control value.[65] If the patient has ascites, the half-life of many of these factors is decreased, and it is difficult to correct the coagulopathy. Prothrombin complex concentrates can be given, but there is an increased risk of precipitating intravascular coagulation and causing DIC if it is not already present. In general, the use of these concentrates is not recommended. Only when the administration of fresh-frozen plasma does not correct the coagulopathy and the patient continues to have serious bleeding should PCCs be considered.

The use of heparin and antifibrinolytic drugs (e.g., EACA) is controversial. EACA has been tried and may be successful, especially with mucosal bleeding from the genitourinary tract; however, acute renal failure may occur. Heparin has not been demonstrated to improve survival and may exacerbate the underlying coagulopathy even if DIC is present. In the few clinical studies that have been done, both controlled and uncontrolled trials have not shown any definite benefit with heparin in severe acute hepatic necrosis. Platelet transfusions may also be necessary if thrombocytopenia occurs secondary to hepatocellular disease and/or hypersplenism.

Antithrombin III concentrates have been evaluated in liver disease with full-blown DIC. Results have been disappointing, with only minor improvement in laboratory abnormalities and no impact on clinical outcomes.[90]

▶ PRINCIPLES OF PHARMACOTHERAPY

- Hemophilia is an inherited bleeding disorder resulting from a congenital deficiency in either factor VIII or IX.
- The goal of therapy for hemophilia is to arrest bleeding when it occurs and to prevent bleeding episodes and their long-term complications.
- Factor concentrates (either plasma derived or recombinant technology products) have largely replaced the use of blood products like cryoprecipitate. Dose and duration of these will depend on the site and severity of bleeding.
- DDAVP can be used in mild cases of hemophilia A or as an adjunct to factor VIII concentrate.
- The goal of therapy on von Willebrand's disease (vWD) is to improve factor VIII levels and to improve bleeding time.
- The use of cryoprecipitate should be reserved for cases of acute bleeding without a type characterization of vWD.
- DDAVP and/or factor VIII concentrate are the agents of choice for the treatment of vWD.
- The optimal approach for patients with disseminated intravascular coagulation remains to be determined. The goal of treatment is to diagnose and treat the underlying disease.
- Prophylactic use of vitamin K_1 can effectively prevent hemorrhagic disease of the newborn.

REFERENCES

1. Bick RL, Murano G. Physiology of hemostasis. Clin Lab Med 1994;14:677–707.
2. Fenton JW, Ofosu FA, Brezniak DV, et al. Understanding thrombin and hemostasis. Hematol Oncol Clin North Am 1993;7:1107–1119.
3. Kottke-Marchant K. Laboratory diagnosis of hemorrhagic and thrombotic disorders. Hematol Oncol Clin North Am 1994;8:809–853.
4. Hassouna HI. Laboratory evaluation of hemostatic disorders. Hematol Oncol Clin North Am 1993;7:1161–1236.
5. Miletich JP. Bleeding time. In: Beutler E, Lichtman MA, Coller BS, Kipps TJ, eds. William's Hematology. New York, McGraw-Hill, 1995: L111–L112.
6. Miletich JP. Prothrombin time. In: Beutler E, Lichtman MA, Coller BS, Kipps TJ, eds. William's Hematology. New York, McGraw-Hill, 1995:L82–L84.
7. Miletich JP. Activated partial thromboplastin time. In: Beutler E, Lichtman MA, Coller BS, Kipps TJ, eds. William's Hematology. New York, McGraw-Hill, 1995:L85–L86.
8. Galanakis DK. Plasma thrombin time and related tests. In: Beutler E, Lichtman MA, Coller BS, Kipps TJ, eds. William's Hematology. New York, McGraw-Hill, 1995:L91–L93.
9. Giannelli F, Green PM. The molecular basis of haemophilia A and B. Baillieres Clin Haematol 1996;9:211–228.
10. DiMichele D. Hemophilia 1996: New approach to an old disease. Pediatr Clin North Am 1996;43:709–736.
11. Hoyer LW. Hemophilia A. N Engl J Med 1994;330:38–47.
12. Lusher JM, Warrier I, Hemophilia A. Hematol Oncol Clin North Am 1992;6:1021–1033.
13. Kurachi K. Furukawa M, Yao S-N, et al. Biology of factor IX. Hematol Oncol Clin North Am 1992;6:991–997.
14. Aledort LM. von Willebrand disease: From the bedside to therapy. Thromb Hemost 1997;78:562–565.
15. Werner EJ. von Willebrand disease in children and adolescents. Pediatr Clin North Am 1996;43:683–707.

16. Roberts HR, Hoffman M. Hemophilia and related conditions: Inherited deficiencies of prothrombin (factor II), factor V, and factors VII to XII. In: Buetler E, Lichtman MA, Coller BS, Kipps TJ, eds. William's Hematology. New York, McGraw-Hill, 1995:1413–1439.
17. Ewenstein BM. von Willebrand's disease. Annu Rev Med 1997;48: 525–542.
18. Larson PJ, High KA. Biology of inherited coagulopathies: Factor IX. Hematol Oncol Clin North Am 1992;6:999–1009.
19. Lozier JN, Brinkhous KM. Gene therapy and the hemophilias. JAMA 1994;271:47–51.
20. Connelly S, Kaleko M. Gene therapy for hemophilia A. Thromb Haemost 1997;78:31–36.
21. Eisensmith RC, Woo SLC. Viral vector-mediated gene therapy for hemophilia B. Thromb Haemost 1997;78:24–30.
22. Kitchens CS. Approach to the bleeding patient. Hematol Oncol Clin North Am 1992;6:983–989.
23. Kasper CK, Lusher JM, The Transfusion Practices Committee. Recent evolution of clotting factor concentrates for hemophilia A and B. Transfusion 1993;33:422–434.
24. Lusher JM, Arkin S, Abildaard CF, Schawartz RS, the Kogenate Previously Untreated Patient Study Group. Recombinant factor VIII for the treatment of previously untreated patients with hemophilia A. N Engl J Med 1993;328:453–459.
25. Bray GL, Gomperts ED, Courter S, et al. A multicenter study of recombinant factor VIII (Recombinate): Safety, efficacy, and inhibitor risk in previously untreated patients with hemophilia A. Blood 1994; 83:2428–2435.
26. Recombinant antihemophilic factor. Med Lett Drugs Ther 1993;35: 51–52.
27. Goldsmith JC. Rationale and indications for continuous infusion of antihemophilic factor (factor VIII). Blood Coagul Fibrinolysis 1996; 7(suppl 1):S3–S6.
28. Morfini M, Messori A, Longo G. Factor VIII pharmacokinetics: Intermittent infusion versus continuous infusion. Blood Coagul Fibrinolysis 1996;7(suppl 1):S11–S14.
29. Martinowitz UP, Schulma S. Continuous infusion of factor concentrates: Review of use in hemophilia A and demonstration of safety and efficacy in hemophilia B. Acta Haematol 1995;94(suppl 1): 35–42.
30. Lethagen S. Desmopressin (DDAVP) and hemostatis. Ann Hematol 1994;69:173–180.
31. Menitove JE, Gill JC, Montgomery RR. Preparation and clinical use of plasma and plasma fractions. In: Beutler E, Lichtman MA, Coller BS, Kipps TJ, eds. William's Hematology. New York, McGraw-Hill, 1995:1649–1663.
32. Rodeghiera F, Castaman G, Manucci PM. Prospective multicenter study on subcutaneous concentrated desmopressin for home treatment of patients with von Willebrand disease and mild hemophilia A. Br J Haematol 1996;92:973–978.
33. Package insert. Stimate® (desmopressin acetate) nasal spray. Rhône-Poulenc Rorer. Collegeville, PA, 1994.
34. Rose EH, Aledort LM. Nasal spray desmopression (DDAVP) for mild hemophilia A and von Willebrand disease. Ann Intern Med 1991;114: 563–568.
35. Nilsson IM, Berntorp E, Löfquist, Petersson H. Twenty-five years' experience of prophylactic treatment in severe haemophilia A and B. J Intern Med 1992;232:25–32.
36. Lovqvist T, Nilson IM, Berntorp E, et al. Haemophilia prophylaxis in young patients: A long-term follow-up. J Intern Med. 1997;241: 395–400.
37. Lusher JM. Prophylaxis in children with hemophilia: Is it the optimal treatment? Thromb Haemost 1997;78:726–729.
38. Aledort LH, Haschmeyer RH, Petterson H, the Orthopaedic Outcomes Study Group. A longitudinal study of orthopaedic outcomes for severe factor-VIII-deficient haemophiliacs. J Intern Med 1994;236: 591–599.
39. Roberts HR, Eberst ME. Current management of hemophilia B. Hematol Oncol Clin North Am 1993;7:1269–1279.
40. Kim HC, McMilan CW, White GC, et al. Purified factor IX using monoclonal immunoaffinity technique: Clinical trials in hemophilia B and comparison to prothrombin complex concentrates. Blood 1992; 79:568–575.
41. Djulbeqovic B, Hannan NM, Bergman GE. Concomitant treatment with factor IX concentrates and antifibrinolytics in hemophila B. Acta Haematol 1995;94(suppl 1):43–48.
42. White GC, Beebe A, Nielsen B. Recombinant factor IX. Thromb Haemost 1997;78:261–265.
43. Bray G. Inhibitor questions: Plasma-derived factor VIII and recombinant factor VIII. Ann Hematol 1994;68:S29–S34.
44. Hay CRM, Colvin BT, Ludlam CA, et al. Recommendations for the treatment of factor VIII inhibitors: From the UK Haemophilia Centre Directors' Organisation Inhibitor Working Party. Blood Coagul Fibrinolysis 1996;7:134–138.
45. Rosendal FR, Nieuwenhuis HM, Berg VD, et al. A sudden increase in factor VIII inhibitor development in multitransfused hemophilia A patients in the Netherlands. Blood 1993;81:2180–2186.
46. Brettler DB. Inhibitors in congential haemophilia. Baillieres Clin Haematol 1996;9:319–329.
47. Gilles JGG, Jacquemin MG, Saint-Remy J-MR. Factor VIII inhibitors. Thromb Haemost 1997;78:641–646.
48. Hoyer LW, Scandella D. Factor VIII inhibitors: Structure and function in autoantibody and hemophilia A patients. Semin Hematol 1994;31: 1–5.
49. Ludlam CA, Morrison AE, Kessler C. Treatment of acquired hemophilia. Semin Hematol 1994;31:16–19.
50. Kessler CM. Factor VIII inhibitors: An algorithmic approach to treatment. Semin Hematol 1994;31:33–36.
51. Brackman MH, Oldenburg J, Schwabb R. Immune tolerance for the treatment of factor VIII inhibitors—Twenty years "Bonn Protocol." Vox Sang 1996;70(suppl 1):30–35.
52. Cohen AJ, Kessler CM. Acquired inhibitors. Bailliere's Clin Haematol 1996;9:331–354.
53. Hedner U, Glazer S. Management of hemophilia patients with inhibitors. Hematol Oncol Clin North Am 1992;6:1035–1045.
54. Kasper CK. The therapy of factor VIII inhibitors. In: Zimmerman TS, Rugerri ZM, eds. Coagulation and Bleeding Disorders: The Role of Factors VIII and von Willebrand Factor. New York, Marcel Dekker, 1989:59–75.
55. Hay CRM, Laurian Y. Induction of tolerance using porcine factor VIII. Vox Sang 1996;70:(suppl 1):68–69.
56. Hedner U. Dosing and monitoring Novoseven treatment. Haemostasis 1996;26(suppl 1):102–108.
57. Lindley CM, Sawyer WT, Macik BG, et al. Pharmacokinetics and pharmacodynamics of recombinant factor VIIa. Clin Pharmacol Ther 1994;55:638–648.
58. Hilgartner MW. Factor replacement therapy. In: Hilgartner MW, Pochedly C, eds. Hemophilia in the Child and Adult. New York, Raven Press, 1989:1–26.
59. Ruggeri ZM. Stucture and function of von Willebrand factor: Relationship to von Willebrand disease. Mayo Clin Proc 1991;66:847–861.
60. Bloom AL. Von Willebrand factor: Clinical features of inherited and acquired disorders. Mayo Clin Proc 1991;66:743–751.
61. Saddler JE. A revised classification of von Willebrand disease. Thromb Haemost 1994;71:520–525.
62. Aledort LM. Treatment of von Willebrand's disease. Mayo Clin Proc 1991;66:841–846.
63. Scott JP, Montgomery RR. Therapy of von Willebrand disease. Semin Thromb Hemost 1993;19:37–47.
64. Mannucci PM, Tenconi PM, Castarman G, Rodeghiero F. Comparison of four virus-inactivated plasma concentrates for treatment of severe von Willebrand disease: A crossover randomized trial. Blood 1992;79:3130–3137.
65. Fresh-Frozen Plasma, Cryoprecipitate, and Platelets Administration Practice Guidelines Development Task Force of the College of American Pathologists. Practice parameters for the use of fresh-frozen plasma, cryoprecipitate, and platelets. JAMA 1994;271:777–781.

66. Hanna WT, Bonna RD, Zimmerman CE, et al. The use of intermediate and high purity factor VIII products in the treatment of von Willebrand disease. Thromb Haemost 1994;71:173–179.
67. Menache D, Aronson DL. New treatment of von Willebrand disease: Plasma derived von Willlebrand factor concentrates. Thromb Haemost 1997;78:566–570.
68. Lusher JM. Response to 1-deamino-8-D-arginine vasopressin in von Willebrand disease. Haemostasis 1994;24:276–284.
69. Bolton-Maggs PHB. The rarer inherited coagulation disorders: A review. Blood Rev 1995;9:65–76.
70. Sharpiro CN. Transmission of hepatitis viruses. Ann Intern Med 1994;120:82–84.
71. Scharrer I. The need for highly purified products to treat hemophilia B. Acta Haematol 1995;94(suppl 1):2–7.
72. Hay CRM, Lozier JN, Lee CA, et al. Porcine factor VIII therapy in patients with congenital hemophilia and inhibitors: Efficacy, patient selection, and side effects. Semin Hematol 1994;31:20–25.
73. Bick RL. Disseminated intravascular coagulation. Objective criteria for diagnosis and management. Med Clin North Am 1994;78: 511–543.
74. Risberg B, Andreasson S, Erickson E. Disseminated intravascular coagglutation. Acta Anaesthesiol Scand 1991;35:S60–S71.
75. Gilbert JA, Scalzi RP. Disseminated intravascular coagulation. Emerg Med Clin North Am 1993;11:465–480.
76. Fourrier F, Chopin C, Huart JJ, et al. Double-blind, placebo-controlled trial of antithrombin III concentrates in septic shock with disseminated intravascular coagulation. Chest 1993;104:883–888.
77. Diaz-Cremades JM, Lorenzo R, Sanchez M, et al. Use of antithrombin III in critical patient. Intensive Care Med 1994;20:577–580.
78. Feinstein DI. Treatment of disseminated intravascular coagulation. Semin Thromb Hemost 1988;14;351–362.
79. Levi M, ten Cate H, van der Poll T, van Deventer SJH. Pathogenesis of disseminated intravascular coagulation in sepsis. JAMA 1993;270: 975–979.
80. Okajima K, Imamura H, Koga S, et al. Treatment of patients with disseminated intravascular coagulation by protein C. Am J Hematol 1990;33:277–278.
81. Cofrancesco E, Boschetti C, Leonardi P, Gianese F, Cortellaro M. Dermatan sulphate for the treatment of disseminated intravascular coagulation (DIC) in acute leukaemia: A randomized, heparin-controlled pilot study. Thromb Res 1994;74:65–75.
82. Okamura T, Niho Y, Itoga T, et al. Treatment of disseminated intravascular coagulation and its prodromal stage with gabexate mesilate (FOY): A multicenter trial. Acta Haematol 1993;90:120–124.
83. Shearer MJ. Vitamin K. Lancet 1995;345:229–234.
84. Loughnan PM, McDougall PN. Does intramuscular vitamin K_1 act as an unintended depot preparation? J Pediatr Child Health 1996;32: 251–254.
85. Greer FR. Vitamin K deficiency and hemorrhage in infancy. Clin Perinatol 1995;22:759–777.
86. Marcus R, Coulston AM. Fat-soluble vitamins: Vitamins A, K, and E. In: Hardman JG, Limbird LE, Molinoff PB, Ruddon RW, Gilman AG, eds. Goodman & Gilman's The Pharmacological Basis of Therapeutics. New York, McGraw-Hill, 1996:1573–1590.
87. Mammen EF. Coagulation defects in liver disease. Med Clin North Am 1994;78:545–554.
88. Castelino DJ, Salem HH. Natural anticoagulants and the liver. J Gastroenterol Hepatol 1997;12:77–83.
89. Violi F, Ferro D, Quintarelli, et al. Clotting abnormalities in chronic liver disease. Dig Dis 1992;10:162–172.
90. Lechner K, Kyrle P. Antithrombin III concentrates—Are they clinically useful? Thromb Haemost 1995;73:340–348.
91. Stead RB. Regulation of hemostasis. In: Goldhaber SZ, ed. Pulmonary Embolism and Deep Vein Thrombosis. Philadelphia, Saunders, 1985:28–40.
92. Lammle B, Griffin JH. Formation of the fibrin clot: The balance of procoagulant and inhibitory factors. Clin Haematol 1985;14:282–342.
93. Castaman G, Rodeghiero F. Current management of von Willebrand's disease. Drugs 1995;50:602–614.

93

Sickle Cell Anemia

Clarence E. Curry, Jr., PharmD, and Eula D. Beasley, PharmD

Although Herrick[1] has generally been credited with the discovery of sickle cell anemia (SCA), Konotey-Ahulu[2] has presented evidence that the problem had been recognized in Africa by Ghanaians long before the earliest description offered in the medical literature after the turn of the twentieth century. Such information suggests that SCA is not a distinctly modern problem, as once thought. Since the time of Herrick's description, SCA has been well characterized through the advances of molecular biology and related disciplines, such as protein chemistry.

It was Nobel laureate Linus Pauling and his coworkers,[3] using moving boundary electrophoresis, who reported that hemoglobin from a patient with SCA had a mobility different from that of hemoglobin from a normal adult. As a result, the hemoglobin of SCA patients was referred to as sickle hemoglobin or hemoglobin S (Hb-S) and the hemoglobin of normal individuals, hemoglobin A (Hb-A). The door had been opened for greater exploration leading to better treatment options.

EPIDEMIOLOGY

A common misconception is that sickle hemoglobin is found only in people of African heritage. However, it also occurs in a wide area including the Mediterranean region, parts of Greece and Italy, as well as India, Iran, and Turkey. Serjeant[4] has noted that sickle hemoglobin is becoming more common in the United Kingdom, France, the Netherlands, Belgium, and Germany. Central America and South America also are affected.

Hemoglobin S is the most frequently found sickle gene among the black population in the United States, where the frequency of sickle cell trait is about 8% and that of sickle cell disease (SCD) is 1 in 400. Hemoglobin C (Hb-C) is found chiefly in west and northern Africa or in descendants of people from this area, with the highest frequency in northern Ghana.[5] Hb-C has a frequency of about 3% in the U.S. population. Other abnormal hemoglobins seen in various areas are hemoglobin E (Sri Lanka, Malaysia, Thailand, Cambodia, Laos, Burma, Indonesia, Vietnam, and the Philippines) and hemoglobin D (India, Pakistan, Afghanistan, and Iran). Of all the sickle hemoglobin genes, Hb-S is the most common.

For years it has appeared that sickle cell trait offered a degree of protection against malarial infection. Abnormal red blood cells (RBCs) are less easily parasitized by *Plasmodium falciparum* than are normal RBCs. Consequently, reports have suggested that persons who are heterozygous for the sickle gene (trait) have a selective advantage in regions (tropical areas) where malaria is hyperendemic.[6] However, later observations have shown that adults with the trait, unlike children, were sick more often from this infection than adults with Hb-C or normal homozygotes.[7] It now appears that the advantage of individuals carrying the trait over those with normal hemoglobin is a limited one, occurring especially during the early childhood years before the child has developed a substantial degree of acquired immunity from his or her own antibody production.[8]

Patients having SCA must inherit two genes for the S hemoglobin. Figure 93–1 illustrates the genetic profiles possible for offspring of parents with normal hemoglobin, sickle cell trait, and SCA. A person with entirely normal hemoglobin is designated AA. A person with the sickle cell trait is designated AS. Sickle cell anemia is represented as SS. When one parent has normal hemoglobin and the other carries the sickle cell trait (example one), the children may have either normal hemoglobin or sickle cell trait. No child from this union would have SCA. When both parents carry the trait (example two), there is a 50% chance a child will carry sickle cell trait, a 25% chance a child will have SCA, and a 25% chance the child will have normal hemoglobin. If one parent has SCA and the other parent has normal hemoglobin (example three), all offspring from their union have a 50% chance of having SCA and a 50% chance of carrying sickle cell trait (example four). The union of two persons with SCA, if able to produce offspring, would produce only children with SCA.[9]

ETIOLOGY

The biochemical defect that leads to the development of hemoglobin S involves the substitution of valine for glutamic acid as the sixth amino acid in the β-polypeptide chain. Hemoglobin C, another abnormal hemoglobin commonly included in the sickle cell disease group, is produced by the substitution of lysine for glutamic acid as the sixth amino acid in the β-chain (Fig. 93–2).

The α-chains of Hb-S, Hb-A, and Hb-C are structurally identical. Therefore, sickling and the related sequelae can be explained on the basis of the chemical difference in the β-chain. When deoxygenated, both Hb-S and Hb-A have similar physical properties in dilute solutions; however, in concentrated solutions, deoxygenated Hb-S is insoluble and forms a gel, whereas deoxygenated Hb-A remains soluble. This solubility difference represents the physiochemical basis for sickling.

A

Hb-A

Position 1 2 3 4 5 6* 7

β-chain valine–histidine–leucine–threonine–proline–glutamate–glutamate

B

Hb-S

Position 1 2 3 4 5 6* 7

β-chain valine–histidine–leucine–threonine–proline–valine–glutamate

C

Hb-C

Position 1 2 3 4 5 6* 7

β-chain valine–histidine–leucine–threonine–proline–lysine–glutamate

FIGURE 93–1. The sixth-position (*) amino acid in the β-chain differentiates **(A)** Hb-A from **(B)** Hb-S and **(C)** Hb-C.

PATHOPHYSIOLOGY

In the pathogenesis of sickle cell disease, three known problems appear to constitute the basis of the various clinical manifestations: impaired circulation, destruction of RBCs, and stasis of blood flow. These three problems probably relate directly to two major disturbances involving RBCs. The first involves damage to the membrane of the RBCs containing hemoglobin S. These cells may lose potassium and water, leading to a dehydrated state that enhances the formation of sickled forms. After continually repeating this process, the RBC membrane probably retains greater quantities of calcium and develops a more rigid form, that of an irreversibly sickled cell (ISC).

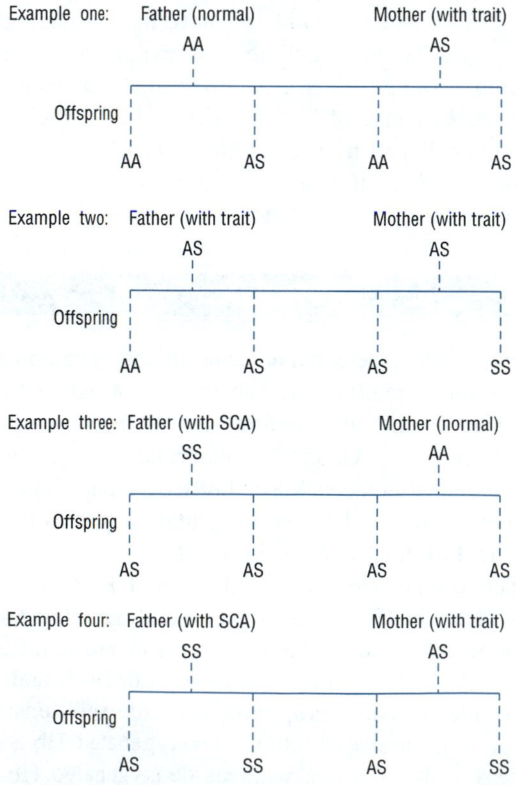

FIGURE 93–2. Inheritance scheme for the sickle gene. A = hemoglobin A (normal) and S = hemoglobin S (sickle hemoglobin).

When the blood of patients with sickle cell disease is deoxygenated, blood viscosity increases. This second disturbance has been related to an alteration of the flow properties of RBCs containing polymerized hemoglobin S. The polymerization process is a manifestation of the β-chain substitution of valine for glutamic acid.[7] Polymerization allows deoxygenated hemoglobin molecules to exist as a semisolid gel. This process is affected by small changes in mean corpuscular hemoglobin concentration (MCHC). Temperature, pH, and the oxygen affinity of the RBCs all contribute to the deoxygenation process. These cells have more difficulty deforming themselves than normal cells and, as a result, remain more rigid, retarding their flow, particularly through the microcirculation. Evidence suggests that significant amounts of intracellular polymerized Hb-S, enough to bring about a change in normal erythrocyte flow, may exist at oxygen saturation levels as high as 80% to 90%[10]; however, such a finding has yet to be specifically related to the actual clinical events in a SCA patient. The presence of sickled RBCs increases blood viscosity and encourages sludging in the capillaries and small venous vessels. Such obstructive events lead to local tissue hypoxia, which tends to accentuate the pathologic process. Other events, such as the elevation of fibrinogen or globulin level, or both, also increase blood viscosity and, thus, would aggravate the hematologic environment in the sickle cell patient (e.g., during infections).[11] The cycle of sickling and unsickling that occurs in response to variations in oxygen tension results in loss of the cell membrane containing hemoglobin. This sickle–unsickle cycle leads to loss of membrane flexibility and to production of the ISC. Membranes of ISCs are permanently deformed regardless of the oxygenation state of the hemoglobin within the cell.

The normal life span of a red blood cell is 120 days. The typical sickled cell survives for about 10 to 20 days. Intravascular destruction of sickle cells may occur at an accelerated rate in this disease. In view of the various stresses of circulation, including rigid deoxygenated cells and repetitive sickle–unsickle cycles, cell fragmentation is a likely result.[12]

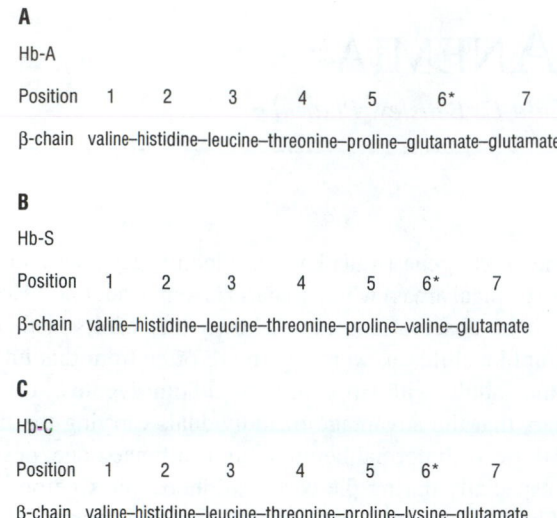

It has been known for a number of years that some cells of patients with sickle cell disease contain increased amounts of hemoglobin F (Hb-F) or fetal hemoglobin. Fetal hemoglobin is the primary hemoglobin present in the fetus from mid to late gestation. It binds oxygen more tightly than hemoglobin A. Fetal hemoglobin does not appear to participate in the gelling of deoxygenated Hb-S. Red blood cells containing Hb-F sickle less readily than cells with Hb-S. In contrast, ISCs exhibit a lower concentration of Hb-F and a higher MCHC. ISCs are also smaller than other red cells of patients with SCA. Increased levels of fetal hemoglobin moderate or even ameliorate the disease in some patients, thereby producing more benign forms of SCA.

The pathogenesis of a number of clinical manifestations associated with sickle cell disease is not easily attributed directly to the sickling phenomenon. Other factors may be responsible. For example, impairment in reticuloendothelial function in SCA may be noted early in the sickle cell disease patient owing to functional asplenia, loss of splenic function with an intact spleen. This defect may be related to the increased susceptibility of many of these patients to infection by encapsulated organisms (particularly pneumococcal disease) and to disseminated intravascular coagulation (DIC).[11] Patients with SCA have a deficient pneumococcal opsonization, although the exact nature of the defect is unclear.[13,14]

CLINICAL PRESENTATION

In the patient who is homozygous for Hb-S, the anemia usually appears from 4 to 6 months after birth. Symptoms are delayed because the infant's RBCs contain mainly fetal hemoglobin (Hb-F). Fetal hemoglobin's oxygen-carrying ability and its lesser propensity to engage in sickling prevents the development of early clinical symptoms. Still, sufficient quantities of Hb-S are present at birth to allow a diagnosis to be made by hemoglobin electrophoresis. As RBC turnover occurs during those early months, RBCs containing Hb-F are replaced by cells containing Hb-S. This replacement process typically leads to attacks of pain frequently accompanied by fever. Pneumonia is often a common initial symptom and splenomegaly a common finding. Many cases initially present with pain and swelling of the hands and feet. This condition is commonly referred to as "hand-and-foot syndrome" or dactylitis. Many states have established newborn screening programs for SCA and other hemoglobinopathies along the lines of the long-standing PKU screening.[15] Newborn screening is an important strategy because it affords the opportunity for earlier preventive and therapeutic methods to be applied. However, it is important to note that commonly used tests (Sickledex, Sickleprep) do not differentiate between patients who have the sickle cell trait and those with sickle cell disease. Hemoglobin electrophoresis is required for confirmation. Also, high levels of fetal hemoglobin may interfere with the screening assay. Alternatively, direct analysis of DNA obtained from amniotic fluid can provide a prenatal diagnosis.

The term *sickle cell disease* (SCD) does not exclusively imply that the patient is homozygous for hemoglobin S (Hb-SS). Sickle cell anemia is a form of SCD in which both abnormal genes code for formation of hemoglobin S; however, varying degrees of anemia may be present in other variants of SCD.

As previously noted, a person who carries sickle cell trait has one normal gene (A) and one abnormal gene (S, C, D). Such a person would not belong in the SCD group. A person with a genotype of AS is often referred to as a heterozygote; however, caution must be exercised because the heterozygous states can be pathologic, especially sickle-C and sickle-thalassemia. β-Thalassemia is often found in conjunction with Hb-S. β^+-Thalassemia usually leads to a milder course than the homozygous SS state. β^0-Thalassemia leads to a course similar to that of the homozygous SS patient. In addition, several haplotypes characterize the β^s-gene, resulting in differing clinical and hematologic courses. Included among these types are the three most commonly found in the United States: the Central Africa Republic (CAR) haplotype, characterized by severe disease; the Atlantic West African Senegal (SEN) haplotype, characterized by mild disease; and the Central West African Benin (BEN) haplotype, characterized by a course intermediate to the other two haplotypes. Although there are a number of other haplotypes seen around the world, the remaining major types include Saudi Arabian (Saudi) and Cameroon (CAM). Both of these types usually result in milder courses.[16]

Hemoglobin disorders can be screened by hemoglobin electrophoresis on cellulose acetate, followed by solubility testing for sickling in all blood samples showing anything other than the usual Hb-A. If such tests suggest the presence of abnormal hemoglobin patterns, confirmation should be sought with such methods as citrate agar electrophoresis, quantitation of hemoglobin fractions, alkali denaturation, and family studies.[17]

Persons with sickle cell trait are usually asymptomatic, although some clinical signs and symptoms have occasionally been associated with sickle cell trait. An impairment of renal function, which probably arises from the sickling of RBCs, tends to promote a more dilute urine. Such patients may be at some risk of dehydration during periods in which the body normally conserves water, such as hot and dry weather. Hematuria has also been noted and probably also relates to sickling within the kidney.

Castro and Scott[18] have shown that a group of persons with sickle cell trait had a small but statistically significant decrease in RBC size and in MCHC; however, the decreases did not affect the blood hemoglobin or hematocrit levels. The cause is unknown. Although some persons with sickle cell trait may experience abnormalities under certain conditions, these instances are not routine and trait carriers are not considered to have clinical disease.

The usual clinical signs and symptoms associated with Hb-SS disease include chronic anemia, fever and pallor, arthralgia, scleral icterus, abdominal pain, weakness, anorexia, fatigue, enlargement of liver and heart, and hematuria. Infants may show enlargement of the spleen. The typical Hb-SS patient exhibits reduced Hgb and increased reticulocyte count. The platelets and leukocytes are usually increased and a peripheral smear demonstrates sickle forms. Contrast this with the picture of Hb-SC disease, which is characterized primarily by mild anemia (hemoglobin levels above 9 g/100 mL), infrequent episodes of pain, persistence of splenomegaly into adult life, and excessive target cells in the peripheral blood smear.

These patients experience delays in growth and sexual maturation (Table 93–1). Both height and weight are usually below average. There is also a tendency toward a reduced level of fertility. Female patients show some menstrual abnormalities more often than normal women.[19] Other typical physical characteristics include a protuberant abdomen with exaggerated lumbar lordosis. There is usually an asthenic appearance with rather long extremities and tapered fingers. The chest is frequently barrel shaped. One report indicates that despite having abnormal tests for bone age, zinc, and somatomedin c, no correlation could be established with growth status. As a result, it was concluded that nutritional factors alone could not explain poor growth in SCD patients.[20]

SICKLE CELL CRISIS

Chronic hemolytic anemia in the SCD patient is periodically interrupted by crises. Crises are more common in childhood than in adulthood for the average patient. Patients with Hb-SS disease experience crises more often on average than patients with Hb-SC disease or some other variants. Fever, infections, dehydration, hypoxia, acidosis, and sudden temperature alterations often precipitate crises. Often, multiple factors are at work in bringing about a crisis. The time between crises is called the steady-state period, and patients not in crisis are said to be in the steady state.[2] Clinically, four types of crises are generally described (Table 93–2).

APLASTIC CRISIS

The bone marrow becomes hypoplastic. There may be associated pain. There is a definite drop in reticulocytes accompanied by a rapidly developing severe anemia. The crisis is often thought to be caused by a viral infection. The presenting patient is most often under the age of 18.

HEMOLYTIC CRISIS

The patient affected shows a rate of hemolysis even greater than that usually present. Hemoglobin and RBC levels fall, often without a change in the number of reticulocytes and with a hyperplastic bone marrow. This crisis may be accompanied by pain and fever. An increase in the icteric state is usually observed. This condition may be confused with glucose-6-phosphate dehydrogenase (G6PD) deficiency particularly during a febrile episode when antipyretics are used.[21]

SEQUESTRATION CRISIS

This crisis is described as a sudden massive enlargement of the spleen and liver, resulting from the sequestration by these organs of blood from the reticuloendothelial system. There is a dramatic fall in hematocrit and hemoglobin concentration, with no evidence of marrow failure and accelerated hemolysis. The trapping of the sickled red cells by the spleen also leads to a drop in circulating blood volume, resulting in hypotension and shock. The condition is most often seen in infants and children because they have intact spleens that have not undergone multiple infarctions and fibrosis. Because repeated infarctions lead to autosplenectomy as the disease progresses, the incidence of this type of crisis declines as adolescence approaches. These crises are a cause of sudden death in young children. It is rarely seen in adult Hb-SS patients but may be seen in adult Hb-SC or sickle cell thalassemia patients.[22]

VASO-OCCLUSIVE (INFARCTIVE) CRISIS

This most common type of crisis has a number of clinical manifestations. Pain usually occurs over the involved areas, but there may be no change in hemoglobin or other laboratory values. Laboratory changes that may be seen include leukocytosis, increased serum fibrinogen, and decreased serum pH and bicarbonate. A study of pain in SCD has concluded that early death is associated with the number of pain episodes in patients older than 20 years. Adult patients

TABLE 93–1. Delayed Growth and Sexual Maturation in Sickle Cell Disease

Growth is delayed in both sexes, in variant as well as homozygous SCA.

Weight is more affected than height; delays are more significant in children > 7 years.

Adolescents with homozygous disease, on the average, experience a 2-year delay in sexual maturation.

No pituitary–hypothalamic axis abnormalities have been demonstrated.

The degree of anemia correlates positively with a delay in growth.

Nutritional factors (intake, requirements, absorption, and utilization) are thought to be important in the delayed growth process. Mechanisms are yet undetermined.

Adapted from Wethers DL. Delayed growth and sexual maturation in SCD. Ann NY Acad Sci 1989;565:137–142.)

TABLE 93–2. Manifestations of Sickle Cell Disease: Crises and Complications

Crisis	Characteristic
Vaso-occlusive	Infarction/pain
Hemolytic	Massive hemolysis
Sequestration	Sequestration of red blood cells
Aplastic	Bone marrow failure
Organ System	**Complication**
Pulmonary	Acute chest syndrome
Neurologic	Various, including cerebrovascular accident
Dermatologic	Chronic ulcers
Cardiovascular	Hypertrophy
Genitourinary	Priapism, hematuria, hyposthenuria
Skeletal	Aseptic necrosis, osteomyelitis
Ocular	Retinal problems
Hepatic	Cholelithiasis

with three or more episodes of pain per year had a higher death rate than those with fewer than three episodes per year.[23] Painful crises may have numerous possible precipitating factors including dehydration, muscular exertion, emotional upset, and changes in climate. The following are the usually observed manifestations:

- *Sickle cell dactylitis (hand-and-foot syndrome).* This condition occurs in infancy and early childhood, in which the dorsal aspects of the hands and feet, as well as the fingers and toes, swell. The episodes are painful and accompanied by erythema. There usually is no permanent damage.
- *Involvement in joints and extremities.* This form of crisis may be caused by areas of infarction over long bones or of periarticular tissues of the larger joints. Often, the pain mimics that of rheumatic fever. Pain may migrate from one site to another. Mild temperature elevations may be noted.
- *Abdominal involvement.* This involvement may simulate an acute abdominal process, suggesting surgical intervention. The episodes are usually related to areas of infarction in abdominal structures. The pain may be severe and episodic in nature. Although the usual duration is about 3 or 4 days, protracted courses are occasionally encountered. Low-grade fever is often present.
- *Hepatic involvement.* This element of crisis is characterized by a rise in the serum bilirubin level well beyond the steady-state value, as some degree of hyperbilirubinemia is common in SCD. It is associated with right upper-quadrant pain. Widespread intrahepatic sickling may occur, leading to hepatocellular necrosis and swelling. Such an extensive occurrence could be fatal. These severe obstructive jaundice processes, as well as episodes of cholelithiasis, must be distinguished early in affected patients. Hepatic crises are seen more often in the older sickle cell patient.
- *Pulmonary involvement.* Lung infarctions occur in both children and adults. Children seem to have pulmonary episodes most often as a result of infection. It may sometimes be very difficult to distinguish between infection and infarction and, indeed, both may be present. Infection is usually caused by pneumococcus; infarction is often related to embolization from sickled RBCs or pieces of necrotic bone marrow tissue.

COMPLICATIONS

Acute chest syndrome is the pulmonary illness that occurs in SCD patients and is characterized by cough, dyspnea, chest pain, fever, pulmonary infiltration, and an equivocal response to antibiotic therapy.[24] Pulmonary infarcts seem more often to involve the lower lobes of the lungs and are a frequent cause of pleural effusions. Pneumonia appears to occur most often in the middle and upper lobes. These pulmonary manifestations can and do occur in the absence of bone, joint, or abdominal pain. There is some degree of disagreement over the predominant cause of acute chest syndrome. Oppenheimer and Esterly[25] reviewed autopsy findings on 36 patients with sickle cell anemia; intimal proliferation and pulmonary infarcts had occurred in more than 20% of the cases. Sprinkle and associates[24] reviewed 100 cases in children and found little evidence of bacterial infection to support the clinical picture seen. These data contrast dramatically with those of Barrett-Conner,[26] who showed pulmonary infarction in only 5% of 66 cases. Furthermore, intravascular fluid overload with pulmonary edema can occasionally simulate sickle cell lung disease in the sickle cell patient hospitalized for other causes.[27] Sudden death can occur after the occlusion of large vessels in the absence of infarction. Pulmonary edema has been a common finding in patients who have died suddenly, the pulmonary capillaries of such patients being overly distended from packed sickled cells.[28]

Neurologic abnormalities can occur in both adults and children. Vaso-occlusive processes occasionally lead to cerebral vascular occlusion in which patients show signs and symptoms similar to those of stroke. These include drowsiness, paralysis, transitory or permanent blindness, aphasia, visual disturbances, spinal cord infarction, and convulsions. The onset is usually sudden, but occasionally may be gradual. Milder symptoms may occur as a result of vascular stasis. Some patients recover rapidly and completely. Others are left with permanent neurologic deficits.

Chronic leg ulcers are a difficult problem and a common finding in many young adults with Hb-SS disease. The inner aspect of the lower leg just above the ankle seems to be the site most often affected. Ulcers are often seen after trauma or infection. They are usually slow to heal (several weeks to a year).

Cholelithiasis is a common occurrence in the SCD patient. It is seen more frequently and at a younger age than in the general population. It is the result of the chronic hemolysis that occurs in increased bilirubin production. Cholecystitis, exemplified by pain in the right iliac fossa, can be confused with abdominal pain crises.[29]

As with any anemia, cardiovascular abnormalities, including cardiac enlargement and various murmurs, occur. Patients complain of various degrees of exertional dyspnea, tachycardia, and palpitation owing to the decreased oxygen-carrying capacity of the system. Effects are most prominent in Hb-SS disease.

Priapism is a very painful complication that develops in certain male patients. It is caused by sickling in the sinusoids of the penis. This produces a sustained painful erection that might last several hours or several days. Impotence has been reported after repeated episodes. An interesting syndrome has been reported to occur in some priapism patients.[30] Called ASPEN (Association of Sickle Cell Disease, Priapism, Exchange Transfusion and Neurological Events), it occurs after partial exchange transfusion to treat priapism and is characterized by severe headache and other neurologic symptoms ranging from seizures to obtundation that requires ventilation.

Destructive bone and joint problems are frequently seen. Aseptic necrosis, particularly of the femoral or humeral heads, causes permanent damage and disability. This problem is seen both in patients with Hb-SS disease and in heterozygous patients. Patients are also susceptible to an increased incidence of osteomyelitis. The organism most often responsible is *Salmonella.*

Ocular problems occur in the form of transient monocular blindness, visual field defects from retinal hemorrhage, retinal detachment, vitreous hemorrhage, venous microaneurysms, and neovascularization in the adult. Patients with Hb-SC disease are most likely to suffer from these disorders.

Renal complications include unilateral hematuria and hyposthenuria. Death from renal disease is unusual except in long-term survivors.

▶ TREATMENT: Sickle Cell Anemia

DESIRED OUTCOME

Although a cure for SCD has been elusive, both longevity and general quality of life can be positively affected by appropriate, comprehensive care. This includes long-standing use of prophylactic and symptomatic general supportive care as well as judicious use of newer more specific therapies aimed at altering hematologic capacity and function. A therapeutic overview is shown in Table 93–3.

GENERAL MANAGEMENT

FOLIC ACID

Folic acid demands are increased in sickle cell patients because there is accelerated erythropoiesis. Low serum folate levels are common and megaloblastic changes have been reported. The incidence of megaloblastic anemia in association with SCD, however, is unknown. Although folic acid supplementation has become standard, there are few controlled data evaluating this therapy. Although it is not clear that folic acid supplementation is essential, there exists at least a theoretical argument for prescribing folate supplementation in all sickle cell patients owing to increased demands. A dose of 1 mg/d is most commonly used and is more than adequate for supplementation.[31,32]

PROPHYLAXIS OF PNEUMOCOCCAL INFECTIONS

Administration of the pneumococcal vaccine alone or in combination with prophylactic penicillin may be of benefit in sickle cell patients. Sickle cell patients are more susceptible to infection caused by encapsulated organisms than the general population owing mainly to impairment of splenic function. There is an especially high risk of pneumococcal infections, with sickle cell patients being 300 to 400 times more likely to develop pneumococcal septicemia or meningitis.[33] Several studies have been conducted to evaluate the efficacy of immunization against pneumococcal infections. Results have varied greatly. Prior to 1983, however, the available pneumococcal vaccine was a 14-valent product. It now contains 23 capsular polysaccharide types. Although there are no controlled studies demonstrating decreased morbidity and mortality from pneumococcal infection with the use of the 23-valent product, it is recommended that all patients with sickle cell disease receive the vaccine at 24 months of age or shortly thereafter.[15] Children should be revaccinated 3 to 5 years after initial immunization.

The use of prophylactic penicillin has been shown to decrease the risk of pneumococcal septicemia and meningitis. Early administration of prophylactic penicillin, with therapy preferably begun before the age of 4 months, is suggested in children with sickle cell anemia. It has not been determined how long prophylactic penicillin therapy should be continued.[15] However, Falletta et al found that prophylactic penicillin therapy could be safely stopped at the age of 5 years in children receiving comprehensive care, who had not had a splenectomy or prior severe pneumococcal infection.[34] In patients in whom penicillin therapy is begun in infancy, it is recommended that it be continued indefinitely until a safe discontinuation time is determined by clinical studies. The initiation of therapy in children older than age 5 who have not received previous prophylaxis is probably not required.[15] Regimens that have been used are shown in Table 93–4.[34–37]

Potential noncompliance is a concern with long-term oral penicillin use. The occurrence of pneumococcal septicemia with some subsequent deaths has been reported in patients who were prescribed penicillin, but were noncompliant.[38]

Another concern in the attempt to decrease pneumococcal infections is the increase in the number of penicillin-resistant pneumococcal strains. Drug-resistant strains are far more common now than they were in the past.[39] This will present new challenges in the sickle cell population. Studies are needed to determine appropriate regimens for prophylaxis against these resistant strains.

TABLE 93–3. Treatment Overview

General management	Folic acid, immunizations (+/– prophylactic antibiotics)
Painful crises	Analgesics, hydration
Priapism	Heat, cold, vasoconstrictors, vasodilators
CNS infarction	Transfusions
Acute chest syndrome	Spirometry, analgesics, oxygen if hypoxic
Prophylaxis in selected patients	Hydroxyurea

TABLE 93–4. Pneumococcal Prophylaxis Regimens

Benzathine penicillin	600,000 U IM q month	Ref. 35
Benzathine penicillin	600,000 U IM q 4 weeks for age 6 mo–6 yr; 1.2 mU q 4 weeks for age > 6 yr	Ref. 36
Penicillin V potassium	125 mg bid orally	Ref. 37
Penicillin V potassium	250 mg bid orally	Ref 34

HAEMOPHILUS INFLUENZAE VACCINE

Routine pediatric immunization should include administration of the hemophilus b conjugate vaccine. This is of particular importance in the sickle cell patient because of increased susceptibility to *Haemophilus influenzae* infections. It is currently recommended that an immunization series be initiated at 2 months of age. Doses should be administered at 2 months, 4 months, and 6 months of age, with a booster at age 12 to 15 months. For children age 15 months to 5 years who have not received prior immunization against *H. influenzae*, a single dose should be administered.

TRANSFUSION THERAPY

Transfusion therapy may be of great benefit in some sickle cell patients. Transfusion therapy has been used to treat life-threatening complications of sickle cell disease. Though the benefits of transfusion therapy are relatively clear-cut in some clinical situations, its use in other situations remains controversial.

Transfusions have yielded favorable benefits in patients with central nervous system infarction. Chronic transfusions decrease the chance of further stroke and halt clinical progression.[40] Stroke recurrence rates in children are often as high as 90%. Reduction in recurrence rates to less than 10% have been achieved with chronic transfusion therapy. The optimal protocol for transfusion therapy has not been determined.[41] In the Stroke Prevention Trial in Sickle Cell Anemia (STOP), blood transfusions were given every 3 to 4 weeks to children who were at high risk for strokes, as determined by transcranial doppler. Transfusion therapy yielded a 90% reduction in the rate of stroke.[42] The optimal length of therapy was not determined in this study. Previous data also lacked concrete guidelines on when therapy could be safely discontinued. Stopping transfusions after 1 to 2 years, however, has resulted in a high risk of recurrence of strokes.[41]

Transfusions are also indicated in patients with symptomatic aplastic crises, severe symptomatic anemia, symptomatic splenic sequestration episodes, and severe acute chest episodes with hypoxia. Patients in whom transfusions may possibly be of use include patients undergoing complicated surgery, or patients with complicated obstetric problems. Patients with refractory leg ulcers, refractory painful episodes, acute severe priapism, or multiorgan failure may also benefit from transfusions.[43]

Most sickle cell patients tolerate their anemia well. A low hemoglobin concentration alone is not justification for transfusion therapy. Transfusion therapy is not merited in patients who have stable anemia that is well tolerated. However, the presence of circulatory instability or other clinical dysfunction would justify the use of transfusions.[41,43]

The risks of transfusion therapy must be weighed against possible benefits. Limitations of transfusion therapy include sensitization to the blood received, transfusion-related infections, and iron overload. Sickle cell patients appear to be at increased risk of alloimmunization versus other patients who receive multiple transfusions. Transfusion-related infections, such as hepatitis, can still occur. Routine testing of all blood products for hepatitis B, although reducing the risk, has not completely prevented the transmission of hepatitis B. Administration of the hepatitis B vaccine to young children with sickle cell disease has been recommended by some pediatricians. Although there is some risk of contracting hepatitis C through transfusions, improved testing has dramatically decreased the chances of developing hepatitis C posttransfusion. Extensive donor screening and blood testing have also reduced the risks of transfusion-associated AIDS.[41]

When iron overload occurs as a result of transfusion therapy, desferoxamine, an iron chelator, may be used. Parenteral administration is required. In most cases, compliance to the regimen is poor.[43]

GELATION INHIBITORS

One therapeutic approach that has gained increased attention is the use of gelation inhibitors. The goal with these agents is to inhibit the gelation of deoxyhemoglobin S. This inhibition can be affected by alteration of the sickle hemoglobin. In addition, because gelation is concentration dependent, decreasing the sickle hemoglobin concentration (e.g., by increasing the concentration of fetal hemoglobin) may markedly delay gelation. Many drugs have been considered as possible gelation inhibitors. Hydroxyurea is the most appealing agent.

A significant decrease in crises was seen in patients on hydroxyurea therapy during a double-blind randomized trial. There was also a significant decrease in the development of chest syndrome. The number of patients who required transfusions was also significantly reduced in the hydroxyurea group.[44] There is also some evidence suggesting that long-term use of hydroxyurea may reverse organ dysfunction.[45] It appears that increasing fetal hemoglobin may not be the only mechanism by which hydroxyurea decreases the incidence of painful crises. Contributing mechanisms may include altering properties of red-cell membranes, increasing water content of red cells, increasing deformity of red cells, or decreasing adhesion of red cells to the endothelium.[44] The question, of course, must be answered regarding which patients should receive hydroxyurea therapy. Steinberg[43] suggests that possible candidates may include patients with frequent painful episodes (at least two or three per year) or patients with a history of at least one or two episodes of acute chest syndrome. Other possible candidates include patients with severe symptomatic anemia and patients with leg ulcers resistant to other therapies. Patient age, motivation, compliance, and accessibility for needed laboratory monitoring may also play a role.

The ideal hydroxyurea regimen has not been determined. In a placebo-controlled, double-blind study, which showed benefits when hydroxyurea was used, doses up to 35 mg/kg/d were used. Doses were started at 15 mg/kg/d and then increased by 5 mg/kg/d every 12 weeks until marrow suppression was present. Therapy was then resumed at a dose 2.5 mg/kg/d lower than the dose associated with marrow depression. Although a benefit of therapy was shown, an ideal regimen was not elucidated.[44] Steinberg[43] suggests a starting dose of 500 mg/d with the dose increased cautiously if the patient is toxicity free. He notes that doses of 1000 to 1500 mg/d are required in most patients to achieve the greatest increases in fetal hemoglobin. Patients on hydroxyurea must be closely monitored for myelotoxicity.[44]

Although the ideal therapeutic end point for hydroxyurea therapy would be achieving a decrease in pain or painful episodes, this alone may not be indicative of success or failure due to the unpredictable nature of painful episodes.[46] Doses of hydroxyurea sufficient to cause mild myelosuppression produce marked increases in the percentage of fetal hemoglobin in most sickle cell patients. It has been suggested that the slight neutropenia induced from the use of hydroxyurea may contribute to the drug's efficacy. A correlation between the neutrophil count and the rate of painful crises has been seen. Because laboratory testing for fetal hemoglobin is expensive and not always readily available, Steinberg suggests that monitoring mean corpuscular volume (MCV) could be a reasonable alternative. MCV generally increases as fetal hemoglobin increases. Failure to see an increase in MCV with hydroxyurea therapy may indicate that the marrow is unable to respond. It might also be indicative of an inadequate hydroxyurea dose or noncompliance. Iron deficiency can also prevent or decrease response.[43] It should be noted that it takes several months for the beneficial effects of hydroxyurea to be seen. It appears that hydroxyurea can be used safely if patients are monitored frequently. Data are at present lacking, however, to determine the safety of long-term therapy.[44]

Another agent that may stimulate fetal hemoglobin is butyrate. In a pilot trial, IV administration of arginine butyrate resulted in an increase in fetal hemoglobin production. Minimal side effects were seen. Further studies of this agent are warranted.[47] Likewise, clotrimazole is being investigated for a possible role in sickle cell treatment. Although the drug may cause a desired decrease in cell density, it is unclear whether it will be clinically useful in the treatment of sickle cell anemia.[43]

PENTOXIFYLLINE

Researchers have reported a significant decrease in the number of painful crises in patients who received pentoxifylline. For example, one study that used a pentoxifylline regimen of 400 mg orally three times per day showed a significant decrease in the number and severity of painful crises. Not all studies, however, have yielded positive results. Although pentoxifylline may find a place in preventive therapy of sickle cell crises, it does not appear to have a role in the actual treatment of a crisis that is already in process.[48]

BONE MARROW TRANSPLANTATION

Bone marrow transplantation (BMT) has yielded remarkable results in the treatment of sickle cell anemia. Allogenic BMT from a matched sibling donor has resulted in cure of the disease. There have been more than 50 successful transplants in children and young adults. Bone marrow transplantation, however, has several limitations. There are a limited number of patients for whom there is an HLA-matched sibling without the disease. In addition, there is a 10% transplant-related mortality rate. Graft rejection and graft-versus-host disease are also a concern, with a reported incidence of up to 20%. The cost of such a procedure may also be prohibitive.[15]

ERYTHROPOIETIN

Erythropoietin, when given in large doses, may have a beneficial effect on fetal hemoglobin. Combination with hydroxyurea has yielded mixed results, however. Additionally, therapy is very costly. Due to limited and conflicting data, erythropoietin therapy is not at present an accepted therapeutic approach.[49]

PRIAPISM

Initial treatment of priapism should involve providing appropriate analgesic therapy and reducing anxiety. Morphine and hydroxyzine may be used to achieve these goals. Hydration should also be initiated. Both ice packs and hot baths have been used in the treatment of priapism. Some have noted that the use of ice packs, however, may be painful. Heat may be beneficial by increasing blood flow; however, it is not effective in all types of priapism. Although transfusions have been used, the usefulness of this therapeutic intervention has not been established.[50]

Both vasoconstrictors and vasodilators have been used in the treatment of priapism. Vasoconstrictors, such as phenylephrine or epinephrine, are proposed to exert their benefit by forcing blood out of the cavernosa into the venous return. Epinephrine use has been associated with increases in heart rate and blood pressure. Additionally, repeated uses of α-adrenergic agents, such as epinephrine, may cause a worsening of the ischemia of the cavernosa. β-Agonists and hydralazine, in contrast, produce relaxation of the smooth muscle of the vasculature. It is suggested that this relaxation allows oxygenated arterial blood to enter the cavernosa. This arterial blood displaces or washes out the damaged sickle cells that are stagnant in the cavernosa.[50] For persistent penile erection, a subcutaneous dose of terbutaline 0.25 to 0.5 mg has been given every 4 to 6 hours. An oral regimen of 2.5 to 5 mg every 4 to 6 hours is another option suggested by the investigators.[51,52] More invasive approaches to the treatment of priapism include aspiration and irrigation of the cavernosa and the use of vascular shunts.[50]

Some therapeutic agents have been used to prevent recurrent attacks of priapism. Stilbesterol is one such agent. The effective dose of stilbesterol, however, varied not only among patients, but also within patients with requirements sometimes fluctuating with time.[53] Levine and Guss[54] reported the successful use of monthly injections of a gonadotropin-releasing hormone analog in a patient who experienced recurrent episodes of painful erections. Resolution of priapism persisted for more than a year with continued therapy.

IDIOPATHIC UNILATERAL RENAL HEMATURIA

In cases of idiopathic unilateral renal hematuria, a high fluid intake should be maintained to prevent clotting and urethral colic. Iron therapy may be needed if blood loss continues. If blood loss is brisk, transfusions may be necessary. Nephrectomy should be considered only in cases involving massive hemorrhaging.

ACUTE CHEST SYNDROME

In patients with acute chest syndrome, frequent use of spirometry has been recommended. The use of incentive spirometry at least every 2 hours has been advocated. In addition, proper management of pain is important. The goal is to provide relief while avoiding analgesic-induced hypoventilation. Appropriate fluid therapy should avoid overhydration, which may worsen respiratory distress. Oxygen therapy should be used for patients who are hypoxic or in acute distress. Transfusions are often used in the treatment of acute lung disease. Although transfusions appear to be effective, conflicting data do exist. Hydroxyurea administration, chronic transfusions, and BMT may be of use in preventing recurrences of acute chest syndrome in selected patients.[55]

MANAGEMENT OF CRISES

VASO-OCCLUSIVE CRISIS

Although hydration and analgesia are the mainstays of treatment for vaso-occlusive (painful) crises, there is no consensus on specific guidelines for their use. Fluid replacement at a rate of 3 to 4 L/d has been recommended. This can be given intravenously if necessary. Oral replacement, however, can be used if feasible.[43] The superiority of a given intravenous fluid has not been established. Overhydration should be avoided because vigorous intravenous fluid therapy has been associated with the development of pulmonary edema in some hospitalized patients.[24]

Despite the common and frequent use of analgesics in sickle cell patients, controlled studies to determine the optimal regimen are lacking. Although meperidine has frequently been used in sickle cell crises, morphine is now considered by many practitioners to be the drug of choice. Morphine has the advantage of having a longer duration of action than meperidine. It is available in a wide variety of formulations. Morphine's use also avoids the possible problems resulting from accumulating normeperidine, a meperidine metabolite. Such accumulation is a potential toxicity to which sickle cell patients are especially prone. Nor-meperidine accumulation can cause anxiety, tremor, and seizures. Morphine does have a metabolite that can accumulate with repetitive doses, especially in renally compromised patients. This metabolite, however, is not associated with the same type of toxicities as is nor-meperidine. Nonetheless, there have been reports of fatal pulmonary failure in sickle cell patients treated with morphine. Hydromorphone is another option in treating severe sickle pain.[56] Care should be exercised in determining dosing regimens that achieve the desired therapeutic effect without producing oversedation or respiratory depression.

Administering analgesics on an as-needed basis does not provide effective pain control. Opioids should be administered on a scheduled basis. Continuous intravenous infusions of narcotics and the use of patient-controlled analgesia are good alternatives.[56,57] Patient-controlled analgesia combines the advantages of providing steady analgesic blood concentrations with the ability to administer additional doses as needed.

Because crises may be precipitated by infection, an infectious etiology should be ruled out in presenting patients. Appropriate empiric therapy should be initiated in patients with high fever or patients who appear critically ill. Sickle cell patients are particularly prone to infection caused by pneumococcus, *H. influenzae,* and *Salmonella* species.

Although hospitalization is necessary for severe crisis, milder cases may be treated on an outpatient basis with rest, hydration, warmth, and oral analgesics.[57] Oral analgesic options include nonsteroidal anti-inflammatory drugs (NSAIDs) or acetaminophen generally in combination with codeine or a codeine derivative. Strong opioids such as morphine or hydromorphone may be necessary for more severe pain.

SEQUESTRATION CRISIS

Splenic sequestration crisis is a major cause of mortality in young sickle cell patients. The sequestration of red cells in the spleen may result in a rapid drop of hematocrit, leading to hypovolemia, shock, and death. Acute treatment includes whole-blood transfusion to correct hypovolemia. Broad-spectrum antibiotic therapy, which includes coverage for pneumococcus and *H. influenzae,* may also be warranted, because infection may precipitate crises. The indications for splenectomy are controversial. Splenic sequestration crises tend to recur, however, and prompt splenectomy remains a treatment option. Splenectomy is probably indicated, even after a single sequestration crisis, if that event is life threatening. Repetitive episodes, even if less serious, also may merit a splenectomy. For children less than 2 years of age, chronic blood transfusions have been recommended to prevent sequestration and allow delay of splenectomy until the age of 2, when risk of postsplenectomy septicemia becomes less.[15,58]

APLASTIC CRISIS

Treatment of aplastic crisis is primarily supportive. Blood transfusions may be needed if the anemia that develops is severe. The patient should also be receiving folic acid supplementation, because folic acid deficiency has been implicated as a cause of aplastic crisis. Although it is possible that a bacterial infection may precipitate aplastic crisis, it is more likely that a virus, probably a parvovirus, is the precipitating factor.[33,58] Consequently, antibiotic therapy generally is not warranted with aplastic crisis.

HEMOLYTIC CRISIS

There is no specific treatment for hemolytic crises. Treatment is supportive and may include blood transfusions.

PHARMACOECONOMIC CONSIDERATIONS

Although drugs are often thought of as the most important factor to consider when making payment and reimbursement decisions, the overall cost of hospital-related care for SCD is considerable, as evidenced by a recent study.[59] Newer therapies such as hydroxyurea and BMT are also especially costly when considered broadly for all patients. However, an Illinois study points out what most caregivers have known: that a small number of patients consume a disproportionate amount of care as a result of severe illness.[60] Undoubtedly the small group of high-use patients reported in the study, when multiplied around the country, suggests much greater expenditures needed per capita than the recurrent cost of new therapies like hydroxyurea or the one-time cost plus follow-up costs of BMT.[61] Although expensive therapies themselves, they have the great potential to keep patients out of emergency and inpatient beds, leading to improved cost effectiveness in the long run. Of course, it is presumed that the affected patients would also enjoy a higher quality of life. A recent report indicates that sickle cell patients who showed positive feelings about themselves, embraced religious or spiritual life values, and had a strong social support system rated their quality of life higher than those who did not.[62]

EVALUATION OF THERAPEUTIC OUTCOMES

In the long-term management of the patient with sickle cell anemia, administration of folic acid is aimed at preventing folate deficiency and megaloblastic changes. Folate levels and MCV values should be monitored. The true efficacy of gelation inhibitors such as hydroxyurea can best be assessed in terms of the decrease in number, severity, and duration of sickle cell pain crises. Fetal hemoglobin concentrations or MCV values may also give some indication of response to therapy. When painful crises do occur, the evaluation of effectiveness of analgesics depends mainly on the subjective assessments made by the patient and health care practitioners. Adequate hydration is important in the resolution of painful crisis. However, caution should be exercised to avoid overhydration, especially in patients predisposed to complications from this therapy such as renal failure patients and patients with cardiac dysfunction. Evaluation of the efficacy of prophylactic immunizations and antibiotics involves monitoring for the occurrence of pneumococcal or *Haemophilus* infections. When infections do occur, appropriate antibiotic therapy should be initiated and the patient monitored for laboratory and clinical improvement. The success of blood transfusions poststroke can be assessed through monitoring for clinical progression or the occurrence of subsequent strokes.

CONCLUSIONS

In the general management of SCA, the goal is to decrease the number of sickle cell crises, to decrease the complications arising from the disease, and to improve the overall quality of life. Gelation inhibitors, especially hydroxyurea, which increase fetal hemoglobin, may decrease the frequency of painful episodes. Studies to determine the optimal regimen for hydroxyurea are still needed. Continued studies on other possible agents that may reduce crises or reverse organ damage are warranted. When vasoocclusive crises occur, hydration and administration of analgesics remain core interventions. General care of SCA patients still includes folate administration and appropriate immunization.

▶ PRINCIPLES OF PHARMACOTHERAPY

- Sickle cell disease is an inherited disorder caused by a defect in the gene for hemoglobin.
- Patients may have one defective gene (sickle cell trait) or two defective genes (sickle cell disease).
- Although most often seen in persons of African ancestry, other ethnic groups are affected.
- Sickle cell disease may cause various kinds of crises, growth retardation, myocardial infarction, aseptic necrosis of joints, and cholelithiasis.
- Folate administration is recommended for sickle cell patients because of the demands of accelerated erythropoiesis.
- Sickle cell patients should receive the pneumococcal vaccine and *Haemophilis influenzae* type b vaccine to decrease the chance of developing infections due to encapsulated organisms.
- Blood transfusions, which increase the percentage of normal hemoglobin, have been shown to be beneficial in decreasing the occurrence of stroke in children with sickle cell disease.
- Hydroxyurea has been shown to decrease the incidence of painful crises when given prophylactically in sickle cell patients. However, the patient population that receives hydroxyurea should be carefully selected and monitored.
- Fluid replacement, at a rate of 3 to 4 L/d, is recommended in treating vaso-occlusive crises. Overhydration should be avoided.
- Analgesic options include parenteral or oral opioids, nonsteroidal anti-inflammatory agents, and acetaminophen. The choice of agent and regimen should be determined based on patient characteristics and the severity of the crisis.

REFERENCES

1. Herrick JB. Peculiar elongated and sickle-shaped red blood corpuscles in case of severe anemia. Arch Intern Med 1910;6:517–521.
2. Konotey-Ahulu FID. The sickle cell diseases: Clinical manifestations including the "sickle cell." Arch Intern Med 1974;133:611–619.
3. Pauling L, Itano HA, Singer SJ, et al. Sickle cell anemia: A molecular disease. Science 1949;110:543–548.
4. Serjeant GR. Geography and the clinical picture of sickle cell disease: An overview. Ann N Y Acad Sci 1989;565:109–119.
5. Cerami A, Washington E. Sickle Cell Anemia. New York, Third Press, 1974.
6. Allison AC. Protection afforded by sickle cell trait against subtertian malarial infections. Br Med J 1954;1:290.
7. Thompson GR. Significance of hemoglobins S and C in Ghana. Br Med J 1962;1:682.
8. Edelstein SJ. The Sickled Cell: From Myths to Molecules. Cambridge, MA, Harvard University Press, 1986.
9. Ferguson AD, Carrington HT, Scott RB. Studies in sickle cell anemia—A clinical review. Med Ann DC 1955;24:517–532.
10. Rodgers GP, Noguchi CT, Schechter AN. Noninvasive techniques to evaluate the vaso-occlusive manifestations of sickle cell disease. Am J Pediatr Hematol Oncol 1985;7:245–253.
11. Rickles F, O'Leary DS. Role of coagulation system in pathophysiology of sickle cell disease. Arch Intern Med 1974;133:635–641.
12. Bensinger TA, Gillete PN. Hemolysis in sickle cell disease. Arch Intern Med 1974;133:624–631.
13. Winkelstein JA. Pneumococcal infections in sickle cell disease. J Pediatr 1977;91:521.
14. Winkelstein JA. The role of complement in the host's defense against *Streptococcus pneumoniae.* Rev Infect Dis 1981;3:289.
15. Buchanan GR. Sickle cell disease: Recent advances. Curr Probl Pediatr 1993;23:219–229.
16. Powars DR. Beta-s-gene-cluster haplotypes in sickle cell. Hematol Oncol Clin North Am 1991;5:476–447, 485–486.
17. Scott RB, Castro O. Sickle cell thalassemia: Interpretation of test results. JAMA 1981;246:81.
18. Castro O, Scott RB. Red blood cell counts and indices in sickle cell trait in a black American population. Hemoglobin 1985;9:65–67.
19. Samuels-Reid J, Scott RB. Characteristics of menstruation in sickle cell disease. Fertil Steril 1985;43:139–141.
20. Finan AC, Elmer MA, Sasanow SR, et al. Nutritional factors and growth in children with sickle cell disease. Am J Dis Child 1988;142: 237–240.
21. Scott RB, Samuels-Reid JH. Sickle cell disease. In: Gellis SS, Kagan BM, eds. Current Pediatric Therapy. Philadelphia, Saunders, 1990:241.
22. Githers JH, Gross GP, Eife RF, et al. Splenic sequestration syndrome at mountain altitudes in sickle/hemoglobin C disease. J Pediatr 1977;90:203–206.
23. Platt OS, Thorington BD, Brambilla DJ, et al. Pain in sickle cell disease: Rates and risk factors. N Engl J Med 1994;325:11–16.
24. Sprinkle RH, Cole T, Smith S, et al. Acute chest syndrome in children with sickle cell disease. Am J Pediatr Hematol Oncol 1986;8: 105–110.
25. Oppenheimer EH, Esterly J. Pulmonary changes in sickle disease. Am Rev Respir Dis 1971;103:853–859.
26. Barrett-Conner E. Acute pulmonary disease in sickle cell anemia. Am Rev Respir Dis 1971;104:159–165.
27. Young RC, Castro O, Baxter RP, et al. The lung in sickle cell disease: A clinical overview of common vascular, infectious and other problems. J Natl Med Assoc 1981;73:19–26.
28. Bromberg PH. Pulmonary aspects of sickle cell disease. Arch Intern Med 1974; 133:652–657.
29. Lachman BS, Lazerson J, Starshak RJ, et al. The prevalence of cholelithiasis in sickle cell disease as diagnosed by ultrasound and cholecystography. Pediatrics 1979;64:601–603.
30. Siegel JF, Rich MA, Brock WA. Association of sickle cell disease, priapism, exchange transfusion, and neurological events: ASPEN syndrome. J Urol 1993;150:1480–1482.
31. Maclver JE, Went NL. Sickle cell anemia complicated by megaloblastic anemia of infancy. Br Med J 1960;1:775–779.
32. Alperin JB. Folic acid deficiency complicating sickle cell anemia. Arch Intern Med 1967;120:298–306.
33. Galloway SJ, Harwood-Nuss AL. Sickle-cell anemia—A review. J Emerg Med 1988;6:213–226.
34. Falletta JM, Woods GM, Verter JI, et al. Discontinuing penicillin prophylaxis in children with sickle cell anemia. J Pediatr 1995;127: 685–690.
35. John AB, Ramlal A, Jackson H, et al. Prevention of pneumococcal infection in children with homozygous sickle cell disease. Br Med J 1984;288:1567–1570.
36. El-Hazmi MAF, Bahakim HM, Al-Swailem AM, et al. Symptom-free intervals in sicklers: Does pneumococcal vaccination and penicillin prophylaxis have a role? J Trop Pediatr 1990;36:56–62.
37. Gaston MH, Vertu JL, Woods G, et al. Prophylaxis with oral penicillin in children with sickle cell anemia. N Engl J Med 1986;314: 1593–1599.
38. Buchanan GR, Siegel JD, Smith SJ, DePasse BM. Oral penicillin prophylaxis in children with impaired splenic function: A study of compliance. Pediatrics 1982;70:926–930.

39. Breiman RF, Butler JC, Tenover FC, et al. Emergence of drug-resistant pneumococcal infections in the United States. JAMA 1994; 271:1831–1835.
40. Piomelli S. Chronic transfusions in patients with sickle cell disease. Am J Pediatr Hematol Oncol 1985;7:51–55.
41. King KE, Ness PM. Treating anemia. Hematol Oncol Clin North Am 1996;10:1305–1319.
42. New treatment prevents strokes in children with sickle cell anemia. News release. National Institutes of Health, Sept. 18, 1997.
43. Steinberg MH. Review: Sickle cell disease: Present and future treatment. Am J Med Sci 1996;312:166–174.
44. Charache S, Terrin ML, Moore RD, et al. Effect of hydroxyurea on the frequency of painful crises in sickle cell anemia. N Engl J Med 1995;332:1317–1322.
45. Claster S, Vichinsky E. First report of reversal of organ dysfunction in sickle cell anemia by the use of hydroxyurea: Splenic regeneration. Blood 1996;88:1951–1953.
46. Epstein F. Pathogenesis and treatment of sickle cell disease. N Engl J Med 1997;337:762–769.
47. Perrine SP, Ginder GD, Faller DV, et al. A short-term trial of butyrate to stimulate fetal-globin-gene expression in the beta-globin disorders. N Engl J Med 1993;328:81.
48. Ambrus JL. Stiff red cell syndrome. A review of the treatment of sickle cell disease with pentoxifylline. J Med 1993;24:1–9.
49. Charache S. Experimental therapy. Hematol Oncol Clin North Am 1996;10:1373–1382.
50. Powars DR, Johnson CS. Priapism. Hematol Oncol Clin North Am 1996;10:1363–1372.
51. Shanta TR. Intraoperative management of penile erection by using terbulatine. Anesthesiology 1989;70:707–709.
52. Shanta TR, Finnerty DP, Rodriquez AL. Treatment of persistent penile erection and priapism using terbutaline. J Urol 1989;141:1427–1429.
53. Serjeant GR, DeCeular K, Maude GH. Stilbesterol and stuttering priapism in homozygous sickle-cell disease. Lancet 1985;1274–1276.
54. Levine LA, Gudd SP. Gonadotropin-releasing hormone analogues in the treatment of sickle cell anemia-associated priapism. J Urol 1993; 150:475–477.
55. Vichinsky E, Styles L. Pulmonary complications. Hematol Oncol Clin North Am 1996;10:1275–1286.
56. Ballas SK. Management of sickle pain. Curr Opin Hematol 1997;4: 104–111.
57. Gonzalez ER, Bahal N, Hansen LA, et al. Intermittent injection vs patient-controlled analgesia for sickle cell crisis pain. Arch Intern Med 1991;151:1373–1378.
58. Evans JPM. Practical management of sickle cell disease. Arch Dis Child 1989;64:1748–1751.
59. Davis H, Moore RM, Gergen PJ. Cost of hospitalizations associated with sickle cell disease in the United States. Public Health Rep 1997; 112:40–43.
60. Woods K, Karrison T, Koshy M, et al. Hospital utilization patterns and costs for sickle cell patients in Illinois. Public Health Rep 1997;112: 44–51.
61. Shechter AN. Sickle cell disease expenditures and outcomes. Public Health Rep 1997;112:38–39.
62. Pippalla RS, Tucker G, Perlin E, et al. An assessment of quality of life in sickle cell patients: World Health Organization quality of life assessment scale (whoqol-100). Presented to the 4th annual meeting of the International Society of Quality of Life Research. Vienna, Austria, November 5–9, 1997.

94

DRUG-INDUCED HEMATOLOGIC DISORDERS

Thomas E. Johns, PharmD, BCPS, and J. William Harbilas, PharmD, BCPS

Hematologic disorders have always been a risk of drug therapy. Granulocytopenia (agranulocytosis) was reported while using one of medicine's early therapeutic agents, sulphanilamide, in 1938.[1] Many drugs, such as antineoplastic agents, cause predictable diseases of the blood as a result of the drug's major pharmacologic effect. This chapter will not address these agents, but will describe idiosyncratic reactions not directly related to the drug's pharmacology. The drug-induced hematologic disorders included are aplastic anemia, agranulocytosis, megaloblastic anemia, thrombocytopenia, and hemolytic anemia. Definitions for most of these diseases have been standardized and will be discussed in their individual sections.[2]

By most reports, idiosyncratic, drug-induced hematologic disorders are rare. Relatively few epidemiologic studies have addressed the actual incidence of these adverse reactions. The latest epidemiologic study was held in Europe and Israel. Summaries of this study have been published and estimated the incidences of aplastic anemia and agranulocytosis to be 0.5 cases per million per year and 3.1 cases per million per year, respectively.[3] Although rare, drug-induced hematologic disorders are important because they are associated with significant morbidity and mortality. Mortality rates of 9% and 46% in cases of drug-induced agranulocytosis and aplastic anemia, respectively, have been described.[3] Older data from Sweden reported similar results for agranulocytosis and aplastic anemia, but also reported incidences of hemolytic anemia and thrombocytopenia of 1.6 cases and 2.7 cases per million per year. According to this report, thrombocytopenia and agranulocytosis were the most common, followed by hemolytic anemia and aplastic anemia. Deaths were estimated at 32% for agranulocytosis, 51% for aplastic anemia, 4% for hemolytic anemia, and 3% for thrombocytopenia.[4] An epidemiologic study held in the United States estimated that 4490 deaths in 1984 were attributable to blood dyscrasias from all causes. Aplastic anemia was the leading cause of death, followed by thrombocytopenia, agranulocytosis, and hemolytic anemia.[5] Like most other adverse drug reactions (ADRs), drug-induced hematologic disorders are more common in the elderly; the risk of death also appears greater with increasing age.[5] The risk of agranulocytosis has been reported to be greater in women than in men.[4,6]

Because of the seriousness associated with drug-induced hematologic disorders, tracking these reactions is needed to predict their occurrence and to estimate their incidence. Reporting during postmarketing surveillance of a drug is usually the method by which the incidence of rare adverse drug reactions (ADRs) is established. The MedWatch program supported by the Food and Drug Administration is one such program. This program relies on health care professionals to submit cases of adverse drug reactions for recording and further study. Many facilities have similar drug-reporting programs to follow adverse drug reaction trends and to help diagnose cases of drug-induced disease. The programs contain a standardized system that accurately establishes the association between a drug and an ADR as being either causal or coincidental. In the case of drug-induced hematologic disorders, these programs can enable practitioners to confirm that an adverse event is indeed the result of drug therapy, because these effects could potentially have many other causes; general guidelines are readily available.[2,7] Because drug-induced blood disorders are dangerous, rechallenging a patient with a suspected agent in an attempt to confirm a diagnosis may not be ethical. *In vitro* studies using the offending agent and cells or plasma from the patient's blood have been described to determine causality.[8] These methods, however, are often expensive and require facilities and expertise that are not generally available. One study demonstrated that only 19% of the cases with suspected drug-induced agranulocytosis could be documented by *in vitro* testing.[9]

The understanding of drug-induced hematologic disorders requires a basic understanding of hematopoiesis. A detailed discussion can be found in Chapter 90. The blood is maintained by pluripotential hematopoietic stem cells (PHSCs) in the bone marrow, which have the ability to self-reproduce. PHSCs are further differentiated to intermediate precursor cells, which are also called "progenitor cells" or "colony-forming cells." These intermediate stem cells are committed to a particular cell line and differentiate into colonies of each type of blood cell in respose to a particular colony-stimulating factor (Fig. 94–1). Some investigators believe that the earlier the drug-induced hematologic disorders occur in the differentiation process, the more severe the disorder will become.[10]

Any cell line can be affected in drug-induced hematologic disorders including the white blood cells (WBCs), red blood cells (RBCs), and platelets. When a drug causes decreases in all three cell lines accompanied by a hypoplastic bone marrow, the result is termed drug-induced aplastic anemia. The decrease in WBC count alone by a medication is termed drug-induced agranulocytosis. Drugs can affect RBCs by causing a number of different anemias including

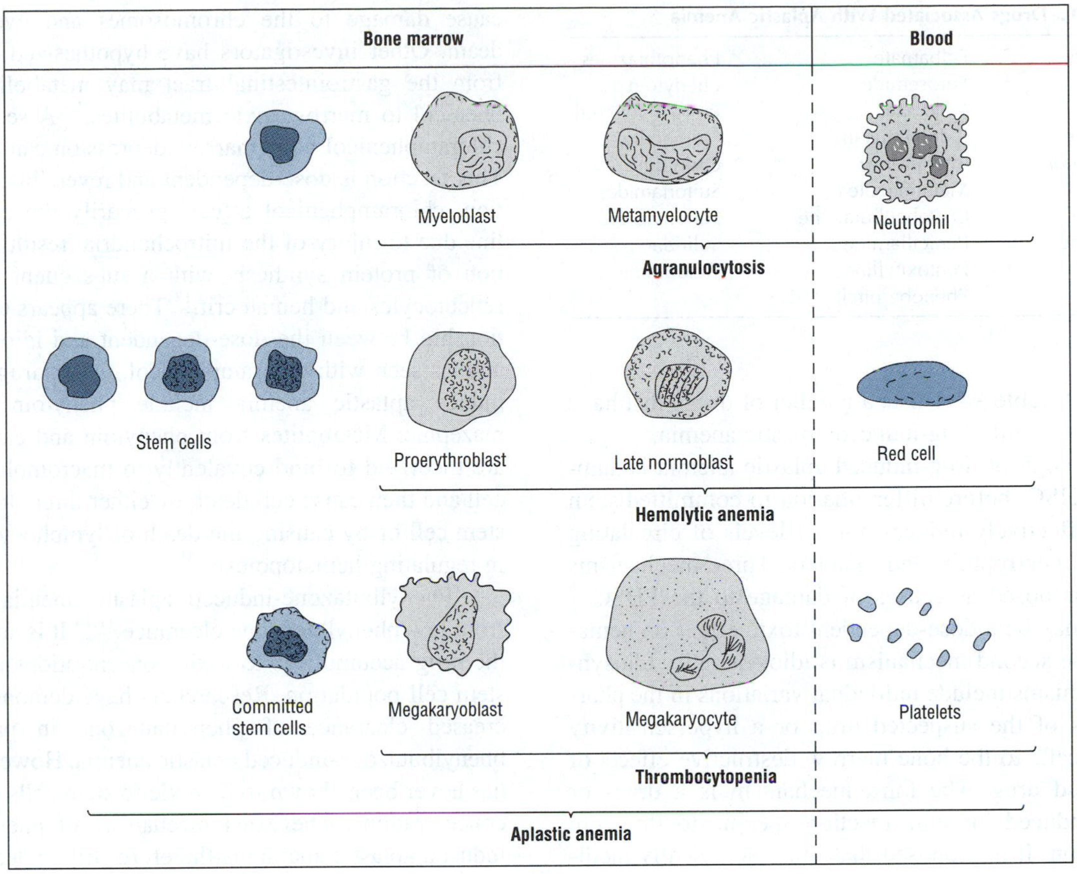

FIGURE 94–1. Differentiation of the stem cell to committed cell lines, illustrating the origins of various drug-induced hematologic disorders.

drug-induced immune hemolytic anemia, drug-induced oxidative hemolytic anemia, or drug-induced megaloblastic anemia. A drug-induced decrease in platelet count is called drug-induced thrombocytopenia. The remainder of this chapter discusses specific aspects of drug-induced hematologic disorders with particular emphasis on the dyscrasias previously stated.

DRUG-INDUCED APLASTIC ANEMIA

Drug-induced aplastic anemia is classified as an acquired form of the disorder and accounts for approximately 50% of cases.[11] It is considered the most serious drug-induced blood dyscrasia due to the high mortality rate, often exceeding 50% of treated cases.[12] It is characterized by pancytopenia (presence of anemia, neutropenia, and thrombocytopenia) with a hypocellular or "fatty" bone marrow and no gross evidence of increased peripheral blood cell destruction.[2] A diagnosis of aplastic anemia can be made by the presence of two of the following criteria: a white blood cell count of 3500/mm^3 or less, a platelet count of 55,000/mm^3 or less, or a hemoglobin value of 10.0 g/dL or less with a reticulocyte count of 30,000/mm^3 or less.[12] Severe aplastic anemia is defined by at least two of the following three peripheral blood findings: neutrophil count of less than 500/mm^3, platelet count of less than 20,000/mm^3, and anemia with a corrected reticulocyte index of less than 1%.[13,14] An extremely poor prognosis has been associated with a neutrophil count of less than 200/mm^3.[14] A bone marrow aspirate and biopsy are required to exclude other causes of pancytopenia including neoplastic infiltration or significant myelofibrosis.[11] There must also be no history of iatrogenic exposure to cytotoxic chemotherapy known to cause transient marrow suppression, or to intensive radiation. The onset of drug-induced aplastic anemia is variable and insidious with symptoms usually appearing on the average about 6.5 weeks after initiation of the offending agent.[15] The disease may appear after the drug has been discontinued. Clinical features of drug-induced aplastic anemia depend on the degree each cell line is suppressed, similar to idiopathic disease. Symptoms of anemia include pallor, fatigue, and weakness, while neutropenia may be characterized by fever, chills, pharyngitis, or other infection. Thrombocytopenia, often the initial clue to diagnosis, is manifested by easy bruisability, petechiae, and bleeding. The incidence of drug-induced aplastic anemia is estimated at 0.5 to 5 cases per 1 million population per year.[3,14,16] Higher rates of occurrence have been seen in patient's taking such drugs as indomethacin, phenylbutazone, and gold

TABLE 94–1. Drugs Associated With Aplastic Anemia

Acetazolamide	Felbamate	Phenothiazines
Aspirin	Furosemide	Phenytoin
Captopril	Gold salts	Propylthiouracil
Carbamazepine	Indomethacin	Quinacrine
Chloramphenicol	Interferon-α	Quinidine
Chloroquine	Methimazole	Sulfonamides
Chlorothiazide	Oxyphenbutazone	Sulfonylureas
Chlorpromazine	Penicillamine	Sulindac
Dapsone	Pentoxifylline	Ticlopidine
Diclofenac	Phenobarbital	

compounds.[12] Table 94–1 lists a number of drugs that have been associated with drug-induced aplastic anemia.

The etiology of drug-induced aplastic anemia is damage to the PHSC, before differentiation to committed stem cells. This effectively reduces normal levels of circulating erythrocytes, neutrophils, and platelets. Three mechanisms have been proposed as causes of damage to the PHSC.[15] First, there may be a dose-dependent toxic effect on hematopoiesis. The second mechanism is idiosyncratic. Idiosyncratic mechanisms include individual variations in the pharmacokinetics of the suspected drug or a hypersensitivity of the stem cells to the bone marrow destructive effects of the implicated drug. The third mechanism is a drug- or metabolite-induced immune reaction specific to the stem cell population. It is proposed that immunologically mediated, tissue-specific organ destruction occurs following exposure to an inciting antigen (drug) that activates cells and cytokines of the immune system leading to death of stem cells.[13] There is no evidence that drug-induced aplastic anemia occurs due to the destruction of the microenvironment of the bone marrow.[11]

The dose-dependent mechanism for development of aplastic anemia is exemplified by the antineoplastic agents. Many of these agents have the ability to suppress one or more cell lines in a reversible manner. The degree of suppression and the cell line involved depends on the nature of the drug and its potential for inhibiting marrow proliferation.

Idiosyncratic drug-induced aplastic anemia may be characterized by (1) dose independence, (2) a latent period prior to onset of anemia, and (3) continuance of marrow injury following drug discontinuation.[17] Drugs that cause drug-induced aplastic anemia in a minority of patients can imply abnormal metabolism or excretion of a drug. Chloramphenicol is the most common drug associated with aplastic anemia with an incidence of about 1 case per 20,000[14] patients treated, although the overall incidence has fallen with decreased use.[17] It is known to cause both a dose-dependent and idiosyncratic reaction. The idiosyncratic mechanism is thought to result from abnormal metabolism of chloramphenicol. The nitrobenzene ring present on chloramphenicol is thought to be reduced to form a nitroso group on the chloramphenicol molecule.[18] The nitroso group then could interact with DNA in the stem cell to cause damage to the chromosomes and eventually cell death. Other investigators have hypothesized that bacteria from the gastrointestinal tract may metabolize chloramphenicol to marrow-toxic metabolites.[19] A second type of chloramphenicol bone marrow depression can also be seen. This reaction is dose-dependent and reversible. In this reaction, chloramphenicol affects primarily the erythroid cell line due to injury of the mitrochondria, resulting in inhibition of protein synthesis with a subsequent reduction in reticulocytes and hematocrit.[18] There appears to be no relationship between the dose-dependent and idiosyncratic reactions seen with chloramphenicol. Other drugs thought to induce aplastic anemia include phenytoin and carbamazepine. Metabolites from phenytoin and carbamazepine are theorized to bind covalently to macromolecules in the cell and then cause cell death by either direct toxicity to the stem cell or by causing the death of lymphocytes involved in regulating hematopoiesis.[20]

Phenylbutazone-induced aplastic anemia may result from low phenylbutazone clearance.[11,15] It is suggested that the drug accumulates to toxic concentrations and kills the stem cell population. Researchers have demonstrated a decreased clearance of phenylbutazone in patients with phenylbutazone-induced aplastic anemia. However, the drug has never been shown to be toxic to stem cells even in high concentrations. The exact mechanism of phenylbutazone-induced aplastic anemia is therefore still unclear.

Genetic predisposition may also influence the development of drug-induced aplastic anemia. Studies in animals and a case report of chloramphenicol-induced aplastic anemia in identical twins suggest a genetic predisposition to development of drug-induced aplastic anemia.[11,18]

Drug-induced aplastic anemia due to the development of an immune reaction has also been speculated. The mechanism could be similar to drug-induced immune agranulocytosis or drug-induced immune hemolytic anemia (discussed later in the chapter). The appearance of antibodies to chloroquine and subsequent bone marrow suppression supports the previous hypothesis.[15] Drugs could also affect the function of suppressor T cells, which in turn could initiate the inhibition of stem cell production.[15] The clinical success of antithymocyte globulin in the treatment of possible drug-induced aplastic anemia may also indicate a drug effect on suppressor T-cell function in drug-induced aplastic anemia.[21] Additional supporting evidence for an immunologic basis as a mechanism of aplastic anemia comes from a recently published retrospective study involving bone marrow transplantation from genetically identical twins into patients with aplastic anemia. Patients receiving their first transplantation who were administered a conditioning regimen prior to first transplantation including total-body radiation, cyclophosphamide, cyclosporine, antilymphocyte globulin, corticosteroids, or some combination were more likely to attain hematologic recovery compared to those who did not receive preconditioning.[22]

▶ TREATMENT: Drug-Induced Aplastic Anemia

The 2-year survival rate for a patient who develops drug-induced aplastic anemia is approximately 62%.[15] As with all cases of drug-induced hematologic disorders, the suspected offending agent must be removed. Early withdrawal of the agent may allow for reversal of the aplastic anemia.[15] Supportive care for drug-induced aplastic anemia includes symptomatic treatment of infection with antibiotics and administration of blood products for bleeding. It must be emphasized that prognosis, response to therapy, and management of drug-induced aplastic anemia is similar to idiopathic disease.[17] A detailed discussion of the management of aplastic anemia is beyond the scope of this chapter. Management of aplastic anemia involves allogeneic bone marrow transplantation, the only curative treatment modality, or pharmacotherapy, which may include use of immunosuppressive agents, androgens, or hematopoietic growth factors.[14] Conflicting data exist regarding the efficacy of immunosuppressive therapy compared to bone marrow transplantation; historical data suggest equal or greater efficacy[14] while more recent data clearly demonstrate the superiority of marrow transplant.[23]

Long-term complications of immunosuppressive therapy include relapse and conversion to other stem cell disorders such as myelodysplastic syndrome, acute myelogenous leukemia, or paroxysmal nocturnal hemoglobinuria, which have occurred with relatively high incidence.[14,23] Immunosuppressive therapy may include use of antithymocyte globulin (ATG), antilymphocyte globulin (ALG), glucocorticoids, or cyclosporine. Antithymocyte globulin has been employed to reverse aplastic anemia in doses of 10 to 20 mg/kg body weight per day by intravenous infusion for 8 to 10 consecutive days.[23,24] Corticosteroids have been used in drug-induced aplastic anemia but their efficacy is questionable.[15] Several investigators have employed cyclosporine for the treatment of aplastic anemia with beneficial results,[25,26] but one prospective study in 12 patients showed no response to cyclosporine.[27] In contrast, patients with severe aplastic anemia treated with ALG, corticosteroids, and cyclosporine observed a survival rate of 92% at 3 years.[28] Granulocyte-macrophage colony-stimulating factor (GM-CSF)[29,30] and interleukin-1[31] have also been investigated in the treatment of aplastic anemia with some success. An additional case report described the use of cyclosporine and filgrastim (G-CSF) in combination in the treatment of aplastic anemia.[32] If long-term bone marrow suppression continues after initial treatment with the previous agents, the only viable option at present is bone marrow transplantation. Some experts believe bone marrow transplantation is the treatment of choice if the patient has a matched donor. In a recent retrospective analysis of 395 patients with aplastic anemia, primary immunosuppressive therapy with ATG was compared to preconditioned bone marrow transplantation. Patients administered ATG also received adjunctive corticosteroids as well as oxymetholone. Eighty-nine percent of patients receiving bone marrow transplantation sustained engraftment while 44% of patients administered immunosuppressive therapy achieved a complete, partial, or minimal response.[23]

DRUG-INDUCED AGRANULOCYTOSIS

Drug-induced agranulocytosis can be defined as a drug-mediated reduction in the mature myeloid cells in the blood (granulocytes and immature granulocytes [bands]) to a total count of 2000/mm^3 or less. Symptoms of agranulocytosis include sore throat, fever, malaise, weakness, and chills. It occurs more frequently in females than males.[33] The overall mortality rate in agranulocytosis is 16%.[34] Mortality in patients with agranulocytosis increases when the patient develops bacteremia or renal failure.[34] The symptoms can appear rapidly, within 7 to 14 days after initiation of the offending agent, or in the case of phenothiazine-induced agranulocytosis, patients can be asymptomatic at the time of diagnosis probably due to a milder form of the disorder.[35] In the large majority of cases the drug-induced agranulocytosis will resolve over time.[35] Table 94–2 provides a list of medications that have been associated with drug-induced agranulocytosis.

A number of different mechanisms may produce drug-induced agranulocytosis. Initially, it was thought that drugs affected only the mature granulocytes, causing a "maturation arrest." In recent years, however, studies have demonstrated a possible toxic effect of drugs on the myeloid colony-forming unit in the bone marrow (either a direct toxic effect or antibody mediated)[36,37]; this may be the most frequent mechanism of drug-induced agranulocytosis.[33] Drug-induced agranulocytosis can be classified into three types.[38] The type I reaction is immune mediated and involves the drug or drug metabolite, antibodies, and neutrophils. A type II reaction is associated with accumulated drug toxicity in hypersensitive individuals. The final type, type III, represents other etiologies induced by a combination of both immune and toxic mechanisms.

TABLE 94–2. Drugs Associated With Agranulocytosis

Acetaminophen	Flucytosine	Penicillamine
Acetazolamide	Fosphenytoin	Pentazocine
Allopurinol	Furosemide	Phenothiazines
p-Aminosalicylic acid	Ganciclovir	Phenytoin
Benzodiazepines	Gentamicin	Primidone
β-Lactam antibiotics	Gold salts	Procainamide
Brompheniramine	Griseofulvin	Propranolol
Captopril	Hydralazine	Propylthiouracil
Carbamazepine	Hydroxychloroquine	Pyrimethamine
Chloramphenicol	Imipenem–cilastatin	Quinine
Chloropropamide	Imipramine	Rifampin
Cimetidine	Isoniazid	Streptomycin
Clindamycin	Levodopa	Sulfonamides
Clomipramine	Lincomycin	Sulfonylureas
Clozapine	Meprobamate	Thiazide diuretics
Colchicine	Methazolamide	Ticlopidine
Dapsone	Methimazole	Tocainide
Desipramine	Methyldopa	Tolbutamide
Doxycycline	Metronidazole	Vancomycin
Ethacrynic acid	Nitrofurantoin	Zidovudine
Ethosuximide	NSAIDs	

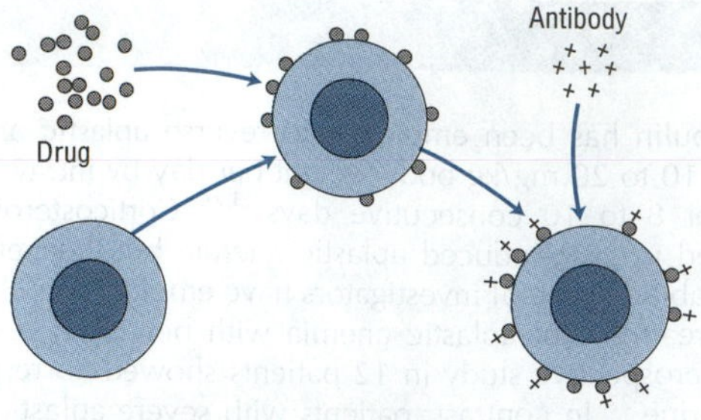

FIGURE 94–2. The drug adsorption mechanism. The drug binds to the membrane of the blood cell. Antibodies are formed to the drug–membrane complex (a hapten). The antibodies then attach to the complex and cell toxicity occurs. *(From Ref. 61, with permission.)*

Drug-induced immune agranulocytosis (type I) has been theorized to develop by one of four different mechanisms.[39] The first type involves drug adsorption on the membrane of the neutrophil. The drug–membrane complex then acts as a hapten to stimulate antibody formation. The antibodies produced attach to the drug–membrane complex causing WBC destruction through complement activation and removal by the phagocytic system (Fig. 94–2). This hapten-type reaction is often seen when drugs are given in large doses. The penicillin derivatives are frequently associated with this type of agranulocytosis. The dose at which this immune-mediated reaction occurs is usually higher than 150 mg/kg/d with the majority of penicillin derivatives but has occurred at lower doses.[37,40,41]

The second type of immune-mediated agranulocytosis is called the "innocent bystander phenomenon." In this reaction, the drug combines with a drug-specific antibody. The complex is nonspecifically adsorbed to the neutrophil membrane, resulting in complement activation. The activated complement then destroys the cell (Fig. 94–3). Quinidine has been associated with this type of reaction.

A similar type of immune response involves a protein carrier that combines with the drug and then attaches to the cell membrane. This in turn causes antibody formation. The antibodies attach to the drug protein carrier–membrane complex and activate complement. The cells are then cleared by the phagocytic system (Fig. 94–4).

The final mechanism for an immune-mediated reaction is the production of autoantibodies to a "spoiled membrane" caused by the offending drug. The drug alters the neutrophil membrane, which induces the formation of autoantibodies (antibodies that attach directly to the neutrophil). These antibodies attach to the neutrophil, causing cellular destruction by the phagocytic system.

The onset of symptoms due to immune-mediated mechanisms is rapid, occurring in 7 to 15 days of drug exposure. In the case of penicillin-induced agranulocytosis, the patient can often be restarted on a lower dose of penicillin after the neutropenia has resolved without any relapse of drug-induced agranulocytosis.[40,41] Due to the rapid onset of symptoms and the dose-related phenomenon, a second mechanism (type II) could possibly be involved with penicillin-induced agranulocytosis. This mechanism involves an accumulation of drug to toxic concentrations in hypersensitive individuals. Researchers have shown with *in vitro* cell cultures that penicillin derivatives in high concentrations inhibit growth of myeloid colony-forming units in patients recovering from drug-induced agranulocytosis.[42] Penicillin derivatives may therefore exert WBC suppression by several mechanisms.

Antithyroid medications such as propylthiouracil and methimazole produce agranulocytosis in about 0.3% to 0.6% of patients.[43,44] The mechanism by which antithyroid agents cause agranulocytosis is unknown, but antibodies to granulocytes have been demonstrated.[45,46] In a study by Cooper and coworkers,[43] agranulocytosis occurred more frequently in older patients (> 40 years old) and occurred within 2 months after initiation of therapy. The investigators also reported a possible dose relationship with methimazole.[43] For patients receiving less than 30 mg/d of methimazole, no agranulocytosis occurred, but in patients

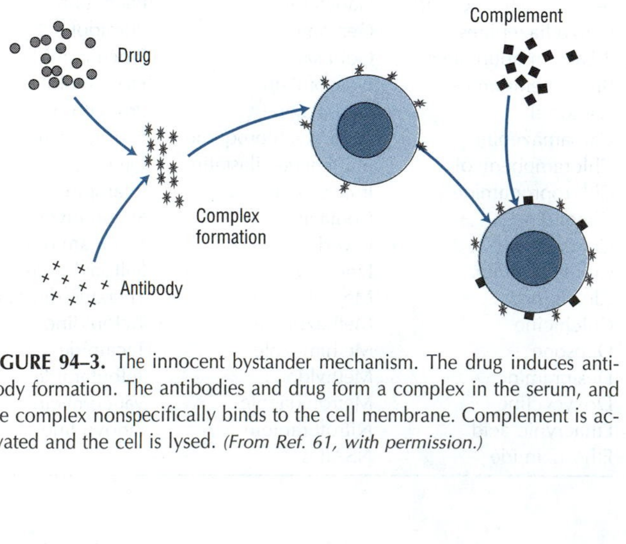

FIGURE 94–3. The innocent bystander mechanism. The drug induces antibody formation. The antibodies and drug form a complex in the serum, and the complex nonspecifically binds to the cell membrane. Complement is activated and the cell is lysed. *(From Ref. 61, with permission.)*

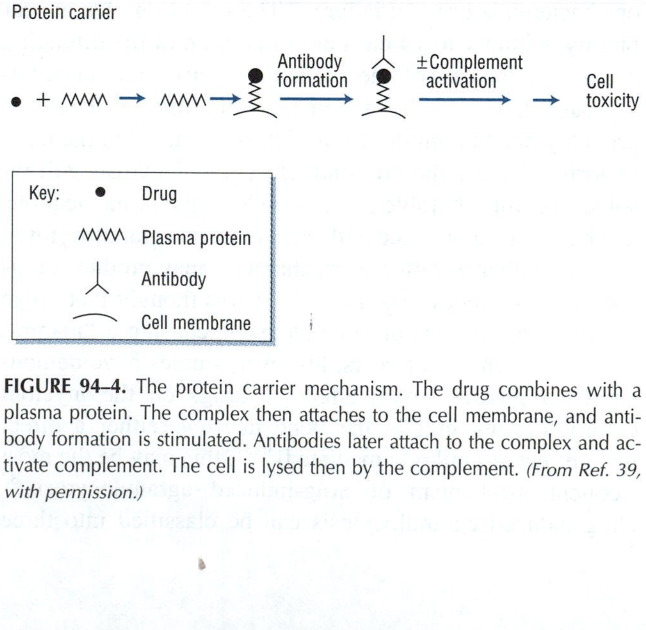

FIGURE 94–4. The protein carrier mechanism. The drug combines with a plasma protein. The complex then attaches to the cell membrane, and antibody formation is stimulated. Antibodies later attach to the complex and activate complement. The cell is lysed then by the complement. *(From Ref. 39, with permission.)*

receiving higher doses, neutropenia was seen.[43] There appeared to be no dose relationship with conventional doses of propylthiouracil. However, another study demonstrated no relationship between age or dose in the incidence of thioamide-induced agranulocytosis.[47]

The phenothiazines as a group are known to cause a type II drug-induced agranulocytosis. The onset of phenothiazine-induced agranulocytosis is approximately 2 to 15 weeks after initiating therapy.[39] Short-term toxicity is not usually seen in patients taking phenothiazines on a chronic basis, although there is one report of acute agranulocytosis in a child who accidentally ingested a large quantity of chlorpromazine.[36] Usually patients have ingested 10 to 20 g of a phenothiazine before the onset of neutropenia. Phenothiazine-induced agranulocytosis occurs most frequently in females older than 50 years of age.[35] The mechanism by which phenothiazines cause the drug-induced agranulocytosis has been primarily studied with chlorpromazine.[35] Chlorpromazine is thought to affect cells in the cell cycle that are in the phase that manufactures enzymes needed for DNA synthesis (G_1 phase) or the phase in which cells are resting and not committed to cell division (G_0 phase).[35] The antipsychotic agents are known to precipitate proteins and may coprecipitate polynucleotides so they can no longer participate in nucleic acid synthesis. Chlorpromazine also increases the loss of macromolecules from the intracellular pools that are essential for cellular replication.[35] When the bone marrow from a patient with phenothiazine-induced agranulocytosis is examined, it initially appears to have no cellularity (aplastic), but over time it becomes highly hyperplastic. It is believed that toxic effects of the phenothiazines are not seen in all patients taking the medications because the majority of patients have enough bone marrow reserve to overcome the toxic effects.[35] Clozapine, an antipsychotic agent, has demonstrated an approximately 10-fold higher incidence of agranulocytosis compared to other antipsychotics.[48] The incidence of clozapine-induced agranulocytosis increases with age and occurs more frequently in female patients.[49] There appear to be no dose-related effects with clozapine-induced agranulocytosis.[49] The agranulocytosis is reversible if detected early in therapy; therefore close monitoring of the WBC count is warranted. An *in vitro* study has suggested that the formation of a free radical metabolite may be responsible for clozapine-induced agranulocytosis.[50] The resulting oxidative stress caused by this metabolite may cause cytotoxicity or an immune reaction.[50]

▶ TREATMENT: Drug-Induced Agranulocytosis

The primary treatment of drug-induced agranulocytosis is the removal of the offending drug. Following discontinuation of the drug, most cases of neutropenia will resolve over time and only symptomatic treatment (such as antimicrobials for infections) is necessary. Sargramostim (GM-CSF) and filgrastim (G-CSF) have been be used to decrease the time period of neutropenia with varying degrees of success.[51–58] The time to recovery of the granulocyte count ranged from 3 to 15 days.[55–58]

DRUG-INDUCED HEMOLYTIC ANEMIA

Following their release from the bone marrow, normal RBCs have a life span of 120 days before they are removed by phagocytic cells of the spleen and liver. The process of destroying red blood cells prematurely is referred to as hemolysis, which can occur due to defective red blood cells or abnormal changes in the intravascular environment. Drugs can promote hemolysis by both processes.

The causes of drug-induced hemolytic anemia can be divided into two categories: immune or metabolic. The first category can be similar to immune-regulated agranulocytosis or it may be due to the suppression of regulator cells, which allows production of autoantibodies. The second category involves the induction of hemolysis by metabolic abnormalities in the RBCs. Patients with drug-induced hemolytic anemia can present with signs of intravascular or extravascular hemolysis. Intravascular hemolysis refers to the lysis of red cells in the circulation and can be caused by trauma, complement fixation to the red cell, and exogenous toxic factors. Extravascular hemolyis refers to the ingestion of RBCs by macrophages in the spleen and liver, a process that requires the existence of surface abnormalities on RBCs, such as bound immunoglobulin.[59] The onset of drug-induced hemolytic anemia is variable and depends on the drug and mechanism of the hemolysis. Table 94–3 provides a list of drugs that have been associated with drug-induced hemolytic anemia.

Drug-induced immune hemolytic anemia is best identified with a laboratory test called the direct Coombs test (DAT or direct antihuman globulin test), which identifies foreign immune globulins either in the patient's serum or on the RBCs themselves. The Coombs test begins with the antiglobulin serum, which is produced by injecting rabbits with preparations of human complement, Fc fragments, or immunoglobulins producing antibodies that are foreign to

TABLE 94–3. Drugs Associated With Hemolytic Anemia

Acetaminophen	Levodopa	Procainamide
α-Interferon	Mefenamic acid	Quinidine
p-Aminosalicylic acid	Melphalan	Quinine
β-Lactam antibiotics	Methadone	Rifampin
Chlopropamide	Methyldopa	Sulfonamides
Chlorpromazine	Methysergide	Streptomycin
Hydralazine	NSAIDs	Tacrolimus
Hydrochlorothiazide	Nomifensine	Tetracycline
Imipenem–cilastatin	Omeprazole	Tolbutamide
Isoniazid	Probenecid	Triamterene

human immunoglobulins and complement. The direct Coombs test is performed by combining the patient's RBCs with the antiglobulin serum. If the patient's RBCs are coated with antibody or complement (as a result of a drug-induced process), the antibodies in the serum (produced by the rabbit) will attach to the Fc regions of the autoimmune globulins on two separate RBCs, creating a lattice formation called agglutination.[60] Agglutination is considered positive for the presence of IgG or complement on the cell surfaces. An indirect Coombs test can identify antibodies in the patient's serum. This test is performed by combining the patient's serum with normal RBCs, then subjecting them to the direct Coombs test. Antibodies that have attached to the normal RBCs will be identified. This process is important in blood bank procedures.

DRUG-INDUCED IMMUNE HEMOLYTIC ANEMIA

The proposed mechanisms by which drugs can cause drug-induced immune hemolytic anemia are similar to the mechanisms that produce drug-induced agranulocytosis. The first mechanism is the adsorption of the drug to the RBC membrane to form a hapten and subsequent antibody formation. The extravascular anemia that follows is usually caused by IgG, and generally there is no complement activation. The anemia usually takes 7 to 10 days to develop, and reverses quickly upon discontinuing the offending drug. The direct Coombs test becomes negative in 2 to 3 months. The penicillin and cephalosporin derivatives given in high doses are mainly associated with this type of immune reaction.[61] Other drugs that have been reported to cause drug-induced immune hemolytic anemia by this process include tetracycline and certain antineoplastic agents (cyclophosphamide, cisplatin, and melphalan).[61] Streptomycin is also associated with this type of reaction and is the only agent that will activate complement.[62]

Drug-induced immune hemolytic anemia has also been described as occurring due to immune complex formation or the "innocent bystander phenomenon." Quinidine and phenacetin are the prototype drugs of this reaction, but many other drugs have been implicated including quinine and several sulfonamides. Drugs that induce this reaction attach to a plasma protein to form a neoantigen, which in turn complexes with drug-specific antibodies (IgG or IgM) that adhere to the RBC membrane. Complement then lyses the RBC membrane.[61] This type of mechanism is associated with acute intravascular hemolysis. Interestingly, the drug–antigen complex is attached to the RBC via a nonimmune-mediated reaction.[60] As soon as complement is activated, the complex can detach and move on to other RBCs in addition to leukocytes or platelets. Because of this low affinity, only a small amount of drug is needed to cause the reaction, and the direct Coombs test is positive for complement only. Red blood cells are essentially victims or "innocent bystanders" of the immunologic reaction. Following discontinuation of the drug, the direct Coombs test will be negative as soon as the drug is cleared from the circulation.

A third type of immune-mediated mechanism has been seen with cephalosporin derivatives. The cephalosporins can combine with nonspecific proteins including albumin, IgG, IgA, and fibrinogen, and adhere to the RBC, causing a positive Coombs test. The binding is not immunologic in origin and hemolytic anemia has not been associated with this reaction (Fig. 94–5). However, the reaction can cause difficulties in cross-matching patients for blood transfusions, due to the nonspecific binding of antibodies to the RBC membrane.[61]

The fourth type of mechanism is also the best known. Methyldopa, as well as a few other drugs, is known to induce true autoantibodies to RBCs; the antibodies can be identified without the presence of the offending drug or its metabolites. This phenomenon is also interesting in that about 20% of patients receiving methyldopa will have a positive Coombs test, but less than 1% of these patients will experience hemolysis. The Coombs test will usually turn positive 3 to 6 months after the beginning of therapy, but hemolysis will develop from 4 to 6 months to more than 2 years after the start of therapy. After the withdrawal

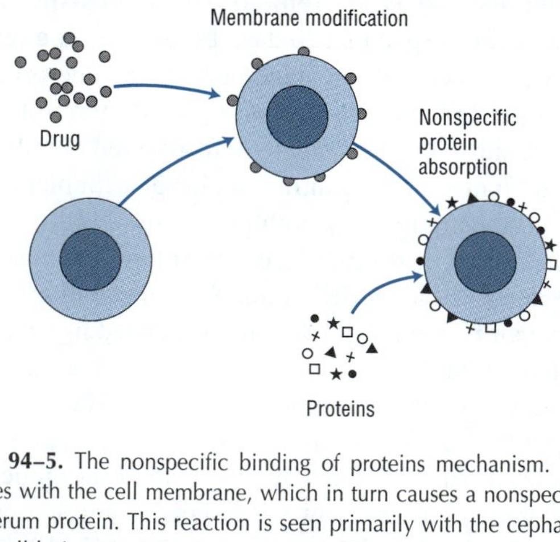

FIGURE 94–5. The nonspecific binding of proteins mechanism. The drug combines with the cell membrane, which in turn causes a nonspecific binding of serum protein. This reaction is seen primarily with the cephalosporins and no cell lysis or toxicity occurs. *(From Ref. 61, with permission.)*

of the drug, the Coombs test can remain positive for many months.[62]

The mechanism by which methyldopa induces antibody production is not completely known, but several hypotheses exist. One hypothesis suggests that methyldopa inhibits suppressor T-cell function, resulting in uncontrolled autoantibody formation by B cells.[63] More recent data, however, have not supported this concept.[64] Another hypothesis suggests the offending drug may bind to immature red cells, altering the membrane antigens and inducing autoantibodies.[65]

Overall, however, the reason that only some patients develop autoantibodies, and that only some of those have hemolytic disease, is not known. In an effort to explain why patients may have a positive Coombs test and no hemolysis, Kelton demonstrated that methyldopa impairs the ability of these patients to remove antibody-sensitized cells.[66] In Coombs-positive patients receiving methyldopa, patients with impairment of the reticuloendothelial system could not clear the RBCs coated with autoantibodies from their bloodstream, and therefore hemolysis did not occur. In patients presenting with hemolysis, no impairment of the reticuloendothelial system was demonstrated. Procainamide has also been reported to cause a positive direct antiglobulin test and hemolytic anemia.[67] Other drugs that have been reported to cause autoimmune hemolytic anemia include levodopa, mefanamic acid, tolmetin, diclofenac, and cimetidine.[61,65]

▶ TREATMENT: Drug-Induced Immune Hemolytic Anemia

The severity of the resulting anemia is usually a function of the rate of hemolysis. Hemolytic anemia caused by drugs via the hapten/adsorption and autoimmune mechanisms tend to be slower in onset and mild to moderate in severity. Conversely, hemolysis prompted via the immune complex (innocent bystander) phenomenon may have a sudden onset, severe hemolysis, and renal failure. The treatment of drug-induced immune hemolytic anemia includes the removal of the offending agent and supportive care. Glucocorticoids are usually unnecessary and practitioners have questioned their efficacy.[65] Intravenous immunoglobulins have been used in severe cases of immune hemolytic anemia, but are not standard therapy.[68]

DRUG-INDUCED OXIDATIVE HEMOLYTIC ANEMIA

Drug-induced oxidative hemolytic anemia is a hereditary condition most often associated with a glucose-6-phosphate dehydrogenase (G6PD) enzyme deficiency but can occur because of other enzyme defects (NADPH methemoglobin reductase or GSH peroxidase). G6PD deficiency is a disorder of the hexose monophosphate shunt, which is responsible for producing NADPH in erythrocytes, which in turn keeps glutathione in a reduced state. Reduced glutathione is a substrate for glutathione peroxidase, an enzyme that removes peroxide from erythrocytes, thus protecting them from oxidative stress.[69] Without reduced glutathione, oxidative drugs may oxidize the sulfhydryl groups of hemoglobin, which are removed prematurely from the circulation, causing hemolysis.

G6PD deficiency is the most common of all enzyme defects, affecting millions of people. The G6PD gene is located on the X chromosome and the disorder is consequently inherited via a sex-linked mode. There are many G6PD variants, but the most common types occur in American and African blacks (about 10% to 11%), people from Mediterranean areas (e.g., Greeks, Sardinians, and Khurdic and Sephartic Jews), and Asians.[62,69] The Mediterranean variety tends to be more severe, and those with this defect also may experience hemolysis from the ingestion of fava beans ("favism").[69]

The degree of hemolysis depends on the severity of the enzyme deficiency and the amount of oxidative stress. However, the dose required for hemolysis to occur is often less than prescribed quantities of the suspected agent.[70] Any drug that places oxidative stress on the RBC will cause drug-induced oxidative hemolytic anemia, but severe hemolysis is rare.[70] An interesting case of drug-induced oxidative hemolytic anemia occurred in a child when dapsone (an oxidizing agent) was transferred through the breast milk of the mother, who was taking the drug.[71] For a list of agents associated with drug-induced oxidative hemolytic anemia refer to Table 94–4.

TABLE 94–4. Drugs Associated With Oxidative Hemolysis

Ascorbic acid	Menadiol	Salazosulphapyridine
Benzocaine	Methylene blue	Sulfacetamide
Chloramphenicol	Naldixic acid	Sulfamethoxazole
Chloroquine	Nitrofurantoin	Sulfanilamide
Dapsone	Nitrofurazone	Sulfapyridine
Diazoxide	NSAIDs	
Furazolindone	Phenazopyridine	

▶ TREATMENT: Drug-Induced Oxidative Hemolytic Anemia

The treatment for drug-induced oxidative hemolytic anemia is removal of the drug. No other therapy is usually necessary since most cases of drug-induced oxidative hemolytic anemia are mild in severity. Patients should be advised to avoid medication capable of inducing the hemolysis.

DRUG-INDUCED MEGALOBLASTIC ANEMIA

Drug-induced megaloblastic anemia is the result of abnormal development of RBC precursors called megaloblasts in the bone marrow. Examination of peripheral blood will show a rise in the mean corpuscular hemoglobin. These megaloblastic changes are due to the direct or indirect effects of the drug on DNA synthesis. The abnormality can be seen in any portion of the replication process including DNA assembly, base precursor metabolism, or RNA synthesis.[72] The antineoplastic agents because of their pharmacologic action on DNA replication are most frequently associated with drug-induced megaloblastic anemia. However, other drugs such as cotrimoxazole, phenytoin, or the barbiturates have also been implicated. Cotrimoxazole has been reported to cause drug-induced megaloblastic anemia with both low and high doses.[73,74] The drug-induced megaloblastic anemia produced by cotrimoxazole is thought to occur most frequently in patients with a partial B_{12} or folate deficiency.[72] Because the drug's affinity for human dihydrofolate reductase is low, patients with adequate stores of these vitamins are probably at low risk of developing drug-induced megaloblastic anemia. Phenytoin, primidone, and phenobarbital have been postulated to cause drug-induced megaloblastic anemia by either inhibiting folate absorption or by increasing the folate catabolism. In both instances, relative deficiency of folate is produced. Table 94–5 provides a list of drugs that have been suggested to produce drug-induced megaloblastic anemia.

▶ TREATMENT: Drug-Induced Megaloblastic Anemia

When drug-induced megaloblastic anemia is related to chemotherapy, no real therapeutic option is available, and drug-induced megaloblastic anemia is an accepted side effect of therapy. If drug-induced megaloblastic anemia occurs due to cotrimoxazole, a trial course of folinic acid 5 to 10 mg up to four times a day may correct the anemia.[73,74] Folic acid supplementation of 1 mg every day will often correct the drug-induced megaloblastic anemia produced by either phenytoin or phenobarbital, but some clinicians suggest that supplementation of folic acid may decrease the effectiveness of the antiepileptic medications.

DRUG-INDUCED THROMBOCYTOPENIA

Thrombocytopenia is defined as a platelet count below 150,000/mm^3. Three types of drug-induced thrombocytopenia have been described: direct toxicity, hapten type, and innocent bystander type immune reaction. Direct toxicity reactions, resulting in suppressed thrombopoiesis, are characterized by a decrease in megakaryocytes in the bone marrow. In contrast, immune reactions result in an increased peripheral destruction of platelets and an increased number of megakaryocytes. Early symptoms of drug-induced thrombocytopenia include increased bruising, petechiae, ecchymosis, and epistaxis. Bleeding from mucous membranes and severe purpura can appear later in the disorder.

TABLE 94–5. Drugs Associated With Megaloblastic Anemia

p-Aminosalicylate	Hydroxyurea	Phenytoin
Azathioprine	6-Mercaptopurine	Primidone
Chloramphenicol	Metformin	Pyrimethamine
Colchicine	Methotrexate	Sulfasalazine
Cyclophosphamide	Neomycin	Triamterene
Cytarabine	Nitrofurantoin	Trimethoprim
5-Fluorodeoxyuridine	Oral contraceptives	Vinblastine
5-Fluorouracil	Phenobarbital	

Drugs that induce thrombocytopenia by their toxic effects are primarily cancer chemotherapy agents, but organic solvents, pesticides, and amrinone have also been implicated. Orally administered amrinone has been shown to cause thrombocytopenia in up to 18.6% of patients.[75] Although investigators have demonstrated an amrinone-dependent antibody, it is believed that because of the rapid onset, the dose-related response, and the absence of anamestic effect, the disorder is indicative of a reaction other than immune mediated, probably toxic.[75] Intravenous amrinone, the only commercially available form in the United States, is associated with a 2% to 4% incidence of thrombocytopenia, reflecting the short-term nature of administration. Amphotericin B has also been implicated in a case of thrombocytopenia. A direct toxic effect on the bone marrow has been proposed because no peripheral destruction of the patient's platelets occurred.[76]

In the majority of patients, drug-induced thrombocytopenia is caused by an immune reaction. The mechanisms are similar to those described earlier in the chapter. The formation of a hapten between the drug and a molecule on the platelet membrane is seen with penicillin derivatives, trimethoprim, and heparin. A list of medications associated with drug-induced thrombocytopenia can be found in Table 94–6. Hapten-mediated thrombocytopenia occurs 7 to 15 days after initiation of the drug and is seen frequently in patients receiving large doses of the medication (penicillin derivatives > 150 mg/kg).[77,78] The recovery period is often short in duration following discontinuation of the suspected drug.[79]

Heparin can cause at least two types of thrombocytopenia.[80] The first is a mild, reversible, nonimmune-mediated reaction that occurs 2 to 4 days after initiation of therapy. The platelet count then slowly returns to normal following the initial decline. This benign condition is thought to result from weak activation of platelets leading to sequestration.[80] The patients develop no major sequelae from the thrombocytopenia.

The second type of heparin-induced thrombocytopenia (HIT), also known as white clot syndrome, is severe and may be associated with a platelet count below 100,000/mm^3 and thrombosis.[80,81] The platelet count generally begins to decline 6 to 12 days after starting heparin therapy or sooner in patients previously treated with heparin. Patients can develop thrombocytopenia and thrombosis even on low-dose heparin[80,82] or with heparin-coated catheters,[83] leading to significant morbidity and mortality. The reaction was historically thought to be mediated by the formation of antibodies to the platelet–heparin complex. Recent evidence suggests a complex interaction between heparin, platelet factor 4 (PF4), platelet membrane Fc receptors, and possibly heparin-like molecules on the surface of endothelial cells (Fig. 94–6). Circulating heparin reacts with PF4 to produce a complex that is seen as antigen. Antibodies (IgG and IgM) react with this heparin–PF4 conjugate to form immune complexes that bind to Fc receptors on the platelet membrane. Platelet activation and aggregation occurs with

TABLE 94–6. Drugs Associated With Thrombocytopenia

Abciximab	Fluconazole	Penicillin
Acetazolamide	Furosemide	Phenothiazines
Allopurinol	Ganciclovir	Phenytoin
Aminoglutethimide	Gold salts	Procainamide
Amphotericin B	Heparin	Quinidine
Amrinone	Hydrochlorothiazide	Quinine
β-Lactam antibiotics	Hydroxychloroquine	Rifabutin
Carbamazepine	Imipenem–cilastatin	Rifampin
Chlorothiazide	Interferon	Sulfonamide antibiotics
Cimetidine	Isoniazid	Sulfonylureas
Colchicine	Low-molecular-weight heparin	Ticlopidine
Desipramine	Meclofenamate	Trimethoprim
Diazepam	Milrinone	Valproic acid
Didanosine	Morphine	Vancomycin
Digitoxin	NSAIDs	
Disopyramide		

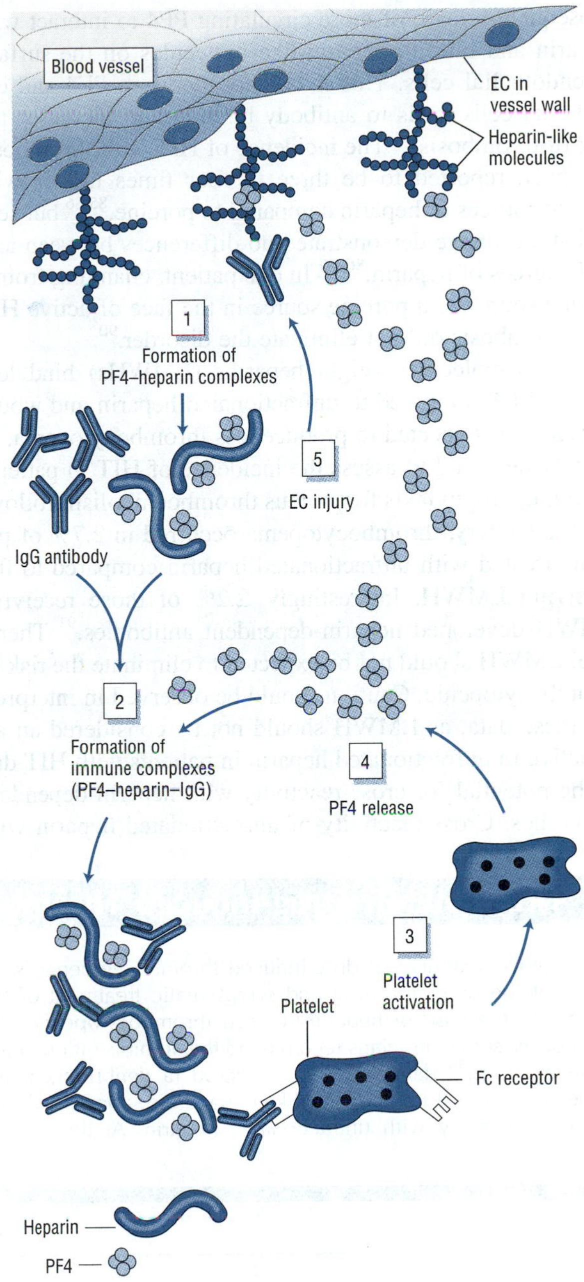

FIGURE 94–6. Proposed explanation for the presence of both thrombocytopenia and thrombosis in heparin-sensitive patients who are treated with heparin. Injected heparin reacts with platelet factor 4 (PF4), which is normally present on the surface of endothelial cells (ECs) or released in small quantities from circulating platelets, to form PF4–heparin complexes (1). Specific IgG antibodies react with these conjugates to form immune complexes (2) that bind to Fc receptors on circulating platelets. Fc-mediated platelet activation (3) releases PF4 from α-granules in platelets (4). Newly released PF4 binds to additional heparin, and the antibody forms more immune complexes, establishing a cycle of platelet activation. PF4 released in excess of the amount that can be neutralized by available heparin binds to heparin-like molecules (glycosaminoglycans) on the surface of ECs to provide targets for antibody binding. This process leads to immune-mediated EC injury (5) and heightens the risk of thrombosis and disseminated intravascular coagulation. *(From Ref. 84, with permission.)*

subsequent release of more circulating PF4 to interact with heparin and bind to heparin-like molecules on the surface of endothelial cells. This interaction between PF4 and endothelial cells leads to antibody binding and increases the risk of thrombosis.[84] The incidence of HIT with thrombosis has been reported to be three to four times higher with bovine sources of heparin compared to porcine,[85,86] but several studies have demonstrated no differences between animal sources of heparin.[86–89] In one patient, changing from a bovine source to a porcine source in the face of active HIT and thrombosis did not eliminate the disorder.[90]

Low-molecular-weight heparins (LMWHs) bind less well to PF4 compared to unfractionated heparin and would therefore be expected to produce less thrombocytopenia. In a study designed to assess the incidence of HIT in patients receiving prophylaxis for venous thromboembolism following hip surgery, thrombocytopenia occurred in 2.7% of patients treated with unfractionated heparin compared to 0% receiving LMWH. Interestingly, 2.2% of those receiving LMWH developed heparin-dependent antibodies.[91] Therefore, LMWH should not be expected to eliminate the risk of thrombocytopenia. Caution should be observed in interpreting these data, as LMWH should not be considered an alternative to unfractionated heparin in patients with HIT due to the potential for cross-reactivity with heparin-dependent antibodies. Cross-reactivity of unfractionated heparin with the heparinoid, danaparoid sodium (ORG 10172), has been demonstrated to occur in 19.6% of patients and 25.5% to 60.6% receiving LMWHs.[92] The clinical relevance of this *in vitro* cross-reactivity has yet to be determined.

The thrombocytopenia induced by gold salts is related to antibody formation to platelets.[93,94] The incidence of gold-induced thrombocytopenia is from 1% to 3% and often has a abrupt and severe onset.[93] The autoantibody formed to the platelet appears to be associated with the human leukocyte antigens (HLAs) which are located on the platelet membrane and on a number of other different cells in the body.[93,94] An interaction between the gold salts and the HLA antigens occurs, causing the platelets to be recognized as nonself, and thus inducing destruction of the platelets. The most commonly reported HLA antigen associated with induction of the autoantibodies is DR-3, but DR-4 may also interact with the antibodies.[93–95] The exact mechanism by which gold causes the formation of the autoantibody to regulated DR-3 and DR-4 antigens has not been elucidated.

The third mechanism described for drug-induced thrombocytopenia is the innocent bystander immune response. The most commonly implicated drug is quinidine, and the drug-induced thrombocytopenia is frequently related to high doses of quinidine.[96] Quinidine may also form a hapten with the platelet membrane to produce thrombocytopenia.[97]

▶ TREATMENT: Drug-Induced Thrombocytopenia

The primary treatment of drug-induced thrombocytopenia is removal of the offending drug and symptomatic treatment of the patient. In the case of heparin-induced thrombocytopenia with thrombosis, some clinicians recommend the administration of antiplatelet drugs,[98] danaparoid,[99,100] ancrod (a defibrinogenating snake venom), or hirudin.[100] Unlike danaparoid, ancrod exhibits no cross-reactivity with unfractionated heparin. At the present time, however, no studies have been performed to demonstrate the efficacy of the antiplatelet agents. In addition, it appears that large doses of steroids have no effect.[101] If the agents named here are unavailable immediately, use of dextran and warfarin should be considered.[100] In gold salt-induced thrombocytopenia, however, some investigators believe prednisone in a dose of 60 mg daily is beneficial in correcting the thrombocytopenia.[93]

▶ PRINCIPLES OF PHARMACOTHERAPY

- Drug-induced hematologic disorders are, in general, rare adverse effects associated with drug therapy.
- Drug-induced hematologic disorders are more common in women and the elderly; the risk of death also appears greater with increasing age.
- Reporting during postmarketing surveillance of a drug is usually the method by which the incidence of rare adverse drug reactions (ADRs) is established.
- The most common drug-induced hematologic disorders include aplastic anemia, agranulocytosis, megaloblastic anemia, thrombocytopenia, and hemolytic anemia.
- Drug-induced hematologic disorders range from mild reductions in affected cell lines to life-threatening reactions associated with significant morbidity and mortality.
- The mechanisms of drug-induced hematologic disorders are thought to be direct toxicity or immunologic in nature.
- Clinicians should be cognizant of agents with the potential of causing hematologic disorders and educate prescribers and patients accordingly.
- Frequent laboratory monitoring may be warranted for agents commonly demonstrating severe hematologic reactions.
- The primary treatment of drug-induced hematologic disorders is removal of the drug in question and symptomatic support of the patient.
- Because drug-induced blood disorders are dangerous, rechallenging a patient with a suspected agent in an attempt to confirm a diagnosis may not be ethical.

REFERENCES

1. Johnston FD. Granulocytopenia following the administration of sulphanilamide compounds. Lancet 1938;2:1044–1047.
2. Council for International Organizations of Medical Sciences. Standardization of definitions and criteria of assessment of adverse drug reactions. Drug-induced cytopenia. Int J Clin Pharmicol Toxicol 1990;29:75–81.
3. Patton WN, Duffull SB. Idiosyncratic drug-induced haematologic abnormalities. Drug Saf 1994;11:445–462.
4. Bottiger LE, Furhoff AK, Holmberg L. Drug-induced blood dyscrasias. A ten-year material from the Swedish Adverse Drug Reaction Committee. Acta Med Scand 1979;205:457–461.
5. Hine LK, Gerstman BB, Wise RP, Song YT. Mortality resulting from blood dyscrasia in the United States. Am J Med 1990;88:151–153.
6. Arneborn P, Palmblad J. Drug-induced neutropenia—A survey for Stockholm 1973–1978. Acta Med Scand 1982;212:289–292.
7. ASHP reports. ASHP guidelines on adverse drug reaction monitoring or reporting. Am J Hosp Pharm 1989;46:336–337.
8. Parent-Mussin DM, Sensebe L, Leqlise MC, et al. Relevance of in-vitro studies of drug-induced agranulocytosis. Report of 14 cases. Drug Saf 1993;9:463–469.
9. Claas FHJ. Drug-induced immune granulocytopenia. Baillieres Clin Immunol Allergy 1987;1:357–368.
10. Niewg HO. Aplastic anemia (panmyelopathy). In: Girdwood RH, ed. Blood Disorders Due to Drugs and Other Agents. Amsterdam, Excerpta Media, 1974.
11. Vincent PC. *In vitro* evidence of drug action in aplastic anemia. Blut 1984;49:3–12.
12. International Agranulocytosis and Aplastic Anemia Study. Risk of agranulocytosis and aplastic anemia. A first report of their relation to drug use with special reference to analgesics. JAMA 1986;256: 1749–1757.
13. Young NS, Maciejewski J. The pathophysiology of acquired aplastic anemia. N Engl J Med 1997;336:1365–1372.
14. Shadduck RK. Aplastic anemia. In: Williams WJ, et al, eds. Hematology, 5th ed. New York, McGraw-Hill, 1995:238–251.
15. Heimpel H, Heit W. Drug-induced aplastic anemia: Clinical aspects. Clin Haematol 1980;9:641–662.
16. Lubran MM. Hematologic side effects of drugs. Ann Clin Lab Sci 1989;19:114–121.
17. Malkin D, Koren G, Saunders EF. Drug-induced aplastic anemia pathogenesis and clinical aspects. Am J Pediatr Hematol Oncol 1990; 12:402–410.
18. Yunis AA, Miller AM, Salem Z, et al. Chloramphenicol toxicity: Pathogenetic mechanisms and the role of the *p*-NO_2 in aplastic anemia. Clin Toxicol 1980;17:359–373.
19. Jimenez JJ, Arimura GK, Abou-Khalil WH, et al. Chloramphenicol-induced bone marrow injury: Possible role of bacterial metabolites of chloramphenicol. Blood 1987;70:1180–1185.
20. Gerson WT, Fine DG, Spielberg SP, et al. Anticonvulsant-induced aplastic anemia: Increased susceptibility to toxic drug metabolites *in vitro*. Blood 1983;61:889–893.
21. Thomas ED, Storb R. Acquired severe aplastic anemia: Progress and perplexity. Blood 1984;64:325–328.
22. Hinterberger W, Rowlings PA, Hinterberger-Fischer M, et al. Results of transplanting bone marrow from genetically identical twins into patients with aplastic anemia. Ann Intern Med 1997;126:116–122.
23. Doney K, Leisenring W, Storb R, et al. Primary treatment of acquired aplastic anemia: Outcomes with bone marrow transplantation and immunosuppressive therapy. Ann Intern Med 1997;126:107–115.
24. Champlin R, Ho W, Gale RP. Antithymocyte globulin treatment in patients with aplastic anemia. N Engl J Med 1983;308:113–118.
25. Litzow MR, Kyle RA. Multiple responses of aplastic anemia to low-dose cyclosporine therapy despite development of a myelodysplastic syndrome. Am J Hematol 1989;32:226–229.
26. Bridges R, Pineo G, Blahey W. Cyclosporin A for the treatment of aplastic anemia refractory to antithymocyte globulin. Am J Hematol 1987;26:83–87.
27. Jacobs P, Wood L, Martell RW. Cyclosporin A in the treatment of severe acute aplastic anaemia. Br J Haematol 1985;61:267–272.
28. Bacigalupo, Broccia G, Codra G, et al. Antilymphocyte globulin, cyclosporin, and granulocyte colony-stimulating factor in patients with acquired severe aplastic anemia (SAA): A pilot study of the EBMT SAA Working Party. Blood 1995;85:1348–1353.
29. Antin JH, Smith BR, Holmes W, et al. Phase I/II study of recombinant human granulocyte-macrophage colony stimulating factor in aplastic anemia and myelodysplastic syndrome. Blood 1988;72:705–713.
30. Vadhan-Raj S, Buescher S, Broxmeyer HE, et al. Stimulation of myelopoiesis in patients with aplastic anemia by recombinant human granulocyte-macrophage colony-stimulating factor. N Engl J Med 1988;319:1628–1634.
31. Walsh CE, Liu JM, Anderson SM, et al. A trial of recombinant human interleukin I in patients with severe refractory aplastic anaemia. Br J Haematol 1992;80:106–110.
32. Bertrand Y, Amri F, Capdeville R, et al. The successful treatment of two cases of severe aplastic anemia with granulocyte-colony stimulating factor and cyclosporine A. Br J Haematol 1991;79:648–652.
33. Heit W, Heimpel H, Fischer A, et al. Drug-induced agranulocytosis: Evidence for the commitment of bone marrow haematopoiesis. Scand J Haematol 1985;35:459–468.
34. Julia A, Olona M, Bueno J, et al. Drug-induced agranulocytosis: Prognostic factors in a series of 168 episodes. Br J Haematol 1991; 79:366–371.
35. Pisciotta V. Drug-induced agranulocytosis. Drugs 1978;15:132–143.
36. Burckart GJ, Snidow J, Bruce W. Neutropenia following acute chlorpromazine ingestion. Clin Toxicol 1981;18:797–801.
37. Neftel KA, Muller MR, Hauser SD, et al. More on penicillin-induced leukopenia. N Engl J Med 1983;308:901.
38. Heit WF. Hematologic effects of antipyretic analgesics: Drug-induced agranulocytosis. Am J Med 1983;75:65–68.
39. Young GA, Vincent PC. Drug-induced agranulocytosis. Baillieres Clin Haematol 1980;9:483–504.
40. Kirkwood CF, Smith LL, Rustagi PK, et al. Neutropenia associated with beta-lactam antibiotics. Clin Pharmacy 1983;2:569–578.
41. Homayouni H, Gross PA, Setia V, et al. Leukopenia due to penicillin and cephalosporin homologues. Arch Intern Med 1979;139:827–828.
42. Neftel KA, Hauser SP, Muller MR. Inhibition of granulopoiesis *in vivo* and *in vitro* by beta-lactam antibiotics. J Infect Dis 1985;152: 90–98.
43. Cooper DS, Goldmiriz D, Lewin AA, et al. Agranulocytosis associated with antithyroid drug. Ann Intern Med 1983;98:26–29.
44. Tajiri J, Noguchi S, Murakami T, et al. Antithyroid drug-induced agranulocytosis. The usefulness of routine white blood cell count monitoring. Arch Intern Med 1990;150:621–624.
45. Toth AL, Mant MJ, Shivji S, et al. Propylthiouracil-induced agranulocytosis: An unusual presentation and a possible mechanism. Am J Med 1988;85:725–727.
46. McIntyre PA, Laleli YR, Hodkinson BA, et al. Evidence for antileukocyte antibodies as a mechanism for drug-induced agranulocytosis. Trans Assoc Am Phys 1971;84:217–225.
47. Werner MC, Romaldini JH, Bromberg N, et al. Adverse effects related to thionamide drugs regimen. Am J Med Sci 1989;297:216–219.
48. Clozaril new drug application, vols 28–31, 36, 39, 48, 50, 52, 84, 98, 99, 100, 103. East Hanover, NJ, Sandoz, 1987.
49. Alvir JM, Lieberman JA, Safferman AZ, et al. Clozapine-induced agranulocytosis. Incidence and risk factors in the United States. N Engl J Med 1993;329:162–167.
50. Fischer V, Haar JA, Greiner L, et al. Possible role of free radical formation in clozapine (Clozaril) induced agranulocytosis. Molec Pharmacol 1991;40:846–853.
51. Frampton JE, Lee CR, and Faulds P. Filgrastim. A review of its pharmacologic properties and therapeutic efficacy in neutropenia. Drugs 1994;48(5):731–760.

52. Willfort A, Lorber C, Kapiotis S, et al. Treatment of drug-induced agranulocytosis with recombinant granulocyte colony-stimulating factor (rh G-CSF). Ann Hematol 1993;66:241–244.
53. Delannoy A. GM-CSF therapy for drug-induced agranulocytosis. J Intern Med 1992;231:269–271.
54. MacDonald AG, Capell HA, Murphy J. Gold-induced aplastic anemia unresponsive to G-CSF. Annal Rheum Dis 1993;52:488.
55. Teitelbaum AH, Bell AJ, Brown SL. Filgrastim (r-metHuG-CSF) reversal of drug-induced agranulocytosis. Am J Med 1993;95:245–246.
56. Nielsen H. Recombinant human granulocyte colony-stimulating factor (rhG-CSF): Filgrastim treatment of clozapine-induced agranulocytosis. J Intern Med 1993;234:529–531.
57. Bjorkholm M, Pisa P, Arver S, Beran M. Haematologic effects of granulocyte-macrophage colony stimulating in a patient with thiamazole-induced agranulocytosis. J Intern Med 1992;232:443–445.
58. Nand S, Bayer R, Prinz R. Granulocyte-macrophage colony stimulating factor for the treatment of drug induced agranulocytosis. Am J Hematol 1991;37:267–269.
59. Tabbara IA. Hemolytic anemias. Diagnosis and management. Med Clin North Am 1992;76:649–669.
60. McKenzie SB. Hemolytic anemias due to extrinsic factors. In: Balado D, ed. Textbook of Hematology, 2nd ed. Baltimore, Williams & Willkins, 1996:245–257.
61. Petz LD. Drug-induced immune haemolytic anaemia. Baillieres Clin Haematol 1980;91:455–482.
62. Jandl JH. Immunohemolytic anemias. In: Strangis JT, ed. Blood, Textbook of Hematology, 2nd ed. Boston, Little, Brown, 1996: 421–518.
63. Kirtland HH, Mohler DN, Horwitz DA. Methyldopa inhibition of suppressor-lymphocyte function. A proposed cause of autoimmune hemolytic anemia. N Engl J Med 1980;302:825–832.
64. Garratty G, Arndt P, Prince HE, Schulman IA. The effect of methyldopa and procainamide on suppressor cell autoantibody production. Br J Haematol 1993;84:310.
65. Packman CH, Leddy JP. Drug-related immune hemolytic anemia. In: Williams WJ, et al, eds. Hematology, 5th ed. New York, McGraw-Hill, 1995:691–697.
66. Kelton JG. Impaired reticuloendothelial function in patients treated with methyldopa. N Engl J Med 1985;313:596–600.
67. Kleinman S, Nelson R, Smith L, et al. Positive direct antiglobulin tests and immune hemolytic anemia in patients receiving procainamide. N Engl J Med 1984;311:809–812.
68. Flores G, Cunningham-Rundles C, Newland AC, et al. Efficacy of intravenous immunoglobin in the treatment of autoimmune hemolytic anemia: Results in 73 patients. Am J Hematol 1993;44:237–242.
69. Beutler E. G6PD deficiency. Blood 1994;84:3613–3636.
70. Gordan-Amith EC. Drug-induced oxidative hemolysis. Clin Haematol 1980;9:587–605.
71. Sanders SW, Zone JJ, Foltz RR, et al. Hemolytic anemia induced by dapsone transmitted through breast milk. Ann Intern Med 1981;96: 465–466.
72. Scott JM, Weir DG. Drug-induced megaloblastic change. Clin Haematol 1980;9:587–605.
73. Magee F, O'Sullivan H, McCann SR. Megaloblastosis and low-dose trimethoprim–sulfamethoxazole. Ann Intern Med 1981;95:657.
74. Kobrinsky NL, Ramsay NK. Acute megaloblastic anemia induced by high-dose trimethoprim–sulfamethoxazole. Ann Intern Med 1981;94: 780–781.
75. Ansell J, Tiarks C, McCue J, et al. Amrinone-induced thrombocytopenia. Arch Intern Med 1984;144:949–952.
76. Chan CP, Tuazon CU, Lessin LS. Amphotericin-B-induced thrombocytopenia. Ann Intern Med 1982;96:332–333.
77. Murphy MF, Riordant T, Minchinton RM, et al. Demonstration of an immune-mediated mechanism of penicillin-induced neutropenia and thrombocytopenia. Br J Haematol 1983;55:155–160.
78. Salamon DJ, Nusbacher J, Stroupe T, et al. Red cell and platelet-bound IgG penicillin antibodies in a patient with thrombocytopenia. Transfusion 1984;24:395–398.
79. Miescher PA, Graf J. Drug-induced thrombocytopenia. Clin Haematol 1980;9:505–519.
80. Johnson RA, Lazarus KH, Henry DH. Heparin-induced thrombocytopenia prospective study. Am J Hematol 1984;17:349–353.
81. Cines DB, Kaywin P, Bina M, et al. Heparin-associated thrombocytopenia. N Engl J Med 1980;303:788–795.
82. Cheng TC. Thrombocytopenia associated with minidose heparin therapy. Postgrad Med 1981;70:73–78.
83. Laster JL, Nichols WK, Silver D. Thrombocytopenia associated with heparin-coated catheters in patients with heparin-associated antiplatelet antibodies. Arch Intern Med 1989;149:2285–2287.
84. Aster RH. Heparin-induced thrombocytopenia and thrombosis. N Engl J Med 1995;332:1374–1376.
85. King DJ, Kelton JG. Heparin-associated thrombocytopenia. Ann Intern Med 1984;100:535–540.
86. Bell WR, Royall RM. Heparin-associated thrombocytopenia: A comparison of three heparin preparations. N Engl J Med 1980;303: 902–907.
87. Green D, Martin GJ, Shoichet SH, et al. Thrombocytopenia in a prospective, randomized, double-blind trial of bovine and porcine heparin. Am J Med Sci 1984;288:60–64.
88. Rao AK, White GC, Sherman L, et al. Low incidence of thrombocytopenia with porcine mucosal heparin. A prospective multicenter study. Arch Intern Med 1989;149:1285–1288.
89. Bailey RT, Ursick JA, Heim KL, et al. Heparin-associated thrombocytopenia: A prospective comparison of bovine lung heparin, manufactured by a new process, and porcine intestinal heparin. Drug Intell Clin Pharm 1986;20:374–378.
90. Guay DR, Richard A. Heparin-induced thrombocytopenia—Association with a platelet aggregating factor and cross-sensitivity to bovine and porcine heparin. Drug Intell Clin Pharm 1984;18:398–401.
91. Warkentin TE, Levine MN, Hirsh J, et al. Heparin-induced thrombocytopenia in patients treated with low-molecular-weight heparin or unfractionated heparin. N Engl J Med 1995;332:1330–1335.
92. Kikta MJ, Keller MP, Humphrey PV, et al. Can low molecular weight heparins and heparinoids be safely given to patients with heparin-induced thromocytopenia syndrome? Surgery 1993;114:705–710.
93. Armstrong RD, Faith A, Panayi GS, et al. Gold-induced thrombocytopenia: Detection of anti-platelet antibody. Clin Rheumatol 1983;2: 183–188.
94. Adachi JD, Bensen WG, Singal DP, et al. Gold induced thrombocytopenia: Platelet associated IgG and HLA typing in three patients. J Rheumatol 1984;11:355–357.
95. Coblyn JS, Weinblatt M, Holdsworth D, et al. Gold-induced thrombocytopenia. A clinical and immunogenic study of twenty-three patients. Ann Intern Med 1981;95:178–181.
96. Kelton JG, Meltzer D, Moore J, et al. Drug-induced thrombocytopenia is associated with increased binding of IgG to platelets both *in vivo* and *in vitro*. Blood 1981;58:524–529.
97. Chong BH, Berndt MC, Koutts J, et al. Quinidine-induced thrombocytopenia and leukopenia: Demonstration and characterization of distinct antiplatelets and antileukocyte antibodies. Blood 1983;62: 1218–1223.
98. Matsuo T, Yamada T, Chikahira Y, et al. Effect of aspirin on heparin-induced thrombocytopenia (HIT) in a patient requiring hemodialysis. Blut 1989;59:393–395.
99. Chong BH, Ismdil F, Cade J, et al. Heparin-induced thrombocytopenia: Studies with a new low molecular weight heparinoid, Org 10172. Blood 1989;73:1592–1596.
100. Hirsh J, Raschke R, Warkentin TE, et al. Heparin: Mechanism of action, pharmacokinetics, dosing considerations, monitoring, efficacy, and safety. Chest 1995;108:258S–275S.
101. Rector TS, Cipolle RJ, Seifert RD, et al. Characteristics of heparin-associated thrombocytopenia. Am J Hosp Pharm 1979;36:1561–1565.

95 LABORATORY TESTS TO DIRECT ANTIMICROBIAL PHARMACOTHERAPY

Michael J. Rybak, PharmD, FCCP, BCPS, and Jeffrey R. Aeschlimann, PharmD

Appropriate antimicrobial therapy for a given infectious disease requires knowledge of the infecting pathogen, host characteristics, and the drug's expected activity against the pathogen. The most fundamental aspect of therapy starts with an appropriate diagnosis. A vast array of laboratory tests are available to assist the clinician in verifying the presence of infection and for monitoring the response to therapy. Although useful, these tests are subject to interpretation and cannot be substituted for sound clinical judgment. Organism susceptibility to a given group of antimicrobials is key to determining the patient's therapy. Host characteristics, however, such as immune status, infection-site location, and body organ function, play a significant role in selecting the most appropriate antimicrobial for a given individual.[1] This chapter reviews the basic laboratory tests available to the clinician to assist in the diagnosis and treatment of infection.

LABORATORY TESTS CONFIRMING THE PRESENCE OF INFECTION

NONSPECIFIC TESTS

Several tests are routinely used to detect the presence of infection. The usefulness of a particular test depends on how sensitive the test is in detecting an infection when an infection truly exists versus the possibility of providing a false-positive result indicating an infection when an alternative explanation exists. Positive results usually prompt the clinician to perform a directed search for the infectious etiology and the specific pathogen using techniques described later in this chapter.

WHITE BLOOD CELL COUNT AND DIFFERENTIAL

An elevation in the total white blood cell (WBC) count is often indicative of systemic infection. The elevation may be mild, rising slightly above the normal range of 5000 to 10,000 cells/mm^3 in non–life-threatening infections or in the elderly, or it may exceed 50,000 cells/mm^3 in cases of overwhelming sepsis. The absolute WBC count remains a nonspecific test because elevations may occur in noninfectious diseases, such as leukemia or rheumatoid arthritis, or during drug therapy (e.g., corticosteroids or lithium). A differential blood cell count is often done to determine the approximate amounts of the various leukocytes (WBCs). Table 95–1 displays a normal differential count for an adult. An excess or a deficiency of all or a particular group may be helpful in determining the etiology of the infection.

White blood cells are divided into two groups, the granulocytes, which have prominent cytoplasmic granules, and the agranulocytes, which lack granules. Polymorphonuclear granulocytes or neutrophils (PMNs) are made up of neutrophils, basophils, and eosinophils. The two other classes of WBCs are the monocytes and lymphocytes. Neutrophils are the most common type of WBCs in the blood. In response to infection, they leave the bloodstream and enter the tissue to interact with and phagocytize the offending pathogen. Mature neutrophils are sometimes referred to as "segs" because of their segmented nucleus, which usually consists of two to five lobes. Immature neutrophils lack this segmented feature and are referred to as "bands." During an acute infection, immature neutrophils, such as bands, are released from the bone marrow into the bloodstream at an increased rate, and they may exceed 10% to 20% of the total WBCs, resulting in a shift from a predominance of mature cells to immature cells. This has been referred to as the so-called "shift to the left" because of the location of these cells in conjunction with mature cells in textbook diagrams.

Leukocytosis is a normal host defense to infection and is an important adjunct to antimicrobial therapy. Unfortunately, bacterial infection is a common complication of neutropenia from cancer chemotherapy. These patients are incapable of increasing their WBCs in response to infection. In fact, susceptibility to infection in these patients is highly dependent on their WBC status. It is well known that patients with neutrophil counts of less than 500 cells/mm^3 are at high risk for the development of bacterial or fungal infections. The absence of leukocytosis also has been reported to occur during acute infection in the elderly and in cases of overwhelming sepsis.[2]

Lymphocytes are cells of the immune system. Two functional types of lymphocytes are the T cell, which is involved in cell-mediated immunity, and the B cell, which produces antibodies when activated. Lymphocytosis is

TABLE 95–1. Normal White Blood Cell Differential in an Adult

Cell Type	Percent (%)
Neutrophils (PMNs[a])	50–70
Immature neutrophils (bands, stabs)	3–5
Metamyelocytes	0–1
Lymphocytes	20–40
Monocytes	0–7
Eosinophils	0–5
Basophils	0–1

[a]PMNs = polymorphonuclear leukocytes.

frequently associated with viral infections.[3] For example, acute Epstein-Barr virus infection (mononucleosis) produces an absolute leukocytosis with a lymphocytic predominance. These lymphocytes are frequently described as being atypical because of their morphologic appearance on microscopic examination.

Lymphopenia, particularly with the helper (or CD-4) subset of T-cell lymphocytes, is characteristic of human immunodeficiency virus (HIV) infection. Malignancies may also adversely affect cellular immunity. Patients with Hodgkin's disease and other types of lymphoma exhibit defective cell-mediated immunity that predisposes them to a variety of infections, notably fungal diseases and infections by the *Listeria* species. Drug treatment with cytotoxic chemotherapy and corticosteroids may also have profound deleterious effects on cell-mediated immunity.[4] Defects in cell-mediated immune function can be demonstrated by a variety of simple laboratory tests, including quantification of lymphocytes on a routine complete blood cell count and skin testing for anergy. A more detailed investigation would include quantitative measurements of T-helper and T-suppressor cells. Monocytosis is less frequently correlated with acute bacterial infection, although its presence has been associated with the response of certain infections (e.g., tuberculosis) to chemotherapy. Eosinophilia may result from parasitic infection.

OTHER TESTS

There are a variety of nonspecific laboratory tests that are useful to support the diagnosis of infection. The inflammatory process initiated by an infection sets up a complex of host responses. Activation of complements, such as C3a and C5a, initiates inflammation and sets off a cascade of changes and the subsequent release of mediators, all of which can be measured and monitored. Serum complement concentrations, and in particular C3, are usually consumed as part of the host defense mechanism and are subsequently reduced during the early stages of an acute infectious process. Acute-phase reactants, such as the erythrocyte sedimentation rate (ESR) and the C-reactive protein, are elevated in the presence of an inflammatory process but do not confirm the presence of infection, because they are often elevated in noninfectious conditions, such as collagen vascular diseases and arthritis. Large elevations in ESR have been associated with infections, such as endocarditis, osteomyelitis, and intra-abdominal infections.[5]

Changes in endothelial membranes and the presence of a foreign pathogen and its endotoxins cause certain cytokines, such as the interleukins (IL) IL-1, IL-6, IL-8, and tumor necrosis factor (TNF)-α, to be released from macrophages and lymphocytes. Fluctuations in cytokine levels occur during the course of an infection, which may be useful in staging and monitoring the response to therapy. Although abnormal levels of TNF have been associated with a variety of noninfectious causes, consistent elevations in TNF are found in patients with serious infections, such as sepsis. Studies of the relationship of circulating mediators to patient outcome have determined the value of endotoxin and cytokine measurements in patients with sepsis. Although the combination of elevations in endotoxin and individual cytokines has correlated well with the mortality rate, measurement of IL-6 was by far the best individual cytokine that predicted patient outcome.[6] Direct and rapid measurement of endotoxin and cytokines at the bedside may be available in the future to assist clinicians in diagnosing, staging, and monitoring serious infections, such as sepsis.[7]

LABORATORY IDENTIFICATION OF PATHOGENS

COLONIZATION VERSUS INFECTION

Pathogens are organisms that are capable of damaging host tissues and that elicit specific host responses and symptoms that are consistent with an infectious process. These organisms are routinely predictable as the cause of the infection in question. On the other hand, the human body contains a vast variety of microorganisms that colonize body systems and make up the so-called "normal" flora. These organisms occur naturally in the tissues of the host and provide some benefits, including defense by occupying space, competing for essential nutrients, stimulating cross-protective antibodies, and suppressing the growth of potentially pathogenic bacteria and fungi (Table 95–2).

Organisms that make up the normal flora can become pathogenic when host defenses become impaired or if they are translocated to other body sites during trauma. The identification of an organism considered to be normal flora in a wound or otherwise sterile body cavity or fluid often becomes a dilemma for the clinician in deciding whether or not a patient is infected and whether or not he or she requires treatment. Such is the case of *Staphylococcus epidermidis* when it is identified in the blood of a hospitalized patient. *S. epidermidis* is considered normal skin flora and commonly colonizes intravenous catheters. In these conditions, the identification of the organism must be taken in light of the patient circumstances (signs and symptoms, laboratory indices supporting infection) and the probability of the organism being responsible for the infection. Often, the simple removal of the catheter may eliminate the organism

TABLE 95–2. Organisms Frequently Regarded as Normal, Colonizing Flora

Skin
Diphtheroids (e.g., *Corynebacterium* sp.)
Propionibacteriaceae
Staphylococci (especially, coagulase-negative strains)
Streptococci
Gastrointestinal Tract
Bacteroides sp.
Clostridium sp.
Diphtheroids
Enterobacteriaceae (e.g., *Escherichia coli, Klebsiella* sp.)
Fusobacterium sp.
Streptococci (anaerobic)
Upper Respiratory Tract
Bacteroides sp.
Haemophilus sp.
Neisseria sp.
Streptococci
Genital Tract
Corynebacterium sp.
Enterobacteriaceae
Lactobacillus sp.
Mycoplasma sp.
Staphylococci
Streptococci

from the bloodstream, thereby preventing misdiagnosis and unnecessary application of antimicrobials.[8]

DIRECT EXAMINATION

Direct examination of tissue or body fluids believed to be infected can provide simple, rapid information to the clinician. Microscopic examination of wet mount specimen preparations can provide valuable information regarding potential pathogens. Applications of this procedure with or without staining preparations include direct examination of sputum, bronchial aspirates, scrapings of mucosal lesions, and urinary sediment. The Gram stain is one of the first differential tests run on a specimen brought to the laboratory for identification. For this procedure, crystal violet is applied as the primary stain with iodine added to enhance the staining process and to form a crystal-violet iodine complex. Alcohol decolorization is the next step in the procedure. Gram-negative cells are decolorized by the addition of alcohol, and they take on a red color when counterstained by safranin. Gram-positive cells are not decolorized by alcohol and retain the crystal-violet color and appear purple. Gram staining in conjunction with microscopic examination may provide a presumptive diagnosis and some indication of the organism's characteristics (gram-positive, gram-negative, gram-variable, bacillus, or cocci). This is extremely useful information for the selection of empiric antibiotic therapy.

Gram stains are routinely performed on cerebral spinal fluid in cases of suspected meningitis, on urethral smears for venereal diseases, and on abscess or effusion specimens. They are helpful in identifying organisms, such as anaerobes, which may not grow on culture and would otherwise be missed. Although Gram stains of sputum are routinely performed where respiratory tract infections are suspected, there is controversy regarding the usefulness of this test since the sputum is often contaminated with mixed or normal flora. The predominance of one particular organism, the overall number of organisms present, the amount of PMNs present, and the presence or absence of a significant amount of squamous epithelial cells (< 10 per low-power field) may improve the significance of the sputum Gram stain specimen.[9] Table 95–3 lists some common infecting pathogens grouped according to Gram stain and other characteristics.

A variety of other staining techniques are used by the clinician and laboratory. In particular, staining procedures are used for those pathogens that are best identified microscopically because of their poor growth characteristics in the laboratory setting. The best examples of these would be the Ziehl-Neelsen stain for acid-fast bacilli, which is used for the identification of mycobacteria, and the India ink, potassium hydroxide (KOH), and Giemsa's stains, which are useful for detecting certain fungi.[9]

CULTURES

Isolation of the etiologic agent by culture is the most definitive method available to the clinician for the diagnosis and eventual treatment of infection. Although suspicion of a specific pathogen or group of pathogens is helpful to the laboratory for the selection of specific cultivating media, the more common procedure for the laboratory is to screen for the presence of any potential pathogen. After receipt of a clinical specimen, the laboratory will inoculate the specimen in a variety of artificial media. Some culture media are designed to differentiate various organisms on the basis of biochemical characteristics or to select specific organisms on the basis of resistance to certain antimicrobials. Other media commonly employed allow for the isolation of more fastidious organisms, such as *Listeria, Legionella,* mycobacteria, or *Chlamydia*. Cultures for viruses are more difficult to perform and are primarily undertaken by larger hospitals or reference laboratories because of the expense of the equipment, personnel, and time involved in processing samples.

When a culture is obtained, careful attention must be taken to ensure that specimens are appropriately collected and transported to the laboratory. Every effort should be made to avoid contamination with normal flora and to ensure that the specimen is placed in the appropriate transport media. Culture specimens should be transported to the laboratory as soon as possible because organisms may perish because of prolonged exposure to air or drying. This is especially important for swab specimen preparations. Transport media may not be ideal for all organisms. Specimens that contain fastidious organisms or anaerobes require special transport media and should be immediately forwarded to the laboratory for processing. Last, the source of the specimen should be clearly recorded and forwarded along

TABLE 95–3. Examples of Important Bacterial Pathogens Classified According to Staining Characteristics, Morphology, and Other Salient Features

Gram-Positive Cocci
- Staphylococci
  - Coagulase-positive *Staphylococcus aureus*
  - Coagulase-negative *S. epidermidis*
- Streptococci
- Anaerobes
  - *Peptostreptococcus*
- *Streptococcus pneumoniae* (diplococcus, pneumococcus)
- Group A, β-hemolytic
  - *Streptococcus pyogenes*
- Group B
  - *Streptococcus agalactiae*
- Group D
  - *Enterococcal* sp.
    - *E. rafinosus*
    - *E. faecalis*
    - *E. durans*
    - *E. faecium*
- Nonenterococcal species
  - *S. bovis*
  - *S. equinus*
- Viridans group
  - *S. sanguis*
  - *S. mitior*
  - *S. mutans*
  - *S. milleri*

Gram-Positive Bacilli
- *Bacillus* sp.
  - *B. cereus*
- *Clostridium* sp.
  - *C. difficile*
  - *C. perfringens*
  - *C. tetani*
- Diphtheroids
  - *Corynebacterium diphtheriae*
  - JK group *Corynebacterium*
  - *Listeria monocytogenes*

Gram-Negative Bacilli
- Anaerobes
  - *Bacteroides fragilis*
  - *Bacteroides* sp.
- Enterobacteriaceae
  - *Citrobacter* sp.
  - *Enterobacter* sp.
  - *Escherichia coli*
  - *Klebsiella* sp.
  - *Serratia* sp.
  - *Morganella* sp.
  - *Proteus* sp.
    - Indole-negative: *P. mirabilis*
    - Indole-positive: *P. vulgaris*
  - *Providencia* sp.
  - *Salmonella* sp.
  - *Serratia* sp.
  - *Shigella* sp.
- *Pseudomonas* sp.
  - *P. aeruginosa*
  - *P. cepacia*
- *Stenotrophomonas maltophilia*

Gram-Negative Cocci
- *Moraxella catarrhalis*
- *Neisseria gonorrhoeae*
- *N. meningitidis*

Mycobacteria (acid-fast bacilli)
- *Mycobacterium avium*–intracellulare complex
  - *M. bovis*
  - *M. fortuitum*
  - *M. tuberculosis*

Fungi
- Yeasts
  - *Candida* sp.
  - *Cryptococcus neoformans*
  - *Aspergillus* sp.
    - *A. fumigatus*

with the culture to the laboratory. This process will aid the laboratory in differentiating true pathogens from the expected, normal flora, and it will help in the selection of the appropriate culture media.

The ability to detect microorganisms in the bloodstream by standard culturing techniques is difficult because of the inherently low yield of organisms diluted by blood, humoral factors with bactericidal activity, and the potential of antimicrobial pretreatment affecting organism growth. Newer automated systems employing the use of media-containing culture bottles and innovative organism detection techniques have improved this situation. Most blood collection bottles dilute the blood specimen 1:10 with growth media to neutralize the bactericidal properties of blood and antimicrobials. The addition of a polyanionic anticoagulant abolishes the effect of complement and antiphagocytic activity in the specimen. Some laboratories also add β-lactamase to their blood collection bottles. Antibiotic-binding resin bottles, such as Bactec 16 B, are also commercially available.

Rapid detection of bacteria or fungi within a few hours of specimen collection is now possible by the use of automated culturing systems, such as Bactec (Becton Dickinson Diagnostic Instruments, Sparks, MD), that use bottles of growth media containing a fluorescent sensor that monitors for the presence of CO_2 as a byproduct of microorganism growth. Culture bottles are monitored every 10 minutes for the presence of CO_2. Computers monitoring the system alert laboratory personnel of positive culture results by both audible and visual alarms. Once detected, a battery of testing can be performed rapidly that allows the clinicians to obtain preliminary information about the organism and shorten the reporting time.[10,11]

The initial identity of the organism can be determined by a variety of testing procedures. General schemes differentiate organisms into primary groups, such as gram-positive and gram-negative bacteria. This can be accomplished through simple Gram staining, as previously described, evaluating organism growth patterns on selective media, testing for the presence or absence of specific enzymes, and chemical characteristics, such as hemolytic and fermentation properties. For example, a non–lactose-fermenting, gram-negative bacilli that is oxidase positive may suggest *Pseudomonas aeruginosa* as opposed to a variety of other potential gram-negative organisms. This preliminary information, which is readily obtainable from the laboratory, may greatly assist the clinician in choosing the appropriate empiric therapy.

Definitive identification of organisms requires more complex testing procedures and devices that can further differentiate the organism on the basis of specific fermentation and biochemical reactive properties. Commercially available automated systems can inoculate the test organism into a series of panels containing a variety of test media, sugars, and other reagents. The system can then photometrically determine the results and compare the findings to a library of organism characteristics to produce a definitive identification.

Viral agents may be detected by direct observation of inoculated culture cells for cytopathic effects or by detection of antigens after incubation by immunofluorescent methods. The culture method is most useful for organisms, such as cytomegalovirus (CMV) or herpes simplex virus, since these viral agents are rapidly propagated in culture cells and are, therefore, easily detected.

DIAGNOSIS OF INFECTION USING IMMUNOLOGIC AND MOLECULAR METHODS

ANTIBODY AND ANTIGEN DETECTION

The use of immunologic methods for the diagnosis and monitoring of human–host immune response to infection has become an indispensable laboratory tool. This is especially important in the detection of microorganisms, such as bacteria, fungi, and viruses, that would otherwise elude or severely delay results from conventional culturing techniques. These methods have the advantage of a rapid turnaround time and an acceptable level of sensitivity and specificity. Some tests (e.g., identification of group A streptococci) are simple to use, can be performed conveniently in the physician's office, and may often be used to decide whether antibiotics are administered for a suspected upper respiratory infection.

The primary immunologic methods involve the detection and quantification of antibodies directed against a specific pathogen or its components (i.e., surface proteins of HIV, such as p24 antigen). The commercial availability of specific monoclonal antibodies in a variety of testing formats has led to an increased use of these methods for direct pathogen detection. Although pathogen antigenic proteins may be increased and, therefore, easily detected during acute infection, detection of past or asymptomatic infection may result in undetectable levels of antigen and, therefore, low antibody titers. Continued advancement in sensitivity (the ability to detect a true positive state) and specificity (the ability to detect a negative state), as well as the use of amplification techniques, will likely improve these tests in the near future. Antibody or antigen detection may be accomplished by a variety of techniques, including immunofluorescence, which has been routinely used for the detection of cytomegalovirus, respiratory syncytial virus, varicella-zoster virus, *Treponema pallidum* (syphilis), *Borrelia burgdorferi* (Lyme's disease), and *Chlamydia trachomatis*. Latex agglutination has been useful for detection of the meningococcal capsular antigens in cerebral spinal fluid of patients suspected of having bacterial meningitis and to aid in the diagnosis of *Legionella pneumophilia*. Enzyme-linked immunosorbent assay or ELISA is one of the most commonly employed methods used for the detection of HIV, herpes simplex virus, respiratory syncytial virus, pneumococcal serum antibody, *Neisseria gonorrhoeae,* and *Haemophilus pylori*.[12]

MOLECULAR TECHNIQUES FOR THE DETECTION OF MICROORGANISMS

HYBRIDIZATION DNA PROBES

Highly sensitive and specific molecular methods are now available for the rapid detection and identification of a variety of pathogens. The two primary molecular techniques commonly employed use nucleic acid hybridization, which involves the binding of a specific DNA or RNA probe to its target or DNA amplification schemes. Probe-based methods require the extraction of DNA or RNA from a clinical specimen (body fluid, tissue, white blood cell) or directly from a microorganism culture. The extract is then tested for the presence of pathogen DNA or RNA using a probe that contains a specific oligonucleic acid–based sequence for the organism. For example, a probe with a sequence of ACTGTT would bind to the complementary organism nucleic acid sequence of TGACAA. Because the probe is labeled with a signal-emitting molecule (radiolabeled, colorometric, or chemoluminescent), a match would be detected. The primary means for detection involves the use of separation of the organism DNA into specific fragments (gel electrophoresis), the mixing of the DNA fragments with the labeled probe (hybridization), transfer and fixation of the mixture to specialized paper or nylon membranes (Southern or Northern blotting), and transfer to radiographic or photographic film for processing. These techniques have been used for many years and are fairly standardized methods for the detection of a variety of organisms.[13]

Hybridization probes are useful for a variety of diagnostic and clinical applications, one of which is the direct examination of organisms in tissue. This allows for the evaluation and documentation of organism infestation, location, distribution, and host response. The use of hybridization probes is particularly helpful for the detection of slow-growing organisms, such as *Mycobacterium tuberculosis, N. gonorrhoeae,* and certain species of fungi. This technique is also used to document the presence or absence of antimicrobial-resistant genes in a cell culture and to track the spread of resistant microorganisms in hospital and outpatient settings.

Although widely employed, the use of hybridization probes is often limited by their lack of sensitivity. Probe amplification methods have become available to improve the sensitivity of these assays. The principle of these probe amplification schemes is to boost the probe's signal-emitting molecule to make it more easily detected. The most advanced signal amplification system available is the branched DNA (bDNA) probe system (Chiron Corp., Emeryville, CA). This system uses multiple probes and multiple signal-emitting molecules (reporters). The target-binding probe contains two hybridization regions. One of these regions is complementary to the target, and the other is capable of binding with the bDNA amplification multimer. The amplification multimer binds multiple reporter molecules (as many as 3000), which provides a significant boost in the probe's signal. Branched DNA probe systems are being developed for rapid detection of hepatitis B and C, HIV-1, and CMV. Because of the system's high specificity and quantitative ability, bDNA probe assays may be useful for therapeutic monitoring, such as in the case of monitoring the response to antiretroviral therapy in acquired immunodeficiency syndrome (AIDS).[14]

NUCLEIC ACID AMPLIFICATION METHODS

Nucleic acid amplification (NAA), now considered by most a standard laboratory tool, has had a tremendous impact on the diagnosis and treatment of infectious diseases. These highly sensitive methods have the ability to detect and quantitate minute amounts of target nucleic acid in a rapid manner. The polymerase chain reaction (PCR) is based on the ability of a DNA polymerase to copy and elongate a targeted strand of DNA. This is accomplished by the use of short oligonucleotide primers (20 to 25 nucleotides long) that correspond to the DNA targeted to be expanded. After an excess of primers and heat-stable DNA, polymerases are added to the targeted DNA mixture, and the targeted DNA is denatured and separated by a process of cycling hot and cool temperatures. The heat-stable DNA polymerase elongates the primers on the two separate strands of DNA, thereby generating two new strands of targeted DNA. The process of cycling is typically repeated 20 to 35 times. Each cycle doubles the amount of DNA originally present at the start of the cycle, thereby exponentially increasing the overall number of DNA copies. In theory, more than one million copies of the original DNA can be generated from as few as 20 cycles.

Although this amplification technique is very sensitive and has tremendous application potential, it is not without problems. The powerful amplification procedure may yield false-positive results when samples are contaminated by nucleic acid left over from previous amplified DNA. Other problems include primer artifact formation and nonspecific hybridization of primers to DNA samples. Several modifications to the original PCR technology have been made over the years to improve the sensitivity and application potential for PCR, including the use of multiple sets of amplification primers, the amplication of two or more target DNA sequences simultaneously, PCR amplication of RNA by converting targeted RNA with reverse transcriptase to complementary DNA templates, which are then suitable for DNA amplification by traditional PCR techniques, and the use of thermostable DNA polymerase.

The cost–benefit ratio of PCR compared to traditional microbiologic methods must be evaluated. Molecular amplification schemes like PCR are likely to find early acceptance in situations where rapid turnaround time is essential to improve patient diagnosis and outcome. Such would be the case for the isolation and detection of fastidious or slow-growing organisms like *M. tuberculosis* and *B. burgdorferi.* Another potential application for this technology is the early detection of multidrug-resistant organisms. Amplification of resistant gene markers would aid in rapid selection of the most appropriate therapy in the treatment of organisms in which days or weeks are traditionally required for culturing and determining basic susceptibility. Examples fitting this description include the rapid detection of isoniazid and rifampin gene markers for *M. tuberculosis,* early detection of the *mec* gene responsible for methicillin resistance in *S. aureus,* and identification of resistant genes responsible for production of β-lactamase capable of destroying specific cephalosporins.[14,15]

EVALUATION OF THE PHARMACODYNAMIC PROPERTIES OF ANTIMICROBIALS

The laboratory evaluation of antimicrobial susceptibility is an important component of the pharmacotherapeutic management of infectious diseases. With the rapid increases in antimicrobial resistance in bacteria, fungi, and viruses, the integration of susceptibility data into empiric treatment choices and subsequent regimen modifications is becoming even more crucial. As well, analysis of organism susceptibility profiles is a mandatory step for many cost-containment strategies, such as antimicrobial streamlining programs or intravenous-to-oral switch protocols.[16]

Although most susceptibility tests used are well characterized and standardized by the National Committee for Clinical Laboratory Standards (NCCLS), there still is much controversy concerning methods, interpretation, and integration of the results into the management of the patient.[17] Often, susceptibility reporting methods can make the pharmacodynamic optimization of antimicrobial therapy potentially difficult. Nevertheless, many investigations have shown that the general susceptibility profile of an infecting organism can correlate with both clinical and microbiologic responses to therapy.

Most standardized and well-accepted test methods evaluate the susceptibility of aerobic, nonfastidious bacteria. In recent years, encouraging progress has been made in the development of sensitive, specific, and reproducible tests for anaerobes, yeasts, mycobacteria, and viruses. As technology continues to advance testing methods, more rapid and accurate procurement of results should help to aid the clinician in the diagnosis and treatment of all infectious diseases. These systems are often very expensive, but the pharmacotherapist can play an important role in the collaborative assessment of the impact of these tests on the overall costs and quality of care for the patient with infection. A discussion of these tests in the upcoming sections should suggest potential areas where pharmacoeconomic evaluation would prove useful.

MINIMUM INHIBITORY CONCENTRATION

The minimum inhibitory concentation (MIC) is the lowest antimicrobial concentration that prevented visible growth of an organism after 24 hours of incubation in a specified growth medium. The MIC allows for quantitative determination of *in vitro* antibacterial activity. Classically, MIC testing via the macrotube method involves the use of liquid growth medium (broth), doubling serial dilutions of antimicrobials in test tubes, and a standard inoculum of bacteria (1 to 5 × 10^5 colony-forming units [CFU]/mL). The tubes (1 to 2 mL) are incubated at ~35°C for 18 to 24 hours and then examined for visible bacterial growth (Fig. 95–1). The MIC allows for testing of the sensitivity of the most resistant subpopulation(s) within a pure culture. Because of the rapid growth rate of most bacteria in a test broth, even a single highly resistant bacterium within the total inoculum should be able to grow sufficiently in the 18- to 24-hour period to cause visible turbidity.[18] Although macrodilution MIC testing is laborious and supply intensive, it does allow for a large inoculum of bacteria to be tested, which can help to detect the smaller numbers of resistant subpopulations or the presence of inducible resistance.[19]

The use of 96-well microtiter plates has allowed for the increased use of broth dilution MIC testing in the clinical laboratory while significantly reducing the amount of labor and media needed. Volumes of 100 to 200 µL or less of media are used, and multichannel pipets, automated systems, or both can allow for the rapid preparation of numerous tests (Fig. 95–2). The microdilution MIC test method is the most common method used in the clinical microbiology laboratory.[20]

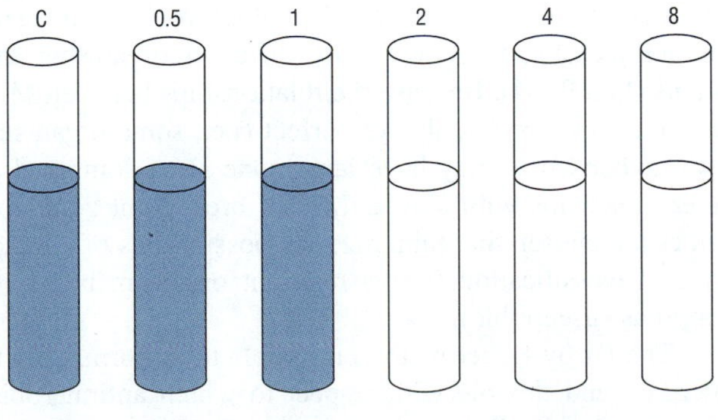

FIGURE 95–1. Macrotube minimum inhibitory concentration (MIC) determination. The growth control (C), 0.5-mg/L, and 1-mg/L tubes are visibly turbid, indicating bacterial growth. The MIC is read as the first clear test tube (2 mg/L).

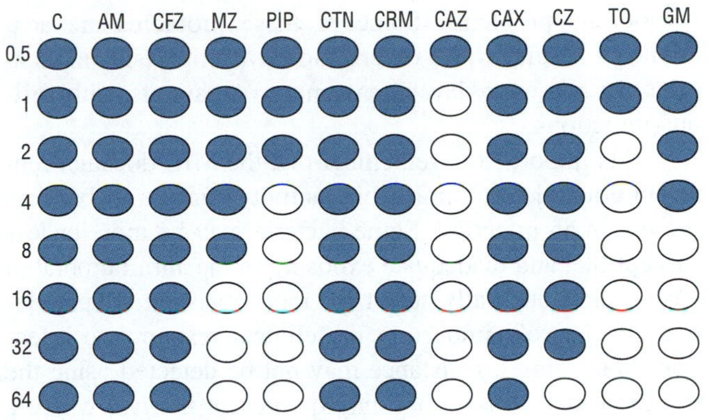

FIGURE 95–2. A prepared microtiter minimum inhibitory concentration (MIC) tray (96 wells). The tray provides a range of MICs from 0.5 to 64 mg/L. The panel represents antibiotics commonly tested against gram-negative pathogens. This tray indicates that the organism is resistant to ampicillin (AM), cefazolin (CFZ), cefotetan (CTN), cefuroxime (CRM), ceftriaxone (CAX), and gentamicin (GM). The isolate is sensitive to mezlocillin (MZ), piperacillin (PIP), ceftazidime (CAZ), and tobramycin (TO). The isolate would be considered intermediately susceptible to ceftizoxime (CZ).

Although microdilution MIC testing is a vast improvement over macrodilution MIC testing, it still has important shortcomings, including decreased flexibility of antimicrobial test panels (especially with premade or premanufactured trays), as well as a decrease in the sensitivity to detect some forms of antimicrobial resistance compared to the macrodilution method. Although the preparation of several serial twofold drug dilutions and inoculation with bacteria are time consuming, expensive, and not feasable for most clinical laboratories, these problems are minimized by the increased automation offered by computer-assisted testing systems.

The MIC can also be determined using solid agar media. This method is considered to be the "gold standard" for the testing of many fastidious or slow-growing organisms, such as *M. tuberculosis*. For agar dilution MIC tests, the antimicrobial to be tested is added to molten agar, often in doubling dilutions similar to broth dilution methods. The molten agar is poured into petri dishes and allowed to harden. After the agar has hardened, samples of bacteria (~10^4 CFU) are applied to the surface of the agar using a pipet or calibrated multipoint prongs (Steers replicator). With the use of this device, up to 36 strains of bacteria may be tested simultaneously on the same plate. After incubation, plates are inspected for growth. As with broth methods, the MIC is the lowest concentration with no visible growth of organism. The use of the agar dilution method is rare in the clinical laboratory. Its use even for difficult to test organisms has decreased in favor of more direct molecular biologic techniques or indirect radiometric or fluorometric tests.

LIMITATIONS AND PROBLEMS WITH MIC TESTING

Although the MIC is the most rigorously tested and standardized *in vitro* test of antimicrobial activity, it is not without its problems. Some of these problems are academic in nature, while others can have important implications for the everyday management of patients with serious infections.

It is important to remember that the MIC does not represent equivalent antimicrobial activity against all bacteria present in an infection. Some bacteria may be more or less susceptible, and inadequate exposure to the antimicrobial *in vivo* could potentially select for more resistant subpopulations, negatively impacting the clinical response to infection. Many times, resistance may not be detected using the inocula tested *in vitro* but may be present *in vivo,* where a much higher inoculum increases the chances for spontaneously resistant mutants.[21]

Many factors can influence the *in vitro* MIC value obtained and its relevance to the *in vivo* situation. The bacterial growth medium used and cation content can significantly affect the activity of many drugs. For example, aminoglycosides are less active against *P. aeruginosa* in a medium supplemented with physiologic concentrations of magnesium and calcium (standardized method) than in a medium without these cations.[17] MIC values of antibiotics highly bound to plasma proteins are often significantly higher in a medium containing human serum, but testing of these drugs in a serum-supplemented medium has not gained widespread acceptance. The bacterial inoculum significantly affects the MIC of some drugs against certain organisms. This is particularly true for most β-lactam antibiotics and gram-negative bacilli, where a 100-fold increase in the size of an inoculum can increase the β-lactam's MIC to such an extent as to make a susceptible organism at a lower inoculum become resistant. Fortunately, standardized guidelines for testing and quality assurance procedures proposed by the NCCLS attempt to minimize the impact of these problems and are followed by most clinical and research laboratories.[22]

Standardization of *in vitro* testing procedures cannot eliminate the impressive differences between *in vitro* testing conditions and the conditions found *in vivo* at the site of infection. The MIC is performed with a small inoculum of logarithmically growing bacteria (compared to that of an infection) in a nutrient-rich, aerobic growth medium at near physiologic pH.[23] In an infection such as an abscess, decreased oxygen tension or an anaerobic environment may be present, as well as a low pH. These conditions have been shown to decrease the activity of antibiotics, such as the aminoglycosides. In sequestered sites of infection, such as the valvular vegetations of endocarditis, organisms may be in a slower or stationary growth phase, which decreases the killing activity of β-lactams and other cell wall active agents. As previously discussed, the high inoculum encountered in such infections would also alter the antimicrobial activity. *In vitro* MIC testing exposes bacteria to a constant concentration of antibiotic, whereas antimicrobial concentrations fluctuate *in vivo,* significant protein binding may occur, and penetration to the site of infection may be minimal.[23] Finally, the potential contribution of the host's immune system to bacterial killing is not routinely assessed via *in vitro* MIC tests.

With the multitude of factors affecting the potential applicability of *in vitro* MIC testing to *in vivo* infections, it is impressive that correlations between susceptibility and clinical outcomes have been observed. Not all patients infected with susceptible organisms, however, will have an adequate clinical or microbiologic response. In these situations of paradoxic antimicrobial therapy failure, the potential confounders mentioned earlier should be considered as possibly being related to observed failure. Data are accumulating that indicate that the combination of *in vitro* susceptibility parameters, such as the MIC, with *in vivo* antimicrobial pharmacokinetic parameters (pharmacodynamic parameters) allow for the better consideration of confounding factors and can result in a better prediction of therapeutic response than organism susceptibility alone.

DISK DIFFUSION ASSAY

The disk diffusion assay method for susceptibility testing (Kirby-Bauer method) was developed in the 1960s by Bauer and coworkers to reduce the labor needed for tube dilution susceptibility testing, and it still is one of the most reliable methods for evaluating qualitative antimicrobial susceptibilities in the clinical laboratory.[24] Up to 12 antibiotic-impregnated disks are placed on an agar plate previously streaked with a standard suspension of bacteria (1 to 2 × 10^8 CFU/mL). The drug diffuses in a concentration gradient from the disk out into the agar. The plate is incubated (18 to 24 hours at 35°C), and bacterial growth occurs only in areas where the drug concentrations are below those required to cause inhibition. The diameters of the zones of inhibition are measured via calipers or automated scanners and compared to standard interpretive zone sizes to determine susceptibility, intermediate susceptibility, or resistance to the antimicrobials tested (Fig. 95–3). Because factors, such as agar composition, incubation temperature, bacterial inoculum, and antibiotic paper disk composition, can influence results, standards for test conditions are defined by the NCCLS.

Interpretive zone sizes are determined by constructing a scattergram of logarithmic MIC values versus zone sizes for antimicrobials against many different organisms and strains (Fig. 95–4). Because the relationships between MIC and zone size are not always perfect (i.e., some organisms with higher MICs may have large zone sizes compared to other organisms with similar MICs), breakpoint zone size values are chosen that minimize the possibilities of a major error in classification (i.e., a resistant organism being reported as susceptible).

The Kirby-Bauer method is simple to perform, easy to interpret, and flexible with respect to which antimicrobial agents to test. Until the development of automated systems, Kirby-Bauer testing was by far the most common method for susceptibility testing in the clinical microbiology labo-

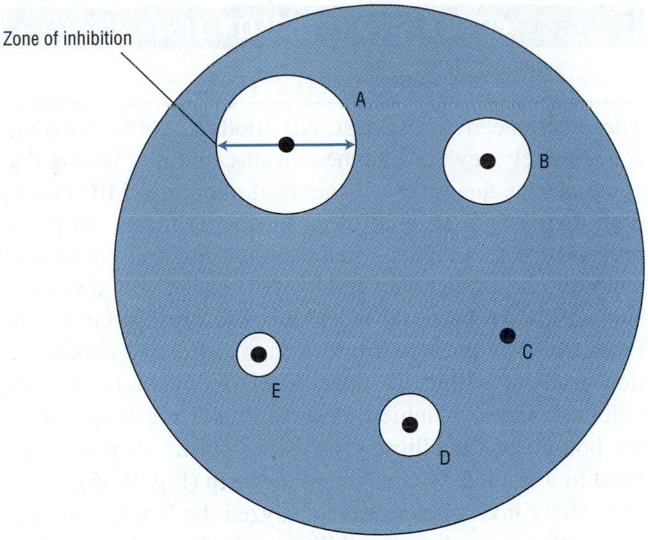

FIGURE 95–3. Disk diffusion susceptibility test. Five disks (A–E) for different drugs were placed on the surface of a seeded agar plate of a test organism and incubated for 18 hours. Antibiotic has diffused from the disk into the agar and is in decreasing concentration with increasing distance from the disk. Antibiotic in the agar inhibited growth of bacteria on the surface according to the susceptibility to the drug. A large zone of inhibition is observed for drug A, indicating that the organism is susceptible to this agent. In contrast, small or nonexistent zones are observed for drugs E and C, respectively, suggesting that the organism is resistant to these drugs. Depending on the established breakpoints for zones of inhibition, the results for B and D indicate that the organism may be susceptible or intermediately susceptible to these drugs.

ratory. A survey of clinical microbiology laboratories indicated that only 27% of laboratories perform disk diffusion as the primary susceptibility test versus 73% for microdilution, automated testing systems, or both—a near reversal of the percentages that were observed in 1983.[20,23] Interestingly, in the late 1990s, some laboratories appear to be reverting back to the old method of Kirby-Bauer susceptibility testing because of the lack of expected benefits associated with automation and the marginal impact on costs.[19] This issue will be explored further in the automated susceptibility testing section.

DETERMINATION AND INTERPRETATION OF QUALITATIVE AND QUANTITATIVE SUSCEPTIBILITIES

The MIC quantifies the activity of an antimicrobial against a bacterial specimen in a standardized *in vitro* test setting. Despite many *in vitro,* animal, and human studies that show correlations between quantitative MICs, dosage regimens, and outcomes, MIC data are qualitatively interpreted as being either sensitive, intermediate to moderately sensitive, or resistant to commonly used antimicrobial agents.[23] Often, this simplification is to allow for quicker and easier interpretation and synthesis of susceptibility data by noninfectious disease practitioners who might not be able to interpret or may have no need for the MIC value.

Many factors are taken into consideration to determine these qualitative susceptibility classifications. Pharmacokinetic properties, such as the peak serum concentration, elimination half-life, and degree of protein binding, are included, as well as the MIC frequency distribution.[17] The establishment of a breakpoint in an area of common MIC values would not be desirable, because a substantial fluctuation in the susceptibility classifications of organisms would occur because of the inherent twofold variability observed during serial dilution MIC testing. The clinical and bacteriologic responses observed for an antimicrobial agent against different strains of bacteria with various MIC values helps to support the clinical relevance of the breakpoints chosen. Most often, the consideration of these factors results in a susceptibility breakpoint of between one-sixteenth to one-fourth of the achievable peak serum concentration.[25]

Pathogens classified as susceptible to an antibiotic are those with the lowest MICs, and they are the most likely to be eradicated during therapy of infections using typical drug doses. Conversely, resistant organisms are bacteria with significantly higher MICs that will cause a less-than-optimal clinical response, even at the highest doses. Organisms that are moderately sensitive or intermediately susceptible are less clearly defined; these organisms appear to be less likely to be effectively treated as compared to a susceptible strain. Treatment of organisms in this range may be successful when maximum doses of a drug are used or when the drug is known to be concentrated in the infected body site. In some cases, the intermediate classification exists because the number of strains with MICs in that range is small and their susceptibility is really indeterminate

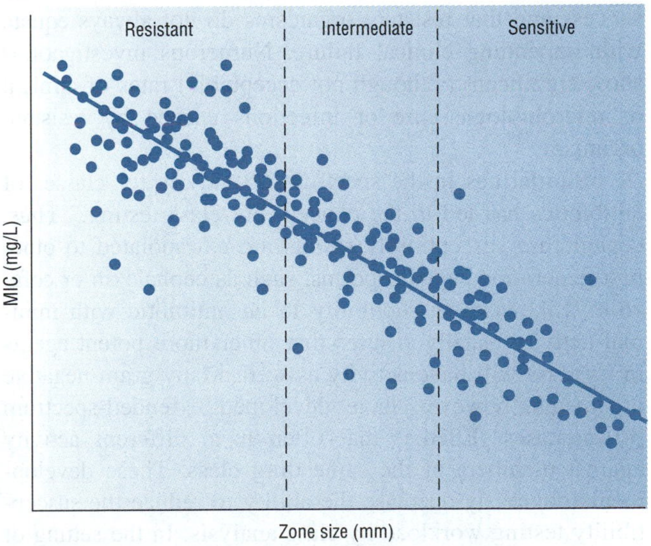

FIGURE 95–4. Scattergram of minimum inhibitory concentrations (MICs) versus Kirby-Bauer disk diffusion zone sizes. Note that although a definite correlation exists, there are also many relationships that are outliers relative to the regression line. The dotted lines indicate where the proposed zone size breakpoints are set.

(i.e., the organism may be either susceptible or resistant). Finally, the intermediate classification serves as a buffer zone to avoid major changes in the interpretation of the MIC value because of the twofold variability in testing.

ISSUES WITH QUALITATIVE SUSCEPTIBILITY TESTING

There are concerns that the "user friendly" breakpoint susceptibility system (susceptible, intermediate, or resistant) could actually oversimplify the decision-making processes in the treatment of infectious diseases.[17] Determination of breakpoint concentrations often does not factor in the impressive alterations in pharmacokinetics in critically ill patients. For example, a critically ill patient may fail antimicrobial therapy of a susceptible organism at the usual doses. If serum concentrations or concentrations at the site of infection were assayed (not commonly done), one might discover suboptimal concentrations, possibly related to poor tissue perfusion. Likewise, a patient with severe vascular insufficiency and a diabetic foot infection may fail a therapy course with normal doses of an antimicrobial and a susceptible organism because of inadequate drug delivery.

Breakpoints are determined by incorporating the peak serum concentration and the drug elimination half-life of the antimicrobial. These parameters alone may not be adequate to describe fully the complex *in vivo* interactions between host, organism, and antimicrobial and, thus, may not be the best parameters to define *in vivo* activity. Some investigators have shown that different outcomes can be achieved for susceptible organisms with different MIC values.[26,27] These reports emphasize that sensitivity does not unequivocally correlate with clinical success and that resistant organisms do not always equate with impending clinical failure. Numerous investigations show significant (although not acceptable) rates of clinical or microbiologic cure of infections caused by resistant organisms.[28]

Similarities in the spectrum of activity for classes of antibiotics has led to the concept of "class testing." Thus, cephalothin susceptibility results are extrapolated to other first-generation cephalosporins, such as cephalexin or cefazolin. Likewise, susceptibility to an antibiotic with minimal activity usually ensures that other more potent agents in its class will have activity as well. Many gram-negative organisms, however, have developed extended-spectrum β-lactamases (ESBLs) that often have different activity against members of the same drug class. These developments obviously decrease the ability to reduce the susceptibility testing workload by class analysis. In the setting of an inadequately responding infection with a common ESBL-producing organism, the possibility of susceptibility to a class antibiotic (if used) but resistance to the antimicrobial agent being used needs to be considered.

OTHER SUSCEPTIBILITY TESTS

EPSILOMETER TEST

The Epsilometer test (E-test; AB Biodisk, Solna, Sweden) is a relatively new development in susceptibility testing that combines the quantitative benefits of microtiter MIC testing with the ease of agar diffusion testing. A plastic strip impregnated with a known, prefixed concentration gradient of antibiotic is placed on an agar plate streaked with a suspension of known bacterial inoculum. The drug instantly diffuses from the plastic strip to form an effective concentration gradient within the agar. After overnight incubation, elliptical zones of inhibition are formed; the point where the bottom of the ellipse crosses the plastic strip is correlated to a printed MIC value on the strip (Fig. 95-5).

Many investigators have analyzed the E-test's correlation with standard susceptibility methods and assessed its potential clinical use. In general, values obtained with E-test methods are comparable or even more consistent and accurate than standard methods. In fact, the E-test method has become the recommended method for susceptibility testing of *Streptococcus pneumoniae*. In addition, good correlation with more laborious agar or broth dilution methods is docu-

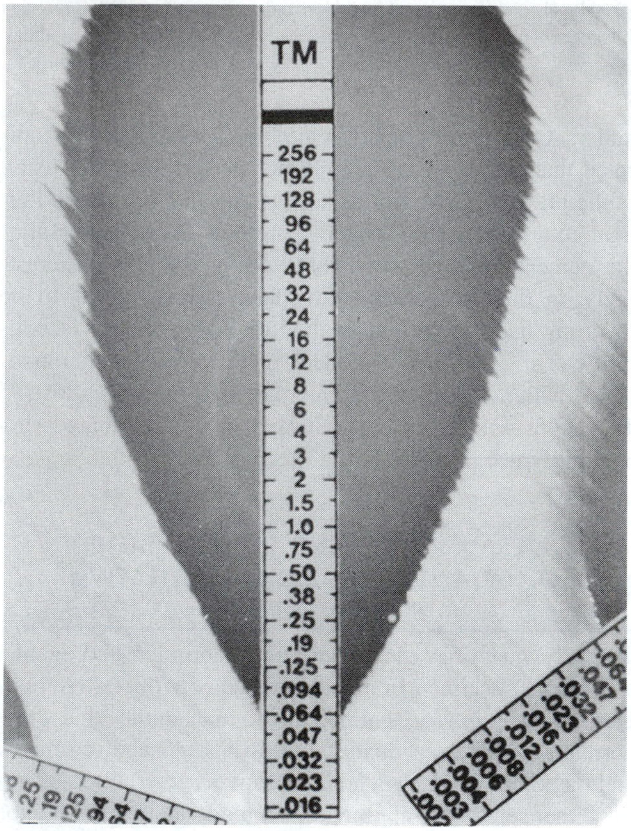

FIGURE 95–5. Photograph of surface of agar plate showing inhibition of bacterial growth surrounding the E-test strip. The minimum inhibitory concentration (MIC) is read at the point where the zone of inhibition intersects the printed scale. *(Photograph courtesy of AB Biodisk, Solna, Sweden.)*

mented for other fastidious or difficult to test organisms, such as *Haemophilus influenzae,* anaerobes, *Bartonella, Flavobacterium, Legionella,* and nutritionally variant streptococci.[29-31] The widespread clinical use of the E-test is limited, however, because of the excessive costs of the test strips in relation to the benefits gained from their use.

SPIRAL GRADIENT MINIMUM INHIBITORY CONCENTRATION DETERMINATIONS

The spiral gradient MIC is peformed using an apparatus that applies a sample of antimicrobial spirally from the center of an agar plate to its periphery. Because of the exponential deposition of the sample, an antimicrobial gradient is formed. Bacterial inocula are streaked radially on the plate, and the distance of growth toward the center is measured after proper incubation. The distance of growth is measured and correlated with an MIC based on predetermined drug concentrations at various distances.[17] This method has proven useful for the testing of anaerobic bacteria and for testing in the research setting, but as with the E-test, its clinical use is limited because of its prohibitively high costs of operation.[19,31]

AUTOMATED ANTIMICROBIAL SUSCEPTIBILITY TESTING

Various degrees of automation have been applied to susceptibility testing. Early advances included automated preparation of microtiter trays, instrument-assisted readers, and computer-assisted result databases.[19] Although these improvements helped to decrease preparation and interpretation times, these methods still required an 18- to 24-hour lag period for bacterial growth to evaluate susceptibility. The availability and increased use of rapid automated susceptibility tests began in the 1980s and continues to increase. In 1991, approximately 15% of clinical microbiology laboratories reported the use of rapid automated test systems.

Rapid antimicrobial susceptibility systems often incorporate the use of microprocessors, robotics, and microcomputers to produce results in as few as 3 hours.[20] Also, these systems allow for rapid identification of organisms through the use of biochemical test batteries. Prior to the Safe Medical Devices Act of 1990, a minimal amount of accuracy and validity testing was needed to market these systems. Since then, premarket approval of any new systems or additions to existing systems is needed from the Food and Drug Administration (FDA) prior to marketing.

There are two rapid susceptibility test systems in common use in clinical microbiology laboratories. The Vitek system (bioMerieux Vitek, Hazelwood, MO) uses technology originally developed for use in spacecraft to identify and test organisms rapidly for antimicrobial susceptibility.[20] This system uses small plastic reagent "cards" that contain 30 or 45 wells for the testing of various antimicrobials or indicator chemicals. Bacterial test suspension (25 μL total, providing ~ 2×10^5 CFU/well) enters the wells by capillary diffusion and growth is monitored automatically via photometric assessment of turbidity every hour for up to 15 hours. When the growth control reaches a specified turbidity level, growth curves for all wells are calculated and compared to the growth control curve for slope normalization. Computerized linear regression and the use of best-fit line coefficients produce an algorithm-derived MIC. The clinical laboratory can control the results output generated (qualitative, quantitative, or both).

The MicroScan WalkAway system (Baxter Diagnostics, Inc., Microscan Division, West Sacramento, CA) is a rapid test system that uses fluorogenic substrate hydrolysis as an indicator of bacterial growth.[20] This system uses standard microdilution test trays and a computer-controlled incubator and reader unit that can perform robotic manipulations, such as reagent addition and tray rotation, to allow for spectrophotometic or fluorometric growth assessments. Bacterial inocula (~6×10^4 CFU/well for gram-negative organisms and ~10^5 CFU/well for gram-positive organisms) are added to the wells, and growth is detected by the production of fluorophores from hydrolysis of amidomethylcoumarin or methyl umbelliferyl fluorogenic substrates. Although this method is a more sensitive assessment of growth compared with turbidity, its indirect nature allows for the possibility of bacterial growth without hydrolysis of the fluorophores; this occurrence is rare, however. As with the Vitek system, growth curves are generated and algorithms applied for the determination of MICs; output is via computer or video display.

With integration and mergers being commonplace in health care systems around the country, an adequate correlation between susceptibility results obtained from these different systems is important to allow for different institutions to compare data reliably. A good correlation between the Vitek and MicroScan WalkAway systems has been shown, with acceptable rates for the categories "very major" and "major discrepancies" shown between the two systems.[32]

Both the Vitek and WalkAway systems contain information management systems that allow for the storage and rapid retreival of susceptibility data. Both systems are also capable of producing chartable patient data reports, antibiograms, and epidemiologic reports. Importantly, these systems can be interfaced with other clinical information systems, such as the pharmacy, infection control, or other laboratory data systems, which may improve clinical outcomes.[33,34]

APPLICATION OF RAPID AUTOMATED SUSCEPTIBILITY TESTING AND IMPACT ON CLINICAL OUTCOMES

Although rapid systems are widely used, there is only minimal data to suggest that they can have an appreciable impact on patient care and outcomes. Rapid testing was associated with a higher likelihood of more appropriate antimicrobial therapy and a change to a more appropriate or less costly therapy in a cohort of 226 patients with bacteremia.[35] Doern and collegues reported that the use of rapid systems allowed for modification of antimicrobial therapy 24 hours sooner in a group of patients with bacteremia.[36] These investigators reported more recently that rapid tests helped to decrease the time to provision of susceptibility and identification results by ~12 hours compared to a procedure simulating the "usual" methods.[37] A significantly lower, infection-related mortality rate was seen in the rapid test group (7%) versus the usual method group (12.7%). Statistically fewer microbiology tests, blood cultures, and other laboratory or clinical tests associated with infections were performed in the rapid group, and mean antimicrobial costs per patient were nearly $300 less than with the usual method group. The mean cost of hospitalization was less for the rapid group (~$15,000) versus the usual group (~$19,000).

PROBLEMS WITH RAPID AUTOMATED SUSCEPTIBILITY SYSTEMS

There are some disadvantages and pitfalls associated with rapid susceptibility systems. Antibiotic test panels or cards are premanufactured in a limited number of combinations, and the number of antibiotics tested per panel is limited; more than one test card may be necessary for some institutions. Compared to the Kirby-Bauer method, flexibility to modify the antimicrobial test battery is extremely compromised.

The growth of fastidious or anaerobic bacteria is such that rapid systems cannot be reliably used; because of this, numerous test methods must be available in the clinical laboratory for the different potential pathogens isolated from clinical specimens. Another potential problem with rapid testing is the unreliable detection of important resistance mechanisms, such as type-1 inducible or chromosomally mediated (derepressed) β-lactamase resistance in *Serratia, Pseudomonas, Enterobacter,* indole-positive *Proteus* and *Providencia,* and *Morganella* species.[20,21] Inducible resistance requires a longer period for detection than that used in rapid systems, while derepressed mutants often occur naturally, but at rates of 1 in 10^{6-7} organisms, which is lower than the number of bacteria tested. Initially, rapid systems also had problems detecting methicillin-resistant *Staphylococcus aureus* (MRSA), but improvements in the media used and in the computerized analysis have improved the ability to detect MRSA substantially.[38] Still, very heterogeneous MRSA (such as 1 MRSA in 10^{6-8} organisms) may not be detected because of the low inoculum used.[20] Regardless of improvements in the rapid systems, it is still recommended to verify the presence of methicillin resistance by other standard and accepted methods.

The substantial initial capital investment for rapid systems, as well as the added and continual costs for disposable trays and maintenance could obviate the cost savings from the decreased manual labor, while producing similar workloads compared to traditional agar dilution testing.[19,39,40]

ADVANCES IN SUSCEPTIBILITY TESTING FOR MYCOBACTERIA, FUNGI, AND VIRUSES

Impressive advances have been made in the past decade in the areas of mycobacterial, fungal, and viral susceptibility testing. The use of radiometric techniques, such as the Bactec system (Becton Dickinson Diagnostic Instruments, Sparks, MD), have revolutionized the analysis of antimicrobial susceptibility in *M. tuberculosis*. Radiometric susceptibility testing involves the incubation of *M. tuberculosis* in liquid media containing ^{14}C-labeled growth substrate. As organisms grow, respiration causes the release of ^{14}C, which is then detected. The growth indices for antimicrobial-containing bottles are compared to those of a control bottle with the calculation of an MIC. The use of this method coupled with the rapid processing of samples has reduced the time to susceptibility result generation to ~2.5 weeks.[41]

Antimicrobial susceptibility testing for *Mycobacterium avium* complex (MAC) is less standardized because of its intrinsic antimicrobial resistance and different colony variants with differing susceptibilities, among other factors. The broth radiometric method for quantitative MIC determination thus far appears to be the most consistent and reproducible method, and it has been advocated for use by leading experts in mycobacteriology.[42] Although data are limited, there appears to be a correlation between *in vitro* susceptibility profiles and clinical response to MAC infection, especially for the macrolide antimicrobials.[42,43] In the future, the use of molecular probes for mycobacterial resistance genes will most likely become a standard for rapid susceptibility determinations, especially in light of the increasing problems with antimicrobial resistance in mycobacteria. Probes or PCR techniques for the *katG* gene, which is needed in order to cause isoniazid (INH) susceptibility, and the *rpoB* gene, which alters the β-subunit of RNA polymerase, causing rifampin resistance have been evaluated in the research laboratory and hold promise for eventual clinical application.[41]

There has been a rapid increase in the prevalence of fungal infections in the 1990s. This increase is related to increases in HIV-infected and AIDS patients, the use of intravenous catheters, and the increase in iatrogenic immunosuppression for organ transplantation and the management of malignancies. An increase in the use of antifungal agents and, not surprisingly, an increase in the detection of antifungal resistance has followed.[44] For many years, no standardized susceptibility tests were available, and there was no way to assess correlations between *in vitro* tests and clinical outcome. Since then, an NCCLS task force has issued guidelines for both macro- and microdilution susceptibility tests that produce a greater than 90% inter- and intralaboratory reproducibility.[45] Studies have been published that show an acceptable correlation of more rapid and less cumbersome test methods, such as microdilution, E-test, and disk diffusion (for fluconazole) with standard macrodilution testing. More importantly, clinical studies show the correlation of these *in vitro* tests for fluconazole susceptibility with outcome in HIV and AIDS patients with oropharyngeal candidiasis and cryptococcal meningitis.[44–47] There is much less or a complete lack of data correlating susceptibility and clinical outcome for itraconazole and amphotericin B, filamentous fungi (such as *Aspergillus fumigatus*), immunosupressed patients without HIV or AIDS, or for patients with candidemia or deep-seated infections.[46] Future research should further define the relationships, if any, for these antifungals and organisms. Routine antifungal testing is not recommended; periodic batch testing for antibiograms and surveillance of resistance or testing of patients with oropharyngeal candidiasis refractory to therapy may be warranted.[44–46]

FUTURE METHODS FOR EVALUATION OF ANTIMICROBIAL ACTIVITY

There are many innovative methods under investigation to provide both qualitative and quantitative assessments of antimicrobial activity. Flow cytometry, a method commonly used to assess human cell lines for abnormalities, has also been studied for its use in bacterial cell analysis. Flow cytometry has the potential to analyze the cellular diversity that is present in bacterial cultures, as well as the gross morphologic effects of antimicrobials on these cells. It also has the potential advantages of (1) rapid determination of susceptibility (one to two cell growth cycles; as quick as 10 minutes for some organisms), (2) better quantification of the subinhibitory and postantibiotic effects of antimicrobials, (3) the ability to investigate cellular changes related to the mechanism of antimicrobial action, and (4) the ability to evaluate the effects of both concentration and time on cellular changes.[48]

DETECTION OF RESISTANCE FACTORS

There are a number of direct resistance detection methods in use. β-Lactamase production can be rapidly and easily detected in the clinical laboratory with the use of nitrocephin disks. Nitrocephin is a chromogenic cephalosporin derivative that changes color upon hydrolysis by β-lactamase. Colonies from a growing bacterial culture can be touched to a disk, with the results of β-lactamase production noted in a few minutes. Although rapid and reliable, this method is limited to the assessment of strains of staphylococci, enterococci, *H. influenzae, M. catarrhalis,* and *N. gonorrhoeae*. The nitrocephin disk also cannot detect β-lactam resistance caused by altered penicillin-binding proteins (PBPs) or by some of the newer ESBLs.[19]

In general, the detection of ESBLs can be difficult. As many as 29% to 75% of strains known to possess ESBL will appear sensitive to cefotaxime or ceftazidime by disk diffusion. This may be a function of test insensitivity, or it may also be related to the breakpoint values being set too high.[21] A double-disk diffusion assay using a β-lactamase inhibitor, such as clavulanate, and various cephalosporins has been shown to more accurately detect the presence of ESBLs (Fig. 95–6). The use of PCR or DNA probes for detection of β-lactamases has been limited to the research setting, as they lack sufficient sensitivity and specificity for routine use in the clinical setting. In the years to come, these molecular biologic techniques should become more refined and more prominent.

Detection of methicillin resistance in *Staphylococcus* is difficult because of the heterogeneous expression of the phenotype. Not all bacteria in a given population will express methicillin resistance (even though they may have the genetic ability to do so); in some cases, only 1 in 10^{4-6} cells may express the resistance phenotype.[40] Methicillin resistance is the result of the *mecA* gene, which encodes for an altered PBP (PBP 2a') with low binding affinity for β-lactams. Screening via oxacillin disks or by oxacillin-containing agar (6 g/mL) were once considered the gold standard for resistance detection prior to the development of PCR and DNA probes specific for *mecA*. The *mecA* PCR test is available for clinical use, is 99% sensitive and specific, and allows for the rapid (within 6 hours) determination of the presence of methicillin resistance. In theory, the presence of a single copy of *mecA* in a clinical isolate could be detected. Many laboratories, however, do not yet use the *mecA* PCR probe because of its high costs. The use of this

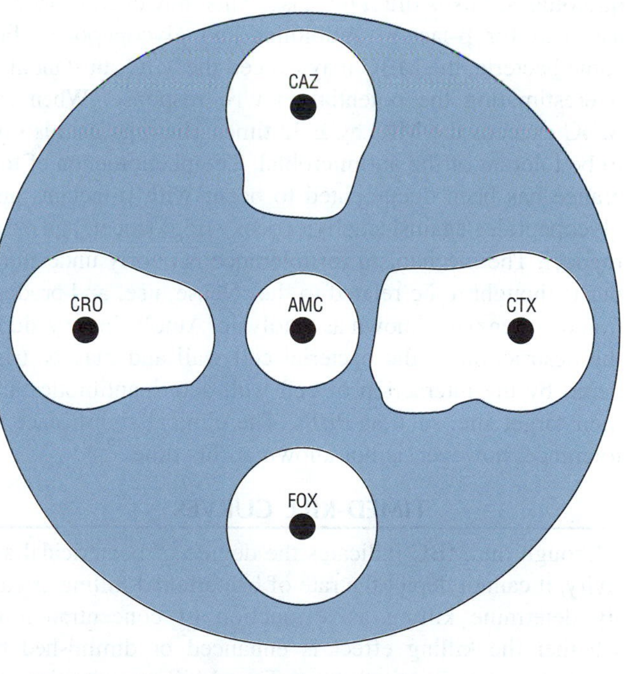

FIGURE 95–6. Double-disk diffusion test for detection of extended-spectrum β-lactamases (ESBLs). The cephalosporins ceftazidime (CAZ), cefotaxime (CTX), cefoxitin (FOX), and ceftriaxone (CRO) are placed on the outside of an agar plate. The disk in the center contains amoxicillin and clavulanate (AMC). The extension in zones observed for ceftazidime, cefotaxime, and ceftriaxone is caused by the clavulanate restoration or augmentation of activity and indicates the presence of ESBL. The cefoxitin zone size is unchanged, indicating that the ESBL present does not hydrolyze this drug.[6]

test could potentially increase, if it can allow for the more rapid discontinuation of empiric vancomycin therapy, especially in hospitals where methicillin resistance is high. In such situations, the cost of the test could be far outweighed by lower antimicrobial costs and the potential for decreased vancomycin resistance.

SPECIAL *IN VITRO* TESTS OF ANTIMICROBIAL ACTIVITY

MINIMUM BACTERICIDAL CONCENTRATION

As previously mentioned, the MIC is the most widely used laboratory parameter used in making decisions on antimicrobial therapy. In some circumstances (e.g. meningitis, endocarditis), however, where bactericidal activity may be more predictive of a favorable infection outcome, it may be of more value to determine the bactericidal activity of a select group of antibiotics. The minimum bactericidal concentration (MBC) is performed in conjunction with the broth microtiter MIC test. After the MIC is determined, an aliquot of the microtiter wells that demonstrates no visible growth are plated onto an antibiotic-free agar and incubated overnight for a period of 24 hours. The MBC is defined as the lowest concentration of drug that kills 99.9% (a 3-log reduction) of the initial organism density.[22] The MIC is often assumed to approximate the MBC, and for certain antibiotic classes, such as the aminoglycosides and the quinolones, this is often the case. This, however, cannot be assumed for β-lactam antibiotics and glycopeptides. For some bacteria, the MBC may exceed the MIC substantially, overestimating the potential *in vivo* response. When the MBC exceeds the MIC by ≥ 32 times, the organism is said to be tolerant of the antimicrobial. The phenomenon of tolerance has been documented to occur with β-lactams and glycopeptides against staphylococci, streptococci, and enterococci. The mechanism for tolerance is poorly understood but is thought to be related to the release, use, and production of an enzyme known as autolysin. Autolysin may aid in the destruction of the bacterial cell wall and may be triggered by the interaction of cell wall active antibiotics and their target site, such as PBPs. The clinical significance of tolerance, however, is not known at this time.[49,50]

TIMED-KILL CURVES

Although the MBC indicates the degree of bactericidal activity, it cannot depict the rate of bactericidal killing or easily determine killing as a function of concentration or whether the killing effect is enhanced or diminished by combination antibiotic therapy. Timed-kill curve testing can yield a wealth of information regarding the antimicrobial's potential. In a simplistic timed-kill curve analysis, a fixed inoculum of a patient's organism is placed in a suitable growth liquid medium and is subsequently exposed to a targeted concentration of antibiotic. The mixture is incubated and sampled repeatedly over a 24-hour period to determine the effect of the antibiotic on the organism. The resulting organism densities over time are then plotted on graph paper. Although timed-kill curve testing is not routinely performed by clinical microbiologic laboratories, it is a useful research tool to identify certain organism and antimicrobial characteristics, such as the effect of organism growth phase (stationary versus exponential), pH, antibiotic protein binding, antibiotic concentration, and the effect of combination therapy.[51]

EFFECT OF CONCENTRATION ON ANTIMICROBIAL KILLING ACTIVITY

The relationship between concentration and antimicrobial killing activity has been documented for most antibiotic classes. Although all antibiotics appear to demonstrate an initial increase in killing activity as a function of antibiotic concentrations that approach or slightly exceed the MIC, a continued linear relationship between antibiotic killing and concentration is not demonstrated for all antibiotics. For example, the β-lactam and glycopeptide antibiotics do not achieve a greater rate of killing once the concentration has exceeded four to five times the MIC. These antibiotics are said to exhibit concentration-independent effects. On the other hand, aminoglycosides and quinolone antibiotics continue to demonstrate increased bactericidal effects as a function of concentration many times above the MIC of the microorganisms in a linear fashion.

The principles of concentration-dependent and independent killing are demonstrated in Figure 95–7. In these timed-kill curve experiments, *Pseudomonas aeruginosa* was exposed *in vitro* to tobramycin, ciprofloxacin, and ticarcillin at concentrations below and above the MIC of the organisms.[52] As demonstrated in the graphs, both tobramycin and ciprofloxacin demonstrate concentration-dependent killing activity achieving greater killing with increasing in-

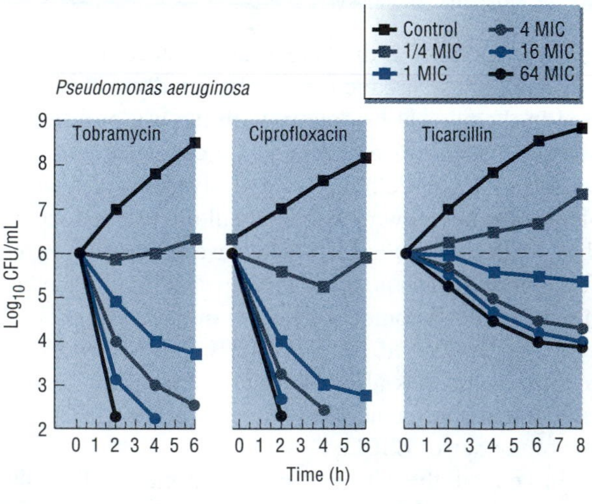

FIGURE 95–7. Killing curves depicting the effect of concentration on antibiotic bactericidal activity. CFU = colony-forming units; MIC = minimum inhibitory concentration. 0.25–64 times the MIC; the organism tested was *P. aeruginosa* ATCC 27853.[52]

crements of concentration. Ticarcillin's maximal killing activity, however, is achieved at four times the MIC. Information regarding the effect of antimicrobial concentration on organism killing is important to determine the most appropriate dosage and administration schemes (such as continuous infusion for concentration-independent effects versus intermittent dosing for concentration-dependent effects) to ensure the optimal outcome for each class of antimicrobial.[52]

POSTANTIBIOTIC EFFECT

The postantibiotic effect (PAE) is the persistent suppression of organism growth (usually measured in hours) after exposure and removal of an antibiotic. Some of the earliest experiments examined the PAE of penicillin on streptococci and staphylococci. Some investigators have reported that the PAE secondary to penicillin against streptococci may be caused by irreversible binding of penicillin to a targeted PBP in the organism's cell wall. The regeneration of new PBPs was necessary for the streptococci to resume normal growth. In general, the PAE experiment is performed by exposing a fixed inoculum of organism to a set concentration of antibiotic (usually some multiple of the MIC). The antibiotic is then removed either by inactivation (such would be the case when a β-lactam is inactivated by the use of β-lactamase) or removal by binding the antibiotic to a resin, centrifugation of the mixture (and removal of the supernatant containing the antibiotic) with resuspension of the organism in an antibiotic-free growth medium or dilution of the antibiotic (1000-fold dilution with antibiotic-free medium) to a concentration that is far below the MIC of the organism. The difference in time that it takes the organism exposed to the antibiotic to grow 10-fold (1-log growth) compared to a separate culture of organism processed the same way and not subjected to the antibiotic is the PAE.[53]

A PAE equal to or greater than 1 hour has been demonstrated for most antibiotics against gram-positive bacteria. Only a select group of antibiotics, such as aminoglycosides and fluoroquinolones, however, consistently demonstrate a significant PAE against gram-negative bacteria. β-Lactams, for example, characteristically do not demonstrate a PAE against gram-negative bacteria. As a general rule, antibiotics that inhibit DNA or protein synthesis (e.g., quinolones and aminoglycosides) demonstrate significant PAEs against gram-negative organisms. An exception to this rule would be the class of compounds known as the carbapenems (imipenem, meropenen, biapenem), which demonstrate PAEs against a select group of gram-negative organisms. A PAE for several compounds is demonstrated in Figure 95–8.

The existence of an *in vivo* PAE has also been well documented in animal studies. *In vivo* PAEs are generally three- or fourfold longer than those reported from *in vitro* studies. One explanation for this discrepancy appears to be related to the contribution of leukocytes that has been termed postantibiotic leukocyte enhancement. Experiments

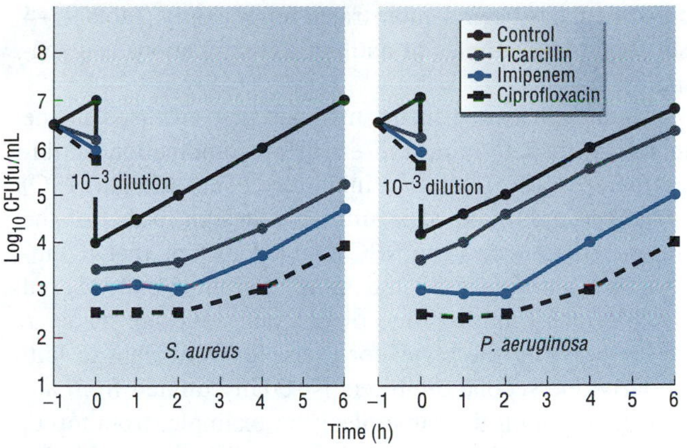

FIGURE 95–8. Postantibiotic effect. In this experiment, a fixed inocula of *S. aureus* and *P. aeruginosa* are exposed to ticarcillin, imipenem, and ciprofloxacin at a set concentration of four times the MIC. The organism and the antibiotic is then diluted 1000-fold to a point where the antibiotic concentration is far below the MIC of the organism. Growth suppression of *S. aureus* following exposure to these three drugs (PAE) occurs for approximately 2 hours. Growth suppression of *P. aeruginosa,* however, is only demonstrated for imipenem and ciprofloxacin. The β-lactam ticarcillin has no effect on the growth of *P. aeruginosa*.[52,53]

in vitro have documented enhanced leukocyte phagocytic activity following antibiotic exposure.[54]

ANTIMICROBIAL COMBINATION TESTING

Antimicrobial combination therapy is often required to treat infections depending on the degree of severity, type of pathogen, or specific infection type. Examples of infections that may require combination therapy include empiric treatment of serious infection before the pathogen or antibiotic susceptibility is known, treatment of infections in neutropenic patients, enteroccocal endocarditis, and treatment of bacteremia, sepsis, or pneumonia caused by *P. aeruginosa*. The combination of antibiotics from different classes may result in activity that is significantly greater than the sum of activity of either agent alone. When this occurs, the combination is said to demonstrate synergy. If the combination of two antibiotics results in an effect that is worse than either agent alone, the combination is said to be antagonistic. Results that are neither synergistic or antagonistic (in between) are said to be indifferent or additive.[58]

Although there is little debate that the combination of a β-lactam and an aminoglycoside is required for treatment of enterococcal endocarditis, the concept of combination therapy is not universally accepted for the treatment of all infections. For example, there is significant debate as to whether the combination of a broad-spectrum β-lactam and an aminoglycoside or the β-lactam alone are most appropriate for the empiric treatment of febrile neutropenic patients.[59,60] *In vitro* antagonism has been demonstrated for several combinations (penicillin plus tetracycline, chloramphenicol and an aminoglycoside), and it has been inconsistently reported for the combination of vancomycin and rifampin or fluoroquinolones and rifampin. *In vivo* antagonism has been demonstrated infrequently. Table 95–4 lists common examples of antibiotic combinations and specific indications.

There are two primary methods that are used in the laboratory to determine the effect of combination antibiotic therapy. The fractional inhibitory concentration (FIC) or checkerboard method is similar in design to that of the microtiter broth or agar MIC method except that it employs two antibiotics on the same microtiter plate. Serial fold dilutions (high to low) of one antibiotic are made in one direction on the plate; for example, from right to left. Similarly, the second antibiotic is serially diluted from another direction on the same plate; for example, from top to bottom. This method of crossing two different antibiotics at various dilutions on the same microtiter plate produces the so-called "checkerboard" of all possible combinations (in twofold dilutions of the MIC) for the two drugs being tested. The test bacteria at a standard inoculum is then added to all wells, and after appropriate incubation, the test results are read in a similar fashion to that of the MIC test. The lowest concentration of drug within each respective row that inhibits growth is plotted on the x and y axis to form an isobologram (Fig. 95–9). The line connecting the respective MICs for each drug is the line of additivity. An inward bowing of the plotted line indicates synergy or additivity. An outward bowing denotes antagonism. Alternatively, the isobologram may be mathematically derived by calculation of the FIC index. The FIC index is calculated as:

$$FIC_{index} = \frac{A}{MIC_A} + \frac{B}{MIC_B}$$

where A or B is the lowest concentration of the drug that is inhibitory in the presence of the second drug, and the MIC is the minimum inhibitory concentration of each drug tested alone. Synergism by the checkerboard method is defined as an FIC index of ≤ 0.5, indifference is defined as an FIC index of > 0.5 to 4.0, and antagonism is defined as an FIC index of > 4.0[61]

The second most common method to determine antibiotic synergism is the timed-kill curve method. It is similar to the timed-kill curve methodology described earlier except that two antibiotics are tested together at a fixed concentration fraction of the MIC for each drug. Synergism in this method is defined as a 100-fold decrease in organism (colony-forming units) count at 24 hours with the combination compared with the reduction in organism count obtained with the most active single agent. Antagonism is defined as an increase in organism count (≥ 100-fold) at 24 hours[62] (Fig. 95–10).

OTHER METHODS

Other methods for testing combination antibiotic therapy include the double-disk diffusion test and the double E-test methods. The double-disk diffusion method is performed by placing two different antibiotic impregnated paper disks onto a solid agar medium plate containing the test organism. The disks are placed in proximity to each other in a way that their zones of inhibition would not be expected to overlap. A synergistic or additive effect is observed when there is an extension of the zones of inhibition between the two drugs.[62] The E-test method is similar to what has been previously described except that two antibiotic E-test strips

TABLE 95–4. Examples of Drug Combinations Frequently Synergistic or Antagonistic *In Vitro* Against Bacteria and Fungi

Drug Combinations	Examples of Organisms
Synergistic	
Aminoglycosides	
+ A broad-spectrum penicillin[a]	Gram-negative bacilli
+ A cephalosporin	Gram-negative bacilli
+ Ampicillin or penicillin G, vancomycin	Enterococci
+ Antistaphylococcal penicillin or vancomycin	Staphylococci
Penicillins	
Nafcillin or oxacillin + rifampin	Staphylococci
Broad-spectrum penicillin[a]	Gram-negative bacilli
+ A third-generation cephalosporin	
Antifungals	
Amphotericin B + flucytosine	*Cryptococcus neoformans*
	Human immunodeficiency virus (HIV)
Antivirals	
Zidovudine + α-interferon	HIV
Antagonistic	
Broad-spectrum penicillin	
+ Imipenem	*Enterobacter cloacae, Pseudomonas aeruginosa, Citrobacter* sp.
+ Chloramphenicol	*Streptococcus pneumoniae*
Aminoglycoside + chloramphenicol	*Enterobacteriaceae*

[a]Mezlocillin, piperacillin, ticarcillin, or azlocillin.

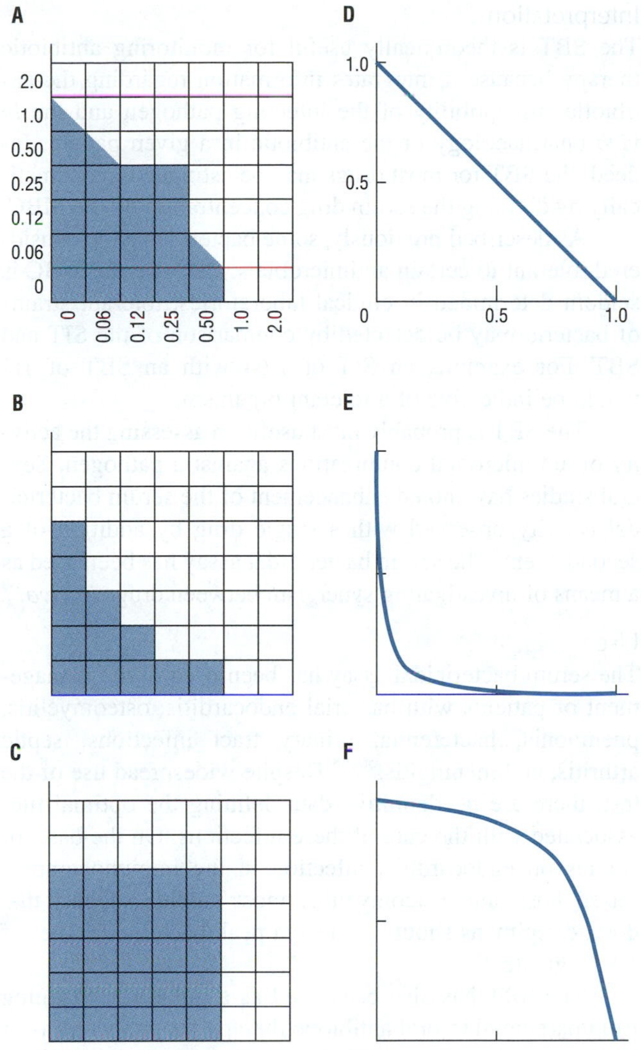

FIGURE 95–9. **(A–C)** Checkerboard dilution technique for the assessment of antimicrobial concentrations. Increasing concentrations of each drug are placed in each of the cells (tubes or wells) as one moves from the lower left corner upward (first drug) or to the right (second drug). Shaded areas depict areas of visible growth after inoculation with test organisms and incubation. The corresponding results are plotted on isobolograms and are plotted as fractions of the minimum inhibitory concentration (MIC) for each drug. Panels **A** and **D**, **B** and **E**, and **C** and **F** depict additivity, synergism, and antagonism, respectively. *(Adapted from Ref. 84.)*

are crossed at the MIC of each antibiotic. Similar to the disk-diffusion method, an extension of the zone of inhibition from either antibiotic alone would be considered additive or synergistic.[63] Other more sophisticated methods to detect synergism are being explored, such as three-dimensional (3-D) models that use 3-D graphing techniques and mathematic equations capable of analyzing and visualizing an entire dose–response surface effect of two antibiotics used in combination. These methods are primarily limited to research laboratory use.[64]

Unfortunately, none of the procedures for testing combination antimicrobials have been adequately examined to determine if the results of these tests are predictive of clinical outcome. In addition, these tests have limitations. For example, the checkerboard method is plagued by reproducibility problems. It can only evaluate the inhibitory effect of two antibiotics, and assessments are made only at one time point (18 or 24 hours). The timed-kill curve method is labor intensive, lacks the ability to detect additive effects using current definitions, is only evaluated at the 24-hour time point, and has no standards for concentrations for which the antibiotics are to be tested. Last, there is a lack of correlation between the two methods for detecting synergism.[65]

Despite these limitations, testing antimicrobial combinations in the clinical laboratory appears to be useful in certain situations, such as in enterococcal infections. Both *Enterococcus faecalis* and *Enterococcus faecium* are inhibited but not killed by penicillin or ampicillin. The combination of penicillin and ampicillin with an aminoglycoside, such as gentamicin, is, however, synergistic and bactericidal. Thus, for infections, except simple cystitis caused by enterococci, the combination of a penicillin or derivative plus an aminoglycoside is recommended. Because enterococci are intrinsically resistant to low levels of aminoglycosides, susceptibility testing with high levels (≥ 500 μg/mL) of gentamicin are used as a predictor for synergism. It is also useful to test certain combinations of antibiotics for their activity against multidrug-resistant strains of bacteria isolated from patients. In these settings, it is hoped that the resistance to one or both antibiotics being tested will become sensitive through a synergistic interaction between the two antibiotics.[65]

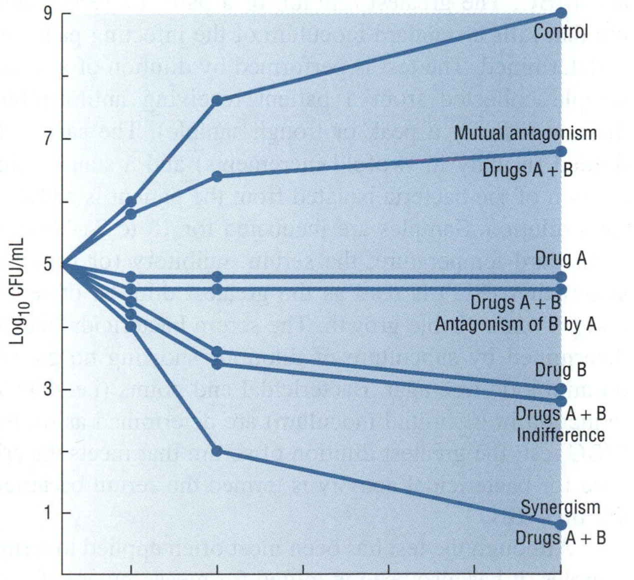

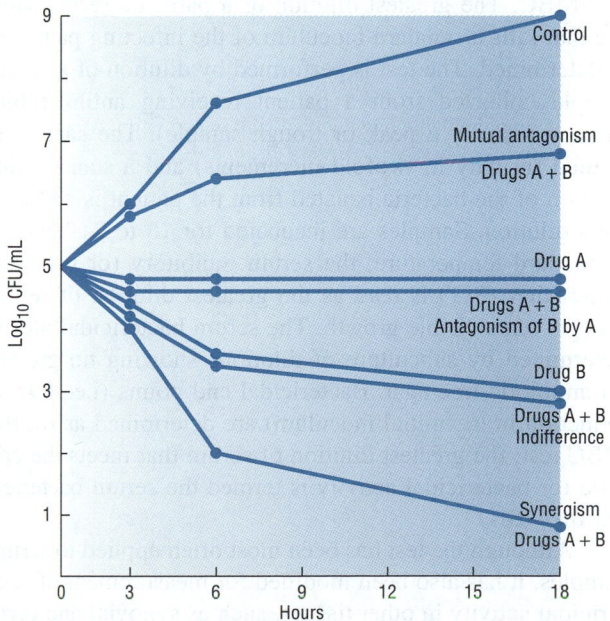

FIGURE 95–10. Timed-kill curve illustrating synergistic, antagonistic, and indifferent effects of two antibiotics tested on fixed concentrations. *(Modified from Rahab JJ. Medicine 1978;57:181, with permission.)*

LABORATORY MONITORING OF ANTIMICROBIAL THERAPY

An understanding of antimicrobial agent disposition *in vivo* is an important component for the selection of therapy and the monitoring of clinical or bacteriologic responses. The clinician needs to recognize the concentrations expected in the bloodstream, as well as the expected delivery of the antimicrobial to the sites where infection can occur. Combining this knowledge with knowledge of expected activity against the infecting organism constitutes a pharmacodynamic approach to the treatment of infections.

Serum concentration monitoring is the most common method used to individualize antimicrobial therapy. The therapeutic window is, however, quite large for most antimicrobial agents, and exact toxic or therapeutic ranges are not well defined. In this context, therapeutic monitoring often is not justified. The clinical benefits of adjusting concentrations to hypothetically "correct" values are unknown, especially in light of the additional costs that concentration monitoring adds to the therapy. There are antimicrobials for which proper monitoring appears to be justified based on either toxicity or efficacy.

METHODS OF ANTIBIOTIC ASSAY

SERUM BACTERICIDAL TITER

Determination of the bactericidal titer of a serum sample from a patient receiving antimicrobial therapy is sometimes used clinically to monitor antimicrobial activity *in vivo*.[66] The test is similar to the determination of the MIC and MBC. The greatest dilution of a patient's serum sample that kills a standard inoculum of the infecting pathogen is determined. The test is performed by dilution of a serum sample collected from a patient receiving antimicrobial therapy (usually a peak or trough sample). The sample is diluted (usually in twofold increments) and a standard inoculum of the bacteria isolated from the patient is added to each dilution. Samples are incubated for 18 to 24 hours at a standard temperature; the serum inhibitory (or bacteriostatic) titer (SIT) is read as the greatest dilution of serum that prevents visible growth. The serum bactericidal titer is determined by subculture of dilutions showing no growth on antibiotic-free agar. Bactericidal end points (i.e., 99.9% reduction in the initial inoculum) are determined as for the MBC test; the greatest dilution of serum that meets the criteria for bactericidal activity is termed the serum bactericidal titer (SBT).

Although the test has been most often applied to serum samples, it has also been modified for measurement of bactericidal activity in other tissues, such as synovial and cerebrospinal fluid, sputum, and urine.[66] It has also been adapted to measure the rate of bacterial killing by performing a timed-kill curve analysis on one or several dilutions of serum.[67,68]

Interpretation

The SBT is theoretically useful for monitoring antibiotic therapy because it integrates information regarding the antibiotic susceptibility of the infecting pathogen and the *in vivo* pharmacology of the antibiotic in a given patient. Indeed, the SBT for most drugs may be estimated mathematically by dividing the serum drug concentration by the MBC.

As described previously, some bacteria may be considered tolerant to certain antimicrobials. Because the MBC is seldom determined in clinical laboratories, tolerant strains of bacteria may be detected by comparison of the SIT and SBT. For example, an SIT of 1:64 with an SBT of 1:2 would be indicative of a tolerant organism.

The SBT is probably most useful in assessing the activity of antimicrobial combinations against a pathogen. Several studies have noted enhancement of the serum bactericidal activity observed with a single drug by addition of a second agent. The serum bactericidal assay has been used as a means of investigating synergism between drugs *in vivo*.[69]

Use

The serum bactericidal assay has been used in the management of patients with bacterial endocarditis, osteomyelitis, pneumonia, bacteremia, urinary tract infections, septic arthritis, and meningitis.[66–68] Despite widespread use of the test, there are no definitive data defining the optimal titer associated with the cure of these infections. On the basis of studies on endocarditis, infection in the immunocompromised host, and osteomyelitis, most studies suggest that dosage regimens should achieve a peak bactericidal titer of 1:8 or greater.[66]

The SBT has also been used as a guide for changing from parenteral to oral antibiotic therapy for endocarditis or bone and joint infection. Use of the test in this setting provides confirmation of adequate oral absorption of antibiotics to allow for prolonged therapy in the outpatient setting.

More recently, serial measurements of the SIT or SBT have been employed in the evaluation of antimicrobial regimens. The reciprocal of the titer is plotted over time, and the area under the bactericidal titer versus time curve (AUBC) is calculated. This area could also be calculated by comparison of the AUBC for the drug compared with the MIC or MBC of a pathogen of interest. This approach seems most useful in studying the combined effects of combination antimicrobial regimens or of drugs with active metabolites.[69]

Limitations

The same technical factors that influence the results of MIC and MBC tests are applicable to the serum bacteriostatic and bactericidal assays. In particular, the use of serum versus broth for making dilutions of the sample may be important, particularly for highly protein-bound drugs. Binding of drugs to serum proteins may be decreased when the sample is diluted in growth medium rather than serum because of dilution of proteins in the original sample. Thus, large dilutions would result in a greater free fraction of bioactive drug because of dilutions of proteins. These and other issues related to the performance and interpretation of the SBT necessitate standardization to make the test of greater clinical value.[67]

MICROBIOLOGIC ASSAY

Bioassay of antimicrobial agents is performed by several methods. The most commonly employed method is a modification of the disk-diffusion technique used for determining antibiotic susceptibility. Paper disks are placed onto or wells are punched into the surface of an agar containing bacteria known to be highly susceptible to the agent to be assayed. A fixed volume (usually 10 μL) of known concentration of the drug to be assayed or sampled is placed on the disks or in the wells. The measured zone of inhibition and the logarithm of drug concentration are plotted; the drug concentration in unknown samples is determined from measurement of the zone size surrounding disks spotted with unknown concentrations of drug. Advantages of this method include its relative ease of performance and low cost for equipment. Disadvantages include possible interference by other antibiotics present in the sample, lack of precision, and slow turnaround time (usually 24 to 48 hours).

FLUORESCENCE POLARIZATION IMMUNOASSAY

The flourescence polarization immunoassay (FPIA) technique involves the application of the principles of fluorescence when molecules are exposed to light. A fluorescein-labeled drug and antibody directed against the drug are added in constant amounts to samples or standards. The antibody–fluorescein-labeled drug complex results in a change in the fluorescence polarization. Changes in fluorescence polarization occur because of competition for antibody between the drug present in the sample and the fluorescein-labeled drug added to the sample; therefore, high drug concentrations in the sample reduce the extent of binding of fluorescein-labeled drug to antibody and, thus, the extent of reduction in fluorescence polarization.

Advantages of this technique include automation through the use of the TDx system (Abbott Laboratories, North Chicago, IL). Disadvantages include the expense for reagents and cost for the purchase of the automated system. In the clinical laboratory setting, FPIA is the most commonly used assay method for the determination of aminoglycoside and vancomycin serum concentrations.

RADIOIMMUNOASSAY

The radioimmunoassay (RIA) technique involves the interaction among the radiolabeled drug, the unlabeled antibiotic, and the antibody directed against the drug. Equilibrium between the antibody and the sources of antigen-radiolabeled drug and drug sample is allowed to occur, and the amount of bound or free radiolabeled drug is determined using standard radiometric methods of detection. Advantages of the system include good precision; disadvantages include the expense of the disposal of radioactive wastes.

HIGH-PRESSURE LIQUID CHROMATOGRAPHY

In the high-pressure liquid chromatography (HPLC) technique, separation of different molecular species is accomplished by passing a mobile solvent phase over a stationary phase. Drugs with a polarity similar to that of the stationary phase will be retained for a time on the chromatography column and then released. These temporarily retained substances are detected using ultraviolet, fluorescence, electrochemical, or radiometric methods. The detector response is proportional to the amount of molecules seen; standard curves containing known drug concentrations are related to the detector response, usually recorded as peak area or peak height. Advantages include a rapid turnaround time, precision, and an ability to detect metabolites. Disadvantages include the cost of instruments and the expertise required.

TIMING OF COLLECTION OF SERUM SAMPLES

In clinical practice, monitoring of antimicrobials is often accomplished by collecting peak and trough samples to assess maximum and minimum antimicrobial concentrations. The samples for the determination of the trough drug concentration should be collected just prior to the next dose. The timing of the peak sample collection appears to be more critical to assure that it provides meaningful data. Generally, the peak concentraion should be obtained after the distribution phase to better characterize the extravascular concentrations, since most interpretive methods use simplified one-compartment pharmacokinetic models. Samples for peak concentration are generally collected 1 hour after the start of a 15- to 45-minute intravenous infusion or 1 hour after an orally administered dose, but there are exceptions. Regardless of sample collection times, it is crucial to record the dosing history and actual dosage given to allow for the proper interpretation of serum concentration data.

Ideally, steady-state pharmacokinetic conditions (approximately four half-lives) should exist before determining serum antibiotic levels. Although this approach can simplify pharmacokinetic interpretation and allow for more accurate dosage adjustments, it may be clinically unsound in the treatment of certain infectious diseases. The achievement of therapeutic serum concentrations early in the course of antibiotic therapy can result in improved survival from some infections[70]; delay in the collection of samples until steady-state pharmacokinetic conditions exist may not be prudent in critically ill patients, as these patients may never achieve a true steady state because of rapidly changing hemodynamics and organ functions. Appropriate methods for the analysis of drug concentration data at non–steady-state conditions should be used to aid in pharmacokinetic parameter estimation and dosage adjustment.

SPECIFIC AGENTS

Target therapeutic ranges for agents where serum level monitoring has been employed for the treatment of infection are listed in Table 95–5. Serum level monitoring of

TABLE 95–5. Suggested Therapeutic Serum Concentrations for Selected Antimicrobial Agents

Drug	Time of Collection	Target Concentrations (mg/L)	Comments
Aminoglycosides[70,71]	Peak (1 h after the start of a 15- to 45-min infusion)	< 5	Urinary tract infections
Traditional dosage regimens			
Gentamicin		> 5	Bacteremia
Tobramycin		> 6	Bacterial pneumonia
		> 12	Endocarditis caused by *Pseudomonas aeruginosa*
	Trough	< 2–3	High trough concentrations are most likely a result and not a cause of nephrotoxicity
Amikacin	Peak	> 15	Urinary tract infections
		> 20	Bacteremia
		> 24	Bacterial pneumonia, other serious infections
	Trough	< 9–10	See comments regarding trough gentamicin/tobramycin concentrations
Single Daily Dosage Regimens[76]			
Gentamicin Netilmicin Tobramycin	8 h postdose	1.5–6	Concentrations above this range associated with nephrotoxicity in one study with netilmicin
Vancomycin[80,81]	Peak (1–2 h after a 30- to 60-min infusion)	20–50	Recommendations should be considered tentative, as definitive data are not available
	Trough	< 10	Therapeutic monitoring is probably not necessary for most patients

aminoglycosides and vancomycin has been extensively studied, although this practice has been challenged.

AMINOGLYCOSIDES

The influence of serum aminoglycoside levels on clinical response in gram-negative infection has been reported in several studies, but one review concluded that the widely disseminated therapeutic ranges for serum levels were poorly supported by this data.[71] Controversy also surrounds the relationship between serum aminoglycoside concentrations and the development of nephrotoxicity and ototoxicity. Early studies suggested that trough concentrations exceeding 2 to 4 mg/L for gentamicin and tobramycin and 10 mg/L for amikacin predisposed patients to nephrotoxicity. More recent analyses of several patient variables have concluded that these other patient factors may be more important and that the development of ototoxicity and nephrotoxicity is more closely related to the total dose and duration of therapy.[72,73] In many of the studies evaluating nephrotoxicity, high serum concentrations were most likely the *result,* not the *cause,* of the reduction in the glomerular filtration rate. Although the clinical benefit of specific levels still remains unproved, the ranges listed in Table 95–5 can be applied based on controlled studies.

Newer regimens of once-daily or extended-interval aminoglycoside administration continue to gain acceptance for use in the clinical setting.[74,75] These regimens attempt to exploit the pharmacodynamics of these agents (concentration-dependent bacterial killing, postantibiotic effect, and reduced adaptive resistance), while attempting to minimize drug toxicity through periods of minimal exposure of target organs to the drug. Traditional methods of serum concentration monitoring using peak and trough concentrations are uninformative for once-daily dosing. Concentrations 24 hours after a dose should be undetectable in most patients, even those with mild renal dysfunction. Newer monitoring strategies use peak samples, with a second sample taken 6 to 12 hours after a dose, although single point methods with serum samples collected between 2 to 8 hours after a dose have also been evaluated.[76]

A plethora of prospective studies evaluating once-daily aminoglycoside dosing and almost as many meta-analyses have been published during this past decade. Most of these studies show either equal rates of efficacy and toxicity or a trend toward improved efficacy and reduced toxicity for once-daily dosage regimens. These clinical studies are fraught with weaknesses and variabilities that make overall interpretation difficult, so any meta-analyses subsequently inherit these scientific study flaws.[77] Additional prospective studies are needed, but they will most likely be plagued by the inherent obstacles of clinical study design and implementation, as well as by a lack of funding because of the generic availability of aminoglycosides.[77,78]

VANCOMYCIN

There are no definitive data that correlate peak or trough serum concentrations with efficacy or toxicity.[79] Although IV administration of vancomycin (particularly early formulations) was associated with the development of ototoxicity and nephrotoxicity, studies in animals show that it is not ototoxic and is minimally nephrotoxic.[80] Furthermore, there are no strong relationships between concentrations and rare episodes of toxicity. The "red man" syndrome reported with IV infusions of vancomycin has not been correlated with serum levels, but it may occur more frequently with infusions of less than 2 hours in duration.[79]

Most dosage regimens used in clinical studies and dosing nomograms provide peak concentrations between 20 and 50 mg/L and trough concentrations of less than 10 mg/L. In light of the known time-dependent killing properties of vancomycin (as opposed to concentration-dependent) and the poor correlation of peak and trough vancomycin concentrations and outcome parameters, a minimization of serum concentration monitoring or a discontinuation of monitoring altogether are probably feasable for most patients.[80,81] The use of empiric dosing nomograms with periodic trough concentration monitoring only in patients on vancomycin for longer durations or in patients with many concurrent known nephrotoxins is one such approach being employed at some institutions.[82]

INTEGRATION OF MINIMUM INHIBITORY CONCENTRATION AND SERUM CONCENTRATION DATA

There has been a considerable advance in our understanding of the role of drug pharmacokinetics and pharmacodynamics in the effective treatment of infectious diseases. Integration of MIC information with antimicrobial pharmacokinetic data has led to the design of regimens that achieve target levels of exposure based on organism susceptibility and the antimicrobial properties of the drug against the particular organism.

For example, a better response would be predicted for a given dose of an antimicrobial with concentration-dependent killing activity against an organism with a lower MIC versus a higher MIC, even if both organisms are considered susceptible. The pharmacodynamic principles behind this are a maximization of the Cpmax-to-MIC ratio and are illustrated in Figure 95–11. The clinical applicability of this principle could be to modify either the dosage of the current aminoglycoside used to achieve the suggested Cpmax:MIC ratio of ≥ 10:1 or to switch to a different aminoglycoside that allows for better optimization of this ratio (such as a switch from gentamicin to tobramycin for an organism with lower tobramycin MIC). The clinical validity of this concept has been shown in studies of susceptible organisms with aminoglycosides and fluoroquinolones.[26,27]

The ratio of overall *in vivo* exposure to an antimicrobial (measured by the area under the plasma concentration versus time curve (AUC) to an organism's susceptibility (the AUC:MIC ratio) is another pharmacodynamic parameter proposed to be used for dosage optimization.[83] For seriously ill patients, a breakpoint AUC:MIC ratio of ≥ 125 was associated with clinical response, while breakpoint AUC:MIC ratios of ≥ 125 and ≥ 250 were associated with stepwise decreases in the time to eradicate the infecting organism.[83]

For β-lactam antimicrobial efficacy, the achievement of concentrations above an organism's MIC for a critical amount of time (time > MIC) appears to be the most important pharmacodynamic parameter.[23,28] The Cpmax:MIC ratio does not appear to be as crucial a factor for response, although the AUC:MIC ratio has also been suggested as a

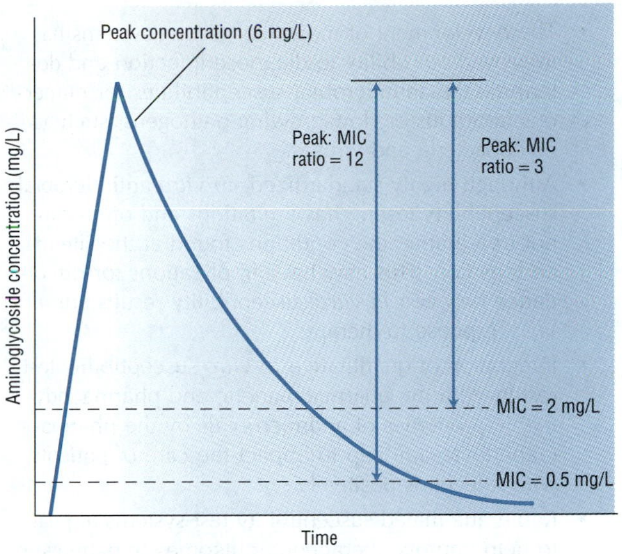

FIGURE 95–11. Illustration of the concept of peak concentration to the minimum inhibitory concentration (MIC) ratio for aminoglycosides. The MIC for the given organism to gentamicin is 2 mg/L, whereas the tobramycin MIC is 0.5 mg/L. Administration of gentamicin would result in a suboptimal peak:MIC ratio (< 10), which could increase the chances for development of resistance or an inadequate response. Administration of tobramycin would result in a peak:MIC ratio of 12, which should improve efficacy. Note that modification of the gentamicin regimen to produce peak serum concentrations of ≥ 20 mg/L (as commonly done with once-daily administration) would also result in a peak:MIC ratio of ≥ 10.

predictor for β-lactam treatment outcome.[23] In the setting of otitis media, for example, a time > MIC of approximately 40% to 50% appears to correlate with rates of response greater than 90%.[28]

Most of the data on pharmacodynamic optimization has been generated in controlled clinical settings. Evaluation of the best and most efficient ways to apply this data to everyday clinical practice is ongoing, and it should result in either the expansion of monitoring for certain antimicrobials or the proposal of nomograms that allow for rapid drug and dose selections that enhance the likelihood for optimal therapy based on the type of infection, patient-specific parameters, and local antimicrobial susceptibility patterns. Such possibilities present exciting opportunities for the pharmacotherapy specialist to become directly involved in the development of multidisciplinary protocols that could improve care for patients with infections in all health care settings.

▶ PRINCIPLES OF PHARMACOTHERAPY

- The pharmacotherapist needs to understand and properly use clinical laboratory tests to help confirm the presence of infection and to acquire knowledge about the host's characteristics (such as immune status).
- Familiarity with normal host flora and typical pathogens will help decide whether a patient is truly infected or merely colonized.

- The development of molecular testing systems has improved our ability to diagnose infection and determine the antimicrobial susceptibilities for numerous fastidious or slow-growing pathogens, such as mycobacteria and viruses.
- Although highly standardized, *in vitro* antimicrobial susceptibility testing has limitations and often cannot truly mimic the conditions found at the site of an infection. This may have implications for discordance between *in vitro* susceptibility results and *in vivo* response to therapy.
- Integration of quantitative *in vitro* susceptibility test results with the pharmacokinetic and pharmacodynamic properties of antimicrobials by the pharmacotherapist can help to impact the care of patients with infections positively.
- Rapid automated susceptibility test systems appear to help improve therapeutic outcomes of patients with infection, especially when linked to other relevant clinical information systems.
- Although not routinely performed in the clinical setting, laboratory tests that determine an antimicrobial's pharmacodynamic properties, such as the effect of concentration, the postantibiotic effect, and the effect of combination antimicrobials are important to consider in the understanding and application of therapy to patients with infection.

REFERENCES

1. Sanders CC. A problem with antimicrobial susceptibility tests. ASM News 1991;57:187–190.
2. Bodey GP. Quantitative relationship between circulating leukocytes and infection in patients with acute leukemia. Ann Intern Med 1966; 64:328–340.
3. Rouse BT, Horohov DW. Immunosuppression in viral infection. Rev Infect Dis 1986;8:850–873.
4. Boumpas DT, Paliogianni F, Anastassiou ED, et al. Glucocorticosteroid action on the immune system: Molecular and cellular aspects. Clin Exp Rheumatol 1991;9:413–423.
5. Sox HC, Liang MH. The erythrocyte sedimentation rate: Guidelines for rational use. Ann Intern Med 1986;104:515–523.
6. Casey LC, Balk RA, Bone RC. Plasma cytokine levels correlate with survival in patients with the sepsis syndrome. Ann Intern Med 1993; 15:771–778.
7. Bone RC, Larson CB. Gram-negative urinary tract infections and the development of SIRS. J Crit Illness 1996;11(suppl):S20-S29.
8. Herwaldt LA, Geiss M, Kao C, Pfaller MA. The positive predictive value of isolating coagulase-negative staphylococci from blood cultures. Clin Infect Dis 1996;22:14–20.
9. Chapin K. Clinical Microscopy. In: Murray PR, Baroon EJ, Pfaller MA, et al., eds. Manual of Clinical Microbiology, 6th ed. Washington, DC, ASM Press, 1995:33–51.
10. Forbes BA, Granato PA. Processing specimens for bacteria. In: Murray PR, Baroon EJ, Pfaller MA, et al., eds. Manual of Clinical Microbiology, 6th ed. Washington DC, ASM Press, 1995:265–281.
11. Smith-Elekes S, Weinstein MP. Blood cultures. Infect Dis Clin North Am 1993;7:221–234.
12. Herrmann JE. Immunoassys for the diagnosis of infectious diseases. In: Rose NE, de Marario EC, Folds JD, et al., eds. Manual of Clinical Laboratory Immunology, 5th ed. Washington, DC, ASM Press, 1997:130–157.
13. Tenover F. DNA hybridization techniques and their application to the diagnosis of infectious diseases. Infect Dis Clin North Am 1993;7: 171–181.
14. Podzorski RP, Persing DH. Molecular detection and identification of microorganisms. In: Rose NE, de Marario EC, Folds JD, et al., eds. Manual of Clinical Laboratory Immunology, 5th ed. Washington, DC, ASM Press, 1997:130–157.
15. Rosenthal N. Tools of the trade-recombinant DNA. N Engl J Med 1994;331:315–317.
16. Hitt CM, Nightingale CH, Quintiliani R, Nicolau DP. Streamlining antimicrobial therapy for lower respiratory tract infections. Clin Infect Dis 1997;24(suppl 2):S231–S237.
17. Ackerman BH, Dello Buono FA. *In vitro* testing of antibiotics. Pharmacotherapy 1996;16(2):201–221.
18. Isenberg DH. Antimicrobial susceptibility testing: A critical evaluation. J Antimicrob Chemother 1988;22(suppl A):73–86.
19. Jorgensen J. Antimicrobial susceptibility testing of bacteria that grow aerobically. Infect Dis Clin North Am 1993;7:393–409.
20. Ferraro MJ. Automated antimicrobial susceptibility testing: What the infectious diseases subspecialist needs to know. Curr Clin Topics Infect Dis 1995;145:103–119.
21. Sanders CC, Thomson KS, Bradford PA. Problems with detection of β-lactam resistance among nonfastidious gram-negative bacilli. Infect Dis Clin North Am 1993;7:411–424.
22. National Committee for Clinical Laboratory Standards (NCCLS). Methods for Dilution Antimicrobial Susceptibility Tests for Bacteria that Grow Aerobically, 3rd ed, approved standard. NCCLS document M7-A3 (ISBN 1-56238-209-8). NCCLS, 771 East Lancaster Avenue, Villanova, PA, 19085, 1993.
23. Craig WA. Qualitative susceptibility tests versus quantitative MIC tests. Diagn Microbiol Infect Dis 1993;16:231–236.
24. Bauer AW, Kirby MM, Sherris JC, et al. Antibiotic susceptibility testing by a standardized, single-disk method. Am J Clin Pathol 1966;45: 493–496.
25. Hessen MT, Kaye D. Principles of selection and use of antimicrobial agents. Infect Dis Clin North Am 1995;9:531–545.
26. Moore RD, Lietman PS, Smith CR. Clinical response to aminoglycoside therapy: Importance of peak concentration to minimal inhibitory concentration. J Infect Dis 1987;155:93–99.
27. Peloquin CA, Cumbo TJ, Nix DE, et al. Evaluation of intravenous ciprofloxacin in patients with nosocomial lower respiratory tract infections. Arch Intern Med 1989;149:2269–2273.
28. Craig WA. The future—Can we learn from the past? Diagn Microbiol Infect Dis 1997;27:49–53.
29. Hsueh PR, Chang JC, Teng LJ, et al. Comparison of E-test and agar dilution method for antimicrobial susceptibility testing of *Flavobacterium* isolates. J Clin Micro 1997;35:1021–1023.
30. Wolfson C, Branley J, Gottlieb T. The E-test for antimicrobial susceptibility testing of *Bartonella henselae*. J Antimicrob Chemother 1996; 38:963–968.
31. Olsson-Liljequist B, Nord CE. Methods for susceptibility testing of anaerobic bacteria. Clin Infect Dis 1994;18(suppl 4):S293–S296.
32. Rittenhouse SF, Miller LA, Utrup LJ, Poupard JA. Evaluation of 500 gram negative isolates to determine the number of major susceptibility interpretation discrepancies between the Vitek and Microscan Walkaway for 9 antimicrobial agents. Diagn Microbiol Infect Dis 1996;26:1–6.
33. Evans RS, Classen DC, Pestotnik SL, et al. Improving empiric antibiotic selection using computer decision support. Arch Intern Med 1994; 154:878–884.
34. Pestotnik SL, Classen DC, Evans RS, Burke JP. Implementing antibiotic practice guidelines through computer-assisted decision support: Clinical and financial outcomes. Ann Intern Med 1996;124:884–890.
35. Trenholme GM, Kaplan RL, Karakusis PH, et al. Clinical impact of rapid identification and susceptibility testing of bacterial blood culture isolates. J Clin Microbiol 1989;27:1342–1345.
36. Doern GV, Scott DR, Rashad AL. Clinical impact of rapid antimicrobial susceptibility testing of blood culture isolates. Antimicrob Agents Chemother 1982;21:1023.

37. Doern GV, Vautour R, Gaudet M, Levy B. Clinical impact of rapid *in vitro* susceptibility testing and bacterial identification. J Clin Microbiol 1994;32:1757–1762.
38. Granato P. The impact of same-day versus traditional overnight testing. Diagn Microbiol Infect Dis 1993;16:237–243.
39. Chambers H. Detection of methicillin-resistant staphylococci. Infect Dis Clin North Am 1993;7:425–433.
40. Berke I, Tierno P. Comparison of efficacy and cost-effectiveness of BIOMIC VIDEO and Vitek antimicrobial susceptibility test systems for use in the clinical microbiology laboratory. J Clin Microbiol 1996; 34:1980–1984.
41. Inderlied CB. Antimycobacterial susceptibility testing: Present practices and future trends. Eur J Clin Microbiol Infect Dis 1994;13: 980–993.
42. Heifets L. Susceptibility testing of *Mycobacterium avium* complex isolates. Antimicrob Agents Chemother 1996;40:1759–1767.
43. Sison JP, Yao Y, Kemper CA, et al. Treatment of *Mycobacterium avium* complex infection: Do the results of *in vitro* susceptibility tests predict therapeutic outcome in humans? J Infect Dis 1996;173:677–683.
44. Pfaller MA, Rex JH, Rinaldi MG. Antifungal susceptibility testing: Technical advances and potential clinical applications. Clin Infect Dis 1997;24:776–784.
45. Rex JH, Pfaller MA, Galgiani JN, et al. Development of interpretive breakpoints for antifungal susceptibility testing: Conceptual framework and analysis of *in vitro–in vivo* correlation data for fluconazole, itraconazole, and candidal infections. Clin Infect Dis 1997;24:235–247.
46. Ghannoum MA. Is antifungal susceptibility testing useful in guiding fluconazole therapy? Clin Infect Dis 1996;22(suppl 2):S161–S165.
47. Witt MD, Lewis RJ, Larsen RA, et al. Identification of patients with acute AIDS-associated cryptococcal meningitis who can be effectively treated with fluconazole: The role of antifungal susceptibility testing. Clin Infect Dis 1996;22:322–328.
48. Pore RS. Antibiotic susceptibility testing by flow cytometry. J Antimicrob Chemother 1994;34:613–627.
49. Voorn GP, Kuyvenhoven J, Goessens WHF, et al. Role of tolerance in treatment and prophylaxis of experimental *Staphylococcus aureus* endocarditis with vancomycin, teicoplanin, and daptomycin. Antimicrob Agents Chemother 1994;38:487–493.
50. Handwerger S, Tomasz A. Antibiotic tolerance among clinical isolates of bacteria. Rev Infect Dis 1985;7:368–386.
51. Amsterdam D. Susceptibility testing of antimicrobials in liquid media. In: Lorian V, ed. Antibiotics in Laboratory Medicine, 4th ed. Baltimore, Williams & Wilkins, 1996:52–111.
52. Craig WA, Ebert SC. Killing and regrowth of bacteria *in vitro:* A review. Scand J Infect Dis Suppl 1991;74:63–70.
53. Craig WA, Gudmundsson S. Postantibiotic effect. In: Lorian V, ed. Antibiotics in Laboratory Medicine, 4th ed. Baltimore, Williams & Wilkins, 1996:296–329.
54. McDonald PJ, Hakendorf P, Pruul H. Postantibiotic leukocyte enhancement: Increased susceptibility of bacteria pretreated with antibiotics to activity of keukocytes. Rev Infect Dis 1981;3:38–44.
55. Craig WA. Post-antibiotic effects in experimental infection models: Relationship to in-vitro phenomena and to treatment of infections in man. J Antimicrob Chemother 1993;31(suppl D):149–158.
56. Ali MZ, Goetz MB. A meta-analysis of the relative efficacy and toxicity of single daily dosing versus multiple daily dosing of aminoglycosides. Clin Infect Dis 1997;24:796–809.
57. Craig WA, Ebert SC. Continuous infusion of B-lactam antibiotics. Antimicrob Agents Chemother 1992;36:2577–2583.
58. Rybak MJ, McGrath BJ. Combination antimicrobial therapy for bacterial infections: Guidelines for the clinician. Drugs 1996;52:390–405.
59. De Jongh CA, Joshi JH, Newman KA, et al. Antibiotic synergism and response in gram-negative bacteremia in granulocytopenic cancer patients. Am J Med 1986;80:96–100.
60. Ramphal R, Gucalp R, Rotstein C, et al. Clinical experience with single agent and combination regimens in the management of infection in the febrile neutropenic patient. Am J Med 1996;100:(suppl 6A): 83S–89S.
61. Elipoulos G, Moellering RC Jr. Antimicrobial combinations. In: Lorian V, ed. Antibiotics in Laboratory Medicine, 4th ed. Baltimore, Williams & Wilkins, 1996:330–397.
62. Moeller O, Holmgren J. A paper disc technique for studying antibacterial synergism. Acta Pathol Microbiol Scand 1969;76:141–145.
63. White RL, Burgess DS, Manduru M, Bosso JA. Comparison of three different *in vitro* methods of detecting synergy: Time-kill, checkerboard, and E test. Antimicrob Agents Chemother 1996;40:1914–1918.
64. Prichard MN, Shipmann C Jr. A three-dimensional model to analyze drug–drug interactions. Antiviral Res 1990;14:181–206.
65. Cappelletty DM, Rybak MJ. Comparison of methodologies for synergism testing of drug combinations against resistant strains of *Pseudomonas aeruginosa*. Antimicrob Agents Chemother 1996;40:677–683.
66. Wolfson JS, Swartz MN. Serum bactericidal activity as a monitor of antibiotic therapy. N Engl J Med 1985;312:968B–975B.
67. Reller LB. The serum bactericidal tests. Rev Infect Dis 1986;8:803–808.
68. Van der Auwera P, Klastersky J. Bactericidal activity and killing rate of serum in volunteers receiving ciprofloxacin alone or in combination with vancomycin. Antimicrob Agents Chemother 1986;30:892–895.
69. Barriere SL, Kapusnik JE, Ely E, et al. Analysis of a new method for assessing activity of combinations of antimicrobials: Area under the bactericidal activity curve. J Antimicrob Chemother 1985;16:49–59.
70. Moore RD, Smith CR, Lietman PS. The association of aminoglycoside plasma levels with mortality in patients with gram-negative bacteremia. J Infect Dis 1984;149:443–448.
71. McCormack JP, Jewesson PJ. A critical reevaluation of the "therapeutic range" of aminoglycosides. Clin Infect Dis 1992;14:320–339.
72. Bertino JS, Booker LA, Franck PA, et al. Incidence of and significant risk factors for aminoglycoside-associated nephrotoxicity in patients dosed by using individualized pharmacokinetic monitoring. J Infect Dis 1993;167:173–179.
73. Parkin N, Whitcomb J, Smith D, et al. The use of a rapid phenotypic HIV-1 drug resistance and susceptibility assay in analyzing the emergence of drug-resistant virus during triple combination therapy. 37th Interscience Conference on Antimicrobial Agents and Chemotherapy. Sept 27–Oct 1, 1997, Toronto, Ontario, Canada. Abstract LB-1.
74. Bates RD, Nahata MC. Once-daily administration of aminoglycosides. Ann Pharmacother 1994;28:757–766.
75. Rotschafer JC, Rybak MJ. Single daily dosing of aminoglycosides: A commentary. Ann Pharmacother 1994;28:797–801.
76. Blaser J, Konig C, Simmen H-P, Thurnheer U. Monitoring serum concentrations for once-daily netilmicin dosing regimens. J Antimicrob Chemother 1994;33:341–348.
77. Bertino JS, Rotschafer JC. Single daily dosing of aminoglycosides—A concept whose time has not yet come. Clin Infect Dis 1997;24: 820–823. Editorial response.
78. Gilbert DN. Meta analyses are no longer required for determining the efficacy of single daily dosing of aminoglycosides. Clin Infect Dis 1997;24:816–819. Editorial response.
79. Healy DP, Sahai JV, Fuller SH, et al. Vancomycin-induced histamine release and "red man syndrome: Comparison of 1- and 2-hour infusions. Antimicrob Agents Chemother 1990;34:550–554.
80. Cantu TG, Yamanaka-Yuen NA, Lietman PS. Serum vancomycin concentrations: Reappraisal of their clinical value. Clin Infect Dis 1994; 18:533–543.
81. Moellering RC Jr. monitoring serum vancomycin levels: Climbing the mountain because it is there? Clin Infect Dis 1994;18:544–546. Editorial.
82. Karam CM, McKinnon PS, Rybak MJ. Outcome assessment of minimizing vancomycin monitoring and dosing adjustments. 37th Interscience Conference on Antimicrobial Agents and Chemotherapy. Sept 27–Oct 1, 1997, Toronto, Ontario, Canada. Abstract LM-20a.
83. Forrest A, Nix DE, Ballow CH, et al. Pharmacodynamics of intravenous ciprofloxacin in seriously ill patients. Antimicrob Agents Chemother 1993;37:1073–1081.
84. Krogstad DS, Moellering RC Jr. Antimicrobial combinations. In: Lorian V, ed. Antibiotics in Laboratory Medicine, 2nd ed. Baltimore, Williams & Wilkins, 1978.

96

ANTIMICROBIAL REGIMEN SELECTION

Betty J. Abate, PharmD, BCPS, and Steven L. Barriere, PharmD, FCCP

Choosing an antimicrobial agent to treat infections is far more complicated than matching a drug to a known or suspected pathogen.[1] Most clinicians generally follow a systematic approach to select an antimicrobial regimen (Table 96–1). Problems arise when this systematic approach is replaced by prescribing broad-spectrum therapy to cover as many organisms as possible. Consequences of not using the systematic approach include the use of more expensive and potentially more toxic agents, which may in turn lead to widespread resistance and difficult to treat superinfections. Another abuse of antimicrobial agents is administration when they are not needed. An example of this is prescribing antibacterials for self-limited, clinical conditions that are most likely viral in origin.

Initial selection of antimicrobial therapy is nearly always empiric, which is the initiation of antimicrobials before the offending organism is identified. Infectious diseases are generally acute, and a delay in antimicrobial therapy may result in serious morbidity or even mortality. An example is the rapidly lethal nature of various forms of meningitis. Thus, empiric antimicrobial therapy selection is based on information gathered from the patient's history and physical examination and results of Gram stains or rapidly performed tests on specimens from the infected site. This information combined with knowledge of the most likely offending organism(s) and an institution's local susceptibility patterns should result in a rational selection of antibiotics to treat the patient.

This chapter outlines a systematic approach for the selection of antimicrobial therapeutic regimens. The principles for selection of antimicrobial prophylactic regimens are discussed in Chapter 112.

CONFIRMING THE PRESENCE OF INFECTION

FEVER

The presence of a temperature greater than the expected 98.6°F (37°C) "normal" body temperature is considered a hallmark of infectious diseases. Body temperature is controlled in the hypothalamus.[2] In addition, the circadian rhythm, a built-in temperature cycle, is also operational. The daily temperature rhythm may vary for each individual. In a healthy person, the internal thermostat is set between the morning low temperature and the afternoon peak as controlled by the circadian rhythm. During fever, the hypothalamus is reset at a higher temperature level.[2]

Fever is defined as a controlled elevation of body temperature above the normal range. The average normal body temperature range taken orally is 98.0 to 98.6°F (36.7 to 37.0°C). Body temperatures obtained rectally are generally 1.0°F (0.6°C) higher, and axillary temperatures are 1.0°F (0.6°C) lower than oral temperatures, respectively. Skin temperatures are also less than the oral temperature but may vary depending on the specific measurement method.

Fever can be a manifestation of disease states other than infection. Collagen vascular (autoimmune) disorders and several malignancies may have fever as a manifestation. A patient with fever and no other, or nonspecific, complaints may have an infection, as well as many other diseases. Fever of unknown or undetermined origin is a diagnostic dilemma and has been reviewed extensively elsewhere.[3]

Many drugs have been identified as causes of fever.[4] Drug-induced fever is defined as persistent fever in the absence of infection or other underlying condition. The fever must coincide temporally with the administration of the offending agent and disappear promptly upon its withdrawal, after which the temperature remains normal.[4] The mechanism of drug-induced fever is believed to be caused by either a hypersensitivity reaction or development of an antigen (drug)–antibody complex that results in the stimulation of macrophages and release of interleuken-1 (IL-1). Although this is not a common drug effect (accounting for no more than 5% of all drug reactions), it should be suspected when obvious reasons for fever are not present. Almost any medication can produce drug-induced fever, but certain ones appear to be responsible more often than others. These include β-lactam antibiotics, anticonvulsants, and a variety of other medications, including allopurinol, hydralazine, nitrofurantoin, sulfonamides and related compounds, phenothiazines, and methyldopa.[4]

Noninfectious etiologies of fever may be referred to as false-positives. Although these certainly may confuse the clinician, even more troublesome are false-negatives: the absence of fever in a patient with signs and symptoms consistent with an infectious disease. Careful questioning of the patient or family should be done to assess the ingestion of any medication that can mask fever. These include aspirin, acetaminophen, nonsteroidal anti-inflammatory agents, and corticosteroids. Similarly, treatment of a disease state with only partially effective therapy may also temporarily reduce fever and other signs of infection. A good example of this is the use of bacteriostatic drugs in a patient with infective endocarditis.

The use of antipyretics should be discouraged during the treatment of infection unless absolutely necessary. The

TABLE 96–1. Systematic Approach for Selection of Antimicrobials

Confirm the presence of infection
Careful history and physical
Signs and symptoms
Predisposing factors
Identification of the pathogen (Chap. 95)
Collection of infected material
Stains
Serologies
Culture and sensitivity
Selection of presumptive therapy considering every infected site
Host factors
Drug factors
Monitor therapeutic response
Clinical assessment
Laboratory tests
Assessment of therapeutic failure

common practice of administering an antipyretic during the treatment of infection may mask a poor therapeutic response. Moreover, elevated body temperature, unless very high (> 105°F), is not harmful and may be beneficial as previously noted.[2] Artificial means of reducing an elevated body temperature (e.g., cooling blankets) are generally unnecessary and may even be dangerous.

SIGNS AND SYMPTOMS

Most infections result in elevated white blood cell (WBC) counts (leukocytosis) because of the mobilization of granulocytes (neutrophils, basophils, eosinophils), lymphocytes, or both to ingest and destroy invading microbes. The generally accepted range of normal values for WBC counts is between 4000 and 10,000 cells/mm^3. Values above or below this range hold important prognostic and diagnostic value.

Bacterial infections are associated with elevated granulocyte counts, often with immature forms (band neutrophils) seen in peripheral blood smears (left-shift). Mature neutrophils are also referred to as segmented neutrophils or polymorphonuclear leukocytes (PMNS). The presence of immature forms is an indication of an increased bone marrow response to the infection. With infection, peripheral WBC counts may be very high, but they are rarely higher than 30,000 to 40,000 cells/mm^3. Since leukocytosis indicates the normal host response to infection, low leukocyte counts after the onset of infection indicate an abnormal response and are generally associated with a poor prognosis of bacterial infection.

The most common granulocyte defect is neutropenia, a decrease in absolute circulating neutrophils. A thorough description of the consequences of neutropenia is discussed in Chapter 112. Relative lymphocytosis, even with normal or slightly elevated total WBC counts, is generally associated with tuberculosis and viral or fungal infections. Increases of monocytes may be associated with tuberculosis or lymphoma and increases in eosinophils may be associated with allergic reactions to drugs or metazoan infections. Many types of infections may be accompanied by a completely normal WBC count and differential.

The classic signs of pain and inflammation may be manifested by swelling, erythema, tenderness, and purulent drainage. Unfortunately, these are only visibly apparent if the infection is superficial or in a bone or joint. The manifestations of inflammation in deep-seated infections, such as meningitis, pneumonia, endocarditis, and urinary tract infection, must be ascertained by examining tissues or fluids. For example, the presence of neutrophils in spinal fluid, lung secretions (sputum), and urine is highly suggestive of a bacterial infection.

Symptoms referable to an organ system must be carefully sought out, for they not only help in establishing the presence of infection, but also aid in narrowing the list of potential pathogens. For example, a febrile patient with complaints of flank pain and dysuria may well have pyelonephritis. In this situation, enteric gram-negative bacilli, especially *Escherichia coli,* are the predominant pathogens. If a febrile patient has no symptoms referable to an organ system, however, but only constitutional complaints, the list of possible infectious diseases is quite long.[3] A febrile individual with cough and sputum production probably has a pulmonary infection. What is not so evident, however, is the etiologic organism in this situation, because it may be caused by bacteria, mycobacteria, viruses, or mycoplasmas.[5] In this situation, attention to the patient's history and background disease states is important. Even more important is a careful examination of the infected material (in this case sputum) to try and ascertain the identity of the pathogen.

INDENTIFICATION OF THE PATHOGEN

Infected body materials must be sampled, if at all possible or practical, before institution of any antimicrobial therapy for two reasons. First, a Gram stain of the material may rapidly reveal bacteria, or an acid-fast stain may detect mycobacteria or actinomycetes. Second, a delay in obtaining infected fluids or tissues until after antimicrobial therapy is started may result in false-negative culture results or alterations in the cellular and chemical composition of infected fluids. This is particularly true in patients with urinary tract infections, meningitis, and septic arthritis.[6]

Blood cultures should nearly always be performed in the acutely ill, febrile patient. Blood culture collection is usually timed to sharp elevations in temperature, suggesting the possibility of microorganisms (or microbial antigens) in the bloodstream. Ideally, blood should be obtained from peripheral sites as two sets (one set consists of an aerobic bottle and one set of an anaerobic bottle) from two different sites approximately 1 hour apart. In selected infections, bacteremia is qualitatively continuous (endocarditis), so cultures may be obtained at any time.[7]

In addition to the infected materials produced by the patient (blood, sputum, urine, stool, wound, or sinus drainage), other less accessible fluids or tissues must be obtained based on localized signs or symptoms (e.g., spinal fluid in meningitis, joint fluid in arthritis). Abscesses and cellulitic areas should also be aspirated.

Once positive Gram stain, culture results, or both are obtained, the clinician must be cautious in determining whether the organism recovered is a true pathogen, a contaminant, or a part of the normally expected flora (see Chap. 95) from the site of specimen collection. This latter consideration is especially problematic with cultures obtained from the skin, oropharynx, nose, ears, eyes, throat, and perineum. These surfaces are heavily colonized with a wide variety of bacteria, some of which may be pathogenic in certain settings. For example, coagulase-negative staphylococci are found in cultures of all the aforementioned sites, yet are seldom regarded as pathogens unless recovered from blood, venous access catheters, or prosthetic devices.

Importantly, cultures of specimens from purportedly infected sites, which are obtained by sampling from or through one of these contaminated areas, may contain significant numbers of the normal flora. In the case of urine cultures, the urinalysis should be used in combination with culture results to assess the presence of WBCs, nitrite, and leukocyte esterase that help confirm infection as opposed to colonization.

Particularly problematic are expectorated sputum specimens that must be carefully evaluated by the determination of the presence of squamous epithelial cells and leukocytes.[5] A predominance of epithelial cells in sputum specimens casts doubt on the pathogenic role of any bacteria recovered, especially when multiple types of organisms are seen on Gram stain. In contrast, the discovery of leukocytes in large numbers with one predominant type of organism is a more reliable indicator of a valid collection. In general, however, sputum evaluation has poor sensitivity and specificity as a diagnostic test.[5]

Caution must also be used in the evaluation of positive culture results from normally sterile sites (blood, cerebrospinal fluid, or joint fluid). The recovery of bacteria normally found on the skin in large quantities (coagulase-negative staphylococci, diphtheroids) from one of these sites may be a result of contamination of the specimen rather than a true infection. These organisms may be pathogenic in certain settings.

Gram-staining techniques, culture methods, and serologic identification, as well as susceptibility testing, are covered in detail in Chapter 95. Emphasis must be placed on the proper collection and handling of specimens and careful assessment of Gram stain or other test results in guiding the clinician toward appropriate selection of initial antimicrobial therapy.[8]

SELECTION OF PRESUMPTIVE THERAPY

To select rational antimicrobial therapy for a given clinical situation, a variety of factors must be considered. These include the severity and acuity of the disease, host factors, factors related to the drugs used, and the necessity for using multiple agents. In addition, there are generally accepted drugs of choice for the treatment of most pathogens (see Appendix 96–1).

The drugs of choice are compiled from a variety of sources and are intended as guidelines rather than specific rules for antimicrobial use. These choices are influenced by local antimicrobial susceptibility data rather than information published by other institutions or national compilations. Each institution usually publishes an annual summary of antibiotic susceptibilities (antibiogram) for organisms cultured from patients. Antibiograms contain both the number of isolates for common species and the percentage susceptible to the antibiotics tested. As a general rule, antibiotics that are active against (inhibit growth) at least 80% of isolates are considered acceptable empiric choices. To further guide empiric antibiotic therapy, some hospitals publish unit-specific antibiograms in unique patient care areas, such as intensive care units or burn units.

Susceptibility of bacteria may differ substantially among hospitals within a community. For example, the prevalence of methicillin-resistant *Staphylococcus aureus* (MRSA) in some centers is quite high, whereas in others the problem may be nonexistent. This particular situation will influence the selection of therapy for possible *S. aureus* infection where either a β-lactam compound or vancomycin would be the choices. The problem of differing susceptibilities is not only limited to gram-positive bacteria but also to gram-negative organisms, and all drug classes are affected.

Empiric therapy is directed at organisms that are known to cause the infection in question. These organisms for different sites of infection are discussed in Chapters 97 to 113. To define the most likely infecting organisms, a careful history and physical examination must be performed. Place of acquisition of infection should be determined, for example, the home (community-acquired), nursing home environment, or hospital-acquired (nosocomial). Nursing home patients may be exposed to potentially more resistant organisms since they are often surrounded by ill patients who may be receiving antibiotics. Other important questions to ask the infected patients regarding the history of the present illness include:

1. Are any other people sick at home, especially children?
2. Are any unusual pets kept in the home such as pigeons?
3. Where are you employed (that is, are they exposed to contaminated meat)?
4. Has there been any recent travel, for example, to endemic areas of fungal infections or developing countries?

HOST FACTORS

Several host factors should be considered when evaluating a patient for antimicrobial therapy. Most important factors include drug allergies, age, pregnancy, genetic or metabolic abnormalities, renal and hepatic function, site of infection, concomitant drug therapy, and underlying disease states.

Allergy to an antimicrobial agent generally precludes its use. Careful assessment of allergy histories must be performed because many patients confuse common adverse drug effects, such as gastrointestinal (GI) disturbance, with true allergic reactions.[9] Among the most commonly cited antimicrobial allergies are those to penicillin, penicillin-related compounds, or both. One can find many authoritative sources that recommend other β-lactam compounds, especially cephalosporins, in this setting, because of suggestive evidence that few patients with a penicillin allergy will react to a cephalosporin. In the absence of complete penicillin skin testing capabilities, a rule of thumb for giving cephalosporins to patients allergic to penicillin is to avoid giving them to patients who give a good history for immediate or accelerated reactions (anaphylaxis, laryngospasm) and to give them cautiously (under close supervision) in patients with a history of delayed reactions, such as a rash.[10] If gram-negative infection is suspected or documented, therapy with a monobactam may be appropriate, since cross-reactivity with other β-lactams is virtually nil.[11]

The patient's age is an important factor, both in trying to identify the likely etiologic agent and in assessing the patient's ability to detoxify or eliminate the drug(s) to be used. The best example of an age determinant of organisms is in bacterial meningitis where the pathogens differ as the patient grows from the neonatal period, through infancy and childhood, and into adulthood.[12] A neonate's hepatic and liver function is not well developed, becomes extremely efficient during infancy and childhood, and slowly wanes with increasing age. Thus, both drug selection and drug dosage must be adjusted based on the age of the patient.

Specific patient groups require additional considerations when using antimicrobials. For example, neonates (especially when premature) may develop kernicterus when given sulfonamides. This results from displacement of bilirubin from serum albumin.[13] Chloramphenicol as a cause of the gray syndrome in babies is well established. The mechanism of this effect is an inability of the newborn's liver to metabolize (and detoxify) the drug, leading to shock and cardiovascular collapse.[14] Thus, serum concentrations of chloramphenicol must be monitored to ensure that concentrations of the drug do not exceed 20 to 25 μg/mL.

Although it is generally believed that the elderly are more predisposed to adverse drug effects, there are no clear-cut explanations for this.[15] An important example is that hepatotoxicity from the antimicrobial agent isoniazid has been documented to increase in frequency with age.[16]

During pregnancy, not only is the fetus at risk for drug teratogenicity, but also the pharmacokinetic disposition of certain drugs may be altered.[17] Penicillins, cephalosporins, and aminoglycosides are cleared from the peripheral circulation more rapidly during pregnancy. This is probably because of the marked increases in intravascular volume, glomerular filtration rate, and hepatic and metabolic activities, especially during late pregnancy. The net result is that maternal serum antimicrobial concentrations may be as much as 50% lower during this period than in the nonpregnant state. Increased dosages of certain compounds may be necessary to achieve therapeutic levels during late pregnancy.

Inherited or acquired metabolic abnormalities will influence the therapy of infectious diseases in a variety of ways. For example, patients with impaired peripheral vascular flow may not absorb drugs given by intramuscular injection. In addition, certain metabolic states may predispose patients to enhanced drug toxicity. For example, patients who are phenotypically slow acetylators of isoniazid are at greater risk for peripheral neuropathy.[18] Patients with severe deficiency of glucose-6-phosphate dehydrogenase (G6PD) may develop significant hemolysis when exposed to drugs, such as sulfonamides, nitrofurantoin, nalidixic acid, antimalarials, dapsone, and perhaps chloramphenicol.[19] Although mild deficiencies are found in blacks, the more severe forms of the disease are generally confined to persons of Eastern Mediterranean origin.

Patients with diminished renal or hepatic function, or both, will accumulate certain drugs unless the dosage is adjusted.[20,21] Recommendations for dosing antibiotics in liver dysfunction are not as formalized as guidelines for renal dysfunction.[21] Antibiotics that should be adjusted in severe liver disease include chloramphenicol, clindamycin, erythromycin, metronidazole, and rifampin. Significant accumulation may occur when both liver and renal dysfunction are present for the following drugs: cefotaxime, nafcillin, piperacillin, and sulfamethoxazole.

Clear-cut identification of the site of the infection or the likely source of a bacteremia can aid in defining the most likely organisms. For example, the overwhelming majority of urinary tract infections are caused by enteric gram-negative bacilli, especially *E. coli.*[22] In contrast, bone and joint infections in children are nearly always caused by *S. aureus.*[23] Bacterial pneumonia in an adult, when acquired in the community, is very likely to be caused by *Streptococcus pneumoniae,* whereas this same infection, when acquired in the hospital, is more likely because of enteric gram-negative bacilli, such as *Enterobacter,* or opportunists, such as *Pseudomonas aeruginosa.*[24] The most common source of bacteremias is the urinary tract, and the majority of the bacteremias from this site are caused by enteric gram-negative bacilli.[22] In contrast, bacteremia from an intravenous catheter site is very likely caused by staphylococci.[25]

Any concomitant therapy the patient is receiving may influence the selection of drug therapy, the dosage, and monitoring. For example, administration of isoniazid to a patient who is also receiving phenytoin may result in phenytoin toxicity. This is caused by an inhibition of phenytoin metabolism by isoniazid. Furthermore, drugs that possess similar adverse-effect profiles may increase the risk for effects, for example, two drugs that cause nephrotoxicity or neutropenia. A list of potentially severe drug–drug interactions is provided in Table 96–2.

Concomitant disease states may influence the selection of therapy. Certain diseases will predispose patients to a particular infectious disease or will alter the type of infecting organism. For example, patients with diabetes mellitus and the resulting peripheral vascular disease often develop infections of the lower extremity soft tissue. Patients with chronic lung disease or cystic fibrosis develop frequent pulmonary infections, which may be caused by somewhat different microorganisms than are found in otherwise normal hosts.

Patients with immunosuppressive diseases, such as malignancies or acquired immunologic deficiencies, are highly predisposed to infections, and the types of organisms may be vastly different from what would be expected. For example, patients undergoing chemotherapy for acute forms of leukemia are often profoundly granulocytopenic and are predisposed to infections caused by staphylococci, enteric gram-negative bacilli, and fungi.[26] In contrast, patients with the acquired immunodeficiency syndrome (AIDS) often become infected with an enormous variety of organisms (Chap. 114). Complicating this assessment is the possibility that the immunosuppressed patient may have been taking prophylactic or suppressive antimicrobial agents such as trimethoprim–sulfamethoxazole for *Pneumocystis carinii* pneumonia, fluconazole for fungal infection, or acyclovir for viral disease.[27]

TABLE 96–2. Major Drug Interactions With Antimicrobials

Antimicrobial	Other Agent(s)	Results of Interaction
Aminoglycosides	Neuromuscular blocking drugs	Increased neuromuscular blockade
	Other nephrotoxins or ototoxins (e.g., cisplatin, amphotericin B, ethacrynic acid, vancomycin, cyclosporine)	Increased nephrotoxicity or ototoxicity
	Penicillins	Inactivation of both drugs (a particular problem in renal failure and when obtaining drug levels)
Sulfonamides	Sufonylureas	Hypoglycemia
	Phenytoin	Increased serum concentration of phenytoin leading to toxicity
	Oral anticoagulants (warfarin derivatives)	Enhanced hypoprothrombinemia
Chloramphenicol	Phenytoin, tolbutamide, ethanol	Increased serum concentration of other agents and enhanced pharmacologic effect or increased toxicity
Metronidazole (also cefamandole, moxalactam, cefoperazone)	Ethanol (including ethanol-containing medications)	Disulfiram-like reaction
Macrolides, azalides	Theophylline	Increased serum theophylline concentration
	Terfenadine, astemizole, cisapride	Cardiac arrhythmias
Fluconazole	Terfenadine, cisapride	Cardiac arrhythmias
	Phenytoin, warfarin	Inhibits metabolism of these drugs
	Rifampin	Enhances metabolism of fluconazole
Itraconazole	Astemizole, terfenadine, cisapride	Cardiac arrhythmias
	Phenytoin, warfarin	Inhibits metabolism of these drugs
	Rifampin	Enhances metabolism of itraconazole
Quinolones (norfloxacin, ciprofloxacin, ofloxacin, lomefloxacin, enoxacin grepafloxacin, levofloxacin, sparfloxacin, trovafloxacin)	Multivalent cations (antacids, iron, sucralfate, zinc), didanosine	Decreased absorption of quinolone
	Theophylline	Inhibits metabolism of theophylline (ciprofloxacin, enoxacin, grepafloxacin)
	Antiarrhythmics	Increased Q/T interval (grepafloxacin and sparfloxacin)
Rifampin	Coumarin anticoagulants	Decreased anticoagulant effect (increased metabolism of drug)
	Quinidine	Decreased effect of quinidine
	Digoxin	Decreased effect of digoxin
	Methadone	Narcotic withdrawal
	Propranolol	Decreased effect of propranolol
	Oral contraceptives	Decreased effect (pregnancy)
	Fluconazole; ketoconazole	Decreased antifungal effect
Tetracyclines	Antacids, iron, calcium	Inhibit intestinal absorption of tetracycline
Penicillins and cephalosporins	Uricosuric agents (probenecid, high-dose aspirin)	Block excretion of β-lactams, causing higher serum levels
	Copper reduction test for glycosuria (Clinitest tablets)	False-positive test for glycosuria (not seen with glucose oxidase method)
Isoniazid	Phenytoin	Increased serum concentrations of both

Immunosuppressive disease states lead to a wide variety of infections (AIDS), while other diseases may predispose the patient to a certain type of infectious disease (recurrent meningococcal infection with complement deficiency). Information from the patient's history regarding underlying disease is vitally important, since the presence of an underlying condition may not only predispose patients to infection, but it also may modify the likely offending pathogen. For example, purulent meningitis in an otherwise healthy adult is almost invariably caused by meningococci or pneumococci, whereas this same infection in a patient with a lymphoma may be caused by *Listeria monocytogenes,* which will infect an immunocompetent patient in only one-third of cases.[28] For a thorough discussion on infection in immunocompromised patients, see Chaps. 111 and 114.

Many factors predisposing to infection are related to disruption of the host's integumentary barriers. For example, trauma, burns, and iatrogenic wounds induced in surgery may lead to a substantial risk of infection, depending on the severity and location of the injury or disruption. For a complete discussion of the various risks involved in surgical procedures see Chap. 112.

DRUG FACTORS

PHARMACOKINETICS

The pharmacokinetic disposition of an agent is an important consideration when choosing antimicrobial therapy. It is desirable, whenever possible, to select agents that will not worsen the underlying dysfunction or will not be dependent on the compromised organ system for detoxification or removal from the body. Estimation of the creatinine clearance using the Cockcroft and Gault equation (see Chap. 3) should be determined for every patient to determine the appropriate dosing interval for drugs primarily eliminated by the kidneys.

PHARMACODYNAMIC CONSIDERATIONS

A great deal of research has been devoted to the study of antimicrobial pharmacodynamics—that is, the relationship between drug concentration and the effects on microorganisms (see Chap. 95).[29] Emerging from these efforts has come a better understanding of the concentration–effect relationships between classes of antimicrobials and selected bacteria.[30] Antimicrobials that produce concentration-dependent bactericidal effects include aminoglycosides and fluoroquinolones. When such concentration-dependent killing is coupled with a prolonged postantibiotic effect (PAE) (a prolonged lag period of growth following a brief exposure to an antimicrobial),[31] it may be possible to modify dosage regimens to take advantage of these effects. An example is the increasing use of high-dose, once-daily aminoglycosides. For these regimens, the drug is given as a single large daily dose (rather than two to three smaller ones).

By contrast, antimicrobials that affect cell wall synthesis (e.g., β-lactams) do not produce concentration-dependent killing nor do they produce prolonged PAE, but rather time-dependent bactericidal effects.[30] Therefore, the most important pharmacodynamic relationship for these antimicrobials is the duration that drug concentrations exceed the MIC. For example, frequent small doses or a continuous infusion of β-lactams appear to be correlated with a good outcome.[32]

TISSUE PENETRATION

The relevance of tissue concentrations of antimicrobials has long been disputed. Since methods to measure the concentrations of antimicrobial agents have become widely used as research tools, a great deal of data have been generated in this area. Some of the difficulties interpreting these data include a lack of correlation with clinical outcomes and poor understanding of whether the antimicrobial agents are present in a biologically active form.[33] An example of the former problem is the recognized efficacy of drugs with low biliary fluid concentrations in the treatment of cholecystitis, cholangitis, or both, and the absence of the enhanced efficacy of drugs whose primary route of elimination is biliary excretion of active drug. An example of the latter difficulty is with penetration to deep infections, such as abscesses, where various factors, such as acid pH, WBC products, and various enzymes, may inactivate even high concentrations of certain drugs. The central nervous system (CNS) is one body site where antimicrobial penetration is relatively well defined and correlations with clinical outcomes are established.[34] Cerebrospinal fluid (CSF) concentrations of antimicrobial agents necessary to eradicate bacterial meningitis have been defined, and drugs that do not reach significant concentrations in the CSF should be avoided in treating meningitis. Apart from the bloodstream, other body fluids where drug concentration data are clinically relevant include urine, synovial fluid, and peritoneal fluid.

Caution must be taken in selecting an antimicrobial agent for clinical use on the basis of tissue or fluid penetration. Apart from CNS penetration data, more attention should be paid to clinical efficacy, antimicrobial spectrum, toxicity, and cost than to comparative data on penetration into a given body site.

The route of administration for an antimicrobial is dependent on the site of infection. Parenteral therapy is warranted when patients have positive blood cultures (except possibly in the case of pyelonephritis) or are being treated for meningitis or febrile neutropenia.[35] Severe pneumonia is often initially treated with intravenous antibiotics and switched to oral therapy as clinical improvement is evident.[5,24,36] Patients treated in the ambulatory setting for upper respiratory tract infections (i.e., pharyngitis, bronchitis, sinusitis, and otitis media), lower respiratory tract infections, skin and soft-tissue infections, uncomplicated urinary tract infections, and selected sexually transmitted diseases may receive oral therapy.

DRUG TOXICITY

It is incumbent on health professionals to avoid toxic drugs whenever possible. Antibiotics associated with CNS toxicities, usually when not dose adjusted for renal function, include penicillins, cephalosporins, quinolones, and imipenem.

Hematologic toxicities are generally manifested with prolonged use of nafcillin (neutropenia), piperacillin (platelet dysfunction), cefotetan (hypoprothrombinemia), chloramphenicol (bone marrow suppression, both idiosyncratic and dose-related toxicity), and trimethoprim (megaloblastic anemia). Reversible nephrotoxicity is classically associated with aminoglycosides and vancomycin. Reversible ototoxicity can occur with aminoglycosides or erythromycin. In the outpatient setting, patients must be cautioned regarding photosensitivity with azithromycin, quinolones, tetracyclines, pyrazinamide, sulfamethoxazole, and trimethoprim. Lastly, all antibiotics have been implicated in causing diarrhea secondary to *Clostridium difficile* (see Chap. 103).[37]

Aside from consideration of drug toxicity, some antimicrobial use requires more intensive risk–benefit analysis. An example of this is the decision to use isoniazid prophylactically to prevent tuberculosis. Because the hepatotoxicity of isoniazid increases in frequency with age, older persons who are candidates for isoniazid prophylaxis (positive skin test) must have additional risk factors for tuberculosis to balance the potential toxic effects. These include evidence of recent skin test conversion, immunosuppression, or previous gastrectomy. Older patients without additional risk factors are more likely to suffer toxicity from isoniazid than derive benefit from its use.[38]

COST

The costs of drug therapy are increasing dramatically, especially as new products, derived from biotechnology, are introduced. Greater attention is being paid to the pharmacoeconomics of drug therapy, where patient outcomes are valued and the costs to arrive at those outcomes are estimated. With increasing numbers of patients enrolled in managed-care organizations, understanding the true cost of antimicrobial therapy is more important than ever. The total cost of antimicrobial therapy includes much more than just the acquisition cost of the drugs.[39]

Many ancillary costs affect the true cost of therapy. These include factors such as storage, preparation, distribution, and administration, as well as all of the costs incurred from monitoring for adverse effects and factors such as length of hospitalization, readmissions, and all directly provided health care goods and services. More difficult to value, but equally as important, are indirect costs, such as patient quality of life issues. Pharmacoeconomic and outcomes analysis are becoming more widely applied and used, in order to derive values such as cost–benefit ratios and the cost effectiveness of various products compared to one another. A detailed review of pharmacoeconomic analyses is beyond the scope of this chapter, but excellent reviews of the subject are available.[40] A great deal more research in this area is needed, and multidisciplinary, collaborative efforts (with the involvement of pharmacy, medicine, nursing, and microbiology) are essential.[41]

Many new oral antimicrobials have been approved including cephalosporins, β-lactam β-lactamase inhibitors, macrolides, and quinolones, that can be used in place of more expensive parenteral therapy. These agents offer extended spectrum killing activity, increased tissue penetration, and excellent safety and pharmacokinetic profiles. Many older, less expensive oral agents also remain appropriate choices. When oral therapy is being considered, the choice between convenient once-a-day expensive agents versus multiple-dose inexpensive agents arises. It is easy to calculate the difference in acquisition cost; however, the overall cost between agents is more difficult to determine. Factors to weigh include safety, effectiveness, tolerability, patient compliance, and potential drug–drug interactions. In some instances, more expensive agents may be warranted to avoid adverse outcomes.[42]

COMBINATION ANTIMICROBIAL THERAPY

In selecting a drug regimen for a given patient, consideration must be given to the necessity of using more than one drug. Combinations of antimicrobials are generally used to: (1) broaden the spectrum of coverage for empiric therapy, (2) achieve synergistic activity against the infecting organism, and (3) prevent the emergence of resistance.

BROADENING THE SPECTRUM OF COVERAGE

Increasing the coverage of antimicrobial therapy is generally necessary in mixed infections where multiple organisms are likely to be present. This is the case in intraabdominal and female pelvic infections in which a variety of aerobic and anaerobic bacteria may produce disease.[43] Traditionally, a combination of a drug active against aerobic gram-negative bacilli, such as an aminoglycoside, and a drug active against anaerobic bacteria, such as metronidazole or clindamycin, is selected. Newer β-lactam compounds, which possess good activity against both of these types of organisms, such as the cephamycins, imipenem, or the β-lactam and β-lactamase inhibitor combinations may be adequate to replace the combination and, thereby, reduce the cost of therapy. The other clinical situation in which an increased spectrum of activity is desirable is with nosocomial infections.[24]

Newer β-lactam agents, such as the third-generation cephalosporins, may be adequate in certain situations in lieu of various combinations. The enhanced gram-negative spectrum of these compounds has been achieved, however, at the expense of gram-positive activity. Thus, most infectious disease consultants would add a drug with good antistaphylococcal activity to the regimen, such as a penicillinase-resistant penicillin or vancomycin. This is especially true in immunosuppressed patients in whom such broad-spectrum coverage is dictated by the likelihood of streptococci, staphylococci, and enteric gram-negative bacilli.[26]

SYNERGISM

Laboratory tests to identify synergy between antibiotic combinations is described in Chapter 95. The achievement of synergistic antimicrobial activity is advantageous for infections caused by enteric gram-negative bacilli in immunosuppressed patients. Traditionally, combinations of aminoglycosides and β-lactams have been used, since these drugs together generally act synergistically against a wide variety of bacteria. The data supporting superior efficacy of synergistic over nonsynergistic combinations is weak, however. At best, it would appear that synergistic combinations produce better results in infections caused by *P. aeruginosa,* in certain infections caused by *Enterococcus* sp., and, perhaps, in patients with profound, persistent neutropenia.[27,44,45]

The most obvious example of the use of synergy is the treatment of enterococcal endocarditis. The causative organism is usually only inhibited by penicillins, but it is rapidly killed by the addition of streptomycin or gentamicin to a penicillin.[44] The necessity for bactericidal activity in the treatment of endocarditis underscores the need for these synergistic combinations.

PREVENTING RESISTANCE

The use of combinations to prevent the emergence of resistance is widely applied but not often realized. The only circumstance where this has been clearly effective is in the treatment of tuberculosis. The prevalence of resistance to a first-line drug, such as isoniazid or rifampin, in a population of organisms may be as high as 1 in 10^6 to 10^8. Since the bacterial load in a patient with active tuberculosis often exceeds this, two drugs are given to reduce the likelihood of encountering resistance to less than 1 in 10.[10,38] There is ample evidence from *in vitro* data and experimental bacterial infections that combinations of drugs with different mechanisms are effective in the prevention of the emergence of resistance. Data from clinical trials, however, are either conflicting or do not convincingly support this concept.[46]

DISADVANTAGES OF COMBINATION THERAPY

Although there are potentially beneficial effects from combining drugs, there also are potential disadvantages. Examples include additive nephrotoxicity from drugs, such as aminoglycosides, amphotericin, and possibly vancomycin.[47] Inactivation of aminoglycosides by penicillins may be clinically significant when excessive doses of penicillin are given to a patient in renal failure.[48]

The combination of two or more antibiotics may result in antagonistic effects (see Chap. 95). Clinically, the effect of antagonism may be evident when one drug induces β-lactamase production and another drug is β-lactamase unstable.[49] Cefoxitin and imipenem are examples of drugs capable of inducing β-lactamases and may result in more rapid inactivation of penicillins when used together.

MONITORING THERAPEUTIC RESPONSE

Once antimicrobial therapy has been instituted, the patient must be monitored carefully for a therapeutic response. Culture and sensitivity reports from specimens sent to the microbiology laboratory must be reviewed, and the therapy changed accordingly. Use of agents with the narrowest spectrum of activity against identified pathogens is recommended. If anaerobes are suspected, even if they are not identified, anaerobic therapy should be continued.

Patient monitoring should include many of the same parameters used to diagnose the infection. The WBC count and temperature should start to normalize. Physical complaints from the patient should also diminish (i.e., decreased pain, shortness of breath, cough, or sputum production). Appetite should improve. Radiologic improvement may lag behind clinical improvement.

Determinations of serum (or other fluid) levels of antimicrobials may be useful in assuring outcome, preventing toxicity, or both. There are only a few antimicrobials that require serum concentration monitoring, and then only in selected situations. These include the aminoglycosides, flucytosine, and chloramphenicol. Achievement of adequate aminoglycoside concentrations within the first few days of therapy of gram-negative infection has been correlated with better therapeutic outcome.[50] In addition, assuring that excessive concentrations of flucytosine or chloramphenicol (in neonates) are avoided will prevent toxicity.

Changes in the distribution volume may have significant impact on the efficacy, safety, or both of therapy. An unexpectedly low volume of distribution (such as in the dehydrated patient) will result in higher, potentially toxic concentrations, whereas a larger than expected volume (such as in patients with edema or ascites) will result in low, potentially subtherapeutic concentrations. The most effective methods use measured serum concentrations of the drugs rather than estimations from renal function tests to assess true drug clearance from the body.

As patients improve clinically, the route of administration should be reevaluated. Streamlining therapy from parenteral to oral (switch therapy) has become an accepted practice for many infections outside the bloodstream and CNS.[36,51] Criteria that should be present include (1) overall clinical improvement, (2) afebrile for 24 to 48 hours, (3) decreased WBC count, and (4) functioning GI tract. Drugs that exhibit excellent oral bioavailability compared to intravenous formulations include amoxicillin, azithromycin, ciprofloxacin, clindamycin, doxycycline, levofloxacin, metronidazole, and trimethoprim–sulfamethoxazole.

FAILURE OF ANTIMICROBIAL THERAPY

A variety of factors may be responsible for an apparent lack of response to therapy.[52] Patients who fail to respond over 2 to 3 days require a thorough reevaluation. It is possible that the diagnosis is not infectious, not nonbacterial in origin, or is a pathogen in a polymicrobial infection that remains unidentified. Other factors include those directly related to drug selection, the host, or the pathogen. Laboratory error in identification, susceptibility testing, or both (presence of inoculum effect or resistant subpopulations) are rare causes of antimicrobial failure.

FAILURES CAUSED BY DRUG SELECTION

Factors directly related to the drug selection include an inappropriate drug selection or dosage or route of administration. Malabsorption of a drug product because of GI disease, such as a short-bowel syndrome, or a drug interaction, such as complexation of fluoroquinolones with multivalent cations resulting in reduced absorption, may lead to potentially subtherapeutic serum concentrations. Accelerated drug elimination is also possible. This may occur in patients with cystic fibrosis or during pregnancy, when more rapid clearance or larger volumes of distribution may result in low serum concentrations, particularly for aminoglycosides. A common cause of failure of therapy is poor penetration into the site of infection. This is especially true for sites such as the CNS, eye, and prostate gland. Drug failure can also result from drugs that are highly protein bound or that are chemically inactivated at the site of infection.

FAILURES CAUSED BY HOST FACTORS

Host defenses must be considered when evaluating a patient who is not responding to antimicrobial therapy. Patients who are immunosuppressed (e.g., granulocytopenia from chemotherapy, or AIDS) may respond poorly to therapy because their defenses are inadequate to eradicate the infection despite seemingly adequate drug regimens. A good example is the poor response of infection in granulocytopenic patients that is seen when their WBC counts remain low during therapy. This contrasts to a much better response when granulocyte counts rise during therapy.[53]

Other host factors are related to the necessity for surgical drainage of abscesses or removal of foreign bodies, necrotic tissue, or both. If these situations are not corrected, they result in persistent infection and, occasionally, bacteremia, despite adequate antimicrobial therapy.

FAILURES CAUSED BY MIRCROORGANISMS

Factors related to the pathogen include the development of drug resistance during therapy.[54] Primary resistance refers to the intrinsic resistance of the pathogens producing the infection. It has become increasingly obvious that, despite the development and introduction of numerous new antimicrobial agents, bacterial resistance has continued to increase, both within and across different bacterial genera.

Most of the newer antibacterial agents developed and licensed in the past 5 years are targeted toward improved activity against gram-negative bacteria. This list includes parenteral and oral fluoroquinolones, carbapenems, β-lactam, β-lactamase inhibitor combinations, and newer fourth-generation cephalosporins. Organisms in which resistance has increased most dramatically include enterococci, pneumococci, and *Mycobacterium tuberculosis.* Enterococci have been isolated with multiple resistance patterns. They may be resistant to β-lactams (by virtue of β-lactamase production, altered penicillin-binding proteins [PBP], or both), vancomycin (via alterations in peptidoglycan synthesis), and high levels of aminoglycosides (via enzymatic degradation). For infections caused by organisms with multiple resistance, the available treatment is suboptimal and may include various combinations of the previously named medications to attack multiple sites of action.[44]

Pneumococci resistant to penicillins, certain cephalosporins, and macrolides are increasingly common. These organisms are generally susceptible to vancomycin and cefotaxime or ceftriaxone. *M. tuberculosis* resistant to one or more first-line antitubercular agents (isoniazid [INH], rifampin, ethambutol, streptomycin, and pyrazinamide) have increased in frequency as well. This has been observed principally in populations of prison inmates and patients with AIDS.

The increase in resistance among these organisms is believed to be caused, in large part, by continued overuse of antimicrobials in the community, as well as in hospitals, and the increasing prevalence of immunosuppressed patients receiving long-term suppressive antimicrobials for the prevention of infections. Note that these resistance patterns are regionally variable, and susceptibility patterns in the community (or hospital) should be monitored closely to promote rational antimicrobial selection.[55]

The emergence of resistance during antimicrobial therapy is reported most frequently in pulmonary or other deep-seated infections caused by *P. aeruginosa.* This occurs in 20% to 30% of cases and with all the available antibacterial agents, including imipenem. This organism and a group of enteric gram-negative bacilli *(Enterobacter aerogenes, Enterobacter cloacae, Citrobacter freundii, Serratia marcescens,* and a few others) can produce a β-lactamase that is capable of hydrolyzing broad-spectrum cephalosporins and, to a lesser extent, penicillins.[55] These enzymes are categorized as Richmond-Sykes type I, and their genetic code is found on the chromosome. Resistant mutants of these aforementioned organisms that produce large quantities of these enzymes may be present within an infection and may be responsible for the emergence of resistance during therapy. The mutants occur at a frequency of 1 in 10^6 to 1 in 10^8 bacteria, the numbers of bacteria commonly encountered in clinical infections.[55] Because only 10^4 to 10^5 bacteria are tested for susceptibility in the microbiology laboratory, however, this potential resistance may not be detected. Treatment of an infection caused by *Enterobacter, Citrobacter, Serratia, or P. aeruginosa* with a third-generation cephalosporin or aztreonam may produce an initial clinical response by eradicating all of the susceptible bacteria in the population. Within a few days, however, the highly resistant subpopulations have a selective advantage and may overgrow the infection site to produce a relapse.[55] These bacteria usually retain susceptibility to aminoglycosides, imipenem, and fluoroquinolones but are resistant to all other β-lactams. It should be obvious that host defenses are extremely important in this scenario. Debilitated patients with pulmonary infections, abscesses, or osteomyelitis are at high risk for drug failure. In these situations, a combination regimen to prevent the emergence of resistance or the use of imipenem or a fluoroquinolone may be warranted for empiric therapy.

ANTIMICROBIAL USE MANAGEMENT

A chapter on antibiotic selection would not be complete without a discussion regarding formulary management. With the vast array of antimicrobials available, institutions must make decisions regarding which antibiotics to include on its formulary. The actual decision to have a formulary remains controversial; however, restricting choices does encourage familiarity with a core of antibiotics for residents and attending physicians. Open formularies allow the use of any commercially available antibiotics empirically with recommended guidelines for changes when culture and sensitivity results are finalized. Many institutions have organized an antibiotic subcommittee to the Pharmacy and Therapeutics Committee, which meets to discuss trends in resistance and review new agents. The subcommittee is generally a multidisciplinary group, including representation from microbiology, infection control, pharmacy, and physicians from several disciplines, including infectious disease. The actual implementation of the guidelines and restrictions recommended by such groups requires the cooperation of the entire medical staff. Education plays a major role in the success of the antibiotic formulary.[56]

Attention must be paid to the literature on antimicrobials to assist in the selection of therapy. The results from prospective, controlled, randomized clinical trials should be evaluated whenever possible when considering appropriate antimicrobial therapy. Results from prelicensing open trials offer only limited information that may be useful in this regard, because patients in these trials are generally not seriously ill, are not infected with multiply resistant bacteria, and other confounding factors found in most clinical situations are excluded by virtue of the study design. Therefore, comparative data in more seriously ill patients is essential for the appropriate application of new agents.[57]

In addition, postmarketing trials may be important if their results demonstrate superiority of one regimen over another, either in efficacy, safety, or cost effectiveness. Appropriate antimicrobial therapy may change as new organisms are discovered, susceptibility patterns change, new drugs become available, and new clinical trial results are published.

▶ PRINCIPLES OF PHARMACOTHERAPY

- Every attempt should be made to obtain specimens for culture and sensitivity testing prior to initiating antibiotics.
- Empiric antibiotic therapy should be based on knowledge of likely pathogens for the site of infection, information from patient history (recent hospitalizations, work-related exposure, travel, pets), and local susceptibility data (when using antibiogram, remember > 80% sensitivity is a good empiric choice).
- Patients with delayed reactions to penicillin (skin rash) can generally receive cephalosporins. Patients with type I hypersensitivity reactions to penicillins (anaphylaxis) should not receive cephalosporins (alternatives include aztreonam, quinolones, sulfa drugs, or vancomycin based on type of coverage indicated).
- Estimated renal function should be calculated for every patient who is to receive antibiotics and the dose interval adjusted accordingly. Hepatic function should be considered for drugs eliminated through the hepatobiliary system, such as clindamycin, erythromycin, and metronidazole.
- All concomitant drugs and nutrient supplements should be reviewed when an antibiotic is added to a patient's therapy.
- Combination antibiotic therapy may be indicated for polymicrobial infections (abdominal, gynecologic infections) to produce synergistic killing (β-lactam plus aminoglycoside versus *P. aeruginosa)* or to prevent the emergence of resistance.
- Positive cultures must be interpreted with caution to distinguish true infection from colonization or contamination.
- Treatment for the specific organisms identified should include an agent(s) with the narrowest spectrum of activity. Improvement on broad-spectrum regimen is not enough reason not to streamline therapy.
- All patients receiving antibiotics should be monitored for efficacy (decreasing temperature and WBC count, diminishing signs and symptoms of infection), toxicity (hypersensitivity: β-lactams, cephalosporins; nephrotoxicity: aminoglycosides, amphotericin; diarrhea: all), and development of superinfection (fungal infection).
- Antibiotic route of administration should be evaluated daily and streamlining from intravenous to oral should be attempted as signs of infection improve for patients with functioning GI tracts (general exceptions are bloodstream and CNS infections).
- Patients not responding to an appropriate treatment in 2 to 3 days should be reevaluated to ensure (1) that infection is the correct diagnosis, (2) therapeutic drug concentrations are being achieved, (3) patient is not immunosuppressed, (4) patient does not have isolated infection (abscess, foreign body), or (5) resistance has not developed.
- Primary literature should be reviewed periodically to determine current opinion on antibiotics of choice.

REFERENCES

1. Hessen TM, Kaye D. Principles of selection and use of antibacterial agents. Infect Dis Clin North Am 1995;9:531–545.
2. Dinarello CA, Cannon JG, Wolff SM. New concepts on the pathogenesis of fever. Rev Infect Dis 1988;10:168–189.
3. Dinarello CA, Wolff SM. Fever of unknown origin. In: Mandell GL, Bennett JE, Dolin R, eds. Principles and Practice of Infectious Diseases, 4th ed. New York, Churchill Livingstone, 1995:530–536.
4. Mackowiak PA, Lemaistre CF. Drug fever: A critical appraisal of conventional concepts. Ann Intern Med 1987;106:728–733.

5. Niederman MS, Bass JB, Campbell GD, et al. Official ATS statement: Guidelines for the initial management of adults with community-acquired pneumonia—Diagnosis, assessment of severity, and initial antimicrobial therapy. Am Rev Resp Dis 1993;148:1418–1426.
6. Greenlee JE. Approach to diagnosis of meningitis. Infect Dis Clin North Am 1990;4:583–598.
7. Washington JA. The microbiological diagnosis of infective endocarditis. J Antimicrob Chemother 1987;20(suppl A):29–36.
8. Wilson ML. General principles of specimen collection and transport. Clin Infect Dis 1996;22:766–777.
9. Weiss ME. Drug allergy. Med Clin North Am 1992;76:857–882.
10. Saxon A. Immediate hypersensitivity reactions to beta-lactam antibiotics. Rev Infect Dis 1983;5(suppl 2):S368–S378.
11. Saxon A, Swabb EA, Adkinson NF. Investigation into the immunologic cross-reactivity of aztreonam with other beta-lactam antibiotics. Am J Med 1985;78(suppl 2A):19–26.
12. Saez-Llorens X, McCraken GH. Bacterial meningitis in neonates and children. Infect Dis Clin North Am 1990;4:623–644.
13. Kantor HI, Sutherland DA, Leonard JT, et al. Effect of bilirubin metabolism in the newborn of sulfisoxazole administered to the mother. Obstet Gynecol 1961;17:494–500.
14. Powell DA, Nahata MC. Chloramphenicol: New perspectives on an old drug. Drug Intell Clin Pharm 1982;16:295–300.
15. Gleckman RA. Antibiotic concerns in the elderly. Infect Dis Clin North Am 1995;9:575–589.
16. Kopanoff DE, Snider DE Jr, Caras GJ. Isoniazid-related hepatitis: A US public health cooperative surveillance study. Am Rev Respir Dis 1978;117:991-1001.
17. Korzeniowski OM. Antibacterial agents in pregnancy. Infect Dis Clin North Am 1995;9:613–639.
18. Relling MV. Polymorphic drug metabolism. Clin Pharm 1989;8: 852–863.
19. Tabbara IA. Hemolytic anemias: Diagnosis and management. Med Clin North Am 1992;76:649–668.
20. Livornese LL, Benz RL, Ingerman MJ, et al. Antibacterial agents in renal failure. Infect Dis Clin North Am 1995;9:591–614.
21. Tschida SJ, Vance-Bryan K, Zaske DE. Anti-infective agents in hepatic disease. Med Clin North Am 1995;79:895–917.
22. Johnson JR, Stamm WE. Urinary tract infections in women: Diagnosis and treatment. Ann Intern Med 1989;111:906–917.
23. Nelson JD. Acute osteomyelitis in children. Infect Dis Clin North Am 1990;4:513–522.
24. Campbell GD, Niederman MS, Broughton WA, et al. Official ATS statement: Hospital-acquired pneumonia in adults: Diagnosis, assessment of severity, initial antimicrobial therapy and preventative strategies. Am J Respir Crit Care Med 1995;153:1711–1725.
25. Richet H, Hubert B, Nitemberg G, et al. Prospective multicenter study of vascular catheter-related complications and risk factors for positive central catheter cultures in ICU patients. J Clin Microbiol 1990;28: 2520–2525.
26. Giamarellou H. Empiric therapy for infections in the febrile, neutropenic, compromised host. Med Clin North Am 1995;79:559–580.
27. USPHS/IDSA guidelines for the prevention of opportunistic infections in persons infected with human immunodeficiency virus: A summary. MMWR 1995;44:1–34.
28. Wispelwey B, Tunkel AR, Scheld WM. Bacterial meningitis in adults. Infect Dis Clin North Am 1990;4:645–660.
29. Levison ME. Pharmacodynamics of antimicrobial agents: Bactericidal and postantibiotic effects. Infect Dis Clin North Am 1995;9:483–495.
30. Drusano GL. Human pharmacodynamics of beta-lactams, aminoglycosides and their combinations. Scand J Infect Dis 1991(suppl);74: 235–248.
31. Spivey JM. The post-antibiotic effect. Clin Pharm 1992;11:865–875.
32. Craig WA, Ebert SC. Continuous infusion of beta-lactam antibiotics. Antimicrob Agents Chemother 1992;36:2577–2583.
33. Nix DE, Goodwin SD, Peloquin CA, et al. Antibiotic tissue penetration and its relevance: Impact of tissue penetration on infection response. Antimicrob Agents Chemother 1991;35:1953–1959.
34. Quagliarello VJ, Scheld WM. Treatment of bacterial meningitis. New Engl J Med 1997;336:708–716.
35. Johnson JR, Lyons MF, Pearce W, et al. Therapy for women hospitalized with acute pyelonephritis: A randomized trial of ampicillin versus trimethoprim/sulfamethoxazole for 14 days. J Infect Dis 1991;163: 325–330.
36. Ramierez JA. Switch therapy in community-acquired pneumonia. Diagn Microbiol Infect Dis 1995;22(1-2):219–223.
37. Kelly CP, Pothoulakis C, Lamont JT. *Clostridium difficile* colitis. N Engl J Med 1994;330:257-262.
38. American Thoracic Society. Treatment of tuberculosis and tuberculosis infection in adults and children. Am J Respir Crit Care Med 1994; 149:1359–1374.
39. Guglielmo BJ, Brooks GF. Antimicrobial therapy—Cost benefit considerations. Drugs 1989;38:473–480.
40. McGhan WF. Pharmacoeconomics and the evaluation of drugs and services. Hosp Formul 1993;28:365–378.
41. Marr JJ, Moffet HL, Kunin CM. Guidelines for improving the use of antimicrobial agents in hospitals: A statement by the Infectious Diseases Society of America. J Infect Dis 1988;157:869–876.
42. Nightingale CH, Quintiliani R. Cost of oral antibiotic therapy. Pharmacother 1997;17:302–307.
43. Landers DV, Wolner-Hanssen P, Paavonen J, et al. Combination antimicrobial therapy in the treatment of acute pelvic inflammatory disease. Am J Obstet Gynecol 1991;164:849–858.
44. Eliopoulos GM. The ten most commonly asked questions about resistant enterococcal infections. Infect Dis Clin Pract 1994;3:125–129.
45. Hilf M, Yu VL, Sharp J, et al. Antibiotic therapy for *Pseudomonas aeruginosa* bacteremia: Outcome correlations in a prospective study of 200 patients. Am J Med 1989;87:540–546.
46. Barriere SL. Bacterial resistance to beta-lactams and its prevention with combination antimicrobial therapy. Pharmacotherapy 1992;12: 391–396.
47. Rybak MJ, Albrecht LM, Boike SC, et al. Nephrotoxicity of vancomycin, alone and with aminoglycoside. J Antimicrob Chemother 1990;25:679–687.
48. Manian FA, Stone WJ, Alford RH. Adverse antibiotic effects associated with renal insufficiency. Rev Infect Dis 1989;10:43–55.
49. Sanders CC, Sanders E Jr. Microbial resistance to newer generation β-lactam antibiotics: Clinical and laboratory implications. J Infect Dis 1985;151:399–406.
50. Moore RD, Smith CR, Lietman PS. Association of aminoglycoside plasma levels with therapeutic outcome in gram-negative pneumonia. Am J Med 1984;77:657–662.
51. Cunha BA. Intravenous-to-oral antibiotic switch therapy. Postgrad Med 1997;101:111–128.
52. Cunha BA, Ortega AM. Antibiotic failure. Med Clin North Am 1995; 79:663–672.
53. Pizzo PA. Management of fever in patients with cancer and treatment-induced neutropenia. N Engl J Med 1993;328:1323–1332.
54. Fraimow HS, Abrutyn E. Pathogens resistant to antimicrobial agents: Epidemiology, molecular mechanisms and clinical management. Infect Dis Clin North Am 1995;9:497–527.
55. Murray BE. The problems and dilemma of antimicrobial resistance. Pharmacotherapy 1992;12(6 part 2):86s–93s.
56. Quintiliani R, Nightingale CH, Crowe HM, et al. Strategic antibiotic decision-making at the formulary level. Rev Infect Dis 1991;13 (suppl 9):S770–S777.
57. Gilbert DN. Guidelines for evaluating new antimicrobial agents. J Infect Dis 1987;156:934–941.

APPENDIX 96–1

Drugs of Choice, First Choice, *Alternative(s)*

GRAM-POSITIVE COCCI

***Streptococcus* (groups A, B, C, G, and *S. bovis*)**

Penicillin G[a] or V[b] or ampicillin

Erythromycin, FGC[c,d] azithromycin, clarithromycin,[e] vancomycin

***Streptococcus pneumoniae*[f]**

Penicillin-sensitive

Penicillin G or V or ampicillin

Erythromycin, FGC,[c,d] cefotaxime or ceftriaxone,[d,g] chloramphenicol[h]

Penicillin-resistant (MIC ≥ 2.0 μg/mL)

Vancomycin (check sensitivities for TGC,[d,o] cefepime,[d] imipenem,[r] grepafloxacin,[j] levofloxacin,[j] sparfloxacin,[j] trovafloxacin[j])

***Streptococcus*, viridans group**

Penicillin G ± gentamicin[i]

Vancomycin ± gentamicin, FGC[c,d]

***Enterococcus faecalis* (generally not as resistant to antibiotics as *Enterococcus faecium*)**

Serious infection (endocarditis, meningitis, pyelonephritis with bacteremia)

Ampicillin (or penicillin G) + gentamicin or streptomycin

Vancomycin with gentamicin or streptomycin

Urinary Tract Infection (UTI)

Ampicillin, amoxicillin, doxycycline,[j] ciprofloxacin,[j] levofloxacin[j]

E. faecium (generally more resistant to antibiotics than *E. faecalis*); no regimen proven efficacious for vancomycin-resistant *E. faecium;* recommend consultation with infectious disease physician

Staphylococcus aureus

Methicillin (oxacillin)-sensitive

PRP[k]

FGC[c,d], trimethoprim–sulfamethoxazole, clindamycin,[l] vancomycin, BLIC,[m] imipenem

Methicillin (oxacillin)-resistant

Vancomycin ± rifampin or gentamicin

Trimethoprim–sulfamethoxazole, doxycycline,[j] either ± rifampin

Teicoplanin (investigational Hoechst Marion Roussel)

GRAM-NEGATIVE COCCI

Moraxella (Branhamella) catarrhalis

Amoxicillin/clavulanate

Trimethoprim–sulfamethoxazole, erythromycin, azithromycin, clarithromycin,[e] doxycycline,[j] SGC,[d,n] TGC,[d,o] TGCpo[d,p]

***Neisseria gonorrhoeae* (also give concomitant treatment for *Chlamydia trachomatis*)**

Uncomplicated infection

Ceftriaxone,[d] cefixime,[d] cefpodoxime[d]

APPG,[q] ciprofloxacin,[j] ofloxacin,[j] cefotaxime,[d] spectinomycin

Disseminated gonnococcal infection

Ceftriaxone[d] + doxycycline[j]

TGC[d,o]

Neisseria meningitidis

Penicillin G

TGC,[d,o] chloramphenicol[h]

GRAM-POSITIVE BACILLI

Clostridium perfringens

Penicillin G ± clindamycin

Clindamycin, metronidazole, doxycycline,[j] cefazolin,[d] imipenem,[r] chloramphenicol[h]

Clostridium difficile

Oral metronidazole

Oral vancomycin, oral bacitracin

GRAM-NEGATIVE BACILLI

***Acinetobacter* sp.**

Imipenem or meropenem either plus amikacin

(ESP,[s] ciprofloxacin,[j] levofloxacin,[j] trovafloxacin,[j] trimethoprim– sulfamethoxazole, ampicillin/sulbactam) any plus amikacin

***Bacteroides fragilis* (and others)**

Metronidazole

BLIC,[u] clindamycin, cephamycin,[d,v] ESP,[s] imipenem[r]

***Enterobacter* sp.**

Imipenem, meropenem, or cefepime any plus AMG[w]

ESP,[s] trimethoprim–sulfamethoxazole, or TGC[d,o] any plus AMG[w] or TGCpo[d,p]

Escherichia coli

FGC[c,d]

AMG,[w] SGC,[d,n] TGC,[d,o] TGCpo[d,p] ampicillin, fluoroquinolone[j,t]

Gardnerella vaginalis

Metronidazole

Clindamycin

Haemophilus influenzae

BLIC,[u] azithromycin, or ampicillin/amoxicillin if β-lactamase negative

TGC,[d,o,r] trimethoprim–sulfamethoxazole, SGC,[d,n] chloramphenicol,[h] erythromycin, clarithromycin,[e] ciprofloxacin,[j,r] imipenem,[r] meropenem,[r] TGCpo[d,p]

Klebsiella pneumoniae

TGC,[d,o] (for UTI: AMG[w])

Trimethoprim–sulfamethoxazole, FGC,[c,d] SGC,[d,n] fluoroquinolone,[j,t] BLIC,[u] ESP,[s] imipenem[r]

***Legionella* sp.**

Erythromycin ± rifampin

Trimethoprim–sulfamethoxazole, ciprofloxacin,[j] ofloxacin,[j] clarithromycin,[e] azithromycin

Pasteurella multocida

Penicillin G

Doxycycline,[j] BLIC,[u] trimethoprim– sulfamethoxazole, ceftriaxone[d,r]

Proteus mirabilis

Ampicillin

Trimethoprim–sulfamethoxazole, most antibiotics except PRP[k]

***Proteus* (indole-positive) (including *Providencia rettgeri, Morganella morganii, Proteus vulgaris*)**

TGC,[d,p] fluoroquinolone[j,t]

Trimethoprim–sulfamethoxazole, BLIC,[u] ESP,[s] aztreonam,[x] imipenem[r]

Providencia stuartii

TGC,[d,o] fluoroquinolone[j,t]

Trimethoprim–sulfamethoxazole, ESP,[s] aztreonam,[x] imipenem[r]

Pseudomonas aeruginosa

ESP[s] or ceftazidime either plus AMG[w]

UTI only: AMG[w]

Ciprofloxacin,[j] aztreonam,[x] imipenem,[r] meropenem[r] any plus AMG[w]

Salmonella typhi

Ciprofloxacin[j] or TGC[d,o]

Trimethoprim–sulfamethoxazole, ampicillin/amoxicillin, chloramphenicol[h]

***Salmonella* (non-typhi)**

Ceftriaxone[d,y]

Trimethoprim–sulfamethoxazole, ampicillin/amoxicillin, ciprofloxacin,[j] chloramphenicol[h]

Serratia marcescens

TGC[d,o] ± gentamicin

Trimethoprim–sulfamethoxazole, ciprofloxacin,[j] ESP,[s] BLIC,[u] aztreonam,[x] imipenem,[r] meropenem[r]

Stentrophomonas (Xanthomonas) maltophilia

Trimethoprim–sulfamethoxazole

Ciprofloxacin,[j] ofloxacin[j]

MISCELLANEOUS MICROORGANISMS

Nocardia

Trimethoprim–sulfamethoxazole (high dose)

Sulfonamide,[z] doxycycline,[j] (imipenem,[r] ceftriaxone[d]/cefuroxime[d]—either plus amikacin), cycloserine[h]

Chlamydia pneumoniae

Doxycycline[j] or erythromycin

Azithromycin, clarithromycin[e]

Chlamydia trachomatis

Doxycycline[j] or azithromycin

Mycoplasma pneumoniae

Erythromycin, azithromycin, clarithromycin[e]

Doxycycline[j]

SPIROCHETES

Treponema pallidum

Penicillin G

Doxycycline,[j] ceftriaxone[d]

***Borrelia burgdorferii* (choice depends on stage of disease)**

Doxycycline[j] or amoxicillin

High-dose penicillin, ceftriaxone,[d] cefotaxime,[d] cefuroxime axetil,[d] azithromycin, clarithromycin[e]

[a]*Either aqueous penicillin G or benzathine penicillin G (pharyngitis only).*
[b]*Only for soft-tissue infections or upper respiratory infections (pharyngitis, otitis media).*
[c]*First-generation cephalosporins. Intravenous (IV): cefazolin; oral (PO): cephalexin, cephradine, or cefadroxil.*
[d]*Some penicillin-allergic patients may react to cephalosporins.*
[e]*Do not use in pregnant patients.*
[f]*S. pneumoniae susceptibility to penicillin is expressed as the following: sensitive (MIC < 0.1 μg/mL), intermediate (MIC 0.1 to 1.0 μg/mL), and resistant (MIC ≥ 2.0 μg/mL). For intermediate strains, cefotaxime or ceftriaxone may be used for meningitis and either high-dose penicillin (≥ 12 MU/day) or cefuroxime may be used for pneumonia. For resistant strains, sensitivites should be used to guide therapy for meningitis and pneumonia. Resistance has been reported to erythromycin, clindamycin, trimethoprom–sulfamethoxazole, clarithromycin, azithromycin, and chloramphenicol. Quinupristin/dalfopristin (an investigational agent available from Rhone Poulenc Rorer ([610-454-3071]) has been sensitive to all strains tested.*
[g]*For the treatment of meningitis.*
[h]*Reserve for serious infection when less toxic drugs are not effective.*
[i]*Gentamicin should be added if tolerance or moderately susceptible (MIC^3 0.1 g/mL) organisms are encountered; streptomycin is used but may be more toxic.*
[j]*Not for use in pregnant patients or children less than 18 years old.*
[k]*Penicillinase-resistant penicillin: nafcillin or oxacillin.*
[l]*Not reliably bactericidal, so should not be used for endocarditis.*
[m]*β-lactamase inhibitor combination. IV: ampicillin/sulbactam; oral: amoxicillin/clavulanate.*
[n]*Second generation cephalosporins. IV: cefuroxime; oral: cefuroxime aextil, cefaclor, cefprozil.*
[o]*Third-generation cephalosporins. IV: cefotaxime, ceftizoxime, ceftriaxone.*
[p]*Third-generation cephalosporins. Oral: cefixime, cefpodoxime, ceftibutin.*
[q]*Aqueous procaine penicillin G.*
[r]*Should only be used in serious infection.*
[s]*Extended-spectrum penicillin: ticarcillin, mezlocillin, or piperacillin.*
[t]*Ciprofloxacin. IV/PO: ofloxacin; IV/PO: levofloxacin; IV/PO: trovofloxacin.*
[u]*β-lactamase inhibitor combination: ampicillin/sulbactam, ticarcillin/clavulanate, piperacillin/tazobactam.*
[v]*Cefoxitin, cefotetan, cefmetazole.*
[w]*Aminoglycosides: gentamicin, tobramycin, amikacin–use per sensitivities.*
[x]*Generally reserved for patients with hypersensitivity reactions to penicillin.*
[y]*Antibiotics should not be given for gastroenteritis, because the carrier state may be prolonged without significant clinical benefit.*
[z]*Sulfisoxazole, sulfadiazine (preferred for central nervous system [CNS] disease), trisulfapyrimidines.*

97
CENTRAL NERVOUS SYSTEM INFECTIONS

Marnie L. Peterson, PharmD, AnhThu D. Hoang, PharmD,
David H. Wright, PharmD, and John C. Rotschafer, PharmD, FCCP

Central nervous system (CNS) infections include a wide variety of clinical conditions and etiologies. Meningitis, meningoencephalitis, encephalitis, brain and meningeal abscesses, and shunt infections are all included under this heading. Central nervous system infections are divided into two categories: septic and aseptic. Septic, or bacterial infections, are the result of hematogenous spread from a primary infection site, parameningeal seeding from a localized infection, or trauma or congenital defects in the CNS. Aseptic infection is a term broadly used to describe chemical irritants, viral, fungal, parasitic, tuberculous, sarcoid, neoplastic, and syphilitic processes of the CNS. This chapter presents relevant aspects of the pathogenesis, pathophysiology, and antimicrobial therapy of CNS infections, specifically meningitis.

EPIDEMIOLOGY

The incidence of acute bacterial meningitis in the United States is approximately 3 cases per 100,000 persons per year.[1] Overall mortality rates for patients with meningitis range from 3% to 33%.[2–5] Adverse neurologic sequelae are frequently associated with meningitis, such as seizures, sensorineural hearing loss, and hydrocephalus. Risk for development of neurologic sequelae depends on the infecting organism. Generally, 10% of patients who survive meningitis may develop neurologic disabilities. Patients surviving gram-negative bacilliary meningitis, however, have a 60% chance of developing complications from their infection.[2–5] Despite the availability of antimicrobial therapy against the most common CNS pathogens, CNS infections continue to be problematic.

ETIOLOGY

Central nervous system infections are caused by a variety of bacteria, fungi, viruses, and parasites. Historically, CNS infections were primarily community-acquired; however, an increasing number are now nosocomial.[5] The last national surveillance study of bacterial meningitis performed in the United States was conducted in 1986 by the Centers for Disease Control (CDC).[6] At that time, *Haemophilus influenzae* was the most commonly identified cause of bacterial meningitis (45%), followed by *Streptococcus pneumoniae* (18%) and *Neisseria meningitidis* (14%). The CDC, however, reported an 82% decrease in the incidence of *H. influenzae* type B between 1985 and 1991 for children less than 5 years old, which coincides with the increased distribution of the HIB vaccine in this age group.[3,7]

Significant and concerning changes in antimicrobial susceptibility have been occurring with the most common bacterial organisms associated with meningitis. Approximately 30% to 40% of *H. influenzae* and 5% to 30% of *S. pneumoniae* are resistant to ampicillin and penicillin, respectively. Undoubtedly, these changes will continue to affect antibiotic management of these bacterial pathogens.

ANATOMY AND PHYSIOLOGY OF THE CENTRAL NERVOUS SYSTEM

MENINGES

The skull and vertebrae protect the CNS from blunt or penetrating trauma (Fig. 97–1). The brain is suspended in these structures by cerebral spinal fluid (CSF) and is surrounded by the meninges. The meninges[8,9] are made up of three separate membranes: dura mater, arachnoid, and pia mater. Dura mater, or pachymeninges, lies directly beneath and is adherent to the skull. The other two membranes are referred to collectively as leptomeninges. Pia mater lies directly over brain tissue. Arachnoid, the middle layer, lies between the dura mater and the pia mater. The subarachnoid space, located between the arachnoid and pia mater, serves as the conduit for CSF. By definition, meningitis is an infection of the subarachnoid space.

CEREBROSPINAL FLUID

Approximately 85% of the CSF is produced within the fourth and lateral ventricles by the choroid plexus (Fig. 97–1). Cerebrospinal fluid volume in the CNS is related to a patient's age. Infants have approximately 40 to 60 mL of CSF, whereas older children have 60 to 100 mL and adults have 110 to 160 mL. Normally, CSF is produced at the rate of approximately 500 mL/day and flows unidirectionally downward through the spinal cord. The CSF is removed by the arachnoid villi and vertebral venus plexus located in the spinal cord and does not recommunicate with the point of production.[9]

The CSF is normally clear with a protein content of < 50 mg/dL, a glucose concentration of approximately 50% to 66% of the simultaneous peripheral serum concentration, a pH of approximately that of blood, and typically contains fewer than ten white blood cells (WBCs) per mm^3, all of which should be mononuclear (Table 97–1).

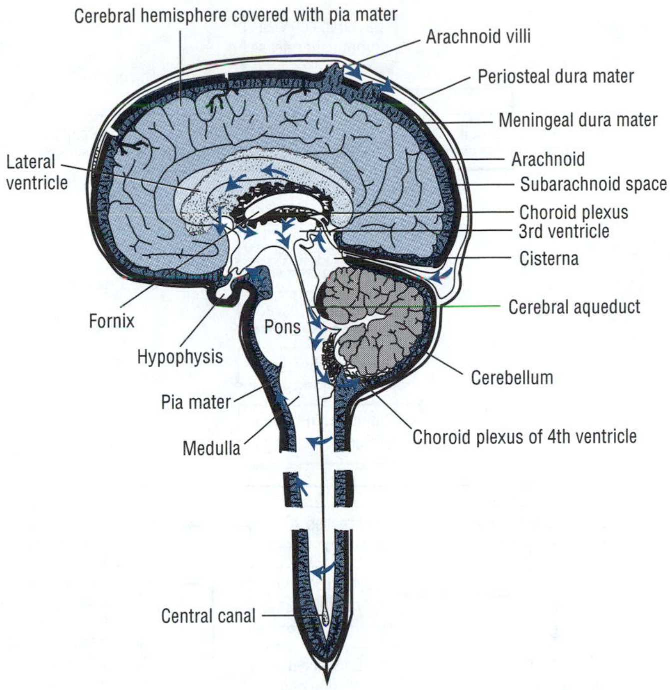

FIGURE 97–1. Diagram of the central nervous system.

BLOOD–BRAIN BARRIER/BLOOD–CEREBROSPINAL FLUID BARRIER

Natural barriers to the exchange of drugs and endogenous compounds among the blood, brain, and CSF are the blood–brain barrier (BBB) and blood–CSF barrier (BCSFB) (Fig. 97–2). The BBB consists of tightly joined capillary endothelial cells. Drug entry into the brain's tissue is accomplished by direct passage through the capillary endothelial cells and further penetration of the glial cells that envelop the capillary structure.[9]

Passage of chemical substances into the CSF is controlled by the BCSFB. This barrier is created by ependymal cells of the choroid plexus, which function as an active transport system similar to the renal tubular epithelial cells. The inflammatory process associated with meningitis inhibits the active transport system of the choroid plexus. Like the active transport system in the kidney, the secretion of substances out of the choroid plexus can also be inhibited by the administration of probenecid.

PATHOPHYSIOLOGY OF THE CENTRAL NERVOUS SYSTEM INFECTION

The critical first step in the acquisition of acute bacterial meningitis is nasopharyngeal colonization of the host by the bacterial pathogen. Bacteria attach themselves to nasopharyngeal epithelial cells with bacterial surface structures called lectins and are phagocytized across nonciliated columnar nasopharyngeal cells into the host's bloodstream.[2] Immunoglobulins (Ig) such as secretory IgA, are found in high concentrations within nasopharyngeal secretions and work to inhibit bacterial colonization.[2]

After accessing the patient's bloodstream, bacteria must overcome the host's defense mechanisms. A common characteristic of most CNS bacterial pathogens is the production of an extensive polysaccharide capsule that is resistant to neutrophil phagocytosis and complement opsonization. Studies with *H. influenzae, Escherichia coli,* and *N. meningitidis* found that strains lacking polysaccharide capsules are unable to cause meningitis. The host possesses defense mechanisms that can effectively counteract the encapsulated bacteria.[2,10] Capsular polysaccharides activate the alternate complement pathway, which promotes phagocytosis and clearance of infecting pathogens. Patients unable to activate the alternative complement pathway, such as asplenic and sickle cell patients, are predisposed to bacterial infections caused by encapsulated microorganisms and are, therefore, at risk for meningitis.

Although the exact site and mechanism of bacterial invasion into the CNS are unknown, studies suggest invasion into the subarachnoid space is accomplished by continuously exposing the CNS to large inocula of bacteria. Bacteremia with inoculum densities of at least 10^3 colony forming units/mL appear to be essential for subarachnoid space invasion.[2] Although several sites of bacterial invasion have been theorized, most plausible are those sites that are highly perfused. The choroid plexus sustains exceptional blood flow rates (approximately 200 mL/g/min) and is consequently, the most likely site of CNS bacterial invasion. Additionally, cells of the choroid plexus possess receptors that facilitate bacterial adherence and allow bacterial transport into the subarachnoid space.[2] Host defense mechanisms within the subarachnoid space are inadequate to combat bacterial pathogens, and bacteria, therefore, replicate

TABLE 97–1. Mean Values of the Components of Normal and Abnormal Cerebrospinal Fluid[15]

Type	Normal	Bacterial	Viral	Fungal	Tuberculosis
WBC (mm^3)	< 10[a]	400–100,000	5–500	40–400	100–1000
Differential	> 90%[a]	> 90 PMN	50[b,c]	> 50[b]	> 80[b,c]
Protein (mg/dL)	< 50	80–500	30–150	40–150	≥ 40–150
Glucose (mg/dL)	2/3 serum	< 1/2 serum	< 30–70	< 30–70	< 30–70

[a]Monocytes.
[b]Lymphocytes.
[c]Initial cerebrospinal fluid (CSF) white blood cell (WBC) count may reveal a predominance of polymorphonuclear neutrophils (PMNs).

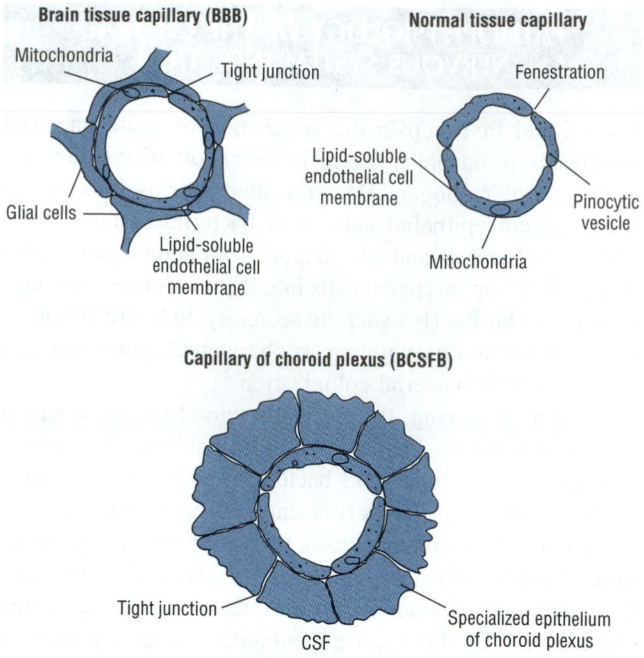

FIGURE 97–2. Schematic representation of a brain tissue capillary, normal tissue capillary, and blood–cerebrospinal fluid barrier capillary. *(From Ref. 104, with permission.)*

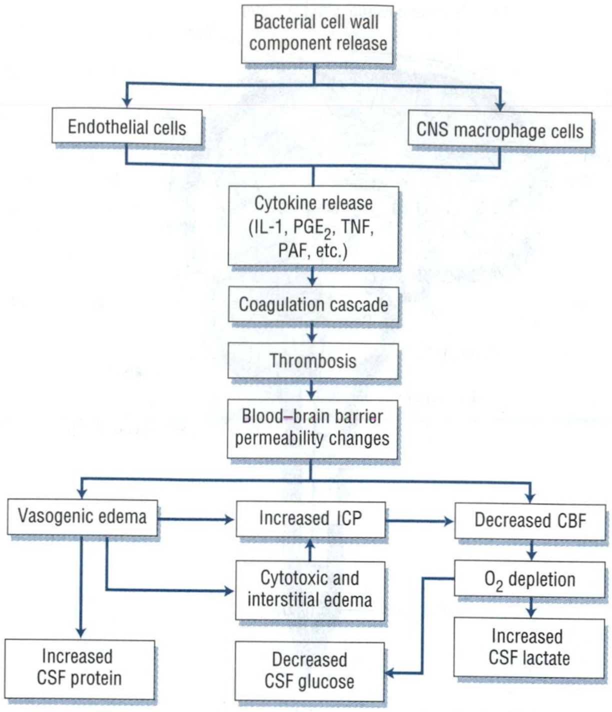

FIGURE 97–3. Hypothetical schema of pathophysiology events that occur during bacterial meningitis. IL-1 = interleukin-1; TNF = tumor necrosis factor; PAF = platelet-activating factor; CBF = cerebral blood flow; CSF = cerebrospinal fluid; PGE_2 = prostaglandin E_2; ICP = intracranial pressure.

freely within the CSF until either bacterial overgrowth occurs or an effective antibiotic regimen is administered that terminates the process.

Bacterial cell death can cause the release of cell wall components, such as lipopolysaccharide (LPS), lipid A (endotoxin), lipoteichoic acid, teichoic acid, and peptidoglycan, depending on whether the pathogen is gram-positive or gram-negative (Fig. 97–3). These cell wall components cause capillary endothelial cells and CNS macrophages to release cytokines (interleukin-1 [IL-1] and tumor necrosis factor [TNF]). Cytokines interact with capillary endothelial cells and CNS leukocytes to release products of the cyclooxygenase–arachidonic acid pathway (prostaglandins and thromboxanes) and platelet-activating factor (PAF). The PAF activates the coagulation cascade, and arachidonic acid metabolites stimulate vasodilation. These events propagate other sequential events and cytokines, which lead to cerebral edema, elevated intracranial pressure, CSF pleocytosis, disseminated intravascular coagulation (DIC), inappropriate antidiuretic hormone secretion (SIADH), decreased cerebral blood flow, cerebral ischemia, and death.[2,10] The delineation of the process of subarachnoid space inflammation has kindled new interest in exploring treatment modalities designed to inhibit the inflammatory process.

CLINICAL PRESENTATION AND DIAGNOSIS

On initial presentation, differentiation of patients with bacterial, viral, or fungal meningitis is virtually impossible. The clinical signs and symptoms of meningitis are variable and dependent on the age of the patient. Adult patients often present with the classic complaints of meningitis, such as photophobia; headache; fever; stiffness of the neck, back, or both; nuchal rigidity; positive Brudzinski's sign (Fig. 97–4), positive Kernig's sign (Fig. 97–5), or both.[11] Later in the course of the disease, the patient may experience seizures, focal neurologic deficits, and hydrocephalus. Conversely, young infants infected with bacterial meningitis may reveal only nonspecific symptoms, such as irritability, altered sleep patterns, vomiting, high-pitched crying, decreased oral intake, or seizures.[12] As a child ages, a more CNS-specific clinical presentation becomes prevalent; changes in activity level, somnolence, confusion, or lethargy are frequently reported.[12] Generally, children less than 2 years of age do not present with the classic meningitis characteristics.[12] It has been estimated that up to 50% of patients diagnosed with meningitis have received prior antibiotic therapy.[4] These patients may present less frequently with fever or mental status changes and may have a longer duration of symptoms.[13]

Diagnosis of bacterial meningitis is usually based on the results of CSF collected soon after meningitis is suspected. Typically, three tubes of CSF are collected via lumbar puncture for chemistry, microbiology, and hematology tests, in that order.[13] Any contamination with skin flora and

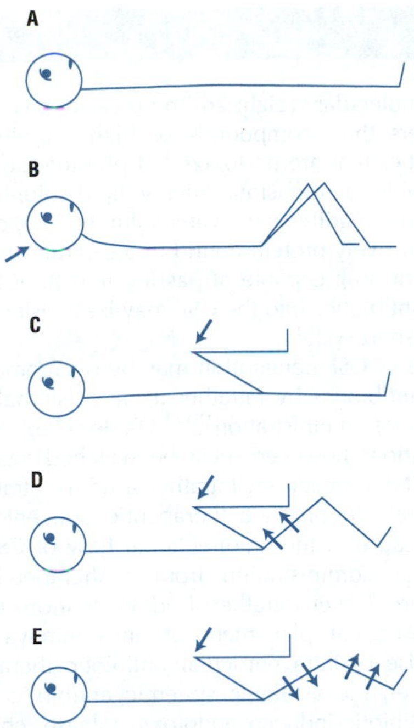

FIGURE 97–4. (A and B) Brudzinski's neck sign. Flexion of the neck by the examiner produces hip and knee flexion (B). (C–E) Brudzinski's leg signs. (C) Examiner passively flexes patient's leg (arrow). (D) The identical contralateral sign: contralateral leg begins to flex (arrows). (E) The reciprocal contralateral sign: the same leg that exhibited the active flexion begins to extend spontaneously, a reflex resembling a little kick (double arrows). *(From Ref. 11, with permission.)*

disinfectant should be minimal after the first tube of CSF is collected. In addition to CSF examination, blood cultures should be performed as meningitis can frequently arise via hematogenous dissemination.

Analysis of CSF chemistries typically include measurement of glucose and total protein concentrations. Elevated CSF protein ≥ 50 mg/dL and a CSF glucose concentration of less than 50% of the simultaneously obtained peripheral value suggest bacterial meningitis (Table 97–1).

Hematologic examination of WBC count and accompanying differential will characteristically reveal the presence of 200 to 10,000 WBC/mm^3 (> 95% polymorphonuclear cells) in bacterial meningitis. In some cases of viral meningitis, however, the initial examination of CSF may reveal a predominance of polymorphonuclear cells.[9,14] The values for CSF glucose, protein, and WBC concentrations found with bacterial meningitis overlap significantly with those for viral, tuberculous, and fungal meningitis.[15] Therefore, CSF WBC counts and glucose and protein concentrations cannot always be relied on to establish or rule out bacterial meningitis. Typical laboratory findings for bacterial, viral, tuberculous, and fungal meningitis are summarized in Table 97–1.[15]

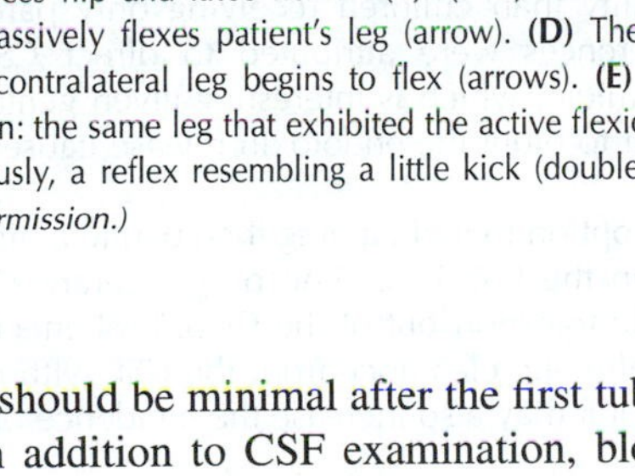

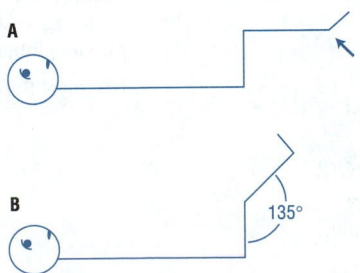

FIGURE 97–5. Kernig's sign. (A) Examiner flexes hip 90 degrees to the trunk and attempts to extend the knees. (B) "Contracture" or extensor spasm at the knee 135 degrees. *(From Ref. 11, with permission.)*

The CSF's pH, lactate, and C-reactive protein concentrations have been suggested as adjunctive diagnostic indicators to distinguish between bacterial and viral meningitis.[12] Since CSF pH and C-reactive protein lack specificity in patients with partially treated or slightly abnormal CSF, they are of questionable diagnostic value.[12,16] The TNF-α has also been identified as a CSF marker for bacterial meningitis.[17] In the case of gram-negative meningitis where CSF may contain measurable concentrations of endotoxin, the limulus lysate assay may be of value. At this time, neither TNF-α nor endotoxin assays are approved for diagnostic use.

Gram stain and aerobic culture of the CSF are the most important laboratory tests performed when attempting to diagnose bacterial meningitis. Recovery of bacterial pathogens from both culture and Gram stain can be greatly influenced by the quantity of CSF available for culture and prior use of antimicrobial therapy.[4] When performed before antibiotic therapy is initiated, Gram stain is both rapid and sensitive and can confirm the diagnosis of bacterial meningitis in 60% to 90% of cases.[8,14] The sensitivity of the Gram stain decreases to 40% to 60% in patients receiving prior antibiotic therapy.[4]

Several rapid diagnostic methods are available for identifying potential bacterial pathogens from CSF.[8,14] Latex fixation, latex coagglutination, and enzyme immunoassay (EIA) tests provide for the rapid identification of *S. pneumoniae,* group B streptococci, *N. meningitidis, H. influenzae* type B, and *E. coli* (K1).[8,14] Rapid identification latex tests work by bringing potential capsular antigens of the pathogen-causing meningitis in contact with a specific antibody, causing an antigen–antibody reaction. This capsular antigen–antibody reaction can be observed visually and quickly without waiting for culture results. In recent years, the widespread introduction of more sensitive latex fixation and coagglutination tests have made counterimmunoelectrophoresis virtually obsolete.[4] The sensitivity and specificity of latex fixation and coagglutination tests can vary with the manufacturer of the antibody, density of antigen present in the CSF, and pathogen being tested. Therefore, no specific product appears to be superior in the identification of all antigens.[8,14]

▶ TREATMENT: Central Nervous System Infections

DESIRED OUTCOME

Mortality associated with bacterial meningitis usually occurs within 24 to 48 hours of onset, and the importance of supportive care, particularly early in the course of treatment, cannot be emphasized enough. Administration of fluids, electrolytes, antipyretics, analgesia, and other supportive measures are indicated as needed for patients presenting with acute bacterial meningitis. Although supportive care is initially important, appropriate antibiotic therapy (empiric or definitive) should be started as soon as possible. Understanding appropriate antibiotic selection and the issues surrounding antibiotic penetration will assist in meeting the goals of treatment, which include ameliorating the signs and symptoms associated with meningitis, eradication of infection, and prevention of the development of neurologic sequelae, such as seizures, deafness, coma, and death.

APPROACH TO TREATMENT

On initial presentation, it is often necessary to employ empiric antibiotic coverage until a pathogen is identified. Based on a patient's profile (that is, allergies, age, concurrent medical condition) and extent of antibiotic CNS penetration, appropriate recommendations can be made (Tables 97–2 and 97–3). Once a causative agent is isolated and identified, therapy should be directed at the most appropriate antimicrobial therapy for the patient (Tables 97–4 and 97–5). The following section discusses issues surrounding the approach to treatment, such as antibiotic penetration within the CNS, duration of antibiotic therapy, and use of adjunctive steroids.

Several factors influence the transfer of antibiotic from capillary blood into the CNS, including inflammation of the meninges, which increases antibiotic penetration (Table 97–3). Antibiotics having low molecular weight are more easily passed through biologic barriers than compounds of higher molecular weight. Only antibiotics that are un-ionized at physiologic or pathologic pH are capable of diffusion. Highly lipid-soluble compounds penetrate more readily than water-soluble compounds. Antibiotics not extensively protein bound in the serum provide a larger free fraction of drug capable of passing into the CSF. Passage of large, polar antibiotics into the CSF may be assisted, however, by a carrier transport system.

Problems of CSF penetration may be overcome by direct instillation of antibiotics by intrathecal, intracisternal, or intraventricular routes of administration[18–23] (Table 97–6). Advantages of direct instillation, however, must be weighed against the risks of invasive CNS procedures. Intrathecal administration of antibiotics is unlikely to produce therapeutic concentrations in the ventricles because of the unidirectional flow of CSF.[19] Although intraventricular administration from a therapeutic standpoint may be preferred over intrathecal administration, the former requires neurosurgical placement of an Ommaya or Rickham reservoir.[20] Use of intraventricular antibiotic therapy is seldom necessary given the available systemic antibiotic therapy. In a review of antibiotic-induced endotoxin release, children receiving both parenteral antibiotics and intrathecal gentamicin had higher CSF endotoxin levels, higher CSF IL-1 β levels, and higher mortality than children receiving only parenteral antibiotics.[24] Differences were attributed to direct CSF administration of gentamicin, which is interesting given gentamicin is generally thought to blunt the endotoxin release caused by β-lactam antibiotics.[24]

Another option to maintaining therapeutic antibiotic concentrations within the CSF is to limit drug clearance by interfering with antibiotic transport out of the CNS. Probenecid will reduce the rate of antibiotic clearance from the CSF with most β-lactam antibiotics, but it may also increase the incidence of adverse drug reactions.

TABLE 97–2. Bacterial Meningitis: Most Likely Bacteria and Empiric Therapy by Age Group

Age Commonly Affected	Most Likely Organisms	Empiric Therapy	Risk Factors for All Ages Groups
Newborn–1 month	Gram-negative enterics[a] Group B streptococcus *Listeria monocytogenes*	Ampicillin + CTX or CTR or AG	Respiratory tract infection Otitis media Mastoiditis Head trauma Alcoholism
1 month–4 years	*Haemophilus influenzae* *Neisseria meningitidis* *Streptococcus pneumoniae*	CTX or CTR ± VM	High-dose steroids Splenectomy Sickle cell disease Immunoglobulin deficiency
5–29 years	*N. meningitidis* *S. pneumoniae* *H. influenzae*	CTX or CTR ± VM	Immunosuppression
30–60 years	*S. pneumoniae* *N. meningitidis*	CTX or CTR ± VM	
> 60 years	*S. pneumoniae* Gram-negative enterics *L. monocytogenes*	Ampicillin + CTX or CTR or AG ± VM	

[a]*Escherichia coli, Klebsiella* sp., *Enterobacter*, sp. common.
CTX = cefotaxime; CTR = ceftriaxone; AG = aminoglycoside; VM, = vancomycin (use should be based on local incidence of penicillin-resistant *S. pneumoniae* and until CTX or CTR minimum inhibitory concentration results are available).

TABLE 97–3. Penetration of Antimicrobial Agents into the Cerebrospinal Fluid

Therapeutic Levels in CSF With or Without Inflammation	
Sulfonamides	Trimethoprim
Chloramphenicol	Isoniazid
Rifampin	Pyrazinamide
Ethionamide	Cycloserine
Metronidazole	
Therapeutic Levels in CSF With Inflammation of Meninges	
Penicillin G	Ampicillin ± sulbactam
Carbenicillin	Ticarcillin ± clavulanic acid
Nafcillin	Mezlocillin
Piperacillin	Cefuroxime
Cefotaxime	Ceftizoxime
Ceftriaxone	Ceftazidime
Imipenem	Aztreonam
Meropenem	Ofloxacin
Vancomycin	Ciprofloxacin
Vidarabine	Ethambutol
Flucytosine	Fluconazole
Pyrimethamine	Ganciclovir
Acyclovir	Foscarnet
Nontherapeutic Levels in CSF With or Without Inflammation	
Aminoglycosides	First-generation cephalosporins
Cefoperozone	Second-generation cephalosporins[a]
Clindamycin[b]	Ketoconazole
Amphotericin B[c]	Itraconazole[c]

[a]Cefuroxime is an exception.
[b]Achieves therapeutic brain tissue concentrations.
[c]Achieves therapeutic concentrations for *Crytococcus neoformans* therapy.
CSF = cerebrospinal fluid.

In exceptional cases, vancomycin may be needed for the treatment of penicillin-allergic patients or in the treatment of patients infected with organisms resistant to first-line antibiotics, such as penicillins and cephalosporins. Although vancomycin appears to distribute well into most tissues of the body, distribution into the CSF is impaired without inflamed meninges. Some authors suggest consideration of intraventricular administration for bacterial meningitis, but only if the patient does not respond clinically to intravenous administration. Congeni and coworkers suggested a daily 5 mg intraventricular dose in addition to continued intravenous administration in this situation.[25] This recommendation has been supported by other investigators.[26] Clinicians should appreciate the pharmacokinetics of vancomycin outside and within the CNS are likely to differ, and the dose and frequency of administration may need to be altered. Considering that vancomycin is a concentration-independent killer, the critical factor is the relationship between the concentration of vancomycin present in the CNS and susceptibility of the infecting bacterial pathogen, not the concentration in the serum. Concentrations of vancomycin in the CNS should be maintained above the minimum inhibitory concentration (MIC)-90 of the likely bacterial pathogens to expect a satisfactory clinical outcome.

Although the length of treatment for bacterial meningitis is generally based on causative organism, there is no universally accepted standard. Traditionally, meningitis caused by *S. pneumoniae, N. meningitidis,* and *H. influenzae* has been successfully treated with 7 to 14 days of antibiotic therapy. In contrast, a longer duration of 14 to 21 days has been recommended for patients infected with *Listeria monocytogenes,* group B streptococci, and enteric gram-negative bacilli because of a high rate of relapse in patients receiving shorter courses. Therapy should be individualized, and some patients may require longer courses.[27–29]

DEXAMETHASONE AS AN ADJUNCTIVE TREATMENT FOR MENINGITIS

In addition to antibiotics, dexamethasone has become a commonly used therapy for the treatment of pediatric meningitis.[30] Corticosteroids inhibit the production of both TNF and IL-1. A series of clinical studies assessing the efficacy of corticosteroid therapy for the initial treatment of bacterial meningitis have reported conflicting results.[31–35] The majority of trials were conducted on small sample populations, each with different pathogenic bacterial causes and treatment modalities. Several meta-analyses have shown significant improvement in markers of active infection, such as CSF glucose concentrations, as well as CSF protein and lactate concentrations, when corticosteroids are administered as an adjunctive treatment.[36,37]

Consistently, trials detected a significantly lower incidence of neurologic sequelae commonly associated with bacterial meningitis when corticosteroids were used. In trials that measured inflammatory mediators, lower levels of TNF, PAF, or IL-1 were detected in patients treated with dexamethasone.[31,32,34] No study, however, has detected a significant difference in time to bacterial eradication. Only one study has detected a significant difference in mortality between patients treated with dexamethasone plus antibiotics and antibiotic therapy alone.[33] Based on these investigations, some authors advocate all infants (> 2 months) and children with suspected bacterial meningitis receive dexamethasone.[3,31,32,34,35,38]

Routine use of dexamethasone in meningitis is not without controversy, and several authors have outlined shortcomings regarding the clinical evidence supporting the use of dexamethasone in pediatric bacterial meningitis.[3,39] A potential concern is that adjunctive dexamethasone therapy might reduce the penetration of antibiotics into the CSF by inhibiting meningeal inflammation. In experimental models of meningitis, steroids have been shown to decrease the CSF concentrations of ampicillin, rifampin, vancomycin, and gentamicin.[35,40] Ceftriaxone penetration into CSF was shown to be unaffected by concurrent dexamethasone administration in pediatric patients.[41]

A fundamental problem with corticosteroid investigations to date is the majority of patients in comparative dexamethasone trials had *H. influenzae* meningitis. While *H. influenzae* was the most commonly identified causative pathogen responsible for bacterial meningitis in the United States in 1986, the incidence of *H. influenzae* meningitis has decreased dramatically because of the introduction of polysaccharide conjugate vaccines.[3,7] At this time, it is unclear whether or not steroids are beneficial in meningitis caused by *S. pneumoniae, N. meningitidis,* and group B streptococci. A retrospective analysis of pediatric patients with pneumococcal meningitis and one unblinded, noncontrolled trial suggested that adjunctive steroids may decrease the neurologic sequelae and mortality associated with *S. pneumoniae* meningitis.[31,42]

The American Academy of Pediatrics suggests the use of dexamethasone be considered for infants and children 2 months of age or older with proven or strongly suspected bacterial meningitis.[38] The commonly used intravenous dose is 0.15 mg/kg every 6 hours for 4 days. Alternatively, prospective, randomized, double-blind studies have found dexamethasone 0.15 mg/kg every 6 hours for 2 days or dexamethasone 0.4 mg/kg every 12 hours for 2 days to be equally effective and potentially less toxic.[35,43] Dexamethasone should be administered prior to the first antibiotic dose and serum hemoglobin and stool guaiac should be monitored for evidence of gastrointestinal (GI) bleeding.[32,34,39,42,43]

TABLE 97–4. Antimicrobial Agents of First Choice and Alternative Choice in Treatment of Meningitis Caused by Gram-positive Microorganisms

Organism	Antibiotic of First Choice[a]	Alternative Antibiotics[a]
Streptococcus pneumoniae		
Penicillin susceptible	Penicillin G 200,000–300,000 units/kg/day, q4h IV max: 4 million units q4h IV	Cefotaxime 200 mg/kg/day q4h IV max: 2 g q4h Ceftriaxone 100 mg/kg/day q24h IV[b] max: adults 2 g q12h Chloramphenicol 100 mg/kg/day q6h max: 1.5 g q6h
Low-level penicillin resistance[c]	Cefotaxime or ceftriaxone	Vancomycin 30–40 mg/kg/day IV
High-level penicillin resistance[d]	Vancomycin ± ceftriaxone	Imipenem 80 mg/kg/day max: 1 g IV q6h
Group B *Streptococcus*	Penicillin	Cefotaxime Ceftriaxone Chloramphenicol
Staphylococcus aureus		
Penicillin resistant	Nafcillin 200 mg/kg/day q4h IV max: 2 g q4h IV	Vancomycin
Methicillin resistant	Vancomycin	—
Staphylococcus epidermidis		
Penicillin resistant	Nafcillin	Vancomycin
Methicillin resistant	Vancomycin	
Listeria monocytogenes	Ampicillin 200–400 mg/kg/day, q6h IV or Penicillin G max: 2 g q4h IV plus aminoglycoside	Trimethoprim 10 mg/kg/day and sulfamethoxazole 50 mg/kg/day, q6h

[a]Recommended doses for adults and pediatric patients with normal renal and/or hepatic function.
[b]Pediatrics.
[c]Incidence of low-level resistance is 10%–20%.
[d]Incidence of high-level resistance is 1%–2%, therapeutic recommendations for this infection have not been clearly defined.

TABLE 97–5. Antimicrobial Agents of First Choice and Alternative Choice in Treatment of Meningitis Caused by Gram-negative Organisms

Organism	Antibiotic of First Choice[a]	Alternative Antibiotics[a]
Neisseria meningitidis (meningococcal)	Penicillin G 200,000–300,000 units/kg/day	Cefotaxime 200 mg/kg/day q4h max: 2 g IV q4h Ceftriaxone 100 mg/kg/day q24h[b] max: adults 2 g IV q12h Chloramphenicol 100 mg/kg/day q6h max: 1.5 g IV q6h
Escherichia coli	Cefotaxime	Ceftriaxone Chloramphenicol
Haemophilus influenzae		
β-lactamase positive	Cefotaxime	Ceftriaxone
β-lactamase negative	Ampicillin 200–400 mg/kg/day q6h IV max: 2 g q4h IV	Cefotaxime Ceftriaxone
Pseudomonas aeruginosa	Ceftazidime 85 mg/kg/day max: 2 g IV q6h plus tobramycin 5–7.5 mg/kg/day IV[c]	Imipenem 80 mg/kg/day max: 1 g IV q6h Piperacillin 200–300 mg/kg/day max: 3 g q4h IV plus tobramycin
Enterobacteriaceae	Cefotaxime	Ceftriaxone Piperacillin plus aminoglycoside Imipenem

[a]Recommended doses for adults and pediatric patients with normal renal and/or hepatic function.
[b]Pediatrics.
[c]Direct central nervous system administration may be added, see Table 97–3 for dosage.

TABLE 97–6. Intraventricular and Intrathecal Antibiotic Dosage Recommendations

Antibiotic	Dose (mg)	Expected CSF Concentration[a] (mg/L)	Reference
Ampicillin	10–50	60–300	95–97
Methicillin	25–100	160–600	95–97
Nafcillin	75	500	95
Cefazolin	1–2 mg/kg (50 mg max)	300	98
Cephalothin	25–100	160–600	95–97
Chloramphenicol	25–100	160–600	96, 97, 99
Gentamicin	1–10	6–60	19, 95–97, 99
Tobramycin	1–10	6–60	100, 101
Vancomycin	5	30	25, 102, 103
Amphotericin B	0.05–0.25 mg/d to 0.05–1 mg 1–3 times weekly	—	21

[a]Assumes adult CSF volume = 150 mL.
CSF = cerebrospinal fluid.

INVESTIGATIONAL ALTERNATIVES

Although discussed here, the use of polymyxin B, monoclonal antibodies, and pentoxifylline are investigational and are not standard therapy at the time of writing. Polymyxin B has been shown to bind to the lipid A portion of LPS, causing an inactivation and interruption of this portion of the inflammatory cascade. Nonsteroidal anti-inflammatory drugs have been shown to inhibit the cyclo-oxygenase pathway of arachidonic acid metabolism and block the ensuing events of this inflammatory process.[10,44] Pentoxifylline, a methylxanthine, indirectly inhibits CNS neutrophil activity and limits neutrophil release of inflammatory mediators, such as TNF.[10,44] Monoclonal antibodies have been developed to the CD18 family of leukocyte receptors, TNF, and the lipid A portion of LPS. During the last 5 years, clinical trials for systemic gram-negative sepsis have raised questions regarding the efficacy and safety of these products, leaving their role in mediating the septic cascade in CNS infections undefined.[10,44]

CAUSATIVE AGENTS

NEISSERIA MENINGITIDIS (MENINGOCOCCUS)

Neisseria meningitidis is most commonly found in children and young adults. The source of infection is usually an asymptomatic carrier. Most cases occur in the winter or spring at a time when viral meningitis is relatively uncommon. Five serogroups of *N. meningitidis* (A, B, C, Y, and W-135) are primarily responsible. Serogroups A and C are usually associated with epidemics of meningitis, while serogroup B is the primary cause of isolated cases of meningitis. Serogroup Y is more frequently associated with pneumonia and is rarely associated with meningitis.

Initially, patients are colonized and, at some point, develop a bacteremia, which most likely occurs prior to hospital admission. Metastatic seeding to the meninges, the most common site, occurs as a result of the bacteremia.[10,44] After the acute phase of meningitis has resolved, there is a unique immune reaction that distinguishes meningococcal meningitis from other bacterial causes. The patient develops a characteristic immunologic reaction of fever, arthritis (usually involving large joints), and pericarditis approximately 10 to 14 days after the onset of disease and despite successful treatment.[45] At this time, examination of the synovial fluid will reveal a large number of polymorphonuclear cells, elevated protein concentrations, normal glucose concentrations, and sterile cultures. The reaction may last a week or longer, and no additional antibiotic therapy is required. Patients, however, may benefit from nonsteroidal anti-inflammatory agents.[45]

Approximately 50% of patients die within the first 24 hours as a result of an acute fulminant course of meningococcemia. Other patients develop a picture of chronic meningococcemia that is characterized by episodes of fever, arthritis, and a morbilliform rash that recurs every 48 to 72 hours.[45]

Seizures and coma are uncommon with meningococcal meningitis. Patients may behave aggressively, however, and are often maniacal. Patients may develop VI, VII, and VIII cranial nerve dysfunction noted by deafness and transiently impaired ocular movements. Deafness unilaterally, or more commonly bilaterally, may develop early or late in the disease course.[45] Hearing loss because of damage to a sensory nerve (sensorineural hearing) is usually permanent, whereas conductive hearing impairment, such as damage to the tympanic membrane, is often reversible. Incidence of sensorineural hearing loss varies with the etiologic organism (*S. pneumoniae,* 31%; *N. meningitidis,* 10.5%; and *H. influenzae,* 6%).[46] Many of the neurologic deficits are transient and resolve within 1 year following meningitis.[47]

Presence of petechiae may be the primary clue that the underlying pathogen is *N. meningitidis.* Approximately 50% of patients with meningococcal meningitis have purpuric lesions, petechiae, or both. Patients may have an obvious or subclinical picture of DIC, which may progress to infarction of the adrenal glands and renal cortex and cause widespread thrombosis.

Aggressive, early intervention with high-dose IV crystalline penicillin G, 50,000 units/kg every 4 hours, is usually recommended for the treatment of *N. meningitidis* meningitis. Chloramphenicol is bactericidal for *N. meningitidis* and may be used in place of penicillin G. Several third-generation cephalosporins (cefotaxime) approved for the treatment of meningitis are acceptable alternatives to penicillin G (Table 97–5).

Cases of meningitis caused by relatively and completely penicillin-resistant meningococci have been reported.[48] The clinical significance of this resistance is unknown since it has not been correlated with any treatment failures. Completely resistant strains produce β-lactamase, whereas relatively resistant strains have an alteration of penicillin-binding protein. These resistance patterns may necessitate a future change away from penicillin as the antibiotic treatment of choice for meningococcal meningitis.

Close contacts of patients contracting *N. meningitidis* meningitis are at an increased risk of developing meningitis. Secondary cases of meningitis usually develop within the first week following exposure, but they may take up to 60 days after contact with the index case.[49] Risk factors in these contacts have been estimated at 200 to 1000 times that of the general population.[50,51] Young children are at the greatest risk of contracting *N. meningitidis;* however, all ages are at risk, especially close contacts exposed via household, daycare, or military contact.

Prophylaxis of contacts should be started without delay and without the aid of culture and sensitivity studies because most secondary cases occur within the first week of the index case contact. Adult patients should receive 600 mg of rifampin orally every 12 hours for four doses. Children 1 month to 12 years of age should receive 10 mg/kg of rifampin orally every 12 hours for four doses, and children younger than 1 month should receive 5 mg/kg orally every 12 hours for four doses.[50] Patients receiving rifampin should be counseled as to the expected red-to-orange color change in urine and other body secretions.

Although not 100% effective, rifampin can eliminate pharyngeal colonization of meningococci.[49] A single dose of ciprofloxacin has been used successfully for meningococcal chemoprophylaxis, but it carries a relative contraindication in children because of the potential to cause cartilage damage.[52,53] A single intramuscular dose of ceftriaxone 125 to 250 mg is a viable alternative to rifampin and may be particularly useful in instances where rifampin cannot be used, such as during pregnancy.[49,50]

Vaccination is of limited value in sporadic cases of meningococcal meningitis that are caused primarily by serogroup B, because the vaccine only contains serogroups A, C, Y, and W-135.[50] Close contacts who are vaccinated should also receive rifampin because there may be a 2-week delay in achieving protective antibody titers after vaccination.[50]

STREPTOCOCCUS PNEUMONIAE (PNEUMOCOCCUS OR DIPLOCOCCUS)

Pneumococci is the most common cause of meningitis in adults and accounts for 12% of meningitis episodes in children 2 months to 10 years. Case fatality rates in children are highest with this organism and approach 20%. Approximately 50% of cases are secondary infections resulting from primary infections involving parameningeal foci, such as the ear or paranasal sinuses. Pneumonia, endocarditis, CSF leak secondary to head trauma, splenectomy, alcoholism, sickle cell disease, and bone marrow transplantation may predispose the patient to the development of pneumococcal meningitis.

Neurologic complications, such as coma and seizures, are common with pneumococcal meningitis; however, bacteremia tends to be less common than *N. meningitidis.*[45] Traumatic tears of the dura, fracture of the cribriform plate or paranasal sinuses, nasal meningoceles, repeated episodes of otitis media, and osteomyelitis of the skull floor are risk factors for recurrent pneumococcal meningitis.

Treatment with IV crystalline penicillin G (50,000 units/kg every 4 hours) in adult patients with normal renal function usually results in a favorable outcome, although there have been increasing reports of penicillin nonsusceptible (MIC 0.12 to 1 mg/L) and penicillin-resistant (MIC ≥ 2 mg/L) *S. pneumoniae* strains in the United States and worldwide.[54–57] Resistant strains are becoming an increasing problem, and meticulous testing of all CSF isolates for penicillin resistance is recommended. Chloramphenicol is bactericidal for *S. pneumoniae* and represents a useful alternative to penicillin G. Several third-generation cephalosporins may also serve as alternatives to penicillin in the treatment of penicillin-sensitive (MIC ≤ 0.6 mg/L) and penicillin nonsusceptible and resistant pneumococcal meningitis. Third-generation cephalosporins containing a 3-methylthiotetrazole substitution (e.g., cefoperazone) should be avoided as the ratio of achievable antibiotic concentrations in CSF to mininum bactericidal concentration (MBC) of the *S. pneumoniae* is too low to be considered curative. Drugs, such as cefotaxime and ceftriaxone, may prove useful as alternatives to penicillin G for penicillin nonsusceptible strains. Treatment failures, however, with third-generation cephalosporins in the management of penicillin-resistant pneumococcal meningitis have been reported.[58,59] The combination of vancomycin and ceftriaxone has been shown to be synergistic for penicillin-resistant pneumococci and has been suggested for initial management until the results of antimicrobial susceptibility testing are available.[60]

Optimal therapy for penicillin resistant strains of pneumococci (MIC ≥ 2 mg/L) has not been clearly defined.[57] Outcome may depend on the serotype of the microorganism (especially type 3), whether the infection is primary or secondary, and the number of WBCs in the CSF.[45] While cefotaxime, ceftriaxone, vancomycin, and imipenem are potentially useful for penicillin-sensitive and nonsusceptible strains of pneumococcus, clear guidelines need to be established for penicillin-resistant strains. Some concern is warranted with the use of imipenem for CNS infections because of the possibility of drug-induced seizures. Vancomycin alone or in combination with ceftriaxone is probably the most effective option at the present time.[54,55,60] Some authors have even suggested direct administration of vancomycin to achieve therapeutic CSF concentrations.[26]

Virtually all serotypes of *S. pneumoniae* exhibiting nonsusceptibility or resistance to penicillin are found in the current 23-serotype pneumococcal vaccine. Clinicians need to universally immunize all patients for which the vaccine is indicated, such as persons 65 years old and older and asplenic or immunocompromised patients.[55,57] Unfortunately, the efficacy of this product in children less than 2 years and immunocompromised adults limits the usefulness of the vaccine as a solution to the problem of penicillin-resistant pneumococci. A new conjugate vaccine in development may change this finding, however.

Chemoprophylaxis with oral penicillin and vaccination for close contacts of an index case with *S. pneumoniae* meningitis are generally not recommended because the risk of acquiring pneumococcal disease is similar to the infection rate in the general population.[50,51] Vaccination and chemoprophylaxis, however, reduces the incidence of pneumococcal septicemia and meningitis in young patients with sickle cell disease.[50]

HAEMOPHILUS INFLUENZAE

In the past, *H. influenzae* was the most common cause of meningitis in children 6 months to 3 years. Since the introduction of effective vaccines, however, the incidence of *H. influenzae* type B disease in the United States has declined.[7] In children older than 3 years and adults, meningitis caused by *H. influenzae* may indicate a parameningeal focus of infection, middle ear infection, paranasal sinus infection, or CSF leakage. Spread of the organism occurs either through draining of these areas via the veins or from bacteremia originating from the local focus of infection.[10,44]

Sterile, subdural effusions are common with *H. influenzae* but are not frequently seen with other causes of meningitis.[45] After an initial defervescence, effusions may provoke fever, seizures, or vomiting, which may necessitate repeated subdural paracentesis. Seizures and coma commonly occur early in the course of the disease. Morbiliform and petechial rashes, which are very uncommon, may resemble the rash seen in meningococcal infection.

Since approximately 30% to 40% of *H. influenzae* are ampicillin resistant, many clinicians use a third-generation cephalosporin or chloramphenicol with ampicillin for initial antimicrobial therapy. If the organism is shown to be sensitive to ampicillin, the patient can then be switched from the third-generation cephalosporin to ampicillin and chloramphenicol can be discontinued. Most clinicians consider third-generation cephalosporins the drugs of choice for meningitis caused by *H. influenzae.* Third-generation cephalosporins (cefotaxime and ceftriaxone) are very active against β-lactamase producing and non–β-lactamase producing strains of *H. influenzae,* are relatively free of toxicity, and do not require serum concentration monitoring. Serum concentration monitoring is required for chloramphenicol to avoid toxicity and subtherapeutic levels.

Secondary cases resulting from close contact with an index case occur within 30 days of the onset of disease. As with meningococcal meningitis, close contacts may be at 200 to 1000 times the risk of the general population for acquiring *H. influenzae* meningitis.[50] Close contacts are usually defined as household members, individuals sharing sleeping quarters, daycare attendees, nursing home residents, and crowded confined populations.[50] The risk of acquiring *H. influenzae* meningitis is low without intimate contact with the index patient's respiratory secretions.[50]

Prophylaxis is to protect close contacts from the index case by eliminating nasopharyngeal and oropharyngeal carriage of *H. influenzae*. Cultures are of no immediate value and may cause a delay in starting effective prophylaxis. Prophylaxis is no longer recommended when the index case is less than 4 years of age and all contacts less than 4 years old are fully immunized.[38,50,61] A "household contact" is anyone (including adults) who has spent 4 hours or more with the index case for at least 5 of the 7 previous days prior to the initiation of therapy. Households with children younger than 12 months (regardless of vaccination status) or with children ages 1 to 3 years who are not adequately vaccinated should all receive rifampin prophylaxis in order to eliminate nasopharyngeal carriage and the subsequent spread of disease to others.[38,50,61] Chemoprophylaxis should be initiated as soon as possible after exposure because the risk of aquisition is greatest within the first week of exposure.[38,50] Prophylaxis is not indicated for persons having casual contact with the index case at work or school and is not indicated for most hospital employees. Index cases should also receive chemoprophylaxis prior to discharge from the hospital because of reports of recolonization after successful antibiotic therapy.[38,50]

Studies conflict regarding recommendations for chemoprophylaxis of daycare center contacts. The American Academy of Pediatrics suggests chemoprophylaxis if two cases are identified within a 60-day period.[38] In addition, if daycare contacts are less than 2 years of age or the number of daycare attendees is small, prophylaxis should be given if one case is identified. Finally, chemoprophylaxis should only be attempted if all children participate or if treated contacts are excluded from attending the center.

Prophylaxis of adults includes 600 mg of rifampin daily for 4 days.[50] Children 1 month to 12 years should receive 20 mg/kg (maximum 600 mg) per day for 4 days, and children less than 1 month should receive 10 mg/kg/d for 4 days.[50] Minocycline is an alternative to rifampin chemoprophylaxis; however, there is a high incidence of drug-induced vestibular dysfunction. Patients receiving *H. influenzae* prophylaxis should be carefully monitored because failures do occur and patients may develop meningitis.

There are several *H. influenzae* type B (HIB) conjugate vaccines available in the United States (HbOC [HibTITER, TETRAMUNE], PRP-OMP [PedvaxHIB], PRP-T [ActHIB, OmniHIB] and PRP-D [ProHIBIT—for use only in children ≥ 12 months]).[61] Vaccination includes a series of doses and is usually begun in children at 2 months of age. In addition to pediatric immunization, the vaccine should also be considered in patients older than 5 years with the following underlying conditions: sickle cell disease, asplenia, and immunocompromising diseases. Refer to Chap. 113, Vaccines, Toxoids, and Other Immunobiologics, for further information on dosing and administration.

GRAM-NEGATIVE MENINGITIS

During the last 20 years, the incidence of gram-negative bacillary meningitis, excluding *H. influenzae,* has been increasing in both children and adults. Enteric gram-negative organisms are the fourth leading cause of meningitis, with only *S. pneumoniae, H. influenzae,* and *N. meningitidis* having a higher incidence.

Gram-negative bacteremia alone is an infrequent cause of meningitis. Several factors can predispose a patient to the development of gram-negative meningitis. Congenital defects involving the CNS, accidental cranial trauma, and neurosurgery alter the anatomic defenses and may predispose the patient to meningitis. Use of antimicrobial agents with exclusive gram-positive activity preoperatively in neurosurgery may also predispose the patient to development of a gram-negative infection. Any form of communication between the skin and subarachnoid space, such as a dermal sinus, greatly increases the risk of gram-negative meningitis. Other risk factors include diabetes, malignancy, urinary tract infection in neonates, cirrhosis, parameningeal infection, strongyloidiasis, spinal anesthesia, and hospitalization in general.

Elderly debilitated patients are also at an increased risk of gram-negative meningitis but usually lack the classic signs and symptoms of the disease. Nuchal rigidity may be difficult to detect because of the presence of cervical arthritis. Presence of a low-grade fever and changes in mental status, without other obvious cause, should prompt consideration of meningitis and a lumbar puncture. Neonates are also at risk for gram-negative meningitis with *E. coli* and *Klebsiella pneumoniae,* which are responsible for 60% to 70% of cases.

Optimal antimicrobial therapies for gram-negative bacillary meningitis have not been fully defined. The treatment of meningitis because of *Pseudomonas aeruginosa* remains a special problem because antibiotics showing good antibacterial activity against *P. aeruginosa,* such as antipseudomonal penicillins and aminoglycosides, penetrate the CSF poorly. Initially, cases of *P. aeruginosa* meningitis should be treated with ceftazidime or piperacillin plus an aminoglycoside, usually tobramycin.[62,63] Since aminoglycosides penetrate the CSF poorly, their inclusion is predominantly to aid in the treatment of extracerebral infection(s). If multidrug-resistant pseudomonas is initially suspected, intraventricular administration of aminoglycoside should be considered along with IV administration. Preservative-free forms of gentamicin and tobramycin are available and should be used for direct administration into the CSF. Intraventricular aminoglycoside dosages should be adjusted to the estimated CSF volume (0.03 mg of tobramycin or gentamicin/mL of CSF and 0.1 mg of amikacin/mL of CSF every 24 hours). The CSF flows unidirectionally with gravity, and most data suggest intraventricular aminoglycoside administration is more likely to produce therapeutic concentrations throughout the CSF than intrathecal administration.[19,63] Ventricular levels of aminoglycoside should be monitored every 2 or 3 days, just prior to the next intraventricular dose, and should approximate 2 to 10 mg/L. Interpretation of drug levels may be difficult to assess because determinations are often contaminated with residual aminoglycoside from the previous dose.

Other gram-negative organisms causing meningitis, excluding *P. aeruginosa,* can most likely be treated with a third-generation cephalosporin, such as cefotaxime, ceftizoxime, ceftriaxone, or ceftazidime. Ceftazidime, however, may not be the best choice of empiric antibiotic for situations where the offending organism is not initially known because CSF antibiotic concentrations greater than ten times the MBC may not be reliably produced for gram-positive organisms. Cefoperazone produces unreliable antibiotic concentrations in the CSF because of high protein binding and should not be a drug of first choice. In adults, daily doses of 8 to 12 g/d of third-generation cephalosporins (2 g twice a day of ceftriaxone) should produce CSF concentrations of 5 to 20 mg/L.

Limitations of third-generation cephalosporins with a 3-methylthiotetrazole substitution, such as cefoperazone, in the treatment of gram-negative meningitis include adverse reactions, such as bleeding diathesis, resistance caused by inducible type 1 β-lactamases, and superinfection resulting from the use of broad-spectrum antibiotics. None of the third-generation cephalosporins are effective for *L. monocytogenes.* Although chloramphenicol is bactericidal against *H. influenzae, N. meningitidis,* and *S. pneumoniae,* it is bacteriostatic against most gram-negative organisms.

Trimethoprim–sulfamethoxazole (TMP/SMX) is useful in the management of the Enterobacteriaceae family, and it may also be useful in the management of *Acinetobacter* sp. and *L. monocytogenes.*[64] One advantage of TMP/SMX is that its penetration into the CSF is not dependent on meningeal inflammation. TMP/SMX is not, however, bactericidal. TMP/SMX produces CSF levels of 1.9 to 5.7 mg/L for the former and 20 to 63 mg/L for the latter when given parenterally in doses of 10 mg/kg/d (trimethoprim) and 50 mg/kg/d (sulfamethoxazole).

Fluoroquinolones are not approved for the treatment of gram-negative bacterial meningitis, and clinical experience is minimal. Fluoroquinolones should only be considered when multidrug-resistant gram-negative rods are suspected.[65]

Cerebrospinal fluid cultures may remain positive for 10 days or more with a regimen that will eventually be curative. Therapeutic efficacy can be monitored through bacterial colony counts every 2 or 3 days, which should progressively decrease over the period of therapy. Therapy for gram-negative meningitis should be continued for 10 days after cultures of CSF become negative.

LISTERIA MONOCYTOGENES

Listeria monocytogenes is a gram-positive diphtheroid-like organism responsible for 3% of all reported cases of meningitis. This disease primarily affects neonates, immunocompromised adults, and the elderly.

Transmission usually involves colonization of the patient's GI tract with the organisms, which then penetrate the gut lumen. If a sufficient cell-mediated immune response (T lymphocyte, macrophages) is not produced, bacteremia, meningitis, meningoencephalitis, or cerebritis may develop.[66] Infection of the CNS may be diffuse or localized, possibly involving the cerebral hemispheres, thalamus, and brain stem. In immunocompromised hosts, approximately 75% of *L. monocytogenes* infections result in transmission into the CNS.[66]

Incidence of *L. monocytogenes* meningitis tends to peak in the summer and early fall. As with gram-negative meningitis, presentation may be subtle and insidious and clinical suspicion should prompt lumbar puncture. *Listeria monocytogenes* produces primarily a mononuclear CSF response.[66] One common laboratory error seen with *L. monocytogenes* is a tendency to misidentify the organism on Gram stain as a diphtheroid or streptococcus.

Treatment of *L. monocytogenes* meningitis with penicillin G or ampicillin may result in only a bacteriostatic effect and possible persistence of infection. Usually the combination of penicillin G or ampicillin with an aminoglycoside results in a bactericidal effect. Patients should be treated for 2 to 3 weeks after defervescence to prevent the possibility of relapse.[66] Combination therapy is usually employed for at least 10 days with the remaining course of therapy completed with penicillin G or ampicillin alone. Trimethoprim–sulfamethoxazole may be an effective alternative as adequate CSF penetration is achieved.

MYCOBACTERIUM TUBERCULOSIS

Mycobacterium tuberculosis var. *hominis* is the primary cause of tuberculous meningitis. Tuberculous meningitis is associated with significant morbidity and mortality and is difficult to diagnose in a timely manner.[67] The most useful diagnostic clue is a history of contact with a known index case of tuberculosis or a prior history of tuberculosis. Although up to 40% of patients may present with evidence of pulmonary involvement with hilar adenopathy, tuberculous meningitis may still exist in the absence of disease in the lung or extrapulmonary sites. The tuberculin skin test (purified protein derivative [PPD]) is also negative in 5% to 50% of cases.[67]

Upon initial examination, CSF usually contains from 100 to 1000 WBC/mm^3, which may be 75% to 80% polymorphonuclear cells.[67,68] Over time, the pattern of WBC in the CSF will shift to lymphocytes and monocytes (Table 97–1). Cerebrospinal fluid glucose may initially be normal, but gradually it decreases as the disease progresses.[67,68] Protein concentration within the CSF may be normal or elevated, with high protein levels shown to correlate with advanced disease.[67–69]

One potentially useful diagnostic sign unique to tuberculous meningitis is paralysis of the VI cranial nerve, which initially is unilateral and then progresses to bilateral.[45] Initial acid-fast bacilli (AFB) smears are approximately 37% sensitive and as high as 87% sensitive following subsequent smears. Sensitivity of the AFB smear is enhanced by the examination of multiple CSF specimens collected on consecutive days. Cultures of CSF are positive in 45% to 90% of cases depending on the quantity of CSF used in the culture, pathogen density, and experience of the laboratory in culturing *M. tuberculosis.* Positive culture results may take up to 8 weeks, providing little help with initial diagnosis.[67,68] The Bactec system, a newer broth-based media with radioactive isotope detectors, has considerably shortened the time to detection and is able to detect organisms in an average of 9 days and determine identification in 5 days.[70] Other methods to shorten the time to detection and increase sensitivity are being developed and include genetic probes and immunoassays (radioimmunoassay ([RIA], enzyme-linked immunosorbent assay [ELISA]).[70]

Unfortunately, the incidence of multiple antibiotic-resistant strains of *M. tuberculosis* has dramatically increased, necessitating the use of up to four and five antibiotics at a time.[71,72] As of 1993, the CDC recommends a regimen of four drugs for empiric treatment of *M. tuberculosis,* unless resistance to isoniazid in the area is less than 4%.[72] This regimen consists of isoniazid, rifampin, pyrazinamide, and ethambutol 15 to 25 mg/kg/d (maximum 2.5 g/d) or streptomycin 15 to 30 mg/kg/d (maximum 1 g/d) for the first 2 months, generally followed by isoniazid plus rifampin for the duration of therapy. Therapy after the first 2 months should be individualized based on susceptibility patterns.[72] Patients with *M. tuberculosis* meningitis should be treated for a duration of 9 months or longer with multiple drug therapy.

Isoniazid, the mainstay in virtually any regimen to treat *M. tuberculosis,* penetrates the CSF with or without meningeal inflammation and achieves concentrations of more than 30 times the MIC of *M. tuberculosis* (MICs of 0.05 to 0.2 mg/L).[66–68] Rifampin's penetration of CSF approximates only 20% of serum concentrations in the presence of meningeal inflammation. *M. tuberculosis* is so exquisitely sensitive to rifampin, however, that its low penetration ratio is of little clinical significance.[67,68,73] The incidence of *M. tuberculosis* resistance to rifampin has also increased, necessitating empiric multiple antibiotic regimens.

Pyrazinamide is a small molecule that penetrates the CSF well in the absence of meningeal inflammation. Streptomycin, an aminoglycoside, penetrates CSF poorly, even in the presence of meningeal inflammation. Ethambutol is a weak antitubercular agent and reaches the CSF in moderate concentrations. Ethambutol's use is also limited by a high incidence of dose-related optic neuritis. Ethionamide and cycloserine are two other agents that are sometimes used to treat tuberculous meningitis. These agents both penetrate the CSF well in the absence of meningeal inflammation.[67,68]

The usual dose of isoniazid in children is 10 to 20 mg/kg/d (maximum 300 mg/d), and adults usually receive 5 to 10 mg/kg/d or a daily dose of 300 mg. Supplemental doses of pyridoxine hydrochloride (vitamin B_6) 50 mg/d are recommended to prevent the peripheral neuropathy associated with isoniazid administration.[67,68] Concurrent administration of rifampin is recommended at doses of 10 to 20 mg/kg/d (maximum 600 mg/d) for children and 600 mg/d for adults.[67,68] The addition of pyrazinamide (children and adults 15 to 30 mg/kg/d; maximum in both 2 g/d) to the regimen of isoniazid and rifampin is recommended.[67,72] Duration of concomitant pyrazinamide therapy should be limited to 2 months in order to avoid hepatotoxicity.

The role of steroids in the management of tuberculous meningitis remains controversial. In some cases, administration of oral prednisone 40 to 60 mg/d or 0.2 mg/kg/d of IV dexamethasone has resulted in a dramatic clearing of sensorium, remission of CSF abnormalities, reduction in fever, and elimination of headaches.[67,68] Concerns regarding the use of steroids include a possible interference with CSF chemistry studies and decreased penetration of antitubercular agents because of a decrease in inflammation. Despite the controversy, the trend toward an improved outcome generally supports their use for tuberculous meningitis.[74]

Tuberculous meningitis has a mortality rate of 10% to 50%, despite early diagnosis and treatment.[67,68] The level of patient consciousness at the start of therapy is the most useful prognostic indicator. Patients who are comatose at the beginning of therapy have a mortality rate of approximately 75%.[68] Other negative prognostic factors include old age, poor nutrition, evidence of miliary disease, high initial CSF protein concentrations, presence of hydrocephalus, and evidence of elevated intracranial pressure.[68] Ten to thirty percent of patients surviving the disease have physical or mental sequelae, including deafness, vertigo, and short-term memory loss.[67,68]

CRYPTOCOCCUS NEOFORMANS

Cryptococcal meningitis is the most common form of fungal meningitis in the United States and is a major cause of morbidity and mortality in immunosuppressed patients. Patients with HIV have a 5% to 10% risk of developing cryptococcus during their lifetime.[75] *Cryptococcus neoformans* is a soil fungus acquired by inhalation of spores from the environment. In immunocompromised hosts, especially neoplastic or AIDS patients, the organisms often disseminate from the lungs. The primary site of dissemination is the meninges, although the skin, prostate, bone, kidneys, eyes, liver, spleen, adrenals, and lymph nodes may also be infected.[76]

Symptoms of cryptococcus meningitis are insidious and may be present for months before the correct diagnosis is made. Fever and a history of headaches are the most common symptoms, although altered mentation and evidence of focal neurologic deficits may be present. Examination of the CSF usually reveals small numbers of WBCs ($< 150/mm^3$), which are primarily lymphocytes (Table 97–1). Diagnosis is based on the presence of a positive CSF, blood, sputum, or urine culture for *C. neoformans.* The CSF cultures are positive in more than 90% of cases. Organisms can be seen microscopically when stained with India ink. An additional rapid test helpful in diagnosis is latex agglutination, which detects the presence of cryptococcal antigens.[76] Latex agglutination is positive in more than 90% of culture-positive cases. A cryptococcal antigen test can be used to follow the prognosis of non-AIDS patients, but cryptococcal antigen titers do not correlate well with treatment efficacy in AIDS patients.[77] Risk factors predictive of a poor outcome include lethargy at presentation, high CSF cryptococcal antigen titer, and low CSF WBC count.[78]

Despite poor penetration into the CSF, amphotericin B has long been the drug of choice for the treatment of acute *C. neoformans* meningitis. Amphotericin B 0.5 to 1 mg/kg/d combined with flucytosine 100 mg/kg/d is more effective than amphotericin alone with successful outcomes in 75% of non-AIDS patients and 50% in AIDS patients.[79] Unfortunately, in the AIDS population, flucytosine is often poorly tolerated, causing bone marrow suppression and GI distress. Amphotericin B alone, although less effective, has been used in AIDS patients with preexisting granulocytopenia.[79,80] Intraventricular amphotericin B with intravenous amphotericin B plus flucytosine have been suggested as initial therapy. Intraventricular amphotericin B, however, is generally reserved for those patients who fail to respond to systemic therapy.[76] Because of the high acute mortality rate of up to 40% and a relapse rate of 50% in AIDS patients receiving therapy, many new agents and regimens are being investigated in this population.[78] A small, noncomparative open study evaluating the safety and efficacy of liposomal amphotericin B (AmBisome) found the product to be well tolerated and moderately effective.[81]

Azole therapy is the most studied alternative regimen for the treatment of *C. neoformans* meningitis in AIDS patients. Fluconazole at doses of 200 mg/d was compared to amphotericin B alone (0.4 mg/kg/d) with no significant difference in overall mortality between groups.[82] Patients receiving fluconazole had a higher 2-week mortality rate and time to CSF conversion.[82] High-dose fluconazole therapy (800 mg/d) was tried as salvage therapy in eight AIDS patients who failed previous antifungal therapy, but success was limited.[83] Itraconazole 200 mg orally twice daily was less effective than amphotericin B plus flucytosine in a small nonblinded study.[84]

Patients with AIDS often require lifelong maintenance or suppressive therapy because of high relapse rates following acute therapy for *C. neoformans.* A large multicenter controlled trial compared fluconazole (200 mg/d) and amphotericin B (1 mg/kg/week) in the prevention of relapse.[85] Two percent of patients receiving fluconazole versus 18% of patients on amphotericin B relapsed. In addition, the amphotericin B group had significantly more frequent bacterial infections, bacteremias, and drug-related toxicity.[85] One study suggested itraconazole (200 mg twice daily) may be a suitable alternative in those patients who are unable to receive fluconazole (400 mg daily) for consolidation therapy (8 weeks of therapy that follows an initial 2 weeks of therapy, which includes amphotericin B plus flucytosine).[86] Therefore, the standard of care for AIDS-associated cryptococcal meningitis is primary therapy, generally using amphotericin B with or without flucytosine or fluconazole alone, followed by maintenance therapy with fluconazole or itraconazole, for the life of the patient.[75]

VIRAL MENINGITIS

Meningitis typically is characterized as being either purulent or aseptic. While purulent meningitis refers to a bacterial etiology, aseptic meningitis historically was defined by a diagnosis of exclusion. Aseptic meningitis is defined as an acute meningeal irritation, usually benign and self-limiting, with complete recovery and sterile pleocytic CSF.[15] At least 70% of aseptic meningitis cases are caused by viruses; however, unusual bacterial organisms, such as *M. tuberculosis, Brucella* sp., and *Borrelia burgdorferi,* can cause aseptic meningitis.[15,87,88] In addition, fungal pathogens, certain drugs, vaccines, and systemic diseases or malignancies have been associated with aseptic meningitis syndrome.[15,87,89]

The epidemiology of viral meningitis in the United States has changed dramatically since the mid-1960s because of the introduction of large-scale polio and mumps immunization programs. Worldwide, mumps and polio are still responsible for a significant percentage of viral meningitis cases; however, in the United States, the incidence of poliomyelitis has decreased from 17.6 cases per 100,000 in 1955 to 0.01 cases per 100,000 in 1972. Similarly, the incidence of mumps has decreased 98% between 1967 and 1985. Eighty-five percent of all viral meningitis cases are caused by nonpolio enteroviruses such as coxsackie B virus, echoviruses, and enteroviruses.[15] Arboviruses, such as St. Louis, Eastern equine, Western equine, and California arboviruses, were responsible for 78 cases of viral meningitis/encephalitis in 20 states in 1993.[56] The remaining 10% of viral meningitis cases are caused by a variety of pathogens, such as adenoviruses, influenzae virus A and B, rotavirus, corona virus, cytomegalovirus, varicella-zoster, herpes simplex, Epstein-Barr virus, and lymphocytic choriomeningitis.[15,87,89] The incidence of aseptic meningitis peaks in late summer and continues into fall.

Viral meningitis is acquired primarily by hematogenous spread or alternatively by neuronal spread of the causing pathogen.[89] After entry into the host, viral replication occurs, resulting in dissemination through the reticuloendothelial system or vasculature. Infection of the capillary endothelial cells and choroid plexus may provide a conduit for CNS infections.[89] Viruses, such as polio, herpes, and varicella-zoster, may also gain access to the CNS by axonal retrograde transmission from peripheral nerve endings.[89] Once a particular virus gains access to the CNS, the course of infection is dependent on the virulence of the particular virus and host immune response. Host response to aseptic CNS infections is mediated by a complex cascade of inflammatory cytokines in a manner similar to purulent meningitis. In contrast to purulent meningitis, host response to viral meningitis is primarily mediated through cytotoxic T-lymphocytes. Although TNF is a prominent mediator in purulent bacterial meningitis, TNF concentrations are not increased in viral meningitis, whereas increases in concentrations of IL-1 and interferon (INF) α and γ occur.[90] Tumor necrosis factor concentrations have been suggested as a diagnostic tool for differentiating between purulent and viral meningitis.[90] While cytokine assays are available for investigational use, they are not routinely used in the clinical diagnosis of viral meningitis.

The clinical syndrome associated with viral meningitis is generally independent of viral etiology and may vary depending on the patient's age. Common signs in adults include headache, mild fever (< 40°C), nuchal rigidity, malaise, drowsiness, nausea, vomiting, and photophobia. Only fever and irritability may be evident in the infant, and meningitis must be ruled out as a cause of fever when no other localized findings are observed in a child. Duration of symptoms generally last 1 to 2 weeks, and specific manifestations outside of the meninges can also occur depending on viral etiology.

Laboratory examination of the CSF usually reveals a pleocytosis with 10 to 1000 WBCs/mm^3, which are primarily lymphocytic; however, 20% to 75% of patients with viral meningitis may have a predominance of polymorphonuclear cells on initial examination of the CSF, especially in enteroviral meningitis.[15] Upon repeat lumbar puncture, 90% of patients initially presenting with a predominance of neutrophils experience a shift to a predominance of mononuclear cells. Other laboratory findings include normal to mildly elevated protein concentrations and normal or mildly reduced glucose concentrations[15] (Table 97–1).

Historically, pathogens responsible for aseptic meningitis were not identified.[91] Poor laboratory recovery of viral pathogens and limited treatment options for aseptic meningitis made the need for specific identification of pathogens questionable. Advances in diagnostic laboratory techniques and the potential for decreased costs associated with longer duration of hospitalization for patients with unconfirmed viral meningitis have led to a reevaluation of the need for confirmatory pathogen diagnosis.[88,91] When clinical signs warrant pathogen identification, appropriate laboratory diagnostic techniques should be undertaken.

Although there are numerous pathogenic causes of viral meningitis, much of the clinical presentation, diagnosis, and treatment is similar. The most commonly isolated viral etiologies are described next.

Nonpolio enteroviruses are unenveloped single-strand RNA viruses. Commonly, the incidence of enteroviral meningitis peaks in late summer and continues into early fall. Enteroviruses are transmitted in the host via the fecal–oral route. Clinical presentation of enteroviral infection is frequently nonspecific and characterized by fever, nausea, vomiting, and malaise; however, GI symptoms may not be present. Following a prodrome of 1 to 2 days, headache, photophobia, and neck stiffness develop. Diagnosis is confirmed by cell culture from the CSF where the incidence of successful isolation has ranged from 40% to 80%.[90] In addition, enterovirus can be isolated from throat swabs (60%) and stool cultures (80%), but they are not necessarily diagnostic because the virus is shed in the stool for 1 to 2 weeks following infection.[91] Treatment for enteroviral meningitis consists of supportive care, fluids, antipyretics, and analgesics. Generally, disease progression is self-limiting, and the patient recovers fully without long-term neurologic complications. An assessment of the potential for long-term neurologic abnormalities in children less than 1 year old with enteroviral meningitis, however, suggests enteroviral meningitis may not be a completely benign disease.

Although arboviruses cause up to 10% of viral meningitis cases, these viruses are most commonly associated with encephalitis.[89] The four most common pathogens are the St. Louis virus, the California virus, and the Eastern and Western equine viruses. Transmission occurs through the bites of ticks and mosquitoes. Typically, an incubation period of 2 to 14 days precedes the onset of clinical symptoms. Infection of the brain tissue results in fever, headache, paralysis, and coma. While many patients have a benign presentation, symptomatic cases are associated with a higher degree of mortality. Mortality rates of 50% to 75% have been reported for Eastern equine virus, while mortality rates for Western equine and St. Louis viruses are 10% to 20%.[89] Treatment is supportive, and in the majority of cases, the disease is self-limiting.[89]

Human immunodeficiency virus (HIV) encephalitis is the most common CNS complication associated with AIDS. Frequently, patients may complain of headache, photophobia, or stiff neck at the time of presumed seroconversion. As the disease progresses, however, neurologic symptoms are frequently reported because of other opportunistic infections. Diagnosis of viral meningitis is difficult because mental status and neurologic exams are not sensitive enough to detect early changes. Direct evidence of HIV meningitis can be obtained through CSF culture, p24 antigen testing, or HIV-RNA testing. Diagnostic workup of other potential copathogens, such as herpes simplex virus (HSV), *Toxoplasma gondii, M. tuberculosis,* and cryptococcus should also be performed.

Both herpes simplex virus types 1 and 2 have been associated with infections of the CNS.[92] Herpes simplex type 1 (HSV1) is associated with meningoencephalitis, whereas herpes simplex type 2 (HSV2) is associated predominantly with meningitis. An HSV2 infection of the meninges is most likely spread hematogenously from an initial site of infection. Sexually active adults acquire herpes simplex meningitis during or after an attack of genital or rectal herpes. Although HSV2 can frequently be cultured from CSF, HSV1 cannot. Diagnosis is usually made by culture or by a fourfold rise in complement-fixing antibody to the virus. It is paramount that the diagnosis be established as early as possible because mortality rates are between 50% and 85% without treatment, and unlike other viral encephalitides, specific and effective therapy is available. Although herpes simplex may be strongly suspected on the basis of local findings after clinical evaluation, only half of these patients will have a diagnosis confirmed by brain biopsy.[92]

Acyclovir has replaced vidarabine as the drug of choice for herpes simplex encephalitis. In patients with normal renal function, acyclovir is usually administered as 10 mg/kg every 8 hours.

Herpes virus resistance to acyclovir has been reported with increasing incidence, particularly from immunocompromised patients with prior or chronic exposures to acyclovir.[93] The alternative treatment for acyclovir-resistant herpes simplex virus is vidarabine. Vidarabine is used intravenously in a dose of 15 mg/kg/d. The drug must be mixed in large volumes of parenteral fluid and infused over a 12-hour period because of its poor solubility in water. In addition, patients receiving vidarabine should be monitored for leukopenia, megaloblastic anemia, thrombocytopenia, and a parkinsonian-like neurologic syndrome.

EVALUATION OF THERAPEUTIC OUTCOMES

Empiric treatment with antibiotics should last 48 to 72 hours or until the diagnosis of meningitis can be ruled out. Continued therapy should be based on assessment of clinical improvement, cultures, and sensitivity testing results. Once a pathogen is identified, antibiotic therapy should be tailored toward the specific pathogen (Tables 97–4 and 97–5). Throughout the course of treatment, various efficacy parameters, such as signs and symptoms, microbiologic findings, and CSF examination should be followed to evaluate the success of meeting the desired outcomes.

SIGNS AND SYMPTOMS

Because of the potential for rapid deterioration associated with meningitis, signs and symptoms of fever, headache, meningism (nuchal rigidity, Brudzinski's sign, or Kernig's sign), vital signs, and signs of cerebral dysfunction should be evaluated every 4 hours for the initial 3 days and then daily thereafter. The Glascow Coma Scale should be used in severely ill patients. When monitoring the signs and symptoms of meningitis, it is important to evaluate the trend in improvement and resolution rather than single evaluations in time.

MICROBIOLOGIC FINDINGS

Cerebrospinal fluid and blood samples (two sets) for Gram stain, cultures, and sensitivity testing should be taken prior to starting antibiotic therapy. If lumbar puncture is delayed, however, antibiotics should be started. Studies show that even 24 hours after initiating antibiotics, up to 38% of CSF cultures were positive.[94] Gram stain results can be obtained immediately and can guide empiric antibiotic treatment. Identification of the organism can be made within 24 to 36 hours, and sensitivities should be available within 48 to 60 hours. Repeat cultures should be performed only when there is no response to therapy or when a relapse of symptoms occurs. A second tube of blood should be taken to allow for latex agglutination tests of antigens to common meningeal pathogens (*H. influenzae, S. pneumoniae, N. meningitidis, E. coli,* and group B streptococcus) if the Gram stain has not been helpful.

CEREBROSPINAL FLUID EXAMINATION

In bacterial meningitis, the CSF WBC count is usually greater than 1000/mm^3, the CSF protein is elevated, and the CSF glucose is often low (< 50 μg/dL or 50% to 60% of a simultaneous blood glucose value). Viral meningitis, in contrast, results in relatively normal CSF protein and glucose levels and typically does not result in greater than 90% polymorphonuclear neutrophils (PMNs) in the CSF (Table 97–1).

▶ PRINCIPLES OF PHARMACOTHERAPY

- In cases of meningitis, initial findings can include
  - *Presenting signs and symptoms:* fever, headache, nuchal rigidity, positive Brudzinski's or Kernig's sign, and altered mental status.
  - *Abnormal CSF chemistries:* elevated WBC (> 100/mm^3), elevated protein (> 50 mg/dL) , and decreased glucose levels (< 40 mg/dL).
- The three most likely pathogens of bacterial meningitis are *Streptococcus pneumoniae, Neisseria meningitidis,* and *Haemophilus influenzae.*
- Three main microbiologic tests that should be obtained include
  - *Gram stain of the CSF:* identifies the organism in 50% to 90% of cases.
  - *CSF cultures:* are positive in 80% of patients.
  - *Blood cultures.*
- Three primary goals of treatment in meningitis include
  - *Amelioration* of signs and symptoms.
  - *Eradication* of infection.
  - *Prevention* of the development of neurologic sequelae, such as seizures, deafness, coma, and death.
- Empiric coverage with an appropriate antibiotic should be started as soon as possible when clinical suspicion of meningitis exists. If there is a delay in doing a lumbar puncture (even 30 to 60 minutes), the first dose of an antibiotic *should not* be withheld. Changes in the CSF after initiation of antibiotics usually take 12 to 24 hours.
- When selecting antibiotics, the clinician must consider the antibiotic's ability to concentrate at the site of infection, as well as the spectrum of antibacterial activity. Empiric choices should be based on age and predisposing conditions.
  - *Ceftriaxone* or *cefotaxime* ± *vancomycin* are reasonable initial choices for empiric coverage of community-acquired meningitis in adult patients.
  - *Listeria monocytogenes* is a common pathogen in infants and elderly. Therefore, *ampicillin* should be empirically added to antimicrobial coverage.

- In contrast to the treatment of other infectious diseases, antibiotic dosages in the treatment of meningitis should be maximized to optimize CNS penetration.
- The duration of antibiotic treatment for meningitis has not been standardized; however, the duration of antibiotic therapy is generally based on the causative organism and the individual case, and it may range from 7 to 21 days.
- Steroid treatment includes dexamethasone 0.15 mg/kg/dose to be given four times daily for 4 days in infants and children older than 2 months of age with proven or strongly suspected bacterial meningitis and adults with a high concentration of bacteria in CSF and evidence of increased intracranial pressure.
- Close contacts and relatives of the index case should be assessed for appropriate prophylaxis, particularly with *N. meningitidis* and *H. influenzae* meningitis.

REFERENCES

1. Segreti J, Harris A, Levin S. Acute bacterial meningitis. In: Klawans HL, ed. Textbook of Neuropharmacology and Therapy, 2nd ed. 1992; 559.
2. Tunkel A, Wispelwey B, Scheld W. Pathogenesis and pathophysiology of meningitis. Infect Dis Clin North Am 1990;4:555–581.
3. Quagliarello VJ, Scheld WM. New perspectives on bacterial meningitis. Clin Infect Dis 1993;17:603–610.
4. Gray LD, Fedorko DP. Laboratory diagnosis of bacterial meningitis. Clin Microbiol Rev 1992;5:130–145.
5. Durand ML, Calderwood SB, Weber DJ, et al. Acute bacterial meningitis in adults: A review of 493 episodes. N Engl J Med 1993; 328:21–28.
6. Wenger J, Hightower A, Group tBMS. Bacterial meningitis in the United States: 1986: Report of a multistate surveillance study. J Infect Dis 1990;162:1316–1323.
7. Adams WG, Deaver KA, Cochi SL, et al. Decline of childhood *Haemophilus influenzae* type b (Hib) disease in the Hib vaccine era. JAMA 1993;269:221–226.
8. Greenlee J. Approach to diagnosis of meningitis, cerebrospinal fluid evaluation. Infect Dis Clin North Am 1990;4:583–598.
9. Greenlee J. Anatomic considerations in central nervous system infections. In: Mandell G, Douglas R, Bennett J, eds. Principles and Practice of Infectious Diseases. New York, Churchill Livingstone, 1990: 732–741.
10. Saez-Llorens X, Ramilo O, Mustafa M, et al. Molecular pathophysiology of bacterial meningitis: Current concepts and therapeutic implications. J Pediatr 1990;116:671–684.
11. Verghese A, Gallemore G. Kernig's and Brudzinski's signs revisited. Rev Infect Dis 1987;9:1187–1192.
12. Lipton JD, Schafermeyer RW. Evolving concepts in pediatric bacterial meningitis. I: Pathophysiology and diagnosis. Ann Emerg Med 1993;22:1602–1612.
13. Rothrock SG, Green SM, Wren J, et al. Pediatric bacterial meningitis: Is prior antibiotic therapy associated with an altered clinical presentation? Ann Emerg Med 1992;21:146–152.
14. Robinson R, Robert H. Acute bacterial meningitis. I: Diagnosis. Dev Med Child Neurol 1990;32:79–86.
15. Maxson S, Jacobs RF. Viral meningitis: Tips to rapidly diagnose treatable causes. Postgrad Med 1993;93:153–166.
16. Hansson LO, Axelsson G, Linne T, et al. Serum C-reactive protein in the differential diagnosis of acute meningitis. Scand J Infect Dis 1993;25:625–630.
17. Glimaker M, Kragsbjerg P, Forsgren M, et al. Tumor necrosis factor-alpha (TNFalpha) in cerebrospinal fluid from patients with meningitis of different etiologies: High levels of TNFalpha indicate bacterial meningitis. J Infect Dis 1993;167:882–889.
18. Klein O, Neu HC. Use of antimicrobial agents to treat central nervous system infection. Neurosurg Clin North Am 1992;3: 323–341.
19. Kaiser A, McGee Z. Aminoglycoside therapy of gram-negative bacillary meningitis. N Engl J Med 1975;293:1215–1220.
20. Ratcheson R, Ommaya A. Experience with the subcutaneous cerebrospinal fluid reservoir. N Engl J Med 1968;279:1026–1031.
21. Wen DY, Bottini AG, Hall WA, et al. The intraventricular use of antibiotics. Neurosurg Clin North Am 1992;3:343–355.
22. Wright P, Kaiser A, Bowmann C, et al. The pharmacokinetics and efficacy of an aminoglycoside administered into the cerebral ventricles in neonates: Implications for further evaluation of this route of therapy in meningitis. J Infect Dis 1981;143:141–147.
23. Thea D, Barza M. Use of antibacterial agents in infections of the central nervous system. Infect Dis Clin North Am 1989;3:553–571.
24. Prins J, van Deventer S, Kuijper E, et al. Clinical relevance of antibiotic induced endotoxin release. Antimicrob Agents Chemother 1994;38:1211–1218.
25. Congeni B, Tan J, Salstrom S. Kinetics of vancomycin after intraventricular and intravenous administration. Pediatr Res 1979;13: 459–463.
26. Luer M, Hatton J. Vancomycin administration into the cerebrospinal fluid: A review. Ann Pharmacother 1993;27:912–921.
27. Segreti J, Harris A. Acute bacterial meningitis. Infect Dis Emerg 1996;10:797–809.
28. Quagliarello V, Scheld W. Treatment of bacterial meningitis. N Engl J Med 1997;336:708–716.
29. Rockowitz J, Tunkel A. Bacterial meningitis. Drugs 1995;50: 838–853.
30. Lebel MH. Dexamethasone therapy of bacterial meningitis. Antibiot Chemother 1992;45:169–183.
31. Girgis NI, Farid Z, Mikhail IA, et al. Dexamethasone treatment for bacterial meningitis in children and adults. Pediatr Infect Dis J 1989;8:848–851.
32. Lebel M, Freij BJ, Syrogiannopoulos G, et al. Dexamethasone therapy for bacterial meningitis: Results of two double-blind, placebo-controlled trials. N Engl J Med 1988;319:964–971.
33. Lebel MH, Hoyt J, Waagner DC, et al. Magnetic resonance imaging and dexamethasone therapy for bacterial meningitis. Am J Dis Child 1989;143:301–306.
34. Odio CM, Faingezicht I, Paris M, et al. The beneficial effects of early dexamethasone administration in infants and children with bacterial meningitis. N Engl J Med 1991;324:1527–1531.
35. Schaad UB, Lips U, Gnehm HE, et al. Dexamethasone therapy for bacterial meningitis in children. Lancet 1993;342:457–461.
36. Yurkowski PJ, Plaisance KI. Prevention of auditory sequelae in pediatric bacterial meningitis: A meta-analysis. Pharmacotherapy 1993; 13:494–499.
37. Havens PL, Wendelberger KJ, Hoffman GM, et al. Corticosteroids as adjunctive therapy in bacterial meningitis. Am J Dis Child 1989; 143:1051–1055.
38. Committee on Infectious Diseases. In: The Redbook. Elk Grove Village, IL, American Academy of Pediatrics 1988:204–210.
39. The Meningitis Working Party of the British Paediatric Immunology and Infectious Diseases Group. Should we use dexamethasone in meningitis? Arch Dis Child 1992;67:1398–1401.
40. Paris MM, Hickey SM, Uscher MI, et al. Effect of dexamethasone on therapy of experimental penicillin- and cephalosporin-resistant

pneumococcal meningitis. Antimicrob Agents Chemother 1994;38: 1320–1324.
41. Gaillard JL, Abadie V, Cheron G, et al. Concentrations of ceftriaxone in cerebrospinal fluid of children with meningitis receiving dexamethasone therapy. Antimicrob Agents Chemother 1994;38:1209–1210.
42. Kennedy WA, Hoyt MJ, McCracken GHJ. The role of corticosteroid therapy in children with pneumococcal meningitis. Am J Dis Child 1991;145:1374–1378.
43. Syrogiannopoulos GA, Lourida AN, Theodoridou MC, et al. Dexamethasone therapy for bacterial meningitis in children: 2- versus 4-day regimen. J Infect Dis 1994;169:853–858.
44. Tunkel A, Scheld M. Pathogenesis and pathophysiology of bacterial meningitis. Clin Microbiol Rev 1993;6:118–136.
45. Weinstein L. Bacterial meningitis. Med Clin North Am 1985;69: 219–229.
46. Dodge P, Davis H, Feigin R, et al. Prospective evaluation of hearing impairment as a sequela of acute bacterial meningitis. N Engl J Med 1984;311:869–874.
47. Pomeroy SL, Holmes SJ, Dodge PR, et al. Seizures and other neurologic sequelae of bacterial meningitis in children. N Engl J Med 1990;323:1651–1656.
48. Van Esso D, Fortanals D, Uriz S, et al. *Neisseria meningitidis* strains with decreased susceptibility to penicillin. Pediatr Infect Dis J 1987; 6:483.
49. Schwartz B. Chemoprophylaxis for bacterial infections: Principles of and application to meningococcal infections. Rev Infect Dis 1991; 13:S170–S173.
50. Lieberman J, Greenberg D, Ward J. Prevention of bacterial meningitis: Vaccines and chemoprophylaxis. Infect Dis Clin North Am 1990;4:703–729.
51. Cuevas LE, Hart CA. Chemoprophylaxis of bacterial meningitis. J Antimicrob Chemother 1993;31:79–91.
52. Gaunt P, Lambert B. Single dose ciprofloxacin for the eradication of pharyngeal carriage of *Neisseria meningitidis*. J Antimicrob Chemother 1988;21:489.
53. Pugsley M, Sworzack D, Horowitz E, et al. Efficacy of ciprofloxacin in the treatment of nasopharyngeal carriers of *Neisseria meningitidis*. J Infect Dis 1987;156:211–213.
54. Appelbaum PC. Antimicrobial resistance in *Streptococcus pneumoniae*: An overview. Clin Infect Dis 1992;15:77–83.
55. Caputo GM, Appelbaum PC, Liu HH. Infections due to penicillin-resistant pneumococci: Clinical, epidemiologic, and microbiologic features. Arch Intern Med 1993;153:1301–1310.
56. Centers for Disease Control. Prevalence of penicillin-resistant *Streptococcus pneumoniae*: Connecticut, 1992–1993. MMWR 1994;43: 216–217, 223.
57. Jacobs MR. Treatment and diagnosis of infections caused by drug-resistant *Streptococcus pneumoniae*. Clin Infect Dis 1992;15:119–127.
58. Jose-Catalan M, Fernandez JM, Vazquez A, et al. Failure of cefotaxime in the treatment of meningitis due to relatively resistant *Streptococcus pneumoniae*. Clin Infect Dis 1994;18:766–769.
59. John CC. Treatment failure with use of a third-generation cephalosporin for penicillin- resistant pneumococcal meningitis: Case report and review. Clin Infect Dis 1994;18:188–193.
60. Friedland IR, Paris M, Ehrett S, et al. Evaluation of antimicrobial regimens for treatment of experimental penicillin- and cephalosporin-resistant pneumococcal meningitis. Antimicrob Agents Chemother 1993;37:1630–1636.
61. Centers for Disease Control. Recommendations for use of *Haemophilus* b conjugate vaccines and a combined diphtheria, tetanus, pertussis, and *Haemophilus* b vaccine. MMWR 1993;42:1–15.
62. Korvick JA, Yu VL. Antimicrobial agent therapy for pseudomonas aeruginosa. Antimicrob Agents Chemother 1991;35:2167–2172.
63. Rodriguez W, Khan W, Cocchetto D, et al. Treatment of *Pseudomonas* meningitis with ceftazidime with or without concurrent therapy. Pediatr Infect Dis J 1990;9:83–87.
64. Wolff MA, Young CL, Ramphal R. Antibiotic therapy for enterobacter meningitis: A retrospective review of 13 episodes and review of the literature. Clin Infect Dis 1993;16:772–777.
65. Wolff M, Boutron L, Singlas E, et al. Penetration of ciprofloxacin into cerebrospinal fluid of patients with bacterial meningitis. Antimicrob Agents Chemother 1987;31:899–902.
66. Rubin R, Hooper D. Central nervous system infection in the compromised host. Med Clin North Am 1985;69:281–296.
67. Leonard J, Dez Prez R. Tuberculous meningitis. Infect Dis Clin North Am 1990;4:769–787.
68. Holdiness M. Management of tuberculosis meningitis. Drugs 1990; 39:224–233.
69. Kent SJ, Crowe SM, Yung A, et al. Tuberculous meningitis: A 30-year review. Clin Infect Dis 1993;17:987–994.
70. Daniel T. The rapid diagnosis of tuberculosis: A selective review. J Lab Clin Med 1990;116:277–282.
71. Block AB, Cauthen GM, Onorato IM, et al. Nationwide survey of drug-resistant tuberculosis in the United States. JAMA 1994;271:665–671.
72. Centers for Disease Control. Initial therapy for tuberculosis in the era of multidrug resistance: Recommendations of the Advisory Council for the Elimination of Tuberculosis. MMWR 1993;42:1–8.
73. Ellard GA, Humphries MJ, Allen BW. Cerebrospinal fluid drug concentrations and the treatment of tuberculous meningitis. Am Rev Resp Dis 1993;148:650–655.
74. Alzeer AH, FitzGerald JM. Corticosteroids and tuberculosis: Risks and use as adjunct therapy. Tubercle Lung Dis 1993;74:6–11.
75. Dismukes WE. Management of cryptococcus. Clin Infect Dis 1993; 17:S507–S512.
76. Sugar A, Stern J, Dupont B. Overview: Treatment of cryptococcal meningitis. Rev Infect Dis 1990;12:S338–S348.
77. Powderly WG, Cloud GA, Dismukes WE, et al. Measurement of cryptococcal antigen in serum and cerebrospinal fluid: Value in the management of AIDS-associated cryptococcal meningitis. Clin Infect Dis 1994;18:789–792.
78. Powderly WG. Therapy for cryptococcal meningitis in patients with AIDS. Clin Infect Dis 1992;14:S54–S59.
79. Bennett J, Dismukes W, Duma R. A comparison of amphotericin B alone and combined with flucytosine in the treatment of cryptococcal meningitis. N Engl J Med 1979;301:126–131.
80. Chuck SL, Sande MA. Infections with *Cryptococcus neoformans* in the acquired immunodeficiency syndrome. N Engl J Med 1989;321: 794–799.
81. Coker RJ, Viviani M, Gazzard BG, et al. Treatment of cryptococcosis with liposomal amphotericin B (AmBisome) in 23 patients with AIDS. AIDS 1993;7:829–835.
82. Saag MS, Powderly WG, Cloud GA, et al. Comparison of amphotericin B with fluconazole in the treatment of acute AIDS-associated cryptococcal meningitis. N Engl J Med 1992;326:83–89.
83. Berry AJ, Finaldi MG, Graybill JR. Use of high-dose fluconazole as salvage therapy for cryptococcal meningitis in patients with AIDS. Antimicrob Agents Chemother 1992;36:690–692.
84. de Gans J, Portegies P, Tiessens G, et al. Itraconazole compared with alphotericin B plus flucytosine in AIDS patients with cryptococcal meningitis. AIDS 1992;6:185–190.
85. Powderly WG, Saag MS, Cloud GA. A controlled trial of fluconazole or amphotericin B to prevent relapse of cryptococcal meningitis in patients with the acquired immunodeficiency syndrome. N Engl J Med 1992;326:793–798.
86. Van Der Horst C, Saag M, Cloud G, et al. Treatment of cryptococcal meningitis associated with the acquired immunodeficiency syndrome. N Engl J Med 1997;337:15–21.
87. Nelsen S, Sealy DP, Schneider EF. The aseptic meningitis syndrome. Am Fam Physician 1993;48:809–815.
88. Dalton M, Newton RW. Aseptic meningitis. Dev Med Child Neurol 1991;33:446–458.
89. Rubeiz H, Roos RP. Viral meningitis and encephalitis. Semin Neurol 1992;12:165–177.

90. Glimaker M. Enteroviral meningitis: Diagnostic methods and aspects on the distinction from bacterial meningitis. Scand J Infect Dis 1992: 1–64.
91. Overall JCJ. Is it bacterial or viral? Laboratory differentiation. Ped Rev 1993;14:251–261.
92. Connolly K, Hammer S. The acute aseptic meningitis syndrome. Infect Dis Clin North Am 1990;4:599–622.
93. Gateley A, Gander R, Johnson P, et al. Herpes simplex virus type 2 meningoencephalitis resistant to acyclovir in a patients with AIDS. J Infect Dis 1990;161:711.
94. Talan D, Hoffman J, Yoshikawa T. Role of empiric parenteral antibiotics prior to lumbar puncture in suspected bacterial meningitis: State of art. Rev Infect Dis 1988;10:365–376.

98

LOWER RESPIRATORY TRACT INFECTIONS

Philip Toltzis, MD, Mark L. Glover, PharmD, and Michael D. Reed, PharmD, FCCP, FCP

Respiratory infections remain the major cause of morbidity from acute illness in the United States, and most likely, they represent the single most common reason patients seek medical attention. These demographic data have far-reaching implications when considering the dramatic changes occurring in methods of health care reimbursement within the United States. This chapter focuses on bacterial and viral infections involving the lower respiratory tract, which includes the tracheobronchial tree and lung parenchyma.

The respiratory tract has an elaborate system of host defenses, including humoral immunity, cellular immunity, and anatomic mechanisms.[1–4] When functioning properly, the host defenses of the respiratory tract are markedly effective in protecting against pathogen invasion and removing potentially infectious agents from the lungs.[2–4] For the most part, infections in the lower respiratory tract occur only when these defense mechanisms are impaired. Examples of impaired defenses would include dysgammaglobulinemia or compromised ciliary function caused by the chronic inflammation that accompanies cigarette smoking. In addition, local defenses may be overwhelmed when a particularly virulent microorganism or excessive inoculum invades lung parenchyma. The majority of pulmonary infections follow colonization of the upper respiratory tract with potential pathogens, which, after achieving sufficiently high concentrations, gain access to the lung via aspiration of oropharyngeal secretions. Less commonly, microbes enter the lung via the blood from an extrapulmonary source or by the inhalation of infected aerosolized particles. The specific type of pulmonary infection caused by an invading microorganism is determined by a variety of host factors, including age, anatomic features of the airway, and specific characteristics of the infecting agent.

The most common infections involving the lower respiratory tract include bronchitis, bronchiolitis, and pneumonia. Lower respiratory tract infections in both children and adults are most commonly a result of either viral or bacterial invasion of lung parenchyma. The diagnosis of viral infections rests primarily on the recognition of a characteristic constellation of clinical signs and symptoms. Since treatment is largely supportive, only occasionally does the diagnosis require laboratory confirmation; this is achieved through serologic tests or the identification of the organism by culture or antigen detection in respiratory secretions. New laboratory techniques employing polymerase chain reaction (PCR) technology are emerging as a means to identify specific pathogens rapidly and accurately.

In contrast, since bacterial pneumonia usually necessitates expedient, effective, and specific antibiotic therapy, its management depends, in large part, on isolation of the etiologic agent by culture from lung tissue or secretions. The pharynx is colonized with many organisms that can potentially cause pneumonia; therefore, culture of expectorated sputum can be misleading unless the specimen is examined to ensure that it has originated from the lower respiratory tract.[5,6] The Gram stain provides the easiest method to distinguish lower from upper respiratory tract secretions; moreover, through determination of the shape and color of the bacteria, the Gram stain frequently narrows the microbiologic differential diagnosis sufficiently to allow accurate initial therapy. Scanned under low power microscopy, Gram-stained expectorated upper respiratory tract secretions contain many irregularly shaped epithelial cells with little evidence of inflammation. Microorganisms of a variety of morphologies are present (Fig. 98–1). In contrast, a lower tract specimen from a patient with bacterial pneumonia usually contains multiple neutrophils per high-powered field and a single or predominant bacterial species. Culture of specimens confirmed to originate from the lower tract by Gram stain provide valuable diagnostic information in the majority of patients with bacterial pneumonia.[7,8]

An appropriate treatment regimen for the patient with an uncomplicated lower respiratory tract infection can usually be established by the history, physical examination, chest radiograph, and properly collected sputum cultures interpreted in light of knowledge of the most common lung pathogens and their antibiotic susceptibility patterns within one's community. More sophisticated or invasive diagnostic methods (such as computerized tomography, bronchoscopy, or lung biopsy)[9–12] should be reserved for very ill patients who are unable to expectorate sputum or are not responding to empiric therapy, or for pulmonary infections occurring in the immunocompromised patient.

BRONCHITIS

Bronchitis and bronchiolitis are inflammatory conditions of the large and small elements, respectively, of the tracheobronchial tree. The inflammatory process does not extend to the alveoli. Bronchitis is frequently classified as acute or chronic. Acute bronchitis occurs in all ages, and chronic bronchitis primarily affects adults. Bronchiolitis is a disease of infancy.

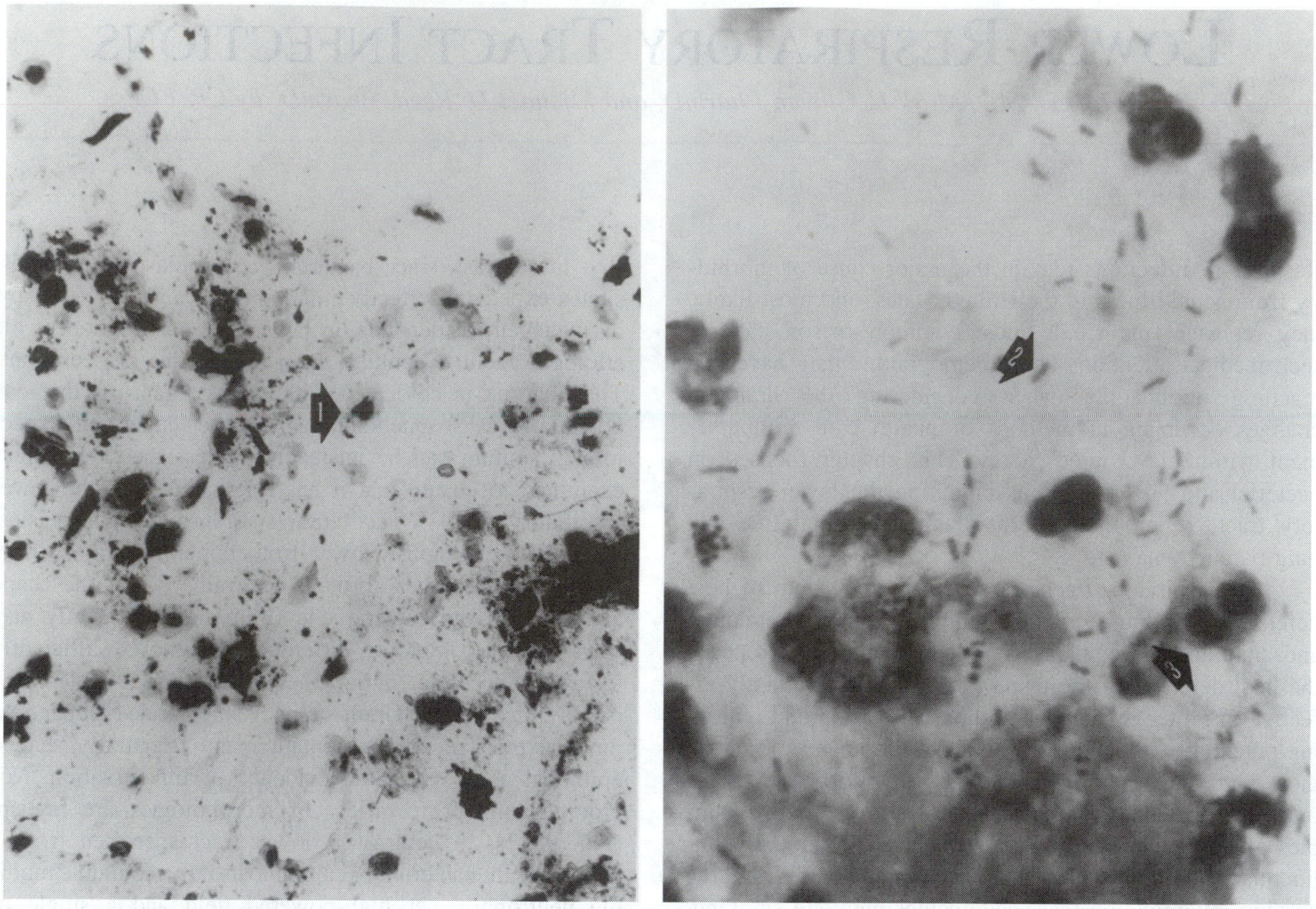

FIGURE 98–1. Gram stain of sputum. *Left panel.* Scanned under low power (10×), this sample contains many irregularly shaped epithelial cells (arrow 1) and no inflammatory cells, indicating that the specimen was derived from the upper respiratory tract. *Right panel.* Under oil emersion (100×), this specimen contains a predominance of gram-negative rods (arrow 2) and many polymorphonuclear cells (arrow 3) per high-power field, confirming that this specimen was derived from the lower respiratory tract. The sample grew *Klebsiella pneumoniae.*

ACUTE BRONCHITIS

EPIDEMIOLOGY

Acute bronchitis most commonly occurs during the winter months, following a pattern very similar to those of other acute respiratory tract infections. Cold, damp climates, the presence of high concentrations of irritating substances, such as air pollution or cigarette smoke, or both of these may precipitate attacks.[13,14]

ETIOLOGY

Respiratory viruses are by far the most common infectious agents associated with acute bronchitis. The common cold viruses, rhinovirus and coronavirus, and lower respiratory tract pathogens, including influenza virus, adenovirus, and respiratory syncytial virus, account for the majority of cases. In children, similar pathogens are observed with the addition of the parainfluenza viruses. While the true incidence remains to be defined, *Mycoplasma pneumonia* also appears to be a frequent cause of acute bronchitis. Additionally, *Chlamydia pneumoniae*[15] and *Bordetella pertussis* (the agent responsible for whooping cough) have been associated with acute respiratory tract infections. Although a variety of bacteria, including *Streptococcus pneumonia, Streptococcus* sp., *Staphylococcus* sp., and *Haemophilus* sp. may be isolated from throat or sputum culture, it is probable that these organisms represent contamination by normal flora of the upper respiratory tract rather than true pathogens. Although a primary bacterial etiology for acute bronchitis appears rare, secondary bacterial infection may be involved.

PATHOGENESIS

Because acute bronchitis is primarily a self-limiting illness and rarely a cause of death, few data are available to describe the pathology. In general, infection of the trachea and bronchi yields hyperemic and edematous mucous membranes with an increase in bronchial secretions. Destruction of respiratory epithelium can range from mild to extensive and may affect bronchial mucociliary function. In addition, the increase in bronchial secretions, which can become thick and tenacious, further impairs mucociliary activity. The probability of permanent damage to the airways as a result of acute bronchitis remains unclear; however, epidemiologic evaluations support the belief that recurrent acute respiratory infections may be associated with increased airway hyperreactivity and possibly the pathogenesis of chronic obstructive lung disease.[13,14,16,17]

CLINICAL PRESENTATION

Acute bronchitis usually begins as an upper respiratory infection. Nonspecific complaints, including malaise and headache, frequently accompany coryza and sore throat. Cough is the hallmark of acute bronchitis and occurs early. The onset of cough may be insidious or abrupt, and the symptoms persist despite the resolution of nasal or nasopharyngeal complaints. Frequently, the cough is initially nonproductive but progresses, yielding mucopurulent sputum. In older children and adults, the sputum is raised and expectorated; in the young child, sputum is often swallowed and can result in gagging and vomiting. Substantial discomfort may result from the coughing. Dyspnea, cyanosis, or signs of airway obstruction are rarely observed unless the patient has underlying pulmonary disease, such as emphysema or chronic obstructive pulmonary disease. Fever, when present, rarely exceeds 39°C and appears most commonly with adenovirus, influenza virus, and *M. pneumonia* infections.

The chest examination in acute bronchitis may reveal rhonchi and coarse, moist rales bilaterally. Chest radiographs are usually normal. The diagnosis is typically made on the basis of a characteristic history and physical examination. Bacterial cultures of expectorated sputum are generally of limited use because of the inability to avoid normal nasopharyngeal flora by the sampling technique. In routine cases, viral cultures are unnecessary and frequently unavailable. Viral antigen detection tests, developed to identify respiratory viral antigens from nasal secretions rapidly, can be obtained in many hospital laboratories and in some practice settings when a specific diagnosis is necessary for clinical or epidemiologic reasons.[18] Cultures or serologic diagnosis of *M. pneumonia* and culture or direct fluorescent antibody detection for *B. pertussis* should be obtained in prolonged or severe cases when epidemiologic considerations would suggest their involvement.[19]

▶ TREATMENT: Acute Bronchitis

DESIRED OUTCOME

In the absence of a complicating bacterial superinfection, acute bronchitis is almost always self-limiting. The goals of therapy, therefore, are to provide comfort to the patient, and, in the unusually severe case, to treat associated dehydration and respiratory compromise.

GENERAL APPROACH TO TREATMENT

The treatment of acute bronchitis is symptomatic and supportive in nature. Reassurance and antipyretics frequently are all that are needed.

NONPHARMACOLOGIC THERAPY

Bed rest for comfort may be instituted as desired. Patients should be encouraged to drink fluids to prevent dehydration and possibly decrease the viscosity of respiratory secretions. Mist therapy, the use of a vaporizer, or both may further promote the thinning and loosening of respiratory secretions.

PHARMACOLOGIC THERAPY

Mild analgesic–antipyretic therapy is often helpful in relieving the associated lethargy, malaise, and fever. Aspirin or acetaminophen (650 mg in adults or 10 to 15 mg/kg per dose in children; maximum daily pediatric dose 60 mg/kg) or ibuprofen (200 to 400 mg in adults or 10 mg/kg per dose in children; maximum daily pediatric dose 40 mg/kg) should be administered every 4 to 6 hours. In children, aspirin should be avoided and acetaminophen used as the preferred agent because of the possible association between aspirin use and the development of Reye's syndrome.[20]

More recently, the use of ibuprofen as an antipyretic has increased. The drug's antipyretic efficacy appears identical to that of aspirin or acetaminophen, although its duration of antipyretic effect may be slightly longer (e.g., 3 to 4 hours for aspirin and acetaminophen versus 5 to 6 hours for ibuprofen). Caution should be exercised in the administration of ibuprofen in very young and elderly patients and individuals with poor renal function. Aspirin and ibuprofen inhibit prostaglandin synthesis and may adversely influence renal function in these predisposed patient populations.

Patients suffering from acute bronchitis frequently medicate themselves with over-the-counter cough and cold remedies containing various combinations of antihistamines, sympathomimetics, and antitussives despite the lack of definitive evidence supporting their effectiveness. In fact, the tendency of these agents to dehydrate bronchial secretions could potentially aggravate and prolong the recovery process. Persistent, mild cough, which may be bothersome, can be treated with dextromethorphan; more severe coughs may require intermittent codeine or other similar agents.[22] In severe cases, cough may be persistent enough to disrupt sleep, and the use of a mild sedative-hypnotic, concomitantly with a cough suppressant, may be desirable; however, antitussives should be used cautiously when the cough is productive. The primary or supplemental use of expectorants is questionable because their clinical effectiveness has not been well established.[21,22]

Routine use of antibiotics in the treatment of acute bronchitis should be discouraged[23]; however, in patients who exhibit persistent fever or respiratory symptoms for more than 4 to 6 days, the possibility of a concurrent bacterial infection should be suspected. When possible, antibiotic therapy should be directed toward anticipated respiratory pathogen(s) (*S. pneumonia, Haemophilus influenzae*). *Mycoplasma pneumonia,* if suspected by history or positive cold agglutinins (titers > 1:32), or if confirmed by culture or serology, may be treated with erythromycin or its analogs (clarithromycin, azithromycin). During known epidemics involving the influenza A virus, amantadine or rimantadine may be effective in minimizing associated symptoms if administered early in the course of the disease.[24]

CHRONIC BRONCHITIS

EPIDEMIOLOGY

Chronic bronchitis is a nonspecific disease that affects primarily adults. Estimates suggest that between 10% and 25% of the adult population 40 or older suffer from chronic bronchitis, resulting in substantial health care dollar expenditures and lost wages.[25–27] This disease is so common that acute bronchitis and acute exacerbations of chronic bronchitis result in approximately 14 million physician visits per year in the United States. Similar to acute bronchitis, cold, damp climates and the presence of elevated airborne concentrations of irritating substances may favor this disease.[25–27] Chronic bronchitis occurs more commonly in men than in women.

ETIOLOGY

Data and experience suggest that chronic bronchitis is a result of several contributing factors; the most prominent of these include cigarette smoking, exposure to occupational dusts, fumes, environmental pollution, and bacterial (and possibly viral) infection. The influence that each of these factors and others, either alone or in combination, contributes to chronic bronchitis is unknown. Cigarette smoke is a well-known airway irritant and is believed by many to be the predominant factor in the etiology of chronic bronchitis. Studies of lungs from smoking and nonsmoking individuals have clearly demonstrated a substantial increase in the number of alveolar macrophages, as well as the presence of bronchial inflammation, in individuals who smoke cigarettes. Although the majority of patients who suffer from chronic bronchitis have a positive smoking history, no history of smoking can be identified in as many as 10% of cases. These findings suggest that additional airway irritants, either alone or more probably in combination, are responsible for the pathogenesis of chronic bronchitis. The only known genetic abnormality leading to chronic obstructive pulmonary disease (COPD) is α-1 antitrypsin deficiency occurring in less than 1% of COPD in the United States.

In addition to the preceding, the influence of recurrent respiratory tract infections during childhood or young adult life on the later development of chronic bronchitis remains obscure. The available data suggest that recurrent respiratory infections at a young age predispose individuals to the development of chronic bronchitis[17,28]; however, it is unclear whether these recurrent respiratory tract infections are a result of unrecognized anatomic abnormalities of the airways or impaired pulmonary defense mechanisms.

PATHOGENESIS

The chronic inhalation of an irritating noxious substance compromises the normal secretory and mucociliary function of bronchial mucosa. In chronic bronchitis, the bronchial wall is thickened and the number of mucous-secreting goblet cells in the surface epithelium of both larger and smaller bronchi is markedly increased.[29] In contrast, goblet cells are generally absent from the smaller bronchi of normal individuals. In addition to the increased number of goblet cells, hypertrophy of the mucous glands and dilation of the mucous gland ducts are also observed.[29] As a result of these changes, chronic bronchitics have substantially more mucus in their peripheral airways, further impairing normal lung defenses. This increased quantity of tenacious secretions within the bronchial tree frequently causes mucous plugging of the smaller airways. Accompanying these changes are squamous cell metaplasia of the surface epithelium, edema and increased vascularity of the basement membrane of larger airways, and variable chronic inflammatory cell infiltration. Continued progression of this pathology can result in residual scarring of small bronchi, augmenting airway obstruction and weakening of bronchial walls.

CLINICAL PRESENTATION

The hallmark of chronic bronchitis is a cough that may range from a mild "smoker's" cough to severe incessant coughing productive of purulent sputum. Coughing may be precipitated by multiple stimuli, including simple, normal conversation. Expectoration of the largest quantity of sputum usually occurs upon arising in the morning, although many patients expectorate sputum throughout the day. The expectorated sputum is usually tenacious and can vary in color from white to yellow-green. As a result, many patients complain of a frequent bad taste in their mouth and halitosis.

The diagnosis of chronic bronchitis is based primarily on clinical assessment and history. Any patient who reports the coughing up of sputum on most days for at least 3 consecutive months each year for 2 consecutive years presumptively has chronic bronchitis.[26,27] The diagnosis of chronic bronchitis is made only when the possibilities of bronchiectasis, cardiac failure, cystic fibrosis, and lung carcinoma have been effectively excluded. In an attempt to be more specific in the diagnosis, some investigators have added lost wages for 3 or more weeks to the criteria. In addition, many clinicians attempt to subdivide their patients into one of three subgroups: (1) those patients with simple chronic bronchitis, (2) those with chronic or recurrent mucopurulent bronchitis (based on the presence of mucopurulent sputum confirmed by microscopic analysis), and (3) those with chronic obstructive bronchitis (based on the clinical history and presence of airway obstruction documented by pulmonary function testing). More recently, an ad hoc international committee comprised of pulmonary and infectious disease physicians developed a classification system that can serve as a practical guide for initial patient assessment and management (Table 98–1) for patients with chronic bronchitis.[27]

Chest auscultation usually reveals inspiratory and expiratory rales, rhonchi, and mild wheezing with an expiratory phase that is frequently prolonged. Normal vesicular breathing sounds are diminished. Depending on the severity of the disease, an increase in the anteroposterior diameter of the thoracic cage (observed as a barrel chest), hyperresonance on percussion with obliteration of the area of cardiac dullness, and depressed diaphragms with limited mobility are often observed. In more advanced stages, cyanosis is common and may be accompanied by a compensatory erythrocytosis. Clubbing of the digits is infrequent, but when observed is usually reflective of advanced disease. In more progressed stages of chronic bronchitis, physical findings associated with cor pulmonale, including cardiac enlargement, hepatomegaly, and edema of the lower extremities, are observed. In general, chronic bronchitics tend to maintain at least normal body weight and are commonly obese. Radiographic studies are of limited value either in the diagnosis or as a means of sequentially following a patient. A decrease in vital capacity and a prolongation of expiratory flow are usually found from pulmonary function studies.

The microscopic and laboratory assessment of sputum is considered an important component in the overall evaluation of patients with chronic bronchitis. A fresh sputum specimen obtained as an early morning sample is preferred. Comparison of the cellular constituents of chronic bronchitic sputum with those of normal sputum can provide insight into the degree of activity of the disease

TABLE 98–1. Useful Classification System for Patients With Chronic Bronchitis and Initial Treatment Options[27]

Baseline Status	Criteria or Risk Factors	Usual Pathogens	Initial Treatment Options
Class I Acute tracheobronchitis	No underlying structural disease	Usually a virus	1st None unless symptoms persist 2nd Amoxicillin or a macrolide/azithromycin
Class II Chronic bronchitis	$FEV_1 > 50\%$ predicted value, increased sputum volume and purulence	*Haemophilus influenzae*, *Hemophilus* sp. *Moraxella catarrhalis*, *Streptococcus pneumoniae* (β-lactam resistance possible)	1st Amoxicillin, or quinolone if prevalence of *H. influenzae* resistance to amoxicillin is > 20% 2nd Quinolone, amoxicillin–clavulanate, azithromycin, tetracycline, or trimethoprim–sulfamethoxazole
Class III Chronic bronchitis with complications	$FEV_1 < 50\%$ predicted value, increased sputum volume and purulence, advanced age, at least four flares/year, or significant comorbidity	Same as class II; also *Klebsiella pneumoniae Pseudomonas aeruginosa*, *K. pneumoniae*, and other gram-negative organisms (β-lactam resistance common)	1st Quinolone 2nd Expanded spectrum cephalosporin, amoxicillin–clavulanate, or azithromycin
Class IV Chronic bronchial infection	Same as for class III plus yearlong production of purulent sputum	Same as class III	1st Oral or parenteral quinolone, carbapenem or expanded spectrum cephalosporin followed by high-dose oral ciprofloxacin or routine dose trovafloxacin

1st = first choices; 2nd = alternate treatment options.
Quinolone: ciprofloxacin, clinafloxacin, grepafloxacin, trovafloxacin.
Tetracycline: tetracycline HCl, doxycycline.
Carbapenem: imipenem/cilistatin, meropenem.
Expanded spectrum cephalosporin: ceftazidime, cefepime.

processes.[25] An increased number of polymorphonuclear granulocytes often suggests continual bronchial irritation, whereas an increased number of eosinophils may suggest an allergic component that should be further investigated. Gram staining of the sputum often reveals a mixture of both gram-positive and gram-negative bacteria, reflecting normal oropharyngeal flora and tracheal colonization by *S. pneumonia, H. influenzae,* and *Moraxella catarrhalis.* The most common bacterial isolates identified from sputum culture in patients experiencing an acute exacerbation of chronic bronchitis are outlined in Table 98–2.

TABLE 98–2. Common Bacterial Pathogens Isolated From the Sputum of Patients With an Acute Exacerbation of Chronic Bronchitis

Pathogen	Estimated Incidence[a]
Haemophilus influenzae[b]	24–26
Haemophilus parainfluenzae	20
Streptococcus pneumoniae[c]	15
Moraxella catarrhalis[b]	15
Klebsiella pneumoniae	4
Serratia marcescens	2
Neisseria meningitidis[b]	2
Pseudomonas aeruginosa	2

[a]Expressed as percent of cultures.
[b]Often β-lactamase positive.
[c]Up to as many as 25% of strains may be intermediate or highly resistant to penicillin.

▶ TREATMENT: Chronic Bronchitis

DESIRED OUTCOME

The goals of therapy for chronic bronchitis are twofold: first, to reduce the severity of the chronic symptoms and second, to ameliorate acute exacerbations and to achieve prolonged infection-free intervals.

GENERAL APPROACH TO TREATMENT

The approach to the treatment of chronic bronchitis is multifactorial. First and foremost, attempts must be made to reduce the patient's exposure to known bronchial irritants (e.g., smoking). Additionally, measures to provide pulmonary toilet can be instituted. Finally, in the face of an acute exacerbation, a trial of antibiotics directed against the most likely underlying pathogens can be started.

NONPHARMACOLOGIC THERAPY

A complete occupational and environmental history for the determination of exposure to noxious, irritating gases, as well as preference toward cigarette smoking must be assessed. Often easier discussed than accomplished, honest yet reasonable attempts should be made with the patient to reduce or eliminate completely the number of cigarettes smoked daily and reduce his or her exposure to second-hand smoke. In an organized, coordinated cessation program, which includes counseling and hypnotherapy, the adjunctive use of nicotine substitutes, such as a nicotine gum or patch, may promote the reduction or complete withdrawal from cigarette smoking. Often just as difficult is the modification of exposure to irritating substances within the home and workplace.

During acute pulmonary exacerbations of the disease, a patient's ability to mobilize and expectorate sputum may be dramatically reduced. In these instances, attempts at postural drainage techniques, with instruction, active participation, or both from a respiratory therapist, may assist in promoting clearance of pulmonary secretions. In addition, humidification of inspired air may promote the hydration (liquefaction) of tenacious secretions allowing for more productive removal. The use of mucolytic aerosols, such as *N*-acetylcysteine and DNAse, is of questionable therapeutic value, particularly considering their propensity to induce bronchospasm and their excessive cost. Oral or aerosolized bronchodilators may benefit some patients during acute pulmonary exacerbations.

PHARMACOLOGIC THERAPY

For those patients that consistently demonstrate clinical limitation in airflow, a therapeutic challenge of bronchodilators (albuterol aerosol) should be considered. Although chronic theophylline administration has been extensively used in the past, this therapy is being employed with decreasing frequency in favor of aerosolized β_2-receptor agonists. Albuterol is most commonly used, one to two puffs of the metered dose inhaler three to four times daily.[26] More recently, the role of aerosolized surfactant has been assessed in patients with stable chronic bronchitis.[30] This preliminary study reveals very encouraging results with surfactant demonstrating improvement in pulmonary function and sputum transport by cilia (i.e., clearance). The role of surfactant as a carrier vehicle for other aerosol medications will most likely be evaluated over the next several years.

A plethora of studies have attempted to describe a beneficial effect of antibiotic administration with acute and chronic treatment of chronic bronchitics.[26,27,31,32] Numerous comparative evaluations, including placebo-controlled studies, have suggested definite clinical benefit, whereas other similar studies have not. The antibiotics most frequently selected (ampicillin, tetracycline [or doxycycline], chloramphenicol, trimethoprim–sulfamethoxazole) possess variable *in vitro* activity against the common sputum isolates *H. influenzae, S. pneumonia, M. catarrhalis,* and *M. pneumonia.*

In general, these conflicting results appear independent of which antibiotic was used or regimen compared. The wide disparity that exists in the results from these studies, combined with the difficulties in recognition and lack of standardized diagnostic criteria for acute exacerbation of chronic bronchitis[31] serves as the basis for the enormous controversy surrounding the use of antibiotics in this condition.[33,34]

Further complicating antibiotic selection is the increasing resistance of the common bacterial pathogens to first-line agents. As many as 30% to 40% of *H. influenzae* and 95% of *M. catarrhalis* produce β-lactamase. Moreover, up to as many as 25% of *S. pneumoniae* isolates demonstrate some resistance to penicillin; approximately 10% of isolates are highly resistant (penicillin minimum inhibitory concentration [MIC] > 2 mg/L) and approximately 15% demonstrate intermediate resistance (penicillin MIC 0.5 to < 2 mg/L). Despite these changes in bacterial susceptibility, it is recommended to initiate therapy with first line agents in less severely affected patients. The scheme outlined in Table 98–1 can be used as an initial guide to the selection of antibiotics based on disease severity (class I through IV). Regardless of which antibiotic is selected, careful attention to predetermined outcome measures should be closely monitored in each patient to determine the success or failure of the therapeutic intervention.[34] Thus, the need to use newer oral antibiotics (cefuroxime, cefixime, amoxicillin-clavulanate, quinolones, or azilides), that possess more potent *in vitro* activity against sputum isolates appears limited as initial therapy, since clinical response often appears independent of the pathogens' *in vitro* susceptibility for many patients.[26,27,32]

An important clinical outcome variable directing future drug selection and criteria for beginning antibiotics in individual patients is to assess the infection-free period when chronic bronchitics are off antibiotics. The actual length of the infection-free time period, as well as the change in the number of physician office visits and hospital admissions with a particular antibiotic regimen, is extremely important to identify, whenever possible, for each patient. The longest infection-free period defines that antibiotic regimen as the "regimen of choice" for the specific patient for future acute exacerbations of their disease. It is important, however, to note that the impact such therapy may have on the disease or its progression, if incorporated as an aggressive targeted strategy over time, is less well characterized.

Antibiotics should be selected that are effective against responsible pathogens, demonstrate the least susceptibility to drug interactions (erythromycin/ciprofloxacin and theophylline), and can be administered in a manner that promotes compliance. Antibiotics commonly used in the treatment of these patients and their respective adult starting doses are outlined in Table 98–3. It is important to note that doses of antibiotics should be adjusted as needed to the desired clinical effect and the lowest incidence of acceptable side effects. A frequent, successful clinical strategy to enhance the duration of symptom-free periods incorporates higher dose antibiotic regimens using the upper limit of the recommended daily antibiotic dose for a period of 10 to 14 days.

Ampicillin is often considered the drug of choice for the treatment of acute exacerbations of chronic bronchitis. Unfortunately, the need for multiple repeat daily doses (four times daily), increased incidence of gastrointestinal side effects, and the increasing incidence of penicillin-resistant β-lactamase producing strains of bacteria (Tables 98–1 and 98–2) have limited the usefulness of this safe and very cost-effective antibiotic. As stated earlier, the proposed classification system outlined in Table 98–1 offers first- and second-line treatment options for acute exacerbations of chronic bronchitis, which is directed by the baseline clinical status of the patient. These treatment recommendations can be used to initiate therapy in patients with class I through IV disease.

The value of the erythromycins when mycoplasma is involved is unquestionable whereas the value, if any, of the newer erythromycin analogs, azithromycin or clarithromycin, as first line agents in the treatment of these patients is not known. Azithromycin should be considered as the macrolide/azilide of choice when considering the drug's *in vitro* antibacterial spectrum of activity, tissue distribution characteristics, and lack of metabolic based drug–drug interactions.[35] In contrast, the fluoroquinolones

TABLE 98–3. Oral Antibiotics Commonly Used for the Treatment of Acute Respiratory Exacerbations in Chronic Bronchitis

Antibiotic	Usual Adult Dose (g)	Dose Schedule (doses/day)
Preferred Drugs		
Ampicillin	0.5–1	4
Amoxicillin	0.5–1	3
Cefprozil	0.5	2
Cefuroxime	0.5	2
Ciprofloxacin	0.5–0.75	2
Clinafloxacin		
Lomefloxacin	0.4	1
Ofloxacin	0.2–0.4	2
Trovafloxacin	0.2	1
Doxycycline	0.1	2
Minocycline	0.1	2
Tetracycline HCl	0.5	4
Amoxicillin–clavulanate	0.5	3
Trimethoprim–sulfamethoxazole	1 DS[a]	2
Supplemental Drugs		
Azithromycin	0.25–0.5	1
Erythomycin	0.5	4
Clarithromycin	0.25–0.5	2
Cefixime	0.4	1
Cephalexin	0.5	4
Cefaclor	0.25–0.5	3

[a]DS, double strength tablet (160 trimethoprim/800 mg sulfamethoxazole).

have emerged as effective alternative agents, particularly when gram-negative pathogens are involved or in more clinically or severely ill patients (Table 98–1). The increasing resistance of selected pathogens to ciprofloxacin may necessitate the use of newer analogs with greater *in vitro* antibacterial activity, including penicillin tolerant or resistant *S. pneumoniae* (trovafloxacin). The increased cost of fluoroquinolones must be carefully weighed against the possible superiority of quinolones in their apparent initial success rate and more prolonged infection-free time period.[26,27]

In the patient whose history suggests recurrent exacerbations of disease that might be attributable to specific events (that is, it is seasonal or related to the winter months), a trial of prophylactic antibiotics might be beneficial. If no clinical improvement is noted over an appropriate time period (2 to 3 months per year for 2 to 3 years), one might elect to discontinue further attempts at prophylactic therapy. Similarly, such patient-specific trials could be performed in individuals experiencing acute exacerbations, focusing on defining the infection-free period. Although less than desirable, this method of clinical assessment might distinguish that subset of patients who will benefit from prophylactic antibiotic therapy from those who will not.

BRONCHIOLITIS

EPIDEMIOLOGY

Bronchiolitis is an acute viral infection of the lower respiratory tract of infants. The disease most commonly affects infants during the first year of life with peak attack rates occurring in children between the ages of 2 and 10 months. Infectious bronchiolitis is unusual in children older than 2 years of age. The occurrence of bronchiolitis peaks during the winter months and persists through early spring. Bronchiolitis remains one of the major reasons infants under 6 months require hospitalization. Estimates suggest that the hospitalization rate for infants younger than 6 months for bronchiolitis approximates 6 per 1000 children per year. The incidence of bronchiolitis appears to be more common in males than females.[13,14,36]

ETIOLOGY

Respiratory syncytial virus is the most common cause of bronchiolitis, accounting for 45% to 60% of all cases. During epidemic periods, the incidence of respiratory syncytial virus-induced bronchiolitis can exceed 80% of cases. Parainfluenza viruses type 3 (10% to 15%), type 1 (5% to 10%), and type 2 (1% to 5%) are the second most common pathogens, constituting as a group nearly 25% of cases. Bacteria serve as secondary pathogens in only a small minority of cases.

CLINICAL PRESENTATION

A prodrome suggesting an upper respiratory tract infection, usually lasting from 2 to 7 days, precedes the onset of clinical symptoms. During this prodromal period, infants may be irritable and restless and have a mild fever. The most common clinical signs of bronchiolitis are cough and coryza. As symptoms progress, infants may experience vomiting, diarrhea, noisy breathing, and an increase in respiratory rate. For those infants presenting to a hospital, examination reveals a rapid pulse and a respiratory rate between 40 and 80 breaths per minute. Breathing is labored with retractions of the chest wall, nasal flaring, and grunting. Chest auscultation reveals wheezing and inspiratory rales. Mild conjunctivitis may be observed in up to one-third of infants, whereas 5% to 10% may have a concurrent otitis media. As a result of limited oral intake because of coughing combined with fever, vomiting, and diarrhea, infants are frequently dehydrated. The increased work of breathing and tachypnea most likely further increases fluid loss. In most cases, this clinical picture persists between 3 and 7 days. Although the hospital course of bronchiolitic children is often variable, substantial clinical improvement is usually observed within the first 2 days, with gradual improvement and resolution over the next 7 to 21 days.

The diagnosis of bronchiolitis is based primarily on history and clinical findings. It is important for the clinician to attempt to differentiate between bronchiolitis and a host of other clinical entities affecting infants, which may produce a similar picture of dyspnea and wheezing. Asthma, congestive heart failure, anatomic airway abnormalities, cystic fibrosis, foreign bodies, and gastroesophageal reflux are the primary disease entities that may present with wheezing on physical examination in children. The isolation of a viral pathogen in the respiratory secretions of a wheezing child establishes a presumptive diagnosis of infectious bronchiolitis. The ability to identify specific viral pathogens is, however, often hindered by the limited availability of special virology laboratories. The proliferation of commercial enzyme-linked immunosorbent assays (ELISA) and fluorescent antibody staining techniques of nasopharyngeal secretions has increased the ability to identify viral antigens within several hours.[37] Identification of respiratory syncytial virus (RSV) by PCR should be routinely available from most clinical laboratories soon.

Multiple clinical laboratory determinations have been used to assist in the management of cases of bronchiolitis. Roentgenographic evaluation of the chest in children with bronchiolitis yields variable findings but may help to distinguish this illness from other entities characterized by wheezing.[17,28] The peripheral white blood cell (WBC) count is usually normal or only slightly elevated. In those children requiring hospitalization, abnormalities in blood gas tensions are frequent and appear to relate to disease severity. Hypoxemia is common and acts to increase the respiratory drive, whereas hypercarbia is seen only in the most severe cases. Despite the presence of moderate degrees of hypoxemia, clinical cyanosis is unusual.

▶ TREATMENT: Bronchiolitis

DESIRED OUTCOME

In the well infant, bronchiolitis is usually a self-limiting illness, and reassurance and antipyretics are usually all that are necessary while waiting for resolution of the underlying viral infection. In-hospital support is necessary for the child suffering from respiratory failure or dehydration; these conditions are potentiated by underlying cardiac and pulmonary disease.

GENERAL APPROACH TO TREATMENT

Almost all otherwise healthy babies with bronchiolitis can be followed as outpatients. Such infants are treated for fever, provided generous amounts of oral fluids, and closely observed for evidence of respiratory deterioration. In severely affected children, the mainstays of therapy for bronchiolitis are oxygen therapy and intravenous fluids. In a subset of patients, aerosolized bronchodilators may have a role. In selected infants, particularly those with underlying pulmonary or cardiac disease or both, with severe acute infection, therapy with the antiviral agent ribavirin may be considered.

PHARMACOLOGIC THERAPY

Aerosolized β-adrenergic therapy appears to offer little benefit for the majority of patients and may even be detrimental.[14,36,38] However, this therapy may offer some benefit to the child with a predisposition toward bronchospasm. In hospitalized patients, bronchodilator therapy may be offered initially but should not be pursued in the absence of a clear-cut clinical benefit. Similarly, controlled trials of corticosteroids have failed to reveal any therapeutic benefit (or harmful effect) when administered to bronchiolitic infants.[36,39] As a result, the routine use of systemically administered corticosteroids is discouraged. Although it has been common practice to place children with bronchiolitis in mist tents, there are no data to document the effectiveness of this practice. Because bacteria do not represent primary pathogens in the etiology of bronchiolitis, antibiotics should not be routinely administered. Despite this, many clinicians frequently administer antibiotics initially while awaiting culture results, because the clinical and radiographic findings in bronchiolitis are often suggestive of a possible bacterial pneumonia.[40]

Ribavirin may offer benefit to a subset of infants with bronchiolitis. Although ribavirin, a synthetic nucleoside, possesses *in vitro* antiviral properties against a variety of RNA and DNA viruses, including influenza A, influenza B, and parainfluenza,[41,42] it is approved only in aerosolized form against RSV.[43,44] Use of the drug requires special equipment (small-particle aerosol generator) and specifically trained personnel for administration via oxygen hood or mist tent. Special care must be taken to avoid drug particle deposition and the resultant clogging of respiratory tubing and valves in mechanical ventilators.

When administered as a small particle aerosol, ribavirin has been shown to diminish systemic and respiratory symptoms, fever, and viral shedding associated with RSV infections in infants. The effectiveness of this agent in routine RSV bronchiolitis appears moderate, however, and clear-cut indications for its use remain to be more fully elucidated.[45] Because of the requirement for special aerosolization equipment and the cost of the drug itself, most experts recommend reserving use of ribavirin for severely ill patients, especially those with chronic lung disease (particularly bronchopulmonary dysplasia), congenital heart disease, prematurity, and immunodeficiency (especially severe combined immunodeficiency and human immunodeficiency virus [HIV] infection). Ribavirin also may be considered in otherwise healthy patients with severe distress because of RSV.[45,46]

PNEUMONIA

EPIDEMIOLOGY

Pneumonia is the most common infectious cause of death in the United States, where it is estimated that approximately 4 million cases are diagnosed annually, at a cost of $23 billion dollars to the health care system. Pneumonia occurs throughout the year, with the relative prevalence of disease resulting from different etiologic agents varying with the seasons. It occurs in persons of all ages, although the clinical manifestations are most severe in the very young, elderly, and chronically ill.

PATHOGENESIS

Microorganisms gain access to the lower respiratory tract by three routes. They may be inhaled as aerosolized particles, or they may enter the lung via the bloodstream from an extrapulmonary site of infection; however, aspiration of oropharyngeal contents, a common occurrence in both healthy and ill persons during sleep, is the major mechanism by which pulmonary pathogens gain access to the normally sterile lower airways and alveoli. When pulmonary defense mechanisms are functioning optimally, aspirated microorganisms are cleared from the region before infection can become established[1–4]; however, aspiration of potential pathogens from the oropharynx can result in pneumonia if lung defenses are impaired. Factors that promote aspiration, such as altered sensorium and neuromuscular disease, may result in an increase in the size of the inoculum delivered to the lower respiratory tract, thereby overwhelming local defense mechanisms. Lung infections with viruses suppress the antibacterial activity of the lung by impairing alveolar macrophage function and mucociliary clearance, thus setting the stage for secondary bacterial pneumonia. Mucociliary transport is also depressed by ethanol and narcotics and by obstruction of a bronchus by mucus, tumor, or extrinsic compression. All of these factors can severely impair the pulmonary clearance of aspirated bacteria.[1–4]

The most prominent pathogens causing community-acquired pneumonia in otherwise healthy adults are *S. pneumonia* (pneumococcus) and *M. pneumonia.* Pneumococcus is the most common cause of bacterial pneumonia in all age groups and accounts for up to 70% of all acute bacterial pneumonias in the United States. *Mycoplasma pneumonia* is believed to account for 10% to 20% of cases. Legionella, *C. pneumoniae,* and a variety of viruses, also cause pneumonia among otherwise healthy persons.[47] Community-acquired pneumonias caused by *Staphylococcus aureus* and gram-negative rods are observed primarily in the elderly, especially those residing in nursing homes, and in association with alcoholism and other debilitating conditions.[48]

Gram-negative aerobic bacilli and *S. aureus* are also the leading causative agents in hospital-acquired pneumonia.[49] Anaerobic bacteria are the most common etiologic agents in pneumonia that follows the gross aspiration of gastric or oropharyngeal contents.

Pneumonia in infants and children is caused by a wider range of microorganisms and, unlike adults, nonbacterial pathogens predominate. Most pneumonias in the pediatric age group are caused by viruses, especially RSV, parainfluenza, and adenovirus. *Mycoplasma pneumonia* is an important pathogen in older children. Beyond the neonatal period, the pneumococcus is the major bacterial pathogen in childhood pneumonia followed by group A streptococcus and *S. aureus. Haemophilus influenza* type B, once a major childhood pathogen, has become an infrequent cause of pneumonia since the introduction of active vaccination against this organism in the late 1980s.

CLINICAL PRESENTATION

BACTERIAL PNEUMONIA

Bacterial pneumonia is most commonly caused by the gram-positive streptococci and staphylococci and gram-negative organisms that normally inhabit the gastrointestinal tract (enterics) and soil and water (nonenterics). In addition, *Legionella multiphilia,* itself a weakly staining gram-negative nonenteric organism, accounts for a small percentage of community- and hospital-acquired bacterial pneumonia. Finally, *Mycobacterium tuberculosis,* an acid-fast staining bacillus, has reemerged as an important cause of pneumonia in urban centers throughout the United States.

Although a wide array of gram-positive and gram-negative organisms can cause pneumonia, they usually present a similar clinical appearance. Typically, the onset of illness is abrupt or subacute, with fever, chills, dyspnea, and productive cough predominating. Pneumococcus, staphylococcus, the enteric gram-negative rods, and occasionally other organisms may produce local irritation or destruction of blood vessels leading to rust-colored sputum or hemoptysis. On physical examination the patient is tachypneic and tachycardiac, frequently with chest wall retractions and grunting respirations. Consolidation of the underlying lung is reflected in diminished breath sounds on auscultation over the affected area accompanied by inspiratory crackles as pus-filled alveoli open during lung expansion. Other signs of localized lung consolidation include dullness to percussion, increased tactile fremitus, whisper pectoriloquy, and egophony. Pleural effusions, both sterile and empyematous, may be associated with many of these entities, evidenced by distant breath sounds and a wide area of dulled percussion.

The chest radiograph and sputum examination and culture are the most useful diagnostic tests in gram-positive and gram-negative bacterial pneumonia. Typically, the chest radiograph reveals a dense lobar or segmental infiltrate. Patchy consolidation occasionally may be seen, however, with virtually all these pathogens. Occasionally, pneumonia resulting from hematogenous spread of the organisms results in a diffuse, alveolar pattern on chest radiograph. Gram stain of the expectorated sputum demonstrates many polymorphonuclear cells per high-powered field in the presence of a predominant organism (see Fig. 98–1), which is reflected in heavy growth of a single species on culture. Other laboratory tests are less sensitive or specific. Blood cultures may be helpful in identifying the offending organism but are positive in only a minority of cases. The complete blood count usually reflects a leukocytosis with a predominance of polymorphonuclear cells; in some instances, particularly pneumococcus, the elevation of the WBC count may be pronounced. Normal or mildly elevated WBC counts, however, do not exclude bacterial pneumonic disease. The patient may also be hypoxic as reflected by low oxygen saturation on arterial blood gas or pulse oximetry.

Although the clinical appearance of the gram-positive and gram-negative pneumonias are similar, there are epidemiologic and clinical clues that render one more likely than the others.

GRAM-POSITIVE BACTERIA

Pneumococcus is the most common community-acquired bacterial pneumonia, accounting for 25% to 70% of cases. It is particularly prevalent and severe in patients with splenic dysfunction, diabetes mellitus, chronic cardiopulmonary or renal disease, or HIV infection. *Staphylococcus aureus* pneumonia occurs in both the community and hospital setting.[49] Community-acquired disease with *S. aureus* is identified most frequently in young infants, patients with early cystic fibrosis, and those recovering from an antecedent respiratory viral infection. *Staphylococcus aureus* is a prominent cause of nosocomial pneumonia and may result from hematogenous spread from a distant source. In both settings, it is characteristically severe and accompanied by the formation of pneumatoceles (air-containing cavities within the lung). Group B streptococcus, while rare in adults, is the most common cause of bacterial pneumonia among neonates, where it typically causes a clinical and radiographic picture nearly indistinguishable from hyaline membrane disease.[50] Group A streptococcus is an uncommon cause of community-acquired pneumonia and frequently occurs after a viral respiratory tract infection. Only occasionally is it associated with streptococcal pharyngitis. The organism is very pyogenic, and the presentation can be severe.

ENTERIC GRAM-NEGATIVE BACTERIA

Community-acquired enteric gram-negative pneumonia is identified most frequently among patients with chronic illness, especially alcoholism and diabetes mellitus. The enteric gram-negative bacteria are also leading causes of nosocomial pneumonia, since the upper respiratory tract becomes rapidly colonized with gram-negative organisms after hospitalization, particularly among critically ill patients and those receiving antibiotics. Outbreaks of nosocomial disease occasionally may be caused by contaminated respiratory therapy equipment. *Klebsiella pneumoniae* is the most frequently encountered pathogen among the gram-negative enteric bacteria, although the relative prominence of these organisms varies from hospital to hospital. The gram-negative bacilli are associated with high mortality, sometimes exceeding 50%; their potential to produce significant morbidity and mortality has also been enhanced by the emergence of highly antibiotic-resistant organisms in some hospital settings.[51]

NONENTERIC GRAM-NEGATIVE BACTERIA

The most prominent nonenteric gram-negative rods associated with pneumonia include *Pseudomonas, Haemophilus,* and *Moraxella.* Like the enteric gram-negative organisms, *Pseudomonas aeruginosa* is a frequent cause of hospital-acquired pneumonia and is particularly prominent among neutropenic and burn patients.[51] In addition, cystic fibrosis patients suffer from chronic, multilobar infections with *P. aeruginosa,* as well as other pseudomonas species; these infections are punctuated with acute exacerbations.[52] *Haemophilus influenza* type B historically has been a prominent pathogen in childhood pneumonia. Since the introduction of the conjugated haemophilus vaccines in the late 1980s, however, there has been a dramatic drop in the incidence of all invasive disease because of this organism in the pediatric age group. Two different clinical presentations of *H. influenza* pneumonia are still seen in adults, however. The most common by far is the bronchopneumonia form, which develops most frequently in patients with underlying chronic lung disease and is believed to represent, in most patients, an exacerbation of chronic bronchitis. In the second form of *H. influenza* pneumonia, segmental or lobar involvement predominates. The course of this illness is more acute, with sudden onset of cough, fever, and pleuritic chest pain. Finally, *M. catarrhalis,* an important cause of otitis media and sinusitis, has been found to be an increasingly important cause of lower respiratory tract infections in immunoincompetent and hospitalized patients.

LEGIONELLA PNEUMOPHILIA

Of the several *Legionella* species known to cause pneumonia in humans, *L. pneumophilia* is by far the most important and accounts for 2% to 15% of all community-acquired pneumonias in North America and Europe.[53] Legionella is a water and soil organism and is most probably transmitted by the inhalation of aerosols containing the organism or by microaspiration of contaminated water. Outbreaks of illness caused by *L. pneumophilia* have been linked to excavation sites and contaminated water from air conditioners and showers. Person-to-person transmission has not been demonstrated. In addition to epidemics, *L. pneumophilia* causes sporadic illness that peaks in summer and fall. Individuals who are male, middle-age or older, immunocompromised, chronic bronchitics, or cigarette smokers are at increased risk.

Infection with *L. pneumophilia* is characterized by multisystem involvement, including rapidly progressive pneumonia. It has a gradual onset, with prominent constitutional symptoms, such as malaise, lethargy, weakness, and anorexia, occurring early in the course of the illness. A dry, nonproductive cough is initially present, which becomes productive of mucoid or purulent sputum over several days. Fevers exceeding 40°C develop in over half of patients and are typically unremitting and associated with a relative bradycardia. Pleuritic chest pain and progressive dyspnea may be seen. Extrapulmonary symptoms remain evident throughout the course of the illness, particularly diarrhea, nausea, and vomiting. Myalgias and arthralgias also occur. Substantial changes in a patient's mental status, often out of proportion to the degree of fever, are seen in approximately one-fourth of patients. Obtundation, hallucinations, grand mal seizures, and focal neurologic findings have also been associated with this illness. Chest roentgenograms initially reveal patchy alveolar infiltrates that may be bilateral. Progression to lobar or multilobar consolidation is frequent, as are small pleural effusions.

Laboratory findings include leukocytosis with a predominance of mature and immature granulocytes in 50% to 75% of patients. Urinalysis may reveal proteinuria, hematuria, and casts; liver function tests may be abnormal. Hyponatremia and hypophosphatemia have also been frequently reported. Because *L. pneumophilia* stains poorly with commonly used stains, routine microscopic examination of sputum is of little diagnostic value. While it exhibits slow growth and has highly selective growth requirements, *L. pneumophilia* has been successfully isolated from tissue using a specialized medium. Direct fluorescent antibody examination of respiratory tract secretions, lung tissue, or pleural fluid is the most rapid means of establishing the diagnosis. The sensitivity of this method approaches 70% for sputum and 90% for lung tissue, and diagnostic specificity is high for both.[53] Commercially available urine antigen tests have been developed for *L. pneumophilia;* these tests are 70% sensitive and remain positive for weeks, even after effective antibiotics have been started. Because these diagnostic tests are unavailable in many clinical laboratories, the diagnosis of Legionnaire's disease often is presumptive and based on a suggestive clinical presentation.

ANAEROBIC PNEUMONIA

Anaerobic pneumonitis is most likely to occur in individuals predisposed to aspiration by impaired consciousness and may be more prevalent in those with periodontal disease or dysphagia. In addition, bronchogenic carcinoma is an associated underlying condition. A variety of gram-positive and gram-negative anaerobic bacteria indigenous to the upper airway may cause pneumonitis when large quantities of oropharyngeal secretions are aspirated into the lower airways. The organisms most frequently implicated are *Peptostreptococcus* sp., *Fusobacteria, Bacteroides melaninogenicus, Bacteroides fragilis,* and *Peptococcus* sp.; polymicrobial infections with anaerobes and aerobes, such as *S. aureus, S. pneumonia,* and gram-negative bacilli, are common.[54]

The course of illness is typically indolent with cough, low-grade fever, and weight loss, although an acute presentation may occur. Rigors are notably absent, and bacteremia is rare. Putrid sputum, when present, is highly suggestive of the diagnosis. Chest radiographs reveal infiltrates typically located in dependent lung segments, and lung abscesses develop in 20% of patients 1 to 2 weeks into the course of the illness.[54,55]

TUBERCULOSIS

Tuberculosis is caused by the acid-fast bacillus *M. tuberculosis.* After years of steady decline, the number of cases of pneumonia caused by *M. tuberculosis* in the United States began to increase in the mid-1980s. The new epidemic is most prominent in urban neighborhoods afflicted with crowded conditions and poor access to health care. Unlike previous eras in which tuberculosis was most frequently seen in elderly men, infection currently is identified in increasing numbers of young minority adults.[56] The reason for the resurgence of tuberculosis is at least partially related to coinfection with HIV; HIV-infected patients are more likely to develop symptomatic disease with its associated fits of coughing than their immunocompetent counterparts, and this enables further spread of infection.[57] Other groups prone to tuberculosis include the homeless, patients in chronic care facilities and homes for the elderly, and recent immigrants from areas of the world in which tuberculosis remains endemic. The reemergence of tuberculosis in the United States has been accompanied by the development of multiple-drug resistance, that is, of mycobacteria that are resistant to two or more of the first-line antituberculous drugs. Infection caused by these organisms is poorly responsive to alternative therapy and is associated with mortality rates exceeding 50% (see Chap. 102).

Tuberculosis is spread person-to-person through the inhalation of droplet nuclei generated by vigorous coughing. The majority of patients who become infected with *M. tuberculosis* remain asymptomatic despite life-long infection and have a normal chest radiograph. Infection in these patients is detected only through routine skin testing. Less frequently, particularly in those with poor immunity, the infection cannot be contained by local macrophages, and the tuberculous burden grows sufficiently to cause clinical manifestations.

Adult disease (from adolescence onward) begins with constitutional complaints followed by a prominent chronic, troublesome cough productive of mucopurulent material. The infection initially appears in the lung apices with little or no hilar adenopathy and, in advanced disease, results in lung necrosis, producing a cavity containing enormous numbers of organisms. With sufficient cough, the cavitary contents are mobilized and aspirated into other areas of the lung, where additional cavities may be formed.

In contrast, pediatric tuberculosis commonly is associated with little cough even in the presence of extensive pulmonary infection. Instead, the child presents with a subacute course of poor appetite, weight loss, lethargy, fever, and sweats. The chest radiograph reveals a widened mediastinum representing enlarged hilar lymph nodes reacting to the tuberculin inoculum. In progressive cases, the nodes impinge upon or erode through a large bronchus, resulting in a dense consolidation of the segment distal to the lesion. Cavitary disease is uncommon.

NONBACTERIAL PNEUMONIA

Viruses, mycoplasma species, chlamydial species, and fungi are recognized causes of pneumonia syndromes in all age groups. The designation atypical pneumonia, distinct from the typical bacterial pneumonia most commonly seen in adults, has been used to describe the illness caused by many of these agents.[58]

MYCOPLASMA PNEUMONIA

Taxonomically, the mycoplasmas are included in their own class labeled Mollicutes. Although their small size and filterability are similar to viruses, the structure of their ribosomal RNA indicates that they have evolved from bacteria, and, unlike any virus, they contain cytoplasm and can replicate in an extracellular environment. They are distinguished from eubacteria by their low genetic content; in addition, the mycoplasmas lack a cell wall and are surrounded instead by a lipid membrane.[58]

Mycoplasma pneumonia causes human disease throughout the year, with a slightly increased incidence in fall and early winter. During the summer months when other causes of pneumonia are less common, *M. pneumonia* is responsible for a greater proportion of cases. Both infection and disease from *M. pneumonia* are common, with two-thirds of children ages 2 to 5 years and 97% of persons older than 17 years of age having detectable serum antibody to the organism. Overall, *M. pneumonia* is responsible for approximately 20% of pneumonia cases, although in enclosed populations, such as military recruits and college dormitory residents, it may cause more than 50%. Infection is spread by close person-to-person contact, and the incubation period is 2 to 3 weeks. *Mycoplasma pneumonia* infections are unusual in children under 5 years of age and show a peak incidence in older children and young adults. Only 3% to 10% of persons infected with *M. pneumonia* develop pneumonia, with the majority of respiratory tract involvement being manifested as pharyngitis and tracheobronchitis. Asymptomatic infection is apparently common.

Mycoplasma pneumonia presents with a gradual onset of fever, headache, and malaise, with the appearance 3 to 5 days after the onset of illness of a persistent, hacking cough that initially is nonproductive. Sore throat, ear pain, and rhinorrhea are often present. Chills are only occasionally seen, and pleuritic pain is uncommon. Lung findings are generally limited to rales and rhonchi; findings of consolidation are rarely present. Nonpulmonary manifestations are extremely common and include nausea, vomiting, diarrhea, myalgias, arthralgias, polyarticular arthritis, skin rashes, myocarditis and pericarditis, hemolytic anemia, meningoencephalitis, cranial neuropathies, and Guillain-Barré syndrome. Systemic symptoms generally clear in 1 to 2 weeks, while respiratory symptoms may persist for up to 4 weeks. Although the course of mycoplasmal pneumonia is usually benign and self-limited, severe respiratory disease may develop in patients with sickle cell disease, agammaglobulinemia, and chronic obstructive lung disease.[58]

Radiographic findings are generally more impressive than the patient's physical findings and include patchy or interstitial infiltrates, which are most commonly seen in the lower lobes. Small unilateral, transient pleural effusions are common, but large effusions and empyema are rare. Roentgenographic abnormalities resolve slowly, and 4 to 6 weeks may be required for complete resolution.

Sputum Gram stain may reveal mononuclear or polymorphonuclear leukocytes, with no predominant organism. Although *M. pneumonia* can be cultured from respiratory secretions using specialized medium, its growth is slow and 2 to 3 weeks may be necessary for culture identification. Indirect evidence of infection by *M. pneumonia* is the presence of elevated levels of serum cold hemagglutinins. These immunoglobulin M (IgM) antibodies develop in approximately half of patients with mycoplasmal pneumonia and can be elevated in other illnesses, especially viral infection. A definitive diagnosis can also be made by demonstrating a fourfold or greater rise in serum antibodies to *M. pneumonia;* however, because this test also requires 2 to 4 weeks for results, the diagnosis of mycoplasmal pneumonia during the acute phase of the illness must be based on the characteristic history, appropriate clinical setting, and typical physical findings.

CHLAMYDIAL PNEUMONIA

Chlamydia pneumoniae, formally designated the "TWAR agent," after the laboratory designations for the first two isolates, is a relatively recently identified pathogen antigenically similar to *Chlamydia psitttaci. Chlamydia pneumoniae* infection is ubiquitous worldwide, but only a small percentage of infections results in clinically apparent pneumonia.[59] Conversely, approximately 5% to 15% of pneumonia is associated with this pathogen. Primary-infection chlamydia pneumonia typically occurs in young adults and is characterized by mild respiratory symptoms with a gradual onset. Constitutional manifestations, particularly fever and headache, are common. The radiographic findings are nonspecific and usually consist of multilobular interstitial infiltrates. Immunity is incomplete, and reinfection with *C. pneumoniae* is common, particularly among the elderly. The definitive diagnosis of *C. pneumoniae*-associated pneumonia depends on identification of the organism in sputum. Culture of this organism is difficult, however, and antigen detection systems, though commercially available, are insensitive.

VIRAL PNEUMONIA

Viruses are not a common cause of pneumonia in adults except in the immunosuppressed. Influenza virus, usually type A, is the most common cause of pneumonia in the adult civilian population, whereas adenoviruses cause most cases in military trainees. In contrast, viruses are by far the most common agents producing pneumonia in infants and young children, with RSV, parainfluenza, and adenovirus producing most cases.

All viral respiratory tract infections occur more commonly in the winter, and rapid person-to-person spread through susceptible populations is typical. Underlying cardiac or pulmonary disease predisposes to an increased incidence and severity of viral lower respiratory tract infection, especially with influenza virus in adults and RSV in children. Radiographic findings are nonspecific and include bronchial wall thickening and perihilar and diffuse interstitial infiltrates. Pleural effusions may be seen, especially in adenovirus and parainfluenza pneumonia.

The clinical pictures produced by respiratory viruses are sufficiently variable and overlap to such a degree that an etiologic diagnosis cannot confidently be made on clinical grounds alone. Although virus isolation in tissue culture is possible, 7 or more days is often required for virus identification; thus, this method usually cannot be relied on for definitive diagnosis during the acute phase of illness. Serologic tests for virus-specific antibodies are often used in the diagnosis of viral infections. The diagnostic fourfold rise in titer between acute and convalescent phase sera may require 2 to 3 weeks to develop. Same-day diagnosis of viral infections is now possible through the use of indirect immunofluorescence tests on exfoliated cells from the respiratory tract. The immunofluorescence technique frequently employs a battery of monoclonal antibodies, including those against influenza A and B, RSV, parainfluenza, and adenovirus to provide rapid diagnosis of a range of viral infections.[37]

PNEUMONIA IN SPECIAL CLINICAL CIRCUMSTANCES

PNEUMONIA IN THE HUMAN IMMUNODEFICIENCY VIRUS-INFECTED PATIENT

Human immunodeficiency virus infects and destroys helper T lymphocytes bearing the CD4 surface molecule; these cells are critical for orchestrating a wide variety of immunologic responses. Their depletion consequently results in the dysfunction of both cell-mediated and humoral immunity. As a result, a broad range of pathogens can cause pneumonia in HIV infection (Table 98–4).[60–62] The HIV-infected patient may be afflicted with pneumonia multiple times in his or her lifetime, particularly in the advanced stages of the disease, and a given episode may be caused by more than one species.

The clinical presentation of pneumonia in HIV-infected persons is frequently not helpful in distinguishing one pathogen from another. The pneumonia usually is subacute in onset and consists of fever, nonproductive cough, and dyspnea. Radiographically, most of these entities produce a multilobular or diffuse pattern. Some practitioners initially treat the HIV-infected patient with pneumonia empirically, covering the most common entities (bacteria and *P. carinii*). More frequently, however, given the wide array of possible pathogens, a specific microbiologic diagnosis is aggressively pursued early in the patient's course through sputum induction or bronchoalveolar lavage to allow a rational choice of an antimicrobial regimen.[60–62] The diagnosis and treatment of HIV-infected patients with pulmonary disease is discussed in detail in Chap. 114.

PNEUMONIA IN THE NEUTROPENIC HOST

Neutropenia in the cancer patient is a common complication of aggressive chemotherapy but occasionally can result from the cancer itself. The risk of infection in the cytopenic

TABLE 98–4. Pulmonary Complications of Human Immunodeficiency Virus Infection[60]

Infections
Viruses
Cytomegalovirus
Herpes simplex virus
Varicella-zoster virus
Respiratory syncytial virus and other common respiratory pathogens (parainfluenza virus, adenovirus)
Measles virus
Bacteria
Pyogenic organisms (especially *Streptococcus pneumoniae, Haemophilus influenzae;* in late disease, *S. aureus,* and gram-negatives)
Mycobacterium tuberculosis
Mycobacterium avium complex and other nontuberculous mycobacteria
Fungi
Histoplasma capsulatum
Coccidioides immitus
Cryptococcus neoformans
Candida sp.
Aspergillus sp.
Parasites
Pneumocystis carinii
Toxoplasma gondii
Cryptosporidia
Strongyloides stercoralis
Malignancies
Kaposi's sarcoma
Non-Hodgkin's lymphoma
Smooth muscle tumors
Lymphocytic interstitial pneumonitis
Nonspecific interstitial pneumonitis
Drug-induced pneumonitis

patient is significantly increased when the absolute neutrophil count falls below 500 cells/mm^3 and the neutropenia persists for longer than 7 days.[63–65] In many patients, the duration of chemotherapy-induced cytopenia can be reduced by the judicious application of colony-stimulating factors.[66,67]

The organisms that cause pneumonia in the cytopenic cancer patient include a broad range of bacteria and fungi. Prominent among these are enteric and nonenteric (particularly pseudomonas) gram-negative rods, streptococci, and staphylococci, as well as the fungi candida, aspergillus, and Mucor.[63–65] The chest radiograph may reveal the lobar pattern typical of bacterial infection in the normal host, or it may exhibit a diffuse pattern; sometimes the pneumonia remains invisible by chest radiograph until the neutropenia resolves. Noninfectious entities may also cause pulmonary symptoms; these include toxicity from radiation or chemotherapy or infiltration of the lung parenchyma by the tumor itself.

NOSOCOMIAL PNEUMONIA

After the urinary tract and the bloodstream, the lungs are the most frequent site of infection acquired in the hospital.[51,68] Nosocomial pneumonia is seen most commonly in critically ill patients. Several factors have been identified that predispose to the development of nosocomial pneumonia, including the severity of illness, duration of hospitalization, and prior antibiotic exposure. The strongest predisposing factor, however, is mechanical ventilation (intubation), which bypasses the natural airway defenses against the migration of upper respiratory tract organisms into the lower tract. This situation is exacerbated by the wide use of H_2-receptor blocking agents in the intensive care unit.[51,69] Such use increases the pH of gastric secretions and may promote the proliferation of microorganisms in the upper gastrointestinal tract. Subclinical microaspirations are events that occur routinely in intubated patients resulting in the inoculation of bacteria-contaminated gastric contents into the lung and a higher incidence of nosocomial pneumonia.

The organisms most commonly associated with nosocomial pneumonia are *S. aureus* and enteric and nonenteric gram-negative bacilli, the organisms that colonize the pharynx of the hospitalized, critically ill patient. The diagnosis of nosocomial pneumonia is usually established by the presence of a new infiltrate on chest radiograph, fever, worsening respiratory status, and the appearance of thick, neutrophil-laden respiratory secretions. In actuality, the diagnosis is often difficult to make in the intensively ill patient with underlying lung pathology that can itself be associated with an abnormal, changing radiograph, such as congestive heart failure or chronic lung disease. Broad-spectrum antibiotics frequently are started empirically even in equivocal circumstances, with bronchoscopy reserved for poorly responsive cases.[68,70]

▶ TREATMENT: Pneumonia

DESIRED OUTCOME

Eradication of the offending organism through the selection of the appropriate antibiotic and complete clinical cure are the goals of therapy for bacterial pneumonia. Therapy should minimize associated morbidity, including either one of both of these: reversible or irreversible disease and drug-induced organ toxicity (e.g., renal, lung, or hepatic dysfunction). Most cases of viral pneumonia are self-limiting, although therapy of influenza pneumonia with specific antiviral agents (amantidine or rimantidine) may hasten recovery. All efforts should focus on the design of the most cost-effective approach to therapy. Whenever possible, the oral (versus parenteral) route for drug administration should be selected, encouraging outpatient management rather than hospitalization.

GENERAL APPROACH TO TREATMENT

The first priority in assessing the patient with pneumonia is to evaluate the adequacy of respiratory function and determine whether there are signs of systemic illness, specifically dehydration or sepsis with resulting circulatory collapse. Oxygen or, in severe cases, mechanical ventilation and fluid resuscitation should be provided as necessary. The second priority is to obtain appropriate sputum samples to determine the microbiologic etiology. In many cases of community-acquired pneumonia, an antibiotic can be selected accurately without sputum sampling, but in complicated cases (for example, the immunocompromised host) samples may have to be obtained through invasive means. Rehydration should be provided to replace losses that may have occurred because of fever, poor intake, associated vomiting, or all of these. Finally, selection of an appropriate antimicrobial must be made based on the patient's probable or documented microbiology, distribution in the respiratory tract, side effects, and cost.

NONPHARMACOLOGIC THERAPY

The supportive care of the patient with pneumonia includes humidified oxygen for hypoxemia, administration of bronchodilators (albuterol) when bronchospasm is present, and chest physiotherapy with postural drainage if there is evidence of retained secretions. Additional therapeutic adjuncts include adequate hydration (intravenously if necessary), optimal nutritional support, and control of fever.

PHARMACOLOGIC THERAPY

The treatment of bacterial pneumonia, like the treatment of most infectious diseases, initially involves the empiric institution of a relatively broad-spectrum antibiotic that is effective against probable pathogens after appropriate cultures and specimens for laboratory evaluation have been obtained. Therapy should be narrowed to cover specific pathogens once the results of cultures are known. Multiple factors that help define the potential pathogens involved include patient age, previous and current medication history, underlying disease(s), major organ function, and present clinical status. These factors must be evaluated to select properly an effective empiric antibiotic regimen, as well as the most appropriate route for drug administration (oral, parenteral). For a more detailed discussion on the principles of antibiotic selection, see Chap. 96.

Numerous antibiotics are available, and the majority have been shown to be effective in the treatment of bacterial pneumonia. Superiority of one compound over another when both demonstrate similar *in vitro* activity and tissue distribution characteristics is difficult to define. Our opinions on appropriate empiric choices for the treatment of bacterial pneumonias relative to a patient's underlying disease are shown in Table 98–5 for adults and Table 98–6 for children. A complete listing of antimicrobial agents for specifically directed therapy is beyond the scope of this chapter and is presented in Chap. 96.

The plethora of commercially available antimicrobial agents with documented bacterial and clinical effectiveness in the treatment of pneumonia often appears endless. These large numbers of frequently expensive drugs mandate critical evaluation for formulary selection and clinical use. Similarities in *in vitro* activity, resistance to bacterial-inactivating enzymes, and overall effectiveness often make rational therapeutic decisions difficult and

TABLE 98–5. Empiric Antimicrobial Therapy for Pneumonia in Adults[a]

Clinical Setting	Usual Pathogen(s)	Presumptive Therapy
Previously healthy, ambulatory patient	Pneumococcus, *Mycoplasma pneumoniae*	Macrolide/azilide,[b] tetracycline[c]
Elderly	Pneumococcus, gram-negative bacilli (such as *Klebsiella pneumoniae*), *Staphylococcus aureus, Haemophilus influenzae*	Ticarcillin/clavulanate, piperacillin/tazobactam, cephalosporin[d]; carbapenem[e]
Chronic bronchitis	Pneumococcus, *H. influenzae, M. catarrhalis*	Amoxicillin, tetracycline,[c] TMP/SMZ,[f] cefuroxime, cefprozil, amoxicillin/clavulanate, macrolide/azilide,[b] quinolone
Alcoholism	Pneumococcus, *K. pneumoniae, S. aureus, H. influenzae,* possibly mouth anaerobes	Ticarcillin/clavulanate, piperacillin/tazobactam, plus aminoglycoside; carbapenem[e]
Aspiration		
Community	Mouth anaerobes	Penicillin or clindamycin
Hospital/residential care	Mouth anaerobes, *S. aureus,* gram-negative enterics	Clindamycin, ticarcillin/clavulanate, piperacillin/tazobactam, plus aminoglycoside
Nosocomial pneumonia	Gram-negative bacilli (such as *K. pneumoniae,* Enterobacter sp., *Pseudomonas aeruginosa), S. aureus*	Ticarcillin/clavulanate, piperacillin/tazobactam, carbapenem[e] or expanded spectrum cephalosporin[g] plus aminoglycoside

[a]See section on treatment of bacterial pneumonia.
[b]Macrolide/azilide: erythromycin, clarithromycin/azithromycin.
[c]Tetracycline: tetracycline Hcl, doxycycline.
[d]Cephalosporin: cefuroxime, ceftriaxone, cefotaxime.
[e]Carbapenem: imipenem/cilistatin, meropenem.
[f]TMP/SMZ, trimethoprim–sulfamethoxazole.
[g]Expanded spectrum cephalosporin: ceftazidime, cefepime.

TABLE 98–6. Empiric Antimicrobial Therapy for Pneumonia in Pediatric Patients[a]

Age	Usual Pathogen(s)	Presumptive Therapy
1 month	Group B streptococcus, *Haemophilus influenzae* (nontypeable), *Escherichia coli, Staphylococcus aureus, Listeria*	Ampicillin/sulbactam, cephalosporin[b] carbapenem[c]
	CMV, RSV, adenovirus	Ribavirin for RSV
1–3 months	*Chlamydia,* possibly *Ureaplasma,* CMV, *Pneumocystis carinii* (afebrile pneumonia syndrome)	Macrolide/azilide,[d] TMP/SMZ
	RSV	Ribavirin
	Pneumococcus, *S. aureus*	Semisynthetic penicillin[e] or cephalosporin[f]
3 months–6 years	Pneumococcus, *H. influenzae,* RSV, adenovirus, parainfluenza	Amoxicillin or cephalosporin[f] Ampicillin/sulbactam, amoxicillin/clavulanate Ribavirin for RSV
6 years	Pneumococcus, *Mycoplasma pneumoniae,* adenovirus	Macrolide/azilide[d] Cephalosporin,[f] amoxicillin/clavulanate

CMV = cytomegalovirus; RSV = respiratory syncytial virus; TMP/SMZ = trimethoprim–sulfamethoxazole.
[a]See section on treatment of bacterial pneumonia.
[b]Third-generation cephalosporin: ceftriaxone, cefotaxime, cefepime. Note that cephalosporins are not active against *Listeria.*
[c]Carbapenem: imipenem/cilistatin, meropenem.
[d]Macrolide/azilide: erythromycin, clarithromycin–azithromycin.
[e]Semisynthetic penicillin: nafcillin, oxacillin.
[f]Second-generation cephalosporin: cefuroxime, cefprozil.
See text for details regarding ribavirin treatment for RSV infection.

even appear random. Some general principles, however, may be applied to guide rational antibiotic choice. First, in community-acquired pneumonia the bacterial causes are relatively constant, even across geographic areas and patient populations. Unfortunately, pathogen resistance to standard antimicrobials is increasing (e.g., penicillin-resistant pneumococci) necessitating careful attention by the clinician to local and regional bacterial susceptibility patterns. Thus, whenever possible based on presumed antibacterial susceptibility, initial therapy should consist of older, less expensive agents, with newer antibiotics reserved for unresponsive illness or special circumstances. The indiscriminate use of recently introduced agents increases health care costs and, in some instances (such as with the widespread use of quinolones), induces resistance among a significant percentage of community-acquired organisms.[71] It must be emphasized, however, that the rapidly evolving epidemiology of bacterial resistance, including the increasing emergence of penicillin-resistant pneumococcus in many areas of the United States and Europe,[73] forces the clinician to be vigilant and knowledgeable about antibiotic sensitivity patterns in each community.

In contrast, antibiotic selection within the hospital environment demands greater care because of constant changes in antibiotic resistance patterns *in vitro* and *in vivo.* Ironically, some β-lactam antibiotics, which were developed to treat multiple antibiotic-resistant hospital-acquired organisms, can themselves induce broad-spectrum bacterial β-lactamases and thereby lead to even greater problems with resistance.[73] These facts underscore the importance of regularly documenting the epidemiology of pathogens and infectious diseases within a specific practice or institution. As a result, an antimicrobial agent for a specific infectious disease favored in one practice site may not be the most desirable selection in another, despite similarities in size and patient profile. Strict and careful control and, possibly, rotation of empiric antibiotics in the hospital environment may help to limit the emergence of resistant organisms. Newer antibiotics developed to treat resistant, hospital-acquired pathogens are, however, costly; therefore, their use must be moderated to some extent in an era where capitated hospital costs and mandated budget cuts will not tolerate careless antibiotic use (see Chap. 96).

The *in vitro* spectrum of antibacterial activity of systemically absorbed fluoroquinolone antibiotics, such as ciprofloxacin, clinafloxacin, enoxacin, grepafloxacin, ofloxacin, pefloxacin, and trovafloxacin, would suggest that these drugs have an important role in the treatment of bacterial infections of the lower respiratory tract. Numerous clinical studies describe the efficacy of these drugs for the treatment of purulent bronchitis, acute exacerbations of chronic bronchitis, pneumonia, and cystic fibrosis. The widespread use of earlier analogs (ciprofloxacin) by primary care physicians has led, however, to pathogen resistance and treatment failures, including, perhaps most important, isolates of *S. pneumonia.* Although newer quinolones are more active against common respiratory tract pathogens than older agents, this experience renders it difficult to recommend their indiscriminate use for routine community-acquired pneumonia. Nevertheless, these drugs may be effective alternative agents for the treatment of community-acquired pneumonia or in the initial treatment of nosocomial pneumonia for hospitalized patients and patients residing in extended-care facilities. The availability of newer analogs with broad spectrums of antibacterial activity, including *S. pneumoniae* and anaerobes (trovafloxacin) further enhances the desirability of a quinolone as a first-line agent, expanding the therapeutic armamentarium for both community-acquired and nosocomially acquired pneumonia. At present, quinolone use in pediatrics remains restricted and limited because of possible fluoroquinolone-induced destructive lesions of growing cartilage primarily of the weight-bearing joints. The need for quinolones for the treatment of selected infections arising in pediatric patients continues, however, and their safety in these patients has served as the foundation for ongoing controlled, clinical efficacy and safety trials in pediatric patients.

Among the more recently introduced classes of oral antibiotics, the newer macrolides possess excellent activity against most *S. pneumonia* and mycoplasma. Azithromycin and clarithromycin appear to offer highly viable alternative agents to erythromycin, particularly in those patients who are intolerant to erythromycin analogs (e.g., gastrointestinal upset) and, for azithromycin, patients who are taking medications that may result in a clinically significant drug–drug interaction with erythromycin (astemizole, terfenadine, carbamazepine, theophylline).[35] Azithromycin offers the added advantage of once daily dosing and short-course therapy because of the drug's extensive tissue distribution characteristics and prolonged elimination half-life.[35]

Numerous investigators have demonstrated that antibiotic concentrations in respiratory secretions in excess of the pathogen minimal inhibitory concentration (MIC) are necessary for successful treatment of pulmonary infections.[74,75] The concept of a blood–bronchus barrier, analogous but dissimilar to the blood–brain barrier, has been used to assess the characteristics of drug penetration into pulmonary secretions. The ability of a drug to penetrate respiratory secretions depends on multiple physicochemical factors, including molecular size, lipid solubility, and degree of ionization at serum and biologic fluid pH. Studies performed in animals and cystic fibrosis patients suggest that larger molecular size favors the accumulation of drugs in bronchial secretions. This finding contrasts with data on drug penetration of other physiologic compartments, such as the cerebrospinal fluid, and may be a result of the trapping of lower molecular weight compounds in mucin pores. Nevertheless, the rate at which a drug may accumulate in certain respiratory secretions would appear to remain an important factor relative to the drug's clinical efficacy in treating pulmonary infections. The un-ionized form of a drug and lipid solubility also appear to favor drug penetration. It should be noted that the pH of the infected bronchi is often more acidic than that of normal tissue and blood.[74–76]

Fewer data are available for assessing the influence of drug protein binding on the rate and amount of respiratory secretion penetration. As the degree of protein binding has been shown to influence a drug's ability to traverse membranes, a similar relationship would be expected within the lung. Thus, it is prudent to assess the pharmacokinetic–pharmacodynamic correlates of drug binding to serum proteins, tissue distribution, and *in vitro* potency when selecting an antimicrobial regimen. These concepts relating to overall drug penetration of respiratory secretions and others have led to the clinical practice of administering certain antibiotics (aminoglycosides) to achieve high peak serum concentrations on the assumption that higher (and possibly more effective) biologic fluid concentrations of the drug will be achieved. Substantial clinical experience supports this practice for treating pulmonary infections with certain antibiotics, although more data are needed to describe the relationships between these variables and clinical response.

Prior to the availability of newer β-lactam and quinolone antibiotics possessing consistently potent activity against multiple gram-negative pathogens, the administration of antibiotics by direct endotracheal instillation was promoted by some investigators.[75,77] This method of drug administration is an attempt to provide increased topical concentrations of antibiotics that do not appear to penetrate respiratory secretions effectively while reducing the likelihood of systemic toxicity. In addition, greater local concentrations of antibiotics, particularly for the polymyxins and aminoglycosides, are believed to overcome partially the substantial decrease in antibiotic bioactivity observed when these agents interact with the purulent material present in infectious foci.[75–77] Despite these potential theoretical advantages, the role of antibiotic aerosols or direct endotracheal instillation in clinical practice remains ill defined.

Sputum is frequently assessed as possibly representing the pharmacodynamic interface for pulmonary infections. It should be noted that sputum represents only one of many pulmonary fluids and secretions, although sputum may serve as a reservoir for pathogen growth. These beliefs have led many investigators to assess antibiotic concentrations in sputum, frequently describing sputum drug concentrations as a ratio of serum to sputum drug concentration. Although sputum drug concentrations provide us with some insight into the characteristics of drug penetration of respiratory secretions, caution should be exercised in the interpretation of these data. Data describing sputum drug concentrations are often difficult to interpret because of differences in analytic techniques, method of sputum sampling, and random nature of sampling times relative to drug dose. Moreover, representation of sputum drug concentrations as a ratio of serum drug concentration can be misleading and most probably should be described relative to absolute drug concentration or apparent area under the drug-concentration curve in sputum. To describe more accurately the distribution characteristics of antimicrobial agents in sputum, research studies should be designed to allow sequential repeated sputum sampling over a dosage interval under both first-dose and steady-state conditions.

PREVENTION

Prevention of some cases of pneumonia is possible through the use of vaccines against selected infectious agents. Inactivated influenza virus vaccines formulated annually to contain antigens representative of expected prevalent strains are widely available and generally well tolerated. Immunization is recommended for individuals likely to experience serious complications from influenza infection, such as patients with underlying heart or lung disease, chronic renal disease, and the elderly. Although it should not replace active immunization, amantadine may be administered for prevention of influenza A infection, beginning as soon as possible after exposure and continuing for at least 10 days. The recommended dose is 5 mg/kg/d in two to three divided doses not to exceed 150 mg/d in children 1 to 9 years old and 200 mg/d in two divided doses in patients 9 years or older. In addition, polyvalent polysaccharide vaccines are available for two of the leading causes of bacterial pneumonia, pneumococcus and *H. influenzae* type B. For a detailed description of the use of these vaccines, the reader is referred to Chapter 113.

EVALUATION OF THERAPEUTIC OUTCOMES

Once therapy has been instituted, appropriate clinical parameters should be monitored to ensure efficacy and safety of the therapeutic regimen. In patients with bacterial infections of the upper or lower respiratory tract, the time to resolution of initial presenting symptoms and the lack of appearance of new associated symptomatology is important to determine. In patients with community-acquired pneumonia or pneumonia from any source of mild to moderate clinical severity, the time to resolution of cough, decreasing sputum production, and fever, as well as other constitutional symptoms of malaise, nausea, vomiting, and lethargy should be noted. If the patient requires supplemental oxygen therapy, the amount and need should also be regularly assessed. A gradual and persistent improvement in the resolution of these symptoms and therapies should be observed. Initial resolution should be observed within the first 2 days progressing to complete resolution within 5 to 7 but usually no more than 10 days. In patients with nosocomial pneumonia or substantial underlying diseases, or both, additional parameters can be followed including the magnitude and character of the peripheral blood WBC count, chest radiograph, and blood gas determinations. Similar to patients with less severe disease, some resolution of symptoms should be observed within 2 days of instituting antibiotic therapy. If within 2 days of starting seemingly appropriate antibiotic therapy, no resolution of symptoms are observed or if the patient's clinical status is deteriorating, the appropriateness of initial antibiotic therapy should be critically reassessed. The patient should be carefully evaluated for deterioration in their underlying concurrent disease(s). Additionally, the caregiver should consider the possibility of changing the initial antibiotic therapy to expand antimicrobial coverage not included in the original regimen (e.g., mycoplasma, legionella, and anaerobes). Further, the possible need for antifungal therapy (amphotericin b) should be considered. Some resolution of symptoms should be observed within 2 days of starting proper antibiotic therapy with complete resolution expected within 10 to 14 days.

▶ PRINCIPLES OF PHARMACOTHERAPY

- In the United States, respiratory infections remain the major cause of morbidity from acute illness and most likely represent the most common reasons patients seek medical attention.
- The majority of pulmonary infections follow colonization of the upper respiratory tract with potential pathogens, whereas less commonly, microbes gain access to the lung via the blood from an extrapulmonary source or by inhalation of infected aerosol particles. The competency of a patient's immune status is an important factor influencing the susceptibility to infection, etiologic cause, and disease severity.
- An appropriate treatment regimen for the patient with uncomplicated lower respiratory tract infection can usually be established by patient history, physical examination, chest radiograph, and properly collected sputum for culture interpreted in light of current knowledge of the most common lung pathogens and their antibiotic susceptibility patterns within one's community.
- Acute bronchitis is most commonly caused by respiratory viruses and almost always is self-limiting with therapy targeting associated symptoms, such as lethargy, malaise, or fever (ibuprofen or acetaminophen); fluids for rehydration; and in some patients, cough suppressants. The routine use of antibiotics should be avoided.
- Chronic bronchitis is a result of several contributing factors; the most prominent of these are cigarette smoking, exposure to occupational dusts, fumes, environmental pollution, and bacterial (and possibly viral) infection. The hallmark of this disease is chronic cough productive of purulent sputum and the persistent presence of microorganisms in the patient's sputum.
- The treatment of acute exacerbations of chronic bronchitis include attempts to mobilize and enhance sputum expectoration (chest physiotherapy, humidification of inspired air), oxygen if needed, aerosolized bronchodilators (albuterol) in select patients with demonstrated benefit and antibiotics.
- Antibiotic selection for the treatment of acute exacerbations of chronic bronchitis is dependent on the drug's inherent activity against presumed and identified pathogens, the patient's severity of disease (see Table 98–1), least propensity for drug–drug interactions, and cost.
- Respiratory syncytial virus is the most common cause of acute bronchiolitis, an infection mostly affecting infants during their first year of life. In the well infant, bronchiolitis is usually a self-limiting viral illness, whereas in the child with underlying respiratory or cardiac disease, or both, he or she may develop severe respiratory compromise (failure) necessitating in-hospital treatment (such as rehydration, oxygen, and in select patients, bronchodilator, ribavirin aerosol, or both).
- The most prominent pathogens causing community-acquired pneumonia in otherwise healthy adults are *S. pneumoniae* (~70%) and *M. pneumoniae* (~ 10% to 20%) whereas the most common pathogens causing hospital-acquired pneumonia (including nursing home residents) are *S. aureus* and gram-negative aerobic bacilli. Anaerobic bacteria are the most common etiologic agents in pneumonia that follows aspiration of gastric or oropharyngeal contents.
- Uncomplicated community-acquired pneumonia can usually be effectively treated with oral antibiotics. Humidified oxygen for hypoxemia, bronchodilators (albuterol) when bronchospasm is present, rehydration fluids, and chest physiotherapy for marked accumulation of retained respiratory secretions may be needed. Antibiotic regimens should be selected based on presumed causative pathogens (see Tables 98–5 and 98–6) and pulmonary distribution characteristics, and they should be adjusted to provide optimal activity against pathogens identified by culture (sputum or blood).

REFERENCES

1. Kolls JK, Nelson S, Summer WR. Recombinant cytokines and pulmonary host defense. Am J Med Sci 1993;306:330–335.
2. Ward PA. Role of compliment, chemokines and regulatory cytokines in acute lung injury. Ann NY Acad Sci 1996;796:104–112.

3. Mason CM, Nelson S. Normal host defenses and impairments associated with the delayed resolution of pneumonia. Sem Resp Infect 1992;7:243–255.
4. Standiford TJ. Cytokines and pulmonary defenses. Curr Opin Pulm Med 1997;3:81–88.
5. Todd JK. Bacteriology and clinical relevance of nasopharyngeal and oropharyngeal cultures. Pediatr Infect Dis 1984;3:159–163.
6. Yungbluth M. The laboratory diagnosis of pneumonia: The role of the community hospital pathologist. Clin Lab Med 1995;15:209–234.
7. Griffen JJ, Meduri GU. New approaches in the diagnosis of nosocomial pneumonia. Med Clin North Am 1994;78:1091–1122.
8. Cook DJ, Brun-Buisson C, Guyatt GH, et al. Evaluation of new diagnostic technologies: Bronchoalveolar lavage and the diagnosis of ventilator associated pneumonia. Crit Care Med 1994;22:1314–1322.
9. Galvin JR, Gingrich RD, Hoffman E, et al. Ultrafast computed tomography of the chest. Radiol Clin North Am 1994;32:775–793.
10. Marik PE, Brown WJ. A comparison of bronchoscopic vs. blind protected specimen brush sampling in patients with suspected ventilator-associated pneumonia. Chest 1995;108:207.
11. Kirtland SH, Corley DE, Winterbauer RH, et al. The diagnosis of ventilator-associated pneumonia: A comparison of histologic, microbiologic, and clinical criteria. Chest 1997;112:445–457.
12. Jimenez P, Saldias F, Meneses M, et al. Diagnostic bronchoscopy in patients with community-acquired pneumonia: Comparison between bronchoalveolar lavage and telescoping plugged catheter cultures. Chest 1993;103:1023–1027.
13. Stark JM. Lung infections in children. Curr Opinion Pediatr 1993;5: 273–280.
14. Everard ML. Bronchiolitis: Origins and optimal management. Drugs 1995;49:885–896.
15. Aldous MB, Grayston JT, Wang SP, et al. Seroepidemiology of *Chlamydia pneumoniae* TWAR infection in Seattle families, 1966–1979. J Infect Dis 1992;166:646–649.
16. Stark JM, Busse WW. Respiratory virus infection and airway hyperreactivity in children. Pediatr Allergy Immunol 1991;2:95–110.
17. Lebowitz MD, Burrows B. The relationship of acute respiratory illness history to the prevalence and incidence of obstructive lung disorders. Am J Epidemiol 1977;105:544–554.
18. Krasinski K, LaCouture R, Holzman RS. Screening for respiratory syncytial virus and assignment to a cohort at admission to reduce nosocomial transmission. J Pediatr 1990;116:894–898.
19. Black S. Epidemiology of pertusis. Pediatr Infect Dis J 1997;16(suppl 4):S85–S89.
20. Visentin M, Salmona M, Tacconi MT. Reye's and Reye-like syndromes: Drug-related diseases? Drug Metab Rev 1995;27:517–539.
21. Hendeles L. Efficacy and safety of antihistamines and expectorants in nonprescription cough and cold preparations. Pharmacotherapy 1993; 13:154–158.
22. Irwin RS, Curley FJ, Bennett FM. Appropriate use of antitussives and protussives: A practical review. Drugs 1993;46:80–91.
23. MacKay DN. Treatment of acute bronchitis in adults without underlying lung disease. J Gen Intern Med 1996;11:557–562.
24. Nicholson KG. Use of antivirals in influenza in the elderly: Prophylaxis and therapy. Gerontology 1996;42:280–289.
25. Chodosh S. Treatment of acute exacerbations of chronic bronchitis: State of the art. Am J Med 1991;91(suppl 6A):87S–92S.
26. American Thoracic Society. Standards for the diagnosis and care of patients with chronic bronchitis. Am J Respir Crit Care Med 1995; 152(suppl):S78–S122.
27. Grossman RF. Acute exacerbations of chronic bronchitis. Hosp Pract 1997;132:85–94.
28. Godfrey S. Bronchioloitis and asthma in infancy and early childhood. Thorax 1996;51(suppl 2):S60–S64.
29. Burrows B. Airway obstructive diseases: Pathogenic mechanisms and natural histories of the disorders. Med Clin North Am 1990;74:547–560.
30. Anzueto A, Jubran M, Ohan JA, et al. Effects of aerosolized surfactant in patients with stable bronchitis: A prospective randomized controlled trial. JAMA 1997;278:957–960.
31. Wilson R, Tillotson G, Ball P. Clinical studies in chronic bronchitis: A need for better definition and classification of severity. J Antimicrob Chemother 1996;37:205–208.
32. Saint S, Bent S, Vittinghoff E, Grady D. Antibiotics in chronic obstructive pulmonary disease exacerbations: A meta analysis. JAMA 1995;273:957–960.
33. Staley H, McDade HB, Paes D. Is an objective assessment of antibiotic therapy in exacerbations of chronic bronchitis possible? J Antimicrob Chemother 1993;31:193–199.
34. Wilson R. Outcome predictors in bronchitis. Chest 1995;108(suppl): 53S–57S.
35. Reed MD, Blumer JL. Azithromycin: A critical review of the first azilde antibiotic and its role in pediatric practice. Pediatr Infect Dis J 1997;16:1069–1083.
36. Klassen TP. Recent advances in the treatment of bronchiolits and laryngitis. Pediatr Clin North Am 1997;44:249–261.
37. Dominguez EA, Taber LH, Couch RB. Comparison of rapid diagnostic techniques for respiratory syncytial and influenza A virus respiratory infections in young children. J Clin Micro 1993;31:2286–2290.
38. Klassen TP, Sutcliff T, Watters LK, et al. Dxamethasone in salbutamol-treated inpatients with acute bronchiolitis: A randomized controlled study. J Pediatr 1997;130:191–196.
39. Springer C, Bar-Yishay E, Uwayyed K, et al. Corticosteroids do not affect the clinical or physiological status of infants with bronchiolitis. Pediatr Pulm 1990;9:181–185.
40. Muller NL, Miller RR. Diseases of the bronchioles: CT and histopathologic findings. Radiology 1995;196:3–12.
41. Patterson JL, Fernandez-Larsson R. Molecular mechanisms of action of ribavirin. Rev Infect Dis 1990;12:1139–1146.
42. Connor E, Morrison S, Lane J, et al. Safety, tolerance, and pharmacokinetics of systemic ribavirin in children with human immunodeficiency virus infection. Antimicrob Agents Chemother 1993;37:532–539.
43. Rodriquez WJ, Kim HW, Brandt CD, et al. Aerosolized ribavirin in the treatment of patients with respiratory syncytial virus disease. Pediatr Infect Dis J 1987;6:159–163.
44. Janai HK, Stuttman HR, Zaleska M, et al. Ribavirin effect on pulmonary function in young infants with respiratory syncytial virus bronchiolitis. Pediatr Infect Dis J 1993;12:214–218.
45. 1997 Redbook: Report of the Committee on Infectious Diseases, 24th ed. Committee on Infectious Diseases, American Academy of Pediatrics, 1997:445.
46. Meert KL, Sarnaik AP, Gelmini MJ, et al. Aerosolized ribavirin in mechanically ventilated children with respiratory syncytial virus lower respiratory tract disease: A prospective, double-blind, randomized trial. Crit Care Med 1994;22:566–572.
47. Bartlett JG, Mundy LM. Community-acquired pneumonia. N Engl J Med 1995;333:1618–1624.
48. Mandell LA. Community-acquired pneumonia: Etiology, epidemiology and treatment. Chest 1995;108(suppl):35S–42S.
49. Mayhall CG. Nosocomial pneumonia: Diagnosis and prevention. Infect Dis Clin North Am 1997;11:427–457.
50. Baker CJ, Edwards MS. Group B streptococcal infections. In: Remington JS, Klein JO, eds. Infectious Disease of the Fetus and Newborn Infant, 4th ed. Philadelphia, WB Saunders, 1995:980–1054.
51. American Thoracic Society. Hospital-acquired pneumonia in adults: Diagnosis, assessment of severity, initial antimicrobial therapy, and preventative strategies. Am J Respir Crit Care Med 1996;153:1711–1725.
52. Reed M. The pathophysiology and treatment of cystic fibrosis. J Pediatr Pharm Pract 1997;2:285–308.
53. Stout JE, Yu VL. Legionellosis. N Engl J Med 1997;337:682–687.
54. Bartlett JG. Anaerobic bacterial pneumonitis. Am Rev Respir Dis 1979;119:19–23.
55. Hickling KG, Howard R. A retrospective survey of treatment and mortality in aspiration pneumonia. Inten Care Med 1988;14:617–622.
56. McCray E, Weinbaum CM, Braden CR, et al. The epidemiology of tuberculosis in the United States. Clin Chest Med 1997;18:99–113.

57. Telzak EE. Tuberculosis and human immunodeficiency virus infection. Med Clin North Am 1997;81:345–360.
58. Lieberman D, Lieberman D. Atypical pathogen pneumonia. Curr Opin Pulm Med 1997;3:111–115.
59. Kauppinen M, Saikku P. Pneumonia due to *Chlamydia pneumoniae*: Prevalence, clinical features, diagnosis, and treatment. Clin Infect Dis 1995;21:S244–S252.
60. Murray JF. Pulmonary complications of HIV infection. Ann Rev Med 1996;47:117–126.
61. Schneider RF, Rosen MJ. Pulmonary complications of HIV infection. Curr Opin Pulm Med 1997;3:151–158.
62. Noskin GA, Glassroth J. Bacterial pneumonia associated with HIV-1 infection. Clin Chest Med 1996;17:713–723.
63. Pizzo PA. Management of fever in patients with cancer and treatment-induced neutropenia. N Engl J Med 1993;328:1323–1332.
64. Hughes WT, Armstrong D, Bodey GP, et al. 1997 guidelines for the use of antimicrobial agents in neutropenic patients with unexplained fever. Clin Infect Dis 1997;25:551–573.
65. Whimbey E, Goodrich J, Bodey GP. Pneumonia in cancer patients. Cancer Treat Rep 1995;79:185–210.
66. ASCO Ad Hoc Colony-Stimulating Factor Guidelines Expert Panel. American Society of Clinical Oncology recommendations for the use of hematopoietic colony-stimulating factors: Evidence-based, clinical practice guidelines. J Clin Oncol 1994;12:2471–2508.
67. ASCO Ad Hoc Colony-Stimulating Factor Guidelines Expert Panel. Update of recommendations for the use of hematopoietic colony-stimulating factors: Evidence-based clinical practice guidelines. J Clin Oncol 1996;14:1957–1960.
68. Gallego M, Valles J, Rello J. New perspectives in the diagnosis of nosocomial pneumonia. Curr Opin Pulm Med 1997;3:116–119.
69. Cook DJ. Stress ulcer prophylaxis: Gastrointestinal bleeding and nosocomial pneumonia: Best evidence synthesis. Scand J Gastroenterol 1995;210(suppl):48–52.
70. Estes RJ, Meduri GU. The pathogenesis of ventilator-associated pneumonia: I. Mechanisms of bacterial transcolonization and airway inoculation. Inten Care Med 1995;21:365–383.
71. Jacoby GA. Prevalence and resistance mechanisms of common bacterial respiratory pathogens. Clin Infect Dis 1994;18:951–957.
72. Appelbaum PC. Epidemiology and *in vitro* susceptibility of drug-resistant *Streptococcus pneumoniae*. Pediatr Infect Dis J 1996; 15(suppl):932–939.
73. Shlaes DM, Gerding DN, John JF, et al. Society for Healthcare Epidemiology of America and Infectious Diseases Society of America Joint Committee on the Prevention of Antimicrobial Resistance: Guidelines for the prevention of antimicrobial resistance in hospitals. Clin Infect Dis 1997;25:584–599.
74. Cunha BA. The antibiotic treatment of community-acquired, atypical, and nosocomial pneumonias. Med Clin North Am 1995;79:581–597.
75. Honeybourne D. Antibiotic penetration in the respiratory tract and implications. Curr Opin Pulm Med 1997;3:170–174.
76. Bodem CR, Lampton LM, Miller DP, et al. Endobronchial pH: Relevance to aminoglycoside activity in gram-negative bacillary pneumonia. Am Rev Resp Dis 1983;127:39–41.
77. Smith AL, Ramsey B. Aerosol administration of antibiotics. Respiration 1995;62(suppl 1):19–24.

99

Upper Respiratory Tract Infections

Monique Richer, PharmD, MA (ed), BCPS, and Michel Deschênes, MD

Otitis media, pharyngitis, croup, and sinusitis are the most common acute upper respiratory tract infections of early childhood. Epiglottitis, otitis media, pharyngitis, and sinusitis also occur in adults. This group of diseases represents one of the most frequent reasons for medical care in North America. Understanding the underlying microbiology, pathophysiology, and predisposing factors, as well as the advent of an armamentarium of new antimicrobial agents, significantly improves their management and outcome, as well as the quality of life of those who suffer from these infections.

OTITIS MEDIA

Otitis media is a nonspecific term describing an inflammation of the middle ear, and it is classified according to clinical presentation.[1] Acute otitis media involves the rapid onset of signs and symptoms of infection in the middle ear.

Otitis media with effusion (accumulation of liquid in the middle ear cavity) differs from acute otitis media in that signs and symptoms of an acute infection are absent. The opacity of the tympanic membrane makes the type of effusion (serous, mucous, purulent) difficult to determine.

Chronic purulent otitis media, characterized by a chronic inflammation of the middle ear and otitis media without effusion are rare conditions and will not be discussed at length in this chapter.

EPIDEMIOLOGY

Acute otitis media is the most frequent diagnosis in infants and children who visit physicians because of illness.[2] Acute episodes are more frequent during the first 3 years of life: by the age of 1 year, 50% of the children will have had one episode of otitis media, and by the age of 3, 60% will have had one episode and 30% will have had at least three episodes.[2,3] Acute otitis media also presents in adults, albeit less frequently.[1]

ETIOLOGY

Several risk factors contribute to the higher incidence and increased frequency of otitis media.[1,2]

SEASON

The frequency of otitis media is greater in winter months and appears to parallel the outbreaks of viral infections of the respiratory tract.[2,4]

MALFORMATIONS

Infants with anatomic problems, such as cleft palate, adenoid hypertrophy, and Down's syndrome, are particularly at risk for the development of acute otitis media and recurrences.

ENVIRONMENTAL FACTORS

A history of recurrent acute otitis media or respiratory tract infections in a sibling doubles the risk of developing acute otitis media. Attending daycare centers and parental smoking increases the risk, while breast feeding appears as a significant protective factor.[2,4–8]

RACE

The incidence of acute otitis media is more predominant in Caucasians than in the American black population.[2] Native Americans and the Inuit represent a population particularly at risk.[2,9] The differences observed among races are attributed to factors such as anatomic differences of the eustachian tube, living conditions, availability of medical care, and the small sample sizes of the groups studied.

AGE AT FIRST EPISODE

The earlier children experience their first episode of otitis media, the greater the risk of developing more severe, persistent, and recurrent episodes. Infants with a first episode before the age of 6 months have a relative risk of 1.5 of acute otitis media in the next 24 months compared with children who have a first episode at an age older than 6 months.[2,4,8]

ANATOMY AND PATHOPHYSIOLOGY

The middle ear is best described as an air-filled cavity that begins at the tympanic membrane and extends to the nasopharynx via the eustachian tube (Fig. 99–1). It is contiguous with air-filled cells of the mastoid, but it also shares the same respiratory mucosa as the nose, nasopharynx, and eustachian tubes.

The eustachian tube lies at a 45 degree angle to the horizontal plane in adults and at a 10 degree angle in infants (Fig. 99–1). Its primary functions with respect to the middle ear are threefold: regulation of atmospheric pressure between both sides of the tympanic membrane, protection

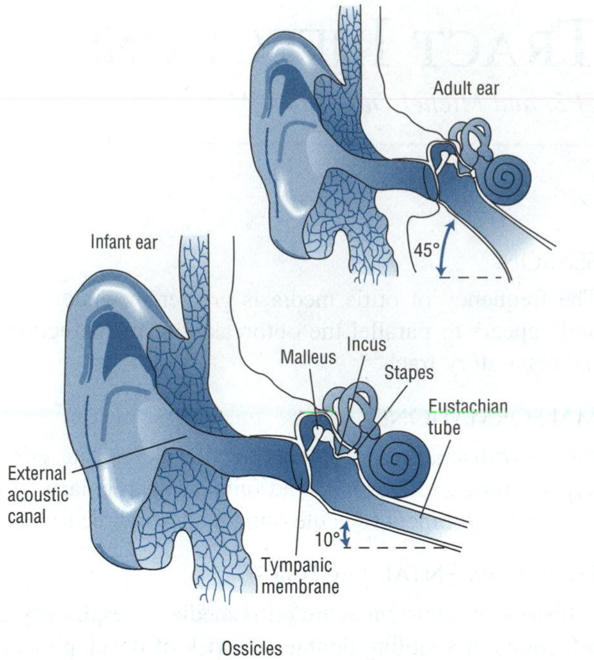

FIGURE 99–1. Anatomy of the middle ear and differences between an infant and adult.

from nasopharyngeal secretions, and draining secretions from the middle ear into the nasopharynx. In infants, this difference in angulation may cause improper drainage of the middle ear as a result of decreased gravitational effects on the eustachian tube. In addition, the muscle responsible for eustachian tube opening, the tensor veli palatini, is less efficient. Thus, abnormal function of the eustachian tubes seems to be the pathogenic basis of middle ear disease, causing reflux transudation of liquid in the middle ear, and finally proliferation of bacteria in these secretions, resulting in acute otitis media.

MICROBIOLOGY

Bacterial cultures from the middle ear effusion of children with acute, symptomatic otitis media have yielded strains of *Streptococcus pneumoniae* (35%), predominantly nontypeable strains of *Haemophilus influenzae* (25%) and *Moraxella catarrhalis* (10%).[9,10] To a lesser extent, *Staphylococcus aureus, Streptococcus pyogenes, Escherichia coli,* and a few other strains (*Pseudomonas aeruginosa* and group B streptococci) have been found. The bacteriology of middle ear effusion has changed little since the mid-1970s, with the exception of the emergence of β-lactam resistance in non–type-B strains of *H. influenzae* (30%) and *M. catarrhalis* (75%).[10,11] Prevalence of β-lactamase production (the most frequent type of resistance) varies from one medical center to another. The bacteriology of otitis media in adults is comparable to children[12] except that the incidence of β-lactamase producing isolates was lower. Anaerobic bacteria, such as *Chlamydia trachomatis,* as well as viruses and *Mycoplasma* have been suspected of playing a role in otitis media.[13,14] Their contribution to the disease process is obscured by the difficulty in isolating these pathogens.

CLINICAL PRESENTATION

Acute otitis media involves the rapid onset of signs and symptoms of inflammation in the middle ear that manifests clinically as one or more of the following: otalgia (denoted by pulling of the ear in some infants), hearing loss (secondary to effusion), and fever. Clinical presentation may include nonspecific symptoms, particularly in young children, such as irritability, lethargy, anorexia, or vomiting. This usually occurs in a child who has had an upper respiratory tract infection for several days. Otitis media may be present, however, without the aforementioned characteristics, which reinforces the need for regular otoscopic examination in the presence of fever.[1,9]

The diagnosis of otitis media is confirmed by the examination of the tympanic membrane. Redness or opacity of the tympanic membrane, the absence of light reflection, bulging, and immobility of the tympanic membrane to pneumatic otoscopy are all indicative of a middle ear effusion and suggestive of otitis media. Redness of the tympanic membrane, however, can also result from crying, sneezing, coughing, or fever. Otorrhea (purulent discharge) through perforation of the tympanic membrane or through tympanostomy tubes is also indicative of otitis media. Evaluation of the mobility of the tympanic membrane by insufflation with a pneumatic otoscope or determined by a tympanometer is considered essential for the proper diagnosis of acute otitis media.[9] The tympanometer uses the reflection of sounds by the eardrum to detect the presence of liquid by the middle ear cavity, which is recognized by a flat tympanogram instead of the normal bell-shaped diagram. In difficult cases, the use of tympanocentesis provides a definitive diagnosis of otitis media and yields identification and susceptibility patterns of the pathogens.

Complications and sequelae of otitis media are categorized as intracranial and intratemporal. The intracranial complications, meningitis, mastoiditis, and brain abscess are infrequent.[2] Intratemporal sequelae, such as eardrum diseases, are more frequent and can result in hearing loss.[2] In 10% of cases, otitis media will result in a persistent effusion in the middle ear.

The difference between acute otitis media and otitis media with effusion is that the child is asymptomatic with the latter. Because of unsuccessful attempts to culture bacteria, it was once thought that the effusion was sterile. Studies have demonstrated the presence of bacteria in approximately 50% of the cases of otitis media with effusion. The bacteria are similar to those isolated in acute otitis media but with a slightly different distribution: *H. influenzae,* 12% to 50%; *S. pneumoniae,* 3% to 40%; and *Staphylococcus epidermidis,* 19% to 37%. *S. aureus* and *M. catarrhalis* are encountered less frequently.[1,15]

▶ TREATMENT: Otitis Media

DESIRED OUTCOME

The goals of treatment of otitis media include the control of pain, the eradication of infection, the prevention of complications, and the avoidance of unnecessary antibiotics.

GENERAL APPROACH TO TREATMENT

Although a significant percentage of children will have cured their acute episode of otitis media with symptomatologic treatment only, oral antibiotic therapy remains the mainstay of therapy. Unfortunately, there are no clinical criteria that can distinguish patients that will require antibiotic therapy. The sharp decrease in suppurative complications of acute otitis media observed with the advent of antibiotic therapy constitutes in itself a sufficient reason for using antibiotics.[10]

NONPHARMACOLOGIC THERAPY

Supportive therapy with analgesics, antipyretics, and local heat is beneficial in the comfort of the child.[15] Although antihistamines and decongestants have been used for the symptomatic relief of acute otitis media, they have not been shown to be efficacious in the resolution of effusion or the relief of symptoms.[9] Topically applied anesthetics for pain relief may be of some value.[9,15]

A frequent nonpharmacologic approach to the treatment of recurrent episodes of otitis media is myringotomy and insertion of tympanostomy tubes. An incision of the tympanic membrane is made under anesthesia, the middle ear effusion is aspirated, and a short biflanged tympanostomy tube is inserted. The insertion of tympanostomy tubes reduces recurrent episodes of otitis media by 50% with an infection-free period of 3 months for most.[16] The insertion of tympanostomy tubes interrupts the cycle of recurrent infections, rapidly restores essential hearing for a short period, and relieves the discomfort that causes irritability in children. The advantages associated with tube placement are not reached without potential risks, primarily, exposure to general anesthesia and permanent scarring of the tympanic membrane.[9]

PHARMACOLOGIC THERAPY

ANTIBIOTIC THERAPY

Selection of the appropriate antibiotic is based on antimicrobial susceptibility, penetration into the middle ear fluid, clinical efficacy, compliance factors, adverse-effects profile, and cost. Amoxicillin, with excellent *in vitro* activity against *S. pneumoniae* and most *H. influenzae* isolates from the middle ear, remains the antibiotic of choice despite the concern about increasing frequency of isolation of β-lactamase producing *H. influenzae* and *M. catarrhalis*.[4,9,10,15] When there is lack of clinical improvement within 24 to 48 hours of the initiation of therapy or documentation of regional resistance to β-lactam agents, β-lactamase–resistant antibiotics should be used. Appropriate choices include trimethoprim–sulfamethoxazole (TMP/SMX), cefixime, cefuroxime axetil, cefaclor, ceftibuten, cefprozil, cefpodoxime proxetil, loracarbef, azithromycin, clarithromycin, and erythromycin–sulfisoxazole.[1,10,17–22] TMP/SMX offers good activity against *H. influenzae*, but its activity against group A *Streptococcus* is poor, and pneumococcal resistance appears to be increasing. *Pneumococcus,* as well as *S. pyogenes,* are showing increasing resistance to both TMP/SMX and the macrolides. The combination of sulfisoxazole with erythromycin also provides coverage for the primary pathogens. In addition, it is a useful alternative for patients who are allergic to penicillin and cephalosporins. Cefaclor has demonstrated good activity against most pathogens. The isolation of resistant strains of *H. influenzae* and *M. catarrhalis* is, however, increasing.[17] Cefuroxime axetil, cefixime, cefprozil, cefpodoxime, and loracarbef are active against most microorganisms isolated in middle ear fluid, notably all β-lactamase–producing strains.[17] Loracarbef and cefixime are less potent than amoxicillin against group A streptococci. The *in vitro* spectrum of activity of azithromycin and clarithromycin includes most pathogens that cause otitis media. Streptococci that are resistant to erythromycin can exhibit cross-resistance to azithromycin.[23] The combination of clarithromycin and its active metabolite has been demonstrated to have synergistic or additive activity against *H. influenzae.*[23] The choice of antibiotic therapy should be guided by *in vitro* and *in vivo* response, compliance, convenience of administration, acceptability, and side effects. Table 99–1 summarizes the recommended doses and dosing schedules of the most frequently used antibiotics for treatment of otitis media. A 10-day course of antimicrobial therapy is recommended. If treatment with a second-line agent fails, tympanocentesis may be indicated to identify the causative agent.

Chronic otitis media with effusion is described as an effusion lasting more than 3 months. A short course of antibiotics appears to be effective in the short-term clearance of the effusion.[24,25] The effect is limited, however, and is of relatively short duration.[24] Improvement of effusion is best seen with insertion of tympanostomy tubes. Tympanostomy should be considered in the following instances: (1) occurrence in young infants because of their inability to communicate symptoms; (2) concurrence of an acute purulent upper respiratory tract infection; (3) the presence of permanent conductive–sensorineural hearing loss; (4) vertigo or tinnitus; (5) the presence of severe atelectasis; (6) changes of the middle ear, such as adhesive otitis or ossicular involvement; (7) presence of effusion for 2 to 3 months or longer; or (8) frequent episodes of effusion, resulting in the accumulation of time of effusion during a period of 6 out of 12 months.[9]

Chemoprophylaxis

Several studies have demonstrated the effectiveness of chemoprophylaxis, but the indications, duration, and selection of the most effective agent are still controversial.[24] The following regimens have been advocated: (1) amoxicillin (20 to 30 mg/kg/d) in one dose at bedtime or in two divided doses every 12 hours, (2) sulfisoxazole (80 to 100 mg/kg/d) every 24 hours, and (3) TMP/SMX (equivalent of 4 mg/kg/d of TMP) every 24 hours. The Food and Drug Administration has not approved TMP/SMX for this indication. Prophylactic therapy appears to have a beneficial but limited effect on recurrent otitis media. It should be initiated during the winter and early spring when recurrences are highest and continued for 3 months or until there is a failure of therapy.[15] The appropriate course of treatment in patients who develop acute otitis media while on prophylaxis is to treat the acute episode with the usual 10 days of antibiotic therapy, using an alternative agent if amoxicillin was used for prophylaxis.

The antipneumococcal vaccines, Pnu-Imune and Pneumovax, contain frequently encountered pneumococcal antigens associated with otitis media. In children older than 2 years, this vaccine has been responsible for an approximately 10% to 20% reduction of acute otitis media (33% in daycare centers).[25] Unfortunately, children less than 2 years of age respond poorly to most polysaccharide vaccines. The *H. influenzae* type B (HIB) polysaccharide vaccine is not useful in the prevention of acute otitis media since nontypeable strains of *H. influenzae* are most frequently implicated.

TABLE 99–1. Dosing Regimen and Cost of Antibiotic Use in Upper Respiratory Tract Infections

Antibiotic(s)	Daily Pediatric Oral Dose	Adult Oral Dose	Regimen	Cost ($)
Amoxicillin	40 mg/kg	250–500 mg	Every 8 h	$
Pivampicillin	40–60 mg/kg	500 mg	Every 12 h	$$
Amoxicillin–clavulanate	40 mg/kg as amoxicillin	250–500 mg	Every 8 h	$$$$
Trimethoprim–sulfamethoxazole	8–10 mg/kg trimethoprim	160/800 mg	Every 12 h	$
Cefaclor	40 mg/kg	250–500 mg	Every 8 or 12 h	$$$
Cefixime	8 mg/kg	400 mg	Every 12 or 24 h	$$$$
Cefpodoxime proxetil	10 mg/kg	100–200 mg	Every 12 or 24 h	$$$$
Cefprozil	7.5–15 mg/kg	250–500 mg	Every 12 or 24 h	$$$$
Ceftibuten	9 mg/kg	400 mg	Every 24 h	$$$$
Cefuroxime axetil	30–40 mg/kg	250–500 mg	Every 12 h	$$$$
Loracarbef	7.5–15 mg/kg	200–400 mg	Every 12 h	$$$$
Erythromycin–sulfisoxazole	40 mg/kg of erythromycin	—	Every 8 or 12 h	$$
Clarithromycin	7.5–15 mg/kg	250–500 mg	Every 12 h	$$$$
Azithromycin	10 mg/kg day 1, 5 mg/kg days 2–5 (OM) 12 mg/kg × 5 days (SP)	500 mg day 1, 250 mg days 2–5	Every 24 h	$$$

OM = otitis media; SP = streptococcal pharyngitis.
$ < $10.
$$ $10–20.
$$$ > $20.
$$$$ > $30.

Clinical Efficacy

Evaluating the efficacies of the antibiotics used in the treatment of otitis media is not straightforward. The majority of clinical trials of antibiotic therapy are comparative and often determine both clinical and bacteriologic outcomes.[19–22] More than a 90% clinical success rate, generally defined as an absence of all presenting signs and symptoms of acute otitis media, can be achieved in the presence of bacteriologic cure (sterile middle ear fluid culture) and a 62% clinical cure can be observed with bacteriologic failure.[26] An 80% clinical success rate was demonstrated in nonbacterial otitis media. It is also important to consider that symptomatic improvement can be observed without antibacterial therapy. A meta-analysis evaluating the complete clinical resolution of otitis media (exclusive of middle ear effusion) reported that the spontaneous rate of resolution without antibiotics or tympanocentesis was 81%.[27] The use of antibiotics increased resolution by 13.7%. Albeit modest, the impact of antibiotic use on clinical resolution was significant. Conversely, symptoms can persist despite effective antibacterial therapy, especially in the presence of viral infections.

Compliance Factors

Most children with otitis media become asymptomatic within 24 to 72 hours of the initiation of therapy. It is, therefore, not surprising that less than 50% of the children treated for otitis media complete the full course of antimicrobials.[28] The number of daily doses to be administered has an impact on the compliance to a therapeutic regimen. Short dosing intervals and the recommended 10-day course of antimicrobial therapy for acute otitis media certainly represent contributory factors to noncompliance, and antibiotics that offer longer dosing intervals are advantageous. In some instances, a shorter course of oral therapy is effective.[29] In this study, tympanocentesis was performed in every patient and may have had an impact on outcome. In a randomized, double-blind clinical trial, rates of improvement, failure, relapse, and reinfection with a single dose of ceftriaxone (50 mg/kg, IM) were comparable to a 10-day course of oral amoxicillin (40 mg/kg/d) in children with acute otitis media.[30]

Although liquid formulations of antimicrobials offer flexibility in dosage adjustment for children, palatability of these preparations impacts on compliance.[31] Fortunately, the majority of the antimicrobial suspensions on the market for children are flavored.

Adverse Effects

The most frequent adverse reactions associated with the use of antimicrobials in the treatment of acute otitis media are gastrointestinal and cutaneous. The incidence of diarrhea is highest with ampicillin (> 20%). The addition of clavulanic acid to amoxicillin increases, in a dose-related manner, the incidence of diarrhea, nausea, and vomiting when compared to amoxicillin alone. Cefixime is reported to cause diarrhea more often than cefaclor (11% to 20%). The incidences of rashes and diarrhea with the newer cephalosporins (cefpodoxime, proxetil, cefprozil, and loracarbef) range from 1% to 3% and are similar to that of other cephalosporins and penicillins. Erythromycin-sulfisoxazole has been associated with abdominal cramping, as well as diarrhea, when the erythromycin component exceeded 40 mg/kg/d. Gastrointestinal disturbances were reported less frequently with azithromycin and clarithromycin than with erythromycin.

The potential for hypersensitivity reactions with β-lactams and sulfonamide-containing antimicrobials is well recognized. The nonallergic rash, well described with aminopenicillins, is reported in approximately 10% of treated patients. Agents containing sulfonamides (TMP/SMX, erythromycin–sulfisoxazole) are known to cause rare hematologic effects and cutaneous reactions that could be as severe as exfoliative dermatitis or Stevens-Johnson syndrome. Cefaclor has been linked to the development of a serum sickness-like illness associated with multiform erythema (1.1%), which is reversible with discontinuation of treatment.

PHARMACOECONOMIC CONSIDERATIONS

The total cost of treating otitis media in the United States is estimated at over 3.5 billion dollars annually.[32] Since the efficacy, antimicrobial activity, and adverse-effect profiles of many of the treatment regimens are comparable, cost of treatment becomes the issue. Table 99–1 lists the average wholesale price for different antimicrobial agents for the 10-day regimen for a 20-kg child as well as for adults. Amoxicillin–clavulanate and the newer molecules offer broader bacterial coverage but are by far more expensive.

EVALUATION OF THERAPEUTIC OUTCOMES

With proper treatment, symptoms of acute otitis media in most children will abate within 24 to 72 hours. It is useful, however, to reexamine the patient at the end of therapy. Even with efficacious antibiotic treatment, effusion of the middle ear may be present and persist in 10% of cases. Otitis media with effusion is classified according to the duration of the effusion: subacute—3 weeks to 3 months, and chronic—longer than 3 months. Middle ear effusion declines exponentially over a period of weeks to months. Thirty-six to 77% of episodes will resolve within 1 month and 9% to 32% of children will have had an episode lasting more than 3 months.[2] The following treatment options could be offered to patients beyond this time: (1) amoxicillin (20 mg/kg/d) or TMP/SMX (4/20 mg/kg/d) continuously while the effusion persists; (2) appropriate antimicrobial therapy of each episode of acute otitis media; or (3) myringotomy and tympanostomy tube placement. If acute otitis media occurs while the patient has tympanostomy tubes, *P. aeruginosa* infection should be considered and appropriate antimicrobial treatment should be initiated. If the effusion persists beyond 2 to 3 months, it is termed otitis media with effusion and should be treated as a chronic otitis media.

If the signs and symptoms of acute otitis media occur within 1 month of the initial episode, it is assumed that the same microorganism caused the infection. Emergence of resistance may be suspected. This new episode should be treated with a different antibiotic, preferably one that is stable to β-lactamase. If the new episode occurs over 1 month after the initial infection in a child who was completely free of signs and symptoms between episodes, the management of the recurrent episode is the same as the first episode. If children exhibit more than four episodes in a 6-month period or six episodes in a 12-month period, these patients can be managed by chemoprophylaxis with antimicrobials, myringotomy and insertion of tympanostomy tubes, or both.

PHARYNGITIS

The evaluation, diagnosis, and treatment of patients with pharyngitis is a common problem for all providers of primary health care. In the United States, approximately 15 million patients annually seek care for the relief of sore throat symptoms. Upper respiratory tract infections account for about 12% of visits to family physicians in Ontario, Canada.[33] Decisions about management often relate to whether or not there is a possibility of group A β-hemolytic streptococcus (GAS) because of the risk of rheumatic heart disease.

Pharyngitis is an inflammation of the pharynx and surrounding lymphoid tissue that may be of viral or bacterial origin. Viruses appear to be the cause of the majority of episodes, often as constituents of the common cold. A significant number are of bacterial origin, however, with group A β-hemolytic streptococci *(S. pyogenes)* being the most prevalent microorganism. It is important to differentiate viral from streptococcal tonsillopharyngitis because of the sequelae of group A β-hemolytic *Streptococcus* (GAS) pharyngitis and its favorable response to antibiotic treatment.

ETIOLOGY AND PATHOPHYSIOLOGY

Microbiologic etiology of acute pharyngitis varies depending on the age of the patients. In children less than 4 years of age, the etiology is usually viral. The peak incidence of GAS is between 4 and 14 years of age.[34] The rarity of this disease in infants younger than 4 years of age has been attributed to the low adherence of GAS to the buccal epithelial cells. Viral sore throats attributed to rhinoviruses and coronaviruses are associated with mild episodes, whereas adenoviruses and herpes simplex viruses, though less prevalent, are attributed to the more severe episodes of pharyngitis.[36]

Epstein-Barr (infectious mononucleosis), influenza, measles, and varicella viruses are capable of producing symptoms of pharyngitis as part of their viradrome. Mononucleosis is a disease transmitted by blood and saliva and is diagnosed mainly in adolescents and young adults.

Bacterial pathogens constitute 10% to 30% of all pharyngitis, and the symptomatology generally overlaps that of viral pharyngitis. The normal pharynx is host to gram-positive and gram-negative cocci and rods, both aerobic and anaerobic in nature. Normal flora is constituted by various bacteria of low pathogenicity. The pathogenic pneumococci (group A, C, G streptococci), *Corynebacterium diphtheriae, Chlamydia pneumoniae, Mycoplasma pneumoniae,* and *H. influenzae* are present in accountable numbers as well. GAS, the most prevalent bacterial pathogen in symptomatic pharyngitis, is responsible for 10% of pharyngitis in adults and 30% in children. Complications of GAS pharyngitis can be infectious (peritonsillar or retropharyngial abscess) or noninfectious (rheumatic fever or glomerulonephritis). The prompt diagnosis and treatment of GAS pharyngitis has decreased the incidence of rheumatic fever but has no effect on the incidence of acute poststreptococcal glomerulonephritis. The endemic incidence of rheumatic fever is 0.3% and can increase to 3% following a streptococcal pharyngitis epidemic.[36] Other groups of streptococci (B, C, and G) have been associated with acute episodes of pharyngitis but are not associated with the development of rheumatic fever or poststreptococcal glomerulonephritis.[26]

Finally, toxigenic strains of *C. diphtheriae* can cause pharyngitis and lead to diphtheria. Like GAS, diphtheria is spread through respiratory secretions and has an incubation period of 2 to 5 days. Fortunately, as a result of immunization programs, diphtheria is rare in North America but the complications associated with this pathogen warrant accurate diagnosis and immediate treatment. The clinical characteristics of diphtheria are a grayish membrane overlaying the tonsils, cervical adenopathy with edema, and a toxic appearance.

When there is a difficulty in establishing a diagnosis, noninfectious causes of pharyngitis should be considered. Allergies, sinusitis, post-nasal drip, and certain malignancies affect the upper respiratory tract or pharynx directly and should be evaluated before initiation of antibiotic therapy. The exposure to irritating substances (e.g., cigarette smoke, environmental pollutants, ingestion of caustic substances, and ingestion of hot foods or liquids) or direct trauma to the pharynx may cause pharyngitis and should not be excluded as primary causes.

CLINICAL PRESENTATION

Symptoms of pharyngitis include a sore throat that is associated with dysphagia and fever. In the presence of a bacterial infection, symptoms appear 1 to 5 days following contact with the microorganism. On physical examination, hyperemia of the pharynx and hypertrophied tonsils can be observed. Occasionally, tonsillar exudates, as well as vesicles, are noted. Examination can further reveal the presence of cervical lymph nodes, as well as a scarlitinous rash. In the majority of cases of acute pharyngitis, however, it is not possible to differentiate, on a clinical basis, between viral and bacterial etiology.[34] In fact, throat findings are similar among those with and without GAS pharyngitis. Consequently, sole reliance on the presence of a red throat would result in up to 80% of those with a negative sore throat culture to be incorrectly diagnosed as having GAS pharyngitis. Pharyngeal or tonsillar exudate has a higher specificity but will miss 75% of GAS cases.

For any symptom or sign, there is a considerable overlap between those with and without GAS pharyngitis. This observation led investigators to develop scoring systems and clinical rules based on a combination of findings to optimize diagnostic accuracy. A sore throat score developed by Centor and associates[27] was derived from a study of 286 consecutive patients over 15 years of age who presented complaining of a sore throat. Four findings independently predicted a positive throat culture for GAS: the presence of a tonsillar exudate, swollen and tender cervical nodes, lack of cough, and a history of fever greater than 38°C (101°F).[37,38]

The sore throat score has proven to have a higher sensitivity than clinical judgment, but its specificity is unsatisfactory for making treatment decisions. This can be corrected by linking the score with explicit decisions about throat culture use (Fig. 99–2).

For patients with none or only one of the clinical findings, the probability of GAS is less than 10%. No throat culture should be taken and no antibiotic should be prescribed to this group. In those with two or three findings, a throat culture should be taken and the treatment decision postponed until culture results are available. Over 70% of the throat cultures in this group will be negative. The third group represents about 10% to 15% of individuals who present with all four characteristics. These individuals have the highest probability of GAS pharyngitis, are likely to be sicker, and sometimes gain the most benefit from relief of symptoms. For these patients, a throat culture should be taken and the decision to initiate antibiotic treatment should be based on clinical grounds. There are some limitations to this scoring system. The scoring system should not be used in those younger than 15 years of age, as children between the ages of 4 and 14 are more susceptible to GAS pharyngitis, or in a community where an outbreak of GAS is occurring.[38] Epidemiologic factors, such as family history, history of contact with patients having a cold or influenza, and time of the year, can provide further information to establish the appropriate diagnosis.

Does the patient meet the following criteria?

- Absence of cough
- History of fever > 38°C (101°F)
- Tonsillar exudate
- Swollen, tender anterior cervical nodes

Number of criteria met	Percent chance of streptococcal infection*	Suggested action
0 1	2–3 3–7	No culture or antibiotic required
2 3	8–16 19–34	Culture all; treat only if culture is positive
4	41–61	Culture all; treat with penicillin on clinical grounds**

* In a community with the usual levels of infection.
** If patient has a high fever, is clinically unwell, and presents early in disease course.

FIGURE 99–2. Determination of sore throat score. This score should not be applied to those younger than 15 years of age or in a community where an outbreak of GAS is occurring. *(Adapted from Ref. 39.)*

The primary purpose of obtaining a throat culture in a patient who presents with signs and symptoms of pharyngitis is to identify the GAS, initiate treatment, and avoid sequelae. Table 99–2 lists the criteria for the identification of individuals with pharyngitis in whom a culture is recommended.

A throat culture obtained from the surface of the tonsils and the posterior pharyngeal wall is the most commonly used test for the identification of GAS. Because the time necessary to obtain results is approximately 24 to 48 hours, rapid streptococcal tests have been developed for the identification of GAS. These tests detect the GAS antigen directly from a throat swab with a specificity of over 90% in the 10 to 70 minutes required for completion (depending on the test).[36] This allows patients to be treated earlier, thus lowering the risk of transmission of GAS. Even though these rapid test kits provide a faster diagnosis than the aerobic culture, they are less sensitive. The recommendation is to perform a throat culture if a negative result is obtained with the rapid test kits. It is important to note that a rapid diagnosis for the prevention of acute rheumatic fever is not essential, since antibiotic therapy can be initiated as late as

TABLE 99–2. Conditions Where a Throat Culture is Recommended in Pharyngitis

Children aged 4–15 years, with an elevated temperature and sore throat as the primary complaint
Close contact with a person with streptococcal pharyngitis
Individuals with a history of rheumatic fever or heart disease
Epidemic of the following pathogens: Group A β-hemolytic streptococcus *Corynebacterium diphtheriae*
Individuals presenting with pharyngitis and one or more of the following signs and symptoms: Fever > 38°C (101°F) Tonsillar exudate Absence of cough Scarlatiniform rash Swollen, tender anterior cervical lymph nodes

9 days after the onset of streptococcal pharyngitis and still be effective.[25]

Tests for antibodies, such as antistreptolysin O (ASO) and antideoxyribonuclease B (anti-DNase B), are useful in confirming a recent GAS infection.[36] These tests can aid in the diagnosis of patients with acute rheumatic fever or acute glomerulonephritis. They are of no immediate value, however, in the diagnosis and management of acute streptococcal infection.

With mononucleosis, a 3- to 5-day prodrome consisting of a sore throat, fever, and asthenia is observed after a 30- to 50-day incubation period. Physical examination usually reveals pharyngitis with tonsillar exudates, palatal petichiae, and posterior cervical adenopathies. In 50% to 75% of cases, splenomegaly can be palpated after 2 weeks of active disease. A macular erythematous rash is present in 10% of cases but increases to 50% in cases where ampicillin has been prescribed. Finally, jaundice can be documented in 5% of patients, whereas elevated liver transaminases (aspartate transaminase [AST], alanine transaminase [ALT]) are reported in 40% of cases.

Diagnosis of mononucleosis is confirmed by blood analysis, which should reveal lymphocytosis and the presence of atypical lymphocytes. A positive Monospot screen (Paul-Bunnell test) for the presence of heterophil (IgM) antibodies confirms the diagnosis of mononucleosis. However, these antibodies are only present in sufficient quantities after 2 weeks of active disease. Possible complications by tonsilar hypertrophy, albeit rare, include upper respiratory airway obstruction, thrombocytopenia, and traumatic or spontaneous spleenic rupture.

▶ TREATMENT: Pharyngitis

DESIRED OUTCOME

The goals of treatment of pharyngitis are to resolve symptoms as quickly as possible, limit spread of infection, and prevent complications, such as rheumatic heart disease. Treatment of pharyngitis varies depending on etiology. The treatment of viral pharyngitis is symptomatic. With a negative throat culture, antibiotics can safely be withheld, as GAS is almost always found on culture in individuals with active infections. When required, antibiotic therapy for GAS infection shortens the clinical course of the disease, prevents acute rheumatic fever, reduces the period of contagion to 24 hours, limits the spread of infection, and reduces the incidence of suppurative complications.[34]

PHARMACOLOGIC THERAPY

Penicillin has long been the drug of choice for pharyngitis caused by GAS.[36,39,40] Despite the development of antimicrobial resistance among most common pediatric pathogens, group A streptococci remains uniformly susceptible to penicillin. Therefore, penicillin remains the drug of choice and is recommended by the Academy of Pediatrics and the American Heart Association. Children younger than 12 years old with GAS pharyngitis should receive penicillin V 250 mg twice daily given orally for 10 days or benzathine penicillin 25,000 to 50,000 U/kg intramuscularly as a single dose.[41,42] The use of the injectable form of penicillin favors compliance but is painful and increases the risk of allergic reactions. For adolescents and adults, penicillin V 500 mg twice daily orally for 10 days should be given. Ampicillin and amoxicillin offer no advantages over penicillin.

For the penicillin-allergic patient, erythromycin estolate 20 to 40 mg/kg/d in two to four divided doses or erythromycin ethylsuccinate 40 to 50 mg/kg/d in two to four divided doses for 10 days are suitable alternatives.[25,42] Resistance of GAS to erythromycin has, however, been observed in the United States in approximately 5% of the strains isolated. New macrolides, like azithromycin, are also effective against GAS and can be used as second-line drugs. Reports have suggested changes to the recommended regimen of 10 days of oral penicillin, such as the use of an alternative agent with a broader antimicrobial spectrum, particularly against penicillinase-producing strains of oral bacteria and a decrease in the duration of therapy. There are insufficient data to support the routine implementation of either of these changes.[40]

EVALUATION OF THERAPEUTIC OUTCOMES

Approximately 10% to 20% of children and adults with GAS pharyngitis who are treated adequately will relapse. Patients who fail to respond to penicillin may harbor a greater number of penicillin-resistant, β-lactamase–producing microorganisms.[35] Other causes besides copathogenicity include lack of compliance and recurrent exposure. A recurrent episode of pharyngitis should be classified as either a relapse (because of the same bacterial strain) or as a reinfection (caused by a new strain). For a relapse, it is appropriate to change the antimicrobial agent. Cephalosporins with activity against β-lactamase–producing bacteria are good alternatives. If a new strain is present, the initial antimicrobial can be reinstated. With persistent recurrent episodes, penicillin for 10 days with rifampin for the last 4 days is suggested.[35]

Tonsillectomy and adenoidectomy in children with recurrent pharyngitis do not significantly decrease the number of GAS infections when compared with controls who did not undergo surgery. The recommended approach in children with severe and recurrent pharyngitis is to delay the surgery hoping for an eventual improvement. If no improvement is seen, tonsillectomy can be considered.

SINUSITIS

Acute sinusitis is a common condition affecting children and adults and is associated with both bacterial and viral infections of the upper respiratory tract. Children have between six and eight common colds per year, depending on age, number of siblings, and type of daycare services. Adults experience approximately two to three common colds per year, and incidence may increase while parenting or working with young children. Of these upper respiratory infections, 0.5% will be complicated by acute sinusitis. Acute sinusitis accounts for 5% of physician visits by young adults.[40]

ETIOLOGY

Studies in which culture specimens were obtained by sinus puncture revealed that the dominant organisms are *S. pneumoniae* (34% in adults, 41% in children) and nontypeable *H. influenzae* (35% in adults, 29% in children). The prevalence of sinusitis because of *M. catarrhalis* is significantly greater among children than among adults (26% versus 2%).[43] Infrequently encountered bacteria include *S. pyogenes, S. aureus,* and anaerobic bacteria. Viruses, such as rhinovirus, influenza virus, adenovirus, and the parainfluenza virus, are isolated in 15% of aspirates and are generally remnants of upper respiratory tract viral infections.

ANATOMY AND PATHOPHYSIOLOGY

The sinuses are four paired, air-filled cavities that are situated around the nasal cavity and adjoin the orbits and anterior cranial fossa (Fig. 99–3). The maxillary and ethmoid sinuses are well developed at birth, whereas the frontal and sphenoid sinuses originate from the ethmoid sinuses and are not fully developed until 10 years of age. The sinuses are contiguous with mucosa of the upper respiratory tract and are lined with ciliated pseudocolumnar epithelium. Small tubular openings called the sinus ostia connect the sinus cavities and facilitate drainage of the sinuses into the nasal cavity through the activity of the ciliated cells.[40]

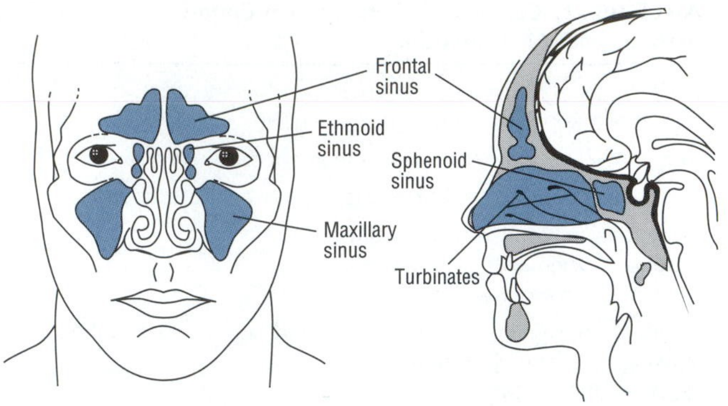

FIGURE 99–3. Anatomy of the sinus cavities.

PATHOGENESIS

Conditions that affect the patency of the sinus ostia, normal function of the mucociliary sinus epithelium, normal immune defenses of the upper respiratory tract, or events that introduce microorganisms into the sinuses predispose to sinus infections. Bacterial and viral infections of the respiratory tract and allergic inflammation are conditions that cause sinus ostia obstruction and lead to the retention of secretions. Preceding viral infection or epithelial damage weakens mucosal defenses and facilitates penetration of bacteria into the sinus mucosa. Although nasal allergies contribute to edema and swelling of the nasal mucosa, little information is available concerning their role in acute sinusitis.

CLASSIFICATION

Sinusitis is classified as acute or chronic primarily on the basis of pathologic findings and duration of infection. Acute sinusitis is defined as any infection process in the sinus that lasts from 1 day to 3 weeks.[44] If the disease persists for 3 months, it is classified as chronic. As well, individuals who experience more than three or four episodes annually or who repeatedly fail to respond to medical therapy may be considered to have chronic disease.[40]

CLINICAL PRESENTATION

The clinical presentation of sinusitis is dependent on the acuteness or chronicity of the infection, as well as the patient's age. Many symptoms of acute sinusitis are nonspecific and may be difficult to differentiate from symptoms of upper respiratory tract infection or allergic rhinitis. The most commonly encountered symptoms include mucopurulent nasal discharge, nasal congestion, facial pain (particularly unilateral), maxillary toothache, and fever.[40]

The persistence of nasal discharge and a cough for more than 10 days following a viral infection of the upper respiratory tract is indicative of sinusitis. The previously clear, thin nasal discharge associated with viral infections may become mucoid or purulent with an increase in both viscosity and quantity. A poor response to decongestants also increases the likelihood of sinusitis.[40] Progression of the cough is the symptom for which parents seek medical attention, even though the child may not appear ill despite a low-grade fever. In children, the presence of malodorous breath (halitosis) in the absence of pharyngitis and poor dental hygiene or morning periorbital swelling with or without pain may be signs of a sinus infection. Headaches caused by sinusitis respond poorly to analgesics. The pain corresponds to the sinuses affected and is described as a feeling of fullness or a dull ache. The incidence of this type of headache in children under 5 years of age is rare because the frontal sinuses are not fully developed.

PREDICTIVE VALUE OF SIGNS AND SYMPTOMS

No single clinical finding is predictive of acute sinusitis. Three symptoms (maxillary toothache, poor response to decongestants, and colored nasal discharge) and two signs (purulent nasal secretions and abnormal transillumination) are the best clinical predictors of acute sinusitis. When four or more of the signs and symptoms are present, the likelihood of sinusitis is high; when fewer than two of the above signs or symptoms are present, acute sinusitis can be ruled out.[45,46] In between these values, the diagnosis is unclear and sinus radiography may be helpful.

In addition to history and physical examination, the diagnosis of sinusitis may require transillumination of maxillary sinuses, radiography of the sinuses for adults and children over 1 year of age, and, occasionally, computed tomography or magnetic resonance imaging. Sinus puncture with aspiration and culture of sinus secretions remains the gold standard for diagnosis; unfortunately, this technique is invasive and impractical.

An interesting and useful laboratory tool is the cytologic examination of fresh nasal secretions. On microscopic examination, a high concentration of polymorphonuclear cells with intracellular bacteria is often observed. Polymorphonucleocytes generally predominate during viral infections, but when present in high numbers in a chronic and profuse rhinorrhea, they are suggestive of sinusitis. A differentiation between chronic sinusitis and allergic rhinitis can be made when eosinophils predominate. If the smear is devoid of eosinophils, chronic sinusitis can be suspected.

Transillumination is helpful in the diagnosis of maxillary and frontal sinusitis. Both the patient and examiner must be in a darkened room. Interpretation of the transillumination of the frontal sinuses is difficult because they are naturally asymmetric. Hence, only maxillary sinuses can be adequately evaluated.[40] The maxillary sinuses are transilluminated when a high-intensity light source, shielded from the examiner, is placed over the midpoint of the inferior orbital rim. Light transmission through the hard palate is assessed by the examiner with the patient's mouth open. Assessment of the symmetry of the blush bilaterally provides clues to the diagnosis. Because of the increased thickness of the soft tissue and bony vault in children 10 years of age and younger, the clinical diagnosis of sinusitis with transillumination is not helpful.

Radiography can confirm the diagnosis of sinusitis. Diagnostic findings include air–liquid levels in sinus cavities, mucosal thickening, and partial or complete opacification of the sinus cavities. When a patient presents with signs and symptoms suggesting sinusitis and abnormal maxillary sinus radiography, bacteria will be present 75% of the time. A normal radiograph in a patient with clinical signs and symptoms of sinusitis, however, does not suggest that the patient is free of disease.

Computed tomography and magnetic resonance imagery are useful in cases of sinusitis that are complicated by intracranial or intraorbital suppuration. They are not otherwise cost-effective and should not be used routinely to diagnose acute sinusitis.

▶ TREATMENT: Sinusitis

DESIRED OUTCOME

Many symptoms of sinusitis will resolve without medical therapy within 48 hours. When they persist, the goals of treatment include symptomatic relief, restoring and improving sinus function, preventing intracranial complications, and eradicating the causative pathogen.

PHARMACOLOGIC THERAPY

Antibiotics are the mainstay of sinusitis therapy, and selection of the appropriate agent is directed against the most likely pathogens. Amoxicillin therapy is considered to be a first-line treatment of acute bacterial sinusitis.[40] Cure rates based on clinical outcome using amoxicillin 500 mg three times daily for 10 days range between 72% and 74%.[47–49] The mean bacterial cure rate was greater than 90%. In adults, TMP/SMX is efficacious but may be ineffective in group A streptococcal infections. It can be considered for first-line therapy in patients allergic to penicillin. Bacteriologic cure rates for amoxicillin–clavulanate, loracarbef, azithromycin, clarithromycin, cefuroxime axetil, cefixime, cefaclor, and erythromycin–sulfisoxazole were comparable.[40] They are considered second-line agents, however, and do not offer a significant advantage for first-line therapy. Dosages and costs are described in Table 99–1. Acute sinusitis is treated for 10 to 14 days, but duration can be extended to 30 days in protracted cases.[50] Rates of antimicrobial resistance (*H. influenzae, M. catarrhalis, S. pneumoniae*) have slowly been increasing in both the community and hospital settings and are causing mounting concern that treatment failure of first-line agents could become common.[40] At present, however, many individuals, even with a proven β-lactamase–producing organism, may respond to amoxicillin alone.

Adverse effects and pharmacoeconomic factors are similar to those described in the section on otitis media.

ADJUNCT THERAPY

Although there are no published placebo-controlled studies of decongestants, these medications are often included in the treatment of acute sinusitis. Nasal spray decongestants, such as phenylephrine hydrochloride (0.5%) or oxymetazoline hydrochloride (0.05%) may facilitate drainage.[51] The use of such agents should not exceed more than 72 hours because of a tolerance effect and possible rebound congestion. Purulent secretions present in the nose should be removed before administration. Topical decongestants should be used with caution in the pediatric population.

Oral decongestants (pseudoephedrine and phenylpropanolamine) reduce nasal blood flow through their α-adrenergic activity. Their use has been shown to improve nasal patency by increasing the functional diameter of the maxillary ostium.[40] Antihistamines are not effective in the management of acute sinusitis, and because of their potential to cause dryness of mucosal membranes (anticholinergic effect), they may interfere with the clearance of purulent mucous secretions. Trials involving the use of an intranasal corticosteroid have shown an increase in ostium patency. This effect has not proven to be consistent in all trials. Since corticosteroids take a long time to act, an episode of acute sinusitis may resolve before their beneficial effects are noticed. Irrigation of the nasal cavity using a saline solution in a squeeze spray bottle may provide symptomatic relief.

EVALUATION OF THERAPEUTIC OUTCOMES

With proper treatment, symptoms of acute sinusitis will abate in 2 to 5 days. It is necessary to stress the importance of continuing antibiotic therapy for 10 days. If treatment failure occurs and the patient has not responded to first-line therapy, second-line therapy can be used. Any agent that is resistant to β-lactamases can be used. Patients with recurrent episodes of acute sinusitis who have been found not to have anatomic anomalies may benefit from second-line therapy. Complications of sinusitis include periorbital cellulitis, particularly in children, as well as meningitis. Finally, unrecognized sinusitis has been cited as a stimulus for poorly controlled asthma. Occult sinusitis should be sought in patients controlled asthma not responding to bronchodilators and corticosteroids.

EPIGLOTTITIS AND LARYNGITIS (CROUP)

Laryngeal dyspnea is frequently encountered in children. The most frequent cause is the infection affecting supra- or subglottic structures. Supraglottic infections include epiglottitis, retropharyngeal abscess, peritonsillar abscess, Ludwig's angina, and acute tonsillitis. Subglottic manifestations (croup) can result in spasmodic laryngitis, as well as viral or bacterial laryngotracheitis. Other etiologies include foreign body aspiration, trauma to the larynx, angioneurotic edema (allergic), and congenital abnormalities.

In order to better understand the manifestations of epiglottitis and croup, it is important to review the anatomic particularities of the upper respiratory tract in children. The epiglottis is one of the main cartilages of the larynx that blocks entry to the glottis during swallowing. In children, the larynx is located higher (the glottis is at the C2–C3 level) and in a position anterior to that in the adult. Unlike adults, the narrowest area of the upper respiratory airway in children is the cricoid ring. Finally, the glottis is of a small caliber (4 × 7 mm). A 1-mm edema of the wall will result in a 35% reduction of the aperture, thereby increasing airway resistance by a factor of 16.

EPIGLOTTITIS

Epiglottitis is a true airway emergency in which acute airway obstruction can occur. It is caused primarily by *H. influenzae* type B (HIB). Epiglottitis is more prevalent in children ages 2 to 6 years, but its incidence has decreased significantly since the advent of the HIB vaccine.[52] The onset of the disease is rapid, and the evolution is often brisk. Respiratory distress, drooling, dysphagia, and dysphonia are the typical signs of the disease (the "four Ds"). Fever is usually high and often manifests as the first symptom. The airway obstruction evolves rapidly and manifests by respiratory distress, an inspiratory stridor, loss of voice, and the presence of intercostal drawing. The typical posture of the child (tripod) with arms at the side, upper body set forward, neck extended with the chin thrust forward, and mouth wide open maximizes the size of the supraglottic airway. One can observe over a period of 2 to 4 hours the signs of upper respiratory airway obstruction, and in half of the cases and sometimes late in the course of the disease, hypersalivation (drooling). Once epiglottitis is suspected, the diagnosis should be confirmed by a person who is prepared for immediate airway intervention. When there is doubt as to the diagnosis, if the condition of the patient permits and the physician is present at bedside, a lateral neck radiography obtained in a sitting position will show an edematous epiglottis in 95% of cases (thumb sign). When the airway has been stabilized, blood gases, as well as blood and epigloteal cultures, can be obtained.

It is important to note that epiglottitis can also manifest itself in adults and usually presents as intense dysphagia progressing over a period of a few days.[53,54] When compared to children, dyspnea appears later in the course of the disease, thus delaying diagnosis.

▶ TREATMENT: Epiglottitis

NONPHARMACOLOGIC THERAPY

The primary concern in the management of epiglottitis is establishing and maintaining the airway. It is important to maintain the patient in a sitting position, to avoid manipulations (for example, blood drawing), and to not attempt a throat exam. If the child presents with imminent respiratory insufficiency, humidified oxygen (FiO_2 of 1.0) in a way best tolerated, with or without manual insufflations, should be administered while preparing for intubation. The optimal treatment consists of transporting the child to the operating room and performing a direct laryngoscopy followed by intubation if epiglottitis is confirmed.

PHARMACOLOGIC THERAPY

After the airway has been established, antibiotic therapy should be instituted and empirically directed against *H. influenzae* type B. The second- or third-generation cephalosporins cefuroxime (50 to 100 mg/kg/d given every 8 hours), cefotaxime (150 to 225 mg/kg/d given every 6 hours), or ceftriaxone (80 to 100 mg/kg/d given every 12 hours) are appropriate and often preferred if the infection is deemed severe. Once the condition improves, the patient is extubated, and oral antibiotic therapy is recommended and continued for a total of 10 days. Corticosteroids (dexamethasone) can be used to decrease laryngeal edema.

Isolation of the hospitalized patient is indicated until 24 hours after initiation of effective therapy. Household contacts, defined as individuals residing in the home of the index patient or nonresidents who spent 4 or more hours with the index patient for at least 5 of the 7 days preceding the day of hospitalization, should receive chemoprophylaxis with rifampin (20 mg/kg/d for 4 days given once a day, maximum 600 mg/d). Management of daycare and nursery school contact groups should be individualized.[26]

LARYNGITIS (CROUP)

Laryngitis (croup) is the most frequent cause of laryngeal dyspnea in children. It is characterized by the presence of stridor and presents most often in the early hours of the night in children less than 3 years of age. In contrast to epiglottitis, a barking cough and an absence of drooling is observed (Table 99–3). Laryngitis can be divided into three groups.

SPASMODIC LARYNGITIS

The etiology is not well defined and could be of viral or allergic origin. The onset is rapid, without a prodrome or fever, and the manifestations resolve rapidly.

VIRAL LARYNGOTRACHEITIS

It is caused primarily by parainfluenza (type 1 and 2).[52] It is preceded by an upper respiratory tract infection and fever (1 to 3 days) and occasionally it progresses toward respiratory distress. This syndrome generally resolves, however, without any specific treatment within 4 days, during which time the symptoms become intermittent with nocturnal exacerbations.

BACTERIAL LARYNGOTRACHEITIS *(PSEUDOMEMBRANOUS LARYNGITIS)*

This is another form of croup that is rare but life threatening. Most cases are caused by a secondary infection following a viral laryngitis, the only primary laryngotracheitis being

TABLE 99–3. Differentiating Clinical Features of Epiglottitis, Viral Croup, and Laryngotracheitis

Feature	Epiglottitis	Viral Croup	Bacterial Croup
Pathogens	HiB	Parainfluenzae virus, RSV	*S. aureus*
Age	2–6 years	6 months–3 years	1 month–6 years
Season	All seasons	Fall–winter	All seasons
Time of day	Anytime	Beginning of night	Anytime
Signs and Symptoms			
Clinical presentation	Toxic, typical posture	Nontoxic, supine	Toxic supine
Progression	Rapid (2–4 hours)	Slow	Slow
Fever	High	Absent or low	Moderate
Stridor	Muffled	Loud	Loud
Barking cough	No	Yes	Yes
Sore throat (dysphagia)	Yes	No	No
Drooling	Yes (50% of cases)	No	No
Laboratory Evaluation			
Leukocytosis	Elevated	Normal	Elevated
Blood culture	+ (70%–90% of cases)	Negative	+ in some cases

HiB = *Hemophilus influenzae* type B; RSV = Respiratory syncytial virus.

caused by diphtheria. The clinical presentation includes copious purulent secretions and, occasionally, the presence of a membranous film in the trachea. Bacteria involved include *S. aureus*, group A β-hemolytic streptococcus, *H. influenzae* B, *M. catarrhalis*, and pneumococcus. Progressive symptoms of stridor, fever, and frequent hoarse cough are usually observed. Contrary to viral laryngitis, this disease evolves toward respiratory distress. A radiograph of the soft tissues of the neck and lungs may reveal an irregularity of the tracheal mucosa (in 10% of cases) or pulmonary infiltrates.

Whatever the cause for laryngitis, it is important to evaluate the severity of the respiratory distress since this will guide the choice of treatment. Severity is determined on physical exam by the presence of stridor, intercostal drawing, vesicular murmur upon pulmonary auscultation, skin coloration, and level of consciousness. The presence of cyanosis, as well as a decrease in the level of consciousness, are indicative of severity. The anterior–posterior view of the soft tissues of the neck on radiography can reveal a narrowing of the air column as a result of subglottic edema. This, however, is not pathognomonic of laryngitis, and the severity of the disease is not well correlated with the amount of subglottic edema.

▶ TREATMENT: Laryngitis

Treatment varies according to the severity (mild, moderate, severe) of the laryngitis. Most cases can be treated as outpatients. Therapeutic options include humidified oxygen, racemic epinephrine, and corticosteroids.

NONPHARMACOLOGIC THERAPY

Humidified oxygen should be administered in the presence of suspected or documented hypoxia ($SaO_2 < 90\%$). Cold humidity can relieve symptoms of laryngitis, although its efficacy has not been proven scientifically. It is believed that it acts by liquefying secretions and soothing the irritated laryngeal mucosa. If the child is in mild respiratory distress, parents can take him or her outdoors for a period of approximately 15 minutes, weather permitting. This is efficacious in relieving less severe symptoms but does not allow for close monitoring of the child. Alternatively, a humidified oxygen tent allows the child to be exposed to cold humidity in a 40% oxygen environment. If the child is cooperative, application of a face mask and nebulizer is an option. This also ensures the delivery of cold humidified air (ice and physiologic saline) while allowing for higher oxygen concentrations (35% to 60% with a flow of 6 to 10 L/minute). Whatever the method used, it is important to keep the child calm and ensure the parents' cooperation.

PHARMACOLOGIC THERAPY

Racemic epinephrine, an α- and β-adrenergic agonist, can be used in moderate to severe laryngitis. Its benefits are derived from its α-receptor activity, which results in vasoconstriction and a decrease in subglottic edema. In addition, its β-receptor effects cause bronchodilation and relieve airway obstruction.

A 0.5-mL dose of 2.25% racemic epinephrine (Vaponefrin) diluted in 2.5 to 3.5 mL of physiologic saline is recommended.[55] Administration by nebulization with a face mask is preferred. A single dose is usually sufficient to relieve the symptoms of obstruction, but additional doses can be administered every 30 minutes if stridor persists while the child is at rest. The time to peak effect is 10 to 30 minutes, and the duration of action is 2 to 3 hours. Contrary to general belief, there is no rebound effect; however, obstructive symptoms can return upon cessation of treatment. A period of observation of a minimum of 3 hours is, therefore, recommended with subsequent reevaluation of the respiratory status.

Corticosteroids are used in moderate to severe laryngitis. Several studies have confirmed the benefits of corticosteroids in laryngitis.[56,57] Their use in hospitalized patients significantly improved the patients' respiratory status in 12 to 24 hours following administration, thereby decreasing the need for intubation and allowing for earlier discharge. Dexamethasone is preferred because of its rapid onset of action (< 2 hours), its peak of action (6 to 8 hours), and its long half-life (36 to 72 hours). A dose–effect relationship has been noted, the optimal dose of dexamethasone being 0.6 mg/kg given orally or intramuscularly (maximum dose of 10 mg). One study showed, however, that, when compared to doses of 0.3 and 0.6 mg/kg, no significant difference in symptom relief was noted when a dose of 0.15 mg/kg of dexamethasone was used.[58] Its pharmacokinetics allow for single-dose administration, although a second identical dose can be administered after 24 hours if respiratory distress persists. At this point, it is recommended that any child requiring the administration of racemic epinephrine be given 0.6 mg/kg of dexamethasone.

Studies have shown the benefit of inhaled steroids. Two milligrams of nebulized budesonide provides short-term clinical effects similar to racemic epinephrine when used in mild to moderate laryngitis. It has an onset of action of 30 minutes and a duration of action of 2 hours.[59–62] The proposed mechanism of action is a topical vasoconstrictive effect on the edematous laryngeal mucosa, thereby reducing capillary permeability. Budesonide offers an interesting alternative in the treatment of laryngitis.

Antibiotics should only be used when the diagnosis of bacterial laryngotracheitis is made, in which case, antibiotics targeting *S. aureus*, streptococcus, and *H. influenzae* B should be used. Cefuroxime is a good first choice, followed by a combination of cloxacillin and cefotaxime, and finally the combination of vancomycin in association with an aminoglycoside. The combined therapy is preferred when laryngitis was contracted in the hospital. Enterobacteria are often implicated if the patient is immunosuppressed. Adjunct therapy includes intubation, which provides adequate humidity and aspirates airway secretions. Bacterial laryngotracheitis is fatal if not recognized early.

▶ PRINCIPLES OF PHARMACOTHERAPY

- The diagnosis of otitis media is confirmed by the examination of the tympanic membrane. Redness or opacity of the tympanic membrane, the absence of light reflection, bulging, and immobility of the tympanic membrane to pneumatic otoscopy are all indicative of a middle ear effusion and suggestive of otitis media.
- Otitis media can be caused by *Streptococcus pneumoniae* (35%), nontypeable strains of *Haemophilus influenzae* (25%), and *Moraxella catarrhalis* (10%).
- Oral antibiotics remain the mainstay of therapy for acute otitis media, and amoxicillin for 10 days is still the drug of choice. In addition to antimicrobial therapy, supportive therapy with analgesics, antipyretics, and local heat have been shown to be beneficial.
- Viruses appear to be the cause of the majority of episodes of pharyngitis, often as constituents of the common cold. A significant number of sore throats are of bacterial origin, with group A β-hemolytic streptococci being the most prevalent microorganism.
- A throat culture obtained from the surface of the tonsils and the posterior pharyngeal wall is the most commonly used test for the identification of GAS.
- Penicillin is the drug of choice for pharyngitis caused by GAS. The recommended duration of therapy is 10 days.
- The predominant organisms causing sinusitis are *S. pneumoniae* and nontypeable *H. influenzae.*
- Three symptoms (maxillary toothache, poor response to decongestants, and history of colored nasal discharge) and two signs (purulent nasal secretions and abnormal transillumination) are the best clinical predictors of acute sinusitis.
- Oral antibiotics remain the mainstay of therapy for acute sinusitis, and amoxicillin (for 10 days) is still the drug of choice. Nasal spray decongestants, such as phenylephrine hydrochloride (0.5%) or oxymetazoline hydrochloride (0.05%), may facilitate drainage.
- Epiglottitis is a true airway emergency in which acute airway obstruction can occur. It is caused primarily by *H. influenzae* type B and should be treated with humidified oxygen and an intravenous cephalosporin, such as cefuroxime or cefotaxime.

REFERENCES

1. Bluestone CD, Klein JO. Otitis media, atelectasis, and eustachian tube dysfunction. In: Bluestone CD, Stool SE, Scheetz MD, eds. Pediatric Otolaryngology. Philadelphia, WB Saunders, 1990:322–334.
2. Infante-Rivard C, Fernandez A. Otitis media in children: Frequency, risk factors, and research avenues. Epidemiol Rev 1993;15:444–465.
3. Rosenfeld RM. An evidence-based approach to treating otitis media. Pediatr Clin North Am 1996;43:1165–1181.
4. Pelton SI. New concepts in the pathophysiology and management of middle ear disease in childhood. Drugs 1996;52(suppl 2):62–66.
5. Owen MJ, Baldwin CD, Swank PR, et al. Relation of infant feeding practices, cigarette smoke exposure, and group child care to the onset and duration of otitis media with effusion in the first two years of life. J Pediatr 1993;123:702–711.
6. Duncan B, Ey J, Holberg CJ, et al. Exclusive breast-feeding for at least 4 months protects against otitis media. Pediatrics 1993;91:867–872.
7. Giebink GS. Preventing otitis media. Ann Otol Rhinol Laryngol 1994;163(suppl):20–23.
8. Klein JO. Current issues in upper respiratory tract infections in infants and children: Rationale for antibacterial therapy. Pediatr Infect Dis J 1994;13(1 suppl 1):S5–S9.
9. Swanson JA, Hoecker JL. Otitis media in young children. Mayo Clin Proc 1996;71:179–183.
10. Médicaments pour le traitement de l'otite moyenne aiguë chez les enfants. La lettre médicale 1994;17:119–121.
11. Carlin SA, Marchant CD, Shurin PA, et al. Host factors and early therapeutic response in acute otitis media. J Pediatr 1991;118:178–183.
12. Celin SE, Bluestone CD, Stephenson J, et al. Bacteriology of acute otitis media in adults. JAMA 1991;266:2249–2252.
13. Del Beccaro MA, Mendelman PM, Inglis AF, et al. Bacteriology of acute otitis media: A new perspective. J Pediatr 1992;120:81–84.
14. Ruuskanen O, Arola M, Heikkinen T, Ziegler T. Viruses in acute otitis media: Increasing evidence for clinical significance. Pediatr Infect Dis J 1991;10:425–427.
15. Berman S. Management of acute and chronic otitis media in pediatric practice. Curr Opin Pediatr 1995;7:513–522.
16. Bluestone CD, Klein JO, Gates GA. "Appropriateness" of tympanostomy tubes: Setting the record straight. Arch Otolaryngol Head Neck Surg 1994;120:1051–1053.
17. Force RW, Nahata MC. Loracarbef: A new orally administered carbacephem antibiotic. Ann Pharmacother 1993;27:321–329.
18. Chocas EC, Paap CM, Godley PJ. Cefpodoxime proxetil: A new, broad-spectrum, oral cephalosporin. Ann Pharmacother 1993;27:1369–1377.
19. Blumer JL, Forti WP, Summerhouse TL. Comparison of the efficacy and tolerability of once-daily ceftibuten and twice daily cefprozil in the treatment of children with acute otitis media. Clin Ther 1996;18:811–820.
20. Khurana CM. A multicenter, randomized, open label comparison of azithromycin and amoxicillin/clavulanate in acute otitis media among children attending daycare or school. Pediatr Infect Dis J 1996;15(9 suppl):S24–S29.
21. Gehanno P, Berche P, Boucot I, et al. Comparative efficacy and safety of cefprozil and amoxicillin/clavulanate in the treatment of acute otitis media in children. J Antimicrob Chemother 1994;33:1209–1218.
22. Aspin MM, Hoberman A, McCarty J, et al. Comparative study of the safety and efficacy of clarithromycin and amoxicillin/clavulanate in the treatment of acute otitis media in children. J Pediatr 1994;125:136–141.
23. Piscitelli SC, Danziger LH, Rodvold KA. Clarithromycin and azithromycin: New macrolide antibiotics. Clin Pharm 1992;11:137–152.
24. Williams RL, Chalmers TC, Stange KC, et al. Use of antibiotics in preventing recurrent acute otitis media and in treating otitis media with effusion: A meta-analytic attempt to resolve the brouhaha. JAMA 1993;270:1344–1351.
25. American Academy of Pediatrics. Report of the Committee on Infectious Diseases. Evanston, IL, American Academy of Pediatrics, 1994.
26. Marchant CD, Carlin SA, Johnson CE, Shurin PA. Measuring the comparative efficacy of antibacterial agents for acute otitis media: The "Pollyanna phenomenon." J Pediatr 1992;120:120–127.
27. Rosenfeld RM, Vertrees JE, Carr J, et al. Clinical efficacy of antimicrobial drugs for acute otitis media: Meta-analysis of 5400 children from 33 randomized trials. J Pediatr 1994;124:355–367.

28. Mattar ME, Markello J, Yaffe SJ. Pharmaceutical factors affecting pediatric compliance. Pediatrics 1975;55:101–108.
29. McLinn S. Double-blind and open label studies of azithromycin in the management of acute otitis media in children: A review. Pediatr Infect Dis J 1995;14(suppl):S62–66.
30. Green SM, Rothrock SG. Single-dose intramuscular ceftriaxone for acute otitis media in children. Pediatrics 1993;91:23–30.
31. Dagan R, Shvartzman P, Liss Z. Variation in acceptance of common oral antibiotic suspensions. Pediatr Infect Dis J 1994;13:686–690.
32. Wandstrat TL, Kaplan B. Pharmacoeconomic impact of factors affecting compliance with antibiotic regimens in the treatment of acute otitis media. Pediatr Infect Dis J 1997;16(2 suppl):S27–29
33. McIsaac WJ, Goel V, Slaughter PM, et al. Reconsidering sore throats: 1. Can Fam Phys 1997;43:485–493.
34. Pichichero ME. Controversies in the treatment of streptococcal pharyngitis. Fam Phys 1990;42:1567–1576.
35. Van Cauwenberge PB, Vander Mijnsbrugge A-M. Pharyngitis: A survey of the microbiologic etiology. Pediatr Infect Dis J 1991;10(suppl): S30–S42.
36. Dajani A, Taubert K, Ferrieri P, et al. Treatment of acute streptococcal pharyngitis and prevention of rheumatic fever: A statement for health professionals. Pediatrics 1995;96;758–764.
37. Centor RM, Witherspoon JM, Dalton HP, et al. The diagnosis of strep throat in adults in the emergency room. Med Decis Making 1981;1: 239–246.
38. McIsaac WJ, Goel V, Slaughter PM, et al. Reconsidering sore throats: 2. Can Fam Phys 1997;43:495–500.
39. Treatment of group A streptococcal pharyngitis. Pediatr Child Health 1997;2(2):97–98.
40. Low DE, Desrosiers M, McSherry J, et al. A practical guide for the diagnosis and treatment of acute sinusitis. Can Med Assoc J 1997;156(6 suppl):S1–S14.
41. Canadian Pharmaceutical Association. Compendium of Products and Pharmaceutical Specialties. Ottawa, Canadian Pharmaceutical Association, 1997.
42. McEvoy GK. American Hospital Formulary Service: Drug Information 1997. Bethesda, MD, American Society of Hospital Pharmacists, 1997.
43. Gwaltney JM, Scheld WM, Sande MA, et al. The microbial etiology and antimicrobial therapy of adults with acute community-acquired sinusitis: A fifteen-year experience at the University of Virginia and review of other selected studies. J Allerg Clin Immunol 1992;90(3 part 2):457–461.
44. Kern EB. Sinusitis. J Allerg Clin Immunol 1984;73:25–31.
45. Williams JW, Simel DL, Roberts L, et al. Clinical evaluation for sinusitis: Making the diagnosis by history and physical examination. Ann Intern Med 1992;117:705–710.
46. Williams JW, Simel DL. Does this patient have sinusitis? Diagnosing acute sinusitis by history and physical examination. JAMA 1993;270: 1242–1246.
47. Casiano RR. Azithromycin and amoxicillin in the treatment of acute maxillary sinusitis. Am J Med 1991;91(suppl 3A):S27–S30.
48. Felstead SJ, Danial R, European Azithromycin Study Group. Short course treatment of sinusitis and other upper respiratory tract infections with azithromycin: A comparison with azithromycin and amoxicillin. J Int Med Res 1991;19:363–372.
49. Karma P, Pukander J, Penttila M, et al. The comparative efficacy and safety of clarithromycin and amoxicillin in the treatment of outpatients with acute maxillary sinusitis. J Antimicrob Chemother 1991;27(suppl A):83–90.
50. Williams JW, Holleman DR, Samsa GP, et al. Randomized controlled trial of 3 vs 10 days of trimethoprim/sulfamethoxazole for acute maxillary sinusitis. JAMA 1995;273:1015–1021.
51. Malow JB, Creticos CM. Nonsurgical treatment of sinusitis. Otolaryngol Clin North Am 1989;22:809–818.
52. Cressman WR, Myer CW. Diagnosis and management of croup and epiglottitis. Pediatr Clin North Am 1994;41:265–276.
53. Strausbaugh LJ. *Haemophilus influenzae* infections in adults: A pathogen in search of respect. Postgrad Med 1997;101:191–192.
54. Farley MM, Stephens DS, Brachman PS, et al. Invasive *Haemophilus influenzae* disease in adults: A prospective population-based surveillance. Ann Intern Med 1992;116:806–812.
55. Folland DS. Treatment of croup: Sending home an improved child and relieved parents. Postgrad Med 1997;101:271–273.
56. Cruz MN, Stewart G, Rosenberg N. Use of dexamethasone in the outpatient management of acute laryngotracheitis. Pediatrics 1995;96(2 part 1):220–223.
57. Geelhoed GC, Macdonald WB. Oral and inhaled steroids in croup: A randomized, placebo-controlled trial. Pediatr Pulmonol 1995;20:355–361.
58. Geelhoed GC, Macdonald WB. Oral dexamethasone in the treatment of croup: 0.15 mg/kg versus 0.3 mg/kg versus 0.6 mg/kg. Pediatr Pulmonol 1995;20:362–368.
59. Godden CW, Campbell MJ, Hussey M, et al. Double blind placebo controlled trial of nebulized budesonide for croup. Arch Dis Child 1997;76:155–158.
60. Fitzgerald D, Mellis C, Johnson M, et al. Nebulized budesonide is as effective as nebulized adrenaline in moderately severe croup. Pediatrics 1996;97:722–725.
61. Klassen TP, Feldman ME, Watters LK, et al. Nebulized budesonide for children with mild-to-moderate croup. N Engl J Med 1994;331: 285–289.
62. Johnson DW, Schuh S, Koren G, et al. Outpatient treatment of croup with nebulized dexamethasone. Arch Pediatr Adolesc Med 1996;150: 349–355.

100

Skin and Soft Tissue Infections

Larry H. Danzinger, PharmD, and Douglas N. Fish, PharmD, BCPS

Infections of the skin and soft tissues are some of the most common infections seen both in and out of the hospital setting. These infections may involve any or all layers of the skin, fascia, and muscle. They may also spread far from the initial site of infection and lead to more severe complications, such as endocarditis, gram-negative sepsis, or streptococcal glomerulonephritis.

The treatment of skin and soft-tissue infections may at times necessitate both medical and surgical management. This chapter presents details of the pathogenesis and management of some of the more important infections involving the skin and soft tissues.

PATHOPHYSIOLOGY

The skin and subcutaneous tissues are normally extremely resistant to infection. Even when high concentrations of bacteria are applied topically or injected into the soft tissue, resultant infections are rare.[1] Several host factors act together to confer protection against skin infections. The surface of the skin is relatively dry and is not conducive to bacterial growth. Also, continuous renewal of the epidermal layer results in the shedding of keratocytes, as well as skin bacteria. In addition, sebaceous secretions are hydrolyzed to form free fatty acids that strongly inhibit the growth of many bacteria and fungi.[1] Conditions that may predispose a patient to the development of skin infections include (1) a high concentration of bacteria (> 10^5 microorganisms), (2) excessive moisture of the skin, (3) occlusion of the blood supply to the skin, (4) availability of proper bacterial nutrients, and (5) damage to the corneal layer allowing for bacterial penetration.[1,2]

The majority of skin and soft-tissue infections result from the disruption of normal host defenses by processes, such as skin puncture, abrasion, or underlying diseases, (e.g., diabetes). The nature and severity of the infection depends on both the type of microorganism present and the site of inoculation. A large percentage of these infections are caused by normal skin flora (Table 100–1). Exposed areas of the body (face, neck) generally have the highest bacterial density and *Staphylococcus epidermidis* is the most common microorganism, whereas moister areas (axilla and groin) are most frequently colonized with gram-negative bacilli.[2]

Common bacterial infections of the skin can be classified as primary or secondary (Table 100–2). Primary bacterial infections usually involve areas of previously healthy skin and are typically caused by a single pathogen. In contrast, secondary infections occur in areas of previously damaged skin and are frequently polymicrobic.

CELLULITIS

Cellulitis is generally an acute, spreading infectious process that initially affects the epidermis and dermis and may subsequently spread within the superficial fascia. Cellulitis is characterized by inflammation with little or no necrosis or suppuration of soft tissue. A variety of bacteria are responsible for the several types of cellulitis most commonly encountered (Table 100–2).

Cellulitis is classically caused by group A β-hemolytic streptococci (usually *Streptococcus pyogenes*) or *Staphylococcus aureus*. Gram-positive cocci, such as *Streptococcus pneumoniae,* or in the newborn, group B streptococci, can also be etiologic agents. *Staphylococcus epidermidis* is an occasional pathogen, particularly in immunocompromised patients (human immunodeficiency virus [HIV] infection, organ transplantation).[3,4] Although less common, cellulitis may also be caused by a wide variety of gram-negative organisms, such as *Escherichia coli, Proteus* sp., and *Klebsiella* sp. Cellulitis as a result of infection by gram-negative organisms is often polymicrobic in nature and may involve anaerobic microorganisms, especially *Bacteroides* and *Peptostreptococcus* (see section on Bacterial Diabetic Foot Infections).[3]

Intravenous drug users (IDUs) are predisposed to a number of infectious complications, including abscess formation and cellulitis at the site of injection. These skin and soft-tissue infections are most frequently located on the upper extremities and are often polymicrobic in nature.[5] *Staphylococcus aureus* or streptococci are the most common pathogenic organisms isolated from these infections (37% to 61% of patients). Anaerobic bacteria are also commonly found (6% to 67% of patients), although the role of these bacteria in the pathogenesis of infection is unclear.[5] Fungal infections (primarily *Candida*) have also been noted to be a cause of skin and soft-tissue infections in IDUs.[6] These various organisms are believed to originate as normal flora of the skin, as well as from the mouth and contaminated needles, syringes, and diluents.[5]

CLINICAL PRESENTATION

Cellulitis is characterized by erythema and edema of the skin. The lesion, which may be extensive, is painful, nonelevated, and has poorly defined margins. Tender lymphadenopathy

TABLE 100–1. Predominant Microorganisms of Normal Skin

Bacteria
Gram positives
- *Staphylococcus epidermidis*
- *Staphylococcus aureus*
- Diphtheroids
  - *Corynebacterium* sp.
  - *Propionibacterium*
- Streptococcal species
- Anaerobic micrococci
- *Bacillus* sp. (soil organism)
- *Micrococcus* sp.

Gram negatives
- *Enterobacteriaceae*

Fungii
Yeast
Pityrosporum ovale
Candida sp.

associated with lymphatic involvement is common. Malaise, fever, chills, and leukocytosis are also commonly present. There is usually a history of an antecedent wound from a minor trauma, abrasion, ulcer, or surgery.

Cellulitis of an incised wound may be caused by any pathogen, but the most aggressively spreading lesions are caused by group A streptococci or *Clostridium perfringens.* These organisms can produce a rapidly evolving cellulitis in a very short time. It is often impossible to differentiate streptococcal and staphylococcal cellulitis.[4] A Gram stain of fluid obtained by injection and aspiration of 0.5 mL of saline (using a small 22-gauge needle) into the advancing edge of the lesion may aid the microbiologic diagnosis but often yields negative results.[7] Diagnosis is usually made on clinical grounds, that is, the appearance of the lesion.

Cellulitis is considered a serious disease because of the propensity of the infection to spread through lymphatic tissue and to the bloodstream. Bacteremia may be present in up to 30% of cases of cellulitis. In older patients, cellulitis of the lower extremities may also be complicated by thrombophlebitis. Other complications of cellulitis may include local abscess, osteomyelitis, and septic arthritis.[3,8]

Acute cellulitis with mixed aerobic and anaerobic flora generally occurs in diabetics, where the skin is adjacent to some site of trauma, at sites of surgical incisions to the abdomen or perineum, or where host defenses have been otherwise compromised (vascular insufficiency). As with other types of cellulitis, warmth, redness, and induration are observed; there may also be gas formation (crepitus). If the cellulitis progresses, it can lead to areas of gangrene. Because these infections often occur in patients with alterations in host defense mechanisms, poor nutrition, or both systemic findings, such as hypotension, dehydration, and altered mental status, are common. Often, needle aspiration of the leading edge of the lesion and subsequent Gram staining and culture are helpful in making a diagnosis.

Haemophilus influenzae cellulitis traditionally occurs most often in young children between 1 and 5 years of age. Most adults have bactericidal antibody, anticapsular antibodies to *H. influenzae,* or both, and they are less often infected. *Haemophilus influenzae* is part of the normal flora of the oropharynx and nasopharynx, and cellulitis often occurs in close association with upper respiratory tract infections. Inclusion of the conjugated *H. influenzae* type B vaccine in routine immunization schedules has resulted in a dramatic reduction in childhood cellulitis in the United States, although infection because of other strains may still occur.[9,10]

Haemophilus influenzae cellulitis typically involves the face, neck, or upper extremities. In young children, the lesions are characteristically blue-red to purple-red with indistinct margins and are surrounded by areas of edema and induration. In adults, the distinctive discolorations may not be present.[9] Fever and leukocytosis are common. Blood cultures are positive for *H. influenzae* in roughly 80% of patients. Aspiration, Gram stain, and culture of the margin of the cellulitis are positive in approximately 50% of all cases.[9]

TABLE 100–2. Bacterial Classification of Important Skin and Soft-Tissue Infections

	Bacterial Classification
Primary Infections	
Cellulitis	Group A streptococcus, *S. aureus, H. influenzae* (children); occasionally other gram-positive cocci or gram-negative bacilli
Gangrenous	Group A streptococci, anaerobic streptococci plus a second organism, as in cellulitis *(Staphylococcus* sp. or gram-negative bacilli, e.g., *Proteus)*
Crepitant cellulitis	*Clostridia* sp., *Bacteroides* sp., anaerobic streptococci, gram-negative bacilli *(Klebsiella, E. coli)*
Impetigo	Group A streptococci, *S. aureus*
Erysipelas	Group A streptococci
Secondary Infections	
Bite wounds	*Pasteurella multocida, S. aureus, Eikenella corrodens,* anaerobic streptococci, *Fusobacterium* sp., *Bacteroides* sp.
Burn wounds	*Pseudomonas aeruginosa, Enterobacter* sp., other gram-negative bacilli, *S. aureus, Streptococcus* sp.
Diabetic foot	*Proteus* sp., *E. coli, S. aureus,* streptococci, *Bacteroides fragilis,* infections *Clostridium* sp., anaerobic streptococci
Decubitus ulcers	Gram-negative bacilli, *Pseudomonas aeruginosa,* various gram-positive and gram-negative anaerobes
Lymphangitis (acute)	Group A streptococci, *S. aureus, Pasteurella multocida*

▶ TREATMENT: Cellulitis

The goal of therapy of acute bacterial cellulitis is successful, rapid eradication of the infection and prevention of further complications. Antimicrobial therapy of bacterial cellulitis depends on the type of bacteria either documented or suspected to be present based on the clinical presentation. In some instances, rapid identification and treatment are imperative (e.g., group A streptococci). Local care of cellulitis includes elevation and immobilization of the involved area to decrease local swelling. Cool sterile saline dressings can decrease the local pain and can be followed later with moist heat to aid in localization of the cellulitis. Surgical intervention (incision and drainage) as a mode of therapy is rarely indicated in the treatment of cellulitis.

As streptococcal cellulitis is usually indistinguishable clinically from staphylococcal cellulitis, administration of a semisynthetic penicillin (nafcillin or oxacillin) is recommended until a definitive diagnosis, by skin or blood cultures, can be made (Table 100–3).[3,8,9] Mild to moderate infections not associated with systemic symptoms may be treated orally with dicloxacillin. If documented to be a mild cellulitis secondary to streptococci, oral penicillin VK or intramuscular (IM) procaine penicillin may be administered. More severe infections, either staphylococcal or streptococcal, should be initially treated with intravenous (IV) antibiotic regimens.[7] The usual duration of therapy for cellulitis is 7 to 10 days.[3,8,9] When treated promptly with appropriate antibiotics, the majority of patients with cellulitis are cured rapidly. Failure to respond to therapy may be indicative of an underlying local or systemic problem or a misdiagnosis.

In penicillin-allergic patients, oral or parenteral erythromycin may be used.[3,9] Alternatively, a first-generation cephalosporin, such as cefazolin (1 to 2 g every 6 to 8 hours), may be used cautiously for patients who have not experienced immediate or anaphylactic penicillin reactions and are negative for a penicillin skin test. In mild cases where an oral cephalosporin can be used, cefadroxil 500 mg twice daily or cephalexin 250 to 500 mg four times daily is recommended. Other oral cephalosporins, such as cefaclor, cefprozil, and cefpodoxime proxetil, are also effective in the treatment of cellulitis but are considerably more expensive.[3] Clarithromycin, azithromycin, and clindamycin may also be effective alternatives for the treatment of cellulitis caused by gram-positive organisms, but they appear to offer no therapeutic advantages and are also relatively expensive. In severe cases when erythromycin or cephalosporins cannot be used because of documented methicillin-resistant staphylococci or severe allergic reactions to β-lactam antibiotics, IV vancomycin should be administered.

Ceftriaxone 50 to 100 mg/kg as a single daily dose is efficacious in the treatment of cellulitis in pediatric patients.[11] The carbapenems (imipenem and meropenem) and the β-lactamase inhibitor combination antibiotics (ampicillin/sulbactam, ticarcillin/clavulanic acid, and piperacillin/tazobactam) also appear to be equivalent to standard therapies in adults.[12–14] The cost of these newer agents without increased efficacy compared to other reliable regimens, however, makes them less desirable. Oral fluoroquinolones have demonstrated efficacy similar to parenteral cephalosporins in the treatment of soft-tissue infections caused by gram-positive organisms.[15–18] The use of fluoroquinolones is of concern, however, because of increasing reports of resistance among gram-positive bacteria, particularly staphylococci. Sensitivity testing is recommended when a fluoroquinolone is to be used. Also, fluoroquinolones are not approved for use in children because of toxicity concerns.

For cellulitis caused by gram-negative bacilli or a mixture of microorganisms, immediate antimicrobial chemotherapy, as determined by Gram stain, is essential (Table 100–3). Surgical excision of necrotic tissue and drainage may also be appropriate. Gram-negative cellulitis may be appropriately treated with an aminoglycoside or first- or second-generation cephalosporin. If gram-positive aerobic bacteria are also present, penicillin G or a semisynthetic penicillin should be added to the regimen. Ceftazidime and the fluoroquinolones are effective in the treatment of cellulitis caused by both gram-negative and gram-positive bacteria.[15–19]

If there is no obvious focus of infection, some internal source should be sought, such as a perforated viscus or a rectal tear, and repaired if possible. As these types of infections are often polymicrobic in nature, antibiotic regimens should be broadened to include agents with good activity against not only gram-negative enteric bacilli, but also anaerobic bacteria. Many different treatment regimens are possible, depending on the bacteriology of the lesion (Table 100–3). Usually an aminoglycoside combined with an antianaerobic cephalosporin, extended spectrum penicillin, or clindamycin will be used. Second- or third-generation cephalosporins have been suggested as single-agent therapy in certain instances.[20,21] Monotherapy with a β-lactam plus a β-lactamase inhibitor combination antibiotic or a carbapenem may also be appropriate in seriously ill patients. Therapy should be 10 to 14 days in duration.

Because gram-negative and mixed aerobic–anaerobic cellulitis can progress quickly to serious tissue invasion, therapeutic intervention should be immediate. If treated early, a quick response can be seen. Unfortunately, because this infection often occurs in patients with compromised immune defenses, the infection may still progress, even with therapeutic intervention. If the infectious process is secondary to a systemic cause (e.g., diabetes), the treatment course can be prolonged and may be associated with high morbidity and mortality.

In mild *H. influenzae* infections in children, oral therapy with either ampicillin or amoxicillin (not recommended for use in infants 4 weeks of age or less) may be used. Treatment should be given for 7 to 10 days. Alternative treatments for penicillin-allergic patients include oral cephalosporins (cefaclor or cefuroxime) or trimethoprim–sulfamethoxazole (TMP/SMX). If the *H. influenzae* is a β-lactamase producer or the patient is allergic to penicillin, then either a cephalosporin or TMP/SMX should be used as first-line therapy.[3,8,9]

Severe *H. influenzae* infections in young children were previously treated with IV ampicillin. Because of the increasing incidence of β-lactamase producing strains resistant to ampicillin, however, it may be advisable to use a third-generation cephalosporin (ceftriaxone or cefotaxime) until results of culture and sensitivity tests are known. Cefuroxime may also be used as an alternative agent in areas where cefuroxime-resistant *H. influenzae* are not common. For children with severe penicillin allergies, chloramphenicol or TMP/SMX may be used.[3,8,9] Chloramphenicol dosing should be guided by serum concentrations. For severe infections, maintenance of chloramphenicol serum concentrations in the range of 10 to 20 μ/mL is associated with a successful outcome and a low incidence of toxicity.[22]

Treatment of *H. influenzae* infections in adults is similar to that in children. Ampicillin or amoxicillin may be used orally for mild infections. For severe infections, a second- or third-generation cephalosporin should be used in areas where β-lactamase producing strains are common. Fluoroquinolones or TMP/SMX may be used in patients with severe penicillin allergy.[3,8,9]

TABLE 100–3. Initial Treatment Regimens for Cellulitis Caused by Various Pathogens

Antibiotic	Adult Dose and Route	Pediatric Dose and Route
Staphylococcal or Unknown Gram-Positive Infection		
Mild infection	Dicloxacillin 0.25–0.5 g PO every 6 h[a,b]	Dicloxacillin 25–50 mg/kg/d PO in four divided doses[a,b]
Moderate–severe infection	Nafcillin or oxacillin 1–2 g IV every 4–6 h[a,b]	Nafcillin or oxacillin 150–200 mg/kg/d (not to exceed 12 g/24 h) IV in four to six equally divided doses[a,b]
Streptococcal (Documented)		
Mild infection	Penicillin VK 0.5 g PO every 6 h[a] or procaine penicillin G 600,000 units IM every 8–12 h[a]	Penicillin VK 125–250 mg PO every 6–8 h, or procaine penicillin G 25,000–50,000 units/kg (not to exceed 600,000 units) IM every 8–12 h[a]
Moderate–severe infection	Aqueous penicillin G 1-2 million units IV every 4–6 h[a]	Aqueous penicillin G 100,000–200,000 units/kg/d IV in four divided doses[a]
Haemophilus influenzae		
Mild infection	Ampicillin 0.5 g PO every 6 h[c] or amoxicillin 0.5 g PO every 8 h[c]	Ampicillin 50–100 mg/kg/d PO in four divided doses[c,d] or amoxicillin 20–40 mg/kg/d PO in three divided doses[c,d]
	or	*or*
	Cefaclor 0.5 g PO every 8 h or cefuroxime axetil 0.5 g PO every 12 h[e]	Cefaclor 20–40 mg/kg/d (not to exceed 1 g) PO in three divided doses[d] or cefuroxime axetil 0.125–0.25 g (tablets) PO every 12 h[d]
Moderate–severe infection	Ampicillin 0.5–1 g IV every 6 h[c]	Ampicillin 50–100 mg/kg/d IV in four divided doses[c,d]
	or	*or*
	Cefuroxime 0.75–1.5 g IV every 8 h or third-generation cephalosporin (ceftriaxone 1 g IV once daily or cefotaxime 1–2 g IV every 6–8 h)[e]	Cefuroxime 75 mg/kg/d IV in three divided doses[d] or a third-generation cephalosporin (ceftriaxone 75–100 mg/kg IV once or twice daily or cefotaxime 200 mg/kg/d IV in three or four divided doses)[d]
Other Single Gram-Negative Aerobes		
Mild infection	Cefaclor 0.5 g PO every 8 h[g] or cefuroxime axetil 0.5 g PO every 12 h[g]	Cefaclor 20–40 mg/kg/d (not to exceed 1 g) PO in three divided doses or cefuroxime axetil 0.125–0.25 g (tablets) PO every 12 h
Moderate–severe infection	Aminoglycoside[f] or IV cephalosporin (first- or second-generation depending on severity of infection or susceptibility pattern)[g]	Aminoglycoside[f] or intravenous cephalosporin (first- or second-generation depending on severity of infection or susceptibility pattern)
Polymicrobic Infection Without Anaerobes		
	Aminoglycoside[f] + penicillin G 0.6–1.0 million units every 4–6 h or a semisynthetic penicillin (nafcillin 1–2 g every 4–6 h) depending on isolation of staphylococci or streptococci[b]	Aminoglycoside[f] + penicillin G 100,000 to 200,000 units/kg/d IV in four divided doses or a semisynthetic penicillin (nafcillin 150–200 mg/kg/d [not to exeed 12 g/24 h] IV in four to six equally divided doses) depending on isolation of staphylococci or streptococci[b]
Polymicrobic Infection With Anaerobes		
Mild infection	Amoxicillin/clavulanic acid 0.5 g PO every 8 h	Amoxicillin/clavulanic acid 20 mg/kg/d PO in three divided doses
	or	
	A fluoroquinolone (ciprofloxacin or levofloxacin) plus clindamycin 0.6–0.9 g PO every 8 h or metronidazole 0.5 g PO every 8 h	
Moderate–severe infection	Aminoglycoside[f] + clindamycin 0.9 g IV every 8 h or metronidazole 0.5 g IV every 8 h	Aminoglycoside[f] plus clindamycin 15 mg/kg/d IV in three divided doses or metronidazole 30–50 mg/kg/d IV in three divided doses
	or	
	Monotherapy with second- or third-generation cephalosporin (cefoxitin 1–2 g IV every 6 h or ceftizoxime 1–2 IV every 8 h)	
	or	
	Monotherapy with imipenem 0.5 g every 6–8 h, meropenem 1g IV every 8 h, or extended-spectrum penicillins with a β-lactamase inhibitor	

[a]For penicillin-allergic patients, use erythromycin 0.5–1 g every 6 h (pediatric dosing 30–40 mg/kg/d in divided doses).

[b]For methicillin-resistant staphylococci, use vancomycin 0.5–1.0 g every 6–12 h (pediatric dosing 40 mg/kg/d in divided doses) with dosage adjustments made for renal dysfunction.

[c]In areas with high incidence of β-lactamase producing strains, a third-generation cephalosporin should be used until sensitivities are available.

[d]For penicillin-allergic children, use trimethoprim–sulfamethoxazole (4 mg/kg twice daily) or chloramphenicol (50 to 100 mg/kg/d in four divided doses).

[e]For penicillin-allergic adults, use trimethoprim–sulfamethoxazole (4–5 mg/kg twice daily) or a fluoroquinolone (ciprofloxacin 200–400 mg IV or 750 mg PO twice daily; ofloxacin 400 mg IV or PO twice daily; levofloxacin 500 mg IV or PO once daily).

[f]Gentamicin or tobramycin, 2 mg/kg loading dose, then maintenance dose determined by serum concentrations.

[g]For penicillin-allergic adults, use a fluoroquinolone.

Infections in IDUs are generally treated similarly to those in other types of patients. It is important that blood cultures be obtained, as 25% to 35% of patients may be bacteremic.[5,23] Also, patients should be assessed for the presence of abscesses; incision, drainage, and culture of these lesions are of extreme importance, when indicated. Seriously ill-appearing patients, or patients with extensive cellulitis or deep-seated infections should receive a parenteral antistaphylococcal penicillin plus an aminoglycoside because of the risk of polymicrobial infections.[5,6,9] In addition, if the patient presents with an infection associated with systemic toxicity and watery, foul-smelling exudate, the suspicion should be high that anaerobes are present, and appropriate therapy instituted. Treatment with either amphotericin B or an azole antifungal agent (fluconazole, itraconazole) is warranted if *Candida albicans* is identified.[6]

ERYSIPELAS

Erysipelas (Saint Anthony's fire) is a distinct type of superficial cellulitis with extensive lymphatic involvement that is almost always caused by *S. pyogenes* (group A streptococci). Other streptococci (in the newborn) and rarely *S. aureus* can cause similar skin lesions.

Erysipelas most commonly occurs in infants, young children, the elderly, and in patients with nephrotic syndrome. This infection also occurs in areas of preexisting lymphatic obstruction or edema. The clinical presentation of erysipelas differs from common cellulitis in that the lesion is sharply circumscribed by an elevated border. The face and scalp are most commonly involved, followed by the hands and genitalia. Fever and leukocytosis are common.

The causative organism usually cannot be cultured from the surface skin lesion but may sometimes be aspirated from the edge of the advancing lesion.[4,7] The microorganism most likely gains access via some small break in the skin. Approximately one-third of patients have had a preceding streptococcal respiratory infection.

▶ TREATMENT: Erysipelas

The goal of treatment of erysipelas is rapid eradication of the infection. Mild to moderate cases of erysipelas are treated with procaine penicillin G 600,000 units IM twice daily or penicillin VK 250 to 500 mg orally four times daily (in children, 25,000 to 90,000 units/kg/day divided into four doses) for 7 to 10 days.[3,8,9] Dramatic improvement is generally expected 24 to 48 hours after treatment has begun. Penicillin-allergic patients can be treated with erythromycin. Strains resistant to erythromycin have been documented so some caution is warranted.[3,8,9] For more serious infections, aqueous penicillin G 2 to 8 million units daily should be administered intravenously, and the patient should be hospitalized.[4,9]

IMPETIGO

Impetigo is another distinctive type of superficial cellulitis caused by group A streptococci (known as streptococcal impetigo or impetigo contagiosa). *Staphylococcus aureus* is the causative agent in approximately 10% of patients. Impetigo is most common during hot, humid weather, which facilitates microbial colonization of the skin. Minor trauma, such as scratches or insect bites, then allows entry of organisms into the superficial layers of skin, and infection ensues. Impetigo occurs most commonly in children. It is also highly communicable and readily spread through close contact, especially among siblings, daycare centers, and schools.[4,9]

Impetigo manifests initially as small, fluid-filled vesicles. These lesions then rapidly develop into pus-filled blisters that readily rupture. The purulent discharges of these lesions dry to form golden-yellow crusts that are quite characteristic of impetigo. Pruritus is common, and scratching of the lesions may further spread infection through excoriation of the skin. Other systemic signs of infection are minimal.

▶ TREATMENT: Impetigo

The goal of therapy for impetigo is rapid eradication of the infection. Penicillin is the antibiotic of choice and should be administered as either a single IM dose of benzathine penicillin G (300,000 to 600,000 units in children, 1.2 million units in adults) or as oral penicillin VK. Penicillin-allergic patients can be treated with oral erythromycin. The duration of therapy is 7 to 10 days. With proper treatment, healing of skin lesions is generally rapid and occurs without residual scarring. Removal of crusts by soaking in soap and warm water may also be helpful in providing symptomatic relief.[3,9,24]

LYMPHANGITIS

Acute lymphangitis refers to an inflammation involving subcutaneous lymphatic channels. This acute process is most frequently caused by group A streptococci, but may occasionally be because of *S. aureus* or *Pasteurella multocida*.[3,25] Lymphangitis usually occurs secondary to puncture wounds, infected blisters, or other skin lesions. Systemic manifestations of infection (fever, chills, malaise, headache, and leukocytosis) often develop rapidly before any sign of infection is evident at the initial site of inoculation or even after the initial lesion has subsided. The systemic symptoms are often more profound than would be expected from examination of the cutaneous lesion. Acute lymphangitis is characterized by the rapid development of fine red linear streaks extending proximally from the initial site of infection toward the regional lymph nodes, which are usually enlarged and tender. Pain and peripheral edema of the involved extremity may often be present.[3,25] Lymphadenitis (acute or chronic inflammation of the lymph nodes) may also occur when microorganisms reach the lymph nodes and elicit an inflammatory response.

Identification of a peripheral lesion associated with proximal red linear streaks directed toward the regional lymph nodes is diagnostic of acute lymphangitis. At times, thrombophlebitis and acute lymphangitis in the lower extremities may be confused, because both are associated with red linear streaking and tender areas; however, in thrombophlebitis, no portal of entry is identifiable. Cultures of the affected lesions often yield negative results, as the infection resides within the lymphatic channels; however, the offending pathogen can often be identified by Gram stain of the initial lesion if done early in the course of the disease.

▶ TREATMENT: Lymphangitis

The goal of therapy for lymphangitis is rapid eradication of infection and prevention of further systemic complications. Penicillin is the antibiotic of choice. Because this infection is potentially serious and rapidly progressive, initial treatment should be with IV penicillin G. Lymphangitis usually responds rapidly to appropriate therapy; signs and symptoms often are markedly decreased or absent within 24 hours of starting antibiotics. Parenteral treatment should be continued for 48 to 72 hours, followed by oral penicillin VK for a total of 10 days.[25,26] Nondrug therapy includes immobilization and elevation of the affected extremity and warm water soaks every 2 to 4 hours.[3] If *S. aureus* is suspected as the causative pathogen, an antistaphylococcal penicillin should be used. For penicillin-allergic patients, erythromycin or clindamycin may be used.

BACTERIAL DIABETIC FOOT INFECTIONS

Disorders of the foot are among the most common complications of diabetes, accounting for approximately 20% of all hospitalizations in diabetic patients at an annual cost estimated at 200 to 350 million dollars.[27,28] Approximately 25% of diabetic patients experience significant soft-tissue infection at some time during the course of their illness. Infection of the lower extremities is also the most common septic problem leading to hospitalization of diabetics. Approximately 55,000 lower extremity amputations, often sequelae of uncontrolled infection, are performed each year on diabetic patients; this represents 50% of all nontraumatic amputations.[28]

PATHOPHYSIOLOGY

Three key factors are involved in the causation of diabetic foot problems: neuropathy, angiopathy and ischemia, and immunologic defects. Any of these disorders can occur in isolation; however, they frequently occur together.

Neuropathic changes to the autonomic nervous system as a consequence of diabetes may affect the motor nerve supply of small intrinsic muscles of the foot, resulting in muscular imbalance, abnormal stresses on tissues and bone, and repetitive injuries.[29] Diminished sensory perception causes an absence of pain and unawareness of minor injuries and ulceration. Also, the sympathetic nerve supply may be damaged and can result in an absence of sweating; this leads to dry cracked skin, which can become secondarily infected.[27]

Atherosclerosis is more common, appears at a younger age, and progresses more rapidly in the diabetic than in the nondiabetic. Diabetics may have problems with both small vessels (microangiopathy) and large vessels (macroangiopathy) that can result in varying degrees of ischemia, ultimately leading to skin breakdown and infection.

Diabetic patients typically have normal humoral immunity, normal levels of immunoglobulins, and normal antibody responses. Patients with diabetes, however, have been documented to have impaired phagocytosis and intracellular microbicidal function compared with nondiabetics, perhaps related to angiopathy and low tissue levels of oxygen.[27] These defects in cell-mediated immunity, thus, make patients with diabetes more susceptible to certain types of infection and impairs the patients' ability to heal wounds adequately.[29]

ETIOLOGY AND CLINICAL PRESENTATION

Diabetic foot infections are polymicrobic in nature with an average of 4.1 to 5.8 isolates per culture (Table 100–4).[30] Previously, the emphasis was on the importance of *S. aureus*, streptococci, and aerobic gram-negative bacilli in causing diabetic foot infections. It is now clear that obligate anaerobes also play a significant part in the bacterial flora of these infections, although their true role has yet to be defined.[30]

TABLE 100–4. Bacterial Isolates From Foot Infections in Diabetic Patients

Organisms of Isolates	Percentage
Aerobes	69
Gram-positive	45
Staphylococcus aureus	13
Streptococcus sp.	11
Enterococcus sp.	8
Coagulase-negative staphylococci	7
Gram-negative	24
Proteus sp.	5
Enterobacter sp.	3
Escherichia coli	3
Klebsiella sp.	2
Pseudomonas aeruginosa	2
Other gram-negative bacilli	7
Anaerobes	31
Peptococcus sp.	8
Peptostreptococcus sp.	5
Bacteroides fragilis group	5
Other *Bacteroides* sp.	4
Clostridium sp.	2
Other anaerobes	7

From Ref. 30.

Superficial cultures from the infected wound are often not reliable. The correlation between superficial cultures and true deep cultures (via biopsy or needle aspiration of drainage or abscess fluid) is poor.[30–32] Therefore, cultures and sensitivity tests should be done with specimens obtained from a deep culture whenever possible. Because of the complex microbiology of these infections, wounds must be cultured for both aerobic and anaerobic specimens.[30–32]

Clinical signs and symptoms of infection of the diabetic foot may not be present secondary to the angiopathy and neuropathy. Infections are often much more extensive than they initially appear. Certain lesions are typical of diabetic foot infections; these include paronychia (infection of the soft tissue adjacent to the nail), infections of the middle foot secondary to painless trauma, toe web space infections, and mal perforans puncture wounds (infection of the sole of the foot over the head of the metatarsals). Diabetic foot infections may be complicated by necrotizing cellulitis, osteomyelitis, or both. Osteomyelitis is one of the most serious complications of foot problems in diabetic patients and may occur in 30% to 40% of infections.[27,28,31,33]

▶ TREATMENT: Bacterial Diabetic Foot Infections

The goal of therapy of diabetic foot infections is preservation of as much normal limb function as possible while preventing additional infectious complications. Up to 90% of these infections can be successfully treated with a comprehensive treatment approach that includes both wound care and antimicrobial therapy.[31] After carefully assessing the extent of the lesion and obtaining necessary cultures, necrotic tissue must be thoroughly debrided with wound drainage and amputation as required. Wounds are kept clean, and dressings changed frequently (two to three times daily). The presence of osteomyelitis must also be assessed via radiograph, bone scan, or both, as appropriate. Because of the relationship between hyperglycemia and immune system defects, glycemic control must be maximized to ensure optimal wound healing. In addition, the patient's activities should initially be restricted to bedrest for leg elevation and control of edema, if present. Finally, appropriate antimicrobials must be initiated.[27,28,31,33]

The majority of mild, uncomplicated infections can be successfully managed on an outpatient basis with oral antimicrobials and good wound care. Many different agents have been studied, including cefaclor, cephalexin, fluoroquinolones, clindamycin, and amoxicillin/clavulanic acid; these agents provide clinical cure rates of 60% to 85% in published studies.[29,32–34] Significant failure rates, relapse rates, or both have been reported by several investigators, however, with the use of oral agents, and the development of resistance was problematic in some infections involving *P. aeruginosa* and staphylococci.[35] Many clinicians consider amoxicillin/clavulanic acid to be the most favorable agent because of its broad spectrum of activity, which includes staphylococci, streptococci, enterococci, many Enterobacteriaceae, and many anaerobes.[32] Fluoroquinolones have been extensively studied as monotherapy, but they are perhaps most appropriately used in combination with metronidazole or clindamycin to provide anaerobic activity.[29,32,36] Oral antimicrobials should be used cautiously in serious infections, especially those complicated by osteomyelitis, extensive ulceration, areas of necrosis, or a combination of these. Therapy should be carefully reevaluated after 48 to 72 hours to assess favorable response.

Initial therapy for patients requiring hospitalization for moderate to severe infections is similar to that for polymicrobic cellulitis with anaerobes (Table 100–3). Monotherapy with broad-spectrum parenteral antimicrobials along with appropriate medical or surgical management, or both, is often effective in treating these infections, including those in which osteomyelitis is present. Monotherapy is particularly attractive because of the potential advantages of convenience, cost, and avoidance of toxicities. Microbiologic and clinical cure rates ranging from 60% to 90% may be expected from any of these agents; selection of a specific regimen is primarily determined by cost. In penicillin-allergic patients, metronidazole or clindamycin plus either a fluoroquinolone, aztreonam, or a third-generation cephalosporin are appropriate choices.[29,32,33] Vancomycin is also frequently used in severe infections because of its excellent activity against gram-positive pathogens. Because these patients may already have some degree of diabetic nephropathy that may place them at higher risk of nephrotoxicity, recommendations have strongly advocated the avoidance of aminoglycoside antibiotics unless no alternative agents are available.[27] When an aminoglycoside is used, care must be taken to avoid further compromising renal function. All antibiotic regimes should be adjusted as necessary for renal dysfunction.

Drug therapy should be appropriately modified according to information from deep tissue culture and the clinical condition of the patient. Infections in diabetic patients often require extended courses of therapy because of impaired host immunity and poor wound healing. Mild infections can be treated with oral agents and should generally be treated for at least 10 to 14 days, while more severe infections dictate initial parenteral therapy and often require up to 21 days or more of antibiotic therapy. In cases of underlying osteomyelitis, treatment should continue for 6 to 12 weeks.[27,29,32,33] After healing of the infection has occurred, a well-designed program for prevention of further infections should be instituted.

INFECTED PRESSURE SORES

The terms *decubitus ulcer, bed sore,* and *pressure sore* are used interchangeably. The decubitus ulcer and the bed sore are types of pressure sores. The term *decubitus ulcer* is derived from the Latin word *decumbere,* meaning "lying down." Pressure sores, however, can develop regardless of a patient's position. Pressure sores are most frequently seen in chronically debilitated persons, the elderly, and persons with serious spinal cord injury. Generally, those patients who are at risk for pressure sores are elderly or chronically ill young patients who are immobilized either in bed or to a wheelchair and who may have altered mental status often associated with incontinence.

PATHOPHYSIOLOGY

Many factors are thought to predispose patients to the formation of pressure sores: paralysis, paresis, immobilization, malnutrition, anemia, infection, and advanced age. Four factors thought to be most critical to their formation are pressure, shearing forces, friction, and moisture; however, there is still debate as to the exact pathophysiology of pressure sore formation.

Pressure is the essential element in the formation of pressure sores. The areas of highest pressure are most often generated over the bony prominences. Studies have shown that when the pressure is relieved intermittently within a 2-hour period, only minimal changes occur in soft tissue and skin structures.[37] Therefore, both the degree of pressure and the length of time that the pressure is applied are important.

Shearing forces are caused by the sliding of adjacent parallel surfaces of soft tissues in an unequal fashion. This situation can occur when the head of a bed is raised, causing the upper torso to slide downward, transmitting pressure to the sacrum and other areas. This effect results in occlusion or distortion of vessels, leading to compromise of the dermis. At the same time, shearing forces are created by sitting and gravity; the posterior sacral skin area can become fixed secondary to friction with the bed. The effects of friction and shearing forces combine, resulting in transmission of force to the deep portion of the superficial fascia and leading to further damage of soft-tissue structures.

Compounding the problems of shearing and friction forces are the macerating effects of excessive moisture in the local environment, resulting from incontinence and perspiration. This factor is of critical importance, because when combined with the other forces, it increases the risk of pressure sore formation fivefold.[38]

CLINICAL PRESENTATION

The persistence of the causative factors (as discussed previously) often results in pressure sore formation. Without treatment, an initial small localized area of ulceration can rapidly progress to 5 to 6 cm within days. The visible ulcer is just a small portion of the actual wound; up to 70% of the total wound is below the skin. A pressure gradient phenomenon is created by which the wound takes on a conical nature; the smallest point is at the skin surface and the largest portion of the defect is at the base of the ulcer (Fig. 100–1).

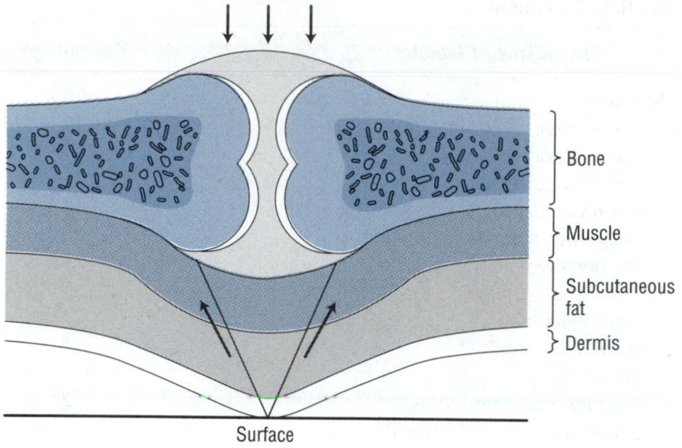

FIGURE 100–1. Distribution of forces involved with sore formation in a conical fashion.

Pressure sores can occur anywhere on the body. More than 95% of all pressure sores are located on the lower part of the body (65% in the region of the pelvis and 3.4% on the lower extremities) (Fig. 100–2). The most common sites

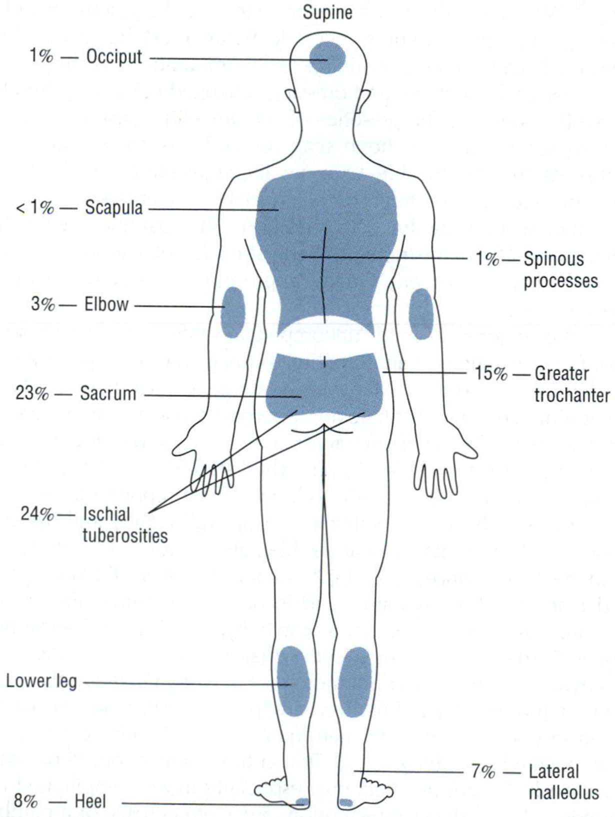

FIGURE 100–2. Supine view of areas where pressure sore formation tends to occur.

on the lower portion of the body are the sacral and coccygeal areas, ischial tuberosities, and greater trochanter.

Numerous systems for classification of pressure sores have been described. The two most frequently used systems are those of Shea[39] and the 1989 National Pressure Ulcer Advisory Panel.[40] These classification systems define the various stages of progression through which a pressure sore may pass (Table 100–5).

Complications of pressure sores are not uncommon and may be life threatening. The most frequently encountered complications are infectious in nature. Pressure sores are routinely colonized by a wide variety of microorganisms; gram-negative aerobes and anaerobes are most often associated with the infections.[41] Systemic infections are not infrequent, with the most common organisms being gram-negative aerobes and anaerobes. Extension to the bone can occur and can lead to osteomyelitis and pyarthroses.

TABLE 100–5. Pressure Sore Classification

Stage	Description
1	Pressure sore is generally reversible, is limited to the epidermis, and resembles an abrasion. It is best described as an irregularly shaped area of soft-tissue swelling with induration and heat.
2	A stage 2 sore may also be reversible; it extends through the dermis to the subcutaneous fat along with extensive undermining.
3[a]	In this instance, the sore or ulcer extends further into subcutaneous fat along with extensive undermining.
4[a]	The sore or ulcer is characterized by penetration into deep fascia involving both muscle and bone.

[a]Stages 3 and 4 lesions are unlikely to resolve on their own and often require surgical intervention.
From Ref. 36.

▶ TREATMENT: Infected Pressure Sores

PREVENTION

Prevention is the single most important aspect in the management of pressure sores. Prevention is far easier and less costly than the intensive care necessary for the healing and eventual closure of pressure sores. Of primary importance, then, is the ability to identify those patients who are at high risk so that preventive measures may be instituted.

Friction and shearing forces can be minimized by proper positioning. Skin care and prevention of soilage are important, with the intent being to keep the surface relatively free of moisture. Patients with problems of incontinence should be frequently cleaned, and efforts should be made to keep the involved areas dry. Natural sheepskin is believed to be useful in minimizing the effects of moisture, shearing forces, and friction. Relief of pressure is probably the single most important factor in preventing pressure sore formation. Relief even for 5 minutes once every 2 hours is believed to give protection against pressure sore formation.[37]

MEDICAL MANAGEMENT

The medical approach to the treatment of pressure sores depends on the stage of the disease. Medical management is generally indicated for lesions that are of moderate size and relatively shallow depth (stage 1 or 2 lesions) and are not located over a bony prominence. Depending on their location and severity, from 30% to 80% of these ulcers will heal without an operation. Generally, medical treatment is not indicated for the management of those ulcers that extend through superficial fascia or into bone (stage 3 and 4 lesions). When the disease becomes this severe, surgical intervention is almost always necessary.

The goal of topical therapy is to clean and decontaminate the ulcer, to promote wound healing by permitting the formation of healthy granulation tissue, or to prepare the wound for an operative procedure. The main factors to be considered for successful topical therapy (local care) are relief of pressure, cleaning measures (debridement), disinfection, and stimulation of granulation tissue. Before any topical agents can be employed effectively, good wound care is necessary.

DEBRIDEMENT

The goals of debridement and cleansing measures are removal of devitalized tissue and reduction of bacterial contamination, which can slow granulation time and, therefore, impede healing. Debridement can be accomplished by surgical, mechanical (wet-to-dry dressing changes, which refers to application of saline-soaked gauze to the wound; after drying, the gauze is removed and with it any adherent necrotic tissue), or chemical means. Chemical debridement is time consuming and is an extremely controversial issue (Table 100–6). None of the available debriding agents has been documented to be superior to wet-to-dry dressings.[42] Surgical debridement rapidly removes necrotic material from the wound, but the associated risks include destruction of surrounding viable tissue, inadvertent enlargement of the ulcer, and possible extension of any existing infection. Another effective mechanical therapy is hydrodebridement—use of the whirlpool (Hubbard tank) to remove necrotic tissue and debris. It is a useful adjunct to both surgical and chemical debridement.

Collagenase is thought by many to be the most effective enzymatic debriding agent.[43,44] Collagenase is able to dissolve undenatured collagen fibers, which anchor necrotic tissue to the surface of the wound, without damaging granulation tissue. Collagenase is effective only within the pH range 6 to 8, so cleansing of the wound with an acidic solution should be avoided. Collagenase is inhibited by many cleansing agents (hexachlorophene, benzalkonium chloride) and many heavy metal-containing antiseptics (silver nitrate, thimerosal).[43] Dakin's solution and buffered (pH 7.0 to 7.5) normal saline solution will not inhibit

TABLE 100–6. Chemical Debriding Agents (Partial List)

Enzymes	Streptokinase/streptodornase (not commercially available)
Sutilains (Travase)	**Elements**
Collagenase (Santyl)	Dextranomer (Debrisan)
Fibrinolysin and desoxyribonuclease (Elase)	Hydrogen peroxide
Trypsin (Granulex)	Silver nitrate
Papin (Panafil)	

enzymatic activity. Generally, collagenase need only be applied to a clean wound once daily, unless the wound is extremely soiled. Adverse reactions to collagenase are rare. It may cause irritation and inflammation of normal skin located at the edges of the wound.

Sutilains (Travase) is a proteolytic enzyme that selectively digests necrotic tissue and has minimal activity in digesting collagen. Sutilains functions optimally in the pH range 6.0 to 6.8.[45] A loose wet dressing should be used and kept moist to allow the best environment for release of the enzyme. The entire dressing process should be repeated every 6 to 8 hours.[43] Sutilains is inactivated by the same agents as collagenase. Adverse reactions reported with the use of sutilains include burning pain, paresthesias, transient dermatitis at the site of application, and occasional bleeding.[43] Sutilains has been documented to improve healing rates in studies in both animals and humans. Other enzymatic debriding agents, such as fibrinolysin and deoxyribonuclease (Elase) and trypsin, are also available but not as commonly used. To date, no specific enzymatic preparation has been shown to be more effective than any other product and use depends on user preference.

Dextranomer (Debrisan) is purported to both clean and debride wounds. It consists of beads composed of hydrophilic dextran molecules cross-linked with O-glycerylene groups. The material is chemically inert and is believed to work by molecular and capillary absorption of fluid from the wound. Dextranomer appears to be effective in cleansing exudative venous stasis and decubitus ulcers. It also appears to increase tissue granulation, decrease wound inflammation, and decrease pus and debris; however, its cost and application techniques limit its usefulness. Few controlled trials are available with which to gauge accurately this drug's efficacy. Application of dextranomer should be preceded by cleansing of the wound, with the site left moist. The site is then packed with dry beads to a depth of one-eighth to one-quarter of an inch and covered with gauze. Two to three times daily, the material should be removed and the application repeated. No major adverse reactions have been reported with the use of dextranomer, although application and removal of the beads may cause intermittent pain, bleeding, blistering, and erythema in some patients. These agents are an aid, not a substitute, for the debridement process.

DISINFECTION

A number of agents have been used to disinfect pressure sores (Table 100–7), as well as other types of open wounds; however, objective clinical trials evaluating their efficacy are lacking. The agents used for disinfection and wound cleansing are classified as soaps, astringents, disinfectants, and topical antibiotics. Disinfectants are used to reduce the bacterial content of open wounds. These agents have not been shown to penetrate tissue well, however, and, as a result, cannot sterilze these infected wounds but may decrease the number of bacteria present to fewer than 100,000 organisms per gram of tissue.[46]

Paradoxically, there is debate as to whether disinfectants help or interfere with wound healing. Lineaweaver and associates[47] reported that many disinfecting agents microscopically cause tissue damage within already existing wounds and, therefore, may delay wound healing. Studies of the effects of various topical antimicrobials and povidone-iodine on wound healing have yielded inconsistent results.[48,49] The role of topical antibiotics (Table 100–7) is still unclear. These products do not penetrate deeper tissue and have not been documented to reduce bacterial counts by significant amounts. Problems with resistance, systemic toxicity, and sensitization further cloud any potential benefit.[46]

Although disinfectants do not sterilize a wound and may interfere with wound healing, they may be of potential benefit.

TABLE 100–7. Disinfecting Agents

Acetic acid	Sodium hypochlorite (Dakin's)
Sodium oxychlorosene	Hydrogen peroxide
Povidone-iodine	Hexachlorophene
Topical antibiotics	Mupirocin ointment
Neomycin	Gentamicin
Chloramphenicol	Bacitracin
Polymyxin B	Metronidazole

These agents can be used to help clean the wound (by decreasing the bacterial counts), but they should be stopped when the wound is clean and granulation appears to be occurring.

GRANULATION/EPITHELIALIZATION

After the pressure sore has been adequately debrided and disinfected, and pressure, friction, and moisture have been kept to a minimum, granulation and reepithelialization begin. An agent that promotes and hastens this process would obviously be desirable. Many agents (Table 100–8) have been suggested, but hardly any evidence of a supportive nature exists.

A different approach to decreasing the time needed for wound healing is aimed at wound dressing materials (Table 100–8). Wound dressing materials should keep the wound moist, allow free exchange of air, act as a physical barrier to bacteria, and prevent physical damage. Two representative types of products are of some interest, DuoDerm and Op-Site (Table 100–8). Hydrocolloid occlusive dressings (DuoDerm) are opaque and impermeable to water and oxygen.[46] This type of dressing absorbs moisture from the wound exudate and forms a gel-like covering over the wound. Op-Site is representative of the polyurethane film class of product. This group is semipermeable, allowing evaporation. One study examined Op-Site, DuoDerm, wet-to-dry dressing, and a control group in pigs.[50] Significantly faster reepithelialization and greater collagen synthesis were noted in the wounds covered with Op-Site and DuoDerm. Both wet-to-dry gauze dressing changes and DuoDerm led to damaged epithelium during removal. The major appeal of these occlusive-type dressings is that they need to be changed only once every several days versus several times daily for the traditional wet-to-dry dressing technique.

Two other product categories are the hydrogel dressings and the synthetic barrier dressings. Hydrogel dressings are nonadhe-

TABLE 100–8. Agents Used to Promote Granulation and Epithelialization[a]

Pharmacologic Agents	Polyurethane Film Dressings	Synthetic Barrier Dressings
Sugar	Op-Site	Hydron
Karaya	Tegaderm	Silicone spray
Insulin	Acu-Derm	Silicone foam
Powdered gelatin	Bioclusive	**Occlusive Dressings**
Gelatin sponge (Gelfoam)	Opraflex	Hydrocolloid occlusive dressing
Benzoyl peroxide	**Hydrogel Dressings**	DuoDerm
Dextranomer	Vigilon	Comfeel ulcer care
Scarlet red	Geliperm	Intact
Mercurochrome		Restore wound care
		IntraSite

[a]Partial listing of wound care products.

sive and oxygen permeable unless covered by a nonpermeable barrier, and they will maintain a moist environment. Synthetic barrier dressings consist of an inert powder and a liquid solvent. When mixed together, a paste is formed that, when applied, will adhere to the wound, maintaining a moist surface. This dressing allows the wound exudate to pass through and then be absorbed by a secondary dressing.

Other nonpharmacologic approaches to shortening the healing time have included the use of oxygen,[51] hydrotherapy,[52] high-frequency, high-intensity sound waves,[53] and electrotherapy.[54] Although more than 2000 agents have either been studied or used in the treatment of pressure sores, few controlled trials have been done that show any single agent to be efficacious. Whichever agent is selected, it must be evaluated on its own merits by the clinician, as limited scientific data are available.

RECOMMENDATIONS

The goal of treatment is to enhance or assist the body's own repair process. The practitioner should not only assess the wound but also the patient's underlying immune status (diabetes mellitus or cancer) and nutritional status. Initially, an attempt should be made to identify the causative or contributing factors that have led to the development of the pressure sore and either eradicate them or substantially lessen their presence. These factors may include pressure, friction, or moisture (excessive sweating or incontinence).

Next, the patient should be evaluated for pain or tenderness at the wound or surrounding tissues. An attempt should be made to alleviate the patient's pain either via drug therapy or by mechanical intervention.

During the initial phase of the evaluation, the wound should be evaluated for the presence or absence of local or systemic infection. The absence or presence of purulent discharge with or without a foul odor may give clues as to the presence of infection.

Treatment of the wound begins with the removal of necrotic tissue via either debridement or surgery, along with elimination of any infection. The goal of therapy is to maintain a "clean and moist" environment. This process may take from days to weeks and include either topical or systemic therapy. Those patients with superficial wounds may require only 2 to 3 days of therapy, while those with severely infected wounds will require a full 10- to 14-day treatment course of antimicrobials.

Unfortunately, there is no one right way to treat patients with pressure sores. Therefore, the patient needs to be continually reassessed and treatment changed accordingly. Some broad, major guidelines can be recommended for the treatment of pressure sores (stages 1 and 2):

1. Relieve pressure.
2. Avoid unnecessary friction and shearing forces.
3. Prevent patient from lying in a moist environment.
4. Use debridement, either pharmacologic or via minor surgical approach.
5. Keep the wound clean by pharmacologic means or through use of a physical barrier.
6. Use occlusive dressing (may also lead to increased healing and simplify the nursing care routine) if possible.

For stages 3 and 4 pressure sores, surgical management is most likely the major approach, with follow-up according to guidelines 1 through 5.

INFECTED BITE WOUNDS

One of the most common problems seen in emergency rooms in the United States is the bite wound. Animal bites have a substantial potential for infectious complications. If left untreated, complications, including soft-tissue infection or osteomyelitis, may occur, possibly requiring extensive debridement or amputation. Approximately 4 million people in this country are bitten by dogs annually. The incidence of other bites (cats, humans, and snakes) remains undetermined. Most of the therapeutic decisions surrounding bite wounds are controversial, since most of the available data are derived from anecdotal case reports.

DOG BITES

In the United States, approximately 2% of the population has been bitten by a dog. Dog bites account for 80% to 90% of all animal bite wounds requiring medical attention. Dog bites commonly occur in individuals less than 20 years of age (52.2% of reported cases) who are most often male (57.8%). More than 70% of bites are to the extremities.[55] Occasionally, facial bites may occur, and these are seen most often in children under 15 and can be a lethal event via exsanguination. From 1979 through 1994, 279 deaths were the result of attacks by dogs.[56]

Health care providers see two distinct groups of patients seeking medical attention for dog bites.[57] The first group of patients presents 8 to 12 hours after the injury. These patients require general wound care, repair of tear wounds, or rabies, tetanus therapies, or both. The second group of patients presents more than 12 hours after the injury has occurred. These patients usually have clinical signs of infection and seek medical attention for infection-related complaints (i.e., pain, purulent discharge, swelling). Those patients at greatest risk of acquiring an infection after a bite have had a puncture wound (usually the hand), have not sought medical attention within 12 hours of the injury, and are older than 50.[58,59]

The infected dog bite is usually characterized by a localized cellulitis and pain at the site of injury. The cellulitis usually spreads proximally from the initial site of injury. If *Pasteurella multocida* is present, a rapidly progressing cellulitis with a gray malodorous discharge may be encountered. Fewer than 20% of patients have a concomitant adenopathy or lymphangitis. Fever is uncommon. Wounds close to bones or joints may lead to infections of these structures.

Infections from dog bite wounds are caused predominantly by organisms documented to be from the dog's oral flora.[59] Studies examining the normal flora of the dog frequently isolate *P. multocida, S. aureus,* coagulase-negative staphylococci, and various unnamed organisms (Ilj and EF-4 are unidentified organisms given numeric designations by the Center for Disease Control and Prevention [CDC]).[60,61] Wound site cultures in both infected and noninfected patients have similar bacteria present, with aerobic organisms (including facultative bacteria) isolated from 74% and anaerobic organisms isolated from 41%.[61,62] The most frequently isolated organisms from infected and noninfected wounds are *S. aureus,* β-hemolytic streptococci, *Streptococcus intermedius, P. multocida, Eikenella corrodens, Capnocytophaga canimursus, Bacteroides* sp., and *Fusobacterium* sp.[62] Cultures obtained from noninfected bite wounds unfortunately have not been of value in predicting the subsequent development of infection. Documentation of the mechanism of injury is important; if possible, an immunization history of the animal should be obtained. It is also important for the patient's tetanus immune status to be determined.

Wounds should be thoroughly irrigated with a sterile saline solution or a chlorhexidine scrub solution. Proper irrigation significantly decreases the rate of subsequent infection.[57] Several management techniques used in the treatment of bite wounds remain controversial; these include the extent and type of debridement,[57] the use of primary closure within 24 hours of the injury,[62] and indications for the use of antibiotics.

The role of prophylactic antimicrobial therapy for the early, noninfected bite wound remains controversial.[55,63] Suggestions concerning the use of prophylactic antibiotics unfortunately are based on minimal data since few clinical trials have been performed. Most reports are of retrospective studies or on observations of complicated cases. A meta-analysis of eight randomized trials of dog bite wounds evaluated the use of antibiotics for prophylaxis for the prevention of infectious complications.[64] The overall occurrence of infectious complications ranged form 3.2% to 45.8%. All studies used oral antibiotics with six of the eight using either penicillin or a penicillinase-resistant penicillin. Five of the eight studies documented a reduced risk for infection in those patients receiving antimicrobial prophylaxis.

Since controlled studies have not definitively shown any benefit for the use of prophylactic antibiotics for noninfected bites, they are not routinely recommended; however, a semisynthetic penicillinase-resistant penicillin orally or amoxicillin should be used for those patients at greater risk for infection (patients older than 50 years of age, puncture wounds, wounds to the hands, and wounds in compromised hosts).[65,66] Amoxicillin/clavulanic acid has been documented as effective in these situations but because of its high cost and increased incidence of side effects some consider it to be of limited use.[57] Tetracycline or TMP/SMX is recommended as an alternative form of therapy for those patients allergic to penicillins. Erythromycin may be considered an alternative for tetracycline in growing children or pregnant women. If erythromycin is selected, then sensitivities should be obtained, because *P. multocida* isolates may be resistant in up to 50% of cases. Prophylactic therapy should be given for 5 days. In addition to irrigation and antibiotics, when indicated, the injured area should be immobilized and elevated.

Infections developing within the first 24 hours of a bite are most often caused by *P. multocida* and should be treated with penicillin or amoxicillin (tetracycline is an alternative for nonpregnant adult penicillin-allergic patients).[65] For severe infections, IV penicillin (1.2 million units every 4 to 6 hours) therapy should be started and followed by oral therapy when the signs of cellulitis have subsided. Treatment should be given for 10 to 14 days. Semisynthetic penicillinase-resistant penicillins should be avoided in these cases because of their poor activity against *P. multocida.* Activity of certain oral cephalosporins (cephalexin, cefaclor, cefadroxil) against this organism *in vitro* has been conflicting.[66] Susceptibilities should be done before prescribing a first- or second-generation cephalosporin where *P. multocida* is considered to be a potential pathogen.

For those infections developing more than 36 to 48 hours after the bite, the risk of *P. multocida* being involved dramatically decreases in likelihood. In these patients, *Staphylococcus* or *Streptococcus* are the most likely causative pathogens. Therapy, in this instance, includes a penicillinase-resistant penicillin (dicloxacillin) or a cephalosporin (cefuroxime axetil) and should be given for a full 10 to 14 days.[65] Results of a Gram stain should be used to confirm the appropriateness of therapy.

The fluoroquinolones are highly active *in vitro* against the aerobic isolates found in these bite wounds; however, in general they have very little activity against the anaerobes isolated in these infections. Their role in the therapy of bite wounds has yet to be defined.

Tetanus does not commonly occur after dog bites; however, it is a theoretical possibility. If the immunization history of a patient with anything other than a clean, minor wound is not known, tetanus-diphtheria (TD) toxoids and tetanus immune globulin (TIG) should be administered.[67] Patients with wounds that do not require immunization with TD toxoid are those who have had three or more immunization doses of TIG within the past 5 years. Patients who have received three or more doses of TIG within the last 10 years or patients who received two doses of TIG within the first 24 hours of injury do not require additional TIG therapy.[67]

Because the rabies virus can be transmitted via saliva, rabies may be a potential complication of a bite. When the symptoms of rabies develop after a bite, the prognosis for survival is poor. Roughly 3% of rabies cases documented in animals were in dogs (the most frequent vectors are skunks, raccoons, and bats).

Once a patient has been exposed to rabies, the treatment objectives consist of thorough irrigation of the wound, tetanus prophylaxis, antibiotic prophylaxis, if indicated, and immunization. Postexposure prophylaxis immunization consists of *both* passive antibody administration and vaccine administration. The only exceptions to antibody administration are patients who have been previously immunized and have the appropriate degree of documented rabies antibody titers.

CAT BITES

Cats are probably the second most common cause of animal bite wounds in the United States, but unfortunately very few data are available on the incidence and infection rate of these bites.[59] The major problems associated with cat bites are puncture wounds and scratches usually located on the lower extremities. Approximately 40% of cat bites and scratches become infected. These infections are frequently caused by *P. multocida,* which has been isolated in the oropharynx of 50% to 70% of healthy cats.[58] Both tularemia *(Pasteurella tularensis)* and rabies have also been transmitted by cat bites.[58]

The management of cat bites is similar to that discussed for dog bites. Antibiotic therapy with penicillin is the mainstay, and therapy is as described for dog bites.

HUMAN BITES

Infected human bites can occur as bites from the teeth or from blows to the teeth (clenched-fist injuries). Human bites are generally more serious than animal bites and carry a higher likelihood of infection. Infectious complications occur in up to 50% of patients with human bites.[68]

Self-inflicted bites most commonly occur on the lips or around the fingernails (from sucking or biting the nails). Bites by others can occur to any part of the body, but most often involve the hands. Bites to the hand are most serious and more frequently become infected. The clenched-fist injury is a traumatic laceration caused by one person hitting another in the mouth and is one of the most serious of bite wounds. The areas most commonly affected by this injury are the third and fourth metacarpophalangeal joints.

Patients with infected bites to the hand may develop a painful, throbbing, swollen extremity. The wound often has a purulent discharge, and the patient complains of a decreased range of motion. In addition to a cellulitis, other complications, such as osteomyelitis, septic arthritis, and tenosynovitis, can occur. Loss of a digit or hand has been reported.

Infections caused by these injuries are similar, and most often are caused by the normal oral flora, which include both aerobic and anaerobic microorganisms. The most frequent aerobic organisms are streptococcal sp., *S. aureus, Streptococcus* sp., *Haemophilus parainfluenzae,* and *Klebsiella pneumoniae.*[69,70] *Eikenella corrodens,* a facultative anaerobe can be isolated from human bite wounds approximately 30% of the time. Other common anaerobic organisms are *Bacteroides* sp., *Fusobacterium* sp., *Peptostreptococcus* sp., and *Peptococcus* sp.[69,70] Anaerobic microorganisms have been isolated in the range of 40% of human bites and 55% of clenched-fist injuries.

Management of bite wounds consists of aggressive irrigation, surgical debridement, and immobilization of the affected area. Primary closure for human bites is not generally recommended. If damage to a bone or joint is suspected, radiographic evaluation should be undertaken. Tetanus toxoid and antitoxin may be indicated.

Patients with noninfected hand bite injuries should be given prophylactic antibiotic therapy. Initial therapy should consist of a penicillinase-resistant penicillin (dicloxacillin) in combination with penicillin. Prophylactic therapy should be given for 3 to 5 days as for dog bites.[71] A first-generation cephalosporin is not recommended, as the sensitivity to *E. corrodens* is variable.[72]

For infected bite wounds, penicillin and a penicillinase-resistant penicillin or amoxicillin/clavulonic acid should be empirically started and changed pending the culture results. Macrolides or tetracyclines may be used as an alternative therapy for the penicillin-allergic patient. Hospitalization for minor wounds is not necessary if surgical repair of vital structures has not been performed. Those patients suffering serious injuries or clenched-fist injuries should be started on IV antibiotics. Duration of therapy for infected bite injuries should be 7 to 14 days.

Antibiotic therapy should always be used in clenched-fist injuries. Therapy should include penicillin (or ampicillin) plus a penicillinase-resistant penicillin until the final cultures are available. Therapeutic failures have been documented when either first-generation cephalosporins or penicillinase-resistant penicillins have been used alone, most likely because of their poor and variable activity against *E. corrodens.*[73,74] Therapy should be continued from 7 to 14 days.[71]

Guidelines for therapy of infections associated with bites are:

1. Determine the time frame of injury to presentation.
2. Determine rabies and tetanus status, and administer rabies and tetanus prophylaxis when necessary.
3. All wounds should be thoroughly cleaned.
4. If the wound looks benign, without infection, or indication of other than local involvement, the patient can be sent home on oral antimicrobial agents (3 to 5 days) based on the type of bite injury.
5. Wounds that are swollen, tender, erythematous, and with lymphadenopathy require hospitalization for observation. In this instance, parenteral antimicrobials along with elevation and splinting of the injured area are the mainstays of therapy (total duration of therapy 7 to 14 days).
6. If improvement is not seen within 24 hours, then aggressive operative debridement is indicated.

▶ PRINCIPLES OF PHARMACOTHERAPY

- Acute cellulitis is usually caused by gram-positive aerobic pathogens, particularly *Staphylococcus aureus* and group A β-hemolytic streptococci and possibly by other gram-positive cocci, enteric gram-negative bacilli, or mixed aerobic–anaerobic pathogens. Infections in other patients (e.g., diabetics, immunocompromised patients, intravenous drug users) may be caused by other pathogens.

- Initial antimicrobial regimens for cellulitis should include agents with activity against staphylococci and streptococci. An antistaphylococcal penicillin (oxacillin or nafcillin) is the drug of choice in most cases; penicillin should be used if the infection is known to be caused by streptococci. Mild infections may be treated with oral therapy, while more severe cases require parenteral therapy. Regimens must be appropriately modified if there is a clinical suspicion of infection because of gram-negative or mixed bacteria.
- Diabetic foot infections are caused by a combination of diabetes-related complications, including neuropathy, angiopathy, and defects in cell-mediated immunity. Appropriate antimicrobial therapy must be combined with proper wound care to achieve optimal patient outcomes.
- Antimicrobial regimens for diabetic foot infections should include coverage for staphylococci, streptococci, enteric gram-negative bacilli, and anaerobes. Mild infections may be treated with oral regimens, including a fluoroquinolone plus clindamycin or metronidazole or amoxicillin/clavulanic acid. Preferred regimens for treatment of severe infections include parenteral monotherapy with second- or third-generation antianaerobic cephalosporins, extended-spectrum penicillins with β-lactamase inhibitors, or carbapenems.
- Prevention is the single most important aspect in the management of pressure sores.
- The main factors for successful topical therapy of pressure sores (local care) are relief of pressure, cleaning measures (debridement), disinfection, and stimulation of granulation tissue. Before any topical agents can be employed effectively, good wound care is necessary.
- Prophylactic antibiotics are not routinely recommended for noninfected dog or cat bites; however, a semisynthetic penicillinase-resistant penicillin orally or amoxicillin should be used for those patients at greater risk for infection, such as patients older than 50 years of age, puncture wounds, wounds to the hands, and wounds in compromised hosts.
- Infections developing within the first 24 hours of a dog bite are caused most often by *P. multocida* and should be treated with 10 to 14 days of injury with penicillin or amoxicillin (tetracycline is an alternative for nonpregnant, adult, penicillin-allergic patients). For those infections developing more than 36 to 48 hours after the bite, *Staphylococcus* or *Streptococcus* are the most likely causative pathogens, and therapy should include a penicillinase-resistant penicillin (dicloxacillin) or a cephalosporin (cefuroxime axetil) and should be given for a full 10 to 14 days.
- Patients with noninfected human bite injuries of the hand should be given prophylactic antibiotic therapy consisting of a penicillinase-resistant penicillin (dicloxacillin) in combination with penicillin (for 3 to 5 days). For infected human bite wounds, penicillin and a penicillinase-resistant penicillin or amoxicillin/clavulonic acid should be empirically started and changed pending the culture results.

REFERENCES

1. Yagupski P. Bacteriologic aspects of skin and soft tissue infections. Pediatr Ann 1993;22:217–224.
2. Ducan WC, McBride ME, Knox JM. Experimental production of infection in humans. J Invest Dermatol 1970;54:319–323.
3. Sadick NS. Current aspects of bacterial infections of the skin. Dermatol Clin 1997;15:341–349.
4. Bisno AL, Stevens DL. Streptococcal infections of skin and soft tissues. New Engl J Med 1996;334:240–245.
5. Orangio GR, Pitlick SD, Latta PD, et al. Soft-tissue infections in parenteral drug abusers. Ann Surg 1984;199:97–100.
6. Bisbe J, Miro J, Latorre, et al. Disseminated candidiasis in addicts who use brown heroin: Report of 83 cases and review. Clin Infec Dis 1992;15:910–923.
7. Hook EW, Hooton TM, Horton C, et al. Microbiologic evaluation of cutaneous cellulitis in adults. Arch Intern Med 1986;146:295–297.
8. Ben-Amitai D, Ashkenazi S. Common bacterial skin infections in childhood. Pediatr Ann 1993;22:225–233.
9. Swartz MN. Cellulitis and subcutaneous tissue infections. In: Mandell GL, Bennett JE, Dolin R, eds. Principles and Practice of Infectious Diseases, 4th ed. New York, Churchill Livingstone, 1995:909–929.
10. Adams G, Deaver KA, Cochi SL, et al. Decline of childhood *Haemophilus influenzae* type b (Hib) disease in the Hib vaccine era. JAMA 1993;269:221–226.
11. Dagan R, Moshe P, Watemberg N, et al. Outpatient treatment of serious community-acquired pediatric infections using once daily intramuscular ceftriaxone. Pediatr Infect Dis J 1987;6:1080–1084.
12. Gould IM, Hudson M, Morris J, et al. Imipenem versus standard therapy in the treatment of serious soft tissue infection. Drugs Exp Clin Res 1988;14(8):555–558.
13. Kulhanjian J, Dunphy M, Hamstra S, et al. Randomized comparative study of ampicillin/sulbactam vs. ceftriaxone for treatment of soft tissue and skeletal infections in children. Pediatr Infect Dis J 1989;8:605–610.
14. Tan JS, Wishnow RM, Talan DA, et al. Treatment of hospitalized patients with complicated skin and skin structure infections: Double-blind, randomized, multicenter study of piperacillin–tazobactam versus ticarcillin–clavulanate. Antimicrob Agents Chemother 1993;37:1580–1586.
15. Gentry LO, Ramirez-Ronda CH, Rodriquez-Noriega E, et al. Oral ciprofloxacin vs. parenteral cefotaxime in the treatment of difficult skin and skin structure infections. Arch Intern Med 1989;148:2579–2583.
16. Gentry LO. Therapy with newer oral β-lactam and quinolone agents for infections of the skin and skin structures: A review. Clin Infect Dis 1992;14:285–297.
17. Gentry LO, Rodriguez-Gomez G, Zeluff BJ, et al. A comparative evaluation of oral ofloxacin versus intravenous cefotaxime therapy for serious skin and skin structure infections. Am J Med 1989;87(suppl 6C):57S–S60.
18. Thadepalli H, Mathai D, Chuah SK, et al. Ciprofloxacin versus ceftazidime in skin and soft tissue infections. J Chemother 1989;1(1):30–34.

19. Dominquez J, Palma F, Vega ME, et al. Brief report: Prospective, controlled, randomized non-blind comparison of intravenous/oral ciprofloxacin with intravenous ceftazidime in the treatment of skin or soft-tissue infections. Am J Med 1989;87(suppl 5A)13:136S–137S.
20. LeFrock J, Blais F, Schell, et al. Cefoxitin in the treatment of diabetic patients with lower extremity infections. Infect Surg 1983;2:361–374.
21. Hughes C, Johnson C, Bamberger D, et al. Treatment and long-term follow-up of foot infections in patients with diabetes or ischemia: A randomized, prospective, double-blind comparison of cefoxitin and ceftizoxime. Clin Ther 1987;10(suppl A):36–49.
22. Feder HM, Osier C, Madefazo EG. Chloramphenicol: A review of its use in clinical practice. Rev Infect Dis 1981;3:479–491.
23. Crane L, Levine D, Aervos M, et al. Bacteremia in narcotic addicts at Detroit Medical Center: Microbiology, epidemiology, risk factors, and empiric therapy. Rev Infect Dis 1986;8:364–373.
24. Baltimore RS. Treatment of impetigo: A review. Pediatr Infect Dis 1985;4:597–601.
25. Swartz MN. Lymphadenitis and lymphangitis. In: Mandell GL, Bennett JE, Dolin R, eds. Principles and Practice of Infectious Diseases, 4th ed. New York, Churchill Livingstone, 1995:936–944.
26. Bass JW. Treatment of skin and skin structure infections. Pediatr Infect Dis J 1992;11:152–155.
27. Lipsky BA, Pecoraro RE, Wheat LJ. The diabetic foot: Soft tissue and bone infection. Infect Dis Clin North Am 1990;4:409–432.
28. Levin ME. Foot lesions in patients with diabetes mellitus. Endocrinol Metab Clin North Am 1996;25:447–462.
29. West NJ. Systemic antimicrobial treatment of foot infections in diabetic patients. Am J Health-Syst Pharm 1995;52:1199–207.
30. Gerding DN. Foot infections in diabetic patients: The role of anaerobes. Clin Infect Dis 1995;20(suppl 2):S283–S288.
31. Caputo GM, Cavanagh PR, Ulbrecht JS, et al. Assessment and management of foot disease in patients with diabetes. New Engl J Med 1994;331:854–860.
32. Grayson ML. Diabetic foot infections: Antimicrobial therapy. Infect Dis Clin North Am 1995;9:143–161.
33. Smith AJ, Daniels T, Bohnen JMA. Soft tissue infections and the diabetic foot. Am J Surg 1996;172(suppl 6A):7S–12S.
34. Parish LC, Aten EM. Treatment of skin and skin structure infections: A comparative study of Augmentin and cefaclor. Cutis 1984;34: 567–570.
35. Eron LJ, Harvey L, Hixon DL, et al. Ciprofloxacin therapy of infections caused by *Pseudomonas aeruginosa* and other resistant bacteria. Antimicrob Agents Chemother 1985;28:308–310.
36. Sesin PG, Paszko A, O'Keefe E. Oral clindamycin and ciprofloxacin therapy for diabetic foot infections. Pharmacother 1990;10:154–156.
37. Goode PS, Allman RM. The prevention and management of pressure sores. Med Clin North Am 1989;73:1511–1524.
38. Reuler JB, Cooney TG. The pressure sore: Pathophysiology and principles of management. Ann Intern Med 1981;94:661–666.
39. Shea JD. Pressure sores—Classification and management. Clin Orthop 1975;112:89–100.
40. National Pressure Ulcer Advisory Panel. Pressure ulcers: Incidence, economics, risk. Consensus Development Conference statement. West Dundee, IL, 1989.
41. Gradon J, Adamsom C. Infections of pressure ulcers: Management and controversies. Infect Dis Clin Pract 1995;1:11–16.
42. Antypas PG. Management of pressure sores. Curr Probl Surg 1980; 17:229–244.
43. Nierman MM. Treatment of dermal and decubitis ulcers. Drugs 1978;15:226–230.
44. Varma AO, Burgatch E, German FM. Debridement of dermal ulcers with collagenase. Surg Gynecol Obstet 1973;136:281–282.
45. Coopwood TB. Evaluation of a topical enzymatic debridement agent—Sutilains ointment. South Med J 1976;69:834.
46. Longe RL. Current concepts in clinical therapeutics: Pressure sores. Clin Pharm 1986;5:669–681.
47. Lineaweaver W, Howard R, Soucy D, et al. Topical antimicrobial toxicity. Arch Surg 1985;120:267–270.
48. Geronemus R, Mertz P, Eaglstein W. Wound healing: The effects of topical antimicrobial agents. Arch Dermatol 1979;115:1311–1314.
49. Dennis D, Luterman A, Ramenofsky F, et al. Does PVP-iodine interfere with wound healing? Infect Surg 1983;4:371–374.
50. Alvarez OM, Mertz AM, Englstein WH. The effect of occlusive dressings on collagen synthesis and re-epithellialization in superficial wounds. J Surg Res 1983;35:142–148.
51. Olenjniczaks S, Zrelinski A. Topical oxygen promotes healing of leg ulcers. Resident Staff Phys 1977;23:165–242.
52. Knight AL. Medical management of pressure sores. J Fam Prac 1988;27:95–100.
53. Paul BJ, Lafratta CW, Dawson AR, et al. Use of ultrasound in the treatment of pressure sores in patients with spinal cord injuries. Arch Phys Med Rehabil 1960;41:438.
54. Wolcott LE, Wheeler PC, Hardwicke HM, et al. Accelerated healing of skin ulcers by electrotherapy: Preliminary clinical results. South Med J 1969;62:795–801.
55. Goldstein E. Bite wounds and infection. Clin Infec Dis 1992;14: 633–640.
56. Anon. Dog bite related fatalities—United States, 1995–1996. MMWR 1997;46:463–467.
57. Callaham ML. Treatment of common dog bites: Infection risk factors. J Am Coll Emerg Phys 1978;7:83–87.
58. Rest JG, Goldstein EJC. Management of human and animal bite wounds. Emerg Med Clin North Am 1985;3:117–126.
59. Goldstein EJC, Citron DM, Finegold SM. Role of anaerobic bacteria in bite wound infections. Rev Infect Dis 1984;6(suppl 1):S177–S183.
60. Baile WE, Stowe EC, Schmitt AM. Aerobic bacterial flora of oral and nasal fluids of canines with reference to bacteria associated with bites. J Clin Microbiol 1978;7:223–231.
61. Wiggins ME, Akelamn E, Weiss AP. The management of dog bites and dog bite infections to the hand. Orthopedics 1994;17:617–623.
62. Goldstein EJC, Citron DM, Finegold SM. Dog bite wounds and infection: A prospective clinical study. Ann Emerg Med 1980;9:508–512.
63. Elenbass RM, McNaoney WK, Robinson WA. Prophylactic oxacillin in dog bite wounds. Ann Emerg Med 1982;11:248–251.
64. Cummings P. Antibiotics to prevent infections in patients with dog bite wounds: A meta-analysis of randomized trials. Ann Emerg Med 1994;23:535–540.
65. Elliot DL, Tolle SW, Goldberg L, et al. Pet-associated illness. N Engl J Med 1985;313:985–995.
66. Goldstein E, Citron DM, Richwals GA. Lack of *in vitro* efficacy of oral forms of certain cephalosporins, erythromycin, and oxacillin against *Pasteurella multocida.* Antimicrob Agents Chemother 1988; 32(2):213–215.
67. Goldstein EJ, Reinhardt JF, Murray PM, et al. Outpatient therapy of bite wounds: Demographic data, bacteriology, and a prospective, randomized trial of amoxicillin/clavulanic acid versus pencillin ± dicloxacillin. Int J Derm 1987;26(2):123–127.
68. Mann RJ, Hoffield TA, Farmer CB. Human bites of the hand: Twenty years of experience. J Hand Surg 1977;2:97–99.
69. Goldstein EJC, Citron DM, Wield B, et al. Bacteriology of human and animal bite wounds. J Clin Microbiol 1978;8:667–672.
70. Peeples E, Boswick JA, Scott FA. Wounds of the hand contaminated by human and animal saliva. J Trauma 1980;20:383–389.
71. Talan D. Infectious disease issues in the emergency department. Clin Infect Dis 1996;23:1–14.
72. Goldstein E, Gombert M, Agyare E. Susceptibility of *Eikenella corrodens* to newer beta-lactam antibiotics. Antimicrob Agents Chemother 1980;18:832–833.
73. Goldstein E, Miller T, Citron D, et al. Infections following clenched-fist injury: A new perspective. J Hand Surg 1978;3:455–459.
74. Goldstein E, Barene M, Miller TA. *Eikenella corrodens* in hand infections. J Hand Surg 1983;8:563–566.

101

INFECTIVE ENDOCARDITIS

Michael A. Crouch, PharmD, BCPS, and Ron E. Polk, PharmD

Endocarditis is an inflammation of the endocardium, which is the membrane lining the chambers of the heart and covering the cusps of the heart valves.[1,2] More commonly, endocarditis refers to infection of the heart valves by various microorganisms. If untreated, endocarditis is usually fatal. With treatment, the average mortality is approximately 20%, although the range in mortality is wide, depending on the presence or absence of various risk factors.[3]

Endocarditis is often referred to as either acute or subacute, depending on the clinical presentation. Acute bacterial endocarditis (ABE) is a fulminating infection associated with high fevers and systemic toxicity; if untreated, death occurs within a few days to weeks. This syndrome most frequently follows infection of previously normal valves by virulent bacteria, such as *Staphylococcus aureus.* Subacute bacterial endocarditis (SBE) is a more indolent infection caused by less invasive organisms, such as viridans streptococci, usually occurring in preexisting valvular heart disease. Infection may also follow surgical insertion of a prosthetic heart valve, resulting in prosthetic valve endocarditis (PVE).[4]

Although endocarditis is caused primarily by bacteria, the clinical presentation does not reliably predict the causative organism. In addition, endocarditis caused by fungi and other atypical microorganisms is becoming more common. Therefore, the more encompassing term *infective endocarditis* (IE) is preferred.

EPIDEMIOLOGY AND ETIOLOGY

Infective endocarditis is an uncommon infection, accounting for approximately 1 out of every 1000 hospital admissions.[1] The male-to-female ratio is 2:1. Overall, the mean age of patients with IE exceeds 50 years; the infection is unusual in children.[5] As the population ages and as valve replacement surgery becomes more common, the mean age of patients with IE increases. An exception is the IV drug abuser, who tends to be a younger male.

Most persons with IE have evidence of risk factors, such as preexisting cardiac valvular abnormalities. Many types of structural heart disease result in turbulence of blood flow that increase the risk for IE. A predisposing factor, however, may be absent in up to 25% of cases.[6] Some of the more important risk factors include:

- Presence of a prosthetic valve.
- Previous bacterial endocarditis.
- Congenital heart disease accompanied by cyanosis (such as single ventricle states).
- Rheumatic heart disease following rheumatic fever.
- Hypertrophic cardiomyopathy.
- Mitral valve prolapse with regurgitation.
- IV drug abuse.

The prevalence of these risk factors within the community will influence the type of IE observed locally. Historically, rheumatic heart disease was the most prevalent risk factor for IE, although this disease has become less common as the overall frequency of acute rheumatic fever has declined. Outbreaks of rheumatic heart disease in different geographic areas of the United States suggest that this risk factor may once again become more common.[2] The risk of IE in persons with mitral valve prolapse and regurgitation is small, but because the condition is prevalent, it is an important contributor to the overall number of cases. Prosthetic valve endocarditis occurs in 1% to 4% of patients undergoing valve replacement surgery.[4] Other predispositions for IE include arteriovenous fistulae (including access for hemodialysis) and various intravascular devices (e.g., central venous catheters), which are associated with nosocomial IE in patients with a prosthetic valve.[7]

Nearly every organism causing human disease has been reported to cause IE (Table 101–1). Three groups of organisms cause most cases: streptococci (55% to 62%), staphylococci (30% to 40%), and enterococci (5% to 18%).[1,8] In general, streptococci cause IE in patients with underlying cardiac abnormalities, such as mitral valve prolapse or rheumatic heart disease. An occurrence of PVE within 1 year of valve surgery (early PVE) is primarily caused by staphylococci (*S. aureus* and coagulase-negative staphylococci) implanted at the time of surgery; whereas, PVE occurring after 1 year has a microbial etiology similar to native valve endocarditis.[3] *Staphylococcus aureus* is the most common cause of IE in IV drug abusers. Nevertheless, there are many exceptions to the preceding generalizations; isolation of the causative pathogen and determination of its antimicrobial susceptibilities offer the best chance for successful therapy.

PATHOPHYSIOLOGY

The development of IE via hematogenous spread, the most common route, requires the sequential occurrence of several factors[1]:

1. *The endothelial surface of the heart must be damaged.* This injury occurs with turbulent blood flow associated with the valvular lesions previously described.
2. *Platelet and fibrin deposition on the abnormal epithelial surface.* These deposits are referred to as nonbacterial thrombotic endocarditis (NBTE).
3. *Bacteremia results in colonization of the endocardial surface.* Bacteremia is the result of trauma to a mucosal surface with a high concentration of resident bacteria, such as the oral cavity and gastrointestinal (GI) tract. Transient bacteremia commonly follows certain dental and GI procedures. Staphylococci, viridans streptococci, and enterococci are most likely to adhere to NBTE, probably because of production of specific adherence factors, such as dextran by some oral streptococci.[9] Gram-negative bacteria rarely adhere to heart valves and are uncommon causes of IE.
4. *After colonization of the endothelial surface, a "vegetation" of fibrin, platelets, and bacteria forms.* The protective cover of fibrin and platelets allows unimpeded bacterial growth to concentrations as high as 10^9 to 10^{10} organisms per gram of tissue. The vegetations may be single or multiple and may vary in size from a few millimeters to centimeters. Bacteria within the vegetation grow slowly and are protected from antibiotics and host defenses.

Turbulent flow and eddy currents from abnormal valvular function injure the endocardium and promote IE "downstream" from the abnormal flow (on the atrial side of mitral regurgitant flow and on the ventricular surface of incompetent aortic valves). Subacute bacterial endocarditis tends to involve the mitral valve; whereas, ABE involves the aortic valve. Formation of vegetations may destroy valvular tissue. Continued destruction may lead to acute heart failure via perforation of the valve leaflet, rupture of the chordae tendineae or papillary muscle, or in the patient with PVE, valve dehiscence. Occasionally, valvular stenosis may occur. Abscesses may develop in the valve ring or in myocardial tissue itself. Even with the resolution of the process, fibrosis of tissue with some residual dysfunction may result.

Vegetations may be friable, and fragments are released downstream. These infected particles, termed septic emboli, can result in an organ abscess or infarction. Septic emboli from right-sided endocarditis commonly lodge in the lung, causing pulmonary abscesses. Emboli from left-sided vegetations commonly affect organs with high blood flow, such as the kidneys, spleen, and brain.

Circulating immune complexes consisting of antigen, antibody, and complement may deposit in organs, producing local inflammation and damage (glomerulonephritis in the kidneys). Other potential pathologic changes that result from immune complex deposition or septic emboli include the development of "mycotic" aneurysms (although the aneurysm is usually bacterial in origin, not fungal), cerebral infarction, splenic infarction and abscess, and skin manifestations, such as petechiae, Osler nodes, and Janeway lesions (as follows).

The pathogenesis of early PVE differs from the hematogenous route; surgery may directly inoculate the valve with bacteria from the patient's skin or operating room personnel. The recently placed, nonendothelialized valve is more susceptible to bacterial colonization than native valves. Bacteria may also colonize the new valve from contaminated bypass pumps, cannulas, and pacemakers, or from a nosocomial bacteremia subsequent to an intravascular catheter.[4,7,10] The mechanism of bacterial colonization and pathogenesis in late PVE is similar to native valve endocarditis.[4,10,11]

TABLE 101–1. Etiologic Agents in Infective Endocarditis

Agent	Percentage of Cases
Streptococci	55–62
Viridans streptococci	30–40
Other streptococci	15–25
Enterococci	5–18
Staphylococci	20–35
Coagulase-positive	10–27
Coagulase-negative	1–3
Gram-negative aerobic bacilli	1.5–13
Fungi	2–4
Miscellaneous bacteria	< 5
Mixed Infections	1–2
"Culture negative"	< 5–24

From Ref.1.

CLINICAL PRESENTATION

The clinical presentation of IE is highly variable (Table 101-2). Fever is the most common finding and is often accompanied by other nonspecific symptoms. The fever may be relatively low grade, particularly in subacute cases. Heart murmurs are found in 85% of patients, with a much lower percentage documented as new or changing murmurs. In patients with SBE, evidence of long-standing infection may include embolic phenomena, such as splenic or renal infarction and skin lesions (*vide infra*). Infective endocarditis usually begins insidiously and gradually worsens. Patients may present with nonspecific findings, such as fatigue, weakness, low-grade fever, anorexia, and weight loss. Arthralgias and myalgias are also common. In contrast, patients with ABE, such as IV drug abusers with *S. aureus,* may appear with classic signs of sepsis.

TABLE 101–2. Clinical Manifestations of Infective Endocarditis

Symptoms	Percentage of Patients	Physical Findings	Percentage of Patients
Fever	80	Fever	90
Chills	40	Heart murmur	85
Weakness	40	Changing murmur	5–10
Dyspnea	40	New murmur	3–5
Sweats	25	Embolic phenomenon	> 50
Anorexia	25	Skin manifestations	18–50
Weight loss	25	Osler nodes	10–23
Malaise	25	Splinter hemorrhages	15
Cough	25	Petechiae	20–40
Skin lesions	20	Janeway lesion	< 10
Stroke	20	Splenomegaly	20–57
Nausea/vomiting	20	Septic complications (pneumonia, meningitis)	20
Headache	20	Mycotic aneurysms	20
Myalgia/arthralgia	15	Clubbing	12–52
Edema	15	Retinal lesion	2–10
Chest pain	15	Signs of renal failure	10–15
Abdominal pain	15		
Delirium/coma	10–15		
Hemoptysis	10		
Back pain	10		

Adapted from Ref. 1.

Other important clinical signs, especially prevalent in subacute illness, may include the following peripheral manifestations ("stigmata") of endocarditis:

- *Osler nodes:* Purplish or erythematous subcutaneous papules or nodules on the pads of the fingers and toes. These lesions are 2 to 15 mm in size and are painful and tender. These nodes are not specific for IE and may be the result of embolic or immunologic phenomena or both.
- *Janeway lesions:* Hemorrhagic, painless plaques on the palms of the hands or soles of the feet. These lesions are also believed to be embolic in origin.
- *Splinter hemorrhages:* Thin, linear hemorrhages found under the nail beds of the fingers or toes. These lesions are not specific for IE and are more commonly the result of traumatic injuries.
- *Petechiae:* Small (usually 1 to 2 mm in diameter), erythematous, painless, hemorrhagic lesions. These lesions appear anywhere on the skin but more frequently on the anterior trunk, buccal mucosa and palate, and conjunctivae. Petechiae are nonblanching and resolve after a few days.
- *Clubbing of the fingers:* Proliferative change in the soft tissues about the terminal phalanges, observed in long-standing bacterial endocarditis.
- *Roth spot:* Retinal infarct with central pallor and surrounding hemorrhage.
- *Emboli:* Embolic phenomena occur in up to one-third of cases and may result in significant complications. Left-sided endocarditis can result in renal artery emboli causing flank pain with hematuria, splenic artery emboli causing abdominal pain, and cerebral emboli, which may result in hemiplegia or alteration in mental status. Right-sided endocarditis may result in pulmonary emboli, causing pleuritic pain with hemoptysis and pneumonia. Splenomegaly is also a frequent finding in patients with prolonged endocarditis.

LABORATORY FINDINGS

Patients with IE typically have laboratory abnormalities; however, none of these changes are specific for endocarditis.[12] A normocytic, normochromic anemia with a low serum iron and low iron-binding capacity is common in SBE. In addition, the white blood cell (WBC) count is normal or slightly elevated, sometimes with a mild left shift. Acute bacterial endocarditis may present with an elevated WBC count, consistent with a fulminate infection. Both SBE and ABE usually have an elevated erythrocyte sedimentation rate.

BLOOD CULTURES

The hallmark of IE is a continuous bacteremia caused by bacteria shedding from the vegetation into the bloodstream.[1,2,12] Three sets of blood cultures, each from separate venipuncture sites, should be collected over 24 hours; more than 95% of patients with IE have positive blood cultures. If there is evidence of cardiac decompensation, several blood cultures should be collected at once, followed by immediate, empiric antimicrobial treatment. In patients with blood cultures initially showing no growth, cultures should be held for up to a month to detect growth of fastidious organisms. This rule also applies to patients who received prior antibiotics, since pathogen growth may be suppressed. In contrast to bacterial valvular infections, only about one-half of fungal endocarditis infections have positive blood cultures. "Culture-negative" endocarditis describes a patient in whom a clinical diagnosis of IE is likely, but blood cultures do not yield a pathogen.[12] This condition is most often a consequence of previous antibiotic therapy.

ECHOCARDIOGRAPHY

Two-dimensional echocardiography, using either the transthoracic (TTE) or transesophageal (TEE) technique, is important to identify and localize valvular lesions in suspected cases of IE.[1,2,13] The TEE technique is more sensitive for detecting vegetations (about 95%) compared to TTE (60% to 65%). A TEE is also helpful in diagnosing IE when blood cultures fail to yield a pathogen or in planning for surgical intervention. The lack of a vegetation on echocardiogram does not exclude endocarditis. On the other hand, a positive test may reveal an unsuspected large vegetation (> 1 cm), a ring abscess, or an intracardiac fistula, which alerts the physician to monitor aggressively for septic emboli and heart failure as well as to evaluate for urgent surgical intervention.[11,13]

DIAGNOSIS

The signs and symptoms of IE are not specific, and the diagnosis is often unclear.[14,15] New diagnostic criteria include major criteria (typical blood culture and positive echocardiogram) and minor criteria (predisposition, fever, vascular phenomena, immunologic phenomena, suggestive echocardiogram, and microbiologic findings).[16] These criteria increase the number of patients diagnosed with definite IE.

PROGNOSIS

Infective endocarditis is usually fatal without appropriate treatment (antimicrobial therapy, surgery, or both); recovery is expected with proper management. Factors associated with increased mortality include (1) congestive heart failure; (2) culture-negative endocarditis; (3) endocarditis caused by resistant organisms, such as fungi and gram-negative bacteria; (4) left-sided endocarditis caused by *S. aureus,* and (5) prosthetic valve endocarditis.[1,3]

▶ TREATMENT: Infective Endocarditis

DESIRED OUTCOMES

The desired outcomes for treatment and prophylaxis of IE are to:

- Relieve the signs and symptoms of the disease.
- Eradicate the causative organism with minimal drug exposure.
- Provide cost-effective antimicrobial therapy, determined by the likely or identified pathogen, drug susceptibilities, hepatic and renal function, drug allergies, and anticipated drug toxicities.
- Prevent IE in high-risk patients with appropriate prophylactic antimicrobials.

GENERAL APPROACH TO TREATMENT

The most important approach in the treatment of IE is the isolation of the infecting pathogen followed by high-dose, bactericidal antibiotics for an extended period.[17,18] Large doses of parenteral antimicrobials are usually necessary to achieve bactericidal concentrations within vegetations. For some pathogens, such as enterococci, the use of synergistic antimicrobial combinations is essential to obtain a bactericidal effect. Combination antibiotics can also decrease the emergence of resistant organisms during treatment (e.g., PVE caused by coagulase-negative staphylococci), and hasten the pace of clinical and microbiologic response (e.g., some streptococcal and staphylococcal infections).

An extended duration of therapy is usually required for adequate treatment of IE, even for susceptible pathogens. Microorganisms are enclosed within valvular vegetations and fibrin deposits; these barriers impair host defenses and protect microbes from phagocytic cells. In addition, the high bacterial concentrations within vegetations may result in an inoculum effect that further resists killing. Many bacteria are also not actively dividing, further limiting the rate of bacteria death. For most patients, 4 to 6 weeks of therapy are required. (Specific treatment recommendations from the American Heart Association for the more common causes of IE are summarized in Tables 101–3 through 101–8.[19])

Pharmacodynamic investigations in the IE animal model allow quantitation of bacterial densities within vegetations over time as a function of antibiotic concentration. These models confirm many of the IE treatment principles observed empirically.[20,21] The effective antibiotic concentration in serum may be many times the minimum bactericidal concentration (MBC) of the infecting pathogen, depending on additional characteristics. The most effective antibiotics have a rapid and homogeneous distribution into the vegetation, kill bacteria rapidly, and are least susceptible to a large inoculum. Aminoglycosides have the most favorable characteristics, followed by β-lactams, and then glycopeptides.[21]

NONPHARMACOLOGIC THERAPY

Surgery is an important adjunct to the management of endocarditis in certain patients and is necessary in at least 25% of cases.[22] The major causes of death in patients with IE are the development of heart failure and infections in vital organs from septic embolization. In most cases, valvectomy and valve replacement are performed to remove infected tissues and restore hemodynamic function. The most important indications for surgery include:[1,4,22]

- Valve dysfunction with heart failure, perivalvular necrosis, aortic dissection, or valve orifice obstruction.
- Persistent bacteremia or other evidence of failure despite appropriate antimicrobial therapy.
- Most cases of early PVE.
- Endocarditis caused by resistant organisms (Enterobacteriaceae, *Pseudomonas,* or fungi).
- Local suppurative complications, such as a myocardial abscess.

Replacement of an infected valve is recommended even in the presence of active and uncontrolled infection. If valvular dysfunction requires surgery, early valve replacement is preferable to waiting for the completion of antimicrobial therapy. Valve replacement surgery, performed during active infection, has a surprisingly low rate of reinfection. The aggressive use of early surgical intervention is particularly important in PVE.[4,10]

PHARMACOLOGIC THERAPY

VIRIDANS STREPTOCOCCCAL ENDOCARDITIS

Viridans streptococci refer to a large number of different species, such as *Streptococcus mutans, Streptococcus sanguis,* and *Streptococcus mitis.* These organisms are the most common cause of IE, especially in cases involving native valves.[18,23] These bacteria are common inhabitants of the human mouth and gingiva. During dental surgery and even when brushing the teeth, these organisms can cause a transient bacteremia, which can result in IE in the susceptible individual. Streptococcal endocarditis is usually subacute, and the response to medical treatment is good. *Streptococcus bovis* is not a viridans streptococcus, but it is included in this group because it is penicillin sensitive and requires the same treatment as virdans streptococci. *Streptococcus bovis* is a group D streptococcus and resides in the GI tract. Infective endocarditis caused by this organism is often associated with GI pathology, especially colon carcinoma.[1]

Antimicrobial regimens for viridans streptococci are well studied and, in uncomplicated cases, response rates exceed 95%. Viridans streptococci are penicillin susceptible, although some are more susceptible than others. Most are exquisitely sensitive to penicillin G and have minimum inhibitory concentrations (MICs) ≤ 0.1 μg/mL.[19,23] Approximately 10% to 20% are moderately susceptible (MIC = 0.1 to 0.5 μg/mL). This difference in *in vitro* susceptibility led to recommendations that the MIC be determined for all viridans streptococci, and the results are used to guide therapy. Although some streptococci are tolerant of the killing effects of penicillin *(vide infra),* this tolerance has not been demonstrated to be clinically important; treatment is identical to nontolerant organisms.[18,19]

Various regimens are recommended for the treatment of uncomplicated endocarditis caused by fully susceptible viridans streptococci (Table 101–3). Two 4-week, single-drug regimens consist of either high-dose parenteral penicillin G or ceftriaxone. Ceftriaxone is a recent addition to the endocarditis treatment guidelines.[19] If a shorter course of therapy is desired, high-dose parenteral penicillin G plus an aminoglycoside is recommended.[19,23] When used in select patients, this combination is equally effective to 4 weeks of penicillin alone. Although streptomycin was listed in the previous guidelines, gentamicin is the preferred aminoglycoside because serum concentrations are easily obtained, clinicians are more familiar with gentamicin use, and the few strains of streptococci resistant to the effects of streptomycin–penicillin *(vide infra)* remain susceptible to gentamicin–penicillin. Other aminoglycosides are not recommended.

The decision of which regimen to use depends on the perceived risk versus benefit. For example, a 2-week course of gentamicin in an elderly patient with renal impairment may be associated with ototoxicity and worsening renal function. On the other hand, a 4-week course of penicillin alone generally entails greater expense, especially if the patient remains in the hospital. Monotherapy with once daily ceftriaxone offers ease of administration, facilitates home health care treatment, and may be cost-effective.[24]

TABLE 101–3. Suggested Regimens for Therapy of Native Valve Endocarditis Due to Penicillin-Susceptible Viridans Streptococci and *Streptococcus bovis* (Minimum Inhibitory Concentration ≤ 0.1 μg/mL)[a]

Antibiotic	Dosage and Route	Duration (wk)	Comments
Aqueous crystalline penicillin G sodium	12–18 million U/24 h IV either continuously or in six equally divided doses	4	Preferred in most patients older than 65 years and in those with impairment of the eighth nerve or renal function
or			
Ceftriaxone sodium	2 g once daily IV or IM[b]	4	
Aqueous crystalline penicillin G sodium	12–18 million U/24 h IV either continuously or in six equally divided doses	2	When obtained 1 h after a 20–30 min IV infusion or IM injection, serum concentration of gentamicin of approximately 3 μg/mL is desirable; trough concentration should be < 1 μg/mL
With gentamicin sulfate[c]	1 mg/kg IM or IV every 8 h	2	
Vancomycin hydrochloride[d]	30 mg/kg per 24 h IV in two equally divided doses, not to exceed 2 g/24 h unless serum levels are monitored	4	Vancomycin therapy is recommended for patients allergic to β-lactams; peak serum concentrations of vancomycin should be obtained 1 h after completion of the infusion and should be in the range of 30 to 45 μg/mL for twice-daily dosing

[a]Dosages recommended are for patients with normal renal function. For nutritionally variant streptococci, see Table 101–7.
[b]Patients should be informed that IM injection of ceftriaxone is painful.
[c]Dosing of gentamicin on a mg/kg basis will produce higher serum concentrations in obese patients than in lean patients. Therefore, in obese patients, dosing should be based on ideal body weight. (Ideal body weight for men is 50 kg + 2.3 kg per inch over 5 feet, and ideal body weight for women is 45.5 kg + 2.3 kg per inch over 5 feet.) Relative contraindications to the use of gentamicin are age greater than 65 years, renal impairment, or impairment of the eighth nerve. Other potentially nephrotoxic agents, such as nonsteroidal anti-inflammatory drugs, should be used cautiously in patients receiving gentamicin.
[d]Vancomycin dosage should be reduced in patients with impaired renal function. Vancomycin given on a mg/kg basis will produce higher serum concentrations in obese patients than in lean patients. Therefore, in obese patients, dosing should be based on ideal body weight. Each dose of vancomycin should be infused over at least 1 h to reduce the risk of the histamine-release "red man" syndrome.
IV = intravenous; IM = intramuscular.
From Ref. 19. Copyright 1995–1997, American Medical Association.

In patients with complicated infection (e.g., extracardiac foci) or when the streptococcus has an MIC of 0.1 to 0.5 μg/mL, combination therapy with an aminoglycoside and penicillin (higher dose preferred) for the first 2 weeks, followed by penicillin alone for an additional 2 weeks is recommended (Table 101–4).[19,23] Some viridans streptococci have biologic characteristics that complicate diagnosis and treatment; an example is nutritional deficiencies that hinder growth in routine culture media.[19] These organisms require special broth supplemented with pyridoxal hydrochloride or cysteine. For patients infected with nutritionally variant streptococci or when the streptococcus has an MIC ≥ 0.5 μg/mL, treatment should follow the enterococcal endocarditis treatment guidelines (as follows).[19]

When a patient has an immediate-type hypersensitivity to penicillin, vancomycin is the drug of choice for IE caused by viridans streptococci. When vancomycin is chosen, the addition of gentamicin is not recommended.[19] First-generation and some third-generation cephalosporins (ceftriaxone) are alternatives in patients with nonimmediate penicillin reactions. The majority of patients who report a penicillin allergy have a negative penicillin skin test and are consequently at low risk of anaphylaxis.[25] The published experience with penicillin is more extensive than with alternative regimens; therefore, a thorough allergy history must be obtained before a second-line therapy is administered.

The rationale for combination therapy for penicillin-susceptible viridans streptococci is that synergy against these organisms is usually observed when cell wall active agents are combined with aminoglycosides *in vitro*.[17–19,23] Synergy results in more rapid sterilization of vegetations in animal models of endocarditis and probably explains the high response rates observed in patients treated for a total of 2 weeks.[19] In contrast, for IE caused by streptococci relatively resistant to penicillin (MIC = 0.1 to 0.5 mg/mL), combination therapy for 2 weeks is recommended, followed by penicillin alone for 2 additional weeks.[19,23] Some authors question the need for combination therapy for such relatively resistant streptococci, emphasizing that few human data suggest that patients with endocarditis caused by these organisms respond less well to penicillin alone.[26]

STAPHYLOCOCCAL ENDOCARDITIS

Endocarditis caused by staphylococci is becoming more prevalent, mainly because of increased IV drug abuse, more frequent use of peripheral and central venous catheters, and increased incidence of valve replacement surgery.[2,4,7,10,27,28] *Staphylococcus aureus* is the most common organism causing IE among IV drug abusers and persons with venous catheters. Coagulase-negative staphylococci (usually *Staphylococcus epidermidis*) are prominent causes of PVE. Staphylococcal endocarditis is not a homogeneous disease; appropriate management requires consideration of several factors, such as (1) Is the organism methicillin resistant? (2) Should combination therapy be used? (3) Is the infection on a native or prosthetic valve? (4) Is the patient an IV drug abuser? (5) Is the infection on the left or right side of the heart?

Any patient who develops staphylococcal bacteremia is at risk for endocarditis. Many investigators have attempted to develop criteria that identify the bacteremic patient likely to have IE.[28] Hospitalized patients with *S. aureus* bacteremia and an identified focus of infection, such as a vascular catheter, have a less than 10% incidence of endocarditis after an appropriate 2-week antimicrobial treatment. This applies only if the patient does not have a prosthetic valve or additional clinical evidence for endocarditis.[27,28] In contrast, patients with outpatient-acquired *S. aureus* bacteremia and no known focus of infection are more likely to have IE, and they may warrant prolonged treatment. These general distinctions are helpful when applied to IV drug abusers, but they may be less accurate in patients with diabetes.[28]

The recommended therapy for patients with left-sided IE caused by methicillin-sensitive *S. aureus* (MSSA) is 4 to 6 weeks of nafcillin or oxacillin, often combined with a short course of gentamicin (Table 101–5). From *in vitro* studies, aminoglycoside antibiotics and penicillinase-resistant penicillins or vancomycin are synergistic for most MSSA. Combinations of a penicillin with an aminoglycoside, in animal models of endocarditis, eradicate organisms from vegetations more rapidly than penicillins alone.[27,28] In human studies, the addition of an aminoglycoside to nafcillin for the first week of therapy hastens the resolution of fever and bacteremia, but it does not affect survival or relapse rates.[29]

If a patient has a mild allergy to penicillin, first-generation cephalosporins are effective alternatives, but they should be avoided in immediate-type hypersensitivity reactions (Table 101–5). The use of cephalosporins, particularly cefazolin, has been controversial for MSSA endocarditis. In the majority of studies, these agents appear effective; however, cefazolin may be more labile to staphylococcal β-lactamase than other cephalosporins, accounting for reported failures.[30] In patients with a history of immediate hypersensitivity to penicillin, vancomycin is the agent of choice. Vancomycin, however, kills *S. aureus* slowly

TABLE 101–4. Therapy for Native Valve Endocarditis Due to Strains of Viridans Streptococci and *Streptococcus bovis* That Are Relatively Resistant to Penicillin G (Minimum Inhibitory Concentration > 0.1 μg/mL and < 0.5 μg/mL)[a]

Antibiotic	Dosage and Route	Duration (wk)	Comments
Aqueous crystalline penicillin G sodium	18 million U/24 h IV either continuously or in six equally divided doses	4	Cefazolin or other first-generation cephalosporins may be substituted for penicillin in patients whose penicillin hypersensitivity is not of the immediate type
With gentamicin sulfate[b]	1 mg/kg IM or IV every 8 h	2	
Vancomycin hydrochloride[c]	30 mg/kg per 24 h IV in two equally divided doses, not to exceed 2 g/24 h unless serum levels are monitored	4	Vancomycin therapy is recommended for patients allergic to β-lactams

[a]Dosages recommended are for patients with normal renal function.
[b]For specific dosing adjustment and issues concerning gentamicin (obese patients, relative contraindications), see Table 101–3 footnotes.
[c]For specific dosing adjustment and issues concerning vancomycin (obese patients, length of infusion), see Table 101–3 footnotes.
IV = intravenous; IM = intramuscular.
From Ref. 19, with permission. Copyright 1995–1997, American Medical Association.

TABLE 101–5. Therapy for Endocarditis Because of *Staphylococcus* in the Absence of Prosthetic Material[a]

Antibiotic	Dosage and Route	Duration	Comments
Methicillin-susceptible Staphylococci			
Regimens for non–β-lactam–allergic patients			
Nafcillin sodium or oxacillin sodium	2 g IV every 4 h	4–6 wk	Benefit of additional aminoglycosides has not been established
With optional addition of gentamicin sulfate[b]	1 mg/kg IM or IV every 8 h	3–5 d	
Regimens for β-lactam–allergic patients			
Cefazolin (or other first-generation cephalosporin in equivalent dosage)	2 g IV every 8 h	4–6 wk	Cephalosporins should be avoided in patients with immediate-type hypersensitivity to penicillin
With optional addition of gentamicin[b]	1 mg/kg IM or IV every 8 h	3–5 d	
Vancomycin hydrochloride[c]	30 mg/kg per 24 h IV in two equally divided doses, not to exceed 2 g/24 h unless serum levels are monitored	4–6 wk	Recommended for patients allergic to penicillin
Methicillin-resistant Staphylococci			
Vancomycin hydrochloride[c]	30 mg/kg per 24 h IV in two equally divided doses, not to exceed 2 g/24 h unless serum levels are monitored	4–6 wk	

[a]For treatment of endocarditis caused by penicillin-susceptible staphylococci (minimum inhibitory concentration ≤ 0.1 μg/mL), aqueous crystalline penicillin G sodium (Table 101–3, first regimen) can be used for 4 to 6 wk instead of nafcillin or oxacillin. Shorter antibiotic courses have been effective in some drug addicts with right-sided endocarditis caused by *Staphylococcus aureus* (see text). See text for comments on use of rifampin.
[b]For specific dosing adjustment and issues concerning gentamicin (obese patients, relative contraindications), see Table 101–3 footnotes.
[c]For specific dosing adjustment and issues concerning vancomycin (obese patients, length of infusion), see Table 101–3 footnotes.
IV = intravenous; IM = intramuscular.
From Ref. 19, with permission. Copyright 1995–1997, American Medical Association.

and is regarded as inferior to penicillinase-resistant penicillins for MSSA. Rifampin as an adjunctive therapy is controversial; however, this agent, added to vancomycin in refractory or complicated infections in patients with left-sided IE, may result in dramatic patient improvement.[27,28,31] Generally, antibiotic therapy should be continued for 4 to 6 weeks. Unfortunately, left-sided IE caused by *S. aureus* continues to have a poor prognosis with a mortality rate of 25% to 40%.[3,19] For reasons discussed in the following section, IV drug abusers have a more favorable response to therapy.

Methicillin-resistant Staphylococcal Endocarditis

During the past decade, greater numbers of staphylococci became resistant to methicillin and isoxazolyl penicillins. At tertiary care hospitals, up to 50% of *S. aureus* and 80% of coagulase-negative staphylococci are methicillin resistant. Vancomycin is the drug of choice for these organisms since most methicillin-resistant *S. aureus* (MRSA) and coagulase-negative staphylococci are susceptible (Table 101–5). By a prospective trial, the addition of rifampin to vancomycin in 42 addicts with IE caused by MRSA did not result in a more rapid rate of sterile blood cultures; rifampin may have even antagonized the effects of vancomycin.[32] By contrast, patients with PVE caused by MRSA, especially coagulase-negative staphylococci, should receive combination antimicrobial therapy (Table 101–6).

Staphylococcus Endocarditis in the Intravenous Drug Abuser

Infective endocarditis in the IV drug abuser is frequently (60% to 80%) caused by *S. aureus,* although other organisms may be common in certain geographic locations.[33] In this setting, the tricuspid valve is often infected, resulting in right-sided IE. Most patients have no history of valve abnormalities, are usually otherwise healthy, and have a good response to medical treatment. Nonetheless, surgery may be required in up to 25% of cases.

Standard treatment for MSSA IE is 4 weeks of monotherapy with a penicillinase-resistant penicillin (Table 101–5). The clinical response, however, in the IV drug abuser with right-sided MSSA endocarditis is usually excellent. Limited data suggest that these patients may be effectively treated with a 2-week course of nafcillin or oxacillin plus an aminoglycoside.[34,35] Short-course vancomycin, in this situation, in place of nafcillin or oxacillin, is ineffective.[36] A more recent trial has suggested that a 2-week regimen of a β-lactamase–stable penicillin alone, without the addition of an aminoglycoside, is as effective as combined therapy in MSSA tricuspid valve endocarditis.[37] Although these data suggest the addition of an aminoglycoside to nafcillin or oxacillin is unnecessary in the IV drug abuser with endocarditis, most clinicians are uncomfortable with a β-lactamase–stable penicillin alone and choose combination therapy if short-course treatment is initiated. Short-course therapy should not be used if left-sided endocarditis is suspected and may be inappropriate in patients with underlying acquired immunodeficiency syndrome (AIDS) or substantial pulmonary complications, such as lung abscess from right-sided IE.[19]

Vancomycin historically was regarded as therapeutically equivalent to penicillins for MSSA infections. A small investigation, however, demonstrated that approximately one-third of IV drug abusers with MSSA IE responded unsatisfactorily to vancomycin,[38] a poorer response rate than penicillinase-resistant peni-

TABLE 101–6. Treatment of Staphylococcal Endocarditis in the Presence of a Prosthetic Valve or Other Prosthetic Material[a]

Antibiotic	Dosage and Route	Duration (wk)	Comments
Regimen for Methicillin-resistant Staphylococci			
Vancomycin hydrochloride[b]	30 mg/kg per 24 h IV in two or four equally divided doses, not to exceed 2 g/24 h unless serum levels are monitored	≥ 6	
With rifampin[c]	300 mg orally every 8 h	≥ 6	Rifampin increases the amount of warfarin sodium required for antithrombotic therapy
With gentamicin sulfate[d,e]	1 mg/kg IM or IV every 8 h	2	
Regimen for Methicillin-susceptible Staphylococci			
Nafcillin sodium or oxacillin sodium	2 g IV every 4 h	≥ 6	First-generation cephalosporins or vancomycin should be used in patients allergic to β-lactam
With rifampin[c]	300 mg orally every 8 h	≥ 6	
And with gentamicin sulfate[d,e]	1 mg/kg IM or IV every 8 h	2	Cephalosporins should be avoided in patients with immediate-type hypersensitivity to penicillin or with methicillin-resistant staphylococci

[a]Dosages recommended are for patients with normal renal function.
[b]For specific dosing adjustment and issues concerning vancomycin (obese patients, length of infusion), see Table 101–3 footnotes.
[c]Rifampin plays a unique role in the eradication of staphylococcal infection involving prosthetic material (see text); combination therapy is essential to prevent emergence of rifampin resistance.
[d]For specific dosing adjustment and issues concerning gentamicin (obese patients, relative contraindications), see Table 101–3 footnotes.
[e]Use during initial 2 wk.
IV = intravenous; IM = intramuscular.
From Ref. 19, with permission. Copyright 1995–1997, American Medical Association.

cillins. This decreased response rate may be related to a slower rate of *in vitro* kill of *S. aureus* by vancomycin compared with nafcillin. This finding is consistent with a prospective study in 42 patients with MRSA IE.[32] Patients treated with vancomycin remained bacteremic for a median duration of 7 days, which is substantially longer than studies with β-lactam therapy. A second, more important reason a penicillin should be used before vancomycin is the increasing prevalence of vancomycin-resistant enterococci (VRE). Frequent, inappropriate use of vancomycin for the treatment of MSSA contributes to selection of VRE.[39,40] These data emphasize the importance of documenting a patient's penicillin allergy prior to initiating vancomycin. If vancomycin is selected, a full 4 weeks of therapy is recommended.

An evolving therapeutic approach for staphylococcal endocarditis in the IV drug abuser is oral antibacterial regimens. A preliminary report compared three oral regimes (dicloxacillin, clindamycin, and penicillin V) for treatment of tricuspid valve MSSA endocarditis in 35 patients (29 with a history of IVDA).[41] All patients demonstrated microbiologic and clinical cure 6 months after a mean 16.4 days of intravenous therapy with nafcillin or clindamycin followed by a mean of 26 days of oral therapy. Another report found a predominantly oral regimen to be effective in 10 addicts with uncomplicated right-sided endocarditis caused by MSSA.[42,43] After a short course of intravenous ciprofloxacin (300 mg q 12h), patients received oral ciprofloxacin for 3 weeks (750 mg every 12 hours). Patients also received oral rifampin (300 mg q 12h) at the start of IV treatment and continued for 28 days. A prospective randomized trial further supports oral ciprofloxacin plus rifampin in the IV drug abuser with right-sided MSSA endocardits.[44] Eighteen (95%) of nineteen patients receiving oral ciprofloxacin (750 mg every 12 hours) and rifampin (300 mg every 12 hours) had a successful outcome. This outcome rate was not statistically different compared to the 22 (88%) out of 25 patients receiving parenteral oxacillin (2 g IV every 4 hours) or vancomycin (1 g IV every 12 hours), plus gentamicin (2 mg/kg every 8 hours for the first 5 days). This trial was limited by the small number of patients; therefore, an important therapeutic difference between oral and IV treatment cannot be excluded. Additional randomized trials with other oral antibacterial regimens are necessary, especially since antibiotic resistance and therapeutic failures in staphylococcal disease have emerged with oral fluroquinolones.[45,46] Currently, oral treatment cannot be routinely recommended for the treatment of IE in the IV drug abuser. Nevertheless, in select cases, oral, abbreviated, and outpatient therapy may be appropriate since costs of hospitalization may be appreciably reduced.

Tolerance

Another consideration in staphylococcal endocarditis is that some organisms exhibit a phenomenon called "tolerance." A tolerant organism is inhibited, but not killed, by an antibiotic normally considered bactericidal.[18] One definition of a tolerant strain is an MBC greater than 32 times the MIC. In contrast, most nontolerant staphylococci have an almost equal MIC and MBC. Bactericidal activity is required for successful treatment of IE; therefore, infections with a tolerant organism may relapse after treatment. When stringent and consistent criteria are used to detect tolerance among *S. aureus,* the frequency of tolerance is actually very low, suggesting this phenomenon is primarily a laboratory finding with little clinical significance.[48] Nevertheless, some animal studies of endocarditis suggest that tolerant strains do not respond as readily to β-lactam therapy.[20,49] The clinical importance of tolerance has not been clearly demonstrated. The American Heart Association guidelines for treatment of IE state the concern for tolerance among staphylococci should not affect antibiotic selection.[19]

Prosthetic Valve Endocarditis

An episode of PVE occurring within 1 year of surgery is usually caused by staphylococci implanted during surgery.[4,10,49] Since this type of IE is a nosocomial infection, methicillin-resistant organisms are common and vancomycin is the cornerstone of therapy. The PVE responds poorly to medical treatment and has a higher mortality compared to native valve endocarditis. This poor response may be caused by an infected sewing ring in addition to the valve, leading to valve dehiscence and incompetence. These events can result in acute heart failure, which may be fatal.[11] Surgery is often an essential component of treatment. Combinations of antimicrobials are recommended because of the high morbidity and mortality associated with PVE and its refractoriness to therapy.[4,10,49] For methicillin-resistant staphylococci (both MRSA and coagulase-negative staphylococci), vancomycin is recommended with rifampin for ≥ 6 weeks (Table 101–6). An aminoglycoside is added for the first 2 weeks if the organism is susceptible. For MSSA, a penicillinase-stable penicillin is administered in place of vancomycin. Combination therapy also decreases the emergence of resistance to rifampin, which frequently occurs when rifampin is used alone. Vancomycin is active *in vitro* for all MRSA; however, some coagulase-negative staphylococci are resistant.[50] Optimum therapy for these unusual organisms is unknown.

ENTEROCOCCAL ENDOCARDITIS

Enterococci are normal inhabitants of the human GI tract and usually are of low virulence.[51] Historically, they were considered group D streptococci, but they have been reclassified into the genus *Enterococcus (E. faecalis and E. faecium). Enterococcus faecalis* is the most common (~90%) clinical isolate of the two species. Enterococci cause 5% to 18% of endocarditis cases and are noteworthy for the following reasons: (1) no single antibiotic is bactericidal; (2) MICs to penicillin are relatively high (1 to 25 mg/mL); (3) intrinsic resistance occurs to all cephalosporins and relative resistance occurs to aminoglycosides (e.g., "low-level" aminoglycoside resistance); (4) combinations of a cell wall active agent, such as a penicillin or vancomycin, plus an aminoglycoside are necessary for killing; and (5) resistance to all available drugs is increasing.[19,53]

Monotherapy with penicillin for IE caused by enterococci results in relapse rates of 50% to 80%; combination therapy is always recommended for susceptible strains.[53] The relapse rate following penicillin–gentamicin therapy for susceptible strains is less than 15%.[3] The killing of enterococci by an aminoglycoside–penicillin combination is the best clinical example of antibiotic synergy. Since the aminoglycoside cannot penetrate the bacterial cell in the absence of the penicillin, enterococci will usually appear to be resistant to aminoglycosides by routine susceptibility testing (low-level resistance). In the presence of an agent that disrupts the cell wall, however, such as penicillin or vancomycin, the aminoglycoside can gain entry, attach to bacterial ribosomes, and cause rapid cell death. An aminoglycoside–vancomycin combination is also synergistic against enterococci and is appropriate therapy for the penicillin-allergic patient.[52]

Enterococcal endocarditis ordinarily requires 4 to 6 weeks of high-dose penicillin G or ampicillin, plus an aminoglycoside for cure (Table 101–7). A 6-week course is recommended for patients with symptoms lasting longer than 3 months, recurrent cases, and mitral valve involvement. Ampicillin has greater *in vitro* activity as compared to penicillin G, although there are no clinical data to document differences in efficacy. Streptomycin has been the most extensively studied aminoglycoside, but gentamicin is presently favored. Other aminoglycosides cannot be routinely substituted. In the treatment of enterococcal endocarditis, relatively low serum concentrations of aminoglycosides appear adequate for successful therapy, such as a gentamicin peak concentration of approximately 3 μg/mL.[52] This low-level peak gentamicin recommendation is debatable.[54] Treatment of enterococcal endocarditis does not have the high success rate seen with IE caused by viridans streptococci, presumably because the organism is more resistant to killing.

Resistance among enterococci to the preceding drugs is increasing.[51,53] Enterococci that exhibit high-level resistance to streptomycin (MIC > 2000 mg/mL) are not synergistically killed by penicillin and streptomycin because the aminoglycoside either no longer binds to the ribosome or is inactivated by an

TABLE 101–7. Standard Therapy for Endocarditis Due to Enterococci[a]

Antibiotic	Dosage and Route	Duration (wk)	Comments
Aqueous crystalline penicillin G sodium	18–30 million U/24 h IV either continuously or in six equally divided doses	4–6	4-wk therapy recommended for patients with symptoms < 3 mo in duration; 6-wk therapy recommended for patients with symptoms > 3 mo in duration
With gentamicin sulfate[b]	1 mg/kg IM or IV every 8 h	4-6	
Ampicillin sodium	12 g/24 h IV either continuously or in six equally divided doses	4-6	
With gentamicin sulfate[b]	1 mg/kg IM or IV every 8 h	4–6	
Vancomycin hydrochloride[b,c]	30 mg/kg per 24 h IV in two equally divided doses, not to exceed 2 g/24 h unless serum levels are monitored	4–6	Vancomycin therapy is recommended for patients allergic to β-lactams; cephalosporins are not acceptable alternatives for patients allergic to penicillin
With gentamicin sulfate[b]	1 mg/kg IM or IV every 8 h	4–6	

[a]All enterococci causing endocarditis must be tested for antimicrobial susceptibility in order to select optimal therapy (see text). This table is for endocarditis because of gentamicin- or vancomycin-susceptible enterococci, viridans streptococci with a minimum inhibitory concentration of > 0.5 μg/mL, nutritionally variant viridans streptococci, or prosthetic valve endocarditis caused by viridans streptococci or *Streptococcus bovis*. Antibiotic dosages are for patients with normal renal function.

[b]For specific dosing adjustment and issues concerning gentamicin (obese patients, relative contraindications), see Table 101–3 footnotes.

[c]For specific dosing adjustment and issues concerning vancomycin (obese patients, length of infusion), see Table 101–3 footnotes.

IV = intravenous; IM = intramuscular.

From Ref. 19, with permission. Copyright 1995–1997, American Medical Association.

aminoglycoside-modifying enzyme, streptomycin adenylase.[53] Since enterococci will appear resistant to aminoglycosides on routine susceptibility testing, the only way to distinguish high-level from low-level resistance is by performing special susceptibility tests using 500 to 2000 μg/mL of the aminoglycoside. High-level streptomycin-resistant enterococci occur with a frequency of 40% to 50%, and high-level resistance to gentamicin is now found in 10% to 50% of isolates. Although most gentamicin-resistant enterococci are resistant to all aminoglycosides (including amikacin), 30% to 50% remain susceptible to streptomycin.[53] High-level gentamicin resistance is mediated by a bifunctional aminoglycoside-modifying enzyme, 6′-acetyltransferase/2″-phosphotransferase, and most strains also possess streptomycin adenylase. These organisms do not commonly cause IE; data on appropriate therapy are sparse, and therapeutic options are few. Case reports indicate that some patients will respond to very high doses of ampicillin as observed in the early trials of penicillin monotherapy.[55]

In addition to isolates with high-level aminoglycoside resistance, β-lactamase–producing enterococci (especially *E. faecium*) are increasingly reported.[51,56,57] Therapy with vancomycin is usually recommended, although penicillin–β-lactamase inhibitor combinations (e.g., ampicillin–sulbactam) appear effective.[56] Vancomycin-resistant enterococci are increasingly reported, mostly for *E. faecium*. Vancomycin resistance occurs when the bacterium replaces the normal vancomycin target, D-alanine, D-alanine, with a peptidoglycan precursor that does not bind vancomycin, D-alanine, D-lactate.[57] Some isolates remain susceptible *in vitro* to tetracyclines, novobiocin, and quinupristin/dalfopristin (Synercid), but these cannot be considered optimal therapy. Quinupristin/dalfopristin appears to be the most promising treatment. Of great concern is that these multiple-drug-resistant enterococci will transmit resistance traits to *S. aureus*.

LESS COMMON CAUSES OF INFECTIVE ENDOCARDITIS

HACEK Group

Gram-negative bacteria from the HACEK group *(Haemophilus parainfluenzae, Haemophilus aphrophilus, Actinobacillus actinomycetemcomitans, Cardiobacterum hominis, Eikenella corrodens,* and *Kingella kingae)* are unusual causes of IE. Usually, this type of IE presents as a subacute illness with large vegetations and emboli.[58] These oropharyngeal organisms are typically slow growing and should be considered as possible causes of culture-negative endocarditis. Ceftriaxone or high doses of ampicillin with gentamicin for 4 weeks is the recommended therapy (Table 101–8).[19] Valve replacement may be required.

Gram-negative Bacilli

Endocarditis caused by gram-negative bacilli is relatively uncommon, although the incidence may be increasing.[58] Patients at higher risk include IV drug abusers and those with prosthetic heart valves. The organism most commonly associated with gram-negative rod endocarditis in IV drug abusers is *Pseudomonas aeruginosa.* Other gram-negative bacilli causing IE include other pseudomonads, *Serratia marcescens, Escherichia coli, Enterobacter, Salmonella,* and *Haemophilus.* Generally, these infections have a poor prognosis, with mortality rates as high as 60% to 80%.[3]

Overall, there is little clinical information to base solid treatment recommendations. For most cases of IE caused by *P. aeruginosa* and Enterobacteriaceae, antibiotics and valve replacement are necessary. Antimicrobial therapy includes the combination of an aminoglycoside and an extended-spectrum β-lactam.[58] One group of investigators reviewed the therapeutic outcome of patients with *Pseudomonas* endocarditis and compared the benefit of combining varying doses of aminoglycosides with or without valve replacement.[59,60] When patients were treated with low-dose aminoglycosides (< 5 mg/kg/d of gentamicin) with or without surgery, the survival rates were 50% and 25%, respectively. When higher doses were used (at least 8 mg/kg/d of gentamicin), the survival rate was 65%; the survival rate increased to 86% when high-dose therapy was combined with surgery. Even at the higher dosage, the frequency of aminoglycoside toxicity was low.

The appropriate regimen for the treatment of gram-negative bacillary endocarditis caused by Enterobacteriaceae depends on the results of *in vitro* susceptibility testing. For *Klebsiella pneumoniae, E. coli,* and *Proteus mirabilis,* a third-generation cephalosporin is frequently combined with an aminoglycoside. Treatment should generally be continued for 6 weeks.

Fungal Endocarditis

Fungi cause between 2% and 4% of endocarditis cases; most patients have undergone recent cardiovascular surgery, are IV drug abusers, have received prolonged treatment with IV catheters or antibiotics, or are immunocompromised.[1,8,61] *Candida* sp. and *Aspergillus* sp. are the most commonly involved, and the mortality rate is high for the following reasons: (1) the large, bulky

TABLE 101–8. Therapy for Endocarditis Due to HACEK Microorganisms (*Haemophilus parainfluenzae, Haemophilus aphrophilus, Actinobacillus actinomycetemcomitans, Cardiobacterium hominis, Eikenella corrodens,* and *Kingella kingae*)[a]

Antibiotic	Dosage and Route	Duration (wk)	Comments
Ceftriaxone sodium[b]	2 g once daily IV or IM[b]	4	Cefotaxime sodium or other third-generation cephalosporins may be substituted
Ampicillin sodium[c]	12 g/24 h IV either continuously or in six equally divided doses	4	
With gentamicin sulfate[d]	1 mg/kg IM or IV every 8 h	4	

[a]Antibiotic dosages are for patients with normal renal function.
[b]Patients should be informed that IM injection of ceftriaxone is painful.
[c]Ampicillin should not be used if laboratory tests show β-lactamase production.
[d]For specific dosing adjustment and issues concerning gentamicin (obese patients, relative contraindications), see Table 101–3 footnotes.
IV = intravenous; IM = intramuscular.
From Ref. 19, with permission. Copyright 1995–1997, American Medical Association.

vegetations that often form; (2) the systemic septic embolization that may occur; (3) the tendency for fungi to invade the myocardium; (4) the poor penetration of vegetations by antifungals; (5) the low toxic:therapeutic ratio of agents, such as amphotericin B; and (6) the lack of consistent fungicidal activity of available antifungal agents.

Since these infections occur infrequently, scant clinical data are available to make solid treatment recommendations. Amphotericin B, with or without flucytosine, along with valve replacement is recommended for *Candida* and *Aspergillus* endocarditis.[61] The usefulness of fluconazole and itraconazole is unknown at this time, although their lack of fungicidal activity suggests a limited role. For most cases of PVE caused by fungi, combined antifungal and surgical therapy is required.

PHARMACOECONOMIC CONSIDERATIONS

Infective endocarditis is a rare disease, but the cost of treatment can be substantial. The long duration of hospitalization that is required to administer IV antimicrobials is the major expense. In selected cases, abbreviated, outpatient, and possibly oral antimicrobial therapy may appreciably reduce the cost of care.

Shorter-course antimicrobial regimens are advocated when possible. For instance, in exquisitely sensitive streptococcal endocarditis (MIC ≤ 0.1), a 2-week regimen of high-dose parenteral penicillin G in combination with an aminoglycoside is equally effective as 4 weeks of penicillin alone.[19,23] Another short-course therapy endorsed (2 weeks) is in the IV drug abuser with uncomplicated right-sided MSSA endocarditis. Treatment with nafcillin or oxacillin, in combination with an aminoglycoside, is likely to be cost effective.

The initiation of outpatient parenteral antibiotics should be considered early in treatment of IE, once the patient is clinically stable and responds favorably to initial antibiotics. Patients considered for outpatient therapy must be hemodynamically stable, be compliant with therapy, have careful medical monitoring, understand the potential complications of the disease, and have immediate access to medical care. Advances in technology allow for the outpatient administration of complex antibiotic regimens that significantly reduce the cost of therapy.[62] Simple regimens, such as single daily doses of ceftriaxone for streptococcal IE, are particularly attractive. Although endocarditis is common in the IV drug abuser and home health care would substantially reduce the cost of treatment, many clinicians are uncomfortable with outpatient IV therapy. Central venous access is required and is not advised in IV drug abusers. Sudden cardiac decompensation in an outpatient setting is also of concern. Oral antimicrombial regimens are an intriguing option in this situation, but limited data preclude their routine use.

EVALUATION OF THERAPEUTIC OUTCOMES

The evaluation of patients treated for IE includes assessment of signs and symptoms, additional blood cultures, *in vitro* microbiologic tests (e.g., MIC, MBC, or serum bactericidal titers [SBTs]), antimicrobial serum concentration determinations, and other tests that evaluate organ function.[63]

SIGNS AND SYMPTOMS

Fever usually subsides within 1 week of initiating therapy.[63] Persistence of fever may indicate ineffective antimicrobial therapy, emboli, infections of intravascular catheters, or drug reactions. In some patients, low-grade fever may persist even with appropriate antimicrobial therapy. With defervescence, the patient should begin to feel better and other symptoms, such as lethargy or weakness, should subside.

BLOOD CULTURES AND BACTERIAL SUSCEPTIBILITY

Blood cultures should be negative within a few days, although microbiologic response to vancomycin may be slower.[63] If bacteria continue to be isolated from blood beyond the first few days of therapy, it may indicate that the antimicrobials are inactive against the pathogen or that the doses are not producing adequate concentrations at the site of infection. After the initiation of therapy, blood cultures should be rechecked, possibly daily, until negative. During the remainder of therapy, frequent blood culturing is not necessary.

For all isolates from blood cultures, MICs and possibly MBCs should be determined.[19,64] The agent currently being used should be tested as well as alternatives that may be required if intolerance, allergy, or resistance occurs. Occasionally, it is useful to determine if synergy exists for antimicrobial combinations, although synergistic regimens can usually be predicted from the literature. Methods for *in vitro* determinations of synergy are summarized in Chapter 97.

SERUM BACTERICIDAL TITER

Serum bactericidal titers (SBTs) (also called Schlicter tests) have been used for many years and in association with a number of infectious diseases.[64,65] The SBT is the greatest dilution of a patient's serum sample, which is obtained while receiving antimicrobial treatment, that kills greater than 99.9% of an inoculum of the infecting pathogen *in vitro* over 18 to 24 hours. The antibiotic in serum accounts for the vast majority of the bactericidal activity; therefore, knowledge of the serum concentration and the MBC for the organism will reliably predict the SBT. The SBT is a rudimentary form of pharmacodynamic modeling since the titer incorporates both the pharmacokinetics of the antibiotic and the MBC.

In animal models of endocarditis, studies suggest that an SBT of 1:8 is predictive of response.[20] In humans with endocarditis, however, the correlation with SBTs and outcome is less clear. A multicenter study found peak and trough SBTs of ≥ 1:64 and ≥ 1:32 were associated with 100% response, respectively, although a lower titer did not predict failure.[66] Serum bactericidal titers ≥ 1:32 are easily achieved for most streptococci causing endocarditis because the MBC is low relative to achievable concentrations of penicillin; however, for enterococci, methicillin-resistant staphylococci, and gram-negative bacilli, high SBTs may be difficult to achieve. Thus, SBTs are of little use in IE caused by streptococci and MSSA (where serum concentrations are high and MBCs are low), but they may be of value for more unusual organisms where the treatment experience is limited.

Serum bactericidal titers have not always predicted outcome because of the failure to consider variables likely to determine response, such as the size of the vegetation, the host defenses, the rates of kill, and the location of the infection (left or right side of the heart). Lack of test standardization is another problem and is addressed in greater detail in Chapter 97. Primary variables include the method of diluting serum (using broth or serum), bacterial inoculum size, timing of collection of the blood sample (peak or trough), and measurement of the test end point.

At present, SBTs have little value in monitoring treatment of common types of IE. This test may be useful when the causative organisms are only moderately susceptible to antimicrobials, when less well-established regimens are used, or when response to therapy is suboptimal and dosage escalation is considered. In addition, an extremely high SBT may suggest that a decrease in antimicrobial dose is acceptable when the patient is at high risk of drug toxicity.

SERUM DRUG CONCENTRATION

Of the agents commonly used for IE, serum concentration determinations are routinely available for aminoglycosides (except streptomycin) and vancomycin.[63] Few data, however, support attaining any specific serum concentrations in patients with IE. In general, serum concentrations of the antimicrobial should exceed the MBC of the organisms, but in practice, this principle is usually not helpful in monitoring patients with endocarditis. Aminoglycoside concentrations rarely exceed the MBC for certain organisms, such as streptococci and enterococci, and concentrations have not been correlated with response, such as aminoglycosides and vancomycin for staphylococci.[67,68] In IE caused by *P. aeruginosa,* however, clinical trials previously discussed suggest that higher aminoglycoside concentrations (15 to 20 μg/mL) improve the outcome of therapy.[59,60] These higher concentrations are justified because of the high mortality associated with IE caused by *P. aeruginosa.* In contrast, when aminoglycosides are given in combination for IE caused by gram-positive cocci, peak serum concentrations are recommended to be on the low side of the traditional ranges (3 μg/mL for gentamicin and tobramycin).

Whether or not extended interval dosing of aminoglycosides has a role in IE is uncertain.[64] Animal models imply large doses of aminoglycosides at infrequent intervals are not optimal for enterococcal endocarditis,[69] but they have an equal and possibly greater efficacy in streptococcal endocarditis.[70,71,72] A small trial in humans also supports extended interval aminoglycosides in the treatment of streptococcal endocarditis.[73] At this time, however, limited human data preclude the routine use of extended interval dosing of aminoglycosides for IE.

ANTICOAGULATION

The use of anticoagulants for patients with native valve endocarditis is ordinarily contraindicated because of increased frequency of subarachnoid hemorrhage or other bleeding complications, possibly from areas of embolic infarction or from mycotic aneurysms. Anticoagulation use is controversial in PVE; however, patients who require anticoagulation for prosthetic valves should probably continue the anticoagulant during endocarditis therapy.[74,75]

PREVENTION

Antimicrobial prophylaxis is used to prevent IE in patients at high risk.[76,77,81] The use of antimicrobials for this purpose requires consideration of (1) cardiac conditions associated with endocarditis, (2) procedures causing bacteremia, (3) organisms likely to cause endocarditis, and (4) pharmacokinetics, spectrum, cost, adverse effects, and ease of administration of available antimicrombial agents. The objective of prophylaxis is to diminish the likelihood of IE in high-risk individuals (Table 101–9) who are undergoing procedures that cause transient bacteremia (Tables 101–10

TABLE 101–9. Cardiac Conditions Associated With Endocarditis

Endocarditis Prophylaxis Recommended
High-risk category
Prosthetic cardiac valves, including biprosthetic and homograft valves
Previous bacterial endocarditis
Complex cyanotic congenital heart disease (e.g., single ventricle states, transposition of the great arteries, tetralogy of Fallot)
Surgically constructed systemic pulmonary shunts or conduits
Moderate-risk category
Most other congenital cardiac malformations (other than above and below)
Acquired valvar dysfunction (e.g., rheumatic heart disease)
Hypertrophic cardiomyopathy
Mitral valve prolapse with valvar regurgitation, thickened leaflets, or both
Endocarditis Prophylaxis Not Recommended
Negligible-risk category (no greater risk than the general population)
Isolated secundum atrial septal defect
Surgical repair of atrial septal defect, ventricular septal defect, or patent ductus arteriosus (without residue beyond 6 mo)
Previous coronary artery bypass graft surgery
Mitral valve prolapse without valvar regurgitation
Physiologic, functional, or innocent heart murmurs
Previous Kawasaki disease without valvar dysfunction
Previous rheumatic fever without valvar dysfunction
Cardiac pacemakers (intravascular and epicardial) and implanted defibrillators

From Ref. 81, with permission. Copyright 1995–1997, American Medical Association.

TABLE 101–10. Dental Procedures and Endocarditis Prophylaxis

Endocarditis Prophylaxis Recommended[a]	Endocarditis Prophylaxis Not Recommended
Dental extractions	Restorative dentistry[b] (operative and prosthodontic) with or without retraction cord[c]
Periodontal procedures, including surgery, scaling, and root planing, probing, and recall maintenance	Local anesthetic injections (nonintraligamentary)
Dental implant placement and reimplantation of avulsed teeth	Intracanal endodontic treatment; postplacement and buildup
Endodontic (root canal) instrumentation or surgery only beyond the apex	Placement of rubber dams
Subgingival placement of antibiotic fibers or strips	Postoperative suture removal
Initial placement of orthodontic bands but not brackets	Placement of removable prosthodontic or orthodontic appliances
Intraligamentary local anesthetic injections	Taking of oral impressions
Prophylactic cleaning of teeth or implants where bleeding is anticipated	Fluoride treatments
	Taking of oral radiographs
	Orthodontic appliance adjustment
	Shedding of primary teeth

[a]Prophylaxis is recommended for patients with high- and moderate-risk cardiac conditions.
[b]This includes restoration of decayed teeth (filling cavities) and replacement of missing teeth.
[c]Clinical judgment may indicate antibiotic use in selected circumstances that may create significant bleeding.
From Ref. 81, with permission. Copyright 1995–1997, American Medical Association.

and 101–11).[81] Although there are no prospective, controlled human trials that demonstrate that prophylaxis in high-risk individuals protects against the development of endocarditis during bacteremia-induced procedures, animal studies suggest a benefit. Retrospective human studies support that a reduction of endocarditis occurs in selected cases following dental surgery when prophylaxis is employed.[78] The mechanism of a beneficial effect in humans is unclear, but antibiotics may decrease the number of bacteria at the surgical site, kill bacteria once introduced into the blood, and prevent adhesion of bacteria to the valve. One study found prophylaxis did not reduce the frequency of bacteremia immediately following tooth extraction compared to a control group, suggesting that a reduction in adhesion or effects after the bacteria adhere to the endocardium are more likely mechanisms.[76,79]

PATIENTS AT RISK

Patients with certain cardiac lesions, particularly those with prosthetic heart valves or a history of bacterial endocarditis, are at high risk for developing IE (Table 101–9). Nevertheless, only 15% to 25% of patients who develop IE are in a definable high-risk category.[76,77] A case-controlled study suggests few cases of infective endocarditis would be preventable with antibiotic prophylaxis, even with 100% effectiveness.[80] Despite the low probability that IE will develop, prophylaxis is recommended for some dental, respiratory, GI, and genitourinary procedures (Tables 101–10 and 101–11) because of the significant morbidity associated with the disease. Patients undergoing valve implant surgery are at a much greater risk for IE than those undergoing dental surgery.

TABLE 101–11. Other Procedures and Endocarditis Prophylaxis

Endocarditis Prophylaxis Recommended

- Respiratory tract
  - Tonsillectomy, adenoidectomy, or both
  - Surgical operations that involve respiratory mucosa
  - Bronchoscopy with a rigid bronchoscope
- Gastrointestinal tract[a]
  - Sclerotherapy for esophageal varices
  - Esophageal stricture dilation
  - Endoscopic retrograde cholangiography with biliary obstruction
  - Biliary tract surgery
  - Surgical operations that involve intestinal mucosa
- Genitourinary tract
  - Prostatic surgery
  - Cystoscopy
  - Urethral dilation

Endocarditis Prophylaxis Not Recommended

- Respiratory tract
  - Endotracheal intubation
  - Bronchoscopy with a flexible bronchoscope, with or without biospy[b]
  - Tympanostomy tube insertion
- Gastrointestinal (GI) tract
  - Transesophageal echocardiography[b]
  - Endoscopy with or without GI biopsy[b]
- Genitourinary tract
  - Vaginal hysterectomy[b]
  - Vaginal delivery[b]
  - Cesarean section
  - In uninfected tissue:
    - Urethral catheterization
    - Uterine dilation and curettage
    - Therapeutic abortion
    - Sterilization procedures
    - Insertion or removal of intrauterine devices
- Other
  - Cardiac catheterization, including balloon angioplasty
  - Implanted cardiac pacemakers, implanted defibrillators, and coronary stents
  - Incision or biopsy of surgically scrubbed skin
  - Circumcision

[a]Prophylaxis is recommended for high-risk patients; optional for medium-risk patients.
[b]Prophylaxis is optional for high-risk patients.
From Ref. 81, with permission. Copyright 1995–1997, American Medical Association.

TABLE 101–12. Prophylactic Regimens for Dental, Oral, Respiratory Tract, or Esophageal Procedures

Situation	Agent	Regimen[a]
Standard general prophylaxis	Amoxicillin	*Adults:* 2 g *Children:* 50 mg/kg orally 1 h before procedure
Unable to take oral medications	Ampicillin	*Adults:* 2 g IM or IV *Children:* 50 mg/kg IM or IV within 30 min before procedure
Allergic to penicillin	Clindamycin *or* Cephalexin[b] or cefadroxil[b] *or* Azithromycin or chlarithromycin	*Adults:* 600 mg *Children:* 20 mg/kg orally 1 h before procedure *Adults:* 2 g *Children:* 50 mg/kg orally 1 h before procedure *Adults:* 500 mg *Children:* 15 mg/kg orally 1 h before procedure
Allergic to penicillin and unable to take oral medications	Clidamycin *or* Cefazolin[b]	*Adults:* 600 mg *Children:* 20 mg/kg IV within 30 min before procedure *Adults:* 1 g *Children:* 25 mg/kg IM or IV within 30 min before procedure

[a]Total children's dose should not exceed adult dose.
[b]Cephalosporins should not be used in individuals with immediate-type hypersensitivity reaction (urticaria, angioedema, or anaphylaxis) to penicillins.
IV = intravenous; IM = intramuscular.
From Ref. 81, with permission. Copyright 1995–1997, American Medical Association.

Such patients should receive parenteral prophylaxis, although the most appropriate agent is unknown.

PROCEDURES CAUSING BACTEREMIA

Bacteremia accompanies many everyday events, such as brushing the teeth and chewing, although certain medical and surgical procedures are more likely to cause a transient bacteremia (Tables 101–10 and 101–11). For dental procedures of the gums and oral structures that cause bleeding, viridans streptococci frequently cause bacteremia, whereas instrumentation and surgery of the GI and genitourinary tracts more often result in enterococcal bacteremia.

ANTIBIOTIC REGIMENS

The American Heart Association has published new guidelines regarding the prevention of IE.[81] A single 2-g dose of amoxicillin is recommended for adult patients at risk, given 1 hour prior to undergoing procedures associated with bacteremia (Table 101–12). These guidelines replace previous recommendations, which were often not followed, at least not for dental surgery.[82,83] The appropriate duration of antimicrobial prophylaxis is not known, but it is believed to be relatively short. Unlike the 1990 guidelines, these new recommendations do not advocate a second dose of amoxicillin following a bacteremia-causing procedure. Alternative

TABLE 101–13. Prophylactic Regimens for Genitourinary Gastrointestinal (Excluding Esophageal) Procedures

Situation	Agent[a]	Regimen[b]
High-risk patients	Ampicillin plus gentamicin	*Adults:* ampicillin 2 g IM or IV plus gentamicin 1.5 mg/kg (not to exceed 120 mg) within 30 min of starting the procedure; 6 h later, ampicillin 1 g IM/IV or amoxicillin 1 g orally *Children:* ampicillin 50 mg/kg IM or IV (not to exceed 2 g) plus gentamicin 1.5 mg/kg within 30 min of starting the procedure; 6 h later, ampicillin 25 mg/kg IM/IV or amoxicillin 25 mg/kg orally
High-risk patients allergic to ampicillin/amoxicillin	Vancomycin plus gentamicin	*Adults:* vancomycin 1 g IV over 1–2 h plus gentamicin 1.5 mg/kg IV/IM (not to exceed 120 mg); complete injection/infusion within 30 min of staring the procedure *Children:* vancomycin 20 mg/kg IV over 1–2 h plus gentamicin 1.5 mg/kg IV/IM; complete injection /infusion within 30 min of starting the procedure
Moderate-risk patients	Amoxicillin or ampicillin	*Adults:* amoxicillin 2 g orally 1 h before procedure, or ampicillin 2 g IM/IV within 30 min of starting the procedure *Children:* amoxicillin 50 mg/kg orally 1 h before procedure, or ampicillin 50 mg/kg IM/IV within 30 min of starting the procedure
Moderate-risk patients allergic to ampicillin/amoxicillin	Vancomycin	*Adults:* vancomycin 1 g IV over 1–2 h; complete infusion within 30 min of starting the procedure *Children:* vancomycin 20 mg/kg IV over 1–2 h; complete infusion within 30 min of starting the procedure

[a]Total children's dose should not exceed adult dose.
[b]No second dose of vancomycin or gentamicin is recommended.
IV = intravenous; IM = intramuscular.
From Ref. 81, with permission. Copyright 1995–1997, American Medical Association.

prophylaxis regimens for patients allergic to penicillins, those unable to take oral medications, and regimens for genitourinary and GI procedures are provided (Tables 101–12 and 101–13).

▶ PRINCIPLES OF PHARMACOTHERAPY

- Infective endocarditis is an uncommon infection usually occurring in persons with preexisting cardiac valvular abnormalities (prosthetic heart valves) or with other specific risk factors (IV drug abuse).
- Three groups of organisms generally cause IE: streptococci (50% to 62%), staphylococci (30% to 40%), and enterococci (5% to 18%).
- The clinical presentation of IE is highly variable and nonspecific, although a fever and murmur are usually present. Classical, peripheral manifestations (Osler nodes) may or may not occur.
- The diagnosis of IE is often unclear. Nonspecific signs, symptoms, and laboratory findings are important but do not reliably determine infection. The two major diagnostic criteria are blood cultures, to identify the infecting pathogen, and a transesophageal echocardiogram (TEE), to determine the presence of a valvular vegetation.
- Isolation of the infecting pathogen and determination of antimicrobial susceptibilities are the most important approach in the treatment of IE. High-dose, bactericidal anti-infectives are necessary for an extended period of time (usually 4 to 6 weeks).
- Surgical replacement of the infected heart valve is an important adjunct to endocarditis treatment in certain situations (e.g., patients with acute heart failure).
- β-Lactam antibiotics, such as penicillin G, nafcillin, and ampicillin, remain the drugs of choice for streptococcal, staphylococcal, and enterococcal endocarditis, respectively. Aminoglycosides are essential to obtain a synergistic bactericidal effect in enterococcal endocarditis. Adjunctive aminoglycosides may also hasten the pace of clinical or microbiologic cure (such as in case of streptococcal and staphylococcal endocarditis) and prevent the emergence of resistant organisms (PVE caused by coagulase-negative staphylococci). Vancomycin is reserved for resistant organisms and patients with immediate β-lactam allergies.
- Patients at high risk of IE, such as persons with prosthetic heart valves, should receive antimicrobial agents prior to a bacteremia-causing procedure (dental extraction). The agent is determined by the likely organism(s) leading to bacteremia and drug-specific parameters.

REFERENCES

1. Scheld WM, Sande MA. Endocarditis and intravascular infections. In: Mandell GL, Dolin R, Bennett JE, eds. Principles and Practice of Infectious Diseases, 4th ed. New York, Churchill Livingstone, 1995; 740–783.
2. Bayer AS. Infective endocarditis. Clin Infect Dis 1993;173:313–320.
3. Gold MJ. Cure rates and long-term prognosis. In: Kaye D, ed. Infective Endocarditis, 2nd ed. New York, Raven Press, 1992:455–464.
4. Threlkel MG, Cobbs CG. Infectious disorders of prosthetic valves and intravascular devices. In: Mandell GL, Dolin R, Bennett JE, eds. Principles and Practice of Infectious Diseases, 4th ed. New York, Churchill Livingstone, 1995:783–793.
5. Saiman L, Prince A, Gersony WM. Pediatric infective endocarditis in the modern era. J Pediatr 1993;122:847–853.
6. Steckelberg JM, Wilson WR. Risk factors for infective endocarditis. Infect Dis Clin North Am 1993;7:9–19.
7. Fang G, Keys TF, Gentry LO, et al. Prosthetic valve endocarditis resulting from nosocomial bacteremia: A prospective, multicenter study. Ann Intern Med 1993;119:560–567.
8. Tunkel AR. Infecting microorganisms. In: Kaye D, ed. Infective Endocarditis, 2nd ed. New York, Raven Press, 1992:85–97.
9. Johnson CM. Adherence events in the pathogenesis of infective endocarditis. Infect Dis Clin North Am 1993;7:21–36.
10. Whitener C, Caputo GM, Weitekamp MR, Karchmer AW. Endocarditis due to coagulase-negative staphylococci: Microbiologic, epidemiologic, and clinical considerations. Infect Dis Clin North Am 1993;7: 81–96.
11. Murphy JG, Foster-Smith K. Management of complications of infective endocarditis with emphasis on echocardiographic findings. Infect Dis Clin North Am 1993;7:153–165.
12. Kaye KM, Kaye D. Laboratory findings including blood cultures. In: Kaye D, ed. Infectious Endocarditis, 2nd ed. New York, Raven Press, 1992:117–124.
13. Mugge A. Echocardiographic detection of cardiac valve vegetations and prognostic implications. Infect Dis Clin North Am 1993;7: 877–898.
14. Lukes AS, Bright DK, Durack DT. Diagnosis of infective endocarditis. Infect Dis Clin North Am 1993;7:1–8.
15. Bush LM, Johnson CC. Clinical syndrome and diagnosis: In: Kaye D, ed. Infectious Endocarditis, 2nd ed. New York, Raven Press, 1992: 99–115.
16. Durack DT, Lukes AS, Bright DK. New criteria for diagnosis of infective endocarditis: Utilization of specific echocardiographic findings. Am J Med 1994;96:200–209.
17. Baldassarre JS, Kaye D. Principles and overview of antibiotic therapy. In: Kaye D, ed. Infectious Endocarditis, 2nd ed. New York, Raven Press, 1992:169–190.
18. Levison ME. *In vitro* assays. In: Kaye D, ed. Infectious Endocarditis, 2nd ed. New York, Raven Press, 1992:151–167.
19. Wilson WR, Karchmer AW, Dajani AS, et al. Antibiotic treatment of adults with infective endocarditis due to streptococci, enterococci, staphylococci, and HACEK microorganisms. JAMA 1995;274: 1706–1713.
20. Tunkel AR, Scheld WM. Experimental models of endocarditis. In: Kaye D, ed. Infectious Endocarditis, 2nd ed. New York, Raven Press, 1992:37–56.
21. Carbon C, Cremieux A-C, Fantin B. Pharmacokinetics and pharmacodynamic aspects of therapy of experimental endocarditis. Infect Dis Clin North Am 1993;7:37–51.
22. Douglas JL, Dismukes WE. Surgical therapy of infective endocarditis on natural valves. In: Kaye D, ed. Infectious Endocarditis, 2nd ed. New York, Raven Press, 1992:397–411.
23. Roberts RB. Streptococcal endocarditis: The viridans and beta hemolytic streptococci. In: Kaye D, ed. Infectious Endocarditis, 2nd ed. New York, Raven Press, 1992:191–208.
24. Francioli PB. Ceftriaxone and outpatient treatment of infective endocarditis. Infect Dis Clin North Am 1993;7:97–116.
25. Weiss ME, Adkinson NF. Beta-lactam allergy. In: Mandell GL, Dolin R, Bennett JE, eds. Principles and Practice of Infectious Diseases, 4th ed. New York, Churchill Livingstone, 1995:272–278.

26. DiNubile MJ. Treatment of endocarditis caused by relatively resistant nonenterococcal streptococci: Is penicillin enough? Rev Infect Dis 1990;12:112–115.
27. Karchmer A. Staphylococcal endocarditis. In: Kaye D, ed. Infectious Endocarditis, 2nd ed. New York, Raven Press, 1992:225–249.
28. Mortara LA, Bayer AS. Staphylococcus aureus bacteremia and endocarditis: New diagnostic and therapeutic concepts. Infect Dis Clin North Am 1993;7:53–68.
29. Korzeniowski O, Sande MA. The National Collaborative Endocarditis Study Group: Combination antimicrobial therapy for *Staphylococcus aureus* endocarditis in patients addicted to parenteral drugs and in non-addicts. Ann Intern Med 1982;97:496–503.
30. Sabath LD. Reappraisal of the antistaphylococcal activities of first-generation (narrow spectrum) and second-generation (expanded spectrum) cephalosporins. Antimicrob Agents Chemother 1989;33: 407–411.
31. Faville RJ, Zaske DE, Kaplan EL, et al. *Staphylococcus aureus* endocarditis: Combined therapy with vancomycin and rifampin. JAMA 1978;240:1963–1965.
32. Levine DP, Fromm BS, Reddy BR. Slow response to vancomycin or vancomycin plus rifampin in methicillin-resistant *Staphylococcus aureus* endocarditis. Ann Intern Med 1991;115:674–680.
33. Sande MA, Lee B, Mills J, Chambers HF. Endocarditis in intravenous drug abusers. In: Kaye D, ed. Infectious Endocarditis, 2nd ed. New York, Raven Press, 1992:345–357.
34. Chambers HF. Short-course combination and oral therapies of *Staphylococcus aureus* endocarditis. Med Clin North Am 1993;7:69–80.
35. Torres-Tortosa M, de Cueto M, Vergara A, et al. Prospective evaluation of a two-week course of intravenous antibiotics in intravenous drug addicts with infective endocarditis. Eur J Clin Microbiol Infect Dis 1994;13:559–564.
36. Chambers HF, Miller T, Newman MD. Right-sided endocarditis in intravenous drug abusers: Two-week combination therapy. Ann Intern Med 1988;109:619–624.
37. Ribera E, Gomez-Jimenez J, Cortes E, et al. Effectiveness of cloxacillin with and without gentamicin in short-term therapy for right-sided *Staphylococcus aureus* endocarditis: A randomized, controlled trial. Ann Intern Med 1996;125:969–974.
38. Small PM, Chambers HF. Vancomycin for *Staphylococcus aureus* endocarditis in intravenous drug users. Antimicrob Agents Chemother 1990;34:1227–1231.
39. Ena J, Dick R, Jones R, et al. The epidemiology of intravenous vancomycin usage in a university hospital. JAMA 1993;269:598–602.
40. Hospital Infection Control Practices Advisory Committee (HICPAC). Recommendations for preventing the spread of vancomycin resistance. Infect Control Hosp Epidemiol 1995;16:105–113.
41. Parker RK, Fossieck BE. Intravenous followed by oral antimicrobial therapy for staphylococcal endocarditis. Ann Intern Med 1980;93: 832–834.
42. Chambers H. Short-course combination and oral therapies of *Staphylococcus aureus* endocarditis. Infect Dis Clin North Am 1993;7: 69–80.
43. Dworkin RJ, Lee BL, Sande MA, Chambers HF. Treatment of right-sided *Staphylococcus aureus* endocarditis in intravenous drug abusers with ciprofloxacin and rifampin. Lancet 1989;2:1071–1073.
44. Heldman AW, Hartert TV, Ray SC, et al. Oral antibiotic treatment of right-sided staphylococcal endocarditis in injection drug users: Prospective randomized comparison with parenteral therapy. Am J Med 1996;101:68–76.
45. Tebas P, Martinez Ruiz R, Roman F, et al. Early resistance to rifampin and ciprofloxacin in the treatment of right-sided *Staphylococcus aureus* endocarditis. J Infect Dis 1991;163:204–205. Letter.
46. Hendershot EF. Fluroquinolones. Infect Dis Clin North Am 1995;9: 715–730.
47. Patton JP. Infective endocarditis: Economic considerations. In: Kaye D, ed. Infective Endocarditis, 2nd ed. New York, Raven Press, 1992: 413–422.
48. Douglas JL, Cobbs CG. Prosthetic valve endocarditis. In: Kaye D, ed. Infective Endocarditis, 2nd ed. New York, Raven Press, 1992: 375–396.
49. Sherris J. Problems in *in vitro* determination of antibiotic tolerance in clinical isolates. Antimicrob Agents Chemother 1986;30:633–637.
50. Voorne GP, Thompson J, Goessens WHF, et al. Role of tolerance in cloxacillin treatment of experimental *Staphylococcus aureus* endocarditis. J Infect Dis 1991;163:640–643.
51. Johnson AP, Uttey AH, Woodford N, George RC. Resistance to vancomycin and teicoplanin: An emerging clinical problem. Clin Microbiol Rev 1990;3:280–291.
52. Murray BE. The life and times of the enterococcus. Clin Microbiol Rev 1990;3:46–65.
53. Eliopolis GM. Enterococcal endocarditis. In Kaye D, ed. Infective Endocarditis, 2nd ed. New York, Raven Press, 1992:209–223.
54. Eliopolis GM. Aminoglycoside resistant enterococcal endocarditis. Infect Dis Clin North Am 1993;7:117–133.
55. Fantin B, Carbon C. Importance of the aminoglycoside dosing regimen in the penicillin-netilmicin combination for treatment of *Enterococcus faecalis*-induced experimental endocarditis. Antimicrob Agents Chemother 1990;34:2387–2391.
56. Lipman ML, Silva J. Endocarditis due to *Streptococcus faecalis* with high-level resistance to gentamicin. Rev Infect Dis 1989;11: 325–328.
57. Wells VD, Wong ES, Murray BE, et al. Infections due to beta-lactamase-producing, high-level gentamicin-resistant *Enterococcus faecalis*. Ann Intern Med 1992;116:285–292.
58. Tailor SA, Bailey EM, Rybak MJ. Enterococcus: An emerging pathogen. Ann Pharmacother 1993;27:1231–1242.
59. Hessen MT, Abrutyn E. Gram-negative bacterial endocarditis. In: Kaye D, ed. Infective Endocarditis, 2nd ed. New York, Raven Press, 1992:251–264.
60. Reyes MP, Brown WJ, Lerner AM. Treatment of patients with *Pseudomonas* endocarditis with high dose aminoglycoside and carbenicillin therapy. Medicine 1978;57:57–67.
61. Reyes MP, Lerner AM. Current problems in the treatment of infective endocarditis due to *Pseudomonas aeruginosa*. Rev Infect Dis 1983;5: 314–321.
62. Moyer DV, Edwards JE. Fungal endocarditis. In: Kaye D, ed. Infective Endocarditis, 2nd ed. New York, Raven Press, 1992:299–312.
63. Karchmer AW. Infective endocarditis. In: Braunwald E, ed. Heart Disease: A Textbook of Cardiovascular Medicine, 5th ed. Philadelphia, WB Saunders, 1997:1077–1104.
64. Santoro J, Ingerman M. Response to therapy: Relapse and reinfections. In: Kaye D, ed. Infective Endocarditis, 2nd ed. New York, Raven Press, 1992:423–433.
65. Levinson ME. *In vitro* assays. In: Kaye D, ed. Infective Endocarditis, 2nd ed. New York, Raven Press, 1992:151–167.
66. MacLowery JD. Perspective: The serum dilution test. J Infect Dis 1989;160:624–629.
67. Weinstein MP, Stratton CW, Ackley A, et al. Multicenter collaborative evaluation of a standardized serum bactericidal test as a prognostic indicator in infective endocarditis. Am J Med 1985;78: 262–269.
68. McCormack JP, Jewesson PJ. A critical reevaluation of the "therapeutic range" of aminoglycosides. Clin Infect Dis 1992;14:320–339.
69. Cantu TG, Yamnanaka-Yuen NA, Lietman PS. Serum vancomycin concentrations: A reappraisal of their clinical value. Clin Infect Dis 1994;18:533–543.
70. Marangos MN, Nicolau DP, Quintiliani R, Nightingale CH. Influence of gentamicin dosing interval on the efficacy of penicillin-containing regimens in experimental *Enterococcus faecalis* endocarditis. J Antimicrob Chemother 1997;39:519–522.
71. Blatter M, Fluckiger U, Entenza J, et al. Simulated human serum profiles of one daily dose of ceftriaxone plus netilmicin in treatment of experimental streptococcal endocarditis. Antimicrob Agents Chemother 1993;37:1971–1976.

72. Francioli PB, Glauser MP. Synergistic activity of ceftiraxone combined with netilmicin administered once daily for treatment of experimental streptococcal endocarditis. Antimicrob Agents Chemother 1993;37:207–212.
73. Gavalda J, Pahissa A, Almirante B, et al. Effect of gentamicin dosing interval on therapy of viridans streptococcal experimental endocarditis with gentamicin plus penicillin. Antimicrob Agents Chemother 1995;39:2098–2103.
74. Francioli P, Ruch W, Stamboulian D, et al. Treatment of streptococcal endocarditis with a single daily dose of ceftriaxone and netilmicin for 14 days: A prospective multicenter study. Clin Infect Dis 1995;21: 1406–1410.
75. Wilson WR, Geraci JE, Danielson GK, et al. Anticoagulant therapy and central nervous system complications in patients with prosthetic valve endocarditis. Circulation 1978;57:1004–1007.
76. Davenport J, Hart RG. Prosthetic valve endocarditis 1976–1987: Antibiotics, anticoagulation and stroke. Stroke 1990;21:993–999.
77. Durack DT. Prevention of infective endocarditis. N Engl J Med 1995; 332:38–44.
78. Greenman RL, Bisno AL. Prevention of bacterial endocarditis. In: Kaye D, ed. Infective Endocarditis, 2nd ed. New York, Raven Press, 1992:465–481.
79. Van der Meer JT, Van Wijk W, Thompson J, et al. Efficacy of antibiotic prophylaxis for prevention of native-valve endocarditis. Lancet 1992;339:135–139.
80. Hall G, Hedstrom SA, Heimdahl A, Nord CE. Prophylactic administration of penicillins for endocarditis does not reduce the incidence of postextraction bacteremia. Clin Infect Dis 1993;17:188–194.
81. Strom BL, Abrutyne E, Berlin JA, et al. Dental and cardiac risk factors for infective endocarditis: A population-based, case-control study. Ann Intern Med 1998;129:761–769.
82. Dajani AS, Taubert KA, Wilson W, et al. Prevention of bacterial endocarditis: Recommendations by the American Heart Association. JAMA 1997;277:1794–1801.
83. Wahl MJ. Myths of dental-induced endocarditis. Arch Intern Med 1994;154(2):137–144.
84. Wehrmacher WH. Myths: Endocarditis. Arch Intern Med 1994;154: 129–130.

102

TUBERCULOSIS

Charles A. Peloquin, PharmD, and Steve C. Ebert, PharmD

Tuberculosis (TB) is a communicable infectious disease caused by *Mycobacterium tuberculosis.*[1,2] It can produce a silent, latent infection, as well as an active disease state. Although TB is far less common today in the United States than it was a century ago, it remains the most prevalent infection on the planet, afflicting roughly one-third of the world's population.[1] *M. tuberculosis* is found almost exclusively in humans and survives only briefly when isolated in the environment. Still, efforts to eliminate TB in the United States and globally have failed.[1,2] Through shifts in the population considered endemic for TB, changes in health care policies, an increase in the number of immunocompromised individuals, and the development of drug resistance, TB staged a recent "comeback" in the United States and remains out of control in many developing nations.[1,2]

EPIDEMIOLOGY

Tuberculosis-like diseases have afflicted man since the beginning of recorded history.[1–3] Mummies from Egyptian tombs, as well as preserved corpses from Incan and Mayan burial sites, have shown evidence of tuberculous infection.[3] While such skeletal evidence is consistent with TB, it has not been possible to determine if *M. tuberculosis, Mycobacterium bovis,* or another related pathogen produced the disease.[3] Tuberculosis was originally termed "phthisis" because of the emaciated features of patients with the disease, and later became known as consumption.[1] Tuberculosis has been most prevalent in urbanized cultures, particularly when overcrowding has occurred.[2,3]

It appears likely that *M. tuberculosis* is a variant of *M. bovis,* which causes a tuberculosis-like disease in livestock, and that it emerged in Europe centuries ago.[3] In Europe and the United States, TB became a major public health problem during the Industrial Revolution, because of increased crowding in urban areas.[3] During the eighteenth and nineteenth centuries, as many as 25% of recorded adult deaths could be attributed to TB.[1–3] Many advances in the prevention of infection, such as pasteurization of milk and isolation of infected persons, are the result of the threat of TB.

Today, TB remains the world's leading infectious killer. Globally, it is estimated that one in every three people is infected with *M. tuberculosis,* and approximately 3 million people die from it each year.[1,2,4] In the United States, approximately 13 million people are infected with *M. tuberculosis,* resulting in 22,813 cases of active disease in 1995 and 21,327 in 1996. Of these new cases of TB, approximately 2000 patients die annually. Prior to 1984, the annual incidence of TB in the United States had declined steadily by about 5% per year (Fig. 102–1). In 1984, however, this decline slowed, and the incidence of TB in the United States actually increased during 1988 to 1992 from 9.3 to 10.5 cases/100,000. Since then, implementation of more stringent screening criteria, infection control practices, and treatment protocols have resulted in a downturn in incidence, with case rates of 8/100,000. Although this represents significant improvement, the eradication of TB in the United States remains a distant goal.[4]

RISK FACTORS FOR INFECTION

LOCATION AND PLACE OF BIRTH

From 1985 to 1992, five states—New York, New Jersey, California, Florida, and Texas—accounted for 92% of the total national increase in cases.[4] The proportion of reported TB patients that are foreign-born has increased each year since 1986, and in 1995, accounted for 36% of all U.S. cases.[4] Many of these patients come from Asia and Latin America, and the five states listed are the primary entry points for these immigrants.

Within the United States, TB cases cluster in urban areas.[4] Since 1985, the frequency of TB in rural populations has remained constant, but it has increased 29% in urban populations. Tuberculosis is concentrated in patients who are the most difficult to treat: underprivileged patients without access to health care and who live in crowded conditions; recalcitrant patients who are noncompliant with treatment protocols; and immune-compromised patients, who are unable to ward off the disease.[2,4]

Close contacts (greater than 40 hours per week) of patients with pulmonary TB are at particularly high risk of infection, with an estimated infection rate of 25% to 30%.[5,6] Although less common, patients with extrapulmonary TB can spread the disease if the infected site is exposed to the environment.

RACE AND ETHNICITY

From 1985 to 1992, TB cases in the United States increased from 9.3 to 10.5 cases/100,000, up 12.9%, even though the incidence of TB in Caucasians decreased by 11.1%. The increase resulted from a rise in incidence of TB in Hispanic Americans by 4.7%; in Asian-Pacific Islanders, by 12%; and in non-Hispanic blacks, by nearly 38%. This represents both TB in immigrants of those races, as well as spread of TB among U.S.-born ethnic minorities.[4] Fortunately, since

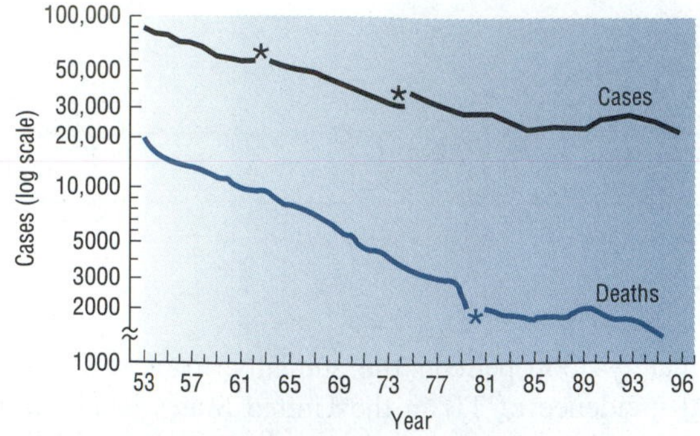

FIGURE 102–1. Tuberculosis cases and deaths in the United States, 1953–1996.

1993, TB control efforts have produced large decreases in the rates of TB in two of these groups. There has been a 19% decrease in Hispanics and a 22.5% decrease in non-Hispanic blacks. The modest 1.5% decrease among Asian-Pacific Islanders probably reflects ongoing activation of latent infection among recent immigrants to the United States. Because the latter represents infections acquired in areas beyond the reach of the United States's TB control efforts, it is likely that improvement in this population will take more time.

AGE, GENDER, AND OCCUPATION

During the 1970s and early 1980s, TB in the United States increasingly had become a disease of the elderly.[3,4] In 1987, this group accounted for 12% of the total population, but 27% of TB cases, with a case rate of 20.6/100,000.[7] Many of these patients were infected in the early 1900s, when TB was much more common. A substantial number of elderly patients, however, are infected de novo, especially those residing in nursing homes. The rate of tuberculous infection in nursing home residents is twice that of the elderly population as a whole, with the risk increasing proportionately with the length of stay.[7]

Despite the high prevalence in the elderly, the greatest increase has occurred in the 25- to 44-year-old age group, especially in minority populations (Fig. 102–2).[4] Because

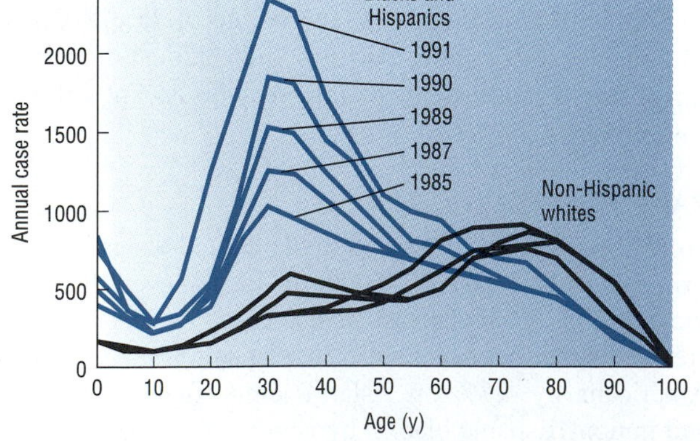

FIGURE 102–2. Tuberculosis rates by age group, for whites and non-white minorities, United States, 1985–1991.

this age group is of child-bearing age, the rate of TB in children has also risen. The differences between whites and nonwhites are even more pronounced at younger ages; 80% of new cases of TB in the United States that occur in persons less than 15 years of age occur in ethnic minorities.[4] It appears, therefore, that the upswing in TB case rates has occurred because of an increased infection rate in certain younger populations, especially those in crowded living conditions with reduced access to health care.

Men have a twofold higher rate for TB than do women. Also, health care workers in hospitals and long-term care facilities may be at risk, especially those involved in respiratory care, such as respiratory therapists and pulmonologists. This has lead to substantial efforts to control the spread of TB in health care facilities.[4,8,9]

COINFECTION WITH HUMAN IMMUNODEFICIENCY VIRUS

A significant contributor to the rise in TB is the human immunodeficiency virus (HIV) epidemic. In 1990, in excess of 5% of HIV-infected patients had been diagnosed with TB, and 39% of patients with TB had concurrent HIV infection.[2,4] When asymptomatic tuberculous infection is considered, the numbers are likely much greater.[10] Overlaps exist between patients at risk for HIV infection and TB. Disproportionately high numbers of TB patients are IV drug abusers, reside in larger cities, such as New York City, have been imprisoned, are less than 44 years of age, or have been hospitalized on wards designated for HIV-infected patients.[2,4] While it does not appear that HIV disease itself increases the risk of tuberculous infection, many of the habits and experiences associated with HIV-infected patients increase their risk for infection.[2,11,12]

RISK FACTORS FOR DISEASE

After infection, the lifetime risk of developing active TB disease is roughly one in ten, with the first 2 years postexposure carrying the greatest risk. Infected children less than 2 years of age and the elderly are considered to have a two to five times greater risk for developing clinical TB as compared to other age groups. For persons with underlying immune suppression (renal failure, cancer, immunosuppressive drug treatment), the risk is estimated at 4- to 16-fold. Finally, the Centers for Disease Control (CDC) estimates that HIV-infected patients with tuberculous infection are more than 100 times more likely to develop active TB.[4,13] Unlike normal hosts, their *annual* risk of disease reactivation is about one in ten. Therefore, all patients with HIV infection should be screened for tuberculous infection and vice versa.

ETIOLOGY

Mycobacterium tuberculosis can cause both a silent infection and the disease known as tuberculosis (TB). Using modern genetic methods for identification, the genus *Mycobacterium* now consists of more than 60 species of aerobic, non–spore-forming, rod-shaped bacteria. A unique feature of the genus is that after staining with carbol-fuchsin, the organisms retain the red pigment despite attempts at decolorization with acid-alcohol, hence the term acid-fast bacilli (AFB).[14] Most strains of mycobacteria are slow growing (generation time approaching 24 hours instead of every 20 to 40 minutes for bacteria), most produce heat-sensitive catalase, and all lack pigment production. Among the mycobacteria, only *M. tuberculosis* is a frequent pathogen for normal human hosts. Certain nontuberculous myconbacteria (NTM), such as *M. kansasii, M. fortuitum,* and *M. avium* complex (MAC) have been shown to be pathogenic in immunocompromised patients, most notably those with acquired immunodeficiency syndrome (AIDS).[2] Treatment of these pathogens is discussed in the chapter on AIDS (Chap. 114).

Mycobacterium tuberculosis is a slender, straight, or slightly curved bacillus, ranging 1 to 4 μm in length.[1,14,15] Because of its waxier outer layer, *M. tuberculosis* does not stain well with Gram stain.[1] The Ziehl-Neelsen or the fluorochrome stains must be used instead.[1] Microscopic examination can detect about 10,000 organisms/mL of specimen, but it cannot differentiate among the various species of mycobacteria or determine if the organisms in the original sample were alive or dead.[1,14,15]

CULTURE AND SUSCEPTIBILITY TESTING

Specialized media are needed to grow mycobacteria.[1,14,15] Direct susceptibility testing involves inoculation of the test media with organisms taken directly from a concentrated, smear-positive specimen, producing susceptibility results in about 3 weeks. Indirect susceptibility testing involves inoculation of the test media with organisms obtained from a previously grown pure culture of the organisms, which can take several weeks longer. Results from this solid agar method, also known as the proportion method, are determined as the ratio of colony counts between drug-containing and drug-free agar.[1,15] In the United States, the critical proportion for designating the strain resistant is 1%. Limitations to the proportion method include the several weeks required to obtain results, drug loss because of adsorption and degradation, and the qualitative nature of the result (susceptible or resistant). The Bactec system (Becton-Dickinson, Sparks, MD) uses liquid media (7H12 broth) and detects live mycobacteria based on the release CO_2.[14] Advantages of the system include reduced incubation time, reduced drug adsorption and degradation in the media, and, when multiple concentrations are tested, a truly quantitative end point.[1,14,15]

Additional newer tests are available to help clinicians in identifying the pathogen. Nucleic acid probes such as the AccuProbe (Gen-Probe, San Diego), use DNA probes to identify the presence of complimentary rRNA for several mycobacterial species.[14,16] DNA fingerprinting using restriction fragment length polymorphism (RFLP) analysis has been used to identify clusters of cases.[1,14,16] Amplification of the genetic material can be achieved through polymerase chain reaction (PCR; Roche Molecular Systems, Branchburg, NJ), amplified *M. tuberculosis* direct test (MTD; Gen-Probe), and strand displacement amplification (SDA; Becton-Dickinson, Sparks, MD).[14,17] Thin layer chromatography (TLC), high performance liquid chromatography (HPLC) for mycolic acid identification, and gas chromatography (GC) for short chain fatty acids (methyl esters) have been used to speciate mycobacterial isolates.[1,14,16]

TRANSMISSION

Mycobacterium tuberculosis is transmitted from person-to-person through microsize droplet nuclei that are dispersed by either coughing or sneezing.[5] The classic studies of Riley and colleagues in the late 1950s demonstrated the ability of air circulated from a hospital ward of patients with TB to cause disease in guinea pigs.[18] When the air was filtered or exposed to ultraviolet radiation, the animals were not infected.[18] It is estimated that 30% of individuals who experience a significant length of direct contact with a person with pulmonary TB will develop tuberculous infection.

A person with cavitary pulmonary TB and a cough may infect roughly one person per month until they are effectively treated, although this number can vary significantly. A person with laryngeal TB can spread organisms even when talking, so the transmission rates can be very high with this form of the disease. While immunocompromised conditions, such as AIDS, do not change the acquisition of the organisms, such newly infected persons have a higher risk for going on to active disease.[2]

PATHOPHYSIOLOGY

IMMUNE RESPONSE

The process by which the immune system recognizes and suppresses mycobacterial proliferation is now being elucidated. The cell types responsible for immunity to mycobacteria are the macrophage and T lymphocytes. T lymphocytes with an α-β T cell receptor (TCR) compose 95% of T lymphocytes and are capable of recognizing both cellular and soluble antigens. The α-β T lymphocytes are further divided into CD4 (helper) and CD8 (cytotoxic/suppresser) lymphocytes. One subset of these CD4 lymphocytes appears to act against mycobacteria (Th-1 cells). These differ from the Th-2 subpopulation of CD4 cells that activate B cells. This subset recognizes the antigen presented by macrophages, is activated by interleukin-12 (IL-12), and is suppressed by IL-4 and IL-10. These lymphocytes secrete interferon γ (IFN-γ), which activates macrophages to destroy mycobacteria. Later, cytolytic T lymphocytes join in destroying cells harboring mycobacteria.[19] A third group of T lymphocytes possesses a γ-Δ TCR. These cells appear to recognize ligands different from those of α-β T cells.[19] Having an immunoregulatory role, they appear to contribute to host resistance to infection. Because the CD4 T cells are depleted by HIV infection, one can see how AIDS patients would have difficulty controlling an *M. tuberculosis* infection.

PRIMARY INFECTION

Primary infection is the result of inhalation of organisms contained in small particles known as droplet nuclei. These particles are small enough (1 to 5 mm) to escape the ciliary epithelial cells of the upper respiratory tract, leading to the deposition of organisms on the alveolar surface. The degree of subsequent progression of infection to clinical disease depends on the initial inoculum size, as well as the state of the host's cell-mediated immune system.[5,20,21] Once implanted, the organisms multiply and are ingested by pulmonary macrophages where they continue to multiply, albeit more slowly. Intracellular organisms then spread to involve regional lymph nodes in the hilar, mediastinal, and retroperitoneal areas. At this point (days 5 to 15), α-β-CD4 lymphocytes are presented with antigen, activate, and secrete IFN-γ, which stimulates macrophages to become bactericidal. Depending on the concentration of antigen present and the inflammatory response evoked, tissue necrosis and calcification of the originally infected site and regional lymph nodes may occur, resulting in the formation of a radiodense area referred to as a Ghon complex.

After this stage of lymph node involvement, the organisms may be held in check or, more frequently, they may spread through the bloodstream to a variety of organ systems. These include other lymph nodes, bone and bone marrow, liver, kidneys, central nervous system, and most commonly, the posterior apical region of the lungs. Seeding of these sites probably occurs because of their relatively high blood flow but limited lymphatic drainage.[20] Nodular infiltrates that may arise in the apices of the lung secondary to this hematogenous spread are referred to as *Simon foci*. By this time (days 15 to 25), macrophages have begun to form granulomas to contain the organisms. In addition, γ-Δ-T lymphocytes may begin to destroy AFB-containing macrophages. This acts to reduce the number of bacteria, but also probably prevents "overstimulation" of the immune system, which could result in autoimmunity.[19]

Concurrent with the proliferation of organisms is the development of delayed hypersensitivity via activation and multiplication of CD4 lymphocytes. When activated, lymphocytes reach an adequate number (usually 1 to 3 months after infection), tissue hypersensitivity results, as evidenced by the presence of a positive tuberculin skin test, and any remaining viable organisms within the body will be contained. It should be noted, however, that the immune-mediated cessation of dissemination (Th-1 response) and the development of cutaneous hypersensitivity are two separate events. Finally, by days 20 to 40, cytolytic T cells begin to destroy macrophages containing AFB. Dissemination is halted, and the remaining mycobacteria reside within granulomas or macrophages that have avoided detection and lysis.[19]

The arrest of mycobacterial proliferation is characterized pathologically by formation of granulomas of two types: proliferative granulomas, which are stable and can effectively limit the spread of the organism, and caseating granulomas, so named for their cheese-like appearance, which have a necrotic center, are relatively unstable, and permit the limited growth of *M. tuberculosis* within them.[5,20,21] Approximately 90% of patients who experience primary disease have no further clinical manifestations other than a positive skin test either alone (70%) or in combination with radiographic evidence of stable granulomas (15% to 20%). Approximately 3% to 5% of patients (usually children, the elderly, or the immunocompromised) experience "progressive primary" disease, which occurs before skin test conversion.[22,23] This form of the disease is characterized by progressive pneumonia originating at the site of the primary infection (usually the lower lobes) and frequently by dissemination, leading to meningitis and often to involvement of the upper lobes of the lung as well.[22,23]

REACTIVATION DISEASE

The remaining 7% to 10% of patients develop reactivation disease, which arises subsequent to the hematogenous spread of the organism, typically within 2 years of exposure.[20] In the United States, development of TB in patients with a positive skin test is statistically more likely to be caused by reactivation than reinfection. Reinfection is uncommon because of the low rate of exposure in this country and because previously sensitized individuals possess some degree of immunity to reinfection. Exceptions to this general trend may include some patients coinfected with HIV living in areas of high transmission of *M. tuberculosis*.

When the mycobacteria reactivate, the apical areas of the lung have been the most common sites for reactivation (85% of cases). For reasons that are not entirely known (waning cellular immunity, loss of specific T-cell clones, blocking antibody), organisms within granulomas emerge and begin multiplying extracellularly.[24] This typically originates as a small lesion that is visualized as an alveolar infiltrate. The resultant inflammatory response produces caseating granulomas, which will eventually liquefy and cavitate as a result of the inflammatory process. Because the host has prior immunity at the time of reactivating disease, the immune response may in fact contribute to the severity of the infection. For example, cavitary pulmonary TB, caused largely by invasion of neutrophils into lung parenchyma, is seen almost exclusively in previously sensitized individuals. The aerobic environment of a cavity enhances growth of the organism; bacterial counts within the cavity may be as high as 10^8 organisms per milliliter of sputum. Fluid within the cavity is easily aerosolized by coughing, which results in the spread of the organism to other areas within the upper and lower respiratory tracts, as well as into the surrounding environment. Partial healing may result from fibrosis of cavities and other infected sites, but the potential exists for breakdown of these areas and subsequent reactivation.[5,20] If left untreated, pulmonary TB will eventually spread to involve the entire respiratory tract, resulting in hypoxia, respiratory acidosis, and death.

EXTRAPULMONARY AND MILIARY TUBERCULOSIS

In some cases, a caseating granuloma at an extrapulmonary site will undergo liquefaction and release tubercle bacilli, resulting in symptomatic disease. Extrapulmonary TB occurs in a limited number of normal hosts, but it is quite common in patients coinfected with HIV (Table 102–1). Because of the unusual presentations, diagnosis is difficult and often delayed. Organs and systems most commonly involved include the central nervous system (meningitis and cranial tuberculomas), peritoneum, genitourinary tract, lymphatic system, skeletal system, pericardium, adrenal glands, and liver.[20] As with the pulmonary form, extrapulmonary TB left untreated may continue to spread and may eventually result in death.

Occasionally, a massive inoculum of organisms may be introduced into the bloodstream, causing widely disseminated disease and granuloma formation known as miliary TB. While primary miliary TB (occurring at the time of initial bacillemia) is most common, some patients may develop miliary TB from a second bacillemia occurring during reactivation. This form of the disease acquired its name from the millet seed-like appearance of the small granulomas viewed on chest radiograph, as well as in films of other soft tissues.[20]

INFLUENCE OF HUMAN IMMUNODEFICIENCY VIRUS INFECTION ON PATHOGENESIS

As antimycobacterial α-β-CD4 lymphocytes multiply in response to tuberculous infection, HIV multiplies within these cells and selectively destroys them. This results in a depletion of the cells with mycobactericidal activity. The impairment of CD4 lymphocyte activity increases the rate and extent of tuberculous infection.[19] Infection with HIV thereby increases the risk that a patient infected with *M. tuberculosis* will develop active disease. As previously mentioned, the risk for developing active TB disease increases over 100-fold in HIV-infected patients compared to an immunocompetent host.[25] For decades, about 90% of all cases of TB in this country have been reactivation disease from previous infection. Based on sophisticated epidemiologic studies using DNA fingerprinting, investigators now estimate that 40% to 50% of all new cases of TB arise from recent infection in certain populations. The presence of HIV infection has been established as a major risk factor for rapid-onset of disease.[26–28]

As suggested, evidence exists that the immune response associated with tuberculous infection may increase HIV replication in both lymphocytes and macrophages, and subsequently accelerate progression of HIV disease. Markers of HIV progression, such as serum β_2-microglobulin concentrations, are higher in HIV-infected patients with tuberculous infection.[29] In addition, HIV-infected patients with tuberculous infection who are not treated progress to AIDS more rapidly than those without infection or those who receive prophylactic antimycobacterial chemotherapy.[30] This has prompted widespread screening for tuberculous infection in HIV-infected patients, and empiric chemoprophylaxis for those in whom infection cannot be ruled out.

CLINICAL PRESENTATION

Tuberculosis can present with generalized symptoms of weight loss, malaise, fever, and night sweats.[1,5,21] As the disease progresses, the patient may develop a persistent cough, which is often productive of sputum. Frequently, the onset of TB is insidious, and the diagnosis may not be considered until a chest radiograph is performed. Typical radiographic findings include patchy or nodular infiltrates in the apical areas of the upper lobes or the superior segment of the lower lobes. As the infection progresses, cavitation is often seen, with or without air-fluid levels. Unfortunately, many patients do not seek medical attention until more dramatic symptoms, such as hemoptysis, occur. At this point, patients typically have large cavitary lung lesions with high mycobacterial burdens. Expectoration or swallowing of sputum containing large numbers of organisms may result in extension of disease involving the upper respiratory or gastrointestinal (GI) tract. Ulceration of the pharynx, larynx, tongue, and oral mucosa, as well as otitis media, gastric ulceration,

TABLE 102–1. Likelihood of Various Clinical Presentations of Tuberculous Infection in Different Patient Groups

Status at Exposure	Asymptomatic Infection	Progressive Primary Infection	Reactivation Pulmonary	Extrapulmonary Disease	Miliary Tuberculosis
< 1 yr old	++	+++	+/–	++	+
1–5 yr	++	++	+/–	++	+
6–10 yr	++	+	+	+	+
11–15 yr	+++	+/–	+	+	+/–
HIV (–) adult	+++	+/–	+	+	+/–
HIV (+) adult	+	++	+	++	+

+++ = predominant feature; ++ = common; + = occasional; +/– = rare.

and perirectal abscess, may occur.[1,5,21] Physical exam is nonspecific but suggestive of progressive pulmonary disease. Dullness to chest percussion suggests consolidation in involved areas of the lung. Rales and increased vocal fremitus are frequently observed on auscultation. In patients in whom impaired oxygenation has developed, cyanosis and clubbing of the digits may be seen. Abnormal laboratory data are usually limited to moderate elevations in the white blood cell (WBC) count with a lymphocyte predominance. Other abnormal values may occasionally be observed but are too infrequent to be useful diagnostically.

The presentation of TB in patients coinfected with HIV varies, depending on the stage of HIV infection (Table 102–2). Because TB is more virulent than other HIV-associated opportunistic infections *(Pneumocystis carinii, M. avium),* it often occurs early in course of immunosuppression.[1,31–33] Tuberculosis in AIDS patients is less likely to involve cavitary disease, be associated with a positive skin test, or be associated with fever. These patients often present with reactivation of latent pulmonary infection, but radiographic findings may be minimal or absent. Patients infected with HIV have a high incidence of extrapulmonary TB, including lymphadenitis, bacteremia, involvement of the central nervous system (CNS), genitourinary tract, bone marrow, and miliary disease. Patients with AIDS also are much more likely to present as the progressive primary form of TB or with involvement of multiple lobes of the lung. Because their symptoms are not specific to TB, the diagnosis is often delayed. Postmortem diagnoses of TB account for roughly 5% of all reported cases.[34]

Clinical features associated with extrapulmonary TB vary, depending on the organ system(s) involved, but typically consist of slowly progressive compromise of organ function with low-grade fever and other constitutional symptoms, as mentioned previously. Patients with genitourinary TB may present with sterile pyuria or culture-negative urinary tract infection, hematuria, abnormal intravenous pyelogram, epididymitis, irregular menses, or infertility. Lymphadenitis often involves the cervical and supraclavicular nodes and may appear as a neck mass with spontaneous drainage. Tuberculous arthritis and osteomyelitis most commonly occur in the elderly and usually affect the lower spine and weight-bearing joints. Abnormal behavior, headaches, or convulsions are suggestive of tuberculous meningitis, often without pulmonary involvement. Involvement of the peritoneum, pericardium, larynx, and adrenal glands also occurs.[21]

TABLE 102–2. Clinical Features of Tuberculosis in HIV-Positive Versus HIV-Negative Patients

	HIV-Negative (Immunocompetent)	HIV-Positive (AIDS)
Onset	Gradual	Abrupt
Presentation	Reactivation	Progressive primary
PPD result	Usually positive	Usually negative
Chest radiograph	Apical infiltrate	Diffuse, lower lobes
Extrapulmonary forms	Occasional	Common
Other pathogens present	Occasional	Common
AFB-positive sputum	Usually	Usually
Response to therapy	Excellent	Good

AFB = acid–fact bacilli; AIDS = acquired immunodeficiency syndrome; HIV = human immunodeficiency virus; PPD = purified protein derivative.

THE ELDERLY

The clinical presentation of TB in the elderly is often atypical in nature, mimicking other respiratory diseases. Many clinical findings are muted or absent altogether. Compared with younger patients, TB in the elderly is associated with fevers and positive skin tests 50% less often, sputum production and hemoptysis 60% less often, and night sweats 80% less often.[35,36] Weight loss appears to be equally prevalent in both groups. In contrast, mental status changes are twice as common in the elderly, and mortality because of TB in the elderly is six times more common than in younger patients.[35] Tuberculosis is a preventable cause of death in the elderly that should not be overlooked.

CHILDREN

Tuberculosis in children is more apt to present in a manner similar to a typical bacterial pneumonia and is termed progressive primary TB.[22,23] Clinical disease often begins 1 to 2 months after exposure and precedes cutaneous hypersensitivity. In contrast to that seen in adults, pulmonary TB in children often involves the lower and middle lobes of the lung.[22,23,37] In addition, dissemination to sites such as lymph nodes, GI and genitourinary tracts, bone marrow, and meninges is fairly common. Because of the delay in recruitment of cellular immunity, cavitary disease is observed infrequently in pulmonary disease of children, and the number of organisms present is typically smaller than in an adult. Because cavitary lesions are uncommon, children do not readily spread the disease to others. Pediatric TB, however, can be rapidly fatal, and it requires the prompt introduction of effective chemotherapy.

DIAGNOSIS

SKIN TESTING

The key to preventing the spread of TB is the identification of those individuals who are infected.[1,21,38] This involves the use of the tuberculin purified protein derivative (PPD) skin test. Populations in whom skin testing is indicated include those listed in Table 102–3. The members of these high-risk groups should be tested for TB infection, and they should also be educated about TB in an effort to reduce transmission.

TABLE 102–3. Candidates for Screening With PPD Skin Test

Individuals	Initial Screening	Retest Periodically	Test If Local Outbreak
HIV-infected	×	If possible	N/A
Hospital employees	×	Annually–semiannually	Yes, if exposed
Nursing home staff	×	Annually	Yes, if exposed
Nursing home residents	×	Probably not	Yes, if exposed
Workers at prisons, homeless shelters, clinics	×	Annually	Yes, if exposed
Immigrants	×	If possible	N/A
Health care students	×	Annually–biannually	Yes, if exposed
General population	No	No	Yes, if exposed

HIV = human immunodeficiency virus; N/A = not applicable; PPD = purified protein derivative.

Because it is quantitative, the Mantoux test is preferred to the Heaf or tine test. The standard 5 tuberculin unit (5 TU) PPD dose is placed intracutaneously on the volar aspect of the forearm with a 26- or 27-gauge needle.[5] This injection should produce a small, raised, blanched wheal. It is important that the injection not be placed too deeply, or it may be washed away by the vasculature. This test should then be read by an experienced professional in 48 to 72 hours, and a record made of the size of induration. In some cases, the test may remain positive as long as 5 days. An area of induration (not erythema) of ≥ 10 mm for most immunocompetent patients at risk for recent infection and ≥ 5 mm for HIV-infected individuals is considered positive.[1,21,38,39] For patients with AIDS or young children with recent exposure to an index case, any extent of induration might be read as positive.

Some have recommended that a control panel of candida, trychophyton, and mumps antigens be placed in HIV-infected individuals to rule out anergy.[1,5,21,38,39] While anergy panels are imperfect tools, they can provide additional information regarding the patient's ability to respond to an antigenic challenge. If the reaction to the anergy panel is positive, there is additional evidence that the patient is immunologically capable of responding to the PPD challenge. As the immune system weakens (or the CD4 counts decrease), the likelihood of a small or undetectable response to antigenic challenge increases. Because of frequent coinfection, patients known to be HIV positive should be tested for TB, and patients with positive TB skin tests should be considered for HIV testing. A further diagnostic work-up in HIV patients is recommended to diagnose or rule-out TB adequately.[21,31,39]

Although three test strengths of PPD-S are available (first strength = 1 TU, intermediate strength = 5 TU, and second strength = 250 TU), the intermediate-strength form is almost invariably used. First-strength PPD-S is sometimes used for testing patients in whom a severe reaction may be expected (patients with known prior positive test), although few data exist to support this practice.[40] Second-strength PPD-S may be used in testing patients with depressed cell-mediated immunity who have had a negative result with the intermediate-strength test but appear likely to have TB on the basis of clinical criteria. Two products, Aplisol and Tubersol, are commercially available, but because of more predictable results, Tubersol appears to be the preferred product.

While the tuberculin skin test alone cannot induce cutaneous hypersensitivity de novo, it may sufficiently enhance the low-level reactivity present in some patients so that conversion of a negative test result to a positive result could occur after repeat testing. This "booster effect" usually occurs in patients with past tuberculous infection, immunization with bacillus Calmette-Guérin (BCG) vaccine, or from infection with NTM.[21,41] In individuals who will be skin tested periodically (annually, semiannually), it is recommended that the initial testing involve a two-stage method (i.e., PPD tests are placed twice within a 1- to 2-week period) to detect boosters.[42] All individuals who initially boost should be further examined for evidence of TB. The clinician should also consider other factors (history of exposure, signs, symptoms) when determining whether a subsequent skin test result is positive, and should not base the decision to treat or not to treat solely on this result. Nonboosters are considered to be without infection, and any subsequent positive skin test should be viewed as indicative of recent infection requiring treatment.[5,41]

False-negative results may be caused by faulty test material (outdated, improperly stored), poor administration technique, observer error, impairment of the host's immune system (cancer, sarcoid, certain viral infections, immunosuppressant drugs, AIDS), and, in up to 20% of patients, with active TB disease.[38] False-positive results are more common when the patients tested have little risk of having the disease and in some patients recently vaccinated with BCG. A BCG vaccination, however, should not lead one to ignore a positive PPD result. Such patients require careful evaluation for active disease, and preventive therapy may be considered.

ADDITIONAL TESTS

Patients who are diagnosed as having tuberculous infection by skin testing, as well as those who present with clinical findings consistent with TB, should undergo diagnostic testing to rule out active disease. Confirmatory diagnosis of a clinical suspicion of TB must be made through chest radiographs and microbiologic examination of sputum or other infected material.

RADIOLOGIC DIAGNOSIS

A chest radiograph should be routinely ordered in patients suspected of having TB to assist in the initial diagnosis and assess the extent of disease in those previously diagnosed. Although no pathognomonic pattern exists, a number of radiographic findings occur that are characteristic of TB. In the reactivation form of the disease, ongoing infection is characterized by patchy infiltrates of the upper segments or apices of the lung with ipsilateral lymph node involvement.[5,21] In advanced cases, cavitation is commonly observed. Granulomas in various stages of development are also seen frequently. In quiescent disease, calcification of granulomas often occurs. Thickening of the pleura and apical scarring are also seen in patients with history of active disease.

Early primary TB in children or AIDS patients is often characterized by a discrete lower lobe lesion with enlarged hilar lymph nodes. Subsequent active disease in the lower lobes of the lung, however, is radiographically indistinct from other pneumonias.[5,22,23] In fact, the finding of an apical infiltrate on chest radiograph, felt to be pathognomonic of TB in an immunocompetent individual, is more likely to be *Pneumocystis carinii* in a patient with advanced HIV infection.[43]

MICROBIOLOGIC DIAGNOSIS

In addition, every attempt should be made to isolate *M. tuberculosis* from the site of infection. As described earlier, examination of sputum is important in providing microbiologic evidence of pulmonary TB.[21] Sputum collected in the morning is considered to have the highest number of organisms per volume and hence the highest yield.[14,15] Daily sputum collections over 3 consecutive days are recommended. For patients unable to expectorate sputum, sputum induction with aerosolized hypertonic saline may produce a diagnostic sample. Alternatively, bronchoscopy or aspiration of gastric fluid may be attempted, although these should probably be avoided in the elderly because of the risks of aspiration.[21] For patients with suspected extrapulmonary TB, sampling of fluid, biopsy of the infected site, or both may be attempted, although the likelihood of a positive AFB smear or culture is low (with the exception of liver and bone marrow biopsies). Blood cultures are also unlikely to be positive, although bacteremia is more common in AIDS patients.[44]

▶ TREATMENT: Tuberculosis

DESIRED OUTCOME

The desired outcomes in the treatment of TB are as follows:

1. Rapid clinical identification of a new case of TB.
2. Immediate isolation of the patient with active disease to prevent the spread of the disease.
3. Successful collection of appropriate samples for smears and cultures.
4. Initiation of specific antituberculosis treatment.
5. Prompt resolution of the signs and symptoms of the disease.
6. Achievement of a noninfectious state in the patient, allowing for the termination of isolation.
7. Adherence to the treatment regimen by the patient.
8. Cure of the patient in as short a period as possible (generally at least 6 months).

Secondary goals are the identification of the index case that infected the patient, the identification of all persons infected by both the index case and the new case of TB, and the completion of appropriate treatments for those individuals.

GENERAL APPROACHES TO TREATMENT

Drug treatment is the cornerstone of TB management. Other interventions are important additions to patient care but do not supplant chemotherapy. Monotherapy can be used only for infected patients who do *not* have active TB (latent infection as shown by positive skin test). Once active disease is present, a minimum of two drugs, and generally three or more must be used simultaneously. The duration of treatment depends on the condition of the host, extent of disease, presence of drug resistance, and tolerance of medical interventions. The shortest duration of treatment is generally 6 months, although 2 to 3 years of treatment may be necessary in extreme cases of multidrug-resistant TB (MDR-TB). Because the duration of therapy is so long and because patients may feel relatively well after a few weeks of treatment, careful follow-up is required. It increasingly has been shown that directly observed therapy (DOT) by a health care worker is cost-effective.[45,46]

PRINCIPLES FOR TREATING INFECTION AND TREATING DISEASE

Asymptomatic patients with tuberculous infection have a bacillary load of approximately 10^3 organisms, compared with 10^{11} organisms in a patient with cavitary pulmonary TB.[5,37,47] As the number of organisms increases, the likelihood of finding naturally occurring, drug-resistant mutants also increases. Naturally occurring mutants are found at rates of 1 in 10^6 to 1 in 10^8 organisms for the antituberculosis drugs. When treating asymptomatic infection with isoniazid (INH) monotherapy, the risk of selecting out INH-resistant organisms is low. The INH mutation rate is about 1 in 10^6, but only about 10^3 organisms are present in the body. In contrast, the risk of selecting out INH-resistant organisms would be unacceptably high in patients with cavitary TB. One can guard against selecting out these INH-resistant mutants by adding another drug, such as rifampin (RIF). The rates for multiple drug mutations occur as an additive function of the individual rates; only 1 in 10^{13} (INH rate of 10^6 + RIF rate of 10^7) organisms would be resistant to both drugs by natural mutation. Since this number is larger than the number of organisms typically found in a cavitary lesion, it is unlikely that many such organisms are present. Therefore, combination chemotherapy is the rule for treating active TB disease; and the patient should be on at least two drugs to which the isolate is susceptible. Rifampin and INH are the antimycobacterial agents most capable of preventing resistance, followed by ethambutol, streptomycin, and pyrazinamide (PZA).[37,47]

Three subpopulations of mycobacteria are proposed to exist within the body, each of which may be best eliminated with certain antimycobacterial agents.[15,37,47] Most numerous (possibly 10^7 to 10^9 organisms) are the extracellular, rapidly dividing bacteria, often within cavities. These are inhibited or killed most readily by INH, followed by RIF, streptomycin, and the other antimycobacterial drugs. A second group (possibly 10^5–10^7 organisms) is comprised of those organisms residing within caseating granulomas; these organisms are usually in a semi-dormant metabolic state but on occasion will increase their activity for short periods of time. It is believed that PZA, through its conversion to pyrazinoic acid in the region of the granuloma, is active against such organisms. Rifampin and INH are also likely to be active against this subpopulation. The final subset is the intracellular mycobacteria present within macrophages (10^4 to 10^6). Debate continues regarding the percentage of such cells that produce an acidic environment, since *M. tuberculosis* appears to block the normal fusion and acidification of the phagosomes with the lysosomes. Rifampin, INH, PZA, and the quinolones are believed to be most active against intracellular *M. tuberculosis.* While these theories appear to explain what happens during the treatment of TB, there is no practical way to quantitate these populations in any given patient.

NONPHARMACOLOGIC THERAPY

These interventions focus on several themes: (1) prevention of the spread of the disease, (2) contact investigation (finding where TB has already spread), and (3) replenishing the weakened (consumptive) patient to a state of normal weight and well-being. The first two are the purview of the public health department. Pharmacists involved in the treatment of TB should verify that the local health department has been notified of a new case of TB. While it is often assumed that the physician or laboratory has already done this, studies have repeatedly shown that up to 37% of cases are not properly reported.[4] Workers in hospitals and other institutions must be very conscious of the potential for spreading TB within their facilities, and appropriate steps need to be taken to prevent this.[8,9] Pharmacists caring for TB patients should learn and follow the institution's infection control guidelines. Debilitated TB patients may require therapy for multiple medical problems, including substance abuse and HIV infection, and some may desperately need nutritional reconstitution. Therefore, pharmacists involved in substance abuse rehabilitation and nutritional support services should become familiar with the particular needs of TB patients.

Other nonpharamacologic interventions include surgery for advanced cases of pulmonary disease, tuberculomas, and certain extrapulmonary lesions. Vaccines against TB include BCG (discussed later) and *M. vaccae.* The latter is an experimental treatment designed to shift the immune response toward the more effective and less destructive Th-1 response. There is no vaccine, however, that can prevent infection by *M. tuberculosis,* which is what is truly needed.

PHARMACOLOGIC THERAPY

Most importantly, the treatment of active TB involves multiple drugs. There are two primary antituberculosis drugs: INH and RIF, with the rest of the drugs playing specific roles. Isoniazid and RIF should be used together whenever possible. Tables 102–4 and 102–5 list these and other drugs by their primary targets: drugs that work primarily against the mycobacterial cell wall and those that work primarily against intracellular targets.[1] It is clear from these data that INH and RIF are much more potent than the other drugs against *M. tuberculosis.* Depending on the dosing strategy, the aminoglycosides (as shown by streptomycin, but including kanamycin and amikacin) can display considerable activity versus *M. tuberculosis.* The remaining drugs are considerably weaker, and their use requires much longer durations of treatment. These parameter estimates are based on published minimum inhibitory concentrations (MIC) and pharmacokinetic data. Using the midpoint of the proposed normal ranges for the maximum serum concentration (Cmax) and typical first-order elimination half-lives, the pharmacodynamic parameters Cmax:MIC ratio, AUC > MIC, and time > MIC were derived.[1] The use of higher doses of the TB drugs to treat moderately resistant organisms has not been systematically studied. Typically, *M. tuberculosis* is either very susceptible or very resistant to a given drug. This contrasts with *M. avium,* where moderately resistant organisms are a frequent occurrence. Theoretically, MIC results could be used to guide dosing in the treatment of moderately resistant *M. tuberculosis,* but this remains to be prospectively studied.[1]

TABLE 102–4. Potency of Antimycobacterial Drugs That Act Primarily Against the Cell Wall

Drug	Cmax:MIC	t > MIC	AUC > MIC
Cycloserine	3.8	22.5	195.5
Ethambutol 25 mg/kg	10.0	13.0	23.4
Ethionamide	1.6	1.5	1.0
Isoniazid			
(f)	40.0	9.0	11.6
(s)	40.0	18.0	19.2
Thiacetazone	1.3	5.5	1.2

AUC = area under the serum concentration time curve; Cmax = maximum serum concentration; f = fast acetylator; MIC = minimum inhibitory concentration; s = slow acetylator; t > MIC = time serum concentrations remain above the MIC.

From Ref. 1, with permission.

DRUG TREATMENTS OF FIRST CHOICE AND ALTERNATIVE TREATMENTS

Treating Latent Infection

The treatment of latent infection can reduce the risk that a patient will progress to active disease. This is not only good for the patient in question, but also prevents additional cases of TB that might have occurred had the patient developed active disease. This early intervention is called prophylaxis, chemoprophylaxis,

TABLE 102–5. Potency of Antimycobacterial Drugs That Act Primarily Against Intracellular Targets

Drug	Cmax:MIC	t > MIC	AUC > MIC
Rifampin	24.0	9.0	39.9
Streptomycin			
(h)	18.8	11.0	274.6
(c)	10.0	8.0	124.5
Aminosalicylate[a]	75.0	4.0	153.7
Ciprofloxacin	5.0	10.5	16.9
Ofloxacin	5.0	15.5	47.4

AUC = area under the serum concentration time curve; c = 12 to 15 mg/kg IV five times per week; Cmax = maximum serum concentration; h = 22 to 25 mg/kg three times per week; MIC = minimum inhibitory concentration; t > MIC = time serum concentrations remain above the MIC.

[a]Despite the high Cmax:MIC ratio, aminosalicylate is known to be a relatively weak agent versus TB. Its mechanism of action is poorly understood but is primarily bacteriostatic. Aminocalicylate may be misclassified as an intracellular agent.

From Ref. 1, with permission.

or preventive treatment, although referring to it as treatment of infection prior to disease development is most accurate. Individuals who qualify for chemoprophylaxis and the appropriate drug regimens are listed in Table 102–6. In particular, children less than 5 years old or HIV-positive patients with recent exposures to infectious cases of TB should be evaluated for active disease. Once this is ruled out, they should be given preventive treatment.[1,22,23,39] In young children, therapy should be continued for 3 months after contact with the source case is broken.[23] If the repeat skin test is negative at that time, treatment can be stopped. Otherwise, treatment for children should be continued for a total of 9 months.[23] Preventive treatment for HIV-positive patients may be continued for 9–12 months.[48]

Isoniazid-preventive therapy (typically given as 300 mg daily to an adult) is the primary treatment for TB infection in the United States.[1] This is effective in about 69% of patients, but it approaches 93% effective when patients adhere to a 52-week regimen.[1,39,49–51] The keys to success are (1) infection caused by an INH-susceptible isolate, (2) adherence to the INH regimen for 6 to 12 months, and (3) a low risk of exogenous reinfection.[1] The 52-week regimens are somewhat more effective than the 24-week regimens (75% versus 65% for all patients, and 93% versus 69% for patients who take more than 80% of the prescribed regimen), but it is difficult to persuade patients to take a medication 3 to 6 months longer than the source patient with active disease.[1,49] Isoniazid doses of 5 to 10 mg/kg of body weight, up to 300 mg per day, are used (Table 102–7).[52] Doses lower than this were found to be less effective.[1,49] Whenever possible, these drugs should be given on an empty stomach, and antacids should be avoided within 2 hours of dosing.

When the isolate from the presumed source case is resistant to INH alone, RIF has been the primary alternative drug.[1,48,49] There are insufficient data, however, with which to assess the efficacy of this approach. Concern has also been expressed over the possibility of selecting for RIF resistance in previously INH-resistant organisms. This seems unlikely and has not been proven to occur in humans. A more conservative approach would be to add another drug, such as PZA or ethambutol (EMB) to the regimen. Of course, this also increases the risk of drug-induced adverse effects. Short course chemoprophylaxis is under study: 3 months of daily RIF (or rifabutin [RBN]) or 2 months of RIF/PZA or RBN/PZA may emerge as viable alternatives.[48]

When the isolate from the presumed source case is resistant to INH and RIF (MDR-TB), there is no alternative regimen proven to be effective.[1] Based on the known or likely susceptibility pattern of the infecting organism, regimens of PZA plus EMB or EMB plus a fluoroquinolone (ciprofloxacin, ofloxacin, levofloxacin, or sparfloxacin), or EMB and a fluoroquinolone have been proposed.[1,39] Since none of these agents are as potent as INH or RIF, it is not known how effective such regimens may be.

Some physicians are hesitant to treat asymptomatic patients, even with positive skin tests, for fear of toxicity caused by INH. It has been documented repeatedly that the risk of infection outweighs the risk for drug toxicity in patients eligible for treatment. In fact, reports suggest that this may even be the case in elderly patients and patients at lower risk for developing TB.[53]

Patients treated with INH may receive pyridoxine (vitamin B_6) 10 to 50 mg daily to reduce the incidence of CNS effects or peripheral neuropathies. Pregnant women, alcoholics, and others with poor diets definitely should receive B_6.

All patients who receive chemoprophylaxis should be monitored monthly for improvement or worsening of symptoms. Any worsening of the clinical condition should prompt a chest radiograph and sputum analysis for AFB.

Treating Active Disease

If available, the drug susceptibility pattern of the source case's isolate should guide the initial drug selection for the new patient.[1] If the source case cannot be identified, the drug resistance pattern in the area where the patient is likely to have acquired TB must be taken into account.[1] If the patient is being evaluated for the retreatment of TB, it is imperative to know what drugs were used previously and for how long.[1] At the National Jewish Medical and Research Center, the patient's drug history calendar is known as a Drug-O-Gram, which shows the start and stop dates of all antimycobacterial drugs on a horizontal bar graph.[1,54] The failure to reconstruct the drug history carefully can seriously compromise any effort at retreatment. Finally, appropriate samples should be sent for culture and susceptibility testing prior to initiating therapy.[1]

It is possible to cure selected cases of TB with just 9 months of INH and RIF treatment. The addition of 2 months of PZA shortens the duration of treatment to 6 months for patients with drug-susceptible TB. Table 102–8[1,5] shows the recommended treatment regimens for drug-susceptible disease. Note that drugs can be given daily or intermittently. When intermittent therapy is used, DOT is essential. Missed doses during an intermittent regimen can seriously compromise the efficacy of the treatment and increase the relapse rate.

Different end points may be reached during the treatment of TB. First, the patient may convert to a negative sputum smear. When this occurs, the patient has less than 10,000 organisms per mL of sputum and is at reduced risk of spreading TB. Such patients can be removed from respiratory isolation, provided that they are careful not to cough on others. It is still advisable that they meet with others only in well-ventilated places, particularly outdoors. The combination of air dilution and ultraviolet radiation from the sun eliminates the risk of spreading TB.

Patients can be smear negative but culture positive. These patients must continue treatment because they still harbor many live organisms. Once the patients are smear and culture negative

TABLE 102–6. Antimicrobial Regimens for Treatment of Tuberculosis Infection in Asymptomatic Patients

Patient Type and Situation	Drug and Regimen
Child with documented recent exposure to an index case of pulmonary tuberculosis	Skin test and INH for 3 months; continue for 12 months if skin test positive
Adult with "positive" PPD skin test and no other confounding factors	INH for 6 months
HIV-infected patient with "positive" PPD skin test or anergic with risk factors for tuberculosis	INH for 9 months, RBN/PZA for 2 months
Positive skin test and documented exposure to INH-resistant TB	RIF for 6 months or RIF/PZA for 2 months
Positive skin test and documented exposure to INH- and rifampin-resistant TB	PZA/ofloxacin for 12 months, EMB/PZA or EMB/levofloxacin for 6 to 12 months

HIV = human immunodeficiency virus; INH = isoniazid; PPD = purified protein derivative; PZA = pyrazinamide; TB = tuberculosis; RIF = rifampin; RBN = rifabutin; and EMB = ethambutol.

TABLE 102–7. Dosing Information

Drug	Route and Frequency	Adult Daily	Adult 2 × Weekly	Pediatric Daily	Pediatric 2 × Weekly	Dose: Renal Failure	CSF Penetration
Amikacin (AK)	IM, IV QD	12–15 mg/kg	25–30 mg/kg[a]	12–15 mg/kg 15–30 mg/kg[a]	(Presumably as adults)	12–15 mg/kg 3 × weekly	20%–40% est.
Aminosalicylic acid (PAS)	Oral, [IV[b]] BID or TID	4 g/dose 8–12 g total 150 mg/kg[a]	Not known divided tid	150 mg/kg[a]	Not known	Unknown; avoid if possible	10%–50%
Capreomycin (CM)	IM, IV QD	12–15 mg/kg	Not known	12–15 mg/kg 15–30 mg/kg[a]	Not known	12–15 mg/kg 3 × weekly	20%–40% est.
Ciprofloxacin (CIPRO)	Oral QD	750–1000 mg	Not known	Not known 8–10 mg/kg?	Not known	Unchanged unless severe	4%–10%
Clofazimine[d] (CFZ)	Oral QD	100–200 mg	Not known	Not known 2–3 mg/kg?	Not known	Unchanged	Not known, est. poor
Cycloserine[e] (CSN)	Oral QD or BID	250–500 mg/dose 750–1000 mg total	Not known	15–20 mg/kg[a]	Not known	250–500 mg 3 × weekly	50%–80%
Ethambutol (EMB)	Oral, [IV[b]] QD	25 mg/kg (2 mo) then 15 mg/Kg	50 mg/kg	25 mg/kg (2 mo) then 15 mg/kg	50 mg/kg	15–25 mg/kg 3 × weekly	5%–65% est.; variable, inflammation
Ethionamide[e] (ETA)	Oral QD or BID	250–500 mg/dose 750–1000 mg total	Not known	15–20 mg/kg	Not known	Unchanged	20%–100% est.
Isoniazid (INH)	Oral, IM, IV[c] QD	300 mg (5 mg/kg)	15 mg/kg 900 mg max[a]	10–20 mg/kg 300 mg max[a]	20–40 mg/kg 900 mg max[a]	Unchanged or reduced to QOD	20%–100%
Kanamycin (KM)	IM, IV QD	12–15 mg/kg	25–30 mg/kg[a]	12–15 mg/kg 15–30 mg/kg[a]	(Presumably as adults)	12–15 mg/kg 3 × weekly	20%–40% est.
Levofloxacin (LEVO)	Oral QD	750–1000 mg	Not known	Not known, 8–10 mg/kg	Not known	~800 mg 3 × weekly	30%–90%
Pyrazinamide (PZA)	Oral QD or BID	15–30 mg/kg 2 g max[a]	35–70 mg/kg 4 g max[a]	15–30 mg/kg, 2 g max[a]	35–70 mg/kg 4 g max[a]	15–30 mg/kg 3 × weekly	50%–100%
Rifabutin (RBN)	Oral QD	300–450 mg	300–450 mg proposed	5–10 mg/kg proposed	Not known	Unchanged in most patients	30%–70%
Rifampin (RIF)	Oral, IV QD	450–600 mg (10 mg/kg)	450–600 mg (10 mg/kg)	10–20 mg/kg 600 mg max[a]	10–20 mg/kg 600 mg max[a]	Unchanged in most patients	5%–20% est.; variable, inflammation
Streptomycin (SM)	IM, IV[c] QD	12–15 mg/kg	25–30 mg/kg[a]	12–15 mg/kg 20–40 mg/kg[a]	25–30 mg/kg[a]	12–15 mg/kg 3 × weekly	20%–40% est.
Thiacetazone (TB-1)	[Oral[b]] QD	150 mg	Not known	2–5 mg/kg proposed	Not known	Not known; avoid if possible	Not known

[a]ATS/CDC 1994 guidelines, which may differ from practice at National Jewish Center.
[b]Available outside of United States; may be imported under IND, an investigational new drug application.
[c]IV route of administration not FDA approved.
[d]Various intermittent clofazimine regimens have been proposed for leprosy, but not MTB or MAC.
[e]Introduce gradually over several days.
CSF = cerebrospinal fluid; est. = estimated; FDA = Food and Drug Administration; MTB = mycobacterium tuberculosis; MAC = mycobacterium avium complex; ATS = American Thoracic Society; CDC = Centers for Disease Control and Prevention.

TABLE 102–8. Regimen Options for the Initial Treatment of Active Tuberculosis Among Children and Adults

TB Without HIV Infection			
Option 1	*Option 2*	*Option 3*	TB With HIV Infection
Administer daily INH, RIF, and pyrazinamide for 8 wk followed by 16 wk of INH and RIF daily or two to three times/wk[a] in areas where the INH resistance rate is not documented to be < 4%. Ethambutol or streptomycin should be added to the initial regimen until susceptibility to INH and RIF is demonstrated. Continue treatment for at least 6 mo and 3 mo beyond culture conversion. Consult a TB medical expert if the patient is symptomatic or smear or culture positive after 3 mo.	Administer daily INH, RIF, pyrazinamide, and streptomycin or ethambutol for 2 wk followed by two times/wk[a] administration of the same drugs for 6 wk (by DOT), and subsequently, with two times/wk administration of INH and RIF for 16 wk (by DOT). Consult a TB medical expert if the patient is symptomatic or smear or culture positive after 3 mo.	Treat by DOT, three times/wk[a] with INH, RIF, pyrazinamide, and ethambutol or streptomycin for 6 mo.[b] Consult a TB medical expert if the patient is symptomatic or smear or culture positive after 3 mo.	Options 1, 2, or 3 can be used, but treatment regimens should continue for a total of 9 mo and at least 6 mo beyond culture conversion.

DOT = directly observed therapy; HIV = human immunodeficiency virus; INH, = isoniazid; RIF = rifampin; TB = tuberculosis.
[a]All regimens administered two times/wk or three times/wk should be monitored by DOT for the duration of therapy.
[b]The strongest evidence from clinical trials is the effectiveness of all four drugs administered for the full 6 mo. There is weaker evidence that streptomycin can be discontinued after 4 mo if the isolate is susceptible to all drugs. The evidence for stopping pyrazinamide before the end of 6 mo is equivocal for the three times/wk regimen, and there is no evidence on the effectiveness of this regimen with ethambutol for less than the full 6 mo.
From Ref. 1, with permission.

consistently, they are on their way to cure. Occasionally, patients will have isolated positive smears or cultures. Tuberculosis patients with positive smears and negative cultures typically have dead organisms in their samples, indicating effective chemotherapy. They may be releasing organisms that were contained in a previously closed cavity. Provided that subsequent smears and cultures remain negative, such patients can complete standard or slightly prolonged treatment courses.

With rare exceptions, patients must complete 6 months or more of treatment. It has been argued that HIV-positive patients should be treated for an additional 3 months and for at least 6 months from the time that they convert to smear and culture negativity.[1,5] When INH and RIF cannot be used, treatment durations become 2 years or more, regardless of immune status.

Ethambutol or streptomycin (SM) are typically added to INH, RIF, and PZA at the start of treatment until susceptibility information is available.[1,5,39,55] This provides a good regimen in the event of INH resistance and at least avoids monotherapy in the event of initial INH and RIF resistance. Adjustments to the original regimen can be made once the susceptibility data is available.[1,55] Specifically, if the organism is drug-susceptible, a regimen of INH and RIF for 6 months, supplemented by 2 months of PZA initially, can be used in immunocompetent patients. If the organism is drug-resistant, careful consideration of the remaining therapeutic options must be made. The aim is to introduce two *or more* active agents that the patient has not received previously. Should any doubt exist as to the correct course of action, TB specialists should be consulted.[1,55]

In the case of retreatment for TB or MDR-TB, no standard regimen can be proposed.[1,55] Each patient's exposure history (known source case or geographic location where infection likely occurred), previous treatment history (including toxicity and adherence issues), and current susceptibility data must be considered simultaneously. In addition to avoiding monotherapy, it is critical to avoid adding just a single drug to a failing regimen.[1,54,55] This leads to the sequential selection of drug resistance, until there are no drugs left to give the patient. The treatment of such patients is best managed by specialists in TB. It is important to realize that it may take several months for a patient with MDR-TB to become culture negative, because the drugs typically used lack the potency of INH and RIF.[1] Therefore, prolonged respiratory isolation may be required.

Drug resistance should be suspected in the following situations:

- Patients who have received prior therapy for TB.
- Patients from geographic areas with a high prevalence of resistance (New York, Mexico, Southeast Asia).
- Patients who are homeless, institutionalized, IV drug abusers, or infected with HIV.
- Patients who still have AFB-positive sputum smears after 2 months of therapy.
- Patients who still have positive cultures after 4 months of therapy.
- Patients who require retreatment.

These patients, along with those in whom therapy is failing and those with a documented exposure to drug-resistant organisms, should be considered to be infected with resistant organisms until proven otherwise. In patients with prior treatment, therapy should be modified to include two additional drugs that have not been used previously. For empiric therapy in suspected drug-resistant TB, at least four drugs should be used (INH, RIF, PZA, EMB, or SM). These regimens may be altered when the susceptibility pattern becomes known. If the index case is known, then the same effective regimen should be employed for the new case. Again, MDR-TB cases should be referred to specialists.

SPECIAL POPULATIONS

Tuberculous Meningitis and Extrapulmonary Disease

In general, INH, PZA, ethionamide (ETA), and cycloserine (CS) penetrate the cerebrospinal fluid (CSF) readily,[56] but RIF, EMB, and SM have variable CNS penetration. Of the quinolones, levofloxacin may be preferred over ofloxacin or ciprofloxacin. Patients with CNS tuberculosis are often treated for longer periods (9 to 12 months).[22] Extrapulmonary TB of the soft tissues can be treated with conventional regimens. Tuberculosis of the bone is typically treated for 9 to 12 months, occasionally with surgical debridement.[1,5,57]

Children

Tuberculosis in children may be treated with regimens similar to those used in adults, although some physicians still prefer to extend treatment to 9 months.[22,23,37,57] Pediatric doses of INH and RIF on a milligram per kilogram basis are higher than those used in adults (see Table 102–7).[52]

Pregnancy

Women with TB should be cautioned against becoming pregnant, as the disease poses a risk to the fetus as well as to the mother. Studies that have examined the incidence of birth defects resulting from various antituberculosis drugs concluded that the risk to infants born to mothers treated with INH or ethambutol was equal to that in normal populations.[56–59] It appears that INH is relatively safe when used during pregnancy, despite its ability to cross the placenta. Supplementation with B vitamins is particularly important during pregnancy. Rifampin is not frequently associated with birth defects, but those seen are occasionally severe, including limb reduction and CNS lesions.[56] Some have proposed that RIF be reserved for cases in which the mother has more advanced disease requiring more aggressive therapy. Pyrazinamide has not been studied in pregnant women. Given the fact that it is similar to INH and ETA in size and general structure, it probably crosses the placenta readily. Data on its potential teratogenicity are not available. Reports on the use of EMB during pregnancy indicate that it is relatively safe.[56–59] Ethambutol does not appear to produce frequent physical or mental aberrations in the developing fetus, and is, therefore, preferable to many other agents.

Streptomycin has been associated with varying degrees of hearing impairment in the newborn, including complete deafness, so the use of this agent must be reserved for situations in which it is an essential component of the therapy in the mother.[56] Fortunately, it appears that the majority of infants exposed to SM in utero have no ill effects from the drug, so there is hope for a favorable outcome in those situations in which it must be used. The other aminoglycosides have also been shown to cross the placenta, presenting similar risks. Although capreomycin (CM) has not been studied, it may be anticipated to act similarly to SM.

Ethionamide may be associated with premature delivery and congenital deformities when used during pregnancy.[56] Mongolism has also been reported in the offspring of mothers who took ETA during pregnancy. Despite occasional reports of ETA's safe use during pregnancy, ETA cannot be recommended in this setting. Para-aminosalicylic acid (PAS) has been used in pregnancy, apparently without ill effect. Cycloserine is known to cross the placenta. The effect that CS may have on the developing fetus, however, is not known. Therefore, CS cannot be generally recommended during pregnancy, although it may have some future role in selected cases.[56]

Ciprofloxacin, ofloxacin, levofloxacin, and the other quinolones, although not shown to be teratogens, have been associated with permanent damage to cartilage in the weight-bearing joints of immature animals, especially dogs and rabbits.[56] While these drugs have not been shown to cause joint problems frequently in humans, other antituberculosis agents should be used during pregnancy.

Pregnant women with active TB should receive INH and RIF for a period of 9 months. If a third drug is necessary, EMB may be added. Therapy with INH for asymptomatic tuberculous infection may be delayed until after pregnancy or, if recent skin test conversion has occurred, started during the second trimester of pregnancy.[56–59] Although most antituberculosis drugs are excreted in breast milk, the amount of drug received by the infant through nursing is insufficient to cause toxicity. Quinolones should be avoided in nursing mothers if possible.

Human Immunodeficiency Virus

Patients with AIDS and other immunocompromised hosts may be managed with chemotherapeutic regimens similar to those used in immunocompetent individuals, although treatment is often extended (9 to 12 months).[1,5,33,57] Prognosis has been particularly poor for HIV-infected patients infected with MDR-TB. Differentiation must be made between infection with *M. tuberculosis* and NTM, such as *M. avium* complex, because the drugs used are different. While awaiting laboratory results, the patient can be empirically treated for TB if there is any doubt about the causative organism. Some patients with AIDS malabsorb their oral medications; this is discussed under therapeutic drug monitoring later.[1]

Renal Failure

Details regarding the excretion of the antimycobacterial drugs can be found in Table 102–7.[52] Antituberculosis drugs that rely on renal clearance for most of their elimination include the aminoglycosides (amikacin [AK], Kanamycin [KM], and SM), the polypeptide CM (and viomycin), EMB, CS, ofloxacin, and levofloxacin. Ciprofloxacin is about 50% cleared by the kidneys.[56] In addition, some of the metabolites of the antituberculosis drugs, particularly those of INH, PZA, and PAS, are cleared primarily by the kidneys. The precise role of these metabolites in the toxicity profiles of their parent compounds is largely unknown, so the danger of their accumulation in renal failure has not been determined.

Isoniazid is primarily excreted through metabolism in the liver.[56] It has been recommended that most patients receive standard doses (300 mg daily) of INH, preferably after hemodialysis. Rifampin can be given in normal daily doses to patients in renal failure after dialysis. Pyrazinamide is converted primarily to pyrazinoic acid and 5-hydroxypyrazinoic acid, which are renally eliminated. Normal doses of PZA (20 to 35 mg/kg) can be administered approximately three times per week following each dialysis session. Patients with decreased renal function may accumulate EMB, as renal elimination accounts for about 80% of the dose. A dose of 15 mg/kg three times per week after dialysis appears reasonable. It is essential that such patients have frequent examinations for visual acuity and red-green color descrimination.

Aminoglycosides and CM (and viomycin) should also be avoided in patients with end-stage renal disease, if possible; otherwise two to three doses per week should be the maximum. Ethionamide and its sulfoxide metabolite are not found in significant quantities in the urine, so dosing is generally unchanged. Para-aminosalicylic acid is converted largely to metabolites prior to renal elimination; these metabolites may accumulate in renal failure. Cycloserine is dependent on renal clearance for elimination and will accumulate in renal failure. Serum concentration monitoring must be performed to avoid dose-related toxicities in renal failure patients.[56,60] Ciprofloxacin is only partially dependent on renal clearance, so it may be the preferred quinolone in this setting.

Hepatic Failure

Antituberculosis drugs that rely on hepatic clearance for most of their elimination from the body include INH, ETA, RIF, PZA, and PAS.[56] Ciprofloxacin is about 50% cleared by the liver. Reports have indicated a decreased clearance of INH and RIF in liver disease, with moderate increases in the half-life of each agent (30%

to 100%). Specific information regarding the effects of hepatic dysfunction on the clearance of ETA are not available. One paper has been published that showed significant accumulation of PZA in icteric TB patients, with concentrations in some patients reaching 300 µg/mL. In another study, PAS pharmacokinetics were not substantially altered in patients with a variety of liver diseases. Ciprofloxacin concentrations are not substantially altered in hepatic disease. Unfortunately, elevations of serum transaminase concentrations may indicate damage to the liver, but transaminase concentrations generally are not correlated with the residual capacity of the liver to metabolize drugs. Additional consideration should be given to avoiding drugs known to produce hepatotoxicity, such as INH, RIF, PZA, and to a lesser degree, ETA, PAS, and rarely, EMB, if the risk of further liver damage outweighs the benefits of the drugs in controlling the mycobacterial infection.[56]

Morbid Obesity

Only limited information on the volume of distribution of most of the antituberculosis drugs is available, so the proper doses of these drugs in morbid obesity is still unclear.[56] Hydrophilic drugs (INH, PZA, the aminoglycosides, CM, EMB, PAS, CS), or those that typically display relatively small volumes (INH, RIF, the aminoglycosides, CM, EMB) should initially be used in doses based on ideal body weight (IBW). These drugs can be expected to remain largely in the vascular space and the extracellular fluid and not attain high concentrations in adipose tissue. Elevated serum concentrations can be avoided by initially prescribing doses of these drugs based on IBW, followed by serum concentration monitoring to confirm that effective concentrations can be maintained in the serum.

DRUG CLASS INFORMATION

This section provides summary information regarding the antimycobacterial drugs. The interested reader is also referred to several other publications that provide additional detail regarding these drugs.[1,5,15,22,37,47,49,56,57,61–71] Credit is given to these authors for providing the information that is summarized here. Please refer to the tables for specific dosing information.

Primary Antituberculosis Drugs

Isoniazid. Isoniazid is highly specific for mycobacteria, with an MIC against *M. tuberculosis* of 0.01 to 0.25 mg/mL. Most NTM are resistant to INH, although *M. kansasii* and *M. xenopi* are susceptible. The most common mechanism of resistance results from mutations in the *katG* gene, leading to the loss of catalase-peroxidase activity and the failure to produce the toxic INH derivatives.

Isoniazid is readily absorbed from the GI tract and from IM injection sites. It can also be given as a short IV infusion over 5 minutes if diluted in about 20 mL of normal saline.[72] Food and antacids may reduce isoniazid's absorption; INH should be given on an empty stomach whenever possible. Hepatic and potentially intestinal *N*-acetyltransferase form the principle metabolite, acetylisoniazid, which lacks antimycobacterial activity. The rate at which humans acetylate isoniazid is genetically determined; slow acetylation is an autosomal recessive trait and is a result of a relative *N*-acetyltranferase deficiency. Fast acetylators are heterozygous or homozygous dominants, with approximately 50% of whites and blacks and 80% to 90% of Asians and Eskimos being rapid acetylators. Slow acetylators may be at an increased risk of hepatotoxicity. The association of acetylator status and risk of hepatotoxicity from clinical trials, however, appears to be weak.

Transient elevations of the serum transaminases occur in 12% to 15% of patients, and usually occurs within the first 8 to 12 weeks of therapy. Overt hepatotoxicity, however, occurs in only 1% of cases. Risk factors for hepatotoxicity include patient age (Table 102–9), preexisting liver disease, pregnancy, and the postpartum state. Moderate consumption of alcohol is probably not a risk factor if it has not resulted in preexisting liver disease.

Isoniazid also may result in neurotoxicity, most frequently presenting as peripheral neuropathy or, in overdose, seizures and coma. Central nervous system effects, such as ataxia, mental status changes, or exacerbation of preexisting convulsive disorders, are also occasionally observed. Isoniazid appears to exert its neurotoxic effect through enhanced elimination of pyridoxine, competitive inhibition with pyridoxine in its action as a cofactor in the synthesis of synaptic neurotransmitters, or both. Patients with pyridoxine deficiency, such as alcoholics, children, and the malnourished, are at increased risk, as are patients who are slow acetylators of INH and those predisposed to neuropathy, such as diabetics. Coadministration of as little as 6 mg of pyridoxine daily will reduce the incidence of these neurotoxic effects from 20% to less than 1%. Isoniazid has been reported to inhibit the metabolism of phenytoin, carbamazepine, primidone, and warfarin. Patients who are being treated with these agents should be monitored closely, and appropriate dose adjustments should be made when necessary.

Rifampin. The introduction of RIF into routine use during the 1970s allowed for true short-course treatment of TB (6 to 9 months). Without RIF, treatment is generally 18 months or longer. Drug resistance to RIF is the one of the most ominous prognostic factors influencing the outcome of therapy, because it is frequently associated with INH resistance and leaves the patient with few good therapeutic options.

Rifampin shows bactericidal activity against *M. tuberculosis* and several other mycobacterial species, including *M. bovis* and *M. kansasii.* Other NTM, including *M. avium* complex, show variable susceptibility to RIF. Rifampin is also active against a broad array of other bacteria. Alteration of the target site on RNA polymerase, primarily through changes in the *rpoB* gene, leads to most forms of RIF resistance.

Rifampin is usually given orally, but it can also be given as a 30 minute IV infusion. Patients with AIDS, diabetes, and other GI problems appear to have difficulty absorbing RIF after oral doses, and this has been associated with therapeutic failures in some cases. Rifampin is metabolized to 25-desacetylrifampin, which retains most of RIF's activity; most of RIF and its metabolite are cleared in the bile.

Elevations in hepatic enzymes have been attributed to RIF in 10% to 15% of patients, with overt hepatotoxicity occurring in less than 1%. More frequent adverse effects of RIF include rash, fever, and GI distress. Allergic reactions to RIF have been reported and occur more frequently with intermittent RIF doses ≥ 900 mg twice weekly. These reactions may take the form of a flu-like syndrome, with development of fever, chills, headache, arthralgias, and, rarely, hypotension and shock. Alternatively, hemolytic anemia or acute renal failure may occur, requiring permanent discontinuation.

Rifampin's potent induction of hepatic enzymes, especially CYP 3A4, may enhance the elimination of many other drugs,

TABLE 102–9. Effect of Age on Incidence of Hepatitis From Isoniazid

Age (yr)	Frequency (%)
0–19	0.3–0.6
20–34	0.3–2.2
35–49	1.2–3.2
50–64	2.3–3.4
> 65	2.3–4.2

most notably the protease inhibitors used to treat HIV. Also, women who use oral contraceptives must use another form of contraception during therapy, because increased clearance of the hormones may lead to unexpected pregnancies. Patient records should be reviewed for potential drug interactions before dispensing RIF.[63] Rifampin may turn urine and other secretions orange-red and may permanently stain some types of contact lenses.

Other Rifamycins. Rifabutin (RBN), used primarily for disseminated *M. avium* infection in AIDS patients, also is quite active against *M. tuberculosis.* A very limited number of RIF-resistant organisms are susceptible to RBN, although most are resistant to all rifamycins. Because RBN is less potent an enzyme inducer than RIF, it may be considered for patients receiving protease inhibitors. Regimens that use mostly intermittent RBN (twice weekly) for TB are being investigated. Rifapentine is a very long acting rifamycin also being studied for TB.

Other First-Line Antituberculosis Drugs

After INH and RIF, all TB drugs are much weaker and, without INH and RIF, cannot effect a cure in less than 2 years. Judicious use of these drugs can, however, shorten the duration of treatment and prevent the development of drug resistance.

Pyrazinamide. Adding PZA to the first 2 months of treatment with INH and RIF shortens the duration to as little as 6 months. The drug can be used daily or intermittently, and it is used almost exclusively for TB. Pyrazinamide is well absorbed after oral doses and is largely converted to pyrazinoic acid (active metabolite) and 5-hydroxypyrazinoic acid, which are subsequently excreted renally. The most common toxicities of pyrazinamide are GI distress and elevations in the serum uric acid concentrations. Most patients are free from gouty symptoms and do not require therapy for this laboratory toxicity. Hepatotoxicity is the major limiting adverse effect, but it is far less common with current dosing regimens.

A fixed combination product (Rifater, Hoechst Marion Roussell) of RIF 120 mg, INH 50 mg, and PZA 300 mg is now available in the United States. It is designed to prevent drug resistance by keeping the self-medicating patient from using only one drug at a time. If the patient is receiving DOT, there is no particular advantage to this product. The typical daily dose of Rifater will be five to six tablets daily. When PZA is discontinued after 2 months of treatment, the combination product Rifamate (INH 150 mg and RIF 300 mg) can be substituted.

Ethambutol. Ethambutol replaced PAS as a first-line agent in the 1960s because it was better tolerated by patients. Ethambutol is used as a fourth drug for TB while awaiting susceptibility data. If the organism is susceptible to INH, RIF, and PZA, EMB can be stopped. Ethambutol is active against most mycobacteria, including *M. tuberculosis* and *M. avium,* but it is generally bacteriostatic.

Ethambutol displays adequate absorption after oral doses, but like RIF, appears to have variable absorption in patients with AIDS, diabetes, cystic fibrosis, and others with GI problems. An IV form is available in Europe and can be obtained from the U.S. manufacturer under an investigational new drug (IND) application. The EMB dose should be reduced to three times per week in patients with renal failure.[73]

Retrobulbar neuritis is the major adverse effect noted in patients treated with EMB. Incidence is dose related, with occurrence rates of 5% or more in patients receiving daily doses of > 30 mg/kg/day. Patients usually complain of a change in visual acuity, the inability to see the color green or both. They should be monitored monthly while on the drug using Snellen wall charts and Ishihara red-green discrimination cards. Ethambutol is sometimes avoided in children because of the difficulty in monitoring visual acuity in this group; however, the drug appears to be safe even in this group.[37,74] Other adverse effects that may be observed include rash, fever, arthralgias, and GI irritation.

Streptomycin. Streptomycin (SM) is one of three aminoglycoside antibiotics (along with amikacin and kanamycin) that are active against mycobacteria. Streptomycin is quite active against MAC and several other mycobacteria, *Enterococci, Brucella, Yersinia,* and various other bacteria. Streptomycin is now available only on special order from Pfizer. Like EMB, SM is used as a fourth drug for TB while awaiting susceptibility data or in cases of MDR-TB.

Although labeled only for IM dosing, SM (and capreomycin) can be safely given as IV infusions (100 mL of dextrose 5% water or normal saline) over 30 minutes, similar to the other aminoglycosides.[75] Streptomycin, like other aminoglycosides, is renally cleared by glomerular filtration and must be given less often in patients with renal dysfunction.

Streptomycin occasionally causes nephrotoxicity, although it tends to be mild and reversible. It also is capable of causing ototoxicity (vestibular and cochlear), which may become permanent with continued use. Streptomycin is said to have more ototoxicity and less nephrotoxicity than other aminoglycosides, but this largely reflects different patterns of use. Streptomycin is given daily or twice weekly (12 to 27 mg/kg) for several months, while other aminoglycosides are typically given in smaller doses every 8 to 24 hours for only 1 to 2 weeks. Toxicity profiles cannot be accurately compared from such divergent practices. Neuromuscular blockade has been reported to occur rarely with SM.

The polypeptides capreomycin and viomycin, and the aminoglycosides kanamycin and amikacin share many features with SM, and the previous discussion also pertains to them. Resistance to amikacin and kanamycin are highly linked, but they are independent of resistance to SM, which is also independent of resistance to capreomycin and viomycin. Therefore, susceptibility tests should guide the selection of these injectable drugs. Aminosidine (paromomycin) is also being studied for use against TB through an IND designed by the University of Illinois in Chicago.

Second-Line Antituberculosis Drugs

Para-aminosalicylic Acid. Para-aminosalicylic acid is a synthetic structural analog of aminobenzoic acid. In the United States, only the enteric-coated, sustained-release granule form (Paser) is available. An IV form is available in Europe; if imported under an IND, it is essential to test for the toxic breakdown product m-aminophenol before administering it to the patient. Both PAS and the acetyl derivative are renally excreted, and this drug is generally avoided in renal failure.

Gastrointestinal disturbances are the most common adverse effects from PAS. With the older dosage forms, nausea, vomiting, abdominal pain, and diarrhea were very common. The new Paser granules have offered significant relief from the nausea, vomiting and abdominal pain; however, diarrhea remains a significant problem. This diarrhea is usually self-limited, with symptoms improving after the first 1 to 2 weeks of therapy. Occasionally, a few doses of an opiod will resolve the problem. It is also important to tell the patient that the empty granules will appear in the stool.

Various types of malabsorption, including steatorrhea, were reported with previous dosage forms of PAS. Hypersensitivity may occur, and rarely, severe hepatitis. Mortality associated with PAS-induced hepatitis may be as high as 21%. Para-aminosalicylic acid may cause a positive direct Coombs' test, which may lead to hemolytic anemia in patients with glucose-6-phosphate dehydrogenase deficiency. Para-aminosalicylic and is known to produce goiter, with or without myxedema, that seems to occur more frequently with concomitant therapy with ethionamide.

Cycloserine. Cycloserine has moderate activity versus *M. tuberculosis* and selected NTMs. It possesses marginal activity against other organisms, such as *Staphylococcus aureus* and some gram-negative bacilli, such as *Escherichia coli*. Cycloserine is well absorbed orally and is best taken on an empty stomach. It is cleared primarily through the kidneys by glomerular filtration, and requires dosage reduction in renal failure. Cycloserine can produce dose-related CNS toxicity, including lethargy, confusion, or unusual behavior. Seizures, although reported, are exceedingly rare. Therapy is vastly improved by maintaining 2-hour postdose serum concentrations between 20 and 35 μg/mL.[60] Most patients reach a maximum dose of 750 mg daily, divided unevenly into two doses. This can be achieved by starting cycloserine 250 mg daily for 2 days, followed by 250 mg increments over 2-day intervals. This dose can be maintained if the patient complains of only occasional, mild CNS effects, such as difficulty concentrating. Serum concentrations can be checked 1 to 2 weeks into therapy. The addition of pyridoxine 50 mg with each 250 mg of cycloserine may improve patient tolerance of cycloserine.

Ethionamide. Ethionamide shares structural features with two other antimycobacterial agents, INH and, more distantly, thiacetazone. Prothionamide, the n-propyl derivative of ethionamide, is used in Europe. Ethionamide is only active against organisms of the genus *Mycobacterium,* and it should be considered primarily bacteriostatic, as it is difficult to achieve serum concentrations that would be bactericidal.

Gastrointestinal toxicity is the dose-limiting adverse effect. The drug should be introduced gradually in 250 mg increments, as described earlier for cycloserine. Rarely will a patient tolerate more than 1000 mg daily in divided oral doses. Ethionamide may be administered with a light snack or prior to bedtime to minimize GI intolerance. Because data are not available regarding the effect of food on the absorption of ETA, minimal amounts of simple carbohydrates should be considered if food must be given with ETA. Ethionamide suppositories, while better tolerated, produce serum concentrations only about 50% of those achieved with oral doses. Little ETA is recovered in the urine, so doses remain the same in renal failure.

Ethionamide has been associated with hepatocellular injury and, rarely, with various CNS effects, such as headache, drowsiness, giddiness, depression, psychosis, peripheral neuritis, and visual disturbances. Other adverse effects include goiter, with or without hypothyroidism (especially when given with PAS), gynecomastia, alopecia, impotence, menorraghia, photodermatitis, and acne. The management of diabetes may also be more difficult in patients receiving ETA.

Clofazimine. Clofazimine is a drug with good activity versus *M. leprae* and weak activity versus *M. tuberculosis* and *M. avium*. It is used in doses of 100 to 200 mg daily in advanced cases of MDR-TB or MAC, especially when therapeutic options are limited.[76] The drug has a terminal elimination half-life weeks long. Gastrointestinal distress and skin discoloration are the most important adverse reactions. Although uncommon, severe GI pain may occur because of deposition of clofazimine crystals within the intestines; this may require surgical correction.

Thiacetazone. Thiacetazone (TB-1) is a weak agent still used in parts of the developing world because of its low cost. Skin reactions, including rash and Stevens-Johnson syndrome, may occur; TB-1 must be permanently discontinued as soon as a rash appears. Similar to trimethoprim–sulfamethoxazole, the incidence of skin reactions is much higher in AIDS patients.[77]

Quinolones. Ofloxacin, levofloxacin, ciprofloxacin, and sparfloxacin have been used in the treatment of TB. They are bactericidal against extracellular *M. tuberculosis* and achieve good intracellular concentrations. These agents are also useful because most are available in both oral and IV dosage forms. Ofloxacin, and now levofloxacin, are generally favored over ciprofloxacin because of its higher serum concentrations in relationship to *in vitro* activity.[78,79] Levofloxacin is twice as active as ofloxacin, and it may emerge as the preferred quinolone for MDR-TB.

Levofloxacin is renally cleared, and should be given only three times weekly to patients on hemodialysis. Ciprofloxacin is both hepatically and renally cleared, and may be preferred in that situation. Adverse effects, including headache, dizziness, confusion, and caffeine-like effects, including insomnia, joint pain, GI distress, and dysuria. Limited experience suggests that these drugs may be used safely in children with MDR-TB. Sparfloxacin, while most active among quinolones in animal models, has dose-limiting adverse effects, including photosensitization and prolongation of the Q-T interval. These toxicities make this agent less attractive compared to levofloxacin or ciprofloxacin. The combination of ofloxacin and PZA has been reported to have a higher than expected incidence of toxicity when used as chemoprophylaxis in patients exposed to MDR-TB. This may be idiosyncratic, or it may represent an interaction, such as competition for renal secretion between ofloxacin and the PZA metabolites. Levofloxacin would be expected to produce the same effects.

β-Lactam and β-Lactamase Inhibitor Combinations. The β-lactams have limited activity against mycobacteria because these organisms produce β-lactamases and because β-lactams fail to enter macrophages.[80] Cefoxitin, a β-lactamase stable cephalosporin, has useful activity against rapidly growing mycobacteria, such as *M. fortuitum* and *M. chelonae*. Combinations of β-lactams with β-lactamase inhibitors have been used in salvage regimens for patients with no other options.

Macrolides/Azalides. The new macrolide, clarithromycin, and azalide, (azithromycin) represent substantial advances in the treatment of *M. avium* complex, but demonstrate limited activity against *M. tuberculosis,* and are not frequently used for TB.

New Drugs and Delivery Systems. The 5-nitroimidazoles, chemically related to metronidazole and tinidazole, and the oxazolidinones may produce useful agents for TB. Also, chemical modification of existing compounds, such as PZA or the quinolones, may produce new TB drugs. Finally, continuing research on the construction of the mycobacterial cell wall and intracellular pathways may lead to agents with unique activity against this genus.

Liposomes have been investigated as delivery systems for various agents against mycobacteria, including INH, RIF, and the aminoglycosides. Liposomes could also be used to deliver β-lactams or other agents that are generally excluded from macrophages. By changing the pharmacokinetic profile of such agents, their use in the treatment of mycobacterial infections could be greatly enhanced.

Corticosteroids. Adjunctive therapy with corticosteroids may be of benefit in some patients with tuberculous meningitis or pericarditis to relieve inflammation and pressure.[81] They should be avoided in most other circumstances, as they detract from the immune response to TB.

Bacille Calmette–Guérin Vaccine. The BCG vaccine is an attenuated, hybridized strain of *M. bovis*. It was originally developed in 1921 and is used as a prophylactic vaccine against TB. Administration of BCG vaccine is compulsory in many developing countries and is officially recommended in many others. Vaccination with BCG produces a subclinical infection resulting in sensitization of T lymphocytes and cross-immunity to *M. tuberculosis*, as well as cutaneous hypersensitivity and, in many cases, a positive tuberculin skin test.

In the published clinical trials, several different BCG preparations were used, and the efficacy of these vaccinations ranged from −56% to 80% (some patients did worse with the vaccine).[1] Trials within the United States and Puerto Rico have shown efficacy rates of 6% to 29%. The primary benefit of BCG vaccination appears to be the prevention of severe forms of TB in children. Data from the BCG trials show that the incidence of tuberculous meningitis and miliary TB is 52% to 100% lower and that the incidence of pulmonary TB is 2% to 80% lower in vaccinated children younger than 15 years of age than in it was unvaccinated controls. Unfortunately, BCG does not appear to be very reliable in preventing disease by *M. tuberculosis* in other segments of the population. Side effects occur in 1% to 10% of vaccinated persons and usually include severe or prolonged ulceration at the vaccination site, lymphadenitis, and lupus vulgaris. It is recommended that pregnant women and patients with impaired immune systems, including those with HIV infection, avoid vaccination. The World Health Organization (WHO) has recommended, however, that in populations where the risk of TB is high, HIV-infected infants who are asymptomatic should receive BCG vaccine at birth or as soon as possible thereafter. Because BCG infection has occurred in AIDS patients given the vaccine, individuals with symptomatic HIV infection should not be vaccinated.[1]

In the United States, BCG vaccination is recommended only for uninfected children who are at unavoidable risk of exposure to TB and for whom other methods of prevention and control have failed or are not feasible.[1]

PHARMACOECONOMIC CONSIDERATIONS

The WHO and the World Bank agree that the control of TB is one of the most cost-effective health interventions any nation can pursue. Early identification of TB cases and the effective use of INH, RIF, PZA (plus EMB or SM) while the isolate is still drug-susceptible should always be the primary goals of public health departments. Contact investigation and treatment of those infected but without disease are important secondary goals to reduce the number of future cases.

Patients who complete all of their treatment for drug-susceptible TB have cure rates approaching 100%. Noncompliance, drug resistance, extrapulmonary disease, and concomitant disease states reduce the overall effectiveness of chemotherapy of TB to about 75%.

The treatment of TB is not particularly expensive, especially if hospitalization is not required.[82] Further, TB is quite curable. Because the various TB drugs each have a role to play in the treatment of TB or MDR-TB, all of the FDA-approved antituberculosis drugs should be on institutional formularies. Centers that see little MDR-TB need not keep stocks of the second-line drugs, provided that they are readily available should the need arise. Because the treatment of MDR-TB is difficult and potentially disastrous, such patients should be referred to centers experienced in their management.[83,84]

EVALUATION OF THERAPEUTIC OUTCOMES

MONITORING OF THE PHARMACEUTICAL CARE PLAN

The most serious problem with TB therapy is patient nonadherence to the prescribed regimens.[85–88] Unfortunately, there is no reliable way to identify such patients a priori. In the study by Brudney and Dobkin, 89% of the patients were noncompliant with therapy.[82] It is critical to the control of TB in the United States that such adherence rates be dramatically improved. The most effective way to achieve this end is with DOT.[45,46,57] Despite criticisms that it will cost more money, it is far cheaper in the long run to prevent the further spread of disease with DOT than to track down and treat additional cases of TB continuously.

It is assumed that the homeless and other underprivileged individuals constitute the group of patients considered "unreliable" and that DOT should be reserved for them; it is also assumed that "responsible" patients cared for by private physicians may be treated with daily, unsupervised therapy. A study conducted in Baltimore, Md, however, compared outcomes (sputum culture conversion to negative at 3 months) in patients with pulmonary TB who were treated by private physicians with outcomes in patients treated via DOT in a city-run clinic. Surprisingly, 3-month culture conversion occurred in only 40% of the private-care patients, compared with 90% in the city clinic-care patients.[89] Clearly, expansion of the use of DOT to nearly all patients with TB may be of benefit.

Patients should have sputum samples sent for AFB stains every few days until smears are negative. This may take 10 to 14 days. Once smear negative, the patient may be removed from isolation and, if symptomatically improved, discharged from the hospital. Once on maintenance therapy, sputum cultures can be performed monthly until negative, which generally occurs within 2 months. If sputum cultures continue to be positive after 2 months, drug susceptibility testing should be repeated, and serum concentrations of the drugs should be checked.

Serum chemistries, including BUN, creatinine, aspartate transaminase (AST) and alanine transaminase (ALT) and a complete blood count with platelets should be performed at baseline and periodically thereafter, depending on the presence of other factors that may increase the likelihood of toxicity (advanced age, alcohol abuse, pregnancy). Hepatotoxicity should be suspected in patients whose transaminases exceed five times the upper limit of normal or whose total bilirubin exceeds 3 mg/dL. At this point, the offending agent(s) should be discontinued. Sequential reintroduction of the drugs with frequent testing of liver enzymes is frequently successful in identifying the offending agent; other agents may be continued. Alternative agents should be selected as needed. Audiometric testing should be performed at baseline and monthly in patients who must receive SM for more than 1 to 2 months. Vision testing should be performed on all patients who must receive EMB. All patients diagnosed with TB should be tested for HIV infection.

THERAPEUTIC DRUG MONITORING

Therapeutic drug monitoring (TDM) or applied pharmacokinetics is the use of serum drug concentrations to optimize therapy.[1,75,88] Non-AIDS patients with drug-susceptible TB generally do well, and TDM should only be used if they are failing appropriate DOT (no clinical improvement after 2 to 4 weeks or smear positive after 4 to 6 weeks). On the other hand, patients with AIDS, diabetes, cystic fibrosis, and various GI disorders fail to absorb these drugs properly and are candidates for TDM. Also, patients with hepatic or renal disease should be monitored, given their potential for overdoses.

In the treatment of MDR-TB, the differences between the Cmax and MIC for the second-line agents are much smaller that with INH and RIF. Therefore, alterations in the absorption of these drugs can have significant impact on the outcome of therapy.[60] Although the optimal serum concentrations for TB are not known, target serum peak concentrations have been proposed.[60] Blood collected at 2 and 6 hours postdose have been used with some success, although they may not be the optimal sampling times for all of the drugs. Long half-life drugs (PZA, CS, levofloxacin) can be sampled at 2 and 10 hours if an estimate of the half-life is desired.[60]

CONCLUSIONS

Good patient compliance is the cornerstone to effective antimycobacterial chemotherapy. Pharmacists should monitor TB therapy with particular interest in drug–drug interactions, drug malabsorption, and the error of adding a single drug to a failing regimen. They should educate patients on the importance of continuing their chemotherapy, despite symptomatic improvement. Pharmacists should become part of a multidisciplinary team (with nurses, physicians, social workers) devoted to successful chemotherapy of TB patients and their families.

▶ PRINCIPLES OF PHARMACOTHERAPY

- Tuberculosis is the most prevalent communicable infectious disease on earth.
- In the United States, TB disproportionately affects ethnic minorities as compared to whites.
- Coinfection with HIV and TB accelerates the progression of both diseases, thus requiring rapid diagnosis and treatment of both diseases.
- Mycobacteria are slow growing organisms; in the laboratory, they require special stains, special growth media, and long periods of incubation.
- Tuberculosis can produce atypical signs and symptoms in infants and immunocompromised hosts, and it can progress rapidly in these patients.
- Latent TB infection can lead to reactivation disease years after the primary infection occurred.
- The patient suspected of having active TB disease must be isolated until the diagnosis is confirmed and they are no longer contagious.
- Isoniazid and rifampin are the two most important TB drugs; organisms resistant to both of these drugs (MDR-TB) are much more difficult to treat.
- Never add a single drug to a failing regimen.
- Directly observed treatment should be used whenever possible to reduce treatment failures and the selection of drug-resistant isolates.

REFERENCES

1. Peloquin CA, Berning SE. Infections due to *Mycobacterium tuberculosis.* Ann Pharmacother 1994;28:72–84.
2. Pitchenik AE, Fertel D. Tuberculosis and nontuberculous mycobacterial disease. Med Clin N Am 1992;76:121–170.
3. Stead WW. The origin and erratic global spread of tuberculosis. Clin in Chest Med 1997;18:65–77.
4. McCray E, Weinbaum CM, Braden CR, Onorato IM. The epidemiology of tuberculosis in the United States. Clin in Chest Med 1997;18: 99–113.
5. Haas DW, Des Prez RM. *Mycobacterium tuberculosis.* In: Mandell GL, Bennett JE, Dolin R, eds. Principles and Practice of Infectious Diseases, 4th ed. New York, John Wiley, 1995:2213–2243.
6. Bloch AB, Rieder HL, Kelley GD, et al. The epidemiology of tuberculosis in the United States. Semin Respir Infect 1989;4:157–170.
7. Bentley DW. Tuberculosis in long-term care facilities. Infect Control Hosp Epidemiol 1990;11:42–46.
8. Fennelly KP. Personal respiratory protection against *Mycobacterium tuberculosis.* Clin Chest Med 1997;18:1–17.
9. Davis YM, McCray E, Simone PM. Personal respiratory protection against *Mycobacterium tuberculosis.* Clin Chest Med 1997;18:19–33.
10. Rosenblum LS, Castro KG, Dooley S, Morgan M. Effect of HIV infection and tuberculosis on hospitalizations and cost of care for young adults in the United States, 1985 to 1990. Ann Intern Med 1994;121: 786–792.
11. Small PM, Shafer RW, Hopewell PC, et al. Exogenous reinfection with multidrug-resistant *Mycobacterium tuberculosis* in patients with advanced HIV infection. N Engl J Med 1993;328:1137–1144.
12. Beck-Sague C, Dooley SW, Hutton MD, et al. Hospital outbreak of multidrug-resistant *Mycobacterium tuberculosis* infections: Factors in transmission to staff and HIV-infected patients. JAMA 1992;268: 1280–1286.
13. Centers for Disease Control. Meeting the challenge of multidrug-resistant tuberculosis: Summary of a conference. MMWR 1992;41 (RR-11):51–71.
14. Heifets L. Mycobacteriology laboratory. Clin Chest Med 1997;18: 35–53.
15. Heifets LB. Drug susceptibility tests in the management of chemotherapy of tuberculosis. In: Heifets LB, ed. Drug Susceptibility

in the Chemotherapy of Mycobacterial Infections. CRC Press, Boca Raton, FL, 1991:89–122.
16. Roberts GD, Böttger EC, Stockman L. Methods for the rapid identification of macybacterial species. Clin Lab Med 1996;16:603–615.
17. Sandin RL. Polymerase chain reaction and other amplification techniques in mycobacteriology. Clin Lab Med 1996;16:617–39.
18. Riley RL, Mills CC, Nyka W, et al. Aerial dissemination of pulmonary tuberculosis: A two-year study of contagion in a tuberculosis ward. Am J Hygiene 1959;70:185–196.
19. Orme IM, Andersen P, Boom WH. T cell response to *Mycobacterium tuberculosis.* J Infect Dis 1993;167:1481–1497.
20. Haque AK. The pathology and pathophysiology of mycobacterial infections. J Thorac Imag 1990;5:8–16.
21. American Thoracic Society. Diagnostic standards and classification of tuberculosis. Am Rev Respir Dis 1990;142:725–735.
22. Peloquin CA, Berning SE. Tuberculosis and multi-drug resistant tuberculosis in children. Pediatr Nurs 1995;21:566–572.
23. Correa AG. Unique aspects of tuberculosis in the pediatric population. Clin Chest Med 1997;18:89–98.
24. Kleinhenz ME, Ellner JJ. Antigen responsiveness during tuberculosis: Regulatory interactions of T cell subpopulations and adherent cells. J Lab Clin Med 1987;110:31–40.
25. Markowitz N, Hansen NI, Wilcosky TC, et al. Tuberculin and anergy testing in HIV-seropositive and HIV-seronegative persons. Ann Intern Med 1993;119:185–193.
26. Alland D, Kalkut GE, Moss AR, et al. Transmission of tuberculosis in New York City: An analysis of DNA fingerprinting and conventional epidemiologic methods. N Engl J Med 1994;330:1710–1716.
27. Small PM, Hopewell PC, Singh SP, et al. The epidemiology of tuberculosis in San Francisco: A population-based study using conventional and molecular methods. N Engl J Med 1994;330:1703–1709.
28. Daley CL, Small PM, Schecter GF, et al. An outbreak of tuberculosis with accelerated progression among persons infected with the human immunodeficiency virus: An analysis using restricted-fragment-length polymorphisms. N Engl J Med 1992;326:231–235.
29. Wallis RS, Vjecha M, Amir-Tahmasseb M, et al. Influence of tuberculosis on human immunodeficiency virus (HIV-1): Enhanced cytokine expression and elevated β2-microglobulin in HIV-1-associated tuberculosis. J Infect Dis 1993;167:43–48.
30. Pape JW, Jean SS, Ho JL, et al. Effect of isoniazid prophylaxis on incidence of active tuberculosis and progression of HIV infection. Lancet 1993;342:268–272.
31. Barnes PF, Bloch AB, Davidson PT, Snider DE. Tuberculosis in patients with human immunodeficiency virus infection. New Engl J Med 1991;324:1644–1650.
32. American Thoracic Society/Centers for Disease Control. Joint statement: Mycobacterioses and the acquired immunodeficiency syndrome. Am Rev Respir Dis 1987;136:492–496.
33. Cohn DL, Dobkin JF. Treatment and prevention of tuberculosis in HIV infection. AIDS 1993;7(suppl 1):S195–S202.
34. Snider DE. Recognition and elimination of tuberculosis. Adv Intern Med 1993;38:169–87.
35. Alvarez S, Shell C, Berk SL. Pulmonary tuberculosis in elderly men. Am J Med 1987;82:602–606.
36. Umeki S. Comparison of younger and elderly patients with pulmonary tuberculosis. Respiration 1989;55:75–83.
37. Starke JR. Multidrug therapy for tuberculosis in children. Pediatr Infect Dis J 1990;9:785–793.
38. American Thoracic Society/Centers for Disease Control. Joint statement: Control of tuberculosis in the United States. Am Rev Respir Dis 1992;146:1623–1633.
39 Centers for Disease Control. Management of persons exposed to multidrug-resistant tuberculosis. MMWR 1992;41:61–71.
40. Sbarbaro JA. Skin testing in the diagnosis of tuberculosis. Semin Respir Infect 1986;1:234–238.
41. Thompson NJ, Glassroth JL, Snider DE, et al. The booster phenomenon in serial tuberculin testing. Am Rev Respir Dis 1979;119:587–597.
42. Rosenberg T, Manfreda J, Hershfield ES. Two-step tuberculin testing in staff and residents of a nursing home. Am Rev Resp Dis 1993;148: 1537–1540.
43. Barnes PE, Steele MA, Young SMM, Vachon LA. Tuberculosis in patients with human immunodeficiency virus infection: How often does it mimic *Pneumocystis carinii* pneumonia? Chest 1992;102:428–432.
44. Bouza E, Diaz-Lopez MD, Moreno S, et al. *Mycobacterium tuberculosis* bacteremia in patients with and without human immunodeficiency virus infection. Arch Intern Med 1993;153:496–500.
45. Fujiwara PI, Larkin C, Frieden TR. Directly observed therapy in New York City. Clin Chest Med 1997;18:135–148.
46. Weis SE. Universal directly observed therapy. Clin Chest Med 1997; 18:155–163.
47. Mitchison DA. Basic mechanisms of chemotherapy. Chest 1979;76 (suppl):771–781.
48. Bishai WR, Chaisson RE. Short-course chemoprophylaxis for tuberculosis. Clin Chest Med1997;18:115–122.
49. Comstock GW, Woolpert SH. Prophylaxis. In: Schlossberg D, ed. Tuberculosis, second edition. Springer-Verlag, New York, 1986:55–59.
50. Comstock GW. Evaluating isoniazid preventive therapy: The need for more data. Ann Intern Med 1981;94:817–819.
51. Snider DE. Decision analysis for isoniazid preventive therapy: Take it or leave it? Am Rev Respir Dis 1988;137:2–4.
52. Peloquin CA, Iseman MD. Antimycobacterial agents. In: Root RK, ed. Clinical Infectious Diseases: A Practical Approach. Oxford University Press, New York, 1999. In press.
53. Stead WW, To T, Harrison RW, et al. Benefit–risk considerations in preventive treatment for tuberculosis in elderly persons. Ann Intern Med 1987;107:843–845.
54. Goble M. Drug-resistant tuberculosis. Semin Respir Infect 1986;1: 220–229.
55. Centers for Disease Control and Prevention. Initial therapy for tuberculosis in the era of multidrug resistance. MMWR 1993;42(RR-7): 1–8.
56. Peloquin CA. Antituberculosis drugs: Pharmacokinetics. In: Heifets LB, ed. Drug Susceptibility in the Chemotherapy of Mycobacterial Infections. CRC Press, Boca Raton, FL, 1991:59–88.
57. American Thoracic Society. Treatment of tuberculosis and tuberculosis infection in adults and children. Am J Respir Crit Care Med 1994; 149:1359–1374.
58. Hamadeh MA, Glassroth J. Tuberculosis and pregnancy. Chest 1992; 101:1114–1120.
59. Vallejo JG, Starke JR. Tuberculosis and pregnancy. Clin Chest Med 1992;13:693–707.
60. Peloquin CA. Using therapeutic drug monitoring to dose the antimycobacterial drugs. Clin Chest Med 1997;18:79–87.
61. Offe HA. Historical introduction and chemical characteristics of antituberculosis drugs. In: Bartmann K, ed. Antituberculosis Drugs. Springer-Verlag, Berlin, 1988:1–30.
62. Kucers A, Bennett N McK, eds. The Use of Antibiotics, 4th ed. JB Lippincott; Philadelphia, 1988.
63. McEvoy GK, ed. AHFS Drug Information. American Soc Health-Systems Pharmacists, Bethesda, MD, 1997.
64. Yu VL, Merigan TC, Barriere S, White NJ, eds. Antimicrobial Chemotherapy. Williams and Wilkins, Baltimore, MD, 1998.
65. Girling DJ. Adverse effects of antituberculous drugs. Drugs 1982; 23:56–74.
66. Holdiness MR. Clinical pharmacokinetics of the antituberculosis drugs. Clin Pharmacokinet 1984;9:511–544.
67. Peloquin CA. Pharmacology of the antimycobacterial drugs. Med Clin N Am 1993;77:1253–62.
68. Blanchard JS. Molecular mechanisms of drug resistance in *Mycobacterium tuberculosis.* Ann Rev Biochem 1996;65:215–239
69. Verbist L. Mode of action of antituberculous drugs: I. Medicon Intl 1974;3:11–23.
70. Verbist L. Mode of action of antituberculous drugs: II. Medicon Intl 1979;3:3–17.

71. Winder FG. Mode of action of the antimycobacterial agents and associated aspects of the molecular biology of the mycobacteria. In: Ratledge C, Stanford J, eds. The Biology of Mycobacteria: Vol 1. Physiology, Identification, and Classification. London, Academic Press, 1982:353–438.
72. Crabbe SJ. Drug infosearch—intravenous isoniazid. P&T 1990;15: 1483–1484.
73. Summers KK, Hardin TC. Treatment of tuberculosis in hemodialysis patients. J Infect Dis Pharmacother 1996;2:37–55.
74. Trébucq A. Should ethambutol be recommneded for routine treatment of tuberculosis in children? A review of the literature. Int J Tuberc Lung Dis 1997;1:12–15.
75. Peloquin CA, Berning SE. Comment: Intravenous Streptomycin. Ann Pharmacother 1993;27:1546–1547. Letter.
76. Garrelts J. Clofazimine: A review of its use in leprosy and *Mycobacterium avium* complex infection. Ann Pharmacother 1991;25: 525–531.
77. Elliott AM, Foster SD. Thiacetazone: Time to call a halt? Tubercle Lung Dis 1996;77:27–29.
78. Berning SE, Madsen L, Iseman MD, Peloquin CA. Long-term safety of ofloxacin and ciprofloxacin in the treatment of mycobacterial infections. Am J Respir Crit Care Med 1995;151:2006–2009.
79. Peloquin CA, Berning SE, Madsen L, Iseman MD. Ofloxacin and ciprofloxacin in the treatment of mycobacterial infections: Development of resistance and drug interactions. J Infect Dis Pharmacother 1995;1:45–65.
80. Zhang Y, Steingrube VA, Wallace RJ. Beta-lactamase inhibitors and the inducibility of the beta-lactamase of *Mycobacterium tuberculosis*. Am Rev Resp Dis 1992;145:657–660.
81. Kaojarern S, Supmonchai K, Phuapradit P, et al. Effect of steroids on cerebrospinal fluid penetration of antituberculous agents in tuberculous meningitis. Clin Pharmacol Ther 1991;49:6–12.
82. Reves R, Burman W, Dalton C, et al. A cost-effectiveness analysis of directly-observed therapy versus self-administered therapy for treatment of tuberculosis. Am J Resp Crit Care Med 1997;155(suppl):A33. Abstract.
83. Goble M, Iseman MD, Madsen LA, et al. Treatment of 171 patients with pulmonary tuberculosis resistant to isoniazid and rifampin. N Engl J Med 1993;328:527–532.
84. Iseman MD. Treatment of multidrug-resistant tuberculosis. N Engl J Med 1993;329:784–791.
85. Bloch AB, Cauthen GM, Onorato IM, et al. Nationwide survey of drug-resistant tuberculosis in the United States. JAMA 1994;271: 665–671.
86. Frieden TR, Sterling T, Pablos-Mendez A, et al. The emergence of drug-resistant tuberculosis in New York City. N Engl J Med 1993;328: 521–526.
87. Brudney K, Dobkin J. Resurgent tuberculosis in New York City: Human immunodeficiency virus, homelessness, and the decline of tuberculosis control programs. Am Rev Resp Dis 1991;144:745–749.
88. Mahmoudi A, Iseman MD. Pitfalls in the care of patients with tuberculosis: Common errors and their association with the acquisition of drug resistance. JAMA 1993;270:65–68.
89. Chaulk CP, Bartlett JG, Chaisson RE. 15 years of directly observed therapy for TB. Program and Abstracts, 32nd Annual Meeting, Infectious Diseases Society of America, Orlando, FL, October 7–9, 1994. Abstract 181.

103

GASTROINTESTINAL INFECTIONS AND ENTEROTOXIGENIC POISONINGS

Laura J. Odell, PharmD, and Tom A. Larson, PharmD, FCCP

Collectively, gastrointestinal (GI) infections are among the more common causes of morbidity and mortality around the world. In underdeveloped and developing countries, dehydrating diarrhea is the leading cause of death in infants and children under 5 years of age. The prevalence of diarrhea is estimated to be 3 to 5 billion cases per year and results in as many as 10 million deaths per year.[1] Developed countries, including the United States, are not isolated from diarrheal illness. Diarrhea is responsible for approximately 10% of hospitalizations in children under 5 years of age or approximately 220,000 admissions per year. Between 300 and 500 children in the United States die every year from dehydration caused by diarrhea.[2–4] These figures underscore the severity of diarrhea in children and the urgency for timely reversal of progressive dehydration.

Children are at increased risk of dying from diarrheal illness because of the high turnover of body fluid proportional to body weight, but other groups are at risk as well. These groups include travelers and campers, immunocompromised patients, such as those people with AIDS, patients in chronic care facilities, and military personnel assigned overseas. More than half of the surveyed U.S. troops during Operation Desert Shield reported at least one episode of diarrhea. Diarrhea interfered with work and resulted in a medical visit in nearly 20%.[5] The elderly are also at increased risk because of decreased immune function, achlorhydria, and colonic dysmotility.

Because of the self-limited nature of infectious diarrhea after appropriate rehydration and the economic burden of identification, the infectious agents often go unidentified. Bacteria, viruses, and protozoans account for the vast majority of infectious diarrhea. This chapter focuses on the bacterial and viral etiologies of GI infections and their treatment.

REHYDRATION THERAPY

Fluid replacement is the cornerstone of therapy for diarrhea regardless of etiology. Infection may require specific antimicrobial therapy in certain cases (Table 103–1). Initial assessment of fluid loss is essential for rehydration. Weight loss is the most reliable means of determining the extent of water loss. If the degree of weight loss is not available, clinical signs, such as changes in skin turgor, sunken eyes, dry mucous membranes, decreased tearing, decreased urine output, altered mentation, and changes in vital signs, can be helpful in determining approximate deficits[6] (Table 103–2). Physical assessment is generally more reliable in young children and infants than in adults.

Glucose-based oral rehydration therapy (ORT) is able to reverse dehydration in most cases of mild-to-moderate diarrhea.[7] Oral rehydration therapy offers the advantages of being inexpensive, noninvasive, and does not require hospitalization to administer. Glucose-based ORT generally does not decrease the duration of diarrhea or stool volume, but it does prevent dehydration, which is responsible for most diarrheal deaths.[8–10] Fluid loss greater than 10% of body water is considered severe. Intravenous (IV) fluid replacement is indicated in patients with uncontrolled vomiting, presence of an ileus, and with severe fluid deficit with toxicity.[8]

The necessary components of ORT solutions include glucose, sodium, potassium, chloride, and water (Table 103–3). Oral rehydration therapy takes advantage of glucose-coupled sodium transport in the small bowel. Glucose enhances sodium, and secondarily, water transport across intestinal walls. Glucose concentrations greater than 5% may produce an osmotic diarrhea, worsening the dehydration.[8] Glutamine has been proposed as an additive because of its function as a metabolic fuel for enterocytes.[11] Rice-based ORT has been shown to reduce stool volume by up to 45% and decrease duration of diarrhea.[10,12,13] Slow rice hydrolysis allows some rice absorption to take place before hydrolysis occurs. Therefore, a larger carbohydrate load can be given with rice solutions, resulting in a greater nutritional advantage without an increased osmotic load in the gut.[12–14] Human breast milk, cow's milk, glycine, soy fiber formulas, and cereal preparations have been used successfully as rehydration substrates.[14–17]

Sodium content should be between 50 and 90 mEq/L for initial rehydration. The American Academy of Pediatrics recommends rehydration with a more electrolyte-concentrated rehydration phase and a subsequent maintenance phase using the more dilute solutions and larger volume.[18] The rehydration phase should provide 50 to 100 mL of ORT per kilogram body weight over 4 to 6 hours. In children with vomiting and diarrhea, ORT may be given as 5 mL every 2 to 5 minutes in a teaspoon or oral syringe. Maintenance rehydration requires sodium concentrations between 40 and 60 mEq/L. Oral rehydration therapy solutions with high sodium content may be alternated with water if a low sodium fluid is not available. The maintenance phase should provide at least 150 mL/kg/d

TABLE 103–1. Antibiotic Selection

Organism	First Choice	Alternatives
Clostridium difficile	Metronidazole	Vancomycin
Campylobacter	Fluoroquinolone	Macrolide, doxycycline
Escherichia coli	TMP/SMX,[a,b] fluoroquinolone	Aminoglycoside, chloramphenicol, cephalosporin
Salmonella	Fluoroquinolone	Cephalosporin, TMP/SMX, chloramphenicol
Shigella	Fluoroquinolone	TMP/SMX, ampicillin, third-generation cephalosporin
Vibrio cholerae	Fluoroquinolone	Doxycycline, TMP/SMX
Yersinia enterocolitica	Fluoroquinolone	TMP/SMX, aminoglycoside, ceftriaxone

Dosing Guidelines[c]

Drug	*Children*	*Adults*
Amikacin (IV)	15–22.5 mg/kg/day divided every 8 h	15 mg/kg/day divided every 8–12 h
Ampicillin (IV, PO)	100–200 mg/kg/day divided every 6 h 50 mg/kg/day divided every 6 h	150–200 mg/kg/day divided every 6 h 250–500 mg every 6 h
Bacitracin (PO)	800–1200 U/kg/day divided every 8 h	25,000 units every 6 h
Cefoperazone (IV)	100–150 mg/kg/day divided every 8–12 h	4–16 g/day divided every 6–12 h
Ceftriaxone (IV)	50–100 mg/kg/day divided every 12–24 h	1–2 g/day divided every 12–24 h
Chloramphenicol (PO)	50–75 mg/kg/day divided every 6 h	50 mg/kg/dose every 6 h
Ciprofloxacin (IV, PO)	NR	200–400 mg every 12 h 500–750 mg every 12 h
Clindamycin (PO, IV)	20–30 mg/kg/day divided every 6 h 25–40 mg/kg/day divided every 6–8 h	150–450 mg every 6 h 150–900 mg every 8 h
Doxycycline (PO)	NR	100 mg every 12–24 h
Enoxacin (PO)	NR	600–800 mg/day divided every 12–24 h
Erythromycin (PO)	30–40 mg/kg/day divided every 6–8 h	250–500 mg every 6 h
Gentamicin (IV)	3–7.5 mg/kg/day divided every 8 h	3–5 mg/kg/day divided every 8 h
Lomefloxacin (PO)	NR	400 mg every 24 h
Metronidazole (PO)	15–35 mg/kg/day divided every 8 h	500 mg every 6 h
Netilmicin (IV)	3–7.5 mg/kg/day divided every 8 h	4–6.5 mg/kg/day divided every 8 h
Norfloxacin (PO)	NR	400 mg every 12 h
Ofloxacin (PO)	NR	200–400 mg every 12 h
TMP/SMX (PO)	8–12 mg/kg/day divided every 12 h	160 mg every 12 h
Tobramycin (IV)	3–6 mg/kg/day divided every 8 h	3–5 mg/kg/day divided every 8 h
Vancomycin (PO)	10–50 mg/kg/day divided every 6 h, max 125 mg per dose	125 mg every 6 h

NR = not recommended.
[a]Fluoroquinolone: ciprofloxacin, ofloxacin, lomefloxacin, enoxacin, norfloxacin (fluoroquinolones are not approved for children).
[b]TMP/SMX, trimethoprim–sulfamethoxazole.
[c]*Compiled from Refs. 26 and 31.*

TABLE 103–2. Signs of Dehydration

% Body Weight Loss as Water	Clinical Signs
Adults and Older Children	
< 4 yr (mild)	Decreased tearing, thirsty, alert, restless
4–8 yr (moderate)	Decreased skin turgor, sunken eyes, tachycardia, reduced urine flow, postural hypotension, dry mucous membranes, thirsty
> 8 yr (severe)	Hypotension, muscle cramps, variable alertness, cold, sweaty, cyanotic, wrinkled skin, usually conscious
Infants and Young Children	
< 5 yr (mild)	Thirsty, alert, restless, moist mucous membranes, normal urine flow, tearing
5–10 yr (moderate)	Thirsty, restless, lethargic, irritable, tachycardia, hypotension, deep respirations, sunken fontanel, sunken eyes, absent tearing, dry mucous membranes, reduced and dark urine
> 10 yr (severe)	Drowsy, limp, cold, sweaty, cyanotic, comatose, tachycardia, tachypnea, very sunken fontanels, hypotension, sunken eyes, absent tears, dry mucous membranes, no urine production

Adapted from Ref. 19.

TABLE 103–3. Comparison of Solutions Used in Oral Rehydration and Maintenance

	Electrolytes (mEq/L)						
Product	***Na***	***K***	***Cl***	***Base***	***Cations***	***Carbohydrate (g/L)***	***Osmolarity (mOsm/L)***
Infalyte (Penwalt)	50	20	40	30	—	20	251
Lytren (Mead Johnson)	50	25	45	30	—	20	583
Pedialyte (Ross)	45	20	35	30	—	25	388
Pedialyte RS (Ross)	75	20	65	30	—	25	314
Ricelyte (Mead Johnson)	50	25	45	34	—	30	200
WHO (Unicef)	90	20	80	30	—	20	333
Resol (Wyeth)	50	20	50	34	4 Ca, 4 mg, 5 PO_4	20	
Rehydralyte (Ross)	75	20	65	30	—	25	
EquaLYTE (Ross)	78.2	22.3	67.6	30.1	—	25	305
Less Desirable Alternatives							
Cola	0–6.5	0–4	—	13	—	100–120	390–750
Gatorade	20–24	3	17	30	—	46–58	305
Grape juice	3	31–34	—	32	—	156	1180
Jell-O (1/2 strength)	6–17	0.2	0–5	—		70–80	600
Kool-Aid	1	1	—	—	—	102	250–590
7-Up	5–7	2	—	—	—	74–102	535

Adapted from package information and Ref. 92.

plus additional replacement for stool losses. Traditional clear fluids, such as soda, apple juice, broth, and Gatorade, are hyperosmolar solutions that may draw free water into the gut lumen and cause hypernatremia. Use of these solutions should be avoided. Guidelines for parenteral fluid replacement of severe fluid loss are shown in Table 103–4.[19]

Early refeeding as tolerated is recommended.[3,6,13,19] Breast milk, soy formula, and cow's milk-based formulas can often be continued. Early initiation of feeding has shortened the course of diarrhea. Initially, easily digested foods, such as bananas, applesauce, and cereal, may be added. Foods high in fiber, sodium, and sugar should be avoided. Lactase deficiency may be exacerbated among known lactase-deficient patients and may persist up to 10 days. After starting rehydration therapy, parents should be instructed to observe the child for a reversal of the signs of dehydration, increased stool consistency, and decreased stool frequency. If ORT is not improving the fluid status and the patient continues to produce frequent large volume watery stools, close supervision with medical support is justified.[20,21]

A variety of pathogens can be responsible for acute infectious diarrhea. Viruses are the most common cause of gastroenteritis in children. Bacterial species that are commonly associated with infectious diarrhea in the United States are *Shigella* sp., *Salmonella* sp., *Campylobacter* sp., *Yersinia* sp., *Escherichia* sp., *Clostridium* sp., and *Staphylococcus* sp. Although not a major cause in North America, *Vibrio* sp. is a leading cause of bacterial gastroenteritis on a global scale.

BACTERIAL INFECTIONS

ENTEROTOXIGENIC (CHOLERA-LIKE) DIARRHEA

CHOLERA *(VIBRIO CHOLERAE)*

EPIDEMIOLOGY AND ETIOLOGY

Cholera has been endemic in the Ganges delta, West Bengal, Bangladesh, and Southern Asia (including Southeast Asia) since at least 1817. A 1994 outbreak of a multidrug resistant strain of cholera among Rwandan refugees resulted in more than 20,000 deaths.[22] In 1991, the cholera epidemic spread into Peru, and as of June 1995, the Pan American Health Organization had received reports of more than 1 million cholera cases in Latin America.[23,24] As international

TABLE 103–4. Parenteral Replacement of Fluid Deficit for Severely Dehydrated (> 10% of Body Weight) Children

		% Replaced During Noted Period		
Type of Dehydration	**Replacement Solution**	***0–12 h***	***12–24 h***	***24–48 h***
Isonatremic (130–150 mEq/L)	D5 1/3 NS	50	50	—
Hyponatremic (< 130 mEq/L)	D5 1/2 NS	75	25	—
Hypernatremic (> 150 mEq/L)	D5 1/4 NS	25	25	50

D5 = dextrose 5%; NS = normal saline (0.9% sodium chloride).
Adapted from Ref. 19.

travel increases, the occurrence of cholera in the United States is increasing as well. Cholera has been reported in all major regions of the United States since 1992.[23]

Vibrio cholerae 01 is the most common serotype associated with causing epidemics and pandemics. A new strain, *V. cholerae* 0139 Bengal, appeared in India in 1992 and spread rapidly through Southeast Asia. Four mechanisms for transmission have been proposed, including animal reservoirs, chronic carriers, asymptomatic or mild disease victims, or water reservoirs. A relatively large inoculum is required to produce clinical disease. The majority of people infected with *V. cholerae* 01 have no symptoms, and only 2% to 5% will develop severe diarrhea, which may cause death within 24 hours.

PATHOPHYSIOLOGY

Most pathology of cholera is thought to result from an enterotoxin (cholera toxin) produced by the bacteria.[1] Cholera toxin stimulates adenylate cyclase, which increases intracellular cAMP and results in increased secretion of fluids and electrolytes. The toxin likely acts along the entire intestinal tract; however, most fluid loss occurs in the duodenum. The net effect of cholera toxin is isotonic secretion (primarily in the small intestine), which exceeds the absorptive capacity of the intestinal tract (primarily the colon).

CLINICAL PRESENTATION

The average incubation period of *V. cholerae* is 1 to 3 days. The clinical presentation can vary from asymptomatic to the most severe typical cholera syndrome. In the most severe state, this disease can progress to death in 2 to 4 hours if not treated. Initial stools generally do not have the "rice water" appearance that is classically seen with cholera.

Most signs and symptoms are a direct result of fluid and electrolyte loss. These frequently include poor skin turgor, sunken eyes, cyanosis, shallow or absent pulses, tachycardia, hypotension, and tachypnea. The presentation generally correlates well with the severity of fluid loss. Fluid collection within the intestines may cause further intravascular depletion without diarrhea.

Hypokalemia is often seen in children, perhaps as a reflection of a greater potassium loss with diarrhea than seen with adults. Altered consciousness, hypoglycemia, muscle weakness and cramping, cardiac arrhythmias, and ileus may be manifestations of electrolyte losses. Other complications include acidosis, renal failure secondary to volume depletion, iatrogenic water intoxication from overrehydration, and aspiration pneumonia.

▶ TREATMENT: Enterotoxigenic Diarrhea

The mainstay of treatment for cholera consists of fluid and electrolyte replacement.[25] Meta-analyses of general studies indicate that rice-based rehydration formulations are the preferred ORT for cholera patients.[13,14] Volume loss can be dramatic, with a few patients losing a liter or more of isotonic fluid every hour. The amounts of water and salts given are dictated by those that are lost. Intravenous therapy is usually required only in severe cases when intractable vomiting prevents sufficient fluid replacement with ORT.

Antibiotics have been shown to shorten the duration of diarrhea, decrease the volume of fluid lost, and shorten the duration of the carrier state.[26] The tetracyclines or fluoroquinolones are considered drugs of choice.[27] When the tetracyclines are not available or desirable, as in pregnancy or young children, trimethoprim–sulfamethoxazole (TMP/SMX) is an appropriate alternative.[6] Other agents, such as chloramphenicol and furazolidone, have also been effective. The new strain, *V. cholerae* 0139, is resistant to furazolidone and TMP/SMX, so a fluoroquinolone becomes the drug of choice.[28] Increasing multiple antibiotic resistance dictates regional antibiotic selection. Antibiotics need only be given for 3 to 5 days in most cases. The available vaccine is an inactivated suspension of *V. cholerae*. Newer vaccines using purified cholera toxin or live attenuated, recombinant strains have been well tolerated and highly immunogenic.[29,30] The World Health Organization (WHO) does not require vaccination for international travel to or from endemic areas since the series of two injections is effective in only 50% of people and immunity wanes in 6 months or less. Common side effects of the cholera vaccine include fever, myalgias, fatigue, and pain at the site of injection.

ESCHERICHIA COLI

EPIDEMIOLOGY AND ETIOLOGY

Escherichia coli is a gram-negative bacillus commonly found in the human GI tract.[31] It is divided into five groups based on mechanisms of diarrheal disease and toxin production: enterotoxigenic *E. coli* (ETEC), enteroinvasive *E. coli* (EIEC), enteropathogenic *E. coli* (EPEC), enteroadhesive *E. coli* (EAEC), and enterohemorrhagic *E. coli* (EHEC).

The most common group is ETEC, which accounts for about half of all cases of *E. coli* diarrhea.[32] Enterotoxigenic *E. coli* is incriminated as being the most common cause of traveler's diarrhea and a common cause of food- and water-associated outbreaks.[1,25] Recently recognized as a common and potentially deadly cause of infectious diarrhea, EHEC can progress into hemolytic uremic syndrome (HUS), which is potentially fatal. In 1993, an isolate of *E. coli*, serotype 0157:H7 was associated with a major outbreak of EHEC diarrhea from undercooked hamburgers served in a fast food restaurant. More than 700 persons in four states were affected, 51 cases of HUS were reported, and four people died.[30] Reports of EHEC enteritis continue to increase.

PATHOPHYSIOLOGY

Enterotoxigenic *E. coli* are capable of producing two plasmid-mediated enterotoxins: heat-labile toxin (HLT) and heat-stable toxin (HST). A cholera-like toxin, HLT has two subunits (A and B) that have similar antigenic properties and action on the gut mucosa. The net effect of this toxin on the mucosa is production of a cholera-like secretory diarrhea. With a rapid onset of action, HST is nonantigenic, has a low molecular weight, and probably acts only on the small intestine.[33] The pathogenicity of EHEC is related to the production of cytotoxins, commonly called shiga-like toxins because of their resemblance to the shiga toxin of *Shigella dysenteriae*.[34]

CLINICAL PRESENTATION

Disease caused by ETEC is characterized by nausea and watery stools, with or without abdominal cramping. Usually, there is no blood or pus in the stool. Signs and symptoms are directly dependent on the extent of fluid loss, which in most cases is subclinical. Most ETEC diarrhea resolves within 24 to 48 hours without complication.

The first human cases of EHEC were reported in 1983 and were caused by contaminated hamburger. Symptoms can be severe, with as many as 11 to 12 bloody stools per day.[34] Cramping and severe abdominal pain are common, nausea occurs in about two-thirds of patients, and vomiting occurs in less than one-third. The white blood cell (WBC) count is elevated and accompanied by a left shift. Death may rarely occur, usually as a result of HUS and postdiarrheal thrombocytopenic purpura (TTP).[30]

▶ TREATMENT: Enterotoxigenic *Escherichia coli* Diarrhea

Most patients do not require specific therapy, although some will have loss of fluid and electrolytes requiring replacement therapy. Most cases respond readily to ORT, and, although antibiotic therapy is seldom necessary, prophylaxis has been shown to prevent the development of ETEC diarrhea effectively.[35] Effective prophylactic agents include tetracycline, TMP/SMX, neomycin, furazolidone, norfloxacin, and ciprofloxacin. Because multidrug-resistant strains of ETEC have developed, many prescribers prefer to reserve antibiotics for the treatment of symptomatic patients.[25,35] Nonantibiotic regimens, including bismuth subsalicylate and cholestyramine, have been recommended as effective prevention or treatment regimens.[36,37] Antibiotic therapy in EHEC diarrhea is controversial and may increase the risk of HUS. Antimotility agents are contraindicated in EHEC and in severe invasive diarrhea.[32]

TRAVELER'S DIARRHEA

Traveler's diarrhea is defined as three or more loose stools per day or any number of loose stools accompanied by abdominal cramping, fever, or vomiting in people traveling to developing countries.[38] Traveler's diarrhea often occurs during the first week of travel and usually resolves in 2 to 3 days. It is rarely life-threatening but is often an inconvenience. Approximately 20% of patients will be bedridden by the illness. Travel destinations are divided into high-, intermediate-, and low-risk areas. High-risk areas include Latin America, Africa, Asia, the Middle East, and some areas of the Caribbean.[38–40] The most common causes of traveler's diarrhea are ETEC, salmonella, and shigella. Other common causes are listed in Table 103–5.

TABLE 103–5. Traveler's Diarrhea

Likely pathogens	ETEC, *Salmonella, Shigella, Campylobacter, Yersinia,* viruses
High-risk areas	Latin America, Africa, Asia, Middle East, some areas of Caribbean
Patients at risk	Patients with achlorhydria, AIDS, secretory IgA deficiency, insulin-dependent diabetes, patients using diuretics
Prevention	Boil water, diarrhea travel kit, antibiotics in high-risk patients, bismuth subsalicylate
Treatment	Fluid replacement, fluoroquinolone, TMP/SMX in Central Mexico, loperamide, bismuth subsalicylate

AIDS = acquired immunodeficiency virus; ETEC = enterotoxigenic *E. coli*; IgA = immunoglobulin A; TMP/SMX = trimethoprim–sulfumethoxazole.
Compiled from Refs. 39 and 40.

Prevention and patient education are important. Although many travelers avoid drinking water, the major source of infection appears to be food. Patients should be educated on the "peel it, boil it, cook it, or forget it" approach to selecting foods for consumption. Education on water filtration devices and the "diarrhea travel kit" is also recommended. The travel kit should contain toilet paper, a thermometer, loperamide, 3 to 5 days of antibiotics, oral rehydration solution salts, and a water purification method.

Treatment may include dietary and fluid modifications, antimotility agents, prophylaxis agents, and antimicrobials. Because most cases of traveler's diarrhea are short lasting and self-limited, oral rehydration solutions are generally not required in otherwise healthy individuals. Flavored mineral water contains glucose and sodium and can be used in mild-to-moderate cases. Clear liquids plus salted crackers can also be used.

Loperamide and bismuth subsalicylate are effective in traveler's diarrhea. Loperamide has been shown to be more effective than bismuth in terms of quicker onset and longer relief of diarrhea. Loperamide should be used with caution in cases of bloody diarrhea or temperature > 38°C.

Ericsson and Dupont presented a discussion of pros and cons of antibiotic prophylaxis.[37] They recommended the use of antibiotics in the following situations:

1. Patients with underlying illness who would likely suffer consequences from even short-term illness (insulin-dependent diabetics, patients on diuretics, people with chronic GI disorders).

2. Situations where short-term illness could ruin the purpose of the trip.
3. Patients who are unable or unwilling to comply with dietary restrictions.

Cons of prophylaxis may include a false sense of security, the cost of prophylactic therapy, side effects of the medication, and risk of emergence of resistant strains of bacteria.

Antimicrobial treatment of diarrhea should be started with onset of symptoms. Antibiotics can shorten the duration of diarrhea from 59 to 93 hours to 16 to 30 hours. Fluoroquinolones are the drugs of choice because of increasing resistance to TMP/SMX. In central Mexico, TMP/SMX is still effective and is the drug of choice for travelers to that area. Antibiotics should be continued for 3 to 5 days. Antibiotics may be used in combination with loperamide in afebrile patients without bloody diarrhea. Bismuth subsalicylate may be preferred in patients with severe vomiting. Metronidazole should be used in patients with diarrhea lasting more than 14 days to treat possible giardiasis or small bowel bacterial overgrowth.[41]

PSEUDOMEMBRANOUS COLITIS (*CLOSTRIDIUM DIFFICILE*)

Pseudomembranous colitis (PMC) was first reported in 1893 and was first associated with antibiotic therapy in 1955. Although described in the preantibiotic era, the incidence has increasingly been associated with antibiotic administration. *Clostridium difficile* is the major cause of antibiotic-associated PMC.[42]

Epidemiology and Etiology

Clostridium difficile is a gram-positive spore-forming anaerobic bacillus. The incidence of intestinal colonization is variable, ranging from 30% to 70% in infants to 3% to 5% in healthy adults.[43,44] *Clostridium difficile* may be found in greater than 10% of hospitalized adults who have received broad-spectrum antibiotics. The relationship between the colonized state and active disease is poorly understood. Many people are colonized with the bacteria yet do not go on to develop PMC.

The exact incidence of PMC within the United States is not known. It occurs most often in high-risk groups, such as the elderly, debilitated patients, cancer patients, surgical patients, or any patient receiving antibiotics. Pseudomembranous colitis has been associated with use of broad-spectrum antimicrobials, including clindamycin, ampicillin, or cephalosporins. Other agents that have been implicated include aminoglycosides, erythromycin, fluoroquinolones, TMP/SMX, and suprisingly, vancomycin and metronidazole, two of the most commonly used antimicrobials for treatment of *C. difficile*.

Pathophysiology

Clostridium difficile colitis is a toxin-mediated disease. Two toxins (A and B) have been described. Toxin A is the major pathogenic factor and has been characterized as an enterotoxin that causes disease through actin disaggregation, intracellular calcium release, and damaging neurons.[43] Toxin B is a nonenterotoxic cytotoxin that causes depolymerization of filamentous actin. The toxins appear to act on mucosal membranes, causing necrosis, inflammation, increased peristalsis, and loss of fluid and electrolytes.

Clinical Presentation

Pseudomembranous colitis is characterized by vomiting, fever, cramping, abdominal pain and tenderness, and profuse greenish diarrhea either during or after antibiotic therapy. Fevers and marked leukocytosis can also occur. Symptoms can start a few days after the start of antibiotic therapy or several weeks after antibiotics have been discontinued. The onset of illness is often abrupt.

The diagnosis of PMC should be suspected in patients with diarrhea who have received antibiotics within the previous 2 months or whose diarrhea began 72 hours or more after hospitalization. Diagnosis can be made in several ways, including endoscopy, demonstration in stool samples of toxin A or B, and stool culture for *C. difficile*.[45] The American College of Gastroenterology published guidelines for diagnosis and treatment of *C. difficile*-associated diarrhea.[46] They recommend that endoscopy be reserved for situations when rapid diagnosis is needed, ileus is present, and a stool is not available, or when other colonic diseases are in the differential.

▶ TREATMENT: Pseudomembranous Colitis

As with all types of diarrhea, supportive care is of primary concern. Fluid and electrolyte losses may be significant. The offending antibiotic should be discontinued if possible or switched to an alternate antibiotic. Antibiotic therapy should be initiated when the diagnosis of *C. difficile* is confirmed or if *C. difficile* is highly likely and the patient is seriously ill or has not responded to 48 to 72 hours of supportive therapy.

The American College of Gastroenterology recommends the use of oral metronidazole as the preferred agent for therapy of PMC in most instances.[46] Metronidazole 250 to 500 mg four times daily for 10 days has been shown to be as effective as vancomycin 500 mg four times daily in terms of duration of diarrhea, frequency of side effects, and post-treatment relapses. Metronidazole can be given intravenously in patients who are unable to take it orally, but treatment failures have occurred. Side effects may include metallic taste, nausea, vomiting, diarrhea, headache, and confusion. Patients should be cautioned against drinking alcohol while taking metronidazole because of the potential for disulfiram-like reactions.

Vancomycin was traditionally considered the gold standard for treatment of PMC. Its use has fallen out of favor partly as a result of concern that overuse will encourage the spread of vanomycin-resistant enterococcus and because metronidazole has been shown to be as effective and less expensive for most patients. Vancomycin 125 to 500 mg orally four times daily is reserved for therapy until one or more of the following conditions are met:

1. Patient has not responded to oral metronidazole.
2. Organism is resistant to metronidazole.
3. Patient is allergic to metronidazole, is unable to tolerate it, or is being treated with ethanol containing solutions.
4. Patient is either pregnant or is under 10 years of age.
5. Patient is critically ill because of *C. difficile* diarrhea or colitis.
6. There is evidence suggesting that the diarrhea is caused by *Staphylococcus aureus.*

Vancomycin should not be given intravenously as the only treatment for *C. difficile* because effective concentrations in the colonic lumen are not achieved.

Relapse after antibiotic treatment occurs in about 15% to 35% of patients and does not appear to be influenced by whether metronidazole or vancomycin was used for treatment or by the dose or duration of treatment of the initial episode.[45-47] Recurrences occur because of the persistence of the spore forms of *C. difficile* which are not killed by antibiotic therapy or reinfection by a new strain. Recurrences usually occur 2 weeks to 2 months after antibiotics are stopped. Retreatment with metronidazole or vancomycin is often successful. Some investigators have found prophylaxis with competing, nonpathogenic organisms, such as *Lactobacillus* sp. or *Saccharomyces* sp., to be helpful in preventing relapse in small numbers of patients.[45,48] It is thought that these organisms help to restore the natural flora in the gut and make patients more resistant to colonization by *C. difficile.*

Bacitracin has been used in doses of 500 mg four times daily for treatment of PMC. It is not recommended, however, because of its unpleasant taste and because resistant strains of *C. difficile* are not uncommon.[45-47] Anion exchange resins have been used with variable success. Cholestyramine binds *C. difficile* toxins and is a treatment option for mild cases, but it should not be used in place of antibiotic therapy in moderate-to-severe cases. Anion exchange resins may bind vancomycin; therefore, concomitant administration should be avoided, or administration of antibiotics and exchange resins should be separated by several hours.[46]

Drugs that inhibit peristalsis, such as diphenoxylate, are contraindicated in PMC. Some patients have become worse after use of these drugs. Slowing of fecal transit time is thought to result in extended toxin-associated damage.

INVASIVE (DYSENTERY-LIKE) DIARRHEA

BACILLARY DYSENTERY (SHIGELLOSIS)

EPIDEMIOLOGY AND ETIOLOGY

The shigellae are gram-negative bacilli belonging to the family Enterobacteriaceae. Four species most often associated with disease are *Shigella dysenteriae* type I, *S. flexneri, S. bovdii,* and *S. sonnei.* The shigellae have worldwide distribution, with regional differences in prevalence of subgroups responsible for disease. For example, in the United States, the common causes of shigellosis are *S. sonnei* and *S. flexneri.* Cases caused by other shigellae are most often acquired during travel to developing countries. Poor sanitation, poor personal hygiene, inadequate water supply, malnutrition, and increased population density are associated with an increased risk of shigella gastroenteritis epidemics, even in developed countries.

The majority of cases result from fecal–oral transmission. A few well-documented food- and water-associated outbreaks have been reported. Peak incidence in the United States is in late summer. An estimated 300,000 cases of shigellosis occur in the United States each year.[49]

Shigellosis is primarily a disease of children, with the highest incidence between ages 6 months and 5 years. Infection among infants is uncommon, and only one-third of all cases occur in adults.

PATHOGENESIS

Ingestion of as few as 10 to 200 viable organisms of the shigella species has been shown to cause disease in healthy adults, explaining the ease with which the disease is transmitted from person to person.[50] The bacteria multiply and spread within the submucosa, but they rarely extend beyond the mucosa. Penetration of the mucosa is coded by large "invasion plasmids" and results in distortion of the crypts, death to gastric epithelium causing focal ulceration, sloughing of mucosal cells, bloody mucoid exudate into the gut lumen, and submucosal accumulation of inflammatory cells with microabscess formation. Microabscesses may eventually coalesce, forming larger abscesses. Infection frequently involves the entire colon. Some *Shigella* sp. produce a cytotoxin, or shiga-toxin, the pathogenic role of which is unclear, although it is thought to damage endothelial cells of the lamina propria, resulting in microangiopathic changes that can progress to HUS. Watery diarrhea commonly precedes the dysentery and may be a result of these toxins.

CLINICAL PRESENTATION

Signs and symptoms are initially nonspecific: nausea, fever, malaise, lower quadrant pain, and hyperactive bowel sounds. Frequent watery stools appear within 48 hours and are followed by bloody diarrhea and dysentery within a few days. Stools are greenish in color and often contain mucus or blood, or both, as well as many leukocytes.

Fluid and electrolyte loss may be significant, particularly in infants and elderly patients. Stool culture will establish *Shigella* sp. as the causative agent. *Shigella*-specific invasion plasmids are now detectable directly from stool without cultivation by amplification of DNA by the polymerase chain reaction, allowing same day, sensitive test results.[51]

If untreated, bacillary dysentery usually lasts about 1 week (range 1 to 30 days). Complications are unusual but may include severe dehydration, generalized seizures, septicemia, toxic megacolon, perforated colon, arthritis, protein-losing enteropathy, and HUS. Mortality is rare, but it may be more likely with *S. dysenteriae* type I.

▶ TREATMENT: Shigellosis

Shigellosis is generally a self-limiting disease. Patients most often become afebrile and completely recover within 4 to 7 days. Approximately 10% experience a recurrence. Fluid and electrolyte losses can usually be replaced with oral therapy, as dysentery is not associated with significant fluid loss. Intravenous replacement is necessary only for those patients with severe illness.

Because diarrhea from shigellosis is self-limited and antibiotic resistance is increasing, some clinicians feel antibiotics should be reserved for the very young and old and those who are severely ill. Since antibiotic therapy has been shown to shorten the period of fecal shedding and attenuate the clinical illness, many clinicians prefer to treat with antibiotics. Tetracyclines, TMP/SMX, and ampicillin were at one time drugs of choice for shigellosis. With an increasing incidence of ampicillin-resistant strains in much of the world, either ciprofloxacin or TMP/SMX have become the treatments of choice.[52,53] Other antibiotics shown to have activity include third-generation cephalosporins, nalidixic acid, azithromycin, other quinolones, and furazolidone.[52–57] Antispasmodics and agents that inhibit intestinal peristalsis should not be used because they may prolong fever and diarrhea and worsen the dysentery. Oral vaccines are under development. These vaccines contain avirulent live organisms, which colonize the gut and stimulate local immune response to the *Shigella* antigen. Preliminary results are encouraging, although an ideal vaccine has not yet been developed.[29]

SALMONELLOSIS

Epidemiology and Etiology

Salmonella sp. are gram-negative bacilli belonging to the family Enterobacteriaceae. The genus *Salmonella* has three species *(S. typhi, S. enteritidis,* and *S. choleraesuis).* Human disease caused by salmonella generally falls into four categories: acute gastroenteritis (enterocolitis), bacteremia, extraintestinal localized infection, and enteric fever (typhoid and paratyphoid fever). Salmonellosis is a disease primarily of infants, children, and adolescents. Children under the age of 5 years account for about 25% of all diagnosed cases.[58] Approximately 1 to 2 million cases of salmonellosis occur in the United States annually.[2] Contaminated food or water has been implicated in the majority of cases. Direct fecal–oral transmission occurs less frequently but is particularly important in children. Foods most often implicated in human salmonellosis are poultry, poultry products, beef, pork, and dairy products. An outbreak of *S. enteritidis* in the Midwest in 1994 affecting over 2000 people was traced to ice cream produced in a single location.[59] Pets, particularly reptiles, have been shown to be a common source of infection.[50,58]

Most reports of outbreaks occur sporadically within households and institutions. It is quite common for family contacts to acquire infection. While the incidence of salmonella infection overall has increased over the past decade, that attributed to *S. typhi* has declined. Conditions that may predispose to infection include those that decrease gastric acidity, antibiotic use, malnutrition, and immunodeficient states.[50]

Pathophysiology

Salmonellae enterocolitis appears to occur secondary to mucosal invasion of microorganisms.[2] The different serotypes have a broad range of invasive potential. Some salmonellae like *S. choleraesuis,* the most invasive, are frequently associated with bacteremia and metastatic localization, whereas others seldom cause disease. There is evidence that an enterotoxin may be produced, perhaps within the enterocyte.[49] Other as yet unclear mechanisms may also play a role.

Clinical Presentation

ENTEROCOLITIS

Most patients experience symptoms within 72 hours of ingestion. Patients often complain of nausea and vomiting followed by abdominal cramps, headache, fever, and diarrhea, although the actual presentation is quite variable. Some patients do not have increased stool frequency, while others have more than one stool per hour. Stools are generally loose and may be mucoid or bloody (dysentery-like), or both. Temperatures usually range between 100 and 102°F, but may be higher. Some evidence suggests that higher fever, greater than or equal to 104°F, is associated with shorter bacterial excretion.[60] Diarrhea and fever usually spontaneously resolve within 1 to 5 days but may last 2 weeks.

Stool cultures inevitably yield the causative organism if obtained early. Recovery of organisms continues to decrease with time, however, so that by 3 to 4 weeks, only 5% to 15% of adult patients are passing salmonella. Infants and children tend to pass bacteria for longer periods than adults. Some patients may continue to shed salmonella for a year or longer. These "chronic carrier" states are rare for serotypes other than *S. typhi.*

BACTEREMIA

Salmonellae can produce bacteremia without classic enterocolitis or enteric fever. Bacteremia rarely occurs in older adults, but it can occur in up to 40% of infants.[50] The clinical syndrome is characterized by persistent bacteremia and prolonged intermittent fever with chills. Stool cultures are frequently negative. This is the most frequent, and highly likely, with serotype *S. choleraesuis* infections (50%). Leukocyte counts are often within the normal range.

LOCALIZED INFECTIONS

Extraluminal infection or abscess formation or both can occur at any site. They may follow any of the other syndromes, or they may be the primary presentation. Metastatic infections have been reported to involve bone, cysts, heart, kidney, liver, lungs, pericardium, spleen, and tumors. The clinical presentation is usually determined by the organ systems involved. Polymorphonuclear leukocyte counts are often elevated.

ENTERIC FEVER (TYPHOID AND PARATYPHOID)

Enteric fever caused by *S. typhi* is called typhoid fever. If caused by any other serotype, it is referred to as paratyphoid fever. The clinical presentations of typhoid fever and paratyphoid fever are generally indistinguishable, although in retrospect, paratyphoid fever tends not to be as severe as typhoid fever. Incubation time can range from 10 to 14 days. The onset of symptoms is gradual. Nonspecific symptoms of fever, dull headache, malaise, anorexia, and myalgias are most common. Initially, fever tends to be remittent, but gradually progresses over the first week to temperatures that are often sustained over 104°F. Other frequently encountered symptoms include chills, nausea, vomiting, cough, weakness, and sore throat. Symptoms slowly subside within 4 weeks.

Physical examination generally reveals an acutely ill patient. An erythematous maculopapular rash, known as rose spots, appears primarily on the abdomen in 15% to 50% of patients. The abdomen may also be tender, particularly in the lower quadrants. Hepatomegaly, splenomegaly, or both may also be present in 50% of the cases, and cervical lymph nodes may be enlarged.

A normochromic anemia may develop rapidly without evidence of GI blood loss, although intestinal bleeding may be contributory. Leukopenia may be caused by a relative decrease in polymorphonuclear leukocytes. White cell counts may range from 1200 to 20,000 cells/mm^3. As many as one-third of the patients have elevated levels of the liver enzymes glutamic–oxaloacetic transaminase and alkaline phosphatase. About 80% of patients have positive blood cultures. Bacteremia persists in about one-third of cases for several weeks if not treated. Intestinal perforation, thrombophlebitis, toxemia with circulatory collapse, intestinal hemorrhage, and pneumonia all contribute to a fatality rate of 1% to 2%. Without treatment, mortality may be 10%.

▶ TREATMENT: Salmonellosis

ENTEROCOLITIS

Antibiotic therapy is not indicated in healthy adults as they have no effect on duration of fever or diarrhea, and frequent use of antibiotics encourages selection of resistant bacterial strains.[61] Use of antidiarrheal drugs should be avoided as these increase the risk of mucosal invasion and complications.[57] When required, the most important part of therapy for salmonella enterocolitis is fluid and electrolyte replacement. The vast majority of patients respond well to ORT. Antibiotic therapy should be used in: (1) neonates or infants less than 6 months since young children have an increased risk of complicated infection; (2) patients with primary or secondary immunodeficiency, such as AIDS or chemotherapy patients; and (3) patients after splenectomy.[2,26] Both TMP/SMX and ciprofloxacin have been used to treat salmonella enterocolitis. Ampicillin, third-generation cephalosporins, and chlorampenicol are other alternatives. Susceptibility testing is recommended because many drug-resistant strains of salmonella have emerged.[26,31]

BACTEREMIA AND LOCALIZED INFECTIONS

Chloramphenicol or ampicillin is most frequently used for the treatment of these syndromes. Trimethoprim–sulfamethoxazole, which is effective in treatment of localized salmonella infections, should be considered when the organism is resistant to both chloramphenicol and ampicillin. When bactericidal activity is desired, as with endocarditis or other intravascular infections, ampicillin is the preferred agent, although floroquinolones and third-generation cephalosporins have also been used. The duration of antibiotic therapy should be dictated by the site; for example, osteomyelitis should be treated for 4 to 6 weeks or longer.

ENTERIC FEVER (TYPHOID AND PARATYPHOID)

Until the 1990s, chloramphenicol was the mainstay of therapy for enteric fever in most areas of the world. Chloramphenicol resistance is quickly rising, however, so that in 1994 to 1995 35% of isolates in Great Britain were resistant.[62] Outbreaks of multidrug-resistant *S. typhi* have been reported in many developing countries, including Pakistan, India, Southeast Asia, and North and South Africa.[53] Resistance is often transferred via plasmids to sulfonamides, tetracycline, and streptomycin. Ampicillin, amoxicillin, and TMP/SMX are sometimes effective, although resistance has been reported with these agents as well. Ciprofloxacin is now used extensively for treatment of typhoid in both developing and developed countries and is the drug of choice for adults in areas where multidrug resistance is common.[63,64] Although quinolones are not recommended in children, use of ciprofloxacin in areas where multidrug-resistant *S. typhi* occurs is acceptable. Ceftriaxone is another alternative.[27,58] Therapy should be continued for 10 to 14 days. Clinical response to antibiotics is often seen within 2 days; however, temperatures slowly normalize within 3 to 5 days.

Although not a recommended standard of practice, some clinicians feel that severely ill patients may have a beneficial response to a short course of corticosteroids. Dexamethasone 1 mg/kg every 6 hours for 24 to 48 hours has been used with some success.[58] Three vaccines against *S. typhi* are licensed in the United States: a heat-phenol–inactivated vaccine (Typhoid Vaccine, USP), an orally administered vaccine (Ty21a, Vivotif), and a parenteral polysaccharide vaccine (Typhim Vi).[65-67] Efficacy ranges from 42% to 77% and immunity persists for 3 to 5 years. Vaccination is recommended for high-risk groups, including household contacts of *S. typhi* carriers, laboratory technicians with repeated exposure, sanitation workers in endemic areas, and travelers to developing countries. The oral typhoid vaccine should not be administered to immunocompromised persons, patients taking antibiotics, or patients with gastroenteritis.

CAMPYLOBACTERIOSIS

EPIDEMIOLOGY AND ETIOLOGY

The *Campylobacter* sp. are flagellated, curved, gram-negative rods. *Campylobacter jejuni* is the species responsible for more than 99% of *Campylobacter*-associated gastroenteritis.[68] The true incidence is difficult to estimate since *Campylobacter* is difficult to culture and is not included in routine stool cultures. *Campylobacter* sp. are thought to be a major cause of diarrhea in children, with an incidence greater than *Salmonella* or *Shigella*.[69] The peak incidence is in young children and young adults. Patients with AIDS are particularly susceptible; the incidence in AIDS patients is 40 times that of the general population.[68] The incidence is also higher in males than females, although the reason for this is unknown. Most reported cases occur during the summer months.

Transmission of infection appears to be by ingestion of contaminated food or water. Mammals, such as livestock, dogs, cats, and birds, including poultry, are believed to be the primary reservoir of *Campylobacter*. Epidemiologic studies suggest that previous exposure confers immunity to the infecting strain.

PATHOPHYSIOLOGY

Campylobacter sp. is susceptible to acid, much like *Salmonella*. Therefore, an inoculum of approximately 800 organisms is required to initiate infection. Conditions in the upper small intestine are favorable for multiplication. Flagella-mediated adherence and tissue invasion by bacteria have been demonstrated in the jejunum, ileum, and colon. Infection results in an acute inflammatory enteritis. *Campylobacter jejuni* can produce an enterotoxin or cytotoxin.[70] Both cytotoxins and enterotoxins may be produced in many strains.

CLINICAL PRESENTATION

The average incubation period of *Campylobacter* is 2 to 4 days. The most common presenting symptoms include diarrhea of varying consistency and severity, abdominal pain, and fever. Nausea, vomiting, headache, myalgias, and malaise may also occur. Bowel movements may be numerous, bloody (dysentery-like), foul-smelling, and range from loose to watery. Cramping and abdominal pain are usually relieved by defecation.

The disease is usually self-limited to about 1 week, but it may persist longer in 10% to 20% of patients. A reactive arthritis may be seen in as many as 5% of cases. Complications, including pseudoappendicitis, thrombophlebitis, abscess, septicemia, peritonitis, empyema, urinary tract infection, and cholecystitis are uncommon but occur more frequently in those who are immunocompromised. *Campylobacter jejuni* has been associated with Guillain-Barré syndrome, but the relationship is not well understood.[68,69,71,72] Diagnosis is made by stool culture, but the bacteria is sometimes identifiable with Gram stain or carbol-fuchsin stain.

▶ TREATMENT: Campylobacteriosis

As with other acute diarrheal illnesses, fluid and electrolyte support is a mainstay of therapy. The majority of *Campylobacter*-induced fluid loss can be managed with ORT. Antibiotic therapy has been shown to shorten the duration of bacteria excretion but not the duration or severity of diarrhea. Antibiotics should be considered in the very young and very old and when the patient has severe bloody diarrhea, continued fever (> 102°F), persistence of symptoms beyond 7 days, worsening symptoms, or a compromised immune system. *Campylobacter* sp. are usually susceptible to erythromycin, tetracycline, chloramphenicol, clindamycin, quinolones, and the aminoglycosides.[68] Ciprofloxicin is the agent of choice, with erythromycin or azithromycin as alternatives.[27] If therapy is delayed beyond 4 days after disease onset, there appears to be no clinical benefit to use of antibiotics. Antimotility drugs may impede the resolution of infection and are not recommended.

YERSINIOSIS

EPIDEMIOLOGY AND ETIOLOGY

Yersinia is an anaerobic gram-negative coccobacillus that is widely distributed in nature. The genus *Yersinia* includes six species known to cause disease in humans. Of these, *Y. enterocolitica* is most likely to be associated with intestinal infection. More than 50 serotypes exist, of these 0:3, 0:8, and 0:9 are most frequently associated with enterocolitis. Peak incidence occurs during the winter months.

The organisms have been isolated from a variety of food sources, including pigs and raw goat and cow milk. Refrigeration does not deter the development of adherence and invasive virulence factors. *Yersinia pestis* is the causative agent of plague and is usually spread by bites from infected animals, such as fleas, rodents, or cats.[73] Plague is rare in the United States. Only ten confirmed cases were reported to the Centers for Disease Control (CDC) in 1993.[74]

PATHOPHYSIOLOGY

Yersinia enterocolitica invades the intestinal epithelium and penetrate the intestinal mucosa.[75] Most strains produce an enterotoxin, but the role of toxin production in causing diarrhea is not well established.

CLINICAL PRESENTATION

These bacteria cause a wide spectrum of clinical syndromes. The majority of cases present with enterocolitis that is mild and self-limiting. Symptoms include vomiting, abdominal pain, diarrhea, and fever. Up to 60% of patients will have blood-streaked stools. Diarrhea resolves after 1 to 4 weeks, but the bacteria excretion may continue for up to 3 months after diarrhea subsides. In older children who can report symptoms, pain symptoms may closely mimic appendicitis. Children under 3 months are at greatest risk of developing bacteremia. Other complications that may occur include peritonitis, cholangitis, intestinal perforation, ileocolic intussusception, and toxic megacolon. Many patients develop a reactive arthritis 1 to 2 weeks after recovery from enteritis. The arthritis usually resolves in 1 to 4 months but may persist in about 10% of cases.[76] Other postinfection complications include erythema nodosum and exudative pharyngitis.

▶ TREATMENT: Yersiniosis

Yersiniosis is generally a self-limited disease, and antibiotic therapy does not alter the disease course. Antibiotics are considered in infants under 3 months because of the risk of bacteremia. *Yersinia enterocolitica* is generally susceptible *in vitro* to third-generation cephalosporins, aminoglycosides, chloramphenicol, tetracycline, TMP/SMX, and quinolones. It is frequently resistant to penicillin G, ampicillin, and first-generation cephalosporins. Suggested antibiotics of choice are shown in Table 103–1. A formalin-inactivated plague vaccine does exist and is effective in preventing flea-borne transmission. The vaccine is recommended for laboratory personnel frequently exposed to *Y. pestis* and people with regular contact with wild rodents or their fleas in endemic areas.[73]

ACUTE VIRAL GASTROENTERITIS

Acute viral gastroenteritis was unknown until the 1970s. Viruses are now recognized as the leading cause of diarrhea in the world, although in many cases an exact pathogen cannot be determined. Viruses that have been recovered from the stools of patients with gastroenteritis include rotavirus, enteric adenovirus, Norwalk virus, calicivirus, astrovirus, and coronavirus.

ROTAVIRUSES

EPIDEMIOLOGY AND ETIOLOGY

Rotavirus is the major cause of severe diarrhea worldwide and accounts for approximately 55,000 hospitalizations in the United States per year, as well as 20 to 40 deaths per year. The fecal–oral route is thought to be the most common mode of transmission.[77] Although infection is most often seen in children aged 3 to 24 months, adults can be infected and may act as a potential reservoir for transmission. Outbreaks are not common among infants; however, this age group may be more susceptible to complications as evidenced by a higher hospitalization rate. Serologic surveys show that nearly all children are infected by age 4 years. Reinfections with rotavirus are common. Rotavirus infection rates peak in the winter, with 70% to 95% of all infections occurring during the 4-month period of November to February.[78]

Rotaviruses are double-stranded wheel-shaped RNA viruses. Rotaviruses cause diarrhea by infecting the small intestinal villi. Changes to villi include shortening of villi, crypt hyperplasia, and mononuclear cell infiltration of the lamina propria. Diarrhea results from decreased absorption across intestinal mucosal surface.[77]

CLINICAL PRESENTATION

The rotavirus incubation period is less than 48 hours. Clinical manifestations of rotavirus infections vary from asymptomatic (which is common in adults) to severe nausea, vomiting, and diarrhea with dehydration. The first infection tends to be the most severe. Symptoms are characterized initially by nausea and vomiting (67% to 90%). Fever occurs in about two-thirds of children. Diarrhea occurs in most patients and lasts from 1 to 9 days. Other signs and symptoms include respiratory symptoms, irritability, lethargy, pharyngeal erythema, rhinitis, red tympanic membranes, and palpable cervical lymph nodes. Dehydration and electrolyte disturbances occur more frequently in children.

Laboratory findings reflect the degree of vomiting, diarrhea, or both. Transient rises in liver enzymes may be seen in 60% of children hospitalized for rotavirus diarrhea. The WBC count is usually normal. Stools rarely contain blood or leukocytes. Rotavirus detection in stool samples is possible with an enzyme immunoassay and a latex agglutination assay, both of which are commercially available.

▶ TREATMENT: Rotaviruses

Treatment of rotavirus-associated vomiting, diarrhea, or both is directed at prevention or correction of dehydration. Bismuth subsalicylate was shown to decrease duration of diarrhea and stool output in two trials conducted in Chile and Peru. Routine use is not recommended because of the self-limited nature of the disease and risk of inadvertent overdosing of bismuth subsalicylate. Antimotility agents are also not recommended. Two pharmaceutical companies are testing a candidate rotavirus vaccine. The candidate vaccines are tetravalent vaccines to be administered at 2, 4, and 6 months of age.

NORWALK AND NORWALK-LIKE AGENTS

EPIDEMIOLOGY

Parvovirus-like agents constitute a group of viruses that can cause acute gastroenteritis. The Norwalk virus was the first of these agents to be described in 1972. Agents of this group are named according to the location of the outbreak of illness or contaminated source, such as Norwalk, Hawaii, Montgomery County, Ditchling, Cockle, Paramatta, Snow Mountain, and Marin County.[79]

As with most viruses, the epidemiology of the Norwalk-like agents is not well understood. The disease commonly affects children and adults, but it is not often associated with disease in neonates and very young children.[80] Outbreaks have been documented in families, health care systems, cruise ships, and college dormitories.[81] Norwalk-like viruses are often spread from person-to-person. Other vectors of transmission include contaminated water supplies, fecal–oral spread, and food-borne outbreaks. A major source of food-borne gastroenteritis is contamination of shellfish beds from raw sewage dumped into the water supply.[82,83]

PATHOPHYSIOLOGY

The pathophysiology of this disease is similar to that caused by the rotavirus agents. Human volunteer studies have shown histopathologic changes appear within 24 hours of viral challenge, and clinical manifestations appear within 48 hours.[79] Brush border enzyme activity may be decreased, resulting in lactose intolerance, but it generally returns to preinfection levels within 2 weeks. The exact mechanisms of virus-induced vomiting or diarrhea are unknown.

CLINICAL PRESENTATION

Norwalk-like viral gastroenteritis is characterized by sudden onset of abdominal cramps with nausea, vomiting, or both. Although adults frequently experience nonbloody diarrhea, children experience vomiting more often than diarrhea. Other complaints are myalgias, headache, and malaise, which are accompanied by fever in about 50% of cases. Signs and symptoms generally last 12 to 48 hours.[58,77]

▶ TREATMENT: Norwalk and Norwalk-like Agents

The disease is generally self-limiting and does not require therapy. On occasion, oral rehydration may be required. Rarely is parenteral hydration necessary.

ENTERIC ADENOVIRUS

Adenovirus is an icosahedral virus previously associated with respiratory, ocular, and genitourinary infections; however, serotypes 40 and 41 have been identified as GI pathogens. Peak incidence is in children less than 2 years of age, and infections occur year-round. Transmission is primarily person-to-person and fecal–oral, and shedding from the gut may be long term. The incubation period is 8 to 10 days. Diarrhea and vomiting often last 1 to 2 weeks. Low-grade fever and respiratory symptoms are also common.[80] Diagnosis can be made by enzyme immunoassay (EIA) that identifies serotypes 40 and 41.

OTHER POTENTIAL VIRAL PATHOGENS

Although less commonly associated with severe GI disease, calicivirus, astrovirus, pestivirus, torovirus, and coronavirus-like particles have been recovered from diarrheal stools. In human immunodeficiency virus (HIV)-infected patients, the presence of diarrhea has been associated with virus in 35% of stool specimens. Astrovirus, picobirnavirus, calicivirus, and adenovirus appear to be the most commonly isolated viral pathogens.[84,85] More specific characteristics of these agents are presented in Table 103–6.

FOOD POISONING

Food poisoning results from the ingestion of food containing pathogenic microorganisms, preformed toxins that were produced by microorganisms, or other toxic compounds. An average of 18,335 cases from 479 outbreaks are reported annually to the CDC, although estimates for actual cases are approximately 12.6 million.[86] A number of bacteria can cause food poisoning (Table 103–7).

TABLE 103–6. Agents Responsible for Acute Viral Gastroenteritis and Diarrhea

Virus	Peak Age of Onset	Time of Year	Duration	Mode of Transmission	Symptoms
Rotavirus	6 mo–2 yr	October to April	3–8 d	Fecal–oral, water, food	Vomiting, diarrhea, fever, abdominal pain, lactose intolerance
Enteric adenovirus	< 2 yr	Year-round	7–9 d	Fecal–oral	Diarrhea, respiratory symptoms, vomiting, fever
Calicivirus	3 mo–6 yr	Peak in winter	4 d	Fecal–oral, water, shellfish	Vomiting, diarrhea
Astrovirus	< 7 yr	Winter	1–4 d	Fecal–oral, water, shellfish	Vomiting, diarrhea, fever, abdominal pain
Pestivirus	< 2 yr	NR	3 d	NR	Mild
Coronavirus-like particles	< 2 yr	Fall and early winter	7 d	NR	Respiratory disease
Enterovirus	NR	NR	NR	NR	Mild diarrhea, secondary organ damage
Norwalk	> 5 yr	Variable	12–24 h	Fecal–oral, food, water, aerosol	Vomiting, diarrhea, abdominal cramps, headache, fever, chills, myalgias

NR = not reported.
Compiled from Refs. 77, 80, and 81.

TABLE 103–7. Food Poisonings

Organism	Time to Symptoms (h)	Principal Foods	Peak Incidence (U.S.A.)	Principal Mechanism of Pathophysiology	Duration	Treatment
Staphylococcus aureus	1–6	Salad, pastries, ham, poultry	Summer	Preformed toxins A–E (heat stable)	12 h	Supportive
Bacillus cereus	1–6	Meats, vegetables, fried rice	None	Preformed toxins	12 h	Supportive
	8–16			Toxin production (in vivo)	24 h	Supportive
Clostridium perfringens (type A)	6–24	Meats, poultry	Fall, winter, spring	Toxin production (in vivo)	24 h	Supportive
Vibrio parahemolyticus	16–72	Shellfish	Spring, summer, fall	Toxin production and tissue invasion	2–7 d	Supportive
Salmonella sp.	16–48	Beef, poultry, water, eggs, dairy products	Summer	Tissue invasion	2–7 d	Supportive
Shigella sp.	16–48	Salad, water	Summer	Tissue invasion	2–7 d	Supportive
EPEC	16–48	Water	None	Tissue invasion	2–7 d	Supportive
Campylobacter	16–48	Poultry, dairy products, clams, water	Spring, summer	Tissue invasion	2–7 d	Supportive
ETEC	16–72	Water	None	Toxin production (in vivo)	1–7 d	Supportive
Vibrio cholerae	16–72	Water		Toxin production (in vivo)	2–12 d	Supportive, antibiotics
Yersinia enterocolitica	16–48	Dairy products		Toxin production and/or tissue invasion	1–30 d	Supportive
Clostridium botulinum	12–72	Canned fruits, vegetables, meats, honey	None	Preformed toxins A, B, and E (children and adults) Toxin production (in vivo) (infants)		Supportive (including mechanically assisted ventilation) Trivalent antitoxin

EPEC = enteropathogenic *E. coli;* ETEC = enterotoxigenic *E. coli.*

Staphylococcal food poisoning results from the ingestion of food contaminated by an enterotoxin produced by certain strains of *Staphylococcus aureus* growing within the food. Enterotoxin production generally results from leaving foods at room temperature, allowing the staphylococci to grow. The syndrome accounts for over 600 infections per year. Symptoms are rapid in onset, generally occurring within 1 to 6 hours of ingestion of toxin-containing foods. The condition is characterized by nausea and vomiting (75%), although abdominal cramps and diarrhea may also be present. Symptoms resolve in less than 12 hours. Oral replacement should be provided in severe cases; antibiotics are not indicated.

Over 6000 cases of salmonellosis are reported each year in the United States, and estimates for actual infection incidence are as high as 4 million cases annually. Proper preparation and handling of potential food vectors is essential in reducing the incidence of illness. Eggs should be stored only short term, held no longer than 2 hours at room temperature, prepared in small batches, thoroughly cooked before serving, and consumed immediately after preparation.[87] Further information regarding GI salmonella infection is presented under "Salmonellosis."

Like salmonella, food-borne shigella disease usually manifests as inflammatory diarrhea. *Shigella* is common in the summer and fall and is spread from person to person via fecal–oral contamination. Treatment is best accomplished with TMP/SMX, a fluoroquinolone, or a third-generation cephalosporin.[86]

Food-borne clostridium infections are related to *Clostridium perfringens,* which manifests with a noninflammatory diarrhea, and *Clostridium botulinum,* which is characterized by neurologic symptoms. *Clostridium perfringens* may present as two distinct syndromes. Type A organisms are seen in Western nations and result in a 24-hour illness characterized by watery diarrhea and epigastric pain. Symptoms generally resolve within 24 hours. Type C organisms can be found in undercooked pork and occur in underdeveloped tropical regions. Type C can produce a toxin-related syndrome called enteritis necroticans, which is a coagulative, transmural necrosis of the intestinal wall. This syndrome can result in intestinal perforation leading to sepsis and mortality in approximately 40% of victims.

Food-borne botulism results from the ingestion of food contaminated with preformed toxins or toxin-producing spores from *C. botulinum. Clostridium botulinum* is relatively rare, only 30 to 50 cases are reported per year in the United States. Botulism is almost always associated with improper preparation or storage of food. Seven distinct toxins (A–G) have been described. The toxins, which are produced by the bacteria and released upon lysis, are the most potent biologic or chemical toxins known to man. The toxin prevents the release of acetylcholine at the peripheral cholinergic nerve terminal. Toxin activity has prompted the use of minute locally injected doses to treat select spastic disorders, such as blepharospasm, hemifacial spasm, and certain dystonias.[88,89]

Food-borne botulism presents as a symmetric descending paralysis without sensory or central nervous system involvement. Symptoms usually begin 18 to 24 hours after ingestion and progress over days to weeks. Other symptoms can include blurred vision, photophobia (90%), dysphagia (76%), generalized weakness (58%), nausea and vomiting (56%), and dysphonia (55%).

Diagnosis is made by culturing *C. botulinum* from the stool. Treatment consists primarily of respiratory support and use of botulinum antitoxin. Respiratory failure may occur prior to involvement of other upper muscle groups. If evaluation is performed within several hours of ingestion, gastric lavage or induction of vomiting is suggested. Cathartics and enemas can also be used to remove residual toxin from the bowel, but they are contraindicated in cases of ileus.

Although the effectiveness of antitoxins is unknown, patients diagnosed with botulism should receive botulinum antitoxin. Botulinum antitoxin is a concentrated preparation of equine globulins obtained from horses immunized with toxins A, B, and E. Because trivalent antitoxin is equine in origin, patients should be tested for hypersensitivity before receiving the product intravenously.

Other agents used experimentally as adjunctive therapy are guanidine, which antagonizes the effect of botulinum toxin at the neuromuscular junction, and 4-aminopyridine, which increases acetylcholine release.[90,91] Newer and more effective methods of treatment and prevention are under development, including a botulinum toxin vaccine consisting of nontoxic botulinum fragments.

Prevention should always be stressed. Botulinum toxins are heat labile and readily destroyed by 10 minutes of boiling. All home-canned foods should be processed according to directions and boiled, not just warmed, prior to consumption.

PHARMACOECONOMIC CONSIDERATIONS OF GASTROINTESTINAL INFECTIONS

Although infectious diarrhea in the United States is often self-limited, the economic impact of GI infections is enormous. As was mentioned at the beginning of this chapter, 20% of soldiers in Operation Desert Shield who experienced diarrhea missed work or required a visit to a physician.[5] Traveler's diarrhea interferes with planned activities or work in 20% of those affected, accounting for unknown dollars lost because of decreased productivity.[38]

Diarrheal illness accounts for 2 to 3.7 million doctor visits and 200,000 hospitalizations per year in children under 5 years of age in the United States. Avendano and associates evaluated the costs of diarrhea episodes resulting in a physician visit in children under 5 years of age.[91] They estimated the total cost per episode to be approximately $290. This extrapolates to a cost of $0.6 to $1.1 billion per year for children under 5 years of age. In 50% of cases, diarrheal illness leads to at least 1 full day of lost activity by the patient or parents of patients. This results in a total projected cost of $23 billion per year in the United States based on estimated medical costs and lost productivity.[1]

▶ PRINCIPLES OF PHARMACOTHERAPY

- Etiologies of infectious diarrhea include bacteria, viruses, and protozoans. Viral infections are the leading cause of diarrhea in the world.
- Fluid and electrolyte replacement is the cornerstone of therapy. Most cases of mild and moderate diarrhea can be treated with oral rehydration therapy.
- The necessary components of oral replacement therapy are glucose, sodium, potassium, chloride, and water.
- Metronidazole is the treatment of choice for *C. difficile* colitis. Vancomycin is an alternative.
- Antimicrobial therapy is often not indicated for enteritis as many cases are mild and self-limited or are viral in nature.
- When antimicrobials are used for enteritis they should be active against the most likely pathogen based on clinical symptoms, epidemiologic patterns, and resistance patterns in the area.
- Food poisoning is responsible for over 12 million cases of diarrhea per year. Common pathogens include *Staphylococcus, Salmonella, Shigella,* and *Clostridium.*
- Patient education and prevention strategies are important in preventing and treating traveler's diarrhea. Prophylaxis with antibiotics is appropriate in certain situations.

REFERENCES

1. Cheney CP, Wong RKH. Acute infectious diarrhea. Gastrointest Emerg 1993;77:1169–1196.
2. Laney DW, Cohen MB. Approach to the pediatric patient with diarrhea. Gastroenterol Clin North Am 1993;22:499–515.
3. Brown KH. Dietary management of acute diarrheal disease: Contemporary scientific issues. Am Inst Nutr 1994;124:1455S–1460S.
4. Glass RI, Lew JF, Gangarosa RE, et al. Estimates of morbidity and mortality rates for diarrheal disease in American children. J Pediatr 1991;118:S27–S33.
5. Hyams KC, Bourgeois AL, Merrell BR, et al. Diarrheal disease during Operation Desert Shield. N Engl J Med 1991;325:1423–1428.
6. Meyers A. Modern management of acute diarrhea and dehydration in children. Am Fam Physician 1995;51:1103–1115.
7. Gavin N, Merrick N, Davidson B. Efficacy of glucose-based oral rehydration therapy. Pediatrics 1996;98:45–51.
8. Anonymous. The management of acute diarrhea in children: Oral rehydration, maintenance, and nutritional therapy. MMWR 1992; 41(RR16):1–20.
9. Lebenthal E, Khin-Maung-U, Rolston DDK, et al. Thermophilic amylase-digested rice-electrolyte solution in the treatment of acute diarrhea in children. Pediatrics 1995;95:198–202.
10. Islam A, Molla AM, Ahmed MA, et al. Is rice based oral replacement therapy effective in young infants? Arch Dis Child 1994;71:19–23.
11. Powell DW, Szauter KE. Nonantibiotic therapy and pharmacotherapy of acute infectious diarrhea. Gastroenterol Clin North Am 1993;22: 683–707.
12. Molina S, Vettorazzi C, Peerson JM. Clinical trial of glucose-oral rehydration solution (ORS), rice dextrin-ORS, and rice flour-ORS for the management of children with acute diarrhea and mild or moderate dehydration. Pediatrics 1995;95:191–197.
13. Fayad IM, Hashem M, Duggan C, et al. Comparative efficacy of rice-based and glucose-based oral rehydration salts plus early reintroduction of food. Lancet 1993;342:772–775.
14. Santosham M, Fayad IM, Hashem M, et al. A comparison of rice-based oral rehydration and "early feeding" for the treatment of acute diarrhea in infants. J Pediatr 1990;16:868–875.
15. Vanderhoof JA, Murray ND, Paule CL, Ostrom KM. Use of soy fiber in acute diarrhea in infants and toddlers. Clin Pediatr 1997;March: 135–139.
16. Goepp JG, Katz SA. Oral rehydration therapy. Am Fam Physician 1993;47:843–848.
17. Gore SM, Fontaine O, Pierce MF. Impact of rice-based oral rehydration solution on stool output and duration of diarrhoea: Meta-analysis of 13 clinical trials. BMJ 1992;304:287–291.
18. Snyder JD. Use and misuse of oral therapy for diarrhea: Comparison of US practices with American Academy of Pediatrics recommendations. Pediatrics 1991;87:28–33.
19. Kallen RJ. The management of diarrheal dehydration in infants using parenteral fluids. Pediatr Clin North Am 1990;37:265–286.
20. Alam NH, Ahmed T, Khatun M, Molla AM. Effects of food with two oral rehydration therapies: A randomized, controlled clinical trial. Gut 1992;33:560–562.
21. Faruque ASG, Mahalanabis D, Islam A, et al. Breast feeding and oral rehydration at home during diarrhoea to prevent dehydration. Arch Dis Child 1992;67:1027–1029.
22. Khan WA, Bennish ML, Seas C, et al. Randomised controlled comparison of single-dose ciprofloxacin and doxycycline for cholera caused by *Vibrio cholerae* 01 or 0139. Lancet 1996;348:296–300.
23. Mahon BE, Mintz ED, Greene KD, et al. Reported cholera in the United States, 1992–1994. JAMA 1996;276:307–312.
24. Blake PA. Epidemiology of cholera in the Americas. Gastroenterol Clin North Am 1993;22:639–659.
25. Afghani B, Stutman HR. Toxin-related diarrheas. Pediatr Ann 1994; 23:549–555.
26. Ashkenazi S, Cleary TG. Antibiotic treatment of bacterial gastroenteritis. Pediatr Infect Dis J 1991;10:140–148.
27. Sanford JP. Guide to Antimicrobial Therapy 1997. Bethesda, MD, Antimicrobial Therapy, 1997:12–13.
28. Dutta D, Bhattacharya SK, Bhattacharya MK, et al. Efficacy of norfloxacin and doxycyline for treatment of *Vibrio cholerae* 0139 infection. J Anitmicrob Chemother 1996;37;575–581.
29. Levine MM, Noriega F. Vaccines to prevent enteric infections. Baillieres Clin Gastroenterol 1993;7:501–517.
30. Dellert SF, Cohen MB. Diarrheal disease: Established pathogens, new pathogens, and progress in vaccine development. Gastroenterol Clin North Am 1994;23:637–654.
31. Isada CM, Kasten BL, Goldman CM, et al. Infectious Disease Handbook 1997–1998, 2nd ed. Lexi-Comp, Inc, Hudson, OH, 1996:136–138.
32. Cantey JR. *Escherichia coli* diarrhea. Gastroenterol Clin North Am 1993;22:609–622.
33. Brook MG, Bannister BA. Diarrhoea-causing *Escherichia coli.* Dig Dis 1993;11:288–297.
34. Slutsker L, Ries AA, Greene KD, et al. *Escherichia coli* 0157:H7 diarrhea in the United States: Clinical and epidemiologic features. Ann Intern Med 1997;126:505–513.
35. Hart CA, Batt RM, Saunders JR. Diarrhoea caused by *Escherichia coli.* Ann Trop Paediatr 1993;13:121–131.
36. Soriano-Brucher HE, Avendano P, O'Ryan M, et al. Use of bismuth subsalicylate in acute diarrhea in children. Rev Infect Dis 1990; 12(S1):S51–S56.

37. Gorbach SL. Bismuth therapy in gastrointestinal diseases. Gastroenterology 1990;99:863–875.
38. Ericsson CD, DuPont HL. Travelers' diarrhea: Approaches to prevention and treatment. Clin Infect Dis 1993;16:616–626.
39. Larson SC. Traveler's diarrhea. Emerg Med Clinics North Am 1997; 15:179–189.
40. Okhuysen PC, Ericsson CD. Travelers' diarrhea: Prevention and treatment. Med Clinics North Am 1992;76:1357–1373.
41. DuPont HL. Travellers' diarrhoea: Which antimicrobial? Drugs 1993; 45:910–917.
42. Pothoulakis C, LaMont JT. *Clostridium difficile* colitis and diarrhea. Gastroenterol Clin North Am 1193;22:623–637.
43. Reinke CM, Messick CR. Update on *Clostridium difficile*-induced colitis: 1. Am J Hosp Pharm 1994;51:1771–1781.
44. Caputo GM, Weitekamp MR, Bacon AE, Whitener C. *Clostridium difficile* infection: A common clinical problem for the general internist. J Gen Int Med 1994;9:528–533.
45. Feteky R, Shah AB. Diagnosis and treatment of *Clostridium difficile* colitis. JAMA 1993;269:71–75.
46. Feteky R. Guidelines for the diagnosis and management of *Clostridium difficile*-associated diarrhea and colitis. Am J Gastroenterol 1997; 92:739–750.
47. Reinke CM, Messick CR. Update on *Clostridium difficile*-induced colitis: 2. Am J Hosp Pharm 1994;51:1892–1901.
48. Elmer GW, Surawicz CM, McFarland LV. Biotherapeutic agents: A neglected modality for the treatment and prevention of selected intestinal and vaginal infections. JAMA 1996;275:870–876.
49. Anonymous. U.S. Food & Drug Administration Center for Food Safety and Applied Nutrition Foodborne Pathogenic Microorganisms and Natural Toxins, 1992.
50. Stutman HR. *Salmonella, Shigella,* and *Campylobacter:* Common bacterial causes of infectious diarrhea. Pediatr Ann 1994;23:538–543.
51. Frankel G, Riley L, Giron JA, et al. Detection of shigella in feces using DNA amplification. J Infect Dis 1990;161:1252–1256.
52. Ashkenazi S, Amir J, Waisman Y, et al. A randomized, double-blind study comparing cefixime and trimethoprim–sulfamethoxazole in the treatment of childhood shigellosis. J Pediatr 1993;123:817–821.
53. Sack RB, Rahman M, Yunus M, Khan EH. Antimicrobial resistance in organisms causing diarrheal disease. Clin Infect Dis 1997;24(suppl 1): S102–S105.
54. Khan WA, Seas C, Dhar U, et al. Treatment of shigellosis: V. Comparison of azithromycin and ciprofloxacin. Ann Int Med 1997;126: 697–703.
55. Eidlitz-Marcus T, Cohen YH, Nussinovitch M, et al. Comparative efficacy of two- and five-day courses of ceftriaxone for treatment of severe shigellosis in children. J Pediatr 1993;123:822–824.
56. Patwari AK. Multidrug resistant *Shigella* infections in children. J Diarrhoeal Dis Res 1994;12:182–186.
57. Varsano I, Eidletz-Marcus T, Nussinovitch M, Elian I. Comparative efficacy of ceftriaxone and ampicillin for treatment of severe shigellosis in children. J Pediatr 1991;118:627–632.
58. Hogan DE. The emergency department approach to diarrhea. Emerg Med Clin North Am 1996;14:673–694.
59. Anonymous. Outbreak of *Salmonella enteritidis* associated with nationally distributed ice cream products—Minnesota, South Dakota, and Wisconsin, 1994. MMWR 1994;43:740–741.
60. El-Radhi AS, Rostila T, Vesikari T. Association of high fever and short bacterial excretion after salmonellosis. Arch Dis Child 1992;67: 531–532.
61. Sanchez C, Garcia-Restoy E, Garau J, et al. Ciprofloxacin and trimethoprim–sulfamethoxazole vs placebo in acute uncomplicated *Salmonella enteritis:* A double-blind trial. J Infect Dis 1993;168: 1304–1307.
62. Rowe B, Ward L, Threlfall EJ. Multidrug-resistant *Salmonella typhi:* A worldwide epidemic. Clin Infect Dis 1997;24(suppl 1):S106–S109.
63. Alam MN, Haq SA, Das KK, et al. Efficacy of ciprofloxacin in enteric fever: Comparison of treatment duration in sensitive and multidrug-resistant *Salmonella.* Am J Trop Med Hyg 1995;53:306–311.
64. Hosek G, Leschinsky D, Irons S, Safranek TJ. Multidrug-resistant *Salmonella* serotype typhimurium—United States, 1996. JAMA 1997; 277:1513.
65. Conrad DA, Jenson HB. New and improved vaccines: Promising weapons against varicella, hepatitis A, and typhoid fever. Postgrad Med 1996;100:113–126.
66. Plotkin SA, Bouveret-LeCam N. A new typhoid vaccine composed of the Vi capsular polysaccharide. Arch Intern Med 1995;155:2293–2299.
67. Levine MM, Noriega F. Vaccines to prevent bacterial enteric infections in children. Pediatr Ann 1993;22:719–725.
68. Allos BM, Blaser MJ. *Campylobacter jejuni* and the expanding spectrum of related infections. Clin Infect Dis 1995;20:1092–1101.
69. Peterson MC. Clinical aspects of *Campylobacter jejuni* infections in adults. Western J Med 1994;161:148–152.
70. Wallis MR. The pathogenesis of *Campylobacter jejuni.* Br J Biomed Sci 1994;51:57–64.
71. Mishu B, Blaser M. Role of infection due to *Campylobacter jejuni* in the initiation of Guillain-Barré syndrome. Clin Infect Dis 1993;17: 104–108.
72. Ketley JM. Pathogenesis of enteric infection by *Campylobacter.* Microbiology 1997;143:5–21.
73. Gage KL, Dennis DT, Tsai TF. Prevention of plague: Recommendations of the advisory committee on immunization practices (ACIP). MMWR; 45(RR14):1–15.
74. Werner SB, Murray R, Reilly K, et al. Human plague—United States, 1993–1994. JAMA 1994;271:1312.
75. San Joaquin VH. *Aeromonas, Yersinia,* and miscellaneous bacterial enteropathogens. Pediatr Ann 1994;23:544–548.
76. Baert F, Peetermans W, Knockaert D. Yersinosis: The clinical spectrum. Acta Clinica Belgica 1994;49:76–85.
77. Lieberman JM. Rotavirus and other viral cases of gastroenteritis. Pediatr Ann 1994;23:529–535.
78. Glass RI, Kilgore PE, Holman RC, et al. The epidemiology of rotavirus diarrhea in the United States: Surveillance and estimates of disease burden. J Infect Dis 1996;174(suppl 1):S5–S11.
79. Caul EO. Viral gastroenteritis: Small round structured viruses, caliciviruses, and astroviruses: I. The clinical and diagnostic perspective. J Clin Pathol 1996;49:874–880.
80. Taterka JA, Cuff CF, Rubin DH. Viral gastrointestinal infections. Gastroenterol Clin North Am 1992;21:303–329.
81. Caul EO. Viral gastroenteritis: Small round structured viruses, caliciviruses, and astroviruses: II. The epidemiological perspective. J Clin Pathol 1996;49:959–964.
82. Aristeguieta C, Koenders I, Windham D, et al. Multistate outbreak of viral gastroenteritis associated with consumption of oysters—Apalachicola Bay, Florida, December 1994–January 1995. JAMA 1995;273:452.
83. Cirino J, Cumberland D, Pollack L, et al. Multistate outbreak of viral gastroenteritis related to consumption of oysters—1993. JAMA 1994;271:183–184.
84. Grohmann GS, Glass RI, Pereira HG, et al. Enteric viruses and diarrhea in HIV-infected patients. N Engl J Med 1993;329:14–20.
85. Smith PD. Infectious diarrheas in patients with AIDS. Gastroenterol Clin North Am 1993;22:535–548.
86. Bishai WR, Sears CL. Food poisoning syndromes. Gastroenterol Clin North Am 1993;22:579–608.
87. Anonymous. Update: *Salmonella enteritidis* infections and grade A shell eggs—United States 1989. MMWR 1990;38(51–52):877–880.
88. Hatheway CL. Toxigenic *Clostridia.* Clin Microbiol Rev 1990;3:66–98.
89. Roblot P, Roblot F, Fauchere JL, et al. Retrospective study of 108 cases of botulism in Poitiers, France. J Med Microbiol 1994;40:379–384.
90. Middlebrook JL. Protection strategies against botulinum toxin. Adv Exper Med Biol 1995;383:93–98.
91. Avendano P, Matson DO, Long J, et al. Costs associated with office visits for diarrhea in infants and toddlers. Pediatr Infect Dis J 1993; 12:897–902.
92. Facts and Comparisons. St. Louis, JB Lippincott. Updated monthly, 1998, 17a.

104

INTRA-ABDOMINAL INFECTIONS

Joseph T. DiPiro, PharmD, FCCP, and David A. Rogers, MD, FACS, FAAP

Intra-abdominal infections are those contained within the peritoneum or retroperitoneal space. The peritoneal cavity extends from the undersurface of the diaphragm to the floor of the pelvis and contains the stomach, most of the small bowel, the large bowel, liver, gallbladder, and spleen. The duodenum, pancreas, kidneys, adrenal, great vessels (aorta and vena cava), and most mesenteric vascular structures reside in the posterior retroperitoneum. These infections may be generalized or localized. They may be contained within visceral structures, such as the liver, spleen, pancreas, or female reproductive organs. Two general types of intra-abdominal infection are discussed throughout this chapter: peritonitis and abscess. Peritonitis is defined as the acute, inflammatory response of peritoneal lining to microorganisms, chemicals, irradiation, or foreign body injury. This chapter deals only with peritonitis of infectious origin.

An abscess is a purulent collection of fluid separated by a more or less well-defined wall from surrounding tissue. It usually contains necrotic debris, bacteria, and inflammatory cells. These processes differ considerably in their presentation and the required approach to treatment.

EPIDEMIOLOGY

Peritonitis may be classified as either primary or secondary. With primary peritonitis, an intra-abdominal focus of disease (such as disruption of an intra-abdominal hollow viscus) is not evident.[1] Bacteria may be transported from the bloodstream to the peritoneal cavity where the inflammatory process begins. In secondary peritonitis, a focal disease process is evident within the abdomen. Secondary peritonitis may involve acute perforation of the gastrointestinal (GI) tract (possibly because of ulceration or ischemia), postoperative peritonitis, or post-traumatic peritonitis (blunt or penetrating trauma). Primary peritonitis is relatively uncommon. It has been reported to occur infrequently in adults, as well as in normal infants and children. Primary peritonitis develops in up to 25% of patients with alcoholic cirrhosis.[2] In fact, it is estimated that 60% of all patients on chronic ambulatory peritoneal dialysis (CAPD) will have at least one episode of peritonitis during the first year.[3] The average incidence of peritonitis in patients undergoing continuous ambulatory peritoneal dialysis is 1.3 to 1.4 episodes per patient per year.[4] Epidemiologic data for secondary intra-abdominal infections is limited. Appendicitis is one of the most common causes of intra-abdominal infection. In 1990, 274,000 appendectomies were performed in the United States for suspected appendicitis.[5]

ETIOLOGY

A major risk factor for primary peritonitis is the presence of a catheter used for peritoneal dialysis that connects the abdominal cavity with the exterior of the body through the abdominal wall. The risk of primary peritonitis is also increased by recent paracentesis, upper GI endoscopy, portacaval anastomosis, arterial or umbilical vein catheterization, and barium enema or sigmoidoscopy.

Table 104–1 summarizes many of the potential causes of bacterial peritonitis. These include inflammatory processes of the GI tract or abdominal organs, mechanical problems, such as bowel obstruction, vascular occlusions that may lead to gangrene of the intestines, and neoplasias that may cause intestinal perforation or obstruction. Other possible causes include those resulting from traumatic injuries or postoperative infections.

Abscesses are the result of chronic inflammation and most often occur without preceding generalized peritonitis. They may be located within one of the spaces of the peritoneal cavity or within one of the visceral organs and may range from a few milliliters to a liter or more in volume. These collections often have a fibrinous capsule and may take from a few days to years to form.

The causes of intra-abdominal abscess somewhat overlap those of peritonitis and, in fact, both may occur sequentially or simultaneously. Appendicitis is the most frequent cause of abscess followed by pancreatitis and lesions of the genitourinary tract (particularly in women). Other potential causes of intra-abdominal abscesses include diverticulitis, lesions of the biliary tract, osteomyelitis of the spine, perforating tumors in the abdomen, trauma, and leaking intestinal anastomosis. For certain diseases, such as appendicitis and diverticulitis, abscesses occur much more frequently than does generalized peritonitis.

MICROFLORA OF THE GASTROINTESTINAL TRACT AND FEMALE GENITAL TRACT

A full appreciation of intra-abdominal infections requires an understanding of the normal microflora within the GI tract. There are striking differences in flora within the various segments of the GI tract (Table 104–2), and this bacterial environment usually determines the severity of infectious processes in the abdomen. Generally, the low gastric pH eradicates bacteria that enter the stomach. With achlorhydria, bacterial counts may rise to 10^5 to 10^7/mL. The normally low bacterial count may increase by 1000- or 10,000-fold with gastric outlet obstruction and gastric cancer, in patients who

TABLE 104–1. Causes of Bacterial Peritonitis

Primary Bacterial Peritonitis
Peritoneal dialysis
Cirrhosis with ascites
Spontaneous peritonitis in children and adults
Secondary Bacterial Peritonitis
Miscellaneous causes
Diverticulitis with perforation
Appendicitis
Inflammatory bowel diseases
Salpingitis
Biliary tract infections
Necrotizing pancreatitis
Neoplasms
Intestinal obstruction
Perforation
Mechanical gastrointestinal problems
Any cause of small bowel obstruction
Vascular causes
Mesenteric arterial or venous occlusion
Mesenteric ischemia without occlusion
Trauma
Blunt abdominal trauma with rupture of intestine
Penetrating abdominal trauma
Iatrogenic intestinal perforation
Peritoneal contamination during abdominal operation
Leakage from gastrointestinal anastomosis

have been on histamine-2 (H_2) receptor antagonists, proton pump inhibitors, or antacids, or in the presence of blood.[6]

The biliary tract (gallbladder and bile ducts) is sterile in most healthy individuals but in certain groups (those older than the age of 70 or those with acute cholecystitis, jaundice, or common bile duct stones), it is likely to be colonized by aerobic gram-negative bacilli (particularly *Escherichia coli* and *Klebsiella* sp.) and enterococci.[7] Patients who have a biliary tract that is colonized with bacteria are at greater risk of intra-abdominal infection.

At the distal ileum, bacterial counts of aerobes and anaerobes are quite high. In the colon, there may be 400 to 500 different types of bacteria with bacterial concentrations often reaching 10^{11}/mL, and anaerobic bacteria outnumber aerobic bacteria by more than 1000 to 1. In fact, up to 50% of the dry mass of stool is bacteria. Fortunately, most colonic bacteria are not pathogens because they cannot survive in environments outside the colon. Perforation of the colon results in the release of very large numbers of anaerobic and aerobic bacteria into the peritoneum. The colonic flora are generally stable unless broad-spectrum antimicrobials have been in use, in which case increases in *Candida* or gram-negative bacteria are noted.

The lower female genital tract is generally colonized by a large number of aerobic and anaerobic bacteria. Anaerobes may number 10^9/mL and often include lactobacilli, eubacteria, clostridia, anaerobic streptococci, and, less frequently, *Bacteroides fragilis.* Aerobic bacteria are most often streptococci and *Staphylococcus epidermidis*, and these may number 10^8/mL.

PATHOPHYSIOLOGY

Intra-abdominal infection results from bacterial entry into the peritoneal or retroperitoneal spaces or from bacterial collections within intra-abdominal organs. In primary peritonitis, the route of bacterial spread is usually not apparent. Bacteria may enter the abdomen via the bloodstream or the lymphatic system by transmigration through the bowel wall or via the fallopian tubes in females. Hematogenous bacterial spread (through the bloodstream) occurs more frequently with tubercular peritonitis or peritonitis associated with cirrhotic ascites. When peritonitis results from peritoneal dialysis, skin surface flora are introduced via the peritoneal catheter.[8] In secondary peritonitis, bacteria most often enter the peritoneum or retroperitoneum as a result of perforation of the GI tract caused by diseases or traumatic injuries. Also, peritonitis or abscess may result from contamination of the peritoneum during a surgical procedure or from lesions of the female genital tract.

The physiologic characteristics of the peritoneal cavity determine the nature of the response to infection or inflammation within it. The peritoneum is lined by a highly per-

TABLE 104–2. Usual Microflora of the Gastrointestinal Tract

Site	Commonly Found Bacteria	Approximate Concentration (No. Organisms/mL) Aerobes	Approximate Concentration (No. Organisms/mL) Anaerobes
Stomach[a]	*Streptococcus, Lactobacillus*	$10–10^2$	Rare
Biliary tract	Normally sterile (*Escherichia coli, Klebsiella,* or enterococci in some patients)	0	0
Proximal small bowel	*Streptococcus* (including enterococci), *E. coli, Klebsiella, Lactobacillus,* diphteroids	10^2	Few
Distal ileum	*E. coli, Klebsiella, Enterobacter,* enterococci, *Bacteroides fragilis, Clostridium,* peptostreptococci	$10^4–10^6$	$10^5–10^7$
Colon	*Bacteroides* sp., peptostreptococci, *Clostridium, E. coli, Klebsiella,* enterococci, *Enterobacter,* and many others	$10^5–10^8$	$10^9–10^{11}$

[a]With achlorhydria, H_2-antagonist therapy, gastric cancer, or gastric outlet obstruction, bacterial counts may rise to 10^5/mL.

meable, serous membrane with a surface area approximately that of skin. The normal peritoneal cavity contains about 50 mL of a serous fluid that is normally sterile, is low in protein and leukocytes, and contains no fibrinogen. These conditions change drastically with peritoneal infection or inflammation, as will be described later.

After bacteria are introduced into the peritoneal cavity, there is an immediate response to contain the insult. Humoral and cellular defenses respond first; then the omentum migrates to the affected area. A limited bacterial inoculum is rapidly handled by defense mechanisms. Under certain conditions the bacterial insult is not contained, and bacteria disseminate throughout the peritoneal cavity, resulting in peritonitis. This is more likely to occur in the presence of a foreign body or where there is (1) a large bacterial inoculum, (2) continuing bacterial contamination, and (3) contamination involving a mixture of organisms that by synergistic action are particularly virulent.

When bacteria become dispersed throughout the peritoneum, the inflammatory process involves the majority of the peritoneal lining. There is an outpouring into the peritoneum of serous fluid containing leukocytes, fibrin, and other proteins that form exudates on the inflamed peritoneal surfaces and begin to form adhesions between peritoneal structures. This process, combined with a paralysis of the intestines (ileus), may result in confinement of the contamination to one or more locations within the peritoneum. Fluid also begins to collect in the bowel, and distention may result. The fluid and protein shift into the abdomen (third-spacing) may be so dramatic that circulating blood volume is decreased, which causes decreased cardiac output and possibly hypotension and shock. The fluid imbalance may be worsened by accompanying fever, vomiting, or diarrhea. A reflex sympathetic response, manifested by sweating, tachycardia, and vasoconstriction may be evident. With an inflamed peritoneum, bacteria and endotoxins are easily absorbed into the bloodstream (translocation), and this may result in septic shock. Other foreign substances that may be present in the peritoneal cavity potentiate peritonitis. These adjuvants, notably feces, dead tissues, barium, mucus, bile, and blood, have detrimental effects on host defense mechanisms, particularly on bacterial phagocytosis.

Many of the manifestations of intra-abdominal infections, particularly peritonitis, result from cytokine activity. Inflammatory cytokines, such as tumor necrosis factor (TNF)-α, interleukin-1 (IL-1), IL-6, and interferon (INF)-γ, are produced in response to bacteria and bacterial products or to tissue injury resulting from the surgical incision.[9] These cytokines produce wide-ranging effects on organs, particularly the liver and heart, as well as on endothelial cells. With uncontrolled activation of these mediators, sepsis may result (see Chap. 109).

Peritonitis often results in mortality because of the effects on major organ systems. As mentioned earlier, fluid shifts and endotoxins may cause hypotension and shock. Fluid loss from the vasculature with generalized peritonitis is similar to that which occurs after a 50% second-degree burn. Hypoalbuminemia may result from protein loss into the peritoneum. Pulmonary function may be compromised because the inflamed peritoneum causes splinting (muscle rigidity caused by pain) that inhibits proper ventilation. Then, atelectasis and pulmonary shunting of blood may result in respiratory distress syndrome and hypoxemia. With fluid loss and hypotension or sepsis, renal perfusion may be compromised and acute renal failure is a potential threat. In addition, endotoxin is hepatotoxic, and exposure during sepsis may lead to hepatic dysfunction.

If the body is successful in localizing peritoneal contamination but fails to eliminate bacteria completely, an abscess results. This collection of necrotic tissue, bacteria, and white blood cells (WBCs) may be at single or multiple sites and may be within one of the spaces of the peritoneal cavity or in one of the visceral organs. The location of the abscess is often related to the site of primary disease. For example, abscesses resulting from appendicitis tend to appear in the right lower quadrant or the pelvis; those resulting from diverticulitis tend to appear in the left lower quadrant or pelvis.

An abscess begins by the combined action of inflammatory cells (such as neutrophils), bacteria, fibrin, and other inflammatory components. Bacteria may release heparinases that cause local thrombosis and tissue necrosis or fibrinolysins, collagenases, or other enzymes that allow extension of the process into surrounding tissues. Neutrophils that have gathered in the abscess cavity die in 3 to 5 days, releasing lysosomal enzymes that liquefy the core of the abscess. A mature abscess may have a fibrinous capsule that isolates bacteria and the liquid core from antimicrobials and immunologic defenses.

In this environment, the oxygen tension is low, anaerobic bacteria thrive, and the size of the abscess may increase. Also, abscesses are hypertonic, resulting in an additional influx of fluid. Hypertonicity promotes the formation of bacterial L forms, which are resistant to antimicrobial agents that disrupt cell walls. This process may continue and stabilize for long periods of time and may not be readily evident to patient or physician. In some instances, the abscess may resolve, and infrequently, it may erode into adjacent organs or rupture and cause diffuse peritonitis. If the abscess erodes through the skin, it may result in a fistula, which connects the bowel to the skin, or a noncommunicating sinus tract.

MICROBIOLOGY OF INTRA-ABDOMINAL INFECTION

Primary bacterial peritonitis is often caused by a single organism. In children, the pathogen is usually *Streptococcus pneumoniae* or a group A streptococcus.[9] When peritonitis occurs in association with cirrhotic ascites, enteric organisms are usually responsible.[10,11] *Escherichia coli* is isolated most frequently, followed by streptococcal sp. (including pneumococcus), *Klebsiella, Bacteroides* sp., *Pseudomonas aeruginosa,* and numerous other organisms. Occasionally, primary peritonitis may be caused by *Mycobacterium tuberculosis.*

Peritonitis in patients undergoing peritoneal dialysis is most often caused by common skin organisms, such as *S. epidermidis, Staphylococcus aureus,* streptococci, and diphtheroids.[10] Occasionally, aerobic gram-negative bacilli may cause infections, particularly in patients undergoing dialysis during hospitalization.

Because of the diverse bacteria present in the GI tract, secondary intra-abdominal infections are often polymicrobial.[12] The mean number of different bacterial species isolated from infected intra-abdominal sites has ranged from 2.5 to 5.0, including an average of 1.4 to 2.0 aerobes and 2.4 to 3.0 anaerobes.[13,14] With proper anaerobic specimen collection, anaerobic organisms are isolated in most patients. In one report of patients with gangrenous and perforated appendicitis, an average of 10.2 different organisms was isolated from each patient, including 2.7 aerobes and 7.5 anaerobes.[15] Purely aerobic or anaerobic infections are uncommon, as are infections caused by fungi. The frequencies with which specific bacteria were isolated in intra-abdominal infections are given in Table 104–3.[16] *Escherichia coli* and *Bacteroides* sp. were most often isolated from the infection site, as well as from blood cultures. With patients who have severe infections, the pattern of bacterial isolates may change and may more commonly include *Candida, Enterococci, Enterobacter,* and *S. epidermidis.*[16]

Some visceral abscesses differ in character from the typical intra-abdominal abscess. Hepatic abscesses may be polymicrobial (involving *E. coli* and anaerobes) or occasionally may be caused by amoeba. Pancreatic abscesses are often polymicrobial, involving enteric bacteria that ascend through the biliary system. Splenic abscesses usually result from hematogenous dissemination of bacteria, such as *S. aureus,* streptococci, and occasionally *Salmonella* or anaerobic organisms.

BACTERIAL SYNERGISM

The size of the bacterial inoculum and the number and types of bacterial species present significantly affect patient outcome. The combination of aerobic and anaerobic organisms appears to increase the severity of infection greatly. In animal studies, combinations of aerobic and anaerobic bacteria were much more lethal than infections caused by the aerobes or anaerobes alone.

TABLE 104–3. Pathogens Isolated From 255 Patients With Intra-abdominal Infections[1]

Aerobic Bacteria	Number of Isolates	Anaerobic Bacteria	Number of Isolates
E. coli	140	*Bacteroides* sp.	305
Klebsiella sp.	33	*Peptostreptococcus*	78
Enterobacter sp.	19	*Fusobacteria*	48
Proteus sp.	15	*Clostridium*	35
Pseudomonas sp.	33	*Prevotella*	27
Streptococcus	184	*Gemella*	26
Enterococcus	35	*Porphyromonas*	18
Staphylococcus	34		
Others	24		

In intra-abdominal infections, facultative bacteria may provide an environment conducive to the growth of anaerobic bacteria.[12] Although many bacteria isolated in mixed infections are nonpathogenic by themselves, their presence may be essential for the pathogenicity of the bacterial mixture.[2] The role of facultative bacteria in mixed infections may include (1) promotion of an appropriate environment for anaerobic growth through oxygen consumption, (2) production of nutrients necessary for anaerobes, or (3) production of extracellular enzymes that promote tissue invasion by anaerobes. *Bacteroides fragilis* has a capsular polysaccharide complex that promotes the formation of intra-abdominal abscesses.[17]

Rat models of intra-abdominal infection have demonstrated that uncontrolled infection with a mix of aerobes and anaerobes leads to a two-stage infectious process. During the first 5 days after intra-abdominal implantation of gelatin capsules containing a mixture of 22 aerobic and anaerobic bacteria, acute generalized peritonitis was observed, and the mortality rate was 39%. After 5 days, mortality from intra-abdominal infection was not observed; however, almost all surviving animals had intra-abdominal abscesses when sacrificed at 2 weeks. During the peritonitis stages, *E. coli* was noted in the bloodstream of most animals, and *E. coli, B. fragilis,* and enterococci were isolated from peritoneal exudates. Bacteremia could not be demonstrated during the abscess stage, but abscesses were found to contain predominantly anaerobic bacteria *(B. fragilis* and *Fusobacterium varium). Escherichia coli* and enterococcus were also isolated from the abscess cavity. These experiments and others support the concept that aerobic enteric bacteria and anaerobic bacteria are pathogens in intra-abdominal infection. Aerobic bacteria, particularly *E. coli,* appear responsible for the early mortality from peritonitis, whereas anaerobic bacteria are major pathogens in abscesses, with *B. fragilis* predominating.

Enterococcus can be isolated from many intra-abdominal infections in humans, but its role as a pathogen is not clear.[18] Antimicrobial regimens that are not effective against enterococcus *in vitro* have been successful in treating intra-abdominal infections. Others have noted that enterococcal infection occurs in the presence of factors, indicating failure of the host's defenses (immunocompromised patients). One report suggested that isolation of enterococcus from an intra-abdominal focus was a predictor of treatment failure in complicated intra-abdominal infections.[19]

CLINICAL PRESENTATION

Intra-abdominal infections have a wide spectrum of manifestations, often depending on the specific disease process, the location and magnitude of bacterial contamination, and concurrent host factors. Peritonitis is usually easily recognized but intra-abdominal abscesses may often continue for considerable periods of time, either going unrecognized or attributed to an unrelated disease process.

Generalized bacterial peritonitis usually commands the immediate attention of the physician, because the patient most often presents in acute distress. The patient lies still, usually on his or her back, possibly with hips slightly flexed. Any movement of the patient, including deep breaths, worsens the generalized abdominal pain, so the patient exhibits voluntary guarding of the abdomen and respirations are shallow and frequent. There is generalized abdominal tenderness on examination and after a short period of time the abdominal muscles become rigid, a product of involuntary guarding; this is called a "board-like abdomen." Bowel sounds are at first faint, then become absent as peristalsis ceases and abdominal distention ensues. Sometimes the patient has nausea often accompanied by vomiting. The secretion of serous fluid into the peritoneal cavity causes the vascular volume to contract. This, as well as the physiologic response to stress, causes a reflex tachycardia. Initially, the patient's temperature is normal but increases to 100 to 102°F within the first few hours and may continue to rise for the next several hours. Because of the fluid loss into the peritoneum and vomiting, the patient may appear dehydrated, and a decreased urine output is noted.

If peritonitis continues untreated, the patient may experience hypovolemic shock from fluid loss into the peritoneum. This may be accompanied by sepsis because the inflamed peritoneum absorbs bacteria and toxins from the suppurative process into mesenteric blood vessels, which initiates production of inflammatory cytokines. Dehydration with hypovolemic shock is the major factor for mortality in the early stage of peritonitis.

Laboratory evaluations usually demonstrate leukocytosis (15,000 to 20,000 WBC/mm^3), with neutrophils predominating and an elevated count of immature neutrophils (bands). The hematocrit and the blood urea nitrogen may be elevated because of the dehydration. Early after the insult, the patient is usually alkalotic because of hyperventilation and vomiting. As the process progresses, the patient may become acidotic from hypovolemia or presence of devitalized tissue, which leads to anaerobic metabolism. At this stage, serum lactic acid will probably be elevated. Abdominal radiographs may be useful, as free air in the abdomen (indicating intestinal perforation) or distention of the small or large bowel is often evident.

The presentation of primary peritonitis can be quite different from that of secondary peritonitis. Primary peritonitis can develop over a period of days to weeks and is evident as an acute febrile illness. Usually the patient has nausea, vomiting (sometimes with diarrhea), abdominal tenderness, and hypoactive bowel sounds, although the abdominal signs are variable. The patient's temperature or WBC count may be only mildly elevated. The cirrhotic patient may have worsening encephalopathy.

Patients with peritonitis related to chronic peritoneal dialysis usually have abdominal pain and tenderness, possibly with nausea and vomiting, but fever is not a consistent finding. In these patients, a cloudy dialysate drainage is often noted as a first sign of peritonitis, indicating the presence of bacteria and inflammatory cells.

With primary peritonitis, routine evaluative procedures should be performed (serum chemistries, complete blood count, abdominal radiographs, blood cultures), and, if possible, the ascitic fluid, which is collected by paracentesis or peritoneal dialysate, should be examined. In the presence of peritonitis, ascitic fluid usually contains greater than 300 leukocytes/mm^3 and bacteria may be evident on Gram stain of a centrifuged specimen; however, in 60% to 80% of patients with cirrhotic ascites, the Gram stain is negative.

Intra-abdominal abscesses pose a difficult diagnostic challenge because the symptoms are often neither specific nor dramatic. The patient may complain of abdominal pain or discomfort, but these symptoms are not reliable. Fever is usually present; often it is low grade, but it can have a high, spiking pattern. The patient may have paralytic ileus and abdominal distention. The abdominal examination is unreliable; tenderness and pain may be present, and a mass may be palpated.

Peritonitis may result from an abscess that ruptures, spreading bacteria and toxins throughout the peritoneum. In other patients, the entry of bacterial toxins into the systemic circulation from the abscess may lead to sepsis and progressive multisystem organ failure (renal, hepatic, or cardiac).

Laboratory studies are generally not helpful in the diagnosis of intra-abdominal abscess, although most patients will have leukocytosis. Some patients may have positive blood cultures, whereas others, particularly diabetics, may have hyperglycemia. The finding of *Bacteroides* or any two enteric bacteria in the bloodstream is often indicative of an intra-abdominal infectious process.

Radiographic methods are used to make the diagnosis of an intra-abdominal abscess. Plain radiographs may show air–fluid levels or may demonstrate the shift of normal intra-abdominal contents by the abscess mass. Gastrointestinal contrast studies may also demonstrate this displacement of abdominal structures. Both of these modalities provide indirect evidence of the abscess presence but are not generally helpful in precisely locating the abscess.

Ultrasound is frequently the first diagnostic method used when the presence of an intra-abdominal abscess is suspected. The procedure may be done at the bedside, which is particularly helpful in the patient in the intensive care unit. The other advantage of this procedure is that it involves no radiation exposure. Limitations of ultrasound include difficulty in distinguishing between an early abscess and loops of the intestine. In some patients, particularly the obese, it is technically impossible to perform the exam.[20]

Computed tomography (CT) scan is frequently used to evaluate the abdomen for the presence of an abscess. Oral radiocontrast agents may be given to allow differentiation of the abscess from the bowel. Intravenous radiocontrast agents will be taken up preferentially in the wall of the abscess, creating a unique radiographic appearance.

Magnetic resonance imaging might be used to locate some intra-abdominal abscesses, particularly in the retroperitoneum but this modality offers no advantage when compared to CT scan and is infrequently used.

The final diagnostic imaging modality is radioactive isotope imaging. Specific techniques include the use of gallium ga-67 citrate, technetium Tc^{99m}, and ^{111}In-labeled leukocytes.[21] These studies require a long period of imaging and are not routinely employed.

Intra-abdominal infection caused by disease processes at specific sites often produces characteristic manifestations that are helpful in diagnosis. For example, a patient with diverticulitis may exhibit stabbing left lower quadrant abdominal pain and constipation. Fever and leukocytosis are often present, and a tender mass is sometimes palpable. With appendicitis, the findings may be inconsistent, but many patients have a sudden onset of periumbilical or epigastric pain, which is usually colicky and shifts to the right lower quadrant. The location of pain may vary, as the appendix can be in many locations in the abdomen. A mass may be palpable on abdominal or rectal examination. The patient's temperature is generally mildly elevated early and then increases. If perforation and diffuse peritonitis were to occur, the manifestations just described would apply. More frequently, however, appendiceal perforation results in a local abscess.

Abscesses in specific locations may produce clues to their existence. Pelvic abscesses may be palpable by pelvic examination. A subdiaphragmatic abscess may result in pleural effusion or dyspnea. Retroperitoneal abscesses may cause lumbar or psoas muscle spasm resulting in lower back pain and may cause the patient to flex the legs at the hip.

The presentation and outcome of any intra-abdominal infection are significantly influenced by patient specific factors. Those who are malnourished, have undergone multiple traumatic injuries, or are at the extremes of age are more likely to succumb to intra-abdominal infection or require an extended period for recovery. In addition to these factors, those with associated diseases, such as diabetes mellitus, malignancies, renal failure, and cirrhosis, are recognized to be immunocompromised and at greater risk for most infectious processes, including intra-abdominal infections. Other risk factors often related to intra-abdominal infection are the use of corticosteroids, particularly in patients with Crohn's disease, and radiation therapy for tumors. Also, use of antimicrobial agents may prevent the prompt diagnosis of abscesses, particularly subphrenic. In some instances, acute intra-abdominal infectious processes may become chronic with the initiation of antimicrobial agents. Geriatric patients with intra-abdominal infection frequently present without the typical signs and symptoms of abdominal pain, nausea, vomiting, diarrhea, and fever.[22]

▶ TREATMENT: Intra-abdominal Infections

DESIRED OUTCOME

The goals of treatment are the correction of intra-abdominal disease processes or injuries that have caused infection and the drainage of collections of purulent material (abscess). For primary and secondary intra-abdominal infections, the infectious process should resolve within a few days. A secondary objective is to achieve a resolution without major organ system complications (pneumonia or renal failure) or adverse drug effects. Ideally, the patient should be discharged from the hospital with full function for self-care and routine daily activities.

GENERAL APPROACH TO TREATMENT

The treatment of intra-abdominal infection most often requires the coordinated use of three major modalities (1) prompt drainage, (2) support of vital functions, and (3) appropriate antimicrobial therapy to treat bacteria not removed by surgery.

Antimicrobials are an important adjunct to drainage procedures in the treatment of intra-abdominal infections; however, the use of antimicrobial agents without surgical intervention is usually inadequate. For some specific situations (e.g., most cases of primary peritonitis), drainage procedures may not be required, and antimicrobial agents become the mainstay of therapy.

In the early phase of serious intra-abdominal infections, much attention should be paid to the maintenance of body organ system functions. With generalized peritonitis, large volumes of intravenous (IV) fluids are required to restore vascular volume, improve cardiovascular function, and maintain adequate tissue oxygenation. Adequate urine output should be maintained to ensure proper renal function. This is done by correcting hypovolemia and restoring cardiac output. Respiratory function can be assisted by a variety of methods, including ventilatory support in severely ill patients. Often, the critically ill patient with intra-abdominal infection will require intensive care monitoring, particularly if there is cardiovascular or respiratory instability. Also, isolation procedures may be required if the infectious process poses a threat to other hospitalized patients.

An additional important component of therapy is parenteral nutrition. Intra-abdominal infections often directly involve the GI tract or disrupt its function (paralytic ileus). The return of GI motility may take days, weeks, and occasionally months. In the interim, parenteral nutrition allows patient recovery and wound healing while maintaining nutritional status.

NONPHARMACOLOGIC TREATMENT

DRAINAGE PROCEDURES

Primary peritonitis is treated with antimicrobials and does not require drainage. Secondary peritonitis requires surgical correction of the underlying pathology. The drainage of the purulent material is the critical element in the management of an intra-abdominal abscess. Without adequate drainage of the abscess, antimicrobial therapy and fluid resuscitation can be expected to fail.

Secondary peritonitis is treated surgically. At the time of laparotomy, attempts are made to correct the cause of the peritonitis. This may include patching a perforated ulcer with omentum, resection of a segment of perforated colon, or resection of a portion of gangrenous small intestine. The goal of all of these procedures is to remove the inflamed or gangrenous viscous and prevent further bacterial contamination. The presence of active inflammation increases the difficulty of the surgical procedure. This results in a higher morbidity and mortality rate than if the same procedures were performed in an elective setting without inflammation.

The presence of active inflammation may make it technically impossible to perform the definitive surgical procedure. In this situation, attempts are made to provide drainage of the infected or gangrenous structures. An example of this situation is empyema of the gallbladder. If it is unsafe or impossible to perform the cholecystectomy, then a tube is placed into the gallbladder. This procedure, cholecystostomy, provides for drainage of the purulent material present in the gallbladder. The gallbladder would then be removed at a subsequent operation.

If an intra-abdominal abscess, separate from any intra-abdominal organ, is discovered during an exploratory laparotomy, then it may be debrided, excised, or drained. If the intra-abdominal abscess involves an abdominal structure, then a resection of part or all of that organ may be required. An example of this situation is an abscess associated with diverticular disease of the colon. Management may include drainage of the abscess and resection of the involved colon. All foreign material, necrotic tissue, feces, blood, or pus should be removed from the operative field, and the peritoneum should be copiously irrigated with 0.9% sodium chloride to decrease the concentrations of bacteria or other noxious substances.

Once an abscess is located, it must be drained. This may be performed surgically or using percutaneous, image-guided techniques.[23,24] Typically, image-guided techniques are done using ultrasound or CT. The management of intra-abdominal abscess with percutaneous catheter drainage may represent the definitive procedure or the patient may require a subsequent procedure to treat the underlying conditions. In this latter circumstance, a significant advantage is obtained by first draining the abscess percutaneously. This allows the surgical procedure to be performed on a patient who is no longer suffering the systemic manifestations of uncontrolled infections.

A number of drainage techniques have been described using endoscopy and laparoscopy.[25,26] These minimal access techniques may offer some advantages when compared to traditional surgery but will probably be used less often than radiologic assisted percutaneous drainage techniques.

The most valuable microbiologic information may be obtained at the time of operation or percutaneous abscess drainage. If pus or fluids are found that are believed to be infected, it is best to aspirate 2 to 3 mL into a syringe, remove any air, and tightly cap the syringe. The specimen should be taken promptly to the microbiology laboratory where a Gram stain should be performed immediately and cultures prepared for identification of aerobic bacteria and anaerobic bacteria. If there is no fluid available for collection, culture swab devices may be applied to the infected area. A swab transported under anaerobic conditions is required, and it should be analyzed as just described.

FLUID THERAPY

Aggressive fluid repletion and management are required for successful treatment of intra-abdominal infections. Fluid therapy is instituted for the purposes of achieving or maintaining proper intravascular volumes and adequate urine output and correcting acidosis. Intravascular volume is often decreased in patients with severe intra-abdominal infections because fluids accumulate in the abdomen; they collect in a third space at the expense of the plasma volume. Loss of fluid through vomiting, diarrhea, or a nasogastric suction tube contributes to dehydration. Intravascular volume can be assessed by blood pressure and heart rate but more accurately by measurement of central venous pressure or pulmonary capillary wedge pressure. When a contracted vascular volume is accompanied by hemorrhage, the hematocrit initially is about normal, but if there is no hemorrhage, the hematocrit is usually elevated as an indication of hemoconcentration. Urine output should be continuously monitored in severely ill patients by use of a transurethral bladder catheter, quantitated hourly, and it should equal or exceed 1 mL/kg body weight per hour.

In patients with peritonitis, hypovolemia is often accompanied by acidosis, so a reasonable IV fluid would be lactated Ringer's, which contains the bicarbonate precursor, lactate, as well as sodium, potassium, and calcium. In the initial hour of treatment, a large volume of solution may need to be administered to restore intravascular volume. Although this volume may frequently approach 4 L, much more fluid may be required to restore vital functions. For a few hours thereafter, fluids may be required at a rate of 1 L/hour. Maintenance fluids should be instituted (after intravascular volume is restored) with 0.9% sodium chloride and potassium chloride (20 mEq/L) or 5% dextrose and 0.45% sodium chloride with potassium chloride (20 mEq/L). The administration rate should be based on estimated daily fluid loss through urine and nasogastric suction, including 0.5 to 1.0 L for insensible fluid loss. Potassium would not routinely be included if the patient is hyperkalemic or has renal failure.

In patients with significant blood loss, blood should be given. This is generally in the form of packed red blood cells. The criteria for blood transfusion are controversial, but a hematocrit of 25% is generally accepted. In the individual patient, the decision is often determined by the overall clinical status and the ability of the patient to compensate for the reduction in oxygen-carrying capacity associated with an acute anemia. Additional blood component therapy with clotting factors or platelets is also based on the needs of the individual patient. Aggressive fluid therapy must often be continued in the postoperative period, as fluid will continue to sequester in the peritoneal cavity causing hypovolemia.

PHARMACOLOGIC TREATMENT

ANTIMICROBIAL THERAPY

The goals of antimicrobial therapy are to (1) control bacteremia and the establishment of metastatic foci of infection, (2) reduce suppurative complications after bacterial contamination, and (3) prevent local spread of existing infection. Once suppuration has occurred (e.g., an abscess has formed), a cure by antibiotic alone is very difficult to achieve; antimicrobials may serve to improve the results that would have been attained with surgery alone.

An empiric antimicrobial regimen should be started as soon as the presence of intra-abdominal infection is suspected. Therefore, they are usually begun before identification of infecting bacteria is complete. Therapy must be initiated based on the likely pathogens. Predominant pathogens, as discussed in the previous section, vary depending on the site of intra-abdominal infection and the underlying disease process. Likely pathogens, those against which antimicrobial agents should be directed, are listed in Table 104–4.

ANTIMICROBIAL EXPERIENCE

Many studies have been conducted evaluating or comparing the effectiveness of antimicrobials for treatment of intra-abdominal infections. Substantial differences in patient outcomes from treatment with a variety of agents have generally not been demonstrated. Trials of antimicrobial therapy for intra-abdominal infection often had serious defects in design, and these defects usually prevented the detection of differences between agents. One investigator found that there was no difference in clinical outcomes between two regimens with disparate activity against intra-abdominal isolates (cefoxitin and imipenem/cilistatin).[27] Ninety-eight percent of isolates were susceptible to imipenem/cilistatin and 72% to cefoxitin.

Important findings regarding selection of antimicrobials from the last 20 years of clinical trials with intra-abdominal infections are:

1. Single-agent regimens (such as second-generation cephalosporins, extended spectrum penicillins, or carbapenems) have been as effective as

TABLE 104–4. Likely Intra-abdominal Pathogens

Type of Infection	Aerobes	Anaerobes
Primary Bacterial Peritonitis		
Children (spontaneous)	Pneumococci, group A *Streptococcus*	—
Cirrhosis	*E. coli, Klebsiella,* pneumococci (many others)	—
Peritoneal dialysis	*Staphylococcus, Streptococcus*	—
Secondary Bacterial Peritonitis		
Gastroduodenal	*Streptococcus, E. coli*	—
Biliary tract	*E. coli, Klebsiella,* enterococci	*Clostridium* or *Bacteroides* (infrequent)
Small or large bowel	*E. coli, Klebsiella* sp., *Proteus* sp.	*Bacteroides fragilis* and other *Bacteroides, Clostridium*
Appendicitis	*E. coli, Pseudomonas*	*Bacteroides* sp.
Abscesses	*E. coli, Klebsiella,* enterococci	*B. fragilis* and other *Bacteroides, Clostridium,* anaerobic cocci
Liver	*E. coli, Klebsiella,* enterococci staphylococci, amoeba	*Bacteroides* (infrequent)
Spleen	*Staphylococcus, Streptococcus*	

combinations of aminoglycosides with antianaerobic agents. This is also true for antimicrobial treatment of acute bacterial contamination from penetrating abdominal trauma.[28,29]

2. Clindamycin and metronidazole appear to be equivalent in efficacy when combined with agents effective against aerobic, gram-negative bacilli (gentamicin or aztreonam).

A number of studies have been conducted in patients with established intra-abdominal infections. A compilation of some notable studies is provided in Table 104–5. Generally, these studies do not demonstrate clinical differences between agents, although it is doubtful that many of the studies would have detected clinically significant differences in patient outcome, because the numbers of patients studied were often too few.

Intra-abdominal infection presents in many different ways and with a wide spectrum of severity. The regimen employed and duration of treatment depend on the specific clinical circumstances (i.e., the nature of the underlying disease process and the condition of the patient). Compromised patients require more aggressive therapies than otherwise healthy patients who experience the same intra-abdominal infection.

RECOMMENDATIONS

For most intra-abdominal infections, the antimicrobial regimen should be effective against both aerobic and anaerobic bacteria.[32] Although it is impossible to provide antimicrobial activity against every possible pathogen, agents with activity against enteric gram-negative bacilli, such as *E. coli* and *Klebsiella,* and anaerobes such as *B. fragilis* and *Clostridia* sp., should be administered. If most of the organisms can be eliminated through drainage or antimicrobials, the synergistic effect may be removed and the patient's defenses may be able to eradicate the remaining organisms.

Table 104–6 presents recommended and alternative regimens for selected situations. These are general guidelines, not rules, because there are many factors that cannot be incorporated into such a table.

Most patients with severe intra-abdominal infections where there is generalized peritonitis or sepsis should be placed on a β-lactam (antianaerobic cephalosporins, with or without metronidazole, or carbapenems) or a penicillin/β-lactamase inhibitor combination. Combinations of an aminoglycoside in with an antianaerobic agent, such as clindamycin or metronidazole, may be used but is considered by some to be obsolete.[1] Gentamicin is the aminoglycoside of choice based on its lower cost. Other aminoglycosides, such as tobramycin, amikacin, and netilmicin, have no advantages in intra-abdominal infections and are generally not drugs of first choice. Aztreonam may be used as an alternative to aminoglycosides.

The dosage for aminoglycosides should be adjusted on the basis of a patient's weight and renal function. Because the enteric gram-negative bacilli are usually very susceptible to aminoglycosides and because aminoglycosides are well distributed into peritoneal fluid,[33] high serum aminoglycoside concentrations are generally not required. Unless relatively resistant bacteria are suspected, a gentamicin or tobramycin peak concentration of 5 to 6 μg/mL will usually be effective. To achieve these serum concentrations, gentamicin or tobramycin dosage may range from 1 to 3 mg/kg per dose given as often as every 6 hours or as infrequently as every 48 hours if the patient has renal failure. Since aminoglycosides have concentration-dependent killing and a relatively long postantibiotic effect for aerobic gram-negative bacilli, once-daily administration is a reasonable alternative and appears to be equivalent to multiple daily dosing.

TABLE 104–5. Some Comparative Studies of Intra-abdominal Infection

Investigators	Agent(s) Tested	Number of Patients Studied	Percent of Patients With Satisfactory Outcome
Solomkin et al., 1990[29]	Imipenem/cilistatin	81	83
	Tobramycin/clindamycin	81	70
Brismar et al., 1992[30]	Imipenem/cilistatin	58	69
	Piperacillin/tazobactam	55	93
Cristou et al., 1996[27]	Cefoxitin	109	82
	Imipenem/cilistatin	104	83
Wilson, 1997[31]	Meropenem	97	92
	Tobramycin/clindamycin	94	86

TABLE 104–6. Recommendations for Initial Antimicrobial Agents for Intra-abdominal Infections

Primary Bacterial Peritonitis		
Cirrhosis	Cefotaxime	1. Add clindamycin or metronidazole if anaerobes are suspected 2. Other third-generation cephalosporins, extended-spectrum penicillins, aztreonam, and imipenem as alternatives 3. Aminoglycoside with antipseudomonal penicillin
Peritoneal dialysis	Regimen based on organism isolated 1. *Staphylococcus:* penicillinase-resistant penicillin or first-generation cephalosporin 2. *Streptococcus:* penicillin G 3. Aerobic gram-negative bacilli: cefotaxime, ceftazidime, or aminoglycoside plus an antipseudomonal penicillin 4. *Pseudomonas aeruginosa*: aminoglycoside plus antipseudomonal penicillin or ceftazidime	1. Alternative for resistant staphylococci is vancomycin 2. Alternative for *Streptococcus* is a first-generation cephalosporin 3. Alternatives for gram-negative bacilli are other third-generation cephalosporins, aztreonam, and extended-spectrum penicillins with β-lactamase inhibitors
Secondary Bacterial Peritonitis		
Perforated peptic ulcer	First-generation cephalosporins	1. Antianaerobic cephalosporins[a] 2. Possibly add aminoglycoside if patient condition is poor
Other	Imipenem/cilistatin, antianaerobic cephalosporins[a], or extended-spectrum penicillins with β-lactamase inhibitor	1. Aminoglycoside with clindamycin or metronidazole, add ampicillin if patient is immunocompromised or if biliary tract origin of infection 2. Aztreonam with clindamycin 3. Antianaerobic cephalosporins or an extended-spectrum penicillin with β-lactamase inhibitor
Abscess		
General	Imipenem/cilistatin, antianaerobic cephalosporins[a], or extended-spectrum penicillins with β-lactamase inhibitor	1. Aztreonam with clindamycin or extended-spectrum penicillins with β-lactamase inhibitor, as alternatives 2. Aminoglycoside with clindamycin or metronidazole, possibly add ampicillin
Liver	As above but add a first-generation cephalosporin	3. Use metronidazole if amoebic liver abscess is suspected
Spleen	Aminoglycoside plus penicillinase-resistant penicillin	4. Alternatives for penicillinase-resistant penicillin are first-generation cephalosporins or vancomycin
Appendicitis		
Normal or inflamed	Antianaerobic cephalosporins[a] (discontinued immediately postoperation)	1. Aminoglycoside with clindamycin or metronidazole
Gangrenous or perforated	Imipenem/cilistatin, antianaerobic cephalosporins[a] or extended-spectrum penicillins with β-lactamase inhibitor	1. Aztreonam with clindamycin, or imipenem alone 2. Aminoglycoside with clindamycin or metronidazole
Acute Cholecystitis	First-generation cephalosporin	Aminoglycoside plus ampicillin if severe infection
Cholangitis	Aminoglycoside with ampicillin with or without clindamycin or metronidazole	Use vancomycin for ampicillin if patient is allergic to penicillin
Acute Contamination from Abdominal Trauma	Antianaerobic cephalosporins[a] or extended-spectrum penicillins	Aminoglycoside with one of the following: clindamycin, metronidazole, or antianaerobic cephalosporins[a]

[a]Cefoxitin, cefotetan, ceftizoxime, and cefmetazole.

When used for intra-abdominal infection, aminoglycosides should be combined with agents that are effective against the majority of *B. fragilis.* Clindamycin or metronidazole would be the agents of first choice but others, such as antianaerobic cephalosporins (cefoxitin, cefotetan, ceftizoxime, or cefmetazole), piperacillin, mezlocillin, and combinations of extended-spectrum penicillins with β-lactamase, would be suitable alternatives. Clindamycin should be administered intravenously in a dosage of 600 or 900 mg every 8 hours. Patients receiving multiple, broad-spectrum antimicrobial agents who are immunocompromised should receive an oral antifungal agent for prevention of fungal overgrowth in the mouth and GI tract. The benefits of systemic antifungal prophylaxis (with fluconazole) have not been established for intra-abdominal infection and should not routinely be used.

With intra-abdominal contamination from the upper GI tract (perforation of a peptic ulcer or biliary tract disease), *B. fragilis* is an uncommon pathogen and other agents may, therefore, be substituted for clindamycin or metronidazole. Alternatives would include ampicillin, penicillin, or first-generation cephalosporins.

Ampicillin may be added to combinations of aminoglycosides and clindamycin or metronidazole to assure antimicrobial coverage for enterococci, although this is controversial.[34] Regimens without activity against enterococci (gentamicin with clindamycin or cephalosporins) are generally effective in treating these infections; however, there are numerous reports of enterococcal superinfection in immunocompromised patients, particularly after cephalosporin use. Enterococcus is the most common gram-positive isolate.[35]

The failure of host defenses may be a critical factor in the pathogenicity of enterococci. In immunocompromised patients or patients with valvular heart disease or a prosthetic heart valve,[36] there is justification to provide specific antimicrobial activity against enterococci. Ampicillin or other penicillins that are active against enterococci (penicillin, piperacillin, mezlocillin) should be used in patients at high risk, patients with persistent or recurrent intra-abdominal infection, patients in shock, or patients who are immunosuppressed, such as after organ transplantation. Ampicillin remains the drug of choice for this purpose because it is most active *in vitro* against enterococci and is relatively inexpensive. Vancomycin is active against most enterococci; however, resistance is increasing, and this agent should be reserved for established infections when first-line therapies cannot be used.

With peritonitis that occurs from chronic peritoneal dialysis (CPD), the antimicrobial regimen used should be tailored to the isolated organism. The selection of a specific agent or combination should be based on culture and susceptibility data. If microbiologic data are unavailable, empiric therapy with a first-generation cephalosporin plus an aminoglycoside is recommended. In less severe infections, a first-generation cephalosporin alone given intraperitoneally may suffice. Infection with staphylococci may be treated with a penicillinase-resistant penicillin (methicillin, nafcillin, oxacillin), first-generation cephalosporins, or vancomycin if the patient is allergic to penicillin or the isolate is resistant to methicillin. For streptococcal infections, penicillin or ampicillin would be preferable to penicillinase-resistant penicillins. Most aerobic gram-negative bacilli may be effectively treated with an aminoglycoside. For infections caused by *P. aeruginosa,* an antipseudomonal penicillin (ticarcillin, piperacillin, mezlocillin, or azlocillin) or ceftazidime may be added.

Patients with peritonitis who are undergoing CPD may receive parenteral, as well as intraperitoneal, antimicrobial agents. Intraperitoneal antimicrobial agents alone are often sufficient, unless severe infection is present. A number of agents may be instilled through peritoneal catheters. Recommended concentrations of antimicrobial agents for intraperitoneal irrigation solutions are 8 mg/L for gentamicin and tobramycin, 1 to 3 mg/L for clindamycin, 50,000 U/L for penicillin G, 125 mg/L for cephalosporins, 100 to 150 mg/L for ticarcillin or carbenicillin, 50 mg/L for ampicillin, 100 mg/L for methicillin, 30 mg/L for vancomycin, and 3 mg/L for amphotericin B.[37]

The usual duration of therapy for peritonitis associated with CPD is 10 to 14 days, but it may extend to 3 weeks. Antimicrobial therapy should be continued until dialysate fluid is clear, cultures are negative for 2 to 3 days, and the patient is asymptomatic. When parenteral agents are administered, the initial dose would be the same as that for patients with normal renal function, while subsequent doses should be much less or given less frequently for renally excreted agents and should account for possible loss through peritoneal dialysis. Serum concentrations should be performed for aminoglycosides and vancomycin. Some studies have demonstrated that in patients with spontaneous bacterial peritonitis associated with cirrhotic ascites, treatment duration may be a short as 5 days when ascitic fluid polymorphonuclear cell counts are used to guide treatment.[38,39]

After acute bacterial contamination, such as with abdominal trauma where GI contents enter the peritoneum, combination antimicrobial regimens are not required. If the patient is seen soon after injury (within 2 hours) and surgical measures are instituted promptly, single-agent regimens, such as antianaerobic cephalosporins or extended-spectrum penicillins, are effective in preventing most infectious complications. Antimicrobials should be begun as soon as possible after injury.

For appendicitis, the antimicrobial regimen used should depend on the appearance of the appendix at the time of operation, which may be normal, inflamed, gangrenous, or perforated. Because the condition of the appendix is unknown preoperatively, it is advisable to begin antimicrobial agents before the appendectomy is performed. Reasonable regimens would be antianaerobic cephalosporins or, if the patient is seriously ill, a combination of aminoglycoside with clindamycin or metronidazole. If, at operation, the appendix is found to be normal or inflamed, postoperative antimicrobials would not be required. If the appendix is gangrenous or perforated, a treatment course of 7 to 10 days with the agents listed in Table 104–6 would be appropriate.

The necessary duration of treatment for intra-abdominal infections is not clearly defined. Acute intra-abdominal contamination, such as after a traumatic injury, may be treated with a very short course (24 hours). For established infections (peritonitis or intra-abdominal abscess), an antimicrobial course of at least 7 days is justified. This allows eradication of bacteria that may remain in the peritoneum after a surgical procedure or bacteria that may enter the peritoneum through healing suture lines. Comparative studies examining shorter courses of therapy (2 or 3 days) have not been conducted to verify that longer courses are essential. Under certain conditions, therapy for longer than 7 days would be justified; for example, if the patient remains febrile or is in poor general condition, when relatively resistant bacteria are isolated, or when a focus of infection in the abdomen may still be present. For some abscesses, such as pyogenic liver abscess, antimicrobials may be required for a month or longer.

Intraperitoneal irrigation of antimicrobial agents for treatment of intra-abdominal infection has often been studied with somewhat conflicting results.[40] Intraoperative antimicrobial irrigation has not been shown to improve patient outcomes in comparison with copious intraoperative irrigation with normal saline. Possibly the most important aspect of peritoneal irrigation is the dilutional effect on bacteria and adjuvants or substances that promote infection (intestinal contents and hemoglobin). As discussed before, investigators have shown that most systemically administered antimicrobials easily cross the peritoneal membrane so that peritoneal fluid concentrations are similar to serum.[33,41] Confined areas, such as abscess, could be expected to attain much lower antimicrobial concentrations.

EVALUATION OF THERAPEUTIC OUTCOMES

Whichever antimicrobial regimen is chosen, the patient should be continually reassessed to determine the success or failure of therapies. The clinician should recognize that there are many reasons for poor outcome of patients with intra-abdominal infection; improper antimicrobial administration is only one. The patient may be immunocompromised, which decreases the likelihood of successful outcome with any regimen. It is impossible for antimicrobials to compensate totally for a nonfunctioning immune system. There may be surgical reasons for poor patient outcome. Failure to identify all intra-abdominal foci of infection or leaks from a GI anastomosis may cause continued intra-abdominal infection. Even when intra-abdominal infection is controlled, accompanying organ system failure, most often renal or respiratory, but possibly hepatic or cardiac, may lead to patient demise.

The outcome from intra-abdominal infection is not determined solely by what transpires in the abdomen. Unsatisfactory outcomes in patients with intra-abdominal infections may result from complications that arise in other organ systems. A complication commonly associated with mortality after intra-abdominal infection is pneumonia.[42,43] In fact, one investigator found that the cause of death in patients with intra-abdominal infection was more likely related to the lower respiratory tract than the abdomen.[42] A high APACHE II score, low serum albumin, and high New York Heart Association cardiac function status were significantly and independently associated with mortality for intra-abdominal infection.[44]

Once antimicrobials are initiated and the other important therapies described earlier are used, most patients should show improvement within 2 to 3 days. Usually, temperature will return to near normal, vital signs should stabilize, and the patient should not appear in distress with the exception of recognized discomfort and pain from incisions, drains, and nasogastric tube. At 24 to 48 hours, aerobic bacterial culture results should return. If a suspected pathogen is not sensitive to the antimicrobial agents being given, the regimen should be changed if the patient has not shown sufficient progress. If the isolated pathogen is extremely sensitive to one antimicrobial and the patient is progressing well, concurrent antimicrobial therapy may often be discontinued. While some investigators have suggested that routine culturing of patients with community-acquired intra-abdominal infections contributes little to their management.[45] Others have suggested that antimicrobial therapy should be based on susceptibility of the flora collected from the operative site since this has been shown to correlate with clinical outcome.[46]

With present anaerobic culturing techniques and the slow growth of these organisms, anaerobes are often not identified until 4 to 7 days after culture, and sensitivity information is difficult to obtain. For this reason there are usually few data with which to alter the antianaerobic component of the antimicrobial regimen. A report indicating that anaerobes were not isolated should not be the sole justification for discontinuing antianaerobic drugs because anaerobic bacteria that were present in the infectious process may not have been properly transported to the microbiology laboratory or other problems may have led to cell death *in vitro*.

Reasons for antimicrobial failure may not always be apparent. Even when antimicrobial susceptibility tests indicate that an organism is susceptible to the antimicrobial *in vitro,* therapeutic failures may occur. Possibly there is poor penetration of the antimicrobial into the focus of infection, or, after initiation of antimicrobial therapy, bacterial resistance may develop. Also, it is possible that an antimicrobial regimen may encourage the development of infection by organisms not susceptible to the regimen being used. Superinfection in patients being treated for intra-abdominal infection is often caused by *Candida,* but enterococci or opportunistic gram-negative bacilli such as *Pseudomonas* or *Serratia* may be involved.

Treatment regimens for intra-abdominal infection can be judged successful if the patient recovers from the infection without recurrent peritonitis or intra-abdominal abscess and without the need for additional antimicrobials. A regimen can be considered unsuccessful if a significant adverse drug reaction occurs, reoperation is necessary, or patient improvement is delayed beyond 1 or 2 weeks.

▶ PRINCIPLES OF PHARMACOTHERAPY

- Most secondary intra-abdominal infections are caused by a defect in the gastrointestinal tract that must be treated by surgical drainage and repair.
- Secondary intra-abdominal infections are usually caused by a mixture of enteric gram-negative bacilli and anaerobes.
- For peritonitis, early and aggressive intravenous fluid and electrolyte therapy is essential.
- Antimicrobial regimens for secondary intra-abdominal infections should include coverage for enteric gram-negative bacilli and anaerobes. Regimens that may be used for treatment of secondary intra-abdominal infections include (a) an aminoglycoside plus clindamycin (or metronidazole), (b) aztreonam plus clindamycin, (c) imipenem/cilistatin, (d) extended spectrum penicillins with β-lactamase inhibitors, or (e) antianaerobic cephalosporins.
- Cultures of secondary intra-abdominal infection sites are generally not useful for directing antimicrobial therapy.
- Antimicrobial regimens should be adjusted to provide excellent activity against any pathogens isolated from blood specimens.
- The duration of antimicrobial treatment has not been well established but should extend 3 to 4 days beyond the return to normal body temperature and white blood cell count.
- Primary peritonitis is generally caused by a single organism (*Staphylococcus aureus* in patients undergoing chronic ambulatory peritoneal dialysis [CAPD] or *Escherichia coli* in patients with cirrhosis).
- Treatment of primary peritonitis for CAPD patients should include an antistaphylococcal antimicrobial, such as a first-generation cephalosporin or vancomycin (usually given by the intraperitoneal route).
- Patients treated for intra-abdominal infections should be assessed for the occurrence of drug-related adverse effects, particularly hypersensitivity reactions (β-lactam antimicrobials), diarrhea (most agents), fungal infections (most agents), and nephrotoxicity (aminoglycosides).

REFERENCES

1. Whittmann DH, Schein M, Condon RE. Management of secondary peritonitis. Ann Surg 1996;224:10–18.
2. Johnson CC, Baldessarre J, Levinson ME. Peritonitis: Update on pathophysiology, clinical manifestations, and management. Clin Infec Dis 1997;24:1035–1047.
3. Saklayen MG. CAPD peritonitis. Incidence: pathogens, diagnosis, and management. Med Clin North Am 1990;74:997–1010.
4. Linblad AS, Novak JW, Nolph KD, et al. The 1987 USA National CAPD Registry report. Trans Am Soc Artif Intern Organs 1988;34:150–156.
5. Graves EJ. Detailed diagnoses and procedures, Nation Hospital Discharge Survey, 1990, National Center for Health Statistics. Vital Health Stat 13 1992;113–225.
6. Ruddell WSF, Axon ATR, Findlay JM, et al. The effect of cimetidine on gastric bacterial flora. Lancet 1980;1:672–674.
7. Toloza EM, Wilson SE. Cholecystitis and cholangitis. In: Fry DE, ed. Surgical Infections. Boston, Little, Brown, 1995:254.
8. Keene WF, Alexander SR, Bailie GR, et al. Peritoneal dialysis—Related peritonitis treatment recommendations: 1996 update. Periton Dialys Internat 1996;16:557–573.
9. Schein M, Wittman DH, Holzheimer R, et al. Hypothesis: Compartmentalization of cytokines in intraabdominal infection. Surgery 1996; 119:694–700.
10. Bhuva M, Ganger D, Jensen D. Spontaneous bacterial peritonitis: An update on evaluation, management, and prevention. Am J Med 1994; 97:169–175.
11. Gilbert J, Kamath PS. Spontaneous bacterial peritonitis: An update. May Clin Proc 1995;70:365–370.
12. McClean KL, Shhehan GJ, Harding GKM. Intraabdominal infection: A review. Clin Infec Dis 1994:19:100–116.
13. Lorber B, Swenson RM. The bacteriology of intra-abdominal infections. Surg Clin North Am 1975;55:1249–1355.
14. Nichols RL. Empiric antibiotic therapy of intraabdominal infections. Rev Infect Dis 1983;5(suppl):590–597.
15. Bennion RS, Baron EJ, Thompson JE, et al. The bacteriology of gangrenous and perforated appendicitis—Revisited. Ann Surg 1990;211: 165–171.
16. Sawyer RG, Rosenlof LK, Adams RB, et al. Peritonitis into the 1990s: Changing pathogens and changing strategies in the critically ill. Am Surgeon 1992;58:82–87.
17. Tzianabos AO, Kasper DL, Onderdonk AB. Structure and function of *Bacteroides fragilis* capsular polysaccharides: Relationship to induction and prevention of abscesses. Clin Infec Dis 1995;20(suppl 2): S132–S140.
18. Montravers P, Andremont A, Massias L, Carbon C. Investigation of the potential role of *Enterococcus faecalis* in the pathophysiology of experimental peritonitis. J Infec Dis 1994;169:821–830.
19. Burnett RJ, Haverstock DC, Dellinger EP, et al. Definition of the role of enterococcus in intraabdominal infection: Analysis of a prospective randomized trial. Surgery 1995;118:721–723.
20. Gazelle GS, Mueller PR. Abdominal abscess: Imaging and intervention. Radiol Clin North Am 1994;32:913–932.
21. Datz FL. Abdominal abscess detection: Gallium, ^{111}In-, and ^{99m}Tc-labeled leukocytes, and polyclonal and monoclonal antibodies. Sem Nuclear Med 1996;XXVI:51–64.
22. Cooper GS, Shlaes DM, Salata RA. Intraabdominal infection: Differences in presentation and outcome between younger patients and the elderly. Clin Infec Dis 1994;19:146–148.
23. Montgomery RS, Wilson SE. Intraabdominal abscesses: Image-guided diagnosis and therapy. Clin Infect Dis 1996;23:28–36.
24. Shuler FW, Newman CN, Angood PB, et al. Nonoperative management for intra- abdominal abscesses. Am Surgeon 1996;62:218–222.
25. Robles PJ, Lancaster B. Laparoscopic drainage of right subphrenic abscess: Report of one case. J Laparoendoscopic Surg 1996;6:55–60.
26. Kim HB, Gregor MB, Boley SJ, Kleinhaus S. Digitally assisted laparoscopic drainage of multiple intraabdominal abscesses. J Laparoscopic Surg 1993;3:477–479.
27. Christou NV, Turgeon P, Wassef R, et al. Management of intra-abdominal infections: The case for intraoperative cultures and comprehensive broad-spectrum antibiotic coverage. Arch Surg 1996;131: 1193–1201.
28. Hooker KD, DiPiro JT, Wynn JJ. Aminoglycoside combinations versus single β- lactams for penetrating abdominal trauma: A meta analysis. J Trauma 1991;31:1155–1160.
29. Solomkin JS, Dellinger EP, Christou NV, et al. Results of a multicenter trial comparing imipenem/cilistatin to tobramycin/clindamycin for intra-abdominal infections. Ann Surg 1990;212:581–591.
30. Brismar B, Malmborg AS, Tunevall G, et al. Piperacillin-tazobactam versus imipenem-cilistatin for treatment of intra-abdominal infections. Antimicrob Agents Chemother 1992;36:2766–2773.
31. Wilson SE. Results of a randomized, multicenter trial of meropenem versus clindamycin/tobramycin for the treatment of intra-abdominal infections. Clin Infec Dis 1997(suppl 2):S197–206.
32. Bohnen JMA, Solomkin JS, Dellinger EP, et al. Guidelines for clinical care: Anti-infective agents for intra-abdominal infection. Arch Surg 1992;127:83–89.
33. Gerding DN, Hall WH. The penetration of antibiotics into peritoneal fluid. Bull NY Acad Med 1975;51:1016–1019.
34. Dougherty SH. Role of enterococcus in intraabdominal sepsis. Am J Surg 1984;148:308–312.
35. Jones RC. Antibiotics in trauma. J Surg Pract 1977;26–30.
36. Barrie PS, Christou NV, Dellinger EP, et al. Pathogenicity of the enterococcus in surgical infections. Ann Surg 1990;212:155–159.
37. Levison ME, Pontzer RE. Peritonitis and other intra-abdominal infections. In: Mardell GL, Douglas RG, Bennett JE, eds. Principles and Practice of Infectious Diseases. New York, John Wiley and Sons, 1985:488.
38. Fong T, Akriviadis ES, Runyon BA, et al. Polymorphonuclear cell count response and duration of antibiotic therapy in spontaneous bacterial peritonitis. Hepatology 1989;9:423–426.
39. Runyon BA, McHutchison JG, Antillon MR, et al. Short-course versus long-course antibiotic treatment of spontaneous bacterial peritonitis. Gastroenterol 1991;100:1737–1742.
40. Schein M, Gecelter G, Freinkel W, et al. Peritoneal lavage in abdominal sepsis: A controlled clinical study. Arch Surg 1990;125:1132–1135.
41. Wittman DH, Schassan HH. Penetration of eight β-lactam antibiotics into peritoneal fluid. Arch Surg 1983;118:205–213.
42. Mustard RA, Bohnen JMA, Rosati C, Schouten D. Pneumonia complicating abdominal sepsis. Arch Surg 1991;126:170–175.
43. Richardson JD, DeCamp MM, Garrison RN, Fry DE. Pulmonary infection complicating intra-abdominal sepsis. Ann Surg 1982;195: 732–737.
44. Christou NV, Barie PS, Dellinger EP, et al. Surgical infection society intra-abdominal infection study. Arch Surg 1993;128:193–199.
45. Dougherty SH. Antimicrobial culture and susceptibility testing has little value for routine management of secondary bacterial peritonitis. Clin Infec Dis 1997;25(suppl 2):S258–S261.
46. Wilson SE, Hopkins JA. Clinical correlates of anaerobic bacteriology in peritonitis. Clin Infec Dis 1995;20(suppl 2):S251–S256.

105

PARASITIC DISEASES

J. V. Anandan, PharmD, BCPS

Parasitic diseases are receiving increasing attention from clinicians in the United States because of the high frequency of travel, inflow of immigrants from wider geographical distribution, and the presence of immunosuppressed populations (acquired immunodeficiency syndrome [AIDS], transplant patients). Migrant farm workers who work and live in substandard hygienic conditions, the large and growing Central and South American immigrant population, and other poorly screened immigrants from Asia, represent significant sources of parasitic infections in the United States.[1–4] Clinicians need to have a heightened awareness for parasitic diseases and how to treat them. Clinical signs and symptoms, together with patient's travel history, should be used with other diagnostic aids in the identification of parasitic diseases. Parasitic infections caused by pathogenic protozoa or helminths affect more than 3 billion people worldwide and impose tremendous health and economic burdens on developing countries.[5]

This chapter covers the major parasitic diseases, including protozoan diseases (amebiasis, malaria), helminthic infections (ascariasis, enterobiasis), and ectoparasitic infestations (head and body lice). Emphasis is placed on diseases more frequently seen in the United States. World distribution of parasites is dependent on the presence of suitable hosts, habitats, and environmental conditions.[4] A human parasite that does not use an intermediate host is likely to be found in any inhabited region of the world, as long as the environmental conditions are suitable. Ascaris (round worm) and trichuris (whip worm) require carelessness of habits for transfer and require time outside the body, where they are exposed to heat and dryness, to reach the infective stage. The distribution of the hookworm is more limited, because the free-living forms are unprotected by resistant shells or cysts. African trypanosomiasis never occurs outside the range of the tsetse flies, malaria beyond the range of the infective *Anopheles* mosquito, and schistosomiasis in the absence of a specific water snail. The prevalence of clonorchiasis (Chinese liver fluke) is an example of the impact of both environmental and geographical factors. Clonorchiasis not only requires simultaneous presence of humans, specific snail species, and certain fish, but also unsanitary conditions that make the eggs accessible to the snails, an association of the snail and fish, and the established local habit of eating raw fish. The ability of some parasites to infect hosts other than humans may perpetuate an infection, even when human habits preclude the possibility of more than occasional access to the human body. In North America, the broad tapeworm (*Diphyllobothrium latus*) would perish if it were not that dogs and other carnivores, such as the brown bear, serve as reservoir hosts.

HOST–PARASITE RELATIONSHIP

The association of two species for the purpose of obtaining food for either one or the other is called symbiosis. Parasitism is defined as a symbiotic relationship in which one species, the host, is injured through the activities of the other. Through evolution, parasites have made specific morphologic adaptations. Adaptation to the host has taken a number of forms: loss of locomotor organelles in the protozoan *Sporozoa*; partial and complete lack of digestive systems in the trematodes and cestodes, respectively; elaboration of proteolytic enzymes to penetrate the host intestinal mucosa by *Entamoeba histolytica,* the cercariae of the blood fluke that penetrate the skin of the host by elaborate enzymes; and finally, the ability to infect an intermediate host to increase reproductive capacity as seen among the cestodes and trematodes.[4] Parasites normally inflict some degree of injury to the host, the extent of which is dependent on such factors as parasite load, nutritional status, and immunologic competence of the host. *Entamoeba coli* is considered commensal because it subsists on the bacterial flora of the gut and does not cause any harm to the host. Unlike *E. coli, Fasciolopsi buski,* the giant intestinal fluke, and *E. histolytica* can produce severe local damage to the intestinal wall. *Ascaris,* the round worm, can perforate the bowel wall, cause intestinal obstruction, and invade the appendix and bile duct. Malarial parasites destroy red cells by multiplying inside them. *Diphyllobothrium latum,* or the broad fishworm, removes vitamin B_{12} from the gastrointestinal (GI) tract, resulting in megaloblastic anemia.[4]

PROTOZOAN DISEASES

MALARIA

Malaria represents the most devastating disease in terms of human suffering and economic implications. It affects the largest number of people in the world, with deaths in excess of 2 million worldwide.[6]

EPIDEMIOLOGY

The exact geographical distribution of the various species is not well documented; however, it is reported that *Plasmodium vivax* is more prevalent in India, Pakistan, Bangladesh, Sri Lanka, and Central America, while *Plasmodium falciparum* is predominantly in Africa, Haiti, Dominican Republic, the Amazon region of South America, and New Guinea. Both *P. falciparum* and *P. vivax* are prevalent in all of

Southeast Asia, South America, Middle East, North Africa, Ethopia, Somalia, and Sudan.[7,8] Most of the infections with *Plasmodium ovale* occur in Africa, and the distribution of *Plasmodium malariae* is considered worldwide.

In the United States, most cases of malaria are reported in immigrants from endemic areas and in American travelers. Blood transfusion has also been cited as a cause of malarial infection.[9] The transmission of malaria from recent immigrants from endemic areas is a real threat because of the presence of two mosquito vectors, *Anopheles albimanus* and *A. freeborni,* in the United States.[8]

ETIOLOGY

Malaria is transmitted by the bite of an infected *Anopheles* mosquito that introduces the sporozoites (tissue parasites) of the plasmodia (*Plasmodium falciparum, P. vivax, P. malariae,* and *P. ovale*) into the bloodstream. The asexual reproduction stage develops in humans, while the sexual stage occurs in the mosquito.[7,8] The sporozoites invade parenchymal hepatocytes, multiply in stages referred to as exoerythrocytic stages, and become hepatic vegetative forms or schizonts. Schizonts rupture to release daughter cells or merozoites, which then infect erythrocytes.

Plasmadium falciparum and *P. malariae* remain in the primary exoerythrocytic stage in the liver for about 4 weeks before invading erythrocytes, while *P. vivax* and *P. ovale* can exist in the liver in the latent exoerythrocytic form for extended periods, and, therefore, infected subjects can experience relapses. The merozoites that invade the erythrocytes develop sequentially into ring forms, trophozoites, schizonts, and finally into merozoites, which can invade other erythrocytes, or develop into gametocytes, which undergo the sexual stage in the *Anopheles* vector. Erythrocytic forms never reinvade the liver without developing into sporozoites in the vector and, therefore, malaria infections from transfusion never result in the exoerythrocytic or liver form.[7,8] *Plasmodium falciparum* can result in high levels of parasitemia because of its ability to invade erythrocytes of all ages, unlike *P. vivax* and *P. ovale,* which only invade young cells.[8]

PATHOLOGY

Patients with malaria usually present with nonspecific fever, headache, malaise, and vomiting.[8] The malarial paroxysm characterized by fever, chills, and rigor can cause vasodilation and orthostatic hypotension. The high fever, marked diaphoresis, and vomiting can lead to serious fluid and electrolyte abnormalities. The erythrocytic phase causes extensive hemolysis, which results in anemia and splenomegaly. The most serious complications are usually associated with *P. falciparum* infections and include hypoglycemia, acute renal failure, pulmonary edema, thrombocytopenia, high-output heart failure, cerebral congestion, and adult respiratory syndrome.[6–8,10–16] It has been postulated that these complications are caused by tissue hypoxia from anemia and alterations in the microcirculation. Hypoxia may be responsible for the loss of capillary endothelial integrity, leading to increased capillary permeability and interstitial edema. *Plasmodium malariae* has been implicated in immune-mediated glomerulonephritis and nephrotic syndrome.[8]

CLINICAL PRESENTATION

The erythrocytic phase of malaria is preceded by a prodrome that includes headache, anorexia, malaise, fatigue, and myalgias. Patients may also have nonspecific complaints, such as abdominal pain, diarrhea, chest pain, and arthralgias. The prodromal period is followed by the paroxysm, manifested as high fever, chills, and rigor.[7] The typical malarial paroxysm is usually followed by a "cold phase," severe pallor, cyanosis of the lips and nail bed, and cutis anserina ("goose flesh").[7–8] These symptoms are replaced by a "hot phase" where the patient's fever may be between 40.5 and 41°C. The hot phase is followed in 2 to 6 hours by a "sweating phase," where the fever resolves, and the patient shows marked fatigue and drowsiness. Other symptoms during this phase will include warm dry skin, tachycardia, cough, severe headache, nausea, vomiting, abdominal pain, and delirium. Lactic acidosis and hypoglycemia have been reported as complications of falciparum malaria.[8–16] Patients are usually asymptomatic between the malarial paroxysms.

To ensure a positive diagnosis, blood smears should be obtained every 12 to 24 hours for 3 consecutive days.[8–13] The presence of parasites in the blood 3 to 5 days after initiation of therapy suggests drug resistance. Advances for detecting malaria parasite have included DNA or RNA probes by polymerase chain reaction and a rapid dipstick test (Parasight F, Becton-Dickinson, Cockeysville, MD).[8,16,17] The dipstick is reported to have a sensitivity of 88% and specificity of 97%, and it is comparable to microscopy.[13,17]

▶ TREATMENT: Malaria

DESIRED OUTCOME

The primary goals in the management of malaria include rapid diagnosis of the *Plasmodia* sp. by blood smears (repeated every 12 hours for 3 days), initiating appropriate antimalarial therapy, and symptomatic treatment of hypoglycemia, pulmonary edema, renal failure, or other complications that are responsible for increased mortality in malaria.

PHARMACOLOGIC THERAPY

In adults, the chemoprophylaxis for all species of *Plasmodia* is chloroquine phosphate 300 mg (base) once weekly, beginning 1 week prior to departure and continued for 4 weeks after leaving an endemic area.[18] The pediatric dose of chloroquine phosphate is 5 mg (base)/kg (maximum 300 mg). When visiting or leaving an area endemic for *P. vivax* or *P. ovale*, primaquine phosphate (Primaquine) 15 mg (base) daily for 14 days beginning the last 2 weeks of chloroquine prophylaxis should be added to the regimen.[7,8,18,19] The pediatric dose of primaquine is 0.3 mg (base)/kg/d for 14 days. Pediatric doses of chloroquine can be calculated based on body weight, the tablets pulverized, and placed in gelatin capsules. Parents can be instructed to suspend the dose in food, simple syrup, or drink.

In areas where chloroquine-resistant *P. falciparum* strains exist, travelers should receive mefloquine (Lariam) for prophylaxis. The adult dose of mefloquine is 250 mg once weekly, beginning 1 week prior to departure and continuing for the full period of exposure, followed by 250 mg for 4 weeks after last exposure.[18,19] The pediatric dose of mefloquine for prophylaxis is the following:

Body weight (kg)	Dose
15–19	1/4 tablet
20–30	1/2 tablet
31–45	3/4 tablet
> 45	1 tablet

An alternative regimen for prophylaxis in chloroquine-resistant areas for those who cannot tolerate mefloquine is to take doxycycline 100 mg daily starting 1 to 2 days prior to departure, during exposure period and continuing for 4 weeks after leaving the endemic area.[8,18] Children over 8 years should receive 2 mg/kg/d (up to 100 mg) of doxycycline. Children under 8 years should not be given doxycycline.[18]

In an uncomplicated attack of malaria (for all plasmodia except chloroquine-resistant *P. falciparum*), chloroquine 600 mg (base) initially, followed by 300 mg (base) 6 hours later, and then 300 mg (base) daily for 2 days is the recommended regimen. In severe illness or when oral therapy is not tolerated, quinidine gluconate 10 mg/kg as a loading dose (maximum 600 mg) in 250 mL normal saline should be administered slowly over 1 to 2 hours followed by continuous infusion of 0.02 mg/kg/min until oral therapy can be started.[7,18,19] In patients who have either received quinine or mefloquine, the loading dose of quinidine should be omitted. Oral quinine (300 mg every 8 hours) should follow the intravenous (IV) dose of quinidine to complete 3 days for all infections, except for *P. falcipraum* acquired in Thailand where a full 7-day course should be given.[7,18] The pediatric dose of IV quinidine gluconate is the same as in adults.[18] The pediatric dose of quinine is 25 mg/kg/d in three divided doses for 3 or 7 days.[18]

In *P. falciparum* (chloroquine-resistant) infections, a single dose of mefloquine 1250 mg should be used. The pediatric dose of mefloquine is 25 mg/kg (> 45 kg) as a single dose.[8,18] Intravenous quinidine gluconate followed by oral quinine should be administered for severe illness as already indicated.[7,8,13,18] A second drug needs to be administered in chloroquine-resistant *P. falciparum* , and this should follow the oral quinidine regimen: either a single dose of three tablets of pyrimethamine/sulfdoxime (Fansidar) on the last day of IV quinidine, tetracycline 250 mg four times daily for 7 days, or clindamycin 900 mg three times daily for 3 to 5 days.[7,8,10–15] Oral tetracycline should overlap oral quinine for 2 to 3 days.[7] The IV quinidine regimen requires close monitoring of the electrocardiogram and other vital signs (hypotension, hypoglycemia).[7,8,13,18] Because falciparum malaria is associated with serious complications, including pulmonary edema, hypoglycemia, jaundice, renal failure, confusion, delirium, seizures, coma, and death, careful monitoring of fluid status and hemodynamic parameters is mandatory.[6–8,10–15] Exchange transfusion may be required in patients with *P. falciparum* malaria where parasitemia occurs in 5% to 15% of patients; this may manifest as mental status changes, pulmonary edema, or renal failure.[6,13] Either peritoneal or hemodialysis may be indicated in renal failure.

An active research program has been initiated to develop a malaria vaccine.[20,21] A vaccine that blocks the entry of sporozoites into the liver cells will prevent malaria at this stage. Immunity to sporozoites does not, however, protect the host against parasites in the erythrocytic cycle.[21] Infective sporozoites of *P. falciparum* are covered by a polypeptide, circumsporozoite protein.[20] Isolation and identification of the gene encoding for this circumsporozoite protein has led to the development of a monoclonal antibody by recombinant DNA technology. This *P. falciparum* sporozoite vaccine is now under investigation.[20]

EVALUATION OF THERAPEUTIC OUTCOMES

When advising potential travelers on prophylaxis for malaria, one needs to be aware of the incidence of chloroquine-resistant *P. falciparum* malaria and the countries where this is prevalent.[7,8,18] Detailed recommendations for prevention of malaria may be obtained by calling the Centers for Disease Control (CDC) (see Appendix 105–1). A number of newer drugs are under active study and include Artemether and WR238605, an 8-aminoquinoline.[7,8,11,13,15,22,23] Halofantrine (Halfan), approved in 1992 as an alternative agent for *P. falciparum* malaria, has poor bioavailability and is not available commerically.[13,18]

Acute *P. falciparum* malaria resistant to chloroquine should be treated with IV quinidine. These patients should have a central venous catheter to follow fluid status and the electrocardiogram should be closely monitored. Hypoglycemia that is associated with *P. falciparum* should be checked and corrected with dextrose infusions.[6] Quinidine infusion should be temporarily slowed or stopped if a QT interval of > 0.6 seconds, an increase in QRS complex of > 50%, or hypotension unresponsive to fluid challenge results. The suggested quinidine levels should be maintained at 3 to 7 mg/L.[7,13] Blood smears should be checked every 12 hours until parasitemia is < 1%. Resolution of fever should take place between 36 to 48 hours after initiation of the IV quinidine therapy, and the blood should be clear of parasites in 5 days.[7,13] If parenteral therapy is required for more than 48 hours, it is suggested that the dose of quinidine be lowered by one-third to one-half.[18]

Travelers to endemic areas for malaria should be advised to remain in well-screened areas, wear clothes that cover most of the body, and sleep in mosquito nets. It is prudent to carry the insect repellent DEET (*N,N*-diethylmetatoluamide) or other insect sprays containing DEET for use in mosquito-infested areas. Readers are urged to check publications from the CDC for the list of countries where chloroquine-resistant *P. falciparum* exists.[7]

AMEBIASIS

EPIDEMIOLOGY AND ETIOLOGY

Because of its worldwide distribution and serious GI manifestations, amebiasis is one of the most important parasitic diseases of humans.[4,24–26] The major causative organism in amebiasis is *Entamoeba histolytica,* which inhabits the colon, and must be differentiated from the *Entamoeba dispar,* which is associated with an asymptomatic carrier state and is considered nonpathogenic. Although *E. histolytica* and *E. dispar* are indistinguishable morphologically, research using monoclonal antibodies has been able to separate the two.[24–26] Invasive amebiasis is almost exclusively the result of *E. histolytica* infection. Fifty million cases of invasive disease are estimated to occur each year worldwide, leading to an excess of 100,000 deaths.[27] In the United States, the incidence of amebiasis is estimated at about 4% in the general population.[25,27] The highest incidence is found in institutionalized mentally retarded patients, sexually active homosexuals, patients with acquired immunodeficiency syndrome (AIDS), the Native American population, and new immigrants from endemic areas (Mexico, India, West and South Africa, and portions of Central and South America).[25–27]

PATHOLOGY

Entamoeba histolytica invades the mucosal cells of colonic epithelium, producing the classic flask-shaped ulcer in the submucosa.[24,25] The trophozoite has a cytolethal effect on cells through a toxin. If the trophozoite gets into the portal circulation, it will be carried to the liver where it produces an abscess and periportal fibrosis. Amebic ulcerations can affect the perineum and genitalia, and abscesses may occur in the lung and brain.[25–28]

CLINICAL PRESENTATION

The most frequent clinical manifestations of the disease are GI, with vague complaints of abdominal discomfort and malaise to severe abdominal cramps, flatulence, and bloody diarrhea with mucus (heme-positive in 100% of cases).[25]

Right upper quadrant pain, hepatomegaly, and liver tenderness, with referred pain to the left or right shoulder, usually suggest an amebic liver abscess. Liver abscesses that are located in the right lobe can spread to the lungs and pleura.[25–27] Pericardial infection, though rare, may be associated with extension of the amebic abscess from the left lobe of the liver. Erosion of liver abscesses also presents as peritonitis.[27–28]

Eosinophilia is usually absent, though mild leukocytosis is not unusual in intestinal amebiasis. [28] A patient with liver abscess, however, will usually present with high fever, significant leukocytosis with left shift, elevated alkaline phosphatase, and liver tenderness on palpation.[25–28]

A review of the patient's history and recent travel cannot be overemphasized. Intestinal amebiasis is diagnosed by demonstrating *E. histolytica* cysts or trophozoites in fresh stool or from a specimen obtained by sigmoidoscopy. Stool examinations should include permanent trichrome stains.[27] Three stool samples obtained 24 hours apart will produce a 60% to 90% yield for *E. histolytica*. Endoscopy with scraping or biopsy may provide more definitive diagnosis where stool examinations do not provide adequate evidence.[25–27]

When amebic liver abcess is suspected from initial physical examination and history, confirmatory diagnostic procedures will include serology and liver scans (using isotopes by ultrasound or computerized tomography).[24,27–29] In rare instances, needle aspiration of the hepatic abscess may be attempted using ultrasound guidance.

▶ TREATMENT: Amebiasis

DESIRED OUTCOME

In amebiasis, the goals of therapy are initially to eradicate the parasite by use of specific amebicides and then to render supportive therapy.

TREATMENT REGIMENS

A number of different regimens have been suggested, depending on the category of amebiasis: asymptomatic cyst passers, intestinal amebiasis, and amebic liver abscess.[24,25] Electrolyte replacement and nutritional support are essential adjunctive treatment modalities. Large hepatic abscess or amebic pericarditis may require needle aspiration or surgery before drug therapy.[25,27] Most regimens require a combination of drugs administered concurrently or sequentially.[18]

HISTORY

A careful history should be taken when one of the differential diagnoses is ulcerative colitis, because corticosteroid administration has the potential to unmask amebiasis and produce toxic megacolon.[25] All patients diagnosed as having inflammatory bowel disease should have a serologic test for amebiasis to avoid the serious consequence that results from administration of corticosteroids.[27]

PHARMACOLOGIC THERAPY

Metronidazole (Flagyl), tetracycline, dehydroemetine, and chloroquine (Aralen) are systemic agents, whereas iodoquinol (Yodaxin), diloxanide furoate (Furamide), and paramomycin (Humatin) are luminal amebicides. A systemic agent may be so well absorbed that only small amounts of the drug stays in the bowel and, as such, may prove ineffective as a luminal agent.[18,25–27,30] A luminal-acting agent on the other hand may be too poorly absorbed to be effective in the tissue. In the asymptomatic cyst passer, it is necessary to eradicate the causative agent from the lumen to prevent intestinal amebiasis or the development of amebic liver abscess. Drug effectiveness must be monitored by stool examination, that is, three or more negative specimens should be obtained from 1 to 3 months after treatment.

Asymptomatic cyst passers and patients with mild intestinal amebiasis should receive one of the following luminal agents: paromomycin 25 to 30 mg/kg/d three times daily for 7 days or iodoquinol 650 mg three times daily for 20 days or diloxanide furoate 500 mg three times daily for 10 days. These regimens have cure rates between 85% to 94%.[25] Diloxanide furoate is only available from the CDC.[18] The pediatric dose for paromomycin is the same as in adults, while the dose of iodoquinol is 30 to 40 mg/kg/d in three doses for 20 days, and diloxanide furoate is 20 mg/kg/d in three doses for 10 days.[18] Paromomycin is the preferred luminal agent in pregnant patients.[18,25,30]

Patients with severe intestinal disease or liver abscess should receive metronidazole 750 mg three times daily for 10 days, followed by a course of one of the luminal agents indicated previously.[18,25,28] In the pediatric patient, the dose of oral metronidazole is 50 mg/kg/d in divided doses to be followed by a luminal agent.[18] Patients who are too ill to take oral metronidazole should receive the drug in equivalent doses by the IV route.[25]

Evaluation of Therapeutic Outcomes

Follow-up in patients with amebiasis should include repeat stool examination, serology, colonoscopy (in colitis), or computed tomography (CT) (in liver abscess) between days 5 and 7, at the end of the course of therapy and monthly for 3 months.[28] Most patients with either intestinal amebiasis or colitis will respond in 3 to 5 days with amelioration of symptoms. Patients with liver abscesses may take from 7 to 10 days to respond; patients not responding during this period may require aspiration of abscesses or exploratory laparotomy.

Sanitation and Preventive Measures

Travelers and tourists visiting an epidemic area should avoid local tap water, ice, salad, and unpeeled fruits. Water can be disinfected by use of iodine (tincture of iodine or commercial sources: Potable Aqua tablet, Wisconsin Pharmacal or Globaline, Wallace & Trernain) or strong chlorine (laundry bleach) solution, but boiled water is probably the safest. An alternative or additional measure may be to carry a portable water purifier (Safewater, Durango, Colorado). Because food handlers in Asia and Latin America may be a source of amebiasis, travelers should avoid eating at food stalls and open markets.

GIARDIASIS

Epidemiology and Etiology

Giardia lamblia (also known as *G. intestinalis* or *G. duodenalis*), an enteric protozoan, is the most common intestinal parasite responsible for diarrheal syndromes throughout the world.[31–33] *Giardia* is the most frequently identified intestinal parasite in the United States with a prevalence rate of 16% in some areas and is usually the first enteric pathogen seen in children in developing countries with prevalence rates between 15% to 20%.[33,34]

There are two stages in the life cycle of *G. lamblia*: the trophozoite and the cyst. *Giardia lamblia,* which is found in the small intestine, gallbladder, and biliary drainage, is a pear-shaped trophozoite with four pairs of flagella. Two nuclei lie in the area of the sucking disk, giving the protozoan a characteristic face-like image.

The distribution of giardiasis is worldwide. Children seem to be more frequently affected than adults. Children in daycare centers may infect parents and other family members.[33] In less developed countries, fecal contamination of the environment, lack of potable water, education, and housing continue to be risk factors for giardiasis among children.

Pathology

Giardiasis results from ingestion of *G. lamblia* cysts in fecally contaminated water or food. The protozoan excysts under the stimulus of low gastric pH to release the trophozoite.[27] Colonization and multiplication of the trophozoite leads to mucosal invasion, localized edema, and flattening of the villi, resulting in malabsorption states in the host.[33,35,36]

Lactose intolerance precipitated by giardiasis can persist even after eradication of the protozoan. Achlorhydria, hypogammaglobulinemia, or deficiency in secretory immunoglobulin A (IgA) are predispositions for giardiasis.[33,34,35]

Clinical Presentation

Following an incubation period of 1 to 2 weeks after ingestion of the *G. lamblia* cysts, symptomatic giardiasis is marked by acute onset of diarrhea, cramp-like abdominal pains, bloating, and flatulence.[33–37] Complaints from patients include malaise, nausea, anorexia, and belching. Signs and symptoms may be confused with other GI conditions.[37] Chronic diarrhea may continue with foul-smelling, copious, light-colored fatty stools and weight loss. Periods of diarrhea may alternate with constipation. Patients will complain of malaise, headache, and abdominal and epigastric discomfort frequently exacerbated by eating. Giardiasis can cause steatorrhea and vitamin B_{12} and fat-soluble vitamin deficiencies if left untreated.[33,34]

Diagnosis of giardiasis is made by examination of fresh stool or a preserved specimen during the acute diarrheal phase. Fresh stool specimens may show the trophozoites, whereas preserved specimens usually yield the cysts. The alternative method is to use the string or Entero-Test (Hedeco, Palo Alto, CA). The Entero-Test consists of a weighted gelatin capsule secured to a nylon string, the free end of which is secured at the mouth while the capsule is swallowed. The string is removed in 4 to 6 hours, and the end, which normally is located in the jejunum, is checked for trophozoites under a microscope.[34] If both the stool exam and string test prove unsuccessful, it may be necessary to attempt duodenal aspiration and biopsy to confirm the diagnosis; this may be more important in AIDS patients or patients with hypogammaglobulinemia.[34] Most clinicians would advocate a clinical trial of the standard therapy before undertaking invasive diagnostic tests.[34] An indirect fluorescent antibody (IFA) that uses a monoclonal antibody to a protein in *Giardia* cyst is commercially available for detection of the *Giardia* antigen (Meridan Diagnostics, Inc., Cincinnati, OH).[33,34]

▶ TREATMENT: Giardiasis

DESIRED OUTCOME

In patients with prolonged diarrhea, including malabsorption, positive history for travel recently to endemic area, or other predisposing circumstances (parents of small children in daycare centers or homosexual life-style), the goal is to identify the parasite by ova and parasites (O&P) examination or one of the antigen detection tests and institute therapy.

PHARMACOLOGIC THERAPY

All symptomatic adults and children over 8 years of age should be treated with metronidazole 250 mg three times daily for 7 days. The alternative drugs include furazolidone 100 mg four times or paromomycin 25 to 30 mg/kg/d in divided doses daily for 1 week.[18,33–36,38] Paromomycin or bacitracin or bacitracin zinc may be safe agents in pregnancy.[18] The pediatric dose for metronidazole is 15 mg/kg/d three times daily for 5 to 7 days.[18] Furazolidone suspension (50 mg/15 mL) is an alternative drug for pediatrics. Quinacrine, which was the drug of choice in giardiasis, has been discontinued by the manufacturer in the United States. A study indicated that albendazole 400 mg daily for 5 days had cure rates of 97% and was equivalent to metronidazole in children.[39]

EVALUATION OF THERAPEUTIC OUTCOMES

Patients with symptomatic giardiasis, positive stool samples, or detection of *Giardia* antigen by IFA or enzyme-linked immunosorbent assay (ELISA), should be treated with metronidazole for 7 days. Metronidazole produces cure rates between 85% and 95%.[33–35] Diarrhea will stop within a few days, although in some patients it may take 1 to 2 weeks. Cyst excretion will cease within days; however, intestinal dysfunction manifested as increased transit time, and radiologic changes (irregular thickening of the folds in the upper small intestine), may take a few months to resolve. Patients who fail initial therapy with metronidazole should receive a second course of therapy. Pregnant patients can receive paromomycin 25 to 30 mg/kg/d in divided doses for 7 days. Metronidazole has been used in the second and third trimester of pregnancy.[33]

Giardiasis can be prevented by good personal hygiene and caution in food and drink consumption. Preventive measures are similar to those discussed in amebiasis (see section on "Sanitation and Preventive Measures").

LEISHMANIASIS

EPIDEMIOLOGY AND ETIOLOGY

This disease is caused by a protozoan belonging to the genus *Leishmania*. The three variations of the disease are visceral leishmaniasis (*kala-azar*, "black fever," or Assam fever), cutaneous leishmaniasis, and mucocutaneous leishmaniasis.[40–42] The visceral form is predominantly caused by *Leishmania donovani,* while the other two forms are caused by other species. Leishmaniasis is a complex disease, but space constraints do not justify an extended discussion here; interested readers are urged to consult other sources.[41,42]

Leishmania exists in two forms: as a flagellated extracellular parasite in the sandfly vector (*Phlebotomus* in the Indian subcontinent and *Lutzomyia* and *Psychodopygus* in North and South America, Africa, or Middle East) and an aflagellar amastigote (intracellular form) in the host.[40–42] The major reservoirs for *Leishmania,* depending on geographical location, are dogs, foxes, squirrels, and rodents. In the United States, a rodent reservoir (*Neotoma micropus*), has been traced to 27 cutaneous leishmaniasis cases in Texas.[43] The sandflies ingest the parasite when they feed on the reservoir animals. After metamorphosis in the gut of the sandfly, the parasite is transferred to the human host when the infected sandfly takes a blood meal. Cutaneous leishmaniasis seen most frequently in the United States would be caused by either *Leishmania braziliensis* or *Leishmania mexicana,* which are endemic to Southern Mexico and Central America.[43,44]

The disease can range from cutaneous ulcers to the mucocutaneous form affecting the nose, oral cavity, and pharynx. The highest incidence is usually seen in the summer months, especially in subjects working near forested areas.[43]

CLINICAL PRESENTATION

Visceral leishmaniasis usually begins as a papule, which may or may not ulcerate. Subsequently, the amastigote disseminates throughout the reticuloendothelial system to include the spleen, liver, bone marrow, and lymphatic nodes. Hypertrophy of the spleen and liver can take place. Visceral (vicerotropic) leishmaniasis usually develops between 6 to 12 months after exposure.[45] Patients may present with high fever, chills, and malaise.

In the cutaneous disease, the initial lesion appears between 2 and 8 weeks following the bite of the infected sandfly and progresses to a raised ulcer that may persist for months and years.[44] The mucocutaneous form, which is usually caused by *L. braziliensis,* will result in mutilating mucosal infections affecting the nose, soft palate, and trachea. Demonstration of amastigote in tissue or bone marrow will confirm the diagnosis of leishmaniasis.[40–42]

▶ TREATMENT: Leishmaniasis

DESIRED OUTCOME

The major goal is to eradicate the amastigote in the tissue and mimimize the ensuing complications of leishmaniasis.

PHARMACOLOGIC THERAPY

All three forms of leishmaniasis are treated with stibogluconate sodium (antimony sodium gluconate-pentavalent antimony-Pentostam), which is obtained from the CDC. In the adult, both the cutaneous and mucocutaneous forms (*L. braziliensis* and *L. mexicana*) are treated with stibogluconate 20 mg /kg/d for 20 to 28 days.[18] The drug may be administered by either the IV or intramuscular (IM) route. Therapy for all forms of leishmaniasis may be repeated.[18] The alternative drug for the visceral and mucocutaneous forms are pentamidine isethionate (Pentam 300) or amphotericin B (Fungizone).[18,40,42] Pediatric patients receive the same dose as adults (see Appendix 105–1 for side effects of drugs). Pentavalent antimony therapy combined with α-interferon or liposomal amphotericin may be alternatives in refractory leishmaniasis.[18]

EVALUATION OF THERAPEUTIC OUTCOMES

The presence of dead amastigotes in tissue and bone marrow, resolution of anemia and leukopenia, and disappearance of splenomegaly and hepatomegaly may be used as monitoring parameters for the disease. Travelers to endemic areas should use insect repellents and sleep in fine-mesh netting to avoid exposure to the sandfly. No effective chemoprophylaxis against leishmaniasis is available.

AMERICAN TRYPANOSOMIASIS

ETIOLOGY

Two distinct forms of the genus *Trypanosoma* occur in humans. One associated with African trypanosomiasis (sleeping sickness) and the other with American trypanosomiasis (Chagas disease).[46–48] *Trypanosoma brucei gambiense* and *Trypanosoma brucei rhodesiense* are the causative organisms for African trypanosomiasis. In Chagas disease, the trypomastigote is found in the bloodstream, and an ovoid unflagellated intracellular form is found in cardiac and other tissues.[46–50]

Trypanosoma cruzi is the agent that causes American trypanosomiasis. American trypanosomiasis is transmitted by a number of species of a reduviid bug (*Triatoma infestans, Rhodrium prolixus*) that live in wall cracks of houses in rural areas of North, Central, and South America. The reduviid bug is infected by sucking blood from animals (opossums, dogs, and cats) or humans infected with circulating trypomastigotes.

CLINICAL PRESENTATION

Acute infection is frequently seen in children, although Chagas' disease in adults can also be present with the acute phase. Unilateral orbital edema (Romana's sign) caused by local inflammation produced by the multiplying parasite may be seen. A local inoculation granuloma or chagoma appearing as a dusty erythematous lesion may be present, indicating the site of entry of the parasite. Fever, hepatosplenomegaly, and lymphadenopathy may also be present.

In chronic disease, patients will present with cardiomyopathy and congestive heart failure. Electrocardiograms will usually be abnormal, demonstrating extrasystoles, first-degree heart block, right bundle branch block, and other serious conduction disturbances.[46,49] Degeneration of the autonomic ganglia in the smooth muscle of the esophagus and colon lead to uncoordinated peristalsis. The end result has been reported to be "mega syndromes" of affected organs.[46] Penetration of central nervous system results in meningeal signs, oculogyric crises, generalized seizures, and coma.[50]

A history to verify the possible exposure to *T. cruzi* should be an important initial diagnostic workup. Recovery of *T. cruzi* would be definitive; however, this is not always possible, especially in chronic disease. Positive serologic tests using indirect hemagglutination test, ELISA, and a complement fixation (CF) test are used.[47] Specimens may be sent to the CDC for testing. False-positive reactions are seen, especially in those exposed to leishmaniasis, syphilis, or malaria.[16]

▶ TREATMENT: American Trypanosomiasis

DESIRED OUTCOME

The primary goal of drug therapy in trypanosomiasis is to reduce the duration and severity of the illness, and possibly to decrease mortality.

PHARMACOLOGIC THERAPY

The drugs that have been used to treat *T. cruzi* infections are nifurtimox (Lampit, Bayer 2502) and benznidazole (Rochagan). Oral nifurtimox is available from the CDC, while benznidazole is only available in Brazil. The adult dose of nifurtimox is 8 to 10 mg/kg/d in divided doses for 120 days. Because pediatric patients tolerate the drug better than adults, the dose for children 1 to 10 years is 15 to 20 mg/kg/d, and, for those 11 to 16 years, it is 12.5 to 15 mg/kg/d in divided doses.[18] Symptomatic treatment for heart failure includes digitalis and diuretics, while the GI complications require surgical revisions and reconstruction.

EVALUATION OF THERAPEUTIC OUTCOMES

American trypanosomiasis (Chagas' disease), which is endemic in all Latin American countries, can be transmitted congentitally, by blood transfusion, and by organ transplantation.[48,50] Treatment with nifurtimox of the acute phase (fever, malaise, edema of face, generalized lymphadenopathy, and heptosplenomegaly) produces only about a 50% cure rate.[47] Treatment of chronic infection with nifurtimox is not recommended. It is essential to identify *T. cruzi*-infected patients by serology and monitor the cardiovascular status of these patients by electrocardiogram periodically. The congestive failure of cardiomyopathic Chagas' disease is treated the same way as cardiomyopathies resulting from other causes.[48,49]

HELMINTHIC DISEASES

The majority of intestinal helminthic infections may not be associated with a clearly defined manifestation of disease, but they can cause significant pathology. One of the factors that determines the pathogenicity of helminths is their population density. Light infections may be fairly well tolerated, whereas high populations of intestinal helminths can result in predictable disease presentations.[51–54] In the United States, these infections are most frequently seen in recent immigrants from Southeast Asia, the Caribbean, Mexico, and Central America.[1,55] There is a higher incidence of helminthic infections in the southern states. Other populations that have a high risk of infestation include institutionalized patients (both young and the elderly), preschool children in daycare centers, residents of Indian reservations, and homosexual individuals. Certain conditions and drugs (fever, corticosteroids, anesthesia) can cause atypical localization of worms.[53,54] Immunocompromised hosts can be overwhelmed by some helminthic infections, such as strongyloidiasis.[52]

NEMATODES

HOOKWORM DISEASE

This is an infection of the small intestine caused by either *Ancylostoma duodenale* or *Necator americanus*. *Necator americanus* is found in the southeastern United States where the temperature and humidity provide the proper environment. *Ancylostoma* is rarely seen in the United States.

The life cycle of both species of hookworm is similar. The adult worms live in the small intestine attached to the mucosa. The females liberate eggs that are eliminated in the feces and develop into larvae. Infective larva enter the host in contaminated food or water or penetrate the skin, where a papular eruption with localized edema and erythema can result.

In the small intestine where the adult worm lives attached to the mucosa, injury is usually caused by mechanical and lytic destruction of tissue. The loss of blood can lead to anemia and hypoproteinemia.[4,53,54,56]

Stool should be examined for eggs and the rhabditiform larvae. Eosinophilia is present in patients with chronic infection (30% to 60%).

▶ TREATMENT: Hookworm Disease

Mebendazole (Vermox), an oral synthetic benzimidazole, is the agent of choice. It is also effective against ascariasis, enterobiasis, and trichuriasis.[18,52,53,55,56] The adult dose for treatment of hookworm infestation is 100 mg twice daily for 3 days. Pediatric patients over 2 years of age should receive the same dose as adults.[18]

ASCARIASIS

Ascariasis is caused by the giant roundworm, *Ascaris lumbricoides*. Female worms range from 20 to 35 cm in length. The worm is found worldwide, but more commonly in areas where sanitation is poor. In the United States, endemic areas include southeastern parts of the Appalachian range and the Gulf Coast states.[52] It is estimated that about four million people in the United States have ascariasis.

CLINICAL MANIFESTATIONS

During the migration of the larvae through the lungs, patients can present with pneumonitis, fever, cough, eosinophilia, and pulmonary infiltrates.[52,55] Other symptoms of ascariasis include abdominal discomfort, abdominal obstruction, vomiting, and appendicitis.[57] Diagnosis is made by demonstrating the characteristic egg in the stool.

▶ TREATMENT: Ascariasis

In both adults and pediatric patients over 2 years of age, the treatment for ascariasis is mebendazole (Vermox) 100 mg twice daily for 3 days. An alternative drug for ascariasis is pyrantal pamoate (Antiminth).[18]

ENTEROBIASIS

Enterobiasis or pinworm infection is caused by *Enterobius vermicularis.* The pinworm is a small thread-like spindle-shaped worm about 1 cm long. It is the most widely distributed helminthic infection in the world. There are estimated to be 42 million cases in the United States.[52] The majority of those infected are children.

There are no significant pathologic changes with the infection. The most common problem is cutaneous irritation in the perianal region, made by the migrating females or presence of eggs. The intense pruritus and scratching can cause dermatitis and secondary bacterial infections. In children, the itching can cause loss of sleep and restlessness.

The most effective method of diagnosing pinworm infections is by the use of perianal swab using Scotch tape. The Scotch tape, which is applied to the perianal region with a tongue depressor, is microscopically examined for eggs.[52,55]

▶ TREATMENT: Enterobiasis

Helminthic drugs are used to eradicate or reduce the parasitic load in patients. The common agents for treatment include pyrantal pamoate, mebendazole, or albendazole (Zentel). The dose of pyrantal pamoate is 11 mg/kg (maximum 1 g) as a single dose, which can be repeated in 2 weeks. The dose of mebendazole for adults and children over 2 years of age is 100 mg as a single dose; this may be repeated in 2 weeks.[18] Following treatment, all bedding and underclothes should be sterilized by steaming or boiling to eradicate the eggs. Bathroom rugs and toilet accessories should also be sterilized.

EVALUATION OF THERAPEUTIC OUTCOMES

Morbidity and disease with intestinal nematodes is related to the intensity of infection or worm burden; subjects with transient exposure have less severe disease. The major adverse effects of intestinal nematodes is malnutrition, fatigue, and diminished work capacity. Treatment with antihelminthic agents results in complete eradication and significant change in the well-being of subjects. Unlike other nematodes, strongyloidiasis can perpetuate itself by autoinfection, and under immunosuppression, the filariform can invade various organs (lungs, central nervous system) to produce disseminated infection that can be fatal.[52,53,55,56]

ECTOPARASITES

A parasite that lives on the outside of the body of the host is called an ectoparasite. It is estimated that there are three million cases of pediculosis in the United States.[58,59] Pediculosis is usually associated with poor personal hygiene, and infections are passed from person-to-person through social and sexual contact. The three types of human lice belong to two genera: *Pediculus,* including the head and body lice, and *Phthirus,* with only one species, the crab louse.[4,58] The human louse is detectable to the human naked eye and measures about 2 to 3 mm long.

LICE

The two species that belong to this group include *Pediculus humanus var. capitis* (head louse) and *P. humanus var. corporis* (body louse). Female lice deposit eggs on the hair. The eggs (or nits) remain firmly attached to the hair, and in about 10 days, the lice hatch to form nymphs, which mature in 2 weeks. Using both their piercing mouth parts and pumping device, the larvae and adults feed on the blood of the host. The body louse and head louse are essentially identical, though they live on different parts of the body. Unlike the head louse, which lives on the hair, the body louse may more frequently be found on clothing of the infected host.

The pubic or crab louse is found on the hairs around the genitals, though they can occur in other areas of the body (e.g., eyelashes, beards, axillae).

CLINICAL PRESENTATION

Patients usually complain of severe pruritus from papular lesions produced by the bite of the louse. Hypersensitivity to foreign material injected by the lice can produce macular swellings and occasionally lead to secondary bacterial infections. As a result of long-standing pediculosis and secondary infections, hyperpigmentation and thickening of the skin can take place, a condition referred to as "vagabond's" disease.[58,59]

▶ TREATMENT: Lice

The goal of therapy is to eradicate the causative organisms and provide symptomatic relief to patients. The agent of choice for all three infections (body, head, and crab lice) is 1% permethrin (Nix).[18,58–60] Permethrin is a derivative of the flowers of the plant *Chrysanthemum cinerariaefolium*. The term *pyrethrin* is usually applied to several esters of chrysanthemic acid and pyrethric acid. Permethrin has both pediculicidal and ovicidal activity against *Pediculus humanus var. capitis*. The cure rate has been reported to be in the range of 97% to 99%.[61–63] Individuals who have a history of ragweed or chrysanthemum allergy should use this compound with caution. The side effects reported with permethrin products include itching, burning, stinging, and tingling.[59,64] Permethrin 1% is applied to the scalp after the hair has been dried following a shampooing. The scalp should be saturated with permethrin liquid, and a towel should be wrapped around the scalp to allow the application to stay on for 10 minutes. The hair should then be rinsed off. A cream rinse of permethrin 1% (Nix-Creme Rinse) is also available and has been shown to be as effective as lindane.[62] Either of these two preparations may also be used for *Phthirus pubis* and *Pediculus humanus* infestations.[18] Other members of the family or sexual partners should also be treated. All bedding and clothes should be sterilized by boiling or steaming to avoid reinfections. Seams of clothes should be examined to verify that all organisms are eradicated. An ocular lubricant (Lacri-Lube S.O.P.), applied twice daily, may be used to remove crab louse infection of the eyelids.

Another alternative for pediculosis is pyrethrin 0.3% combined with 3% piperonyl butoxide and 1.2% petroleum distillate (R&C, RID).[58,59,63] The same directions for permethrin should be followed when applying this preparation. For the relief of pruritus, a soothing lotion of calamine liniment or lotion with 0.1% menthol may be used.

SCABIES

Scabies is caused by the itch mite *Sarcoptes scabei,* which not only affects humans but also animals. Mange in domestic animals is caused by the same organism. Infection usually affects the interdigital and popliteal folds, axillary folds, the umbilicus, and scrotum.[59,65]

CLINICAL PRESENTATION

Patients will complain of severe itching, inability to sleep, and may have excoriations in the interdigital web spaces, wrists, elbows, buttocks, groin, and scalp. Excoriations may lead to secondary bacterial infections. The diagnosis is made by looking for burrows formed by the mite and taking skin scrapings, which will demonstrate the mite on a wet mount.

▶ TREATMENT: Scabies

Because these infections cause a great deal of discomfort and distress to patients and families, the goal of therapy is to eradicate the infestations rapidly, institute symptomatic treatment, and provide counseling and reassurance. The treatment of choice is permethrin 5% (Elimite) cream.[18,60,62,64] To initiate the treatment, the skin should be scrubbed thoroughly in a warm soapy bath, using a soft brush to remove all scabs. The lotion is then applied to the whole body, avoiding the face, mucous membranes, and eyes. The application should be left on for 8 to 14 hours before bathing.[18] A single application has been demonstrated to eradicate 91% of scabies in subjects.[62,66,67] All close contacts should be checked and treated appropriately.

Other agents used to treat scabies are γ-benzene hexachloride 1% lotion (Kwell, Lindane) and crotamiton 10% (Eurax). These should be used in patients who have hypersensitivity to permethrin preparations. Topical corticosteroids and antihistamines may be used to decrease pruritus.

Evaluation of Therapeutic Outcomes

Permethrin (1% to 5%) for pediculosis and scabies is the preferred agent and remains the safest agent, especially in infants and children.[62,64] One application of permethrin is consistently effective in eradicating more than 90% of all infections. Pruritus may persist for 2 to 4 weeks, however, because of the remnants of mite parts in the skin.

▶ PRINCIPLES OF PHARMACOTHERAPY

- All deaths from malaria are preventable. The primary reasons for deaths are the failure to take chemoprophylaxis, a delay in seeking medical care, and misdiagnosis.[74]
- Falciparum malaria, primarily affecting travellers to Africa, which may be resistant to chloroquine, should be treated with quinidine. The estimated median cost of treating one case of severe *P. falciparum* infection is $12,516 compared to $56 for a 23-day full prophylactic course of mefloquine.[74]
- Either chloroquine or quinidine may be used for malaria during pregnancy.[7,8,13]
- Patients with severe intestinal disease or liver abscess should receive metronidazole 750 mg tid × 10 days, followed by a full course of a luminal agent (either diloxanide furoate or iodoquinol).
- Paromomycin 25 to 30 mg/kg tid × 7 days is the preferred luminal agent for amebiasis in pregnant patients.[18,25,27]
- If three stools for ova and parasites are negative for giardiasis, consider treating empirically with metronidazole 250 mg tid × 5 days. Alternatives are small bowel sampling (Entero test) and endoscopy for biopsy; if these are negative, consider other diagnoses.
- The treatment of choice for leishmaniasis is sodium stibogluconate: 20 mg/kg/d × 20 to 28 days.[77] An alternative therapy is amphotericin B lipid complex 1 to 3 mg/kg/d for 5 days.[76]
- Patient history, including blood transfusions and serology should be reviewed to establish diagnosis of trypanosomiasis (Chagas' disease).
- All cardiac manifestations, which are chronic symptoms of Chagas' disease, are treated with standard regimens for cardiomyopathies (diuretics, digoxin and antiarrhythmic drugs).[47,49]
- Either mebendazole 100 mg bid × 3 days or albendazole 400 mg daily (approved in the United States for neurocysticercosis) are approriate therapy for all helminthic infestations (except for pinworms where a single dose repeated after 2 weeks is the therapy).[18]
- The drug of choice for both pediculosis and scabies is permethrin (Nix, and Elimite, respectively). An alternate therapy for pediculosis is ivermectin (Mectizan) 200 mg/kg as a single oral dose.[63]

REFERENCES

1. Ciesielski SD, Seed JR, Ortiz JC, et al. Intestinal parasites among North Carolinia migrants farmworkers. Am J Public Health 1992;82:1258–1262.
2. Gilson GJ, Harner KA, Abrams J, et al. Chagas disease in pregnancy. Obstet Gynecol 1995;86(4 Pt 2):646–647.
3. Paxton LA, Slutsker L, Schultz LJ, et al. Imported malaria in Montagnard refugees settling in North Carolina: Implication for prevention and control. Am J Trop Med Hyg 1996;54:54–57.
4. Markell EK, Voge M. Medical Parasitology, 6th. ed. Philadelphia, WB Saunders, 1991.
5. Warren KS. Tropical medicine or tropical health: The Heath Clark lectures, 1988. Rev Infect Dis 1990;12:142–156.
6. Hamer DH, Wyler DJ. Cerebral malaria. Semin Neurol 1993;13:180–188.
7. Zucker JR, Campbell CC. Malaria: Principles of prevention and treatment. Infect Dis Clin North Am 1993;7:547–567.
8. Krogstad DJ. Plasmodium species (malaria). In: Mandell GL, Dolin R, Bennett JE, eds. Principles and Practice of Infectious Diseases, 4th ed. New York, Churchill Livingstone, 1995:2415–2427.
9. Herwaldt BL, Juranek DD. Laboratory-acquired malaria, leishmaniasis, trypanosomiasis, and toxoplasmosis. Am J Trop Med Hyg 1993; 48:313–323.
10. Gopdeuk V, Thuma P, Brittenham G, et al. Effect of iron chelation therapy on recovery from deep coma in children with cerebral malaria. New Engl J Med 1992;327:1473–1477.
11. Looareesuwan S, Kyle DE, Viravan C, et al. Treatment of patients with recrudescent falciparum malaria with sequential combination of artesunate and mefloquine. Am J Trop Med Hyp 1992;47:794–799.
12. Kremsner PG, Winkler S, Brants C. Curing of chloroquine-resistant malaria with clindamycin. Am J Trop Med Hyg 1993;49:650–654.
13. White NJ. The treatment of malaria. N Engl J Med 1996;335:800–806.
14. Looareesuwan S, Charoenpan P, Ho M, et al. Fatal *Plasmodium falciparum* malaria after inadequate response to quinine treatment. J Infect Dis 1990;161:577–580.
15. Hien TT, Day NPJ, White NJ, et al. A controlled trial of artemether or quinine in Vietnamese adults with severe *Falciparum malaria.* N Engl J Med 1996;335:76–83.
16. Golden RF, Hill DR. Serodiagnosis of parasitic infection of the central nervous system. Semin Neurol 1993;13:219–233.
17. Humar A, Ohrt C, Kain KC, et al. PARASIGHT F test compared with the polymerase chain reaction and microscopy for the diagnosis of *Plasmodium falciparum* malaria in travellers. Am J Trop Med Hyg 1997;56:44–48.
18. Anon. Drugs for parasitic infections. Med Lett 1995;37:99–108.
19. Wyler DJ. Malaria chemoprophylaxis for the traveller. New Engl J Med 1993;329:31–37.
20. Stoute JA, Slaoui M, Ballou WR, et al. A preliminary evaluation of the recombinant circumsporozoite protein vaccine against *Plasmodium falciparum* malaria. N Engl J Med 1997;336:86–91.
21. Nussenzweig RS, Zavala F. A malaria vaccine based on a sporozoite antigen. N Engl J Med 1997;336:128–130.
22. Van Hensbroek MB, Onyiorah E, Jaffar S, et al. A trial of artemether or quinine in children with cerebral malaria. N Engl J Med 1996;335:69–75.
23. Hoffman SL. Artemether in severe malaria—Still too many deaths. N Engl J Med 1996;335:124–126.
24. Aucott JN, Ravdin JI. Amebiasis and nonpathogenic intestinal protozoa. Infect Dis Clin North Am 1993;7:467–485.
25. Ravadin JI, Petri WA. *Entamoeba histolytica* (amebiasis). In: Mandell GL, Dolin R, Bennett JE, eds. Principles and Practice of Infectious Diseases, 4th ed. New York, Churchill Livingstone, 1995:2395–2408.

26. Irusen EM, Jackson TFHG, Simjee AE. Asymptomatic intestinal colonization by pathogenic *Entamoeba histolytica* in amebic liver abscess: Prevalence, response to therapy and pathogenic potential. Clin Infect Dis 1992;14:889–893.
27. Ravadin JI. State-of-the-art clinical practice: Amebiasis. Clin Infect Dis 1995;20:1453–1466.
28. Wolfe M. Intestinal and genital infections. Amebiasis. In: Strickland GT, ed. Hunter's Tropical Medicine, 7th ed. Philadelphia, WB Saunders, 1991:550–565.
29. Filice C, Di-Perri G, Strosselli M, et al. Outcome of hepatic amebic abscesses managed with three different therapeutic strategies. Dig Dis Sci 1992;37:240–247.
30. Rosenblatt JE. Antiparasitic agents. Mayo Clin Proc 1992;67:276–287.
31. Mutz ED, Hudson-Wragg M, Mshar P, et al. Foodborne giardiasis in a corporate setting. J Infect Dis 1993;167:250–253.
32. Quick R, Paugh K, Addiss D, et al. Restaurant-associated outbreak of giardiasis. J Infect Dis 1992;166:673–676.
33. Hill DR. *Giardia lamblia*. In: Mandell GL, Dolin R, Bennett JE, eds. Principles and Practice of Infectious Diseases, 4th ed. New York, Churchill Livingstone, 1995:2487–2493.
34. Hill DR. Giardiasis: Issues in diagnosis and management. Infect Dis Clin North Am 1993;7:503–525.
35. Farthing MJ. Gardiasis. Gastroenterol Clin North Am 1996;25:493–515.
36. Farthing MJ. Diarrhoeal disease: Current concepts and future challenges. Pathogenesis of giardiasis. Trans R Soc Trop Med Hyg 1993; 87(suppl 3):17–21.
37. Gunasekaran TS, Hassall E. Giardiasis mimicking inflammatory bowel disease. J Pediatr 1992;120:424–426.
38. Jernigan JA, Pearson RD. Antiparasitic agents. In: Mandell GL, Dolin R, Bennett JE, eds. Principles and Practice of Infectious Diseases, 4th ed. New York, Churchill Livingstone, 1995:458–492.
39. Hall A, Nahar Q. Albendazole as a treatment of infections with *Giardia duodenalis* in children in Bangladesh. Trans R Soc Trop Med Hyg 1993;87:84–86.
40. Evans TG. Leismaniasis. Infect Dis Clin North Am 1993;7:527–546.
41. Chulay JD. Cutaneous leismaniasis of the new world. In: Strickland GT, ed. Hunter's Tropical Medicine, 7th ed. Philadelphia, WB Saunders, 1991:652–655.
42. Pearson RD, De Queiroz-Sousa A. Leishmania species: Visceral (Kala-Azar), cutaneous, and mucosal leismaniasis. In: Mandell GL, Dolin R, Bennett JE, eds. Principles and Practice of Infectious Diseases, 4th ed. New York, Churchill Livingstone, 1995:2428–2442.
43. McHugh CP, Melby PC, LaFon G. Leismaniasis in Texas: Epidemiology and clinical aspects of human cases. Am J Trop Med Hyg 1996; 55:547–555.
44. Herwaldt BL, Stokes SL, Juranek DD. American cutaneous leishmaniasis in U.S. travelers. Ann Intern Med 1993;118:779–784.
45. Centers for Disease Control. Viscerotropic *Leishmaniasis* in persons returning from Operation Desert Strom—1990–1991. MMWR 1992; 41:131–134.
46. Garcia-Zapata MTA, McGreevy PB, Marsden PD. American trypanosomiasis. In: Strickland GT, ed. Hunter's Tropical Medicine, 7th ed. Philadelphia, WB Saunders, 1991:628–637.
47. Kirchhoff LV. Chagas disease: American trypanosomiasis. Infect Dis Clin North Am 1993;7:487–502.
48. Kirchhoff LV. American trypanosomiasis (Chagas' disease): A tropical disease now in the United States. New Engl J Med 1993;329:639–644.
49. Hager JM, Rahimtoola SH. Chagas heart disease in the United States. New Engl J Med 1991;325:763–768.
50. Villanueva MS. Trypanosomiasis of the central nervous system. Semin Neurol 1993;13:209–218.
51. Mahmoud AAF. Diseases due to helminths: Introduction. In: Mandell GL, Dolin R, Bennett JE, eds. Principles and Practice of Infectious Diseases, 4th ed. New York, Churchill Livingstone, 1995:2525–2526.
52. Mahmoud AF. Intestinal nematodes (roundworms). In: Mandell GL, Dolin R, Bennett JE, eds. Principles and Practice of Infectious Diseases, 4th ed. New York, Churchill Livingstone, 1995:2526–2531.
53. Liu LX, Weller PF. Strongloidiasis and other intestinal nematode infections. Infect Dis Clin North Am 1993;7:655–682.
54. Kappas KD, Lundgren RG, Juranek DD. Intestinal parasitism in the United States: Update on a continuing problem. Am J Trop Med Hyg 1994;50:705–713.
55. Schwartzman JD. Intestinal nematodes that migrate through lungs (Ascariasis). In: Strickland GT, ed. Hunter's Tropical Medicine, 7th ed. Philadelphia, WB Saunders, 1991:696.
56. Pearson RD, Guerrant RL. Intestinal nematodes that migrate through skin and lung. In: Strickland GT, ed. Hunter's Tropical Medicine, 7th ed. Philadelphia, WB Saunders, 1991:700.
57. De Silva NR, Guyatt HL, Bundy DA. Morbidity and mortality due to ascaris-induced intestinal obstruction. Trans R Soc Trop Med Hyg 1997;91:31–36.
58. Wilson BB. Lice (Pediculosis). In: Mandell GL, Dolin R, Bennett JE, eds. Principles and Practice of Infectious Diseases, 4th ed. New York, Churchill Livingstone, 1995:2558–2560.
59. Hogan DJ, Schachner L, Tanglertsampan C. Diagnosis and treatment of childhood scabies and pediculosis. Pediatr Clin North Am 1991;38: 941–957.
60. Anon. Facts and Comparisons Publication. St. Louis, JB Lippincott, 1997:584a–585a.
61. Stichele RHV, Dezeure EM, Bogaert MG. Systematic review of the clinical efficacy of topical treatments for head lice. Br Med J 1995; 311:604–608.
62. Brown S, Becher J, Brady W. Treatment of ectoparasitic infections: Review of the English-Language literature 1882–1992. Clin Infect Dis 1995;20(suppl 1):S104–S109.
63. Anon. Drugs for head lice. Med Lett 1997;39:6–7.
64. Taplin D, Meinking TL. Safety of permethrin vs lindane for treatment of scabies. Arch Dermatol 1996;132:959–962.
65. Orkin M, Maibach HI. Scabies therapy—1993. Semin Dermatol 1993; 12:22–25.
66. Anon. Permethrin for scabies. Med Lett 1990;32:21–22.
67. Elgart ML. A risk-benefit assessment of agents used in the treatment of scabies. Drug Saf 1996;14:386–393.
68. Goldsmith RS. Antiprotozoal drugs. In: Katzung BG, ed. Basic and Clinical Pharmacology, 6th ed. Los Altos, CA, Appleton & Lange, 1994:780–803.
69. Goldsmith RS. Clinical pharmacology of antihelmintic drugs. In: Katzung BG, ed. Basic and Clinical Pharmacology, 6th ed. Los Altos, CA, Appleton & Lange, 1994:804–822.
70. Webster LT Jr, Tracy JW. Drugs used in the chemotherapy of protozoal infections. In: Hardman JG, Limbird LE, Molinoff PB, Ruddon RW, Gilman AG, eds. The Pharmacological Basis of Therapeutics, 9th ed. New York, Pergamon Press, 1996:965–985, 987–1008.
71. Webster LT Jr, Tracy JW. Drugs used in the chemotherapy of helminthiasis. In: Hardman JG, Limbird LE, Molinoff PB, Ruddon RW, Gilman AG, eds. The Pharmacological Basis of Therapeutics, 9th ed. New York, Pergamon Press, 1996:1009–1026.
72. Cook GC. Adverse effects of chemotherapeutic agents used in tropical medicine. Drug Saf 1995;13:31–45.
73. Anon. Malaria in an immigrant and travellers—Georgia, Vermont, and Tennessee, 1996. MMWR 1997;46:536–539.
74. Sundar S, Agrawal NK, Murray HW, et al. Short-course, low-dose amphotericin B lipid complex therapy for visceral leishmaniasis unresponsive to antimony. Ann Intern Med 1997;127:133–137.
75. Herwaldt BL, Berman JD. Recommendations for treating leishmaniasis with sodium stibogluconate (Pentostam) and review of pertinent clinical studies. Am J Trop Med Hyg 1992;46:296–306.

APPENDIX 105–1
Antiparasitic Drugs

Drug	Indications	Side Effects	Comments	References
Albendazole (Zentel)	Giardiasis, ascariasis	GI: Abdominal pain, nausea, diarrhea, increase in liver function enzymes	Not recommended in children < 2 years old	18, 39, 69, 71
Chloroquine phosphate (Aralen, Nivaquine) 250- and 500-mg tablets; 50 mg/mL (as HCl); 5-mL ampules	Malaria	GI: Nausea, vomiting, diarrhea CNS: Dizziness, headache, blurring of vision, confusion, fatigue Dermatologic: Pruritis	Administer oral does after meals IV route: Recommened ECG monitoring *Contraindication:* Patients with psoriasis or porphyria	13, 18, 19, 30, 38, 68, 70, 72
Dehydroemetine Dihydrochloride[a] 30 mg/mL; 2-mL ampule	Amebiasis	GI: Nausea, vomiting, diarrhea Cardiac: Hypotension, arrhythmias, cardiac failure Other: Muscular pains, paralysis, death Cumulative toxicity: Doses > 650 mg	Prolongation: QT, PR, QRS, ST segment on ECG (may be indication to stop therapy) *Contraindication:* Cardiac and renal disease	18, 25, 28, 68
Diloxanide furoate[a] (Furamide) 500-mg tablet	Amebiasis	GI: Nausea, flatulence Dermatologic: Pruritus		18, 30, 38, 70, 72
Furazolidone (Furoxone) 100-mg tablet Suspension: 50 mg/5 mL	Giardiasis; alternative to metronidazole	GI: Nausea, vomiting Hypersensitivity: Hypotension, fever, arthralgia, uticaria Other: Headache	Disulfiram-like reaction with alcohol; avoid in G6PD[b] deficiency; may cause hemolysis; changes color of urine to brown	18, 30, 33, 34, 38, 68
Halofantrine (Halfan)	*P. falciparum* malaria	GI: abdominal pain, diarrhea Cardiac: Prolongation of QT interval	Should *not* be taken with fatty meals *Contraindication:* Preexisting condition defects	13, 18, 68, 70
Iodoquinol (Yodoxin) 210-mg tablet	Amebiasis	GI: Abdominal pain, diarrhea Dermatologic: Rash	May interfere with thyroid function test *Contraindication:* Patients with iodine intolerance	18, 25, 68, 70, 72
Mebendazole (Vermox) 100-mg chewable tablet	Ascariasis, trichuriasis, hookworm, pinworm	GI: Abdominal pain, diarrhea CNS: Headache, dizziness Other: Pyrexia, neutropenia	Drug should be taken with meals *Contraindication:* Pregnancy *Drug interaction:* Can increase serum levels of theophylline	18, 30, 52, 68, 70, 72
Mefloquine (Lariam) 250-mg tablet	*P. falciparum* malaria	Incidence 17% GI: Nausea, vomiting, abdominal pain, diarrhea Cardiac: Sinus bradycardia CNS: Vertigo, dizziness, confusion, hallucinations, psychosis, convulsions Dermatologic: Itching, skin rash	Patients given doses in excess of 12 mg/kg should be carefully monitored as the side effects are does related	7, 8, 13, 18, 30, 38, 68, 70, 72
Metronidazole (Flagyl) Oral: 250 mg, 500-mg tablets IV	Amebiasis, giardiasis	GI: Nausea, anorexia, vomiting, diarrhea, abdominal cramping, glossitis, metallic taste CNS: Dizziness, vertigo, headache, paresthesias	Avoid alcohol; alcohol ingestion will cause the disulfiram reaction: abdominal distress, vomiting, hypotension *Contraindication:* First trimester of pregnancy	18, 30, 33, 34, 37, 38, 68, 72
Nifurtimox[a] (Lampit, Bayer 2502)	South American trypanosomiasis	GI: Anorexia, nausea CNS: Peripheral neuritis, psychosis Hematologic: Hemolysis in G6PD[b] deficiency patients	Monitor pulmonary function and hematologic parameters	18, 38, 46–48, 68
Primaquine phosphate 26.3-mg tablet	Malaria *(Plasmodium vivax) (P. ovale)*	GI: Nausea, abdominal pain CNS: Mental depression	In G6PD[b] deficiency can cause hemolysis	18, 30, 38, 68, 70

continued

APPENDIX 105–1 *(continued)*
Antiparasitic Drugs

Drug	Indications	Side Effects	Comments	References
Pyrantel pamoate (Antiminth) 50-mg/mL suspension	Pinworm, hookworm	GI: Anorexia, nausea, abdominal cramps, diarrhea CNS: Headache, dizziness	—	18, 30, 38, 69, 71
Pyrimethamine (Daraprim) 25-mg tablet	Malaria (see pyrimethamine-sulfadoxime)	GI: Abdominal pain, vomiting, glossitis Hematologic: Megaloblastic anemia, hemolytic anemia	Recommended that folinic acid 1–5 mg/d be concurrently administered; can cause hemolysis in patients with G6PD[b] deficiency	13, 18, 38, 68, 70
Pyrimethamine 25 mg *plus* sulfadoxime 500 mg (Fansidar)	*P. falciparium* resistant malaria	For pyrimethamine see above GI: Nausea, abdominal pain, stomatitis Hematologic: Agranulocytosis, aplastic anemia, leukopenia	Combination has been reported to cause the Stevens-Johnson syndrome; patients should be advised to call their physician/pharmacist if a skin rash or other reactions are seen	8, 13,18,19, 30, 38, 68, 70
Quinidine gluconate 500-mg base/mL; 10 mL	Acute malaria	GI: Nausea, vomiting, diarrhea Cardiac: Hypotension, widening of QRS and QT on ECG, heart block	Administration of IV quinidine requires close monitoring; should normally monitor ECG and all vital signs	8, 13, 18, 38, 68, 70
Quinine sulfate 325 mg, 650-mg tablets	Acute malaria	Cinchonism: Flushing dizziness, nausea, vomiting, diarrhea (levels over 10 mg/mL) Cardiac: Hypotension, widening of QRS complex Hematologic: Hemolysis, leukopenia, thrombocytopenia	When drug is administered IV, it should be administered by slow infusion (600 mg over 8 h); close monitoring of vitals and ECG required *Avoid use:* IM administration	8, 13, 18, 19, 30, 38, 68, 70
Sodium stibogluconate (Pentostam)[a]	Leishmaniasis	GI: Nausea, vomiting, abdominal pain, pancreatitis, increase LFTs Musculoskeleton: Myalgia, fatigue Cardiac: T-wave inversion, bradycardia Hematologic: Leukopenia, thrombocytopenia	Highly toxic, requires careful monitoring of vitals and ECG, caution in patients with liver or cardiac problems	18, 68, 70, 72, 75

[a]Investigational drugs obtained from The Centers for Disease Control, Parasitic Disease Drug Service, Atlanta, GA 30333. (707) 488-7760 (business hours: 8:00 AM–4:30 PM est), (404) 639-2888 (night, weekend, or holiday—for emergency calls only). Readers may also call local state health offices for specific information on travel information and parasitic diseases.

[b]G6PD/glucose-6-phosphate dehydrogenase.

Internet: CDC International Travel Information: http://www.cdc.gov/travel/travel.htm.[74]

CNS = central nervous system; ECG = electrocardiogram; GI = gastrointestinal; LFTs = liver function tests.

106

URINARY TRACT INFECTIONS AND PROSTATITIS

Timothy A. Mullenix, PharmD, MS, and Randall A. Prince, PharmD

Infections of the urinary tract represent a wide variety of syndromes, including urethritis, cystitis, prostatitis, and pyelonephritis. Urinary tract infections (UTIs) are one of the most commonly occurring bacterial infections in medicine today and account for 7 million patient visits annually.[1] It is estimated that 20% of all women will suffer a symptomatic URI at some point in their lives with many having multiple recurrences.[2] Infections in men occur much less frequently until the age of 50, at which point the incidence rates in men and women are similar.

An UTI may be defined as the presence of microorganisms in the urinary tract that cannot be accounted for by contamination. The organisms present have the potential to invade the tissues of the urinary tract and adjacent structures. Infection may be limited to the growth of bacteria in the urine, which frequently may not produce symptoms. An UTI may present as several syndromes associated with an inflammatory response to microbial invasion and can range from asymptomatic bacteriuria to pyelonephritis with bacteremia or sepsis.

Generally speaking, UTIs may be classified by several methods. Typically, they have been described by anatomic site of involvement. Lower tract infections include cystitis (bladder), urethritis (urethra), prostatitis (prostrate gland), and epididymitis. Pyelonephritis is an infection involving the kidneys and represents upper tract infection.

Also, UTIs may be designated as uncomplicated or complicated. Uncomplicated infections occur in individuals who lack structural or functional abnormalities of the urinary tract that interfere with the normal flow of urine or voiding mechanism. These infections occur in females of childbearing age who are otherwise normal, healthy individuals. Male infections are generally not classified as uncomplicated because these infections are rare, and most often represent a structural or neurologic abnormality.

Complicated UTIs are the result of a predisposing lesion of the urinary tract, such as a congenital abnormality or distortion of the urinary tract, a stone, indwelling catheter, prostatic hypertrophy, obstruction, or neurologic deficit that interferes with the normal flow of urine and urinary tract defenses. Complicated infections occur in both genders and frequently involve the upper and lower urinary tract.

Recurrent UTIs are characterized by multiple symptomatic infections with asymptomatic periods occurring between each episode. These infections are either caused by reinfection or relapse. Reinfections are caused by a different organism than originally isolated and account for the majority of recurrent UTIs. Relapse is the development of repeated infections with the same initial organism and usually indicates a persistent infectious source.

Asymptomatic bacteriuria is a common finding, particularly among the elderly, when there is significant bacteriuria (> 10^5 bacteria/mL of urine) in the absence of symptoms. Symptomatic bacteriuria or acute urethral syndrome consists of symptoms of frequency and dysuria in the absence of significant bacteriuria. This syndrome has been commonly associated with chlamydia infections (see Chap. 107).

Significant bacteriuria is a term used to distinguish the presence of microorganisms that represent true infection versus contamination of the urine as it passes through the distal urethra prior to collection. Historically, bacterial counts equal to or greater than 100,000 organisms/mL of urine in a clean catch specimen were judged to indicate true infection.[3]

Counts less than 100,000, however, may represent true infection in certain situations, for example, with concurrent antibacterial drug administration, rapid urine flow, low urinary pH, or upper tract obstruction.[4] Table 106–1 lists the clinical definitions of significant bacteriuria that are dependent on the clinical setting and the method of specimen collection.[3] These criteria allow for more appropriate specificity and sensitivity in documenting infection under differing clinical circumstances.

EPIDEMIOLOGY

The prevalence of UTIs varies with age and gender. In newborns and infants up to 6 months of age, the prevalence of bacteriuria is about 1% and is more common in boys. Most of these infections are associated with structural or functional abnormalities of the urinary tract and have been correlated to the lack of circumcision.[5] Between the ages of 1 and 5 years, UTIs occur more frequently in females. The prevalence of bacteriuria in females and males of this age group is 4.5% and 0.5%, respectively.[6] Infections occurring in preschool boys usually are associated with congenital abnormalities of the urinary tract. These infections are difficult to recognize because of the age of the patient, but they often are symptomatic. In addition, it is believed that the majority of renal damage associated with UTI develops at this age.[6]

Through grade school and before puberty, the prevalence of UTI is about 1%, with 5% of females reported to

TABLE 106–1. Diagnostic Criteria for Significant Bacteriuria

≥ 10^2 CFU coliforms/mL or ≥ 10^5 CFU noncoliforms/mL in a symptomatic female
≥ 10^3 CFU bacteria/mL in a symptomatic male
≥ 10^5 CFU bacteria/mL in asymptomatic individuals on two consecutive specimens
Any growth of bacteria on suprapubic catheterization in a symptomatic patient
≥ 10^2 CFU bacteria/mL in a catheterized patient

CFU = colony-forming units.

have significant bacteriuria prior to leaving high school. This percentage increases dramatically to 1% to 4% after puberty in nonpregnant females, primarily as a result of sexual activity. It is estimated that one in five women will suffer a symptomatic UTI at some point in their lives. Many women have recurrent infections, with a significant proportion of these women having a history of childhood infections. In contrast, the prevalence of bacteriuria in adult men is very low (< 0.1%).[7]

In the elderly, the ratio of bacteriuria in women and men is altered dramatically and is approximately equal in persons over the age of 65.[8] The overall incidence of UTI increases substantially in this population with the majority of infections being asymptomatic. The rate of infection increases further for those elderly residing in nursing homes, particularly those patients who are frequently hospitalized. The increase is probably the result of a number of factors, including obstruction from prostatic hypertrophy in males, poor bladder emptying as a result of prolapse in females, fecal incontinence in demented patients, neuromuscular disease including strokes, and increased urinary instrumentation (catheterization).

ETIOLOGY

The microbiologic etiology of UTIs usually originates from bowel flora of the host. While virtually every organism has been associated with UTIs, certain organisms predominate as a result of specific virulence factors. The most common cause of uncomplicated UTIs is *Escherichia coli,* which accounts for 85% of community-acquired infections. Additional causative organisms in uncomplicated infections include *Staphylococcus saprophyticus* (5% to 15%), *Klebsiella pneumoniae, Proteus* sp., *Pseudomonas aeruginosa,* and *Enterococcus* sp. (5% to 10%).

Staphylococcus epidermidis is frequently isolated from the urinary tract, it should usually be considered a contaminant initially. Repeat cultures should be performed to help confirm the organism as a real pathogen.

Organisms isolated from individuals with complicated infections are more varied and are generally more resistant than those found in uncomplicated infections. *Escherichia coli* is a frequently isolated pathogen, but it accounts for less than 50% of infections. Other frequently isolated organisms include *Proteus* sp., *K. pneumoniae, Enterobacter* sp., *P. aeruginosa, Staphylococci,* and *Enterococci. Enterococcus fecalis* represents the second-most frequently isolated organism in hospitalized patients.[9] In part, this finding may be related to the extensive use of third-generation cephalosporin antibiotics, which are not active against the enterococci. *Enterococcus fecalis* resistance to vancomycin has become more widespread and has become a major therapeutic, as well as infection control issue.[10]

Staphylococcus aureus infections may arise from the urinary tract, but they are more commonly a result of bacteremia producing metastatic abscesses in the kidney. *Candida* sp. are common causes of UTI in the critically ill and chronically catheterized patient.

The majority of UTIs are caused by a single organism; however, in patients with stones, indwelling urinary catheters, or chronic renal abscesses, multiple organisms may be isolated. Depending on the clinical situation, the recovery of multiple organisms may represent contamination and a repeat evaluation should be done.

PATHOPHYSIOLOGY

ROUTE OF INFECTION

In general, organisms gain entry into the urinary tract via three possible routes: the ascending, hematogenous (descending), and lymphatic pathways. The female urethra is usually colonized with bacteria believed to originate from the fecal flora. The short length of the female urethra and its proximity to the perirectal area make colonization of the urethra likely. Other factors that promote urethral colonization include the use of spermicides and diaphragms as methods of contraceptives.[1] Although there is evidence in females that bladder infections follow the colonization of the urethra, the mode of ascent of the microorganisms is not completely understood. Massage of the female urethra and sexual intercourse have been shown to allow bacteria to reach the bladder.[11] Once bacteria have reached the bladder, the organisms quickly multiply and can ascend the ureters to the kidneys. This sequence of events is more likely to occur if vesicoureteral reflux is present. The fact that UTIs are more common in females than males because of the anatomic differences in location and length of the urethra tends to support to the ascending route of infections as the primary acquisition route.

Infection of the kidney by hematogenous spread of microorganisms usually occurs as the result of dissemination of organisms from a distant primary infection in the body. Infections via the descending route are uncommon and involve a relatively small number of invasive pathogens. Bacteremia caused by *S. aureus* may produce renal abscesses. Additional organisms include *Candida* sp., *Mycobacterium tuberculosis, Salmonella* sp., and *Enterococcus* sp. Of particular interest, it is difficult to produce experimental pyelonephritis by intravenously administering common gram-negative organisms, such as *E. coli* and *P. aeruginosa.* Overall, less than 5% of documented UTIs result from hematogenous spread of microorganisms.

There appears to be little evidence supporting a significant role for renal lymphatics in the pathogenesis of UTIs. There are lymphatic communications between the bowel and kidney, as well as the bladder and kidney. There is no evidence, however, that microorganisms are transferred to the kidney via this route.

Once bacteria reach the urinary tract, three factors determine the development of infection: the size of the inoculum, the virulence of the microorganism, and the competency of the natural host defense mechanisms. The majority of UTIs reflect a failure in host defense mechanisms.

HOST DEFENSE MECHANISMS

The normal urinary tract is generally resistant to invasion by bacteria and is very efficient in rapidly eliminating microorganisms that reach the bladder. The urine under normal circumstances is capable of inhibiting and killing microorganisms. The factors thought to be responsible include a low pH, extremes in osmolality, high urea concentration, and high organic acid concentration. Bacterial growth is further inhibited in males by the addition of prostatic secretions.[12]

The introduction of bacteria into the bladder stimulates micturition with increased diuresis and efficient emptying of the bladder. These factors are critical in preventing the initiation and maintenance of bladder infections. Patients who are unable to void urine completely are at greater risk of developing UTIs and frequently have recurrent infections. Also, patients with even small residual amounts of urine in their bladder respond less favorably to treatment than patients who are able to empty their bladders completely.[13]

An important virulence factor of bacteria is their ability to adhere to urinary epithelial cells, resulting in colonization of the urinary tract, bladder infections, and pyelonephritis. Various factors are present in the bladder that act as antiadherence mechanisms, thus preventing bacterial colonization and infection. The epithelial cells of the bladder are coated with a urinary mucus or slime called glycosaminoglycan. This thin layer of surface mucopolysaccharide is hydrophilic and strongly negatively charged. When bound to the uroepithelium, it attracts water molecules and forms a layer between the bladder and urine. The antiadherence characteristics of the glycosaminoglycan layer are nonspecific and, when removed by dilute acid solutions, result in rapid bacterial adherence.[14]

In addition, the Tamm-Horsfall protein is a glycoprotein produced by the ascending limb of Henle and distal tubule, which is secreted into the urine and contains mannose residues. These mannose residues bind *E. coli* that contain small surface projecting organellae on its surface called pili or fimbriae. Type 1 fimbriae are mannose sensitive, and this interaction prevents the bacteria from binding to similar receptors present on the mucosal surface of the bladder. Other factors that possibly prevent adherence of bacteria include immunoglobulins (Ig) G and A. Investigators have documented both systemic and local kidney Ig synthesis in upper tract infections. The role of Igs in preventing bladder infection is less clear. Patients with reduced urinary levels of secretory IgA are, however, at increased risk of infections of the urinary tract.[12]

Once bacteria have actually invaded the bladder mucosa, an inflammatory response is stimulated with the mobilization of polymorphonuclear leukocytes (PMNs) and resulting phagocytosis. Polymorphonuclear leukocytes are primarily responsible for limiting the tissue invasion and controlling the spread of infection in the bladder and kidney. They do not play a role in preventing bladder colonization or infections and actually have been implicated in contributing to renal tissue damage.

BACTERIAL VIRULENCE FACTORS

Pathogenic organisms have differing degrees of pathogenicity (virulence), which play a role in the development and severity of infection. Bacteria that adhere to the epithelium of the urinary tract are associated with colonization and infection. The mechanism of adhesion of gram-negative bacteria, particularly *E. coli,* is related to bacterial fimbriae that are rigid hair-like appendages of the cell wall.[15] These fimbriae adhere to specific glycolipid components on epithelial cells. The most common type of fimbriae is type 1, which binds to mannose residues present in glycoproteins. Glycosaminoglycan and Tamm-Horsfall protein are rich in mannose residues that readily trap those organisms that contain type 1 fimbriae and are then washed out of the bladder.[16] Other fimbriae are mannose resistant and are more frequently associated with pyelonephritis, such as P fimbriae, which bind avidly to specific glycolipid receptors on uroepithelial cells. These bacteria are resistant to washout or removal by glycosaminoglycan and are able to multiply and invade tissue, especially the kidney. In addition, polymorphonuclear leukocytes, as well as secretory IgA antibodies, contain receptors for type 1 fimbriae, which facilitates phagocytosis, but they lack receptors for P fimbriae.

Other virulence factors include the production of hemolysin and aerobactin.[15] Hemolysin is a cytotoxic protein produced by bacteria that lyse a wide range of cells, including erythrocytes, PMNs, and monocytes. *Escherichia coli* and other gram-negative bacteria require iron for aerobic metabolism and multiplication. Aerobactin facilitates the binding and uptake of iron by *E. coli;* however, the significance of this property in the pathogenesis of UTIs remains unknown.

PREDISPOSING FACTORS TO INFECTION

The normal urinary tract is typically resistant to infection and colonization by pathogenic bacteria. In patients with underlying structural abnormalities of the urinary tract, the typical virulence factors previously discussed are usually lacking. There are several known abnormalities of the urinary tract system that interfere with its natural defense mechanisms, the most important of which is obstruction.

Obstruction can inhibit the normal flow of urine, disrupting the natural flushing and voiding effect in removing bacteria from the bladder and resulting in incomplete emptying. Common conditions that result in residual urine volumes include prostatic hypertrophy, urethral strictures, calculi, tumors, bladder diverticula, and drugs, such as anticholinergic agents. Additional causes of incomplete bladder emptying include neurologic malfunctions associated with stroke, diabetes, spinal cord injuries, tabes dorsalis, and other neuropathies.

Vesicoureteral reflux represents a condition in which urine is forced up the ureters to the kidneys. Urinary reflux is not only associated with an increased incidence of UTIs and pyelonephritis, but it is also associated with renal damage.[17] Reflux may be the result of a congenital abnormality or more commonly the result of bladder overdistention from obstruction.

Other risk factors include urinary catheterization, mechanical instrumentation, pregnancy, and the use of spermicides and diaphragms.

CLINICAL PRESENTATION

CLINICAL FINDINGS

The presenting signs and symptoms of UTIs in adults are easily recognized. Unfortunately, a large portion of patients with significant bacteriuria are asymptomatic. These patients may be normal healthy patients, elderly patients, children, pregnant patients, and patients with indwelling catheters. The typical manifestations of lower tract infections include dysuria, urgency, frequency, nocturia, and suprapubic heaviness. Women will frequently report gross hematuria. Systemic symptoms, including fever, are typically absent in this setting.

The manifestations of upper tract infections classically involve systemic symptoms, including flank pain, costovertebral tenderness, abdominal pain, fever, nausea, vomiting, and malaise. Lower tract symptoms may or may not precede upper tract infections but often occur 1 to 2 days prior to systemic symptoms. It is important to note that attempts at differentiating upper tract from lower tract infections on the basis of symptoms alone are not reliable.

Elderly patients frequently do not experience specific urinary symptoms, but they will present with altered mental status, change in eating habits, or gastrointestinal symptoms. In addition, patients with indwelling catheters or neurologic disorders will commonly not have lower tract symptoms, while flank pain and fever may be recognized. Many of the aforementioned patients will, however, frequently develop upper tract infections with bacteremia with no or minimal urinary tract symptoms.

Acute bacterial prostatitis (ABP) presents as other acute infections. Common symptoms include perineal, sacral, or suprapubic pain; fever; urinary retention; and other urinary tract symptoms (frequency, dysuria, nocturia). Digital palpation of the prostate via the rectum typically reveals a swollen, tender, warm, and indurated prostate.

In contrast to acute bacterial prostatitis, manifestations of chronic bacterial prostatitis (CBP) are more variable. Presenting symptoms include the vague description of voiding difficulties, such as frequency, dysuria, and urgency, along with low back pain and perineal and suprapubic discomfort. Many patients are asymptomatic, but most have varying degrees of voiding discomfort. Although the physical examination is frequently unremarkable, the prostate gland may feel boggy, indurated, or normal.

LABORATORY FINDINGS

Symptoms alone are unreliable for the diagnosis of bacterial UTIs. The key to the diagnosis of UTI is the ability to demonstrate significant numbers of microorganisms in an appropriate urine specimen to distinguish contamination from infection. The type and extent of laboratory examination required depends on the clinical situation.

Examination of the urine is the cornerstone of laboratory evaluation for UTIs. There are three acceptable methods of urine collection. The first is the midstream clean-catch method. After cleaning the urethral opening area in both men and women, 20 to 30 mL of urine is voided and discarded. The next part of the urine flow is collected and should be processed immediately (refrigerated as soon as possible). Specimens that are allowed to sit at room temperature for several hours may result in falsely elevated bacterial counts. The midstream clean catch is the preferred method for the routine collection of urine for culture. When a routine urine specimen cannot be collected or contamination occurs, alternative collection techniques must be used.

The two acceptable alternative methods include catheterization and suprapubic bladder aspiration. Catheterization may be necessary for patients who are uncooperative or are unable to void urine. If catheterization is performed carefully with aseptic technique, the method yields reliable results. Note, however, that introduction of bacteria into the bladder may result, and the procedure is associated with infection in 1% to 2% of patients. Suprapubic bladder aspiration involves inserting a needle directly into the bladder and aspirating the urine. This procedure bypasses the contaminating organisms present in the urethra, and any bacteria found using this technique are generally considered to represent significant bacteriuria. Suprapubic aspiration is a safe and painless procedure that is most useful in newborns, infants, paraplegics, seriously ill patients, and others when infection is suspected and routine procedures have provided confusing or equivocal results.

The diagnosis of UTI is based on the isolation of significant numbers of bacteria from a urine specimen. Microscopic examination of a urine sample is an easy to perform and reliable method for the presumptive diagnosis of bacteriuria. The examination may be performed by preparing a Gram stain of unspun or centrifuged urine. The presence of at least one organism per oil-immersion field in a properly collected uncentrifuged specimen correlates well with ≥ 100,000 bacteria/mL of urine. For detecting smaller numbers of organisms, a centrifuged specimen is more sensitive. Such examinations detect > 10^5 bacteria/mL with a sensitivity > 90% and a specificity > 70%.[18] Counts of less than 30,000, however, are usually not reliably recognized by these methods.[19]

Microscopic examination of the urine for leukocytes is also used to determine the presence of pyuria. The presence of pyuria in a symptomatic patient correlates with significant bacteriuria.[20] Pyuria is defined as a white blood cell (WBC) count of greater than 10 WBC/mm^3 of urine. A count of 5 to 10 WBC/mm^3 is accepted as the upper limit of normal. It should be emphasized that pyuria is nonspecific and signifies only the presence of inflammation and not necessarily infection. Thus, patients with pyuria may or may not have infection. Sterile pyuria has long been associated with urinary tuberculosis, as well as chlamydial and fungal urinary infections.

Hematuria, microscopic or gross, is frequently present in patients with UTI but is nonspecific. Hematuria may indicate the presence of other disorders, such as renal calculi, tumors, or glomerulonephritis. Proteinuria is commonly found in the presence of infection.

Several biochemical tests have been developed for screening urine for the presence of bacteria. A common dipstick test detects the presence of nitrite in the urine, which is formed by bacteria that reduce nitrate normally present in the urine. False-positive tests are uncommon. False-negative tests are more common and are frequently caused by the presence of gram-positive organisms or *Pseudomonas aeruginosa* that do not reduce nitrate.[21] Other causes of false tests include low urinary pH, frequent voiding, and dilute urine.

The leukocyte esterase (LE) dipstick test is a rapid screening test for detecting the presence of pyuria. Leukocytes esterase is found in primary neutrophil granules and indicates the presence of WBCs. The LE test is a sensitive and highly specific test for detecting more than 10 WBC/mm^3 of urine. When the LE test is used with the nitrite test, the range of reported sensitivity and specificity is 70% to 100% and 60% to 98%, respectively, for the detection of bacteriuria.[22] These tests are very useful in the outpatient evaluation of uncomplicated UTIs.

The most reliable method of diagnosing UTI is by quantitative urine culture. Urine in the bladder is normally sterile, therefore, it is statistically possible to differentiate contamination of the urine from infection by quantifying the number of bacteria present in a urine sample. This criterion is based on a properly collected midstream clean-catch urine specimen. Patients with infection usually have greater than 10^5 bacteria/mL of urine. It should be emphasized that as many as one-third of women with symptomatic infection have less than 10^5 bacteria/mL. A significant portion of patients with UTIs, either symptomatic or asymptomatic, also have less than 10^5 bacteria/mL of urine.

Several laboratory methods are used to quantify bacteria present in the urine. The most accurate method is the pour-plate technique. This method is unsuitable for a high-volume laboratory because it is expensive and time consuming. The streak-plate method is an alternative that involves using a calibrated loop technique to streak a fixed amount of urine on an agar plate. This method is used most commonly in diagnostic laboratories because it is simple to perform and less costly.

Once identification and quantification have been completed, the next step is to determine the susceptibility of the organism. There are several methods by which bacterial susceptibility testing may be performed (see Chap. 95). Knowledge of bacterial susceptibility and achievable urine concentration of the antibiotics puts the clinician in a better position to select an appropriate agent for treatment.

Several methods have been evaluated to determine the location of infection within the urinary system and differentiate upper tract involvement from lower tract. The most direct method is a ureteral catheterization procedure as described by Stamey and colleagues.[23] The method involves the passage of a catheter into the bladder and then into each ureter where quantitative cultures are obtained. History and physical examination were of little value in predicting the site of infection. Although this method provides direct quantitative evidence for UTI, it is invasive, technically difficult, and expensive. The Fairley bladder washout technique is a modification of the Stamey procedure, which involves Foley catheterization only.[24] After the catheter is passed, bladder samples are obtained and the bladder is washed out with culture samples taken at 10, 20, and 30 minutes. The procedure has shown that up to 50% of patients have renal involvement, regardless of signs and symptoms. Others have found 10% to 20% of tests to be equivocal.[25]

Noninvasive methods of localization may be more acceptable for routine use; however, they have limited clinical value. Patients with pyelonephritis having abnormalities in urinary concentrating ability. The use of concentrating ability for localization of UTIs is, however, associated with a high false-positive and false-negative response and is not useful clinically.[21] The antibody coated bacteria (ACB) test is an immunofluorescent method that detects bacteria coated with Ig in freshly voided urine. The sensitivity and specificity of this test to localize the site of infection has been reported to average 88% and 76%, respectively.[25] Because of the high incidence of false-positive and false-negative results, ACB testing is not routinely used in the management of UTIs.

Some clinicians have observed that therapeutic outcome may be useful in separating patients with lower and upper tract infections. This statement is based on the assumption that virtually all patients with uncomplicated lower tract infections can be cured with a short course of antibiotic therapy. Those patients who do not respond or relapse do so because of upper tract involvement. It is rarely necessary to localize the site of infection to direct the clinical management of the patient.

▶ TREATMENT: Urinary Tract Infections

DESIRED OUTCOME

The goals of treatment of UTIs are three: (1) prevent or treat systemic consequences of infection, (2) eradicate the invading organism, and (3) prevent the reoccurrence of infection.

MANAGEMENT

The management of a patient with a UTI includes initial evaluation, selection of an antibacterial agent and duration of therapy, and follow-up evaluation. The initial selection of an antimicrobial agent for the treatment of UTI is primarily based on the severity of the presenting signs and symptoms, the site of infection, and whether the infection is determined to be uncomplicated or complicated. Other considerations include side-effect potential, cost, and the comparative inconvenience of different therapies.

Various pharmacologic factors may affect the action of antibacterial agents. Certainly the ability of the agent to achieve appropriate concentrations in the urine is of utmost importance. Factors that affect the rate and extent of excretion through the kidney include the patient's glomerular filtration rate and whether or not the agent is actively secreted. Filtration depends on the molecular size and degree of protein binding of the agent. Agents, such as sulfonamides, tetracyclines, and aminoglycosides, enter the urine via filtration. As the glomerular filtration rate is reduced, the amount of drug that enters the urine is reduced. Most β-lactam agents and quinolones are not only filtered but also are actively secreted into the urine. For this reason, these agents achieve high urinary concentrations, despite unfavorable protein-binding characteristics or the presence of renal dysfunction.

The ability to eradicate bacteria from the urine is directly related to the sensitivity of the microorganism and the achievable concentrations of the antimicrobial agent in the urine. Unfortunately, most susceptibility testing is directed at achievable concentrations in the blood. There is a poor correlation between achievable blood levels of antimicrobial agents and the eradication of bacteria from the urine.[26] In the treatment of lower tract infections, plasma concentrations of antibacterial agents may not be important; however, achieving appropriate plasma concentrations appears critical in patients with bacteremia and renal abscesses.

There are a number of nonspecific therapies that have been advocated in the treatment and prevention of UTIs. Fluid hydration has been used to produce rapid dilution of bacteria and removal of infected urine by increased voiding. A critical factor appears to be the amount of residual volume remaining after voiding. As little as 10 mL of residual urine can significantly alter the eradication of infection.[13] Paradoxically, increased diuresis also may promote susceptibility to infection by diluting the normal antibacterial properties of the urine. Often in clinical practice, the concentrations of antimicrobial agents in the urine are so high that dilution has little effect on efficacy.

The antibacterial activity of the urine is related to the low pH, which is the result of high concentrations of various organic acids. Large volumes of cranberry juice have been found to increase the antibacterial activity of the urine and prevent the development of UTIs.[27] Apparently, the cranberry juice content of fructose and other unknown substances acts to interfere with adherence mechanisms of some pathogens, thereby preventing infection. Acidification of the urine by cranberry juice does not appear to play a significant role. The use of other agents to acidify the urine (ascorbic acid) to hinder bacterial growth is usually unable to achieve significant acidification clinically. Therefore, attempts to acidify urine with systemic agents are not recommended.

Urinary analgesics, such as phenazopyridine hydrochloride (Pyridium), are frequently used by many clinicians. If the pain or dysuria present in an UTI is a consequence of infection, then urinary analgesics have little clinical role as most patients' symptoms respond quite rapidly to appropriate antibacterial therapy.

PHARMACOLOGIC THERAPY

Ideally, the antimicrobial agent chosen should be well tolerated, well absorbed, achieve high urinary concentrations, and have a spectrum of activity limited to the known or suspected pathogen(s). Table 106–2 lists the most common agents used in the treatment of UTIs along with comments concerning their general use. Table 106–3 presents an overview of various therapeutic options for outpatient therapy of UTI. Table 106–4 describes empiric treatment regimens for selected clinical situations.

The therapeutic management of UTIs is best accomplished by first categorizing the type of infection: acute uncomplicated cystitis, symptomatic bacteriuria, asymptomatic bacteriuria, complicated UTIs, recurrent infections, and prostatitis.

ACUTE UNCOMPLICATED CYSTITIS

Acute uncomplicated cystitis is the most common form of UTI. These infections typically occur in women of childbearing age and are often related to sexual activity. Although the presence of dysuria, frequency, urgency, and suprapubic discomfort are frequently associated with lower tract infection, a significant number of patients have upper tract involvement as well.[28] These infections are predominantly caused by *E.coli* and antimicrobial therapy should initially be directed against this organism. Other common causes include *S. saprophyticus* and occasionally *K. pneumoniae* and *Proteus mirabilis*. Because the causative organisms and their susceptibility are generally known, many clinicians advocate a cost-effective approach to management. This approach includes a urinalysis and initiation of empiric therapy without a urine culture[28] (Fig. 106–1).

The goal of treatment for uncomplicated cystitis is to eradicate the causative organism and reduce the incidence of recurrence caused by relapse or reinfection. The ability to reduce the chance of recurrence is dependent on the agent's efficacy in eradicating the uropathogenic bacteria from the vaginal and gastrointestinal reservoir. In the past, conventional therapy consisted of an effective oral antibiotic administered for 7 to 14 days. It is now apparent, however, that acute cystitis is a superficial mucosal infection that can be eradicated with much shorter courses of therapy. Single-dose therapy provides high urinary concentrations for 12 to 24 hours and is highly effective in eliminating bacteria in patients with uncomplicated cystitis. Cure rates have ranged from 65% to 100% using single doses of sulfisoxazole (2 g), trimethoprim–sulfamethoxazole (two double-strength tablets), amoxicillin (3 g) and fosfomycin (3 g).[29] Advantages of single-dose therapy include less expense, greater compliance, fewer side effects, and less potential for the development of resistance. Clinicians should not assume that all antimicrobial agents are effective as single-dose agents. For example, a 2 g oral dose of cefaclor produced a 57% failure rate in lower tract infections.[30] Data suggest trimethoprim–sulfamethoxazole is the most efficacious agent in single-dose therapy. The fluoroquinolones and fosfomycin have also been used successfully. The efficacy of these agents is probably related to observations that *E. coli* causing community-acquired

TABLE 106–2. Commonly Used Antimicrobial Agents in the Treatment of Urinary Tract Infections

	Comments
Oral Therapy	
Sulfonamides	These agents have generally been replaced by more agents because of resistance.
Trimethoprim–sulfamethoxazole	This combination is highly effective against most aerobic enteric bacteria except *Pseudomonas aeruginosa*. High urinary tract tissue levels and urine levels are achieved, which may be important in complicated infection treatment. Also effective as prophylaxis for recurrent infections.
Penicillins Ampicillin Amoxicillin Amoxicillin/clavulanic acid Carbenicillin indanyl	Ampicillin is the standard penicillin that has broad-spectrum activity. Increasing *Eschericha coli* resistance has limited its use in acute cystitis. It is the drug of choice for enterocci sensitive to penicillin. Amoxicillin clavulanate is preferred for resistance problems. Carbenicillin indanyl is only indicated for the treatment of UTIs.
Cephalosporins Cephalexin Cephradine Cefaclor Cefadroxil Cefuroxime Cefixime Cefzil Cefpodoxime	There are no major advantages of these agents over other agents in the treatment of UTIs, and they are more expensive. They may be useful in cases of resistance to amoxicillin and trimethoprim–sulfamethoxazole. These agents are not active against enterococci.
Tetracyclines Tetracycline Doxycycline Minocycline	These agents have been effective for initial episodes of UTIs. Resistance develops rapidly, however, and their use is limited. These agents also lead to candidal overgrowth. They are primarily useful for treating chlamydial infections.
Quinolones Ciprofloxacin Ofloxacin Norfloxacin Levofloxacin	The newer quinolones have a greater spectrum of activity that includes *P. aeruginosa.* These agents are effective for pyelonephritis and prostatitis. Avoid in pregnancy and children.
Nitrofurantoin	This agent is effective as both a therapeutic and prophylactic agent in patients with recurrent UTI. Its main advantage is lack of resistance, even after long courses of therapy. Adverse effects may limit use (GI intolerance, neuropathies, pulmonary reactions).
Azithromycin	Single-dose therapy for chlamydial infections.
Methanamine hippurate/mandalate	These agents are reserved for prophylactic therapy or suppressive use between episodes of infection.
Fosfomycin	Single-dose therapy for uncomplicated infections.
Parenteral Therapy	
Aminoglycosides Gentamicin Tobramycin Netilmicin Amikacin	Gentamicin and tobramycin are equally effective; gentamicin is less expensive. Tobramycin has better pseudomonal activity, which may be important in serious systemic infections. Amikacin is generally reserved for multiresistant bacteria.
Penicillins Ampicillin Ampicillin/sulbactam Ticarcillin/clavulanate Piperacillin Piperacillin/tazobactam	These agents are generally equally effective for susceptible bacteria. The extended-spectrum penicillins are more active against *P. aeruginosa* and enterococci. Often they are preferred over cephalosporins. They are very useful in renally impaired patients or when an aminoglycoside is to be avoided.
Cephalosporins First, second, and third generation	Second- and third-generation cephalosporins have a broad spectrum of activity against gram-negative bacteria, but they are not active against enterococci and have limited activity against *P. aeruginosa*. Ceftazidime and cefepime are active against *P. aeruginosa.* They are useful for nosocomial infections and urosepsis because of susceptible pathogens.
Imipenem/cilastin Meropenem	These agents have a broad spectrum of activity, including gram-positive, gram-negative, and anaerobic bacteria. They are active against *P. aeruginosa* and enterococci but may be associated with candidal superinfections.
Aztreonam	A monobactam that is only active against gram-negative bacteria, including some strains of *P. aeruginosa*. Generally useful for nosocomial infections when aminoglycosides are to be avoided and in penicillin-sensitive patients.
Quinolones Ciprofloxacin Ofloxacin Levofloxacin Sparfloxacin	These agents have broad-spectrum activity primarily against gram-negative pathogens, including *P. aeruginosa* and other resistant organisms. They provide urine and high-tissue concentrations and are actively secreted in reduced renal function.

GI = gastrointestinal; UTI = urinary tract infection.

TABLE 106–3. Overview of Outpatient Antimicrobial Therapy for Lower Tract Infections in Adults

Indications	Antibiotic	Dose[a]	Interval	Duration
Lower tract infections	Trimethoprim–sulfamethoxazole	2 DS tablets	Single dose	1 day
Uncomplicated	(TMP/SMX)	1 DS tablet	bid	3 days
	Ciprofloxacin	250 mg	bid	3 days
	Norfloxacin	400 mg	bid	3 days
	Ofloxacin	200 mg	bid	3 days
	Levofloxacin	250 mg	qd	3 days
	Lomefloxacin	400 mg	qd	3 days
	Enoxacin	200 mg	bid	3 days
	Amoxicillin	6 × 500 mg	Single dose	1 day
		500 mg	bid	3 days
	Amoxicillin/clavulanate	500 mg	tid	3 days
	Trimethoprim	100 mg	bid	3 days
	Nitrofurantoin	100 mg	qid	3 days
	Fosfomycin	3 g	Single dose	1 day
Complicated	TMP/SMX	1 DS tablet	bid	7–10 days
	Trimethoprim	100 mg	bid	7–10 days
	Norfloxacin	400 mg	bid	7–10 days
	Ciprofloxacin	250–500 mg	bid	7–10 days
	Ofloxacin	200–400 mg	bid	7–10 days
	Lomefloxacin	400 mg	qd	7–10 days
	Levofloxacin	250 mg	qd	7–10 days
	Amoxicillin/clavulanate	500 mg	tid	7–10 days
Recurrent Infections	Nitrofurantion	50 mg	qd	6 mo
	Trimethoprim	100 mg	qd	6 mo
	TMP/SMX	1/2 ss tablet	qd	6 mo
Acute urethral syndrome	TMP/SMX	1 DS	bid	3 days
Failure of TMP/SMX	Azithromycin	1 g	Single dose	
	Doxycycline	100 mg	bid	7 days
Acute pyelonephritis	TMP/SMX	1 DS tablet	bid	14 days
	Ciprofloxacin	500 mg	bid	14 days
	Ofloxacin	400 mg	bid	14 days
	Norfloxacin	400 mg	bid	14 days
	Levofloxacin	250 mg	qd	14 days
	Lomefloxacin	400 mg	qd	14 days
	Enoxacin	400 mg	bid	14 days
	Amoxicillin/clavulanate	500 mg	tid	14 days

[a]Dosing intervals for normal renal function.
DS = double strength; SS = single strength.

TABLE 106–4. Empiric Treatment of Urinary Tract Infections and Prostatitis

Diagnosis	Pathogens	Treatment	Comments
Acute uncomplicated cystitis	*Escheriche coli* *Staphylococcus saprophyticus*	1. TMP/SMX × 3 days 2. Quinolone × 3 days	Short-course therapy more effective than single dose
Pregnancy	As above	1. Amp/clav × 7 days 2. Cephalosporin × 7 days 3. TMP/SMX × 7 days	Avoid TMP/SMX during third trimester
Acute pyelonephritis			
Uncomplicated	*E. coli*	1. TMP/SMX × 14 days 2. Quinolone × 14 days	Can be managed as outpatient
Complicated	*E. coli, Proteus mirabilis Klebsiella pneumoniae, Pseudomonas aeruginosa, Enterococcus fecalis*	1. Quinolone × 14 days 2. Extended-spectrum penicillin plus aminoglycoside	Severity of illness will determine duration of IV therapy. Culture results should direct therapy. Oral therapy may complete 14 days of therapy
Prostatitis	*E. coli, K. pneumoniae, Proteus* sp., *P. aeruginosa*	1. TMP/SMX × 4-6 wk 2. Quinolone × 4–6 wk	Acute prostatis may require IV therapy initially. Chronic prostatitis may require longer treatment periods or surgery

Amp/clav = amoxicillin/clavulanate; TMP/SMX = trimethoprim–sulfamethoxazole.

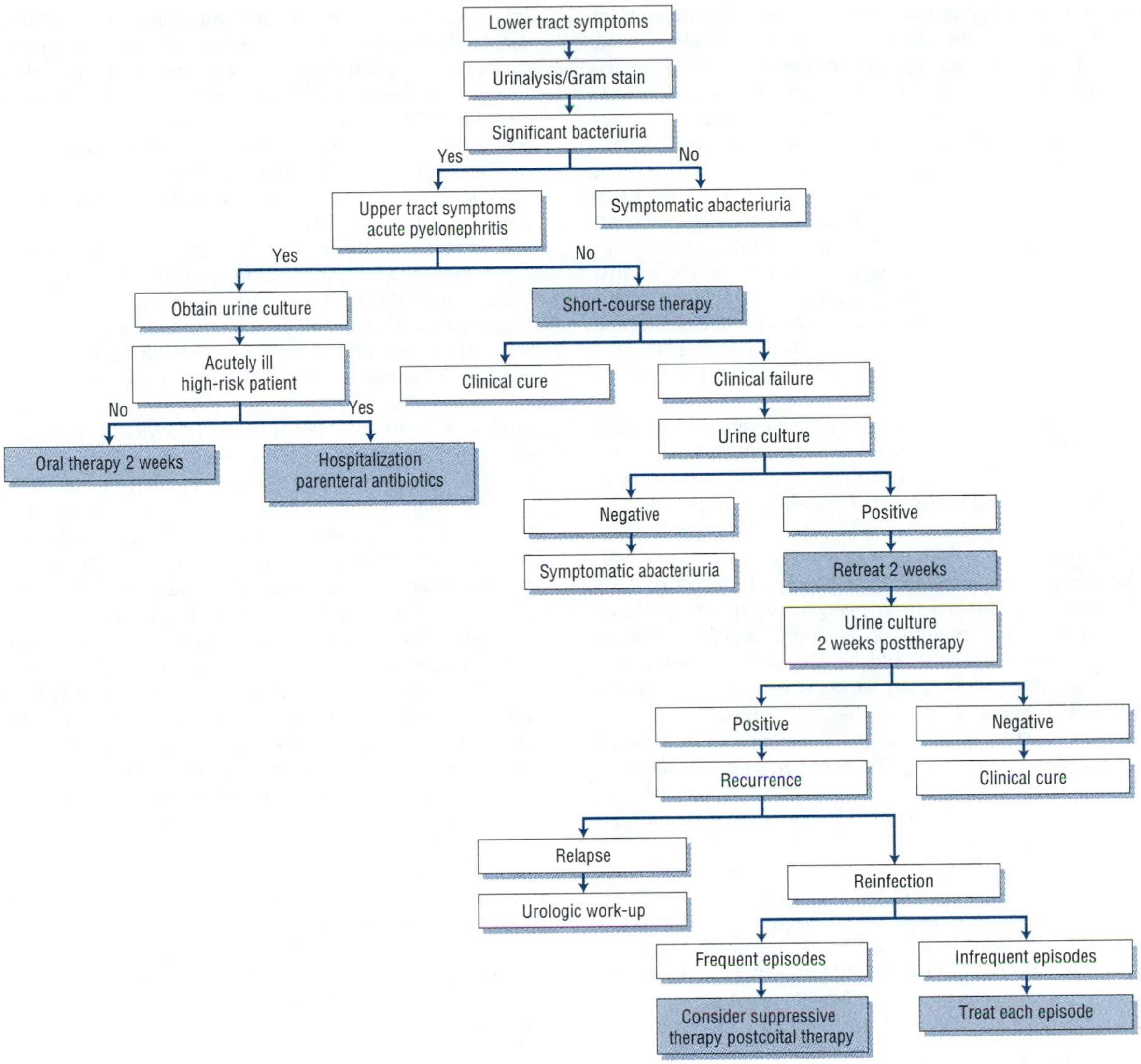

FIGURE 106–1. Management of urinary tract infections in females.

UTIs are increasingly resistant to ampicillin, amoxicillin, and sulfonamides. In addition, oral β-lactam antibiotics are eliminated more rapidly and do not achieve high renal tissue concentrations as compared to trimethoprim–sulfamethoxazole and are less successful in eradicating uropathogens from the vaginal and gastrointestinal reservoirs.

Three-day courses of trimethoprim–sulfamethoxazole or a fluoroquinolone have been shown superior to single-dose therapies.[31] The use of amoxicillin, sulfonamides, and nitrofurantoin is not recommended because of the high incidence of resistant *E. coli*. For most adult females, short-course therapy has become the treatment of choice for uncomplicated lower UTIs. Short-course therapy is not appropriate for those patients who have had previous infections caused by resistant bacteria, male patients, or others with complicated UTIs. If symptoms do not respond or recur, a urine culture should be obtained and conventional therapy with a suitable agent instituted.

SYMPTOMATIC ABACTERIURIA

Symptomatic abacteriuria or acute urethral syndrome represents a clinical syndrome in which females present with dysuria and pyuria, but the urine culture reveals less than 10^5 bacteria/mL of urine. Acute urethral syndrome is estimated to account for more than half of the complaints of dysuria seen in the community today. These women are most likely to be infected with small numbers of coliform bacteria including *E. coli, Staphylococcus* sp., or *Chlamydia trachomatis*. Additional causes include *Neisseria gonorrhoeae, Gardnerella vaginalis,* and *Ureaplasma urealyticum.*

Most patients presenting with pyuria will, in fact, have infection that requires treatment. Single-dose or short-course therapy with trimethoprim–sulfamethoxazole has been used effectively, and prolonged courses of therapy are not necessary for the majority of patients. If single-dose or short-course therapy is ineffective, a culture should be obtained. If the patient reports recent sexual activity, therapy for *C. trachomatis* should be considered. Chlamydial treatment should consist of a 1 g dose of azithromycin or doxycycline 100 mg bid for 7 days. Often concomitant treatment of all sexual partners is required to cure chlamydial infections and prevent reacquisition.

ASYMPTOMATIC BACTERIURIA

Asymptomatic bacteriuria represents those patients who, in the absence of urinary symptoms, are found to have two consecutive urine cultures with > 10^5 of the same organism. The majority of patients with asymptomatic bacteriuria are elderly and female. Another group of patients frequently presenting with asymptomatic bacteriuria are pregnant women. Although this group of patients typically will respond to treatment, relapse and reinfection are very common and chronic asymptomatic bacteriuria is difficult to eradicate.

The management of asymptomatic bacteriuria is dependent on the age of the patient and whether or not they are pregnant. In children, because of a greater risk of developing renal scarring and long-standing renal damage, treatment should consist of conventional courses of therapy as that for symptomatic infection. The greatest risk of renal damage occurs during the first 5 years of life.[32] In the nonpregnant female, therapy is controversial; however, treatment has little effect on the natural course of infections.

Two groups characterize asymptomatic bacteriuria in the elderly: those with persistent bacteriuria and those with intermittent bacteriuria. Most clinicians feel that asymptomatic bacteriuria in the elderly is a benign disease and does not warrant treatment. Most data indicate that the patient without urinary tract obstruction is not destined to develop progressive renal damage. Investigators who have demonstrated an association between bacteriuria and decreased survival, however, have questioned this approach. In this setting, there is no apparent urgency in initiating therapy, so two cultures should be obtained to confirm the presence of bacteriuria. Treating ambulatory, nonhospitalized elderly women is effective in eliminating bacteria for at least 6 months and may protect against the development of symptomatic bacteriuria; however, only 50% of patients remained free of bacteria after 1 year.[33]

Several studies in hospitalized elderly subjects, however, have not found antimicrobial therapy to be efficacious.[34,35] A number of questions remain unanswered; for example, the effect of eradication of bacteriuria on life expectancy, the cost-effectiveness and risk: benefit ratio of therapy, and the effect on morbidity. Certainly, with the information available and the high adverse reaction rate in the elderly, vigorous treatment and screening programs cannot be advocated.

COMPLICATED URINARY TRACT INFECTIONS

ACUTE PYELONEPHRITIS

The presentation of high-grade fever and severe flank pain should be treated as acute pyelonephritis, and aggressive management is warranted. Severely ill patients with pyelonephritis should be hospitalized and intravenous antimicrobials administered initially. Although more mild cases may be managed with orally administered antibiotics in an outpatient setting, symptoms of nausea, vomiting, and dehydration may require hospitalization.

At the time of presentation, a Gram stain of the urine should be performed along with a urinalysis, culture, and sensitivity tests. The Gram stain should indicate the morphology of the infecting organism(s) and help direct the selection of an appropriate antibiotic. The precise identity and susceptibility of the infecting organism(s) will be unknown initially, warranting empiric therapy.

The goals of treatment include the achievement of therapeutic concentrations of an antimicrobial agent in the bloodstream and urinary tract to which the invading organism is susceptible and sufficient therapy to eradicate residual infection in the tissues of the urinary tract.

In the mild-to-moderate symptomatic patient in which oral therapy is considered, an effective agent should be administered for at least a 2-week period. Although the sulfonamides and ampicillin or amoxicillin have been the primary choices for the treatment of gram-negative bacillary infections, they are no longer considered reliable agents in this setting.[31] Reports of increasing resistance to *E. coli* have tempered their use. In addition, treatment with trimethoprim–sulfamethoxazole (one double strength tablet twice daily) for 2 weeks was superior to ampicillin, despite the organism being susceptible to both agents.[29] Oral antibiotics that are highly active against the probable pathogens and are sufficiently bioavailable are preferred. Agents, such as trimethoprim–sulfamethoxazole and the fluoroquinolones, are the agents of choice. If a Gram stain reveals gram-positive cocci, *Enterococcus fecalis* should be considered and treatment directed against this potential pathogen (ampicillin). Close follow-up of outpatient treatment is mandatory to assure success.

In the seriously ill patient, parenteral therapy should be administered initially. Therapy should provide a broad spectrum of coverage and should be directed toward bacteremia or sepsis, if present. A number of antibiotic regimens have been used as empiric therapy, including ampicillin plus gentamicin; parenteral trimethoprim–sulfamethoxazole and fluoroquinolones; the extended-spectrum cephalosporins; aztreonam; the β-lactamase inhibitor combinations (BLIC) (ampicillin/sulbactam, ticarcillin/ clavulanate, and piperacillin/tazobactam); or imipenem. If the patient has been hospitalized in the last 6 months, has a urinary catheter, or is a nursing home resident, the possibility of *Pseudomonas aeruginosa* and enterocccci, as well as, mutiply resistant organisms should be considered. In this setting, ceftazidime, ticarcillin/clavulanate, piperacillin, aztreonam or imipenem in combination with an aminoglycoside is recommended. The rationale for combination therapy is that in experimental animals, 3 days of aminoglycoside combination therapy followed by nonaminoglycoside single-agent therapy for 7 days resulted in a 100% cure rate.[36] If the patient responds to initial combination therapy, the aminoglycoside may be discontinued after 3 days. Although the aminoglycoside therapy is stopped, renal tissue concentrations of the aminoglycoside will persist for days. Based on sensitivity data, the patient can then be maintained or switched to a less expensive single agent, and ultimately an appropriate oral agent may be used.

Effective therapy should stabilize the patient within 12 to 24 hours. A significant reduction in urine bacterial concentrations should occur in 48 hours. If bacteriologic response has not occurred, an alternative agent should be considered based on susceptibility testing. If the patient fails to respond clinically within 3 to 4 days or has persistently positive blood or urine cultures, further investigation is needed to exclude bacterial resistance, possible obstruction, papillary necrosis, intrarenal or perinephric abscess, or some other disease process. Usually by the third day of therapy, the patient is afebrile and significantly less symptomatic. In general, after the patient has been afebrile for 24 hours, parenteral therapy may be discontinued, and oral therapy instituted to complete a 2-week course. Follow-up urine cultures should be obtained 2 weeks after completion of therapy to ensure a satisfactory response and detect possible relapse.

URINARY TRACT INFECTIONS IN MALES

The management of UTIs in males is distinctly different and often more difficult than in females. Infections in male patients are considered to be complicated because they are caused by endogenous bacteria in the presence of functional or structural abnormalities that disrupt the normal defense mechanisms of the urinary tract. The incidence of infections in males less than 60 years of age is much less than that in females. During the adult years, the occurrence of infection can be directly related to some manipulation of the urinary tract. The most common causes are instrumentation of the urinary tract, catheterization, and renal and urinary stones. Uncomplicated infections are rare, but they may occur in young males as a result of homosexual activity, lack of circumcision, and having sex with partners who are colonized with uropathogenic bacteria. As the patient ages, the most common cause of infection is related to bladder outlet obstruction because of prostatic hypertrophy. In addition, the prostate gland may become infected and provide a nidus for recurrent infection in males.

The conventional view is that therapy in males requires prolonged treatment (Fig. 106–2). A urine culture should be obtained before treatment because the cause of infection in men is not as predictable as in women. Single-dose or short-course therapy is not recommended in this setting. Considerably fewer data are available comparing various antimicrobial agents in males as compared to females. If gram-negative bacteria are presumed, trimethoprim–sulfamethoxazole or the quinolone antimicrobials should be considered because these agents achieve high renal tissue, urine, and prostatic concentrations.

Initial therapy should be for 10 to 14 days. Factors associated with treatment success are isolation of a single organism, the absence of significant obstruction or anatomic abnormalities, a normal functioning urinary tract, and the absence of prostatic involvement. Parenteral therapy may be required in certain situations, such as in severely ill patients, the presence of acute prostatitis, or epididymitis, and in patients who cannot tolerate oral medications. A comparison of 2-week versus 6-week therapy in males with recurrent infections who were given trimethoprim–sulfamethoxazole had cure rates of 29% and 62%, respectively.[37] Others have advocated longer treatment periods in males as well.[38] Follow-up cultures at 4 to 6 weeks after treatment are important in males to ensure bacteriologic cure. Many patients will require longer periods of treatment and possible alterations in antibiotics, depending on culture and sensitivity results and clinical response.

RECURRENT INFECTIONS

Recurrent episodes of UTI account for a significant portion of all UTIs. Of those patients suffering from recurrent infections, 80% can be considered reinfections. That is, the recurrence of infection by an organism different than that isolated from the preceding infection. These patients are most commonly female and recurrence develops in about 20% of them with cystitis. Reinfections can be divided into two groups: those with less than two or three episodes per year and those who develop more frequent infections.

Management strategies depend on predisposing factors, number of episodes per year, and patient's preference. Factors that have commonly been associated with recurrent infections include sexual intercourse and diaphragm or spermicide use for birth control. Therapeutic options include self-administered therapy, postcoital therapy, and continuous low-dose prophylaxis. In those patients with infrequent infections (less than three infections per year), each episode should be treated as a separately occurring infection. Short-course therapy is appropriate in this setting.

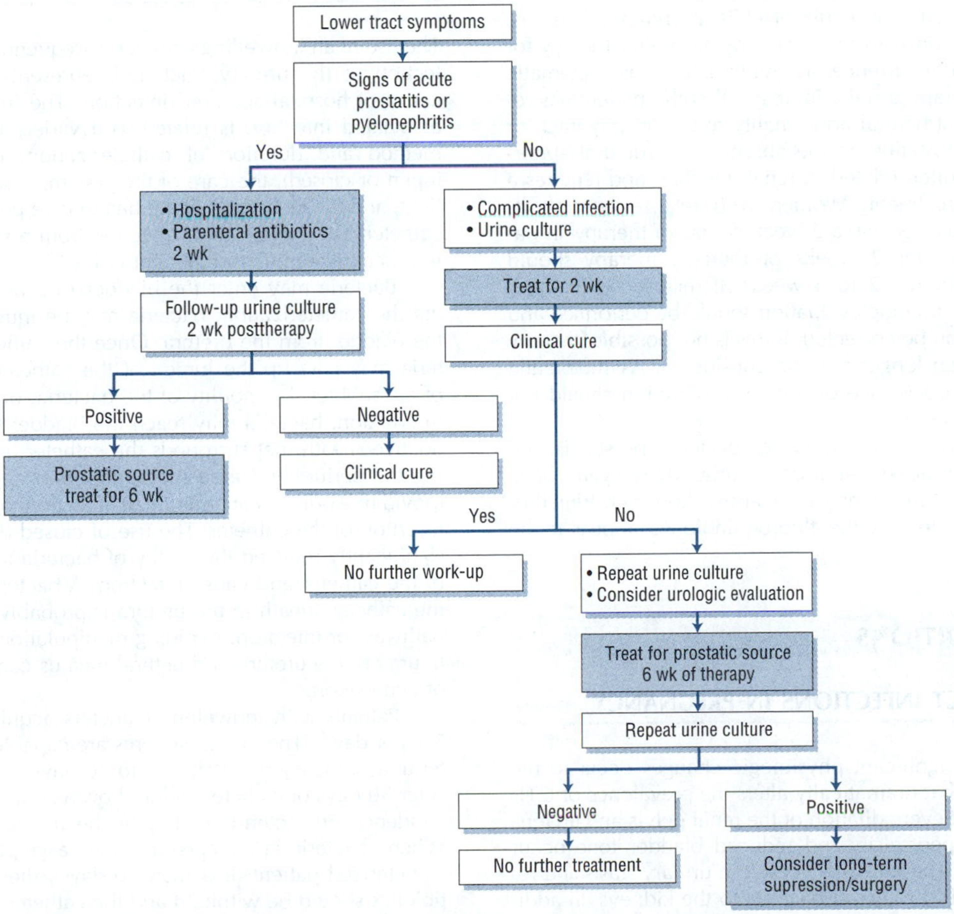

FIGURE 106–2. Management of urinary tract infections in males.

Many women have been successfully treated with self-administered short-course therapy at the onset of symptoms.[39]

In those patients with more frequent symptomatic infections and no apparent precipitating event, long-term prophylactic antimicrobial therapy may be instituted. Prophylactic therapy has been found to reduce the frequency of symptomatic infections in elderly men, women, and children. In women, most studies have shown a reinfection rate of two to three per patient year reduced to 0.1 to 0.2 per patient year with treatment.[40] Before prophylaxis is initiated, patients should be treated conventionally with an appropriate agent. Trimethoprim–sulfamethoxazole (one-half of a single strength tablet), trimethoprim (100 mg daily), a fluroquinolone (one tablet), or nitrofurantoin (50 or 100 mg daily) have all been found to reduce the rate of reinfection as single-agent therapy.[11] Full-dose therapy with these agents is unnecessary, and single daily doses can be used. Therapy is generally prescribed for a period of 6 months, during which time urine cultures are followed monthly. If symptomatic episodes develop, the patient should receive a full course of therapy with an effective agent and should be restarted on prophylactic therapy.

In those women who experience symptomatic reinfections in association with sexual activity, voiding after intercourse may help prevent infection. Also, single-dose prophylactic therapy with trimethoprim–sulfamethoxazole taken after intercourse has been found to reduce the incidence of recurrent infection significantly.[41]

In postmenopausal women with recurrent infections, the lack of estrogen results in changes of the bacterial flora of the vagina, resulting in increased colonization with uropathogenic *E. coli*. Topically administered estrogen cream has been reported to reduce the incidence of infections in this population.[42]

The remaining 20% of recurrent UTIs are relapses. That is, persistence of infection with the same organism after therapy for an isolated UTI. The recurrence of symptomatic or asymptomatic bacteriuria after therapy usually indicates that the patient has renal involvement, a structural abnormality of the urinary tract, or chronic bacterial prostatitis. In the absence of structural abnormalities, relapse is often related to renal infection and requires a long duration of treatment. Women who relapse after short-course therapy should receive a 2-week course of therapy. In patients who relapse after 2 weeks of therapy, therapy should be continued for another 2 to 4 weeks. If relapse occurs after 6 weeks of therapy, urologic evaluation should be performed and any obstructive lesion be corrected. If this is not possible, therapy for 6 months or even longer may be considered. Asymptomatic adults who have no evidence of urinary obstruction should not receive long-term therapy.

In males, relapse usually indicates bacterial prostatitis, the most common cause of persistent bacteriuria. Many agents have been used for long-term therapy of relapses; however, trimethoprim–sulfamethoxazole and the fluoroquinolones appear to be highly effective.

SPECIAL CONDITIONS

URINARY TRACT INFECTIONS IN PREGNANCY

During pregnancy, significant physiologic changes occur to the entire urinary tract that dramatically alters the prevalence of UTIs and pyelonephritis. Severe dilation of the renal pelvis and ureters, decreased ureteral peristalsis, and reduced bladder tone occur during pregnancy.[43] These changes result in urinary stasis and reduced defenses against reflux of bacteria to the kidneys. In addition, hormonal changes, primarily hyperestrogenism, have been suggested to predispose women to infection. These changes increase the incidence of bacteriuria resulting in symptomatic infections, especially during the third trimester.

Asymptomatic bacteriuria occurs in 4% to 7% of pregnant patients. Of these, 20% to 40% will develop acute symptomatic pyelonephritis during pregnancy. If untreated, asymptomatic bacteriuria has the potential to cause significant adverse effects, including prematurity, low birth weight, and stillbirth.[44] As pyelonephritis is associated with significant adverse events during pregnancy, routine screening tests for bacteriuria be should performed at the initial prenatal visit and again at 28 weeks' gestation. In those patients with significant bacteriuria, symptomatic or asymptomatic, treatment is recommended in order to avoid possible complications. Organisms associated with bacteriuria are the same as those seen in uncomplicated UTIs with *E. coli* isolated most frequently.

Therapy should consist of an agent administered for 7 days that has a relatively low adverse effect potential and is safe for the mother and baby. The administration of a sulfonamide, amoxicillin, amoxicillin/clavulanate, cephalexin, or nitrofurantion is effective in 70% to 80% of patients. Tetracyclines should be avoided because of teratogenic effects, and sulfonamides should not be administered during the third trimester because of the possible development of kernicterus and hyperbilirubinemia. In addition, the available fluoroquinolones should not be given because of their potential to inhibit cartilage and bone development in the newborn. A follow-up urine culture 1 to 2 weeks after completing therapy and then monthly until gestation is complete is recommended.

CATHETERIZED PATIENTS

The use of an indwelling catheter is frequently associated with infection of the urinary tract and represents the most common cause of hospital-acquired infection. The incidence of catheter-associated infection is related to a variety of factors, including method and duration of catheterization, the catheter system (open or closed), the care of the system, susceptibility of the patient, and the technique of the health care personnel inserting the catheter. The incidence of infection from a single catheterization in a healthy ambulatory patient is 1%.[45]

Bacteria may enter the bladder in a number of ways. During the catheterization, bacteria may be introduced directly into the bladder from the urethra. Once the catheter is in place, bacteria may pass up the lumen of the catheter via the movement of air bubbles, by motility of the bacteria, or by capillary action. In addition, bacteria may reach the bladder from around the exudative sheath that surrounds the catheter in the urethra. Cleaning the periurethral area thoroughly and applying an antiseptic (povidine–iodine) can minimize infection occurring during the insertion of the catheter. The use of closed drainage systems has significantly reduced the ability of bacteria to pass up the lumen of the catheter and cause infection. A bacterium passing around the catheter sheath in the urethra is probably the most important pathway for infection. Avoiding manipulation of the catheter and trauma to the urethra and uethral meatus can minimize this path of acquisition.

Patients with indwelling catheters acquire UTIs at a rate of 5% per day.[45] The closed systems are capable of preventing bacteriuria in most patients for up to 10 days with appropriate care. After 30 days of catheterization, however, there is a 78% to 95% incidence of bacteriuria, despite the use of a closed system.[45] When bacteriuria occurs in the asymptomatic, short-term catheterized patient (less than 30 days), the use of systemic antibiotics should be withheld and the catheter removed as soon as possible. If the patient becomes symptomatic, the catheter should be removed and treatment as described for complicated infections started. The optimal duration of therapy is not known. In the long-term catheterized patient (more than 30 days), bacteriuria is inevitable.[45] The administration of systemic antibiotics active against the infecting organism will sterilize the urine; however, reinfection occurs rapidly in over 50% of patients. In addition, the recolonization of the urine is with resistant organisms. Symptomatic patients must be treated because they are at risk of developing pyelonephritis and bacteremia. Bacteria have been found to adhere to the catheter and produce a biofilm consisting of bacterial glycocalices, Tamm-Horsfall protein, and apatite and struvite salts, which act to protect the bacteria from antibiotics.[46] Recatheterization with a new, sterile unit should be performed in those symptomatic patients, if the existing catheter has been in place for more than 2 weeks.

Various methods have been proposed to prevent the development of bacteriuria and infection in the patient with an indwelling catheter (Table 106–5). The success of these methods depends on the type of catheter and length of time it is in place. The use of constant bladder irrigation with antiseptic or antibacterial solutions has been investigated and found to reduce the incidence of infection in those with open drainage systems, but they have no advantage in those with closed systems. The use of prophylactic systemic antibiotics in patients with short-term catheterization has been found to reduce the incidence of infection over the first 4 to 7 days.[47] In long-term catheterized patients, however, antibiotics only postpones the development of bacteriuia and leads to the emergence of resistant organisms.

TABLE 106–5. Guidelines of Urinary Catheter Care

Use catheters only when absolutely necessary and remove as soon as possible.
Insert catheters aseptically and maintain by trained personnel only.
A sterile closed drainage system is mandatory.
Obtain urine for culture by aspirating the catheter with a 21-gauge needle after the catheter is prepared with povidone-iodine.
Maintain downhill, unobstructed flow with the collection bag always below the level of the bladder. Empty bag at frequent intervals.
Replace indwelling catheters when obstruction or concretions are demonstrated.
Separate catheterized patients from each other whenever possible.
Administer prophylactic antibiotics during catheter insertion and removal to patients predisposed to bacterial endocarditis (e.g., prosthetic valve patients).

PROSTATITIS

Bacterial prostatitis is defined as inflammation of the prostate gland and surrounding tissue as a result of infection. It may be classified as either acute or chronic. By definition, pathogenic bacteria and significant inflammatory cells must be present in prostatic secretions and urine to make the diagnosis of bacterial prostatitis. Prostatitis rarely occurs in young males, but it is commonly associated with recurrent infections in persons older than 30 years. As many as 50% of all males develop some form of prostatitis at some period in their life.[48] The acute form is typically an acute infectious disease characterized by a sudden onset of fever, tenderness, and urinary and constitutional symptoms. Chronic prostatitis presents with few symptoms related to the prostate, but rather symptoms of urinating difficulty, low back pain, perineal pressure, or a combination of these. It represents a recurring infection, with the same organism that results from incomplete eradication of bacteria from the prostate gland.

PATHOGENESIS AND ETIOLOGY

The exact mechanism of bacterial infection of the prostate is not well understood. The possible routes of infection are the same as those for UTIs. Reflux of infected urine into the prostate gland is thought to play a important role in causing infection. Studies suggest that intraprostatic reflux of urine occurs commonly and results in direct inoculation of infected urine into the prostate.[49] In addition, intraprostatic reflux of sterile urine can result in a chemical prostatitis and may be the cause of nonbacterial prostatitis. Sexual intercourse may contribute to infection of the prostate gland, since prostatic secretions from men with chronic prostatitis and vaginal cultures from their sexual partners grew identical organisms.[50] Other known causes of bacterial prostatitis include indwelling urethral and condom catheterization, urethral instrumentation, and transurethral prostatectomy in patients with infected urine.

A number of physiologic factors are believed to contribute to the development of prostatitis. Functional abnormalities found in bacterial prostatitis include altered prostate secretory functions. Prostatic fluid obtained from normal males contains prostatic antibacterial factor (PAF). This heat stable, low molecular weight cation is a zinc-complexed polypeptide that is bactericidal to most urinary tract pathogens.[51] The antibacterial activity of PAF is directly related to the zinc content of prostatic fluid. Prostate fluid zinc levels and PAF activity also appear diminished in patients with prostatitis, as well as the elderly.[49] Whether these changes are a cause or effect of prostatitis remains to be determined.

The pH of prostatic secretions in patients with prostatitis has also been reported to be altered.[52] Normal prostatic secretions have a pH in the range of 6.6 to 7.6. With increasing age, the pH tends to become more alkaline. In patients with inflammation of the prostate, prostatic secretions may have an alkaline pH in the range of 7 to 9. These changes suggest a generalized secretory dysfunction of the prostate, which not only may affect the pathogenesis of prostatitis, but it also may influence the mode of therapy.

Gram-negative, enteric organisms are the most frequent pathogens in acute bacterial prostatitis.[49] *Escherichia coli* is the predominate organism occurring in 75% of cases. Other gram-negative organisms frequently ioslated include *K. pneumoniae, P. mirabilis,* and less frequently *P. aeruginosa, Enterobacter* sp., and *Serratia* sp. Occasionally, cases of gonococcal and staphylococcal prostatitis occur, but they are infrequent.

Escherichia coli most commonly causes chronic bacterial prostatitis with other gram-negative organisms isolated less frequently. The importance of gram-positive organisms in chronic bacterial prostatitis remains controversial. *Staphylococcus epidermidis, S. aureus,* and diphtheroids have been isolated in some studies.

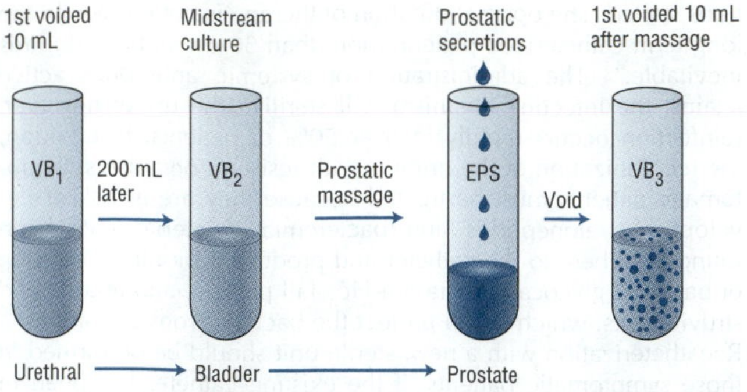

FIGURE 106–3. Segmented cultures of the lower urinary tract in men.

CLINICAL PRESENTATION

Acute bacterial prostatitis presents as other acute infections. Common symptoms include high fever, chills, malaise, myalgia, localized pain (perineal, rectal, sacrococcygeal), and other urinary symptoms (frequency, urgency, dysuria, nocturia, retention). Digital palpation of the prostate via the rectum may reveal a swollen, tender, warm, tense, or indurated gland. Massage of the prostate will express a purulent discharge, which will readily grow the pathogenic organism. Prostatic massage is contraindicated in ABP, however, because of the risk of inducing bacteremia and associated local pain. The diagnosis of ABP can be made from the patient's clinical presentation and the presence of significant bacteriuria. As with other UTIs, the infecting organism can be isolated from a midstream specimen.

In contrast, CBP is more difficult to diagnose and treat. Chronic bacterial prostatitis is typically characterized by recurrent UTIs with the same pathogen and is the most common cause of recurrent UTI in males. Although examination of the prostate gland often reveals a normal gland, most will have prostatic enlargement. The patient's clinical presentation can vary widely. Presenting symptoms include the vague description of voiding difficulties, such as frequency, urgency, and dysuria. In addition, symptoms of low back pain and perineal and suprapubic discomfort are present. Many adults, however, are asymptomatic.

Because physical examination of the prostate is often normal, urinary tract localization studies are critical to the diagnosis of CBP. The method of quantitative localization culture, as described be Meares and Stamey, remains the diagnostic standard[53] (Fig. 106–3). The method compares the bacterial growth in sequential urine and prostatic fluid cultures obtained during micturition. The first 10 mL of voided urine is collected (voiding bladder 1 or VB_1) and constitutes urethral urine. After approximately 200 mL of urine has been voided, a 10 mL midstream sample is collected (VB_2). This specimen represents bladder urine. After the patient voids, the prostate is massaged and expressed prostatic secretions (EPS) are collected. After prostatic massage, the patient voids again and 10 mL of urine is collected (VB_3).

The diagnosis of bacterial prostatitis is made when the number of bacteria in EPS is ten times that of the urethral sample (VB_1) and midstream sample (VB_2). If no EPS is available, the urine sample following massage (VB_3) should contain a bacterial count tenfold greater than that of VB_1 or VB_2. If significant bacteriuria is present, ampicillin, cephalexin, or nitrofurantoin should be given for 2 to 3 days to sterilize the urine prior to performing the localization study.

▶ TREATMENT: Prostatitis

The goals in the management of bacterial prostatitis are the same as those for UTIs in general. Acute bacterial prostatitis responds well to appropriate antimicrobial therapy that is directed at the most commonly isolated organisms. Prostatic penetration of antimicrobials occurs because the acute inflammatory reaction alters the cellular membrane barrier between the bloodstream and the prostate. The majority of patients can be managed with oral antimicrobial agents, such as trimethoprim–sulfamethoxazole and the fluoroquinolones (ciprofloxacin, levofloxacin, ofloxacin). Other effective agents in this setting include cephalosporins and β-lactam and β-lactamase combinations. Although intravenous therapy is rarely necessary for total treatment, intravenous to oral sequential therapy with trimethoprim–sulfamethoxazole or the fluoroquinolones would be appropriate. The conversion to an oral antibiotic can be considered after the patient is afebrile for 48 hours or after 3 to 5 days of intravenous therapy. The total course of antibiotic therapy should be 4 weeks in order to reduce the risk of development of chronic prostatitis.

Chronic bacterial prostatitis often presents a more vexing situation because cures are rarely obtained. In the past, it was recognized that despite high serum concentrations of antibacterial drugs in excess of the minimal inhibitory concentrations of the infecting organisms, bacteria persisted in prostatic fluid. The failure to eradicate sensitive bacteria was thought to be related to the inability of antibiotics to reach sufficient concentrations in the prostatic fluid and cross the prostatic epithelium.

Several factors that determine antibiotic diffusion into prostatic secretions were delineated from the canine model. Lipid solubility is a major determinant in the ability of drugs to diffuse from plasma across epithelial membranes. The degree of ionization in plasma also affects the diffusion of drugs. Only un-ionized molecules can cross the lipid barrier of prostatic cells and the drug's pK_a directly determines the fraction of unchanged drug.

The pH gradient across the membrane has an influence on tissue penetration as well. A pH gradient of at least one pH unit between separate compartments allows for ion trapping. As the un-ionized drug crosses the epithelial barrier into prostatic fluid, it becomes ionized, thus allowing less drug to diffuse back across the lipid barrier. In early studies with the canine model, the prostatic pH was reported to be acidic (6.4).[49] More recent studies in man, however, have reported that the pH of prostatic secretions from an inflamed prostate is actually basic (8.1 to 8.3).[49]

The choice of antibiotics in CBP should include those agents that are capable of reaching therapeutic concentrations in the prostatic fluid and that possess the spectrum of activity to be effective. Agents that achieve therapeutic prostatic concentrations include trimethoprim and the fluoroquinolones. Sulfamethoxazole penetrates poorly and probably contributes very little to trimethoprim. The fluoroquinolones appear to provide the best therapeutic options in the management of CBP. Trimethoprim–sulfamethoxazole is also effective. Therapy should be continued for 4 to 6 weeks initially. Longer treatment periods may be necessary in some cases. If therapy fails with these regimens, chronic suppressive therapy may be used or surgery considered.

PHARMACOECONOMIC CONSIDERATIONS

The cost-effective management of UTIs requires a knowledge of its pathogenesis and causative organisms associated with the various clinical syndromes described in this chapter. The costs associated with managing a UTI include direct costs, such a laboratory tests, medication, and health care visits. The indirect costs include lost work time and general quality of life issues, such as disease or therapy adverse effects.

Direct costs are those associated with diagnosis, treatment, and follow-up. Reported percentages for these costs in cystitis are physician consultation 23%, laboratory costs 64%, and pharmaceuticals 13%.[54] The cost of pharmaceuticals varies according to the agents used and the duration of therapy. When trimethoprim–sulfamethoxazole and amoxicillin have been compared, trimethoprim–sulfamethoxazole results in a higher cure rate, lower relapse, fewer symptoms, and lower costs.[55] The fluoroquinolones have also been found to be highly effective agents but are generally more expensive. The outcome and total cost are dependent on whether therapy is empiric or definitive (based on a culture diagnosis for acute infection).

▶ PRINCIPLES OF PHARMACOTHERAPY

- Urinary tract infections can be classified as uncomplicated and complicated. Uncomplicated refers to an otherwise healthy female who lacks structural or functional abnormalities of the urinary tract. Most often, complicated infections are associated with a predisposing lesion of the urinary tract; however, the term may be used to refer to all other infections, except for those in the otherwise healthy adult female.
- Significant bacteriuria has traditionally been defined as bacterial counts of greater than 100,000 (10^5)/mL of urine. Many clinicians, however, have challenged this as a too general statement. Indeed, significant bacteriuria in patients with symptoms of a urinary tract infection may be defined as greater than 10^2 organisms/mL.
- The most frequent mechanism of infections is via the ascending route with organisms that originate from the fecal flora.
- Eighty-five percent of uncomplicated urinary tract infections are caused by *Escherichia coli* and the remainder primarily by *Staphylococcus saprophyticus, Proteus* sp., and *Klebsiella* sp. Complicated infections are more frequently associated with gram-negative organisms and *Enterococcus fecalis.*
- The key to the diagnosis of urinary tract infections is the ability to demonstrate significant numbers of microorganisms in an appropriate urine specimen. The extent of laboratory examination depends on the clinical situation.
- The goals of treatment of urinary tract infections are to prevent or treat systemic consequences of infections, eradicate the invading organism, and prevent the reoccurrence of infection.
- Uncomplicated urinary tract infections can be most effectively managed with short-course (3 to 5 days) therapy with either trimethoprim–sulfamethoxazole or a fluoroquinolone. Complicated infections require longer treatment periods (2 weeks) with one of these agents.
- Acute bacterial prostatitis can be managed with many agents that have activity against the causative organism. Chronic prostatitis requires an agent that is not only active against the causative organism, but also concentrates in the prostatic secretions. Therapy with trimethoprim–sulfamethoxazole or a fluoroquinolone are preferred for 4 to 6 weeks.

REFERENCES

1. Bacheller CD, Bernstein JM. Urinary tract infections. Med Clin North Am 1997;81:719–729.
2. Plumridge RJ, Golledge CL. Treatment of urinary tract infection: Clinical and economic considerations. Pharmacoeconomics 1996;9: 295–306.
3. Johnson CC. Definitions, classification, and clinical presentation of urinary tract infections. Med Clin North Am 1991;75:241–252.

4. Platt R. Quantitative definition of bacteriuria. Am J Med 1983;75: 44–52.
5. Stull TL, LiPuma JJ. Epidemiology and natural history of urinary tract infections in children. Med Clin North Am 1991;75:287–298.
6. Smellie JM. Reflections of thirty years of treating children with urinary tract infections. J Urol 1991;146:665–668.
7. Sobel JD, Kaye D. Urinary tract infections. In: Mandell GL, Bennett JE, Dolin R, eds. Principles and Practice of Infectious Diseases, 4th ed. New York, Churchill Livingstone, 1995:662–690.
8. Baldassarre JS, Kaye D. Special problems in urinary tract infections in the elderly. Med Clin North Am 1991;75:375–390.
9. Turck M, Stamm WE. Nosocomial infection of the urinary tract. Am J Med. 1981;70:651–654.
10. Boyce JM. Vancomycin-resistant Enterococcus: Detection, epidemiology, and control measures. Infect Dis Clin North Am 1997;11: 367–384.
11. Nicolle LE, Harding GKM, Preiksaitis J, et al. The association of urinary tract infection with sexual intercourse. J Infect Dis 1982;146: 579–583.
12. Stamey TA, Fair WR, Timothy MM, et al. Antibacterial nature of prostatic fluid. Nature 1968;218:444–447.
13. Shand DG, Nimmon CC, O'Grady F, et al. Relation betwen residual urine volume and response to treatment of urinary infection. Lancet 1970;1:1305–1306.
14. Parsons CL, Schrom SH, Hanno P, et al. Bladder surface mucin: Examination of possible mechanisms for its antibacterial effect. Invest Urol 1978;6:196–200.
15. Sobel JD. Bacterial etiologic agents in the pathogenesis of urinary tract infections. Med Clin North Am 1991;75:253–273.
16. Orskov I, Ferencz A, Orskov F. Tamm-Horsfall protein or uromucoid is the normal urinary slime that traps type-1 fimbriated *Escherichia coli.* Lancet 1980;1:887.
17. Measley RE, Levison ME. Host defense mechanisms in the pathogenesis of urinary tract infection. Med Clin North Am 1991;75:275–286.
18. Jenkins RD, Fenn JP, Matsen JM. Review of urine microscopy for bacteriuria. JAMA 1986;255:3397.
19. Pezzlo M. Detection of urinary tract infections by rapid methods. Clin Microbiol Rev 1988;2:268–280.
20. Stamm WE. Measurement of pyuria and its relation to bacteriuria. Am J Med 1983;75(suppl 1):53–58.
21. Pappas PG. Laboratory in the diagnosis and management of urinary tract infections. Med Clin North Am 1991;75:313–325.
22. Pels RJ, Bor DH, Woolhandler S, et al. Dipstick urinalysis screening of asymptomatic adults for urinary tract disorders. JAMA 1989;262: 1221–1224.
23. Stamey TA, Govan DE, Palmer JM. The localization and treatment of urinary tract infections: The role of bactericidal urine levels as opposed to serum levels. Medicine 1965;44:1–36.
24. Fairley KF, Bond AG, Brown RB, et al. Simple test to determine the site of urinary tract infection. Lancet 1967;2:427–428.
25. Thomas VC, Forland M. Antibody-coated bacteria in urinary tract infection. Kidney Int 1982;21:1–7.
26. Stamey TA, Fair WR, Timothy MM, et al. Serum versus urinary antimicrobial concentrations in cure of urinary tract infections. N Engl J Med 1974;291:1159–1163.
27. Avorn J, Monane M, Gurwitz JH, et al. Reduction of bacteriuria and pyuria after ingestion of cranberry juice. JAMA 1994;271:751–754.
28. Johnson JR, Stamm WE. Urinary tract infection in women: Diagnosis and treatment. Ann Intern Med 1989;11:906–917.
29. Norrby SR. Short term treatment of uncomplicated lower urinary tract infections in women. Rev Infect Dis 1990;12:458–467.
30. Greenberg RN, Sanders CV, Lewis AS, et al. Single dose therapy for urinary tract infection with cefaclor. Am J Med 1981;71:841–845.
31. Stamm WE, Hooton TM. Management of urinary tract infections in adults. N Engl J Med 1993;329:1328–1334.
32. Sherbotie JR, Cornfield D. Management of urinary tract infections in children. Med Clin North Am 1991;75:327–338.
33. Boscia JA, Kobasa WD, Knight RA, et al. Therapy versus no therapy for bacteriuria in elderly ambulatory non-hospitalized women. JAMA 1987;257:1067–1071.
34. Nicolle LE, Mayhew WJ, Bryan L. Prospective, randomized comparison of therapy and no therapy for asymptomatic bacteriuria in institutionalized women. Am J Med 1987;83:27–33.
35. Nicolle LE, Bjornson J, Harding GKM, et al. Bacteriuria in elderly institutionalized men. N Engl J Med 1983;309:1420–1425.
36. Bergeron MG, Beauchamp D, Poirier A, et al. Continuous vs. intermittent administration of antimicrobial agents: Tissue penetration and efficacy *in vivo*. Rev Infect Dis 1985;3:84–97.
37. Gleckman R, Crowley M, Natsios GA. Therapy of recurrent invasive urinary tract infection in men. N Engl J Med 1979;301:878–880.
38. Lipsky GA. Urinary tract infections in men: Epidemiology, pathophysiology, diagnosis, and treatment. Ann Intern Med 1989;110: 138–150.
39. Wong ES, McKevitt M, Running K, et al. Management of recurrent urinary tract infections with patient-administered single dose therapy. Ann Intern Med 1985;102:302–307.
40. Nicolle LE, Ronald AR. Recurrent urinary tract infection in adult women: Diagnosis and treatment. Infect Dis Clin North Am 1987; 1:793–806.
41. Stapleton A, Latham RH, Johnson C, et al. Post-coital antimicrobial prophylaxis for recurrent urinary tract infection. JAMA 1990;264: 703–706.
42. Raz R, Stamm WE. A controlled trial of intravaginal estriol in postmenopausal women with recurrent urinary tract infections. N Engl J Med 1993;329:753–756.
43. Andriole VT, Patterson TF. Epidemiology, natural history, and managment of urinary tract infection in pregnancy. Med Clin North Am 1991;75:359–373.
44. McGrady GA, Daling JR, Peterson DR. Maternal urinary tract infection and adverse fetal outcomes. Am J Epidemiol 1985;121:377–381.
45. Warren JW. The catheter and urinary tract infection. Med Clin North Am 1991;75:481–493.
46. Ohkawa M, Sugata T, Sawaki M, et al. Bacterial and crystal adherence to the surfaces of indwelling urethral catheters. J Urol 1990;143: 717–721.
47. Stamm WE. Catheter-associated urinary tract infection: Epidemiology, pathogenesis, and prevention. Am J Med 1991;91:(supp 3B)65s–71s.
48. Schaefer AJ. Urinary tract infection in men: State of the art. Infection 1994;22(suppl 1):S19–S21.
49. Meares EM. Prostatitis. Med Clin North Am 1991;75:405–424.
50. Stamey TA. Urinary infections in males. In: Pathogenesis and Treatment of Urinary Tract Infections. Baltimore, Williams & Williams, 1980:342–429.
51. Fair WR, Couch J, Wehner M. Prostatic antibacterial factor: Identity and significance. Urology 1976;7:169–177.
52. Pfau A, Perlberg S, Shapiro A. The pH of prostatic fluid in health and disease: Implications of treatment in chronic bacterial prostatitis. J Urol 1978;119:384–387.
53. Meares EM, Stamey TA. Bacteriologic localization patterns in bacterial prostatitis and urethritis. Invest Urol 1968;5:492–518.
54. Patton JP, Nash DB, Abrutyn E. Urinary tract infection: Economic considerations. Med Clin North Am 1991;75:495–513.
55. MacDonald TM, Collins D, McGilchrist MM, et al. The utilization and economic evaluation of antibiotics prescribed in primary care. J Antimicrob Chemother 1995;35:191–204.

107

SEXUALLY TRANSMITTED DISEASES

Leroy C. Knodel, PharmD

Over the years, the spectrum of sexually transmitted diseases (STDs) has broadened from the classic venereal diseases—gonorrhea, syphilis, chancroid, lymphogranuloma venereum, and granuloma inguinale—to include a variety of pathogens known to be spread by sexual contact (Table 107–1).[1,2] Because of the large number of infected individuals, the diversity of clinical manifestations, the changing drug susceptibility patterns of some pathogens, and the high frequency of multiple STDs occurring simultaneously in infected individuals, the diagnosis and management of patients with STDs are much more complex than even a decade ago.

Despite a higher reported incidence of all major STDs in men, the complications of STDs generally are more frequent and severe in women. In particular, serious effects on maternal and infant health during pregnancy are well documented. Damage to reproductive organs, increased risk of cancer, complications associated with pregnancy, and transmission of disease to the fetus or newborn are associated with several STDs. As a result of the physiologic, psychosocial, and economic consequences of STDs and because of the increasing prevalence of some viral STDs, such as human immunodeficiency virus (HIV) and genital herpes, for which curative therapy is not available, there has been a resurgence of interest in STD research and the primary prevention of these diseases.[3]

With the exception of the acquired immunodeficiency syndrome (AIDS), which is reviewed in detail in Chapter 114, the most frequently occurring STDs in the United States are discussed in this chapter. For other less common STDs, only recommended treatment regimens are presented. The most current information on the epidemiology, diagnosis, and treatment of STDs provided by the Centers for Disease Control (CDC) can be obtained at their website on the Internet (http://www.cdc.gov/).

Numerous interrelated factors contribute to the epidemic nature of sexually transmitted diseases. Sociocultural, demographic, and economic factors together with patterns of sexual behavior, host susceptibility to infection, changing properties of the causative pathogens, disease transmission by asymptomatic individuals, and environmental factors are important determinants of the frequency and distribution of STDs in the United States and worldwide.[2,3]

Age is one of the most important demographic determinants of STD incidence. Overall, two-thirds of STD cases each year occur in persons in their teens and twenties, the peak years of sexual activity. With increasing age, the incidence of most STDs decreases exponentially. In sexually active teenagers, STD rates are highest in the youngest, suggesting that physiologic differences may contribute to increased susceptibility.[2,4]

Age-specific rates of STDs are higher in men than in women; however, reported rates may not represent true gender differences, but rather may reflect greater ease of detection in men. In recent years, the ratio of male-to-female cases for most STDs has declined, possibly reflecting improvements in the diagnosis of STDs in asymptomatic women or changes in female sexual behavior following the availability of improved methods of contraception.[2,4] Although some racial disparity exists for rates of STD infection, it is possible that this is a reflection of socioeconomic differences.

Epidemiologic data have shown that the single greatest risk factor for contracting STDs is the number of sexual partners. As the number of sexual partners increases, the risk of being exposed to someone infected with an STD increases. Sexual preference also plays a major role in the transmission of STDs. For all major STDs, rates are disproportionately greater in homosexual men than in heterosexuals. Also, a number of less common STDs, including several caused by enteric protozoans and bacterial pathogens, occur primarily in homosexual men. The major risk factors for homosexual men appear to be related to the greater number of sexual partners and the practice of unprotected anal–genital, oral–genital, and oral–anal intercourse. In addition, prostitution and illicit drug use continue to be associated with a higher incidence of most STDs.[2,4,5]

Some of the most serious sequelae of STDs are associated with congenital or perinatal infections. The majority of neonatal infections are acquired at birth, after infant passage through an infected cervix or vagina. Neonatal *Chlamydia trachomatis, Neisseria gonorrhoeae,* and herpes simplex virus (HSV) infections are associated with this type of spread. For pregnant women with syphilis, infection is usually transmitted transplacentally, producing a congenital infection. Depending on the organism, neonatal infections can manifest in a variety of ways. Ophthalmia neonatorum can result from chlamydial or gonorrheal infections, while syphilis and herpes infections can produce more severe complications, including neurologic impairment. Neonatal herpes infections also are associated with a high mortality.[5]

Other than complete abstinence, the most effective way to prevent STD transmission is by maintaining a mutually monogamous sexual relationship between uninfected partners. Short of this, use of barrier contraceptive methods,

TABLE 107–1. Sexually Transmitted Diseases

Disease	Pathogen
Bacterial	
Gonorrhea	*Neisseria gonorrhoeae*
Syphilis	*Treponema pallidum*
Chancroid	*Haemophilus ducreyi*
Granuloma inguinale (donovanosis)	*Calymmatobacterium granulomatis*
Salmonellosis	*Salmonella* sp.
Shigellosis	*Shigella* sp.
Campylobacter infection	*Campylobacter jejuni*
Bacterial vaginosis	*Gardnerella vaginalis, Mycoplasma hominis, Bacteroides* sp., *Mobiluncus* sp.
Group B streptococcal infections	Group B streptococcus
Chlamydial	
Nongonococcal urethritis	*Chlamydia trachomatis*
Lymphogranuloma venereum	*C. trachomatis*
Viral	
Acquired immunodeficiency syndrome (AIDS)	Human immunodeficiency virus
Herpes genitalis	Herpes simplex virus
Viral hepatitis	Hepatitis A–D viruses
Condylomata acuminata	Human papilloma virus
Molluscum contagiosum	Poxvirus
Cytomegalovirus infection	Cytomegalovirus
Mycoplasmal	
Nongonococcal urethritis	*Ureaplasma urealyticum*
Protozoal	
Trichomoniasis	*Trichomonas vaginalis*
Amebiasis	*Entamoeba histolytica*
Giardiasis	*Giardia lamblia*
Fungal	
Candidiasis	*Candida albicans*
Parasitic	
Scabies	*Sarcoptes scabiei*
Pediculosis	*Phthirus pubis*
Enterobiasis	*Enterobius vermicularis*

such as the male and female condoms, diaphragm, cervical cap, vaginal sponges, and vaginal spermicides alone or in combination, have been shown to provide varying degrees of protection from a number of STDs. When used correctly and consistently, male latex condoms with or without spermicide are more effective than natural skin condoms in protecting against STD transmission, including HIV, gonorrhea, chlamydia, HSV, and hepatitis B.[4–8] When lubrication is desired with latex condoms, water-based products, such as K-Y Jelly, are recommended because oil-based agents (e.g., petroleum jelly) can weaken latex condoms and reduce their effectiveness. The female condom is a lubricated polyurethane sheath with a diaphragm-like ring on each end. When inserted into the vagina, it may act as a mechanical barrier to disease transmission. The female condom may provide an alternative protective device for women with male sexual partners who do not desire to use a condom. Limited data suggest that the female condom blocks penetration of viruses, including HIV; for nonviral STDs, only protection from trichomoniasis transmission has been studied and documented. Use of nonoxynol-9, a vaginal spermicide with cytolytic activity, has been shown to reduce the risk for acquiring cervical gonorrhea and chlamydia when used alone. While *in vitro* data suggest that nonoxynol-9 possesses some activity against HIV, there is no evidence that it prevents transmission of the virus or provides any additional benefit in preventing HIV transmission when used in conjunction with latex condoms. Some evidence exists that diaphragms may protect against cervical gonorrheal, chlamydial, and trichomonal infections. Although vaginal spermicides and diaphragms may confer some protection to women, their effect on preventing disease transmission to men has not been evaluated.[6–8]

The varied spectrum of clinical syndromes produced by common STDs is determined not only by the etiologic pathogen(s), but also by differences in male and female anatomy and reproductive physiology. For a number of STDs, the signs and symptoms overlap sufficiently to prevent accurate diagnosis without microbiologic confirmation. Frequently, symptoms are minimal or absent despite the presence of infection. Common clinical syndromes associated with STDs are listed in Table 107–2.[4]

GONORRHEA

EPIDEMIOLOGY AND ETIOLOGY

Neisseria gonorrhoeae is a gram-negative diplococcus estimated to cause up to 1 million infections per year in the United States.[8] Although the number of reported cases of

TABLE 107–2. Selected Syndromes Associated With Common Sexually Transmitted Pathogens

Syndrome	Commonly Implicated Pathogens	Common Clinical Manifestations[a]
Urethritis	*Chlamydia trachomatis*, herpes simplex virus, *Neisseria gonorrhoeae, Trichomonas vaginalis, Ureaplasma urealyticum*	Urethral discharge, dysuria
Epididymitis	*C. trachomatis, N. gonorrhoeae*	Scrotal pain, inguinal pain, flank pain, urethral discharge
Cervicitis/vulvovaginitis	*C. trachomatis, Gardnerella vaginalis*, herpes simplex virus, human papilloma virus, *N. gonorrhoeae, T. vaginalis*	Abnormal vaginal discharge, vulvar itching/irritation, dysuria, dyspareunia
Genital ulcers (painful)	*Haemophilus ducreyi*, herpes simplex virus	Usually multiple vesicular/pustular (herpes) or papular/pustular *(H. ducreyi)* lesions that may coalesce; painful, tender lymphadenopathy[b]
Genital ulcers (painless)	*Treponema pallidum*	Usually single papular lesion
Genital warts	Human papilloma virus	Multiple lesions ranging in size from small papular warts to large exophytic condylomas
Pharyngitis	*C. trachomatis* (?), herpes simplex virus, *N. gonorrhoeae*	Symptoms of acute pharyngitis, cervical lymphadenopathy, fever[c]
Proctitis	*C. trachomatis*, herpes simplex virus, *N. gonorrhoeae, T. pallidum*	Constipation, anorectal discomfort, tenesmus, mucopurulent rectal discharge
Salpingitis	*C. trachomatis, N. gonorrhoeae*	Lower abdominal pain, purulent cervical or vaginal discharge, adnexal swelling, fever[d]

[a]For some syndromes, clinical manifestations may be minimal or absent.
[b]Recurrent herpes infection may manifest as a single lesion.
[c]Most cases of pharyngeal gonococcal infection are asymptomatic.
[d]Salpingitis increases the risk of subsequent ectopic pregnancy and infertility.

gonorrhea in the United States has declined each year since 1989, a substantial number of infections remain unreported.[9,11] Humans are the only known natural host of this intracellular parasite. Because of its rapid incubation period and the large number of infected individuals with asymptomatic disease, gonorrhea is difficult to control.[8–10]

The risk of a female acquiring a cervical infection after a single episode of vaginal intercourse with an infected male may be as high as 60%, and the risk increases with multiple exposure. While the risk of disease transmission from an infected female to an uninfected male is less, it still is as high as 30% following a single act of coitus. No data are available on the risk of transmission after other types of sexual contact.[7,9]

PATHOPHYSIOLOGY

On contact with a mucosal surface lined by columnar, cuboidal, or noncornified squamous epithelial cells, the gonococci attach to cell membranes by means of surface pili and are then pinocytosed. The virulence of the organism is mediated primarily by the presence of pili and other outer membrane proteins. Once mucosal damage is established, polymorphonuclear leukocytes invade the tissue, submucosal abscesses form, and purulent exudates are secreted.[9,10]

CLINICAL PRESENTATION

Infected individuals may be symptomatic or asymptomatic, have complicated or uncomplicated infections, and may have infections involving several anatomic sites. Urethritis is the most common presenting manifestation in males, and it usually develops within 2 to 8 days of exposure. Dysuria and urinary frequency are seen initially, followed in 1 to 2 days by a profuse, purulent urethral discharge. In approximately 25% of cases, the discharge is scant and only minimally purulent, making it almost indistinguishable from nongonococcal urethritis (NGU). Because most men seek treatment from discomforting symptoms, complications resulting from extension of the infection in males, such as epididymitis, prostatitis, inguinal lymphadenopathy, and urethral stricture, rarely are seen today. The majority of symptomatic patients who are not treated become asymptomatic within 6 months, with only a few becoming asymptomatic carriers of the disease.[9,10,12]

The most common site of gonococcal infection in women is the endocervical canal. Anterior spread of infected vaginal secretions produces urethritis. The incubation period is more variable in females, but symptoms typically appear within 10 days following exposure. Symptoms are relatively nonspecific and include dysuria, urinary frequency, abnormal vaginal discharge, and abnormal uterine bleeding. Diagnosis based on symptoms alone is confounded because infection with other organisms may produce similar manifestations. The majority of gonococcal urethral or cervical infections in females are either asymptomatic or produce minimal symptoms.[9,10,12]

Other sites of gonococcal infection include the rectum, oropharynx, and eye. Anorectal gonococcal infections are common in females and homosexual males. In homosexuals, rectal intercourse is the primary cause, whereas most infections in women are caused by perineal contamination with vaginal discharge. Many patients with anorectal gonorrhea have minimal, if any, symptoms. When present, symptoms range from mild pruritis to severe rectal pain, tenesmus, and a mucopurulent rectal discharge.[9,10,12]

Like rectal infections, pharyngeal infections are more common in females and homosexual males. Symptoms can mimic pharyngitis or tonsillitis, although patients are typically asymptomatic. Gonococcal conjunctivitis is rare and usually results from autoinoculation via the fingers from an anogenital infection.[9,10,12] As a result of the nonspecific signs and symptoms, many women do not seek treatment until after the development of serious complications, such as pelvic inflammatory disease (PID). Approximately 15% of women with gonorrhea develop PID. Left untreated, PID can be an indirect cause of infertility and ectopic pregnancies. In 0.5% to 3.0% of patients with gonorrhea, the gonococci invade the bloodstream and produce disseminated disease. Disseminated gonorrhea infection (DGI) is three times more common in women than in men. The usual clinical manifestations of DGI are tender necrotic skin lesions, tenosynovitis, and monarticular arthritis. Occasionally, mild hepatitis, myocarditis, and endocarditis occur; very rarely, gonococcal meningitis is reported.[4,9,12–14]

DIAGNOSIS

Diagnosis of gonococcal infections can be made by Gram-stained smears, culture, or newer methods based on the detection of cellular components of the gonococcus (enzymes, antigens, DNA, or lipopolysaccharide) in clinical specimens. Various stains have been used to identify gonococci microscopically, with the Gram stain most widely used in clinical practice. Gram-stained smears are positive for gonococci when gram-negative diplococci of typical kidney bean morphology are identified within polymorphonuclear leukocytes. In the presence of equivocal smears (extracellular gonococcal forms that can be nonpathogenic, commensal *Neisseria,* or gram-negative diplococci of atypical morphology), a culture is mandatory. In urethral smears from men with symptomatic urethritis, the smear is highly sensitive and specific, and culture is considered optional. Gram-stained smears are specific but insensitive for endocervical, rectal, cutaneous, and asymptomatic male urethral infections. In these situations, culture is the most reliable means of diagnosis.[9,13,15] Because of the presence of nonpathogenic *Neisseria* in the pharynx of most people, the Gram stain is not useful in the diagnosis of pharyngeal infection.[9,12]

Culture is considered the most reliable means of diagnosing gonococcal infections. Anatomic sites to be cultured depend on the individual's sexual preferences and body areas exposed. In women, because the urethra and other sites are rarely the sole locus of infection, cervical cultures produce the highest yield and are frequently performed in conjunction with rectal cultures. Urethral cultures are recommended in women who have had hysterectomies and heterosexual men. In homosexual males, anorectal cultures generally produce the highest yields, and pharyngeal and urethral cultures are considered optional.[9,13,15]

Because technical constraints and cost preclude the use of culture techniques in most office settings and clinics, alternative methods of diagnosis have been developed, including enzyme immunoassay, DNA probe techniques and nucleic acid amplification techniques employing polymerase chain reaction (PCR) and ligase chain reaction (LCR). In most cases, the tests do not have increased sensitivity or specificity over either Gram stain for symptomatic gonococcal urethritis in men or culture in women with endocervical infections. For gonococcal infections other than symptomatic urethritis in males, however, these tests may prove a more rapid means of diagnosis than culture. Of particular clinical importance is the high sensitivity of DNA probe and PCR methods for detecting *N. gonorrhoeae* in first-void urine samples of infected individuals and the extension of this technology to allow detection of multiple STDs from a single specimen.[13,15,16]

▶ TREATMENT: Gonorrhea

Neisseria gonorrhoeae have demonstrated susceptibility to a variety of antibiotics. The development of chromosomally-mediated and plasmid-mediated resistance has resulted, however, in an increasing number of isolates resistant to former first-line antibiotics, such as penicillin, ampicillin, amoxicillin, and tetracycline. While still used in some countries because they are cheap, easy to use, and well tolerated, these antibiotics are no longer recommended as either first-line or alternative regimens by the CDC.[17–19]

All gonorrhea treatment regimens recommended by the CDC consist of various oral or parenteral cephalosporins and fluoroquinolones given as a single dose (Table 107–3).[14] Coexisting chlamydial infection, which is documented in up to 60% of individuals with gonorrhea, constitutes the major cause of postgonococcal urethritis, cervicitis, and salpingitis in patients treated for gonorrhea.[13] As a result, concomitant treatment with doxycycline or azithromycin is recommended in all patients treated for gonorrhea. Alone, none of the single-dose regimens recommended for gonorrhea in the CDC guidelines is effective against chlamydia.[14] Azithromycin (2 g) as a single dose is highly effective in treating both gonorrhea and chlamydia, however. Concerns over gastrointestinal (GI) adverse effects, as well as cost, preclude its routine use at this time.[17] Ceftriaxone, the only parenteral agent included in CDC recommended first-line agents for the treatment of gonorrhea, is administered intramuscularly (IM) as a single 125-mg dose. Unfortunately, vials containing less than 250 mg are unavailable, and ceftriaxone remains an expensive alternative to oral antibiotic alternatives.[14,17]

Although oral therapy offers a promising alternative to the expense and pain associated with parenteral therapy, it may not be preferred for all cases of gonorrhea. Of the regimens of choice, only ceftriaxone is effective in eradicating both gonor-

TABLE 107–3. Treatment of Gonorrhea

Type of Infection	Recommended Regimen[a]	Alternative Regimen
Uncomplicated urethral, endocervical, rectal, proctitis, or epididymitis infection in adults[b,c]	Ceftriaxone 125 mg IM once; *or* ciprofloxacin 500 mg PO once; *or* cefixime 400 mg PO once; *or* ofloxacin 400 mg PO once *plus* A treatment regimen for presumptive *C. trachomatis* coinfection (see Table 107–5)	Spectinomycin 2 g IM once; *or* ceftizoxime 500 mg IM once; *or* cefotetan 1 g IM once; *or* Cefoxitin 2 g IM once; *or* Cefuroxime axetil 1 g PO once; *or* Cefpodoxime proxetil 200 mg PO once; *or* Lomefloxacin 400 mg PO once; *or* Enoxacin 400 mg PO once; *or* Norfloxacin 800 mg PO once *plus* A treatment regimen for presumptive *C. trachomatis* coinfection (see Table 107–5)
Gonococcal infections in pregnancy	Ceftriaxone 125 mg IM once[d,e] *plus* Erythromycin base 500 mg PO four times daily for 7 days	Spectinomycin 2.0 g IM once *plus* A treatment regimen for presumptive *C. trachomatis* coinfection (see Table 107–5)
Disseminated gonococcal infection in adults (> 45 kg)[e–h]	Ceftriaxone 1 g IM or IV every 24 h	Ceftizoxime 1 g IV every 8 h *or* Cefotaxime 1 g IV every 8 h until all symptoms resolve *or* Spectinomycin 2 g IM every 12 h
Disseminated gonococcal infection in infants[i]	Ceftriaxone 25–50 mg/kg IV or IM once daily for 7 days *or* Cefotaxime 25 mg/kg IV or IM twice daily for 7 days	
Uncomplicated urethritis, vulvovaginitis, cervicitis, pharyngitis, or proctitis infection in children (< 45 kg)	Ceftriaxone 125 mg IM once[j]	Spectinomycin 40 mg/kg IM once (not to exceed 2 g)
Gonococcal conjunctivitis	Ceftriaxone 1 g IM once[k]	
Ophthalmia neonatorum	Ceftriaxone 25–50 mg/kg IV or IM once (not to exceed 125 mg)	
Infants born to mothers with gonococcal infection (prophylaxis)	Ceftriaxone 25–50 mg/kg IV or IM (not to exceed 125 mg)	

[a]Recommendations are those of the CDC.
[b]Treatment failures are usually caused by reinfection and necessitate patient education and sexual partner referral; additional treatment regimens for gonorrhea and chlamydial infections should be administered. Epididymitis should be treated for 10 days (see Table 107–5).
[c]Patients allergic to β-lactams should receive a quinolone. Persons unable to tolerate a β-lactam (penicillin or cephalosporin) or a quinolone should receive spectinomycin.
[d]Another recommended IM or PO cephalosporin also may be used.
[e]The fluoroquinolones, doxycycline, and erythromycin ethylsuccinate are contraindicated during pregnancy.
[f]Patients treated with one of the recommended regimens should be treated with doxycycline or azithromycin for possible coexistent chlamydial infection.
[g]Patients with gonococcal meningitis should be treated for 10 to 14 days and those with endocarditis for at least 4 wk with ceftriaxone 1–2 g IV every 12 h.
[h]Treatment regimen should be continued for 24–48 h after improvement begins and switched to cefixime 400 mg PO twice daily or ciprofloxacin 500 mg two times a day to complete a week of therapy.
[i]Treatment for 10–14 d is required if meningitis is present.
[j]Patients with bacteremia or arthritis should receive ceftriaxone 50 mg/kg (max 1 g) IM or IV once daily for 7 days. Patients with meningitis should be treated for 10–14 days, with a daily dose of ceftriaxone not to exceed 2 g.
[k]The eye should be lavaged one time with saline solution.

rhea and incubating syphilis. Since the overall incidence of concomitant infection with both gonorrhea and syphilis appears low in most areas, selection of ceftriaxone based on this criterion should be considered only in areas where the incidence of syphilis infection is high.[17] Resistance to the broad-spectrum cephalosporins recommended for the treatment of gonorrhea has not been reported. The development of high-level resistance to fluoroquinolones has, however, resulted in a small, but increasing number of treatment failures.[17–19] This appears to be a particular problem in Asia and Western Pacific nations, although outbreaks of resistant infection are reported in many parts of the United States. Both ciprofloxacin 250 and 500 mg are safe and effective for gonorrhea at all sites, but the 500-mg dose is recommended to minimize development of quinolone resistance. Ofloxacin is useful in eradicating both *N. gonorrhoeae* and *C. trachomatis;* however, different dosage regimens are required for each pathogen, and it is unknown if the lower, multiple daily dosing regimen used in chlamydial infections is effective in eradicating gonorrheal infections.[14,17,18]

Spectinomycin is still the preferred alternative for patients unable to tolerate the recommended cephalosporin or fluoroquinolone regimens. Although some resistance to spectinomycin is reported, its limited use appears to have prevented widespread resistance from developing. Unlike ceftriaxone and the fluoroquinolones, spectinomycin has only limited efficacy in treating pharyngeal infections.

Pregnant women infected with *N. gonorrhoeae* should be treated with either a cephalosporin or spectinomycin since fluoroquinolones are contraindicated.[14,18] Although not extensively studied, other effective alternative treatment regimens include single doses of the parenteral antibiotics cefotaxime, cefotetan, cefoxitin, ceftizoxime, netilmicin, imipenem/cilastin, and aztreonam. Orally administered alternatives to antibiotics recommended in the CDC guidelines include cefuroxime axetil, cefpodoxime proxetil, a number of fluoroquinolones, and the combination of rifampin and erythromycin stearate. None of these antibiotics, however, offers important advantages over other more commonly used and recommended agents.[14,17,18]

Ceftriaxone is the recommended therapy for DGI, gonococcal meningitis, endocarditis, and any type of gonococcal infection in children. Parenteral therapy is suggested for children primarily because oral regimens have not been studied adequately. In cases of DGI, patients should be hospitalized and treated initially with either ceftriaxone, ceftizoxime, or cefotaxime. Although marked improvement is usually noted within 48 hours of initiating therapy, treatment should be continued as an outpatient with a 7-day course of either cefixime or ciprofloxacin. Children and pregnant or lactating women should not receive ciprofloxacin because of the concern for bone and joint disorders. In homosexual males with DGI, ceftriaxone is preferred because of its efficacy in treating coexisting rectal, pharyngeal, and urethral infections.[14,18]

Gonococcal ophthalmia is highly contagious in adults and neonates and requires IM ceftriaxone therapy. Single-dose therapy is adequate for gonococcal conjunctivitis. Topical antibiotics are not sufficiently effective when used alone for ocular infections and are not necessary with appropriate systemic therapy. Infants with either type of ophthalmologic infection should be evaluated for signs of DGI.[14,18]

Treatment of gonorrhea during pregnancy is essential to prevent ophthalmia neonatorum. Gonococcal infection in newborns results primarily from passage through an infected birth canal, but it also can be transmitted in utero. Ophthalmia neonatorum is the most common ophthalmic infection in newborns (1.6% to 12%), although membranes of the vagina, pharynx, or rectum also can become colonized. Conjunctival involvement usually develops within 7 days of delivery and is characterized by intense, bilateral conjunctival inflammation with chemosis. If not promptly treated, corneal ulceration and blindness can develop. Because neonatal prophylaxis with topical ocular antimicrobials is required by law in most states, gonococcal ophthalmia neonatorum is rare in the United States. The American Academy of Pediatrics recommends that either silver nitrate (1%), tetracycline (1%), or erythromycin (0.5%) be instilled in each conjunctival sac immediately postpartum. Approximately 2% of infants at risk of infection fail treatment with recommended ophthalmic antibiotics. As a result, infants born to infected mothers should also receive an IM or intravenous (IV) injection of ceftriaxone 50 mg/kg for 7 days. Of the three topical agents, tetracycline and erythromycin are used most frequently because they possess some activity against chlamydia, another important cause of ophthalmia neonatorum. Silver nitrate produces a chemical conjunctivitis that may make assessment of therapeutic efficacy difficult, although the chemical reaction usually disappears within 3 to 5 days.[14,18,20,21]

EVALUATION OF THERAPEUTIC OUTCOMES

Although it had been suggested that follow-up cultures should be obtained at least 3 days after treatment, combination gonorrhea and chlamydial therapy rarely results in treatment failures, and routine follow-up of patients treated with a regimen included in the CDC guidelines is not recommended. Persistence of symptoms following any treatment requires culture of the site(s) of gonorrheal infection, as well as susceptibility testing if gonococci are isolated. In most cases, the presence of gonococci indicates reinfection rather than treatment failure and reflects the need for improved patient education and sex partner referral. Persistence of symptoms can also be caused by other infectious causes, such as *C. trachomatis.*[14]

SYPHILIS

EPIDEMIOLOGY AND ETIOLOGY

Although syphilis was the fifth most frequently reported communicable disease in the United States in 1995, the incidence of this disease has declined by nearly 50% since 1990. The demographics of the disease have remained virtually unchanged, however, with a disproportionately higher rate among blacks and Hispanics in comparison to whites.[11] In addition to being highly contagious, syphilis is of major concern because, if left untreated, it can progress to a chronic systemic disease that can be fatal or seriously disabling.[12,13,22–27]

Syphilis is usually acquired by sexual contact with infected mucous membranes or cutaneous lesions, although on rare occasions it can be acquired by nonsexual personal contact, accidental inoculation, or blood transfusion. The causative organism of syphilis is *Treponema pallidum,* a spirochete. The risk of acquiring syphilis from an infected individual after a single sexual encounter is approximately 50%. After sexual contact, the organism penetrates the intact mucous membrane or a break in the cornified epithelium and spirochetemia occurs.[24–27]

Evidence of a strong association between syphilis and HIV infection has been noted. While complex and incompletely understood, it appears that syphilis, similar to other sexually transmitted genital ulcer diseases, can increase the risk of acquiring HIV in exposed individuals. Also, immunologic defects in HIV-infected individuals can modify the serologic response to syphilis. In particular, the possibility of delayed seroreactivity, markedly elevated serologic titers, and increased false-positive results could complicate the diagnosis, as well as assessment of treatment efficacy, in HIV-positive individuals infected with syphilis. Further, anecdotal evidence suggests compromised immune function may result in an accelerated progression of syphilis requiring more aggressive antibiotic therapy in comparison to an immunocompetent host.[12,23–25,27]

CLINICAL PRESENTATION

PRIMARY SYPHILIS

After exposure and an incubation period of 10 to 90 days (average 21 days), a painless lesion or chancre appears at the site of inoculation. Classically, the chancre is single, but multiple lesions are reported in up to 30% of infections.[24] The chancre usually begins as a dull red macule that subsequently develops into a papule that erodes and ulcerates. Although chancres vary markedly in appearance, most are rounded or oval in shape, indurated, and well marginated. Oral and anorectal chancres are common in homosexual males and frequently have an atypical appearance. All chancres are highly infectious, although they are generally painless lesions unless secondarily infected or located at extragenital sites. Even without treatment, chancres persist only for 1 to 8 weeks before spontaneously healing. During this stage, painless, nonsuppurative inguinal lymphadenopathy is not uncommon. Because syphilitic chancres can be confused with other infectious etiologies, appropriate diagnostic testing is important.[22,24–26]

SECONDARY SYPHILIS

The secondary stage of syphilis develops 2 to 6 weeks after the onset of the primary stage in untreated or inadequately treated patients. This stage is characterized by a variety of mucocutaneous eruptions, resulting from widespread hematogenous and lymphatic spread of *T. pallidum.* Skin lesions can either be generalized or localized to a small portion of the body and, with the exception of follicular lesions, are nonpruritic. Often lesions appear on the palms of the hands and the soles of the feet. Because few dermatologic conditions are characterized by palm and sole manifestations, involvement of these areas is highly suggestive of syphilis. In addition to the skin lesions, mild and transitory malaise, fever, pharyngitis, headache, anorexia, and arthralgia are common. Generalized lymphadenopathy also is seen in the majority of patients. In untreated individuals, signs and symptoms of secondary syphilis disappear in 4 to 10 weeks; however, lesions may recur at any time within 4 years if the patient remains untreated.[22,24–26]

LATENT SYPHILIS

By definition, persons with a positive serologic test for syphilis but with no other evidence of disease have latent syphilis. Latent syphilis is further divided into early and late latency. During early latency the patient is considered potentially infectious because of the risk of spontaneous mucocutaneous relapses. The U.S. Public Health Service defines early latency as 1 year from the onset of infection, although a longer interval, such as 2 to 4 years, is proposed by others. With the exception of pregnancy where the mother may pass the disease to the fetus, late latency is considered noninfectious, although the patient remains a host.[14,22,27]

Most untreated patients with late latent syphilis have no further sequelae; however, approximately 25% to 30% progress to either neurosyphilis or late syphilis with clinical manifestations other than neurosyphilis. Treatment of all patients with latent syphilis is essential since there is no way to predict which patients will have progression of their disease.[22,24]

NEUROSYPHILIS AND LATE SYPHILIS OTHER THAN NEUROSYPHILIS

If left untreated, syphilis can slowly produce an inflammatory reaction in virtually any organ in the body. Manifestations of this progression of the disease were previously referred to as tertiary syphilis.[24] More recently, these clinical manifestations are differentiated into two subgroups based on the presence or absence of CNS involvement—neurosyphilis or late syphilis with clinical manifestations other than neurosyphilis. Most typically, evidence of disease progression is not apparent until 10 to 25 years following the initial infection.[22,24–27]

Classically, neurosyphilis was used to describe the approximately 20% of patients experiencing disease progression from the latent stage and manifesting with signs of general paresis, eighth cranial nerve deafness, optic atrophy and blindness, progressive dementia, meningovascular complications, or tabes dorsalis. The term since then is used to encompass any patient with cerebrospinal fluid (CSF) abnormalities consistent with central nervous system infection.[24–27] It is estimated that approximately 40% of patients with primary or secondary syphilis exhibit such abnormalities, although most remain asymptomatic.[27] Persistence of CSF abnormalities into late latency is associated with a greater risk of progression to symptomatic neurosyphilis. Because of the availability of effective antibiotic therapy, the manifestations of severe late syphilis are rare, particularly for patients with intact immune systems. Although data are conflicting, some investigators have suggested that HIV-infected patients are at greater risk of developing symptomatic neurosyphilis.[24–26]

Rarely seen, the most common manifestations of disease progression from late latency are benign gumma formation and cardiovascular syphilis. The gumma, a nonspecific granulomatous lesion, is the classic lesion of late syphilis and develops in 50% of patients with disease progression. These chronic, destructive lesions characteristically infiltrate the skin, bone, soft tissue, and liver, but can be found in any organ or tissue. Gummas of critical organs, such as the heart or brain, can be fatal. Cardiovascular syphilis is characterized by aortitis and aortic insufficiency. Syphilitic aortic aneurysms also are common.[22,25,26]

CONGENITAL SYPHILIS

In pregnant women with syphilis, *T. pallidum* can cross the placenta at any time during pregnancy. Fetal infection is not likely to occur, however, if exposure takes place during the first 20 weeks of pregnancy. After this period, transplacental infections can occur, resulting in fetal death, prematurity, or congenital syphilis. Symptoms can be seen during the first months of life (early congenital syphilis) or later in childhood or adolescence (late congenital syphilis). Manifestations of early congenital syphilis resemble those of secondary syphilis, although those of late congenital syphilis correspond to the tertiary stage in adults.[12,22]

DIAGNOSIS

Because *T. pallidum* is difficult to culture *in vitro*, diagnosis is based primarily on microscopic examination of serous material from a suspected syphilitic lesion or on results from serologic testing. In primary syphilis, diagnosis is established by the presence of *T. pallidum* on dark-field microscopic examination of material from cutaneous lesions and enlarged lymph nodes in patients with secondary syphilis. In incubating syphilis, confirmation is frequently by dark-field microscopic examination, because serologic tests can be unreactive early in the disease.[22,29–31] Another method of direct microscopic examination, the direct fluorescent antibody test (DFA-TP), which uses monoclonal or polyclonal antibodies specific for *T. pallidum,* has greater specificity and sensitivity than dark-field examination and does not require the immediate examination of fresh specimens.[31]

Serologic tests used in the diagnosis of syphilis are categorized as nontreponemal or treponemal. Commonly used nontreponemal tests include the Venereal Disease Research Laboratory (VDRL) slide test and rapid plasma reagin (RPR) card test. Nontreponemal tests, which are inexpensive and easily performed, rely on the detection of reagin, a heterogeneous group of antibodies. A positive nontreponemal test can indicate the presence of any stage of syphilis or congenital syphilis, although incubating syphilis and very early primary syphilis produce a negative reaction; however, because they are nonspecific tests, false-positive reactions occur, making them inappropriate to confirm the diagnosis alone. Transiently positive results can be seen in patients with acute febrile illnesses, after immunizations, and during pregnancy. Chronic false-positive results are commonly associated with heroin addiction, aging, chronic infections, connective tissue diseases, and malignant disease. In some cases, false-positive reactions are familial and are related to abnormal serum globulin levels.[12,22,29–31]

Nontreponemal tests are used primarily as screening tests; however, because reaginic antibody titers also can be quantitated by testing serial dilutions of the patient's serum for reactivity, they are useful in following the progression of the disease, recovery after therapy, and possible reinfection. Since antibody titers vary to some extent between tests, it is important that sequential serologic testing be performed using the same method each time. In patients successfully treated for primary and secondary syphilis, nontreponemal tests will almost always return to seronegativity. If these tests are going to return to negative in patients with early latent syphilis, they will do so within the first 4 years after adequate therapy; patients with disease of longer duration usually remain seropositive for life. In addition to its use in serologic testing, the VDRL is often used on cerebrospinal fluid (CSF) to diagnose neurosyphilis.

In some patients with secondary syphilis, a prozone phenomenon occurs that produces a negative VDRL despite the presence of high reaginic antibody titers. This is corrected by diluting the patient's serum prior to testing.[12,22,29–31] For HIV-positive individuals with syphilis, the reactivity of nontreponemal tests can vary depending on the stage of the HIV infection. In the early stages, reaginic titers higher than in non–HIV-infected patients have been seen, resulting in the prozone phenomenon. During the later stages of HIV infection, however, when immune function deteriorates to a greater extent, serologic responses can be reduced or delayed. As a result, the diagnosis of syphilis in HIV-infected individuals can be more difficult.[24,31]

In diagnosing all stages of syphilis, treponemal tests are more sensitive than nontreponemal tests. Because these tests are technically more demanding and are more expensive, however, they are used primarily as confirmatory rather than as screening tests. The fluorescent treponemal antibody absorption (FTA-ABS) test is the most frequently used treponemal test. In the FTA-ABS test, the *T. pallidum* antigen is used to detect specific antibodies to treponemal organisms. The FTA-ABS test becomes positive earlier than nontreponemal tests in primary syphilis. After adequate antibiotic therapy for any stage of syphilis, the FTA-ABS test usually remains reactive for life, and, therefore, is not useful in assessing serologic response to therapy, relapse, or reinfection. In suspected neurosyphilis when the VDRL for CSF is negative, testing of CSF with the FTA-ABS is sometimes recommended. While less specific than the VDRL for CSF involvement, the FTA-ABS appears highly sensitive.[27] Other serologic tests specific for the treponemal antibody are the *T. pallidum* hemagglutination assay (TPHA) and the microhemagglutination assay for antibodies to *T. pallidum* (MHATP).[29–31] There are PCR-based tests being investigated, particularly in situations where serologic testing has poor sensitivity and specificity (congenital syphilis, early primary syphilis, neurosyphilis).[13,31]

▶ TREATMENT: Syphilis

Treatment recommendations from the CDC are presented in Table 107–4.[14] Parenteral penicillin G is the treatment of choice for all stages of syphilis. Because *T. pallidum* multiplies slowly, single doses of short- or intermediate-acting penicillins do not provide the prolonged, low-level exposure to penicillin required for eradication of the treponeme. As a result, benzathine penicillin G is the only penicillin effective for single-dose therapy.[12–14,24–28]

The recommended treatment for syphilis of less than 1 year's duration is benzathine penicillin G 2.4 million units as a single dose. Although the relapse rate for this regimen is less than 3%, some advocate that 2.4 million units be administered once a week for 2 consecutive weeks. In patients with syphilis of greater than 1 year's duration and normal CSF examination, benzathine penicillin G is administered weekly for three successive doses. Although not specifically recommended by the CDC, this three-dose regimen is used by some experts to treat HIV-infected patients with syphilis of less than 1 year's duration based on data suggesting a greater risk of treatment failure with single-dose therapy.[26] Some experts even prefer to treat all patients with syphilis of less than 1 year's duration with the three-dose regimen since single-dose therapy is not consistently effective in eradicating Treponemes from the CSF; this is of primary concern in patients with undiagnosed CSF involvement.[28]

Patients with abnormal CSF findings should be treated as having neurosyphilis. Preferred regimens for neurosyphilis provide treatment over 10 to 14 days with parenteral penicillin G administered every 4 hours. Benzathine penicillin G alone in standard weekly doses or procaine penicillin G in doses under 2.4 million units do not consistently provide treponemicidal levels in the CSF and have resulted in treatment failures.[14,24–29]

Since *T. pallidum* resistance to penicillin has not emerged, the primary need for alternative drugs in treating syphilis is for penicillin-allergic patients. Alternative regimens recommended for penicillin-allergic patients are doxycycline 100 mg orally twice daily or tetracycline or erythromycin (stearate, ethyl succinate, or base) 500 mg orally four times daily for 2 to 4 weeks, depending on the duration of syphilis. Although neither the tetracyclines nor erythromycin have been evaluated as extensively as

TABLE 107–4. Drug Therapy and Follow-Up of Syphilis

Stage/Type of Syphilis	Recommended Regimen[a]	Follow-Up Serology
Primary, secondary, or latent syphilis of less than 1 year's duration (early latent syphilis)	Benzathine penicillin G 2.4 million units IM in a single dose[b]	Quantitative nontreponemal tests at 3 and 6 mo for primary and secondary syphilis; at 6 and 12 mo for early latent syphilis[c]
Syphilis of more than 1 year's duration (includes late latent syphilis of unknown duration and late syphilis other than neurosyphilis)	Benzathine penicillin G 2.4 million units IM once a week for 3 successive weeks	Quantitative nontreponemal tests at 6 and 12 mo for late latent syphilis[d]
Neurosyphilis	Aqueous crystalline penicillin G 12–24 million units IV (2–4 million units every 4 h) for 10–14 days[e] *or* Aqueous procaine penicillin G 2.4 million units IM daily plus probenecid 500 mg PO four times daily, both for 10–14 days[e]	CSF[f] examination every 6 mo until the cell count is normal; if it has not decreased at 6 mo or is not normal by 2 years, retreatment is suggested
Congenital syphilis	Aqueous crystalline penicillin G 50,000 units/kg IV every 12 h during the first 7 d of life and every 8 h thereafter for 10–14 days *or* Procaine penicillin G 50,000 units/kg IM daily for 10–14 days	Quantitative nontreponemal tests every 2–3 mo until nonreactive (6–12 mo)
Penicillin-allergic patients[g] Primary, secondary, or latent syphilis of less than 1 year's duration	Doxycycline 100 mg PO two times daily for 2 wk *or* Tetracycline 500 mg PO four times daily for 2 wk *or* Erythromycin 500 mg PO four times daily for 2 wk	Same as for non–penicillin-allergic patients
Syphilis of more than 1 year's duration (except neurosyphilis)	Doxycycline 100 mg PO two times a day for 4 wk *or* Tetracycline 500 mg PO four times daily for 4 wk	Same as for non–penicillin-allergic patients

[a]Recommendations are those of the CDC.
[b]Some experts recommend multiple doses of benzathine penicillin G or other supplemental antibiotics in addition to benzathine penicillin G in HIV-infected patients with primary or secondary syphilis; HIV-infected patients with early latent syphilis should be treated with the recommended regimen for syphilis of more than 1 year's duration.
[c]More frequent follow-up (1, 2, 3, 6, 9, and 12 mo) recommended for HIV-infected patients.
[d]Minimal data exist on which to base specific follow-up recommendations for late syphilis.
[e]CSF, cerebral spinal fluid.
[f]Some experts administer benzathine penicillin G 2.4 million units IM after completion of the neurosyphilis regimens to provide a total duration of therapy comparable to that used for late syphilis in the absence of neurosyphilis.
[g]For nonpregnant patients. Pregnant patients should be treated with penicillin after desensitization.

penicillin G in the treatment of syphilis, some evidence suggests higher treatment failure rates in erythromycin-treated patients. Alternative treatment regimens should be used only in cases of documented penicillin allergy and, given concerns regarding patient compliance with these regimens, follow-up serologic testing is of particular importance.[12–14,24–29]

Other antibiotics used successfully in treating syphilis include various β-lactam antibiotics; however, none offer significant advantages over benzathine penicillin G. While ceftriaxone is considered effective in eradicating incubating syphilis when given as a single 125-mg dose, higher doses and more frequent administration appear necessary for more advanced syphilis, and treatment failures are reported in HIV-infected patients.[14,22,23,25,26]

For pregnant patients, penicillin is the treatment of choice at the dosage recommended for that particular stage of syphilis. To assure treatment success and prevent transmission to the fetus, some experts advocate an additional IM dose of benzathine penicillin G 2.4 million units 1 week after completion of the recommended regimen. This may be particularly beneficial in women diagnosed and treated during the third trimester or those with secondary syphilis. In women allergic to penicillin, safe and effective alternatives are not available; therefore, skin testing should be performed to confirm a penicillin allergy. It is recommended that women with positive skin tests undergo penicillin desensitization and receive the appropriate treatment regimen for their stage of disease.[14]

The majority of patients treated for primary and secondary syphilis experience the Jarisch-Herxheimer reaction after treatment. This benign, self-limiting reaction is characterized by flu-like symptoms, such as transient headache, fever, chills, malaise, arthralgia, myalgia, tachypnea, peripheral vasodilation, and aggravation of syphilitic lesions. The exact mechanism of the reaction is unknown, although proposed etiologies, including immunologic mechanisms and release of endotoxin or other toxic treponemal products, are not substantiated.[19,20] The Jarisch-Herxheimer reaction is independent of the drug and dose used and should not be confused with penicillin allergy. It usually begins within 2 to 4 hours of initiating therapy, peaks at 8 hours, and is complete within 12 to 24 hours. Most reactions can be managed symptomatically with analgesics, antipyretics, and rest. Steroids and antihistamines have been administered prior to initiation of syphilitic therapy but are of limited value.[12,14,22,27]

EVALUATION OF THERAPEUTIC OUTCOMES

The CDC recommendations for serologic follow-up of patients treated for syphilis are given in Table 107–4.[14] Quantitative nontreponemal tests should be performed at 3 and 6 months in all patients treated for primary and secondary syphilis and at 6 and 12 months for early and late latent disease. In general, the time to reach seronegativity is proportional to the duration of the disease. Specific testing recommended for other stages of syphilis is included in Table 107–4. Despite adequate therapy, some patients may remain seropositive based on nontreponemal test results. In these cases, stabilization of low reaginic titers is indicative of adequate therapy. For women treated during pregnancy, monthly quantitative nontreponemal tests are recommended until the adequacy of therapy is established. Women who do not demonstrate a fourfold decrease in titer over a 3-month period or who show a fourfold increase in titer between tests should be retreated.[14,22,23,27]

CHLAMYDIA TRACHOMATIS

EPIDEMIOLOGY AND ETIOLOGY

Nearly 500,000 cases of *C. trachomatis* genital infection were reported to the CDC in 1995, ranking it as the most frequently reported infectious disease in the United States.[11] Similar to other STDs, gross underreporting is believed to exist, in part because of the large number of individuals who are treated presumptively without confirmatory microbiologic testing and the large number of individuals with asymptomatic infections. As a result, it is estimated that as many as 4 million Americans contract chlamydial infections each year at a cost of greater than $2.4 billion.[32–35] Chlamydial infections represent the most common cause of NGU, accounting for up to 50% of such infections.[33]

PATHOPHYSIOLOGY

Chlamydia trachomatis is an obligate intracellular parasite that shares properties of both viruses and bacteria. Like viruses, chlamydiae require cellular material from host cells for replication; however, unlike viruses, chlamydiae maintain their cellular identity throughout development. Although *C. trachomatis* lacks a cell wall peptidoglycan, its major outer membrane is similar to gram-negative bacteria. At least 15 serovars (subspecies) of *C. trachomatis* exist, of which only the lymphogranuloma venereum strains produce potentially invasive infections. The remaining serovars are involved primarily with superficial infection of epithelial cells.[33,35–38]

Specific data on the risk of transmissibility of chlamydia after exposure are not available. It is estimated that coinfection with chlamydia occurs in up to 60% of individuals with gonorrhea.[13] As a result, chlamydia is the most common cause of postgonococcal urethritis in heterosexuals. All individuals diagnosed with *N. gonorrhoeae* should be assumed to have *C. trachomatis* present also.[38] In addition to genital infections, ocular and pharyngeal infections occur. Such infections occur most frequently secondary to vaginal delivery through an infected birth canal and from orogenital contact, respectively.[32,34,36,38]

CLINICAL PRESENTATION

In males, the most common symptoms of chlamydial genital tract infections are dysuria, urinary frequency, and a mucoid urethral discharge occurring 7 to 21 days after exposure. The discharge is usually less profuse and more mucoid or watery than the urethral discharge associated with gonorrhea. Typically, it is more obvious in the morning. In many cases, the discharge is not noticeable, and crusting of the meatus or staining of undergarments may be the only sign. In up to 50% of infected heterosexual males, no signs or symptoms are present. *Chlamydia trachomatis* is responsible for approximately 50% of all cases of acute epididymitis reported in the United States annually.[33,35] Rectal infections occur in men practicing receptive anal intercourse, and while these infections are usually asymptomatic, they can produce complications, such as proctitis or proctocolitis.[32,33,36,37]

The majority of women with chlamydial infections are asymptomatic. In women with urethral infections, dysuria and frequency are uncommon. When symptomatic, the most common manifestation of infection is endocervicitis with a mucopurulent discharge. On exam, the cervix tends to be friable and ectopic. Chlamydia has been recognized as a major cause of PID and its associated complications, such as infertility and ectopic pregnancy.[32–34,36]

Similar to gonorrhea, chlamydia may be transmitted to an infant during contact with infected cervicovaginal secretions. Nearly two-thirds of infants acquire chlamydial infection after endocervical exposure, with the primary morbidity associated with seeding of the infant's eyes, nasopharynx, rectum, or vagina. In exposed infants, neonatal conjunctivitis develops in up to 50% and pneumonia develops in up to 16%. Inclusion conjunctivitis in newborns is usually self-limited, but it can result in scarring and micropanus of the cornea. Interstitial pneumonitis occurring secondary to carriage in the nasopharynx is typically mild, but it can be severe and require hospitalization.[33,34,36,37,39]

DIAGNOSIS

Because of the high rate of asymptomatic disease and the relative lack of specificity of symptoms when present, laboratory confirmation of chlamydial infection is important. Cell culture is the reference standard against which all other diagnostic tests are measured. Because chlamydiae are obligate intracellular parasites, specimens for culture must be obtained from endocervical (women) or urethral (men) epithelial cell scrapings rather than from urine or urethral discharges. Although tissue culture techniques have close to a 100% specificity, their sensitivity is reported to be as low as 70%, in part because of problems of improper specimen collection, transport, or processing. Because of the technical demands, expense, and length of time until results are available (3 to 7 days), culture is not as widely used for diagnostic purposes today. However, culture remains the diagnostic standard in medicolegal cases such as sexual assault and child abuse because of its high specificity and ability to detect only viable organisms.[13,15,32,33,40] Serologic tests are of limited value in diagnosing genital chlamydial infections and are used primarily as a research tool.

Tests that detect chlamydial antigens and nucleic acid provide more rapid results, are technically less demanding to perform, are less costly, and, in some situations, have greater sensitivity than culture. The most commonly used nonculture tests for detection of *C. trachomatis* are the enzyme immunoassay (EIA), DNA hybridization probe, and the direct fluorescent monoclonal antibody (DFA) test. In comparison to culture, these tests have reduced sensitivities and slightly reduced specificities overall. While the DFA test can be conducted in a short period of time, its sensitivity is highly dependent on skilled personnel in preparing the specimen for viewing under a fluorescent microscope and in interpreting the results. This test is frequently used as a confirmatory test for positive results seen with other nonculture tests. Most commercially available tests used to detect *C. trachomatis* use EIA techniques that detect chlamydial lipopolysaccharide (LPS) antigen. Some EIA methods, however, are not specific for *C. trachomatis,* and false-positive results are reported with other chlamydia species as well as with some gram-negative bacteria. The sensitivity and specificity of the test are generally lower when urine specimens are used.[33,35,40–43]

Rapid office tests that employ EIA technology for diagnosing chlamydial infections are widely available, and most provide results in 30 minutes. These tests are generally much less sensitive and specific than laboratory-performed EIA, and they are subject to a high false-positive rate because of the cross-reactivity of LPS from other microorganisms. As a result, a positive rapid office test should only be considered presumptive, and test results should be confirmed by a laboratory-based method. Another frequently used office diagnostic test is the leukocyte esterase test (LET), a urine dipstick test for detecting pyuria. Used primarily as a screening test, a positive test occurs in the presence of infection caused by chlamydia, gonorrhea, and a number of other microorganisms. As a result, all positive test results require further testing to determine the etiology of the urethritis.[33,35]

The greatest advances in the detection of chlamydial infection involved the development of various nucleic acid detection methods. The DNA hybridization probe test is probably the most common test used in public health laboratories in the United States. Overall, the sensitivity and specificity of the DNA probe tests are greater than with EIA. Of all the advances in the diagnosis of *C. trachomatis* infections, the development of DNA amplification tests (PCR or LCR) hold the greatest promise. These tests are highly sensitive and specific for detecting infection in both urogenital specimens and urine. Because of their ability to detect as little as a single gene copy in a specimen, nucleic acid residues that persist following successful antibiotic therapy of a chlamydial infection can result in a false-positive test for several weeks following eradication of the organism.[33,35,40–43]

▶ TREATMENT: Chlamydia

A number of antimicrobials including rifampin, tetracyclines, macrolides, ofloxacin, and sulfonamides, display good *in vitro* and *in vivo* activity against *C. trachomatis.* In most clinical trials, cure rates exceeding 90% are reported for these agents. With the exception of sulfonamides, all of these antimicrobials also appear to have good efficacy against *Ureaplasma urealyticum,* the second most common cause of NGU.[29,32,34,35,38,44–47]

Azithromycin 1 g orally as a single dose or doxycycline 100 mg orally twice daily are the regimens of choice for the treatment of chlamydial infections (Table 107–5).[32] Although tetracycline has an efficacy comparable to doxycycline, it is no longer included in treatment recommendations because of concerns about compliance with its four times daily dosage schedule. Because of its prolonged serum and tissue half-life, azithromycin is the only single-dose therapy shown to be effective in treating *C. trachomatis.*[29,32,38,44] Despite a higher acquisition cost than generic doxycycline, azithromycin may be a more cost-effective alternative in patient populations where compliance is a problem.[29,38,47,48] Unlike the capsule dosage form that should be taken on an empty stomach, the single 1 g azithromycin dose packet for oral suspension can be taken without regard to meals.

Ofloxacin is the only fluoroquinolone with established efficacy in *C. trachomatis* infections and is considered an alternative to both doxycycline and azithromycin. Ofloxacin is dosed twice daily for 7 days like doxycycline, but it is more expensive. Although ciprofloxacin has activity against *C. trachomatis* and *U. urealyticum,* dosages as high as 2 g per day have not consistently eradicated chlamydial infections.[29,34,35,44,46,48]

For pregnant women with chlamydial urogenital infections, treatment can significantly reduce the risk of pregnancy complications and transmission to the newborn. Since the use of doxycycline and ofloxacin are contraindicated during pregnancy, erythromycin base or erythromycin ethyl succinate are the recommended treatments (Table 107–5).[32,34,38,48] Erythromycin stearate is probably effective also, although it has not been adequately evaluated. Patients intolerant of the recommended erythromycin dosage should be treated with half of the daily dose for 2 weeks instead of 1 week.[32,34] Amoxicillin 1.5 g daily for 7 to 10 days appears to be as effective as erythromycin and is associated with a lower incidence of adverse effects; however, it is uncertain whether infections are actually eradicated or just suppressed.[32,34,45] Although not recommended for use during preg-

TABLE 107–5. Treatment of Chlamydial Infections

Infection	Recommended Regimen[a]	Alternative Regimen
Uncomplicated urethral, endocervical, or rectal infection in adults	Doxycycline 100 mg PO two times daily for 7 days *or* Azithromycin 1 g once[b]	Ofloxacin 300 mg PO two times daily for 7 days[c] *or* Erythromycin base 500 mg PO four times daily for 7 days *or* Erythromycin ethyl succinate 800 mg PO four times daily for 7 days *or* Sulfisoxazole 500 mg four times daily for 10 days
Urogenital infections during pregnancy	Erythromycin base 500 mg four times PO daily for 7 days	Erythromycin base 250 mg PO four times daily for 14 days *or* Erythromycin ethyl succinate 800 mg PO four times daily for 7 days (or 400 mg PO four times daily for 14 days) *or* Amoxicillin 500 mg PO three times daily for 7 days[d]
Conjunctivitis of the newborn	Erythromycin suspension 50 mg/kg/d PO in four divided doses for 10–14 days	
Pneumonia in infants	Erythromycin suspension 50 mg/kg/d PO in four divided doses for 10–14 days	
Acute epididymo-orchitis	Ceftriaxone 250 mg IM[e] *plus* Doxycycline 100 mg PO two times daily for 10 days	

[a]Recommendations are those of the CDC.
[b]Data regarding the use of azithromycin in children ≤ 15 years old are not established.
[c]Ofloxacin is contraindicated during pregnancy and should not be used in patients ≤ 17 years old.
[d]Only if gastrointestinal intolerance to erythromycin; limited data exist for efficacy.
[e]The efficacy of ceftriaxone 125 mg or azithromycin has not been studied and is unknown.

nancy, azithromycin has been shown to produce high cure rates without adverse fetal effects in a small number of subjects.[34,49] Like erythromycin, azithromycin is in pregnancy category B and is probably an acceptable agent for use during pregnancy. It is recommended that post-treatment cultures be obtained for pregnant patients treated for chlamydial infections to ensure eradication of the infection.[34]

Chlamydia trachomatis transmission during perinatal exposure can result in infections of the eye, oropharynx, lungs, urogenital tract, and rectum of the neonate or infant. Despite their efficacy in preventing gonococcal ophthalmia, topical erythromycin, tetracycline, and silver nitrate are associated with an unacceptably high infection rate when used to prevent chlamydial ophthalmia. Additionally, topical therapy has no effect on nasal carriage or colonization of other parts of the infant's body, so the potential for other infections, including pneumonia, still remains.[29,34,48] Because of the high percentage of treatment failures, topical therapy should not be used to treat ophthalmia due to *C. trachomatis*. Instead, oral erythromycin 50 mg/kg/d in four divided doses for 10 to 14 days is recommended.[14,48]

EVALUATION OF THERAPEUTIC OUTCOMES

Treatment of chlamydial infections with the recommended regimens is highly effective, therefore, post-treatment laboratory testing is not routinely recommended unless symptoms persist or there are other specific concerns (e.g., pregnancy). When post-treatment tests for chlamydia are positive, they usually represent noncompliance, failure to treat sexual partners, or laboratory error, rather than inadequate therapy or resistance to therapy. Infants with pneumonitis should receive follow-up testing since erythromycin is only 80% effective and a second course of therapy may be necessary.[14,32,33,38,42,43]

GENITAL HERPES

EPIDEMIOLOGY AND ETIOLOGY

Genital herpes infections represent the most common cause of genital ulceration seen in the United States. It is estimated that approximately 31 million Americans have genital herpes, and this number is increasing by approximately 500,000 each year.[5,50] Whether these figures represent increased prevalence or greater recognition as a result of improved diagnostic capabilities is uncertain. Because of its morbidity, recurrent nature, and potential for complications, as well as its ability to be transmitted asymptomatically, genital herpes has received increasing attention.[13,50–61]

PATHOPHYSIOLOGY

Herpes comes from the Greek word meaning "to creep" and is used to describe two distinct but antigenically related serotypes of herpes simplex virus. Herpes simplex virus type 1 (HSV-1) is most commonly associated with oropharyngeal disease, and herpes simplex virus type 2 (HSV-2) is most closely associated with genital disease; however, each virus is capable of causing infections clinically indistinguishable in both anatomic areas.[51,52,54]

Humans are the sole known reservoir for HSV. Infection is transmitted via inoculation of virus from infected secretions onto mucosal surfaces (e.g., urethra, oropharynx, cervix, conjunctivae) or through abraded skin. Evidence that the virus survives for a limited time on environmental surfaces suggests the possibility of fomitic transfer as a nonvenereal route of transmission.[51,54]

The cycle of HSV infection occurs in five stages: primary mucocutaneous infection, infection of the ganglia, establishment of latency, reactivation, and recurrent infection. After viral inoculation, HSV infection is associated with cytoplasmic granulation, ballooning degeneration of cells, and production of mononucleated giant cells. Initially, the cellular response is predominantly polymorphonuclear, followed by a lymphocytic response. Replication occurs with viral spread to contiguous cells and peripheral sensory nerves. Latency then is established in sensory or autonomic nerve root ganglia. Latency appears to be lifelong, interrupted only by reactivation of the viral infection. It is unclear what factors are important in maintaining latency, but immune responses and emotional and physical stresses appear important in reactivating latent virus.[51,55,56,59]

CLINICAL PRESENTATION

The clinical manifestations of first episodes of genital herpes usually appear within 2 to 14 days after exposure. The signs and symptoms are influenced by many factors, including previous exposure to HSV, previous genital herpes infection, viral type, and host factors, such as age and site of infection. On the basis of retrospective studies, it is estimated that up to 50% of genital HSV infections are asymptomatic, and these infections may represent the most common source of transmission of genital and neonatal herpes infections. As a result, identification of individuals with asymptomatic disease may prove beneficial in the control of genital herpes transmission.[13,51,55,56,59,61] In terms of the natural history of genital herpes infection and its treatment, it is important to distinguish between first-episode primary, first-episode nonprimary, and recurrent infections.

FIRST-EPISODE INFECTIONS

First-episode primary infections are classified as infections occurring in persons lacking antibody to either type of HSV. These infections are characterized by a prolonged duration of systemic and local symptoms, sometimes requiring hospitalization. More than 50% of patients with primary infections experience flu-like symptoms of fever, headache, malaise, and myalgias. Systemic symptoms gradually resolve over the course of a week. Local symptoms include development of pustular or ulcerative lesions on the external genitalia. Lesions usually begin as papules or vesicles that rapidly spread over the genitalia. Clusters of the lesions coalesce into large areas of ulceration, which over 2 to 3 weeks, crust, reepithelialize, or both. Genital lesions are described as painful by more than 90% of infected men and women. Development of new lesions is fairly common during the first 10 days of a primary infection. Other local symptoms can include itching, dysuria, vaginal or urethral discharge, and tender inguinal adenopathy; the latter is usually the last symptom to resolve. Viral shedding lasts approximately 11 to 12 days.[13,51,55,58,59,61]

First-episode nonprimary genital herpes is defined as an infection in individuals who have clinical or serologic evidence of prior HSV (usually HSV-1) infection at another body site. These infections tend to be milder than true primary infections, with a lower incidence of constitutional symptoms and a shorter duration of disease reported. Viral shedding usually lasts about 7 days.[13,54,55,56,58,61] Some data suggest that immunity produced by a prior HSV-1 infection also may reduce the risk of acquiring infection as a result of HSV-2.[52]

RECURRENT INFECTIONS

In contrast to first-episode primary and first-episode nonprimary infections, recurrent infections are infrequently associated with systemic manifestations. Recurrent infection is localized to the genital area and is milder and of a shorter duration (8 to 12 days). Viral shedding lasts approximately 4 days. Approximately 50% of patients with genital herpes experience a prodrome prior to the appearance of recurrent lesions. This typically consists of a mild tingling or itching sensation hours to a few days prior to the appearance of vesicles. In a few patients, symptoms of sacral neuralgia are seen.[13,55–58,61]

As with a first-episode infection, symptoms of recurrent infection tend to be more severe in women, primarily as a result of the greater genital surface area involved. Also, recurrent genital infections caused by HSV-2 tend to be more severe than those associated with HSV-1 infection. Approximately 80% to 90% of patients with a first-episode HSV-2 genital infection experience a recurrence within 12 months compared with approximately 50% to 60% infected with HSV-1.[54,58] The median number of recurrences is estimated at four per year when infection is caused by HSV-2 versus only one per year for HSV-1 infections. Symptoms of first-episode and recurrent infections tend to be more severe and prolonged in immunocompromised patients than in immunocompetent patients. In addition, immunocompromised patients are more susceptible to initial genital infection and subsequent recurrences, as well as generalized systemic infection.[55,56,58,59,61]

COMPLICATIONS

Complications from genital herpes infections result from both genital spread and autoinoculation of the virus and occur most commonly with primary first episodes. Lesions at extragenital sites, such as the eye, rectum, pharynx, and fingers, are not uncommon. Central nervous system involvement is occasionally seen and may take several forms, including an aseptic meningitis, transverse myelitis, or sacral radiculopathy syndrome.[29,54,55,56,58,59]

A major concern is the effect of genital herpes on neonates exposed during pregnancy. Neonatal herpes is associated with a high mortality and significant morbidity. It is transmitted to the newborn primarily through exposure to HSV in the birth canal but, in rare cases, also is transmitted transplacentally. The risk of transmission during birth appears much greater for first-episode primary infections than for recurrent infections. Neonatal herpes infection has a case-fatality rate of approximately 50%, with a large proportion of surviving infants experiencing significant morbidity.[13,29,54,55,59]

DIAGNOSIS

Confirmation of a genital herpes infection can be made only with laboratory testing. Tissue culture is the most specific (100%) and sensitive method (80% to 90%) of confirming the diagnosis of first-episode genital herpes; however, culture is relatively insensitive in detecting HSV in ulcers in the latter stages of healing and in recurrent infections as a result, in part, of reduced viral load. Viral culture is expensive and time consuming, and improper collection or transport of specimens can result in false-negative results. In most situations, HSV isolation on tissue culture takes 24 to 96 hours. Following isolation, it is recommended that typing of the virus be performed because of prognostic implications (HSV-1 is associated with a lower rate of asymptomatic and symptomatic recurrence). In instances in which rapid detection is necessary, such as an impending birth, other detection methods may be more useful. Amplified culture techniques that combine cell culture for 24 hours and HSV-specific antibodies have sensitivities and specificities only slightly less than those of culture.[52,53–55,60–63]

The Tzanck test is a rapid detection method in which cells from suspected lesions are stained and examined for the presence of characteristic multinucleated giant cells. While easy to perform and inexpensive, the specificity and sensitivity are low.[15,61,62] Antigen detection methods, such as direct immunofluorescence, immunoperoxidase staining, and EIA, provide more rapid results than culture and are less expensive.

The majority of patients infected with either HSV-1 or HSV-2 develop circulating antibodies to HSV antigens; however, commercially available serologic assays for detection of HSV antibodies are often overused and have only limited use in the diagnosis of genital herpes.

While the diagnosis of genital herpes can be confirmed only by laboratory tests, less stringent diagnostic criteria (e.g., characteristic physical findings or clinical history) frequently are used in clinical practice. A presumptive diagnosis of genital herpes commonly is made based on the presence of dark-field-negative, vesicular, or ulcerative genital lesions. A prior history of similar lesions or recent sexual contact with an individual with similar lesions also is useful in making the diagnosis. Other STDs, including chancroid, lymphogranuloma venereum, and granuloma inguinale, and causes, such as trauma, allergic reactions, and bacterial or fungal infections, are considered in the differential diagnosis.

▶ TREATMENT: Genital Herpes

The most achievable goals in the management of genital herpes are to relieve symptoms and shorten the clinical course, prevent complications, prevent recurrences, and decrease disease transmission. Although research has focused primarily on the treatment of active infection and suppression of recurrences, increasing emphasis is being placed on various approaches, including immunotherapy that might provide protection from disease transmission or possibly eliminate established latency.[58]

Palliative and supportive measures are the cornerstone of therapy for patients with genital herpes. Pain and discomfort usually respond to warm saline baths or the use of analgesics, antipyretics, or antipruritics; good genital hygiene can prevent the development of bacterial superinfection. Specific chemotherapeutic approaches to treating genital herpes include antiviral compounds, topical surfactants, photodynamic dyes, immune modulators, vaccines, and interferons. Few of these have undergone extensive evaluation, however, and only the antiviral agents have demonstrated any consistent clinical efficacy.[29,53–63] Although the CDC recommendations for the treatment of genital herpes include only acyclovir (Table 107–6), two related antiviral agents, valacyclovir and famciclovir, have been marketed for the management of genital HSV.[14] Valacyclovir, a prodrug of acyclovir, and famciclovir, a prodrug of penciclovir, possess improved pharmacokinetic profiles over acyclovir, allowing them to be dosed less frequently. Their overall efficacy in treating genital HSV infection, however, appears comparable to acyclovir.[48,54]

FIRST-EPISODE INFECTIONS

Oral and IV formulations of acyclovir have demonstrated efficacy in reducing viral shedding, duration of symptoms, and time to healing of first-episode genital herpes infections, with maximal benefits seen when therapy is initiated at the earliest stages of infection. In contrast, topical acyclovir therapy, when used alone or in combination with oral therapy, is considered of little or no benefit in most patients. Oral acyclovir 200 mg five times daily for 7 to 10 days or when clinical resolution occurs is the treatment of choice for outpatients with first-episode genital herpes. Some evidence suggests that larger doses given less frequently (400 mg three times daily) may be just as efficacious.[14] In patients with severe symptoms or complications necessitating hospitalization, parenteral acyclovir may be beneficial; however, the IV regimen has been associated with renal, GI, bone marrow, and central nervous system toxicity, particularly in patients with renal dysfunction receiving high doses. No acyclovir regimen is known to prevent latency or alter the subsequent frequency and severity of recurrences in humans.[54–56,58,59]

The recommended dosage of valacyclovir in first-episode genital HSV is 1 g twice daily for 10 days. The usual dosage of famciclovir to treat first-episode infections has ranged from 250 to 750 mg three times daily for 5 days; final Food and Drug Administration (FDA) labeling approval for this indication is anticipated. Although the valacyclovir and famciclovir dosage regimens are more convenient and offer the potential for greater patient compliance when compared to acyclovir, no therapeutic advantages over acyclovir are apparent at this time.[54]

RECURRENT INFECTIONS

The role of antiviral agents in the treatment of most recurrent genital herpes episodes is controversial. Because signs and symptoms of recurrent infections are generally milder and of shorter duration

TABLE 107–6. Treatment of Genital Herpes

Type of Infection	Recommended Regimen[a,b]	Alternative Regimen
First clinical episode of genital herpes[c]	Acyclovir 200 mg PO five times daily for 7–10 days or until clinical resolution occurs	Acyclovir 5–10 mg/kg IV every 8 h for 5–7 days or until clinical resolution occurs[d]
First clinical episode of herpes proctitis	Acyclovir 400 mg PO five times daily for 10 days or until clinical resolution occurs	Acyclovir 5–10 mg/kg IV every 8 h for 5–7 days or until clinical resolution occurs[d]
Recurrent infection Treatment	Acyclovir 200 mg PO five times daily *or* 400 mg PO three times daily, *or* 800 mg PO twice daily for 5 days initiated within 48 h of onset of lesions[e]	
Suppression	Acyclovir 400 mg PO twice daily[f]	Acyclovir 200 mg PO three to five times daily

[a]Recommendations are those of the CDC.
[b]HIV-infected patients may require more aggressive therapy.
[c]Primary or nonprimary first episode.
[d]Only for patients with severe symptoms or complications that necessitate hospitalization.
[e]Treatment should be limited to patients with severe symptoms. Treatment is most beneficial when instituted at the earliest sign of recurrence (prodrome); therapy initiated 48 h or more after the onset of symptoms has no effect.
[f]Indicated only for patients with frequent or severe recurrences. Although safety and efficacy are documented in patients receiving daily therapy for as long as 5 yr, it is recommended that therapy be discontinued after 1 yr of continuous suppressive therapy to assess the patient's rate of recurrent episodes.

than those of first-episode infections in immunocompetent hosts, demonstration of clinically important therapeutic benefits is difficult. Management of recurrent episodes can take two approaches—episodic or chronic suppressive therapy.[54,56,58]

Episodic therapy is initiated early during the course of the recurrence, preferably at the onset of prodromal symptoms, but no more than 48 hours after symptom onset. In most patients, appreciable effects on symptomatology are not seen. Patients with prolonged episodes of recurrent infection or severe symptomatology are most likely to benefit from episodic therapy. Recommended acyclovir dosages are given in Table 107–6. Because of the relative mildness and brevity of recurrent infections, parenteral administration of acyclovir is not justifiable.[55,56,58,59] For the treatment of recurrent infection, the recommended dosage of valacyclovir is 500 mg twice daily for 5 days, and the recommended dosage of famciclovir is 125 mg twice daily for 5 days.[61]

Because of the cost and potential for adverse effects, available antiviral agents are not recommended for routine use as suppressive therapy in all patients with recurrent genital herpes. Patients with frequent (greater than six per year) and physically or psychologically distressing recurrences, however, are candidates for suppressive therapy. Continuous therapy with oral acyclovir has been shown to reduce the frequency and severity of recurrences in 70% to 90% of patients experiencing frequent recurrences. In some patients experiencing breakthrough recurrences while taking acyclovir, resistant HSV isolates have been identified. While there is some concern for the development of resistant strains with suppressive therapy, clinical trials have found no evidence of cumulative toxicity or significant resistance in patients treated continuously with acyclovir for up to 6 years.[29,48,54–56,59,64]

Results from several controlled trials indicate the superiority of continuous acyclovir suppression for 1 year versus intermittent or weekend suppressive therapy.[29,54–56] Although the CDC guidelines recommend a dosage of 400 mg twice daily, a regimen of 200 mg twice daily is reported to be almost as effective.[60] Large single daily doses of acyclovir are associated with a greater risk of breakthrough recurrences than multiple daily doses and are not recommended. Topical acyclovir has no role in the prophylaxis of recurrent infections in most patients.[53,56,57] Neither valacyclovir nor famciclovir are approved by the FDA for chronic suppressive therapy. Preliminary data suggest, however, that a famciclovir regimen of either 125 or 250 mg twice daily is effective and well tolerated.[60]

SELECTED POPULATIONS

Immunocompromised patients are at greatest risk for severe and recurrent HSV infections and have been shown to benefit from therapy with all three formulations of acyclovir. As with the immunocompetent host, effects are more pronounced with the IV and oral dosage forms. Both IV and oral acyclovir have been used to prevent reactivation of infection in patients seropositive for HSV who undergo transplantation procedures or induction chemotherapy for acute leukemia. Immunocompromised individuals, such as patients with AIDS, who fail treatment or prophylaxis with recommended doses of acyclovir, frequently demonstrate improved response with higher doses. If acyclovir-resistance is suspected or confirmed, alternative antivirals, such as foscarnet or vidarabine, are usually effective. Their use is associated, however, with a greater risk of serious adverse effects.[29,50,56,58,59,60]

The safety of acyclovir therapy during pregnancy is not established, although there is no evidence of teratogenic effects in humans. Because of the high maternal and infant morbidity associated with first-episode primary genital infections at or near term, the use of systemic acyclovir has been advocated as being appropriate; however, the effectiveness of such therapy is unknown. The use of acyclovir to treat or suppress recurrent episodes near term is more controversial, primarily because of the lack of data demonstrating significant benefits in this situation.[48,50,53–56,65–67]

With the increasing prevalence of genital herpes worldwide, the potential exists for widespread use and misuse of the nucleoside analogs acyclovir, valacyclovir, and famciclovir, resulting in development of resistant HSV isolates. *In vitro* resistance to these three agents is usually mediated by alterations in viral thymidine kinase; the majority of resistant isolates are either thymidine kinase deficient or have altered thymidine kinase. The incidence and clinical implications of HSV resistance require further study, particularly with respect to immunocompromised hosts in whom resistance may develop with greater frequency and be of greater clinical importance. Unlike acyclovir, valacyclovir, and famciclovir, foscarnet and vidarabine do not require the presence of thymidine kinase to be effective.[29,54,56,59,60]

Numerous agents for the prophylaxis and treatment of genital herpes infections are being studied. Neither topical nor systemic interferons have demonstrated consistent beneficial effects in genital HSV infections; however, a reduction in pain and time to healing of lesions have been reported with an interferon preparation incorporated into a gel containing nonoxynol-9.[59] Other treatments under investigation include cidofovir and immune modulators, such as imiquimod.[61] Agents that can eliminate ganglionic latency and prevent recurrent HSV infections are not expected to be available in the near future. Much more promising for the near future are vaccines under development. Unfortunately, safety concerns with live attenuated virus vaccines has resulted in research focused primarily on recombinant protein vaccines that have exhibited relatively poor immunogenicity. Similarly, use of heterologous vaccines (bacillus Calmette-Guérin and influenza vaccines) to stimulate the immune system in patients with recurrent genital herpes have proven of no significant benefit.[68,69]

EVALUATION OF THERAPEUTIC OUTCOMES

Available antiviral compounds are of greatest benefit in patients experiencing first-episode primary infections, immunocompromised patients, and patients with frequent or severe recurrent infections. Antivirals, however, are palliative and not curative. Patients receiving suppressive therapy should be monitored closely for adverse drug effects and have therapy withdrawn periodically to observe any changes in their intrinsic pattern of recurrence. Although recurrence rates after discontinuation of antiviral therapy are generally similar to pretreatment rates, changes in severity of symptoms sometimes occur. Use of suppressive therapy has the additional benefit of significantly reducing asymptomatic viral shedding that potentially results in a reduced risk of disease transmission to infected sexual partners.[70,71]

TRICHOMONIASIS

EPIDEMIOLOGY AND ETIOLOGY

Trichomonas vaginalis, a flagellated, motile protozoan is responsible for an estimated 2.5 to 3 million cases of trichomoniasis annually in the United States. Humans are host to two other *Trichomonas* species, *T. tenax* and *T. hominis,* but *T. vaginalis* is the only species thought to be pathogenic.[5,13,72–75] Although infection by nonsexual contact is reported, it is uncommon. Contamination of inanimate objects and spread of infection via communal bathing or contact with infected bath or toilet articles is possible since *T. vaginalis* can survive for short periods on moist surfaces. Neonatal infections also represent another possible nonvenereal route of disease transmission.[72–76]

Coinfection with other STDs is not unusual in patients diagnosed with trichomoniasis. Women infected with *T. vaginalis* are three times more likely to have gonorrhea than those who do not have trichomoniasis; approximately 20% of men with gonococcal urethritis also have trichomoniasis.[74] In patients treated appropriately for genital *C. trachomatis* or *Ureaplasma urealyticum* infection, persistent urethritis can result from coexisting trichomonal infection.[13,72,73,75]

PATHOPHYSIOLOGY

Trichomonads are isolated from the vagina, urethra, and Skene's gland in 90% to 95% of infected women. Infrequently, they are recovered from the endocervix. Extragenital sites are epidemiologically important, because infection can persist and result in reinfection of the vagina if local therapy alone is used.[29] This may account for the higher relapse rates reported for local versus systemic therapy.[77] After attachment to the vaginal or urethral mucosa, trichomonads usually elicit an inflammatory response that manifests as a discharge containing large numbers of polymorphonuclear leukocytes.[73–75,78,79]

CLINICAL PRESENTATION

Trichomonal infections are much more common in women than in men. This may in part be because of the reported greater transmissibility of the organism from men to women. The incubation period of trichomoniasis is 3 to 28 days, with as many as 50% of infected women remaining asymptomatic.[73,79] When symptomatic, females can present with mild-to-severe vaginal discharge, vulvar pruritis, dyspareunia, and dysuria. Symptoms frequently worsen during menstruation when the pH of the vagina is optimal for growth of trichomonads. Vaginal discharge is noted in approximately 50% to 75% of infected women and classically has been described as malodorous, foamy, and yellow-green in color; however, more typically the discharge is grayish and only mildly odoriferous. In up to 50% of women, severe pruritis is noted.[73,75,76,79,80]

On examination of symptomatic women, the vulva and surrounding areas may be diffusely erythematous and excoriated as a result of scratching. Secondary infection of excoriated areas is not uncommon. The vagina is often erythematous, and surface erosions of the cervix are seen in up to 90% of women ("strawberry" vagina and cervix). Tender inguinal lymphadenopathy and lower abdominal pain occur infrequently. In a small percentage of patients, there may be no abnormal findings on vaginal examination. There is no evidence that trichomonads spread beyond the cervix to cause PID or disseminated disease; however, it is suggested that cervical erosion secondary to trichomoniasis may contribute to malignant transformation.[73–75,79]

Trichomoniasis may be responsible for causing premature rupture of the membranes and preterm delivery.[13,29] It also can be transmitted to neonates after passage through an infected birth canal. Although the risk is low (5%) and most cases of neonatal infections are self-limited, persistent vaginal or urethral infections should be treated.[14,73,77,79]

The majority of trichomonal infections in men are asymptomatic, largely because of the smaller number of organisms usually present.[13] It is likely that differences in pathogenicity of trichomonads in men and women reflect differences in the microenvironment of the vagina and urethra.[78] The most common site of infection in men is the urethra, and when symptoms are present, urethral discharge is seen most commonly, followed by pruritis and dysuria. The discharge can range from mucoid to purulent. For most men, trichomonal urethritis is associated with a high spontaneous cure rate. Complications of infection in men are uncommon, although some cases of prostatitis and epididymitis have been attributed to *T. vaginalis.*[72,75,79]

DIAGNOSIS

Trichomonas vaginalis produces nonspecific symptoms also consistent with bacterial vaginosis, and as a result, laboratory diagnosis is required. Because *T. vaginalis* requires a pH range of 4.9 to 7.5 for survival, a vaginal discharge pH of greater than 5.0 usually indicates the presence of either *T. vaginalis* or *Gardnerella vaginalis,* a common cause of bacterial vaginosis. The simplest and most reliable means of diagnosis is a wet-mount examination of the vaginal discharge.[72,75,78,79] Trichomoniasis is confirmed if characteristic pear-shaped, flagellating organisms are observed. The wet mount is only about 75% to 80% sensitive in detecting the presence of trichomonads, with lower sensitivities reported in men and in women with low-grade, subacute, or chronic infections.[73–75,80]

Although the presence of trichomonads may be reported on a Papanicolaou (Pap) smear, the sensitivity of this cytologic technique is less than for wet mount and also is associated with a number of false-positive results. Stained smears of cervical specimens have been used in diagnosis, but they are less sensitive and more time consuming than the wet mount and, therefore, are not recommended. Culture techniques for trichomonads are highly specific and more sensitive than the wet mount, but they are not useful in rapid diagnosis since up to 48 hours or longer may be necessary for growth. Cultures may be necessary, however, to confirm the diagnosis in the absence of a positive wet mount or determine the antimicrobial susceptibility in intractable cases.[13,72–75,79,80]

In males, demonstration of trichomonads in urethral specimens or urine sediment by wet mount is difficult, and diagnosis depends largely on culture. Specimens from males should be taken prior to first voiding, as the small number of trichomonads in males may be reduced by micturition.[13,75,79]

▶ TREATMENT: Trichomoniasis

Metronidazole is the only antimicrobial agent available in the United States that is consistently effective in *T. vaginalis* infections. In only a few cases have *T. vaginalis* isolates been resistant to standard metronidazole doses. In these instances, longer courses of therapy or doses higher than those routinely recommended as initial therapy will usually produce a cure.[14,72,73,75–77]

Treatment recommendations for *Trichomonas* infections are given in Table 107–7.[14] The standard therapy for trichomoniasis is metronidazole 2 g orally as a single dose; cure rates are comparable to the recommended alternative regimen of 500 mg twice daily for 7 days. When sexual partners are treated simultaneously, cure rates greater than 95% are reported.[13,73] If sexual partners are not treated concurrently, cure rates are in the range of 80% to 90%. In limited clinical testing, a single 1.5-g dose of metronidazole also has produced a high cure rate comparable to the 2-g dose.[73,74,75,79,81]

Advantages of single-dose therapy over the multidose alternative regimen include better patient compliance, lower total dose, lower cost, and shorter exposure of the patient's GI and urogenital anaerobic bacterial flora to the drug. As a result of the latter, the likelihood of developing pseudomembranous colitis or symptomatic candidal vulvovaginitis is decreased.[73,74,80] Because high doses of metronidazole have mutagenic effects in bacteria and oncogenic effects in mice, a reduced time of exposure in humans may be beneficial. There is no conclusive evidence for either of these effects in humans after short-term, low-dose metronidazole therapy.[74,77,80] Gastrointestinal complaints (e.g., anorexia, nausea, vomiting, diarrhea) are more common with the single 2-g dose, occurring in 5% to 10% of treated patients. Some patients also complain of a bitter metallic taste in the mouth. Patients intolerant of the single 2-g dose because of GI adverse effects usually tolerate the multidose regimen.[73–75,80,82]

TABLE 107–7. Treatment of Trichomoniasis

Type	Recommended Regimen[a]	Alternative Regimen
Symptomatic and asymptomatic infections	Metronidazole 2.0 g PO in a single dose[b]	Metronidazole 500 mg PO two times daily for 7 days[c]
Treatment in pregnancy	No treatment recommended unless symptoms are severe[d]	
Neonatal infections[e]	Metronidazole 10–30 mg/kg/d for 5–8 days	

[a]Recommendations are those of the CDC.
[b]Treatment failures should be treated with metronidazole 500 mg PO two times daily for 7 days. Persistent failures should be managed in consultation with an expert. Metronidazole 2 g PO daily for 3–5 days has been effective in patients infected with *Trichomonas vaginalis* strains mildly resistant to metronidazole, but experience is limited. Higher doses also have been used.
[c]Metronidazole labeling approved by the FDA does not include this regimen. Dosage regimens for treatment of trichomoniasis included in the product labeling are the single 2 g dose; 250 mg three times daily for 7 days; and 375 mg two times daily for 7 days. The 250- and 375-mg dosage regimens are not included in the CDC recommendations.
[d]Metronidazole is contraindicated in the first trimester of pregnancy and generally should be avoided throughout pregnancy. If used, a single 2-g dose administered after the first trimester of pregnancy is recommended by the CDC; however, a 7-day regimen is preferred by some since they produce lower peak serum concentrations.
[e]Only infants with symptomatic trichomoniasis or with urogenital trichomonal colonization that persists beyond the fourth week of life.

To achieve maximal cure rates and prevent relapse with the single 2-g dose of metronidazole, simultaneous treatment of infected sexual partners is necessary. In women treated with the alternative 7-day course, however, relapse rates are not appreciably different regardless of whether or not sexual partners are treated. It is speculated that in men spontaneous resolution of trichomonal infection or a reduction in the number of trichomonads below the inoculum necessary to transmit disease may occur during the 7 days of a female's therapy.[73,75,79,80]

Patients who fail to respond to an initial course of metronidazole therapy usually respond to a second course. In these cases, sexual partners also should be retreated. For some *T. vaginalis* strains, higher dosages (2 to 7.5 g daily for 3 to 14 days) are effective. Good response rates also are reported for metronidazole 2 to 3 g orally plus a single 500-mg tablet administered intravaginally for 7 to 14 days. One report described the successful use of intravaginal nonoxynol-9 in treating a trichomonal infection resistant to metronidazole. Use of IV metronidazole may be warranted for rare cases of intolerance to oral medication.[13,73,75,80,82]

Patients taking metronidazole should be instructed to avoid alcohol ingestion during therapy and for 1 to 2 days after completion of therapy because of a possible disulfiram-like effect. Metronidazole can potentiate the hypoprothrombinemic effects of warfarin, but a clinically significant effect is unlikely with single-dose regimens. Because metronidazole is secreted in breast milk, it is recommended that breast feeding be interrupted for at least 24 hours after maternal ingestion of a single 2-g dose.[14,75,77,79,80,82]

No satisfactory treatment is available for pregnant women with *Trichomonas* infections. Metronidazole is contraindicated during the first trimester of pregnancy, and many experts recommend avoiding its use throughout pregnancy. Metronidazole easily crosses the placenta, and fetal blood levels are comparable to maternal levels. A clear association between teratogenic effects and maternal ingestion during pregnancy has not been shown; on the basis of limited data, short courses of metronidazole administered during the second and third trimesters do not appear to increase the incidence of teratogenicity, prematurity, or fetal death. In pregnant patients with severe symptoms not responsive to local palliative treatment, a single 2-g dose of metronidazole may be required.[14,29,73,75,77,79,80,82]

Various local therapies for trichomoniasis also have been proposed for pregnant patients, particularly as a treatment option during the first trimester. Clotrimazole vaginal suppositories, 100 mg at bedtime for 1 to 2 weeks, relieve symptoms in many women and produce cure rates of 50% or greater.[29,73,76,80] An alternative therapy is gentle douching with 2 tablespoons of vinegar in a quart of warm water once or twice daily until symptoms improve, then less frequently thereafter. This therapy generally provides some symptomatic improvement but few cures. Although once recommended, povidone–iodine douches should be avoided during pregnancy because of the risk of fetal thyroid suppression.[75,77,79]

Several 5-nitroimidazole antibiotics related to metronidazole (tinidazole, nimorazole, ornidazole, carnidazole) are being investigated worldwide for the treatment of trichomoniasis. None appears superior to metronidazole in treating susceptible strains of *T. vaginalis.* Some of these antibiotics, however, may prove beneficial in infections exhibiting resistance to metronidazole.[74,75,79,82]

EVALUATION OF THERAPEUTIC OUTCOMES

Follow-up is considered unnecessary in patients who become asymptomatic after treatment with metronidazole. When patients remain symptomatic, it is important to determine if reinfection has occurred. In these cases, a repeat course of therapy, as well as identification and treatment or retreatment of infected sexual partners, is recommended. In situations where reinfection can be excluded, a relative resistance to metronidazole should be assumed and an alternative, multidose metronidazole regimen should be prescribed. Culture and sensitivity are warranted for infections unresponsive to alternative metronidazole regimens.

OTHER SEXUALLY TRANSMITTED DISEASES

Several STDs other than those previously discussed occur with varying frequency in the United States and throughout the world. While an in-depth discussion of these diseases is beyond the scope of this chapter, recommended treatment regimens are given in Table 107–8.[14]

CONCLUSIONS

More than 20 different diseases have been identified for which sexual transmission is epidemiologically important. For most STDs, curative drug therapies are available;

TABLE 107–8. Treatment Regimens for Miscellaneous Sexually Transmitted Diseases

Infection	Recommended Regimen[a]	Alternative Regimen
Chancroid *(Haemophilus ducreyi)*	Azithromycin 1 g PO in a single dose *or* Ceftriaxone 250 mg IM in a single dose *or* Erythromycin 500 mg PO four times daily for 7 days	Amoxicillin 500 mg plus clavulanic acid 125 mg three times daily for 7 days *or* Ciprofloxacin 500 mg PO two times daily for 3 days
Lymphogranuloma venereum	Doxycycline 100 mg PO two times daily for 21 days	Erythromycin 500 mg PO four times daily for 21 days *or* Sulfisoxazole 500 mg PO four times daily for 21 days or equivalent sulfonamide course
Condylomata acuminata		
External genital/perianal warts	Cryotherapy (liquid nitrogen or cryoprobe) *or* Podofilox 0.5% solution applied twice daily for 3 days followed by 4 days of no therapy; cycle is repeated as necessary for a total of four cycles[b] *or* Podophyllin 10%–25% in compound tincture of benzoin applied to lesions and washed off in 1–4 hours; repeat weekly for up to six applications[c] *or* Trichloroacetic acid 80%–90% applied to warts; repeat weekly for up to six applications *or* Electrodesiccation[d] or electrocautery	

[a]Recommendations are those of the CDC.
[b]Genital warts only.
[c]Because podophyllin is systemically absorbed and is toxic, use of large amounts should be avoided. Use of podophyllin is contraindicated in pregnancy.
[d]Electrodessication is contraindicated in patients with cardiac pacemakers or for lesions proximal to the anal verge.
[e]Some experts caution against vaginal use; care must be taken to ensure that the treated area is dry before removing the speculum.

however, therapeutic approaches to viral STDs, such as genital herpes, provide only palliation and suppression of symptoms. Technologic advances in laboratory medicine have resulted in improved and more rapid diagnostic capabilities for many STDs. These advances are of particular importance for individuals with undiagnosed, asymptomatic disease who comprise a vast reservoir for continued disease transmission. Sexually active persons can reduce their risk of transmitting or acquiring an STD by avoidance of unsafe sexual practices, maintaining a mutually monogamous sexual relationship, or proper use of physical and chemical barriers during intercourse. In the future, vaccines providing protection from common STDs may have a significant effect on reducing the incidence of these infections.

▶ PRINCIPLES OF PHARMACOTHERAPY

- Sexually transmitted diseases (STDs) are the most common infectious diseases in the United States, with nearly two-thirds of all cases occurring in individuals under the age of 25 years.
- Individuals diagnosed with one STD are at a high risk of having a second or third coincident STD.
- For hormonal and anatomic reasons, STDs generally are more easily transmitted to and more difficult to diagnose in women. Similarly, serious or life-threatening complications of undiagnosed or inadequately treated STDs are much more likely to occur in women, including pelvic inflammatory disease, infertility, ectopic pregnancy, and cervical cancer.
- A high percentage of cases of many STDs are asymptomatic or minimally symptomatic, which adds to the difficulty in controlling their transmission.
- With the exception of viral STDs, such as genital herpes, human papilloma virus, or HIV, most STDs are easily cured with available antibiotics.
- The Centers for Disease Control and Prevention guidelines for treatment of STDs should be followed (available on the internet at www.cdc.gov).
- Single-dose therapies are preferred for the treatment of STDs to improve patient compliance, but they may not be economically feasible in some settings.
- Treatment failures for many STDs are generally a result of reinfection or noncompliance with multidose antibiotic regimens rather than a lack of efficacy of recommended regimens.
- Infection with many common STDs appears to facilitate the transmission of HIV.
- Other than abstinence or a monogamous sexual relationship between two uninfected individuals, barrier methods of contraception, such as latex condoms, diaphragms, and spermicides, offer the only available methods for providing some degree of protection from transmission of some STDs.

REFERENCES

1. Krieger JN. Biology of sexually transmitted diseases. Urol Clin North Am 1984;11:15–25.
2. Holmes KK, Bell TA, Berger RE. Epidemiology of sexually transmitted diseases. Urol Clin North Am 1984;11:3–13.
3. Handsfield HH. Sex, science, and society: A look at sexually transmitted diseases. Postgrad Med 1997(May);101(5):268–273, 277–278.
4. Adimora AA, Hamilton H, Holmes KK, Sparling PF. Sexually Transmitted Diseases, 2nd ed, Companion Handbook. New York, McGraw-Hill, 1994;1–9.
5. Donovan P. Testing Positive: Sexually Transmitted Disease and the Public Health Response. New York, Alan Guttmacher Institute, 1993; 4–25.
6. McCree DH. The use of condoms and spermicides in preventing STDs. Pharm Times 1996(May);62(5):85, 88, 92–94, 97, 99.
7. Stratton P, Alexander NJ. Prevention of sexually transmitted infections: Physical and chemical barrier methods. Infect Dis Clin North Am 1993;7:841–859.
8. Krieger JN. New sexually transmitted diseases treatment guidelines. J Urol 1995;154:209–213.
9. Zenilman JM. Gonorrhea: Clinical and public health issues. Hosp Pract (Off Ed). 1993(Feb 28);28(2A):29–35, 39, 40, 43–45.
10. Adimora AA, Hamilton H, Holmes KK, Sparling PF. Sexually Transmitted Diseases, 2nd ed, Companion Handbook. New York, McGraw-Hill, 1994:25–40.
11. Anonymous. Summary of notifiable diseases, United States, 1995. MMWR Morb Mortal Wkly Rep 1996;44(53):1–87.
12. Siegel MA. Syphilis and gonorrhea. Dent Clin North Am 1996;40: 369–383.
13. Anderson JR. Genital tract infections in women. Med Clin North Am 1995;79:1271–1298.
14. Anonymous. 1993 sexually transmitted diseases treatment guidelines: Centers for Disease Control and Prevention. MMWR Morb Mortal Wkly Rep 1993;42(RR-14):1–102.
15. Woods GL. Update on laboratory diagnosis of sexually transmitted diseases. Clin Lab Med 1995;15:665–684.
16. Mahony JB. Multiplex polymerase chain reaction for the diagnosis of sexually transmitted diseases. Clin Lab Med 1996;16:61–71.
17. Moran JS, Levine WC. Drugs of choice for the treatment of uncomplicated gonococcal infections. Clin Infect Dis 1995;20(suppl 1): S47–S65.
18. Bignell C. Antibiotic treatment of gonorrhoea—Clinical evidence for choice. Genitourin Med 1996;72:315–320.
19. Fox KK, Knapp JS, Holmes KK, et al. Antimicrobial resistance in *Neisseria gonorrhoeae* in the United States, 1988–1994: The emergence of decreased susceptibility to the fluoroquinolones. J Infect Dis 1997;175:1396–1403.
20. Hammerschlag MR. Neonatal conjunctivitis. Pediatr Ann 1993;22: 346–351.
21. O'Hara MA. Ophthalmia neonatorum. Pediatr Clin North Am 1993; 40:715–725.
22. Hutchinson CM, Hook EW III. Syphilis in adults. Med Clin North Am 1990;74:1389–1416.
23. Hook EW III, Marra CM. Acquired syphilis in adults. N Engl J Med 1992;326:1060–1069.
24. Tramont EC. Syphilis in adults: From Christopher Columbus to Sir Alexander Fleming to AIDS. Clin Infect Dis 1995;21:1361–1371.
25. Goens JL, Janniger CK, de Wolf K. Dermatologic and systemic manifestations of syphilis. Am Fam Physician 1994;50:1013–1020.
26. Flores JL. Syphilis—A tale of twisted treponemes. West J Med 1995;163:552–559.
27. Anon. Syphilis. USP DI Update (Vols I, II). Rockville, MD, The United States Pharmacopeial Convention, 1997;434–444.
28. Sanchez MR. Infectious syphilis. Semin Dermatol 1994;13:234–242.

29. Quinn TC, Zenilman J, Rompalo A. Sexually transmitted diseases: Advances in diagnosis and treatment. Adv Intern Med 1994;39: 149–196.
30 Johnson PC, Farnie MA. Testing for syphilis. Dermatol Clin 1994; 12:9–17.
31. Larsen SA, Steiner BM, Rudolph AH. Laboratory diagnosis and interpretation of tests for syphilis. Clin Microbiol Rev 1995;8:1–21.
32. Anonymous. Recommendations for the prevention and management of *Chlamydia trachomatis* infections, 1993: Centers for Disease Control and Prevention. MMWR Morb Mortal Wkly Rep 1993;42 (RR-12):1–39.
33. Black CM. Current methods of laboratory diagnosis of *Chlamydia trachomatis* infections. Clin Microbiol Rev 1997;10:160–184.
34. Weinstock H, Dean D, Bolan G. *Chlamydia trachomatis* infections. Infect Dis Clin North Am 1994;8:797–819.
35. Heath CB, Heath JM. Chlamydia trachomatis infection update. Am Fam Physi 1995;52:1455–1461.
36. Martin DH. Chlamydial infections. Med Clin North Am 1990;74: 1367–1388.
37. Westrom LV. *Chlamydia trachomatis*—Clinical significance and strategies of intervention. Semin Dermatol 1990;9:117–125.
38. Majeroni BA. Chlamydial cervicitis: Complications and new treatment options. Am Fam Phys 1994;49:1825–1829.
39. Bell TA, Stamm WE, Wang SP, et al. Chronic *Chlamydia trachomatis* infections in infants. JAMA 1992;267:400–402 [Erratum, JAMA 1992;267:2188].
40. Schubiner H, LeBar W. *Chlamydia trachomatis* infections in women. Curr Probl Dermatol 1996;24:25–33.
41. Hook EW, Spitters C, Reichart CA, et al. Use of cell culture and rapid diagnostic assay for *Chlamydia trachomatis* screening. JAMA 1994; 272:867–870.
42. LeBar WD. Keeping up with the new technology: New approaches to diagnosis of *Chlamydia* infection. Clin Chem 1996;42:809–812.
43. Skolnik NS. Screening for *Chlamydia trachomatis* infection. Am Fam Phys 1995;51:821–826.
44. Nickel P, Naher H. Nongonococcal urethritis. Curr Probl Dermatol 1996;24:97–104.
45. Levine WC, Berg AO, Johnson RE. Development of sexually transmitted diseases treatment guidelines, 1993. Sex Transm Dis 1994; 21(suppl 2):S96–S101.
46. Tartaglione TA, Hooton TM. The role of fluoroquinolones in sexually transmitted disease. Pharmacother 1993;13:189–201.
47. Nuovo J, Melnikow J, Paliescheskey M, et al. Cost-effectiveness analysis of five different antibiotic regimens for the treatment of uncomplicated *Chlamydia trachomatis* cervicitis. J Am Board Fam Pract 1995;8:7–16.
48. Anon. Drugs for sexually transmitted diseases. Med Lett Drugs Ther 1995;37:117–122.
49. Bush MR, Rosa C. Azithromycin and erythromycin in the treatment of cervical chlamydial infection during pregnancy. Obstet Gynecol 1994; 84:61–63.
50. Conant MA, Berger TG, Coates TJ, et al. Genital herpes: An integrated approach to management. J Am Acad Dermatol 1996;35: 601–605.
51. Kinghorn GR. Genital herpes: Natural history and treatment of acute episodes. J Med Virol 1993;(suppl 1):33–38.
52. Corey L. The current trends in genital herpes: Progress in prevention. Sex Transm Dis 1994;21(suppl 2):S38–S44.
53. Mertz GJ. Epidemiology of genital herpes infections. Infect Dis Clin North Am 1993;7:825–839.
54. White C, Wardropper AG. Genital herpes simplex infection in women. Clin Dermatol 1997;15:81–91.
55. Prober CG. Herpetic vaginitis in 1993. Clin Obstet Gynecol 1993; 36:177–187.
56. de Ruiter A, Thin RN. Genital herpes: A guide to pharmacologic therapy. Drugs 1994;47:297–304.
57. Mindel A. Long-term clinical and psychological management of genital herpes. J Med Virol 1993;(suppl 1):39–44.
58. Clark JL, Tatum NO, Noble SL. Management of genital herpes. Am Fam Phys 1995;51:175–182.
59. Lavoie SR, Kaplowitz LG. Management of genital herpes infection. Semin Dermatol 1994;13:248–255.
60. Mertz GJ. Management of genital herpes. Adv Exp Med Biol 1996; 394:1–10.
61. McDonald LL, Stites PC, Buntin DM. Sexually transmitted diseases update. Dermatol Clin 1997;15:221–232.
62. Hoffman IF, Schmitz JL. Genital ulcer disease: Management in the HIV era. Postgrad Med 1995(Sept);98(3):67–70, 73–76, 79–82.
63. Thin RN. Diagnosis of genital herpes simplex infections. Curr Probl Dermatol 1996;24:50–56.
64. Fife KH, Crumpacker CS, Mertz GJ, et al. Recurrence and resistance patterns of herpes simplex virus following cessation of ≤ 6 years of chronic suppression with acyclovir. J Infect Dis 1994;169:1338–1341.
65. Blanchier H, Huraux J-M, Huraux-Rendu C, Sainte-Croix le Baleur A. Genital herpes and pregnancy—Preventive measures. Eur J Obstet Gynecol Reprod Biol 1994;53:33–38.
66. Baker DA. Herpes and pregnancy: New Management. Clin Obstet Gynecol 1990;33:253–257.
67. Whitley RJ. Neonatal herpes simplex virus infections. J Med Virol 1993;(suppl 1):13–21.
68. McKenzie R, Straus SE. Therapeutic immunization for recurrent herpes simplex virus infections. Adv Exp Med Biol 1996;394:67–83.
69. Adimora A, Sparling PF, Cohen MS. Vaccines for classic sexually transmitted diseases. Infect Dis Clin North Am 1994;8:859–876.
70. Beutner KR. Genital herpes. Curr Probl Dermatol 1996;24:132–139.
71. Wald A, Corey L, Cone R, et al. Frequent genital herpes simplex virus 2 shedding in immunocompetent women: Effect of acyclovir treatment. J Clin Invest 1997;99:1092–1097.
72. Krieger JN. Trichomoniasis in men: Old issues and new data. Sex Transm Dis 1995;22:83–96.
73. Heine P, McGregor JA. *Trichomonas vaginalis:* A reemerging pathogen. Clin Obstet Gynecol 1993;36:137–144.
74. Moldwin RM. Sexually transmitted protozoal infections. Urol Clin North Am 1992;19:93–101.
75. Adimora AA, Hamilton H, Holmes KK, Sparling PF. Sexually Transmitted Diseases, 2nd ed, Companion Handbook. New York, McGraw-Hill, 1994:212–222.
76. Goode MA, Grauer K, Gums JG. Infectious vaginitis: Selecting therapy and preventing recurrence. Postgrad Med 1994(Nov 1);96(6): 85–88, 91, 93–96, 98.
77. Murphy PA, Jones E. Use of oral metronidazole in pregnancy: Risks, benefits, and practice guidelines. J Nurse Midwif 1994;39:214–220.
78. Graves A, Gardner WA. Pathogenicity of *Trichomonas vaginalis.* Clin Obstet Gynecol 1993;36:145–152.
79. Sobel JD. Vaginal infections in adult women. Med Clin North Am 1990;74:1573–1602.
80. Sweet RL, Gibbs RS. Infectious Diseases of the Female Genital Tract, 3rd ed. Baltimore: William & Wilkins, 1995: 343–347.
81. Spence MR, Harwell TS, Davies MC, Smith JL. The minimum single oral metronidazole dose for treating trichomoniasis: A randomized, blinded study. Obstet Gynecol 1997;89:699–703.
82. Schwebke JR. Metronidazole: Utilization in the obstetric and gynecologic patient. Sex Transm Dis 1995;22:370–376.

108

BONE AND JOINT INFECTIONS

Edward P. Armstrong, PharmD, BCPS, FASHP, and Victor A. Elsberry, PharmD, BCNSP

Bone and joint infections are comprised of two disease processes known respectively as osteomyelitis and septic or infectious arthritis. As such, they are unique and separate infectious entities, with different signs and symptoms and infecting organisms. Introduction of oral antibiotic therapy has had a dramatic impact on antibiotic regimens used to treat these diseases. In spite of advances in therapy, however, these infections continue to cause significant morbidity from residual damage and chronic recurring infections. Both infectious processes continue to be a serious problem from a diagnostic, as well as a management, viewpoint. Emphasis on initiating antibiotic therapy as soon as possible is important in reducing long-term complications.

EPIDEMIOLOGY

Osteomyelitis is generally an uncommon disease. One classic publication reported that 247 patients had osteomyelitis in a prominent American teaching hospital during a 4-year period.[1] Acute hematogenous osteomyelitis has an estimated annual incidence of 4.5 per 100,000 population.[2] Osteomyelitis caused by contiguous spread, including postoperative, direct puncture, and that associated with adjacent soft-tissue infections, comprises 47% of infections. Hematogenous osteomyelitis comprises 19% of infections, and osteomyelitis occurring in patients with significant peripheral vascular disease comprises 34% of infections. Reviewing osteomyelitis cases based on duration of disease, it is observed that acute disease constitutes 56% of patients and that chronic osteomyelitis, defined as having a previous hospitalization for the same infection, constitutes 44% of patients.

Infectious or septic arthritis is an inflammatory reaction within the joint space. Distinct from osteomyelitis, septic arthritis is a more common disease and is known to be one of the most common causes of new cases of arthritis. One series in children from a referral hospital reported 30.8 cases per year for 5 years.[3] Another study reported 97 cases of nongonococcal infections during an 18-year period and noted a slightly higher incidence of gonococcal infections.[4]

ETIOLOGY

HEMATOGENOUS OSTEOMYELITIS

The most common method of classifying osteomyelitis is based on the route in which the infecting organism reaches the bone. Infection that results from spread through the bloodstream is termed *hematogenous osteomyelitis.* When the organism reaches the bone from an adjoining soft-tissue infection, it is termed *contiguous osteomyelitis.* Osteomyelitis that results from direct inoculation, such as from trauma, puncture wounds, or surgery, generally is also classified under the contiguous osteomyelitis category. Patients with peripheral vascular disease are at risk for development of osteomyelitis, and these patients are often separated into a third distinct category because of their unique management features.

Osteomyelitis may also be classified based on the duration of the disease. Acute osteomyelitis describes infections of recent onset, usually several days to 1 week, while chronic infections are those of a longer duration. Some authors describe chronic infections as those with symptoms for more than 1 month before therapy, and other authors define chronic infections as relapse of an initial infection. Yet a third system sometimes used to classify osteomyelitis has been developed.[5] It is a staging system based on the anatomic location of the infection (medullary or superficial) and the physiologic status of the patient (otherwise healthy, systemic immunologic compromise, local immunologic compromise). This classification system may be useful when comparing patients between different studies and attempting to categorize the severity of infection.

INFECTIOUS ARTHRITIS

Infectious arthritis may occur from many different types of microorganisms. Most infecting organisms are known to produce an infection in a single joint, termed *monarticular infections;* however, infections also may involve two or more joints.[6] As with osteomyelitis, joint infections also may be classified according to the mechanisms by which the infecting organism reaches the joint. Infectious arthritis may result from the spread of an adjacent bone infection, direct contamination of the joint space, or hematogenous dissemination. Hematogenous spread of the disease comprises the majority of infections; spread from osteomyelitis and direct inoculation are much less frequent.[7] Infectious arthritis most commonly occurs in patients older than age 30; 20% of cases occur in children.[8]

PATHOPHYSIOLOGY

HEMATOGENOUS OSTEOMYELITIS

Hematogenous osteomyelitis is classically described as a disease of children because most cases occur in patients younger than 16 years of age.[9] Table 108–1 summarizes the

TABLE 108–1. Types of Osteomyelitis, Age Distribution, Common Sites, and Risk Factors

Type of Osteomyelitis	Typical Age (yr)	Site(s) Involved	Risk Factors
Hematogenous	Less than 1	Long bones and joints	Prematurity, umbilical catheter or venous cutdown, respiratory distress syndrome, perinatal asphyxia
	1–20	Long bones (femur, tibia, humerus)	Infection (pharyngitis, cellulitis, respiratory infections), sickle cell disease, puncture wounds to feet
	Older than 50	Vertebrae	Diabetes mellitus, blunt trauma to spine, urinary tract infection
Contiguous	Older than 50	Femur, tibia, mandible	Hip fractures, open fractures
Vascular insufficiency	Older than 50	Feet, toes	Diabetes mellitus, peripheral vascular disease, pressure sores

primary characteristics of osteomyelitis. Less commonly, these infections occur in older patients. One exception, vertebral osteomyelitis, involves the vertebrae and occurs most frequently in patients older than 50 years of age.

Unique features of the anatomy and physiology of some bones appears to predispose them to become infected.[10] The vascular structure within the long bones appears to predispose the bone for hematogenous infections to begin within the metaphyses (Fig. 108–1). The nutrient arteries of the long bones divide within the medullary canal of the bone into small arterioles.[11] These end in hairpin turns near the growth plate and flow into veins, of much wider diameter, that drain the medullary cavity. An infection in hematogenous disease is initiated within the bend of the arterioles. There is considerable slowing of blood flow passing through the hairpin turns within the arterioles and then into the wider venous structures. This sludging of blood flow allows bacteria present within the bloodstream to settle and initiate an inflammatory response. In addition to these structural features, there also appears to be less active phagocytosis within the metaphysis. A lack of reticuloendothelial cells within this area of the bone may allow bacteria to settle and establish an infection. After the bacteria settle in the bone, avascular necrosis may occur from occlusion of the nutrient vessels and release of bacterial enzymes.

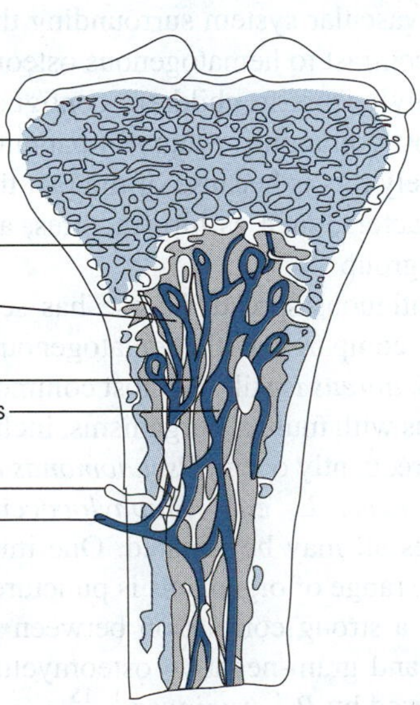

FIGURE 108–1. Cross-section of normal bone.

In addition to these anatomic and functional features, there is some evidence that trauma is associated with developing an infection in specific bones. Children who develop hematogenous osteomyelitis may report some type of trauma as an etiologic event. Animal data also indicate that traumatized bone is more likely to become infected than normal bone.

Once the infection is initiated, exudate begins to form within the bone, which produces increased pressure. The age of the patient largely determines the next stage in the pathophysiology. In children older than 12 to 18 months, the infection that started in the metaphysis of a long bone will be prevented from spreading into the joint because of the growth plate; however, the exudate will often expand laterally through the thin outer cortex of the bone and raise the loose periosteum. The periosteum is thick and not easily broken, and the resulting pus usually remains subperiosteal. If there is significant periosteal damage, a soft-tissue abscess may develop. Impairment of blood flow to the outer portion of the cortical bone may occur, producing dead bone that separates from healthy bone, termed *sequestra.* The elevated periosteum remains viable because its blood supply, derived from the overlying muscle, is unaffected. The raised periosteum will continue to produce bone; however, this new bone is now separated from the cortex because the periosteum has been raised from the infection. This new bone is termed *involucrum.*

In adults, the periosteum is tightly bound, and the cortex is thick. These anatomic features generally cause the infections to remain intramedullary. As expected, subperiosteal abscess formations are less common in this population. The infection may spread to adjacent bone structures through the Haversian and Volkmann canals. Chronic osteomyelitis is more likely to occur if large segments of bone become avascular and necrotic.

Neonatal patients also have unique characteristics. In these patients, there are blood vessels that spread through the cortex of the metaphyses and up into the epiphyses. This allows an infection that may have started within the metaphyseal area to spread easily to involve the epiphyses and then into the joint. Therefore, in infants, not only can the infection spread to involve the periosteum and the shaft as in children, but the infection also may spread to involve the joint.

Hematogenous osteomyelitis also is known to have a predilection for certain bones. The specific bones most likely to be involved also depend on the age of the patient. Children most commonly develop infections within the femur, tibia, humerus, and fibula. Vertebral infections are more common in patients older than 50 years of age. Neonatal infections commonly involve multiple bones.

The bacteriology of hematogenous osteomyelitis is unique compared with osteomyelitis caused by other routes of infection. A single organism is responsible for the vast majority of hematogenous infections. *Staphylococcus aureus* is isolated from 60% to 90% of the hematogenous infections in children. In one report of children with acute osteomyelitis during a 7-year period, *S. aureus, Haemophilus influenzae* type B, and *Pseudomonas aeruginosa* were responsible for 45%, 21%, and 10%, respectively, of the 75 cases for which organisms were identified.[12] Neonatal osteomyelitis has a wider spectrum in infecting organisms.[13] The three most common etiologic agents are *S. aureus,* group B streptococcus, and *Escherichia coli.* The infections from *S. aureus* and *E. coli* have been linked to complications occurring during pregnancy or delivery, and they are most frequently involved in multiple bone infections.

Vertebral osteomyelitis has several unique features. Vertebral osteomyelitis most commonly occurs in adults. The highest incidence is noted in patients in their fifties and sixties. The lumbar and thoracic regions are the locations of the majority of infections. Hematogenous infections are most likely to develop in the vascular areas near the subchondral plate region of the vertebral body. Staphylococci cause approximately 60% of these infections; however, gram-negative organisms now play a significant role. It is presumed that these gram-negative organisms, particularly *E. coli,* most likely originate within the urinary tract. *Escherichia coli* vertebral infections have been associated with urinary tract infections, positive urine cultures, and bacteremias. *Mycobacterium tuberculosis* also is known to cause infections in the spine.[11] Skin and respiratory tract infections are other foci of infections known to lead to vertebral infections.

A unique category of osteomyelitis patients are those individuals with a history of intravenous (IV) drug abuse. More than 50% of the osteomyelitis infections in this group of patients are found in the vertebral column. Less than 20% of infections are located in either the sternoarticular or pelvic girdle. Infections are much less frequent within the extremities. A very unusual feature of osteomyelitis in the IV drug–abusing population is the spectrum of organisms. Gram-negative organisms are responsible for 88% of infections. *Pseudomonas aeruginosa,* either singly or in combination with other organisms, is cultured in 78% of all infections. *Klebsiella, Enterobacter,* and *Serratia* also may be found but less commonly. In addition, staphylococcal and streptococcal organisms may be cultured.

Patients with sickle cell anemia and related hemoglobinopathies have a much higher rate of infection with *Salmonella* compared to other populations.[14] *Salmonella* species are responsible for two-thirds of the infections in these patients. It is believed that bowel infarctions from the sickle cell disease may facilitate salmonellae entry into the bloodstream from the colon and spread hematogenously to the bone. Osteomyelitis in patients with sickle cell disease may occur in any bone, but it is observed to be most common in the medullary cavity of long or tubular bones. Because of the difficulty in separating bone pain during a sickle cell crisis from that of an infection, osteomyelitis may be relatively advanced in these patients when the diagnosis is made. Although salmonellae are cultured most frequently, staphylococci and other gram-negative organisms also may be isolated.

CONTIGUOUS-SPREAD OSTEOMYELITIS

This category of osteomyelitis includes those infections caused by direct entrance of organisms from a source outside of the body or progressive spread of an infection from tissue adjacent to the bone.[14] Penetrating wounds (e.g., trauma), open fractures, or various invasive orthopedic procedures may result in direct inoculation of organisms into the bone. More than 80% of cases of postoperative osteomyelitis are known to occur following open reductions of fractures. Specifically, these infections occur most commonly after internal fixation of a hip fracture or femoral or tibial shaft fracture. Although less common, osteomyelitis also may occur following craniotomies, disc surgery, and repair of degenerative arthritis.

Osteomyelitis secondary to an adjoining soft-tissue infection comprises another very important group of contiguous infections, and most often involves the fingers and toes. Less commonly, infections may spread from infected teeth to involve the mandible or occur secondary to sinus infections by spreading through the mucosal lining of the sinuses into the vascular system surrounding the bone.

In contrast to hematogenous osteomyelitis, which most commonly occurs in children, contiguous-spread osteomyelitis most commonly occurs in patients older than age 50. Most likely this is because of the fact that important predisposing factors, such as hip fractures, are more common in this age group.

Contiguous-spread disease has several important differences compared with hematogenous osteomyelitis. Although *S. aureus* is still the most common organism isolated, infections with multiple organisms, including gram-negative bacilli, frequently occur. *Pseudomonas aeruginosa, Proteus, Streptococcus, E. coli, Staphylococcus epidermidis,* and anaerobes all may be isolated. One important exception to this wide range of organisms is puncture wounds of the feet. There is a strong correlation between puncture wounds of the feet and gram-negative osteomyelitis, especially infections caused by *P. aeruginosa.*[14,15]

Patients with osteomyelitis in association with severe vascular insufficiency are extremely difficult to manage.[16]

TABLE 108–2. Characteristics of Acute Infectious Arthritis

Feature	Finding
Peak incidence	*Children* less than 16 years *Adults* greater than 50
Clinical findings	Fever of 38–40°C in children; painful swollen joint in the absence of trauma Physical exam: effusion, restriction of joint motion, tenderness and warmth of joint
Most commonly affected joints	Knee, hip, ankle, elbow, wrist, and shoulder
Laboratory findings:	
Erythrocyte sedimentation rate	Elevated in 90% of cases
White blood cell count	Elevated in 30%–60% of cases
Left shift	Seen in two-thirds of patients
Blood culture	Positive in 40% of cases
Needle aspiration of joint	Gram stain diagnostic in 30%–50% of cases. Synovial fluid cultures are positive in 60%–80% of cases. Synovial fluid differential reveals 90% polymorphonuclear leukocytes. Synovial fluid glucose decreased relative to serum glucose. Lactic acid levels elevated in nongonococcal infectious arthritis but not in gonococcal infectious arthritis

As anticipated, most of these patients have diabetes mellitus or severe atherosclerosis, and they develop their infections from contiguous-spread mechanisms. Generally, these patients are between the ages of 50 and 70 years when they develop osteomyelitis. Frequently, patients with vascular disease develop osteomyelitis in their toes and fingers, and there is usually an adjacent area of infection, such as cellulitis or dermal ulcers. Many diabetic patients who develop osteomyelitis also have other complications, such as neuropathy and nephropathy.

Another important characteristic of osteomyelitis in association with vascular insufficiency is the spectrum of infecting organisms. Infections in these patients almost always include multiple organisms. The mixed floral infections often include *Staphylococcus* and *Streptococcus* or the combination of *Staphylococcus, Streptococcus,* and Enterobacteriaceae. *Enterococcus* and anaerobic organisms also may be seen.

Anaerobic organisms also play a role in osteomyelitis. When anaerobes are grown from cultures, they usually are found in association with other organisms, including aerobic bacteria. The two most common predisposing factors in patients who have anaerobic osteomyelitis are previous fractures (48%) and diabetes mellitus (11%).[17] The anaerobic infections in association with diabetes mellitus occur almost always within the feet. *Bacteroides fragilis* and *B. melaninogenicus* comprise the majority of anaerobic isolates.

INFECTIOUS ARTHRITIS

Distinct from osteomyelitis, infectious arthritis is usually acquired by hematogenous spread.[18] The synovial tissue is very vascular and does not have a basement membrane, so organisms in the blood can easily reach the synovial fluid. Table 108–2 summarizes the characteristics of acute infectious arthritis. Some organisms, such as *Neisseria gonorrhoeae,* are especially likely to infect a joint during bacteremia. In addition, organisms also may gain access to the joint from a deep penetrating wound, an intra-articular steroid injection, arthroscopy, prosthetic joint surgery, and contiguous osteomyelitis expansion into the joint.

Table 108–3 summarizes the risk factors associated with adult infectious arthritis. Trauma also appears to be a risk factor in facilitating microorganism entry into the synovial space. Unlike children, adults often have significant systemic diseases that predispose them to infectious arthritis, such as diabetes mellitus, immunosuppressive states (cancer, liver disease), or preexisting arthritis. Intravenous drug abusers also are prone to develop septic arthritis. Arthritis, joint trauma, and surgery are other important risk factors, because chronic inflammation or trauma makes the joint more susceptible to infection.[19] In addition, rheumatoid arthritis patients may be prone to bacterial infection because of an inherent phagocytic defect, as well as concomitant corticosteroid therapy. Hormonal factors appear to play a role in *N. gonorrhoeae* infectious arthritis. Women are more prone to develop disseminated gonococcal infections than men. The second and third trimesters of pregnancy and during menstruation appear to be the times of greatest risk for developing gonococcal bacteremia.

After bacteria gain access to the joint, the organisms begin to multiply and produce a persistent purulent effusion within the joint. If this joint effusion is present beyond 7 days, chronic and sometimes irreversible damage may occur. Purulent effusions may promote cartilage destruction by increasing leukocyte enzyme activity. In conjunction with the development of the effusion, almost all patients will develop a hot, swollen, painful joint. The proteolytic enzymes within the effusion and pressure necrosis may lead to cartilage and bone damage.

TABLE 108–3. Risk Factors for Adult Infectious Arthritis[a]

Systemic corticosteroid use
Preexisting arthritis
Arthrocentesis
Distant infection
Diabetes mellitus
Trauma
Other diseases

[a]More than one factor may be present.
From Ref. 53.

Staphylococcus aureus is the single most common infecting organism; it is found in 40% of cases of nongonococcal bacterial arthritis. Streptococcal infections account for 33% of cases and gram-negative organisms comprise 23% of infections. Overall, *E. coli* is the most common of the gram-negative organisms; however, *P. aeruginosa* is the most frequent organism in IV drug abusers.

Infants under 1 month of age may have infectious arthritis because of a broad range of organisms, with *S. aureus, Streptococcus,* and gram-negative organisms being most common. *Staphylococcus aureus, H. influenzae* type B, and *Streptococcus* are the most common pathogens in children less than 5 years of age. Other countries, however, may observe a lower frequency of *S. aureus* infections.[20] Within the adult population, *S. aureus* is responsible for the vast majority of nongonococcal infections. The most common cause of bacterial arthritis in adults less than 30 years of age is *N. gonorrhoeae,* which are the most common infections in women. Although less common, nonbacterial causes of osteomyelitis and septic arthritis include fungi and viruses.

CLINICAL PRESENTATION

OSTEOMYELITIS

The specific signs and symptoms seen in osteomyelitis vary depending on the route by which the organism reached the bone and the age of the patient. Most patients with hematogenous osteomyelitis complain of significant tenderness of the infected area, pain, swelling, fever, chills, decreased motion, and malaise. Although this presentation is classic, some patients with hematogenous disease may only have mild tenderness and a low-grade fever. Although hematogenous neonatal osteomyelitis infections may rapidly spread to involve the joint, often there are few systemic symptoms present. A joint effusion, present in 60% to 70% of neonatal infections, decreased limb motion, and edema over the affected area may be the only signs from which to make a diagnosis.

A commonly described diagnostic dilemma is pyogenic vertebral osteomyelitis. Many patients complain of nonspecific symptoms, such as severe back pain, fever or night sweats, and weight loss. Other patients may note a gradual onset in symptoms with a possible low-grade fever and complaints of continuous back pain. The pain is typically described as being present at rest and increasing in severity with movement. Of great concern is that if the infection extends and compresses the spinal cord, neurologic symptoms may develop.[21]

Signs and symptoms of osteomyelitis caused by spread of infection from a contiguous focus depend on the precipitating cause. If the infection follows surgery or bone trauma, the symptoms of the infection are usually noted within 1 month. The most frequent symptom is simply pain in the area of infection. Less commonly, patients also may develop a fever and elevated white blood cell (WBC) count. On physical examination, a patient with contiguous-spread osteomyelitis may have an area of localized tenderness, warmth, edema, and erythema over the infected site. Patients with significant vascular insufficiency usually have local symptoms, such as pain, swelling, and redness. Less commonly, patients with vascular disease also may have a fever and elevated WBC count.

INFECTIOUS ARTHRITIS

Because the differences in the clinical presentation and microbiologic characteristics of infectious arthritis are major, it is useful to separate this disease into nongonococcal and gonococcal bacterial arthritis. Patients with nongonococcal bacterial arthritis almost always present with a fever, and 50% of the patients will have an elevated WBC count. The average initial synovial WBC count is 100,000 cells/mm^3 or greater in nongonococcal bacterial disease.

Nongonococcal bacterial arthritis almost always involves only a single joint.[6] The knee is the most commonly involved joint, but infections also may occur in the shoulder, wrist, hip, ankle, interphalangeal, and elbow joints. Usually, the initial focus of infection that acted as the source for bacterial or microbial entrance can be identified. Common routes for bacterial entrance include infections of the respiratory tract, skin, and urinary tract. Blood cultures are important in these patients because they may be positive in 50% of patients.

In contrast to the other forms of infectious arthritis, the most frequent initial sign of disseminated gonococcal infections is a migratory polyarthralgia. In addition, two-thirds of patients also will complain of fever, dermatitis, and tenosynovitis (inflammation of the tendon sheath). Unique to gonococcal disease, 50% of these patients will have polyarthritis. Small papules on the trunk or extremities are the most frequent skin lesions seen in these infections, but only 30% to 40% of patients with disseminated gonococcal infection present with the classic hot, swollen, purulent joint. The mean synovial WBC count in gonococcal arthritis is usually 50,000 cells/mm^3 or more.

Another type of infectious arthritis occurs following prosthetic joint surgery. Because joint operations are being performed more frequently, more cases are now occurring. Fortunately, the risk of developing a joint infection following surgery is low. Because these are clean operations, the risk of developing a postoperative infection is estimated to be less than 5%. Infections are observed, however, more commonly after surgical revision of prosthetic joints. As anticipated, the candidates for this surgical procedure are usually elderly and have a history of either osteoarthritis or rheumatoid arthritis. When patients develop infectious arthritis following joint surgery, they often state that they have experienced some pain in the area. With an infection present, their erythrocyte sedimentation rate is usually elevated, although a leukocytosis often is absent. Infections that result from postoperative contamination usually become apparent within 1 year of surgery. If an infection occurs after this period, it is usually the result of hematogenous spread rather than from the surgery itself. Staphylococci continue to comprise the most common infecting organisms. *Staphylococcus epidermidis* is responsible for 40% of prosthetic joint infections, and *S. aureus* is responsible for 20% of infections.[22] Multiple organisms and anaerobic bacteria, however, also may be seen in some infections.

RADIOLOGIC AND LABORATORY TESTS

The evaluation of a patient who may potentially have osteomyelitis has several unusual aspects. Radiographs of the involved area should be obtained; however, bone changes characteristic of osteomyelitis are not seen for at least 10 to 14 days after the onset of the infection.[23] Radiologists may note soft-tissue swelling before any bone changes become obvious. Bone lesions do not appear on roentgenogram films until 10 days after infection because more than 50% of the bone matrix must be removed before the lesions can be detected. As an aide to improve the diagnosis, bone scanning is commonly used.[24] Technetium and gallium scanning may be positive as early as 1 day after the onset of symptoms, well before any radiographic changes may be seen.

Despite the seriousness of osteomyelitis, often there are few laboratory abnormalities. Often, the erythrocyte sedimentation rate and the WBC count are the only laboratory abnormalities. The degree of abnormality of these two laboratory findings does not correlate with the disease outcome; however, they are useful for monitoring therapy.

Once a clinical assessment of osteomyelitis is suspected, it is important to establish a bacteriologic diagnosis by culture of the infected bone. Accurate culture information is especially important as a guide for treatment of osteomyelitis. Bone aspiration is valuable in determining an accurate bacteriologic diagnosis. In addition, performing a bone aspiration will determine whether or not there is an abscess present. If an abscess is located, the pus is cultured and a Gram stain is performed. If an abscess is found, drainage will be needed and the fluid cultured. Aspirates of subperiosteal pus or metaphyseal fluid yield a pathogen in 70% of cases. Cultures should be done for both aerobic and anaerobic bacteria. A Gram stain of the aspirate may be useful in initiating empiric antibiotic therapy. This allows a more appropriate choice of antibiotics from the first day of therapy, rather than waiting several days while culture results are pending.

If a specimen is obtained from a previously undrained or unopened wound abscess, the pathogen usually can be identified. In chronic osteomyelitis, however, identification may be more difficult. Open wounds and draining sinuses frequently are contaminated with other organisms and, thus, provide inaccurate culture information. A comparison between sinus tract cultures and cultures obtained during surgery from 40 patients with chronic osteomyelitis demonstrated that less than half the sinus tract cultures contained the operative pathogen.[25] Therefore, because of the inaccuracies with sinus tract cultures, they cannot be relied on to reflect the pathogen. Cultures of loculated pus aspirates in the area of orthopedic devices removed from infected bone can be trusted, however, to identify the infecting organism. The preferable time to obtain culture material in a patient with chronic draining sinus is at the time of open surgical debridement.

In addition to performing cultures from the involved bone, it also is important to obtain cultures from any site believed to be the source of a bacteremia. In addition, it is important to obtain blood cultures. Approximately 50% of patients with hematogenous osteomyelitis will have positive blood cultures.

When evaluating the possibility of a patient having infectious arthritis, immediate joint aspiration with subsequent analysis of the synovial fluid is extremely important. The presence of purulent fluid usually indicates the presence of a septic joint. The synovial fluid WBC count is usually 50,000 to 200,000 cells/mm^3 when an infection is present. Approximately half of the patients with an infected joint will have a low synovial glucose level, usually less than 40 mg/dL.

Gram stains of joint fluid demonstrate bacteria in 50% of patients with septic arthritis; however, such stains may be positive in only 25% of patients with gonococcal arthritis infections. Synovial fluid cultures usually are positive in patients with nongonococcal infections. Both blood and joint fluid should be cultured aerobically and anaerobically in a patient suspected of having an infected joint. Blood cultures are positive in one-half of patients with nongonococcal infections, but in only 20% of those with gonococcal infections. Pharyngeal, rectal, cervical, or urethral smears and cultures should be performed if a disseminated gonococcal infection is considered. As with osteomyelitis, most patients will have an elevated erythrocyte sedimentation rate.

Radiographs of infected joints often reveal distention of the joint capsule with soft-tissue swelling in the adjacent space. Magnetic resonance imaging may be helpful in identifying an infected hip. In patients who have developed an infected prosthetic joint, loosening of the prosthesis may be seen radiographically.

▶ TREATMENT: Bone and Joint Infections

DESIRED OUTCOME

The goals of treatment are resolution of the infection and prevention of long-term sequlae. The ultimate outcome of osteomyelitis depends on the acute or chronic nature of the disease and how rapidly appropriate therapy is initiated. Patients with acute osteomyelitis have the best prognosis. One study of 58 patients with acute osteomyelitis who had surgery as indicated and received injectable antibiotics for a median duration of 12 weeks had a cure rate of 83%.[26]

In contrast, patients with chronic osteomyelitis have a much poorer prognosis.[27] Dead bone and other necrotic material from the infection act as a bacterial reservoir and make the infection very difficult to eliminate. Adequate surgical debridement to remove all the dead bone and necrotic material combined with prolonged administration of antibiotics provide the best chance to obtain a cure. The inability to remove all the dead bone may allow residual infection and require suppressive antibiotics to control the infection.

In comparison, many patients who develop infectious arthritis recover with no long-term sequelae. Gonococcal arthritis usually resolves rapidly with antibiotics; however, patients with staphylococcal arthritis have a higher incidence of joint damage. Individuals at greatest risk for long-term sequelae are those patients who have symptoms present for more than 7 days before starting therapy, infections occurring within the hip joint, and infections caused by gram-negative organisms. Common, long-term residual effects following infectious arthritis are limited joint motion and persistent pain. Shortening of the affected extremity is another well-known complication. One study noted that more than half the children who subsequently developed residual joint damage were believed normal at the time of hospital discharge.[28]

GENERAL APPROACH TO TREATMENT

Following completion of the steps needed to determine the infecting organism, the most important treatment modality of acute osteomyelitis is the administration of appropriate antibiotics in adequate doses for a sufficient length of time. It is important to stress that early antibiotic therapy may avoid the need for surgery.[29] A delay in treatment may allow bone necrosis to occur and make eradication of the infection much more difficult. In these patients, recurrent exacerbations of the infection may result if all necrotic tissue is not removed surgically and all microorganisms eliminated.

If the patient does not respond by having a decrease in fever, local swelling, redness, and pain following the initiation of adequate antibiotic therapy in a patient with hematogenous osteomyelitis, the patient should undergo surgical debridement of the infected area. It is important to emphasize the priority of starting antibiotics after the cultures have been obtained. One study reported no treatment failures in eliminating the infection if injectable antibiotics were started within 48 hours from the onset of symptoms in children with osteomyelitis.[30]

PHARMACOLOGIC THERAPY

ANTIBIOTIC BONE CONCENTRATION

Antibiotics used in the management of acute osteomyelitis are generally given in high doses (adjusted for weight, renal function, hepatic function, or both) so that adequate antimicrobial concentrations are reached within the infected bone. Empirically, 8 to 12 g/d of a penicillinase-resistant penicillin (nafcillin or oxacillin), ampicillin, or cephalosporin, or a similar large dose of another parenteral antibiotic is used in the initial management of adults with osteomyelitis. These dosing recommendations are, however, empiric; the relationship between a specific dose of a given antibiotic and its resultant concentration within the infected bone is largely unknown.[31] Semisynthetic penicillins, cephalosporins, clindamycin, and the aminoglycosides can be detected in bone homogenates soon after their administration.

DURATION OF ANTIBIOTIC THERAPY

The specific length of antibiotic therapy needed in the management of osteomyelitis is not clearly defined. Dich and coworkers[32] observed a failure rate of 19% in children treated with injectable antibiotics for 3 weeks or less. For those patients treated for more than 3 weeks, there was only 1 failure in 48 children. This study also found that the same results are achieved in patients treated for longer than 3 weeks with parenteral antibiotic therapy regardless of whether or not they receive subsequent oral antibiotics. Another trial in children with acute osteomyelitis also supported the minimum 3-week duration.[33] Thus, with the data indicating a minimum of 3 weeks of antibiotic therapy, the standard treatment for osteomyelitis has been parenteral antibiotics for 4 to 6 weeks. Although these data were determined in children, the duration of therapy recommendations are used in adults as well.

A modification of this recommendation has been used in some patients. Children receiving an appropriate oral antibiotic regimen and adults receiving an oral fluoroquinolone antibiotic, such as ciprofloxacin, for a duration of 6 weeks have been treated successfully. Monitoring the patient's clinical signs and symptoms and their erythrocyte sedimentation rate are important parameters in order to assess therapy. If signs or symptoms are still present at 6 weeks, therapy should be extended.

ORAL ANTIBIOTIC THERAPY

One of the most significant changes in the management of osteomyelitis is the use of oral antibiotics to complete therapy. Table 108–4 identifies criteria for the use of oral outpatient antibiotic therapy for osteomyelitis. Two primary populations have benefited from oral treatment. Children responding to initial parenteral therapy may be excellent candidates to receive follow-up oral therapy with an agent such as dicloxacillin, cephalexin, or ampicillin, depending on their culture and sensitivity results.[34,35] Although more controversial, the other population to benefit from oral therapy is adults with an infecting organism sensitive to a fluoroquinolone. These two populations now no longer routinely require expensive and complicated courses of long-term parenteral antibiotics.

The use of oral antibiotics has been well studied in children. Several studies documenting the effectiveness of oral therapy used injectable antibiotics initially and then switched to oral antibiotics when there was a decrease in the signs of inflammation and the erythrocyte sedimentation rate, or when the patient was afebrile for 3 days.[35] If pus was obtained on the initial needle aspirate or if a reduction in fever, local swelling, and tenderness did not occur despite adequate rest, immobilization, and intensive antibiotic therapy, the patients underwent surgical drainage.

The patients enrolled in oral antibiotic trials generally had disease of recent onset, identification of the infecting organism, enforced compliance, and surgery as indicated. In patients who meet these criteria, oral antibiotics appear to offer a great advantage in the treatment of osteomyelitis. Patients not meeting these criteria are more likely to develop chronic osteomyelitis with resultant recurrent exacerbations of the infection if oral therapy is attempted.

TABLE 108–4. Criteria for Oral Outpatient Therapy for Osteomyelitis

Confirmed osteomyelitis
Organism identified
Antibiotic sensitivity determined
Suitable oral agent available
Compliance assured
Suitable candidates:
Children with good clinical response to IV therapy
Adults without diabetes mellitus or peripheral vascular disease

Ciprofloxacin is effective in the treatment of osteomyelitis caused by gram-negative strains, such as *Enterobacter cloacae* and *Serratia marcescens*. Many strains of streptococci are relatively resistant. Its activity against gram-negative bacilli allows patients to be treated orally and avoids the potential toxic complications of 4 to 6 weeks of aminoglycoside therapy.[36–42] Another benefit with this agent is that it may be administered on an every 12-hour schedule. An important limitation of the drug, however, is that it should not be used in children younger than 16 to 18 years of age or in pregnant women because of its potential to cause cartilage damage. Other limitations of ciprofloxacin are that it has poor coverage against anaerobic organisms and staphylococci and that *P. aeruginosa* may develop resistance.[43]

There has been concern raised with staphylococci resistance to fluoroquinolones.[41] Methicillin-resistant *S. aureus* infections do not respond well to ciprofloxacin; however, resistance may also be troublesome for methicillin-sensitive strains. It is now recommended that when ciprofloxacin is to be used to treat osteomyelitis with mixed etiologies that include *S. aureus,* ciprofloxacin should be combined with an antistaphylococcal drug.[42,43]

ANTIBIOTIC SELECTION

A critical component in the management of osteomyelitis is the selection of appropriate antibiotics. Empiric therapy must be selected on the basis of the most likely infecting organism while the results of culture and sensitivity data are pending. Empiric therapy recommendations are summarized in Table 108–5. Dosages expressed in terms of milligrams per kilogram per day are generally given in divided doses every 6 to 8 hours (three to four times a day).

Because *S. aureus,* streptococci, and *E. coli* are the most common infecting organisms in newborns, an IV dosage of 40 mg/kg/d (given in two divided doses) of cefazolin is appropriate. For children 5 years of age or younger, *S. aureus, H. influenzae* type B, and streptococci are the most common infecting organisms. Appropriate therapy in this age group is cefuroxime IV 100 mg/kg/d. For children older than five years, *S. aureus* is the most likely infecting organism, and either nafcillin 100 mg/kg/d IV or cefazolin 100 mg/kg/d IV are recommended. If patients are allergic to penicillins or cephalosporins, vancomycin or clindamycin may be used for *S. aureus* coverage. Children with osteomyelitis usually can be successfully treated with 4 weeks of parenteral therapy.

An oral regimen may be an alternative to the previous recommendation in many cases of osteomyelitis in children. Children in whom the infecting organism is identified, who have undergone surgery if needed, and have had a good clinical response to IV therapy may be candidates for the alternate oral antibiotic regimen. It is recommended that parenteral antibiotic therapy be initiated and continued until there has been a resolution in the erythema, swelling, and tenderness, and until the patient is afebrile. Dicloxacillin, cloxacillin, and cephalexin (100 mg/kg/d) are effective oral agents. Patients should be monitored with periodic WBC counts, erythrocyte sedimentation rates, and radiographic findings. When oral antibiotics are used, the total duration of oral and injectable therapy is usually at least 4 to 6 weeks. As previously stated, because of the risk of cartilage damage, fluoroquinolones should not be used in children.

Hematogenous osteomyelitis in adults is most frequently caused by *S. aureus* and, thus, is appropriately treated with 8 to 12 g/d of a penicillinase-resistant penicillin, such as nafcillin. A similar dose of a first-generation cephalosporin, clindamycin 2.4 g/d or vancomycin 2 g/d (with normal renal function), may be used in those individuals allergic to penicillin; however, if the infection is located within the vertebrae, *E. coli* must be considered, and, thus, depending on the culture and sensitivity data, a switch to a cephalosporin may be needed.[44] After institution of appropriate antibiotic therapy, the antimicrobial agent should be continued for at least 4 to 6 weeks total (parenteral plus oral).

Special Populations

Osteomyelitis in a patient with a hemoglobinopathy, such as sickle cell anemia, is commonly caused by either *Salmonella* or *S. aureus.* Thus, empiric antibiotics of first choice are a penicillinase-resistant penicillin plus ampicillin. Alternatives to ampicillin are a third-generation cephalosporin, chloramphenicol, or ciprofloxacin (in adults).

Bone infections in patients with a history of IV drug abuse require coverage for gram-negative organisms; therefore, empiric

TABLE 108–5. Empiric Treatment of Osteomyelitis

Patient Subtype	Likely Infecting Organism	Antibiotic[a]
Newborn	*Staphylococcus aureus,* streptococci, *Escherichia coli*	Cefazolin 40 mg/kg/d IV (divided in two doses)
Children 5 years or younger	*S. aureus, H. influenzae* type B, streptococci	Cefuroxime 100 mg/kg/d IV
Children older than 5 years	*S. aureus*	Nafcillin 100 mg/kg/d IV *or* cefazolin 100 mg/kg/d IV
Adults	*S. aureus*	Nafcillin 2 g IV every 4 h *or* cefazolin 2 g IV every 8 h
Intravenous drug abusers	*Pseudomonas*	Ciprofloxacin 750 mg PO twice daily *or* ceftazidime 2 g IV every 8 h plus tobramycin 5 mg/kg/d IV
Postoperative or post-trauma patients	Gram-positive and gram-negative organisms	Nafcillin 2 g IV every 4 h plus ceftazidime 2 g IV every 8 h *or* ticarcillin/clavulanate 3.1 g IV every 4 h
Patients with vascular insufficiency	Gram-positive and gram-negative organisms	Nafcillin 2 g IV every 4 h *or* cefazolin 2 g IV every 8 h plus ceftazidime 2 g IV every 8 h
	If anaerobes suspected	Cefotetan 2 g IV every 12 h *or* clindamycin 900 mg IV every 8 h plus ceftazidime 2 g IV every 8 h

[a]Dosage should be adjusted for some agents in patients with renal dysfunction, hepatic dysfunction, or both.

treatment with ceftazidime 2 g IV every 8 hours plus an aminoglycoside is indicated. If compliance can be assured, these patients are excellent candidates to receive oral ciprofloxacin 750 mg twice daily. Antibiotic therapy in these patients should be continued for at least 4 to 6 weeks.

As previously discussed, bone infections occurring after surgery or from contiguous spread of an adjacent soft-tissue infection may be caused by several microorganisms. *Staphylococcus aureus* is the single most common organism, but multiple organisms may be involved. To provide the required broad-spectrum coverage, nafcillin 2 g IV every 4 hours plus ceftazidime 2 g IV every 8 hours should be used as initial therapy. An alternative single agent is ticarcillin/clavulanate potassium 3.1 g IV every 4 hours; however, there is less experience with this agent. The antibiotic regimen may require modification after culture and sensitivity information is evaluated. Based on the culture and sensitivity data, ciprofloxacin may be an appropriate oral alternative for these patients. Frequently, the antibiotics must be continued for 6 weeks to obtain a cure, and surgery often is required to remove any infected or devitalized tissue.

Patients with established vascular insufficiency who subsequently develop osteomyelitis are extremely difficult to manage.[45,46] Impaired blood flow to the extremities impedes the healing process. Infections in these patients include a wide range of organisms, including *S. aureus, Streptococcus,* anaerobes, and gram-negative organisms. Broad-spectrum therapy with a penicillinase-resistant penicillin in combination with ceftazidime is the preferred initial therapy. If anaerobes are suspected, an antianaerobic cephalosporin or clindamycin plus ceftazidime may be substituted. Ampicillin may need to be added to the regimen to provide coverage against *Enterococcus.* In spite of aggressive antibiotic therapy along with surgical debridement, however, these patients continue to have very low cure rates. Amputation of the involved area may be required to obtain a cure of the infection.

Home Antibiotic Therapy

Because the management of bone and joint infections frequently requires prolonged parenteral antibiotics, newer antibiotic regimens are being evaluated. Administration of antibiotics in the home environment and the use of antibiotics with extended elimination half-lives are being studied. Although acute osteomyelitis is one of the more common infectious diseases that may be treated with home IV antibiotics, not all patients are acceptable candidates for home administration. Patients must be screened to include only those patients who are receiving a stable treatment program, who are interested and are motivated in participating, and who have good venous access, as well as those who have support from family members or neighbors and have home facilities for storage and refrigeration.[47] Young, otherwise healthy patients may be able to use a peripheral IV catheter; however, a central IV catheter may be required if venous access difficulties occur. Certain exclusion criteria also must be considered. Complications of other preexisting diseases, such as diabetic retinopathy, intention tremor, disabling inflammation or degenerative joint disease, coagulopathies, or various neurologic disorders may prevent individuals from receiving home antibiotics.[48] Histories of alcoholism and IV drug abuse also are important exclusion criteria. Patients fluent in only a foreign language or those who are illiterate or hard of hearing may have to be excluded if a qualified guardian is unavailable. In addition to meeting these initial screening criteria, patients must successfully complete a thorough training program before hospital discharge. Aseptic technique, proper catheter care, and correct administration techniques must be documented. Once a patient is receiving therapy in the home environment, continued monitoring of their antimicrobial therapy is important. It is vital to ensure compliance with the antimicrobial regimen.

In addition, the specific antibiotic regimen characteristics must be considered in evaluating a patient for home antibiotics.[49] Some features that may be important include microbiologic culture and sensitivity data, the number of required daily antimicrobial doses, antibiotic stability data, and requirements for unique monitoring for the specific antimicrobial regimen, such as serum creatinine and peak and trough concentration measurements with aminoglycosides.[50] Although an organism may be sensitive to several antimicrobial agents, one antibiotic may provide practical benefits over other agents. Patients who have an infecting organism sensitive to one of the longer-acting (less frequently dosed) cephalosporins and who are resistant to less expensive agents (cefazolin) may benefit from the newer antibiotics.[51] It is important, however, to monitor for the development of resistant strains and superinfections.

Infectious Arthritis

The three most important therapeutic maneuvers in the management of infectious arthritis are appropriate antibiotics, joint drainage, and joint rest. Initial smears of the synovial fluid may be useful in initially selecting appropriate antibiotic therapy. If bacteria are not observed on the Gram stain in a patient who has a purulent joint effusion, antibiotics should still be initiated because of the high risk of an infection being present. A delay in initiating antibiotics significantly increases the likelihood for long-term complications.

The specific antibiotic selected depends on the most likely infecting organism. In infants less than 1 month old, the infecting organisms vary widely and empiric therapy must, thus, provide broad-spectrum coverage. A penicillinase-resistant penicillin, such as nafcillin or oxacillin (50 mg/kg/d), plus an aminoglycoside is appropriate. Children less than 5 years of age may be infected with *H. influenzae,* for which ampicillin therapy is indicated. The substitution of cefuroxime may be required if the patient is located in a geographical area with a high level of ampicillin resistance.

In children older than 5 years of age and in adults, initial therapy with a penicillinase-resistant penicillin is appropriate to provide the necessary coverage against *S. aureus*. Therapy should be changed to vancomycin if the *S. aureus* is resistant to methicillin. As with osteomyelitis, IV drug abusers require coverage for *P. aeruginosa* and, therefore, combination therapy with an aminoglycoside is needed. The antibiotics selected are usually administered parenterally. Antibiotics administered by this route achieve sufficient concentrations within the synovial fluid, and, thus, intra-articular antibiotic injections are not necessary. Although studies to define clearly the appropriate length of therapy have not been conducted, 2 to 3 weeks of antibiotic therapy is generally adequate in nongonococcal infections. Joint fluid cultures are usually no longer positive after 7 days of antibiotics.

Disseminated gonococcal infections often respond quickly to antibiotics. Ceftriaxone 1 g/d for 7 to 10 days is the treatment of choice. After culture and sensitivity results are available, and the organism is sensitive, therapy can be switched on the fourth day to either oral amoxicillin, doxycycline, or tetracycline to complete the 7- to 10-day course of antibiotic therapy. Clinical resolution of signs and symptoms is usually rapid.

Closed-needle aspiration is recommended for all infected joints except the hip. Joint drainage may be repeated daily for 5 to 7 days until effusions no longer reaccumulate. Open drainage is required in hip infections since closed-needle aspiration is difficult.[52] During the initial phase of the infection, weight bearing, such as walking, on the joint should be avoided. Passive range-of-motion exercises should be initiated when the pain begins to subside in order to maintain joint mobility.

PHARMACOECONOMIC CONSIDERATIONS

Cost and outcome issues are important in osteomyelitis and infectious arthritis. If long-term sequalae develop, such as impaired joint motion, draining sinus tracts, or amputations, patient quality of life may be significantly diminished. Cost and quality of life issues have clearly played a major role in evaluating other treatment alternatives (oral therapy or home antibiotic treatment) rather than requiring patients to remain hospitalized to receive 4 to 6 weeks of parenteral antibiotics.[49] More recently, a Markov model compared different treatments in non–insulin-dependent diabetes mellitus patients who had foot infections and suspected osteomyelitis.[16] This study found that a 10-week course of culture-guided oral antibiotics after surgical debridement may be as effective and less costly than other treatment approaches, such as immediate amputation.

EVALUATION OF THERAPEUTIC OUTCOMES

Patients with bone and joint infections must be monitored closely. Table 108–6 summarizes a pharmaceutical care monitoring protocol. An assessment of a therapy's success or failure is based on the patient's clinical findings and laboratory values. The clinical signs of inflammation, such as swelling, tenderness, pain, redness, and fever, should resolve with appropriate therapy. Initially, the clinical signs are assessed daily until improvement, then periodically thereafter. Elevations in WBC count also should gradually decline. The WBC count is usually obtained once or twice per week until it returns to the normal range. The erythrocyte sedimentation rate is usually determined weekly. Elevations in the erythrocyte sedimentation rate may not return to normal for several weeks of therapy. If, by the end of the 4- to 6-week antibiotic course, the clinical findings of osteomyelitis are no longer present and the erythrocyte sedimentation rate is within normal limits, the patient may be considered a clinical cure. Patients may relapse, however, after initially appearing to be cured. No relapse for 1 year is generally considered a complete cure.

If a patient fails to resolve the clinical signs and symptoms of inflammation after appropriate empiric antibiotics, surgical debridement may be needed. In addition, the patient may have a resistant infecting organism that may require a modification of the antibiotic therapy. It is especially important to note the infecting organism and its sensitivity pattern. Follow-up cultures at subsequent debridements may be useful to assess the antibiotic therapy.

Despite apparently adequate surgery and antibiotics, some patients may fail therapy and have recurrent relapses in their infection. This scenario is more common in the population with chronic osteomyelitis. These patients may require long-term oral antibiotics in order to keep the infection under control.

TABLE 108–6. Monitoring Protocol

Parameter	Frequency	Notes
Culture and sensitivity	At initiation of treatment	
White blood cell count	One to two times/wk until within normal range	
Erythrocyte sedimentation rate	Weekly	May not decrease to normal range until several weeks of therapy
Clinical signs of inflammation (redness, pain, swelling, tenderness, fever)	Daily during initiation of therapy	
Compliance of outpatient therapy	Reinforce before starting oral therapy and with each health care visit	Compliance is critical if treatment is to be successful

▶ PRINCIPLES OF PHARMACOTHERAPY

- The most common cause of osteomyelitis (particularly that acquired by hematogenous spread) and infectious arthritis is *Staphylococcus aureus.*
- Culture and susceptibility information are essential as a guide for antimicrobial treatment of osteomyelitis.
- Joint aspiration and examination of synovial fluid are extremely important to evaluate the possibility of infectious arthritis.
- The most important treatment modality of acute osteomyelitis is the administration of appropriate antibiotics in adequate doses for a sufficient length of time.
- Antibiotics should be started as soon as cultures have been obtained.
- Antibiotics used in the management of acute osteomyelitis are generally given in high doses so that adequate antimicrobial concentrations are reached within infected bone.
- The standard duration of antimicrobial treatment for osteomyelitis is 4 to 6 weeks.
- Oral antimicrobial therapy may be used for osteomyelitis to complete a parenteral regimen in children who have had a good clinical response to IV antibiotics or in adults without diabetes mellitus or peripheral vascular disease, when the organism is susceptible to the oral antimicrobial, a suitable oral agent is available, and compliance is assured.
- The three most important therapeutic maneuvers in the management of infectious arthritis are appropriate antibiotics, joint drainage, and joint rest.

REFERENCES

1. Waldvogel FA, Medoff G, Swartz MN. Osteomyelitis: A review of clinical features, therapeutic considerations and unusual aspects. N Engl J Med 1970;282:198–206, 260–266, 316–322.
2. Peltola H, Vahuanen V. A comparative study of osteomyelitis and purulent arthritis with special reference to aetiology and recovery. Infection 1984;12:75–79.
3. Fink CW, Nelson JD. Septic arthritis and osteomyelitis in children. Clin Rheum Dis 1986;12:423–435.
4. Goldenberg DL, Reed JI. Bacterial arthritis. N Engl J Med 1985;312: 764–771.
5. Mader JT, Ortiz M, Calhoun JH. Update on the diagnosis and management of osteomyelitis. Clin Podiatr Med Surg 1996;13:701–724.
6. Smith JW, Piercy EA. Infectious arthritis. Clin Infect Dis 1995;20: 225–231.
7. Stimmler MM. Infectious arthritis: Tailoring initial treatment to clinical findings. Postgrad Med 1996;99:127–139.
8. Goldenberg DK, Cohen AS. Acute infectious arthritis: A review of patients with nongonococcal joint infections (with emphasis on therapy and prognosis). Am J Med 1976;60:369–377.
9. Dirschl DR, Almekinders LC. Osteomyelitis: Common causes and treatment recommendations. Drugs 1993;45:29–43.
10. Lew DP, Waldvogel FA. Osteomyelitis. N Engl J Med 1997;336:999–1007.
11. Sonnen GM, Henry NK. Pediatric bone and joint infections. Pediatr Clin North Am 1996;43:933–947.
12. Faden H, Grossi M. Acute osteomyelitis in children: Reassessment of etiologic agents and their clinical characteristics. Am J Dis Child 1991;145:65–69.
13. Barton LL, Villar RG, Rice SA. Neonatal group B streptococcal vertebral osteomyelitis. Pediatrics 1996;98(3 Pt 1):459–461.
14. Haas DW, McAndrew MP. Bacterial osteomyelitis in adults: Evolving considerations in diagnosis and treatment. Am J Med 1996;101:550–561.
15. Puffingarger WR, Gruel CR, Herndon WA, Sullivan JA. Osteomyelitis of the calcaneus in children. J Pediatr Orthop 1996;16:224–230.
16. Eckman MH, Greenfield S, Mackey WC, et al. Foot infections in diabetic patients: Decision and cost-effectiveness. JAMA 1995;273:712–720.
17. Raff MJ, Melo JC. Anaerobic osteomyelitis. Medicine 1978;57:83–103.
18. Norman DC, Yoshikawa TT. Infections of the bone, joint, and bursa. Clin Geriatr Med 1994;10:703–718.
19. Kaandorp CJE, van Schaardenburg D, Krijnen P, et al. Risk factors for septic arthritis in patients with joint disease. Arthritis Rheum 1995;38: 1819–1825.
20. Yagupsky P, Bar-Ziv Y, Howard CB, Dagan R. Epidemiology, etiology, and clinical features of septic arthritis in children younger than 24 months. Arch Pediatr Adolesc Med 1995;149:537–540.
21. Ozuna RM, Delamarter RB. Pyogenic vertebral osteomyelitis and post-surgical disc space infections. Orthop Clin North Am 1996;27:87–94.
22. Inman RD, Gallegos RV, Brause BD, et al. Clinical and microbial features of prosthetic joint infection. Am J Med 1984;77:47–53.
23. Roy DR. Osteomyelitis. Pediatr Rev 1995;16:380–385.
24. Sutter CW, Shelton DK. Three-phase bone scan in osteomyelitis and other musculoskeletal disorders. Am Fam Physician 1996;54:1639–1647.
25. Mackowiak PA, Jones SR, Smith JW. Diagnosis value of sinus tract cultures in chronic osteomyelitis. JAMA 1978;239:2772–2775.
26. Glover SL, McKendrick MW, Padfield C, et al. Acute osteomyelitis in a district general hospital. Lancet 1982;1:609–611.
27. Eckardt JJ, Wirganowicz PZ, Mar T. An aggressive surgical approach to the management of chronic osteomyelitis. Clin Orthop 1994;298: 229–239.
28. Howard JB, Highgenboten CL, Nelson JD. Residual effects of septic arthritis in infancy and childhood. JAMA 1976;236:932–935.
29. Hamdy RC, Lawton L, Carey T, et al. Subacute hematogenous osteomyelitis: Are biopsy and surgery always indicated? J Pediatr Orthop 1996;16:220–223.
30. Jacobs JC. Acute osteomyelitis medical management in children. NY State J Med 1978;78:1273–1278.
31. Xue IB, Davey PG, Phillips G. Variation in postantibiotic effect of clindamycin against clinical isolates of *Staphylococcus aureus* and implications for dosing of patients with osteomyelitis. Antimicrob Agents Chemother 1996;40:1403–1407.
32. Dich VQ, Nelson JD, Haltalin KC. Osteomyelitis in infants and children. Am J Dis Child 1975;129:1273–1278.
33. Syrogiannopoulos GA, Nelson JD. Duration of antimicrobial therapy for acute suppurative osteoarticular infections. Lancet 1988;1:37–40.
34. Lane-O'Kelly A, Moloney AC. Acute haematogenous osteomyelitis—Evaluation of management in the 1990s. Ir J Med Sci 1995;164:285–288.
35. Peltola H, Unkila-Kallio L, Kallio MJT. Simplified treatment of acute staphylococcal osteomyelitis of childhood. Pediatrics 1997;99:846–850.
36, Gentry LO, Rodriguez GG. Oral ciprofloxacin compared with parenteral antibiotics in the treatment of osteomyelitis. Antimicrob Agents Chemother 1990;34:40–43.
37. Mader JT, Cantrell JS, Calhoun J. Oral ciprofloxacin compared with standard parenteral antibiotic therapy for chronic osteomyelitis in adults. J Bone Joint Surg Am 1990;72:104–110.
38. Gentry LO, Rodriguez-Gomez G. Ofloxacin versus parenteral therapy for chronic osteomyelitis. Antimicrob Agents Chemother 1991;35: 538–541.
39. Dan M, Siegman-Igra Y, Pitlik S, Raz R. Oral ciprofloxacin treatment of *Pseudomonas aeruginosa* osteomyelitis. Antimicrob Agents Chemother 1990;34:849–852.
40. Gentry LO. Oral antimicrobial therapy for osteomyelitis. Ann Intern Med 1991;114:986–987.
41. Trucksis M, Hooper DC, Wolfson JS. Emerging resistance to fluoroquinolones in staphylococci: An alert. Ann Intern Med 1991;114:424–426.
42. Wispelwey B, Scheld WM. Ciprofloxacin in the treatment of *Staphylococcus aureus* osteomyelitis: A review. Diagn Microbiol Infect Dis 1990;13:169–171.
43. Lew DP, Waldvogel FA. Quinolones and osteomyelitis: State-of-the-art. Drugs 1995;49(suppl 2):100–111.
44. Sapico FL. Microbiology and antimicrobial therapy of spinal infections. Orthop Clin North Am 1996;27:9–13.
45. LeFrock JL, Joseph WS. Bone and soft-tissue infections of the lower extremity in diabetics. Clin Podiatr Med Surg 1995;12:87–103.
46. HaVan G, Siney H, Danan JP, et al. Treatment of osteomyelitis in the diabetic foot: Contribution of conservative surgery. Diabetes Care 1996;19:1257–1260.
47. McAllister JC. The role of the pharmacist in home health care. Drug Intell Clin Pharm 1985;19:282–284.
48. Goldenberg RI. Pitfalls in the delivery of outpatient intravenous therapy. Drug Intell Clin Pharm 1985;19:293–296.
49. Mauceri AA. Treatment of bone and joint infections utilizing a third-generation cephalosporin with an outpatient drug delivery device. Am J Med 1994;97(suppl 2A):14–22.
50. Reed MD. Evaluation of antibiotics for home care programs. Drug Intell Clin Pharm 1985;19:288–290.
51. Gentry LO. Antibiotic therapy for osteomyelitis. Infect Dis Clin North Am 1990;4:485–499.
52. Broy SB, Schmid FR. A comparison of medical drainage (needle aspiration) and surgical drainage (arthrotomy or arthroscopy) in the initial treatment of infected joints. Clin Rheum Dis 1986;12:501–522.
53. Esterhai JL, Gelb I. Adult septic arthritis. Orthop Clin North Am 1991;22:504.

109

SEPSIS AND SEPTIC SHOCK

Thomas C. Hardin, PharmD, FCCP, and Joseph T. DiPiro, PharmD, FCCP

Sepsis and septic shock are significant causes of patient morbidity and mortality. In the late 1980s, sepsis was the 13th leading cause of death and accounted for nearly $10 billion in health care expense in the United States annually.[1,2] Estimates suggested an incidence of 400,000 cases of sepsis, 200,000 cases of septic shock, and 100,000 deaths each year from these serious infectious processes.[3] From 1979 to 1987, septicemia discharges increased by 139%, with the greatest increase occurring in those 65 years of age or older. The percentage of infectious disease diagnoses that included septicemia increased from 9.2% to 25.2%.[1] Factors contributing to the increasing incidence of sepsis and septic shock include increased use of cytotoxic and immunosuppressive therapies, increased use of invasive devices (intravascular catheters), the aging of the population, and an increased frequency of infection with antibiotic-resistant organisms. Even with a growing understanding of the pathophysiology of sepsis and a wider range of potent antibacterials, antifungals, and antivirals, the success of the health care community in the management of sepsis has been disappointing. Reported mortality rates for patients with gram-negative sepsis range from 20% to 80%.[3] Sepsis and associated sequelae continue to be the leading causes of death in intensive care units. New pharmacotherapeutic approaches aimed at improving patient outcomes associated with these conditions are under investigation. While the emphasis within the medical care system is often seen as shifting toward disease prevention and the outpatient management of chronic diseases, there remains a vital need for clinicians to comprehend the pathophysiology and appreciate the management options available for acutely ill patients with sepsis or septic shock.

DEFINITIONS

Differentiation of the terms associated with sepsis and septic shock are important to the understanding of the events that occur when microorganisms, most commonly bacteria, invade the bloodstream.[4] Bacteremia or fungemia may be transient, continuous, or intermittent. Transient bacteremia or fungemia can resolve quickly without complications. Continuous bacteremia or fungemia infer a sustained presence of bacteria or fungi in the blood (endocarditis). Intermittent bacteremia or fungemia are often associated with the presence of abscesses or focal tissue infections that seed the blood periodically.

Septicemia is an imprecise term classically associated with severe clinical signs and symptoms characteristic of systemic toxicity considered secondary to bloodstream invasion by microorganisms or associated toxins. *Sepsis* is a term used to describe the physiologic events that occur within the host in response to an infection. Because of widespread confusion with the use of these terms and the need to provide a flexible classification scheme for patient identification and treatment in both clinical and research settings, a joint committee of the American College of Chest Physicians and the Society of Critical Care Medicine standardized the terminology related to sepsis in 1992 (Table 109–1).[5] The criteria for the new terms provide specific physiologic variables that can be used to categorize a patient as having bacteremia, systemic inflammatory response syndrome (SIRS), sepsis, severe sepsis (consistent with the older term *sepsis syndrome*), septic shock, or multiple organ dysfunction syndrome (MODS), suggesting an important continuum of severity.[6] Introduction of the term SIRS is consistent with the knowledge that a physiologically similar systemic inflammatory response can be seen in the absence of identifiable infection. Noninfectious causes of SIRS include pancreatitis, severe trauma and burns, and hemorrhagic shock. Figure 109–1 represents the general relationship of infection, sepsis, and SIRS. It is important to note that progression from sepsis to MODS can occur in the absence of an intervening period of septic shock. Although it has been suggested that the terms septicemia and sepsis syndrome be abandoned, they are still widely used in clinical medicine.

The concept of a compensatory anti-inflammatory response syndrome (CARS) has been described.[7,8] This balancing compensatory anti-inflammatory response is consistent with the understanding that the human body is capable of mounting a range of physiologic responses to infection or injury.[9] It is when this localized balanced response is lost that the patient becomes systemically ill. As illustrated in Figure 109–2, when there is a systemic spillover of excessive proinflammatory mediators (tumor necrosis factor-α [TNF-α], interleukin-1β [IL-1β], IL-6), the patient presents with SIRS and possibly MODS, although with systemic spillover of excessive anti-inflammatory mediators (IL-4, IL-10, IL-11, IL-13, TGF-β), suppression of the host immune system will predominate.[7,10] The clinical consequences of this immune suppression are not fully understood.

EPIDEMIOLOGY AND ETIOLOGY

While almost any microorganism can be associated with the clinical development of sepsis, the most common etiologic pathogens are gram-negative bacteria, gram-positive bacteria, and fungi.

TABLE 109–1. Definitions Related to Sepsis

Condition	Definition
Infection	Microbial phenomenon characterized by inflammatory response to the presence of microorganisms or invasion of normally sterile host tissue by the microorganisms
Bacteremia	Presence of viable bacteria in the bloodstream
Fungemia	Presence of viable fungi in the bloodstream
Systemic inflammatory response syndrome (SIRS)	Systemic inflammatory response to a variety of severe clinical insults that is considered secondary to the widespread effects of proinflammatory cytokine mediators (TNF-α, IL-1, IL-6). The response is manifested by two or more of the following conditions: T > 38°C or < 36°C; HR > 90 beats/min; RR > 20 breaths/min or $Paco_2$ < 32 torr; WBC > 12,000 cells/mm³, < 4000 cells/mm³, or > 10% immature (band) forms
Sepsis	The systemic inflammatory response syndrome that is secondary to infection—most commonly by bacteria or fungi—but also occasionally because of infection by viruses or parasites
Severe sepsis	Sepsis associated with organ dysfunction, hypoperfusion, or hypotension. Hypoperfusion and perfusion abnormalities may include, but are not limited to, lactic acidosis, oliguria, or acute alteration in mental status
Septic shock	Sepsis with hypotension, despite aggressive fluid resuscitation, along with the presence of perfusion abnormalities (listed earlier). Patients who are on inotropic or vasopressor agents may not be hypotensive at the time perfusion abnormalities are measured
Multiple organ dysfunction syndrome (MODS)	Presence of altered organ function in an acutely ill patient such that homeostasis cannot be maintained without clinical intervention
Compensatory anti-inflammatory response syndrome (CARS)	Compensatory physiologic response to systemic inflammatory response syndrome that is considered secondary to the actions of anti-inflammatory cytokine mediators (IL-4, IL-10, IL-11, IL-13, TGF-β)

HR = heart rate; IL = interleukin; RR = respiratory rate; T = temperature; TNF-β = transforming growth factor β; TNF-α = tumor necrosis factor α.
From Ref. 5.

GRAM-NEGATIVE BACTERIAL SEPSIS

Considered the most important cause of sepsis, gram-negative bacterial infection has increased greatly in the last 20 years. A greater proportion of patients with gram-negative bacteremia develop clinical sepsis than do patients bacteremic with other organisms, and sepsis secondary to gram-negative rods results in the highest mortality rate when compared to other organisms.[11] Summaries of gram-negative sepsis show that *Escherichia coli* is the most commonly isolated pathogen in sepsis.[11] Other common gram-negative pathogens include *Klebsiella* sp., *Serratia* sp., *Enterobacter* sp., and *Proteus* sp. *Pseudomonas aeruginosa,* although not considered a predominant endogenous flora, is found widely in the environment and is the most frequent cause of sepsis fatality. Normally, these commensal organisms are not aggressive pathogens, but when the body's colonization immunity breaks down, these organisms extend beyond normal sites and often progress from colonization to clinical illness. Normal host flora inhibit the overgrowth of potentially pathogenic organisms. With the administration of antimicrobial agents having broad spectra of activity, the protective flora are presumably removed, thus allowing overgrowth of more virulent species. Additionally, the integrity of the gastrointesinal (GI) mucosa as a mechanical barrier is critical. The infectious implications of trauma, penetrating wounds, small surface ulcerations, mechanical obstructions, and ischemic necrosis of the bowel carry a high risk of subsequential gram-negative infection that often progresses to sepsis.

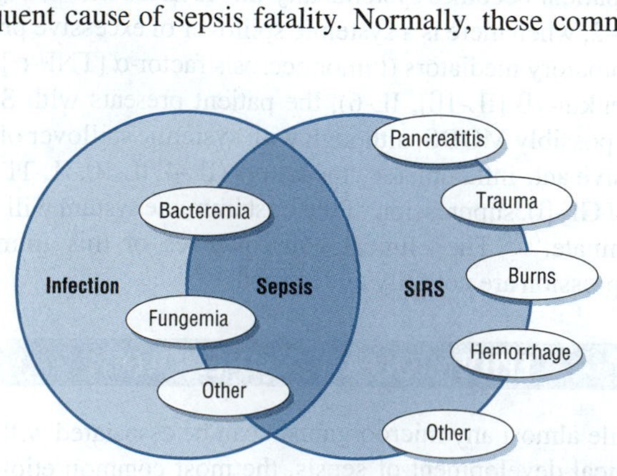

FIGURE 109–1. Relationship of infection, sepsis, and systemic inflammatory response syndrome (SIRS).[5]

The mortality rate reported in gram-negative sepsis is high. The major factor associated with the outcome of gram-negative sepsis appears to be the severity of any underlying condition. Patients with rapidly fatal conditions, such as acute leukemia, aplastic anemia, and > 70% of the body's surface burn injury, have a significantly worse prognosis than those with nonfatal underlying conditions, such as diabetes mellitus or chronic renal insufficiency.[11] Patient age does not appear to be an independent determinant of septic mortality in gram-negative sepsis.

GRAM-POSITIVE BACTERIAL SEPSIS

Gram-positive organisms are becoming more frequent pathogens in nosocomially acquired infections. These infections are commonly caused by *Staphylococcus aureus* and coagulase-negative staphylococci *(Staphylococcus epi-*

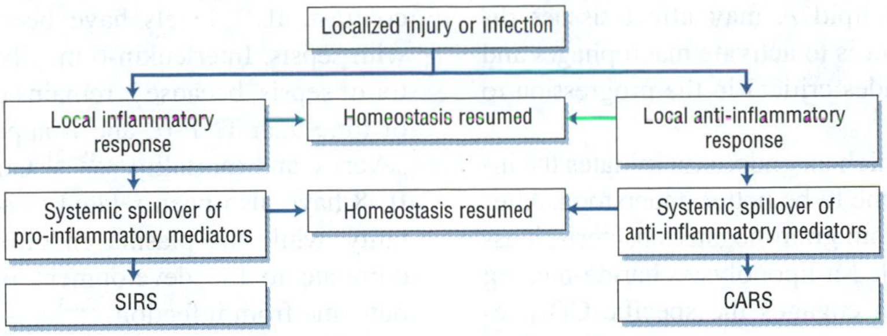

FIGURE 109–2. Relationships between systemic inflammatory response syndrome (SIRS) and compensatory anti-inflammatory response syndrome (CARS) following infection or injury.[10]

dermidis), and they are most often related to infected intravascular devices, such as artificial heart valves and stents and the use of intravenous (IV) and intra-arterial catheters. While the report of a single blood or tissue culture being positive for coagulase-negative staphylococci may often be considered a contaminant and clinically innocuous, severe life-threatening sepsis secondary to *S. epidermidis* has been described. Bacteremia secondary to *Streptococcus pneumoniae* is not common, but it has been reported to be associated with an overall mortality rate of over 25%. Factors related to a higher mortality include shock, respiratory insufficiency, preexisting renal failure, and the presence of a rapidly fatal underlying disease. The rates of nosocomial enterococcal bacteremia and associated sepsis are also increasing. Enterococci *(S. faecium, S. faecalis,* and *S. durans)* appear most commonly in blood cultures following a prolonged hospitalization and treatment with broad-spectrum cephalosporins.

ANAEROBIC, POLYMICROBIAL, AND MISCELLANEOUS BACTERIAL SEPSIS

Usually, anaerobes are considered low-risk organisms for the development of sepsis. If present, anaerobes are commonly found together with other pathogenic bacteria. Polymicrobial bacteremias usually involve the same organisms seen with single organism bacteremia, and the reported mortality rates are similar to sepsis caused by a single organism. Although some clinicians believe the particular combination of organisms present in polymicrobial sepsis may provide clues to the source of infection, in up to 25% of cases, no clear source for the infection can be identified. A number of other less common pathogens have been reported as causes of bacteremia and clinical sepsis. These include meningococcus, gonococcus, rickettsia, chlamydia, and spirochetes.[11]

FUNGAL SEPSIS

Candida sp. (especially *C. albicans, C. krusii, C. parapsilosis,* and *C. glabrata),* are common causes of fungal sepsis in hospitalized patients. Risk factors include abdominal surgery, poorly controlled diabetes mellitus, prolonged granulocytopenia, broad-spectrum antibiotic treatment, corticosteroid treatment, prolonged hospitalization, central venous catheter, total parenteral nutrition, hematologic malignancy, and chronic, indwelling bladder (Foley) catheter. The rates of nosocomial candidemia have been increasing, possibly because of the use of broad-spectrum antibiotics and the advancements in critical care, allowing for longer survival of critically ill patients. Mortality for candidemia has been reported to be as high as 52%. Other fungi identified as causes of sepsis include *Cryptococcus, Coccidioides, Fusarium,* and *Aspergillis.*

VIRAL SEPSIS

Viremia is common to many viral illnesses, but it does not usually lead to the development of clinical sepsis. Development of hypotension and disseminated intravascular coagulation (DIC) may occur with unusual viruses, such as ebola virus and lassa fever virus, and may be seen occasionally with influenza A, arbovirus, and possibly severe measles.[11]

PATHOPHYSIOLOGY

The pathophysiologic sequelae resulting from the interaction of the invading pathogen and the human host are diverse, complex, and incompletely understood.[3,11,12] Definitive relationships between infection and progression to septic shock have been difficult to demonstrate. Furthermore, clinical and histopathologic changes attributed to infection may be similar to those of coexisting conditions. Finally, observations from work with animal models of sepsis are difficult to apply to humans because of potential marked differences in responses.

The pathophysiologic focus of gram-negative sepsis has been on the lipopolysaccharide component of the gram-negative cell wall. Commonly referred to as endotoxin, this substance is unique to the outer membrane of the gram-negative cell wall and is generally released with bacterial lysis. The lipopolysaccharide molecule consists of three distinct regions. The outermost component, referred to as *O-antigen,* has diverse antigenicity, depending on bacterial species. The middle region, referred to as the *core,* has less antigenic diversity. *Lipid A* is the innermost region and is found in both aerobic and anaerobic gram-negative bacilli. Lipid A is highly immunoreactive and is considered responsible for most of the toxic effects observed with gram-negative sepsis. Although lipid A may affect tissues directly, its predominant effect is to activate macrophages and trigger inflammatory cascades critical in the progression to sepsis and septic shock.[10,12]

The mechanism by which an endotoxin initiates the inflammatory process has come to be better understood. After the endotoxin is released from gram-negative bacteria, it associates with a protein called a lipopolysaccharide-binding protein. This complex then engages the specific CD_{14} receptor on the surface of the macrophage, leading to activation and release of cytokine mediators.

Although not specifically identified, constituents of gram-positive bacterial, fungal, viral, and parasitic pathogens are also considered capable of initiating the cascades of events leading to sepsis and septic shock, including the release of TNF-α and other cytokines.

Sepsis involves a complex interaction of proinflammatory and anti-inflammatory mediators.[10,12–14] Primary proinflammatory mediators include TNF-α, IL-1β, and IL-6, which are released by activated macrophages, as well as IL-8, platelet activating factor (PAF), leukotrienes, and thromboxane A_2. Important anti-inflammatory mediators include IL-1 receptor antagonist (IL-1ra), IL-4, and IL-10. The net effect of a given mediator can vary depending on the state of activation of the target cell, the presence of other mediators near the target cell, and the ability of the target cell to release mediators that can augment or inhibit the primary mediator.[12]

The TNF-α is considered the primary mediator of sepsis, although this is probably not altogether accurate since sepsis involves the actions of many other cytokines and cells.[12,13,15] Evidence supporting an important role for TNF-α includes, however, the observations that endotoxin injected in healthy humans results in the detection of free TNF-α in plasma and the development of many symptoms associated with gram-negative infection; in meningococcemia, increased morbidity and mortality are associated with high plasma concentrations of TNF-α; and anti-TNF-α monoclonal antibodies injected into animals have a protective effect, particularly when the antibody was administered prior to the endotoxin challenge. The TNF-α release leads to activation of other cytokines (IL-1β and IL-6) associated with cellular damage.[10,12] In addition, TNF-α stimulates the release of cyclo-oxygenase-derived arachidonic acid metabolites (thromboxane A_2 and prostaglandins) that contribute to vascular endothelial damage.

Measurement of endotoxin and cytokine levels in plasma has been proposed to detect sepsis in its early stages or quantify the severity of sepsis.[16–21] The TNF-α has received much attention because it is elevated in the plasma of most patients with sepsis. Septic patients, however, are not the only ones who have elevated TNF-α levels. The TNF-α levels may be increased in patients with a variety of diseases and in many healthy people.[12] There is a correlation of TNF-α levels with the severity of sepsis, and high TNF-α levels are found in patients with septic shock. In contrast, IL-1 levels have been inconsistently associated with sepsis. Interleukin-6 may be a more consistent predictor of sepsis, because it remains elevated for a longer period of time than TNF-α, and it appears to be related to sepsis severity and mortality.[17,19–21] Circulating concentrations of IL-8 have also been related to severity of sepsis and mortality, while the plasma endotoxin concentration does not correlate to the development of gram-negative sepsis or outcome from infection.[22,23]

Through the actions of the mediators mentioned previously, a variety of cells become activated, initiating cascades believed to be detrimental to the host (as outlined in Fig. 109–3).[12,13,15,24] Initially, macrophages become activated and produce inflammatory cytokines. These cytokines then influence a wide range of cells, including endothelial cells, lymphocytes, hepatocytes, neutrophils, and platelets. A primary mechanism of injury with sepsis is mediated by endothelial cells that respond to and produce a variety of cytokines. When injured, endothelial cells allow circulating cells (granulocytes) and plasma constituents to enter inflamed tissues, which may result in organ damage. In addition, endothelial cells can cause vasodilation through the action of nitric oxide on vascular smooth muscle. Pulmonary dysfunction may result from the destructive mechanisms (proteolytic enzymes and reactive oxygen species) of neutrophils that are attracted to lung tissue through the action of IL-8 (and other chemoattractants).

Additional signs and symptoms are associated with the activation of the complement and Hageman factor. While the activation of a complement can occur by the classic (antigen–antibody activation) pathway, activation through the alternate pathway seems to be more important in sepsis. The pathophysiologic consequences of activated components of complement result in the generation of anaphylatoxins and other substances that augment or exaggerate the inflammatory response. Stimulation of leukocyte chemotaxis, phagocytosis with lysosomal enzyme release, increased aggregation and adhesion of platelets and neutrophils, and the production of toxic superoxide radicals are attributed, in part, to complement activation. Among these responses is the release of histamine from mast cells and the resultant increase in capillary permeability and the "third-spacing" of fluid in interstitial spaces. Disseminated intravascular coagulation, a frequent complication of gram-negative sepsis, is primarily attributed to the activation of factor XII (Hageman factor) by endotoxin. The subsequent activation and use of coagulation factors II, V, VIII, and platelets far exceed the rate of synthesis, resulting in an inability to maintain hemostasis. Paradoxic bleeding may occur because of the consumption of clotting factors and the rapid lysis of clots resulting from the simultaneously activated plasminogen (fibrinolytic system). Fibrin breakdown results in circulating soluble peptides called fibrin degradation products. Complications of DIC are varied and depend on the target organ affected and severity of the coagulopathy.

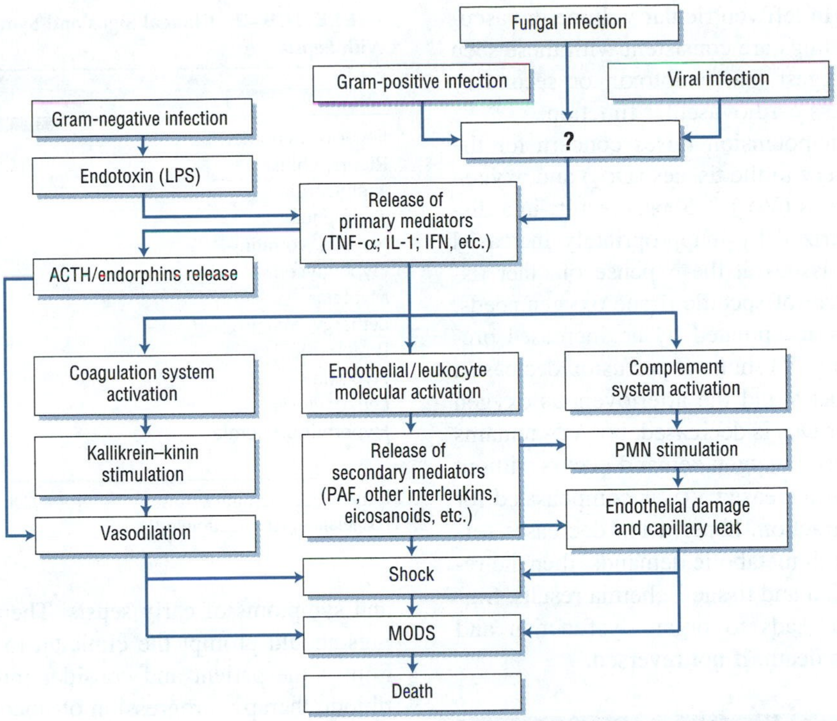

FIGURE 109–3. Cascades of sepsis.[24]

Another important complication of sepsis is acute respiratory distress syndrome (ARDS).[25] This is a functional lung injury, characterized by diffuse alveolar damage, where the alveolocapillary membrane is damaged, leading to noncardiogenic pulmonary edema through increased vascular permeability.[25,26] The result is that air spaces fill with fluid, and there is deterioration of gas exchange of the lung, impaired compliance, and refractory hypoxemia. This has been defined as acute lung injury with detection of bilateral pulmonary infiltrates on the frontal chest radiograph, a pulmonary artery wedge occlusion pressure (PAWP) of ≤ 18 mm Hg (or no clinical evidence of elevated left atrial pressure on the basis on chest radiograph and other clinical data), and a ratio of Pa_{O_2} to $Fi_{O_2} \leq 200$ (regardless of the level of positive end-expiratory pressure).[27] Approximately one-fourth of patients with gram-negative sepsis develop ARDS, and this carries an associated mortality rate of 60% to 90%.[28]

Shock is the most ominous complication associated with gram-negative sepsis. Severe hypotension associated with sepsis appears to be caused in part, by the release of vasoactive peptides, such as bradykinin and serotonin, and by endothelial cell damage leading to the extravasation of fluids into interstitial spaces. In 1951, Waisbren's classic description of a "shock-like picture" associated with gram-negative bacteremia suggested two clinically distinct syndromes.[29] Approximately one-half of the patients evaluated exhibited manifestations of acute bacterial infections (fever, bounding rapid pulses, wide pulse pressure, warm flushed skin, hypotension). This state, characterized by a high cardiac output and peripheral vasodilation, was referred to as "warm shock," occurring earlier in the progression of sepsis and associated with a better prognosis. In contrast, the remaining group exhibited hypotension with cold, clammy skin and lethargy (low cardiac output, peripheral vasoconstrictive state). This condition was referred to as "cold shock," occurring late in the progression of sepsis and associated with a poor prognosis. Although this clinical description of the spectrum of presentation seen with septic shock is consistent with that observed clinically and aids in the understanding of the underlying pathology, these terms are not widely used for classification of septic shock.

The hallmark of the hemodynamic effect of sepsis is the hyperdynamic state characterized by high cardiac output and an abnormally low systemic vascular resistance (SVR).[30] A low cardiac output appears to reflect inadequate maintenance of the circulating volume. Evidence suggests that myocardial function is impaired. In one dramatic study, Suffredini and coworkers injected small doses of endotoxin from *E. coli* into normal volunteers to study the cardiovascular effects compared to controls who received saline.[31] In subjects receiving endotoxin, the cardiac index before volume loading increased by 53%, the heart rate increased by 36%, and the SVR decreased by 46%. After volume loading, the ejection fraction decreased by 1% from the baseline value in subjects receiving endotoxin, but increased by 14% in controls. Left ventricular end-diastolic and end-systolic indices increased by 14% and 24%, respectively. Finally, left ventricular performance as measured by the ratio of the peak systolic pressure to the end-systolic volume index was depressed in subjects receiving endotoxin and increased in the control group. The conclusions drawn from these data suggest that endotoxin depresses left ventricular function independent of changes in left ventricular volume or vascular resistance. These findings are consistent with those seen in septic shock and suggest that endotoxin or secondary mediators directly depress cardiovascular function.

Sepsis associated hypotension raises concern for the balance of oxygen delivery to the tissues (Do_2) and oxygen consumption by the tissues (Vo_2).[32] Sepsis results in a distributive shock characterized by inappropriately increased blood flow to selected tissues at the expense of other tissues, which is independent of specific tissue oxygen needs. This perfusion defect is accentuated by an increased precapillary atrioventricular (AV) shunt. If perfusion decreases, oxygen extraction increases and the arteriovenous oxygen gradient widens. Cellular Do_2 is decreased, but Vo_2 remains unaffected. When increased oxygen demand occurs without increased blood flow, the increased Vo_2 is compensated for by increased oxygen extraction. If perfusion decreases sufficiently in the face of high metabolic demands, then the reserve Do_2 can be exceeded and tissue ischemia results. Significant tissue ischemia leads to organ dysfunction and failure, and ultimately to death, if not reversed.

TABLE 109–2. Clinical Signs and Symptoms Associated With Sepsis

Early Sepsis	Late Sepsis
Fever or hypothermia	Lactic acidosis
Rigors, chills	Oliguria
Tachycardia	Leukopenia
Tachypnea	DIC
Nausea, vomiting	Myocardial depression
Hyperglycemia	Pulmonary edema
Myalgias	Hypotension (shock)
Lethargy, malaise	Hypoglycemia
Proteinuria	Azotemia
Hypoxia	Thrombocytopenia
Leukocytosis	ARDS
Hyperbilirubinemia	GI hemorrhage
	Coma

ARDS = adult respiratory distress syndrome; DIC = disseminated intravascular coagulation; GI = gastrointestinal.

CLINICAL PRESENTATION

Table 109–2 lists the clinical features characteristic of sepsis, although a number of these findings are not limited to infectious processes. The initial clinical presentation of patients with systemic infection can be referred to as signs and symptoms of early sepsis. The presence of these findings should prompt the clinician to pursue further evaluation of the patient and consider initiation of systemic antibiotic therapy. Progression of uncontrolled sepsis leads to clinical evidence of organ system dysfunction as represented by the signs and symptoms attributed to late sepsis. The pathogenesis for many of these findings was discussed earlier. The distinction between early and late sepsis is arbitary, and it is recognized that sepsis represents a spectrum of clinical findings.[33,34]

▶ TREATMENT: Sepsis and Septic Shock

The primary goals of therapy for patients with sepsis include (1) timely diagnosis and identification of pathogen; (2) rapid elimination of the source of infection; (3) early initiation of aggressive antimicrobial therapy; (4) appropriate provision of cardiovascular and pulmonary support, to include fluid resuscitation, use of vasopressors, and mechanical ventilation; and (5) consideration of metabolic and other supportive therapies.

DIAGNOSIS AND IDENTIFICATION OF PATHOGEN

The initial evaluation of the infected patient should start with a careful physical examination and collection of specimens to be sent for culture. Generally, at least two sets of blood samples should be sent for aerobic and anaerobic culture, and samples of urine and sputum should also be sent for culture. Aspiration of any area suggestive of infection may be needed. If the patient is confused, complains of severe headache, or experiences a seizure, then a lumbar puncture is indicated, assuming intracranial pressure is not increased and there are no focal cranial lesions identified by computed tomography (CT) scan. Ideally, all culture samples should be collected prior to the initiation of any systemic antimicrobial therapy. Further specific laboratory tests may be indicated based on clinical findings. Additionally, the evaluation should include a careful history with special attention focused on any underlying conditions that could influence the etiology of the infection. A history of recent travel, injury, or animal exposure may be important. Any history of recent infection or antimicrobial use may prove useful in the choice of initial empiric therapy.

ELIMINATION OF SOURCE OF INFECTION

Should a clear source of infection be identified, prompt efforts to remove or eliminate the source should be initiated. Often gram-positive bacterial and fungal bloodstream infections are associated with infected intravascular catheters, and if suspected, these catheters should be removed and cultured. Urinary tract catheters may be associated with gram-negative bacterial and fungal infections of the genitourinary tract, and these should be removed in situations where association with sepsis is suspected. Suspicion of soft tissue (cellulitis or wound infection) or bone involvement should lead to aggressive debridement of the affected area. Evidence of an abscess or sepsis associated with any intra-abdominal pathology should prompt surgical consultation.

ANTIMICROBIAL THERAPY

Aggressive, early antimicrobial therapy is critical in the management of septic patients.[11,24,34,35] Because of the inherent problems associated with the timely identification of the infecting organism or organisms, empiric antimicrobial regimens are usually started initially. The empiric regimen selected should be based on the clinician's judgment of likely pathogens and the latest antibiotic susceptibility and resistance profile for the local institution.[36] An attempt should be made to cover all likely pathogens in the context of the clinical setting. A seriously ill patient should be treated with IV antibiotics because intramuscular (IM) and oral absorption may be erratic because of changes in regional blood flow associated with sepsis. Empiric therapy for an immunocompromised patient should consist of antimicrobial combinations likely to be synergistic. Loading doses for antibiotics other than aminoglycosides are unnecessary. Aminoglycosides should be dosed aggressively (> 2 mg/kg/dose) initially to achieve high-serum concentrations within the first 24 hours of treatment. Dosage adjustment based on assessment of serum concentrations can be made later, if needed. Patients should be monitored carefully, and therapy adjusted, if needed, based on changes in renal function. Once the pathogen is identified, a change to more specific antimicrobial therapy should be made.

The optimal choice of antimicrobial therapy for sepsis is not often clear.[4,24,35] There have been few controlled trials evaluating comparative antibiotic regimens in the treatment of sepsis, and generally, the studies have been designed to show equal efficacy, rather than superiority. The development of new antibiotics with an expanded spectra of activity and enhanced *in vitro* activities provide the clinician with a wide range of potential choices. Unfortunately, even with these expanded choices, the mortality associated with sepsis remains high.

When serious gram-negative sepsis is suspected, the use of combination antibiotics is usually recommended in order to provide additive or synergistic effects, to expand the spectrum of coverage, and to reduce the emergence of resistant bacterial subpopulations. On the other hand, a few studies comparing monotherapy with standard combination regimens in selected clinical situations have demonstrated equal efficacy. For example, ceftazidime alone appears equivalent to an antipseudomonal penicillin plus aminoglycoside combination in febrile neutropenic patients. It is critical, however, to pay particular attention to local resistance patterns when considering monotherapy, especially with *P. aeruginosa,* where monotherapy is more likely to be successful in nonneutropenic patients, patients who are not otherwise immunocompromised, and against highly susceptible isolates. Nevertheless, most clinicians still empirically start critically ill patients on combination therapies and adjust treatment once organisms and sensitivities are known.

Table 109–3 is a list of antibiotics that can be used in the treatment of sepsis. As stated earlier, the selection of specific agents should be based on individual institution sensitivity patterns. In the nonneutropenic patient with a community-acquired urinary tract infection, a third-generation cephalosporin, fluoroquinolone, or antipseudomonal penicillin, each with or without an aminoglyoside, should be considered. In a patient with a nonurinary tract, community-acquired infection, a third- or fourth-generation cephalosporin plus metronidazole, piperacillin/tazobactam, ampicillin/sulbactam, or ticarcillin/clavulanate regimen should be considered. If antipseudomonal activity is desired, ceftazidime or cefepime should be used; otherwise use of cefotaxime, ceftriaxone, or ceftizoxime is acceptable. Again, concurrent aminoglycoside therapy could be added if the clinician desires a potentially synergistic antibiotic regimen for the patient. Imipenem or meropenem may be indicated if resistance patterns prohibit use of other, less expensive therapies. New fluoroquinolones with expanded gram-positive, gram-negative, and anerobic activity, such as trovofloxacin, may prove useful in the future for empiric coverage.[37] Vancomycin should be added whenever the risk of methicillin-resistant staphylococci is significant. For septic patients with nosocomially-acquired infections, aggressive therapy with activity against *P. aeruginosa* and *Enterobacter* sp. should be instituted. Acceptable regimens include the combination of piperacillin/tazobactam plus an aminoglycoside, ticarcillin/clavulanic acid plus an aminoglycoside, imipenem or meropenem with or without an aminoglycoside, and ceftazidime or cefepime plus metronidazole and an aminoglycoside. In patients where the use of aminoglycosides may be too risky, a combination of a fluoroquinolone with a β-lactam can be cautiously considered, but synergistic activity between a fluoroquinolone and a β-lactam is not uniformly observed. Again, if the chance of methicillin-resistant staphylococci is high, vancomycin should be added.

When considering the use of aminoglycosides, the clinician is reminded that amikacin is less susceptible than gentamicin and tobramycin to plasmid-mediated enzyme inactivation and has proved a valuable alternative in situations of suspected or established resistance to gentamicin and tobramycin. *In vitro,* tobramycin appears somewhat more active (based on concentrations achievable in serum relative to usual minimum inhibitory concentration [MIC]) than gentamicin against *P. aeruginosa.* Gentamicin, however, appears more active than tobramycin against *Serratia* sp. Overall, amikacin appears most active against the *Klebsiella–Enterobacter–Serratia* group. It is not clear whether or not these differences observed *in vitro* have clinical significance.

Although aminoglycosides have been traditionally administered using doses of 1.5 to 2 mg/kg every 8 hours for gentamicin and tobramycin and 5 to 7.5 mg/kg every 8 to 12 hours for amikacin, there has been widespread acceptance of administering aminoglycosides in a single daily dose of 4 to 7 mg/kg for gentamicin and tobramycin and 10 to 15 mg/kg for amikacin.[38–41] The basis for single daily dosing is dependent on the well-defined, concentration-dependent killing of gram-negative bacteria by aminoglycosides, the prolonged postantibiotic effect against a number of important gram-negative bacterial pathogens, and the reported saturable, or rate-limited, uptake of aminoglycosides into proximal renal tubular cells.[42] In light of the growing literature to support the use of single daily dosing of aminoglycosides in most patients, this dosing technique is not universally accepted.[43] Because of insufficient clinical data, single daily administration of high dose aminoglycosides should not be used in pediatric patients, burn victims, pregnant patients, patients with preexisting or progressing renal dysfunction, and patients requiring aminoglycosides for synergy against gram-positive pathogens.

There is marked variability in aminoglycoside pharmacokinetic parameters between individual patients, and this leads to variable serum concentrations relative to the dose administered.[44] Therefore, appropriate monitoring of aminoglycoside serum concentrations becomes imperative. Early (within the first 24 hours of therapy) attainment of high peak concentrations is associated with improved outcome and reduced mortality for serious gram-negative infections.[45] Additionally, breakthrough bacteremias are associated with subtherapeutic aminoglycoside serum concentrations.[45] Nephrotoxicity and ototoxicity from aminoglycosides is considered secondary to accumulation of the drug within the body. This aminoglycoside accumulation is reflected clinically by an increasing trough serum concentration. With traditional dosing, gentamicin and tobramycin peak concentrations in the range of 6.0 to 10.0 μg/mL are generally associated with optimal response, although amikacin peak concentrations of 20 to 40 μg/mL are desirable.[46] Target trough concentrations should be less than 2 μg/mL for gentamicin and tobramycin, and less than 7 μg/mL for amikacin. When single daily dosing of aminoglycosides is employed, recommendations for serum concentration monitoring vary.[39] While there are several published nomograms and monitoring schemes, an aminoglycoside trough concentration that is undetectable is consistently desired.[38,47] The trouble with only monitoring a trough in many patients is that if an undetectable value is obtained, it is not known how long the concentration has been undetectable, and the dosing regimen cannot be satisfactorily assessed. One consistent method of assessing aminoglycoside serum concentrations for single daily dose administration is to obtain a concentration approximately 30 to 60 minutes after the dose and another concentration 8 to 10 hours later. With two concentration points, extrapolation to actual peak and trough concentrations will be possible using accepted pharmacokinetic equations.

The average duration of therapy in the normal host with sepsis is 10 to 14 days.[11,24,34] Once the patient is hemodynamically stable, has been afebrile for 48 to 72 hours, has a normalizing

TABLE 109–3. Options for Parenteral Antibiotic Therapy in the Management of Sepsis[a]

Antibiotic (Trade Name)	Adult Dose	Pediatric Dose	Comments
Aminoglycosides			
Gentamicin (generic)	1–1.5 mg/kg q 8 h 4–7 mg/kg q 24 h	2–2.5 mg/kg q 8 h	Active against gram-negative aerobes only; single daily dose not recommended in pediatrics
Tobramycin (generic)	See gentamicin		See gentamicin
Amikacin (generic)	5–7.5 mg/kg q 8–12 h 10–15 mg/kg q 24 h	5–7.5 mg/kg q 8 h	See gentamicin
Penicillins			
Penicillin G (generic)	2–4 million units q 4 h	25–50,000 units/kg q 4–6 h	Use generally limited to streptococcal infections
Ampicillin (generic)	2 g q 4–6 h	25–50 mg/kg q 6 h	Use is limited because of widespread resistance
Oxacillin (generic)	2 g q 4 h	25–50 mg/kg q 6 h	Use limited to staphylococcal infections
Nafcillin (generic)	See oxacillin		See oxacillin
Ticarcillin (Ticar)	3 g q 4 h	75 mg/kg q 6 h	Broad gram-negative activity
Piperacillin (Piperacil)	4 g q 6 h	75 mg/kg q 6 h	See ticarcillin
Mezlocillin (Mezlin)	4 g q 6 h	75 mg/kg q 6 h	See ticarcillin
β-lactamase Inhibitor Combinations			
Ampicillin/sulbactam (Unasyn)	3 g q 6 h	See ampicillin	Covers staphylococci and anaerobes
Ticarcillin/clavulanate (Timentin)	3.1 g q 4–6 h	See ticarcillin	Expanded gram-negative, staphylococci, and anaerobic activity
Piperacillin/tazobactam (Zosyn)	3.375–4.5 q 6 h	See piperacillin	See piperacillin
Cephalosporins			
Cefotaxime (Claforan)	1–2 g q 6–8 h	50 mg/kg q 6 h	Broad gram-negative and gram-positive; not *Pseudomonas*
Ceftriaxone (Rocephin)	1–2 g q 24 h	50–75 mg/kg q 24 h	See cefotaxime
Ceftizoxime (Ceftizox)	1–2 g q 6–8 h	50 mg/kg q 6 h	See cefotaxime
Ceftazidime (various)	1–2 g q 8 h	50 mg/kg q 8 h	Very good against *Pseudomonas;* weak gram-positive
Cefepime (Maxipime)	1–2 g q 8–12 h	50 mg/kg q 8 h	Antipseudomonal and antistaphylococcal
Fluoroquinolones			
Ciprofloxacin (Cipro)	400 mg q 8–12 h	Relative contraindication	Good antipseudomonal and other gram-negatives
Ofloxacin (Floxin)	400 mg q 12 h	Relative contraindication	Antipseudomonal activity less than ciprofloxacin
Levofloxacin (Levoquin)	500 mg q 24 h	Relative contraindication	Active stereoisomer of ofloxacin
Carbapenems			
Imipenem/cilastatin (Primaxin)	500 mg q 6 h	10–15 mg/kg q 6 h	Very broad spectrum to include anaerobes and pseudomonas
Meropenem (Merem)	500 mg q 8 h	10–15 mg/kg q 8 h	See imipenem
Monobactam			
Aztreonam (Azactam)	1–2 g q 8 h	50 mg/kg q 6 h	Use limited to gram-negative aerobes only
Others			
Vancomycin (generic)	1 g q 12 h	10 mg/kg q 6 h	Use should be limited to methicillin-resistant staphylococci
Metronidazole (generic)	500 mg q 6–8 h	15 mg/kg q 12 h	Excellent antianaerobic activity
Clindamycin (Cleocin)	600 mg q 8 h	10 mg/kg q 6–8 h	Good antianaerobic activity; some gram-positive activity
Cotrimoxazole (various)	160/800 mg q 12 h	4/20 mg/kg q 12 h	Good gram-negative activity; not antipseudomonal

[a]Doses listed are for normal renal function.

white blood cell (WBC) count, and is able to take oral medications, then a "step-down" from parenteral to oral antibiotics can be considered for the duration of therapy. Treatment may continue considerably longer if the infection is persistent. In the neutropenic patient, therapy is usually continued until the patient is no longer neutropenic and has been afebrile for at least 72 hours.

Suspected systemic mycotic infection leading to sepsis should be empirically treated with parenteral amphotericin B.[48] The initial amphotericin B dose should be 0.5 to 1 mg/kg infused daily over a period of 2 to 4 hours based on patient tolerance. In order to reduce the nephrotoxicity associated with amphotericin B therapy, infusion of 250 to 500 mL of normal saline before and after the amphotericin B dose is suggested. If the patient suffers from infusion-related fever, chills, and rigors, pretreatment with acetaminophen and diphenhydramine may be useful. Parenteral meperidine can be used to stop rigors, but it is not recommended as a pretreatment.[49] If the patient demonstrates evidence of worsening renal failure during amphotericin B therapy, a change to either amphotericin B lipid complex (ABLC), amphotericin B colloidal dispersion (ABCD), or liposomal amphotericin B should be considered.[50] Once the fungal pathogen is identified, parenteral fluconazole, dosed 400 to 800 mg daily, can be used if the fungus is susceptible.[48,51]

When sepsis is caused by a systemic viral infection, the choice of therapy is dependent on the suspected or documented etiology. Parenteral antivirals that may be employed include acyclovir, ganciclovir, foscarnet, and ribavirin. Aerosol administration of ribavirin may be indicated in serious illness secondary to respiratory syncytial virus.

FLUID THERAPY

Septic patients have enormous fluid requirements as a result of peripheral vasodilation and capillary leakage.[35,52] Rapid restoration of the intravascular fluid volume to improve cardiac output and expand circulating blood volume is, therefore, an essential therapeutic intervention in the initial management of sepsis and septic shock. The goal of fluid therapy is to maintain a systolic blood pressure greater than 90 mm Hg and prevent hypoperfusion to tissues and vital organs.[34] In its early stages, hypotension associated with sepsis is responsive to volume replacement. Several liters of fluid may be required to keep pace with capillary leakage in order to maintain an adequate intravascular volume. A patient in septic shock may require 10 or more liters of fluid within a 24-hour period to maintain intravascular volume and support blood pressure. With progression of illness, the blood pressure becomes less responsive to the parenteral administration of large fluid volumes.

Controversy exists about whether it is better to administer crystalloids or colloids in patients with septic shock.[53] Isotonic crystalloids, such as 0.9% NaCl (normal saline) or lactated Ringer's solution, distribute into interstitial and intravascular spaces. These fluids do effectively restore volume loss and are less expensive than colloid products. Approximately 25% of the infused volume of crystalloid remains in the intravascular space, while the balance distributes to extravascular spaces. While this expansion of the extravascular space is considered beneficial because it aids vascular capacitance, overexpansion can result in excessive edema and compromised gas exchange in the lungs and peripheral tissues. An increased incidence of transitory pulmonary edema has been demonstrated with crystalloid volume expansion compared with volume expansion using colloid products, but it is not clear if there are significant long-term sequelae. Iso-oncotic colloid solutions (5% albumin, plasma protein fractions, and 6% hetastarch) offer the advantage of more rapid restoration of intravascular volume with less volume infused. The use of colloid solutions and blood products may be particularly important if there is significant blood loss associated with sepsis or if the patient had severe preexisting anemia.[52] Drawbacks to the routine use of colloid solutions are the lack of significant expansion of the interstitial space and the very high cost associated with these products. Another disadvantage to the use of colloids during the acute phases of systemic inflammation associated with sepsis is the leakage of oncotically active particles into the interstitial space and the possibility of prolonging tissue edema.

The patient's response to fluid therapy should be frequently monitored by evaluation of the heart rate and blood pressure, as well as clinical parameters, such as urinary output and mental status. Invasive hemodynamic monitoring is often indicated to assess adequately cardiac index (CI), central venous pressure (CVP), and pulmonary artery wedge pressure (PAWP). Maintenance of the PAWP in a range of 15 to 18 mm Hg should provide sufficient left ventricular filling pressure without excessive risk of developing pulmonary edema.[35] The measurement of serum lactate can provide an excellent assessment of tissue perfusion. An increased serum lactate indicates inadequate tissue perfusion, resulting in cellular anaerobic metabolism and lactate production.

INOTROPE AND VASOACTIVE DRUG SUPPORT

Vasopressor and inotropic therapy are indicated when fluid resuscitation is insufficient to maintain tissue perfusion.[35,54] Common agents to consider include dopamine, dobutamine, norepinephrine, phenylephrine, and epinephrine, and the comparative receptor activities of these drugs are summarized in Table 109–4.[55] Dopamine, an α- and β-adrenergic agent with dopaminergic activity, is often the initial choice in sepsis because of combined vasopressor and inotropic effects. Although low-dose dopamine (1 to 5 μg/kg/min) may maintain renal perfusion, higher doses (10 to 20 μg/kg/min) are frequently required to support blood pressure in septic patients. Doses as high as 50 μg/kg/min have been employed in patients with severe circulatory collapse, but they are generally unnecessary.

Dobutamine is a β-adrenergic inotropic agent considered by many clinicians to be the preferred drug for improvement of cardiac output and oxygen delivery, particularly in early sepsis before significant peripheral vasodilation has occurred. When used, dobutamine is infused in dosages of 2 to 20 μg/kg/min to achieve a target CI above 2.4 $L/min/m^2$.

Norepinephrine, a potent α-adrenergic agent with some β-adrenergic activity, can be useful in septic shock when the clinician desires potent vasoconstriction of peripheral vascular beds. Dosages of 2 to 100 μg/min are usually effective, but the dose can be titrated higher in order to achieve a systolic blood pressure of > 90 mm Hg. Low-dose dopamine is often used at 3 to 5 μg/kg/min. concurrently with norephinephrine to maintain renal perfusion.[56]

Phenylephrine, a selective α_1-agonist administered in doses of 20 to 200 μg/min, may be useful in some patients, with refractory hypotension, but reported experience in septic shock is limited. Epinephrine, a nonspecific α- and β-drenergic agonist capable of increasing CI and producing significant peripheral vasoconstriction in doses of 0.04 to 1 μg/kg/min, can be used when other vasoactive agents fail to produce the desired response.

The nonadrenergic inotropic agent, amrinone, may be tried in a dose of 5 to 10 μg/kg/min if severe myocardial failure appears resistant to the adrenergic agents.

The following suggestions are offered as a reasonable approach to the selection of vasopressor and inotropic therapy in sepsis and septic shock. In a septic patient without marked hypotension, dobutamine (an inotrope without significant peripheral vascular effects) can be used. The goal is to maintain systolic

TABLE 109–4. Receptor Activity of Cardiovascular Agents Commonly Used in Septic Shock

Agent	α_1	α_2	β_1	β_2	Dopaminergic
Dopamine	++/+++	?	++++	++	++++
Dobutamine	+	+	++++	++	0
Epinephrine	++++	++++	++++	+++	0
Norepinephrine	+++	+++	+++	+/++	0
Phenylephrine	++/+++	+	?	0	0

α_1 = α_1-adrenergic receptor; α_2 = α_2-adrenergic receptor; β_1 = β_1-adrenergic receptor; β_2 = β_2-adrenergic receptor; 0 = no activity; ++++ = maximal activity; ? = unknown activity.

From Ref. 55.

blood pressure above 90 mm Hg by supporting cardiac output. This strategy often is successful and reduces the possibility of impaired organ perfusion through pharmacologic peripheral vasoconstrictive effects. Alternatively, dopamine in moderate doses (5 to 10 μg/kg/min) can also be used as an initial agent because of its selective effect on increasing cardiac output with its minimal effect on the systemic vascular resistance. For the septic patient with significant hypotension (mean arterial pressure [MAP] < 60 mm Hg) and a low systemic vascular resistance index (SVRI) (< 500 dynes/cm^5/m^2) that are unresponsive to fluids and inotropic agents, an agent with α-adrenergic activity should be used, such as dopamine in doses of 10 to 20 μg/kg/min. If dopamine does not produce the desired hemodynamic response, norepinephrine, often combined with low-dose dopamine, can be tried. The α-agonist phenylephrine can be employed either with other agents or as single-agent therapy when the SVR is markedly decreased and unresponsive to other medications.

PULMONARY SUPPORT

Hypoxia is common in septic patients, even those without pulmonary infection.[32] The acute lung injury associated with sepsis is related to the generalized systemic inflammatory state with activation and subsequent sequestration of neutrophils in the pulmonary microvasculature leading to progressive endothelial injury.[34] This leads to leakage of fluid into the interstitial space. As the septic patient is supported with aggressive fluid therapy, fluid accumulation in these tissues increases further, producing a significant ventilation–perfusion mismatch and progressive hypoxia. Oxygen therapy is indicated to maintain oxygen saturation greater than 90%, and with progressive pulmonary insufficiency, the patient may require assisted ventilation. In up to 40% of cases of severe sepsis, particularly with gram-negative infections, the patient will develop ARDS, mainfested by severe hypoxia, pulmonary edema, vascular congestion, increased extravascular lung water, decreased lung compliance, and diffuse pulmonary infiltrates on chest radiograph.[57] Acute respiratory distress syndrome can be determined by a ratio of Po_2 to the fraction of inspired oxygen (Fio_2) < 200 with diffuse pulmonary infiltrates evident on chest radiograph and absence of left ventricular failure (PAWP < 18 mm Hg). The management of patients with ARDS is primarily supportive. Uncontrolled reports suggest that IV methylprednisolone, in doses of 75 mg to 250 mg q 6 hours, may improve survival in severely ill patients with refractory late ARDS.[58,59] Other agents have been evaluated as interventions in ARDS, including exogenous surfactant, acetylcysteine, and cyclo-oxygenase inhibitors, but none consistently improves outcome.[24,35,54]

The imidazole antifungal ketoconazole reduced the progression to ARDS and increased survival in a small study of septic surgical patients, possibly because of its inhibitory effects on alveolar macrophage production of leukotriene B_4 and thromboxane A_2.[60] Nitric oxide (NO), an endogenous vasodilator also known as endothelium-derived relaxing factor, is under investigation for use in ARDS.[61,62] Nitric oxide is believed to protect endothelial cells from injury induced by free radicals released from activated neutrophils. Early work with inhaled administration of NO in patients with ARDS suggest improved arterial oxygenation and reduced pulmonary artery pressures.[63] Additional work is needed to define any role for these agents in the management of sepsis.

OTHER SUPPORTIVE THERAPIES

The corticosteroids have been the subject of much controversy in the management of septic patients. Because of their suppressive effect on the activation of polymorphonuclear leukocytes, complement activation, release of TNF, and the activation of the coagulation system, the administration of corticosteroids would appear potentially useful in altering the progressive cascades of sepsis. The counterpoint is that the inhibitory effects of corticosteroids on the host immune system will inhibit resolution of the infectious process and be detrimental to patient outcome. Two meta-analyses of this issue concluded that there is no evidence to support the use of corticosteroids in patients with sepsis or septic shock.[64,65]

The use of heparin in patients with DIC has been suggested based on the understanding that DIC represents a hypercoagulable condition. While heparin has been shown to control this coagulopathy, there is no evidence that heparin prolongs the survival of patients who experience DIC. Heparin therapy for DIC is discouraged by most clinicians.[66] Hemorrhage is best managed by the replacement of clotting factors, platelets, and packed red blood cells.

The nutritional needs of the septic patient must also be addressed. Sepsis is a hypermetabolic state characterized by alterations in carbohydrate, lipid, and protein metabolism.[67] Nonprotein caloric requirements range from 25 to 40 kcal/kg/d, and overfeeding of carbohydrates should be avoided to reduce the ventilatory requirements of the patient. Hyperglycemia associated with insulin-resistance is common, and management of elevated serum glucose may not be satisfactory with insulin therapy alone. The use of increased amounts of lipid to meet nonprotein caloric needs while reducing carbohydrate administration may be useful in this setting. Protein requirements are increased to 1.5 to 2.5 g/kg/d, and there is some evidence that administration of increased amounts of branched-chain amino acids may be beneficial in septic patients.[68] Whenever possible, enteral feeding is preferred over parenteral nutritional support.

Animal models of sepsis indicate that β-endorphins are released in response to the stress of sepsis. These endogenous opiates are thought to contribute to myocardial depression and progressive hypotension. Naloxone, an antagonist to opiates and the β-endorphins, has been shown to support systolic blood pressure in septic animals. Results of human trials have been inconsistent. In light of the fact that there are no data to indicate a survival benefit or that the hemodynamic benefit is prolonged, the use of naloxone is not recommended.[54] Additionally, should naloxone be used, it would interfere with the use of narcotic analgesics that may be indicated for pain relief in many patients.

IMMUNOTHERAPY

Evaluation of immunologic interventions for sepsis has been one of the most active areas of clinical investigation over the past decade. A wide variety of strategies have been used to reverse or control the inflammatory process initiated with sepsis, including antibody against lipopolysaccharide (endotoxin), IL-1 receptor antagonist, PAF antagonist, anti-TNF-α antibody, and polyclonal immunoglobulin.[69–71] One of the first interventions to gain attention was direct inhibition of the effects of endotoxin with specific monoclonal antibodies. Recognition of the major role that endotoxin plays in the inflammatory progression of gram-negative sepsis and the similarity of lipid A among gram-negative bacterial species supported the search for specific therapeutic modalities directed at lipid A. Studies conducted with monoclonal antibodies (E5, HA-1A) that bind to the lipid A portion of the endotoxin molecule have failed to demonstrate beneficial effects when administered to patients with clinical evidence of sepsis when treated, suggesting that the window of time to reduce the initiation of the sepsis cascades because of endotoxin had passed by the time treatment was initiated.

Additional approaches include inhibition of inflammatory cytokines by antibodies that bind the cytokines, competitive inhibitors of cytokine receptor binding, or soluble receptors that interact with the cytokine but do not lead to activation of target cells. An example is the use of antibodies that bind to TNF-α. Administration of anti-inflammatory cytokines, such as IL-4, IL-10, proinflammatory cytokines, such as interferon-γ, and use of pentoxiphylline, known to reduce cytokine production and release from leukocytes, are under investigation.[11,69,72] While the hope and enthusiasm that ushered in clinical investigations of immunotherapeutic interventions for sepsis were based on the sound understanding of the pathophysiology involved, overall results of these evaluations have been disappointing. Nevertheless, this work has led to an increased appreciation and knowledge of the systemic complexity of sepsis and septic shock that will hopefully lead to successful therapeutic interventions in the future.

▶ PRINCIPLES OF PHARMACOTHERAPY

- The etiologies of sepsis and septic shock include not only gram-negative bacterial pathogens, but also increasingly common are gram-positive bacterial and fungal pathogens.
- Sepsis represents a complex pathophysiology, resulting from important interactions between the pathogen and host, progressing to a systemic inflammatory state mediated by disregulation of proinflammatory and anti-inflammatory mediators.
- Timely diagnosis and identification of the pathogen is critical to successful management of the septic patient.
- If possible, treatment of sepsis should begin with the removal or drainage of any source of infection.
- Prompt, aggressive initiation of broad-spectrum, parenteral antibiotic therapy is required. Antibiotic selection should be based on clinical presentation, site of infection, and suspected pathogens.
- Significant fluid leaks from the vasculature occur with sepsis, and administration of large volumes of fluid are required. Crystalloid solutions, such as normal saline, are generally recommended.
- Hemodynamic support using inotropic agents and vasopressors should be initiated in patients who cannot maintain acceptable blood pressure with aggressive fluid therapy alone.
- Supplemental oxygen and assisted ventilatory support may be required in many patients with progressive sepsis and acute respiratory distress syndrome.
- Patients with sepsis are usually hypermetabolic and may require up to 40 kcal/kg/d of nonprotein calories and 2 g/kg/d of protein to support their nutritional needs.
- The role of immunotherapy in sepsis is not defined, and such interventions remain investigational.

REFERENCES

1. Centers for Disease Control and Prevention. Increase in national hospital discharge survey cases for septicemia—United States, 1979–1987. MMWR 1990;39:31–34.
2. Centers for Disease Control and Prevention, National Center for Health Statistics. Mortality patterns—United States, 1990. Mo Vital Stat Report 1993;41:5.
3. Parillo JE, Parker MM, Natanson C. Septic shock in humans: Advances in the understanding of pathogenesis, cardiovascular dysfunction, and therapy: NIH conference report. Ann Intern Med 1990;113:227–242.
4. Bone RC. The sepsis syndrome: Definition and general approach to management. Clin Chest Med 1996;17:175–181.
5. American College of Chest Physicians/Society of Critical Care Medicine Consensus Conference. Definitions for sepsis and organ failure and guidelines for the use of innovative therapies in sepsis. Crit Care Med 1992;20:864–874.
6. Rangel-Frausto MS, Pittet D, Costigan M, et al. The natural history of systemic inflammatory response syndrome (SIRS): A prospective study. JAMA 1995;273:117–123.
7. Bone RC. Sir Isaac Newton, sepsis, SIRS, and CARS. Crit Care Med 1996;24:1125–1128.
8. Vincent JL. Dear SIRS, I'm sorry to say that I don't like you. . . . Crit Care Med 1997;25:372–374.
9. Bone RC. Immunologic dissonance: A continuing evolution in our understanding of the systemic inflammatory response syndrome (SIRS) and the multiple organ dysfunction syndrome (MODS). Ann Intern Med 1996;125:680–687.
10. Bone RC. Toward a theory regarding the pathogenesis of the systemic inflammatory response syndrome: What we do and do not know about cytokine regulation. Crit Care Med 1996;24:163–172.
11. Young LS. Sepsis syndrome. In: Mandell GL, Bennett JE, Dolin R, eds. Principles and Practice of Infectious Diseases, 4th ed. New York, Churchhill Livingstone, 1995;690–704.
12. Bone RC. The pathogenesis of sepsis. Ann Intern Med 1991;115:457–469.
13. Wenzel RP, Pinsky MR, Ulevitch RJ, Young Y. Current understanding of sepsis. Clin Infect Dis 1996;22:407–413.
14. Hack CE, Hart M, Strack RJM, et al. Interleukin-8 in sepsis: Relation to shock and inflammatory mediators. Infect Immun 1992;60:2835–2842.
15. Parillo JE. Pathogenic mechanisms of septic shock. N Engl J Med 1993;328:1471–1477.
16. Damas P, Canivet J, De Groote D, et al. Sepsis and serum cytokine concentrations. Crit Care Med 1997;25:405–412.
17. Damas P, Ledoux D, Nys M, et al. Cytokine serum level during sepsis in human IL-6 as a marker of severity. Ann Surg 1992;215:356–362.
18. Damas P, Reuter A, Gysen P, et al. Tumor necrosis factor and interleukin-1 serum levels during severe sepsis in humans. Crit Care Med 1989;17:975–978.
19. Casey LC, Balk RA, Bone RC. Plasma cytokine and endotoxin levels correlate with survival in patients with sepsis syndrome. Ann Intern Med 1993;119:771–778.
20. Steinmetz HT, Herbertz A, Bertram M, Diehl V. Increase in interleukin-6 serum level preceding fever in granulocytopenia and correlation with death from sepsis. J Infect Dis 1995;171:225–228.
21. Calandra T, Gerain J, Heumann D, et al. High circulating levels of interleukin-6 in patients with septic shock: Evolution during sepsis, prognostic value, and interplay with other cytokines. Am J Med 1991;91:23–29.
22. Marty C, Misset B, Tamion F, et al. Circulating interleukin-8 concentrations in patients with multiple organ failure of septic and nonseptic origin. Crit Care Med 1994;22:673–679.

23. Guidet B, Barakett V, Vassal T, et al. Endotoxemia and bacteremia in patients with sepsis syndrome in the intensive care unit. Chest 1994; 106:1194–1201.
24. Saez-Llorens X, McCracken GH. Sepsis syndrome and septic shock in pediatrics: Current concepts of terminology, pathophysiology, and management. J Pediatr 1993;123:497–508.
25. Kollef MH, Schuster DP. The acute respiratory distress syndrome. N Engl J Med 1995;332:27–37.
26. Sessler CN, Bloomfield GL, Fowler AA. Current concepts of sepsis and acute lung injury. Clin Chest Med 1996;17:213–235.
27. Bernard GR, Artgas A, Brigham KL, et al. The American–European Consensus Conference on ARDS: Definitions, mechanisms, relevant outcomes and clinical coordination. Am J Resp Crit Care Med 1994; 149:818–824.
28. Martin MA, Silverman HJ. Gram-negative sepsis and the adult respiratory distress syndrome. Clin Infect Dis 1992;14:1213–1228.
29. Waisbren BA. Bacteremia due to gram-negative bacilli other than *Salmonella*. Arch Intern Med 1951;88:467–488.
30. Bunnell E, Parrillo JE. Cardiac dysfunction during septic shock. Clin Chest Med 1996;17:237–248.
31. Suffredini AF, Fromm RE, Parker MM, et al. The cardiovascular response of normal humans to the administration of endotoxin. N Engl J Med 1990;321:280–287.
32. Chittock DR, Russell JA. Oxygen delivery and consumption during sepsis. Clin Chest Med 1996;17:263–278.
33. Conboy K, Welage LS, Walawander MA, et al. Sepsis syndrome associated sequelae in patients at high risk for gram-negative sepsis. Pharmacother 1995;15:66–77.
34. Parillo JE, Parker MM, Natanson C. Septic shock in humans: Advances in the understanding of pathogenesis, cardiovascular dysfunction, and therapy: NIH conference report. Ann Intern Med 1991;113: 227–242.
35. Wiessner WH, Casey LC, Zbilut JP. Treatment of sepsis and septic shock: A review. Heart Lung 1995;24:380–392.
36. Anderson MR, Blumer JL. Advances in the therapy for sepsis in children. Ped Clin North Am 1997;44:179–205.
37. Thadepalli H, Reddy U, Chuah SK, et. al. *In vivo* efficacy of trovafloxacin (CP-99,217), a new quinolone, in experimental intra-abdominal abscesses caused by *Bacteroides fragilis* and *Escherichia coli.* Antimicrob Agents Chemother 1997;41:583–586.
38. Nicolau DP, Freeman CD, Belliveau PP, et al. Experience with a once-daily aminoglycoside program administered to 2,184 adult patients. Antimicrob Agents Chemother 1995;39:650–655.
39. Preston SL, Briceland LL. Single daily dosing of aminoglycosides. Pharmacother 1995;15:297–316.
40. Hatala R, Dinh T, Cook DJ. Once-daily aminoglycoside dosing in immunocompetent adults: A meta-analysis. Ann Intern Med 1996;124: 717–725.
41. Hatala R, Dinh T, Cook DJ. Single daily dosing of aminoglycosides in immunocompromised adults: A systemic review. Clin Infect Dis 1997; 24:810–815.
42. Gilbert DN. Once daily dosing of aminoglycoside therapy. Antimicrob Agents Chemother 1991;35:339–405.
43. Bertino JS, Rotschafer JC. Single daily dosing of aminoglycosides—A concept whose time has not yet come. Clin Infect Dis 1997;24: 820– 823. Editorial response.
44. Fry DE. The importance of antibiotic pharmacokinetics in critical illness. Am J Surg 1996;172(suppl 6A):20S–25S.
45. Moore RD, Lietman PS, Smith CR. The association of aminoglycoside plasma levels with mortality in patients with gram-negative bacteremia. J Infect Dis 1984;149:443–448.
46. Moore RD, Lietman PS, Smith CR. Clinical response to aminoglycoside therapy: Importance of the ratio of peak concentration to minimum inhibitory concentration. J Infect Dis 1987;155:93–97.
47. Bailey TC, Little JR, Littenberg B, et al. A meta-analysis of extended-interval dosing versus multiple daily dosing of aminoglycosides. Clin Infect Dis 1997;24:786–795.
48. Sarosi GA, Davies SF. Therapy for fungal infections. Mayo Clin Proc 1994;69:1111–1117.
49. Goodwin SD, Cleary JD, Walawander CA, et al. Pretreatment regimens for adverse events related to infusion of amphotericin B. Clin Infect Dis 1995;20:755–761.
50. Hiemenz JW, Walsh TJ. Lipid formulations of amphotericin B: Recent progress and future directions. Clin Infect Dis 1996;22(suppl 2): S166–S178.
51. Edwards JE, Bodey GP, Bowden RA, et al. International conference for the development of a consensus on the management and prevention of severe candidal infections. Clin Infect Dis 1997;25:43–59.
52. Ognibene FP. Hemodynamic support during sepsis. Clin Chest Med 1996;17:279–287.
53. Weil MH, Rockow EE. A guide to volume repletion. Emerg Med 1984;16:101.
54. Weikert LF, Bernard GR. Pharmacotherapy of sepsis. Clin Chest Med 1996;17:289–305.
55. Rudis MI, Basha MA, Zarowitz BJ. Is it time to reposition vasopressors and inotropes in sepsis? Crit Care Med 1996;24:525–537.
56. Schaer GL, Fink MP, Parilto JE. Norepinephrine alone versus norepinephrine plus low-dose dopamine: Enhanced renal blood flow with combination pressor therapy. Crit Care Med 1985;13:492–496.
57. Kollef MH, Shuster DP. The acute respiratory distress syndrome. N Engl J Med 1995;332:27–37.
58. Hooper RG, Kearl RA. Established adult respiratory distress syndrome successfully treated with corticosteroids. South Med J 1996;89: 449–451.
59. Biffl WL, Moore FA, Moore EE, et al. Are corticosteroids salvage therapy for refractory acute respiratory distress syndrome? Am J Surg 1995;170:591–596.
60. Yu M, Tomasa G. A double-blind, prospective, randomized trial for ketoconazole, a thromboxane synthetase inhibitor, in the prophylaxis of the adult respiratory distress syndrome. Crit Care Med 1993;21: 1635–1642.
61. Payen D, Bernard C, Beloucif S. Nitric oxide in sepsis. Clin Chest Med 1996;17:333–350.
62. Fink MP, Payen D. The role of nitric oxide in sepsis and ARDS: Synopsis of a roundtable conference held in Brussels on 18–20 March 1995. Inten Care Med 1996;22:158–165.
63. Rossaint R, Falke KJ, Lopez F, et al. Inhaled nitric oxide for the adult respiratory distress syndrome. N Engl J Med 1993;328:339–405.
64. Cronin L, Cook DJ, Carlet J, et al. Corticosteroid treatment for sepsis: A critical appraisal and meta-analysis of the literature. Crit Care Med 1995;23:1430–1439.
65. Lefering R, Neugebauer AEM. Steroid controversy in sepsis and septic shock: A meta-analysis. Crit Care Med 1995;23:1294–1303.
66. Staudinger T, Locker GJ, Frass M. Management of acquired coagulation disorders in emergency and intensive-care medicine. Sem Thromb Hemostasis 1996;22:93–104.
67. Page CP, Hardin TC, Melnik G. Nutritional assessment and support: A primer, 2nd ed. Baltimore, Williams & Wilkins, 1994.
68. Garcia-de-Lorenzo A, Ortiz-Leyba C, Planas M, et al. Parenteral administration of different amounts of branch-chain amino acids in septic patients: Clinical and metabolic aspects. Crit Care Med 1997;25: 418–424.
69. Ralston DR, St. John RC. Immunotherapy for sepsis. Clin Chest Med 1996;17:307–317.
70. Schedel I, Dreikhkausen U, Nentwig B, et al. Treatment of gram-negative septic shock with an immunoglobulin preparation: A prospective, randomized clinical trial. Crit Care Med 1991;19:1104–1113.
71. Bone RC, Balk RA, Fein AM, et al. A second large controlled clinical study of E5, a monoclonal antibody to endotoxin: Results of a prospective, multicenter, randomized, controlled trial. Crit Care Med 1995;23:994–1006.
72. Doche WD, Randow F, Syrbe U, et al. Monocyte deactivation in septic patients: Restoration by IFN-γ reatment. Nature Med 1997;3: 678–681.

110

INVASIVE FUNGAL INFECTIONS

Peggy L. Carver, PharmD

For many years, fungal infections were classified as either superficial "nuisance diseases," such as athlete's foot or vulvovaginal candidiasis, or as relatively rare infections confined primarily to endemic areas of the country. When invasive fungal infections were encountered, amphotericin B was the only consistently effective, systemically active agent available for the treatment of systemic mycoses. Advances in medical technology, including organ and bone marrow transplantation, cytotoxic chemotherapy, the widespread use of indwelling intravenous (IV) catheters, and the increased use of potent, broad-spectrum antimicrobial agents have all contributed to the dramatic increase in the incidence of fungal infections worldwide. Fungal infections have emerged as a major cause of death among cancer patients and transplant recipients.[1] In addition, patients with acquired immunodeficiency syndrome (AIDS) experience substantially more frequent and severe forms of cryptococcosis, histoplasmosis, coccidioidomycosis, and mucocutaneous (esophageal, oral, and vulvovaginal) candidiasis.[1–3]

Problems remain in the diagnosis, prevention, and treatment of fungal infections. Unlike the available diagnostic techniques for most bacterial pathogens, there remains a host of unresolved issues regarding standardization of susceptibility testing methods, *in vitro* and *in vivo* models of infection, the utility of monitoring antifungal plasma concentrations, and the development and identification of resistant pathogens.[4–6]

MYCOLOGY

Fungi are eucaryotic organisms with a defined nucleus enclosed by a nuclear membrane; a cytoplasmic membrane containing lipids, glycoproteins and sterols, mitochondria, Golgi apparatus, ribosomes bound to endoplasmic reticulum; and a cytoskeleton with microtubules, microfilaments, and intermediate filaments. Fungi have rigid cell walls composed of chitin, cellulose, or both, that stain with Gomori methenamine silver or periodic acid-Schiff reagent. Most fungi, except *Candida,* are too weakly gram-positive to be seen well on Gram's stain. *Cryptococcus neoformans* has a polysaccharide capsule surrounding the cell wall.[7]

Morphologically, pathogenic fungi can be grouped as either filamentous molds or unicellular yeasts. *Molds* grow as multicellular branching, thread-like filaments (hyphae) that are either septate (divided by transverse walls) or coenocytic (multinucleate without cross walls) (Fig. 110–1). On agar media, molds grow outward from the point of inoculation by extension of the tips of filaments, and then branch repeatedly, interweaving to form fuzzy, matted growths called *mycelium. Yeasts* are oval or spherically shaped unicellular forms that generally produce pasty or mucoid colonies on agar media, similar to those observed with bacterial cultures. Yeasts have rigid cell walls that reproduce by budding, a process in which daughter cells arise from pinching off a portion of the parent cell.

Fungi reproduce by forming spores asexually via mitosis to produce motile sporangiospores or nonmotile conidia (singular, conidium), or they reproduce sexually through meiosis to produce ascospores, basidiospores, oospores, or zygospores. Although terms such as *spore* and *conidia* should no longer be used interchangeably, some newer literature and much of the older medical literature continue to confuse these terms.

In the past, clinical identification and naming of fungi was based on observations of the fruiting structures (often the asexual form) associated with the development of conidia. In more recent years, complete life cycles of many clinically relevant fungi have been elucidated, and additional names have been added to describe their sexual forms. Many microbiology laboratories and clinicians, however, continue to use the older names assigned to the asexual forms since most fungi isolated in the clinical laboratory are found in the asexual form, and the human diseases resulting from the pathogen are often based on this name. For example, *Blastomyces dermatitidis,* the etiologic agent of human blastomycosis, was named in 1898 based on its asexual (conidial) characteristics. In 1968, the life cycle of the fungus was found to include a meiotic stage that produces ascospores. A new name, *Ajellomyces dermatitidis,* was chosen to describe the sexual (ascomycetous) form; however, since the form isolated in clinical microbiology laboratories is *B. dermatitidis,* this name is retained for clinical use.

Many pathogenic fungi, termed *dimorphic fungi,* exist as either a yeast or a mold, depending on pathogen, site of growth (in the host or in the laboratory setting), and temperature. Usually, yeasts are the parasitic form that invade human or animal host tissue, while molds are the free-living form found in the environment. For example, *Histoplasma capsulatum* exists as a yeast in humans and as a mold in the laboratory.[7,8]

SUSCEPTIBILITY TESTING OF ANTIFUNGAL AGENTS

Most laboratories do not routinely perform susceptibility tests on fungal isolates, but standardized methods for performing these tests are being developed.[5,9]

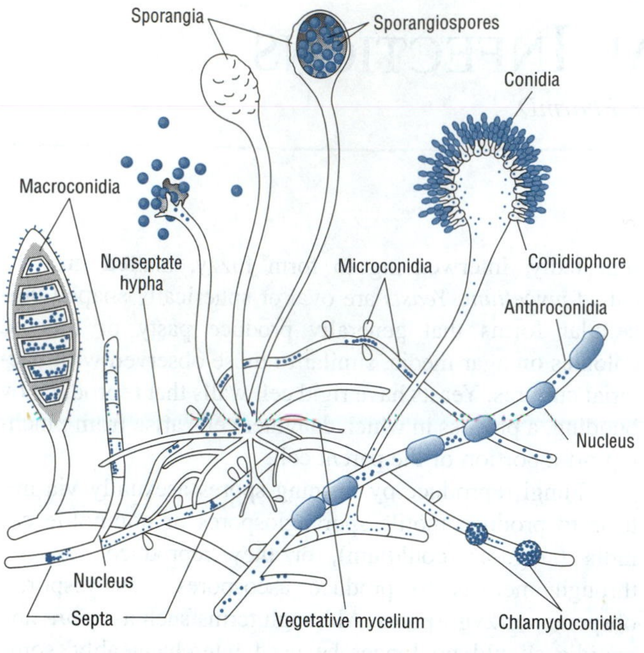

FIGURE 110–1. Forms of molds. The tube-like hyphae form their basic structure. Examples of spores and conidia and of the structures that bear them are shown. *(From Ref. 73, with permission.)*

PLASMA CONCENTRATION MONITORING OF ANTIFUNGAL AGENTS

Routine monitoring of plasma concentrations of antifungal agents to assess efficacy or toxicity of these agents is generally not available. Correlations between plasma concentrations of antifungal agents and therapeutic outcomes have been poorly studied. Data demonstrating the emergence of azole-resistant *Candida albicans* in HIV-infected patients and the decreased bioavailability of ketoconazole and itraconazole in selected patient populations have, however, prompted new studies addressing these issues.[5,10]

PATHOGENESIS AND EPIDEMIOLOGY

Systemic mycoses caused by primary or pathogenic fungi include histoplasmosis, coccidioidomycosis, cryptococcosis, blastomycosis, paracoccidioidomycosis, and sporotrichosis. Primary pathogens can cause disease in both healthy and immunocompromised individuals, although disease is generally more severe or disseminated in the immunocompromised host. In contrast, mycoses caused by opportunistic fungi, such as *C. albicans, Aspergillus* sp., *Trichosporon, Torulopsis (Candida) glabrata, Fusarium, Alternaria,* and *Mucor,* are generally found only in the immunocompromised host.[7]

Most fungal infections are acquired as a result of accidental inhalation of airborne conidia. For example, *H. capsulatum* is found in soil contaminated by bat, chicken, or starling excreta, and *C. neoformans* is associated with pigeon droppings. Although some fungi, including *C. albicans, C. neoformans,* and *Aspergillus* sp., are ubiquitous pathogens with worldwide distribution, other fungi have regional distributions associated with specific geographical environments.[7]

Systemic fungal infections are a major cause of morbidity and mortality in the immunocompromised patient.[7] Fungal infections account for 20% to 30% of fatal infections in patients with acute leukemia, 10% to 15% of fatal infections in patients with lymphoma, and 5% of fatal infections in patients with solid tumors. The frequency of fungal infections among transplant recipients ranges from 0% to 20% for kidney and bone marrow transplant recipients to 10% to 35% for heart and 30% to 40% for liver transplant recipients.

Approximately 2% to 4% of all hospitalized patients develop a nosocomial infection. Of these, bacteria comprise the most common etiologic agent.[7] Fungi, however, are becoming increasingly significant nosocomial pathogens. Although only limited data exist documenting the incidence and prevalence of nosocomial fungal infections, the Centers for Disease Control (CDC) reported via its National Nosocomial Infections System (NNIS) that in 1990, fungi accounted for 9.9% of all bloodstream isolates. *Candida* sp. (primarily *C. albicans*) accounted for 78.3% of all nosocomial fungal infections.[8,11,12]

Nosocomially acquired fungal infections may arise from either exogenous or endogenous flora. Endogenous flora may include normal commensals of the skin, gastrointestinal (GI), genitourinary, or respiratory tract. *Candida albicans* is found as a normal commensal of the gastrointestinal tract in 20% to 30% of humans.[8,13]

A complex interplay of host and pathogen factors influences the acquisition and development of fungal infections. Intact skin or mucosal surfaces serve as primary barriers to infection. Desiccation, epithelial cell turnover, fatty acid content, and low pH of the skin are believed to be important factors in host resistance. Bacterial flora of the skin and mucous membranes compete with fungi for growth. Alterations in the balance of normal flora caused by the use of antibiotics or alterations in nutritional status can allow the proliferation of fungi, such as *Candida,* increasing the likelihood of systemic invasion and infection.[7]

The growth of fungi within tissues is restrained by a number of mechanisms. For example, serum has fungistatic activity against *Candida* in part because of transferrins, the human iron-binding proteins, that deprive microbes of the iron needed for synthesis of respiratory enzymes. Serum also contains globulins, which cause a nonimmunologic clumping of *Candida,* facilitating their elimination by inflammatory cells.[7,8]

Tissue reaction in the presence of fungi varies with fungal species, site of proliferation, and duration of infection. Phagocytosis by neutrophils and macrophages is the earliest mechanism that prevents the establishment of fungi. Consequently, patients with decreased neutrophil counts or decreased neutrophil function are at higher risk of infections, particularly those caused by *Candida* and *Aspergillus.*

Some mycoses are characterized by a low-grade inflammatory response that does not eliminate the fungi. Fungal cells can sometimes persist within macrophages without being killed, perhaps because of resistance to the effects of lysosomal enzymes.[7]

DIAGNOSIS

The diagnosis of invasive fungal infections is generally accomplished by careful evaluation of clinical symptoms, results of serologic tests, and histopathologic examination and culture of clinical specimens. Skin tests are generally not useful diagnostically because they do not distinguish between active and past infection. They remain useful as screening tools and in epidemiologic studies to determine endemic areas. It is beyond the scope of this chapter to discuss the relative merits of each of the immunologic tests used in the diagnosis of invasive fungal infections. Interested readers are, however, referred to several excellent reviews concerning this topic.[6,14,15]

▶ TREATMENT: Invasive Mycoses

Strategies for the prevention of invasive mycoses can be broadly classified as prophylaxis, early empirical therapy, empirical therapy, and secondary prophylaxis or suppression.[16] In patients undergoing cytotoxic chemotherapy, antifungal therapy is directed primarily at the prevention or treatment of infections caused by *Candida* and *Aspergillus*.

Prophylactic therapy with topical, oral, or IV antifungal agents is administered prior to and throughout the period of granulocytopenia (absolute neutrophil count < 1000/ L). The potential benefits of prophylactic therapy must be weighed against the potential risks inherent in each regimen. Perfect[17] has suggested that each clinician consider at least six criteria before justifying antifungal prophylaxis: (1) safety, (2) efficacy, (3) cost, (4) consequence, (5) prevalence, and (6) resistance.

Early empirical therapy is the administration of systemic antifungal agents at the onset of fever and neutropenia.

Empirical therapy with systemic antifungal agents is administered to granulocytopenic patients with persistent or recurrent fever despite the administration of appropriate antimicrobial therapy.

Secondary prophylaxis (or suppressive therapy) refers to administration of systemic antifungal agents (generally prior to and throughout the period of granulocytopenia) to prevent relapse of a documented invasive fungal infection that was treated during a previous episode of granulocytopenia. Although these treatment classifications have also been applied to the treatment of fungal infections in AIDS, patients with AIDS rarely acquire systemic infections caused by *Candida* or *Aspergillus* sp. unless they become granulocytopenic because of disease or drugs. The use of antifungal prophylaxis is much less widely studied in this population, although studies have suggested that early antifungal prophylaxis may decrease the incidence of invasive cryptococcal disease. Suppressive therapy is generally necessary following acute therapy for histoplasmosis, coccidioidomycosis, and cryptococcosis because of the high rates of relapse when antifungal therapy is discontinued.

PROPHYLAXIS OF HUMAN IMMUNODEFICIENCY VIRUS-INFECTED PATIENT

Fluconazole has been shown to prevent cryptococcosis and local *Candida* infections, including esophagitis, but overall mortality was not improved.[18] Because of the high costs of long-term prophylaxis, improved therapeutic regimens available for treating cryptococcal meningitis, and increasing reports of fluconazole resistance among *Candida* isolates from AIDS patients, many clinicians prefer not to use fluconazole prophylaxis in AIDS patients. For some patients with very low CD4 counts, however, some clinicians feel it is cost-effective to use fluconazole prophylaxis to prevent cryptococcosis.[18,19]

HISTOPLASMOSIS

In humans, histoplasmosis is caused by inhalation of dust-borne microconidia of the dimorphic fungus *Histoplasma capsulatum.* Although there exist two dimorphic varieties of *H. capsulatum,* the small-celled (2 to 5 m) form (var. *capsulatum*) occurs globally, while the large-celled (8 to 15 m) form (var. *duboisii*) is confined to the African continent and Madagascar. *Histoplasma capsulatum* was originally named on the basis of intrahistiocytic plasmodia-like organisms recovered from tissues; however, the pseudoencapsulated appearance proved to be an artifact caused by cytoplasmic shrinkage from the rigid cell wall during tissue fixation. In tissues stained by conventional techniques, *H. capsulatum* appears as an oval or round, narrow-pore, budding, unencapsulated yeast.[3,20]

EPIDEMIOLOGY

Although histoplasmosis is found worldwide, certain areas of North and Latin America are recognized as endemic areas; in the United States, most disease is localized along the Ohio and Mississippi river valleys, where > 90% of residents may be affected. *Histoplasma capsulatum* is found in nitrogen-enriched soils, particularly those heavily contaminated by avian or bat guano, that accelerate sporulation. Blackbird or pigeon roosts, chicken coops, and sites frequented by bats, such as caves, attics, or old buildings, serve as "microfoci" of infections. Although birds are not infected because of their high body temperature, bats (mammals) may be infected and pass yeast forms in their feces, allowing the spread of *H. capsulatum* to new habitats.[3,20]

PATHOPHYSIOLOGY

At ambient temperatures, *H. capsulatum* grows as a mold. The mycelial phase consists of septate branching hyphae with terminal micro- and macroconidia that range in size from 2 to 14 μm in diameter. When soil is disturbed, these conidia become aerosolized and reach the bronchioles or alveoli.[20,21]

Animal studies have demonstrated that within 2 to 3 days after reaching lung tissue, the conidia germinate, releasing yeast forms that begin multiplying by binary fission. During the next 9 to 15 days, organisms are ingested but not destroyed by large numbers of macrophages that are recruited to the infected site, resulting in small infiltrates. Infected macrophages migrate to the mediastinal lymph nodes and other sites within the mononuclear phagocyte system, particularly the spleen and liver. At this time, the onset of specific T cell immunity in the nonimmune host activates the macrophages, rendering them capable of fungicidal activity. Tissue granulomas form, many of which develop central caseation and necrosis over the next 2 to 4 months. Over a period of several years, these foci become encapsulated and calcified, often with viable yeast trapped within the necrotic tissue.[20,21]

Cellular immunity, as measured by histoplasmin skin test reactivity, wanes in the absence of occasional reexposure. Although exposure to heavy inoculae may overcome these immune mechanisms, resulting in severe disease, reinfection occurs frequently in endemic areas. In the immune individual, the reactions of acquired immunity begin 24 to 48 hours after the appearance of yeast forms, resulting in milder forms of illness and little proliferation of organisms. Although viable organisms may be found within granulomas years after initial infection, the organisms appear to have little ability to proliferate within the fibrous capsules, except in immunocompromised patients.[20,21]

CLINICAL PRESENTATION

The outcome of infection with *H. capsulatum* depends on a complex interplay of host, pathogen, and environmental factors. Host factors include the degree of immunosuppression and the presence of immunity (from prior infection). Environmental factors include inoculum size, exposure within an enclosed area, and duration of exposure. In the vast majority of patients, low-inoculum exposure to *H. capsulatum* results in asymptomatic infection. Patients exposed to a higher inoculum during an acute primary infection or reinfection may experience an acute, self-limited illness with flu-like pulmonary symptoms, including fever, chills, headache, myalgia, and a nonproductive cough. A small percentage of patients will present with arthritis, erythema nodosum, pericarditis, or mediastinal granuloma, which may require the addition of anti-inflammatory agents to their therapy.[20,21]

Chronic pulmonary histoplasmosis generally presents as an opportunistic infection imposed on a preexisting structural abnormality, such as lesions resulting from emphysema. Patients demonstrate chronic pulmonary symptoms and apical lung lesions that progress with inflammation, calcified granulomas, and fibrosis. Patients with early, noncavitary disease often recover without treatment. Progression of disease over a period of years, seen in 25% to 30% of patients, is associated with cavitation, bronchopleural fistulas, extension to the other lung, pulmonary insufficiency, and often death.[21]

In patients exposed to a large inoculum and in immunocompromised hosts, successful containment of the organism within macrophages may not occur, resulting in a progressive illness characterized by yeast-filled phagocytic cells and an inability to produce granulomas. This disease, termed *disseminated histoplasmosis,* is characterized by persistent parasitization of macrophages. The clinical severity of the diverse forms of disseminated histoplasmosis (Table 110–1) generally parallels the degree of macrophage parasitization observed.[20]

Acute (infantile) disseminated histoplasmosis is characterized by massive involvement of the mononuclear phagocyte system by yeast-engorged macrophages. Classically, this severe type of infection is seen in infants and young children and (rarely) in adults with Hodgkin's disease or other lymphoproliferative disorders. In infants or children, acute disseminated histoplasmosis is characterized by unrelenting fever, anemia, leukopenia or thrombocytopenia, enlargement of the liver, spleen, and visceral lymph nodes, and GI symptoms, particularly nausea, vomiting, and diarrhea. The chest roentgenogram often demonstrates remnants of the initiating acute pulmonary lesion. Untreated disease is uniformly fatal in 1 to 2 months. A less severe "subacute" form of the disease, which occurs in both infants and immunocompetent adults, is characterized by focal destructive lesions in various organs, weight loss, weakness, fever, and malaise. Untreated disease is generally fatal in approximately 10 months.[20]

Most adults with disseminated histoplasmosis demonstrate a mild, chronic form of the disease. Untreated patients are often ill for 10 to 20 years, demonstrating long asymptomatic periods interrupted by relapses of clinical illness, characterized primarily by weight loss, weakness, and fatigue. Chronic disseminated histoplasmosis can be seen in patients with lymphoreticular neoplasms (Hodgkin's disease) and patients undergoing immunosuppressant chemotherapy for organ transplantation or for rheumatic diseases. Although central nervous system (CNS) involvement occurs in 10% to 20% of patients with severe underlying immunosuppressive conditions, focal organ involvement is uncommon. The disease is characterized by the development of focal granulomatous lesions, often with bone marrow involvement resulting in thrombocytopenia, anemia, and leukemia. Fever, hepatosplenomegaly, and GI ulceration are common.[20]

TABLE 110–1. Clinical Manifestations and Therapy of Histoplasmosis

Type of Disease and Common Clinical Manifestations	Approximate Frequency (%)[a]	Therapy / Comments
Nonimmunosuppressed Host		
Acute Pulmonary Histoplasmosis		
Asymptomatic histoplasmosis	50–99	*Asymptomatic disease:* No therapy generally required.
Self-limited disease	1–50	*Self-limited disease:* AmB[b] 0.3–0.5 mg/kg/day × 2–4 weeks (total dose 500 mg) *or* ketoconazole 400 mg orally daily × 3–6 months may be beneficial in patients with severe hypoxia following inhalation of large inoculae. Antifungal therapy generally not useful for arthritis, or pericarditis. NSAIDs[c] or corticosteroids may be useful in some cases. *Mediastinal granulomas:* Most lesions resolve spontaneously. Surgery or antifungal therapy with AmB 40–50 mg/d × 2–3 weeks *or* ketoconazole 400 mg/d orally × > 30 months may be beneficial in some cases.
Immunosuppressed Host		
Inflammatory/fibrotic histoplasmosis	0.02	*Fibrosing mediastinitis:* Antifungal therapy generally not helpful; surgery may be of benefit if disease is detected early; late disease may not respond to therapy. *Sarcoid-like:* NSAIDs or corticosteroids may be of benefit for some patients.
Chronic Pulmonary Histoplasmosis	0.05	Antifungal therapy generally recommended for immunosuppressed patients with either persistent cavitation, cavitary wall thickness > 2 mm, or progressive symptoms (including weight loss, cough, sputum production, low grade fever). Itraconazole 200–400mg PO QD or ketoconazole 400 mg/d orally for 1 yr; Relapses common
Disseminated Histoplasmosis	0.02–0.05	*Disseminated histoplasmosis:* Untreated mortality 83%–93%; Relapse 5%–23% in non–AIDS patients.
Acute (infantile)		*Nonimmunosuppressed patients:* ketoconazole 400 mg/d orally × 6–12 months *or* AmB 35 mg/kg IV
Subacute		Immunosuppressed patients (non–AIDS) *or* plus endocarditis or CNS disease: AmB ≥ 35 mg/kg
Chronic (adult-type)		*Non–AIDS:* Life threatening: AmB 0.5–0.75 mg/kg/d IV
Progressive disease of AIDS	25–50[d]	*AIDS patients:* AmB 15–30 mg/kg (1–2 g over 4–10 weeks) *or* itraconazole 200 mg PO QD; followed by chronic suppressive therapy with itraconazole 200 mg PO QD

[a]As a percentage of all patients presenting with histoplasmosis.
[b]AmB = amphotericin B.
[c]NSAIDs = nonsteroidal anti-inflammatory drugs.
[d]As a percentage of AIDS patients presenting with histoplasmosis as the initial manifestation of their disease.
Compiled from Refs. 20 and 27.

Adult patients with AIDS demonstrate an acute form of disseminated disease that resembles the syndrome seen in infants and children. Progressive disseminated histoplasmosis (PDH) can occur as the direct result of initial infection or because of the reactivation of dormant foci. In endemic areas, 50% of AIDS patients demonstrate PDH as the first manifestation of their disease. Progressive disseminated histoplasmosis is characterized by fever (75% of patients), weight loss, chills, night sweats, enlargement of the spleen, liver, or lymph nodes, and anemia. Pulmonary symptoms occur in only one-third of patients and do not always correlate with the presence of infiltrates on chest roentgenogram. A clinical syndrome resembling septicemia is seen in approximately 25% to 50% of patients.[20,21]

DIAGNOSIS

Detection of single, yeast-like cells 2 to 5 µm in diameter with narrow-based budding in direct exam or histologic study of blood smears or tissues should raise strong suspicion of infection with *H. capsulatum,* since colonization does not occur as with *Aspergillus* or *Candida* infection. Identification of mycelial isolates from clinical cultures can be made by conversion of the mycelium to the yeast form (requires 3 to 6 weeks) via commercially available exoantigen test kits, or it can be made by the more rapid (2 hours) and 100% sensitive DNA probe. In patients with suspected disseminated or chronic cavitary histoplasmosis, two to three blood, sputum, and bone marrow cultures and stains should be obtained using the lysis centrifugation technique, and the cultures held for 14 to 21 days for optimal yield of *H. capsulatum.* In patients with acute self-limited histoplasmosis, extensive testing to verify the diagnosis may not be necessary.[14,20,21]

In most patients, serologic evidence remains the primary method in the diagnosis of histoplasmosis. Results obtained from commercially available complement fixation (CF), immunodiffusion (ID), and latex agglutination (LA) antibody tests are used alone or in combination. In general, the use of histoplasmin skin tests are of little value except in epidemiologic studies, since histoplasmin reactivity waxes in the absence of occasional reexposure. In addition, histoplasmin skin testing may result in a false increase in the CF titer for mycelial antigen (CF-M) to *H. capsulatum*. A fourfold rise in the CF titer is usually indicative of recent infection, although some patients with severe disease or profound immunosuppression may demonstrate a weaker antibody response. Since the ID test is not as sensitive as CF, it should be used to assess the importance of weakly reactive results obtained by CF rather than as a screening procedure. Radioimmunoassay (RIA), which measures immunoglobulin M (IgM) and IG antibodies against a histoplasmin extract, is the most sensitive test, but it may show a large number of false-positive reactions in patients living in an endemic area.[14,20,21]

In the AIDS patient with PDH, the diagnosis is best established by bone marrow biopsy and culture, which yield positive cultures in > 90% of patients, although blood cultures and histopathologic exam and culture of pulmonary tissue, sputum, skin, and lymph nodes may also be helpful. Detection of *H. capsulatum* polysaccharide antigen (HPA) in urine, blood, or cerebrospinal fluid (CSF) by enzyme-linked immunosorbent assay (ELISA) or modified radioimmunoassay assay are promising new techniques for the rapid diagnosis of histoplasmosis. The HPA (RIA) levels have also been used successfully to monitor the course of therapy and detect relapses in patients with AIDS, and the clearance of antigen from serum and urine correlates with clinical efficacy during maintenance therapy with itraconazole. Unfortunately, these tests are not yet available for clinical use.[14,21,22]

▶ TREATMENT: Histoplasmosis

NON–HUMAN IMMUNODEFICIENCY VIRUS-INFECTED PATIENT

Recommended therapy for the treatment of histoplasmosis is summarized in Table 110–1. In general, asymptomatic patients and patients with fibrosing mediastinitis or sarcoid-like disease do not benefit from antifungal therapy. Patients with mild, self-limited disease, chronic disseminated disease, or chronic pulmonary histoplasmosis who have no underlying immunosuppression can usually be treated with either oral ketoconazole or IV amphotericin B.

HUMAN IMMUNODEFICIENCY VIRUS-INFECTED PATIENT

In AIDS patients, intensive primary antifungal therapy (induction and consolidation therapy) is followed by lifelong suppressive (maintenance) therapy. In patients with underlying immunosuppression, including AIDS patients with progressive disseminated histoplasmosis, amphotericin B remains the drug of choice for induction therapy, although The British Society for Antimicrobial Chemotherapy recommends oral itraconazole 400 mg daily for 6 weeks as an alternative to amphotericin B. Amphotericin B dosages of 50 mg/d (up to 1 mg/kg/d) should be administered to a cumulative dose of 15 to 35 mg/kg (1 to 2 g) and until negative fungal cultures are achieved.[21–24]

EVALUATION OF THERAPEUTIC OUTCOMES

Response to therapy should be measured by resolution of radiologic, serologic, and microbiologic parameters and by improvement in signs and symptoms of infection. Although investigators are limited by the lack of standardized criteria to quantify the extent of infection, degree of immunosuppression, or treatment response, response rates (based on resolution or improvement in presenting signs and symptoms) of > 80% have been reported in case series in AIDS patients receiving varied dosages of amphotericin B. Rapid responses are reported, with the resolution of symptoms in 25% and 75% of patients by day 3 and day 7 of therapy, respectively.

Once the initial course of therapy for histoplasmosis is completed, lifelong suppressive therapy with oral azoles or amphotericin B (1 to 1.5 mg/kg weekly or biweekly) is recommended, because of the frequent recurrence of infection.[24,25] Relapse rates in AIDS patients not receiving maintenance therapy range from 50% to 90%. Limited data suggest that oral fluconazole 200 to 400 mg/d is successful in preventing relapse of disease. Itraconazole 200 mg orally twice daily for 3 to 12 weeks was successful in 39 of 42 (93%) AIDS patients, and only one patient was removed from the trial because of toxicity (hypokalemia). Oral thrush, however, was reported in six patients, three of whom had undetectable serum concentrations of itraconazole. Itraconazole may soon be recognized as the drug of choice for maintenance therapy because of the drug's ease of administration and favorable safety profile. Patients failing suppressive therapy with itraconazole may benefit from plasma concentration monitoring of itraconazole.[20–24]

BLASTOMYCOSIS

North American blastomycosis is a systemic fungal infection caused by *Blastomyces dermatitidis* a dimorphic fungus that infects primarily the lungs. Patients, however, may present with a variety of pulmonary and extrapulmonary clinical manifestations. Pulmonary disease may be acute or chronic and can mimic infection with tuberculosis, pyogenic bacteria, other fungi, or malignancy. Blastomycosis can disseminate to virtually every other body organ, and approximately 40% of patients with blastomycosis present with skin, bone and joint, or genitourinary tract involvement without any evidence of pulmonary disease.[26]

EPIDEMIOLOGY

Blastomycosis was renamed "North American blastomycosis" in 1942 when Conant and Howell named a similar fungus endemic to South America *Blastomyces braziliensis* and the disease it caused "South American blastomycosis." The disease had previously been called paracoccidioidomycosis. Although the disease is now recognized to be endemic to the southeastern and south central states of the United States (especially those bordering on the Mississippi and Ohio river basins), and the midwestern states and Canadian provinces bordering on the Great Lakes, numerous cases of North American blastomycosis have been diagnosed in Africa, northern parts of South America, India, and Europe. Endemic areas have primarily been defined by analysis of sporadic cases and epidemics or clusters of disease, since the lack of a dependable skin or laboratory test makes widescale epidemiologic testing to determine the incidence of infection unfeasible at present.[26] Although initial review of sporadic cases suggested that males with outdoor occupations that exposed them to soil were at greatest risk for blastomycosis, more recent data suggest that there is no sex, age, or occupational predilection for blastomycosis.[26]

Although *B. dermatitidis* is generally considered to be a soil inhabitant, attempts to isolate the organism in nature have frequently been unsuccessful. *Blastomyces dermatitidis* has been isolated from soil containing decayed vegetation, decomposed wood, and pigeon manure, frequently in association with warm moist soil of wooded areas that is rich in organic debris.[21,26]

PATHOPHYSIOLOGY AND CLINICAL PRESENTATION

Pulmonary infection probably occurs by inhalation of conidia, which convert to the yeast form in the lung. A vigorous inflammatory response ensues, with neutrophilic recruitment to the lungs followed by the development of cell-mediated immunity and the formation of noncaseating granulomas.[11,21,26]

Acute pulmonary blastomycosis is generally an asymptomatic or self-limited disease characterized by fever, shaking chills, and productive, purulent cough, with or without hemoptysis, in immunocompetent individuals. The clinical presentation may be difficult to differentiate from other respiratory infections, including bacterial pneumonia, on the basis of clinical symptoms alone. Sporadic (nonepidemic) cases of pulmonary blastomycosis may present as a more chronic or subacute disease, with low-grade fever, night sweats, weight loss, and productive cough that resembles tuberculosis rather than bacterial pneumonia.[21,26]

Chronic pulmonary blastomycosis is characterized by fever, malaise, weight loss, night sweats, chest pain, and productive cough. Patients are often thought to have tuberculosis. Unlike patients with chronic pulmonary histoplasmosis, patients with chronic pulmonary blastomycosis often have evidence of disseminated disease that may appear 1 to 3 years after the primary pneumonia has resolved. Reactivation of disease may occur in the lungs or as the foci of new infection in other organs. In approximately 40% of patients, however, dissemination is not accompanied by reactivation of pulmonary disease. The most common sites for disseminated disease include the skin and bony skeleton, although less commonly the prostate, oropharyngeal mucosa, and abdominal viscera are involved. Central nervous system disease, while exceedingly uncommon, is associated with the highest mortality rate.[21,26]

DIAGNOSIS

The simplest and most successful method of diagnosing blastomycosis is by direct microscopic visualization of the large, multinucleated yeast with single, broad-based buds in sputum or other respiratory specimens, following digestion of cells and debris with 10% potassium hydroxide, since, like *Histoplasma,* colonization does not occur with *Blastomyces.*[14,26] Histopathologic examination of tissue biopsies and culture of secretions should also be used to identify *B. dermatitidis,* although it may require up to 30 days to isolate and identify a small inoculum. Unfortunately, no reliable skin test exists to determine the incidence and prevalence of disease in endemic populations. Reliable serologic diagnosis of blastomycosis has long been hampered by the lack of specific and standardized reagents, and unfortunately, serologic response does not always correlate with clinical improvement, although some investigators have noted that a decline in the number of precipitins or CF titers may offer evidence of a favorable prognosis in patients with established disease.[21,26]

▶ TREATMENT: Blastomycosis

NON–HUMAN IMMUNODEFICIENCY VIRUS-INFECTED PATIENT

In patients with mild pulmonary blastomycosis, the clinical presentation of the patient and the toxicity of the antifungal agents are the main determinants of whether or not to administer antifungal therapy. Regardless of whether or not the patient receives treatment, however, they must be followed carefully for many years for evidence of reactivation or progressive disease.[21,26] Some authors recommend ketoconazole therapy for the treatment of self-limited pulmonary disease, with the hope of preventing late extrapulmonary disease; however, data supporting the efficacy of these regimens are lacking.[21,26] Ketoconazole appears to be as effective as amphotericin B for non–life-threatening, nonmeningeal, mild-to-moderate blastomycosis in immunocompetent hosts. In a prospective, randomized, multicenter study conducted by the National Institute of Allergy and Infectious Diseases (NIAID) Mycoses

Study Group,[27] high-dose (800 mg/d) oral therapy with ketoconazole was associated with a significantly higher cure rate than low-dose (400 mg/d) therapy (100% vs 79%, respectively) in 80 patients with blastomycosis. The increased frequency of adverse effects (primarily intolerable nausea and vomiting) associated with high-dose therapy, however, prompted the NIAID's recommendation of low-dose ketoconazole therapy for patients with nonmeningeal, non–life-threatening disease. The cure rate observed with low-dose therapy compares favorably with reported cure rates of 66% to 93% among patients treated with amphotericin B. The dosage of ketoconazole should be increased to 600 to 800 mg orally per day in the absence of a favorable clinical response.[27] Patients with CNS disease, progressive or life-threatening disease, or those experiencing toxicity while on ketoconazole should receive amphotericin B (40 to 50 mg/d) until clinical improvement is observed, followed by administration three times weekly until a total dose of 1.5 to 2 g is achieved.

All patients with chronic pulmonary blastomycosis and those with extrapulmonary disease require therapy. Ketoconazole 400 mg orally per day for 6 months cures more than 80% of patients with chronic pulmonary and nonmeningeal disseminated blastomycosis. Amphotericin B is more efficacious but more toxic, and, therefore, is reserved for noncompliant patients and patients with overwhelming or life-threatening disease, CNS infection, and treatment failures.[21,26–28] Patients with genitourinary tract disease should be treated initially with 600 to 800 mg/d of ketoconazole because of the low concentrations of drug achieved in the urine and prostate tissue.

Patients should be monitored carefully for signs of clinical failure, and those who fail or are unable to tolerate itraconazole therapy or develop CNS disease should be treated with amphotericin B for a total dose of 30 to 35 mg/kg.[21,26–28]

HUMAN IMMUNODEFICIENCY VIRUS-INFECTED PATIENT

For unclear reasons, blastomycosis is an uncommon opportunistic disease among immunocompromised individuals, including AIDS patients; however, blastomycosis may occur as a late (CD4+ lymphocytes < 200/mm^3) and frequently fatal complication of HIV infection. In this population, overwhelming disseminated disease with frequent involvement of the CNS is common.[28] Following induction therapy with amphotericin B (total dose of 1 g), HIV-infected patients should receive chronic suppressive therapy with an oral azole antifungal.[26,28] Despite its higher cost, itraconazole has become the drug of choice for non–life-threatening histoplasmosis (mild-to-moderate disease) in HIV-infected patients.[23,26]

COCCIDIOIDOMYCOSIS

EPIDEMIOLOGY

Coccidioidomycosis is caused by infection with *Coccidioides immitis,* a dimorphic fungi found in the southwestern and western United States, as well as parts of Mexico and South America. In North America, the endemic regions encompass the semiarid regions of the southwestern United States from California to Texas known as the Lower Sonoran Zone, where there is scant annual rainfall, hot summers, and sandy, alkaline soil. *Coccidioides immitis* grows in the soil as a mold, and mycelia proliferate during the rainy season. During the dry season, resistant arthroconidia form and become airborne when the soil is disturbed.

Although generally considered to be a regional disease, coccidioidomycosis has increased in importance in recent years because of the increased tourism and population in endemic areas, the increased use of immunosuppressive therapy in transplantation and oncology, and the AIDS epidemic. Although there is no racial, hormonal, or immunologic predisposition for acquiring primary disease, these factors affect the risk of subsequent dissemination of disease.[29]

PATHOPHYSIOLOGY

When individuals come in contact with contaminated soil during ranching, dust storms, or proximity to construction sites or archaeological excavations, arthroconidia are inhaled into the respiratory tree, where they transform into spherules, which reproduce by cleavage of the cytoplasm to produce endospores. The endospores are released when the spherules reach maturity. Similar to histoplasmosis, an acute inflammatory response in the tissue leads to infiltration of mononuclear cells, ultimately resulting in granuloma formation.[29]

CLINICAL PRESENTATION

Initial or primary infection with *C. immitis* almost always involves the lungs. Although approximately one-third of the population in endemic areas is infected, the average incidence of symptomatic disease is only approximately 0.43%. Sixty percent of subjects are asymptomatic or have nonspecific symptoms that are often indistinguishable from ordinary upper respiratory infections, including fever, cough, headache, sore throat, myalgias, and fatigue. A fine diffuse rash may appear during the first few days of the illness. "Valley fever" is a syndrome characterized by erythema nodosum and erythema multiforme of the upper trunk and extremities in association with diffuse joint aches or fever. Valley fever occurs in approximately 25% of patients although, more commonly, a diffuse mild erythroderma or maculopapular rash is observed. Patients may have pleuritic chest pain and peripheral eosinophilia. Radiographic features tend to be quite variable; hilar adenopathy with alveolar infiltrates, tissue excavation of an infiltrate (resulting in a thin-walled cavity), or small pleural effusions are all commonly seen. The development of erythema nodosum is thought to indicate the development of hypersensitivity to *C. immitis.*[29]

Some patients present with an acute pneumonia as the primary manifestation of disease. They have a productive cough that may be blood-streaked, and single or multiple soft or dense homogeneous hilar or basal infiltrates on chest roentgenogram. The disease usually lasts a few days to a few weeks and usually resolves spontaneously without therapy, although it can be fatal, particularly in patients who are immunocompromised.[29]

Although most primary pneumonias follow a benign course, pulmonary coccidioidomycosis can also develop into a chronic, persistent pneumonia complicated by hemoptysis, pulmonary scarring, and the formation of cavities or bronchopleural fistulas. Necrosis of pulmonary tissue with drainage and cavity formation occurs commonly in coccidioidal pneumonia. Most parenchymal cavities close spontaneously or form dense nodular scar tissue that may become superinfected with bacteria or spherules of *C. immitis.* These patients often have persistent cough, fevers, and weight loss. Primary disease lasting more than 6 weeks is termed persistent pulmonary coccidioidomycosis. Rarely, chronic pulmonary (also known as chronic progressive) pneumonia occurs, in which patients usually experience persistent cough, weight loss, chest pain, and intermittent fevers and hemoptysis. *Coccidioides immitis* can often be cultured from the sputum for a period of several years. Chest radiographs usually demonstrate apical fibronodular lesions or slowly progressive cavitation.[29]

Disseminated infection with *C. immitis* occurs in less than 1% of infected patients. The most common sites for dissemination are the skin, lymph nodes, bone, and meninges, although the spleen, liver, kidney, and adrenal gland may also be involved.[29] Occasionally, miliary coccidioidomycosis occurs, with rapid, widespread dissemination, often in concert with positive blood cultures for *C. immitis.* Patients with AIDS frequently present with miliary disease. Coccidioidomycosis in AIDS patients appears to be caused by reactivation of disease in most patients.[29,30]

Risk factors for severe, disseminated infection include race (blacks, Hispanics, Native Americans, and Filipinos) and pregnancy, although these data have been disputed by several investigators. Older data suggest that race-related differences in the incidence of severe disease exist, while newer studies suggest that an exposure to dust containing high inocula of *C. immitis* played a more important role. Pregnancy may lead to a general depression in cell-mediated immunity (particularly during the third trimester) or to an increase in sex hormones that stimulate the growth of the fungus. Immunocompromised hosts, particularly patients with AIDS and those receiving corticosteroids or immunosuppressive agents, are also at an increased risk for disseminated disease.[30] For unclear reasons, males appear to be at higher risk than females for disseminated disease, as are neonates and patients with type B or AB blood type. Surprisingly, the risk of disseminated disease does not appear to increase with age or the presence of diabetes mellitus.[29,30]

Central nervous system infection with *C. immitis* is a particularly devastating complication that develops in approximately 16% of patients with disseminated coccidioidomycosis.[30] Left untreated, coccidioidal meningitis is invariably fatal within 1 to 2 years. Early diagnosis is important, since early treatment appears to correlate with improved outcome. Patients may present with meningeal disease without previous symptoms of primary pulmonary infection, although disease usually occurs within 6 months after the primary infection. Signs of meningeal irritation common in bacterial meningitis are often absent. The signs and symptoms of coccidioidal meningitis are often subtle and nonspecific, including headache, weakness, changes in mental status (lethargy and confusion), neck stiffness, low-grade fever, weight loss, and occasionally hydrocephalus. Space occupying lesions are rare, and the main areas of involvement are the basilar meninges. Analysis of the CSF generally reveals a lymphocytic pleocytosis with elevated protein and a decreased glucose. Although serum is usually positive for coccidioidal CF antibodies, the coccidioidal skin test is often negative.[29,30]

Infection of the genitourinary system is an increasingly recognized site of disseminated disease. Although patients tend to have chronic disease at these sites, including endometritis, prostatitis, epididymitis, and coccidioidouria, these do not necessarily indicate disseminated disease or a poor prognostic sign. Therapy is generally not necessary, except in the AIDS population, in whom chronic suppressive therapy is usually required.[29,30]

DIAGNOSIS

A number of tests have been developed to detect past or present infection with *C. immitis.* Most patients develop a positive skin test within 3 weeks of the onset of symptoms. Baseline evaluation of skin test reactivity and serology is essential in order to assess cell-mediated immunity. Patients who develop early positive skin test reactivity or whose coccidioidin skin test reactivity turns from negative to positive during therapy have an improved prognosis versus patients whose skin test reactivity develops later or does not change during therapy.[29,30] Patients with disseminated coccidioidomycosis whose skin tests are persistently negative are more likely to require prolonged therapy, and they are more likely to relapse after completion of therapy. The coccidioidal skin test also affects serologic tests for histoplasmosis but not those for coccidioidomycosis.[30]

Antibody production can be used to follow the course of disease because most patients produce antibodies in response to infection with *C. immitis.* Early infection is characterized by the development of the IgM antibody, which peaks within 2 to 3 weeks of infection then declines rapidly. The IgM antibody can be detected by either tube precipitin or immunodiffusion techniques.[29,30]

The IgG antibody levels rise between 4 and 12 weeks after infection and decrease slowly over months to years, and IgG can be detected in many body fluids, including serum, CSF, and pleural fluid by CF and ID techniques. Higher titers (> 1:16 or 1:32) occur more frequently with severe disease. Titers can be followed serially to evaluate the efficacy of antifungal therapy.[29]

Recovery of *C. immitis* from infected tissues or secretions for direct examination and culture provides an accurate and rapid method of diagnosis. Since the spherule–endospore phase of coccidioidomycosis found in tissue is not infective, transmission of coccidioidomycosis from person to person does not occur. The mycelial–arthroconidia phase of *C. immitis* is extremely infective, however, and laboratory-acquired disease because of inhalation of aerially transmitted infective arthroconidia has been documented in more than 200 cases. In the past, inoculation of laboratory animals to produce spherule-containing abscesses was used to diagnose coccidioidomycosis definitively. This has largely been replaced by detection of antigen from an extract of the mold phase. Direct microscopic examination and histopathologic studies of infected tissues will reveal the large, mature endosporulating spherules. Young spherules without endospores may be confused, however, with other fungi. Silver stains of body fluids or tissue biopsies are also helpful.[6,29]

▶ TREATMENT: Coccidioidomycosis

Therapy for coccidioidomycosis is difficult, and the results are unpredictable. The efficacy of antifungal therapy for coccidioidomycosis is often less certain than that for other fungal etiologies, such as blastomycosis, histoplasmosis, or cryptococcus, even when *in vitro* susceptibilities and the sites of infections are similar. The refractoriness of coccidioidomycosis may relate to the ability of *C. immitis* spherules to release hundreds of endospores, maximally challenging host defenses.[29,30] Fortunately, only about 5% of infected patients require therapy. Candidates for therapy include those with severe primary pulmonary infection or increasing CF antibody titers (particularly 1:16 to 1:32), immunocompromised patients, and those with persistent (> 6 weeks) fever, prostration, or worsening pulmonary disease. Any patient with evidence of disseminated disease should receive therapy.[30]

Although most patients with symptomatic primary pulmonary disease recover without therapy, severe infections should probably be treated, particularly in patients with high CF titers, in whom incipient or occult dissemination is likely. Almost all patients with disease located outside the lungs should receive antifungal therapy. Amphotericin B is usually administered in IV dosages of 1 to 1.5 mg/kg/d, tapering to 1 to 1.5 mg/kg three times a week to a total dose of 0.5 to 1.5 g over 2 to 4 weeks, based on clinical response.[30] Some patients will require higher doses or more prolonged therapy; a minimum of 2 to 3 g of amphotericin B is probably necessary for the treatment of persistent pulmonary infection or miliary coccidioidomycosis. Approximately 50% to 75% of patients treated with amphotericin B for nonmeningeal disease achieve a sustained remission, and therapy is usually curative in patients with infections localized strictly to skin and soft tissues without extensive abscess formation or tissue damage. The efficacy of local injection into joints or the peritoneum, as well as intra-articular or intradermal administration, remains poorly studied. Amphotericin B appears to be most efficacious when cell-mediated immunity is intact (as evidenced by a positive coccidioidin or spherulin skin test or low CF antibody titer). Controlled trials that document these clinical impressions are lacking, however.[30]

The introduction of the azole antifungal agents (miconazole, ketoconazole, fluconazole, itraconazole) into practice has offered alternative therapy to amphotericin B. Miconazole was the first systemic azole to be used for the treatment of coccidioidomycosis. Miconazole in an IV dosage of 0.6 to 1.2 g three times daily was efficacious in a series of patients with skin and soft-tissue or chronic pulmonary coccidioidomycosis who were unresponsive to amphotericin B. Although less toxic than amphotericin B, relapses following therapy are common. The role of miconazole in relation to other antifungal agents is unsettled and requires further comparative trials. The advent of orally available, less toxic alternatives, such as ketoconazole, fluconazole, and itraconazole makes these studies unlikely to be performed.[18,30,31]

Ketoconazole, the first orally available azole, demonstrates variable absorption, particularly in patients with increased gastric pH because of H_2-receptor antagonists, antacids, or diseases (achlorhydria or AIDS). Several noncomparative, open evaluations of ketoconazole for the treatment of progressive coccidioidomycosis have suggested that ketoconazole at a dosage of 400 mg orally per day is efficacious in patients with infiltrative pulmonary disease, soft-tissue infection, or skeletal involvement. The efficacy, however, of ketoconazole in treatment of primary pulmonary coccidioidomycosis, vertebral osteomyelitis, and meningitis has not been established. Dosages of 200 to 400 mg daily produce response rates in all forms of disease (with the exception of meningitis) comparable to those observed for amphotericin B or miconazole, even in patients unresponsive to other forms of therapy. Soft-tissue infections improve more frequently following lower dosages of ketoconazole than do skeletal or pulmonary infections; however, relapse rates of 25% are disturbing. Dosages greater than 400 mg daily appear to be more toxic but no more efficacious than lower dosages.[18,30,31]

Itraconazole has been used effectively for the treatment of chronic coccidioidal meningitis. The usual dosage is 400 mg PO qd, given as two daily doses, although higher amounts have been required in some patients. Ketoconazole cannot be routinely recommended for the treatment of coccidioidal meningitis because of its poor CNS penetration following oral administration.[18,30–33]

Fluconazole has become the drug of choice for the treatment of coccidioidal meningitis.[18,30–33] A minimum dose of 400 mg PO qd leads to a clinical response in most patients and has been shown to obviate the need for intrathecal amphotericin B. It is also clear, however, that fluconazole only leads to remission rather than curing the infections, and thus, suppressive therapy must be continued for life.

CRYPTOCOCCOSIS

EPIDEMIOLOGY

Cryptococcosis is a noncontagious, systemic mycotic infection caused by the ubiquitous encapsulated soil yeast *Cryptococcus neoformans*, which is found in soil, particularly in pigeon droppings, although disease occurs throughout the world, even in areas where pigeons are absent. Infection is acquired by inhalation of the organism. The incidence of cryptococcosis has risen dramatically in recent years, reflecting the increased numbers of immunocompromised patients, including those with malignancies, diabetes mellitus, chronic renal failure, and organ transplants, or those receiving immunosuppressive agents. The AIDS epidemic has also contributed to the increased numbers of patients; cryptococcosis is the fourth most common infectious complication of AIDS and the second most common fungal pathogen.[34]

Although *C. neoformans* produces no toxins and evokes only a minimal inflammatory response in tissue, the polysaccharide capsule appears to allow the organism to resist phagocytosis by the host. The capsular polysaccharide of *C. neoformans* appears to comprise the major virulence factor for this pathogen. Four serotypes of *C. neoformans* (A through D) have been identified, which vary in their polysaccharide content, virulence, geographical foci, and response to antifungal therapy. Serotypes A and D are commonly associated with pigeon droppings and other environmental sites, and generally require shorter therapy than infections caused by serotypes B or C, which have been found only in infected humans and animals. Serotypes B and C appear more resistant to antifungal agents *in vitro*. Patients with AIDS are almost always infected with serotypes A and D, even in areas endemic for serotypes B and C. There is no particular geographical area of endemic focus for *C. neoformans*.

Cell-mediated immunity appears to play a major role in host defense against infection with *C. neoformans;* 29% to 55% of patients with cryptococcal meningitis have a predisposing condition. Many patients with disseminated cryptococcosis demonstrate defects in cell-mediated immunity. The predilection of *C. neoformans* for the CNS appears to be caused by the lack of immunoglobulins and complement and the excellent growth media afforded by CSF.[34]

CLINICAL PRESENTATION

Primary cryptococcosis in humans almost always occurs in the lungs, although the pulmonary focus usually produces a subclinical infection. Symptomatic infections are usually manifested by cough, rales, and shortness of breath that generally resolve spontaneously. Disease may remain localized in the lungs or it may disseminate to other tissues, particularly the CNS, although the skin can also be affected. Hematogenous spread generally occurs in the immunocompromised host although it has also been seen in individuals with intact immune systems. Cryptococcemia is the most common symptomatic extraneural infection associated with *C. neoformans*. Cryptococcemia can be documented in 5% to 22% of non–AIDS patients, and CNS involvement of *C. neoformans* can be found in 18% to 50% of AIDS patients. In the non–AIDS patient, the symptoms of cryptococcal meningitis are nonspecific. Headache, fever, nausea, vomiting, mental status changes, and neck stiffness are generally observed. Less common symptoms include visual disturbances (photophobia and blurred vision), papilledema, seizures, and aphasia. In AIDS patients, fever and headache are common, but meningismus and photophobia are much less common than in non–AIDS patients. Approximately 10% to 12% of AIDS patients have asymptomatic disease, similar to the rate observed in non–AIDS patients. Cryptococcal disease is present in 7.5% to 10% of AIDS patients. Therefore, patients with evidence of extraneural cryptococcosis should be evaluated for CNS disease.[34]

DIAGNOSIS

Examination of CSF in patients with cryptococcal meningitis generally reveals an elevated opening pressure, CSF pleocytosis (usually lymphocytes), leukocytosis, a decreased CSF glucose, an elevated CSF protein, and a positive cryptococcal antigen. Antigens to *C. neoformans* can be detected by latex agglutination. The test is rapid, specific, and extremely sensitive, but false negatives can occur. False-positive tests can result from cross-reactivity with rheumatoid factor and *T. beigelii. Cryptococcus neoformans* can be detected in approximately 60% of patients by India ink smear of CSF, and it can be cultured in more than 96% of patients. Occasionally, large volumes of CSF are required in order to confirm the diagnosis. The CSF parameters in patients with AIDS are similar to those seen in non–AIDS patients with the exception of a decreased inflammatory response to the pathogen, resulting in a strikingly low number of leukocytes in CSF and extraordinarily high cryptococcal antigen titers.[6,34]

▶ TREATMENT: Cryptococcosis

NON–HUMAN IMMUNODEFICIENCY VIRUS-INFECTED PATIENT

Prior to the introduction of amphotericin B, cryptococcal meningitis was an almost uniformly fatal disease; approximately 86% of patients died within 1 year. The use of large (1 to 1.5 mg/kg) daily doses of amphotericin B resulted in cure rates of approximately 64%. When amphotericin B is combined with flucytosine, a smaller dose of amphotericin B can be employed because of the *in vitro* and *in vivo* synergy between the two antifungal agents (Table 110–2). Resistance develops to flucytosine in up to 30% of patients treated with 5-flucytosine alone, limiting its usefulness as monotherapy. In a randomized, comparative trial, amphotericin B in a dosage of 0.3 mg/kg/d plus oral flucytosine 150 mg/kg/d for 6 weeks was as effective as amphotericin B administered alone at a dosage of 0.4 mg/kg/d for 6 weeks, followed by 0.8 mg/kg every other day for 4 weeks. Combination therapy resulted in cure or improvement in 16 of 24 (67%) patients as compared to 11 of 27 (41%) patients treated with amphotericin B alone. In addition, the combination therapy resulted in less nephrotoxicity, fewer relapses, and more rapid sterilization of CSF cultures. This study has been criticized, however, for the low dosage of amphotericin B used in the amphotericin-B-alone arm of the study, which resulted in lower cure rates than those reported in earlier studies employing higher dosages. In addition, flucytosine toxicity (primarily bone marrow suppression) was observed in approximately one-third of patients.[34]

TABLE 110–2. Therapy of Cryptococcosis[a,b]

Type of Disease and Common Clinical Manifestations	Therapy / Comments
Nonimmunocompromised Host	Comparative trials for AmB vs azoles not available
Cutaneous disease	Asymptomatic disease: Drug therapy generally not required
Acute Cryptococcocal Meningitis	AmB IV 0.3 mg/kg/day + 5-FC 150 mg/kg/day x 6 wk 4 wk of therapy for patients with no underlying disease, no immunosuppression, and uncomplicated course of disease
Recurrent or progressive disease not responsive to AmB	AmB IV 0.5–0.75 mg/kg/day +/– IT AmB 0.5 mg two to three times weekly
HIV-infected Patient	
Prophylactic therapy	None *or* FLU 200 mg PO QD
Treatment	
Acute disease	AmB IV 0.7 mg/kg/day + 5-FC 100 mg/kg/day PO QD × 2 wk *(induction therapy)* followed by FLU 400 mg PO QD *or* ITRA 400 mg PO QD × 8 wk *(consolidation therapy)*, then *suppressive therapy*
Suppressive therapy	FLU 200 mg PO QD

[a]When more than one therapy is listed, they are listed in order of preference
[b]See text for definitions of induction, consolidation, suppressive therapy, and prophylactic therapy
AmB = amphotericin B; IT = intrathecal; 5-FC = flucytosine; FLU = fluconazole; ITRA = itraconazole.
Compiled from Refs. 34–38.

In a follow-up study,[35] a 4-week regimen of combination therapy was as effective as the 6-week regimen in patients with no underlying disease who were not receiving immunosuppressive therapy and had an uncomplicated course of disease. Unfortunately, these criteria exclude most patients with cryptococcal meningitis. Peak serum flucytosine concentrations > 100 mg/L were associated with greater toxicity. In patients with impaired renal function, serum concentrations of flucytosine should be monitored and adjusted accordingly.[35]

Ketoconazole has been used successfully in the treatment of cutaneous cryptococcosis, but it is not useful in the treatment of CNS disease, probably because of its poor penetration into the CNS. Despite low CSF concentrations of amphotericin B (2% to 3% of those observed in plasma), the use of intrathecal amphotericin B is not recommended for the treatment of cryptococcal meningitis except in patients who fail to respond to amphotericin B alone. Intraventricular therapy should be reserved for very ill patients or those with recurrent or progressive disease despite aggressive therapy with IV amphotericin B. The dosage of amphotericin B employed is usually 0.5 mg administered via the lumbar, cisternal, or intraventricular (via an Ommaya reservoir) route two or three times weekly. Side effects of intrathecal amphotericin B include arachnoiditis and paresthesias. Intrathecal amphotericin B therapy should be administered in combination with IV amphotericin B.[3,36]

ACUTE DISEASE IN HUMAN IMMUNODEFICIENCY VIRUS-INFECTED PATIENT

Fluconazole is beneficial for both acute and chronic maintenance therapy for cryptococcal meningitis. Amphotericin B 0.4 to 0.5 mg/kg IV daily was compared to oral fluconazole 200 mg daily. Although the overall 10-week mortality was the same in both groups, the time until the CSF culture became negative was longer, and there were more deaths in the first 2 weeks of therapy in the fluconazole group.[37] A smaller study performed at the same time showed the superiority of higher dose amphotericin B (0.7 mg/kg IV daily for 2 weeks, followed by 0.7 mg/kg three times weekly for 8 weeks) combined with flucytosine over fluconazole.[18,31] In later trials,[38] amphotericin B 0.7 mg/kg IV daily for 2 weeks (with or without oral flucytosine 100 mg/kg/d), followed by consolidation therapy with either itraconazole 400 mg PO qd or fluconazole 400 mg PO qd led to markedly improved outcomes in comparison to the results published earlier. This study also confirmed the benefit of flucytosine added to amphotericin B for induction therapy and the slight superiority of fluconazole over itraconazole for consolidation therapy.

Another approach used in the treatment of cryptococcal meningitis in AIDS patients is to add flucytosine to fluconazole.[18,31] In patients treated with fluconazole 400 mg PO qd plus flucytosine 150 mg/kg/d, CSF became culture negative more quickly than in other trials using fluconazole 200 mg PO qd as primary therapy.[18,31,37]

SUPPRESSIVE (MAINTENANCE) THERAPY FOR CRYPTOCOCCAL MENINGITIS IN HUMAN IMMUNODEFICIENCY VIRUS-INFECTED PATIENT

Relapse of *C. neoformans* meningitis occurs in approximately 50% of AIDS patients after completion of primary therapy. Persistence of asymptomatic urinary *C. neoformans* has been documented in a high percentage of AIDS patients despite seemingly adequate courses of therapy for primary meningeal disease. The prostate appears to act as a sequestered reservoir of infection in these patients, resulting in systemic relapse. Fluconazole is recommended for chronic suppressive therapy of cryptococcal meningitis in AIDS patients. The AIDS Clinical Trials Groups (ACTG) 026 study demonstrated that oral fluconazole 200 mg daily was superior to IV administration of amphotericin B 1 mg/kg weekly in preventing relapse. In addition, the fluconazole-treated group showed a lower incidence of adverse drug reactions and bacterial infections.[36]

EVALUATION OF THERAPEUTIC OUTCOMES

Once the CNS is involved, the usual course is weeks to months of progressive deterioration with 80% of untreated patients dying within the first year. The prognosis of cryptococcal meningitis depends largely on the underlying predisposing factors of the host. Although cryptococcal antigen is positive in 90% of patients with cryptococcal meningitis, fewer than half of the patients with cryptococcal meningitis develop antibody to capsular polysaccharide. Those who produce antibody have a slightly improved prognosis. In contrast, the presence of headache is a favorable symptom, presumably because it leads to an earlier diagnosis. A favorable outcome is also associated with a normal mental status upon diagnosis, and a CSF white blood cell (WBC) count of > 20/mm^3. A poor outcome is predicted, however, by the presence of one or more underlying diseases (including hematopoietic disorders and AIDS), corticosteroid or immunosuppressive therapy, pretreatment serum cryptococcal antigen titers of 1:32, and post-therapy serum antigen titers of 1:8. In non–AIDS patients, the cryptococcal antigen titer can be followed during therapy to assess response to antifungal therapy. In AIDS patients, decreasing titers are not necessarily predictive of success, and titers rarely become negative at the completion of therapy.[18,31]

CANDIDA INFECTIONS

Candida sp. are yeasts that exist primarily as small (4 to 6 μm), unicellular, thin-walled, ovoid cells that reproduce by budding. On agar media, they form smooth, white, creamy colonies resembling staphylococci. Although there are more than 150 species of *Candida,* eight species are regarded as clinically important pathogens in human disease, including *C. albicans, C. tropicalis, C. parapsilosis, C. krusei, C. stellatoidea, C. guilliermondi, C. lusitaniae,* and *Ciglabrata.*[8,11,39] Yeast forms, hyphae, and pseudohyphae may be found in clinical specimens. A rapid presumptive identification of *C. albicans* can be made by incubation of the organism in serum; formation of a germ tube within 1 to 2 hours offers a positive identification of *C. albicans.* A negative germ tube test does not rule out the possibility of *C. albicans,* but further biochemical tests must be performed in order to differentiate between other nonalbicans species.[8]

EPIDEMIOLOGY

Candida albicans is a normal commensal of the skin, female genital tract, and the entire GI tract of humans. Therefore, the mere presence of hyphae or pseudohyphae in a clinical specimen is not sufficient for the diagnosis of invasive disease. Thus, the majority of infections with *C. albicans* are acquired endogenously, although human-to-human transmission can also occur. Oral candidiasis in the newborn is probably acquired during passage through the birth canal, and balanitis in the uncircumcised male may be acquired through contact with a female with vaginal candidiasis.[8,39] Although the term *fungemia* refers to the presence of fungi in the blood, the most commonly isolated organism is *C. albicans.* Candidiasis may cause mucocutaneous or systemic infection, including endocarditis, peritonitis, arthritis, and infection of the CNS.

PATHOPHYSIOLOGY

The role of an intact integument is crucial in the prevention of mucocutaneous or hematogenous candidiasis. Once *Candida* invades the dermis or enters the bloodstream, polymorphonuclear leukocytes (PMNs) play a major role in the defense of the patient, since PMNs are capable of damaging pseudohyphae and can phagocytize and kill blastoconidia.[8,39] In addition to neutrophils, lymphocytes, monocytes, macrophages, complement, and eosinophils play a role in the prevention of infection. The complex role of each of these components in the pathogenesis of infections with *Candida* has been reviewed by Odds.[39] Adherence of *C. albicans* is important in the pathogenesis of oral candidiasis and subsequent colonization of the GI tract. Because evidence suggests that the GI tract is often the portal of entry for *Candida* in disseminated disease, factors that alter the adherence of *Candida* are crucial in the development of local and systemic infection. *Candida tropicalis* adheres to intravascular catheters at a higher rate than *C. albicans,* a factor that may help to account for the increased incidence of systemic infections caused by this pathogen.

MUCOCUTANEOUS CANDIDIASIS

Mucocutaneous candidiasis can generally be divided into several categories: oropharyngeal candidiasis (thrush), esophageal candidiasis, GI candidiasis, and vaginal candidiasis. Mucocutaneous candidiasis is generally caused by *C. albicans,* although other species of *Candida* (including *C. glabrata, C. tropicalis,* and *C. krusei*) are occasionally implicated. Oral candidiasis is often the first sign of infection in patients with AIDS; as many as 50% of AIDS patients with oral candidiasis who are not treated with antiretroviral therapy will develop an opportunistic infection within 3 months of the development of oral candidiasis.

CHRONIC MUCOCUTANEOUS CANDIDIASIS

Chronic mucocutaneous candidiasis refers to a collection of syndromes characterized by chronic or recurrent infections of the skin, nails, and mucous membranes by *C. albicans.* Most patients exhibit abnormalities in cell-mediated immunity. Although fungal infections in these patients generally respond to treatment with conventional antifungal agents, relapses are common after treatment is stopped. Ketoconazole, itraconazole, and fluconazole have been used successfully as long-term therapy for this syndrome.[11]

ORAL CANDIDIASIS (THRUSH)

A variety of local and systemic factors are generally necessary for the development of oral candidiasis. Precipitating factors include age, mucosal damage, presence of host immune deficiencies (including malignancies, diabetes mellitus, and AIDS), nutritional deficiencies, radiation therapy, antineoplastic agents, and use of local or systemic antibiotics or corticosteroids. Oral candidiasis occurs in as many as 5% of all newborn infants, > 35% of patients with acute leukemia or those receiving chemotherapy for solid tumors, patients undergoing organ transplantation, and approximately 10% of all hospitalized, debilitated, elderly patients.[8,39]

Oral candidiasis is characterized by the presence of creamy, white plaques on the tongue and buccal mucosa that generally leave a painful, raw, ulcerated surface when scraped. The diagnosis of oral candidiasis is based on the clinical appearance of the lesions and by scraping of lesions, using either 10% potassium hydroxide digestion of this material to reveal the presence of pseudohyphae and yeast forms or the presence of gram-positive staining yeast forms.[8]

Although oral candidiasis is generally not life-threatening, it causes discomfort and, in immunocompromised patients, can spread to the esophagus, causing ulcerations and mucosal perforation. Colonization of the GI tract with *C. albicans* increases the risk of invasive disease, particularly in patients with decreased numbers of neutrophils secondary to the administration of chemotherapy or immunosuppressive agents. When suspensions of *C. albicans* are administered into the GI tract, they can migrate across intact endothelium by a process known as *persorption*. Ulceration of the GI tract secondary to chemotherapy may facilitate migration of *Candida* into the bloodstream. In addition a variety of factors, including endotoxin, chemotherapy, and administration of adrenal corticosteroids, can interfere with the elimination of *Candida* via the reticuloendothelial system. It is important to note that patients with defects in cell-mediated immunity (patients with chronic mucocutaneous candidiasis or AIDS) are generally predisposed to mucosal but *not* systemic infections with *Candida.*[39]

▶ TREATMENT: Thrush

NON-HUMAN IMMUNODEFICIENCY VIRUS-INFECTED PATIENT

Topical (local) therapy with a variety of antifungal agents, including nystatin suspension and clotrimazole troches, are generally efficacious in the prophylaxis and therapy of oral candidiasis (Table 110–3). The optimal dosage or agent has not been clearly defined. Nystatin has been used as a "swish and swallow" regimen in dosages ranging from 0.5 million units (MU) four times daily to 1.5 MU six times daily. Some investigators, however, have found nystatin therapy to be no more beneficial than a placebo in the treatment of oral candidiasis or the prevention of systemic infection with *C. albicans.*

The comparative efficacy of topical and systemic agents is also controversial. Although most agents have proven efficacious in controlled studies compared with a placebo, few comparative trials are available to assess the relative efficacy of these agents. In oncology patients, ketoconazole in dosages of 200 to 400 mg daily is as efficacious as nystatin in dosages of 0.5 to 3 MU four times daily for the treatment of oral candidiasis, but it is superior in the prevention of candidiasis at other mucocutaneous sites (*Candida* esophagitis and vaginal candidiasis) and in the prevention of systemic candidal infections.[31,40,41] Fluconazole 100 mg orally appears to be as efficacious as ketoconazole 400 mg daily, clotrimazole troches 10 mg five times daily, or amphotericin B 400 mg (as 200-mg tablets plus 200-mg suspension) administered

TABLE 110–3. Therapy of Candidiasis[a]

Type of Disease and Common Clinical Manifestations	Therapy / Comments[b]
Chronic mucocutaneous candidiasis	KETO 100–200 mg PO QD *or* FLU 100 mg PO QD *or* ITRA 100–200 mg PO QD
Oral candidiasis (thrush)	
Treatment:	
Acute disease	Non–AIDS: FLU 100 mg PO QD *or* KETO 400 mg PO QD *or* ITRA 200 mg PO QD AIDS: generally not recommended because of development of resistant isolates
Resistant isolates	FLU 400–800 mg PO QD *or* ITRA-S 200–400mg PO QD *or* AmB-S 100 mg topically QID × 2 weeks
Esophageal candidiasis	FLU 100–200 mg PO QD *or* KETO 100–200mg PO QD *or* AmB 10–15 mg IV QD
Vaginal candidiasis	
Acute therapy	Topical agents (miconazole, clotrimazole) PV QD × 1–3 days *or* FLU 150 mg PO × 1 dose *or* KETO 100–200 mg PO
Suppression of recurrent infections	FLU 100 mg PO QD
Invasive candidiasis	
Prophylaxis	FLU 100 mg PO QD *or* KETO 400 mg PO QD *or* ITRA 200 mg PO QD
Treatment	Nonimmunocompromised host: FLU 400 mg IV/PO QD *or* AmB 0.5 mg/kg/d IV Immunocompromised host: AmB 0.5–0.75 mg/kg/day (total dosages of 0.5–1 g) *or* Lipid formulation of AmB 3–5 mg/kg/day (in patients who fail therapy with traditional AmB)
Candiduria	AmB bladder wash (50 mg in 500 mL of sterile water) can be instilled twice daily into the bladder via a three-way catheter) *or* FLU 100 mg PO QD

[a]Therapy is generally the same for AIDS/non–AIDS patients except where indicated.
[b]When more than one therapy is listed, they are listed in order of preference.
AIDS = acquired immunodeficiency disease syndrome; AmB = amphotericin B; AmB-S = amphotericin B oral solution; IT = intrathecal; 5-FC = flucytosine; FLU = fluconazole; ITRA = itraconazole; ITRA-S = itraconazole oral solution; KETO = ketoconazole.
Compiled from Refs. 18, 31, and 40.

four times daily in the prophylaxis or therapy of oropharyngeal candidiasis.[40,41]

HUMAN IMMUNODEFICIENCY VIRUS-INFECTED PATIENT

In the AIDS patient, nystatin therapy is often poorly tolerated or inefficacious in the prevention or treatment of oral candidiasis (Table 110–3). The recurrent nature of oral candidiasis and the propensity for the development of esophageal candidiasis in this population suggests that topical agents may not be sufficient. Fluconazole in dosages of 100 mg daily is superior to ketoconazole 200 mg daily, and dosages of 100 mg daily are superior to clotrimazole 10 mg five times daily. Although fluconazole has become the drug of choice for the treatment of oral thrush in AIDS patients, most authorities advocate the use of topical preparations for initial therapy since they are less costly, are associated with few side effects and drug interactions, and pose a lower risk for the development of resistance.[18,31,42]

ESOPHAGEAL CANDIDIASIS

Candida esophagitis is most commonly associated with the treatment of malignancies and AIDS patients, although it occasionally occurs in patients with no known underlying risk factors. Patients generally complain of pain and difficulty in swallowing, a feeling of obstruction, and occasionally substernal chest pain. Patients may occasionally have no symptoms until obstruction, bleeding, or perforation of the esophagus occurs.[8]

Although a definitive diagnosis is made by endoscopy with brush biopsy, a barium swallow can often reveal a characteristic "shaggy mucosa" appearance. Although the need for endoscopy is controversial, in patients with AIDS, a variety of bacterial, viral, and protozoal pathogens can also cause similar symptoms and may be present in association with *C. albicans.* Although the presence of oral thrush is often used as a marker for esophageal candidiasis, based on the theory that esophageal disease arises from the "spread" of oral disease, as many as 20% to 50% of cancer patients with esophageal candidiasis have no associated oral candidiasis.[8]

The treatment of *Candida* esophagitis has not been well studied, particularly in patients with AIDS. Anecdotal evidence suggests that topical agents, such as nystatin and clotrimazole, are generally not efficacious because of a lack of contact time with the mucosa. Generally, systemic antifungal agents are required in this setting. Ketoconazole 200 to 400 mg daily has proven efficacious in small, noncomparative trials. A multicenter trial in predominantly AIDS patients demonstrated fluconazole 100 to 200 mg daily to be superior to ketoconazole 100 to 200 mg orally daily.[43] The decreased efficacy of ketoconazole in this population may be caused by the hypochlorhydria observed in some AIDS patients, resulting in a decreased absorption of ketoconazole. A lack of response to antifungal therapy can be a result of altered absorption of drugs, such as ketoconazole, or an inaccurate diagnosis. In patients who do not respond to oral therapy with ketoconazole or fluconazole, a low dose (10 to 15 mg) of IV amphotericin B is often successful.[18,31]

VAGINAL CANDIDIASIS

Vulvovaginal candidiasis is characterized by the presence of a thick, curd-like vaginal discharge, intense pruritus, and the presence of masses of epithelial cell, hyphae, and pseudohyphae on potassium hydroxide (KOH) smear of the vaginal discharge. Vulvovaginal candidiasis is a common infection in women; approximately one-fourth of women in their childbearing years develop an infection.[8] Factors thought to predispose toward the development of vulvovaginal candidiasis include the use of hormonal contraceptives, pregnancy, obesity, debilitation, diabetes, and drug therapy with systemic corticosteroids, antineoplastic agents, and systemic antibiotics. Women with AIDS may be more susceptible to the development of recurrent vaginal infections with *C. albicans,* although studies have disputed this finding.[44]

Although treatment with 7-day topical regimens have been traditionally employed, studies have demonstrated success using 1- and 3-day topical regimens. Topical preparations are well tolerated, efficacious, and often less expensive than oral preparations, as they are available over the counter. A number of European studies have documented the efficacy of single oral doses (150 mg) of fluconazole. Not surprisingly, many women prefer oral therapy with fluconazole or ketoconazole (200 to 400 mg daily) to topical therapy in the management of vaginal infections with *C. albicans.* Fluconazole has been associated with birth defects, however, and even the single-dose therapy should not be used in pregnant women.[18,31]

HEMATOGENOUS CANDIDIASIS

EPIDEMIOLOGY

The term *systemic candidiasis* has been used in the literature to describe any candidal infection that invades beyond the membranes of the skin or mucosa. This term does not differentiate hematogenously disseminated candidiasis (in a neutropenic transplant patient) from infections arising from the urinary tract. Accordingly, some clinicians have proposed that systemic candidiasis be eliminated, and the term *hematogenous candidiasis* be used to describe the clinical circumstances in which hematogenous seeding to deep organs, such as the eye, brain, heart, and kidney, occurs in a patient.[18,31] Specific anatomic reference should be made to the site of the infection. For example, *Candida* infection of the peritoneum would be termed *Candida* peritonitis.

Hematogenous candidiasis is reported in significantly higher frequency because of the increased numbers of immunosuppressed patients, including those with lymphoreticular or hematologic malignancies, diabetes, immunodeficiency diseases, or those receiving immunosuppressive therapy with high-dose corticosteroids, immunosuppressants, antineoplastic agents, or broad-spectrum antimicrobial agents.[2,8,18,31] Patients who have undergone surgery (particularly surgery of the GI tract) are increasingly susceptible to disseminated candidal infections.[45,46] Data from the CDC's National Nosocomial Infection Survey implicated fungi as the cause of 7.9% of nosocomial pathogens implicated as a cause of infection. *Candida* species accounted for 79% of these nosocomial fungi.[18,31]

Pathophysiology

Candida is generally acquired via the GI tract, although organisms may also enter the bloodstream via indwelling IV catheters. Risk factors for hematogenous disease include prior therapy with antibiotics, the presence of indwelling urinary or IV catheters, recent surgery, concomitant bacterial infections, extensive burns, and the administration of total parenteral nutrition. In the postoperative group, patients undergoing organ transplants, heart surgery, or GI tract surgery are at the greatest risk of infection.[8,12,46] A case-controlled study in patients with acute lymphocytic leukemia found previous bacteremia, prolonged neutropenia, prolonged fever, prolonged administration of antimicrobial agents, treatment with multiple antimicrobial agents, and a relatively high concentration of *Candida* in the stool to be significant risk factors for candidemia. In a logistic regression analysis, however, only administration of vancomycin, imipenem, or both was identified as an independent risk factor for candidemia. Further analysis showed that administration of vancomycin promoted proliferation of *Candida* in the GI tract and that this proliferation was associated with an increased risk of candidemia.[18,31]

Recognition of the role of the GI tract in invasive *Candida* infections has led to efforts to decrease infections by prophylactic administration of topical or systemically absorbed antifungal agents in immunocompromised patients. This literature was reviewed by Reents and coworkers,[40] who concluded that the use of systemically absorbable agents, such as azole antifungal agents, appears to decrease the risk of invasive fungal infections. Concerns have been raised by numerous investigators, however, regarding the potential for selection of intrinsically resistant pathogens or the development of resistant strains with widespread use of these agents. For example, although administration of oral fluconazole appears to decrease the incidence of invasive *Candida* infections in patients undergoing bone marrow transplantation, some centers have reported an increase in the number of infections caused by *C. krusei,* a species of *Candida* that is intrinsically resistant to fluconazole.[40,47,48]

Dissemination of *C. albicans* can result in infection in single or multiple organs, particularly the kidney, brain, myocardium, skin, eye, bone, and joints. Three distinct presentations of disseminated *C. albicans* have been recognized. In the first (and most common) type, patients present with the acute onset of fever, tachycardia, tachypnea, and occasionally chills or hypotension. The clinical presentation is generally indistinguishable from that seen with sepsis of bacterial origin. The second group of patients develops intermittent fevers and are ill only when febrile. A third group of patients manifests progressive deterioration of their condition with or without fever.[11,39] In most patients, multiple, micro-, and macroabscesses are formed. Infection of the liver and spleen is becoming recognized as a particularly common and difficult to treat site of infection that characteristically occurs in patients undergoing chemotherapy for acute leukemia or lymphoma. Hepatosplenic candidiasis, which has been termed *chronic systemic candidiasis* by some investigators in order to distinguish this syndrome from acute, disseminated disease, is often manifested only as fever while the patient remains neutropenic (< 1000 WBC/mm^3). As the WBC count increases to > 1000 cells/mm^3, imaging studies can detect the presence of abscess or microabscesses in the liver and spleen, often found with acute suppurative and granulomatous reactions. Infection may persist for months and ultimately cause the patient's death despite aggressive systemic therapy with antifungal agents.[2]

Diagnosis

The diagnosis of hematogenous candidiasis remains a major stumbling block in the treatment of infectious diseases. Although a variety of serologic tests have been proposed for the detection of *Candida* protein antigens, serum antibodies to *Candida*, and antibodies to cell wall components such as mannan, no test has demonstrated reliable accuracy in the clinical setting for the diagnosis of disseminated infection with *Candida.*[6,8] The problem is often confounded by the absence of positive blood cultures; only 25% to 45% of neutropenic patients with disseminated candidiasis at autopsy have a positive blood culture with *C. albicans* prior to death. The interpretation of positive surveillance cultures of the skin, mouth, sputum, feces, or urine is hampered by their occurrence as commensal pathogens and in distinguishing colonization from invasive disease. Patients with positive blood cultures for *C. tropicalis* should, however, receive serious consideration as candidates for systemic antifungal therapy.

▶ TREATMENT: Hematogenous Candidiasis

NONIMMUNOCOMPROMISED PATIENT

The clinical management of suspected or documented candidemia poses significant clinical dilemmas (Table 110–3).[41,49,50] Fraser and colleagues[45] documented the high rate of mortality in nonneutropenic patients with fungal blood cultures. Mortality was highest in patients with sustained positive blood cultures, those who did not receive antifungal therapy, and those infected with nonalbicans strains of *Candida*. This study clearly documented the importance of early recognition and treatment of positive fungal blood cultures. Administration of fluconazole 400 mg daily is as efficacious as IV amphotericin B 0.5 to 0.6 mg/kg/d in nonneutropenic patients with blood cultures with *C. albicans*.[41,51] Few data are available for assessing the role of fluconazole as empiric therapy for fungemia or for isolates other than *C. albicans*. Since fluconazole has poor activity against *Aspergillus* sp. and some non-albicans strains of *Candida,* amphotericin B remains the therapy of choice in patients with suspected fungemia.

In some patients, particularly those patients with a relatively intact immune system and in whom candidemia is clearly associated with the presence of an indwelling venous catheter, removal of the catheter will result in spontaneous resolution. Withholding treatment of catheter-associated candidemia may be considered in patients who meet the following criteria: (1) no unexplained fever, (2) improving clinical course, (3) no recurrence of candidemia following removal of the IV catheter, and (4) no clinical evidence consistent with disseminated candidiasis.[11]

IMMUNOCOMPROMISED PATIENTS

In immunocompromised patients, the presence of candidemia has been associated with evidence of disseminated disease in > 70% of patients and a 70% to 80% fatality rate. Therapy should include removal of the catheter and administration of systemic antifungal therapy.[2] The optimal agent, dose, and duration of therapy is unclear, and patients must be carefully monitored with serial blood cultures and careful physical examinations, particularly of the retina. Most clinicians recommend amphotericin B in total dosages of 0.5 to 1 g administered over approximately 1 to 2 weeks in patients with *Candida* endophthalmitis and in all neutropenic patients with candidemia.[8,11,41] Longer courses of therapy may be needed in some patients.[11] The decision to add flucytosine to therapy with amphotericin B remains controversial; although *in vitro* studies document synergy with these agents against *C. albicans*, the *in vivo* efficacy has not been well studied at this time. Similarly, the clinical use of combinations of azole antifungal agents (ketoconazole, fluconazole, itraconazole) with amphotericin B or flucytosine is also under investigation.

Many clinicians advocate early institution of empiric IV amphotericin B in patients with neutropenia and persistent (> 5 to 7 days) fever.[41] Only two prospective randomized studies have examined the use of this practice. Pizzo and coworkers[52] evaluated neutropenic patients with fever of unknown origin after receiving broad-spectrum antimicrobial therapy with cephalothin, carbenicillin, plus gentamicin. After 1 week, patients were randomly assigned to discontinue antimicrobial therapy, continue antimicrobial therapy until resolution of fever and granulocytopenia, or continue antimicrobial therapy with the addition of amphotericin B (0.5 mg/kg/d). The results clearly favored administration of amphotericin B. The European Organization for Research on Treatment of Cancer (EORTC) conducted a prospective, randomized trial to evaluate the efficacy of empiric amphotericin B 1.2 mg/kg every other day or 0.6 mg/kg/d in febrile neutropenic cancer patients. The investigators concluded that empiric amphotericin B reduced the early mortality from fungal infection but appeared to have little effect on established infections, particularly in patients with progressive underlying diseases. Empiric therapy with amphotericin B was of particular benefit in patients who did not receive antifungal prophylaxis, those who were severely granulocytopenic, febrile patients with a clinically documented infection, and patients older than 15 years of age.[41,49,50]

Although empiric amphotericin B is clearly indicated for some patients, the potential toxicities (particularly nephrotoxicity) of this agent preclude its routine use in all patients. Suggested criteria for the empiric use of amphotericin B include (1) fever of 5 to 7 days duration that is unresponsive to antibacterial agents, (2) neutropenia of > 7 days duration, (3) no other obvious cause for fever, (4) progressive debilitation, (5) chronic adrenal corticosteroid therapy, and (6) indwelling intravascular catheters. In patients who fail therapy with amphotericin B, lipid formulations of amphotericin B may be used (3 to 5 mg/kg/d).[41,49,50]

CANDIDURIA

Within the urinary tract, most common lesions are either *Candida* cystitis or hematogenously disseminated renal abscesses. *Candida* cystitis often follows catheterization or therapy with broad-spectrum antimicrobial therapy. The diagnosis of *Candida* cystitis may be problematic because of the frequent presence of *Candida* pseudohyphae and yeast cells in urine specimens secondary to urethral colonization. The usefulness of urine colony counts or antibody coating techniques is of questionable value. The recovery of 10,000 organisms or visualization of both yeast and pseudohyphae from fresh midstream urine or from bladder urine obtained by single catheterization (not indwelling) is suggestive of genitourinary candidiasis.[8] In most patients, the infection is asymptomatic and clears spontaneously without specific antifungal therapy.

Initial therapy of candidal cystitis should focus on removal of urinary catheters whenever possible. If this is not feasible, local irrigation may be used. Amphotericin B (50 mg in 500 mL of sterile water) can be instilled twice daily into the bladder via a three-way catheter. Minimal quantities (< 3%) of amphotericin B are absorbed systemically from the bladder.[3] Alternatively, oral therapy with flucytosine or fluconazole can be considered for short courses of therapy; high urinary concentrations are achieved following oral administration. Flucytosine, however, may have serious hematopoietic side effects and resistance rapidly develops when the drug is used alone.[3] Although fluconazole is excreted as active drug in high concentrations in the urine, studies evaluating its use for *Candida* urinary tract infections have yielded conflicting results, in part because of the difficulties in differentiating colonization from infection and in controlling the role played by indwelling catheters.

ASPERGILLOSIS

EPIDEMIOLOGY

Aspergillus is an ubiquitous mold that grows well on a variety of substrates, including soil, water, decaying vegetation, moldy hay or straw, and organic debris. Although over 300 species of *Aspergillus* have been characterized, three species are most commonly pathogenic: *A. fumigatus, A. flavus,* and *A. niger.* The varying degrees of pathogenicity of each species depend on their relative geographical prevalence, conidial size and shape, thermotolerance, and production of mycotoxins. For example, transport of *A. fumigatus* conidia into the lungs is facilitated by their smaller diameter in comparison to *A. flavus* and *A. niger.*[53]

The term *aspergillosis* may be broadly defined as a spectrum of diseases attributed to allergy, colonization, or tissue invasion caused by members of the fungal genus *Aspergillus.* A single satisfactory classification system for these disease entities is difficult because different populations of patients may develop the same type of infection. For example, osteomyelitis may result from local trauma or hematogenous dissemination in an immunocompromised host. Colonization in normal hosts can lead to allergic diseases ranging from asthma to allergic bronchopulmonary aspergillosis or, rarely, invasive disease.[53,54]

PATHOPHYSIOLOGY

Aspergillosis is generally acquired by inhalation of airborne conidia that are small enough (2.5 to 3 μm) to reach alveoli or the paranasal sinuses. Each conidiophore releases 10^4 conidia that remain suspended for long periods and are viable for months in dry locations. Although monitoring of hospital air for *Aspergillus* conidia has been advocated by some authors, guidelines for interpreting results do not exist. The use of high-efficiency particulate air (HEPA) filters in operating rooms and laminar flow rooms and removal of immunocompromised patients from hospital renovation sites may be helpful in preventing infection in this population. Although the fate of *Aspergillus* conidia in the GI tract has not been closely studied, limited evidence suggests that this route may provide an important portal of entry for disseminated infections in humans.[53,54]

SUPERFICIAL INFECTION

Superficial or locally invasive infections of the ear, skin, or appendages can often be managed with topical antifungal therapy. Skin infections in patients with burn wounds, while uncommon, may progress to deep tissue invasion despite the use of topical or parenteral antifungal agents. Risk factors for deep infection include extensive thermal injuries, malnutrition, cirrhosis, and previous infection with *Pseudomonas aeruginosa.*[54]

ALLERGIC BRONCHOPULMONARY ASPERGILLOSIS

Allergic manifestations of *Aspergillus* range in severity from mild asthma to allergic bronchopulmonary aspergillosis (BPA). Bronchopulmonary aspergillosis, which is almost always caused by *A. fumigatus,* is characterized by severe asthma with wheezing, fever, malaise, weight loss, chest pain, and a cough productive of blood-streaked sputum. Following recurrent episodes of severe asthma, the disease usually progresses to fibrosis and bronchiectasis with granuloma formation. When *Aspergillus* conidia become trapped in the viscous mucus of asthmatic patients, BPA develops. The fungus grows, releasing toxins and antigens. The resulting host sensitization results in a variety of immune reactions. Early in the course of disease, an IgE-mediated (type I) immune reaction results in bronchospasm, eosinophilia, and immediate skin reactivity. The ensuing fibrosis and pulmonary infiltrates appear to be mediated by circulating or precipitating antibody complexes of IgG antibody, followed by granuloma formation and mononuclear infiltration because of a type IV delayed hypersensitivity reaction. Therapy is aimed at minimizing the quantity of antigenic material released in the tracheobronchial tree. Management of acute asthma attacks minimizes trapping of *Aspergillus* by bronchial secretions, and administration of parenteral corticosteroids clears lung infiltrates. Antifungal therapy is generally not indicated in the management of allergic manifestations of aspergillosis, although some patients have demonstrated a decrease in their corticosteroid dose following therapy with itraconazole.[53–55]

ASPERGILLOMA

In the nonimmunocompromised host, *Aspergillus* infections of the sinuses most commonly occur as saprophytic colonization (aspergillomas or "fungus balls") of previously abnormal sinus tissue. Infection is usually localized in the maxillary sinus and is rarely associated with local invasion of adjacent bone or brain tissue. Treatment consists of removal of the aspergilloma. Sinus aspergillosis can also present as allergic sinusitis with nasal drainage of brownish mucous plugs. Therapy with corticosteroids and surgery is generally successful. In the immunocompromised host, subacute, chronic, or fulminant invasive disease can be seen, and a combination of antifungal and surgical therapy is generally required.[53–55]

Pulmonary aspergillomas are fungus balls arising in preexisting cavities because of tuberculosis, histoplasmosis, lung tumors, or radiation fibrosis, although occasionally no previous pulmonary disease is present. Patients generally experience chest pain, dyspnea, and sputum production. Hemoptysis is observed in 50% to 80% of patients, probably because of ulceration of the epithelial lining of the cavity with formation of granulation tissue, and approximately 10% of patients have hemorrhage severe enough to cause death. Although *Aspergillus* can only be cultured in 50% to 60% of patients, precipitating antibodies are positive in virtually 100% of patients. Invasive disease rarely occurs, and therapy for this disease is controversial. Concern regarding the risk of severe hemorrhage has led some clinicians to use aggressive surgical excision of aspergillomas or pulmonary resection in patients with hemoptysis. Complications, including bronchopulmonary fistulas, hemorrhage, empyema, and persistent air space problems, have, however, led to the recommendation that surgical intervention be reserved for patients with severe (> 500 mL/24 hours) hemoptysis. Mild-to-moderate hemoptysis should be managed conservatively. Although IV amphotericin B is generally not useful in eradicating aspergillomas, intracavitary instillation of amphotericin B has been employed successfully in a limited number of patients. Hemoptysis generally ceases when the aspergilloma is eradicated.[53–55]

INVASIVE ASPERGILLOSIS

Although exposure to *Aspergillus* conidia is nearly universal, impaired host defenses are required for the development of invasive disease. Phagocytes (neutrophils, monocytes, macrophages) rather than antibodies or lymphocytes constitute the primary host defense system against invasive disease with aspergillosis. Macrophages prevent germination of conidia and also eradicate conidia, providing the first line of defense against invasive disease. Administration of corticosteroids appears to impair the killing of conidia by macrophages and impair mobilization of neutrophils. Neutrophils halt hyphal growth and dissemination and kill mycelia, constituting a second line of defense. Prolonged neutropenia appears to be the most important predisposing factor to the development of invasive aspergillosis, accounting for the high frequency of disease in patients with acute leukemia. Complement provides a source of chemotactic factor, and facilitates neutrophil damage to hyphae and monocyte killing of conidia. Complement is not necessary for the attachment or ingestion of conidia by human alveolar macrophages.[53–55]

Until recently, aspergillosis was an uncommon fungal infection in patients with AIDS. It has been suggested that AIDS patients are at less risk for aspergillosis than other fungal infections since the primary cellular defect in AIDS patients is in the T lymphocytes, whereas neutrophils and macrophages constitute the primary lines of defense to infection with aspergillosis. Until recently, aspergillosis has been reported as a late complication of disease in AIDS patients with additional risk factors for aspergillosis, such as corticosteroid use, neutropenia, previous *Pneumocystis carinii* or cytomegalovirus pneumonia, marijuana smoking, or the use of broad-spectrum antibiotics. One study reported, however, that approximately 50% of patients with aspergillosis had no classic risk factors. The majority of these patients had CD4+ counts < 50/mm^3. Although some patients diagnosed early in their infection responded to treatment, most have not responded to therapy with amphotericin B 0.5 mg/kg/d or itraconazole 200 to 600 mg daily.[56,57]

Invasive disease with *Aspergillus* can arise de novo or from any of the allergic or colonizing forms of aspergillosis. Predisposing factors to the development of invasive aspergillosis include glucocorticoid therapy, particularly following chronic administration or with higher dosages (30 to 200 mg of prednisone daily), cytotoxic agents, and recent or concurrent therapy with broad-spectrum antimicrobial agents. Patients with chronic hepatitis, alcoholism, diabetes mellitus, chronic granulomatous disease, leukopenia (< 1000 cells/mm^3), leukemia (particularly acute lymphocytic or myelogenous leukemia), lymphoma, and acute rejection of an organ transplant are also at a higher risk of invasive disease. Although rare, invasive aspergillosis has been reported in apparently normal hosts.[53–55]

Clinical Presentation

Although the lung is the most common site of invasive disease, the liver, spleen, brain, heart, GI tract, pericardium, and other body sites are involved in a substantial minority of cases. In neutropenic patients with *Aspergillus* pneumonia, hyphae invade the walls of bronchi and surrounding parenchyma, resulting in an acute necrotizing, pyogenic pneumonitis. As a result, patients often present with classic signs and symptoms of acute pulmonary embolus: pleuritic chest pain, fever, hemoptysis, friction rub, and wedge-shaped infiltrate on chest radiographs. Invasion of blood vessels causes thrombosis with resultant infarction, necrosis, and dissemination to other tissues and organs in the body. Survival beyond 2 or 3 weeks is uncommon. If bone marrow function returns, cavitation of the pulmonary lesion generally occurs and the spread of infection may be halted.[53–55]

Diagnosis

The diagnosis of aspergillosis is complicated by the presence of *Aspergillus* as a normal commensal in the human GI tract and respiratory secretions. Though suggestive of infection, the presence of hyphae in a smear or biopsy specimen is not diagnostic. Demonstration of *Aspergillus* by repeated culture and microscopic examination of tissue provides the most firm diagnosis.[6,14,53–55] The appearance of *Aspergillus* in tissues varies with increasing host resistance from the normal vegetative hyphae found with necrotic tissue and exudate in the alveoli of immunocompromised hosts to the compact tangled filaments ("granules") observed in fungal balls. Identification of *Aspergillus* is generally based on the appearance of 2 to 4 m wide septate hyphae that are dichotomously branched at 45-degree angles. Sporulation is rarely observed in tissue.[1,6,14]

In the immunocompromised host, aspergillosis is characterized by vascular invasion leading to thrombosis, infarction, and necrosis of tissue. Abundant hyphae in radially branching clusters can be observed in tissue. In contrast, vascular invasion is uncommon, and there are sparse numbers of hyphae in patients with chronic granulomatous disease. Although growth on Sabouraud dextrose or brain–heart infusion agar may be used for primary culture, bronchoscopy or bronchoalveolar lavage cultures are positive in only 40% of histopathologically identified specimens.[8] Blood or bone marrow cultures are rarely positive for *Aspergillus*.

Many clinicians have treated positive respiratory cultures of *Aspergillus* as a common contaminant and argued that a minimum of two to three positive cultures is necessary before antifungal therapy is indicated. Any positive culture, however, may be indicative of true infection in the immunocompromised host. In a large series (98 patients) reported by the National Institutes for Health, 82% of patients had positive fungal cultures at some point during the course of their terminal illness. Despite these vigorous culturing methods, only 34% of patients had one antemortem culture positive for *Aspergillus* and only 9% had more than one positive culture.[53] Isolation of *Aspergillus* from respiratory tract cultures correlated with proven aspergillosis in 100% of patients with acute leukemia, 94% of neutropenic patients, and 65% of patients receiving adrenal corticosteroids, but only 40% of patients receiving parenteral antibiotics.[58] Aspergillosis has been correlated with isolation of *Aspergillus* from nasal cultures.[59]

Serologic tests (immunoprecipitation, ID, and counterimmunoelectrophoresis) to detect antibody production to *Aspergillus* are generally helpful only in the diagnosis of allergic BPA and aspergilloma. Unfortunately, their usefulness in invasive aspergillosis is limited because of the inability of these patients to elaborate antibodies. Although serum precipitins are positive in 70% to 80% of patients with invasive pulmonary aspergillosis, the specificity and predictive value of single antibody titers is relatively low. Serum antigen detection has shown promise in animal models of *Aspergillus* infection; however, results cannot be directly extrapolated to humans since these models employed IV injection of *Aspergillus* rather than acquisition via the respiratory tract, as occurs in human hosts. Thus far, data from human studies suggest that serum antigen detection by radioimmunoassay may be valuable in the detection of pulmonary or disseminated infection, but less so in localized or sinus infections. These tests appear useful, however, in determining the prognosis of disease and response to antifungal therapy.[8,53]

▶ TREATMENT: Invasive Aspergillosis

Therapy for invasive aspergillosis is far from optimal at this time, in part because of the difficulties in establishing a diagnosis, and in part because of a lack of truly effective antifungal agents. Administration of amphotericin B appears to decrease mortality from > 90% to approximately 45%. These data, however, are difficult to interpret since many patients were diagnosed postmortem or amphotericin B therapy was not administered until the patient had very advanced disease. Mortality from pulmonary aspergillosis in bone marrow transplant recipients exceeds 94% regardless of therapy.[54] Although early diagnosis and administration of antifungal therapy may result in higher response rates, correction of underlying immune deficits (in particular, return of neutrophil counts) is of paramount importance in eradication of infection.[53,60]

Until the diagnosis of aspergillosis can be more rapidly and definitively determined, empiric therapy must be instituted when invasive disease is suspected. In patients at highest risk for invasive disease (acute leukemia and bone marrow transplant recipients), the most important predisposing factors include prolonged severe neutropenia (< 100 cells/mm^3 for > 1 week), graft rejection, chronic administration of corticosteroids, and tissue damage from preexisting infection. In these patients, antifungal therapy should be instituted in any of the following conditions: (1) persistent fever or progressive sinusitis unresponsive to antimicrobial therapy; (2) an eschar over the nose, sinuses, or palate; (3) the presence of characteristic radiographic findings, including wedge-shaped infarcts, nodular densities, and new cavitary lesions; or (4) any clinical manifestation suggestive of orbital or cavernous sinus disease or an acute vascular event associated with fever. Isolation of *Aspergillus* sp. from nasal or respiratory tract secretions should be considered confirmatory evidence in any of the previously mentioned clinical settings.[53–55]

NON–HUMAN IMMUNODEFICIENCY VIRUS-INFECTED PATIENT

The optimal dosage or duration of amphotericin B therapy for the treatment of invasive aspergillosis has not been determined.[54,61,62] Since *Aspergillus* is only moderately susceptible to amphotericin B, full doses (1 to 1.5 mg/kg/d) are generally recommended, with response measured by defervescence and radiographic clearing. The use of granulocyte transfusions or recombinant colony-stimulating factors to stimulate granulocyte production remains controversial, and controlled trials are lacking at this time. Although the addition of flucytosine, rifampin, or both is advocated by some authors, controlled clinical studies verifying the efficacy of these combination therapies are lacking. Amphotericin B (1 mg/kg/d) with flucytosine decreases mortality in neutropenic patients with pulmonary aspergillosis who did not receive a bone marrow transplant, but relapse is common. Response to therapy may be difficult to determine, since residual disease may remain for long periods of time and cavities may remain long after a patient becomes asymptomatic. Although liposomal preparations of amphotericin B appear less toxic than standard preparations, only limited data regarding their relative efficacy are available at this time.[54,61–63]

Although earlier azole antifungal agents (miconazole and ketoconazole) possessed poor *in vitro* activity against *Aspergillus* sp., newer triazoles have demonstrated improved activity both *in vitro* and in animal models of infection.[55] Itraconazole (100 to 500 mg daily for 11 to 192 days) has shown therapeutic benefit in patients with pulmonary, skeletal, and pericardial aspergillosis, particularly in those patients who are less immunocompromised.[54,55,64] The wide range of dosages, durations of therapy, and degree of immunosuppression in these trials makes selection of an appropriate regimen difficult. Jennings and Hardin[55] reviewed the role of itraconazole for aspergillosis and recommended that itraconazole be reserved as a second-line agent for patients intolerant or not responding to high-dose amphotericin B. If itraconazole is used, a loading dose of 200 mg three times daily with food for 2 to 3 days should be employed, followed by itraconazole 200 mg twice daily with food for a minimum of 6 months. Although early studies employing relatively low dosages (50 to 100 mg daily) of fluconazole demonstrated some activity against less invasive forms of aspergillosis, including chronic pulmonary disease and aspergillomas, data regarding the use of higher dosages (> 100 mg daily) in patients with invasive disease are not available.

The use of prophylactic antifungal therapy to prevent primary infection or reactivation of aspergillosis during subsequent courses of chemotherapy is controversial.[55,60] Studies assessing the utility of IV administration of amphotericin B in low doses (0.1 mg/kg/d) as prophylactic therapy or with higher dosages of 0.5 to 0.6 mg/kg/d as empiric therapy for invasive fungal infections in patients with granulocytopenia have not included sufficient numbers of patients to enable detection of differences in the number of *Aspergillus* infections.[55] The prophylactic use of intranasal amphotericin B aerosol sprays (5 or 10 mg daily in three divided doses) appeared beneficial in small studies in humans and animal models. A larger randomized trial found, however, that amphotericin B sprays reduced colonization of the nasal mucosa without any reduction in the frequency of invasive pulmonary infections with aspergillosis. Since failure of amphotericin B sprays may be because of the ability of small airborne conidia to access the alveolar spaces directly and establish infection, use of aerosolized forms of amphotericin B capable of reaching the alveolar spaces may be required.[55,65]

In granulocytopenic patients who recover from an episode of invasive aspergillosis, the risk of relapse of aspergillosis during subsequent courses of chemotherapy is > 50%. Secondary prophylaxis of aspergillosis with empiric administration of high-dose amphotericin B decreases the risk of relapse. Amphotericin B 1 mg/kg/d is started 24 to 48 hours prior to the start of chemotherapy and continued throughout the period of granulocytopenia. Some investigators recommend the addition of flucytosine (dosed to achieve peak serum concentrations of 30 to 60 μg/mL) to the amphotericin B regimen.[16] Although the use of itraconazole (alone or in combination with amphotericin B or flucytosine) may be beneficial in this patient population, little is known regarding its efficacy in this setting. If itraconazole is administered, serum levels should be monitored to assess absorption, since poor absorption of drug has been documented in this patient population.[16,64]

ANTIFUNGAL THERAPY

AMPHOTERICIN B

Amphotericin B remains the therapy of choice for many systemic fungal infections despite a lack of controlled clinical trials documenting the optimal dosage, duration of therapy, or relative efficacy of this agent in comparison to newer azole antifungal agents, such as ketoconazole, itraconazole, or fluconazole.[3,61,62]

Recommendations for the administration of amphotericin B are largely empiric and, in general, have not been tested in a controlled fashion. Most clinicians recommend administration of a 1-mg test dose of amphotericin B in 25 to 50 mL of 5% dextrose in water or as an aliquot of the initial daily dose infused over 1 to 2 hours in order to detect the rare patient likely to experience an anaphylactic reaction to the drug. If tolerated, the remaining daily dose is prepared in a concentration of 0.1 mg/mL of 5% dextrose and infused over 2 to 4 hours. Amphotericin B is usually administered in gradually increasing dosages; most guidelines suggest daily increments of 5 mg or 0.1 mg/kg until the maximum daily dose of 0.5 to 0.75 mg/kg daily is achieved. Many clinicians, however, advocate the rapid escalation of doses in patients with documented infections or highly suspicious clinical symptoms; often therapy is instituted with 0.25 mg/kg on the first day of therapy, followed by full-dose therapy on subsequent days of treatment.[3]

Infusion of amphotericin B over 2 hours is safe and may result in a lower incidence of fever and chills. The use of rapid infusions of amphotericin B should be avoided in patients with renal impairment because they may be unable to tolerate the increased intracellular potassium released secondary to high serum concentrations of amphotericin B.[3]

The optimal total dosage or duration of amphotericin B therapy has not been determined for most fungal infections. For most deep-seated infections, therapy is often continued for 6 to 12 weeks. In severe infections, however, those caused by less susceptible pathogens (*Aspergillus* or *C. tropicalis*), infections in sites that are difficult to penetrate, or in immunocompromised hosts, the daily dosage of amphotericin B may range up to 1 mg/kg and total dosages of 2 to 4 g of amphotericin B may be administered over a period of months to years.

The side effects of amphotericin B are generally categorized as acute (infusion-related) or long-term. Shaking chills, fever, myalgias, arthralgias, and headache are reported in > 50% of patients receiving amphotericin B. Evidence suggests that some of the infusion-related side effects may be caused by induction of prostaglandins. A variety of premedications are routinely used in an effort to decrease the incidence and severity of these reactions; however, few have been studied in a controlled fashion. Administration of oral ibuprofen (10 mg/kg) 30 minutes prior to administration of amphotericin B has been shown to reduce the incidence of chills from 87% to 49%. Meperidine has also been successful in terminating fever and chills in a randomized, double-blind trial. In another study, the administration of IV hydrocortisone (25 mg) at the beginning of amphotericin B infusions was significantly more effective than aspirin and diphenhydramine in reducing the incidence of fever, chills, and vomiting. Larger doses of hydrocortisone do not appear to offer any additional benefit.[3]

Thrombophlebitis is commonly reported in patients receiving amphotericin B therapy, probably as a result of the acidic pH of the reconstituted solution. Methods to reduce the problem include infusion into distal hand veins or in central venous lines in patients receiving long-term therapy, use of dilute solutions (< 0.1 mg/mL), and the addition of 500 to 1000 units of heparin per liter of solution. The efficacy of heparin in reducing the incidence of phlebitis has not been studied in a controlled fashion.[3]

The relatively nonselective affinity of amphotericin B for ergosterol versus cholesterol is thought to provide the basis for many of the long-term side effects of amphotericin B. The most significant side effect of amphotericin B administration is renal toxicity. Although the exact mechanism of this adverse effect is unclear, amphotericin B appears to alter membrane permeability and activate an intrarenal tubuloglomerular feedback mechanism that alters proximal and distal tubule delivery of ions, resulting in a decreased glomerular filtration and renal blood flow. Hypokalemia and hypomagnesemia may occur in association with decreased renal function, and the administration of supplemental potassium and magnesium may be required. Reversible impairment of renal function occurs within the first 2 weeks of amphotericin B therapy in up to 80% of patients. Irreversible renal dysfunction, while rare, occurs in some patients. It is unclear whether this effect is related to the total cumulative dosage of amphotericin B or individual patient susceptibility. Amphotericin B can also produce a reversible renal tubular acidosis in patients receiving total dosages of 0.5 to 1 g or more.[3] In an effort to decrease the incidence of nephrotoxicity, clinicians have tried several therapeutic modalities, including sodium loading, alternate-day therapy, and mannitol administration.

Amphotericin B can also produce a normochromic, normocytic anemia that is thought to result from a direct inhibition of erythrocyte or erythropoietin production. Hemoglobin concentrations generally return to normal within 2 to 3 months following discontinuation of amphotericin B. Thrombocytopenia has been rarely reported.

Combination therapy with amphotericin B and flucytosine may result in enhanced bone marrow suppression. The increased toxicity may result from enhanced cellular penetration of flucytosine or accumulation of flucytosine resulting from amphotericin B-induced renal dysfunction. Serum concentrations of flucytosine should be monitored carefully to maintain peak concentrations (2 hours after oral administration) of < 100 g/mL.[18]

The association between increased pulmonary toxicity with the concomitant use of amphotericin B and granulocyte transfusions remains controversial. Nevertheless, slow administration of amphotericin B and avoidance of concomitant administration of amphotericin B and granulocytes is recommended in order to minimize the potential interaction.

LIPOSOMAL AMPHOTERICIN B

Interest has been focused on the use of liposomally encapsulated preparations of amphotericin B. In these preparations, amphotericin B is incorporated into the phospholipid bilayer membrane, rather than in the enclosed aqueous phase. The preparation consists of both sheets and multilamellar spherical liposomes, ranging in size from 0.5 to 6 μm. The sheets contain more amphotericin B than do the spheres. The optimal preparation and sterol composition of these compounds is still not known (Table 110–4).[61,66–69]

TABLE 110–4. Pharmacology of Liposomal Preparations of Amphotericin B

	Deoxycholate Amphotericin	Amphotericin B Lipid Complex	Amphotericin B Colloid Dispersion	Liposomal Amphotericin
Brand name (manufacturer)	Fungizone (Bristol Myers Squibb, Lyphomed)	Abelcet (Liposome)	Amphocil (Sequus)	Ambisome (Fujisawa/Nexstar)
Molecular weight	416	306	531	706
Size (nm)	< 10	1600–11,000	120–140	80–120
Drug formulation	Micelles	Lipid complex	Colloid dispersion	Lyophilized powder
Appearance	Suspension	Ribbons, sheets	Disks	Small unilamellar vesicles
mol % amphotericin	34	35	50	< 10
Protein binding (%)	High 90	Low 12	High 99	High 99.8
Water solubility	Poor	Excellent	Poor	Poor
Dosage (mg/kg/day)	0.3–1	5	7	5
CSF penetration (CSF/serum)	Poor (< 10%)	Excellent (> 80%)	Poor (< 10%)	Poor (< 10%)
Elimination half-life (h)	20	30	8	21–64

CSF = cerebrospinal fluid.
Compiled from Refs. 8, 31, and 61.

The majority of liposomally encapsulated drug appears to be cleared by the reticuloendothelial system; amphotericin B is taken up by macrophages in the lung, liver, spleen, bone marrow, and circulating monocytes in plasma. In the lung, liposome-loaded monocytes migrate to alveoli to become alveolar macrophages. Although larger doses of these preparations are required to achieve similar pharmacologic effects as the desoxycholate form of amphotericin B, the toxicity appears to be much lower. Other clinical studies have used 30 mol% of amphotericin B in the same phospholipid, which provides a formulation with only sheets and ribbons, rather than spherical particles.[61,66]

The use of liposomal preparations of amphotericin B has resulted in decreased toxicity in animal models of infection and in early human clinical trials. Although preliminary studies appear encouraging, controlled clinical trials evaluating the safety and efficacy of liposomal preparations of amphotericin B are incomplete.[67]

FLUCYTOSINE

Flucytosine (also known as 5-flucytosine or 5-FC) is a fluorinated pyrimidine analog that is highly water soluble. Flucytosine is transported into the cell and transformed into 5-fluorouracil (an antimetabolite) by cytosine deaminase, which then inhibits DNA synthesis by incorporation into RNA. Patients with creatinine clearances > 40 mL/min should receive 100 to 150 mg/kg daily in four divided doses. The dosage should be reduced by 50% in patients with a creatinine clearance of 25 to 50 mL/min, and by 75% in patients with a clearance of 13 to 25 mL/min. Peak serum concentrations (2 hours after an oral dose) should be monitored in all patients (particularly those with a creatinine clearance of < 10 mL/min) to maintain peak serum concentrations < 100 mg/L.[4,70]

Flucytosine is generally associated with very few side effects in patients with normal renal, GI, and hematologic function, although rash, GI discomfort, diarrhea (5% to 10%), and reversible elevations in hepatic enzymes are occasionally observed. In patients with renal dysfunction or with concomitant amphotericin B therapy, leukopenia, thrombocytopenia, and (rarely) enterocolitis may occur. Although studies have suggested that little or no conversion of flucytosine to 5-fluorouracil occurs *in vitro,* serum concentrations of > 1000 ng/mL (therapeutic for the treatment of malignancies) have been documented in some patients. Investigators have theorized that flucytosine may be secreted into the GI tract, deaminated by intestinal bacteria, and reabsorbed as 5-fluorouracil.[70]

Flucytosine is used in the treatment of cryptococcosis, candidiasis, and chromomycosis. The rapid development of resistance to flucytosine, however, precludes its use as single-agent therapy except perhaps in the treatment of chromomycosis. Mechanisms for drug resistance may include loss of deaminase and decreased permeability to the drug.[70]

The introduction of the azole antifungal agents has rapidly expanded the armamentarium of agents useful in the treatment of systemic fungal infections. Clotrimazole, an early imidazole antifungal, proved inadequate for the treatment of systemic infections because it was found to induce its own metabolism rapidly after oral or IV administration. Its use is now largely confined to topical therapy, primarily for the treatment of vulvovaginal candidiasis and in the treatment and prophylaxis of mucocutaneous candidiasis. N-Substitution of imidazoles, such as miconazole, clotrimazole, and ketoconazole has resulted in the triazole antifungal agents itraconazole and fluconazole. Although these agents have the same mechanism of action and spectrum of activity as imidazoles, they appear to interact much less with human cytochrome P-450. Consequently, they have less effect on human sterol metabolism.[64]

AZOLE ANTIFUNGAL AGENTS

MICONAZOLE

Miconazole was the first systemically available imidazole antifungal agent (Table 110–5). Miconazole is poorly soluble in aqueous solutions and is, therefore, administered in a polyethoxylated castor oil vehicle (Cremaphor EL) for IV administration. This vehicle appears to be responsible for many of the adverse effects associated with miconazole therapy, which include phlebitis and pruritis in more than 20% of patients; nausea, fever, and chills in 10% to 20%; and vomiting and anemia in > 5%. With higher dosages of the drug, thrombocytosis, rouleaux formation of erythrocytes, and hyperlipidemia are reported. Rapid infusions of miconazole have resulted in cardiorespiratory arrest and anaphylactoid reactions, which are theorized to result from massive histamine release triggered by the solvent vehicle.

Although miconazole has been widely used for a variety of systemic fungal infections, including cryptococcosis, coccidioidomycosis, candidiasis, and paracoccidioidomycosis, its IV use has been largely supplanted by newer azoles. At this time, it remains the drug of choice for the treatment of infections caused by *Pseudallescheria boydii.* Miconazole is generally administered in dosages of 600 to 3600 mg daily in three or four doses as an IV infusion over 30 to 60 minutes. Miconazole is widely used in topical formulations for the treatment of vulvovaginal candidiasis and superficial skin infections.[18,31]

KETOCONAZOLE

Ketoconazole is a well-tolerated, orally available imidazole with a broad spectrum of activity against most fungal pathogens with the exception of *Aspergillus* sp. Ketoconazole is poorly soluble in aqueous fluids; it is soluble only in acidic (pH < 3) media. Consequently, the dissolution and absorption of ketoconazole is impaired in patients with elevated gastric pH. Patients with achlorhydria because of drugs (antacids or H_2-receptor antagonists) or disease (including AIDS patients) may not adequately absorb the drug. In addition, sucralfate appears to interfere with the absorption of ketoconazole when they are administered simultaneously. This

TABLE 110–5. Pharmacology of Azole Antifungal Agents

Feature	Miconazole	Ketoconazole	Itraconazole	Fluconazole
Water solubility	Poor	Poor	Poor	Excellent
Protein binding (%)	High 90	High 99	High 99.8	Low 12
CSF penetration (CSF/serum)	Poor (< 10%)	Poor (< 10%)	Poor (< 10%)	Excellent (> 80%)
Affinity for mammalian cyst P-450	High	High	Low	Low
Elimination half-life (h)	20	8	21–64	30
Excretion in urine (%)	< 5	< 5	< 1	80
Reduction of dose in renal failure	Not necessary	Not necessary	Not necessary	> 50 mL/min: no reduction 20–50 mL/min: reduce by 50% 10–20 mL/min: reduce by 75%
Oral bioavailability (%) with meal without meal	< 10%	~75[a] (See text)	99.8[a] 40[a] (capsule)	90[b]
Influence of food on oral bioavailability	Not applicable	Variable	Increase (capsule) decrease (solution)	None
Effect of gastric pH on oral bioavailability	Not applicable	Decrease	Decrease	None
Dosage formulations	IV 20 mg/mL IV solution in 1% Cremophor EL	Oral 200 mg tabs	Oral 100 mg capsules	IV/oral 50-, 100-, 150-, 200-mg tablets, 2 mg/mL IV solution, 50 mg or 200 mg/5 mL suspension
Usual daily dose	200–2400 mg	200–800 mg	100–400 mg	100 to 800 mg
Dosing regimen	Every 8 h	Once daily	≤ 200 mg: once daily > 200 mg: twice daily	once daily

[a]As compared to aqueous oral solution.
[b]As compared to IV solution.
CSF = cerebrospinal fluid.
Compiled from Refs. 18 and 31.

interaction can be avoided by separating the doses by 2 hours. For unclear reasons, some bone marrow transplant patients have also demonstrated a decreased absorption of ketoconazole. In achlorhydric patients, ketoconazole may be dissolved in 0.1 N HCl and the solution sipped through a straw (to avoid erosion of tooth enamel). Alternatively, administration of oral glutamic acid capsules (360 to 720 mg) may be employed to increase absorption.[18,31]

The most common adverse effect of ketoconazole is dose-related GI discomfort. Nausea, vomiting, and anorexia have been reported in over 20% of patients receiving 200 mg daily; the incidence rises to > 50% of patients when the dosage is increased to 400 mg daily. As many patients experience GI discomfort with ketoconazole, administration with food is generally recommended.

Ketoconazole inhibits adrenal steroid synthesis by reversible, dose-dependent inhibition of the cytochromes P450-dependent 11-β-hydroxylation of steroids. Although precipitation of adrenal crisis is exceedingly rare, patients should be considered potentially unable to mount an adrenal stress response. Administration of ketoconazole as a single (rather than multiple) daily dose appears to minimize adrenal axis suppression. Gynecomastia, decreased libido, oligospermia, azospermia, and impotence secondary to decreased testosterone synthesis have been reported in men following high (> 600 mg) daily dosages and during prolonged administration of lower dosages. Ketoconazole is teratogenic in rats and should not be used in pregnant women.[27,18,31]

ITRACONAZOLE

Itraconazole is an investigational triazole antifungal with a broad spectrum of antifungal activity. Despite its marked structural similarity to ketoconazole, itraconazole differs in several important respects. Itraconazole appears to have greater specificity against fungal versus mammalian cytochrome P450, resulting in greater potency and a decrease in P450-mediated side effects. In addition, itraconazole possesses excellent *in vitro* activity against *Aspergillus* and *Sporothrix* sp.

Like ketoconazole, itraconazole depends on the availability of low gastric pH for dissolution and absorption. Administration with food appears to enhance significantly the bioavailability of itraconazole capsules, while it decreases the bioavailability of the oral solution. Since itraconazole exhibits pH-dependent dissolution and absorption, absorption is impaired in patients receiving antacids or H_2-receptor antagonists and in patients with achlorhydria. Plasma concentrations of itraconazole following a single oral dose in HIV-infected patients are approximately 50% lower than concentrations observed in healthy volunteers.[18,31,64]

Adverse effects of itraconazole appear to be similar to those observed with ketoconazole, but they occur with lower frequency. Gastrointestinal disturbances (primarily nausea, vomiting, epigastric pain, and diarrhea) have been the most common complaints, occurring in up to 20% of patients. Although there are no data in humans, itraconazole, similar to the other azoles, is potentially teratogenic and should be avoided in pregnant women.[18,31,64]

FLUCONAZOLE

Fluconazole is a recently marketed triazole antifungal agent with markedly different pharmacologic features than previously marketed azole antifungals. The small molecular weight, low protein binding, and increased water solubility of fluconazole results in rapid, essentially complete absorption of drug following oral administration.

Fluconazole is excreted primarily (> 80%) as unchanged drug in the urine, with the remainder of the dose excreted as glucuronide and N-oxide metabolites in the urine and as unchanged drug in the feces.

Side effects of fluconazole suggest that the drug is well tolerated in most patients. Gastrointestinal complaints are the most frequently reported, followed by headaches and rash. Unlike ketoconazole, fluconazole does not inhibit testicular or adrenal steroidogenesis in healthy volunteers or hospitalized patients. Reversible alopecia occurs not infrequently and usually appears after several months of treatment with higher doses of fluconazole. Fluconazole has been associated with several well-described cases of fetal malformations and should not be used in pregnant women.[18,31,64]

DRUG INTERACTIONS WITH AZOLE ANTIFUNGAL AGENTS

Drug interactions with azole antifungals can generally be placed into two broad categories: (1) decreases in azole bioavailability because of chelation or secondary to increases in gastric pH and (2) interactions other with cytochromes P450-metabolized drugs. Drug interactions in the second category may result in increases or decreases in both the azole antifungal, the interacting drug, or in both drugs.[18,31]

Simultaneous administration of sucralfate and ketoconazole (and probably itraconazole but not fluconazole) results in a significant decrease in oral bioavailability, probably via a chelation interaction at acidic pHs. This interaction can be avoided by separation of doses by 2 hours.

The interaction of azole antifungal agents with other cytochromes P450-metabolized drugs is well recognized. The azoles appear to be metabolized almost entirely via the cytochrome P450 IIIA4 subfamily. As expected, they interact with other drugs metabolized partly or wholly via this enzyme pathway. Decreases in the metabolism of warfarin and cyclosporine because of administration of IV miconazole results in increased plasma concentrations and toxicity of both drugs. Although older agents, such as miconazole, have been poorly studied, numerous clinically significant interactions have been documented with ketoconazole, itraconazole, and fluconazole with a variety of other drugs (Tables 110–6 and 110–7). In most cases, the azole interferes with the metabolism of the other cytochromes P450-metabolized drug.

Particularly noteworthy are the interactions between azoles and cisapride, terfenadine, astemizole, or loratidine. Cisapride, terfenadine, and astemizole are metabolized almost entirely via the cytochrome P450 IIIA4 subfamily; inhibition of metabolism by azoles results in accumulation of the cardiotoxic parent drug. Torsades de pointes and fatal arrhythmias have been described as consequences of the interactions between azoles (ketoconazole and itraconazole) and terfenadine. Although no published reports are available, the manufacturer reports similar toxicities in patients receiving cisapride and itraconazole, ketoconazole, fluconazole, or miconazole (manufacturer's package insert for cisapride, September 1995). Syncope and torsades de pointes has been reported in a patient receiving erythromycin (which also inhibits cytochrome P450 IIIA4), ketoconazole and astemizole (manufacturer's package insert for astemizole, July 1993).

The interaction between ketoconazole and cyclosporine has been exploited in order to reduce drug costs associated with administration of cyclosporine following organ transplantation. Relative to ketoconazole and itraconazole, fluconazole appears to be intermediate in its ability to inhibit human cytochromes P450. The magnitude of fluconazole-induced inhibition of cyclosporine metabolism appears, however, to depend on the dosage of fluconazole.

Predictably, drugs, such as rifampin, rifabutin, isoniazid, phenytoin, and carbamazepine, which are known to induce the activity of cytochromes P450, result in increased metabolism of the azole antifungals and may result in therapeutic

TABLE 110–6. Effects of Concomitantly Administered Drugs on Azole Antifungal Drug Concentrations

Drug Affecting Azole Concentration	Azole Antifungal Drug Concentration[a]		
	Ketoconazole	*Itraconazole*	*Fluconazole*
Alterations in Cytochromes P450			
Carbamazepine	None known[b]	↓	None known
Phenytoin	↓	↓	None known
Isoniazid	↓	None known	None known
Rifampin	↓	↓	↓
Rifabutin	None known	↓	No effect[c]
Inhibition of Absorption from the Gastrointestinal Tract			
Sucralfate	↓	None known	No effect
H_2 receptor antagonists	↓	↓	No effect
Omeprazole	↓	↓	No effect
Antacids	↓	↓	No effect
Didanosine (DDI)	None known	↓	None known

[a]Reductions in plasma azole concentrations have led to therapeutic failure for some fungal infections.
[b]None known: Interaction has not been studied in human subjects; caution should be used in using this combination until further information is available.
[c]No effect: Drug combination has been studied in human subjects, and no clinically significant pharmacokinetic or pharmacodynamic interaction was detected.

TABLE 110–7. Effects of Azole Antifungal Drugs on Serum Concentrations of Concomitantly Administered Drugs

Drug Affected by Azole	Azole Antifungal Drug		
	Ketoconazole	*Itraconazole*	*Fluconazole*
Alterations in Cytochromes P450			
Warfarin	↑[a]	↑	↑[a]
Cyclosporine	↑[a]	↑[a]	↑[a]
Phenytoin	↑[a]	None known[c]	↑[a]
Triazolam, alprazolam, midazolam	↑	None known	None known
Diltiazem	↑	None known	None known
Lovastatin	None known	None known	↑
Zidovudine	None known	None known	↑
Carbamazepine	None known	None known	↑[a]
Terfenadine	↑[b]	↑[b]	No effect[d]
Astemizole	↑[b]	↑[b]	None known
Loratidine	↑	None known	None known
Cisapride	↑[b]	↑[b]	↑
Alterations in Cytochromes P450			
Oral hypoglycemics	↑	None known	↑
Isoniazid	↓[a]	None known	None known
Rifampin	↓[a]	None known	None known
Rifabutin	None known	None known	↑
FK 506	None known	None known	↑[a]
Quinidine	↑	None known	None known
Unknown Mechanisms			
Digoxin	None known	↑[a]	None known

[a]Clinically significant interaction; serum concentrations of drug, clinical status of patient, or both should be monitored.
[b]Life-threatening interaction causing arrhythmias; avoid use of combination.
[c]None known: Interaction has not been studied in human subjects; however, caution should be exercised in using this combination until further information is available.
[d]No effect: Drug combination has been studied in human subjects, and no clinically significant pharmacokinetic or pharmacodynamic interaction was detected.
Compiled from Refs. 18 and 31.

failures. Increased dosages of azole antifungals may be required in patients receiving these combinations of drugs.[18,31]

RESISTANCE TO ANTIFUNGAL AGENTS

Resistance to azole antifungal agents has been intensively studied, which is caused in part by the increase in the number of fluconazole-resistant *Candida* strains isolated from AIDS patients. This issue has been reviewed.[18,31,71,72]

Resistance to miconazole was noted only rarely. A single case report documented resistance in a strain of *C. albicans* isolated from a patient who had received miconazole per nephrostomy tube for 2 months for chronic *Candida* urinary tract infection.

Even though ketoconazole was used widely for the treatment of mucocutaneous candidiasis, resistant strains appeared very rarely. In patients with the uncommon syndrome of chronic mucocutaneous candidiasis, however, the chronic use of ketoconazole was associated with the emergence of ketoconazole-resistant *C. albicans.* It appears likely that resistance developed in this specific population of patients because of two factors: the chronic use of ketoconazole and the inability of patients with this syndrome to eradicate the organism by normal host defense mechanisms.

Fluconazole-resistant *C. albicans* have been noted almost entirely in AIDS patients and usually only after CD4 counts are < 50/μL and after fluconazole has been used chronically for repeated episodes of thrush over months to years. It appears that resistance develops in a step-wise progression in patients who have repeated episodes of thrush with one or several persisting strains of *C. albicans. In vitro* susceptibility testing shows a progressive decrease in susceptibility to fluconazole, and this has been correlated with clinical failure. This type of resistance has not yet become a problem in hospitalized patients treated with short courses of fluconazole or in those in whom fluconazole has been used for prophylaxis.[71,72]

In the last few years, among hospitalized patients, there is increasing evidence for a shift toward isolation of other resistant species, such as *Candida glabrata* and *C. krusei,* that have moderate or high-level resistance to fluconazole. This phenomenon has been especially common among patients in whom fluconazole has been used extensively.

Resistance has not been described widely with itraconazole. This may be partly related to the fact that the drug has been used primarily for treatment of endemic mycoses and not candidiasis. Even in patients never treated with itraconazole, however, *C. albicans* strains that are resistant to fluconazole also show decreased susceptibility to itraconazole.

The most commonly reported mechanisms of azole resistance among *C. albicans* isolates include reduced permeability of the fungal cell membrane to azoles, alteration in the target fungal enzymes (cytochromes P450) resulting in decreased binding of the azole to the target site, and overproduction of the fungal cytochrome P450 enzymes.[18,31,71] Studies have also suggested the presence of efflux pumps capable of actively pumping azoles from the target pathogen, thereby conferring multidrug resistance to azole antifungals.[18,31]

Torulopsis glabrata is intrinsically more resistant than *C. albicans* to ketoconazole. Several strains of *T. glabrata* have been well-characterized in terms of the mechanism of ketoconazole resistance. Decreased permeability to azoles has been described, but other strains show enhanced activity of the P450 cell membrane enzymes as well. *Candida krusei* is inherently resistant to fluconazole, but it appears to be more susceptible to the other azoles. Decreased uptake of fluconazole into the fungal cell has been noted for several *C. krusei* strains.[18,31,71,72]

▶ PRINCIPLES OF PHARMACOTHERAPY

- Systemic mycoses may be caused by pathogenic fungi, including histoplasmosis, coccidiomycosis, cryptococcosis, blastomycosis, paracoccidiomycosis, and sporotrichosis, or opportunistic fungi, such as *Candida albicans, Aspergillus* sp., *Trichosporon, Candida glabrata, Fusarium, Alternaria,* and *Mucor.*

- The diagnosis of fungal infection is generally accomplished by careful evaluation of clinical symptoms, results of serologic tests, and histopathologic examination and culture of clinical specimens.
- Histoplasmosis is caused by *Histoplasma capsulatum* and is endemic in parts of the central United States along the Ohio and Mississippi river valleys. Although most patients experience asymptomatic infection, some may experience chronic, disseminated disease.
- Asymptomatic patients with histoplasmosis are not treated, although non–AIDS patients with evident disease are treated with either oral ketaconazole or intravenous amphotericin B; AIDS patients are treated with amphotericin B, then receive lifelong suppression.
- Blastomycosis is caused by *Blastomyces dermatitidis* and is generally an asymptomatic, self-limited disease; however, reactivation can lead to chronic disease. Although treatment for self-limited disease is controversial, patients with chronic pulmonary disease or extrapulmonary disease should be treated with ketoconazole, and those with CNS, progressive, or life-threatening disease should receive amphotericin.
- Coccidiomycosis is caused by *Coccidioides immitis* and is endemic in some parts of the southwest United States. It may cause nonspecific symptoms, acute pneumonia, chronic pulmonary, or disseminated disease. Primary pulmonary disease (unless severe) is often not treated, while extrapulmonary disease is treated with amphotericin B, and meningitis is treated with fluconazole.
- Cryptococcus is caused by *Cryptococcus neoformans* and occurs primarily in immunocompromised patients. Nonimmunocompromised patients with acute meningitis are treated with amphotericin B with flucytosine. Patients infected with HIV require long-term treatment with fluconazole or itraconazole.
- A variety of *Candida* sp. (including *C. albicans, C. glabrata, C. tropicalis, C, krusei*) may cause diseases, such as mucocutaneous, oral, esophageal, vaginal, and hematogenous candidiasis, as well as candiduria.
- Ketoconazole, fluconazole, and itraconazole have been used successfully to treat mucocutaneous, oral, and esophageal candidiasis. Vaginal candidiasis may be treated with topical miconazole or clotrimazole or oral fluconazole or ketoconazole. Invasive candidiasis may be treated with fluconazole or amphotericin B.
- Aspergillosis may be caused by a variety of *Aspergillus* sp. that may cause superficial infections, pneumonia, allergic bronchopulmonary aspergillosis, or invasive infection. Treatment with amphotericin B is generally instituted but often not successful.

REFERENCES

1. Rinaldi MG. Problems in the diagnosis of invasive fungal diseases. Rev Infect Dis 1991;13:493–495.
2. Bodey GP. Fungal infections in cancer patients. Annals NY Acad Sci 1988;544:431–442.
3. Gallis HA, Drew RH, Pickard WW. Amphotericin B: 30 years of clinical experience. Rev Infect Dis 1990;12:308–329.
4. Galgiani JN. Susceptibility of *Candida albicans* and other yeasts to fluconazole: Relation between *in vitro* and *in vivo* studies. Rev Infect Dis 1990;12(suppl 3):S272–S275.
5. National Committee for Clinical Laboratory Standards. Reference method for broth dilution antifungal susceptibility testing of yeasts: Proposed standard. December 1992;12:25: Document M27-P.
6. de Repentigny L. Serodiagnosis of candidiasis, aspergillosis, and cryptococcosis. Clin Infect Dis 1992;14(supp 1):S11–S22.
7. Bennett JE. Mycoses. Introduction. In: Mandell GL, Bennett JE, Dolin R, eds. Principles and Practice of Infectious Diseases, 4th ed. New York, Churchill Livingstone Inc., 1995:2288–2289.
8. Bennett JE. Pathogenic fungi. In: Sherris JC, ed. Medical Microbiology, 2nd ed. New York, Elsevier, 1991:440.
9. Ghannoum MA. Is antifungal susceptibility testing useful in guiding fluconazole therapy? Clin Infect Dis 1996;22(suppl 2):S161–S165.
10. Pfaller MA, Rinaldi MG. Antifungal susceptibility testing: Current state of technology, limitations, and standardization. Infect Dis Clin North Am 1993;7:435–444.
11. Edwards JE. Candida species. In: Mandell GL, Bennett JE, Dolin R, eds. Principles and Practice of Infectious Diseases, 4th ed. New York, Churchill Livingstone Inc., 1995:2289–2306.
12. Beck-Sague C, Jarvis WR. Secular trends in the epidemiology of nosocomial fungal infections in the United States, 1980–1990. National Nosocomial Infections Surveillance System. J Infect Dis 1993;167:1247–51.
13. Vazquez JA, Sanchez V, Dmuchowski C, et al. Nosocomial acquisition of *Candida albicans:* An epidemiologic study. J Infect Dis 1993; 168:195–201.
14. Kaufman L. Laboratory methods for the diagnosis and confirmation of systemic mycoses. Clin Infect Dis 1992;14(suppl 1):S23–S29.
15. Kappe R, Seeliger HP. Serodiagnosis of deep-seated fungal infections. Curr Top Med Mycol 1993;5:247–280.
16. Walsh TJ, Lee JW. Prevention of invasive fungal infections in patients with neoplastic diseases. Clin Infect Dis 1993;17(suppl 2):S468–S480.
17. Perfect JR. Antifungal prophylaxis: To prevent or not. Am J Med 1993;94:233–234.
18. Kauffman CA, Carver PL. Antifungal Agents in the 1990s: Current status and future developments. Drugs 1997;53:539–549.
19. USPHS/IDSA Prevention of opportunistic infections working group. USPHS/IDSA guidelines for the prevention of opportunistic infections in persons infected with human immunodeficiency virus: Disease-specific recommendations. Clin Infect Dis 1995;21(suppl 1):S32–S43.
20. Bullock WE. *Histoplasma capsulatum.* In: Mandell GL, Bennett JE, Dolin R, eds. Principles and Practice of Infectious Diseases, 4th ed. New York, Churchill Livingstone Inc., 1995:2340–2353.
21. Bradsher RW. Histoplasmosis and blastomycosis. Clin Infect Dis 1996;22(suppl 2):S102–S111.
22. Drew RH. Pharmacotherapy of disseminated histoplasmosis in patients with AIDS. Ann Pharmacother 1993;27:1510–1518.
23. Dismukes WE, Bradsher RW, Cloud GC, et al. Itraconazole therapy for blastomycosis and histoplasmosis. Am J Med 1992;93:489–497.
24. Wheat J, Hafner R, Korzun AH, et al. Itraconazole treatment of disseminated histoplasmosis in patients with the acquired immunodeficiency syndrome. Am J Med 1995;98:336–342.
25. Wheat J, Hafner R, Wulfsohn M, et al. Prevention of relapse of histoplasmosis with itraconazole in patients with acquired immunodeficiency syndrome. Ann Intern Med 1993;118:610–616.
26. Chapman SW. Blastomyces dermatitidis. In: Mandell GL, Bennett JE, Dolin R, eds. Principles and Practice of Infectious Diseases, 4th ed. New York, Churchill Livingstone Inc., 1995:2353–2365.

27. National Institute of Allergy and Infectious Diseases Mycoses Study Group. Treatment of blastomycosis and histoplasmosis with ketoconazole: Results of a prospective randomized clinical trial. Ann Intern Med 1985;103:861–872.
28. Pappas PG, Pottage JC, Powderly WG, et al. Blastomycosis in patients with the acquired immunodeficiency syndrome. Ann Intern Med 1992;116:847–853.
29. Stevens DA. Coccidioides immitis. In: Mandell GL, Bennett JE, Dolin R, eds. Principles and Practice of Infectious Diseases, 4th ed. New York, Churchill Livingstone Inc., 1995:2365–2374.
30. Galgiani JN, Ampel NM. Coccidioidomycosis in human immunodeficiency virus-infected patients. J Infect Dis 1990;162:1165–1169.
31. Kauffman CA, Carver PL. Use of azoles for systemic antifungal therapy. Adv Pharmacol 1997;39:143–189.
32. Graybill JR, Stevens DA, Galgiani JN, et al. Itraconazole treatment of coccidioidomycosis. Am J Med 1990;89:282–290.
33. Galgiani JN, Catanzaro A, Cloud GA, et al. Fluconazole therapy for coccidioidal meningitis. Ann Intern Med 1993:119:28–35.
34. Bennett JE, Dismukes WE, Duma RJ, et al. A comparison of amphotericin B alone and combined with flucytosine in the treatment of cryptococcal meningitis. New Engl J Med 1979;301:126–131.
35. Dismukes WE, Cloud G, Gallis HA, et al. Treatment of cryptococcal meningitis with combination amphotericin B and flucytosine for four as compared with six weeks. New Engl J Med 1987;317:334–341.
36. Powderly WG, Saag MS, Cloud GA, et al. A controlled trial of fluconazole or amphotericin B to prevent relapse of cryptococcal meningitis in patients with the acquired immunodeficiency syndrome. N Engl J Med 1992;326:793–798.
37. Saag MS, Powderly WG, Cloud GA, et al. Comparison of amphotericin B with fluconazole in the treatment of acute AIDS-associated cryptococcal meningitis: The NIAID Mycoses Study Group and the AIDS Clinical Trials Group. N Engl J Med 1992;326:83–89.
38. van der Horst CM, Saag MS, Cloud GA, et al. Treatment of cryptococcal meningitis associated with the acquired immunodeficiency syndrome. N Engl J Med 1997;37:15–21.
39. Odds FC. Pathogenesis of candidosis. In: *Candida* and Candidosis: A Review and Bibliography, 2nd ed. London: Bailliere Tindall, 1988: 236.
40. Reents S, Goodwin SD, Singh V. Antifungal prophylaxis in immunocompromised hosts. Ann Pharmacother 1993;27:53–60.
41. Edwards DE. International conference for the development of a consensus on the management and prevention of severe candidal infections. Clin Infect Dis 1997;25:43–59.
42. Sangeorzan JA, Bradley SF, He X, et al. Epidemiology of oral candidiasis in HIV-infected patients: Colonization, infection, treatment, and emergence of fluconazole resistance. Am J Med 1994;97:339–346.
43. Laine L, Dretler RH, Conteas CN, et al. Fluconazole compared with ketoconazole for the treatment of *Candida* esophagitis in AIDS: A randomized trial. Ann Intern Med 1992;117:655–660.
44. White MH. Is vulvovaginal candidiasis an AIDS-related illness? Clin Infect Dis 1996;22(suppl 2):S124–S127.
45. Fraser VJ, Jones M, Dunkel J, et al. Candidemia in a tertiary care hospital: Epidemiology, risk factors, and predictors of mortality. Clin Infect Dis 1992;15:414–421.
46. Wey SB, Mori M, Pfaller MA, et al. Risk factors for hospital-acquired candidemia: A matched case-control study. Arch Intern Med 1989; 149:2349–2353.
47. Winston DJ, Chandrasekar PH, Lazarus HM, et al. Fluconazole prophylaxis of fungal infections in patients with acute leukemia: Results of a randomized placebo-controlled, double-blind, multicenter trial. Ann Intern Med 1993;118:495–503.
48. Goodman JL, Winston DJ, Greenfield RA, et al. A controlled trial of fluconazole to prevent fungal infections in patients undergoing bone marrow transplantation. N Engl J Med 1992;326:845–851.
49. Pfaller MA. Nosocomial candidiasis: Emerging species, reservoirs, and modes of transmission. Clin Infect Dis 1996;22(suppl 2):S89–S94.
50. Uzun O, Anaissie EJ. Problems and controversies in the management of hematogenous candidiasis. Clin Infect Dis 1996;22(suppl 2):S95–S101.
51. Rex JH, Bennett JE, Sugar AM, et al. A randomized trial comparing fluconazole with amphotericin B for the treatment of candidemia in patients without neutropenia. N Engl J Med 1994;331:1325–1330.
52. Pizzo PA, Robichaud KJ, Gill FA, Witebsky FG. Empiric antibiotic and antifungal therapy for cancer patients with prolonged fever and granulocytopenia. Am J Med 1982;72:101–111.
53. Andriole VT. Infections with *Aspergillus* species. Clin Infect Dis 1993;17(suppl 2):S481–S486.
54. Denning DW, Stevens DA. Antifungal and surgical treatment of invasive aspergillosis: Review of 2,121 published cases. Rev Infect Dis 1990;12:1147–1181.
55. Jennings TS, Hardin TC. Treatment of aspergillosis with itraconazole. Ann Pharmacother 1993;27:1206–1211.
56. Lotholary O, Meyohas M, Dupont B, et al. Invasive aspergillosis in patients with acquired immunodeficiency syndrome: Report of 33 cases. Am J Med 1993;95:177–187.
57. Stansell JD. Pulmonary fungal infections in HIV-infected persons. Semin Respir Infect 1993;8(2):116–123.
58. Yu VL, Muder RR, Poorsattar A. Significance of isolation of *Aspergillus* from the respiratory tract in diagnosis of invasive pulmonary aspergillosis. Am J Med 1986;81:249–254.
59. Aisner J, Murillo J, Schimpff SC, Steere AC. Invasive aspergillosis in acute leukemia: Correlation with nose cultures and antibiotic use. Ann Intern Med 1979;90:4–9.
60. Perfect JR, Klotman ME, Gilbert CC, et al. Prophylactic intravenous amphotericin B in neutropenic autologous bone marrow transplant recipients. J Infect Dis 1992;165:891–897.
61. Hiemenz JW, Walsh TJ. Lipid formulations of amphotericin B: Recent progress and future directions. Clin Infect Dis 1996;22(suppl 2): S133–S144.
62. Gallis HA. Amphotericin B: A commentary on its role as an antifungal agent and as a comparative agent in clinical trials. Clin Infect Dis 1996;22(suppl 2):S145–S147.
63. Ambisome data—Liposomal AmB in neutropenic patients. ICAAC abstract, 1997.
64. Como JA, Dismukes WE. Oral azole drugs as systemic antifungal therapy. N Engl J Med 1994;330:263–272.
65. Jeffery GM, Beard ME, Ikram RB, et al. Intranasal amphotericin B reduces the frequency of invasive aspergillosis in neutropenic patients. Am J Med 1991;90:685–691.
66. Mills W, Chopra R, Linch DC, et al. Liposomal amphotericin B in the treatment of fungal infections in neutropenic patients: A single-centre experience of 133 episodes in 116 patients. Br J Haematol 1994;86: 754–760.
67. Berenguer J, Munoz P, Parras F, et al. Treatment of deep mycoses with liposomal amphotericin B. Eur J Clin Microbiol Infect Dis 1994;13: 504–507.
68. de Marie S, Janknegt R, Bakker-Woudenberg IA. Clinical use of liposomal and lipid-complexed amphotericin B. J Antimicrob Chemother 1994;33:907–916.
69. Moreau P, Milpied N, Fayette N, et al. Reduced renal toxicity and improved clinical tolerance of amphotericin B mixed with intralipid compared with conventional amphotericin B in neutropenic patients. J Antimicrob Chemother 1992;30:535–541.
70. Francis P, Walsh TJ. Evolving role of flucytosine in immunocompromised patients: New insights into safety, pharmacokinetics, and antifungal therapy. Clin Infect Dis 1992;15:1003–1018.
71. Rex J, Rinaldi MG, Pfaller MA. Resistance of *Candida* species to fluconazole. Antimicrob Agents Chemother 1995;39:1–8.
72. Graybill JR. The future of antifungal therapy. Clin Infect Dis 1996; 22(suppl 2):S166–S178.
73. Ryan KJ. Pathogenic fungi. In: Sherris JC, ed. Sherris Medical Microbiology, 3rd ed. Norwalk, CT, Appleton & Lange, 1994:574.

111

INFECTIONS IN IMMUNOCOMPROMISED PATIENTS

Douglas N. Fish, PharmD, BCPS

An immunocompromised host is a patient with intrinsic or acquired defects in host defenses that predispose to infection. Advances in modern medicine are creating more immunocompromised hosts than ever before. Historically, many of these patients died from their underlying diseases. More aggressive therapy of underlying diseases and improved supportive care has led to often dramatic improvements in survival. Because aggressive therapy often renders these patients profoundly immunosuppressed for long periods, however, opportunistic infections remain important causes of morbidity and mortality. This chapter focuses on risk factors for infection, common pathogens and infection sites, and prevention and management of suspected or documented infections in hematology and oncology patients (including bone marrow transplant [BMT] patients), and solid organ transplant recipients. Infectious complications associated with human immunodeficiency virus (HIV) infection are discussed in Chapter 114.

RISK FACTORS FOR INFECTION

GRANULOCYTOPENIA

Granulocytopenia is an abnormal reduction in the number of granulocytes (primarily neutrophils) circulating in peripheral blood. Although exact definitions of granulocytopenia often vary, an absolute neutrophil count (ANC) of < $1000/mm^3$ indicates a reduction sufficient to predispose patients to infection.[1,2] The ANC is the sum of the absolute numbers of both mature neutrophils (polymorphonuclear cells, [PMNs], also called "polys," or "segs") and immature neutrophils (bands). The absolute number of polys and bands is determined by dividing the percentage of these cells (obtained from the white blood cell [WBC] differential) by 100 and multiplying the quotient obtained by the total number of WBCs.

The degree or severity of granulocytopenia is an important risk factor for infection.[1] All granulocytopenic patients are considered to be at risk for infection; however, those with an ANC of < $500/mm^3$ are at greater risk than those with ANCs of 500 to $1000/mm^3$. Most treatment guidelines use an ANC of < $500/mm^3$ as the critical value in making therapeutic decisions regarding the management of infections.[1–3] Risk of infection and death is greatest among patients with < $100/mm^3$ granulocytes.[1,2]

In addition to the degree of granulocytopenia, the rate of neutrophil decline and duration of neutropenia are important risk factors for infection.[1–3] In patients with chemotherapy-induced neutropenia, the rapidity of ANC decline increases the risk for infection. Patients whose ANCs are falling rapidly and are expected to be < $500/mm^3$ within 24 hours are already considered to be severely neutropenic and are treated accordingly. Infection risk also increases as the duration of neutropenia increases; patients with severe neutropenia of > 7 to 10 days' duration are considered to be at especially high risk.[2,4] The duration of chemotherapy-induced neutropenia varies considerably among subsets of cancer patients according to intensity of treatment; BMT patients may have no detectable granulocytes in peripheral blood for up to 3 to 4 weeks.

Bacteria and fungi commonly cause infections in neutropenic patients. Gram-negative bacilli (*Escherichia coli, Klebsiella pneumoniae, Pseudomonas aeruginosa*) and gram-positive cocci (*Staphylococcus aureus, S. epidermidis,* streptococci) are the most common causes of infection. Patients who are neutropenic for extended periods of time and receive broad-spectrum antibiotics are at risk for fungal infection, usually due to *Candida* or *Aspergillus* sp. Viral infections, although not as common as bacterial and fungal infections, may also cause severe infection in the granulocytopenic patient.[5] Successful treatment of infections in neutropenic patients is dependent on resolution of neutropenia.[1–4]

Although not readily quantifiable, abnormalities may exist in granulocyte function as well as cell numbers. Defects in phagocyte function may be caused by underlying disease (e.g., leukemias) or its treatment (e.g., corticosteroids, antineoplastic agents, radiation).[6] Leukemic patients with relapsing disease are at increased risk of infection, even in the absence of neutropenia.[1]

IMMUNE SYSTEM DEFECTS

In addition to granulocytopenia, defects in T-lymphocyte and macrophage function (cell-mediated immunity), B-cell function (humoral immunity), or both predispose patients to infection. Cellular immune dysfunction is the result of underlying disease or immunosuppressive drug therapy; these defects result in a reduced ability of the host to defend against intracellular pathogens. Patients with Hodgkin's disease and transplant patients receiving immunosuppressive drugs, such as cyclosporine, tacrolimus, mycophenolate, corticosteroids, antineoplastic agents, or azathioprine, are at risk for a variety of bacterial, fungal, viral, and protozoal infections (Table 111–1). While some of these pathogens are associated with asymptomatic or mild disease in normal hosts, they can cause disseminated, life-threatening infections in immunocompromised hosts.

TABLE 111–1. Risk Factors and Common Pathogens in Immunocompromised Patients

Risk Factor	Patient Conditions	Common Pathogens
Neutropenia	Acute leukemia Chemotherapy	Bacteria: *Escherichia coli, Klebsiella pneumoniae, Pseudomonas aeruginosa, Staphylococcus aureus, Staphylococcus epidermidis* Fungi: *Candida, Aspergillus, Zygomycetes* Viruses: Herpes simplex
Impaired cell-mediated immunity	Lymphoma Immunosuppressive therapy (steroids, cyclosporine, chemotherapy)	Bacteria: *Listeria, Nocardia, Legionella, Mycobacterium* Fungi: *Cryptococcus neoformans, Candida, Aspergillus, Histoplasma capsulatum* Viruses: Cytomegalovirus, varicella zoster, herpes simplex Protozoal: *Pneumocystis carinii*
Impaired humoral immunity	Multiple myeloma Chronic lymphocytic leukemia Splenectomy Immunosuppressive therapy (steroids, chemotherapy)	Bacteria: *Streptococcus pneumoniae, Haemophilus influenzae, Neisseria meningitidis*
Loss of protective barriers		
Skin	Venipuncture, bone marrow aspiration, urinary catheterization, vascular access devices, radiation	Bacteria: *S. aureus, S. epidermidis, Bacillus* sp. Fungi: *Candida*
Mucous membranes	Respiratory support equipment, endoscopy, chemotherapy, radiation	Bacteria: *S. aureus, S. epidermidis,* Enterobacteriaceae, streptococci, *P. aeruginosa, Bacteroides* sp. Fungi: *Candida* Viruses: Herpes simplex
Surgery	Solid organ transplantation	Bacteria: *S. aureus, S. epidermidis,* Enterobacteriaceae, *P. aeruginosa, Bacteroides* sp. Fungi: *Candida* Viruses: Herpes simplex
Alteration of normal microbial flora	Antimicrobial therapy Chemotherapy Hospital environment	Bacteria: Enterobacteriaceae, *P. aeruginosa, Legionella, S. aureus, S. epidermidis* Fungi: *Candida, Aspergillus*
Blood products, donor organs	Bone marrow transplantation Solid organ transplantation	Fungi: *Candida* Viruses: Cytomegalovirus, Epstein-Barr virus, hepatitis B, hepatitis C Protozoal: *Toxoplasma gondii*

Compiled from Refs. 4, 5, 8, and 30.

Defects in humoral immune function are frequently caused by underlying disease. Patients with multiple myeloma and chronic lymphocytic leukemia have progressive hypogammaglobulinemia.[7] Splenectomy performed as a part of the staging process for Hodgkin's disease places patients at risk for infectious complications. Disease states in which humoral immune dysfunction occur predispose the patient to serious, life-threatening infection with encapsulated organisms, such as *Streptococcus pneumoniae, Haemophilus influenzae,* and *Neisseria meningitidis.*

DESTRUCTION OF PROTECTIVE BARRIERS

Loss of protective barriers is a major factor predisposing immunocompromised patients to infection. Damage to skin and mucous membranes by surgery, venipuncture, intravenous (IV) and urinary catheters, radiation, and chemotherapy disrupts major host defense systems, leaving patients at high risk for infection. Chemotherapy-induced mucositis may erode mucous membranes of the oropharynx and gastrointestinal (GI) tract and establish a medium for subsequent infection by bacteria, herpes simplex, and *Candida.* Medical and surgical procedures, such as transplant surgery, indwelling IV catheter placement, bone marrow aspiration, biopsies, and endoscopy further damage the integument and predispose patients to infection. Infections resulting from disruption of protective integumental barriers are usually a result of skin flora, such as *S. aureus, S. epidermidis,* and various streptococci.[4,8]

ENVIRONMENTAL CONTAMINATION/ALTERATION OF MICROBIAL FLORA

Infections in immunocompromised patients are caused by organisms either colonizing the host or acquired from the environment. Microorganisms may easily be transferred from patient-to-patient on the hands of hospital personnel unless strict infection control guidelines are followed. Contaminated equipment, such as nebulizers or ventilators, and contaminated water supplies have been responsible for outbreaks of *P. aeruginosa* and *Legionella pneumophila* infections, respectively. Foods, such as fruits and green leafy vegetables, that are often heavily colonized with gram-negative bacteria and fungi are also sources of microbial contamination and subsequent infection in immunocompromised hosts.[8,9]

Most infections in patients with cancer are caused by organisms colonizing body sites, such as the skin, oropharynx, and GI tract.[8–10] The GI tract is the most common site from which infections in immunocompromised hosts originate. Periodontitis, pharyngitis, esophagitis, colitis, perirectal cellulitis, and bacteremias are predominantly caused by normal flora of the gut; bloodstream infections are thought to arise from microbial translocation across injured GI mucosa.[8,11] Normal flora may also be significantly disrupted and altered; oropharygeal flora rapidly changes to primarily gram-negative bacilli in hospitalized patients. The incidence and rapidity of oropharyngeal gram-negative colonization has been correlated with the severity of the underlying disease; 100% of seriously ill patients are colonized with gram-negative bacilli within 1 week of hospital admission, compared with 18% of less severely ill patients.[10] Many cancer patients may already be colonized with gram-negative bacilli upon admission, perhaps the result of frequent hospitalizations and clinic visits. In hospitalized cancer patients, 50% of infections, however, are caused by colonizing organisms acquired after admission.[9]

Although hospitalization and severity of illness are risk factors for colonization by gram-negative bacilli, administration of broad-spectrum antimicrobial agents has the greatest impact on flora of immunocompromised hosts. Use of these agents disrupts the delicate balance of GI tract flora and predisposes patients to infection with more virulent pathogens. Antineoplastic drugs (e.g., cyclophosphamide, doxorubicin, fluorouracil) and acid-suppressive therapy (e.g., H_2-receptor antagonists, antacids) may also result in changes in GI flora and possibly predispose patients to infection.[12]

Numerous factors, such as underlying disease, immunosuppressive drug therapy, and antimicrobial administration, determine the immunocompromised host's risk of developing infection. Several risk factors are present concomitantly in many patients (Table 111–1).

INFECTIONS IN NEUTROPENIC CANCER PATIENTS

Infection remains the leading cause of autopsy-determined death in neutropenic cancer patients (ANC < 1000/mm^3); 6% to 30% of deaths are caused by infection.[13,14] Patients with profound neutropenia are at greatest risk for systemic infection. Areas of impaired or damaged host defenses, such as the oropharynx, lungs, skin, sinuses, and GI tract, are common sites of infection. These local infections may also progress to cause systemic infection and bacteremia.[9] Febrile episodes in granulocytopenic cancer patients can be attributed to microbiologically or clinically documented infection in only about 30% to 40% of cases.[3,4,15]

ETIOLOGY

Table 111–1 lists organisms commonly infecting immunocompromised patients. About 55% to 60% of bacteremic episodes in cancer patients are the result of gram-positive organisms, compared to only 9% to 18% of episodes documented during the 1970s and 1980s.[4,16] This shift is thought to have been caused by the frequent use of indwelling IV catheters (e.g., Hickman, Broviac) and broad-spectrum antibiotics with excellent gram-negative activity but relatively poor gram-positive coverage.[4,7,8,15,17,18] *Staphylococcus aureus* and coagulase-negative staphylococci (especially *S. epidermidis)* are the most common organisms, but *Bacillus* sp. and *Corynebacterium jeikeium* may also cause indwelling catheter infections.[4,5] Viridans streptococci have also emerged as important pathogens, particularly in patients with chemotherapy-induced mucositis of the oropharynx.[4,15,19] Although gram-positive infections are associated with somewhat lower mortality rates compared to gram-negative infections (15% versus 30% to 75%, respectively), gram-positive infections may also cause severe complications, such as disseminated intravascular coagulation (DIC) and adult respiratory distress syndrome (ARDS).[4,5,15] Prevention and timely treatment of gram-positive infections are clearly of great importance in the management of neutropenic cancer patients.

Gram-negative infections remain important causes of morbidity and mortality in immunocompromised cancer patients, and the relative frequency of infection due to specific pathogens has been shifting among gram-negative infections as well. *Escherichia coli* and *Klebsiella* sp. remain the most common isolates at many centers. The frequency of infections resulting from other organisms, however, such as *Enterobacter, Serratia,* and *Citrobacter,* has been reportedly increasing.[4,5,14] *Enterobacter* sp. have emerged as important causes of bacteremias; the use of broad-spectrum antibiotics, particularly third-generation cephalosporins, is thought to have played a major role in this trend. Infections due to *Enterobacter, Serratia,* and *Citrobacter* may be difficult to treat because of the ease of β-lactamase induction and the more frequent development of resistance to multiple antibiotics.[4,5,15] Infections caused by *P. aeruginosa* appear to have decreased in frequency during the past decade; however, morbidity and mortality associated with these infections remain very high.[3,8,14] In addition, the frequency of infection caused by difficult to treat organisms, such as *Stenotrophomonas (Xanthomonas) maltophilia* and *Burkholderia (Pseudomonas) cepacia,* appears to be increasing at many centers, probably because of selective pressures of broad-spectrum antimicrobial use.[4,5,8,14,15] Although the GI tract is a common site of bacterial infection, severe infections caused by anaerobic organisms are relatively infrequent.[20] Anaerobes are most frequently found in mixed infections, such as perirectal cellulitis and mucositis-associated oropharyngeal infections.[4]

In addition to bacterial infections, neutropenic cancer patients are at risk for invasive fungal infections. Patients with extended periods of profound neutropenia who have been receiving broad-spectrum antibiotics, corticosteroids, or both are at the highest risk for invasive fungal infection. A large international autopsy study revealed that 12% to 25% of patients with hematologic malignancies had deep fungal infections not diagnosed prior to the time of death. Approximately 65% of these infections were the result of *Candida* sp., and another 30% were caused by *Aspergillus* species.[21]

Candida albicans is the most common fungal pathogen in neutropenic cancer patients, accounting for approximately 50% of all fungal isolates. Because candidal species are normal flora, alteration of body host defenses is an important risk factor for the development of these infections. Oral thrush is the most common clinical manifestation of fungal infection, occurring in up to 60% of all patients.[5] Mucous membranes damaged from chemotherapy and radiation serve as areas of candidal surface colonization and subsequent entry into the bloodstream; disease may then disseminate throughout the body. Organs, such as the liver, spleen, kidney, and lungs, are commonly involved in disseminated disease.[5,21] Hepatosplenic candidiasis, also known as chronic disseminated candidiasis, is an important infection in patients with hematologic malignancies.[22] *Candida* is isolated from the blood in less than 25% of these patients; therefore, histopathologic identification from biopsy specimens is often required.[3] Other species of *Candida,* such as *C. tropicalis, C. parapsilosis,* and *C. krusei,* are being isolated with increasing frequency. An increase has also been noted in infections caused by *Torulopsis glabrata, Trichosporon* sp., *Fusarium* sp., and *Curvularia.*[3,5,8]

Infections resulting from *Aspergillus* sp. are acquired via inhalation of airborne spores. After colonizing the lungs, *Aspergillus* invades the lung parenchyma and pulmonary vessels, resulting in hemorrhage, pulmonary infarcts, and a high mortality rate. *Aspergillus* sp. may also cause sinusitis in neutropenic patients. Prolonged granulocytopenia has been shown to be the primary risk factor for invasive pulmonary aspergillosis in neutropenic patients with acute leukemia; use of corticosteroids may also predispose patients to disease.[5,23] Invasive aspergillosis should be suspected in those neutropenic cancer patients colonized with *Aspergillus* who remain persistently febrile despite a week or more of broad-spectrum antibiotic therapy.[2,3,5,23]

Chemotherapy-induced mucous membrane damage may predispose neutropenic cancer patients to the reactivation of herpes simplex virus (HSV), manifesting as gingivostomatitis or recurrent genital infections. Untreated oropharyngeal HSV infections may spread to involve the esophagus and often coexist with candidal infections. Clinical disease resulting from HSV occurs most often in patients with serologic evidence (e.g., serum antibodies to HSV) of prior infection. Both HSV-seropositive BMT patients and HSV-seropositive leukemics receiving intensive chemotherapy are at high risk for recurrent HSV disease during periods of immunosuppression.[24,25]

Pneumocystis carinii and *Toxoplasma gondii* are the most common parasitic pathogens in immunocompromised cancer patients. Patients with hematologic malignancies (acute lymphocytic leukemia, lymphoma, Hodgkin's disease) and those receiving high-dose corticosteroids as part of chemotherapy regimens are considered to be at the greatest risk of infection.[5,25,26] Routine use of trimethoprim–sulfamethoxazole (TMP/SMX) prophylaxis has, however, substantially reduced the incidence of these infections.[25,26]

Because the majority of infecting organisms in cancer patients are from the host's own flora, some centers have employed routine surveillance cultures in an attempt to identify causes of fever and suspected infection prospectively. In a typical surveillance culture program, cultures of the nose, mouth, axillae, and perirectal area are performed twice weekly, and culture results correlated with the clinical status of the patient. Because these cultures are costly and of low diagnostic yield, the utility of surveillance culture programs is felt to be limited. Surveillance cultures are, however, useful as research tools and in certain clinical situations; these would include patients with prolonged profound neutropenia and in institutions with high rates of antimicrobial resistance or problems with virulent pathogens, such as *P. aeruginosa* or *A. flavus.* Recommendations are that surveillance cultures should be limited to the anterior nares for detecting colonization with methicillin-resistant *S. aureus* and *Aspergillus* and to the rectum for detecting *P. aeruginosa,* multiple-antibiotic–resistant gram-negative rods, *Candida,* or *Salmonella.*[2–4]

CLINICAL PRESENTATION

Because neutropenic cancer patients are at high risk for serious infections, frequent clinical assessments and physical examinations must be performed to search for possible signs of infection. The most important clinical finding in the neutropenic patient is the presence of fever. Fever in this setting is variously defined as a single oral temperature of $\geq$ 38.3°C, multiple oral temperatures of $\geq$ 38.0°C persisting for over 1 hour, or three oral temperatures of $>$ 38.0°C during a 24-hour period in the absence of other causes.[2–4] Because of the significant morbidity and mortality associated with infection in the neutropenic cancer patient, fever should be considered to be the result of infection until proven otherwise. The site of infection can be documented clinically or microbiologically in only 30% to 40% of febrile neutropenic cancer patients.[3,4,15] Other causes of fever unrelated to infection in this patient population include reactions to blood products, chemotherapeutic agents, and other drugs, including biologics, cell lysis, and the underlying malignancy itself.

At the appearance of fever, the patient should be carefully evaluated for other signs and symptoms of infection. The usual clinical signs and symptoms of infection may, however, be absent or altered in neutropenic patients because of their relative reduction in leukocytes and inability to mount an appropriate inflammatory response. For example, cough, sputum production and purulence, and dysuria, frequency, urgency, and pyuria were noted less commonly in granulocytopenic patients with pneumonia and urinary tract infections, respectively.[27] Even patients with bacteremia commonly exhibit no signs of infection other than fever.[4,27] At the onset of fever, at least two sets of blood cultures should be obtained, including cultures both from peripheral veins and vascular access devices. These cultures should be evaluated for bacteria and fungi. Urine cultures should be obtained if a urinary catheter is in place or the urinalysis is abnormal. Other cultures (e.g., diarrheal stools, sputum) should be obtained as clinically indicated. Because the lungs are a common site of systemic infection in this patient population, a chest radiograph should be performed at the onset of febrile episodes.[2–4]

▶ TREATMENT: Infections in Neutropenic Cancer Patients

FEBRILE EPISODES IN NEUTROPENIC CANCER PATIENTS

The goals of antimicrobial drug use in neutropenic patients (including BMT recipients) include prevention of bacterial, fungal, viral, and protozoal infections during periods of neutropenia and effective treatment of established infections to reduce patient morbidity and mortality and allow for administration of optimal neoplastic therapy. All of these goals must be achieved at the lowest possible toxicity and cost. Guidelines for management of febrile episodes and documented infections in neutropenic patients are presented in Figure 111–1.[2] These guidelines were first adopted by the Infectious Diseases Society of America (IDSA) in 1990 and revised in 1997. Although many controversies remain regarding optimal management of these patients, the IDSA guidelines remain the basis for antimicrobial management of febrile neutropenia.

Because fever in the neutropenic cancer patient is considered a result of infection until proven otherwise, high-dose, parenteral, broad-spectrum, bactericidal, empiric antibiotic therapy should be initiated at the onset of fever or at the first signs or symptoms of infection. Withholding antibiotic therapy until isolation of an organism results in unacceptably high mortality rates.[28] In immunosuppressed patients, undiagnosed infection can rapidly disseminate and result in death if left untreated or if treated improperly. Failure to initiate appropriate antibiotic therapy for *P. aeruginosa* bacteremia at the onset of fever in granulocytopenic cancer patients resulted in mortality rates of 15% and 70% within 12 and 48 hours, respectively.[29] Empiric antibiotic therapy has been able to reduce early morbidity and mortality by at least 50% compared to the pre-1970s.[14,28] Therapy must be appropriate, however, and promptly initiated.

The goal of empiric antibiotic therapy is to protect the neutropenic patient from early death because of undiagnosed infection. The optimal antibiotic regimen for empiric therapy in febrile neutropenic cancer patients remains controversial; however, because of their frequency and relative pathogenicity, *P. aeruginosa,* other gram-negative bacilli, and *S. aureus* remain the primary targets of empiric antimicrobial therapy. Although *P. aeruginosa* infections appear to have decreased in frequency, adequate antipseudomonal antibiotic coverage must still be included in empiric regimens because of the high mortality associated with this pathogen.[2–4,15,30]

At least five different types of empiric antibiotic regimens are in use: (1) monotherapy with antipseudomonal β-lactam, aztreonam, or carbapenem; (2) aminoglycoside plus an antipseudomonal penicillin (e.g., piperacillin), an antipseudomonal cephalosporin (ceftazidime, cefepime), or carbapenem (imipenem/cilastatin, meropenem); (3) double antipseudomonal β-lactam therapy; (4) addition of vancomycin to β-lactam regimens; and (5) fluoroquinolone (ciprofloxacin) in combination with antipseudomonal β-lactam, aminoglycoside, or vancomycin.[2–4,15,30] Each of these regimens is associated with both advantages and disadvantages, which are summarized in Table 111–2. There is no overwhelming evidence that any one of these regimens is superior to the others. The overall response to empiric antibiotic regimens in febrile neutropenic cancer patients is about 75% to 90%, regardless of whether or not a pathogen is isolated.[15]

In designing optimal empiric antibiotic regimens, clinicians must consider infection patterns and antimicrobial susceptibility trends in their respective institutions. Also, patient factors, such as drug allergies and concomitant nephrotoxins, must be considered. Regardless of initial antibiotic selection, empiric regimens must be appropriately revised on the basis of documented infections, susceptibilities of bacterial isolates, development of more defined clinical signs and symptoms of infection, or a combination of these. The IDSA guidelines recommend three general empiric antibiotic regimens, selected as shown in Figure 111–2. Other alternative regimens may also be appropriate, however, based on specific patient characteristics.

β-LACTAM MONOTHERAPY

Several β-lactam antibiotics have been evaluated as monotherapy for the management of febrile episodes in neutropenic cancer patients. These include antipseudomonal cephalosporins (cefoperazone, ceftazidime, cefepime), antipseudomonal penicillins (ticarcillin/clavulanic acid, piperacillin, mezlocillin), and carbapenems (imipenem/cilastatin, meropenem).[2] Although the ureidopenicillins (e.g., piperacillin, mezlocillin) have good activity against *E. coli, K. pneumoniae,* and *P. aeruginosa,* response rates in febrile neutropenic cancer patients have been only about 50%, much lower than the 75% to 90% response rates usually noted.[14] Regimens with ceftazidime, cefepime, and the carbapenems have been much more successful.[30,31,32] A landmark early study compared ceftazidime monotherapy with a three-drug combination (cephalothin, gentamicin, carbenicillin) in 550 episodes of fever and neutropenia.[31] Ceftazidime monotherapy was as effective as combination therapy in initial empiric management (first 72 hours); 78% of febrile patients with undocumented infections were managed successfully with one antibiotic, and no morbidity or mortality resulted from adding other antimicrobial agents only when clinically indicated. Ceftazidime monotherapy was more recently compared with the combination of piperacillin plus tobramycin in 876 febrile episodes.[15] Both regimens were similar in efficacy, even in patients with prolonged, profound neutropenia. Similar favorable results have been reported with cefepime and the carbapenems.[30,32–34]

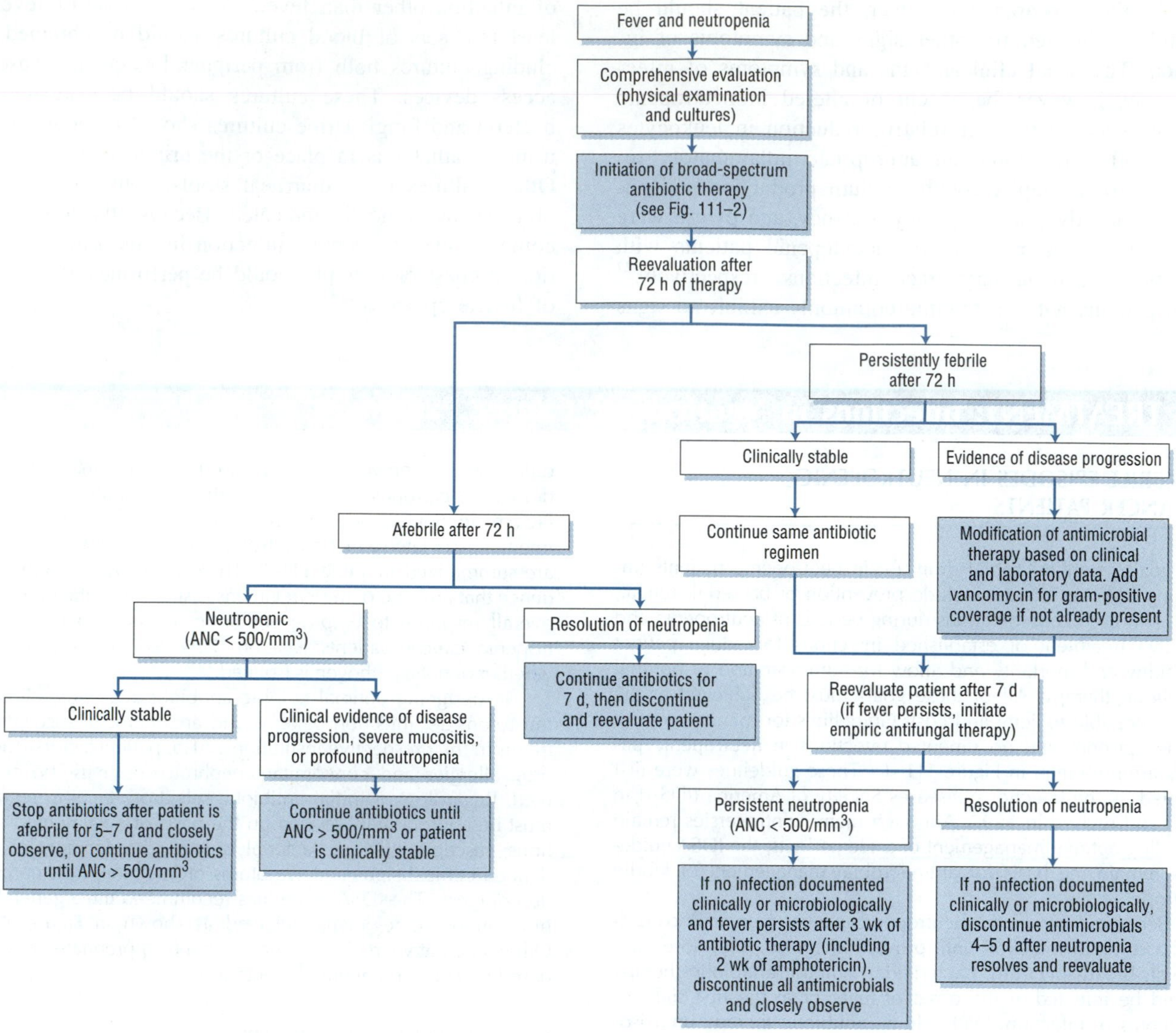

FIGURE 111–1. Management of febrile episodes in neutropenic cancer patients. ANC = absolute neutrophil count. (*Adapted from Ref. 2, with permission.*)

The use of monotherapy has many potential advantages and disadvantages (Table 111–2). Perhaps the most common concerns are those regarding the selection of resistant strains of organisms, such as *P. aeruginosa, Enterobacter* sp., and *Serratia* sp., through β-lactamase induction.[2,4,15,35] Activity against gram-positive organisms, such as coagulase-negative staphylococci, methicillin-resistant *S. aureus,* and enterococci, is poor with single β-lactams. Also, colonization and superinfection with both gram-positive and gram-negative organisms may occur more often with β-lactam monotherapy than when β-lactams are administered in combination with an aminoglycoside.[2]

Use of monotherapy may not be appropriate in institutions with high rates of gram-positive infections or infections caused by gram-negative pathogens such as *P. aeruginosa* and *Enterobacter* sp. Imipenem/cilastatin and meropenem, however, are less susceptible to inducible β-lactamases and may often be effectively used in these institutions. Monotherapy should be limited to patients with an ANC of 500 to 1000/mm^3 or only for brief periods of more severe neutropenia[2]; however, patients with more severe, protracted neutropenia may also be successfully treated with monotherapy.[2,4,15,31]

AMINOGLYCOSIDE PLUS ANTIPSEUDOMONAL β-LACTAM

Regimens consisting of an aminoglycoside plus an antipseudomonal penicillin, antipseudomonal cephalosporin, or carbapenem have traditionally been the most commonly used for empiric treatment of febrile neutropenia, although many such regimens may have inadequate gram-positive activity (Table 111–2). This relative lack of activity remains a concern because of the increasing incidence of gram-positive infections. The choice of aminoglycoside and β-lactam for inclusion in empiric regimens should be based on institutional epidemiology and antimicrobial susceptibility patterns. If *P. aeruginosa* is a common institutional pathogen, use of empiric tobramycin or amikacin should be considered since they are generally more active than gentamicin against this organism. Piperacillin and ceftazidime are the best studied drugs in this clinical situation.

Combinations of broad-spectrum β-lactams and aminoglycosides often provide synergistic activity against bacteria commonly infecting neutropenic patients. The exact role of synergy in the

TABLE 111–2. Comparative Advantages and Disadvantages of Various Antibiotic Regimens for Empiric Therapy of Febrile Neutropenic Cancer Patients

Regimen	Potential Advantages	Potential Disadvantages
β-Lactam monotherapy (ceftazidime 1–2 g every 8 h, cefepime 1–2 g every 8 h, or imipenem/cilastatin 0.5 g every 6 h)[a]	Efficacy apparently comparable to combination regimens, decreased drug toxicities, ease of administration, less expensive	Possibly less efficacy in profound neutropenia or prolonged neutropenia, limited gram-positive activity, no potential for additive/synergistic effects, increased selection of resistant organisms, increased colonization and superinfection rates
Antipseudomonal β-lactam plus aminoglycoside (piperacillin 4 g every 6 h or ceftazidime 1–2 g every 8 h + tobramycin)[a,b]	Traditional regimen, best studied; broad-spectrum coverage, optimal therapy of *Pseudomonas aeruginosa,* rapidly bactericidal, synergistic activity, decreased bacterial resistance, reduction of superinfections	Limited gram-positive activity, potential for nephrotoxicity, need for therapeutic monitoring of aminoglycoside concentrations
Double β-lactam combination (piperacillin 4 g every 6 h + ceftazidime 1–2 g every 8 h)[a]	Efficacy comparable to β-lactam/aminoglycoside regimens without nephrotoxicity risk	Limited gram-positive activity, possibility of antagonism, selection of resistant gram-negative organisms, may prolong duration of neutropenia, expensive
Empiric regimens containing vancomycin (ceftazidime 1–2 g every 8 h + vancomycin 0.5–1 g every 6–12 h)[a]	Early effective therapy of gram-positive infections	No apparent decrease in morbidity or mortality related to gram-positive infection, increased risk of selection for vancomycin-resistant enterococci, risk of toxicities, excessive cost, need for therapeutic monitoring of vancomycin concentrations
Fluoroquinolones (ciprofloxacin 0.4 g every 12 h + ceftazidime 1–2 g every 8 h, tobramycin,[b] or vancomycin 0.5–1 g every 6–12 h)[a]	Efficacy similar to other regimens when used in combination therapy, no cross-resistance with β-lactams, safe, possibility for oral administration; may be useful in patients with renal impairment in whom aminoglycosides are undesired	Marginal gram-positive activity, less efficacious as monotherapy, resistance may develop rapidly

[a]Dosing guidelines in patients with normal renal function.
[b]Tobramycin, 2 mg/kg loading dose, then maintenance dose determined by serum concentrations.
Adapted from Refs. 2, 3, 4, 15, and 30.

outcome of febrile neutropenic patients treated with empiric antibiotic therapy, however, remains somewhat controversial, particularly in light of the efficacy of single-drug regimens. Data from the European Organization for Research in the Treatment of Cancer (EORTC) demonstrate that response to combinations of β-lactam plus aminoglycoside is primarily related to the activity of the β-lactam agent; thus, the need for synergy with highly active agents, such as ceftazidime, is unclear.[4,15] Nevertheless, synergistic combinations of antibiotics appear to be beneficial in patients with persistent profound neutropenia. In one series, 44% of patients receiving a synergistic combination responded to treatment, whereas no responses were noted in patients receiving nonsynergistic antibiotic combinations.[36]

Aminoglycoside toxicity may be a concern in patients receiving these regimens because they may already be receiving other nephrotoxic drugs, such as cisplatin and cyclosporine. Administration of aminoglycosides in large single daily doses (once-daily dosing [ODD]) may be as effective, less costly, and no more toxic than conventional dosing methods.[37] Four randomized, prospective trials involving approximately 800 patients have now been conducted to evaluate the efficacy of ODD in febrile neutropenia. A review of these studies failed to find significant differences in either efficacy or toxicity between ODD versus traditional dosing of aminoglycosides.[38] Although ODD regimens appear to be safe and efficacious in these patients, there is not yet sufficient data to recommend ODD for routine use at this time.

DOUBLE β-LACTAM THERAPY

Double β-lactam therapy remains a controversial regimen for empiric management of febrile episodes in neutropenic patients. Several combinations of antipseudomonal β-lactams have been studied; all have included a penicillin (e.g., piperacillin) in combination with a cephalosporin (e.g., ceftazidime).[2] Combinations of broad-spectrum β-lactams are as effective as aminoglycoside/antipseudomonal β-lactam regimens.[2] Although double β-lactam combinations may be less toxic than aminoglycoside-containing regimens, these regimens are expensive and have relatively poor activity against gram-positive organisms. Also, theoretical concerns exist regarding possible antibiotic antagonism and the emergence of resistant organisms.[4,15,39] Double β-lactam regimens are not commonly used at most institutions.

EMPIRIC REGIMENS CONTAINING VANCOMYCIN

There has been considerable debate over the inclusion of vancomycin in initial empiric therapy of febrile neutropenia. This controversy continues because of the increasing incidence of gram-positive infections in these patients. One approach is to include vancomycin in the initial empiric antibiotic regimen, thereby providing early effective treatment of possible gram-positive infections. A second approach is to withhold vancomycin from initial empiric regimens, later adding the drug if gram-positive organisms are isolated from cultures or if there is no response to initial therapy. Support for both of these approaches can be found in the medical

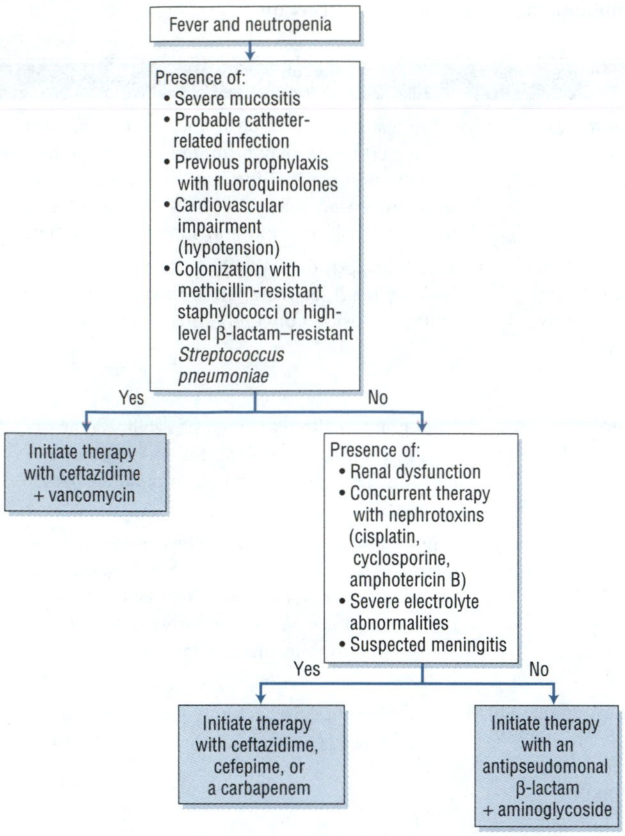

FIGURE 111–2. Guide to selection of initial empiric antibiotic therapy in neutropenic cancer patients. (*Adapted from Ref. 2.*)

literature.[2–4,15] Several prospective studies, however, indicate that there is no advantage to adding vancomycin to initial empiric regimens routinely.[40] In addition to increased costs of therapy, there is overwhelming evidence that the selection of vancomycin-resistant enterococci (VRE) is associated with excessive vancomycin use.[41]

Vancomycin is recommended for inclusion in initial empiric regimens only in patients at high risk of gram-positive infection, particularly because of methicillin-resistant *S. aureus* and coagulase-negative staphylococci.[2–4,15,30] These patients include those with evidence of infection of central venous catheters and other indwelling lines, severe mucositis, or pneumonitis in hospitals with high rates of methicillin-resistant staphylococcal infections. Empiric vancomycin use may also be justified in institutions employing empiric antibiotic regimens without good activity against streptococci (e.g., ciprofloxacin) and in patients known to be colonized with methicillin-resistant staphylococci or *S. pneumoniae* with high-level resistance to β-lactams. Lastly, empiric use of vancomycin may be recommended in patients with hypotension or other evidence of cardiovascular impairment.[2] Vancomycin use should be discouraged in patients not meeting these above criteria.[41] If vancomycin therapy is initiated and cultures remain negative after 72 hours, the drug should be discontinued.[4]

FLUOROQUINOLONE PLUS AMINOGLYCOSIDE, β-LACTAM, OR VANCOMYCIN

Because the fluoroquinolone antibiotics have broad-spectrum activity (particularly versus gram-negative pathogens), rapid bactericidal activity, and favorable pharmacokinetic and toxicity profiles, these agents have been investigated as empiric therapy in febrile neutropenic cancer patients. Ciprofloxacin is the preferred quinolone for use in this clinical situation because of its better activity against *P. aeruginosa*. Response rates of quinolone-containing combination regimens are comparable to those obtained with the other regimens previously described.[2,4,30] Quinolones are not recommended for monotherapy, however, because of their relatively poor activity against gram-positive pathogens and variable response rates in clinical studies.[2,4,30] Quinolones should also not be used as empiric therapy in patients who previously had received quinolones as infection prophylaxis because of the risk of drug resistance.[2,4] Although fluoroquinolones are not generally considered first-line empiric therapy, they may be useful as one component of combination regimens in patients with poor renal function.

ORAL ANTIBIOTIC THERAPY FOR INPATIENT AND OUTPATIENT MANAGEMENT OF FEBRILE NEUTROPENIA

Because of the excellent spectrum of activity and favorable pharmacokinetics of newer oral antibiotics, particularly the fluoroquinolones, conversion of IV therapy to oral therapy is possible and may allow for less expensive hospitalizations and earlier patient discharges. Studies have shown that carefully selected neutropenic patients may be safely switched from broad-spectrum parenteral therapy to oral antibiotics (usually ciprofloxacin) with response rates comparable to patients remaining on IV therapy.[42,43] Patient selection criteria often included defervescence within 72 hours after initiation of parenteral therapy, hemodynamic stability, absence of positive cultures or discernable site of infection, and ability to take oral medications. Many of these patients were able to complete their course of therapy at home.[2,42,43] Oral ofloxacin has also been studied as initial therapy of febrile neutropenic episodes; there was no difference in efficacy compared to patients receiving initial therapy with parenteral β-lactam/aminoglycoside regimens.[42,43]

The availability of oral antibiotics with broad spectrums of activity has even made possible the treatment of febrile neutropenia completely in the outpatient setting. Studies have demonstrated that patients undergoing chemotherapy with an expected duration of neutropenia of less than 7 days, or those with prolonged neutropenia but who are without fever and clinically stable, may safely self-administer antibiotics at home on first becoming febrile without examination by a physician or laboratory evaluation.[42,43] Fluoroquinolones, either as monotherapy or in combination with clindamycin or amoxicillin/clavulanate for enhanced gram-positive coverage, have been most commonly studied. Oral cephalosporins, such as cefixime, may also be suitable for outpatient treatment.[2] Careful patient selection is obviously required for such management strategies; important patient characteristics include a history of medication compliance, good caregiver support, and close proximity to medical care in the event of failure to respond to home therapy.

ANTIMICROBIAL THERAPY AFTER INITIATION OF EMPIRIC THERAPY

After the administration of 72 hours of empiric antimicrobial therapy, the clinical status and culture results of febrile neutropenic patients should be reevaluated to determine whether or not therapeutic modifications are necessary. Additions or modifications to the initial antimicrobial regimen will likely be required in patients with ANCs < 500/mm^3 for greater than a week. Modifications of antimicrobial therapy should be based on clinical and laboratory data; antibiotic therapy should be optimized based on culture results. During periods of neutropenia, however, patients should generally continue to receive broad-spectrum therapy because of the risk of secondary infections or breakthrough bacteremias when antimicrobial coverage is too narrow.[2–4,15,30]

INITIATION OF ANTIFUNGAL THERAPY

A high percentage of febrile patients who die during prolonged neutropenia have evidence of invasive fungal infection on autopsy, even though many had no evidence of fungal disease before death.[21] Persistence of fever or development of a new fever during broad-spectrum antibiotic therapy may indicate the presence of fungal infection in approximately 33% of patients.[44] The lack of rapid, sensitive diagnostic tests for fungi and the high morbidity and mortality associated with waiting for isolation of fungal organisms justify the empiric addition of antifungal therapy in this clinical setting.[44] Therefore, empiric antifungal therapy should be initiated after 4 to 5 days of broad-spectrum antibiotic therapy to prevent fungal superinfection or treat undiagnosed fungal infection.

The optimal empiric antifungal regimen is not presently known. Amphotericin B or fluconazole are, however, the antifungals most commonly used. *Aspergillus* is particularly common in patients with hematologic malignancies and BMT patients; therefore, amphotericin B is usually preferred in these patients.[4,21,23] Concerns regarding the emergence of azole-resistant fungi have also prevented fluconazole and itraconazole from replacing amphotericin B as the gold standard in persistently febrile neutropenic patients in spite of the high rate of amphotericin B toxicities.[4,21,23] Lipid-associated and liposomal amphotericin B products are promising in this setting because of their apparently reduced toxicities[45]; however, data in this setting are limited, and their role in the empiric therapy of febrile neutropenia is unknown at this time.[4]

Antifungal therapy should be continued for at least 2 weeks in the absence of signs and symptoms of active fungal disease, but many clinicians continue empiric antifungal therapy until resolution of granulocytopenia. In addition to fungal infections, other causes of persistent fever of unknown origin include resistant bacterial infection, tissue necrosis as a result of underlying tumor, nonbacterial and nonfungal infection (e.g., viral, mycobacterial, parasitic), and drug or blood product administration.

INITIATION OF ANTIVIRAL THERAPY

Febrile neutropenic patients with vesicular or ulcerative skin or mucosal lesions should be carefully evaluated for infection resulting from herpes simplex or varicella zoster virus (VZV). If viral infection is presumed or documented, these patients should receive aggressive acyclovir therapy to aid healing of primary lesions and prevent disseminated disease. Routine use of antiviral agents in the management of patients without mucosal lesions or other evidence of viral infection is not generally recommended.[2,4]

MANAGEMENT OF CATHETER INFECTIONS

Cancer patients are at high risk for development of catheter-related infections (incidence of 9% to 80%, depending on the series), most often because of *S. aureus* or coagulase-negative staphylococci.[2,3] The diagnosis of catheter-related bacteremia is made when blood cultures from both peripheral blood and the catheter itself are positive. Three types of infections have been identified: exit-site infection, subcutaneous tunnel infection, and catheter-related bacteremia/fungemia.[44] Indwelling catheters are invaluable for providing continued vascular access in these patients; attempts at controlling infections with antimicrobial therapy should be made in most cases prior to removing the catheter. Indications for catheter removal include subcutaneous tunnel infection, failure of bacteremia to clear within 72 hours after initiation of antibiotic therapy, persistence of fever, septic emboli, hypotension associated with catheter use, a nonpatent catheter, or bacteremia caused by *Bacillus* sp., *Corynebacterium jeikeium, P. aeruginosa,* and fungus (*Candida* sp.).[2,46] Removal of catheters in patients with fungemia may be adequate to achieve resolution of fungal infection; however, 10 to 14 days of antifungal therapy with amphotericin B or fluconazole may avoid development of fungal abscesses or disseminated disease. When multilumen catheters are involved, administration of antimicrobial agents should be rotated among the ports to ensure eradication of the infecting organism from all catheter sites.

DURATION OF THERAPY

The optimal duration of antimicrobial therapy in the neutropenic cancer patient remains controversial. Decisions regarding discontinuation of empiric antimicrobial therapy often are more difficult and complex than those regarding initiation of therapy (Fig. 111–1). One point on which most authorities agree, however, is that the most important determinant of the total duration of antibiotic therapy is the patient's ANC.[2–4] If the ANC is $\geq 500/mm^3$, the patient is afebrile for 48 to 72 hours and clinically stable, and no pathogen has been isolated, antibiotics may be discontinued after 7 days of therapy. Patients with ANCs of $< 500/mm^3$ should be maintained on antibiotics until resolution of neutropenia, even if afebrile.[2,47] Prolonged antibiotic use has been associated with superinfections resulting from resistant bacteria and fungi, and increases the risk of antibiotic-related toxicities.[4] If patients are clinically stable but the ANC is still $< 500/mm^3$, antibiotics may be discontinued after a total of 5 to 7 afebrile days. Patients, however, who remain profoundly neutropenic (ANC of $< 100/mm^3$), have mucosal lesions, or have unstable vital signs should continue to receive antibiotics until the ANC has increased to $\geq 500/mm^3$ or the patient is clinically stable. Patients who are persistently neutropenic and febrile, but who are clinically stable with negative blood cultures, may often be successfully discontinued from antimicrobial therapy. These patients, however, must be carefully monitored as reinstitution of antibiotics is necessary in approximately 50% of cases.[2–4] Patients with documented infections should receive antimicrobial therapy until the infecting organism is eradicated and signs and symptoms of infection have resolved (at least 10 to 14 days of therapy).

COLONY-STIMULATING FACTORS

Because resolution of granulocytopenia is the most important determinant of patient outcome from both febrile episodes and documented infections, many studies have evaluated hematopoietic colony-stimulating factors (CSFs) (sargramostim, granulocyte-macrophage colony-stimulating factor [GM-CSF], filgrastim, granulocyte colony-stimulating factor [G-CSF], and macrophage colony-stimulating factor [M-CSF]) as adjunct therapy to antimicrobial treatment of febrile neutropenic cancer patients.[48–50] These studies consistently found that the use of CSFs reduces the total duration and severity of chemotherapy-related neutropenia. Compared to placebo, however, these studies failed to demonstrate consistent benefits of CSFs related to important outcome variables, such as total febrile days, days of hospitalization, infectious complications, or mortality.[48–50] An expert panel of the American Society of Clinical Oncology (ASCO) has concluded that there is no clear support for the routine use of CSFs in febrile neutropenic patients.[48] The ASCO panel further concluded that the use of CSFs may be useful in patients with pneumonia, fungal sepsis, multiorgan dysfunction, hypotension, or other factors likely to cause rapid clinical deterioration. It was clearly stated, however, that even under these severe circumstances the benefits of CSF therapy were not substantiated. Although CSFs are not recommended for routine therapy of febrile neutropenia, clinical judgment may be exercised in determining which patients may likely benefit from judicious use of these expensive agents.

▶ TREATMENT: Prophylaxis

INFECTIONS IN NEUTROPENIC CANCER PATIENTS

Efforts are routinely made to prevent infectious complications in neutropenic patients through a number of environmental modifications and prophylactic antimicrobial regimens. The goal of antimicrobial prophylaxis in cancer patients is to decrease the number and severity of systemic infections during prolonged periods of neutropenia.

GENERAL MEASURES

Since about 50% of pathogens infecting neutropenic cancer patients are acquired in the hospital,[9] efforts at reducing acquisition of infectious organisms from the environment is a basic component in controlling nosocomial infection rates. Neutropenic patients should be placed in reverse isolation (isolation to protect patients from contracting infections after exposure to others) with strict adherence to infection control guidelines by hospital personnel. Proper, meticulous handwashing by hospital personnel is a simple, yet very effective infection control measure. Fresh fruits and vegetables are frequently colonized with bacteria and fungi; therefore, most centers exclude these foods from the diets of neutropenic patients.[8]

To reduce the risk of infection caused by airborne pathogens, such as *Aspergillus* sp., laminar air flow rooms are in use at some cancer centers. Laminar air flow rooms work by directing filtered air away from the patient, thus minimizing the risk of infection from airborne or environmental pathogens. When laminar air flow rooms are combined with dietary restrictions, infection control practices, and nonabsorbable antibiotics, rates of infection in neutropenic cancer patients are reduced by at least 50%.[51] Laminar air flow rooms are expensive, however, and use of these protective environments has not been shown to improve overall survival in BMT recipients.[8]

BACTERIAL INFECTIONS

Early attempts at pharmacologic reduction of flora colonizing the GI tract used combinations of nonabsorbable antibiotics, including gentamicin, nystatin, vancomycin, polymyxin B, and colistin. If anaerobic flora are preserved within the GI tract, risk of infection and subsequent bacteremia from virulent gram-negative bacilli is decreased; this is referred to as *colonization resistance.* These combinations of nonabsorbable antibiotics, however, destroy resident anaerobic flora as well as aerobic gram-negative rods. Therefore, colonization resistance is not preserved, and patients may be at risk for gram-negative infections because of translocation of virulent pathogens, such as *P. aeruginosa,* into the bloodstream.[52]

Although clinical trials have demonstrated that oral nonabsorbable antibiotics successfully reduce infections, these regimens are not routinely recommended for infection prophylaxis.[8] This is because of several problems associated with these regimens, including unpalatability, high cost, and frequent adverse effects (e.g., nausea, vomiting, diarrhea). Poor compliance inherent with these regimens may lead to abrupt discontinuation of antibiotics, which in turn may allow rapid repopulation of the GI tract with more virulent organisms and subsequent infection. Use of nonabsorbable antibiotic regimens has also been associated with the development of resistance to aminoglycosides among gram-negative bacilli, making the aminoglycosides useless as treatment alternatives for the ensuing infections.[8]

Recognition of the value of preservation of colonization resistance has prompted numerous studies of orally administered absorbable antibiotics, particularly TMP/SMX and the fluoroquinolones. Unlike nonabsorbable regimens, these antibiotics theoretically provide protection against systemic infections in addition to preserving colonization resistance and being well tolerated. Data from most placebo-controlled studies indicate that TMP/SMX significantly reduces infection rates in cancer patients.[2] Although TMP/SMX is also effective as prophylaxis against *P. carinii,* its lack of activity against *P. aeruginosa* is worrisome, particularly in institutions where pseudomonal infections are frequent. Other concerns with TMP/SMX prophylaxis include selection of resistant organisms, predisposition to development of fungal infections, and delay in bone marrow recovery resulting in prolonged neutropenic episodes.[8]

Numerous studies have shown that oral fluoroquinolones are more effective than placebo, nonabsorbable antibiotics, and TMP/SMX in preventing gram-negative infections in neutropenic cancer patients.[8] There are, however, several limitations to their injudicious use. In particular, quinolone prophylaxis has clearly led to an increase in the frequency of gram-positive infections. As a result, combination of a quinolone with a second agent providing enhanced gram-positive activity (e.g., rifampin, penicillin, or a macrolide) may be required for effective prophylaxis.[53,54] Quinolone prophylaxis has also been associated with the development of resistant gram-negative organisms.[8] In addition, quinolone prophylaxis has apparently not changed infectious mortality among cancer patients in spite of efficacy in preventing gram-negative infections. Last, patients experiencing breakthrough infection during quinolone prophylaxis should not be subsequently placed on a quinolone for empiric therapy, thus removing a valuable class of drugs from the available list of alternatives. The exact role of the fluoroquinolones remains unclear at this time.

The use of antibacterial prophylaxis remains somewhat controversial because of poor patient tolerance, lack of consistent efficacy, potential for development of resistant bacteria, high cost, and lack of impact on patient survival.[3,4] Prophylaxis, however, is generally indicated for patients expected to be profoundly neutropenic for greater than 1 week, such as BMT patients. Additional risk factors that may also provide justification for prophylaxis include extensive mucous membrane or skin lesions, presence of indwelling catheters, need for instrumentation, or severe periodontal disease.[2] Granulocyte recovery eliminates the need for continued prophylaxis, and recovery may be facilitated via use of CSFs.[48–50] In contrast to their unclear role in the treatment of febrile neutropenia, CSFs have been formally recommended by the ASCO for prevention of febrile neutropenia in high-risk patients. Such patients include those receiving chemotherapy regimens that produce a high rate of febrile neutropenia (> 40% incidence) or those with active tissue infection at the time of chemotherapy, history of febrile neutropenia with previous courses of chemotherapy, or underlying bone marrow compromise.[48]

FUNGAL INFECTIONS

Because most neutropenic patients are at risk for mucocutaneous candidal infections that may disseminate and cause serious systemic illness, antifungal prophylaxis is administered during high-risk periods. Antifungal agents administered for both local effects (nystatin suspension, clotrimazole troches) and systemic activity (ketoconazole, fluconazole, itraconazole) have been employed to prevent fungal infections. Although the choice of antifungal prophylaxis agents remains controversial, azole compounds (clotrimazole, ketoconazole, fluconazole, itraconazole) appear to be more effective and better tolerated than nystatin suspension.[55] Fluconazole prophylaxis (400 mg/d) has been particularly well studied and has been shown to reduce the incidence of both superficial and systemic fungal infections, as well as significantly decrease the mortality from fungal infections in BMT recipients.[55,56] The use of fluconazole prophylaxis has resulted in emergence of *C. krusei* and *Torulopsis glabrata* infections.[56,57] Routine fluconazole prophylaxis (400 mg/d) should, therefore, be limited to patients undergoing BMT.[58] Prophylaxis against fungal infection has also been shown to be beneficial in leukemic patients, although the choice of either fluconazole, itraconazole, or amphotericin B should be determined by the types of fungal isolates at individual institutions.[58]

Strategies being investigated for *Aspergillus* prophylaxis in neutropenic patients include the oral azole itraconazole, reduced doses of amphotericin B, and intranasal/aerosolized amphotericin B.[59] None of these interventions can be routinely recommended in clinical practice.

OTHER INFECTIONS

The use of TMP/SMX in cancer patients at risk for *P. carinii* pneumonia has substantially reduced the incidence of this infection.[8] Acyclovir prophylaxis is employed in most centers to reduce risk of HSV reactivation in patients with acute leukemia undergoing intensive chemotherapy.[24] Varicella vaccine provides good protection (90%) in leukemic children and may also be useful in seronegative adults, although the vaccine has been less well studied in this population.

EVALUATION OF THERAPEUTIC OUTCOMES

Close monitoring of febrile neutropenic patients, including both clinical and laboratory data, is essential for early detection and treatment of infectious complications. In addition, because many of the drugs that may be used in this setting have significant toxicity potential (aminoglycosides, amphotericin B), careful attention must be paid to the prevention and management of drug-related adverse effects. The reader is referred to individual chapters within this book for more detailed discussions of monitoring parameters related to specific types of infections (e.g., pneumonia, urinary tract infections).

INFECTIONS IN BONE MARROW TRANSPLANT PATIENTS

Along with graft-versus-host disease (GVHD), infection remains a major barrier to successful bone marrow transplantation. Recipients of BMT share risk factors discussed previously with other cancer patients. These patients, however, are at enhanced risk of infection because of prolonged periods of neutropenia. In addition, patients receiving allogeneic transplants have added immune system insults imposed by immunosuppressive drug therapy for the prevention and treatment of GVHD. Pretransplant conditioning regimens (high-dose chemotherapy and total body irradiation), as well as GVHD itself, often disrupt protective barriers, such as mucous membranes, skin, and the GI tract, placing patients at further risk of infection. Patients experiencing marrow graft failure have extended periods of profound neutropenia, often resulting in death due to infectious causes. Sargramostim (GM-CSF) is approved by the Food and Drug Administration (FDA) for marrow graft failure in both autologous and allogeneic transplants.

ETIOLOGY AND CLINICAL PRESENTATION OF INFECTIONS

After the administration of intensive conditioning regimens to eliminate malignant cells and prevent rejection of donor marrow, patients may remain profoundly neutropenic for 3 to 4 weeks. During this period, they are at risk for the same types of infectious complications noted in other granulocytopenic cancer patients (e.g., bacterial and fungal infections) and should be managed accordingly (Table 111–1). Regimens for the treatment of specific infections are given in Table 111–3.

In addition to bacterial and fungal infections, BMT recipients also are at risk for serious HSV infections manifesting as severe gingivostomatitis, esophagitis, genital lesions, and, rarely, pneumonia during the first month post-transplant. Clinical disease is more common in patients with serologic evidence (e.g., serum antibodies) of prior exposure and latent HSV infection pretransplant. Therefore, reactivation of latent disease during periods of immunosuppression is the most common etiology of HSV infection. Without prophylaxis, up to 80% of HSV-seropositive patients experience mucocutaneous disease after intensive chemotherapy, compared to less than 25% of seronegative patients.[25,46] The HSV infections often coexist with candidal infection and mucositis secondary to chemotherapy, radiation, or both. Painful swallowing associated with these conditions makes it difficult for patients to take oral medications and maintain adequate nutritional intake. Because of the considerable morbidity associated with reactivation of HSV post-transplant, the HSV serologic status of patients should be determined prior to transplant.

Recipients of BMT remain at high risk for infection after bone marrow engraftment has occurred. Significant defects in neutrophil function and cell-mediated and humoral immunity, persisting for several months post-transplant, predispose patients to infectious complications. Acute and chronic GVHD result in prolonged periods of immunosuppression and increased infection rates.

Bone marrow transplant patients are at high risk for cytomegalovirus (CMV) infections during the early postengraftment period. These range in severity from asymptomatic viral shedding (urine, throat, lungs) to life-threatening disseminated disease and interstitial pneumonia.

As with HSV, patients seropositive for CMV pretransplant are at high risk for recurrent disease during periods of immunosuppression; about 70% of seropositive patients

TABLE 111–3. Infectious Complications After Bone Marrow and Solid Organ Transplantation: Syndromes of Disease and Treatment Guidelines

Pathogen	Syndromes of Disease	Treatment
Bacterial		
Gram-negative aerobic rods (Enterobacteriaceae, *Pseudomonas aeruginosa, Haemophilus influenzae*)	Blood, urinary tract, pulmonary, abdomen	*Empiric*: Ceftazidime 1–2 g every 8 h + tobramycin[a,b]; piperacillin 3–4 g every 6 h + tobramycin[a,b] *Definitive*: According to culture and sensitivity results
Gram-positive cocci (*Staphylococcus aureus, Staphylococcus epidermidis, Streptococcus pneumoniae, Enterococcus fecaelis*)	Skin, blood, urinary tract, pulmonary, abdomen	*Empiric*: Nafcillin 1 g every 4–6 h; vancomycin 0.5–1 g every 6–12 h *Definitive*: According to culture and sensitivity results
Legionella sp.	Pulmonary	Erythromycin 0.5–1 g every 6 h
Listeria monocytogenes	Central nervous system	Ampicillin 1–2 g every 4–6 h with gentamicin[a]; TMP/ SMX 4 mg/kg every 12 h[c]
Nocardia sp.	Skin, pulmonary, central nervous system	Sulfadiazine 1 g every 4–6 h; TMP/SMX 4 mg/kg every 12 h[c]
Fungal		
Candida sp.	Blood, urinary tract, mucous membranes, skin	Clotrimazole 10 mg five times daily; nystatin 100,000 units every 6 h; ketoconazole 200 mg daily; fluconazole 100–200 mg daily; amphotericin B 0.5–0.7 mg/kg/day ± 5-flucytosine 100–150 mg/kg/d divided every 6 h
Aspergillus sp.	Skin, pulmonary, central nervous system	Amphotericin B 1 mg/kg/day ± 5-flucytosine; itraconazole 200–400 mg daily
Cryptococcus neoformans	Skin, pulmonary, central nervous system	Amphotericin B 0.5 mg/kg/day ± 5-flucytosine; fluconazole 400 mg daily
Zygomycetes (Mucor)	Rhinocerebral disease	Amphotericin B 1 mg/kg/day
Viral		
Herpes simplex virus	Skin, central nervous system, mucous membranes, pulmonary	Acyclovir 5–10 mg/kg every 8 h; foscarnet 40 mg/kg every 8 h
Cytomegalovirus	Pulmonary, blood, urinary tract, GI tract	Ganciclovir 5 mg/kg every 12 h; foscarnet 60 mg/kg every 8 h; hyperimmune globulins 100–500 mg/kg every 1–2 wk
Varicella zoster virus	Skin, disseminated disease	Acyclovir 10 mg/kg every 8 h, foscarnet 40 mg/kg every 8 h
Epstein-Barr virus	Lymphoproliferative disease	No effective treatment
Papovaviruses (BK, JC)	Skin, central nervous system	No effective treatment
Protozoal/parasitic		
Pneumocystis carinii	Pulmonary	TMP/SMX 15–20 mg/kg/day divided every 6 h[c]; atovaquone 750 mg every 12 h; pentamidine 4 mg/kg daily; dapsone 100 mg daily + TMP 15–20 mg/kg/day divided every 6 h; clindamycin 450–600 mg every 6 h + primaquine 15 mg daily
Toxoplasma gondii	Central nervous system	Pyrimethamine 50–100 mg daily + sulfadiazine 1 g every 4–6 h[d]; pyrimethamine 50–100 mg daily + clindamycin 450–600 mg every 6 h[d]
Strongyloides stercoralis	Pulmonary, central nervous system	Thiabendazole 25 mg/kg every 12 h (max 3.0 g/day)

[a]Tobramycin or gentamicin 2 mg/kg loading dose, then maintenance dose determined by serum concentrations.
[b]For penicillin-allergic adults, use ciprofloxacin 0.4 g every 12 h plus an aminoglycoside.
[c]Based on the trimethoprim component of the combination.
[d]Folinic acid (5–10 mg/d) often recommended in conjunction with pyrimethamine-containing regimens for prevention of bone marrow toxicity.
TMP/SMX = trimethoprim–sulfamethoxazole.

develop recurrent CMV disease after transplantation.[25,46,60] Other risk factors for CMV disease in BMT patients include advanced age, human lymphocyte antigen (HLA) mismatch, total body irradiation, multiagent conditioning regimens, and presence of GVHD.[46] Patients without evidence of latent CMV infection (CMV seronegative) pretransplant may develop primary CMV disease after receiving bone marrow or blood products from CMV-seropositive donors. Onset of both primary and recurrent CMV infection is 1 to 2 months post-transplant; patients receiving allogeneic transplants are at highest risk for CMV disease.[25,46]

The most serious clinical manifestation of CMV disease and the leading cause of infectious death in BMT recipients is interstitial pneumonia (IP), which is associated with an 85% mortality rate if untreated.[25,46] This clinical syndrome manifests as fever, dyspnea, hypoxia, nonproductive cough, and diffuse pulmonary infiltrates. Up to 40% of allogeneic BMT patients will develop IP, of which up to 40% of cases are the result of CMV.[25,46] Interstitial pneumonia also may be caused by other infectious (*P. carinii,* varicella zoster virus) and noninfectious causes (pulmonary damage by radiation and chemotherapy).

During the late transplant period (beginning about 4 months post-transplant), infections remain a major problem in patients suffering from chronic GVHD. Additional immunosuppressive therapy for treatment of GVHD places these patients at added risk for infection. Infections common during the late transplant period include those caused by encapsulated organisms, such as *S. pneumoniae* and *H. influenzae;* infections resulting from staphylococci and gram-negative bacilli are less common.[25,46] Patients not suffering from chronic GVHD generally have few infections in this period.

Up to 50% of all patients surviving up to 10 months post-transplant develop an infection caused by VZV. Infection with VZV is most common in patients receiving allogeneic transplants with acute or chronic GVHD.[25] Both primary (varicella) or recurrent disease (herpes zoster) usually present as skin lesions, most of which remain contained to local areas; however, 30% to 45% of these infections may disseminate to other cutaneous areas or body organs, causing mortality as high as 50%.[25,46]

▶ PROPHYLAXIS AND MANAGEMENT: Infection in Bone Marrow Transplant Recipients

The goals of antimicrobial drug use in BMT patients include (1) prevention of bacterial, fungal, viral, and protozoal infections during periods of neutropenia and postengraftment and (2) effective treatment of established infections. The overall goal of prophylaxis and treatment of infection in BMT patients is the prevention of infectious morbidity and mortality. These goals must be achieved at the lowest possible toxicity and cost. Prophylactic therapy should be specifically aimed at pathogens known to cause a high incidence of infection within the BMT population, the specific institution, or both. In addition, prophylactic therapy should be limited to those regimens proven to be effective through well-designed clinical trials.

BACTERIAL INFECTIONS

Prophylaxis of infections in BMT patients is in many ways similar to that used in other neutropenic patients. Selective decontamination with oral antimicrobials is commonly used; considerations are the same as those previously discussed. Fluoroquinolones have become the most frequently used agents, often combined with another agent (e.g., macrolides, rifampin) for enhanced gram-positive activity.[25,53,54] These regimens are usually begun within 72 hours of beginning the chemotherapy conditioning regimens and continued throughout the neutropenic period. Patients who become febrile while receiving prophylaxis should be managed according to general guidelines for febrile neutropenic patients.

Because of the high incidence of gram-positive infections following transplantation, some centers employ prophylactic parenteral vancomycin. Studies of this practice have produced conflicting data, and there are also concerns regarding the selection of vancomycin-resistant enterococci. Prophylactic vancomycin use is not recommended.[25]

VIRAL INFECTIONS

Prophylaxis of recurrent HSV infection has been evaluated in a number of clinical studies using various dosage regimens of acyclovir.[24] Depending on the series, 0% to 10% of HSV-seropositive patients receiving acyclovir experienced viral shedding, clinical symptoms of viral reactivation, or both compared to 60% to 80% of patients receiving placebo. Acyclovir doses commonly used for prophylaxis are 250 mg/m^2 (5 mg/kg) IV every 8 to 12 hours or 200 to 400 mg orally four to five times daily.[24,25] Intravenous therapy will eventually be necessary in most patients because of the development of severe mucositis from conditioning regimens. Oral acyclovir, however, is effective and considerably less expensive in those patients who can take oral medications. Although the duration of antiviral prophylaxis differs between centers, acyclovir is usually begun at the time of the conditioning regimen and continued for about 6 weeks or until resolution of neutropenia. Besides preventing recurrence of HSV disease, acyclovir prophylaxis also may reduce the incidence of CMV reactivation.[61] High-dose oral acyclovir given for 6 months post-transplant also significantly reduces reactivation of VZV infections; however, routine use of long-term acyclovir is controversial and not generally used.[46] Patients developing active HSV or VZV infection should be treated with high-dose acyclovir (10 mg/kg IV every 8 hours).

Acyclovir-resistant HSV has occasionally been reported in BMT patients receiving acyclovir prophylaxis. Foscarnet is the drug of choice for treatment of acyclovir-resistant HSV. Foscarnet, however, has not been well studied for HSV prophylaxis.[25]

Prevention of CMV disease has been extensively studied in BMT patients because of the severe potential morbidity and mortality. If possible, CMV-seronegative patients should receive donor marrow and supportive blood products from seronegative donors only; however, CMV-seropositive patients do not appear to be at additional risk by receiving blood or marrow from seropositive donors.[25] Although acyclovir has relatively poor *in vitro* activity versus CMV, a decrease in CMV infection and an improvement in overall survival was reported in HSV- and CMV-seropositive allogeneic BMT recipients receiving IV acyclovir.[61] Therefore, acyclovir prophylaxis is commonly used in many transplant centers.

Ganciclovir has also been studied for prophylaxis because of its superior activity against CMV compared to acyclovir. Although administration of prophylactic ganciclovir to CMV-seropositive patients may significantly decrease the occurrence of CMV disease, studies found no clear survival benefit, and ganciclovir-related bone marrow suppression was frequently problematic. Ganciclovir prophylaxis for all seropositive patients is not recommended at present.[25] Perhaps a more appropriate role for ganciclovir is in early or preemptive therapy, in which ganciclovir is administered at first isolation of CMV from the blood or bronchoalveolar lavage (BAL) fluid. Preemptive therapy was evaluated in one study and shown to reduce significantly the occurrence of CMV disease (including CMV pneumonia), as well as improve survival significantly up to 180 days post-transplant.[62] Because CMV viremia and BAL cultures have been shown to be highly predictive of subsequent CMV disease, preemptive ganciclovir therapy may be considered for these patients. Ganciclovir-associated bone marrow suppression is a concern in allogeneic BMT recipients. Colony-stimulating factors are beneficial in this setting, providing benefits similar to those noted in neutropenic AIDS patients receiving ganciclovir therapy for CMV retinitis.

Pharmacologic prevention of CMV disease with either intravenous immunoglobulin (IVIG) or hyperimmune CMV-IVIG has also been studied; however, results have been variable and inconclusive.[25,63] Because the benefit of immunoglobulins for CMV prophylaxis in BMT patients is controversial and associated with considerable expense, they are not recommended. This, however, will likely continue to be an area of intense evaluation.

Ganciclovir is the drug of choice in the treatment of active CMV infection in BMT patients (Table 111–3). Foscarnet is effective in the treatment of severe CMV disease in AIDS patients and may also be of benefit for treatment or prevention of infections in BMT patients. Foscarnet may be used as an alternative to ganciclovir because of its relative lack of bone marrow toxicity. Foscarnet-related nephrotoxicity may be problematic, however, especially in the post-transplant period when patients may be receiving other nephrotoxic agents. Use of cidofovir is also limited by risk of nephrotoxicity, and this agent has not been well studied in BMT patients.

Numerous single-agent treatments, such as vidarabine, interferon, and ganciclovir, have been employed unsuccessfully as treatment for CMV IP. The combination of high-dose IVIG and ganciclovir may, however, decrease the mortality of this syndrome from 85% to only 30% to 50%.[64,65] The potential for ganciclovir-associated bone marrow suppression in patients just recovering from granulocytopenia remains a concern, especially in patients with unstable renal function. Ganciclovir plus IVIG, however, is the treatment regimen of choice in this life-threatening infection.[25,63]

FUNGAL INFECTIONS

Fluconazole prophylaxis, as previously discussed for neutropenic patients, is safe and efficacious for prevention of mucocutaneous and disseminated candidal infections in BMT patients. Fluconazole prophylaxis is usually continued throughout the period of granulocytopenia. The variable activity of fluconazole against nonalbicans species of *Candida* may be problematic in this population, as is lack of activity against *Aspergillus*. The use of low-dose amphotericin B (0.15 to 0.25 mg/kg/d) is occasionally used in institutions with high rates of *Aspergillus* infection after BMT. This practice is controversial, however, and not well studied.[8,25,58] Fluconazole and other azole antifungals may cause significant elevations in serum cyclosporine concentrations and predispose to cyclosporine toxicities; this interaction should be closely monitored in BMT patients receiving these agents concurrently.[58]

PROTOZOAL INFECTIONS

Pulmonary infection with *P. carinii* is a relatively infrequent complication of BMT. Mortality rates in this population, however, are approximately 60% and are especially high in patients with GVHD.[25] Prophylactic use of TMP/SMX (one double-strength tablet three times/week or one single-strength tablet daily) is commonly employed in this setting. Toxoplasmosis is not a common infection in BMT patients; nevertheless, its occurrence should also be prevented by TMP/SMX prophylaxis.

USE OF COLONY-STIMULATING FACTORS

Several studies have evaluated the use of filgrastim (G-CSF) and sargramostim (GM-CSF) in BMT patients in an effort to speed bone marrow recovery, reduce the period of neutropenia, and decrease infectious complications. Although the time to neutrophil recovery was consistently decreased, these studies failed to show significant differences in infection rates, transplant-related mortality, or overall survival. The use of CSFs appears to be safe, but their use in BMT patients has not been formally recommended because of lack of clear benefits.[48]

EVALUATION OF THERAPEUTIC OUTCOMES

Close monitoring of BMT patients, including both clinical and laboratory data, is essential for early detection and treatment of infectious complications. In addition, because many of the drugs that may be commonly used in this setting have significant toxicity potential in BMT patients (e.g., ganciclovir, amphotericin B, TMP/SMX), careful attention must be paid to the prevention and management of drug-related adverse effects. Monitoring parameters related to specific types of infections (e.g., pneumonia, urinary tract infections) should be applied as appropriate. The reader is referred to other chapters within this book for more specific information.

INFECTIONS IN SOLID ORGAN TRANSPLANT RECIPIENTS

Since the introduction of cyclosporine in 1980, solid organ transplantation has become an established mode of treatment for end-stage diseases of the kidney, liver, heart, lungs, and pancreas. Both patient and allograft survival rates greatly exceed those of the past. Reasons for improved survival include improvements in immunosuppressive drug therapy, candidate selection, transplant surgery techniques, and more experience in the management of complications (including infection) in these patients. Major hindrances to successful transplantation and extended long-term survival include problems with allograft dysfunction and rejection and infectious complications. Despite advances in diagnostic techniques and antimicrobial therapy, infection remains an important cause of morbidity and mortality.

RISK FACTORS

Many of the risk factors for infection discussed at the beginning of this chapter are present in solid organ transplant patients (Table 111–1). The most important risk factor in this population is the immunosuppressive drug therapy that patients receive for prevention and treatment of allograft rejection. Risk of infection is dependent on specific immunosuppressive drug regimens and on the dose and duration of immunosuppression. Most opportunistic infections in transplant patients occur during the first 6 months post-transplant when the intensity and total cumulative doses of immunosuppressive therapy are very high.[66,67]

Since the introduction of cyclosporine-containing regimens, the incidence, types, and severity of infectious complications associated with these regimens have been compared with those of past regimens.[68,69] Rates of infection and resulting mortality from infectious complications are generally believed to be lower with cyclosporine/prednisone compared with azathioprine/prednisone.[68,69] This is probably because of the selective effect of cyclosporine on cell-mediated immunity. The risk of *P. carinii* pneumonia may be higher, however, in renal transplant patients receiving cyclosporine regimens.[70] Data from clinical trials suggest that tacrolimus may also be associated with lower rates of serious bacterial and viral infections than are seen with cyclosporine-based immunosuppressive regimens.[67,71] This may be because of a steroid-sparing effect of tacrolimus that enables patients to be maintained on greatly reduced doses of corticosteroids; in many cases, steroids are completely unnecessary.[71,72] When evaluating published literature on infection patterns after solid organ transplantation, one must always consider the organ being transplanted and the nature of the immunosuppressive drug regimens in use at reporting centers.

Immunosuppressive drugs, often in escalated doses, are also used to treat episodes of graft rejection. Drugs used to treat rejection include immunoglobulins directed against T cells (e.g., anti-thymocyte globulin [ATG]), murine monoclonal antibodies (muromonab, OKT3), and high-dose IV or oral corticosteroids. Rejection episodes often occur during the post-transplant period when the overall cumulative dose or net state of immunosuppression is highest (2 to 4 months).[67] Therefore, patients already at risk for infection are placed at even higher risk if additional immunosuppressive therapy is needed to treat one or more episodes of graft rejection. When infections occur, immunosuppressive drug therapy must be carefully evaluated because, in many cases, immunosuppression may have to be reduced in order for the patient to survive the infectious episode.

Risk of increased infectious complications from immunosuppressive therapy used to treat rejection episodes is also determined, at least in part, by the specific therapy employed. The many drug combinations used to prevent and treat allograft rejection, however, make it difficult to determine the contribution of each specific agent to the overall infection risk. Use of ATG appears to be associated with significantly higher infection rates, particularly CMV infections.[73] Although the risk of infection with muromonab use is less well defined, patients receiving this agent may have increased rates of viral (HSV, CMV) and *P. carinii* infections.[74,75] Because much of the data concerning muromonab for treatment of rejection are from patients failing standard antirejection therapy (steroids ± ATG), however, prior immunosuppression may have played a role in infection development. High-dose corticosteroids are often used in the treatment of rejection and place patients at further risk for infections.

ETIOLOGY

As in cancer patients, microorganisms infecting organ transplant patients are present pretransplant or acquired from exogenous sources. All transplant recipients are at risk for mucocutaneous candidiasis from species colonizing body sites. Invasive fungal infection may also occur in 30% to 40% of heart, lung, pancreas, and liver transplant recipients; rates are highest following liver transplantation and are associated with mortality rates of up to 60%.[76,77] Abdominal surgery, especially the demanding operations required for liver transplantation, has been shown to predispose patients to serious fungal disease, most likely as a consequence of entering an area highly colonized with *Candida* sp.[75] Liver and lung transplant recipients are also at particularly high risk for serious gram-negative bacterial infections as a result of the technically difficult surgical procedures.[67]

Organisms present as latent tissue infections may reactivate and cause clinical disease post-transplant after the administration of immunosuppressive drug therapy. Disease resulting from infection reactivation has been noted with viral (HSV I and II, CMV, VZV, Epstein-Barr virus [EBV]), protozoal *(Toxoplasma gondii, P. carinii),* and mycobacterial *(Mycobacterium tuberculosis)* organisms. Serologic or immunologic tests are performed prior to transplantation to assess the risk for infection because of reactivation and identify other subclinical infections (hepatitis B, *Legionella*). Many patients with reactivated disease have no clinical symptoms; often the only evidence of active infection is a rise in antibody titer from the pretransplant baseline, a positive culture, or histologic evidence. Reactivation of latent infection may also result in severe, life-threatening disease in immunosuppressed hosts.

Exogenous sources of infection in transplant patients include environmental contamination and transmission of microorganisms via transplanted organs and blood products. Environmental sources of infection are similar to those noted in other immunocompromised hosts, such as cancer patients. Airborne pathogens, especially fungi, such as *Aspergillus* and *Cryptococcus neoformans,* may cause infections in transplant patients. Transplant patients are also at risk for common nosocomial infections and infections occurring as hospital outbreaks *(P. aeruginosa* and *Legionella).* Optimal prevention and management of nosocomial infections in transplant patients requires knowledge of current epidemiology of infections and susceptibility patterns in the institution.

Infections transmitted via donor organs or blood products are major causes of morbidity and mortality in transplant patients. Infections that may be transmitted in this manner include HSV, *T. gondii,* and hepatitis B and C. The most important infections transmitted from the donor, however, are caused by CMV. These infections may cause serious disease (pneumonia, hepatitis, hematologic disorders, chorioretinitis), as well as predisposing patients to other opportunistic infections and contributing to allograft dysfunction.[67] In contrast to reactivation disease, transplant patients contracting primary CMV disease are at increased risk for serious, life-threatening infections.[67,78] The most important source of primary CMV infection in transplant patients is the donor organ. Efforts are made to avoid transplanting organs from CMV-seropositive donors into CMV-seronegative recipients because of the potentially severe consequences. With the scarcity of suitable organs and the rapidity with which transplant decisions must often be made, however, this is not always possible. The consequences of transplanting an organ from a CMV-seropositive donor into an already CMV-seropositive recipient are less clear. Evidence exists that CMV reinfection (as well as reactivation) syndromes may occur in these patients.[79] Organs from donors seropositive for *T. gondii* or HSV are generally not withheld from seronegative patients. Organs from known HIV-infected donors, however, are not used for transplantation. It has been recommended that asymptomatic HIV-seropositive individuals with a $CD4^+$ lymphocyte count greater than 400/mm^3 may be considered for liver, heart, or lung transplantation without prohibitively high risk of acceleration of HIV disease.[80] Patients developing primary EBV infections after transplant are more likely to have clinical symptoms and develop lymphoproliferative disease, including lymphoma, than are patients with reactivated disease.[81]

In addition to transmission from donor organs, primary CMV disease may also be transmitted from seropositive blood products, although this is a much less common mode of infection transmission. Risk of such transmission increases with the administration of large numbers of blood products.

Table 111–3 contains information on microbiology, clinical presentation, and treatment of infections in solid organ recipients. Although opportunistic viral, fungal, and protozoal infections may commonly occur, bacterial infections remain the most frequent infectious complications after transplantation in all allograft recipients.

TIMING OF INFECTIONS AFTER TRANSPLANTATION

Although risk of infection with specific pathogens varies with the type of transplant, the time course of infections is similar in all transplant recipients. The overall risk of infection is greatest during the first 6 months post-transplant when the greatest number of risk factors are present. Both daily doses and cumulative doses of immunosuppressive drugs are at high levels, and additional agents may be necessary for treatment of rejection episodes.[67]

The time course for infections can be divided into three periods post-transplant. During the first month post-transplant, patients are at risk for infections already present and brought forward from the pretransplant period (e.g., hepatitis B); postoperative infections, such as surgical wound and catheter infections; infection resulting from colonized donor organs (pneumonia following lung transplant); and reactivation of HSV.[67] From 2 to 6 months post-transplant, risk is highest for viral infections, including CMV, EBV, and hepatitis B and C. The combination of these "immunomodulating" viruses plus sustained immunosuppressive therapy leads to a high risk for opportunistic infections with pathogens such as *P. carinii, Aspergillus,* and *Nocardia asteroides.*[67,78] After 6 months, the patient is at risk for persistent infections (particularly viral) from earlier post-transplant periods, reactivation of VZV and *C. neoformans,* and routine infections affecting the general population.[67] In addition, patients who have required additional immunosuppression therapy for acute or chronic rejection are at continued high risk for opportunistic infections *(Aspergillus, P. carinii).*[67] Although Figure 111–3 illustrates infection patterns after kidney transplantation, this infection time course can be applied to other types of solid organ transplants. The relative incidence and importance of a particular pathogen will vary, however, according to the type of transplant.

TYPES OF INFECTIONS AND CLINICAL PRESENTATION

Transplant patients are at risk for infections occurring at a variety of sites, including skin, surgical wound, urinary tract, lungs, blood, abdomen, and central nervous system; however, most infections occur at or near the site of the transplanted organ. For example, heart and heart and lung transplant recipients are most often infected within the lungs or thoracic cavity. Urinary tract infections remain an important cause of morbidity in renal transplant patients, especially in the early post-transplant period. Administration of prophylactic antibiotics, such as TMP/SMX, to these patients has, however, reduced the incidence and severity of urinary tract infections.[82] Serious, life-threatening bacterial and fungal infections originating from the abdomen and GI tract are most common after liver transplantation and are related to variables such as length of surgery and surgical procedures performed.[75] Risk of bacteremia, usually originating from the gut, is highest in liver transplant patients. Renal transplant recipients appear to be at the lowest risk of infections and infectious deaths, while patients receiving heart and lung transplants are at the highest risk of infection-related morbidity and mortality.[67,83]

Clinical presentation of infection in transplant patients is variable and depends on the infecting organism, site of infection, host immune status, time after transplantation, and dose and duration of immunosuppressive therapy. History of prior exposure is important, because primary disease is usually more symptomatic and severe than disease caused by reactivation. As in neutropenic patients, fever is

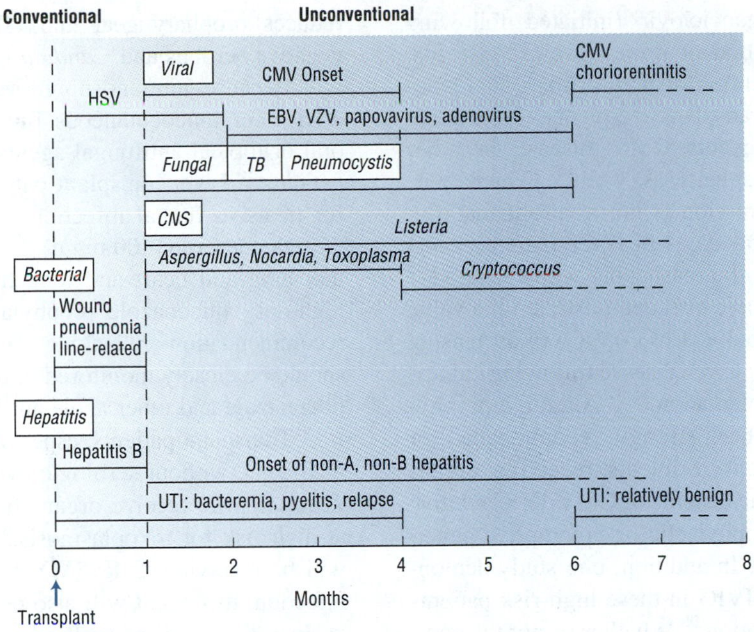

FIGURE 111–3. Timetable for the occurrence of infection in the renal transplant patient. CMV = cytomegalovirus; HSV = herpes simplex virus; EBV = Epstein-Barr virus; VZV = varicella zoster virus; TB = tuberculosis; CNS = central nervous system; UTI = urinary tract infection. *(From Ref. 98, with permission.)*

the single most important clinical sign indicating the presence of infection.[67] At the onset of fever, patients should be evaluated for other signs and symptoms of infection, especially at sites near the surgical incision and transplanted organ. Signs of allograft dysfunction may be related to infection; distinguishing fever resulting from allograft rejection versus infection is often difficult and must be determined via allograft biopsy. Noninfectious sources of fever may include drug therapy and medical or surgical problems, such as embolic events and ischemic injury. Febrile responses to infection may be blunted by the administration of high-dose corticosteroids.

In contrast to febrile neutropenic patients, the threshold for initiating empiric antimicrobial therapy is higher in febrile transplant patients. As seen in Table 111–3, appropriate therapy for the large numbers of pathogens that may cause infections in transplant patients varies greatly from organism to organism. Therefore, careful attempts at definitive diagnosis of suspected infections must be made. If comprehensive workup reveals no source of infection, careful observation of the febrile transplant patient (rather than empiric therapy) is a common practice. Surveillance cultures may be useful during the first 3 months for detecting CMV and HSV infections.[66] Management and monitoring of documented infections, such as urinary tract infections, pneumonias, and intra-abdominal infections, are similar to that in other types of patients.

PREVENTION

The goals of antimicrobial drug use in solid organ transplant recipients include (1) prevention of infectious complications in the immediate postoperative period; (2) prevention of late infectious complications associated with prolonged periods of immunosuppression; and (3) effective treatment of established infections in order to prevent graft dysfunction and rejection and decrease patient morbidity and mortality. All of these goals must be achieved at the lowest possible toxicity and cost.

Prevention of infection in the transplant patient can be accomplished in a number of ways. First, risk of environmental contamination should be minimized. Patients should be protected from institutional infectious outbreaks. Transplant patients should receive the pneumococcal vaccine once and the influenza vaccine yearly; however, their immunologic responses to these vaccines may be blunted by immunosuppressive therapy.[66,84]

Because the most important source of primary CMV disease is an infected donor organ, CMV-seronegative patients should not receive organs or blood products from seropositive donors if possible. A number of pharmacologic strategies have also been studied in an attempt to prevent CMV infection. Prophylactic ganciclovir (usually 5 mg/kg every 12 hours) has been evaluated in solid organ transplantation and demonstrated to be effective in reducing the incidence of both primary and reactivated CMV disease.[85] Ganciclovir prophylaxis may also significantly reduce reactivation of CMV disease in seropositive patients receiving ALG for treatment of acute rejection.[86] High-dose oral acyclovir has been shown to reduce the incidence of CMV infection and disease effectively following renal transplantation.[87] Trials, however, have demonstrated that acyclovir is less efficacious in high-risk renal transplant patients (donor-positive, recipient-negative for CMV serum antibodies) and other nonrenal transplant types.[85,88,89] Preemptive ganciclovir (initiated following isolation of CMV from blood or urine) is more effective than acyclovir in the prevention of both primary and reactivation disease in liver transplant recipients. Preemptive ganciclovir effectively prevents CMV disease in other types of solid organ transplants as well.[85] Ganciclovir-related bone marrow suppression is not as problematic in solid organ transplant recipients as in BMT patients; most studies reported the drug to be reasonably well tolerated.[85]

A number of studies have also demonstrated the value of CMV hyperimmune globulin (CMV-IVIG) in decreasing the incidence and severity of CMV disease following kidney, heart, lung, and liver transplantation.[85,87] Although prophylaxis with CMV-IVIG has been strongly recommended for CMV-seronegative transplant recipients receiving organs from seropositive donors, the benefits of CMV-IVIG relative to other therapies (e.g., prophylactic or preemptive ganciclovir) are not well known. In addition, one study demonstrated no benefit of CMV-IVIG in these high-risk patients undergoing liver transplantation.[90] Whether or not the combination of CMV-IVIG plus ganciclovir offers advantages over the use of either agent alone, either for primary prophylaxis or treatment of established CMV disease, is also unclear in solid organ transplantation.[84] The lack of data clearly indicating the most optimal regimen for prevention of CMV disease is strikingly illustrated in a review in which a summary of practices at five major U.S. transplant centers revealed a wide array of different prophylactic and preemptive regimens in use.[85]

Although the use of prophylactic acyclovir in HSV-seropositive patients undergoing bone marrow transplantation is well accepted, prophylaxis in solid organ transplant recipients remains controversial. Acyclovir is being used at some centers because of the high incidence of clinical HSV infection, including pneumonias, after transplantation.[91]

Prophylactic antimicrobial agents are of benefit to transplant patients in certain clinical situations. Antibiotic prophylaxis, with agents such as cefazolin begun perioperatively and continued for less than 24 hours, is considered to reduce wound infection rates effectively following renal transplantation.[84,92] Surgical prophylaxis is considered mandatory in liver, heart, and lung transplant patients because of the high risk of perioperative bacterial infections. In addition, post-transplant antibiotic prophylaxis has been shown to be effective in decreasing the number of bacterial infections in renal transplant patients.[82] Prophylactic TMP/SMX has been a traditionally used agent because it is inexpensive and well tolerated; other antibiotics, such as the fluoroquinolones, are also being evaluated.[84] Administration of oral low-dose TMP/SMX (one double-strength tablet daily) for 6 to 12 months for prevention of *P. carinii* infection following heart and lung transplantation is common, although the efficacy and optimal duration are still somewhat controversial.[93] Selective bowel decontamination with nonabsorbable antibiotics in combination with a low bacterial diet (no fresh fruits and vegetables) effectively reduces oropharyngeal and GI colonization with gram-negative aerobes and *Candida* in liver transplant patients.[94]

Because immunosuppressed transplant recipients are at risk for mucocutaneous fungal infections, prophylactic oral or topical antifungal agents may be indicated in these patients.[56] Liver transplant patients are clearly at high risk for invasive fungal infections and should be prophylaxed with fluconazole (400 mg/d).[58,95] It has also been suggested that lung and heart and lung transplant recipients receive high-dose fluconazole prophylaxis, although data for this recommendation are lacking.[58] Cyclosporine concentrations should be closely monitored in transplant patients receiving fluconazole and other azole antifungal agents.[58]

Transplant patients, especially heart and heart and lung recipients, without serologic evidence of prior exposure to *T. gondii* who receive organs from seropositive donors are at high risk for toxoplasmosis.[67,96] Many of these patients will be receiving TMP/SMX for prophylaxis of *P. carinii* infection; this agent will also provide effective prophylaxis against *T. gondii,* as well as against *Nocardia asteroides.* Although prophylaxis is not routinely given at all centers, this therapy may be justified in high-risk patients because of the delays in diagnosis and serious infections associated with toxoplasmosis.[97]

The use of prophylactic isoniazid (INH) therapy for transplant patients with evidence of exposure to *M. tuberculosis* (those with a positive purified protein derivative skin test) remains controversial. Risk of reactivation and development of clinical tuberculosis is enhanced with post-transplant immunosuppression. Some clinicians believe, however, that the risk of INH-induced hepatotoxicity, especially in liver transplant recipients, outweighs the benefits of treatment.

EVALUATION OF THERAPEUTIC OUTCOMES

Close monitoring of transplant recipients, including both clinical and laboratory data, is essential for early detection and treatment of potentially severe opportunistic infections.

▶ PRINCIPLES OF PHARMACOTHERAPY

- An *immunocompromised host* is a patient with defects in host defenses that predispose to infection. Risk factors include granulocytopenia, immune system defects (including immunosuppressive drug therapy), compromise of natural host defenses, environmental contamination, and changes in normal flora of the host.
- Immunocompromised patients are at high risk for a variety of bacterial, fungal, viral, and protozoal infections. Infection is documented in only 30% to 40% of febrile episodes in neutropenic patients.

- Risk of infection in granulocytopenic patients is associated with both the severity and duration of neutropenia. Patients with severe neutropenia (ANC < 500/mm^3) for greater than 7 to 10 days are considered to be at high risk of infection.
- Fever (> 38°C) is the most important clinical finding in neutropenic patients. Fever should be considered to be caused by infection until proven otherwise.
- Initial antimicrobial regimens for treatment of febrile neutropenia must have good activity against *Pseudomonas aeruginosa.* Regimens that may be used for initial treatment include monotherapy with an antipseudomonal β-lactam or carbapenem; antipseudomonal β-lactam plus aminoglycoside; double β-lactam therapy with antipseudomonal agents; one of the above regimens plus vancomycin; or fluoroquinolone plus antipseudomonal β-lactam, aminoglycoside, or vancomycin.
- Neutropenic patients who remain febrile after 72 hours should be clinically reevaluated to determine whether antimicrobial modifications are necessary. Common modifications to regimens include addition of vancomycin (if not already present), and antifungal therapy (fluconazole or amphotericin B).
- The optimal duration of therapy for febrile neutropenia is controversial. The decision to discontinue antimicrobials is based on resolution of granulocytopenia, persistent fever, culture results, and clinical stability of the patient.
- Prophylactic antimicrobials are commonly administered to cancer patients with anticipated prolonged neutropenia, as well as to both bone marrow and solid organ transplant recipients. Common prophylactic regimens may include antibacterial, antifungal, antiviral, or antiprotozoal agents, or a combination of these, selected according to risk of infection with specific pathogens in each patient population. Optimal prophylactic regimens are controversial for most types of infection.
- Patients undergoing bone marrow transplantation are at an extremely high risk of infection because of prolonged neutropenia following intensive chemotherapy ± irradiation, while solid organ transplant recipients are at risk because of prolonged administration of immunosuppressive drugs. Fungal *(Aspergillus)* and viral (CMV) infections are particularly troublesome in these patients and prophylactic regimens directed against these pathogens are commonly used.
- Immunocompromised patients must be continuously assessed for evidence of infection and response to antimicrobial therapy. Because a large number of antimicrobials may be used, including many with significant toxicities, the occurrence of drug-related adverse effects must also be carefully assessed.

REFERENCES

1. Bodey GP, Buckley M, Sathe YS, Freireich EJ. Quantitative relationships between circulating leukocytes and infection in patients with acute leukemia. Ann Intern Med 1966;64:328–340.
2. Hughes WT, Armstrong D, Bodey GP, et al. 1997 Guidelines for the use of antimicrobial agents in neutropenic patients with unexplained fever. Clin Infect Dis 1997;25:551–573.
3. Pizzo PA. Management of fever in patients with cancer and treatment-induced neutropenia. N Engl J Med 1993;328:1323–1332.
4. Giamarellou H. Empiric therapy for infections in the febrile, neutropenic, compromised host. Med Clin North Am 1995;79:559–580.
5. Koll BS, Brown AE. Changing patterns of infections in the immunocompromised patient with cancer. Hematol Oncol Clin North Am 1993;7:753–769.
6. Mandell LA. Effects of antimicrobial and antineoplastic drugs on the phagocytic and microbicidal function of the polymorphonuclear leukocyte. Rev Infect Dis 1982;4:683–697.
7. Bodey GP. Infections in cancer patients: A continuing association. Am J Med 1986;81(suppl 1A):11–26.
8. Hathorn JW. Critical appraisal of antimicrobials for prevention of infections in immunocompromised hosts. Hematol Oncol Clin North Am 1993;7:1051–1099.
9. Schimpff SC, Young VM, Greene WH, et al. Origin of infection in acute nonlymphocytic leukemia: Significance of hospital acquisition of potential pathogens. Ann Intern Med 1972;77:707–714.
10. Johanson WG, Pierce AK, Sanford JP. Changing pharyngeal bacterial flora of hospitalized patients. N Engl J Med 1969;281:1137–1140.
11. Vartivarian SE. Virulence properties and nonimmune pathogenic mechanisms of fungi. Clin Infect Dis 1992;14(suppl 1):530–535.
12. Bonten MJM, Gaillard CA, van der Geest S, et al. The role of intragastric acidity and stress ulcus prophylaxis on colonization and infection in mechanically ventilated ICU patients: A stratified, randomized, double-blind study of sucralfate versus antacids. Am J Respir Crit Care Med 1995;152:1825–1834.
13. Talcott JA, Finberg R, Mayer RJ, Goldman L. The medical course of cancer patients with fever and neutropenia. Arch Intern Med 1988; 148:2561–2568.
14. Hathorn JW, Rubin M, Pizzo PA. Empirical antibiotic therapy in the febrile neutropenic cancer patient: Clinical efficacy and impact of monotherapy. Antimicrob Agents Chemother 1987;31:971–977.
15. De Pauw BE, Donnelly JP. Controversies in the antibacterial treatment of patients with neutropenia: A matter of comprehension or apprehension. Cancer Invest 1997;15:37–46.
16. Awada A, Van der Auwera P, Meunier F, et al. Streptococcal and enterococcal bacteremia in patients with cancer. Clin Infect Dis 1992;15: 33–48.
17. Bow EJ, Loewen R, Vaughan D. Reduced requirement for gram-negative antibiotic therapy in febrile, neutropenic patients with cancer who are receiving antibacterial chemoprophylaxis with oral quinolones. Clin Infect Dis 1996;20:907–912.
18. Cruciani M, Rampazzo R, Malena M, et al. Prophylaxis with fluoroquinolones for bacterial infections in neutropenic patients: A meta-analysis. Clin Infect Dis 1996;23:795–805.
19. Bochud PY, Eggiman PH, Calandra TH, et al. Bacteremia due to viridans streptococcus in neutropenic patients with cancer: Clinical spectrum and risk factors. Clin Infect Dis 1994;18:25–31.
20. Brown EA, Talbot GH, Provencher M, Cassileth P. Anaerobic bacteremia in patients with acute leukemia. Infect Control Hosp Epidemiol 1989;10:65–69.
21. Bodey GP, Bueltmann B, Duguid W, et al. Fungal infections in cancer patients: An international autopsy survey. Eur J Clin Microbiol Infect Dis 1992;11:99–109.
22. Thaler M, Pastakia B, Shawker TH, et al. Hepatic candidiasis in cancer patients: The evolving picture of the syndrome. Ann Intern Med 1988;108:88–100.

23. Anaissie E. Opportunistic mycoses in the immunocompromised host: Experience at a cancer center and review. Clin Infect Dis 1992; 14(suppl 1):S43–S48.
24. Whitley RJ, Gnann JW Jr. Acyclovir: A decade later. 10 years later. N Engl J Med 1992;327:782–789.
25. Momin F, Chandrasekar PH. Antimicrobial prophylaxis in bone marrow transplantation. Ann Intern Med 1995;123:205–215.
26. Sepkowitz KA, Brown AE, Telzak EE, et al. *Pneumocystis carinii* pneumonia among patients without AIDS at a cancer hospital. JAMA 1992;267:832–838.
27. Sickles EA, Greene WH, Wiernik PH. Clinical presentation of infection in granulocytopenic patients. Arch Intern Med 1975;135: 715–719.
28. Schimpff S, Satterlee W, Young VM, Serpick A. Empiric therapy with carbenicillin and gentamicin for febrile patients with cancer and granulocytopenia. N Engl J Med 1971;284:1061–1065.
29. Bodey GP, Jadeja L, Elting L. *Pseudomonas* bacteremia: Retrospective analysis of 410 episodes. Arch Intern Med 1985;145:1621–1629.
30. Kibbler CC. Neutropenic infections: Strategies for empirical therapy. J Antimicrob Chemother 1995;36(suppl B):107–117.
31. Pizzo PA, Hathorn JW, Hiemenz J, et al. A randomized trial comparing ceftazidime alone with combination antibiotic therapy in cancer patients with fever and neutropenia. N Engl J Med 1986;315:552–558.
32. Winston DJ, Ho WG, Bruckner DA, Champlin RE. Beta-lactam antibiotic therapy in febrile, granulocytopenic patients: A randomized trial comparing cefoperazone plus piperacillin, ceftazidime plus piperacillin, and imipenem alone. Ann Intern Med 1991;115:849–859.
33. Fish DN, Singletary TJ. Meropenem: A new carbapenem antibiotic. Pharmacotherapy 1997;17:644–669.
34. Ramphal R, Gucalp R, Rotstein C, et al. Clinical experience with single agent and combination regimens in the management of infection in the febrile neutropenic patient. Am J Med 1996;100(suppl 6A): 83S–89S.
35. Chow JW, Fine MJ, Shlaes DM, et al. *Enterobacter* bacteremia: Clinical features and emergence of antibiotic resistance during therapy. Ann Intern Med 1991;115:585–590.
36. DeJongh CA, Joshi JH, Newman KA, et al. Antibiotic synergism and response in gram-negative bacteremia in granulocytopenic cancer patients. Am J Med 1986;80(suppl C):96–100.
37. Gilbert DN. Once-daily aminoglycoside therapy. Antimicrob Agents Chemother 1991;35:399–405.
38. Hatala R, Dinh TT, Cook DJ. Single daily dosing of aminoglycosides in immunocompromised adults: A systematic review. Clin Infect Dis 1997;24:810–815.
39. Gutmann L, Williamson R, Kitzis M-D, Acar JF. Synergism and antagonism in double β-lactam antibiotic combinations. Am J Med 1986;80(suppl 5C):21–29.
40. EORTC International Antimicrobial Therapy Cooperative Group and the National Cancer Institute of Canada—Clinical Trials Group. Vancomycin added to empirical combination antibiotic therapy for fever in granulocytopenic cancer patients. J Infect Dis 1991;163:951–958.
41. Centers for Disease Control and Prevention. Recommendations for preventing the spread of vancomycin resistance: Recommendations of the Hospital Infection Control Practices Advisory Committee (HICPAC). MMWR 1995(Sept 22);44(No. RR-12):1–13.
42. Rolston KVI, Rubenstein EB, Freifeld A. Early empiric antibiotic therapy for febrile neutropenia patients at low risk. Infect Dis Clin North Am 1996;10:223–237.
43. Escalante CP, Rubenstein EB, Rolston KVI. Outpatient antibiotic therapy for febrile episodes in low-risk neutropenic patients with cancer. Cancer Invest 1997;15:237–242.
44. Pizzo PA, Robichaud KJ, Gill FA, Witebsky FG. Empiric antibiotic and antifungal therapy for cancer patients with prolonged fever and granulocytopenia. Am J Med 1982;72:101–111.
45. White MH, Anaissie EJ, Kusne S, et al. Amphotericin B colloidal dispersion vs. amphotericin B as therapy for invasive aspergillosis. Clin Infect Dis 1997;24:635–642.
46. Sable CA, Donowitz GR. Infections in bone marrow transplant recipients. Clin Infect Dis 1994;18:273–284.
47. Pizzo PA, Robichaud KJ, Gill FA, et al. Duration of empiric antibiotic therapy in granulocytopenic patients with cancer. Am J Med 1979; 67:194–200.
48. American Society of Clinical Oncology. American Society of Clinical Oncology recommendations for the use of hematopoietic colony-stimulating factors: Evidence-based, clinical practice guidelines. J Clin Oncol 1994;12:2471–2508.
49. Geller RB. Use of cytokines in the treatment of acute myelocytic leukemia: A critical review. J Clin Oncol 1996;14:1371–1382.
50. Dix SP, Gilmore CE. Cytokine therapy after bone marrow transplantation. Pharmacotherapy 1996;16:593–608.
51. Schimpff SC. Infection prevention during profound granulocytopenia: New approaches to alimentary canal microbial suppression. Ann Intern Med 1980;93:358–361.
52. Deitch EA, Winterton J, Berg R. Effect of starvation, malnutrition, and trauma on the gastrointestinal tract flora and bacterial translocation. Arch Surg 1987;122:1019–1024.
53. Gilbert C, Meisenberg B, Vredenburgh J, et al. Sequential prophylactic oral and empiric once-daily parenteral antibiotics for neutropenia and fever after high-dose chemotherapy and autologous bone marrow support. J Clin Oncol 1994;12:1005–1011.
54. Kern WV, Hay B, Kern P, et al. A randomized trial of roxithromycin in patients with acute leukemia and bone marrow transplant recipients receiving fluoroquinolone prophylaxis. Antimicrob Agents Chemother 1994;38:465–472.
55. Reents S, Goodwin SD, Singh V. Antifungal prophylaxis in immunocompromised hosts. Ann Pharmacother 1993;27:53–60.
56. Goodman JL, Winston DJ, Greenfield RA, et al. A controlled trial of fluconazole to prevent fungal infections in patients undergoing bone marrow transplantation. N Engl J Med 1992;326:845–851.
57. Wingard JR, Merz WG, Rinaldi MG, et al. Increase in *Candida krusei* infection among patients with bone marrow transplantation and neutropenia treated prophylactically with fluconazole. N Engl J Med 1991; 325:1274–1277.
58. Edwards JE Jr, Bodey GP, Bowden RA, et al. International conference for the development of a consensus on the management and prevention of severe candidal infections. Clin Infect Dis 1997;25:43–59.
59. Beyer J, Schwartz S, Heinemann V, Siegert W. Strategies in prevention of invasive pulmonary aspergillosis in immunocompromised or neutropenic patients. Antimicrob Agents Chemother 1994;38:911–917.
60. Meyers JD, Flournoy N, Thomas ED. Risk factors for cytomegalovirus infection after human marrow transplantation. J Infect Dis 1986;153:478–488.
61. Meyers JD, Reed EC, Shepp DH, et al. Acyclovir for prevention of cytomegalovirus infection and disease after allogeneic marrow transplantation. N Engl J Med 1988;318:70–75.
62. Schmidt GM, Horak DA, Niland JC, et al. A randomized, controlled trial of prophylactic ganciclovir for cytomegalovirus pulmonary infection in recipients of allogeneic bone marrow transplants. N Engl J Med 1991;324:1005–1011.
63. Barnes RA. Immunotherapy and immunoprophylaxis in bone marrow transplantation. J Hosp Infect 1995;30(suppl):223–231.
64. Schmidt GM, Kovacs A, Zaia JA, et al. Ganciclovir/immunoglobulin combination therapy for the treatment of human cytomegalovirus-associated interstitial pneumonia in bone marrow allograft recipients. Transplantation 1988;46:905–907.
65. Emanuel D, Cunningham I, Jules-Elysee K, et al. Cytomegalovirus pneumonia after bone marrow transplantation successfully treated with the combination of ganciclovir and high-dose intravenous immune globulin. Ann Intern Med 1988;109:777–782.
66. Dummer JS. Infectious complications of transplantation. Cardiovasc Clin 1988;20(2):163–178.
67. Kontoyiannis DP, Rubin RH. Infection in the organ transplant recipient: An overview. Infect Dis Clin North Am 1995;9:811–822.

68. Najarian JS, Fryd DS, Strand M, et al. A single institution, randomized, prospective trial of cyclosporine versus azathioprine-antithymocyte globulin for immunosuppression in renal allograft recipients. Ann Surg 1985;201:142–157.
69. Hofflin JM, Potasman I, Baldwin JC, et al. Infectious complications in heart transplant patients receiving cyclosporine and corticosteroids. Ann Intern Med 1987;106:209–216.
70. Hardy AM, Wajszczuk CP, Suffredini AF, et al. *Pneumocystis carinii* pneumonia in renal-transplant recipients treated with cyclosporine and steroids. J Infect Dis 1984;149:143–147.
71. Hooks MA. Tacrolimus, a new immunosuppressant—A review of the literature. Ann Pharmacother 1994;28:501–511.
72. The U.S. Multicenter FK506 Liver Study Group. A comparison of tacrolimus (FK506) and cyclosporine for immunosuppression in liver transplantation. N Engl J Med 1994;331:1110–1115.
73. Pass RF, Whitley RJ, Diethelm AG, et al. Cytomegalovirus infection in patients with renal transplants: Potentiation by antithymocyte globulin and an incompatible graft. J Infect Dis 1980;142:9–17.
74. Singh N, Dummer JS, Kusne S, et al. Infections with cytomegalovirus and other herpes viruses in 121 liver transplant recipients: Transmission by donated organ and the effect of OKT3 antibodies. J Infect Dis 1988;158:124–131.
75. Kusne S, Dummer JS, Singh N, et al. Infections after liver transplantation: An analysis of 101 consecutive cases. Medicine 1988;67:132–143.
76. Hibberd PL, Rubin RH. Clinical aspects of fungal infection in organ transplant recipients. Clin Infect Dis 1994;19(suppl 1):S33–S40.
77. Singh N, Gayowski T, Wagener MM, et al. Invasive fungal infections in liver transplant recipients receiving tacrolimus as the primary immunosuppressive agent. Clin Infect Dis 1997;24:179–184.
78. Dummer JS, White LT, Ho M, et al. Morbidity of cytomegalovirus infection in recipients of heart or heart–lung transplants who received cyclosporine. J Infect Dis 1985;152:1182–1191.
79. Chou S. Neutralizing antibody responses to reinfecting strains of cytomegalovirus in transplant recipients. J Infect Dis 1990;160:16–21.
80. Rubin RH, Tolkoff-Rubin NE. The impact of infection on the outcome of transplantation. Transplant Proc 1991;23:2068–2074.
81. Ho M, Miller G, Atchison RW, et al. Epstein-Barr virus infections and DNA hybridization studies in posttransplantation lymphoma and lymphoproliferative lesions: The role of primary infection. J Infect Dis 1985;152:876–886.
82. Tolkoff-Rubin NE, Cosimi AB, Russell PS, Rubin RH. A controlled study of trimethoprim-sulfamethoxazole prophylaxis of urinary tract infection in renal transplant recipients. Rev Infect Dis 1982;4:614–618.
83. Dummer JS, Montero CG, Griffith BP, et al. Infections in heart–lung transplant recipients. Transplantation 1986;41:725–729.
84. Rubin RH, Tolkoff-Rubin NE. Antimicrobial strategies in the care of organ transplant recipients. Antimicrob Agents Chemother 1993;37:619–624.
85. Patel R, Snydman DR, Rubin RH, et al. Cytomegalovirus prophylaxis in solid organ transplant recipients. Transplantation 1996;61:1279–1289.
86. Hibberd PL, Tolkoff-Rubin NE, Conti D, et al. Preemptive ganciclovir therapy to prevent cytomegalovirus disease in cytomegalovirus antibody-positive renal transplant recipients: A randomized controlled trial. Ann Intern Med 1995;123:18–26.
87. Dickinson BI, Gora-Harper ML, McCraney SA, et al. Studies evaluating high-dose acyclovir, intravenous immune globulin, and cytomegalovirus hyperimmuneglobulin for prophylaxis against cytomegalovirus in kidney transplant recipients. Ann Pharmacother 1996;30:1452–1462.
88. Singh N, Yu VL, Mieles L, et al. High-dose acyclovir compared with short-course preemptive ganciclovir therapy to prevent cytomegalovirus disease in liver transplant recipients. Ann Intern Med 1994;120:375–381.
89. Goral S, Ynares C, Dummer S, et al. Acyclovir prophylaxis for cytomegalovirus disease in high-risk renal transplant recipients: Is it effective? Kidney Int 1996;50(suppl 57):S62–S65.
90. Snydman DR, Werner BG, Dougherty NN, et al. Cytomegalovirus immune globulin prophylaxis in liver transplantation: A randomized, double-blind, placebo-controlled trial. Ann Intern Med 1993;119:984–991.
91. Smyth RL, Higenbottam TW, Scott JP, et al. Herpes simplex virus infection in heart–lung transplant recipients. Transplantation 1990;49:735–739.
92. Barone GW, Hudec WA, Sailors DM, et al. Prophylactic wound antibiotics for combined kidney and pancreas transplants. Clin Transplantation 1996;10:386–388.
93. Kramer MR, Stoehr C, Lewiston NJ, et al. Trimethoprim-sulfamethoxazole prophylaxis for *Pneumocystis carinii* infections following heart–lung and lung transplantation—How effective and for how long? Transplantation 1992;53:586–589.
94. Wiesner RH, Hermans PE, Rakela J, et al. Selective bowel decontamination to decrease gram-negative aerobic bacterial and *Candida* colonization and prevent infection after orthotopic liver transplantation. Transplantation 1988;45:570–574.
95. Menichetti F. Prevention of candidiasis in the immunocompromised host: What are the best strategies? Int J Infect Dis 1997;1(suppl 1):S52–S55.
96. Luft BJ, Naot Y, Araujo FG, et al. Primary and reactivated toxoplasma infection in patients with cardiac transplants. Ann Intern Med 1983;99:27–31.
97. Wreghitt TG, Hakim M, Cory-Pearce R, et al. The impact of donor-transmitted CMV and *Toxoplasma gondii* disease in cardiac transplantation. Trans Proc 1986;18:1375–1376.
98. Rubin RH, Wolfson JS, Cosimi AB, Tolkoff-Rubin NE. Infection in the renal transplant recipient. Am J Med 1981;70:405–411.

112

Antimicrobial Prophylaxis in Surgery

Stephen W. Janning, PharmD, and Michael J. Rybak, PharmD, FCCP, BCPS

Approximately 23 million surgical procedures are performed annually in the United States. The reported postoperative infection rate is about 6%.[1] This number increases by 50% when data captured by postdischarge wound surveillance are included.[2] Surgical site infections (SSIs) prolong hospital stays at an estimated direct cost of more than $1.5 billion per year and account for almost one-quarter of all nosocomial infections.[1] Prophylactic antibiotics have been shown to decrease the risk of infection for many different procedures and, thus, represent an important component of optimal management of the surgical patient.

By definition, *prophylactic antibiotics* are administered prior to contamination of previously sterile tissues or fluids. The goal is to *prevent* an infection from developing. Eradication of a preexisting distal infection lowers the postoperative infection risk, but it does not constitute a prophylactic regimen. In fact, surgical prophylaxis is often prescribed concurrently under these circumstances because of spectrum and timing issues (see section on Timing of Antibiotics). Similarly, the prevention and management of postoperative complications (non-SSI), such as catheter-related urinary tract infections and atelectasis, are important and occasionally require antibiotics, but that is not the goal of surgical prophylaxis.

Antibiotics that are given when there is a strong possibility, as yet unproved, of established infection are termed *presumptive.* Examples include acute cholecystitis and acute appendicitis of less than 24 hours' duration. If no signs of perforation or infection are found during surgery, then only perioperative antibiotics are indicated. Operative findings of a gangrenous gallbladder or a perforated appendix, for example, mean that an established infection is present and *therapeutic antibiotics* are required.[3]

Surgical site infections are classified as either incisional or deep. Incisional SSI is diagnosed when purulent or culture positive drainage is isolated from any structure above the fascia in proximity to the initial wound. Deep SSIs are characterized by purulent drainage from subfascial drains, wound dehiscence, or abscess formation and involve adjacent sites manipulated during surgery. Both types, by definition, occur by postoperative day 30. This period extends to 1 year in case of deep infection associated with prosthesis implantation. Although culture and sensitivity testing of drainage material can yield important information, a negative culture does not rule out SSI.[4]

RISK FACTORS FOR SURGICAL SITE INFECTION

The incidence of SSI depends on numerous factors specific to either the procedure itself or the individual patient. The traditional classification system developed by the National Research Council (NRC) stratifying surgical procedures by infection risk is reproduced in Table 112–1.[5] According to the NRC data, the risk of SSI depends on the microbiology of the surgical site, presence of established infection, risk of contaminating previously sterile tissue during surgery, and perioperative events.[5,6] In general, the procedure classification determines whether or not antibiotics are indicated. It should be emphasized that the NRC wound classification for a specific procedure is determined intraoperatively and is influenced by surgical findings (e.g., gangrenous gallbladder) and events (e.g., major technique breaks).[3]

INTRINSIC PATIENT RISK

While the NRC classification adequately categorizes the SSI risk for specific procedures, it does not account for underlying patient risk factors. Many underlying disease states and conditions are known to increase SSI risk. Several, such as diabetes mellitus, chronic immunosuppressed states, and extremes in age, cannot be modified and will always influence SSI risk assessment. Others factors, such as recent corticosteroid use, prolonged hospitalization, and perhaps obesity, can be minimized by simply delaying or scheduling elective procedures properly.[4] Preexisting distal infections increase SSI rates and should be resolved prior to surgery whenever possible. Underlying malnutrition is associated with an increased rate of postoperative complications, including SSI. Attempts to improve the outcome in this population with perioperative total parenteral nutrition have not shown any benefit.[7]

INDIVIDUALIZATION FOR SURGICAL SITE INFECTION

Two large epidemiologic studies have been published that objectively quantify SSI risk based on both patient and procedure specific factors. The Study on the Efficacy of Nosocomial Infection Control (SENIC) analyzed more than 100,000 surgery cases in order to identify and validate risk factors for SSI.[8] Abdominal operations, operations lasting > 2 hours, contaminated or dirty procedures by NRC classification, and more than three underlying medical diagnoses were associated with an increased incidence of SSI. When the NRC

TABLE 112–1. National Research Council Wound Classification, Risk of Surgical Wound Infection, and Indication for Antibiotics

Classification	SWI Rate (%)	Criteria	Antibiotics
Clean	< 2	No acute inflammation or transection of gastrointestinal, oropharyngeal, genitourinary, biliary, or respiratory tracts. Elective case, no technique break	Not indicated unless high-risk procedure[a] (? high-risk patient)
Clean-contaminated	< 10	Controlled opening of aforementioned tracts with minimal spillage/minor technique break. Clean procedures performed emergently or with major technique breaks	Prophylactic antibiotics indicated
Contaminated	20	Acute, nonpurulent inflammation present. Major spillage/technique break during clean-contaminated procedure	Prophylactic antibiotics indicated
Dirty	40	Obvious preexisting infection present (abscess, pus, or necrotic tissue present)	Therapeutic antibiotics required

[a]High-risk procedures include implantation of prosthetic materials and other procedures where surgical wound infection is associated with high morbidity (see text).
SWI = surgical wound infection.

classification was stratified by the number of SENIC risk factors present, the infection rates varied by as much as a factor of 15 within the same operative category (Table 112–2).[2]

The National Nosocomial Infections Surveillance System (NNIS) published the results of a similar analysis of more than 84,000 cases that simplifies and refines the SENIC system.[9] Intrinsic patient risk was quantified using the American Society of Anesthesiologists (ASA) preoperative assessment score (Table 112–3).[10] An ASA score of ≥ 3 was associated with increased SSI risk. Other risk factors identified include operations classified as contaminated or dirty by the NRC and procedures lasting longer than *T* hours, where *T* varies according to the specific procedure performed (for example, greater than 2 hours for a cholecystectomy). Again, the SSI rate was linked to the number of risk factors present and varied considerably within NRC class (Table 112–4).

Appropriate antimicrobial prophylaxis during surgery is best established by the results of randomized clinical trials. Studies do not stratify according to overall SSI risk. Recognition of high-risk patients will help identify situations when antibiotic prophylaxis should be used for clean procedures. Future studies, particularly those involving clean procedures, should be prospectively stratified so that high-risk patients who might benefit from prophylaxis can be identified. Data collected in this fashion are now emerging, although the numbers studied are relatively small.[11]

TABLE 112–2. Surgical Wound Infection Incidence (%) Stratified by National Research Council Wound Classification and SENIC Risk Factors[a]

No. of SENIC Risk Factors	Clean	Clean-Contaminated	Contaminated	Dirty
0	1.1	0.6	N/A	N/A
1	3.9	2.8	4.5	6.7
2	8.4	8.4	8.3	10.9
3	15.8	17.7	11.0	18.8
4	N/A	N/A	23.9	27.4

[a]The Study on the Efficacy of Nosocomial Infection Control (SENIC) risk factors include abdominal operation, operations lasting > 2 hours, contaminated or dirty procedures by National Research Council (NRC) classification, and more than three underlying medical diagnoses.
Adapted from Ref. 2.

REDUCING SURGICAL SITE INFECTION RISK

Although appropriate antibiotics are crucial in lowering SSI risk for many surgical procedures, other effective measures can also be taken. Prolonged hospitalization is associated with colonization of (and, occasionally, infection with) nosocomial bacteria, which increases the incidence of SSI. For this reason, elective surgery is often postponed if the patient is hospitalized for an unrelated medical problem. Eradicating nasal carriage of *Staphylococcus aureus,* which is present in 20% to 30% of the population, by applying mupirocin ointment has also been attempted to reduce SSI risk, but it is not recommended.[12] Shaving the incision site with a razor the day before surgery is associated with higher infection rates. Clipping the operative site just prior to the procedure is preferred. Preoperative showering with an antiseptic soap may also lower infection rates.[4]

Recognizing the importance of maintaining sterile technique was a major advance in the evolution of surgery. Enhancing the sterility of the operating room by using ultraviolet light or a laminar air flow system has been attempted, but it does not consistently reduce the infection

TABLE 112–3. American Society of Anesthesiologists Physical Status Classification

Class	Description
1	Normal healthy patient
2	Mild systemic disease
3	Severe systemic disease that is not incapacitating
4	Incapacitating systemic disease that is a constant threat to life
5	Not expected to survive 24 hours with or without operation

From Ref. 10.

TABLE 112–4. SSI Rates by Traditional Wound Classification and Risk Index

NRC Classification	G[a]	No. of Risk Factors[b]	% of Operations	SSI Rate (%)
Clean (n = 49,333)	0.47	0	40	1.0
		1	46	2.3
		2	10	5.4
Clean-contaminated (n = 30,479)	0.40	0	59	2.1
		1	35	4.0
		2	6	9.5
Contaminated (n = 3101)	0.44	1	40	3.4
		2	47	6.8
		3	13	13.2
Dirty-infected (n = 1778)	0.43	1	35	3.1
		2	52	8.1
		3	13	12.8

[a]Goodman-Kruskal correlation coefficient.
[b] See text.
NRC = National Research Council; SSI = surgical site infection.
From Ref. 9.

risk. Unnecessary prolongation of the surgical procedure results in a higher incidence of SSI, possibly because of subtherapeutic antibiotic concentrations.[13] Placement of open (Penrose) drains instead of closed suction drains (Jackson-Pratt) increases SSI rates. Strict control of blood glucose levels in the perioperative period may also lower SSI risk.[14]

MICROBIOLOGY

Because the premise for surgical prophylaxis is protection from infection, the type of antibiotic prophylaxis required depends on the most likely anticipated pathogens. Organisms involved in SSI are either acquired from the patient's normal flora (endogenous) or from contamination during the surgical procedure (exogenous). Based on the type of procedure, NRC classification (Table 112–1) and body location, resident flora can be anticipated (Table 112–5) and appropriate antibiotic choices can be made.

The ability of an organism to cause SSI depends on a variety of factors that includes the virulence of the organism, number of organisms involved, and general condition of the host immune system. The majority of organisms that make up the commensal flora are generally not pathogenic and, in fact, serve the host as a form of protection against more invasive organisms that would otherwise colonize the tissue site. These opportunistic organisms, although more problematic to the host in large numbers, are kept in check by the normal flora. Therefore, loss of these protective flora via antibiotics can upset the balance and allow pathogenic bacteria to proliferate and increase infectious risk. Normal flora can become pathogenic when translocated to a normally sterile tissue site or fluid during surgical procedures. Examples of this phenomenon would be the translocation of *S. aureus* or *Staphylococcus epidermidis* from the surface of the skin to deeper tissues and *Escherichia coli* from the colon to the peritoneal cavity, bloodstream, or urinary tract.

Studies in animals and healthy volunteers have shown that the number of organisms acquired during bacterial contamination of the surgical wound is important in determining the incidence of secondary infection.[15,16] In the past, animal models of infection have demonstrated that more than 1,000,000 *S. aureus* per square centimeter or gram of tissue are required to produce infection in a small clean wound site. Less than 100,000 of *Streptococcus pyogenes* per square centimeter or gram are required, however, to produce infection because of its more virulent nature.[16,17]

Compromises in host defenses reduce the number of bacteria required to establish infection. Obviously, any alteration of normal host defenses through surgical intervention (breach of skin or mucous membrane barriers, prosthetic devices) may potentiate the ability of organisms to cause infection. Loss of specific immune factors, such as complement activation, tissue-derived inhibitors, cell-mediated response (T cell), and granulocytic or phagocytic function (neutrophils, macrophages), can greatly increase the risk of SSI.[18,19] In addition, vascular occlusive states from the surgical procedure or those occurring from hypovolemic shock, the use of vasopressors, or both can greatly affect the blood flow to the surgical site, diminishing much of the host's ability to defend against microbial invasion.[20] The presence of traumatized tissue, hematomas, and foreign material also enhances the potential infection.[20,21] When a foreign body is introduced during a surgical procedure, fewer than 100 bacterial colony-forming units (CFUs) are required to cause a wound infection.[21] Experiments with polytetrafluoroethylene tissue cages and vascular grafts have demonstrated the ability of *S. aureus* to produce wound infections when given a suitable niche sequestered from normal host defenses.[17,21,22] Studies carried out with *S. aureus* contaminated sutures in the skin of healthy volunteers demonstrated a 10,000-fold reduction in the amount of organism required to establish a wound infection compared to a wound induced without sutures.[15]

TABLE 112–5. Most Likely Pathogens and Specific Recommendations for Surgical Prophylaxis[a]

Type of Operation	Likely Pathogens	Recommended Prophylaxis Regimen	Comments
Gastroduodenal	Enteric gram-negative bacilli, gram-positive cocci, oral anaerobes	Cefazolin 1 g × one IV	Hish-risk patients only
Biliary tract	Enteric gram-negative bacilli, enterococci, clostridia	Cefazolin 1 g × one IV	Bactobilia does not correlate well with pathogens
Colorectal	Anaerobes, enteric gram-negative bacilli	PO: neomycin 1 g + erythromycin base 1 g at 1 PM, 2PM, + 11 PM 1 day preoperation plus mechanical bowel preparation IV: cefoxitin or cefotetan 1 g × one IV	Benefit of oral plus IV is controversial
Appendectomy	Anaerobes, enteric gram-negative bacilli	Cefoxitin or cefotetan 1 g × one IV	3–5 days of therapeutic antibiotics postoperative if established infection present
Urologic	*Escherichia coli*	Cefazolin 1 g IV or oral antibiotic with comparable spectrum (where appropriate) × one	Only beneficial in high-risk cases (preexisting bacteriuria, high infection rate)
Cesarean section	Enteric gram-negative bacilli, anaerobes, group B streptococci, enterococci	Cefazolin 2 g × one IV	Give after cord is clamped
Hysterectomy	Same as Cesarean section	*Vaginal:* cefazolin 1 g × one IV, may repeat q8h × two doses hysterectomy *Abdominal:* cefazolin 1 g × one IV	Beneficial in abdominal hysterectomy regardless of risk, ?lower SSI rate with cefotetan
Head and neck	*S. Aureus*, streptococci, oral anaerobes	Clindamycin 600 mg IV or cefazolin 2 g IV at induction and q8h × two more doses	Addition of gentamicin to clindamycin is controversial, ampicillin/sulbactam also studied
Cardiac	*S. aureus, S. epidermidis,* corynebacterium, enteric gram-negative bacilli	Cefazolin 1 g q8h IV × 48 hours beginning at induction	Second-generation cephalosporins have been advocated; controversial shorter courses also studied
Vascular	*S. aureus, S. epidermidis,* enteric gram-negative bacteria	Cefazolin 1 g IV at induction and q8h × two more doses	Abdominal and lower extremity procedures have highest infection rate
Orthopedic	*S. aureus, S. epidermidis*	*Joint replacement:* Cefazolin 1 g × one IV preoperatively, then q8h × two more doses *Hip fracture repair:* Same except continue for 48 hours total	Open fractures assumed contaminated with gram-negative bacilli; aminoglycosides often used—see text
Neurosurgery	*S. aureus, S. epidermidis*	Cefazolin 1 g × one IV	Use in CSF shunting procedure is controversial

[a]One-time doses are optimally infused at induction of anesthesia except as noted. Repeat doses may be required for long procedures.
CSF = cerebrospinal fluid.
Compiled from Refs. 3, 26, and 41. See text for details and further references.

RESISTANT MICROORGANISMS

All organisms have the potential to become antibiotic resistant. Resistant organisms causing surgical infections can be acquired from the hospital setting prior to the surgical intervention through recolonization of the host with antibiotic resistant hospital flora. Epidemiologic studies have indicated that nosocomial acquired multiresistant organisms are largely transmitted to patients via the hands of hospital personnel.[23] The concomitant use of antibiotics also increases the colonization of patients with hospital flora. The other major route for acquisition of resistant hospital flora occurs by direct introduction during the surgical intervention.

According to the NNIS, the five most common pathogens encountered in surgical wounds are *S. aureus,* enterococci, coagulase-negative staphylococci, *E. coli,* and *Pseudomonas aeruginosa.*[24] Although the degree of resistance among these pathogens differs from one institution to another, the increased frequency of these resistant pathogens being implicated in surgical infections is of concern. Since the cephalosporins have been considered the workhorse for prophylactic antibiotics, cephalosporin-resistant organisms, such as methicillin-resistant *S. aureus,* coagulase-negative staphylococci, and gram-negative bacilli, represent the bulk of the problematic organisms.

An alarming increase in vancomycin-resistant enterococci (VRE), particularly *Enterococcus faecium,* has been reported by the Centers for Disease Control (CDC).[24,25] Risk factors for the colonization of VRE include critically injured patients, patients with severe underlying diseases, immunosuppression, intensive care unit patients, transplant patients, and patients who have had intra-abdominal or cardiothoracic surgical procedures, indwelling catheters, central venous lines, and prolonged courses of antimicrobials, including vancomycin.[25,26] The CDC has published recommendations to control the spread of VRE, including the restriction of routine prophylaxis with vancomycin.[25] Vancomycin may be substituted for cefazolin in institutions where methicillin-resistant *S. aureus* are prevalent.[27] Caution must be observed with the routine use of vancomycin as a prophylactic agent since there are a number of drawbacks associated with this antibiotic, including the lack of broad-spectrum coverage, potential for resistance development, and increased prevalence of adverse reactions, including infusion-related problems.[27] The emergence of *S. aureus* displaying intermediate resistance (minimum inhibitory concentration [MIC] $\geq 8\ \mu g/mL$) further underscores the need to limit routine use of vancomycin for prophylaxis (see Antimicrobial Selection).[28,29]

In cases involving methicillin-sensitive *S. aureus*, cefazolin failure has been reported in patients undergoing cardiac surgery. It has also been proposed that the β-lactamase expressed by some strains of methicillin-sensitive *S. aureus* hydrolyzes cefazolin more readily than cefuroxime or cefamandole. Although this information is disturbing, two large comparative trials have demonstrated the equivalence of cefazolin with these second-generation cephalosporins.[30,31] Cefazolin remains a mainstay in cardiovascular surgical procedures.[30–32] Lastly, an increased frequency of fungal infections in surgical patients has drawn increasing concern. The increased incidence of fungal infections in surgical patients is likely to be the result of overzealous use of broad-spectrum antibiotics. There are no recommendations for the use of prophylactic antifungal agents at this time.[33,34]

TIMING OF ANTIBIOTICS

The basic principles for the use of antimicrobial surgical prophylaxis include (1) antimicrobials should be delivered to the targeted tissue site prior to the initial incision and (2) bactericidal antibiotic tissue concentrations should be maintained throughout the length of the surgical procedure. Animal and human models have demonstrated the efficacy of a single dose of an antibiotic when administered just prior to bacterial contamination.[35,36] Considerable debate exists, however, over the importance of administering subsequent postoperative doses.[36,37] It is difficult to predict the exact moment of bacterial contamination during a procedure, however, the greatest risk probably occurs during the closing of the wound. Studies in patients undergoing cardiac surgery have demonstrated a higher infection rate among patients with undetectable antibiotic serum concentrations at the close of surgery.[38]

The question of whether single or multiple perioperative doses are required to ensure adequate protection depends on a number of factors. The ideal prophylactic antibiotic should rapidly achieve tissue concentrations well above the MIC of the potential contaminating pathogens and maintain therapeutic concentrations throughout the procedure after a single preoperative dose. Therefore, antimicrobials with long half-lives would theoretically be preferable to ensure sustained tissue concentrations. Antimicrobials with short serum half-lives may require multiple dosing at frequent dosing intervals, especially if the surgery is prolonged or in instances of massive blood loss. Studies examining serum concentrations secondary to intravenous (IV) administration of antibiotics with different pharmacokinetic profiles have demonstrated variability in achieved and sustained antimicrobial concentrations.[13]

Under ideal conditions, the antibiotic chosen for surgical prophylaxis would achieve its highest tissue concentrations at the time of initial skin incision during surgery. Antibiotics administered too early or after skin incision would likely achieve subtherapeutic concentrations, putting the patient at high risk of infection.[13,37] In a study examining the timing of antibiotics in 2847 patients receiving prophylaxis, Classen and associates[37] evaluated patients who received prophylaxis early (2 to 24 hours), preoperative (0 to 2 hours prior to surgery), perioperative (up to 3 hours after incision), and postoperatively (> 3 hours after incision). The risk of infection was lowest (0.6%) for those patients who received preoperative prophylaxis, moderate (1.4%) for those who received perioperative antibiotics, and greatest for those who received postoperative antibiotics (3.3%) or preoperative antibiotics too early (3.8%). The results indicated that the risk of infection increased dramatically with each hour postsurgical incision until antibiotics are administered (Fig. 112–1).[37] For these reasons, prophylactic antibiotics should not be prescribed to be given "on call to OR," nor should concurrent therapeutic antibiotics be relied on to provide adequate protection. In both situations, the chance for improperly timed doses is high.

Additional considerations in the selection and timing of antibiotic administration should include the underlying disease states of the patient with regard to circulation, metabolism, and elimination of antibiotics. Patients with thermal burn and spinal cord injuries have been shown to eliminate certain classes of antibiotics, primarily the aminoglycosides and β-lactams, at unusually high rates compared to controls.[39–41] Individuals undergoing cardiac bypass may have altered antibiotic disposition and may require special consideration.[42–44]

ANTIMICROBIAL SELECTION

The choice of the prophylactic antimicrobial depends on a multitude of factors, including the type of surgical procedure, most likely pathogenic organisms, safety and efficacy of the antimicrobial, track record for success based on pub-

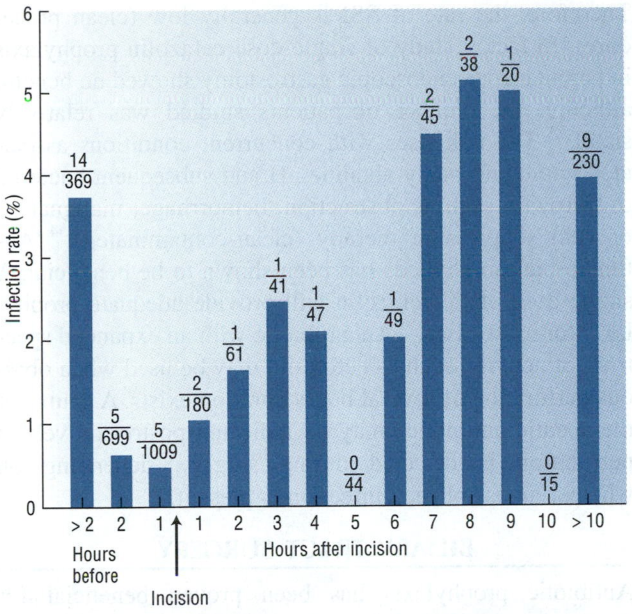

FIGURE 112–1. Rates of surgical wound infections (SWI) corresponding to the temporal relation between antibiotic administration and the start of surgery. The number of infections and the number of patients for each hourly interval appear as the numerator and denominator, respectively, of the fraction for that interval. The trend toward higher rates of infection for each hour that antibiotic administration was delayed after the surgical incision was significant (z score = 2.00; $P < .05$ by the Wilcoxon test). *(From Ref. 37, reprinted with permission of The New England Journal of Medicine. Copyright 1992, Massachusetts Medical Society.)*

lished literature, and costs. Although most surgical infections involve the patient's own flora, the selection of the antimicrobial must also take into account the susceptibility patterns of nosocomial-derived pathogens associated with the specific institution. Typically, gram-positive coverage is included in the choice of surgical prophylaxis since organisms, such as *S. aureus* and *S. epidermidis,* are commonly encountered as skin flora. The decision to broaden coverage to gram-negatives and anaerobic organisms is site specific (upper respiratory tract, gastrointestinal tract, genitourinary tract, Table 112–5) and depends on whether the operation will transect a hollow viscous or mucous membrane containing resident flora.[45]

Although a variety of antimicrobial prophylactic administration routes (oral, topical, intramuscular) are advocated, IV is favored because of its reliability in achieving suitable tissue concentrations.[13] As previously mentioned, the cephalosporin class of compounds is by far the most often prescribed class of agents for surgical prophylaxis. This is justified by the antimicrobial spectrum, the favorable pharmacokinetic profile, the low incidence of unwanted side effects, and the pharmacoeconomic advantages. First-generation cephalosporins, such as cefazolin, are the preferred choice (as good as second- or third-generation cephalosporins) for surgical prophylaxis, including most clean surgical procedures.[32] Although there are some reports of failure with cefazolin in cardiac procedures associated with methicillin-sensitive *S. aureus,* the majority of concern is because of the increasing incidence of methicillin-resistant *S. aureus* (MRSA) infections.[32,46,47] Vancomycin would seem to be a logical alternative to cefazolin in institutions with a high incidence of MRSA; however, its narrow spectrum of coverage, increased potential for toxicities, resistance development, and cost should limit its use to those procedures at highest risk or for patients with significant β-lactam hypersensitivity. The likelihood of the patient being already colonized with MRSA as a result of prior exposure may also be a factor when selecting prophylactic antibiotics. If preexisting colonization is doubtful, then vancomycin may not be necessary, even if the institution has a high incidence of MRSA. If the risk of MRSA is low and a β-lactam hypersensitivity exists, clindamycin can be used for many procedures instead of cefazolin in order to further limit vancomycin use. In cases where broader gram-negative and anaerobic coverage is desired, the antianaerobic cephalosporins, such as cefoxitin, cefotetan, and cefmetazole, are appropriate. Although third-generation cephalosporins (e.g., ceftriaxone) have been advocated for prophylaxis because of the increased gram-negative coverage and prolonged half-lives, inferior gram-positive, anaerobic coverage, and high cost discourage widespread use of these agents for prophylaxis.[32,45,47] As previously mentioned, the side effects of cephalosporins are relatively minor in comparison to the overall benefit from their routine use. Side effects encountered include allergic reactions ranging from minor skin manifestations at the site of infusion, rash, and pruritus to anaphylaxis. Cross-reactivity from penicillins to cephalosporins is approximately 5%. Therefore, caution should be used when administering cephalosporin agents to individuals with history of a penicillin anaphylactic reaction.

The overall incidence of pseudomembranous colitis secondary to cephalosporins is infrequent and generally manageable with a short course of oral metronidazole. Although the incidence is relatively low, bleeding abnormalities secondary to cephalosporin use have been reported.[48] The primary hematologic effect appears to be an inhibition of normal platelet function and the coagulation cascade. These effects are reflected by changes in bleeding times and increases in prothrombin time and activated partial thromboplastin time. The mechanism is thought to be related to α-carboxyl substitution on the β-lactam molecule or the methylthiotetrazole (NMTT) side chain of some agents, particularly cefamandole and cefotetan. Most data indicate that patients at greatest risk have received multiple doses of these agents and have underlying risk factors, such as vitamin K-deficient hypoprothrombinemia.[49] Infusion-related side effects, such as thrombophlebitis and hypotension, particularly with vancomycin, can usually be controlled by adequate dilution and slower administration rates.[50–52]

Because prophylactic antibiotic use represents a major potential for antibiotic resistance development and usually accounts for most of the antibiotic budget, curtailing inappropriate prophylactic use has become a focal point for most institutions. Inappropriate antibiotic prophylaxis includes the use of broader spectrum antimicrobials when a specific targeted spectrum is preferred, continuing prophylaxis beyond the standard recommendations of one to three doses of antibiotic coverage, and use of more costly antibiotics when equivalent, less expensive agents are available.

The most effective tools for control of prophylactic antibiotics are knowledge of the institution's postsurgical infection rate for each type of procedure, bacterial epidemiology studies, protocols that focus on control of problem pathogens, and institution-based antibiotic susceptibility data broken down for each surgical area within the hospital. With this information in hand, formulary selection, criteria for use, and policies governing surgical prophylaxis can be drafted with surgical attending staff involvement.

The goal of antimicrobial prophylaxis in surgery is the prevention of SSI. Proper prophylactic regimens are not designed to prevent postoperative infections at other sites (see Evaluation of Therapeutic Outcomes). Unfortunately, the incidence of these other infectious complications is often reported along with SSI rates in the surgical prophylaxis literature. The reader is advised to evaluate the data critically before accepting efficacy claims based on these reports. Inadequate sample size is also common in the literature, especially when clean procedures are studied.

RECOMMENDATIONS FOR ANTIBIOTIC PROPHYLAXIS IN SPECIFIC TYPES OF SURGERY

Traditionally, recommendations for surgical prophylaxis have been grouped according to which tissues will be manipulated during surgery. This is a logical approach because although many different surgical procedures can be performed at a given location, features such as endogenous flora and the pharmacokinetics, pharmacodynamics, and spectrum of selected antimicrobials are constant (see section on Antimicrobial Selection). The reader is reminded that prophylactic regimens are best evaluated through the results of properly conducted clinical trials. In the absence of data specific to the procedure in question, regimens appropriate for the anatomic site involved should suffice. Subsequent modifications are based on intraoperative findings or events.

A comprehensive review of the surgical prophylaxis literature is beyond the scope of this chapter. What follows is a brief discussion of the issues pertinent to the types of surgical procedures most frequently encountered. Specific recommendations are summarized in Table 112–5. The reader is also referred to the reviews published by the Surgical Infection Society[3] and the American Society of Hospital Pharmacists Commission on Therapeutics.[47] The latter document includes a comprehensive bibliography with primary references.

GASTROINTESTINAL SURGERY

Because of their relative acidity, the stomach and the duodenum normally contain insignificant numbers of bacteria. Therefore, the rate of SSI is generally low (clean procedure). In fact, a study of single-dose cefazolin prophylaxis in percutaneous endoscopic gastrostomy showed no benefit, although the number of patients studied was relatively small.[53] The risk rises with concurrent conditions associated with abnormally alkaline pH and subsequent bacterial overgrowth, such as obstruction, hemorrhage, malignancy, or acid suppression therapy (clean-contaminated).[54] Antimicrobial prophylaxis has been shown to be beneficial. A single dose of IV cefazolin will provide adequate prophylaxis for most cases.[55] An antibiotic with an expanded spectrum of activity, such as cefoxitin, may be used when obvious perforation of several hours duration exists. A course of therapeutic antibiotics may be indicated postoperatively if perforation is detected during surgery, depending on whether an established infection is present.

BILIARY TRACT SURGERY

Antibiotic prophylaxis has been proven beneficial for surgery involving the biliary tract. The bile is normally sterile and in the absence of any other underlying risk factors, the SSI rate is low. Bile contamination (bactobilia), however, occurs with many concurrent conditions, such as acute cholecystitis, biliary obstruction, and advanced age. Bactobilia is associated with a higher frequency of SSI.[56] The most frequently encountered organisms include *E. coli, Klebsiella,* and enterococci. *Pseudomonas* is an uncommon finding in the absence of cholangitis. The correlation between bactobilia in surgical specimens and subsequent pathogens implicated in SSI is poor and may explain the lack of a detectable difference in comparative studies involving antibiotics with different spectrums.[57] Single-dose prophylaxis with cefazolin is recommended. Several comparative studies using second- and third-generation cephalosporins exist, but they have not demonstrated any advantage over cefazolin to date.[56] Most cholecystectomies are now performed with a laparoscope. Since this is theoretically less invasive, lower SSI risk is presumed. Controlled trials of prophylactic antibiotics in this setting are lacking, but early evidence suggests that prophylaxis may be unnecessary.[58] In the interim, when prophylaxis is desired, a single dose of cefazolin should suffice.

Some surgeons use presumptive antibiotics for cases of acute cholecystitis or cholangitis and defer surgery until the patient is afebrile in an attempt to decrease infection rates further, but this practice is controversial. Detection of an active infection during surgery (gangrenous gallbladder, suppurative cholangitis) is an indication for therapeutic postoperative antibiotics. In either case, antibiotics with additional antianaerobic activity (e.g., cefoxitin or cefotetan) are indicated.[59]

COLORECTAL SURGERY

Bacterial counts in fecal material present in the colon frequently exceed 10^9 g. Anaerobes and gram-negative aerobes predominate, although gram-positive aerobes are also important (Table 112–5). Therefore, the risk of SSI in the absence of an adequate prophylactic regimen is substantial. Reducing this bacteria load with a thorough bowel preparation regimen (4 L of polyethylene glycol solution administered orally the day before surgery) is the single most important method to prevent SSI.

Effective antibiotic prophylaxis reduces SSI risk even further. Specific recommendations are listed in Table 112–5. Several oral regimens designed to reduce bacterial counts in the colon have been studied. The combination of 1 g of neomycin plus 1 g of erythromycin base given orally 19, 18, and 9 hours preoperatively is the most commonly used regimen in the United States. Optimally, the bowel preparation regimen should be completed before the oral antibiotics are started. This is of particular concern since most of these procedures are now performed electively on a "same day surgery" basis. The preparation regimen is administered to the patient at home on the day prior to hospital admission and, thus, cannot be monitored closely. Administration of the antibiotics while the bowel preparation is still ongoing may compromise efficacy, although this has not yet been studied.

Neomycin is poorly absorbed and provides high intralumen concentrations effective against most gram-negative aerobes. Oral erythromycin is partially absorbed, but still produces concentrations in the colon sufficient to suppress the involved anaerobes. If surgery is postponed, the antibiotics must be redosed to maintain efficacy. It is worth noting that elective colorectal surgery is the only procedure where oral antibiotics have consistently been shown to provide effective prophylaxis.[60] Patients who cannot take oral medications should receive parenteral antibiotics (Table 112–5). Whether or not perioperative parenteral antibiotics, in addition to the standard preoperative oral antibiotic regimen, will lower SSI rates further still is controversial.[61,62] Intravenous antibiotics are required for colostomy reversal, since enterally administered antibiotics will not reach the distal segment to be reanastomosed. Postoperative antibiotics are unnecessary in the absence of any untoward events or findings during surgery.

APPENDECTOMY

Appendectomy is one of the most frequently performed abdominal procedures. A multitude of different antibiotic regimens with activity against gram-positive and gram-negative aerobes plus anaerobes have been studied and found to be effective in reducing the incidence of SSI. A cephalosporin with antianaerobic activity, such as cefoxitin or cefotetan, is recommended as first-line therapy.[63] Selection of an antibiotic with an unnecessarily broad spectrum (*Pseudomonas*) does not further reduce SSI risk,[64] but it may increase cost of therapy and promote resistance. Single-dose therapy is adequate as long as the appendix is not found to be gangrenous or perforated during surgery.[63] One report suggests superiority of cefotetan versus cefoxitin when both were given as a single dose, possibly because of their different half-lives, but more studies are needed.[65] Established intra-abdominal infections require appropriate therapeutic postoperative antibiotics.

UROLOGIC PROCEDURES

The most important risk factor for development of a SSI after urologic surgery is the presence of preoperative bacteriuria. It is, therefore, imperative to test for bacteriuria prior to the procedure and to administer therapeutic antibiotics as necessary. As long as the urine is sterile preoperatively, the risk of SSI after urologic procedures is very low, and the benefit of prophylactic antibiotics in this setting is controversial.[66] This is further obscured by the frequent presence of urinary catheters in the postoperative period and the subsequent risk of bacteriuria independent of any risk accrued from the surgery itself. Specific recommendations are listed in Table 112–5. *Escherichia coli* is the most frequently encountered organism. Routinely expanding the spectrum by using a third-generation cephalosporin or a fluoroquinolone does not lower SSI rates any further and is not recommended. Single-dose therapy is adequate: Regimens as long as 3 weeks have been reported, but this is probably unnecessary. Urologic procedures requiring an abdominal approach, such as a nephrectomy or cystectomy, require prophylaxis appropriate for a clean-contaminated abdominal procedure.[3]

CESAREAN SECTION

Cesarean section is the most frequently performed surgical procedure in the United States. Previously, antibiotics were felt to be beneficial only in patients considered at high risk, such as in emergency cases, premature rupture of membranes, or those who did not receive prenatal care. Several large trials and a meta-analysis have, however, documented the efficacy of antibiotics for all women undergoing cesarean section regardless of underlying risk factors. Prophylactic antibiotics are given to avoid SSI and prevent endometritis. Several types of bacteria have been implicated (Table 112–5). Despite this, cefazolin remains the drug of choice. Providing a broader spectrum by using cefoxitin against anaerobes or piperacillin for better coverage against *Pseudomonas* or enterococci, for example, does not lower postoperative infection rates any further in comparative studies.

Unlike most surgical procedures, a single 2-g dose of cefazolin has been found to be superior to a 1-g dose and is, thus, recommended.[67] Another distinctive feature is that unlike most operations (see section on Timing), antibiotics are given *after* the incision is made. Administering the antibiotic just after the umbilical cord is clamped avoids exposing the infant to the drug and may actually lower rates of neonatal sepsis. Longer durations of therapy do not result in lower infection rates.

HYSTERECTOMY

The incidence of SSI after hysterectomy depends on the type of procedure performed. Because of the polymicrobial flora normally present at the operative site (Table 112–5), vaginal hysterectomies are associated with a high rate of postoperative infection when performed without the benefit of prophylactic antibiotics. As with cesarean sections, cefazolin is the drug of choice in spite of the involved microbiology.[68] Single-dose therapy should be adequate, but most reports used a 24-hour regimen.

Abdominal hysterectomy is not associated with bacterial contamination from the vaginal flora, and SSI rates are correspondingly lower. Prophylactic antibiotics, however, are still recommended regardless of underlying risk factors. Both cefazolin and antianaerobic cephalosporins (e.g., cefoxitin, cefotetan) have been studied extensively.[69,70] Although a comparative trial showed lower SSI rates with cefotetan compared to cefazolin,[70] at this point, it is unclear which is superior. In either case, a course not exceeding 24 hours' duration is sufficient, and, in fact, single-dose therapy has been effective.[70] As with other procedures, perioperative events and findings may require the use of therapeutic antibiotics after surgery. Antibiotics have not been shown to be beneficial in tubal microsurgery, but more studies are needed.[71]

HEAD AND NECK SURGERY

The use of prophylactic antibiotics during head and neck surgery depends on the type of procedure performed. Many, such as parotidectomy or a simple tooth extraction, are clean procedures by NRC definition and are associated with very low rates of SSI. As expected, surgical prophylaxis has not been proven to be beneficial in these circumstances.[72] Head and neck procedures involving an incision through a mucosal layer (and therefore breaching primary immune system barriers), however, carry a high risk of SSI. The normal mouth flora is polymicrobic (see Table 112–5) as are SSIs after head and neck surgery. Anaerobes and gram-positive aerobes predominate. Specific recommendations for prophylaxis are listed in Table 112–5. A meta-analysis proposed that a 24-hour regimen of clindamycin is the regimen of choice,[73] although cefazolin is also recommended. While typical doses of cefazolin are ineffective for anaerobic infections, the 2-g dose recommended produces concentrations high enough to be inhibitory to these organisms. A combination of clindamycin plus gentamicin has also been described. It is unclear whether or not the addition of an aminoglycoside further reduces SSI risk since clindamycin alone has been shown to be effective. Topical therapy with clindamycin and β-lactamase inhibitor combinations has been described, though early data do not suggest lower SSI rates compared to parenteral clindamycin alone.[74]

CARDIAC SURGERY

Although most cardiac surgeries are technically clean procedures, prophylactic antibiotics have been shown to lower rates of SSI. The substantial morbidity associated with SSI after cardiac surgery and the use of prosthetic implants further justify routine prophylaxis. The usual pathogens are skin flora (see Table 112.5) and, rarely, gram-negative enteric organisms. Cefazolin has been extensively studied and is considered the drug of choice.[75] Several studies and a meta-analysis have been published that advocate preferential use of a second-generation cephalosporin (cefuroxime, cefamandole) instead of cefazolin.[76] The significance of these findings is controversial, however, because of numerous problems with study design, and cefazolin remains the standard of care (see section on Resistant Microorganisms). In fact, cefazolin has been shown to be as effective as the second-generation cephalosporins in two studies.[30,31] The accepted duration of prophylactic antibiotics after cardiac surgery is 48 hours. There is some evidence that 24 hours is sufficient.[77] Extending therapy for 3 to 5 days does not lower SSI rates further.[75,77]

It may be necessary to use vancomycin in hospitals with a high incidence of SSI with MRSA. The need for vancomycin should be evaluated carefully as previously discussed. Vancomycin is also frequently used presumptively when sternal wounds are to be explored surgically for possible mediastinitis. This is a reasonable approach, since this constitutes a failure of the previous prophylactic regimen. Subsequent antibiotic therapy is guided by intraoperative findings.

NONCARDIAC VASCULAR SURGERY

As with cardiac surgery, most vascular surgery is considered clean by NRC criteria. Similarly, SSI in this setting results in extensive morbidity and mortality, especially when a prosthetic graft is involved. Prophylactic antibiotics are beneficial, especially in procedures involving the abdominal aorta and the lower extremities. Again, *Staphylococci* and gram-negative enterics are the most likely pathogens. Twenty-four hours of prophylaxis with IV cefazolin is adequate.[78] Patients requiring prosthesis implantation may ultimately benefit from antibiotic-coated grafts, but controlled trials are needed.

ORTHOPEDIC SURGERY

Although most orthopedic surgery is clean by definition, prophylactic antibiotics have been shown to be beneficial in cases involving implantation of prosthetic material (pins, plates, artificial joints).[79,80] Late-occurring infectious complications in particular result in substantial morbidity (and often require prosthesis removal for definitive management), further justifying prophylaxis. The most likely pathogens mirror those of other clean procedures and include staphylococci and, infrequently, gram-negative aerobes. Again, cefazolin is the best studied antibiotic and is, thus, the drug of choice. Rates of SSI after total joint replacement are reduced with 24 hours of prophylactic antibiotics. They are also indicated for hip fracture surgery, but the accepted duration is 48 hours. Antibiotic-impregnated cement and beads have been used to lower SSI rates, but conclusive data are lacking.[81] This technique has also been used therapeutically. Patients suffering open (compound) fractures are especially susceptible to infection since contamination is almost always present. The use of antibiotics is presumptive under these circumstances. Cefazolin is often combined with an aminoglycoside in this setting, but controlled trials are lacking.[82] The duration of therapy is highly variable and depends on surgical findings during debridement and results of intraoperative cultures.[83] Established joint infections or osteomyelitis requires an extended course of therapeutic antibiotics.

NEUROSURGERY

The use of prophylactic antibiotics in neurosurgery is controversial. The rates of SSI after these clean operations are very low, but they are associated with significant morbidity and mortality. Consequently, in contrast to the other clean procedures discussed previously, data demonstrating the benefit of prophylactic antibiotics in this setting are equivocal. A review and meta-analysis concluded that single doses of cefazolin or, where required, vancomycin (see section on Antimicrobial Selection) appear to lower SSI risk after craniotomy.[84,85] Conversely, studies performed on shunting procedures do not consistently show lower infection rates with antibiotic prophylaxis, although a meta-analysis suggests efficacy.[86]

PHARMACOECONOMIC CONSIDERATIONS

Several investigators have attempted some sort of financial analysis when reporting the results of comparative trials.[78,87] Detailed studies of the pharmacoeconomics of antimicrobial prophylaxis in surgery are lacking, however. Most of the analyses available only address drug charges or costs and do not address other important outcomes (such as SSIs and adverse effects from the antibiotics) and their related costs. Future efforts in this area should consider these factors. This will be particularly important as the role of prophylaxis for clean procedures is further defined (see Individualizing Risk for Surgical Site Infection).

EVALUATION OF THERAPEUTIC OUTCOMES

As stated previously, the goal of antibiotic prophylaxis in surgery is the prevention of SSI. To assess the outcome, SSI must be differentiated from other postoperative infections or complications. Leukocytosis and fever are common in the immediate postoperative period, but typically resolve with prompt ambulation, timely removal of invasive devices, prevention or resolution, or both, of atelectasis through optimal respiratory care, and effective analgesia. The emergence of distal infections, such as pneumonia, does not constitute a failure of surgical prophylaxis. Unnecessarily prolonged prophylactic regimens will, however, contribute to the selection of resistant organisms and make these infections more difficult to treat.

The appearance of the surgical site is the most important determinant of SSI. Redness, warmth, and tenderness or pain accompanied by drainage of pus from any portion of the incision is consistent with SSI. By definition, any surgical site that requires incision and drainage by the surgeon is considered infected regardless of appearance. Failure of an incision to heal, wound dehiscence, or both are also common with SSI, although surgical technique and nutritional factors are also important.

The timing of the appearance of symptoms of SSI is also important when evaluating therapeutic outcomes of surgical prophylaxis. As stated previously, only a portion of SSIs will be evident during acute hospitalization. Surgical site infections may not become evident until up to 30 days later, or in the case of prosthesis implantation, up to 1 year later. As a result, the true incidence of SSI can only be determined in conjunction with proper postdischarge surveillance. All studies investigating the efficacy of surgical prophylaxis must include adequate postdischarge wound surveillance data to report the success of any regimen fully.

▶ PRINCIPLES OF PHARMACOTHERAPY

Antimicrobial prophylaxis remains an important component of optimal surgical care. When prescribed properly, the incidence of SSIs can be substantially reduced with minimal risk to the patient. The following principles of therapy need to be considered when designing appropriate regimens for surgical prophylaxis:

- The goal of antimicrobial prophylaxis in surgery is the prevention of surgical site infections (SSIs). It is not intended to clear distal infections or prevent other nosocomial infections.
- Prophylaxis with antimicrobials is adjunctive. A definitive surgical procedure employing optimal aseptic technique is the best defense against SSI.
- The choice of antibiotics depends on intrinsic patient risk, type of surgical procedure, and intraoperative events. First-generation cephalosporins (cefazolin) remain the mainstay for antimicrobial prophylaxis for the vast majority of procedures (with the exception of some types of abdominal surgery).
- Proper timing of prophylactic antibiotics is crucial. Optimally, they should be given within 1 hour of incision. Giving antibiotics "on call to OR" or relying on concurrent therapeutic antibiotics results in improperly timed doses and contributes to increased SSI risk.
- Prolonged regimens using unnecessarily broad-spectrum antibiotics increase costs and adverse effects without lowering SSI rates further.
- Postdischarge surveillance is necessary to determine true SSI incidence.
- The use of vancomycin for surgical prophylaxis should be limited to cases where either a serious β-lactam hypersensitivity exists or there is a high likelihood preexisting colonization with resistant organisms.
- Single-dose prophylaxis appears to be effective for many types of surgery.

REFERENCES

1. Wenzel RP. Preoperative antibiotic prophylaxis. N Engl J Med 1992; 326:337–339.
2. Weigelt JA, Dryer D, Haley RW. The necessity and efficiency of wound surveillance after discharge. Arch Surg 1992;127:77–82.
3. Page CP, Bohnen JMA, Fletcher JR, et al. Antimicrobial prophylaxis for surgical wounds: Guidelines for clinical care. Arch Surg 1993; 128:79–88.
4. Nichols RL. Surgical wound infection. Am J Med 1991;91(suppl 3B): 54S–64S.
5. National Academy of Sciences—National Research Council. Postoperative wound infections: The influence of ultraviolet irradiation of the operating room and of various other factors. Ann Surg 1964; 160:32–135.
6. Cruse PJE, Foord R. A five-year prospective study of 23,649 surgical wounds. Arch Surg 1973;107:206–210.
7. The Veterans Affairs Total Parenteral Nutrition Cooperative Study Group. Perioperative total parenteral nutrition in surgical patients. N Engl J Med 1991;325:525–532.
8. Haley RW, Culver DH, Morgan WM, et al. Identifying patients at high risk of surgical wound infection: A simple multivariate index of patient susceptibility and wound contamination. Am J Epidemiol 1985; 121:206–215.
9. Culver DH, Horan TC, Gaynes RP, et al. Surgical wound infection rates by wound class, operative procedure, and patient risk index. Am J Med 1991;91(suppl 3B):152S–157S.
10. Owens WD, Felts JA, Spitznagel EL. ASA physical status classifications: A study of consistency of ratings. Anesthesiology 1978;49: 239–243.
11. Lewis RT, Weigand FM, Mamazza J, et al. Should antibiotic prophylaxis be used routinely in clean surgical procedures. A tentative yes. Surgery 1995;118:742–747.
12. Boyce JM. Preventing staphylococcal infections by eradicating nasal carriage of *Staphylococcus aureus:* Proceeding with caution. Infect Control Hosp Epidemiol 1996;17:775–779.
13. Condon RW, Wittman DH. The use of antibiotics in general surgery. Curr Probl Surg 1991;28:802–907.
14. Zerr KJ, Furnary AP, Grunkemeier GL, et al. Glucose control lowers the risk of wound infection in diabetics after open heart operation. Ann Thorac Surg 1997;63:356–361.
15. Elek SD, Conen PE. The virulence of *Staphylococcus pyogenes* for man: A study of the problems of wound infection. Br J Exp Pathol 1958;38:573–586.
16. Burke JF. Identification of the sources of staphylococci contaminating the surgical wound during operation. Ann Surg 1963;158:898–904.
17. Kaiser AB, Kernodle DS, Parker RA. Low-inoculum model of surgical wound infection. J Infect Dis 1992;166:393–399.
18. Meakins JL, Pietsch JB, Bubenick O, et al. Delayed hypersensitivity: Indicator of acquired failure of host defenses in sepsis and trauma. Ann Surg 1977;186:241–250.
19. Christou NV, McLean APH, Meakins JL. Host defense in blunt trauma: Interrelationships of kinetics of anergy and depressed neutrophil function, nutritional status and sepsis. J Trauma 1980;20: 833–841.
20. Richet HM, Chidiac C, Prat A, et al. Analysis of risk factors for surgical wound infections following vascular surgery. Am J Med 1991; 91:(suppl 3b):170S–172S.
21. Zimmerli W, Waldvogel FA, Vaudaux P, et al. Pathogenesis of foreign body infection: Description and characteristics of an animal model. J Infect Dis 1987;146:487–497.
22. Arbeit RD, Dunn RM. Expression of capsular polysaccharide during experimental focal infection with *Staphylococcus aureus.* J Infect Dis 1987;156:947–952.
23. Schaberg D. Major trends in the microbial etiology of nosocomial infection. Am J Med 1991;91(suppl 3B):72S–75S.
24. Jarvis WR, Martone WJ. Predominant pathogens in hospital infections. J Antimicrob Chemother 1992;29(suppl A):19–24.
25. Centers for Disease Control and Prevention. Recommendations for preventing the spread of vancomycin resistance: Hospital Infection Control Practice Advisory Committee. Infect Control Hosp Epidemiol 1995;16:105–113.
26. Handwerger S, Raucher B, Altarac D, et al. Nosocomial outbreak due to *Enterococcus faecium* highly resistant to vancomycin, penicillin, and gentamicin. Clin Infect Dis 1993;16:750–755.
27. Ena J, Dick RW, Jones RN, et al. The epidemiology of intravenous vancomycin usage in a university hospital: A 10 year study. JAMA 1993;269:598–602.
28. Centers for Disease Control and Prevention. Reduced susceptibility of *Staphylococcus aureus* to vancomycin. United States. MMWR 1997; 46:765–766.
29. Centers for Disease Control and Prevention. Interim guidelines for prevention and control of *Staphylococcus aureus* infection associated with reduced susceptibility to vancomycin. MMWR 1997;46: 626–635.
30. Townsend TR, Reitz BA, Bilker WB, Bartlett JG. Clinical trial of cefamandole, cefazolin, and cefuroxime for antibiotic prophylaxis in cardiac operations. J Thorac Cardiovasc Surg 1993;106:664–670.
31. Curtis JJ, Boley TM, Walls JT, et al. Randomized, prospective comparisons of first and second generation cephalosporins as infection prophylaxis for cardiac surgery. Am J Surg 1993;166:734–737.
32. Abramowicz M, ed. Antimicrobial prophylaxis in surgery. Med Lett 1995;37:79–82.
33. Fraser VJ, Jones M, Dunkel J, et al. Candidemia in a tertiary care hospital: Epidemiology, risk factors and predictors of mortality. Clin Infect Dis 1992;15:414–421.
34. Pittet D, Monod M, Suter PM, et al. Candida colonization and subsequent infections in critically ill surgical patients. Ann Surg 1994;220: 751–758.
35. Burke JF. The effective period of preventive antibiotic action in experimental incisions and dermal lesions. Surgery 1961;50:161–168.
36. DiPiro JT, Cheung RPF, Bowden TA, Mansberger JA. Single dose systemic antibiotic prophylaxis of surgical wound infections. Am J Surg 1986;152:552–559.
37. Classen DC, Evans RS, Pestotnik SL, et al. The timing of prophylactic administration of antibiotics and the risk of surgical wound infection. N Engl J Med 1992;326:281–286.
38. Goldman DA, Hopkins CC, Karchmer AW. Cephalothin prophylaxis in cardiac valve surgery: A prospective, double-blind comparison of two-day and six-day regimen. J Thorac Cardiovasc Surg 1977;73: 470–479.
39. Sawchuk RJ. Drug absorption and disposition in burn patients. In: Benet LZ, Massoud N, Gambertoglio JG, eds. Pharmacokinetic Basis for Drug Treatment. New York, Raven Press, 1984:333–348.
40. Rybak MJ, Albrecht LM, Berman J, et al. Vancomycin pharmacokinetics in burn patients and intravenous drug abusers. Antimicrob Agents Chemother 1990;34:792–795.
41. Segal JL, Gray DR, Gordon SK, et al. Gentamicin disposition in humans with spinal cord injury. Paraplegia 1985;23:47–55.
42. Miller KW, McCoy HG, Chan KHK, et al. Effect of cardiopulmonary bypass on cefazolin disposition. Clin Pharmacol Ther 1980;27: 550–556.
43. Klamerus KJ, Rodvold KA, Silverman NA, Levitsky S. Effect of cardiopulmonary bypass on vancomycin and netilmicin disposition. Antimicrob Agents Chemother 1988;32:631–635.
44. Jungbluth GL, Pasko MT, Beam TR, Jusko WJ. Ceftriaxone disposition in open-heart surgery patients. Antimicrob Agents Chemother 1989;33:850–856.
45. Alexander JW, Dellinger PE. Surgical infections and choice of antibiotics. In: Sabiston DC, ed. Textbook of Surgery, 14th ed. Philadelphia, WB Saunders, 1990:221–236.

46. Kernodole DS, Classen DC, Burke JP, et al. Failure of cephalosporins to prevent *Staphylococcus aureus* surgical wound infections. JAMA 1990;263:961–966.
47. ASHP Commission on Therapeutics. ASHP therapeutic guidelines on antimicrobial prophylaxis in surgery. Clin Pharm 1992;11:483–513.
48. Sattler FR, Weitekamp MR, Ballard JO. Potential for bleeding with the new beta lactam antibiotics. Ann Intern Med 1986;105:924–931.
49. Babiak LM, Rybak MJ. Hematological effects associated with beta-lactam use. Drug Intell Clin Pharm 1986;20:833–836.
50. Romanelli VA, Howie MB, Myerowitz PD, et al. Intraoperative and postoperative effects of vancomycin administration in cardiac surgery patients: A prospective, double-blind, randomized trial. Crit Care Med 1993;21:1124–1131.
51. Polk RE. Anaphylactoid reactions to glycopeptide antibiotics. J Antimicrob Chemother 1991;27(suppl B):17–29.
52. O'Sullivan TL, Ruffing MJ, Lamp KC, et al. Prospective evaluation of red man syndrome in patients receiving vancomycin. J Infect Dis 1993;168:773–776.
53. Sturgis TM, Yancy W, Cole JC, et al. Antibiotic prophylaxis in percutaneous endoscopic gastrostomy. Am J Gastroenterol 1996;91: 2301–2304.
54. LoCicero J, Nichols RL. Sepsis after gastroduodenal operations: Relationship to gastric acid, motility, and endogenous microflora. South Med J 1980;73:878–880.
55. Lewis RT, Goodall RG, Marien B, et al. Efficacy and distribution of single- dose preoperative antibiotic prophylaxis in high-risk gastroduodenal surgery. Can J Surg 1991;34:117–122.
56. Meijer WS, Schmitz PIM, Jeekel J. Meta-analysis of randomized controlled clinical trials of antibiotic prophylaxis in biliary tract surgery. Br J Surg 1990;77:283–290.
57. Garibaldi RA, Skolnick D, Maglio S, et al. Postcholecystectomy wound infection: The impact of prophylactic antibiotics on the epidemiology of infections. Ann Surg 1986;204:650–654.
58. Watkin DS, Wainwright AM, Thompson MH, Leaper DJ. Infection after laparoscopic cholecystectomy: Are antibiotics really necessary? Eur J Surg 1995;161:509–511.
59. Lee WJ, Chang KJ, Lee CS, Chen M. Surgery in cholangitis: Bacteriology and choice of antibiotic. Hepatogastroenterology 1992;39: 347–349.
60. Bartlett JG, Condon RE, Gorbach SL, et al. Veterans administration cooperative study on bowel preparation for elective colorectal operations: Impact of oral antibiotic regimen on colonic flora, wound irrigation cultures and bacteriology of septic complications. Ann Surg 1978;188:249–254.
61. Condon RE, Bartlett JG, Greenlee H, et al. Efficacy of oral and systemic antibiotic prophylaxis in colorectal operations. Arch Surg 1983;118:496–502.
62. Stellato TA, Gordon NH, Danziger LH. Addition of parenteral cefoxitin to regimen of oral antibiotics for elective colorectal operations. Ann Surg 1991;213:375–376. Letter.
63. Bauer T, Vennits B, Holm B, et al. Antibiotic prophylaxis in acute nonperforated appendicitis. Ann Surg 1989;209:307–311.
64. Lau WY, Fan ST, Chu KW, et al. Randomized, prospective, and double-blind trial of new β-lactams in the treatment of appendicitis. Antimicrob Agents Chemother 1985;28:639–642.
65. Liberman MA, Greason KL, Frame S, Ragland JJ. Single-dose cefotetan or cefoxitin versus multiple-dose cefoxitin as prophylaxis in patients undergoing appendectomy for acute nonperforated appendicitis. J Am Coll Surg 1995;180:77–80.
66. Childs SJ, Wells WG, Mirelman S. Antibiotic prophylaxis for genitourinary surgery in community hospitals. J Urol 1983;130:305–308.
67. Faro S, Martens MG, Hammill HA, et al. Antibiotic prophylaxis: Is there a difference? Am J Obstet Gynecol 1990;162:900–909.
68. Hemsell DL, Bawdon RE, Hemsell PG, et al. Single-dose cephalosporin for prevention of major pelvic infection after vaginal hysterectomy: Cefazolin versus cefoxitin versus cefotaxime. Am J Obstet Gynecol 1987;156:1201–1205.
69. Hemsell DL, Johnson ER, Hemsell PG, et al. Cefazolin for hysterectomy prophylaxis. Obstet Gynecol 1990;76:603–606.
70. Hemsell DL, Johnson ER, Hemsell PG, et al. Cefazolin is inferior to cefotetan as single dose prophylaxis for women undergoing elective total abdominal hysterectomy. Clin Infect Dis 1995;20:677–684.
71. Letterie GS, Hibbert M. The role of antibiotic prophylaxis for tubal microsurgery. Arch Gynecol Obstet 1993;253:193–196.
72. Tabet JC, Johnson JT. Wound infection in head and neck surgery: Prophylaxis, etiology, and management. J Otolaryngol 1990;19:197–200.
73. Velanovich V. A meta-analysis of prophylactic antibiotics in head and neck surgery. Plast Reconstruc Surg 1991;87:429–435.
74. Grandis JR, Vickers RM, Rihs JD, et al. Efficacy of topical amoxicillin plus clavulanate/ticarcillin plus clavulanate and clindamycin in contaminated head and neck surgery: Effect of antibiotic spectra and duration of therapy. J Infect Dis 1994;170:729–732.
75. Ariano RE, Zhanel GG. Antimicrobial prophylaxis in coronary bypass surgery: A critical appraisal. DICP Ann Pharmacother 1991;25: 478–484.
76. Kreter B, Woods M. Antibiotic prophylaxis for cardiothoracic operations: A metaanalysis of thirty years of clinical trials. J Thorac Cardiovasc Surg 1992;104:590–599.
77. Nooyen, SMH, Overbeek BP, de la Riviere AB, et al. Prospective randomized comparison of single-dose versus multiple dose cefuroxime for prophylaxis in coronary artery bypass grafting. Eur J Microbiol Infect Dis 1994;13:1033–1037.
78. Edwards WH, Kaiser AB, Tapper S, et al. Cefamandole versus cefazolin in vascular surgical wound infection prophylaxis: Cost effectiveness and risk factors. J Vasc Surg 1993;18:470–476.
79. Pollard JP, Hughes SPF, Scott JE, et al. Antibiotic prophylaxis in total hip replacement. B Med J 1979;1:707–709.
80. Hill C, Mazas F, Flamant R, Evrard J. Prophylactic cefazolin versus placebo in total hip replacement. Lancet 1981;1:795–797.
81. Wininger DA, Fass RJ. Antibiotic-impregnated cement and beads for orthopedic infections. Antimicrob Agents Chemother 1996;40: 2675–2679.
82. Patzakis MJ, Wilkins J, Wiss DA. Infection following intramedullary nailing of long bones. Clin Orthop 1986;212:182–191.
83. Dellinger EP, Caplan ES, Weaver LD, et al. Duration of preventive antibiotic administration for open extremity fractures. Arch Surg 1988; 123:333–339.
84. Haines SJ. Efficacy of antibiotic prophylaxis in clean neurosurgical operations. Neurosurgery 1989;24:401–405.
85. Barker FG. Efficacy of prophylactic antibiotics for craniotomy: A meta-analysis. Neurosurgery 1994;35:484–492.
86. Haines SJ, Walters BC. Antibiotic prophylaxis for cerebrospinal fluid shunts: A meta-analysis. Neurosurgery 1994;34:87–93.
87. Blair EA, Johnson JT, Wagner RL, et al. Cost analysis of antibiotic prophylaxis in clean head and neck surgery. Arch Otolaryngol Head Neck Surg 1995;121:269–271.

113

VACCINES, TOXOIDS, AND OTHER IMMUNOBIOLOGICS

Joseph S. Bertino, Jr., PharmD, FCCP, and Daniel T. Casto, PharmD, FCCP

The discovery and introduction of vaccines, toxoids, and immunoglobulins has resulted in a significant decline in worldwide morbidity and mortality because of their respective diseases. In addition, they have been shown to be generally safe and cost-effective.[1–3] This chapter is aimed at introducing the reader to three groups of agents: vaccines, toxoids, and immune sera (together known as immunobiologics). These groups will be defined, and related agents will be dealt with concurrently in an attempt to illustrate total immunotherapy. Obscure agents and agents used only by the military have been eliminated from this discussion in the interest of brevity. The process of inducing or providing immunity artificially by administering an immunobiologic agent is known as immunization. The term *immunization* is considered more specific than the term *vaccination.*

PRODUCTS TO PRODUCE IMMUNIZATION

Vaccines and toxoids are separate and distinct products. Both types of products, however, act to induce active immunity; that is, immunity generated by a natural immunologic response to an antigen. Vaccines are derived from the infecting organism itself. Viral vaccines can be either live attenuated or killed. Killed viral vaccines may consist of whole or split viral particles or specific viral fragments (subunits), as in the case of hepatitis B vaccine. Bacterial vaccines are generally killed whole bacteria or specific bacterial wall antigens. Live attenuated vaccines induce an immunologic response more consistent with that occurring with natural infection. Because the organisms in live attenuated vaccines multiply in the body after injection, they may confer lifelong immunity with one dose (as does a primary natural infection); however, this is not an absolute (as evidenced by the need for an additional dose of measles vaccine some time after the initial dose in infancy). Killed vaccines, on the other hand, do not induce permanent immunity and require additional doses at varying time intervals (booster doses).

Toxoids are inactivated bacterial toxins that are generally combined with aluminum salts (alum) to enhance their antigenicity by prolonging antigen absorption. These adjuvants also increase local tissue irritation when injected. Toxoids retain the ability to stimulate the formation of antitoxin.

Immune sera are sterile solutions containing antibody derived from human (immune globulin) or equine (horse; antitoxin) sources. Immune globulins are derived from donor pools of blood plasma and are processed using cold ethanol fractionation in order to inactivate any potentially infecting agent. Antitoxins are made by immunizing animals with an antigen and then harvesting the antibodies (antitoxins) made against the antigens. These sera are indicated for induction of passive immunity (temporary immunity to infection as a result of the administration of antibodies not produced by the host). Human immune sera is preferred because of its lower incidence of serum sickness and other allergic reactions as compared to equine derived sera (see section on Other Immunobiologics).

In addition to the active component in an immunobiologic, other active and inert ingredients are often present. Suspending agents, such as water, saline, or complex fluids containing proteins or antigens, are used as the vehicle for the immunobiologic agent. Preservatives, stabilizers, and antibiotics are often added to help maintain sterility. Finally, adjuvants to enhance immunologic response are used (aluminum salts). It must be kept in mind that patients may respond with allergic reactions, not to the immunobiologic agent itself, but to the other components of the pharmaceutical preparation. Different manufacturers of the same immunobiologic may have different active and inert ingredients in their product.[4]

Certain vaccines manufactured by various companies are considered interchangeable. Hepatitis B vaccine produced by two different companies (Merck & Co., Inc., West Point, PA, and SmithKline Beecham, Collegeville, PA) are considered interchangable.[3] Both human diploid cell vaccine and rabies vaccine adsorbed are fully interchangeable with intramuscular (IM) use only. Diphtheria, pertussis, and tetnaus (DPT), oral polio, and inactivated polio vaccines are interchangeable between manufacturers. Finally, all licensed *H. influenzae* type b conjugate vaccines are considered interchangeable with the primary series being three doses of vaccine.

In general, vaccines and toxoids must be kept refrigerated, as breaking the "cold chain" may result in loss of potency. Certain vaccines, such as measles-mumps-rubella (MMR), may also be frozen. Immune sera generally should be kept refrigerated and not frozen except for lyophilized intravenous (IV) human immune globulin, which can be stored at room temperature. Certain vaccines, such as yellow fever and oral polio vaccine (OPV), are very sensitive to increased temperature. While some vaccines may be stored below 0°C, toxoids in general tend to aggregate upon freezing, leading to increased adverse local effects. On the other hand, some vaccines when stored under incorrect conditions may not be easily distinguished from potent vaccine.

FACTORS AFFECTING RESPONSE TO IMMUNIZATION

Various factors are known to affect response to vaccines and toxoids.[4] Viability of the antigen is an important factor (live attenuated versus killed) as previously discussed. Total dose is also important, as there seems to exist a threshold dose above which no further increase in antibody titer is seen.[4] The use of split doses or multiple reduced doses of a vaccine (such as those used in patients with allergies to some immunobiologic component as both a desensitization and immunization program), however, may result in inadequate protection. In such instances, serologic testing should be performed to ascertain whether or not protection to the antigen had been attained. The interval between immunization doses, the number of doses given, or both may change immune response to an agent. For hepatitis B vaccine, giving the third dose (in a three-dose series) at 12 months (after the first dose) has been shown to result in increased antibody titers, as compared to giving the third dose at 6 months.[5] Alternatively, additional doses of influenza vaccine have been shown to be minimally effective in immunocompetent, non–human immunodeficiency virus (HIV)-infected patients, HIV-infected patients, and patients with acquired immunodeficiency syndrome (AIDS)-related complex (ARC).[6] Generally, intervals longer than those recommended between vaccine doses do not reduce immune response.[7]

The route and site of administration of the immunobiologic is also important. This is best illustrated by the hepatitis B vaccine, which elicits a satisfactory antibody response when given in the deltoid muscle but not consistently when administered in the gluteal area.[8] Injections should be administered in a site where there is little likelihood of site damage. Immunobiologics containing adjuvants should be given into muscle mass because they can cause irritation when given subcutaneously or intradermally.

VACCINE ADMINISTRATION

Subcutaneous injections should be administered into the thigh of infants and in the deltoid area of older children and adults. A five-eights to three-quarter inch, 23- to 25-gauge needle should be used, being careful not to administer the dose intradermally or intramuscularly. For IM injection, the anterolateral aspect of the upper thigh (infants and toddlers) or the deltoid muscle of the upper arm (children and adults) should be used. The buttock should not be used because of the potential for inadequate immunologic response and because of the potential risk of injury to the sciatic nerve. When the buttock must be used (as for large doses of immune globulin), only the upper, outer quadrant should be used with the needle being inserted anteriorly. Intradermal injections should be administered on the volar surface of the forearm except for human cell rabies vaccine (HDCV), which should be given into the deltoid area to reduce reactions. A three-eights to three-quarter inch, 25- or 27-gauge needle should be used, with care being taken to not inject the immunobiologic substance into the subcutaneous tissue.

Jet injectors are considered safe and effective for multiple-person immunization despite the fact that the nozzle tip is used over and over again. No reports exist in the United States of transmission of blood-borne pathogens (HIV or hepatitis B or C) with the use of jet injectors.[3] Generally, it is suggested that if a jet injector is used, if contamination of the nozzle is noted, the device should be cleaned or the tip changed. In addition, the swabbing of the nozzle with alcohol or acetone between patients is routinely suggested.

For orally administered vaccines (typhoid or oral polio), the general recommendation is to readminister the vaccine at the same visit if the vaccine is regurgitated within 5 to 10 minutes of administration. If the second dose is not retained, neither dose should be counted, and the vaccine should be readministered at the next visit.

Questions often arise concerning the simultaneous administration of vaccines. In general, inactivated vaccines can be simultaneously administered at separate sites. If single-site administration must be done, the thigh muscle is the preferred site of injection. If two or more killed antigens cannot be administered simultaneously, they may be administered with no regard to spacing between doses. Killed and live antigens may be administered simultaneously or, if they cannot be administered simultaneously, at any interval between doses with the exception of cholera (killed) and yellow fever (live) vaccine, which should be given at least 3 weeks apart. Simultaneous administration of live attenuated vaccines should be avoided if possible, unless specified (MMR). Theoretically, live vaccines should be given at least 1 month apart (however, the OPV may be given at the same time as the MMR vaccine). The data on simultaneous administration of live attenuated viral vaccines should be prefaced with the knowledge that simultaneous administration of these vaccines has been performed with no resultant decrease in immunity to any of the agents used, when compared to single vaccine administration alone. Oral polio vaccine and oral typhoid vaccine (both live vaccines) may be administered simultaneously. Live viral vaccines may interfere with purified protein derivative (PPD) response and, thus, tubercular testing should be postponed 4 to 6 weeks after live virus vaccine administration.

The simultaneous administration of immune globulin (general or disease specific) and live attenuated vaccines (but not inactivated vaccines) may inhibit host antibody response because of impairment of viral replication. Guidelines state that there is a dose relationship between administration of immune globulin and inhibition of immune response to a vaccine (Table 113–1). Whole blood and other

TABLE 113–1. Suggested Intervals Between Administration of Immune Globulin Preparations for Various Indications and Vaccines Containing Live Measles Virus[a]

Indication	Dose (Including mg IgG/kg)	Suggested Interval Before Measles Vaccination (mo)
Tetanus (TIG)	250 units (10 mg IgG/kg) IM	3
Hepatitis A (IG)		
Contact prophylaxis	0.02 mL/kg (3.3 mg IgG/kg) IM	3
International travel	0.06 mL/kg (10 mg IgG/kg) IM	3
Hepatitis B prophylaxis (HBIG)	0.06 mL/kg (10 mg IgG/kg) IM	3
Rabies prophylaxis (HRIG)	20 IU/kg (22 mg IgG/kg) IM	4
Varicella prophylaxis (VZIG)	125 units/10 kg (20–40 mg IgG/kg) IM (max 625 units)	5
Measles prophylaxis (IG)		
Normal contact	0.25 mL/kg (40 mg IgG/kg) IM	5
Immunocompromised contact	0.50 mL/kg (80 mg IgG/kg) IM	6
Blood transfusion		
Red blood cells (RBCs), washed	10 mL/kg (negligible IgG/kg) IV	0
RBCs, adenine-saline added	10 mL/kg (10 mg IgG/kg) IV	3
Packed RBCs (Hct 65%)[b]	10 mL/kg (60 mg IgG/kg) IV	6
Whole blood (Hct 35–50%)[b]	10 mL/kg (80–100 mg IgG/kg) IV	6
Plasma/platelet products	10 mL/kg (160 mg IgG/kg) IV	7
Replacement of humoral immune deficiencies	300–400 mg/kg IV[c] (as IGIV)	8
Treatment of:		
ITP[d]	400 mg/kg IV (as IGIV)	8
ITP[d]	1000 mg/kg IV (as IGIV)	10
Kawasaki disease	2 g/kg IV (as IGIV)	11

[a]This table is not intended for determining the correct indications and dosage for the use of immune globulin preparations. Unvaccinated persons may not be fully protected against measles during the entire suggested interval and additional doses of immune globulin measles vaccine for both may be indicated following measles exposure. The concentration of measles antibody in a particular immune globulin preparation can vary by lot. The rate of antibody clearance following receipt of an immune globulin preparation can also vary. The recommended intervals are extrapolated from an estimated half-life of 30 days for passively acquired antibody and an observed interference with the immune response to measles vaccine for 5 months following a dose of 80 mg IgG/kg.
[b]Assumes a serum IgG concentration of 16 mg/mL.
[c]Measles vaccination is recommended for children with HIV infection but is contraindicated in patients with congenital disorders of the immune system.
[d]Immune (formally, idiopathic) thrombocytopenic purpura.
IGIV = immune globulin intravenous.
From Ref. 57.

blood products containing antibodies may interfere with the response to the MMR vaccine. For women who have experienced a birth and have received a blood product in the last trimester or anti-RhoD immuneglobulin (IG) at the time of delivery, vaccination with MMR should be done immediately, with antibody testing at least 3 months later to determine response. In any patient, if vaccination with MMR and immune globulin administration must be done, separate injection sites are recommended with seroconversion to the viral antigens confirmed at 3 months and reimmunization if necessary. Immune globulin does not interfere with the response to oral vaccines or yellow fever vaccine.

Simultaneous administration of killed vaccines along with immune globulins is not contraindicated. Different sites are recommended, however, for killed vaccine and immune globulin administration. It is not recommended to increase the dose or number of vaccines used in this circumstance.

IMMUNIZATION OF SPECIAL POPULATIONS

NEONATES, INFANTS, AND PREGNANT WOMEN

The age of the recipient is another important determining factor in vaccine and toxoid response. In the first few months of life, passive immunity (temporary immunity to infection as a result of the acquisition of antibodies via maternal–fetal passage) both protects an infant and prevents adequate vaccine and toxoid response to certain agents.

Premature infants should be vaccinated at the same chronologic age using the same schedule and precautions as full-term infants. Full recommended doses of vaccines should be used regardless of age or birthweight. Hepatitis B vaccine should be administered if the infant weighs 2000 g, or it should be held until the infant is 2 months of age. Breast fed infants should be vaccinated according to standard pediatric schedules.

Pregnant women present a particularly difficult problem in deciding on vaccination. In general, administration of live attenuated vaccines should not be done during pregnancy, and inactivated vaccines should not be given until the second trimester; however, inactivated vaccines have not been shown to be teratogenic during the first trimester.[9,10] Administration of the rubella vaccine during pregnancy is not a reason to interrupt pregnancy routinely.[10] Diptheria and tetanus vaccination should be carried out with the use of a booster dose or a complete series of vaccines in unimmunized women. Hepatitis B, oral polio, influenza, and pneumococcal vaccines are all recommended in pregnant women, if indicated.

IMMUNOCOMPROMISED HOSTS

Vaccination in compromised hosts (those with chronic disease, such as diabetes, connective tissue disease, or alcoholics, or those with cancer or HIV disease) must be individualized based on the disease state and its treatment. The Centers for Disease Control (CDC) has classified persons with immunocompromised conditions into three groups[11]:

1. Persons with a condition that causes limited immune deficiency (renal disease, diabetes, liver disease, asplenia).
2. Individuals who are severely immunocompromised but not as a result of HIV infection (congenital immunodeficiency, drug- or radiation-induced disease, hematologic or solid tumor).
3. Persons with HIV infection.

Patients with chronic pulmonary, renal, hepatic, or metabolic disease who are not receiving immunosuppressants may receive both live attenuated and killed vaccines and toxoids to induce active immunity. These patients may often need higher doses of vaccines or more frequent dosing to induce immunity. Generally, immunization should be considered early in the course of the disease in an attempt to induce immunity at a point when the disease is less severe.

Those patients with active malignant disease may receive killed vaccines or toxoids but should not be given live vaccines. In addition, OPV should not be administered to household contacts of these patients. The MMR vaccine is not contraindicated for close contacts, however. Live virus vaccines may be administered to persons with leukemia who have not received chemotherapy for at least 3 months. Vaccines should be timed to avoid coinciding with the start of chemotherapy or radiation therapy (at least 2 weeks in advance of the start of these therapies). If vaccines cannot be given at least 2 weeks or more before the start of these therapies, immunization should be postponed until 3 months after the therapy has been completed. Passive immunization with immune globulin may be used in place of active immunization, regardless of the history of immunization.

Glucocorticoids may cause suppressed responses to vaccines. When steroid therapy duration is $\leq$ 2 weeks (low-to-moderate dose, that is < 20 mg or 2 mg/kg/d, whichever is less), then no contraindication to immunization exists.[11] In addition, long-term, alternate-day steroid therapy with short-acting agents, maintenance physiologic doses, topical, aerosol, intra-articular, bursal, or tendon injections are not considered contraindications to immunization. If patients have been receiving high-dose corticosteroids or have had a course lasting $\geq$ 2 weeks, then a 3-month period of time should pass before immunization with live virus vaccines.

The patient with HIV infection requires special consideration. Responses to live and killed antigens is generally suboptimal and decreases as the disease progresses because HIV produces defects in cell-mediated immunity and humoral immunity. This results in increased morbidity for measles infection. Consequently, a measles vaccine (given as MMR) is recommended in all child and adult patients regardless of HIV status using standard schedules. There is no suggestion that serious adverse events are seen more frequently in these individuals. Enhanced inactivated polio vaccine (eIPV) should be used as an alternative to OPV in these patients; however, full response may not be assured. If OPV is inadvertently administered to a household contact, close contact between the immunized individual and the patient should be avoided for 30 days. Pneumococcal vaccine is recommended for HIV-infected persons $\geq$ 2 years of age. Children younger than 2 years should receive *Haemophilus influenzae* vaccine according to the recommended schedule for nonimmunocompromised children. Vaccination with DPT is also recommended. There is no suggestion that larger doses or more frequent vaccine dosing is of benefit. Other killed vaccines may be used without concern for increased risk. Live typhoid vaccine should be avoided. Yellow fever vaccine may be used if absolutely necessary, but it may pose a theoretical risk of encephalitis.

MISCONCEPTIONS ABOUT THE USE OF IMMUNIZATION

There are very few contraindications to the use of vaccines except as those outlined earlier. These contraindications include a history of anaphylactic reactions to the vaccine or a component of the vaccine, immunosupression (as specified for each group), pregnancy (for MMR), and administration of immunoglobulin or blood products. For agents such as DPT, a history of encephalopathy or a hypotonic–hyporesponsive episode with a previous dose and fever of $\geq$ 40.5°C within 48 hours of a previous dose are contraindications. Generally, history of mild-to-moderate local reactions, mild acute illnesses, concurrent antibiotic use, prematurity, family history of adverse events, diarrhea, and breast feeding are not contraindications to immunization.

OBTAINING AN IMMUNIZATION HISTORY

An immunization history should be obtained from every patient, regardless of the reason for the health care visit. Ideally, any history provided by the patient from memory should be verified by reviewing the patient's personal, written "shot record" or a database that contains the complete immunization history. If an official, written record is not available, patient characteristics (military service, travel history, occupation) may provide clues as to the immunization history. Serologic testing for immunity against certain diseases can provide specific information, but it is routinely employed for only a few selected diseases (measles, rubella, hepatitis A and B, varicella) and selected circumstances (employment in a health care facility). In the event a written record does not exist, one should be generated at the time of initiation of immunization. Patients without a written record should be considered susceptible and an immunization program started and completed unless a serious adverse reaction occurs (more commonly to DPT or Td). As a general rule, the risks associated with overimmunization are minimal relative to the risks associated with contracting vaccine-preventable diseases.[3]

VACCINE DELIVERY

Shortfalls in vaccine coverage exist in both the adult and pediatric populations.[12,13] Among children, those of preschool age historically have been the most neglected.[14] Entry into public school is contingent on receipt of certain required immunizations, resulting in vaccine coverage rates above 97% in children 6 years and older. The lack of a similar enforcement mechanism in younger patients, however, has contributed to exceptionally low immunization rates (< 50%), particularly in children less than 2 years of age. From 1989 to 1991, the United States experienced a national measles epidemic, largely caused by inadequately immunized preschool-aged children. Additionally, other segments of the population (adolescents and senior citizens) have been identified as needing better vaccine coverage.[13,15]

In many instances, unvaccinated individuals have been seen by health care providers, but they have not received the indicated vaccines either because of oversight, inappropriate "contraindications" to vaccination, or a reluctance to administer multiple vaccines at the same visit. These missed opportunities to immunize patients have been shown to occur in patients of all ages and in a variety of practice settings.[16,17]

According to the CDC, every health care visit, regardless of its purpose, should be viewed as an opportunity to review a patient's immunization status and administer needed vaccines. Immunization is perhaps the most cost-effective medical practice available. Pharmaceutical care should encompass assessment of individuals' vaccine needs, administration of indicated agents, and documentation of immunization histories. The outcome measurement of what percentage of patients in a particular practice site are completely immunized is extremely important because the benefits of optimal vaccine use extend beyond the individual patient to the public as a whole.

COMBINATION VACCINES

The problem of numerous vaccine injections is being addressed through the development of combination vaccines. Combining several antigens that normally would be administered as separate entities can reduce the number of injections required. Several combination vaccines have been approved for use in the United States, each of which has a HIB conjugate as one of its components[3,18,19] (Table 113–2). While each of these products is useful in decreasing the number of injections a child may require, each also has limitations.

TABLE 113–2. HIB-Containing Combination Vaccines

Trade Name	Manufacturer	Antigen Content
Tetramune	Wyeth-Lederle	HbOC + DPT
TriHIBit	Pasteur Merieux	PRP-T + DTaP
Comvax	Merck	PRP-OMP + Hepatitis B

NATIONAL VACCINE INJURY COMPENSATION ACT

In 1986, the National Vaccine Injury Compensation Act (NVICA) was passed by the U.S. Congress.[20] The act consists of four parts. Part A outlines compensation for vaccine-related injuries, per a Vaccine Injury Table, and limits the size of compensatory awards to injured individuals. Part B is the "no-fault" provision, which frees the manufacturer from liability for damage if adequate warnings for vaccine use are provided. Part C provides that adverse reactions to vaccines must be reported to the Food and Drug Administration (FDA) by health care providers and vaccine manufacturers within 7 days of their occurrence. Part D gives legal recourse against the Secretary of the Department of Health and Human Services for not performing duties as outlined by the act.[21] The bill also instituted mandatory record keeping by health care providers in the permanent medical record. Specifically, the manufacturer and lot number of the vaccine, date of administration, and name, address, and title of the person giving the vaccine must be recorded. Additionally, the Act mandates that health care providers report to their local health department or the FDA any occurrence of the adverse events listed in Table 113–3. This table is subject to periodic review and modification. To facilitate reporting of any adverse events suspected of being vaccine-related, the Vaccine Adverse Event Reporting System (VAERS) was established. The VAERS toll-free telephone number for obtaining information or report forms is 1-800-822-7967.[22]

USE OF VACCINES AND TOXOIDS

The recommended schedules for routine immunization of children and adults are shown in Appendixes 113–1 and 113–2. Appendix 113–3 lists the minimum age for initial vaccination and minimum interval between vaccine doses. Many states require children to be fully immunized prior to entering elementary school; however, optimal protection is achieved by giving the recommended vaccines at the recommended ages, which means special attention should be devoted to children under 2 years of age. Adults and adolescents also require vaccination, and are often unaware of this need. All adults should be fully immunized against diphtheria, tetanus, measles, mumps, and rubella. Certain high-risk individuals should be vaccinated against other agents as outlined in Appendix 113–2.

TABLE 113–3. Reportable Events Following Immunization[a]

Vaccine/Toxoid	Event	Interval From Vaccination
Tetanus in any combination; DTaP, DPT, DPT-HIB, DT, Td, TT	Anaphylaxis or anaphylactic shock	7 d
	Brachial neuritis	28 d
	Any sequela (including death) of above	No limit
	Events described in manufacturer's package events insert as contraindications to additional doses of vaccine	See package insert
Pertussis in any combination; DTaP, DPT, DPT-HIB, P	Anaphylaxis or anaphylactic shock	7 d
	Encephalopathy (or encephalitis)	7 d
	Any sequela (including death) of above events	No limit
	Events described in manufacturer's package insert as contraindications to additional doses of vaccine	See package insert
Measles-mumps-rubella in any combination; MMR, MR, M, R	Anaphylaxis or anaphylactic shock	7 d
	Encephalopathy (or encephalitis)	15 d
	Any sequela (including death) of above events	No limit
	Events described in manufacturer's package insert as contraindications to additional doses of vaccine	See package insert
Rubella in any combination; MMR, MR, R	Chronic arthritis	42 d
	Any sequela (including death) of above events	No limit
	Events described in manufacturer's package insert as contraindications to additional doses of vaccine	See package insert
Measles in any combination; MMR, MR, M	Thrombocytopenic purpura	30 days
	Vaccine-strain measles viral infection in an immunodeficient recipient	6 mo
	Any sequela (including death) of above events	No limit
	Events described in manufacturer's package insert as contraindications to additional doses of vaccine	See package insert
Oral polio (OPV)	Paralytic polio	
	In a nonimmunodeficient recipient	30 d
	In an immunodeficient recipient	6 mo
	In a vaccine-associated community case	No limit
	Vaccine-strain polio viral infection	
	In a nonimmunodeficient recipient	30 d
	In an immunodeficient recipient	6 mo
	In a vaccine-associated community case	No limit
	Any sequela (including death) of above events	No limit
	Events described in manufacturer's package insert as contraindications to additional doses of vaccine	See package insert
Inactivated polio (IPV)	Anaphylaxis or anaphylactic shock	7 d
	Any sequela (including death) of the above events	No limit
	Events described in manufacturer's package insert as contraindications to additional doses of vaccine	See package insert
Hepatitis B	Anaphylaxis or anaphylactic shock	7 d
	Any sequela (including death) of the above events	No limit
	Events described in manufacturer's package insert as contraindications to additional doses of vaccine	See package insert
Haemophilus influenzae type B	Early onset HIB disease	7 d
	Any sequela (including death) of the above events	No limit
	Events described in manufacturer's package insert as contraindications to additional doses of vaccine	See package insert

[a]Effective March 1997.
From Ref. 124, with permission.

TOXOIDS AND THEIR IMMUNOBIOLOGICS

DIPHTHERIA TOXOID ADSORBED AND DIPHTHERIA ANTITOXIN

Diphtheria toxoid adsorbed is a sterile suspension of modified toxins of *Corynebacterium diphtheriae*, which induce immunity against the exotoxin of this organism. Two strengths of diphtheria toxoid are available in the United States: the pediatric strength (D) and the adult strength (d), which contains less antigen because of the higher rate of adverse effects seen when the pediatric strength is used in adult patients. The widespread use of diphtheria toxoid has essentially eliminated diphtheria from the United States.

Primary immunization with D is indicated for children over 6 weeks of age. The usual dose is 0.5 mL IM at rotating sites. Generally, the toxoid is given in combination with tetanus toxoid and pertussis vaccine (as DPT) at ages 2, 4, and 6 months of age. Additional doses are given at 15 to 18 months and again at 4 to 6 years of age.[23] Completing the primary D immunization series usually induces immunity of at least 10 years' duration immunity in 90% of persons. Booster doses should be given every 10 years. Adverse effects of diphtheria toxoid include mild to moderate tenderness, erythema, and induration at the injection site. Rarely do systemic reactions occur.[21]

If primary immunization is given to an immunosuppressed patient, an additional dose of D should be administered 1 month following the return to normal immune status. Diphtheria toxoid D may be administered to persons with mild febrile illnesses and with other live or killed vaccines.[24]

For nonimmunized adults, a complete three-dose series of diphtheria toxoid should be administered with the first two doses given at least 4 weeks apart and the third dose given 6 to 12 months after the second. The combined preparation, diphtheria-tetanus (Td) is recommended in adults since it contains less diphtheria toxoid than DT or DPT and is associated with fewer reactions to the diphtheria component. It also includes the recommended tetanus toxoid, but it omits the pertussis component, which is not used in patients > 7 years old. All adults should receive booster doses of Td every 10 years.

Diphtheria antitoxin (DA) is a sterile antitoxin derived from hyperimmunized horses and is indicated for immediate use in patients with diphtheria. It should be stored at 2 to 8°C but may be frozen without affecting potency. It is rarely indicated for diphtheria prophylaxis. The DA vaccine is given IM or IV in a dosage related to the site and size of the diphtheric membrane, severity of illness, and duration of illness. Sensitivity testing by performing an intradermal or scratch test and a conjunctival test should be performed before administration. These tests do not rule out systemic allergic reactions in 100% of the cases.

The usual dose of DA is 20,000 to 40,000 U for pharyngeal disease, 40,000 to 60,000 U for nasopharyngeal lesions, and 80,000 to 120,000 U for extensive disease of 3 or more days. When given IV, the dose should be diluted 1:20 in 0.9% saline or dextrose 5% in water and infused at 1 mL/min after being warmed to 32 to 34°C.

Adverse reactions to DA include anaphylactic reactions in 7% of patients, serum sickness occurring 12 days postadministration, or both. Serum sickness may be accelerated (7 to 12 days) in persons previously sensitized. Fortunately, the widespread use of diphtheria toxoid has greatly reduced the incidence of the disease and, thus, the use of DA.

TETANUS TOXOID, TETANUS TOXOID ADSORBED, AND TETANUS IMMUNE GLOBULIN

Tetanus toxoid and tetanus toxoid adsorbed (adsorbed onto aluminum hydroxide, phosphate, or potassium sulfate to increase antigenicity) are sterile suspensions of the toxoid derived from *Clostridium tetani*. Both toxoids are used to promote active immunity against tetanus; however, tetanus toxoid adsorbed (T) is the preferred agent, because it illicits a greater immune response and is associated with fewer adverse reactions.

Although single doses of T in a nonimmunized individual do not produce sufficient antibody response, a series of three 0.5-mL doses results in protection for 90% of vaccinees. Primary vaccination provides protection for at least 10 years. Additional doses of T (combined with diphtheria toxoid Td) are recommended as part of traumatic wound management if a patient has not received a dose of T over the preceding 5 years. For minor or clean wounds, no dose is given. These recommendations are summarized in Table 113–4 In certain situations, tetanus immune globulin (TIG) should also be given. It can be administered with T, provided separate syringes and separate injection sites are used.

In children, primary immunization against tetanus is usually offered in conjunction with diphtheria and pertussis vaccination (using DPT or DTaP). A 0.5-mL dose is recommended at 2, 4, 6, and 15 to 18 months of age, but the first dose can be administered as early as 6 weeks of age.[24] In children ≥ 7 years old and adults who have not previously been immunized, a series of three 0.5-mL doses of Td are administered IM initially. The first two doses are given 1 to 2 months apart, and the third dose is recommended 6 to 12 months after the second dose. Boosters are recommended every 10 years, and unless there is contraindication to diphtheria toxoid, Td should be used. Tetanus toxoid may be simultaneously given with other killed and live vaccines, and if indicated, it may be given to immunosuppressed patients.

Adverse reactions to tetanus toxoid include mild-to-moderate local reactions at the injection site, such as warmth, erythema, and induration. Rarely, fever, malaise,

TABLE 113–4. Summary Guide to Tetanus Prophylaxis in Routine Wound Management[a]

	Clean, Minor Wounds		All Other Wounds[b]	
	Td[c]	*TIG*[d]	*Td*[c]	*TIG*[d]
Uncertain or < 3	Yes	No	Yes	Yes
> 3[e]	No[f]	No	No[g]	No

[a]Refer also to text on specific vaccines or toxoids for contraindications, precautions, dosages, side effects, adverse reactions, and special considerations. Important details are in the text and in the ACIP recommendations on diphtheria, tetanus, and pertussis (DTP).
[b]Such as, but not limited to, wounds contaminated with dirt, feces, and saliva; puncture wounds; avulsions; and wounds resulting from missiles, crushing, burns, and frostbite.
[c]Td, tetanus and diphtheria toxoids, adsorbed (for adult use). For children < 7 years old, DPT (DT, if pertussis vaccine is contraindicated) is preferred to tetanus toxoid alone. For persons ≥ 7 years old, Td is preferred to tetanus toxoid alone.
[d]TIG, tetanus immune globulin.
[e]If only three doses of fluid toxoid have been received, a fourth dose of toxoid, preferably an adsorbed toxoid, should be given.
[f]Yes, > 10 years since last dose.
[g]Yes, > 5 years since last dose. (More frequent boosters are not needed and can accentuate side effects.)
From Ref. 10.

aches and pains, or neurologic disorders have been reported. In general, major local reactions occur within 2 to 8 hours after administration to patients with high serum tetanus antitoxin levels. This type of reaction suggests a high level of protection. Local reactions do not limit the use of the toxoid for further dosing. While safe use during pregnancy has not been definitely established, tetanus toxoid has been administered to pregnant women for the prevention of neonatal tetanus. Generally, waiting until the second trimester is suggested.

Tetanus immune globulin is a sterile, concentrated, nonpyrogenic solution of immunoglobulins prepared from hyperimmunized humans. It is used to provide passive immunity to tetanus following the occurrence of traumatic wounds in nonimmunized or suboptimally immunized persons (see Table 113–4). A dose of 250 to 500 U IM should be administered. When administered with tetanus toxoid adsorbed (TTA), separate sites for administration should be used. Also, TIG is used for the treatment of tetanus. In this setting, a single dose of 3000 to 6000 U IM is administered.[25]

Adverse effects of TIG include pain, tenderness, erythema, and muscle stiffness at the injection site, which may persist for several hours. Rarely do systemic reactions occur. Intravenous administration has been associated with severe adverse reactions and is not recommended.

VACCINES AND THEIR IMMUNOBIOLOGICS

BACILLUS CALMETTE-GUÉRIN VACCINE

The increased incidence of TB has led the CDC to recommend greater use of Bacillus Calmette-Guérin (BCG) vaccine.[26] All available BCG vaccines are derived from a live attenuated strain of *Mycobacterium bovis*. Since many brands are available throughout the world, and since subculture of *M. bovis* can alter the immunologic properties, immunogenicity varies, however, with the brand of vaccine. In the United States, the Tice strain of *M. bovis* is used to produce the vaccine. This heterogeneity of BCG vaccine immunogenicity and the fact that the majority of TB prevention trials with the vaccine have examined different at-risk populations in different geographical areas, have led to some questions concerning the efficacy of BCG vaccine in TB prevention. Multiple meta-analysis of these BCG trials have led to the conclusion that the vaccine is efficacious (> 80%) in preventing serious illness in children. Data are not conclusive, however, in clarifying vaccine efficacy for preventing pulmonary TB in adolescents and adults, or in health care workers. Additionally, the protective effects of BCG vaccine based on different vaccine strains, the age of initial vaccination, or the use of vaccine in HIV-infected individuals are still indeterminate.

The CDC has issued guidelines recommending which persons are candidates for BCG vaccine.[26] These guidelines cover children, high- and low-risk health care workers, and persons with HIV infection. When using BCG vaccine, a negative Mantoux skin test should be assured before vaccination because of the difficulty in using the skin test for a prolonged period of time following immunization.

In the pediatric population, generally, acquisition of tuberculosis (TB) in a child is a result of exposure from infected adults who often reside in the same household. Vaccination with BCG should be considered for an infant or child who has a negative tuberculin skin test but is continually exposed to an untreated or ineffectively treated patient with infectious pulmonary TB, especially if the infection is caused by isoniazid- and rifampin-resistant strains of *M. tuberculosis*.

While infection control measures are paramount in reducing the transmission of TB in health care facilities, there are certain situations in which use of BCG may be considered. Other important considerations in the use of BCG in health care workers is the potential interference with diagnosing a newly acquired TB infection in a vaccinated person. Generally, BCG vaccination of health care workers should be considered when infection control precautions have been implemented but have not been effective in preventing the spread of TB, especially multidrug-resistant strains. Vaccination with BCG should not be required for employment or assignment of health care workers in specific work areas. In areas where the TB risk is low, vaccination of health care workers with BCG is unnecessary.

In HIV-infected persons, the data are inconsistent to address safety issues with this live vaccine. In addition, the efficacy of BCG vaccine in HIV-infected persons is unknown. Therefore, even in high-risk groups, such as children with continuous household exposure and health care workers in the high-risk category, BCG vaccination is not recommended by the CDC, although the World Health Organization (WHO) does recommend BCG use in asymptomatic HIV-positive children in a high-risk situation. In addition, the vaccine is contraindicated in persons who are immunocompromised because of leukemia, lymphoma, and generalized malignancy, and in those who are receiving corticosteroids, alkylating agents, antimetabolites, or radiation therapy.

Adverse effects of the vaccine are usually local in nature. These include moderate axillary or cervical lymphadenopathy and induration and subsequent pustule formation at the injection site (with intradermal use) persisting for up to 3 months. Permanent scarring generally does occur. When subcutaneous injection is used, higher rates of local reactions are seen, including muscle soreness, erythema, and purulent drainage. For the treatment of BCG adenitis (adherent or fistulated lymph nodes), treatment ranges from no treatment to surgical drainage and administration of anti-TB drugs, or both. These local reactions are approximately 15-fold more common in children < 1 year of age versus children 1 to 20 years. Little incidence data are available in older age groups. More uncommon are severe reactions, including suppurative lymphadenitis, caseous lesions at the injection site (occurring within 5 months of vaccination), and disseminated BCG infection. Occasional reports of erythema multiforme in adults have been reported. Vaccination with BCG has not been shown to cause harm to the fetus, however, it is not recommended during pregnancy.[26]

It is generally believed that BCG induces a positive Mantoux TB test. Some individuals who receive BCG, however, may have no induced reactivity to the TB skin test. Tuberculin reactivity develops 6 to 12 weeks after vaccination. Tuberculin reactivity induced by BCG does not persist longer than 10 years after immunization. In addition, the presence or size of a postvaccination-positive TB skin test reaction does not predict protection by BCG. Tuberculin skin testing is not contraindicated for persons who have been vaccinated with BCG, and the skin test results of such persons are used to support or exclude the diagnosis of *M. tuberculosis* infection. A diagnosis of *M. tuberculosis* infection and the use of preventive therapy should be considered for any BCG-vaccinated person who has a tuberculin skin test reaction of > 10 mm of induration, especially if any of the following circumstances are present: (1) the vaccinated person is a contact of another person who has infectious TB, particularly if the infectious person has transmitted *M. tuberculosis* to others; (2) the vaccinated person was born or has resided in a country in which the prevalence of TB is high; or (3) the vaccinated person is exposed continually to populations in which the prevalence of TB is high (some health care workers, employees and volunteers at homeless shelters, and workers at drug-treatment centers). Studies have demonstrated that persons who are infected with HIV have decreased tuberculin skin test responses after BCG vaccination compared to uninfected persons.

Vaccination with BCG should be reserved for persons who have a reaction of < 5 mm induration after skin testing with 5 TU of PPD tuberculin. The Tice strain of BCG is administered percutaneously; 0.3 mL of the reconstituted vaccine is usually placed on the skin in the lower deltoid area (the upper arm) and delivered through a multiple-puncture disk. Infants < 30 days of age should receive one-half the usual dose, prepared by increasing the amount of diluent added to the lyophilized vaccine. If the indications for vaccination persist, these children should receive a full dose of the vaccine after they are 1 year of age, if they have an induration of < 5 mm when tested with 5 TU of PPD tuberculin. Normal reactions to the vaccine are characterized by the formation of a bluish-red pustule within 2 to 3 weeks after vaccination. After approximately 6 weeks, the pustule ulcerates, forming a lesion approximately 5 mm in diameter. Draining lesions resulting from vaccination should be kept clean and bandaged. Scabs form and heal usually within 3 months after vaccination. Tuberculin reactivity resulting from BCG vaccination should be documented. A vaccinated person should be tuberculin skin tested 3 months after BCG administration, and the induration size documented. Vaccinated persons whose skin test results are negative (< 5 mm of induration) and who are enrolled in ongoing periodic skin testing programs (health care workers) should continue to be included in ongoing testing programs if their skin test results are < 5 mm induration. Those vaccinees who have positive tuberculin skin test reactions (> 5 mm of induration) after vaccination should not be retested except after exposure to a case of infectious TB; an increase in induration (> 10 mm increase for persons < 35 years of age and > 15 mm increase for persons > 35 years of age) from a previous to the current skin test may indicate a newly acquired *M. tuberculosis* infection.

While the major use of BCG vaccine has been as immunoprophylaxis of tuberculosis, other uses of the agent in neoplastic disease have been studied. In these circumstances, the agent has been used in various dosages and routes of administration. Specific protocols are generally followed. This form of immunotherapy in neoplastic disease has been met with limited success.

HEPATITIS A VACCINE

Two interchangeable vaccines are available for use in the United States to induce active immunity, Havrix (Smith Kline Beecham) and Vaqta (Merck & Co., Inc.). Available vaccines are killed whole virus vaccines that are propagated through the use of cell culture in human fibroblasts. The live virus is then formalin-inactivated and adsorbed to aluminum. Havrix is formulated with 2-phenoxyethanol as a preservative, while Vaqta contains no preservatives. For Havrix, the final vaccine potency (per dose) is expressed as enzyme-linked immunosorbent assay (ELISA) units (ELU). For Vaqta, the antigen content is expressed as units (U) of hepatitis A antigen. These vaccines should be stored and shipped at temperatures of 2 to 8°C and not frozen. Storage at 37°C for 1 week does not, however, affect immunogenicity.

The CDC has issued guidelines on active and passive immunization against hepatitis A virus (HAV), and the reader is referred to this publication for a complete discussion of the material that follows.[27]

A number of groups have been determined to be at risk for HAV infection and, thus, the CDC has suggested that they receive active immunization with hepatitis A vaccine. These groups include (1) travelers to areas that are not developed (even if the traveler is staying in a nice hotel), (2) men who have sex with men, (3) persons working with primates, (4) persons who have clotting factor disorders, (5) illegal drug users, (6) persons with chronic liver disease, (7) food handlers where the vaccine is cost-effective, and (8) children in highly endemic areas. Other groups who may not be at risk but who may serve to expose large numbers of people to HAV include those working in a daycare center, those working in a home for the disabled, and those working in food service. The CDC has stated that in order to eradicate HAV effectively, children < 2 years of age would ideally be vaccinated.

While no lower limit of anti-HAV titer has been defined to prevent HAV infection, *in vitro* data suggest that anti-HAV levels of > 20 mIU/mL (measured with an enzyme immunoassay) or > 10 mIU/mL (measured with a modified radioimmunoassay) may be protective.

Both commercially available hepatitis A vaccines are highly immunogenic over a wide age and weight range. In persons ≥ 18 years of age, Havrix (1440 ELU dose) anti-HAV levels of > 20 mIU/mL were seen in 88% of adults within 15 days of the first dose and in 99% to 100% after 30 days. After a second dose, all persons had seroconversion with high geometric mean antibody titers (GMTs) for anti-HAV. Results with Vaqta were similar, with 95% seroconversion 1 month after a 50 U dose and 100% conversion 1 month after a second dose 6 months later. In children and adolescents, both commercially available vaccines have been shown to be highly immunogenic with 100% seroconversion 1 month after two doses were given at 0 and 6 months.

ROUTE OF ADMINISTRATION, VACCINATION SCHEDULE, AND DOSAGE

The vaccine should be administered intramuscularly into the deltoid muscle. Havrix is licensed in three formulations, with the formulation and number of doses differing according to the vaccinee's age. For persons 2 to 18 years of age, 360 ELU (0.25 mL) per dose in a three-dose schedule (0, 1, and 6 months) or 720 ELU (0.5 mL) per dose in a two-dose schedule (0 and 6 to 12 months) is recommended. For persons > 18 years of age, 1440 ELU (1 mL) per dose in a two-dose schedule (0 and 6 to 12 months) is recommended. Vaqta is licensed in two formulations, and the formulation and number of doses differ according to the person's age. For persons 2 to 17 years of age, 25 U (0.5 mL) in a two-dose schedule (0 and 6 to 18 months) is recommended, while for persons > 17 years of age, 50 U per dose in a two-dose schedule (0 and 6 months) is used. Because seroconversion rates are so high, obtaining anti-HAV titers is not recommended.

The vaccine has been shown to be highly effective in the prevention of hepatitis A infections, particularly in children and adolescents.[27] In addition, some data exist to suggest that in outbreak settings, vaccination of susceptible individuals with HAV results in a substantial decrease in hepatitis A infections.[27]

Unlike hepatitis B vaccine, factors such as body size, age, smoking status, and sex do not appear to affect the development of seroconversion. The vaccine can be given with immune globulin and although the levels of anti-HAV are blunted, they still are 100-fold higher than levels considered to be protective.

There is only limited data about the persistence of protective levels of anti-HAV since the vaccine has only been available for a limited time period. It is estimated, however, that protective levels of anti-HAV may be present for 20 years or longer.[27] In addition, the effect of immune memory on the duration or protection is unknown.

Adverse effects of HAV have been mild and generally local in nature. Within 3 days of injection, injection site soreness, redness, or pain is reported in approximately 50%, and headache in 5% to 10%. Adverse effect rates may be less in children than adults. Although the vaccine is an inactivated virus and its potential risk to the fetus is low, its use in pregnancy is not recommended. The vaccine may be used in immunocompromised individuals with safety.

HEPATITIS B VACCINE

The first commercially available hepatitis B vaccine (Heptavax) was derived from plasma of carefully screened and monitored human, high-titer hepatitis B carrier donors. In 1986, a recombinantly produced hepatitis B vaccine (Recombivax-HB) was introduced in the United States followed by an additional recombinant vaccine introduced in 1989 (Engerix-B). These recombinant vaccines have been shown to be approximately equally effective (albeit they produce lower GMTs) as compared to human-derived vaccine. Hepatitis B vaccine is an inactivated vaccine, consisting of hepatitis B surface antigen (HBsAg) subunit particles, and it does not include the preS1 or preS2 particles. The vaccine induces only anti-hepatitis B surface antibody (anti-HBs) in recipients.[28,29]

Clinical trials in healthy individuals have demonstrated antibody conversion rates of approximately 90% after completion of the three-dose series[29] and a protective effect in vaccinees subsequently exposed to hepatitis B virus (HBV).[4] The 10% of subjects who are considered unprotected fall into the categories nonresponders (anti-HBs < 2.1 mIU/mL) and hyporesponders (anti-HBs < 10 mIU/mL). Of persons who do not develop protective levels of anti-HBs, approximately 50% are nonresponders and 50% hyporesponders. Lack of development of a protective response is seen in older individuals, with nonresponse rates increasing with increasing age (over 50 years of age).[30] Other factors that have been identified as leading to poor vaccine response include increased body mass index, being a smoker, and male gender.[31–33] Smoking status is the most important factor in determining nonresponse in normal individuals. Nonsmokers have an approximate sevenfold increased chance of developing protective levels of anti-HBs as do smokers.[31] When protective antibody concentrations are induced, this protective response lasts 6 to 10 years in 40% to 75% of patients.[33] While the two available vaccines are considered equivalent in inducing protection to hepatitis B, some data suggest that Recombivax-HB may lead a higher failure rate than Engerix-B.[31–35] (The true significance of this is still unclear.) A normal immune response has also been seen in patients with Down's syndrome.[30] Response rates in hemodialysis and immunocompromised patients have been lower, requiring higher vaccine dosages to achieve protective levels. The vaccine protects against all hepatitis B serotypes, including delta viroid, but does not cross-react with other hepatitis viruses (hepatitis A, C, E, G).

In the preexposure setting, the vaccine has been recommended for persons with occupational risk (health care workers, public safety workers), persons in training for health care fields, clients and staff of institutions for the developmentally disabled, hemodialysis patients, recipients of clotting factor concentrate, household contacts and sex partners of hepatitis B carriers, adoptees from countries where hepatitis B is endemic, international travelers (those spending more than 6 months in areas with high rates of hepatitis B infection or high-risk, short-term travelers), injecting drug users, sexually active homosexual/bisexual men, sexually active heterosexual men and women, and inmates of long-term correctional facilities.[28–30] In addition, the American Academy of Pediatrics recommends universal immunization of all newborns.[29]

Hepatitis B vaccine is also used with hepatitis B immune globulin (HBIG) in the postexposure setting. Persons for whom this regimen is recommended include susceptible individuals having percutaneous or permucosal exposure to blood containing HBsAg, sexual contacts of HBsAg carriers who will continue to be exposed, and infants born to mothers who are HBsAg carriers.[30,35,36] The HBIG does not interfere with the induction of neutralizing antibody, and the combination has been shown to be more protective than when two doses of HBIG alone have been given (85% to 90% efficacy versus 70% to 75%).[37]

For neonates born to mothers who are not positive for HBsAg, the primary vaccination series is 5 μg of Recombivax-HB or 10 μg of Engerix-B. The first dose should be given at 0 to 2 days of age, the second dose at 1 to 2 months of age, and the third dose at 6 to 18 months of age. An alternative schedule of the three doses administered at 2, 4, and 6 to 18 months of age may be used. In addition, the appropriate pediatric dose of either brand of hepatitis B vaccine may be used at 2, 4, and 6 months of age for primary immunization.[38] This schedule corresponds more closely with the immunization schedule for other vaccines in infancy. In infants born to HBsAg positive mothers, immunization should proceed on a different dosing regimen. In addition to administration of HBIG, vaccination with 5 μg of Recombivax-HB or 10 μg of Engerix-B should be given at 12 hours after birth (but no more than 7 days after birth), 1 month, and 6 months of age. These infants should be tested for anti-HBs at 9 months of age or later. A fourth dose of vaccine should be administered to infants who are anti-HBs nonresponders or hyporesponders (this is very uncommon) and are HBsAg negative. These children should be tested 1 month after the fourth dose for anti-HBs. If titers of > 10 mIU/mL are still not achieved, two additional doses, 1 month apart, may be given with testing for anti-HBs 1 month after the last dose.

For children less than 11 years old who are not born to mothers who are HBsAG positive, 5 μg of Recombivax-HB or 10 ug of Engerix-B should be administered at 0, 1, and 6 months. Children and adolescents ages 11 to 19 years should receive 5 μg or Recombivax-HB or 20 μg of Engerix-B at 0, 1, and 6 months. An alternate four-dose schedule (0, 1, 2, and 12 months) may be used for Engerix-B. Future studies will examine the use of more convenient dosage schedules for adolescents.

Adults ≥ 20 years of age should receive 10 μg of Recombivax-HB or 20 μg of Engerix-B at 0, 1, and 6 months. An alternative schedule of 20 μg at 0, 1, 2, and 12 months may be used for Engerix-B only. Data have suggested that a two-dose schedule may be as effective in inducing protective antibody response as a three-dose schedule for healthy adults.[39]

Hemodialysis patients are considered poor responders to hepatitis B vaccine, thus, the dose of vaccine is escalated in this population. These patients should receive either 40 μg of Recombivax-HB or 40 μg of Engerix-B in a 0, 1, and 6 month schedule. Anti-HBs should be determined and if the value is < 10 mIU/mL, one to three booster doses should be administered. In addition, these persons should be tested yearly and boosted with a single dose of 40 μg if anti-HBs < 10 mIU/mL.[30]

The preferred site of administration is the deltoid muscle in adults (immunogenicity is significantly lower in adults who receive injection in the buttock) and the anterolateral thigh in infants.

Patients who should receive postvaccination serologic testing include immunocompromised patients (because of any cause), persons at occupational risk of exposure, and infants born to HBsAG positive mothers. Data have questioned the cost-effectiveness of postvaccination anti-HBs testing in health care workers.[32]

Approximately 5% to 15% of normal persons will not mount a sufficient antibody titer. In some instances, this may be because of measuring the anti-HBs level too long after the last vaccination in the primary series. Generally, while measurement of anti-HBs is suggested 1 to 6 months after the last dose of vaccine, in reality, measurement of anti-HBs 1 to 3 months after the last dose is probably wiser.[34] Data in gay men suggest that 15% to 25% respond (with development of protective anti-HBs levels) to a single additional dose of vaccine with 30% to 50% responding to three additional doses.[40] These data were generated, however, for the plasma-derived vaccine.

Our data suggest that three doses of 40 μg Recombivax-HB results in development of protective antibody response in 100% of normal hypo- and nonresponders.[41] Thus, our suggestion (and what we believe cost-effective) in a person who has not mounted a protective anti-HBs titer after a standard vaccine series is to administer a standard dose at 0, 1, and 2 months with anti-HBs testing 1 to 2 months after the last dose. Approximately 65% of non- and hyporesponders will develop a protective anti-HBs titer with this regimen. If a protective anti-HBs titer is still lacking, 40 μg of Recombivax-HB should be administered at 0, 1, and 2 months with an anti-HBs titer obtained 1 to 2 months after the last dose. If this strategy does not work, we do not recommend any additional doses of vaccine. Non- and hypo-response may be determined genetically (on the HLA locus); however, the data to assure this are limited.

The need for booster doses of vaccine has not been established.[42] Of persons who develop protective antibody (≥ 10 or more sample ratio units by radioimmunoassay or positive antibody by enzyme immunoassay), 10% to 15% will have lost detectable antibody within 4 years with 40% to 75% of patients having a protective antibody level after 6 to 10 years. Protection against serious infection and liver inflammation appears to persist.[43–45] Controversy continues, however, for individuals with normal immune function. Some authors recommend checking antibody status 3 to 5 years after initial vaccination and administering a single booster dose if antibody concentration is less than 10 mIU/mL. Other authors note that data suggest that protection is in force for at least 7 to 9 years, and thus, they do not recommend repeat doses before then.[28,46] World Health Organization information suggests that no cases of hepatitis B have been reported in individuals who have mounted a protective level of anti-HBs after a vaccine series, even with the progression of time. Immune memory may play a function in this regard. Further studies are needed to elucidate this, and thus, no booster doses are recommended for normal individuals.

The same dosage schedule used for primary immunization is used in the postexposure setting. The hepatitis B vaccine series should be initiated as soon as possible after HBIG administration. Table 113–5 illustrates the specifics of vaccine use.

Side effects following vaccine administration have been minimal, with soreness at the injection site being the primary complaint in approximately 25% of vaccinees. Arthralgias and neurologic side effects are exceedingly rare.[30] The incidence of Guillain-Barré syndrome temporally related to administration of the vaccine does not appear to be above the expected case rate in adults, and no etiologic association with the vaccine has been made. The vaccine does not adversely or therapeutically affect hepatitis B carriers or persons who are already antibody positive.[47]

HEPATITIS B IMMUNE GLOBULIN

Hepatitis B immune globulin is used for postexposure, and rarely preexposure, prophylaxis for hepatitis B infection. The product is prepared from pooled plasma obtained from a small group of healthy donors who have high titers of hepatitis B surface antibody (anti-HBs) as a result of hyperimmunization with hepatitis B vaccine. Immune serum globulin is not indicated for hepatitis B postexposure prophylaxis.

Indications for the use of HBIG include passive immunization following exposure to hepatitis B virus via percutaneous, permucosal, or oral ingestion routes (needlesticks, accidental splash, sexual contact, mouth pipetting) and for infants born to mothers who are hepatitis B carriers. It has also been used for preexposure prophylaxis in the dialysis setting. With the advent of hepatitis B vaccine and the use of erythropoietin, however, a decline in the incidence of hepatitis B in dialysis units has been noted, and thus, HBIG is not generally recommended.

Reports on the use of HBIG have confirmed a significant protective effect of this product (70% to 75% efficacy) and, in general, superior efficacy when compared to standard immune globulin.[30,47–51] There is evidence, however, that HBIG may prolong the incubation period in situations where protective efficacy is not achieved.[52]

The timing of HBIG prophylaxis regarding both frequency of dosing and proximity to the time of exposure has not been completely defined. It is recommended by the CDC that HBIG be given as soon as possible after acute exposures (percutaneous, permucosal, oral ingestion), preferably within 24 hours. It is not recommended that HBIG be given beyond 14 days after acute exposure.

TABLE 113–5. Recommendations for Hepatitis B Prophylaxis Following Percutaneous Exposure

	Treatment When Source Is Found to Be		
Exposed Person	*HBsAg Positive*	*HBsAg Negative*	*Unknown or Not Tested*
Unvaccinated	Administer HBIG × 1[a] and initiate hepatitis B vaccine	Initiate hepatitis B vaccine	Initiate hepatitis B vaccine
Previously Vaccinated			
Known responder	Test exposed person for anti-HBs 1. If adequate, no treatment 2. If inadequate, hepatitis B vaccine booster dose	No treatment	No treatment
Known nonresponder	HBIG × 2 or HBIG × 1, plus one dose of hepatitis B vaccine	No treatment	If known high-risk source, may treat as if source were HBsAg positive
Response unknown	Test exposed person for anti-HB[b] 1. If inadequate HBIG × 1, plus hepatitis B vaccine booster dose 2. If adequate, no treatment	No treatment	Test exposed person for anti-HBs[b] 1. If inadequate, hepatitis B vaccine booster dose 2. If adequate, no treatment

[a]Hepatitis B immune globulin (HBIG) dose 0.06 mL/kg intramuscularly.
[b]Adequate anti-HBs is ≥ 10 mIU.
From Ref. 42.

Variations in the recommendations reflect the relative risk associated with the type of exposure that exists.[53] Generally, the use of HBIG (single dose) with initiation of the hepatitis B vaccine series is thought to be 70% to 95% effective in preventing infection with hepatitis B.[54]

HAEMOPHILUS INFLUENZAE TYPE B VACCINES

Haemophilus influenzae type B (HIB) is responsible for thousands of cases of serious illnesses (meningitis, epiglottitis, pneumonia, sepsis, septic arthritis). The incidence of HIB disease has declined by about 95%, however, since the introduction of vaccines based on the organism's capsular substance, polyribosylribitol phosphate (PRP).[55]

The first HIB vaccines introduced consisted of purified PRP; however, they lacked immunogenicity in the highest risk patients—those under the age of 18 months. The HIB vaccines in use are conjugate products, consisting either of a polysaccharide or oligosaccharide of PRP covalently linked to a protein carrier (Table 113–6). The protein carrier is important because it provides for T-lymphocyte dependent immunologic response, whereas earlier HIB vaccines that consisted of only unconjugated PRP elicited a response that was T-cell independent. T-cell involvement in the response provides for: (1) a greater antibody response, regardless of the age of the patient receiving the vaccine, (2) immunologic response at an earlier age (including infants), and (3) a booster effect on subsequent exposure to the HIB capsule, whether through revaccination or natural exposure.

The HIB conjugate vaccines are stable at 2 to 8°C and should not be frozen. They are indicated for routine use in all infants and children less than 5 years of age. All of the conjugate products are more immunogenic than the earlier nonconjugated vaccines, but only three of the four commercially available products are sufficiently immunogenic for use in infants. Additionally, these three products differ in their immunogenicity and schedule of administration. The primary series of HIB vaccination consists of a 0.5-mL IM dose at ages 2, 4, and 6 months, if HbOC (HibTITER) or PRP-T (OmniHIB) is used. If PRP-OMP is being used, the primary series consists of doses given at 2 and 4 months of age. Although use of one product for the entire primary series is desirable, data suggest that adequate protection is achieved even when different products are used during the initial doses. Following the primary series, a booster dose is recommended at age 12 to 15 months. Any of the four HIB conjugate products, including PRP-D (ProHIBit), are suitable for the booster dose, regardless of which conjugate was used for the primary series of doses.[3,56,57]

Schedules become more complex for infants who do not begin their HIB immunization at the recommended age. For infants 7 to 11 months who have not been vaccinated, three doses of HbOC, PRP-OMP, PRP-T should be given: two doses, spaced 8 weeks apart, and then a booster dose at age 12 to 18 months (but at least 8 weeks since dose two). For unvaccinated children ages 12 to 14 months, two doses should be given, with an interval of 2 months between them. In a child older than 15 months, a single dose of any of the four conjugate vaccines is indicated.[58,59]

Vaccines for HIB are recommended for routine use only in patients up through the 59 month of age. Beyond this age, most individuals will have natural immunity to HIB infection. Patients with certain underlying conditions (HIV infection, IgG_2 subclass deficiency, sickle cell disease, splenectomy, bone marrow transplants, and those receiving chemotherapy for malignancies) are, however, at higher than normal risk for HIB infection, and use of the vaccine in these patients should be considered. Antibody response is less in individuals with these conditions, and based on limited data, two doses of HIB vaccine are recommended.

Adverse reactions to the HIB vaccine are uncommon. Erythema and induration at the injection site occur in approximately 10% to 12% of children and resolve within 24 hours. Fever, diarrhea, and vomiting are occasionally reported. Fever of greater than 38°C is reported in 2.4% of children.

INFLUENZA VIRUS VACCINE

The Advisory Committee on Immunization Practices makes yearly recommendations concerning the composition of influenza virus vaccine. These are published in Morbidity and Mortality Weekly Report annually. The reader is suggested to refer to these annual guidelines as a supplemental update to this chapter.

Influenza virus vaccine (IVV) is an inactivated (killed), trivalent whole or split virus vaccine. Available preparations generally contain 45 μg of antigen, in 15-μg trivalent units per 0.5 mL.

TABLE 113–6. *Haemophilus Influenzae* Vaccines Available in the United States

Manufacturer	Abbreviated Name	Trade Name	Protein Carrier
Connaught Labs	PRP-D	ProHIBit	Diphtheria toxoid
Lederle-Praxis	HbOC[a]	HIBTITER	CRM_{197} (diphtheria toxin)
Merck	PRP-OMP[b]	PedvaxHIB	Outer membrane protein (from *Neisseria meningitidis*)
Pasteur Merieux	PRP-T[c]	ActHIB/OmniHIB	Tetanus toxoid

Note: PRP-D is *not* recommended for infants = 12 months of age. HbOC, PRP-OMP, and PRP-T are suitable for use in infants, beginning at about 2 months of age.
[a]Available as Tetramune, a combination vaccine containing DPT.
[b]Available as Comvax, a combination vaccine containing Hepatitis B vaccine.
[c]Can be given as a combination vaccine by mixing it in the same syringe with Tripedia brand of DTaP.
From Ref. 58.

Influenza is classified as type A or B, with influenza A further subtyped based on hemaglutinin (H) and neuraminidase (N) surface antigens. Influenza A causes significant disease in humans, and the virus is subject to mutation by a phenomenon known as antigenic drift and shift, resulting in the development of different influenza strains. Influenza B, also a significant cause of human disease, is less likely to mutate. The antigenic composition of IVV is determined from year-to-year by the predominant circulating strains worldwide and generally, changes on a yearly basis.

Efficacy and reactogenicity for IVV may be related to the dose of the antigen and the immune status of the individual.[60] Split virus vaccine is felt to be less reactogenic than whole virus vaccine, particularly in children.[61] Antigenic superiority of whole versus split virus vaccine is controversial. In patients who are immunologically "unprimed" (previously unexposed to the antigen), whole and split virus vaccines are likely to induce equal rises in antibody titer.[62,63] In "primed" individuals, however, split virus vaccine may be more effective than whole.[65]

Response to IVV is generally measured in terms of antibody response and, more importantly, efficacy. High-risk, nursing home patients who are vaccinated are significantly less likely to develop influenza, be hospitalized (50% to 60% reduction), develop radiologically proven pneumonia, or die (80% reduction). While IVV has been shown to be cost-effective,[65] not all individuals respond with a significant antibody titer rise and, thus, acquire full protection. Even in those patients who do not develop protective titers, however, IVV is effective in preventing lower respiratory tract infections and secondary complications of the disease. Younger individuals (ages 16 to 25 years) generally have a lower antibody response to a single dose than those 26 years or older.[66] These differences have led to vaccine dose standardization to facilitate response in the majority of subjects. Antibody titers that generally decline at least twofold by 6 months postvaccination are not changed significantly by the use of booster doses.[66] Patients who are HIV positive may have an inadequate response to a one- or two-dose IVV regimen (less than 50%). Individuals with HIV should be vaccinated, however.[67]

Indications for split and whole virus influenza vaccines are (1) adults and children with chronic cardiovascular or pulmonary diseases, (2) residents of nursing home facilities, (3) health care personnel dealing with high-risk patients, (4) healthy adults ≥ age 65 years, (5) adults and children with chronic metabolic disease, (6) women who will be in the second or third trimester during the influenza season, (7) household members (including children) of persons in high-risk groups, and (8) HIV-infected patients. In addition, groups that can transmit influenza to high-risk people should be vaccinated. These groups include health care personnel, employees of nursing homes or chronic care facilities who have patient contact, and providers of home care to high-risk patients and household members (including children) of persons in high-risk groups. Individuals who should not be vaccinated are those with anaphylactic hypersensitivity to eggs or other components of the vaccine or adults with febrile illness (until the fever abates).

Split or whole virus IVV is given as a single 0.5-mL IM injection to persons older than 12 years of age. Because the availability of split virus vaccine is greater, it is the more commonly used vaccine. In persons 3 to 12 years of age, one or two 0.5-mL doses of split virus vaccine given 1 month apart are recommended. For ages 6 to 35 months, 0.25 mL of the split virus vaccine is administered.[67] Two doses are given to children less than 9 years of age who are receiving influenza vaccine for the first time. Influenza vaccine may be administered simultaneously with most other vaccines, especially childhood vaccines. The optimal time period for IVV administration is October through mid-November.

Adverse reactions to the vaccine include local tenderness or low-grade fever in 3% to 5% beginning 6 to 12 hours postimmunization and lasting 1 to 2 days. Treatment with salicylates or acetaminophen is recommended. Immediate allergic reactions are rare but may occur in patients with hypersensitivity to eggs. Guillain-Barré syndrome was only associated with the 1976 swine influenza vaccine and has not been associated with subsequent vaccines.

MEASLES VACCINE

The measles vaccine is a live attenuated viral vaccine that produces a subclinical, noncommunicable infection. Approximately 95% of vaccine recipients seroconvert after a single dose, and most are protected for life.[66] Most persons failing to respond to the initial dose of measles vaccine will seroconvert following a second dose, and this forms the basis for the two-dose vaccine strategy that was implemented in the United States in 1989. The second dose is not harmful to individuals who seroconverted after the first dose, because it merely reinforces their immunity. There is an important genetic role in the immune response to the measles vaccine because persons lacking HLA-DRB1*13 alleles often fail to respond.[68]

The measles vaccine is administered subcutaneously as a 0.5-mL dose in the arm (or in the thigh if the patient is less than 15 months of age). The vaccine is routinely administered for primary immunization to persons 12 to 15 months of age, usually as the MMR vaccine. The measles vaccine is not administered earlier than 12 months (except in certain outbreak circumstances) because persisting maternal antibody that was acquired transplacentally late in gestation can neutralize the vaccine virus and deprive the opportunity for immune response. A second dose of MMR is recommended prior to entry into elementary school or junior high school.[3,68] The second dose of vaccine results in seroconversion in 95% of those individuals who were first-dose nonresponders and also reinforces immunity in those who had a measurable response to the first dose.[69]

Measles-containing vaccine should not be given to pregnant women or immunosuppressed patients. The one exception is HIV-infected patients, who are at very high risk for severe complications if they develop measles. Persons with HIV who have never had measles or been vaccinated against it should be given measles-containing vaccine, unless there is evidence of severe immunosuppression (CD4+ counts < 500 in children 1 to 5 years old or < 200 in patients ≥ 6 years old).[70]

Measles vaccine should not be given within 6 weeks (preferably 3 months) of IM immune globulin administration or within 8 months of IGIV that is given as replacement therapy for humoral immune deficiencies.[3] It is also recommended not to give the vaccine within 1 month of any other live vaccine except mumps, rubella, and oral polio. Historically, persons with a history of anaphylactic reaction to egg protein were considered to be at high risk for serious reactions to measles vaccine, a product derived from chick embryo fibroblasts. As a precaution, skin testing of egg-allergic persons and possible egg-desensitization was recommended prior to measles vaccination. Skin test results poorly predict adverse reactions, however, and the risk of measles vaccination to egg-allergic patients has been shown to be exceedingly low. Therefore, individuals in need of measles vaccine should receive it, regardless of the history of egg allergy.[71] A history of serious neomycin hypersensitivity remains a contraindication to measles vaccine use, as each 0.5-mL dose contains 25 μg of neomycin. Finally, mild febrile illness and upper respiratory tract infections are not contraindications to vaccination.

Measles vaccination is indicated in all persons born after 1956 or in those who lack documentation of wild virus infection either by history or antibody titers. Persons who received killed measles vaccine alone, were given live vaccine within 3 months of receiving killed vaccine, or who have received a vaccine of unknown type between 1963 and 1967 should be revaccinated. Revaccination should be considered for students entering college, because of outbreaks on college campuses. It is also important to vaccinate health care workers who have low antibody titers because of the possibility of becoming infected by patients and transmitting the disease to other compromised individuals. If two doses are needed (the person has never been vaccinated), they should be given at least 1 month apart. Following vaccination, antibodies may be detected within 2 to 3 weeks in patients 12 months of age or older.

For postexposure prophylaxis, the vaccine is effective if given within 72 hours of exposure. In addition, immune globulin may be administered at a dose of 0.25 mg/kg IM (maximum dose, 15 mL), if given within 6 days of exposure. In children under 1 year of age, postexposure vaccination may be given as early at 6 months of age, but it should be repeated at 12 to 15 months of age.

The measles vaccine has an excellent safety record. The most common side effect following vaccination is fever, which occurs in 5% to 15% of vaccinees. Transient rash (generalized) may also occur in about 5% of vaccine recipients. These reactions generally appear 5 to 12 days postvaccination and last 2 to 5 days. Febrile seizures rarely occur, and there is no association between MMR vaccination and development of a subsequent seizure disorder. Other adverse effects, such as headache, cough, sore throat, eye pain, malaise, and transient thrombocytopenia, occur less frequently. Local reactions at the injection site, while rare, may occur in subjects who have previously been vaccinated with killed vaccine. Live measles vaccine may suppress a positive tuberculin skin test for up to 6 weeks postadministration.[66,71]

MENINGOCOCCAL POLYSACCHARIDE VACCINE

Meningococcal polysaccharide vaccine (MPV) containing purified capsular polysaccharide antigen from *Neisseria meningitidis* is licensed for use in the United States. The vaccine is a quadrivalent product, containing serogroups A, C, Y, and W-135.[72]

The MPV is indicated in high-risk populations, such as those exposed to the disease, those in the midst of uncontrolled outbreaks, travelers to an area with epidemic or hyperendemic meningococcal disease, or individuals who have terminal complement component deficiencies or asplenia. Routine vaccination of all individuals is not recommended in the United States because serogroup B, which is poorly immunogenic and not contained in the current vaccine, causes the majority of disease. The vaccine should not be given to pregnant women unless there is a substantial risk of infection.

Meningococcal polysaccharide vaccine is administered subcutaneously as a single 0.5-mL dose. Subjects should be over 2 years of age because of the difficulty younger patients have responding to polysaccharide antigens. Younger children may produce sufficient antibody levels against serogroup A, however, if given two doses 3 months apart.[72] Antibody levels thought to be protective are attained within 10 to 14 days. Revaccination may be reconsidered in 2 to 3 years in high-risk children, who are less than 4 years old, on initial vaccination because of rapid antibody decline.[72] The vaccine shows documented effectiveness in preventing meningococcal disease in 85% to 95% of recipients for serotypes A and C. Efficacy of the vaccine for serotypes Y and W-135 is presumed but not documented. Adverse effects of MPV include fever and erythema at the injection site lasting 1 to 2 days. Occasionally, headache occurs.

MUMPS VACCINE

The mumps vaccine is a lyophilized live attenuated vaccine prepared from chick embryo cultures. Each 0.5-mL dose of the vaccine also contains 25 μg of neomycin. The vaccine is available alone or in combination with a measles and rubella vaccine.

The mumps vaccine is used to produce active immunity while producing a subclinical, noncommunicable infection. A single dose induces antibody formation in 97% of children older than 12 months of age and 93% of adults. Clinical efficacy approaches 75% to 90%.[74] Although protection may last a lifetime, outbreaks have been reported in previously vaccinated young adults, suggesting the possibility of waning immunity.[75]

The vaccine is usually given in conjunction with measles and rubella vaccines (as MMR) and is administered as a 0.5-mL subcutaneous injection in the upper arm. Dosing recommendations coincide with those for measles vaccine, with the first dose being administered at age 12 to 15 months, and the second one prior to entry into elementary school (or alternatively, prior to entry into junior high school). If the vaccine is given before 12 months of age, revaccination is necessary and should be given after reaching 1 year of age. The vaccine is also indicated in previously unvaccinated adults, in those who have previously been vaccinated with killed mumps vaccine (an older product no longer available), and in those with an uncertain history of wild virus infection. Postexposure vaccination is of no benefit.[75]

Mumps vaccine should not be given to pregnant women or immunosuppressed patients. Additionally, conception should be avoided for 3 months following vaccination. In patients with a history of anaphylaxis to eggs, the same schema as in the case of measles should be used. The vaccine should not be given within 6 weeks (preferably 3 months) of administration of immune globulin. Finally, the vaccine should not be given to neomycin-sensitive individuals.

Serious adverse reactions to the vaccine are rarely reported. Parotitis, rash, pruritus, and purpura rarely occur. Local reactions, including soreness, burning, and stinging, may occur at the injection site. Although aseptic meningitis has been epidemiologically linked with a mumps vaccine containing the Urabe strain of mumps virus, no such link has been established with vaccine containing the Jeryl Lynn strain, which is in use in the United States.[71]

PERTUSSIS VACCINE

Whole cell pertussis vaccine is a suspension of killed, whole *Bordetella pertussis* organisms. It is usually administered in combination with diphtheria and tetanus toxoids (as DPT). The primary immunization series for pertussis vaccine consists of four 0.5-mL IM doses given at ages 2, 4, 6, and 15 to 18 months, and a booster dose is recommended at age 4 to 6 years. The efficacy of pertussis vaccine is approximately 80%. Because disease-related risks decline and vaccine-related side effects increase after age 7, whole-cell pertussis vaccine is not recommended for use beyond this age.[76]

Significant controversy has surrounded whole-cell pertussis vaccine because of adverse effects that occur frequently after its use. Local reactions (pain, redness, and swelling at the site of injection) and febrile reactions occur after approximately 50% of doses. More worrisome events that reportedly have a temporal relationship to pertussis vaccine administration include prolonged crying (3%), unusual high-pitched cry (0.1%), convulsions (0.06%), and acute encephalopathy (0.0001% to 0.001%).[77] Although numerous attempts to determine whether or not there is risk of lasting brain damage following receipt of pertussis vaccine, experts have not been able to reach consensus. If such a risk exists, however, it appears to be exceptionally small.[78]

When defending pertussis vaccine use despite its frequent side effects, advocates frequently cite the increased incidence of pertussis that occurred in Great Britain following decreased use of vaccine.[79,80] Advocates also stress the decline in mortality resulting from pertussis in the United States and England prior to and following vaccine institution. Between 1926 and 1930, there were 36,013 whooping cough deaths in the United States. Finally, 1984 data suggest a significant decrease in pertussis among household contacts ages 6 months to 9 years vaccinated with three or more doses of the vaccine versus nonvaccinated individuals.[81] Use of the vaccine has reduced the number of reported cases one-hundred fold or more.

The American Academy of Pediatrics and the Immunization Practices Advisory Committee continue to recommend routine use of pertussis vaccine.[82] There are only two absolute contraindications to pertussis administration: an immediate anaphylactic reaction to a previous dose, or encephalopathy within 7 days of a previous dose with no evidence of other cause. A convulsion within 3 days, persistent inconsolable screaming (for 3 or more hours) within 2 days, hypotonic–hyporesponsive episode within 48 hours, and a temperature of 40.5°C or greater, unexplained by another cause, within 48 hours of receiving pertussis-containing vaccine once were considered contraindications but are now identified as precautions. None of these events has been proved to cause permanent sequelae. The decision of whether or not to administer additional doses of pertussis vaccine to patients who have experienced one of these events should be based on the possible risks of the disease (i.e., during a pertussis outbreak).

Whether or not patients with a seizure disorder should receive pertussis vaccine has been a matter of debate; but a history of a seizure disorder is not itself a contraindication. In patients with a recent onset of seizures, vaccine should be withheld until it is determined whether or not a neurologic disorder is evolving; if not, pertussis vaccine may be continued.

Concern over the side effects of whole cell pertussis vaccine prompted a search for safer agents and the development of so-called acellular pertussis products. Several acellular pertussis vaccines have been approved by the FDA, and still others are under clinical study. As with whole cell vaccine, the acellular pertussis vaccines are combined with tetanus and diphtheria toxoids, as DTaP.

Acellular pertussis vaccines contain selective components of the *B. pertussis* organism, rather than the intact, killed microbe. All acellular vaccines contain pertussis toxin (PT), and some contain one or more additional bacterial components (filamentous hemagglutinin [FHA], pertactin [a 69Kd outer membrane protein], and fimbrae types 2 and 3). Each of the approved acellular pertussis vaccines contains less endotoxin than whole cell vaccine and is associated with fewer side effects. Therefore, acellular pertussis vaccines can be viewed as safer than whole cell products. Erythema, swelling, pain, fever, and drowsiness occur less frequently. Because most vaccine-associated seizures are actually febrile convulsions, the lessened febrile response also may result in fewer vaccine-associated seizures. There is no evidence that the rare, more serious adverse effects occur less often though. The same cautions and contraindications to the use of whole cell pertussis vaccine are applicable to the acellular vaccines.[83]

Available acellular pertussis products have a clinical efficacy that is at least equivalent to whole cell pertussis vaccine. Based on this and improved safety, recommendations suggest the use of acellular rather than whole cell vaccine (as DTaP) whenever possible. Not all products have gained approval for the entire series of doses though. It is advisable to consult the manufacturer's recommendations for dosing prior to use of any DTaP product.

POLIOVIRUS VACCINES

Two types of trivalent poliovirus vaccines are licensed for distribution in the United States. An inactivated vaccine, developed by Salk, was licensed for use in 1955. In 1987, an enhanced-potency inactivated polio vaccine (IPV) was introduced, and this has replaced the original inactivated vaccine. Since 1962, a live attenuated, oral polio vaccine (OPV), developed by Sabin, has been the primary immunizing agent for poliovirus infection. Recommendations, however, indicate that IPV may be the preferred vaccine in the future.[84,85]

The OPV is administered in a series of 0.5-mL oral doses. In children, OPV immunization generally begins at 6 to 12 weeks of age, commonly with the first DPT immunization. Doses are recommended at 2, 4, and 6 to 18 months, with a booster at 4 to 6 years of age. The OPV closely parallels natural infection, stimulating humoral antibody and secretory IgA in lymphatic tissues surrounding the intestinal tract within 7 to 10 days of ingestion. Virus replicates within the gastrointestinal tract and can be found in pharyngeal secretions and stool for several weeks. This shedding of virus can result in immunization of some contacts of vaccinees, as well as risk of infection in contacts with compromised immune status. Immunity is achieved in 95% of vaccine recipients.

There are no immediate side effects of OPV. Rarely, vaccine-associated paralytic poliomyelitis (VAPP) will develop in vaccinees (1 out of 6.2 million doses) or contacts (1 out of 7.6 million doses). Individuals with primary immune deficiency are at increased risk for this adverse reaction, and for this reason, OPV is not recommended for persons who are immunodeficient or for normal individuals who reside in a household with an immunocompromised person. The OPV should not be given during pregnancy because of a small, theoretical risk to the fetus.[86,87]

Primary immunization with IPV consists of a series of 0.5-mL IM injections. Doses are recommended at 2, 4, and 12 to 18 months, with a booster dose at 4 to 6 years of age. If interruption of the series occurs, a sufficient immune response can be obtained by administration of only those doses that had been omitted. Following immunization, humoral antibodies are induced in 95% of recipients. The duration of protection following immunization has not been definitively determined. There are no serious side effects attributable to IPV, and the only contraindication is pregnancy, in which case IPV should be given only if there is a clear need (e.g., women who will be traveling or living in an area with endemic or epidemic poliovirus).

Primary poliomyelitis immunization is recommended for all children and young adults up to age 18. Primary immunization of adults over the age of 18 is not routinely recommended since a high level of immunity already exists in this age group and the risk of exposure in developed countries is small. Unimmunized adults who are at increased risk for exposure because of travel, residence, or occupation should, however, receive poliovirus vaccine. Because the risk of vaccine-induced paralysis following OPV is slightly greater in adults than in children, IPV is the recommended product. Patients who are HIV positive should receive IPV.

Incompletely immunized adults or children should complete the series of IPV or OPV regardless of the interval since initiation of primary immunization. Booster doses of OPV or IPV are recommended for children before entering school. Adults do not routinely need a booster dose unless there is an increased risk of exposure (travel) in which case, a single dose of OPV or IPV should be given.

It appears that poliomyelitis has been eradicated in the United States. There have been no confirmed cases because of wild-type poliovirus since 1982. Each year approximately 8 to 10 cases of paralytic disease are reported to the CDC, but these are caused by vaccine strains of the virus. Because of the absence of natural polio in the United States, many authorities feel there is little justification for continued preferential use of OPV, with its associated risk of VAPP. Discontinuation of all polio vaccines is not yet practical because polio remains a problem in other regions of the world, and imported cases could still cause outbreaks in the United States.

The CDC has suggested that sequential use of IPV and OPV is the preferred regimen for immunizing children. For the first two doses, IPV is recommended, and OPV is preferred for the third and fourth doses. This regimen is believed to minimize the risk of VAPP, which is greatest following the first dose of OPV in a previously unimmunized person. The initial doses of IPV are thought to provide systemic immunity, and the subsequent OPV doses stimulate local (gastrointestinal) antibody production. Although this sequential use of poliovirus vaccines is being promoted as the preferred regimen, giving all doses as OPV or IPV is also acceptable. Reluctance to implement an all-IPV national policy has been based on concern over the large number of IM injections that infants already require. When a combination product containing IPV and DPT becomes commercially available, IPV will likely become the preferred product.

PNEUMOCOCCAL VACCINE

Pneumococcal vaccine (Pneumovax 23 and Pnu-Immune 23) is a mixture of highly purified capsular polysaccharides from 23 of the 83 most prevalent or invasive types of *Streptococcus pneumoniae* seen in the United States. The serotypes included are 1, 2, 3, 4, 5, 6B, 7F, 8, 9N, 9V, 10A, 12F, 14, 15B, 17F, 18C, 19A, 20, 22F, 23F, and 33F. These 23 types represent 85% to 90% of all blood isolates and 85% of pneumococcal isolates from other generally sterile sites seen in the United States. Each 0.5-mL dose of vaccine contains 25 μg of each polysaccharide type dissolved in isotonic saline solution (for a total of 575 μg of polysaccharide) and 0.25% phenol as preservative. Significant cross-reactivity with other pneumococcal capsular antigens not represented in the vaccine does not occur.[88]

Pneumococcal vaccine efficacy has been debated in the literature. In nonbacteremic disease, while prelicensure trials in young healthy gold miners in South Africa showed reduction in disease rates,[89] in the postmarketing period, randomized clinical trials performed in elderly persons with chronic disease did not confirm these findings.[88] A meta-analysis of various trials also has not confirmed protection in nonbacteremic disease with pneumococcal vaccine.[88] In addition, the vaccine has not been shown to be effective for the prevention of sinusitis or acute otitis media in children.

For invasive disease, reduction rates of 56% to 81% have been shown with the vaccine. In adults, vaccine efficacy was shown for persons with chronic disease and immunocompromised individuals ≥ 65 years of age. A meta-analysis of nine randomized controlled trials concluded that the vaccine was efficacious in reducing the frequency of bacteremic pneumococcal pneumonia among adults in low-risk groups. Cost-effectiveness has also been shown.[88] The vaccine is only effective for the serotypes included.

Pneumococcal vaccine induces type-specific antibodies (T-cell independent mechanisms) with a twofold rise within 2 to 3 weeks in ≥ 80% young healthy adults. No correlation of antibody levels and protection has been defined. Antibody levels to these strains remain elevated for at least 5 years. In certain individuals, these levels decline within 10 years. Children may be protected for only 3 to 5 years. Elderly individuals and patients with chronic disease may have lower antibody levels produced with the vaccine. Children < 2 years of age do not respond adequately to the vaccine.

A number of other groups have reduced antibody production with the vaccine. These include immunocompromised patients (leukemia, lymphoma, multiple myeloma), dialysis patients, and AIDS patients. Asymptomatic HIV-infected patients respond sufficiently to the vaccine. Patients with Hodgkin's disease respond to the vaccine better before splenectomy, chemotherapy, or radiation therapy.

Pneumococcal vaccine is recommended for the following immunocompetent persons[88]:

1. Persons ≥ 65 years of age. If an individual received vaccine more than 5 years earlier and was less than age 65 at the time of administration, revaccination should be given.
2. Persons ages 2 to 64 years with a chronic illness.
3. Persons ages 2 to 64 with functional or anatomic asplenia. When splenectomy is planned, pneumococcal vaccine should be given at least 2 weeks prior to surgery. Revaccination is recommended at ≥ 5 years in subjects > 10 years old and ≥ 3 years in subjects ≤ 10 years old.
4. Persons ages 2 to 64 years living in environments where the risk of invasive pneumococcal disease or its complications are increased. This does not include daycare center employees and children.

Pneumococcal vaccine is recommended for immunocompromised persons ≥ 2 years of age with: (1) HIV infection, (2) leukemia, (3) lymphoma, (4) Hodgkin's disease, (5) multiple myeloma, (6) generalized malignancy, (7) chronic failure or nephrotic syndrome, (8) patients receiving immunosuppressive therapy including corticosteroids, and (9) organ and bone marrow transplant recipients. A single revaccination should be given if 5 years or more has passed since receipt of the first dose in subjects older than 10 years of age. In subjects 10 years of age or older, revaccination should be given 3 years after the previous dose.

While the safety of pneumococcal vaccine during the first trimester or pregnancy has not been evaluated, no adverse effects have been seen in newborns whose mothers received the vaccine during pregnancy.[88]

Pneumococcal vaccine safety is well documented. Local reactions occur frequently within the first 48 hours and are generally mild. Local erythema and induration (30%), local discomfort (40%), and local swelling (3%) are the side effects most commonly observed. Revaccination has been associated with no more local adverse effects than after the first dose.[88,90] Rarely, severe systemic reactions can occur, and they consist of weakness, myalgia, headache, photophobia, chills, and fever. Guillain-Barré syndrome has not been reported. In patients with HIV infection, pneumococcal vaccine may cause a transient increase in viral replication, however, the importance of this is unknown.

The vaccine should be administered intramuscularly or subcutaneously as a single 0.5-mL dose. The vaccine may be given simultaneously as influenza vaccine (in separate arms) and with DPT or poliovirus vaccine.

RABIES VACCINE

Human diploid cell vaccine (HDCV) and rabies vaccine adsorbed (RVA) are killed vaccines used for preexposure and postexposure rabies virus prophylaxis. Transmission of rabies can occur via percutaneous, permucosal, or airborne exposure to the rabies virus. Circumstances favoring such transmission include animal bites or attacks and contamination of scratches, cuts, abrasions, or mucous membranes with saliva or other infectious material (brain tissue). Unprovoked attacks and daytime attacks by nocturnal animals are considered highly suspect. Common wild animal transmitters include skunks, foxes, and raccoons. Dog rabies is very common in certain foreign countries (India, African nations). Rodents, rabbits, and hares are rarely infected. There have been four reports of person-to-person transmission via corneal transplant.[91] Reports of rabid animals have increased over the past decade in the United States.

Preexposure indications for using HDCV or RVA include persons whose vocation or avocation place them at high risk for rabies exposure, for example, veterinarians, animal handlers, laboratory workers in rabies research laboratories, and field personnel (trappers, hunters, cave explorers). Travelers who will be in a country or area of a country where there is a constant threat of rabies, whose stay is likely to extend beyond 1 month, and who may not have readily available medical services (Peace Corps workers, missionaries) should also be considered for preexposure prophylaxis. The population at large need not be vaccinated.[91,92] The vaccine is not recommended for persons who are immunocompromised because of inadequate response. If the vaccine is used in immunocompromised persons, it should be given by the IM route only and antibody titers should be checked postimmunization.

Postexposure prophylaxis should be given after percutaneous or permucosal exposure to saliva or other infectious material from a high-risk source. Each case needs to be considered individually. Consideration needs to be given to the geographical area, species of animal, circumstances of the incident, and type of exposure. Local or state health departments may be able to provide guidelines.

The HDCV for preexposure prophylaxis is administered in three doses of 1.0 mL IM or 0.1 mL intradermally on days 0 and 7 and once between days 21 and 28.[93] For intradermal prophylaxis HDCV must be given using the specific intradermal dosage form and syringe. Although the literature suggests that intradermal vaccine gives protective titers in an equal number of patients compared to IM dosing,[93–95] field reports suggest that intradermal HDCV may give a nonprotection rate of 7.5%.[96] This observation has lead the New York State Department of Health to recommend the routine use of IM HDCV. [97] If intradermal injection is used, it is suggested that rabies antibody titers be checked 30 days after the last dose of vaccine. Rabies vaccine adsorbed may be used intramuscularly but not intradermally for preexposure prophylaxis. Pregnancy is not a contraindication if the risk of rabies is great.

An IM booster dose every second year is recommended for persons who will have continued exposure. Some authors recommend testing rabies antibody with booster doses deferred if the rapid fluorescent focus inhibition test (RFFIT) is > 1:5. Intradermal boosters doses, although recommended by some groups,[2] is not recommended by the New York State Department of Health.[97] Suboptimal responses have been documented in persons receiving chloroquine chemoprophylaxis for malaria,[98] and, thus, the vaccine should be administered 1 month prior to the institution of chloroquine therapy. If this is not possible, IM HDCV or RVA should be used. For individuals who have received the duck-embryo vaccines in the past, a single IM booster dose of HDCV or RVA may be used.

Preexposure prophylaxis does not eliminate the need for postexposure prophylaxis. The regimen for postexposure prophylaxis is determined by whether or not a person has previously received HDCV or RVA. Persons previously immunized with HDCV or RVA or those who have received postexposure prophylaxis previously should receive two 1.0-mL IM doses of HDCV or RVA on postexposure days 0 and 3. Rabies immune globulin should not be given to this group. Individuals who have not been previously immunized should receive the recommended regimen of rabies immune globulin (see later section) and five doses of HDCV or RVA, 1.0-mL IM on days 0, 3, 7, 14, and 28 after exposure.[92,99,100] The intradermal route should not be used for postexposure prophylaxis.

Intramuscular vaccine should be given in the deltoid muscle in adults and the anterolateral thigh in children. The gluteal region should not be used.

Adverse reactions to HDCV and RVA are not uncommon. Approximately 20% will experience pain, erythema, swelling, and itching at the injection site. Another 20% may have headache, nausea, abdominal pain, muscle aches, dizziness or a combination of these.[101] Systemic allergic reactions ranging from hives to anaphylaxis occur in an estimated 11 out of 10,000 vaccinees.[101] It is recommended that persons exposed to rabies who do have adverse reactions continue the vaccine series in a setting with medical support services. In persons receiving booster doses of HDCV an immune complex-like disease has been seen 2 to 21 days later in up to 7% of vaccinees. The incidence of serum sickness-like reactions 7 to 14 days later with RVA booster doses is < 1%.

Antibody conversion occurs in virtually 100% of HDCV or RVA recipients. The CDC considers titers of 1:5 by RFFIT testing as being protective. The WHO uses a value of 0.5 IU/mL as evidence of protective antibody. Persons who are receiving corticosteroids or other immunosuppressant agents and who receive postexposure prophylaxis should have their antibody status determined. Cholorquine or mefloquine may weaken the antibody response to HDCV when it is administered intradermally. In patients receiving these agents, the IM route is recommended.

RABIES IMMUNE GLOBULIN

Human rabies immune globulin is an immunoglobulin used in conjunction with rabies vaccine as part of postexposure rabies management for previously unvaccinated individuals. The product is derived from plasma obtained from donors who have been hyperimmunized with rabies vaccine and have high titers of circulating antibody.

In persons who have not been previously immunized against rabies, rabies immune globulin is given simultaneously with rabies HDCV or RVA to provide optimal coverage in the interval before immune response to the vaccine occurs. The efficacy of this regimen has been clearly demonstrated. In situations where a vaccine has been used alone, mortality rates of 50% to 60% have been observed. Mortality after the combination vaccine and rabies immune globulin regimens is an exceedingly rare event; however, failures have been reported when the wound was not infiltrated with rabies immune globulin.[102]

Rabies immune globulin does not interfere with vaccine-induced antibody formation. Its use is not recommended beyond 8 days after initiation of the vaccine series nor in persons previously immunized to rabies, however.

Human rabies immune globulin is administered in a dose of 20 IU/kg (0.133 mL/kg), half to be given intramuscularly and the other half infiltrated around the wound site. This product should never be administered by the intravenous route. Because other antibodies in the rabies immune globulin may interfere with the response to live virus vaccines (MMR), it is recommended that these immunizations be delayed for 3 months.

Side effects are rare but may include local soreness at the wound or IM injection site and mild temperature elevations. Caution is advised when administering this product to persons with known systemic allergies to immune globulin or thimerosal. Pregnancy is not a contraindication for its use.

RUBELLA VACCINE

Rubella vaccine contains lyophilized live attenuated rubella (German measles) virus grown in human diploid cell culture. The vaccine is available alone or in combination with measles or mumps vaccine, or both. Each 0.5-mL dose also contains 25 μg of neomycin.

Rubella vaccine induces antibodies to the virus that are thought to be protective against wild-virus infection. Following a single 0.5-mL subcutaneous dose, 95% of children 1 year of age become rubella antibody positive within 2 to 6 weeks.[103] The duration of immunity has not been established, and booster doses are not recommended. A second dose is recommended, however, at the same time measles vaccine is administered (as a second dose of MMR). The vaccine is indicated for children older than 1 year of age, persons 12 years or older without evidence of wild-virus infection, women of childbearing potential for whom serologic testing is unavailable, and persons at a substantial risk for exposure. The vaccine should not be given to immunosuppressed individuals nor used within 6 weeks (preferably 3 months) of immune globulin administration. Additional immune globulin should not be given within 14 days of vaccine. The vaccine should not be given to neomycin-sensitive patients.[104]

Adverse effects of the rubella virus vaccine tend to increase with the age of the recipient. Symptoms are similar to wild-virus infection and include lymphadenopathy, rash, urticaria, fever, malaise, sore throat, headache, myalgias, and paresthesias of the extremities. These occur 11 to 20 days after vaccination and last 1 to 5 days. Joint symptoms occur at 1 to 10 weeks in 20% to 40% of adult women, and their incidence is greater in adolescent women than in children. Overt arthritis occurs in less than 1% of recipients. Symptoms last 1 to 3 days and rarely recur. The vaccine may cause suppression of tuberculin skin tests for up to 6 weeks postvaccination. While the vaccine virus may be excreted in nose and throat secretions, it is not contagious.

While the vaccine has been shown to be safe to the fetus, its use in pregnancy is discouraged. Women should be counseled not to become pregnant for 3 months following vaccination. Termination of pregnancy is not indicated in women who are accidentally given the vaccine.

VARICELLA VACCINE

Live attenuated varicella vaccine contains the Oka-Merck strain of varicella virus, which was attenuated by propagation through several different cell culture lines. Varicella vaccine (VAR) is a lyophilized product that must be kept frozen and protected from light. Once reconstituted, it must be administered subcutaneously within 30 minutes. Each 0.5-mL dose contains a minimum of 1350 plaque forming units of virus, as well as 12.5 mg of hydrolyzed gelatin and trace amounts of neomycin, fetal bovine serum, and residual components from cell culture.[105]

The VAR vaccine is safe and immunogenic in healthy children and adults. A single dose results in seroconversion in greater than 94% of healthy children, and over 90% have persisting antibodies 1 year later. Studies in normal, healthy adults have shown lower seroconversion rates (as low as 80%) following a single dose, but this increases to 95% when a two-dose regimen is used. In clinical studies, Var vaccine has been 70% to > 95% effective in preventing chickenpox. Vaccinated individuals who develop chickenpox typically experience milder disease, with less fever and fewer skin lesions, many of which do not vesiculate.[106] Similarly, the secondary spread of virus following vaccination occurs at a low rate and has resulted in mild disease, confirming attenuation of the virus.[107]

The duration of protection provided by VAR is unknown, but it is of concern since chickenpox typically is more severe in adults than children. Although antibody titers may decline with time, VAR stimulates both humoral and cell-mediated immune response. Humoral and cell-mediated immunity persists for a minimum of 6 years in vaccinated children, suggesting that protection is long-lasting.[108] Additionally, children who are immunized against varicella and then exposed to wild-virus experience an immunologic boost.[109] As VAR use becomes more widespread, the circulation of wild-virus can be expected to diminish, and the opportunity for immunologic boosting because of natural exposure will also decline. It is not known if booster doses will be needed under these circumstances. Long-term studies assessing the duration of VAR's protective effect and the advisability of booster doses are ongoing.

The varicella vaccine is recommended for all children at 12 to 18 months of age. It is also recommended for patients above this age, if they have not already had chickenpox. Individuals who are 12 months to 12 years of age require one dose. Persons 13 years and older should receive two doses, separated by 4 to 8 weeks. Because VAR is a live vaccine, it is contraindicated in immunosuppressed or pregnant patients. It is also contraindicated in individuals with a history of anaphylactic reaction to any component of the vaccine. Persons who have received blood, plasma, or immune globulin products within the past 5 months should not receive VAR, because of concern that passively acquired antibody will interfere with response to the vaccine. Although adverse events associated with salicylate use after vaccination have been reported, VAR recipients are recommended to avoid salicylates for 6 weeks postvaccination because of the association of salicylate use and Reye's syndrome following varicella infection.[105,110]

The VAR vaccine has an excellent safety record. Pain, local swelling, and erythema at the injection site occurs in up to 25% of patients, fever in 4% to 10%, and mild upper respiratory symptoms in a smaller number. A varicella-like rash occurs in approximately 4% of vaccinees, accompanied by few if any systemic symptoms. The rash may be localized at the injection site or generalized. Lesions are usually few in number (2 to 10) and often papular rather than vesicular. Transmission of vaccine virus to susceptible close contacts has occurred, but it is not common, and the risk of transmission correlates with the number of vaccine-induced lesions. Presumed vaccine-related secondary cases have proved to be mild, owing to attenuation of the vaccine virus.

Acquisition of either wild-virus or the vaccine strain of varicella renders an individual susceptible to zoster (shingles) at a later date because of reactivation of latent virus. Data indicate that following VAR, zoster occurs less frequently than following natural infection.

VARICELLA ZOSTER IMMUNE GLOBULIN

Varicella zoster immune globulin (VZIG) is used for passive immunization of susceptible immunodeficient patients exposed to varicella zoster (VZ) infection. It is prepared by Cohn cold ethanol fractionation from plasma found in routine screening of normal volunteer blood donors to contain high titers of VZ antibody. On the average, VZIG has been found to contain 10 to 20 times more VZ antibody than immune globulin (IG).[105]

Postexposure prophylaxis with VZIG should be considered in certain children and adults who are at very high risk of complications or death if they contract varicella. Criteria for VZIG use in children are listed in Table 113–7. A positive history of varicella infection eliminates the need for VZIG. A negative history for infection is not, however, a valid indicator of need, as 75% to 95% of persons with negative or unknown varicella infection histories are serologically positive for VZ antibodies. Positive serologic tests on immunocompromised patients can be misleading as VZ antibody may be transiently acquired from blood products. In such cases, it is best to consult with the regional Red Cross Blood Distribution Center regarding the appropriate course of action.

TABLE 113–7. Conditions Warranting Consideration of Varicella Zoster Immune Globulin (VZIG) After Varicella Zoster Virus Exposure

Neoplastic diseases
Primary or acquired immunodeficiency
Immunosuppressive treatment
Pregnancy
Newborn of mother who had onset of chickenpox within 5 days before delivery or within 48 hours after delivery
Premature infant > 28 weeks' gestation whose mother has no history of chickenpox
Premature infant < 28 weeks' gestation or < 1000 g, regardless of maternal history of chickenpox

Abstracted from Ref. 105.

Varicella can cause congenital malformation early and, rarely, late in pregnancy. While VZIG may attenuate maternal infection, its efficacy in preventing intrauterine infection has not been demonstrated. There is an increased risk of serious infection and an associated 30% mortality in infants whose mothers develop varicella 4 days prior to or 2 days after delivery or whose onset of infection is between 5 and 10 days of age. Normal, full-term infants exposed postnatally are not at increased risk for complications. Use of VZIG perinatally is, therefore, aimed at the critical period for complications (see Table 113–7).[110]

The efficacy of VZIG has been measured by three parameters: clinical attack rates, severity of illness, and incidence of subclinical disease. Clinical attack rates in immunocompromised children after VZIG have varied from 33% to 50%, as compared to normal attack rates of 80% to 90% after household exposures without prophylaxis. The severity of illness has been significantly affected with VZIG, however, and the majority of cases have been mild, with complications occurring in only 7%. Subclinical infections commonly occur after VZIG. In one study, 33% of leukemic patients had evidence of subclinical infection after VZIG as compared to a 5% incidence after natural infections.

For maximum effectiveness, VZIG must be given within 48 hours and not more than 96 hours following exposure. Because this agent may only attenuate infection, patients who receive VZIG may still have a period of communicability, and VZIG may prolong the incubation period to 28 days.

Varicella zoster immune globulin is distributed by the American Red Cross Services. Contact with the distribution centers must be made within 72 hours of exposure and specific criteria met in order for the product to be released.

Administration of VZIG is by the IM route (never IV) at doses of 125 U/10 kg of body weight up to 625 U (five vials) for patients more than 40 kg. The dose for newborn infants is 125 U. Side effects include local soreness at the site of injection. Although VZIG should be avoided in persons with bleeding diathesis, there are no other contraindications for the use of this product. Duration of antibody protection is not known, but it is felt to be at least one half-life of the immune globulin or approximately 3 weeks.

OTHER IMMUNOBIOLOGICS

CYTOMEGALOVIRUS IMMUNE GLOBULIN

Cytomegalovirus immune globulin intravenous (CMV-IGIV) contains IgG antibodies obtained from healthy persons with high titers of antibodies to cytomegalovirus (CMV).[111] The agent is available commercially.

Attenuation of primary CMV disease associated with kidney transplantation in seronegative recipients of seropositive kidneys is the only indication for CMV-IGIV.[112] It is dosed using a tapering schedule. Dosage is 150 mg/kg preoperatively or within 72 hours postoperatively; 100 mg/kg at 2, 4, 6, and 8 weeks; and 50 mg/kg at weeks 12 and 16. These doses are for all ages. The use of CMV-IVIG has resulted in 50% of CMV-related syndromes.[112] It has been investigated for use with gancyclovir in treating CMV infection in liver and bone marrow transplant patients. Data are preliminary in this area, and its routine use is not recommended.

Adverse effects of CMV-IGIV are seen in less than 5% of recipients and include flushing, chills, muscle cramps, back pain, chest tightness, fever, nausea, vomiting, hypotension, and tachycardia. Anaphylaxis rarely occurs. Since CMV-IVIG contains other antibodies, it has been suggested that vaccination with live viral vaccines be withheld until 3 months after CMV-IVIG administration.

IMMUNE GLOBULIN

Immune globulin is available as both intramuscular (IGIM) and intravenous preparations (IGIV). The IGIM preparation, or the Cohn fraction II, is prepared from pooled plasma of several thousand donors by cold ethanol fractionation.[113] It typically contains greater than 95% IgG and trace amounts of IgM, IgA, and other plasma proteins. Because IG is harvested from a large donor pool, it contains a wide spectrum of IgG antibodies to the pathogens prevalent in the area from which the donors were obtained. In the fractionation process, high molecular weight IgG aggregates are formed, which can activate complement in the absence of antigen and precipitate anaphylactoid reactions. For this reason, IGIM is unsuitable for IV administration. Intramuscular IG typically contains 15% to 18% protein and not less than 90% IgG.

A number of IV preparations of IG are commercially available in the United States.[114] Generally, these preparations contain greater than 90% IgG monomers and trace to small amounts of IgA.[115] These agents are rendered suitable for intravenous use because their anticomplement activity is removed. These products are available as lyophilized powders or solutions.

When administered either IV or IM, IG distributes in approximately 5% of the body weight of the recipient.[114] The plasma half-life of IG averages 18 to 32 days. This range of half-life is probably attributable to the variation in the half-life of IgG subclasses. Peak serum concentrations occur relatively immediately with IGIV whereas IGIM produces peak concentrations within 2 days. After the initial period of equilibration, circulating IgG levels are superimposable between IV and IM equivalent dosages. No dosage adjustment is necessary in patients with renal or hepatic insufficiency, or both, dialysis patients, or geriatric patients. Serum IgG levels increase approximately 250 mg% for each 100 mg/kg of IGIV infused.[116,117]

Immune globulin is indicated in a wide variety of circumstances to provide passive immunity to individuals.[114] The indications for IGIM differ from that for IGIV. Intramuscular IG is indicated for providing passive immunity in hepatitis A infections, as an alternative to HBIG in hepatitis B exposures (however, HBIG is significantly more effective), hepatitis C (but not hepatitis E), measles, VZ, and primary immunodeficiency diseases. Intramuscular IG is not indicated for prevention of rubella, mumps or poliomyelitis. Table 113–8 lists the suggested dosages for IGIM in various disease states.

There are many approved indications and other nonapproved indications for IGIV. Dosages vary based on the preparation used.[116,118]

- *Primary immunodeficiency states:* In primary immunodeficiency states, monthly doses of between 100 and 800 mg/kg are administered, with the average dose being 200 to 400 mg/kg. The immunodeficiency states for which IGIV is indicated include both antibody deficiencies and combined immune deficiencies. In patients with immune deficiency who are candidates for IGIV, those with IgA deficiency should receive Gammagard brand since it has the lowest amount of IgA. Significant reactions can occur in patients with low intrinsic levels of IgA given IGIV with greater amounts of IgA. Intravenous IG is indicated in patients with HIV, however, the data to support its use are better in the pediatric population. With the advent of availability of new antiretroviral agents and combination therapies, the usefulness of IGIV may be even more limited.

TABLE 113–8. Indications and Dosage of Intramuscular Immune Globulin in Infectious Diseases

Primary immunodeficiency states	1.2 mL/kg IM then 0.6 mL/kg IM every 2–4 wk
Hepatitis A exposure	0.02 mL/kg IM within 2 wk
Hepatitis A prophylaxis	0.02 mL/kg IM if exposure < 3 mo 0.06 ml/kg if exposure > 3 mo, every 4–6 mo
Hepatitis B	0.06 mL/kg IM (HBIG is preferred in known exposures) as soon as possible
Non-A/non-B hepatitis	0.06 mL/kg IM as soon as possible (questionable effectiveness)
Measles	0.25 mL/kg IM within 6 days (maximum dose = 15 mL)
Rubella	0.55 mL/kg, single dose
Primary immunodeficiency states	1.2 mL/kg IM then 0.6 mL/kg IM every 2–4 wk

HBIG = hepatitis B immune globulin.

- *Idiopathic thrombocytopenic purpura:* For the treatment of idiopathic (or immune) thrombocytopenic purpura (ITP), doses of 400 mg/kg daily for 2 to 5 days are indicated. Some manufacturers recommend 1 g/kg for 1 to 2 days. Adults tend to respond less well than children to IGIV. Intravenous IG is acceptable for treatment of both chronic and acute ITP, and IGIV has been used in ITP associated with pregnancy without adverse effects on the fetus.[116] It should be noted that corticosteroids are the drugs of choice for adult ITP. In thrombotic thrombocytopenia purpura, IGIV is reported to be effective in patients who do not respond to plasmaphresis. Other platelet disorders in which IGIV may be useful include neonatal immune, thrombocytopenia, perinatal autoimmune thrombocytopenia, drug-induced thrombocytopenia, thrombocytopenia secondary to infection, and transfusion refractory thrombocytopenia; however, the data to support these indications are minimal.
- *Chronic lymphocytic leukemia (CLL):* IGIV is used as a prophylaxis measure in CLL patients who have had a serious bacterial infection. Doses of 400 mg/kg every 3 to 4 weeks are used.
- *Kawasaki disease (mucocutaneous lymph node syndrome):* This disease, which generally occurs in children, carries the hallmark of development of coronary artery abnormalities. Generally, it is recommended by the American Academy of Pediatrics that if the strict criteria for Kawasaki disease is met, an IGIV dose of 400 mg/kg/d for 4 consecutive days be used or preferable 2 g/kg as a single dose. The dose should be administered within 10 days of disease onset. Aspirin should also be administered.[115]
- *Bone marrow transplant:* IGIV is approved for reducing graft-versus-host disease and infections in patients over the age of 20. Patients receive 500 mg/kg 7 and 2 days before transplantation and weekly up to 3 months after. At 100 days post-transplant, patients receive a monthly dose of IGIV for 1 year. Infection (CMV, fungal, bacterial, and interstitial pneumonia) decreased from 51% to 34%.[119] Intravenous IG is not indicated in patients < 20 years of age.
- *Varicella zoster:* Another approved indication for IGIV is in the prophylaxis of varicella zoster if VZIG is not available.

A number of other proposed uses of IGIV can be identified. It is important to note that generally these are not approved indications and are not generally accepted in the medical community for routine treatment. These uses include:

- *Neonatal sepsis:* Neonatal sepsis can cause significant morbidity within 24 hours of birth. While group B streptococcus and *Escherichia coli* remain the primary infecting organisms, other bacteria and fungi may be associated with sepsis. Intravenous IG appears to be effective in neonates < 34 weeks' gestational age or < 1500 g. Doses of 500 to 900 mg/kg have been used.[116,118] Routine use is not recommended; however, IGIV may be useful in neonates with recurrent infections.
- *Autoimmune diseases:* IGIV may be effective in self-limited immunoregulatory diseases but less effective in chronic diseases, such as systemic lupus erythematosus. Definite conclusions about the use of IGIV cannot be made in this category.
- *Cystic fibrosis:* Only one study exists that has examined the use of IGIV in this disease. No firm recommendations can be made on its use.[116]
- *Intractable epilepsy:* In patients who have confirmed IgG deficiency, IGIV may be useful. Otherwise, it is not indicated.[115]
- *Thermal injury:* Not indicated.
- *Cytomegalovirus infection:* The use of CMV-IVIG is recommended versus the use of IGIV.

Other diseases for which IGIV has been used in an uncontrolled setting include Guillain-Barré syndrome, myasthenia gravis, epilepsy, amyotrophic lateral sclerosis, rheumatoid arthritis, and factor VIII inhibition because of autoantibody. In addition, data suggest the efficacy of IGIV in severe IgA nephropathy and Henoch-Schonlein purpura.[120]

Adverse effects of IG vary with the route of administration. Following IGIM, pain, tenderness, and muscle stiffness persisting for hours or days are seen. Repeat courses may cause sensitization with resultant allergic reactions. With IGIV, adverse effects are seen in less than 1% of immunocompetent patients and in less than 10% of others. Most adverse effects are related to the rate of the infusion. Infusion should be given at a rate of 0.01 to 0.02 mL/kg/min for 30 minutes and then, if no reactions occur, increased to 0.02 to 0.04 mL/kg/min. While infusion rate recommendations vary slightly depending on the preparation, the guidelines presented can be followed for the various IV preparations.

RH_O(D) IMMUNE GLOBULIN

Rh_o(D) immune globulin (RDIG) is a sterile solution of immunoglobulins prepared from human sera with high titers of Rh_o(D) antibody. Plasma or serum used to prepare RDIG is negative for hepatitis B surface antigen.

Rh_o(D) immune globulin suppresses the antibody response and formation of anti-Rh_o(D) in Rh_o(D)-negative, D^u-negative women exposed to Rh_o(D)-positive blood. Administration of RDIG prevents the future chance of erythroblastosis fetalis in subsequent pregnancies with a Rh_o(D)-positive fetus. When administered within 72 hours of delivery of a full-term infant, RDIG reduces active antibody formation from 12% to 1% to 2%. Reduced antibody formation is less when it is given after 72 hours postpartum. Additionally, smaller doses of RDIG are used after abortion, miscarriage, amniocentesis, or abdominal trauma. In addition, RDIG is also used in the case of a premenopausal woman who is Rh_o(D)-negative or D^u-negative and has inadvertently received Rh_o(D)-positive or D^u-positive blood or blood products.

The dosage of RDIG varies with the indication. A standard dose of 300 μg is given within 72 hours of a term delivery. Occasionally, where the fetus is known to be Rh_o(D)-positive, a 300-μg dose is given at 28 weeks' gestation and within 72 hours after delivery. For postpregnancy termination occurring up to 13 weeks' gestation, one microdose (50 μg) vial is given within 72 hours. For pregnancy termination after 13 weeks, one standard dose (300 μg) is given within 72 hours. In other circumstances, such as in abdominal trauma, amniocentesis, or transfusion accidents, the dosage (number of standard dose vials) is based on the estimated packed red blood cell volume of the fetal/maternal hemorrhage divided by 15. Rh_o(D) immune globulin is administered intramuscularly only.

When considering RDIG for use, one must be certain of the mother's Rh_o(D) and D^u antigen status; RDIG should not be given to individuals positive for either of these antigens or to those with anti-Rh_o(D) antibodies. Occasionally, a large fetal bleed of Rh_o(D)- or D^u-positive blood may make cross-matching of the mother difficult. In these cases, RDIG should only be given if previous tests have shown the mother to be Rh_o(D)-negative and D^u-negative with no anti-Rh_o(D) antibody.

Adverse reactions to RDIG include injection site tenderness and fever.

VACCINES FOR TRAVEL

Persons who are planning travel to underdeveloped parts of the world where unsanitary conditions or unusual disease exposures exist need to be evaluated for additional vaccines or immunobiologics. The yearly publication *Health Information for International Travel*[121] published by the CDC, provides country-specific information on required and recommended immunization for travel. The following sections review five vaccines commonly used for foreign travel to prevent cholera, typhoid, Japanese encephalitis, tick-borne encephalitis, and yellow fever. Based on the nature of the travel, other vaccines previously discussed may need to be considered. These include polio, tetanus, rabies, hepatitis A and B, measles, and meningococcal vaccines.

CHOLERA VACCINE

The available vaccine for cholera consists of a suspension of killed whole cell *Vibrio cholerae* bacteria from two bacterial strains: Ogawa and Inaba.

Cholera vaccine is approximately 25% to 50% effective in reducing the incidence of disease but does not prevent transmission of infection. The vaccine provides greater efficacy in persons who have previously had the disease. The duration of antibody following vaccination is 3 to 6 months, as compared to 3 years following natural infection. Frequent booster doses (every 6 months) are, therefore, needed to sustain protection. The vaccine may be used in immunocompromised individuals.[122,123]

The primary use of cholera vaccine is in travelers who will be visiting highly endemic areas under less than adequate hygienic conditions. The risk of cholera to tourists is exceedingly low and, therefore, does not warrant routine vaccination.[121,122]

The primary immunization series in adults consists of two 0.5-mL IM or subcutaneous doses administered 1 week to 1 month apart. Doses in children under 10 years are modified accordingly: 0.2 mL for ages 6 months to 4 years and 0.3 mL for ages 5 to 10 years. The intradermal route may be used in individuals ≥ 5 years of age with a 0.2 mL dose. Similar sized booster doses are recommended every 6 months.[121,122]

Side effects are common and consist of local reactions (pain, erythema, induration, tenderness), fever, malaise, and headache. The systemic reactions, such as fever, malaise, and headache, occur in < 1% of individuals and may last 1 to 2 days. Serious reactions, including neurologic complications, are rare. No data are available on its use in pregnancy, but it is not felt to be contraindicated. The only contraindication is a history of previous severe systemic reaction to the vaccine. A 3-week interval between administrations of cholera and yellow fever vaccine is recommended because of reported decreased antibody response with their simultaneous administration. There is no evidence, however, that protection is affected by simultaneous administration, and when necessary, it may be done.[122,123]

JAPANESE ENCEPHALITIS VIRUS VACCINE

Japanese encephalitis (JE) is an arboviral infection spread by mosquitoes. It affects 50,000 people annually in Asia and Oceania, causing viral encephalitis. Transmission is seasonal, with the highest times of transmission occurring in the summer and early fall. While the risk for the most travelers is quite low, the risk for individuals depends on the season, location, and duration of travel. It is estimated that the risk of acquiring JE is less than one person per one million travelers; however, this may be a low estimate.[123]

Monovalent inactivated JE virus vaccine has been commercially available in the United States since 1992. Three doses are needed to provide protective levels of neutralizing antibodies. The vaccine is more immunogenic when administered in a 0-, 7-, 30-day schedule rather that in a 0-, 7-, 14-day regimen (GMTs higher at 6 months for the 30-day schedule). Duration of antibody protection is unknown. Protective titers have been reported for up to 3 years after primary immunization. Additionally, single booster doses given 1 year after primary immunization have resulted in substantial rises in antibody titers.

Adverse reactions include pain and tenderness at the injection site (20%) and systemic side effects, such as fever, headache, malaise, rash, chills, dizziness, myalgia, nausea, vomiting, and abdominal pain in 10%.[123] In addition, there are sporadic reports of hypersensitivity reactions to the vaccine. The manifestations of this type of reaction includes urticaria, angioedema, and respiratory distress. These reactions generally have occurred after a median of 12 hours after the first dose of vaccine with 88% of reactions within 3 days. After a second dose, these hypersensitivity reactions may occur 3 to 14 days after injection.

The JE virus vaccine is recommended for U.S. expatriates residing in areas where JE is endemic or epidemic. The vaccine is not routinely recommended for travelers to Asia.

The JE vaccine is administered to individuals ≥ 3 years of age as 1 mL doses given subcutaneously on days 0, 7, and 30. The 0-, 7- and 14-day schedule can be used if time is a constraint. In addition, a 0, 7 schedule can be used if absolutely necessary, and it will provide protection for 80% of persons. The last dose should be administered at least 10 days before traveling to observe for adverse reactions. For children ages 1 to 2 years, 0.5 mL of vaccine are administered subcutaneously using the schedules already listed. No data are available in children < 1 year of age. Booster doses are recommended every 36 months with 1 mL booster doses being given to children who are ≥ 3 years of age, even if they received 0.5 mL as initial dose. Pregnant women who travel to an epidemic or endemic area should be vaccinated. No data are available for immunocompromised patients. The JE vaccine can be administered simultaneously with the DPT vaccine. No data are available for concurrent administration with other vaccines or antimalarial agents.

TICK-BORNE ENCEPHALITIS

Tick-borne encephalitis (TBE) is a viral infection of the central nervous system (CNS) caused by certain vector ticks. While there are no vaccines or specific immune globulins available in the United States, they are available in Europe. A killed virus vaccine is available that provides protection within 24 hours and lasts for 4 weeks. For long-term protection, a three-dose series given over many months is indicated.[122]

TYPHOID VACCINE

Typhoid vaccine consists of a saline suspension of killed *Salmonella typhi* bacteria. It is recommended for travelers to underdeveloped areas where there is poor sanitation and typhoid is often endemic. It is also recommended for use in household contacts of *S. typhi* carriers. The vaccine is 50% to 90% effective, depending, in part, on levels of existing natural immunity and size of inocula exposures.[121,122] Hence, careful selection of food and water is still a very important part of disease prevention.

Three vaccines are available in the United States. Primary vaccination with oral Ty21a vaccine consists of a single capsule (swallowed whole) taken every other day for a total of four doses. The dose should be taken with cool liquid (not alcohol or milk) 1 hour before a meal. The capsules should be kept refrigerated, if frozen, they should be allowed to thaw in the refrigerator. Capsules can be kept at 80° F for up to 48 hours, but this is not recommended. This vaccine is not recommended in children < 6 years of age. Booster doses are given as a complete series every 5 years. This vaccine is a live attenuated vaccine and should not be administered within 24 hours of a dose of mefloquine (but not chloroquine). The vaccine should not be administered to patients with immunodeficiencies. It can be administered with immunoglobulin. Side effects to the vaccine include nausea, vomiting, fever, headache, and rash. Urticaria is rare.

Primary vaccination with the heat-phenol inactivated parenteral vaccine is as follows. The recommended primary immunization schedule for adults is two 0.5-mL subcutaneous doses given 4 or more weeks apart or, where time does not permit, three 0.5-mL doses given weekly. For children 6 months to 10 years of age, 0.25 mL given subcutaneously in the same schedule as for adults is recommended. A single booster dose (0.5 mL subcutaneously [ages ≥ 10 years] or 0.1 mL intradermally [ages ≥ 6 months]) is recommended every 3 years for persons traveling to or remaining in endemic areas. If a period longer than 3 years has passed since immunization, a single booster dose is still recommended. An unproven alternative for booster doses is the use of an oral vaccine (four dose) booster series. The intradermal dose is not recommended for primary immunization. This is the least preferred vaccine because of the adverse effect profile. Side effects are common and include local reactions (pain, induration, and erythema at the injection site), malaise, headache, and fever starting within 24 hours of receiving the vaccine and lasting 1 to 2 days, usually responsive to mild analgesia.

Primary immunization using the Vi capsular polysaccharide vaccine is accomplished by giving 0.5 mL once IM (in the deltoid or vastus lateralis) in patients ≥ 2 years of age. Booster doses are recommended every 2 years. The most common side effect is injection site pain, erythema, and induration within 48 hours of injection. The incidence of adverse effects is less than with other parenteral typhoid vaccines.

Both parenteral vaccines can be administered to immunocompromised persons since they are inactivated. None of the vaccines should be given to febrile individuals. Pregnancy is not an absolute contraindication to use of any of the vaccines, but the benefits versus the risks must be weighed.

YELLOW FEVER VACCINE

Live, attenuated, yellow fever virus vaccine is recommended for persons who will be traveling or living in areas where yellow fever infection occurs (parts of Africa and South America) and is required for entry into certain countries.[121,122] Vaccination should also be considered for laboratory workers who may be exposed to the virus. The reconstituted vaccine is thermolabile, and unused portions must be discarded 1 hour after reconstitution.

The recommended dose is 0.5 mL subcutaneously given once with similar booster doses recommended every 10 years. The vaccine, however, has been shown to be highly immunogenic with antibodies persisting for at least 40 years and perhaps for life. Mild side effects consisting of headache, myalgias, and low-grade fever 1 to 2 weeks after vaccination occur in less than 10% of vaccinees; treatment should be symptomatic. Immediate hypersensitivity reactions are rare (one per million doses) and occur primarily in persons who have anaphylactic reactions to eggs. Neurologic accidents are rare (20 cases to date) and have occurred primarily in infants less than 6 months of age in whom the vaccine is not recommended. The French Neurotropic Vaccine (Dakar strain) was associated with meningoencephalitis in children and is no longer manufactured. This has not occurred with the 17D strain.

On theoretical grounds, the vaccine should be avoided during pregnancy unless travel to a high-risk area is imperative. It may be given to breast feeding mothers. The vaccine may be used in immunocompromised patients if the risk of infection in an endemic area outweighs the potential vaccine risk. Additionally, it should not be given to infants less than 4 months of age and in general, should be used only if a child is 9 months of age or older. Children 4 to 9 months must be considered on an individual basis. It is contraindicated in persons with a history of an anaphylactic reaction to eggs. Where the history is in question, intradermal testing consisting of 0.02-mL doses of vaccine and normal saline control applied to the volar surface of the forearm should be done. The demonstration of an erythematous, urticarial wheal and negative control constitutes a positive response and contraindicates vaccination. This intradermal testing may be sufficient to produce antibodies, however, serologic testing should be done to confirm this.

Yellow fever vaccine may be simultaneously administered with all other vaccines except cholera, with which a 3-week interval between vaccines is recommended. Simultaneous administration of immune globulin does not interfere with the immune response to this agent.

REFERENCES

1. Willems JS, Sanders CR. Cost-effectiveness and cost-benefits analysis of vaccines. J Infect Dis 1981;144:486–493.
2. Koplan JP, Axnick MW. Benefits, risks and costs of viral vaccines. Prog Med Virol 1982;28:180–191.
3. Advisory Committee on Immunization Practices. General recommendations on immunization. MMWR 1994;43(RR-1):1–38.
4. Edsall G. Immunoprophylaxis of bacterial diseases. In: Gell PGH, Coombs RRA, Lachmann PJ, eds. Clinical Aspects of Immunology. Oxford, Blackwell Scientific, 1975:1601.
5. Jilg W, Schmidt M, Deinhardt F. Prolonged immunity after late booster doses of hepatitis B vaccine. J Infect Dis 1988;157:1267–1269.
6. Miotti P, Nelson KE, Dallabetta GA, et al. The influence of HIV infection on antibody response to a two-dose regimen of influenza vaccine. JAMA 1989;262:779–783.
7. Immunization Practices Advisory Committee. General recommendations on immunization. MMWR 1989;38:205–228.
8. Centers for Disease Control. Suboptimal response to hepatitis B vaccine given by injection into the buttock. MMWR 1985;34:105–113.
9. Immunization Practices Advisory Committee. Guide for Adult Immunization 1990, 2nd ed. Philadelphia, American College of Physicians, 1990:19–35.
10. Centers for Disease Control. Adult immunization: Recommendations of the Immunization Practices Advisory Committee. MMWR 1991; 40:1–94.
11. Advisory Committee on Immunization Practices. Use of vaccines and immune globulins in persons with altered immunocompetence. MMWR 1993;42(RR-4):1–19.
12. Centers for Disease Control. Physician vaccination referral practices and vaccines for children—New York, 1994. MMWR 1995; 44:3–6.
13. Fedson DS. Adult immunization: Summary of the National Vaccine Advisory Committee Report. JAMA 1994;272:1133–1137.
14. Centers for Disease Control. State and national vaccination coverage levels among children aged 19–35 months—United States, April–December 1994. MMWR 1995;44:613–623.
15. Centers for Disease Control. Immunization of adolescents: Recommendations of the Advisory Committee on Immunization Practices, the American Academy of Pediatrics, the American Academy of Family Physicians, and the American Medical Association. MMWR 1996;45(RR-13):1–19.
16. Williams WW, Hickson MA, Kane MA, et al. Immunization policies and vaccine coverage among adults: The risk for missed opportunities. Ann Intern Med 1988;108:616–625.
17. Szilagyi PG, Rodewald LE, Humiston SG, et al. Missed opportunities for childhood vaccinations in office practices and the effect on vaccination status. Pediatrics 1993;91:1–7.
18. Centers for Disease Control. FDA approval for infants of a *Haemophilus influenzae* type B conjugate and hepatitis B (recombinant) combined vaccine. MMWR 1997;46:107–109.
19. Centers for Disease Control. Approval of a *Haemophilus* B conjugate vaccine combined by reconstitution with an acellular pertussis vaccine. MMWR 1996;45:993–995.
20. Bartell LH, Charney SA. National Vaccine Injury Compensation Act: A viable alternative to litigation? J Pharm Pract 1989;2:36–44.
21. Middaugh JP. Side effects of diphtheria-tetanus toxoid in adults. Am J Public Health 1979;69:246–249.
22. Centers for Disease Control. Vaccine Adverse Event Reporting System—United States. MMWR 1990;39:730–733.
23. Peter G. Diphtheria. In: 1997 Red Book: Report of the Committee on Infectious Diseases, 4th ed. Elk Grove Village, Il, American Academy of Pediatrics, 1997:191–195.
24. Centers for Disease Control. Recommendation of the Immunization Practices Advisory Committee: Diphtheria, tetanus and pertussis: Guidelines for vaccine prophylaxis and other preventive measures. MMWR 1981;30:392–396, 401–407.
25. Peter G. Tetanus. In: 1997 Red Book: Report of the Committee on Infectious Diseases, 24th ed. Elk Grove Village, Il, American Academy of Pediatrics, 1997:518–523.
26. A Joint Statement by the Advisory Council for the Elimination of Tuberculosis and the Advisory Committee on Immunization Practices. The role of BCG vaccine in the prevention and control of tuberculosis in the United States. MMWR 1996;45(No. RR-4):1–27.
27. Advisory Committee on Immunization Practices. Prevention of hepatitis A through active or passive immunization. MMWR 1996; 45(RR-15):1–38.
28. Advisory Committee on Immunization Practices. Hepatitis B virus: A comprehensive strategy for eliminating transmission in the United States through universal childhood vaccination. MMWR 1991;40 (RR-13):1–25.
29. Committee on Infectious Diseases. Universal hepatitis B immunization. Pediatrics 1992;89:795–800.
30. Centers for Disease Control, Recommendations for protection against viral hepatitis. MMWR 1985;34:313.
31. Roome AJ, Walsh SJ, Cartter ML, Hadler JL. Hepatitis B vaccine responsiveness in Connecticut public safety personnel. JAMA 1993; 270:2931–2934.
32. Alimonos KA, Murray J, Nafziger AN, Bertino JS Jr. Prediction of Response to Hepatitis B Vaccine in Health Care Workers: Whose Titers of Antibodies to Hepatitis B Surface Antigen Should Be

Determined After a 3 Dose Series and What Are the Implications of Cost-effectiveness. Clin Infect Dis 1998;26:566–571.
33. Wood RC, MacDonald KL, White KE, et al. Risk factors for lack of detectable antibody following hepatitis B vaccination of Minnesota health care workers. JAMA 1993;270:2935–2939.
34. Margolis HS, Presson AC. Host factors related to poor immunogenicity of hepatitis B vaccine in adults. JAMA 1993;270:2971–2972.
35. Treadwell TL, Keeffe EB, Lake J, et al. Immunogenicity of two recombinant hepatitis B vaccines in older individuals. Am J Med 1993; 95:584–588.
36. Tada H, Mosohiko Y, Mishira J, et al. Combined passive and active immunization for preventing perinatal transmission of hepatitis B virus carrier state. Pediatrics 1982;70:613–619.
37. Seef L, Koff D. Passive and active immunoprophylaxis of hepatitis B. Gastroenterol 1984;86:958–981.
38. Anon. Smithkline Beecham's Engerix-B new dosing schedule gets go-ahead from FDA committee: AAP/ACIP flexible dose recommendations okayed for all HBV vaccines. Pink Sheet 1994;56:(5)12.
39. Gelin BG, Greenberg RN, Hart RH, et al. Immunogenicity of two doses of yeast recombinant hepatitis B vaccine in healthy older adults. J Infect Dis 1997;175:1494–1497.
40. Hadler SC, Francis DP, Maynard JE, et al. Long-term immunogenicity and efficacy of hepatitis B vaccine in homosexual men. N Engl J Med 1986;315:209–214.
41. Bertino JS Jr, Tirrell P, Greenberg R, et al. A comparative trial of standard or high dose recombinant hepatitis B vaccine versus a vaccine containing S subunit, PreS1 and Pre S2 particles for revaccination of healthy adult nonresponders. J Infect Dis 1997;337:256–260.
42. Centers for Disease Control. Recommendations of the Immunization Practices Advisory Committee: Hepatitis B virus: A comprehensive strategy for eliminating transmission in the United States through universal childhood vaccination. MMWR 1992;40:1–25.
43. Troisi C, Heiberg D, Hollinger F. Normal immune response to hepatitis B vaccine in patients with Down's syndrome: A basis for immunization guidelines. JAMA 1985;254:3196–3199.
44. Wainwright RB, McMahon BJ, Bulkow LR, et al. Duration of immunogenicity and efficacy of hepatitis B vaccine in a Yupik Eskimo population. JAMA 1989;261:2362–2366.
45. Lo KJ, Lee SD, Tsai YT, et al. Long-term immunogenicity and efficacy of hepatitis B vaccine in infants born to HBeAG-positive HBsAG-carrier mothers. Hepatology 1988;8:1647–1650.
46. Lanphear BP. Hepatitis B immunoprophylaxis: Developing a cost-effective program in the hospital setting. Infect Control Hosp Epidemiol 1990;11:47–50.
47. Dienstag JL, Stevens CO, Bhan AK, et al. Hepatitis B vaccine administered to chronic carrier of hepatitis B surface antigen. Ann Intern Med 1982;96:575–579.
48. Prince AM. Hepatitis B immune globulin: Final report of a controlled multicenter trial of efficacy in prevention of dialysis-associated hepatitis. J Infect Dis 1978;137:131–144.
49. Seef LB. Type B hepatitis after needle-stick exposure: Prevention with hepatitis B immune globulin. Ann Intern Med 1978;88:285–293.
50. Frosner G, Frosner H, Dienhardt F, et al. Failure of hyperimmune serum globulin, given several days after exposure, to protect against hepatitis B. Lancet 1977;2:1023.
51. Masuko K, Mitsui T, Iwano K, et al. Factors influencing postexposure immunoprophylaxis of hepatitis B virus infection with hepatitis B immune globulin. Gastroenterology 1985;88:151–155.
52. Grady GF, Lee VA. Hepatitis B immune globulin—prevention of hepatitis from accidental exposure among medical personnel. N Engl J Med 1975;293:1067–1070.
53. Perillo R, Campbell C, Strang S, et al. Immune globulin and hepatitis B immune globulin: Prophylactic measures for intimate contacts exposed to acute type B hepatitis. Arch Intern Med 1984;144:81–85.
54. Centers for Disease Control. Update on hepatitis B prophylaxis. MMWR 1987;36:353–360
55. Centers for Disease Control. Update: Vaccine side effects, adverse reactions, contraindications, and precautions: Recommendations of the Advisory Committee on Immunization Practices (ACIP). MMWR 1996;45(RR-12):1–25.
56. American Academy of Pediatrics. *Haemophilus influenzae* infections. In: Peter G, ed. 1997 Red Book: Report of the Committee on Infectious Diseases, 24th ed. Elk Grove Village, Il, American Academy of Pediatrics, 1997:220–230.
57. Centers for Disease Control. General recommendations on immunization: Recommendations of the Advisory Committee on Immunization Practices. MMWR 1994;43(RR-1):1–38.
58. Anon. *Haemophilus influenzae* infections. In: Peter G, ed. 1997 Red Book: Report of the Committee on Infectious Diseases, 24th ed. Elk Grove Village, Il, American Academy of Pediatrics, 1997: 220–230.
59. Centers for Disease Control. Recommended childhood immunization schedule—United States, January–December 1997. MMWR 1997; 46:35–40.
60. LaMontagne JR, Noble GR, Quinnan GV, et al. Summary of clinical trials of inactivated influenza vaccine—1978. Rev Infect Dis 1983;5: 723–736.
61. Gross RA, Ennis FA. Influenza vaccine: Split product versus whole virus types—How do they differ? N Engl J Med 1977;296: 567–568.
62. Waldman RH, Mann JJ, Small PA Jr. Immunization against influenza: Prevention of illness in man by aerosolized inactivated vaccine. JAMA 1969;207:520–524.
63. Hobson D, Curry RL, Beare AS. Hemoglutinin-inhibiting antibody titers as a measure of protection against influenza in man. In: Perkins FT, Regamey RH, eds. Symposia Series in Immunological Standardization, No. 20. Basel, S. Karger AG, 1973:164–168.
64. Quinnan GV, Schooley R, Dolin R, et al. Serologic responses and systemic reactions in adults after vaccination with monovalent A/USSR/77 and trivalent A/USSR/77, A/Texas/77, B/Hong Kong/72 influenza vaccines. Rev Infect Dis 1983;5:748–757.
65. Riddiough MA, Sisk JE, Bell JC. Influenza vaccination cost-effectiveness and public policy. JAMA 1983;249:3189–3195.
66. Peter G. Measles. In: 1997 Red Book: Report of the Committee on Infectious Diseases, 23rd ed. El Grove Village, Il, American Academy of Pediatrics, 1994:44–357.
67. Advisory Committee on Immunization Practice. Prevention and control of influenza. MMWR 1996;46(RR-9):1–32.
68. Hayney MS, Poland GA, Jacobson RM, et al. The influence of the HLA-DBR1*13allele on measles vaccine response. J Investig Med 1996;44:261–263.
69. Cote TR, Sivertson D, Horan JM, et al. Evaluation of a two-dose measles, mumps, and rubella vaccination schedule in a cohort of college athletes. Pub Health Rep 1993;108:431–435.
70. Centers for Disease Control. Measles pneumonitis following measles-mumps-rubella vaccination of a patient with HIV infection, 1993. MMWR 1996;45:603–606.
71. Centers for Disease Control. Recommendations of the Advisory Committee on Immunization Practices (ACIP). Update: Vaccine side effects, adverse reactions, contraindications, and precautions. MMWR 1996;45(RR-12):1–35.
72. Centers for Disease Control. Control and prevention of meningococcal disease and control and prevention of serogroup C meningococcal disease: Evaluation and management of suspected outbreaks: recommendations of the Advisory Committee on Immunization Practices (ACIP). MMWR 1997;46(RR-5):1–21.
74. Centers for Disease Control. Mumps prevention. MMWR 1989;38: 388–400.
75. Peter G. Mumps. In: 1997 Red Book: Report of the Committee on Infectious Diseases, 24th ed. Elk Grove Village, Il, American Academy of Pediatrics, 1997:366–369.
76. Centers for Disease Control. Diphtheria, tetanus, and pertussis: Recommendations for vaccine use and other preventive measures: Recommendations of the Immunization Practices Advisory Committee (ACIP). MMWR 1991;40(RR-10):1–28.

77. Cody CL, Baraff LJ, Cherry JD, et al. The nature and rate of adverse reactions associated with DTP and DT immunization in infants and children. Pediatrics 1981;68:650–660.
78. Institute of Medicine. DPT vaccine and chronic nervous system dysfunction: A new analysis. Washington, DC, National Academy Press, 1994.
79. Johnstone T. Whooping cough in the United States and Britain. N Engl J Med 1983;309:108–109. Letter.
80. Fulginitti VA. Pertussis vaccine. Am J Dis Child 1984;183:890–891.
81. Centers for Disease Control. Pertussis—United States, 1982–1983. MMWR 1984;33:573–575.
82. Peter G. Pertussis. In: 1997 Red Book: Report of the Committee on Infectious Diseases, 24th ed. Elk Grove Village, Il, American Academy of Pediatrics, 1997:394–407.
83. Centers for Disease Control. Pertussis vaccination: Use of acellular pertussis vaccines among infants and young children: Recommendations of the Advisory Committee on Immunization Practices (ACIP). MMWR 1997;46(RR-7):1–25.
84. Centers for Disease Control. Poliomyelitis prevention in the United States: Introduction of a sequential vaccination schedule of inactivated poliovirus vaccine followed by oral poliovirus vaccine: Recommendations of the Advisory Committee on Immunization Practices (ACIP). MMWR 1997;46(RR-3):1–25.
85. Peter G. Poliovirus infections. In: 1997 Red Book: Report of the Committee on Infectious Diseases, 24th ed. Elk Grove Village, Il, American Academy of Pediatrics, 1997:424–433.
86. Centers for Disease Control. Poliomyelitis prevention: Enhanced potency inactivated poliomyelitis vaccine—Supplementary statement. MMWR 1987;36:795–798.
87. Centers for Disease Control. Poliomyelitis prevention in the United States: Introduction of a sequential vaccination schedule of inactivated poliovirus vaccine followed by oral poliovirus vaccine: Recommendations of the Advisory Committee on Immunization Practices (ACIP). MMWR 1997;46(RR-3):1–25.
88. Recommendations of the Immunization Practices Advisory Committee. Prevention of pneumococcal disease. MMWR 1997:46(RR-8); 1–31.
89. Smit P, Oberholzer D, Hayden-Smith S, et al. Protective efficacy of pneumococcal polysaccharide vaccines. JAMA 1977;238:2613–2626.
90. Hilleman M, Carlson A, McLean A, et al. *Streptococcus pneumoniae* polysaccharide vaccine: Age and dose responses, safety, persistence of antibody, revaccination, and simultaneous administration of pneumococcal and influenza vaccines. Rev Infect Dis 1981; 3:S31–S42.
91. Advisory Committee on Immunization Practices. Rabies Prevention—United States, 1984. MMWR 1984;33:393–402, 407–408.
92. Advisory Committee on Immunization Practices. Rabies prevention. MMWR 1991;40(RR-3):1–19.
93. Bernhard KW, Roberts MA, Samner J, et al. Human diploid cell rabies vaccine: Effectiveness of immunization with small intradermal or subcutaneous doses. JAMA 1982;247:1138–1142.
94. Bernard KW, Mallonnee J, Wright JC, et al. Preexposure immunization with intradermal human diploid cell rabies vaccine. JAMA 1987;257:1059–1063.
95. Fishbein DB, Pacer RE, Holmes DF, et al. Rabies preexposure prophylaxis with human diploid cell rabies vaccine: A dose- response study. J Infect Dis 1987;156:50–55.
96. Trimarchi CV, Safford M Jr. Poor response to rabies vaccination by the intradermal route. JAMA 1992;268:874.
97. State of New York, Department of Health Memorandum, Public Health Series H-28, PH-11, Series 92–93. Rabies control update. November 25, 1992.
98. Pappaioanou M, Fishbein D, Dressen D, et al. Antibody response to pre-exposure human diploid cell rabies vaccine given concurrently with chloroquine. N Engl J Med 1986;314:280–284.
99. Nicholson KG, Turner GS, Aoki EY. Immunization with a human diploid cell strain of rabies virus vaccine: Two-year results. J Infect Dis 1978;137:783–788.
100. Bahmanyar M, Fayaz A, Nour-Salehi S, et al. Successful protection of humans exposed to rabies infection: Post-exposure treatment with the new human diploid cell rabies vaccine and antirabies serum. JAMA 1976;236:2751–2754.
101. Centers for Disease Control. Systemic allergic reactions following immunization with human diploid cell rabies vaccine. MMWR 1984; 33:185.
102. Wilde H, Sirikawin S, Sabcharoen A, Kingnate D, et al. Failure of postexposure treatment of rabies in children. J Infect Dis 1997;22: 228–232.
103. Centers for Disease Control. Rubella vaccine: Recommendations of the Immunizations Practice Advisory Committee (ACIP). MMWR 1990;39(RR-15):1–18.
104. Peter G. Rubella. In: 1997 Red Book: Report of the Committee on Infectious Diseases, 24th ed. Elk Grove Village, Il, American Academy of Pediatrics, 1997:456–462.
105. Centers for Disease Control. Prevention of varicella: Recommendations of the Advisory Committee on Immunization Practices (ACIP). MMWR 1996;45(RR-11):1–36.
106. Watson BM, Piercy SA, Plotkin SA, Starr SE. Modified chickenpox in children immunized with the Oka/Merck varicella vaccine. Pediatrics 1993;91:17–22.
107. Krause PR, Klinman DM. Efficacy, immunogenicity, safety, and use of live attenuated chickenpox vaccine. J Pediatr 1995;127: 518–525.
108. Watson B, Gupta R, Randall T, Starr S. Persistence of cell-mediated and humoral immune responses in healthy children immunized with live attenuated varicella vaccine. J Infect Dis 1994;169:197–199.
109. Johnson C, Rome LP, Stancin T, et al. Humoral immunity and clinical reinfections following varicella vaccine in healthy children. Pediatrics 1989;84:418–421.
110. Peter G. Varicella-zoster infections. In: 1997 Red Book: Report of the Committee on Infectious Diseases, 23rd ed. Elk Grove Village, Il, American Academy of Pediatrics, 1994:573–585.
111. Snydman DR, Werner BG, Heinze-Lacey B. Use of cytomegalovirus immune globulin to prevent cytomegalovirus disease in renal transplant recipients. N Engl J Med 1987;312:1049–1054.
112. Young FE, Nightingale SL. FDA's newly designated treatment INDs. JAMA 1988;260:224–225.
113. Cohn E, Strong L, Hues W. Preparation and properties of serum plasma proteins. IV: A system for the separation into fractions of the protein and lipoprotein components of biological tissues and fluids. J Am Chem Soc 1946;68:459–675.
114. Berkman SA, Lee ML, Gale RP. Clinical uses of intravenous immunoglobulins. Ann Intern Med 1990;112:278–292.
115. Anon. ASHP Commission on Therapeutics. ASHP therapeutic guidelines for intravenous immune globulin. Clin Pharm 1992;11: 117–136.
116. Morell A, Schurch B, Ryser D, et al. *In vivo* behaviour of g-globulin preparations. Vox Sang 1980;38:272–283.
117. Ochs HD, Fischer SH, Wedgwood RJ, et al. Comparison of high-dose and low-dose intravenous immunoglobulin therapy in patients with primary immunodeficiency diseases. Am J Med 1984;76:78–82.
118. Miles' Gamimune N IVIG gains BMT and pediatric HIV infection indication. Pink Sheet 1994;56(No. 1):6.
119. Rostoker G, Desvaux-Belghiti D, Pilatte Y, et al. High-dose immunoglobulin therapy for severe IgA nephropathy and henoch-schonlein purpura. Ann Intern Med 1994;120:476–484.
120. Siber GR, Snydman DR. Use of immune globulins in the prevention and treatment of infections. Curr Clin Top Infect Dis 1992:12:1–40.
121. Centers for Disease Control. Health Information for International Travel, 1996.
122. Thompson RF. Travel and routine immunizations: A practical guide for the medical officer. 1996 edition, Shoreland Medical Marketing Inc., Milwaukee, WI.
123. Advisory Committee on Immunization Practices. Inactivated Japanese encephalitis virus vaccine. MMWR 1993;42(RR-1):1–15.
124. Anon. Active and passive immunization. In: Peter G, ed. 1997 Red Book: Report of the Committee on Infectious Diseases, 24th ed. Elk Grove Village, Il, American Academy of Pediatrics, 1977:1–71.

Appendix 113–1

Immunization Schedules in Children

Recommended Childhood Immunization Schedule
United States, January–December 1997

Vaccines[a] are listed under the routinely recommended ages. Bars indicate range of acceptable ages for vaccination. Shaded bars indicate *catch-up vaccination:* at 11–12 years of age, hepatitis B vaccine should be administered to children not previously vaccinated, and varicella vaccine should be administered to children not previously vaccinated who lack a reliable history of chickenpox.

Age ▶ Vaccine ▼	Birth	1 mo	2 mo	4 mo	6 mo	12 mo	15 mo	18 mo	4–6 yr	11–12 yr	14–16 yr
Hepatitis B[b,c]	Hep B-1										
			Hep B-2		Hep B-3					Hep B[c]	
Diphtheria, Tetanus, Pertussis[d]			DTaP or DPT	DTaP or DPT	DTaP or DPT		DTaP or DPT[d]		DTaP or DPT	Td	
Haemophilus influenzae type B[a]			HIB	HIB	HIB[e]		HIB[e]				
Polio[f]			Polio[f]	Polio			Polio[f]		Polio		
Measles-Mumps-Rubella[g]							MMR		MMR[g] or	MMR[g]	
Varicella[h]							Var			Var[h]	

[a]This schedule indicates the recommended age for routine administration of currently licensed childhood vaccines. Some combination vaccines are available and may be used whenever administration of all components of the vaccine is indicated. Providers should consult the manufacturers' package inserts for detailed recommendations.

[b]*Infants born to HBsAg-negative mothers* should receive 2.5 µg of Merck vaccine (Recombivax HB) or 10 µg of SmithKline Beecham (SB) vaccine (Engerix-B). The second dose should be administered ≥ 1 mo after the first dose.

Infants born to HBsAg-positive mothers should receive 0.5-mL hepatitis B immune globulin (HBIG) within 12 hr of birth, and either 5 µg of Merck vaccine (Recombivax HB) or 10 µg of SB vaccine (Engerix-B) at a separate site. The second dose is recommended at 1–2 mo of age and the third dose at 6 mo of age.

Infants born to mothers whose HBsAg status is unknown should receive either 5 µg of Merck vaccine (Recombivax HB) or 10 µg of SB vaccine (Engerix-B) within 12 hr of birth. The second dose of vaccine is recommended at 1 mo of age and the third dose at 6 mo of age. Blood should be drawn at the time of delivery to determine the mother's HBsAg status; if it is positive, the infant should receive HBIG as soon as possible (no later than 1 wk of age). The dosage and timing of subsequent vaccine doses should be based on the mother's HBsAg status.

[c]Children and adolescents who have not been vaccinated against hepatitis B in infancy may begin the series during any childhood visit. Those who have not previously received three doses of hepatitis B vaccine should initiate or complete the series during the 11–12 year old visit. The second dose should be administered at least 1 mo after the first dose, and the third dose should be administered at least 4 mo after the first dose and at least 2 mo after the second dose.

[d]DTaP (diphtheria and tetanus toxoids and acellular pertussis vaccine) is the preferred vaccine for all doses in the vaccination series, including completion of the series in children who have received ≥ 1 dose of whole-cell DPT vaccine. Whole-cell DPT is an acceptable alternative to DTaP. The fourth dose (DtaP or DPT) may be administered as early as 12 mo of age, provided 6 mo have elapsed since the third dose, and if the child is considered unlikely to return at 15–18 mo of age. Td (tetanus and diphtheria toxoids, absorbed, for adult use) is recommended at 11–12 years of age if at least 5 years have elapsed since the last dose of DPT, DTaP, or DT. Subsequent routine Td boosters are recommended every 10 years.

[e]Three *H. influenzae* type B (HIB) conjugate vaccines are licensed for infant use. If PRP-OMP (PedvaxHIB [Merck]) is administered at 2 and 4 mo of age, a dose at 6 mo is not required. After completing the primary series, any HIB conjugate vaccine may be used as a booster.

[f]Two poliovirus vaccines are currently licensed in the US: inactivated poliovirus vaccine (IPV) and oral poliovirus vaccine (OPV). The following schedules are all acceptable by the ACIP, the AAP, and the AAFP, and parents and providers may choose among them:

1. IPV at 2 and 4 mo; OPV at 12–18 mo and 4–6 yr
2. IPV at 2, 4, 12–18 mo, and 4–6 yr
3. OPV at 2, 4, 6–18 mo, and 4–6 yr

The ACIP routinely recommend schedule 1. IPV is the only poliovirus vaccine recommended for immunocompromised persons and their household contacts.

[g]The second dose of MMR is routinely recommended at 4–6 yr of age or at 11–12 yr of age but may be administered during any visit, provided at least 1 mo has elapsed since receipt of the first dose and that both doses are administered at or after 12 mo of age.

[h]Susceptible children may receive varicella vaccine (Var) at any visit after the first birthday, and those who lack a reliable history of chickenpox should be immunized during the 11–12 year old visit. Children ≥ 13 years of age should receive two doses, at least 1 mo apart.

Approved by the Advisory Committee on Immunization Practices (ACIP), the American Academy of Pediatrics (AAP), and the American Academy of Family Physicians (AAFP).

APPENDIX 113–2

Immunization Schedules in Adults

Age Group (yr)	Vaccine/Toxoid[a]					
	Td[b]	*Measles*	*Mumps*	*Rubella*	*Influenza*	*Pneumococcal Polysaccharide*
18–24	X	X	X	X		
25–64	X	X[c]	X[c]	X		
≥ 65	X				X	X

[a]Refer also to sections in text on specific vaccines or toxoids for indications, contraindications, precautions, dosages, side effects, adverse reactions, and special considerations.
[b]Td, tetanus and diphtheria toxoids, adsorbed (for adult use), which is a combined preparation containing < 2 flocculation units of diphtherai toxoid.
[c]Indicated for persons born after 1956.
From Ref. 10, with permission.

APPENDIX 113–3

Minimum Age for Pediatric Vaccination

Vaccine	Minimum Age for First Dose[a]	Minimum Interval from Dose 1 to 2[a]	Minimum Interval from Dose 2 to 3[a]	Minimum Interval from Dose 3 to 4[a]
DPT (DT)[a]	6 wk[c]	4 wk	4 wk	6 mo
Combined DPT-HIB	6 wk	1 mo	1 mo	6 mo
DTaP[b]	15 mo			6 mo
HIB (primary series)				
HbOC	6 wk	1 mo	1 mo	[d]
PRP-T	6 wk	1 mo	1 mo	[d]
PRP-OMP	6 wk	1 mo	[d]	
OPV	6 wk[c]	6 wk	6 wk[f]	
IPV[e]	6 wk	4 wk	6 mo[f]	
MMR	12 mo[g]	1 mo		
Hepatitis B	Birth	1 mo	2 mo[h]	

DPT = diphtheria-pertussis-tetanus; DTaP = diphtheria-tetanus-acellular pertussis; HIB = *Haemophilus influenzae* type B conjugate; IPV = inactivated poliovirus vaccine; MMR = measles-mumps-rubella; OPV = live oral polio vaccine.
[a]These minimum acceptable ages and intervals may not correspond with the optimal recommended ages and intervals for vaccination.
[b]DTaP can be used in place of the fourth (and fifth) dose of DPT for children who are at least 15 mo of age. Children who have received all four primary vaccination doses before their fourth birthday should receive a fifth dose of DPT (DT) or DTaP at 4–6 years of age before entering kindergarten or elementary school and at least 6 mo after the fourth dose. The total number of doses of diphtheria and tetanus toxoids should not exceed six each before the seventh birthday.
[c]The American Academy of Pediatrics permits DPT and OPV to be administered as early as 4 weeks of age in areas with high endemicity and during outbreaks.
[d]The booster dose of HIB vaccine that is recommended following the primary vaccination series should be administered no earlier than 12 mo of age and at least 2 mo after the previous dose of HIB vaccine.
[e]See text to differentiate conventional inactivated poliovirus vaccine from enhanced-potency IPV.
[f]For unvaccinated adults at increased risk of exposure to poliovirus with < 3 months but > 2 months available before protection is needed, three doses of IPV should be administered at least 1 mo apart.
[g]Although the age for measles vaccination may be as young as 6 mo in outbreak areas where cases are occurring in children < 1 year of age, children initially vaccinated before the first birthday should be revaccinated at 12–15 months of age, and an additional dose of vaccine should be administered at the time of school entry or according to local policy. Doses of MMR or other measles-containing vaccines should be separated by at least 1 mo.
[h]This final dose is recommended no earlier than 4 months of age.
From Ref. 57, with permission.

114

HUMAN IMMUNODEFICIENCY VIRUS INFECTION

Courtney V. Fletcher, PharmD, Thomas N. Kakuda, PharmD, and Ann C. Collier, MD

The acquired immunodeficiency syndrome (AIDS) was first recognized by the medical community as a distinct clinical entity in 1981. This syndrome was initially described in a cohort of young homosexual males and characterized by profound immunologic deficits, *Pneumocystis carinii* pneumonia (PCP), and Kaposi's sarcoma (KS).[1,2] A retrovirus, human immunodeficiency virus type 1 (HIV-1) (formerly called lymphadenopathy-associated virus [LAV] or human T lymphotropic virus type III [HTLV-III]) is the major cause of AIDS.[3,4] A second retrovirus, HIV-2, has also been recognized to cause AIDS, although it is far less prevalent than HIV-1. These retroviruses are transmitted by sexual contact and by contact with contaminated blood or blood products. Several risk behaviors for acquisition of HIV infection have been identified, most notably the practice of anorectal intercourse and the sharing of blood-contaminated needles by injection-drug users. Transmission of HIV between heterosexuals and from childbearing women to their offspring is an increasing problem worldwide.[5] The development of serologic tests to detect the presence of antibodies to HIV-1 in the blood was a major advance and important for both prevention and treatment strategies. More recently, tests have been developed to quantitate HIV-1 and can provide a means for monitoring the course of disease. Statistics on the prevalence and incidence of this disease worldwide remain grim, and all treatments to date have been unsuccessful in eradicating HIV from infected persons. However, highly active antiretroviral therapy (HAART) has been able to suppress HIV, delay the onset of AIDS, and prolong patient survival. The purpose of this chapter is to provide a discussion of the epidemiology and manifestations of HIV infection, therapeutic strategies directed at inhibiting the virus, and management of HIV-associated opportunistic infections.

EPIDEMIOLOGY

The total number of reported cases of AIDS in the United States (meeting the surveillance definition of the Centers for Disease Control and Prevention [CDC]) at the end of June 1997 was 612,078; 379,258 (more than half) of these individuals have already died. AIDS is the second leading cause of death in the United States among men between the ages of 25 and 44. Each year, approximately 60,000 new cases of HIV infection are reported in the United States and of these, an estimated 1000 cases are perinatally acquired newborn infections.[5] HIV infection, however, is a worldwide epidemic. The World Health Organization (WHO) estimates that 30.6 million people are infected with HIV worldwide with approximately 5.8 million additional infections occurring each year, a rate of 16,500 infections per day. Women account for a growing proportion (41%) of those newly infected. Children account for 1.1 million of the estimated 30.6 million infected.[6] By the year 2000, an estimated 40 million persons worldwide will have been infected with HIV. Three-fourths of these infections will be acquired through heterosexual transmission.[7]

AIDS cases in the United States conform to the CDC surveillance case definition and are reported by health care providers to a public health department. The CDC case definition was first established in 1981 and has undergone modifications in 1985, 1987, and 1993. The latest version expands the definition of AIDS to include not only persons with serious symptomatic disease, but also all HIV-infected people who have < 200 CD4 lymphocytes/μL or a percentage of CD4 lymphocytes < 14% of the total lymphocytes.[8] Table 114–1 presents the classification system for adult HIV infection and a listing of the clinical conditions included in the 1993 definition.

ETIOLOGY

The origin of HIV is still unknown, but it has been suggested that the virus originated among primates in sub-Saharan Africa. This hypothesis proposes that the primate retrovirus evolved into a strain capable of infecting humans and was transmitted through cultural practices. The earliest known human infection with HIV has been traced to central Africa in 1959.[9] Modern transportation, promiscuity, and drug abuse have been blamed for the rapid spread of the virus to the United States and throughout the world.

HIV is a member of the lentivirinae (lenti = slow) subfamily of retroviruses. Lentiviruses are characterized by their indolent infectious cycle. There are two related but distinct types of HIV, HIV-1 and HIV-2, both of which are associated with causing AIDS. HIV-1 is divided into two major groups based on genetic sequencing, M (major) and O (outlier or other). Subtypes (clades) of HIV-1 group M are identified as A–J.[10] HIV-1 subtype B has been primarily responsible for the epidemic in North America and Western

TABLE 114–1. Centers for Disease Control and Prevention 1993 Revised Classification System for HIV Infection in Adults and AIDS Surveillance Case Definition

CD4 + T-cell Categories (Absolute Number and Percentage)	(A) Asymptomatic, Acute (Primary) HIV or PGL[a]	(B) Symptomatic, Not (A) or (C) Conditions	(C) AIDS-indicator Conditions
≥ 500/μL or ≥ 29%	A1	B1	C1
200–499/μL or 14%–28%	A2	B2	C2
< 200/μL or < 14%	A3	B3	C3

AIDS-indicator Conditions

Candidiasis of bronchi, trachea, or lungs
Candidiasis, esophageal
Cervical cancer, invasive
Coccidiodomycosis, disseminated or extrapulmonary
Cryptococcosis, extrapulmonary
Cryptosporidiosis, chronic intestinal (duration > 1 mo)
Cytomegalovirus disease (other than liver, spleen, or nodes)
Cytomegalovirus retinitis (with loss of vision)
Encephalopathy, HIV-related
Herpes simplex: chronic ulcer(s) (duration > 1 mo); or bronchitis, pneumonitis, or esophagitis
Histoplasmosis, disseminated or extrapulmonary
Isosporiasis, chronic intestinal (duration > 1 mo)
Kaposi's sarcoma
Lymphoma, Burkitt's
Lymphoma, immunoblastic
Lymphoma, primary, of brain
Mycobacterium avium complex or *M. kansasii,* disseminated or extrapulmonary
Mycobacterium tuberculosis, any site (pulmonary or extrapulmonary)
Mycobacterium, other species or unidentified species, disseminated or extrapulmonary
Pneumocystis carinii pneumonia
Pneumonia, recurrent
Progressive multifocal leukoencephalopathy
Salmonella septicemia, recurrent
Toxoplasmosis of brain
Wasting syndrome due to HIV

[a]PGL = persistent generalized lymphadenopathy.

Europe. This chapter will focus on HIV-1 because this is the predominant strain likely to be encountered in the United States.

DETECTION OF HIV AND SURROGATE MARKERS OF DISEASE PROGRESSION

When HIV-1 infection is suspected, whether owing to symptoms or high-risk behavior, it should be confirmed by laboratory methods. The current most commonly used screening method in the United States is an enzyme-linked immunosorbent assay (ELISA, EIA), which detects antibodies against HIV-1. The ELISA test is both highly sensitive and specific, greater than 99% and 98% respectively, but false positives can occur in multiparous women, recent recipients of influenza or hepatitis B vaccine, patients with multiple blood transfusions or hematologic malignancy, or those on chronic hemodialysis. False negatives may occur if the patient is newly infected and the test is performed before antibody production is detectable.[11] The median time to develop antibodies is 2 months from initial exposure, with greater than 95% of individuals developing antibodies within 6 months; therefore, the ELISA test is optimally performed after 2 months for detection purposes, but may be done earlier to document seroconversion.[12] Convenient methods for obtaining an ELISA sample have been developed, including an oral collection device (OraSure) and an over-the-counter home fingerstick blood-collection test system (Home Access).[13,14] Positive ELISAs are repeated in duplicate and if one or both tests are reactive, a confirmatory test is performed for final diagnosis. Several confirmatory tests exist, including Western blot assay, indirect immunofluorescence assay (IFA), or radioimmunoprecipitation assay (RIPA). A positive confirmatory test with a reactive ELISA indicates an established HIV-1 infection. If the confirmatory test is negative, the patient is most likely not infected. An indeterminate result can be resolved by using another confirmatory test, retesting the individual after 3 to 6 months, culturing the blood for virus, or performing a viral-load assay.[11]

The viral load (or viral burden) test quantifies the degree of viremia by measuring the amount of viral RNA. There are three commonly used methods for determining the amount of HIV RNA: reverse transcriptase-coupled polymerase chain reaction (RT-PCR), branched DNA (bDNA) signal amplification, and nucleic acid sequence–based assay (NASBA).[15–17] RT-PCR and bDNA are more widely used than the NASBA technique. Irrespective of the method used, viral load is reported as the number of viral RNA copies per milliliter. Each assay has its own lower limit of sensitivity, and results can vary from one assay method to the other; therefore, it is recommended that the same assay method be used consistently within patients. Reductions in viral load are often reported in base 10 logarithm. For example, if a patient initially presents with a viral load of 100,000 copies/mL (10^5 copies/mL) and subsequently has a viral load of 10,000 copies/mL (10^4 copies/mL), the decrease in viral load is 1 $\log_{10}$. Viral load assays have greater than 99% specificity and can be used to detect most strains of HIV. More importantly, viral load can be used as a prognostic factor to monitor disease progression and the effects of treatment.[18] The

Multicenter AIDS Cohort Study measured viral load in 181 HIV-positive men and followed them for as long as 11 years. Only 8% of patients with fewer than 4530 copies/mL progressed to AIDS within 5 years, whereas the 5-year progression rate for those with initial viral loads above 36,270 copies/mL was 62%. The mortality rates within 5 years were 5% and 49%, respectively. Those with viral loads between 4531 and 13,020 progressed to AIDS at a rate of 26%, with a mortality rate of 10%; and those with viral loads from 13,021 to 36,270 progressed to AIDS at a rate of 49%, with a mortality rate of 25%. Clearly, a higher level of viremia at the onset is associated with poorer prognosis.[19]

Because HIV attacks and destroys cells bearing the CD4 receptor, the number of CD4 lymphocytes in the blood has been proposed as a surrogate marker of disease progression. The normal adult CD4 lymphocyte count ranges from 500 to 1600 cells/μL or 40% to 70% of all lymphocytes. CD4 counts in children are age-dependent, with younger children having higher CD4 counts. Depletion of CD4 cells has been associated with the development of opportunistic infection and other AIDS malignancies.[20] Viral load is a better predictor of disease progression than the absolute CD4 lymphocyte count, but prognosis is much more accurate when the two are used together.[18]

Other previously used laboratory markers of disease progression include HIV p24 antigen, β_2-microglobulin, and serum neopterin. The first marker widely available for quantifying HIV was the serum p24 antigen. The HIV p24 antigen is clinically useful for diagnosing patients with acute primary HIV infection who have not yet developed antibodies when HIV RNA is not immediately available. However, in patients with established HIV infection, it is not as sensitive or predictive of clinical course as plasma HIV RNA assays. β_2-Microglobulin is a protein present on all nucleated cells. It is a nonspecific indicator of mononuclear cell destruction, and levels greater than 5 mg/L in HIV-infected persons have been associated with greater risk for developing an opportunistic infection or AIDS progression.[21] Neopterin is produced during guanosine triphosphate metabolism and is a nonspecific indicator of monocyte or macrophage activation. Levels of neopterin greater than 15 ng/mL have been detected in AIDS patients.[22] Both β_2-microglobulin and neopterin have limited clinical use because of their nonspecificity and lack of predictive value.

TRANSMISSION OF HIV

Infection with HIV occurs through three primary modes: sexual, parenteral, and perinatal. Sexual intercourse, primarily receptive anal and vaginal intercourse, is the most common vehicle for transmission of infection.[7] HIV can be found in semen and cervical secretions, and exposure to either of these infected body fluids may transmit the virus.[23] Male-to-male transmission of HIV currently accounts for 38% of cases in the United States. Women infected by their male partner is increasingly becoming more common.[5] No sexual act between individuals can be considered absolutely safe. The probability of HIV transmission from heterosexual or homosexual intercourse has been estimated at 0.1 to 0.2 per sexual contact.[24] In general, the risk is increased when the index partner is in an advanced stage of disease.[25] Persons at highest risk for heterosexual transmission include persons with ulcerative sexually transmitted diseases, individuals with multiple sex partners, and sexual partners of injection-drug users. Data suggest that male-to-female sexual transmission is 7 to 9 times more efficient than female-to-male sexual transmission.[26] Risk of transmission is elevated when women experience vaginal bleeding during intercourse.[25] Individuals with genital ulcers such as from syphilis, chancroid, or herpes are at a fourfold greater risk of contracting HIV. Gonorrhea, chlamydia, and trichomoniasis increase the risk two- to threefold.[27] Sexual partners of circumcised males are less likely to acquire HIV infection when compared with sex partners of uncircumcised males, suggesting that the absence of the foreskin has a protective effect for the partner.[25] Infections can also occur from artificial insemination with infected semen.[28] The risk of acquiring HIV infection from oral intercourse is less well established, but cases have been reported.[29] Casual contact with AIDS patients or persons with HIV is not a significant risk factor for HIV transmission.[30] Prevention of sexual transmission in adults has primarily been focused on encouraging the use of condoms, reducing high-risk behavior (anal intercourse and promiscuity), and the treatment of sexually transmitted diseases. A combined approach has been advocated for successful prevention. Abstinence is encouraged among adolescents.[31] Future interventions under development such as HIV vaccines and topical vaginal microbicides may further limit the spread of sexually transmitted HIV.

Parenteral transmission of HIV broadly encompasses infections due to contaminated blood exposure such as from needlesticks, intravenous injection with used needles, receipt of blood products, or organ transplants. The use of contaminated needles or other injection-related paraphernalia by drug abusers has been the main cause of parenteral transmissions and currently accounts for one-fourth of AIDS cases reported in the United States. Cases in which receipt of infected blood transfusion, blood components, or organ transplant was involved currently portray only 1% of reports.[5] This low incidence is attributable to blood- and organ-donor screening and viral inactivation procedures for many clotting factors. These preventive measures have reduced the estimated risk for receiving tainted blood or blood products to 1 in 493,000.[32] The transmission of HIV from a human bite is rare but has occurred.[33] Likewise, there has been only one possible case of transmission involving mucous membrane exposure to contaminated blood.[34] Health care workers have a small but definite occupational risk of contracting HIV through accidental injury. Most cases of occupationally acquired HIV have been the result of a percutaneous needlestick injury. Studies indicate that the risk of HIV infection following this route is approximately 0.3%. Significant risk factors for seroconversion include deep injury, injury with a device visibly contaminated with blood, and exposure from a source who later died of AIDS.[35] Guidelines for health care and public safety workers have been developed to minimize the hazard of occupational exposure.[36]

The question of saliva exposure often arises in the context of bodily fluids that may transmit HIV. Thus far, there have been no reports of HIV acquisition attributable to saliva exposure. Levels of HIV in saliva from HIV-infected individuals are low and virus is infrequently isolated. Moreover, saliva inhibits HIV-1 infectivity.[34] Saliva commingled with blood, however, poses a risk.

Perinatal infection, or vertical transmission, is the most common cause (> 90%) of pediatric HIV infection.[7,37] Most infections occur during or near to the time of birth and therefore treatment of the HIV-1 infected mother is important. The risk of mother-to-child transmission is 15% to 35% without antiretroviral therapy. Factors that increase the likelihood of vertical transmission include ruptured membranes exceeding 4 hours in duration, CD4 percentage below 29%, birth weight less than 2500 g, hard drug use during pregnancy, and a high maternal viral load.[38,39] Breast feeding can also transmit HIV-1. The risk involved with breast feeding is 7% to 22%; therefore, in countries where safe and available alternatives to breast feeding exist, HIV-infected mothers are strongly recommended not to breast feed.[40]

PATHOGENESIS

The life cycle of HIV (Fig. 114–1) is complicated but useful to understand since the strategies employed in the treatment of HIV target various points in this cycle. Once HIV enters a human body, the outer glycoprotein (gp160) expressed on the virus allows HIV to bind to CD4 receptors, proteins present on the cell surface of T-helper (Th) lymphocytes, monocytes, macrophages, and dendritic cells. The glycoprotein gp160 consists of two subunits, gp120 and gp41. The gp120 subunit has high affinity for the CD4 receptor and is responsible for the initial binding of the virus to the CD4 cell.[41] Most strains of HIV primarily infect the Th lymphocytes (CD4 lymphocytes); those that do not infect monocytes or macrophages are called T-tropic viruses, and those viruses that can infect monocytes or macrophages are called M-tropic. The M-tropic virus is predominantly detected during the early course of infection, whereas the T-tropic virus emerges over time.[42] The third hypervariable region of gp120, termed the V3 loop, is apparently responsible for this tropism. Once initial binding occurs, the intimate association of HIV with the cell is further enhanced by chemokine coreceptors. There are two major chemokine receptors involved in HIV infection, CXCR4 (formerly fusin) and CCR5, but other receptors such as CCR2b and CCR3 may also play a role. CXCR4 is the coreceptor responsible for enhancing the infectivity of T-tropic strains of HIV, whereas CCR5 is the main coreceptor for M-tropic strains.[43,44] Genetic defects in

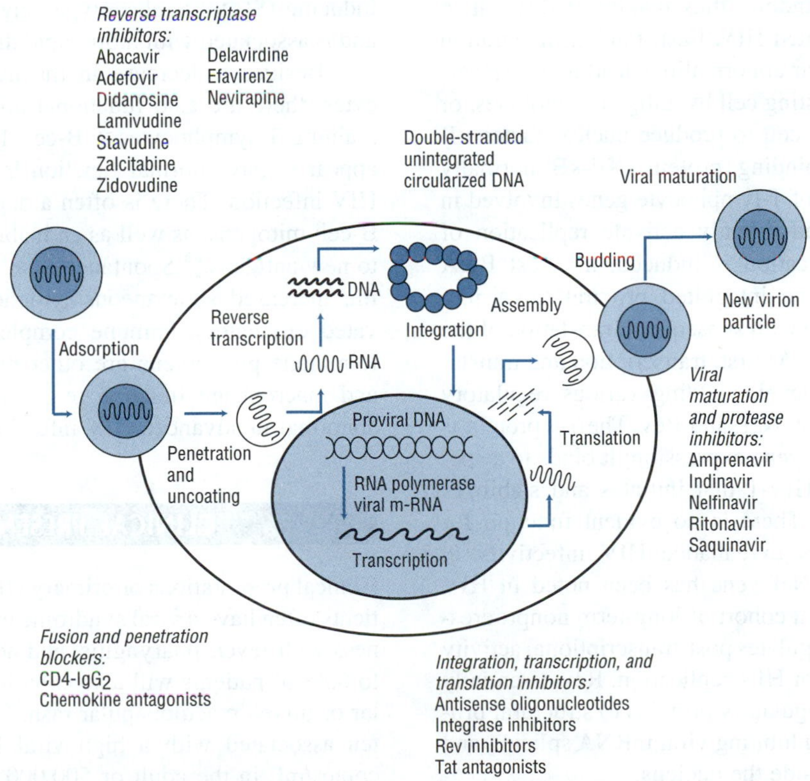

FIGURE 114–1. Life cycle of HIV with potential targets where replication may be interrupted and known or putative antiretroviral agents. *(Reprinted with permission, © Courtney V. Fletcher, 1998.)*

the expression of chemokine receptors appear to protect some individuals from developing AIDS despite their being exposed to the virus.[45] Attachment of HIV to the cell promotes fusion and internalization (adsorption) of the virus—a process mediated by the gp41 subunit.[46]

After internalization, the virus is uncoated in preparation for replication. The genetic material of the virus is positive-sense, single-strand RNA (ssRNA); the virus must transcribe this RNA into DNA to optimally replicate in human cells (transcription normally occurs from DNA to RNA—HIV works backward, hence the name retrovirus). To do so, HIV is equipped with a unique enzyme, RNA-dependent DNA polymerase (reverse transcriptase). Reverse transcriptase first synthesizes a complementary strand of DNA using the viral RNA as a template. The RNA portion of this RNA–DNA hybrid is then partially removed by ribonuclease H (RNase H), allowing reverse transcriptase to complete the synthesis of a double-stranded DNA (dsDNA) molecule. Unfortunately, the fidelity of reverse transcriptase is poor and many mistakes are made during the process.[47] These errors in the final DNA product contribute to the rapid mutation of the virus. Following reverse transcription, the final dsDNA product migrates into the nucleus and is integrated into the host cell chromosome by integrase, another enzyme unique to HIV.

The integration of HIV into the host chromosome is troublesome for several reasons. First, HIV can establish a chronic and persistent infection, particularly in certain cells of the immune system, such as the memory T lymphocyte.[48] Second, integration is random, thus making it difficult to target and extract integrated HIV. Last, random integration of HIV may cause cellular abnormalities leading to cancer.

Activation of the resting cell by antigens, cytokines, or other factors induces the cell to produce nuclear factor κB (NF-κB), an enhancer-binding protein. NF-κB normally regulates the expression of T-lymphocyte genes involved in growth but can also inadvertently activate replication of HIV-1. When HIV replication is induced, the host RNA polymerase transcribes the integrated proviral DNA into messenger RNA (mRNA) with subsequent translation of the mRNA into viral proteins. At first, transcription and translation are done at a low level, yielding various regulatory HIV-1 proteins such as Tat, Nef, and Rev. The Tat protein is a potent amplifier of HIV gene expression; it binds to a specific RNA sequence of HIV-1 that initiates and stabilizes transcription elongation. There is no evident function for Nef, although it appears to enhance HIV infectivity *in vitro*.[49] Deletion of the Nef gene has been noted in HIV strains that have infected a cohort of long-term nonprogressors.[50] The Rev protein regulates post-transcriptional activity and like Tat is essential for HIV replication. Rev essentially shifts synthesis of HIV regulatory proteins to structural proteins, such as gp160, by inhibiting viral mRNA splicing and exporting the mRNA outside the nucleus.

Assembly of new virion particles occurs in a stepwise manner beginning with the coalescence of HIV proteins beneath the host cell lipid bilayer. The nucleocapsid is subsequently formed with viral ssRNA and other components packaged inside. Proper packaging of the viral ssRNA is aided by a nucleocapsid protein designated as NCp7. NCp7 is a basic protein with two highly conserved sequences of amino acids that each form a triple-loop zinc finger motif unique to retroviruses. Once packaged, the virion then buds through the plasma membrane, acquiring the lipid bilayer of the host along with some host proteins. After the virus buds, the maturation process begins. Within the virion an enzyme, HIV protease, begins cleaving a large precursor polypeptide (*gag* and *gag-pol*) into functional proteins that are necessary to produce a complete virus. Without protease, the virion is immature and unable to adequately infect cells.[51] Protease inhibitors such as saquinavir, ritonavir, indinavir, and nelfinavir are potent, highly effective inhibitors of this enzyme.

HIV-1 exhibits a very high turnover rate, with an estimated 10 billion new viruses produced each day. More than 99% of these viruses are produced in newly infected cells.[52–54] Ultimately, most infected cells will be destroyed from a number of mechanisms, including cell lysis by newly budding virions, accumulation of unintegrated viral DNA, interference of protein synthesis, syncytia formation, or apoptosis. Uninfected cells may also be destroyed through syncytia formation or the apoptosis pathway. Syncytia formation occurs when viral proteins on the surface of the infected cell act as ligands for receptors expressed on uninfected cells. Uninfected cells clump onto the infected cell and then fuse into a giant multinucleated cell. The syncytium-inducing (SI) virus phenotype may develop later in disease and is associated with more rapid disease progression.[55]

Besides a decrease in the number of CD4 lymphocytes, there are also functional abnormalities with the remaining T lymphocytes.[55] B-cell lymphocytes also do not appear to have normal function in patients with advanced HIV infection. There is often a depressed response to pure B-cell mitogens, as well as an inability to mount a response to new antigens.[56] Spontaneous secretion of immunoglobulin, increased spontaneous lymphocyte proliferation, elevated circulatory immune complexes, and numerous autoimmune phenomena are other manifestations. Monocyte and macrophage function (e.g., chemotaxis) may also be abnormal in advanced HIV infection.[57]

CLINICAL PRESENTATION

Clinical presentations of primary HIV infection vary, but patients often have a viral syndrome or mononucleosis-like illness with fever, pharyngitis, and adenopathy.[31] About 40% to 60% of patients will also exhibit an erythematous macular or mixed maculopapular rash.[58] Primary infection is often associated with a high viral load (exceeding 50,000 copies/mL in the adult or 500,000 copies/mL in the child) and development of an immune response that for a period of time suppresses, but may not eliminate, viral replication.[59] During this period, HIV is trapped by follicular dendritic

TABLE 114–2. Centers for Disease Control and Prevention 1994 Revised Classification System for HIV Infection in Children Less Than 13 Years of Age

Immunologic Categories	< 12 Mo Cells/μL (%)[a]	1–5 Yr Cells/mL (%)[a]	6–12 Yr Cells/μL (%)[a]
1. No evidence of suppression	≥ 1500 (≥ 25%)	≥ 1000 (≥ 25%)	≥ 500 (≥ 25%)
2. Evidence of moderate suppression	750–1499 (15%–24%)	500–999 (15%–24%)	200–499 (15%–24%)
3. Severe suppression	< 750 (< 15%)	< 500 (< 15%)	< 200 (< 15%)

Immunologic Categories	N: No Signs/Symptoms	A: Mild Signs/Symptoms	B: Moderate Signs/Symptoms	C: Severe Signs/Symptoms
1. No evidence of suppression	N1	A1	B1	C1
2. Evidence of moderate suppression	N2	A2	B2	C2
3. Severe suppression	N3	A3	B3	C3

[a]Percentage of total lymphocytes.

cells in lymphoid tissue and replicates in the germinal center. The plasma HIV RNA levels fall substantially at that point and symptoms gradually resolve.[60] The clinically latent period, however, is not virologically latent because HIV replication and immune system deterioration are ongoing. A persistent decrease in CD4 lymphocytes is the most obvious and measurable aspect of this immune-system destruction. Plasma viral load, on the other hand, will appear to have stabilized at a particular level or "set-point."[19] Approximately 5% of infected individuals will develop AIDS within 3 years, and 20% within 5 years; the median time from initial infection with HIV to the development of an opportunistic infection or AIDS is 10 years.[61] Since 1995, however, the incidence of opportunistic infections has decreased partly owing to better recognition, prophylactic therapies, and the use of HAART.[5] It is becoming more apparent that what determines progression to AIDS and morbidity is the viral set-point.[18,19]

Most patients with advanced HIV infection are anergic. Patients with AIDS have inadequate immune responsiveness to specific antigens and eventually lose the ability to respond to nonspecific mitogens.[62] Characteristically, they also have a moderate anemia (hemoglobin of 7 to 12 g/dL), moderate transient leukopenia (1000 to 3000 cells/μL), and moderate thrombocytopenia. Antiplatelet antibodies are sometimes detectable. Lymphocyte counts are frequently below 1500 cells/μL with a disproportionate decrease in T lymphocytes compared with B lymphocytes. Following lymphopenia, there is a CD8 lymphocytosis with depletion of CD4 lymphocytes and the appearance of atypical lymphocytes. The abnormalities discussed appear more pronounced in patients who have had opportunistic infections than in persons who present only with Kaposi's sarcoma.

HIV-related illnesses in children often present with unexplained physical signs such as hepatomegaly, failure to thrive and weight loss, unexplained fever, splenomegaly, unexplained lymphadenopathy, low birth weight (in prenatally exposed infants), eczema, and parotitis. Laboratory findings include anemia, hypergammaglobulinemia, altered mononuclear cell function, and altered T-cell subset ratios. Of note, the normal range for CD4 cell counts in young children is much different than in adults (Table 114–2). Bacterial infections, including streptococcus pneumonia, *Salmonella* species, and mycobacterium tuberculosis may be more prevalent in children with AIDS than in adults with the disease. Kaposi's sarcoma is rare in children. Children with HIV infection may develop lymphocytic interstitial pneumonitis without evidence of *P. carinii* or other pathogens on lung biopsy. Some children present with progressive, unexplained, neurologic deterioration, including late-onset seizures, loss of developmental milestones, cessation of brain growth, and diffuse, unexplained encephalopathy. A history of recurrent or persistent bacterial, viral, or fungal infections, which may be chronic, and initially subclinical or slowly progressive, has been observed. Included in this group are children with recurrent bacterial sepsis, meningitis, and chronic otitis media, and children with chronic oral candidiasis and presumed disseminated histoplasmosis.[63,64] The CDC's current pediatric AIDS surveillance definition (Table 114–2) excludes children with congenital or perinatally acquired cytomegalovirus or other identified causes of congenital immunodeficiency. Management of the HIV-infected child involves similar principles as the adult: antiretroviral therapy, treatment and prophylaxis of opportunistic infections, and supportive care.[65]

▶ TREATMENT: HIV Infection

DESIRED OUTCOME

The goal of antiretroviral therapy is to achieve the maximum suppression of HIV replication. This is commonly interpreted to be a plasma HIV-RNA level that is less than the lower limit of quantitation. As the methods of quantitation become more sensitive it will be important to know whether there is a long-term difference in AIDS-associated complications and survival if replication is suppressed below 500 copies/mL versus 50 copies/mL. The weight of available data indicate that the regimen likely to achieve maximum suppression for most patients is one that consists of two nucleoside reverse transcriptase inhibitors and a protease inhibitor.[66,67] Figure 114–2 illustrates various combinations of these agents.

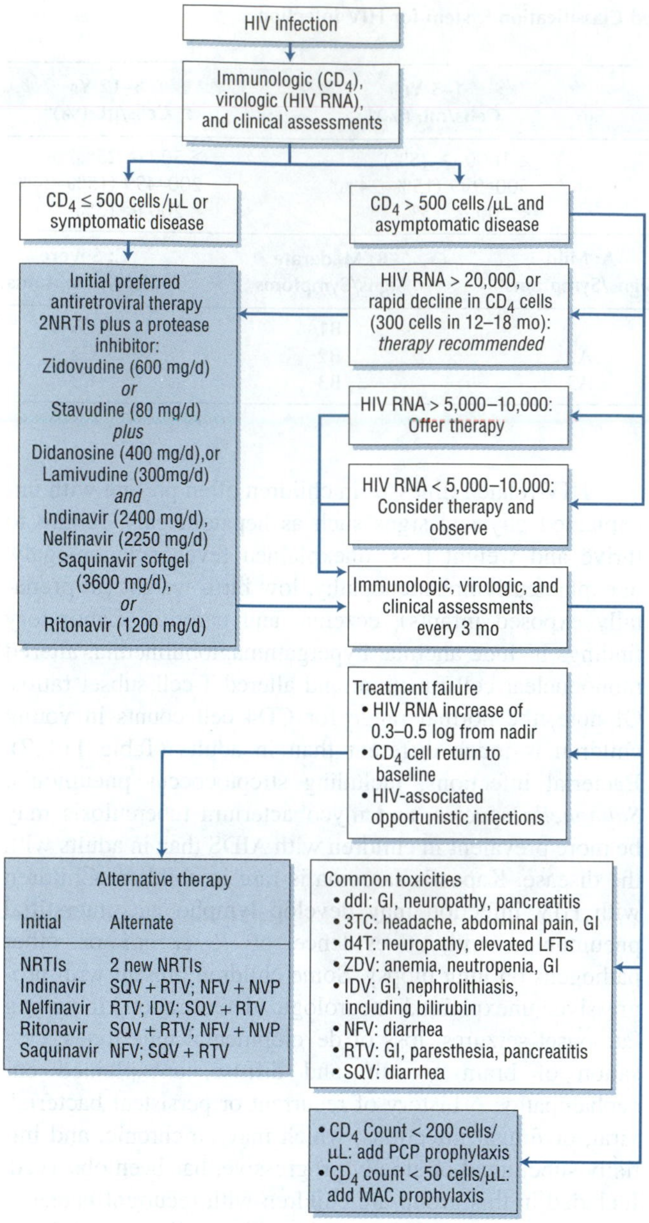

FIGURE 114–2. HIV management: state of the art. NRTIs = nucleoside/nucleotide reverse transcriptase inhibitors; SQV = saquinavir; RTV = ritonavir; NFV = nelfinavir; NVP = nevirapine; IDV = indinavir; ddI = didanosine; 3TC = lamivudine; d4T = stavudine; ZVD = zidovudine; PCP = *Pneumocystis carinii* pneumonia; MAC = *Mycobacterium avium* complex. *(Reprinted with permission, © Courtney V. Fletcher, 1998.)*

TREATMENT DURING PREGNANCY

Treatment guidelines have also been developed for HIV-infected pregnant women and prevention of vertical transmission.[68] Therapy is warranted particularly in light of the dramatic reduction in transmission seen with zidovudine monotherapy (ACTG protocol 076).[39,69] Unfortunately, little is known about the use of antiretrovirals in pregnant women and the effect these drugs may have on the developing fetus. Although there are no data to indicate any adverse consequences of the administration of zidovudine to pregnant women during the second and third trimester and their newborns for 6 weeks, long-term monitoring of the women and their children who participated in ACTG protocol 076 is ongoing. The NIH Treatment Principles recommend women receive optimal therapy regardless of pregnancy status. Although this recommendation is appropriate in theory, it is more difficult in practice because few of the other available agents have been evaluated in a controlled study of maternal-to-fetal transmission. However, given the compelling evidence for a potent antiviral effect, pregnant women should be treated similarly to a nonpregnant adult; and, if possible, zidovudine should be used for both the mother and the infant.[66–68]

POSTEXPOSURE PROPHYLAXIS

Protection of health care worker from accidental exposure to HIV is an important concern. The CDC has issued provisional guidelines governing treatment for occupational HIV exposure. Postexposure prophylaxis (PEP) with a triple drug regimen consisting of two nucleoside reverse transcriptase inhibitors and a protease inhibitor is recommended for percutaneous blood exposure involving significant risk (large volume of blood or blood from patients with advanced AIDS). Others have endorsed the use of two nucleoside reverse transcriptase inhibitors and nevirapine because nevirapine is widely distributed in tissue including the central nervous system, inhibits an early stage of replication (reverse transcription), reaches therapeutic levels after a single dose, and rapidly decreases HIV viral load. Two nucleoside reverse transcriptase inhibitors may be offered to the health care worker with lower risk of exposure such as those involving either the mucous membrane or skin. Treatment is not necessary if the source of exposure is urine or saliva. The optimal duration of treatment is unknown but at least 4 weeks of therapy is advocated. Treatment should ideally be initiated within 1 to 2 hours.[36] A similar treatment approach should be initiated for postcoital and postinjection-drug use prophylaxis.[71]

GENERAL APPROACH TO TREATMENT

In mid-1997 the National Institutes of Health Office of AIDS Research convened a panel to define the scientific principles that might serve as a guide for the clinical use of antiretroviral agents.[71] The 11 principles presented below are an amalgamation of knowledge of the life cycle of HIV, the consequences of HIV replication, clinical trials of antiretroviral agents, and scientific opinion.

1. Ongoing HIV replication leads to immune-system damage and progression to AIDS. HIV infection is always harmful, and true long-term survival free of clinically significant immune dysfunction is unusual.
2. Plasma HIV RNA levels indicate the magnitude of HIV replication and its associated rate of CD4 cell destruction, whereas CD4 cell counts indicate the extent of HIV-induced immune damage already suffered. Regular, periodic measurement of plasma HIV RNA levels and CD4 cell counts is necessary to determine the risk of disease progression in an HIV-infected individual and to determine when to initiate or modify antiretroviral treatment regimens.
3. Because rates of disease progression differ among individuals, treatment decisions should be individualized by level of risk indicated by plasma HIV RNA levels and CD4 cell counts.
4. The use of potent combination antiretroviral therapy to suppress HIV replication to below the levels of detection of sensitive plasma HIV RNA assays limits the potential for selection of antiretroviral-resistant HIV variants, the major factor limiting the ability of antiretroviral drugs to inhibit virus replication and delay disease progression. Therefore, maximum achievable suppression of HIV replication should be the goal of therapy.

5. The most effective means to accomplish durable suppression of HIV replication is the simultaneous initiation of combinations of effective anti-HIV drugs with which the patient has not been previously treated and that are not cross-resistant with antiretroviral agents with which the patient has been treated previously.
6. Each of the antiretroviral drugs used in combination therapy regimens should always be used according to optimum schedules and dosages.
7. The available effective antiretroviral drugs are limited in number and mechanism of action, and cross-resistance between specific drugs has been documented. Therefore, any change in antiretroviral therapy increases future therapeutic constraints.
8. Women should receive optimal antiretroviral therapy regardless of pregnancy status.
9. The same principles of antiretroviral therapy apply to both HIV-infected children and adults, although the treatment of HIV-infected children involves unique pharmacologic, virologic, and immunologic considerations.
10. Persons with acute primary HIV infections should be treated with combination antiretroviral therapy to suppress virus replication to levels below the limit of detection of sensitive plasma HIV RNA assays.
11. HIV-infected persons, even those with viral loads below detectable limits, should be considered infectious and should be counseled to avoid sexual and drug-use behaviors that are associated with transmission or acquisition of HIV and other infectious pathogens.

The extent to which these principles will stand the test of time is unknown; new information on the pathogenesis of HIV accrues constantly. The field of antiretroviral therapy is also rapidly evolving. Several of the clinical trials used in formulating the principles of therapy enrolled small numbers of participants and had limited follow-up. Eleven agents are now FDA approved and more are certain to come. Health care professionals involved in care of the HIV-infected person must always consult the most current literature with respect to the principles and strategies for therapy. With these caveats, Figure 114–2 presents the state-of-the-art for treatment of the HIV-infected individual at the time of the writing of this chapter. Treatment is recommended for all HIV-infected persons with symptomatic disease, CD4 lymphocyte counts < 500 cells/μL, or with plasma HIV RNA > 20,000 copies/mL (by RT-PCR) or > 10,000 copies/mL (by bDNA) regardless of the CD4 count.[66] A more aggressive treatment approach recommends treatment if viral load becomes > 5000 copies/mL.[67] The available data do not permit an absolute treatment threshold to be established based on plasma HIV RNA level. Therefore, the relative merits of a cautious approach that delays therapy for patients with values > 5000 copies/mL, and considers therapy for patients with values between 5000 and 10,000 copies/mL, is as valid as an aggressive approach of offering therapy to any patient who requests it and is committed to lifelong medication compliance.

PHARMACOLOGIC THERAPY

Conceptually, there are three primary methods of therapeutic intervention against HIV: inhibition of viral replication, vaccination to stimulate a more effective immune response, and restoration of the immune system with immunomodulators. HIV vaccines and therapeutic approaches for restoring the immune system are reviewed elsewhere and will not be discussed in this chapter.[72,73]

ANTIRETROVIRAL AGENTS

Inhibiting viral replication with HAART has been the most clinically successful strategy in the treatment of HIV infection. Thus far, there have been two primary groups of drugs used: reverse transcriptase inhibitors and protease inhibitors (Table 114–3). Reverse transcriptase inhibitors are of two types, those that are chemical derivatives of purine- and pyrimidine-based nucleosides and nucleotides (nucleoside/nucleotide reverse transcriptase inhibitors or NRTIs) and those that are not (nonnucleoside reverse transcriptase inhibitors or NNRTIs). Nucleoside reverse transcriptase inhibitors include thymidine analogs such as stavudine (d4T) and zidovudine (AZT or ZDV); cytosine analogs such as lamivudine (3TC)

TABLE 114–3. Pharmacologic Parameters of Antiretroviral Compounds

Drug	*In Vitro* Susceptibility (IC_{50} range)	F (%)	V_d (L/kg)	$T_{1/2}$ (h)	CL/F (L/h)	Adult dose[a]	Plasma C_{max}/C_{min} (μM)	Ratio fetal:maternal conc.	Ratio CSF:plasma conc.
Nucleoside reverse transcriptase inhibitors									
Didanosine	0.01–10 μM	40	1.00	1.4	26.9	200 mg bid	4/0.02	0.3–0.5	0.22
Lamivudine	0.015–0.321 μg/mL[b]	86	1.3	5	23.1	150 mg bid	7.5/0.22	> 0.7	0.12
Stavudine	0.009–4 μM	82	0.53	1.6	40	40 mg bid	4/0.004	> 0.7	0.02
Zalcitabine	0.03–0.5 μM	85	0.53	2	12	0.75 mg tid	0.05/0.001	0.3–0.5	0.2
Zidovudine	0.03–0.13 μg/ml	64	1.6	1.1	112	200 mg tid 300 mg bid	2/0.2	> 0.7	0.6
Nonnucleoside reverse transcriptase inhibitors									
Delavirdine	0.05–0.1 μM[b]	85	1.0	4.7	4	400 mg tid	35/14	?	0.004
Nevirapine	0.010–0.1 μM	50	1.21	25	2.6	200 mg bid[c]	5.5/3.0	1	0.45
Protease inhibitors									
Indinavir	0.025–0.1 μM[b]	60	1.2	1.5	43	800 mg q8h	13/0.25	?	0.03–0.94
Nelfinavir	0.009–0.06 μM	?	2	2.6	37.4	750 mg tid	5.6/0.7	?	—
Ritonavir	0.0038–0.154 μM	60	0.41	3–5	8.8	600 mg bid[c]	16/5	?	—
Saquinavir[d]	0.001–0.03 μM	12	10	3	80	1200 mg tid	0.4/0.15	?	—

[a]Dose adjustment may be required for weight, renal or hepatic disease, and drug interactions.
[b]Range given is for IC_{90} (concentration necessary to inhibit 90% of viral replication).
[c]Initial dose escalation recommended to minimize side effects.
[d]Soft-gel formulation.
Abbreviations: IC_{50} = concentration necessary to inhibit 50% of viral replication; F = bioavailability; V_d = distribution volume; $T_{1/2}$ = elimination half-life; CL = total body clearance; C_{max} = maximum plasma concentration; C_{min} = minimum plasma concentration; CSF = cerebrospinal fluid.

and zalcitabine (ddC); the inosine derivative didanosine (ddI); and the adenosine derivatives abacavir (ABV) and lodenosine (FddA). Adefovir dipivoxil (bis-POM PMEA) is an adenosine-derived nucleotide reverse transcriptase inhibitor. Nucleoside and nucleotide reverse transcriptase inhibitors require phosphorylation to the 5′-triphosphate moiety to be active. Because HIV does not encode viral kinases, the compounds must be phosphorylated intracellularly by host cell kinases and phosphotransferases. Thymidine analogs (ZDV and d4T) are preferentially phosphorylated in activated cells compared with didanosine, zalcitabine, and lamivudine, which are phosphorylated independent of cellular activation.[74] Following prodrug activation, the 5′-triphosphate moiety acts in two ways: (1), it prematurely terminates DNA elongation due to the modified 3′-hydroxyl group; and (2), it competes with natural deoxynucleotides for reverse transcriptase. Hydroxyurea (hydroxycarbamide), a ribonucleotide reductase inhibitor, theoretically depletes intracellular deoxynucleotides and has been used in combination with nucleoside reverse transcriptase inhibitors with some success.[75] Presumably, the reduction of endogenous triphosphates by hydroxyurea shifts the competition for reverse transcriptase in favor of the exogenous triphosphate (i.e., nucleotide reverse transcriptase inhibitor). Although nucleoside and nucleotide reverse transcriptase inhibitors are specific for HIV reverse transcriptase, their adverse effects may in part be owing to some inhibition of human DNA polymerase. A specific discussion of the pharmacology and effects of nucleoside reverse transcriptase inhibitors can be found elsewhere.[76–80]

Nonnucleoside reverse transcriptase inhibitors are a chemically heterogeneous group of agents that bind noncompetitively to reverse transcriptase close to its catalytic site of polymerase activity. Unlike nucleoside reverse transcriptase inhibitors, nonnucleoside reverse transcriptase inhibitors do not require intracellular activation, do not compete with endogenous deoxynucleoside triphosphates, and do not have strong antiviral activity against HIV-2. Nonnucleoside reverse transcriptase inhibitors used clinically include nevirapine (NVP), delavirdine (DLV), and efavirenz (EFV). The clinical utility of nonnucleoside reverse transcriptase inhibitors has been somewhat limited by the development of rapid resistance owing to mutations in the reverse transcriptase enzyme, especially with monotherapy.

The protease inhibitors are a potent class of antiretrovirals that include saquinavir (SQV), ritonavir (RTV), indinavir (IDV), and nelfinavir (NFV). The pharmacology, pharmacokinetics, safety, and efficacy of these drugs are reviewed elsewhere.[81] Briefly, protease inhibitors block the maturation process, thereby resulting in the production of immature, noninfectious virions.[51]

PIVOTAL DEVELOPMENTS IN TREATMENT STRATEGIES

The pharmacotherapy of HIV infection has rapidly changed over the years as newer agents became available and treatment paradigms evolved. The current use of antiretroviral agents is built on several developments in our understanding of these compounds.

The antiretroviral properties of zidovudine were discovered in 1985. The drug was used therapeutically for HIV-1 infection 1 year later and approved by the FDA in March 1987. Zidovudine was the first antiretroviral agent to demonstrate a survival benefit in patients infected with HIV. The first controlled study of zidovudine randomized 282 individuals with AIDS or AIDS-related complex (ARC) to receive either zidovudine (1500 mg/day) or placebo.[82] In this trial, zidovudine therapy reduced the probability of development of an opportunistic infection (23% vs 43%, $P < .001$) and significantly improved survival. After 12 weeks of treatment, the concentration of HIV p24 antigen was statistically lower in the zidovudine recipients compared with placebo and mean CD4 lymphocyte count was higher (68 cells/μL vs 33 cells/μL, $P < .0001$). This study was the first to demonstrate that an antiretroviral agent, in this case a nucleoside inhibitor of reverse transcriptase, could alter the clinical course of HIV infection. Furthermore, the trial established four key requirements for antiretroviral therapy that remain objectives today: (1) improved survival; (2) a decrease in the incidence of opportunistic infections; (3) a reduction in viral burden; and (4) an increase in CD4 lymphocytes.

Subsequently, zidovudine when used alone transiently delayed the onset of AIDS-defining events in both symptomatic and asymptomatic HIV-infected individuals.[83,84] A European–Australian Collaborative Group study of zidovudine (1000 mg/day) in asymptomatic persons with HIV infection and > 400 CD4 cells/μL demonstrated a delay in overall disease progression over a period of approximately 2 years.[85] The Concorde trial evaluated the survival and/or progression of disease benefits of immediate zidovudine use compared with deferred therapy in asymptomatic individuals.[86] This study demonstrated a delay in the clinical progression to AIDS or severe ARC at short-term follow-up periods. However, the overall results indicated no delay in disease progression after a longer period of time (3 years). The duration of the benefits of zidovudine therapy was also evaluated in a long-term follow-up of ACTG protocol 019. During follow-up of up to 4.5 years, zidovudine use in this population remained associated with a significant decrease in the risk of progression to AIDS or death. This prolonged follow-up, however, clearly demonstrated that the effect of zidovudine was not permanent because benefit decreased with increased duration of use.[87] Last, the results from the third part of ACTG 019 protocol, which evaluated zidovudine therapy in persons with CD4 cells > 500 cells/μL, demonstrated similar efficacy results to those in persons with < 500 CD4 cells/μL.[88] Since these initial studies, the dosing of zidovudine has been refined to reflect the intracellular half-life of triphosphorylated zidovudine; zidovudine is now dosed 600 mg/d given either tid or bid.

One of the most important accomplishments in the development of antiretroviral therapies was the demonstration that zidovudine reduced the rate of HIV-1 maternal-to-fetal transmission. ACTG protocol 076 randomized 477 HIV-infected pregnant women (14 to 34 weeks' gestation) to either zidovudine or placebo. The zidovudine regimen consisted of antepartum zidovudine (100 mg five times daily) plus a continuous infusion of zidovudine during labor (2 mg/kg IV over 1 hour followed by 1 mg/kg/h), and zidovudine for the newborn (2 mg/kg orally q6h for 6 weeks). The HIV transmission rate was 25.5% among those that received placebo, but was 8.3% when the mothers and their babies received zidovudine. This difference corresponds to a two-thirds reduction in the risk of maternal-to-infant HIV transmission. Adverse reactions associated with zidovudine therapy in the study were minimal: hemoglobin concentrations were significantly lower at birth in infants whose mothers received zidovudine, but this difference disappeared by 12 weeks of age; there was no difference in minor or major structural abnormalities in the two groups.[69]

Two more nucleoside reverse transcriptase inhibitors, didanosine and zalcitabine, became available in 1991 and 1992, respectively. Although both drugs are active alone, several studies indicate that the combination of two nucleoside reverse transcriptase inhibitors has a synergistic effect and provides better immunologic and virologic improvements than zidovudine used alone.[89–91] ACTG protocol 175 was a randomized, double-blind, placebo-controlled study comparing four treatment arms: zidovudine (200 mg tid), didanosine (200 mg bid), zidovudine plus didanosine, and zidovudine plus zalcitabine (0.75 mg tid). The study enrolled 2467 HIV-infected adults (1067 antiretroviral-naive patients and 1400 with previous therapy) with CD4 counts between 200 and 500 cells/μL. The median duration of treatment was 118 weeks. The primary endpoint for this study was a greater than 50% decline in CD4 count, development of AIDS, or death.

Of patients receiving zidovudine monotherapy, 32% progressed to the primary endpoint compared with 22% on didanosine monotherapy or 18% and 20% for zidovudine plus didanosine, and zidovudine plus zalcitabine, respectively. When zidovudine was used alone, the incidence of AIDS-defining events was 16% compared with 11% to 12% in the other three arms. The mortality rate in the zidovudine-only group was 9% compared with 7% in the zidovudine plus zalcitabine group and 5% in the two didanosine-containing arms. Mean CD4 counts at week 8 were substantially higher in the group receiving zidovudine and didanosine (63 cells/μL) than didanosine alone (49 cells/μL), zidovudine plus zalcitabine (41 cells/μL), or zidovudine alone (14 cells/μL) in treatment-naive patients.[89] Viral-load data from a subset of patients revealed a mean decrease in viral load of 0.26 $\log_{10}$ copies/mL for zidovudine monotherapy, 0.65 for didanosine monotherapy, 0.93 for zidovudine and didanosine, and 0.89 for zidovudine with zalcitabine after 8 weeks. A higher baseline viral load, less suppression of viral load by treatment, and syncytium-inducing virus were significantly associated with an increased risk for progression of disease.[90] Taken together, ACTG protocol 175 demonstrated that the combined regimen of zidovudine and didanosine or zalcitabine was superior to zidovudine monotherapy in immunologic and virologic parameters, particularly in patients with no previous antiretroviral therapy. Additionally, didanosine alone was found to be better than zidovudine alone.

Data from combination trials in children (ACTG 152) and patients with advanced disease (CPCRA 007, NuCombo) show similar results.[92,93] Collectively, evidence from the trials of combination nucleoside reverse transcriptase inhibitor regimens strongly support the following conclusions: (1) clinical progression of disease can be delayed with treatment; (2) combination therapy is more effective than monotherapy in producing favorable immunologic and virologic responses; (3) patients are more likely to respond to combination therapy when CD4 counts are higher and baseline viral load is lower; and (4) patients never treated (naive) are more likely to have better response than experienced patients.

During 1994 and 1995 two more nucleoside reverse transcriptase inhibitors, stavudine and lamivudine, respectively, became available. The combination of zidovudine and lamivudine was evaluated in a randomized, double-blind, placebo-controlled study (NUCA 3001) comparing zidovudine 200 mg q8h plus lamivudine 150 (low-dose) or 300 mg (high-dose) q12h with zidovudine or lamivudine 300 mg q12h monotherapy in patients who had received little or no previous therapy with zidovudine. Sustained virologic improvement was noted in patients receiving combination therapy. At week 24, the mean decrease in HIV RNA of the two combination regimens were 0.9 and 0.99 $\log_{10}$ copies/mL for low-dose lamivudine and high-dose lamivudine, respectively. Lamivudine alone reduced viral load 0.42 $\log_{10}$ copies/mL, which was more than the reduction seen with zidovudine alone (0.25 $\log_{10}$ copies/mL). In this study, mean CD4 cell count increased 61 cells/μL after 52 weeks in patients on zidovudine and low-dose lamivudine, which was similar to the 60 cells/μL increase seen with zidovudine and lamivudine 300 mg q12h. Those on zidovudine monotherapy had a mean decrease of 53 cells/μL after 52 weeks.[94]

The first protease inhibitor to become available was saquinavir in the hard-gel capsule formulation in December of 1995. The efficacy of saquinavir was demonstrated in a study (ACTG protocol 229) of 295 patients with extensive zidovudine experience, advanced disease, and CD4 cell counts between 50 and 300 cells/μL.[95] These patients were randomized to receive one of three regimens: zidovudine and zalcitabine; zidovudine and saquinavir; or zidovudine, zalcitabine, and saquinavir. The proportion of responders (i.e., those patients maintaining a 1 $\log_{10}$ reduction in plasma HIV RNA for at least 4 weeks) in the triple therapy group was 28% compared with 12% in the zidovudine and zalcitabine group and 6% in the saquinavir and zidovudine group. Higher doses of saquinavir (3600 mg/d and 7200 mg/d) were subsequently shown to substantially reduce plasma HIV RNA and increase CD4 cell counts without added toxicity.[96] An enhanced oral formulation (soft-gel capsule) of saquinavir became available in late 1997, which delivers approximately eight to nine times the drug exposure of the former formulation.

Two more protease inhibitors, ritonavir and indinavir, were licensed in March 1996. A multi-center study (M94-247) of 1090 patients with advanced HIV disease was the first to demonstrate a reduction in both mortality and AIDS-defining clinical events with a protease inhibitor. Patients were required to be on an antiretroviral regimen, which could have consisted of up to two nucleoside reverse transcriptase inhibitors, and were randomized to receive either ritonavir 600 mg bid or placebo. The mean CD4 cell count at baseline was 32 cells/μL. After 6 months, the cumulative mortality rate among patients who received ritonavir was 5.8% compared with 10.1% for those patients randomized to placebo. Furthermore, the 6-month cumulative incidence of clinical disease progression or death was 17% for patients who received ritonavir compared with 34% for patients randomized to placebo.[97]

The potent virologic and immunologic effect of triple therapy with zidovudine, lamivudine, and indinavir was shown in a double-blind, placebo-controlled study (protocol 035) of zidovudine-experienced, lamivudine-naive patients randomized to receive either indinavir monotherapy, zidovudine in combination with lamivudine, or all three drugs.[98] Reduced mortality with indinavir was confirmed in ACTG protocol 320, which compared a regimen of zidovudine, lamivudine, and indinavir to zidovudine and lamivudine.[99] A total of 1156 lamivudine and protease inhibitor–naive patients with < 200 CD4 cells/μL were enrolled in this multicenter, randomized, placebo-controlled study. Progression of disease to AIDS or death was lower in the group given indinavir compared with placebo (6% and 11%, respectively). Moreover, indinavir reduced the incidence of mortality by half: mortality was 3.1% in the two-drug regimen and 1.4% in the three-drug regimen. The effects of treatment were similar regardless of whether the CD4 count was below 50 or between 51 and 200 cells/μL.

The fourth protease inhibitor, nelfinavir, was introduced in March 1997. In a multicenter, double-blind, randomized trial (study 511), 297 antiretroviral-naive patients were randomized to receive zidovudine, lamivudine, and placebo; zidovudine, lamivudine, and nelfinavir 500 mg tid; or zidovudine, lamivudine, and nelfinavir 750 mg tid. Of patients on the regimen of zidovudine, lamivudine, and nelfinavir 750 mg tid, 88% had viral load < 1200 copies/mL (the lower limit of quantitation) at week 24 compared with 75% and 36% of patients in the nelfinavir 500 mg tid arm and placebo arm, respectively. The mean increase in CD4 counts after 24 weeks was approximately 120 cells/μL for both arms containing nelfinavir compared with a mean CD4 count increase of approximately 80 cells/μL in the placebo arm. The durability of response for patients receiving nelfinavir was still evident after 1 year. Patients receiving nelfinavir 750 mg tid remained a mean 1.98 $\log_{10}$ copies/mL below their initial baseline with 79% below the lower limit of quantitation (< 500 copies/mL). Treatment with 500 mg tid and placebo was associated with a mean drop in viral load of 1.94 and 1.87 $\log_{10}$ copies/mL, respectively; the percentage of patients with undetectable viral load (< 500 copies/mL) were 58% and 53%, respectively. CD4 counts increased steadily over the course of treatment, with a mean increase of 198 cells/μL at 12 months in patients receiving nelfinavir 750 mg tid, compared with 191 cells/μL for nelfinavir 500 mg tid, and 127 cells/μL for zidovudine and lamivudine alone.[100]

The first nonnucleoside reverse transcriptase inhibitor to be approved was nevirapine in June 1996. The combination of nevirapine (200 mg daily for 2 weeks then 400 mg daily), zidovudine, and didanosine demonstrated an 18% greater mean absolute increase in CD4 count ($P = .001$) and 0.25 $\log_{10}$ greater reduction in plasma viral load ($P = .028$) than the combination of zidovudine, didanosine, and nevirapine placebo after a 48-week study period. No difference in disease progression between the two groups, however, could be demonstrated in this study ($P > .2$).[101] A second nonnucleoside reverse transcriptase inhibitor, delavirdine, has shown modest and transient reductions in plasma HIV-RNA when combined with nucleoside reverse transcriptase inhibitors.[102] This agent was approved in April 1997.

EVALUATION OF THERAPEUTIC OUTCOMES

Following the initiation of therapy, patients are usually monitored at 3 month intervals with immunologic (CD4 count), virologic (viral load), and clinical assessments. There are two general indications to change therapy: significant toxicity or treatment failure. Each of the available antiretroviral agents has its own set of drug-limiting adverse reactions; fortunately alternatives with nonoverlapping adverse effects are available. For example, the patient who experiences significant peripheral neuropathy on the combination of didanosine and stavudine could be changed to a combination of zidovudine and lamivudine. Specific criteria to indicate treatment failure have not been established through controlled clinical trials. As a general guide, the following events should prompt consideration for changing therapy:

1. Less than a 1 log reduction in HIV RNA 1 month after the initiation of therapy, or a failure to achieve maximal suppression of HIV replications within 4 to 6 months
2. A persistent decline in the CD4 cell count or a return to the pretreatment value or an increase in HIV RNA of 0.3 to 0.5 $\log_{10}$ copies/mL from nadir
3. Clinical disease progression, usually the development of a new opportunistic infection

THERAPEUTIC FAILURE

HIV has been shown to develop resistance to antiretroviral drugs. A thorough discussion of the genotypic and phenotypic alterations in the viral population as a consequence of therapy is beyond the scope of this chapter but has been reviewed elsewhere.[103] The full implications of the emergence of mutations associated with resistance to these compounds are not known; suffice is to state that resistance will likely be associated with decreased efficacy and clinical progression of disease. Thus, in selecting alternative agents for the patient failing therapy, the health care provider must consider the available information on mutation patterns, potential for cross-resistance, and clinical implications. Few clinical data are available to indicate what alternative treatment strategies should be employed for patients who fail their initial regimen. The guiding principles (numbers 5 and 7) are to change to at least two new antiretroviral drugs that are not cross-resistant with agents the patient has received previously. Figure 114–2 presents some examples of alternative regimens.

INFECTIOUS COMPLICATIONS OF HIV

HIV itself does not produce most of the morbidity and mortality associated with AIDS. Rather, opportunistic infections, many caused by organisms that are common in the environment, are responsible for almost 90% of deaths.[104] These opportunistic diseases often represent the reactivation of quiescent infections and thus are overt manifestations of the loss of cell-mediated immunity. The development of certain opportunistic infections is directly or indirectly related to the level of CD4 lymphocytes (Fig. 114–3) and can be predicted with some degree of accuracy.[20] Until the immunosuppression induced by HIV can be prevented, the prevention and management of opportunistic infections will remain an essential component of the comprehensive care of HIV-infected individuals.

Surveillance data indicate that the incidence of certain opportunistic infections in HIV-infected persons in the United States has been changing. The incidence of *Pneumocystis carinii* pneumonia, toxoplasmic encephalitis, cryptococcal meningitis, esophageal candidiasis, herpes zoster, and *Mycobacterium avium* complex (MAC) appear to have decreased.[105] However, these declines have primarily been observed among homosexual men and not among injecting-drug users. Potent antiretroviral regimens and prophylactic strategies for opportunistic infections are major factors associated with these decreases. Nevertheless, opportunistic diseases continue to be relatively frequent complications of HIV disease and seem to be occurring at more advanced stages of immunosuppression than in the past. The most

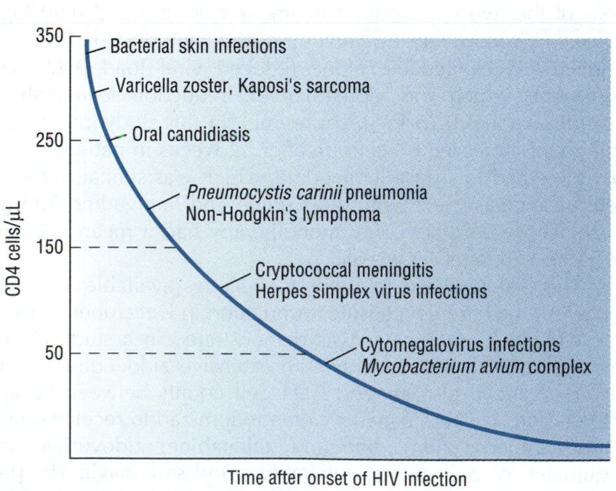

FIGURE 114–3. Natural history of opportunistic infections associated with HIV infection. (*Reprinted with permission, © Courtney V. Fletcher, 1998.*)

TABLE 114–4. Therapies for Common Opportunistic Pathogens in HIV-Infected Individuals

Clinical Disease	Selected Initial Therapies for Acute Infection in Adults	Common Drug or Dose-Limiting Adverse Reactions
Fungi		
Candidiasis, oral	Fluconazole 200 mg PO single dose or 100 mg PO for 5 days	Elevated liver function tests, hepatotoxicity, nausea and vomiting
	or	
	Nystatin 500,000 units PO swish 4–6 times daily for 7–10 days,	Taste, patient acceptance
	or	
	Clotrimazole 10 mg (1 troche) PO 5 times daily for 7–10 days	
Candidiasis, esophageal	Fluconazole 200 mg PO or IV on the first day then 100 mg/d for 10–14 days	Elevated liver function tests, hepatotoxicity, nausea and vomiting
	or	
	Ketoconazole 400 mg/d PO for 10–14 days	Elevated liver function tests, hepatotoxicity, rash, nausea and vomiting
Pneumocystis carinii pneumonia	Trimethoprim-sulfamethoxazole IV or PO 12–20 mg/kg/d as TMP component in 3–4 divided doses for 21 days[a]	Skin rash, fever, leukopenia thrombocytopenia
	or	
	Pentamidine iv 3–4 mg/kg/d for 21 days[a]	Azotemia, hypoglycemia, hyperglycemia
	Mild Episodes	
	Atovaquone suspension 750 mg (5 mL) PO twice daily with meals for 21 days[a]	Rash, elevated liver enzymes, diarrhea
Cryptococcal meningitis	Amphotericin B IV 0.5–1.0 mg/kg/d for minimum of 2 weeks *with or without*	Nephrotoxicity, hypokalemia, anemia, fever, chills
	flucytosine 100–150 mg/kg/d PO in 4 divided doses	Bone marrow suppression, elevated liver enzymes
	followed by	
	Fluconazole 100–200 mg/d, PO[a]	Same as above
Histoplasmosis	Amphotericin B 0.5–1 mg/kg/d IV for 6–8 weeks[a]	Same as above
	or	
	Itraconazole 200–400 mg/d PO for 3 months[a]	Elevated liver function tests, hepatotoxicity, nausea and vomiting, hypertension
Coccidioidomycosis	Amphotericin B 0.5–1 mg/kg/d IV for ≥ 6–8 wk[a]	Same as above
Protozoa		
Toxoplasmic encephalitis	Pyrimethamine 200 mg PO once then 50–100 mg/d	Bone marrow suppression
	plus	
	Sulfadiazine 1–1.5 g PO four times daily	Allergy, rash, drug fever
	and	
	Folinic acid 10–20 mg PO daily for a minimum of 28 days[a]	
Isosporiasis	Trimethoprim-sulfamethoxazole: 1–2 double-strength tablets (160 mg TMP and 800 mg SMZ) PO twice daily for 2–4 weeks	Same as above
Bacteria		
Organisms associated with T-cell defects		
Mycobacterium avium complex	Clarithromycin 500 mg PO twice daily, *plus* ethambutol 15 mg/kg/d PO to a maximum of 1000 mg/d, *and*	Gastrointestinal intolerance, Optic neuritis, peripheral neuritis
	Rifabutin 300 mg/d[a]	Rash, gastrointestinal intolerance, neutropenia, discolored urine, uveitis
Salmonella enterocolitis or bacteremia	Ciprofloxacin 500–750 mg PO twice daily for 14 days	Gastrointestinal intolerance
	or	
	Trimethoprim (160 mg)-sulfamethoxazole (800 mg): 1 tablet PO twice daily for 14 days	Same as above

continued

TABLE 114–4. Therapies for Common Opportunistic Pathogens in HIV-Infected Individuals *(continued)*

Clinical Disease	Selected Initial Therapies for Acute Infection in Adults	Common Drug or Dose-Limiting Adverse Reactions
Organisms associated with B-cell defects		
Campylobacter enterocolitis	Ciprofloxacin 500 mg PO twice daily for 7 days	Same as above
	or	
	Erythromycin 250–500 mg PO four times daily for 7 days	Gastrointestinal intolerance, colitis, ototoxicity
Shigella enterocolitis	Ciprofloxacin 500 mg PO twice daily for 5 days	Same as above
Viruses		
Mucocutaneous herpes simplex	Acyclovir 1–2 g/d PO in 3–5 divided doses for 7–10 days	Gastrointestinal intolerance
	or	
	Valacyclovir, 500 mg PO q12h for 7–10 days	Gastrointestinal intolerance
	or	
	Famciclovir, 500 mg PO q12h for 7–10 days	Headache, gastrointestinal intolerance
Varicella zoster	Acyclovir 30 mg/kg/d IV in 3 divided doses *or* 4 g/d PO for 7–10 days	Obstructive nephropathy, CNS symptomatology
	or	
	Valacyclovir, 1 g PO q8h for 7–10 days	
	or	
	Famciclovir, 500 mg PO q8h for 7–10 days	Obstructive nephropathy, CNS symptomatology
Cytomegalovirus	Ganciclovir 7.5–10 mg/kg/d in 2 or 3 divided doses for 14 days[a]	Neutropenia, thrombocytopenia
	or	
	Foscarnet 180 mg/kg/d in 2 or 3 divided doses for 14 days[a]	Nephrotoxicity, hypo or hypercalcemia, hypo- or hyperphosphatemia, anemia
Cytomegalovirus retinitis	Ganciclovir intraocular implant	

[a]Maintenance therapy is recommended.

common opportunistic diseases and their frequencies found before death in 1883 patients with AIDS between 1990 and 1994 were *Pneumocystis carinii* pneumonia, 45%; *Mycobacterium avium* complex, 25%; wasting syndrome, 25%; bacterial pneumonia, 24%; cytomegalovirus (CMV) disease, 23%; and candidiasis, 22%.[106] These data indicate the need for continued research on preventative strategies.

The spectrum of infectious diseases observed in HIV-infected individuals and recommended first-line therapies are shown in Tables 114–4 and 114–5. An exhaustive review of all opportunistic infections associated with HIV infection is beyond the scope of this chapter. The major opportunistic infections include *Pneumocystis carinii* pneumonia, candidal esophagitis (discussed elsewhere in this text), central nervous system toxoplasmosis, cryptococcosis, mycobacterial disease, and herpes group virus infections. The following discussion will emphasize these pathogens and will provide an overview of the epidemiology, diagnosis, clinical manifestations, and results of treatment for these infections. Readers desiring more specific information, for either the diseases or agents mentioned, will need to consult additional references.

PNEUMOCYSTIS CARINII

Pneumocystis carinii pneumonia (PCP) is the most common life-threatening opportunistic infection in patients with AIDS. Early in the AIDS epidemic approximately 60% of patients with AIDS had PCP as their AIDS-defining event and 80% experienced PCP at some point during their lifetime.[107] The advent of effective prophylaxis for PCP has decreased the relative incidence of PCP. However, PCP prophylaxis has not eliminated the disease because of persons unaware of their HIV infection, breakthrough PCP in those receiving prophylaxis, and variable compliance with prophylaxis. The taxonomy of the organism is unclear, having been classified as both protozoan and fungal. Recent evidence based on genomic sequences suggests that *P. carinii,* however, is a fungus.[108] Exposure to *P. carinii* is widespread: 80% of the population have developed serum antibodies by age 2 or 3 years.[109] The organism appears to reside without consequence in the human unless the host becomes immunologically compromised; immunosuppression allows the organism to multiply, giving rise to clinical disease. A report of a cluster of PCP in the elderly without a specific underlying immunosuppressive illness suggests a potential for other patients being at risk for this disease.[110]

CLINICAL PRESENTATION

PCP in patients with AIDS differs in clinical presentation from patients with other immunosuppressive conditions, such as malignant neoplasms. In AIDS patients, the presentation is often more subacute. Characteristic symptoms include fever and dyspnea; clinical signs are tachypnea with or without rales or rhonchi, and a nonproductive or mildly productive cough. Chest radiographs may show florid or subtle infiltrates or occasionally be normal. Infiltrates are usually interstitial and bilateral. Arterial blood gases may

TABLE 114–5. Therapies for Prophylaxis of First Episode Opportunistic Diseases in Adults and Adolescents

Pathogen	Indication	First Choice
I. Standard of Care		
Pneumocystis carinii	CD4+ count < 200/µL *or* oropharyngeal candidiasis *or* unexplained fever ≥ 2 weeks	Trimethoprim-sulfamethoxazole (TMP-SMZ), 1 DS tablet PO qd
Mycobacterium tuberculosis		
Isoniazid-sensitive	TST reaction ≥ 5 mm *or* prior positive TST result without treatment *or* contact with case of active tuberculosis	Isoniazid, 300 mg PO *plus* pyridoxine, 50 mg PO qd × 12 mo, *or* isoniazid, 900 mg PO *plus* pyridoxine, 50 mg PO twice weekly × 12 mo
Isoniazid-resistant	Same; high probability of exposure to isoniazid-resistant tuberculosis	Rifampin, 600 mg PO qd × 12 mo
Toxoplasma gondii	IgG antibody to *Toxoplasma* and CD4+ count < 100/µL	TMP-SMZ, 1 DS tablet PO qd
Mycobacterium avium complex	CD4+ count < 50/µL	Azithromycin, 1200 mg PO once weekly or clarithromycin, 500 mg PO bid
Streptococcus pneumoniae	All patients	Pneumococcal vaccine, 0.5 mL IM × 1
Varicella zoster virus (VZV)	Significant exposure to chickenpox or shingles for patients who have no history of either condition or, if available, negative antibody to VZV	Varicella zoster immune globulin (VZIG), 5 vials (1.25 mL each) IM, administered ideally within 48 h of exposure, but ≤ 96 h
II. Generall Recommended		
Hepatitis B virus	All susceptible (anti-HBc-negative) patients	Engerix B, 20 µg IM × 3 or Recombivax HB, 10 µg IM × 3
Influenza virus	All patients (annually, before influenza season)	Whole or split virus, 0.5 mL IM/yr
III. Indicated for Use Only in Selected Circumstances		
Candida species	CD4+ count < 50/µL	Fluconazole, 100–200 mg PO qd
Bacteria	Neutropenia	Granulocyte-colony-stimulating factor (G-CSF), 5–10 µg/kg SC qd × 2–4 wk *or* granulocyte-macrophage colony-stimulating factor (GM-CSF), 250 µg/m^2 IV over 2 h qd × 2–4 wk
Cryptococcus neoformans	CD4+ count < 50/µL	Fluconazole, 100–200 mg PO qd
Histoplasma capsulatum	CD4+ count < 100/µL, endemic geographic area	Itraconazole, 200 mg PO qd
Cytomegalovirus	CD4+ count < 50/µL and CMV-antibody positivity	Oral ganciclovir, 1 g PO tid

show minimal hypoxia (Pa_{O_2} 80 to 95 mm Hg), but in more advanced disease may be markedly abnormal. The onset of PCP is often insidious, occurring over a period of weeks, although more fulminant presentations can occur. The diagnosis of PCP is usually made by identification of the organism in induced sputum or in specimens obtained from bronchoalveolar lavage. Less commonly, transbronchial biopsy is used for diagnosis.

▶ TREATMENT: *Pneumocystis carinii* Pneumonia

Untreated PCP has a mortality of nearly 100%. Treatment with agents such as trimethoprim-sulfamethoxazole (TMP-SMZ or cotrimoxazole) or parenteral pentamidine is associated with a 60% to 100% response rate. Historically, pentamidine was the drug of choice for PCP until the 1970s, when Hughes compared the efficacy and tolerance of TMP-SMZ and pentamidine in children with PCP.[111] Both agents were found to be equally efficacious, but TMP-SMZ was less toxic. TMP-SMZ became the regimen of choice for treatment and subsequently prophylaxis of PCP in patients with and without HIV.[112]

TMP-SMZ, when used for the treatment of PCP, is usually given in doses of 15 to 20 mg/kg/d (based on the TMP component) as three to four divided doses. Doses of 12 to 15 mg/kg/d may be as effective and perhaps reduce the incidence of toxicity. TMP-SMZ is usually initiated by the intravenous route, although oral therapy (because oral absorption is high) may suffice in mildly ill and reliable patients or to complete a course of therapy after a response has been achieved with intravenous administration. If oral therapy is used, it would be prudent to document absorption with serum concentrations of TMP or SMZ, because gastrointestinal disturbances or a malabsorption syndrome are known to alter drug absorption in patients with AIDS. Target concentrations for TMP are between 5 and 8 µg/mL.

For treatment of HIV-associated PCP, pentamidine isethionate is administered intravenously usually in doses of 4 mg/kg/d, although a pilot study has reported successful treatment with 3 mg/kg/d.[113,114] The elimination half-life ranges from 6 to 10 hours, and renal elimination accounts for the majority of drug clearance.[115] Aerosolized pentamidine has also been used for the treatment of PCP. Comparative studies with intravenous pentamidine indicate that aerosolized pentamidine treatment is associated with a slower clinical response, higher rates of therapeutic failure, and PCP relapse.[115,116]

The efficacy of TMP-SMZ or pentamidine for treatment of an initial episode of PCP in HIV-infected individuals is similar, with published response rates between 60% and 80%. Although comparative studies between the two regimens are few, one prospective, randomized trial found that oxygenation improved more quickly and survival was better in those that received TMP-SMZ.[117] The optimum length of therapy for treatment of PCP with either agent is not known, but 21 days is commonly recommended. Clinical improvement in patients with AIDS is often slower than in non–AIDS patients. One study demonstrated improvement in chest radiograph or gallium scan in only two-thirds of patients at the end of treatment.[118] Thus, the lack of prompt clinical improvement is not necessarily an indication of no response. In fact, patients frequently may worsen before they improve. However, continued worsening after 4 days or lack of improvement after 7 to 10 days is an indication for a change in therapy, regardless of which agent was started initially. There are no data regarding the utility of concurrent therapy with both TMP-SMZ and pentamidine, and this approach is not recommended.

Adverse reactions to both TMP-SMZ and pentamidine are common and range between 20% and 85% in this setting. The more common adverse reactions seen with TMP-SMZ are rash, fever, leukopenia, elevated serum transaminases, and thrombocytopenia. Mild rashes should be watched closely for progression to more severe reactions, but are not an absolute contraindication to continuing therapy. The incidence of these adverse reactions is higher in HIV-infected individuals than in those not infected with HIV.[119] For pentamidine, side effects include hypotension, tachycardia, nausea, vomiting, severe hypoglycemia or hyperglycemia, pancreatitis, irreversible diabetes mellitus, elevated transaminases, nephrotoxicity, leukopenia, and cardiac arrhythmias. Some of these reactions appear infusion-rate related (hypotension, tachycardia) and can be minimized by infusing pentamidine over 1 hour or more. The overall incidence of adverse reactions to pentamidine appears similar between individuals infected with HIV and those not infected. Dosage modification or pharmacokinetic monitoring can reduce somewhat the toxicity of both pentamidine and TMP-SMZ.[118] Dose reductions of pentamidine from 4 to 3 mg/kg/d appear successful in minimizing further rises in serum creatinine. Maintenance of serum TMP concentrations between 5 and 8 μg/mL may help prevent severe myelosuppression.

The early addition of adjunctive corticosteroid therapy to anti-PCP regimens has been shown to decrease the risk of respiratory failure and improve survival in patients with AIDS and moderate to severe PCP ($Pao_2 < 70$ mm Hg or A-a gradient > 35 mm Hg).[120,121] The adverse effects associated with corticosteroid therapy in these patients were minimal, primarily an increased incidence of herpetic lesions, although some concerns exist about the potential for reactivation of tuberculosis. The optimal dose and duration of corticosteroid therapy have not been identified. The regimen currently recommended is 40 mg of prednisone orally twice daily during days 1 through 5; 40 mg once daily on days 6 through 10; and 20 mg once daily on days 11 through 21, or for the duration of therapy.[122] Methylprednisolone at 75% of the prednisone dose can be used if parenteral therapy is necessary. In general, adjunctive corticosteroid therapy should be initiated when antipneumocystis therapy is started, because the data supporting the use of corticosteroids are based on initiation within the first 24 to 72 hours of the start of antipneumocystis therapy.

Alternative therapies for PCP include dapsone plus trimethoprim, clindamycin plus primaquine, atovaquone, and trimetrexate. Dapsone should not be used alone for the treatment of PCP.[123] The combination of dapsone plus trimethoprim compared with TMP-SMZ was found to have similar efficacy in a small controlled trial of patients with AIDS and first episode PCP.[124] Treatment failures were 7% and 10%, respectively, for the dapsone–trimethoprim group versus the TMP-SMZ group. However, major adverse reactions (neutropenia and elevation of liver function tests) were significantly more common in the TMP-SMZ group and necessitated a change to alternate therapy more frequently. The group that received dapsone-trimethoprim had a higher incidence of methemoglobinemia, a known complication of dapsone. The existence of a drug interaction between dapsone and trimethoprim resulting in increased concentrations of each in the presence of the other may have contributed to the incidence of methemoglobinemia.[125]

Oral administration of dapsone-trimethoprim does appear to represent a satisfactory alternative for mild to moderately ill patients with PCP. Candidates for this regimen should be screened for glucose-6-phosphate dehydrogenase deficiency before therapy is initiated; individuals deficient in this enzyme should not receive dapsone. Malaise, fatigue, cyanosis, and decreased hemoglobin are suggestive of methemoglobinemia and methemoglobin concentrations should be obtained.

The combination of clindamycin (600 mg tid) and primaquine (30 mg qd) had efficacy similar to oral TMP-SMZ and dapsone-trimethoprim in a study of 181 patients with mild or moderate PCP.[126] The clindamycin-primaquine regimen was associated with potentially serious adverse reactions including rash, neutropenia, anemia, and methemoglobinemia. Atovaquone was found to be less effective than TMP-SMZ in a study of 322 patients with AIDS and mild or moderately severe PCP; however, treatment-limiting adverse reactions were less in the atovaquone recipients.[127] Trimetrexate has been useful for "salvage" therapy in patients who do not respond or cannot tolerate standard PCP therapies. The use of trimetrexate is complicated by myelosuppression, and simultaneous leucovorin must be administered during treatment and for 48 to 72 hours after trimetrexate is administered. In an open trial of trimetrexate-leucovorin, the survival rate appeared equivalent to that of TMP-SMZ and pentamidine, although relapse rates were high.[128]

PCP PROPHYLAXIS

HIV-infected individuals who have had PCP are at high risk for recurrent PCP if no prophylactic measures are taken. Even though the treatment of PCP is becoming increasingly successful, the mortality rate from first episode PCP is still between 5% to 20%, and therapy is often complicated by adverse reactions. Prevention of PCP is clearly a preferable strategy to treatment. A retrospective study of 100 HIV-infected individuals found that the circulating CD4 lymphocyte counts were < 200 cells/μL within 60 days before 46 of 49 episodes of PCP.[104] The relative risk of PCP in 1665 HIV-infected participants who did not have AIDS was 4.9 in those with CD4 lymphocyte counts < 200/μL.[129] These data indicate that HIV-infected adults with a CD4 count < 200 cells/μL or whose CD4 cells are < 20% of total lymphocytes are at high risk to develop PCP and are especially likely to benefit from prophylactic therapy. Prophylactic therapy for PCP is necessary despite treatment with antiretroviral agents. Currently, in the United States, PCP prophylaxis is recommended for all HIV-infected individuals who have already had previous PCP. Prophylaxis is also recommended for any HIV-infected person who has a CD4 lymphocyte count < 200 cells/μL or whose CD4 cells are < 20% of total lymphocytes, or who has had unexplained fever (> 100°F) for > 2 weeks, or a history of oropharyngeal candidiasis.[130] Patients on PCP prophylaxis whose CD4 counts increase above 200 cells/μL owing to antiretroviral therapy should not discontinue PCP prophylaxis at this point.

TMP-SMZ is the preferred therapy for both primary and secondary prophylaxis of PCP in adults and adolescents. TMP-SMZ has been found to be more effective than aerosolized pentamidine as secondary prophylaxis, is less expensive, and appears to confer cross-protection against toxoplasmosis and many bacterial infections. The earliest controlled study of TMP-SMZ for PCP prophylaxis in patients with AIDS used a regimen of 160-mg TMP and 800-mg SMZ orally, given twice daily with 5 mg of leucovorin given once daily.[131] No patient (0 of 30) developed PCP while taking TMP-SMZ. Additionally, the use of TMP-SMZ was associated with an increase in the mean survival time compared with those patients who received no prophylaxis. The addition of leucovorin to the TMP-SMZ regimen was an attempt to reduce the incidence of adverse reactions (primarily neutropenia and rash). The effectiveness of leucovorin for this use is unknown, however, because there was no group who received TMP-SMZ without leucovorin and 50% of patients who received the TMP-SMZ plus leucovorin combination still experienced some type of adverse reaction. This study established that PCP prophylaxis in patients with AIDS had a high degree of efficacy. Subsequently, a study of TMP-SMZ versus aerosolized pentamidine in 310 adults with AIDS recently recovered from an episode of PCP found 1-year estimated recurrence rate of 3.5% for TMP-SMZ but 18.5% for aerosolized pentamidine.[132] Results of an evaluation comparing TMP-SMZ, dapsone, and aerosolized pentamidine for primary PCP prophylaxis in 843 patients with HIV infection and < 200 CD4 cells indicate that all three treatment strategies have similar efficacy.[133] However, the lowest rates of PCP breakthrough among all subgroups were in those individuals currently taking TMP-SMZ. TMP-SMZ and dapsone were more effective than aerosolized pentamidine in patients with fewer than 100 CD4 cells. These data provide additional support for the selection of TMP-SMZ as the first-line agent for PCP prophylaxis. The recommended dose in adults and adolescents is one double-strength tablet daily, although other regimens, such as one double-strength tablet thrice weekly or one single-strength tablet daily, have been used in an attempt to reduce the incidence of adverse reactions and improve compliance.

TMP-SMZ is also the recommended drug of choice for PCP prophylaxis in children.[134] As previously described, the normal range for CD4 lymphocytes is very different for children than for adults. Both the absolute CD4 count and CD4 cells as a percentage of the total should be determined. A CD4 percentage less than 25% is an indication of immunosuppression. The utility of TMP-SMZ for prophylaxis is well established for children not HIV-infected receiving myelosuppressive therapy.[135] The TMP-SMZ regimen recommended (although other acceptable alternatives exist) is 150 mg/m^2/d of TMP and 750 mg/m^2/d of SMZ given in divided doses twice daily, three times weekly on consecutive days (Monday, Tuesday, Wednesday).[135] The total daily dose of TMP-SMZ in children should not exceed 320 mg of TMP with 1600 mg of SMZ. PCP prophylaxis in HIV-exposed/infected children is strongly recommended as follows: (1) all HIV-exposed infants beginning between 4 and 6 weeks of age and continuing to 12 months of age if infection status is unknown; (2) all HIV-infected infants beginning at 4 to 6 weeks of age to 12 months of age; and (3) all HIV-infected children greater than 1 year with severe immunosuppression.[134]

Alternative prophylactic regimens if TMP-SMZ cannot be tolerated include dapsone, dapsone plus pyrimethamine and leucovorin, aerosolized pentamidine, and atovaquone. A study of primary PCP prophylaxis in 843 HIV-infected patients found lower failure rates with TMP-SMZ and dapsone compared with aerosolized pentamidine.[133] Dapsone failures were more common with the 50 mg/d than the 100 mg/d dose. A dapsone plus pyrimethamine regimen would likely confer protection against toxoplasmosis but not against most bacterial pathogens. Aerosolized pentamidine has shown efficacy in the prevention of PCP. A three arm study of HIV-infected persons found that recipients of 300 mg of pentamidine via a Respirgard II nebulizer every 4 weeks had fewer confirmed episodes of PCP as compared to those who received 30 mg every 2 weeks or 150 mg every 2 weeks.[136] A placebo-controlled study demonstrated that aerosolized pentamidine (300 mg every 28 days) was 60% to 70% effective in preventing first episode PCP.[137] The most frequent adverse event related to aerosolized pentamidine use is cough. Pretreatment with a bronchodilator is widely used and may help alleviate this problem. Additional issues to be considered with the use of aerosolized pentamidine include potential for upper lobe pneumonia, presumably secondary to decreased drug deposition in these areas; late breakthrough disseminated disease (extrapulmonary pneumocystosis)[138]; and cost, because aerosolized pentamidine is considerably more expensive than TMP-SMZ. Other agents, which could be considered for prophylaxis of PCP when neither TMP-SMZ, dapsone, nor aerosolized pentamidine can be administered, include pyrimethamine-sulfadoxine, pyrimethamine-clindamycin, and clindamycin-primaquine. Insufficient data prevent a clear recommendation of the role of these regimens in the prophylaxis of PCP.

TOXOPLASMA GONDII

The seroprevalence of *Toxoplasma gondii* in HIV-infected individuals from major urban areas of the United States varies from 10% to 45%, but is considerably higher in countries such as France. The parasite is passed to humans from raw or undercooked meat and by contact with feces from infected cats. *T. gondii* can infect any organ of the body and cause an acute infection; it has a predilection for the brain and the eye. Once infected, the organism can replicate forming tissue cysts that persist for the life of the host. Many individuals will not have symptoms of disease. Immunosuppression, however, allows the release of tachyzoites from tissue cysts that produce a necrotic foci of infection, most often the brain. In the patient with AIDS, *T. gondii* is an important opportunistic pathogen, responsible for most focal intracerebral lesions.[139] A retrospective study suggested that 30% of AIDS patients seropositive for *T. gondii* will ultimately develop toxoplasmic encephalitis.[140]

CLINICAL PRESENTATION

The clinical signs and symptoms of toxoplasmosis are most frequently associated with involvement of the CNS, and less commonly the lungs and eyes, although any organ can be affected. Clinical presentation often includes fever, headache, seizures (in approximately 10% to 25% of patients), focal neurologic abnormalities (in approximately 60% to 90%), and mental status changes. Brain biopsy is required to make a definitive diagnosis of toxoplasmic encephalitis, although presumptive diagnosis is commonly made in *T. gondii* seropositive patients with typical CNS lesions. Characteristic radiographic abnormalities found by computerized axial tomography (CAT) or magnetic resonance imaging (MRI) have also been useful in the diagnosis of CNS toxoplasmosis.

▶ TREATMENT: CNS Toxoplasmosis

The initial treatment of CNS toxoplasmosis is usually empiric. Brain biopsy in the patient with AIDS may be complicated by potential morbidity, location of lesion(s), or thrombocytopenia. Anti-*Toxoplasma* therapy is usually initiated in patients with AIDS who are seropositive for *Toxoplasma* and have clinical symptoms suspicious for toxoplasmosis and characteristic findings on neuroradiographic studies (multiple ring-enhancing lesions). In this setting, brain biopsy is usually not undertaken unless the patient fails to respond clinically or radiologically to 10 to 14 days of therapy, or clinically deteriorates. Brain biopsy is an initial consideration in the *T. gondii* seronegative patient or in patients with atypical lesions.

The combination of pyrimethamine and sulfadiazine is considered the most effective regimen for acute therapy of AIDS-related CNS toxoplasmosis.[141] This regimen works synergistically by sequentially inhibiting two steps in folic acid synthesis of the proliferative form of *T. gondii.* There is no widespread agreement on the optimal doses of pyrimethamine and sulfadiazine. Pyrimethamine loading doses of 75 mg orally on the first day, followed by 25 mg/d thereafter have been commonly used. The erratic concentrations of pyrimethamine found in patients with AIDS and toxoplasmic encephalitis at lower doses (25 mg/d) have prompted some investigators to use larger doses.[142] Loading doses of 100 to 200 mg followed by daily oral doses of 1 to 1.5 mg/kg/d (50 to 100 mg/d) have been recommended.[143] The usual dose of sulfadiazine is 1 to 1.5 g every 6 hours (4 to 8 g/d). Folinic acid, in doses of 10 to 20 mg/d (although doses as high as 50 mg/d have been used) is usually added to the combination to reduce the pyrimethamine-induced bone marrow toxicity. Acute therapy with this combination should be continued for at least 3 weeks, but 6 weeks of treatment is recommended for more severely ill patients. Response rates (combined partial and complete) of approximately 85% have been observed following a minimum of 4 weeks of therapy. Adverse reactions, primarily bone marrow suppression associated with pyrimethamine and sulfadiazine hypersensitivity reactions, may limit therapy in as many as 40% of AIDS patients.[142] A regimen of pyrimethamine (50 mg daily) plus clindamycin (2400 mg daily) for 6 weeks followed by reduced-dose maintenance therapy was less effective (disease progression risk 1.8 times higher) than pyrimethamine-sulfadiazine.[141] The combination of pyrimethamine plus clindamycin does appear to be less toxic than that of pyrimethamine plus sulfadiazine. Other investigational alternative regimens include TMP-SMZ, and pyrimethamine and leucovorin plus either clarithromycin, azithromycin, atovaquone, or dapsone.

The discontinuation of pyrimethamine-sulfadiazine after successful initial therapy is associated with a relapse rate that may approach 100%.[144] Thus, lifelong maintenance therapy/secondary prophylaxis is recommended for AIDS patients to prevent recrudescence of the disease. Again, there is no general agreement on the doses of pyrimethamine and sulfadiazine to be used but it is likely that lower doses may be satisfactory if patients have had a favorable outcome from primary therapy. A regimen of pyrimethamine (25 to 75 mg/d with folinic acid) plus of sulfadiazine (500 to 1000 mg qid) has been recommended.[134] Pyrimethamine plus clindamycin can also be considered for maintenance therapy, but this regimen may be associated with a higher relapse rate. A further advantage to the combination of pyrimethamine plus sulfadiazine is that an additional agent for prophylaxis of PCP is unnecessary, which is not the case with the pyrimethamine plus clindamycin combination.[145]

TOXOPLASMA PROPHYLAXIS

Only limited information about primary prophylaxis of *T. gondii* in the HIV-infected person is available from carefully controlled prospective studies. However, data from several sources do suggest that it may be possible to prevent reactivation of latent toxoplasmosis. Regimens that have been found to have some efficacy in the primary prophylaxis of toxoplasmosis include TMP-SMZ, pyrimethamine plus dapsone, and pyrimethamine plus sulfadoxine (Fansidar). A double-blind placebo-controlled comparison of clindamycin and pyrimethamine was halted prematurely because adverse reactions (primarily diarrhea and rash) were significantly higher in the clindamycin group.[146] Pyrimethamine alone offers little if any protection. Prophylaxis for *T. gondii* is recommended for all HIV-infected persons with IgG antibody to *Toxoplasma* and CD4 count < 100/μL. The preferred regimen is TMP-SMZ.

CRYPTOCOCCUS NEOFORMANS

Infection with *Cryptococcus neoformans* occurs in up to 7% of individuals with AIDS in the United States.[147] Infections are probably originally contracted through inhalation, and the respiratory tract is believed to be the first infected site. Cryptococcal infection is the fourth most common infection in patients with AIDS and is the most common life-threatening fungal infection.

CLINICAL PRESENTATION

The usual clinical presentation of cryptococcal infection is meningitis, although recognition of pneumonia and disseminated disease may be increasing. The clinical features of cryptococcal meningitis may be subtle, nonspecific, and not localized to the CNS.[147] Fever, headache, and malaise are the most frequent symptoms. Meningeal features, mental status changes, and other focal neurologic signs occur in only a minority of patients. The diagnosis of cryptococcal meningitis should always be considered when HIV-infected individuals with advanced disease or low CD4 lymphocyte counts present with nonspecific symptoms or pulmonary or CNS findings.

Methods for diagnosis of cryptococcal infection includes serum and cerebrospinal fluid (CSF) testing for cryptococcal antigen, and fungal cultures. Detection of cryptococcal antigen in serum and CSF is the most sensitive and specific test; an antigen titer > 1:8 should be regarded as evidence for infection. Identification of *C. neoformans* on India ink examination of the CSF or from culture may also be used to confirm the diagnosis when antigen is unavailable. Factors suggestive of a poor prognosis in patients with cryptococcal meningitis include alteration in mental status, CSF antigen > 1:1024, a low CSF leukocyte count, and age > 35 years.

▶ TREATMENT: *Cryptococcus neoformans*

The goals of therapy for cryptococcal meningitis in patients with AIDS are to induce a remission and maintain a high quality of life. The standard therapeutic approach has been amphotericin B for both acute and maintenance therapy, though the introduction of azole compounds has changed the therapeutic approach for clinically stable patients. One retrospective evaluation supports the effectiveness of amphotericin B for the treatment of cryptococcal meningitis in patients with AIDS and the value of long-term suppressive therapy.[147] The addition of flucytosine to the amphotericin B regimen was not found to enhance survival in this retrospective evaluation of patients with AIDS, which is in marked contrast to data on this combination in non–AIDS patients with cryptococcal meningitis.[148] Early uncontrolled evaluations of the triazole compound, fluconazole, suggested efficacy of this drug for cryptococcal infections in AIDS patients.[149] The combination of amphotericin B and flucytosine, however, was found superior to fluconazole in one small, randomized trial in patients with AIDS and cryptococcal meningitis.[150] The largest controlled clinical trial of amphotericin B (mean daily dose 0.4 mg/kg) plus flucytosine at physician's discretion, versus fluconazole for cryptococcal meningitis, in 194 patients with AIDS found treatment was successful in 40% of the amphotericin recipients and in 34% of fluconazole.[151] The death rate in the first 2 weeks of treatment was 18% in the fluconazole arm and 14% in the amphotericin arm. The death rate after 2 weeks was 4% and 6%, respectively, in the fluconazole and amphotericin groups. The median time to sterilization of CSF cultures was 42 days in amphotericin B recipients and 64 days in those who received fluconazole. These data suggest that while fluconazole is effective for treatment of cryptococcal meningitis, amphotericin B is more effective because of its lower rates of early death and disease progression. Most patients with cryptococcal meningitis should probably receive amphotericin B in an intravenous dose of at least 0.5 mg/kg/d for a minimum of 2 weeks as acute therapy. Flucytosine in doses of 100 to 150 mg/kg/d can be considered for combination with amphotericin B; serum concentrations should be monitored and peak levels kept below 100 μg/mL to minimize hematologic adverse reactions. A recent trial did not find that the addition of flucytosine to an amphotericin B regimen of 0.7 mg/kg/d for 2 weeks significantly improved mortality, clinical course, or CSF culture status at 2 weeks.[152]

Once the acute treatment of cryptococcal meningitis is completed, maintenance therapy is necessary to prevent relapse. A retrospective review found that long-term suppressive therapy with either ketoconazole or amphotericin B was associated with improved survival in patients with AIDS.[147] Placebo-controlled trials of 100 to 200 mg/d of fluconazole, as well as controlled trials versus 1 mg/kg/wk of amphotericin B, have been conducted to prevent recurrence of cryptococcal disease in patients who completed acute therapy.[153,154] Compared with patients receiving amphotericin B maintenance therapy, the probability of remaining relapse free at 1 year was higher for fluconazole recipients (97% vs 78%) and the rate of serious drug toxicity was lower (7% vs 31%). Fluconazole is superior to either placebo, amphotericin, or itraconazole for maintenance therapy and is the drug of choice to prevent relapse of cryptococcal meningitis.

CRYPTOCOCCUS PROPHYLAXIS

In addition to treatment strategies, investigations are underway to determine whether fungal infections can be prevented. Results of a controlled trial of fluconazole (200 mg/d) versus clotrimazole troches (10 mg five times daily) suggest that after a median follow-up of 35 months, fluconazole recipients had a significant benefit in terms of reduced rate of invasive fungal infection (primarily cryptococcosis) and esophageal candidiasis.[155] For example, there was a total of 32 invasive fungal infections, 17 of which were cryptococcosis. Two cases occurred in fluconazole recipients, whereas 15 developed in clotrimazole recipients. The benefit of fluconazole therapy was greater for patients with < 50 CD4 cells/μL. The 2-year cumulative risk of cryptococcosis was 1.6% in the fluconazole group and 9.9% in the clotrimazole group ($P = .02$), in contrast to risks of 0.8% and 4.3%, respectively in patients with higher CD4 counts. There was, however, no survival difference between the two groups. Despite fluconazole therapy, 10.6% of recipients developed proved or presumed candidiasis, raising the possibility of emergence of resistance to fluconazole. Drug-resistant candidiasis caused by *Candida albicans* and *Candida krusei* has been observed in patients infected with HIV who are receiving fluconazole. The central question of whether the benefit of fluconazole and other agents for prophylaxis of fungal infections outweighs the risks, including resistance, remains to be clearly delineated. At present, routine antifungal prophylaxis of cryptococcosis is not recommended.

MYCOBACTERIUM INFECTIONS

Mycobacterium tuberculosis infection is a well-recognized and treatable complication of HIV infection and AIDS. A discussion of the clinical presentation and treatment is found elsewhere in this book.

Infections with nontuberculous mycobacterial organisms especially *Mycobacterium avium* complex (MAC) were recognized early in the AIDS epidemic. Disseminated MAC infections are among the most common systemic bacterial infections, reportedly occurring in up to 40% of patients with AIDS.[156,157] MAC is the index diagnosis of

AIDS in approximately 3% to 4% of HIV-infected individuals. The major risk factor for MAC is advanced immunosuppression; the mean CD4 lymphocyte count in patients with disseminated MAC is usually < 50 cells/μL, and infection is rare in individuals with >100 cells/μL. The organism is a common water and soil saprophyte; the routes of acquisition in patients with AIDS are thought to be gastrointestinal and/or respiratory. In patients with advanced HIV disease, MAC causes a widely disseminated infection. Local colonization can also occur and precede disseminated disease, although culture of sputum or gastrointestinal tract have a poor predictive value for subsequent disseminated MAC.

CLINICAL PRESENTATION

The clinical syndrome associated with MAC includes high spiking fevers, diarrhea, night sweats, malaise, weight loss, anemia, and neutropenia. Persistent diarrhea and abdominal pain, a malabsorption syndrome, and extrahepatic biliary obstruction are manifestations associated with MAC gastrointestinal infection. Diagnosis of MAC infection is usually based on culture of the organisms from the blood, although biopsies of the liver, bone marrow, and lymph nodes are also highly sensitive and specific. Diagnosis of disseminated MAC in advanced HIV disease suggests a poor long-term prognosis without therapy.

▶ TREATMENT: *Mycobacterium avium* Complex Infections

Unfortunately, MAC is resistant to the standard drugs used for tuberculosis like isoniazid and pyrazinamide. Multiple agents such as rifampin, rifabutin (ansamycin), clofazimine, imipenem, amikacin, ethambutol, ciprofloxacin, clarithromycin, and azithromycin have varying degrees of *in vitro* anti-MAC activity.[158] Controversy formerly existed as to whether treatment for MAC is beneficial, but recent data have been supportive that an aggressive therapeutic approach decreases symptoms and prolongs survival. One indication of the benefit of antimycobacterial therapy for MAC comes from a prospective evaluation of the treatment of MAC bacteremia in 367 patients with AIDS and CD4 cells ≤ 50/μL.[159] In this study, treatment was initiated within 60 days of positive mycobacterial culture; the treatment regimen was left to the discretion of the physician. MAC bacteremia was found to be associated with an increased risk of death and those patients who were treated had a longer median survival (263 vs 139 days, *P* < .001) than those who were not. A role for clarithromycin in the treatment of MAC is derived from a randomized, double-blind study of 154 patients with HIV infection, positive blood cultures for MAC, and symptomatic MAC disease.[160] After 6 weeks of clarithromycin therapy, mycobacterial quantitative blood cultures were significantly decreased; there was no difference in the reduction between the three regimens (500, 1000, and 2000 mg bid). Patients receiving 500 mg bid had a longer survival (median 249 days) and a lower death rate in the first 12 weeks than patients receiving 1000 mg or 2000 mg bid.

The largest randomized comparison of MAC treatment regimens evaluated rifabutin, ethambutol, and clarithromycin versus rifampin, ethambutol, clofazimine, and ciprofloxacin in 187 patients with AIDS.[161] Compared with the four-drug regimen, the recipients of the three-drug regimen had a significantly higher rate of bacteremia clearance (69% vs 29%) and better reduction in symptoms (fever or chills, night sweats, fatigue or malaise, nausea or anorexia, diarrhea, abdominal pain). Most important, the three-drug regimen of rifabutin, ethambutol, and clarithromycin improved the median survival by 65% (8.6 months vs 5.2 months).

There are several important issues regarding therapy of MAC, most notably whom to treat, which drugs to use and for how long, and how to assess response to therapy. A U.S. Public Health Service Task Force has constructed a series of recommendations to address these issues.[162] First, treatment regimens should contain at least two antimycobacterial agents. Second, every regimen should contain either clarithromycin or azithromycin. Of these agents, clarithromycin (500 mg bid) is the preferred agent for MAC treatment based on greater clinical experience. For the second agent numerous choices are available, although ethambutol (15 mg/kg/d) is preferred by many experts. Many clinicians would add a third and some a fourth drug to this regimen. Among the alternatives available for the third drug, only rifabutin (300 mg/d) has been shown to add a significant microbiologic benefit. The use of clofazimine at present is discouraged because of data indicating that its use may be associated with decreased survival.[163] Clinical responses usually occur within 2 to 8 weeks of the start of therapy. If a clinical and microbiologic response is observed, therapy should continue for the duration of the patient's life.

MAC PROPHYLAXIS

Disseminated MAC infection contributes significantly to morbidity and mortality in the HIV-infected person; therapy is not uniformly successful, and a high-risk population can be identified. Therefore, a basis for prophylaxis of MAC exists and guidelines have been published.[162] Two trials of rifabutin for prophylaxis have been conducted in patients with AIDS and CD4 cell counts < 200/μL.[164] In both, rifabutin significantly reduced the incidence of MAC bacteremia, 17% for placebo versus 8% for rifabutin in the first, and 18% for placebo versus 9% for rifabutin in the second. These data indicate that rifabutin can decrease by about 50% the incidence of MAC bacteremia. The dose of rifabutin used is 300 mg qd, and prophylactic therapy should continue for the patient's lifetime unless disseminated MAC develops. Clarithromycin and azithromycin have both been reported to reduce the risk of disseminated MAC. In a double-blind placebo-controlled study, 682 persons with AIDS and CD4 lymphocyte counts < 100 were randomized to receive clarithromycin, 500 mg bid, or placebo.[165] MAC bacteremia developed nearly three times as often in placebo as in clarithromycin recipients. There were 19 (6%) breakthrough MAC infections in the clarithromycin group versus 53 (16%) in the placebo arm (*P* < .001). Clarithromycin-resistant strains of MAC were detected in some patients. During about 10 months of follow-up, 32% of the patients who received clarithromycin died compared with 41% (*P* = .026) in the placebo group. Azithromycin has also been shown to have a protective benefit against MAC infection. A three-arm trial evaluated azithromycin (1200 mg weekly), rifabutin (300 mg daily), or the combination in 693 HIV-infected persons with < 100 CD4 cells/μL.[166] The incidence of disseminated MAC infection at 1 year was 7.6% for azithromycin, 15.3% for rifabutin, and 2.6% for the combination. MAC isolates resistant to azithromycin were found in 11% of the patients who failed azithromycin prophylaxis. Dose-limiting adverse reactions, primarily gastrointestinal, were more common in the azithromycin plus rifabutin group. There was no difference in survival among the three regimens.

PROPHYLAXIS

MAC prophylaxis is now strongly recommended for all HIV-infected adults and adolescents with a CD4 count < 50 cells/μL.[134] The first-line choices are either azithromycin or clarithromycin. Persons considered for prophylaxis should be evaluated to be sure they do not have active disease due to MAC or *M. tuberculosis*.

HERPES VIRUS INFECTIONS

HERPES SIMPLEX VIRUS

Herpes simplex viruses (HSV) types 1 and 2 cause significant morbidity in patients with AIDS. Seropositivity for HSV is widespread among adults with AIDS, and clinical disease is usually the result of reactivation of latent virus. The manifestations of HSV disease observed in persons with AIDS include orolabial, genital, or anorectal mucocutaneous disease; esophagitis; and less commonly encephalitis. Ulcerative HSV lesions present for longer than 1 month in an individual with laboratory evidence for HIV infection, or no other apparent cause for immunodeficiency, are considered an AIDS-defining condition.

Anorectal lesions are the most common clinically evident HSV disease causing morbidity in homosexual men with AIDS, and likely reflect the common risk factors for acquisition (sexual contact) of both HSV and HIV. Chronic perianal HSV lesions were among the first opportunistic infections associated with AIDS.[167] Symptoms include pain, itching, and painful defecation. The clinical presentation of anal, orolabial, and genital herpes in the patient with AIDS is similar to that in other immunosuppressed individuals. The severity of the episode can range from mild to severely destructive. The severity of mucocutaneous HSV disease increases with progressive immunosuppression. Other HSV manifestations such as encephalitis are rare in the patient with AIDS, but are life threatening. Differentiation from other central nervous system infections such as those caused by *C. neoformans* or *T. gondii* is important, and prompt treatment is essential.

Acyclovir is the drug of choice for treatment of HSV disease. For mild to moderate mucocutaneous disease, oral acyclovir in doses of 200 mg five times daily or 400 mg tid are used, although regimens of 400 mg five times daily have occasionally been described as clinically necessary. Intravenous acyclovir (15 mg/kg/d) should be used in those settings where absorption of oral drug is questionable, or oral tolerance is unlikely (HSV esophagitis) or perhaps when severe mucocutaneous disease is present. Treatment of mucocutaneous disease should be continued until all lesions have crusted. Intravenous acyclovir (30 mg/kg/d) should also be used for viscerally disseminated disease and for HSV encephalitis. Famciclovir and valacyclovir are alternatives to oral acyclovir.

Recurrent HSV disease is common in many patients with AIDS following discontinuation of therapy. These individuals can often be managed with low-dose suppressive oral acyclovir therapy, as have other immunosuppressed patients at risk for frequently recurring HSV diseases.[168] Regimens commonly used include acyclovir 200 mg qid, 400 mg bid, or 800 mg qd.

Acyclovir-resistant HSV has been isolated from patients with AIDS.[169] The primary mechanism of resistance appears to be a deficiency in viral thymidine kinase. Strategies that have been employed for management of severe, acyclovir-resistant HSV infections include increasing the dose of acyclovir, discontinuation of acyclovir, or use of an alternative antiviral agent. Vidarabine and foscarnet, because they do not require phosphorylation by thymidine kinase, are examples of potential alternative agents.[170,171] A randomized comparison of foscarnet and vidarabine indicates that foscarnet is more effective and associated with fewer adverse reactions than vidarabine.[172]

VARICELLA-ZOSTER VIRUS

Most adults with AIDS have been previously infected with varicella-zoster virus (VZV) and thus are not susceptible to primary infection (chickenpox) but may develop recurrent infection (zoster). The prevalence of zoster in HIV-infected individuals appears higher than in other age-matched immunocompetent persons and seems to reliably herald the loss of cell-mediated immunity and progression to AIDS.[173,174]

Zoster usually begins as radicular pain followed by localized erythematous rash and characteristic vesicles. Zoster will usually remain confined to a limited number of dermatomes, but complications such as widespread cutaneous involvement and disseminated visceral zoster may occur. As with the treatment of HSV infections, acyclovir is the drug of choice for VZV infections. Although an oral acyclovir regimen of 4 g/d has been shown effective for the treatment of zoster in immunocompetent adults, the drug has not been fully evaluated in immunocompromised patients such as those with AIDS.[175] For practical reasons, oral acyclovir, valacyclovir, or famciclovir are often used for localized zoster. However, careful monitoring for signs of progression of zoster is essential. AIDS patients with disseminated cutaneous or visceral zoster should receive treatment with intravenous acyclovir in doses of 30 mg/kg/d for at least 7 days or until all lesions are crusted. Acyclovir-resistant VZV infections have been reported in patients with AIDS.[176]

CYTOMEGALOVIRUS

Cytomegalovirus (CMV) is the most common life-threatening viral infection in patients with AIDS. Like other herpes group viruses, infection with CMV is ubiquitous; seropositivity among homosexual men with AIDS approaches 100%.[177] There are numerous manifestations of CMV infection including retinitis, esophagitis, hepatitis, gastrointestinal involvement, and less commonly radiculopathy, encephalitis, and pneumonitis. CMV end-organ disease occurs in up to 44.9% of AIDS patients, particularly when their CD4 cell count is below 50/μL. The incidence, however, appears to be decreasing in the era of HAART.[178]

CMV retinitis, the most commonly recognized CMV disease associated with AIDS, occurs in approximately 29% to 32% of patients with AIDS.[179] CMV retinitis is usually associated with a painless progressive loss of vision. Patients may initially complain of blurry vision, loss of visual acuity or "floaters." CMV retinitis usually begins unilaterally, but bilateral involvement may occur. Untreated, CMV retinitis invariably leads to blindness. The diagnosis of CMV retinitis is made by funduscopic examination and identification of characteristic findings. Lesions characteristic of CMV retinitis include a fluffy white perivascular exudate frequently associated with hemorrhage. Early diagnosis and treatment are crucial to prevent further visual deterioration.

The first approved agent of treatment for CMV diseases was ganciclovir. Structurally ganciclovir differs from acyclovir by only a single hydroxyl side chain, but it is 30 to 50 times more active *in vitro* against CMV. The use of ganciclovir therapy has traditionally been divided into two phases, induction and maintenance, because high relapse rates are found after discontinuation of the drug following successful completion of a 2- to 3-week course of initial therapy. Induction regimens are typically 7.5 to 10 mg/kg/d intravenously in two or three equally divided doses for 14 days or longer if there is a slow clinical response. Maintenance therapy is usually 5 to 6 mg/kg once daily, although doses of 10 mg/kg have been used, 5 to 7 days a week for an indefinite period of time. Initial response rates for retinal CMV disease range from 60% to 90%.[180,181] Unfortunately, even with intravenous maintenance therapy, relapse of CMV retinitis is common and occurs at a median of approximately 55 to 80 days.

Despite the poor oral bioavailability of ganciclovir (6% to 9%), oral regimens have been evaluated as a possible alternative to long-term intravenous maintenance administration. Two randomized trials have evaluated intravenous or oral ganciclovir as maintenance therapy for CMV retinitis. In both studies, oral ganciclovir maintenance therapy was associated with a slightly more rapid rate of disease progression. The differences in mean time to progression ranged from 5 to 11 days.[182,183] The convenience of oral administration, however, may favor use of oral drug in certain individuals. The recommended dose of oral ganciclovir for maintenance therapy of CMV retinitis is 1000 mg tid taken with food. CMV isolates resistant to ganciclovir have been recovered from immunocompromised patients; the incidence and prevalence remain to be determined.[184]

Neutropenia and thrombocytopenia are the most common drug- or dose-limiting adverse reactions associated with use of intravenous ganciclovir. Up to 50% of patients with AIDS receiving ganciclovir (alone) may need a dose reduction or interruption of therapy as a result of hematologic toxicity. The combination of zidovudine and ganciclovir is poorly tolerated by HIV-infected individuals owing to additive hematologic toxicity.[185] Filgrastim (G-CSF), erythropoietin, or sargramostim (GM-CSF) offers some potential amelioration of the adverse hematologic effects of ganciclovir. Intravitreal administration has also been used as salvage therapy in an attempt to circumvent these adverse reactions.[179]

Sustained-release intraocular ganciclovir implants represent another strategy developed not only to overcome systemic toxicity but to preclude the need for intravitreal injections.[186] Twenty-six patients (30 eyes) were enrolled in an evaluation of immediate therapy with a ganciclovir intraocular implant intended to release 1 μg/h of ganciclovir over an 8-month period, or deferred treatment until progression of retinitis. The median time to progression of retinitis was 15 days in the deferred group but was 226 days ($P <$ .00001) in the immediate-implant recipients. This small study presents compelling evidence that the ganciclovir implant has efficacy for the treatment of CMV retinitis.

Further evidence of efficacy was demonstrated by the ganciclovir-implant study group.[187] One-hundred and seventy three patients representing 222 eyes were randomized to receive either ganciclovir implant 1 μg/h (75 eyes), 2 g/h (71 eyes), or intravenous ganciclovir (76 eyes). Median progression to CMV retinitis was similar in the 1 and 2 μg/h implant groups, 221 days and 191 days, respectively; however, median time to progression in the patients treated with intravenous ganciclovir was 71 days ($P < .001$). Intravenous ganciclovir was associated with an almost threefold risk of progression compared with ganciclovir implants. Ganciclovir implants, however, do not protect patients from CMV occurring elsewhere, including the initially uninvolved eye. Intravenous ganciclovir cuts by half the risk of CMV retinitis in the initially uninvolved eye. Extraocular involvement of CMV did not occur in patients receiving intravenous ganciclovir compared with 10.3% of patients who received an implant only. Therefore, patients having an implant should also receive systemic therapy such as oral ganciclovir.

Foscarnet is a pyrophosphate analog with both anti-HIV and anti-CMV activity. Controlled trials to evaluate immediate versus delayed foscarnet therapy of CMV retinitis in HIV-infected individuals found immediate foscarnet therapy more effective than delayed therapy in preventing progression of CMV disease.[188] Furthermore, prolonged survival and an anti-HIV effect (as assessed by a decline in HIV or p24 antigen) was observed.[189] An unblinded randomized trial comparing ganciclovir with foscarnet therapy of CMV retinitis was conducted in 234 patients with AIDS.[190] Both drugs were administered in standard 14-day induction regimens followed by maintenance therapy. Ganciclovir and foscarnet were equally effective in delaying the progression of CMV disease. The median time to progression of retinitis was 56 days in the ganciclovir groups and 59 days in the foscarnet group. There was a difference, however, in survival between these two groups. Median survival was 8.5 months for ganciclovir recipients, whereas it was 12.6 months for those who received foscarnet. The explanation for this survival difference is unknown. It is conceivable that the difference in mortality was owing to the anti-HIV effect of foscarnet. Adverse reactions that necessitated a switch in therapy were more common among the foscarnet recipients. The choice of therapy for CMV retinitis is largely dictated by the adverse reaction profiles of the two agents, convenience, concomitant medications being taken by the patient, and underlying disease states.

Although foscarnet appears less likely to cause neutropenia than ganciclovir, it has a variety of potential adverse effects. The most common side effects are renal insufficiency and metabolic disturbances (both increases and decreases) in calcium and phosphorus. Other adverse reactions include anemia, thrombocytopenia, infusion-site reactions, nausea and vomiting, penile ulcerations, and seizures. Hydration has been demonstrated to reduce the incidence of serum creatinine elevations from 66% in a nonhydrated control group to 13% in hydrated individuals.[191] Foscarnet, like ganciclovir, is currently administered in two phases, induction and maintenance. Induction doses are 180 mg/kg/d intravenously in two or three divided doses for 14 days, followed by maintenance therapy in doses of 90 to 120 mg/kg intravenously once daily; foscarnet doses must be adjusted in individuals with renal insufficiency.

Other approaches to the treatment of CMV disease include the combination of ganciclovir and foscarnet, and cidofovir. In patients who have relapsed CMV retinitis, the ganciclovir-foscarnet combination was compared with retreatment with either drug alone.[192] The median times to retinitis progression were foscarnet, 1.3 months; ganciclovir, 2.0 months; and ganciclovir-foscarnet, 4.3 months. Adverse events among the three groups were similar. However, the combined use of ganciclovir-foscarnet had the greatest negative impact on quality of life most likely because of the time-intensive and complex administration requirements. Cidofovir is a nucleotide analogue shown to delay the progression of CMV retinitis. In a study of 64 patients with AIDS and previously untreated CMV retinitis, the median time to progression was 21 days in the deferred-therapy group versus 64 days in those who received low-dose cidofovir.[193] While cidofovir has certain advantages over ganciclovir and foscarnet including its less frequent dosing schedule, the drug is nephrotoxic and can cause irreversible damage to the proximal renal tubules. Cidofovir must be given with aggressive IV hydration and concomitant probenecid, although these efforts only reduce, not prevent, nephrotoxicity. Also of concern is the finding that cidofovir did not show a significant effect on CMV viremia at the 3-week assessment point in the trial previously mentioned; this finding is in contrast to ganciclovir or foscarnet, which both suppress CMV viremia.

Various strategies have been evaluated to determine whether CMV disease in HIV-infected individuals can be prevented. High-dose oral acyclovir has been shown effective in reducing the incidence of CMV infection and disease in bone marrow and renal transplant recipients but not in patients infected with HIV.[194–196] Valacyclovir is an oral prodrug of acyclovir that achieves three to four fold higher concentrations following an equivalent dose. Valacyclovir given 2 g qid reduced the relative risk of CMV disease by 33% compared with acyclovir given either as 3.2 g or 800 mg per day.[196] The delay in developing disease was also longer in the valacyclovir-treated group. A randomized, double-blind, placebo-controlled study of oral ganciclovir (1000 mg q8h) in CMV-seropositive patients with AIDS found that oral ganciclovir significantly reduced the incidence of CMV disease.[197] CMV disease occurred in 26% of placebo recipients versus 14% of ganciclovir recipients ($P < .001$). However, there was no difference in survival between the two groups: The 1-year mortality rate was 26% for placebo versus 21% for ganciclovir recipients. A study of oral ganciclovir for prevention in patients with a slightly higher CD4 lymphocyte count did not find any protective benefit. Currently, prophylaxis with oral ganciclovir should be considered in HIV-infected adults and adolescents who have a CD4 cell count < 50 cells/μL; ganciclovir prophylaxis is not a recommended standard of care.

CMV infection of the gastrointestinal tract can involve sites ranging from the esophagus and stomach to the colon and rectum. In one series of AIDS patients with gastrointestinal tract infection, the colon was the most common site of infection, followed by the stomach or esophagus.[198] CMV colitis may be characterized by abdominal pain, fever, weight loss, and diarrhea, symptoms quite common among patients with HIV disease even in the absence of CMV infection. Characteristic symptoms of CMV esophagitis are dysphagia and substernal chest pain. Barium contrast studies may demonstrate abnormalities but will not distinguish between other etiologic agents such as candida or HSV, both of which are more common. The definitive diagnosis of CMV gastrointestinal infection requires endoscopy and biopsy with histologic identification of CMV inclusions or in situ antigen detection.

The therapy of CMV gastrointestinal disease has been more controversial. Few randomized, controlled trials have been conducted. A small randomized comparison of ganciclovir and foscarnet for AIDS-associated gastrointestinal disease found both therapies equally effective.[199] Judged by endoscopy, 83% of foscarnet recipients and 85% of ganciclovir recipients showed a response. Survival, however, was poor, at less than 40 weeks for both groups. Although patients were not randomized to receive maintenance therapy or not, it is interesting that there was no difference in the time to progression of disease between those who did and did not. Symptomatic CMV gastrointestinal disease warrants treatment and it appears that ganciclovir and foscarnet are equivalent. The role of maintenance therapy is less clear.

CONCLUSION

Irrefutable progress has been made in the management of HIV: Disease progression can be delayed, survival can be prolonged, and the risk of maternal-to-fetal HIV transmission can be reduced. Thirteen antiretroviral agents are now available for clinical use, and additional compounds are likely to follow. However, therapy is still suboptimal in that complete suppression of viral replication has not been achieved. There remain significant deficits in our understanding of the virologic and immunologic processes associated with HIV infection and the clinical pharmacology of anti-HIV compounds. Critical issues include the need for simpler and more potent regimens, emergence of drug-resistant viral isolates, and the inexorably progressive nature of HIV infection in some patients despite antiretroviral therapy. There is a clear need for more selective and potent inhibitors of HIV. The medical management of opportunistic infections associated with HIV disease has also changed dramatically since the recognition of AIDS early in the 1980s and has improved survival. The approach to PCP is most illustrative. The transition from an era marked by only treatment of established disease to one where primary and secondary prophylaxis based on CD4 lymphocyte count are standards of care reflects progress both in understanding the risk factors for opportunistic infections and in pharmacologic therapy. Collectively, three important lessons have been learned from the treatment of HIV and associated opportunistic infections: the need for prospective immunologic and virologic monitoring and early recognition of HIV infection; the use of potent combinations of antiretroviral agents to maximally inhibit viral replication; and primary and secondary prophylaxis of opportunistic infections. Emphasis on these principles coupled with carefully controlled investigations of novel agents and therapeutic strategies will continue to offer definite benefit and improve the quality of life for HIV-infected individuals and will yield an advantage over this pernicious virus that causes AIDS.

▶ PRINCIPLES OF PHARMACOTHERAPY

- Infection with HIV causes a spectrum of diseases, the end-stage manifestation of which is AIDS.
- Ongoing replication of HIV has a primary role in the onset and progression of disease.
- The replication of HIV can be suppressed with a potent combination of antiretroviral agents, which, for a period of time, can prevent further progression of disease.
- General principles for the management of opportunistic infections include prospective monitoring, primary prophylaxis, treatment, and secondary prophylaxis.

ACKNOWLEDGMENTS

We thank Teresa A. Tartaglione for her invaluable contributions to this chapter in the first and second editions of this textbook. We also acknowledge grant support (RO1 AI 33835, UO1 41089, UO1 38858, UO1 AI27551, UO1 AI 27661, AI 27757, and AI 27664) from the National Institute of Allergy and Infectious Disease.

REFERENCES

1. Centers for Disease Control. *Pneumocystis* pneumonia— Los Angeles. MMWR 1981;30:250–252.
2. Centers for Disease Control. Kaposi's sarcoma and *Pneumocystis* pneumonia among homosexual men—New York City and California. MMWR 1981;30:305–308.
3. Barre-Sinoussi F, Chermann JC, Rey F, et al. Isolation of a T-lymphotropic retrovirus from a patient at risk for acquired immunodeficiency syndrome (AIDS). Science 1983;220:868–871.
4. Gallo RC, Salahuddin SZ, Popovic M, et al. Frequent detection and isolation of cytopathic retroviruses (HTLV-III) from patients with AIDS and at risk for AIDS. Science 1984;224:500–503.
5. Centers for Disease Control. HIV/AIDS Surveillance Report 1997;9: 1–37.
6. United Nations Program on HIV/AIDS. Report on the global HIV/AIDS epidemic. 1997.
7. Quinn T. Global burden of the HIV pandemic. Lancet 1996;348:99–106.
8. Centers for Disease Control. 1993 revised classification system for HIV infection and expanded surveillance case definition for AIDS among adolescents and adults. MMWR 1993;41(RR-17):1–19.
9. Nahmias AJ, Weiss J, Yao X, et al. Evidence for human infection with an HTLV-III LAV-like virus in Central Africa, 1959. Lancet 1986;1:1279–1280.
10. Workshop Report from the European Commission and the Joint United Nations Programme on HIV/AIDS. HIV-1 subtypes: Implications for epidemiology, pathogenicity, vaccines and diagnostics. AIDS 1997;11:17–36.
11. Nuwayhid NF. Laboratory tests for detection of human immunodeficiency virus type 1 infection. Clin Diagn Lab Immunol 1995;2:637–645.
12. Horsburgh CR Jr, Ou CY, Jason J, et al. Duration of human immunodeficiency virus infection before detection of antibody. Lancet 1989;2:637–639.
13. Gallo D, George JR, Fitchen JS, et al. Evaluation of a system using oral mucosal transudate for HIV-1 antibody screening and confirmatory testing. JAMA 1997;277:254–258.
14. Frank AP, Wandell MG, Headings MD, et al. Anonymous HIV testing using home collection and telemedicine counseling. Arch Intern Med 1997;157:309–314.
15. Mulder J, McKinney N, Christopherson C, et al. A rapid and simple PCR assay for quantitation of HIV-1 RNA in plasma: Application to acute retroviral infection. J Clin Microbiol 1994;32:292–300.
16. Pachl C, Todd JA, Kern DG, et al. Rapid and precise quantification of HIV-1 RNA in plasma using a branched DNA signal amplification assay. J Acquir Immune Defic Syndr 1994;8:446–454.
17. Van Gemen B, Kievits T, Schukkink R, et al. Quantification of HIV-1 RNA in plasma using NASBA during a primary HIV-1 infection. J Virol Methods 1993;43:177–188.
18. Mellors JW, Muñoz A, Giorgi JV, et al. Plasma viral load and CD_4+ lymphocytes as prognostic markers of HIV-1 infection. Ann Intern Med 1997;126:946–954.
19. Mellors JW, Rinaldo CR Jr, Gupta P, et al. Prognosis in HIV-1 infection predicted by the quantity of virus in plasma. Science 1996;272: 1167–1170.
20. Centers for Disease Control. Public Health Service Task Force on antipneumocystis prophylaxis in human immunodeficiency virus–infected individuals. MMWR 1989;38:1–9.
21. Anderson RE, Lang W, Shiboski S, et al. Use of β_2-microglobulin level and CD4 lymphocyte count to predict development of acquired immunodeficiency syndrome in persons with human immunodeficiency virus infection. Arch Intern Med 1990;150:73–77.
22. Reddy MH, Grieco MM. Neopterin and alpha and beta interleukin 1 levels in sera of patients with human immunodeficiency virus infection. J Clin Microbiol 1989;27:1919–1923.
23. Liuzzi G, Chirianni A, Clementi M, et al. Analysis of HIV-1 load in blood, semen and saliva: Evidence for different viral components in a cross-sectional and longitudinal study. AIDS 1996;10:F51–F56.
24. Anderson RM, May RM. Epidemiological parameters of HIV transmission. Nature 1988;333:514–519.
25. Seidlin M, Vogler M, Lee E, et al. Heterosexual transmission of HIV in a cohort of couples in New York City. AIDS 1993;7:1247–1254.
26. Padian NS, Shiboski SC, Glass SO, et al. Heterosexual transmission of human immunodeficiency virus (HIV) in northern California: Results from a ten-year study. Am J Epidemiol 1997;146:350–357.
27. Wasserheit JN. Epidemiological synergy: Interrelationships between human immunodeficiency virus infection and other sexually transmitted diseases. Sex Transm Dis 1992;19:61–77.

28. Chaisson MA, Stoneburner RL, Joseph SC. Human immunodeficiency virus transmission through artificial insemination. J Acquir Immune Defic Syndr 1990;3:69–72.
29. Bratt GA, Berglund, T, Glantzberg BL, et al. Two cases of oral-to-genital HIV-1 transmission. Int J STD AIDS 1997;8:522–525.
30. Friedland GH, Saltzman BR, Rogers MF, et al. Lack of transmission of HTLV-III/LAV infection to household contacts of patients with AIDS or AIDS-related complex with oral candidiasis. N Engl J Med 1986;314:344–349.
31. Schacker T, Collier AC, Hughes J, et al. Clinical and epidemiologic features of primary HIV infection. Ann Intern Med 1996;125:257–264.
32. Schreiber GB, Busch MP, Kleinman SH, et al. The risk of transfusion-transmitted viral infections. N Engl J Med 1996;26:1685–1690.
33. Vidmar L, Poljak M, Tomazic J, et al. Transmission of HIV-1 by human bite. Lancet 1996;347:1762–1763.
34. Centers for Disease Control. Transmission of HIV possibly associated with exposure of mucous membrane to contaminated blood. MMWR 1997;46:620–623.
35. Cardo DM, Culver DH, Ciesielski CA, et al. A case-control study of HIV seroconversion in health care workers after percutaneous exposure. N Engl J Med 1997;337:1485–1490.
36. Bell DM, Gerberding JL, eds. Human immunodeficiency virus (HIV) postexposure management of health care workers. Am J Med 1997; 102(5B):5B-1S–5B-126S.
37. World Health Organization. Global AIDS Surveillance. Weekly Epidemiological Record 1997;72:17–24.
38. Landesman SH, Kalish LA, Burns DN, et al. Obstetrical factors and the transmission of human immunodeficiency virus type 1 from mother to child. N Engl J Med 1996;334:1685–1690.
39. Sperling RS, Shapiro DE, Coombs RW, et al. Maternal viral load, zidovudine treatment, and the risk of transmission of human immunodeficiency virus type 1 from mother to infant. N Engl J Med 1996; 335:1621–1629.
40. Dunn DT, Newell ML, Ades AE, et al. Risk of human immunodeficiency virus type 1 transmission through breastfeeding. Lancet 1992; 340:585–589.
41. Dalgleish AG, Beverly PCL, Clapham PR, et al. The CD4 (T4) antigen is an essential component of the receptor for the AIDS retrovirus. Nature 1984;312:763–767.
42. Cocchi F, DeVico A, Garzino-Demo A, et al. Identification of RANTES, MIP-1α and MIP-1β as the major HIV-suppressive factors produced by CD8+ T cells. Science 1995;270:1811–1815.
43. Feng Y, Broder CC, Kennedy PE, et al. HIV-1 entry cofactor: Functional cDNA cloning of a seven-transmembrane, G protein-coupled receptor. Science 1996;272:872–877.
44. Doranz BJ, Rucker J, Yi Y, et al. A dual-tropic primary HIV-1 isolate that uses fusin and the β-chemokine receptors CKR-5, CKR-3, and CKR-2b as fusion cofactors. Nature 1996;85:1149–1158.
45. Dean M, Carrington M, Winkler C, et al. Genetic restriction of HIV-1 infection and progression by a deletion allele of the CKR5 structural gene. Science 1996;273:1856–1861.
46. Bedinger P, Moriarty A, von Borstel RC Jr, et al. Internalization of the human immunodeficiency virus does not require the cytoplasmic domain of CD4. Nature 1988;334:162–165.
47. Preston BD, Poiesz BJ, Loeb LA, et al. Fidelity of HIV-1 reverse transcriptase. Science 1988;242:1168–1171.
48. Michie CA, McLean A, Alcock C, et al. Lifespan of human lymphocyte subsets defined by CD45 isoforms. Nature 1992;360:264–265.
49. Chowers MY, Spina CA, Kwoh TJ, et al. Optimal infectivity *in vitro* of HIV-1 requires an intact nef gene. J Virol 1994;68:2906–2914.
50. Deacon NJ, Tsykin A, Soloman A, et al. Genomic structure of an attenuated quasi species of HIV-1 from a blood transfusion donor and recipients. Science 1995;270:988–991.
51. Kohl NE, Emini EA, Schlief WA, et al. Active human immunodeficiency virus protease is required for viral infectivity. Proc Natl Acad Sci USA 1988;85:4686–4690.
52. Ho DD, Neumann AU, Perelson AS, et al. Rapid turnover of plasma virions and CD4 lymphocytes in HIV-1 infection. Nature 1995;323: 123–126.
53. Wei X, Ghosh SK, Taylor ME, et al. Viral dynamics in human immunodeficiency virus type 1 infection. Nature 1995;373:117–122.
54. Perelson AS, Neumann AU, Markowitz M, et al. HIV-1 dynamics *in vivo:* Virion clearance rate, infected cell life-span, and viral generation time. Science 1996;271:1582–1586.
55. Pantaleo G, Graziosi C, Fauci A. New concepts in the immunopathogenesis of human immunodeficiency virus infection. N Engl J Med 1993;328:327–335.
56. Lane HC, Masur H, Edgar LC, et al. Abnormalities of B-cell activation and immunoregulation in patients with the acquired immunodeficiency syndrome. N Engl J Med 1983;309:453–458.
57. Smith P, Ohura K, Masur H, et al. Monocyte function in the acquired immunodeficiency syndrome: Defective chemotaxis. J Clin Invest 1984;74:2121–2128.
58. LeBoit PE. Dermatopathologic findings in patients infected with HIV. Dermatol Clin 1992;10:59–71.
59. Piatak M Jr, Saag MS, Yang LC, et al. High levels of HIV-1 in plasma during all stages of infection determined by competative PCR. Science 1993;259:1749–1754.
60. Niu MT, Stein DS, Schnittman SM, et al. Primary human immunodeficiency virus type 1 infection. J Infect Dis 1993;168:1490–1501.
61. Mu-oz A, Wang MC, Bass S, et al. Acquired immunodeficiency syndrome (AIDS)-free time after human immunodeficiency virus type 1 (HIV-1) seroconversion in homosexual men. Am J Epidemiol 1989; 130:530–539.
62. Edelman AS, Zolla-Pazner S. AIDS: A syndrome of immune dysregulation, dysfunction, and deficiency. FASEB J 1989;3:22–30.
63. Wykoff RF, Pearl RF, Saulsbury FT, et al. Immunologic dysfunction in infants infected through transfusions with HTLV-III. N Engl J Med 1985;312:294–296.
64. Falloon J, Eddy J, Wiener L, et al. Human immunodeficiency virus infection in children. J Pediatr 1989;114:1–29.
65. Working Group on Antiretroviral Therapy and Medical Management of HIV Infected Children. Guidelines for the use of antiretroviral agents in pediatric HIV infection. http://www.hivatis.org
66. Panel on Clinical Practices for Treatment of HIV Infection. Guidelines for the use of antiretroviral agents in HIV-infected adults and adolescents. http://www.hivatis.org
67. Carpenter CCJ, Fischl MA, Hammer SM, et al. Antiretroviral therapy for HIV infection— 1997. JAMA 1997;277:1962–1969.
68. United States Public Health Service. USPHS recommendations for use of antiretroviral drugs during pregnancy for maternal health and reduction of perinatal transmission of human immunodeficiency virus type 1 in the United States. http://www.hivatis.org
69. Connor EM, Sperling RS, Gelber R, et al. Reduction of maternal–infant transmission of human immunodeficiency virus type 1 with zidovudine treatment. N Engl J Med 1994;331:1173–1180.
70. Katz MH, Gerberding JL. Postexposure treatment of people exposed to the human immunodeficiency virus through sexual contact or injection-drug use. N Engl J Med 1997;336:1097–1100.
71. NIH Panel to Define Principles of Therapy of HIV Infection. Report of the NIH panel to define principles of therapy of HIV infection. http://www.hivatis.org
72. Graham BS, Wright PF. Candidate AIDS vaccines. N Engl J Med 1995;333:1331–1339.
73. Piscitelli SC, Minor JR, Saville W, et al. Immune-based therapies for treatment of HIV infection. Ann Pharmacother 1996;30:62–76.
74. Gao W-Y, Agbaria R, Driscoll JS, et al. Divergent anti-human immunodeficiency virus activity and anabolic phosphorylation of 2′,3′-dideoxynucleoside analogs in resting and activated human cells. J Biol Chem 1994;269:12633–12638.
75. Montaner JSG, Zala C, Conway B, et al. A pilot study of hydroxyurea among patients with advanced human immunodeficiency virus (HIV) disease receiving chronic didanosine therapy: Canadian HIV trials network protocol 080. J Infect Dis 1997;175:801–806.

76. Acosta EP, Page LM, Fletcher CV. Clinical pharmacokinetics of zidovudine. An update. Clin Pharmacokinet 1996;30:251–262.
77. Perry JA, Balfour CM. Didanosine. An update on its antiviral activity, pharmacokinetic properties and therapeutic efficacy in the management of HIV disease. Drugs 1996;52:928–962.
78. Perry CM, Faulds D. Lamivudine. A review of its antiviral activity, pharmacokinetic properties and therapeutic efficacy in the management of HIV infection. Drugs 1997;53:657–680.
79. Lea AP, Faulds D. Stavudine: A review of its pharmacodynamic and pharmacokinetic properties and clinical potential in HIV infection. Drugs 1996;51:846–864.
80. Adkins JC, Peters DH, Faulds D. Zalcitabine. An update of its pharmacodynamic and pharmacokinetic properties and clinical efficacy in the management of HIV infection. Drugs 1997;53:1054–1080.
81. Kakuda TN, Struble KA, Piscitelli SC. Protease inhibitors for the treatment of HIV infection. Am J Health Syst Pharm 1998;55:233–254.
82. Fischl MA, Richman DD, Grieco MH, et al. The efficacy of azidothymidine (AZT) in the treatment of patients with AIDS and AIDS-related complex. N Engl J Med 1987;317:185–189.
83. Volberding PA, Lagakos SW, Koch MA, et al. Zidovudine in asymptomatic human immunodeficiency virus infection: A controlled trial in persons with fewer than 500 CD4-positive cells per cubic millimeter. N Engl J Med 1990;322:941–949.
84. Fischl MA, Richman DD, Hansen N, et al. The safety and efficacy of zidovudine (AZT) in the treatment of midly symptomatic human immunodeficiency virus type I (HIV) infection: A double-blind, placebo-controlled trial. Ann Intern Med 1990;112:727–737.
85. Cooper DA, Gatell JM, Kroon S, et al. Zidovudine in persons with asymptomatic HIV infection and CD4 cell count greater than 400 per cubic millimeter. N Engl J Med 1993;329:297–303.
86. Concorde Coordinating Committee. MRC/ANRS randomized double-blind controlled trial of immediate and deferred zidovudine in symptom-free HIV infection. Lancet 1994;343:871–881.
87. Volberding PA, Lagakos SW, Grimes JM, et al. The duration of zidovudine benefit in persons with asymptomatic HIV infection. JAMA 1994;272:437–442.
88. Volberding PA, Lagakos SW, Grimes JM, et al. A comparison of immediate with deferred zidovudine therapy for asymptomatic HIV-infected adults with CD4 cell counts of 500 or more per cubic millimeter. N Engl J Med 1995;333:401–407.
89. Hammer SM, Katzenstein DA, Hughes MD, et al. A trial comparing nucleoside monotherapy with combination therapy in HIV-infected adults with CD4 counts from 200 to 500/μL. N Engl J Med 1996;335:1081–1090.
90. Katzenstein DA, Hammer SM, Hughes MD, et al. The relation of virologic and immunologic markers to clinical outcomes after nucleoside therapy in HIV-infected adults with 200 to 500 CD4 cells per cubic millimeter. AIDS Clinical Trials Group Study 175 Virology Study Team. N Engl J Med 1996;335:1091–1098.
91. Delta Coordinating Committee. Delta: A randomized double-blind controlled trial comparing combinations of zidovudine plus didanosine or zalcitabine with zidovudine alone in HIV-infected individuals. Lancet 1996;348:283–291.
92. Saravolatz LD, Winslow DL, Collins G, et al. Zidovudine alone or in combination with didanosine or zalcitabine in HIV-infected patients with the acquired immunodeficiency syndrome or fewer than 200 CD4+ cells per cubic millimeter. N Engl J Med 1996;335:1099–1106.
93. Englund JA, Baker CJ, Raskino C, et al. Zidovudine, didanosine, or both as the initial treatment for symptomatic HIV-infected children. N Engl J Med 1997;336:1704–1712.
94. Eron JJ, Benoit SL, Jemsek J, et al. Treatment with lamivudine, zidovudine or both in HIV-positive patients with 200-500 CD4+ cells per cubic millimeter. N Engl J Med 1995;333:1662–1669.
95. Collier AC, Coombs RW, Schoenfeld DA, et al. Treatment of human immunodeficiency virus infection with saquinavir, zidovudine, and zalcitabine. N Engl J Med 1996;334:1011–1017.
96. Schapiro JM, Winters MA, Vierra M, et al. The effect of high dose saquinavir on viral load and CD4+ T-cell counts in HIV-infected patients. Ann Intern Med 1996;124:1039–1050.
97. Cameron DW, Heath-Chiozzi M, Kravcik S, et al. Prolongation of life and prevention of AIDS complications in advanced HIV immunodeficiency with ritonavir: Update, 11th International Conference on AIDS, Vancouver, BC, July 7–12, 1996.
98. Gulick RM, Mellors J, Havlir D, et al. Treatment with indinavir, zidovudine, and lamivudine in adults with human immunodeficiency virus infection and prior antiretroviral therapy. N Engl J Med 1997;337:734–739.
99. Hammer SM, Squires KE, Hughes MD, et al. A controlled trial of two nucleoside analogues plus indinavir in persons with human immunodeficiency virus infection and CD4 cell counts of 200 per cubic millimeter or less. AIDS Clinical Trials Group 320 Study Team. N Engl J Med 1997;337:725–733.
100. Saag M, Knowles M, Chang Y, et al. Durable effect of Viracept (nelfinavir mesylate, NFV) in triple combination therapy, 37th Interscience Conference on Antimicrobial Agents and Chemotherapy, Toronto, Ont, Sept 28–Oct 1, 1997.
101. D'Aquilla RT, Hughes MD, Johnsons VA, et al. Nevirapine, zidovudine, and didanosine compared with zidovudine and didanosine in patients with HIV-1 infection. Ann Intern Med 1996;124:1019–1030.
102. Davey RT Jr, Chaitt DG, Reed GF, et al. Randomized, controlled phase I/II trial of combination therapy with delavirdine (U-90152S) and conventional nucleosides in human immunodeficiency virus type-1 infected patients. Antimicrob Agents Chemother 1996;40:1657–1664.
103. De Clercq E. Development of resistance of human immunodeficiency virus (HIV) to anti-HIV agents—how to prevent the problem. Int J Antimicrob Agents 1997;9:21–36.
104. Masur H, Ognibene FP, Yarchoan R, et al. CD4 counts as predictors of opportunistic pneumonias in human immunodeficiency virus (HIV) infection. Ann Intern Med 1989;111:223–231.
105. Moore RD, Chaisson RE. Natural history of opportunistic disease in an HIV-infected urban clinical cohort. Ann Intern Med 1996;124:633–642.
106. Chan ISF, Neaton JD, Saravolatz LD, et al. Frequencies of opportunistic diseases prior to death among HIV-infected persons. AIDS 1995;9:1145–1151.
107. Control Centers for Disease. AIDS Weekly Surveillance Report. 1989.
108. Davey RT Jr, Masur H. Recent advances in the diagnosis, treatment, and prevention of *Pneumocystis carinii* pneumonia. Antimicrob Agents Chemother 1990;34:499–504.
109. Santamauro JT, Stover DE. *Pneumocystis carinii* pneumonia. Med Clin North Am 1997;81:299–318.
110. Jacobs JL, Libby DM, Winters RA, et al. A cluster of *Pneumocystis carinii* pneumonia in adults with predisposing illness. N Engl J Med 1991;324:246–250.
111. Hughes WT, Feldman S, Chaudary S, et al. Comparison of pentamidine isethionate and trimethoprim-sulfamethoxazole in the treatment of *Pneumocystis carinii* pnemonia. J Pediatr 1978;92:285–291.
112. Masur H. Prevention and treatment of *Pneumocystis* pneumonia. N Eng J Med 1992;327:1853–1860.
113. Conte JE Jr, Hollander H, Golden JA, et al. Inhaled pentamidine or reduced dose intravenous pentamidine for *Pneumocystis carinii* pneumonia: A pilot study. Ann Intern Med 1987;107:495–498.
114. Conte JE, Chernoff D, Feigal DW, et al. Intravenous or inhaled pentamidine for treating *Pneumocystis carinii* pneumonia in AIDS. Ann Intern Med 1990;113:203–209.
115. Conte JE, Upton RA, Phelps RT, et al. Use of a specific and sensitive assay to determine pentamidine pharmacokinetics in patients with AIDS. J Infect Dis 1987;156:923–929.
116. Soo Hoo GW, Mohsenifar Z, Meyer R. Inhaled or intravenous pentamidine therapy for *Pneumocystis carinii* pneumonia. Ann Intern Med 1990;113:195–202.
117. Sattler FR, Cowan R, Nielsen DM, et al. Trimethoprim-sulfamethoxazole compared with pentamidine for treatment of *Pneumocystis*

carinii pneumonia in the acquired immunodeficiency syndrome. Ann Intern Med 1988;109:280–287.
118. Wharton JM, Coleman DL, Wofsy CB, et al. Trimethoprim-sulfamethoxazole or pentamidine for *Pneumocystis carinii* pneumonia in the acquired immunodeficiency syndrome. Ann Intern Med 1986; 105:37–44.
119. Wofsy WB. Use of trimethoprim-sulfamethoxazole in the treatment of *Pneumocystis carinii* pneumonitis in patients with acquired immunodeficiency syndrome. Rev Infect Dis 1987;9 (suppl 2):S184–S194.
120. Bozzette SA, Sattler FR, Chiu J, et al. A controlled trial of early adjunctive treatment with coricosteriods for *Pneumocystis carinii* pneumonia in the acquired immunodeficiency syndrome. N Engl J Med 1990;323:1451–1457.
121. Gagnon S, Boota AM, Fischl MA, et al. Corticosteriods as adjunctive therapy for severe *Pneumocystis carinii* pneumonia in the acquired immunodeficiency syndrome. N Engl J Med 1990;323:1444–1450.
122. The National Institutes of Health–University of California Expert Panel for Coricosteriods as Adjunctive Therapy for *Pneumocystis carinii* Pneumonia. Consensus statement on the use of corticosteriods as adjunctive therapy for *Pneumocystis* pneumonia in the acquired immunodeficiency syndrome. N Engl J Med 1990;323:1500–1504.
123. Mills J, Leoung G, Medina I, et al. Dapsone treatment of *Pneumocystis carinii* pneumonia in the acquired immunodeficiency syndrome. Antimicrob Agents Chemother 1988;32:1057–1060.
124. Medina I, Mills J, Leoung G, et al. Oral therapy for *Pneumocystis carinii* pneumonia in the acquired immunodeficiency syndrome: A controlled trial of trimethoprim-sulfamethoxazole versus trimethoprim-dapsone. N Engl J Med 1990;323:776–782.
125. Lee BL, Medina I, Benowitz NL, et al. Dapsone, trimethoprim, and sulfamethoxazole plasma levels during treatment of *Pneumocystis* pneumonia in patients with the acquired immunodeficiency syndrome (AIDS). Evidence of drug interactions. Ann Intern Med 1989; 110:606–611.
126. Safrin S, Finkelstein DM, Feinberg J, et al. Comparison of three regimens for treatment of mild to moderate *Pneumocystis carinii* pneumonia in patients with AIDS. Ann Intern Med 1996;124:792–802.
127. Hughes W, Leoung G, Kramer F, et al. Comparison of atovaquone (566C80) with trimethoprim-sulfamethoxazole to treat *Pneumocystis carinii* pneumonia in patients with AIDS. N Engl J Med 1993;328: 1521–1527.
128. Allegra CJ, Chabner BA, Tuazon CU, et al. Trimetrexate for the treatment of *Pneumocystis carinii* pneumonia in patients with the acquired immunodeficiency syndrome. N Engl J Med 1987;317:978–985.
129. Phair J, Munoz A, Detels R, et al. The risk of *Pneumocystis carinii* pneumonia among men infected with human immunodeficiency virus type 1. N Engl J Med 1990;322:161–165.
130. Centers for Disease Control. Recommendation for prophylaxis against *Pneumocystis carinii* pneumonia for adults and adolescents infected with human immunodeficiency virus. MMWR 1992;41:1–11.
131. Fischl MA, Dickinson GM, La Voie L. Safety and efficacy of sulfamethoxazole and trimethoprim chemoprophylaxis for *Pneumocystis carinii* pneumonia in AIDS. JAMA 1988;259:1185–1189.
132. Hardy WD, Feinberg J, Finkelstein DM, et al. A controlled trial of trimethoprim- sulfamethoxazole or aerosolized pentamidine for secondary prophylaxis of *Pneumocystis carinii* pneumonia in patients with the acquired immunodeficiency syndrome. AIDS Clinical Trials Group protocol 021. N Engl J Med 1992;327:1842–1848.
133. Bozzette SA, Finkelstein DM, Spector SA, et al. A randomized trial of three antipneumocystis agents in patients with advanced human immunodeficiency virus infection. NIAID AIDS Clinical Trials Group. N Engl J Med 1995;332:693–699.
134. Centers for Disease Control. USPHS/IDSA guidelines for the prevention of opportunistic infections in persons infected with human immunodeficiency virus. MMWR 1997;46:1–46.
135. Hughes WT, Kuhn S, Chaudhary S, et al. Successful chemoprophylaxis for *Pneumocystis carinii* pneumonitis. N Engl J Med 1977;297: 1419–1426.
136. Leoung GS, Feigal DW, Montgomery BA, et al. Aerosolized pentamidine for prophylaxis against *Pneumocystis carinii* pneumonia. N Engl J Med 1991;324:696–697.
137. Hirschel B, Lazzarin A, Chopard P, et al. A controlled study of inhaled pentamidine for primary prevention of *Pneumocystis carinii* pneumonia. N Engl J Med 1991;324:1079–1083.
138. Northfelt DW, Clement MJ, Safrin S. Extrapulmonary pneumocystosis: Clinical features in human immunodeficiency virus infection. Medicine 1990;69:392–398.
139. Tuazon CU. Toxoplasmosis in AIDS patients. J Antimicrob Chemother 1989;23(suppl A):77–82.
140. Grant IH, Gold JWM, Rosenblum M, et al. *Toxoplasma gondii* serology in HIV-infected patients: The development of central nervous system toxoplasmosis. AIDS 1990;4:519–521.
141. Katlama C, Wit SD, O'Doherty E, et al. Pyrimethamine-clindamycin vs. pyrimethamine-sulfadiazine as acute and long-term therapy for toxoplasmic encephalitis in patients with AIDS. Clin Infect Dis 1996;22:268–275.
142. Weiss LM, Harris C, Berger M, et al. Pyrimethamine concentrations in serum and cerebrospinal fluid during treatment of acute *Toxoplasma* encephalitis in patients with AIDS. J Infect Dis 1988;157:580–583.
143. Wong SY, Remington JS. Toxoplasmosis in the setting of AIDS. In: Broder SMTJ, Bolognesi D, eds. Textbook of AIDS Medicine. Baltimore, Williams & Wilkins, 1994.
144. Luft BJ, Remington JS. Toxoplasmic encephalitis. J Infect Dis 1988; 157:1–6.
145. Herald A, Flepp M, Chave J-P, et al. Treatment for cerebral toxoplasmosis protects against *Pneumocystis carinii* pneumonia in patients with AIDS. Ann Intern Med 1991;115:760–763.
146. Jacobson MA, Besch CL, Child C, et al. Toxicity of clindamycin as prophylaxis for AIDS-associated toxoplasmic encephalitis. Lancet 1992;339:333–334.
147. Chuck SL, Sande MA. Infections with *Cryptococcus neoformans* in the acquired immunodeficiency syndrome. N Engl J Med 1989;321: 794–799.
148. Bennett JE, Dismukes WE, Duma RJ, et al. A comparison of amphotericin B alone and combined with flucytosine in the treatment of cryptococcal meningitis. N Engl J Med 1979;301:126–131.
149. Robinson PA, Knirsch AK, Joseph JA. Fluconazole for life-threatening fungal infections in patients who cannot be treated with conventional antifungal agents. Rev Infect Dis 1990;12(suppl 3):S349–S363.
150. Larsen RA, Leal MAE, Chan LS. Fluconazole compared with amphotericin B plus flucytosine for cryptococcal meningitis in AIDS. Ann Intern Med 1990;113:183–187.
151. Saag MS, Powderly WG, Cloud GA, et al. Comparison of amphotericin B with fluconazole in the treatment of acute AIDS-associated cryptococcal meningitis. N Engl J Med 1992;326:83–89.
152. van der Horst CM, Saag MS, Cloud GA, et al. Treatment of cryptococcal meningitis associated with the acquired immunodeficiency syndrome. National Institute of Allergy and Infectious Diseases Mycoses Study Group and AIDS Clinical Trials Group. N Engl J Med 1997;337:15–21.
153. Bozzette SA, Larsen RA, Chiu J, et al. A placebo-controlled trial of maintenance therapy with fluconazole after treatment of cryptococcal meningitis in the acquired immunodeficiency syndrome. N Engl J Med 1991;324:580–584.
154. Powderly WG, Saag MS, Cloud GA, et al. A controlled trial of fluconazole or amphotericin B to prevent relapse of cryptococcal meningitis in patients with the acquired immunodeficiency syndrome. N Engl J Med 1992;326:793–798.
155. Powderly WG, Finkelstein DM, Feinberg J, et al. A randomized trial comparing fluconazole with clotrimazole troches for the prevention of fungal infections in patients with advanced human immunodeficiency virus infection. N Engl J Med 1995;332:700–705.
156. Horsburgh CR Jr. *Mycobacterium avium* complex infection in the acquired immunodeficiency syndrome. N Engl J Med 1991;324:332–338.

157. Benson CA, Ellner JJ. *Mycobacterium avium* complex infection and AIDS: Advances in theory and practice. Clin Infect Dis 1993;17:7–20.
158. Peloquin CA. *Mycobacterium avium* complex infection. Pharmacokinetic and pharmacodynamic considerations that may improve clinical outcomes. Clin Pharmacokinetics 1997;32:132–144.
159. Chin DP, Reingold AL, Stone EN, et al. The impact of *Mycobacterium avium* complex bacteremia and its treatment on survival in AIDS patients—a prospective study. J Infect Dis 1994;170:578–584.
160. Chaisson RE, Benson CA, Dube MP, et al. Clarithromycin therapy for bacteremic *Mycobacterium avium* complex disease. Ann Intern Med 1994;121:905–911.
161. Shafran SD, Singer J, Zarowny DP, et al. A comparison of two regimens for the treatment of *Mycobacterium avium* complex bactermia in AIDS: Rifabutin, ethambutol, and clarithromycin versus rifampin, ethambutol, clofazimine, and ciprofloxacin. N Engl J Med 1996;335:377–383.
162. Masur H. Recommendations on prophylaxis and therapy for disseminated *Mycobacterium-avium* complex disease in patients infected with the human immunodeficiency virus. N Engl J Med 1993;329:898–904.
163. Horsburgh CR. Advances in the prevention and treatment of *Mycobacterium avium* disease. N Engl J Med 1996;335:428–430.
164. Nightingale SD, Cameron DW, Gordin FM, et al. Two controlled trials of rifabutin prophylaxis against *Mycobacterium avium* complex infection in AIDS. N Engl J Med 1993;329:828–833.
165. Pierce M, Crampton S, Henry D, et al. A randomized trial of clarithromycin as prophylaxis against disseminated *Mycobacterium avium* complex infections in patients with advanced acquired immunodeficiency syndrome. N Engl J Med 1996;335:383–391.
166. Havlir DV, Dube MP, Sattler FR, et al. Prophylaxis against disseminated *Mycobacterium avium* complex with weekly azithromycin, daily rifabutin, or both. N Engl J Med 1996;335:392–398.
167. Siegel FP, Lopez C, Hammer BS, et al. Severe acquired immunodeficiency in male homosexuals, manifested by chronic perianal ulcerative herpes simplex lesions. N Engl J Med 1981;305:1439–1444.
168. Wade JC, Newton B, Flournoy N, et al. Oral acyclovir for prevention of herpes simplex virus reactivation after marrow transplantation. Ann Intern Med 1984;100:823–828.
169. Erlich KS, Mills J, Chatis P, et al. Acyclovir-resistant herpes simples virus infections in patients with the acquired immunodeficiency syndrome. N Engl J Med 1989;320:293–296.
170. Fletcher CV, Englund JA, Bean B, et al. Continuous infusion high-dose acyclovir for serious herpesvirus infections. Antimicrob Agents Chemother 1989;33:1375–1378.
171. Erlich KS, Jacobson MA, Koehler JE, et al. Foscarnet therapy for severe acyclovir-resistant herpes simplex virus type-2 infections in patients with the acquired immunodeficiency syndrome. Ann Intern Med 1989;110:710–713.
172. Safrin S, Crumpacker C, Chatis P, et al. A controlled trial comparing foscarnet with vidarabine for acyclovir-resistant mucocutaneous herpes simplex virus in the acquired immunodeficiency syndrome. N Engl J Med 1991;325:551–555.
173. Rogers MF, Morens DM, Stewart JA, et al. National case control study of Kaposi's sarcoma and *Pneumocystis carinii* pneumonia in homosexual men: Part 2, laboratory results. Ann Intern Med 1983;99:151–158.
174. Melbye M, Grossman RJ, Goedert JJ, et al. Risk of AIDS after herpes zoster. Lancet 1987;1:728–731.
175. Huff JC, Bean B, Balfour HH Jr, et al. Therapy of herpes zoster with oral acyclovir. Am J Med 1988;85(suppl 2A):84–89.
176. Jacobson MA, Berger TG, Fikrig S, et al. Acyclovir-resistant varicella-zoster virus infection after chronic oral acyclovir therapy in patients with the acquired immunodeficiency syndrome. Ann Intern Med 1990;112:187–191.
177. Quinnan GV, Masur H, Rook AH, et al. Herpes virus infections in the acquired immunodeficiency syndrome. JAMA 1984;252:72–77.
178. Jacobson MA, Zegans M, Pavan PR, et al. Cytomegalovirus retinitis after initiation of highly active antiretroviral therapy. Lancet 1997;349:1443–1445.
179. Smith CL. Local therapy for cytomegalovirus retinitis. Ann Pharmacother 1998;32:248–255.
180. Fletcher CV, Balfour HH Jr. Evaluation of ganciclovir for cytomegalovirus disease. Ann Pharmocother 1989;23:5–12.
181. Buhles WC, Mastre BJ, Tinker AJ, et al. Ganciclovir treatment of life-or-sight-threatening cytomegalovirus infection: Experience in 314 immunocompromised patients. Rev Infect Dis 1988;10(suppl 3): S495–S504.
182. Drew LW, Ives D, Lalezari JP, et al. Oral ganciclovir as maintenance treatment for cytomegalovirus retinitis in patients with AIDS. N Engl J Med 1995;333:615–620.
183. The Oral Ganciclovir European and Australian Cooperative Study Group. Intravenous versus oral ganciclovir: European/Australian comparative study of efficacy and safety in the prevention of cytomegalovirus retinitis recurrence in patients with AIDS. AIDS 1995; 9:471–477.
184. Erice A, Chou S, Biron KK, et al. Progressive disease due to ganciclovir-resistant cytomegalovirus in immunocompromised patients. N Engl J Med 1989;320:289–293.
185. Hochster H, Dieterich D, Bozzette S, et al. Toxicity of combined ganciclovir and zidovudine for cytomegalovirus disease associated with AIDS. Ann Intern Med 1990;113:111–117.
186. Martin DF, Parks DJ, Mellow SD, et al. Treatment of cytomegalovirus retinitis with an intraocular sustained-release ganciclovir implant. Arch Ophthalmol 1994;112:1531–1539.
187. Musch DC, Martin DF, Gordon JF, et al. Treatment of cytomegalovirus retinitis with a sustained-release ganciclovir implant. N Engl J Med 1997;337:83–90.
188. Palestine AG, Polis MA, de Smet MD, et al. A randomized controlled trial of foscarnet in the treatment of cytomegalovirus retinitis in patients with AIDS. Ann Intern Med 1991;115:665–673.
189. Polis MA, de Smet MD, Bard BF, et al. Increased survival of a cohort of patients with acquired immunodeficiency syndrome and cytomegalovirus retinitis who received sodium phosphonoformate (foscarnet). Am J Med 1993;94:175–180.
190. Studies of the Ocular Complications of AIDS Research Group. Mortality in patients with the acquired immunodeficiency syndrome treated with either foscarnet or ganciclovir for cytomegalovirus retinitis. N Engl J Med 1992;326:213–220.
191. Deray G, Katlama C, Dohin E. Prevention of foscarnet nephrotoxicity. Ann Intern Med 1990;113:332.
192. The Studies of Ocular Complications of AIDS Research Group in Collaboration with the AIDS Clinical Trials Group. Combination foscarnet and ganciclovir therapy vs monotherapy for the treatment of relapsed cytomegalovirus retinitis in patients with AIDS. Arch Ophthamol 1996;114:23–33.
193. Studies of Ocular Complications of AIDS Research Group in Collaboration with the AIDS Clinical Trials Group. Parenteral cidofovir for cytomegalovirus retinitis in patients with AIDS: The HPMPC peripheral cytomegalovirus retinitis trial. Ann Intern Med 1997;126:264–274.
194. Meyers JD, Reed EC, Shepp DH, et al. Acyclovir for prevention of cytomegalovirus infection and disease after allogeneic marrow transplantation. N Engl J Med 1988;318:70–75.
195. Fletcher CV, Englund JA, Edelman CK, et al. Pharmacologic basis for high-dose oral acyclovir prophylaxis of cytomegalovirus disease in renal allograft recipients. Antimicrob Agents Chemother 1991;35: 938–943.
196. Feinberg JE, Hurwitz S, Cooper D, et al. A randomized, double-blind trial of valaciclovir prophylaxis for cytomegalovirus disease in patients with advanced human immunodeficiency virus infection. J Infect Dis 1998;177:48–56.
197. Spector SA, McKinley GF, Lelezari JP, et al. Oral ganciclovir for the prevention of cytomegalovirus disease in persons with AIDS. N Engl J Med 1996;334:1491–1497.
198. Dietrich DT, Chachoua A, LaFleur F, et al. Ganciclovir treatment of gastrointestinal infections caused by cytomegalovirus in patients with AIDS. Rev Infect Dis 1988;10(suppl 3):S532–S537.
199. Blanshard C, Benhamou Y, Dohin E, et al. Treatment of AIDS-associated gastrointestinal cytomegalovirus infection with foscarnet and ganciclovir: A randomized comparison. J Infect Dis 1995;172:622–628.

115
CANCER TREATMENT AND CHEMOTHERAPY

Amy Wells Valley, PharmD, BCPS, and Carol McManus Balmer, PharmD

Cancer is a group of more than 100 different diseases, characterized by uncontrolled cellular growth, local tissue invasion, and distant metastases.[1] It is second only to cardiovascular disease in causes of mortality in Americans. Over 1.2 million cases of cancer are diagnosed annually, and cancer claims approximately 560,000 lives in the United States each year.[2] The estimated incidence of common cancers and cancer-related deaths is illustrated in Figure 115–1. The four most common cancers are prostate, breast, lung, and colorectal cancer. The most common cause of cancer-related deaths in the United States is lung cancer, which claims approximately 160,000 lives each year. These cancers are discussed in further detail in the chapters that follow.

The role of the pharmacist in the management of the cancer patient can be very diverse. Thorough knowledge of antineoplastic drug pharmacology and pharmacokinetics is essential to prevent and manage many drug-induced toxicities. Supportive-care issues such as nutritional support, pain management, infection, and nausea and vomiting require application of both clinical and pharmacologic principles. Provision of drug information is another critical role for the oncology pharmacist. This service is provided to other health professionals and to patients and their families. Experienced pharmacists are well equipped to fulfill these roles and make valuable contributions to patient care in the oncology setting.

This chapter (1) introduces the basic concepts of carcinogenesis, tumor growth, and cancer treatment; (2) provides general information on the pharmacology and clinical use of the antineoplastic agents; and (3) presents an overview of supportive care issues in the oncology patient.

ETIOLOGY OF CANCER

CARCINOGENESIS

The mechanism by which cancers occur is not completely understood. A cancer, or neoplasm, is thought to develop from a cell in which the normal mechanisms for control of growth and proliferation are altered. Current evidence supports the concept of carcinogenesis as a multistage process that is genetically regulated (Fig. 115–2).[3–5] The first step in this process is *initiation,* which requires exposure of normal cells to carcinogenic substances. These carcinogens produce genetic damage that, if not repaired, results in irreversible cellular mutations. This mutated cell has an altered response to its environment and a selective growth advantage, giving it the potential to develop into a clonal population of neoplastic cells. During the second phase, known as *promotion,* carcinogens or other factors alter the environment to favor growth of the mutated cell over normal cells. The primary difference between initiation and promotion is that promotion is a reversible process. In fact, because it is reversible, the promotion phase may be the target of future chemoprevention strategies, including changes in life-style and diet. At some point, however, the mutated cell becomes cancerous (conversion or transformation). Depending on the type of cancer, months to years may elapse between the two carcinogenic phases and the development of a clinically detectable cancer. The final stage of neoplastic growth, called *progression,* involves further genetic changes leading to increased cell proliferation. The critical elements of this phase include tumor invasion into local tissues and the development of metastases.

Substances that may act as carcinogens or initiators include chemical, physical, and biologic agents.[3,6] Exposure to chemicals may occur by virtue of occupational and environmental means, as well as life-style habits. The association of aniline dye exposure and bladder cancer is one such example. Benzene is known to cause some leukemias. Some drugs and hormones used for therapeutic purposes are also classified as carcinogenic chemicals (Table 115–1).[6] Physical agents that act as carcinogens include ionizing radiation and ultraviolet light. These types of radiation induce mutations by forming free radicals that damage deoxyribonucleic acid (DNA) and other cellular components. Viruses are biologic agents that have been associated with certain cancers. The Epstein–Barr virus is believed to be an important factor in the initiation of African Burkitt's lymphoma. Likewise, infection with hepatitis B virus is known to be a major cause of hepatocellular cancer. All the previously mentioned carcinogens, as well as age, gender, diet, growth factors, and chronic irritation, are among the factors considered to be promoters of carcinogenesis.[3,6]

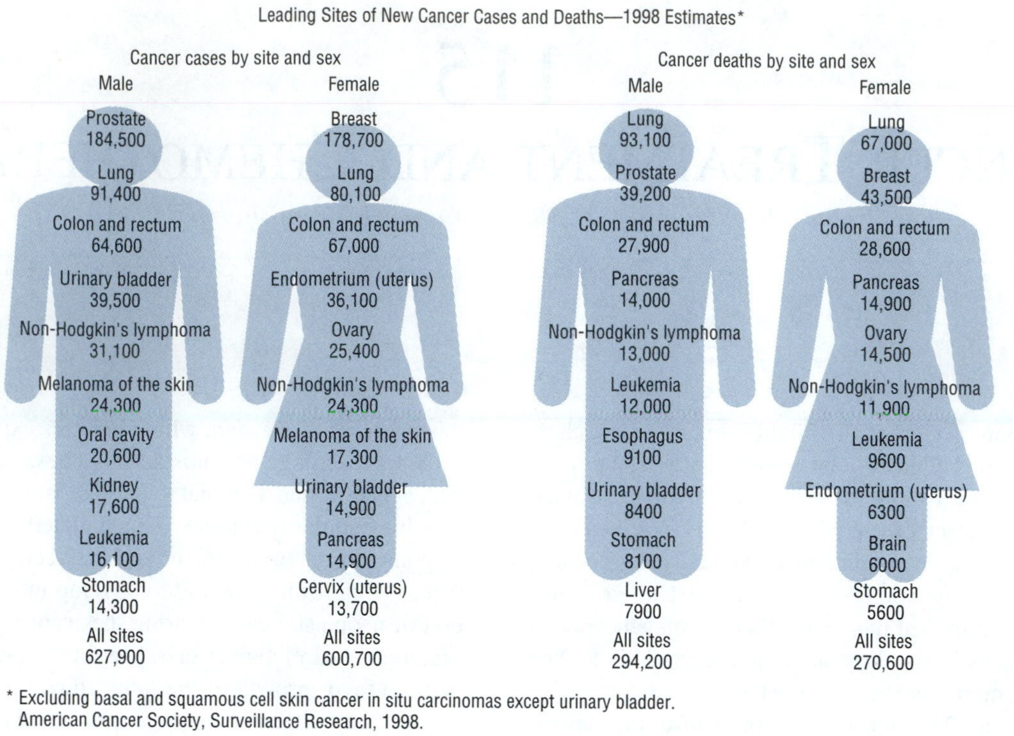

Leading Sites of New Cancer Cases and Deaths—1998 Estimates*
Cancer cases by site and sex
Male
Prostate 184,500
Lung 91,400
Colon and rectum 64,600
Urinary bladder 39,500
Non-Hodgkin's lymphoma 31,100
Melanoma of the skin 24,300
Oral cavity 20,600
Kidney 17,600
Leukemia 16,100
Stomach 14,300
All sites 627,900
Female
Breast 178,700
Lung 80,100
Colon and rectum 67,000
Endometrium (uterus) 36,100
Ovary 25,400
Non-Hodgkin's lymphoma 24,300
Melanoma of the skin 17,300
Urinary bladder 14,900
Pancreas 14,900
Cervix (uterus) 13,700
All sites 600,700
Cancer deaths by site and sex
Male
Lung 93,100
Prostate 39,200
Colon and rectum 27,900
Pancreas 14,000
Non-Hodgkin's lymphoma 13,000
Leukemia 12,000
Esophagus 9100
Urinary bladder 8400
Stomach 8100
Liver 7900
All sites 294,200
Female
Lung 67,000
Breast 43,500
Colon and rectum 28,600
Pancreas 14,900
Ovary 14,500
Non-Hodgkin's lymphoma 11,900
Leukemia 9600
Endometrium (uterus) 6300
Brain 6000
Stomach 5600
All sites 270,600
* Excluding basal and squamous cell skin cancer in situ carcinomas except urinary bladder.
American Cancer Society, Surveillance Research, 1998.

FIGURE 115–1. 1998 Cancer incidences (left) and deaths (right) in the United States for males and females. *(From Ref. 2.)*

GENETIC BASIS OF CANCER

Recent explorations into the etiology of cancer have centered on the role of genes in the multistage cancer process.[3,6,7] There are two major classes of genes involved in carcinogenesis: oncogenes and tumor-suppressor genes. The effects of oncogenes and tumor-suppressor genes on normal cellular function are illustrated in Figure 115–3. Oncogenes develop from normal genes, called proto-oncogenes, and may have important roles in all phases of carcinogenesis. Proto-oncogenes are present in all cells and are essential regulators of normal cellular functions, including the cell cycle. Genetic alteration of the proto-oncogene through point mutations, insertions, deletions, or chromosomal translocations activates the oncogene. These genetic alterations may be caused by carcinogenic agents such as radiation, chemicals, or viruses or they may be inherited. Once

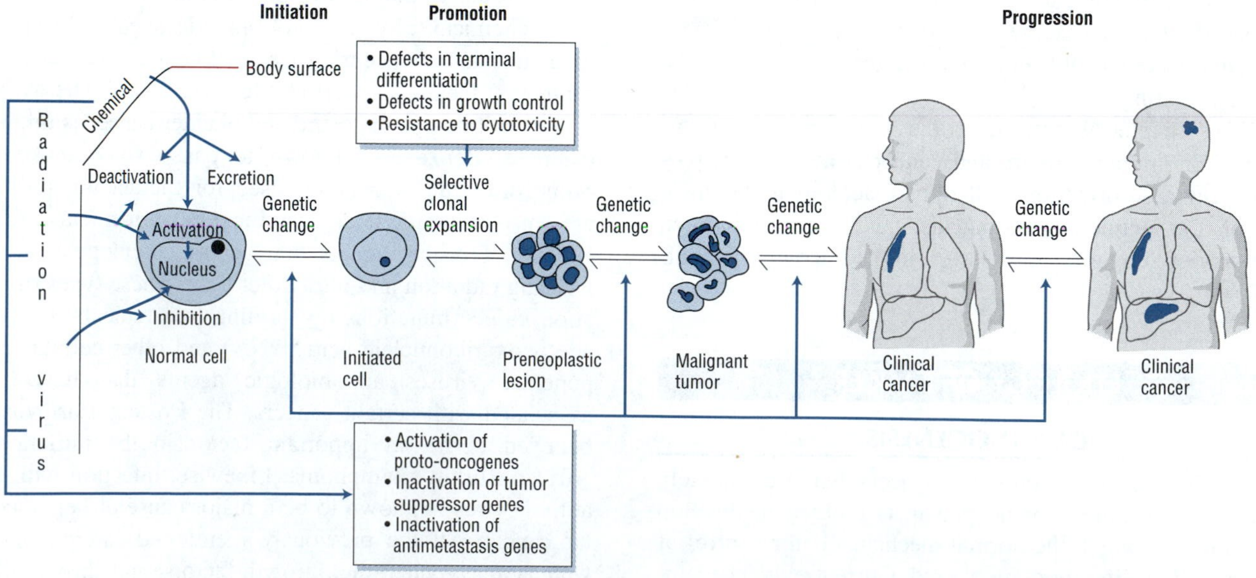

FIGURE 115–2. Multistage model of carcinogenesis. *(Adapted from Shields PG, Harris CC. Principles of carcinogenesis: Chemical. In: DeVita VT Jr, Hellman S, Rosenberg SA, eds. Cancer: Principles and Practice of Oncology, 4th ed. Philadelphia, Lippincott, 1993:201, with permission.)*

TABLE 115–1. Selected Drugs and Hormones That Are Known to Cause Cancer in Humans

Drug or Hormone	Type of Cancer Caused
Alkylating agents (e.g., chlorambucil, mechlorethamine, melphalan, nitrosoureas)	Leukemia
Anabolic steroids	Liver
Analgesics containing phenacetin	Renal, urinary bladder
Anthracyclines (e.g., doxorubicin)	Leukemia
Antiestrogens (tamoxifen)	Endometrium
Coal tars (topical)	Skin
Estrogens	
Nonsteroidal (diethylstilbesterol)	Vagina/cervix, endometrium, breast, testes
Steroidal (estrogen replacement therapy, oral contraceptives)	Endometrium, breast, liver
Epipodophyllotoxins (etoposide, teniposide)	Leukemia
Immunosuppressive drugs (cyclosporine, azathioprine)	Lymphoma, skin
Oxazaphosphorines (cyclophosphamide, ifosfamide)	Urinary bladder, leukemia

Compiled from Refs. 5, 6, and 10.

activated, the oncogene produces either excessive amounts of the normal gene product or an abnormal gene product. The result is dysregulation of normal cell growth and proliferation, which imparts a distinct growth advantage to the cell and increases the probability of neoplastic transformation. An example is the *myc* family of oncogenes. The normal gene product of *myc* acts as a signal for cellular proliferation. As an oncogene, the gene product is overexpressed or amplified, resulting in excessive cellular proliferation. Examples of other oncogenes and their classification by mechanism are listed in Table 115–2.

In contrast, tumor-suppressor genes regulate and inhibit inappropriate cellular growth and proliferation.[4,7] Gene loss or mutation results in loss of control over normal cell growth (see Fig. 115–3). Two common examples of tumor-suppressor genes are the retinoblastoma (Rb) and *p*53 genes. Mutation of *p*53 is one of the most common genetic changes associated with cancer, estimated to occur in half of all malignancies.[7] The normal gene product of *p*53 is responsible for negative regulation of the cell cycle, allowing the cell cycle to halt for repairs, corrections, and responses to other external signals. Inactivation of *p*53 by various mechanisms removes this checkpoint, allowing mutations to occur. Mutation of *p*53 has been linked to a variety of malignancies, including brain tumors (astrocytoma); carcinomas of the breast, colon, and lung; and osteosarcoma. Another important function of *p*53 may be in modulation of cytotoxic drug effects. Loss of *p*53 has been associated with antineoplastic drug resistance.

Oncogenes and tumor-suppressor genes provide the stimulatory and inhibitory signals that ultimately regulate the cell cycle.[7] These signals converge on a molecular system in the nucleus known as the cell cycle clock (see Fig. 115–3). The function of the clock in normal tissue is to integrate the signal input and to determine if the cell cycle

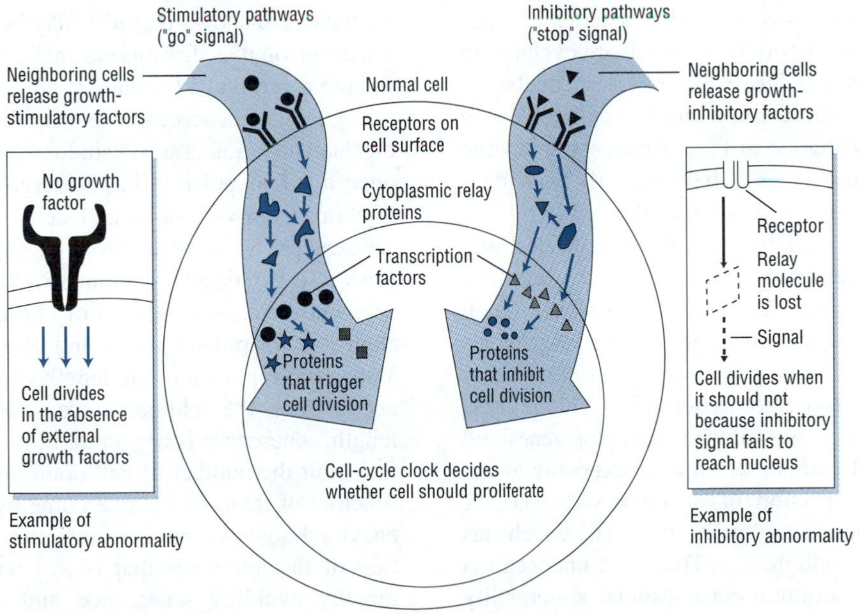

FIGURE 115–3. The effects of oncogenes and tumor-suppressor genes on cellular function. Signaling pathways in normal cells relay growth-controlling messages from the outer surface to the nucleus, where the cell-cycle clock receives these messages and decides whether the cell should divide. In cancer cells, genetic mutations can either activate oncogenes, resulting in excessive stimulation (too many "go" signals) or inactivate tumor-suppressor genes, resulting in loss of cell-cycle inhibition (no "stop" signals). Examples of abnormal stimulatory or inhibitory processes are provided in the boxes. *(Adapted from Ref. 7, with permission.)*

TABLE 115–2. Oncogenes and Tumor-Suppressor Genes

Oncogenes		
Genes for growth factors or their receptors		
PDGF	Codes for platelet-derived growth factor	Involved in gliomas, osteosarcoma
erb-B	Codes for epidermal growth factor	Involved in glioblastoma, breast cancer
erb-B2	Codes for a growth factor receptor Also called *HER-2* or neu	Involved in breast, salivary gland, and ovarian cancers
Genes for cytoplasmic relays in stimulatory signaling pathways		
Ki-ras		Involved in lung, ovarian, colon, pancreatic cancers
N-ras		Involved in leukemias
Genes for transcription factors that activate growth-promoting genes		
c-myc		Involved in leukemias and breast, gastric, and lung cancers
N-myc		Involved in neuroblastoma and glioblastoma
L-myc		Involved in lung cancer
Genes for other molecules		
Bcl-2	Codes for a protein that blocks apoptosis	Involved in low-grade lymphomas
Bcl-1	Codes for cyclin D1, a cell-cycle clock stimulator Also called *PRAD-1*	Involved in breast, head, and neck cancers
Tumor-Suppressor Genes		
Genes for proteins in the cytoplasm		
APC		Involved in colon and gastric cancers
NF-1	Codes for a protein that inhibits the stimulatory *Ras* protein	Involved in neurofibroma, leukemia, and pheochromocytoma
NF-2		Involved in meningioma, ependymoma, and schwannoma
Genes for proteins in the nucleus		
MTS1	Codes for the p16 protein, a cell-cycle brake	Involved in a wide range of cancers
RB	Codes for the pRB protein, a master brake of the cell cycle	Involved in retinoblastoma, osteosarcoma, and bladder, small-cell lung, prostate, and breast cancers
p53	Codes for the *p53* protein, which can halt cell division and induce apoptosis	Involved in a wide range of cancers
Genes for protein whose cellular location is unclear		
BRCA1		Involved in breast and ovarian cancers
BRCA2		Involved in breast cancer
VHL		Involved in renal cell cancer

Adapted from Ref. 7.

should proceed. The clock is composed of a series of interacting proteins, the most important of which are cyclins and cyclin-dependent kinases (CDKs). Cyclins (especially cyclin D1) and CDKs promote entry into the cell cycle and are known to be overexpressed in several cancers, including breast cancer.[7,8] Inhibitors of CDK have recently been identified as important negative regulators of the cell cycle.[8]

When the normal regulatory mechanisms for cellular growth fail, backup defense systems may be activated. The secondary defenses include apoptosis (programmed cell death or suicide) and cellular senescence (aging). Apoptosis (pronounced "ay-puh-TOE-sis") is a normal mechanism of cell death required for tissue homeostasis.[6,8,9] This process is regulated by oncogenes and tumor-suppressor genes and is also a mechanism of cellular death after exposure to cytotoxic agents. Overexpression of oncogenes responsible for apoptosis may produce an "immortal" cell, which has increased potential for malignancy. The *bcl*-2 oncogene is an example. The most common chromosomal abnormality found in lymphoid malignancies is the t(14;18) translocation. The *bcl*-2 proto-oncogene is normally located on chromosome 18. Translocation of this proto-oncogene to chromosome 14 in proximity to the immune globulin heavy gene leads to overexpression of *bcl*-2, which decreases apoptosis and confers a survival advantage to the cell. Studies have also shown that *p*53 may be a regulator of apoptosis. Loss of *p*53 disrupts normal apoptotic pathways, imparting a survival advantage to the cell.

Cellular senescence is another important defense mechanism.[7] Laboratory studies have demonstrated that once a cell population has undergone a preset number of doublings, growth stops and cells die. This is known as senescence. Subsequent research has determined that this process is regulated by telomeres. Telomeres are the DNA segments or caps at the end of chromosomes. They are responsible for protecting the end of the DNA from damage. With each replication, the length of the telomeres is shortened. Once the telomeres are shortened to a particular length, senescence is triggered. In this way, telomeres count and limit the number of cell doublings. In cancer cells, the function of telomeres is overcome by overexpression of an enzyme known as telomerase. Telomerase replaces the portion of the telomeres that is lost with each cell division, thereby avoiding senescence and permitting an infinite number of cell doublings. Telomerase is a new target for antineoplastic drug development.

As information regarding the role of oncogenes and tumor-suppressor genes accumulated, it became evident that a single mutation was probably not sufficient to initiate cancer. Scientists postulated that combinations of mutations

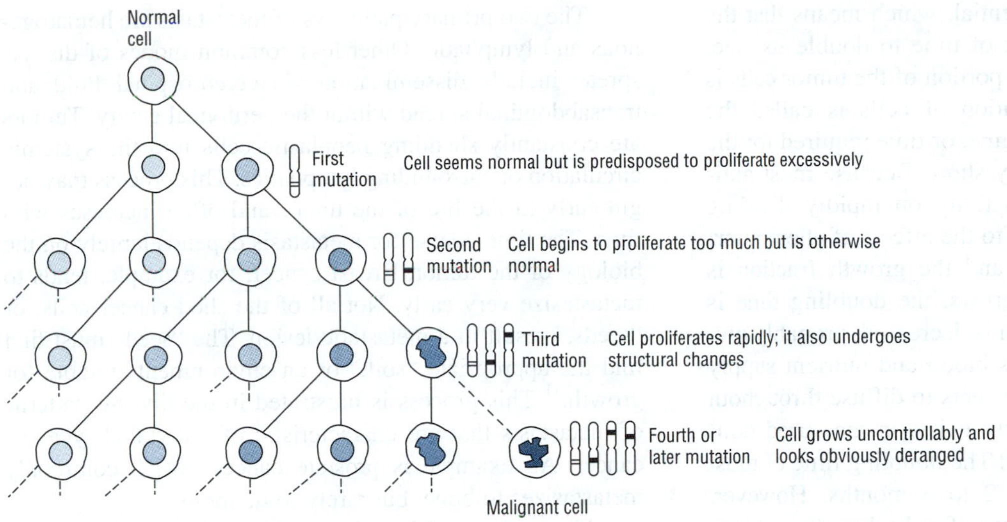

FIGURE 115–4. Emergence of a cancer cell from a normal cell is thought to occur through a process known as clonal evolution. First, one daughter cell inherits or acquires a cancer-promoting mutation and passes the defect to its progeny and all future generations. At some point, one of the descendants acquires a second mutation, and a later descendant acquires a third, and so on. Eventually, some cell accumulates enough mutations to cross the threshold to cancer. *(From Cavanee WK, White RL. The genetic basis of cancer. Sci Am 1995;72–79, with permission.)*

were required for carcinogenesis and that each mutation was inherited by the next generation of cells (Fig. 115–4). Thus, in an established tumor there may be several detectable genetic mutations. Early mutations are found in both premalignant lesions and established tumors, whereas later mutations are found only in the established tumor. This theory of sequential genetic mutations resulting in cancer has been best demonstrated in colon cancer and in brain tumors.[4] In colon cancer, the initial genetic mutation is believed to be loss of the APC (adenomatous polyposis coli) gene, which results in formation of a small benign polyp. Oncogenic mutation of the *ras* gene is often the next step, leading to enlargement of the polyp. Loss of the *p*53 gene and another gene, believed to be the deleted in colorectal cancer (DCC) gene, complete the transformation into a malignant lesion.

Identification of genes and other proteins involved in carcinogenesis has several important clinical implications. In the future, they may be used in cancer screening to identify individuals at increased risk for cancer and in cancer treatment to design new anticancer agents and gene therapies. If the presence of these genes is found to reliably predict the clinical course of a cancer or response to certain cancer therapies, then genetic analysis may become an important prognostic and treatment decision tool.

PRINCIPLES OF TUMOR GROWTH

The study of tumor growth forms the foundation for many of the basic principles of modern cancer chemotherapy. The growth of most tumors is illustrated by the Gompertzian tumor growth curve (Fig. 115–5).[6,10] Gompertz was a German insurance actuary who described the relationship between age and expected death. This mathematical model also approximates tumor cell proliferation. In the early

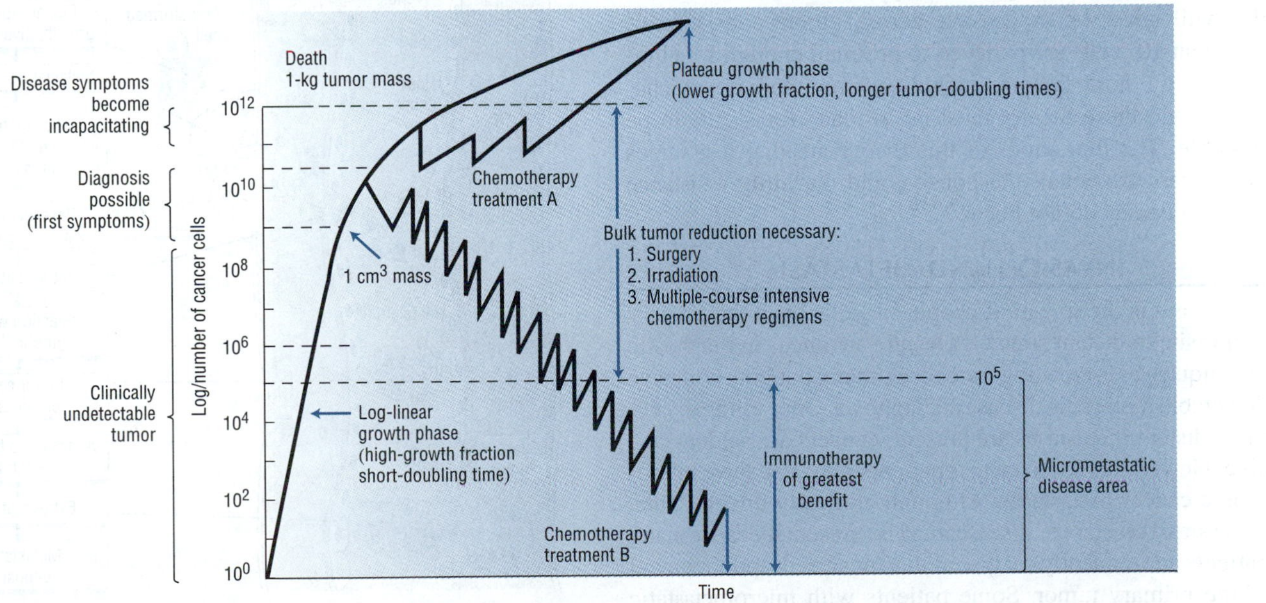

FIGURE 115–5. Gompertzian kinetics tumor-growth curve. Relationship to symptoms, diagnosis, and various treatment regimens. *(From Buick RN. Cellular basis of chemotherapy. In: Dorr RT, Von Hoff DD eds. Cancer Chemotherapy Handbook, 2nd ed. New York, Elsevier, 1994:8, with permission.)*

stages, tumor growth is exponential, which means that the tumor takes a constant amount of time to double its size. During this early phase, a large portion of the tumor cells is actively dividing. This population of cells is called the *growth fraction.* The doubling time, or time required for the tumor to double in size, is very short. Because most anticancer drugs have a greater activity on rapidly dividing cells, tumors are most sensitive to the effects of chemotherapy when the tumor is small and the growth fraction is high. However, as the tumor grows, the doubling time is slowed.[1,6,10] The growth fraction is decreased, probably owing to the tumor outgrowing its blood and nutrient supply or the inability of blood and nutrients to diffuse throughout the tumor mass. Wide variability exists in measured doubling times for different cancers. The doubling time of most solid tumors is approximately 2 to 3 months. However, some tumors have doubling times of only days (e.g., high-grade lymphomas) and others have even longer doubling times (e.g., some salivary gland tumors).[6]

The impact of tumor burden is also illustrated by Figure 115–5. It takes 10^9 cancer cells (1-g mass, 1 cm in diameter) for a tumor to be clinically detectable by palpation or radiography. Such a tumor has undergone approximately 30 doublings in cell number. It only takes 10 additional doublings for this 1-g mass to reach 1 kg in size. A tumor possessing 10^{12} cancer cells (1-kg mass) is considered lethal. Thus, a tumor is clinically undetectable for most of its life span. Tumor burden also relates to response to chemotherapy. The cell kill hypothesis states that a certain percentage of cancer cells (not a certain number of cells) will be killed with each course of chemotherapy. For example, if a tumor consists of 1000 cancer cells and the chemotherapy regimen kills 90% of the cells, then 10% or 100 cancer cells would remain. The second chemotherapy course kills another 90% of cells, and again only 10% or 10 cells remain. According to this hypothesis, the tumor burden will never reach absolute zero. Tumors consisting of less than 10^4 cells are believed to be small enough for elimination by host factors, including immunologic mechanisms, and these factors must be in place for a cure to be possible. The limitations of this theory are that it assumes all cancers are equally responsive and that drug resistance and metastases do not occur.[1,6,10]

INVASION AND METASTASIS

Metastasis is the spread of neoplastic cells from the primary tumor site to distant sites.[6,11] Despite advances in diagnostic techniques and screening for cancer, many patients will have detectable metastatic disease at diagnosis. Once clinically evident distant metastases are present, cancers are seldom curable. Newly diagnosed cancer patients may also have microscopic cancer metastases. Although clinically undetectable, these small clusters of disease must be present, because many patients subsequently relapse at distant sites despite removal of the primary tumor. Some patients with micrometastatic disease may be cured with systemic chemotherapy.

The two primary pathways of metastasis are hematogenous and lymphatic. Other less common modes of disease spread include dissemination via cerebrospinal fluid and transabdominal spread within the peritoneal cavity. Tumors are constantly shedding neoplastic cells into the systemic circulation or surrounding lymphatics. This process may begin early in the life of the tumor and often increases with time. The time course for metastasis depends largely on the biology of the tumor. Breast cancer, for example, tends to metastasize very early. Not all of the shed cancer cells, or "seeds," result in a metastatic lesion. The "seed" must first find the appropriate "soil," or an environment suitable for growth.[11] This process is illustrated in the diverse patterns of metastasis that are characteristic of individual types of cancer. An example is prostate cancer, which commonly metastasizes to bone, but rarely to the brain.

The process of invasion and metastasis involves several essential steps (Fig. 115–6). After neoplastic transformation, the malignant cells and surrounding host tissue secrete substances that stimulate the formation of new blood vessels to provide oxygen and nutrients. This process is known as *angiogenesis* or *neovascularization.* Tumor cells must then detach from the primary mass and invade surrounding blood and lymph vessels. The tumor cells or cell aggregates detach and embolize through these vessels, but most do not survive circulation. The disseminated cells must then attach to the vascular endothelium. The cells may proliferate within the lumen of the vessel, but most commonly extravasate into the surrounding tissue. The local microenvironment may provide growth factors that potentiate the proliferation of the metastasis. At every step of the

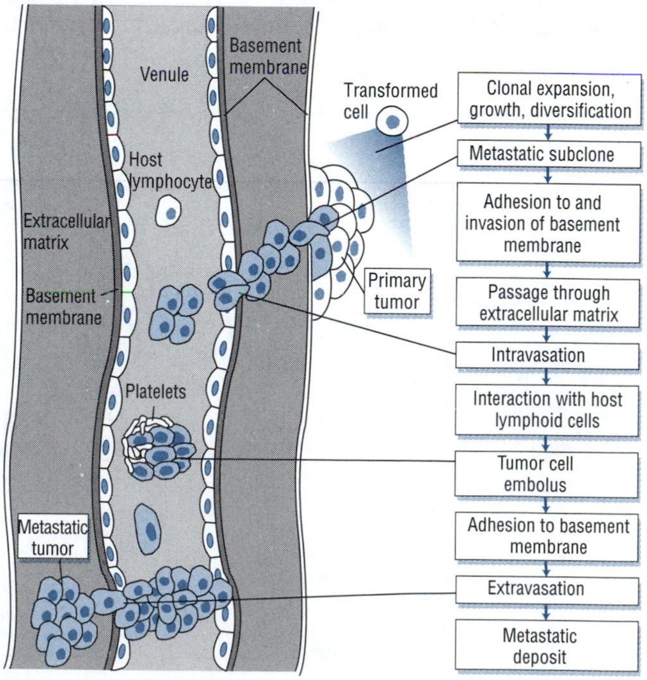

FIGURE 115–6. The process of developing a cancer metastasis.

way, the potential metastatic cell must fight the host immune system. Last, the metastasis must again initiate angiogenesis to ensure continued growth and proliferation. Because angiogenesis has been recognized as a critical element in primary tumor growth as well as metastasis, it has become a target for development of new anticancer agents.

PATHOLOGY OF CANCER

TUMOR CHARACTERISTICS

Tumors may be either benign or malignant. Benign tumors are noncancerous growths that are often encapsulated, localized, and indolent. Cells of benign tumors resemble the cells from which they developed. These masses seldom metastasize and, once removed, they rarely recur. In contrast, malignant tumors invade and destroy the surrounding tissue. The cells of malignant tumors are genetically unstable, and loss of normal cell architecture results in cells that are atypical of their tissue or cell of origin. These cells lose the ability to perform their usual functions. This loss of structure and function is defined as anaplasia. In contrast to benign tumors, malignant tumors tend to metastasize and, consequently, recurrences are common after removal or destruction of the primary tumor.

TUMOR ORIGIN

Tumors may arise from any of four basic tissue types: epithelial tissue, connective tissue (i.e., blood, bone, and cartilage), muscle tissue, and nerve tissue. Although some malignant cells are atypical of their cells of origin, the involved cells usually retain enough of their parent's traits to identify their origin. Benign tumors are named by adding the suffix -oma to the name of the cell type. Hence, adenomas are benign growths of glandular origin, or growths that exhibit a glandular pattern. A list of common tumor nomenclature by tissue type is presented in Table 115–3.[6]

Some cancers are preceded by cellular changes that are abnormal, but not yet malignant. Detection of these early changes could potentially prevent the occurrence of a cancer. Precancerous lesions may be described as consisting of either hyperplastic or dysplastic cells. Hyperplasia is an increase in the number of cells in a particular tissue or organ, which results in an increased size of the organ. It should not be confused with hypertrophy, which is an increase in the size of the individual cells. Hyperplasia occurs in response to a stimulus and reverses when the stimulus is removed. Dysplasia is defined as an abnormal change in the size, shape, or organization of cells or tissues. Hyperplasia and dysplasia may precede the appearance of a cancer by several months or years.

Malignant cells are divided into those of epithelial origin or the other tissue types. Carcinomas are malignant growths arising from epithelial cells. Malignant growths of muscle or connective tissue are called sarcomas. Therefore, an adenocarcinoma is a malignant tumor arising from glandular origin. Another term used frequently in the description of malignancy is the term *carcinoma in situ.* In this instance, the cancer is limited to the epithelial cells of origin; it has not yet invaded the basement membrane. Carcinoma *in situ* is a preinvasive stage of malignancy, and most tumors have progressed well beyond this stage at diagnosis. Like all classification systems, there are exceptions to these rules. Malignancies of hematologic origin are classified separately. Leukemias and lymphomas are discussed in later chapters.

TABLE 115–3. Tumor Classification by Tissue Type

Tissue of Origin	Benign	Malignant
Epithelial		
Surface epithelium	Papilloma	Carcinoma (squamous, epidermoid)
Glandular	Adenoma	Adenocarcinoma
Connective tissue		
Fibrous tissue	Fibroma	Fibrosarcoma
Bone	Osteoma	Osteosarcoma
Smooth muscle	Leiomyoma	Leiomyosarcoma
Striated muscle	Rhabdomyoma	Rhabdomyosarcoma
Fat	Lipoma	Liposarcoma
Lymphoid tissue and hematopoietic cells		
Bone marrow elements		Leukemias
Lymphoid tissue		Hodgkin's disease, non-Hodgkin's lymphoma
Plasma cell		Multiple myeloma
Neural tissue		
Glial tissue	"Benign" gliomas	Glioblastoma multiforme, astrocytoma
Nerve sheath	Neurofibroma	Neurofibrosarcoma
Melanocytes	Pigmented nevus (mole)	Malignant melanoma
Mixed tumors		
Gonadal tissue	Teratoma	Teratocarcinoma

Adapted from Ref. 6.

TABLE 115–4. Recommendations for Early Detection of Cancer in an Asymptomatic Person

Disease	Test or Procedure	Sex	Age (yr)	Frequency
Breast cancer	Breast self-exam	F	20 & over	Monthly
	Clinical breast exam	F	20–40	Every 3 years
			40 & over	Every year
	Mammography	F	40 & over	Every year
Cervical cancer	Pap test and pelvic exam	F	18 & over; under 18 if sexually active	Every year[a]
Colon and rectum cancer	Fecal occult blood test	M & F	50 & over	Every year
	Flexible sigmoidoscopy and digital rectal exam OR	M & F	50 & over	Every 5 years
	Colonoscopy and digital rectal exam OR	M & F	50 & over	Every 10 years
	Double-contrast barium enema and digital rectal exam	M & F	50 & over	Every 5–10 years
Endometrial (uterus) cancer	Endometrial tissue sample	F	At menopause if at high risk[b]	At discretion of physician
Prostate cancer	Digital rectal exam	M	50 & over	Every year[c]
	Prostate-specific antigen (PSA) and blood test	M	50 & over	Every year[c]
Cancer-related medical exam	Health counseling and physical exam[d]	M & F	20–40	Every 3 years
			40 & over	Every year

[a]After three negative annual examinations, the Pap test may be done at less frequent intervals, as determined by the physician.
[b]High risk includes patients with history of infertility, obesity, failure to ovulate, abnormal uterine bleeding, or estrogen or tamoxifen therapy.
[c]Beginning at age 50, men with a life expectancy of at least 10 years should discuss the need for PSA testing and digital rectal exam with their health care provider. Testing may begin at an earlier age for high-risk men (African-Americans and men with strong family history).
[d]To include examination for cancers of the mouth, thyroid, testicles, skin, lymph nodes, prostate, and ovaries.
From The American Cancer Society Recommendations for the Early Detection of Cancer in Asymptomatic People, Revised 10/97.

DIAGNOSIS AND STAGING

SCREENING

Because cancers are most curable with surgery or radiation before they have metastasized, early detection and treatment have obvious potential benefit. In addition, small tumors are more responsive to chemotherapy, as discussed previously. Early diagnosis is difficult for many cancers because they do not produce clinical signs or symptoms until they have become large or have metastasized. Lack of effective screening methods for some cancers and inaccessibility of some anatomic sites further complicate the process. Education of the public on the early warning signs of common cancers is extremely important to facilitate early detection. For some cancers, effective screening procedures do exist. The Pap smear test, for example, has been proven to be an effective tool to detect cervical cancer in its early stages. Self-examination of the breasts in women and of the testicles in men may lead to early diagnosis of cancers in these organs. The American Cancer Society has published guidelines for routine screening examinations. These recommendations are listed in Table 115–4.[12,13]

DIAGNOSIS

The presenting signs and symptoms of cancer vary widely and depend on the type of cancer. The presentation in adults may include one of cancer's seven warning signs (Table 115–5), as well as pain and loss of appetite.[14] The warning signs of cancer in children are different and reflect the types of tumors more common in this patient population (Table 115–6).[15] Even with increased public awareness, the fear of a cancer diagnosis can deter patients from seeking medical attention. The definitive diagnosis of cancer relies on the procurement of a sample of the tissue or cells suspected of malignancy and pathologic assessment of this sample. This sample can be obtained by numerous methods, including

TABLE 115–5. Cancer's Seven Warning Signs

Change in bowel or bladder habits
A sore that does not heal
Unusual bleeding or discharge
Thickening or lump in breast or elsewhere
Indigestion or difficulty in swallowing
Obvious change in wart or mole
Nagging cough or hoarseness

If YOU have a warning signal, see your doctor!

TABLE 115–6. Cancer's Warning Signs in Children

Unexplained or persistent lump
Unexplained or persistent limp
Unexplained normocytic anemia
Unexplained thrombocytopenic bruising
Unexplained weight loss
Abdominal mass
Unexplained persistent headache and/or vomiting on awakening

Adapted from Ref. 15.

biopsy, exfoliative cytology, or fine-needle aspiration. A tissue diagnosis is essential, because many benign conditions can masquerade as cancer. Definitive treatment should not begin without a pathologic diagnosis.

STAGING

In addition to tissue diagnosis, tumors should be staged to determine the extent of disease before any definitive treatment is initiated.[16] The process is dictated by knowledge of the biology of the tumor and signs and symptoms elicited in the history and physical examination. Staging provides information on prognosis and guides treatment selection. Once treatment is begun, the initial staging workup is usually repeated to evaluate the effectiveness of the treatment. Uniform staging criteria are imperative in clinical research aimed at evaluating cancer treatment regimens. Staging has been valuable in learning more about the biology of various tumor types. A staging workup may involve x-rays, computed tomography (CT) scans, magnetic resonance imaging (MRI), ultrasounds, bone-marrow biopsies, bone scans, lumbar puncture (LP), and a variety of laboratory tests, including appropriate tumor markers. Some cancers produce antigens, or other substances, that are characteristic of that particular cancer. These so-called tumor markers are often nonspecific and may be elevated in patients with more than one type of cancer, or in nonmalignant diseases. As a result, tumor markers are generally more useful for monitoring response and detecting recurrence than as diagnostic tools. Examples are the measure of human chorionic gonadotropin (HCG) and α-fetoprotein (AFP) in patients with testicular cancer, or prostate-specific antigen (PSA) in prostate cancer.

The most commonly applied staging system for solid tumors is the TNM classification, where T = tumor, N = node, and M = metastases. A numerical value is assigned to each letter to indicate the size or extent of disease. The designated rating for tumor describes the size of the primary mass and ranges from T_1 to T_4. Carcinoma *in situ* is designated T_{is}. Nodes are described in terms of the extent and quality of nodal involvement (N_0 to N_3). Metastases are scored depending on their presence or absence (M_0 or M_1). To simplify the staging process, most cancers are classified according to extent of disease by a numerical system involving stages I through IV. In this system, stage I is localized tumor, stages II and III represent local and regional extension of disease, and stage IV denotes the presence of distant metastases. The assigned TNM rating translates into a particular stage classification. For example, in general, a $T_3N_1M_0$ tumor is a moderate- to large-sized primary mass, with regional lymph node involvement and no distant metastases, and for most cancers is stage III. The criteria for classifying disease extent are quite specific for each different type of cancer. For some tumors, alternative alphabetical systems (stage A, B, C, or D) are used in clinical practice. An example of the staging system for colon cancer is outlined in Table 115–7.[16]

TABLE 115–7. TNM Staging Classification System for Colorectal Cancer

Primary Tumor (T)					
TX	Primary tumor cannot be assessed				
T_0	No evidence of primary tumor				
T_{is}	Carcinoma *in situ*				
T_1	Tumor invades submucosa				
T_2	Tumor invades muscularis propria				
T_3	Tumor invades through the muscularis propria into the subserosa or into nonperitonealized pericolic or perirectal tissues				
T_4	Tumor perforates the visceral peritoneum or directly invades other organs or structures				
Regional Lymph Nodes (N)					
NX	Regional lymph nodes cannot be assessed				
N_0	No regional lymph node metastasis				
N_1	Metastasis in one to three pericolic or perirectal lymph nodes				
N_2	Metastasis in four or more pericolic or perirectal lymph nodes				
N_3	Metastasis in any lymph node along the course of a named vascular trunk				
Distant Metastasis (M)					
MX	Presence of distant metastasis cannot be assessed				
M_0	No distant metastasis				
M_1	Distant metastasis				
Stage	**Grouping**			**Dukes**	**Modified Astler–Collier**
Stage 0	T_{is}	N_0	M_0		
Stage IA	T_1	N_0	M_0	A	A
Stage IB	T_2	N_0	M_0	A	B1
Stage II	T_3	N_0	M_0	B	B2
	T_4	N_0	M_0	B	B2, B3
Stage III	Any T	N_1	M_0	C	C1–3
	Any T	N_2	M_0	C	C1–3
	Any T	N_3	M_0	C2	
Stage IV	Any T	Any N	M_1	D	D

From Ref. 16.

▶ TREATMENT: Modalities of Cancer Treatment

Four primary modalities are employed in the approach to cancer treatment: surgery, radiation, chemotherapy, and immunotherapy.[17] The oldest of these is surgery, which plays a major role in the diagnosis and treatment of cancer. Surgery remains the treatment of choice for many solid tumors diagnosed in the early stages. Radiation therapy was first used for cancer treatment in the late 1800s and remains a mainstay in the management of cancer. Although very effective for treating many types of cancer, surgery and radiation are local treatments. These modalities are likely to produce a cure in patients with truly localized disease. However, because the majority of patients with cancer have metastatic disease at diagnosis, localized therapies often fail to completely eliminate the cancer. In addition, systemic diseases such as leukemia cannot be treated with a localized modality. Chemotherapy (including hormonal therapy) accesses the systemic circulation and can theoretically treat the primary tumor, as well as any metastatic disease. The 1990s have seen rapid advances in biotechnology and the application of immunologic principles to cancer treatment. Immunotherapy provides another means to deliver systemic anticancer therapy. This modality usually involves stimulating the host's immune system to fight against the cancer. Many of the agents in this category are naturally occurring cytokines, which have been produced with recombinant-DNA technology. Agents used in immunotherapy include tumor vaccines, levamisole, interferons (IFNs), interleukins (ILs), and monoclonal antibodies.

Many cancers appear to be eliminated by surgery or radiation. However, the high incidence of later recurrence implies that the primary tumor began to metastasize before it was removed. These early metastases are too small to detect with currently available diagnostic tests and are known as micrometastases. Adjuvant therapy is defined as the use of systemic agents to eradicate micrometastatic disease following localized modalities such as surgery or radiation or both. The hope is that systemic therapy given in this setting will reduce subsequent recurrence rates and prolong long-term survival. Thus, adjuvant therapy is given to patients with potentially curable malignancies, who have no clinically detectable disease after surgery or radiation. Because adjuvant therapy is given at a time that the cancer is undetectable, its effectiveness cannot be measured by response rates. Instead, it is evaluated by recurrence rates and survival. Adjuvant therapy has been most extensively studied in the management of breast cancer. Chemotherapy may also be given in the neoadjuvant preoperative setting. The goal in this instance is to make other treatment modalities more effective by reducing tumor burden, as well as destroying micrometastases. For example, in head and neck cancer, neoadjuvant chemotherapy is employed in an attempt to shrink large tumors and make them more amenable to later surgical resection.

The management of most types of cancer involves the use of combined modalities. Breast cancer is a good example of the use of a combined-modality approach. The primary tumor is removed surgically, and radiation therapy is delivered to the remaining breast (after lumpectomy) or to the axilla (if there is marked lymph node involvement). Adjuvant chemotherapy and/or hormonal therapy is then administered to eradicate any micrometastatic disease.

▶ TREATMENT: Principles of Chemotherapy

PURPOSES OF CHEMOTHERAPY

The era of modern cancer chemotherapy was born in 1941, when Goodman and Gilman first administered nitrogen mustard to patients with lymphoma.[18] Since that time, numerous antineoplastic agents have been developed, and a variety of chemotherapy regimens have been investigated in every type of cancer. A list of tumors and their responsiveness to chemotherapy is provided in Table 115–8.[10,19] Cancer chemotherapy may be indicated as a primary, palliative, adjuvant, or neoadjuvant treatment modality. Treatment with cytotoxic drugs is the primary curative modality for a few diseases, including leukemias, choriocarcinomas, and testicular cancer. Most solid tumors are not curable with chemotherapy alone, either because of the biology of the tumor or because of advanced disease at presentation. Chemotherapy in this setting is often initiated for palliative purposes. It is often possible to decrease tumor size or retard growth enough to reduce untoward symptoms caused by the tumor. Adjuvant and neoadjuvant chemotherapy are defined in the previous section.

RESPONSE CRITERIA

The response to chemotherapy and other treatment modalities may be described as a cure, complete response, partial response, stable disease, or progression.[19] These terms are used routinely in oncology to define the response to chemotherapy and other treatment modalities. A cure implies that the patient is entirely free of disease and has the same life expectancy as a cancer-free individual. Although there is no way to be absolutely certain that an individual patient is cured, a stable plateau in the survival curve after cancer treatment is taken as evidence of cure. For most cancers, the survival curves have plateaued by approximately 5 years. Thus, 5 years of survival without disease recurrence is equated with a cure. However, there are some malignancies, such as breast cancer and melanoma, for example, in which patients are still at significant risk for relapse after 5 years.

Complete response (CR) means complete disappearance of all cancer and no evidence of new disease for at least 1 month after treatment. The terms "cure" and "CR" are not synonymous. Although an individual must have a CR to be cured, many individuals who achieve a CR will eventually relapse. A *partial response* (PR) is defined as a 50% or greater decrease in the tumor size or other objective disease markers, and no evidence of any new disease for at least 1 month. Overall objective response rates for a given treatment are determined by adding the CR and PR rates. A patient whose tumor size neither grows nor shrinks significantly has stable disease. Despite the small changes in tumor size, some patients may experience subjective improvement in the symptoms caused by their cancer. Though clinically important, this does not indicate an objective response. Recently, the term *clinical benefit response* has been coined and is used to refer to patients who have clinical benefit as measured by decreases in pain or analgesic consumption, or improved quality of life or performance status. Progression of disease is defined as a 25% increase in the tumor size or the development of any new

TABLE 115–8. The Role of Chemotherapy in the Treatment of Cancer

Chemotherapy used alone with curative intent	
Acute lymphocytic leukemia	Acute nonlymphocytic (myelogenous) leukemia
Burkitt's lymphoma	Diffuse large-cell lymphoma
Hodgkin's disease	Testicular cancer
Choriocarcinoma (gestational trophoblastic neoplasm)	
Chemotherapy used as adjuvant therapy with curative intent	
Breast cancer (early stage)	Colorectal cancer
Ewing's sarcoma	Osteosarcoma
Wilm's tumor	Ovarian cancer
Chemotherapy used as neoadjuvant therapy	
Anal carcinoma[a]	Bladder cancer
Breast cancer (locally advanced)[a]	Cervical cancer
Esophageal cancer	Head and neck cancers[a]
Osteosarcoma[a]	Soft-tissue sarcoma[a]
Chemotherapy used to palliate symptoms in advanced disease	
Bladder cancer	Brain tumors
Breast cancer[a]	Carcinoid tumors
Cervical cancer	Chronic lymphocytic leukemia
Chronic myelogenous leukemia[a]	Colorectal cancer (metastatic)
Endometrial cancer	Esophageal cancer
Gastric cancer	Head and neck cancers
Hairy cell leukemia[a]	Kaposi's sarcoma
Low-grade lymphomas	Metastatic melanoma
Multiple myeloma[a]	Neuroblastoma[a]
Non–small-cell lung cancer	Osteosarcoma
Ovarian cancer[a]	Pancreatic cancer
Prostate cancer	Small-cell lung cancer[a]
Soft-tissue sarcoma	
Chemotherapy has little or no effect on palliation	
Hepatocellular cancer	Renal cell carcinoma
Thyroid cancer	

[a]Significant increase in survival is achieved.
Compiled from Refs. 6, 10, and 17.

lesions while receiving treatment. These response definitions are applicable to solid tumors, but diseases such as the leukemias and multiple myeloma are not characterized by discrete, measurable masses. Responses in these diseases are measured by elimination of abnormal cells (e.g., return to normal hematology parameters and normal bone marrow in leukemia), return of tumor markers to normal levels (e.g., normal serum protein electrophoresis in multiple myeloma), disappearance of pleural or peritoneal effusions, or improved function of affected organs (e.g., improved renal function after obstructive uropathy).

FACTORS AFFECTING RESPONSE TO CHEMOTHERAPY

These include tumor burden, tumor-cell heterogeneity, drug resistance, dose intensity, and patient-specific factors. The significance of tumor burden has been discussed earlier. Tumors consist of a heterogeneous population of cell types. Because of the genetic instability of cancer cells compared to normal cells, mutations commonly occur during cell division. Large tumors have undergone multiple cell divisions and, hence, multiple cell mutations resulting in genetically varied cell populations.[1,6,10,19] In 1979, Goldie and Coldman proposed that these cytogenetic changes were not completely random and were highly associated with the development of the ability to resist drug action.[1,6,10] The probability of developing resistant cell populations increases as tumor size increases. It is believed that a small percentage of resistant cancer cells may survive initial chemotherapy. This resistant population later proliferates and eventually becomes the dominant cell type. This explains the relative frequency of an initial response to chemotherapy, followed by progressive tumor regrowth despite continuing the same treatment regimen.

Drug resistance may be either an acquired or inherited property of a neoplastic cell. Mechanisms of drug resistance include decreased activation of prodrugs, decreased uptake of drugs secondary to alterations in drug transport systems, changes in the target enzymes, alterations in the cell's ability to repair drug-induced damage, and increased drug inactivation.[1,6,10] Research in the area of drug resistance currently focuses on pleiotropic drug resistance or multidrug resistance (MDR).[1,10,20] When some cancer cells are exposed to increasing concentrations of a specific antineoplastic agent *in vitro*, they become resistant to this agent. Surprisingly, these same cells also become resistant to other structurally unrelated antineoplastic agents, that is, they are multidrug resistant. Cytotoxic agents derived from natural products, such as the anthracyclines, actinomycin D, mitomycin C, the vinca alkaloids, the epipodophyllotoxins, and the taxanes, have been shown to produce MDR. The resistant cancer cells have been shown to possess a membrane-associated protein known as P170 or P-glycoprotein, which appears to enhance the export of toxins, such as chemotherapy agents, out of the cell (Fig. 115–7). The gene that encodes for P-glycoprotein is known as the MDR1 gene. Expression of this gene is amplified in cells that are resistant to the natural products listed previously. P-glycoprotein is also found in high concentrations in tumors that are traditionally resistant to chemotherapy (e.g., renal cell and non–small-cell lung cancers) and thus may also be an important mechanism of intrinsic or inherited drug resistance. Several drugs have been investigated as possible inhibitors of this efflux pump, such as the calcium channel blockers, quinidine, cyclosporine, and the phenothiazines. Another efflux pump, known as the multidrug resistance–associated protein (MRP) has also recently been identified. Other potential mechanisms of drug resistance include inactivation of chemotherapy agents by glutathione metabolism, upregulation of target enzymes like topoisomerases or dihydrofolate reductase,

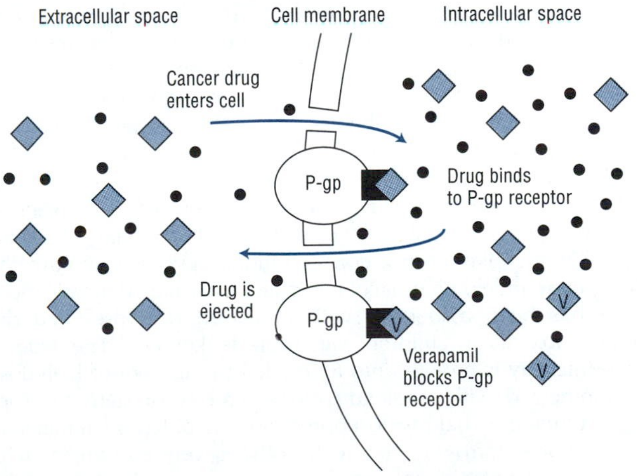

FIGURE 115–7. P-glycoprotein (P-gp) is a membrane-associated protein that acts as a drug efflux pump. Anticancer agents enter the cell, bind to the P-gp receptor, and are ejected. Some agents that modify multidrug resistance, like verapamil, block the P-gp receptor, allowing the anticancer agent to remain in the cell.

TABLE 115–9. Performance Status Scales

Description: Karnofsky Scale	Karnofsky Scale (%)	Zubrod Scale (ECOG)[a]	Description: ECOG Scale
No complaints; no evidence of disease	100	0	Fully active, able to carry on all predisease activity
Able to carry on normal activity; minor signs or symptoms of disease	90		
Normal activity with effort, some signs or symptoms of disease	80	1	Restricted in strenuous activity, but ambulatory and able to carry out work of a light or sedentary nature
Cares for self; unable to carry on normal activity or to do active work	70		
Requires occasional assistance but is able to care for most personal needs	60	2	Out of bed more than 50% of time; ambulatory and capable of self-care, but unable to carry out any work activities
Requires considerable assistance and frequent medical care	50		
Disabled; requires special care and assistance	40	3	In bed more than 50% of time; capable of only limited self-care
Severely disabled; hospitalization indicated, although death not imminent	30		
Very sick; hospitalization necessary; requires active supportive treatment	20	4	Bedridden; cannot carry out any self-care; completely disabled
Moribund; fatal processes progressing rapidly	10		
Dead	0		

[a]ECOG, Eastern Cooperative Oncology Group.
Adapted from Ref. 26.

and decreased apoptosis after exposure to chemotherapy.[20,21] The latter mechanism can be mediated by *bcl*-2 oncogene overexpression or loss of the *p*53 gene, as discussed in the oncogene section.

The relationship between dose and response has been extensively explored in the arena of cancer chemotherapy. Dose is believed to be a critical factor in determining response for many types of cancers. Dose intensity is defined as the dose delivered to the patient over a specified period of time.[1,22] The delivery of optimal dose intensity is compromised by the toxicities of the oncologic drugs. Treatment cycles are commonly delayed owing to inadequate recovery from drug toxicity, especially myelosuppression. Subsequent doses of chemotherapy are often reduced to prevent or reduce the severity of these toxicities. The impact of this issue on patient outcome has been proven in studies showing reduced rates of response and survival in individuals receiving less than optimal chemotherapy doses.[22] The development of drug- and toxicity-specific chemoprotective agents may aid in the application of dose-intensity principles.[23] The colony-stimulating factors avert neutropenia and permit delivery of dose-intensive regimens that are usually compromised by this toxicity. Monitoring of antineoplastic drug concentrations may also improve the therapeutic index. Pharmacokinetic and pharmacodynamic modeling has been associated with improved responses and decreased toxicity in children with acute leukemia.[24] The issue of dose intensity is brought into a new light in the era of high-dose chemotherapy with autologous bone marrow or stem cell support. Although lethal myelosuppression is avoided by administration of bone marrow or stem cells, other severe end-organ toxicities emerge as antineoplastic doses are increased.

Patient-specific factors create unpredictable variability in response to chemotherapy. The biology of cancer is strongly affected by host characteristics and genetics. Interindividual variations in drug absorption or metabolism, for example, may lead to sub- or supertherapeutic levels of antineoplastic agents and their metabolites.[25] As a result, both drug efficacy and drug toxicity can be affected. Underlying nononcologic disease states may also affect response to treatment by limiting treatment options. The overall functional status of a patient may be assessed using performance status scales, such as the Karnofsky and ECOG scales (Table 115–9).[19,26] These scales can be used to predict patient tolerance of chemotherapy, as well as to assess the effects of chemotherapy on the patient's level of activity and quality of life. In many cancers, performance status is the most important prognostic indicator.

COMBINATION CHEMOTHERAPY

Although single-agent therapy is sometimes employed, more commonly the approach to chemotherapy involves administration of multiple agents.[1,17,19] This approach is based on the Goldie–Coldman hypothesis, which addresses the issue of tumor cell heterogeneity and the inevitable development of drug resistance. Combination chemotherapy is employed to target as many types of cells in the tumor as possible. Selection of agents for combination chemotherapy regimens involves consideration of drug-specific factors such as mechanism of action, antitumor activity, and toxicity profile. Drugs that possess minimally overlapping mechanisms of action and toxicities are combined, when possible. Myelosuppressive combinations are sometimes alternated with nonmyelosuppressive combinations to allow bone marrow recovery, but still gain additive antitumor effects. The selected agents should each have significant activity against the tumor that is to be treated. If a synergistic reaction is known to exist for two agents, they may be combined in various treatment regimens.

CELL CYCLE

Both cancer cells and normal cells reproduce themselves in a series of steps known as the cell cycle. Figure 115–8 depicts the cell cycle and the phases of activity for commonly used antineoplastic agents.[10] The first phase is mitosis (M). Mitosis lasts for approximately 30 to 60 minutes and during this phase, cell division occurs. After mitosis, the cell may enter a dormant phase (G_0), or proceed to the first gap phase (G_1). G_0 is the largest variable in the cell cycle, and during this resting phase, the cell is not actively committed to cell division. Some stimulus results in the cell entering the first gap phase (G_1). During G_1, the cell prepares for DNA synthesis by manufacturing necessary enzymes. DNA synthesis (S) occurs next, and this phase lasts 10 to 20 hours. The percentage of cells in the S phase can be measured by flow cytometry and is an indicator of the rate of tumor cell proliferation. Tumors with a high percentage of S-phase cells are aggressively growing. The synthesis phase is followed by a second gap or premitotic phase (G_2), lasting 2 to 10 hours. During this second gap, the cell prepares for mitosis by producing ribonucleic acid (RNA) and specialized proteins, as well as the mitotic spindle apparatus. The cycle then begins again with the M phase. Most normal human cells exist in the G_0 phase, and most cancer cells are not sensitive to the effects of chemotherapy when in this stage. The cell cycle is regulated by external mitogens, including lymphokines, hormones, and growth factors. As mentioned earlier, some of the genes that regulate the cell cycle are known to be proto-oncogenes and tumor-suppressor genes.

All cancer cells do not proliferate faster than normal cells; some cancer cells reproduce more rapidly, and others are more indolent. Many anticancer drugs target rapidly proliferating cells (both normal and cancerous cells) and these agents may act at selective or multiple sites of the cell cycle. Agents with major activity in a particular phase of the cell cycle are known as cell cycle phase–specific agents. The antimetabolites exert their major effect during the S phase. Cell cycle phase–specific agents may also be active to a lesser extent in other phases of the cycle. Cell cycle phase–nonspecific agents are those with significant activity in multiple phases. The alkylating agents, such as nitrogen mustard, are an example. In many cases, the cytotoxic effect of a drug may result from interactions with other intracellular activities and is not related to specific cell cycle events. Hormonal agents are an example of this type of drug.

Knowledge of cell cycle specificity has been applied to the scheduling of chemotherapy administration. By definition, phase-specific agents exert their major activity when cells are in a particular phase of the cell cycle. At any given time, the heterogeneous cell populations within a tumor are at various stages in the cell cycle. By giving phase-specific agents as a continuous infusion or in multiple repeated fractions, it is theoretically possible to target more cells by allowing them to progress to the drug-sensitive phase. Thus, phase-specific agents are also termed *schedule dependent.* In contrast, cell cycle phase–nonspecific drugs are active at many stages and, consequently, are not schedule dependent. The activity of this group of drugs is dependent on the magnitude of the dose, and these drugs are termed *dose dependent.*

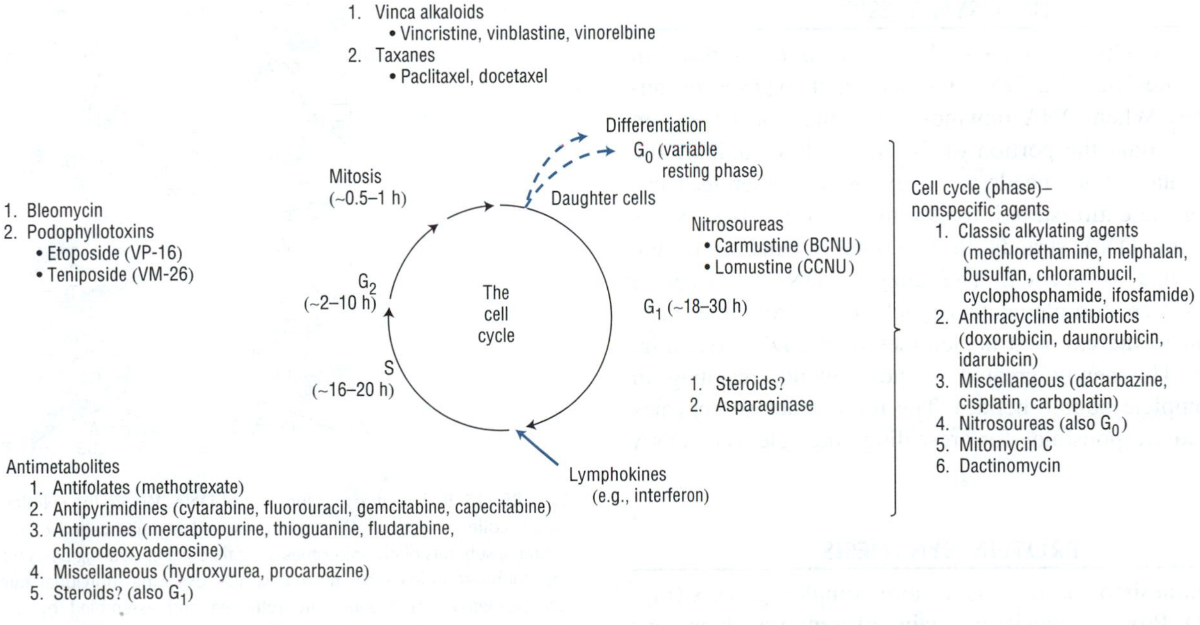

FIGURE 115–8. Cell cycle activity for anticancer drugs. Cell cycle (phase)–specific agents appear to be most active during a particular phase, but may also be active in another phase. Cell cycle (phase)–nonspecific agents may have greater activity in one phase than another, but not to the degree of cell cycle (phase)–specific agents. In many cases, it is likely that drug cytotoxicity involves multiple intracellular sites of action and may not be linked to specific cell-cycle events.

MOLECULAR BIOLOGY

Because many antineoplastic agents interfere with the cellular synthesis of DNA, RNA, and proteins, it is important to review the basic principles of molecular biology.[27,28] Each normal human cell contains 46 chromosomes, which are composed of DNA (deoxyribonucleic acid) (Fig. 115–9). Hereditary information is carried by DNA in units called genes. A single chromosome can contain 20,000 genes. Genes code for specific proteins that regulate cellular activity and inherited traits. The genetic information is encoded in DNA by precise sequencing of subunits known as nucleotides. Each nucleotide consists of a sugar (deoxyribose), phosphoric acid, and a base. Four bases exist in DNA: adenine, thymine, guanine, and cytosine. Adenine and guanine are purine-type bases; thymine and cytosine are pyrimidine-type bases (Fig. 115–10). These nucleotides are connected linearly to form a chain. Each DNA molecule is made up of two chains of nucleotides, which wind around each other to form a double helix (see Fig. 115–9). The two strands are held together by chemical bonding between the bases. The bonding process is very specific; adenine binds only with thymine, and guanine binds only with cytosine. This is known as complementary base-pairing. RNA (ribonucleic acid) is important in the DNA-directed synthesis of proteins or enzymes. RNA differs from DNA in that it is composed of a single strand of nucleotides; the sugar is ribose, and the base uracil is substituted for thymine. There are three known types of RNA: messenger RNA (mRNA), transfer RNA (tRNA), and ribosomal RNA (rRNA).

DNA SYNTHESIS

During the DNA synthesis phase, which takes place in the cell nucleus, the DNA unwinds and exposes its nucleotides. When DNA unwinds for replication or protein synthesis, only the portion of the molecule containing the needed nucleotides needs to be exposed. Rather than unwinding the entire strand, topoisomerase I and II enzymes cleave the DNA strands to facilitate unwinding of the section that is needed. The enzyme DNA polymerase matches free complementary nucleotides from the environment to the exposed nucleotides of the DNA (see Fig. 115–9). The newly created strands rewind, resulting in two complete double helices. The topoisomerase enzymes are also responsible for resealing the cleaved DNA strands.

PROTEIN SYNTHESIS

The synthesis of proteins is a more complex process (Fig. 115–11). Proteins consist of chains of amino acids in very specific sequences. As in DNA synthesis, the double helix must unwind. However, in protein synthesis, only the portion of the DNA molecule that codes for the desired pro-

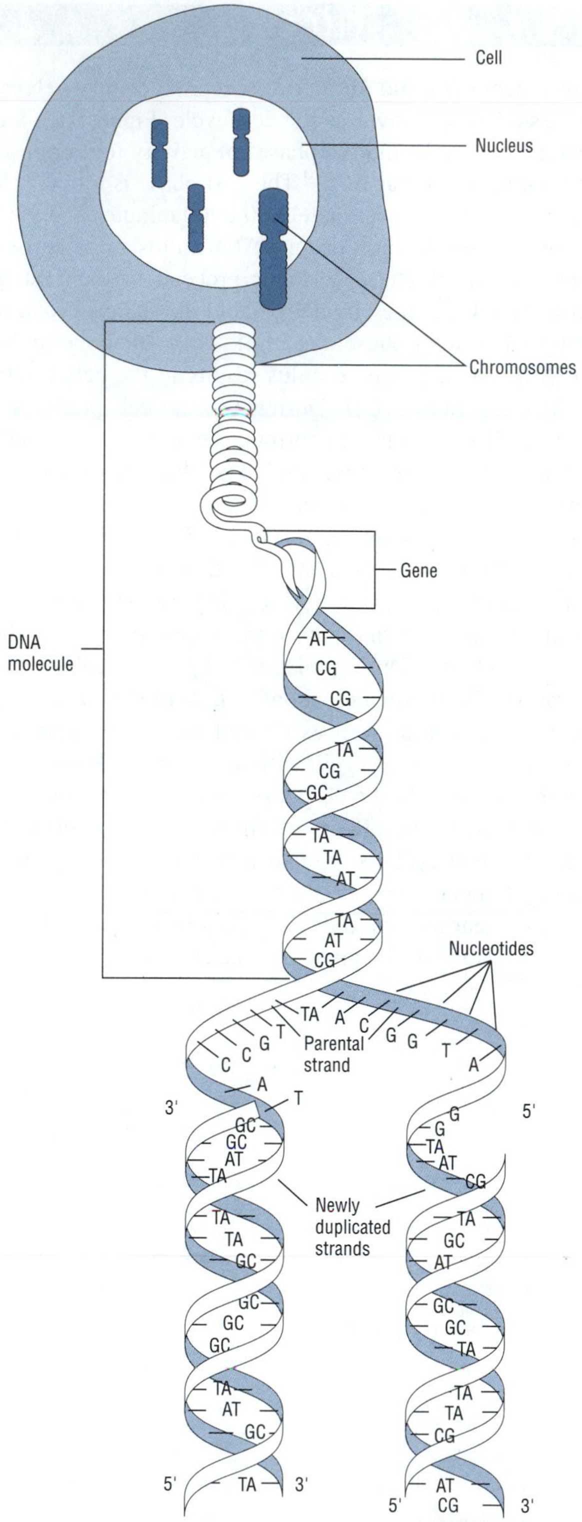

FIGURE 115–9. Structure and function of DNA. Within the cellular nucleus, tightly coiled strands of DNA are packaged in units called chromosomes. Working subunits of chromosomes are called genes. During DNA replication, the double-stranded DNA helix unwinds, exposing individual nucleotides. Complementary nucleotides are retrieved and assembled by DNA polymerases to form new strands of DNA.

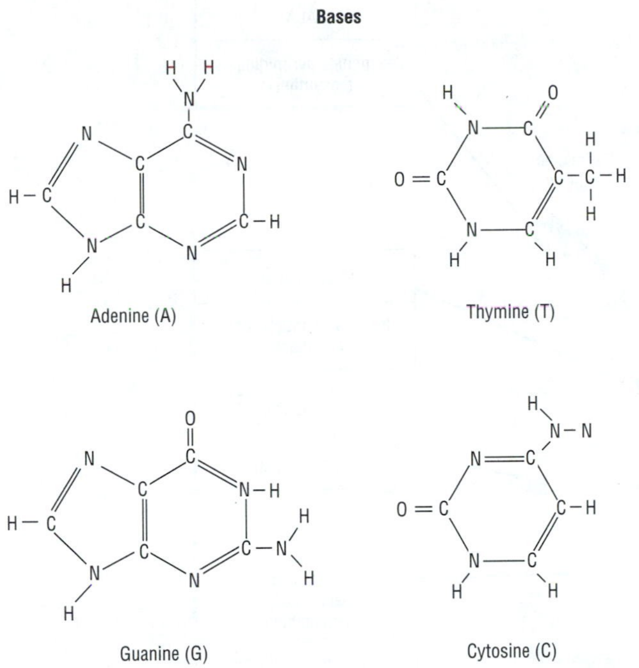

FIGURE 115–10. Structures of DNA constituents.

tein is exposed. The enzyme RNA polymerase matches free complementary RNA nucleotides to the exposed DNA nucleotides, and the resultant chain of nucleotides is called mRNA. This process is called transcription. The mRNA travels to ribosomes in the cytoplasm, where protein synthesis occurs. Each three nucleotides of the mRNA chain compose a codon, whose sequence is specific for a particular amino acid. The codon is recognized by tRNA, which then carries the amino acid to the ribosome, where it is added to the growing peptide chain. This process is known as translation. The completed protein is then ready for its intended use as an enzyme or as a structural component.

CLINICAL PHARMACOLOGY OF ANTICANCER AGENTS

Agents used in cancer chemotherapy are commonly categorized by their mechanism of action or by their origin. The alkylating agents exert their effects on DNA and protein synthesis by binding to DNA and preventing the unwinding of the DNA molecule. The antimetabolites resemble naturally occurring nuclear structural components ("metabolites"), such as the nucleotide bases, or inhibit enzymes involved in the synthesis of DNA and proteins. Antitumor antibiotics gain their name from their source of derivation; they are fermentation products of *Streptomyces* species. Figure 115–12 depicts the sites of activity of common categories of antineoplastic agents.[18] The following section discusses these classes of agents and the most commonly used cytotoxic agents in the treatment of cancer. The clinical uses of these agents are summarized in Table 115–10.

ANTIMETABOLITES

FLUORINATED PYRIMIDINES

Fluorouracil

Fluorouracil (5-FU) is a fluorinated analog of the naturally occurring pyrimidine uracil and was originally synthesized in the late 1950s (Fig. 115–13).[23,29] It is a prodrug and must be metabolized to the nucleotide form, fluorodeoxyuridine monophosphate (FdUMP), to be active. In the presence of folates, FdUMP binds tightly to and interferes with the function of thymidylate synthase. This enzyme is required for synthesis of thymidine, one of the four essential building blocks of DNA. Another metabolite of 5-FU, the triphosphate nucleotide, is incorporated into RNA and interferes with its function. Interference with both thymidine formation and RNA function is important in producing the cytotoxic effects of 5-FU. Although 5-FU nucleotides can also be incorporated directly into DNA and may affect its stability, the contribution to cell damage remains

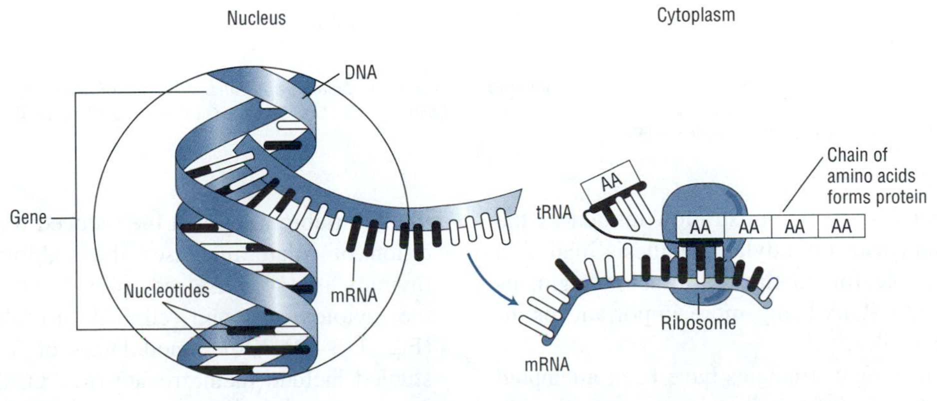

FIGURE 115–11. Protein synthesis. When a specific protein is needed, the portion of DNA responsible for that protein unwinds, exposing the necessary nucleotide sequence. Complementary nucleotides are assembled to form messenger RNA (mRNA), which travels to ribosomes in the cytoplasm. There, transfer RNA (tRNA) matches amino acids to the nucleotide sequence on the mRNA. The amino acids are assembled to form proteins.

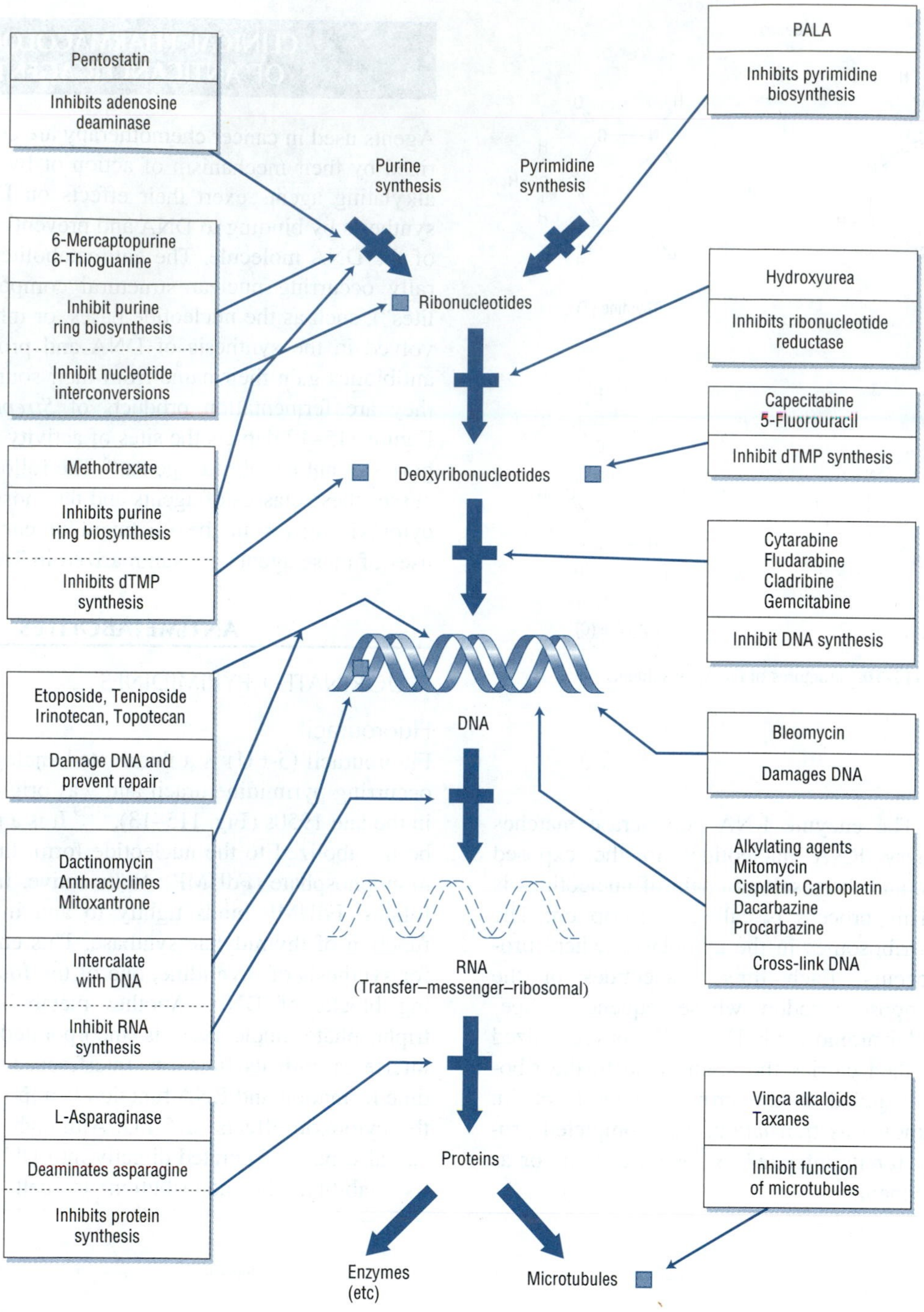

FIGURE 115–12. Mechanisms of action of commonly used antineoplastic agents. *(Adapted from Calabresi P, Chabner BA. Chemotherapy of neoplastic diseases. In: Hardman JG, Limbird LE, Molinoff PB, Ruddon RW, Gilman AG eds. Goodman & Gilman's The Pharmacologic Basis of Therapeutics, 9th ed. New York, McGraw-Hill, 1996:1226.)*

unclear.[29–31] The method of administration influences the mechanism of action, with thimidylate-synthesis inhibition playing more of a role for continuous-infusion regimens and incorporation into RNA being more important for intermittent-bolus schedules.[32]

Several pharmacologic strategies have been attempted to increase the cytotoxicity of 5-FU against tumor cells and to decrease its toxicity to normal cells. The most successful of these attempts at biochemical modulation are combinations of fluorouracil and the reduced folate leucovorin. Addition of folate increases the stability of the FdUMP–thymidylate synthase complex, and, in turn, increases the cytotoxicity and clinical usefulness of the drug (Fig. 115–14). Other modulators of 5-FU that have been studied include methotrexate (MTX), dipyridamole, interferon, phosphonoacetyl-*l*-aspartate (PALA), and uracil.[31] New modulation strategies focus on inhibition of the enzyme dihydropyrimidine dehydrogenase (DPD), which is

TABLE 115–10. Selected Clinical Uses of Anticancer Agents

Agent	Approved Indications	Other Clinical Uses
Antimetabolites		
Capecitabine	Breast cancer	Colorectal cancer
Cladribine	Hairy cell leukemia	Low-grade NHL
Cytarabine	ANLL, ALL, CML[a], CNS leukemia (IT)	NHL
Fludarabine	CLL	Low-grade NHL, Waldenstrom's macroglobulinemia
Fluorouracil	Colorectal, breast, gastric, and pancreatic cancers	Esophageal, head and neck, and cervical cancers, cataract surgery
Gemcitabine	Pancreatic cancer, NSCLC	Bladder, head and neck, and ovarian cancers
6-Mercapturine	ALL	
Methotrexate	ALL, CNS leukemia (IT), GTN	NHL, bladder, breast, gastric, head and neck cancers, osteosarcoma, BMT, rheumatoid arthritis, SLE
Pentostatin	Hairy cell leukemia	
6-Thioguanine	ANLL	
Plant Alkaloids		
Docetaxel	Breast cancer	NSCLC, SCLC, gastric, head and neck, and ovarian cancers, melanoma, soft-tissue sarcomas
Etoposide	Testicular cancer, SCLC	ANLL, HD, NHL, NSCLC, gastric cancer, BMT, KS
Irinotecan	Colorectal cancer	NSCLC, cervical, gastric, and ovarian cancers
Paclitaxel	Breast and ovarian cancers, KS	NSCLC, SCLC, bladder, esophageal, head and neck, and testicular cancers
Teniposide	ALL	
Topotecan	Ovarian cancer	SCLC
Vincristine	ALL	HD, NHL, myeloma, SCLC, brain tumors, breast cancer, KS, soft-tissue sarcoma, osteosarcoma, neuroblastoma, Wilm's tumor
Vinblastine	HD, NHL, testicular cancer, KS	NSCLC , bladder, breast, prostate, and renal cell cancers
Vinorelbine	NSCLC	HD, breast, ovarian, and prostate cancers
Alkylating Agents		
Busulfan	CML	BMT
Carmustine	Brain tumors, myeloma, HD, NHL	BMT, melanoma
Chlorambucil	CLL, NHL, HD	
Cyclophosphamide	NHL, CLL, CML,[a] ANLL, ALL, myeloma, neuroblastoma, breast and ovarian cancers, retinoblastoma	HD, NSCLC, SCLC, bladder and endometrial cancers, BMT, soft-tissue sarcoma, SLE
Dacarbazine	Melanoma, HD	Soft-tissue sarcoma, brain tumors
Ifosfamide	Testicular cancer	NSCLC, SCLC, NHL, soft-tissue sarcoma
Mechlorethamine	HD, CML,[a] CLL,[a] NSCLC[a]	NHL (topically in cutaneous T-cell NHL)
Melphalan	Myeloma, ovarian cancer[a]	BMT, melanoma (regional limb perfusion)
Procarbazine	HD	Brain tumors, NSCLC
Thiotepa	Breast and ovarian[a] cancers, intracavitary effusions,[a] bladder cancer (BI)	BMT
Antitumor Antibiotics		
Bleomycin	Testicular cancer, HD, NHL, squamous cell cancer of the head and neck, cervix, skin, penis, or vulva	KS
Dactinomycin	Wilm's tumor, soft-tissue sarcoma, GTN, testicular cancer	
Daunorubicin	ANLL, ALL, KS (liposomal)	
Doxorubicin	ALL, ANLL, NHL, HD Wilm's tumor, bladder, breast, gastric, ovarian, and thyroid cancers, neuroblastoma, SCLC, osteosarcoma, soft-tissue sarcoma, KS (liposomal)	NSCLC, myeloma, endometrial cancer
Idarubicin	ANLL	

(continued)

TABLE 115–10. Selected Clinical Uses of Anticancer Agents (Continued)

Agent	Approved Indications	Other Clinical Uses
Mitomycin C	Gastric and pancreatic[a] cancers	Bladder (BI), breast, colorectal, and esophageal cancers, NSCLC, pterygium
Mitoxantrone	ANLL, prostate cancer	NHL, HD, breast cancer
Heavy Metal Compounds		
Carboplatin	Ovarian cancer	NSCLC, SCLC, bladder, head and neck, and testicular cancers
Cisplatin	Bladder, ovarian, and testicular cancers	NHL, NSCLC, SCLC, cervical, endometrial, esophageal, and gastric cancers, melanoma, osteosarcoma
Immune Therapies		
Aldesleukin	Renal cell cancer, melanoma	
Interferon-α	KS, hairy cell leukemia, melanoma, hepatitis B and C condyloma acuminata	CML, NHL, myeloma, renal cell cancer
Rituximab	NHL	
Other		
All-*trans*-retinoic acid	APL	
L-Asparaginase	ALL	
Estramustine	Prostate cancer	
Hydroxyurea	CML, melanoma,[a] ovarian,[a] and head and neck[a] cancers, sickle cell anemia	

[a]Although an FDA-approved indication, the drug is no longer used for this disease.
ALL = acute lymphocytic leukemia; ANLL = acute nonlymphocytic leukemia; APL = acute promyelocytic leukemia; BI = bladder instillation; BMT = bone marrow transplantation; CLL = chronic lymphocytic leukemia; CML = chronic myelogenous leukemia; GTN = gestational trophoblastic neoplasm; HD = Hodgkin's disease; IT = intrathecal; KS = Kaposi's sarcoma; NHL = non-Hodgkin's lymphoma; NSCLC = non–small-cell lung cancer; SCLC = small-cell lung cancer; SLE = systemic lupus erythematosus.

responsible for breakdown of 5-FU. DPD inihibitors may increase or prolong systemic exposure to 5-FU, and even permit oral dosing of this agent.

Pharmacokinetics. Fluorouracil is distributed rapidly throughout the body and also is cleared rapidly from the plasma. Ninety percent of its elimination is accounted for by metabolism, mainly by the enzyme DPD. Deficiency of this enzyme has been associated with increased toxicity (and potentially efficacy) of 5-FU. Catabolism takes place primarily in the liver and in the kidneys, although lung tissue is also an important site of 5-FU metabolism. Because some of the clearance of 5-FU is extrahepatic and only small amounts of drug are excreted unchanged in the urine, dose adjustment is not known to be necessary in hepatic or renal dysfunction.

Toxicity. Clinical toxicity of 5-FU is a function of the schedule, dose, and route of administration. It is most typically administered either as an intravenous bolus or as continuous intravenous infusion. Higher total doses are tolerated by continuous infusion compared with bolus regimens. The toxicity pattern differs by the schedule of administration. The dose-limiting toxicity after bolus administration is myelosuppression, which especially affects white blood cells (WBCs) and platelets. In continuous-infusion regimens, and in combination regimens with leucovorin, mucosal damage is dose limiting, and myelosuppression is less prominent. Diarrhea and stomatitis secondary to mucosal damage can be life threatening, with elderly women at greatest risk.[33] Severe diarrhea necessitates dose reduction on subsequent cycles of 5-FU. Conventional antidiarrheal agents, such as loperamide, and also octreotide are useful in the treatment of 5-FU–induced diarrhea. Oral cryotherapy, consisting of ice chips in the mouth for 30 minutes before and during bolus 5-FU administration, can decrease the incidence of mucositis. Dermatologic toxicities, including hyperpigmentation, alopecia, photosensitivity, and nail banding, can also occur. Ocular toxicity manifests as excessive tearing, itching, and burning, all of which are well-recognized effects. Application of ocular ice packs before and during the 5-FU bolus administration may decrease the severity of this toxicity.[34] Nausea and vomiting are generally mild and easily controlled with antiemetics. Major organ toxicity has been increasingly recognized with 5-FU administration. Cardiac toxicity, most commonly manifested as myocardial ischemia, occurs in about 2% of patients receiving 5-FU and may exceed 5% in patients receiving high-dose continuous infusions.[35] Recently, mild and reversible hepatic toxicity has been noted in nearly 40% of patients receiving 5-FU and levamisole as adjuvant therapy for colorectal cancer. Asymptomatic elevations of alkaline phosphatase are the most common abnormalities.[36]

Capecitabine

Capecitabine is the first orally active pyrimidine analog approved by the FDA. Despite the similarity of its name to cytidine derivatives such as cytarabine and gemcitabine, capecitabine is an analog of uracil, rather than cytidine (see Fig. 115–13). It is a fluoropyrimidine carbamate and is a prodrug of 5-fluorouracil. Because capecitabine is converted to 5-FU, it shares the same mechanisms of antineoplastic

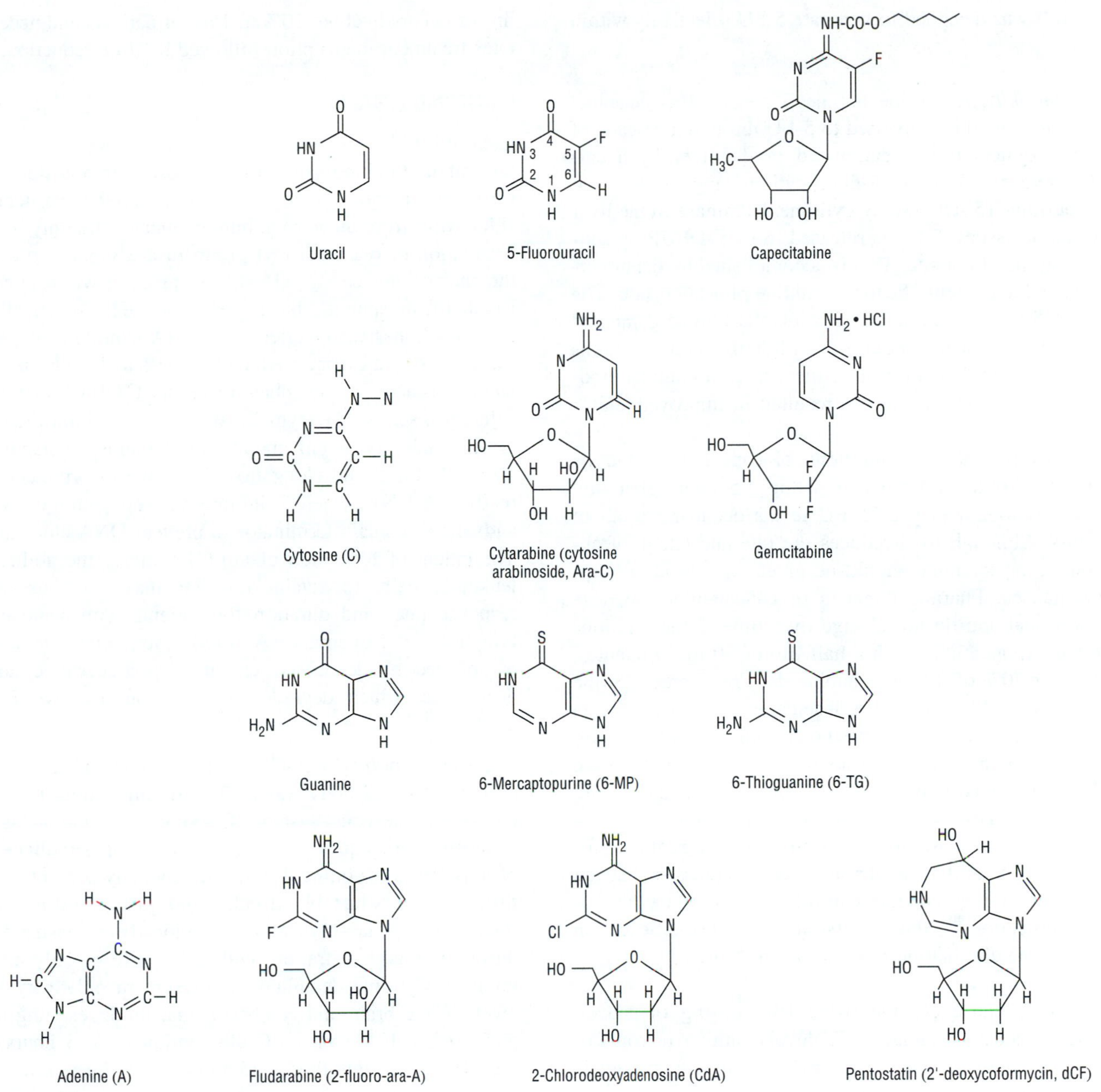

FIGURE 115–13. Structures of natural purines and pyrimidines and their structural analogs.

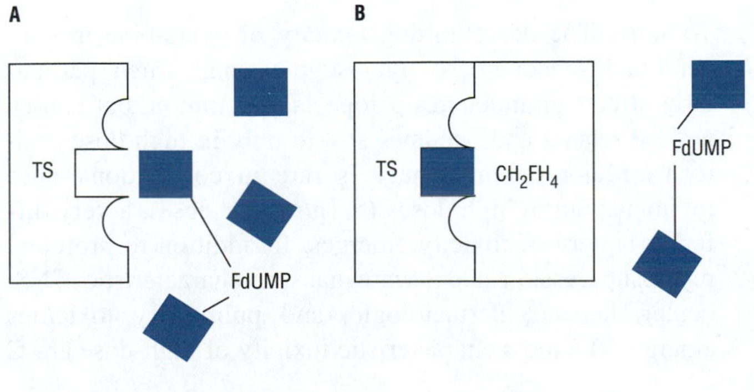

FIGURE 115–14. Interaction of leucovorin and 5-fluorouracil. (**A**) Binding of fluorodeoxyuridine monophosphate (FdUMP) to thymidylate synthase (TS) in the absence of folate cofactor. In the absence of the folate cofactor, which is supplied by leucovorin, FdUMP binds poorly to the enzyme TS. Therefore, DNA synthesis is not adequately inhibited, resulting in poor cytocidal outcome. (**B**) Binding of FdUMP to TS in presence of folate cofactor. In the presence of the folate cofactor, a very stable ternary complex is formed, made up of FdUMP, TS, and the folate cofactor methylenetetrahydrofolate (CH_2FH_4 folate.) By binding available TS and making it unavailable for DNA synthesis, the cytocidal outcome is significantly enhanced. *(Adapted from Bertino JR, Knobf T, Remington JS. Leucovorin: Interaction of leucovorin with 5-fluorouracil. Burroughs Wellcome, monograph WE-49, 1985:1–6.)*

action. It was designed to generate 5-FU selectively within tumors.[37]

Pharmacokinetics. Capecitabine is absorbed as an intact molecule, which is converted to 5-FU through a cascade of three enzymes. It is metabolized in the liver by a carboxyesterase to 5′-deoxy-5-fluorocytidine, then 5′-deoxy-5-fluorouridine (5′-DFUR) by cytidine deaminase in the liver and tumor tissues. 5-FU is released from 5′-DFUR by activation at the tumor site. This is accomplished by the tumor-associated angiogenic factor thymidine phosphorylase. The ratio of 5-FU concentration in colorectal tumors compared with healthy tissue is about 3:1, with higher concentrations in primary tumors than in liver metastases. In animal models, this tumor selectivity has resulted in improved antitumor efficacy.[38]

Peak plasma concentrations of capecitabine and its main metabolites are reached within 1.5 hours after oral administration, with peak 5-FU levels occurring at about 2 hours. Although food reduces the rate and extent of absorption, capecitabine should be given with food to minimize nausea. Pharmacokinetics of capecitabine are dose proportional and do not change over time. Concentrations decline exponentially with a half-life of 30 to 60 minutes, with over 70% of the capecitabine dose recovered in urine as drug-related species.[39] Because capecitabine depends on the liver for metabolism, it has been studied in patients with mild to moderate liver dysfunction. Area-under-the-curve (AUC) and maximum concentrations of capecitabine are decreased in these patients, but 5-FU concentrations are not affected. Initial dose modifications are not required for patients with mild to moderate liver dysfunction, but the manufacturer recommends careful monitoring in this patient population.[40] The effects of renal insufficiency on capecitabine elimination have not been studied.

Toxicity. Because chronic twice-daily dosing of capecitabine produces sustained 5-FU levels, similar to continuous intravenous infusions of 5-FU, the toxicity pattern is similar to that of 5-FU infusions. Myelosuppression and alopecia are uncommon, but diarrhea can be severe. The usual onset of diarrhea is approximately 1 month, but it may begin from 1 day to nearly a year after initiation of capecitabine therapy. As with 5-FU, the elderly are at greater risk for severe diarrhea and its complications. Diarrhea can usually be managed with antidiarrheals such as loperamide. Severe diarrhea necessitates interruption of capecitabine therapy until the diarrhea resolves, with attention to hydration and electrolyte status, and dose reduction. Nausea is common but is usually mild.[37]

Another toxicity similar to continuous 5-FU infusion is hand–foot syndrome (palmar–plantar erythrodysesthesia), which can be dose limiting. More than half of patients on capecitabine will experience some degree of painless or painful erythema and swelling of the hands and/or feet that can desquamate, blister, or ulcerate. Severe hand–foot syndrome occurs in about 10% to 15% of patients and necessitates treatment interruption followed by dose reduction.[37]

CYTIDINE ANALOGS

Cytarabine

Cytarabine (arabinosyl cytosine, cytosine arabinoside, ara-C) is an arabinose analog of cytosine. Arabinose nucleosides differ from the normal human nucleosides only by the orientation of one hydroxyl group in the sugar portion of the nucleoside (see Fig. 115–13). Cytarabine was originally isolated from sponges, but is now produced synthetically.

Ara-C has many effects on DNA synthesis. It penetrates cells by a carrier-mediated process and is phosphorylated to its active triphosphate form (ara-CTP) within tumor cells by a series of enzymatic steps. Once within the cell, ara-CTP inhibits the enzyme DNA polymerase, which is responsible for strand elongation. It is also incorporated directly into DNA, where it inhibits the replication of DNA and acts as a chain terminator to prevent DNA elongation. The extent of formation of ara-CTP and/or the ability of leukemic cells to retain ara-CTP may correlate with response rates and duration for patients with acute nonlymphocytic leukemias (ANLLs). Activation of ara-C is opposed by deaminase enzymes, particularly cytidine deaminase, which degrades ara-C to an inactive form, ara-U.[29,30,41]

Pharmacokinetics. Ara-C is water soluble and distributes rapidly into total body water after administration. It enters the central nervous system (CNS) readily and achieves concentrations equal to 20% to 40% of simultaneous plasma levels. Cytidine deaminase is widely present in the liver, plasma, white blood cells, and gastrointestinal (GI) tract; however, ara-C disappears rapidly from plasma after intravenous administration, with a half-life of only a few minutes. Cytidine deaminase is present in only very low levels in the brain and cerebral spinal fluid, resulting in a prolonged half-life of ara-C elimination (2 to 3 hours) in the CNS after intrathecal administration. Increased concentrations of deaminase enzymes present in tumor cells may account for the resistance of some cancers to the antitumor effects of ara-C. Cytarabine is well absorbed after subcutaneous injection, but has very low oral bioavailability, because it is rapidly destroyed by enzymes in the gastrointestinal tract.[29,41]

Toxicity. The dose-limiting toxicity of cytarabine in conventional schedules is myelosuppression, which particularly affects granulocytes. Alopecia is common, but nausea is dose related and becomes severe only in high-dose regimens. Major organ damage is rare in conventional-dose regimens, but at high doses (> 1g/m^2 per dose), a very different pattern of toxicity emerges. In addition to profound myelosuppression and severe nausea, characteristic CNS, ocular, hepatic, dermatologic, and pulmonary toxicities emerge. The most characteristic toxicity of high-dose ara-C

(HDAC) regimens is CNS damage, typically manifesting as a cerebellar syndrome of dysarthria, nystagmus, and ataxia, often with dysdiadochokinesia and dysmetria. Cerebral dysfunction, with generalized encephalopathy and seizures, may accompany the cerebellar syndrome or occur independently. CNS toxicity has been documented in up to 40% of patients receiving HDAC, although severe toxicity is estimated to occur in 10% to 14%.[41] Cerebellar toxicity is usually reversible, resolving over several days after cytarabine discontinuation, but may be permanent, and is occasionally fatal. Risk of CNS toxicity is strongly correlated with advanced age and renal dysfunction. These two factors are probably related, because renal impairment is more common in aged populations. It is probable that renal insufficiency permits accumulation of high levels of ara-CTP, which is believed to be neurotoxic. A combination of dose reduction and once-daily rather than twice-daily dosing is recommended in patients with renal insufficiency (Table 115–11). Hepatic dysfunction, high cumulative doses, and administration schedule may also increase the risks of neurotoxicity.[42–44] Intrathecal administration of cytarabine can also produce CNS dysfunction, particularly when administered in conjunction with high systemic ara-C doses or cranial irradiation.

Other toxicities characteristic of HDAC are chemical conjunctivitis, which can be prevented or managed by application of steroid eye drops or saline eye washes; intrahepatic cholestasis; and dermatologic toxicity consisting most characteristically of palmar–plantar or acral erythema.[29,41] Pulmonary toxicity may be related to a capillary-leak syndrome. Respiratory distress and noncardiogenic pulmonary edema typically present suddenly, a few days to a month after treatment with HDAC. These symptoms may be particularly common in pediatric patients and are more frequently fatal.[45]

Gemcitabine

Gemcitabine (difluorodeoxycytidine, LY-188011) is a fluorine-substituted deoxycytidine analog related structurally to cytarabine.[41,46,47] Its activation and mechanism of action are similar to those of cytarabine, with phosphorylation to the active diphosphate and triphosphate forms necessary for antitumor effect. Gemcitabine is incorporated into DNA, where it causes inhibition of DNA polymerase activity. It also inhibits ribonucleotide reductase, blocking conversion of ribonucleotides to their deoxy forms and inhibiting de novo nucleotide production. Gemcitabine demonstrates important differences from ara-C in schedule dependency and activity, probably owing to differences in clinical pharmacology. With comparable exposure, gemcitabine achieves intracellular concentrations about 20 times higher than does ara-C, secondary to increased permeation of cell membranes, and greater affinity for the activating enzyme deoxycytidine kinase. Parent gemcitabine is eliminated very

TABLE 115–11. Empiric Dose Modifications in Patients With Renal and Hepatic Disease[a]

Agent	Organ Dysfunction	Suggested Dose Modification
Methotrexate Cisplatin	Renal impairment	In proportion to lowered creatinine clearance (normal 60 mL/min/m²)
Carboplatin	Renal impairment	See Table 115–15 for dosing guideline
Cyclophosphamide	Renal failure (creatinine clearance < 25 mL/min)	50% decrease
Bleomycin	Renal failure (creatinine clearance < 25 mL/min)	50%–75% decrease
Cytarabine (high dose > 1g/m²)	Renal impairment	For creatinine 1.5–1.9 mg/dL, reduce dose 50% For creatinine > 2.0 mg/dL, reduce dose by 95%
Cladribine Fludarabine Pentostatin Hydroxyurea Topotecan	Renal impairment	In proportion to lowered creatinine clearance
Streptozotocin	Renal impairment	50%–75% decrease
Doxorubicin Daunorubicin Vincristine Vinblastine Vinorelbine	Hepatic dysfunction	For bilirubin > 1.5 mg/dL, reduce dose by 50% For bilirubin > 3.0 mg/dL, reduce dose by 75%
Docetaxel Idarubicin Irinotecan Mitoxantrone	Hepatic dysfunction	Consider dose reductions; no published guidelines available
Paclitaxel	Hepatic dysfunction	Reduce by ≥ 50% for moderate to severe increases in bilirubin or transaminases

[a]Only approximate guidelines can be given. See text for explanations and limitations.
Compiled from Ref. 1 and package inserts.

rapidly from the plasma by deamination, with a terminal half-life of only 8 to 14 minutes, but the gemcitabine that is incorporated into DNA has a prolonged intracellular half-life. Gemcitabine's stereoconfiguration causes another normal base pair to be added subsequent to the fraudulent gemcitabine base pair in the DNA strand. This "masked chain termination" protects the gemcitabine from excision. The gemcitabine deamination product, difluorodeoxyuridine (dFdU) demonstrates a long terminal phase of 14 to 24 hours and is eliminated primarily by the kidneys.

Toxicity. Gemcitabine's dose-limiting side effect is myelosuppression, predominantly neutropenia. Elevations in liver transaminases are common. Although these hepatic abnormalities rarely necessitate stopping treatment, gemcitabine should be used with caution in patients with impaired liver function. Mild proteinuria and hematuria are reported in about half of patients, but are rarely clinically significant. However, caution is recommended in patients with impaired renal function, because a few cases of renal failure of uncertain etiology have been reported in patients receiving gemcitabine. Generalized rashes occur in about 25% of patients. The rashes are typically erythematous, pruritic, and maculopapular and develop 2 to 3 days after drug administration. They are reversible, respond to local therapy, and only rarely require discontinuation of drug. Fevers and flu-like symptoms, which usually occur within 6 to 12 hours of drug administration, are also common, especially following administration of the first dose. Nausea and vomiting are mild, but peripheral edema may be clinically important. In contrast to cytarabine, gemcitabine is not known to be neurotoxic.[41,46,47]

PURINES AND PURINE ANTIMETABOLITES

6-Mercaptopurine and 6-Thioguanine

Some of the oldest and newest anticancer agents are synthetic analogs of the naturally occurring purines guanine and adenine (see Fig. 115–13). 6-Mercaptopurine (6-MP) was the first purine analog to be used in cancer chemotherapy since its introduction for treatment of acute lymphocytic leukemia (ALL) about 40 years ago. Thioguanine (6-TG) is the 2-amino analog of 6-mercaptopurine. These two purine analogs are believed to act similarly, although the true mechanism of their cytotoxicity is still unclear. Neither agent is active in its administered form but both are rapidly converted to ribonucleotides that inhibit purine biosynthesis and also undergo various purine interconversion reactions needed to supply purine precursors for synthesis of nucleic acids. Although both compounds may be incorporated into DNA as "false" purines, this is believed to be a major mechanism of action only for 6-thioguanine. Clinical cross-resistance is generally observed between these two agents and probably results from decreased activation within resistant cells.[29,30,48]

Pharmacokinetics. The pharmacokinetics of the two drugs are similar as well. Both compounds are rapidly activated and distributed into most peripheral compartments, although neither enters the CNS in therapeutically useful concentrations following conventional doses. 6-MP demonstrates rapid clearance after oral administration, secondary to extensive first-pass metabolism. Oral bioavailability of both drugs is variable and incomplete and is reduced by food intake. Variability in absorption can result in significant differences in systemic exposure to a given dose of 6-MP and has been suggested as a prognostic consideration affecting the risk of relapse in children with ALL.[48] Despite this unreliable oral absorption, 6-MP and 6-TG are currently available commercially for oral use only. An intravenous formulation of 6-MP is being studied.[49]

After conventional doses, both 6-MP and 6-TG are eliminated primarily by metabolism in the liver and other tissues, although renal excretion of intact drug may become significant when high doses of 6-MP are administered.[49] Metabolites are eliminated renally, and consideration should be given to decreasing doses in patients with hepatic or renal disease, although criteria for dose adjustment have not been defined.

An important difference between these agents is the pathway of metabolic inactivation. 6-MP depends on the enzyme xanthine oxidase for an initial oxidation step. Because of this dependence, metabolism is markedly decreased by concomitant administration of the xanthine oxidase inhibitor allopurinol, and serious toxicity may result. This drug interaction is of major clinical significance, and oral 6-MP doses must be reduced by at least 50% when allopurinol is administered together with 6-MP. Because xanthine oxidase is not involved in the elimination of 6-TG, no interaction with allopurinol occurs, and no dose reduction is necessary.[29,48]

Toxicity. Both 6-MP and 6-TG are relatively well tolerated. Gastrointestinal toxicity occurs more commonly with 6-MP than 6-TG, but even with 6-MP, it occurs in less than one-third of patients. Bone marrow suppression is mild with typical oral doses of 6-MP, but is dose limiting for 6-TG. Chronically administered 6-MP produces hepatic injury in 6% to 40% of patients, which most typically manifests as jaundice after 1 to 2 months of treatment. Hepatic toxicity is dose related and is more common in adults than children. 6-TG has also caused hepatocellular damage, as well as rare hepatic veno-occlusive disease (VOD).[48–50]

Fludarabine Monophosphate

Fludarabine monophosphate (FAMP) is an analog of the purine adenine that incorporates two structural changes from the parent molecule (see Fig. 115–13). The arabinose analog of adenine (ara-A or vidarabine) was first developed in an attempt to design new antineoplastics using the same structural alterations that resulted in the effective anticancer drug cytarabine. Ara-A demonstrated some antineoplastic activity, as well as antiviral activity, but was rapidly inactivated by deaminase enzymes. It is marketed as an antiviral drug. The fluorinated analog, fludarabine or F-ara-A, proved to be both resistant to deamination and to have significant antitumor activity.[48,51]

Pharmacology and Pharmacokinetics. Fludarabine monophosphate is rapidly dephosphorylated in plasma to F-ara-A by first-pass metabolism, then enters cells, where it is rephosphorylated to its pharmacologically active triphosphate form (F-ara-ATP) by the enzyme deoxycytidine kinase. The intracellular accumulation of F-ara-ATP results in inhibition of DNA synthesis. Like cytarabine, fludarabine interferes with DNA polymerase, causing chain termination. Unlike ara-C, fludarabine is incorporated into RNA, resulting in inhibited transcription. It is inactivated by deaminase enzymes. The dephosphorylated form is eliminated with a terminal half-life of about 10 hours. Renal excretion accounts for the major clearance of metabolites, and renal failure predisposes patients to increased toxicity. Guidelines for dose modification (see Table 115–11) are not yet available.[51]

Toxicity. Although high doses of fludarabine were extremely effective in inducing remissions in patients with acute nonlymphocytic leukemia (ANLL) during phase I trials, its use was limited by a syndrome of delayed CNS toxicity, characterized by blindness, paralysis, and coma. Fortunately, fludarabine is effective at lower doses in patients with chronic lymphocytic leukemia (CLL) (25 mg/m^2/d × 5 days), at which serious CNS toxicity is rare. About 15% of patients treated with this dose of fludarabine experience some degree of neurotoxicity, most commonly somnolence, mild peripheral neuropathy, paresthesias, and mild visual disturbances.[52] The usual dose-limiting toxicity at these lower doses is myelosuppression. Fludarabine is also known to be immunosuppressive, with associated opportunistic infections. Pulmonary toxicity consistent with interstitial pneumonitis has been documented, with a usual onset after several courses of therapy, and is slowly reversible. Tumor lysis syndrome may occur secondary to effective cell kill. Prophylactic use of allopurinol, hydration, and alkalinization of urine are recommended in patients with large tumor burdens during initiation of fludarabine therapy. Nausea and vomiting are mild and easily controlled.[48,51]

Cladribine

Cladribine (2-chlorodeoxyadenosine, 2-CDA) is another recently developed purine nucleoside analog. Cladribine is resistant to inactivation by adenosine deaminase. Like fludarabine, the drug is sequentially phosphorylated intracellularly by deoxycytidine kinase. The triphosphate form of this agent is incorporated into DNA, resulting in inhibition of DNA synthesis and early chain termination. Cladribine's antitumor activity is unusual in that it affects both actively dividing and resting cancer cells. This drug also appears to be involved in induction of apoptosis.[48,53]

Pharmacokinetics. In contrast to the other purine nucleoside analogs, cladribine is well absorbed following oral administration, with a bioavailability of approximately 50%, although it is not currently available in an oral preparation. After subcutaneous dosing, the drug is 100% bioavailable. The terminal elimination half-life approaches 7 hours. The metabolic fate of cladribine is unknown, although approximately 20% of the drug is eliminated unchanged in the urine.[48,53]

Toxicity. The dose-limiting toxicity of cladribine is myelosuppression. Like fludarabine, cladribine possesses immunosuppressive effects that place patients at risk for serious opportunistic infections. The most common toxicity noted in clinical trials was culture-negative fever, usually beginning on the fifth to seventh day of therapy.[48,53]

Pentostatin

Pentostatin, or deoxycoformycin, is an unrelated purine analog that is a potent inhibitor of adenosine deaminase, the enzyme responsible for breakdown of adenosine and deoxyadenosine. Triphosphate forms of the nucleosides accumulate intracellularly, inhibiting ribonucleotide reductase, and ultimately causing a relative deficiency of other deoxyribonucleotides that are needed for normal DNA and RNA synthesis. Other mechanisms may also be involved in pentostatin's cytotoxicity. Pentostatin has a large volume of distribution following intravenous administration. It crosses the blood–brain barrier, reaching concentrations within the cerebrospinal fluid (CSF) that are about 10% of serum concentrations, and is cleared from the CSF slowly compared with systemic clearance. Pentostatin is eliminated largely unchanged in the urine and may require dose adjustment in patients with impaired renal function (see Table 115–11).[54]

Toxicity. In the doses currently recommended (4 mg/m^2 every 2 weeks), the most common toxicities of pentostatin are nausea and vomiting, which are delayed in onset. Symptoms usually begin 12 to 24 hours after drug administration and may persist for 2 to 3 days, making several days of antiemetic therapy advisable. Reversible elevation of liver transaminases is very common, with rare incidence of severe hepatotoxicity. Nephrotoxicity was common in earlier higher-dose studies, but is rare at approved doses. Similarly, severe neurotoxicity is uncommon with standard-dose therapy. Mild to moderate paresthesias, lethargy, and transient confusion are the most common neurologic effects. They occur in about 15% of patients and are usually transient and reversible.[52,54]

Methotrexate

The folate vitamins are essential cofactors in many reactions important for the synthesis of DNA. They carry one-carbon groups in transfer reactions that are required for purine and thymidylic acid synthesis and, in turn, for formation of DNA and for cell division. Structurally, the folates consist of a multiring pteridine group, attached to para-aminobenzoic acid, with one or more glutamic acid groups attached. Natural folates circulating in the blood have a single glutamic acid group, but within cells they are converted to polyglutamates, which are more efficient cofactors and which are preferentially retained inside the cells.[29,30,55,56]

Dietary folates must be chemically reduced to their tetrahydro forms, with four hydrogens on the pteridine ring, to be active. The enzyme responsible for this reduction is dihydrofolate reductase, and it is this enzyme whose actions methotrexate and other antifolates inhibit. The result of this inhibition is depletion of intracellular pools of reduced folate (tetrahydrofolates) essential for thymidylate and purine synthesis. Lack of either thymidylate or purines prevents synthesis of DNA. The effects of antifolate drugs on normal and probably cancerous cells may be counteracted by supplying reduced folates exogenously. The reduced folate used clinically for "rescue" is leucovorin (folinic acid). Leucovorin bypasses the metabolic block induced by antifolate drugs (Fig. 115–15).[55,56]

The folic acid analog MTX is the most widely used and best understood of all drugs in the broad category of "antimetabolites." It has activity in many different cancer types and also has several nononcology applications. MTX has been in clinical use for more than 40 years, since its original success for remission induction in childhood acute leukemias in the 1950s. It differs from folic acid by substitution of an amino group for a hydroxyl group on the pteridine ring, and in an additional methyl group.[55,56]

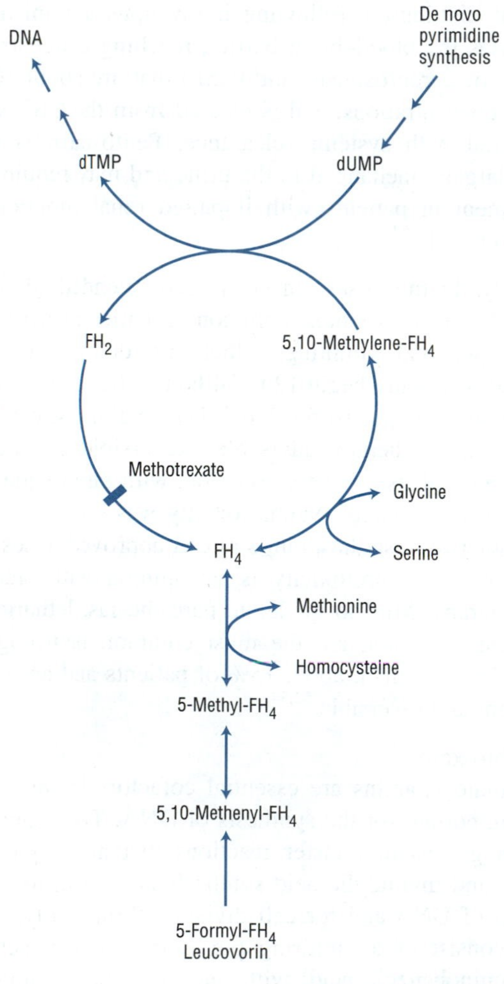

FIGURE 115–15. The folate cycle, the site of action of methotrexate, and the activation and entry "bypass" site of leucovorin. *(From Bleyer WA. Clinical pharmacology and therapeutic drug monitoring. Am Assoc Clin Ther Drug Monit-Toxicology 1985;6[11];1–14, with permission.)*

Clinical Pharmacology. Like physiologic folates, methotrexate is transported intracellularly by an active transport system. In high doses, passive diffusion becomes important in transport and may therefore overcome tumor cell resistance based on limited or saturated active transport systems. Resistance to the antifolates can also occur by several other mechanisms. The most clinically significant of these, in addition to impaired transport, are increased production of the target enzyme dihydrofolate reductase and inherently slow rates of thymidylate synthesis, which make cells less susceptible to the effects of antifolate drugs. Like impaired transport mechanisms, increased production of dihydrofolate reductase may also be overcome by administering high doses of MTX.

Other, less well-documented causes of resistance are decreased affinity of the enzyme for methotrexate or lack of polyglutamation of MTX within tumor cells.[55,56] MTX, like naturally occurring folates, is normally polyglutamated within cells. These polyglutamated forms of MTX are not readily extruded from cells and are at least as potent as and likely less rapidly reversible than MTX itself as dihydrofolate reductase inhibitors. Malignant cells may achieve greater MTX polyglutamate levels than normal cells, which may provide relative protection of normal cells from MTX-induced damage.[56]

Pharmacokinetics. The pharmacokinetics of methotrexate have been well characterized. Bioavailability of oral doses is variable and incomplete. Low doses (up to 30 mg/m^2) are completely absorbed. At higher doses, absorption is significantly less and varies from 12% to 77%. MTX is rapidly distributed into total body water and is 40% to 50% bound to plasma proteins. Other organic acids such as sulfonamides can displace MTX from binding sites, although the clinical significance of this interaction is not proven. Distribution of MTX into abnormal fluid accumulations, such as ascites or pleural effusions, can have important clinical effects. These "third-space" fluids act as depots from which MTX is slowly released. This may result in prolonged exposure to concentrations above those required to cause both tumor cell effects and toxicity to normal cells. Careful monitoring of serum MTX levels is needed and prolonged duration of leucovorin rescue may be required in these patients. In conventional oral or parenteral doses, levels of MTX achieved in the CNS are low, and direct instillation into the CNS is necessary for therapeutic effects. High-dose MTX regimens (greater than 1 g/m^2) produce therapeutic CNS levels and may avoid the need for intrathecal or intraventricular administration.

Methotrexate is metabolized to 7-hydroxy-methotrexate (7-OH-MTX) by the liver, to diamino-methylpteroic acid

TABLE 115–12. Methotrexate Toxicities

	Myelotoxicity	Nephrotoxicity	Hepatotoxicity	Mucositis	Pulmonary Toxicity	Neurotoxicity
Intermediate IV (50–100 mg/m²)	+++	+	+ (transaminasemia)	++	±	—
High-dose IV with leucovorin (100–12,000 mg/m²)	+	+++ (requires urinary alkalinization and hydration)	++ (transaminasemia)	++	±	++
Low-dose PO daily dose (5–25 mg/m²)	—	—	+++ (up to 25% cirrhosis)	—	±	—
Low-dose PO pulse therapy (5–25 mg/m²)	—	—	++ (rarely cirrhosis)	—	±	—
Intrathecal	—	—	—	—	—	++ (acute, subacute, and chronic)

+ = low risk; ++ = moderate risk; +++ = high risk; ± = inconclusive association.
From Ref. 55, with permission.

(DAMPA) by intestinal bacteria during enterohepatic cycling, and intracellularly to methotrexate polyglutamates. DAMPA usually accounts for less than 5% of an administered dose. Both MTX and its metabolites are eliminated renally, by glomerular filtration and tubular secretion. At high doses, concentrations in the renal tubules may exceed MTX solubility and result in renal damage from crystallization. The distribution half-life is 0.45 to 2 hours, and the distribution half-life ranges from 3 to 5 hours in patients with normal renal function. A terminal-phase half-life of 8 to 26 hours represents redistribution from deep tissue sites. Elimination may be greatly prolonged in patients with renal insufficiency, mandating dose reduction and careful therapeutic drug monitoring (Table 115–12).[57] Presence of third-space fluids (as described above) or gastrointestinal obstruction, which can increase enterohepatic cycling, can also delay elimination.[55–57]

Both DAMPA and 7-OH-MTX have only very modest cytotoxic potential and do not contribute significantly to MTX's antineoplastic effects. However, 7-OH-MTX concentrations may exceed those of the parent drug and may alter MTX's therapeutic and toxic effects. 7-OH-MTX may decrease elimination of MTX by competing for tubular secretion. It is less soluble in the urine than is MTX and may contribute to crystallization damage in high-dose regimens. 7-OH-MTX may also compete with MTX for polyglutamation within cells.[57]

Accurate and readily available assays for MTX levels in the serum have made therapeutic drug monitoring of MTX a practical and useful tool. The threshold for cytotoxic effects of MTX is approximately 5×10^{-8} *M*. Toxicity and, it appears, efficacy are related not only to achievement of therapeutic drug concentrations but, more importantly, to duration of time that concentrations are above this threshold level. With MTX doses requiring leucovorin rescue (generally greater than 100 mg/m²), leucovorin must be administered until levels fall below this cytotoxic threshold (Fig. 115–16). Several excellent reviews are available that detail the appropriate therapeutic monitoring of MTX and determination of leucovorin rescue regimens.[55–57] Therapeutic drug monitoring is not only useful for prevention and management of potential toxicity but has also been established as an effective means of increasing the likelihood of therapeutic success, by individualizing doses based on target parameters. This has been best applied in the treatment of children with ALL.[57]

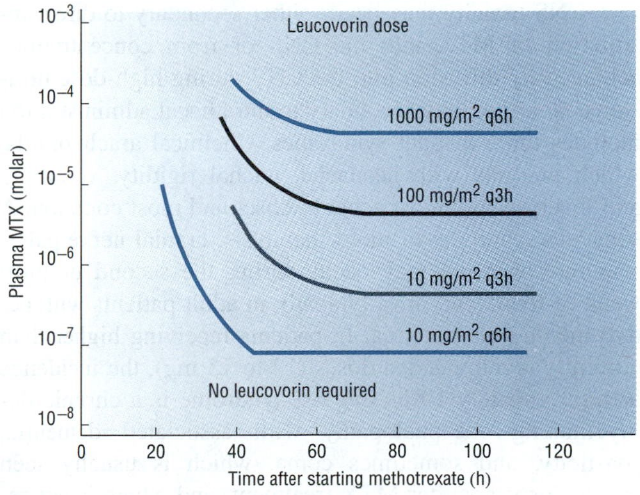

FIGURE 115–16. Leucovorin dosing based on monitored serum methotrexate (MTX) levels. Note that the level for discontinuation of leucovorin in this nomogram is 1.0×10^{-7} *M*. The actual value recommended may be lower, depending on the MTX assay used, patient age, prior or concurrent therapy, whether or not the patient has had a bone marrow transplant, and other factors. *(From Bleyer WA. New vistas for leucovorin in cancer chemotherapy. Cancer 1989;63:995–1007, with permission.)*

Toxicity. The normal cells most sensitive to MTX damage are the rapidly growing cells of the bone marrow and the gastrointestinal mucosa, making myelosuppression and mucositis the most common dose-limiting toxicities. Toxicity is dose and schedule dependent (see Table 115–12).[55] Mucositis usually precedes myelosuppression and occurs 3 to 7 days after drug administration. Stomatitis is the most common manifestation of mucosal damage, but diarrhea may also occur. Mucosal ulceration can be life threatening and requires dose interruption. Granulocytes and platelets are the most sensitive blood cells to MTX's effects. Myelosuppression and mucositis can both be prevented with leucovorin rescue, but cannot be reversed with leucovorin after they have occurred.[55–57]

Major organ toxicity from MTX includes hepatic, renal, neurologic, and pulmonary damage. Hepatic toxicity, which manifests as portal fibrosis and occasionally cirrhosis, is common in patients treated with chronic low-dose oral daily regimens, such as those used for psoriasis. "Pulse" dosing decreases the risk of severe toxicity and has largely replaced chronic daily dosing. Hepatic damage is uncommon with intermittent intravenous dosing, even with high-dose regimens. Nephrotoxicity, as discussed above, is a result of exceeding drug solubility in the renal tubules during high-dose MTX infusions. It can be prevented by alkaline hydration with bicarbonate solutions to maintain the urine pH above 7 for 1 to 2 days after drug administration to increase the solubility of methotrexate in urine. Vigorous hydration can also alter the disposition of MTX and reduce the frequency of high MTX concentrations and toxicity in high-dose MTX regimens. Pulmonary toxicity is a much less common, but potentially fatal, complication. It generally presents as fever, dry cough, dyspnea, and chest pain. It is not clearly dose related and is variably responsive to corticosteroids.[45,56,58]

CNS toxicity may occur either secondary to direct instillation of MTX into the CNS or from concentrations achieved by diffusion into the CNS during high-dose infusions. Neurotoxicity secondary to intrathecal administration includes three distinct syndromes. Chemical arachnoiditis, which presents with headache, nuchal rigidity, vomiting, and fever, is both most acute in onset and most common. A subacute syndrome of motor paralysis, cranial nerve palsy, seizures, or coma may occur during the second or third week of treatment, most typically in adult patients with active meningeal leukemia. In patients receiving higher than currently recommended doses (12 to 15 mg), the incidence is approximately 10%. The last syndrome is a chronic demyelinating encephalopathy with associated dementia, spasticity, and sometimes coma, which is usually seen months or years after MTX treatment, and which is not reversible. Most patients who develop encephalopathic symptoms have also received cranial irradiation. CNS toxicity may also occur with high-dose intravenous regimens. The etiology of CNS toxicity from MTX is not known, but it is not preventable with leucovorin.[44,55,56]

Other toxicities from MTX include mild nausea and vomiting, photosensitivity, eye discomfort, and hypersensitivity reactions, which can include anaphylaxis.[59] It is highly teratogenic, especially when administered during the first trimester of pregnancy.[55,56]

Drug Interactions. Several pharmacokinetic and pharmacodynamic drug interactions with MTX are of clinical importance. The most clinically important interactions are those with cisplatin, probenecid, and nonsteroidal anti-inflammatory drugs (NSAIDs). Cisplatin is an established nephrotoxin that may decrease the elimination of methotrexate, even when patients fail to show laboratory evidence of renal insufficiency. Probenecid also delays methotrexate elimination by inhibiting renal tubular transport. Therapeutic as well as toxic effects of methotrexate may be increased. Aspirin and other NSAIDs may decrease elimination by effects on renal function.[57,60]

PLANT ALKALOIDS

VINCRISTINE, VINBLASTINE, AND VINORELBINE

Vincristine, vinblastine, and vinorelbine are natural alkaloids derived from the periwinkle (vinca) plant. They act as mitotic inhibitors, or "spindle poisons." Although the alkaloids are very similar structurally (Fig. 115–17), they have different activities and patterns of toxicity.

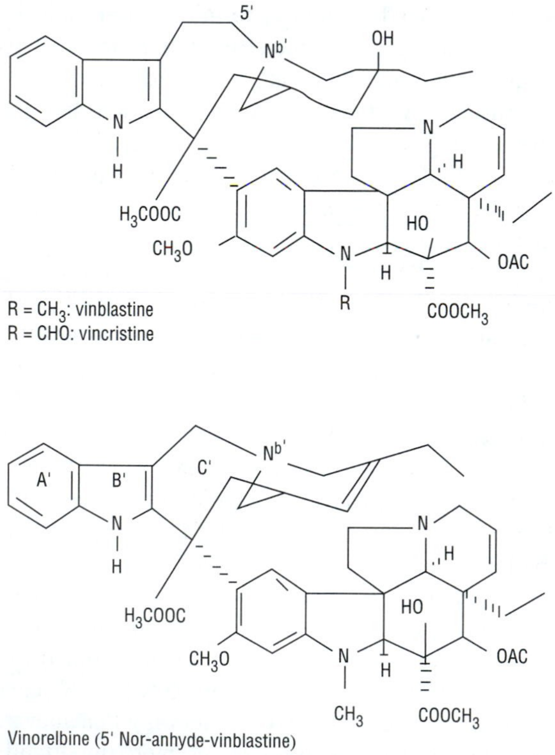

FIGURE 115–17. Structures of vinca alkaloids.

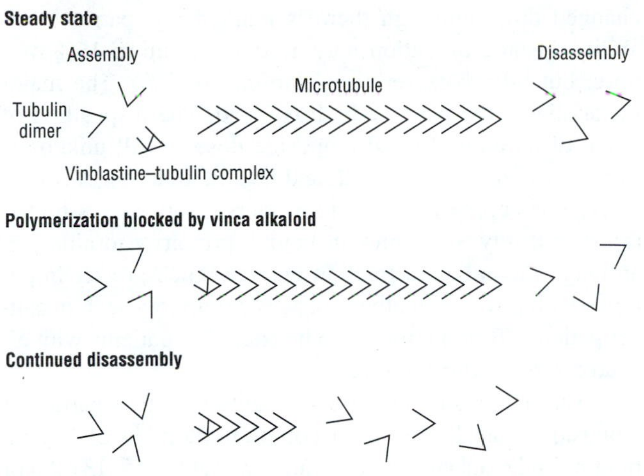

FIGURE 115–18. Mechanism of action of vinca alkaloids. *(From Pratt WB, Ruddon RW. The Anticancer Drugs. New York, Oxford University Press, 1979: 225, with permission.)*

Clinical Pharmacology. The vinca alkaloids are believed to function as antineoplastic agents by binding to tubulin, the structural protein that polymerizes to form microtubules. These are the hollow tubes that make up the mitotic spindle and that are also important in nerve conduction and neurotransmission. Vincas disrupt the normal balance between polymerization and depolymerization of microtubules. The result is inhibition of assembly of the microtubules (Fig. 115–18). This interferes with formation of the mitotic spindle and causes cells to accumulate in the mitosis phase of the cell cycle. Resistance to the vinca alkaloids develops from P-glycoprotein–mediated multidrug resistance, or secondary to alterations in tubulin, which lead to decreased drug binding.[29,30,60,61]

Pharmacokinetics. Oral absorption of vincristine and vinblastine is unpredictable, and so they are administered intravenously.[62] Vinorelbine exhibits 40% bioavailability, and an oral formulation is under investigation. The vincas bind tightly to blood elements, especially platelets, and do not enter the CNS in significant amounts. All three drugs are hepatically metabolized and are eliminated primarily by biliary excretion. Dose modification is required in patients with biliary obstruction (see Table 115–11). Vincristine has the slowest elimination, with a terminal half-life of approximately 85 hours, compared to 27 hours for vinorelbine and 24 hours for vinblastine. The long half-life of vincristine may partially explain why its maximum tolerated dose is lower than that of other vincas.[29,60]

Toxicity. The dose-limiting toxicity of vincristine is neurotoxicity. This is probably an extension of its therapeutic effects, because microtubules are involved in nerve conduction as well as in formation of the mitotic spindle. The neuropathy is usually distal and symmetrical and affects both sensation and motor function. Depressed deep tendon reflexes are the earliest objective signs of neurotoxicity, and paresthesias of the fingers and toes are the most common clinical manifestations. These changes are generally reversible and are not reasons to discontinue therapy unless they are disabling. Cranial nerves may also be affected and their damage may present as hoarseness, facial palsies, or jaw pain. Autonomic neuropathy also occurs, usually manifesting as constipation or colicky abdominal pain, but occasionally as orthostatic hypotension. Although vincristine doses are traditionally capped at 2 mg to decrease the risk of neurotoxicity, the justification for this is controversial.[63] Vincristine generally is not myelosuppressive and is therefore frequently used in combination regimens with myelosuppressive drugs. It may produce inappropriate antidiuretic hormone secretion (SIADH). Vinblastine and vinorelbine dosing, in contrast, is limited by myelosuppression. Neurotoxicity is not common from vinblastine, but when it occurs, it most commonly manifests as muscle aching.[44] The incidence of neurotoxicity from vinorelbine is intermediate between that of vincristine and vinblastine. All three agents are vesicants and may cause tissue damage if extravasated. No antidote has been demonstrated to be effective in humans, but hyaluronidase use is supported by animal data.[64]

ETOPOSIDE AND TENIPOSIDE

Etoposide (VP-16) and teniposide (VM-26) are semisynthetic podophyllotoxin derivatives. Podophyllin is extracted from the mayapple or mandrake plant and, like the vincas, binds to tubulin and interferes with microtubule formation. Unlike the parent compound, however, the cell damage produced by etoposide and teniposide is caused by strand breakage, which they produce by inhibiting the enzyme topoisomerase II.[29,30,60,65]

Pharmacology. Topoisomerases are essential enzymes involved in maintaining DNA topologic structure during replication and transcription. As shown in Figure 115–19, DNA topoisomerase enzymes relieve torsional strain during DNA unwinding by producing strand breaks: They cleave DNA strands and form intermediates with the strands, which makes a gap through which DNA strands can pass, then

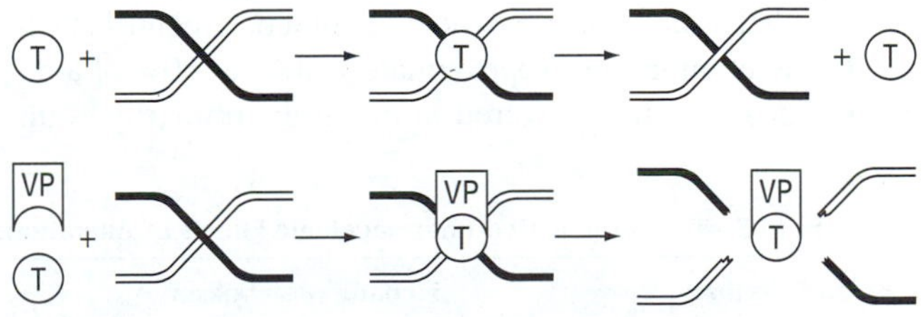

FIGURE 115–19. Topoisomerase II (T) interaction with DNA and etoposide (VP). T normally interacts with DNA to produce breakage–cleavage reactions required for normal cellular function (*upper panel*). The epipodophyllotoxins seem to cause DNA strand breakage by forming a complex with DNA and T (*lower panel*). *(From Bender RA, Hamel E, Hande KR. Plant alkaloids. In: Chabner BA, Collins JM eds. Cancer Chemotherapy: Principles and Practice. Philadelphia, Lippincott, 1990:253–275, with permission.)*

reseal the breaks. Topoisomerase I produces single-strand breaks whereas topoisomerase II produces double-strand breaks. Etoposide and teniposide both form complexes with topoisomerase II and DNA, which inhibit strand rejoining after breakage. Teniposide differs from etoposide by the addition of a sulfur-containing group in place of a methyl group on its sugar ring. It is several times more potent than etoposide in stimulating DNA cleavage. Resistance to either etoposide or teniposide drugs may be caused by cellular differences in topoisomerase II levels, by increased cell ability to repair strand breaks, or by increased levels of P-glycoproteins. They are usually clinically cross-resistant. Etoposide and teniposide are cell cycle phase specific and arrest cells in the S or early G_2 phase.[29,30,60,65] As a result, activity is dramatically greater when these agents are administered in divided doses over several days than in large single doses.[66] Chronic daily administration of oral etoposide and prolonged low-dose infusional schedules are being studied to take advantage of this schedule dependency.[65]

Pharmacokinetics. Etoposide and teniposide are not soluble in water. Etoposide is formulated in a polyethylene glycol (PEG) solution for parenteral administration, and teniposide is solubilized for parenteral use in a formulation containing polyoxyethylated castor oil (Cremophor EL). These formulations result in concentration-dependent stability and contribute to hypotension with rapid infusions and to hypersensitivity reactions. Etoposide phosphate is a water-soluble derivative that is rapidly converted to etoposide. This formulation permits bolus dosing and treatment at high drug concentrations. It is pharmacokinetically and biologically equivalent to etoposide. Etoposide is available for oral use in liquid-filled gelatin capsules. Oral bioavailability is dose dependent. Mean bioavailabilities of 76% to 86% have been reported after administration of a 100-mg oral dose, compared with 45% to 48% following a 400-mg dose. At both dose levels, interpatient variability is marked, producing a range of bioavailability that can have serious clinical consequences if either significantly more or less drug is absorbed than predicted.[65]

Etoposide has a volume of distribution of approximately 25% of body weight and low CNS penetration. It is known that both renal and hepatic function contribute to etoposide elimination. Approximately 40% to 60% of a delivered dose can be recovered in the urine, primarily as unchanged drug, although there is marked interpatient variability. Fecal elimination may account for up to 16% of a dose, but biliary excretion is minimal (< 2%). The major metabolite is the inactive hydroxy acid. The disposition of much of an administered etoposide dose is still unknown. In patients with normal renal and hepatic function, terminal half-life is approximately 4 to 8 hours. Etoposide is highly (approximately 95%) protein bound, primarily to albumin, although the unbound fraction may be much greater in patients with low serum albumin, as is commonly seen in cancer patients. Binding may also be altered in patients with elevated serum bilirubin levels.[65,66]

The pharmacologic effects resulting from a particular etoposide dose depend on a complex interplay of protein binding and renal and hepatic function (Table 115–13). All of these are important in dosing considerations in cancer patients. Unfortunately, no validated guidelines for dose changes in patients with abnormal renal or hepatic function or hypoalbuminemia currently exist. One guideline of a 30% dose reduction in patients with serum creatinine levels above 1.5 mg/dL has been recommended, but has not been prospectively validated. Pharmacologic effects may or may not be increased in patients with impaired hepatic function, depending on the binding status, so no dosing guidelines can be given.[67]

Teniposide is even more highly protein bound than is etoposide (> 97%). Teniposide has a lower systemic clearance, a longer elimination half-life of about 9 hours, and less urine elimination of parent drug than etoposide. Renal elimination accounts for only about 10% of teniposide clearance; therefore, renal insufficiency is unlikely to be important in dose considerations. Hepatic metabolism is the predominant route of teniposide elimination, but dose modification guidelines are not available for patients with impaired hepatic function. As with etoposide, serum albumin and factors that affect protein binding must also be taken into consideration in dosing decisions.[65,66]

Drug interactions with drugs that affect hepatic function and protein binding may be clinically significant in patients receiving etoposide or teniposide. This has been best described with anticonvulsants.[66]

Toxicity. Both etoposide and teniposide are well-tolerated drugs. Their dose-limiting toxicity is myelosuppression. Nausea and vomiting are usually mild, although more likely after oral administration of etoposide than parenteral. Alope-

TABLE 115–13. Anticipated Pharmacologic Effects of Alterations in Etoposide Excretion, Metabolism, and Protein Binding

Renal Excretion	Hepatic Metabolism	Protein Binding	Anticipated Pharmacologic Effect
Normal	Normal	Decreased[a]	None
Decreased	Normal	Normal	Increased
Normal	Decreased	Normal	Increased
Decreased	Normal	Decreased[a]	Increased
Normal	Decreased	Decreased[a]	None (?)
Decreased	Decreased	Decreased[a]	Increased

[a]For example, hypoalbuminemia, hyperbilirubinemia.
Adapted from Ref. 67.

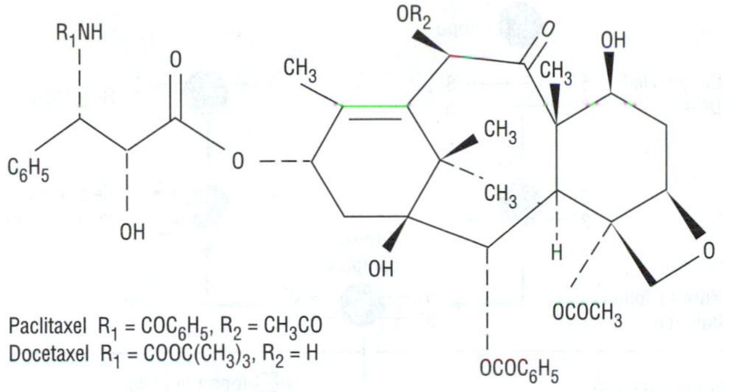

FIGURE 115–20. The chemical structures of paclitaxel and docetaxel.

cia is common, and mucositis may be limiting at high doses. Orthostatic hypotension can occur with either drug, but is generally preventable by a slow infusion time over 30 minutes to 1 hour. Etoposide phosphate may be administered as a rapid bolus without producing cardiovascular effects. Hypersensitivity reactions have occasionally been reported, although the mechanism of these reactions is not established.[59,65] Major organ toxicity is rare, although etoposide has occasionally been implicated as a cause of hepatotoxicity.

Secondary leukemias associated with etoposide and teniposide use have recently been recognized. Most of the secondary leukemias have been acute nonlymphocytic leukemias identified in children receiving these agents for treatment of acute lymphocytic leukemia. These iatrogenic leukemias typically occur after a short latency period between drug administration and diagnosis of the leukemia (< 5 years) and do not demonstrate a preleukemic or myelodysplastic phase, in contrast to leukemias induced by alkylating agents. Like those leukemias, however, the leukemias secondary to etoposide and teniposide are characterized by low response rates to treatment and short remission durations.[65]

PACLITAXEL AND DOCETAXEL

Paclitaxel and docetaxel are novel taxane plant alkaloids with antimitotic activity (Fig. 115–20). Paclitaxel (Taxol) was isolated from the bark of the Pacific yew tree, *Taxus brevifolia,* in 1971. Development of the drug was hindered by inadequate drug supplies. The yew is a slow-growing plant, and once the bark is harvested, the tree dies. The bark from more than 2000 trees was required to produce 1 kg of paclitaxel. The complex taxane ring structure proved difficult to synthesize. Commercial paclitaxel is now produced semisynthetically from the needles of the European yew, *Taxus baccata.* The search for more readily available and renewable resources than yew tree bark also led to the discovery of docetaxel (Taxotere). Docetaxel is a semisynthetic taxoid extracted from 10-deacetyl baccatin III, a noncytotoxic precursor found in the renewable needle biomass of yew plants.[60,61,68,69]

Clinical Pharmacology. Paclitaxel and docetaxel both act by binding to tubulin but, unlike the vincas, do not interfere with tubulin assembly. Instead, the taxanes promote microtubule assembly and interfere with microtubule disassembly. This is accomplished by induction of tubulin polymerization, resulting in formation of stable, but nonfunctional, microtubules. Preliminary studies indicate that docetaxel is twice as potent as paclitaxel in binding to tubulin.[61,68,69]

Pharmacokinetics. The taxanes are widely distributed after administration and bind extensively to plasma and tissue proteins. As expected, this results in large volumes of distribution for both agents and plasma protein binding that exceeds 90%. Elimination half-lives range from 1.3 to 8.6 hours for paclitaxel and 11.4 to 18.5 hours for docetaxel and are not dose dependent.[61,68,69] Elimination is primarily through hepatic metabolism and biliary excretion; less than 10% of parent drug is found unchanged in the urine. The optimal dose for patients with hepatic impairment has not been established, but dose reduction is necessary in patients with moderate or severely elevated bilirubin or serum aminotransferase concentrations.[61]

Toxicity. The dose-limiting side effect of the taxanes is myelosuppression, particularly neutropenia. Anemia and thrombocytopenia are uncommon. For paclitaxel, the incidence of neutropenia may be related to the duration of infusion, with longer durations producing more profound neutropenia. For docetaxel, neutropenia is not schedule dependent. Both drugs also produce cumulative neurotoxicity, predominantly peripheral neuropathy. Although no uniformly effective treatment exists for established neuropathy, there are some encouraging early reports using the chemoprotectant amifostine for prevention of this disabling toxicity.[70] Other common shared toxicities include mucositis, total alopecia, none to mild nausea and vomiting, and hypersensitivity reactions. The hypersensitivity reactions were noted early in the development of paclitaxel, occurring in 30% to 60% of patients. The duration of infusion was prolonged to 24 hours and a prophylactic regimen of corticosteroids and H_1- and H_2-receptor antagonists was adopted (Table 115–14). Subsequently, the incidence of serious reactions was reduced to 2% to 4%. Recent case series have described safe and effective use of a single-dose dexamethasone regimen given just prior to paclitaxel administration.[71] The hypersensitivity reactions may be due, in part, to the

TABLE 115–14. Prophylactic Regimens for Patients Receiving Taxanes

Paclitaxel (Taxol)
Dexamethasone 20 mg PO at 12 and 6 h OR 20 mg IV 30–60 min prior to paclitaxel
Diphenhydramine 50 mg IV 30–60 min prior to paclitaxel
Cimetidine 300 mg or ranitidine 50 mg IV 30–60 min prior to paclitaxel
Docetaxel (Taxotere)
Dexamethasone 8 mg PO bid × 5 d, starting 24 h prior to docetaxel

Cremophor EL (castor oil and absolute ethanol) vehicle used in its formulation. Docetaxel is much more water soluble than paclitaxel and is formulated in a polysorbate 80 vehicle. However, docetaxel is also associated with hypersensitivity reactions in 18% of patients, suggesting that the taxane ring structure, rather than the vehicle, may be the cause of hypersensitivity.[61,69]

Docetaxel, but not paclitaxel, causes cumulative fluid retention, which may result in edema, weight gain, and pleural effusions. A corticosteroid regimen is recommended in conjunction with docetaxel to prevent fluid retention and hypersensitivity reactions (see Table 115–14). Docetaxel also commonly causes dermatologic reactions, which usually consist of a maculopapular rash affecting the hands and feet, with occasional desquamation.[61,69]

Toxicities unique to paclitaxel include myalgias and cardiac toxicity. Cardiac rhythm disturbances were noted in early clinical trials of paclitaxel, and routine telemetry monitoring was initiated. Asymptomatic bradycardia is the most common adverse cardiac effect, although heart block and ventricular arrhythmias can also occur. However, serious cardiac effects are uncommon, and routine cardiac monitoring is no longer recommended. Cardiotoxicity is more likely in individuals with a prior history of cardiac disease.[61,68]

Drug Interactions. Studies of paclitaxel in combination with cisplatin indicate that administration of paclitaxel after cisplatin results in a 25% reduction in paclitaxel clearance and more severe neutropenia than when paclitaxel precedes cisplatin. Toxicity of doxorubicin–paclitaxel regimens are also affected by sequence of drug administration. Since taxane metabolism is mediated by hepatic P450 enzymes (CYP3A4), agents that interact with these enzymes can alter taxane pharmacokinetics and clinical effects.

IRINOTECAN AND TOPOTECAN

Camptothecin, a plant alkaloid derived from *Camptotheca acuminata,* is a potent inhibitor of DNA topoisomerase I. Although camptothecin showed significant activity in preclinical testing, clinical trials failed to show activity, and the drug produced severe, unpredictable toxicity. The camptothecin analogs irinotecan (CPT-11) and topotecan were synthesized in an attempt to reduce toxicity and improve therapeutic effects.

Clinical Pharmacology. Irinotecan and topotecan are novel plant alkaloids in that they are the first topoisomerase I inhibitors. Topoisomerase enzymes have been described above (see Etoposide and Teniposide). Topoisomerase I inhibitors act by stabilizing DNA single-strand breaks and inhibiting religation (Fig. 115–21).[60,72–75]

Pharmacokinetics. Irinotecan is rapidly converted by carboxylesterases to an active metabolite known as SN-38, which has 250- to 1000-fold greater antitumor activity than irinotecan. Irinotecan, SN-38, and topotecan undergo

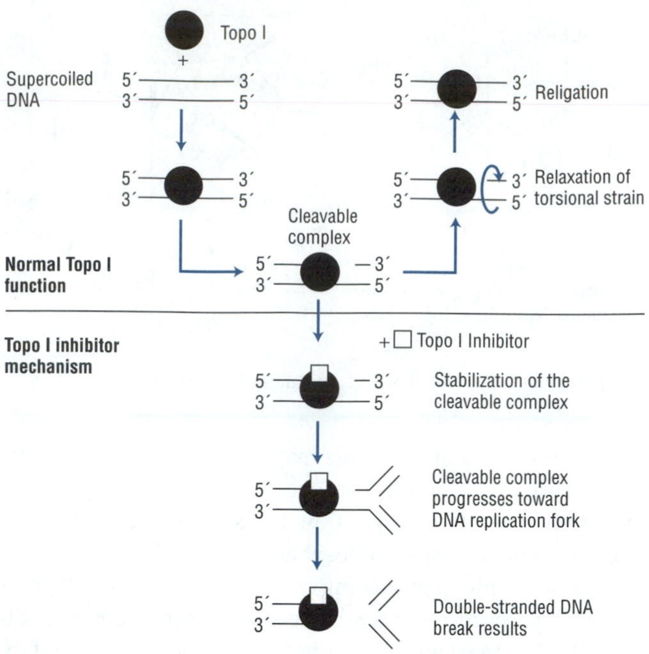

FIGURE 115–21. Topoisomerase I (Topo 1) function (*top*) and mechanism of topoisomerase I inhibitors (*bottom*).

pH-dependent hydrolysis of the E-ring lactone to an open-ringed hydroxy acid (Fig. 115–22). Only the closed lactone form, which is favored in an acidic environment, exerts antitumor effects. The preferred diluent for these agents is 5% dextrose, which has a more acidic pH than saline and slows hydrolysis of the lactone ring. However, once administered systemically, hydrolysis occurs rapidly; at equilibrium approximately 50% of drug exists in the closed lactone form. The major route of elimination of irinotecan and SN-38 is biliary excretion. Although no specific guidelines for dosage modification exist, increased total bilirubin levels have been associated with increased concentrations of irinotecan and SN-38. These alterations in excretion have been correlated with increased gastrointestinal toxicity and myelosuppression. Dosage reductions should be considered in patients with elevated total bilirubin.[72] In contrast, topotecan undergoes renal excretion, with 45% of the drug eliminated in the urine in the first 24 hours. Dosage reductions are recommended for renal insufficiency (see Table 115–11).[72,74,75]

Toxicity. The dose-limiting toxicity of irinotecan and topotecan agents is myelosuppression. Neutrophils are most profoundly affected, and neutropenia is often accompanied by mild to moderate thrombocytopenia. For irinotecan, diarrhea can also be dose limiting, with grade 4 diarrhea occurring in 20% of patients. The diarrhea has two different presentations—either an acute onset occurring during or immediately after irinotecan administration or a delayed onset occurring several days later. The acute form is believed to be a cholinergic process, a result of inhibition of acetylcholinesterase by irinotecan, but not SN-38. It is of-

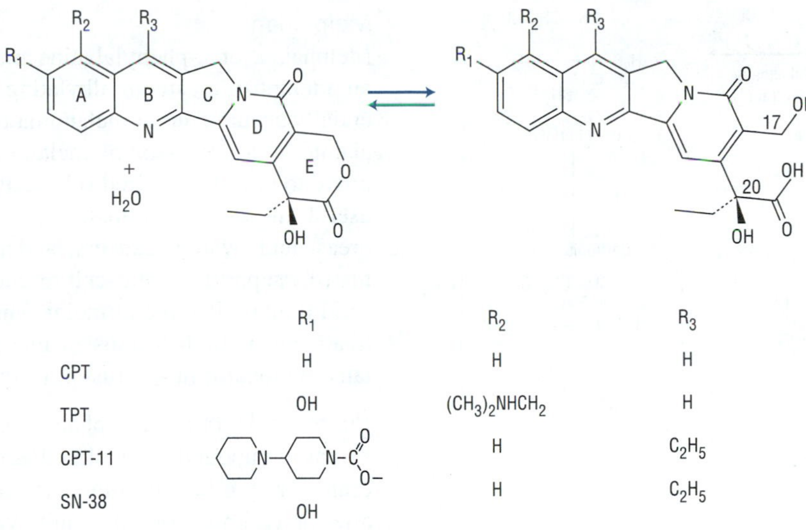

FIGURE 115–22. Structure of camptothecin (CPT), topotecan (TPT), irinotecan (CPT-11), and SN-38 lactone and the hydroxy acid form.

ten accompanied by facial flushing, diaphoresis, and abdominal cramping and responds to atropine 0.25 to 1 mg IV. The chronic form is a secretory diarrhea, which may result in life-threatening dehydration. Prompt initiation of high-dose loperamide at the first sign of diarrhea has reduced the incidence of grade 4 diarrhea to 2% of courses. Loperamide 4 mg should be given orally at the onset of diarrhea or abdominal cramping and continued at a dose of 2 mg every 2 hours until no bowel movement has occurred for 12 hours. Diarrhea is not commonly observed with topotecan and is mild when it occurs. Nausea and vomiting from irinotecan can be severe, but are easily prevented with serotonin-receptor antagonist and corticosteroid premedication. In contrast, nausea and vomiting from topotecan are mild. Side effects common to both agents include alopecia, rash, low-grade fevers, malaise, mucositis, and mild elevations in liver function tests.[72–75]

ALKYLATING AGENTS

The alkylating agents are among the oldest and most useful of antineoplastic drugs. Their clinical use evolved from observed shrinkage of lymph nodes in victims of sulfur mustard gas warfare during World War I. On the possibility that similar agents might be useful in overgrowths of lymphoid tissues such as lymphomas, less reactive derivatives were synthesized. Their effectiveness as anticancer agents was confirmed by clinical trials in the middle 1940s.[76]

All of the alkylating agents are highly reactive compounds that work through the covalent bonding of alkyl groups or substituted alkyl groups with nucleophilic groups of cell components. Some of these nucleophilic groups are phosphates or amino, carboxyl, sulfhydryl, or imidazole groups of proteins and nucleic acids. The most common site of binding for alkylating agents is the 7-nitrogen group of guanine. These covalent reactions can result in cross-linking between two DNA strands or between bases in the same strand of DNA. Reactions between DNA and RNA and between drug and proteins may also occur, but the main insult that results in cell death is inhibition of DNA replication. Because the alkylating agents can damage DNA during any phase of the cell cycle, they are considered cell cycle nonphase specific. However, their greatest effect is seen in rapidly dividing cells.[29,76] The several chemical classes of alkylators (e.g., nitrogen mustard derivatives, nitrosoureas, aziridines, sulfonic acid esters) differ in their spectrum of activity, pharmacologic characteristics, and toxicity patterns, but all alkylators are cytotoxic, mutagenic, teratogenic, carcinogenic, and myelosuppressive. Resistance to these agents can occur from increased DNA repair capabilities or from decreased entry into cells. Various degrees of clinical cross-resistance among the alkylators exist.[29,30,60,76]

NITROGEN MUSTARD DERIVATIVES

The best understood and most commonly used alkylating agents are the nitrogen mustard derivatives: mechlorethamine, melphalan, chlorambucil, cyclophosphamide, and ifosfamide.

Mechlorethamine

Mechlorethamine (also referred to as "nitrogen mustard" or HN_2) was the first mustard derivative to be used extensively. It is a bifunctional alkylating agent, that is, it has two reactive groups. A schematic of the alkylation reaction of mechlorethamine is illustrated in Figure 115–23. Mechlorethamine is a highly unstable compound in aqueous solutions and is degraded within minutes in the body to its alkylating intermediate. This also creates practical problems in patient care, because parenteral solutions must be freshly prepared and administered immediately after use. Because of this rapid degradation, the pharmacokinetics of mechlorethamine are not well characterized. Almost no intact drug

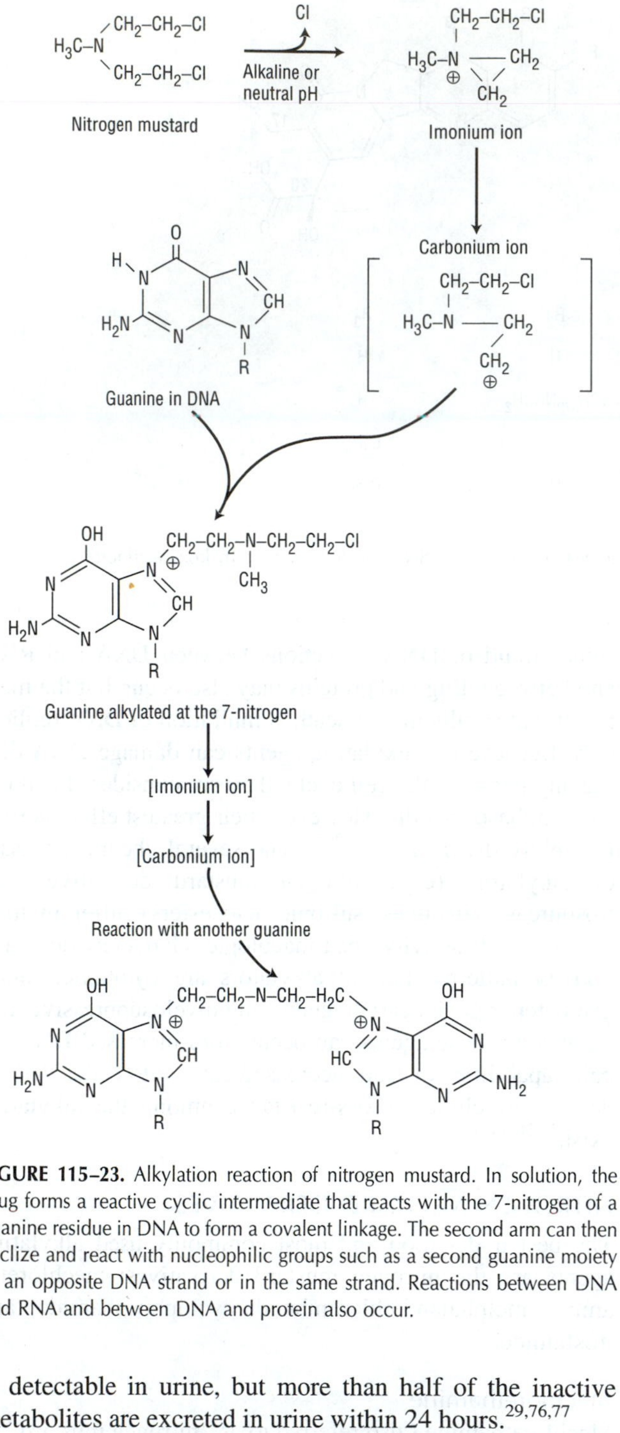

FIGURE 115–23. Alkylation reaction of nitrogen mustard. In solution, the drug forms a reactive cyclic intermediate that reacts with the 7-nitrogen of a guanine residue in DNA to form a covalent linkage. The second arm can then cyclize and react with nucleophilic groups such as a second guanine moiety in an opposite DNA strand or in the same strand. Reactions between DNA and RNA and between DNA and protein also occur.

is detectable in urine, but more than half of the inactive metabolites are excreted in urine within 24 hours.[29,76,77]

Toxicity. Myelosuppression affecting all blood cell lines is the dose-limiting toxicity. Nausea and vomiting are severe and occur very soon after systemic drug administration. It is a vesicant and can be neutralized in tissue after extravasation or on skin or other surfaces with solutions of sodium thiosulfate, an electron-rich compound that binds with and inactivates the reactive groups of nitrogen mustard.[64] The most serious long-term consequences of this agent are development of second cancers, especially when it is used in combination with radiation therapy, and sterility.[76]

Melphalan

Melphalan, or L-phenylalanine mustard, was developed in an attempt to create an alkylating agent that would preferentially accumulate in melanoma tumor cells, since phenylalanine is a precursor of melanin. The compound did not prove to have the desired selectivity for melanocytes, but is useful in several tumors, especially multiple myeloma, breast and ovarian cancers, and in high doses with bone marrow support or stem-cell rescue for treatment of various solid tumors. Parenteral melphalan is also administered for treatment of limb lesions in malignant melanoma by isolated regional limb-perfusion techniques.[76]

Pharmacokinetics. Melphalan is less reactive than the parent compound, mechlorethamine, and can be given orally, or by infusion of the parenteral form. Bioavailability after oral administration is quite variable, but approximates 70%. It is decreased by food. Following intravenous administration, melphalan is distributed into total body water and eliminated with a half-life of 1 to 2 hours. The disposition half-life is affected by the hydration status of the patient. Spontaneous degradation is believed to be the main route of elimination. Although only about 15% of an administered intravenous dose is detectable in urine within 24 hours, toxicity of intravenous melphalan may be increased in patients with renal dysfunction and may require dose reduction. Dose considerations are affected by variations in the percentage of unbound drug in plasma.[76,77]

Toxicity. Dose-limiting toxicity of melphalan is myelosuppression, which is characterized by damage to marrow stem cells, resulting in slow recovery of blood counts, and sometimes cumulative marrow damage. It does not usually cause nausea, vomiting, or alopecia in conventional low daily doses. Hypersensitivity reactions have been documented in fewer than 5% of patients receiving intravenous melphalan, but have not been reported with oral use. In high doses administered as part of marrow transplant regimens, gastrointestinal toxicity with mucositis, nausea, vomiting, and diarrhea become dose limiting, and alopecia is also reported.[29,76,77]

Chlorambucil

Chlorambucil is a nitrogen mustard derivative with selective cytotoxicity for lymphocyte cell lines. It is available only for oral use and is more rapidly and completely absorbed than melphalan, although its absorption is also decreased by food. Elimination is mainly by metabolic degradation, and the half-life is about 1.5 hours. An active metabolite, phenylacetic acid mustard, may contribute to both therapeutic and toxic effects. Chloramubucil is well tolerated, with dose-limiting myelosuppression and little nausea. Chronic therapy has been associated with a high incidence of secondary acute leukemias.[76,77]

Cyclophosphamide and Ifosfamide

Cyclophosphamide is the most widely used of the nitrogen mustard derivatives and of all the alkylating agents. Ifosfamide is closely related in structure, clinical use, and toxicity. Neither agent is active in its parent form and must be activated by mixed hepatic oxidase enzymes to the alkylating moieties. The active metabolite of cyclophosphamide is probably phosphoramide mustard. Another metabolite, 4-hydroxycyclophosphamide, is cytotoxic, but is not an alkylating agent, and probably acts as a transport form to deliver phosphoramide mustard into cells. Another metabolite of both cyclophosphamide and ifosfamide, acrolein, does not have antitumor activity, but may be responsible for some of the toxicity seen with these drugs. Ifosfamide undergoes hepatic activation to its active alkylating metabolite, ifosfamide mustard, and to acrolein, but this activation process occurs more slowly than with cyclophosphamide.[29,76,78]

Pharmacokinetics. Characterization of the pharmacokinetic behavior of these compounds is complicated by the existence of multiple active and inactive metabolites. Cyclophosphamide is well absorbed orally, with a systemic availability approaching 100%, although it is variable among patients. The terminal-phase half-life is about 7 hours, and the major metabolic site is the liver. About 15% of unchanged drug and most of the metabolites are eliminated in the urine. Empiric dose reductions have been recommended in patients with creatinine clearances below 30 mL/min. Although cyclophosphamide is largely metabolized, there has been no consistent pattern of altered metabolism in patients with hepatic dysfunction, and dose reductions are not known to be necessary. Significant amounts of an administered cyclophosphamide dose can be cleared by dialysis. It does not enter the CNS in significant concentrations.[76,77]

Pharmacokinetics of ifosfamide are similar. Because of the slower rate of activation, ifosfamide must be used in greater doses (approximately three to four times) than the cyclophosphamide dose required to achieve similar alkylating activity. More unchanged drug is excreted in the urine (20% to 50%) than is true for cyclophosphamide. The half-life is schedule dependent and is about 6 hours if divided daily doses are administered, but increases to 16 hours with single large doses. Unchanged drug is detectable in the CNS in significant quantities, but only very small amounts of the active metabolites are detectable. It is unlikely that ifosfamide will therefore be active in CNS tumors, but this limited penetration may account for its CNS toxicity.[76–78]

Toxicity. Myelosuppression occurs with both agents and is dose limiting for cyclophosphamide. White blood cells are particularly sensitive to these drugs, but platelets are uncommonly reduced to hazardous levels, making these drugs relatively platelet sparing. Recovery from leukopenia is rapid, indicating little stem-cell damage. Myelosuppression from ifosfamide is much less severe with divided daily doses than with a single large dose. Emetogenicity is dose dependent; in high-dose regimens, both agents are severe emetogens. The nausea and vomiting from cyclophosphamide, but not ifosfamide, is characterized by a delay in onset of up to 8 hours. Alopecia is also dose related.[76,78]

The classic toxicity of these drugs, and the dose-limiting toxicity for ifosfamide, is hemorrhagic cystitis. This is a syndrome of blood loss from the bladder mucosa accompanied by symptoms of frequency and irritation, which can cause fibrosis of the bladder, massive hemorrhage, and occasionally bladder carcinoma. The toxic metabolite common to both cyclophosphamide and ifosfamide, acrolein, is believed to produce this cystitis by binding to critical thiols in the bladder wall. Damage, proportional to dose and to duration of exposure, may be minimized by hydration with frequent voiding to decrease acrolein contact with the bladder mucosa. Patients receiving conventional doses of cyclophosphamide should be counseled to drink 3 L of fluids on the day of cyclophosphamide administration, and for 2 days after dosing. In most cases, this will successfully prevent mucosal damage. However, with ifosfamide, hydration is typically inadequate prevention. The sulfhydryl compound "mesna" (*m*ercapto *e*thane *s*ulfonate *s*odium [*Na*]) must be used in conjunction with ifosfamide. The sulfhydryl groups of mesna bind preferentially to acrolein, forming a nontoxic complex that can be voided from the bladder, preventing mucosal acrolein attachment and damage. Mesna does not interfere with the cytotoxic activity of cyclophosphamide or ifosfamide. When ifosfamide is administered in fractionated daily doses, mesna is given before and at 4 and 8 hours after the ifosfamide dose, in doses equal to 20% of the ifosfamide dosage. For high-dose cyclophosphamide regimens ($> 2\ g/m^2$/dose), hyperhydration, mesna, or continuous bladder irrigations have been used successfully to prevent hemorrhagic cystitis.[78,79]

Although bladder toxicity is most characteristic of these compounds, damage to the renal tubules may also occur. Nephrotoxicity has been best documented in children receiving ifosfamide and in patients receiving high-dose cyclophosphamide regimens.[80] Toxicity may be mediated by a similar mechanism to bladder toxicity, or through the effects of the ifosfamide metabolite, chloroacetaldehyde. Although mesna may be able to detoxify the toxic metabolites within the bladder, it may not reach the renal tubules in a high enough concentration to provide adequate protection.[80,81]

One toxicity that is common with ifosfamide but does not occur with cyclophosphamide is CNS toxicity, which typically presents as decreased level of arousal, with occasional progression to somnolence, coma, and death. Confusion, hallucinations, and seizures may also occur. CNS toxicity is less severe with fractionated doses of ifosfamide than with single large doses. Increased amounts of the chloroacetaldehyde metabolite have been associated with the occurrence of CNS toxicity.[44,78] Rare toxicities from cyclophosphamide include pulmonary fibrosis and cardiac toxicity, especially in bone marrow transplant doses. Inappropriate antidiuretic hormone release (SIADH) may also occur from cyclophosphamide therapy.[76]

NITROSOUREAS

The nitrosoureas are alkylating agents characterized by lipophilicity and ability to cross the blood–brain barrier. Carmustine or *b*is*c*hloroethyl*n*itroso*u*rea (BCNU), lomustine (CCNU), and a closely related methylnitrosourea, streptozotocin, are commercially available. BCNU is available as an intravenous preparation and recently as a drug-impregnated wafer (Gliadel) for direct application to brain tumors. The nitrosoureas decompose to reactive alkylating metabolites as well as to isocyanate compounds that have several effects on reproducing cells and that may be involved in the toxicity of these drugs.[29,30,60,76]

Pharmacokinetics. The nitrosoureas are extensively and rapidly biotransformed after administration, and the degradation products demonstrate a prolonged elimination, perhaps from binding to cellular components. Metabolites and a small percentage of intact drug are excreted in urine. Because of the lipophilic nature of these compounds, they enter the CNS readily and achieve concentrations of about 30% of simultaneous plasma levels. Lomustine is administered orally and is well absorbed. Some enterohepatic circulation may occur. Streptozotocin disposition is similar to that of the other nitrosoureas.[29,76,77]

Toxicity. Myelosuppression is the dose-limiting toxicity of the nitrosoureas in conventional doses. The myelosuppression is unusually delayed and prolonged, and complete recovery typically takes 6 to 8 weeks. Thrombocytopenia occurs earlier and is generally more pronounced than leukopenia. Streptozotocin, however, is not myelosuppressive. All of these compounds, particularly streptozotocin, cause severe nausea and vomiting. They are also renal toxins and produce dose-related damage, which consists of glomerulosclerosis, severe tubular loss, and interstitial fibrosis. Renal toxicity correlates with cumulative doses. Carmustine commonly causes facial flushing and pain along the vein during infusion, which may be related to the alcohol vehicle.[76]

In long-term treatment or in the high doses used with bone marrow transplantation, pulmonary toxicity of carmustine can be dose limiting. Incidence may be as high as 30% in patients with brain tumors treated with carmustine as a single agent. Patients typically present with shortness of breath, tachypnea, and nonproductive cough and may improve clinically with administration of corticosteroids. Histologic damage is usually characterized as interstitial pneumonitis and fibrosis. Lomustine has also occasionally produced pulmonary damage.[45,76]

As mentioned earlier, carmustine is also available in a biodegradable polymer formulation for local application to residual brain tumor tissue. The drug-impregnated wafers are inserted into the cavity left following tumor resection. Drug is released as the polymer dissolves, resulting in prolonged drug exposure at the site of any residual tumor. This method of carmustine administration is not associated with any significant local or systemic toxicities.[82]

OTHER ALKYLATING AGENTS

Thiotepa

Thiotepa is the only member of the aziridine group of alkylating agents currently in clinical use. The aziridines are analogs of the closed-ring intermediates of the nitrogen mustards and are believed to alkylate through opening of the aziridine ring. Thiotepa, or triethylenethiophosphoramide, is poorly absorbed from the gastrointestinal tract, is lipid soluble, achieves therapeutic levels in the CNS, and is primarily excreted unchanged in the urine. It is administered intravesically, intravenously, or, occasionally, intrathecally. Bone marrow depression may occur even after bladder instillation. Paresthesias can occur when thiotepa is administered intrathecally in hypertonic solutions, so sterile water rather than saline is the recommended diluent for CNS administration. However, because of the ready entry of thiotepa and its active metabolite into the CNS after systemic administration, there is no pharmacokinetic advantage to intrathecal injection.[76,77]

Busulfan

The last of the classic alkylating agents to be discussed is busulfan, an alkyl alkane sulfonate. Busulfan, like other alkylators, is toxic to the bone marrow, but, unlike the other agents, produces greater myelosuppressive damage to myeloid than lymphoid cells. This relative specificity has made it a useful agent for treatment of chronic myelogenous leukemia. It is not active against solid tumors in conventional doses, but has activity in high-dose alkylating regimens used in bone marrow transplantation. Busulfan is well absorbed orally in low doses, and the intact drug disappears very rapidly from the plasma. Metabolites are excreted in the urine. Pharmacokinetics of high-dose busulfan are age dependent, with lower systemic exposure in children than adults. In contrast to most cytotoxic drugs, busulfan enters the CSF readily after systemic administration, achieving concentrations at least equal to those in plasma, and persisting in the CSF for several hours.[76,83]

Toxicity. The most common toxicity of busulfan is an extension of its therapeutic effects—bone marrow suppression. It appears to damage bone marrow stem cells and can produce prolonged myelosuppression. Busulfan also causes skin hyperpigmentation, especially at skin creases and, occasionally, addisonian symptoms. Nausea and vomiting are uncommon at standard doses, but may occur in high-dose regimens. Neurotoxicity characterized by generalized tonic–clonic seizures is associated with high-dose regimens administered as preparation for bone marrow transplantation, but can be prevented by prophylactic anticonvulsant administration. High doses of busulfan are also believed to contribute to the occurrence of hepatic veno-occlusive disease (VOD) in bone marrow transplant patients, although the cause of VOD is multifactorial.[83] The most classic toxicity of busulfan is pulmonary fibrosis, or "busulfan lung." Clinical incidence is estimated at 4% of patients overall, although the incidence of subclinical damage is probably much higher. The mechanism of pulmonary damage is unknown, but increased epithelial sensitivity to the drug may be a factor. The best established risk factor is duration of busulfan treatment, with an average time to onset of more than 3 years of busulfan therapy. Radiation exposure also increases risk. Onset of symptoms is insidious and characteristically includes development of nonproductive cough, shortness of breath, weight loss, and sometimes fevers. Chest x-ray usually shows a reticular pattern in the lung bases, and histologically, interstitial pulmonary fibrosis is prominent. No treatment has been proven effective by controlled trials but, anecdotally, corticosteroids may be helpful. The mean survival after diagnosis, however, is only 5 months.[45,83]

NONCLASSIC ALKYLATING AGENTS

Several other cytotoxic agents appear to act as alkylators, although their structures do not include the classic alkylating groups. They are capable of binding covalently to cellular components and include procarbazine, dacarbazine, and altretamine. In addition, some antitumor antibiotics have been proposed to function as alkylators.[29,30,60,84]

Procarbazine

Procarbazine was originally synthesized as a monoamine oxidase (MAO) inhibitor but was shown in routine screening to have antitumor activity. It is a prodrug and must be converted to cytotoxic intermediates, probably by liver cytochrome P450. These intermediates are believed to have alkylating activity, although several other cellular-damaging effects have been detected. Ultimately, procarbazine inhibits DNA, RNA, and protein synthesis.[29,84,85]

Pharmacokinetics. Pharmacokinetic information for procarbazine is incomplete despite its many years of use. Procarbazine is administered orally and is rapidly and completely absorbed. A "first-pass" effect is likely. It is rapidly metabolized, with metabolites eliminated primarily in the urine. Procarbazine enters the CNS very readily and achieves concentrations comparable to those in plasma.[84,85]

Toxicity. The most common toxicities of procarbazine administration are protracted myelosuppression and gastrointestinal symptoms of anorexia, nausea, and vomiting. Tolerance often occurs to these gastrointestinal symptoms with continued use. Occasional neurotoxic and hypersensitivity reactions also occur. Procarbazine is highly toxic to reproductive organs and commonly produces sterility, particularly in males. It is highly mutagenic and carcinogenic, and together with mechlorethamine, is associated with an increased risk of secondary malignancies after MOPP [*m*echlorethamine, *O*ncovin (vincristine), *p*rednisone, and *p*rocarbazine] therapy for treatment of Hodgkin's disease.[84,85] There are also several drug–drug and drug–food interactions of potential consequence. Because procarbazine is an MAO inhibitor, therapy with tricyclic antidepressants, sympathomimetic drugs, and foods containing high levels of tyramine, such as red wines, aged cheeses, yogurt, and bananas, can precipitate acute hypertensive reactions. A disulfiram-like reaction can occur with alcohol, and the effects of other CNS depressants may be potentiated.[85]

Dacarbazine

Dacarbazine, or dimethyl triazeno imidazole carboxamide (DTIC), is a nonclassic alkylating agent. It was synthesized in an attempt to make purine antimetabolites, as an analog of the carboxamide intermediate in purine synthesis, but it does not interfere with formation of purines. Its exact mechanism of action is unknown, but the parent molecule does undergo demethylation to active intermediates that can alkylate nucleic acids *in vitro*. In cell culture, dacarbazine also inhibits DNA, RNA, and protein synthesis. It appears to be active in all phases of the cell cycle and may cause delays in the G_2 phase.[29,60,84,85]

Pharmacokinetics. Dacarbazine is not well absorbed orally and is administered by intravenous infusion. It disappears from the plasma biphasically with an α-phase half-life of about 19 minutes and a β-phase half-life of 5 hours. About half of an administered dose is recoverable in urine as parent drug; tubular secretion is believed to be involved. Hepatobiliary excretion may also occur, but effects of renal and hepatic dysfunction on drug elimination are not defined. Dacarbazine penetrates poorly into the CNS. It decomposes in the presence of light, but this is not clinically relevant in usual administration schedules.[84,85]

Toxicity. Toxicity to dacarbazine is characterized by severe nausea and vomiting, which tends to decrease with successive doses on multiple-day schedules, and mild to moderate myelosuppression. It also produces a flu-like syndrome, which occurs near the end of dacarbazine treatment and persists for several days; burning pain along the injection path; and photosensitivity. Hepatic toxicity has been reported, with rare instances of VOD.[85]

ANTITUMOR ANTIBIOTICS

ANTHRACENE DERIVATIVES

The anthracene derivatives are very useful anticancer drugs with a broad spectrum of anticancer activity. The most widely used and best understood of the group is doxorubicin, also commonly known by its earliest trade name, Adriamycin or "Adria," although it is now available from several manufacturers. Other members of the anthracene group include daunorubicin (daunomycin), idarubicin, the investigational agent epirubicin, and mitoxantrone. All of these agents except mitoxantrone are anthracyclines and share a common, four-membered anthracene ring complex with an attached aglycone or sugar portion. The ring complex is a chromophore and accounts for the intense colors of these compounds. Doxorubicin differs from its parent compound daunorubicin by the addition of a hydroxyl group on the attached sugar, and it is sometimes consequently referred to as hydroxydaunorubicin. A hydroxyl group on epirubicin is in the epi conformation compared with doxorubicin (epi-doxorubicin), and idarubicin is demethoxydaunorubicin. Mitoxantrone is an anthracenedione rather than an anthracycline and has no sugar group attached to the three-membered anthracene ring complex.[29,60,86,87]

Doxorubicin, Daunorubicin, and Idarubicin

The mechanism of action of the anthracyclines is not yet completely defined. It is known that they bind tightly to double-stranded DNA and that binding is essential for their cytotoxic action. Traditionally they have been considered intercalating agents, that is, compounds that insert between base pairs of DNA, causing deformation and local uncoiling of the DNA. Although it is well established that the planar groups of the anthracene ring complex do intercalate with DNA, this is not believed to be the direct mechanism of cytotoxicity. The anthracycline intercalators cause protein-associated breaks from interference with the actions of topoisomerase II (see Etoposide and Teniposide section).[60,86,87]

Another consideration in the mechanism of anthracycline-induced cytotoxicity is that of free radical formation. The anthracyclines can undergo electron reductions to reactive compounds that can damage DNA and cell membranes. Free radicals formed from reduction of the anthracyclines donate electrons to oxygen to make superoxide, which can react with itself to make hydrogen peroxide. Cleavage of this produces the highly reactive and destructive hydroxyl radical. This last step is believed to require iron, and the anthracyclines are potent iron binders. Iron–anthracycline complexes can bind to DNA and react rapidly with hydrogen peroxide to produce the hydroxyl radicals that actually cleave DNA. Human cells have natural defenses against oxygen radical damage, specifically enzymes that can convert the radicals to less reactive compounds, or that can repair DNA damage. Differences in distribution of these defensive enzymes may account for characteristic sites of toxicities of the anthracyclines. For example, cardiac muscle has low levels of defensive enzymes and high levels of enzymes that activate anthracyclines (see Toxicity discussion). Oxygen radical formation is firmly established as a cause of toxicity such as cardiac damage and extravasation injury, but is less likely as a cause of tumor-cell kill.[86–88] Other potential mechanisms of cytotoxicity include interactions with helicases, enzymes that separate double-stranded DNA, and interactions with the cell membranes.[88]

Resistance to the anthracyclines is usually secondary to P-glycoprotein–dependent multidrug resistance, which causes active pumping of drug from the cells. Altered topoisomerase II activity or altered free-radical chemistry may also be clinically important mechanisms of resistance to the anthracyclines.[86–88]

Pharmacokinetics. The most important factor in the pharmacokinetic behavior of doxorubicin is its extensive tissue binding. Doxorubicin distributes rapidly to all body tissues except those of the CNS and binds primarily to DNA, accounting for its very large volume of distribution of about 1000 L/m^2. It is only slowly released from tissues, with a half-life of 30 hours. Doxorubicin has been detected in tissue even months after administration. It is metabolized to doxorubicinol, an active metabolite, and 50% is excreted in bile. Less than 10% is eliminated in the urine, although this is enough to discolor the urine a characteristic orange-red color. Ability of the liver to metabolize the drug is much greater than the rate of release of drug from tissues and brings into question the validity of empiric guidelines for dose modification based on elevated liver function tests (see Table 115–11). Elevated bilirubin levels in association with primary liver cancer have recently been confirmed to alter doxorubicin pharmacokinetics and pharmacodynamics. The presence of large or diffuse liver metastases may alter anthracycline pharmacokinetics, even in the absence of bilirubin elevations. There is some evidence that aspartate aminotransferase levels may be more useful than bilirubin in adjustment of anthracycline doses. Until dosing guidelines can be validated, dose modification in patients with elevated bilirubin remains the accepted, but cautious, recommendation.[86–89]

Daunorubicin's pharmacokinetics are similar to those of doxorubicin. It is rapidly and extensively metabolized to daunorubicinol. The elimination is believed to be biphasic, with terminal half-lives of 15 to 20 hours for daunorubicin and about 30 hours for daunorubicinol. As with doxorubicin, tissue binding is extensive, but similar empiric dose modifications should be considered in patients with hepatic dysfunction (see Table 115–11).[86–89]

Idarubicin is more lipophilic than the other anthracyclines and is taken up into cells more rapidly. Its primary metabolite, idarubicinol, is as active as the parent drug. The concentration of idarubicinol in plasma is typically more than double that of the parent compound. Elimination is poorly defined. Renal excretion is greater than for doxorubicin, but accounts for < 5% of idarubicin elimination and about 10% of idarubicinol. The role of hepatic elimination also has been questioned, and much of the elimination is uncertain. The half-life of idarubicin is 15 to 20 hours, but that of idarubicinol is 40 to 60 hours. An oral formulation is under investigation.[88–90]

Toxicity. Although the anthracyclines are very active drugs, they are also very toxic. The most common dose-limiting toxicity in the short term is myelosuppression. They also cause moderate to severe dose-related nausea and vomiting, alopecia, and mucositis. Mucositis may be dose limiting in doxorubicin infusion protocols.[86,87] Recently, secondary acute myeloid leukemia with chromosome translocations similar to epipodophyllotoxin-associated leukemia has been recognized in patients receiving anthracyclines in combination with alkylating agents.[87] However, the anthracyclines are most famous for their cardiac toxicity and for extravasation injuries.

The manifestations of anthracycline-induced cardiac damage are acute, subacute, chronic, and late-onset toxicities. Acute toxicity consists primarily of rhythm disturbances, especially nonspecific ST-T wave changes, sinus tachycardia, and increased frequency of ventricular premature beats. Typically, these occur within the first 24 hours after drug administration. They are usually self-limited and do not appear to increase the risks of future cardiac events. A rare subacute pericarditis–myocarditis syndrome of fever, pericarditis, and congestive heart failure can also occur at low cumulative doses and may be fatal.[86,87,91]

More serious than the acute cardiac changes is the risk of chronic congestive cardiomyopathy, which effectively limits the cumulative dose of anthracycline that can be administered. Cardiomyopathy is believed to be secondary to free radical formation within the heart muscle, which results in damage to the sarcoplasmic reticulum and gradual loss of myofibrils from the cells. Damage to the sarcoplasmic membrane results in loss of its ability to bind calcium and disrupts the link between electrical excitation and muscle contraction. Clinical evidence of cardiac damage is clearly dose related and depends on the extent of myofibril loss. Although there is a real but very low incidence in patients with cumulative doxorubicin dose less than 550 mg/m^2, the incidence approaches 50% in doses that are double that, in bolus dosing (Fig. 115–24). Risk is greater and deterioration occurs at lower cumulative doses in patients with previous cardiac irradiation. The elderly, the very young, females, and those with preexisting hypertension or cardiac disease are also at increased risk.[86,87,91] Recent data on long-term cancer survivors who received anthracyclines as part of their chemotherapy show that these individuals are at risk for a late cardiotoxicity characterized by left ventricular dysfunction and arrhythmias.

Incidence of congestive cardiomyopathy is also closely associated with dose schedule. The risk estimates

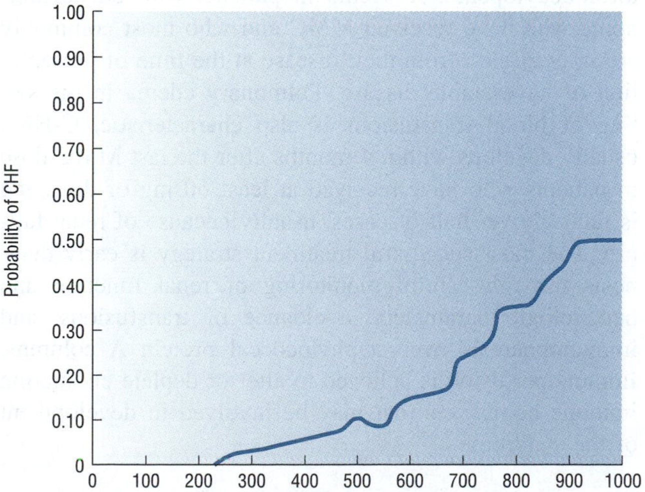

FIGURE 115–24. Risk of cardiac toxicity with cumulative doxorubicin dose. CHF = congestive heart failure. *(From Von Hoff DD, Layard MW, Basa P, et al. Risk factors for doxorubicin-induced congestive heart failure. Ann Intern Med 1979;91:710–717, with permission.)*

outlined above and in Figure 115–24 refer to traditional doxorubicin dosing, that is, 60 mg/m^2 by intravenous bolus every 3 to 4 weeks. It has been established that cardiac damage correlates with peaks of drug concentration achieved, rather than with total exposure to the drug (AUC, area under the concentration–time curve). Administering the same total dose in small weekly doses or by continuous infusion over 2 to 4 days markedly improves the cardiology risk–benefit ratio of doxorubicin administration, but continuous infusion leads to more severe stomatitis. Serial endomyocardial biopsies or evaluations of left ventricular ejection fraction may be useful in assessing the extent of cardiac muscle injury. This information is used to determine the risk of continuing anthracycline therapy in patients who are responding to treatment, but approaching the recommended maximum dose, especially in those with coexisting risk factors. Unfortunately, the appearance of cardiac toxicity may be delayed until months or years after completion of therapy, which decreases the utility of prospective monitoring.[86,87,91]

Although many different pharmacologic interventions to prevent cardiac damage have been attempted, the only FDA-approved agent is dexrazoxane (ICRF-187). The carboxylamine metabolite of dexrazoxane is a potent chelator of divalent ions, including iron in its ferric state. Anthracycline complexation with iron is known to be essential for the free radical formation that initiates cardiac damage. Dexrazoxane's ability to disrupt the iron–anthracycline complex and prevent reactive radical formation may be responsible for its cardioprotective effects. It is indicated for reducing the incidence and severity of doxorubicin-induced cardiomyopathy. FDA approval for its use is currently limited to women with breast cancer who have received a cumulative dose of 300 mg/m^2 of doxorubicin who are expected to benefit from continued doxorubicin therapy. Formulation of anthracyclines in liposomal delivery systems (see later discussion) may also decrease cardiotoxicity of these compounds, because liposomes are not taken up as readily by cardiac tissue as free drug.[23,91,92]

Daunorubicin and doxorubicin have similar potential for cardiac toxicity, but, because of the limited use of daunorubicin and the rarity of high cumulative doses in the leukemic population, clinically important cardiomyopathy is uncommonly seen. Doses of 900 to 1000 mg/m^2 are approximately equivalent in risk to doxorubicin doses of 550 mg/m^2. Idarubicin may be less cardiotoxic than doxorubicin or daunorubicin in equivalent doses.[87,91]

The other classic toxicity of the anthracycline drugs is tissue damage on extravasation. Deep ulceration with tissue necrosis may occur and progress over many weeks. Ulcers typically have raised red edges and necrotic centers and heal very slowly if at all. Drug may be detected in the ulcer tissue for months after extravasation. At present, no effective remedy exists to prevent or reverse tissue damage, although application of ice to the extravasation site is the current standard of care. Topical application of dimethylsulfoxide (DMSO) to the extravasation site is inconsistently useful in animal models and anecdotally useful in humans, but DMSO has not been studied systematically and is not considered standard treatment for anthracycline extravasation.[64,86,87,93] Doxorubicin may also cause a "flare" reaction that presents during or immediately after injection, with redness and urticaria extending up the vein. It is self-limiting and usually subsides within 30 minutes. Doxorubicin may also reactivate skin damage in sites of previous radiation therapy, the so-called radiation recall reaction.

Both doxorubicin and daunorubicin are available in liposomal formulations. Within liposomes, anthracyclines are protected from systemic degradation and can be delivered in higher amounts to target tissues. The toxicity profiles of these formulations differ from the parent compounds in that the risks of cardiac toxicity and extravasation injuries are lessened.[94–96]

Mitoxantrone

The anthracenedione mitoxantrone was synthesized in an attempt to develop compounds with comparable antitumor activity to doxorubin but with a better safety profile. The mechanisms of action of mitoxantrone are similar to the anthracyclines and include intercalation with production of single- and double-stranded DNA breaks, but its potential for free radical formation is much less than that of the anthracycline drugs. Pharmacokinetics are characterized by extensive tissue binding and slow elimination, with metabolism and biliary excretion accounting for most of the known elimination. Perhaps because of the decreased tendency for free radical formation, the risks of cardiac toxicity and ulceration after extravasation, although still present, are markedly reduced. Other nonmarrow toxicities of mitoxantrone are also markedly less than the traditional anthracyclines. Nausea and vomiting, mucositis, and alopecia are substantially less common and severe than with doxorubicin. Mitoxantrone's intense blue color produces a blue-green discoloration of urine and may give a blue tint to sclera and skin. In high doses, hyperbilirubinemia may be dose limiting.[86,87]

OTHER ANTITUMOR ANTIBIOTICS

Mitomycin C

Mitomycin C (MMC) is an antitumor antibiotic first produced as a fermentation product from *Streptomyces caespitosus* in the late 1950s. It is believed to function as an alkylating agent. MMC itself is a prodrug and must be activated by reduction reactions to the alkylating species. Ultimately, strand breakage and inhibition of DNA synthesis occur. MMC activation may also result in the production of superoxide free radicals, which can contribute to the cytotoxic effects by causing lipid peroxidation or nucleic acid damage.[29,30,60,97]

Pharmacokinetics. Plasma concentrations of MMC decline in a biexponential manner, with a distribution half-life of less than 10 minutes and a terminal half-life of 0.5 to 1.5 hours. Only 1% to 20% of drug is recoverable from urine, and the liver is believed to be the main site of biotransformation. Hepatic dysfunction, however, does not alter MMC pharmacokinetics, and it is possible that MMC is cleared from the plasma by a biodegradation process.[97] Very little MMC is absorbed into the systemic circulation after intravesical administration.

Toxicity. The dose-limiting toxicity of MMC is cumulative myelosuppression, which is characteristically delayed in onset and prolonged in duration. Recovery may take up to 8 weeks. Anorexia, nausea and vomiting, and alopecia are uncommon and generally mild.[97] Extravasation may result in severe tissue necrosis, which is characterized by delayed presentation, sometimes weeks or months after injection, and which may be remote from the injection site. No antidote for this damage is of established efficacy in humans, but application of topical DMSO is useful in animal models.[64,93]

MMC also produces serious major organ toxicity, consisting of pulmonary damage and, more frequently, the hemolytic uremia syndrome (HUS). Pulmonary toxicity typically presents with insidious onset of dyspnea, cough, and fatigue, although acute respiratory decompensation may occur, particularly when MMC is administered with vincas. Pulmonary function tests show a restrictive defect, and chest x-ray commonly shows a diffuse reticular pattern. Known risk factors are previous or concurrent thoracic radiation and exposure to high oxygen concentrations, but it is not known to be dose related. Mortality of MMC-induced pulmonary damage is high, although corticosteroids may produce dramatic responses and, anecdotally, may decrease the risk of pulmonary toxicity when administered concurrently with MMC therapy.[45,97]

Cancer-associated HUS (C-HUS) consists of microangiopathic hemolytic anemia, renal dysfunction, and thrombocytopenia. It occurs in patients with adenocarcinoma who have received MMC and who most commonly are in remission from their disease at the time of presentation or have stable disease. Pulmonary edema in the setting of blood transfusions is also characteristic. C-HUS usually develops within 4 months after the last MMC dose in patients who have received at least 60 mg of drug and is fatal in over half of cases, usually because of renal failure. The most successful treatment strategy is early diagnosis through careful monitoring of renal function and hematologic parameters, avoidance of transfusions, and immunopheresis over staphylococcal protein A columns. Immunoperfusion is believed to alter or deplete circulating immune complexes that may be involved in development of the syndrome.[97,98]

Actinomycin D

Actinomycin D (Act-D, DACT, or dactinomycin) is an antitumor antibiotic isolated from *Streptomyces* species.[29,30,60,97]

Pharmacology and Pharmacokinetics. Actinomycin D contains a chromophore ring and, like the anthracene derivatives, inserts itself either between bases of a single DNA strand (intercalation) or between bases in nonpaired strands (pseudointercalation). Binding to DNA inhibits RNA and protein synthesis. Act-D accumulates in tissues by passive diffusion and is susceptible to P170-glycoprotein–mediated resistance. Plasma elimination is slow, with a half-life of 36 hours, likely secondary to extensive tissue binding. Only about 35% of drug is accounted for by urinary and fecal excretion.[97]

Toxicity. Myelosuppression is common and is usually the dose-limiting toxicity, although severe nausea and vomiting may be acutely dose limiting. Diarrhea, mucositis, and alopecia are also common. Actinomycin D is a severe vesicant if extravasated. No antidote to extravasation damage from this drug is known. It may also cause inflammatory radiation recall reactions in previously irradiated sites.[64,97]

Bleomycin

Bleomycin or "bleo" is one of the most widely used of the antitumor antibiotics. It is a mixture of peptides from fungal *Streptomyces* species, and as such, its strength is expressed in units of drug activity. One unit is roughly equal to 1 mg of polypeptide protein.[99] The predominant peptide is bleomycin A_2, which makes up approximately 70% of the commercial product. Bleomycin's cytotoxicity is secondary to DNA strand breakage, or scission, which it produces via free radical formation. Cytotoxicity depends on binding of an iron–bleomycin complex to DNA. There is some evidence that intercalation between opposing DNA strands might occur. The bleomycin–iron complex then reduces molecular oxygen to free oxygen radicals, which primarily cause single-strand breaks in the DNA. Bleomycin has greatest effect on cells in the G_2 phase of the cell cycle and in mitosis.[29,30,60,99]

Pharmacokinetics. Bleomycin is taken up slowly by cells and is inactivated within cells by the enzyme aminohydrolase. This enzyme is widely distributed but is present in only low concentrations in the skin and the lungs, perhaps accounting for the predominant toxicities of bleomycin in those sites. The presence of hydrolase enzymes in the cytosol is probably the primary mechanism of resistance to bleomycin as well. Cells can also become resistant by repairing the DNA breaks produced by bleomycin, and resistance has been correlated with increased repair capacity. Bleomycin is eliminated renally; 45% to 70% of the dose is excreted in the urine within 24 hours. Half-life of elimination is 2 to 4 hours in patients with normal renal function and may increase to more than 20 hours in the presence of renal failure. Clearance may also be decreased in patients receiving concurrent cisplatin. Increased toxicity, especially pulmonary toxicity, has been associated with renal impairment. Dose reduction proportional to the degree of impairment is recommended in patients with severely compromised renal function (i.e., creatinine clearance less than 25 to 35 mL/min), although no validated guidelines exist (see Table 115–11).[60,99] Following intracavitary (such as intrapleural) administration, cavitary levels are about 10 to 20 times higher than corresponding plasma levels, although nearly half of an intracavitary dose eventually reaches the systemic circulation.[100]

Toxicity. Unlike most antineoplastic agents, bleomycin is not myelosuppressive and, consequently, is frequently given in combination with agents that are toxic to bone marrow. Nausea and vomiting are also mild. Bleomycin does produce fevers within hours to 2 days of administration in 25% to 50% of patients, which may be prevented or managed with antipyretics. Rarely, high fevers occur, which can produce tachypnea, hypotension, delirium, and even death. Although these reactions have sometimes been characterized as anaphylactic reactions, they probably are not true hypersensitivity reactions. They are believed to be caused by the direct release of pyrogens in unusually sensitive patients. Patients with lymphoma who have preexisting disease-related fevers are most susceptible to these hyperpyrexial episodes. Administering a test dose (1 U) of bleomycin before the first dose has only limited utility in predicting which patients are at risk for this reaction.[59,99]

The most important toxicities of bleomycin are to the lungs and the skin. Characteristic pulmonary toxicity is interstitial pneumonitis, which can progress to fibrosis and cause death from hypoxia. It is related both to high single doses (greater than 30 U) and to cumulative dose, with an incidence of about 3% up to a total dose of 450 U, and 10% in patients receiving higher doses. Advanced age, preexisting pulmonary disease, previous chest irradiation, exposure to high oxygen concentrations, and renal impairment also increase risk. The clinical features are usually dyspnea with pulmonary infiltrates. Deterioration may be sudden and severe and may occur months after completing therapy. Chest radiograph findings are nonspecific, and lung biopsy is required for definitive diagnosis. Measurement of carbon monoxide–diffusing capacity has been recommended as a means of monitoring toxicity and predicting risk, although the utility of this is controversial. Treatment of pulmonary damage is drug discontinuation, but pulmonary symptoms may continue to progress after discontinuation. The value of corticosteroids has not been proven. In patients who survive bleomycin pneumonitis, the pulmonary symptoms may reverse with long-term follow-up.[45,60,99]

Mucocutaneous toxicity is less serious than pulmonary damage, but more common. It includes mild stomatitis; hyperpigmentation over the elbows, knees, and small joints of the hands; thickening of the nail beds; alopecia; and a syndrome of skin erythema and edema.[60,99]

HEAVY METAL COMPOUNDS

CISPLATIN

Cisplatin is a platinum complex with a broad spectrum of antitumor activity and remarkable usefulness in cancer treatment. Recognition of its cytotoxic activity was the result of a serendipitous observation that bacterial growth in culture was altered when an electric current was delivered to the media through platinum electrodes. The growth change was noted to be similar to that produced by alkylating agents and radiation, and it was found that a platinum–chloride complex, now known as cisplatin, generated by the current was responsible for the changes. In clinical trials, cisplatin was found to have desirable efficacy but unacceptable serious toxicity, especially gastrointestinal and renal toxicities. Later, successful attempts were made to improve the therapeutic index by hydration and vigorous antiemetic therapy, which led to cisplatin's approval for commercial use in the late 1970s.[29,30,60,85,101]

Clinical Pharmacology. The main cytotoxic target of cisplatin is believed to be DNA, although the type of DNA lesion produced by platinum compounds is not conclusively established. Cytotoxicity in culture and probably *in vivo* depends on platinum binding to DNA and the formation of intrastrand cross-links between neighboring guanines. These intrastrand links cause a major bending of the DNA and may cause cellular damage by distorting the normal DNA conformation and preventing bases that are normally paired from lining up with each other. Interstrand cross-links also occur, although with much lower frequency than intrastrand links. It is known that *cis* forms of platinum compounds are much more cytotoxic than those in a *trans* configuration. Although the reasons for this are not clearly established, it may be related to the ability to form strand linkages.[85,101]

The cytotoxic form of cisplatin is the aquated species, that is, that in which the two chloride groups have been replaced by hydroxyl groups or water molecules (Fig. 115–25). This reaction occurs readily in low concentrations of chloride, such as the concentrations present within cells, and produces a positively charged compound that can react with DNA. The aquated species is responsible for both the efficacy and toxicity of cisplatin. Resistance to the therapeutic effects of cisplatin may occur through several mechanisms. Transmembrane transport of drug may be altered, the ability to repair DNA damage may be increased, or cisplatin may be neutralized by intracellular glutathione or sulfhydryl-containing proteins.[29,60,85,101,102]

Pharmacokinetics. Assessment of cisplatin pharmacokinetics following intravenous infusion is complicated by the existence of three major compartments, which include free or unbound drug, protein-bound drug, and drug bound to erythrocytes. It is characterized by a triphasic removal pattern. The first two phases represent removal of free drug, with elimination half-lives of 20 to 30 minutes and of about 1 hour. This elimination is primarily renal and represents a combination of glomerular filtration and tubular secretion. Protein-bound drug is removed much more slowly, with a terminal half-life of 1 to 3 days. Although renal excretion is important in elimination of protein-bound drug, protein catabolism and biliary excretion also contribute. In addition to depending on renal function for its elimination, cisplatin is also nephrotoxic; thus dose reduction is recommended in patients with preexisting or therapy-induced renal dysfunction (see Table 115–11). Clearance has been demonstrated to decrease and exposure to drug (AUC) to increase with successive cisplatin courses, even in the absence of significant changes in creatinine clearance. These changes correlate with increased drug toxicity and make guidelines for dose changes based on serum creatinine or creatine clearance undependable.[60,85,101,103]

Cisplatin is also administered regionally, especially in the peritoneal cavity. Peak peritoneal-cavity concentrations of free drug exceed plasma levels by at least 20-fold. This regional pharmacokinetic advantage may be increased by simultaneous intravenous infusion of the sulfhydryl compound sodium thiosulfate (see later discussion).[60,93,103]

Toxicity. Cisplatin is a highly toxic antineoplastic agent, with potential for serious nephrotoxicity, ototoxicity, peripheral neuropathy, emesis, and anemia. The significant efficacy of cisplatin against many tumor types makes it a valuable agent despite these toxicities, many of which can be prevented or managed with aggressive supportive care measures.

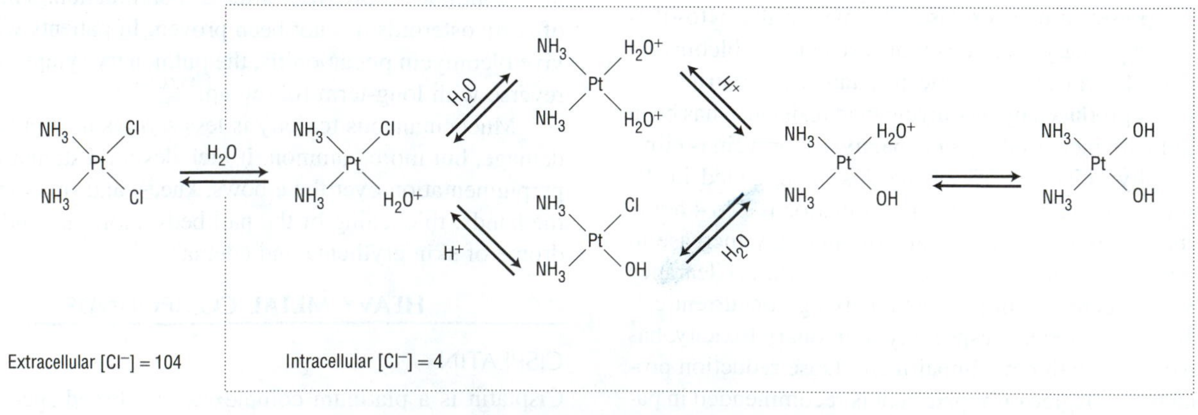

FIGURE 115–25. The aquation reaction of cisplatin. *(From Loehrer PJ, Einhorn LH. Cisplatin. Ann Intern Med 1984;100:705, with permission.)*

Nephrotoxicity and emesis were previously the most common dose-limiting toxicities of cisplatin administration, but these have been problems amenable to preventive measures. The proximal tubules are most sensitive to cisplatin-induced damage, but distal tubular function is also affected. Nephrotoxicity is characterized clinically by reduced glomerular filtration rates (GFRs); electrolyte losses, especially potassium and magnesium; or renal failure, which may occur acutely even in the first day after drug administration. Hypomagnesemia and reduced filtration rate are most characteristic of the acute phase of toxicity. Reduction in creatinine clearance, which may not produce elevated serum creatinine, occurs chronically. Renal damage from cisplatin is often slowly reversible, although hypomagnesemia and reduced creatinine clearance may persist in one-third or more of patients for many years. Risk of nephrotoxicity correlates with high single doses, cumulative doses, dehydration, preexisting renal impairment, and administration of other renal toxins.[77,101,104–106]

The incidence of nephrotoxicity can be decreased by careful diuresis and by aggressive hydration with chloride-containing solutions, which help to keep the cisplatin in the renal tubules in the nonaquated and therefore nontoxic form. Drug administration in hypertonic saline solutions is not clearly established as superior to providing large amounts of chloride via hydration fluids and is probably not necessary at conventional cisplatin doses. Diuretics, especially mannitol and furosemide, have been used to increase urine flow and reduce contact time of the cisplatin with the renal tubule. It is possible that mannitol may protect the kidney by delaying cisplatin binding onto renal tubular proteins. Furosemide has not been convincingly shown to decrease nephrotoxicity, but diuretics are useful in patients with cardiovascular compromise.[103–105] Sodium thiosulfate has also been used to decrease nephrotoxicity in combination with both intraperitoneal and systemic administration of cisplatin. Sodium thiosulfate accumulates in the renal tubules in high concentrations, where it rapidly neutralizes the cytotoxic activity of cisplatin. In the concentrations achieved in plasma, the half-life of the neutralization reaction is much slower; therefore thiosulfate does not interfere with the therapeutic effect of the drug. It is not effective in ameliorating any toxicity except nephrotoxicity. Some newer chemoprotective agents have been studied in attempts to decrease the nephrotoxic potential of cisplatin. Amifostine (WR-2721) is a thiol ester that can protect normal tissues against radiotherapy and alkylating agent–induced damage. It is moderately effective in prevention of cisplatin nephrotoxicity and its effects are most beneficial in high-risk patients.[23,106]

Cisplatin is one of the most severe emetogens known among marketed antineoplastic agents. Acute nausea and vomiting are nearly universal without prophylactic interventions, but can be prevented or limited with aggressive antiemetic therapy. Regimens containing corticosteroids and serotonin-receptor antagonists have been very successful in controlling acute cisplatin-induced emesis. About 60% of patients receiving cisplatin will also experience delayed nausea and vomiting, 2 to 4 days after drug administration, which is less easily prevented by conventional antiemetic therapy and which can have a serious impact on fluid and nutritional status.[107]

Neuropathy, which includes ototoxicity, peripheral neuropathy, and, rarely, ocular toxicity, has emerged as a dose-limiting toxicity of cisplatin with current effective management of renal damage and emesis. Ototoxicity most commonly affects the high-frequency hearing ranges and may be associated with loss of outer hair cells from the cochlea. Hearing loss is usually permanent, but associated vestibular toxicity generally reverses over time. Concurrent ifosfamide administration may exacerbate cisplatin-induced hearing loss. Effective means of preventing these toxicities are not known.[44,85,101]

Peripheral neuropathy is characteristically distal, in a "stocking-and-glove" distribution, and may begin and progress after cisplatin is discontinued. The dorsal root ganglia is the neural structure most sensitive to cisplatin damage. The most common symptoms include paresthesia and mild to severe pain. Peripheral neuropathy is associated with cumulative doses and is usually reversible, although complete resolution may take more than a year.[44,85,101] Chemoprotectors such as amifostine may limit neural damage.[106]

Although significant granulocytopenia or thrombocytopenia are unusual from cisplatin administration, normocytic, normochronic anemia is common. This anemia may respond to erythropoietin treatment. Hemolytic anemia also occurs.[60,85,101] Other toxicities of cisplatin include disturbances in color perception, hypersensitivity reactions, Raynaud's phenomenon, hypercholesterolemia, and rare hepatic toxicity.[60,85,101]

CARBOPLATIN

Carboplatin is a structural analog of cisplatin in which the chloride groups of the parent compound are replaced by a carboxycyclobutane moiety. It shares the same mechanism of action as cisplatin, although it generates an aquated reactive form much more slowly than cisplatin. The spectrum of activity is similar, and cross-resistance between the two agents is common. Carboplatin differs markedly from cisplatin, however, in its pharmacokinetics and toxicity.[60,85,101]

Pharmacokinetics. Many pharmacokinetic differences between carboplatin and cisplatin may be accounted for by differences in plasma protein binding. Carboplatin binds to plasma protein more slowly and less extensively than does cisplatin, resulting in a much longer plasma half-life of unbound carboplatin platinum in comparison with cisplatin. Carboplatin's pharmacokinetics are linear, with a steady-state volume of distribution approximately equal to total body water, and clearance of ultrafilterable carboplatin platinum is more than double that of creatinine clearance. The reduced protein binding also results in a much larger percentage of carboplatin than cisplatin being excreted in urine (60% to 80%).[85,101] In patients with compromised renal function, doses of carboplatin must be reduced to limit myelosuppressive toxicity. Several guidelines for dose modification in patients with impaired renal function have been developed,[108,109] but the most widely used dosage schema uses a target AUC and renal function parameters to estimate the carboplatin dose.[110] This schema was developed by Calvert and colleagues and is referred to as the "Calvert formula" (Table 115–15). Estimated or measured creatinine clearance is typically used to represent glomerular filtration rate (GFR) in this formula, but may underpredict the GFR. Similar dose guidelines have been developed for children.[111]

Toxicity. Unlike cisplatin, whose dose-limiting toxicities include nephrotoxicity and neurotoxicity, carboplatin administration is limited by hematologic toxicity. It causes suppression of white blood cells, but more particularly, platelets, with characteristic delayed recovery that can prevent retreatment more often than every 4 weeks. In contrast, however, its potential to cause renal damage, peripheral neuropathy, and ototoxicity is much less than that of comparable cisplatin doses, and it has proven to be a very useful alternative to cisplatin therapy in patients with preexisting compromise to these organs or at high risk of damage. The emetogenic potential of carboplatin is also substantially less than that of cisplatin, although it is still a moderate to severe emetogen.[85,101]

MISCELLANEOUS AGENTS

HYDROXYUREA

Hydroxyurea is a drug that falls broadly into the category of antimetabolites but is not a nucleoside analog. It inhibits ribonucleotide reductase, the enzyme required to convert ribonucleotides into the deoxyribonucleotide forms required for both DNA synthesis and repair. Consequently, hydroxyurea stops DNA synthesis without interfering with formation of RNA or protein. Cells accumulate in the S phase because DNA synthesis is inhibited, and only abnormally short DNA strands are produced.[29,60,112]

TABLE 115–15. Carboplatin Dose Modifications in Patients With Impaired Renal Function

Dose =	AUC × (GFR + 25)
where	
Dose =	Total dose in milligrams
AUC =	Desired area under the curve in mg/mL × min: Target AUC is 5–7 for single-agent carboplatin. Target AUC is 4–5 for carboplatin in combination with other myelosuppressive drugs.
GFR =	Glomerular filtration rate (not normalized for surface area). Estimated or measured creatinine clearance is usually substituted for true GFR, but may underestimate carboplatin dose.
25 =	Average nonrenal clearance for adults

From Ref. 110.

Pharmacokinetics. Hydroxyurea is well absorbed orally and is administered by that route, with peak concentrations achieved in 1 to 2 hours. The main route of elimination is renal excretion, although the percentage detected in urine varies markedly from patient to patient. Guidelines for dose reduction in patients with impaired renal function are not available, but hydroxyurea should be used cautiously in these patients. It distributes rapidly to tissues and enters both the CNS and "third-space" fluids readily.[29,60,112]

Toxicity. Toxicity is primarily marrow suppression of rapid onset, which is sometimes a desired therapeutic effect of the drug. It produces significant nausea, vomiting, anorexia, and mucositis, particularly in high-dose regimens. Chronic therapy produces skin hyperpigmentation, erythema especially of the face and hands, and rashes. Radiation recall reactions may occur.[60,112]

L-ASPARAGINASE

L-Asparaginase is unique among antineoplastics in its unusual mechanism of action, pattern of toxicity, and source. It is an enzyme produced by bacteria. It is commercially available in two forms, both of *Escherichia coli* origin. The first is an unconjugated form of the enzyme, available under the trade name Elspar, which is sometimes called native protein. L-Asparaginase has also recently been marketed as pegaspargase (Oncospar), in which polyethylene glycol (PEG) has been covalently conjugated to L-asparaginase.

Clinical Pharmacology. L-Asparagine is a nonessential amino acid that can be synthesized by most mammalian cells, except for those of certain human malignancies, which lack or have very low levels of the synthetase enzyme required for L-asparagine formation. L-Asparagine is degraded by the enzyme L-asparaginase, which depletes existing supplies and inhibits protein synthesis, with secondary block of nucleic acid synthesis. Malignant cells of lymphocyte origin are most likely to lack the capacity to synthesize new supplies of asparagine and are therefore most affected by L-asparagine depletion. Increased L-asparagine synthetase activity within tumor cells causes resistance to L-asparaginase treatment.[29,60,113]

Pharmacokinetics. The metabolic fate and elimination of L-asparaginase are not known but are believed to be mediated, at least in some patients, by antibody reactions with the L-asparaginase protein. The half-life of elimination of the native protein form of L-asparaginase is slightly longer than 1 day. Conjugation with PEG reduces uptake by the reticuloendothelial system and antibody formation in response to the protein, resulting in significant prolongation of the half-life to about 6 days. PEG protection of L-asparaginase permits both lower doses and less frequent drug administration. Clearance of either preparation is markedly accelerated in patients who develop hypersensitivity to the drug. Peak levels after intramuscular administration of native asparaginase are approximately half of levels after equal doses given intravenously. Asparaginase distributes within the intravascular space and achieves low but useful levels within the CNS. No L-asparaginase activity is detectable in urine.[60,113]

Toxicity. Toxicity of L-asparaginase consists primarily of hypersensitivity reactions to the antigenic protein and reactions that are effects of its therapeutic inhibition of protein synthesis. Hypersensitivity reactions occur in about 25% of patients receiving unconjugated L-asparaginase and are most common in those receiving intravenous doses, single-agent therapy, or repeated courses of treatment. True anaphylaxis occurs in 5% to 9% of patients, is fatal in about 1%, and requires allergic precautions during administration. Skin testing may be helpful in selecting patients at high risk for reactions, but is not uniformly predictive of allergic reactions, which occasionally occur even on first drug administration. PEG–asparaginase, which is less immunogenic than the native form, is indicated in patients who have experienced hypersensitivity reactions to conventional L-asparaginase. Hypersensitivity reactions are still common in patients receiving the PEG conjugated form of L-asparaginase but are rarely severe.[113]

Inhibition of protein synthesis results in several toxicities, particularly hemorrhage or thrombosis from impaired synthesis of clotting factors and/or naturally occurring anticoagulants, such as protein C and antithrombin III. Hyperglycemia secondary to decreased insulin synthesis is also common and can be abrupt in onset. Pancreatic toxicity may manifest as acute pancreatitis and occasionally progresses to hemorrhagic pancreatitis. Liver toxicity is common, with increases in transaminases, bilirubin, alkaline phosphatase, and hypoalbuminemia, and is sometimes dose limiting. Cerebral dysfunction, which most typically manifests as somnolence or confusion but which may progress to coma, occurs in about 25% of patients. This may be secondary to low amino acid levels within the CNS. Nausea occurs in more than half of patients. L-Asparaginase, however, does not produce myelosuppression, mucositis, or alopecia. The incidence of nonhypersensitivity-related adverse reactions is not affected by conjugation of L-asparaginase with PEG.[113]

One drug interaction with L-asparaginase is of established clinical significance. L-Asparaginase administered after methotrexate can stop both methotrexate's therapeutic and toxic actions, perhaps by interfering with protein synthesis and the entry of cells into the S phase, which are important for methotrexate's cytotoxic effects. This effect has been used to an advantage in some combination regimens.[60,113]

ALL-*TRANS*-RETINOIC ACID

All-*trans*-retinoic acid (ATRA, tretinoin) is a naturally occurring derivative of vitamin A (retinol). Vitamin A and its metabolites, collectively referred to as the retinoids, are known to play important roles in numerous biologic processes, including cellular differentiation. The promotion of normal differentiation of squamous cells prompted extensive investigation of the retinoids as chemoprevention agents in several malignancies, including head and neck cancer and lung cancer. The retinoids also stimulate differentiation of erythroid and myeloid progenitor cells. Because leukemias are often defined as a failure of normal hematopoietic differentiation, the retinoids have also been studied as potential antileukemic agents. This section focuses on that application.

Clinical Pharmacology. All-*trans*-retinoic acid has recently been reported to produce high complete-remission rates in patients with acute promyelocytic leukemia (APL). In the past few years, researchers have discovered that the genetic defect characteristic of APL seems to be a 15;17 chromosomal translocation. The gene for nuclear retinoic acid receptor α (RAR-α) is located on chromosome 17, and the translocation is associated with production of an abnormal RAR-α fusion protein. Administration of ATRA reverses the effects of abnormal RAR-α and promotes terminal myeloid differentiation. Unlike standard chemotherapeutic agents, which produce rapid antileukemic effects, the response to ATRA is delayed, usually occurring at 1 to 2 months.[114,115]

Pharmacokinetics. Following oral administration, peak plasma concentrations occur at 1 to 2 hours, but vary significantly among patients. This retinoid is heavily protein bound to albumin. Unlike its stereoisomer *cis*-retinoic acid, ATRA is rapidly cleared from the systemic circulation, with a half-life of approximately 1 hour. ATRA undergoes hydroxylation by P450 enzymes. Its metabolites are conjugated and secreted via the biliary system into the gastrointestinal tract, where they may undergo enterohepatic recycling. Over time, plasma concentrations of ATRA markedly diminish, and this effect may be associated with loss of clinical response in APL.[115]

Toxicity. The most commonly reported adverse effect is headache, which usually responds to mild analgesics. However, intracranial hypertension (pseudotumor cerebri) has also been reported. These patients present with severe headache, nausea, and papilledema and may require serial lumbar punctures, high-dose corticosteroids, and narcotic analgesics. Other toxicities are common to vitamin A derivatives in general and affect the skin and mucous membranes (xerostomia, cheilitis, skin desquamation), the eyes (dryness, blepharoconjunctivitis, corneal erosion), musculoskeletal system (myalgias, arthralgias, bone pain), and hypertriglyceridemia. Dry skin and mucous membranes respond well to topical emollients. Tolerance usually develops to headache and musculoskeletal symptoms with continued dosing. ATRA does not accumulate in the liver, as does vitamin A, and chronic liver damage has not been reported. However, reversible elevations in serum transaminases and bilirubin may occur. ATRA also shares the teratogenic properties of the retinoids, and all patients should be counseled to avoid pregnancy.[114,115]

Hyperleukocytosis (white blood count > 20,000/mm^3) occurs in up to 50% of APL patients who receive ATRA. This requires no specific intervention if unaccompanied by other symptoms and often indicates a positive response to ATRA therapy. However, hyperleukocytosis may also be an early indicator of the "retinoic-acid syndrome," a syndrome that occurs in up to 25% of patients and is characterized by fever and respiratory distress in addition to hyperleukocytosis. Patients may develop pulmonary infiltrates, pleural or pericardial effusions, weight gain, edema, and hypotension. The clinical scenario is comparable to the capillary-leak syndrome seen with administration of some cytokines such as interleukin-2. This syndrome usually occurs during the first 2 to 3 weeks of ATRA administration but has occurred as early as the second day of therapy. Progressive respiratory deterioration may require mechanical ventilation. Multiorgan failure and death have occurred in up to one-third of affected patients. The most effective known treatment is early institution of high-dose corticosteroids (dexamethasone 10 mg every 12 hours for 3 days).[114,115]

ESTRAMUSTINE

Estramustine is an unusual drug that structurally combines an alkylating agent, nor-nitrogen mustard, with the hormone estradiol. It was designed about 35 years ago for management of prostate cancer patients with the intent that the estradiol portion of the molecule would facilitate uptake of the alkylating agent into hormone-sensitive prostate cancer cells. Despite the inclusion of a known alkylator, estramustine does not function *in vivo* as an alkylating agent. Estrogens are released after its administration, but all of estramustine's pharmacologic effects cannot be attributed to estrogenic hormones. In the mid-1980s a new mechanism of action was demonstrated for this agent, redefining it as an antimicrotubule agent. Estramustine binds covalently to microtubule-associated proteins (MAPs) that are part of the structural support for microtubules. The binding of estramustine to MAPs causes the separation of MAPs from the microtubules, inhibiting microtubule assembly and eventually causing disassembly of the microtubules.[61] It has its greatest clinical utility in combination regimens with other microtubule agents.

Pharmacokinetics. Estramustine is administered orally and is well absorbed, with a bioavailability of at least 75%. Milk and calcium-containing antacids can decrease absorption. Metabolites of both nor-nitrogen mustard and estradiol are excreted into the bile, feces, and urine. Drug disposition is believed to be primarily nonrenal.[61]

Toxicity. Nausea and vomiting are the dose-limiting effects of oral estramustine. Despite the presence of the alkylating moiety, myelosuppression is very uncommon. Although the estrogenic component of estramustine is not believed to contribute significantly to its cytotoxic effects, it does contribute to toxicity. Most patients develop gynecomastia and nipple tenderness. Cardiovascular effects that are attributable to the estrogenic component are the most serious adverse effects. Edema with worsening symptoms of congestive failure occurs, with rarer complications of thromboembolism, myocardial infarction, and cerebrovascular events.[61]

ENDOCRINE THERAPIES

Endocrine manipulation is an option for management of cancers from tissues whose growth is under gonadal hormonal control, especially breast, prostate, and endometrial cancers.[116] These cancers may regress if the "feeding" hormone is eliminated or antagonized. Major organ system toxicity is uncommon from hormonal treatment, making it the least toxic of systemic anticancer therapies. The clinical applications and toxicity of individual agents are detailed in the breast and prostate cancer chapters.

Corticosteroids are also useful anticancer agents because of their lymphocytotoxic effects. Their primary use is in management of hematologic malignancies, especially lymphomas, lymphocytic leukemias, and the plasma cell cancer multiple myeloma. In addition to their cytotoxic effects, corticosteroids have many other applications in supportive care of cancer patients as outlined in Table 115–16. The corticosteroids have diverse toxicities in chronic or high-dose use but are generally well tolerated in short-term therapy.[117]

All steroid hormones share the same four-ring cyclopentane-perhydrophenanthrene structural nucleus, and all are derived from cholesterol. Despite their greatly diverse actions, all steroid hormones are believed to act by a similar mechanism (Fig. 115–26). Hormones diffuse passively across cell membranes and are trapped by protein receptors in the cytoplasm. The hormone–receptor complex is then "activated" and transferred into the nucleus, where it binds to DNA and ultimately alters gene expression. These gene alterations in turn change protein synthesis and, through this, change cell function and produce the hormone's biologic effects. The secretion of steroid hormones is under hypothalamic and pituitary control.[116,117]

TABLE 115–16. Application of Corticosteroids in Supportive Care of Cancer Patients

Nausea and vomiting
Cerebral edema secondary to brain metastases or cranial irradiation
Spinal cord compression
Hypercalcemia
Transfusion reactions
Appetite stimulation
Radiation or drug-induced pneumonitis
Prevention and treatment of anaphylactic reactions
Graft-versus-host disease after bone marrow transplantation
Pain secondary to nerve compression or edema
Decrease fluid retention from docetaxel

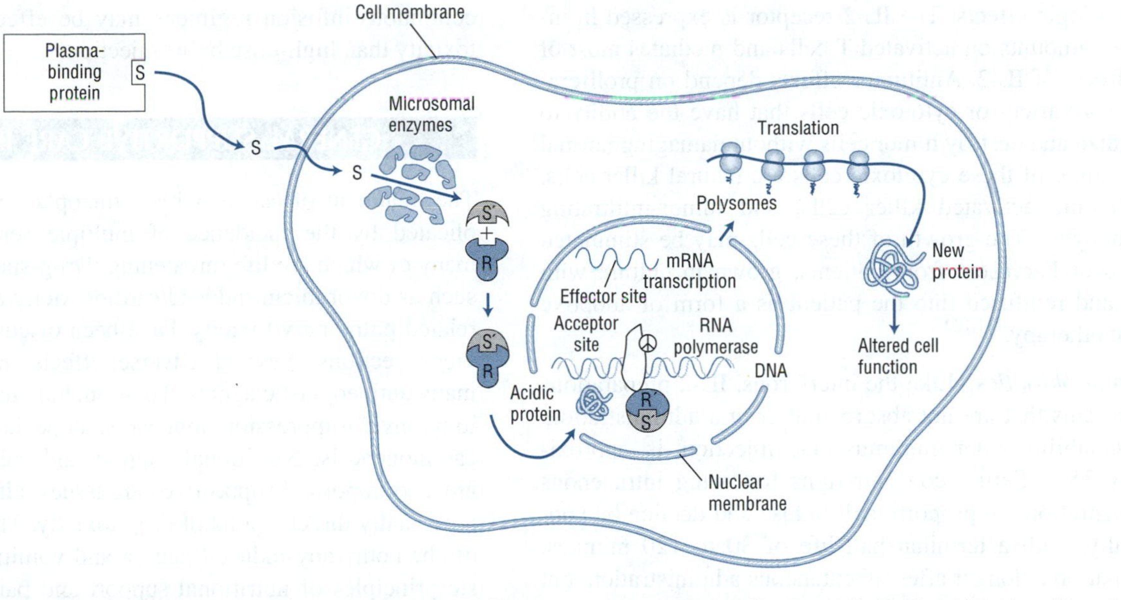

FIGURE 115–26. Schematic representation of the mechanism of steroid hormone action. Hormones diffuse into cells (S), bind to receptors (R), and are translocated to the nucleus, where they bind to DNA and alter expression of specific genes and, in turn, change protein production and alter cell function. *(From Lipman ME, Eil C. Steroid therapy of cancer. In: Chabner BA ed. Pharmacologic Principles of Cancer Treatment. Philadelphia, Saunders, 1982:132–182, with permission.)*

BIOLOGIC RESPONSE MODIFIERS

INTERFERONS

The interferons (IFN) are a family of proteins produced by nucleated cells and now also by means of recombinant-DNA technology, which have antiviral, antiproliferative, and immunoregulatory activities. They are classified as α-, β-, or γ-interferons based on antigenic, biologic, and pharmacologic properties. Many subtypes of IFN-α are known. IFN-α-2a and -α-2b are each single-species recombinant products and are very similar both structurally and biologically. These are the only interferons approved for anticancer indications.

The mechanism of IFN-α's antitumor action remains speculative. Although IFN administration increases the activity of various cytotoxic cells within the immune system, direct antiproliferative effects certainly play a role as well. These actions may be an extension of IFN's antiviral actions, in which a protein kinase is activated, which in turn alters the activity of other factors needed for protein synthesis. IFN-α also inhibits ornithine decarboxylase production, which may result in overall cell cycle slowing. Interferons can inhibit new blood vessel formation in tumors and can increase the expression of antigens on tumor-cell surfaces, making them more easily recognized by the cells of the immune system, and can inhibit or block certain oncogenes.[118–120]

Pharmacokinetics. The interferons are not absorbed orally, because they are proteins destroyed by digestive enzymes. The bioavailability of IFN-α after intramuscular or subcutaneous administration is nearly complete, however. Total body clearance is nearly double normal creatinine clearance, suggesting that renal secretion and catabolism or extrarenal elimination occur. Little or no IFN is excreted into the urine, and hepatic metabolism of IFN-α is minor. Animal data indicate that proteolytic degradation in renal tubules may be the major method of elimination. The half-life of plasma elimination is 4 to 5 hours, but biologic effects may persist for several days, permitting convenient three-times-weekly dosing schedules.[118,120]

Toxicity. The most characteristic toxicity of IFN is an acute flu-like syndrome of fever, chills, malaise, myalgias, and headache, which responds to pretreatment with antipyretic analgesics. Tolerance to the flu-like effects develops over several days to weeks but does not develop to fatigue, which is dose related and is the most common dose-limiting toxicity of IFN-α. Gastrointestinal toxicities, myelosuppression, increased liver function tests, and neurologic toxicities (vertigo, decreased mental status, confusion, depression, paresthesias) are rarely troublesome at low doses, but increase in incidence and severity as doses increase. Permanent major-organ toxicity is rare. Drug interactions with IFN use may be clinically important and may be a result of inhibition of cytochrome P450 enzymes.[118–120]

INTERLEUKIN-2 (ALDESLEUKIN)

Interleukin-2 (aldesleukin), formerly known as T-cell growth factor, is a lymphokine now produced recombinantly that has diverse immunologic effects. IL-2 promotes B- and T-cell proliferation and differentiation and initiates a cytokine cascade with multiple interacting immunologic effects. The IL-2 receptor is expressed in increased amounts on activated T cells and mediates most of the effects of IL-2. Antitumor effects depend on proliferation of a variety of cytotoxic cells that have the ability to recognize and destroy tumor cells without damaging normal cells. Some of these cytotoxic cells are natural killer cells, lymphokine activated killer cells, and tumor-infiltrating lymphocytes. The growth of these cells may be stimulated *in vivo* or harvested from patients, grown in culture with IL-2, and reinfused into the patient as a form of adoptive immunotherapy.[121,122]

Pharmacokinetics. Like the interferons, IL-2 preparations are proteins that are not absorbed after oral administration. Bioavailability after intramuscular injection is approximately 35%. Serum concentrations following intravenous administration are proportional to dose and decline biexponentially, with a terminal half-life of 30 to 120 minutes. Elimination is longer after subcutaneous administration, but peak concentrations achieved are 10 to 100 times lower than those immediately after intravenous bolus. Clearance is estimated at 120 mL/min, suggesting that renal tubular filtration is the major means of elimination.[121]

Toxicity. The toxicity of IL-2 is related to dose, route, and duration of therapy, but, in general, IL-2 is toxic therapy that requires vigorous supportive care in conventional-dose regimens. Low doses may be well tolerated, even in outpatient administration.

The most common dose-limiting toxicities are hypotension, fluid retention, and renal dysfunction. IL-2 decreases peripheral vascular resistance with peripheral vasodilation and tachycardia, which produce hypotension. A characteristic vascular or capillary-leak syndrome results in fluid retention often greater than 10% of body weight, which in turn can cause respiratory compromise. These toxicities require administration of vasopressors, judicious use of fluid support and diuretics, and supplemental oxygen in most patients. Patients with underlying cardiovascular or renal abnormalities are more susceptible to these adverse effects.[121,122]

In addition to the hemodynamic and renal effects, most patients treated with IL-2 in full doses experience thrombocytopenia, anemia, eosinophilia, reversible cholestasis, and skin erythema with burning and pruritus. Neuropsychiatric changes, hypothyroidism, and bacterial infections, particularly staphylococcal infections, are also common.[121–124] In general, the toxicities from IL-2 therapy are reversible and can be managed or prevented by careful prospective monitoring and pharmacologic supportive care. Although many of the IL-2 adverse effects can be ameliorated by corticosteroid administration, it is possible that steroids decrease the antitumor effects of IL-2. Their concurrent use is not recommended at present. A variety of dose regimens and schedules have been evaluated to decrease the toxicity associated with IL-2 administration. Prolonged low-dose regimens and continuous-infusion regimens may be effective, with less toxicity than high-dose bolus injection.

GENERAL SUPPORTIVE CARE ISSUES

The treatment of cancer with antineoplastic drugs is complicated by the incidence of multiple serious toxicities, many of which are life threatening. Drug-specific toxicities, such as doxorubicin-induced cardiotoxicity and bleomycin-related pulmonary toxicity, have been discussed in the previous sections. Several adverse effects are common to many antineoplastic agents. These include nausea and vomiting, myelosuppression, mucositis, alopecia, infertility, and carcinogenesis. Nutritional support and pain management are also important supportive care issues, although they are not usually direct results of drug toxicity. The management of chemotherapy-induced nausea and vomiting and the basic principles of nutritional support and pain management are discussed in detail in other sections of this text.

Because many antineoplastic drugs affect DNA synthesis, any cell with a high turnover rate will be more sensitive to the toxic effects of chemotherapy. Cancer cells do not necessarily proliferate faster than normal cells. Normal tissues that consist of rapidly proliferating cells are targets for the toxicities of many anticancer drugs.[10] The bone marrow, intestinal mucosa, and hair follicles are such tissue sites where drug effects are manifested.

MYELOSUPPRESSION

Although not seen with all antineoplastic agents, myelosuppression is the most common dose-limiting side effect of cytotoxic agents. Bone marrow suppression does not usually occur immediately after chemotherapy administration. Blood components that have already been produced must be consumed before the effect is evident. WBCs, especially granulocyte precursors, are most significantly affected because of their rapid proliferation and short life span (6 to 12 hours). Platelets (5- to 10-day life span) are also affected, but to a much lesser degree than granulocytes. Erythrocytes, with a 120-day life span, are affected the least. Usual nadirs, or lowest blood cell counts, occur at 10 to 14 days following chemotherapy administration, with recovery by 3 to 4 weeks. There are some exceptions to this general rule. The nitrosoureas and mitomycin C exhibit a delayed pattern of nadir (4 to 6 weeks) and recovery (6 to 8 weeks). Planned courses of chemotherapy may have to be delayed while waiting for the granulocyte count to return to normal. For a patient to safely receive another cycle of chemotherapy, a WBC count $\geq 3000/mm^3$ or an absolute neutrophil count (ANC) of $\geq 1500/mm^3$ and a platelet count of $\geq 100{,}000/mm^3$ is usually required.

Myelotoxicity is a desired therapeutic effect in leukemia patients during induction chemotherapy. However, myelosuppression is an undesirable side effect during chemotherapy for other malignancies. If undesirable myelosuppression has occurred with prior courses of chemotherapy, the doses of the offending agent(s) in subsequent courses may be reduced. However, dosage reduction may also compromise antitumor response. The magnitude of dose reduction is dictated by the degree of myelosuppression incurred and the incidence and severity of infection or bleeding. Empiric dosage reductions may be made or hematopoietic growth factors initiated for the first chemotherapy treatment if the patient has a low baseline WBC or platelet count, has diminished bone marrow reserve, has impaired drug-elimination capabilities, or is to receive a combination of several drugs that cause myelosuppression. Patients who have received multiple prior courses of other myelotoxic chemotherapy regimens or extensive radiation therapy, especially to the pelvis, may have a decreased bone marrow reserve. They are more sensitive to the myelosuppressive effects of chemotherapy, and normal doses may produce profound marrow toxicity. The pharmacokinetic profile of a myelosuppressive agent is also important in determining the appropriate dose. For example, the anthracyclines produce bone marrow suppression as an acute dose-limiting toxicity, and these agents depend on biliary excretion as their primary route of elimination. A patient with biliary obstruction may have compromised elimination of anthracyclines and is at increased risk for severe bone marrow suppression.

NEUTROPENIA

When the ANC falls below 500, infection risk increases.[125,126] The ANC may be calculated by multiplying the percentage of neutrophils (segmented plus banded neutrophils) by the total WBC count. The risk of infection is also directly proportional to the duration of neutropenia. Other risk factors for infection include alteration in the integrity of physical defense barriers and the functional integrity of WBCs. The patient's underlying cancer, as well as treatment with cytotoxic drugs and radiation, can affect neutrophil function. The diagnosis of infection in the neutropenic patient is complicated by the lack of WBCs. Usual signs and symptoms of infection, such as pus, abscesses, and infiltrates on chest x-ray, depend on the presence of WBCs. The only reliable indication of infection in these patients is fever. Definitive culture results may take days, and a septic neutropenic cancer patient can die within hours if not treated. Therefore, the basic approach to the management of the febrile neutropenic cancer patient is prompt initiation of empiric antibiotics. The antibiotics are chosen based on reliable coverage of the most likely organisms, antibiotic sensitivities at the institution, the patient's signs and symptoms (if present), side-effect profiles, and cost.[126] The most common source of infection in these patients is self-infection with body flora, which includes both gram-positive and gram-negative bacteria. Although most early infections are caused by bacteria, fungi become important pathogens as the course of neutropenia is prolonged. Traditionally, all febrile neutropenic cancer patients have received intravenous antibiotics in the hospital setting until full recovery of neutrophils. However, it is possible to identify patients at low risk for infectious complications who may be candidates for alternative treatment strategies, including early discharge from the hospital and outpatient oral or intravenous antibiotics.[127,128]

Numerous methods have been explored to prevent infections in cancer patients.[129–132] Colony-stimulating factors (CSFs) are commonly employed for this reason.[130–134] These hormones are naturally occurring proteins that are essential for the normal growth and maturation of blood cell components (Fig. 115–27). The CSFs have the ability to enhance the production and also the function of their target cells. Two agents, G-CSF (granulocyte colony-stimulating factor) and GM-CSF (granulocyte–macrophage colony-stimulating factor) are commercially available in the United States. Several interleukins (IL-1, IL-3, IL-6, IL-11) and other growth factors (macrophage CSF [M-CSF], and stem-cell factor [S-CSF]) are currently being investigated in clinical trials. G-CSF (filgrastim, Neupogen) specifically stimulates the production of neutrophilic granulocytes. GM-CSF (sargramostim, Leukine) promotes the proliferation of granulocytes (neutrophils and eosinophils), as well as monocytes/macrophages. Although GM-CSF has been shown to stimulate megakaryocytes, in vitro, no consistent effect on platelet production has been defined in clinical trials. Both agents initially enhance demargination and mobilization of mature cells from the marrow and then provide constant stimulation on stem cell progenitors. The two CSFs have contrasting effects on neutrophil migration: G-CSF enhances this process, whereas GM-CSF inhibits it. The clinical implications of this difference are unknown. Another effect unique to GM-CSF is an increase in neutrophil adhesion to capillary endothelial cells. This process may account for some of the side effects seen more commonly with GM-CSF. Several host sources have been employed in the recombinant-DNA technology used to produce CSFs, including bacteria (*E. coli*), yeast, and mammalian cells (Chinese hamster ovary or CHO cells) (Table 115–17). Products derived from yeast or mammalian sources are glycosylated to varying degrees, as are naturally occuring CSFs, whereas those derived from *E. coli* are nonglycosylated. This difference has not been shown to result in any clinically significant effects.

The CSFs reduce the incidence, magnitude, and duration of neutropenia following a variety of myelosuppressive chemotherapy regimens.[130–134] These effects have been accompanied by a decrease in febrile days, fewer infections, and fewer days on antibiotics. An unexpected benefit in some G-CSF studies has been a decrease in the incidence of mucositis. Growth factors have also permitted the administration of subsequent chemotherapy courses on schedule, resulting in enhanced dose intensity. Whether the increased

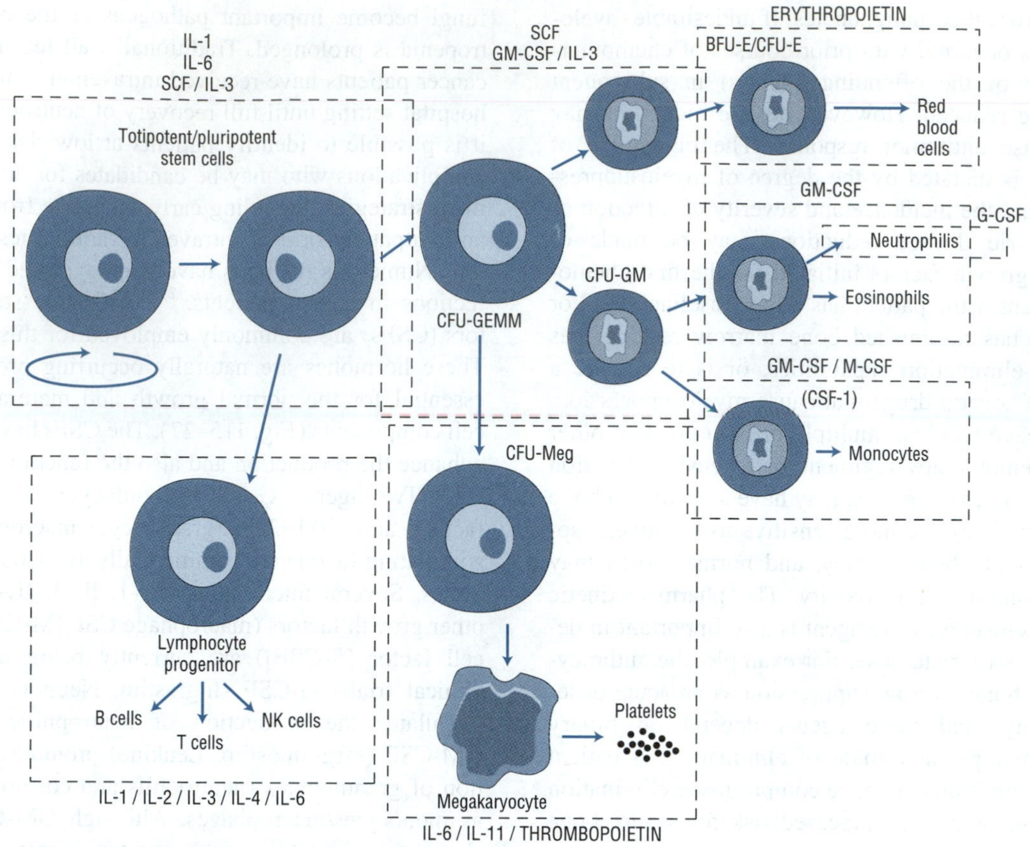

FIGURE 115–27. Regulation of hematopoietic cell development. A self-sustaining pool of marrow stem cells differentiates under the influence of specific growth factors to form a variety of myeloid and lymphoid cells. SCF = stem cell factor; GM-CSF = granulocyte–macrophage colony-stimulating factor; G-CSF = granulocyte colony-stimulating factor; M-CSF = macrophage colony-stimulating factor; and IL-1, IL-2, IL-3, IL-4, IL-6, IL-11 = interleukins 1–6, and 11, respectively. *(Adapted from Hillman RS. Hematopoietic agents: Growth factors, minerals and vitamins. In: Hardman JG, Limbird LE, Molinoff PB, Ruddon RW, Gilman AG eds. Goodman & Gilman's The Pharmacologic Basis of Therapeutics, 9th ed. New York, McGraw-Hill, 1996:1312.)*

dose intensity provided by the CSFs will translate into improved tumor response remains to be demonstrated. Although there is experience with both G-CSF and GM-CSF in prevention of febrile neutropenia after administration of standard doses of chemotherapy, at this time only G-CSF is FDA approved for this indication. One exception is in the induction treatment of acute leukemia in patients over the age of 55, in whom both GM-CSF and G-CSF have demonstrated a modest reduction in the duration of neutropenia, sometimes accompanied by decreased infectious complications. These beneficial effects, however, have not resulted in improved response rates or overall survival.[134]

Only a few studies have addressed the role of CSFs in the treatment of established neutropenia.[133,134] These initial studies suggest no or only minimal clinical benefit from use of CSFs. Future studies will determine the true cost effectiveness of this strategy. Both CSFs have also proven effective in acceleration of hematopoietic engraftment and in treatment of graft failure following bone marrow transplantation. Other uses for the CSFs include peripheral blood

TABLE 115–17. Granulocyte Colony-stimulating Factor (G-CSF) and Granulocyte–Macrophage Colony-stimulating Factor (GM-CSF) Products and Sources

CSF	Generic Name	Brand Name	Manufacturer	Recombinant-DNA Source
G-CSF	Filgrastim	Neupogen	Amgen	*Escherichia coli*
	Lenograstim	Neutrogin[b] Investigational	Chugai-Rhone Poulenc	CHO[a] cells
GM-CSF	Sargramostim	Leukine	Immunex	*Saccharomyces cerevisiae* Yeast
	Molgramostim	Leucomax[b]	Schering-Plough/Sandoz	*E. coli*

[a]Chinese hamster ovary.
[b]Available outside the United States.

stem cell mobilization, neutropenia in AIDS patients, myelodysplastic syndromes, congenital neutropenia, and aplastic anemia. The American Society of Clinical Oncology has developed evidence-based clinical practice guidelines to promote appropriate use of the CSFs.[133,134]

At currently recommended doses, the CSFs are well tolerated. Side effects are more commonly seen with GM-CSF and may be related to the drug's ability to enhance binding of neutrophils to endothelial cells or to activation of monocytes/macrophages, which may stimulate the release of cytokines, such as IL-1 and tumor necrosis factor.[130] The most common toxicity of the CSFs is bone pain (20% to 25% of patients), which can be treated with acetaminophen or NSAIDs. Bone pain was the most significant toxicity seen in clinical trials with G-CSF. Other side effects of G-CSF include an increase in lactate dehydrogenase, alkaline phosphatase, and uric acid levels. Additional toxicities of GM-CSF include constitutional symptoms, such as low-grade fever, myalgias, arthralgias, lethargy, and mild headache. GM-CSF may also produce an elevation in liver transaminase enzymes. At higher doses of GM-CSF, pleural and pericardial effusions, capillary-leak syndrome, and thrombus formation may occur. A first-dose reaction described after GM-CSF administration has been reported more commonly with the *E. coli*–derived product (molgramostim), which is investigational. This reaction is more common after intravenous infusion and consists of dyspnea, facial flushing, hypotension, hypoxia, and tachycardia. Both G-CSF and GM-CSF may produce mild erythema at subcutaneous injection sites, as well as a generalized maculopapular rash with either subcutaneous or intravenous administration.

For prophylaxis of chemotherapy-induced neutropenia, CSF therapy should begin not sooner than 24 hours after the last dose of chemotherapy and be continued until the ANC exceeds a safe level following the expected chemotherapy nadir. In the setting of bone marrow transplantation, CSFs should not begin sooner than 24 hours after the last dose of chemotherapy or 12 hours after the last radiotherapy treatment. The recommended starting dose of G-CSF with standard chemotherapy is 5 μg/kg/d. Doses of 5 to 10 μg/kg/d are used in bone marrow transplantation. The recommended dose of yeast-derived GM-CSF is 250 $\mu g/m^2$/d. Both agents are most commonly administered as a subcutaneous injection but continuous intravenous or subcutaneous infusions and short intravenous infusions have also been used. The optimal dose, route, and method of administration are currently unknown. Because of the high cost associated with CSF use, alternative regimens are being explored. These regimens attempt to decrease the total amount of CSF used by either delaying the start of CSFs (e.g., to day 3 after chemotherapy), decreasing the dose (e.g., to 3 μg/kg/d G-CSF), or decreasing the duration of CSF therapy. Specifically, the posttreatment target ANC of 10,000/mm^3 recommended by product information is often reduced to an ANC of greater than 2000 or 5000/mm^3 in clinical practice. Standardized doses of 300 μg or 480 μg of G-CSF and 500 μg of GM-CSF, based on product vial sizes, are often used to minimize waste.

THROMBOCYTOPENIA

Chemotherapy-induced thrombocytopenia puts the patient at risk for significant bleeding. To date, platelet transfusions remain the mainstay of management. Recently, interleukin-11 (oprelvekin) has been approved by the FDA based on a decreased need for platelet transfusions and numbers of platelet transfused after chemotherapy.[135,136] Other CSFs, such as interleukins-1, -3, and -6, have also been studied, but significant impacts on platelet counts within an acceptable adverse-effect profile have not been demonstrated.[137] The recent discovery and development of thrombopoietin (megakaryocyte growth and development factor) may represent the most significant factor in the future of thrombocytopenia treatment.[138–140]

ANEMIA

Anemia, a common finding in cancer patients, often has multiple contributing factors, including anemia of chronic disease, chronic gastrointestinal blood loss, chemotherapy and radiation therapy, and bone marrow invasion by the tumor. Chemotherapy-induced anemias may be owing to a direct effect on the bone marrow, but some anticancer drugs have the potential to cause other types of anemia. Cisplatin-induced anemia is a common finding and may be due to stem cell damage, but hemolysis has also been documented.[101] Previously, the only option for the treatment of chemotherapy-related anemia was red blood cell transfusions. This intervention is still the mainstay of management, but the availability of human recombinant erythropoietin has provided another option.[141] Recent studies have documented the efficacy of erythropoietin in the anemia of malignancy and in treating chemotherapy-induced anemias.[141,142] Erythropoietin in doses of 100 to 150 U/kg given subcutaneously three times per week results in increases in hematocrit, decreases in transfusion requirements, and improved quality of life. Studies are underway to identify those patients most likely to benefit from this agent. Several early indicators of response have been derived, including an increase in hemoglobin of 0.5 g/dL above baseline, a decline in ferritin, or an increase in the absolute reticulocyte count after 2 to 4 weeks of therapy. The surrogate end points help to identify nonresponders early so that therapy may be modified or discontinued, as indicated.[141]

MUCOSITIS

The gastrointestinal (GI) mucosa is composed of epithelial cells with a high mitotic index and rapid turnover rate, making it a common site of chemotherapy-induced toxicity.[107,143,144] The subsequent inflammation, or mucositis, can lead to painful ulcerations, local infection, and inability to eat, drink, or swallow. Disruption of the GI mucosal barrier may also provide an avenue for systemic microbial invasion. The time course for development and resolution of mucositis often parallels that of neutropenia. Agents most commonly associated with mucositis include 5-fluorouracil (5-FU), doxorubicin, and methotrexate. The most effective means of preventing mucositis is through good oral hygiene. Patients at high risk for this toxicity (with poor dentition, high-dose chemotherapy, or radiation therapy involving the oropharynx) should be evaluated by a dentist prior to chemotherapy and should be instructed to rinse their mouths frequently with baking soda and salt water or chlorhexidine (Peridex) rinses following chemotherapy.[107] For patients receiving 5-FU treatment, the use of ice (oral cryotherapy) may decrease the risk for mucositis by decreasing drug delivery to the oral mucosa.[107,143] Once mucositis has developed, treatment is mainly supportive, including use of topical or systemic analgesics and oral hygiene (including the rinses described). Viscous lidocaine, diphenhydramine liquid, and dyclonine are topical anesthetics commonly employed. Severe cases of mucositis may lead to dehydration and require intravenous hydration. Local infections due to *Candida* species and herpes simplex viruses are common in these patients. Suspicious lesions should be cultured, and appropriate antifungal and/or antiviral treatment should then be instituted. Antifungal therapy may be delivered topically for mild infections (thrush), using clotrimazole (Mycelex) troches or nystatin (Nilstat, others) oral suspension. For more severe oral or esophageal fungal infections, systemic treatment with oral ketoconazole (Nizoral), fluconazole (Diflucan), or intravenous amphotericin B is indicated.[107,143]

Mucosal damage can occur at any point along the entire length of the GI tract. In the lower portion of the GI tract, this damage is usually manifested as diarrhea (mild to life threatening in nature) and abdominal pain. Support with intravenous fluids and electrolyte supplementation should be initiated promptly in severe cases. Once infectious causes have been ruled out, diarrhea can safely be treated with antispasmodics like Lomotil or loperamide (Immodium). The somatostatin analog octreotide has also been used successfully to treat severe cases of 5-FU–induced diarrhea.[107]

ALOPECIA

Although not a life-threatening side effect of chemotherapy, the toxicity that many patients find most distressing is alopecia. Alopecia from chemotherapy is usually temporary, and the degree of hair loss varies widely.[145] The loss of hair is not limited to the scalp; any area of the body may be affected. Hair loss usually begins 1 to 2 weeks after chemotherapy, and regrowth may begin before the chemotherapy courses are completed. Cryotherapy (local application of ice) and scalp tourniquets have both been investigated as methods of preventing alopecia. Both techniques produce vasoconstriction, resulting in decreased exposure of hair follicles to the chemotherapy agents. These techniques have not been found to be uniformly effective and are contraindicated in patients with cancers that may metastasize to the scalp, such as leukemia and lymphoma.

EXTRAVASATION

Certain antineoplastic agents, which have the ability to cause severe tissue damage if they escape from the vasculature, are called *vesicants.*[60,93,146] These agents include the anthracyclines, actinomycin D, the vinca alkaloids, mitomycin C, and nitrogen mustard. The anthracyclines are the most notorious agents, and most extensively investigated. The tissue damage may result in prolonged pain, tissue sloughing, infection, and loss of mobility. Prompt initiation of the appropriate interventions is important to minimize morbidity. Unfortunately, most information on extravasation management is anecdotal; few controlled clinical studies have been conducted to determine optimal intervention strategies. Therefore, prevention has become the focus of extravasation management. The most important method of prevention is good administration technique,[146] but even then, extravasations may occur. The vein selected for administration should be on the distal portion of the arm. The large veins of the forearm are desirable because if a drug does extravasate, there is adequate soft-tissue coverage to protect crucial structures like nerves and tendons, and joint function is not risked. Peripherally administered vesicants should be given slowly via intravenous injection (IV push) through the side-arm of a running IV. The person administering the vesicant should verify needle stability and adequate blood return after each 1 to 2 mL of drug is injected. Vesicants should not be administered by intravenous infusion unless the patient has a central venous catheter. For extravasation of vesicants, one of the most important interventions is the application of ice packs to the affected area. One exception to this rule is the vinca alkaloids, which are better managed with application of heat. Only a few antidotes to vesicant agents are employed clinically. Sodium thiosulfate is used to neutralize nitrogen mustard extravasations, and hyaluronidase has been shown to improve the outcome after vinca alkaloid extravasation. Topical application of dimethyl sulfoxide (DMSO) may be an effective method for managing anthracycline and mitomycin C extravasations.[64,93]

INFERTILITY

Advances in the treatment of some cancers, such as Hodgkin's disease and testicular cancer, have produced long-term survivors and the opportunity to examine the late consequences of chemotherapy administration. Infertility and secondary cancers have emerged as important late effects. The gonadal toxicities of chemotherapy have not received much attention in the past because they are not life threatening. High rates of fertility deficits and sexual dysfunction have been noted for both men and women.[147,148] In men, the antitumor drugs have been shown to produce severe oligospermia or azoospermia as well as infertility. Serum testosterone levels are only rarely altered. The recovery of spermatogenesis after completion of chemotherapy is unpredictable. Men receiving combination chemotherapy appear to have more long-lasting adverse effects on fertility than men receiving single-agent therapy. Age, total dose, duration of therapy, and type of drug are other important variables. In women, toxic effects on the ovaries result clinically in amenorrhea, vaginal epithelial atrophy, and menopausal symptoms. These effects are related to dose and age. Younger patients appear to be more resistant to the effects on the ovaries. As with men, the recovery of fertility is unpredictable, but women younger then 25 years of age appear to have the best outcomes. The effects of the alkylating agents on fertility have been extensively studied. This group of drugs exerts profound and consistently detrimental effects on reproductive function. Less is known about commonly used agents such as doxorubicin, taxanes, and platinum compounds. Patients with potentially curable tumors, who desire to have children in the future, should be informed about the risk for infertility and sperm or oocyte banking options.

SECONDARY MALIGNANCIES

Secondary cancers induced by chemotherapy and radiation pose a serious long-term complication.[149] Although many types of solid tumors have been reported as chemotherapy-induced malignancies, ANLL is the most common secondary cancer. ANLL has been reported following successful treatment of Hodgkin's disease, acute leukemias, non-Hodgkin's lymphomas, multiple myeloma, breast cancer, and advanced ovarian cancer. For curable cancers, the relatively small risk for occurrence of secondary malignancies is far outweighed by the benefits of survival in large numbers of patients. However, for cancers such as ovarian cancer, the risk of leukemia is not offset by improved survival in chemotherapy recipients. The issue of secondary malignancies is of particular concern in patients receiving adjuvant chemotherapy. As with the late complication of infertility, the group of antineoplastic agents primarily associated with secondary cancers is the alkylating agents. Etoposide, teniposide, and the anthracyclines have also been linked to secondary leukemias. Solid tumors as secondary malignancies occur more commonly after treatment with radiation than with chemotherapy,

SAFETY AND HANDLING ISSUES

As discussed previously, the cytotoxic drugs used to treat cancer are carcinogenic, mutagenic, and teratogenic. Consequently, these drugs should be handled with care to avoid inadvertent exposure of health care professionals.[150] All pharmacies should have written standard procedures for handling these drugs, and all personnel should be oriented to these procedures. The most common avenue of exposure is via inhalation of aerosolized drug. Individuals preparing chemotherapy should work in a Class II biologic safety cabinet and wear gowns and powder-free disposable latex gloves. The gowns should be made of lint-free, low-permeability fabric with a solid front, long sleeves, and tight-fitting elastic cuffs. Negative-pressure techniques should be employed in drug preparation to minimize aerosolization. Health care workers administering these agents should take similar precautions to avoid exposure. Kits for cleaning up chemotherapy spills should be located in all areas of the institution in which chemotherapy is handled. Cytotoxic waste should be disposed of properly, and patients should be informed of proper methods of disposing of potentially contaminated body excreta and cytotoxic waste.

CANCER PREVENTION

DIET

The relationship between diet and cancer is the subject of intense investigation. Although controversy exists over the true role of dietary factors in carcinogenesis, some general recommendations have been developed by the National Cancer Institute (Table 115–18).[151] Consumption of a high-fat diet appears to increase the risk for breast, colorectal, and prostate cancers. The average American consumes 36% to 38% of daily calories as fat. A decrease in fat intake to less than 30% of daily calories may decrease the risk for developing cancer, as well as heart disease. Obese individuals have been shown to have increased risk of several cancers, including colorectal, breast, biliary, and uterine. The inverse relationship between dietary fiber and colon cancer has received much attention. The American diet is typically low in fiber (11 g/d). High fiber intake (20 to 30 g/d) may decrease the risk of colon cancer. A high alcohol intake has been shown to increase the risk for many upper aerodigestive tract malignancies, especially in smokers.

TABLE 115–18. American Cancer Society Dietary Recommendations

Choose most of the foods you eat from plant sources
- Eat five or more servings of fruits and vegetables daily
- Eat other foods from plant sources, such as breads, cereals, grain products, rice, pasta, or beans several times each day

Limit your intake of high-fat foods, particularly from animal sources
- Choose foods low in fat
- Limit consumption of meats, especially high-fat meats

Be physically active: achieve and maintain a healthy weight
- Be at least moderately active for 30 minutes or more most days of the week
- Stay within your healthy weight range

Limit consumption of alcoholic beverages, if you drink at all

From Ref. 151, with permission.

CHEMOPREVENTION

This is defined as the systemic use of natural or synthetic products to reverse, suppress, or prevent carcinogenesis. Several agents have been studied in chemoprevention. There is evidence that vitamins and trace elements such as vitamin A and related retinoids, vitamins C and E, and selenium may prevent, halt, or reverse the carcinogenic process. These vitamins are present in fresh fruits and vegetables. The known effects of these agents on the cancer process have resulted in several trials to determine their effectiveness as chemoprotective agents.[152,153] To date, the most encouraging results have been in the area of oral leukoplakia and squamous cell head and neck cancer. Oral leukoplakia is a white, patchy, premalignant lesion of the oral mucosa associated with tobacco use and is also related to carcinogenesis at other sites within the aerodigestive tract. Patients with smoking-related malignancy have acquired a so-called field cancerization defect, meaning that any part of the aerodigestive tract exposed to the tobacco carcinogens is at risk for development of cancer. For example, patients cured of head and neck cancer commonly present several years later with a second primary cancer of the upper aerodigestive tract. Clinical trials of vitamin A and the retinoids have shown significant activity against oral leukoplakia and the development of second primary tumors in patients with head and neck cancer. In addition to smoking cessation, patients cured of their head and neck malignancy should be considered candidates for chemoprevention. In contrast, β-carotene has been not been found to be of benefit in prevention of lung cancer; in fact one large trial suggested it caused an increased risk of cancer.[154] These results emphasize the importance of evaluating chemoprevention strategies in a systematic fashion before they are used widely in clinical practice.

Hormonal therapy may represent another effective mechanism of chemoprevention. It is known that certain hormones play a role in the initiation, promotion, and progression of malignancy. For example, estrogen is known to stimulate breast cancer cell growth and testosterone stimulates prostate cancer growth. The antiestrogen tamoxifen effectively blocks this stimulatory effect in breast cancer. A large clinical trial sponsored by the National Surgical Adjuvant Bowel and Breast Project (NSABP) assessed tamoxifen's efficacy in breast cancer prevention in high-risk individuals. The trial was stopped prematurely in 1998 after demonstrating a 45% reduction in the risk of developing breast cancer among patients receiving tamoxifen compared with placebo.[155] However, there was also a mild increase in risk for endometrial cancer and thromboembolic disease. The ultimate role and appropriate patients for tamoxifen prevention remain to be determined. The nationwide Prostate Cancer Prevention Trial is assessing the efficacy of the 5-α-reductase inhibitor finasteride, which inhibits the conversion of testosterone to its active form, dihydrotestosterone, in preventing prostate cancer. The results of these trials will provide valuable information on the utility of hormonal manipulation on cancer prevention.

TOBACCO

In 1990, almost 413,000 deaths (20% of all deaths) in the United States were caused by smoking-related illnesses.[156] Cigarette smoking remains the most preventable cause of premature death in the United States. For many types of cancer, the underlying etiology is unknown. One notable exception is lung cancer; cigarette smoking is the major cause of this disease.[157] More than 90% of all cases of lung cancer are diagnosed in smokers. Tobacco smoking also increases the relative risk for development of many other types of cancer, including cancers of the mouth, pharynx, larynx, esophagus, and bladder. Passive inhalation of exhaled tobacco byproducts and cigarette smoke represents a significant risk factor for lung cancer in the nonsmoking population. Smokeless tobacco has been connected to the development of oral cancers. Abstinence from chewing and smoking tobacco is believed to be a major factor in the prevention of these malignancies.

SUN EXPOSURE

The association between sun exposure and skin neoplasms is also well established. The incidence of both nonmelanomatous skin cancer and melanoma has steadily increased in past decades, paralleling the increase in recreational sun exposure.[158] During this same time period, protection from the ultraviolet light exposure normally provided by the ozone layer has been compromised. Fair-skinned individuals who sunburn easily are particularly at high risk. Melanoma and skin cancers can be largely prevented by minimizing exposure to the sun and by applying strong sunscreens and sunblocks to sun-exposed areas (SPF-15).

REFERENCES

1. Kaufman D, Chabner BA. Clinical strategies for cancer treatment: The role of drugs. In: Chabner BA, Longo DL, eds. Cancer Chemotherapy and Biotherapy: Principles and Practice. Philadelphia, Lippincott–Raven, 1996:1–16.
2. Cancer facts and figures—1998. American Cancer Society, Atlanta, 1998.
3. Pitot HC. The molecular biology of carcinogenesis. Cancer 1993;72: 962–970.
4. Cavanee WK, White RL. The genetic basis of cancer. Sci Am 1995; 72–79.
5. Yuspa SH, Shields PG. Etiology of cancer: Chemical factors. In: DeVita VT Jr, Hellman S, Rosenberg SA, eds. Cancer: Principles and Practice of Oncology, 5th ed. Philadelphia, Lippincott–Raven, 1997: 185–202.
6. Cotran RS, Kumar V, Robbins SL. Neoplasia. In: Cotran RS, Kumar V, Robbins SL, eds. Pathologic Basis of Disease. Philadelphia, Saunders, 1994:241–303.
7. Weinberg RA. How cancer arises. Sci Am 1996;275:62–70.
8. Hirama T, Koeffler HP. Role of cyclin-dependent kinase inhibitors in the development of cancer. Blood 1995;86:841–854.

9. Stewart BW. Mechanisms of apoptosis: Integration of genetic, biochemical, and cellular indicators. J Natl Cancer Inst 1994;86: 1286–1296.
10. Buick RN. Cellular basis of chemotherapy. In: Dorr RT, Von Hoff DD, eds. Cancer Chemotherapy Handbook, 2nd ed. New York, Elsevier, 1994:3–14.
11. Fidler IJ. Molecular biology of cancer: Invasion and metastasis. In: DeVita VT Jr, Hellman S, Rosenberg SA, eds. Cancer: Principles and Practice of Oncology, 5th ed. Philadelphia, Lippincott-Raven, 1997: 135–154.
12. Fink DJ, Mettlin CJ. Cancer detection: The cancer-related checkup guidelines. In: Murphy GP, Lawrence W, Lenhard RE, eds. American Cancer Society Textbook of Clinical Oncology, 2nd ed. Atlanta, American Cancer Society, 1995:178–193.
13. American Cancer Society. New Guidelines for the Early Detection of Prostate Cancer (97-500M-No. 3021-CC). American Cancer Society, Atlanta, 1997.
14. Seven warning signs of cancer. American Cancer Society, Atlanta.
15. Fernbach DJ, Vietti TJ, eds. Clinical Pediatric Oncology, 4th ed. St. Louis, Mosby-Year Book, 1991:1–10.
16. Beahrs OH, Henson DE, Hutter RVP, Kennedy BJ, eds. American Joint Committee on Cancer. Manual for Staging of Cancer, 4th ed. Philadelphia, Lippincott, 1992.
17. Fleming ID, Brady LW, Cooper MR. Basis for major current therapies for cancer. In: Murphy GP, Lawrence W, Lenhard RE, eds. American Cancer Society Textbook of Clinical Oncology, 2nd ed. Atlanta, American Cancer Society, 1995:96–134.
18. Calabresi P, Chabner BA. Chemotherapy of neoplastic diseases. In: Hardman JG, Limbird LE, Molinoff PB, Ruddon RW, Gilman AG, eds. Goodman & Gilman's The Pharmacologic Basis of Therapeutics, 9th ed. New York, McGraw-Hill, 1996:1225–1232.
19. Haskell CM. Principles and modalities of cancer treatment. In: Haskell CM, ed. Cancer Treatment, 3rd ed. Philadelphia, Saunders, 1990:21–43.
20. Fisher GA, Sikic BI. Clinical studies with modulators of multidrug resistance. Hematol Oncol Clin North Am 1995;9:363–382.
21. Safa AR. Multidrug resistance. In: Schilsky RL, Milano GA, Ratain MJ, eds. Principles of Antineoplastic Drug Development and Pharmacology. New York, Dekker, 1996:457–486.
22. Hryniuk WM. Dose intensity. In: Schilsky RL, Milano GA, Ratain MJ, eds. Principles of Antineoplastic Drug Development and Pharmacology. New York, Dekker, 1996:263–280.
23. Dorr RT, Huber SL. New chemoprotectants: Developing a strategic plan. Monograph. Bala Cynwyd, PA, Meniscus Ltd, 1996:1–17.
24. Rodman JH, Relling MV, Stewart CF, et al. Clinical pharmacokinetics and pharmacodynamics of anticancer drugs in children. Semin Oncol 1993;20:18–29.
25. Collins JM. Pharmacokinetics and clinical monitoring. In: Chabner BA, Longo DL, eds. Cancer Chemotherapy and Biotherapy: Principles and Practice. Philadelphia, Lippincott–Raven, 1996:17–29.
26. Fischer DS, Knobf MT, Durivage HJ, eds. The Cancer Chemotherapy Handbook. St. Louis, Mosby-Year Book, 1993:499.
27. Rosenthal N. DNA and the genetic code. N Engl J Med 1994;331: 39–41.
28. Klausner R, Collins F. Understanding gene testing. U.S. Department of Health and Human Services, Public Health Service, National Institutes of Health, National Cancer Institute, NIH Publication No. 96-3905, December 1995.
29. Pratt WB, Ruddon RW, Ensminger WD, Maybaum J. The Anticancer Drugs, 2nd ed. New York, Oxford University Press, 1994:69–107.
30. Chabner BA, Allegra CJ, Curt GA, et al. Antineoplastic agents. In: Hardman JG, Limbird LE, Molinoff PB, Ruddon RW, Gilman AG, eds. Goodman & Gilman's The Pharmacologic Basis of Therapeutics, 9th ed. New York, McGraw-Hill, 1996:1233–1288.
31. Grem JL. 5-Fluoropyrimidines. In: Chabner BA, Longo DL, eds. Cancer Chemotherapy and Biotherapy: Principles and Practice. Philadelphia, Lippincott–Raven, 1996:149–212.
32. Sobrero AF, Aschele C, Bertino JR. Fluorouracil in colorectal cancer—A tale of two drugs: Implications for biochemical modulation. J Clin Oncol 1997;15:368–381.
33. Stein BN, Petrelli NJ, Douglass HO, et al. Age and sex are independent predictors of 5-fluorouracil toxicity. Cancer 1995;75:11–17.
34. Loprinzi CL, Wender DB, Veeder MH, et al. Inhibition of 5-fluorouracil-induced ocular irritation by ocular ice packs. Cancer 1994; 74:945–948.
35. Anand AJ. Fluorouracil cardiotoxicity. Ann Pharmacother 1994;28: 374–378.
36. Moertel CG, Fleming TR, Macdonald JS, et al. Hepatic toxicity associated with fluorouracil plus levamisole adjuvant therapy. J Clin Oncol 1993;11:2386–2390.
37. Xeloda^{R} (capecitabine) Product Information. Roche Laboratories, Inc, 1998.
38. Schuller J, Cassidy J, Reigner BG, et al. Tumor selectivity of Xeloda in colorectal cancer patients. Proc Ann Meet Am Soc Clin Oncol 1997;16:A797. Abstract.
39. Twelves C, Budman DR, Creaven PJ, et al. Pharmacokinetics and pharmacodynamics of capecitabine in two phase 1 studies. Proc Ann Meet Am Soc Clin Oncol 1996;15:A1509. Abstract.
40. Reigner BG, Jones RG, Cassidy J, et al. Hepatic dysfunction due to liver metastasis does not affect the bioactivation of Xeloda^{R}. Proc Ann Meet Am Soc Clin Oncol 1998;17:A863. Abstract.
41. Chabner BA. Cytidine analogs. In: Chabner BA, Longo DL, eds. Cancer Chemotherapy and Biotherapy: Principles and Practice. Philadelphia, Lippincott–Raven, 1996:213–234.
42. Baker WJ, Royer GL Jr, Weiss RB. Cytarabine and neurologic toxicity. J Clin Oncol 1991;9:679–693.
43. Smith GA, Damon LE, Rugo HS, Ries CA, Linker CA. High-dose cytarabine dose modification reduces the incidence of neurotoxicity in patients with renal insufficiency. J Clin Oncol 1997;15: 833–839.
44. Tuxen MK, Hansen SW. Neurotoxicity secondary to antineoplastic drugs. Cancer Treat Rev 1994;20:191–214.
45. Kreisman H, Wolkove N. Pulmonary toxicity of antineoplastic therapy. Semin Oncol 1992;19:508–520.
46. Gucchelaar HJ, Richel DJ, van Knapen A. Clinical, toxicological and pharmacological aspects of gemcitabine. Cancer Treat Rev 1996;22: 15–31.
47. Noble S, Goa KL. Gemcitabine. A review of its pharmacology and clinical potential in non-small cell lung cancer and pancreatic cancer. Drugs 1997;54:447–472.
48. Hande KR, Garrow GC. Purine antimetabolites. In: Chabner BA, Longo DL, eds. Cancer Chemotherapy and Biotherapy: Principles and Practice. Philadelphia, Lippincott–Raven, 1996:235–252.
49. Pinkel D. Intravenous mercaptopurine: Life beings at 40. J Clin Oncol 1993;11:1826–1831.
50. Perry MC. Chemotherapeutic agents and hepatotoxicity. Semin Oncol 1992;19:551–565.
51. Kolesar JM, Morris AK, Kuhn JG. Purine nucleoside analogs: Fludarabine, pentostatin and cladribine. Part 1: Fludarabine. J Oncol Pharm Prac 1996;2:160–181.
52. Cheson BD, Vena DA, Foss FM, Sorensen JM. Neurotoxicity of purine analogs: A review. J Clin Oncol 1994;12:2216–2228.
53. Morris AK, Kolesar J, Kuhn JG. Purine nucleoside analogs: Fludarabine, pentostatin and cladribine. Part 3: Cladribine. J Oncol Pharm Prac 1997;3:94–109.
54. Kolesar J, Morris AK, Kuhn JG. Purine nucleoside analogs: Fludarabine, pentostatin and cladribine. Part 2: Pentostatin. J Oncol Pharm Prac 1996;2:211–224.
55. Chu E, Allegra CJ. Antifolates. In: Chabner BA, Longo DL, eds. Cancer Chemotherapy and Biotherapy: Principles and Practice. Philadelphia, Lippincott–Raven, 1996:109–148.
56. Bertino JR, Kamen BA, Romanini A. Folate antagonists. In: Holland JF, Frei E III, Bast RC Jr, et al, eds. Cancer Medicine, 4th ed. Philadelphia, Williams & Wilkins, 1997:907–922.

57. Madden T, Eaton VE. Methotrexate. In: Schumacher GE, ed. Therapeutic Drug Monitoring. Norwalk, CT, Appleton & Lange, 1995: 527–552.
58. Relling MV, Fairclough D, Ayers D, et al. Patient characteristics associated with high-risk methotrexate concentrations and toxicity. J Clin Oncol 1994;12:1667–1672.
59. Weiss R. Hypersensitivity reactions. Semin Oncol 1992;19:458–477.
60. Dorr RT, VonHoff DD. Drug monographs. In: Dorr RT, Von Hoff DD eds. Cancer Chemotherapy Handbook, 2nd ed. Stamford, CT, Appleton & Lange, 1994:129–978.
61. Rowinsky EK, Donehower RC. Antimicrotubule agents. In: Chabner BA, Longo DL, eds. Cancer Chemotherapy and Biotherapy: Principles and Practice. Philadelphia, Lippincott–Raven, 1996:263–296.
62. Jones SF, Burris HA. Vinorelbine: A new antineoplastic drug for the treatment of non-small cell lung cancer. Ann Pharmacother 1996;30: 501–506.
63. McCune JS, Lindley C. Appropriateness of maximum dose-guidelines for vincristine. Am J Health Syst Pharm 1997;54:1755–1758.
64. Dorr RT. Antidotes to vesicant chemotherapy administration. Blood Rev 1990;4:41–60.
65. Pommier YG, Fesen MR, Goldwasser F. Topoisomerase II inhibitors: The epipodophyllotoxins, m-AMSA, and the ellipticine derivatives. In: Chabner BA, Longo DL, eds. Cancer Chemotherapy and Biotherapy: Principles and Practice. Philadelphia, Lippincott–Raven, 1996:435–462.
66. McLeod HL, Evans WE. Clinical pharmacokinetics and pharmacodynamics of epipodophyllotoxins. Cancer Surv 1993;17:253–268.
67. Stewart CF. Use of etoposide in patients with organ dysfunction: Pharmacokinetic and pharmacodynamic considerations. Cancer Chemother Pharmacol 1994;34(suppl):S76–S83.
68. Kohler DR, Goldspiel BR. Paclitaxel (Taxol). Pharmacotherapy 1994;14:3–34.
69. Cortes JE, Pazdur R. Docetaxel. J Clin Oncol 1995;13:2643–2655.
70. DiPaola R, Rodriguez R, Recio A, et al. A phase I study of amifostine and paclitaxel in patients with advanced malignancies. Proc ASCO 1996;15:1556. Abstract.
71. Markman M, Kennedy A, Webster K, et al. Simplified regimen for the prevention of paclitaxel-associated hypersensitivity reactions (letter). J Clin Oncol 1997;15:3517.
72. Takimoto CH, Arbuck SG. Camptothecins. In: Chabner BA, Longo DL, eds. Cancer Chemotherapy and Biotherapy: Principles and Practice. Philadelphia, Lippincott–Raven, 1996:463–484.
73. Wiseman LR, Markham A. Irinotecan. A review of its pharmacological properties and clinical efficacy in the management of advanced colorectal cancer. Drugs 1996;52:606–623.
74. Creemers GJ, Lund B, Verweij J. Topoisomerase I inhibitors: Topotecan and irenotecan. Cancer Treat Rev 1994;20:73–96.
75. Dennis MJ, Beijnen JH, Grochow LB, van Warmerdam LJ. An overview of the clinical pharmacology of topotecan. Semin Oncol 1997;24(suppl 5):S5–S18.
76. Tew K, Colvin M, Chabner BA. Alkylating agents. In: Chabner BA, Longo DL, eds. Cancer Chemotherapy and Biotherapy: Principles and Practice. Philadelphia, Lippincott–Raven, 1996:297–332.
77. Lind MJ, Ardiet C. Pharmacokinetics of alkylating agents. Cancer Surv 1993;17:157–188.
78. Schoenike SE, Dana WJ. Ifosfamide and mesna. Clin Pharm 1990;9:179–191.
79. West NJ. Prevention and treatment of hemorrhagic cystitis. Pharmacotherapy 1997;17:696–706.
80. Jones DP, Chesney RW. Renal toxicity of cancer chemotherapeutic agents in children: Ifosfamide and cisplatin. Curr Opin Pediatr 1995; 7:208–213.
81. Patterson WP, Reams GP. Renal toxicities of chemotherapy. Semin Oncol 1992;19:521–528.
82. Brem H, Piantadosi S, Burger PC, et al. Placebo-controlled trial of safety and efficacy of intraoperative controlled delivery by biodegradable polymers of chemotherapy for recurrent gliomas. The Polymer–Brain Tumor Treatment Group. Lancet 1995;345:1008–1012.
83. Buggia I, Locatelli F, Regazzi MB, Zecca M. Busulfan. Ann Pharmacother 1994;28:1055–1062.
84. Friedman HS, Averbach SD, Kurtzberg J. Nonclassic alkylating agents. In: Chabner BA, Longo DL, eds. Cancer Chemotherapy and Biotherapy: Principles and Practice. Philadelphia, Lippincott–Raven, 1996:333–356.
85. Colvin M. Alkylating agents and platinum antitumor compounds. In: Holland JF, Frei E III, Bast RC Jr, et al, eds. Cancer Medicine, 4th ed. Philadelphia, Williams & Wilkins, 1997:949–975.
86. Myers C. Anthracyclines and DNA intercalators. In: Holland JF, Frei E III, Bast RC Jr, et al, eds. Cancer Medicine, 4th ed. Philadelphia, Williams & Wilkins, 1997:977–988.
87. Doroshow JH. Anthracyclines and anthracenediones. In: Chabner BA, Longo DL, eds. Cancer Chemotherapy and Biotherapy: Principles and Practice. Philadelphia, Lippincott–Raven, 1996:409–434.
88. Booser DJ, Hortobagyi GN. Anthracycline antibiotics in cancer therapy: Focus on drug resistance. Drugs 1994;47:223–258.
89. Robert J, Gianni L. Pharmacokinetics and metabolism of anthracyclines. Cancer Surv 1993;17:219–252.
90. Robert J. Clinical pharmacokinetics of idarubicin. Clin Pharmacokinet 1993;24:275–288.
91. Shan K, Lincoff M, Young JB. Anthracycline-induced cardiotoxicity. Ann Intern Med 1996;125:47–58.
92. Seifert CF, Nesser ME, Thompson DF. Dexrazoxane in the prevention of doxorubicin-induced cardiotoxicity. Ann Pharmacother 1994; 28:1063–1072.
93. Dorr RT. Pharmacologic management of vesicant chemotherapy extravasations. In: Dorr RT, Von Hoff DD, eds. Cancer Chemotherapy Handbook, 2nd ed. Stamford, CT, Appleton & Lange, 1994:109–118.
94. Patel J. Liposomal doxorubicin: Doxil^R. J Oncol Pharm Pract 1996; 2:201–210.
95. Gill PS, Espina BM, Muggia F, et al. Phase I/II clinical and pharmacokinetic evaluation of liposomal daunorubicin. J Clin Oncol 1995; 13:996–1003.
96. Gill PS, Wernz J, Scadden DT, et al. Randomized phase III trial of liposomal daunorubicin versus doxorubicin, bleomycin, and vincristine in AIDS-related Kaposi's sarcoma. J Clin Oncol 1996;14: 2353–2364.
97. Verweij J, Schellens JHM, Loo TL, Pinedo HM. Antitumor antibiotics. In: Chabner BA, Longo DL, eds. Cancer Chemotherapy and Biotherapy: Principles and Practice. Philadelphia, Lippincott–Raven, 1996:395–408.
98. Lesesne JB, Rothschild N, Erickson B, et al. Cancer-associated hemolytic-uremic syndrome: Analysis of 85 cases from a national registry. J Clin Oncol 1989;7:781–789.
99. Lazo JS, Chabner BA. Bleomycin. In: Chabner BA, Longo DL, eds. Cancer Chemotherapy and Biotherapy: Principles and Practice. Philadelphia, Lippincott–Raven, 1996:379–394.
100. Andrews CO, Gora ML. Pleural effusions: Pathophysiology and management. Ann Pharmacother 1994;28:894–902.
101. Reed E, Dabholkar M, Chabner BA. Platinum analogs. In: Chabner BA, Longo DL, eds. Cancer Chemotherapy and Biotherapy: Principles and Practice. Philadelphia, Lippincott–Raven, 1996:357–378.
102. Gosland M, Lum B, Schimmelpfennig J, Baker J, Doukas M. Insights into mechanisms of cisplatin resistance and potential for its clinical reversal. Pharmacotherapy 1996;16:16–39.
103. Calvert H, Judson I, Van Der Vijgh WJF. Platinum complexes in cancer medicine: Pharmacokinetics and pharmacodynamics in relation to toxicity and therapeutic activity. Cancer Surv 1993;17: 189–218.
104. Pinzani V, Bressolle F, Haug IJ, et al. Cisplatin-induced renal toxicity and toxicity-modulating strategies: A review. Cancer Chemother Pharmacol 1994;35:1–9.

105. Anand AJ, Bashey B. Newer insights into cisplatin nephrotoxicity. Ann Pharmacother 1993;27:1519–1525.
106. Foster-Nora JA, Siden R. Amifostine for protection from antineoplastic drug toxicity. Am J Health Syst Pharm 1997;54:787–800.
107. Valley AW. Gastrointestinal complications of cancer chemotherapy. In: Finley R, Balmer CM, eds. Concepts in Oncology Therapeutics, 2nd ed. Bethesda, American Society of Health-Systems Pharmacists 1998.
108. Egorin MJ, Van Echo DA, Olman EA, et al. Prospective validation of a pharmacologically based dosing schema for *cis*-diamminedichlorplatinum (II) analog diammine-cyclobutanedicarboxylato-platinum. Cancer Res 1985;45:6502–6506.
109. Chatelut E, Canal P, Brunner V, et al. Prediction of carboplatin clearance from standard morphological and biological patient characteristics. J Natl Cancer Inst 1995;87:573–580.
110. Calvert AH. Dose optimisation of carboplatin in adults. Anticancer Res 1994;14:2273–2278.
111. Newell DR, Pearson ADJ, Balmanno K, et al. Carboplatin pharmacokinetics in children: The development of a pediatric dosing formula. J Clin Oncol 1993;11:2314–2323.
112. Donehower RC. Hydroxyurea. In: Chabner BA, Longo DL, eds. Cancer Chemotherapy and Biotherapy: Principles and Practice. Philadelphia, Lippincott–Raven, 1996:253–261.
113. Chabner BA. Enzyme therapy: L-Asparaginase. In: Chabner BA, Longo DL, eds. Cancer Chemotherapy and Biotherapy: Principles and Practice. Philadelphia, Lippincott–Raven, 1996:485–492.
114. Parkinson DR, Pluda JM, Cazenave L, et al. Investigational anticancer drugs. In: Chabner BA, Longo DL, eds. Cancer Chemotherapy and Biotherapy: Principles and Practice. Philadelphia, Lippincott–Raven, 1996:518–519.
115. Frankel SR, Eardley A, Heller G, et al. All-*trans*-retinoic acid for acute promyelocytic leukemia. Ann Intern Med 1994;120: 278–286.
116. Swain SM, Lippman ME. Endocrine therapies of cancer. In: Chabner BA, Longo DL, eds. Cancer Chemotherapy and Biotherapy: Principles and Practice. Philadelphia, Lippincott–Raven, 1996:59–108.
117. Schwartzman RA, Cidlowski JA. Corticosteroids. In: Holland JF, Frei E III, Bast RC Jr, et al, eds. Cancer Medicine, 4th ed. Philadelphia, Williams & Wilkins, 1997:1087–1102.
118. Balmer CM. Clinical use of biologic response modifiers in cancer treatment: An overview. Part I: The interferons. DICP, Ann Pharmacother 1990;24:761–767.
119. Dorr RT. Interferon-alpha in malignant and viral diseases: A review. Drugs 1993;45:177–211.
120. Witt PL, Lindner DJ, D'Cunha J, Borden EC. Pharmacology of interferons: Induced proteins, cell activation, and antitumor activity. In: Chabner BA, Longo DL, eds. Cancer Chemotherapy and Biotherapy: Principles and Practice. Philadelphia, Lippincott–Raven, 1996:585–608.
121. Bruton JK, Koeller JM. Recombinant interleukin-2. Pharmacotherapy 1994;14:635–656.
122. Whittington R, Faulds D. Interleukin-2: A review of its pharmacological properties and therapeutic use in patients with cancer. Drugs 1993;46:446–514.
123. Guleria AS, Yang JC, Topalian SL, et al. Renal dysfunction associated with the administration of high-dose interleukin-2 in 199 consecutive patients with metastatic melanoma or renal carcinoma. J Clin Oncol 1994;12:2714–2722.
124. Pockaj BA, Topalian SL, Steinberg SM, et al. Infectious complications associated with interleukin-2 administration: A retrospective review of 935 treatment courses. J Clin Oncol 1993;11:136–147.
125. Pizzo PA. Empirical therapy and prevention of infection in the immunocompromised host. In: Mandell GL, Bennet JE, Dolin R, eds. Mandell, Douglas and Bennett's Principles and Practice of Infectious Disease, 4th ed. New York, Churchill Livingstone, 1995: 2686–2696.
126. Hughes WT, Armstrong D, Bodey GP, et al. 1997 Guidelines for the use of antimicrobial agents in neutropenic patients with unexplained fever. Clin Infect Dis 1997;25:551–573.
127. Buchanan GR. Approach to the treatment of the febrile cancer patient with low-risk neutropenia. Hematol Oncol Clin North Am 1993;7: 919–936.
128. Malik IA, Khan WA. Feasibility of outpatient management of fever in cancer patients in low-risk neutropenia: Results of a prospective, randomized trial. Am J Med 1995;98:224–231.
129. Hathorn JW. Critical appraisal of antimicrobials for prevention of infections in immunocompromised hosts. Hematol Oncol Clin North Am 1993;7:1051–1099.
130. Demetri GD. Hematopoietic growth factors: Current knowledge, future prospects. Curr Prob Cancer 1992;16:179–259.
131. Nemunaitis J. A comparative review of the colony-stimulating factors. Drugs 1997;54:709–729.
132. Vose JM, Armitage JO. Clinical applications of hematopoietic growth factors. J Clin Oncol 1995;13:1023–1035.
133. ASCO Ad Hoc Colony-Stimulating Factor Guideline Expert Panel. American Society of Clinical Oncology recommendations for the use of hematopoietic colony-stimulating factors: Evidence-based, clinical practice guidelines. J Clin Oncol 1994;12:2471–2508.
134. ASCO Ad Hoc Colony-Stimulating Factor Guideline Expert Panel. Update of recommendations for the use of hematopoietic colony-stimulating factors: Evidence-based, clinical practice guidelines. J Clin Oncol 1996;14:1957–1960.
135. Isaacs C, Robert N, Bailey FA, et al. Randomized placebo-controlled study of recombinant human interleukin-11 to prevent chemotherapy-induced thrombocytopenia in patients with breast cancer receiving dose-intensive cyclophosphamide and doxorubicin. J Clin Oncol 1997;15:3368–3377.
136. Tepler I, Elias L, Smith JW II, et al. A randomized placebo-controlled trial of recombinant human interleukin-11 in cancer patients with severe thrombocytopenia due to chemotherapy. Blood 1996;87:3607–3614.
137. Kaushansky K. The thrombocytopenia of cancer: prospects for effective cytokine therapy. Hematol Oncol Clin North Am 1996;10:431–455.
138. Kaushansky K. The primary regulator of platelet production. Blood 1995;86:419–431.
139. Fannucchi M, Glaspy J, Crawford J, et al. Effects of polyethylene glycol-conjugated recombinant human megakaryocyte growth and development factor on platelet counts after chemotherapy for lung cancer. N Engl J Med 1997;336:404–409.
140. Vadhan-Raj S, Murray LJ, Bueso-Ramos C, et al. Stimulation of megakaryocyte and platelet production by a single dose of recombinant human thrombopoietin in patients with cancer. Ann Intern Med 1997;126:673–681.
141. Cazzola M, Mercuriali F, Brugnara C. Use of recombinant human erythropoietin outside the setting of uremia. Blood 1997;89:4248–4267.
142. Del Mastro L, Venturini M, Lionetto R, et al. Randomized phase III trial evaluating the role of erythropoietin in the prevention of chemotherapy-induced anemia. J Clin Oncol 1997;15:2715–2721.
143. Berger AM, Kilroy TJ. Oral complications. In: DeVita VT Jr, Hellman S, Rosenberg SA, eds. Cancer: Principles and Practice of Oncology, 5th ed. Philadelphia, Lippincott–Raven, 1997:2714–2724.
144. National Institutes of Health Consensus Development Conference Statement. Oral complications of cancer therapies: Diagnosis, prevention, and treatment. U.S. Department of Health and Human Services, April 17–19, 1989.
145. Siepp CA. Hair loss. In: DeVita VT Jr, Hellman S, Rosenberg SA, eds. Cancer: Principles and Practice of Oncology, 5th ed. Philadelphia, Lippincott–Raven, 1997:2757–2758.
146. Cancer chemotherapy guidelines: Recommendations for the management of vesicant extravasation, hypersensitivity, and anaphylaxis. Oncology Nursing Society, 1992.

147. McInnes S, Schilsky RL. Infertility following cancer chemotherapy. In: Chabner BA, Longo DL, eds. Cancer Chemotherapy and Biotherapy: Principles and Practice. Philadelphia, Lippincott–Raven, 1996:31–44.
148. Lenz KL, Valley AW. Infertility after chemotherapy: A review of the risks and strategies for prevention. J Oncol Pharm Pract 1996;2: 75–100.
149. Carcinogenesis: A late complication of cancer chemotherapy. In: Chabner BA, Longo DL, eds. Cancer Chemotherapy and Biotherapy: Principles and Practice. Philadelphia, Lippincott–Raven, 1996:45–58.
150. ASHP technical assistance bulletin on handling cytotoxic and hazardous drugs. Am J Hosp Pharm 1990;47:1033–1049.
151. American Cancer Society 1996 guidelines on diet, nutrition, and cancer prevention. American Cancer Society, 1996.
152. Lippman SM, Benner SE, Hong WK, et al. Cancer chemoprevention. J Clin Oncol 1994;12:851–873.
153. Kelloff GJ, Hawk ET, Karp JE, et al. Progress in clinical chemoprevention. Semin Oncol 1997;24:241–252.
154. Siegfried JM. Biology and chemoprevention of lung cancer. Chest 1998;113(suppl):40S–45S.
155. Goldberg KB, ed. Prevention trial shows 45% reduction in breast cancer incidence in women at high risk who took tamoxifen. Clin Cancer Lett 1998;21:1, 7.
156. Boring CC, Squires TS, Tong T, et al. Mortality trends for detected smoking-related cancers and breast cancer: United States, 1950–1990. MMWR 1993;42:857–866.
157. Blum A. Curtailing the tobacco pandemic. In: Devita VT Jr, Hellman S, Rosenberg SA, eds. Cancer: Principles and Practice of Oncology, 4th ed. Philadelphia, Lippincott, 1993:480–491.
158. Balch CM, Houghton A, Peters LJ. Cutaneous melanoma. In: Devita VT Jr, Hellman S, Rosenberg SA, eds. Cancer: Principles and Practice of Oncology, 4th ed. Philadelphia, Lippincott, 1993:1612–1661.

116

Breast Cancer

Celeste M. Lindley, PharmD, MS, FCCP, BCPS

INCIDENCE AND MORTALITY TRENDS

Breast cancer is the most common site of cancer and is second only to lung cancer as a cause of cancer death in American women. Estimates are that 180,300 new cases of breast cancer will be diagnosed and that 43,900 women will die of breast cancer in 1998.[1] These projections are based on the Surveillance, Epidemiology, and End Results (SEER) program of the National Cancer Institute (NCI). Since 1973, the SEER program has collected cancer incidence, mortality, and survival data each year for residents in nine metropolitan areas (or entire states), comprising about 10% of all the cancers diagnosed in the United States.

A great deal of public and health professional concern currently surrounds the increasing incidence of breast cancer. The Connecticut Tumor Registry demonstrated a 1% per year increase in breast cancer incidence between 1940 and 1980. SEER program estimates also show an increase of about 1% per year from 1973 to 1980.[2] In 1980, the breast cancer incidence rate started to rise more sharply. Between 1980 and 1987, cancer incidence rate grew from 84.4 to 112.4 per 100,000. This represents an increase of 32.5% according to SEER data or more than 4% per year. After reaching a peak in 1987, breast cancer incidence rates plateaued in subsequent years (Fig. 116–1).

The increased incidence of breast cancer is believed to be a result of three factors.[3] Approximately 30% of the increase is owing to the slow, but steady increase in breast cancer that has been observed over the last 50 years. It is likely that this gradual increase is related to dietary, body habitus, hormonal, and reproductive factors that will be discussed in detail in the upcoming section on epidemiology. About 60% of the increase is attributable to the detection of cases that were present in the population, but were often not detected without the use of mammographic screening and regular examinations. Approximately 10% of the new cases occur because women are living longer and the mortality from other causes is decreasing.

The increase in breast cancer incidence in the 1980s is characterized by an increase in the detection of small-sized lesions as well as carcinoma *in situ*.[4] As shown in Figure 116–2, the incidence rate for invasive cancers smaller than 1 cm grew from 9 per 100,000 in 1982 to 36 per 100,000 in 1988. The number of cancers 1 to 1.9 cm detected increased from 40 per 100,000 in 1982 to 84 per 100,000 in 1988. On the other hand, the rate of detection for tumors 2 to 2.9 cm remained about the same from 1982 to 1989, while the number of large cancers found at diagnosis (those of 3 cm) decreased. Although not reflected in the SEER data, the rate of detection of carcinoma *in situ* increased greatly from 4 per 100,000 in 1973 to a high of 15 per 100,000 in 1987. Ductal carcinoma *in situ,* which often manifests solely as microcalcifications seen on screening mammography, has been estimated to account for 10% to 20% of all breast cancer diagnoses in screened populations.[5] Increased public awareness and increased use of screening mammography are largely responsible for increased detection of breast cancers in the small or localized stage.

It is well recognized that breast cancer in the early stages is potentially curable in the majority of patients and that metastatic breast cancer is incurable. Thus, increased detection of localized and small breast cancer seen in the 1980s should have an impact on mortality rate from breast cancer. One recent report found that the age-adjusted mortality rate for breast cancer increased by approximately 10% between 1970 and 1994 among women 55 years of age or older with a recent plateau, but decreased by almost 25% among younger women during the same time period.[6] The decline in mortality for women less than 55 years of age has been attributed to the use of adjuvant systemic therapy following primary local-regional therapy. These investigators concluded that the decrease among younger women and the increase among older women has left population-wide mortality from breast cancer essentially unchanged. However, researchers from the National Cancer Institute recently announced that between 1990 and 1994, age-adjusted mortality rates from breast cancer for U.S. women decreased about 1.8% per year.[7]

EPIDEMIOLOGY AND ETIOLOGY

The two variables most strongly associated with the occurrence of breast cancer are gender and age. Although one commonly thinks of breast cancer as a disease confined to women, approximately 1400 cases of male breast cancer were projected to be diagnosed in the United States in 1998.[1] Although male gender had been considered a poor prognostic factor in some investigations, it is now believed that higher mortality rates in men are attributable to more advanced disease at the time of diagnosis. When stage and other known prognostic factors are controlled for, men do not fare differently from their female counterparts. Similarly, treatment of male breast cancer is not different from treatment of breast cancer in females.

The incidence of breast cancer increases with advancing age. Perhaps the most frequently quoted breast cancer

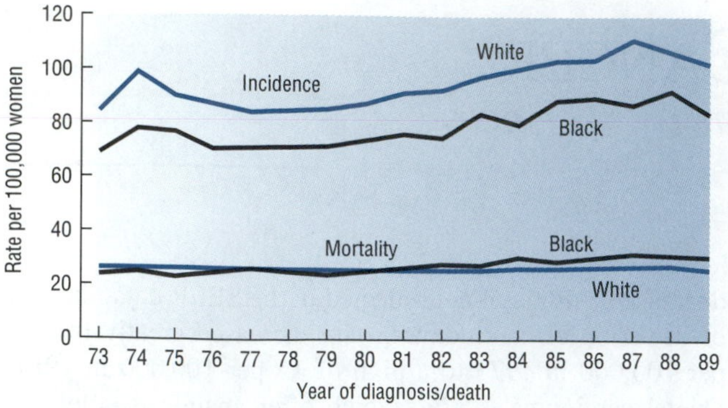

FIGURE 116–1. Breast cancer incidence and mortality rates by race, SEER, 1973–1989.

statistic is that one in eight women will develop breast cancer during their lifetime.[3] It should be emphasized that this is a cumulative lifetime risk of developing the disease from birth to age 110 and the estimates are weighted by the probability of surviving through each decade of life. Women over 90 contribute very little to the overall risk statistic because their numbers are so small. The "one in eight women" statistic has created fear of a breast cancer epidemic, with some women assuming that it translates to one in eight women being diagnosed with breast cancer each year. Feuer, et al. have developed a more useful method of presenting the risk data based on age intervals.[3] As demonstrated in Table 116–1, the risk of developing breast cancer before the age of 40 is 1 in 217. It is apparent from this table that although the cumulative probability of developing breast cancer increases with increasing age, more than half of the risk occurs after age 60.

Aside from female gender and age, a number of additional risk factors have been identified. Complex experimental and epidemiologic evidence points to an association between breast cancer and endocrine factors, environment, and genetics. Although the exact nature of the association is unclear, the majority of factors recognized as increasing a woman's risk above the average are related to one or more of these influences. The strength of the association between a given risk factor and the development of breast cancer is indicated by a "relative risk ratio" or "odds ratio." These are derived from epidemiologic studies and case control or cohort studies, where the incidence of disease among persons possessing a characteristic in question is divided by the incidence of disease among otherwise similar persons without the characteristic. Computation of "relative risk ratios" through epidemiologic research is complex and inexact. This area of research is hindered by many fundamental methodologic problems such as selection bias, recall bias, incomplete data, and, most important, the presence of confounding factors. A large number of case control and cohort studies that examine the relationship between certain factors and risk of developing breast cancer have been conducted and often have yielded conflicting results. However, it is important to review established and probable risk factors for cancer and to continue to conduct research in this area. Through these efforts, the etiology of breast cancer can be further elucidated, women who would benefit from intensified surveillance or prophylactic treatment may be identified, and recommendations for modifiable risk factors that will ultimately reduce the incidence of breast cancer can be established.

An understanding of the relationship between age and the incidence of breast cancer is particularly relevant when one discusses "risk factors" or factors other than age that increase a woman's probability of developing breast cancer. The "relative risk" (RR) of developing breast cancer for an individual woman in a defined risk group is usually multiplied by the probability of a woman developing breast cancer during her lifetime, and this figure is taken as the cumulative lifetime risk of that individual developing breast cancer. However, the risk of developing breast cancer is age dependent. Thus, a more meaningful way to counsel patients regarding their risk of developing breast cancer based on the presence of a known risk factor incorporates an age-specific incidence rate, not cumulative lifetime risk. For example, if a 40-year-old woman with a strong family history of breast cancer is thought to have a "relative risk ratio" of 2.0, her risk of developing breast cancer by the age of 50 is only 3.17% (2 × 1.58) not 25.14% (2 × 12.57) (see Table 116–1). It is also important to note that recognized risk factors are not "additive" in a simple mathematical sense and that the observed cumulative lifetime risk associated with nongenetic risk factors has rarely exceeded 30% (1 in 3) in any study regardless of the number and significance of individual risk factors. Finally, it should be emphasized that over 60% of women with breast cancer have no identifiable major risk factor, indicating that the search for the etiology of this disease is largely incomplete.[5]

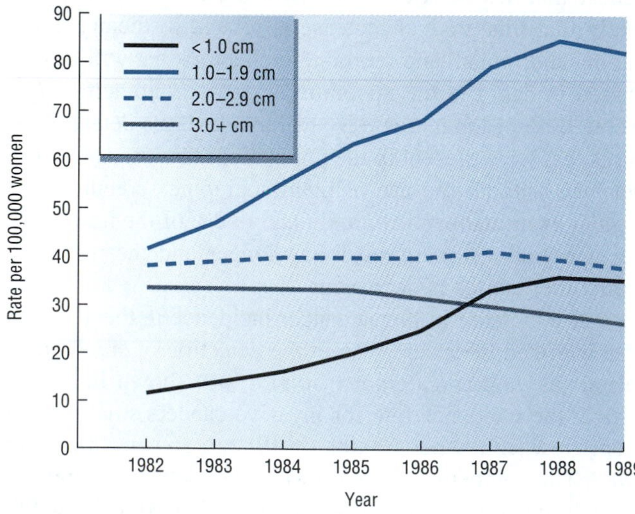

FIGURE 116–2. Breast cancer incidence rates by size at diagnosis, SEER, 1982–1989.

TABLE 116–1. Risk of Developing Breast Cancer in SEER Areas, Women, All Races 1987–1988

Age Interval	Probability (%) of Developing Invasive Breast Cancer During the Interval
Before 40	0.46 or 1 in 217
40–50	1.58 or 1 in 63
50–60	2.41 or 1 in 41
60–70	3.59 or 1 in 28
70–80	4.13 or 1 in 24
70–death	7.08 or 1 in 14
From birth to death	12.57 or 1 in 8

From Ref. 3.

ENDOCRINE FACTORS

A number of endocrine factors have been linked to the incidence of breast cancer.[8] Many of these relate to the total duration of menstrual life. Early menarche, generally defined as menstruation beginning before age 12, has been shown by a number of investigators to increase the cumulative lifetime risk of breast cancer development compared to menarche at age 16 or greater. Conversely, early age of natural menopause has been shown to result in a reduction of risk. Similarly, investigators have reported that bilateral oophorectomy prior to age 35 reduces the relative risk of developing breast cancer.

Nulliparity and a late age at first birth (greater or equal to 30 years) have been reported to increase the lifetime risk of developing breast cancer twofold. Women who have their first child after the age of 35 have a slightly higher risk than a nulliparous woman. It has been suggested that the period between the onset of menses and the age of first pregnancy provides a "window of initiation" for the development of breast cancer. This is a time when an unbalanced hormonal environment reacts with the abundant and highly responsive breast tissue. Investigators have postulated that international differences in age of menarche, age at menopause, and childbearing may account for a substantial part of the international differences in the incidence of breast cancer. In underdeveloped countries where the incidence of breast cancer is low compared to the United States, a late onset of menarche is the rule and frequently there is a decreased interval between puberty and first pregnancy followed by several pregnancies and early menopause.

A large number of investigators have evaluated the relationship between exogenous hormones and development of breast cancer. Postmenopausal estrogen replacement therapy has been the subject of several recent meta-analyses. A report from investigators from the Harvard School of Public Health concluded that women who have used estrogens in the past are not at an increased risk of breast cancer, but that current use may be associated with a 40% increased risk (i.e., RR = 1.4). This meta-analysis also suggested that long-term use might lead to a slight increase in risk.[9] Another meta-analysis has suggested that the combined results from multiple studies provide evidence that menopausal therapy (consisting of 0.625 mg or less of conjugated estrogen per day) does not increase breast cancer risk.[10] A study from the Centers for Disease Control and Prevention reported that the risk did not appear to increase until after at least 5 years of estrogen use.[11] These data are encouraging and suggest that a large effect of hormone therapy on breast cancer risk may be excluded and that the use of low doses of estrogen for short periods as replacement therapy in postmenopausal women is relatively safe. The important question is how the benefits of estrogen replacement therapy (lowered cardiovascular mortality, decreased bone loss, relief of menopausal symptoms) weigh against the risks (increased endometrial cancer, if used without progesterone, and slight increase in breast cancer). The Women's Health Initiative, a study sponsored by the National Cancer Institute, will randomize 80,000 women to take or not take postmenopausal estrogen replacement therapy and should provide important answers regarding the benefits and risks associated with this therapy.

The use of postmenopausal estrogen replacement therapy in women with a history of breast cancer is generally considered contraindicated. Because of the association of estrogen and risk of breast cancer, many physicians believe that patients with a strong family history or other risk factors for breast cancer should not receive postmenopausal estrogen replacement therapy. This dogma has recently been challenged in the medical literature.[12] Proponents of estrogen replacement therapy in patients with successfully treated operable breast cancer often state that the benefits of replacement therapy in terms of cardiovascular risk reduction and reduction of morbidity and mortality from osteoporosis and subsequent fractures outweigh an unknown but potential increased risk of breast cancer development. At the current time, there is not enough information to state confidently that estrogen replacement therapy has any significant impact, positive or negative, on prognosis in women with a personal or family history of breast cancer and all recommendations are based on speculation and circumstantial evidence.

There are more than 20 epidemiologic studies of the potential carcinogenic effect of oral contraceptives, most of which have not shown a relationship between birth control pills and breast cancer incidence. However, results are conflicting and assessment of the studies necessitates consideration of the particular oral contraceptive products involved, daily and cumulative doses of the hormones administered, and the latency for development of breast cancer. A review and meta-analyses suggest that, overall, there has been no increase in the risk of breast cancer for women who had ever received oral contraceptive drugs; however, women who had used these agents for a prolonged period of time or prior to a first pregnancy were at a higher risk (RR = 1.5 to 2) of developing breast cancer until the age of 45 years.[13] It should be pointed out that early use of oral contraceptives may be associated with early menarche and may result in late age of first birth, both of which are recognized risk factors for breast cancer. Although it is not entirely possible to rule out a promotional effect of oral contraceptives on breast cancer development in young patients, most experts believe that the safety and benefits of low-dose oral contraceptives currently outweigh the potential risks and that changes in the prescribing practice for the use of oral contraceptives are not warranted. Oral contraceptives are known to reduce the risk of ovarian cancer by about 40% and the risk of endometrial cancer by 60%.[5]

GENETIC FACTORS

Both personal and family history influence a woman's risk of developing breast cancer. A past medical history for breast cancer is associated with the relative risk of 5.0 for the development of a contralateral breast cancer. Cancer of the uterus and ovary have also been associated with an increased risk of the development of breast cancer. Breast cancer is observed as part of cancer family syndromes in association with other tumors. Only 5% of breast cancer patients are thought to have a pedigree consistent with hereditary breast cancer.

A topic that bears some discussion because of its prevalence in the general population is the relationship of fibrocystic breast disease to the development of invasive breast cancer. As many as 85% of American women have "lumpy breasts" and may bear a clinical diagnosis of fibrocystic breast disease or benign breast disease. The relative risk of breast cancer in patients with a history of fibrocystic breast disease has ranged from 1.5 to 2.0 in reported studies. However, fibrocystic disease involves a heterogeneous group of pathologic changes associated with various degrees of breast cancer risk. Thus, a clinical diagnosis of fibrocystic or benign breast disease has little practical significance for counseling patients regarding individual risk of breast cancer. A useful system for classifying benign breast disease was recently adapted by the American College of Pathologists.[14] Benign breast conditions were classified as nonproliferative or proliferative, and on the basis of review of more than 10,000 breast biopsies, relative risks of breast cancer were determined. Women with proliferative disease were found to have a relative risk of 1.9 and the subcategory of women with atypical hyperplasia had a relative risk of 4.4. Nonproliferative breast disease was not associated with an excess risk of breast cancer. Approximately 78% of the reviewed biopsies were found to have nonproliferative breast disease, and of those demonstrating proliferation, only 3.6% were "atypical." These data suggest that in the majority of women, benign breast disease or fibrocystic disease is most often not associated with proliferation and the women are not at an increased risk for developing breast cancer. However, it must be noted that "lumpy breasts" may lead to a delay in diagnosis of breast cancer owing to the inability of the patient or physician to detect a true malignant lesion.[14]

It has been recognized for some time that a family history of breast cancer is associated rather strongly with a woman's own risk for developing the disease. Empirical estimates of the risks associated with particular patterns of family history of breast cancer indicate the following[15]:

1. Having any first-degree relative with breast cancer increases a woman's risk of breast cancer 1.5- to 3-fold, depending on age.
2. The higher relative risk is associated with breast cancer with onset younger than age 45 in one or more first-degree relatives.
3. Having multiple first-degree relatives affected has been inconsistently associated with elevated risks.
4. Having a second-degree relative affected increases a woman's risk of developing breast cancer by approximately 50% (relative risk 1.5).
5. Affected family members on the maternal side and the paternal side contribute similarly to the risk.

Although certain patterns of family history are associated with substantial elevations in the risk of breast cancer, these high-risk patterns occur infrequently in the general population (Table 116–2). The percentage of all breast cancers in the population that can be attributed to family history range between 6% and 12%. Thus, it appears that genetically transmitted susceptibility contributes to their etiology of breast cancer in a sizable minority of patients.

In the early 1990s, pedigree analysis of 23 high-risk families for breast and ovarian cancer provided evidence for a rare autosomal dominant allele.[5,16] From these families, a gene on the long arm of chromosome 17 (17q21) was identified as abnormal in a large percentage of these hereditary breast and ovarian cancer patients. Isolation of the BRCA1 gene was initially reported in 1994. Already a second breast cancer gene, called BRCA2, has been mapped to chromosome 13. From these data, a woman with a strong family history of breast or ovarian cancer, or both, who carries a germ line mutation of BRCA1 faces roughly an 85% lifetime risk of breast cancer and 60% risk of ovarian cancer. Carriers of the BRCA2 mutation have similar risks for breast cancer but much lower risks for ovarian cancer. An interesting and exciting development in this area concerns genetic counseling for women in high-risk families. Now that BRCA1 and BRCA2 germ line mutations can be identified, many women in high-risk and lower-risk groups are seeking genetic testing. This has resulted in a large number of issues that are currently unresolved. Perhaps of most importance, the risk of breast and ovarian cancer in BRCA1 and BRCA2 carriers was derived from studies of high-risk families and may not apply to all carriers of these mutations. It has been reported that Jewish people of Eastern European decent (Ashkenazi Jews) have an unusually high (2%) carrier rate of germ line mutations in BRCA1 and

TABLE 116–2. Established and Probable Risk Factors for Breast Cancer

Risk Factor	Comparison Category	Risk Category	Typical Relative Risk
Family history of breast cancer	No first-degree relatives affected	Mother affected before the age of 60	2.0
		Mother affected after the age of 60	1.4
		Two first-degree relatives affected	4–6
		Breast cancer in one or more second-degree relatives	1.36
		Ovarian cancer in one or more first-degree relatives	1.59
Age at menarche	16 yr	11 yr	1.3
Age at birth of first child	Before 20 yr	20–24 yr	1.3
		25–29 yr	1.6
		≥ 30 yr	1.9
Age at menopause	45–54 yr	After 55 yr	1.5
		Before 45 yr	0.7
		Oophrectomy before 35 yr	0.4
Benign breast disease	No biopsy or aspiration	Proliferation only	1.5
		Atypical hyperplasia	3.5
		Lobular carcinoma in situ	7.2
Obesity	10th percentile	90th percentile	
		Age, 30–49 yr	0.8
		Age ≥ 50 yr	1.2
Oral contraceptive use	Never used	Ever use	1.0
		≥ 4 yr before first pregnancy	1.7
Postmenopausal estrogen replacement	Never used	Current use all ages	1.4
		15+ years	1.3
		Past use	1.0
Alcohol use	Nondrinker	1 drink/day	1.10
		2 drinks/day	1.25
		3 drinks/day	1.50

Adapted from Ref. 8.

BRCA2 compared to the normal U.S. population. A recent study that examined carriers of BRCA1 and BRCA2 in Ashkenazi Jews in the Washington, DC, area found that over 2% of the population carried these germ line mutations and that they confer increased risks of breast, ovarian, and prostate cancer compared to the SEER data from the general population.[17] However, the risks of these cancers, and breast cancer in particular, fell well below previous estimates based on subjects from high-risk families; the risks were 50% for breast cancer and 16% for ovarian cancer, rather than the 85% and 60% estimates on the basis of studies in patients who were BRCA positive and had strong family histories for these cancers. In addition, Ashkenazi families with breast cancer have a far higher probability of being carriers of the BRCA1 mutation (48%) than non-Ashkenazi families with breast cancer (17%), which suggests that the BRCA1 mutation is a more important predictor of breast carrier development in Ashkenazi families than non-Ashkenazi families. These observations taken together underscore the role of other modifying factors in determining whether a given BRCA mutation causes cancer. Furthermore, new genes are still being discovered that contribute to the risk of breast cancer through different mechanisms. Without facts about these other variables, it is difficult, if not impossible, to predict one's likelihood of developing disease based on the presence of a specific mutation. The question of who should receive screening for BRCA is unresolved. The probability of being a carrier of the gene is related to ethnicity and family history. Important factors in family history include the number of affected and unaffected family members, age at which cancer is diagnosed, and the presence of ovarian cancer. Current estimates are that if breast and ovarian cancer occur concurrently in one or more family members, the risk of a BRCA1 mutation increases 20-fold.

To date, there are no clear recommendations for carriers of BRCA1 and BRCA2 from high-risk families. Bilateral total mastectomy does reduce the risk of breast cancer occurrence; however, both breast and ovarian cancer have been reported in patients who have had prophylactic removal of these organs.[15,16] Current recommendations for BRCA carriers who do not opt for surgical prophylaxis is mammography every 6 months. Because no effective screening for ovarian cancer exists, most experts recommend bilateral oophorectomy at completion of childbearing and estrogen replacement therapy until the age of 50 years. Estrogen replacement therapy provides approximately one-third of physiologic estrogen concentrations and, although controversial, most feel that the benefits in terms of cardiovascular disease and osteoporosis outweigh the risk of cancer.

Most importantly, isolation and cloning of BRCA1 and BRCA2 should ultimately lead to a greater understanding of the biology of malignant transformation of mammary epithelium, and to major advances in diagnostics and therapeutics benefiting all breast cancer patients. It is hoped that an improved basic understanding of the molecular mechanisms involved in breast cancer development and the discovery of novel approaches to reverse or prevent these processes will ultimately lead to the ability to cure this extremely common and often fatal disease.

ENVIRONMENTAL AND LIFE-STYLE FACTORS

The observation that breast cancer incidence rates vary 10-fold between countries suggests that environmental factors play an important role in the etiology of breast cancer. Perhaps the most compelling evidence is derived from studies of Asian women who migrated from Japan to the San Francisco Bay area. Although the incidence of breast cancer in Asian women is quite low (10 to 15 per 100,000 women), the incidence of breast cancer in Asian women who were U.S. born, or who migrated from Asia to the United States, gradually increases to equal that of the white population in the same area.[5]

Diet is an obvious environmental factor, and possible relations between fat or cholesterol intake and steroid hormone metabolism have led to an emphasis on dietary fat as a possible etiologic agent. International studies demonstrate a positive correlation between age-adjusted cancer mortality rate and national per capita fat intake.[18] The correlation is stronger in postmenopausal than in premenopausal women. Studies in laboratory animals provide further evidence of a relationship between dietary fat intake and breast cancer.[19] Despite these compelling indirect data, case control and prospective studies performed in the United States have generally failed to show an association between dietary fat and breast cancer risk. There was no relation between the relative risk of breast cancer and calorie-adjusted total fat, saturated fat, linoleic acid, or cholesterol intake. In fact, the relative risk of developing breast cancer among the women with the highest quintile of total fat intake was 0.85 compared with women in the lowest quintile. However, the difference in fat intake among women in these two extremes was only 25%.[20] Practically, this suggests that women who reduce fat intake in the context of the usual American diet are not likely to reduce their breast cancer risk. The possible benefits of lowering fat intake to levels substantially below 30% of caloric intake will need to be tested in randomized trials.

Additional dietary factors that have been investigated include micronutrients and food-derived heterocyclic amines. Many of the studies that have examined the relative risk for breast cancer for high fat intake have also examined the association between breast cancer and intake of fiber, beta-carotene, and vitamins C, E, and A. The relationship between vitamin A and breast cancer risk is unclear. In contrast, most studies support some benefit from beta-carotene, vitamin C, and/or dietary fiber.[18] It should be cautioned that these studies are limited by very small numbers of breast cancer cases, as well as the many difficulties inherent in cohort and case control studies. Experimental and epidemiologic evidence suggests an association between breast cancer and the Western diet, which typically includes a high amount of cooked meats and fat, as well as a high caloric intake. One group of compounds that may play a role in human breast cancer is heterocyclic amines found in commonly cooked beef, fish, and chicken. At least 19 heterocyclic amines with mutagenic activity have been identified in grilled, broiled, and fried meat and fish. Among these, 10 have been examined for long-term carcinogenicity and all were proven to be positive.[21] Experimental studies examining the interaction between heterocyclic amines and other dietary factors with respect to mammary carcinogenesis are warranted.

Both body weight and height are associated with breast cancer. Indices of obesity are related to breast cancer risks in a complex way that differs by age and menopausal status. Most studies of premenopausal women show either no relationship with body weight or slightly declining breast cancer risks with increasing body weight. One plausible biologic mechanism to explain this phenomenon is reduced ovarian activity in obese women. Most studies in postmenopausal women, however, show increasing breast cancer risks with increasing body weight. Not only obesity but the distribution of body fat also may play an independent role in breast cancer. Upper body (central or abdominal) adiposity increases the risk of breast cancer independent of overall obesity. This association has been proposed to be caused by the excess levels of free-circulating estrogen resulting from the conversion of androstenedione to estradiol in peripheral adipose tissue in conjunction with suppressed levels of circulating sex hormone binding globulin in women with central adiposity.[22]

Reports of more than 50 epidemiologic investigations of the relationship between alcohol and breast cancer have appeared in the literature. A recent meta-analysis[23] of these studies indicates both a modest positive association between alcohol and breast cancer and a dose–response relationship. Data suggest that risk increases with consumption of alcohol in general, regardless of the beverage type. Several factors, including age, weight, and estrogen usage, have been shown to modify this relation in some studies. The mechanism of the alcohol–breast cancer hypothesis may include increased levels of estradiol or other reproductive steroid hormones; altered hepatic mechanism of carcinogens; production of cytotoxic protein products; diminished immunologic surveillance; impaired DNA repair; or possibly an influencing effect of alcohol on cell membrane integrity and/or metabolism of conjugers.[23] A series of methodologic issues in the study of alcohol and breast cancer are apparent from the meta-analysis, and these include inherent errors in alcohol assessment, the relatively small relative risk demonstrated, the presence of confounding variables in women who drink alcohol, and the lack of consistency of positive findings for the relationship between alcohol and the development of breast cancer. In addition, animal studies have yielded mixed results regarding the influence of alcohol on the incidence of breast cancer. Although a causal relationship between alcohol consumption and breast cancer has not been proven in a prospective trial, the weight of the epidemiologic and preclinical evidence suggests that a relationship, direct or indirect, may exist.

Radiation is associated with an increased risk of breast cancer in survivors of the atomic bomb, in patients given radiation for postpartum mastitis, in women receiving multiple fluoroscopes during therapy for tuberculosis, and in animal models. Interestingly, this risk appears to be confined to exposure to radiation prior to the age of 40, which again suggests that a "window of initiation" for breast cancer occurs at a relatively early age. Exposure to diagnostic x-rays including annual screening mammography does not impart a sufficient dose of radiation for clinical concern. A critical reassessment of benefits versus risks from screening mammography found recently that for a woman beginning annual screening mammography at age 50 and continuing to age 75, the benefit exceeds the radiation risk by a factor of 100. Even for a woman who begins annual screening at age 35 and continues until age 75, the benefit of reduced mortality is projected to exceed the radiation risk by a factor of more than 25.[24]

Cigarette smoking and augmentation mammoplasty do not appear to increase the risk of breast cancer. Blood pressure medications, reserpine, and other drugs that increase prolactin levels have not been shown to increase the risk of breast cancer. Caffeine also has no predisposing effect on breast cancer, but may play a role in exacerbation of benign breast disease. The role of environmental carcinogens has not been systematically evaluated.

CLINICAL PRESENTATION

A painless lump is the initial sign in more than 90% of women with breast cancer. The typical malignant mass is solitary, unilateral, solid, hard, irregular, and nonmobile. In approximately 10% of cases, stabbing or aching pain is the first symptom. Less commonly, nipple discharge, retraction, or dimpling may herald the onset of the disease. In more advanced cases, prominent skin edema, redness, warmth, and induration of the underlying tissue may be observed.

It should be emphasized that the breast is a complex organ composed of skin, subcutaneous tissue, fatty tissue, and branching ductal and glandular structures. Various diseases that affect these structures can produce a palpable mass. In addition, the physiologic changes associated with the menstrual cycle can cause abnormalities of the breast that produce a three-dimensional mass. The foremost common causes of breast masses in young women are fibroadenoma, fibrocystic disease, carcinoma, and fat necrosis.

Approximately 80% of women first detect some breast abnormalities themselves, underscoring the importance of breast self-examination. In the United States, it is increasingly common for breast cancer to be detected during routine screening mammography in asymptomatic women. It is widely accepted that the smaller the mass, the higher the likelihood of cure, and the more conservative the treatment options offered to the patient. Thus, as the number of breast cancer cases found by screening mammography increases, overall survival of breast cancer patients is expected to improve significantly.

Breast cancer that is confined to a localized breast lesion is often referred to as *early, primary, localized,* or *curable.* Unfortunately, as is discussed shortly, breast cancer cells often spread by contiguity, lymph channels, and through the blood to distant sites. As discussed in subsequent sections, this often occurs early in the breast cancer growth, and deposits of tumor cells form in distant sites (micrometastases) that cannot be detected with current diagnostic methods and equipment. When breast cancer cells can be detected clinically or radiologically in sites distant from the breast, the disease is referred to as *advanced* or *metastatic* breast cancer. Tissues most commonly involved with metastases are lymph nodes (other than axillary or internal mammary), skin, bone, liver, lungs, and brain. Symptoms of bone pain, difficulty breathing, abdominal enlargement, jaundice, and mental status changes may herald the clinical presentation of metastatic breast cancer. Approximately 10% of women have signs and symptoms of distant metastases when they first seek treatment. In virtually all of them, a breast mass has been present for several months to years. In addition, approximately one-half of all patients who initially are treated for localized disease develop signs and symptoms of metastatic breast cancer, most commonly 3 to 5 years following local potentially curative therapy with surgery, radiation, and systemic adjuvant therapy.

DIAGNOSIS

Initial workup for a woman presenting with a lesion or symptoms suggestive of breast cancer should include a careful history, physical examination of the breast, three-dimensional mammography, and potentially other breast imaging techniques such as ultrasound. Most (80% to 85%) breast cancers can be visualized on a mammogram as a mass, a cluster of calcifications, or a combination of both. The detection of a mass smaller than 2 mm is considered ideal, but realistically, it is difficult to detect tumors smaller than 5 mm. Large, noncalcified masses may be difficult to detect in the dense glandular breast, which is common in premenopausal women. The threshold for the detection of a cancer is variable and depends on the radiographic abnormality, the fat–to–glandular tissue ratio of the breast, the technical quality of the examination, and the diligence and expertise of the radiologist.

Interpretations of mammography obtained either for screening or to evaluate a new breast mass generally fall into one of three categories: (1) the radiologist notes nothing suspicious for malignancy; (2) something of concern is seen and follow-up or further testing is advised; and (3) something clearly suspicious is present and a biopsy is indicated. A detailed discussion of abnormal mammogram radiographic findings and their significance is beyond the scope of this chapter; however, excellent references are available.[25,26] However, it should be noted that well-circumscribed x-ray masses are benign in 98% of cases; such lesions may not require a biopsy, but may be followed radiographically at 6-month intervals. Masses interpreted as "suspicious and a biopsy should be performed" have a 20% to 30% probability of malignancy. Masses interpreted as "highly suspicious radiographically" are malignant in 75% to 90% of cases. The overall probability of malignancy when a biopsy is performed on a nonpalpable mammographic abnormality ranges from 20% to 35%.[27]

Breast biopsy is indicated for a mammographic abnormality that suggests malignancy or for a palpable mass on physical examination. The type of biopsy depends on the mass size and characteristics. Excisional biopsy is the standard biopsy technique for clinically benign lesions or for malignant lesions less than 2 cm in diameter. This term indicates the complete removal of the abnormal tissue. Excisional biopsy may be performed with either a local or general anesthesia. It is usually done as an outpatient operative procedure.

Mammographically, and less commonly ultrasonographically, guided needle biopsy is a promising technique for the diagnosis of breast lesions. This procedure is associated with minimal discomfort and anxiety, few complications, and no disfigurement and could represent significant cost-savings when compared to conventional surgical excisional biopsy. Needle biopsies have included both core needle biopsy (which removes a core of tissue) and fine-needle aspiration (which removes cells from the suspicious site). These procedures require experienced mammographers and cytopathologists. Numerous studies have shown that the accuracy of core needle biopsy is at least equal to that of traditional localization and open-surgical excisional breast biopsy. The accuracy of fine-needle aspiration is quite good in experienced hands, but its limitations include false negatives (range 1% to 10%) and specimens with insufficient material for diagnosis (1% to 10%). Results of a fine-needle aspiration can be used as the basis for mastectomy when the physical examination and mammographic abnormality coincide with the cytologic diagnosis. It should be pointed out that excisional biopsy, as well as needle localization biopsy, with fine needle or core, is used only to establish the diagnosis. Following confirmation of malignancy, subsequent surgical procedures are performed to assure complete removal of the abnormal tissue.[5]

STAGING AND PROGNOSIS

Few malignant diseases illustrate the importance of stage (anatomic extent of disease) at the time of diagnosis and

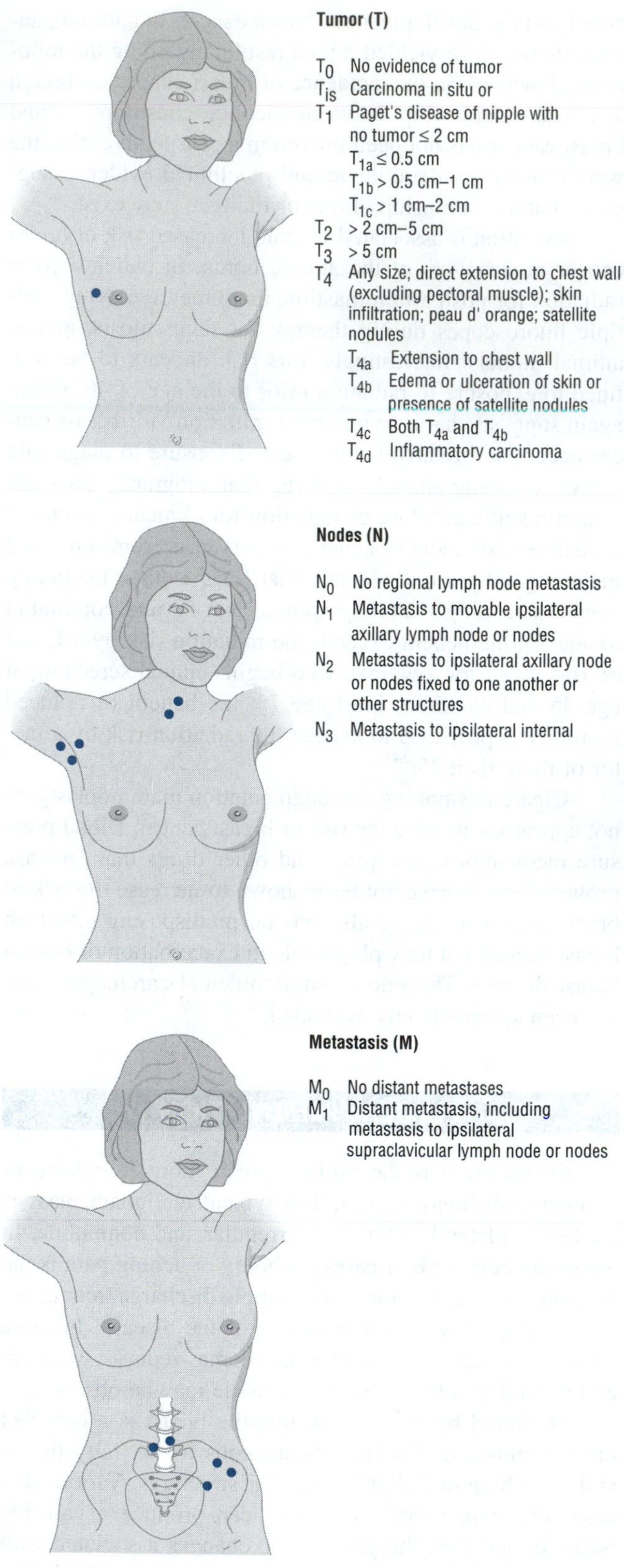
Tumor (T)
T_0 No evidence of tumor
T_{is} Carcinoma in situ or
T_1 Paget's disease of nipple with
no tumor ≤ 2 cm
T_{1a} ≤ 0.5 cm
T_{1b} > 0.5 cm–1 cm
T_{1c} > 1 cm–2 cm
T_2 > 2 cm–5 cm
T_3 > 5 cm
T_4 Any size; direct extension to chest wall (excluding pectoral muscle); skin infiltration; peau d' orange; satellite nodules
T_{4a} Extension to chest wall
T_{4b} Edema or ulceration of skin or presence of satellite nodules
T_{4c} Both T_{4a} and T_{4b}
T_{4d} Inflammatory carcinoma
Nodes (N)
N_0 No regional lymph node metastasis
N_1 Metastasis to movable ipsilateral axillary lymph node or nodes
N_2 Metastasis to ipsilateral axillary node or nodes fixed to one another or other structures
N_3 Metastasis to ipsilateral internal
Metastasis (M)
M_0 No distant metastases
M_1 Distant metastasis, including metastasis to ipsilateral supraclavicular lymph node or nodes

FIGURE 116–3. TNM four-stage system (see Table 116–3.) *(Adapted from Stockdale FE. Breast cancer. In: Rubenstein E, Federman DD, eds. Scientific American Medicine. New York, Scientific American, 1991:1–17.)*

overall survival more clearly than breast cancer. Stage is defined on the basis of the primary tumor size (T_{1-4}), presence and extent of lymph node involvement (N_{1-3}), and presence or absence of distant metastases (M) (Fig. 116–3 and Table 116–3). Although many possible combinations of T and N are possible within a given stage, simplistically, stage 0 represents carcinoma *in situ* or disease that has not invaded the basement membrane. Stage I represents small primary tumor without lymph node involvement, and the majority of stage II disease involves regional lymph nodes. Stages 0, I, and II are often referred to as *early breast cancer.* It is in these early stages that the disease is curable. Stage III, also referred to as *locally advanced disease,* usually represents a large tumor with extensive nodal involvement in which either node or tumor is fixed to the chest wall. Stage IV disease is characterized by the presence of metastases to organs distant from the primary tumor. Stages III and IV are often referred to as *advanced disease.* Although a small number of patients with stage III disease may be cured, most patients with locally advanced breast cancers are incurable with currently available standard treatment approaches.

The approximate percentage of patients presenting with each stage of breast cancer and an estimate of their 5-year disease-free survival (DFS) are shown in Table 116–4. Five-year DFS is not synonymous with cure and 10-year DFS rates are on average 20% lower for each stage. It is important to recognize that many subsets exist within each stage. Both detection and treatment approaches for breast cancer are evolving at a rapid rate, and therefore these estimates may vary among reference sources. Current estimates suggest that the majority of women present with early breast cancer and that the majority of these women are cured with today's treatment approaches. As is discussed in subsequent sections, adjuvant (postsurgery) systemic therapy has improved absolute survival rates by up to 10% in selected populations of patients with early breast cancer (stages I and II). Combined modality approaches with neoadjuvant chemotherapy (before surgery), surgery and/or radiation, followed by adjuvant chemotherapy have resulted in benefits of a similar magnitude in patients with locally advanced breast cancer (stage III). Unfortunately, a still significant percentage of women with early breast cancer and locally advanced breast cancer eventually experience recurrence, usually manifested in lungs, bone, liver, skin, or brain following treatment of the primary disease.[5]

TABLE 116–3. Stages of Primary Breast Cancer[a]

	T	N	M
Stage 0	T_{is}	N_0	M_0
Stage I	T_1	N_0	M_0
Stage IIA	T_0	N_1	M_0
	T_1	N_1	
	T_2	N_0	
Stage IIB	T_2	N_1	M_0
	T_3	N_0	
Stage IIIA	T_0	N_2	M_0
	T_1	N_2	
	T_2	N_2	
	T_3	N_1, N_2	
Stage IIIB	T_4	Any N	M_0
	Any T	N_3	
Stage IV	Any T	Any N	M_1

[a]See Figure 116–3.
Adapted from Stockdale FE. Breast cancer. In: Rubenstein E, Federman DD, eds. Scientific American Medicine. New York, Scientific American, 1991:1–17.

TABLE 116–4. Estimated Stage at Presentation and 5-Year Disease-Free Survival (DFS): Breast Cancer 1994

	Percent of Total Cases	5-Year DFS[a] (%)
Stage I	40	70–90
Stage II	40	50–70
Stage III	15	20–30
Stage IV	5	0–10[b]

[a]With current conventional local and systemic therapy.
[b]Patients in stage IV are rarely free of disease; however, 10% to 20% of these patients may survive with minimal disease for 5 to 10 years.

PATHOLOGY

The pathologic evaluation of breast lesions serves to establish the histologic diagnosis and to confirm the presence or absence of other factors believed to influence prognosis. These nonhistologic prognostic factors include the presence of necrosis, lymphatic or vascular invasion, nuclear grade, hormone receptor status, proliferative index, amount of aneuploidy, presence or absence of oncogenes, presence or absence of mutations in the tumor suppressor *p53* gene, and, perhaps, presence or absence of elevated growth factor levels, as well as enzymes (cathepsin D), proteins, and angiogenesis factors.

INVASIVE CARCINOMA

Invasive breast cancers are a histologically heterogeneous group of lesions. Most breast carcinomas are adenocarcinomas and are classified on the basis of their microscopic appearance as either ductal or lobular corresponding to the ducts and lobules of the normal breast. The various histologic types of breast cancer have different prognoses, but it is not known whether their response to therapy differs, since patients in therapeutic trials are not typically stratified according to histologic type. The five most common types of invasive breast cancer are briefly described.

Invasive or *infiltrating ductal carcinoma* is the most common histology. The other histologic patterns can occur alone or with infiltrating ductal carcinoma. These tumors are generally referred to as infiltrating ductal carcinoma "not otherwise specified" and account for approximately 75% of all invasive breast cancers. These tumors commonly spread to the axillary lymph nodes and their prognosis is poorer than for other histologic types (specifically tubular, medullary, mucinous/colloid). *Infiltrating lobular carcinoma* accounts for only 5% to 10% of breast tumors. Typical presentation is an area of ill-defined thickening in the breast, in contrast to a prominent lump characteristic of infiltrating ductal carcinoma. A greater proportion of infiltrating lobular carcinomas are multicentric tumors, either in the same or opposite breast, as compared with infiltrating ductal carcinoma. Overall, infiltrating lobular carcinoma and infiltrating ductal carcinoma have similar likelihoods of axillary node involvement and similar prognosis, yet the sites of metastases tend to differ. Ductal carcinoma more frequently metastasizes to the bone or to the liver, lung, or brain, whereas lobular carcinoma metastasizes more commonly to meningeal and serosal surfaces and other unusual sites.

The three most common special types of invasive cancer are *tubular, medullary,* and *mucinous. Medullary carcinoma* is a well-defined lesion with a characteristic microscopic appearance that includes a well-circumscribed border, intense infiltration with small lymphocytes, and other factors. It accounts for 5% to 7% of all breast carcinomas and is believed to have a better prognosis than infiltrating ductal carcinoma. *Mucinous (or colloid) carcinoma* constitutes about 3% of all breast carcinomas and is characterized by the abundant accumulation of extracellular mucin around clusters of tumor cells. It is slow growing and can be bulky. When the tumor is predominantly mucinous, the prognosis tends to be more favorable. *Tubular carcinoma* accounts for about 2% of all breast cancers and is a type of carcinoma in which tubule formation is conspicuous on pathology. Axillary metastases are uncommon and the prognosis is considerably better than for infiltrating ductal carcinomas. Histologies rarely reported include adenocystic carcinoma, carcinosarcomas, and papillary carcinoma. In some pathology reports, infiltrating ductal carcinoma may include small areas containing these special tumor types.

Special situations seen clinically and histologically include Paget's disease of the breast and inflammatory breast cancer. Paget's disease of the breast occurs in 1% to 4% of all patients with breast cancer. Clinically, the patient presents with a relatively long history of eczematous changes in the nipple with itching, burning, oozing, bleeding, or some combination of these. The nipple changes are associated with an underlying carcinoma in the breast that is usually palpable. The histology of the tumor type is either ductal carcinoma *in situ* (DCIS) or invasive ductal carcinoma. Prognosis is related to the histologic type of the associated tumor.

Inflammatory breast cancer is characterized clinically by prominent skin, edema, redness and warmth, visible erysipeloid margin, and induration of the underlying tissue. Biopsies of the involved skin reveal cancer cells in the dermal lymphatics. Prognosis of patients with inflammatory breast cancer is poor, even if the disease is apparently localized.[5]

NONINVASIVE CARCINOMA

As with invasive carcinoma, the noninvasive lesions may be divided broadly into ductal and lobular categories. Evidence supports that the development of malignancy is a multistep process and that invasive breast cancer has a preinvasive phase. During the carcinoma *in situ* phase, normal epithelial cells undergo genetic alterations that result in malignant transformation. Transformed epithelial cells proliferate and pile up within lobulars or ducts, but lack the required genetic alterations that enable the cells to penetrate the basement membrane. Therefore, carcinoma *in situ* is diagnosed when malignant transformation of cells has occurred but the basement membrane is intact by light microscopy.

The widespread use of screening mammography and subsequent biopsy coupled with recognition of noninvasive breast carcinoma by pathologists has resulted in a significant increase in the diagnosis of *in situ* breast cancer during the past decade. Its incidence has risen from 1% to 5% in the early 1970s to 9% to 17% in the late 1980s.[5] The natural history of these disorders is not well described in the literature and, thus, the debate continues regarding carcinoma *in situ*: Is carcinoma *in situ* preinvasive cancer or simply a marker of unstable epithelium that represents an increased risk for the development of subsequent aggressive cancer? Although a detailed discussion of the biology and appropriate management of noninvasive breast cancer is beyond the scope of this chapter, some of the more salient characteristics of DCIS and lobular carcinoma *in situ* (LCIS) are described below and the reader is referred to a number of excellent reviews for a more comprehensive discussion.[5,28,29]

DCIS is seen more frequently than LCIS at a rate of about 6 to 3:1. Most DCIS cases diagnosed currently are small nonpalpable lesions, unlike its presentation in years prior to mammography as a palpable mass in over half of cases. Today, most cases of DCIS are found by biopsies performed for clustered calcifications seen on screening mammography. There are four distinct histologic patterns of DCIS, which probably represent successive steps in its evolution toward invasive carcinoma. The biologic characteristics are consistent with its role as a direct precursor to invasive carcinoma, which appears to develop in the majority of cases if left untreated within 10 years of diagnosis. The peak incidence of DCIS is 51 to 59 years, which closely parallels that of invasive carcinoma. Treatment of DCIS is dependent on its presentation, size, and pathology. The patient and physician have the following options: (1) excision with negative margins, preferably 1 to 2 cm; (2) excision followed by breast irradiation; and (3) traditional total mastectomy with reconstruction. It is important to note, however, that in all cases, carcinoma *in situ* is treated as cancer. Mastectomy had been the standard treatment of DCIS for several decades. The combined data from 1061 women who underwent mastectomy for DCIS, reported in 14 published studies, with follow-up ranging from

2 to more than 15 years, show an overall local recurrence rate of only 0.75% and overall cancer mortality rate of less than 1%. Breast conservation, that is, wide local excision followed by irradiation of breast tissue, may be an effective alternative to mastectomy. The recently completed NASBP B17 trial randomized 808 women with DCIS to receive lumpectomy alone or lumpectomy with radiation.[30] The results of this trial demonstrated an advantage for radiation plus lumpectomy in terms of fewer local recurrences. Although radiation following lumpectomy does not appear to change the survival of patients with DCIS, it significantly reduces the incidence of local recurrences and enhances the breast preservation rate in these women. If more than one area of the breast is involved with DCIS, a mastectomy is the preferred option. It has also been suggested that breast conservation may not be appropriate for younger women whose lifetime risk of breast cancer is high given a diagnosis of DCIS. Axillary dissection is generally not indicated. There is currently no proven benefit for the use of cytotoxic chemotherapy or hormonal manipulation in this disease. Follow-up of women who have been treated for DCIS should be as comprehensive as that of a woman with invasive carcinoma to facilitate early detection of any subsequent malignancy.

LCIS is a microscopic diagnosis, not a gross abnormality. Therefore, it is always nonpalpable and it is virtually impossible to make the diagnosis of LCIS by clinical examination. Unlike DCIS, LCIS does not demonstrate calcifications on mammography and, in fact, is not associated with mammographic abnormalities. LCIS is most frequently diagnosed in biopsy specimens that were obtained because of symptoms or mammography findings consistent with benign lesions. Multicentricity is common (> 30%) with LCIS and the opposite breast is affected in up to 50% of patients. It is unclear whether LCIS proceeds to invasive carcinoma or serves as a marker for a high probability of invasive carcinoma developing elsewhere in the breast. Thus, the management of LCIS is very controversial. Some authorities favor a program of breast examination, periodic physician examination, and mammography as management of LCIS. In selected patients who are particularly anxious about the development of cancer, bilateral total mastectomies and prompt reconstruction represent a reasonable approach. Radiation, systemic chemotherapy, or hormonal therapy have no role in the management of LCIS.

PATHOLOGY

The natural history of breast cancer varies between patients, with some having an extremely aggressive disease that progresses rapidly, whereas others follow a more indolent course. The ability to predict which patients have a better disease prognosis is extremely important in designing treatment recommendations to maximize quantity and quality of life. A number of potential pathologic prognostic factors have been identified and intense research in this area is ongoing.

Tumor size and the presence and number of involved axillary lymph nodes are established primary factors in assessing the risk for breast cancer recurrence and subsequent metastatic disease. Table 116–5 shows the 5-year relapse rate according to size of primary tumor and axillary node involvement from results of three investigations.[31–33] These data clearly demonstrate that the major factor that influences the likelihood of recurrence is the presence of positive axillary nodes. However, regardless of axillary node studies, the size of the primary tumor remains an independent prognostic factor for disease recurrence. In axillary node–negative patients, a tumor size of less than 2 cm is associated with a very favorable prognosis. However, there does not appear to be a large difference between prognosis in patients with large (greater than 5 cm) tumors and negative nodes compared to patients with 2- to 5-cm tumors and negative nodes. Thus, the size of the primary tumor in patients with negative axillary lymph nodes may not provide as much information regarding prognosis as in node-positive patients. The number of affected nodes is directly related to disease recurrence. Estimates are that 35% of patients with one to three positive nodes will relapse within 5 years compared to 75% of patients with greater than or equal to four positive nodes.[34,35]

Aside from the stage (TNM) of the disease, hormone receptor studies have received the most attention in the characterization of primary breast cancer. Hormone receptors are used clinically as indicators of prognosis and to predict response to hormone therapy. Hormone receptors are cytoplasmic proteins that transmit signals to the nucleus of the cell for growth and proliferation. The hormone receptors clinically useful in discussions of breast cancer include the estrogen receptor (ER) and the progesterone receptor (PR). The presence of these proteins in the primary tumor (or less often metastases) is routinely measured by enzyme-linked immunochemical assays and radioassays (enzyme-linked immunosorbent assay [ELISA]). Concentrations of hormone receptors less than 3 fentamoles per

TABLE 116–5. Five-Year Relapse Rate (%) Based on Size of Primary Tumor and Axillary Nodal Status

	Size of Primary Tumor (cm)		
Axillary Status	< 2	2–5	> 5
Axillary nodes negative			
Fisher et al.[31]	12	24	27
Nemoto et al.[32]	13	19	25
Valagussa et al.[33]	8	24	19
Axillary nodes positive			
Fisher et al.[31]	50	60	79
Nemoto et al.[32]	39	50	65
Valagussa et al.[33]	37	64	74

milligram of cytosol protein are considered negative, 3 to 10 fentamoles per milligram of cytosol protein are "intermediate," and concentrations of hormone receptors greater than 10 fentamoles per milligram of cytosol protein are positive. The level (i.e., quantitative) of hormone receptor and the methodology used to assess hormone receptors are important for predictive ability. Although the estrogen receptor has received the most attention to date, more recent data suggest that the presence of the progesterone receptor protein is required for the functional effects of the estrogen receptor protein to occur. This is evidenced by data that have found that response to hormonal manipulation and prognosis are highly correlated with the presence of both positive estrogen receptor protein and positive progesterone receptor protein. Hormone receptors are most valuable in predicting response to hormone therapy. Approximately 70% to 80% of patients who are ER positive and PR positive will respond to hormonal manipulation. ER-negative patients rarely respond to hormonal manipulation. Patients who are ER negative and PR positive lie somewhere in between.

Approximately 50% to 70% of patients with primary or metastatic breast cancer have hormone receptor–positive tumors. The median level and frequency of hormone receptor–positive tumors are higher in postmenopausal patients compared with premenopausal patients. This difference is likely responsible for the different recommendations for adjuvant and metastatic treatment of breast cancer between premenopausal and postmenopausal patients discussed in later sections of this chapter. A number of prominent authorities in breast cancer research have suggested that breast cancer in postmenopausal women is substantively different than that occurring in premenopausal women. Breast cancer is predominantly a disease of the elderly. When it occurs in younger patients, the course of the disease is more aggressive. This is observed with many of the other common tumor types. Hormone receptor positivity, more common in postmenopausal women, is associated with a superior response to hormone therapy and a longer disease-free interval between primary and subsequent metastatic disease, and overall a more favorable prognosis. The presence of hormone receptors in tumors has been associated with a favorable disease-free interval and perhaps an overall survival difference of 5% to 10% (compared to hormone receptor–negative patients). However, the value of hormone receptors as a prognostic factor is being eroded by increasing knowledge of newer prognostic factors such as epidermal growth factor receptor, proliferative capacity, nuclear grade, and expression of the HER-2/neu oncogene.[36–40]

The rate of tumor cell proliferation also has prognostic significance in breast cancer recurrence. Rate of cell proliferation can be determined with either the tritiated thymidine-labeling index (TLI) or DNA flow cytometry, which determines the percentage of tumor cells actively dividing (S-phase fraction). Both techniques have shown that patients with rapidly proliferating tumors have a decreased DFS compared to patients with slowly proliferating tumors.[38] S-phase fraction has been disappointing as a predictor of response to cytotoxic chemotherapy. Flow cytometry can also detect abnormal DNA content, or aneuploidy, in breast cancer cells. Although there are conflicting reports regarding the clinical significance of ploidy status, a number of studies report that patients with aneuploid tumors have significantly shorter relapse-free survival times than do patients with diploid tumors.[38]

Nuclear grade and tumor (histologic) differentiation are known, independent prognostic indicators. Several histologic grading systems have been developed and shown to have prognostic value in the evaluation of breast cancer. Fisher et al.[39] have shown a 5-year survival of 93% for patients with good nuclear grade compared with 79% for patients with poor nuclear grade. However, interobserver lack of concordance between pathologist grading has thwarted the use of this prognostic indicator in clinical trials.

A number of additional potential prognostic factors have been identified in the past 5 years. These include overexpression of the erbB-2 (or HER-2/neu) oncogene, cathepsin D, angiogenic growth factors, mutations in the tumor suppresser *p*53 gene, and others. Research in this area is proceeding at a rapid rate and the reader is referred to several excellent reviews for more detailed information.[36–40] A number of the new potential prognostic factors have been shown to be strongly correlated with established risk factors. For example, ER-positive tumors are commonly HER-2 negative and cathepsin D negative as well, thus making it difficult to discern from clinical trials the relative importance of potential prognostic factors. Thus, it is unclear at the present time which of these serve as independent prognostic factors. Identification of these numerous factors and correlations between these and known prognostic factors that affect clinical outcome is of interest because each correlation allows basic mechanistic insights into disease processes. Practically, they allow prediction of probable clinical outcomes that can guide therapeutic decision making. Several of these new prognostic factors, specifically the HER-2 oncogene overexpression and *p*53 mutations, have shown early promise as predictors of efficacy of adjuvant chemotherapy.

Although there is a growing understanding of the prognostic significance of individual factors, the topic of how to practically use multiple prognostic factors in concert is largely unexplored. The development of decision-making systems for clinical applications will require improvements in the areas of (1) standardization of methodologies and interlaboratory quality control for prognostic factor determinations, (2) definition of a limited set of prognostic markers that are independently predictive, and (3) staging systems that integrate this information.

▶ TREATMENT: Breast Cancer

EARLY BREAST CANCER

LOCAL-REGIONAL THERAPY

The majority of patients presenting with breast cancer today have either an *in situ* tumor, a small tumor with negative lymph nodes (stage I), or a small stage II cancer. Surgery alone can cure most, if not all, patients with *in situ* cancers and approximately half of all patients with stage II cancers. The choice of surgical procedures has changed drastically over the past 50 years. This is in part due to our changing understanding of the biology of breast cancer and in part owing to a series of well-conducted trials performed over this time period.

The Halstedian theory and concept of tumor growth, formulated at the end of the 19th century, held that breast cancer was a local-regional disease that spread to involve larger contiguous areas of the breast, chest wall, and adjacent lymph nodes. This hypothesis gave rise to emphasis throughout most of the 20th century on the Halsted radical mastectomy, the hallmark of an approach holding that cure of early diseases could best be achieved with expansive, meticulously performed surgical procedures. The *radical mastectomy* involves removal of the breast and both major and minor pectoralis muscles. The axillary nodes on the same side (ipsilateral) as the breast lesion are also removed. Substantial morbidity is associated with this procedure. Muscle resection decreases strength and range of motion, and removal of axillary lymph nodes can produce edema of the arm and resected breast area. This procedure was often followed by external beam radiation therapy to the involved area.

During the 1960s, it was recognized that breast cancer is often microscopically disseminated at the time of initial diagnosis. The evolutionary concept that breast cancer is not only a local, but also a systemic disease has resulted in major changes in local and systemic therapy. In 1980, the Commission on Cancer of the American College of Surgeons reported that there had been an apparent gradual shift from a radical to modified radical mastectomy since December of 1972.[41] The modified radical mastectomy, also termed *total mastectomy with axillary lymph node dissection,* is not as precisely defined or standardized as the radical mastectomy. The pectoralis minor muscle may be excised, divided, or left intact, and more importantly there may be variation in the extent of axillary lymph node dissection ranging from sampling to full dissection. It was recognized during this time period that a major factor in prognosis was involvement of axillary lymph nodes rather than the type of initial surgical procedure performed.

Results of a large trial conducted in the United States by the National Surgical Adjuvant Breast and Bowel Project (NSABP) repudiated the Halsted theory and supported the alternative systemic hypothesis. NSABP B-04 published in 1977 randomized almost 2000 women among three treatment regimens: radical mastectomy, simple mastectomy with local-regional irradiation, and simple mastectomy and removal of nodes if they later became clinically positive.[42] Forty percent of patients who underwent the radical mastectomy had pathologically positive lymph nodes; thus, it can be assumed that 40% of patients in the other two groups had positive axillary nodes that were not removed. Despite the disparity in local-regional treatment, no significant difference in treatment failure, distant metastases, or overall survival was observed through more than 14 years of follow-up.

With negation of the primacy radical mastectomy, the NSABP instituted a second trial (B-06) in which patients with stage I or II breast cancer, with tumor size 4 cm or less, were treated with either modified radical mastectomy or lumpectomy with or without radiation therapy.[43] Lumpectomy followed by radiation resulted in a 5-year survival of 85% compared to 76% for modified radical mastectomy with consistent findings at the 8-year results of the study. This study also found that radiation therapy reduced the probability of local tumor recurrence by approximately 30% in patients treated with lumpectomy. The local failure rate of modified radical mastectomy was 8.1% compared to 7.2% for lumpectomy alone and 1.1% for lumpectomy and radiation therapy. Neither the rate nor development of distant metastases nor contralateral breast cancer was different in the treatment groups.

The National Institutes of Health (NIH) Consensus Conference on the Treatment of Early Stage Breast Cancer addressed the roles of modified radical mastectomy versus breast conservation and concluded that primary therapy for breast cancer stages I and II should be *breast conservation.*[44] Breast conservation consists of lumpectomy, also referred to as segmental mastectomy or partial mastectomy, and is defined as excision of the primary tumor and adjacent breast tissue, followed by radiation therapy to reduce the risk of local recurrence. Sampling of axillary lymph nodes is recommended for completeness of staging and prognostic information. The reason given for favoring breast conservation therapy is that it achieved similar results to more extensive surgical procedures with cosmetically superior results.

The majority of patients with breast cancer can be treated by lumpectomy and radiation therapy. Several factors should be considered in selecting patients for breast conservation therapy. Multiple sites of cancer within the breast and the inability to attain negative pathologic margins on the excised breast specimen are predictive for an increased risk of recurrence with breast-conserving therapy and indications for mastectomy. Preexisting collagen vascular disease is a contraindication for the use of breast-conserving radiation and surgery. Although local recurrence following breast-conservation therapy is not associated with increased mortality, it is distressing to the patient and requires surgical removal of the breast. In addition, reconstructive therapy is often not feasible in a breast that has previously received irradiation. Another major consideration in selecting patients for breast-conserving therapy is the expected cosmetic result. Although the size of the tumor is not an important consideration for breast cancer recurrence, the relationship of the size of the tumor to the total breast volume is an important cosmetic consideration. If the volume of the tissue removed is large in a woman with small breasts, better results can often be obtained with mastectomy and reconstruction. Despite the desire of the patient and the willingness of the surgeon to avoid mastectomy, in some circumstances, a lumpectomy will approximate so closely a mastectomy that both the patient and the physician will agree that preservation of a very limited amount of breast tissue would not justify the inconvenience of radiation therapy. Aside from the probability of local recurrence and the ability to achieve a satisfactory cosmetic result, consideration must be given to the availability of an external beam radiation facility and the patient's willingness to comply with the prescribed course of radiotherapy. In most instances, external beam radiation therapy used in conjunction with breast-conserving procedures involves 4 to 6 weeks of radiation therapy directed to the breast tissue (total of 5000 cGy administered as 200-cGy doses daily to eradicate residual disease). Complications associated with radiation therapy to the breast are minor and include reddening and erythema of the breast tissue and subsequent shrinkage of total breast mass beyond that predicted on the basis of breast tissue removal.

Simple or total mastectomy involves removal of the entire breast without resection of the underlying muscle or axillary nodes. The major disadvantage of this procedure is that axillary nodal status is not determined and, thus, important prognostic information may be lost. This procedure is used in patients with carcinoma *in situ*, in whom there is a 1% incidence of axillary node involvement, or in cases of local recurrence following breast-conservation therapy. However, the importance of determining axillary lymph node involvement is being challenged by the identification of new prognostic pathologic factors that bear concordance with axillary nodal status and with the new and evolving recommendations for systemic adjuvant therapy for all patients regardless of nodal status. Thus, simple mastectomy may be a reasonable alternative for women who wish to avoid the inconvenience of radiation therapy and preserve their option for breast reconstruction in the future. The NSABP B-04 and B-06 trials are most commonly credited with the finding that breast conservation is an appropriate primary therapy for the majority of women with stages I and II disease and is preferable in that it provides survival rates equivalent to those of modified radical mastectomy. However, these trials were no less important for the valuable information they provided regarding the natural history of the disease and the identification of pathologic prognostic factors associated with early cancer spread. The preponderance of information available regarding predicting women most likely to benefit from systemic adjuvant therapy was derived from pathologic evaluation of the archives of these trials.

SYSTEMIC ADJUVANT THERAPY

Systemic adjuvant therapy is defined as the administration of systemic therapy following definitive therapy (surgery, radiation, or a combination of these) when there is no evidence of metastatic disease, but a high likelihood of disease recurrence. The concept of breast cancer being a systemic disease and the rationale of adjuvant chemotherapy was based on a series of laboratory and clinical investigations conducted during the 1960s and 1970s that were directed primarily toward achieving a better understanding of tumor metastases. The laboratory findings, clinical abnormalities, and biologic hypothesis that lead to recognition of breast cancer as a systemic disease and documented the value of adjuvant chemotherapy are illustrated in Table 116–6. The very earliest adjuvant trials in breast cancer consisted of perioperative administration of alkylating agents with the intent of eradicating micrometastases that were disseminated at the time of surgical excision of the tumor. Large numbers of collaborative research groups have conducted stepwise series of studies designed to identify appropriate candidates for systemic adjuvant therapy, as well as optimal regimens and duration of systemic adjuvant therapy. Several hundred randomized clinical trials evaluating various systemic adjuvant modalities have been reported. Most published results confirmed that chemotherapy, hormonal therapy, or a combination of the two result in advantages in DFS or overall survival for all treated patients, or more commonly for patients in specific prognostic subgroups (nodal involvement, menopausal status, hormonal receptor status, growth fraction, nuclear grade). The huge amount of data generated by these trials has resulted in a great deal of controversy, with different conclusions being reached by various experts.

A number of factors make interpretation of results of systemic adjuvant therapy trials difficult. These include differences in the patient populations studied, the variation in natural history of breast cancer, the absence of information regarding pathologic prognostic factors in many studies, and differences in treatment approach and methods of analysis. It is important to remember that the goal of systemic adjuvant therapy is cure. Therefore, patients in these studies must be followed for long periods of time before results can be determined. In addition, because the majority

TABLE 116–6. Laboratory Findings, Clinical Observations, and Biologic Hypothesis of Breast Cancer as a Systemic Disease and the Value of Adjuvant Chemotherapy

- By the time cancer becomes clinically detectable, it is advanced (about 30 doublings) and has had ample opportunity to establish distant micrometastases.
- There is no orderly pattern of tumor cell dissemination, and the bloodstream is of considerable importance in tumor spread.
- Operable breast cancer is often a systemic disease and variations in local-regional therapy have not substantially affected survival. Only by control of distant disease can there be an improvement in the outcome of breast cancer patients.
- Likelihood of disease recurrence is related to size of tumor mass and axillary node involvement at diagnosis.
- Recurrence of breast cancer following local-regional therapy is most commonly at sites distant from the breast.
- Tumor growth fraction is inversely related to tumor population site. Therefore, optimal kinetic conditions to achieve cure with chemotherapy exist in the setting of micrometastatic disease.
- Efficacy of chemotherapy is dose dependent and optimal doses of combination chemotherapy can be more safely and effectively administered in the adjuvant setting as opposed to the setting of advanced disease.

of patients with early breast cancer (50% to 90%) in the various trials are cured with local-regional therapy alone, large numbers of patients are required to show a statistically significant difference that can be attributed to systemic adjuvant therapy. For these reasons, combined analysis, or meta-analysis, of all breast cancer trials has been conducted and is the most frequently referred to information regarding systemic adjuvant therapy. This effort, organized by the Early Breast Cancer Trialists' Collaborative Group, is based on a worldwide collaboration involving 133 randomized trials conducted between 1957 and 1985 with 31,000 recurrences of disease, and 24,000 deaths among 75,000 women. The most recent publication of this overview was in 1992.[45] The majority (70%) of women in these trials were node positive. Data on hormone receptor status and many of the newer pathologic prognostic factors were not available in many of the trials.

The 10-year results of the overview are described in Table 116–7. As can be seen in this table, in women less than 50 years of age, adjuvant chemotherapy alone reduces the annual odds of recurrence by 37%, and the annual odds of death by 27%. This is in contrast to tamoxifen alone, which reduced the annual odds of recurrence by 27% and the annual odds of death by 17%.

When one compares the results of trials that compared tamoxifen plus chemotherapy versus chemotherapy alone, or chemotherapy and tamoxifen versus tamoxifen alone, it is apparent that tamoxifen offered very little benefit in women age 50 years or younger. An interesting theory with some laboratory and clinical support holds that tamoxifen antagonizes the beneficial effects of chemotherapy in women age 50 years or younger. Chemotherapy acts by inhibiting DNA synthesis and thereby causing death of tumor cells, whereas tamoxifen is believed to have a static effect on tumor cell growth. The growth inhibitory effect of tamoxifen may thereby diminish the cytotoxic effect of chemotherapy, resulting in subsequent recurrence of disease in women who received the two agents together. This has led to controversy regarding the optimal way to administer chemo–endocrine therapy in the adjuvant setting with some experts favoring sequential use (chemotherapy followed by tamoxifen), whereas others continue to use concurrent (chemotherapy plus tamoxifen) therapy.

TABLE 116–7. Ten-Year Results of the Overview Analysis

		Reduction in Annual Odds of (± 1 Standard Deviation)	
	No. Patients	***Recurrence***	***Death***
Women < 50 yr			
Tamoxifen	8578	12 ± 4	6 ± 5
Tamoxifen alone vs no treatment	2216	27 ± 7	17 ± 10
Tamoxifen + chemotherapy vs chemotherapy	6362	7 ± 4	3 ± 5
Chemotherapy	3362	36 ± 5	25 ± 5
Chemotherapy alone vs no treatment	2976	37 ± 5	27 ± 6
Chemotherapy + tamoxifen vs tamoxifen	386	32 ± 16	23 ± 6
Ovarian ablation	1817	26 ± 6	25 ± 7
Ablation alone vs no treatment	878	30 ± 9	28 ± 9
Ablation + chemotherapy vs chemotherapy	939	21 ± 9	19 ± 11
Women > 50 yr			
Tamoxifen	21,262	29 ± 2	20 ± 2
Tamoxifen alone vs no treatment	13,114	30 ± 2	19 ± 3
Tamoxifen + chemotherapy vs chemotherapy	8148	28 ± 3	20 ± 4
Chemotherapy	7677	23 ± 3	12 ± 4
Chemotherapy alone vs no treatment	3745	22 ± 4	14 ± 5
Chemotherapy + tamoxifen vs tamoxifen	3932	26 ± 5	10 ± 7

Adapted from Gelber RD, Goldhirsch A, Coates AS. Adjuvant therapy for breast cancer: Understanding the overview. J Clin Oncol 1993;11:580–585.

Interestingly, results of the meta-analysis suggest that ovarian ablation has approximately the same magnitude of effects in women age 50 years or younger as chemotherapy. These findings have renewed interest in adjuvant ovarian ablation in women age 50 years or younger. It is incorrect to infer from the overview that chemotherapy and ovarian ablation are equivalent. These are "indirect comparisons" between the results of the chemotherapy trials and ovarian ablation trials. Patient selection factors and other aspects of the early ablation trials may have differed from those in the more recent chemotherapy trials, so these trials are not comparable. The relative value of chemotherapy and ovarian ablation must be evaluated in direct comparison using randomized trials.

Of note, premenopausal women treated with adjuvant chemotherapy often develop amenorrhea. The potential therapeutic importance of chemotherapy-induced amenorrhea has been recognized for many years, leading some to speculate that the effects of adjuvant chemotherapy are mediated by the endocrine effects of ovarian ablation. Supporting this view is the observation that chemotherapy-induced amenorrhea is associated with superior DFS in some adjuvant trials, although not in others. An alternative hypothesis is that amenorrhea is merely a marker that identifies patients for whom the chemotherapy is more effective. Although this debate is difficult to resolve precisely, it seems likely that patients with hormonally responsive cancers will benefit from both the cytotoxic effects of chemotherapy and the estrogen deprivation of ovarian ablation.

In women 50 years of age or older, adjuvant tamoxifen reduces the annual odds of recurrence by 30% and the annual odds of death by 19%. Chemotherapy alone offers smaller benefits in this group, reducing the annual odds of recurrence and death by 22% and 14%, respectively. In the trials that compared tamoxifen plus chemotherapy to tamoxifen alone, the combination was found to be superior for both recurrence (28%) and death (20%). Between the ages of 50 and 69, direct comparisons show that chemotherapy plus tamoxifen is superior to chemotherapy alone for both recurrence and mortality and better than tamoxifen alone for recurrence.

The overview also demonstrated that the proportional benefits of chemotherapy in node-negative and node-positive patients are comparable, combination chemotherapy is superior to single agents, and adjuvant treatment duration of 12 to 24 months is no more effective than 6 months of treatment. Indirect comparisons showed that long-term tamoxifen (2 to 5 years) is significantly more effective than tamoxifen treatment programs of shorter duration and that tamoxifen doses greater than 20 mg/d are not associated with better responses than 20-mg daily doses.

Proportional reductions in the annual odds of recurrence or death describe the treatment benefit only in those who might have had recurrences or those who died during the observation period. It is important to consider that the underlying risk of death or recurrence varies in breast cancer patients and, therefore, the absolute benefits of adjuvant therapy will also vary accordingly. For example, in a group of untreated axillary node–positive patients, perhaps 50% or more would be expected to die within 10 years. A 25% reduction in the annual odds of death amounts to about 12 fewer deaths per 100 treated patients at the end of 10 years or an absolute increase in the 10-year survival from 50% to 62%. However, the absolute benefits of treatment are much smaller in node-negative patients with a favorable prognosis. For example, if 25% of a group of node-negative patients were expected to die within 10 years, a 25% reduction in the annual odds of death amounts to about 6 fewer deaths per 100 treated patients at the end of 10 years or an absolute increase in the 10-year survival from 75% to 81%. Therefore, the benefit of adjuvant therapy expressed as a reduction in the annual odds of recurrence or death must be put into perspective with the likelihood of death without treatment.

Despite the very large number of clinical trials conducted in women with early-stage breast cancer, optimal therapy has not been defined. To assist in identifying optimal treatment guidelines, all women with early-stage breast cancer are encouraged to participate in randomized cooperative group clinical trials. Current estimates are that fewer than 5% of women in the United States and Europe with early breast cancer are enrolled in cooperative group research studies. This is unfortunate because optimal treatment cannot be defined in the absence of data derived from well-designed, well-conducted clinical investigations. From a practical standpoint, it is also unfortunate that this leaves the medical oncologist, as well as the patient, with a dilemma in selecting treatment outside of the context of clinical trials. To assist in these situations, the NIH conducted consensus conferences in

1985 and 1990 on the treatment of early stage breast cancer. In February 1998, an international group of researchers met at St. Gallen in Switzerland for the Sixth International Conference on Adjuvant Therapy of Primary Breast Cancer.[46] At the conclusion of the conference, a consensus panel of experts reviewed and modified its previous guidelines and recommendations for selection of adjuvant systemic therapies in specific patient populations outside of the framework of clinical trials (Table 116–8). Criteria used to construct Table 116–8 included risk of relapse, predicted response, results of treatment from randomized clinical trials and patient preferences concerning risks and benefits of effective therapy. Patient populations are defined based on risk of relapse. The panel defined minimal/low risk as patients with all of the following: negative lymph nodes, tumor < 1 cm, ER positive, grade 1, and age ≥ 35 years. High risk node negative patients have one of the following: tumor > 2 cm, ER negative grade 2–3, age < 35 years. Intermediate risk includes all patients that fall outside of criteria for minimal or high risk. Node positive patients are by definition at high risk. Elderly patients are listed separately since specific considerations are required regarding toxicity and competing cause of morbidity and mortality. Therapies for which high level evidence of benefit has been demonstrated are noted in bold text and therapies that are still investigational or require special consideration are noted as described in the footnotes.

The absolute benefits of adjuvant therapy are primarily related to the patient's risk of metastases and ultimately cancer death. Although it is recognized that the risk of recurrence is greater in node-positive compared to node-negative women, the proportional reduction in odds of death is similar. Data from the overview and newer data published in the past 5 years suggest that the benefits of therapy are sufficient to justify the use of adjuvant chemotherapy for all premenopausal women (except those at minimal/low risk), regardless of hormone receptor status, and adjuvant tamoxifen for all hormone receptor–positive postmenopausal women. Adjuvant chemotherapy is similarly justified in postmenopausal women who are hormone receptor negative. A question that remains is the benefits of combined chemohormonal therapy. Recent data from the NSABP (B-20) and the International Breast Cancer Study Group support the addition of chemotherapy to tamoxifen in lymph node–negative or –positive, estrogen receptor–positive patients.[47,48] Therefore, although benefits of chemotherapy are less in the postmenopausal and node-negative subsets of patients, essentially all women with stage I and II breast cancer derive some benefit from chemotherapy. As previously discussed, tamoxifen is indicated in all postmenopausal hormone receptor–positive patients. The decision to add tamoxifen in premenopausal women with positive hormone receptors following chemotherapy depends on the age of the patient and whether or not permanent ovarian failure followed cytotoxic chemotherapy. In patients with positive receptors who resume menses, there is likely a small benefit derived from the addition of tamoxifen therapy. However, some patients and clinicians may choose to forgo a possible survival benefit in favor of avoidance of menopause and its attendant risks, especially in very young patients. Node-negative patients with primary breast tumors of less than 1 cm have an excellent prognosis and there is general agreement that the absolute benefits of adjuvant therapy may be too small to justify its use outside the clinical trial. The National Comprehensive Cancer Network (NCCN) recently developed practice guidelines for the treatment of breast cancer. Figure 116–4 illustrates the NCCN guidelines for adjuvant treatment of stage I–IIIA breast cancer following total mastectomy or

TABLE 116–8. Adjuvant Treatment for Patients With Node-Negative (A) and Node-Positive (B) Breast Cancer[a]

A. Node Negative			
Patient Group	***Minimal/Low Risk***	***Intermediate Risk***	***High Risk***
Premenopausal, ER or PR positive	**None or tamoxifen**	**Tamoxifen ± chemotherapy[b]** Ovarian ablation[c] GnRH analogue[c]	**Chemotherapy + tamoxifen[b]** Ovarian ablation[c] GnRH analogue[c]
Premenopausal, ER and PR negative	Not applicable	Not applicable	**Chemotherapy[d]**
Postmenopausal, ER or PR positive	**None or tamoxifen**	**Tamoxifen ± chemotherapy[b]**	**Tamoxifen + chemotherapy[b]**
Postmenopausal, ER and PR negative	Not applicable	Not applicable	**Chemotherapy[d]**
Elderly	**None or tamoxifen**	**Tamoxifen ±** chemotherapy	**Tamoxifen** If no ER and PR expression: chemotherapy

B. Node Positive	
Patient Group	***Treatments***
Premenopausal, ER or PR positive	**Chemotherapy + tamoxifen** **Ovarian ablation** (or GnRH analogue) ± tamoxifen[c] Chemotherapy ± ovarian ablation or (GnRH analogue) ± tamoxifen[c]
Premenopausal, ER and PR negative	**Chemotherapy[d]**
Postmenopausal, ER or PR positive	**Tamoxifen + chemotherapy[b]**
Postmenopausal, ER and PR negative	**Chemotherapy[d]**
Elderly	**Tamoxifen** If no ER and PR expression: **chemotherapy**

[a]ER = estrogen receptor; PR = progesterone receptor; GnRH = gonadotropin releasing hormone. Bold entries are treatments accepted for routine use or baseline in clinical trials.

[b]The addition of chemotherapy is considered an acceptable option based on evidence from clinical trials. Considerations about a low relative risk of relapse, age, toxic effects, socioeconomic implications, and information on patient's preference might justify the use of **tamoxifen alone.**

[c]Indicates treatments still being tested in randomized clinical trials.

[d]The addition of tamoxifen following chemotherapy might be considered for patients whose tumors are classified as ER and PR negative but which exhibit minimal/trace levels of either ER or PR.

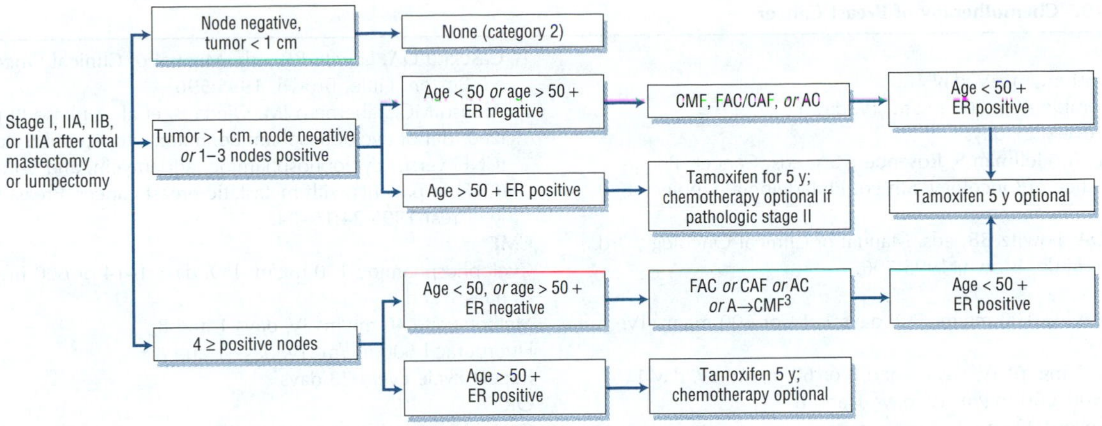

The NCCN guidelines are a statement of consensus of its authors regarding their views of currently accepted approaches to treatment. Any clinician seeking to apply or consult any NCCN guideline is expected to use independent medical judgment in the context of individual clinical circumstances to determine any patient's care or treatment. The National Comprehensive Cancer Network makes no warranties of any kind whatsoever regarding their content, use or application and disclaims any responsibility for their application or use in any way.

The NCCN Breast Cancer Practice Guidelines are a work in progress that will be refined as often as new significant data becomes available; 1997, 1998, and 1999 versions of the NCCN Breast Cancer Practice Guidelines are available.

FIGURE 116–4. NCCN Breast Cancer (Invasive) Guidelines for Adjuvant Treatment, Version 1, November 1996, Oncology Supplement, with permission. (Copyrighted by the National Comprehensive Cancer Network. All rights reserved. These guidelines and illustrations may not be reproduced in any form without the express written permission of the NCCN.)

lumpectomy. These more recent guidelines reflect the increasing trend toward the use of chemotherapy in postmenopausal (age over 50), as well as the well established premenopausal (< 50) patient, hormonal therapy in all hormone receptor–positive women regardless of age or menopausal status, and the combination of both chemotherapy and hormonal therapy.

Intensive research efforts are directed toward identifying those characteristics of the primary tumor (pathologic prognostic factors) that may predict for a higher or lower likelihood of metastases and death in node-negative patients. Although a multitude of prognostic factors are being investigated, no single factor or combination of factors sufficiently identifies those at risk of metastases or is sufficiently standardized to be reproducibly applicable to all patients. Furthermore, it cannot be assumed that patients with a poor prognosis have the same or greater likelihood of benefiting from adjuvant therapy. Certainly, decisions regarding adjuvant therapy, particularly in node-negative patients, should be individualized based on the estimated risk of relapse and death, the expected benefits of treatment, the toxicity of treatment, and the impact of therapy on quality of life. There is an increasing trend in clinical decision making to take hormone receptor status, nuclear grade, and tumor size into consideration in recommending adjuvant therapy. HER-2 is gaining acceptance as a predictor of poor prognosis and indicator of benefit from systemic adjuvant therapy. For a more in-depth discussion of the issues and controversies regarding adjuvant therapy of breast cancer, the reader is referred to several excellent references.[49–51] Adjuvant therapy of breast cancer is an emerging treatment; therefore, the most up-to-date information will be found only in the primary literature.

Adjuvant Chemotherapy

Cytotoxic drugs that have been used alone and in combination as adjuvant therapy in breast cancer include doxorubicin, cyclophosphamide, methotrexate, fluorouracil, melphalan, prednisone, and vincristine. The most common combination chemotherapy regimens employed in the adjuvant setting are listed in Table 116–9.

Combination chemotherapy regimens used in the adjuvant setting are essentially the same as regimens used for metastatic breast cancer. One important exception exists with respect to adjuvant treatment of breast cancer at the current time. In the past several years a number of recently marketed agents, the most notable being the taxanes paclitaxel and docetaxel, have demonstrated significant single-agent activity in metastatic breast cancer. Combination therapy with a taxane and anthracycline, cyclophosphamide, cisplatin, flurouracil, vinorelbine, and so on has shown high activity in phase II trials in treatment of metastatic disease. Some of these newer combinations are being investigated in randomized clinical trials in the adjuvant setting. However, it would be premature to move these newer combination regimens into the adjuvant setting in routine clinical practice at the current time.

The basic principle of adjuvant therapy for any cancer type is that the regimen with the highest response rate in advanced disease is the optimal regimen for use in the adjuvant setting. Early administration of effective combination chemotherapy at a time when the tumor burden is low should increase the likelihood of cure and minimize the emergence of drug-resistant tumor cell clones. Doxorubicin has historically been referred to as the most active single agent in the treatment of metastatic breast cancer. This has led to the assumption that doxorubicin-containing regimens are associated with a higher cure rate than non–doxorubicin-containing regimens when used in the adjuvant setting. An indirect comparison of the effects of adjuvant chemotherapy in 12 trials that used doxorubicin-containing regimens with results of trials in which cyclophosphamide, methotrexate, fluorouracil (CMF)-type regimens were used failed to show any significant advantage for the doxorubicin regimens.[52] However, significant overall survival advantage for patients randomized to the doxorubicin arm was observed in at least one of these studies, which most clearly demonstrated the value of doxorubicin in patients with four or more positive lymph nodes. In addition, several of these trials have demonstrated a DFS benefit. Additional follow-up is required to definitively evaluate the benefit of doxorubicin over non-doxorubicin in conventional dose adjuvant combination chemotherapy regimens. However, doxorubicin-containing regimens, or the sequential administration of doxorubicin alone for four cycles followed by CMF for eight cycles, are preferred by many oncologists for high-risk adjuvant patient groups.

Although the optimal duration of adjuvant chemotherapy administration is unknown, it appears to be on the order of 12 to

TABLE 116–9. Chemotherapy of Breast Cancer

AC

Doxorubicin 60 mg/m^2 IV, day 1
Cyclophosphamide 400–600 mg/m^2 IV, day 1
Repeat cycle every 21 days

1. In: DeVita VT, Hellman S, Rosenberg SA, eds. Cancer: Principles & Practice of Oncology, 5th ed. Philadelphia, Lippincott, 1997:1557.
2. Casciato DA, Lowitz BB, eds. Manual of Clinical Oncology, 3rd ed. Boston, Little, Brown, 1995:596.

CAF (FAC)

Cyclophosphamide 100 mg/m^2 PO, days 1–14 or 600 mg/m^2 IV, day 1
Doxorubicin 25 mg/m^2 IV, days 1 and 8 or 60 mg/m^2 IV, day 1
Fluorouracil 500–600 mg/m^2 IV, days 1 and 8
Repeat cycle every 28 days

1. Facts and Comparisons. May 1996:643a.
2. Chemotherapy Sourcebook, 2nd ed. 1996:845.
3. Smalley RV, Carpenter J, Bartolucci A, Vogel C, Krauss S. A comparison of cyclophosphamide, adriamycin, 5-fluorouracil (CAF) and cyclophosphamide, methotrexate, 5-fluorouracil, vincristine, prednisone (CMFVP) in patients with metastatic breast cancer. Cancer 1977;40:625–632.

OR

Cyclophosphamide 500 mg/m^2 IV, day 1
Doxorubicin 50 mg/m^2 IV, day 1
Fluorouracil 500 mg/m^2 IV, day 1[a]
Repeat cycle every 21 days

1. Finley RS. Neoplastic disorders. In: Young LL, Koda-Kimble MA, eds. Applied Therapeutics: The Clinical Use of Drugs, 6th ed. Vancouver, Applied Therapeutics, 1995:90–116.
2. Lindley CM. Breast cancer. In: DiPiro JT, Talbert RL, Yee GC, et al., eds. Pharmacotherapy, 3rd ed. Stanford, Appleton & Lange, 1996:2485.

CFM (CNF, FNC)

Cyclophosphamide 500–600 mg/m^2 IV, day 1
Fluorouracil 500–600 mg/m^2 IV, day 1
Mitoxantrone 10–12 mg/m^2 IV, day 1
Repeat cycle every 21 days

1. Casciato DA, Lowitz BB, eds. Manual of Clinical Oncology, 3rd ed. Boston, Little, Brown, 1995:596.
2. Alonso MC, Tabernero JM, Ojeda B, et al. A phase III randomized trial of cyclophosphamide, mitoxantone, and 5-fluorouracil (CNF) versus cyclophosphamide, adriamycin, and 5-fluorouracil (CAF) in patients with metastatic breast cancer. Breast Cancer Res Treat 1995;24:15–24.

CMF

Cyclophosphamide 100 mg/m^2 PO, days 1–14 or 600 mg/m^2 IV, days 1 and 8
Methotrexate 40 mg/m^2 IV, days 1 and 8
Fluorouracil 600 mg/m^2 IV, days 1 and 8
Repeat cycle every 28 days

OR

Cyclophosphamide 600 mg/m^2 IV, day 1
Methotrexate 40 mg/m^2 IV, day 1
Fluorouracil 600 mg/m^2 IV, day 1
Repeat cycle every 21 days

1. Chemotherapy Sourcebook, 2nd ed. 1996:1146.
2. Hall PD, Lesher BA, Hall RK. Adjuvant therapy of node-negative breast cancer. Ann Pharmacother 1995;29:292.

NFL

Mitoxantrone 12 mg/m^2 IV, day 1
Fluorouracil 350 mg/m^2 IV, days 1–3, given after leucovorin
Leucovorin 300 mg IV, over 1 hour, days 1–3

OR

Mitoxantrone 10 mg/m^2 IV, day 1
Fluorouracil 1000 $mg/m^2/d$ C1, days 1–3, given after leucovorin
Leucovorin 100 mg/m^2 IV, over 15 minutes, days 1–3
Repeat cycle every 21 days

1. Hainsworth JD, Andrews MB, Johnson DH, et al. Mitoxantrone, fluorouracil, and high-dose leucovorin: An effective, well-tolerated regimen for metastatic breast cancer. J Clin Oncol 1991;9:1732.

Sequential DOX-CMF

Doxorubicin 75 mg/m^2 IV, every 21 days for 4 cycles followed by 21 or 28 days CMF for 8 cycles

16 weeks. Chemotherapy is usually initiated within 3 weeks of surgical removal of the primary tumor. The use of "neoadjuvant chemotherapy" or "primary chemotherapy" prior to surgery and radiation, as discussed in the section on locally advanced breast cancer (stage III), is predominantly confined to clinical trials in stage I and II breast cancer at the current time. "Dose intensity" and "dose density" appear to be critical factors in achieving optimal outcomes in adjuvant breast cancer therapy. *Dose intensity* is defined as the amount of drug administered per unit of time and is typically reported in milligrams per square meter of body surface per week ($mg/m^2/wk$). Dose intensity may be increased by increasing dose, decreasing time, or both. *Dose density* is equivalent to the concept of increasing dose intensity, but not by increasing the numerator of the fraction $mg/m^2/time$, as occurs with dose escalation, but by decreasing the denominator of time. Retrospective analysis and prospective randomized trials support the importance of dose intensity and dose density in the treatment of breast cancer.[54] The Cancer and Leukemia Group B (CALGB) compared three dose intensities of cyclophosphamide, doxorubicin, and fluorouracil (CAF) in a randomized study and clearly established that the lower dose therapy was less effective. Another cooperative group study found that a dose dense doxorubicin-based regimen administered over 16 weeks demonstrated results superior to the CAF regimen. Bonadonna et al. reported that sequential use of doxorubicin followed by CMF is superior to the same drugs in alternations, perhaps because the dose intensity of each regimen is increased over the time it is given.[53] A dose dense regimen of doxorubicin, paclitaxel, and cyclophosphamide reported a remarkable low relapse rate of 17% at 36 months' median follow-up in a group of women at high risk of relapse (median node involvement > 8).[54] Thus, evidence is accumulating to support dose intensity and dose density in adjuvant chemotherapy of breast cancer. The relative importance of dose intensity versus dose density is unclear. It is similarly unclear what subset of patients benefit from administration of high-dose or dose-intense regimens.[54]

A major focus in clinical investigation is the use of more high-dose chemotherapy regimens as adjuvant therapy. Because bone marrow suppression is the dose-limiting toxicity for most chemotherapeutic agents, high-dose chemotherapy regimens followed by colony-stimulating factors (CSFs) or reinfusion of autologous bone marrow and/or peripheral blood progenitor cells have been developed. Trials to define the specific usefulness of high-dose regimens, as well as autologous stem cell transplantation in conjunction with dose-intense regimens, are justified given the positive response rates seen in the metastatic breast cancer setting and the very poor prognosis associated with stage II disease with 4 to 9 and, particularly, 10 or more positive axillary lymph nodes. Several cooperative groups are conducting trials of high-dose chemotherapy versus conventional adjuvant therapy, although none of the trials have shown a significant difference to date. However, use of high-dose chemotherapy outside

TABLE 116–9. (Continued)

1. Bonadonna G, Zambetti M, Valagussa P. Sequential or alternating doxorubicin and CMF regimens in breast cancer with more than three positive nodes. JAMA 1995;273:542–543.

VATH

Vinblastine 4.5 mg/m^2 IV, day 1
Doxorubicin 45 mg/m^2 IV, day 1
Thiotepa 12 mg/m^2 IV, day 1
Fluoxymesterone 10 mg PO tid
Repeat cycle every 21 days

1. Skeel RT. Carcinoma of the breast. In: Skeel RT, Lachant NA, eds. Handbook of Cancer Chemotherapy, 4th ed. Boston, Little, Brown, 1995:283.
1. Chemotherapy Sourcebook, 2nd ed. 1996:848.

Vinorelbine
Doxorubicin

Vinorelbine 25 mg/m^2 IV, days 1 and 8
Doxorubicin 50 mg/m^2 IV, day 1
Repeat cycle every 21 days

1. Spielman M, Dorval T, Turpin F, et al. Phase II trial of vinorelbine/doxorubicin as first-line therapy of advanced breast cancer. J Clin Oncol 1994;12:1764–1770.

Single-Agent Regimens

Anastrozole

Anastrozole 1 mg PO daily

1. Anastrozole, a potent and selective aromatase inhibitor, versus megestrol acetate in postmenopausal women with advanced breast cancer: Results of overview analysis of two phase III trials. J Clin Oncol 1996;14:2000–2011.

Docetaxel

Docetaxel 60–100 mg/m^2 IV, over 1 hour, every 21 days
Concomitant dexamethasone 8 mg PO bid for 5 days, begin 1 day before docetaxel

1. Taxotere® (docetaxel) product information. Rhone Poulenc Rorer: Collegeville, PA. May 1996.

Gemcitabine

Gemcitabine 725 mg/m^2 IV, over 30 minutes, weekly for 3 weeks, followed by 1-week rest
Repeat cycle every 28 days

1. Carmichael J, Possinger K, Phillip P, et al. Advanced breast cancer: A phase II trial with gemcitabine. J Clin Oncol 1995; 13:2731–2736.
2. Carmichael J, Walling J. Phase II activity of gemcitabine in advanced breast cancer. Semin Oncol 1996;23(suppl 10):77–86.

Megestrol

Megestrol 40 mg PO qid

1. Bozdar A, Jonat W, Howell A, et al. Anastrozole, a potent and selective aromatase inhibitor, versus megestrol acetate in postmenopausal women with advanced breast cancer: Results of overview analysis of two phase III trials. J Clin Oncol 1996;14:2000–2011.

Paclitaxel[b]

Paclitaxel[b] 250 mg/m^2 IV, over 3 or 24 hours, every 21 days
OR
Paclitaxel[b] 175 mg/m^2 IV, over 3 hours, every 21 days

1. Seidman AD, Tiersten A, et al. Phase II trial of paclitaxel by 3 hour infusion as initial and salvage chemotherapy for metastatic breast cancer. J Clin Oncol 1995;13:2575–2581.
2. Taxol® (Paclitaxel) product information. Bristol Myers: Illinois, April 1994.

Tamoxifen

Tamoxifen 20 mg PO daily

1. Nolvadex® (Tamoxifen) product information. Zeneca Pharmaceuticals.

Vinorelbine

Vinorelbine 30 mg/m^2 IV, every 7 days

1. Fumoleau P, Delozier T, Extra JM, et al. Vinorelbine in the treatment of breast cancer. Semin Oncol 1995;22:(suppl 5):22.
2. Navelbine® (Vinorelbine) product information. Glaxo Wellcome: Research Triangle Park, December 1994.

[a]Also given day 8 with FAC.

of a clinical trial is rapidly being adopted by the oncology community and although the impact of high-dose therapy on survival and quality of life is unknown, breast cancer is the most common indication for high-dose chemotherapy in North America.[54]

The short-term toxic effects of chemotherapy used in the adjuvant setting are generally well tolerated. Although a number of investigators have demonstrated a reduction in quality of life, most patients are able to maintain a reasonable level of function and emotional and social well-being during treatment.[55] In general, supportive therapy of the patient receiving systemic adjuvant chemotherapy has improved in the past decade. Increased attention to the impact of symptoms on quality of life may account for some of this improvement. In addition, serotonin-antagonist antiemetics have become available to assist in managing chemotherapy-induced nausea and vomiting, and CSFs are often helpful in preventing febrile neutropenia, particularly in elderly patients or patients receiving high-dose and dose-intense chemotherapy regimens. However, a number of side effects are common with the regimens employed and patients should be appropriately counseled regarding the likelihood of alopecia, weight gain, and fatigue. Patients who are menstruating will experience a cessation of menses that may or may not return. Along with cessation of menses are accompanying signs and symptoms of menopause. Deep vein thrombosis has been reported in women receiving combination chemotherapy regimens.[56] A recent study estimated that about 1 to 10 of 10,000 patients treated for 6 months with cyclophosphamide-based regimens might be expected to have leukemia within 10 years of diagnosis of breast cancer.[57]

Cardiomyopathy induced by doxorubicin occurs less than 1% of the time in women whose total dose is less than 320 mg/m^2 of body surface area.[58] Toxicities associated with the chemotherapy regimens employed in the experimental autologous bone marrow transplant and/or peripheral blood progenitor cell transplant programs are likely to be greater than those incurred with the standard adjuvant chemotherapy regimens described.

A final note before leaving the topic of adjuvant chemotherapy in stage I and II breast cancer: As discussed previously, the magnitude of survival benefit for chemotherapy appears to be small, with an absolute odds reduction in mortality of only 5% at 10 years for patients with negative axillary lymph nodes and 10% for patients with positive axillary lymph nodes. In addition, there is currently no means to identify patients who will attain this survival benefit. However, two investigators have reported that most patients with breast cancer would accept severe toxicity from treatment to achieve as little as a 1% to 5% improvement in survival.[59,60] Therefore, in the absence of the ability to predict who will benefit, it is likely that all patients with stage I and II breast cancer will opt for adjuvant chemotherapy treatment.

Adjuvant Endocrine Therapy

Hormonal therapies that have been studied in the treatment of primary or early breast cancer include oophorectomy, ovarian irradiation, tamoxifen, and luteinizing hormone–releasing hormone (LHRH) agonists.

Tamoxifen is currently the adjuvant hormonal therapy of choice. Tamoxifen has been used in the adjuvant setting for three decades. Tamoxifen is antiestrogenic in breast cancer cells, but it appears to have estrogenic properties in other tissues and organs.[61,62] Although its major mechanism of action has been attributed to its ability to block hormone receptors, studies have shown that the drug is capable of stimulating the production of transforming growth factor β, an inhibitory growth factor that could in fact inhibit the growth of estrogen receptor-positive and -negative cancer cells. In the laboratory, tamoxifen has also been shown to reduce angiogenesis. It does this presumably by decreasing local stimulatory growth factors, thus creating a hostile environment for tumor cells. Women receiving adjuvant tamoxifen therapy have a reduced incidence of development of contralateral breast cancer compared to women not receiving adjuvant tamoxifen therapy.[45] This, coupled with evidence of tamoxifen's beneficial estrogenic effects on the cardiovascular system and bone density, has led to tamoxifen being the hormonal agent of choice, not only in the adjuvant setting but in the treatment of metastatic disease as well.

The optimal dose of tamoxifen appears to be 20 mg/d. Owing to the long biologic half-life of tamoxifen, this can be administered as a single daily dose. Adjuvant tamoxifen therapy is generally initiated shortly after surgery or as soon as pathology results are known and the decision to administer tamoxifen as adjuvant therapy is made. An exception to this may be in women who receive combined chemo–endocrine therapy in whom, for the reasons described earlier, tamoxifen therapy is postponed until chemotherapy is completed. The optimal duration of tamoxifen therapy in the adjuvant setting has not been defined. Although most current recommendations suggest 5 years of tamoxifen therapy, there is a growing trend in practice toward continuing tamoxifen for more than 5 years. Data currently do not exist to support the use of prolonged courses of tamoxifen (> 5 years) in the adjuvant setting. However, a number of studies are ongoing that will provide this information within the next 5 years. As discussed in a subsequent section, tamoxifen is currently being studied for its value as a chemopreventive agent in women at high risk for developing breast cancer (see section on Prevention and Early Detection). Women with a personal history of breast cancer are clearly at high risk for the development of a subsequent breast cancer. If the results of the chemoprevention trials under way are positive, it may become standard to continue the administration of adjuvant tamoxifen therapy for life.

Tamoxifen is usually well tolerated. Symptoms of estrogen withdrawal (hot flashes and vaginal bleeding) are the most troublesome but decrease in frequency and intensity over time.

Nonspecific CNS symptoms such as depression, irritability, headache, insomnia, lethargy, and dizziness have been rarely observed in women taking tamoxifen. Thromboembolic disease (i.e., deep vein thrombosis and pulmonary embolism) has been reported to occur occasionally, although a causal relationship is not well established. Currently available data from adjuvant trials indicate a possible increase in, but low overall incidence of, thromboembolic disorders (1% to 3%) with the use of tamoxifen. Ocular effects, including corneal changes, optic neuritis, retinopathy, and macular edema have been associated with very high-dose tamoxifen (> 180 mg/d) but are rarely seen in patients receiving 30 mg/d. When used in the metastatic setting, a flare of bone pain and hypercalcemia occasionally occur, particularly in patients with bone metastases. This does not occur in the adjuvant setting. Of particular importance are concerns about carcinoma of the liver and endometrium in women receiving tamoxifen.[63] Proliferation of the endometrium, an estrogenic effect of tamoxifen, appears to be dose dependent and related to the duration of therapy. The incidence of endometrial cancer has been highest in patients receiving doses of 40 mg/d for at least 2 years. However, the results of six trials using tamoxifen doses of 20 mg/d, continuously for 5 years, found a twofold increase (i.e., 1 per 1000 to 2 per 1000 tamoxifen-treated women per year) in endometrial cancer in women receiving tamoxifen compared to women receiving placebo.[63] This twofold increase in risk of endometrial cancer is similar in magnitude to that associated with postmenopausal estrogen replacement therapy. Arguments are made that this risk is acceptable because the endometrial cancer induced by tamoxifen is low stage and low grade, is easily treated with surgery or other means, and does not pose a life-threatening risk to women. A number of new antiestrogens are in development that reportedly lack tamoxifen's estrogenic effects on the uterus. There have been no reports of liver cancer in patients receiving tamoxifen 20 mg/d and only two in patients receiving 40 mg/d. The carcinogenic potential of tamoxifen is of some concern in the adjuvant and chemoprevention settings. Annual gynecologic exams and education regarding the importance of immediately reporting vaginal bleeding to primary physicians for further evaluation are important counseling points to women receiving adjuvant tamoxifen therapy. These would not be concerns in the metastatic breast cancer setting owing to the short length of survival associated with metastatic breast cancer.

LOCALLY ADVANCED BREAST CANCER (STAGE III)

Locally advanced cancer of the breast refers to breast carcinomas with significant primary tumor and nodal disease but in which distant metastases cannot be documented. This stage of breast cancer has been shown to be poorly controlled by surgery alone and to have a poor prognosis. Patients may present with a wide spectrum of disease, ranging from large tumors to skin or chest wall involvement, sometimes associated with advanced regional lymph node tumor involvement. Many patients with stage III breast cancer have disease that is technically unresectable at diagnosis. Inflammatory breast cancer with pathologic evidence of dermal lymphatic tumor permeation with clinical findings of diffuse erythema in duration and edema of at least 30% of the breast usually without a palpable mass is a special type of locally advanced breast cancer.

Local-regional therapy of locally advanced breast cancer consists of surgery, radiation, or a combination of the two. The reported local recurrence rate ranges from 6% to 40% with mastectomy alone, and with radiation alone 25% to 50%. Survival with either modality is about 40% to 50% at 5 years and 30% at 10 years.[5] Radiation therapy can be effective in controlling these locally advanced cancers, but doses greater than those used to treat early stage tumors are required. Whereas 5000 cGy is effective in irradicating microscopic amounts of tumor in breast-conservation techniques, doses in excess of 6000 cGy are required for gross tumor. These higher doses of radiation therapy are associated with moderate to severe arm edema, brachial plexopathy, and adverse cosmetic effects such as breast retraction and telangiectasia. The results from a number of trials suggest that there is no advantage for mastectomy over primary radiation therapy in patients with stage III disease. The benefit of combining mastectomy and postoperative radiation for patients with locally advanced breast cancer is controversial. Retrospective studies of patients treated with a combination of mastectomy and radiation have shown excellent local tumor control (local-regional recurrence 10% to 20%) in 5 years compared with mastectomy or radiation alone (15% to 40%), but demonstration of a definitive impact on survival is lacking. Addition of radiation to mastectomy to improve local tumor control must be balanced against the possible increase and likelihood of complications. Unfortunately, similar to early breast cancer, distant metastases are the ultimate cause of death.

In the early 1980s, reports began to appear in the literature describing improvement in local-regional tumor control, DFS, and, in some instances, overall survival with combinations of multiagent chemotherapy, surgery, and radiation.[5] The natural history of locally advanced breast cancer suggested that even when local-regional control was accomplished, systemic relapse and death from breast cancer were eventually observed in the majority of patients. This led to interest in the use of "neoadjuvant" or "primary" chemotherapy in locally advanced breast cancer. Neoadjuvant or primary chemotherapy is the administration of systemic chemotherapy prior to a definitive local-regional procedure. Early aggressive systemic therapy has been used to control micrometastases, reduce tumor bulk, and allow for more limited procedures for local control. Primary or neoadjuvant chemotherapy followed by surgery with radiation therapy or both, and adjuvant systemic therapy has become the treatment choice for locally advanced breast cancer, including inflammatory breast cancer. Most tumors respond with more than a 50% decrease in tumor size; approximately 70% of patients experience downstaging through neoadjuvant chemotherapy. Breast conservation is possible for many patients with locally advanced breast cancer, and almost all patients initially are rendered disease free.

Although it is clear that neoadjuvant chemotherapy should be the initial choice of treatment for patients with locally advanced breast cancer, it is unclear what the optimal sequence of subsequent therapies should be, whether one or two local treatment modalities are necessary, and whether the addition of hormonal therapy to chemotherapy has significant benefit. The use of neoadjuvant treatment strategies for early breast cancer is currently under evaluation. One of the research directions to improve the survival of patients with locally advanced breast cancer is dose intensification of neoadjuvant or postoperative (adjuvant) chemotherapy. Several reports of open phase II trials have suggested an early benefit in DFS, but no definite survival benefits have been reported. However, comparative trials are necessary to assess the relative value of dose intensification in this group of patients.

METASTATIC BREAST CANCER (STAGE IV)

The goal of therapy with early and locally advanced breast cancer is to cure the disease. However, breast cancer is currently incurable once it has advanced beyond a local-regional disease. The goal of treatment of metastatic breast cancer is to improve symptoms and quality of life. Thus, it is important to choose therapy with good activity while minimizing toxicities. Treatment of metastatic breast cancer with either cytotoxic or endocrine therapy often results in regression of disease and improvements in quality of life. In patients who respond to therapy, duration of survival is also increased. The choice of therapy for metastatic disease is based on the site of disease involvement and presence or absence of certain characteristics. For example, patients who experience a long DFS following local-regional therapy, or have disease that is primarily located in the bone or soft tissue, or are late premenopausal or postmenopausal will likely respond to endocrine therapy. The most important factor predicting response to endocrine therapy is the presence of estrogen and progesterone receptors in the primary tumor tissue. Fifty percent to sixty percent of ER-positive patients and 75% to 80% of ER- and PR-positive patients will respond to hormonal therapy, while those with ER- and PR-negative tumors have a less than 10% response rate. Thus, the largest factor determining choice of endocrine versus cytotoxic chemotherapy is the presence of hormone receptors in the primary breast tumor. Site of disease is also important in that numerous studies have shown that endocrine therapy is more likely to be effective in patients with bone and soft tissue metastases. Visceral involvement (e.g., liver) and central nervous system involvement are generally nonresponsive to hormonal therapy and seldom respond to chemotherapy. Endocrine therapy is the treatment of choice for patients who are hormone receptor positive and exhibit the first sign of metastatic disease in soft tissue, bone, or pleura owing to the equal probability of response to hormonal compared to chemotherapy and the lower toxicity profile of endocrine therapy.

Patients who respond to initial endocrine therapy often respond to a second hormonal manipulation. Response rate is lower and duration of response is shorter with second hormonal manipulations. Patients are sequentially treated with endocrine therapy until they have progressive symptoms resulting from advancing metastatic disease, at which time cytotoxic chemotherapy can be given. Combinations of hormonal therapies or chemotherapy plus hormones are not employed in the setting of metastatic breast cancer. Women with hormone receptor–negative tumors, with rapidly progressive lung, liver, or bone marrow involvement, or having failed initial endocrine therapy are not likely to benefit from endocrine therapy and are usually treated initially with cytotoxic chemotherapy.

ENDOCRINE THERAPY

In general, there is little evidence that the response or survival benefit from one endocrine therapy is superior to that achieved with other therapies. Antiestrogens, aromatase inhibitors, progestins, estrogens, and androgens, as well as surgical procedures including oophorectomy, adrenalectomy, and hypophysectomy, have been shown to be equivalent in many randomized trials in patients with metastatic breast cancer. Because most endocrine therapies are equally effective, the choice of a particular one is based primarily on toxicity (Table 116–10). In women who received tamoxifen as adjuvant therapy, tamoxifen is still usually the preferred initial agent when metastases are present. An exception to this occurs when the patient is receiving adjuvant tamoxifen at the time or within 1 year of occurrence of metastatic disease. In these cases, either a progestin or an aromatase inhibitor is generally employed.

Tamoxifen is generally considered to be the agent of choice in both premenopausal and postmenopausal women with metastatic breast cancer who are also hormone receptor positive. Tamoxifen is usually administered in doses of 10 mg twice daily or 20 mg once daily. There is no advantage for higher doses of tamoxifen. Moreover, long-term administration of very high doses of tamoxifen (e.g., 12 months of 60 to 100 mg/m^2 twice daily) have been associated with decreased visual acuity and retinopathy.

A dose schedule of tamoxifen 20 mg/d reaches a steady-state concentration after about 4 minutes of therapy at about week 16. The half-life of a single dose of tamoxifen is 9 to 12 hours, but after chronic dosing is 7 days. Serum tamoxifen concentrations can be detected 6 weeks after discontinuation of therapy. Thus, the maximum beneficial effects of tamoxifen are not observed for at least 2 months following initiation of therapy and it is unlikely that symptoms of metastatic disease will return if patients miss several doses. The toxicities of tamoxifen are described in the Adjuvant Endocrine Therapy section of this chapter. The only additional toxicity that one might expect to find in the setting of metastatic breast cancer is a tumor flare or hypercalcemia, which occurs in approximately 5% of patients following the initiation of any endocrine therapy and is not an indication to discontinue tamoxifen therapy. It is generally accepted that this is a positive indication that the patient will respond to endocrine therapy.

No difference has been found in two randomized trials of the overall response rate between tamoxifen and oophorectomy in premenopausal women. However, the secondary response rate to oophorectomy after tamoxifen treatment was somewhat higher than to tamoxifen after primary oophorectomy (33% vs 11%).[64] This has been interpreted by some experts as suggesting that tamoxifen does not completely antagonize estrogen production, particularly in premenopausal women. Ovarian ablation (surgically

TABLE 116–10. Endocrine Therapies Used for Metastatic Breast Cancer

Class	Drug	Dose	Side Effects
Antiestrogens	Tamoxifen Toremifene	10–20 mg PO bid 60 mg qd	Disease flare, hot flashes, nausea, vomiting, edema, thromboembolism, endometrial cancer
LHRH analogs	Leuprolide Goserelin	7.5 mg SC q28d 3.6 mg SC q28d	Amenorrhea, hot flashes, occasional nausea
Progestins	Medroxyprogesterone acetate Megestrol acetate	400–1000 mg IM qwk	Weight gain, hot flashes, vaginal bleeding, edema, thromoembolism
Aromatase inhibitors	Anastrazole Letrozole Aminoglutethimide	1 mg qd 2.5 mg qd 250 mg PO qid w/hydrocortisone 40 mg/d	Lethargy, rash, postural dizziness, ataxia, nystagmus, nausea
Estrogens	Ethinylestradiol Conjugated estrogens	1 mg PO tid 2.5 mg PO tid	Nausea/vomiting, fluid retention, hot flashes, anorexia, thromboembolism, hepatic dysfunction
Androgens	Fluoxymesterone	10 mg PO bid	Deepening voice, alopecia, hirsutism, facial/truncal acne, fluid retention, menstrual irregularities, cholestatic jaundice

or chemically) is still commonly used in some parts of the United States and is considered by many specialists to be the endocrine therapy of choice in premenopausal women. The mortality rate with surgical oophorectomy is low, usually less than 2% to 3% in appropriately selected patients. Chemical castration with LHRH analogs is increasingly used in lieu of oophorectomy in premenopausal women. In postmenopausal patients, response rate to surgical oophorectomy was inferior to tamoxifen and, thus, oophorectomy is not employed in this group.

Medical castration with LHRH analogs has been used in premenopausal metastatic breast cancer patients and induces remission in about one-third of unselected cases. The mechanism of action of LHRH analogs in breast cancer is thought to result from downregulation of LHRH receptors in the pituitary. Decreased levels of luteinizing hormone subsequently lead to a decrease in estrogen to castrated levels. Thus, the effect of LHRH analogs on circulating estrogen levels in premenopausal breast cancer simulates oophorectomy. The two agents available in the United States are leuprolide and goserelin. Both of these agents are administered as a subcutaneous injection every 4 weeks and are associated with minimal side effects including amenorrhea, hot flashes, and occasional nausea. Studies of oophorectomy, tamoxifen, or LHRH analogs as first-line therapy in premenopausal patients with metastatic breast cancer are necessary to determine the definitive choice for initial therapy. Combination endocrine therapy with tamoxifen or an aromatase inhibitor plus an LHRH analog is also under investigation. The rationale behind this combination is that tamoxifen and aromatase inhibitors interfere with peripheral estradiol production and the LHRH analog interferes with ovarian estradiol production.

A number of antiestrogens are currently in development for the treatment of breast cancer.[65,66] The goal of these newer compounds is to maintain the beneficial effects of tamoxifen's antagonism at breast cells, as well as its estrogenic properties on bone density and lipid profile, while avoiding the estrogenic effect of tamoxifen on the endometrium. There are currently two types of antiestrogens in development, the triphenylethylenes, which include toremifene, droloxifene, idoxifene, and raloxifene, and the pure antiestrogens. The pure antiestrogens differ from the triphenylethylene (tamoxifen-like) antiestrogens in their chemical structure, pharmacology, and biologic activity. Toremifene was approved in May of 1997 for the treatment of metastatic breast cancer in postmenopausal women with estrogen receptor positive or unknown tumors. Efficacy data were based on three trials in a total of 1500 postmenopausal metastatic breast cancer patients comparing 60 mg of toremifene to either 20 mg or 40 mg of tamoxifen. The primary efficacy variables included response rate and time to progression. Survival was also determined. Two of the three studies showed similar results for all effectiveness end points, although one study did show a longer time to progression for tamoxifen. Incidences of adverse effects were comparable between the two medications. Data to support the use of toremifene in the adjuvant setting, or in premenopausal women, are currently lacking. Data are insufficient to allow evaluation of the long-term toxicity of toremifene, and it is still unknown if toremifene will differ from tamoxifen with respect to endometrial cancer and bone mineralization. Cross-resistance to toremifene has been demonstrated in patients with tamoxifen-refractory disease. Therefore, at the current time, toremifene appears to be an alternative to tamoxifen in postmenopausal patients with positive or unknown hormone receptor status with metastatic breast cancer. Costs of the two products are equivalent.

Raloxifene, also a member of the triphenylethylene-type of antiestrogen, received approval in December 1997 for prevention of osteoporosis in postmenopausal women. The manufacturer of raloxifene refers to this agent as a selective estrogen receptor modulator based on its estrogenic agonist activity in the skeleton and on lipid metabolism and estrogen antagonist action in the breast and uterus. This product is being marketed as an alternative to hormone replacement therapy for patients concerned about breast and endometrial cancer. Conjugated estrogen administration is associated with increased risk of breast cancer, endometrial hypoplasia, and endometrial cancer. Preliminary data indicate that raloxifene is not associated with development of breast or endometrial cancer. The role of raloxifene in the treatment of patients with metastatic breast cancer is currently unknown.

Antiestrogens bind to estrogen receptors and prevent receptor-mediated gene transcription and are therefore used to block the effect of estrogen on the end target. In postmenopausal and castrated women, the main source of estrogen is derived from the peripheral conversion of androstenedione, produced by the adrenal gland, into estrone and estradiol. This conversion requires the aromatase enzyme. Aromatase also catalyzes the conversion of androgens to estrogens in the ovary in premenopausal women and in extraglandular tissue, including the breast itself, in postmenopausal women. Therefore, aromatase inhibitors would effectively reduce the level of circulating estrogens, as well as that in the target organ. Aminoglutethimide is the prototype aromatase inhibitor. Aminoglutethimide has been compared to tamoxifen, adrenalectomy, and hypophysectomy in randomzied trials. In general, response rates are equivalent, but in several trials, aminoglutethimide appeared to be more effective than tamoxifen.[67] Aminoglutethimide has been demonstrated to produce secondary response rates equivalent or superior to progestational agents and surgical procedures in women who have become refractory to tamoxifen. Although effective, a significant limitation of aminoglutethimide is its toxicity profile. Aminoglutethimide inhibits the adrenal conversion of cholesterol to pregnenolone, resulting in a decrease in androstenedione and, thus, glucocorticosteroids. For this reason, aminoglutethimide has been traditionally administered concurrently with hydrocortisone, 40 mg/d divided into three doses at 3 PM, 6 PM, and 10 PM. The rationale behind this dosage administration of hydrocortisone is that it mimics the natural cortisol production and thereby prevents the suppression of hypothalamic–pituitary axis. Side effects of aminoglutethimide include nystagmus, ataxia, lethargy, dizziness, nausea, and rash. Although aminoglutethimide has historically been very effective in the treatment of women with metastatic breast cancer, its use has been considered third-line owing to its toxicity profile.

In 1997, two nonsteroidal aromatase inhibitors, anastrozole and letrozole, were introduced to the U.S. market.[68] Both have far greater selectivity and higher potency for the aromatase enzyme than aminoglutethimide. Additional agents are in development. The major advantage of these newer compounds is their reduced toxicity profile, which consists mainly of nausea, hot flashes, and mild fatigue. Supplemental corticosteroids are not necessary with these newer agents. The new inhibitors have been compared with megesterol as second-line therapy in postmenopausal women with positive or unknown hormone receptor status who have failed tamoxifen. Response rates throughout these studies have varied widely between 10% to 30% and have typically shown similar antitumor activity as megesterol. In one study, a higher response rate and an improved time to treatment failure were documented for letrozole.[69] Toxicity patterns showed more nausea, vomiting, and hot flashes with the aromatase inhibitor and more weight gain and fluid retention with progestone. Studies that have compared anastrozole and letrozole to tamoxifen or toremifene in first-line therapy of patients with metastatic disease have not been conducted to date.

Progestins such as megesterol acetate (Megace) and medroxyprogesterone acetate (Provera) have been compared with tamoxifen in randomized trials and have been found to yield equal response rates. Although there were no direct comparisons of these two forms of progestational therapy, they appear to be equally effective. Medroxyprogesterone acetate is more frequently used in Europe and megesterol acetate in the United States. A number of recent trials have suggested that progestins may be an alternative to first-line therapy with tamoxifen. The most common dose used for medroxyprogesterone is 160 mg/d, and weight gain, occurring in 20% to 50%, is the most common side effect. Patients experiencing weight gain may have fluid retention, but fluid retention is not totally responsible for total weight gain. In cachectic cancer patients, the weight gain may be desirable, but this is not uniformly true of all patients with metastatic breast cancer. Additional side effects associated with progestins include vaginal bleeding in 5% to 10% of patients either while patients are taking the progestational agent or when it is discontinued, and somewhat less than a 10% incidence of hot flashes.

Estrogens and androgens are used rarely today because these agents are more toxic than the other hormonal agents discussed thus far. Approximately one-third of patients placed on estrogens will discontinue them because of side effects, the most important of which are vomiting and fluid retention. Less common side effects include areolar hyperpigmentation, breast tenderness and engorgement, vaginal discharge, incontinence, hot flashes, and phlebitis. All the effective androgens have masculinizing effects, including hirsutism and acne, in more than 50% of patients. In addition to their toxicities, the mechanism by which these agents exert a therapeutic effect in breast cancer is unknown. Approximately 20% response rates were reported in clinical trials conducted in the 1960s and 1970s in unselected groups of breast cancer patients. Given the recent availability of the aromatase inhibitors, use of androgens and estrogens will likely become obsolete.

CYTOTOXIC THERAPY

Cytotoxic chemotherapy will eventually be required in most patients with metastatic breast cancer. Patients with hormone receptor–negative tumors require chemotherapy as initial therapy of symptomatic metastases. Patients who initially respond to hormonal manipulations will eventually cease to respond and go on to require chemotherapy. Combination chemotherapy results in an objective response in approximately two-thirds of patients previously unexposed to chemotherapy. The majority of patients have partial responses, and complete disappearance of disease occurs in fewer than 20% of patients treated. The median duration of response is 5 to 12 months, but some patients will have an excellent response to an initial course of chemotherapy and may live 5 to more than 10 years without evidence of disease. In general, median survival of patients after treatment with commonly used drug combinations for metastatic breast cancer is 14 to 33 months. The median time to response has ranged from 2 to 3 months in most studies, but this period is dependent in large part on the site of measurable disease. The median time to appearance of response is between 3 and 6 weeks in patients whose disease is primarily in the skin and lymph nodes, 6 and 9 weeks for patients with metastatic lung involvement, 15 weeks with hepatic involvement, and nearly 18 weeks in patients with bone involvement. Thus, it is oftentimes the case that an immediate response to therapy is not apparent and, in general, once a chemotherapy regimen has been initiated, it is continued until there is unequivocal evidence of progressive disease.

There are no well-defined clinical characteristics or established tests to identify patients likely to benefit from chemotherapy. Factors associated with an increased probability of response that have been identified include a good performance status, a limited number (one to two) of disease sites, and patients who respond to chemotherapy or hormonal therapy with a long disease-free interval. Patients whose disease progresses during chemotherapy have a lower probability of response to a different type of chemotherapy. However, this is not necessarily true for patients who are given chemotherapy after some interval during which they have received no chemotherapy. Patients who do not respond to endocrine therapy are as likely to respond to chemotherapy as patients who are treated with chemotherapy as their initial treatment modality. Age, menopausal status, and receptor status have not been associated with favorable or unfavorable response to chemotherapy. Although, in general, site of disease is not a predictor of response to chemotherapy, patients with visceral disease involvement typically respond poorly to chemotherapy, as well as hormonal therapy.

A number of chemotherapeutic agents have demonstrated activity in the treatment of breast cancer, including doxorubicin, cyclophosphamide, fluorouracil, methotrexate, mitoxantrone, vinblastine, mitomycin-C, thiotepa, and melphalan. The objective response rates reported with these drugs as single-agent therapy range from 20% to 40%. The drug discovery program of the National Cancer Institute and the pharmaceutical industry have recently provided oncologists with a wide array of new chemotherapeutic agents that have considerable potential for breast cancer treatment. Foremost among these new agents are paclitaxel and docetaxel, which have impressive single-agent response rates of up to 50% to 60% in patients with metastatic breast disease who have not received prior chemotherapy for metastatic disease.[70] In the spring of 1994, paclitaxel (Taxol) was approved by the FDA for single-agent treatment of metastatic breast cancer for patients who had relapsed following therapy with a doxorubicin-containing regimen. The recommended dose of paclitaxel is 175 mg/m^2 every 21 days, which is considerably higher than the dose used for treatment of ovarian cancer, the other disease for which paclitaxel has obtained FDA approval for use. Efforts are now being directed toward optimizing dose and schedule of single-agent paclitaxel in the metastatic setting. Recent reports describe a dose-dense regimen of 175 mg/m^2/wk (6 weeks, rest 2 weeks) with exceptional response rates.[71] Docetaxel (Taxotere) has also demonstrated high single-agent activity against metastatic breast cancer. It was approved by the FDA in the winter of 1995 for treatment of metastatic breast cancer for patients with relapse following therapy with doxorubicin-containing regimens. The approved dose is 60 to 100 mg/m^2 administered every 3 weeks. Impressive overall response rates of 54% to 68% were reported in four studies of docetaxel 100 mg/m^2 as first-line chemotherapy. Although randomized controlled studies comparing doses in the 60 to 100 mg/m^2 range have not been performed, a dose–response relationship with docetaxel has been demonstrated indirectly and, therefore, the importance of maintaining dose intensity with this agent is recognized. Myelosuppression is the major dose-limiting toxicity of docetaxel. Nonhematologic toxicities include fatigue, mucosal toxicity, mild to moderate nausea/vomiting, diarrhea, and neurosensory complaints. Although randomized comparative data are not yet available, docetaxel seems to be associated with less neuropathy, myalgia, and hypersensitivity than paclitaxel; but febrile neutropenia, fluid retention, and skin reactions appear to occur more frequently with the newer taxane. The median cumulative docetaxel dose to the onset of fluid retention is 400 mg/m^2 in nonpremedicated patients. Recent data demonstrate that the prophylactic use of dexamethasone 8 mg orally, twice a day for 3 to 5 days, starting 24 hours before docetaxel infusion can significantly delay the onset and reduce the severity of fluid retention.

Vinorelbine (Navelbine), a microtubule interactive agent, has also shown impressive response rates in metastatic breast cancer.[72] Vinorelbine was approved by the FDA in December 1994 for the treatment of non–small cell lung cancer. It is not yet approved for breast cancer; however, response rates in patients with advanced breast cancer to weekly IV doses of 30 mg/m^2 of vinorelbine range from 30% to 50% with an overall 5% complete response rate in the phase I and II studies reported. As has been observed with paclitaxel and docetaxel, patients with less prior treatment fare better than those who are more heavily pretreated. Importantly, paclitaxel, docetaxel, and vinorelbine display evidence of not being cross-resistant with anthracyclines, which are currently considered first-line in treatment of metastatic breast cancer.

Combination chemotherapy regimens have been associated with higher response rates than single-agent therapy in the treatment of metastatic breast cancer. The chemotherapy regimens frequently used first-line in the metastatic setting are similar to the ones previously described for the adjuvant setting. As discussed above, the taxanes and vinorelbine have demonstrated unusually high activity as single agents in metastatic disease. Initial clinical trials of new cytotoxic agents involve patients who have experienced disease progression after treatment with the best available therapy. If the new drugs prove efficacious in these very poor-prognosis patients, trials will progress to patients with no prior treatment. Docetaxel, paclitaxel, and vinorelbine are currently moving into first-line treatment of metastatic breast cancer, oftentimes in combination with anthracyclines. When cytotoxic drugs are used in combination, it is important to consider the dose–response relationship and the toxicity profiles of the agents involved. It often is necessary to reduce the dose of drugs given in combination to avoid excessive toxicity, which may also inadvertently result in the administration of suboptimal doses. The emerging role of the taxanes and their optimal integration into new combination treatment strategies for patients with metastatic breast cancers is a major focus of research. Specific information regarding the most promising combination regimens and their attendant toxicities can be found only in the primary literature. In addition to determining the combination chemotherapy regimen of first, second, and third choice, other issues that remain to be determined in the management of metastatic breast cancer with systemic chemotherapy include optimal duration of treatment. Recognizing that complete response is not frequently observed, typically patients will receive one chemotherapy regimen until evidence of disease progression, at which time a second regimen may be initiated.

There is an undeniable dose–response effect for most of the drugs used to treat breast cancer. Research innovations designed to improve the efficacy of combination chemotherapy have included the use of high doses of drugs. Very high doses of single agents or combinations have been used with autologous bone marrow or peripheral blood progenitor cell support to circumvent dose-limiting myelosuppression. Autologous bone marrow transplantation was developed as a treatment for solid tumors responsive to, but not currently cured by, chemotherapy. Metastatic breast cancer has been the model for solid tumors in a number of large autologous bone marrow transplant research programs. Peripheral blood progenitor cells have largely replaced autologous bone marrow cells in most transplant programs owing to their lower cost, greater convenience, and shortened time to engraftment. A recent review of the results of these programs suggests that patients with refractory metastatic disease have a high response rate, but the duration of response is brief.[54,73] However, patients with metastatic breast cancer who obtain a complete response or a near complete response to conventional combination chemotherapy regimens may derive a far greater benefit from participation in high-dose chemotherapy with stem cell support. From the limited data available, it would appear that approximately 10% to 20% of patients with metastatic breast cancer who receive high-dose chemotherapy with stem cell support following a complete or near complete response to conventional chemotherapy may in fact be cured of their disease or at least derive the benefit of a prolonged disease-free interval. Current controversy surrounds when to administer high-dose therapy in the small percentage of patients with metastatic disease who are complete responders to conventional chemotherapy (i.e., immediately following response to conventional therapy or at relapse).[73] Ongoing work in this field includes the use of multicycle high-dose therapy, modulation of drug resistance, and use of maintenance therapy with biologic agents.

RADIATION THERAPY

Radiation is an important modality in the treatment of symptomatic metastatic disease. The most common indication for the treatment with radiation therapy is painful bone metastases or other localized sites of disease refractory to systemic therapy. Approximately 90% of patients treated for painful bone metastases will obtain significant pain relief. Radiation is also an important modality in the palliative treatment of metastatic brain lesions and spinal cord lesions, which respond poorly to systemic therapy, as well as eye or orbit lesions and other sites where significant accumulation of tumor cells occurs.

PREVENTION AND EARLY DETECTION

Current efforts at breast cancer prevention are directed toward the identification and removal of risk factors. Unfortunately, a number of risk factors associated with development of breast cancer do not lend themselves to modification. For example, family history of breast cancer or personal history of breast or other gynecologic malignancies cannot be modified. Isolation and cloning of breast cancer susceptibility genes now allows screening of women with histories suggestive of "breast cancer families" and identification of appropriate candidates for prophylactic bilateral mastectomy. There are currently no absolute indications for prophylactic bilateral mastectomy. This surgery is considered for women at very high risk for the development of breast cancer, particularly if the women's breasts are difficult to evaluate by both physical examination and mammography, and they have persistent disabling fears that they will have the disease.

In the past 5 years, there has been increasing interest in "chemoprevention" of breast cancer. This includes interventions directed at inhibiting neoplastic development through pharmacologic measures. Two important agents being studied in research on breast cancer chemoprevention are retinoids and tamoxifen. Retinoids (all vitamin A [Retinol] and its isomer derivatives and synthetic analogs) are biologic regulators of orderly epithelial cell development and are therefore potentially ideal agents for controlling abnormal epithelial proliferation that occurs in carcinogenesis. The agent that is currently receiving the most attention as a chemoprevention agent is tamoxifen. As previously described, tamoxifen is useful as an adjunct after treatment of primary breast cancer, especially in postmenopausal women. In randomized trials of tamoxifen as an adjuvant treatment for breast cancer, women who received tamoxifen were also found to have a reduced incidence of contralateral primary breast carcinomas.

The NSABP recently conducted a trial in the United States that compared 5 years of tamoxifen therapy to placebo in 16,000 women aged 35 and older who are at increased risk for breast cancer (the Breast Cancer Prevention Trial [BCPT]). This trial is the first large chemoprevention trial conducted in the United States and generated a great deal of controversy. Controversy largely surrounded the unknown benefit of tamoxifen therapy as a chemoprevention agent, and the potential for toxicity associated with its administration. Tamoxifen has been repeatedly shown to be a relatively safe drug with an acceptable toxicity profile when used to treat patients with breast cancer. However, its estrogenic effects on the uterus and possibly the coagulation system renders it not without risk and of no known benefit in healthy high-risk women. On April 21, 1998, the NSABP Chairman issued a press release announcing that the BCPT shows a 45% reduction in breast cancer incidence among the high-risk participants who were assigned to receive tamoxifen (20 mg/d). Investigators released the initial study results about 14 months earlier than expected and notified the 13,388 participants of the finding, so that those women who were taking placebo could consider taking tamoxifen. According to the press release, there were 85 cases of invasive breast cancer in women receiving tamoxifen compared to 154 cases in women assigned to placebo. Breast cancer that developed in women receiving tamoxifen was usually hormone receptor negative. Endometrial cancer (n = 33) and thromboembolic disorders (n = 21) were more common in the tamoxifen group than the placebo group (n = 14; n = 25, respectively). Although these early reports are promising, questions remain regarding the ability of tamoxifen to prevent breast cancer mortality in the long term, which women are most likely to benefit, the optimal age of initiation, duration of use, and risks associated with tamoxifen use for greater than 5 years. The ultimate benefit and risks associated with use of tamoxifen as a chemoprevention agent in breast cancer await publication of the full results of the BCPT, as well as the two chemoprevention trials that are ongoing in European countries.

The rationale for early detection of breast cancer is based on the clear relationship between stage of breast cancer at diagnosis and the probability for cure. Thus, if all breast cancer could be detected at a very early stage of the disease (i.e., small primary tumor and negative lymph nodes), then more patients with the disease could be cured. Screening guidelines for early detection of breast cancer have been put forward by the American Cancer Society, the U.S. Preventive Task Force, and the National Cancer Institute (Table 116–11).[74,75] Currently, the American Cancer Society recommends that all women over the age of 20 perform monthly breast self-examinations. There is evidence to support this recommendation, and at least one investigator has demonstrated that women who perform breast

TABLE 116–11. Guidelines for Early Detection of Breast Cancer

	U.S. Preventive Task Force	American Cancer Society	National Cancer Institute
Breast self-exam (BSE)	NR	Monthly (20+)	NR
Clinical breast exam (CBE)	Annual 50–69 with mammography	Every 3 years (20–40)	Every 3 years (20–40) Annual (40+)
Mammogram	NR (40–49) 1–2 years (50–69)	Annual (40+)	NR (40–49) Annual (50+)

NR = not recommended.

self-examinations were generally diagnosed with an earlier stage of the disease and had a higher 5-year survival rate when compared to women who did not perform self-examinations.[76] However, the results of a recently reported randomized clinical trial in 267,040 women, conducted by the NCI in Shanghai, found that the group of women trained and performing monthly breast self-exams did not have earlier stage disease at diagnosis and underwent more biopsies for benign conditions, compared to the group who were not trained to perform monthly breast self-exams.[77] Although the results of this study have dampened enthusiasm, most U.S. experts continue to promote the value of breast self-exam as an effective screening procedure. Numerous brochures are available that outline the current methodology for performing breast examinations. It is generally agreed that for this to be an effective screening tool, the examination should be thorough and conducted at approximately the same time in a woman's monthly cycle. Recommendations for breast examination by a physician (clinical breast exam) vary among the three groups. A large majority of breast cancers are discovered by patients during regular self-examinations. Therefore, the value of the clinical breast exam recommendation for women who perform regular self-examinations is questionable. However, since many women fail to perform monthly self-examinations, an annual physician examination may be of value to them.

Clearly, the largest area of controversy in screening recommendations for breast cancer surrounds annual mammography. Most, if not all, guidelines recommend annual mammography for women 50 years old and older. Nearly 75% of all breast cancer occurs in women 50 years of age or greater and it has been conclusively demonstrated that regular use of screening mammography can reduce mortality from breast cancer by 20% to 40% in this age group. Controversy regarding the use of screening mammography is confined to women less than 50 years of age. The American Cancer Society recommends that a baseline mammography be performed between 35 and 40 years of age, and that screening mammography occur every 1 to 2 years in the 40- to 50-year age group. However, in December 1993, the National Cancer Institute (NCI) withdrew its support of the use of screening mammography in women less than 50 years of age. This was based on a report of the NCI's International Workshop on Screening for Breast Cancer held in February 1993.[78] Data from eight major randomized control trials of breast cancer screening performed over the previous 30 years were reviewed and it was concluded that no benefit from screening women between the ages of 40 and 49 years was apparent 5 to 7 years after enrollment into any of these studies. Possible reasons for these findings include the much lower incidence of breast cancer in women 40 to 49 years of age, as well as the increased density of breast tissue found in menstruating women, which renders detection of lesions by mammography more difficult.

Opponents of screening women less than 50 years of age suggest that multiple studies have failed to prove a benefit. However, proponents for screening women 40 to 49 years of age claim that the studies were not designed to detect a difference of a 25% to 30% decrease in mortality. A recent review of these trials concluded that none of these trials included in the NCI analysis had enough statistical power to be able to provide clear proof of benefit for screening women ages 40 to 49 years because none of the trials involved sufficient numbers of women in these age groups.[79] These authors suggest that the conclusion from these trials is that a benefit from screening was demonstrated that lacked statistical significance. Five of the eight trials with all their performance and design flaws (insufficient numbers of women ages 40 to 49 years, poor-quality mammography, single-view mammography, 2-year screening interval, high contamination rate, and high intervention threshold) suggest a benefit, which indicates the benefit would be significant if the number of women in these trials had been sufficiently large to permit statistical significance. The debate regarding the value of screening mammography in women less than 50 years of age continues among various health care providers and is the source of great confusion for the health care consumer.

The NIH conducted another Consensus Development Panel to address cancer screening for women ages 40 to 49 in January 1997.[80] The NIH Consensus Statement on Breast Cancer Screening of Women Ages 40 to 49 contains two reports: a majority report and a minority report. Although consensus was initially achieved by the entire panel at the end of the consensus conference, 2 of the 12 panel members subsequently differed on the draft document in the weeks that followed and ultimately did not agree entirely with the majority statement. It should be emphasized that the press release of the panel's report in January 1997 created a great deal of public and political pressure on the NCI to reverse its conclusion, which, once again, found that data currently available do not warrant a universal recommendation for mammography for all women in their 40s. The panel went on to state that "each woman should decide for herself whether to undergo mammography . . . her decision may be based, not only on objective analysis of the scientific evidence and consideration of her individual medical history, but also on how she perceives and weighs each potential risk and benefit, the value she places on each, and how she deals with uncertainty."[80] The report further states that information should be developed and provided to women in their 40s regarding potential benefits and risks to enable each woman to make the most appropriate decision. Educational materials for physicians were also recommended in the report. The two panel members writing the minority report believed that risks of mammography were overemphasized by the majority and concluded that the data did support the recommendation for mammography screening for all women in this age group and that survival benefit and diagnosis at an earlier stage outweighed the potential risks.

Significant advances in the safety and efficacy of screening mammography have occurred during the past two decades. This has allowed superior visualization of breast and breast tissue with a concurrent reduction in the dose of radiation that is delivered. Approximately 10% of all palpable masses are not detected by mammography. This is most commonly observed in premenopausal women and is felt to be directly related to the increased density of breast tissue in this estrogen-rich environment. Radiation from yearly mammograms during the ages 40 to 49 has been estimated as possibly causing one additional death per 10,000 women.[80] As women age, incidence for developing mammography-related breast cancer is lower because of the lower carcinogenic effects of radiation in older women. Although the safety and efficacy of screening mammography in terms of image quality and dosimetry are very acceptable, the American College of Radiology (ACR) has recognized for some years the need for greater quality control in mammography. A voluntary accreditation program developed by this organization and adopted by various state and federal agencies has greatly improved the overall quality of mammography in the majority of facilities in this country. Many of the details of the accreditation process have recently been adopted for use by governmental agencies, culminating in the Mammography Quality Standards of 1992. This act, which essentially codifies the ACR program, assures that all mammographic facilities will now be required to achieve a common high standard of quality assurance. Responsibility for operation of the act has been given to the FDA. As of October 1, 1994, all facilities that offer mammography must be FDA-certified to remain open. Passage of this landmark legislation, as well as provision of appropriate levels of funding to conduct this program, represents an important contribution to the health of women.

EVALUATION OF THERAPEUTIC OUTCOMES

The desired therapeutic outcome of adjuvant therapy of breast cancer differs significantly from that of metastatic disease. Adjuvant therapy—chemotherapy, hormonal therapy, or both—is administered with curative intent. The rationale behind adjuvant therapy in breast cancer is that breast cancer, even when diagnosed in early stages when clinical evidence of distant spread is not apparent, is a systemic disease that spreads early to distant sites. Adjuvant therapy is intended to eradicate these micrometastases and thus cure the patient of breast cancer. Therefore, the overall goal of adjuvant therapy is to cure the disease, which is something that cannot be fully evaluated for years following initial diagnosis and treatment. In addition, because there is no clinical evidence of disease at the time adjuvant therapy is administered, assessment of disease response is not possible. Instead, a predetermined number of cycles of adjuvant therapy and/or years of hormonal therapy is administered. Oftentimes, adjuvant chemotherapy is associated with significant toxicity. Maintaining dose intensity has been demonstrated to be important in the cure of disease and, therefore, optimizing supportive care measures such as antiemetics and growth factors is highly recommended.

Palliation is the therapeutic outcome in treatment of metastatic breast cancer. In general, the least toxic therapies are used initially with increasingly aggressive therapies applied in a sequential fashion and in a manner that does not significantly compromise the quality of the patient's life. Tumor response to a particular treatment regimen may be measured by clinical chemistry such as liver enzyme elevation in a patient with hepatic metastases, or imaging techniques such as bone scans or chest x-rays. However, assessment of the patient's clinical status and symptom control is often adequate to evaluate response to the therapy administered. In the patient with metastatic breast cancer, it is common to initiate hormonal therapy or chemotherapy and continue administration until signs and symptoms of disease progress or new signs and symptoms present. Optimizing quality of life is the therapeutic end point in the treatment of patients with metastatic breast cancer. A number of valid and reliable tools are available for objective assessment of quality of life in patients with breast cancer.

CONCLUSIONS

Breast cancer is the most commonly occurring cancer in women in the United States and is second only to lung cancer as the most common cancer cause of death. The incidence of breast cancer has been increasing during the past 50 years and has increased rapidly since the early 1980s. It is unclear whether the recent increase in the incidence of breast cancer reflects a true increase in the new cases of this disease or, instead, increased detection of the disease by screening mammography. The etiology of breast cancer is unknown; however, a number of factors have been identified that increase a woman's chances of developing the disease. These risk factors, as well as information regarding the biology of the disease, suggest that a complex interplay between hormones, genetic factors, and environmental and life-style influences all contribute to the etiology of this disease. The recent identification of the BRCA1 and BRCA2 genes, tumor suppresser genes important in the development of inherited and perhaps sporadic breast and ovarian cancer, holds promise in identifying patients at high risk, as well as improving our basic understanding of the causes of breast and ovarian cancer.

The majority of breast cancers are diagnosed in early stages before the disease has disseminated to sites distant from the breast. Treatment consists of local management, as well as systemic adjuvant therapy with either chemotherapy, hormonal therapy, or a combination of these. Breast-conservation therapy, which consists of complete removal of the tumor (lumpectomy), combined with breast irradiation and axillary lymph node sampling, is currently the preferred method of treatment for most patients with localized breast cancer. Patients who are not candidates for breast conservation or who do not choose this local therapy will generally receive the modified radical mastectomy.

It is apparent from clinical and laboratory experiments and observation that the spread of breast cancer via the bloodstream occurs early in the course of the disease. This results in patients relapsing with systemic metastatic disease following local curative therapy. The likelihood of later development of metastatic disease is related to the size of the primary tumor, presence of lymph node involvement and number of nodes affected, and a number of additional pathologic prognostic factors, which include proliferative capacity, nuclear grade, hormone receptor status, and presence or absence of oncogenes and other protein products. Systemic adjuvant therapy is commonly administered to patients with localized breast cancer following surgical procedures to diminish the risk of or delay disease recurrence. Specific recommendations for adjuvant therapy are determined by stage of the disease, age of the patient, presence of hormone receptors in the primary tumor, as well as other pathologic prognostic factors. Adjuvant therapy treatment recommendations have been developed by an NIH consensus conference, as well as an international consensus group, and these treatment recommendations continue to evolve as new data become available.

Advanced breast cancer includes locally advanced breast cancer (stage III) and metastatic breast cancer (stage IV). Treatment of stage III breast cancer generally consists of a combination of surgery, radiation, and chemotherapy administered in an aggressive approach. Although response rates and survival have improved, there is still much progress to be made in stage III breast cancer. Metastatic breast cancer is, in the majority of cases, incurable. The only exception to this is that some promising long-term response rates have been observed in a subset of patients with metastatic disease who have a complete or near complete response to conventional chemotherapy and then receive high-dose chemotherapy with stem cell support. Unfortunately, this represents a small number of the total population of patients with metastatic breast cancer. Metastatic breast cancer is treated with endocrine therapy or combination chemotherapy. Patients who are hormone receptor positive will generally receive initial endocrine therapy followed by combination chemotherapy when endocrine therapy fails. Patients who are hormone receptor negative or have disease involving the liver or central nervous system will generally receive combination chemotherapy as first-line therapy of metastatic disease. Combination chemotherapy will result in an objective response in approximately 70% of patients previously unexposed to chemotherapy. The majority of patients have partial response, and complete disappearance of disease occurs in fewer than 20% of patients treated. Median duration of response is 5 to 12 months; although some patients will have an excellent response to an initial course of chemotherapy and may live 5 to 10 years without evidence of disease. In general, survival of patients after treatment with commonly used drug combinations for metastatic breast cancer is a median of 14 to 33 months. Response to second- and third-line combination chemotherapy has been on the order of 20% to 40%. This is in large part dependent on previous chemotherapy regimens the patient has received. The availability of paclitaxel, docetaxel, and vinorelbine offers the promise of more successful second- and third-line treatment of metastatic breast cancer in the future.

Current efforts at breast cancer prevention are directed toward the identification and removal of risk factors. In addition, two agents, the retinoids and tamoxifen, are being evaluated for their ability to prevent breast cancer. Any statement regarding the value of these modalities awaits the results of ongoing clinical trials. Early detection of breast cancer remains an important modality for decreasing breast cancer mortality. The rationale for early detection of breast cancer is based on the clear relationship between stage of breast cancer at diagnosis and the probability of a cure. Screening guidelines for early detection of breast cancer have been developed by the American Cancer Society, the U.S. Preventive Task Force, and the National Cancer Institute. Although all these agencies agree that annual clinical breast exam and screening mammographies should be performed in women older than 50, controversy exists regarding the value of screening women in the 40 to 50 age group. This controversy has, unfortunately, created a great deal of confusion in the general public.

Intensive research efforts are ongoing in all aspects of breast cancer etiology, detection, prevention, and treatment. Efforts in the past have resulted in substantial reduction in mortality in selected patient subsets. The information obtained in the next decade will hopefully result in the knowledge required to significantly reduce mortality from breast cancer for all women.

▶ PRINCIPLES OF PHARMACOTHERAPY

- Breast cancer is most commonly diagnosed in early stages, when it is a highly curable malignancy.
- Local therapy of early stage breast cancer consists of either modified radical mastectomy or lumpectomy plus external beam radiation therapy.
- Adjuvant systemic therapy with tamoxifen (20 mg/d) for 5 years reduces the risk of breast cancer recurrence by 50% and risk of death by 25% in all estrogen receptor–positive women.
- Adjuvant systemic therapy with combination chemotherapy reduces mortality from breast cancer in all patient subsets but is of greatest benefit in estrogen receptor–negative premenopausal patients.
- Initial therapy of metastatic breast cancer in women with hormone receptor–positive tumors should consist of hormonal therapy.

- Women with metastatic breast cancer who are hormone receptor positive and respond to an initial hormonal manipulation will usually respond to a second hormonal manipulation.
- Twenty-five percent to fifty percent of women with metastatic breast cancer will respond to chemotherapy regimens; doxorubicin- and taxane-containing regimens are the most active.
- The goal of adjuvant chemotherapy is curative, whereas the goal of chemotherapy in the metastatic setting is palliative; therefore, the importance of dose intensity in the adjuvant setting is greater than in the metastatic setting.
- Although experts do not agree on the benefits of annual screening mammography in women less than 50 years of age, a large number of national and international studies have demonstrated a 20% to 40% reduction in breast cancer mortality from annual or biannual screening mammography in women aged 50 to 70 years.
- Tamoxifen has been demonstrated to reduce the incidence of breast cancer by approximately 45% in high-risk women by the NSABP in the Tamoxifen Chemoprevention Trial.

REFERENCES

1. Lanids SH, Murray T, Bolden S, Wingo PA. Cancer Statistics 1998. CA Cancer J Clin 1998;48:6–29.
2. Miller BA, Ries LAG, Hankey BF, et al, eds. Cancer Statistics Review: 1973–1990 (NIH Pub. 93-2789). Bethesda, MD, National Cancer Institute, 1993.
3. Feuer EJ, Wun LM, Boring CC, et al. The lifetime risk of developing breast cancer. J Natl Cancer Inst 1993;85:892–897.
4. Miller BA, Feuer EJ, Hankey BF. Recent incidence trends for breast cancer in women and the relevance of early detection: An update. CA Cancer J Clin 1993;43:27–41.
5. Abeloff MD, Lichter AS, Niederhuber JE, Pierce LJ, Aziz DC. Breast. Management of specific malignancies. In: Clinical Oncology. Churchill Livingstone, 1995:1617–1714.
6. Bailar JC, Gornik HL. Cancer undefeated. N Engl J Med 1997;336:1569–1574.
7. Ries LAG, Kosary CL, Hankey BF, et al, eds. SEER Cancer Statistics Review, 1973–1994: Tables and Graphs (NIH Pub. 97-2789). Bethesda, MD, National Cancer Institute, 1997.
8. Harris JR, Lippman ME, Veronesi U, Willett W. Breast cancer. Part 1. N Engl J Med 1992;327:319–328.
9. Colditz GA, Stampfer MJ, Willett WC. Prospective study of estrogen replacement therapy and risk of breast cancer in postmenopausal women. JAMA 1990;264:2648–2653.
10. Dupont WD, Page DL. Menopausal estrogen replacement therapy and breast cancer. Arch Intern Med 1991;151:67–72.
11. Steinberg KK, Thacker SB, Smith SJ, et al. A meta-analysis of the effect of estrogen replacement therapy on the risk of breast cancer. JAMA 1991;265:1985–1990.
12. DiSaia PJ. Hormone-replacement therapy in patients with breast cancer. Cancer 1993;71:1490s–1500s.
13. Romieu I, Berlin JA, Colditz G. Oral contraceptives and breast cancer: Review and meta-analysis. Cancer 1990;66:2253–2263.
14. Harris JR, Morrow M, Bonadonna G. Cancer of the breast. In: DeVita VT Jr, Hellman S, Rosenberg SA, eds. Cancer: Principles of Oncology, 4th ed. Philadelphia, Lippincott, 1993:1264–1324.
15. Thompson WD. Genetic epidemiology of breast cancer. Cancer 1994;74:279–287.
16. Weber BL, Abel JK, Brody LC, et al. Familial breast cancer. Cancer 1994;74:1013–1020.
17. Struewing JP, Hartge P, Wacholder S, et al. The risk of cancer associated with specific mutations of BRCA1 and BRCA2 among Ashkenazi Jews. N Engl J Med 1997;336:1401–1408.
18. Byers T. Nutritional risk factors for breast cancer. Cancer 1994;74:288–295.
19. Howe GR. Dietary fat and breast cancer risks. Cancer 1994;74:1078–1084.
20. Howe GR, Friedenreich CM, Jain M, Miller AB. A cohort study of fat intake and risk of breast cancer. J Natl Cancer Inst 1991;83:336–340.
21. Nagao M, Ushijima T, Wakabayashi K, et al. Dietary carcinogens and mammary carcinogenesis. Cancer 1994;74:1063–1069.
22. Schapira DV, Kumar NB, Lyman GH. Obesity, body fat distribution and sex hormones in breast cancer patients. Cancer 1991;67:2215–2218.
23. Longnecker MP. Alcohol consumption in relation to risk of breast cancer. Cancer Causes Control 1994;5:73–82.
24. Feig SA, Ehrlich SM. Estimation of radiation risk from screening mammography: Recent trends and comparison with expected benefits. Radiology 1990;174:639–647.
25. McKenna RJ. The abnormal mammogram radiographic findings, diagnostic optional, pathology, and stage of cancer diagnosis. Cancer 1994;79:244–255.
26. Baines CJ, Miller AB, Kopans DB. Canadian national breast screening study: Assessment of technical quality by external review. Am J Radiol 1990;155:743–747.
27. Kopans DB. The Breast Imaging Report. Philadelphia, Lippincott, 1989:351–353.
28. Frykberg ER, Bland KI. Overview of the biology and management of ductal carcinoma *in situ* of the breast. Cancer 1994;74:350–361.
29. Frykberg ER, Ames FC, Bland KI. Current concepts for management of early (*in situ* and occult invasive) breast carcinoma. In: Bland KI, Copeland EM, eds. The Breast: Comprehensive Management of Benign and Malignant Diseases. Philadelphia, Saunders, 1991:731–751.
30. Fisher B, Constantio J, Redmond C, et al. Lumpectomy compared with lumpectomy and radiation therapy for the treatment of intraductal breast cancer. N Engl J Med 1993;328:1581–1586.
31. Fisher B, Slack NH, Bross IDJ. Cancer of the breast: Size of neoplasm and prognosis. Cancer 1969;24:1071–1080.
32. Nemoto T, Vana T, Bedwani RN, et al. Management and survival of female breast cancer. Cancer 1980;45:2917–2924.
33. Valagussa P, Bonadonna G, Veronesi U. Patterns of relapse and survival in operable breast carcinoma with positive and negative axillary nodes. Tumori 1978;64:241–258.
34. McGuire WL, Clark GM. Prognosis in breast cancer. Recent Results Cancer Res 1989;115:170–174.
35. Osborne CK. Prognostic factors in breast cancer. Princ Pract Oncol Updates 1990;4:1–11.
36. Mansour EG, Ravdin PM, Dressler L. Prognostic factors in early breast cancer. Cancer 1994;74:381–400.
37. Dhingra K, Hortobagyi GN. Critical evaluation of prognostic factors. Semin Oncol 1996;23:436–445.
38. Hedley DW, Clark GM, Cornelisse CJ, et al. Consensus review of the clinical utility of DNA cytometry in carcinoma of the breast. Cytometry 1993;14:482–485.
39. Fisher B, Redmond C, Fisher E, et al. Relative worth of estrogen or progesterone receptor and pathologic characteristics of differentiation as indicators of prognosis in node-negative breast and Bowel Project Protocol B-06. J Clin Oncol 1988;6:1076–1087.

40. Gasparini G, Pozza F, Harris AL. Evaluating the potential usefulness of new prognostic and predictive indicators in node-negative breast cancer patients. J Natl Cancer Inst 1993;85:1206–1219.
41. Nemoto T, Vana J, Bedwani RN, et al. Management and survival of female breast cancer: Results of a national survey by the American College of Surgeons. Cancer 1980;45:2917–2924.
42. Fisher B, Redmond C, Fisher ER, et al. Ten-year results of a randomized clinical trial comparing radical mastectomy and total mastectomy with or without radiation. N Engl J Med 1985;312:674–681.
43. Fisher B, Redmond C, Poisson R, et al. Eight-year results of a randomized clinical trial comparing total mastectomy and lumpectomy with or without irradiation in the treatment of breast cancer. N Engl J Med 1989;320:822–828.
44. NIH Consensus Conference. Treatment of early-stage breast cancer. JAMA 1991;265:391–395.
45. Early Breast Cancer Trialists' Collaborative Group T. Systemic treatment of early breast cancer by hormonal, cytotoxic, or immune therapy: 133 randomized trials involving 31,000 recurrences and 24,000 deaths among 75,000 women. Lancet 1992;339:1–15.
46. Goldhirsch A, Glick JH, Gelber RD, et al. Meeting highlights: International consensus panel on the treatment of primary breast cancer. J Natl Cancer Inst 1998(90):1601–1608.
47. Fisher B, Dignam J, Wolmark N, et al. Tamoxifen and chemotherapy for lymph node-negative, estrogen receptor-positive breast cancer. J Natl Cancer Inst 1997;89:1673–1682.
48. International Breast Cancer Study Group. Effectiveness of adjuvant chemotherapy in combination with tamoxifen for node-positive postmenopausal breast cancer patients. J Clin Oncol 1997;15:1385–1394.
49. Hortobagyi GN, Buzdar AU. Current status of adjuvant systemic therapy for primary breast cancer: Progress and controversy. CA Cancer J Clin 1995;45:199–226.
50. Shapiro CL, Henderson IC. Adjuvant therapy of breast cancer. Hematol Oncol Clin North Am 1994;8:213–231.
51. Piccart MJ, Biganzoli L, Roy JA. Adjuvant systemic therapy for breast cancer. Curr Opin Oncol 1996;8:478–484.
52. Henderson JC. Adjuvant systemic therapy for early breast cancer. Cancer 1994;74:401–409.
53. Buzzoni R, Bonadonna G, Valagussa P, Zambetti M. Adjuvant chemotherapy with doxorubicin plus cyclophosphamide, methotrexate, and fluorouracil in the treatment of resectable breast cancer with more than three positive axillary nodes. J Clin Oncol 1991;9:2134–2140.
54. Burtness B. High-dose chemotherapy for breast cancer. PPO Updates 1997;11:1–13.
55. Winer EP. Quality-of-life research in patients with breast cancer. Cancer 1994;74:410–415.
56. Levine MN, Gent M, Hirsh J, et al. The thrombogenic effect of anticancer drug therapy in women with stage II breast cancer. N Engl J Med 1988;318:404–407.
57. Curtis RE, Boice JD Jr, Stovall M, et al. Risk of leukemia after chemotherapy and radiation treatment for breast cancer. N Engl J Med 1992;326:1745–1751.
58. Henderson IC, Sloss JL, Jaffe N, et al. Serial studies of cardiac function in patients receiving adriamycin. Cancer Treat Rep 1978;62:923–929.
59. Slevin ML, Stubbs L, Plant HJ, et al. Attitudes to chemotherapy: Comparing views of patients with cancer: Attitudes of doctors, nurses, and the general public. BMJ 1990;300:1458–1460.
60. Lindley C, Vasa S, Sawyer WT, Winer EP. Quality of life and preferences for treatment following systemic adjuvant therapy for early stage breast cancer. J Clin Oncol 1998;16:1380–1387.
61. Love RR, Mazess RB, Barden HS, et al. Effects of tamoxifen on bone mineral density in postmenopausal women with breast cancer. N Engl J Med 1992;326:852–856.
62. Love RR, Wiebe DA, Newcomb PA, et al. Effects of tamoxifen on cardiovascular risk factors in postmenopausal women. Ann Intern Med 1992;115:860–864.
63. Nayfield SG, Karp JE, Ford LG, et al. Potential role of tamoxifen in prevention of breast cancer. J Natl Cancer Inst 1991;83:1450–1459.
64. Ingle JN, Krook JE, Green SJ, et al. Randomized trial of bilateral oophorectomy versus tamoxifen in premenopausal women with metastatic breast cancer. J Clin Oncol 1986;4:178–185.
65. Howell A, Downey S, Anderson E. New endocrine therapies for breast cancer. Eur J Cancer 1996;32A:576–588.
66. Baker VL, Jaffe RB. Clinical uses of antiestrogens. Obstet Gynecol Surv 1995;51:45–59.
67. Lipton A, Harvey HA, Santen RJ, et al. Randomized trial of aminoglutethimide versus tamoxifen in metastatic breast cancer. Cancer Res 1982;42:3434s–3435s.
68. Brodie AMH, Njar VCO. Aromatase inhibitors and breast cancer. Semin Oncol 1996;23:10–20.
69. Letrozole Product Information.
70. D'Andrea GM, Seidman A. Docetaxel and paclitaxel in breast cancer therapy: Present status and future prospects. Semin Oncol 1997; 24(suppl 13):S13-27–S13-44.
71. Akerley W, Sikov W, Cummings F, et al. Weekly high-dose paclitaxel in metastatic and locally advanced breast cancer: A preliminary report. Semin Oncol 1997;24(suppl 17):S17-87–S17-90.
72. Hortobagyi GN. New cytotoxic agents for the treatment of breast cancer. Oncology 1996;10(suppl 6):21–29.
73. Peters WP, Dansey R. New concepts in the treatment of breast cancer using high-dose chemotherapy. Cancer Chemother Pharmacol 1997; 40(suppl):S88–S93.
74. Leitch AM, Dodd GD, Costanza M, et al. American Cancer Society Guidelines for the Early Detection of Breast Cancer: Update 1997. CA Cancer J Clin 1997;47:150–153.
75. Guide to Clinical Preventive Sciences, 2nd ed. Report of the U.S. Preventive Services Task Force. Washington, DC, Department of Health and Human Services, 1995.
76. Huguley CM, Brown RL, Greenberg RS, Clark WS. Breast self-examination and survival from breast cancer. Cancer 1988;62:1389–1396.
77. Thomas DB, Gao DL, Self SG, et al. Randomized trial of breast self-examination in Shanghai: Methodology and preliminary results. J Natl Cancer Inst 1997;89:355–365.
78. Fletcher SW, Black W, Harris R, et al. Report of the international workshop on screening for breast cancer. J Natl Cancer Inst 1993;85: 1644–1656.
79. Kopans DB, Halpern E, Hulka CA. Statistical power in breast cancer screening trials and mortality reduction among women 40–49 years of age with particular emphasis on the National Breast Screening Study of Canada. Cancer 1994;74:1196–1203.
80. National Institues of Health Consensus Development Panel. National Institutes of Health Consensus Development Conference Statement: Breast Cancer Screening for Women Ages 40–49, January 21–23, 1997. J Natl Cancer Inst 1997;89:1015–1026.

117
LUNG CANCER

Sally A. Felton, PharmD, and Rebecca S. Finley, PharmD, MS

Lung cancer is a major cause of morbidity and mortality that has reached epidemic proportions in many industrialized countries and is the most frequently fatal malignancy in the world. The American Cancer Society estimates that 171,500 new cases of lung cancer will be diagnosed in the United States during 1998, resulting in approximately 160,100 deaths.[1] Despite major advances in the understanding and management of lung cancer, the overall 5-year survival rate for all types of lung cancer remains a dismal 13%.[1]

Lung cancer is estimated to account for 13% of all newly diagnosed cancers in adults.[1] It remains the leading cause of cancer death in men aged 35 years and older (accounting for 32% of all cancer deaths in men) and the leading cause of cancer death in women (25% of all cancer deaths).[1] In 1987, for the first time, lung cancer surpassed breast cancer as the primary cause of cancer death among American women.[1] The incidence of lung cancer increases with age; the peak age of diagnosis is between 55 and 65 years. Among patients 40 years of age and older, the likelihood that a solitary pulmonary nodule seen on chest x-ray is a carcinoma is high and this probability increases proportionally with age. Patients with lung cancer may undergo surgery, chemotherapy, radiation, or multimodality therapy, depending on the histologic type of their tumor, its size and location, and the presence of metastases at diagnosis.

ETIOLOGY

Lung carcinomas arise from pluripotent epithelial cells which are capable of expressing a variety of phenotypes.[2] The natural history of lung cancer begins with exposure of these cells to carcinogens, which causes chronic inflammation eventually leading to genetic and cytologic changes that progress to carcinoma.[3] Hereditary phenotypes that influence activation or detoxification of carcinogens may influence the risk of lung cancer, and there appears to be genetic susceptibility in some individuals that is significant only if they smoke.[3,4] Activation of proto-oncogenes, inhibition or mutation of tumor suppressor genes, and production of autocrine growth factors also contribute to cellular proliferation and malignant transformation.[5,6] Under normal circumstances, cell surface peptidases produced by epithelial cells are capable of degrading and regulating these growth factors; however, these enzymes are expressed at low or undetectable levels by most lung cancer cells, thus facilitating uncontrolled growth.[7] As in many other malignant diseases, further elucidation of molecular attributes of lung cancer are likely to provide insight regarding improved preventive, diagnostic, prognostic, and therapeutic strategies.

Numerous studies have established the relationship between tobacco exposure and lung cancer. The American Cancer Society estimates that cigarette smoking is responsible for about 83% of all lung cancer cases, and studies have established a dose–response relationship between the number of cigarettes smoked, the number of years an individual has smoked, the tar and nicotine content of cigarettes, and the development of lung cancer.[3] Likewise, smokers with obstructive airway disease or chronic bronchitis have a three- to fivefold greater risk of developing lung cancer than smokers with normal pulmonary function.[7,8] Mattson et al. estimated that a 35-year-old man who smokes 25 cigarettes per day or more has a 13% risk of dying of lung cancer before age 75.[9] The increased rate of lung cancer deaths among women has also been attributed to increased smoking.[1] Cessation of smoking is associated with a gradual decrease in the risk, but a long period of time (more than 6 years) is necessary before an appreciable diminution of the risk occurs.[10] However, the high number of lung cancers in ex-smokers emphasizes the need to prevent individuals from ever smoking. Passive exposure to cigarette smoke is believed to contribute to the increased risk of lung cancer in non-smokers living with smokers.[3] Other carcinogens also increase the risk of lung cancer and may act synergistically with cigarette smoking.[3] Occupational or environmental exposure to asbestos, chloromethyl ethers, various heavy metals, polcyclic aromatic hydrocarbons, and radon has also been associated with the development of lung cancer.[3] In addition, the incidence of lung cancer is higher in urban than in rural areas, and air pollution has been implicated as a possible causative agent.[11] Observational epidemiologic data have suggested that intake of β-carotene and carotene (vitamin A) is inversely associated with lung cancer risk.[12,13] The first prospective randomized chemoprevention trial with antioxidants in a large, well-nourished population was reported in 1994.[14] This trial randomized more than 29,000 middle-aged male smokers to receive dietary supplementation with β-carotene, α-tocopherol, or both for 6 years. Interestingly, the trial failed to detect any significant protective effect of either vitamin and, in fact, there were significantly more new cases of lung cancer in the group treated with β-carotene. Other prospective trials have also failed to demonstrate significant positive effects of carotenoids, vitamin C, or vitamin E against lung cancer.[3] Conversely, several other trials and case-control studies have shown a significant difference in relative risk related to intake of one of these antioxidants.[3,11] Clearly, additional studies are necessary to define the role of antioxidants in lung cancer prevention.

HISTOLOGIC CLASSIFICATION

The World Health Organization lung cancer classification is accepted worldwide (Table 117–1).[15] Four major cell types of carcinomas (squamous cell carcinoma, adenocarcinoma, and large cell and small cell carcinomas) account for more than 90% of all lung tumors. Histologic confirmation of cell type is usually made by light microscopy and is essential in treatment planning because of differences in the natural histories, clinical features, and response to therapy of the various types. Several additional biologic and cytogenetic characteristics (e.g., secretion of peptide hormones, autocrine growth factor receptors, specific mutations, or chromosomal deletions of lung tumors) are currently being evaluated for their prognostic significance. In terms of management strategy and overall prognosis, adenocarcinoma, squamous cell and large cell carcinomas are frequently grouped together and referred to as non–small cell lung cancer (NSCLC).

Although once the most common type of NSCLC, squamous cell (or epidermoid) carcinoma now accounts for less than 30% of all lung cancers and is distinguished histologically by evidence of squamous differentiation.[3] This tumor tends to be central in origin, arising from metaplastic bronchial epithelium, and frequently extends into the bronchial lumen, resulting in obstruction. Squamous cell carcinomas (along with small [SCLC] cell lung cancers) have a much higher incidence among smokers and among males, and there appears to be a strong dose–response relation to tobacco exposure.[3] Although they can grow rapidly, most squamous cell carcinomas tend to be slow growing and confined to the lungs (especially early in the disease course). Such tumors may eventually metastasize to the hilar and mediastinal lymph nodes, liver, adrenal glands, kidneys, bone, and gastrointestinal tract.

Adenocarcinoma is now the most common type of lung cancer in North America, accounting for about 40% of cases. This is partly due to the increased incidence of lung cancer in women, who tend to have more adenocarcinomas then epidermoid cancers. Interestingly, it does not have a dose–response relation to tobacco exposure.[3] These tumors are usually located in the peripheral sections of the lung and are distinguished pathologically by a glandular or papillary pattern and mucin production.[3] Adenocarcinomas may present as a single nodule, multifocal nodules, or rapidly progressing, bilateral, diffuse processes. However, they are likely to metastasize at an early stage (often before the diagnosis of the primary tumor) and spread widely to distant sites including the contralateral lung, liver, bone, adrenal glands, kidneys, and central nervous system.

Large cell carcinomas are anaplastic tumors that show no evidence of differentiation. These tumors account for only about 15% of all lung cancers.[3] The large cell carcinomas tend to be large and bulky tumors arising in the periphery of the lung, tend to have a propensity to metastasize in a pattern quite similar to adenocarcinomas, and are associated with a similar poor prognosis.

Small cell carcinomas account for about 25% of all lung tumors, and epidemiologic evidence suggests that it is the most rapidly increasing type of lung cancer, especially in women.[16] Almost all cases are associated with a history of smoking. They are distinguished by a proliferation of neoplastic cells with round to oval nuclei. These tumors tend to arise in the central portion of the lung but may also be found in the lung periphery. SCLC is a very aggressive and rapidly growing tumor with about 60% to 70% of patients initially presenting with disseminated disease outside of the hemithorax.[3] These tumors commonly express neuroendocrine differentiation that may account for some of the paraneoplastic syndromes frequently associated with this disease. SCLC secretes gastrin-releasing peptide that acts as an autocrine growth factor.[17] Secretion of other peptide hormones, cytogenetic abnormalities, and amplification and increased expression of oncogenes are also common. This disease has a propensity to metastasize to the lymph nodes, opposite lung, liver, adrenal glands and other endocrine organs, bone, bone marrow, and central nervous system.

Lung tumors frequently exhibit more than one histology and it is now evident that all types of lung cancer share a common pluripotent stem cell. Studies of lung cancer cells have also shown that cell lines may spontaneously change phenotype, which may explain the mixed histology.[7] Occasionally patients also have multiple lung nodules arising in different lobes or the contralateral lung. This is referred to as *synchronous tumors,* and the nodules may be of similar or different cell types. This usually worsens the patient's overall prognosis.

TABLE 117–1. World Health Organization Classification of Lung Cancer

- I. Benign
- II. Dysplasia and carcinoma *in situ*
- III. Malignant
  - A. Squamous cell carcinoma (epidermoid)
  - B. Small cell carcinoma
    1. Oat cell
    2. Intermediate cell
    3. Combined oat cell
  - C. Adenocarcinoma
    1. Acinar
    2. Papillary
    3. Bronchoalveolar
    4. Mucus secreting
  - D. Large cell carcinoma
    1. Giant cell
    2. Clear cell

From Ref. 3.

CLINICAL PRESENTATION

Location and extent of the tumor will determine the presenting signs and symptoms. If the lesion is in the central portion of the bronchial tree, it is likely to cause symptoms at an earlier stage than a lesion in the periphery of the lung, which may remain asymptomatic until the lesion is quite large or has spread to other areas. The most common initial signs and symptoms include cough, dyspnea, chest pain, sputum production, and hemoptysis. Unfortunately, many patients with lung cancer also have chronic pulmonary and/or cardiovascular diseases (usually related to smoking), and such symptoms may go unnoticed or be attributed to the concomitant disease. Many patients also exhibit systemic symptoms such as anorexia, weight loss, and fatigue that are suggestive of a malignancy.[3,18] Other signs and symptoms that may be associated with the primary tumor or its spread within the thorax are listed in Table 117–2. Such symptomatology may occur at the tumor's initial presentation or at any point during its recurrence or progression.

Disseminated disease also may be responsible for extrapulmonary signs and symptoms such as neurologic deficits resulting from central nervous system metastases, bone pain or pathologic fractures secondary to bone metastases, or liver dysfunction resulting from tumor involvement in the liver.

Paraneoplastic syndromes are signs and symptoms that occur at sites away from the primary tumor or its metastases and are not associated with "direct" tumor involvement. They may be due to the production of biologically active substances (e.g., peptide hormones) or antibodies, or other undefined mechanisms. Paraneoplastic syndromes occur more frequently with lung cancer than with any other tumor. These syndromes may be the first signs of a tumor and may prompt the search for an underlying malignancy. Paraneoplastic syndromes that commonly occur in association with lung cancers include cachexia, hypercalcemia, syndrome of inappropriate hormone secretion, and Cushing's syndrome.[3,18]

TABLE 117–2. Common Signs and Symptoms of Lung Cancer

Local signs and symptoms associated with primary tumor or regional spread within the thorax
Cough
Hemoptysis
Dyspnea
Rust-streaked or purulent sputum
Chest, shoulder, or arm pain
Wheeze and stridor
Superior vena caval obstruction
Pleural effusion or pneumonitis
Dysphagia (secondary to esophageal compression)
Hoarseness (secondary to laryngeal nerve paralysis)
Horner's syndrome
Phrenic nerve paralysis
Pericardial effusion/tamponade
Tracheal obstruction
Extrapulmonary signs and symptoms associated with metastatic involvement
Bone pain and/or pathologic fractures
Liver dysfunction
Neurologic deficits
Spinal cord compression
Paraneoplastic syndromes
Weight loss
Cushing's syndrome
Hypercalcemia
Syndrome of inappropriate antidiuretic hormone (SIADH)
Pulmonary hypertrophic osteoarthropathy
Clubbing
Anemia
Eaton–Lambert myasthenic syndrome

SCREENING

At the time of initial diagnosis, many patients with lung cancer have advanced disease and unfortunately the prognosis is poor. In an attempt to detect lung tumors earlier and improve the cure rate, screening studies have been conducted in high-risk populations (e.g., men over age 40 who smoke).[19–21] Chest x-rays and sputum cytology have been the most commonly used screening techniques in these studies. Although several of these studies have demonstrated that lung cancers may be detected at an earlier stage, actual mortality rates are not affected.[20,21] Furthermore, chest x-rays and sputum cytology are associated with false-positive results in approximately 5% and 0.5% of these high-risk individuals, respectively, leading to unnecessary and costly workups and anxiety.[22] Currently, no biochemical markers (tumor markers) have been identified with sufficient sensitivity and specificity to reliably screen for early lung cancer.

DIAGNOSIS

Once signs and symptoms of lung cancer have been recognized, chest x-rays and computed tomography (CT) scans are the most valuable diagnostic tests. Chest x-ray is the primary method of lung cancer detection and may also be useful in measuring tumor size, establishing gross lymph node enlargement, and aiding in detection of other tumor-related findings such as pleural effusion, lobar collapse, and metastatic bone involvement of ribs, spine, and shoulders. CT is helpful in all of the above as well as in evaluation of parenchymal lung abnormalities, detection of masses only suspected on the chest x-ray, and assessment of mediastinal and hilar lymph nodes.

Clinical characteristics of a lung nodule may also help to differentiate benign from malignant nodules and thus determine when invasive diagnostic tests are warranted. For example, benign lesions usually have sharp borders, whereas malignant lesions usually have irregular or radiating borders.

When there is clinical and radiologic evidence of a tumor, pathologic confirmation must be established. This may be accomplished by examination of sputum cytology and/or tumor biopsy by fiberoptic bronchoscopy, percutaneous needle biopsy, or open-lung biopsy. All patients must also have a thorough history and physical examination with emphasis on detecting signs and symptoms of the primary tumor, regional spread of the tumor, distant metastases, and paraneoplastic syndromes. The physical examination also aids in determining whether or not a patient may be able to withstand aggressive surgery or chemotherapy.

Unfortunately, by the time the tumor is diagnosed, dissemination has already occurred in many patients. Determination of the extent (or stage) of the tumor involvement is important because it will aid in the selection of treatment, and estimation of the probability of cure and survival, as well as facilitating comparison of the individual patient to large-scale clinical trials.

STAGING

NON–SMALL CELL LUNG CANCER

The American Joint Committee [23] has established a TNM staging classification for lung cancer based on the primary tumor size and extent (T), regional lymph node involvement (N), and the presence or absence of distant metastases (M). Table 117–3 outlines this staging system. For comparison of various therapeutic modalities, a more simple stage grouping system is also used in which stage I refers to tumors confined to the lung without lymphatic spread, stage II refers to large tumors with ipsilateral peribronchial or hilar lymph node involvement, stage III includes other lymph node and regional involvement, and stage IV includes any tumor with distant metastases.[23]

The primary tumor is assessed with chest x-rays and fiberoptic bronchoscopy whereas lymphatic spread is usually assessed by mediastinoscopy, gallium-67 citrate scanning, or CT.[3] If the history and physical examination or other routine clinical studies (e.g., CBC, liver functions tests) suggest the possibility of metastatic disease, then special scans (e.g., bone, brain, or liver) or biopsies (e.g., bone marrow or liver) may be necessary for staging.[3]

TABLE 117–3. Tumor (T), Node (N), Metastasis (M) Staging for Lung Cancer

T_X	Positive malignant cell; no lesion seen
T_1	≤ 3 cm surrounded by lung or visceral pleura
T_2	> 3 cm or involvement of main bronchus 2 cm or more distal to the carina, or invasion of visceral pleura, or associated atelectasis or obstructive pneumonitis extending to hilar region
T_3	Direct invasion of chest wall, diaphragm, mediastinal pleura, or parietal pericardium; or tumor in main bronchus less than 2 cm distal to the carina; or associated atelectasis or obstructive pneumonitis of the entire lung
T_4	Invasion of mediastinum, heart, great vessel, trachea, esophagus, vertebral body, carina; or tumor with a malignant pleural effusion
N_0	No regional lymph node involvement
N_1	Metastasis in ipsilateral peribronchial and/or ipsilateral hilar lymph node(s), including direct extension
N_2	Metastasis in ipsilateral mediastinal and/or subcarinal lymph node(s)
N_3	Metastasis in contralateral mediastinal, contralateral hilar, ipsilateral or contralateral scalene, or supraclavicular lymph node(s)
M_0	No distant metastases
M_1	Distant metastases

Stage Groupings

Stage IA	T_1	N_0	M_0
Stage IB	T_2	N_0	M_0
Stage IIA	T_1	N_1	M_0
Stage IIB	T_2	N_1	M_0
	T_3	N_0	M_0
Stage IIIA	T_1–T_3	N_2	M_0
	T_3	N_1	M_0
Stage IIIB	Any T	N_3	M_0
	T_4	Any N	M_0
Stage IV	Any T	Any N	M_1

From Ref. 23.

SMALL CELL LUNG CANCER

A two-stage classification established by the Veterans Administration Lung Cancer Study Group is widely used in the United States to stage small cell lung cancer (SCLC).[18] Limited disease is classified as disease confined to one hemithorax and to the regional lymph nodes. All other disease is classified as extensive. Approximately 70% of patients initially present with extensive disease. Because of this high frequency of disseminated disease at diagnosis (bone 38%, liver 22% to 28%, bone marrow 17% to 23%, CNS 8% to 14%), radionuclide scans of the bone and liver, CT scans of the brain, and bone marrow biopsies are generally recommended prior to initiation of therapy.[18] In addition, any suspicious signs or symptoms detected during the physical examination should be carefully investigated.

▶ TREATMENT: Lung Cancer

NON–SMALL CELL LUNG CANCER

Currently only surgery and, to a lesser extent, radiation therapy offer an opportunity for long-term survival in a significant percentage of patients; although, only about 30% of unselected patients have localized disease (stage I or II) that is amenable to local therapy.[3] Curative therapy in this disease is determined by the anatomic stage of the disease (it must be localized with no evidence of distant metastases) and the ability of the patient to withstand the therapy. If untreated, most patients die within 1 year of diagnosis.

SURGERY

Surgical resection is the treatment of choice for patients with clinical stage I and II disease (disease that by all evidence is stage I or II before surgical dissection of mediastinal lymph nodes). Overall, over 50% of patients with stage I and 35% of patients with stage II disease who undergo surgical resection survive 5 years without disease recurrence.[3] The single most important prognostic factor in patients undergoing curative resection is the presence or absence of lymph node involvement. In one series of 216 patients who had clinical stage I disease before surgery, only 125 patients were found to have stage I disease after surgery and pathologic examination of lymph nodes.[24] Therefore, it is apparent that mediastinal lymph node dissection at the time of surgery is of great importance. In patients with T_1N_0 tumors, various groups have reported 5-year survival rates exceeding 70%.[3] Stage II disease (N_1) has a poorer prognosis with a 5-year survival rate of only about 35%.[3] Pneumonectomy (versus lobectomy) is indicated in patients found to have lymph node involvement (stage II) at the time of surgery, and such patients may benefit from postoperative radiation therapy or radiation plus chemotherapy.[3] Even if no residual disease is evident at surgery, 50% of patients die within 2 years as a result of recurrent disease.[3]

The size of the tumor in stage I and II disease also has prognostic importance. In patients with stage I disease (old staging system), Martini and Beattie reported a 5-year survival rate of 80% when the primary tumor was 3 cm or less but only 50% when the tumor was larger than 3 cm.[24] It has been suggested that pneumonectomy, rather than lobectomy, also may reduce the rate of local recurrences in patients with larger stage I tumors.[25]

Management of stage IIIA tumors is more controversial. Although most are technically resectable, the prognosis is poorer, with 5-year survival rates ranging from 20% to 40% depending on tumor size and lymph node involvement.[3] For patients with locally advanced NSCLC (stages IIIA and IIIB), trials in recent years suggest that chemotherapy with or without radiation, followed by surgery, improves local and regional control and survival over radiation alone followed by surgery.[3]

RADIATION

Radiation therapy is considered an alternative modality in patients with stage I or II disease who decline surgery or are considered high surgical risks because of concomitant illness or restrictive pulmonary reserve.[3] In addition, radiation therapy may also be used when the tumor is not resectable because of fixation to a major blood vessel, the trachea, or the esophagus. The 2- and 5-year survival rates appear to be highest for patients whose tumors would otherwise be considered resectable.[26] Although local control of tumor growth may be achieved in up to 60% of patients with stage III disease, the overall 5-year survival is only about 6%.[3] When radiation therapy is given after surgery, it may reduce the incidence of local recurrences; however, it does not appear to improve survival because distant metastases still occur.[3]

In situations in which radiation is used with curative intent, relatively higher doses and large treatment volumes are required and there are significant risks to the normal tissue surrounding the tumor (see Complications and Supportive Care).

CHEMOTHERAPY

Because many patients with NSCLC are inoperable at diagnosis (e.g., locally advanced stage IIIB or metastatic disease stage IV), and because systemic dissemination occurs in the majority of patients who are initially surgically resected or radiated for potential cure, there is clearly a definite need for effective systemic therapy (i.e., chemotherapy) in this disease.

METASTATIC OR RECURRENT DISEASE

Historically, the response rates for chemotherapy in NSCLC have been disappointingly low, and until recently the use of chemotherapy was considered controversial. However, data have consistently shown that patients who respond to chemotherapy are likely to have a survival benefit over nonresponders.[3] Nonetheless, response rates were low and overall survival poor for early chemotherapy regimens used in NSCLC. Improved response rates and survival with newer chemotherapy agents and combinations have led most experts to agree that most patients with stage IV disease should receive at least one chemotherapy regimen.[3] Despite significant advances, chemotherapy for stage IV NSCLC is not curative, although it frequently prolongs survival and decreases symptoms. Several comparative trials have also demonstrated improved survival for patients receiving chemotherapy versus those receiving best supportive care.[27–29] One of these also demonstrated decreased overall costs of patient management with chemotherapy.[28,30] Meta-analyses of these and other studies have confirmed this conclusion.[31–34]

Several factors have been suggested as having prognostic importance in terms of response and survival in patients receiving chemotherapy. These factors include the patient's initial performance status, weight loss, and extent of disease.[3,35] Among these factors, an initial favorable performance status of the patient appears to be the most consistent factor predicting a better response and improved survival.[3,35] There is no evidence of the usefulness of chemotherapy in persons with a Karnofsky performance status of less than 50%.[3] Patients with an unfavorable prognosis (weight loss, poor performance status, elevated lactate dehydrogenase [LDH] and/or significant concomitant diseases) should be given supportive care and palliative radiation when necessary.

Direct comparison of response rates between clinical trials is difficult and interpretation of the results requires careful analysis of the methodology. Two factors that must be considered are the method of patient selection and the criteria for response that were used. As previously mentioned, several factors are believed to have prognostic significance, and it is necessary to know the status of such factors (e.g., performance status, extent of disease prior to therapy) in the study population when comparing clinical trials. Likewise, it is important to know if patients with an unfavorable prognosis were intentionally excluded from the trial. In addition, to compare results of clinical trials it is imperative that both trials use the same response criteria. In most series a complete response (CR) is defined as the complete disappearance of all evidence of the tumor whereas a partial response (PR) is defined as a reduction in measurable tumor mass of greater than 50% lasting longer than 1 month. Because many lung tumors do not have definite margins to measure, the term *objective response* is used to describe disease when there has been a definite decrease in the size of the lesion without appearance of any new lesions.[3]

Single-agent chemotherapy has generally demonstrated objective response rates of 5% to 25% with no significant effect on overall survival. When responses do occur after single-agent chemotherapy, the duration of the response is usually quite brief (2 to 4 months) and complete responses are rare.[3] Among the most active single agents in NSCLC are cisplatin, carboplatin, docetaxel, etoposide, gemcitabine, ifosfamide, irinotecan, mitomycin, paclitaxel, topotecan, vinblastine, and vinorelbine. Numerous investigational agents, including LY231514, a thymidylate synthase inhibitor; marimastat, a matrix metalloproteinase inhibitor; tirapazamine, a cytotoxic targeting hypoxic cells; and amrubicin, a synthetic anthracycline compound, are currently being evaluated as single agents or in combination therapy in phase II and III clinical trials.

Combination chemotherapy has been used in the management of NSCLC since the late 1960s, and although response rates

TABLE 117–4. Traditional Combination Chemotherapy in Non–Small Cell Lung Cancer

Combination	Dosages	Schedule	Overall Response Rate (%)	Reference
CE				
DDP	60–100 mg/m² IV day 1	Repeat course every 3–4 wk	19–30	3
ETOP	80–120 mg/m² IV days 1, 2, and 3			
DDP/VIND				
DDP	120 mg/m² IV days 1 and 29	Repeat every 6 wk	30	3
VIND	3 mg/m² IV every week × 6 wk	Then repeat course every 2 wk		
MVP				
MT	8 mg/m² IV days 1 and 29		43	36
VIND	3 mg/m² IV days 1, 8, 29, and 36			
DDP	80 mg/m² IV days 1 and 29			
ICE				
IFOS	1.5 g/m² IV days 1, 2, and 3	Repeat every 3 wk	43	3
CARBO	300–350 mg/m² day 1			
ETOP	60–100 mg/m² days 1, 2, and 3			

DDP = cisplatin; ETOP = etoposide; VIND = vindesine; MT = mitomycin; IFOS = ifosfamide; CARBO = carboplatin.

for combination therapy generally have been better than those for single-agent therapy, consistent improvement in overall survival rates has been more difficult to demonstrate. The introduction of cisplatin is hailed as the most significant development in combination therapy in NSCLC. Today it is included in the most widely studied and recommended regimens. Table 117–4 describes some of the platinum-containing regimens studied in NSCLC.

Active regimens that have commonly reported response rates exceeding 30% have used various combinations of cisplatin, ifosfamide, mitomycin, and vinblastine, vinorelbine, or vindesine (Table 117–4). Evidence suggests that the dose of cisplatin may have impact on response. Single-agent cisplatin trials in NSCLC demonstrated higher response rates for increasing doses, and a meta-analysis of 100 chemotherapy regimens showed that cisplatin 100 mg/m² (in combination with other agents) had higher response rates than trials using 70 mg/m². Cisplatin dose escalations above 100 mg/m² resulted in increased toxicity without any additional survival benefit.[3]

At present, new chemotherapeutic agents in four distinct classes have shown single-agent activity of greater than 20% in NSCLC (Table 117–5). The plant alkaloids (vinorelbine), taxanes (antimicrotubule agents; paclitaxel and docetaxel), antimetabolites (gemcitabine), and topoisomerase 1 inhibitors (topotecan and irinotecan) are being extensively studied in various combinations, with platinum compounds (cisplatin or carboplatin), with and without concurrent or sequential radiation therapy and/or postinduction surgery (multimodality therapy). The earlier studies of these compounds focused primarily on response rates, while the newer studies focus on improved survival rates (disease free, overall), quality of life, toxicity (short and long term), and cost ef-

TABLE 117–5. Single-Agent Studies of New Chemotherapy Agents for Non–Small Cell Lung Cancer

Reference	Evaluable/Total Patients (Stage)	Regimen	Overall Response Rates (%)	Median Survival Duration (wk)	Median 1-Year Survival (%)
Vinorelbine					
LeChevalier (37, 38)	199/206 (IIIA 20, IIIB 65, IV 97)	30 mg/m² weekly	14	31	30
Depierre (39)	119	30 mg/m² weekly	16	32	(2 yr = 5)
Paclitaxel					
Murphy (40)	25/25 chemo-naive	200 mg/m² over 24 h every 3 wk	24	40	38
Chang (41)	24/24 chemo-naive	250 mg/m² over 24 h every 3 wk	21	24	41.7
Docetaxel					
Francis (42)	29/29 (IIIB 17%, IV 83%)	100 mg/m² every 3 wk	31	37	39
Fossella (43)	39/41 chemo-naive (IIIB 10%, IV 90%)	100 mg/m² every 3 wk	33	14	NR
Fossella (44, 45)	42/44 (prior DDP) (IIIB 9%, IV 91%)	100 mg/m² every 3 wk	21	43	39
Gandara (46)	80/80 (prior DDP)	100 mg/m² every 3 wk	15	28	25
Gemcitabine					
Abratt (47)	76/84 (IIIA 17.8%, IIIB 40.5%, IV 41.7%)	Dose escalation trial with initial doses = 1000–1250 mg/m² weekly × 3 wk, off 1 wk, then repeat	20	NR	NR
Gatzemier (48)	151/161 chemo-naive (IIIA 4.3%, IIIB 31.3%, IV 64.6%)	1250 mg/m² every week × 3, off 1 wk, then repeat	22	11.5	16
IRINOTECAN					
Fukuoka (49)	72/72 chemo-naive	100 mg/m²	31.9	42	NR

NR = not reported.

TABLE 117–6. Combination Regimens of Newer Agents for Non–Small Cell Lung Cancer

Reference	Evaluable/Total Patients (Stage)	Regimen	Overall Response Rates (%)	Median Survival Duration (wk)	1-Year Survival (%)
Paclitaxel + Platinum					
Langer (51)	53/54 (IIIB 4, IV 50)	Paclitaxel 135–215 mg/m² over 24 h Carboplatin AUC = 7.5 (+ G-CSF added at cycle 2)	62 (9 CR)	53	54
Bonomi (52)	560/574 (IIIB 108, IV 466)	Cisplatin 75 mg/m² day 1 plus etoposide 100 mg/m² every week × 3	12	33	31.6
		vs			
		Paclitaxel 135 mg/m² over 24 h plus cisplatin 75 mg/m²	26.5	41	36.9
		vs			
		Paclitaxel 250 mg/m² over 24 h plus cisplatin 75 mg/m² (+ G-CSF)	32.1	43	39.1
Docetaxel + Cisplatin or Vinorelbine					
LeChevalier (53)	24 chemo-naive (IIIB and IV)	Docetaxel 75 mg/m² plus cisplatin 100 mg/m² on days 1, 21, and 42 every 6 wk	25	NR	NR
Early (54)	17 (IIIB and IV)	Vinorelbine 15–37.5 mg/m² over 10 min followed by Docetaxel 50 mg/m² every 2 wk (+ G-CSF)	29	NR	NR
Gemcitabine + Cisplatin					
Abratt (55)	50/53	Gemcitabine 1000 mg/m² weekly × 3 wk, every 28 d plus cisplatin 100 mg/m² day 15	52	52	61
Crino (56)	48/48 (IIIA 1, IIIB 21, IV 26)	Gemcitabine 1000 mg/m² weekly × 3 weeks, every 28 d plus cisplatin 100 mg/m² day 2	54	61.5	NR
Vinorelbine + Cisplatin					
LeChavalier (37, 38)	192/206 (IIIA 23, IIIB 58, IV 102)	Vinorelbine 30 mg/m² weekly plus cisplatin 120 mg/m² days 1 and 29, then every 6 wk	30	40	35
		vs			
	183/200 (IIIA 21, IIIB 49, IV 109)	Vindesine 3 mg/m² every week × 6 wk, then every 2 wk plus cisplatin 120 mg/m² days 1 and 29, then every 6 wk	19	32	27
		vs			
	199/206 (IIIA 20, IIIB 65, IV 97)	Vinorelbine 30 mg/m² weekly	14	31	30
Depierre (39)	208/240 (121 III and IV)	Vinorelbine 30 mg/m² weekly plus cisplatin 80 mg/m² every 3 wk	43	33	(2 yr = 10)
		vs			
	(199 III and IV)	Vinorelbine 30 mg/m² weekly	16	32	(2 yr = 5)

AUC = area-under-the-curve.

fectiveness.[50] Results from numerous recently published trials combining these new chemotherapeutic agents with platinum-based regimens have suggested improved 1-year survival rates in advanced NSCLC of 30% to 40% versus 15% to 25% with the previously used platinum-based regimens (Table 117–6).

Direct comparisons of results between studies requires critical assessment of the inclusion and exclusion criteria and study design. The importance of subsets within stage III locally advanced NSCLC (stage IIIA minimally bulky disease and stage IIIB bulky disease) and whether pathologic documentation of stage IIIA (N_2) disease is required. A mixture of subsets with minimal and bulky disease, with or without documented N_2 disease, may have contributed to the wide ranges reported in 3- to 5-year survival rates and differences observed between study arms in many of the early phase I and II trials. Currently, phase III large-scale randomized trials with detailed subset selection and disease documentation are ongoing to evaluate the efficacy of various combinations of chemotherapy, radiation, and surgery. Clinicians must refrain from extrapolating the results of the currently published trials into their general daily practice and should continue to refer patients to carefully designed randomized trials to define the optimal therapy for the various subsets within NSCLC.

Vinorelbine (Navelbine) is a semisynthetic, vinca alkaloid. Single-agent activity has been demonstrated in advanced NSCLC, with response rates of up to 33%, median survival of 40 weeks, and 1-year survival rates of 24% to 30%.[37–39] The combination of vinorelbine plus cisplatin has demonstrated superior efficacy to either agent alone, and to vindesine plus cisplatin in randomized phase III trials.[36–39,57]

Neutropenia is the dose-limiting toxicity for vinorelbine therapy. Thrombocytopenia and grade 3 and 4 anemia have occurred in less than 1% and 10% of patients, respectively. Mild to moderate nonhematologic adverse effects include nausea and vomiting, peripheral neuropathy, and transient elevations in liver function tests. Vinorelbine is easily administered in the outpatient oncology setting by peripheral or central venous access over 6 to 10 minutes, followed by a 75- to 100- mL intravenous flush. Longer infusions of vinorelbine have been associated with an increased frequency of peripheral injection site reactions.[58] Based on the survival advantage and minimal added toxicity of vinorelbine combined with cisplatin, this regimen may be considered the standard against which future combination chemotherapy regimens should be measured. Thus, the Southwest Oncology Group (SWOG 9509) is currently conducting a randomized phase III trial of cisplatin plus vinorelbine versus carboplatin plus paclitaxel in chemo-naive patients with advanced NSCLC.

The taxanes, paclitaxel (Taxol) and docetaxel (Taxotere), are antimicrotubular agents that bind to the microtubules and promote and stabilize microtubular assembly, resulting in the inhibition of mitosis and cell death. Paclitaxel as a single agent and in combination regimens has been evaluated in patients with advanced NSCLC with promising results. Regimens have included paclitaxel administered 1-hour, 3-hour, and 24-hour continuous infusion schedules at low doses (175 mg/m^2) and high doses (250 mg/m^2) with granulocyte colony-stimulating factor (G-CSF) support. Neutropenia is the dose-limiting toxicity of paclitaxel, but nonhematologic adverse reactions occur with differing frequencies based on the duration of infusion.[59] Hypersensitivity reactions (possibly owing to the Cremophor EL base) were frequent in the early phase I trials, leading to the current recommendations for pretreatment with corticosteroids and histamine H_1 and H_2 antagonists. Paclitaxel, owing to its aqueous insolubility, is formulated in Cremophor EL and dehydrated alcohol, requiring additional infusion related costs for non-PVC administration systems.

Bonomi and colleagues[52] at the Eastern Cooperative Oncology Group (ECOG) reported the preliminary results from 560 evaluable patients enrolled in a three-arm randomized trial with improved 1-year survival rates of 37% and 39% in the cisplatin plus paclitaxel 175 mg/m^2/24 hour infusion and the cisplatin plus paclitaxel 250 mg/m^2/24 hour infusion with G-CSF support versus the standard regimen arm of cisplatin plus etoposide, which yielded a lower 1-year survival rate of 31%. No difference in efficacy was observed between the low- and high-dose paclitaxel arms; however, the high-dose arm resulted in significantly greater toxicity (neutropenia and peripheral neuropathy).

Langer and colleagues[51] at ECOG reported the results from a phase II trial of 53 patients with stage IIIB or IV NSCLC treated with paclitaxel (135 to 215 mg/m^2) via 24-hour continuous infusion plus carboplatin (AUC 7.5) on day 2 infused every 3 weeks. The regimen resulted in significant myleosuppression, with grade 3 or 4 neutropenia in 57% of patients after the first cycle, necessitating the addition of G-CSF for the second and subsequent cycles. Significant thrombocytopenia and anemia were also reported in 47% and 33% of patients, respectively. Despite initially high response rates of 62% and an encouraging 1-year survival rate of 54%, the 2-year and 3-year survival rates remain dismal at 15% and 4%, respectively.[60,61] A subsequent trial by Langer and colleagues[60] compared a 1-hour versus 24-hour infusion of paclitaxel plus carboplatin, using identical dosage escalations. The 1-hour regimen resulted in an increased rate of peripheral neuropathy and minimal myelosuppression; but the response rate decreased to 27% (overall survival rates are not yet available). The shorter (< 3 hour) infusions of paclitaxel are easily administered in the outpatient oncology setting and rarely require G-CSF support, making them more patient friendly and cost effective to administer than the 24-hour infusions. However, the results of ongoing cooperative trials in advanced NSCLC will be required to clarify the most appropriate infusion schedule and the role of paclitaxel in combination with platinum compounds and the other newer agents.

Docetaxel (Taxotere) is a highly active semisynthetic taxoid, without the schedule-dependent efficacy and toxicity issues associated with paclitaxel administration. The majority of clinical trials have used docetaxel dosages ranging from 75 to 100 mg/m^2 infused intravenously over 1 hour every 3 weeks. Initial response rates from 25% to 38% have been reported in chemo-naive patients with advanced NSCLC.[42,43] In addition, docetaxel has demonstrated activity in platinum-refractory NSCLC with response rates of 15% to 17%.[44–46] The potential role of docetaxel as an active second-line agent in platinum-refractory NSCLC is unique among the currently available cytotoxic agents.

Phase I and II trials have defined neutropenia as the dose-limiting toxicity for docetaxel. Nonhematologic adverse effects include hypersensitivity reactions, fluid retention syndrome (cumulative effect resulting in peripheral edema and pleural effusions), rash, asthenia, mucositis, alopecia, and peripheral neuropathy. Patients should be premedicated with an oral corticosteroid regimen beginning 24 hours prior to the docetaxel infusion and continuing for a total of 3 to 5 days to reduce the incidence and severity of fluid retention. Numerous cooperative trials are ongoing to evaluate the efficacy and toxicity of docetaxel in combination with carboplatin, cisplatin, vinorelbine, gemcitabine, irinotecan, and thoracic radiation therapy. To date, a randomized comparison trial of docetaxel versus paclitaxel in advanced NSCLC has not been reported.

Gemcitabine (Gemzar) is a nucleoside analog (antimetabolite) that is phosphorylated intracellularly by deoxycytidine kinase.[61] It has an increased membrane permeability and affinity for deoxycytidine kinase, yielding higher intracellular concentrations of the active metabolite and prolonged inhibition of DNA, as compared to its structurally related predecessor cytarabine. Phase I and II trials of gemcitabine have demonstrated antitumor activity against a variety of solid tumors, including lung, breast, ovarian, and pancreatic cancers. Gemcitabine has been shown in numerous phase I and II trials to exhibit schedule dependent toxicity.[62–65] The weekly regimen, using a 30-minute intravenous infusion of gemcitabine (days 1, 8, and 15) for 3 weeks followed by a 1-week rest period administered every 4 weeks (28 days per cycle), allows maximally tolerated dosages to be administered with acceptable toxicity in the outpatient oncology setting.[65,66] Dose-limiting toxicity (DLT) for this regimen was thrombocytopenia and reversible hepatotoxicity. The overall toxicity profile of gemcitabine is modest with mild myelosuppression, nausea and vomiting, rash, flu-like symptoms, fatigue, and anorexia. The proven single-agent efficacy and minimal toxicity of gemcitabine in phase I and II trails make it a viable agent for inclusion in combination chemotherapy regimens.

Irinotecan (Camptosar) and topotecan (Hycamtin) are potent inhibitors of topoisomerase 1, the nuclear enzyme responsible for maintaining DNA topologic structure. Inhibition of topoisomerase 1 stabilizes single-strand DNA breaks and prevents religation (resealing), resulting in DNA dysfunction.[67] Irinotecan (CPT-11) has demonstrated single-agent response rates in advanced NSCLC of 35% in early phase I and II trials, with dose-limiting toxicities of neutropenia and severe diarrhea.[49] Combination chemotherapy utilizing irinotecan plus cisplatin and vindesine have yielded preliminary response rates of 40% to 54%; however, 1-year survival rates are not yet available.[68,69] Early trials of concurrent irinotecan and chest irradiation therapy resulted in dose-limiting esophagitis, diarrhea, and unexpected severe pneumonitis precluding further investigation. Clearly, the significant toxicities associated with irinotecan therapy must be carefully evaluated in concert with long-term survival data to define its role in the treatment of NSCLC.

Tumor response to chemotherapy is generally evaluated at the end of the second cycle, and at the end every second cycle thereafter. Patients with stable disease (SD) or with objective tumor response (CR, PR) should continue with the same chemotherapy regimen. The chemotherapy regimen should be discontinued if progressive disease (PD) is documented, and an alternative regimen or investigational protocol should be considered.

LOCALLY ADVANCED DISEASE

Because of the poor long-term survival rates following surgery alone or surgery followed by radiation therapy in locally advanced disease (stage III) and because recurrence at distant sites is a major problem,[70] chemotherapy is now used with other modalities with curative intent. When administered prior to surgery (neoadjuvant), the goals of chemotherapy are to (1) deliver chemotherapy to the tumor site prior to destruction of the local vasculature by surgery and/or radiation; (2) reduce the size of the tumor to increase the likelihood of successful local therapy (e.g., complete surgical resection); and (3) eradicate undetectable micrometastases. In addition, neoadjuvant chemotherapy may allow for less extensive resections and therefore conservation of normal lung tissue.[4] Conversely, potential disadvantages of neoadjuvant chemotherapy include (1) a risk that toxicities resulting from the chemotherapy may decrease the patient's ability to tolerate subsequent surgery and/or radiation; (2) a risk that if the tumor does not respond to the chemotherapy it will continue to grow and become unresectable; and (3) a significant prolongation of the duration of treatment.

The foregoing rationale coupled with the identification of newer chemotherapy regimens with apparent increased activity in NSCLC stimulated several pilot studies of neoadjuvant chemotherapy in patients with locally advanced disease.[71] The highest response rates have been observed with regimens that include cisplatin 100 mg/m^2. Results of these studies indicated that most patients with stage III disease were able to tolerate two or three courses of aggressive chemotherapy followed by definitive surgery and/or radiation. Although several of these studies reported encouraging response rates (> 50%), survival advantages could not be appropriately addressed in these nonrandomized trials. The Cancer and Leukemia Group B (CALGB) randomized 155 evaluable patients with unresectable NSCLC to receive either radiation alone or two courses of cisplatin and vinblastine followed by radiation. Forty-three percent of patients receiving radiation alone responded versus 56% of patients receiving the combined modality. At a median follow-up of 19 months, the median survival for combined modality therapy was 16.5 months versus 8.5 months for radiation alone, thus demonstrating a survival advantage for the combination.[72] Follow-up at 5 years continued to show this survival advantage.[73] It is important to note that this study and a similar trial reported by Sause et al.[74] included only fully ambulatory patients with less than 5% weight loss and no malignant pleural effusions prior to treatment. Therefore, these results may not be applicable for patients with poor prognostic disease characteristics. A meta-analysis of 11 trials including 1780 patients receiving chest radiation with or without cisplatin-based chemotherapy also indicated that mortality was reduced by 13% in patients randomized to receive chemotherapy.[75] Overall, evidence strongly suggests that chemotherapy with or without radiation increases the likelihood that tumors may be completely resected and is superior to radiation alone followed by surgery.

Other investigators have evaluated the use of concomitant radiation and chemotherapy in patients with locally advanced unresectable NSCLC. This strategy allows for micrometastases to be treated at the earliest possible time and maximizes the additive effects of radiation and chemotherapy. A wide range of median survival durations have been reported and it is not clear that overall survival is improved using the concomitant strategy.[3] This is likely due to the variability of radiation therapy regimens that have been employed and the inherent toxicities of the concurrent regimens.

SMALL CELL LUNG CANCER

CHEMOTHERAPY

In contrast to NSCLC, the use of aggressive combination chemotherapy regimens in SCLC has demonstrated a four- to five-fold increase in median survival. Without treatment, survival is generally less than 5 to 7 weeks for patients with metastatic disease (extensive-disease SCLC) and less than 12 weeks for patients with regional disease (limited-disease SCLC). Because SCLC has the propensity to disseminate early on in the disease, surgery is almost never indicated, except possibly in the rare patient who presents with a small, isolated lesion. A number of factors have been identified that appear to have prognostic importance in SCLC.[76,77] Patients who initially present with limited disease and are treated with aggressive chemotherapy regimens demonstrate a significantly longer median survival than patients presenting with extensive disease treated with the same regimens.[18,78] Patients presenting with a better (i.e., ambulatory) performance status and no weight loss also appear to have an improved prognosis.[18,79] Females appear to have a better prognosis than males, as do patients under age 60 to 70 years.[78,79] Patients with normal pretreatment serum lactate dehydrogenase (LDH) are also more likely to have limited disease, higher complete response rates, and longer median survivals.[79,80] A simple prognostic model for SCLC has been developed and verified, using LDH levels in concert with performance status and extent of disease.[81] In addition, LDH levels have been shown to be an independent prognostic factor for SCLC, correlating with disease stage, response to therapy, and survival.[77,80] A recent European study has shown that serum neuron-specific endolase (S-NSE), a biologic marker, may be substituted for LDH levels in the simple prognostic model for SCLC.[82]

A number of cytotoxic agents have demonstrated significant single-agent activity in chemotherapy-naive patients with limited- and extensive-disease SCLC; however, activity in recurrent or refractory SCLC is marginal. Among the more commonly used agents in the United States are cisplatin, carboplatin, cyclophosphamide, ifosfamide, doxorubicin, etoposide (VP-16), teniposide (VM-26), and vincristine. Newer agents currently being investigated for a potential role in the treatment of SCLC include docetaxel, gemcitabine, irinotecan, paclitaxel, topotecan, and vinorelbine. These newer single-agent regimens are described in Table 117–7. Of note, a recent single-agent phase II trial of paclitaxel in heavily pretreated patients with drug-resistant SCLC limited disease = 9, extensive disease = 15) reported PRs in seven patients (29%) and SD in five patients, with a median survival of 100 days, thus indicating the need for continued evaluation of paclitaxel in combination chemotherapy regimens.[83] Recently it has also been reported that topotecan produces responses and improves symptoms in up to 25% to 38% of patients who initially fail or relapse following conventional regimens.[85,86]

COMBINATION CHEMOTHERAPY

Combination chemotherapy is clearly superior to single-agent therapy and the best results are generally observed when three or

TABLE 117–7. Selected Single-Agent Trials of Newer Agents in Small-Cell Lung Cancer

Reference	Evaluable/Total Patients (Stage)	Drug Regimen/Dose	Overall Response Rates (%)	Median Survival Duration (wk)	1-Year Survival (%)
Smit (83)	21/24 (9 LD) (15 ED) Drug resistant	Paclitaxel 175 mg/m² IV over 3 h q 3 wk	29 (7 PR) (+ 5 SD)	14	NR
Ettinger (84)	32/36 (36 ED) (Res. + Sens.)	Paclitaxel 250 mg/m² over 24 h q 3 wk × 4 cycles	34 (11 PR) (+ 6 SD)	43	NR
		Followed by salvage chemo for non-CRs:	*+ salvage* 53		
		DDP 60 mg/m² IV day 1 + ETOP 120 mg/m² IV days 1, 2, and 3	(2 CR) (15 PR)		
Ardizzoni (85)	92/101 (47 Drug res.) (45 Drug sens.)	Topotecan 1.5 mg/m² IV q days 1 through 5, q 3 wk	Drug res. 6.4 (1 CR) (2 PR)	33	NR
			Drug sens. 37.8 (6 CR) (11 PR)	48	NR
Perez-Soler (86)	28/32 Drug res. (ETOP + DDP)	Topotecan 1.25 mg/m² IV q days 1 through 5, q 3 wk (cycle 2, ↓ 1.0 mg/m²)	11 (3 PR) (+ 5 SD)	20	NR
Eckardt (87) (Abstract) *Pooled analysis*	168 Drug sens.	Topotecan 1.5 mg/m² IV q days 1 through 5, q 3 wk	18 (10 CR) (20 PR)	30	21
Masuda (88)	15/16 (5 LD) (10 ED) (Res. + Sens.)	Irinotecan 100 mg/m² IV over 90 min q wk (median 7 cycles, range 2–13)	47 (7 PR) (7 SD)	27	NR
Cormier (89)	26/29 ED Chemo-naive	Gemcitabine 1000 mg/m² IV q wk × 3 wk, every 28 d (patients 1–17) *followed by:* Gemcitabine 1250 mg/m² IV q wk × 3 wk, q 28 d (patients 18–26)	27 (1 CR) (6 PR) (12 SD)	52	NR
DePierre (90) (Abstract)	30 Chemo-naive	Vinorelbine 30 mg/m² IV q wk × 10 wk	26.7 (8 PR) (7 SD)	NR	NR
Furuse (91)	24/24 Drug sens.	Vinorelbine 25 mg/m² IV q wk × ≥ 4 wk	12.5 (3 PR) (9 SD)	NR	NR

Drug res. = Drug-resistant tumors, progressing during first-line therapy or within 3 months from response to chemotherapy; Drug sens. = Drug-sensitive tumors, progressing after 3 months from response to chemotherapy; ED = extensive disease; LD = limited disease; CR = complete response; PR = partial response; DDP = cisplatin; ETOP = etoposide.

more active agents are combined. In recent years it has been observed that aggressive chemotherapy regimens appear to produce higher response rates, longer median survivals, and a higher percentage of long-term survivals.[18] Some of the more frequently used regimens have been: (1) CAV—cyclophosphamide + doxorubicin (A) + vincristine (V); (2) CAE—C-A-etoposide (E); and (3) CE (PE)—cisplatin (P) + E; (4) (V)ICE—ifosfamide (I) (with mesna IV and/or oral) + carboplatin + etoposide (E) ± vincristine (V).[92] Several of these and other popular regimens are described in Table 117–8. Overall response rates (80% to 90% versus 60% to 80%) and survival durations (12 to 20 months vs 7 to 11 months) are generally superior in patients with limited disease versus those with extensive disease (Table 117–9). The 2-year disease-free survival rate for patients with limited stage disease at diagnosis is 15% to 40%; however, 2-year disease-free survival is uncommon in patients with extensive disease. Unfortunately, when the disease recurs, it is usually less sensitive to chemotherapy. Restaging to determine the effects of chemotherapy is usually done after two to three cycles of treatment. At this point therapy is continued for patients with a complete or partial response (CR or PR) or stable disease (SD) and discontinued or changed to a non–cross-resistant regimen in patients demonstrating evidence of progressive disease (PD).

Induction followed by maintenance chemotherapy for limited and extensive SCLC was evaluated in a randomized trial

TABLE 117–8. Selected Combination Chemotherapy Regimens for Small-Cell Lung Cancer

Reference	Evaluable/Total Patients and Characteristics	Drug Regimen/Dose	Overall Response Rates (CR + PR)	Median Survival Duration (mo)	2-Year Survival (%)
Roth (93)		Arm A: **EP** Cisplatin 20 mg/m²/d IV Days 1–5 ETOP mg/m²/d IV days 1 through 5 Every 3 wk × 4 cycles	61% (CR 10%)	4.3	NR
		vs			
		Arm B: **CAV** CTX 1000 mg/m²/d IV day 1 DOX 40 mg/m²/d day 1 VCR 1 mg/m²/d day 1 Every 3 wks × 6 cycles	51% (CR 7%)	4.0	NR
		vs			
		Arm C: **CAV/EP** CAV on day 1 followed by EP on days 22 through 26 Every 6 wk × 3 cycles	59% (CR 7%)	5.2	NR
Maksymiuk (94)	552 (LD + ED)	Arm A: **EP** Cisplatin 30 mg/m²/d followed by ETOP 130 mg/m²/d (IV) Days 1–3 every 4 wk × 2 cycles; then CAV every 4 wk × 4 cycles, finally CR/PR received TRT and PCI	84% (CR 52%)	15 (LD 20)	26 (LD 42)
Loehrer (95)	163/171 Untreated/ED (84 VP)	**VP** Cisplatin 20 mg/m²/d ETOP 100 mg/m²d (IV) Days 1 through 4, q 3 wk × 4 cycles	67% (20% CR)	7.3	5 (3 yr = 0)
		vs			
	(87 VIP)	**VIP** Cisplatin 20 mg/m²/d ETOP 75 mg/m²/d (IV) IFOS 1.2 g/m²/d Days 1 through 4, + mesna, every 3 wk × 4 cycles	73% (21% CR)	9.1	13 (3 yr = 5)
Faylona (96)	42/46 Previously Tx (LD 9) (ED 33)	**VIP** IFOS 1.2 gm/m²/d (IV) + mesna days 1 through 4 Cisplatin 20 mg/m²/d (IV) Days 1 through 4 ETOP (PO) 37.5 mg/m²/d Days 1 through 21 (22); ↓ 1 through 14 (20), q 4 wk × 4 cycles	55% (14% CR) (40% PR)	7.2	NR NR
Hainsworth (97)	79 Untreated (LD 41) (ED 79)	**TCE** Paclitaxel 200 mg/m²/d IV over 1 h, day 1 CBDCA-AUC 6.0, day 1 ETOP 50/100 mg/d alt. PO, days 1 through 10, q 21 d × 4 cycles	LD 98% (CR 71%) ED 84% (CR 21%)	LD > 16 ED 10	NR
Wolff (98)	35 ED Untreated	**ICE** IFOS 3750–5000 mg/m²/d IV over 24 h (CIV) Day 1 + mesna CDBCA 300 mg/m²/d day 1 ETOP 50 mg/d PO days 1 through 14 or 1 through 21	ED 83% (CR 23%) (PR 60%)	8.3	14

(continued)

TABLE 117–8. Selected Combination Chemotherapy Regimens for Small Cell Lung Cancer (Continued)

Reference	Evaluable and Total Patients and Characteristics	Drug Regimen/Dose	Overall Response Rates (CR + PR)	Median Survival Duration (mo)	2-Year Survival (%)
Thatcher (99)	89 (LD 73) (ED 14)	**(V)ICE** IFOS 5000 mg/m^2/d day 1 + mesna CBDCA 300 mg/m^2/d day 1 ETOP 120 mg/m^2/d (IV) days 1 and 2 followed by 240 mg/m^2/d (PO) day 3 VCR 1 mg/d day 1	LD 84% (CR 60%) ED 71% (29%)	LD 16.6 ED 13.4	LD 32 ED 21

CTX = cyclophosphamide; ADR = doxorubicin or Adriamycin; VCR = vincristine; ETOP = etoposide; CBDCA = carboplatin; IFOS = ifosfamide; CIV = continuous intravenous infusion;

with 585 evaluable patients who received the CAE (cyclophosphamide, doxorubicin, and etoposide) regimen for 5 cycles versus 12 cycles.[100] The extended chemotherapy regimen did not significantly improve long-term survival (median survival 325 days; limited disease 396 days and extensive disease 267 days, with a 3.2% overall survival in both arms at 5 years). In addition, patients who received the extended duration (12 cycles) of chemotherapy experienced an increased incidence of acute toxicity and second malignancies. The Eastern Cooperative Oncology Group (ECOG) demonstrated an overall median survival of approximately 20 months, in a comparative study of concurrent once versus twice daily thoracic radiation plus only 4 cycles of cisplatin plus etoposide (CE) chemotherapy.[101] This trial demonstrated the greatest overall median survival for SCLC seen to date in a cooperative trial group, which further supports the recommendation for a short course of induction therapy. These data have been confirmed by several randomized trials, comparing induction with or without maintenance chemotherapy regimens versus supportive care, with the majority reporting similar survival outcomes.[18] At this time, it is reasonable and cost effective to administer chemotherapy for approximately 4 to 6 cycles in SCLC patients who respond (CR, PR) to initial chemotherapy.

DOSE INTENSITY

Experimental animal and human tumor data have suggested that the amount of drug administered over a unit of time may be critical to the degree of tumor cell kill.[102] This influence of dose intensity has been evaluated in many types of human cancer, particularly those like SCLC that are initially responsive to chemotherapy, but not usually curable with conventional therapies. Randomized trials using dose-intensive (high-dose) CAE, CAVE, CE, and CEEP (CTX, epirubicin, etoposide, cisplatin) versus standard dosage regimens failed to significantly improve overall survival,[103–107] although in the subset of patients with limited-stage SCLC, several studies reported positive results.[108,109] A meta-analysis of 60 reported clinical trials failed to establish a consistent dose-intensity–outcome correlation for most SCLC chemotherapy regimens.[109] As expected, toxicities (including granulocytopenia, febrile neutropenia, and weight loss) were significantly increased in the patients who received the dose-intensive treatment regimens. At present, dose-intensive chemotherapy should be reserved for clinical trials, in patients with limited-stage SCLC, and for the evaluation of newer agents used in combination chemotherapy regimens and should not be used in routine oncology practice.

TABLE 117–9. Responses to Optimal Chemotherapy Regimens Based on Stage of Disease

	Limited Disease	Extensive Disease
Overall response (CR + PR)	80%–95%	60%–85%
Complete Response	50%–60%	15%–30%
Median survival (mo)	12–20	7–11
2-Year disease-free survival	15%–40%	Rare

CR = complete response; PR = partial response.
Adapted from Ref. 18.

ALTERNATING NON–CROSS-RESISTANT REGIMENS

Because the duration of response is usually brief (less than 1 year) for patients achieving a complete response, it appears that drug-resistant cells continue to grow during treatment and eventually constitute a major portion of the tumor. The Goldie–Coldman theory[110] predicts that the cycling of two active, non–cross-resistant chemotherapeutic regimens may overcome this problem. Although theoretically it would seem ideal to administer all the drugs simultaneously, the treatment-related toxic effects would be prohibitive. A number of phase III clinical trials have used alternating, non–cross-resistant regimens in the management of SCLC, but most have failed to demonstrate substantial benefits.[111,112] Examples of such regimens include cyclophosphamide, methotrexate, and lomustine alternating with vincristine, doxorubicin, and procarbazine; vincristine, doxorubicin, and cyclophosphamide alternating with etoposide; cyclophosphamide, doxorubicin, and etoposide alternating with vincristine, methotrexate, lomustine, and procarbazine; and cyclophosphamide, doxorubicin, and vincristine alternating with cisplatin and etoposide. It should be noted, however, that in many of these trials the second regimen was not cross-resistant and subtherapeutic doses were administered.[113] However, in at least one large trial of patients with extensive-disease SCLC, the National Cancer Institute of Canada demonstrated a higher overall response rate (n = 285, 80% vs 63%, $P < .002$) and longer progression-free survival and overall survival (9.6 vs 8.0 months, $P = .03$) for patients randomized to receive six cycles of CAV alternating with CE versus CAV only.[114] By contrast, Fukuoka et al. compared CAV versus CE versus alternating cycles of CAV/CE in limited- and extensive-stage SCLC patients.[115] There was no difference in survival between the regimens for patients with extensive-stage SCLC, but a significant overall survival advantage was demonstrated in the patients with limited-stage SCLC receiving the alternating CAV/CE regimens versus either the CE or CAV regimens (16.8 months CAV/CE vs 11.7 months CAV [$P = .023$] and 12.4 months CE arms [$P = .14$], respectively). Thus, the limited-disease SCLC patients appear to have a greater response rate to alternating non–cross-resistant regimens than do the extensive-disease patients. The relatively recent availability of new classes of cytotoxins such as the taxanes and the topoisomerase 1 inhibitors provides new opportunities for exploring alternating strategies.

COMBINATION CHEMOTHERAPY PLUS COLONY-STIMULATING FACTOR

The majority of the chemotherapy regimens are associated with a significant degree of toxicity, especially granulocytopenia, which increases the risk of serious infections; therefore, aggressive SCLC regimens have been combined with a colony-stimulating factor such as filgrastim (G-CSF, Neupogen) or sargramostim (granulocyte macrophage colony-stimulating factor [GM-CSF], Leukine) to reduce the incidence and severity of infectious complications. When patients receiving CAE therapy were randomized to receive either filgrastim or placebo, those receiving the CSF experienced shorter durations of severe neutropenia (5.2 vs 1.8 days) and fewer febrile neutropenic episodes and required fewer days of antibiotics or hospitalization.[116]

BONE MARROW OR PERIPHERAL BLOOD STEM-CELL TRANSPLANT

High-dose chemotherapy followed by bone marrow (ABMT) or peripheral blood stem-cell transplant (PBSCT) has been evaluated in numerous small phase I and II trials in patients with limited- or extensive-disease SCLC, with inconsistent results.[18,117–120] To date, only one randomized phase III trial has been published.[118] Eligible patients were less than 65 years of age, with a good performance status and no serious concurrent medical conditions. One hundred one patients initially received conventional chemotherapy with methotrexate, cyclophosphamide, vincristine, doxorubicin plus prophylactic cranial irradiation (PCI) for three cycles, followed by two cycles of cisplatin and etoposide. Patients were then restaged; those ($n = 45$) with either limited disease in CR or PR and those with extensive disease in CR were randomized to receive either an additional cycle of conventional chemotherapy with carmustine, cyclophosphamide, etoposide, or the same agents at high dosages followed by ABMT. There was a significant increase in DFS in the patients receiving high-dose chemotherapy plus ABMT (28 weeks vs 10 weeks; $P = .002$) measured from the time of randomization. However, no significant difference was noted in the median overall survival, measured from the date of the first cycle of induction chemotherapy (68 weeks vs 55 weeks respectively, including 4 deaths due to complications attributed to high-dose plus PBSCT therapy; $P = .13$).

Because there exists a small, but definite, cure rate in SCLC, extensive research efforts to evaluate potential new treatment modalities is crucial. Thus, further evaluation of high-dose chemotherapy + PBSCT continues to be investigated in select cohorts of younger SCLC patients with good performance status and minimal concurrent disease states.

RADIOTHERAPY

Small cell lung cancer is considered a very radiosensitive tumor, and radiotherapy has been used in combination with chemotherapy to treat tumors limited to the thoracic cavity. The rationale for combined-modality therapy is that radiotherapy and chemotherapy together will fight bulk disease within the chest primary tumor site and that chemotherapy will fight systemic metastases.[18] This combined-modality therapy may decrease the incidence and delay the onset of local tumor recurrences.[121] In most randomized trials, combined modality therapy has only modestly improved the overall duration of survival (e.g., 1 to 4 months) and 2-year survival (7% vs 17%) over that achieved with chemotherapy alone. A meta-analysis of 13 randomized studies including over 2100 patients with limited-stage SCLC reported that chemotherapy plus radiation significantly reduced the death rate by 14% and improved the 3-year survival by 5.4%.[122] Both of these results were statistically significant. The optimal dose and scheduling of radiation therapy (standard versus accelerated hyperfractionated thoracic irradiation) in combination with chemotherapy is not yet defined. However, it appears that radiation therapy given concurrently or alternating with chemotherapy is more likely to produce favorable responses versus administration of radiation after completion of chemotherapy.[18,123] Unfortunately, many such studies of combined-modality therapy also have been associated with increased morbidity when compared to chemotherapy alone or radiation after chemotherapy. When radiation therapy is combined with radiosensitizing drugs like doxorubicin, the incidence of radiation esophagitis and pneumonitis may increase.[124] Clinical trials currently under way are evaluating various dosages and schedules of radiation therapy in combination with a variety of chemotherapeutic agents in an attempt to maximize tumor control with an acceptable degree of toxicity.

BRAIN METASTASES

Central nervous system metastases are present in about 10% of patients initially and occur at some point in the disease process in 20% to 30% of patients.[18] For this reason, prophylactic cranial irradiation has been commonly recommended in all patients achieving a complete response to chemotherapy. In a review of randomized trials evaluating prophylactic whole-brain irradiation, Bleehan et al. reported that the incidence of brain metastases was 20% in patients not receiving prophylactic whole-brain irradiation compared with 6% in patients who did receive it.[125] Neurologic and cognitive impairment and abnormalities on brain CT scans have been reported in long-term survivors following prophylactic cranial irradiation (PCI).[18,126,127] This has led to increased controversy regarding whether patients achieving a complete response should receive PCI. Some experts now recommend to withhold cranial radiation until brain metastases manifest, whereas others recommend PCI, but only in lower dose fractions (200 to 300 cGy versus 400 cGy) after chemotherapy has been completed.[18,128] In patients with persistent disease, despite chemotherapy, the tumor may continue to seed the CNS, thereby negating any effects of prophylactic irradiation and denying the patients a future chance of palliative irradiation for acute symptoms.[129] In patients with intracranial metastases, therapeutic cranial irradiation usually controls the CNS disease and patients generally die from progressive systemic disease. Adrenocorticosteroids (to decrease intracranial pressure) and anticonvulsants (to prevent seizures) are routinely administered to patients with CNS metastases.

Topotecan crosses the intact blood–brain barrier, and the concentration of drug in the cerebrospinal fluid is about 40% of plasma levels.[130–132] Several trials using intravenous topotecan have now reported reduction in the size of cerebral metastases.[133,134] As this agent becomes more widely used in the treatment of newly diagnosed SCLC, it will be important to evaluate whether or not it has impact on the frequency of brain metastases later in the disease.

COMPLICATIONS AND SUPPORTIVE CARE

Patients with lung cancer frequently have many concurrent medical problems. Such problems may be related to the primary tumor and its metastases (see Clinical Presentation), the antitumor therapy, or concomitant diseases.

Many of the chemotherapy regimens used in the management of lung cancer are intensive and are associated with a wide variety of toxic effects. Nausea and vomiting may be severe (especially in the cisplatin-containing regimens) and may require aggressive acute and delayed antiemetic regimens. Patients experiencing protracted nausea and vomiting may require intravenous hydration and nutritional support. Myelosuppression is often the dose-limiting toxic effect associated with these combinations. Granulocytopenia following many of the more aggressive regimens places patients at high risk of serious infections. Other toxic effects associated with these regimens include mucositis, peripheral neuropathies, nephrotoxicity, and ototoxicity.

Likewise, patients receiving radiation therapy may experience complications including fatigue, esophagitis, radiation pneumonitis, and cardiac toxicity. When combined with chemotherapy these toxicities are often enhanced.[135] The patient's baseline performance status and the degree of pulmonary dysfunction (e.g., chronic obstructive pulmonary disease from years of tobacco use/smoking) must be considered in the decision of radiation dosage and fractionation.

It is readily apparent that many patients with lung cancer receive complex pharmacologic regimens that may include chemotherapeutic agents, antiemetics, antibiotics, analgesics, anticoagulants, bronchodilators, corticosteroids, anticonvulsants, and cardiovascular agents. Such regimens necessitate intensive therapeutic monitoring to avoid drug-related toxic effects and to optimize patient outcomes.

CONCLUSIONS

Lung cancer is currently the leading cause of cancer death in the United States. Ironically, the American Cancer Society has estimated that up to 83% of all cases of lung cancer could be prevented if cigarette smoking were eliminated. Unfortunately, even with application of the current best diagnostic and therapeutic strategies, the overall cure rate is only about 10%.

Surgery and radiation therapy to a lesser extent offer the only chance of cure for patients with NSCLC; however, the majority of patients are inoperable at diagnosis. Unfortunately, the response rates to combination chemotherapy in this disease are disappointingly low, and it is controversial whether such therapy offers significant benefit to the patient in terms of quality of life or survival. Research endeavors continue to look for new, effective agents and regimens in NSCLC in the hope of improving response rates and survival.

By contrast, combination chemotherapy has demonstrated dramatic response rates and clearly improved survival in patients with small cell lung cancer; however, the percentage of long-term survivors remains low. Research endeavors in SCLC continue to look for new agents, improved combinations, and new modalities that will enhance the cure rate.

Despite progress over the past decade in the management of advanced lung cancer, the only clear-cut hope for control of this devastating disease lies in the elimination of cigarette smoking.

▶ PRINCIPLES OF PHARMACOTHERAPY

- Lung cancer is the leading cause of cancer deaths in both men and women in the United States. The overall 5-year survival rate for all types of lung cancer is only about 13%. Cigarette smoking is responsible for about 83% of all lung cancers.
- Four major histologic types account for > 90% of all lung cancers; these include adenocarcinoma, large cell and squamous cell carcinoma, and small cell lung cancer. Small cell cancer is the most rapidly growing and, in general, the most sensitive to cytotoxic chemotherapy.
- Although early-detection strategies have been very effective in reducing mortality of other common cancers such as cervical and breast cancers, efforts to detect lung tumors at an earlier stage (e.g., sputum cytology or chest x-rays) have not reduced the mortality rates associated with lung cancer.
- Many lung cancers go undetected until they are advanced because individuals who have a long history of cigarette smoking are unlikely to notice the early symptoms of cough or dyspnea. It is often symptoms associated with large tumors or metastatic disease that prompt medical attention.
- Surgery is the treatment of choice for non–small cell lung cancers (NSCLC) that are early stage (stage I or II). If the tumor is deemed inoperable owing to its anatomic location or if the patient is a poor surgical risk, radiation therapy may be used, although 5-year survival rates are usually inferior to those with surgery.
- For patients with locally advanced NSCLC (stage III), recent evidence suggests that chemotherapy with or without radiation followed by surgery improves survival over radiation followed by surgery.
- Although, historically, NSCLC has not been considered to be amenable to cytotoxic chemotherapy, regimens developed in recent years have demonstrated improved response and survival rates. Several randomized trials have demonstrated that combination chemotherapy was superior to best supportive care. Patients who are most likely to benefit from chemotherapy include those with a good baseline performance status, no (or minimal) weight loss prior to treatment, and less extensive disease spread. Regimens that have demonstrated the highest response rates include cisplatin plus ei-

ther etoposide, vinorelbine, paclitaxel, docetaxel, or gemcitabine.

- No single regimen is considered the standard. The most appropriate chemotherapy regimen for a patient with NSCLC should be selected based on the patient's ability to tolerate the expected toxicities and consideration of whether concomitant radiation will be administered (and how that will impact toxicities). For example, single-agent vinorelbine is an acceptable alternative for elderly or debilitated patients who cannot tolerate the side effects of cisplatin.
- Combination chemotherapy will prolong the survival of most patients with SCLC. Patients with limited disease are more likely to have a complete response to chemotherapy and longer survival than those who have extensive disease at the time of diagnosis. Patients with no weight loss and a better performance status at diagnosis also have an improved prognosis.
- The most widely used chemotherapy regimens for SCLC include cyclophosphamide, doxorubicin, and etoposide; cisplatin and etoposide; and ifosfamide, carboplatin, and etoposide.
- Despite very high response rates to chemotherapy, most patients with SCLC eventually have disease progression and die from this disease. Alternative strategies such as alternating non–cross-resistant chemotherapy regimens or high-dose chemotherapy with stem cell transplantation have not improved long-term survival rates in most studies.
- Radiation therapy to the involved lung field given concurrently or alternating with chemotherapy appears to improve survival; however, it may also significantly increase the risk of toxicities, including myelosuppression and esophagitis.
- Over the past decade, supportive care therapies such as hematopoietic growth factors to attenuate myelosuppression and 5-HT_3 antagonist antiemetics have drastically improved patients' abilities to tolerate the toxicities associated with cytotoxic regimens commonly used to treat lung cancer.

REFERENCES

1. Landis SH, Murray T, Bolden S, Wingo PA. Cancer statistics, 1998. CA Cancer J Clin 1998;48:6–29.
2. Linnoila I. Pathology of non–small cell lung cancer. Hematol Oncol Clin North Am 1990;4:1027–1051.
3. Ginsberg RJ, Vokes EE, Raben A. Non–small cell lung cancer. In: DeVita VT, Hellman S, Rosenberg SA, eds. Cancer. Principles and Practice of Oncology, 5th ed. Philadelphia, Lippincott–Raven, 1997: 858–911.
4. Sellers TA, Bailey-Wilson JE, Elston RC, et al. Evidence for Mendelian inheritance in the pathogenesis of lung cancer. J Natl Cancer Instit 1990;82:1272.
5. Minna J, Battey J, Birrer M, et al. Genetic changes involved in the pathogenesis of human lung cancer including oncogene activation, chromosomal deletions, and autocrine growth factor production. In: Fortner JG, Rhoads JE, eds. Accomplishments in Cancer Research 1987. Philadelphia, Lippincott, 1988:155–182.
6. Aaronson SA. Growth factors and cancer. Science 1991;254:1146–1153.
7. Miller YE, Franklin WA. Molecular events in lung carcinogenesis. Hematol Oncol Clin North Am 1997;11:215–234.
8. Islam SS, Schottenfeld D. Declining FEV_1 and chronic productive cough in cigarette smokers: A 25-year prospective study of lung cancer incidence in Tecumseh, Michigan. Cancer Epidemiol Biomarkers Prev 1994;3:289–298.
9. Mattson ME, Pollack ES, Cullen JW. What are the odds that smoking will kill you? Am J Public Health 1987;77:425–431.
10. Damber LA, Larson LG. Smoking and lung cancer with special regard to type of cancer: A case-control study in north Sweden. Br J Cancer 1986;53:673–681.
11. Menck HR, Casagrande JT, Henderson BE. Industrial air pollution. Possible effect on lung cancer. Science 1974;183:210–212.
12. Menkes MS, Comstock GW, Vulleumier JP, et al. Serum beta-carotene, vitamin A and E, selenium and the risk of lung cancer. N Engl J Med 1986;315:1250–1254.
13. Ziegler RG, Mason TJ, Stemhagen A, et al. Carotenoid intake, vegetables, and the risk of lung cancer among white men in New Jersey. Am J Epidemiol 1986;123:1080–1093.
14. The Alpha-Tocopherol, Beta Carotene Cancer Prevention Study Group. The effect of vitamin E and beta carotene on the incidence of lung cancer and other cancers in male smokers. N Engl J Med 1994;330:1029–1035.
15. Sobin LH. The World Health Organizations Histological Classification of Lung Tumors: A comparison of the first and second editions. Cancer Detect Prev 1982;5:391–406.
16. El-Torky M, El-Zeky F, Hall JC. Significant changes in the distribution of histologic types of lung cancer. Cancer 1990;65:2361–2367.
17. Cuttitta F, Carney DN, Mulshine J, et al. Bombensin-like peptides can function as autocrine growth factors in human small-cell lung cancer. Nature 1985;316:823–826.
18. Ihde DC, Pass HI, Glatstenin E. Small cell lung cancer. In: DeVita VT, Hellman S, Rosenberg SA, eds. Cancer. Principles and Practice of Oncology, 5th ed. Philadelphia, Lippincott–Raven, 1997:911–949.
19. Fontana RS, Sanderson DR, Woolner LB, et al. Lung cancer screening: The Mayo Program. J Occup Med 1986;28:746–750.
20. Melamed MR, Flehinger BJ, Zaman MB, et al. Screening for early lung cancer. Results of the Memorial Sloan-Kettering Study in New York. Chest 1984;86:44–53.
21. Tockman MS. Survival and mortality from lung cancer in a screened population. The Johns Hopkins Study. Chest 1986;89(suppl):324S–325S.
22. Eddy DM. Screening for lung cancer. Ann Intern Med 1989;111: 232–237.
23. American Joint Committee on Cancer (AJCC): Manual for Staging of Cancer, 4th ed. Philadelphia, Lippincott, 1997:127–137.
24. Martini R, Beattie EJ. Results of surgical treatment in stage I lung cancer. J Thorac Cardiovasc Surg 1977;74:499–506.
25. Klingman RR, DeMeester TR. Surgical approach to non–small cell lung cancer. Stage I and II. Hematol Oncol Clin North Am 1990;4: 1079–1091.
26. Seagren SL. Radical radiation therapy for lung cancer. Hematol Oncol Clin North Am 1990;4:1093–1109.
27. Cormesir Y, Bergeron D, LaForge J, et al. Benefits of polychemotherapy in advanced non–small-cell bronchogenic carcinoma. Cancer 1982;50:845–849.
28. Rapp E, Pater J, Willan A, et al. Chemotherapy can prolong survival in patients with advanced non–small cell lung cancer: Report of a Canadian multicenter randomized trial. J Clin Oncol 1988;6: 633–641.
29. Cartei G, Cartei F, Cantone A, et al. Cisplatin–cyclophosphamide–mitomycin combination chemotherapy with supportive care versus

supportive care alone for treatment of metastatic non–small-cell lung cancer. J Natl Cancer Instit 1993;85:794–800.
30. Jaakimainen L, Goodwin J, Pater J, et al. Counting the costs of chemotherapy in a National Cancer Institute of Canada randomized trial in non–small cell lung cancer. J Clin Oncol 1990;8:1301–1309.
31. Souquet PJ, Chauvin F, Boissel JP, et al. Polychemotherapy in advanced non–small cell lung cancer: A meta-analysis. Lancet 1993; 342:19–21.
32. Grilli R, Oxman AD, Julian JM. Chemotherapy for advanced non–small cell lung cancer: How much benefit is enough? J Clin Oncol 1993;11:1866–1872.
33. Marino P, Pampallona S, Prestoni A, et al. Chemotherapy versus supportive care in advanced non–small cell lung cancer: Results of a meta-analysis of the literature. Chest 1994;106:861–865.
34. Non–Small Cell Lung Cancer Collaborative Group. Chemotherapy in non–small cell lung cancer: A meta-analysis using updated data on individual patients from 52 randomized clinical trials. BMJ 1995; 311:899–909.
35. O'Connell JP, Kris MG, Gralla RJ, et al. Frequency and prognostic importance of pretreatment clinical characteristics in patients with advanced non–small cell lung cancer treated with combination chemotherapy. J Clin Oncol 1986;4:1604–1614.
36. Fukouka M, Masuda N, Furuse K, et al. A randomized trial in inoperable non–small cell lung cancer: Vindesine and cisplatin versus mitomycin, vindesine, and cisplatin versus etoposide and cisplatin alternating with vindesine and mitomycin. J Clin Oncol 1991;9:606–613.
37. LeChevalier T, Brisgand D, Douillard J, et al. Randomized study of vinorelbine and cisplatin versus vindesine and cisplatin verses vinorelbine alone in advanced non–small-cell lung cancer: Results of a European multicenter trial including 612 patients. J Clin Oncol 1994: 12;360–367.
38. Data on file, Glaxo Wellcome Inc. (THRS/92/0047/129/W3(5)).
39. Depierre A, Chastang CI, Quiox E, et al. Vinorelbine versus vinorelbine plus cisplatin (P) in non–small-cell lung cancer: A randomized trial. Ann Oncol 1994;5:37–42.
40. Murphy WK, Fossella FV, Winn RJ, et al. Phase II study of Taxol in patients with untreated advanced non–small cell lung cancer. J Natl Cancer Instit 1993;85:384–388.
41. Chang AY, Kim K, Glick J, et al. Phase II study of Taxol, merbarone, and piroxantrone in stage IV non–small cell lung cancer; the Eastern Cooperative Oncology Group Results. J Natl Cancer Instit 1993;85: 388–392.
42. Francis PA, Rigas JR, Kris MG, et al. Phase II trial of docetaxel in patients with stage III and IV non–small-cell lung cancer. J Clin Oncol 1994;12:1232–1237.
43. Fossella FV, Lee JS, Murphy WK, et al. Phase II study of docetaxel for recurrence of metastatic in non–small-cell lung cancer. J Clin Oncol 1994;12:1238–1244.
44. Fossella FV, Lee JS, Shin DM, et al. Phase II study of docetaxel for advanced or metastatic platinum-refractory non–small-cell lung cancer. J Clin Oncol 1995;13:645–651.
45. Fosella FV, Lee JS, Kau SW, et al. Docetaxel (D) for platinum-refractory non–small cell lung cancer (NSCLC): Comparison of phase II results to historical controls (HC). Proc Am Soc Clin Oncol 1997; 16:A-1682. Abstract.
46. Gandara DR, Vokes E, Green M, et al. Docetaxel (Taxotere) in platinum-treated non–small cell lung cancer (NSCLC): Confirmation of prolonged survival in a multicenter trial. Proc Am Soc Clin Oncol 1997;16:A-1632. Abstract.
47. Abratt RP, Bezwoda WR, Falkson G, et al. Efficacy and safety profile of gemcitabine in non–small-cell lung cancer: A phase II study. J Clin Oncol 1994;12:1535–1540.
48. Gatzemier U, Shepherd FA, LeChevalier T, et al. Activity of gemcitabine in patients with non–small-cell lung cancer: A multicentre, extended phase II study. Eur J Cancer 1996;32:243–248.
49. Fukuoka M, Niitao H, Suzuki H, et al. A phase II study of CPT-11, a new derivative of camptothecin for previously untreated non–small cell lung cancer. J Clin Oncol 1992;10:16–20.
50. Outcomes Working Group HSRC, American Society of Clinical Oncology. Outcomes of cancer treatment for technology assessment and cancer treatment guidelines. J Clin Oncol 1996;14:671–679.
51. Langer C, Leighton J, Comis RL, et al. Paclitaxel and carboplatin in combination in the treatment of advanced non–small-cell-lung cancer: A phase II toxicity, response, and survival analysis. J Clin Oncol 1995;13:1860–1870.
52. Bonomi P, Kim K, Chang A, et al. Phase III trial comparing etoposide (E), cisplatin (C) versus Taxol (T) with cisplatin-G-CSF (G) versus Taxol-cisplatin in advanced non-small cell lung cancer. The Eastern Cooperative Oncology Group (ECOG) trial. Proc Am Soc Clin Oncol 1996;15:382. Abstract.
53. LeChevalier T, Belli L, Monnier A, et al. Phase II study of docetaxel (Taxotere®) and cisplatin in advanced non–small-cell lung cancer (NSCLC): An interim analysis. Proc Am Soc Clin Oncol 1995;14: 350. Abstract 1059.
54. Early E, Miller VA, Grant SC, et al. Phase I/II trial of docetaxel (DTX) and vinorelbine (VNR) with filgrastim (G-CSF) in patients (PTS) with advanced non–small cell lung cancer (NSCLC). Proc Am Soc Clin Oncol 1997;16:467. Abstract.
55. Abratt RP, Bezwoda WR, Goedhals L, Hacking DJ. Weekly gemcitabine with monthly cisplatin: Effective chemotherapy for advanced non–small-cell lung cancer. J Clin Oncol 1997;15:744–749.
56. Crino L, Scagliotti G, Marangolo F, et al. Cisplatin-gemcitabine combination in advanced non–small-cell lung cancer: A phase II study. J Clin Oncol 1997;15:297–303.
57. Worniak AJ, Crowley JJ, Balcerzak SP. Randomized phase III trial of cisplatin (CDDP) vs CDDP plus navelbine (NVB) in treatment of advanced IV non–small-cell lung cancer (NSCLC): Report of a Southwestern Oncology Group study (SWOG 9308). Proc Am Soc Clin Oncol 1996;15:A1110. Abstract.
58. Rittenberg CN, Gralla RJ, Rehmeyer TA. Assessing and managing venous irritation associated with vinorelbine tartrate (Navelbine). Oncol Nurs Forum 1995;22:707–710.
59. Rowinsky EK, Donehower RC. Antimicrotubule agents. In: Chabner BA, Longo DL, eds. Cancer Chemotherapy and Biotherapy, Principles and Practice, 2nd ed. Philadelphia, Lippincott–Raven, 1996:263–296.
60. Langer CJ, Rosvold E, Millenson M, et al. Paclitaxel by 1 or 24 hour infusion combined with carboplatin in advanced non–small cell lung cancer (NSCLC): A comparative analysis. Proc Am Soc Clin Oncol 1997;16:A-1625. Abstract.
61. Gemzar package insert, Indianapolis: Eli Lilly and Company; 1996 May.
62. O'Rourke TJ, Brown TD, Havlin K, et al. Phase I clinical trial of gemcitabine given as an intravenous bolus on 5 consecutive days. Eur J Cancer 1994;30:417–418.
63. Tanis B, Clavel M, Guastalla J, et al. Phase I study of gemcitabine (difluorodexycytidine, dFdC (LY188011)) administered in a two-weekly schedule. Proc Am Assoc Cancer Res 1990;31:1239. Abstract.
64. Abbruzzese JL, Grunewald R, Weeks EA, et al. A phase I clinical, plasma, and cellular pharmacology study of gemcitabine. J Clin Oncol 1991;9:491–498.
65. Kaye SB. Gemcitabine: Current status of phase I and II trials. J Clin Oncol 1994;12:1527–1531.
66. Fossella FV, Lippman SM, Shin DM, et al. Maximum-tolerated dose defined for single-agent gemcitabine: A phase I dose-escalation study in chemotherapy-naive patients with advanced non–small cell lung cancer. J Clin Oncol 1997;15:310–316.
67. Takimoto CH, Arbuck SG. The camptothecins. In: Chabner BA, Longo DL, eds. Cancer Chemotherapy and Biotherapy, Principles and Practice, 2nd ed. Philadelphia, Lippincott–Raven, 1996:463–484.
68. Masuda N, Fukuoka M, Takada M, et al. CPT-11 in combination with cisplatin for advanced non–small cell lung cancer. J Clin Oncol 1992;10:1775–1780.
69. Shinkai T, Arioka H, Kunikane H, et al. A phase I study of CPT-11 and cisplatin in combination with fixed dose of vindesine in meta-

static non–small cell lung cancer (NSCLC). Proc Am Soc Clin Oncol 1993;12:328. Abstract.
70. Stanley KE, Cox JD, Petrovich Z, et al. Patterns of failure with inoperable carcinoma of the lung. Cancer 1981;47:2725–2729.
71. Vokes EE. Sequential combined modality therapy for stage III non–small cell lung cancer. Hematol Oncol Clin North Am 1990;4:1133–1142.
72. Dillman RO, Seagren SL, Propert KJ, et al. A randomized trial of induction chemotherapy plus high-dose radiation versus radiation alone in stage III non–small-cell lung cancer. N Engl J Med 1990;323: 940–945.
73. Dillman RO, Seagren SL, Propert KJ, et al. Randomized trial of induction chemotherapy plus radiation therapy vs RT alone in stage III non–small cell lung cancer (NSCLC): Five-year follow-up of CALGB 84-33. Proc Am Soc Clin Oncol 1993;12:329.
74. Sause W, Scott C, Taylor C, et al. Preliminary analysis of phase III trial in regionally advanced unresectable non–small cell lung cancer. Proc Am Soc Clin Oncol 1994;13:325. Abstract.
75. Pignon JP, Stewart RL, Souhami R, et al. A meta-analysis using individual patient data from randomized clinical trials of chemotherapy in non-small cell lung cancer: (3) Survival in the locally advanced setting. Proc Am Soc Clin Oncol 1994;13:334. Abstract.
76. Armstrong JG. Long-term outcome of small cell lung cancer. Cancer Treat Rev 1990;17:1–13.
77. Lassen U, Osterlind K, Hansen M, et al. Long-term survival in small-cell lung cancer; posttreatment characteristics in patients surviving 5 to 18+ years—An analysis of 1,714 consecutive patients. J Clin Oncol 1995;13:1215–1220.
78. Spiegelman D, Maurer L, Ware J, et al. Prognostic factors in small-cell carcinoma of the lung: An analysis of 1251 patients. J Clin Oncol 1989;7:334–354.
79. Albain K, Crowley JJ, LeBlanc M, Livingston RB. Determinants of improved outcome in small-cell lung cancer: An analysis of the 2,580-patient Southwest Oncology Group database. J Clin Oncol 1990;8:1563–1574.
80. Sagman U, Feld R, Evans WK, et al. The prognostic significance of pretreatment serum lactate dehydrogenase in patients with small-cell lung cancer. J Clin Oncol 1991;9:954–961.
81. Sagman U, Leblanc M, Maki E, et al. Verification of a multi-centre prognostic model for small-cell lung carcinoma (SCLC). For the Consensus Group for Prognostic Factors. Proc Am Soc Clin Oncol 1993;12:337. Abstract 1125.
82. Jorgensen LG, Osterlind K, Genolla J, et al. Serum neuron-specific enolase (S-NSE) and the prognosis in small-cell lung cancer (SCLC). A combination multivariable analysis on data from nine centers. Br J Cancer 1996;74:463–467.
83. Smit EF, Fokkema E, Biesma B, et al. A phase II study of paclitaxel in heavily pretreated patients with small-cell lung cancer. Br J Cancer 1998;77:347–351.
84. Ettinger D, Finkelstein DM, Sarma RP, et al. Phase II study of paclitaxel in patients with extensive-disease small-cell lung cancer, ECOG. J Clin Oncol 1995;13:1430–1435.
85. Ardizzani A, Hansen H, Dombernowsky P, et al. Topotecan, a new active drug in the second-line treatment of small-cell lung cancer: A phase II study in patients with refractory and sensitive disease. J Clin Oncol 1997;15:2090–2096.
86. Perez-Solar R, Glisson BS, Lee JS, et al. Treatment of patients with small-cell lung cancer refractory to etoposide and cisplatin with the topoisomerase I poison topotecan. J Clin Oncol 1996;14:2785–2790.
87. Eckardt J, Depierre A, Ardizzoni A, et al. Pooled analysis of topotecan (T) in the second-line treatment of patients (pts) with sensitive small-cell lung cancer (SCLC). Proc Am Soc Clin Oncol 1997;17: 1624. Abstract.
88. Masuda N, Fukuoka M, Kusunoki Y, et al. CPT-11: A new derivative of camptothecin for the treatment of refractory or relapsed small-cell lung cancer. J Clin Oncol 1992;10:1225–1229.
89. Cormier Y, Eisenhauer E, Muldal A. Gemcitabine is an active new agent in previously untreated extensive small-cell lung cancer, a study of the National Cancer Institute of Canada clinical trials group. Ann Oncol 1994;5:283–285.
90. DePierre A, LeChevalier T, Quoix E, et al. Phase II study of Navelbine (NVB) in small-cell lung cancer (SCLC). Proc Am Soc Clin Oncol 1995;14:A1050. Abstract.
91. Furuse K, Kubota K, Kawahara M, et al. Phase II study of vinorelbine in heavily pretreated small cell lung cancer. Oncology 1996;53: 169–172.
92. Goren MP, Anthony LB, Hande KR, et al. Pharmacokinetics of an intravenous-oral versus intravenous-mesna regimen in lung cancer patients receiving ifosfamide. J Clin Oncol 1998;16:616–621.
93. Roth BJ, Johnson DH, Einhorn LH, et al. Randomized study of cyclophosphamide, doxorubicin, and vincristine versus etoposide and cisplatin versus alternation of these two regimens in extensive small-cell lung cancer: A Phase III trial of the Southeastern Cancer Study Group. J Clin Oncol 1992;10:282–291.
94. Maksymiuk AW, Jett JR, Earle JD, et al. Sequencing and schedule effects of cisplatin plus etoposide in small-cell lung cancer: Results of a North Central Cancer Treatment Group Randomized Clinical Trial. J Clin Oncol 1994;12:70–76.
95. Loehrer PJ, Ansari R, Gonin R, et al. Cisplatin plus etoposide with and without ifosfamide in extensive small-cell lung cancer: A Hoosier Oncology Group Study. J Clin Oncol 1995;13:2594–2599.
96. Faylona EA, Loehrer PJ, Ansari R, et al. Phase II study of daily oral etoposide plus ifosfamide plus cisplatin for previously treated recurrent small-cell lung cancer: A Hoosier Oncology Group Trial. J Clin Oncol 1995;13:1209–1214.
97. Hainsworth JD, Gray JR, Stroup SL, et al. Paclitaxel, carboplatin, and extended-schedule etoposide in the treatment of small-cell lung cancer: Comparison of sequential Phase II trials using different dose-intensities. J Clin Oncol 1997;15:3464–3470.
98. Wolff AC, Ettinger DS, Neuberg D, et al. Phase II study of ifosfamide, carboplatin, and oral etoposide chemotherapy for extensive-disease small-cell lung cancer: An Eastern Cooperative Oncology Group pilot study. J Clin Oncol 1995;13:1615–1622.
99. Thatcher N. Ifosfamide/carboplatin/etoposide (ICE) regimen in small-cell lung cancer. Lung Cancer 1993;9(suppl 1):551–567.
100. Giaccone G, Dalesio O, McVie GJ. Maintenance chemotherapy in small-cell-lung cancer: Long-term results of a randomized trial, EORTC. J Clin Oncol 1993;11:1230–1240.
101. Johnson DH, Kim K, Sauuse W, et al. Cisplatin (p) and etoposide (e) + thoracic radiotherapy (trt) administered once or twice daily (bid) in limited stage IIs) small-cell lung cancer (SCLC): Final report of intergroup trial 0096. Proc Am Soc Clin Oncol 1996;15:374. Abstract.
102. Schabel FM, Griswold DP, Corbett TH, et al. Increasing the therapeutic response rates to anticancer drugs by applying the basic principles of pharmacology. Cancer 1984;54:1160–1167.
103. Johnson DH, Einhorn LH, Birch R, et al. A randomized comparison of high-dose versus conventional-dose cyclophosphamide, doxorubicin, and vincristine for extensive stage small cell lung cancer. J Clin Oncol 1987;5:1731–1738.
104. Figuerdo AT, Hryniuk WM, Straufmanis I, et al. Co-trimoxazole prophylaxis during high-dose chemotherapy of small cell lung cancer. J Clin Oncol 1985;2:54–64.
105. Ihde DC, Johnson BE, Mulshine JL, et al. Randomized trial of high dose versus standard dose etoposide and cisplatin in extensive stage small cell lung cancer. Proc Am Soc Clin Oncol 1987;6:181.
106. Pujol JL, Douillard JY, Riviere A, et al. Dose-intensity of a four-drug chemotherapy regimen with or without recombinant human granulocyte-macrophage colony-stimulating factor in extensive-stage small-cell lung cancer: A multicenter randomized Phase III study. J Clin Oncol 1997;15:2082–2089.
107. Ihde DC, Mulshine JL, Kramer BS, et al. Prospective randomized comparison of high-dose etoposide and cisplatin chemotherapy in patients with extensive-stage small-cell lung cancer. J Clin Oncol 1994;12:2022–2034.

108. Arriagada R, Le Chevalier T, Pignon JP, et al. Initial chemotherapeutic doses and survival in patients with limited small-cell lung cancer. N Engl J Med 1993;325:1848–1852.
109. Klasa RJ, Murray N, Coldman AJ. Dose-intensity meta-analysis of chemotherapy regimens in small-call carcinoma of the lung. J Clin Oncol 1991;9:499–508.
110. Goldie JH, Coldman AJ, Gudauskas GA. Rationale for the use of alternating non–cross resistant chemotherapy. Cancer Treat Rep 1982; 66:439–449.
111. Goodman GE, Crowley JJ, Blasko JC, et al. Treatment of limited small-cell lung cancer with etoposide and cisplatin alternating with vincristine, doxorubicin, and cyclophosphamide versus concurrent etoposide, vincristine, doxorubicin, and cyclophosphamide and chest radiotherapy: A Southwest Oncology Group Study. J Clin Oncol 1990;8:39–47.
112. Wolf M, Pritsch M, Drings P, et al. Cyclic-alternating versus response-oriented chemotherapy in small-cell lung cancer: A German multicenter randomized trial of 321 patients. J Clin Oncol 1991;9: 614–624.
113. Greco FA, Johnson DH, Hainsworth JD, Wolff SN. Chemotherapy of small-cell lung cancer. Semin Oncol 1985;4(suppl 6):31–37.
114. Evans WK, Feld R, Murray N, et al. Superiority of alternating non–cross-resistant chemotherapy in extensive small cell lung cancer. Ann Intern Med 1987;107:451–458.
115. Fukuoka M, Furuse K, Saijo N, et al. Randomized trail of cyclophosphamide, doxorubicin, and vincristine versus cisplatin and etoposide versus alteration of these regimens in small-cell lung cancer. J Natl Cancer Inst 1991;83:855–861.
116. Crawford J, Ozer H, Stoller R, et al. Reduction by granulocyte colony-stimulating factor of fever and neutropenia induced by chemotherapy in patients with small-cell lung cancer. N Engl J Med 1991;325: 164–170.
117. Sandler AB. Current management of small cell lung cancer. Semin Oncol 1997;24:463–476.
118. Humblet Y, Symann M, Bosly A, et al. Late intensification chemotherapy with autologous bone marrow transplant in selected small-cell carcinoma of the lung: A randomized study. J Clin Oncol 1987;5:1864–1873.
119. Elias AD, Ayash L, Frei E III, et al. Intensive combined modality therapy for limited stage small-cell lung cancer. J Natl Cancer Inst 1993;85:559–566.
120. Leyvraz S, Rosti G, Lange A, et al. Early intensification chemotherapy for the treatment of small-cell lung cancer (SCLC). Proc Am Soc Clin Oncol 1997;16:1626. Abstract.
121. Wilson HE, Stanley K, Vincent RG, et al. Comparison of chemotherapy alone versus chemotherapy and radiation therapy of extensive small cell carcinoma of the lung. J Surg Oncol 1983;23:181–184.
122. Johnson DH, Arriagada R, Ihde DC, et al. Meta-analysis of randomized trials evaluating the role of thoracic radiotherapy in limited-stage small cell lung cancer. Proc Am Soc Clin Oncol 1992;11:288. Abstract.
123. Murray N, Coy P, Pater JL, et al. Importance of timing for thoracic irradiation in the combined modality treatment of limited-stage small-cell-lung cancer. J Clin Oncol 1993;11:336–344.
124. Phillips TL. Acute and late effects of multi therapy on normal tissues. Cancer 1977;40:489–494.
125. Bleehen NM, Bunn PA, Cox JD, et al. Role of radiation therapy in small anaplastic carcinoma of the lung. Cancer Treat Rep 1983;67: 11–19.
126. Fleck JF, Einhorn LH, Lauer RC, et al. Is prophylactic cranial irradiation indicated in small-cell lung cancer? J Clin Oncol 1990;8:209–214.
127. Johnson BE, Becker B, Goff WB, et al. Neurologic, neuropsychologic, and cranial computed tomography scan abnormalities in 2–10 year survivors of small cell lung cancer. J Clin Oncol 1985;3:1659–1667.
128. Shaw EG, Su JQ, Eagan RT, et al. Prophylactic cranial irradiation in complete responders with small-cell lung cancer: Analysis of the Mayo Clinic and North Central Cancer Treatment Group data bases. J Clin Oncol 1994;12:2327–2332.
129. Kristensen CA, Kristjansen P, Hansen HH. Systemic chemotherapy of brain metastases from small-cell lung cancer: A review. J Clin Oncol 1992;10:1498–1502.
130. Blaney SM, Cole DE, Balis FM, et al. Plasma and cerebrospinal fluid pharmacokinetic study of topotecan in nonhuman primates. Cancer Res 1993;53:725–727.
131. Sung C, Blaney SM, Cole DE, et al. A pharmacokinetic model of topotecan clearance from plasma and cerebrospinal fluid. Cancer Res 1994;54:5118–5122.
132. Baker. Clin Pharmacol Ther 1994;55:189.
133. Ardizzoni A, Wanders J, Hansen H, et al. Activity of topotecan in the treatment of small-cell lung cancer patients with brain metastases. Proc Eur Assoc Neur Oncol 1996; Abstract.
134. Manegold C, von Pawel J, Gatzemeier U, et al. Activity of topotecan (Hycamtin®) in patients with SCLC brain metastases after failure of first-line therapy. Proc Eur Assoc Neur Oncol 1996; Abstract.
135. Payne DG, Feld R. Concurrent radiotherapy and chemotherapy in lung cancer at the Princess Margaret Hospital. Antibiot Chemother 1988;41:96–101.

118

Colorectal Cancer

Lisa E. Davis, PharmD, FCCP, BCPS, and Motria M. Horodysky, PharmD, BCPS

Colorectal cancer involves the colon, rectum, and the anal canal. It is one of the three most common cancers occurring in adult men and women in the United States, and accounts for about one out of eight cancer diagnoses. In 1998, an estimated 131,600 new cases will be diagnosed, of which 95,600 will involve the colon and 36,000 the rectum.[1]

For both adult men and women, colorectal cancer is the third leading cause of cancer-related deaths in the United States. An estimated 56,500 deaths will occur during 1998.[1] Mortality associated with colorectal cancer has decreased during the past 30 years; the rate of decline is greatest for females.

Mortality rates associated with colorectal cancer in the United States are comparable to those of other industrialized areas in North America, certain areas of Northern and Western Europe, Australia, and New Zealand. Deaths attributed to cancer of the colon or rectum in less developed areas such as South America and rural Africa are less frequent than in the United States.

Multiple factors are associated with the development of these malignancies, including acquired and inherited genetic susceptibility, environmental elements, and life-style. Overall, approximately 37% of affected individuals undergo a surgical procedure alone intended for cure. An additional 35% can potentially be cured by undergoing surgery followed by radiation therapy, chemotherapy, or both. Curability is influenced primarily by extent of tumor invasion into adjacent tissues or organs and presence of metastatic disease. Five-year survival rates are close to 93% and 88% for persons with early stages of colon and rectal cancer, respectively. Once tumor has spread regionally to adjacent organs or lymph nodes, survival rates drop to 67% for colon cancer and 56% for cancer of the rectum. Five-year survival for individuals with metastatic disease is approximately 7%.

Treatment modalities include surgery, radiation therapy, chemotherapy, and immunotherapy. Surgery is the most important and definitive procedure associated with cure; radiation therapy can be used to improve curability following surgical resection and to reduce symptoms and complications associated with advanced disease. Chemotherapy alone or with immunotherapy (levamisole) is used in adjuvant treatment regimens. Chemotherapy, either a single agent or a combination of agents, can be used for advanced stages of disease. Although the efficacy of a standard postoperative monitoring program for patients with resected colorectal cancer has not been established, elements of such a program may include physical examination, colonoscopy, chest and abdominal imaging studies, serum carcinoembryonic antigen (CEA) measurements, liver function tests, and fecal occult blood testing.

EPIDEMIOLOGY

Worldwide, the highest incidence rates occur in highly industrialized areas such as North America, certain areas of Northern and Western Europe, Australia, and New Zealand. Less developed areas such as South America and rural Africa report the lowest incidence rates of colorectal cancer. Rates have increased substantially, however, in previously lower-risk countries such as Japan and China, as well as among persons migrating from low-risk areas to the United States.

The incidence of colon cancer is greatest among males, who have an age-adjusted incidence rate of 35.1 per 100,000, as compared to females in whom the rate is 27.9 per 100,000.[2] Cancer of the rectum occurs less frequently. The overall incidence of colon and rectal cancers in the United States has declined since 1985. This decline is greater in the female population than for males. Trends for incidence and mortality rates among white males and females in the United States can be compared in Figure 118–1. These rates are somewhat higher for black males and females.

The median age at diagnosis is about 69 years.[3] Fewer than 3% of affected persons are under the age of 40. An individual's risk, however, increases with increasing age. Sixty-two percent of cases develop in adults greater than 60 years of age. Hispanics and African-Americans have a younger mean age at diagnosis and tend to present with later-stage disease at diagnosis than do non-Hispanic whites.

Approximately 1 of every 10 cancer deaths is due to cancer of the colon or rectum. Roughly 56,500 deaths were estimated in 1998, despite a decline in overall combined mortality for both colon and rectal cancer observed during the last 20 years by 25% for women and 13% for men. Differences exist, however, among specific racial and gender populations. The greatest decline has been experienced within white females, whereas mortality rates among black males continues to rise. These trends in mortality are similar to those of other countries such as Spain, Italy, Portugal, and Greece between 1975 and 1988.[4] Factors contributing to the overall decline in mortality are unclear but may reflect the impact of decreasing incidence rates, better treatment, a decrease in treatment-related complications, changes in dietary habits, screening programs, polyp removal, and possibly other contributing factors such as nonsteroidal anti-inflammatory drug (NSAID) use.

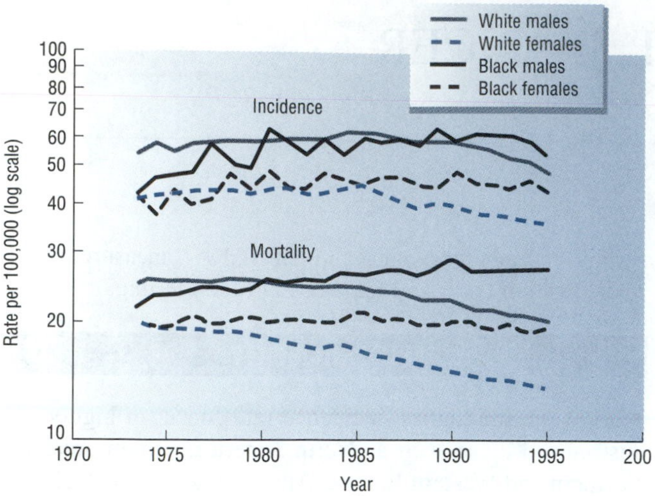

FIGURE 118–1. SEER incidence and mortality rates (age adjusted and age specific) of colon and rectum cancer, 1973–1995. *(From Ref. 2.)*

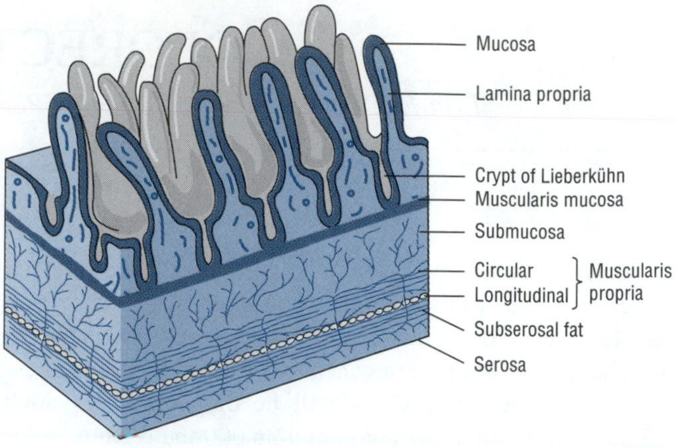

FIGURE 118–3. Cross-section of bowel wall.

PATHOGENESIS

ANATOMY AND BOWEL FUNCTION

The large intestine consists of the cecum; ascending, transverse, descending, and sigmoid colon; and the rectum (Fig. 118–2). In adults it extends approximately 1.5 m and has a diameter ranging from 8 cm in the cecum to 2 cm in the sigmoid colon. The function of the large intestine is to receive 500 to 2000 mL of ileal contents per day. Absorption of fluid and solutes occurs in the right colon or the segments proximal to the middle of the transverse colon, with movement and storage of fecal material in the left colon and distal segments of the colon. Mucus secretion from goblet cells into the intestinal lumen lubricates the mucosal surface and facilitates movement of the dehydrated feces. It also serves to protect the luminal wall from bacteria and colonic irritants such as bile acids.

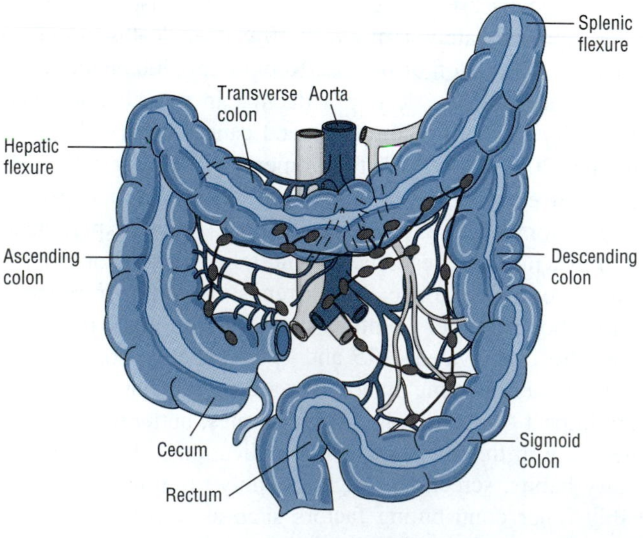

FIGURE 118–2. Colon and rectum anatomy.

Four major tissue layers, from the lumen outward, form the large intestine: the mucosa, submucosa, muscularis externa, and serosa (Fig. 118–3). Embedded in the submucosa and muscularis externa is a rich lymphatic capillary system. Lymphatic channels do not extend into the mucosa. The muscularis externa consists of circular smooth muscle and three outer longitudinal smooth muscle bands. Contraction of these muscle groups moves colonic material toward the anal canal. The outermost layer of the colon, the serosa, secretes a fluid that allows the colon to slide easily over nearby structures within the peritoneum. The serosa covers only the anterior and lateral aspects of the upper third of the rectum. The lower third lies completely extraperitoneal and is surrounded by fibrofatty tissue as well as adjacent organs and structures.

The surface epithelium of the colonic mucosa undergoes continual renewal, and complete replacement of epithelial cells occurs every 4 to 8 days. Cell replication normally takes place within the lower third of crypts, the tubular glands located within the intestinal mucosa. The cells then mature and differentiate to either goblet or absorptive cells as they migrate toward the bowel lumen. The total number of epithelial cells remains relatively constant as the number of cells migrating from the crypts is balanced by the rate of exfoliation of cells from the mucosal surface. This two-phase process is critical to the malignant transformation of the epithelial cells.

ETIOLOGY

Numerous studies suggest that the development of colorectal cancer can be caused or promoted by dietary or environmental factors that affect the bowel.[5,6] An understanding of these processes has formed the basis for several interventional and preventive trials, which are discussed later in this chapter. Key areas of study include dietary fat, fiber, and micronutrient intake.

Epidemiologic studies of worldwide incidence of colorectal cancer suggest that economic development and dietary habits strongly influence its development. Inhabitants of affluent societies are more likely to have more fat and less fiber in their diets. In Western countries, fat consumption typically accounts for approximately 40% of total caloric intake.[7] Although prospective studies thus far have failed to support a direct causal relationship between dietary fat consumption and cancer, numerous studies suggest that a relationship exists between dietary fat intake and colorectal cancer risk.[8] Whether the source of the fat is important is unclear, because most of the fat in many of these studies was derived from ingested animal meat. Results from case-control studies are somewhat inconsistent but also provide evidence supporting a relationship between dietary fat intake and colorectal cancer. In addition, animal studies demonstrate an influence of type, timing, and amount of dietary fat consumed on carcinogenesis.[7] Administration of high-fat substances (e.g., corn oil boluses) to human volunteers is correlated with increased colonic crypt cell proliferation rates as well as increased fecal concentrations of bile acids.

The role of dietary fat in cancer development is most likely due to its influence on fecal bile acid concentrations. The release of bile acids is stimulated following ingestion of dietary fat. These acids are then converted by colonic flora to secondary bile acids, which are associated with bowel mucosal irritation and cell proliferation responses and may promote tumor growth.[9] In general, the data suggest that dietary fat consumption plays a greater role in tumor promotion than in initiation.

Dietary fiber is the part of ingested plant material that is not processed by normal human digestive enzymes. Fibers are frequently classified as either water soluble (pectins, gums, mucilages) or insoluble (celluloses, hemicellulose, lignins). Numerous studies clearly demonstrate an inverse association between dietary fiber intake and colorectal cancer development. However, comparative and case-control studies of dietary fiber intake among countries with dissimilar incidences of colorectal cancer fail to demonstrate the role of dietary fiber alone. Accurate interpretation of these results is further hampered by the inconsistent definition and categorization of dietary fiber. Furthermore, an inverse correlation between dietary fat and fiber intake exists within most diets.[7] Thus, it is difficult to ascertain the true contribution of this dietary constituent alone toward cancer development. Postulated protective effects of dietary fiber include dilution of carcinogens in the bowel, reduction of fecal pH, and enhanced bowel transit. These effects may also reflect an associated concomitant reduction in dietary fat intake. Fiber from fruit and vegetable sources may be more desirable than cereal fiber.[10]

Several life-style factors have also been shown to affect colorectal cancer risk, including postmenopausal hormone use, alcohol intake, physical inactivity and obesity, tobacco use, serum lipid levels, occupational exposure, and dietary intake of various micronutrients and macronutrients.[5,6] Postmenopausal hormone replacement therapy is associated with a 30% to 35% decrease in colon cancer risk.[11] The risk is reduced in postmenopausal women receiving both estrogen only and combined estrogen and progestin therapy, but appears to increase after hormone replacement therapy is discontinued. The data suggest that estrogen exerts its protective effect during the later stages of carcinogenesis. Although a prospective study of oral contraceptive use suggests a protective effect, other studies do not support this association.[12] Alcohol use and physical inactivity, both occupational and recreational, are positively linked to colon cancer risk. High levels of dietary folate are associated with decreased colon and rectal cancer risk, whereas study results of calcium intake are less consistent. Micronutrients that have been demonstrated through several studies to decrease colorectal cancer risk include selenium, vitamin C, vitamin E, and β-carotene; however, the benefit of dietary supplementation does not appear to be substantial.

CLINICAL RISK FACTORS

Several clinical conditions and genetic disorders increase one's risk of developing colorectal cancer. Chronic ulcerative colitis, particularly when it involves the entire large intestine, predisposes individuals to colorectal cancer at a rate that is up to 30 times higher than average.[5,6,13] The risk is even greater for young individuals and increases for all affected individuals with extent of bowel involvement and disease duration. Although a precise causative link has not been established, chronic underlying inflammation may be a significant predisposing factor. The progressive dysplastic changes that the bowel mucosa undergo are similar to those observed in adenomatous polyps. Similarly, patients with Crohn's disease are also at increased risk, although the relative risk is slightly lower than that of patients with ulcerative colitis. This difference may be related to the decreased length of bowel affected by the chronic inflammatory process in individuals with Crohn's disease. Overall, persons diagnosed with either disease constitute approximately 1% to 2% of all new cases of colorectal cancer each year.

Although most cases of colorectal cancer are sporadic in nature, 10% to 20% of cases are thought to be hereditary. First-degree relatives of patients diagnosed with colorectal cancer have an increased risk of the disease that is at least two to four times that of persons in the general population without a family history.[14] The two most common forms of hereditary cancer are familial adenomatosis polyposis (FAP) and hereditary nonpolyposis colorectal cancer (HNPCC). FAP is an autosomal dominant trait that accounts for 0.5% of all colorectal cancers. The disease is manifested by hundreds to thousands of tiny sessile adenomatous polyps that carpet the colon and rectum, typically arising during adolescence.[15] The risk of developing colorectal cancer for individuals with untreated FAP is virtually 100%; most will develop colorectal cancer by their fourth decade of life.[16]

HNPCC, also referred to as Lynch syndrome I or II, is an autosomal dominantly inherited syndrome that accounts for 5% to 10% of colon cancer cases. In contrast to FAP, adenomatous polyps generally number only up to 100 and tend to be located primarily in the proximal (cecum, ascending, transverse) colon. Type I or Lynch syndrome I is characterized by the aggregation of colorectal cancer at an early age within a particular family, whereas type II (Lynch syndrome II, family cancer syndrome) represents multiple colon and extracolonic adenocarcinomas as well. Typical extracolonic sites include endometrial carcinoma and carcinomas of the breast, stomach, ovary, pancreas, small bowel, and urinary tract. The age at onset of colorectal cancer is typically before or around 40 years of age. Approximately 50% of patients with HNPCC are diagnosed with colorectal cancer by age 80.[17]

PATHOLOGY

The development of a colorectal neoplasm is a multistep process of several genetic and phenotypic alterations of normal bowel epithelium structure and function.[8,18] Since the majority of colorectal cancers develop sporadically, efforts have been directed toward identifying these alterations, determining if they develop in any type of sequential order, and learning whether discovery of the presence of such changes may lead to improved cancer detection and/or treatment outcomes.

A genetic model has been proposed for colorectal tumorigenesis that describes a process of transformation from adenoma to carcinoma.[19,20] An overview of the model is depicted in Figure 118–4. The adenoma–carcinoma sequence of tumor development reflects a sequential series of mutations within colonic epithelium, each of which results in

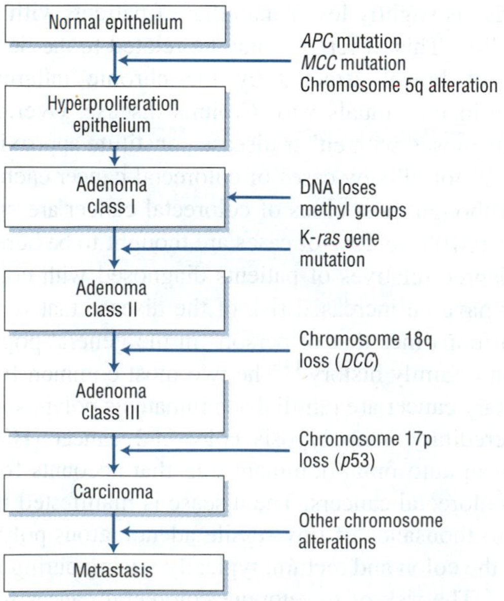

FIGURE 118–4. Adenoma–carcinoma sequence. *(Modified from Ref. 20, with permission.)*

cellular replication or enhanced invasiveness. Key elements of this process include hyperproliferation of epithelial cells to form a small benign neoplasm or adenoma in conjunction with cellular gene mutations. These mutations occur early and frequently in sporadic cases of both adenomas and colorectal cancer.[16,21] Genetic changes include mutational activation of oncogenes as well as inactivation of tumor suppressor genes. Both types of genetic alterations are required to produce the malignant tumor.

Oncogenes are mutated forms of normal cellular genes, or protooncogenes, that induce many of the aberrant features of malignant cells. Activating mutations of *ras* protooncogenes, primarily involving the K-*ras* and N-*ras* genes, occur frequently in colorectal cancer.[22] The *ras* family of genes is responsible for encoding proteins involved in signal transduction. Although the effects of these mutated genes are not completely understood, their activation is believed to be important in tumor progression.

Tumor suppressor genes are normal cellular genes that are capable of transforming normal cells to cancerous cells through their deletion or inactivation. One of the earliest genetic changes in colorectal tumorigenesis involves the mutation or loss of the adenomatous polyposis coli (*APC*) gene, a tumor suppressor gene, localized on the long arm of chromosome 5q21. The *APC* gene encodes for a protein that binds to β- and γ-catenin that belong to a family of proteins associated with intracellular adhesion.[18] The catenins also bind to the cytoplasmic domain of E-cadherin, an important molecule responsible for cell–cell adhesion. These activities among others are believed to be involved in regulation of cell shape and cell-to-cell communication and may affect cell cycle regulation or apoptosis. These alterations lead to abnormal epithelial proliferation and differentiation of cells. Inactivation of the *APC* gene is the single gene defect responsible for FAP and is frequently seen in sporadic colorectal cancer cases.

Mutational inactivations of two additional important tumor-suppressor genes, *p53*, located on chromosome 17p, and the *DCC* (deleted in colorectal carcinoma) gene, located on chromosome 18q, occur later during the adenoma–carcinoma sequence. Normal *p53* gene expression is responsible for apoptosis, an irreversible cell process resulting in cell death. Loss of *p53* activity through mutation is the most common genetic abnormality associated with human tumors and may contribute toward their growth advantage by allowing for uninhibited cellular proliferation, despite damaged DNA.[23] The protein encoded by the normal *DCC* gene is believed to share similar structural features to certain types of cell-adhesion molecules, and as such may interact with various proteins to control cell–cell interaction and cellular proliferation. Loss of specific cell-adhesive properties could contribute toward tumor invasion and metastasis.

A distinct group of genetic traits has also been identified for individuals with HNPCC. "Replication errors" occur frequently and represent widespread alterations in the length of a series of repeated nucleotides, or microsatellites, within tumor DNA.[21] Mutations of those genes that appear to recognize and regulate DNA replication errors, or "mismatch-repair genes," *MSH2, MLH1, PMS1, PMS2,* and *MSH6,* contribute to microsatellite instability and colorectal tumorigenesis.[18,24] Although mutations of *MLH1* and *MSH2* account for most cases of HNPCC where mutations have been documented, mutations of *PMS2* and *MSH6* have also been implicated. Failure to repair DNA mismatches may cause further mutations that may result in oncogene activation or tumor suppressor gene inactivation. Tumor progression may then be facilitated through a link between DNA repair defects and mutations of critical growth regulatory genes. Inactivation of a receptor for type II transforming growth factor-β (TGF-β), a protein that has antiproliferative effects on colonic epithelial cell growth, has been demonstrated in cells with replication errors.[25]

Adenocarcinomas account for more than 90% of tumors of the large intestine.[5] Other histologic types such as mucinous adenocarcinoma, signet ring adenocarcinoma, carcinoid simplex, and carcinoid tumors occur less frequently. Adenocarcinomas are assigned one of three tumor grade designations based on the degree of cellular differentiation, the degree to which the tumor resembles the structure, and function of its cell of origin. The most differentiated adenocarcinomas, or grade I tumors, generally resemble adenomas, whereas grade III tumors are considered "high grade," the most undifferentiated, and have frequently lost the characteristics of mature normal cells. Features of well-differentiated tumors include relatively normal tubule and glandular formation and low numbers of mitoses. Poorly differentiated or high-grade tumors contain few or no glandular structures and have an increased nuclear-to-cytoplasmic ratio, large nuclei, and dark staining due to increased DNA content. Poorly differentiated tumors are associated with a worse prognosis than those that are better differentiated.[26,27]

Mucinous adenocarcinomas possess the same basic structure as adenocarcinomas but differ in that they secrete an abundant quantity of extracellular mucus. They account for only about 10% of colorectal carcinomas but tend to be most frequent in patients with HNPCC and patients with coexisting ulcerative colitis.[17] Signet-ring adenocarcinomas have a characteristic appearance due to the displacement of the nucleus to one side by large vacuoles of intracellular mucin. Patients tend to present with a more advanced stage of disease and have a highly invasive tumor. Both mucinous and signet-ring adenocarcinoma histologies confer a poor prognosis.

DNA content of the tumor is also related to overall prognosis.[5] This is easily and reliably measured with flow cytometry. Tumors with DNA content equal to normal are referred to as *diploid;* tumors with abnormal DNA content are referred to as *aneuploid.* Aneuploid tumors are more likely to recur following primary resection, and patients with aneuploid tumors have decreased survival compared to patients with diploid tumors.

The frequencies at which cancer occurs in the various areas of the colon vary. The proportion of tumors occurring in the right (cecum, ascending, and transverse colon) side of the colon has increased during the past 30 years with fewer occurring in the rectum and left (descending and sigmoid colon) side. For example, the percentage of colon cancer cases detected in the ascending colon/cecum in 1990 increased to 36.3% from 28.6% in 1971.[3] About 33.7% of tumors arise in the sigmoid colon area. Seventeen percent are detected in the area of the transverse colon and splenic flexure, and 7.7% develop in the descending colon. In addition, the tendency for tumors to shift to the proximal (right) side increases with increasing patient age.[28] Whether this is due to more frequent and better access to the proximal area of the bowel or rather a shift in the biology of the disease is unknown. The implications of this phenomenon suggest that fewer lesions are accessible to sigmoidoscopy, a standard screening program procedure that only allows evaluation of the more distal (left) colon.

MANIFESTATIONS AND COMPLICATIONS

The signs and symptoms associated with colorectal cancer can be extremely varied, subtle, and nonspecific. Patients with early-stage colorectal cancer are often asymptomatic and usually found as a result of screening studies. Although rectal bleeding and abdominal pain are the most common signs, any change in bowel habits (e.g., constipation, diarrhea, alteration in size or shape of stool), vague abdominal discomfort, or distention may all be warning signs of a malignant process.

Colorectal lesions tend to involve the bowel in a circular rather than longitudinal fashion, thereby narrowing and compressing the lumen. The presence or absence of symptoms is therefore often related to the location and size of the primary tumor and extent of disease involvement.[29] Tumors of the cecum and ascending colon are usually not associated with significant changes in bowel habits; although, watery diarrhea sometimes develops. In contrast, obstructive symptoms and changes in bowel habits frequently develop with tumors located in the transverse and descending colon. This is where the stool is the driest.

Nausea, vomiting, and abdominal discomfort are often secondary signs of a larger underlying problem such as obstruction, perforation, and/or bleeding. Bleeding may be acute or chronic and most commonly appears as bright, red blood mixed with stool. Iron deficiency anemia, presenting as weakness and occasionally high-output congestive heart failure, frequently develops as a result of chronic occult blood loss.

Approximately 20% to 25% of patients with colorectal cancer present with metastatic disease.[2,3] Metastatic spread occurs as a result of direct tumor invasion of adjacent tissues or by lymphatic or hematogenous spread. The venous drainage of the colon and rectum influences the pattern of metastases most commonly seen. The most common site of metastasis is the liver, often the only site of metastatic disease in 40% of patients, followed by the lungs and then bones, specifically the sacrum, coccyx, pelvis, and lumbar vertebrae. Hepatomegaly, obstruction, weight loss, and jaundice are indicative of liver metastases, which are present in 5% to 10% of patients at presentation. Other evidence of widespread disease may include leg edema due to lymph node involvement, thrombophlebitis, fistula formation, jaundice, weight loss, or pain, especially in the lower back or radiating down the legs.[28] Pain associated with hepatic metastases is sometimes localized in the right upper quadrant of the abdomen, right posterior chest, or right shoulder, and characterized as a continuous ache.

PREVENTION AND SCREENING

Cancer prevention efforts can be considered as either primary or secondary. Primary prevention strategies are aimed at preventing the development of colorectal cancer in a population at risk. Secondary prevention approaches are undertaken to prevent subsequent malignancy in a population that has already manifested an initial disease process.[30] The basis for primary prevention depends on identification of etiologic factors followed by eradication or alteration of their effects on carcinogenesis. Primary prevention also includes life-style and diet modification. Several primary preventive measures have undergone or are currently undergoing study; some of the most promising strategies are listed in Table 118–1. A daily dietary fiber intake of at least 39 g could be associated with a 31% reduction in colorectal cancer risk in North American males.[31] A 50% reduction in dietary fat intake may reduce the incidence of colon cancer in the United States by as much as 67%.[8] However, the results of large prospective trials are needed to confirm the extent of risk reduction that might be achieved through dietary fat and fiber modification.

Studies of aspirin and other NSAIDs have demonstrated the potential use of these agents for decreasing colorectal cancer incidence or mortality.[30] These agents, through their inhibition of cyclooxygenase and free radical formation, appear to modulate carcinogenesis. Cyclooxygenase-2 levels are elevated in human colon cancer cells and may act as a promotor of neoplasia by increasing the expression of *bcl-2*. A number of large cohort and case-control trials have demonstrated that regular use (≥ 2 doses/wk) of aspirin or other NSAIDs reduces colorectal cancer risk or mortality by 30% to 50%.[30] Data from randomized trials are limited, although follow-up data from the Physician's Health Study suggest a lack of association between aspirin use and the incidence of colorectal cancer.[34] Factors that may account for these differing results include uncontrolled confounding cancer risk factors, aspirin or NSAID dose, treatment duration, and length of follow-up. Although the bulk of epidemiologic evidence suggests that regular use of aspirin and other NSAIDs may have a protective effect, the evidence to date is not conclusive. In addition, any beneficial effect may not be apparent until at least 10 years of regular use.

Aspirin, sulindac, and other NSAIDs have also been demonstrated to reduce adenoma development and induce adenoma regression in patients with FAP.[30,35] However, these effects are incomplete and therefore inadequate to replace surgical resection. Other secondary prevention measures include procedures that range from colonoscopic removal of precancerous polyps (colonoscopic polypectomy) to total colectomy for individuals with FAP or in other high-risk settings.[16,36]

Although results of numerous trials of dietary modifications and chemopreventative agents suggest that they play an important role in colorectal cancer prevention, clinical application of much of these data is hampered by the lack of definitive associations between intermediate biomarkers commonly employed in chemoprevention trials (tritiated thymidine incorporation for colonic epithelial proliferation; abnormal crypts, microadenomas, protein kinase C) and frank cancer development. Furthermore, the potential benefit of confounding components of diets rich in fruits and vegetables such as fiber, selenium, vitamins C and E, and carotenoids, on colorectal carcinogenesis remains a challenge to elucidate.

Based on the recognized incidence of colorectal cancer, identification of high-risk individuals, and the high rate of curability associated with localized lesions, cancer

TABLE 118–1. Prevention Strategies for Colorectal Cancer

Intervention	Proposed Beneficial Effects
Fiber supplementation[8,31,32]	Decreases fecal bile acids; decreases bowel transit time; binds to fecal mutagens; dilutes fecal material
Dietary fat reduction[8]	Decreases fecal bile acids; may reduce consumption of carcinogenic heterocyclic amines associated with meat preparation techniques
Calcium supplementation[6]	Reduces the colonic epithelial cell proliferative response to fatty acids and bile acids
Aspirin and nonsteroidal anti-inflammatory drugs[30]	Decreases colonic cell cyclooxygenase-2 levels; reduces cyclooxygenase-mediated free radical formation; may interfere with cellular membrane processes; may inhibit growth factor synthesis in response to tumor promoters; may influence cell-cycle phase transitions
Difluoromethylornithine[33] (DFMO)	Inhibits ornithine decarboxylase, which reduces polyamine synthesis, thereby suppressing cellular growth and inhibiting carcinogenesis

TABLE 118–2. American Cancer Society Screening Recommendations for Colorectal Cancer[a]

- Annual occult fecal blood testing starting at age 50 years with:
  Flexible sigmoidoscopy every 5 years *or*
  Colonoscopy every 10 years *or*
  Double-contrast barium enema every 5 to 10 years
- A digital rectal examination should be performed at the same time as the sigmoidoscopy, colonoscopy, or barium enema

[a]Average-risk individuals.
From Ref. 37, with permission.

screening recommendations have been established. The current American Cancer Society guidelines for average-risk individuals are outlined in Table 118–2. More rigorous screening recommendations have been established for high-risk individuals.[38–40]

The digital rectal examination has been a traditional part of the annual physical examination in patients older than 40 years of age and accounts for the detection of approximately 10% of all cancers that are within reach of 7 to 10 cm of the anus. By itself, the digital rectal examination has not been shown an effective screening tool, but should be used in combination with other screening examinations.[40] The use of fecal occult blood tests results further in an increased number of asymptomatic individuals with early stages of disease discovered.[41] Three major methods are available to detect occult blood in the feces: guaiac dye or derivative, heme-porphyrin, and immunochemical methods. Guaiac-based tests utilize paper impregnated with a guaiac resin that contains α-guaiaconic acid, a phenolic compound that responds to peroxidases in the blood. When a solution containing hydrogen peroxide is poured over paper that has previously been exposed to absorbed peroxidases from blood in the stool, the phenolic compound is oxidized and a blue colorization develops.

The sensitivity of the test, a positive result in the setting in which blood is present, can be influenced by several factors. Because hemoglobin is degraded by bacteria in the stool, test sensitivity is diminished when samples are stored or when the lesion is located in the proximal area of the bowel. Although the sensitivity can be improved by rehydrating the stool sample, the procedure is more costly and time consuming and the specificity of the test is reduced. Ascorbic acid ingestion in excess of 250 mg/d, failure to ingest a high-residue diet for several days prior to testing, and assays of dry stools may also yield false-negative results.[41] Conversely, foods containing pseudoperoxidase or peroxidase activity can cause a false-positive reaction: rare red meat and uncooked fruits and vegetables such as broccoli, turnips, cauliflower, cantaloupe, and radishes. These foods should be avoided for 3 days prior to and during testing. Other sources of potential false-positive results include the use of iron supplements, rectal medications, or any medications that may potentially alter the integrity of the gastrointestinal lining. Anti-inflammatory agents should be avoided for 7 days prior to and during testing. Because tumors bleed intermittently, multiple stool specimens should be sampled to minimize false-negative results.

Heme-porphyrin and immunochemical assays were developed to reduce the rate of false-positive results associated with fecal guaiac blood tests. The heme-porphyrin assay quantifies the conversion of heme to fluorescent porphyrins. Because it also measures fecal heme that has been degraded by bacteria, test sensitivity is not altered significantly by the site of bleeding or fecal storage. Immunochemical tests react with the globin moiety of hemoglobin and are therefore affected less by dietary influences. However, test sensitivity is influenced by bleeding site and stool storage. Both of these assays are more complex and labor intensive to perform. Several comparative trials of fecal occult blood tests have been performed.[40,41] The HemeSelect, Hemoccult II SENSA, and FlexSure OBT appear to provide the best combination of sensitivity and specificity. A two-step approach in which a combination of the HemeSelect and the Hemoccult II SENSA tests are both used improves overall screening sensitivity without compromising test specificity.

The limitations associated with fecal occult blood screening remain an issue of active concern. Many early-stage tumors do not bleed, and therefore the false-negative rates are approximately 70% for cancer and 90% for polyps. Between 1% and 5% of unselected individuals will have a positive test result and approximately 2% to 17% of those individuals will be found to have colorectal cancer.[41] Even though false-positive rates are only between 2% and 10%, a false-positive result can prove to be very expensive and inconvenient for a patient due to the follow-up tests required for a positive result. Nevertheless, studies evaluating the effects of fecal occult blood screening tests have established that their use is associated with a reduction in mortality due to colorectal cancer by approximately 33%.[41,42]

Sigmoidoscopy is useful for examining the lower 35% to 60% of the bowel, depending on the instrument, and thus increases the detection rate by approximately two- to threefold. A 60-cm flexible sigmoidoscope can be used to reach the splenic flexure in order to detect 50% to 60% of cancers but it requires more operator training, is associated with increased risk, and patient tolerance is less than with the 35-cm instrument.[43] Studies suggest that screening sigmoidoscopy, according to currently recommended guidelines, could effectively reduce mortality from colorectal cancer by about 60% to 80%.[44,45] These data, however, have yet to be validated through randomized, prospective trials.

A colonoscope facilitates examination of the bowel to the cecum in the majority of patients and allows for simultaneous removal of premalignant lesions. Although it allows for greater visualization of the colon, colonoscopies involve greater risk and inconvenience to patients and are therefore not routinely included in current screening practices for average-risk individuals.[40] A double-contrast barium enema produces an image of the entire colon in most examinations, and small polyps and mucosal lesions are outlined by the retained barium. The combination of double-contrast barium enema with flexible sigmoidoscopy provides a sensitivity of 98% for colorectal malignancies.[40] Because it takes approximately 10 years for normal mucosa to evolve into an invasive carcinoma, the use of double-contrast barium enemas in routine screening practices for average-risk individuals is recommended only every 5 to 10 years. It may be useful, however, for certain high-risk individuals due to its ability to identify small abnormalities of the mucosa.[39] Promising future screening approaches include the analysis of stool samples or other body tissues or fluids for the presence of specific chromosomal point mutations, such as K-*ras,* or microsatellite instability.[24,46]

WORKUP AND DIAGNOSIS

When a patient is suspected of having colorectal carcinoma, a careful history and physical examination should be performed. The patient history should include a past medical history and family history, especially noting the presence of inflammatory bowel disease, colorectal cancer, polyps, and cancers of the breast, ovary, and endometrium. A complete physical examination includes careful abdominal examination for the presence of masses or ascites, a rectal examination, and an assessment for possible hepatomegaly and lymphadenopathy. In all women, a breast and pelvic examination is recommended, especially in women with a history of breast, ovarian, or endometrial cancer.

An unexplained anemia in an older patient requires surveillance of the entire large bowel, especially the right colon. Red blood cell indices (e.g., hemoglobin, hematocrit, mean corpuscular volume, reticulocyte count) and a workup of iron status (e.g., serum ferritin, serum iron, and total iron-binding capacity) may be useful to confirm acute or chronic blood loss and/or iron-deficiency anemia. An evaluation of the entire large bowel is undertaken with either colonoscopy or sigmoidoscopy and an double-contrast barium enema. A barium enema may be preferred in situations in which a partially obstructing lesion prohibits passage of the endoscope; however, it should be avoided if complete obstruction or perforation of the bowel is suspected. A characteristic finding indicative of colon cancer seen on barium enema is an apple core-shaped lesion with tumor involving the circumference of the bowel. When possible, the endoscope is used to collect tissue for a histologic evaluation and provide a preliminary diagnosis following the procedure.

Baseline laboratory tests should be obtained and include a complete blood cell (CBC) count, platelet count, prothrombin time (PT), activated partial thromboplastin time (aPTT), liver function tests, and serum CEA. Abnormal liver function tests may suggest liver involvement with tumor. However, patients with metastatic disease to the liver may have normal liver function tests, and abnormal liver function tests are not always indicative of metastatic disease.

CEA belongs to a group of cell-surface glycoproteins, termed "oncofetal proteins," which are expressed during embryonic development and reexpressed on the cell surfaces of many carcinomas, particularly those of the gastrointestinal tract. Although the function of CEA is not well understood, it is proposed to be a cellular adhesion molecule and possibly contribute toward tumor invasion and metastasis. The concentration of CEA can be measured in the blood and can therefore potentially serve as a "marker" for colorectal cancer. Approximately 28% of patients with stage A and 45% of patients with stage B colorectal cancer will have an elevated serum CEA level at time of diagnosis.[47] Elevated concentrations are even more frequent in patients with metastatic disease. It is important to recognize, however, several concomitant disease states that can artificially elevate CEA: alcoholic and chronic hepatitis, diverticulitis, renal failure, cholelithiasis, fibrocystic breast disease, and smoking.[48,49] Although CEA measurement is too insensitive and nonspecific to be used as a screening test for early-stage colorectal cancer, it may be useful for monitoring colorectal cancer response to treatment, particularly if the pretreatment concentration is elevated.[47,48] The CEA test also has preoperative prognostic implications because it has been shown to correlate with the size and degree of differentiation of the carcinoma.[49] Elevated preoperative CEA levels correlate with a poor survival, regardless of tumor stage upon diagnosis. After a potentially curative resection, CEA levels should return to normal within 1 month. Persistently elevated CEA levels may indicate residual disease.

Radiographic imaging studies help evaluate the extent of disease involvement. A chest x-ray should be performed to rule out the presence of metastatic spread to the lungs. A bone scan can also be helpful in evaluating the extent of disease involvement in a symptomatic patient. A computed tomography (CT) scan or ultrasound of the abdomen is often performed to evaluate hepatic and retroperitoneal involvement and occult abdominal and pelvic disease, and to determine the depth of tumor penetration into the bowel wall and/or invasion to adjacent organs. Detection of lymph node involvement with either study is limited by the difficulty of distinguishing inflammatory or reactive lymph nodes from those infiltrated with tumor. Because peritoneal seeding, small distant lymph node metastasis, or liver metastasis in colon cancer may not be adequately detected by CT scan, an occasional patient may need to undergo a laparotomy in order to confirm metastatic disease. This is infrequent, however, because most patients eventually undergo surgical resection for colorectal cancer unless the procedure is contraindicated.

Intrarectal or transrectal ultrasonography is a technique that is becoming more widely available for the evaluation of patients with rectal cancer. It is excellent for detecting the depth of tumor penetration and, like pelvic CT scans, is fair to good in determining lymph node involvement.[48] Cystoscopy or intravenous pyelography studies are rarely indicated except for very large rectal tumors found on examination, if the patient exhibits symptoms, or if a CT scan suggests bladder involvement. Intraluminal and hepatic MRI studies may also provide useful information.

Immunodetection of tumors using tumor-directed antibodies is receiving greater recognition as an imaging technique for the early detection and imaging of colorectal cancers. Several tumor-associated proteins have been identified within or on the surface membrane of colorectal malignant cells to which monoclonal antibodies have been targeted.[50] Of these, CEA and TAG-72 antigen have undergone the greatest amount of study. Radiolabeled monoclonal antibodies directed against these antigens have been used in clinical studies for both external immunoscintography as well as intraoperative localization of tumor. OncoScint CR/OV, an indium-111–labeled monoclonal antibody targeted to the TAG-72 antigen, is an FDA-approved diagnostic imaging agent available for determining the location and extent of extrahepatic disease in patients with colorectal cancer. CEA-Scan arcitumomab (IMMU-4^{99m}Tc Fab′ RAID), a radiolabeled murine monoclonal immunoglobulin directed against the human CEA molecule, and HumaSPECT-Tc (^{99m}Tc 88BV59), a radiolabeled human monoclonal immunoglobulin that recognizes a tumor-associated antigen (CTAA 16.88, CTA #1), can also provide useful information regarding the presence, extent, and location of colorectal cancer.[51,52] The use of these agents is generally reserved for those patients who have completed standard diagnostic imaging tests but may still require additional information regarding the extent of disease. However, they may play an important role in identifying metastatic or recurrent disease in individuals with negative standard radiographic studies. Although these approaches are helpful for addressing some of the limitations of current radiographic techniques, they are limited somewhat by the heterogeneity associated with antigen expression at different sites of tumor within individual patients.[53]

STAGING

The purpose of the staging examinations is to describe precisely the malignancy at a point in its natural history that is germane to patient treatment options and overall prognosis. Traditionally, the Dukes classification, originally published in 1932, has been used in the staging of colorectal cancers.[54] Since then, it has undergone several modifications; a modified Astler–Coller version is used more extensively.[55] Prognosis and survival data associated with each stage of disease in this classification system have been collected extensively. However, because multiple staging systems exist and have been used for various clinical trials, the literature is often difficult to evaluate. Therefore, in an effort to standardize the staging system for colorectal cancer, the American Joint Committee on Cancer (AJCC) and the International Union Against Cancer (IUAC) jointly agreed to use and recommend the TNM classification system. This classification takes three aspects of cancer growth—T (*t*umor size), N (lymph *n*ode involvement), and M (presence or absence of *m*etastases)—into account for determining the disease stage. The TNM classification allows for various subdivisions within each of the three categories.[56] A schematic representing the relationship between both staging systems can be found in Figure 118–5.

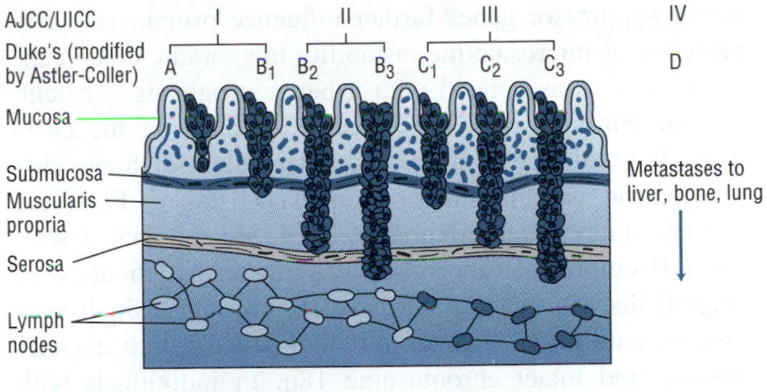

FIGURE 118–5. Staging system for colorectal cancer.

The stage of colorectal cancer upon diagnosis, identified primarily by depth of tumor invasion of the bowel wall and presence or absence of involved lymph nodes, is the most important independent prognostic factor for survival and disease recurrence. A comparison of the stage of disease upon presentation and relative survival rates for individuals with colon and rectum cancer is provided in Table 118–3. The stage of disease also provides the basis for determining the most appropriate initial treatment. However, additional clinical and pathologic variables may affect the prognosis of patients with colorectal cancer. Consideration of these factors plays an important role in determining optimal strategies for treatment as well as appropriate follow-up. The patient's overall health status will also influence treatment tolerability and therapeutic options. Clinical factors present at time of diagnosis that are associated with a poor prognosis and decreased survival include bowel obstruction or perforation, rectal bleeding, high preoperative CEA level, distant metastases, and location of the primary tumor in the rectum or rectosigmoid area.[5,47]

Pathologic variables associated with a negative influence on prognosis include depth of muscular invasion; venous, lymphatic, or perineural invasion; number of involved lymph nodes; high proliferation indices; increased aneuploidy; sialyl Lewis antigen (CA 19-9); mucinous or signet-ring histology; and poor tumor differentiation. Data from recent and ongoing studies demonstrate that *p53* overexpression and genetic alterations on certain oncogenes and

TABLE 118–3. Colon and Rectum Cancer Disease Stage and Survival Rates (SEER Data, 1989–1994)

Tumor Stage at Diagnosis	Patients Presenting (%)		5-Year Relative Survival (%)	
	Colon	*Rectum*	*Colon*	*Rectum*
Localized	35	42	93.6	87.1
Regional	38	35	69.3	57.7
Metastatic	22	16	9.2	6.0
Unstaged	5	8	62.7[a]	60.5[a]

[a]All stages.
From Ref. 2.

tumor suppressor genes further influence prognosis.[57] The presence of microsatellite instability in sporadic colon cancer lesions is associated with a better prognosis.[58] Allelic loss of chromosome 18q, which is located on the *DCC* gene, is predictive of mortality, independent of tumor differentiation, vascular invasion, and TNM stage.[59] Five-year survival rates of approximately 93% are associated with stage II colorectal cancer; survival rates for patients with stage II disease and allelic loss of chromosome 18q drop to approximately 54%, similar to that of patients with stage III disease and intact chromosome 18q. In individuals with stage III disease, the presence of chromosome 18q allelic loss is associated with a 5-year disease-free survival rate of 38%, compared to 76% among individuals without loss of heterozygosity.[60] High expression of thymidylate synthase (TS) in resected tumor specimens is also associated with a poorer prognosis. Although the 10-year overall survival for individuals with TS-positive tumors was no different from that with TS-negative tumors, survival in a subset of patients who received chemotherapy was only 42.9% for TS-positive tumors compared to 85.7% for TS-negative tumors.[61] These factors may provide important clues as to which patients with intermediate-stage disease should receive additional therapy after surgical resection.

TREATMENT MODALITIES

SURGERY

Surgical removal of the primary tumor is the treatment of choice for most patients with colorectal cancer. Patients with advanced, metastatic colorectal cancer may also require surgery for palliation of bleeding, obstruction, or localized abdominal pain due to a bulky tumor mass.[48] The surgical approach for colon cancer generally involves a complete resection of the tumor with an appropriate margin of tumor-free bowel and a regional lymphadenectomy. In the elective setting, a temporary colostomy is rarely required.[5] A total colectomy may, however, be indicated for selected patients with FAP or chronic ulcerative colitis. An ongoing study is comparing laparoscopic colectomy with standard colectomy in an attempt to reduce morbidity and surgical complications as well as reduce costs. Surgery for rectal cancer depends on the region of tumor involvement.[62] A low anterior resection is the procedure of choice in patients with lesions in the mid- to upper rectum.[63] Patients with lesions in the lower portion of the rectum may require an abdominoperineal resection if either the amount of unaffected bowel is insufficient for a resection far enough away from the tumor or too close to areas that cannot permit an anastomosis. Newer surgical techniques have been developed in an attempt to retain function of the rectal sphincter and still achieve complete tumor resection. Individuals who are not candidates for sphincter-sparing resections or have extensive local spread of tumor will require an abdominoperineal resection. This involves removal of the distal sigmoid, rectosigmoid, rectum, and anus with the establishment of a permanent sigmoid colostomy. Fewer than one-third of patients will require a permanent colostomy for rectal cancer.[62] The American Cancer Society, United Ostomy Association, and the International Association of Enterostomal Therapy offer ostomy rehabilitation services. Surgery for colorectal cancer is associated with a morbidity and mortality rate of 8% to 15% and 1% to 2%, respectively.[48] Other complications associated with colorectal surgery can include infection, anastomotic leakage, obstruction, adhesion formation, and malabsorption syndromes. Additional complications unique to surgery for rectal cancer include urinary retention, incontinence, impotence, and locoregional recurrence.

RADIATION THERAPY

Radiation therapy (XRT) can be administered in conjunction with curative surgical resection and in the setting of advanced or metastatic disease. In patients undergoing surgery, XRT is used to reduce local tumor recurrence. Symptom reduction is the primary goal of XRT for patients with advanced or metastatic disease. XRT is given prior to or following surgery and can be delivered using a variety of dosing regimens, administration schedules, and techniques that expose different amounts of body surface area.[5,62,64]

Retrospective data suggest that preoperative XRT may be used to reduce the initial size of the tumor to such an extent that the tumor could be reclassified to a lower stage, or "downstaged," and therefore rendered more resectable. This might then lead to improved patient survival or require that a less extensive surgical procedure be performed. Preoperative XRT is also administered to reduce the amount of tumor seeding that can occur during surgery; however, this approach is more likely to affect a greater area than is necessary.[62] Postoperative administration of XRT may more adequately treat a defined area, but is associated with more toxicity due to a greater amount of bowel being present in the treatment field.

Adverse effects associated with XRT can be acute or chronic. Acute effects primarily include hematologic depression, dysuria, diarrhea, abdominal cramping, and proctitis. Chronic symptoms that sometimes persist for months following discontinuation of XRT may involve persistent diarrhea, proctitis, or enteritis, small bowel obstruction, perineal tenderness, and impaired wound healing.

CHEMOTHERAPY

Since the mid-1950s, 5-fluorouracil (5-FU) has been the most active and widely used chemotherapeutic agent for colorectal cancer. Biochemical modulation is an alternative approach to single-agent 5-FU therapy that involves the addition of another agent in an attempt to modify or change its activity in order to improve response rates and, ultimately, patient survival. Examples of biochemical modulating agents used for colorectal cancer of greatest interest include leucovorin, interferon-α (IFN-α), methotrexate, trimetrexate, and *N*-(phosphonacetyl)-L-aspartate (PALA). Most recently, topoisomerase I inhibitors, thymidylate synthase inhibitors, 5-FU prodrugs and degradation modulators, and platinum analogs have undergone substantial study.[65] The pharmacology of the key agents used for colorectal cancer is discussed briefly in the next sections.

5-FLUOROURACIL AND 5-FLUORO-2′-DEOXYURIDINE

The most common fluorinated pyrimidine used clinically, 5-FU, is a member of the only group of cytotoxins whose development is based on rational predicted biochemical action. The same cytotoxic effect as with 5-FU is produced by 5-fluoro-2′-deoxyuridine (FUDR, Floxuridine) through its conversion in a single-step reaction by deoxyuridine kinase to an active metabolite, 5-fluorodeoxyuridine-5′-monophosphate (FdUMP).

As a prodrug, 5-FU undergoes anabolism to two primary products, 5-fluorouridine-5′-triphosphate (FUTP) and FdUMP, to exert its antitumor effects (Fig. 118–6).[65,66] FUTP is incorporated into RNA, thereby impairing protein synthesis. FdUMP forms a tight but reversible covalent bond with thymidylate synthase (TS) in the presence of methylenetetrahydrofolate (CH_2-THF), one of the intracellular metabolites of folinic acid. TS is the key enzyme necessary for synthesis of thymidylate through conversion of deoxyuridine monophosphate (dUMP) to 2′-deoxythymidine-5′-monophosphate (dTMP). The lack of available TS therefore reduces the rate of DNA synthesis, replication, and repair. When combined with folinic acid, the antitumor effects of 5-FU are enhanced through stabilization of the ternary complex of TS, FdUMP, and CH_2-THF. The degree of TS activity and duration of TS inhibition may be predictive for tumor response to 5-FU therapy.[67] These findings may help identify which patients will benefit from 5-FU therapy for colorectal cancer.

Used alone and in combination, 5-FU forms the basis for many chemotherapy regimens used in the adjuvant setting and metastatic treatment of colorectal cancer. 5-FU is typically administered as an intravenous (IV) bolus injection, generally once weekly or daily for 5 days each month, or via a continuous IV infusion. Although the duration of continuous IV infusions is usually 5 days, it can extend for several weeks. FUDR can be administered intravenously but intrahepatic use is more common. It is preferable to 5-FU for intrahepatic administration because a much greater percentage of FUDR is removed from the systemic circulation with one pass through the liver.

Clinical studies comparing efficacy of bolus and continuous infusion schedules consistently appear to favor continuous infusion of 5-FU. This is consistent with evidence that suggests that the duration of infusion may be an important determinant of the biologic activity of 5-FU.[68] The primary cytotoxic effect associated with bolus 5-FU is on RNA synthesis, whereas interference with DNA is the predominant effect of continuous 5-FU infusion.

Toxicity patterns also differ based on the dose, route, and schedule of 5-FU administration. Leukopenia is the primary dose-limiting toxicity of IV bolus 5-FU, although diarrhea, stomatitis, and nausea and vomiting can also occur.[68,69] The incidence and severity of stomatitis can be significantly reduced with the use of oral cryotherapy.[65] In this approach, the patient is required to chew and hold ice chips in the mouth during the period between 5 minutes prior to and 30 minutes following the bolus injection of 5-FU. The basis for

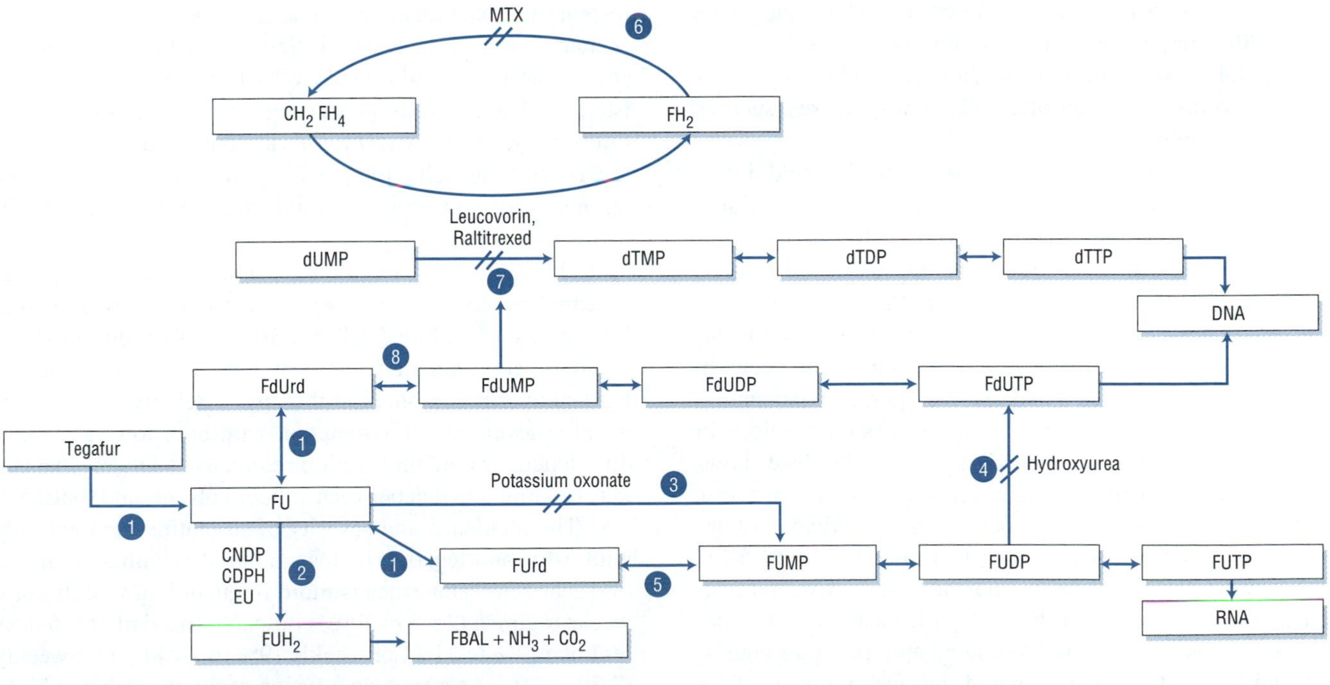

FIGURE 118–6. Metabolic pathways and sites of 5-Fluorouracil: (1) thymidine/uridine phosphorylase; (2) dihydrouracil dehydrogenase; (3) orotate phosphoribosyl-transferase; (4) ribonucleotide reductase; (5) uridine kinase; (6) dihydrofolate reductase; (7) thymidylate synthase; and (8) thymidine kinase. (CNDP = 3-cyano-2,6-dihydropyridine; CDPH = 5-chloro-2,4-dihydroxypyridine; EU = eniluracil.) *(Adapted from Zhang AG, Harstrick A, Rustum YM. Mechanisms of resistance to fluoropyrimidines. Semin Oncol 1992;19:5.)*

the protective effects of this procedure is based on the premise that local vasoconstriction caused by the ice chips temporarily reduces blood flow to the oral mucosa, thereby reducing drug exposure to the oral mucosa.

Although continuous IV infusion 5-FU is generally well tolerated, dose-limiting toxicities can be substantial. A distinct toxicity, palmar–plantar erythrodysesthesia ("hand–foot syndrome") and stomatitis occur most frequently with this route of administration.[68–70] Hand–foot syndrome occurs in 24% to 40% of patients receiving extended continuous IV infusions and is characterized by painful swelling and erythroderma of the soles of the feet, palms of the hands, and distal fingers. This type of skin toxicity is fully reversible upon interruption of therapy or dose reduction, and is not life threatening; however, it can be significant and acutely disabling. The incidence of stomatitis, diarrhea, and hematologic toxicity is not substantial at standard doses but increases with increasing doses of 5-FU. In a meta-analysis of six randomized trials, no significant difference was noted in the incidence of mucositis, diarrhea, nausea and vomiting, or alopecia between continuous and bolus intravenous 5-FU administration.[68,69]

LEVAMISOLE

Levamisole (Ergamisol) is a synthetic, oral anthelmintic drug with immunomodulatory properties. Some of its stimulatory effects on the immune system include T-cell activation, augmentation of macrophage activity, and enhancement of the chemotactic response of polymorphonuclear cells and monocytes. Despite its synergy with 5-FU *in vitro*, levamisole alone does not produce direct cytotoxicity at levels achieved clinically. Although the mechanism of its synergistic effect with 5-FU is unknown, various mechanisms have been proposed.[71] Effects of levamisole or its metabolites may be related to its immune effects, biochemical modulation independent of immunomodulatory activity, or possibly inhibition of cellular phosphatases, such as tyrosine phosphatase.[72]

Toxicities due to levamisole are generally mild, infrequent, and clinically tolerable. Levamisole is associated with taste abnormalities (described as metallic and occasionally associated with an altered sense of smell), arthralgias, and myalgias.[73] Central nervous system (CNS) toxicities expressed as anxiety, irritability, somnolence, depression, insomnia, agitation, confusion, or cerebellar ataxia occur in fewer than 5% of patients and resolve upon discontinuation of therapy. Significant hematologic depression develops in less than 1% of patients receiving levamisole alone; however, agranulocytosis has been reported which, in a few cases, has been fatal. The most common toxicities of levamisole plus 5-FU are similar to those seen with 5-FU alone and include leukopenia, diarrhea, stomatitis, and nausea and vomiting. Up to 40% of patients treated with levamisole plus 5-FU show laboratory abnormalities consistent with hepatic toxicity noted by elevations in liver function enzymes (alkaline phosphatase, transaminases, or serum bilirubin) or CT-documented fatty infiltration of the liver.[74] These laboratory changes are mild, rarely symptomatic, and reversible on discontinuation of therapy.

LEUCOVORIN CALCIUM

The administration of leucovorin (folinic acid, citrovorum factor) increases intracellular concentrations of reduced folate, which stabilizes the ternary complex between FdUMP and TS. As a result, there is a reduction in the availability of free TS, which catalyzes the conversion of dUMP to dTMP, a rate-limiting step in DNA synthesis. Inhibition of TS activity is more complete and prolonged, thereby enhancing 5-FU cytotoxicity.

Leucovorin is generally nontoxic in therapeutic doses, although hypersensitivity reactions, such as anaphylaxis and urticaria, have been reported. The combination of 5-FU with either low-dose (20 mg/m^2) or high-dose (20 to 500 mg/m^2) leucovorin, however, produces greater toxicity to the gastrointestinal epithelium, the primary dose-limiting toxicity. An increase in the incidence and severity of stomatitis (25% to 30%) and diarrhea is most commonly observed.[75,76] Serious toxic effects develop in 3% to 6% of patients.[77,78] The dose-limiting toxicity for low-dose leucovorin is usually neutropenia and stomatitis as compared to diarrhea with high-dose 5-FU plus leucovorin regimens.[79]

Severe diarrhea develops in 25% of patients receiving high-dose leucovorin regimens, and has resulted in a 5% mortality rate due to diarrhea-related events or cardiovascular collapse.[75] Early treatment of diarrhea-related dehydration with bowel rest, IV fluids, and discontinuation of chemotherapy until resolution of all symptoms is recommended. Loperamide and diphenoxylate can also be used for symptomatic treatment. For those patients who do not respond to these treatment measures, the use of octreotide acetate should be considered. Several studies have demonstrated the safety and efficacy of octreotide acetate, administered subcutaneously at a dosage of 100 μg two or three times daily, or 50 to 150 μg/h via continuous IV infusion, for controlling refractory, 5-FU–induced diarrhea.[65] The optimal dose and route of administration of octreotide remains to be defined.

Occasionally, stomatitis and conjunctivitis develop. Significant hematologic toxicity is uncommon, although severe leukopenia (white blood cells [WBCs] $< 2000/mm^3$) has been noted in approximately 20% of patients treated with 5-FU/leucovorin combination therapy.[76] Seizures have infrequently developed in association with both low- and high-dose leucovorin administration regimens.[65] The mechanism may be similar to that between anticonvulsants and folic acid.

The incidence and severity of stomatitis vary not only with 5-FU and leucovorin dosage but also with administration schedule.[79] Diarrhea is more frequent in a weekly for 6 weeks regimen (23% to 40%) compared to a daily for 5 days regimen (9% to 11%) or weekly (9% to 14%) and biweekly (2.2% to 16%) continuous infusion regimens utilizing high-dose leucovorin and 5-FU.[69] The incidence of stomatitis and diarrhea using a daily for 5 days regimen of high-dose leucovorin ranges from 15% to 31% and 23.2% to 45%, respectively. A significant increase in leukopenia and stomatitis was noted in the daily for 5 days low-dose leucovorin plus 5-FU arm compared to a weekly arm of 5-FU plus low-dose leucovorin administered as an intravenous bolus or continuous infusion (7.9% to 29% versus 1.4% to 4%) and (9.9% to 28% versus 0%), respectively.[69] More treatment-related deaths due to sepsis occur with the daily for 5 days low-dose leucovorin plus 5-FU, which could be explained by higher doses of 5-FU given as intravenous bolus infusions. Continuous or intermittent administration of 5-FU permits use of higher doses of 5-FU to be administered with significantly less myelosuppression, stomatitis, and diarrhea. Increased dose intensity may account for the higher response rates observed with prolonged infusions of 5-FU.[69]

IRINOTECAN

Irinotecan (CPT-11, Camptosar) is a water-soluble camptothecin derivative that inhibits topoisomerase I, an enzyme necessary for DNA replication. Irinotecan itself is a weak inhibitor of topoisomerase I and therefore must be converted to an active metabolite, 7-ethyl-10-hydroxy camptothecin (SN-38), which is 100- to 1000-fold more potent than the parent drug.[80]

The most common adverse effects of irinotecan are diarrhea, neutropenia, nausea and vomiting, asthenia, and alopecia; diarrhea and neutropenia are dose limiting.[81–85] Two distinct patterns of diarrhea have been described. Early-onset diarrhea occurs during or within 2 to 6 hours after irinotecan administration and is characterized by lacrimation, diaphoresis, abdominal cramping, flushing, and/or diarrhea. These cholinergic symptoms, thought to be due to inhibition of acetylcholinesterase, respond to atropine 0.25 to 1 mg given intravenously or subcutaneously. More commonly, late-onset diarrhea appears 1 to 12 days or more after irinotecan administration and may last for 3 to 5 days.[81,85] A few patients have required hospitalization or discontinuation of therapy, and fatalities have been reported.[85] Aggressive intervention with high-dose loperamide therapy should consist of 4 mg taken at the first sign of soft or watery stools, followed by 2 mg orally every 2 hours until symptom free for 12 hours. This regimen can be modified to 4 mg every 4 hours taken during the night.[81] Of note, a significant correlation has been identified between the severity of diarrhea, CPT-11, and SN-38 area under the concentration-versus-time curve (AUC).[80,81] Bone marrow suppression due to irinotecan is not cumulative and affects primarily the neutrophils, with a median nadir of 8 to 15 days and prompt recovery. The incidence of febrile neutropenia and sepsis requiring hospitalization is more common at higher dosage levels.[81,82,85] The use of granulocyte colony-stimulating factors is generally not required unless the patient has persistent myelosuppression despite a dose reduction. An idiosyncratic pulmonary-induced toxicity and drug interaction with phenothiazines has been reported with irinotecan. Discontinuation of irinotecan has resulted in symptomatic improvement of dyspnea, pulmonary infiltrates, and/or fever.[82] At this time however, routine pulmonary function testing is not recommended. Akathisia has been observed in patients premedicated with prochlorperazine 30 minutes prior to irinotecan, and has lasted 24 to 48 hours following the infusion.[81]

INTERFERON

Several potential mechanisms by which IFNs modulate 5-FU activity and metabolism have been identified.[5,65] *In vivo* data have demonstrated that the administration of IFN-α alters the pharmacokinetics of 5-FU, causing a dose-dependent decrease in 5-FU clearance, an increased 5-FU half-life, and a 30% increase in 5-FU area under the concentration-versus-time curve. This may be due to an inhibition of dihydropyrimidine dehydrogenase (DPD), the key enzyme responsible for regulating 5-FU degradation.[86] IFN-α has also been shown to decrease thymidine kinase activity, inhibit thymidine incorporation into DNA, and decrease the rate of thymidine phosphorylation. IFN-α may also increase FdUMP formation, thereby elevating intracellular levels of FdUMP and enhancing TS inhibition.[62]

The toxicities related to IFN-α and 5-FU include flu-like symptoms that resolve either spontaneously or upon dose reduction or discontinuation of the IFN. Lethargy has also been problematic and can be dose limiting for some individuals. Stomatitis and leukopenia can develop and may require a reduction in the dose of 5-FU.

METHOTREXATE

Methotrexate (Mexate) blocks purine nucleotide synthesis, which results in increased intracellular phosphoribosyl-l-pyrophosphate (PRPP), a substrate that promotes an increase in 5-FU conversion to the synthesis of 5′-FdUMP and 5′-FUTP.[5] Studies in cell cultures and animals demonstrate enhanced cytotoxic activity when 5-FU is administered sequentially following methotrexate. In randomized trials of patients with metastatic disease, sequential methotrexate plus 5-FU can produce response rates in individuals who have previously failed 5-FU itself.[87] Common toxicities include mucositis and leukopenia.

TRIMETREXATE

Trimetrexate (Neutrexin) is a nonclassical antifolate that leads to inhibition of thymidylate synthase and reduced protein synthesis via a mechanism of action similar to that of methotrexate. Trimetrexate offers several advantages to the use of methotrexate: (1) increased lipophilicity; (2) activity does not require activation by folylpolyglutamate synthase (FPGS); (3) does not compete with leucovorin for intracellular uptake; (4) has a broader spectrum of *in vitro* and *in vivo* activity; and (5) possesses increased efficiency in methotrexate-resistant cells.[88] Dose limiting toxicities of trimetrexate include primarily leukopenia and thrombocytopenia; in combination with 5-FU and leucovorin, diarrhea becomes dose-limiting.

PALA

PALA (*N*-(phosphonacetyl)-L-aspartate) inhibits pyrimidine synthesis by blocking aspartate carbamyl transferase, an enzyme that competes with and depletes uridine and cytidine nucleotide stores. As a result, the ratio of FUTP to uridine triphosphate (UTP) is increased, thereby increasing the incorporation of FUTP into RNA.[65] The addition of PALA to a 5-FU–containing regimen does not alter the toxicity profile of 5-FU; however, a syndrome of ascites, hyperbilirubinemia, and hypoalbuminemia with elevated liver function tests has been reported in patients receiving combination 5-FU and PALA.[89]

▶ TREATMENT: Colorectal Cancer

PRIMARY TREATMENT OF COLORECTAL CANCER

Adjuvant therapy in colorectal cancer is administered after complete tumor resection in an attempt to eliminate residual local or metastatic microscopic disease, thereby decreasing tumor relapse and improving patient survival. Adjuvant radiation therapy plus chemotherapy is considered standard treatment for patients with stage II/III rectal cancer, and adjuvant chemotherapy is standard therapy for patients with stage III colon cancer.[90] The approach to adjuvant therapy requires different treatment strategies for colon and rectal cancer because the natural history and patterns of recurrence following resection are uniquely different. Because tumors arising in the rectum are technically more difficult to resect with wide circumferential margins, local recurrences occur more frequently than with colon cancers. Therefore, radiation therapy is an important aspect of adjuvant therapy for rectal cancer to reduce risk of local tumor recurrence.

The stage of disease is the most important prognostic factor for risk of relapse and survival and is therefore the primary determinant for the selection of patients into adjuvant treatment trials. Because greater than 90% of patients with stage I colorectal cancer are cured by surgical resection alone, adjuvant therapy is not indicated.[5] Also, by definition, adjuvant therapy is not given to patients with metastatic disease. The administration of agents with proven activity at maximally tolerated doses is most effective when the tumor burden is minimal and tumor growth kinetics is optimal. An additional factor, the risk-to-benefit ratio for therapy, must be favorable for individuals who remain asymptomatic for their natural life expectancy after tumor resection.

Although numerous trials have been conducted to improve the results of curative surgery, this chapter focuses on prospective randomized controlled trials with adequate long-term follow-up. In order for adjuvant therapy to be beneficial for a specific malignancy, clinical trials need to demonstrate a significant improvement in the rates of local recurrence, survival, or quality of life. Once a benefit of adjuvant therapy has been established, additional trials need to evaluate the optimal duration of treatment.

ADJUVANT THERAPY FOR COLON CANCER

The presence of lymph node involvement with tumor places patients with stage III colon cancer at highest risk for relapse. The value of adjuvant therapy is less clear for patients with stage II colon cancer. Although there is no lymph node involvement, these tumors can penetrate through the muscle wall, into surrounding structures, or through the visceral peritoneum. Even though the relative 5-year survival rates are more favorable than for stage III disease, an intermediate risk of relapse still exists due to the invasive nature of stage II disease. Thus far, analyses of clinical trial results have been unable to identify patients with stage II colon cancer who clearly benefit from adjuvant therapy. However, the status of chromosome 18q, thymidylate synthase expression, and perhaps other genetic markers provides important prognostic information for patients with stage II disease and may soon help identify a subset of patients for whom adjuvant therapy should be administered.

RADIATION THERAPY

There is currently no definitive role for adjuvant XRT in colon cancer because most recurrences are extrapelvic and occur in the abdomen.[5,64] Although local recurrence and debilitating pelvic pain is uncommon, a subset of patients with T_4 tumors located in the cecum, hepatic and spenic flexures, and sigmoid are at increased risk of local recurrence and may benefit from postoperative radiation therapy and chemotherapy. Early phase II trials using effective doses of whole abdominal XRT were limited by considerable toxicity.[64] However, the results of a recent study reported by the Southwest Oncology Group employing tolerable doses of whole abdominal XRT plus continuous infusion 5-FU followed by maintenance continuous infusion 5-FU are promising. To date, postoperative local XRT may reduce the risk of local recurrence and improve 5-year survival in select patients.[5]

SINGLE-AGENT CHEMOTHERAPY

Alkylating agents such as nitrogen mustard and thiotepa were the first chemotherapeutic drugs used in the adjuvant setting in the late 1950s.[5] Their use, however, failed to improve results associated with surgery alone, primarily due to suboptimal drug doses and schedules, and flaws in study design. During the 1970s, interest centered around the use of single-agent chemotherapy with 5-FU and FUDR, based on their activity against metastatic colorectal cancer, and immunotherapy. In 1988, a meta-analysis of adjuvant therapy was published evaluating 25 randomized controlled trials with approximately 10,000 patients.[91] A small but statistically significant difference in overall survival was noted with 5-FU–based regimens. Results should be interpreted with caution because the doses and schedules of 5-FU were not indicated or were of lower intensity compared to current standards.

COMBINATION CHEMOTHERAPY

5-FU and Levamisole

In 1990, the National Institutes of Health Consensus Development Conference recommended that the use of 5-FU and levamisole be considered standard therapy for patients with surgically treated stage III colon cancer. In a study sponsored by the Mayo Clinic and the North Central Cancer Treatment Group (NCCTG), surgery alone was compared with postoperative levamisole and postoperative levamisole plus 5-FU in patients with surgically treated stage II and stage III colorectal cancer.[92] 5-FU, 450 mg/m^2/d, was administered by IV bolus injection for 5 consecutive days, starting within 21 to 35 days following surgery. Starting 1 month later, patients received 5-FU, 450 mg/m^2, as a single IV bolus injection each week for 48 weeks. Levamisole was administered 50 mg orally every 8 hours each day for 3 consecutive days. Each 3-day cycle was repeated every 2 weeks and continued for 1 year. Although the combination of levamisole and 5-FU significantly reduced recurrence rates, it did not confer a statistically significant survival advantage. A potential survival benefit for patients with stage III disease was, however, identified through subset analysis of the data. Results of a larger Intergroup trial, first published in 1990 and later updated in 1995 after a median follow-up of 6.5 years, demonstrated that the combination of 5-FU plus levamisole following surgical resection for stage III colon cancer reduced the recurrence rate by 40% and the death rate by 33%.[73] Levamisole alone provided no significant reduction in either recurrence or deaths. Toxicities from postoperative levamisole or levamisole plus 5-FU were clinically tolerable. This combination appears to be cost-effective adjuvant therapy for stage III colon cancer, with an estimated cost of $1565 compared to $2094 per year of life saved.[93,94]

However, recommendations for patients with stage II colon cancer remain inconclusive. Based on a median follow-up of 7 years, the combination of 5-FU plus levamisole did not reduce the risk of recurrence or overall survival in patients with stage II colon cancer.[95] Compared to patients with stage III colon cancer, the relative reduction in recurrence was similar, although the absolute reduction was less than 10%. In a recent analysis of four National Surgical Adjuvant Breast Project (NSABP) adjuvant chemotherapy trials, a comparable relative reduction in recurrence rates and mortality was observed in patients with both Dukes B and C colon cancer.[96]

5-FU and Leucovorin

Based on the observation that 5-FU plus leucovorin substantially improves response rates associated with 5-FU alone for metastatic disease, this combination has been undergoing extensive study in the adjuvant setting. Since the mid-1980s, several randomized trials have evaluated the efficacy of 5-FU plus leucovorin as adjuvant therapy for patients with stage II or III colon cancer (Table 118–4). In each of the studies, rates of recurrence and survival improved substantially for patients receiving 5-FU plus either high-dose or low-dose leucovorin compared to surgery alone. In addition, these studies attempted to determine the optimal duration of adjuvant chemotherapy. However, in 1990, once emerging results of the Intergroup trial documented significant efficacy of adjuvant 5-FU plus levamisole for patients with stage III colorectal cancer, surgery-alone arms were terminated from ongoing trials comparing 5-FU plus leucovorin versus surgery.

In light of previous data confirming the efficacy of postoperative adjuvant 5-FU, semustine (methyl-CCNU), and vincristine (MOF), patients with stage II and III colorectal cancer were randomized to receive either MOF chemotherapy or weekly 5-FU plus high-dose leucovorin (500 mg/m^2) for 1 year.[5,77] The benefit of adding high-dose leucovorin to 5-FU produced a significant survival advantage in terms of both disease-free survival and overall survival (Table 118–4). Final results of data originally reported in 1993 have been recently published evaluating the combination of 5-FU (425 mg/m^2/d) and low-dose leucovorin (20 mg/m^2/d) administered for 6 months following surgery in high-risk stage II and III patients with colon cancer.[97] Although the study was prematurely discontinued, based on a median follow-up of 6 years, postoperative intensive 5-FU with low doses of leucovorin administered for 6 months also substantially reduced tumor relapse rates and improved survival. The International Multicentre Pooled Analysis of Colon Cancer Trials (IMPACT) analyzed pooled data from three ongoing trials comparing surgery alone to adjuvant 5-FU (370 to 400 mg/m^2) plus high-dose leucovorin (200 mg/m^2) administered for 6 months in patients with stage II and III colon cancer.[78] Fifty-six percent of patients were diagnosed with stage II disease. The recurrence and death rates were reduced by 35% and 22%, respectively. The results of this polled analysis indicate comparable benefit can be achieved using an intense 6-month course of adjuvant 5-FU plus high-dose leucovorin.

TABLE 118–4. Selected Trials of Adjuvant Chemotherapy Regimens for Stages II and III Colon Cancer

Reference	No. Patients	Regimen	Duration (mo)	DFS (%)	OS (%)	End Point (yr)
Intergroup 0035[73]	929	5-FU + LEV	12	61	60	6.5
		LEV	12	45	40	
		Surgery alone		44	47	
NSABP C-03[77]	519	5-FU + HD-LV	6	73	84	3
	522	MOF		64	77	
IMPACT trial[78]	736	5-FU + HD-LV	6	71	83	3
	757	Surgery alone		62	78	
Intergroup[97]	158	5-FU + LD-LV	6	74	74	5
	151	Surgery alone		58	63	
NSABP C-04[98]	2151[a]	5-FU + HD-LV	6	64	74	5
		5-FU + LEV	12	64	73	
		5-FU + HD-LV + LEV[b]		60	69	
NCCTG/Canada[99]	222	5-FU + LEV	6	60	59	5
	223	5-FU + LD-LV + LEV	6	63	69	
	220	5-FU + LEV	12	65	64	
	226	5-FU + LD-LV + LEV	12	58	61	
INT-0089[100]	3759[a]	5-FU + LD-LV	6	63	71	4
		5-FU + HD-LV	6	62	70	
		5-FU + LD-LV	6	62	70	
		5-FU + LEV	12	58	67	
		5-FU + HD-LV	6	62	70	
		5-FU + LEV	12	58	67	
		5-FU + LD-LV	6	62	70	
		5-FU + LD-LV + LEV	6	63	73	

DFS = disease-free survival; OS = overall survival; 5-FU = 5-fluorouracil; LD-LV = low-dose leucovorin (20 mg/m^2); HD-LV = high-dose leucovorin (200–500 mg/m^2); LEV = levamisole; MOF = semustine, vincristine, 5-fluorouracil.

[a]Total number of patients; specific numbers per group not reported.

[b]HD-LV for 6 months, LEV administered for 12 months.

Most recently, three large trials have been conducted in an attempt to determine whether the combination of 5-FU plus leucovorin is superior to the standard 5-FU plus levamisole regimen or a combination of all three agents in high-risk patients with stage II and III colon cancer.[98–100] In addition, these trials also attempted to assess the impact of 6 versus 12 months of adjuvant chemotherapy on efficacy. In the NSABP C-04 trial, patients with stage II and III colon cancer were randomized into one of three study arms consisting of 5-FU plus high-dose leucovorin (FU-LV) for 6 months, 5-FU plus levamisole (FU-LEV) for 12 months, and the combination of 5-FU plus high-dose leucovorin and levamisole (FU-LV-LEV) in patients 6 to 12 months.[98] Based on a median follow-up of 5 years, preliminary results indicate no significant difference in disease-free and overall survival exists among the three groups, although a slight advantage was noted for the FU-LV arm. A second trial conducted by the NCCTG and the Canada Clinical Trials group randomized patients to receive 6 or 12 months of standard 5-FU plus levamisole or 5-FU plus low-dose leucovorin and levamisole, resulting in four treatment arms.[99] With a median follow-up of 5 years, there was no significant improvement in relapse rates or survival between a 12- and 6-month course of the three drugs or a 12-month course of 5-FU plus levamisole. A third adjuvant trial (INT-0089) randomized high-risk stage II and III patients with colon cancer to receive 12 months of 5-FU plus levamisole or 6 months of 5-FU plus low-dose leucovorin, 5-FU plus high-dose leucovorin, or 5-FU plus low-dose leucovorin and levamisole.[100] With a median follow-up in excess of 4 years, 6 months of 5-FU plus leucovorin appeared as effective as the standard 12-month 5-FU plus levamisole regimen. No difference in response rates was observed between the low-dose and high-dose leucovorin arms. Regardless of the leucovorin dose, a slight trend toward improved overall survival was observed in both leucovorin arms compared to 5-FU plus levamisole. The addition of levamisole did not appear to significantly add to the efficacy of 5-FU plus leucovorin.

Differences in the toxicity profile and patient compliance may help determine the optimal adjuvant chemotherapy regimen. Grade 3 toxicities, consisting of diarrhea, granulocytopenia, and stomatitis, usually occurred during the first month of therapy. Toxicities were most prevalent in the low-dose leucovorin arms with or without levamisole. Patients receiving levamisole experienced slightly greater toxicity compared to those receiving high-dose leucovorin. The incidence of diarrhea occurred more frequently in the high-dose leucovorin arm, followed by low-dose leucovorin with or without levamisole, and was least with levamisole alone. Granulocytopenia and stomatitis were more commonly observed with low-dose leucovorin compared to high-dose leucovorin or levamisole, although the addition of levamisole to the low-dose leucovorin arm further augmented the risk of granulocytopenia and stomatitis. A similar pattern of increased toxicity was observed with the addition of levamisole to low and high doses of leucovorin.[98,99] A preliminary analysis of toxicity based on patient age indicates a greater risk of myelosuppression in patients older than 70 years compared to those between the ages of 40 and 70 years and less than 40. Results from other studies suggest that an increased incidence of neutropenia and stomatitis in women, particularly elderly women, is associated with a decrease in 5-FU clearance.[100,102]

Over the last 10 years, studies of 5-FU plus levamisole or 5-FU plus leucovorin have demonstrated a 30% to 40% reduction in relapse rates in patients with stage III colon cancer. Recent results of preliminary studies demonstrate that 6 months of adjuvant 5-FU plus low- or high-dose leucovorin appear to be as effective, and possibly more effective, than 12 months of 5-FU plus levamisole in patients with stage III colon cancer. At this time, patients with stage III colon cancer should be considered for either 5-FU plus levamisole, 5-FU plus either low- or high-dose leucovorin, or a regimen under investigation in clinical trials. The addition of levamisole to the combination of 5-FU plus leucovorin does not appear to be of additional benefit and may increase toxicity. The impact of adjuvant therapy on patients with stage II colon cancer is currently unknown, although high-risk individuals will probably benefit from adjuvant therapy. Those individuals should be offered adjuvant chemotherapy in the setting of a randomized clinical trial based on individual clinical, pathologic, and biologic prognostic factors. Optimal dosing, administration schedule, and duration of therapy have yet to be determined. Although the efficacy and toxicity associated with each of the regimens are relatively similar, the costs of leucovorin doses ranging from 20 to 500 mg/m^2 are significantly different. Treatment toxicities, overall treatment costs, and the effect of treatments on overall quality of life will also play a role in influencing therapeutic decisions. Current recommendations for adjuvant treatment of colon cancer which incorporate guidelines developed by the National Comprehensive Cancer Network (NCCN) are summarized in Table 118–5.

5-FU and Interferon

Based on promising results in the metastatic setting, modulation of 5-FU by leucovorin and interferon-α in the adjuvant setting is

TABLE 118–5. Recommendations for Adjuvant Therapy for Colon Cancer

Stage: *Pathologic/Duke*	Stage: *TNM*	Treatment Options
0	I	None
A	I	None
B_1	I	None
B_2	II	Clinical trial; 5-FU + LV (LD or HD)[a] × 6 months or 5-FU + LEV[b] × 12 months for high-risk patients
B_3	II	5-FU + LEV[b] × 12 months or 5-FU + LV (LD or HD)[a] × 6 months; 5-FU + LV + XRT[c]; clinical trial
C_1–C_2	III	5-FU + LEV[b] × 12 months or 5-FU + LV (LD or HD)[a] × 6 months; clinical trial
C_3	III	5-FU + LEV[b] × 12 months or 5-FU + LV (LD or HD)[a] × 6 months; 5-FU + LV + XRT[c]; clinical trial

[a]Begin 3–5 weeks following surgery; 5-FU 425 mg/m^2 IVP + LV 20 mg/m^2 IVP on days 1–5, repeated every 4–5 weeks × 6 months OR 5-FU 370–400 mg/m^2 IVP + LV 200 mg/m^2 IVP on days 1–5, repeated every 5 weeks × 6 months OR 5-FU 500 mg/m^2 IVP + LV 500 mg/m^2 IVP weekly during 6 of every 8 weeks × 1 year.
[b]Begin 3–5 weeks following surgery; 5-FU 450 mg/m^2 IVP daily × 5 days, then weekly starting at day 28 × 1 yr; LEV 50 mg PO tid daily × 3 days, repeated every 2 weeks × 1 year.
[c]National Comprehensive Cancer Network (NCCN)-specific recommendation.
Compiled from Refs. 63, 73, 77, 78, 92, 93, 97, 98, and 100.

being evaluated in an ongoing NSABP C-05 trial.[103] Patients are randomized into one of two groups: 5-FU plus leucovorin or 5-FU in combination with leucovorin and interferon-α. Preliminary analysis will be available in the near future.

PERIOPERATIVE PORTAL VEIN AND INFUSIONAL CHEMOTHERAPY

Because the liver is the site of recurrence in approximately 40% of patients, infusion of chemotherapy via the portal vein provides an additional adjuvant treatment approach. The rationale for this is based on a belief that intraoperative manipulation of the tumor provides emboli of tumor that travel directly into the portal vein circulation, ultimately developing into hepatic micrometastasis.[5] Historically, 5-FU has been the most common agent used for hepatic portal vein infusion. Because greater than 80% of a dose of 5-FU administered systemically is metabolized by the liver, direct hepatic infusion of 5-FU provides high local concentrations of the drug at the most common site of recurrence and minimizes systemic toxicity. Perioperative portal vein chemotherapy administration might then destroy cells before they can establish tumor growth.

An early trial evaluated the effect of a postoperative infusion of 1 g of 5-FU infused via the portal vein daily for 7 days as compared to no further therapy following surgical resection in patients with stages I to III colorectal cancer. Heparin was also infused to reduce thrombosis.[104] Those patients who received 5-FU and heparin experienced a significant benefit in the reduction of hepatic metastasis and a dramatic improvement in survival. Results from a larger trial of patients with stages I to III colon cancer, who were randomized to receive either a continuous infusion of 5-FU 600 mg/m^2/d for 7 days with heparin via the portal vein or no therapy following surgical resection, have been updated.[105] Although there was no significant difference in hepatic metastases between the two groups, a modest but statistically significant improvement in disease-free survival (68% versus 60%) and overall survival (76% versus 71%) was observed in the chemotherapy group. Results of other trials evaluating 5-FU portal vein infusions also suggest that mortality and recurrence rates are significantly decreased.[74,106] However, some studies failed to demonstrate a consistent reduction in the number of metastatic liver lesions. Complications are generally mild and include nausea, vomiting, hematologic depression, hepatotoxicity, and infection. The efficacy of perioperative chemotherapy is currently being evaluated in high-risk patients with stage B_2, B_3, and C (stage II and III) colon cancer. In the Intergroup trial (INT-0136), patients are randomized to receive either surgery alone or a 7-day 600-mg/m^2/d 5-FU continuous infusion beginning 24 hours after surgery.[74] Upon completion, patients with stage B_2 disease receive no additional treatment whereas patients with stage B_3 and C colon cancer are scheduled to receive 12 months of 5-FU plus levamisole, beginning 4 weeks postoperatively. At this time, the value of portal vein infusion of 5-FU for colon cancer remains unproven and controversial because it is unclear as to whether any benefits are due to the specific administration technique or perioperative chemotherapy in general.

IMMUNOTHERAPY

A variety of agents with immunomodulating effects have undergone or are currently under study in adjuvant treatment regimens, including bacillus Calmette–Guérin (BCG), levamisole, autologous tumor cell vaccines, IFN-α, and monoclonal antibodies. The nonspecific immunomodulators, BCG and levamisole, have not shown a specific benefit in preventing tumor recurrence.[5,107]

Passive immune therapy with monoclonal antibodies involves the administration of preformed antibodies to patients with cancer. Monoclonal antibodies exert direct antitumor effects and initiate antibody-dependent cytotoxicity (ADCC) on antibody-coated tumor cells.[107] Early results from some studies of specific immunomodulators, such as autologous tumor cell vaccines and monoclonal antibodies, suggest that they may help reduce the rates of tumor recurrence and perhaps influence survival.[5] A recent study evaluated the effect of a murine IgG_{2a} antibody directed against the 17-1A antigen on disease recurrence and patient survival following curative surgery for stage III colorectal cancer.[108] Patients were randomized to receive 5 monthly intravenous infusions of 17-1A antibody or postoperative observation alone. After a median follow-up of 7 years, a reduction in the recurrence rate by 23% and the overall death rate by 32% was observed in the antibody-treated group. Patients in whom distant metastases developed as the first site of relapse appeared to benefit most. Although the most common toxicities were gastrointestinal and general flu-like symptoms, they were infrequent. Anaphylactic reactions were rare and could be managed with intravenous steroids. Additional studies evaluating edrecolomab (Panorex) as a single agent in combination with 5-FU–based regimens in the adjuvant setting are also ongoing. Based on these results, the use of monoclonal antibodies in adjuvant treatment regimens appears promising and may provide an alternative to the use of chemotherapeutic agents.

Another novel approach involves the vaccination of patients with anti-idiotypic monoclonal antibodies with increased specificity for the antigen-binding site of antibodies, resulting in enhanced immunogenicity compared to the tumor antigen.[107] Serial administration of an anti-idiotypic vaccine directed against the 17-1A antigen has been evaluated postoperatively in patients with Dukes B and C colon cancer with positive evidence of humoral and cellular responses and minimal toxicity.

ADJUVANT THERAPY FOR RECTAL CANCER

Rectal cancer involves those tumors found below the peritoneal reflection in the most distal 15 cm of the large bowel and, as such, is very distinct from colon cancer in that it has a propensity for both local and distant recurrence. The higher incidence of local failure and poorer overall prognosis associated with rectal cancer is due to anatomic limitations in excising adequate radial margins around the rectal tumor. The local recurrence rate following surgery alone is approximately 25% for patients with stage II and 50% for patients with stage III disease. Because treatment with surgery, radiation therapy, or systemic chemotherapy at the time of the recurrence is often suboptimal, adjuvant therapy after tumor resection is an important aspect of treatment of the primary tumor.

RADIATION THERAPY

The goal of adjuvant radiation therapy for rectal cancer is to decrease local tumor recurrence after surgery, to increase the probability of sphincter preservation in patients with clinically resectable disease, and to improve the rate of resectability in patients with locally advanced or unresectable disease. In general, pre- or postoperative XRT administered in conventional doses effectively decreases local recurrence rates for rectal cancer by up to 50% compared to rates with surgery alone.[62,64,74] Prospective data for postoperative XRT are limited but suggest that this approach decreases local failure. Preoperative XRT may be more likely to improve survival; however, data regarding this approach are mostly retrospective. Recently published prospective trials of pre- and postoperative XRT have confirmed a reduction in local recurrence rates.[109–112] In addition, the first trial to demonstrate a survival advantage using an intensive short course of high-dose preoperative XRT in patients with resectable rectal cancer has been reported.[111,112] A 5-year survival rate of 58% was observed in patients who received preoperative XRT in five fractions over a 1-week period of time compared to 48% in patients who underwent surgery only. This study is important because it renews the debate regarding the value of preoperative XRT and the necessity of using adjuvant chemotherapy in rectal cancer. In Europe, patients receive intensive short courses of preoperative XRT; adjuvant chemotherapy is considered investigational. In a practical sense, a short-intensive course of preoperative XRT is more convenient and less expensive for the patient compared to the usual postoperative XRT regimen in the United States, which consists of 45 to 55 Gy of irradiation delivered in small fractions of 1.8 to 2.0 Gy over 6 weeks. To date, only one prospective randomized trial comparing preoperative and postoperative XRT has been published. Currently, three randomized trials using conventional doses and techniques for delivering XRT along with concurrent 5-FU–based chemotherapy have been designed to address this question.[112] Until survival results of the Swedish trial can be confirmed, postoperative delivery of XRT in adjuvant regimens will remain the standard approach in the United States for rectal tumors.

XRT PLUS CHEMOTHERAPY

Combination regimens of XRT and systemic chemotherapy have been developed to improve the results of adjuvant therapy for rectal cancer. Similar to adjuvant therapy for colon cancer, 5-FU provides the basis for chemotherapy regimens for rectal cancer. In addition, 5-FU also sensitizes rectal tumor cells to the cytotoxic effects of XRT. Although postoperative systemic chemotherapy alone can reduce disease recurrence in distant sites and increase survival, local recurrence rates are not improved. Systemic chemotherapy in combination with XRT, however, reduces local tumor recurrence and improves patient survival in high-risk patients.[113–115] Results from the Gastrointestinal Tumor Study Group (GITSG) and the North Central Cancer Treatment Group (NCCTG) studies form the basis for the current recommendations that all patients receive combined modality adjuvant therapy for stage II or III rectal cancer.[90,113–116]

The GITSG trial was designed to evaluate patients with stage II or III rectal cancer who were randomized into one of four groups: (1) observation only (control), (2) postoperative XRT alone, (3) postoperative chemotherapy consisting of 5-FU and semustine (methyl-CCNU) for 18 months, or (4) postoperative combination of XRT and chemotherapy.[113] The XRT was administered over 4 to 5.5 weeks. Despite a substantial number of protocol violations and a median follow-up of only 80 months, the study finished earlier than anticipated due to the statistically significant results favoring the combined modality treatment. The patients receiving the combination therapy had a reduction in both local (11% versus 24%) and distant (26% versus 34%) recurrence rates as compared to the control group. Local and distant recurrence rates for patients receiving chemotherapy or XRT were similar between groups. Although overall survival did not differ significantly among the four treatment groups at the time of initial data analysis, a subsequent reestimate of survival probabilities at a median follow-up of 94 months demonstrated that the combination treatment was associated with a 24% survival advantage over the control group.[115] As expected, combined modality therapy resulted in severe hematologic toxicity, enteritis, and diarrhea as compared to either chemotherapy or XRT alone.

The NCCTG trial evaluated postoperative XRT with or without combination chemotherapy of 5-FU and semustine in a similar population of 204 patients with rectal cancer.[114] The decision to consider XRT as the control group was based on the acknowledgment that, in many centers, XRT alone was considered standard therapy. The failure of the GITSG trial to demonstrate a significant advantage for combination therapy over XRT alone might be attributed to the relatively low XRT doses employed and the high deviation rate (39%) from the XRT treatment protocol.

The postoperative treatment, XRT or XRT plus 5-FU, was both preceded and followed by one cycle of 5-FU plus semustine. This was the first randomized trial in which one cycle of combination chemotherapy was given before and after XRT in addition to the administration of 5-FU during XRT. This is sometimes referred to as a "sandwich" treatment regimen. The use of combined chemotherapy and XRT significantly affected local recurrence, relapse-free survival, and overall survival as compared to XRT alone. Patients receiving combined therapy experienced a 42% recurrence rate at 5 years compared to a 63% recurrence rate in the XRT-only group for an overall relative reduction by 34%. Similarly, reductions of 46% and 37% in local and distant recurrence rates were seen in the combined group compared to XRT alone. An improvement of 36% and 29% in disease-free and overall survival at 5 years was observed in the combined group.

Acute complications such as severe hematologic toxicity (leukopenia and thrombocytopenia), enteritis, and diarrhea were commonly observed in the combined group. Hematologic toxicity was more noticeable during postradiation chemotherapy, despite reduced doses. Although small bowel complications were uncommon, four deaths were reported as a result of complications due to small bowel obstruction, fistulas, septicemia resulting from perforation, and hemorrhage. There was a 6% incidence of primary cancers, equally divided between the XRT and combined groups. Due to the leukemogenic potential associated with semustine and results from prospective comparative trials that demonstrate that it does not contribute to overall treatment efficacy, semustine is not included in current standard adjuvant treatment regimens outside of clinical trials.[93] This regimen without semustine represents the current standard adjuvant regimen for rectal cancer.

Based on preclinical studies that suggest continuous infusions of 5-FU provide more effective radiosensitization than intravenous bolus injections, a third trial was undertaken to compare protracted intravenous 5-FU infusion to intermittent bolus injections.[116] Six hundred sixty patients with stage II or III rectal cancer received either administration regimen during postoperative pelvic XRT with either 5-FU plus semustine or 5-FU alone both before and after XRT. With a median follow-up of 46 months, both disease-free and overall survival were significantly improved among the patients receiving protracted 5-FU infusion. The incidence of leukopenia (WBCs < 2000/mm^3) was greater in the 5-FU bolus group, whereas diarrhea was more frequent in the protracted infusion group. Longer follow-up of these results is needed to determine whether or not this regimen will replace the current standard adjuvant therapy for rectal cancer.

Combined data from the GITSG, NSABP, and Intergroup trials indicate that survival benefits can be achieved with the addition of chemotherapy to postoperative XRT.[113–117] Preliminary results from the NSABP R-02 trial have shown a significant reduction in local recurrence with the addition of postoperative XRT to chemotherapy.[118] Final analysis of this trial evaluating the contribution of pelvic XRT to systemic adjuvant chemotherapy is still pending. Based on the NCCN colorectal cancer guidelines, no adjuvant therapy is recommended for patients with stage A and B_1 rectal cancer (T_1 or T_2, and N_0 lesions).[63] Patients with stage B_2 or C rectal cancer should receive pre- or postoperative chemotherapy plus XRT surgery, consisting of either an anterior–posterior or low anterior resection, depending on tumor location. A summary of these guidelines can be found in Table 118–6.

Further work is needed to establish the best combination of surgery, XRT, and chemotherapy because neither modality alone provides satisfactory efficacy for both disease recurrence and survival from rectal cancer. Interest in preoperative adjuvant therapy has resurfaced based on advances in both imaging techniques (transrectal ultrasound and MRI) and more accurate preoperative staging of rectal tumors. Studies evaluating the contribution of levamisole and leucovorin to the efficacy of adjuvant therapy for rectal cancer are also ongoing.

TABLE 118–6. Recommendations for Adjuvant Therapy for Rectal Cancer[a]

Stage: Pathologic/Duke	Stage: TNM	Treatment Options
A_1	I	None
B_1	I	None
B_2, C_1–C_2	II	Preoperative chemotherapy[b] + XRT, postoperative 5-FU + LV × 4 cycles; postoperative 5-FU ± LV × 2 cycles followed by protracted 5-FU infusion or bolus 5-FU + leucovorin + XRT, then 5-FU ± LV × 2 cycles
B_3, C_3	II, III	Preoperative chemotherapy[b] + XRT, surgery with intraoperative brachytherapy,[c] followed by 5-FU + LV × 4 cycles; postoperative 5-FU ± LV × 2 cycles followed by protracted 5-FU infusion or bolus 5-FU + leucovorin + XRT, then 5-FU ± LV × 2 cycles

[a]Total duration of therapy is approximately 6 months.
[b]Preoperative chemotherapy: bolus 5-FU, with or without leucovorin.
[c]National Comprehensive Cancer Network (NCCN)-specific recommendation.
Compiled from Refs. 63, 116, and 117.

TREATMENT OPTIONS FOR METASTATIC DISEASE

Several recent advances have been made in developing efficacious treatment options for metastatic colorectal cancer. Whereas surgery and radiation therapy are most often used to manage isolated sites of tumor, chemotherapy is most useful for patients with disseminated disease and is the primary treatment modality for unresectable metastatic colorectal cancer. Upon disease progression following standard initial therapy consisting of 5-FU plus leucovorin, continuous infusion 5-FU, or intrahepatic therapy for selected patients, general options include irinotecan, supportive care, or a clinical trial. The site(s) of tumor involvement and presence of symptoms help to define an appropriate initial management strategy. A general management scheme is described in Figure 118–7. In general, treatment options are similar for metastatic cancer of the colon and rectum.

SURGERY

Surgical resection of isolated hepatic and pulmonary metastases in patients with colorectal cancer can be accomplished and may offer selected patients an opportunity to experience extended disease-free survival.[119,120] Retrospective and prospective investigations have confirmed that curative resection of isolated hepatic metastases improves median survival.[119,120] Patients with no significant general medical risk factors, fewer than four hepatic lesions, CEA levels less than 200 ng/mL, small tumor size, lack of extrahepatic tumor, and adequate surgical margins have the best opportunity for an improved long-term outcome. For these patients, 5-year survival rates are approximately 30% to 40%. Since modalities other than surgical resection have not consistently improved survival in patients with isolated hepatic metastases and operative morbidity and mortality risks are acceptable, this approach should be considered for patients with potentially

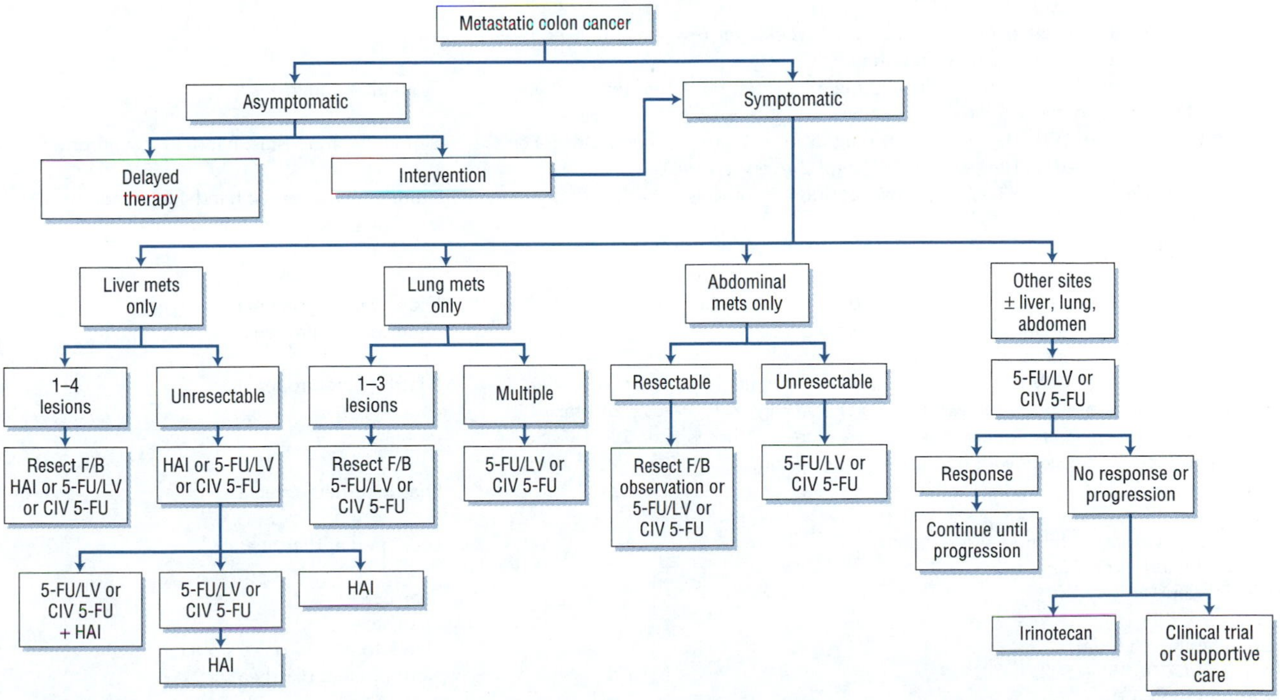

FIGURE 118–7. Algorithm for the methodic approach to the patient with metastatic colorectal cancer. (5-FU = 5-fluorouracil; HAI = hepatic intraarterial infusion; CIV = continuous intravenous infusion).*(Adapted from Ref. 63 and Kemeny N, Lokich JJ, Anderson N, et al. Recent advances in the treatment of advanced colorectal cancer. Cancer 1993;71:16.)*

resectable disease. Although resection of pulmonary metastases has been studied to a lesser extent, patients with three or fewer metastases confined to the lungs and a normal prethoracotomy CEA level are most likely to benefit from pulmonary metastectomy; overall 5-year survival rates have ranged from 30% to 40%.[119–121]

CHEMOTHERAPY

5-FU continues to be incorporated into most chemotherapy regimens used against metastatic colorectal cancer. Despite evidence that suggests that continuous IV infusion schedules are more effective than IV bolus injections of 5-FU, effective treatment regimens may involve either method of administration. 5-FU is most often administered with leucovorin to improve tumor response rates; trials are under way to evaluate the effectiveness of new agents and alternate approaches toward biochemical modulation of 5-FU. Irinotecan provides an effective alternative to 5-FU plus leucovorin and ongoing trials are evaluating its role in initial treatment for metastatic disease as well as in combination with 5-FU. A summary of potentially useful agents for metastatic colorectal cancer can be found in Table 118–7.

5-FU

Intravenous 5-FU Bolus Injection. Typical regimens consist of 5-FU at a dose of 450 to 500 mg/m^2/d for 5 consecutive days as an IV bolus injection administered over 5 to 10 minutes. This is repeated every 4 to 5 weeks. Alternatively, 5-FU may be administered as a bolus IV injection in doses ranging up to 600 mg/m^2 administered weekly for 6 out of 8 weeks.[70,122] In general, response rates that should be anticipated for IV bolus 5-FU schedules are approximately 10% to 20%.[123] Unfortunately, no significant improvement in either disease-free or overall survival has been gained with IV bolus 5-FU. However, a small survival benefit (12 to 18 versus 6 to 8 months) has been documented for patients receiving weekly 5-FU IV bolus injections who were able to achieve an objective response.[5]

Continuous Intravenous 5-FU Infusion. The relatively low response rates achieved with bolus 5-FU administration can perhaps be explained based on our understanding of tumor cell and drug kinetics.[68,70] Slow-growing colorectal cancer cells are found primarily in the resting or G_0 phase of the cell cycle. Because 5-FU primarily kills actively dividing tumor cells and has a short plasma half-life, many susceptible tumor cells may not be exposed to 5-FU for an adequate period of time. A variety of continuous IV infusion regimens have therefore been developed to increase the duration of drug exposure and hopefully improve efficacy. Some of these schedules include 8- to 24-hour, 4- to 5-day, and most recently 24-hour infusions (1000 mg/m^2/d for 4 days repeated every 28 days).[122] Protracted continuous infusions have used 5-FU at doses of 250 to 300 mg/m^2 IV over 24 hours

TABLE 118–7. Chemotherapeutic Options for Metastatic Colorectal Cancer

Regimen	Major Dose-limiting Toxicity
Initial or Second-line Therapy	
5-FU + low-dose leucovorin[76,77,124]	
5-FU 370–425 mg/m^2 IVP + leucovorin 20 mg/m^2 IVP on days 1–5, repeated at 4 and 8 weeks and every 5 weeks thereafter	Stomatitis, mucositis
5-FU 500–600 mg/m^2 IVP + leucovorin 20–25 mg/m^2 IV weekly for 6 weeks, followed by a 2-week rest period prior to repeating the cycle	Diarrhea
5-FU + high-dose leucovorin[69,75,76,79,124]	
5-FU 500 mg/m^2 IVP + leucovorin 500 mg/m^2 IV weekly for 6 weeks, followed by a 2-week rest period prior to repeating the cycle	Diarrhea
5-FU 370–400 mg/m^2 IVP + leucovorin 200 mg/m^2 IVP on days 1–5, repeated at 4 and 8 weeks, and every 5 weeks thereafter	Stomatitis, mucositis
5-FU 300–400 mg/m^2 IVP + leucovorin 200 mg/m^2/d as 2-hr CIV, then 22-hr 5-FU 300–600 mg/m^2/d; administered on days 1 and 2 every 2 weeks	Stomatitis, mucositis; hand–foot syndrome
5-FU 2600 mg/m^2/d as 24-hr CIV + leucovorin 500 mg/m^2/d as 2–24-hr CIV, repeated weekly	Stomatitis, mucositis; hand–foot syndrome
Second-line Therapy	
Irinotecan	
125 mg/m^2 IV weekly for 4 weeks, followed by 2-week rest period	Diarrhea, neutropenia
350 mg/m^2 IV every 3 weeks	Diarrhea, neutropenia
Trimetrexate + 5-FU + leucovorin[128]	
Trimetrexate 110 mg/m^2 IV over 1 hour on day 1; 24 hours later: leucovorin 200 mg/m^2 IV over 1 hour, followed by 5-FU 500 mg/m^2 IV bolus plus oral leucovorin, 15 mg every 6 hours for 7 doses, starting 6 hours after 5-FU. Cycle repeated weekly × 6, followed by a 2-week rest period	Diarrhea, neutropenia
Mitomycin C + 5-FU[129]	Diarrhea, neutropenia
Investigational	
Thymidylate synthase inhibitors (Raltitrexed)	Leukopenia, diarrhea
Oral fluorinated pyrimidines	
UFT (Ftorafur)	Diarrhea
S-1	Diarrhea
Capecitabine (Xeloda)	Hand–foot syndrome, stomatitis
Eniluracil (776C85) + 5-FU	Neutropenia, diarrhea
BOF-A2 (Emitefur)	
Oxaliplatin (Eloxatine, L-OHP) + 5-FU ± leucovorin	Peripheral sensory neuropathy, diarrhea, stomatitis

IVP = intravenous bolus injection; CIV = continuous intravenous infusion.

each day for up to 10 weeks without a substantial amount of toxicity.[5,70] Currently, 300 mg/m^2/d is the maximally tolerated dose for long-term continuous infusion 5-FU. Several phase II trials of patients receiving continuous infusions of 5-FU for up to 12 weeks have reported improved response rates of up to 31% to 53%.[70] Although only a small number of patients were studied, comparative investigations have shown statistically greater overall response rates with continuous infusion as compared to IV bolus 5-FU (30% to 44% versus 7% to 22%).[5,70] Dose intensification may account for some differences seen in efficacy. As yet, however, these increased response rates have not translated into significant survival advantages.

A recently published meta-analysis of six randomized trials evaluating more than 1200 patients with advanced colorectal cancer compared the efficacy and toxicity profile of intravenous continuous infusion of 5-FU with bolus administration.[68] A significantly higher tumor response rate (22% versus 14%) and a slight increase in overall survival was observed in patients receiving 5-FU by continuous intravenous infusion.

Continuous infusion of 5-FU is one of the most efficacious methods of dose intensification, based on the assumption that a dose–response relationship exists for colorectal cancer. The maximum cumulative 5-FU dose that can be administered via continuous IV infusion in a 28-day period is approximately 4000 to 7400 mg/m^2 as compared to 2400 to 2500 mg/m^2 with IV bolus 5-FU.[122] Technologic advancement in venous access devices and portable infusion pumps has made continuous IV infusion of 5-FU both possible and practical. Future clinical trials need to address whether the efficacy of infusional 5-FU may be further enhanced with the addition of leucovorin based on comparable response rates observed with continuous-infusion 5-FU and biochemical modulation strategies containing 5-FU plus leucovorin. For now, however, the current trend favors IV bolus schedules because of inexpensive cost, ease of administration, and documented efficacy.

Biochemical Modulation of 5-FU

5-FU PLUS LEUCOVORIN (HIGH VERSUS LOW DOSE). Numerous studies have evaluated various doses of leucovorin in an attempt to improve the response rates and survival of single-agent 5-FU given via IV bolus or continuous IV infusion. Response rates of 14% to 58% have been observed with a variety of doses of 5-FU with leucovorin doses between 20 and 500 mg/m^2.[69] Leucovorin can be given by IV bolus, prolonged infusion, and orally. The administration sequence and timing of leucovorin may be important factors in evaluating the efficacy of biochemical modulation with leucovorin. A schedule for administering leucovorin prior to 5-FU is the most effective approach to enable the level of intracellular-reduced folates to accumulate prior to 5-FU administration. Prolonged exposure of low levels of leucovorin increase the intracellular concentration of reduced long-chain polyglutamates, which in turn stabilize the FdUMP–thymidylate synthase complex, resulting in increased 5-FU cytotoxicity. However, the maximum tolerated dose of 5-FU when given in combination with leucovorin is lower than that when given alone. In addition, a qualitative alteration of the toxicity pattern has been noted.

In a phase III trial conducted by the GITSG, a 5-day course of IV bolus 5-FU (500 mg/m^2) repeated every 4 weeks was compared to a combination of 5-FU (600 mg/m^2) and low-dose (25 mg/m^2) or high-dose (500 mg/m^2) leucovorin, administered for 6 out of 8 weeks.[75] The 5-FU and low-dose leucovorin regimen was no more effective than 5-FU alone (19% versus 12% response rate), whereas a 30% response rate was observed in patients who received weekly 5-FU and high-dose leucovorin. Conflicting results were published by the Mayo Clinic and NCCTG, which found 5-FU (425 mg/m^2/d by IV bolus injection for 5 days, repeated every 4 to 5 weeks) and low-dose leucovorin (20 mg/m^2) to be more effective than either 5-FU alone or 5-FU (370 mg/m^2/d for 5 days) with high-dose leucovorin (200 mg/m^2/d) (43%, 10%, and 26% response rate, respectively).[76] These results were confirmed.[124] Although the low-dose leucovorin regimen was more effective than the high-dose regimen, the difference in response could be attributed to the higher doses of 5-FU that were administered in combination with low-dose leucovorin. In a study of patients with nonmeasurable metastatic disease, the addition of either low- or high-dose leucovorin increased survival from 7.7 to 12.0 and 12.2 months, respectively.[76] Other studies, however, have noted a trend toward survival benefit with high-dose leucovorin only.[75] A direct comparison of the GITSG and NCCTG trials was unable to identify a significant difference in tumor response rates (28% versus 33%) or median survival (10 months for each group) between patients receiving high-dose or low-dose leucovorin.[79]

A meta-analysis of nine randomized clinical studies comparing weekly and monthly 5-FU plus leucovorin published in 1992 and later reviewed by a second author in 1997, confirmed that the addition of leucovorin to 5-FU provided a treatment benefit in terms of objective tumor response only (23% versus 11%).[69,124] Despite the improvement in response rates, there was no significant improvement in survival (11.5 versus 11 months) noted in any of the trials, with the exception of one trial of low-dose leucovorin that was not used in the original meta-analysis.[76] The lack of survival benefit might be explained by the short duration of tumor response, large number of patients who did not respond to treatment, or crossover administration of 5-FU plus leucovorin in patients who failed single-agent 5-FU. The two most frequently used regimens in advanced colorectal cancer are weekly 5-FU administered via intravenous bolus infusion at the midpoint of a 2-hour infusion of high-dose leucovorin and the administration of low-dose leucovorin followed by 5-FU, both given as intravenous bolus infusions, daily for 5 days every 4 to 5 weeks.

The control arm for many studies of 5-FU plus leucovorin was single-agent 5-FU administered in doses ranging from 370 to 500 mg/m^2/d for 5 days, with a cycle repeated every 3 to 5 weeks. In one trial, the response rate for single-agent 5-FU (500 mg/m^2) was 24% compared to historical controls of 10% to 15%.[69,125] The response rates and median survival for daily regimens of 5-FU plus low- or high-dose leucovorin appear comparable. Higher response rates of 24% to 54% have been noted in biweekly regimens of 5-FU administered first as an IV bolus infusion followed by a 22-hour continuous infusion in combination with high doses of leucovorin administered over 2 hours.[69] The higher dose intensity of 5-FU administered in the biweekly regimen over a comparable period of time makes it difficult to compare this regimen with daily 5-FU plus leucovorin regimens. In addition, high response rates (39% to 58%) have also been observed in previously untreated and treated patients receiving weekly 5-FU as a continuous 24-hour infusion in combination with high doses of leucovorin given over 2 to 24 hours. Median survival rates have not changed significantly since the pivotal trials were published, although weekly continuous infusions of 5-FU plus leucovorin have produced a prolongation in survival, in some cases by greater than 22 months.[69,75,76,79,124] Four clinical trials have been conducted to evaluate 5-FU and the *l*-isomer of leucovorin in an attempt to improve efficacy compared to the usual *d,l*-isomer preparation.[69] Continuous or intermittent administration of 5-FU ± *l*-leucovorin every 3 weeks compared to intravenous bolus infusion of 5-FU ± *l*-leucovorin every 4 weeks may also permit higher doses of 5-FU to be administered with significantly less myelosuppression, stomatitis, and diarrhea. This increase in dose intensity may account for the higher response rates observed with prolonged infusions of 5-FU. Comparative randomized trials with standard regimens of 5-FU plus low and high doses of leucovorin need to confirm these observations.

Phase III trials evaluating 5-FU and leucovorin for metastatic colorectal cancer have been criticized because doses of 5-FU used in control groups have been below the maximum-tolerated dose.[75] As a result, the addition of leucovorin may appear to produce a greater antitumor effect when in fact it is being compared to a suboptimal control group. Thus, the dose of 5-FU must also be evaluated.

5-FU plus low-dose leucovorin is currently recommended as standard systemic treatment for metastatic colorectal cancer based on response rates, toxicity, lower estimated drug costs, and quality of life indices such as performance status, weight gain, and symptoms.[69,76,93,124] However, the weekly schedule of high-dose leucovorin plus 5-FU may be more convenient for the patient in terms of fewer scheduled clinic appointments, less interference with work schedules, and ease in dose adjustments based on toxicity. The optimal dose and schedule of administration of 5-FU in combination with leucovorin for metastatic disease still remains to be defined.

5-FU AND IFN-α ± LEUCOVORIN. Although most published studies in metastatic colorectal cancer have employed a variety of intermediate doses of IFN-α, the most common administration schedule is 9 to 10 × 10^6 units SQ given three times weekly.[5,65] The routes of 5-FU administration have also varied. One of the most common 5-FU dosing regimens involves a 5-day continuous infusion of 5-FU 750 mg/m^2/d followed by a weekly IV bolus at the same dose. Overall response rates between 26% and 63% have been reported with IFN-α and 5-FU in previously untreated patients with metastatic disease, a few of which were complete responses. Complete responses to IFN-α in patients previously treated for advanced disease have not been reported. Compared to 5-FU alone, patients who received 5-FU in combination with IFN-α required dose reductions because of greater toxicities, including dose-limiting bone marrow suppression (leukopenia and neutropenia), diarrhea, neurologic toxicities, flu-like symptoms, stomatitis, and alopecia.

Slightly lower response rates have been documented in two larger studies comparing 5-FU plus IFN-α to 5-FU alone (19% versus 30%) and 5-FU plus leucovorin (21% versus 18%).[126,127] The studies were again hampered by significant toxicity resulting in treatment interruption, discontinuation, and death due to sepsis. Promising activity was reported in a phase II study evaluating 5-FU, leucovorin, and IFN-α in previously untreated patients with good performance status and measurable metastatic disease.[103] IFN-α dosed at 5 × 10^6 units/m^2 via SQ injection was administered on days 1 to 7, and on days 2 to 6; 5-FU 370 mg/m^2/d IV bolus injection was infused 1 hour following a 30-minute IV infusion of leucovorin 500 mg/m^2/d. IFN-α was administered immediately prior to leucovorin on concomitant days of therapy and cycles were repeated at 3-week intervals. An overall response rate of 54% was achieved, and included some complete responses. After a median follow-up of 19 months, disease-free recurrence and overall survival were 8 and 16 months, respectively. Although 5-FU doses were escalated to 425 mg/m^2/d, only 40% of patients could tolerate the higher doses. Dose-limiting toxicity occurred in 61% of patients and 26% of patients required a significant IFN-α dose reduction because of flu-like symptoms.

In summary, the combination of 5-FU and IFN-α at current doses and administration schedule provides no improvement in efficacy, produces significant toxicity, and does not improve survival compared to standard 5-FU plus leucovorin regimens. As a result, this combination is currently not recommended as standard therapy. However, current trials are exploring double biochemical modulation strategies of 5-FU in combination with lower doses and different administration schedules of IFN-α and leucovorin.

5-FU + PALA. As a single agent, PALA (*N*-(phosphonacetyl)-L-aspartate) is inactive against human malignancies; however, the combination of 5-FU and PALA has undergone extensive clinical testing.[65] Controlled studies have failed to show any significant advantage of PALA with 5-FU compared to 5-FU alone, although complete and partial responses have been reported in previously untreated patients with advanced disease.[5,65] Early trials employed a weekly regimen of high dose PALA 250 mg/m^2 infused over 24 hours followed by a 24-hour infusion of 5-FU in doses ranging from 2600 to 3400 mg/m^2. Toxicity of PALA is similar to that of 5-FU alone, although the syndrome of ascites, hyperbilirubinemia, and hypoalbuminemia that can develop with this combination occurs more frequently in patients who are experiencing a response.[89] Currently, lower doses of PALA are being evaluated in combination with 5-FU plus leucovorin in an attempt to optimize both RNA and DNA synthesis inhibition.

Topoisomerase I Inhibitors

Irinotecan is currently approved by the FDA for patients with metastatic colorectal cancer who have recurred or progressed following 5-FU therapy. Efficacy has been evaluated using a variety of intravenous dosing schedules ranging from 100 to 150 mg/m^2 weekly, 150 to 250 mg/m^2 biweekly, 125 mg/m^2 weekly for 4 weeks, followed by a 2-week rest period, to 300 to 350 mg/m^2 IV every 3 weeks.[81–85] In each of these regimens, neutropenia and diarrhea are the dose-limiting toxicities. The most common administration schedule in the United States is the weekly regimen for 4 consecutive weeks followed by a rest period, with therapy repeated every 6 weeks based on patient tolerability. Objective response rates of 19% to 32% in chemotherapy-naive and 13% to 27% in previously treated patients with metastatic colorectal cancer with disease progression or recurrence following 5-FU–based therapy have been observed in phase II studies.[81,82,85] Overall response rates in chemotherapy-naive patients are similar to those with 5-FU plus leucovorin. Higher response rates have also been observed in patients with lung (39% to 40%) compared to liver (15% to 29%) metastases, which might be explained by differences in tissue distribution or drug metabolism of its active metabolite, SN-38.[81,82] Prior exposure to 5-FU does not appear to influence response rates or duration of response to irinotecan. A Phase III trial comparing irinotecan 300–350 mg/m^2 IV every 3 weeks to supportive care alone in patients with metastatic disease who failed 5-FU showed improved 1-year survival (36.2% versus 13.8%) and quality of life.[83] A comparison of irinotecan to continuous infusion 5-FU in a similar population also demonstrated improved survival with irinotecan.[84] Therefore, irinotecan should be considered standard therapy for patients who have failed prior treatment with 5-FU based regimens.

Topotecan and 9-aminocamptothecin (9-AC) have also demonstrated promising antitumor activity against colorectal carcinomas in preclinical studies; however, tumor response rates in phase I and II clinical trials have not been meaningful.[65] It is unlikely that either agent plays a significant role in colorectal cancer management.

Ongoing clinical trials are evaluating irinotecan as first-line therapy for metastatic colorectal cancer; its use in various combinations with other active agents, including 5-FU; in adjuvant treatment regimens; and to better define optimal dosing schedules.

Combination Chemotherapy

Attempts to improve response rates to chemotherapy by combining 5-FU with either cisplatin or methotrexate have been generally disappointing, although both cisplatin and methotrexate have some activity against colorectal cancer. Response rates are higher when cisplatin is administered with continuous IV infusion 5-FU as compared to bolus IV 5-FU, but they are not significantly better than those of 5-FU alone.[123] Furthermore, myelosuppression, primarily of the granulocytic cell line, also appears to be enhanced by the combination of cisplatin and IV bolus 5-FU. The timing between sequential administration of methotrexate and 5-FU appears to be an important determinant of efficacy. Intervals of as much as 24 hours between methotrexate and 5-FU administration, as well as duration of 5-FU infusions, have been studied. It is unclear, however, whether this combination provides any therapeutic advantage to the combination of 5-FU and leucovorin.

5-FU + Trimetrexate. Although results from phase I and II trials of single-agent trimetrexate in colorectal cancer have been disappointing, the combination of 5-FU, leucovorin, and trimetrexate (Neutrexin) appears promising. The rationale for this combination is based on an attempt to maximize the accumulation of 5-phosphoribosyl-1-pyrophosphate (PRPP), which promotes the conversion of 5-FU to FUMP. Two multicenter phase II trials have evaluated trimetrexate in untreated patients with metastatic colorectal cancer.[128] Trimetrexate was administered on day 1, followed 24 hours later by leucovorin and 5-FU. The cycle was repeated weekly for 6 weeks followed by a 2-week rest period. Several additional doses of oral leucovorin were given in an attempt to decrease the incidence of severe neutropenia. Objective response rates of 39% to 50% and a median survival duration of 53 weeks were comparable to 5-FU plus leucovorin. Furthermore, response rates of 40% were seen in patients who received prior adjuvant therapy. Diarrhea was the dose-limiting toxicity with this combination, in contrast to myelosuppression, which is dose limiting for single-agent trimetrexate. Randomized clinical trials need to confirm the efficacy of trimetrexate in combination with 5-FU plus leucovorin in both chemotherapy-naive and previously treated patients with metastatic colorectal cancer.

5-FU + Mitomycin C. Mitomycin C in combination with 5-FU plus leucovorin has also been used to induce response rates in patients with metastatic disease, primarily rectal cancer. A study of patients with progressive disease following 5-FU/leucovorin reported a partial response rate of 17% with a median duration of response of 9.5 months.[129] The regimen consisted of 5-FU, leucovorin, and a bolus injection of mitomycin C, 10 mg/m^2. Although a small number of patients participated, this combination may represent a viable option for refractory disease.

Investigational Agents

At present, the combination of 5-FU plus leucovorin is the standard systemic regimen for metastatic colorectal cancer, providing overall response rates of 25% to 40% with no or little effect on improving overall survival. Newer chemotherapeutic agents, such as thymidylate synthase inhibitors, oral 5-FU analogs and prodrugs, biochemical modulators of 5-FU, platinum analogs, and matrix metalloproteinase inhibitors, have been developed in an attempt to improve antitumor efficacy and reduce treatment toxicities.

Other investigational treatments include targeting specific proteins or metabolic pathways; using *ras* inhibitors that inhibit farnesyl transferase; protein kinase C inhibitors; cyclin-dependent kinase inhibitors; and growth factor–receptor inhibitors. In addition, monoclonal antibodies directed against tumor-associated antigens, biologic modifier therapy cytokines (rIFN-α and rIL-2), vaccines against CEA, mutant *ras,* mutant *p53,* antiangiogenesis agents, and gene therapy techniques represent some of the technologic advances aimed toward metastatic colorectal cancer.[80,107]

Thymidylate Synthase Inhibitors. Raltitrexed (ZD1694, Tomudex) is a quinazoline water-soluble, folate analog that acts as a potent and selective inhibitor of thymidylate synthase (TS).[130] Raltitrexed is transported by a reduced-folate carrier into the cell and is rapidly metabolized by folylpolyglutamate synthase (FPGS) to higher-chain polyglutamates, which are 60- to 100-fold more potent than the parent compound. The intracellular polyglutamates bind to the folate substrate site of TS and accumulate, resulting in sustained TS inhibition and cell death. Other folate-based TS inhibitors—BW1843U89, LY231514, ZD9331, AG331, and AG337 (Thymitaq, Nolatrexed)—are currently in early clinical development and differ from raltitrexed in chemical structure, degree of lipophilicity, method of entry into the cell, degree of polyglutamation, dosing schedule, route of administration, and toxicity profile.[80,130] In comparison to 5-FU, these specific TS inhibitors are more selective, potent, and may be less toxic. Potential mechanisms for drug resistance may include decreased FPGS activity, resulting in an impaired ability to form polygutamates; increased tissue TS proteins and activity; and impaired intracellular uptake.[130]

Clinical trials of single-agent raltitrexed dosed at 3 mg/m^2 IV every 3 weeks have produced similar objective response rates compared to 5-FU plus leucovorin in previously untreated patients with metastatic colorectal cancer (14% to 20% versus 15% to 18%).[131–133] The low response rates of 5-FU plus leucovorin compared to original trials might be explained by differences in patient characteristics and time to assessment of response. Time to progression and overall survival were also comparable between the two arms, approximately 10 to 12 months, with the exception of one trial where the results favored 5-FU plus leucovorin. The most frequent grade 3 or 4 toxicities associated with raltitrexed are transient leukopenia, asthenia, nausea and vomiting, diarrhea, and an asymptomatic but reversible elevation of serum transaminases.[131–133] The incidence of grade 3 or 4 leukopenia, and mucositis or diarrhea, was significantly reduced compared to that with 5-FU plus leucovorin. However, a higher incidence of reversible grade 3 or 4 hepatic transaminase elevations was observed with raltitrexed. Fewer patients receiving raltitrexed required dose reduction due to toxicity. Palliation of symptoms, noted by improvement in performance status and/or weight gain, was similar in both groups.

Determination of FPGS, tissue TS expression, and *p53* status, as well as posttreatment polyglutamates and TS expression, may help identify patients who would be most likely to benefit from TS inhibitors, as well as aid in dosage adjustments.[80,130] In addition, *in vitro* studies have demonstrated synergistic activity with raltitrexed and 5-FU or irinotecan. Many questions, such as the possibility of cross-resistance between 5-FU and raltitrexed, the development of a more efficacious dosing schedule, and comparisons of raltitrexed to other 5-FU–based regimens or in combination with other agents, remain unanswered. With the exception of cost, raltitrexed appears to have a more convenient dosing schedule, similar efficacy, and a favorable toxicity profile compared to 5-FU plus leucovorin. At present, however, the role of raltitrexed in the treatment of metastatic colorectal cancer remains unanswered.

Oral Fluorinated Pyrimidines. Extensive understanding of the pharmacology of 5-FU has led to the investigation of agents that would prolong *in vivo* 5-FU exposure and enhance antitumor effects without the use of continuous intravenous infusions. Key strategies include administration of 5-FU prodrugs and inhibitors of 5-FU catabolism. Potential advantages of oral forms of 5-FU include prolonged 5-FU exposure at lower peak concentrations, patient convenience, lower treatment costs, and decreased toxic effects. Figure 118–6 compares the pharmacology of these agents to 5-FU.

CAPECITABINE. Capecitabine (Xeloda) is an oral, tumor-activated and tumor-selective fluoropyrimidine carbamate. As a prodrug, it passes through the intestines as an intact molecule and is converted to 5-FU through three sequential conversion steps: first by hepatic carboxylesterase, next, by hepatic and tumor cytidine deaminase, and finally by thymidine phosphorylase, which is present in greatest concentrations at the tumor site.[130,134] These activation steps lead to an approximate threefold increase in tumor and 1.4-fold increase in hepatic 5-FU levels. Because capecitabine first passes through the intestines as an intact molecule, the incidence of diarrhea is significantly reduced. A randomized, multicenter phase II trial evaluated three dosing schedules of capecitabine administered on a continuous or intermittent infusion schedule as a single agent or in combination with leucovorin.[134] The most promising regimen consisted of capecitabine, 2510 $mg/m^2/d$, given orally in two divided doses on an intermittent schedule for 2 weeks on and 1 week off. The objective response rate was 30% with a 30-week time to progression. Hand–foot syndrome and stomatitis were the most common toxicities observed. Additional trials of capecitabine in metastatic colorectal cancer are warranted. Pretreatment measures of thymidine phosphorylase may be useful to identify potential responders of capecitabine therapy.[135]

UFT. UFT (Ftorafur), a combination of uracil and tegafur in a 4:1 molar ratio, is an oral prodrug of 5-FU that is converted to 5-FU by thymidine/uridine phosphorylase in the liver, resulting in increased and sustained 5-FU exposure.[80,130] Tegafur is an oral 5-FU prodrug that has been used in Japan for gastrointestinal malignancies for many years but gained little interest in the United States after the 1970s because of substantial toxicities. Uracil acts as a substrate for dihydropyrimidine dehydrogenase (DPD), thereby inhibiting 5-FU degradation to dihydrofluorouracil.[130] The addition of leucovorin further optimizes the activity of 5-FU from UFT by enhancing TS inhibition.

Pooled data from Japanese phase II trials of single-agent UFT in doses of 300 to 600 mg/d, administered orally in 2 or 3 divided doses for 28 days, reveal a 25% response rate in previously treated and untreated patients with colorectal cancer.[136] Phase II trials of UFT in combination with low and high doses of leucovorin reported objective response rates of 25% and 42%, respectively, which is similar to that of 5-FU plus leucovorin.[124,137,138] UFT dosed at 300 to 350 $mg/m^2/d$ in combination with leucovorin, 15 to 150 mg/d, was administered orally in 3 divided doses every 8 hours for 28 days, followed by a 1-week rest period. The dose-limiting toxicity of UFT in combination with leucovorin was prolonged diarrhea, which resulted in treatment delay and dose reduction. In contrast to 5-FU plus leucovorin, however, no grade 3 or 4 neutropenia, mucositis, or hand–foot syndrome was observed, although patients did experience less severe grades of mucositis, fatigue, nausea, and vomiting. Because of documented activity and a favorable toxicity profile, ongoing trials are comparing the safety and efficacy of UFT plus oral leucovorin with 5-FU plus leucovorin in both metastatic and adjuvant settings.

ENILURACIL. Dihydropyrimidine dehydrogenase (DPD) is the rate-limitng enzyme responsible for 5-FU catabolism to dihydrofluorouracil, which is further catabolized to CO_2, urea, and α-fluoro-β-alanine.[80,139] Patients with normal DPD activity excrete greater than 80% of a dose of 5-FU as α-fluoro-β-alanine, with a 5-FU elimination half-life that is variable but generally shorter than 15 minutes.[130] In contrast, patients with deficient or lower levels of DPD eliminate greater than 90% of a dose of 5-FU as unchanged drug, with a mean elimination half-life greater than 2.5 hours. These individuals also develop extreme toxicities following 5-FU administration.[130,139] Several studies have demonstrated in a variety of tumor types that an inverse correlation exists between tumor DPD expression and tumor response to therapy. Although found primarily in the liver, the presence of intestinal DPD probably contributes to the wide variability in oral 5-FU absorption, and the circadian pattern of its activity might account for the variability in 5-FU systemic clearance among individuals. DPD inactivation increases the oral bioavailability and reduces systemic clearance of 5-FU to produce comparable systemic levels achieved with IV 5-FU.

Eniluracil (776C85, 5-Ethynyluracil) is a potent inactivator of DPD by first binding with it in a reversible manner and then irreversibly inactivating the enzyme. It is administered with oral 5-FU in a 10:1 ratio. In a phase I study conducted to determine the bioavailability, pharmacokinetic disposition, efficacy, and toxicity of oral 5-FU in patients treated with eniluracil, patients with refractory solid tumors were randomized to receive either oral or IV 5-FU, 10 $mg/m^2/d$, given on day 2, or eniluracil 3.7 $mg/m^2/d$ orally on days 1 and 2.[139] Patients then received escalating doses of 5-FU 10 to 25 $mg/m^2/d$ orally for 5 days with eniluracil 3.7 $mg/m^2/d$ orally for 7 days every 4 weeks. As a single agent, eniluracil did not demonstrate antitumor activity, although an improvement in oral bioavailability, increase in serum half-life, and decrease in systemic clearance of 5-FU was comparable to that seen with IV administration. Interpatient variability in the bioavailability of oral 5-FU significantly improved with eniluracil. Additional phase II studies of a prolonged 28-day administration schedule of oral eniluracil and 5-FU, with or without leucovorin, have documented responses in patients with metastatic colorectal cancer.[140,141] The most common dose-limiting toxicity of oral 5-FU plus eniluracil using the multiple 5-day dosing regimen was myelosuppression, primarily neutropenia. In contrast, diarrhea was dose limiting with the prolonged 28-day administration of eniluracil and 5-FU.[139–142] Other nonhematologic toxicities included grade 1 or 2 nausea and vomiting and a varied severity of elevated serum transaminases and bilirubin. Ongoing clinical trials are evaluating the combination of 5-FU plus eniluracil given as a 5-day schedule every 3 to 4 weeks, a 28-day schedule of twice-daily administration followed by a 1-week rest period, and in patients with 5-FU refractory colorectal cancer.

S-1. S-1 is a fixed oral formulation consisting of UFT, 5-chloro-2,4-dihydroxypyridine (CDHP), and potassium oxonate in a molar ratio of 1:0.4:1.[130] CDHP is a potent inhibitor of DPD, approximately 200-fold greater than uracil, and potassium oxonate blocks 5-FU phosphorylation in the gastrointestinal tract via phosphoribosyl transferase, resulting in the inhibition of RNA processing and function. Early animal trials have shown superior antitumor activity and a favorable toxicity profile compared to 5-FU or UFT alone, particularly when given for prolonged periods of time. In a recent phase I trial, the maximum tolerated dose of S-1 was 45 mg/m^2 administered orally twice daily; diarrhea was the dose-limiting toxicity.[143]

BOF-A2. BOF-A2 (Emitefur) consists of a 1:1 molar ratio of 1-ethoxymethyl 5-FU (EM-FU), a slow-release or "masked" formulation of 5-FU that requires activation by hepatic microsomes, and 3-cyano-2,6-dihydropyridine (CNDP), a potent inhibitor of DPD that is approximately 2000-fold more potent than uracil. Most of the preclinical and phase I/II trials have been conducted in Japan, although a recent phase I trial of BOF-A2 plus leucovorin demonstrated some activity in 5-FU–resistant patients.[144] BOF-A2 is currently being evaluated in regimens involving two to three-times daily oral administration for 14 consecutive days, followed by a 7-day rest period.

Platinum Analogs. Oxaliplatin (Eloxatin, *L*-OHP) is a new diaminocyclohexane–platinum coordination complex with a mechanism of action similar to that of cisplatin.[80] Both drugs bind to two close or adjacent guanine or adenine base pairs leading to the formation of DNA adducts or cross-links, which result in the inhibition of DNA synthesis.[145] Although cisplatin and carboplatin have limited activity against colorectal cancer, oxaliplatin produces DNA adducts that differ somewhat and may more effectively inhibit DNA synthesis.

In phase II trials of oxaliplatin administered as a single agent, 130 mg/m^2 IV over 2 to 6 hours every 3 weeks, objective response rates of 27% have been observed in chemotherapy-naive patients and 10% to 11% in patients with 5-FU–resistant metastatic colorectal cancer.[80] The most common toxicities include a cumulative, dose-limiting, and reversible peripheral sensory neuropathy and nausea and vomiting. Unlike cisplatin, renal and ototoxicity are not observed. Its efficacy in combination with 5-FU, particularly chronomodulated 5-FU, and leucovorin is most notable. The chronomodulated regimen takes advantage of the diurnal variation associated with several key enzymes involved in 5-FU metabolism, and delivers drugs in a schedule that provides peak drug levels at times when the tumor is most susceptible.[146] Significant efficacy was observed with intravenous oxaliplatin 20 to 25 mg/m^2/d and 5-FU 600 to 1000 mg/m^2/d plus leucovorin 300 mg/m^2/d given for 4 to 5 days every 2 to 3 weeks, as noted by response rates of 59% to 69% in untreated patients and 40% to 67% in previously treated patients with metastatic colorectal cancer.[147–149] Median survivals were 15 to 21 months and 15 to 19 months, respectively. Toxicities in the chronomodulated arm included dose-limiting diarrhea and stomatitis and cumulative grade 1 or 2 sensory peripheral neuropathy and nausea and vomiting.[147–149] Chronomodulation allowed for an increase in median dose intensity of 5-FU and significantly decreased the incidence and severity of bone marrow suppression, neurotoxicity, and stomatitis.

In summary, the combination of oxaliplatin with 5-FU plus leucovorin has produced a greater than 20% improvement in efficacy compared to that seen with 5-FU plus leucovorin or other 5-FU combinations, especially in previously treated patients.[75,76,125] However, larger numbers of patients are needed to determine whether the response rates and improvement in survival can be maintained. The increase in 5-FU dose intensity using chronomodulation and favorable toxicity profile of this combination make oxaliplatin an exciting drug for further study in colorectal cancer.

Matrix Metalloproteinase Inhibitors. Matrix metalloproteinases are zinc-containing enzymes responsible for extracellular matrix protein turnover and remodeling.[80] Tumor spread is facilitated by the presence of these enzymes, which are activated and expressed to a greater degree during tumor progression and metastasis. Matrix metalloproteinase-9 (MMP-9) may facilitate colorectal cancer invasion and metastases, and its production may provide important information about the tumor's metastatic potential.[150] Marimastat (BB-2516) inhibits a broad spectrum of matrix metalloproteinases and has a reasonable pharmacokinetic profile, including oral bioavailability.[151] It is currently being studied in a variety of human tumors, including colorectal cancer, to determine whether it can reduce tumor progression or metastases.

Regional Therapeutic Approaches

Hepatic Artery Infusion. The rationale for hepatic artery infusion (HAI) is based on the principle that normal liver hepatocytes and early micrometastases obtain their primary blood supply from the portal vein. In contrast, tumors in the liver are thought to receive most of their blood supply via the hepatic artery.[120,152] FUDR and 5-FU have undergone the most study for infusion via the hepatic artery either via continuous infusion or IV bolus injection. The majority of hepatic arterial infusions have been directed at patients with unresectable liver metastases.[5,120,121]

The pharmacokinetic properties of FUDR in particular provide for rapid systemic clearance and high liver drug extraction. Delivery of FUDR via the hepatic artery therefore results in increased local drug concentrations at the tumor site that may translate into improved response rates. 5-FU is used less frequently because of a much lower hepatic extraction rate. Also, because approximately 80% of the administered FUDR dose is metabolized by the liver, systemic toxicity due to exposure of normal extrahepatic tissues is minimized.[123]

Early trials of HAI revealed objective response rates ranging from 30% to 80%, many of which were observed in previously treated patients.[120] The greatest problems encountered were related to complications of external catheters such as arterial thrombosis, catheter dislodgement, bleeding, bulky pump equipment limiting patient mobility, and hospitalization. The availability of implantable, portable infusion devices has significantly decreased complications and renewed interest in hepatic arterial infusional chemotherapy.[119,120] As a result, randomized trials comparing HAI with systemic therapy in patients with liver metastases were initiated in the 1980s. Their results have been summarized in several general reviews.[5,119,120]

FUDR via HAI has been compared to IV infusion of 5-FU and FUDR. The dose is typically 0.3 mg/kg/d administered as a continuous 24-hour infusion for a total of 14 days. This is in contrast to a comparable IV dose equal to 0.125 mg/kg/d. Heparin, in doses ranging from 10,000 to 17,500 units/50 mL of solution, is often added to the HAI mixture in an attempt to decrease the incidence of arterial thromboses. Prospective randomized studies have consistently demonstrated significantly higher response rates of 40% to 60% with HAI as compared to 10% to 20% response rates observed with IV therapy.[5,119,120] Median survival rates also are slightly higher for patients receiving HAI as compared to systemic therapy (17 to 20 versus 11 to 12 months). In addition, a general trend toward a superior 2-year survival rate appears to exist for patients who receive HAI, whether it is administered initially or following failure with systemic therapy. Patients with minimal liver involvement and lack of extrahepatic disease are most likely to benefit from therapy. Studies evaluating HAI therapy must be interpreted with caution, however, because complicating features such as crossover treatment design and presence of extrahepatic disease may account for differences in response rates and survival. However, significant improvement in survival was noted in two trials that did not allow treatment crossover.[120]

The primary limitations of HAI include development and/or progression of extrahepatic disease and treatment toxicities. Common toxicities include gastric ulceration and hepatobiliary toxicity. The degree of hepatobiliary toxicity ranges from an elevation in hepatic enzymes resulting in a chemical hepatitis to sclerosing cholangitis (bile duct strictures). Elevation of liver function enzymes occurs in 26% to 79% of patients and is manifested by an elevation of transaminase enzymes or increased serum bilirubin levels, noted in 25% of patients. Bile duct toxicity resulting in biliary sclerosis occurs in less than 10% of patients with careful monitoring and is thought to result from ischemia and inflammation. It is most often seen with higher doses (≥ 0.3 mg/kg/d) and prolonged infusions (≥ 2 weeks) and should be suspected when alkaline phosphatase and bilirubin levels are elevated. Hepatobiliary toxicity often resolves on discontinuation of therapy within 2 to 4 weeks, although permanent damage to the biliary tree has been reported.[5,119,120] Various approaches have been suggested in an attempt to limit hepatobiliary toxicity and include regimens alternating FUDR with 5-FU, decreasing the FUDR dose, or combining FUDR with dexamethasone.[5,120] Gastritis and gastrointestinal ulceration have been reported in 8% to

21% of patients and are reversible upon discontinuation of therapy. They are believed to occur because of perfusion of chemotherapy into the stomach and duodenum via small vessels branching from the hepatic artery.[120] This toxicity may be ameliorated by surgical ligation of the blood vessels supplying the stomach and duodenum or H_2-antagonist therapy. Because of toxicities associated with HAI, most patients require some transient interruption of therapy, a decrease in dosage, or discontinuation of therapy. Rest periods between therapy have also been recommended in an attempt to prevent or minimize toxicity. Although increased response rates and a trend toward improved survival have been reported, the costs and toxicities with this approach are significant. Until more data become available, HAI should be reserved for palliative treatment of isolated liver metastases and in patients who have failed systemic therapy.

Hepatic Arterial Chemoembolization. The largest experience with hepatic arterial chemoembolization has been seen in patients with metastatic carcinoid tumors or primary hepatocellular carcinomas. Most recently, small trials have been expanded to include hepatic metastases caused by colorectal cancer.[120,152,153] Hepatic arterial chemoembolization delivers high concentrations of cytotoxic agents directly to the tumor and results in the embolization or devascularization of the liver, which blocks perfusion of the tumor and eliminates its blood supply. This procedure involves the instillation of a mixture that incorporates chemotherapeutic agents, radioactive contrast dye, and/or an embolic agent directly into the hepatic artery. Agents and doses most commonly studied have included doxorubicin (40 to 60 mg), mitomycin (10 to 20 mg), and cisplatin (100 to 150 mg), which are usually dissolved in approximately 10 to 15 mL of a radiographic contrast dye. Addition of an embolic agent to the mixture, such as a gelatin sponge (Gelfoam), polyvinyl alcohol particles, bovine collagen, or iodized poppyseed oil (Lipiodol, Ethiodol), results in either a temporary or permanent occlusion of the hepatic artery. Although approximately 80% of patients in one trial experienced a response, the number of patients with colorectal cancer who have undergone this procedure thus far is relatively low. In addition, patients still have eventual disease progression and response durations are measured only in months. Review articles describing the procedure, complications, and patient selection criteria have been published.[152,153] Other novel organ-targeted approaches for colorectal cancer that are under current investigation include HAI of newer agents; leucovorin with IFN-α, FUDR, or monoclonal antibodies; direct intralesional chemotherapy using ethanol or cisplatin; and cryosurgery via ultrasound-guided cryoprobe placement.[120]

MONITORING THERAPEUTIC OUTCOMES

The goal of monitoring is to evaluate whether the patient is receiving any benefit from the management of the disease or to detect recurrence. Similarly, follow-up examinations help to determine whether preventive interventions or screening studies effectively reduce an individual's risk for developing colorectal cancer or presenting with an advanced stage of disease. During treatment for active disease, patients should undergo monitoring for measurable tumor response, progression, or new metastases; these tests may include chest CT scans or x-rays, abdominal or pelvic CT scans or x-rays, and CEA measurements every 2 to 3 months if the CEA is or was previously elevated.[47] In addition, a CBC and selected serum chemistries should be routinely evaulated to monitor anticipated treatment toxicities and any new symptoms as indicated.

Symptoms of recurrence such as pain syndromes, changes in bowel habits, rectal or vaginal bleeding, pelvic masses, anorexia, and weight loss develop in less than 50% of patients.[154] A greater percentage of recurrences are detected in asymptomatic patients due to increased serum CEA levels that lead to further examination. Although the value of CEA monitoring for asymptomatic disease recurrence is questioned by some due to the related expense and emotional stress associated with false-positive elevations, CEA monitoring plays an important role in postoperative follow-up studies for most individuals.[49] Patients who undergo curative surgical resection, with or without adjuvant therapy, require close follow-up based on the premise that early detection and treatment of recurrence could still render them cured.[155] In addition, early treatment for asymptomatic metastatic colorectal cancer may be superior to observation only in improving median survival and prolonging the asymptomatic interval.[156] Although specific tests and the time intervals at which they should be performed are somewhat controversial, general guidelines have been reported (Table 118–8). The NCCN colorectal cancer practice guidelines recommend specific surveillance examinations based on the stage of disease at presentation.[63] Individuals with rectal cancer who undergo potentially curative low anterior resections should undergo close surveillance for local recurrence and metachronous lesions.[157] Although radiolabeled monoclonal antibodies for tumor immunodetection may be useful in selected individual case situations, their incorporation into postoperative surveillance

TABLE 118–8. General Guidelines for Follow-up after Curative Resection

Procedure or Test	Frequency
History and physical exam Fecal occult blood testing CEA	Every 3–4 months for 3 years, then every 6 months for 2 years, then annually
Colonoscopy or sigmoidoscopy + barium enema	Annually for several years, then every 2–3 years if no adenomas are detected
Breast and pelvic examination, mammogram	Per age-specific guidelines for women
Chest x-ray	Annually
Liver function tests Chest, abdominal, or pelvic CT scan Liver ultrasound Liver–spleen scan Bone scan Laparotomy	As indicated by above findings; chest and abdominal CT scans every 2 months for 2 years, then annually for patients with resected pulmonary or hepatic metastases

Compiled from Refs. 5, 156, and 157.

TABLE 118–9. Current Recommendations for Treatment of Cancer of the Colon and Rectum

Stage I (Duke A)	Surgical resection of primary tumor and regional mesenteric lymph nodes
Stage II (Duke B)	
Colon	Surgery as above; selected patients may benefit from adjuvant 5-FU + leucovorin/5-FU + levamisole
Rectum	Surgery + postoperative protracted infusion 5-FU or bolus 5-FU + leucovorin, followed by 5-FU ± leucovorin radiosensitization, followed by 5-FU ± leucovorin
Stage III (Duke C)	
Colon	Surgery + adjuvant 5-FU + leucovorin/5-FU + levamisole
Rectum	Surgery + postoperative protracted infusion 5-FU or bolus 5-FU + leucovorin, followed by 5-FU ± leucovorin radiosensitization, followed by 5-FU ± leucovorin
Stage IV (Duke D)	Radiation therapy, systemic chemotherapy, hepatic chemotherapy, surgical resection of isolated pulmonary or hepatic metastases, symptom management

guidelines will depend on the results of clinical trials that evaluate their sensitivity, specificity, and cost effectiveness in those settings.

Recommendations for the general management of colorectal cancer are reviewed in Table 118–9. The goals of adjuvant therapy for both stage III colon cancer and stages II and III rectal cancer are to reduce local and distant recurrence and improve patient survival. These end points represent the key therapeutic outcomes for which treatments should be evaluated. Although the pathologic stage is used clinically to determine prognosis, newer assays are being developed in an attempt to predict patient survival, to identify patients whose disease is most likely to respond to specific chemotherapeutic agents, and to identify those individuals who will benefit most from therapy.[74] Increased expression of TS and amplification of TS-specific genes are associated with poorer response to 5-FU, 5-FU resistance, and decreased survival.[158] However, further studies are needed before the use of these assays can be routinely incorporated into clinical practice.

Although some regimens may not provide a substantial improvement in overall patient survival, an improvement in disease-free survival may still be a viable therapeutic outcome. Treatment approaches for metastatic colorectal cancer are assessed by their ability to produce a partial tumor response (generally considered as at least a 50% reduction in the tumor mass) or a complete response (total absence of any remaining measurable tumor). Some measurable tumor response is usually necessary for any treatment to improve disease-free or overall patient survival. In the absence of the ability of a specific treatment to improve survival, important outcome measures should include the effects of the treatment on patient symptoms, daily activities and performance status, and other quality-of-life indicators. Because metastatic colorectal cancer is incurable, a specific decision regarding an individual patient's care will ultimately be required; this should be based on a careful assessment of the balance between risks associated with treatment (or lack thereof) and benefits of treatment. Effort should also be made to ensure that the costs of screening, diagnostic tests, treatments, and follow-up procedures for colorectal cancer are consistent with their value in improving patient outcomes.

▶ PRINCIPLES OF PHARMACOTHERAPY

- Maintaining a diet with high-fiber and low-fat intake is an important strategy to reduce colorectal cancer risk. Hormone replacement therapy reduces risk in postmenopausal women, and aspirin and other NSAIDs have been shown to reduce colorectal cancer incidence and mortality, although choice of optimal agent(s), doses, and duration of administration are undefined.
- Effective colorectal cancer screening programs incorporate regular physical examinations including digital rectal exam, fecal occult blood testing, and regular visualization of the bowel via sigmoidoscopy or colonoscopy, starting at age 50 for average-risk individuals.
- The stage of colorectal cancer upon diagnosis—determined by depth of bowel invasion, lymph node involvement, and presence of metastases—is the most important prognostic factor for disease recurrence and survival. Newer prognostic factors include tumor *p53* status, chromosome 18q allelic loss, and tumor thymidylate synthase expression, which may also be important determinants of tumor response to specific chemotherapeutic agents and help identify those individuals likely to benefit from adjuvant therapy.
- Surgical removal of tumor is the treatment of choice for patients with resectable colorectal cancer. Adjuvant chemotherapy, consisting of 5-FU plus leucovorin or 5-FU plus levamisole, should be offered to patients with stage III colon cancer and considered for patients with stage II disease at high risk for tumor recurrence. Because of the risk of local recurrence for individuals with rectal cancer, adjuvant chemotherapy consisting of 5-FU or 5-FU plus leucovorin, plus chemosensitized radiation therapy, should be administered to patients with stage II and III rectal cancer. Postoperative surveillance programs should include regular physical examination, fecal occult blood testing, serum CEA determinations, CBC and serum chemistries, chest x-ray, and colonoscopy or sigmoidoscopy plus barium enema. Women should undergo regular mammography and breast and pelvic examinations.

- Tumor resection for metastatic colorectal cancer is generally reserved for selected individuals with fewer than 3 solitary pulmonary metastases or 4 solitary hepatic lesions. Patients with isolated unresectable hepatic metastases are candidates for systemic or hepatic intra-arterial chemotherapy, although neither has been shown to significantly improve overall survival.
- Intravenous 5-FU forms the basis for chemotherapy regimens for initial treatment of metastatic colorectal cancer. Effective regimens incorporate 5-FU as a bolus or short infusion in combination with low-dose (20 mg/m^2) or high-dose (200 to 500 mg/m^2) leucovorin administered 5 days weekly, once weekly, or biweekly. 5-FU can also be administered as a continuous IV infusion, alone or in combination with leucovorin, administered weekly or continuously in a protracted manner. Dose-limiting toxicities associated with low-dose leucovorin regimens consist primarily of stomatitis and mucositis, whereas diarrhea is most often dose limiting for high-dose leucovorin regimens. Stomatitis and a hand–foot syndrome occur most frequently with continuous 5-FU infusions. Selection of a specific regimen should be based on anticipated side effects, patient convenience, and cost considerations.
- Patients with tumor progression during active treatment for metastatic colorectal cancer are candidates for irinotecan or alternate therapies of biochemically modulated 5-FU. Promising combinations include 5-FU plus trimetrexate and leucovorin and experimental agents, including specific thymidylate synthase inhibitors, oral fluorinated pyrimidines, and oxaliplatin plus chronomodulated 5-FU and leucovorin. Potential advantages for the use of oral fluorinated pyrimidines include oral administration, reduced treatment costs, and possibly fewer treatment-related side effects.
- Novel therapies under investigation for colorectal cancer include matrix metalloproteinase, farnesyl transferase, protein kinase C, growth factor and cyclin-dependent kinase inhibitors, monoclonal antibodies, tumor vaccines, and gene therapy techniques.
- Although treatments for metastatic colorectal cancer may not substantially improve patient disease-free or overall survival, they can be highly beneficial in reducing patient symptoms and their effects on daily activities and general sense of well-being.

REFERENCES

1. Landis SH, Murray T, Bolden S, Wingo PA. Cancer statistics, 1998. CA Cancer J Clin 1998;48:6–29.
2. Ries LAG, Kosary CL, Hankey BF, et al, eds. SEER Cancer Statistics Review, 1973–1995. Bethesda, National Cancer Institute, 1998.
3. Steele GD. The national cancer data base report on colorectal cancer. Cancer 1994;74:1979–1989.
4. Coleman MP, Esteve J, Damiecki P, et al. Trends in cancer incidence and mortality. IARC Sci Publ 1993;121:1–806.
5. Cohen AM, Minsky BD, Schilsky RL. Cancer of the colon. In: DeVita VT, Hellman S, Rosenberg SA, eds. Cancer: Principles and Practice of Oncology, 5th ed. Philadelphia, Lippincott, 1997:1144–1197.
6. Kroser JA, Bachwich DR, Lichtenstein GR. Risk factors for the development of colorectal carcinoma and their modification. Hematol Oncol Clin North Am 1997;11:547–577.
7. Burnstein MJ. Dietary factors related to colorectal neoplasms. Surg Clin North Am 1993;73:13–29.
8. Wilmink AB. Overview of the epidemiology of colorectal cancer. Dis Colon Rectum 1997;4:483–493.
9. Peipins LA, Sandler RS. Epidemiology of colorectal adenomas. Epidemiol Rev 1994;16:273–297.
10. Trock B, Lanza E, Greenwald P. Dietary fiber, vegetables, and colon cancer: Critical review and meta-analyses of the epidemiologic evidence. J Natl Cancer Inst 1990;82:650–661.
11. Grodstein F, Martinez ME, Platz EA, et al. Postmenopausal hormone use and risk for colorectal cancer and adenoma. Ann Intern Med 1998;128:705–712.
12. Martinez ME, Grodstein F, Giovannucci E, et al. A prospective study of reproductive factors, oral contraceptive use, and risk of colorectal cancer. Cancer Epidemiol Biomarkers Prev 1997;6:1–5.
13. Eckbom A, Helmick C, Zack M, Adami HO. Ulcerative colitis and colorectal cancer: A population-based study. N Engl J Med 1990; 323:1228–1233.
14. Fuchs CS, Giovannucci EL, Colditzs GA, et al. A prospective study of family history and the risk of colorectal cancer. N Engl J Med 1994;331:1669–1674.
15. Lynch HT, Watson P, Smyrk T, et al. Colon cancer genetics. Cancer 1992;70:1300–1312.
16. Rustgi AK. Hereditary gastrointestinal polyposis and nonpolyposis syndromes. N Engl J Med 1994;331:1694–1702.
17. Lynch HT, Smyrk TC, Watson P, et al. Genetics, natural history, tumor spectrum, and pathology of hereditary nonpolyposis colorectal cancer: An updated review. Gastroenterology 1993;104:1535–1549.
18. Hoops TC, Traber PG. Molecular pathogenesis of colorectal cancer. Hematol Oncol Clin North Am 1997;11:609–633.
19. Vogelstein B, Fearon ER, Hamilton SR, et al. Genetic alterations during colorectal-tumor development. N Engl J Med 1988;319:525–532.
20. Fearon ER, Vogelstein B. A genetic model for colorectal tumorigenesis. Cell 1990;61:759–767.
21. Aaltonen LA, Peltomäki P, Leach FS, et al. Clues to the pathogenesis of familial colorectal cancer. Science 1993;260:812–816.
22. Fearon ER, Vogelstein B. A genetic model for colorectal tumorigenesis. Cell 1990;61:759–767.
23. Cho KR, Vogelstein B. Genetic alterations in the adenoma–carcinoma sequence. Cancer 1992;70:1727–1731.
24. Aaltonen LA, Salovaara J, Kristo P, et al. Incidence of hereditary nonpolyposis colorectal cancer and the feasibility of molecular screening for the disease. N Engl J Med 1998;338:1481–1487.
25. Markowitz S, Wang J, Myeroff L, et al. Inactivation of the type II TGF-β receptor in colon cancer cells with microsatellite instability. Science 1995;268:1336–1338.
26. Dukes CE. The classification of cancer of the rectum. J Pathol 1932; 35:323–332.
27. Spratt JS, Spuitt HJ. Prevalence and prognosis of individual clinical and pathological variables associated with colorectal carcinoma. Cancer 1967;20:1976–1985.
28. Cooper GS, Yuan Z, Landefeld CS, et al. A national population-based study of incidence of colorectal cancer and age. Cancer 1995;75: 775–781.
29. Silverman AL, Desai TK, Dhar R, et al. Clinical features, evaluation and detection of colorectal cancer. Gastroenterol Clin North Am 1988; 17:713–725.
30. Kahn MJ, Morrison DG. Chemoprevention for colorectal carcinoma. Hematol Oncol Clin North Am 1997;11:779–794.

31. Howe GR, Bentino E, Castelleto R, et al. Dietary intake of fiber and decreased risk of cancers of the colon and rectum: Evidence from the combined analysis of 13 case-control studies. J Natl Cancer Inst 1992;84:1887–1896.
32. Reddy BS, Engle A, Simi B, et al. Effect of dietary fiber on colonic bacterial enzymes and bile acids in relation to colon cancer. Gastroenterology 1990;50:3595–3599.
33. Meyskins FL, Gerner EW. Development of difluoromethylornithine as a chemoprevention agent for the management of colon cancer. J Cell Biochem 1995;22(suppl):126–131.
34. Stürmer T, Glyn RJ, Lee IM, et al. Aspirin use and colorectal cancer: Post-trial follow-up data from the physician's health study. Ann Intern Med 1998;128:713–720.
35. Giardiello FM, Hamilton SR, Krush AJ, et al. Treatment of colonic and rectal adenomas with sulindac in familial adenomatous polyposis. N Engl J Med 1993;328:1313–1316.
36. Winawer SJ, Zauber AG, Ho MN, et al. Prevention of colorectal cancer by colonoscopic polypectomy. N Engl J Med 1993;329:1977–1981.
37. Cancer Facts and Figures—1998. Atlanta, American Cancer Society, 1998.
38. Burke W, Petersen G, Lynch P, et al. Recommendations for follow-up care of individuals with an inherited predisposition to cancer: I. Hereditary nonpolyposis colon cancer. JAMA 1997;277:915–919.
39. Markowitz AJ, Winawer SJ. Screening and surveillance for colorectal carcinoma. Hematol Oncol Clin North Am 1997;11:579–608.
40. Winawer SJ, Fletcher RH, Miller L, et al. Colorectal cancer screening: Clinical guidelines and rationale. Gastroenterology 1997;112: 594–642.
41. Ransohoff DF, Lang CA. Screening for colorectal cancer with the fecal occult blood test: A background paper. Ann Intern Med 1997;126: 811–822.
42. Mandel JS, Bond JH, Church TR, et al. Reducing mortality from colorectal cancer by screening for fecal occult blood. Minnesota Colon Cancer Control Study [Erratum appears in N Engl J Med 1993;329: 672]. N Engl J Med 1993;328:1365–1371.
43. Ferrante JM. Colorectal cancer screening. Med Clin North Am 1996;80:27–43.
44. Selby JV, Friedman GD, Quesenberry CP, Weiss NS. A case-control study of screening sigmoidoscopy and mortality from colorectal cancer. N Engl J Med 1992;326:653–657.
45. Newcomb PA, Norfleet RG, Storer BE, et al. Screening sigmoidoscopy and colorectal cancer mortality. J Natl Cancer Inst 1992;84: 1572–1575.
46. Sidransky D, Tokino T, Hamilton SR, et al. Identification of *ras* oncogene mutations in the stool of patients with curable colorectal tumors. Science 1992;256:102–105.
47. American Society of Clinical Oncology. Clinical practice guidelines for the use of tumor markers in breast and colorectal cancer. J Clin Oncol 1996;14:2843–2877.
48. Bertagnolli MM, Mahmoud NN, Daly JM. Surgical aspects of colorectal carcinoma. Hematol Oncol Clin North Am 1997;11:655–677.
49. Moertel CG, Fleming TR, Macdonald JS, et al. An evaluation of the carcinoembryonic (CEA) test for monitoring patients with resected colon cancer. JAMA 1993;240:943–947.
50. Cohen A. Preoperative evaluation of patients with primary colorectal cancer. Cancer 1992;70:1328–1332.
51. Moffat FL, Pinsky CM, Hammershaimb L, et al. Clinical utility of external immunoscintigraphy with the IMMU-4 technetium-99m Fab′ antibody fragment in patients undergoing surgery for carcinoma of the colon and rectum: Results of a pivotal, phase III trial. J Clin Oncol 1996;14:2295–2305.
52. Serafini An, Klein JL, Wolff BG, et al. Radioimmunoscintigraphy of recurrent, metastatic, or occult colorectal cancer with technetium 99m-labeled totally human monoclonal antibody 88VB59: Results of pivotal, phase III multicenter studies. J Clin Oncol 1998;16:1777–1787.
53. Kuhn JA, Thomas G. Monoclonal antibodies and colorectal carcinoma: A clinical review of diagnostic applications. Cancer Invest 1994; 12:314–323.
54. Dukes CE. The classification of cancer of the rectum. J Pathol 1932;35:2310–2314.
55. Thompson WM, Trenkner SW. Staging colorectal carcinoma. Radiol Clin North Am 1994;32:25–37.
56. American Joint Committee on Cancer. In: Beahrs OH, Henson D, Hutter RVP, et al, eds. Manual for Staging of Cancer, 4th ed. Philadelphia, Lippincott, 1992.
57. Skibber JM, Curley SA, Lotan R. Colon tumor markers for prognosis and therapy. Cancer Bull 1994;46:331–335.
58. Mohiuddin M, Ahmed MM. Critical issues in the evolving management of rectal cancer. Semin Oncol 1997;24:732–744.
59. Jen J, Kim H, Plantadosi S, et al. Allelic loss of chromosome 18q and prognosis in colorectal cancer. N Engl J Med 1994;331:213–221.
60. Ogunbiyi OA, Goodfellow PJ, Herfarth K, et al. Confirmation that chromosome 18q allelic loss in colon cancer is a prognostic indicator. J Clin Oncol 1998;16:427–433.
61. Yamachika T, Nakanishi H, Tsukamoto T, et al. A new prognostic factor for colorectal carcinoma, thymidylate synthase, and its therapeutic significance. Cancer 1998;82:70–77.
62. Cohen Am, Minsky BD, Schilsky RL. Cancer of the rectum. In: DeVita VT, Hellman S, Rosenberg SA, eds. Cancer: Principles and Practice of Oncology, 5th ed. Philadelphia, Lippincott, 1997:1197–1234.
63. NCCN Colorectal Cancer Practice Guidelines. Oncology 1996; 10(suppl 11):140–170.
64. Minsky BD. The role of adjuvant radiation therapy in the treatment of colorectal cancer. Hematol Clin North Am 1997;11:679–697.
65. Meropol NJ, Creaven PH, Petrelli NJ. Metastatic colorectal cancer: Advances in biochemical modulation and new drug development. Semin Oncol 1995;22:509–524.
66. Zaniboni A. Adjuvant chemotherapy in colorectal cancer with high-dose leucovorin and fluorouracil: Impact on disease-free survival and overall survival. J Clin Oncol 1997;15:2432–2441.
67. Peters GJ, van der Wilt CL, van Groeningen CJ, et al. Thymidylate synthase inhibition after administration of fluorouracil with or without leucovorin in colon cancer patients: Implications for treatment with fluorouracil. J Clin Oncol 1994;12:2035–2042.
68. The Meta-Analysis Group in Cancer. Efficacy of intravenous continuous infusion of fluorouracil compared with bolus administration in advanced colorectal cancer. J Clin Oncol 1998;16:301–308.
69. Machover D. A comprehensive review of 5-fluorouracil and leucovorin in patients with metastatic colorectal carcinoma. Cancer 1997; 80:1179–1187.
70. Kemeny N. Current approaches to metastatic colorectal cancer. Semin Oncol 1994;21(suppl 7):67–75.
71. Stevenson HC, Green I, Hamilton JM, et al. Levamisole: known effects on the immune system, clinical results and future applications to the treatment of cancer. J Clin Oncol 1991;9:2052–2066.
72. Kovach JS, Svingen PA, Schaid DJ. Levamisole potentiation of fluorouracil antiproliferative activity mimicked by orthovanadate, an inhibitor of tyrosine phosphatase. J Natl Cancer Inst 1992;84:515–519.
73. Moertel CG, Fleming TR, Macdonald JS, et al. Fluorouracil plus levamisole as effective adjuvant therapy after resection of stage III colon carcinoma: A final report. Ann Intern Med 1995;122:321–326.
74. Vaughn DJ, Haller DG. The role of adjuvant chemotherapy in the treatment of colorectal cancer. Hemotol Clin North Am 1997;11:699–719.
75. Petrelli N, Douglass HO, Herrera L, et al. The modulation of fluorouracil with leucovorin in metastatic colorectal carcinoma: A prospective randomized phase III trial. J Clin Oncol 1989;7:1419–1426.
76. Poon MA, O'Connell MJ, Moertel CG, et al. Biochemical modulation of fluorouracil: Evidence of significant improvement of survival and quality of life in patients with advanced colorectal carcinoma. J Clin Oncol 1989;7:1407–1418.
77. Wolmark N, Rockette H, Fisher B, et al. The benefit of leucovorin-modulated fluorouracil as postoperative adjuvant therapy for primary

colon cancer: Results from National Surgical Adjuvant Breast and Bowel Project Protocol C-03. J Clin Oncol 1993;11:1879–1887.

78. International Multicentre Pooled Analysis of Colon Cancer Trials (IMPACT) Investigators. Efficacy of adjuvant fluorouracil and folinic acid in colon cancer. Lancet 1995;345:939–944.
79. Gerstner J, O'Connell MJ, Wieand HS, et al. A prospectively randomized clinical trial comparing 5-FU combined with either high or low dose leucovorin for the treatment of advanced colorectal cancer. Proc Am Soc Clin Oncol 1991;10:134.
80. O'Reilly S, Rowinsky EK. Experimental chemotherapeutic agents for the treatment of colorectal carcinoma. Hematol Clin North Am 1997;11:721–758.
81. Rothenberg ML, Eckardt JR, Kuhn JG, et al. Phase II trial of irinotecan in patients with progressive or rapidly recurrent colorectal cancer. J Clin Oncol 1996;14:1128–1135.
82. Conti JA, Kemeny NE, Saltz LB, et al. Irinotecan is an active agent in untreated patients with metastatic colorectal cancer. J Clin Oncol 1996;14:709–715.
83. Cunningham D, Pyrhönen S, James RD, et al. Randomized trial of irontecan plus supportive care versus supportive care alone after fluorouracil failure for patients with metastatic colorectal cancer. Lancet 1998;352:1413–1418.
84. Rougier, Van Cutsem Bajetta E, et al. Randomized trial of irinotecan versus fluorouracil by continuous infusion after fluorouracil failure in patients with metastatic colorectal cancer. Lancet 1998;352:1407–1412.
85. Rougier P, Douillard JY, Culine S, et al. Phase II study of irinotecan in the treatment of advanced colorectal cancer in chemotherapy-naive patients and patients pretreated with fluorouracil-based chemotherapy. J Clin Oncol 1997;15:251–260.
86. Milano G, Fischel JL, Etiennne MC, et al. Inhibition of dihydropyrimidine dehydrogenase by α-interferon: Experimental data on human tumor cell lines. Cancer Chemother Parmacol 1994;34:147–152.
87. Advanced Colorectal Cancer Meta-Analysis Project. Meta-analysis of randomized trials testing the biochemical modulation of fluorouracil by methotrexate in metastatic colorectal cancer. J Clin Oncol 1994; 12:960–969.
88. Blanke CD, Kasimis B, Schein P, et al. Phase II study of trimetrexate, fluorouracil, and leucovorin for advanced colorectal cancer. J Clin Oncol 1997;15:915–920.
89. Kemeny N, Seiter K, Martin D, et al. A new syndrome: Ascites, hyperbilirubinemia, and hypoalbuminemia after biochemical modulation of fluorouracil with *N*-phosphoacetyl-*L*-aspartate (PALA). Ann Intern Med 1991;115:946–951.
90. National Institutes of Health Consensus Development Conference. Adjuvant therapy for patients with colon and rectal cancer. JAMA 1990;264:1444–1450.
91. Buyse M, Zeleniuch-Jacquotte A, Chalmers TC. Adjuvant therapy of colorectal cancer—Why we still don't know. JAMA 1988;259:3571–3578.
92. Laurie JA, Moertel CG, Fleming TR, et al. Surgical adjuvant therapy of large bowel carcinoma: An evaluation of levamisole and combination of levamisole and 5-fluorouracil. J Clin Oncol 1989;7:1447– 1456.
93. Moertel CG. Chemotherapy for colorectal cancer. N Engl J Med 1994;330:1136–1142.
94. Brown ML, Nayfield SG, Shibley LM. Adjuvant therapy for stage III colon cancer: Economics returns to research and cost-effectiveness of treatment. J Natl Cancer Inst 1994;86:424–430.
95. Moertel CG, Fleming TR, Macdonald JS, et al. Intergroup study of fluorouracil plus levamisole as adjuvant therapy for stage II/Dukes' B2 colon cancer. J Clin Oncol 1995;13:2936–2943.
96. Mamounas EP, Rockette H, Jones J, et al. Comparative efficacy of adjuvant chemotherapy in patients with Dukes' B vs. Dukes' C colon cancer: Results from four NSABP adjuvant studies (C01, C02, C03, C04). Proc Am Soc Clin Oncol 1996;15:205.
97. O'Connell MJ, Mailliard J, Kahn MJ, et al. Controlled trial of fluorouracil and low dose leucovorin given for 6 months as postoperative adjuvant therapy for colon cancer. J Clin Oncol 1997;15:246–250.
98. Wolmark N, Rockette H, Mamounas EP, et al. The relative efficacy of 5-FU + leucovorin (FU-LV) + levamisole (FU-LEV), and 5-FU + leucovorin + levamisole (FU-LV-LEV) in patients with Dukes' B and C carcinoma of the colon: First report of NSABP C-04. Proc Am Soc Clin Oncol 1996;15:205.
99. O'Connell MJ, Laurie JA, Kahn M, et al. Prospectively randomized trial of postoperative adjuvant chemotherapy in patients with high-risk colon cancer. J Clin Oncol 1998;16:295–300.
100. Haller DG, Catalano PJ, Macdonald JS, et al. Fluorouracil (FU), leucovorin (LV) and levamisole (LEV) adjuvant therapy for colon cancer: Four year results of INT-0089. Proc Am Soc Clin Oncol 1997; 16:265.
101. Zalcberg J, Cunningham D, Rath U, et al. Modulated 5-FU: Female gender and increasing age are associated with significantly more grade 3 or 4 leukopenia and mucositis. Proc Am Soc Clin Oncol 1996; 15:201.
102. Weinerman B. Increased incidence of toxicity in elderly females treated with 5FU, leucovorin. Proc Am Soc Clin Oncol 1996;15:225.
103. Grem JL, Robson ME, Binder RA, et al. Phase II study of fluorouracil, leucovorin, and interferon alfa-2a in metastatic colorectal carcinoma. J Clin Oncol 1993;11:1737–1745.
104. Taylor I, Machin D, Mullee M, et al. A randomized controlled trial of adjuvant portal vein cytotoxic perfusion in colorectal cancer. Br J Surg 1985;72:359–363.
105. Wolmark N, Rockette H, Petrelli N, et al. Long-term results of the efficacy of perioperative portal vein infusion of 5-FU for treatment of colon cancer: NSABP C-02. Proc Am Soc Clin Oncol 1994;13: 194.
106. Piedbois P, Buyse M, Gray R, et al. Portal vein infusion is an effective adjuvant treatment for patients with colorectal cancer. Proc Am Soc Clin Oncol 1995;14:192.
107. Eck SL. Future directions for the treatment of colorectal cancer. Hematol Clin North Am 1997;11:795–810.
108. Riethmüller G, Holz E, Schlimok G, et al. Monoclonal antibody therapy of Dukes' C colorectal carcinoma: Seven-year outcome of a multicenter randomized trial. J Clin Oncol 1998;16:1788–1794.
109. Medical Research Council Rectal Cancer Working Party. Randomised trial of surgery alone versus radiotherapy followed by surgery for potentially operable locally advanced rectal cancer. Lancet 1996;348: 1605–1610.
110. Medical Research Council Rectal Cancer Working Party. Randomised trial of surgery alone versus surgery followed by radiotherapy for mobile cancer of the rectum. Lancet 1996;348:1610–1614.
111. Swedish Cancer Rectal Trial. Improved survival with preoperative radiotherapy in resectable rectal cancer. N Engl J Med 1997;336: 980–987.
112. Swedish Cancer Rectal Trial. Correction to improved survival with preoperative radiotherapy in resectable rectal cancer. N Engl J Med 1997;336:1539.
113. Gastrointestinal Tumor Study Group. Prolongation of the disease-free interval in surgically treated rectal carcinoma. N Engl J Med 1985;312:1465–1472.
114. Krook JE, Moertel CG, Gunderson LL, et al. Effective surgical adjuvant therapy for high-risk rectal carcinoma. N Engl J Med 1991;324: 709–715.
115. Douglass HO, Moertel CG, Mayer RJ, et al. Survival after postoperative combination treatment of rectal cancer. N Engl J Med 1986; 315:1294–1295.
116. O'Connell MJ, Martenson JA, Wieand HS, et al. Improving adjuvant therapy for rectal cancer by combining protracted infusion fluorouracil with radiation therapy after curative surgery. N Engl J Med 1994;331:502–507.
117. Tepper JE, O'Connell MJ, Petroni GR, et al. Adjuvant postoperative fluorouracil-modulated chemotherapy combined with pelvic radiation therapy for rectal cancer: Initial results of Intergroup 0114. J Clin Oncol 1997;15:2030–2039.
118. Rockette H, Deutsch M, Petrelli N, et al. Effect of postoperative radiation therapy (RTX) when used with adjuvant chemotherapy in

Dukes' B and C rectal cancer: Results from the NSABP R-02. Proc Am Soc Clin Oncol 1994;13:193.
119. VanderMeer TJ, Callery MP, Meyers WC. The approach to the patient with single and multiple liver metastases, pulmonary metastases, and intra-abdominal metastases from colorectal carcinoma. Hematol Clin North Am 1997;11:721–758.
120. Busch E, Kemeny MM. Colorectal cancer: Hepatic-directed therapy—The role of surgery, regional chemotherapy, and novel modalities. Semin Oncol 1995;22:494–508.
121. Girard P, Ducreux M, Baldeyrou P, et al. Surgery for lung metastases from colorectal cancer: Analysis of prognostic factors. J Clin Oncol 1996;14:2047–2053.
122. Leichman CG. Prolonged infusion of fluorinated pyrimidines in gastrointestinal malignancies: A review of recent clinical trials. Cancer Invest 1994;12:166–175.
123. Vaughn DJ, Haller DG. Nonsurgical management of recurrent colorectal cancer. Cancer 1993;71:4278–4292.
124. Poon MA, O'Connell MJ, Wieand HS, et al. Biochemical modulation of fluorouracil with leucovorin: Confirmatory evidence of improved therapeutic efficacy in advanced colorectal cancer. J Clin Oncol 1991;9:1967–1972.
125. Advanced Colorectal Cancer Meta-Analysis Project. Modulation of fluorouracil by leucovorin in patients with advanced colorectal cancer: Evidence in terms of response rate. J Clin Oncol 1992;10:896–903.
126. Corfu-A Study Group. Phase III randomized study of two fluorouracil combinations with either interferon alfa-2a or leucovorin for advanced colorectal cancer. J Clin Oncol 1995;13:921–928.
127. Hill M, Norman A, Cunningham D, et al. Royal Marsden phase III trial of fluorouracil with or without interferon alfa-2b in advanced colorectal cancer. J Clin Oncol 1995;13:1297–1302.
128. Blanke CD, Messenger M, Taplin SC. Trimetrexate: A review and current clinical experience in advanced colorectal cancer. Semin Oncol 1997;24(5 suppl 18):57–63.
129. Conti JA, Kemeny NE, Saltz LB, et al. Continuous infusion fluorouracil/leucovorin and bolus mitomycin-C as a salvage regimen for patients with advanced colorectal cancer. Cancer 1995;75:769–774.
130. Rustum YM, Harstrick A, Cao S, et al. Thymidylate synthase inhibitors in cancer therapy: Direct and indirect inhibitors. J Clin Oncol 1997;15:389–400.
131. Seitz JF, Cunningham D, Rath U, et al. Final results and survival data of a large randomised trial of tomudex in advanced colorectal cancer confirm comparable efficacy to 5-fluorouracil and leucovorin (5-FU + LV). Proc Am Soc Clin Oncol 1996;15:201.
132. Harper P. Tomudex study group. Advanced colorectal cancer (ACC): Results from the latest raltitrexed "Tomudex" comparative study. Proc Am Soc Clin Oncol 1997;16:228a.
133. Pazdur R, Vincent M. Raltitrexed (Tomudex) versus 5-fluorouracil and leucovorin (5-FU + LV) in patients with advanced colorectal cancer (ACC): Results of a randomized, multicenter, North American trial. Proc Am Soc Clin Oncol 1997;16:228a.
134. Findlay M, Van Cutsem E, Kocha W, et al. A randomized phase II study of Xeloda (capecitabine) in patients with advanced colorectal cancer. Proc Am Soc Clin Oncol 1997;16:227a.
135. Ishikawa T, Sawada N, Sekiguchi F, et al. Xeloda (capecitabine), a new oral fluoropyrimidine carbamate with an improved efficacy profile over other fluoropyrimidines. Proc Am Soc Clin Oncol 1997; 1997;16:226a.
136. Ota K, Taguchi T, Kimura K. Report on nationwide pooled data and cohort investigation in UFT phase II study. Cancer Chemother Pharmacol 1988;22:333–338.
137. Pazdur R, Lassere Y, Rhodes V, et al. Phase II trial of uracil and tegafur plus oral leucovorin: An effective oral regiment in the treatment of metastatic colorectal carcinoma. J Clin Oncol 1994;12:2296–2300.
138. Saltz LB, Leichman CG, Young CW, et al. A fixed-ratio combination of uracil and ftorafur (UFT) with low does leucovorin: An active oral regimen for advanced colorectal cancer. Cancer 1995;75:782–785.
139. Baker SD, Khor SP, Adjei AA, et al. Pharmacokinetic, oral bioavailability, and safety study of fluorouracil in patients treated with 776C85, an inactivator of dihydropyrimidine dehydrogenase. J Clin Oncol 1996;14:3085–3096.
140. Schilsky R, Bukowsky R, Burris H, et al. A phase II study of a five day regimen of oral fluorouracil (5-FU) plus GW776 (776C85) with or without leucovorin (LV) in patients with metastatic colorectal cancer. Proc Am Soc Clin Oncol 1997;16:271a.
141. Baker SD, Diasio R, Lucas VS, et al. Phase I and pharmacologic study of oral 5-fluorouracil on a chronic 28-day schedule in combination with the dihydropyrimidine dehydrogenase inactivator 776C85. Proc Am Soc Clin Oncol 1996;15:486.
142. Schilsky RL, Burris H, Ratain M, et al. Phase I clinical and pharmacologic study of 776C85 plus fluorouracil in patients with advanced colorectal cancer. Proc Am Soc Clin Oncol 1996;15:485.
143. Peters GJ, Van Groeningen CJ, Schomage JH, et al. Phase I clinical and pharmacokinetic study of S-1, an oral 5-fluorouracil (5-FU)-based antineoplastic agent. Proc Am Soc Clin Oncol 1997;16:227a.
144. Matei C, Hoff PM, Brito R, et al. Phase I trial of BOF-A2 plus leucovorin in advanced colorectal cancer (CRC): Antitumor activity in fluorouracil-resistant patients. Proc Am Soc Clin Oncol 1998;17:230a.
145. Soulie P, Raymond E, Misset JL, et al. Oxaliplatin: Update on an active and safe DACH platinum complex. Platinum and other metal coordination compounds. Cancer Chemother 1996;165–174.
146. Lévi F, Zidani R, Vannetzel JM, et al. Chronomodulated versus fixed-infusion rate-delivery of ambulatory chemotherapy with oxaliplatin, fluorouracil, and folinic acid (leucovorin) in patients with colorectal cancer metastases: A randomized multi-institutional trial. J Natl Cancer Inst 1994;86:1608–1617.
147. Bertheault-Cvitkovic F, Jami A, et al. Biweekly intensified ambulatory chronomodulated chemotherapy with oxaliplatin, fluorouracil, and leucovorin in patients with metastatic colorectal cancer. J Clin Oncol 1996;14:2950–2958.
148. Lévi F, Misset JL, Brienze S, et al. A chronopharmacologic phase II clinical trial with 5-fluorouracil, folinic acid, and oxaliplatin using an ambulatory multichannel programmable pump. High antitumor effectiveness against metastatic colorectal cancer. Cancer 1992;69: 893–900.
149. Lévi F, Dogliotti L, Perpoint B, et al. A multicentre phase II trial of intensified chronotherapy with oxaliplatin (L-OHP), 5-fluorouracil, and folinic acid (FA) in patients with previously untreated metastatic colorectal cancer (MCC). Proc Am Soc Clin Oncol 1997;16:266a.
150. Zeng ZS, Huang Y, Cohen AM, et al. Prediction of colorectal cancer relapse and survival via tissue RNA levels of matrix metalloproteinase-9. J Clin Oncol 1996;14:3133–3140.
151. Rasmussen HS, McCann PP. Matrix metalloproteinase inhibition as a novel anticancer strategy: A review with special focus on batimastat and marimastat. Pharmacol Ther 1997;75:69–75.
152. Soulen MC. Chemoembolization of hepatic malignancies. Oncology 1994;8:77–84.
153. Tellez C, Benson AB, Lyster MT, et al. Phase II trial of chemoembolization for the treatment of metastatic colorectal carcinoma to the liver and review of the literature. Cancer 1998;82:1250–1259.
154. Steele G. Standard postoperative monitoring of patients after primary resection of colon and rectum cancer. Cancer 1993;71:4225–4235.
155. Markowitz AJ, Winawer SJ. Screening and surveillance for colorectal carcinoma. Hematol Oncol Clin North Am 1997;11:579–608.
156. Nordic Gastrointestinal Tumor Adjuvant Therapy Group. Expectancy or primary chemotherapy in patients with advanced asymptomatic colorectal cancer: A randomized trial. J Clin Oncol 1992;10:904–911.
157. Stotland BR, Siegelman ES, Morris JB, et al. Preoperative and postoperative imaging for colorectal cancer. Hematol Oncol North Am 1997;11:635–654.
158. Johnston PG, Fisher ER, Rocketter HE, et al. The role of thymidylate synthase expression in prognosis and outcome of adjuvant chemotherapy in patients with rectal cancer. J Clin Oncol 1994;12:2640–2647.

119

PROSTATE CANCER

Jill M. Kolesar, PharmD, BCPS, and Barry R. Goldspiel, PharmD, BCPS, FASHP

Prostate cancer is the most frequent cancer among American men and represents the second leading cause of cancer-related deaths in all males.[1] In the United States alone, it is estimated that 184,500 new cases of prostatic carcinoma will be diagnosed and more than 39,200 men will die from this disease in 1998.[1] Although prostate cancer incidence increased during the late 1980s and early 1990s owing to widespread prostate specific antigen (PSA) screening, recent data suggest a continuing decline in prostate cancer incidence.[1]

Localized prostate cancer can be cured by surgery or radiation therapy; however, advanced prostate cancer is not yet curable. Treatment for advanced prostate cancer can provide significant disease palliation for many patients for several years after diagnosis. The endocrine dependence of this tumor is well documented, and hormonal manipulation to decrease circulating androgens remains the basis for the treatment of advanced disease.

EPIDEMIOLOGY AND ETIOLOGY

Table 119–1 summarizes the possible factors associated with prostate cancer.[2–4] The only widely accepted risk factors for prostate cancer are age, race–ethnicity, and family history of prostate cancer.[3] The disease is rare under the age of 40, but the incidence sharply increases with each subsequent decade.[3] The incidence of clinical prostate cancer varies across geographic regions. Scandinavian countries and the United States report the highest incidence of prostate cancer, whereas in Japan and other Asian countries the disease is relatively rare.[5] African-American men have the highest rate of prostate cancer in the world, and in the United States, overall 5-year survival is approximately 15% less for African-Americans compared to Caucasians.[1] Both hormonal and genetic differences may contribute to the altered susceptibility to prostate cancer in these populations.[3] Testosterone, commonly implicated in the pathogenesis of prostate cancer, is 15% higher in African-American men when compared to Caucasian males. Additionally, African-American men may be exposed to higher levels of estrogen and testosterone in utero. Activity of 5-α-reductase, the enzyme that converts testosterone to its more active form, dihydrotestosterone (DHT), in the prostate, is decreased in Japanese men compared to African-Americans and Caucasians.[3]

In addition to hormonal differences, genetic variations in the androgen receptor exist. Activation of the androgen receptor is inversely correlated to CAG repeat length. Shorter CAG repeat sequences have been found in African-Americans; this may in part account for the increased risk of prostate cancer for African-American men.[3]

A positive family history for prostate cancer is associated with a two- to threefold risk elevation. Three other factors, the age of the man at risk, the age of the affected relative, and the number of relatives diagnosed with prostate cancer, modify the magnitude of the excess risk. In general, younger age (< 65) of the man at risk, younger age of affected relatives, and increased number of relatives with prostate cancer increase the risk of prostate cancer beyond two- to threefold.[3] Carter and colleagues[2] have demonstrated that familial clustering of prostate cancer can be explained by Mendelian inheritance of a rare, autosomal dominant allele, which accounts for 9% of all prostate cancer and 45% of disease reported in men under the age of 55.[2] A genomewide scan has identified a major prostate cancer susceptibility locus on chromosome 1.[6]

Other factors thought to be associated with prostate cancer include occupational exposure, diet, benign prostatic hyperplasia (BPH), and vasectomy.[3] Workers exposed to alkaline batteries come into contact with cadmium, a trace mineral that may be antagonistic to zinc. Zinc is found in very high levels in the prostate and is required in several enzymes involved in DNA and RNA repair and synthesis. Farm and rubber-industry workers may also be at increased risk for prostate cancer.

A number of epidemiologic studies support an association between high fat intake and risk of prostate cancer. A strong correlation between national per capita fat consumption and national prostate cancer mortality has been reported, and prospective case-control studies suggest that a high-fat diet doubles the risk of prostate cancer.

Other dietary factors implicated in prostate cancer include retinol, carotenoids, and vitamin D consumption.[3] Retinol, or vitamin A, intake, especially in men older than 70, is correlated with an increased risk of prostate cancer, whereas intake of its precursor, β-carotene, has a protective effect. The antioxidant vitamin E may also decrease the risk of prostate cancer. Men who developed prostate cancer in one cohort study had lower levels of 1,25(OH)$_2$-vitamin D than matched controls, although a prospective study did not support this.[3] Clearly, dietary risk factors require further evaluation, but because fat and vitamins are modifiable risk factors, dietary intervention may be promising in prostate cancer prevention.

Vasectomy has emerged as a possible risk factor for prostate cancer.[7,8] A number of case-control studies have shown an increased incidence of prostate cancer in men

TABLE 119–1. Risk Factors Associated With Prostate Cancer

Factor	Possible Relationship
Probable Risk Factors	
Age	Median incidence in men greater than 50 years old
Race	African-Americans have higher incidence and death rate
Genetic	Familial prostate cancer inherited in an autosomal dominant manner
	Mutations in *p53*, Rb, E-cahedrin, α-catenin, androgen receptor, KIA1, microsatellite instability, loss of heterozygocity at 10q, 16q, 8p, and 17p
	Candidate prostate cancer gene locus identfied on chromosome 1
Possible Risk Factors	
Environmental	Clinical carcinoma incidence varies worldwide
	Latent carcinoma similar between regions
	Nationalized males adopt intermediate incidence rates between that of the United States and their native country
Occupational	Increased risk associated with cadmium exposure
Diet	Increased risk associated with high-meat and -fat diets
	Decreased intake of 1,25-dihydroxyvitamin D, vitamin E, and β-carotene increases risk
Hormonal	Does not occur in eunuchs
	Low incidence in cirrhotic patients
	Up to 80% are hormonally dependent
	African-Americans have 15% increased testosterone
	Japanese have decreased 5-α-reductase activities
	Polymorphic expression of the androgen receptor
Vasectomy	Relative risk: 1.56–1.85

Compiled from Ref. 9.

who have had vasectomies, although similarly designed studies have also shown no association. A prospective cohort study of U.S. health professionals reported an age-adjusted relative risk of 1.56 in men with recent vasectomies and a relative risk of 1.85 in men who had vasectomies more than 20 years ago.[7] Although the relationship between vasectomy and prostate cancer is not definitive, further evaluation appears warranted because of the large number of vasectomies that are performed annually. The precise relationship between benign prostatic hyperplasia and prostate carcinoma is unclear, although some evidence suggests a 5.1 to 11.5 times higher incidence.[9]

Smoking has not been associated with an increased risk of prostate cancer; however, smokers with prostate cancer have an increased mortality resulting from the disease when compared to nonsmokers with prostate cancer (relative risk 1.5 to 2.0).[3]

PATHOPHYSIOLOGY

MOLECULAR GENETICS

E-cadherin gene inactivation via hypermethylation has been reported frequently in prostate cancer.[4] E-cadherin is a prognostic marker in prostate cancer, with aberrant E-cadherin expression associated with high-grade tumors and poor outcome in terms of disease progression and overall survival.[4] P-cadherin expression is absent in most prostate cancers; however, in prostate cancers where P-cadherin is expressed, PSA is characteristically absent.[10] The cadherin–catenin pathway may be inactivated by gene mutations or hypermethylation and is thought to be an early event in prostate carcinogenesis.

In cells with DNA damage, *p*53 is thought to function by halting cell-cycle progression, resulting in cell death via apoptotic pathways. The loss of functional *p*53 may result in replication of damaged DNA and subsequently unregulated cell growth. Point mutations in *p*53 thought to be caused by environmental toxins have been identified in 42% of prostate carcinomas. Mutations were present in stages B to D, although not in latent prostate carcinomas studied.[11] Rb mutations, also thought to be important in cell-cycle regulation, have been reported in prostate cancer patients.[4] Abnormal *p*53 and Rb, as measured by immunohistochemistry, may be independent predictors of survival. In one study,[12] 15-year survival was 38% in patients with abnormal *p*53 compared to 87% for those with normal *p*53.

KAI1, or Kang ai, which is Chinese for anticancer, is an antimetastatic gene. The gene codes for a protein belonging to a family of leukocyte surface glycoproteins that function in cell–cell interactions and cell–extracellular matrix interactions and that is downregulated, without mutation, during the progression of prostate cancer.[13]

Mutations in the androgen receptor gene, altering the hormone-binding activity, have been reported in metastatic androgen-independent prostate cancer.[14] Mutated androgen receptors are activated not only by testicular androgens but also by several androgens, steroids, and nonsteroidal antiandrogens. Androgen receptor mutations are speculated to explain the antiandrogen withdrawal syndrome.[15]

A significant number of latent prostatic carcinomas in Japanese men contain an inactivating mutation in the androgen receptor, whereas no such mutations were found in latent carcinomas of white American men.[16] It appears that the stage in which an androgen receptor mutation occurs (latent vs metastatic), as well as the functional significance of the mutation, can alter the clinical course of prostate cancer. Additional genetic analysis has identified mutations in H-*ras* in less than 4% of American prostate carcinomas and up to 25% of Japanese carcinomas. Mutations in late stage clinical carcinoma were identified in Ha-*ras*; however, latent prostate carcinoma had mutations in K-*ras*, possibly indicating a protective mutation.[4]

Although the molecular characterization of prostate cancer is evolving, this area of study represents a major advance in our understanding of disease pathology and may represent future avenues for diagnosis, staging, and treatment of prostate cancer.

RATIONALE FOR HORMONAL MANAGEMENT

The prostate gland is a solid, rounded, heart-shaped organ positioned between the neck of the bladder and the urogenital diaphragm (Fig. 119–1). The organ consists of single anterior, posterior, and median lobes with two lateral lobes. The posterior lobe is palpable by anterior rectal examination at 2 to 5 cm from the anal verge. Within the four morphologically defined areas of the prostate gland, 95% of the carcinomas arise from the glandular epithelium of the peripheral zone.[17] In contrast, benign prostatic hyperplasia arises from the central or periurethral regions of the prostate gland.

Normal growth and differentiation of the prostate depends on the presence of androgens, specifically DHT.[18] The testes and the adrenal glands are the major sources of circulating androgens. Hormonal regulation of androgen synthesis is mediated through a series of biochemical interactions between the hypothalamus, pituitary, adrenal glands, and testes (Fig. 119–2). Luteinizing hormone–releasing hormone (LH-RH) released from the hypothalamus stimulates the release of luteinizing hormone (LH) and follicle-stimulating hormone (FSH) from the anterior pituitary gland. Luteinizing hormone complexes with receptors on the Leydig cell testicular membrane and stimulates the production of testosterone and small amounts of estrogen. FSH acts on the Sertoli cells within the testes to promote the maturation of LH receptors and to produce an androgen-binding protein. Circulating testosterone and estradiol influence the synthesis of LH-RH, LH, and FSH by a negative-feedback loop operating at the hypothalamic and pituitary level.[18,19] Prolactin, growth hormone, and estradiol appear to be important accessory regulators for prostatic tissue permeability, receptor binding, and testosterone synthesis. However, a precise relationship between these hormones and prostate growth has not been defined.[18]

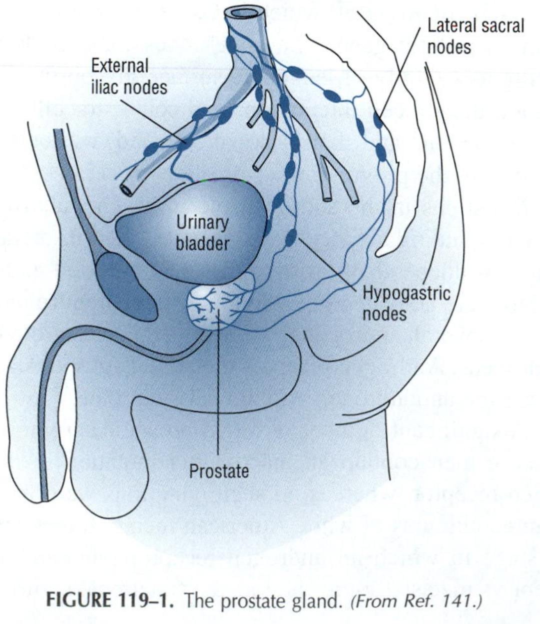

FIGURE 119–1. The prostate gland. *(From Ref. 141.)*

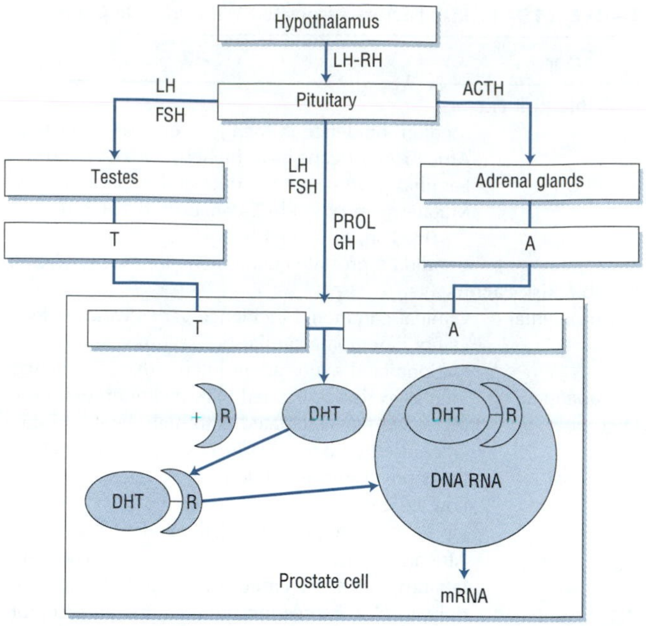

FIGURE 119–2. Hormonal regulation of the prostate gland. LH-RH = luteinizing hormone–releasing hormone; LH = luteinizing hormone; FSH = follicle-stimulating hormone; PROL = prolactin; ACTH = adrenocorticotropic hormone; GH = growth hormone; A = androgens; T = testosterone; R = receptor; DHT = dihydrotestosterone.

Testosterone, the major androgenic hormone, accounts for 95% of the androgen concentration. The primary source of testosterone is the testes; however, 3% to 5% of the testosterone concentration is derived from direct adrenal cortical secretion of testosterone or C19 steroids such as androstenedione.[18,20]

Only 2% of total plasma testosterone is present in the physiologically active unbound state. The remaining testosterone is reversibly bound to a steroid hormone–binding globulin. The unbound testosterone or androgen precursors penetrate the prostatic cell by passive diffusion and are converted to DHT by 5-α-reductase.[21] DHT subsequently binds with a specific cytoplasmic receptor. This DHT–receptor complex is then transported to the nucleus of the cell, where transcription and ultimately translation of stored genetic material occurs.[18]

Huggins and Hodges[22] observed that both normal and malignant prostatic tissue contains a high level of acid phosphatase, suggesting that prostatic malignancy represents an overgrowth of prostate tissue. They then demonstrated that a decrease in serum acid phosphatase along with symptomatic relief occurred in patients with metastatic prostate cancer treated with either estrogens or orchiectomy therapies known to reduce circulating androgens.[22] Androgen ablation is used in the treatment and palliation of advanced prostate cancer because prostatic epithelium undergoes atrophy when the normal physiologic effect of androgens is reduced.[19]

Hormonal manipulations to ablate or reduce circulating androgens can occur through several mechanisms[19,23,24] (Table 119–2). The organs responsible for androgen production can be surgically removed (orchiectomy, hypophysectomy, adrenalectomy). Hormonal pathways that modulate prostatic growth can be interrupted at several steps (see Fig. 119–2). Interference with LH-RH or LH can reduce testosterone secretion by the testes (estrogens, LH-RH agonists, progestogens, and cyproterone acetate). Estrogen administration reduces androgens by directly inhibiting LH release, by acting directly on the prostate cell, or by decreasing free androgens by increasing steroid-binding globulin levels.[19]

The isolation of the naturally occurring hypothalamic decapeptide hormone, gonadotropin hormone–releasing hormone, or LH-RH has provided another group of effective agents for advanced prostate cancer treatment.[23–25] The physiologic response to LH-RH depends on both the dose and the mode of administration. Intermittent pulsed LH-RH administration, which mimics the endogenous release pattern, causes sustained release of both LH and FSH, whereas high-dose or continuous intravenous administration of LH-RH inhibits gonadotropin release due to receptor downregulation.[25] Structural modification of the naturally occurring LH-RH and innovative delivery has produced a series of LH-RH agonists that cause a similar downregulation of pituitary receptors and a decrease in testosterone production.[23–25]

Androgen synthesis can be inhibited in the testes or in the adrenal gland. Aminoglutethimide inhibits the desmolase–enzyme complex in the adrenal gland, thereby preventing the conversion of cholesterol to pregnenolone. Pregnenolone is the precursor substrate for all adrenal-derived steroids including androgens, glucocorticoids, and mineralocorticoids.[26] Ketoconazole, an imidazole antifungal agent, causes a dose-related, reversible reduction in serum cortisol and testosterone concentration by inhibiting both adrenal and testicular steroidogenesis.[27] As a secondary mechanism to its antiandrogen action, megestrol acetate inhibits the synthesis of androgens. This inhibition appears to occur at the adrenal level, but circulating levels of testosterone also are reduced, suggesting that inhibition at the testicular level also may occur.[28]

Antiandrogens inhibit the formation of the DHT–receptor complex and thereby interfere with androgen-mediated action at the cellular level.[29–31] Megestrol acetate, a progestational agent, also is available and has antiandrogen actions.[28] Finally, the conversion of testosterone to DHT may be inhibited by 5-α-reductase inhibitors.[32]

TABLE 119–2. Hormonal Manipulations in Prostate Cancer

Androgen source ablation	Antiandrogens
Orchiectomy	Flutamide
Adrenalectomy	Bicalutamide
Hypophysectomy	Nilutamide
LH-RH or LH inhibition	Cyproterone acetate[b]
Estrogens	Progestogens
LH-RH agonists	5-α-Reductase inhibition
Progestogens[a]	Finasteride[b]
Cyproterone acetate[b]	
Androgen synthesis inhibition	
Aminoglutethimide	
Ketoconazole	
Progestogens[a]	

[a]Minor mechanisms of action.
[b]Investigational compounds or use.

PATHOLOGY

The normal prostate is composed of acinar secretory cells arranged in a radial shape and surrounded by a foundation of supporting tissue. The size, shape, or presence of acini is almost always altered in the gland that has been invaded by prostatic carcinoma. Adenocarcinoma, the major pathologic cell type, accounts for more than 95% of prostate cancer cases.[33] Much rarer tumor types include small-cell neuroendocrine cancers, sarcomas, and transitional-cell carcinomas.

Prostate cancer can be systematically graded according to the histologic appearance of the malignant cell and then grouped into well, moderately, or poorly differentiated grades.[34,35] Gland architecture is examined and then rated on a scale of 1 (well differentiated) to 5 (poorly differentiated). Two different specimens are examined and the score for each specimen is added. Groupings for total Gleason score are 2 to 4 for well differentiated; 5 or 6 for moderately differentiated; and 7 to 10 for poorly differentiated. Poorly differentiated tumors grow rapidly (poor prognosis), whereas well-differentiated tumors grow slowly (better prognosis).

Metastatic spread can occur by local extension, lymphatic drainage, or hematogenous dissemination.[36] Lymph node metastases are more common in patients with large, undifferentiated tumors that invade the seminal vesicles. The pelvic and abdominal lymph node groups are the most common sites of lymph node involvement (see Fig. 119–1). Skeletal metastases from hematogenous spread are the most common sites of distant spread. Typically, the bone lesions are osteoblastic or a combination of osteoblastic and osteolytic. The most common site of bone involvement is the lumbar spine. Other sites of bone involvement include the proximal femurs, pelvis, thoracic spine, ribs, sternum, skull, and humerus. The lung, liver, brain, and adrenal glands are the most common sites of visceral involvement; however, these organs are not usually involved initially. About 25% to 35% of patients will have evidence of lymphangitic or nodular pulmonary infiltrates at autopsy. The prostate is a rare site for metastatic involvement from other solid tumors.

CLINICAL PRESENTATION

Whereas prostatic carcinoma may be asymptomatic in patients with localized disease, most patients with signs and symptoms have advanced disease at presentation. In patients with locally invasive disease, the most common complaints arise from ureteral dysfunction or impingement. Patients complain of alterations in micturation manifested by urinary frequency, hesitancy, and dribbling.[33,36] New-onset impotence or less firm penile erections in an elderly male may indicate prostate cancer.

Most commonly, patients with advanced disease present with back pain and stiffness due to osseous metastases.[37] Eventually, spinal cord lesions may lead to cord compression if not properly treated.[37] Rarely, pathologic fractures can occur. Lower extremity edema can occur as a result of lymphatic obstruction. Anemia and weight loss are nonspecific signs of advanced disease.

SCREENING

For cancer screening to be beneficial, it must reliably and cost effectively detect cancer in an early stage, when intervention would improve patient outcome. Whether prostate cancer screening fits these criteria has generated considerable controversy.[38] Evidence from randomized clinical trials addressing whether screening reduces prostate cancer mortality may not be available for 10 to 15 years. In the interim, clinicians are faced with the dilemma of whether to screen or not to screen, as well as how best to treat early-stage prostate cancer.

DIGITAL RECTAL EXAMINATION

Digital rectal examination (DRE) has been recommended since the early 1900s for the detection of prostate cancer. The primary advantage of DRE is its specificity, reported at > 85%, for prostate cancer. Other advantages of DRE include low cost, safety, and ease of performance. However, DRE is relatively insensitive and is subject to interobserver variability. DRE as a single screening method has poor compliance and has had little effect on preventing metastatic prostate cancer in one large case-control study.[39]

PROSTATE-SPECIFIC ANTIGEN

Prostate-specific antigen (PSA) is a prostate-specific glycoprotein produced only in the cytoplasm of benign and malignant prostate cells.[40,41] PSA functions as a serine protease, which liquefies seminal fluid after ejaculation. In addition to its biologic activity, PSA may also enhance cellular growth by its ability to cleave insulin-like growth factor–binding proteins. Cleavage activates insulin-like growth factor (IGF), which can then bind to IGF receptors and stimulate growth in the prostate.[41]

Unlike acid phosphatase, PSA levels are not influenced by ambient conditions or subject to diurnal variation, but are influenced by sedentary conditions. Therefore, it is recommended that all PSA measurements be made on sera collected from ambulatory patients.[41] PSA levels not only rise with prostatic manipulation such as transrectal ultrasound (TRUS) and/or biopsy but remain above normal for several weeks thereafter. PSA has a serum half-life of 2 to 3 days.[41]

PSA is widely used for prostate cancer screening in the United States, with simplicity its major advantage and low specificity its primary limitation. PSA may be elevated in men with acute urinary retention, acute prostatitis, prostatic ischemia, infarction, as well as benign prostatic hyperplasia (BPH), a nearly universal condition in men at risk for prostate cancer. PSA elevations between 4.1 and 10 ng/mL cannot distinguish between BPH and prostate cancer, limiting the utility of PSA alone for the early detection of prostate cancer.[40,41] Additionally, only 38% to 48% of men with clinically significant prostate cancer have a serum PSA outside the reference range.[40]

Neither DRE nor PSA is sensitive or specific enough to be used alone as a screening test.[40] Though the relative predictability of DRE and PSA is similar, the tumors identified by each method are different. Catalona and associates[42] confirmed that the combination of a rectal examination plus PSA determination is a better method of detecting prostate cancer than rectal examination alone.

Efforts to increase PSA specificity include the use of free PSA measurements, age- and race-specific PSA levels, PSA density, and PSA velocity.[40,43] An increase in serum PSA with increasing age in the absence of clinically detectable prostate cancer has been documented by a number of investigators.[40,43] The proposed age-specific PSA reference ranges (upper limit defined by the 95th percentile) for Caucasian and African-American men are provided in Table 119–3.[41,44]

COST EFFECTIVENESS

Prostate cancer screening remains highly controversial because the survival benefits and the associated costs are not well defined.[45] Available cost-utility studies estimate that the cost per crude or quality-adjusted life-year gained

TABLE 119–3. Diagnostic Algorithm for Prostate Cancer

PSA[a]	DRE[b]	Diagnostic Action
≤ Age-specific range[c]	Neg	Annual PSA and DRE
> Age-specific range[c]	Neg	TRUS: Biopsy-visible lesions. Sextant biopsy of remaining prostate, with two cores containing transition zone tissue
Any value	Pos	TRUS: Biopsy-palpable and -visible lesions; sextant biopsy of remaining prostate

[a]Tandem-R or IM_x PSA.
[b]Digital rectal exam.
[c]

	Normal PSA Range (ng/mL)	
Age Range (yr)	Caucasian	African-American
40–49	0–2.5	0–2.0
50–59	0–3.5	0–4.0
60–69	0–4.5	0–4.5
70–79	0–6.5	0–5.5

Compiled from Refs. 41 and 44.

from prostate cancer screening ranges from \$3000 to \$729,000.[45–48] The Polaroid Medical Department conducted a prostate cancer screening program consisting of a DRE and PSA in all male employees over the age of 49. The entire program cost was \$72,130; 12 prostate cancers were discovered, two by abnormal DRE alone, eight by elevated PSA alone, and two by the combination of the two tests. Polaroid concluded that prostate cancer screening was both effective and cost efficient.[49]

CURRENT SCREENING RECOMMENDATIONS

The American Cancer Society (ACS) currently recommends that DRE and PSA be offered annually to men beginning at age 50 years with at least a 10-year life expectancy and to younger men (45 years old) who are considered to be at high risk for prostate cancer development (strong familial predisposition or African-American).[50] The ACS defines an abnormal PSA value to be above 4.0 ng/mL. If both tests are normal, no further diagnostic action is required; however, if either is abnormal, further workup by transrectal ultrasonography (TRUS) is indicated.

Two ongoing national randomized trials will provide important data to help resolve the prostate cancer screening controversies. The first is the PLCO (prostate, lung, colon, and ovarian) trial, which is designed to test the efficacy of prostate cancer screening in 74,000 men age 60 to 74.[39] The second is the Prostate Cancer Intervention Versus Observation (PIVOT) Trial, which is a randomized study comparing radical prostatectomy to expectant management. These trials, when complete, will likely provide key information regarding the costs and benefits of prostate cancer screening and the most appropriate early management.[51]

DIAGNOSIS

Transperianal or transrectal prostate biopsy is necessary to confirm a prostate cancer diagnosis and to grade the tumor specimen. TRUS-guided biopsies of hypoechoic areas may help define extraprostatic extension.[36] For patients with visceral or lytic metastases, these lesions should be biopsied, because this presentation is common for one of the variant histologies (small-cell neuroendocrine) that requires a treatment strategy different than for adenocarcinomas.[52]

Table 119–4 summarizes the diagnostic staging workup. When DRE is performed, prostatic carcinoma is classically characterized by a rock-hard nodule or mass in the gland, whereas in benign prostatic hypertrophy (BPH), the gland is smooth and rubbery. Recent studies have demonstrated that elevated PSA values may predict for pelvic lymph node and bone involvement.[40,41] If these findings are confirmed, it might be possible to avoid some staging tests (pelvic lymph node dissection, bone scans) in some patients.

STAGING

The information obtained from the diagnostic tests is used to stage the patient. There are two commonly recognized staging classification systems (Table 119–5). The formal international classification system (TNM), adopted by the International Union Against Cancer (UICC) in 1974, was updated in 1992 in an effort to provide congruence with the classical American Urologic System (AUS) staging system for prostate cancer.[53] The AUS classification is the most commonly used staging system in the United States (Table 119–5). Patients are assigned to stages A through D and corresponding subcategories based on size of the tumor (T), local or regional extension, presence of involved lymph node groups (N), and presence of metastases (M).[53] Some studies classify patients who have progressed after hormonal therapy as stage D_3.[36,53] Based on National Cancer Database figures from 1993 including over 84,400 prostate cancer diagnoses, 25%, 49%, 15%, and 12% are initially diagnosed as Stage 0 to I, II, III, and IV, respectively.[54] Localized prostate cancer (stages 0 to I and II) was diagnosed more frequently (74% vs 65%) and advanced disease (stages III and IV) was diagnosed less frequently (26% vs 34%) when comparing the 1990 to the 1986 incidence rates.

TABLE 119–4. Diagnostic and Staging Workup for Prostate Cancer

Initial tests	Digital rectal examination (DRE) Prostate-specific antigen (PSA) Transrectal ultrasonagraphy (TRUS) if either DRE positive or PSA elevated Biopsy
Staging tests	Gleason score on biopsy specimen Bone scan Complete blood count Liver function tests Serum phosphatases (acid/alkaline) Excretory urogram Chest x-ray

Additional staging tests (depends on T classification, PSA, and Gleason score)	Skeletal films
	Lymph node evaluation
	  Pelvic CT scan
	  Indium-111-labeled capromab pendedite scan
	  Bipedal lymphangiogram
	Transrectal MRI

PROGNOSIS

The prognosis for patients with prostate cancer depends on the histologic grade, the tumor size, and local extent of the primary tumor.[34,35] The most important prognostic criterion appears to be the histologic grade, because the degree of differentiation ultimately determines the stage of disease. Poorly differentiated tumors are highly associated with both regional lymph node involvement and distant metastases.[34,35] Other prognostic factors that are being explored include DNA content, cell proliferative activity, epidermal growth factor, transforming growth factor-α, EGF receptor, ERBB2 oncogene, *ras* oncogene, RB1 tumor-suppressor gene, and *p*53 tumor-suppressor gene.[55]

TABLE 119–5. Staging and Classification Systems for Prostate Cancer

AUS[a] Stage (A–D)	AJC-UICC[b] Classification (TNM)
A (occult, nonpalpable)	$T_XN_XM_X$ (cannot be assessed)
	$T_0N_0M_0$ (nonpalpable)
A_1: Focal A_2: Diffuse	T_0: Focal or diffuse
B (confined to prostate)	$T_1N_0M_0$, $T_2N_0M_0$
B_1: Single nodule in one lobe, < 1.5 cm	T_1 (Clinically inapparent tumor not palpable or visible by imaging) T_{1a}: Tumor incidental histologic finding in 5% or less of tissue resected T_{1b}: Tumor incidental histologic finding in 5% or more of tissue resected T_{1c}: Tumor identified by needle biopsy (e.g., because of elevated PSA)
B_2: Diffuse involvement of whole gland, > 1.5 cm	T_2: (Tumor confined within the prostate[c]) T_{2a}: Tumor involves half of a lobe or less T_{2b}: Tumor involves more than half a lobe, but not both lobes T_{2c}: Tumor involves both lobes
C (localized to periprostatic area)	$T_3N_0M_0$, $T_4N_0M_0$
C_1: No seminal vesicle involvement, < 70 g	T_3: (Tumor extends through the prostatic capsule[d]) T_{3a}: Unilateral extracapsular extension T_{3b}: Bilateral extracapsular extension T_{3c}: Tumor invades the seminal vesicle(s)
C_2: Seminal vesicle involvement, > 70 g	T_4: (Tumor is fixed or invades adjacent structures other than the seminal vesicles) T_{4a}: Tumor invades any of bladder neck, external sphincter, or rectum T_{4b}: Tumor invades levator muscles and/or is fixed to the pelvic wall
D (metastatic disease)	Any T, N_{1-4}, M_0, or N_{0-4}, M_1
D_1: Pelvic lymph nodes or ureteral obstruction	N_1: Metastasis in a single lymph node, 2 cm or less in greatest dimension
D_2: Bone, distant lymph node, organ, or soft tissue metastases	N_2: Metastasis in single lymph node more than 2 cm but not more than 5 cm in greatest dimension; or multiple lymph node metastases, none more than 5 cm in greatest dimension N_3: Metastasis in lymph node more than 5 cm in greatest dimension M_{1a}: Nonregional lymph node(s) M_{1b}: Bone(s) M_{1c}: Other site(s)

[a]American Urologic System.
[b]American Joint Committee–International Union Against Cancer.
[c]Note: Tumor found in one or both lobes by needle biopsy, but not palpable or visible by imaging, is classified as T_{1c}.
[d]Note: Invasion into the prostatic apex or into (but not beyond) the prostatic capsule is not classified as T_3 but as T_2.
From Ref. 53, with permission.

During 1986 to 1993, 5-year overall survival rates were estimated at 90% for whites and 75% for African-Americans.[1] For this same period, the survival rates for localized disease (100%), regional disease (95%), and distant disease (31%) in white males were higher than the survival rates for localized disease (91%), regional disease (85%), and distant disease (26%) in African-American males.[1] A 6.3% decline in age-adjusted mortality has been documented for the period 1991 to 1995.[56] Ten-year cancer-specific survival is estimated as 95% for stage A_1, 80% for stages A_2 to B_2, 60% for stage C, 40% for stage D_1, and 10% for stage D_2.[57] It is estimated that more than 85% of patients with stage A_1 can be cured, whereas fewer than 1% of patients with stage D_2 will be cured.

▶ TREATMENT: Prostate Cancer

DESIRED OUTCOME

Localized prostate cancer is curable, and treatment modalities (surgery and radiation) should be performed with an effort to reduce any postprocedure complications (impotence, stricture, and incontinence).[36,58] Advanced prostate cancer (stage D) is not currently curable, and treatment should focus on providing symptom relief and maintaining quality of life.[59]

GENERAL APPROACH TO TREATMENT

The initial treatment for prostate cancer depends primarily on the disease stage.[36,52] Figure 119–3 shows the National Comprehensive Cancer Network (NCCN) consensus-based practice guidelines for initial prostate cancer management.[52] All of the treatment options were considered "Category 1" by the panel of experts that developed these guidelines; this means that the rec-

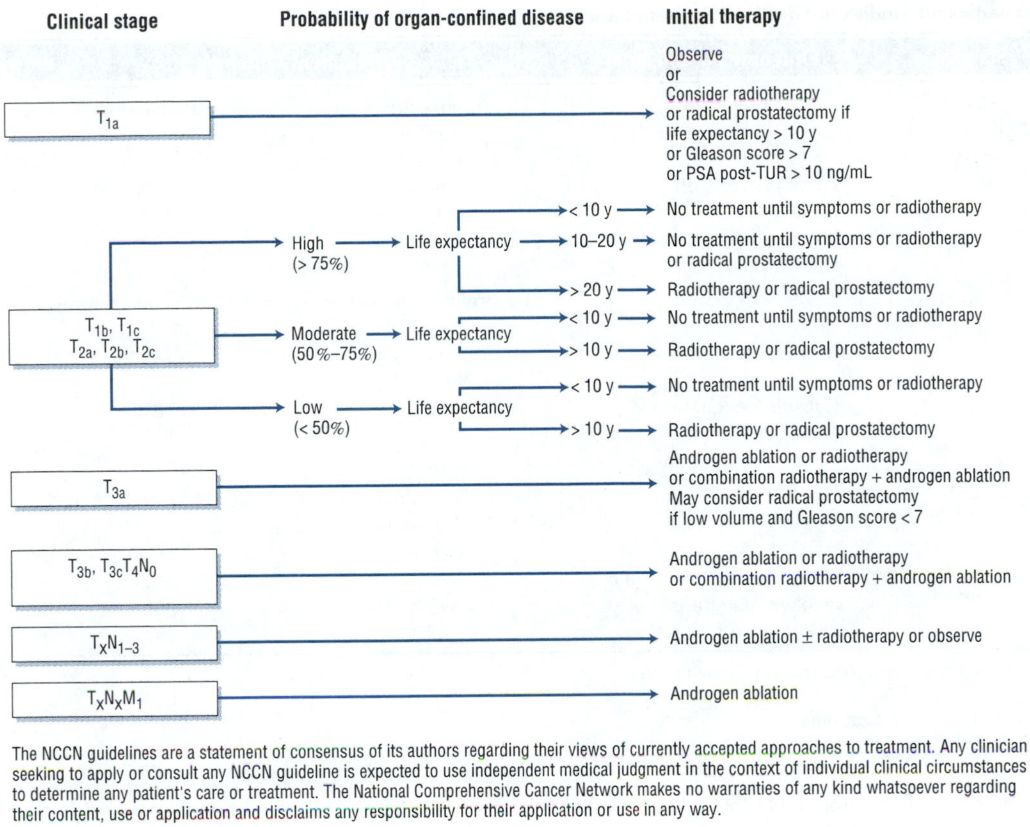

FIGURE 119–3. Initial therapy for prostate cancer. *(Copyrighted by the National Comprehensive Cancer Network. All rights reserved. These guidelines and illustrations may not be reproduced in any form without the express written permission of the NCCN.)*

ommendations were uncontested and generally accepted by all panel members.

Patients with incidental carcinoma found at the time of a transurethral resection for BPH (stage A_1 or T_{1a} or T_{1b}) usually require only careful observation because the 10-year survival rate for these patients is very high.[58] The patient's life expectancy and the probability of having organ-confined disease, as judged by clinical stage, PSA levels, and Gleason score, may alter the treatment decision for patients with stage T_1 or T_2 prostate cancer.[36,52,60] More aggressive therapy is used when the patient's life expectancy exceeds 10 years.[36,52] Patient preference is also important to consider.

Radical prostatectomy and radiation therapy are generally considered therapeutically equivalent for localized prostate cancer.[52,61] Complications from radical prostatectomy include blood loss, stricture formation, incontinence, lymphocele, fistula formation, anesthetic risk, and impotence.[58,61] Nerve-sparing radical prostatectomy can be performed in many patients; 50% to 80% regain sexual potency within the first year.[62] Acute complications from radiation therapy include cystitis, proctitis, hematuria, urinary retention, penoscrotal edema, and impotence (30% incidence).[36,58] Chronic complications include proctitis, diarrhea, cystitis, enteritis, impotence, urethral stricture, and incontinence.[36,58] PSA is a useful marker to follow disease reactivation after either radical prostatectomy or radiation therapy.

There are ongoing studies to define the best treatment for patients with stage B_2 or C disease.[36,58] The failure rate for stage C patients is much higher than for either stage A or B, and better diagnostic techniques have demonstrated that some stage C patients have occult disease dissemination at presentation. Although external beam radiotherapy has been the primary treatment option, some investigators feel there is also a role for androgen deprivation prior to definitive local treatment (neoadjuvant hormonal therapy).[21]

Neoadjuvant androgen-ablative therapy has been used to reduce tumor size or "downstage" disease prior to definitive radical prostatectomy or radiation therapy[63–65] (Table 119–6). These studies demonstrate that neoadjuvant therapy can decrease the local progression rate after radiation therapy or increase the chance to find organ-confined disease at surgery in clinical stage T_1 and T_2 prostate cancers.[64,66] However, the follow-up period in these studies was not long enough to evaluate the effects on progression-free and overall survival. Flutamide (in combination with an LH-RH agonist) has been approved for use prior to and during the period of radiation therapy for patients with stage B_2 or C prostate cancer. However, despite these encouraging results, the optimal duration of neoadjuvant therapy and optimal regimen need to be defined.[66]

Cryosurgery[67] or brachytherapy (interstitial radiotherapy)[68] has been used for localized prostate cancer; however, there is not long enough follow-up to recommend these modalities over radical prostatectomy or radiotherapy as primary therapy.

The treatment of patients with localized prostate cancer remains less than optimal because many of the studies used inadequate methods to define the patient populations treated and assess outcomes.[69,70] No intermediate end points, including PSA levels, are known to be valid surrogate markers, so investigation using compounds such as indium-111-labeled capromab pendedite[71] to help determine disease extent should continue.[69]

There is controversy about the best approach to treating patients with stage D prostate cancer because therapy is palliative and cure is not possible. Patients with stage D_0 prostate cancer may be carefully watched, and appropriate local therapy (surgery or radiation) may be instituted when symptoms appear. The

TABLE 119–6. Neoadjuvant Studies in Localized Prostate Cancer

Reference	Stage(s)	Outcome Parameter(s)	Treatment Outcome		Significance
63	Large T_2, T_3, T_4 No bone mets. (B_2–C)		Goserelin + flutamide[a] + radiation $N = 226$	Radiation $N = 230$	
		Local progression[b]	46%	71%	$P < .001$
		Distant mets.[b]	34%	41%	$P = .09$
		Progression-free survival[b]	36%	15%	$P < .001$
		Overall survival[b]	No difference		$P = .7$
65	$T_{2b}N_XM_0$ (B_2)		Leuprolide + flutamide + radical prostatectomy[c] $N = 138$	Radical prostatectomy $N = 144$	
		Capsule penetration	47%	78%	$P < .001$
		Tumor at urethral margin	6%	17%	$P < .01$
		Tumor at inked margin	18%	48%	$P < .001$
64	T_1,T_2,T_3		Goserelin + flutamide[c] + radical prostatectomy $N = 69$	Radical prostatectomy[d] $N = 72$	
		Pathologic organ confined	73%	56%	
		Positive margins	17%	36%	
		PSA disease-free rate	89%	84%	

[a]Given for 2 months before radiation, then for 2 months during radiation.
[b]Evaluated at 5 years.
[c]Given for 3 months prior to radical prostatectomy.
[d]Nonrandomized control group.

majority of these patients will develop metastatic disease and will then require systemic therapy.[58] Stage D_1 patients may be treated in a similar fashion; however, some clinicians feel that early hormonal intervention in these cases is warranted based on the observations that stage D_2 patients with minimal disease have better overall survival with hormonal therapy compared to those patients with a large tumor burden.[72]

The major initial treatment modality for advanced prostate cancer (stage D_2) is androgen-ablative pharmacotherapy using either orchiectomy or LH-RH agonists either alone or combined with antiandrogens.[19,58] Estrogens have been used also; however, the primary estrogen, diethylstilbesterol (DES), was withdrawn from the U.S. market in 1997. Secondary hormonal manipulations, cytotoxic chemotherapy, or supportive care is used for the patient who progresses after initial therapy.

ORCHIECTOMY

Bilateral orchiectomy rapidly reduces circulating androgens to castrate levels (< 50 ng/dL).[58] Unfortunately, many patients are not surgical candidates owing to their advanced age, and other patients find this procedure psychologically unacceptable.[58] Orchiectomy is probably the preferred initial treatment in patients with impending spinal cord compression or ureteral obstruction.

LUTEINIZING HORMONE–RELEASING HORMONE AGONISTS

Currently available LH-RH agonists include leuprolide,[23] leuprolide depot,[23,73] and goserelin acetate implant.[24,74] Leuprolide acetate is administered once daily, whereas leuprolide depot and goserelin acetate implant can be administered either once monthly, once every 12 weeks, or once every 16 weeks (leuprolide depot: 4 months). The leuprolide depot formulation contains leuprolide acetate in coated pellets. The dose is administered intramuscularly and the coating dissolves at different rates to allow sustained leuprolide levels throughout the dosing interval. Goserelin acetate implant contains goserelin acetate dispersed in a plastic matrix of *d,l*-lactic and glycolic acid copolymer and is administered subcutaneously. Hydrolysis of the copolymer material provides continuous release of goserelin over the dosing period.

Several randomized trials have demonstrated that leuprolide and goserelin are effective agents when used alone in patients with advanced prostate cancer.[23,24] Response rates around 80% have been reported, with a lower incidence of adverse effects compared to estrogens.[23,24,75] There are no direct comparative trials of the currently available LH-RH agonists, so the choice between the two is usually made by cost and by patient and physician preference.

The most common adverse effects reported with LH-RH agonist therapy include a disease "flare up" during the first week of therapy, hot flashes, erectile impotence, decreased libido, and injection site reactions.[23,24] Corresponding to the initial increase in both LH and FSH, the disease "flare" manifests clinically as either increased bone pain or increased urinary symptoms.[23,24] This "flare" reaction usually resolves after 2 weeks and has a similar onset and duration pattern for the depot LH-RH products.[73,74,76]

If LH-RH agonists are used as initial therapy, similar response rates to orchiectomy and estrogen administration can be expected. There is a lower incidence of cardiovascular-related adverse effects associated with LH-RH therapy than with estrogen administration. Patients should be counseled to expect worsening symptoms during the first week of therapy, and caution should be exercised when initiating LH-RH agonist therapy in patients with widely metastatic disease involving the spinal cord or having the potential for ureteral obstruction, because irreversible complications may occur.

ANTIANDROGENS

Three antiandrogens, flutamide,[29,77] bicalutamide,[31,78,79] and nilutamide,[30,80,81] are currently available (Table 119–7).

Antiandrogens have been used as monotherapy in previously untreated patients. Flutamide has a response rate of 50% to 87%,[29,77] bicalutamide has a response rate of 54% to 70%,[82,83] and nilutamide has a response rate of approximately 40%.[84] Objective responses are manifested as decreased bone pain, de-

TABLE 119–7. Antiandrogens

Antiandrogen	Usual Dose	Adverse Effects
Flutamide	750 mg/d	Gynecomastia Hot flushes Gastrointestinal disturbances (diarrhea) Liver function test abnormalities Breast tenderness Methemoglobinemia
Bicalutamide	50 mg/d	Gynecomastia Hot flushes Gastrointestinal disturbances (diarrhea) Liver function test abnormalities Breast tenderness
Nilutamide	300 mg/d for 1st month then 150 mg/d	Gynecomastia Hot flushes Gastrointestinal disturbances (nausea or constipation) Liver function test abnormalities Breast tenderness Visual disturbances (impaired dark adaptation) Alcohol intolerance Interstitial pneumonitis

creased prostate size, decreased PSA, and/or improved performance status. However, for advanced prostate cancer, all currently available antiandrogens are indicated only in combination with androgen-ablation therapy; flutamide and bicalutamide are indicated in combination with an LH-RH agonist, and nilutamide is indicated in combination with orchiectomy.[30,31,77]

The most common antiandrogen-related adverse effects are listed in Table 119–7. In the only randomized comparison of bicalutamide plus an LH-RH agonist versus flutamide plus an LH-RH agonist, diarrhea was more common in flutamide-treated patients.[85] Antiandrogens can reduce the symptoms from the flare phenomenon associated with LH-RH agonist therapy.

COMBINED HORMONAL BLOCKADE

Although up to 80% of patients with advanced prostate cancer will respond to initial hormonal manipulation, almost all patients will relapse within 2 to 4 years after initiating therapy.[58] Two mechanisms have been proposed to explain this tumor resistance.[86] The tumor could be heterogeneously composed of cells that are hormone dependent and hormone independent, or the tumor could be stimulated by extratesticular androgens that are converted intracellularly to DHT. The rationale for combination hormonal therapy is to interfere with multiple hormonal pathways to completely eliminate androgen action. In clinical trials, combination hormonal therapy, sometimes also referred to as "maximal androgen deprivation" or "total androgen blockade," has been used. The combination of LH-RH agonists or orchiectomy with antiandrogens is the most extensively studied combined androgen-deprivation approach.

Labrie et al.[87] provided information for the initial reports combining an LH-RH agonist with flutamide and have subsequently provided follow-up for 363 patients. Response rates, the main end point of these studies, have been greater than 90% in previously untreated patients.[87] However, response rates less than 35% have been observed with this combination in patients previously treated with initial hormonal manipulation.

These studies, although quite encouraging, have been criticized for lack of a concurrent control arm and for using response rather than survival as the final end point. For these reasons, the National Cancer Institute (NCI) sponsored a randomized, placebo-controlled, double-blind, multicenter trial comparing leuprolide with leuprolide plus flutamide 250 mg orally three times a day in newly diagnosed patients with stage D prostate cancer.[72,87]

Both median progression-free survival (16.5 vs 13.9 months) and overall median survival (35.6 vs 28.3 months) were significantly longer in the 303 evaluable patients treated with leuprolide plus flutamide than in the 300 evaluable patients treated with leuprolide alone. The best response to combination therapy was observed in patients with minimal disease (no disease in ribs, long bones, or soft tissue other than lymph nodes) and a good performance status. An update of this trial has demonstrated that median survival was 61 months in the combination arm and 41 months in the leuprolide-alone arm in patients with minimal disease.[88] The addition of flutamide to leuprolide reduced the symptoms from the flare phenomenon associated with LH-RH agonist therapy. Patients in both groups experienced common adverse effects associated with LH-RH agonist treatment. Diarrhea was the only additional adverse effect attributable to flutamide administration.

Several other studies comparing combined androgen blockade to conventional medical or surgical castration have been performed[80,85,89–92] (Table 119–8). In studies with LH-RH agonists, the results have varied, with no consistent benefit demonstrated for combined androgen therapy.

When orchiectomy alone was compared to antiandrogen (nilutamide) in addition to orchiectomy, Janknegt et al. reported a survival advantage of more than 7 months.[80] However, a recently completed NCI intergroup trial involving 1371 evaluable stage D_2 prostate cancer patients failed to show any significant survival benefits for the combination of orchiectomy plus flutamide over orchiectomy alone.[92] Like other studies of combined androgen blockade, overall survival was longest in patients with minimal disease. Diarrhea, elevated liver function tests, and anemia were more common in those patients who received flutamide.

A meta-analysis of 22 randomized trials in 5710 patients comparing maximal androgen blockade to conventional medical or surgical castration failed to show any additional survival benefit for maximal androgen blockade.[93]

In one of the few combination androgen-deprivation studies comparing two different antiandrogens (bicalutamide vs flutamide), the time to treatment failure (the main study end point), time to progression (as defined by appearance of new or worsening bone or extraskeletal lesions), and time to death were equivalent, suggesting that the two treatments are equally effective.[94]

Although some investigators now consider combined androgen ablation to be the initial hormonal therapy of choice for newly diagnosed patients, the clinician is left to weigh the costs of combined therapy against potential benefits in light of conflicting results in the randomized trials.[19] For those trials that did show an advantage for combined androgen blockade, whether these effects are testosterone-deprivation method specific (orchiectomy vs LH-RH agonist), antiandrogen specific (flutamide vs bicalutamide vs nilutamide), or patient selection specific is not clear. The lack of randomized comparisons of the individual agents and therapies does not help answer this question, nor assist the clinician in deciding which specific combination to use. Thus far, studies have demonstrated a major benefit in patients with minimal disease.[19,72,92] So this may be the ideal population for combined androgen ablation. Further carefully designed studies, which use survival, time to progression, quality of life, patient preference, and cost as end points, should be conducted.

TABLE 119–8. Summary of Randomized Combined Androgen Blockade Trials

Reference	Treatment	*N*	Disease-free Survival (mo)		Overall Median Survival (mo)	
72	Leuprolide	300	13.9		28.3	
	Leuprolide + flutamide	303	16.5	*P* = .039	35.6	*P* = .035
89	Orchiectomy	133	16.8		27.6	
	Goserelin + flutamide	129	16.5	NS	22.7	NS
91	Orchiectomy	148			27.1	
	Goserelin + flutamide	149			34.4	*P* = .02
92	Goserelin	282			26.9	
	Goserelin + flutamide	287			29	NS
80	Orchiectomy	208	14.7		29.8	
	Orchiectomy + nilutamide	202	20.8	*P* = .0041	37.1	*P* = .0041
88	Orchiectomy	681	19		30	
	Orchiectomy + flutamide	690	20	NS	32	NS
85	Goserelin + bicalutamide	404	0.9 (0.75–1.08)[a]		0.87 (0.754–1.03)[a]	
	Goserelin + flutamide	409				

[a]Reported as the hazard ratio for goserelin + bicalutamide compared to goserelin + flutamide.
NS = not significant.

There is still considerable debate concerning when to start hormonal-deprivation therapy in patients with advanced prostate cancer.[95,96] The original recommendation to start therapy when symptoms appeared was based on the Veterans Administration Cooperative Urologic Research Group (VACURG) trials, in which no overall survival difference was demonstrated in patients that either started DES initially or crossed over to active treatment when symptoms appeared; the excess mortality was attributed to estrogen administration.[97,98] Because LH-RH agonists and antiandrogens are considered suitable alternatives with less cardiovascular toxicity, it is not clear whether delaying therapy is justified. Reanalysis of the original VACURG data[98] and recent combined androgen-deprivation trials[72,91,99] demonstrate a survival advantage for young, good-performance-status, minimal-disease patients treated initially with hormonal therapy, suggesting that early intervention before symptoms appear may be appropriate.[95] The issue of when best to start hormonal therapy is the subject of several clinical trials.[95,100,101]

ESTROGENS

Although DES is no longer available, the use of estrogens for androgen ablation has an important historical perspective relative to prostate cancer management.[97,102] Other available estrogenic substances, such as ethinyl estradiol, conjugated estrogens, chlorotrianisene, and polyestradiol phosphate, cost more than DES and have not been as extensively studied.[19]

SECONDARY TREATMENTS

Secondary or salvage therapies for patients who progress after their initial therapy depend on what was used for initial management[52,103] (Fig. 119–4). For patients initially diagnosed with localized prostate cancer, radiotherapy can be used in the case of failed radical prostatectomy. Alternatively, androgen ablation can be used in patients who progress after either radiation therapy or radical prostatectomy.

Secondary hormonal manipulations, such as adding an antiandrogen to a patient who incompletely suppresses testosterone secretion with an LH-RH agonist, or withdrawing antiandrogens in a patient receiving combination therapy, or using agents that inhibit androgen synthesis, can be attempted in patients initially treated with one hormonal modality. Supportive care, chemotherapy, or local radiotherapy can be used in pa-

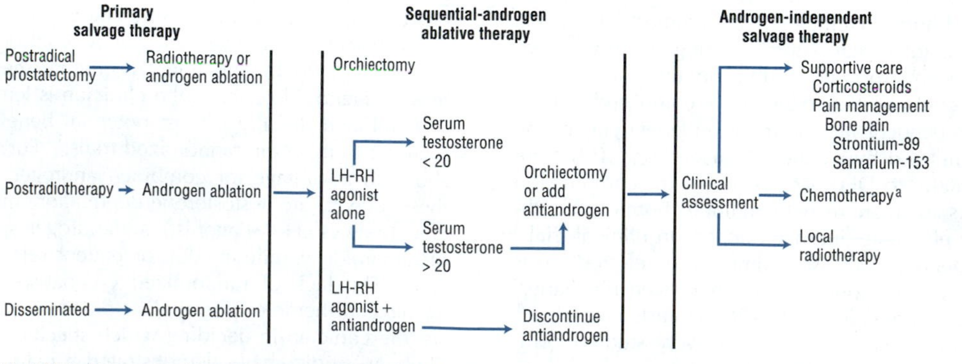

FIGURE 119–4. Secondary therapy for prostate cancer. *(Adapted from Ref. 52.) (Copyrighted by the National Comprehensive Cancer Network. All right reserved. These guidelines and illustrations may not be reproduced in any form without the express written permission of the NCCN.)*

tients who have failed all forms of androgen-ablation manipulations, because these patients are considered to have androgen-independent disease.

For patients who initially received an LH-RH agonist alone, castrate testosterone levels should be documented. Patients with inadequate testosterone suppression (> 20 ng/dL) can be treated by adding an antiandrogen or performing an orchiectomy. If castrate testosterone levels have been achieved, the patient is considered to have androgen-independent disease, and palliative androgen-independent salvage therapy can be used.

If the patient initially received combined androgen blockade with an LH-RH agonist with an antiandrogen, then androgen withdrawal would be the first salvage manipulation. Objective and subjective responses have been noted following the discontinuation of flutamide,[104] bicalutamide,[79,105,106] or nilutamide[107] in patients receiving these agents as part of combined androgen ablation with an LH-RH agonist. Mutations in the androgen receptor have been demonstrated that allow antiandrogens such as flutamide, bicalutamide, nilutamide (or their metabolites) to become agonists and activate the androgen receptor.[14,108,109] Patient responses to androgen withdrawal manifest as significant PSA reductions and improved clinical symptoms. Androgen withdrawal responses lasting 3 to 14 months have been noted in up to 35% of patients, and predicting response seems to be most closely related to longer androgen exposure times.[15] Incomplete cross-resistance has been noted in some patients who received bicalutamide after they had progressed while receiving flutamide.[79] Adding an agent that blocks adrenal androgen synthesis, such as aminoglutethimide, at the time that androgens are withdrawn may produce a better response than androgen withdrawal alone.[110] Because of the potential for response immediately after antiandrogen withdrawal, a sufficient observation and assessment period (usually 4 to 6 weeks) is usually required before a patient can be enrolled on a clinical trial evaluating a new agent or therapy for advanced prostate cancer.

Androgen synthesis inhibitors, such as aminoglutethimide[26] or ketoconazole,[27,58] can provide symptomatic relief for a short time in approximately 50% of patients with progressive disease despite previous androgen-ablation therapy. Adverse effects during aminoglutethimide therapy occur in approximately 50% of patients.[26] Central nervous system effects that include lethargy, ataxia, and dizziness are the major adverse reactions. A generalized morbiliform, pruritic rash has been reported in up to 30% of patients treated. The rash is usually self-limiting and resolves within 5 to 8 days with continued therapy. Adverse effects from ketoconazole include gastrointestinal intolerance, transient rises in liver and renal function tests, and hypoadrenalism.

After all hormonal manipulations are exhausted, the patient is considered to have androgen-independent disease. At this point, palliative supportive therapy is appropriate.[52,111] Palliation can be achieved by pain management, using radioisotopes such as strontium-89[112] or samarium-153 lexidronam[113] for bone-related pain, analgesics, corticosteroids, or local radiotherapy.[111] Chemotherapy with approved agents that have demonstrated palliative activity or in the context of a clinical research trial is another option.

Despite extensive testing of both single agents, combination chemotherapy regimens, and combination chemotherapy/hormonal regimens, no currently approved antineoplastic agent or combinations prolong survival in patients with advanced prostate cancer.[103] This might partially be because the majority of chemotherapy trials have been done in patients with hormone-refractory prostate cancer when the expected resistance rate is high. Recently, PSA reductions and/or clinical improvements, such as quality of life, improved pain, and reduced analgesic requirements, have been adopted as accepted end points for trials evaluating chemotherapy agents in prostate cancer patients.[114,115] Androgen ablation is usually continued when chemotherapy is initiated.[58,116]

Single agents with modest activity in prostate cancer include cyclophosphamide, estramustine, 5-fluorouracil, methotrexate, dacarbazine, mitoxantrone, doxorubicin, and cisplatin.[114,115,117] If disease stabilization is included as a favorable response, response rates up to 46% have been reported.[114,115,117] Several trials have evaluated the various combination regimens containing the most active single agents.[114,115,118–120] Cisplatin plus etoposide is an effective therapy for patients with the small-cell neuroendocrine histology.[52]

Both estramustine combined with vinblastine[118,120–122] and mitoxantrone combined with prednisone are active combination regimens for refractory prostate cancer.[123] Although estramustine as a single agent[122,124] produced similar response rates to other available chemotherapy agents, development of estramustine combinations (such as estramustine plus vinblastine or estramustine plus paclitaxel) continued when its mechanism of action was discovered to involve microtubule proteins, rather than alkylation.[120,122]

Estramustine and vinblastine combinations have been evaluated in several trials.[120,122] Response is manifested as objective tumor regression (partial response rate up to 50%), PSA declines, pain relief, and delay in bone scan progression. The toxicities of estramustine combined with vinblastine are nausea, gynecomastia, fatigue, and fluid retention.

Mitoxantrone plus prednisone is another combination regimen that can palliate hormone-refractory prostate cancer.[123] One hundred sixty-one patients with hormone-refractory prostate cancer with pain were randomized to receive either prednisone 10 mg/d alone or this same prednisone dose with mitoxantrone. The primary end point was a palliative ("clinical benefit") response as assessed by a pain scale and analgesic requirements. Quality of life was assessed with a series of linear analog health-assessment scales and the Prostate Cancer-Specific Quality of Life Instrument.

Palliative responses were noted in 29% of patients in the mitoxantrone plus prednisone group and 12% of patients in the prednisone-alone group ($P = .01$). The duration of palliative response was greater and quality of life scores for pain, physical activity, constipation, and mood were better in patients who received mitoxantrone plus prednisone. Overall survival was the same in both groups. Patients treated with mitoxantrone plus prednisone experienced tolerable adverse effects; however, five patients did develop some cardiac-related adverse effects. Mitoxantrone plus corticosteroids is an FDA approved therapy for hormone-refractory prostate cancer.

Other possible chemotherapeutic regimens suggested by the NCCN guidelines and clinical trials include ketoconazole plus doxorubicin, estramustine plus etoposide, or estramustine plus paclitaxel.[52]

Although it would seem rational that prostate cancer is a heterogeneous disease composed of cells sensitive to hormonal therapy, chemotherapy, both therapies, or neither therapy, attempts to combine endocrine therapy and chemotherapy to produce an additive effect have not produced significant response rates. When orchiectomy was compared to DES plus cyclophosphamide in a prospective randomized trial in patients with stage D prostate cancer, the response rate, median survival, and time to progressive disease were similar between the two treatment groups.[125] Likewise, Osborne et al. demonstrated a higher initial response rate for patients treated with hormonal therapy plus chemotherapy; however, overall median survival was similar.[126] Furthermore, in a randomized trial involving 419 prostate cancer patients with bone metastases, subgroup analysis demonstrated that orchiectomy plus estramustine produced a longer time to progression compared to orchiectomy alone in patients less than 73 years old.[127]

Fluoxymesterone has been used in some trials designed to test androgen-priming strategies to get the cells to cycle more rapidly and therefore be more susceptible to the effects of cytotoxic chemotherapy. However, the response rates have been inconsistent and spinal cord compression has occurred in some patients, and so it appears that the risks of androgen priming outweigh the benefits.[126]

Whenever possible, cytotoxic chemotherapy for hormone refractory prostate cancer should be offered to the patient as part of the clinical trial.[103] To make the results of a clinical trial applicable to the majority of hormone-refractory prostate cancer patients, the patient populations need to be clearly defined with regard to disease extent and hormone sensitivity.[128] Likewise, responses should be quantified by accepted disease-regression measures. If surrogate markers, such as PSA changes, are used, the response needs to be described in terms of the percent decline, the number of times the decline is documented, and the period during which the decline is maintained.[128,129] Quality-of-life end points are also appropriate outcome parameters to measure.[59]

Many new drugs are being developed for prostate cancer management.[114,115,130–132] Of the investigational compounds, suramin, a growth factor antagonist, has advanced the furthest in clinical trial development.[115,133,134] The first 38-patient trial demonstrated a 42-week median survival and significant PSA declines (greater than 75%).[134] Other efforts include agents with novel anticancer targets and mechanisms (apoptosis inhibitors, growth factor inhibitors, and antimetastasis agents), targeted therapy (vaccines, monoclonal antibodies, or growth receptor antibodies), oncogene regulation (farnesyl transferase inhibitors), matrix metalloproteinase inhibitors, and gene therapy.

CHEMOPREVENTION EFFORTS

Prostate cancer is a significant health concern with few modifiable risk factors. Because androgens are involved in prostate cancer development, it would seem that prolonged administration of drugs that block androgens may prevent subclinical disease from becoming clinically apparent.[135,136] In testing prevention strategies for prostate cancer prevention, valid surrogate markers need to be identified. Currently, PSA, nuclear morphology, apoptotic bodies, proliferation indices, microvessel density, and genetic expression, as intermediate end points to monitor cancer prevention efforts, are under investigation.[136,137] As part of an NCI chemoprevention effort, a large double-blind, randomized trial comparing finasteride 5 mg/d for 7 years to placebo has been initiated.[135,136] This trial has met its target accrual goal of 18,000 participants 55 years of age or older with a normal PSA and digital rectal examination. All patients will be biopsied after 7 years, or sooner if prostate cancer is diagnosed before this time point. Long-term follow-up is needed before any conclusions can be drawn. In addition to determining whether this intervention will reduce the prostate cancer incidence, it will also provide information about the epidemiology, risk factors, natural history, screening, and diagnosis of prostate cancer and will collect important quality-of-life data. Other potential prostate cancer prevention efforts include tyrosine kinase inhibitors, differentiation inducers, and angiogenesis inhibitors.[136]

ECONOMIC CONSIDERATIONS

The main economic concerns for prostate cancer treatment focus on the use of combined hormonal blockade for advanced disease. Table 119–9 lists the costs for the initial hormonal therapies for stage D_2 prostate cancer. Using a societal perspective and data from the original leuprolide plus flutamide versus leuprolide alone trial[72] to calculate the incremental cost per life-year gained, Hillner et al. concluded that combined androgen blockade has an incremental cost effectiveness of $25,300 per life-year gained, which is within current accepted benchmarks.[138] The cost dropped to $13,700 per life-year gained in patients with minimal disease.

TABLE 119–9. Comparative Costs of Hormonal Therapy for Advanced Prostate Cancer

Drug	Dose	Average Wholesale Price per Month of Therapy
Leuprolide depot	7.5 mg/mo	$566.85
Leuprolide depot	22.5 mg/12 wk	$1700.63
Leuprolide depot	30 mg/16 wk	$2267.50
Goserelin implant	3.6 mg every 28 d	$439.24
Goserelin implant	10.8 mg/12 wk	$1317.74
Flutamide	750 mg/d	$315.70
Bicalutamide	50 mg/d	$319.74
Nilutamide	300 mg/d for 1st mo then 150 mg/d	$467.16 then $233.58
		Average Wholesale Price per 3 Months of Therapy
Combined Androgen Blockade		
Leuprolide depot 22.5 mg/12 wk		
+ flutamide	750 mg/d	$2647.97
+ bicalutamide	50 mg/d	$2659.85
+ nilutamide	150 mg/d	$2401.37 ($2634.95 1st month)
Goserelin depot 10.8 mg/12 wk		
+ flutamide	750 mg/d	$2265.08
+ bicalutamide	50 mg/d	$2270.96
+ nilutamide	150 mg/d	$2018.48 ($2252.06 1st month)

Compiled from Ref. 142.

In a follow-up study, this same group used physician focus group estimates to generate quality-of-life factors and incorporated these factors into an economic model.[139] The incremental cost per quality-adjusted life-year gained seemed reasonable when data from the original combined androgen blockade were used[72]: $25,000 for patients with minimal disease and $18,000 for patients with severe disease. However, these incremental costs increased dramatically to $53,700 for patients with minimal disease and $41,000 for patients with severe disease when the same model was applied to survival data from a meta-analysis.

Because there is considerable debate about the value of using combined androgen blockade for advanced prostate cancer, continued economic assessments of this therapy will be crucial to help policymakers and physicians decide on the most appropriate therapy. It will also become very important to incorporate economic analyses into chemotherapy trials because these efforts move toward including clinical benefit response as a main end point.

EVALUATION OF THERAPEUTIC OUTCOMES

Clinical trials in prostate cancer should include homogeneous populations[140] and adequate staging criteria. Age-adjusted overall survival and disease-free survival should be the ultimate outcome measures; although standardized subjective and objective response criteria should also be included. Objective parameters include assessment of the primary tumor size, evaluation of involved lymph nodes, and the response of tumor markers to treatment. There is still no agreement about which surrogate marker(s), such as PSA, is(are) most useful and how to best quantify the changes in these surrogates to predict a meaningful response.[40,129] Efforts to better identify markers, such as PSA or indium-111-labeled capromab pendetide scanning to predict or diagnose recurrence, may improve overall outcome.[71] Clinical benefit responses can be documented by evaluating performance status changes, weight changes, and analgesic requirements. Quality-of-life assessments should be included in all clinical trials.[59]

FUTURE DIRECTIONS

Prostate cancer occurs in older males and is curable when local disease is present. Efforts are under way to better define screening and early detection approaches and how best to use PSA as a screening, diagnostic, and therapeutic monitoring test. Proper staging at initial patient presentation is essential because the therapy intensity will depend on the disease stage. Patients with localized prostate cancer can be effectively managed with surgery or radiation therapy. For patients with advanced disease, there are many treatment options. Androgen-ablative therapy is very effective for symptom palliation. Initial androgen-ablative measures include orchiectomy or a luteinizing hormone–releasing hormone agonist. Combined androgen blockade using an antiandrogen with either orchiectomy or an LH-RH agonist is routinely used despite equivocal studies and its cost. The effects of androgen ablation seem most pronounced in patients with minimal disease. Studies are still ongoing to define the best initial therapy, to determine when to start initial therapy, to identify which patient subpopulation might benefit best from a given treatment modality, and to identify which surrogate markers should be used to monitor disease activity.

Secondary therapies, including alternate hormonal therapies, antiandrogen withdrawal in a patient receiving combined androgen blockade, chemotherapy, local radiotherapy, or supportive care can provide disease palliation. Continued efforts to develop new agents with novel mechanisms of action that prolong survival are ongoing. Further insight into the molecular basis for prostate cancer development may provide new therapeutic approaches.

▶ PRINCIPLES OF PHARMACOTHERAPY

- Prostate cancer is the most frequent cancer in U.S. men. African-American ancestry, family history, and increased age are the primary risk factors for prostate cancer.
- Mutations in E-cadherin, *p*53, and the androgen receptor are important in prostate carcinogenesis and may affect treatment outcomes.
- Prostate specific antigen (PSA) is a useful marker for detecting prostate cancer at early stages, predicting outcome for localized disease, defining disease-free status, and following response to androgen-deprivation therapy or chemotherapy for advanced-stage disease.
- Prostate cancer screening is controversial. The American Cancer Society currently recommends that digital rectal examination and PSA be offered annually to men beginning at age 50 years with at least a 10-year life expectancy and to younger men (45 years old) who are considered to be at high risk for prostate cancer development (strong familial predisposition or African-American).
- The prognosis for prostate cancer patients depends on the histologic grade, the tumor size, and disease stage. More than 85% of patients with stage A_1 disease but less than 1% of those with stage D_2 can be cured.
- Localized prostate cancer is curable by surgery or radiation therapy. Advanced prostate cancer (stage D) is not currently curable, and treatment should focus on providing symptom relief and maintaining quality of life.
- Androgen-deprivation therapy, such as using an LH-RH plus an antiandrogen, can be used prior to radiation therapy for patients with locally advanced (stage B_2 or C) prostate cancer to improve outcomes over radiation therapy alone.
- Androgen-deprivation therapy, with either orchiectomy, an LH-RH agonist alone, or an LH-RH plus an antiandrogen (combined hormonal blockade), can be used to provide palliation for patients with advanced (stage D_2) prostate cancer. The effects of androgen deprivation seem most pronounced in patients with minimal disease at diagnosis.
- Antiandrogen withdrawal, for patients having progressive disease while receiving combined hormonal blockade with an LH-RH plus an antiandrogen, can provide additional symptomatic relief. Mutations in the androgen receptor have been documented that cause antiandrogen compounds to act like receptor agonists.
- Chemotherapy, with regimens such as mitoxantrone plus corticosteroids (prednisone), or estramustine plus vinblastine, have been shown to provide a

clinical benefit response in patients with hormone-refractory prostate cancer. Patients with hormone-refractory prostate cancer should be considered for entry on clinical trials investigating new therapies for prostate cancer.

REFERENCES

1. Landis S, Murray T, Bolden S, Wingo PA. Cancer statistics, 1998. CA Cancer J Clin 1998;48:6–29.
2. Carter BS, Beaty TH, Steinberg GD, et al. Mendelian inheritance of familial prostate cancer. Proc Natl Acad Sci USA 1992;89: 3367–3372.
3. Giovannucci E. How is individual risk for prostate cancer assessed? Hematol Oncol Clin North Am 1996;10:537–548.
4. Isaacs WB, Bova SG, Morton RA, et al. Molecular genetics and chromosomal alterations in prostate cancer. Cancer 1995;75:2004–2012.
5. Ross R, Coetzee GA, Reichardt J, et al. Does the racial-ethnic variation in prostate cancer have a hormonal basis? Cancer 1995;75: 1778–1882.
6. Smith JR, Freije D, Carpten JD, et al. Major susceptibility locus for prostate cancer on chromosome 1 suggested by a genome-wide search. Science 1996;274:1371–1374.
7. Giovannucci E, Ascherio A, Rimm EB, et al. A prospective cohort study of vasectomy and prostate cancer in US men. JAMA 1993; 269:873–877.
8. Slattery ML, West DW. Smoking, alcohol, coffee, tea, caffeine, and theobromine: Risk of prostate cancer in Utah (United States). Cancer Causes Control 1993;4:559–563.
9. Pienta KJ, Esper PS. Risk factors for prostate cancer. Ann Intern Med 1993;118:793–803.
10. Soler AP, Harner GD, Knudsen KA, et al. Expression of P-cadherin identifies prostate-specific-antigen-negative cells in epithelial tissues of male sexual accessory organs and in prostatic carcinomas. Implications for prostate cancer biology. Am J Pathol 1997;151:471–478.
11. Chi SG, deVere RW, White FJ. p53 in prostate cancer: Frequent expressed transition mutations. Natl Cancer Inst 1994;86:926–933.
12. Theodorescu D, Broder SR, Boyd JC, Mills SE, Frierson HF Jr. p53, bcl-2 and retinoblastoma proteins as long-term prognostic markers in localized carcinoma of the prostate. J Urol 1997;158:131–137.
13. Dong JT, Suzuki H, Pin SS, et al. Down-regulation of the KAI1 metastasis suppressor gene during the progression of human prostatic cancer infrequently involves gene mutation or allelic loss. Cancer Res 1996;56:4387–4390.
14. Taplin ME, Bubley GJ, Shuster TD, et al. Mutation of the androgen receptor gene in metastic androgen independent prostate cancer. N Engl J Med 1995;332:1334–1342.
15. Kelly WK, Slovin S, Scher HI. Steroid hormone withdrawl syndromes. Pathophysiology and clinical significance. Urol Clin North Am 1997;24:421–431.
16. Takahashi H, Furusato M, Allsbrook WC, et al. Prevalence of androgen receptor gene mutations in latent prostatic carcinomas from Japanese men. Cancer Res 1995;55:1621–1624.
17. Balducci L, Pow-Sang J, Friedland J, Diaz JI. Prostate cancer. Clin Geriatr Med 1997;13:283–306.
18. McConnell JD. Physiologic basis of endocrine therapy for prostatic cancer. Urol Clin North Am 1991;18:1–13.
19. Garnick MB. Hormonal therapy in the management of prostate cancer: From Huggins to the present. Urology 1997;49:5–15.
20. Lalani N, Lanaido ME, Abel PD. Molecular and cellular biology of prostate cancer. Cancer Metastasis Rev 1997;16:29–66.
21. Garnick M, Fair W. First international conference on neoadjuvant hormonal therapy of prostate cancer: Overview consensus statement. Urology 1997;39(suppl 3):1–4.
22. Huggins C, Hodges CV. Studies on prostatic cancer. 1. The effect of castration, of estrogen, and of androgen injection on serum phosphatases in metastatic carcinoma of the prostate. Cancer Res 1941;1: 293–297.
23. Plosker GL, Brogden RN. Leuprorelin. A review of its pharmacology and therapeutic use in prostatic cancer, endometriosis and other sex hormone-related disorders. Drugs 1994;48:930–967.
24. Brogden RN, Faulds D. Goserelin. A review of its pharmacodynamic and pharmacokinetic properties and therapeutic efficacy in prostate cancer. Drugs Aging 1995;6:324–343.
25. Conn PM, Crowley WF. Gonadotropin-releasing hormone and its analogues. N Engl J Med 1991;324:93–103.
26. Crawford ED, Ahmann FR, Davis MA, et al. Aminoglutethimide in metastatic adenocarcinoma of the prostate. Prog Clin Biol Res 1987; 243A:283–288.
27. Trump DL, Havlin KH, Messing EM, et a. High-dose ketoconazole in advanced hormone-refractory prostate cancer: Endocrinologic and clinical effects. J Clin Oncol 1989;7:1093–1098.
28. Geller J. Megestrol acetate plus low-dose estrogen in the management of advanced prostatic carcinoma. Urol Clin North Am 1991;18:83–91.
29. Labrie F. Mechanism of action and pure antiandrogenic properties of flutamide. Cancer 1993;72:3816–3827.
30. Dole EJ, Holdsworth MT. Nilutamide: An antiandrogen for the treatment of prostate cancer. Ann Pharmacother 1997;31:65–75.
31. Blackledge GR, Cockshott ID, Furr BJ. Casodex (bicalutamide): Overview of a new antiandrogen developed for the treatment of prostate cancer. Eur Urol 1997;31(suppl 2):30–39.
32. Rittmaster RS. Finasteride. N Engl J Med 1994;330:120–125.
33. Gittes RF. Carcinoma of the prostate. N Engl J Med 1991;324:236–245.
34. Bostwick DG. Grading prostate cancer. Am J Clin Pathol 1994;102 (suppl 1):S38–S56.
35. Gleason DF. Histologic grade, clinical stage, and patient age in prostate cancer. Natl Cancer Inst Monogr 1988;7:15–18.
36. Garnick MB. Prostate cancer: Screening, diagnosis, and management. Ann Intern Med 1993;118:804–818.
37. Osborn JL, Getzenberg RH, Trump DL. Spinal cord compression in prostate cancer. J Neurooncol 1995;23:135–147.
38. Collins MM, Barry MJ. Controversies in prostate cancer screening. Analogies to the early lung cancer screening debate. JAMA 1996; 276:1976–1979.
39. Gohagan JK, Prorok PC, Kramer BS, Hayes RB, Cornett JE. The prostate, lung, colorectal, and ovarian cancer screening trial of the National Cancer Institute. Cancer 1995;75:1869–1873.
40. Roach M, Small EJ. Using the serum prostate specific antigen (PSA) to screen for and manage prostate cancer. Principles and Practice of Oncology Updates 1997;11:1–14.
41. Oesterline JE. Prostate specific antigen: Its role in diagnostics and staging of prostate cancer. Cancer 1995;75(suppl):1795–1804.
42. Catalona WJ, Smith DS, Ratliff TL, et al. Measurement of prostate-specific antigen in serum as a screening test for prostate cancer. N Engl J Med 1991;324:1156–1161.
43. Pannek J, Partin A. Prostate-specific antigen: What's new in 1997? Oncology (Huntingt) 1997;11:1273–1278.
44. Morgan TO, Jacobsen SJ, McCarthy EF, et al. Age specific reference ranges for serum prostate-specific antigen in black men. N Engl J Med 196;335:304–310.
45. Benoit RM, Naslund MJ. The economics of prostate cancer screening. Oncology (Huntingt) 1997;11:1533–1543.
46. Coley C, Barry M, Fleming C, et al. Early detection of prostate cancer: Part II: Estimating the risks, benefits, and costs. Ann Intern Med 1997;126:468–479.
47. Krahn M, Mahoney J, Eckman M, et al. Screening for prostate cancer: A decision analytic view. JAMA 1994;272:773–780.

48. Thompson IM, Optenberg SA. An overview cost-utility analysis of prostate cancer screening. Oncology (Huntingt) 1995;9:141–145.
49. Kantrowitz W, Doyle J, Semeraro J, Krane RJ. Prostate cancer screening in a large corporation population. J Occup Environ Med 1995;37:1193–1198.
50. Society AC. Prostate Cancer Detection Guidelines, 1997.
51. Wilt TJ, Brawer MK. Early intervention or expectant management for prostate cancer. The Prostate Cancer Intervention Versus Observation Trial (PIVOT): A randomized trial comparing radical prostatectomy with expectant management for the treatment of clinically localized prostate cancer. Semin Urol 1995;13:130–136.
52. Millikan R, Logothetis C. Update of the NCCN Guidelines for Treatment of Prostate Cancer. Oncology (Huntingt) 1997;11:180–193.
53. Montie JE. Staging of prostate cancer: Current TNM classification and future prospects for prognostic factors. Cancer 1995;75(suppl): 1814–1818.
54. Mettlin C, Murphy G, Ho R, Menck H. The national cancer database report on longitudinal observations on prostate cancer. Cancer 1996; 77:150–159.
55. Visakorpi T, Kallioniemi OP, Kaivula T, Isola J. New prognostic factors in prostatic carcinoma. Eur Urol 1993;24:438–449.
56. Hoeksema M, Law C. Cancer mortality rates fall: A turning point for the nation. J Natl Cancer Inst 1996;88:1706–1707.
57. Scardino PT, Weaver R, Hudson MA. Early detection of prostate cancer. Hum Pathol 1992;23:211–222.
58. Catalona WJ. Management of cancer of the prostate. N Engl J Med 1994;331:996–1003.
59. Fossa SD. Quality of life in advanced prostate cancer. Semin Oncol 1996;23:32–34.
60. Partin AW, Kattan MW, Subong EN, et al. Combination of prostate-specific antigen, clinical stage, and Gleason score to predict pathological stage of localized prostate cancer. A multi-institutional update [published erratum appears in JAMA 1997;278:118]. JAMA 1997; 227:1445–1451.
61. Chodak GW, Thisted RA, Gerber GS, et al. Results of conservative management of clinically localized prostate cancer. N Engl J Med 1994;330:242–248.
62. Walsh PC, Partin AW, Epstein JI. Cancer control and quality of life following anatomical radical retropubic prostatectomy: Results at 10 years. J Urol 1994;152:1831–1836.
63. Pilepich M, Krall J, al-Saraff M, et al. Androgen deprivation with radiation therapy compared with radiation therapy alone for locally advanced prostatic carcinoma: A randomized comparison trial of the Radiation Therapy Oncology Group. Urology 1995;45:616–623.
64. Fair WR, Cookson MS, Stroumbakis N, et al. The indications, rationale, and results of neoadjuvant androgen deprivation in the treatment of prostatic cancer: Memorial Sloan-Kettering Cancer Center results. Urology 1997;49:46–55.
65. Soloway M, Sharafi R, Wajsman Z, et al. Randomized prospective study comparing radical prostatectomy alone versus radical prostatectomy preceded by androgen blockade in clinical stage B2 (T2bNxMo) prostate cancer. The Leupron Depot Neoadjuvant Prostate Cancer Study Group. J Urol 1995;154:424–428.
66. Roach M. Neoadjuvant total androgen suppression and radiotherapy in the management of locally advanced prostate cancer. Semin Urol 1996;14:32–38.
67. Wong WS, Chinn DO, Chinn M, Chinn J, Tom WL. Cryosurgery as a treatment for prostate carcinoma: Results and complications. Cancer 1997;79:963–974.
68. D'Amico AV, Coleman CN. Role of interstitial radiotherapy in the management of clinically organ-confined prostate cancer: The jury is still out. J Clin Oncol 1996;14:304–315.
69. Schellhammer P, Cockett A, Boccon-Gibod L, et al. Assessment of endpoints for clinical trials for localized prostate cancer. Urology 1997;49:27–38.
70. Wasson JH, Cushman CC, Bruskewitz RC, et al. A structured literature review of treatment for localized prostate cancer. Prostate Disease Patient Outcome Research Team. Arch Fam Med 1993;2: 487–493.
71. Troyer JK, Beckett ML, Wright GL Jr. Detection and characterization of the prostate-specific membrane antigen (PSMA) in tissue extracts and body fluids. Int J Cancer 1995;62:552–558.
72. Crawford ED, Eisenberger MA, McLeod DG, et al. A controlled trial of leuprolide with and without flutamide in prostatic carcinoma. N Engl J Med 1989;321:419–424.
73. Sharifi R, Bruskewitz RC, Gittleman MC, et al. Leuprolide acetate 22.5 mg 12-week depot formulation in the treatment of patients with advanced prostate cancer. Clin Ther 1996;18:647–657.
74. Fernandez del Moral P, Dijkman GA, Debruyne FM, Witjes WP, Kolvenbag GJ. Three-month depot of goserelin acetate: Clinical efficacy and endocrine profile. Dutch South East Cooperative Urological Group. Urology 1996;48:894–900.
75. Garnick MR, Glode LM. Leuprolide versus diethylstilbestrol for metastatic prostate cancer. N Engl J Med 1984;311:1281–1286.
76. Debruyne F, Dijkman G, Lee D, et al. A new long acting formulation of the leuteinizing hormone-releasing hormone analogue, goserelin: Results of studies in prostate cancer. J Urol 1996;155:1352–1354.
77. Brogden RN, Chrisp P. Flutamide. A review of its pharmacodynamic and pharmacokinetic properties and therapeutic use in advanced prostate cancer. Drugs Aging 1991;1:104–115.
78. Soloway M, Schellhammer P, Smith J, et al. Bicalutamide in the treatment of advanced prostate carcinoma: A phase II multicenter trial. Urology 1996;47:33–37.
79. Scher H, Leibertz C, Kelly W, et al. Bicalutamide for advanced prostate cancer: The natural history versus treated history of disease. J Clin Oncol 1997;15:2928–2938.
80. Janknegt RA, Abbou CC, Bartoletti R, et al. Orchiectomy and nilutamide or placebo as treatment of metastatic prostatic cancer in a multinational double-blind randomized trial. J Urol 1993;149:77–82.
81. Janknegt RA. Total androgen blockade with the use of orchiectomy and nilutamide (Anandron) or placebo as treatment of metastatic prostate cancer. Anandron International Study Group. Cancer 1993; 72:3874–3877.
82. Kaisary A. Current clinical studies with a new nonsteroidal antiandrogen, Casodex. Prostate 1994;5(suppl):27–33.
83. Bales G, Chodak G. A controlled trial of bicalutamide versus castration in patients with advanced prostate cancer. Urology 1996;47:38–43.
84. Decensi A, Bocardo F, Guarneri D, et al. Monotherapy with nilutamide, a pure nonsteroidal antiandrogen, in untreated patients with metastatic carcinoma of the prostate. J Urol 1991;146:377–381.
85. Schellhammer P, Sharifi R, Block N, et al. A controlled trial of bicalutamide versus flutamide, each in combination with luteinizing hormone-releasing hormone analogue therapy, in patients with advanced prostate cancer. Casodex Combination Study Group. Urology 1995; 45:745–752.
86. Labrie F, Dupont A, Simard J, Luu-The V, Belanger A. Intracrinology: The basis for the rational design of endocrine therapy at all stages of prostate cancer. Eur Urol 1993;2:94–105.
87. Labrie F, Dupont A, Cusan L, et al. Combination therapy with flutamide and medical (LH-RH agonist) or surgical castration in advanced prostate cancer: 7-Year clinical experience. J Steroid Biochem Molec Biol 1990;37:943–950.
88. Eisenberger M, Crawford ED, Blumenstein B, et al. National Cancer Institute Integroup Study 0036. Prognostic factors in stage D2 prostate cancer; important implications for future trials: Results of a cooperative intergroup study (INT 0036). Semin Oncol 1994;21:613–619.
89. Iversen P, Rasmussen F, Klarskov P, Christensen IJ. Long-term results of Danish Prostatic Cancer Group Trial 86. Goserelin acetate plus flutamide versus orchiectomy in advanced prostate cancer. Cancer 1993;72:3851–3854.
90. Tyrell CJ, Altwein JE, Klippel F, et al. Multicenter randomized trial comparing Zoladex with Zoladex plus flutamide in the treatment of advanced prostate cancer. Survival update. International Prostate Cancer Study Group. Cancer 1993;72:3878–3879.

91. Denis LJ, Carnelro de Moura JL, Bono A, et al. Goserelin acetate and flutamide versus bilateral orchiectomy: A phase III EORTC trial (30853). EORTC GU Group and EORTC Data Center. Urology 1993;42:119–129.
92. Eisenberger M, Crawford ED, McLeod D, et al. A comparison of bilateral orchiectomy (orch) with or without flutamide in stage D2 prostate cancer (PC) (NCI INT-0105 SWOG/ECOG). Proc ASCO 1997;16:2a. Abstract.
93. Prostate Cancer Trialists' Collaborative Group. Maximum androgen blockade in advanced prostate cancer: An overview of 22 randomised trials with 3283 deaths in 5710 patients. Lancet 1995;346:265–269.
94. Schellhammer P, Sharifi R, Block N, et al. A controlled trial of bicalutamide versus flutamide, each in combination with luteinizing hormone-releasing hromone analogue therapy, in patients with advanced prostate carcinoma: Analysis of time to progression. Cancer 1996;78: 2164–2169.
95. Mazeman E, Bertrand P. Early versus delayed hormonal therapy in advanced prostate cancer. Eur Urol 1996;30(suppl 1):40–3. Discussion 49.
96. Labrie F. Endocrine therapy of prostate cancer: Optimal form and timing. J Clin Endocrinol Metab 1995;80:1066–1071.
97. The Veterans Administration Cooperative Urological Research Group. Carcinoma of the prostate: Treatment comparisons. J Urol 1967; 98:516–522.
98. Byar DP, Corle DK. Hormone therapy for prostate cancer: Results of the Veterans Administration Cooperative Urologic Research Group studies. Natl Cancer Inst Monogr 1988;7:165–170.
99. Denis L, Murphy GP. Overview of phase III trials on combined androgen treatment in patients with metastatic prostate cancer. Cancer 1993;72:3888–3895.
100. Crawford ED, DeAntonio EP, Labrie F, Schroder FH, Geller J. Endocrine therapy of prostate cancer: Optimal form and appropriate timing. J Clin Endocrinol Metab 1995;80:1062–1066.
101. Cookson MS, Sarosdy MF. Hormonal therapy for metastatic prostate cancer: Issues of timing and total androgen ablation. South Med J 1994;87:1–6.
102. Blackard CE. The Veterans' Administration Cooperative Urological Research Group. Studies of carcinoma of the prostate: A review. Cancer Chemother Rep 1975;59:225–227.
103. Waselenko JK, Dawson NA. Management of progressive metastatic prostate cancer. Oncology (Huntingt) 1997;11:1551–1560. Discussion 1560–1563, 1567–1568.
104. Scher HI, Kelly WK. Flutamide withdrawal syndrome: Its impact on clinical trials in hormone refractory prostate cancer. J Clin Oncol 1993;11:1566–1572.
105. Small E, Srinivas S. The androgen withdrawal syndrome: Experience in a large cohort of unselected patients with advanced prostate cancer. Cancer 1995;76:1428–1434.
106. Nieh PT. Withdrawal phenomenon with the antiandrogen casodex. J Urol 1995;153:1070–1072.
107. Huan SD, Gerridzen RG, Yau JC, Stewart DJ. Antiandrogen withdrawal syndrome with nilutamide. Urology 1997;49:632–634.
108. Klocker H, Culig Z, Hobisch A, Cato AC, Bartsch G. Androgen receptor alterations in prostatic carcinoma. Prostate 1994;25:266–273.
109. Scher HI, Kolvenbag GJ. The antiandrogen withdrawal syndrome in relapsed prostate cancer. Eur Urol 1997;31(suppl 2):3–7. Discussion 24–27.
110. Sartor O, Cooper M, Weinberger M, et al. Surprising activity of flutamide withdrawal, when combined with aminoglutethimide, in treatment of hormone-refractory prostate cancer. J Natl Cancer Inst 1994;86:222–227.
111. Esper PS, Pienta KJ. Supportive care in the patient with hormone refractory prostate cancer. Semin Urol Oncol 1997;15:56–64.
112. Crawford ED, Kozlowski JM, Debruyne FM, et al. The use of strontium 89 for palliation of pain from bone metastases associated with hormone-refractory prostate cancer. Urology 1994;44:481–485.
113. Resche I, Chatal JF, Pecking A, et al. A dose-controlled study of ^{153}Sm-ethylenediaminetetramethylenephosphonate (EDTMP) in the treatment of patients with painful bone metastases. Eur J Cancer 1997;33:1583–1591.
114. Kreis W. Current chemotherapy and future directions in research for the treatment of advanced hormone-refractory prostate cancer. Cancer Invest 1995;13:296–312.
115. Siu LL, Moore MJ. Other chemotherapy regimens including mitoxantrone and suramin. Semin Urol Oncol 1997;15:20–27.
116. Hussain M, Wolf M, Marshall E, Crawford ED, Eisenberger M. Effects of continued androgen-deprivation therapy and other prognostic factors on response and survival in phase II chemotherapy trials for hormone-refractory prostate cancer: A Southwest Oncology Group report. J Clin Oncol 1994;12:1868–1875.
117. Tannock IF. Is there evidence that chemotherapy is of benefit to patients with carcinoma of the prostate? J Clin Oncol 1985;3:1013–1021.
118. Seidman AD, Scher HI, Petrylak D, Dershaw DD, Curley T. Estramustine and vinblastine: Use of prostate specific antigen as a clinical trial end point for hormone refractory prostatic cancer. J Urol 1992; 147:931–934.
119. Eisenberger MA. Chemotherapy for prostate cancer. Natl Cancer Inst Monogr 1988;7:151–163.
120. Hudes G. Estramustine-based chemotherapy. Semin Urol Oncol 1997; 15:13–19.
121. Hudes GR, Greenberg R, Krigel RL, et al. Phase II study of estramustine and vinblastine, two microtubule inhibitors, in hormone-refractory prostate cancer. J Clin Oncol 1992;10:1754–1761.
122. Perry CM, McTavish D. Estramustine phosphate sodium. A review of its pharmacodynamic and pharmacokinetic properites, and therapeutic efficacy in prostate cancer. Drugs Aging 1995;7: 49–74.
123. Tannock IF, Osoba D, Stockler MR, et al. Chemotherapy with mitoxantrone plus prednisone or prednisone alone for symptomatic hormone-resistant prostate cancer: A Canadian randomized trial with palliative end points [see comments]. J Clin Oncol 1996;14:1756–1764.
124. Iversen P, Rasmussen F, Asmussen C, et al. Estramustine phosphate versus placebo as second line treatment after orchiectomy in patients with metastatic prostate cancer. DAPROCA study 9002. Danish Prostatic Cancer Group. J Urol 1997;157:929–934.
125. Murphy GP, Beckley S, Brady MF, et al. Treatment of newly diagnosed metastatic prostate cancer patients with chemotherapy agents in combination with hormones versus hormones alone. Cancer 1983;51:1264–1272.
126. Osborne CK, Blumenstein B, Crawford ED, et al. Combined versus sequential chemo-endocrine therapy in advanced prostate cancer: Final results of a randomized southwest oncology group study. J Clin Oncol 1990;8:1675–1682.
127. Janknegt RA, Boon TA, van de Beek C, Grob P. Combined hormono/ chemotherapy as primary treatment for metastatic prostate: A randomized, multicenter study of orchiectomy alone versus orchiectomy plus estramustine phosphate. The Dutch Estracyt Study Group. Urology 1997;49:411–420.
128. Scher HI, Mazumdar M, Kelly WK. Clinical trials in relapsed prostate cancer: Defining the target. J Natl Cancer Inst 1996; 88:1623–1634.
129. Kelly WK, Slovin S, Scher HI. Clinical use of posttherapy prostate-specific antigen changes in advanced prostate cancer. Semin Oncol 1996;23:8–14.
130. Roth BJ. New therapeutic agents for hormone-refractory prostate cancer. Semin Oncol 1996;23:49–55.
131. Warner JA, Heston WDW. Future developments of nonhormonal systemic therapy for prostatic carcinoma. Urol Clin North Am 1991; 18:25–33.
132. Sanda MG. Biological principles and clinical development of prostate cancer gene therapy. Semin Urol Oncol 1997;15:43–55.
133. Eisenberger MA, Sinibaldi V, Reyno L. Suramin. Cancer Pract 1995; 3:187–189.
134. Myers C, Cooper M, Stein C, et al. Suramin: A novel growth factor antagonist with activity in hormone-refractory metastatic prostate cancer. J Clin Oncol 1992;10:881–889.

135. Brawley OW, Thompson IM. Chemoprevention of prostate cancer. Urology 1994;43:594–599.
136. Karp JE, Chiarodo A, Brawley O, Kelloff GJ. Prostate cancer prevention: Investigational approaches and opportunities. Cancer Res 1996;56:5547–5556.
137. Aquilana JW, Lipsky JJ, Bostwick DG. Androgen deprivation as a strategy for prostate cancer prevention. J Natl Cancer Inst 1997;89: 689–696.
138. Hillner BE, McLeod DG, Crawford ED, Bennett CL. Estimating the cost effectiveness of total androgen blockade with flutamide in M1 prostate cancer. Urology 1995;45:633–640.
139. Bennett CL, Matchar D, McCrory D, et al. Cost-effective models for flutamide for prostate carcinoma patients: Are they helpful to policy makers? Cancer 1996;77:1854–1861.
140. Scher HI, Steineck G, Kelly WK. Hormone-refractory (D3) prostate cancer: Refining the concept. Urology 1995;46:142–148.
141. Spirnak JP, Kesnick. Urol Clin North Am 1984;11:224.
142. Drug Topics: Annual Pharmacists' Reference (Redbook). Oradell, NJ, Medical Economics, 1998.

120

MALIGNANT LYMPHOMAS

Val R. Adams, PharmD, and Ashley K. Morris, PharmD, BCPS, BCOP

Lymphomas are a heterogeneous group of malignancies that arise from malignant transformation of immune cells that reside predominantly in lymphoid tissues. They most commonly present as a solid tumor, but can in some cases be found in peripheral blood. The differing histology of lymphoma cells has led to classification of Hodgkin's disease (Reed–Sternberg cells) or non-Hodgkin's lymphoma (B- or T-cell lymphocyte markers). Non-Hodgkin's lymphomas are further classified by their natural clinical course (indolent versus aggressive). Chemotherapy is the mainstay of treatment in patients with lymphoma, especially those with widespread disease. Overall cure rates are high for many subtypes of lymphomas, even when patients present with advanced disease.

HODGKIN'S DISEASE

Thomas Hodgkin first described the mysterious disease of the lymph system that bears his name more than 150 years ago. Hodgkin's disease is a form of lymphoma, the cause of which is still unknown, and is invariably fatal if left untreated. Studies have demonstrated the orderly spread of this disease. Hodgkin's disease is classified into four histologic subtypes that differ in their natural history and treatment. The stage of Hodgkin's disease influences prognosis as well as therapy. The pathologic stage represents the best approximation of extent of disease and is based on histopathologic examination of the specimen obtained from biopsy of appropriate tissue during staging laparotomy. Dramatic advances have been made in the understanding and treatment of Hodgkin's disease during the past three decades. Today, many newly diagnosed patients with Hodgkin's disease will be cured. This extraordinary success has not been without cost. The treatment programs are intense, technically demanding, and associated with significant acute toxicity and long-term complications. The long-term effects of standard chemotherapy regimens have been more fully documented in recent years and could shape therapy in the future.

INCIDENCE AND EPIDEMIOLOGY

It has been estimated that nearly 7100 new cases of Hodgkin's disease will be diagnosed in the United States in 1998, which represents less than 1% of all known cancers. It is also expected that there will be 1400 deaths associated with Hodgkin's disease during the same time period. This disease occurs slightly more frequently in males than in females (52% vs 48%).[1] Once thought to be only a disease of the young, it is now recognized that Hodgkin's disease exhibits a bimodal distribution in industrialized countries.[2,3] The first peak occurs between the ages of 15 and 34 and the second in those older than 55. In recent years, there has been an increased incidence seen in the younger age bracket and a declining incidence in those over 40, which may be owing to more accurate diagnosis of lymphoid malignancies in this age group.[4] When only deaths caused by Hodgkin's disease are considered, the 10-year survival rates for stage I, II, III, and IV disease are 84%, 78%, 62%, and 42%, respectively. Overall survival for all stages combined at 10 years is 65%.[5]

ETIOLOGY

The etiology of Hodgkin's disease has not been fully elucidated. Infection has been considered a potential cause ever since the disease was first described. Viruses have emerged as the leading candidates for an infectious etiology. Studies have suggested an increased risk of Hodgkin's disease in patients who have had mononucleosis caused by the Epstein-Barr virus (EBV). Reed–Sternberg cells (which are large, bilobate, multinuclear cells associated with Hodgkin's disease) have been found in mononucleosis patients. Both serologic and molecular methods have now linked EBV to Hodgkin's disease.[6]

BIOLOGY AND HISTOPATHOLOGY

Lymphocytes, the principal cellular component of lymphoid tissue, are widely distributed throughout the body and in aggregated centers. The bone marrow and thymus are the primary organs of lymphopoiesis, with secondary sites being the lymph nodes, spleen, lamina propria of the gastrointestinal tract, and Waldeyer's ring.

Hodgkin's disease is unique among the lymphomas because only a very small percentage of cells from the involved tissue are malignant; the vast majority of cells are normal reactive hematopoietic cells. The exact cellular origin of the malignant cell has yet to be determined. It is believed that the Reed–Sternberg cell and its variants are derived from either B lymphocytes or a macrophage/reticulum cell lineage. More recent availability of monoclonal antibodies and molecular genetic analysis has greatly improved our understanding of the immunohistology and histopathology of

Hodgkin's disease. Although the BCL-2 oncogene has been identified in Hodgkin's tissue samples (which would indicate a B-cell origin), there is evidence to suggest that the t (14:18) chromosomal translocation is associated with a bystander normal lymphocyte and not the Reed–Sternberg cell.[6] Alterations in the expression of *p*53, a tumor-suppressor gene, have been observed in all types of Hodgkin's disease except lymphocyte-predominance disease. An explanation for the apparent multilineage origin of the Reed–Sternberg cell is that the malignant cell represents an *in vivo* clonal population that occurs in response to viral stimuli (EBV) that promotes fusion of the interdigitating reticular cell, B cells, T cells, or both lymphocytes.[6]

CLASSIFICATION

Lukes, Butler, and Hicks introduced a histopathologic classification of Hodgkin's disease (known as the Lukes–Butler classification) that was modified at the Rye conference in 1965 and is today called the Rye classification.[7,8] This classification is still widely accepted by both pathologists and clinicians, although a new classification system has been proposed recently. In 1994, the International Lymphoma Study Group published the Revised European–American Classification of Lymphoid Neoplasms called the REAL classification.[9] The Rye classification divides Hodgkin's disease into four subtypes: lymphocyte predominance, nodular sclerosis, mixed cellularity, and lymphocyte depletion; the REAL classification makes a distinction between nodular lymphocyte-predominance Hodgkin's disease and lymphocyte-rich classic Hodgkin's disease. The subtypes in these classification systems are based on characteristics of the Reed–Sternberg cell and the surrounding cells and connective tissue. They differ somewhat in natural history and response to treatment. With the introduction of extensive staging, sophisticated megavolt (MeV) radiotherapy, and effective combination chemotherapy, the true prognostic value of these subtypes is much less clear.

LYMPHOCYTE-PREDOMINANCE TYPE

Lymphocyte-predominance Hodgkin's disease (LPHD) has characteristic benign-appearing lymphocytes that have a diffuse growth pattern. LPHD is generally associated with localized, indolent disease. The lymph nodes are usually partially to completely destroyed. Reed–Sternberg cells are uncommon, whereas the predominant cell appears to be a B lymphocyte. Fibrosis is also uncommon. This subtype can account for 9% of all Hodgkin's disease, is slightly more common in males than females, and may represent a more favorable prognosis.[4]

NODULAR SCLEROSIS TYPE

Nodular sclerosis Hodgkin's disease (NSHD) has two features that distinguish it from all other forms: the presence of the lacunar cell, which is a variant of the Reed–Sternberg cell, and the presence of a capsule that divides the lymphoid tissue into distinct nodules. Actually, Reed–Sternberg cells are rare. This subtype can represent up to 56% of all Hodgkin's disease and is equally divided between females and males.[4] NSHD is associated with a more favorable prognosis because it is often localized, although involvement of the mediastinum is common.

MIXED CELLULARITY TYPE

Mixed cellularity Hodgkin's disease (MCHD) occupies a position between the lymphocyte-predominance and lymphocyte-depletion subtypes with regard to the number of neoplastic cells present. It can be mistaken for high-grade non-Hodgkin's lymphoma. Reed–Sternberg cells are more common in this subtype. Diffuse fibrosis is uncommon. This subtype can account for 28% of all Hodgkin's disease, is slightly more common in males than females, and is associated with an intermediate prognosis.[4]

LYMPHOCYTE-DEPLETION TYPE

Lymphocyte-depletion Hodgkin's disease (LDHD) is associated with an abundance of Reed–Sternberg cells and their variants. It also can be easily mistaken for high-grade non-Hodgkin's lymphoma. Diffuse fibrosis and necrosis are commonly seen. This subtype accounts for 7% of all Hodgkin's disease, is more common in males than females, is often widespread at the time of diagnosis, and may be associated with a less favorable prognosis.[4] This category is also most commonly associated with the acquired immunodeficiency syndrome (AIDS) for which the prognosis is very poor.

CLINICAL PRESENTATION

Most patients with lymphomas present with some form of adenopathy. The clinical presentations of Hodgkin's disease and the non-Hodgkin's lymphomas have some striking differences (Table 120–1). It is generally not possible to differentiate between the various lymphomas by the physical characteristics of the lymph node itself, but the distribution can offer useful information.

Patients with Hodgkin's disease may have adenopathy that waxes and wanes for an average of 5 months before diagnosis. This adenopathy is usually localized to the cervical region and is painless and rubbery. Adenopathy of the inguinal and axillary regions may be present at diagnosis but is less common, whereas involvement of Waldeyer's ring and the epitrochlear nodes occurs in roughly 1% of patients (Fig. 120–1).[10] Other common sites of nodal involvement include the mediastinal, hilar, and retroperitoneal regions. Up to 40% of patients with Hodgkin's disease may also present with constitutional symptoms (B symptoms) including fever, night sweats, and weight loss.[10] Pruritis is also commonly noted in patients with Hodgkin's disease, but its presence does not appear to have significant prognostic value.

TABLE 120–1. Clinical Features of the Lymphomas

	Hodgkin's Disease	Non-Hodgkin's Lymphoma
Lymph node disease	Centripetal	Centrifugal
Contiguous spread	Common	Uncommon
Mediastinal disease	50%	20%[a]
Abdominal disease	Uncommon	Common
Bone marrow	Uncommon involvement	Common
Liver involvement	Uncommon (if present, spleen usually involved)	Common in follicular, uncommon in diffuse
Extranodal disease	Uncommon	Gastrointestinal tract, Waldeyer's ring, testes, epitrochlear nodes, brain
Systemic "B" symptoms	40%	20%

[a]With the exception of T-cell lymphoblastic lymphoma.

DIAGNOSIS AND STAGING

The diagnosis and pathologic classification of Hodgkin's disease can be made only by biopsy of the enlarged node and histopathologic examination under a microscope. Full evaluation of extent of disease, or staging, is necessary with Hodgkin's disease. Staging determines appropriate treatment of the disease and provides useful information regarding prognosis. In addition, specific knowledge of the involved sites of disease can be used to determine response. Presence of advanced-stage, extensive B symptoms, and massive mediastinal involvement implies a poorer prognosis for a given patient.

The Ann Arbor staging classification, which was developed at the 1970 Ann Arbor conference, has proven to be a good workable scheme.[11] At the Cotswolds meeting in 1989, the Ann Arbor classification was modified to account for new diagnostic techniques (e.g., computed tomography [CT] and magnetic resonance imaging [MRI]) and the realization that prognosis is associated with the bulk of the disease and the number of involved nodal sites (Table 120–2).[12] After careful staging, roughly half the patients have localized disease (stages I, II, and II_E) and the remainder have advanced disease, of which 10% to 15% are stage IV. One of the most important factors to remember is that Hodgkin's disease appears to follow a predictable pattern of nodal spread that is not seen with the non-Hodgkin's lymphomas.

Diagnostic and staging procedures are based on recommendations made at the Ann Arbor and Cotswolds conferences and new scientific advances.[11,12] Clinical staging begins with a thorough history to evaluate possible symptoms, including fever, night sweats, and weight loss. A complete physical exam is done to determine nodal and extranodal involvement. Laboratory tests assess bone marrow, renal, and hepatic function. As stated previously, a true diagnosis can be made only with an adequate surgical biopsy, not aspiration. A chest roentgenogram and thoracic CT are necessary to evaluate mediastinal involvement. Abdominal involvement is evaluated using the lower extremity lymphangiogram and abdominal CT. With the advent of the abdominal CT, some experts now question the usefulness of the lymphangiogram. Skeletal films are used to evaluate the thoracic and lumbar vertebrae, pelvis, and proximal extremities. A bone marrow biopsy is especially helpful in patients who have constitutional symptoms or have an elevated alkaline phosphatase, hypercalcemia, or unexplained anemia.

Other diagnostic procedures including intravenous pyelogram, whole-lung tomography, pelvic CT, gallium scanning, isotope scanning, and MRI are now reserved for special situations or until a true definitive use can be determined.

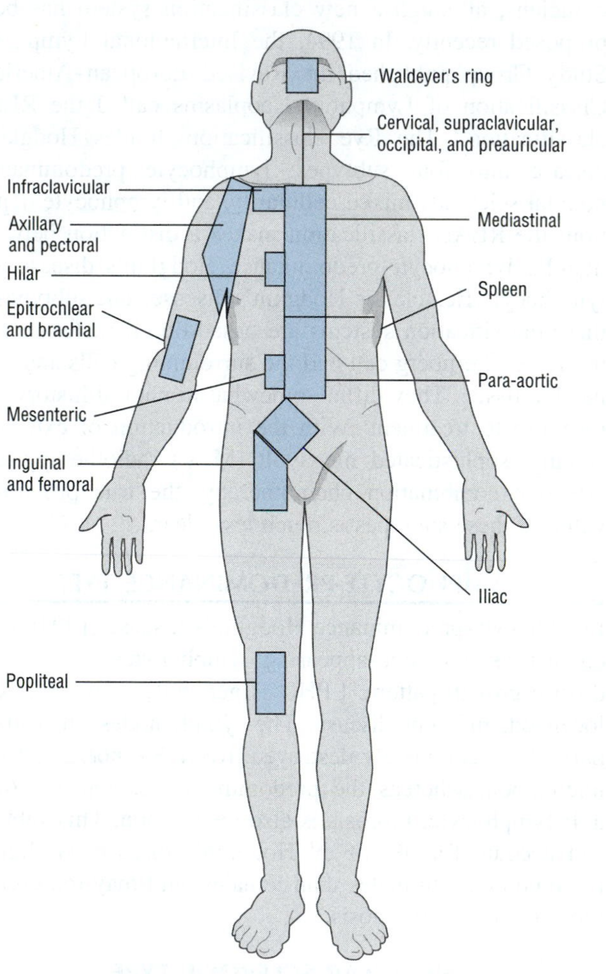

FIGURE 120–1. Schematic representation of the anatomic regions used in the staging of Hodgkin's disease. *(From Rosenberg SA. Staging of Hodgkin's disease [Letter to the Editor]. Radiology 1966;87:146, with permission.)*

TABLE 120–2. The Cotswolds Staging Classification of Hodgkin's Disease

Stage I	Involvement of a single lymph node region or structure (I) or of a single extralymphatic organ or site (I_E)
Stage II	Involvement of two or more lymph node regions on the same side of the diaphragm (II) or localized involvement of an extralymphatic organ or site and of one or more lymph node regions on the same side of the diaphragm (II_E). The number of nodal regions involved should be indicated by a subscript (e.g., II_2)
Stage III	Involvement of lymph node regions on both sides of the diaphragm (III), which may also be accompanied by localized involvement of an extralymphatic organ or site (III_E) or by involvement of the spleen (IIIS) or both ($IIIS_E$). III_1: with or without splenic, hilar, celiac, or portal node involvement. III_2: with para-aortic, iliac, or mesenteric node involvement
Stage IV	Diffuse or disseminated involvement of one or more extralymphatic organs or tissues with or without associated lymph node enlargement
	A—No symptoms
	B—Fever, night sweats, weight loss (> 10%)
	X—Bulky disease
	> one-third the width of the mediastinum
	> 10 cm maximal dimension of nodal mass
	E—Involvement of extralymphatic tissue on one side of the diaphragm by limited direct extension from an adjacent, involved lymph node region
	S—Involvement of the spleen
	CS—Clinical stage
	PS—Pathologic stage

Adapted from Refs. 11 and 12.

Staging can be based on clinical or pathologic findings. Clinical staging (CS) is based on the history, physical exam, initial diagnostic biopsy, laboratory tests, and radiologic findings. Pathologic staging (PS) is based on the biopsy findings of strategic sites (muscle, bone, skin, spleen, abdominal nodes) using an invasive procedure such as a laparoscopy or laparotomy. Those patients with extranodal disease (muscle, skin, bone, Waldeyer's ring) contiguous to involved nodes are classified with the subscript "E" in the Cotswolds staging system.[12]

Laparotomy remains a controversial area in the staging of Hodgkin's disease. Its primary purpose is to determine the presence and extent of abdominal involvement in patients presenting with supradiaphragmatic Hodgkin's disease. Laparotomy should be performed only in patients with clinical evidence of early-stage disease and when treatment with radiation therapy alone is being considered. Laparotomy should not be performed in patients with large bulky mediastinal disease because these patients will require combined-modality therapy including radiation and chemotherapy for appropriate management of their disease. In addition, patients presenting with clinically advanced disease should not undergo staging laparotomy because they will require combination chemotherapy. Laparotomy is not without risk; the overall mortality rate can range from 0.5% to as high as 6% with morbidity rates exceeding 25%.[13] The argument in favor of performing laparotomy is that 20% to 30% of clinically staged IA and IIA patients and 35% of clinically staged IB and IIB patients will be found to have splenic or upper abdominal involvement during laparotomy.[14,15]

More recent efforts focus on the determination of prognostic factors in clinically staged patients that predict the likelihood of occult abdominal involvement.[14,15] Select subgroups of CS I to II patients, including CS IA females, CS IIA females age 26 or younger, and CS IA males with lymphocyte-predominance histology, are at lowest risk of occult abdominal involvement (6% to 9%). Therefore, they can be safely treated with radiation therapy alone. The remainder of patients with CS IIA and all CS IB to IIB patients are at substantial risk for subdiaphragmatic Hodgkin's disease and should undergo staging laparotomy or be treated with combination chemotherapy.[14,15] As the ability to detect subdiaphragmatic disease with noninvasive diagnostic techniques improves and the predictive value of prognostic indicators is validated, the use of laparotomy will decrease.

▶ TREATMENT: Hodgkin's Disease

The current goal in the treatment of Hodgkin's disease is to maximize curability while minimizing short- and long-term treatment-related complications. The development of effective therapies for all stages of Hodgkin's disease remains one of the most remarkable achievements in modern cancer care. This has been brought about by the introduction of modern linear accelerators providing radiation beams in the range of < 10 MeV, effective combination chemotherapy regimens, and new methods of combining these two modalities.

RADIATION THERAPY ALONE

Radiation therapy alone is still the cornerstone of treatment for most patients with localized Hodgkin's disease (stages IA and IIA). The types of fields used are shown in Figure 120–2. Therapeutic doses of radiation, to involved sites, range from 40 to 44 Gy, which are fractionated with daily treatments of 1.5 to 2 Gy (depending on field size and patient tolerance).[10] Treatment of adjacent uninvolved areas, which typically require a minimum of 30 to 35 Gy, may also be an important factor in treatment outcome with radiation therapy alone. A recent meta-analysis conducted by Specht and colleagues indicates that more extensive radiotherapy may reduce the risk of treatment failure at 10 years (31% vs 43%) in patients with early-stage Hodgkin's disease, although there was no apparent improvement in overall 10-year survival.[16]

STAGES IA AND IIA (SUPRADIAPHRAGMATIC)

Patients with stage IA or IIA supradiaphragmatic (above the diaphragm) disease can be successfully treated with radiation

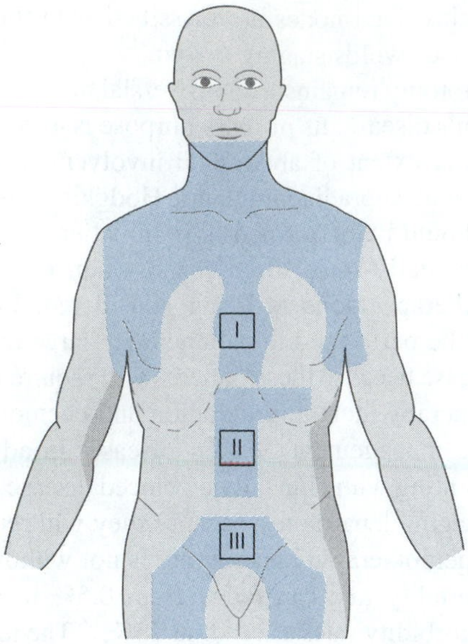

FIGURE 120–2. Radiation fields (shaded areas) commonly employed in Hodgkin's disease. I = mantle; II = para-aortic–splenic pedicle; III = pelvic. I + II = subtotal nodal irradiation. I + II + III = total nodal irradiation. *(From Eyre HJ, Farver ML. Hodgkin's disease and non-Hodgkin's lymphomas. In: Holleb AI, Fink, DJ, Murphy GP, eds. Textbook of Clinical Oncology. Atlanta, GA, American Cancer Society, Inc., 1991:382, with permission.)*

therapy alone. Mantle irradiation using doses ranging from 40 to 44 Gy are employed. This may be followed with treatment of the para-aortic splenic pedicle field alone, or include the area below the bifurcation of the aorta including the iliac nodes (which is called the spade field), with radiation doses ranging from 30 to 40 Gy. Treatment of these additional uninvolved areas is called extended-field radiotherapy. Extended-field radiotherapy (also called subtotal nodal irradiation) is still considered by many to be the treatment of choice for stage IA and IIA disease (see Fig. 120–2). This treatment produces disease-free survival rates ranging from 65% to 85% and overall survival rates ranging from 75% to 93%,[17–20] although some data indicate that there is no difference in both disease-free survival and overall survival when involved-field (IF) (mantle) radiation is given versus extended-field radiation.[10,16] These studies also revealed pelvic relapse rates of less than 5%, which suggests that total nodal irradiation may not be necessary.

Extended-field radiotherapy has been compared to chemotherapy with mechlorethamine, vincristine, procarbazine, and prednisone (MOPP) and was found to be superior in the treatment of pathologic stage I to IIA Hodgkin's disease.[21] Overall survival was 93% in the radiotherapy arm versus 56% in the MOPP arm. Likewise, freedom from progression (FFP) and relapse-free survival were 76% versus 64% and 70% versus 71%, respectively. However, it should be noted that poorer results were obtained with MOPP than expected.

Because laparotomy is associated with complications, the European Organization for Research and Treatment of Cancer (EORTC) tested its value in a randomized controlled trial (H6F—favorable prognosis).[22] Patients with supradiaphragmatic CS I or II Hodgkin's disease without bulky disease or B symptoms were enrolled (n = 262). The study randomized patients to receive radiation or have a laparotomy and then receive radiation and/or chemotherapy as deemed appropriate. There was no difference in FFP or overall survival rates at 6 years, with or without laparotomy (78% vs 83% and 91% vs 85%, respectively). Therefore, laparotomy is not necessary to treat patients with radiation if they have a favorable prognosis and CS I or II disease.

STAGES IB AND IIB

About 15% to 20% of patients with stage I or II disease will present with B symptoms. Data from Stanford University and the Joint Center for Radiation Therapy indicate that subtotal nodal irradiation provides the same overall survival rate as combined-modality therapy (radiation + chemotherapy).[23] After 7 years, the overall survival and freedom-from-relapse (FFR) rates were 88% versus 89% and 86% versus 74% (P = .02) for combined-modality therapy and subtotal nodal irradiation, respectively. Although radiation provides the same survival rate, many clinicians use combined-modality therapy to reduce the relapse rate (discussed under Combined-Modality Treatment). Standard treatment for stage IB or IIB is controversial; either subtotal irradiation or combined-modality therapy is recommended.

STAGES IA AND IIA (SUBDIAPHRAGMATIC)

Nodal involvement below the diaphragm is seen in only 10% of stage I and II patients. Patients who do not have splenic involvement (60% of patients) can receive extended-field or total nodal irradiation (see Fig. 120–2). With these approaches, the outcome will be similar to patients treated for supradiaphragmatic disease.[24]

STAGE IIIA

Only a subset of patients with stage IIIA disease should be considered for radiation therapy alone. Thirty percent of patients belong to a subgroup classified as $IIIA_1$ (limited spleen, celiac, splenic, or portal nodes). These patients have a favorable disease outcome and respond well to total nodal irradiation. The disease-free and overall survival rates compare favorably to earlier-stage disease.[25] Twenty-year disease-free survival is 65%. However, more recent retrospective data suggest that patients with stage $IIIA_1$ disease may be better managed with combined-modality therapy or combination chemotherapy alone.[26] Patients with bulky mediastinal and stage $IIIA_2$ disease are discussed in a later section because radiation therapy alone is not considered treatment of choice.

CHEMOTHERAPY

One of the initial combination chemotherapy regimens introduced in the early 1960s that was shown to produce cures in advanced Hodgkin's disease was the MOPP regimen (Table 120–3).[27] MOPP chemotherapy has been the mainstay of treatment for patients with stage III and IV advanced Hodgkin's disease. According to the 20-year follow-up of the National Cancer Institute (NCI)'s data, MOPP has produced complete remissions (disappearance of all measurable disease) in 84% of patients and has a 10-year cure rate of 54%. Forty-six percent of the original patients are still alive at a median of 14 years (19% died from other illness).[28] This is in contrast to single-agent therapy, with which remissions occur less rapidly and are not as durable. Several other trials reviewed by Longo have reported similar results, with complete response rates ranging from 80% to 95% and cure rates ranging from 55% to 65%.[29] These studies indicate that patients should receive two cycles of therapy beyond that required to produce a complete response; a minimum of six cycles should be administered. Maintenance therapy has not been shown to increase survival and may contribute to the long-term complications seen with therapy. The delivery of full or nearly full doses of chemotherapy is extremely important (dose intensity). Dose reduction within the various studies is probably the single most important factor explaining the differences in response rates between in-

TABLE 120–3. Combination Chemotherapy Regimens for Hodgkin's Disease

Drug	(mg/m^2)	Route	Days
MOPP			
Mechlorethamine	6	IV	1, 8
Vincristine	1.4	IV	1, 8
Procarbazine	100	PO	1–14
Prednisone	40	PO	1–14
ABVD			
Doxorubicin	25	IV	1, 15
Bleomycin	10	IV	1, 15
Vinblastine	6	IV	1, 15
Dacarbazine	375	IV	1, 15
ChlVPP			
Chlorambucil	6	PO	1–14
Vinblastine	6	IV	1, 8
Procarbazine	100	PO	1–14
Prednisone	40	PO	1–14
MOPP/ABVD			
Alternating months of MOPP and ABVD			
MOPP/ABV Hybrid			
Mechlorethamine	6	IV	1
Vincristine	1.4	IV	1
Procarbazine	100	PO	1–7
Prednisone	40	PO	1–14
Doxorubicin	35	IV	8
Bleomycin	10	IV	8
Vinblastine	6	IV	8

Adapted from Ref. 29.

stitutions administering seemingly similar regimens.[29] Dosage reductions based on toxicity may be made, but significant reductions can alter response and survival.[28]

MOPP VARIATIONS AND OTHER ALTERNATIVE REGIMENS

Ever since MOPP therapy was created and the efficacy confirmed, researchers have been modifying the regimen in an attempt to improve efficacy and possibly decrease toxicity. Some MOPP variations and other commonly used regimens are shown in Table 120–3.[29] MVPP (vinblastine substituted for vincristine), CVPP (cyclophosphamide substituted for mechlorethamine), BCVPP (carmustine, cyclophosphamide, vinblastine, procarbazine, and prednisone), and ChlVPP (chlorambucil substituted for mechlorethamine, vinblastine substituted for vincristine) are attractive alternatives to MOPP because they offer equal efficacy and differing or less severe toxicities. ChlVPP is especially attractive because of its equivalent activity and less severe emetogenicity and neurotoxicity. The various combination chemotherapy regimens appear to produce initial complete response rates in over 80% of the patients treated and result in a 55% to 65% cure rate for advanced Hodgkin's disease.

One of the first alternative regimens was ABVD (doxorubicin, bleomycin, vinblastine, dacarbazine) developed by Bonadonna (Table 120–3). ABVD was initially shown to be effective in MOPP failures[30] and was later compared directly to MOPP in advanced disease and produced an 82% complete response rate in contrast to a 67% complete response rate with MOPP. Despite these differences in response, no major differences in 5-year survival were noted.[31] The difference in response is most likely related to excessive dosage reductions that occurred in the MOPP arm. Improved failure-free survival was demonstrated with ABVD in a subgroup with poor prognostic factors.

ALTERNATING AND HYBRID REGIMENS

The Goldie–Coldman hypothesis regarding spontaneous mutation rates and the development of resistant clones can explain many clinical findings related to cancer chemotherapy, including chemotherapy failure.[32] This hypothesis has led to the investigation of combining non–cross-resistant drug combinations.[33] One of the key requirements in such a concept is that each regimen possess equal activity. A major reason for using alternating or hybrid regimens is to decrease cumulative toxicities. In alternating and hybrid regimens such as MOPP and ABVD, the risks of sterility, secondary leukemia, and cardiotoxicity are reduced because of the lower cumulative doses of procarbazine, nitrogen mustard, and doxorubicin administered. In addition, the potential for pulmonary toxicity from bleomycin should also be reduced.

Several trials have been performed to evaluate various ways of administering non–cross-resistant MOPP and ABVD regimens. The results of selected trials representing different approaches are summarized in Table 120–4. In a randomized trial, investigators at the Milan Cancer Institute reported that MOPP alternating with ABVD was superior to MOPP alone.[34] However, some investigators have questioned the conclusions from that study because of the high dropout rate in the alternating regimen (22%) and the dose attenuation of the MOPP regimen. In a Cancer and Leukemia Group B (CALGB) study, no difference in efficacy was observed between the patients treated with the ABVD regimen versus those treated with an MOPP alternating with ABVD regimen.[31] The major conclusion from these trials is that regimens that alternate MOPP and ABVD appear to provide minimal if any improvement over MOPP or ABVD alone.

TABLE 120–4. Randomized Trials Evaluating Various Methods of Delivering Both MOPP and ABVD

Regimen	CR (%)	FFP (%)	OS (%)	Reference
MOPP vs	74	36 (8 yr)	64 (8 yr)	Milan Cancer Institute[34]
MOPP alternating w/ABVD	89	65 (8 yr)	84 (8 yr)	
ABVD vs	82	61 (5 yr)	73 (5 yr)	Cancer and Leukemia Group B (CALGB)[31]
MOPP alternating w/ABVD	83	65 (5 yr)	75 (5 yr)	
MOPP alternating w/ABVD vs	51	67 (5 yr)	81 (5 yr)	National Cancer Institute of Canada[35]
MOPP/ABV hybrid	54	71 (5 yr)	83 (5 yr)	
MOPP alternating w/ABVD vs	91	67 (10 yr)	74 (10 yr)	Milan Cancer Institute[36]
MOPP/ABV hybrid	89	69 (10 yr)	72 (10 yr)	
Sequential MOPP then ABVD vs	75	54 (8 yr)	71 (8 yr)	Intergroup trial[38]
MOPP/ABV hybrid	83	64 (8 yr)	79 (8 yr)	

ABV = doxorubicin, bleomycin, vinblastine; ABVD = doxorubicin, bleomycin, vinblastine, dacarbazine; MOPP = mechlorethamine, vincristine, procarbazine, and prednisone.

Several trials have also evaluated the combination of MOPP and ABVD in a monthly cycle (known as hybrid regimens). The National Cancer Institute of Canada[35] compared the MOPP/ABVD alternating regimen to the MOPP/ABV (doxorubicin, bleomycin, vinblastine) hybrid regimen (omitting the dacarbazine and increasing doxorubicin dosage from 25 mg/m^2 to 35 mg/m^2), and the Milan Cancer Institute[36] compared the MOPP/ABVD alternating regimen to the MOPP/ABV hybrid regimen. Neither of these studies reported a difference in freedom from progression or overall survival. However, both studies reported that patients treated with the hybrid regimen were more likely to develop neutropenic fever and stomatitis. It has also been reported that the MOPP/ABV hybrid regimen is more toxic than the ABVD regimen.[37] Finally, the last approach that has been attempted to improve efficacy is the sequential use of MOPP and ABVD. An intergroup trial reported that sequential MOPP and ABVD was inferior to the MOPP/ABV hybrid regimen in terms of response and survival.[38] The same study also reported a higher rate of secondary malignancies in the patients who received sequential therapy.

None of the alternating, hybrid, or sequential regimen trials have clearly demonstrated an advantage over fully dosed four-drug (MOPP or ABVD) regimens. Until further data are available, these more complex regimens should not replace well-established four-drug regimens.

EARLY-STAGE HODGKIN'S DISEASE

Although combination chemotherapy regimens were initially developed for patients with advanced or relapse disease, current trials are focusing on the use of chemotherapy as initial therapy in patients with pathologic or clinical stage I or II Hodgkin's disease. Current standards recommend treatment with radiation alone, or combined-modality therapy, both of which result in high response rates and cures. Treatment decisions are based on response rates as well as acute and chronic toxicities. To avoid the need for laparotomy and its associated toxicity, systemic chemotherapy and radiation can be used. Various factors can help predict the likelihood of occult abdominal involvement, such as B symptoms and large mediastinal involvement.[14,15,39] However, secondary solid tumors can be seen in 13% of patients treated with combined-modality therapy at 15 years. Because incidence of secondary leukemia is approximately 3% with MOPP and 1% with ABVD, chemotherapy alone is being investigated in low-stage disease. To establish the efficacy of chemotherapy, it has been compared to radiation. Longo and colleagues[40] found that radiation was equivalent to six cycles of MOPP in patients with stage I or II disease without bulky mediastinal disease. However, another study[41] comparing subtotal nodal irradiation to six cycles of MOPP found MOPP to be inferior and associated with increased acute toxicity. A pilot study has evaluated ABVD to treat stage I and II disease and reported an overall survival of 95% at 42 months and a progression-free survival (PFS) rate of 84%.[42] Further randomized, long-term studies are needed to confirm the equivalent efficacy between chemotherapy and radiation for early-stage disease. They also need to show an overall decrease in toxicity, particularly secondary tumors.

COMBINED-MODALITY TREATMENT

Controversy remains as to the true role radiotherapy plays when added to chemotherapy for the treatment of Hodgkin's disease. In settings where radiation therapy alone demonstrated poor results (disease with large mediastinal involvement, bulky disease, stage IIIA$_2$ disease, stage IV disease), chemotherapy alone or a combination of chemotherapy and radiation therapy remain the only other options. Patients with large mediastinal adenopathy are at increased risk for relapse following treatment with chemotherapy alone.[29]

Loeffler and colleagues conducted a meta-analysis of chemotherapy versus combined-modality treatment trials in intermediate- or advanced-stage Hodgkin's disease.[43] Studies that compared standard chemotherapy to the same chemotherapy plus radiation showed that although the addition of radiation improved tumor control, no overall survival advantage could be detected after 10 years of follow-up. These trials included approximately equal numbers of early-stage and advanced-stage patients. This meta-analysis also evaluated studies that compared prolonged chemotherapy treatments (additional cycles of the same chemotherapy or a different regimen) and standard chemotherapy combined with radiation therapy. Surprisingly, there was no difference in tumor control rates, but there was a survival advantage favoring the prolonged chemotherapy group. The majority of patients in the latter trials had advanced disease. There were several limitations of this meta-analysis. There were limited data regarding presence of bulky mediastinal disease and cause of death. There were also differences in trial design, type and number of cycles of chemotherapy, and dose and field size of radiation therapy. Overall, data from this analysis suggest that combined-modality therapy should be reserved for patients with nodular sclerosis Hodgkin's disease, for patients without stage IV disease, and for patients with bulky nodal involvement.

Newer approaches are being tried in an effort to decrease the overall extent of therapy given to patients with early-stage disease. Horning and colleagues compared six cycles of modified chemotherapy with VBM (vinblastine, bleomycin, and methotrexate) in combination with IF radiation therapy to subtotal nodal and splenic irradiation (STLI) in patients with pathologic stage IA to IIB or IIIA Hodgkin's disease.[44] Freedom from progression at 5 years favored IF + VBM (95%) as compared to STLI (70%). There was no difference in overall survival. Ten-year follow-up showed FFP of 98% versus 78% (P = .01) for patients receiving VBM plus IF compared to STLI alone.[45] A similar trial was conducted in patients with favorable clinical stage I to IIA Hodgkin's disease using the same treatment comparisons. With a median follow-up of 4 years, FFP was 87% for the combination compared to 92% for STLI. Further studies need to be done to determine the role of modified combination chemotherapy with involved field radiation in the management of early-stage Hodgkin's disease.

In another meta-analysis, Specht and associates indicated that the addition of chemotherapy to radiotherapy can reduce the risk of failure by one-half at 10 years, but does not significantly improve survival.[16] The primary conclusion from this analysis is that less intensive primary treatment, particularly a reduction in radiotherapy fields, appears to achieve similar survival rates as more intensive treatment.

The patients most likely to benefit from combined-modality therapy are those patients with early-stage disease and massive mediastinal involvement (mediastinal masses larger than one-third the greatest chest diameter on x-ray). Normally, up to 75% of these patients can expect to relapse if treated with radiation alone. The rationale for combined-modality therapy in this setting is clear. Neither radiation therapy nor chemotherapy alone is particularly successful. One group randomized 94 patients with massive mediastinal involvement to receive CVPP alone or in combination with mantle irradiation.[46] At 7 years, in the chemotherapy-alone arm, there was only a 34% disease-free survival rate compared to 75% for the combination arm. In the group with a favorable prognosis, CVPP alone was as effective as CVPP with the addition of involved field radiotherapy.

Combination chemotherapy appears the optimal therapy for most patients with stage IIIA disease. Only in specific settings, such as large mediastinal involvement, does standard combined-modality therapy show benefit in early-stage disease (stage I or II).

SALVAGE CHEMOTHERAPY

Patients who relapse after radiation therapy alone have a good chance of being cured with combination chemotherapy.[29] MOPP or one of its variants can cure 55% to 65% of patients treated for advanced Hodgkin's disease. The remaining 35% to 45% of patients will either not respond initially or will relapse after achieving a complete response.[29] For patients who relapse after an initial complete response to MOPP, reinduction is possible. The NCI has reported on their long-term follow-up of MOPP-retreated patients.[47] Patients with long initial remissions had a 45% disease-free survival rate at 10 years. However, it is doubtful if a regimen that was unable to cure when used as first-line therapy should be used for salvage when other effective regimens with less chance of cross-resistance are available. The choice of salvage treatment, then, should be guided by the estimation of the patient's tolerance for a particular set of agents. Examples of salvage regimens and their response data can be found in the review of chemotherapy in Hodgkin's disease by Longo.[29] Although about 40% of patients will achieve a complete response, only 10% to 15% of those treated will be cured by their salvage regimen.

Patients who relapse after salvage chemotherapy are candidates for high-dose therapy with stem cell rescue. High-dose therapy should also be considered in patients who relapse within 12 months of initial remission or in those who are refractory to first-line chemotherapy. Bone marrow transplantation (BMT) in Hodgkin's disease is fully reviewed in Chapter 125.

COMPLICATIONS

A variety of acute and chronic toxicities may occur as a result of staging procedures or treatment for Hodgkin's disease.[13,48] Immunologic dysfunction may result from the Hodgkin's disease process itself, but further impairment may be induced following staging laparotomy and splenectomy, radiation therapy, and/or chemotherapy. This impairment in cellular immunity predisposes the patient to infection with encapsulated organisms. Therefore, vaccination against *Pneumococcus, Haemophilus influenzae* type B, and *Meningococcus* is recommended 10 to 14 days prior to initiation of therapy for Hodgkin's disease.

Radiation therapy commonly causes anorexia, xerostomia, odynophagia, skin burns, and changes in taste perception, which are usually transient and seldom produce significant morbidity. Hypothyroidism and myelosuppression can also be seen. More serious toxic effects involving the mantle and the heart can occur during radiation therapy for Hodgkin's disease. Radiation pneumonitis and fibrosis, pericarditis, and cardiomyopathy have been reported. Neurologic complications of radiotherapy may include rare spinal cord transections with overlap of mantle and para-aortic fields or Lhermitte syndrome (consisting of numbness and tingling caused by head flexion) in up to 15% of patients. Pelvic irradiation may cause infertility in males and females. In addition, growth retardation may result from radiotherapy in pediatric patients. As the techniques for radiation therapy improve, the significant complications associated with its use will continue to be reduced.

Side effects of chemotherapy can be acute or long term. Acute toxic effects seen with the treatment of Hodgkin's disease are similar to those seen with most combination regimens. Myelosuppression is the major dose-limiting toxicity of most of these regimens. Hematopoietic growth factors (e.g., granulocyte colony-stimulating factor [G-CSF], granulocyte-macrophage colony-stimulating factor [GM-CSF]) can decrease the neutropenia associated with these regimens and allow for the delivery of optimal drug doses on schedule.

Nausea and vomiting are frequently seen with the use of dacarbazine, doxorubicin, and mechlorethamine, although the severity of this complication has been diminished with the use of 5-HT_3 (serotonin) antagonists. A significant number of patients experience neurotoxicity secondary to vincristine. Other acute adverse effects include alopecia, dermatitis, mucositis, phlebitis, malaise and fatigue, and renal dysfunction. Bleomycin or nitrosoureas may cause pneumonitis, and doxorubicin may lead to the development of cardiomyopathy. Patients receiving radiation with chemotherapy have a higher risk of all the aforementioned toxicities than patients not receiving radiation.

Long-term complications of radiation therapy, chemotherapy, and combined-modality therapy have become more evident as the curability and long-term survival of Hodgkin's disease patients have improved. Gonadal dysfunction and secondary malignancies have become important considerations in the treatment of this malignancy. Almost all men and up to 50% of premenopausal women treated with six full cycles of regimens containing alkylating agents will become sterile. This appears to be a dose-related phenomenon. For men, there does not appear to be a safe nonsterilizing dose of nitrogen mustard or chlorambucil, so if fertility is a major concern, ABVD may be the best alternative.

Now that 10-, 15-, and 20-year survival data are available, evaluation of secondary malignancies can be made.[48] The most commonly observed secondary malignancies include a variety of solid tumors, non-Hodgkin's lymphomas, acute leukemias, and associated myelodysplastic syndromes. The occurrence of solid tumors is most strongly associated with prior radiation therapy. The overall risk of developing acute leukemia (most commonly acute nonlymphocytic leukemia) ranges from 3% to 6% but may be significantly higher in certain subsets of patients. There is a higher risk of developing acute leukemia in patients treated with MOPP compared with ABVD; combined-modality therapy further increases the risk of developing secondary leukemias.

An international collaborative group of cancer registries and hospitals recently reported on 163 cases of leukemia in 29,552 patients with Hodgkin's disease.[49] This is the largest report of its kind. They presented their results in terms of relative risk rather than percent chance of developing acute leukemia. Chemotherapy alone produced a relative risk of leukemia of 9 when compared to radiation therapy alone. For patients treated with more than six cycles of combination chemotherapy containing mechlorethamine or procarbazine, the risk of leukemia was 14 times higher than for radiation alone. For patients in this series treated with chemotherapy and radiation, the relative risks were 7.7, or roughly equal to that of chemotherapy alone. The incidence of leukemia peaked at 5 years following chemotherapy, with development lasting for at least 8 years after completion of therapy. Future trials must focus on maintaining high cure rates in Hodgkin's disease while decreasing the number and severity of long-term complications.

CURRENT RECOMMENDATIONS

With radiation therapy, chemotherapy, and salvage BMT, more than 75% of patients with advanced Hodgkin's disease can now be cured. Although the special circumstances of the patient, available resources, technologies, and the skill of the practitioners influence specific treatment recommendations, the following general recommendations can be made (Table 120–5).

For patients with laparotomy-staged, supradiaphragmatic stage IA or IIA disease, mantle radiation with para-aortic fields should be used. If exploratory laparotomy or radiation is not desirable, combination chemotherapy can be recommended. Patients who have laparotomy-staged IB or IIB disease may be treated with subtotal nodal radiation therapy. Again, if a laparotomy has not been performed, stage IB or IIB disease may be best treated with combination chemotherapy. Ongoing trials in early-stage disease are evaluating the role of combination chemotherapy alone, modified chemotherapy regimens or shorter courses of standard chemotherapy combined with radiation therapy, and limited radiation field sizes.

TABLE 120–5. General Treatment Recommendations for Hodgkin's Disease[a,b]

Clinical Stage[c]		Pathologic Stage	
IA	Extended-field radiation	IA[d]	Extended-field radiation
IB	Combination chemotherapy	IB	Extended-field radiation
IIA	Extended-field radiation	IIA[d]	Extended-field radiation
IIB	Combination chemotherapy	IIB	Extended-field radiation
IIIA	Combination chemotherapy	$IIIA_1$	Extended-field radiation or combination chemotherapy
		$IIIA_2$	Combination chemotherapy
IIIB	Combination chemotherapy	IIIB	Combination chemotherapy
IVA	Combination chemotherapy	IVA	Combination chemotherapy
IVB	Combination chemotherapy	IVB	Combination chemotherapy

[a]Patients should be considered for clinical trials when possible.
[b]In general, patients with large mediastinal adenopathy are best treated with chemotherapy followed by radiation to the mediastinum.
[c]Staging laparotomy should be considered for patients with clinical stage IA or IIA disease. Patients with large mediastinal adenopathy, extensive B symptoms, or obvious clinical stage III disease should not undergo surgical staging because radiation alone is not the treatment of choice for these patients.
[d]Selected patients may do well with mantle radiation alone.

Radiation therapy alone may not be appropriate for stage IIIA disease, except in the instance of pathologic stage $IIIA_1$ disease with few splenic nodes. For all other (clinical or pathologic) stage III patients and stage IV patients, combination chemotherapy is the recommended treatment. The chemotherapy regimen selected should be based on expected toxicity, which varies between regimens. Based on the recent CALGB data (discussed earlier) and issues related to sterility, ABVD is a reasonable initial regimen (although the cardiopulmonary toxicities of doxorubicin and bleomycin cannot be taken lightly). If fertility is not an issue, the MOPP alternative ChlVPP may be the best choice. It is very well tolerated and does not generally cause alopecia or neuropathy. Its leukemogenic effects are likely less than those seen with MOPP, but higher than with ABVD. Intolerable nausea and vomiting and neurotoxicity usually lead to larger dosage reductions of MOPP than with ABVD, which can compromise efficacy. Alternating MOPP/ABVD or MOPP/ABV hybrid may be used although neither has been definitively proven to provide benefit over standard four-drug regimens. In addition, MOPP/ABV hybrid has been shown to cause more significant toxicity, including a higher rate of secondary malignancies, when compared to ABVD. The routine use of radiation therapy following combination chemotherapy (combined-modality therapy) cannot be recommended with currently available data. Only in the instance of large bulky mediastinal disease is this appropriate.

Early-stage patients who relapse after radiation therapy alone respond well to combination chemotherapy. Patients with advanced disease who fail or have relapsed following combination chemotherapy may be treated with conventional salvage therapy or with salvage chemotherapy followed by high-dose therapy with bone marrow support (Chap. 125). The decision to use salvage chemotherapy alone versus high-dose therapy with stem cell support is dependent on the patient's risk factors for relapse following salvage chemotherapy.

EVALUATION OF THERAPEUTIC OUTCOMES

Appropriate pharmacotherapeutic monitoring and intervention provide for the optimal care of the lymphoma patient. Disease response to therapy is the primary end point of treatment; however, many other positive outcomes are also of importance. Effective supportive care is necessary for maintaining the patient's quality of life and compliance with therapy.

Prior to initiation of therapy for Hodgkin's disease, patients should receive appropriate vaccinations and continue to be monitored for the development of infection. Prophylactic antibiotics may be given if indicated. Education regarding mouth care should be given to patients receiving radiation therapy and those who develop mucositis from chemotherapy. In selected patients with bulky or advanced disease, measures to prevent tumor lysis syndrome should be taken during initial therapy. This includes the administration of allopurinol and adequate hydration with or without urinary alkalinization. Serum potassium, phosphorus, calcium, and uric acid should be monitored as well as renal function.

If the patient is receiving chemotherapy, appropriate doses should be determined for each agent in the selected regimen. Doses of individual agents should be adjusted for renal or hepatic impairment, if necessary. If the chemotherapeutic regimen includes doxorubicin or bleomycin, the cumulative dose should be noted and the patient should be monitored for cumulative toxicities associated with these agents (cardiomyopathy and pneumonitis/pulmonary fibrosis, respectively). Adequate antiemetic coverage should be provided and adjusted according to response. The complete blood count should be routinely monitored because myelosuppression, especially neutropenia, can result from therapy. Monitoring for signs or symptoms of infection should be performed with initiation of broad-spectrum antibiotics in patients with febrile neutropenia. Hematopoietic growth factors should be given prophylactically following subsequent cycles of therapy for patients who have developed febrile neutropenia. Familiarity with the prevention and management of additional chemotherapeutic adverse effects, such as neuropathy with vincristine or hypersensitivity with bleomycin, is essential. Education of patients regarding expected adverse events and corresponding strategies for prevention and treatment is paramount.

NON-HODGKIN'S LYMPHOMA

The non-Hodgkin's lymphomas are a heterogeneous group of lymphoproliferative disorders that affect people from early childhood to late adulthood. Advances in molecular biology techniques and our understanding of the human immune system have led to major progress in understanding the pathogenesis and treatment of the lymphomas. Non-Hodgkin's lymphomas are classified into prognostic groups that differ in morphologic appearance, natural history, clinical presentation, as well as approach and response to treatment. The use of extensive combination chemotherapeutic regimens has shown dramatic improvement in survival and cure in patients with a disease that once was considered incurable. The 5-year survival rate for patients with non-Hodgkin's lymphomas has increased from 31% to 54% over the past 30 years.[50] Further improvement in survival is anticipated with the continued expansion of our therapeutic armamentarium, including high-dose chemotherapy and biologic therapy.

INCIDENCE AND EPIDEMIOLOGY

Non-Hodgkin's lymphoma is the sixth most common cause of newly diagnosed cancer in the United States and accounts for nearly 5% of all cancers. An estimated 55,400 new cases will be diagnosed in 1998 (56% male and 44% female), and it is estimated that 24,900 people will die from non-Hodgkin's lymphomas during this same period. Although the average age of patients at the time of diagnosis is about 42 years, non-Hodgkin's lymphoma can occur at any age. The incidence of lymphoma has increased by more than 65% since the early 1970s. The increase in non-Hodgkin's lymphomas is in part a result of the increasing number of patients with AIDS and its well-established association with the development of aggressive lymphoma. The incidence of indolent lymphoma is also on the rise.[1]

ETIOLOGY

The etiology of non-Hodgkin's lymphoma is still unknown. A relationship has been demonstrated with immunodeficient states, autoimmune disorders, infectious agents, and physical chemical exposure and the development of non-Hodgkin's lymphoma.

An increased incidence of lymphoma is seen in many congenital and acquired immunodeficiency states, supporting the role of immune dysregulation in the etiology of lymphoma. Patients with congenital immunodeficiency disorders (Wiskott–Aldrich syndrome, ataxia, telangiectasia), acquired immunodeficiency disorders (AIDS, acquired hypogammaglobulinemia, graft-versus-host disease), and chronic pharmacologic immunosuppression (organ transplantation, especially renal) are predisposed to the development of lymphoma, namely diffuse aggressive B-cell lymphomas with central nervous system (CNS) involvement. Other diseases that predispose a patient to the development of lymphoma include Klinefelter's syndrome and Chediak–Higashi syndrome. A hereditary influence has also been suggested as a possible cause of lymphoma, because patients with inherited immunodeficiency diseases and families of patients with immunologic disorders show an increased incidence of non-Hodgkin's lymphoma.[50,51]

Autoimmune diseases (Hashimoto's thyroiditis, Sjögren's syndrome) cause chronic inflammation in the mucosa-associated lymphoid tissue (MALT), which predisposes patients to subsequent lymphoid malignancies. Other autoimmune diseases such as systemic lupus erythematosus and rheumatoid arthritis have also been associated with the development of non-Hodgkin's lymphoma; however, the use of immunosuppressive agents in these diseases makes the pathologic cause less clear.[50,51]

Certain infections have been associated with the development of lymphoma. There is a strong association between infections with EBV and the development of Burkitt's lymphoma in Africa. However, this association with EBV and the diagnosis of Burkitt's lymphomas in the United States does not appear to be as strong.[52] Human T-cell leukemia/lymphoma virus (HTLV-1), a C-RNA type retrovirus, is strongly associated with an aggressive form of T-cell lymphoma, known as adult T-cell leukemia/lymphoma (ATL/L).[50] HTLV-1 is endemic in southwestern Japan, the Caribbean, and the southeastern United States. Recently it has been discovered that gastric infection with *Helicobacter pylori,* a gram-negative bacteria that leads to chronic gastritis, is associated with MALT and predisposes patients to lymphoid malignancies.[50,52,53]

A number of physical agents have also been associated with the development of non-Hodgkin's lymphoma. Phenoxyherbicide and organophosphate exposure has been correlated with the development of lymphoma. Other chemical solvents and dyes can increase the risk of developing lymphoma as much as fourfold. People exposed to radiation from nuclear explosions have an increased incidence of lymphoma. There is also an increased risk of non-Hodgkin's lymphoma in patients who have been treated with chemotherapy and radiation for Hodgkin's disease.[51]

GENETIC LESIONS

Chromosomal translocations have become a hallmark of lymphomas. The mechanisms leading to the translocations are unknown, but they almost always involve the antigen receptor gene rearrangement. In B cells the translocation involves the J and switching region of the immunoglobulin

TABLE 120–6. Chromosomal Translocations in Non-Hodgkin's Lymphoma (NHL)

Tumor[a]	Chromosomal Translocation	Proto-oncogene	Partner Gene	Biologic Function
B-cell NHL				
LPL	t(9;14)(p13;q32)	PAX-5	Ig_H	Transcription factor
FL, DLCL	t(14;18)(q32;q11)	BCL-2	Ig_H	Regulation of apoptosis
	t(2;18)(p11;q11)	BCL-2	Ig_κ	Regulation of apoptosis
	t(18;22)(q11;q11)	BCL-2	Ig_λ	Regulation of apoptosis
DLCL	t(3;-)(q27;-)	BCL-6	Ig_H , Ig_L	Transcription factor
BL	t(8;14)(q24;q32)	c-MYC	Ig_H	Transcription factor
	t(2;8)(p11;q24)	c-MYC	Ig_κ	Transcription factor
	t(8;22)(q24;q11)	c-MYC	Ig_λ	Transcription factor
MCL	t(11;14)(q13;q32)	BCL-1 CCND1	Ig_H	Transcription factor, cell cycle regulator
T-cell NHL				
CD30$^+$ ALCL	t(2;5)(p23;q35)	ALK	NPM	ALK—nucleolar phosphoprotein NPM—tyrosine kinase

[a]LPL = lymphoplasmacytic lymphoma; FL = follicular lymphoma; DLCL = diffuse large-cell lymphoma; BL = Burkitt's lymphoma; MCL = mantle cell lymphoma; ALCL = anaplastic large-cell lymphoma.

Compiled from Refs. 50 and 54.

gene, which is then combined with a *proto-oncogene.* In T cells, the T-cell receptor is commonly involved and is paired with a *proto-oncogene.* These proto-oncogenes then alter normal cell growth functions (Table 120–6).[50,54] Additionally, *p*53, a tumor-suppressor gene that is involved in apoptosis, is mutated or deleted in small lymphocytic lymphoma, Burkitt's lymphoma, adult T-cell leukemia/lymphoma, and transformed lymphoma. Clinically, detection of translocations, such as BCL-2 in follicular lymphomas, can be used to detect residual tumor cells, which predict relapse. Continued research on these and other chromosomal abnormalities will further contribute to our understanding of the development, treatment, and prevention of lymphoma.[50,54]

HISTOPATHOLOGY AND CLASSIFICATION

The non-Hodgkin's lymphomas are neoplasms derived from the monoclonal proliferation of malignant B or T lymphocytes and their precursors. Figure 120–3 shows the anatomic location of normal differentiation of lymphocytes and where the postulated lymphoma originates. Lymphomas of B-cell origin are more common than T-cell lymphomas. The proliferation of the malignant cells results in the replacement of the normal cells and architecture of lymph nodes or bone marrow with a relatively uniform population of lymphoid cells.[50] In 1956, Rappaport and coworkers[55] proposed a classification scheme based on the architecture of the lymph node and cytologic differentiation of the predominant cell. The classification by Rappaport was once the most widely used and valuable scheme for clinicopathologic studies. However, this system was limited because it included some imprecise terms ("histiocytic" for a tumor derived from transformed lymphoid cells). With the advancement in the understanding of the immune system and chromosomal mutations, new classifications were proposed that attempted to classify the lymphomas more precisely. An international study that compared six classification systems led to the Working Formulation.[56] This classification system served as a common language and aided in the translation between the different classification systems. The Working Formulation has been the most commonly used system since its validation in 1988, but owing to improved understanding of lymphomas, a new classification system has recently been set in place. In 1995 the Revised European–American Classification of Lymphoid Neoplasms (REAL) was published by the International Lymphoma Study Group.[9,57] The REAL classification system categorizes lymphoid malignancies into three major categories: B-cell neoplasms, T-cell and natural killer (T/NK)-cell neoplasms, and Hodgkin's disease. This classification scheme includes both lymphomas and lymphoid leukemias because there is no distinction between the solid and circulating forms of these diseases. The Working Formulation and the REAL classification system are compared in Table 120–7.[50,57]

Lymphomas are characterized as being either nodular (also called follicular) or diffuse, depending on the presence or absence of clusters of malignant cells, by cell size (lymphocytic [small cells] or histiocytic [large cells]), and the site of origin. Nodular lymphomas form circumscribed aggregates that may involve only a portion of the node or the entire lymph node, causing total effacement of the nodal architecture. In contrast, the diffuse non-Hodgkin's lymphomas develop from the medullary cord region of the lymph node, which relates to the secretory compartment of the B-lymphocyte system. Lymphoid neoplasms derived from T lymphocytes are much less common. Malignant transformation of T lymphocytes, found predominantly in the paracortical region of the lymph node, gives rise to mycosis fungoides/Sézary syndrome (Fig. 120–3) and approximately one-quarter of the diffuse aggressive non-Hodgkin's lymphomas.[50]

TABLE 120–7. Comparison of the Working Formulation and the REAL Classification

Working Formulation	REAL Classification	
	B-Cell Neoplasm	*T-Cell Neoplasm*
Low Grade		
Small lymphocytic (SL)	B-cell CLL/PLL/SLL Marginal zone/MALT Mantle cell	T-cell CLL/PLL LGL ATL/L(chronic and smoldering types)
Plasmacytoid	Lymphoplasmacytic-immunocytoma Marginal zone/MALT B-cell CLL/PLL/SLL	
Follicular, small cleaved cell (FSC)	Follicle center, follicular, grade I Mantle cell Marginal zone/MALT	
Follicular mixed, small cleaved and large cell (FM)	Follicle center, follicular, grade II Marginal zone/MALT	
Intermediate Grade		
Follicular, large cell (FL)	Follicle center, follicular, grade III	
Diffuse, small cleaved cell (DSC)	Mantle cell Follicle center, diffuse small cell Marginal zone/MALT	T-cell CLL/PLL LGL ATL/L Angioimmunoblastic Angiocentric
Diffuse mixed, small and large cell (DM)	Large B-cell lymphoma (rich in T cells) Follicle center, diffuse small cell Lymphoplasmacytoid Marginal zone/MALT Mantle cell	Peripheral T cell, unspecified ATL/L Angioimmunoblastic Angiocentric Intestinal T-cell lymphoma
Diffuse, large cell (DL)	Diffuse large B-cell lymphoma	Peripheral T cell, unspecified ATL/L Angioimmunoblastic Angiocentric Intestinal T-cell lymphoma
High Grade		
Immunoblastic, large cell	Diffuse large B-cell lymphoma	Peripheral T cell, unspecified ATL/L Angioimmunoblastic Angiocentric Intestinal T cell Anaplastic large cell
Lymphoblastic	Precursor B lymphoblastic	Precursor T lymphoblastic
Small noncleaved cell		
Burkitt's	Burkitt's	
Non-Burkitt's	High-grade B cell, Burkitt-like diffuse large B cell	Peripheral T cell, unspecified

Compiled from Refs. 50 and 57.

Lymphomas of both T-cell and B-cell origin are clinically classified as indolent (untreated survival measured in years), aggressive (untreated survival measured in months), or highly aggressive (untreated survival measured in weeks) tumors.[50,57]

INDOLENT LYMPHOMAS AND LEUKEMIAS

Indolent lymphomas can present in a variety of ways and can be subclassified as disseminated, extranodel, or nodal disease. In the past they have been termed "favorable" because of the long period of time from diagnosis to time of mortality, but they are considered incurable. *Indolent disseminated lymphomas/leukemias* include B-cell small lymphocytic lymphoma (B-SLL), its circulating counterpart chronic lymphocytic leukemia (B-CLL), prolymphocytic leukemia (PLL), lymphoplasmacytic lymphoma (LPL), and splenic marginal zone lymphoma. At the time of diagnosis, tumor cells can usually be found in the bone marrow and peripheral blood, with or without tumor in spleen, or at an extranodal site. Indolent lymphomas are characterized by the predominance of small lymphocytes with low-grade histologic features. There is typically a minor population of large cells, and these lymphomas eventual transform into an aggressive lymphoma. A small number of patients with B-SLL show an emergence and proliferation to larger lymphoid cells, indicating a progression to a diffuse large-cell lymphoma. This transformation is known as Richter syndrome.[50,57]

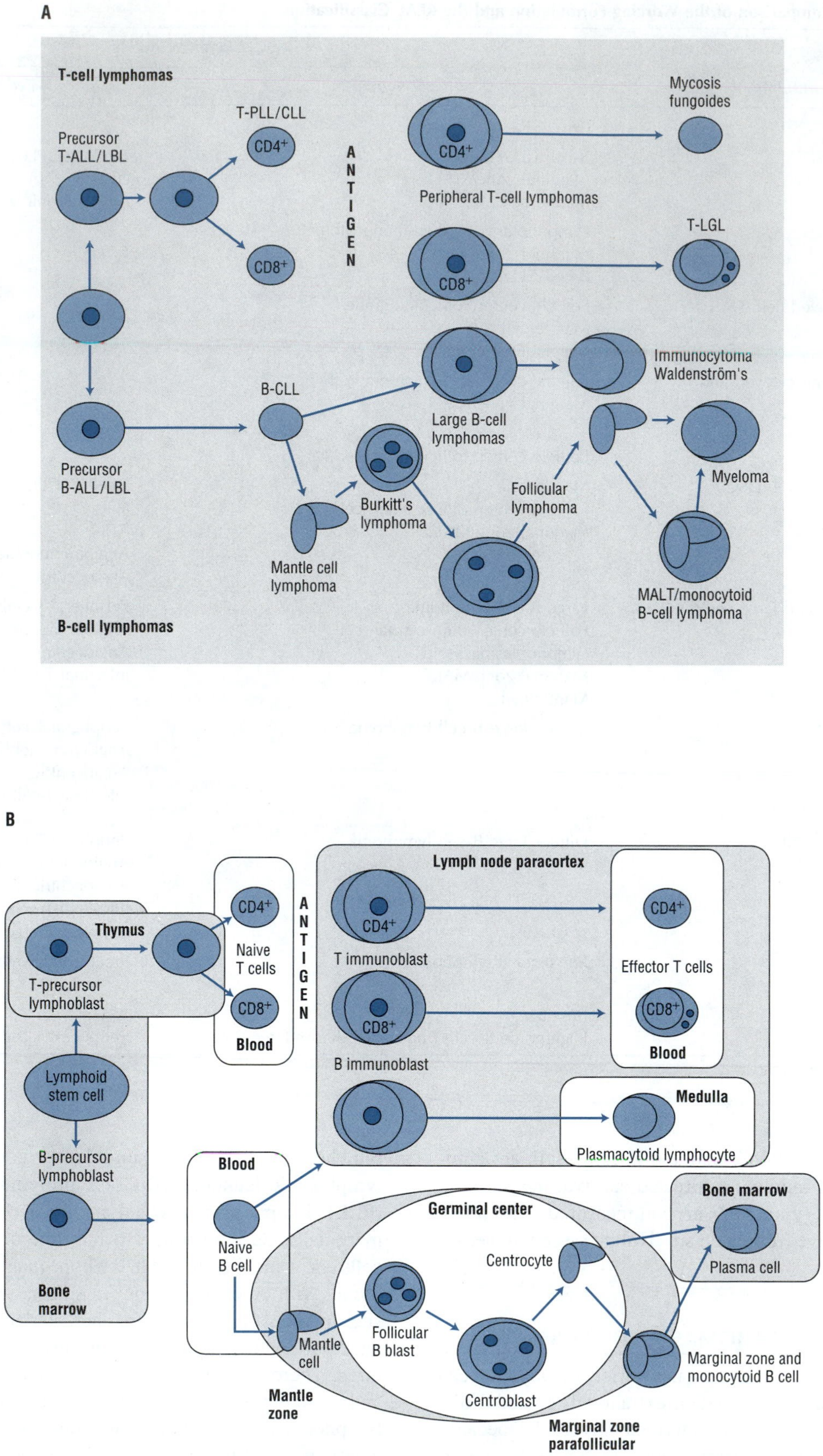

FIGURE 120–3. **A.** Shows where different lymphomas are proposed to occur and the associated tissue where they originate. **B.** Indicates normal lymphocyte maturation and the tissues where the process occurs. *(From Ref. 50.)*

Indolent extranodal lymphomas consist of extranodal MALT lymphoma and the cutaneous T-cell lymphoma, also termed mycosis fungoides. MALT lymphomas constitute 50% of all gastric lymphomas and typically present with a small lymphocyte infiltration, marginal zone B cells, large basophilic blast cells, monocytoid B cells, and plasma cells. Gastric MALT lymphomas have been highly correlated with *H. pylori* infection. These lymphomas also transform into diffuse large B-cell lymphomas. Mycosis fungoides is a CD4+ T-cell neoplasm, which presents in the skin and also in the T-cell portion of lymph nodes, but rarely is found in the bone marrow. These malignant cells can produce cytokines, which stimulate the production of immunoglobulins. Because the neoplastic cells isolated from these tumors cannot be grown *in vitro*, little is known about the molecular biology.[50,54,57]

Indolent nodal lymphomas consist of nodal marginal zone B-cell lymphoma, mantle cell lymphoma (MCL), and follicle center lymphoma (follicular lymphoma). Patients typically present with involvement of lymph nodes, bone marrow, spleen, and liver; however, they rarely present with localized extranodal disease. Nodal marginal zone B-cell lymphoma appears exactly like the extranodal MALT lymphoma except that there is no extranodal involvement. This type of lymphoma is rare and occurs most frequently in patients with Sjögren's syndrome. MCL comprises approximately 5% of all non-Hodgkin's lymphomas in the United States and is composed of small to medium-size lymphocytes with irregular or cleaved nuclear features. This lymphoma progresses differently from other indolent lymphomas because it does not rapidly transform into a large-cell lymphoma, although recurrent disease is associated with an increased population of large cells. Follicular lymphoma consists of a mixture of cleaved follicle center cells (centrocytes) and large noncleaved follicle center cells (centroblasts). The size of the centroblasts and the percent of centroblasts vary in a continuum, with a larger percent of centroblasts correlating with more aggressive disease. Although it is a continuum, pathologist have developed a grading system (grade I, II, or III) that relates to the aggressiveness of the tumor. In the old Working Formulation, all three grades had their own classification (Table 120–7), with grades I and II being low grade and grade III being intermediate. The new REAL classification system groups them together because of their similar histology and our inability to cure these lymphomas when they present at advanced stages. Greater than 80% of indolent or low-grade lymphomas are follicular and 35% to 40% of all non-Hodgkin's lymphomas are follicular. Transformation to diffuse large B-cell lymphoma occurs in 40% to 60% of patients.[50,54,57]

AGGRESSIVE LYMPHOMAS

Aggressive lymphomas are fatal in a matter of months if left untreated because they have a high proliferating fraction. However, with combination chemotherapy, aggressive lymphomas are curable. In general, their histologic appearance shows that they are slightly larger than their circulating B- or T-cell counterparts that are antigen dependent (Fig. 120–3). Aggressive lymphomas are diffuse large B-cell lymphomas or peripheral T-cell lymphomas. Diffuse large B-cell lymphomas are the most common and account for 60% to 70% of aggressive lymphomas and 30% to 40% of all non-Hodgkin's lymphomas in the United States and Europe. They are composed of centroblasts, immunoblasts, or a mixture (the most common presentation). In the Working Formulation, diffuse large-cell and large-cell immunoblasts were considered separately, but the REAL classification has combined them because of the difficulty in differentiating the two and their similar clinical behavior and our approach to therapy. Most diffuse large B-cell lymphomas arise de novo, but some arise from transformation of indolent lymphomas, which have a worse prognosis. Peripheral T-cell lymphomas are composed of several variants including unspecified, angioimmunoblastic T-cell, nasal type (angiocentric), T/NK-cell, intestinal T-cell, and hepatosplenic γ-δ T-cell lymphomas. These tumors constitute approximately 10% to 15% of all non-Hodgkin's lymphomas and present as a mixture of small and large cells. The difference in cell morphology represents the fact that the cells are in different states of transformation.[50,57]

HIGHLY AGGRESSIVE LYMPHOMAS AND LEUKEMIAS

Highly aggressive lymphomas and leukemias are composed of primitive cells and have a large population of proliferating cells. At the time of patient presentation, neoplastic cells are commonly found in the bone marrow, peripheral blood, and CNS. The four highly aggressive lymphomas/leukemias recognized in the REAL system include precursor B-lymphoblastic leukemia/lymphoma (B-LBL), precursor T-lymphoblastic leukemia/lymphoma (T-LBL), Burkitt's lymphoma, and adult T-cell lymphoma/leukemia (ATL/L). B-LBL is the most common highly aggressive lymphoma/leukemia followed by T-LBL, and both can present as solid tumor, leukemia, or both. Although B-LBL is the most common type in this group, it most commonly presents as leukemia, whereas T-LBL more commonly presents as a solid tumor. The lymphocytes of B-LBL and T-LBL are slightly larger than small lymphocytes but are smaller than large B-cell lymphoma. They have a similar morphology and therefore require immunophenotyping to distinguish between them. Burkitt's lymphoma cells are monomorphic, moderately sized lymphocytes with round nuclei. A starry sky pattern is usually present. They can usually be easily determined by their morphology and histologic characteristics; however, some tumors involving larger cells that resemble diffuse large B-cell lymphoma are commonly referred to as Burkitt's-like. In children and HIV-positive patients these tumors behave like Burkitt's lymphoma, but in adults they represent a variant of diffuse large B-cell lymphoma. ATL/L is comprised of CD4+ T cells from patients that have been infected with HTLV-1. The histology varies, and usually a mixture of large and small cells is seen. Multinucleated giant cells resembling Reed–Sternberg cells can occasionally be seen. Cells with hyperlobated nuclei are commonly seen in the peripheral blood. Most patients with this malignancy are adults who have antibodies to HTLV-1. With the exception of ATL/L, all of the highly aggressive lymphomas/leukemias are more common in children than in adults.[50,57]

CLINICAL PRESENTATION

Patients with non-Hodgkin's lymphoma present with a wide variety of symptoms, which depend on the site of involvement and whether tumor involvement is nodal or extranodal. Sites of involvement and dissemination of the malignant cells can, in some cases, be predicted based on the cell of origin and the fact that the tumor frequently disseminates to areas where the normal counterparts of the lymphoma cells are located. For example, lymphomas of B-cell origin involve areas of the lymphoid system normally populated by B lymphocytes, such as lymph nodes, spleen, and bone marrow. T-cell lymphomas commonly disseminate to various extranodal sites, such as the skin and lungs. In contrast to Hodgkin's disease, the bone marrow is commonly involved in non-Hodgkin's lymphoma.

Clinical presentation also is dependent on the type of non-Hodgkin's lymphoma and the stage of disease at presentation. Low-grade lymphomas usually arise in middle-aged or older individuals (median age, 55 years) and are uncommon in individuals before the age of 40. The majority of patients present with advanced stages of disease, often the result of bone marrow involvement (found in 30% to 70% of patients), although privileged sites, such as the CNS and testes, are rarely affected. Low-grade lymphomas usually have an indolent clinical course, and many patients report a history of waxing and waning adenopathy over a period of months to years prior to diagnosis. In contrast, the intermediate- and high-grade lymphomas occur over a broader age range and are more aggressive in their clinical behavior. Patients present at various stages of disease. Although bone marrow involvement is not as common, occurring in only 10% to 30% of patients (except lymphoblastic lymphoma, in which bone marrow is affected in 50% of patients), the lymphoma tends to rapidly disseminate and often involves extranodal and privileged sites.

In general, patients may have either localized or generalized adenopathy, with the involved nodes being painless, rubbery, and discrete, and usually located in the cervical and supraclavicular regions as in Hodgkin's disease. The liver or spleen may be enlarged in patients with generalized adenopathy. Patients with mesenteric or gastrointestinal involvement may present with signs and symptoms of nausea, vomiting, obstruction, abdominal pain, a palpable abdominal mass, or gastrointestinal bleeding. Patients with bone marrow involvement may have symptoms related to anemia (fatigue, pallor, tachycardia, dyspnea on exertion), neutropenia (recurrent infections), or thrombocytopenia (easy bruising, epistaxis, petechiae). Non-Hodgkin's lymphoma has a greater tendency to involve the testes, epitrochlear nodes, and Waldeyer's ring than Hodgkin's disease. The incidence of solitary brain lymphoma is increasing, especially in patients with AIDS. Infrequently, patients with non-Hodgkin's lymphoma may present with acute renal failure from retroperitoneal adenopathy causing ureteral obstruction or from metabolic abnormalities such as hyperuricemia with uric acid nephropathy.[51]

In contrast to Hodgkin's disease, only 20% of patients with non-Hodgkin's lymphoma have the constitutional symptoms of fever, night sweats, and weight loss of greater than 10%. The clinical features of Hodgkin's disease and non-Hodgkin's lymphomas are compared in Table 120–1.[50,58]

DIAGNOSIS AND STAGING

As with Hodgkin's disease, the diagnosis of non-Hodgkin's lymphoma must be established by pathologic review of tissue obtained by biopsy. An entire involved lymph node should be removed for evaluation of its architecture (diffuse or follicular). This procedure should be done carefully to prevent distortional artifact of the architecture, which could lead to an inaccurate diagnosis. Needle biopsy of the node prevents architecture evaluation and is not adequate in the diagnosis of non-Hodgkin's lymphoma. When adenopathy is not present, diagnosis may be established by biopsy of cutaneous lesions, bone marrow biopsy and aspiration in patients with unexplained myelosuppression, liver biopsy in patients with hepatomegaly or elevated liver function transaminases, or biopsy of involved extranodal organs, such as bone, Waldeyer's ring, lung, and testis.

Further diagnostic procedures and staging are not indicated in patients whose age or underlying medical problems limit treatment to palliative therapy. Otherwise, the extent of the investigative workup required prior to therapy is determined by the histopathology and available treatment for the subtype of non-Hodgkin's lymphoma.[50,58,59]

Clinical staging always begins with a thorough history and physical examination. Patients should be questioned about the presence or absence and extent of fever, night sweats, and weight loss. A detailed history of lymphadenopathy should also be obtained, including when and where the lymph nodes were first noted, and their rate of growth. A complete physical examination is performed to assess the extent of disease involvement, with special attention given to all nodal areas. All patients should have a complete blood count, serum chemistries including liver and renal profiles, a chest x-ray, and bone marrow aspiration and biopsy. Bone marrow biopsy from each posterior iliac crest should be performed early in the evaluation of all patients because a positive result establishes stage IV disease and eliminates the need for more extensive and invasive tests.[50,58,59]

Lumbar puncture to evaluate the cerebrospinal fluid (CSF) is recommended as part of the initial staging in patients who are at risk for CNS involvement, including patients with lymphoblastic lymphoma and small noncleaved cell lymphoma (Burkitt's and non-Burkitt's). Evaluation of the CSF is also recommended for patients with diffuse large-cell lymphomas (DLCL) with bone marrow, epidural, or testicular involvement, because these sites are correlated with CNS involvement.[50,59]

Various radiologic studies are used in the staging of non-Hodgkin's lymphoma, but recommendations for their use are somewhat controversial. Abdominal CT is useful and always recommended in the evaluation of the upper abdominal lymph nodes, including mesenteric, splenic, and hepatic nodes. The use of chest CT is not as well established and is usually unnecessary if chest x-rays are normal. Exceptions to this are in cases where chest radiotherapy is to be given alone or to rule out mediastinal disease in patients with stage I disease.[60] Lymphangiography is the most sensitive test for evaluating the para-aortic, iliac, and retroperitoneal nodes and allows easy follow-up of abnormal nodes, but an advance in stage with a positive lymphangiogram is infrequent. The use of lymphangiography varies among institutions and may not be necessary unless less invasive studies, such as the abdominal CT, are negative.[50,59] MRI has not been shown superior to CT, and its use is not routinely recommended.[60] Other tests, such as liver–spleen scan, bone scan, upper gastrointestinal series, and intravenous pyelogram, are useful in patients with organ symptomatology or serum chemistry abnormalities.[50,59]

Staging laparotomy is reserved for patients with CS I disease, where the discovery of intra-abdominal disease would mandate a change in therapy from localized radiation therapy to combination chemotherapy.[50] Most patients will have documented advanced disease by less invasive studies

TABLE 120–8. Risk Factors and Survival According to the International Non-Hodgkin's Lymphoma Prognostic Factors Project

All Patients	Patients ≤ 60 Years of Age
Age ≥ 60 years of age	LDH > normal
LDH > normal	Performance status ≥ 2
Performance status ≥ 2	Ann Arbor stage III or IV
Ann Arbor stage III or IV	
Extranodal involvement > 1 site	

Risk Group	Number of Risk Factors	5-Year Survival Rate (%)
Patients of all ages		
Low	0,1	73
Low–intermediate	2	51
High–intermediate	3	43
High	4,5	26
Patients ≤ 60 years of age		
Low	0	83
Low–intermediate	1	69
High–intermediate	2	46
High	3	32

LDH = lactic dehydrogenase.
Adapted from Ref. 61.

and it is of little value in stages II, III, and IV non-Hodgkin's lymphoma because treatment is essentially the same.

The Ann Arbor staging classification developed for the clinical staging of Hodgkin's disease is also used to stage patients with non-Hodgkin's lymphoma (see Table 120–2). Staging reveals that the majority of patients have advanced disease (stages III and IV). In fact, truly localized disease is usually seen in only three histologic subtypes (diffuse mixed, diffuse large-cell, and immunoblastic lymphoma), in which approximately 50% of patients will present with stage I or II disease.[58,59] Stage is a more important prognostic factor in Hodgkin's disease than in non-Hodgkin's lymphoma. In addition to stage of disease, the prognosis of non-Hodgkin's lymphoma also depends on the histologic subtype and the presence of a variety of clinical factors (Table 120–8).[61]

▶ TREATMENT: Non-Hodgkin's Lymphoma

The primary goals in the treatment of non-Hodgkin's lymphoma are to relieve symptoms and cure the patient of disease whenever possible, and to do this with acceptable toxicity. The treatment strategy depends on many factors including patient's age, concomitant disease, histologic subtype, and stage of disease. With the introduction and improvement of megavoltage radiotherapy, intensive combination chemotherapy regimens, and high-dose chemotherapy with stem cell rescue, complete remission and cure can be achieved in many patients with aggressive and highly aggressive lymphomas.

Traditionally, both the clinical behavior and degree of aggressiveness have been used to classify non-Hodgkin's lymphomas. The terms *good-risk* and *favorable* have been applied to low-grade or indolent lymphomas by virtue of their relatively slow growing behavior. Patients with an indolent lymphoma usually have a relatively long survival (median survival 7 to 10 years), with or without aggressive chemotherapy. Although these lymphomas are responsive to a wide range of therapeutic approaches, the survival curves never plateau, thus indicating that patients are rarely cured of their disease.

In contrast, the aggressive and highly aggressive lymphomas have been termed *unfavorable* owing to their fast growing behavior and short survival (measured in weeks to months), if appropriate therapy is not initiated. Although these unfavorable lymphomas are generally more aggressive than indolent lymphomas, in certain instances they can be cured. Thus, the terminology for the non-Hodgkin's lymphomas represents a paradox, where "good" is bad and "bad" is good in terms of the likelihood for cure.

Different lymphoma histologies can be seen within an individual lymph node or at a separate anatomic site. For example, a follicular pattern may be observed in one area and a diffuse pattern in another. Indolent lymphomas also have the ability to progress over time to an aggressive lymphoma. In these situations, treatment should be based on the more aggressive subtype.

Therapeutic approaches to non-Hodgkin's lymphoma include radiation therapy, chemotherapy, and biologic agents. The role of radiation therapy in the treatment of non-Hodgkin's lymphoma differs from its role in the treatment of Hodgkin's disease. Although the disease is responsive to radiation therapy, only a small percentage of patients with non-Hodgkin's lymphoma are amenable to remission induction and cure with local and/or regional irradiation. This is because truly localized disease at diagnosis is rare. Radiation therapy is used more commonly in advanced disease, but mainly as a palliative measure to control local bulky disease.

Effective chemotherapy for non-Hodgkin's lymphoma ranges from single-agent therapy in the indolent lymphomas to aggressive, complex combination chemotherapy regimens in the aggressive and highly aggressive lymphomas. The most active agents used in the treatment of non-Hodgkin's lymphoma include the alkylating agents (e.g., cyclophosphamide, chlorambucil), bleomycin, doxorubicin, etoposide, methotrexate, vincristine, and corticosteroids (e.g., prednisone, dexamethasone). The rationale for intensive combination chemotherapy regimens is based, in part, on the somatic mutation theory of Goldie and Coldman,[32,33] discussed in Chapter 115, Cancer Treatment and Chemotherapy.

Appropriate therapy for non-Hodgkin's lymphoma depends on the tumor histology and the stage of disease. In general, the therapeutic approach can be divided into limited disease and advanced disease. Limited disease includes those patients with localized disease (Ann Arbor stages I and II). Advanced disease is defined as all Ann Arbor stage III or IV patients, and also frequently includes Ann Arbor stage II patients with one or more of the poor prognostic features listed in Table 120–8.[61]

LIMITED DISEASE (STAGES I AND II)

INDOLENT LYMPHOMAS

Indolent disseminated lymphomas/leukemias include B-cell small lymphocytic lymphoma (B-SLL), its circulating counterpart chronic lymphocytic leukemia (B-CLL), prolymphocytic leukemia (PLL), lymphoplasmacytic lymphoma, and splenic marginal zone lymphoma. Treatment of these lymphomas is similar to that of chronic lymphocytic leukemia,[58] which is discussed in Chapter 123, Chronic Leukemias.

Indolent extranodal lymphomas consist of extranodal MALT lymphomas, which have only recently been described and categorized with the REAL classification system. They primarily occur in the gastrointestinal tract, namely the stomach, where they are associated with *H. pylori*. They also occur in the lung, thyroid, and salivary gland. There are no long-term, randomized, controlled trials evaluating MALT lymphomas. When they present in the stomach, as many as 67% may respond to antibiotics used to treat *H. pylori*.[53] The use of surgery, radiation, or chemotherapy in unresponding MALT lymphomas or those occurring outside of the stomach has not been well studied. Small studies have reported good response using all the aforementioned therapies.[62] A retrospective study that evaluated radiation in MALT tumors of the thyroid reported a 70% 5-year survival, which was better than the 55% survival for non-MALT lymphoma histologies.[63]

Indolent nodal lymphomas consist of nodal marginal zone B-cell lymphoma, MCL, and follicle center lymphoma (follicular lymphoma). Localized disease is uncommon and accounts for approximately 10% of patients. Although only a small percentage of patients have early-stage disease, it is important to identify these patients owing to the potential for cure with therapy.[58]

Radiation therapy is the standard treatment for early-stage indolent lymphomas. Involved field, extended-field, and total nodal irradiation have been used. Carefully staged patients with either stage I or contiguous stage II disease treated with radiation therapy can achieve high disease-free survival rates at 10 years. In a retrospective study from Stanford University, 44% of patients with stage I or II follicular lymphoma treated with radiation therapy were FFR after 10 years of follow-up.[61] To determine if total lymphoid irradiation or involved field irradiation changed relapse rates or survival rates, they grouped patients as (1) receiving radiation to one side of the diaphragm, which includes involved and extended-field irradiation and (2) receiving irradiation on both sides of the diaphragm, which includes total lymphoid and subtotal lymphoid irradiation. A significant improvement in FFR was seen in patients in group 2 as compared with group 1. However, overall survival was similar regardless of the extent of radiation fields. At 10 years, the FFR rates were 36% and 67% for groups 1 and 2, respectively. The reason the FFR did not translate into an improved survival is unclear, although the death rate from secondary malignancies was higher in patients in group 2 (12% vs 5%). Both involved field and total nodal irradiation appear potentially curative, and only 10% of patients relapsed who were FFR at 10 years.[64] Unlike treatment for Hodgkin's disease, there are no data to support the use of extended-field irradiation to clinically uninvolved contiguous lymph node chains. This is owing to the fact that in non-Hodgkin's lymphoma, the spread of disease is frequently noncontiguous and less certain than the usual contiguous spread seen in Hodgkin's disease.[58]

The role of adjuvant chemotherapy in the management of localized stage I or II disease is unclear. Radiation plus chlorambucil has not been shown superior to radiation alone in a randomized trial with a maximum follow-up of 18 years.[65] A recent nonrandomized study reported from the MD Anderson group indicates that the combination of COP (cyclophosphamide, vincristine, prednisone) or CHOP-Bleo (CHOP is in Table 120–9, plus bleomycin) and radiation improves FFR rates and survival compared to other studies.[50,66] Currently, the role of combined chemotherapy and radiation therapy remains unresolved.

AGGRESSIVE LYMPHOMAS

Aggressive lymphomas include diffuse large B-cell lymphomas or peripheral T-cell lymphomas. Diagnosis of stage I or II occurs in 15% to 20% of patients. Aggressive lymphomas usually have a slightly worse 5-year survival rate than indolent lymphomas.

Radiation therapy was the first therapeutic approach used to produce long-term survival in patients with localized aggressive lymphoma. The efficacy of radiation therapy in these patients depends on the extent of disease, the aggressiveness of the staging procedures (e.g., laparotomy), and the number of unfavorable prognostic factors (see Table 120–8).[61] The 10-year relapse-free survival has been reported as 91% and 35% for patients with

TABLE 120–9. CHOP Regimen

Drug	Dose (mg/m^2)	Route	Treatment Days
Cyclophosphamide	750	IV	1
Doxorubicin	50	IV	1
Vincristine	1.4	IV	1
Prednisone	100	PO	1-5
One cycle is 21 days			

Adapted from Ref. 77.

stage I and II disease, respectively.[67] Therefore, radiation therapy is considered effective for stage I disease. However, accurate diagnosis of stage I disease requires a staging laparotomy, which is rarely performed. Staging laparotomy has been associated with various surgical complications and may lead to delays in therapy, which is important considering that these tumors are aggressive and have the potential for rapid growth and dissemination. For this reason, investigators began to evaluate the role of combination chemotherapy in addition to radiation therapy in patients with localized aggressive lymphoma not undergoing laparotomy. Several randomized trials have confirmed a significant improvement in treatment outcome with the use of combined-modality therapy compared with radiation therapy alone.[50] One study reported the 5-year disease-free survival to be 45% with radiation alone and 76% for combined-modality therapy.[50] Subsequently, the question was raised as to whether combined-modality therapy is superior to the use of chemotherapy alone. A Southwest Oncology Group (SWOG) study randomized 401 patients to three cycles of CHOP chemotherapy and radiotherapy or eight cycles of CHOP. Overall survival at 4 years was 87% for the CHOP/radiation therapy arm versus 75% for the CHOP-alone arm (P = .01).[68] The Eastern Cooperative Oncology Group (ECOG) treated 210 patients with eight cycles of CHOP chemotherapy, then randomized them to radiation therapy or observation. The disease-free survival after a median of 6 years was 73% versus 58% for the CHOP/radiation therapy arm and CHOP-alone arm, respectively. However, in the ECOG trial, the difference in overall survival (73% vs 58%, P = .06) was only marginally significant.[69] Therefore, the current recommendations are that combined-modality therapy be given. The optimal number of chemotherapy cycles still remains unresolved. The aforementioned trials seem to indicate that fewer cycles of CHOP chemotherapy given with radiation therapy are as effective as eight cycles of CHOP without radiation therapy. However, they have not been compared in a controlled randomized trial. It is also unclear if there is a superior chemotherapy regimen. Chemotherapy regimens that contain doxorubicin, such as CHOP or BACOP (bleomycin, doxorubicin, vincristine, prednisone), appear superior to non–doxorubicin-containing regimens.[50] The two large trials listed above used CHOP, but excellent results also have been obtained with a reduced-dose ProMACE-MOPP (prednisone, methotrexate, doxorubicin, cyclophosphamide, etoposide, MOPP) regimen in combination with involved field radiation. The current recommended therapy for stage I or II aggressive lymphoma is three cycles of CHOP followed by involved field radiation. In the presence of poor prognostic features, patients should be treated in the same manner as patients with advanced disease.[50]

HIGHLY AGGRESSIVE LYMPHOMAS

Lymphoblastic lymphoma and small noncleaved cell lymphoma (Burkitt's lymphoma) are much more common in children and young adults than in older adults. These lymphomas are extremely aggressive owing to their rapid tumor-doubling times, and prompt initiation of appropriate therapy is required. Acute leukemia-like protocols are used in the treatment of both lymphoblastic lymphoma and small noncleaved cell lymphoma, and include high-dose induction, consolidation, and maintenance regimens, along with CNS prophylaxis. Treatment of limited and advanced disease is essentially the same.[58]

ADVANCED DISEASE (STAGES III AND IV)

INDOLENT LYMPHOMAS

The management of stage III and IV indolent lymphomas remains controversial, as standard therapeutic approaches have not been shown to be curative despite the high complete remission rates. Therapeutic options for these patients are diverse and include radiation therapy, biologics, single-agent chemotherapy, combination chemotherapy, and combined-modality therapy. Although complete remission can be achieved in 60% to 90% of patients with various treatments, the median disease-free interval is typically 17 to 24 months. After relapse, patients are re-treated and again high remission rates are achieved. Unfortunately, the response rates and duration of response both decrease with each re-treatment. Five-year survival rates exceed 80%, but fall to approximately 50% by 10 years. Two different treatment approaches exist and are described as conservative or aggressive. Patients treated with the conservative approach receive no therapy until they become symptomatic; they then receive palliative chemotherapy or radiation therapy. With the aggressive approach, patients typically receive aggressive combination chemotherapy and/or radiation therapy early in the disease course, even if they are asymptomatic. Controversy over these therapeutic approaches exists because all therapy for indolent stage III and IV disease is palliative and no improvement in the overall survival with a given therapeutic approach has been shown.[50,58]

Watch and Wait

Because various treatment regimens have not produced convincing data supporting improved survival, it has been suggested that initial therapy be withheld from patients who are asymptomatic. This "watchful waiting" strategy was first proposed by Horning and Rosenberg.[50,70] Selected patients were followed without initial therapy until they became symptomatic. The median time until therapy was required was 31 months. The 10-year survival was 73%, which does not differ significantly from patients who receive therapy at the time of diagnosis. Of interest, disease progression was significantly more rapid for patients with follicular lymphoma grade II (16.5 months) compared with the other indolent lymphomas (48 to 72 months). In addition, complete remissions following chemotherapy appear to be more durable in follicular lymphoma grade II (approximately 7 years) than in follicular lymphoma grade I (4.5 years). Therefore, watchful waiting may not be appropriate for patients with follicular mixed histologies. In follicular lymphoma grade III, the data are less clear because no prospective controlled clinical trials have been conducted in this group. In the Working Formulation, this type of lymphoma was classified as intermediate. However, because long-term follow-up of these patients indicates that there is no plateau of the survival curve, grade III has been grouped with grade I and II as an indolent lymphoma. Treatment has traditionally been combination chemotherapy with regimens containing doxorubicin and cyclophosphamide, and the watch and wait approach with this lymphoma has not been studied.[50,58]

Advantages of treatment deferral include prevention of exposure to agents that may induce drug resistance, prevention of drug-induced toxicity, possible spontaneous regression, administration of appropriate palliative therapy when the disease progresses, and potential evolution to a potentially curable lymphoma. Potential disadvantages of withholding treatment include disease progression in threatening sites, which may compromise palliative therapy, and evolution of the disease to a lymphoma that is more aggressive and more resistant to therapy.[50] If a watch and wait approach is taken, patients should be evaluated every 2 months and therapy initiated if patients become symptomatic or have involvement of a visceral organ or bone marrow. It is also important to keep in mind that the median time to require treatment is approximately 3 years, with approximately 20% of patients not requiring therapy for up to 10 years.[58]

Radiation

Total lymphoid irradiation alone has been used for stage III indolent lymphoma, with 5-year disease-free survival ranging from 40% to 83%. Patients with five or fewer sites involved had a better prognosis. Most patients had their relapses in nonirradiated sites, suggesting that extended treatment fields might have produced increased disease-free survival.[71] Total-body irradiation therefore has been investigated, but results have not been found superior to those for total lymphoid irradiation or chemotherapy alone.[50]

Radiation has also been combined with chemotherapy. A randomized trial that compared total lymphoid irradiation with or without CVP (cyclophosphamide, vincristine, prednisone) found no difference in disease-free survival at 8 years.[71] Therefore, this approach is not recommended.

Systemic Chemotherapy

The oral alkylating agents alone or in combination have been a mainstay of treatment. Daily chlorambucil (0.1 to 0.2 mg/kg) or cyclophosphamide (1.5 to 2.5 mg/kg) adjusted to maintain a platelet count above 100,000/mm^3 and a white blood cell count above 3000/mm^3 can induce a slow remission, with a complete remission rate of 13% to 46%.[58,71] Median duration of remission ranges from 12 to 35 months or longer, and toxicity is minimal. However, a high rate of secondary acute myelogenous leukemia (AML) is a concern. Cyclophosphamide, chlorabucil, and CVP have been compared to more aggressive chemotherapy regimens like CHOP. Although complete remission rates are higher with the combination chemotherapy, no significant change has been seen in overall survival.[72]

Fludarabine and cladribine have also been used as initial therapy for advanced indolent lymphoma. Overall response rates range from 50% to 88% for cladribine with the median response duration of 10 to 36 months or longer.[72] Similarly, the overall response rate with fludarabine as initial therapy has been reported to be 65%, with a median disease-free relapse of 13.6 months.[73] Although these agents produce high response rates, they have not been shown to prolong overall survival. They are not associated with secondary AML, but can cause bone marrow suppression resulting in infectious complications.

Combination Chemotherapy and Interferon

Several studies have evaluated interferon-α in combination with conventional chemotherapy or as maintenance therapy. Interferon-α-2b (IFN-α-2b) was recently approved to be used in combination with an anthracyline-containing regimen in aggressive follicular lymphoma patients with a large tumor burden. The study that resulted in FDA approval treated 130 patients with CHVP (cyclophosphamide, doxorubicin, teniposide, and prednisone), and 135 patients with CHVP and IFN-α-2b. The study administered CHVP monthly for six cycles, then every 2 months for six more cycles, and patients on the IFN arm received 5 million units of IFN-α-2b three times a week for 18 months. The progression-free interval was 2.9 years and 1.5 years for the interferon group and control group, respectively. With a median follow-up of 6.1 years, the median survival for the CHVP-alone arm was 5.5 years, while the median survival for the IFN-α-2b group had not yet been reached.[74] A recently published study found that 3 million units of IFN-α-2b three times a week for 3 months in combination with CVP resulted in a significantly prolonged PFS compared to CVP alone (6-year PFS—60% vs 24%). However, no difference in overall survival has been seen at the time of this publication.[75] The role for IFN as maintenance therapy has also been assessed. The Groupe d'Etude des Lymphomes de l'Adulte has reported a study in which 242 patients with advanced follicular lymphoma were randomized to receive induction chemotherapy with or without maintenance IFN-α. They report a prolonged relapse-free period and overall survival for the maintenance IFN-α group (34.1 vs 18.6 months; $P = .001$ and 83.1 vs 61.1 months; $P = .009$, respectively).[76] These studies strongly suggest that IFN during induction and/or maintenance can prolong the time to relapse and overall survival, although it is unclear if this is applicable for all lymphoma subtypes or just follicular lymphomas.[50] It appears the prolongation of progression-free survival is similar to the duration of IFN therapy.

An important feature of low-grade lymphoma is its propensity to evolve to a more aggressive intermediate- or high-grade lymphoma. The actuarial risk of histologic transformation appears to increase over time, from a 10% risk reported at 5 years, to a 40% risk at 10 years. This transformation occurs with equal frequency in both treated and untreated patients.[77] Rapid disease progression and short median survival (less than 1 year) are common following transformation. The use of combination chemotherapy may eradicate the aggressive clone, although these patients remain at risk for relapse with either a low-grade or more aggressive lymphoma.

AGGRESSIVE LYMPHOMAS

Among the heterogeneous group of non-Hodgkin's lymphomas, the most important therapeutic advances have been made with intensive chemotherapy regimens for the aggressive lymphomas. There are several important points to consider in the treatment of these lymphomas. First, the aggressive non-Hodgkin's lymphomas are potentially curable diseases, even when they are widely metastatic. Therefore, unlike with the patient with an indolent non-Hodgkin's lymphoma, "watch and wait" is not an option. These tumors, when left untreated, are almost universally fatal within 2 years. Second, intensive combination chemotherapy should be used because it is uncommon to achieve a complete remission with single-agent therapy and long-term survival is not possible without induction of a complete remission. In other words, the treatment regimen with the highest likelihood of cure should be administered first, because durable responses with salvage therapy (other than high-dose chemotherapy) are less likely. Third, dosage and administration schedules for these intensive regimens, which are often accompanied by severe toxic effects, must be rigidly adhered to. Dose reduction or prolongation of the interval between cycles can be associated with rapid regrowth of the tumor and the inability to produce cure. Patients receiving greater than 70% of planned dose intensity (measured in mg/m^2/wk) have a better prognosis than those receiving less than 70% of the planned dose intensity.[78] Last, the use of long-term maintenance therapy following a complete response has not been shown to improve survival. Two cycles of chemotherapy following attainment of a complete response are usually recommended, with the majority of current regimens lasting 6 to 9 months. There are exceptions, however, such as MACOP-B, which requires only 12 weeks of therapy. This heterogeneous group of lymphomas can all be treated the same, but peripheral T-cell lymphomas do not respond as well as aggressive lymphomas of B-cell lineage.

Advanced-stage large-cell lymphoma was considered an incurable disease some 20 to 25 years ago. Initial combination regimens using CVP produced a plateau on the survival curve of just 10%, with a median survival of less than 1 year. Based on the activity of single-agent doxorubicin, McKelvey and associates[77] developed the CHOP regimen (Table 120–9). Other first-generation regimens that contained four or five chemotherapy agents such as CHOP-Bleo, BACOP, and COMLA (cyclophosphamide, vincristine, methotrexate, leucovorin, cytarabine) were also developed around this time. CHOP gained widespread popularity because it had the highest complete remission rate (67%).[58]

However, relapses after treatment with CHOP were common within the first 2 years, and durability of the complete responses were questioned. A review of the Southwest Oncology Group's (SWOG) 12-year experience with CHOP-based regimens in over 400 patients reported a complete remission rate of 53%, with an overall survival of 30%.[79] Overall, these first-generation regimens produce complete remissions in 45% to 55% of patients, and about one-third of all patients appear to be cured with their use.[58]

In the late 1970s, various therapeutic approaches taken by investigators led to the development of the second-generation chemotherapy regimens. These regimens are characterized by the use of six or more antineoplastic agents, including both myelosuppressive and nonmyelosuppressive agents. The myelosuppressive agents are cycled more frequently, generally every 3 weeks, and the nonmyelosuppressive agents are administered during weeks of cytopenias. The additional chemotherapy agents used in these regimens are frequently cell-cycle active and/or marrow sparing, are generally non–cross-resistant to the myelosuppressive agent, and provide continuous tumor suppression even during periods of cytopenia. COP-BLAM (cyclophosphamide, vincristine, prednisone, bleomycin, doxorubicin, procarbazine), M-BACOD (high-dose methotrexate = 3 g/m^2, bleomycin, doxorubicin, cyclophosphamide, vincristine, dexamethasone), m-BACOD (moderate-dose methotrexate = 200 mg/m^2), and ProMACE-MOPP are examples of second-generation regimens.[58] The ProMACE-MOPP flexitherapy combination is based in part on the Norton–Simon hypothesis[80] on the development of drug resistance. To achieve the maximal probability of cure, ProMACE is administered for a flexible number of cycles until the rate of tumor response appears to slow, and then therapy is switched to MOPP. After the rate of response to MOPP slows, or a complete response is achieved, patients are switched back to ProMACE for consolidation.[81] Overall, the second-generation regimens achieve complete response rates of 61% to 74%, and approximately 53% to 63% of patients are cured (Table 120–10). However, treatment with these regimens resulted in increased toxicity and cost. These regimens appear to be superior to the first-generation regimens. However, a randomized comparative trial comparing CHOP, a first-generation regimen, to m-BACOD, a second-generation regimen, showed no difference in complete response rates or overall survival.[82]

The Goldie–Coldman hypothesis[32,33] and the Hryniuk and Bush dose-intensity hypothesis[83] have aided in the design of the third-generation treatment regimens. These new chemotherapy regimens focus on alterations in schedules (the use of many drugs and early exposure to non–cross-resistant agents) and doses (increasing relative dose intensity) rather than sequencing non–cross-resistant regimens. Hryniuk and Bush[83] observed that the treatment outcome of patients with metastatic breast cancer was related to the dose intensity (amount of drug delivered per unit time) of the treatment regimens. In summary, the best chance for cure can be achieved by administration of more drugs at higher doses as frequently as possible. The importance of dose intensity in the treatment outcome of patients with non-Hodgkin's lymphoma has been reviewed.[78]

Initial trials with third-generation treatment regimens, MACOP-B, ProMACE-CytaBOM, COP-BLAM III, and F-MACHOP, reported complete remission rates of 50% to 86% and cure rates of 51% to 70% (see Table 120–10).[84,85] These regimens use multiple agents at higher doses over a short treatment period. For example, the MACOP-B regimen emphasizes dose intensity, with treatment duration of only 12 weeks. During treatment, myelosuppressive agents and nonmyelosuppressive agents are alternated and administered weekly. The COP-BLAM III regimen differs from the other regimens in that it uses a prolonged infusion of vincristine and bleomycin and dose escalation of doxorubicin and cyclophosphamide, allowing maximum dose intensity.[84,85]

The third-generation regimens initially appeared to be superior to the first- and second-generation regimens. However, these observations came from single-institution studies and nonrandomized multicenter comparative trials that had short lengths of follow-up and did not control for differences in patient populations. SWOG conducted some phase II studies to confirm that third-generation regimens were superior to first- and second-generation regimens. The results of these studies did not corroborate the single-institutional findings.[86] Therefore, SWOG initiated an intergroup trial with ECOG to more accurately determine if there was a response or survival difference between CHOP and third-generation combination chemotherapy regimens (m-BACOD, ProMACE-CytaBOM, and MACOP-B). To date, three multicenter studies that compared CHOP to more aggressive regimens have been completed and all were unable to detect differences in complete remission or overall survival (Table 120–11).[86,87] Additionally, two Italian multicenter studies have not been able to detect a difference between second- and third-generation regimens.[86] Therefore, first-, second-, or third-generation regimens may be considered equally efficacious as first-line therapy. However, CHOP is associated with less toxicity and cost, which makes it considered the standard treatment regimen by most clinicians.

TABLE. 120–10. Responses to Second- and Third-Generation Lymphoma Regimens

Regimen[a]	No. of Patients	CR (%)	Long-term Survival (%)[b]	Author
Second Generation				
COP-BLAM	33	73	55	Laurence
M-BACOD	81	72	63	Skarin
m-BACOD	134	61	63	Shipp
ProMACE-MOPP	99	74	53	Fisher
Third Generation				
MACOP-B	126	84	69	Klimo
ProMACE-CytaBOM	94	86	—	Longo
COP-BLAM III	43	86	70	Boyd
F-MACHOP	56	77	60	Guglielmi

[a]COP-BLAM = cyclophosphamide, vincristine, prednisone, bleomycin, doxorubicin, procarbazine; M/m-BACOD = high-dose/moderate-dose methotrexate, bleomycin, doxorubicin, cyclophosphamide, vincristine, dexamethasone; ProMACE-MOPP = prednisone, methotrexate, doxorubicin, cyclophosphamide, etoposide, MOPP; MACOP-B = methotrexate, doxorubicin, cyclophosphamide, vincristine, prednisone, bleomycin; ProMACE-CytaBOM = prednisone, methotrexate, doxorubicin, cyclophosphamide, etoposide, cytarabine, bleomycin, vincristine; COP-BLAM III = cyclophosphamide, vincristine, prednisone, bleomycin, doxorubicin, procarbazine; F-MACHOP = fluorouracil, methotrexate, cytarabine, cyclophosphamide, doxorubicin, vincristine, prednisone; CR = complete response.

[b]Two to three years.

Compiled from Refs. 84 and 85.

TABLE 120–11. Randomized Studies Comparing CHOP to Other Regimens

Regimen[a]	No. of Patients	CR (%)	4–6-yr OS[b]	Research Group—Year
CHOP	174	61	48	ECOG—1992
m-BACOD	151	55	49	
CHOP	76	57.5	42	Spanish Cooperative Group—1996
ProMACE-CytaBOM	72	62	42	
CHOP	111	59	51	Australian/New Zealand Cooperative Group—1994
MACOP-B	125	51	56	
CHOP	225	44	42	SWOG—996
m-BACOD	223	48	40	
ProMACE-CytaBOM	233	56	46	
MACOP-B	218	51	41	

[a]Regimens detailed in previous table.
[b]No significant difference between treatment arms: CR = complete response; OS = overall survival.
Compiled from Refs. 86 and 87.

Approximately 33% of non-Hodgkin's lymphoma patients are over the age of 70 years, which is considered a poor prognostic factor. Some feel that it has been considered a poor prognostic indicator because many clinicians treat the elderly with reduced dose or less aggressive chemotherapy regimens. Over the last 5 years, more rigorous studies involving this patient population have been performed. A recently reported multicenter trial by Tirelli and colleagues[88] randomized 120 patients over the age of 70 years to a less aggressive chemotherapy regimen containing etoposide, mitoxantrone, and prednimustine (VMP) or CHOP. After 2 years the progression-free survival and overall survival were 25% versus 55% ($P = .002$) and 30% versus 65% ($P = .004$) for VMP and CHOP, respectively. There was significantly more alopecia and neurologic and gastrointestinal toxicity for the CHOP arm. Toxic deaths occurred in one VMP-treated patient and two CHOP-treated patients. The results of this study indicate that CHOP at full dose should be considered the treatment of choice in the elderly.

An increased incidence of non-Hodgkin's lymphoma was seen early in the AIDS epidemic. In 1985 the Centers for Disease Control included the appearance of B-cell non-Hodgkin's lymphoma in the diagnostic criteria for AIDS.[89] The National Cancer Institute estimates that as many as 19.4% of AIDS patients will develop non-Hodgkin's lymphoma. Lymphomas occurring in immunodeficiency states are predominantly of B-cell origin and nearly 80% are classified as highly aggressive, either immunoblastic or small noncleaved cell subtypes. The majority of patients present with Ann Arbor stage III or IV disease. Involvement of extranodal sites of disease, especially the bone marrow, CNS, gastrointestinal tract, and liver, is seen in 75% to 95% of patients. Primary CNS lymphoma has been reported in up to 20% of patients with AIDS-associated lymphomas, and survival in these patients is generally poor (2 to 5 months).[90] The total number of $CD4^+$ lymphocytes may also be an important predictor of survival. A median survival is approximately 24 months in patients with a CD4 count greater than 100 cells/mm^3, in contrast to a median survival of 4 months in those with CD4 counts less than 100 cells/mm^3.[91]

The treatment of patients with AIDS-associated lymphomas presents a therapeutic challenge. Because of the immunocompromised state of these patients at the time of diagnosis, the risk of both morbidity and mortality following myelosuppressive therapy are high, primarily owing to the occurrence of opportunistic infections. For a patient with good immune function and without a history of an opportunistic infection, standard-dose chemotherapy may be appropriate. A lower-dose chemotherapy regimen, or even a decision to withhold therapy, may be more appropriate for severely immunocompromised patients. The results of treatment with standard chemotherapy regimens, including CHOP, BACOP, m-BACOD, and MACOP-B, have been disappointing. Complete response rates range from 30% to 50%, relapse frequently occurs, and the median duration of survival ranges from only 4 to 7 months.[89] The most common causes of death are uncontrolled lymphoma and opportunistic infection. The use of intensive "leukemia-like" regimens normally employed in the treatment of small noncleaved cell lymphoma results in particularly high mortality rates. The current approach to therapy is the use of reduced doses of standard chemotherapy regimens or standard-dose combination chemotherapy with concurrent administration of a colony-stimulating factor. Central nervous system prophylaxis and *Pneumocystis carinii* prophylaxis should be incorporated into either approach. A randomized multicenter trial that evaluated the efficacy of reduced-dose m-BACOD compared with standard-dose m-BACOD plus GM-CSF found no difference in efficacy but a lower rate of hematologic toxicity with the reduced dose. Therefore, reduced-dose m-BACOD should be considered standard of care for the treatment of HIV-related non-Hodgkin's lymphoma.[92]

The treatment of primary CNS lymphoma usually consists of whole-brain radiation.[89] Despite complete response rates up to 70%, survival duration remains short (2 to 5 months). Again, opportunistic infection is the most common cause of death, especially because the majority of patients with CNS lymphoma are severely immunocompromised at the time of diagnosis.

Some observations can be made concerning the treatment of advanced aggressive grade lymphomas: (1) the incidence of complete remission and of long-term survival has been improved greatly with the use of combination chemotherapy regimens; (2) a rapid response to chemotherapy (i.e., a complete response achieved in the first three treatment cycles) is associated with a more durable remission compared with patients requiring longer treatment; (3) relapse usually occurs within the first 2 years of induction of a complete remission (although relapses up to 7 years are reported), such that the vast majority of 2- to 3-year disease-free survivors are probably cured; and (4) though the best regimen has not yet been identified, the available studies have confirmed the importance of dose intensity. With the advent of the colony-stimulating factors (e.g., G-CSF, GM-CSF), this goal may be more easily achieved and allow for the safer use of even further dose-intensified regimens.

HIGHLY AGGRESSIVE LYMPHOMAS

As mentioned previously, the treatment of limited and advanced-stage lymphoblastic and small noncleaved cell lymphoma is essentially the same.[50,58]

SALVAGE CHEMOTHERAPY

INDOLENT LYMPHOMAS

The majority of patients with stage I or II indolent lymphomas are cured of their disease, although this constitutes only a small portion of all indolent lymphoma patients. Complete remission can be achieved in 60% to 90% of patients with stage III or IV disease, but the median disease-free interval is typically 17 to 24 months. After relapse, patients are re-treated and again high remission rates are achieved. Similar to the high number of initial therapy options, there is a high number of salvage treatment options. Any of the first-line options that have not been used can be used as salvage therapies. Additional salvage therapies not included in the list of initial treatment options include combination chemotherapy regimens and biologic therapy. The most promising chemotherapy regimens not used as initial therapy include the combination of fludarabine, an anthracycline, and a steroid. Zinzani and colleagues[93] report that a combination of fludarabine, mitoxantrone, and prednisone results in a complete response rate of 35% and overall response rate of 83%. Although these response rates are very high, the projected relapse-free survival in this trial at 33 months was 32% for patients attaining a complete remission and 18% for those achieving a partial response. As stated in the initial treatment section, treatment does not cure these patients, but rather palliates their symptoms. Additionally, there is no evidence that salvage chemotherapy improves the overall survival. High-dose chemotherapy with an allogeneic or autologous transplant has been used as salvage therapy, but this is still very controversial and needs further study.[58]

Biologic response modifiers are emerging as important agents in salvage therapy of non-Hodgkin's lymphoma. Interferons and monoclonal antibodies have been evaluated individually or in combination with each other or with chemotherapy.[58,94,95] The most promising results of these agents have been seen in the follicular lymphomas.

Monoclonal antibodies, a form of specific immunotherapy, are directed against specific cell surface proteins. Rituximab (Rituxan) is a chimeric monoclonal antibody directed at CD20 expressed on B-cell tumors. The FDA recently approved this compound as the first monoclonal antibody to treat non-Hodgkin's lymphoma. The pivotal open-label multicenter study that led to its approval enrolled 166 patients with relapsed or recurrent indolent lymphoma.[94] Rituximab therapy with 375 mg/m^2 weekly for 4 weeks resulted in an overall response of 48% and a complete remission of 6%. A recently reported phase II trial that treated 37 patients with relapsed low-grade or follicular lymphomas with 375 mg/m^2 weekly for 4 weeks showed a 46% clinical response rate.[95] Side effects were commonly seen with only the first infusion and included grade 1 to 2 fever, chills, respiratory symptoms, and occasional hypotension.[94,95] Rituximab is currently approved for use in patients with relapsed or refractory indolent or follicular, CD20-positive, B-cell lymphoma.[94] Because it is effective in chemotherapy-resistant tumors and has different toxicities than other chemotherapy agents, it is being evaluated in combination with other chemotherapy agents earlier in treatment. Other therapeutic approaches that remain under study include antibodies directed to tumor-specific immunoglobulins (anti-idiotype antibodies) or other tumor-related proteins. Another approach that continues to be researched is the conjugation of monoclonal antibodies to radioisotopes, toxins, and chemotherapy agents.

Interferon has been the most extensively studied biologic agent. As a single agent, recombinant IFN-α yields objective response rates of approximately 40% in low-grade lymphoma and 10% to 15% in intermediate- and high-grade lymphoma.[58] The majority of responses are partial, with a median duration of 6 to 12 months. Responses are similar in previously treated and untreated patients. The most effective dose and schedule have not been determined, although lower doses appear to achieve similar results compared with higher doses.[51,59] Interferon will most likely be limited to maintenance therapy for indolent lymphomas as already discussed. Further clinical trials are needed to ultimately define the role of biologic response modifiers in the treatment of non-Hodgkin's lymphoma.

AGGRESSIVE LYMPHOMAS

Though long-term remissions for aggressive non-Hodgkin's lymphoma are possible with intensive treatment regimens, 20% to 30% of patients do not enter a complete remission with these therapies. Of those patients achieving a complete response, 20% to 40% subsequently relapse and die within a few months. Patients who relapse following a complete response to chemotherapy are more likely to respond to salvage therapy than patients with resistant or partially responding disease. Unfortunately, second-line salvage therapies are not capable of consistently inducing remission in relapsed or refractory non-Hodgkin's lymphoma. A possible reason for the failure of salvage regimens may be the use of nearly all effective agents in the primary treatment regimens. Several clinical trials are now evaluating the utility of newer investigational agents, alone and in combination, or the use of commercially available agents in high doses, with or without stem cell rescue.

A variety of conventional-dose salvage chemotherapy regimens have been used in patients with relapsed or refractory non-Hodgkin's lymphoma. Most patients who relapse or have resistant disease will receive a salvage regimen. Following this regimen, selected patients will receive high-dose chemotherapy and hematopoietic stem cell support. The best salvage regimen is undefined owing to a lack of controlled randomized studies in this area. Many regimens have been developed that usually incorporate drugs not used in the initial therapy. Some of the more common salvage regimens include MIME (mitoguazone, ifosfamide, methotrexate, etoposide), DHAP (cisplatin, high-dose cytarabine, dexamethasone), and ESHAP (etoposide, methylprednisolone, high-dose cytarabine, cisplatin).[85,96] Investigators at MD Anderson recently compared the outcomes of two studies, one that treated 122 patients with DHAP and one that treated 116 patients with ESHAP. The patients had similar characteristics, but different outcomes. The overall response rates and complete response rates were 43% versus 56% and 16% versus 31% for DHAP and ESHAP, respectively.[97] This study is far from definitive, but is compelling in favor of ESHAP. Results of selected trials are listed in Table 120–12.[85,96] Generally speaking, complete responses are obtained in 20% to 35% of patients, the median remission duration is 1 to 2 years, and only 5% to 10% of patients will have long-term disease-free survival.[58]

To improve this situation, investigators have evaluated the role of high-dose chemotherapy and/or radiation with bone marrow (BMT) or peripheral blood progenitor cell (PBPC) transplant. Initial studies reported an improvement in the outlook for

TABLE 120–12. Conventional Salvage Regimens

Regimen[a]	N	CR (%)	Median Duration of Response (mo)
MINE	123	32	15
DHAP	74	32	24
ESHAP	88	38	20

[a]MIME = mitoguazone, ifosfamide, methotrexate, and etoposide; DHAP = cisplatin, high-dose cytarabine, and dexamethasone; ESHAP = etoposide, methylprednisolone, high-dose cytarabine, and cisplatin; CR = complete response.
Adapted from Ref. 97.

patients failing primary treatment. The first reports of high response rates and long-term survival in a small proportion of patients with Burkitt's lymphoma following high-dose chemotherapy and autologous BMT reached the literature in the late 1970s. Since that time, various studies have been published using different high-dose regimens followed by PBPC, autologous, allogeneic, or syngeneic BMT. Survival rates are similar regardless of the source of hematopoietic stem cells. BMT has been used at various stages of disease in patients with non-Hodgkin's lymphoma (e.g., initial, consolidation, or salvage therapy). Results in over 500 autologous BMT patients have documented long-term survival rates between 20% and 70%. Non-Hodgkin's lymphoma, namely diffuse large cell lymphoma, has become one of the most common diseases to be treated with autologous BMT.[50,58] A thorough review of BMT can be found in Chapter 125.

CURRENT RECOMMENDATIONS

With radiation therapy, chemotherapy, biologics, and bone marrow transplantation, many patients with non-Hodgkin's lymphoma can be cured. Although specific treatment recommendations are influenced by the special circumstances of the patient, available resources, technologies, and the skill of the practitioners, general recommendations presented in Table 120–13 can be made.

TABLE 120–13. Treatment Recommendations

Category	Option
Indolent lymphoma	
Stage I or II	Radiation
Stage III or IV	Watch and wait or combination chemotherapy ± interferon-α
Aggressive lymphoma	
Stage I or II	CHOP + radiation
Stage III or IV	CHOP
Highly aggressive lymphoma	Combination chemotherapy + CNS prophylaxis ± radiation

EVALUATION OF THERAPEUTIC OUTCOMES

Establishing the correct diagnosis and stage for lymphomas is critical if an appropriate care plan is to be created. Pathologic evaluation of tissue, presenting symptoms, and corresponding laboratory work and additional procedures are all necessary to select appropriate treatment and establish a prognosis.

For non-Hodgkin's disease, medical decisions revolve around the histology and stage of disease. Management can vary from "watch and wait" to immediate initiation of combination chemotherapy with the expectation that patients will receive subsequent high-dose chemotherapy with hematopoietic stem cell support. Keep in mind that with many histologies and stages, appropriate treatment can cure many patients with non-Hodgkin's lymphoma.

Combination chemotherapy remains the mainstay of treatment for most patients with non-Hodgkin's lymphoma, and maintaining dose intensity is an important predictor of a positive outcome. Patients who receive full doses of chemotherapy on time do significantly better than those who do not. However, it must be understood that chemotherapy is not a benign treatment. It often is rigorous and toxic and demands full cooperation of the patient and treatment team. Although the toxicities vary with different treatment regimens, they are bothersome to the patient.

To optimize chemotherapy administration, toxicity management is important. From a pharmaceutical care standpoint, the pharmacist must identify, monitor, treat, and proactively prevent or minimize treatment-related toxicity. A thorough understanding of the patient's medical history and review of systems (from a physical examination standpoint) are essential. Pertinent laboratory data and review of other procedures will help establish a baseline to use for monitoring purposes. Major organ and system toxicities that need to be followed include hematology (blood work), neurology, skin, pulmonary, gastrointestinal, renal, and cardiac. Long-term toxicities and complications including secondary malignancies must also be addressed when treatment decisions are made.

Myelosuppression is a constant concern with aggressive chemotherapy treatment of non-Hodgkin's lymphoma. The risk of neutropenic fever with infection is a real threat, and appropriate patient education and monitoring are critical. Treatment-related anemia must also be monitored.

Nutritional assessment should also be undertaken. Patients may require enteral and/or parenteral nutritional supplementation during their treatment to maintain their physical state and keep up their performance status.

The primary patient outcome to be identified is tumor response. Physical examination and other diagnostic procedures will be necessary to determine response. Complete response is the desired outcome, for only with a complete response will the patient have a chance for cure. Patients typically receive two cycles of chemotherapy beyond achieving a complete response, with a minimum of six cycles of treatment.

Patients are generally monitored at 3- to 6-month intervals for the first year or two following treatment, with longer intervals instituted when appropriate.

CONCLUSIONS

Approximately 25 years ago, lymphomas were considered a fatal disease. Today, at least half of patients with certain types of lymphoma are cured. Although all of the malignant lymphomas may be responsive to chemotherapy and/or radiation, only Hodgkin's lymphomas and the aggressive or highly aggressive lymphomas are curable at this time. Our current capacity to cure these patients is the result of many factors, including development of an accurate and reproducible classification system; a more uniform approach to the staging of lymphoma; and advances in the treatment strategies, especially the use of aggressive combination chemotherapy. The goal for the future is to develop treatment modalities to achieve cure in a larger number of patients, including those with indolent non-Hodgkin's lymphomas, while at the same time avoiding excessive treatment-related morbidity and mortality. The use of high-dose chemotherapy with stem cell and/or progenitor cell support allows for the administration of more dose-intensified chemotherapy regimens. The colony-stimulating factors represent a way to maintain dose intensity, which is important in curable lymphomas. They also represent a way to decrease morbidity resulting from neutropenic fever. A better understanding of the pathogenesis of non-Hodgkin's lymphoma through continued research in molecular biology and immunology will allow further exploration of other treatment modalities, including immune modulation with the biologic response modifiers and monoclonal antibodies.

▶ PRINCIPLES OF PHARMACOTHERAPY

- Lymphomas are common malignancies that are potentially curable.
- Prognosis for malignant lymphomas is based on histology, stage, patient age, performance status, extensive B symptoms, and LDH.
- Radiation therapy alone is the treatment of choice for early-stage Hodgkin's disease.
- Combination chemotherapy is the treatment of choice for advanced Hodgkin's disease.
- Treatment of choice for indolent lymphomas range from watch and wait to aggressive chemotherapy.
- The CHOP chemotherapy regimen is the treatment of choice for stage III and IV aggressive lymphomas.
- Managing toxicity is crucial to ensure dose intensity for malignant lymphomas, which correlates directly to patient outcome.

REFERENCES

1. Cancer Facts and Figures—1998. Atlanta, GA, American Cancer Society, 1998.
2. MacMahon B. Epidemiological evidence of the nature of Hodgkin's disease. Cancer 1957;10:1045–1054.
3. Gutensohn NM. Social class and age at diagnosis of Hodgkin's disease: New epidemiologic evidence for the "two-disease hypothesis." Cancer Treat Rep 1982;66:689–695.
4. Glaser SL, Swartz WG. Time trends in Hodgkin's disease incidence. Cancer 1990;66:2196–2204.
5. Kennedy BJ, Loeb V, Peterson VM, et al. National survey of patterns of care for Hodgkin's disease. Cancer 1985;56:2547–2556.
6. Haluska FG, Brufsky AM, Canellos GP. The cellular biology of the Reed–Sternberg cell. Blood 1994;84:1005–1019.
7. Lukes RF, Butler JJ, Hicks ED. Natural history of Hodgkin's disease as related to its pathological picture. Cancer 1966;19:319.
8. Lukes RJ, Craver LF, Hall TC, et al. Report of the Nomenclature Committee. Cancer Res 1966;26:1311.
9. Harris NL, Jaffe ES, Stein H, et al. A revised European–American classification of lymphoid neoplasms: A proposal from the International Lymphoma Study Group. Blood 1994;84:1361–1392.
10. Kaplan HS. Hodgkin's Disease, 2nd ed. Cambridge, Harvard University Press, 1980.
11. Carbone PP, Kaplan HS, Musshoff K, et al. Report of the committee on Hodgkin's disease staging classification. Cancer Res 1971;31:1860–1861.
12. Lister TA, Crowther D, Sutcliffe SB, et al. Report of a committee convened to discuss the evaluation and staging of patients with Hodgkin's disease: Cotswolds Meeting. J Clin Oncol 1989;7:1630–1636.
13. Hohl RJ, Schilsky RL. Nonmalignant complications of therapy for Hodgkin's disease. Hematol Oncol Clin North Am 1989;3:331–343.
14. Liebenhaut M, Hoppe R, Efron B, et al. Prognostic indicators of laparotomy findings in clinical stage I–II supradiaphragmatic Hodgkin's disease. J Clin Oncol 1989;7:81.
15. Mauch P, Larson D, Osteen R, et al. Prognostic factors for positive surgical staging in patients with Hodgkin's disease. J Clin Oncol 1990;8:257–265.
16. Specht L, Gray RG, Clarke M, et al. Influence of more extensive radiotherapy and adjuvant chemotherapy on long-term outcome of early-stage Hodgkin's disease: A meta-analysis of 23 randomized trials involving 3888 patients. J Clin Oncol 1998;16:830–843.
17. Mauch P, Tarbell N, Weinstein, et al. Stage IA and IIA supradiaphragmatic Hodgkin's disease: Prognostic factors in surgically staged patients treated with mantle and para-aortic irradiation. J Clin Oncol 1988;6:1576–1583.
18. Hoppe RT, Coleman CN, Cox RS, et al. The management of stage I–II Hodgkin's disease with irradiation alone or in combined modality therapy: The Stanford experience. Blood 1982;59:455–465.
19. Hellman S, Mauch P. Role of radiation therapy in the treatment of Hodgkin's disease. Cancer Treat Rep 1982;66:915–923.
20. Zagars G, Rubin P. Hodgkin's disease stage IA and IIA: A long-term follow-up study on the gains achieved by modern therapy. Cancer 1985;56:1905–1912.
21. Biti GP, Cimino G, Cartoni C, et al. Extended-field radiotherapy is superior to MOPP chemotherapy for the treatment of pathologic stage I–IIA Hodgkin's disease: Eight-year update of an Italian Prospective Randomized Study. J Clin Oncol 1992;10:378–382.
22. Carde P, Hagenbeek A, Hayat M, et al. Clinical staging versus laparotomy and combined modality with MOPP versus ABVD in early-stage Hodgkin's disease: The H6 twin randomized trials from the European Organization for Research and Treatment of Cancer Lymphoma Cooperative Group. J Clin Oncol 1993;11:2258–2272.
23. Crnkovich MJ, Leopold K, Hoppe RT, et al. Stage I to IVB Hodgkin's disease: The combined experience at Stanford University and the Joint Center for Radiation Therapy. J Clin Oncol 1987;5:1041–1049.
24. Krikorian JG, Portlock CS, Mauch PM. Hodgkin's disease presenting below the diaphragm: A review. J Clin Oncol 1986;4:1551–1562.
25. Hoppe RT, Cos RS, Rosenberg SA, et al. Prognostic factors in pathologic stage III Hodgkin's disease. Cancer Treat Rep 1982;66:743–749.
26. Marcus KC, Kalish LA, Coleman CN, et al. Improved survival in patients with limited stage IIIA Hodgkin's disease treated with combined radiation therapy and chemotherapy. J Clin Oncol 1994;12:2567–2572.
27. DeVita VT, Simon RM, Hubbard SM, et al. Curability of advanced Hodgkin's disease with chemotherapy: Long-term follow-up of MOPP-treated patients at the National Cancer Institute. Ann Intern Med 1980;92:587–595.

28. Longo DL, Young RC, Wesley M, et al. Twenty years of MOPP therapy for Hodgkin's disease. J Clin Oncol 1986;4:1295–1306.
29. Longo DL. The use of chemotherapy in the treatment of Hodgkin's disease. Semin Oncol 1990;17:716–735.
30. Santoro A, Bonfante V, Bonadonna G. Salvage chemotherapy with ABVD in MOPP-resident Hodgkin's disease. Ann Intern Med 1982; 96:139–143.
31. Canellos GP, Anderson JR, Propert K, et al. Chemotherapy of advanced Hodgkin's disease with MOPP, ABVD, or MOPP alternating with ABVD. N Engl J Med 1992;327:1478–1484.
32. Goldie JH, Coldman AJ. The genetic origin of drug resistance in neoplasms, implications for systemic therapy. Cancer Res 1984;44: 3643–3653.
33. Goldie JH, Coldman AJ, Gudauskas GA. Rationale for the use of alternating non-cross-resistant chemotherapy. Cancer Treat Rep 1982; 66:439–449.
34. Bonadonna G, Valagussa P, Santoro A. Alternating non-cross-resistant combination chemotherapy with ABVD or MOPP in stage IV Hodgkin's disease: A report of eight year results. Ann Intern Med 1986;104:739–746.
35. Connors JM, Klimo P, Adams G, et al. Treatment of advanced Hodgkin's disease with chemotherapy-comparison of MOPP/ABV hybrid regimen with alternating courses of MOPP and ABVD: A report from the National Cancer Institute of Canada Clinical Trials Group. J Clin Oncol 1997;15:1638–1645.
36. Viviani S, Bonadonna G, Santoro A, et al. Alternating versus hybrid MOPP and ABVD combinations in advanced Hodgkin's disease: Ten-year results. J Clin Oncol 1996;14:1421–1430.
37. Duggan D, Petroni G, Johnson J, et al. MOPP/ABV versus ABVD for advanced Hodgkin's disease—A preliminary report of CALGB 8952 (with SWOG, ECOG, NCIC). Proc Am Soc Clin Oncol 1997; 16:12a.
38. Glick JH, Young ML, Harrington D, et al. MOPP/ABV hybrid chemotherapy for advanced Hodgkin's disease significantly improves failure-free and overall survival: The 8-year results of the Intergroup trial. J Clin Oncol 1998;16:19–26.
39. Mauch PM. Controversies in the managment of early stage Hodgkin's disease. Blood 1994;83:318–329.
40. Longo D, Glatstein E, Duffey P, et al. Radiation therapy versus combination chemotherapy in the treatment of early-stage Hodgkin's disease: Seven year results of a prospective randomized trial. J Clin Oncol 1991;9:906–917.
41. Biti GP, Cimino G, Cartoni C, et al. Extended-field radiotherapy is superior to MOPP chemotherapy for the treatment of pathologic stage I–IIA Hodgkin's disease: Eight-year update of an Italian prospective randomized study. J Clin Oncol 1992;10:378–382.
42. Rueda A, Alba E, Ribelles, et al. Six cycles of ABVD in the treatment of stage I and II Hodgkin's lymphoma: A pilot study. J Clin Oncol 1997;15:1118–1122.
43. Loeffler M, Brosteanu O, Hasenclever D, et al. Meta-analysis of chemotherapy versus combined modality treatment trials in Hodgkin's disease. J Clin Oncol 1998;16:818–829.
44. Horning S, Hoppe R, Hancock S, et al. Vinblastine, bleomycin, and methotrexate: An effective adjuvant in favorable Hodgkin's disease. J Clin Oncol 1988;6:1822.
45. Horning SJ, Hoppe RT, Mason J, et al. Stanford–Kaiser Permanente G1 study for clinical stage I to IIA Hodgkin's disease: Subtotal lymphoid irradiation versus vinblastine, methotrexate, and bleomycin chemotherapy and regional irradiation. J Clin Oncol 1997;15: 1736–1744.
46. Pavlovsky S, Maschio M, Santarelli MT, et al. Randomized trial of chemotherapy versus chemotherapy plus radiotherapy for stage I–II Hodgkin's disease. J Natl Cancer Inst 1988;80:1466–1473.
47. Longo DL, Duffey PL, Young RC, et al. Conventional-dose salvage combination chemotherapy in patients relapsing with Hodgkin's disease after combination chemotherapy: The low probability of cure. J Clin Oncol 1992;10:210–1218.
48. Zarrabi MH, Rosner F. Second neoplasms in Hodgkin's disease: Current controversies. Hematol Oncol Clin North Am 1989;3: 303–318.
49. Kaldor JM, Day NE, Clarke A, et al. Leukemia following Hodgkin's disease. N Engl J Med 1990;322:7–13.
50. Shipp MA, Mauch PM, Harris NL. Non-Hodgkin's lympomas. In: DeVita VT Jr, Hellman S, Rosenberg SA, eds. Cancer Principles and Practice of Oncology, 5th ed. Philidelphia, Lippincott–Raven, 1997: 2165–2220.
51. Potter M. Pathogenetic mechanisms in B-cell non-Hodgkin's lymphomas in humans. Cancer Res 1992;52(suppl):5522s–5528s.
52. List AF, Greco FA, Vogler LB. Lymphoproliferative diseases in immunocompromised hosts: The role of Epstein-Barr virus. J Clin Oncol 1987;5:1673–1689.
53. Neubauer A, Thiede C, Morgner A, et al. Cure of *Helicobacter pylori* infection and duration of remission of low-grade gastric mucosa–associated lymphoid tissue lymphoma. J Natl Cancer Inst 1997;89: 1350–1355.
54. Gaidano G, Carbone A. Diagnostic and prognostic implications of genetic lesions in non-Hodgkin's lymphoma. Eur J Cancer 1996;32A: 1477–1482.
55. Rappaport H, Winter WJ, Hicks EB. Follicular lymphoma: A reevaluation of its position in the scheme of malignant lymphoma based on a survey of 253 cases. Cancer 1956;9:792–821.
56. Simon R, Durrleman S, Hoppe RT, et al. The non-Hodgkin lymphoma pathologic classification project: Long-term follow-up of 1153 patients with non-Hodgkin lymphomas. Ann Intern Med 1988;109: 939–945.
57. Pittaluga S, Bijnens L, Teodorovic I, et al. Clinical analysis of 670 cases in two trials of the European Organization for the Research and Treatment of Cancer Lymphoma Cooperative Group subtyped according to the revised European–American Classification of Lymphoid Neoplasms: A comparison with the Working Formulation. Blood 1996;87:4358–4367.
58. Fisher RI, Oken MM. Clinical practice guidelines: Non-Hodgkin's lymphoma. Cleve Clin J Med 1995;62(suppl 1):S16–S42.
59. Fleming ID, Cooper JS, Henson DE, et al. Non-Hodgkin's lymphoma. In: American Joint Committee on Cancer: Manual for Staging of Cancer, 4th ed. Philadelphia, Lippincott, 1992:257–261.
60. Skillings JR, Bramwell V, Nicholson R, et al. A prospective study of magnetic resonance imaging in lymphoma staging. Cancer 1991;67: 1838–1843.
61. The International Non-Hodgkin's Lymphoma Prognostic Factors Project. A predictive model for aggressive non-Hodgkin's lymphoma. N Engl J Med 1993:329:987–994.
62. Zucca E, Roggero E. Biology and treatment of MALT lymphoma: The state-of-the-art in 1996. A workshop at the 6th International Conference on Malignant Lymphoma. Mucosa-Associated Lymphoid Tissue. Ann Oncol 1996;7:787–792.
63. Laing RW, Hoskin P, Hudson VB, et al. The significance of MALT histology in thyroid lymphoma: A review of patients from the BNLI and Royal Marsden Hospital. Clin Oncol 1994:6;300–304.
64. Mac Manus MP, Hoppe RT. Is radiotherapy curative for stage I and II low-grade follicular lymphoma? Results of a long-term follow-up study of patients treated at Stanford University. J Clin Oncol 1996; 14:1282–1290.
65. Kelsey SM, Newland AC, Hudson GV, Jelliffe AM. A British National Lymphoma Investigation randomised trial of single agent chlorambucil plus radiotherapy versus radiotherapy alone in low grade, localised non-Hodgkin's lymphoma. Med Oncol 1994;11:19–25.
66. Seymour JF, McLaughlin P, Fuller LM, et al. High rate of prolonged remissions following combined modality therapy for patients with localized low-grade lymphoma. Ann Oncol 1996;7:157–163.
67. Hallahan DE, Farah R, Vokes EE, et al. The patterns of failure in patients with pathological stage I and II diffuse histiocytic lymphoma treated with radiation therapy alone. Int J Radiat Oncol Biol Phys 1989;17:767–771.

68. Miller TP, Dahlberg S, Cassady JR, et al. Three cycles of CHOP (3) plus radiotherapy (RT) is superior to eight cycles of CHOP (8) alone for localized intermediate and high grade non-Hodgkin's lymphoma (NHL): A Southwest Oncology Group study. Proc Am Soc Clin Oncol 1996;15:411.
69. Glick JH, Kim K, Earle J, et al. An ECOG randomized phase III trial of CHOP vs. CHOP + radiotherapy (XRT) for intermediate grade early stage non-Hodgkin's lymphoma (NHL). Proc Am Soc Clin Oncol 1995;14:391.
70. Horning SJ. Natural history of and therapy for the indolent non-Hodgkin's lymphomas. Semin Oncol 1993;20(suppl 5):75–88.
71. Vose JM. Classification and clinical course of low-grade non-Hodgkin's lymphomas with an overview of therapy. Ann Oncol 1996; 7(suppl 6):S13–S19.
72. Hoffman MA. Cladribine for the treatment of indolent non-Hodgkin's lymphoma. Semin Oncol 1996;33(suppl 1):40–44.
73. Solal-Celigny P, Brice P, Brousse N, et al. Phase II trial of fludarabine monophosphate as first-line treatment in patients with advanced follicular lymphoma: A multicenter study by the Groupe d'Etude des Lymphomes de l'Adulte. J Clin Oncol 1996;14:514–519.
74. Intron A package insert. Schering 1997.
75. Arranz R, Garcia-Alfonso P, Sobrino P, et al. Role of interferon alfa-2b in the induction and maintenance treatment of low-grade non-Hodgkin's lymphoma: Results from a prospective, multicenter trial with double randomization. J Clin Oncol 1998;16:1538–1546.
76. Cole B, Solal-Celigny P, LePage E. Interferon alpha for the treatment of advanced follicular lymphoma: An analysis of quality-of-life-adjusted survival. Blood 1995;86:440a.
77. McKelvey EM, Gottleib JA, Wilson HE, et al. Hydroxyldaunomycin (Adriamycin) combination chemotherapy in malignant lymphoma. Cancer 1976;38:1484–1493.
78. Lepage E, Gisselbrecht C, Haioun C, et al. Prognostic significance of received relative dose intensity in non-Hodgkin's lymphoma patients: Application to LNH-87 protocol. The GELA (Groupe d'Etude des Lymphoomes de l'Adulte). Ann Oncol 1993;4:651–656.
79. Coltman CA, Dahlberg S, Jones SE, et al. CHOP is curative in 30% of patients with large cell lymphomas: A 12-year Southwest Oncology Group follow-up. In: Skarin AT, ed. Advanced in Cancer Chemotherapy: Update on Treatment for Diffuse Large-cell Lymphoma. New York, Park Row, 1986:71–78.
80. Norton L, Simon R. Tumor size, sensitivity to therapy and design of treatment schedules. Cancer Treat Rep 1977;61:1307–1317.
81. Carrion JR, Delgado JR, Dominguez S, et al. ProMACE-C-MOPP in aggressive non-Hodgkin's lymphoma. Long-term results in 45 patients treated in a single institution. Acta Oncol 1991;30:823–829.
82. Gordon LI, Harrington D, Anderson J, et al. Comparison of a second-generation combination chemotherapeutic regimen (m-BACOD) with a standard regimen (CHOP) for advanced diffuse non-Hodgkin's lymphoma. N Engl J Med 1992;327:1342–1349.
83. Hryniuk W, Bush H. The importance of dose intensity in chemotherapy of metastatic breast cancer. J Clin Oncol 1984;2:1281–1288.
84. Urba WJ, Duffey PL, Longo DL. Treatment of patients with aggressive lymphomas: An overview. J Natl Cancer Inst Monogr 1990; 10:29–37.
85. Salles G, Shipp MA, Coiffier B. Chemotherapy of non-Hodgkin's aggressive lymphomas. Semin Hematol 1994;31:46–49.
86. Fisher RI. Cyclophosphamide, doxorubicin, vincristine, and prednisone versus intensive chemotherapy in non-Hodgkin's lymphoma. Cancer Chemother Pharmacol 1997;40(suppl):S42–S46.
87. Montserrat E, Garcia-Conde J, Vinolas N, et al. CHOP vs. ProMACE-CytaBOM in the treatment of aggressive non-Hodgkin's lymphomas: Long-term results of a multicenter randomized trial (PETHEMA: Spanish Cooperative Group for the Study of Hematological Malignancies Treatment, Spanish Society of Hematology). Eur J Haematol 1996;57:337–383.
88. Tirelli U, Errante D, Van Glabbeke M, et al. CHOP is the standard regimen in patients > or = 70 years of age with intermediate-grade and high-grade non-Hodgkin's lymphoma: Results of a randomized study of the European Organization for Research and Treatment of Cancer Lymphoma Cooperative Study Group. J Clin Oncol 1998;16:27–34.
89. Freter CE. Acquired immunodeficiency syndrome–associated lymphoma. J Natl Cancer Inst Monogr 1990;10:45–54.
90. Pluda JM, Yarchoan R, Jaffe ES, et al. Development of non-Hodgkin's lymphoma in a cohort of patients with severe human immunodeficiency virus (HIV) infection on long-term antiretroviral therapy. Ann Intern Med 1990;113:276–282.
91. Kaplan LD, Abrams DI, Feigal L, et al. AIDS-associated non-Hodgkin's lymphoma in San Francisco. JAMA 1989;261:719–724.
92. Kaplan LD, Straus DJ, Testa MA, et al. Low-dose compared to standard-dose m-BACOD chemotherapy for non-Hodgkin's lymphoma associated with human immunodeficiency virus infection. N Engl J Med 1997;336:1641–1648.
93. Zinzani PL, Bendandi M, Magagnoli M, et al. Fludarabine-mitoxantrone combination-containing regimen in recurrent low-grade non-Hodgkin's lymphoma. Ann Oncol 1997;8:379–383.
94. Rituxan package insert, IDEC Pharmaceuticals and Genentech, Inc., 1997.
95. Maloney DG, Grillo-Lopez AJ, White CA, et al. IDEC-C2B8 (Rituximab) anti-CD20 monoclonal antibody therapy in patients with relapsed low-grade non-Hodgkin's lymphoma. Blood 1997;90: 2188–2195.
96. Buzzoni R, Colleoni M, Bajetta E, et al. Effective salvage chemotherapy in relapsed or refractory non-Hodgkin's lymphoma. Ann Oncol 1993;4:251–253.
97. Rodriguez-Monge EJ, Cabanillas F. Long-term follow-up of platinum-based lymphoma salvage regimens. The M.D. Anderson Cancer Center experience. Hematol Oncol Clin North Am 1997;11:937–947.

121
OVARIAN CANCER

William Zamboni, PharmD, BCPS, FASHP, and Barry R. Goldspiel, PharmD, BCPS, FASHP

Ovarian cancer is the sixth most common noncutaneous malignancy diagnosed in women.[1] Overall, it is the fourth leading cause of cancer-related death and most common death from gynecologic malignancy in this group.[1] In the United States alone, it has been estimated that 25,400 new cases of ovarian cancer will be diagnosed and more than 14,500 females would die from this disease in 1998.[1] Based on SEER data collected from 1986 to 1992, 5-year survival in white females for all stages approximates 47%; however, survival dramatically increases to 93% in patients with localized disease.[1] Unfortunately, most patients have disseminated disease at diagnosis because symptoms usually do not appear until late in the disease course.[1] Overall survival is slightly higher for whites (47%) than for African-Americans (42%) as is survival for patients with localized disease (whites: 93% vs blacks: 88%).[1] Surgery is an integral part of ovarian cancer management. Chemotherapy, mostly with taxane plus platinum combinations, plays an important role for adjuvant therapy of localized and advanced disease.

EPIDEMIOLOGY AND RISK FACTORS

Ovarian cancer usually occurs in postmenopausal Caucasian women during the sixth decade.[2–4] The most important risk factor appears to be genetics. The risk for developing ovarian cancer markedly increases in women with a family history involving two or more first-degree relatives.[4–6] The risk for ovarian cancer is decreased in women who have had several pregnancies, especially in women who first became pregnant before age 25, and is increased in nulliparous women or women who first became pregnant after age 35, suggesting that uninterrupted ovulation may be a contributing factor.[3,4] Women of North American or North European descent are at a higher risk for ovarian cancer development compared to other nationalities. Prolonged oral contraceptive use or breast-feeding lowers the risk for developing ovarian cancer.[3,7] A higher risk has been associated with environmental exposure to asbestos or talc.[3,5]

Several hereditary ovarian cancer syndromes have been described, which include the development of breast and ovarian cancers or ovarian, endometrial, and nonpolyposis colon cancers.[2,4,8] These syndromes tend to occur at an earlier age than the usual development for each of the individual malignancies and account for about 5% of the total ovarian cancer incidence.[4,8]

A number of genetic abnormalities have been detected in patients with ovarian cancer.[9,10] These include alterations in the *BRCA1, BRCA2, p21, HER2/neu, p53,* and Rb gene function and loss of heterozygosity at chromosomes 6, 11, and 17. Although it is still too early for this information to be clinically useful, understanding the molecular basis for ovarian cancer development might help to discover methods for early detection and chemoprevention.

PATHOLOGY

Most ovarian tumors (85% to 90%) are derived from the epithelial surface of the ovary.[2,3] The histologic types (percent incidence) of epithelial ovarian cancer are serous cystadenocarcinoma (≈ 40%), endometrioid (≈ 15%), mucinous cystadenocarcinoma (≈ 12%), clear cell (≈ 6%), and undifferentiated carcinoma (≈ 17%).[3,11] Epithelial ovarian cancers can be classified as benign, malignant, or borderline (low malignant potential). The remaining ovarian tumors are derived from germ, sex chord, and stromal cell origin.[11]

CLINICAL PRESENTATION

The majority of women with ovarian cancer have no symptoms until the malignancy has spread outside the pelvis.[3,11] Patients with early ovarian cancer can present with nonspecific, vague abdominal symptoms such as nausea, discomfort, dyspepsia, flatulence, bloating, fullness, early satiety, and digestive disturbances.[3,11] These symptoms can easily be confused with symptoms that happen normally throughout the menstrual cycle. Late symptoms can include pain, abdominal distention, ascites, and abdominal or pelvic masses.[3,11] A palpable ovary in a postmenopausal woman should be promptly evaluated, because functional cysts do not usually occur in this age group.[11]

DIAGNOSIS

The diagnostic workup for suspected ovarian cancer includes a careful physical examination including a thorough breast examination, a Pap smear, and a rectovaginal examination.[5,11,12] A careful family history should be taken, especially noting the rate and pattern of relatives with malignancies.

A complete blood count, chemistry profile including liver and renal function tests, and a CA-125 assay should be performed.[3,5] CA-125 is an antigen common to most nonmucinous epithelial ovarian cancers and is detected in the laboratory by using OC-125, a monoclonal antibody directed at this antigen.[13,14] CA-125 is a useful tumor marker in that it is found in more than 80% of ovarian tumors and rising (or falling) titers correlate with disease extent.[13,14] Normal CA-125 values are less than 35 U/mL.[13,14]

Refractory disease is often associated with a CA-125 level that does not return to normal[14] or that remains elevated after completion of chemotherapy.[13,14] A new elevation in the CA-125 level may be the first sign of relapse.[14]

Other diagnostic tests should include a chest x-ray, an intravenous pyelogram, cystoscopy, proctoscopy, and a barium enema. Depending on clinical evaluation, computed tomography (CT), magnetic resonance imaging (MRI), or ultrasound may be indicated. An upper GI series is indicated in patients with gastrointestinal symptoms or with bowel obstruction.

The approach to diagnosing an adnexal mass discovered on pelvic examination depends on several factors including the patient's reproductive age, adnexal mass size, menopausal status, and symptoms.[15] Exploratory laparotomy is indicated in premenarchal women, women with masses greater than 8 cm, women with masses that increase or persist through several menstrual cycles or that are fixed to peritoneal surfaces, women with bilateral masses, or women with intra-abdominal pain or ascites.[15]

SCREENING

Ovarian cancer would be an ideal malignancy for early screening efforts because greater than 65% of cases are currently diagnosed with advanced disease.[16–18] However, for screening efforts to be successful, suitable sensitive, specific, cost-effective screening tests with an adequate positive predictive value must be available. Also, there must be a detectable preclinical phase, and the disease must be amenable to therapy.[16–18] Three screening tests have been used to detect ovarian cancer: bimanual rectovaginal pelvic examination; CA-125 determination; and transvaginal ultrasonography (TVS).[5,18] Bimanual rectovaginal pelvic examination is inadequate for screening purposes because it lacks useful sensitivity and specificity.[16–18] CA-125 is elevated in only 50% of stage I cases and a significant number of women with benign ovarian disease have abnormal CA-125 values.[16–18] TVS is not specific enough to use as the sole screening modality.

The following screening guidelines were developed at a National Institutes of Health (NIH) consensus conference[19]:

- All women should have a comprehensive family history taken focusing on all the known ovarian cancer risk factors. Rectovaginal pelvic exam should be performed as part of ordinary medical care.
- For women without a family history of ovarian cancer or with a family history of ovarian cancer in one relative, routine screening with ultrasound or CA-125 is not recommended because current evidence does not support any benefit. Participation in ovarian cancer screening trials would be appropriate.
- In women with a family history of ovarian cancer in two or more relatives, the risk for developing ovarian cancer is 7%. No conclusive data support the thinking that screening in these patients will produce additional benefit. However, since this situation carries a 3% risk of having a hereditary ovarian cancer syndrome, these women should be counseled by a gynecologic oncologist or other qualified specialist regarding their individual risk.
- Women from families with hereditary ovarian cancer syndromes have a 40% lifetime risk of developing ovarian cancer. While no data indicate that screening will reduce mortality, annual rectovaginal pelvic examination, CA-125 determinations, and TVS are recommended in these women until age 35 or when childbearing is complete. Prophylactic bilateral oophorectomy should then be considered to reduce the overall risk.

With regard to possible ovarian cancer development, current recommendations for follow-up care for individuals with BRCA1 and/or possibly BRCA2 mutations include genetic counseling and annual or semiannual transvaginal ultrasound with color flow Doppler and serum CA-125 beginning at age 25 to 35.[20] There is not enough information yet to recommend for or against prophylactic oophorectomy or prophylactic use of oral contraceptives in BRCA1 carriers. Participation in ongoing ovarian cancer screening trials should be encouraged.

STAGING

The stage of ovarian cancer depends on the extent of disease found at surgical exploration (Table 121–1). Epithelial ovarian cancer spreads by peritoneal surface shedding and lymphatic dissemination (Fig. 121–1).[5,11] At diagnosis, 22% of ovarian cancers are localized, 10% present with regional metastases, and 60% present with distant metastases.[1] A careful and accurate surgical staging

TABLE 121–1. FIGO[a] Staging for Epithelial Ovarian Cancer

I: Confined to the ovaries
- IA: One ovary, no ascites, intact capsule
- IB: Both ovaries, no ascites, intact capsule
- IC: Ruptured capsule, capsular involvement, positive peritoneal washings, or malignant ascites

II: Ovarian tumor with pelvic extension
- IIA: Extension to uterus or tubes
- IIB: Extension to other pelvic organs (bladder, rectum, or vagina)
- IIC: Pelvic extension, plus findings for IC

III: Tumor outside the pelvis or with positive nodes
- IIIA: Microscopic seeding outside true pelvis
- IIIB: Gross deposits ≤ 2 cm
- IIIC: Gross deposits > 2 cm or positive nodes

IV: Distant organ involvement, including liver parenchyma or pleural space

[a]International Federation of Gynecologic Oncologists.

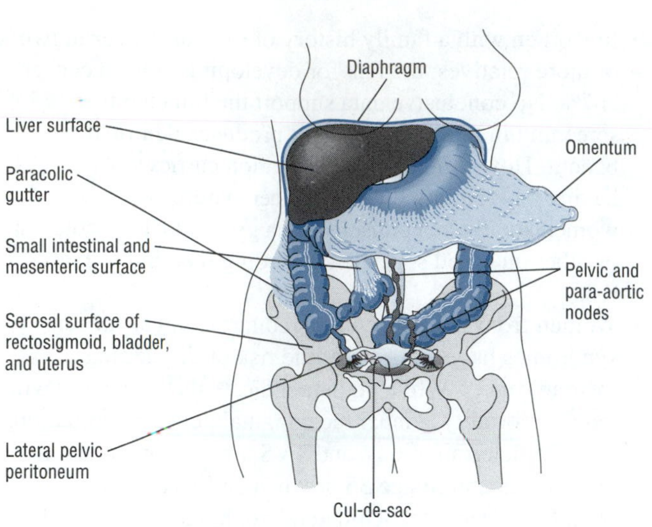

FIGURE 121–1. Staging laparotomy for ovarian cancer.

laparotomy is necessary to properly stage the patient; it is therefore recommended that a gynecologic–oncologic surgeon[21] do this procedure to prevent understaging.[22] Total abdominal hysterectomy, bilateral salpingo-oophorectomy, and partial omentectomy are performed.[5,11,12] A careful examination of all serosal surfaces is done and biopsies of any grossly involved areas are taken. Ovarian capsule rupture, if present, is noted. Ascites is collected and peritoneal washings are done. Integral to the initial surgical staging procedure, the surgeon attempts to debulk as much gross tumor as possible because the amount of residual disease in patients with stage III ovarian cancer correlates with survival.[5]

PROGNOSIS

The prognosis for patients with epithelial ovarian cancer is related to disease stage, pathologic grade, and cell histology. Patients with well-differentiated stage IA or IB tumors have a 5-year survival of greater than 90% with no additional benefit derived from adjuvant therapy.[3,5,12,19,23] With adjuvant therapy, patients with any poorly differentiated stage I, stage IC, or stage II disease have an 80% 5-year survival rate.[3,5,12,24] Survival in patients with stage III disease is poorer than in earlier stages and is directly related to the size of residual tumors present after debulking surgery. Patients with implants under 0.5 cm have a median survival of 40 months, those with implants 0.5 to 2 cm have a median survival of 18 months, and those with residual tumor greater than 2 cm have a median survival of 6 to 12 months.[3,25–27] The 5-year survival rate for stage IV patients is only 5% to 10%.[3] Patients with borderline ovarian cancer have an excellent prognosis, with a 5-year survival rate of 93% and a 10-year survival rate of 91%.[3]

▶ TREATMENT: Ovarian Cancer

Ovarian cancer management is based on the histologic type, pathologic grade, and the stage of disease at initial presentation (Fig. 121–2). In general, the treatment of patients with ovarian cancer initially involves surgical debulking at the time of staging laparotomy followed by adjuvant chemotherapy.[28] However, the effect of debulking on outcome in stage IV disease patients is unclear.[29] Second-line therapy is recommended if residual disease is found after adjuvant chemotherapy. Although response rates are high, many patients with ovarian cancer still die from their disease, so it is appropriate to enter patients with any disease stage into clinical research studies.

TREATMENT BY STAGE

LOCAL/LIMITED DISEASE (STAGES I AND II)

About one-third of ovarian cancer patients present with localized disease (stage I or II) at initial diagnosis.[5,19] In patients with apparent early-stage disease, comprehensive surgical staging is of upmost importance because approximately one-third of patients will have metastatic disease that is not apparent on gross total resection.[5,30] During laparotomy, the patient should undergo comprehensive staging, total abdominal hysterectomy, and bilateral salpingo-oophorectomy.[28] Women with stage IA, grade I ovarian tumors who wish to preserve ovarian and reproduction function can undergo a unilateral salpingo-oophorectomy without significant risk of decreased survival.[5,28,31] The beneficial effects of adjuvant chemotherapy in localized disease depend on the stage and the disease subtype. Postoperative adjuvant chemotherapy is not required in grade 1, stage IA or IB ovarian cancer, whereas patients with grade 2 or 3, stage IA or IB, and stage IC ovarian cancer benefit from adjuvant chemotherapy.[5,11,19,28] All patients with stage II disease should receive adjuvant treatment.[11,19,23,28] For localized ovarian cancer (stage I or II), the recommended adjuvant regimen is paclitaxel plus cisplatin or carboplatin given for 3 to 6 cycles.[28]

ADVANCED DISEASE (STAGES III AND IV)

The majority of women with ovarian cancer present with stage III or IV disease.[3,5] The approach to the treatment of advanced ovarian cancer is initial surgical debulking followed by adjuvant/consolidative paclitaxel plus cisplatin or carboplatin for six cycles[28] (Fig. 121–2). Overall survival is a function of the initial disease stage (stage III vs IV) and the amount of residual disease left after surgical debulking.

PRIMARY CYTOREDUCTIVE SURGERY

The surgical removal of ovarian tumors should be as complete as possible to increase the likelihood of response to chemotherapy. The amount of residual disease after debulking is also a strong prognostic factor. Stage III disease patients with optimal debulking (< 1 to 2 cm of residual tumor) have a 4-year survival rate of approximately 30%.[2,3,5] Patients with stage III or IV disease who have undergone suboptimal debulking (> 2 cm of residual tumor) have less than a 10% chance of long-term survival.[5,25,27]

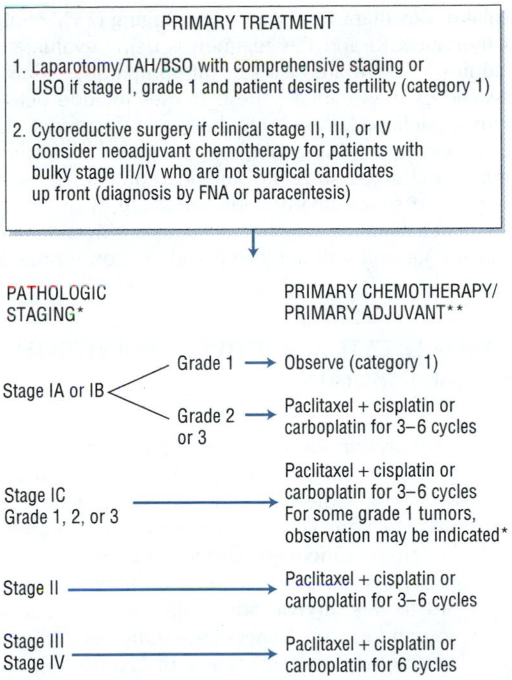

FIGURE 121–2. Initial management of epithelial ovarian cancer. TAH = total abdominal hysterectomy; BSO = bilateral salpingo-oophorectomy; USO = unilateral salpingo-oophorectomy. *Clear-cell pathology is considered high grade regardless of the stage. **Acceptable regimens include (1) cisplatin, 75 mg/m^2, + paclitaxel, 135 mg/m^2, over 24 h *or* carboplatin, AUC 7.5, + paclitaxel, 175 mg/m^2, over 3 h for six cycles for stage III or stage IV disease and for three to six cycles for lower-stage disease; (2) whole-abdominopelvic RT for low-bulk disease (category 3). *(From Ref. 28, with permission. See Figure 121–3 for National Comprehensive Cancer Network guidelines.)*

PRIMARY/ADJUVANT CHEMOTHERAPY

Systemic chemotherapy following optimal surgical debulking is the cornerstone of first-line treatment of advanced epithelial ovarian cancer. A summary of chemotherapeutic regimens used as the initial treatment of newly diagnosed ovarian cancer can be found in Table 121–2. For many years, the "standard" chemotherapy for newly diagnosed patients was a platinum analog (cisplatin or carboplatin) plus a DNA alkylating agent (cyclophosphamide)–containing regimen.[27,32] However, regimens containing paclitaxel in combination with a platinum analog are now recommended for first-line therapy.[15,28]

Cisplatin and carboplatin have been used as single-agent and in combination therapy in previously untreated stage III and IV ovarian cancer.[33] Combination chemotherapy regimens containing cisplatin achieved higher response rates and overall survival than regimens without cisplatin.[3,12,34] In addition, a meta-analysis comparing treatment with platinum analogs either as single agents or in combination regimens reported a greater overall response and longer survival in the combination treatment group.[34] However, there is still controversy whether doxorubicin addition to platinum-containing regimens confers a survival advantage over the same regimen given without doxorubicin.[35] Also, a meta-analysis of 11 clinical studies comparing cisplatin and carboplatin as single agents or in combination regimens reported no significant survival advantage for either platinum analog.[34] The substitution of carboplatin for cisplatin in combination with cyclophosphamide has shown equal efficacy and may have more acceptable toxicity.[34,36,37]

Cisplatin has also been studied in combination with carboplatin. In a phase II study, patients with advanced ovarian cancer received low doses (50 mg/m^2) of cisplatin plus moderate doses (300 mg/m^2) of carboplatin.[38] The overall response rate was 71%, with 57% achieving a complete response (CR). This platinum analog combination may be a practical alternative to high-dose cisplatin in the initial treatment of advanced ovarian cancer.

Dose intensity, or the amount of drug delivered over a specified time interval (expressed as mg/m^2/wk) may be an important factor in determining treatment outcomes with platinum-based regimens in patients with ovarian cancer.[39] However, a retrospective review of 45 randomized trials found no correlation between cisplatin dose and treatment outcome.[34] In addition, a prospective randomized trial in patients with suboptimally debulked stage III (> 1-cm residual masses) and any stage IV disease randomized patients to receive cyclophosphamide 500 mg/m^2 IV plus either

TABLE 121–2. Initial Chemotherapeutic Regimens for Epithelial Ovarian Cancer

Drugs	Dose(s)	Cycle Frequency	Ref.
Cisplatin	100 mg/m^2 IV day 1	q28d	37
Carboplatin	400–800 mg/m^2 IV day 1	q28–35d	33
Cisplatin Cyclophosphamide	50–100 mg/m^2 IV day 1 500–1000 mg/m^2 IV day 1	q21–28d	26,27,32
Carboplatin Cyclophosphamide	200–300 mg/m^2 IV day 1 500–1000 mg/m^2 IV day 1	q28d	36,37
Cisplatin Carboplatin	50 mg/m^2 IV day 1 300 mg/m^2 IV day 1	q28d	38
Cisplatin Doxorubicin Cyclophosphamide	50–60 mg/m^2 IV day 1 40–50 mg/m^2 IV day 1 500–750 mg/m^2 IV day 1	q28d	27,32
Paclitaxel Cisplatin	135 mg/m^2 IV (24-h infusion) day 1 75 mg/m^2 IV day 1	q21d	48
Paclitaxel Carboplatin	175 mg/m^2 IV (3-h infusion) day 1 Dosed to AUC 7.5 on day 1	q21d	28,49
Cyclophosphamide Paclitaxel Cisplatin Filgrastim	750 mg/m^2 IV day 1 250 mg/m^2 IV (24-h infusion) day 1 75 mg/m^2 IV day 2 10 µg/kg SC start day 3	q21d	51

cisplatin 50 mg/m^2 IV (n = 235) or 100 mg/m^2 IV (n = 223) every 3 weeks.[40] Patients in the cisplatin 50-mg/m^2 group received eight cycles and patients in the cisplatin 100-mg/m^2 group received four cycles (same total cisplatin dose). Clinical and pathologic response rates, response duration, and survival were similar in both groups. Hematologic and gastrointestinal effects, febrile episodes, septic events, and renal toxicities were significantly more common and severe in the patients receiving the higher cisplatin dose. Similarly, Kaye et al.[41] reported no survival difference in patients receiving six cycles of cylophosphamide plus cisplatin either 100 mg/m^2 IV or 50 mg/m^2 IV. Neurotoxicity persisted in more patients in the high-dose arm (10 of 31) compared to the low-dose arm (1 of 24). Likewise, dose-intensity analyses with carboplatin have demonstrated equivocal results.[42,43] Accumulating evidence seems to indicate that the dose–response curve for the platinum compounds levels off within the clinically useful dosage range.[42] In addition, it is not clear that providing higher cumulative platinum doses confers any survival advantage over the standard cisplatin 75-mg/m^2 IV dose.[42]

The combination of cyclophosphamide and cisplatin or carboplatin was once the first-line adjuvant therapy of choice in women with advanced-stage ovarian cancer.[26,27,32] However, paclitaxel alone and in combination has shown significant activity in ovarian cancer.[44–47] McGuire et al.[48] reported that the combination of paclitaxel (135 mg/m^2 over 24 hours) and cisplatin (75 mg/m^2) achieved better response rates and survival outcomes compared to cyclophosphamide (750 mg/m^2) and cisplatin (75 mg/m^2) in patients with newly diagnosed suboptimally debulked stages III and IV ovarian cancer. The objective response in the paclitaxel–cisplatin group was 73%, with 51% complete responses; in the cyclophosphamide–cisplatin group, the objective response was 60%, with 31% complete responses (P= .01). The median progression-free survival was 18 months and 13 months, and the median survival was 38 months and 24 months for the paclitaxel–cisplatin and cyclophosphamide–cisplatin treated groups, respectively (P < .001 for both comparisons). Neutropenia, alopecia, and peripheral neuropathy were more severe in the paclitaxel–cisplatin group. Similar trials have reported favorable results with paclitaxel plus carboplatin combinations.[11] Based on this information, the National Comprehensive Cancer Network (NCCN) Ovarian Cancer Practice Guidelines (Fig. 121–2) recommend the combination of paclitaxel and cisplatin as McGuire et al. administered, or paclitaxel 175 mg/m^2 as a 3-hour infusion in combination with carboplatin dosed at an area under the plasma concentration–time curve (AUC) of 7.5 mg/mL/min as first-line adjuvant treatment.[28,49]

The duration of consolidative chemotherapy has been evaluated in several studies. In a study by Hainsworth et al.,[27] the administration of a cisplatin-containing regimen repeated at 4-week intervals for 6 months produced results comparable to prolonged treatment. In advanced ovarian cancer, the administration of 5 cycles of cyclophosphamide, cisplatin, and doxorubicin was equally effective and less toxic as compared to 10 cycles of chemotherapy.[50] Six to 9 cycles of chemotherapy have become the standard approach and result in clinical response rates of approximately 60% to 70% and 5-year survival rates of 10% to 20%. In addition, because approximately 50% of patients with a confirmed pathologic response will ultimately relapse,[2,3,11] chemotherapy may be extended for 2 or 3 cycles beyond best response.[5,16] The NCCN guidelines recommend 3 to 6 cycles of treatment for lower stage tumors, and at least 6 cycles of treatment for patients with stage III or IV disease.[28]

Many questions still need to be answered about initial therapy for advanced stages of ovarian cancer. Ongoing clinical trials are addressing whether some of the paclitaxel-containing regimens are better than current regimens for early-stage disease. Results with a three-drug regimen, cyclophosphamide, paclitaxel, and cisplatin plus filgrastim, seem encouraging (75% clinical CR, 36% pathologic CR) and this regimen is being evaluated in ongoing studies.[51] There are also several comparative trials for advanced-stage ovarian cancer. These studies include determining the optimal paclitaxel dose, schedule, and treatment duration; comparing paclitaxel plus cisplatin to paclitaxel plus carboplatin in optimally debulked stage III patients; comparing these same combinations in suboptimally debulked stage III or stage IV patients; and determining whether dose intensification aided by growth factor support will achieve higher response rates and improve survival.

SECONDARY CYTOREDUCTIVE SURGERY/INTERVAL SURGICAL DEBULKING

Operative reexploration (or secondary laparotomy) was once an integral part of the management of advanced ovarian carcinoma.[52] However, the role of secondary cytoreduction (or interval debulking) after consolidative chemotherapy is currently unclear. A Gynecologic Oncology Group symposium debated the role of secondary cytoreduction.[53] Several conflicting studies exist with regard to the survival advantages of secondary cytoreduction. A nonrandomized Gynecologic Oncology Group study evaluated 112 International Federation of Gynecology and Obstetrics (FIGO) stage I or II ovarian cancer patients who underwent initial surgical staging and then underwent a restaging operation following adjuvant therapy.[54] In this study, only 5% of the patients who were asymptomatic prior to surgery had disease confirmed by second-look laparotomy, as compared to half of the patients who were symptomatic prior to second-look laparotomy. These data suggest that second-look laparotomy may not be warranted in asymptomatic patients with early-stage disease. To support this conclusion, the National Cancer Institute (NCI) consensus conference recommends that second-look operations should be performed only when the results will change management or as part of a clinical trial.[19]

Recent information suggests that interval surgical debulking may improve outcomes. In a randomized trial, van der Burg et al.[55] performed interval debulking surgery on 140 stage IIb to IV, suboptimally debulked (> 1 cm of residual disease) ovarian cancer patients after receiving three cycles of cisplatin plus cyclophosphamide. Patients then received an additional three cycles of these same drugs after surgery. Patients randomized to the nonsurgical treatment arm received six cycles of chemotherapy. Interval debulking surgery significantly prolonged overall and progression-free survival and reduced the death risk by 33%. The additional surgery was not associated with excessive morbidity.

The overall effect of interval debulking is influenced by several factors, including initial response to chemotherapy, the amount of residual disease before and after second-look surgery, and the presence of microscopic residual disease. Ongoing trials will help define which patients should benefit most from interval debulking surgery.

RECURRENT/REFRACTORY DISEASE

Approximately 20% to 50% of patients without evidence of residual disease on second-look laparotomy will relapse.[2,3,5] Patients who were sensitive to the initial chemotherapy and whose response lasted longest have the greatest likelihood of achieving a response to retreatment with the same first-line regimen or to second-line treatment.[56] In addition, patients with recurrent or refractory disease after initial chemotherapy historically have had a poor overall prognosis. Improved outcomes have been achieved in recurrent and refractory ovarian cancer with the use of high-

TABLE 121–3. Chemotherapeutic Regimens for Relapsed or Refractory Epithelial Ovarian Cancer

Drugs	Dose(s)	Cycle Frequency	Ref.
Altretamine	260 mg/m^2 PO (total daily dose divided in four doses) × 14–21 d	q28d	76,77
Paclitaxel	135–250[a] mg/m^2 IV[b] day 1	q21d	47,62,63,116,117
Carboplatin	400–800 mg/m^2 IV day 1	q28–35d	33
Paclitaxel	135 mg/m^2 IV[a] day 1		48
Cisplatin	75 mg/m^2 IV day 1	q21d	
Paclitaxel	250[a] mg/m^2 IV[c] day 1		
Cyclophosphamide	1000 mg/m^2 IV day 2	q21d	118
Topotecan	1.5 mg/m^2 IV qd × 5 d	q21d	66
Tamoxifen	20 mg PO bid	Continuous	57
Etoposide	50 mg/m^2 PO qd × 21 d	q28d	78

[a]Filgrastim used with 250 mg/m^2 dose.
[b]3- or 24-h infusion.
[c]24-h infusion.

dose chemotherapeutic agents such as cisplatin, carboplatin, and paclitaxel and the use of combination regimens containing these agents. In addition, the camptothecin analog, topotecan, has shown antitumor activity in patients with relapsed-refractory ovarian cancer.[56] A summary of chemotherapeutic regimens used in the treatment of recurrent or refractory ovarian cancer can be found in Table 121–3.

The NCCN guidelines for salvage therapy for recurrent or refractory disease include several treatment options (Fig. 121–3).[28] Patients with prior low-stage, low-grade disease who had never received chemotherapy should be treated as if they are newly diagnosed advanced-stage patients, undergoing surgical debulking and adjuvant chemotherapy with the combination of paclitaxel and cisplatin or carboplatin. The NCCN guidelines suggest that tamoxifen would be an appropriate therapy in patients with stage I or II ovarian cancer with a rising CA-125 as their only manifestation of disease progression.[28,57]

For patients who have previously received chemotherapy, the recommended treatment depends on the time frame in which patients relapsed. Patients who progressed during primary therapy or within 6 months after receiving initial therapy would be appropriate for clinical trial referral or supportive care therapy, or can be treated with second-line salvage chemotherapy.[28] Patients who relapse more than 6 months after stopping chemotherapy should receive paclitaxel alone, a platinum alone, or paclitaxel in combination with a platinum analog. Patients with small-volume refractory disease may receive chemotherapy or whole abdominopelvic radiotherapy. Patients who had a long disease-free interval with a locally recurrent tumor might benefit from a second cytoreductive surgery.

A useful guideline when treating a patient with refractory or relapsed disease is to administer a salvage regimen for two courses and then evaluate for response.[56] If no response is observed, then an alternative salvage regimen may be selected. In the case of topotecan, evidence may suggest continuation of treatment for four cycles and then evaluate for response.

The choice of retreatment with platinum-containing chemotherapy depends on the time frame in which the disease recurs.[3,5]

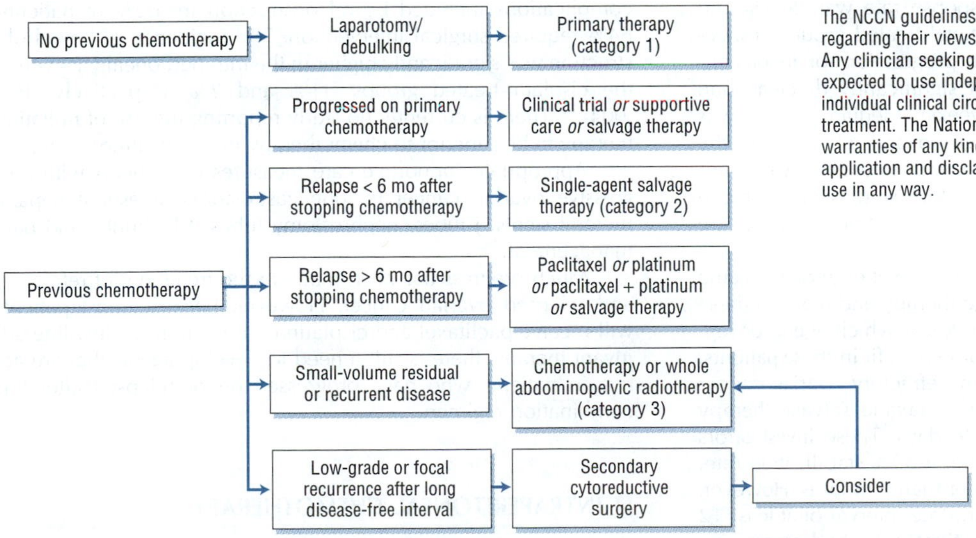

The NCCN guidelines are a statement of consensus of its authors regarding their views of currently accepted approaches to treatment. Any clinician seeking to apply or consult any NCCN guideline is expected to use independent medical judgment in the context of individual clinical circumstances to determine any patient's care or treatment. The National Comprehensive Cancer Network makes no warranties of any kind whatsoever regarding their content, use or application and disclaims any responsibility for their application or use in any way.

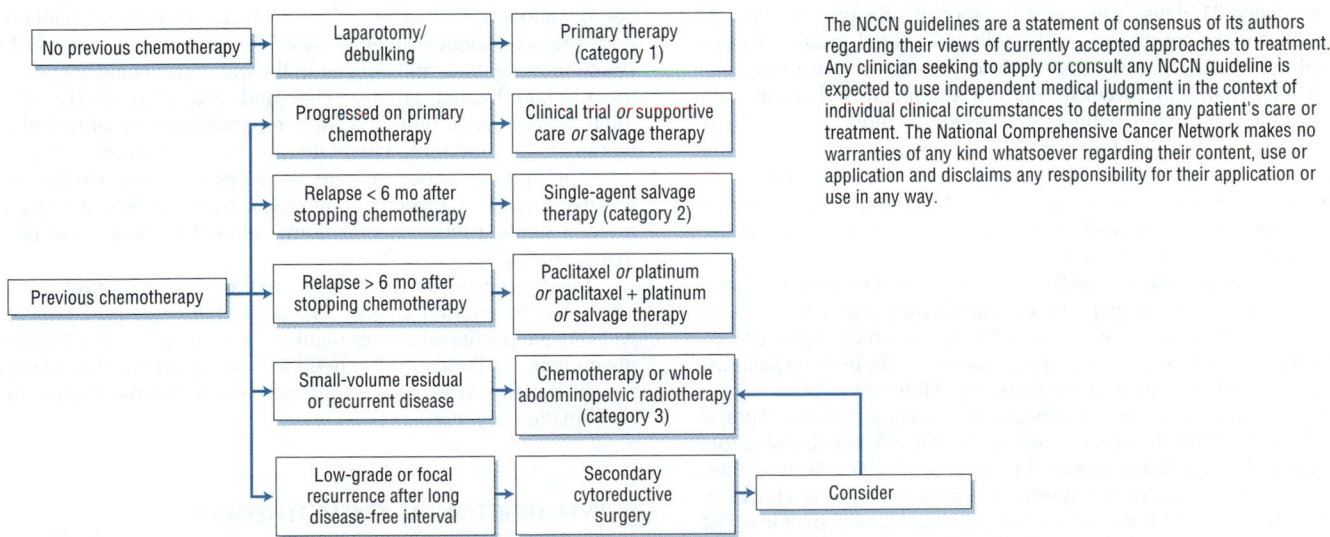

FIGURE 121–3. Management of recurrent/relapsed/progressive epithelial ovarian cancer. The following categories are used in the NCCN guidelines: Category 1 = recommendations that are uncontested and generally accepted by all authorities in the field; Category 2 = recommendations that are somewhat controversial; Category 3 = recommendations that caused real disagreements among members of the NCCN panel. *(From Ref. 28, with permission. Copyrighted by the National Comprehensive Cancer Network. All rights reserved. These guidelines and illustrations may not be reproduced in any form without the express written permission of the NCCN.)*

Patients with disease that is refractory to the initial platinum-containing chemotherapy or that recurs within 6 months after treatment (often termed "platinum-refractory") are unlikely to benefit from additional standard-dose platinum. However, patients in whom the disease recurs more than 6 months after the initial treatment (termed "platinum-sensitive") have a response rate of 27% to 59% with a second-line platinum regimen.[58] Some investigators feel that these same principles can be applied to patients initially treated with paclitaxel-containing regimens as well.

Cisplatin has shown a steep dose–response curve in ovarian carcinoma, where increasing the dose of cisplatin may achieve greater antitumor response.[39,59] The major cisplatin toxicities when administered at doses of 50 to 100 mg/m^2 per cycle are nausea, vomiting, electrolyte disturbances including prolonged magnesium wasting, and nephrotoxicity. Increasing the dose of cisplatin to 200 mg/m^2 per cycle results in myelosuppression and significant, long-lasting neurotoxicity.[59] Amifostine, a thiol chemoprotective agent, can reduce the cumulative hematologic, renal, and neural toxicities associated with cylophosphamide plus cisplatin in ovarian cancer patients.[60] However, the most cost-effective use of amifostine has not yet been determined.

Paclitaxel has shown significant activity in platinum-resistant–refractory ovarian cancer.[45,47,61–64] Dose-intense paclitaxel regimens (250 mg/m^2 over 24 hours every 21 days plus filgrastim support) appear to produce higher objective response rates compared to conventional-dose regimens.[62,65]

Topotecan is an analog of the plant alkaloid 20(S)-camptothecin and has been approved by the Food and Drug Administration for the treatment of metastatic ovarian cancer.[66–69] Topotecan is non–cross-resistant with platinum-based chemotherapy. Preclinical studies suggest that low-dose protracted schedules of administration achieve the greatest antitumor response.[70] Topotecan has demonstrated efficacy in phase II trials as second-line and salvage therapy in patients who have relapsed after or progressed during platinum-based therapy.[66–69] A randomized phase III trial compared topotecan and paclitaxel in patients with advanced ovarian cancer who had failed one platinum-based regimen.[66] Patients were randomized to receive topotecan 1.5 mg/m^2/d as a 30-minute infusion for 5 days repeated every 21 days or paclitaxel 175 mg/m^2 as a 3-hour infusion every 21 days. The overall response rate was 20.5% and 13.2% for the topotecan- and paclitaxel-treated groups, respectively (P = .12). The median time to progression for topotecan-treated patients (32 weeks) was not significantly different than for paclitaxel-treated patients (20 weeks). Median survival was 61 weeks in the topotecan-treated group and 43 weeks in the paclitaxel-treated group. Topotecan is well tolerated, with minimal nonhematologic toxicities.[66–69] Future studies of topotecan in combination with paclitaxel and/or the platinum analogs are needed in this clinical setting.

Since many patients will receive paclitaxel or another taxane derivative as initial therapy or salvage therapy and many of these patients will relapse, it is important to know which agents or regimens can then be used to provide some benefit in these patients. Kavanagh et al.[71] treated 33 platinum-refractory ovarian cancer patients who also had progressed after taxane salvage therapy with carboplatin 300 mg/m^2 every 28 days. These investigators noted a 21% partial response (PR) rate, a 39% stabilization rate, and a median response duration greater than 7 months. However, all responding patients had a platinum-free interval of at least 12 months. Muggia et al.[72] treated 35 patients who had progressive disease after at least one platinum-based regimen or paclitaxel-based regimen with liposomal doxorubicin and noted a 25.7% response rate (CR + PR).

A phase II study evaluated topotecan 1.5 mg/m^2/d as a 30-minute infusion for 5 days repeated every 21 days in patients with progressive or recurrent disease after treatment with paclitaxel in combination with cisplatin or carboplatin.[73] In this group of patients, 81% relapsed within 6 months and 48% of patients had tumors larger than 5 cm after treatment with paclitaxel and cisplatin. An interim analysis showed a 13% and 14% response rate among first-line and second-line failures, respectively. As data mature, more information will be revealed on the stability of topotecan response in this setting.

Other agents that have shown an overall 15% to 25% response rate include etoposide, ifosfamide, 5-fluorouracil, tamoxifen, vinorelbine, gemcitabine, docetaxel, and altretamine.[5,57,74] Altretamine (hexamethylmelamine) is a chemotherapeutic agent that undergoes metabolic activation to form alkylating intermediates.[75] Altretamine has shown activity in resistant–refractory advanced ovarian cancer.[76,77] In this setting, altretamine has achieved objective response rates of up to 33% and disease stabilization in 8% to 78% of patients. Altretamine is approved as single-agent therapy at doses of 260 mg/m^2/d administered in four divided doses for 14 to 21 days given every 28 days. When administered in combination with other bone marrow suppressive agents, the dose is reduced to 150 mg/m^2/d for 14 days repeated every 28 days. Oral etoposide, an attractive option owing to the ease of administration, has a response rate of 25%, 35%, and 32% in patients with platinum-resistant, platinum-sensitive, or paclitaxel-resistant ovarian cancer, respectively.[78] Liposomal doxorubicin is also currently being evaluated in relapsed ovarian cancer.[56,72] Tamoxifen has also been used in the salvage setting and usually produces responses in patients with positive estrogen receptors.[57,79]

The use of radiation therapy in the treatment of ovarian cancer is controversial. The two forms of radiation therapy used in ovarian cancer are external beam whole abdominal irradiation and intraperitoneal isotopes (such as ^{32}P). Radiation therapy has been used as adjuvant therapy in patients with no residual disease and as consolidation therapy in patients with minimal residual disease.

Abdominal irradiation[80,81] and intraperitoneal isotopes[82,83] have not shown improvements in response and have been associated with greater toxicity. Ovarian cancer patients treated with abdominopelvic radiation were analyzed for posttreatment complications.[81] The incidence of acute complications associated with treatment were vomiting (61%) and diarrhea (68%). Serious late complications included bowel obstruction in 4.2% of patients; 64% required surgical intervention. The incidence of bowel obstruction was significantly higher in the intraperitoneal ^{32}P– versus the cisplatin-treated groups (11% and 2%, respectively; P = .004).[83] There is currently no study reporting the use of radiation therapy to be superior to chemotherapy in any treatment setting.

Appropriate supportive care measures for patients with progressive ovarian cancer include gastrostomy, intestinal bypass, ureteral stents, j-tubes, nephrostomy tubes, VP shunts, and pain management.[28]

Much progress has been made in the treatment of refractory and relapsed ovarian cancer. However, because most patients will receive paclitaxel and cisplatin combinations as first-line adjuvant therapy, there is still a need to develop agents that are active in patients who have progressed on or relapsed after this combination regimen.

INTRAPERITONEAL CHEMOTHERAPY

Significant advances have occurred in understanding the advantages, limitations, and administration methods of IP chemotherapy for ovarian cancer treatment.[84–86] The theoretical advantage of IP administration is increasing the intensity and duration of tumor exposure while decreasing the systemic exposure

TABLE 121–4. Intraperitoneal Chemotherapeutic Regimens for Ovarian Cancer

Drugs	Dose(s)	Cycle Frequency	Ref.
Cisplatin	50–100 mg/m^2 IP[a] day 1	q21–28d	85,88
Cisplatin Cyclophosphamide	100 mg/m^2 IP day 1 600 mg/m^2 IV day 1	q21d	88
Etoposide Cisplatin Sodium Thiosulfate	200–350 mg/m^2 IP day 1 100–200 mg/m^2 IP day 1 12–16 g/m^2 IV day 1	q28d	89,90
Cisplatin Cytarabine	100–150 mg/m^2 IP day 1 600–1200 mg/m^2 IP day 1	q28d	91
Paclitaxel	125 mg/m^2 IP day 1	q28d	94
Mitoxantrone	20–30 mg/m^2 IP day 1	q28d	92

[a]IP = intraperitoneally.

and possible toxicity.[84,85] Studies have shown potential value in IP administration for initial, consolidation, and salvage therapy. Data suggest that patients with small-volume tumors (< 2 cm) are best suited for IP administration as initial therapy or as salvage therapy in relapsed disease.[84,85,87] Drugs that have been given IP include cisplatin, carboplatin, cytarabine, etoposide, doxorubicin, mitoxantrone, paclitaxel, 5-fluorouracil, melphalan, and methotrexate.[85,87] A summary of IP chemotherapeutic regimens can be found in Table 121–4.

A phase III trial in women with previously untreated, stage III ovarian carcinoma with residual tumors of < 2 cm were randomized to receive cyclophosphamide 600 mg/m^2 in combination with IP cisplatin 100 mg/m^2 or IV cisplatin 100 mg/m^2.[88] Median survival was significantly longer in the IP cisplatin–treated group (49 months) compared to the IV cisplatin–treated group (41 months). In addition, moderate-to-severe tinnitus, hearing loss, and neuromuscular toxicities were significantly more frequent in the IV cisplatin–treated group. These data suggest that IP cisplatin is more effective and less toxic than IV cisplatin. However, further studies are needed to confirm the advantage of IP cisplatin compared to IV cisplatin.

The combination of IP cisplatin, IP etoposide, and IV sodium thiosulfate has been evaluated in patients with newly diagnosed stage III and IV ovarian cancer.[89] The complete response rate in evaluable patients was 48% in the IP group and 52% in the IV group. There was no difference in response rates between the groups as a function of size of residual disease (< 1 or > 1 cm). At a median follow-up of 46 months, there was no difference between IP and IV therapy with regard to time to recurrence (12 and 14 months, respectively) or survival (44% and 50%, respectively). Both regimens were well tolerated with similar hematologic and nonhematologic toxicities.

Intraperitoneal therapy has also been evaluated in patients with relapsed and refractory ovarian cancer. Intraperitoneal cisplatin and carboplatin have achieved documented complete responses in relapsed patients initially treated with systemic platinum-containing regimens.[90,91] In addition, mitoxantrone IP and paclitaxel IP have been used as single agents in advanced-stage relapsed disease.[92,93] Mitoxantrone IP is associated with a high incidence of severe abdominal pain, abdominal adhesions, and bowel obstructions that required surgical treatment.[92] Large volumes of 0.9% sodium chloride can reduce the severity and frequency of local mitoxantrone IP–related adverse effects.[92] The dose-limiting toxicity (DLT) of paclitaxel IP is abdominal pain at doses greater than 125 mg/m^2.[94] Peritoneal cavity exposure after IP paclitaxel is approximately 30 times higher than plasma exposure.[93,94]

Several studies have evaluated factors that influence the response to IP therapy.[90,95] A retrospective study evaluated the results of IP cisplatin with etoposide or cytarabine as salvage therapy.[90] Of patients with microscopic disease at the time of IP therapy, 41% achieved a surgically defined complete response, whereas only 29% of patients with macroscopic disease (largest residual tumor mass less than 0.5 cm in diameter) had a surgically defined complete response. Patients whose largest residual tumor mass was greater than 1 cm had less than a 5% complete response rate. This is consistent with data showing a 1- to 2-cm depth of penetration of IP cisplatin into tumor or normal tissue.[96] An objective response rate of less than 10% is anticipated for IP cisplatin in patients who have failed to demonstrate at least a partial response to initial systemic cisplatin.[95] Thus, IP cisplatin should not be used in cisplatin-refractory patients. The primary toxicity associated with IP cisplatin was bone marrow suppression.

Complications from IP therapy may be related to catheter function, infection, or bowel problems.[85,87] Mechanical obstruction to fluid inflow has been reported in approximately 5% of patients.[85,87] Most commonly this results from fibrin sheath formation around the catheter tip.[86] In some cases, peritoneal adhesions obstruct fluid entry into the abdominal cavity, causing uneven distribution of the chemotherapeutic agent. Infectious complications, such as superficial cellulitis around the catheter entry site, deep tissue infections, and peritonitis, are the most prevalent IP-related complications and are reported in approximately 10% of patients.[85–87,93] Bowel-related complications (approximate 3% incidence) include obstruction, ileus, and perforation.[85,86] IP administration may also result in a false CA-125 elevation.[85]

Currently, IP chemotherapy outcomes for ovarian cancer treatment have been very encouraging, but additional well-designed comparative trials are needed to define the role of IP versus systemic chemotherapy. The NCCN guidelines consider intraperitoneal therapy an investigational approach to ovarian cancer management.

AUTOLOGOUS MARROW OR PERIPHERAL BLOOD PROGENITOR CELL TRANSPLANTATION

The use of high-dose myeloablative chemotherapy followed by bone marrow or peripheral blood progenitor cell rescue has been used as salvage therapy in hematologic and solid tumor malignancies. The most common ablative regimens used in ovarian cancer contain platinum analogs (i.e., cisplatin or carboplatin), alkylating agents (i.e., melphalan, thiotepa, or cyclophosphamide), and/or etoposide.[97–101]

Shpall et al.[97] evaluated the use of IP cisplatin and high-dose systemic cyclophosphamide and thiotepa followed by autologous bone marrow support in advanced ovarian cancer. Of patients evaluated, 75% had pathologically documented partial response (i.e., > 75% reduction in tumor mass). Legros et al.[100] treated poor-prognosis ovarian cancer patients with either high-dose melphalan or high-dose carboplatin plus cyclophosphamide followed by autologous stem-cell transplantation after receiving cisplatin induction therapy and second-look operations. They reported an overall 60% 5-year survival rate and a 73% 5-year survival rate in patients with a pathologic complete response at second-look laparotomy. In patients with persistent or recurrent ovarian cancer treated with high-dose chemotherapy plus autologous stem-cell transplantation, tumor bulk and cisplatin sensitivity were the most important prognostic factors.[101]

Based on favorable survival data in 100 patients with small-volume disease reported at an American Cancer Society meeting in March 1997, a high-priority, 275-patient, NCI-sponsored trial has been initiated in patients with stage III ovarian cancer with less than 1 cm of residual disease. This study will compare standard-dose chemotherapy to high-dose chemotherapy plus peripheral blood progenitor cell transplantation. However, until results from this and other ongoing trials are available, the role of bone marrow or peripheral blood progenitor cell transplantation in the initial and subsequent treatment of advanced refractory ovarian cancer is unclear and should be considered an investigational approach.[28]

BORDERLINE OVARIAN CANCER

Borderline (low malignant potential) ovarian cancers account for approximately 15% of all epithelial ovarian cancers; the majority (75%) are stage I at the time of diagnosis.[9,102] These tumors must be recognized, because their prognosis and treatment are clearly different from those of malignant invasive carcinomas. Trimble and Trimble reviewed 953 patients with a mean follow-up of 7 years and found a survival rate of 92% for advanced-stage tumors with the usual cause of death being benign disease complications (e.g., small-bowel obstruction) and therapy-related complications. Malignant transformation was rarely the cause of death. In one series, the 5-, 10-, 15-, and 20-year survival rates of patients with all stages of low-malignant-potential tumors were 97%, 95%, 92%, and 89%, respectively.[102]

In patients with stage I or II disease, no additional chemotherapy or radiation treatment is indicated for a completely resected tumor of low malignant potential.[103,104] In the presence of bilateral ovarian cystic neoplasms or a single ovary involvement, partial oophorectomy or a unilateral salpingo-oophorectomy can be performed if childbearing potential is to be maintained. When childbearing is not a consideration, a total abdominal hysterectomy and bilateral salpingo-oophorectomy is appropriate therapy because most clinicians favor removing the remaining ovarian tissue, which is at risk for recurrence of a borderline tumor or rarely developing invasive carcinoma.

Patients with advanced disease should undergo a total hysterectomy, bilateral salpingo-oophorectomy, omentectomy, node sampling, and aggressive cytoreductive surgery. However, there is little evidence that adjuvant chemotherapy or radiotherapy improves outcome.[102,104] There have been no controlled studies comparing postoperative treatment with no treatment.

NONEPITHELIAL OVARIAN CANCER

OVARIAN STROMAL TUMORS

Ovarian stromal tumors normally have an indolent natural history and rarely occur bilaterally. They are managed by unilateral salpingo-oophorectomy and usually do not require additional treatment.[2,5,11] Stage II stromal tumors require more extensive surgery owing to the lack of effective adjuvant therapy. Because this tumor is relatively rare, the role of chemotherapy is unclear.

OVARIAN GERM-CELL TUMORS

Ovarian-derived germ-cell tumors are rare and may have a mixed histology. Thus, treatment should be directed toward the most malignant component of the tumor. Surgery alone has not been very effective, producing 2-year survival rates of 13% to 16%.[105] Combination chemotherapy has produced high cure rates and improved prognosis in patients with germ-cell tumors.[105]

Endodermal sinus and dysgerminoma are two subtypes of germ-cell tumors. Endodermal sinus tumors are aggressive tumors that usually occur unilaterally. Without chemotherapy, most patients die from their disease; thus patients with all stages of disease should receive combination chemotherapy. The most common combination chemotherapeutic regimens used are vincristine, dactinomycin, and cyclophosphamide and cisplatin and bleomycin in combination with vincristine or etoposide.[105] Dysgerminoma tumors have a high cure rate and are highly sensitive to radiation therapy; however, the sterility associated with abdominal irradiation has resulted in systemic chemotherapy becoming first-line therapy. The treatment of choice for newly diagnosed disease is a platinum-containing regimen.[105–107] The combination of bleomycin, etoposide, and cisplatin (BEP) demonstrated a 97% remission rate at 10 to 54 months in 35 patients with germ-cell tumors.[108] Also, two Gynecologic Oncology Group trials demonstrated that 89 of 93 patients with stages I, II, and III disease with completely resected tumors were disease free after three BEP cycles.[106–108] Patients with recurrent or refractory disease after cisplatin-based chemotherapy can be treated with radiation therapy.[105]

PHARMACOECONOMIC CONSIDERATIONS

The majority of economic analyses in ovarian cancer management have focused on whether paclitaxel combinations are cost-effective initial treatment regimens because the combination of paclitaxel and cisplatin has been shown to increase the median survival of newly diagnosed patients with advanced-stage disease compared to the combination of cisplatin and cyclophosphamide.[48] Incremental costs per life-year gained of $20,355 (Canadian dollars),[109] $19,820 (inpatient) or $21,222 (outpatient),[110] $32,213 (Canadian dollars),[111] and $19,603[112] have been calculated for patients treated with paclitaxel plus cisplatin compared to cyclophosphamide plus cisplatin. In addition, Messori et al.[113] reported a $18,200 cost per quality-adjusted life-year gained. The results of these studies suggest that the additional cost for the combination of paclitaxel and cisplatin compares favorably to costs for other medical interventions that are considered cost effective.

EVALUATION OF TREATMENT OUTCOMES

When applied mainly to clinical trials, CR is defined as complete resolution of all disease and is further categorized either as a pathologic or clinical complete response.[3,5,11] A pathologic CR is defined as no detectable disease on second-look laparotomy. A clinical CR is defined as no detectable disease by radiologic imaging techniques. The recent NIH consensus conference on ovarian cancer concluded that second-look laparotomy should be performed only in clinical trials.[19] Partial response (PR) is defined as a greater than 50% decrease in all measurable disease. Stable disease is defined as disease maintenance without progression. In addition, general definitions for response duration and survival apply to ovarian cancer. Disease-free survival is defined from the point of achieving a complete response to the time of disease recurrence. Recent studies have evaluated percent CA-125 declines as a surrogate marker for response.[114]

Localized ovarian cancer is highly curable by surgery and, if appropriate, chemotherapy. The goals of therapy should be to maintain the patient's quality of life and, if possible and desired, preserve reproductive capabilities. Newly diagnosed advanced ovarian cancer is highly responsive to surgical debulking and subsequent consolidative chemotherapy; however, cure rates are much lower than with localized disease. The goals of therapy in advanced ovarian carcinoma are to cure the disease, to extend disease-free survival, and to prolong overall survival. Patients with recurrent or refractory disease are generally not curable and have a poor long-term prognosis. Thus, the primary direction of therapy may be symptom management, quality of life maintenance, and treatment-related toxicity minimization.[115]

FUTURE DIRECTIONS

Although the number of women in the United States dying from ovarian cancer continues to increase, substantial treatment progress has been made. However, there are still several therapeutic questions that need to be asked and problems that need to be solved. New approaches to the treatment of advanced primary as well as recurrent and refractory ovarian cancer, such as agents to overcome resistance, should be studied. The optimum adjuvant and consolidation treatment modalities should be determined. The role of IP chemotherapy in all stages of disease is unclear as is the most appropriate salvage therapy. Answering these therapeutic questions and solving these therapeutic problems may prolong the long-term survival in patients with local and advanced ovarian cancer.

▶ PRINCIPLES OF PHARMACOTHERAPY

- Ovarian cancer usually occurs in postmenopausal women in the sixth decade of life; the risk of developing ovarian cancer is increased in women with a family history involving two or more first-degree relatives.
- Patients with local disease have a 5-year survival rate greater than 90%; however, most patients present with disseminated disease, because symptoms do not appear until late in the disease course, and have a 5-year survival rate of 5% to 10%.
- CA-125 is an antigen common to most nonmucinous epithelial ovarian carcinoma and is a useful marker for ovarian cancer; rising or falling CA-125 titers correlate with the disease extent.
- Ovarian cancer management is based on the histologic type, pathologic grade, and disease stage at initial presentation. In general, the treatment of patients with ovarian cancer involves surgical debulking at the time of staging laparotomy and primary or adjuvant chemotherapy.
- The beneficial effects of adjuvant chemotherapy in the treatment of local disease depend on the stage and disease subtype. Postoperative adjuvant chemotherapy is not required in stage IA or IB grade 1, whereas patients with stage IA or IB grade 2 or 3, and stage IC do require adjuvant chemotherapy. All patients with stage II disease require adjuvant treatment. Paclitaxel plus cisplatin or carboplatin for three to six cycles is the current recommended adjuvant therapy for these patients.
- Survival of patients with advanced ovarian cancer is a function of stage at initial diagnosis and the amount of residual after surgical debulking. Patients with stage III disease treated with optimal debulking (< 1 to 2 cm of residual tumor) have a 4-year survival rate of 30%, whereas patients with stage III or IV disease who have undergone suboptimal debulking (> 2 cm of residual disease) have less than a 10% long-term survival.
- Current recommended treatment of advanced ovarian cancer (stage III or IV) is based on initial surgical debulking followed by paclitaxel plus cisplatin or carboplatin for six cycles.
- Approximately 20% to 50% of patients without evidence of disease on second-look laparotomy will relapse. In addition, patients who were initially sensitive to chemotherapy and whose response lasted the longest have the greatest likelihood of achieving a response to retreatment with the initial treatment regimen or treatment with salvage therapy.
- Patients with disease that is refractory to the initial platinum-containing chemotherapy or that recurs within 6 months after treatment (termed

"platinum-refractory") are unlikely to benefit from standard-dose platinum therapy. However, patients who relapse more than 6 months after the initial platinum-containing regimen (termed "platinum-sensitive") have a response rate of 27% to 59% with a standard-dose second-line platinum regimen.

- The NCCN guidelines recommend retreatment with either paclitaxel, platinum, or the combination of paclitaxel and a platinum compound if disease recurs more than 6 months after the initial treatment with paclitaxel in combination with a platinum analog. Treatment options for patients with refractory disease or disease recurrence within 6 months after treatment include topotecan, altretamine, oral etoposide, liposomal doxorubicin, tamoxifen, referral for a clinical trial, or supportive care therapy.

REFERENCES

1. Landis S, Murray T, Bolden S, Wingo PA. Cancer Statistics, 1998. CA Cancer J Clin 1998;48:6–29.
2. Makar APH, Trope CG. Endometrial and ovarian malignancies: Epidemiology, etiology, and prognostic factors. Acta Obstet Gynecol Scand 1992;71:331–336.
3. Leung Y, DePetrillo AD. Etiology, epidemiology, risk and prognostic factors, screening, and imaging of gynecologic cancers. Curr Opin Oncol 1993;5:869–876.
4. Daly MB. The epidemiology of ovarian cancer. Hematol Oncol Clin North Am 1992;6:729–738.
5. Cannistra SA. Cancer of the ovary [published erratum appears in N Engl J Med 1994;330:448]. N Engl J Med 1993;329: 1550–1559.
6. Koch M, Gaedke H, Jenkins H. Family history of ovarian cancer patients: A case control study. Int J Epidemiol 1989;17:782.
7. Woutersz TB. Benefits of oral contraception: Thirty years' experience. Int J Fertil 1991;3:26–31.
8. Lynch HT, Watson P, Lynch JF, et al. Hereditary ovarian cancer: Heterogeneity in age at onset. Cancer 1993;71(suppl 2):573–581.
9. Taylor RR, Tenerillo MG, Nash JD, Park RC, Birrer MJ. The molecular genetics of gyn malignancies. Oncology 1994;8:63–70.
10. Lancaster JM, Wiseman RW. Recent advances in the molecular genetics of hereditary breast and ovarian cancer. Prog Clin Biol Res 1997;396:31–51.
11. Ozols RF, Vermorken JB. Chemotherapy of advanced ovarian cancer: Current status and future directions. Semin Oncol 1997;24:S2-1–S2-9.
12. Hand R, Fremgen A, Chmiel JS, et al. Staging procedures, clinical management, and survival outcome for ovarian carcinoma. JAMA 1993;269:1119–1122.
13. Kenemans P, Yedema CA, Bon GG, von Mensdorff-Pouilly S. CA 125 in gynecologic oncology—a review. Eur J Obstet Gynecol Reprod Biol 1993;49:115–124.
14. Hempling RE. Tumor markers in epithelial ovarian cancer. Obstet Gynecol Clin North Am 1994;21:41–61.
15. Young RC, Perez CA, Hoskins WJ. Cancer of the ovary. In: Devita VT, Hellman S, Rosenberg SA, eds. Cancer—Principles and Practice of Oncology. Philadelphia, Lippincott, 1993:1226–1263.
16. Mackey SE, Creasman WT. Ovarian cancer screening. J Clin Oncol 1995;13:783–793.
17. van Nagell JR, DePriest PD, Gallion HH, Pavlik EJ. Ovarian cancer screening. Cancer 1993;71:1523–1528.
18. Carlson KJ, Skates S, Singer DE. Screening for ovarian cancer. Ann Intern Med 1994;121:124–132.
19. NIH Consensus Conference. Ovarian cancer. Screening, treatment, and follow-up. NIH Consensus Development Panel on Ovarian Cancer [see comments]. JAMA 1995;273:491–497.
20. Burke W, Daly M, Garber J, et al. Recommendations for follow-up care of individuals with an inherited predisposition to cancer. II. BRCA1 and BRCA2. Cancer Genetics Studies Consortium. JAMA 1997;277:997–1003.
21. Nguyen HN, Averette HE, Hoskins W, et al. National survey of ovarian carcinoma. Part V. The impact of physician's specialty on patients' survival. Cancer 1993;72:3663–3670.
22. Boente MP, Yek K, Hogan VM, Ozols RF. Current status of staging laparotomy in colorectal and ovarian cancer. Cancer Treat Res 1996;82:337–357.
23. Young RC, Walton LA, Ellenberg SS, et al. Adjuvant therapy in stage I and stage II epithelial ovarian cancer: Result of two prospective randomized trials. N Engl J Med 1990;322:1021–1027.
24. Kawai M, Kikkawa F, Hattori S, et al. Long-term follow-up of patients with epithelial carcinoma of the ovary. Int J Gynaecol Obstet 1994;44:259–266.
25. Louie KG, Ozols RF, Myers CE, et al. Long-term results of a cisplatin-containing combination chemotherapy regimen for the treatment of advanced ovarian carcinoma. J Clin Oncol 1986;4: 1579–1585.
26. Omura GA, Brady MF, Homesley HD, et al. Long-term follow-up and prognostic factor analysis in advanced ovarian carcinoma: The Gynecologic Oncology Group experience. J Clin Oncol 1991;9: 1138–1150.
27. Hainsworth JD, Grosh WW, Burnett LS, et al. Advanced ovarian cancer: Long-term results of treatment with intensive cisplatin-based chemotherapy of brief duration. Ann Intern Med 1988;108: 165–170.
28. Morgan RJ Jr, Copeland L, Gershenson D, et al. Update of the NCCN Ovarian Cancer Practice Guidelines. Oncology (Huntingt) 1997;11:95–105.
29. Goodman HM, Harlow BL, Sheets EE, et al. The role of cytoreductive surgery in the management of stage IV epithelial ovarian carcinoma. Gynecol Oncol 1992;46:367–371.
30. Hoskins W, Rice L, Rubin S. Ovarian cancer surgical practice guidelines. Society of surgical oncology practice guidelines: Ovarian cancer. Oncology (Huntingt) 1997;11:896–900, 903–904.
31. Miyazaki T, Tomoda Y, Ohta M, et al. Preservation of ovarian function and reproductive ability in patients with malignant ovarian tumors. Gynecol Oncol 1988;30:329–341.
32. Neijt JP, ten Bokkel Huinink WW, van der Burg ME, et al. Randomized trial comparing two combination chemotherapy regimens (CHAP-5 v CP) in advanced ovarian carcinoma. J Clin Oncol 1987; 5:1157–1168.
33. Taylor AE, Wiltshaw E, Gore ME, Fryatt I, Fisher C. Long-term follow-up of the first randomized study of cisplatin versus carboplatin for advanced epithelial ovarian cancer. J Clin Oncol 1994;12: 2066–2070.
34. Group AOCT. Chemotherapy in advanced ovarian cancer: An overview of randomized clinical trials. BMJ 1991;303:884–893.
35. A'Hern RP, Gore ME. Impact of doxorubicin on survival in advanced ovarian cancer. J Clin Oncol 1995;13:726–732.
36. Alberts DS, Green S, Hannigan EV, et al. Improved therapeutic index of carboplatin plus cyclophosphamide versus cisplatin plus cyclophosphamide: Final report by the Southwest Oncology Group of a phase III randomized trial in stages III and IV ovarian cancer [published erratum appears in J Clin Oncol 1992;10:1505] J Clin Oncol 1992;10:706–717.
37. Swenerton K, Jeffrey J, Stuart G, et al. Cisplatin-cyclophosphamide versus carboplatin-cyclophosphamide in advanced ovarian cancer: A randomized phase III study of the National Cancer Institute of Canada Clinical Trials Group. J Clin Oncol 1992;10:718–726.

38. Segelov E, Stuart-Harris R, Bell D, et al. A phase II study of carboplatin and cisplatin in advanced ovarian cancer. Eur J Gynaecol Oncol 1994;15:277–282.
39. Levin L, Hryniuk WM. Dose intensity analysis of chemotherapy regimens in ovarian carcinoma. J Clin Oncol 1987;5:756–767.
40. McGuire WP, Hoskins WJ, Brady MF, et al. Assessment of dose-intensive therapy in suboptimally debulked ovarian cancer: A Gynecologic Oncology Group study. J Clin Oncol 1995;13:1589–1599.
41. Kaye SB, Paul J, Cassidy J, et al. Mature results of a randomized trial of two doses of cisplatin for the treatment of ovarian cancer. Scottish Gynecology Cancer Trials Group. J Clin Oncol 1996;14: 2113–2119.
42. McGuire WP. How many more nails to seal the coffin of dose intensity? Ann Oncol 1997;8:311–313. Editorial.
43. Jakobsen A, Bertelsen K, Andersen JE, et al. Dose-effect study of carboplatin in ovarian cancer: A Danish Ovarian Cancer Group study. J Clin Oncol 1997;15:193–198.
44. McGuire WP. Taxol: A new drug with significant activity as a salvage therapy in advanced epithelial ovarian carcinoma. Gynecol Oncol 1993;51:78–85.
45. Rowinsky EK, Donehower RC. Paclitaxel (Taxol) [published erratum appears in N Engl J Med 1995;333:75]. N Engl J Med 1995; 332:1004–1014.
46. Kohler DR, Goldspiel BR. Paclitaxel (Taxol). Pharmacotherapy 1994;14:3–34.
47. Einzig AI. Review of phase II trials of Taxol (paclitaxel) in patients with advanced ovarian cancer. Ann Oncol 1994;5:S29–S32.
48. McGuire WP, Hoskins WJ, Brady MF, et al. Cyclophosphamide and cisplatin compared with paclitaxel and cisplatin in patients with stage III and stage IV ovarian cancer. N Engl J Med 1996; 334:1–6.
49. Ozols RF. Carboplatin and paclitaxel in ovarian cancer. Semin Oncol 1995;22:78–83.
50. Hakes TB, Chalas E, Hoskins WJ, et al. Randomized prospective trial of 5 versus 10 cycles of cyclophosphamide, doxorubicin, and cisplatin in advanced ovarian carcinoma. Gynecol Oncol 1992;45: 284–289.
51. Kohn EC, Sarosy GA, Davis P, et al. A phase I/II study of dose-intense paclitaxel with cisplatin and cyclophosphamide as initial therapy of poor-prognosis advanced-stage epithelial ovarian cancer. Gynecol Oncol 1996;62:181–191.
52. Walton L, Ellenberg SS, Major F Jr, et al. Results of second-look laparotomy in patients with early-stage ovarian carcinoma. Obstet Gynecol 1987;70:770–773.
53. Potter ME. Secondary cytoreduction in ovarian cancer: Pro or con? Gynecol Oncol 1993;51:131–135.
54. Schilder RJ, Boente MP, Corn BW, et al. The management of early ovarian cancer. Oncology (Huntingt) 1995;9:171–182. Discussion 185–187.
55. van der Burg ME, van Lent M, Buyse M, et al. The effect of debulking surgery after induction chemotherapy on the prognosis in advanced epithelial ovarian cancer. Gynecological Cancer Cooperative Group of the European Organization for Research and Treatment of Cancer [see comments]. N Engl J Med 1995;332:629–634.
56. Dunton CJ. New options for the treatment of advanced ovarian cancer. Semin Oncol 1997;23:S5-2–S5-11.
57. Hatch KD, Beecham JB, Blessing JA, Creasman WT. Responsiveness of patients with advanced ovarian carcinoma to tamoxifen. A Gynecologic Oncology Group study of second-line therapy in 105 patients. Cancer 1991;68:269–271.
58. Markman M, Rothman R, Hakes T, et al. Second-line platinum therapy in patients with ovarian cancer previously treated with cisplatin. J Clin Oncol 1991;9:389–393.
59. Rothenberg ML, Ozols RF, Glatstein E, et al. Dose-intensive induction therapy with cyclophosphamide, cisplatin, and consolidative abdominal radiation in advanced-stage epithelial ovarian cancer [see comments]. J Clin Oncol 1992;10:727–734.
60. Kemp G, Rose P, Lurain J, et al. Amifostine pretreatment for protection against cyclophosphamide-induced toxicities: Results of a randomized control trial in patients with advanced ovarian cancer. J Clin Oncol 1996;14:2101–2112.
61. Eisenhauer EA, ten Bokkel Huinink WW, Swenerton KD, et al. European–Canadian randomized trial of paclitaxel in relapsed ovarian cancer: High-dose versus low-dose and long versus short infusion. J Clin Oncol 1994;12:2654–2666.
62. Kohn EC, Sarosy G, Bicher A, et al. Dose-intense taxol: High response rate in patients with platinum-resistant recurrent ovarian cancer. J Natl Cancer Inst 1994;86:18–24.
63. Trimble EL, Adams JD, Vena D, et al. Paclitaxel for platinum-refractory ovarian cancer: Results from the first 1,000 patients registered to National Cancer Institute Treatment Referrral Center 9103. J Clin Oncol 1993;11:2405–2410.
64. Thigpen JT, Blessing JA, Ball H, Hummel SJ, Barrett RJ. Phase II trial of paclitaxel in patients with progressive ovarian carcinoma after platinum-based chemotherapy: A Gynecologic Oncology Group study. J Clin Oncol 1994;12:1748–1753.
65. Kavanaugh JJ, Kudelka AT, Edwards RS, et al. A randomized crossover trial of parenteral hydroxyurea v. high dose Taxol in cisplatin/carboplatin resistant epithelial ovarian cancer. Proc Am Soc Clin Oncol 1993;12:259. Abstract.
66. ten Bokkel Huinink W, Gore M, Carmichael J, et al. Topotecan versus paclitaxel for the treatment of recurrent epithelial ovarian cancer [see comments]. J Clin Oncol 1997;15:2183–2193.
67. Swisher EM, Mutch DG, Rader JS, Elbendary A, Herzog TJ. Topotecan in platinum- and paclitaxel-resistant ovarian cancer. Gynecol Oncol 1997;66:480–486.
68. Markman M. Topotecan: An important new drug in the management of ovarian cancer. Semin Oncol 1997;24:S5–S11.
69. Creemers GJ, Bolis G, Gore M, et al. Topotecan, an active drug in the secon-line treatment of epithelial ovarian cancer: Results of a large European phase II study [see comments]. J Clin Oncol 1996; 14:3056–3061.
70. Stewart CF, Zamboni WC, Crom WR, et al. Topoisomerase I interactive drugs in children with cancer. Invest New Drugs 1996;14: 37–47.
71. Kavanagh J, Tresukosol D, Edwards C, et al. Carboplatin reinduction after taxane in patients with platinum-refractory epithelial ovarian cancer. J Clin Oncol 1995;13:1584–1588.
72. Muggia FM, Hainsworth JD, Jeffers S, et al. Phase II study of liposomal doxorubicin in refractory ovarian cancer: Antitumor activity and toxicity modification by liposomal encapsulation. J Clin Oncol 1997;15:987–993.
73. Gordon A, Bookman M, Malmstrom H, et al. Efficacy of topotecan in advanced epithelial ovarian cancer after failure of platinum and paclitaxel: International Topotecan Study Group Trial. Proc Annu Meet Am Soc Clin Oncol 1996;15. Meeting abstract.
74. McGuire WP. Primary treatment of epithelial ovarian malignancies. Cancer 1993;71:1541–1550.
75. Lee CR, Faulds D. Altretamine. A review of its pharmacodynamic and pharmacokinetic properties, and therapeutic potential in cancer chemotherapy. Drugs 1995;49:932–953.
76. Manetta A, MacNeill C, Lyter JA, et al. Hexamethylmelamine as a single second-line agent in ovarian cancer. Gynecol Oncol 1990;36: 93–96.
77. Rosen GF, Lurain JR, Newton M. Hexamethylmelamine in ovarian cancer after failure of cisplatin-based multiple-agent chemotherapy. Gynecol Oncol 1987;27:173–179.
78. Rose P, Blessing J, Mayer A, Homesley H. Prolonged oral etoposide as second-line therapy for platinum-resistant and platinum-sensitive ovarian carcinoma. A Gynecologic Oncology Group Study. J Clin Oncol 1998;16:405–410.
79. Gelmann EP. Tamoxifen for the treatment of malignancies other than breast and endometrial carcinoma. Semin Oncol 1997;24:S1-65–S1-70.

80. Chiara S, Conte P, Franzone P, et al. High-risk early-stage ovarian cancer. Randomized clinical trial comparing cisplatin plus cyclophosphamide versus whole abdominal radiotherapy. Am J Clin Oncol 1994;17:72–76.
81. Fyles AW, Dembo AJ, Bush RS, et al. Analysis of complications in patients treated with abdomino-pelvic radiation therapy for ovarian carcinoma. Int J Radiat Oncol Biol Phys 1992;22: 847–851.
82. Soper JT, Berchuck A, Dodge R, Clarke-Pearson DL. Adjuvant therapy with intraperitoneal chromic phosphate (^{32}P) in women with early ovarian carcinoma after comprehensive surgical staging. Obstet Gynecol 1992;79:993–997.
83. Vergotte IB, Vergote-De Vos LN, Abeler VM, et al. Randomized trial comparing cisplatin with radioactive phosphorus or whole-abdomen irradiation as adjuvant treatment of ovarian cancer. Cancer 1992;69: 741–749.
84. Markman M. Intraperitoneal chemotherapy in the treatment of ovarian cancer. Ann Med 1996;28:293–296.
85. Schneider JG. Intraperitoneal chemotherapy. Obstet Gynecol Clin North Am 1994;21:195–212.
86. Brandner P, Neis KJ. Use of an implantable catheter system for intraperitoneal chemotherapy in ovarian cancer. Artif Organs 1994;18: 328–330.
87. Markman M. Intraperitoneal therapy for treatment of malignant disease principally confined to the peritoneal cavity. Crit Rev Oncol Hematol 1993;14:15–28.
88. Alberts DS, Liu PY, Hannigan EV, et al. Intraperitoneal cisplatin plus intravenous cyclophosphamide versus intravenous cisplatin plus intravenous cyclophosphamide for stage III ovarian cancer. N Engl J Med 1996;335:1950–1955.
89. Kirmani S, Braly PS, McClay EF, et al. A comparison of intravenous versus intraperitoneal chemotherapy for the initial treatment of ovarian cancer. Gynecol Oncol 1994;54:338–344.
90. Markman M, Reichman B, Hakes T, et al. Responses to second-line cisplatin-based intraperitoneal therapy in ovarian cancer: Influence of a prior response to intravenous cisplatin. J Clin Oncol 1991;9: 1801–1805.
91. Piver MS, Recio FO, Baker TR, Driscoll D. Evaluation of survival after second-line intraperitoneal cisplatin-based chemotherapy for advanced ovarian cancer. Cancer 1994;73:1693–1698.
92. Markman M, Hakes T, Reichman B, et al. Phase II trial of weekly or biweekly intraperitoneal mitoxantrone in epithelial ovarian cancer. J Clin Oncol 1991;9:978–982.
93. Markman M, Francis P, Rowinsky E, Hoskins W. Intraperitoneal paclitaxel: A possible role in the management of ovarian cancer? Semin Oncol 1995;22:84–87.
94. Markman M, Francis P, Rowinsky E, et al. Intraperitoneal Taxol (paclitaxel) in the management of ovarian cancer. Ann Oncol 1994;5: S55–S58.
95. Markman M, Berek JS, Blessing JA, et al. Characteristics of patients with small-volume residual ovarian cancer unresponsive to cisplatin-based IP chemotherapy: Lessons learned from a Gynecologic Oncology Group phase II trial of IP cisplatin and recombinant alpha-interferon. Gynecol Oncol 1992;45:3–8.
96. Los G, Mutsaers PH, Vijgh WJ. Direct diffusion of *cis*-diamminedichloroplatinum(II) in intraperitoneal rat tumors after intraperitonal chemotherapy: A comparison with systemic chemotherapy. Cancer Res 1989;49:3380–3384.
97. Shpall EJ, Clarke-Pearson D, Soper JT, et al. High-dose alkylating agent chemotherapy with autologous bone marrow support in patients with stage III/IV epithelial ovarian cancer. Gynecol Oncol 1990;38:386–391.
98. Shpall EJ, Jones RB, Bearman S. High-dose therapy with autologous bone marrow transplantation for the treatment of solid tumors. Curr Opin Oncol 1994;6:135–138.
99. Mulder PO, Willemse PH, Aalders JG, et al. High-dose chemotherapy with autologous bone marrow transplantation in patients with refractory ovarian cancer. Eur J Cancer Clin Oncol 1989;25: 645–649.
100. Legros M, Dauplat J, Fleury J, et al. High-dose chemotherapy with hematopoietic rescue in patients with stage III to IV ovarian cancer: Long-term results [see comments]. J Clin Oncol 1997;15: 1302–1308.
101. Stiff PJ, Bayer R, Kerger C, et al. High-dose chemotherapy with autologous transplantation for persistent/relapsed ovarian cancer: A multivariate analysis of survival for 100 consecutively treated patients [see comments]. J Clin Oncol 1997;15:1309–1317.
102. Trimble CL, Trimble EL. Management of epithelial ovarian tumors of low malignant potential. Gynecol Oncol 1994;55:S52–S61.
103. Leake JF. Tumors of low malignant potential. Curr Opin Obstet Gynecol 1992;4:81–85.
104. Trope C, Kaern J, Vergote IB, Kristensen G, Abeler V. Are borderline tumors of the ovary overtreated both surgically and systemically? A review of four prospective randomized trials including 253 patients with borderline tumors. Gynecol Oncol 1993;51:236–243.
105. Williams SD. Chemotherapy of ovarian germ cell tumors. Hematol Oncol Clin North Am 1991;5:1261–1269.
106. Segelov E, Campbell J, Ng M, et al. Cisplatin-based chemotherapy for ovarian germ cell malignancies: The Australian experience. J Clin Oncol 1994;12:378–384.
107. Williams S, Blessing JA, Liao SY, Ball H, Hanjani P. Adjuvant therapy of ovarian germ cell tumors with cisplatin, etoposide, and bleomycin: A trial of the Gynecologic Oncology Group. J Clin Oncol 1994;12:701–706.
108. Gershenson DM. Update on malignant ovarian germ cell tumors. Cancer 1993;71:1581–1590.
109. Covens A, Boucher S, Roche K, et al. Is paclitaxel and cisplatin a cost-effective first-line therapy for advanced ovarian carcinoma? Cancer 1996;77:2086–2091.
110. McGuire W, Neugut AI, Arikian S, Doyle J, Dezii CM. Analysis of the cost-effectiveness of paclitaxel as alternative combination therapy for advanced ovarian cancer. J Clin Oncol 1997;15:640–645.
111. Elit LM, Gafni A, Levine MN. Economic and policy implications of adopting paclitaxel as first-line therapy for advanced ovarian cancer: An Ontario perspective. J Clin Oncol 1997;15:632–639.
112. Messori A, Trippoli S, Becagli P, Tendi E. Pharmacoeconomic profile of paclitaxel as a first-line treatment for patients with advanced ovarian carcinoma. A lifetime cost-effectiveness analysis. Cancer 1996; 78:2366–2373.
113. Messori A, Cecchi M, Becagli P, Trippoli S. Pharacoeconomic profile of paclitaxel as a first-line treatment for patients with advanced ovarian carcinoma. A lifetime cost-effectiveness analysis. Cancer 1997;79:2264–2266. Letter.
114. Rustin GJ, Nelstrop AE, McClean P, et al. Defining response of ovarian carcinoma to initial chemotherapy according to serum CA 125. J Clin Oncol 1996;14:1545–1551.
115. Montazeri A, McEwen J, Gillis CR. Quality of life in patients with ovarian cancer: Current state of research. Support Care Cancer 1996; 4:169–179.
116. Sarosy G, Kohn E, Stone DA, et al. Phase I study of taxol and granulocyte colony-stimulating factor in patients with refractory ovarian cancer. J Clin Oncol 1992;10:1165–1170.
117. Seewaldt VL, Greer BE, Cain JM, et al. Paclitaxel (Taxol) treatment for refractory ovarian cancer: Phase II clinical trial. Am J Obstet Gynecol 1994;170:1666–1670.
118. Reed E, Sarosy G, Kohn E, et al. Phase I study of paclitaxel and cyclophosphamide in reccurrant adenocarcinoma of the ovary. Proc Gynecol Oncol 1996;61:349–353.
119. Ozols RF, Schwartz PE, Eifel PJ. Ovarian cancer, fallopian tube carcinoma, and peritoneal carcinoma. In: Devita VT, Hellman S, Rosenberg SA, eds. Cancer—Principles and Practice of Oncology, 5th ed. Philadelphia, Lippincott, 1997:1502–1539.

122
ACUTE LEUKEMIAS

Steven P. Smith, PharmD, BCPS, and Susan E. Beltz, PharmD

The leukemias are heterogenous hematologic malignancies characterized by unregulated proliferation of the blood-forming cells of the bone marrow. These immature proliferating leukemia cells (blasts) physically "crowd out" or inhibit normal cellular maturation in bone marrow, resulting in anemia, granulocytopenia, and thrombocytopenia. Leukemic blasts may also leave the bone marrow and infiltrate a variety of tissues such as lymph nodes, skin, liver, spleen, kidney, and the central nervous system.

The term "leukemia" was coined by Virchow to describe the "white blood" of some patients that he saw under the microscope in 1845.[1] Historically, leukemia has been classified as acute or chronic based on differences in cell of origin and cell line maturation, patient life expectancy, clinical presentation, rapidity of progression of the untreated disease, and response to therapy. Using these categories, four major leukemias are recognized: acute lymphocytic leukemia (ALL), acute nonlymphocytic leukemia (ANLL), chronic lymphocytic leukemia (CLL), and chronic myeloid leukemia (CML). Acute leukemias are characterized by undifferentiated, immature cells that autonomously proliferate. Chronic leukemias also autonomously proliferate, but the cells are more differentiated and mature.[1] Untreated, the acute leukemias are rapidly progressive, resulting in death in 2 to 3 months.

INCIDENCE AND EPIDEMIOLOGY

Approximately 12,500 new cases of acute leukemias are diagnosed per year in the United States, accounting for 1% of the total cancer incidence: 9400 cases of ANLL and 3100 cases of ALL. The incidence has been relatively stable for two decades. An estimated 7900 deaths per year, and 1.4% of all cancer deaths, are due to acute leukemias. The acute leukemias are an uncommon cause of cancer-related death after age 35, but they are the leading cause of cancer-related deaths in persons under age 35.[1,2] In adults, acute and chronic leukemias occur at equal rates. More than 90% of the cases of acute and chronic leukemia occur in adults. There are approximately 2.5 cases of ANLL and 1.3 cases of ALL per 100,000 individuals. The median age of patients with ANLL is 65 years while the median age for the ALL population is age 10 years.[1,2] The incidence of ANLL rises with age from 1 in 100,000 individuals under age 40 to 15 per 100,000 over age 75.[1] Acute leukemia is slightly more common in males than in females. In the United States, acute leukemia is more common among whites than blacks.[1,3]

Despite the low incidence rate, the acute leukemias are the most common malignancy in children less than 15 years of age.[4–6] In contrast to adult leukemias, of the 2200 new cases each year, 1300 of them are ALL.[2] ANLL accounts for only 15% to 20% of all childhood leukemias, and the chronic leukemias account for less than 5%.[5] The annual incidence of the childhood acute leukemias is 44 and 25 per million in white and black children under 15 years of age, respectively. Childhood ALL has a slight male dominance and peaks at age 4 years.[6] ANLL in children has not displayed any gender or racial preference and occurs throughout childhood without any peak age periods. Acute leukemia during the first 4 weeks of life (congenital leukemia) is usually ANLL.[6]

Chemotherapy has dramatically improved the outlook of patients with acute leukemia. Over 80% of children and young adults with acute leukemia achieve an initial complete remission from their disease. Overall, only 50% to 75% of adults achieve an initial complete remission.[1,6] Long-term survival in children ranges from 30% to 90% depending on the type of leukemia and patient risk factors.[4] The prognosis of adult acute leukemia is generally worse than that of childhood leukemia, with only 20% to 40% of patients becoming long-term survivors.[1,6]

ETIOLOGY

The exact cause of the acute leukemias is not known. A multifactorial process is likely, involving genetics, environmental factors, toxins, immunologic status, and viral exposures. Table 122–1 summarizes the major factors that have been linked to acute leukemias.[1–3,7,8] In pediatric ALL, a number of environmental factors have been investigated as possible causes: exposure to ionizing radiation, toxic chemicals, diagnostic radiography materials, herbicides and pesticides; maternal use of alcohol, contraceptives, diethylstilbestrol, or cigarettes; parental exposure to drugs or chemicals; and chemical contamination of groundwater.[6] Although there have been several reports of the possible link of electromagnetic fields of high-voltage power lines to the development of leukemia, a recent report by Linet and colleagues provides little evidence to support this association.[9] This study was a blinded comprehensive case-control study of 638 children with ALL and 620 controls. The magnetic field in each child's bedroom was measured and the distance from the home to any power lines was determined, but no correlation to the occurrence of childhood ALL

TABLE 122–1. Conditions Associated With an Increased Frequency of Acute Leukemia

Drugs	Kostman's syndrome
Alkylating agents	Neurofibromatosis
Epipodophyllotoxins	**Chemical**
Genetic Conditions	Benzene
Down's syndrome	**Radiation**
Bloom's syndrome	Ionizing radiation
Fanconi's anemia	**Virus**
Kleinfelter's syndrome	HTLV-1
Ataxia telangiectasia	**Social Habits**
Langerhans' cell histiocytosis	Cigarette smoking
Schwachman's syndrome	Maternal marijuana use
Severe combined immunodeficiency	Maternal ethanol use

could be made. In most patients who develop leukemia, a causative agent cannot be identified.

PATHOGENESIS

A basic understanding of normal hematopoiesis is needed before one can understand the pathogenesis of leukemia. The reader is referred to Chapter 90 for a detailed discussion of hematopoiesis. Normal hematopoiesis consists of multiple, well-orchestrated steps of cellular development. A pool of pluripotent stem cells undergoes differentiation, maturation, and proliferation to form the mature blood cells seen in the peripheral circulation. These pluripotent stem cells initially differentiate to form two distinct stem cell pools. The myeloid stem cell gives rise to six types of blood cells (erythrocytes, platelets, monocytes, basophils, neutrophils, and eosinophils); while the lymphoid stem cell differentiates to form circulating B and T lymphocytes.[10] Leukemia may develop at any stage and within any cell line. Figure 122–1 illustrates sites along the development of the myeloid cell at which myeloid leukemias could arise.

Two features are common to both ANLL and ALL. Both arise from a single leukemic cell that proliferates (monoclonality). Secondly, there is a failure to maintain a relative balance between proliferation and differentiation, so that the cells do not differentiate past a particular stage of hematopoiesis but then proliferate uncontrollably. Proliferation and differentiation are under genetic control, and when the balance between the two is altered in favor of proliferation, leukemia occurs. New antileukemia drug therapies are being developed that are specifically targeted to restore differentiation.[1]

ANLL affects the hematopoietic cell population and probably arises from a defect in the pluripotent stem cell or a more committed myeloid precursor resulting in partial differentiation and proliferation of immature precursors of the myeloid blood-forming cells.[3] In older patients, trilineage leukemic involvement is seen because the cell of origin is probably a very early stem cell. In younger patients, a more differentiated stem cell becomes malignant, allowing maturation of some granulocytic and erythroid populations. These two forms of ANLL exhibit different patterns of resistance to chemotherapy, with resistance more evident in the elderly population of ANLL.[12] The French–American–British (FAB) classification system outlined in Table 122–2 identifies eight different morphologic subtypes of ANLL. As an example, in acute promyelocytic leukemia (APL), the leukemia cells mature and differentiate up to the stage of the promyelocyte, but no further. They then proliferate as promyelocytes without differentiation or maturation into mature neutrophils.[13]

ALL is a disease characterized by proliferation of immature lymphoblasts. In this type of acute leukemia, the defect is probably at the level of the lymphopoietic stem cell or a very early lymphoid precursor.[1,6] Markers on the cell

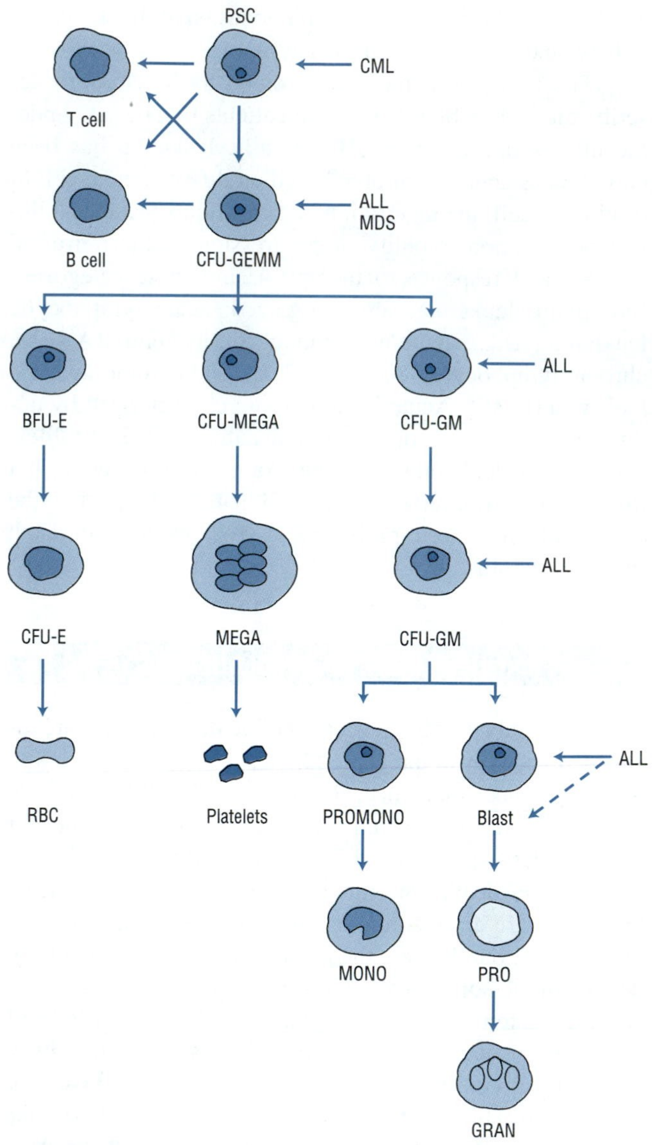

FIGURE 122–1. Cells of origin for acute nonlymphocytic leukemia (ANLL). ANLL may develop at different levels of differentiation and maturation of the myeloid cell line. Acute lymphocytic leukemia (ALL) is synonymous with ANLL in this figure. The sites of development of chronic myelogenous leukemia (CML) and myelodysplastic syndrome (MDS) are also indicated. *(Adapted from Ref. 11, with permission.)*

TABLE 122–2. Morphologic (FAB) Classification of Acute Nonlymphocytic Leukemia

Subtype		Frequency of FAB Subtype[a] Adults (%)	Children < 2 yr (%)	Children > 2 yr (%)
M_1	Acute myeloblastic leukemia with minimal differentiation	15	17	25
M_2	Acute myeloblastic leukemia with maturation	25		27
M_3	Acute promyelocytic leukemia	10		5
M_4	Acute myelomonocytic leukemia	25	30	26
M_{5a}	Acute monoblastic leukemia without differentiation	5	52	16
M_{5b}	Acute monoblastic leukemia with differentiation	5		
M_6	Acute erythroleukemia	5		2
M_7	Megakaryocytic leukemia	10		5–7

FAB = French–American–British.
[a]Percentages should be compared vertically and not horizontally.
Adapted from Refs. 1 and 7.

surface or membrane of the lymphoblast can be used to classify ALL (Table 122–3). Advances in the use of monoclonal antibodies for surface markers led to the recognition of subclasses of B- and T-cell lineages.[4] ALL may also be described by cytogenetic abnormalities. Chromosomes may be too many (hyperploidy) or too few (hypoploidy) or exhibit specific translocations.[4,14]

Leukemic cells have a growth advantage over normal cells, leading to a "crowding out" phenomenon in the bone marrow. This growth advantage is not due to more rapid proliferation as compared with normal cells, but is probably due to a factor produced by leukemic cells that inhibits normal cellular proliferation and differentiation, or to a lower rate of leukemic cell loss compared with normal blood cells (loss of programmed cell death).[12]

The exact genetic alterations that lead to leukemia have only recently become evident. The defect may be activation of a normally suppressed gene to create an oncogene that signals unregulated proliferation, differentiation, or survival. All normal cells are programmed to die at some time, but in cancer cells, the appropriate programmed signal is interrupted, leading to continued survival and replication. There are four types of genetic defects that lead to inappropriate proliferation and differentiation. The leukemia genes may send (1) a growth stimulation signal from the cell membrane to the nucleus, (2) a signal to enhance transcription of DNA to RNA, (3) a signal for differentiation, or (4) a signal to prevent programmed death. One example of a genetic defect leading to acute leukemia is the *ras* gene. This gene is involved in cell signal pathways for proliferation and differentiation. Point mutations in the *ras* gene lead to unregulated proliferation and differentiation. Thirty percent of ANLL patients demonstrate a defect in the *ras* gene. It is less common in ALL.[15]

TABLE 122–3. Morphologic (FAB) Classification of Acute Lymphocytic Leukemia

Subtype	Cells of Origin	Frequency of FAB Subtype[a] Adults (%)	Children (%)
L_1	Early pre-B cell Pre-B cell B cell T cell	30	85
L_2	Early pre-B cell Pre-B cell B cell T cell	65	14
L_3	B cell	5	1

FAB = French–American–British.
[a]Percentages should be compared vertically and not horizontally.
Adapted from Refs. 1 and 6.

A second genetic cause of leukemia is the loss or mutation of genes that suppress cancer development.[15] These genes are referred to as tumor suppressor genes. The tumor suppressor gene *p*53 is found in some hematologic malignancies. Alterations in *p*53 are found in 5% to 10% of ANLL patients and 3% of childhood ALL patients.[12] Some forms of ALL have a *p*53 frequency of 50%.[16] Normal *p*53 allows cells to stop in the G_1 phase of the cell cycle. Mutant *p*53 does not stop the cells in G_1, but allows cells to proliferate unregulated, a characteristic of leukemia. The net effect of these genetic changes is to give either the leukemia cell a proliferative advantage over normal hematopoietic cells or to prevent normal differentiation and cell death of the leukemia cell.[15] Certain antileukemia drugs such as doxorubicin can actually induce normal *p*53 production.[17]

Another example of a genetic defect leading to acute leukemia is the *ras* gene. This gene is involved in cell signal pathways for proliferation and differentiation. Point mutations in the *ras* gene lead to unregulated proliferation and differentiation. Thirty percent of ANLL patients demonstrate a defect in the *ras* gene. It is less common in ALL.[15]

In one form of ANLL, APL, there is a specific chromosomal aberration that leads directly to the cessation of cell differentiation.[13] In APL, there is a reciprocal translocation between chromosomes 15 and 17. The rearrangement leads to formation of an oncogenic retinoic acid receptor gene. Normally the retinoic acid receptor gene codes for a protein that serves as a receptor for retinoids—vitamin

A analogs—that promote differentiation of the promyelocyte to its mature myeloid form. The oncogenic retinoic acid receptor gene codes instead for a protein that impairs differentiation of the promyelocyte and impairs programmed cell death.[13]

CLINICAL PRESENTATION

SIGNS AND SYMPTOMS

The signs and symptoms of acute leukemia are nonspecific and can be attributed to replacement of normal functional blood cells with immature dysfunctional leukemic cells and to leukemic infiltration of a specific organ or site.[1] Anemia often manifests as fatigue, malaise, and pallor. Less commonly, palpitations or dyspnea on exertion may be noted. Granulocytopenia may present as fever with or without frank infection. Thrombocytopenia may manifest as simple petechiae or frank bleeding or bruising, often involving the gums, skin, or gastrointestinal tract. Menorrhagia may be seen in premenopausal women. As leukemic infiltrates may involve any organ, unusual presenting symptoms such as gum hypertrophy, loss of vision, the presence of an abnormal mass, or bone pain may also be observed. Leukemic meningitis occurs at presentation in less than 5% of patients. Seizures, headache, diplopia, nausea, or vomiting may be reported or the patient with meningeal involvement may be asymptomatic. As is frequently seen with many types of cancer, mild weight loss may be present. About 10% of cases of acute leukemia can be diagnosed by routine blood analysis without any significant history of physical findings.[1,3,14]

PHYSICAL AND LABORATORY FINDINGS

Physical findings are compatible with anemia (pallor, tachycardia, cardiac murmurs); granulocytopenia (infection, fever); thrombocytopenia (bruising, frank bleeding, petechiae, ecchymoses, purpura, menorrhagia); and leukemic infiltration (lymphadenopathy, splenomegaly, hepatomegaly, sternal tenderness). Petechiae and ecchymoses are more common in ANLL. Bone pain, hepatomegaly, and splenomegaly are more common in ALL. Lymphadenopathy is rare in ANLL but is common in ALL. Other physical findings related to leukemia cell infiltration include gingival hypertrophy, cranial palsies, and skin infiltration. Skin or soft-tissue infiltration by myeloid leukemia creates a chloroma, so named because intracellular enzymes create a greenish discoloration similar to chlorophyll.[1–3]

Anemia and decreased reticulocytes are nearly always present because of decreased red blood cell production. The anemia is usually normocytic and normochromic.[3] The platelet count is reduced (less than 50,000) in nearly all patients. The white blood cell (WBC) count is normal or elevated in about 85% of patients with ALL; in some patients, the white blood cell count is greatly elevated (over 50,000/μL).[3,6] Hyperleukocytosis can be life threatening, especially in ANLL, because blasts can occlude small vessels in the brain, heart, lungs, or elsewhere.[3] A high white blood cell count is often associated with T-cell ALL.[1,3] In adults with ANLL, the white blood cell count at the time of diagnosis will be elevated in one-third, normal in one-third, and low in one-third. The peripheral blood smear usually demonstrates a decrease in normal granulocytes, with an increase in blasts.[1,3]

Serum uric acid is mildly elevated in about one-half of patients with adult leukemia. Occasionally, patients may present with renal failure secondary to uric acid nephropathy. Serum calcium imbalances may be noted. In patients with mild renal failure, hypocalcemia may be seen, and is usually accompanied by hyperphosphatemia. Hypercalcemia is often due to ectopic parathyroid hormone production by leukemic cells, or rapid destruction of large numbers of leukemic cells. Hyperkalemia may also occur secondary to rapid cell kill.[1,3]

APL or M_3 ANLL is characterized by many of the same signs and symptoms as other types of ANLL. One important difference is the propensity of APL to cause disseminated intravascular coagulation. This syndrome is characterized by thrombocytopenia, hypofibrinoginemia, depletion of clotting factors, and a bleeding diathesis. The unusual laboratory values are helpful to identify this subtype of ANLL so that therapy specific for it may be instituted (discussed later in the chapter).

Marrow biopsy and aspirate is necessary to establish a diagnosis and follow disease progression and response to therapy. At diagnosis, the marrow is usually hypercellular with a predominance of blasts. Leukemia is diagnosed if more than 30% of the marrow cells are blasts. If the percentage is below 5%, then the marrow is considered normal. If the marrow has between 5% and 30% leukemic blasts, the term "myelodysplastic syndrome" is used. This condition is considered a preleukemic state that will eventually evolve into frank ANLL.[3]

RISK FACTORS

Many clinical and laboratory features at diagnosis have been associated with response to treatment. Identification of these risk factors may allow the oncologist to better understand the disease and to tailor treatment according to the predicted response. Such factors aid to identify patients most likely to attain a complete remission, maintain that remission, and experience long-term survival. For example, if a patient has many clinical and laboratory features that are associated with a good response to chemotherapy ("good risk"), then the oncologist may choose to give less intensive therapy to reduce the risk of long-term toxic effects. Conversely, if a patient is not likely to respond well to therapy ("high risk" or "poor risk"), then the oncologist may choose to give more intensive chemotherapy.

In adults with ALL, recent studies have identified several risk factors that correlate with prognosis (Table 122–4).

TABLE 122–4. Prognostic Factors in Acute Lymphocytic Leukemia

Factor	Risk for Leukemic Relapse: Low	Risk for Leukemic Relapse: High
Morphology[a]	L_1	L_2, L_3
Immunologic phenotype	Early pre-B cell	Null cell,T cell, pre-B cell, B cell
Philadelphia chromosome	Absent	Present
Cytogenetics	Normal karyotype	Abnormal karyotype
Myeloid markers	Absent	Present
WBC count at diagnosis	< 10,000/mm^3	> 50,000/mm^3
Hemoglobin	< 7 g/dL	> 10 g/dL
Platelets[a]	> 100,000/mm^3	< 30,000/mm^3
Patient age[a]	3–7 yr	< 1 or > 10 yr
Patient gender[a]	Female	Male
Race	White	Black
CNS leukemia	Absent	Present
Node/liver[a]/spleen enlargement	Absent	Massive
Mediastinal mass[a]	Absent	Present
Time to remission[a]	< 14 d	> 14 d

[a]Factors with greatest relative importance.
Compiled from Refs. 1, 6, and 19.

As most patients with ALL achieve a complete clinical remission, these factors refer to the risk of leukemic relapse rather than the risk of not achieving a complete remission. Adult patients generally have a poorer prognosis than children. Several characteristics of the disease, drug activity, and patient tolerance of treatment make for a poorer outcome in adult ALL (Table 122–5).

Similar prognostic factors apply in childhood ALL (Table 122–4). The most important factors appear to be WBC count at presentation, gender, presence of a mediastinal mass, no evidence of disease in day-14 bone marrow, age, platelet count, liver size, and morphologic type. Race does not appear to be as significant a risk factor as once thought, probably as a result of better treatment. Researchers at St. Jude Children's Research Hospital (SJCRH) recently reported on a retrospective review of treatment outcome for black children compared to white children over a 30-year period. Pui and colleagues found that black children had a significantly poorer rate of survival than white children during the first 20-year treatment period (1962 to 1983). During the second era (1984 to 1992), black children had statistically equivalent survival rates when treated with contemporary protocol–based regimens.[21]

In order to create a standard of comparison, a definition of "standard risk" ALL was developed: patients aged 1 to 9 with a presenting WBC count of 50,000/mm^3 or less.[22] The risk category of a patient may be modified by consideration of additional prognostic factors including DNA index (ratio of leukemia cell to normal cell DNA concentrations), cytogenetics, early response to treatment, immunophenotype, and CNS involvement.[22]

Over the past decade, molecular genetics has become an important tool for the diagnosis, prognosis, and treatment of acute leukemias. Flow cytometry is a technique used to assess leukemia cell chromosome number or "ploidy." Hyperploidy (more than 50 chromosomes per cell) is a good risk factor. Hypoploidy (less than 45 chromosomes per cell) is considered a bad risk factor.[4,14] Recently, technically difficult cytogenetic analysis has been replaced by fluorescence *in situ* hybridization (FISH), because it allows for quick, sensitive analysis of samples that might be inadequate for karyotyping.[23] FISH is a process in which specific genes in an intact cell are visualized using fluorescent-labeled probes. Identifying chromosomal translocations is important because they have been linked to rearrangement and altered regulation of cellular oncogenes.[6]

It was once thought that the presence of any chromosomal translocation in the leukemic cells was an adverse prognostic factor. A study of 139 children with ALL revealed that the outcome for patients with a chromosomal translocation is not inferior to the group lacking a

TABLE 122–5. Features of Adult ALL that Contribute to Poorer Prognosis Compared to Childhood ALL

Disease Biology
1. Increased frequency of cytogenetic abnormalities
2. Increased incidence of expression of myeloid antigens
3. Less frequent early pre-B immunophenotype
4. Decreased formation of methotrexate polyglutamates
5. Increased incidence of specific resistance mechanisms (e.g., P-glycoprotein)
6. Increased incidence of high WBC count at presentation
7. Slower response to therapy
8. Increased frequency of mediastinal masses

Treatment Tolerance
1. Poorer tolerance by the bone marrow to treatment
2. Increased extramedullary intolerance (e.g., heart, liver)
3. Poorer tolerance to specific drugs (e.g., asparaginase)
4. Poorer compliance with intensive protocols

Adapted from Ref. 20.

TABLE 122–6. Prognostic Significance of Common Chromosomal Abnormalities in Acute Leukemias

Chromosomal Abnormality	Prognosis	Comments
Acute Lymphocytic Leukemia		
t(1;19)	Poor	Associated with high WBC count, black race, Philadelphia chromosome
t(9;22)	Poor	Associated with high WBC count and older age
t(4;11)	Poor	Associated with infant ALL and AML
t(8;14)	Poor	Predominantly in males, L_3 morphology, bulky extramedullary disease
t(12;21)	Good	Event-free survival 91% at 5 yr
Acute Myelogenous Leukemia		
t(8;21)	Good	M_2 morphology, Auer rods
t(15;17)	Good	Acute promyelocytic leukemia
t(9;11)	Good	Associated with M_4 or M_5 morphology, infant AML, CNS leukemia, coagulopathy
inv 16	Good	Associated with M_4 Eo morphology and CNS leukemia
t(1;22)	Poor	Associated with M_7 morphology, infant AML
inv 3	Poor	M_1 morphology, thrombocytosis
del 5	Poor	$M_{2,4,5,6}$ morphology, older patients
del 7	Poor	$M_{2,4,5,6}$ morphology, older patients

t(x,y) = translocation of chromosomes; inv = inversion of chromosomes; del = deletion of chromosomes.
Compiled from Refs. 1, 4, 14, 16, and 23.

translocation.[24] The more important consideration is the specific rearrangement. Several specific chromosomal translocations have been identified and are now being routinely used in risk assessment and, subsequently, to direct therapy (Table 122–6).

Prognostic factors in adult ANLL have recently been defined. The most important patient factor is age, with younger patients more likely to achieve a complete remission than older patients (over age 70).[1,3] The lower complete remission rate in older patients appears to result from increased frequency of fatal infectious and bleeding complications as well as chemotherapy resistance.[3] The duration of remission is also shorter in older patients compared to younger ones. Other patient-specific prognostic factors include concurrent infection and any major organ impairment.[3] FAB morphologic subtype may be a factor, with types M_0, M_5, M_6, and M_7 having the worst outcome.[1,3] Patients with extramedullary disease, CNS involvement, or underlying myelodysplastic syndrome have a worse prognosis.[1,3] Certain cytogenetic abnormalities are also known to worsen the response rate and survival of patients with ANLL (Table 122–6).[1,6,23] In addition, patients who develop a "secondary" leukemia after treatment of another malignancy usually have a very poor response to antileukemic chemotherapy, depending upon the cytogenetic abnormality that develops.[1]

Prognostic factors associated with pediatric ANLL have been reported. Unfortunately, there are few factors that can be consistently identified and predictive of outcome from therapy. Factors that reduce the chances of a complete remission include an initial WBC count greater than 100,000/mm^3, FAB classification M_1 without Auer rods present, certain chromosome abnormalities (Table 122–6), ANLL evolving from myelodysplastic syndrome, and having ANLL secondary to prior chemotherapy or radiation therapy.[7] Remission duration may be influenced negatively by the same factors as well as age under 2 years and having FAB classifications M_4 or M_5.[7]

▶ TREATMENT: Acute Leukemia

DESIRED OUTCOME

The short-term goal of treatment for acute leukemia is to rapidly achieve a complete clinical and hematologic remission. In the absence of a complete remission, a rapid and fatal outcome is inevitable. Complete remission is defined as the disappearance of all clinical and bone marrow evidence (normal cellularity with less than 5% blasts) of leukemia, with restoration of normal hematopoiesis. Partial remission is a significant response to treatment, although evidence of residual disease (5% to 25% blasts) in the bone marrow remains.

After a complete remission is achieved, the goal is to maintain the patient in continuous complete remission. As discussed later, the occurrence of leukemic relapse in the bone marrow usually removes any hope of cure of the disease. Most patients who will die from acute leukemia die within the first 5 years; the survival curve (percentage alive versus time) beyond the fifth year after therapy does not continue to decline as rapidly. When the survival curve achieves a plateau, the patients still alive are likely to be cured.

ACUTE LYMPHOCYTIC LEUKEMIA

Successful treatment in acute lymphocytic leukemia (ALL) was first developed in children. Although treatment results with adult ALL are worse than those with childhood ALL, recent use of aggressive therapy in adult ALL has increased the complete remission rate to 65% to 85% and the proportion of 5-year disease-free survivors to 20% to 30%.[1] Therapy for ALL has historically been

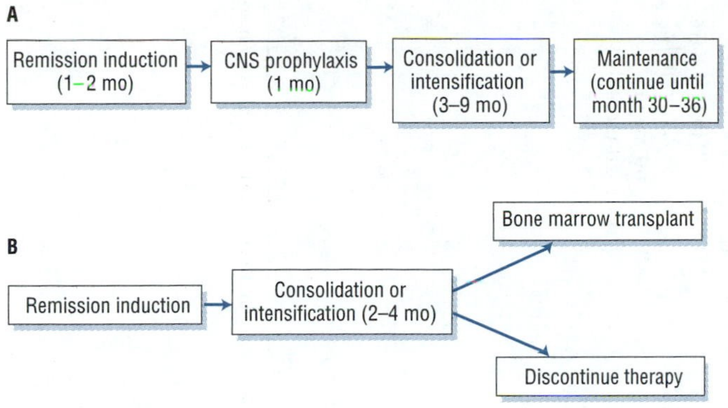

FIGURE 122–2. Treatment algorithm for **(A)** acute lymphocytic and **(B)** nonlymphocytic leukemias.

divided into four phases: (1) remission induction, (2) central nervous system prophylaxis, (3) consolidation therapy, and (4) maintenance therapy (Fig. 122–2). Recently, more complex regimens have been explored, and the lines between phases of therapy are less clear. All patients still receive some form of initial induction therapy to yield a complete remission. Some form of postremission therapy is needed to treat microscopic disease and may include some intensive inpatient therapy (consolidation or intensification therapy) followed by less aggressive outpatient therapy (maintenance). Central nervous system prophylaxis is needed at some time during therapy in all ALL patients to prevent leukemic meningitis. Tables 122–7 and 122–8 illustrate several representative treatment regimens for adult and pediatric ALL.

REMISSION INDUCTION THERAPY

The goal of remission induction is to rapidly induce a complete clinical and hematologic remission. The combination of vincristine and prednisone forms the foundation for induction therapy. Together these two drugs induce complete remission in about 50% of adults with ALL. The addition of an anthracycline (daunorubicin or doxorubicin) to vincristine and prednisone increases the complete remission rate to 83% and carries a treatment-related mortality rate of only 3% to 17%.[1,3,29–31] The addition of a fourth agent to the combination of vincristine, prednisone, and an anthracycline does not dramatically improve the response rate.[32] As seen in Table 122–7, the dosing of prednisone and vincristine is fairly similar from regimen to regimen, but the doses of daunorubicin or asparaginase are diverse. Other agents that are sometimes included in remission induction regimens are cyclophosphamide, cytarabine, mercaptopurine, methotrexate, and mitoxantrone, although it appears that they do not contribute significantly to the efficacy of the remission induction regimen.[33]

Few prospective studies have compared remission induction regimens. The value of adding more drugs to the basic three- or four-drug regimen is unclear. Equally unclear is the value of higher doses of the standard combination of drugs for remission induction. Some data suggest that high-dose methotrexate with cyclophosphamide and cytarabine may improve response and survival in patients with B-cell ALL, and that higher doses of cytarabine or cyclophosphamide may be indicated for patients with T-cell ALL.[20,32–34] Other investigators have explored induction without vincristine and prednisone, using instead high-dose cytarabine and high-dose mitoxantrone. Compared to historical controls receiving vincristine, prednisone, doxorubicin, and cyclophosphamide, the complete response rate was not statistically better, but time to complete response and failure with resistant disease during induction were reduced.[35]

In pediatric ALL, therapy is based upon the risk of relapse. Initially, vincristine and prednisone were used alone until Ortega and associates demonstrated that the complete response rate could be improved with asparaginase three times a week given along with daily prednisone and weekly vincristine.[36] In standard-risk patients, this three-drug combination yields a remission rate near 99%.[14] Three clinically useful sources of asparaginase exist: *Escherichia coli* (gram-negative bacteria), *Erwinia caratovora* (plant parasite), and PEG-*L*-asparaginase (asparaginase covalently conjugated to polyethylene glycol). Only *E. coli* asparaginase and PEG-asparaginase are commercially available. Conventional *E. coli* asparaginase can cause severe hypersensitivity reactions depending upon dose, frequency of administration, and route of administration. PEG-asparaginase has less immunogenicity and a longer half-life, allowing administration every 14 days instead of every other day.[37]

High-risk patients, on the other hand, have a lower remission rate. The risk-based approach to the treatment of pediatric ALL has led investigators to intensify the induction regimen for high-risk patients. It has been suggested that most treatment failures in childhood ALL result from inadequate initial reduction of the leukemic clone and the acquisition of drug resistance by residual lymphoblasts.[38] This is the basis upon which many trials have incorporated four-drug induction remission regimens and aggressive intensification or consolidation regimens in the management of higher-risk patients. Many centers now add an anthracycline such as doxorubicin or daunorubicin to the basic glucocorticoid, vincristine, and asparaginase induction regimen backbone. Other agents that have been used up front in remission induction therapy include cyclophosphamide, methotrexate, cytarabine, and teniposide. Examples of remission induction regimens can be found in Table 122–8.

Historically, prednisone has been the primary glucocorticoid used in pediatric ALL regimens. Some protocols are exploring the role of dexamethasone in place of prednisone. Dexamethasone has an increased duration of biologic activity, higher cerebrospinal fluid (CSF)-to-plasma ratio, and greater lymphotoxic activity on a molar basis than prednisone.[39,40] One study has illustrated that dexamethasone is associated with better prevention of CNS relapse.[41]

Given that the majority of children with ALL will achieve a complete remission by day 28 (usually > 95%), the utility of this as a prognostic indicator is now negligible. Subsequently, day-14 marrow response has been evaluated for its prognostic significance of both early relapse and relapse after discontinuation of therapy.[42] Steinherz and colleagues have recently reported that marrow aspiration on day 7 of therapy provides even more useful information than that done on day 14.[43] A recent trial in Germany stratified patients into postremission therapy arms based on blast count found in peripheral blood after a 7-day exposure to prednisone and one intrathecal dose of methotrexate, because these patients have been found to have a significantly worse prognosis.[44]

CENTRAL NERVOUS SYSTEM PROPHYLAXIS

After patients achieve complete remission, they usually receive central nervous system (CNS) prophylaxis. This phase may overlap with or be incorporated into induction, consolidation, or maintenance. The rationale for CNS prophylaxis is based on two observations. First, many chemotherapeutic agents do not readily cross the blood–brain barrier. Second, many patients with ALL with no evidence of CNS involvement at diagnosis experience a relapse of their leukemia in the CNS. The CNS relapse rate without prophylaxis in adult ALL patients is approximately 21% to 50% and in children it exceeds 50%.[3,7,31,33] Current treatment approaches have reduced the incidence to 10% to 15%.[33] These observations indicate that the CNS is a potential

TABLE 122–7. Representative Chemotherapy Regimens for Adult Acute Lymphocytic Leukemia

Remission Induction		CNS Prophylaxis		Consolidation		Maintenance
Drug and Dose	*Days*	*Prophylaxis*	*Days*	*Drug and Dose*	*Days*	*Drug, Dose, and Timing*
German or Hoelzer Regimen (Adult)[25]						
PRED (PO) 60 mg/m^2	1–28	Cranial irradiation		DEX (PO) 10 mg/m^2	1–28	MP (PO) 60 mg/m^2 qd
VCR (IV) 1.5 mg/m^{2a}	1, 8, 15, 22	MTX (IT) 10 mg/m^{2b}	31, 38, 45, 52	VCR (IV) 1.5 mg/m^{2a}	1, 8, 15, 22	and
DNR (IV) 25 mg/m^2	1, 8, 15, 22			DOX (IV) 25 mg/m^2	1, 8, 15, 22	MTX (PO/IV) 20 mg/m^2 weekly, weeks 10–18 and 29–130
ASP (IV) 5000 U/m^2	1–14					
CTX (IV) 650 mg/m^{2c}	29, 43, 57			CTX (IV) 650 mg/m^{2c}	29	
Ara-C (IV) 75 mg/m^2	31–34, 38–41, 45–48, 52–55			Ara-C (IV) 75 mg/m^2	31–34, 38–41	
				TG (PO) 60 mg/m^2	29–42	
MP (PO) 60 mg/m^2	29–57					
CALGB 8811 (Adult)[26]						
Course I				**Course II: Early Intensification**		**Course V**
CTX (IV) 1200 mg/m^2	1			MTX (IT) 15 mg	1	VCR (IV) 2 mg day 1 monthly
DNR (IV) 45 mg/m^2	1, 2, 3			CTX (IV) 1000 mg/m^2	1	
VCR (IV) 2 mg	1, 8, 15, 22			MP (PO) 60 mg/m^2	1–14	PRED (PO) 60 mg/m^2 days 1–5 monthly
PRED (PO) 60 mg/m^2	1–21			Ara-C (SC) 75 mg/m^2	1–4, 8–11	
ASP (SC) 6000 U/m^2	5, 8, 11, 15, 18, 22			VCR (IV) 2 mg	15, 22	MTX (PO) 20 mg/m^2 days 1, 8, 15, 22 monthly
				ASP (SC) 6000 U/m^2	15, 18, 22, 25	
Induction chemotherapy for patients ≥ 60 yr old, use:						MP (PO) 60 mg/m^2 days 1–28 monthly
CTX 800 mg/m^2	1					
DNR 30 mg/m^2	1–3					
PRED 60 mg/m^2	1–7					
		Course III		**Course IV: Late Intensification**		
		Cranial irradiation		DOX (IV) 30 mg/m^2	1, 8, 15	
		MTX (IT) 15 mg	1, 8, 15, 22, 29	VCR (IV) 2 mg	1, 8, 15	
		MP (PO) 60 mg/m^2	1–70	DEX (PO) 10 mg/m^2	1–14	
		MTX (PO) 20 mg/m^2	36, 43, 50, 57, 64	CTX (IV) 1000 mg/m^2	29	
				TG (PO) 60 mg/m^2	29–42	
				Ara-C (SC) 75 mg/m^2	29–32, 36–39	

Ara-C = cytarabine; ASP = asparaginase; CALGB = Cancer and Leukemia Group B; CNS = central nervous system; CTX = cyclophosphamide; DEX = dexamethasone; DNR = daunorubicin; DOX = doxorubicin; MP = mercaptopurine; MTX = methotrexate; PRED = prednisone; TG = thioguanine; VCR = vincristine.

[a]Maximum single dose, 2 mg.

[b]Maximum single dose, 15 mg.

[c]Maximum single dose, 1000 mg.

TABLE 122–8. Representative Chemotherapy Regimens for Pediatric Acute Lymphocytic Leukemia

Remission Induction			Consolidation		Maintenance
Drug and Dose	*Timing*	CNS Prophylaxis	*Drug and Dose*	*Days*	*Drug, Dose, and Timing*
Children's Cancer Group 1882 (Pediatric)[27]					
PRED (PO) 60 mg/m^2/d	28 d	Cranial irradiation	**Consolidation I**		**Interim Maintenance**
VCR (IV) 1.5 mg/m^2/wk	4 wk	MTX	CTX (IV) 1 g/m^2	0, 28	VCR (IV) 1.5 mg/m^2/d, days 0, 10, 20, 30, 40
DNR (IV) 25 mg/m^2/wk	4 wk		Ara-C (SC/IV) 75 mg/m^2/d	1–4, 8–11, 29–32, 36–39	MTX (IV) 100 mg/m^2/d, days 0, 10, 20, 30, 40
ASP (IM) 6000 U/m^2/3 × weekly 9 doses			MP 60 mg/m^2 PO	0–13, 28–41	ASP (IM) 15,000 U/m^2/d, days 1, 11, 21, 31, 41
			VCR 1.5 mg/m^2/d	14, 21, 42, 49	
			ASP (IM) 6000 U/m^2/d	14, 16, 18, 21, 23, 25, 42, 44, 46, 49, 51, 53	
			Reinduction–Reconsolidation I, II		**Maintenance (3-month cycles)**
			VCR 1.5 mg/m^2/d	0, 7, 14, 42, 49	VCR (IV) 1.5 mg/m^2/d, days 0, 28, 56
			DEX 10 mg/m^2/d PO QD	0–20, then taper	PDN 60 mg/m^2/d, days 0–4, 28–32, 56–60
			DOX 25 mg/m^2/d	0, 7, 14	MP 75 mg/m^2/d, days 0–83
			ASP (IM) 6000 U/m^2	3, 5, 7, 10, 12, 14, 42, 44, 46, 49, 51, 53	MTX 20 mg/m^2/d PO, days 7, 14, 21, 28, 35, 42, 49, 56, 63, 70, 77
			CTX (IV) 1 g/m^2	28	
			Ara-C (SC/IV) 75 mg/m^2/d	29–32, 36–39	
			TG (PO) 60 mg/m^2/d	28–41	
POG 8602 (Pediatric)[28] (ALinC14)					**Overlapping VCR/PRED Pulse Therapy**
PRED (PO) 40 mg/m^2/d (Maximum dose 60 mg/d)	1–29	MTX (IT), Ara-C, HCT	MTX (IV) 1 g/m^2 (with leucovorin rescue)	49, 70, 91,112, 133, 154	Weeks 8, 17, 25, 41, 57, 73, 89, 105:
VCR (IV) 1.5 mg/m^2/wk	1, 8, 15, 22		Ara-C (IV) 1 g/m^2	49, 70, 91,112, 133, 154	VCR (IV) 1.5 mg/m^2/wk × 2 doses
ASP (IM) 6000 U/m^2	1, 3, 5, 8, 10, 12				PRED (PO) 40 mg/m^2/d × 7 days
MP (PO) 75 mg/m^2/d	29–43				**Maintenance**
					Weeks 25–156:
					MP (PO) 75 mg/m^2/d
					MTX (IM) 20 mg/m^2/wk

Ara-C = cytarabine; ASP = asparaginase; CTX = cyclophosphamide; DEX = dexamethasone; DNR = daunorubicin; DOX = doxorubicin; HCT = hydrocortisone, MP = mercaptopurine; MTX = methotrexate; PRED = prednisone; TG = thioguanine; VCR = vincristine.

sanctuary for leukemic cells and that undetectable leukemic cells are present in the CNS in many patients. CNS involvement is more common in ALL than ANLL. CNS involvement at the time of diagnosis is relatively uncommon (5% to 10%) in ALL.[1] Factors that have been associated with an increased risk of CNS involvement at diagnosis include a high initial white blood cell count, rapid leukemic cell proliferation rate (high S-fraction), high plasma lactic dehydrogenase, T-cell phenotype, and B-cell phenotype.[6,33]

The goal of CNS prophylaxis is to eradicate residual but undetectable leukemic cells present in the CNS after remission induction. Leukemic meningitis is more easily prevented than treated. Once CNS relapse has occurred, patients are at increased risk of bone marrow relapse and death from refractory leukemia. It is important to note that the benefit of CNS prophylaxis is not apparent until after 2 years of continuous complete remission. Although CNS prophylaxis has been shown to significantly decrease the risk of CNS relapse in adults, survival in the CNS prophylaxis group was not significantly longer compared with patients not given CNS prophylaxis.[45,46]

Although CNS prophylaxis has not been shown to improve survival in adults with ALL, some form of CNS prophylaxis is usually included in ALL treatment protocols. CNS prophylaxis usually includes cranial irradiation and intrathecal methotrexate to eradicate undetectable leukemia in the cranial region and spinal column, respectively. Cranial irradiation is typically given in 2-Gy fractions to a total dose of 18 to 24 Gy. Methotrexate 10 to 15 mg is given intrathecally once or twice weekly for four to six doses. In some protocols, intrathecal cytosine arabinoside (20 to 100 mg), hydrocortisone (10 to 35 mg), and methotrexate (12 to 15 mg) are given together for CNS prophylaxis.[33]

Initial trials in childhood ALL in the 1960s established cranial irradiation and intrathecal methotrexate as the standards for prevention of CNS relapse. Subsequent efforts have examined the need for radiation because of its potential long-term sequelae. Cranial irradiation has been associated with neuropsychological

TABLE 122–9. Intrathecal Therapy in Pediatric ALL

Age (yr)	Cytarabine (mg)	Methotrexate (mg)	Hydrocortisone (mg)
≥ 1	16	8	8
≥ 2	20	10	10
3–8	24	12	12
≥ 9	30	15	15

ALL = acute lymphocytic leukemia.
Adapted from Ref. 28.

deficits, endocrine dysfunction, greater susceptibility to brain tumors (in children exposed at age 5 or less), short stature, and obesity.[14] Furthermore, it has been reported that about 50% of children receiving cranial irradiation will develop a "somnolence syndrome" characterized by some degree of lethargy, irritability, or low-grade fever at a median onset of 4 to 8 weeks.[5] Adults typically experience somnolence, headache, meningismus, transient paraplegia, arachnoiditis, or injection-site infections.[33]

In the 1980s, trials were conducted examining intrathecal chemotherapy alone or combined with radiation therapy at lower doses than previously used in children. The majority of children with good-prognosis ALL can be treated with age-adjusted doses of either intrathecal methotrexate or triple intrathecal chemotherapy (methotrexate, cytarabine, and hydrocortisone).[47,48] Most treatment protocols now reserve cranial irradiation for patients with overt CNS leukemia at diagnosis or for patients with certain prognostic factors placing them at higher risk of CNS relapse (WBC count > 100,000/mm^3, T-cell ALL with WBC count > 50,000, Philadelphia chromosome–positive ALL, and infants).[5] The doses of intrathecal chemotherapy used in pediatric ALL patients must be individualized based on age due to differences in the volume of cerebrospinal fluid at various ages (Table 122–9).

Trials in adults were also performed to reduce radiation therapy's role. Patients who receive high-dose methotrexate (100 to 300 mg/kg/d monthly for 12 months) may have a CNS relapse rate as low as 8.3%, and with high-dose cytarabine (2 g/m^2 every 12 hours for 12 doses) with systemic methotrexate (200 to 800 mg/m^2) the rate is 11%.[49,50] Recent prospective studies have demonstrated that intravenous high-dose methotrexate alone (usually greater than 1000 mg/m^2 per dose as a short infusion) or intermediate-dose methotrexate (range, 50 to 1000 mg/m^2 per dose, but usually 500 to 1000 mg/m^2 per dose as a long infusion) with intrathecal triple chemotherapy can offer equal protection against CNS relapse as well as standard cranial irradiation and intrathecal methotrexate.[6]

The selection of a CNS prophylaxis regimen must consider efficacy, toxicity, and risk of CNS disease. Patients with low risk of ALL relapse may be adequately treated with only intrathecal therapy. Those with high-risk ALL may need a combination of intrathecal and systemic chemotherapy. Because few randomized studies have compared different CNS regimens in ALL, it is not possible to recommend any one regimen over another. Based on the experience with childhood ALL, CNS prophylaxis should be included in treatment protocols for both childhood and adult ALL and should include intrathecal methotrexate either alone or combined with cranial irradiation, or intravenous infusions of intermediate-dose methotrexate with intrathecal triple chemotherapy, or intravenous high-dose methotrexate or high-dose cytarabine alone.

CONSOLIDATION THERAPY

Consolidation therapy in adult ALL is started after a complete remission has been achieved, and refers to continued intensive chemotherapy in an attempt to eradicate clinically undetectable disease. Many regimens usually incorporate either non–cross-resistant drugs different from the induction regimen or else high-dose chemotherapy.[32] The specific benefit of any one consolidation therapy is difficult to demonstrate because of the overall complexity of therapy in ALL. Randomized trials have been equivocal in demonstrating a survival benefit.[31,33] The two adult regimens listed in Table 122–7 offer two different approaches to consolidation with similar results. The German regimen mostly imitates the induction regimen, but substitutes dexamethasone for prednisone (better CNS penetration to prevent leukemic meningitis), doxorubicin for daunorubicin, and thioguanine for mercaptopurine.[25] The CALGB (Cancer and Leukemia Group B) trial uses a consolidation regimen far more complicated than the induction regimen. The latter includes different drugs and higher doses, at least with the cyclophosphamide dose.[26] The outcome from these distinctly different trials are similar. The German investigators found a median survival of 27.5 months and an estimated 5-year survival of 39%.[25] The CALGB study reported a short follow-up time (median, 43 months) so that only 3-year estimates were available; however, the results included a median survival of 36 months and an overall survival of 39% for those 30 to 59 years old.[26] A consolidation phase in adult ALL therapy appears necessary, although specific questions remain about drug selection, duration of therapy, dosing, and timing of administration.

A phase of dose-intensified chemotherapy usually follows induction in pediatric ALL therapy, especially in patients with recognized poor-risk factors. No specific chemotherapy combination is considered standard of care. Table 122–8 lists two pediatric trials with distinctly different consolidation approaches. Clinical trials incorporating consolidation in the treatment of high-risk ALL have reported long-term survival for 65% to 70% of patients.[6]

MAINTENANCE THERAPY

Many patients relapse shortly after completion of remission induction and consolidation therapy, presumably because of residual disease. Maintenance therapy allows long-term drug exposure to slowly dividing cells, allows the immune system time to eradicate leukemia cells, and promotes apoptosis (programmed cell death).[14,31] The goal of maintenance therapy is therefore to further eradicate residual leukemic cells and prolong remission duration. Although maintenance therapy is clearly beneficial in childhood ALL, the possible benefit in adults has only recently been suggested. In some adult ALL trials that included induction and consolidation, but omitted maintenance, the disease-free survival at 2 years was only 18% to 35% compared to a survival rate of almost 40% in trials that included maintenance.[1,51–53]

Maintenance therapy usually consists of mercaptopurine and methotrexate, at doses that produce minimal myelosuppression, with or without intermittent "pulses" of vincristine and prednisone, or occasionaly an anthracycline or cyclophosphamide.[3] The typical doses for these agents in this phase are listed in Tables 122–7 and 122–8. The optimal duration of maintenance therapy in adults and children is unknown, but most treatment programs continue maintenance therapy for at least 30 months. Most recently, clinicians have begun to make decisions about maintenance therapy based upon what subtype of ALL is found. Common pre–B-cell ALL does benefit from conventional maintenance therapy with methotrexate and mercaptopurine. Patients with B-cell ALL or Philadelphia chromosome–positive ALL probably gain greater benefit from intensive induction and consolidation and little from maintenance.[33]

An additional issue in maintenance therapy of pediatric ALL has been interpatient variability in the pharmacokinetics of oral methotrexate and mercaptopurine. Slow absorbers and rapid eliminators are at higher risk of treatment failure because of decreased exposure to methotrexate or mercaptopurine.[54–56] Futhermore, patients who take their oral methotrexate and mercaptopurine on an evening versus a morning schedule appear to have a superior outcome.[57,58] To account for the interpatient variability, some clinicians titrate the dose of either agent to maintain a WBC count of 1500 to 4000/mm^3. Some protocols circumvent bioavailability and poor compliance problems altogether by parenteral administration of methotrexate. The importance of these pharmacokinetic issues in adults is less well defined.

In an effort to determine the long-term outcome of the duration and intensity of maintenance therapy, the Childhood ALL Collaborative Group recently published findings from a large meta-analysis involving 12,000 randomized children from 42 trials initiated prior to 1987.[59] The analysis revealed that longer maintenance, pulses of vincristine and prednisone, and the inclusion of one or two intensive reinduction courses significantly reduced total number of deaths or relapse. However, only intensive reinduction could improve overall survival.

ALL IN THE ELDERLY

One-third of all ALL cases occur in patients over age 60 but no specific treatment recommendations can be made. The response to therapy and durability of response seem less than in younger adults or children. Older patients have a higher incidence than younger patients of the Philadelphia chromosome and a lower occurrence of T-cell ALL.[31] Recent trials that included patients over age 60 demonstrated that the 3-year survival rate could be up to 20%.[34] For example, in CALGB 8811 (Table 122–7), 9% of the patients were over age 60. The complete remission rate was approximately 65%, but the 3-year survival was only 17%.[26] In general, older patients have a lower complete remission rate and, when achieved, the duration of remission is shorter than with younger patients.

ACUTE NONLYMPHOCYTIC LEUKEMIA

Acute nonlymphocytic leukemia (ANLL) accounts for the majority of acute leukemia in adults and occurs with increasing frequency in elderly patients. It accounts for only 20% of the acute leukemias in children but is responsible for 30% of leukemia-related mortality.[60] With recent advances in chemotherapy and supportive care, 60% to 80% of all patients achieve complete remission and 15% to 30% become long-term survivors.[1,61] In children, the long-term survival with chemotherapy may be 30% to 45%.[6] Overall, the median duration of remission is 1 to 2 years.[61] In patients over age 60, the median duration of remission is shorter than 1 year. In contrast to ALL, all of the active drugs in ANLL are marrow suppressive, with the exception of all-*trans*-retinoic acid (ATRA). As a result, patients with ANLL, particularly elderly patients (over age 60), are at greater risk for treatment-related fatal infectious and bleeding complications.

Treatment of ANLL, unlike that of ALL, usually only consists of induction and intensive postremission therapy (IPRT) (see Fig. 122–2). Central nervous system prophylaxis is not routinely given for ANLL because the risk of CNS relapse is lower than in patients with ALL. Several representative chemotherapeutic regimens for treatment of ANLL are presented in Table 122–10.

REMISSION INDUCTION THERAPY

As with ALL, the goal of remission induction for ANLL is to rapidly induce a complete remission. Compared with ALL, fewer patients with ANLL achieve complete remission. The lower complete remission rate in ANLL is related in part to differences in the toxicity of the drugs in remission induction regimens. In ALL, several active agents are relatively nonmyelosuppressive (prednisone, vincristine, *L*-asparaginase), whereas in ANLL, every active agent (except all-*trans*-retinoic acid) is myelosuppressive. As a result, patients with ALL may achieve complete remission without severe and prolonged marrow hypoplasia. In contrast, because the complete remission rate in ANLL is related to the intensity of the remission induction regimen, the drugs used in ANLL are given at doses that uniformly cause severe marrow hypoplasia. One reason for the lower complete remission rate in ANLL compared with ALL is the inability to give optimal doses of chemotherapy because of marrow toxicity. With continued improvement of supportive care for patients undergoing chemotherapy, more intensive treatment regimens are being given in an effort to reduce the high rate of leukemic relapse and increase the proportion of long-term survivors.

The most active single agents in ANLL are the anthracycline antibiotics (daunorubicin, doxorubicin, and idarubicin) and the antimetabolite cytarabine. The complete remission rate with a combination of cytarabine and an anthracycline is 60% to 80%.[61–63] The remission rate is lower (approximately 50%) in patients over age 60.[61] Several trials have attempted to improve upon conventional "7 + 3" therapy (7 days of cytarabine

TABLE 122–10. Representative Chemotherapy Regimens for Adult Acute Nonlymphocytic Leukemia

Remission Induction	Intensive Postremission Therapy	Maintenance Therapy
Southeastern Cancer Study Group[62]		
Cytarabine 100 mg/m^2/d continuous infusion, days 1–7 Idarubicin 12 mg/m^2/d, days 1–3	Cytarabine 100 mg/m^2 every 12 h for 10 doses Thioguanine 100 mg/m^2 PO every 12 h for 10 doses Idarubicin 15 mg/m^2/d on day 1 (3 courses)	None
CALGB[63]		
Cytarabine 200 mg/m^2/d, days 1–7 continuous infusion Daunorubicin 45 mg/m^2/d, days 1–3	Cytarabine 3 g/m^2 every 12 h, days 1, 3, 5 (4 courses)	Cytarabine 100 mg/m^2 SC every 12 h, days 1–5 Daunorubicin 45 mg/m^2 day 1 (4 courses)
Boston Group[64]		
Daunorubicin 45 mg/m^2/d, days 1–3 Cytarabine 100 mg/m^2/d, days 1–7 continuous infusion	Cycles 1, 3: Daunorubicin 60 mg/m^2/d, days 1–2 Cytarabine 200 mg/m^2/d, days 1–5 continuous infusion	
Cytarabine 2 g/m^2 every 12 h, days 8–10	Cycle 2: Cytarabine 2 g/m^2 every 12 h, days 1–3 Etoposide 100 mg/m^2/d, days 4–5	

CALB = Cancer and Leukemia Group B.

100 mg/m^2/d continuous infusion and 3 days of daunorubicin 45 mg/m^2 bolus), but have shown no improvement by (1) increasing cytarabine to 10 days, (2) shortening cytarabine to 5 days, (3) substituting doxorubicin for daunorubicin, (4) adding thioguanine, or (5) increasing cytarabine to 200 mg/m^2/d continuous infusion.[3]

Idarubicin has been one significant advance in adult ANLL induction therapy in recent years. Some studies have shown a significant improvement in complete remission rate over daunorubicin. In the Southeastern Cancer Study Group trial comparing these two drugs, complete remission was achieved in 69% of patients receiving idarubicin/cytarabine compared to 55% of patients receiving conventional daunorubicin/cytarabine. Median survival in this study was not significantly improved (297 versus 277 days for idarubicin and daunorubicin, respectively).[62] In a similar study with similar complete remission rates, the median time of survival was significantly longer, with survival reaching 328 to 508 days with idarubicin/cytarabine versus 277 to 435 days for daunorubicin/cytarabine.[65] Idarubicin has replaced daunorubicin as the anthracycline of choice for remission induction in adult ANLL in many protocols.

The third regimen in Table 122–10 illustrates another maneuver to improve the complete remission rate in adults. Mitus and colleagues added high-dose cytarabine to conventional 7 + 3 therapy.[64] The remission rate after induction therapy in this trial was 89%, which is higher than that achieved in the Southeastern Cancer Study Group or the CALGB trial reported in Table 122–10. The validity of this result, and the possible impact of substituting idarubicin for daunorubicin in the therapy reported by Mitus and associates, remains to be confirmed by other trials.

Another approach used by clinicians is to employ high-dose cytarabine (1 to 3 g/m^2/dose given every 12 hours for 6 to 12 doses total) in induction chemotherapy. Two recent trials using high-dose cytarabine with an anthracycline reported no improvement in the complete remission rate, but disease-free survival was statistically better.[66,67] This approach should only be considered in patients under age 55 because of increased neurotoxicity in older individuals without any improvement in remission rate or survival.

Recently the National Comprehensive Cancer Network (NCCN) published guidelines for the treatment of ANLL. The classic 7 + 3 regimen may be a disservice to patients under age 60 because the long-term durability is less than some recent studies that employed high-dose cytarabine in induction.[68] The NCCN committee actually recommended more aggressive chemotherapy compared to historical approaches, using high-dose cytarabine with an anthracycline if the patient was under age 60 in order to improve survival. In patients over age 60 or with a generally poor performance status, then conventional 7 + 3 should be used.

Most patients achieve a complete remission after one or two courses of chemotherapy. Patients who require additional chemotherapy to achieve a complete remission have been reported to have a poor prognosis, even if remission is ultimately achieved.

As with adult ANLL, the most effective remission regimens for children have included an anthracycline with cytarabine with or without thioguanine, yielding a remission rate of 70% to 85%. Recent trials have examined the combination of non–cross-resistant drugs used simultaneously in an effort to overcome possible induction failure due to selection and growth of drug-resistant clones arising by spontaneous mutation. A recent trial compared cytarabine, daunorubicin, etoposide, thioguanine, and dexamethasone with standard 7 + 3 therapy with cytarabine and daunorubicin and found them to be equally effective.[69]

INTENSIVE POSTREMISSION THERAPY

Although most adults with ANLL achieve a complete remission, the duration of remission is short (4 to 8 months) if no further treatment is given. Relapse is presumably due to the presence of residual but clinically undetectable leukemic cells after remission induction therapy. The goal of intensive postremission therapy (IPRT) is to eradicate these residual leukemic cells and to prevent the emergence of drug-resistant disease. The need for IPRT is based on postmortem analysis and cell kinetic data suggesting that nearly 10^9 residual leukemic cells remain after effective remission induction therapy.[3]

In the treatment of ANLL, IPRT is often referred to as consolidation or intensification. Consolidation is instituted after a complete remission is achieved but involves the administration of drugs that the patient has not previously received. Intensification therapy is defined as the administration of one or two courses of high doses of the same drugs used for remission induction, immediately after a complete remission is achieved. Intensification may be started early (within a few months of achievement of remission) or late (complete remission longer than 6 to 12 months). As consolidation and intensification are sometimes defined differently by different investigators, both phrases are referred to as IPRT throughout this section. IPRT may be defined as the administration of high-dose combination chemotherapy to a patient in complete remission in an attempt to eradicate clinically undetectable disease.

Most centers incorporate some form of IPRT into ANLL therapy. No consensus exists regarding the best drugs, doses, or duration of treatment. The three regimens in Table 122–10 offer three distinctly different approaches to postremission therapy. The Southeastern group used a consolidation regimen similar to the induction regimen, in terms of dose intensity and drug selection.[62] The median duration of remission in the idarubicin patients was 433 days. CALGB compared three doses of cytarabine: 100 mg/m^2, 400 mg/m^2, and 3 g/m^2.[63] At 4 years, the disease-free survival for all patients was 21%, 25%, and 39% for the three doses, respectively. Disease-free survival was statistically superior for the 3-g/m^2 dose compared to the other two doses for all patients combined and for patients under age 60. For patients over age 60, disease-free survival at 4 years did not differ among the three consolidative regimens. Finally, in the study from Boston, IPRT included a combination of standard-dose cytarabine and daunorubicin for two cycles with a combination of intensified cytarabine with etoposide given in between.[64] Many of the patients later underwent bone marrow transplant (BMT). The overall survival at 5 years was 55%.

It is not clear whether the same agents (cytarabine and an anthracycline) given for remission induction should be used for IPRT in higher doses or whether different agents altogether should be given. If leukemic relapse is caused by a resistant cell line, then the use of agents different from and non–cross-resistant with drugs used in induction would appear to be beneficial.

High-dose cytarabine appears to be a key part of IPRT today, especially if not used in induction therapy. How many g/m^2 of cytarabine to give, how many doses per cycle, or how many cycles of cytarabine to give remain unanswered questions. The only generally accepted practice is that induction alone is insufficient and that some form of IPRT prolongs survival. The NCCN guidelines recommend four cycles of high-dose cytarabine for patients under 60 and with good cytogenetics. If over age 60, then use a dose-reduced high-dose cytarabine regimen or enroll in a clinical trial. Patients with unfavorable cytogenetics, underlying myelodysplastic syndrome, or secondary ANLL should be referred for a bone marrow transplant.[68]

Children with ANLL should also receive IPRT if a stem cell transplant is not available. The event-free survival is again about 30% to 40%. Drugs given for pediatric ANLL usually include cytarabine, asparaginase, thioguanine, vincristine, azacytidine, cyclophosphamide, daunorubicin, doxorubicin, mercaptopurine, methotrexate, etoposide, amsacrine, or dexamethasone. A survival advantage has been shown for those patients who have a HLA-compatible sibling donor and who go on to receive an allogeneic transplantation, yielding a 5-year disease-free survival rate of 50% to 54%.[69,70] There appears, however, to be no survival advantage for autologous transplant over intensive chemotherapy for ANLL in first remission (event-free survival at 3 years of 36% to 38%).[71]

ANLL IN THE ELDERLY

Many older patients tolerate ANLL induction and consolidation as well as younger patients, but often therapy fails because of fatal infections and bleeding. Patients over age 60 tend to have more cytogenetic abnormalities, underlying myelodysplasia, and a poorer performance status, all of which compromise the long-term success of therapy.[72] The complete remission rate varies from as low as 31% to as high as 65%.[73,74] Concern exists about the value of chemotherapy and decreased quality of life when treating older patients. Three approaches have been examined: (1) no therapy, (2) standard anthracycline/cytarabine induction, and (3) low-dose cytarabine. Löwenberg and colleagues prospectively randomized patients to either a conventional chemotherapy arm or an observation arm on which patients could receive modest doses of chemotherapy for symptom palliation. The chemotherapy group survived a median of 21 weeks versus 11 weeks for the observation group. The quality of life of each group was similar, each spending approximately 50% of the study time in the hospital.[75] Chemotherapy may prolong survival without significantly decreasing the quality of life for elderly patients.

Standard anthracycline/cytarabine therapy has been tried in older patients with less positive results than in younger patients.[72–74] The complete response rate may be only near 33% compared to twice that for younger patients. The mortality rate during induction, usually due to infections, is approximately 20%.[75,76] For the patients who achieve a remission, the median disease-free survival is less than 1 year. The studies performed in elderly ANLL patients demonstrate less frequent complete remissions and less durable remissions compared to younger patients.[75,76] An alternative standard-dose chemotherapy regimen investigated has been mitoxantrone and etoposide; this yielded a complete response rate of 55% in a case series of 67 patients.[77]

A third approach uses low-dose cytarabine 10 mg/m^2 subcutaneously for up to 6 weeks. Low-dose cytarabine is believed to work as a differentiating agent that promotes the normal development of a leukemic blast to a normal myeloid cell. Although the experience with low-dose cytarabine is limited, the complete remission rate, the duration of remission, and survival may be comparable to that achieved by conventional chemotherapy in this age group. In one trial, patients were randomized between low-dose cytarabine and conventional chemotherapy and no difference was found in survival or remission duration. Patients receiving chemotherapy had more infections and required more blood product transfusions.[78] In contrast, in a case series using only low-dose subcutaneous cytarabine, the complete response rate was 23% compared to perhaps 65% with conventional chemotherapy in younger patients.[78] This low-dose regimen yielded a median duration of remission of 9.9 months, but even those who maintained remission had a median survival of only 19.5 months.[79] Compared to younger patients with ANLL, in this study the remissions in elderly ANLL patients were less frequent and durable.

No specific recommendations can be made to treat ANLL in the elderly. Some patients will tolerate conventional chemotherapy, but identifying such patients is difficult. Low-dose cytarabine appears to be an option that can induce a remission in some cases, can be given at home, and is less toxic, but it probably does not lead to long-term survival.

ACUTE PROMYELOCYTIC LEUKEMIA

Acute promyelocytic leukemia (APL) is one subclass of ANLL that makes up 10% of all cases. It has historically been diagnosed by the distinctive cytoplasmic granules seen on light microscopy. Treatment has been the same as other subclasses of ANLL. Most recently, the genetic abnormality and pathophysiology of the disease have become better understood. Concurrently, a new treatment modality has been developed, that of differentiation therapy with all-*trans*-retinoic acid (ATRA), which allows induction of remission without life-threatening pancytopenia.[18] The pharmacology, pharmacokinetics, and toxicity of ATRA are reviewed in Chapter 115.

In APL, differentiation and maturation are arrested at the level of the promyelocyte. Examination of the chromosomes reveals a translocation between numbers 15 and 17. Chromosome 15 carries the gene for the retinoic acid receptor. Normal binding of retinoids to this receptor leads to cell proliferation and differentiation, among other functions. The retinoic acid–receptor gene clusters on chromosome 17 near a second gene named PML. The fusion of the these two genes leads to production of a protein that presumably impairs differentiation. The discovery of the 15/17 translocation now provides a cytogenetic marker of the disease. It is a prognostic marker in favor of response to ATRA.[18]

ATRA was first reported in 1987 to induce remission in patients with APL.[80] Subsequently over 1500 patients worldwide have been treated with this new therapy and it has recently obtained FDA approval.[18] ATRA is usually given orally in a dose of 45 mg/m^2 as a single dose or divided into two doses, given after a meal. Depending on the clinical situation, it may be given prior to or after chemotherapy. The complete remission rate can be as high as 95% in patients with the 15/17 translocation. The time to achieve remission may be 1 to 3 months. ATRA does not cross the blood–brain barrier; therefore, leukemic meningitis should be treated with conventional intrathecal chemotherapy. ATRA is usually only given for initial induction because continuous use leads to autoinduction of cytochrome P450 enzymes, enhanced metabolism, and declining blood concentrations. An alternative explanation of why ATRA's activity wanes over time is that leukemic cells overexpress cellular retinoic acid–binding proteins that bind and trap ATRA in the cell, thus lowering plasma concentrations necessary to promote differentiation. The median duration of remission when ATRA is given alone is only 3.5 months.[18] As a result, ATRA induction is followed now with conventional chemotherapy consolidation.

Several clinical trials have now reported positive results with ATRA. The results are summarized in Table 122–11. The complete remission rate is usually quite high (85% to 95%). Disease-free survival, event-free survival, or overall survival are

TABLE 122–11. Results From Clinical Trials With All-*Trans*-Retinoic Acid in Untreated Patients

Authors	Trial Design	CR Rate (%)	DFS (> 2 yr) (%)
Fenaux et al[81]	Randomize against chemotherapy	91	79[a]
Kanamaru et al[82]	Historical controls	89	75
Tallman et al[83]	Randomize against chemotherapy	72	67
Frankel et al[84]	Historical controls	86	
		Med OS	31 mo

CR = complete response; DFS = disease-free survival; Med OS = median overall survival.

[a]Statistically better than comparative group.

usually also better than historical or current controls receiving chemotherapy alone. The efficacy can be shown for newly diagnosed patients or those with prior chemotherapy administration. In general, the four trials also showed less life-threatening toxicity than conventional chemotherapy. The major adverse reactions to ATRA included headache, skin and mucous membrane reactions, bone pain, and nausea.

When ATRA is started, rapid onset of differentiation of promyelocytes occurs, which can lead to leukocytosis and/or retinoic acid syndrome. The retinoic acid syndrome (fever, respiratory distress, interstitial pulmonary infiltrates, and weight gain) may be fatal in one-third of cases. In order to avoid this problem, chemotherapy may be combined with ATRA during induction. Various guidelines regarding the initial WBC count have been used to signal the need for chemotherapy, such as a WBC count of 3000, 5000, or 10,000/mm^3. All investigators agree that if the WBC count exceeds 20,000/mm^3, then a patient needs combination therapy. In addition, other investigators add chemotherapy to ATRA if the WBC count rises more than 4000/mm^3 over the first 2 days of ATRA therapy.[85]

ATRA induces remission in most patients with newly diagnosed or relapsed APL. It is safer than conventional induction chemotherapy, except for the retinoic acid syndrome. The rapid evolution in understanding APL and the role of ATRA should enable more patients to achieve a rapid remission without the complications of conventional chemotherapy.

RELAPSE

Most adult patients with acute leukemia who achieve complete remission eventually experience a leukemic relapse. In children, the relapse rate in ANLL is approximately the same as adults, but less frequent in pediatric ALL. Relapse usually occurs in the bone marrow, but may also occur in the CNS or other extramedullary sites. Treatment and outcome depend primarily on whether relapse occurred during or after completion of treatment. Duration of the initial remission is probably the most important factor associated with the ability to achieve a second remission.[1] After the first relapse, the median survival is 6 to 8 months, with only 7% of patients alive at 3 years.[86]

About one-half of patients with ALL or ANLL who experience a leukemic relapse while receiving chemotherapy achieve a second complete remission with chemotherapy, but remission duration usually lasts only several months, and long-term survivors are uncommon. Some patients with ALL who relapse after chemotherapy is discontinued, however, can experience prolonged survival with chemotherapy. There is no consensus regarding appropriate drugs for reinduction or consolidation after relapse has occurred. Bone marrow transplantation may be undertaken if the patient is a suitable candidate (see Chap. 125).

Salvage therapy for ALL has involved similar drugs used during initial induction administered on different schedules. The VAD regimen reported by the MD Anderson group used a 4-day continuous infusion of vincristine and doxorubicin with intensive dexamethasone therapy. IPRT followed for 24 to 30 months. Overall, 39% of patients achieved a remission and 20% were disease free at 2 years.[87] Another reported regimen uses prednisone, intermediate-dose cytarabine, mitoxantrone, and etoposide in relapsed or refractory ALL. Seventy percent achieved remission with a median survival of 7 months.[88] Combinations with high-dose cytarabine or methotrexate are also commonly employed.

Several agents, including high-dose cytarabine, etoposide, intermediate- or high-dose methotrexate, *L*-asparaginase, carboplatin, mitoxantrone, and idarubicin have been useful in the treatment of relapsed or resistant ANLL. If the relapse occurs 6 months or more beyond the initial remission, then induction with the original chemotherapy may be successful. Single-agent therapy with high-dose cytarabine can yield a complete response rate of 12% to 70%. High-dose cytarabine with etoposide can produce a response rate of 70%.[86] Most recently, the combination of mitoxantrone, etoposide, and cytarabine has yielded a complete remission rate of 60%.[89] Some patients went on to bone marrow transplantation as postremission therapy. The patients who received conventional chemotherapy as consolidation had a median survival of only 7 months. Finally, in an effort to incorporate newer agents active in ANLL into treatment protocols, fludarabine has been combined with cytarabine and granulocyte colony-stimulating factor (G-CSF) to treat relapsed patients. From 28 patients, the complete response rate was 22%.[90]

In childhood ALL, the combination of vincristine, prednisone, asparaginase, and daunorubicin produces complete remissions in approximately 80% to 90% of patients treated for an initial bone marrow relapse.[6] Unfortunately, second remissions are not as durable as first remissions. The duration of second remission is highly dependent upon whether the relapse occurs while therapy is ongoing. Prolonged second remissions (those exceeding 2 years) can be achieved with aggressive chemotherapy in up to 40% of patients who relapse after elective termination of therapy as compared to only 10% to 30% of patients who relapse on therapy.[6] Data suggest that allogeneic hematopoietic stem cell transplantation is the treatment of choice following ALL in second remission, offering 5-year leukemia-free survival of 40% compared to 17% for salvage chemotherapy alone.[91] Autologous transplantation of ALL in second remission appears to offer no survival advantage over postinduction conventional chemotherapy.[92]

For pediatric patients with relapsed ANLL, the chances for prolonged remission with aggressive chemotherapy alone are far more dismal than in ALL, with lower than 10% survival at 1 year.[93] Fortunately, either allogeneic or autologous bone marrow transplantation in second remission may offer long-term survival for 30% to 40% of children.[93]

Of recent interest is the improved understanding of leukemic cell resistance. One mechanism identified has been the P-glycoprotein, a membrane-bound protein capable of removing certain antineoplastics from the intracellular space into the extracellular space. Antileukemic drugs affected by this resistance mechanism include vincristine, doxorubicin, daunorubicin, etoposide, and teniposide. This protein is encoded by the MDR gene (multidrug-resistance gene). Certain substances have been recognized as antagonists of the P-glycoprotein, among them cyclosporine and its analogs. Considerable research is now under way to develop compounds that, when administered with conventional drugs such as daunorubicin or etoposide, would overcome resistance to these agents.[94]

BONE MARROW TRANSPLANTATION

For both ALL and ANLL, bone marrow transplantation (BMT) is yet another viable treatment option once remission is induced. The specific role of either allogeneic or autologous BMT in the treatment of acute leukemia is still being developed; however, its acceptance for high-risk patients and patients in relapse is fairly high. The reader is referred to Chapter 125 for specific details regarding BMT techniques, toxicities, and supportive care.

A number of confounding variables make comparison of chemotherapy and BMT in acute leukemia difficult. For example, the remission induction regimen used is usually different between studies or even within a single study. Conventional consolidation may or may not be given after induction and before BMT. The BMT preparative regimen used can vary from study to study. The source of stem cells, the application of purging techniques to the marrow, the use of colony-stimulating factors, and advances in supportive care all influence the comparison of chemotherapy and BMT. Not all patients are equally eligible for allogeneic BMT, because only 30% of the patients will have an HLA-matched sibling donor. The use of HLA-matched unrelated donor marrow has broadened the pool of donors but increases the risk of transplant-related complications such as graft-versus-host disease (GVHD). Eligibility for bone marrow transplant is frequently limited by age (e.g., under age 50), while the median age for ANLL patients is 62 to 64 years old. Last, the timing of transplantation can vary from study to study. In some studies, patients are transplanted immediately after initial remission and, in other studies, transplanted at the point of early relapse or in second or later remission. The difficulties in comparing chemotherapy alone to BMT arise from a lack of consensus on what constitutes the best chemotherapy and best BMT care.

ACUTE NONLYMPHOCYTIC LEUKEMIA

In the treatment of ANLL, allogeneic BMT has been compared to chemotherapy in patients in first complete remission. In general, disease-free survival and overall survival are longer with BMT. At 4 to 5 years beyond transplantation, 48% to 66% of BMT patients are alive compared to 13% to 21% of patients receiving conventional chemotherapy.[95] Chemotherapy has never been shown superior to BMT but, in some studies, BMT has been statistically better than chemotherapy.[95] Leukemic relapse is less with BMT. In BMT patients, the risk is 13% to 34% compared with 60% to 88% of patients receiving chemotherapy, and this difference has been statistically significant in some studies.[95] In children in first complete remission, if a matched sibling donor is available, then BMT is the preferred IPRT. The 5-year disease-free survival rate is 50% to 54%.[69,70] Autologous bone marrow transplantation offers no advantage over conventional chemotherapy, with an event-free survival at 3 years of 36% to 38%.

Patients who relapse after an initial remission should be offered allogeneic BMT if a donor is available. A recent comparison of allogeneic BMT with autologous BMT or high-dose cytarabine revealed no clinical benefit between the three in disease-free or overall survival after first complete remission, except for patients with recognized high-risk cytogenetics.[96]

Autologous BMT is available to a larger number of patients because the patient serves as the donor and because patients up to age 60 can undergo such a transplant, unlike allogeneic transplants. Most clinicians agree that autologous marrow should be harvested early in remission, when any possible leukemic burden will be low. Results indicate that long-term survival is similar with autologous BMT compared to allogeneic BMT. Whether to purge the autologous marrow of leukemic cells remains an unresolved issue. The survival rate is approximately equal with purged or unpurged marrow regardless of phase of disease. Purged marrow has not been shown clinically superior to unpurged marrow, but many patients still receive purged marrow. The general consensus at this time is that ANLL patients in second or later remission who do not qualify for an allogeneic BMT should be offered autologous BMT as soon as possible after achieving remission.[97]

According to the recently published NCCN guidelines, the decision to proceed to BMT depends on cytogenetics. If the patient has a low-risk cytogenetic profile and is under age 60, then high-dose cytarabine for four cycles is preferred over autologous or allogeneic BMT. If the patient has a poor-risk cytogenetic profile and is under age 60, then allogeneic or matched unrelated donor transplant should be considered early after remission induction. Autologous marrow can be used if a hematologic and cytogenetic remission was achieved. For patients over age 60 years, BMT is not recommended, and either enrollment into a clinical trial or conventional high-dose cytarabine should be considered. For the ANLL patient in early relapse, if a sibling or matched unrelated donor is available, then BMT is the primary therapy because conventional chemotherapy will offer little help. If the relapse occurred late, then BMT can be used as postremission consolidation after conventional induction therapy.[68]

The newest source of stem cells is cytokine-mobilized peripheral blood progenitor cells (PBPCs). Giving cytokines to the patient, syngeneic donor, or an allogeneic donor can generate a pool of stem cells collected by pheresis and reinfused after the patient receives chemotherapy. Recent experience has demonstrated that neutropenia and thrombocytopenia are of a short duration compared to marrow transplants. In the autologous setting, PBPC transplants may allow leukemia patients over age 55 to be transplanted. In the allogeneic setting, the incidence of GVHD does not appear worse.[1,3]

ACUTE LYMPHOCYTIC LEUKEMIA

Allogeneic BMT has also been employed in the treatment of ALL. As a general approach, allogeneic BMT is equivalent to IPRT for patients in first remission and superior to chemotherapy once a relapse has occurred. Horowitz and colleagues conducted a retrospective review of 484 patients in first remission who received conventional IPRT and 250 patients in first remission who received an allogeneic BMT.[98] The 5-year probability of leukemia-free survival was 38% for patients receiving chemotherapy and 44% for patients undergoing BMT. This difference was not statistically significant. The probability of relapse was higher for the chemotherapy group (59%) than for the BMT group (26%). BMT patients died more often from transplant-related complications such as GVHD, interstitial pneumonitis, or infection. Because the initial remission is usually easily achieved in ALL and no benefit to BMT has been demonstrated in immediate postremission BMT, allogeneic BMT is not recommended in first remission for most patients.

Once a relapse has occurred, an allogeneic BMT should be performed if a donor is available. According to data from the International Bone Marrow Transplant Registry, the 5-year disease-free survival for adult patients undergoing allogeneic BMT in second or later remission is 30% and the probability of relapse is 50%, based on a population of over 750 reported patients.[98] A study specifically done in children demonstrated that in second remission ALL, an allogeneic BMT could reduce the risk of relapse at 5 years from 80% to 45% regardless of prognostic risk factors.[91] The risk of leukemic relapse after BMT increases if BMT is delayed to later remissions. Five-year survival is 40% with allogeneic BMT but only 17% with salvage chemotherapy.[91]

A number of risk factors have been identified that may determine who with ALL should be transplanted while in first remission. Transplantation during first remission should be considered for patients with an L_3 marrow, Philadelphia chromosome–positive cytogenetics and certain other cytogenetic findings, a WBC count over 35,000, age over 35, an initial marrow recovery greater than 4 weeks, relapse that occurs during chemotherapy, or having B-cell ALL.[99]

Autologous BMT has not been applied as often in ALL. As with ANLL, various purging techniques have been tried, and the value of purging remains debatable. When used in first remission, autologous BMT yields an overall survival of 20% to 65%. In second or later remission the survival is 18% to 38%.[3] Compared to conventional postremission chemotherapy, autologous BMT offers no survival advantage after an initial remission is achieved. After a relapse occurs, autologous BMT does lead to longer disease-free survival than could be gained from conventional chemotherapy. Compared to allogeneic BMT for patients in second remission or later, overall survival is similar or worse, but the relapse rate is greater with autologous BMT (79% versus 56%).[3] Autologous BMT remains an option for patients after relapse when a suitable donor is not available.

USE OF HEMATOPOIETIC GROWTH FACTORS IN ACUTE LEUKEMIA

Neutropenia with risk of serious infection is one of the most critical complications of acute leukemia therapy. In patients with solid tumors receiving myelosuppressive chemotherapy, the hematopoietic growth factors (HGFs) have reduced infectious morbidity. In acute leukemia patients, use of these drugs has only recently become acceptable, and both G-CSF and granulocyte-macrophage colony-stimulating factor (GM-CSF) are now approved to treat neutropenia after antileukemia chemotherapy. Specific discussion of these drugs can be found in Chapter 115.

The original package inserts listed myeloid malignancies as contraindications to the use of G-CSF or GM-CSF. Myeloid blast cells carry receptors for G-CSF or GM-CSF, and the fear initially existed that using these factors would stimulate regrowth of the myeloid leukemia. Subsequent studies have shown this not to be true. When using HGFs with ANLL therapy, refractory or relapse leukemia has not been more frequent than in historical or concurrent control groups. Several studies now show that the duration of neutropenia can be reduced by up to 4 to 8 days after using an HGF. This reduction in the period of neutropenia has not, however, consistently reduced infectious morbidity. Overall mortality has also not been been reduced in the studies reported, except for one.[100]

Researchers at St. Jude Children's Research Hospital have found similar results for the use of HGFs in children. In a large randomized trial of 164 patients with ALL (aged 2 months to 17 years), patients received either G-CSF (10 μg/kg/d SQ) or placebo after remission induction therapy.[101] G-CSF failed to significantly lower the rate of hospitalization for febrile neutropenia, increase the likelihood of event-free survival at 3 years, or decrease the number of severe infections. Patients treated with G-CSF did have shorter median hospital days (6 compared to 10 days) and fewer documented infections. Unfortunately, this did not translate to a reduction in total costs of supportive care.[101]

The use of HGFs in elderly ANLL patients has received particular attention because complications related to prolonged neutropenia are the major causes of failure to achieve remission. One randomized, blinded, placebo-controlled trial used yeast-derived GM-CSF with induction and consolidation chemotherapy in ANLL patients over age 55 years. There was a statistically significant improvement in overall survival with GM-CSF, but the difference was only marginal, and the survival rate in the placebo arm was unusually low. The incidence and mortality from infections as well as duration of neutropenia were also reduced with GM-CSF.[102] An economic analysis of this trial revealed a $12,513 cost savings per case, mostly from reduction in serious infections that resulted in extended hospital stays in the placebo group.[103] As a further result of this trial and others, the American Society of Clinical Oncology's *Guidelines for the Use of Hematopoietic Colony-stimulating Factors* has recommended HGFs after initial induction therapy in patients over age 55 as acceptable clinical practice.[104] In contrast, the use of GM-CSF in young or middle-aged ANLL patients does not reduce the frequency of infections, use of antibiotics, or length of hospital stay according to one recent trial.[105]

A number of unanswered questions remain. Which HGF should be used, at what dose, starting on what day after chemotherapy, and continuing for how long? Should the marrow be examined for leukemia prior to starting an HGF? Some clinicians stop HGFs after the absolute neutrophil count (ANC) exceeds 1500 for 3 days, but is this threshold of the ANC too high or too low?

The role of HGFs in care of the ALL patient is also being defined. Chemotherapy given to this population is often given frequently with little time in between courses. HGFs might need to be given with chemotherapy to support the neutrophil count. HGFs are not typically given with chemotherapy, but in this population, it is difficult not to administer an HGF without overlapping with chemotherapy. Large studies in ALL patients have not been performed, but preliminary results indicate that G-CSF given during ALL therapy can reduce the depth and duration of neutropenia, but not the incidence of febrile neutropenia. Perhaps most importantly, the HGFs may allow chemotherapy in ALL to be given on time.[106,107] Given during induction or consolidation chemotherapy, G-CSF does not worsen the marrow suppression. An improvement in survival or a reduction in infectious morbidity and mortality have not been demonstrated when a colony-stimulating factor is used with ALL chemotherapy.[107]

SUPPORTIVE CARE

The most common and significant toxic effect of antileukemic agents is marrow suppression. With the exception of prednisone, *L*-asparaginase, and vincristine, antineoplastic agents used to treat acute leukemias cause a rapid fall in peripheral platelet and white blood cell counts. During ANLL remission induction therapy, daily monitoring of the complete blood count and the absolute neutrophil count is necessary to determine when red cell and platelet transfusions are needed and when neutropenia is achieved. Less frequent monitoring than daily may be sufficient during ALL induction. Marrow hypoplasia usually reaches its lowest point (nadir) after 1 to 2 weeks of beginning therapy and lasts for another 1 to 2 weeks. During this period of hypoplasia, infectious and bleeding complications are major causes of death in leukemic patients. As typical signs and symptoms of infection may be absent in the neutropenic host, frequent monitoring of vital signs and daily physical examination are important. Infection control strategies often include routine hand washing; dietary restrictions; reverse isolation and laminar-airflow rooms; routine surveillance cultures; fungal, pneumocystis, and bacterial prophylaxis; and the empiric use of broad-spectrum antibiotics (see Chap. 111). The NCCN guidelines, in contrast to those of many institutions, do not recommend prophylactic antimicrobials unless there is a documented recurrent problem at the institution.[68] Patients are often seen by a dentist prior to induction therapy to identify and treat potential infectious sources in the mouth. Chlorhexidine mouthwash may be used to maintain good oral hygiene.

Acute leukemia patients, particularly those with an initial elevated white blood cell count, should receive allopurinol prior to and during chemotherapy to prevent the development of urate nephropathy from rapid destruction of white cells. In adults, 300 mg of allopurinol once daily, started 1 to 2 days prior to chemotherapy, is usually adequate. Children should receive 10 mg/kg/d of allopurinol on the same schedule. Once marrow hypoplasia ensues, allopurinol may be discontinued. Tumor lysis syndrome may lead not only to hyperuricemia but also to hyperkalemia, hyperphosphatemia, and hypocalcemia. Hypercalcemia has been observed in some patients secondary to ectopic parathyroid production by leukemia cells.

Hematologic support consists primarily of platelet and packed red cell transfusion. Platelet transfusions are often given for peripheral counts below 5000/μL or clinical signs of bleeding. Transfusions of packed red cells for a hematocrit under 20%, profound fatigue, or chest pain may also be indicated. Promyelocytic leukemia can release procoagulants that can cause disseminated intravascular coagulation, necessitating heparin therapy. Because of the gastrointestinal toxic effects of chemotherapy, parenteral nutrition should be used liberally. Patients are frequently receiving infusions of antibiotics, fluids, hyperalimentation, and blood products simultaneously. In order to provide the total support needed for these patients, a multiple-lumen central venous access device such as a Hickman catheter is placed at the start of therapy.

EVALUATION OF THERAPEUTIC OUTCOMES

Appropriate development of a pharmaceutical care plan for the acute leukemia patient begins with establishing the diagnosis and prognosis for the patient. Examination of the bone marrow will identify the diagnosis and genetic abnormalities. According to the NCCN practice guidelines, cytogenetics offers more prognostic information than the FAB system and should be a mandatory part of the initial workup.[68] Initial information from the physical examination and laboratory reports will provide other information to allow the pharmacist to determine the patient's prognosis.

The diagnosis and prognosis determine which chemotherapeutic agents are selected and for how long. High-risk patients will be directed toward bone marrow transplantation for postremission therapy. Patients without high-risk factors will receive conventional therapy.

During induction and postremission therapy, monitoring focuses on reducing infectious and hemorrhagic complications. A coagulation screening panel will identify patients with ongoing disseminated intravascular coagulation who may need heparin.[68] Human leukocyte antigen typing should be done on all patients targeted for bone marrow transplant, especially patients under age 55 with unfavorable cytogenetics.[68] Intense monitoring of hematologic and chemistry laboratory values, microbiology reports, and the patient's physical condition are necessary to identify infections early. Frequent culturing and early institution of antibiotics will prevent infectious deaths. Close monitoring of the patient's condition and laboratory values also allows appropriate blood product support as well as nutritional support.

During therapy, the pharmacist can be an important agent in patient education. Patients should receive information regarding acute and chronic toxicities of the chemotherapy being administered as well as possible treatments for those toxicities. The pharmacist can be an important resource for information regarding antibiotics, antiemetics, nutritional support, HGF, and other supportive care issues.

The chief outcome to be identified initially is the establishment of remission. The return of hematologic values to normal and a repeat bone marrow biopsy that demonstrates no evidence of disease serve as documentation that remission has been achieved. Monitoring guidelines for induction or consolidation are similar. After the appropriate postremission therapy has been completed, the patient may return monthly for 1 year and then every 3 months, to check hematologic values. If no evidence of disease exists after 5 years from the diagnosis and the patient has been in continuous complete remission, the patient is considered cured.

Several late sequelae from leukemia therapy have been recognized. CNS irradiation may lead to several different neurologic problems; most common are cortical atrophy and other endocrine dysfunctions resulting in obesity, short stature, precocious puberty, and osteoporosis. Intellectual function and perceptual motor function can be disturbed. Growth hormone production from the pituitary in children may reduce the rate of growth. Secondary gliomas after cranial radiation have been reported. Long-term cardiomyopathy with symptomatic congestive heart failure has been observed months or years later in some patients receiving anthracyclines during acute leukemia therapy, especially after high cumulative doses.[108] Most recently has been the observation that secondary ANLL can occur in pediatric ALL patients after receiving etoposide or teniposide.[7] Pharmacists caring for leukemia patients after acute therapy is completed should monitor for these effects and initiate any supportive care. The long-term consequences of BMT are discussed in Chapter 125.

▶ PRINCIPLES OF PHARMACOTHERAPY

- Although not a common malignancy in patients over age 35, the acute leukemias are the most common malignancy in children and the leading cause of cancer-related death in patients under age 35.
- The genetic alterations leading to acute leukemia are quickly being discovered and offer targets for future drug therapy. In contemporary practice, the t(15;17) is a specific indicator for initiation of all-*trans*-retinoic acid in acute promyelocytic leukemia.
- Therapeutic choices for both ALL and ANLL are now based on specific risk factors, such as age or WBC count at time of diagnosis in ALL. For both ALL and ANLL, cytogenetic reports offer significant information regarding risk stratification.
- For children with ALL, the foundation of therapy is vincristine, prednisone, and asparaginase. An anthracycline is sometimes added. For adults with ALL, vincristine, prednisone, and an anthracycline are given and asparaginase is sometimes added.
- Because the risk of CNS relapse is so great in ALL, all patients receive prophylaxis, but the choice of therapy can include radiation therapy and single-agent intrathecal administration, triple-drug intrathecal chemotherapy alone, or a combination of systemic chemotherapy and intrathecal single-agent chemotherapy.
- Postremission ALL therapy is given for up to 3 years to erradicate microscopic disease.
- ANLL therapy usually includes induction therapy with an anthracycline and cytarabine. Postremission therapy can include either conventional chemotherapy or bone marrow transplantation.
- Recent understanding of the pathophysiology of APL development has led to the use of ATRA. Remission can be induced without marrow suppression.
- HGFs can now be safely and effectively used with myelosuppressive chemotherapy for acute leukemias. The benefits may include reduced incidence of serious infections and reduced hospital stays.

- Acute leukemia is a life-threatening illness for most patients. In pediatric ALL, long-term survival can be 60% to 80%. In pediatric ANLL, fewer than 50% of patients achieve long-term survival. In adults with ALL, fewer than half survive 5 years. In adult ANLL, only 20% to 40% can expect to live beyond 5 years.

REFERENCES

1. Scheinberg DA, Maslak P, Weiss M. Acute leukemias In: Devita VT, Hellman S, Rosenberg SA, eds. Cancer Principles and Practice of Oncology, 5th ed. Philadelphia, Lippincott, 1997:2293–2321.
2. Landis SH, Murray T, Bolden S, Wingo PA. Cancer Statistics, 1998. CA Cancer J Clin 1998;48:6–27.
3. Schiffer CA. Acute myeloid leukemia in adults. In: Holland JF, Frei E, Bast RC, et al, eds. Cancer Medicine, 4th ed. Philadelphia, Williams & Wilkins, 1997:2617–2649.
4. Pui CH, Evans WE. Acute lymphoblastic leukemia. N Engl J Med 1998;339:605–615.
5. Weinstein HJ, Tarbell NJ. Leukemias and lymphomas of childhood. In: Devita VT, Hellman S, Rosenberg SA, eds. Cancer Principles and Practice of Oncology, 5th ed. Philadelphia, Lippincott-Raven, 1997: 2145-2165.
6. Margolin JF, Poplack DG. Acute lymphoblastic leukemia. In: Pizzo PA, Poplack DG, eds. Principles and Practice of Pediatric Oncology, 3rd ed. Philadelphia, Lippincott-Raven, 1997:409–462.
7. Golub TR, Weinstein HJ, Grier HE. Acute myleogenous leukemia. In: Pizzo PA, Poplack DG, eds. Principles and Practice of Pediatric Oncology, 3rd ed. Philadelphia, Lippincott-Raven, 1997:463–482.
8. Sandler DP, Ross JA. Epidemiology of acute leukemia in children and adults. Semin Oncol 1997;24:3–16.
9. Linet MS, Hatch E, Kleinerman RA, et al. Residential exposure to magnetic fields and acute lymphoblastic leukemia in children. N Engl J Med 1997;337:1–7.
10. Smith SP, Yee GC. Hematopoiesis. Pharmacotherapy 1992;12:11S–19S.
11. Griffin JD, Lowenberg B. Clonogenic cells in acute myeloblastic leukemia. Blood 1986:68:1185.
12. Russell NH. Biology of acute leukaemia. Lancet 1997;349:118–122.
13. Grignani F, Fagioli M, Alcalay M, et al. Acute promyelocytic leukemia: From genetics to treatment. Blood 1994;83:10–25.
14. Pui CH. Childhood leukemias. N Engl J Med 1995;332:1618–1630.
15. Cline MJ. The molecular basis of leukemia. N Engl J Med 1994;330: 328–336.
16. Inamura J, Miyoshi I, Koeffler HP. *P*53 in hematologic malignancies. Blood 1994;84:2412–2421.
17. Prokocimer M, Rotter V. Structure and function of *p*53 in normal cells and their aberrations in cancer cells: Projection on the hematologic cell lineages. Blood 1994;84:2391–2411.
18. Warrell RP, de Thé H, Wang Z, Degos L. Acute promyelocytic leukemia. N Engl J Med 1993;329:177–189.
19. Schiffer CA. Acute lymphocytic leukemia in adults. In: Holland JF, Frei E, Bast RC, et al. eds. Cancer Medicine, 4th ed. Philadelphia, Williams & Wilkins, 1997:2667–2680.
20. Copelan EA, McGuire EA. The biology and treatment of acute lymphoblastic leukemia in adults. Blood 1995;85:1151–1168.
21. Pui CH, Boyett JM, Hancock ML, et al. Outcomes of treatment for childhood cancer in black as compared with white children. JAMA 1995;273:633–637.
22. Smith M, Arthur D, Camitta B, et al. Uniform approach to risk classification and treatment assignment for children with acute lymphoblastic leukemia. J Clin Oncol 1996;14:18–24.
23. Rubnitz JE, Crist WM. Molecular genetics of childhood cancer: Implications for pathogenesis, diagnosis, and treatment. Pediatrics 1997;100:101–108.
24. Rubin CM, LeBeau MM, Mick R, et al. Impact of chromosomal translocations on prognosis in childhood acute lymphoblastic leukemia. J Clin Oncol 1991;9:2183–2192.
25. Hoelzer D, Thiel E, Löffler H, et al. Prognostic factors in a multicenter study for treatment of acute lymphoblastic leukemia in adults. Blood 1988;71:123–131.
26. Larson RA, Dodge RK, Burns CP, et al. A five-drug remission induction regimen with intensive consolidation for adults with acute lymphoblastic leukemia: Cancer and Leukemia Group B study 8811. Blood 1995;85:2025–2037.
27. Nachman J, Sather HN, Gaynon PS, et al. Augmented Berlin–Frankfurt–Munster therapy abrogates the adverse prognostic significance of slow early response to induction chemotherapy for children and adolescents with acute lymphoblastic leukemia and unfavorable presenting features: A report from the Children's Cancer Group. J Clin Oncol 1997;15:2222–2230.
28. Land VJ, Shuster JJ, Crist WM, et al. Comparison of two schedule of intermediate-dose methotrexate and cytarabine consolidation therapy for childhood B-precursor cell acute lymphoblastic leukemia: A Pediatric Oncology Group study. J Clin Oncol 1994;12:1939–1945.
29. Gottleib AJ, Weinberg V, Ellison RR, et al. Efficacy of daunorubicin in the therapy of adult acute lymphocytic leukemia: A prospective randomized trail by Cancer and Leukemia Group B. Blood 1984;64: 267–274.
30. Kantarjian HM. Adult acute lymphocytic leukemia: Critical review of current knowledge. Am J Med 1994;97:176–184.
31. Laport GF, Larson RA. Treatment of adult acute lymphoblastic leukemia. Semin Oncol 1997;24:70–82.
32. Preti A, Kantarjian HM. Management of adult acute lymphocytic leukemia: Present issues and key challenges. J Clin Oncol 1994;12: 1312–1322.
33. Hoelzer D. Treament of acute lymphoblastic leukemia. Semin Hematol 1994;31:1–15.
34. Ong ST, Larson RA. Current management of acute lymphoblastic leukemia in adults. Oncology 1995;9:433–441.
35. Weiss M, Maslak P, Feldman E, et al. Cytarabine with high-dose mitoxantrone induces rapid complete remissions in adult acute lymphoblastic leukemia without the use of vincristine or prednisone. J Clin Oncol 1996;14:2480–2485.
36. Ortega JA, Nesbit ME, Donaldson MH, et al. *L*-asparaginase, vincristine, and prednisone for induction of first remission in acute lymphocytic leukemia. Cancer Res 1977;37:535–539.
37. Ettinger LJ, Kurtzberg J, Voute PA, et al. An open-label multicenter study of polyethylene glycol-*L*-asparaginase for the treatment of acute lymphoblastic leukemia. Cancer 1998;75:1176–1181.
38. Rivera GK, Raimondi SC, Hancock ML, et al. Improved outcome in childhood acute lymphoblastic leukaemia with reinforced early treatment and rotational combination chemotherapy. Lancet 1991;337: 61–66.
39. Gaynon PS, Lustig RH. The use of glucocorticoids in acute lymphoblastic leukemia of childhood. Molecular, cellular, and clinical considerations. J Pediatr Hematol Oncol 1995;17:1–12.
40. Ito C, Evans WE, McNinch L, et al. Comparative cytotoxicity of dexamethasone and prednisolone in childhood acute lymphoblastic leukemia. J Clin Oncol 1996;14:2370–2376.
41. Jones B, Freeman AI, Shuster JJ, et al. Lower incidence of meningeal leukemia when prednisone is replaced by dexamethasone in the treatment of acute lymphocytic leukemia. Med Pediatr Oncol 1991;19: 269–275.
42. Miller DR, Leikin S, Albo V, et al. Prognostic factors and therapy in acute lymphoblastic leukemia of childhood: CCG-141. A report from the Children's Cancer Study Group. Cancer 1983;51:1041–1049.
43. Steinherz PG, Gaynon PS, Breneman JC, et al. Cytoreduction and prognosis in acute lymphoblastic leukemia: The importance of early

marrow response. Report from the Children's Cancer Group. J Clin Oncol 1996;14:389–398.
44. Reiter A, Schrappe M, Ludwig WD, et al. Chemotherapy in 998 unselected childhood acute lymphoblastic leukemia patients. Results and conclusions on the multicenter trial ALL-BFM 86. Blood 1994;84:3122–3133.
45. Omura GA, Moffitt S, Vogler WR, et al. Combination chemotherapy of adult acute lymphoblastic leukemia with randomized central nervous prophlaxis. Blood 1987;55:199–204.
46. Omura GA, Raney M. Long-term survival in adult acute lyphoblastic leukemia: Follow-up of a Southeastern Cancer Study Group trial. J Clin Oncol 1985;3:1053–1058.
47. Pullen J, Boyett J, Shuster J. Extended triple intrathecal chemotherapy trial for prevention of CNS relapse in good-risk and poor-risk patients with B-progenitor acute lymphoblastic leukemia: A Pediatric Oncology Group study. J Clin Oncol 1993;11:839–849.
48. Tubergen DG, Gilchrist GS, O'Brien RT, et al. Prevention of CNS disease in intermediate-risk acute lymphoblastic leukemia: Comparison of cranial radiation and intrathecal methotrexate and the importance of systemic therapy. A Children's Cancer Group report. J Clin Oncol 1993;11:520–526.
49. Wiernik PH, Dutcher JP, Paietta, et al. Long-term follow-up of treatment and potential cure of adult acute lymphocytic leukemia with MOAD: A non-anthracycline containing regimen. Leukemia 1993;7: 1236–1241.
50. Cortes J, O'Brien SM, Pierce S, et al. The value of high-dose systemic chemotherapy and intrathecal therapy for central nervous system prophylaxis in different risk groups of adult acute lymphoblastic leukemia. Blood 1995;86:2091–2097.
51. Cuttner J, Mick R, Budman DR, et al. Phase III trial of brief intensive treatment of adult acute lymphoblastic leukemia comparing daunorubicin and mitoxantrone. A CALGB study. Leukemia 1991;5: 425–431.
52. Cassileth PA, Anderson JW, Bennett JM, et al. Adult acute lymphocytic leukemia: The Eastern Cooperative Oncology Group experience. Leukemia 1992;6(suppl 2):178–181.
53. Dekker AW, van't Veer MB, Sizoo W, et al. Intensive postremission chemotherapy without maintenance therapy in adults with acute lymphoblastic leukemia. J Clin Oncol 1997;15:476–482.
54. Borsi JD, Moe PJ. Systemic clearance of methotrexate in prognosis in acute lymphoblastic leukemia in children. Cancer 1987;60:3020–3024.
55. Koren G, Ferrazini G, Sulhlt D, et al. Systemic exposure to mercaptopurine as a prognostic factor in acute lymphoblastic leukemia in children. N Engl J Med 1990;323:17–21.
56. Bostrom B, Erdmann G. Cellular pharmacology of 6-mercaptopurine in acute lymphoblastic leukemia. Am J Pediatr Hematol Oncol 1993; 15:80–86.
57. Rivard GE, Infante-Rivard C, Hoyoux C, et al. Maintenance chemotherapy for childhood acute lymphoblastic leukemia: Better in the evening. Lancet 1985;2:1264–1266.
58. Schmiegelow K, Glomstein A, Kristinsson J, et al. Impact of morning versus evening schedule for oral methotrexate and 6-mercaptopurine on relapse risk for children with acute lymphoblastic leukemia. J Pediatr Hematol Oncol 1997;2:102–109.
59. Richards S, Gray R, Peto R, et al. Childhood ALL Collaborative Group. Duration and intensity of maintenance chemotherapy in acute leukemia: Overview of 42 trials involving 12,000 randomised children. Lancet 1996;347:1783–1788.
60. Hurwitz CA, Mounce K, Grier HE. Treatment of patients with acute myelogous leukemia: Review of clinical trials of the past decade. J Pediatr Hematol Oncol 1997;17:185–197.
61. Mastrianni DM, Tung NM, Tenen DG. Acute myelogenous leukenia: Current treatment and future directions. Am J Med 1992;92:286–295.
62. Vogler WR, Velez-Garcia E, Weiner RS, et al. A phase III trial comparing idarubicin and daunorubicin in combination with cytarabine in acute myelogenous leukemia: A Southeastern Cancer Study Group study. J Clin Oncol 1992;10:1103–1111.
63. Mayer RJ, Davis RB, Schiffer CA, et al. Intensive postremission chemotherapy in adults with acute myeloid leukemia. N Engl J Med 1994;331:896–903.
64. Mitus AJ, Miller KB, Schenkein DP, et al. Improved survival for patients with acute myelogenous leukemia. J Clin Oncol 1995;13:560–569.
65. Berman E, Heller G, Santorsa J, et al. Results of a randomized trial comparing idarubicin and cytosine arabinoside with daunorubicin and cytosine arabinoside in adult patients with newly diagnosed acute myelogenous leukemia. Blood 1991;77:1666–1674.
66. Weick JK, Kopecky KJ, Appelbaum FR, et al. A randomized investigation of high-dose versus standard-dose cytosine arabinoside with daunorubicin in patients with previously untreated acute myeloid leukemia: A Southwest Oncology Group study. Blood 1996;88: 2841–2851.
67. Bishop JF, Matthews JP, Young GA, et al. A randomized study of high-dose cytarabine in induction in acute myeloid leukemia. Blood 1996;87:1710–1717.
68. National Comprehensive Cancer Network Acute Leukemia Practice Guidlines Committee. NCCN acute leukemia practice guidelines. Oncology 1996;11(suppl):205–221.
69. Wells RJ, Woods WG, Buckley JD, et al. Treatment of newly diagnosed children and adolescents with acute myeloid leukemia: A Children's Cancer Group study. J Clin Oncol 1994;12:2367–2377.
70. Nesbit ME, Buckley JD, Feig SA, et al. Chemotherapy for induction of remission of childhood acute myeloid leukemia followed by marrow transplantation or multiagent chemotherapy: A report from the Children's Cancer Group. J Clin Oncol 1994;12:127–135.
71. Ravindranath Y, Yeager AM, Chang MN, et al. Autologous bone marrow transplantation versus intensive consolidation chemotherapy for acute myeloid leukemia in childhood. N Engl J Med 1996;334: 1428–1434.
72. Baudard M, Marie JP, Cadiou M, Zittoun R. Acute myelogenous leukaemia in the elderly: Retrospective study of 235 consecutive patients. Br J Haematol 1994;86:82–91.
73. Ryan DH, Kopecky KJ, Head D, et al. Analysis of treatment failure in acute nonlymphocytic leukemia patients over fifty years of age. Am J Clin Oncol 1992;15:69–75.
74. Heyll A, Aul C, Gogolin F, et al. Results of conventional-dose cytosine, arabinoside and idarubicin in elderly patients with acute myeloid leukemia. Ann Hematol 1994;68:279–283.
75. Löwenberg B, Zittoun R, Kerkhofs H, et al. On the value of intensive remission-induction chemotherapy in elderly patients of 65+ years with acute myeloid leukemia: A randomized phase III study of the European Organization for Research and Treatment of Cancer Leukemia Group. J Clin Oncol 1989;7:1268–1274.
76. Buchner T, Hiddemann W, Loffler H, et al. Treatment of AML in the elderly: Full dose versus reduced dose induction treatment. Blood 1995;86:434a.
77. Bow EJ, Sutherland JA, Kilpatrick MG, et al.Therapy of untreated acute myeloid leukemia in the elderly: Remission-induction using a non-cytarabine-containing regimen of mitoxantrone and etoposide. J Clin Oncol 1996;14:1345–1355.
78. Tilly H, Castaigne S, Bordessoule D, et al. Low-dose cytarabine versus intensive chemotherapy in the treatment of acute nonlymphocytic leukemia in the elderly. J Clin Oncol 1990;8:272–279.
79. Powell BL, Capizzi RL, Muss HB, et al Low-dose Ara-C therapy for acute myelogenous leukemia in elderly patients. Leukemia 1989; 3:23–28.
80. Meng-er H, Yu-chun Y, Shu-rong C, et al. All-trans retinoic acid with or without low dose cytosine arabinoside in acute promyelocytic leukemia. Chin Med J 1987;100:949–953.
81. Fenaux P, Le Deley MC, Castaigne S, et al. Effect of all transretinoic acid in newly diagnosed acute promyelocytic leukemia. Results of a multicenter randomized trial. Blood 1993;82:3241–3249.

82. Kanamaru A, Takemoto Y, Tanimoto M, et al. All-trans retinoic acid for the treatment of newly diagnosed acute promyelocytic leukemia. Blood 1995;85:1202–1206.
83. Tallman MS, Anderson JW, Schiffer CA, et al. All-*trans*-retinoic acid in acute promyelocytic leukemia. N Engl J Med 1997;337:1021–1028.
84. Frankel SR, Eardley A, Heller G, et al. All-trans retinoic acid for acute promyelocytic leukemia. Ann Intern Med 1994;120:278–286.
85. Fenaux P, Chomienne C. Biology and treatment of acute promyelocytic leukemia. Curr Opin Oncol 1996;8:3–12.
86. Hiddemann W, Büchner T. Treatment strategies in acute myeloid leukemia (AML). Blut 1990;60:163–171.
87. Kantarjian HM, Walters RS, Keating MJ, et al. Experience with vincristine, doxorubicin, and dexamethasone (VAD) chemotherapy in adults with refractory acute lymphocytic leukemia. Cancer 1989;64:16–22.
88. Milpied N, Gisselbrecht C, Harousseau J, et al. Successful treatment of adult acute lymphoblastic leukemia after relapse with prednisone, intermediate-dose cytarabine, mitoxantrone, and etoposide (PAME) chemotherapy. Cancer 1990;66:627–631.
89. Archimbaud E, Thomas X, Leblond V, et al. Timed sequential chemotherapy for previously treated patients with acute myeloid leukemia: Long-term follow-up of the etoposide, mitoxantrone, and cytarabine-86 trial. J Clin Oncol 1995;13:11–18.
90. Visani G, Tosi P, Zinzani PL. FLAG (fludarabine, high dose cytarabine, and G-CSF): An effective and tolerable protocol for the treatment of "poor risk" acute myeloid leukemia. Leukemia 1994;8:1842–1846.
91. Barrett AJ, Horowitz MH, Pollock BH, et al. Bone marrow transplants from HLA-identical siblings as compared with chemotherapy for children with acute lymphoblastic leukemia in a second remission. N Engl J Med 1994;331:1253–1258.
92. Pui CH. Acute lymphoblastic leukemia. Pediatr Clin North Am 1997;44:831–846.
93. Ebb DH, Weinstein HJ. Diagnosis and treatment of childhood acute myelogenous leukemia. Pediatr Clin North Am 1997;44:847–862.
94. Arceci RJ. Clinical significance of p-glycoprotein in multidrug resistance malignancies. Blood 1993;81:2215–2222.
95. Long GD, Blume KG. Allogeneic bone marrow transplantation for acute myeloid leukemia. In: Forman SJ, Blume KG, Thomas ED, eds. Bone Marrow Transplantation. Boston, Blackwell Scientific, 1994: 607–617.
96. Cassileth P, Harrington D, Paietta E, et al. Comparison of autologous bone marrow transplant with high-dose cytarabine in adult acute myeloid leukemia in first remission: An ECOG intergroup study. Proc ASCO 1997;16:89a. Abstract #311.
97. Yeager AM. Autologous bone marrow transplantation for acute myeloid leukemia. In: Forman SJ, Blume KG, Thomas ED, eds. Bone Marrow Transplantation. Boston, Blackwell Scientific, 1994: 709–730.
98. Horowitz MM, Messerer D, Hoelzer D, et al. Chemotherapy compared with bone marrow transplantation for adults with acute lymphoblastic leukemia in first remission. Ann Intern Med 1991;115: 13–18.
99. Chao NJ, Forman SJ. Allogeneic bone marrow transplantation for acute lymphocytic leukemia. In: Forman SJ, Blume KG, Thomas ED, eds. Bone Marrow Transplantation. Boston, Blackwell Scientific, 1994:618–628.
100. Gilmore CE, Dix SP. Colony-stimulating factors in the supportive care of patients with acute myelogenous leukemia. Hosp Pharm 1997;32:669–676, 690.
101. Pui CH, Boyett JM, Hughes WT, et al. Human granulocyte colony-stimualting factor after induction chemotherapy in children with acute lymphoblastic leukemia. N Engl J Med 1997;336:1781–1787.
102. Rowe JM, Anderson JW, Mazza JJ, et al. A randomized placebo-controlled phase III study of granulocyte-macrophage colony-stimulating factor in adult patients (> 55 to 70 years of age) with acute myelogenous leukemia: A study of the Eastern Cooperative Oncology Group (E1490). Blood 1995;86:457–462.
103. Bennett CL, Golub R, Waters TM, et al. Economic analyses of phase III cooperative cancer group clinical trials: Are they feasible? Cancer Invest 1997;15:227–236.
104. American Society of Clinical Oncology. Update of recommendations for the use of hematopoietic colony-stimulating factors: Evidence-based clinical practice guidelines. J Clin Oncol 1996;14:1957–1960.
105. Löwenberg B, Boogaerts MA, Daenen SMGJ, et al. Value of different modalities of granulocyte-macrophage colony-stimulating factor applied during or after induction therapy of acute myeloid leukemia. J Clin Oncol 1997;15:3496–3506.
106. Scherrer R, Geissler K, Kyrle PA, et al. Granulocyte colony-stimulating factor (G-CSF) as an adjunct to induction chemotherapy of adult acute lymphoblastic leukemia (ALL). Ann Hematol 1993;66: 283–289.
107. Ottman OG, Hoelzer D, Gracien E, et al. Concomitant granulocyte colony-stimulating factor and induction chemoradiotherapy in adult lymphoblastic leukemia: A randomized phase III trial. Blood 1995; 86:444–450.
108. Lipshultz SE, Colan SD, Gelber RD, et al. Late cardiac effects of doxorubicin therapy for acute lymphoblastic leukemia in childhood. N Engl J Med 1991;324:808–815.

123
CHRONIC LEUKEMIAS

Timothy R. McGuire, PharmD, and Peter W. Kazakoff, PharmD

Chronic leukemia includes at least four disease entities: chronic myelogenous leukemia (CML), chronic lymphocytic leukemia (CLL), prolymphocytic leukemia, and hairy cell leukemia. Because CML and CLL occur far more frequently, this chapter will deal with these two cancers, which represent about 40% to 50% of all new cases of leukemias occurring in the United States during 1998.[1]

CHRONIC MYELOGENOUS LEUKEMIA

Chronic myelogenous leukemia, also known as chronic granulocytic leukemia, is one of a group of hematologic cancers known as myeloproliferative disorders and results from the malignant transformation of a pluripotent stem cell. This malignant transformation leads to the clonal proliferation and accumulation of both progenitor and mature myeloid and lymphoid cells.[2,3] The clinical course of CML has multiple phases, beginning as an indolent chronic phase in which signs and symptoms can be controlled with conventional chemotherapy, then followed by an acute phase known as blast crisis that, similar to acute leukemia, leads to rapid clinical deterioration and death of the patient. An accelerated phase can usually be identified in the interval between chronic phase and blastic phase, and although the definition of the accelerated phase is vague, it is generally recognized as the stage at which CML becomes more resistant to maintenance chemotherapy.[3]

CML was first described in 1845, but the extensive research into the genetic and molecular aspects of the disease began with the discovery of the Philadelphia chromosome (Ph) in 1960 by Nowell and Hungerford. Research in the 1980s identified the molecular changes that occur as a result of the Ph and an oncogenic protein product resulting from the Ph was identified and implicated in the pathophysiology of CML.[4]

INCIDENCE AND ETIOLOGY

It is estimated that about 4300 new cases of CML occurred in the United States in 1998, representing about 15% to 20% of all leukemias.[1] CML is predominantly a neoplasm of middle-aged adults, with the median age at diagnosis in the fifth decade of life. A "juvenile" variant of CML that occurs in young children is rare and will not be discussed in this chapter.[3]

Although ionizing radiation and heavy occupational exposure to benzene are known to cause CML, it is rare for a newly diagnosed patient to give a history of exposure to a known risk factor. There was a 20- to 25-fold increase in the incidence of all leukemias in atomic bomb survivors. The incidence of leukemia was highest in those who were youngest at the time of exposure, with more CML cases than acute lymphocytic leukemia cases.[5] There are only case reports of CML after radiotherapy for malignancies or ankylosing spondylitis.[3] There are no known oncogenic viruses associated with CML.

PATHOPHYSIOLOGY

MOLECULAR BIOLOGY

Philadelphia chromosome was the first karyotypic abnormality specifically implicated in the pathogenesis of cancer; its discovery has resulted in extensive research into the molecular biology of CML.[3,4] This chromosomal abnormality is characteristic of CML and is present in 90% to 95% of patients with a presumptive diagnosis of the disease. It can also occur in up to 20% of adults and 5% of children with acute lymphocytic leukemia, and 5% of adults and children with acute myelogenous leukemia.[3]

Ph, identified as a shortened long arm of chromosome 22, is found in granulocyte and erythrocyte progenitors, macrophages, megakaryocytes, and some lymphocytes.[3] This anomaly is the consequence of breaks in chromosomes 9 and 22, resulting in a transposition that relocates the 3′ end of the c-*abl* proto-oncogene from its normal site on chromosome 9 at band 34 to the 5′ end of the breakpoint cluster region *(bcr)* on chromosome 22 at band 11.[3] This reciprocal translocation is usually symbolized as t(9;22)(q34;q11) and results in the formation of the hybrid *bcr-abl* fusion gene (Fig. 123–1). Through this chromosomal translocation, the c-*abl* proto-oncogene is able to escape the normal genetic controls on its expression and is activated into a functional oncogene, directing the transcription of an 8.5-kilobase mRNA molecule that is translated into a 210-kilodalton protein. This protein, known as $p210^{BCR\text{-}ABL}$ is unique and has higher tyrosine phosphokinase activity than the 145-kilodalton protein translated by the mRNA of the normal c-*abl* gene. The higher kinase activity of $p210^{BCR\text{-}ABL}$ may be essential in the development of CML because the phosphorylation of tyrosine residues on growth factor receptors are believed to be a critical intracellular signal in cell proliferation and inhibition of programmed cell death (apoptosis). This stimulation of cell proliferation and inhibition of apoptosis leads to accumulation of the malignant clone. The $p210^{BCR\text{-}ABL}$ protein

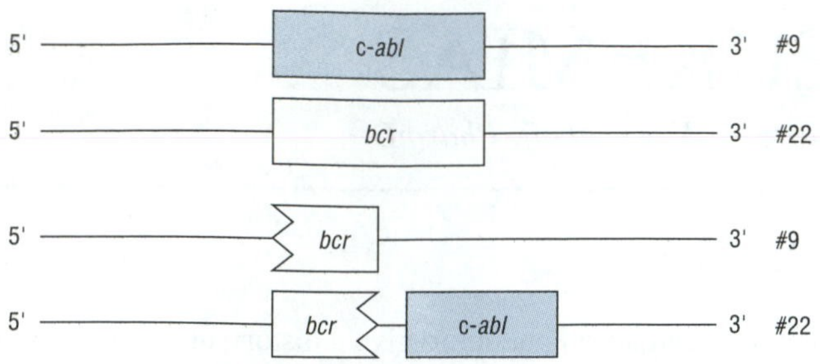

FIGURE 123–1. Diagram of the chromosomal translocation that results in the Philadelphia chromosome. This abnormality is encountered in 90% to 95% of patients who have chronic myelogenous leukemia.
(Reproduced from Ref. 84, with permission.)

has also been shown to transform hematopoietic cells *in vitro* and to induce a CML-like myeloproliferative disorder in mice after infection of their bone marrow with a retrovirus that encodes the p210$^{BCR\text{-}ABL}$ protein.[6]

NATURAL HISTORY

Advances in understanding the cellular events associated with CML has led to the development of a multistep model of disease pathogenesis, beginning with a period of monoclonal hematopoiesis, followed by the chronic phase and ending with the blastic phase.

It is generally accepted that carcinogenesis begins with the transformation of a single cell. In CML, this alteration gives the transformed progenitor cell an inheritable selective growth advantage, leading to the proliferation of a neoplastic, monoclonal population of pluripotent stem cells.[7] These cells initially lack the Ph but soon the disease evolves into a Ph-positive chronic phase. The Ph can be found in both myeloid and lymphoid cells, suggesting that the transformed cell of CML is a totipotent stem cell.[3,7]

Granulocytosis, usually present in CML, results from the increased growth rate of the transformed clone and disruption of normal hematopoietic cell maturation. Disrupted maturation leads to additional divisions by CML progenitor cells before reaching a nonproliferative stage; the resulting number of circulating granulocytes may be many times higher than normal. Immature CML progenitors are also less responsive to cellular and molecular controls that inhibit growth and proliferation in normal hematopoietic cells, such as the induction of apoptosis. Later in the clinical course of CML, cytopenias may occur corresponding to fibrotic changes in the bone marrow.[3]

The silent monoclonal growth phase of CML evolves into the clinically recognized chronic phase when the malignant cells acquire Ph. The chronic phase is not simply a period of increasing granulocytosis; it is common for the white blood cell count to oscillate, and the immature myeloid cells begin to lose the ability to differentiate into mature functioning cells.[7] At this stage therapeutic intervention can effectively control the expansion of these clonal cells and normalize the white blood cell count.[3] As CML progresses, the genetic instability of the malignant clone increases, and chromosomal abnormalities other than Ph begin to occur. Clinical evidence of the accelerated phase of CML begins to emerge as the patient's white blood cell count becomes increasingly difficult to manage. The rate of progression of CML is subject to wide variability; in some instances blastic phase can erupt without any apparent accelerated phase. The relative mass of the chronic-phase cell populations, genetic predetermination, and differences in either genetic stability or proliferative state of the leukemic cells are possible explanations for this variability.[3,8]

The final stage of CML, known as the acute phase or blastic phase, is marked by the presence of rapidly proliferating blast cells that have lost the ability to differentiate into nonproliferating cells.[3,8] The proliferative advantage of blast cells over normal hematopoietic cells is even greater than that of chronic phase leukemic cells. CML in blastic phase is relatively resistant to treatment. This poor response to chemotherapy is not exclusively owing to drug resistance but also results from the high proliferative rate of blastic phase CML and the replacement of malignant cells eliminated by chemotherapy.[9] The increased proliferative rate of blastic phase CML is the consequence of a number of factors, one of which may be the high levels of cytokines produced by CML cells. For example, interleukin-1 β is produced in large quantities by CML cells in culture and antibodies against interleukin-1 β have been shown to inhibit the clonal expansion of blastic phase CML cells *in vitro*. Interleukin-1 β may also indirectly stimulate blastic phase CML cells by inducing endothelial cells and fibroblasts to secrete hematopoietic growth factors.[10]

PHILADELPHIA CHROMOSOME–NEGATIVE CML

In about 5% to 10% of patients diagnosed with CML, the Ph cannot be identified. These patients can be divided into two populations: the first group (Ph–, *bcr+*), in whom the *bcr-abl* fusion gene and p210$^{BCR\text{-}ABL}$ can be demonstrated with molecular techniques; and the second group of patients, in whom there is no evidence of karyotype or fusion gene product (Ph–, *bcr–*). Ph–, *bcr+* CML is indistinguishable from Ph-positive CML in its clinical course. These similarities have led investigators to consider Ph–, *bcr+* CML and its Ph-positive counterpart to be the same disease entity and subject to the same therapeutic strategies.[11] Patients in the other group (Ph–, *bcr–*) have no evidence of either the karyotype or fusion gene but early in the disease display many of the same clinical signs and symptoms of classical CML. This variant has a somewhat different clinical course than Ph+, *bcr+* and Ph–, *bcr+* CML in that it tends to occur in older patients, there is a male predominance, and there are a greater number of cytogenetic abnormalities. Ph–, *bcr–* patients also seem to respond more poorly to treatment and transform to blastic phase more rapidly. Because of the very small number of CML patients who are Ph–, *bcr–*, it is difficult to assess the true nature of *bcr–* CML and how to appropriately classify this disease.[12]

CLINICAL PRESENTATION AND PROGNOSIS

The diagnosis of CML is usually made during the chronic phase following an abnormal peripheral blood smear. Occasionally the blood sample is obtained during a routine physical examination or more commonly after the patient presents with symptoms such as weight loss, fatigue, malaise, night sweats, and fever. Splenomegaly and hepatomegaly are found in 30% to 40% of patients. Typical laboratory findings of the peripheral blood during the chronic phase include leukocytosis, thrombocytosis, basophilia, and abnormal leukocyte alkaline phosphatase levels. In one series of newly diagnosed CML, the most common feature of the peripheral blood was a highly elevated WBC count (> 100,000/μL) occurring in about 70% of patients.[3,13]

Before the advent of modern therapeutic strategies, CML patients had a median survival after diagnosis of about 3 years with only about 20% of patients alive at 5 years. With the use of current therapies, including single-agent and combination chemotherapy, interferon, and bone marrow transplantation (BMT), 5-year survival ranges between 40% and 70%.[14] To date only allogeneic BMT has been able to cure patients by permanently eliminating the Ph-positive clone.

Due to the wide variability in survival among CML patients, there is disagreement in the use of prognostic systems. Two commonly used systems are those by Sokal et al.[15] and the newer synthesis staging system proposed by Kantarjian et al.[13] The synthesis system identifies poor prognostic characteristics from both chronic phase and accelerated phase CML. A summary of the synthesis system is given in Table 123–1. The clinical prognostic factors include age, spleen size, platelet number, and percent blasts at diagnosis. Though these factors in general have prognostic importance, they often fail to accurately identify the risk for disease progression in an individual patient. Recently, Ben-Yehuda et al. reported that methylation of the *bcr-abl* region indicated disease of long standing and thus at high risk for progression to blastic phase.[16] Should this methylation assay be as predictive as the preliminary results suggest, it would be a valuable tool in identifying a high-risk group in whom aggressive intervention would be required.

TABLE 123–1. Synthesis Prognostic System for CML

Stage	Definition	Estimated % Survival		
		1 Year	*2 Year*	*4 Year*
I	0 or 1 element from A	94	87	62
II	2 elements from A	94	78	46
III	≥ 3 elements from A	91	68	25
IV	≥ 1 element from B	71	57	25

List A	List B
• Age ≥ 60 years	• Cytogenetics: clonal evolution
• Spleen ≥ 10 cm below costal margin	• Blasts in blood ≥ 15%
• Blasts ≥ 3% in blood or 5% in marrow	• Blasts + promyelocytes ≥ 30% in blood
• Basophils ≥ 7% blood or ≥ 3% marrow	• Basophils ≥ 20% in blood
• Platelets ≥ 700 × 10^3/μL	• Platelets < 100 × 10^3/μL

Adapted from Ref. 13.

The accelerated phase is clinically the least distinct of the three phases of CML and may be difficult to recognize in some patients. Hematologic signs and symptoms reflect a progression in myeloproliferative acceleration and the approach of fatal blast crisis. Physical symptoms of acceleration include a resurgence of splenic enlargement, unexplained fever, and persistent bone pain. WBC counts and other signs and symptoms begin to be increasingly difficult to control with conventional oral chemotherapeutic agents.

The prognosis for patients not eligible for BMT is poor.[3] The clinical course of CML terminates in blastic phase in which patients have peripheral blood and bone marrow findings very similar to acute leukemia. The one laboratory parameter that is used by most clinicians to confirm this phase is the presence of greater than 30% blasts in the bone marrow or peripheral blood.[3] The median survival for patients in blastic phase is 4 to 6 months, with most treatment options providing no survival advantage.

▶ TREATMENT: Chronic Myelogenous Leukemia

Cure of CML can be achieved only by eradication of the Ph-positive cells. Conventional cytotoxic chemotherapy can be used in chronic-phase CML to attain hematologic remission, which is defined as normalization of WBC count. However, conventional chemotherapy in chronic phase has no significant cytogenetic effects and has only marginally improved median survival in CML. Interferon can produce hematologic and cytogenetic responses that lead to longer median survivals but it has been unable to eliminate the malignant clone, as evidenced by recurrence of the Ph clone after stopping interferon therapy.[3] Cytogenetic remission has been defined as the elimination of Ph from bone marrow, whereas major cytogenetic response is defined as fewer than 35% Ph-positive cells in the bone marrow. Though bone marrow aspirates are the conventional method of determining response, it may be possible to use polymerase chain reaction (PCR) in peripheral blood buffy coat to measure *bcr* gene rearrangements to monitor disease status.[17] To date, only through allogeneic BMT has the Ph-positive malignant clone been permanently eliminated. Table 123–2 illustrates the effect of various treatment modalities on median survival in CML.[15]

CONVENTIONAL CHEMOTHERAPY

Although many chemotherapeutic agents have been used to treat chronic-phase CML, two have been employed most frequently, busulfan (Myleran) and hydroxyurea (Hydrea). These agents can be taken orally, are inexpensive, have a reasonable side-effect

TABLE 123–2. Effect of Various Treatment Modalities on Survival in CML

Therapy	Survival in Months
No treatment	37 (mean)
Splenic irradiation	42 (mean), 28 (median)
Busulfan	35–47
Hydroxyurea	48–69
Combination chemotherapy	45–55
Bone marrow transplantation	40%–70% alive at 5 years[a]
Interferon-α	50%–60% alive at 5 years

[a]Only therapy to eliminate Ph clone.
Adapted from Ref. 14.

profile, and are able to rapidly normalize elevated WBC counts in chronic-phase CML. Although both agents produce predictable declines in WBC count and hematologic remissions in 70% to 80% of chronic-phase CML patients, busulfan and hydroxyurea have very little effect on Ph-positive cells in bone marrow.[3] Despite the fact that busulfan has historically been considered the drug of choice, results from a randomized study of nearly 500 CML patients by the German CML Study Group showed that hydroxyurea treatment provided a significant survival advantage of about 1 year over busulfan therapy.[18] More intense combination chemotherapy has not been shown to provide any improvement in survival over single-agent therapy (see Table 123–2).

Hydroxyurea inhibits the enzyme ribonucleotide reductase, leading to suppression of DNA synthesis and the elimination of cells in the S phase of the cell cycle and the synchronization in the G_1 or pre-DNA synthesis phase.[19] Hydroxyurea is administered either daily or intermittently. In the daily schedule, hydroxyurea is initiated at 50 mg/kg/d in divided doses until the WBC count falls below 10,000/μL. At this point, the dose can be decreased to a maintenance level of 20 mg/kg/d, or temporarily discontinued and reinitiated at the daily maintenance dose when the WBC count begins to climb. With hydroxyurea therapy, the WBC count rarely continues to fall if the drug is discontinued. Because prolonged daily administration of hydroxyurea has been associated with adverse dermatologic effects, an intermittent maintenance dose of 20 mg/kg twice daily (40 mg/kg/d) 2 days each week has been proven effective in controlling the WBC count while minimizing cutaneous toxicity.[19] Occasional dose adjustments may be required in both maintenance dose schedules.

Because of toxicity, busulfan may not be the preferred drug for the initial treatment of CML. Initial doses of busulfan are 4 to 8 mg/d; this regimen is continued until WBC count approaches 20,000/μL, then discontinued. The WBC count will continue to fall after the drug is discontinued and appropriate WBC counts can be maintained for several weeks without continuous drug therapy. Toxicities include prolonged myelosuppression, pulmonary fibrosis, and skin hyperpigmentation. Patients who have received busulfan therapy followed later with allogeneic BMT appear to have a greater incidence of complications.[20] For this reason, and because of the possibility of inducing drug resistance in the malignant clone, busulfan is no longer considered first-line therapy in patients who are candidates for BMT. A comparison of hydroxyurea and busulfan can be seen in Table 123–3.

INTERFERONS

The interferons are a family of glycoproteins involved in many of the functional aspects of the hematopoietic system. Recombinant DNA technology has provided new methods by which sufficient quantities of these cytokines can be produced for therapeutic use. Interferon-alfa (IFN-α) and interferon-beta (IFN-β) bind to the same cell-surface receptor on target cells, whereas interferon-gamma (IFN-γ) binds to a separate receptor. Although all have been studied in the treatment of chronic-phase CML, IFN-α has been most intensely investigated in the management of CML and is FDA approved for this indication.[3,21] IFN-α was first isolated from leukocytes after viral exposure; two recombinant forms are presently marketed: IFN-α-2a (Roferon) and IFN-α-2b (Intron A). Fibroblasts are the primary source of IFN-β, and although this form has potent inhibitory activity on CML cells *in vitro*, no effect has been shown in normalizing blood counts *in vivo*.[22] IFN-γ, originally found in T lymphocytes, has been used in combination with IFN-α in the treatment of chronic-phase CML, with disappointing results.[23]

The exact mechanism of IFN-α activity in CML is not known. One proposed mechanism for IFN-α in the treatment of CML is the binding of IFN-α to its receptor, thus initiating a cascade of biochemical processes that can result in direct cytotoxicity to leukemic cells. For example, synthesis of the enzyme 2′-5′-oligoadenylate-synthetase is enhanced by IFN-α receptor binding and results in the activation of RNAse, which may lead to the degradation of CML growth factor and oncogene transcripts required for growth of the malignant clone.[3,24] Leukemic cells have a reduced expression of cell-surface molecules such as histocompatibility antigens that allow them to escape surveillance by the immune system. It has been suggested that IFN-α binding corrects this abnormality by increasing histocompatibility antigen expression, resulting in the recognition of CML cells as "foreign" and leading to the removal of the malignant clone by immune mechanisms.[24] Perhaps the most important site of action of IFN-α occurs in the bone marrow microenvironment. A reduced expression of cell-adhesion molecules on CML progenitor cells may be responsible for their propensity to enter the circulation rather than adhering to the bone marrow stroma as do normal cells. This decreased adhesion could also be a mechanism by which the leukemic cells escape normal hematopoietic regulation. In co-culture experiments performed with bone marrow–derived stromal cells and CML cells, it was found that cell adhesion was increased sixfold in the presence of IFN-α over control.[3,25] Finally, there is evidence from patient data and *in vitro* experiments that IFN-α suppresses the production of IL-1 and IL-8 (both are elevated in the serum of CML patients) and increases the production of tumor necrosis factor-α; these effects can result in inhibition of leukemic cell proliferation.[26]

The enthusiasm regarding the use of human IFN-α in the treatment of chronic-phase CML is based on the observation that

TABLE 123–3. Comparison of Hydroxyurea and Busulfan in Chronic-Phase CML

Effect of Therapy	Hydroxyurea	Busulfan
Rate of WBC decline	Rapid	Slower
Myelosuppression	Uncommon at usual dose	Common
Side-effect profile	Mild—Skin	Severe—Lung
Effect on platelet count	No effect	Decreased
Effect on splenomegaly	Significant reversal	Significant reversal
Effect on Ph-positive marrow	None	After prolonged myelosuppression
BMT-eligible patients	Recommended	Not recommended

WBC = white blood cell.

some patients achieve cytogenetic response (a decrease or loss of Ph-positive cells), which leads to prolonged survival.[27] Studies performed with the two forms of recombinant IFN-α (IFN-α-2a and IFN-α-2b) have demonstrated similar results. Long-term follow-up results from MD Anderson Cancer Center in early chronic-phase CML patients (< 12 months from diagnosis to treatment) with partially pure human IFN-α, recombinant IFN-α-2a, and IFN-α-2b showed complete hematologic remissions (normalization of blood count) in 70% to 80% of patients. Major cytogenetic response (suppression of Ph-positive metaphases to < 35% of total) occurred in 20% to 40%, and a major durable cytogenetic response in 10% to 25% of patients. Median survival was 65 months, with 60% of patients alive at 5 years.[28] Separate studies done in Italy and Spain resulted in hematologic remission rates of about 50% to 70% with about 30% to 50% of patients obtaining some form of cytogenetic response.[29,30] The doses used in all studies ranged from 2×10^6 U/m^2 to 5×10^6 U/m^2 administered daily either subcutaneously or intramuscularly.[28–30] Several small studies have used three-times-weekly dosing.[31–34] As discussed later, this reduction in dose may reduce response rates.

It is difficult to compare IFN-α studies because of variation in prior therapy, IFN-α dosing, and disease status at the time of treatment. Patients who achieve any cytogenetic response exhibit a distinct survival advantage over those with no decrease in the percentage of Ph-positive cells. Patients who have undergone pretreatment with other agents, have been diagnosed greater than 1 year prior to the start of therapy, or are in accelerated-phase CML may respond poorly to IFN-α. The optimal dose schedule appears to be 5×10^6 U/m^2/d; doses above 5×10^6 U/m^2/d are unlikely to improve response rates and may increase the incidence of toxicities.[3,27]

The importance of IFN-α dose may be illustrated by a randomized study of IFN-α versus hydroxyurea in which the average dose was below 5×10^6 U/m^2/d. Hehlmann et al.[35] reported equivalent survival rates in patients receiving IFN-α versus those receiving hydroxyurea, results that were contradictory to conventional wisdom. These results may be explained by the lower major hematologic and cytogenetic responses in the IFN-α arm compared to studies that used maximum daily doses.[27,36] Reductions in major cytogenetic responses have also been reported in studies where the average daily dose was below 5×10^6 U/m^2/d.[29,31,33,34,37,38] There is one study evaluating the dose of 2×10^6 U/m^2 three times per week that reported response rates approaching those seen with maximal daily doses.[31] A relatively common IFN-α dosing regimen used to treat CML patients is 5×10^6 U/m^2 daily until hematologic remission, followed by maintenance using three-times-weekly dosing.

Table 123–4 describes IFN-α trials and the relationship between dose and response. Data in this table suggest that the three-times-daily dosing has generally led to lower hematologic and cytogenetic remissions. However, other explanations for the response differences are also possible, including differences in baseline prognostic factors, differences in adjunctive therapies, and frequency of assessing cytogenetic response.[39] Unfortunately, prognostic assessment is not always performed and there is great variability in the frequency of evaluating response. Without controlled studies that show similar results with the lower dosing regimens, they cannot be recommended as optimal therapy.[40]

A recent cost-utility analysis performed in Europe and converted into U.S. dollars showed that the use of low dose IFN-α would cost less than $20,000 per quality-adjusted life-year (QALY) gained compared to $50,000 to $100,000 with higher-dose regimens.[41] The use of IFN-α in CML is justifiable on a cost-utility basis if the lower dosing regimens are found to be equivalent. Another study performed in the United States, and thus using U.S. costs, found that the incremental cost effectiveness of IFN-α was $34,800 per QALY. The dosing regimen of IFN-α used to develop the cost-effectiveness model was 5×10^6 U/m^2/d until a complete hematologic response was achieved then to three-times-weekly maintenance dosing.[42]

Adverse effects of IFN-α therapy may limit the administration of the optimal dose of IFN-α and consist of both short-term constitutional effects and potentially dose-limiting long-term effects. The most predictable early toxicity is a flu-like syndrome characterized by fever, chills, myalgias, headache, and anorexia. These dose-dependent effects are a result of IFN-α–induced leukocytosis and release of cytokines. This acute flu-like syndrome can be ameliorated by starting IFN-α dosing at 50% of the final dose during the first week, giving the drug at bedtime, and coadministering acetaminophen or indomethacin. Reduction of initial WBC counts to around 10,000/μL with hydroxyurea may also reduce these symptoms.[3] Despite these methods of ameliorating toxicity, the flu-like syndrome is an important source of morbidity, occasionally requiring termination of therapy. Cardiovascular toxicities (tachycardia, hypotension) are seen in about 15% of patients in the first 1 to 2 weeks. Long-term adverse effects include weight loss, alopecia, neurologic effects (paresthesias, cognitive impairment, depression), and immune-mediated complications (hemolysis, thrombocytopenia, nephrotic syndrome, systemic lupus erythematosus, hypothyroidism), which can be dose limiting in 10% to 25% of patients.[3]

To date, there have not been sufficient clinical data on combining IFN-α with cytotoxic chemotherapy to draw any important conclusions. In several small studies, IFN-α has been used in combination with busulfan, intensive chemotherapy regimens, hydroxyurea, and cytosine arabinoside (Ara-C). Results

TABLE 123–4. Interferon-α Dose–Response in Early Chronic-Phase Chronic Myelogenous Leukemia

Study	IFN-α Dose[a]	No. Patients	CHR (%)[b]	MCR (%)[c]
Kantarjian[27]	5×10^6 U/m^2/d	274	80	58
Mahon[36]	5×10^6 U/m^2/d	52	81	44
Hehlmann[35]	2×10^6 U/m^2/d	133	31	10
Ohniski[37]	4×10^6 U/m^2/d	80	39	17
Ozner[38]	3.2×10^6 U/m^2/d	107	22	29
Italian Group[29]	4.3×10^6 U/m^2/d	218	—	19
Schofield[31]	2×10^6 U/m^2/tiw[d]	27	70	33
Freund[33]	5×10^6 U/tiw	10	33	0
Anger[34]	3×10^6 U/tiw	9	22	20

[a]IFN = interferon.
[b]CHR = complete hematologic response.
[c]MCR = Major cytogenetic response: complete + partial.
[d]tiw = three times per week.

from IFN-α–busulfan studies reported cytogenetic responses at least as frequently as with IFN-α alone, but at the price of myelosuppression as a dose-limiting toxicity.[3,43] Three cycles of intensive chemotherapy consisting of daunorubicin, Ara-C, vincristine, and prednisone followed by daily maintenance IFN-α resulted in significant cytogenetic responses. These responses proved to be transient in most patients and survival rates were equivalent to patients treated with IFN-α alone.[28]

The combination of hydroxyurea and IFN-α has some promise in treating CML. Hydroxyurea was started first at a dose of 50 mg/kg/d and titrated to keep WBC counts at a normal level; IFN-α was then initiated at a dose of 5×10^6 U/m^2/d. The incidence of cytogenetic response was not significantly different from IFN-α therapy alone. In this small study the investigators reported a 82% complete hematologic remission rate and a 62% cytogenetic response compared to 58% complete hematologic remission rate and 48% cytogenetic response in an IFN-α alone group.[30] The advantage of this combination is the rapid normalization of blood counts and differentials, a lower incidence of IFN-α–induced symptoms associated with leukocytosis, and higher complete hematologic remission rates.

Favorable outcomes have resulted from a combination of low-dose Ara-C and IFN-α. This combination has been studied in early chronic-phase CML by Guilhot et al.,[44] and in late chronic-phase and accelerated-phase CML by the MD Anderson follow-up study group.[28] In all the following studies, the dose of IFN-α was 5×10^6 U/m^2 daily. Patients with early chronic-phase CML were given Ara-C at 10 mg/m^2 subcutaneously for 10 days of each month or at 15 mg/m^2 subcutaneously daily in divided doses for 2 weeks during the first cycle then for 7 days of each month thereafter. These regimens were compared with IFN-α therapy alone. This group found no difference in complete hematologic remission rates, which approached 80%, between the IFN-α–low-dose Ara-C and IFN– alone groups. Major cytogenetic responses occurred in 33% of IFN-α–treated patients and in 45% of combination-therapy patients; complete cytogenetic response was 14% versus 23%. In late chronic phase, complete hematologic remission rates were 28% for IFN-α–treated patients and 55% in combination-therapy patients; cytogenetic response was 5% versus 15%. Accelerated-phase patients had similar response rates, although this study had a small number of patients in accelerated phase.[28] In a study recently published, 745 previously untreated patients in chronic phase were randomized to receive hydroxyurea (50 mg/kg) and IFN-α (5×10^6 U/m^2), or the same combination plus Ara-C at 20 mg/m^2 for 10 days repeated monthly.[45] The trial was prematurely terminated because of a demonstrated survival advantage in the Ara-C arm. Major cytogenetic response was 41% for the IFN-α–Ara-C group versus 24% for the IFN-α group.

NONPHARMACOLOGIC THERAPY

Nondrug therapy for CML includes leukopheresis and splenectomy. Leukopheresis can be used to maintain safe WBC counts when pregnancy prevents the use of potentially teratogenic chemotherapy. Leukopheresis may be used when WBC counts become high enough (> 100,000/μL) to cause symptoms of hyperleukocytosis and rapid reduction of WBC count is required. Leukopheresis is accompanied by allopurinol (300 mg/m^2/d) and, when possible, hydroxyurea (1000 mg/m^2 every 8 hours).[3]

Because splenomegaly is often a painful consequence of the disease, splenectomy has occasionally been a useful therapeutic intervention in CML. However, controlled studies have shown that splenectomy does not delay the appearance of blastic phase, does not provide any augmentation of chemotherapy, and does not improve survival.[46] If performed before allogeneic BMT, splenectomy may speed hematopoietic recovery, but may also increase the incidence of graft-versus-host disease (GVHD).[47] The role of splenectomy is limited and should be reserved for symptomatic relief in patients unresponsive to other treatments (chemotherapy, radiation).[3]

TREATMENT IN BLASTIC PHASE

The terminal phase of CML, known as blastic phase, presents as one of two different forms. In about two-thirds of cases, the blast cells are of myeloid origin; the remaining instances are of a lymphoid phenotype, nearly always represented as a B-lymphocyte form.[3] Different acute leukemia induction protocols are used in each form of the blastic phase.

The more common myeloid form has been most responsive to high-dose Ara-C. The usual protocol for this treatment is Ara-C 3000 mg/m^2 every 12 hours for up to 12 doses. This regimen has resulted in complete responses of 25% to 40%.[3] Bauder et al. investigated the addition of amsacrine to Ara-C.[48] The dose of Ara-C was reduced to 500 to 1000 mg/m^2 every 12 hours as a 2-hour infusion on days 1 through 6, with amsacrine given at 120 mg/m^2 once daily (also as a 2-hour infusion) on days 5 to 7. Complete response rates were in the range of 40%, with a median survival of 37 weeks compared to 7 weeks for partial responders and resistant-disease patients. Prolonged bone marrow aplasia occurred in all patients, leading to nearly a 20% mortality from infection.

The most effective treatment of the lymphoid form of blastic phase is a combination vincristine–prednisone regimen; the dose of vincristine is usually 2 mg intravenously each week and prednisone 60 mg/m^2/d. The addition of doxorubicin to this protocol may enhance complete response to around 50%. As with the myeloid form, complete responders survive longer than resistant patients, although survival is usually less than 1 year.[3]

BONE MARROW TRANSPLANTATION

After reviewing all of the treatment modalities used for CML, the clinician is left with the fact that with conventional chemotherapy CML is invariably fatal. The only therapeutic option that can result in cure, achieved only through eradication of the Ph-positive clone, is allogeneic BMT. BMT is discussed in detail in Chapter 125. We will cover special aspects of BMT that relate to the treatment of CML.

Approximately 60% of CML patients in chronic phase undergoing BMT from an HLA- identical sibling donor can be cured of their disease. Results with this type of transplant can be optimized by transplanting patients within the first year of diagnosis, with 5-year survival rates approaching 80%.[49] In patients with a HLA-matched sibling donor, BMT must be considered the treatment of choice and should be performed shortly after diagnosis. Unfortunately, fewer than 30% of patients diagnosed with CML will have this ideal donor, and alternative forms of transplantation must be considered. Studies have demonstrated that related one-antigen-mismatch transplants have survival rates that approach HLA-matched transplants. The mortality associated with the higher incidence of severe acute graft-versus-host disease (GVHD) and graft rejection is offset by a reduction in relapse rates as a result of graft-versus-leukemia effect. However, the use of one-antigen-mismatched related donors increases the donor pool by only 5% to 10%. Attempts to use related donors with two to three antigen mismatch has led to high mortality from graft rejection and acute GVHD. Another potential donor is an unrelated individual who is HLA matched. The results from the National Marrow Donor Program are promising, with about 40% of patients alive and in remission at 2 years.[50] A recent decision analysis indicated that patients who are candidates for unrelated transplant, similar to patients undergoing HLA-matched sibling transplants, should be transplanted within the first year of diagnosis to optimize outcomes.[51] Early transplant in patients with an adequate donor is also supported by a study by Beelen et al, which reported that using IFN-α prior to allogeneic BMT is deleterious to outcomes. There was a higher graft failure rate and slower engraftment time in patients receiving IFN-α therapy before transplant, leading to reduced 5-year survival rates.[52]

One method of reducing the morbidity and mortality associated with acute GVHD in patients undergoing allogeneic BMT is by T-cell depletion of the donor marrow. Unfortunately, this increases the relapse rates in CML patients owing to the loss of a graft-versus-leukemia effect. Soiffer et al. used low-dose IL-2 (2 to 6×10^5 U/m^2/d) starting a median of 60 days after transplant in a group of patients without acute GVHD. IL-2 effectively stimulated immune-related tumor surveillance, leading to significantly lower rates of disease relapse without high rates of severe acute GVHD.[53] Immunostimulants like IL-2 hold promise in reducing relapses in patients with minimal residual disease.

The importance of detecting the *bcr-abl* fusion gene product after BMT has been controversial. A large study has clarified this issue in patients undergoing allogeneic BMT for CML. Radich et al. studied 346 patients and collected 634 blood samples for polymerase chain reaction (PCR) analysis of *bcr-abl.* This group found that a positive PCR 3 months or 36 months after transplant did not predict for relapse of their CML but a positive PCR at 6 or 12 months was highly predictive. With this tool it may be possible to identify patients who are at high risk for relapse after transplant and treat them with IFN-α or IL-2 in an attempt to suppress or irradicate residual disease.[54]

Patients who relapse after allogeneic BMT can be placed back into remission with lymphocyte infusions from the bone marrow donor. Durable remission occurs in the vast majority of patients, with nearly 90% remaining Ph negative at 2 years. Patients who have either a cytogenetic or chronic-phase relapse respond better than those who relapse into an accelerated phase or blast crisis. Nearly all patients who achieved remission also developed either acute or chronic graft-versus-host disease, suggesting that the effect of donor lymphocyte infusion in achieving a second remission is a result of a graft-versus-leukemia effect.[40,55]

The use of autologous BMT has received attention as a result of the observation that there is a reduction in the Ph clone in marrow harvested in chronic phase and stored prior to transplantation. Recently, the use of IFN-α to obtain a cytogenetic remission followed by peripheral blood progenitor cell transplantation has resulted in high survival without relapse. Although this report is encouraging, interpretation must be cautious given the short follow-up.[56] It will require longer follow-up to determine if patients who undergo autologous transplantation after achieving IFN-α–induced cytogentic complete response have a high risk of relapse.

In general, relapse rates remain very high with autologous transplantation, and methods for successfully purging CML marrow have been elusive because of the similarity between CML cells and normal stem cells. It is likely that purging CML cells would also eliminate normal marrow stem cells required for bone marrow engraftment. New molecular methods of purging such as the *in vitro* use of antisense oligonucleotide directed against *bcr-abl* mRNA may be more successful. Antisense oligonucleotides with sequences that are "antisense" and complementary to mRNA for the p210$^{BCR-ABL}$ have been shown to suppress leukemic cell growth by 95% with no effect on the growth of normal and immature bone marrow cells.[57]

CHRONIC LYMPHOCYTIC LEUKEMIA

Chronic lymphocytic leukemia is a lymphoproliferative disorder resulting in a progressive accumulation of functionally incompetent lymphocytes. CLL is an indolent disease that usually results from malignant transformation of a B lymphocyte with subsequent clonal proliferation. CLL is one of the most common forms of leukemia in the United States but is rare in Japan and China.[1] It is estimated that about 7,300 new cases of CLL will be diagnosed in the U.S. in 1998. Occasional family clusters have been recognized, and first-degree relatives of patients with CLL are at three times the risk compared to the general population of developing a lymphoid malignancy. CLL is a disease of the elderly, with a median age of onset in the sixth decade of life, although about 10% of CLL occurs in patients less than 50 years of age. There is a male predominance of approximately 2:1. Etiologic factors have not been identified in CLL, and there are no data supporting either radiation or viral oncogenesis.[58,59]

CLINICAL PRESENTATION AND STAGING

The diagnosis of CLL is often made after the patient complains of various constitutional symptoms (fatigue, fever). These symptoms result from reduction in normal hematopoiesis and the production of dysfunctional lymphocytes.[3,60] Often an abnormal CBC is characterized by high numbers of mature-looking small lymphocytes. A lymphocytosis is nearly always present, and a bone marrow aspirate usually shows an infiltration of mature-appearing lymphocytes making up 30% of nucleated cells. Diagnosis can be confirmed by analyzing phenotypic characteristics of the peripheral blood lymphocytes. If there is a monoclonal B lymphocytosis, this is often sufficient to confirm the diagnosis.[60] Rarely, it becomes difficult to differentiate between CLL and a leukemic phase of indolent non-Hodgkin's lymphoma, which explains the occasional misdiagnosis of these disease entities. In about 60% of patients there is lymphadenopathy, usually in the cervical, axilliary, or inguinal areas. Intra-abdominal nodes may also be palpable, and about 50% of patients have spleen and liver enlargement. In addition to these relatively common presentations, lymphoid infiltrates can uncommonly be detected at other anatomic sites, including skin, lung, gastrointestinal tract, and central nervous system.[3,60]

A number of laboratory abnormalities can be identified at the time of diagnosis. As stated above, lymphocytosis in the peripheral blood and lymphocytic infiltration of the bone marrow are usually seen at diagnosis. Frequently, anemia, thrombocytopenia, and neutropenia are evident either

TABLE 123–5. Rai Staging System and 10-Year Survival

	Lymph[a]	Lymphadenopathy	Organomegaly[b]	Hgb[c]	Platelets[d]
Low Risk (median survival, 7–10 yr)					
Stage 0	+	–	–	–	–
Intermediate Risk (median survival, 5–6 yr)					
Stage I	+	+	–	–	–
Stage II	+	+/–	+	–	–
High Risk (median survival, 2–3 yr)					
Stage III	+	+/–	+/–	+	–
Stage IV	+	+/–	+/–	+/–	+

[a]$> 15 \times 10^9$/L blood lymphocytes.
[b]Enlarged liver and spleen.
[c]Hemoglobin < 11 g/dL.
[d]Platelets $< 100{,}000 \times 10^9$/L.

at the time of diagnosis or some time during the course of the disease. The underlying reason for these cytopenias is not clear but most likely results from infiltration of the bone marrow by malignant lymphocytes. Other potential causes of cytopenias include autoimmune consumption of red blood cells and platelets and excessive T-suppressor cell or diminished T-helper cell function.[3,61] Hypogammaglobulinemia is often present at diagnosis and develops in nearly all patients as the disease progresses. Unlike the Ph in CML, there are no cytogenetic markers for CLL. Although no single chromosomal rearrangement identifies CLL, more than 50% of patients with CLL have abnormal karyotypes. A number of the chromosomal rearrangements have predictive value in determining prognosis for a given patient.[3,61]

There is a wide variability in survival times, with some patients dying within a year of diagnosis and others living two decades with CLL. The Rai staging system has helped to design appropriate management strategies for CLL.[61] Table 123–5 gives the staging system and median survival time for each stage. The staging system attempts to measure tumor burden. For example, the difference between stage I CLL and stage II CLL is the involvement of abdominal organs rather than more superficial lymph nodes. Prognosis is poorer with increasing stage, and it can be concluded that duration of survival is related to tumor burden at diagnosis. There remains variability in disease course within each stage so that one patient may have an indolent course with long survival time whereas another patient may have more aggressive disease and have relatively short survival time.[61]

The Rai staging system has been combined into a risk classification, with low risk being stage 0, intermediate risk being stage I and II, and high risk being stage III and IV.[62]

▶ TREATMENT: Chronic Lymphocytic Leukemia

There are no curative treatments for CLL and therapy is designed to improve quality of life.[3] Without a method to cure this disease, it is not surprising that managment of CLL patients is highly variable. Some clinicians delay drug therapy after diagnosis to obtain several weeks of baseline information on signs and symptoms of the disease.[3,63] The decision on whether drug therapy should be initiated after this baseline period is based on several parameters. If there are signs and symptoms of progressive disease, worsening of blood dyscrasias, autoimmune complications, symptomatic splenomegaly, bulky lymph nodes, severe lymphocytosis (greater than 100,000 to 200,000/μL), and increased infectious complications, treatment is instituted.

Most stage 0 patients do not require treatment and are usually managed with close observation. In patients with stage I or II disease, management is controversial because studies performed in this group of patients have not found a consistent survival benefit from drug therapy.[3,64] The use of cytotoxic chemotherapy in early-stage CLL may be reserved for patients who have disease characteristics consistent with more aggressive disease such as short lymphocyte doubling times and diffuse lymphocytic infiltrates in the bone marrow biopsy. In stage III and IV disease, treatment is required with the intention of achieving a partial or complete remission. Median survival times for patients who achieve some form of remission exceeds 4 years, whereas those who do not achieve remission have a median survival of less than 2 years.[3,64] Usually drug therapy is begun with chlorambucil and corticosteroids; chlorambucil can be replaced with cyclophosphamide without compromising response rates. Splenic radiation or splenectomy is often recommended in patients with stage III and IV disease to reduce symptoms and to improve autoimmune blood dyscrasia.[3,64]

CORTICOSTEROID THERAPY

Prednisone has been studied alone and combined with chlorambucil. Response rates are low when prednisone is used alone, rarely resulting in complete remission. When combined with chlorambucil, response rates can approach 70% with about 40% complete responses. Prednisone is particularly helpful when treating patients with autoimmune thrombocytopenia and anemia, both relatively frequent complications of CLL. Splenomegaly, anemia, and thrombocytopenia often improve under corticosteroid therapy.[3]

CYTOTOXIC CHEMOTHERAPY

Chlorambucil with prednisone continues to be a common initial treatment for CLL. The use of this combination is based on a small study that showed that prednisone added to chlorambucil was better than chlorambucil alone.[65] However, subsequent experience suggests that the addition of prednisone does not significantly increase response rates but is important in decreasing the morbidity associated with autoimmune blood dyscrasias.[3] Chlorambucil is dosed either on a daily basis or intermittently every 2 to 4 weeks. One study showed that chlorambucil given intermittently reduced marrow toxicity without compromising response rates.[66]

Cyclophosphamide gives a similar response to chlorambucil and can be used in patients who have difficulty tolerating chlorambucil or in whom response is not optimal. Some patients refractory to chlorambucil will respond to cyclophosphamide. Cyclophosphamide is less commonly used because of its risk of hemorrhagic cystitis with prolonged treatment.[3]

Inadequate initial response to chemotherapy or the development of refractory disease after chronic treatment results in subsequent response rates that are half those seen with chlorambucil and prednisone in newly diagnosed patients. In these patients, more intensive combination chemotherapy resulted in response rates that range between 30% and 40% with median durations of response of less than 1 year.[3] The new purine nucleoside analogs, fludarabine, 2-chlorodeoxyadenosine (2-Cda), and 2-deoxycoformycin (pentostatin), have an important role in the management of patients who have become resistant to chlorambucil and may increasingly become initial therapy for patients who have not received chemotherapy.

The largest experience with fludarabine has been in patients refractory to standard chlorambucil and prednisone. Keating et al.[67] described the outcome of 369 patients with previously treated CLL; treatment with fludarabine produced about a 30% complete remission rate, and a 15% partial remission rate for an overall response rate of 45%. More recently Sorensen et al. reported similar results with fludarabine in patients with refractory CLL.[68] In general, responses of significant duration occurred in patients with lower-stage disease. Patients receiving prior alkylating therapy who do not respond to the purine nucleosides have a poor survival. With the superior response rates in patients with refractory disease, fludarabine has been investigated in chemotherapy-naive patients, resulting in response rates of about 80%.[69] This high response rate has been confirmed in a randomized study comparing fludarabine to combination chemotherapy (CAP). The fludarabine arm produced an overall response of 71% versus 60% for combination therapy.[70] Fludarabine treatment also led to improvement in the duration of complete and partial remissions. Additional randomized trials are ongoing but the superior effect on remission duration suggests that fludarabine may become first-line therapy. There continues to be concern about the drug's high cost and its potent effects on $CD4^+$ lymphocytes and resulting infectious risk.[3,71]

Pentostatin and 2-Cda inhibit adenosine deaminase, leading to lethal accumulation of deoxyadenosine in lymphocytes. Pentostatin has only moderate activity in CLL, with under 30% of patients achieving a response. It is unlikely that pentostatin alone will have a significant role in the treatment of CLL[72]; 2-Cda does have good activity in CLL, with overall response rates in the range of 45% in previously treated patients.[73] Despite equivalent overall response to fludarabine, complete remission with 2-Cda was only 4%, much lower than that reported with fludarabine therapy.[67] A small study in previously untreated patients suggested similar activity as with fludarabine, with an overall response rate of 85% and complete response rate of 25%.[74] Larger studies are required to investigate 2-Cda in previously treated CLL to determine if complete remission rates are comparable to fludarabine.

Juliusson et al. have reported on four patients who responded to 2-Cda after failing fludarabine therapy, suggesting non–cross-resistance between these two agents.[75] This observation led to a study in 28 fludarabine-resistant CLL patients. Only two patients had a partial remission with 2-Cda without normalization of anemia or thrombocytopenia. It is unlikely that patients who fail fludarabine therapy will benefit from 2-Cda.[76]

ALLOGENEIC BONE MARROW TRANSPLANTATION

Experience regarding BMT in CLL is limited. Review of the literature and International Bone Marrow Registry shows that a total of 26 patients have been treated with BMT for refractory CLL (24 allogeneic, 2 syngeneic). Median age of the patients was 38 years. The conditioning regimens used contained cyclophosphamide and total body irradiation. Of the 22 patients who could be evaluated for disease status, 19 achieved complete remission. Despite this high complete remission rate, only two patients were free from disease after transplant as measured by molecular studies.[77]

Clearly, intensification of CLL therapy is an area of growing interest. Though this modality of treatment holds some promise, difficuties will arise given the advanced age of most CLL patients. The median age of onset of 60 years of age eliminates allogeneic transplant as an acceptable option for most CLL patients. The role of dose intensification of conventional chemotherapy has yet to be determined in CLL but is likely to be of moderate application given the morbidity and mortality associated with aggressive chemotherapy in an elderly population.

BIOLOGIC RESPONSE MODIFIERS

The mechanism by which IFN-α has its beneficial effects on B-cell malignancies (hairy cell leukemia, CLL, and B-cell lymphomas) is not well understood. It may involve the disruption of tumor necrosis factor-α stimulation of the B-lymphocyte clone. This is supported by the preliminary observation that tumor necrosis factor-α antibodies can produce effects similar to IFN-α in patients with CLL.[78]

The current role of IFN-α is limited. Unlike low-grade non-Hodgkin's lymphoma or hairy cell leukemia, in which IFN-α responses range from 50% to 90%, the response in advanced CLL is well under 20%.[79] In one study, there was a 50% response with low-dose IFN-α (2×10^6 U/m^2 three times per week) in patients with untreated low-risk CLL.[3] The relevance of this finding is unclear given the good quality of life and long-term survival of these patients. It is estimated that it would take 10 to 15 years to determine if IFN-α offered a survival benefit in patients with newly diagnosed CLL.

A potentially useful application of low-dose IFN-α is following cytotoxic chemotherapy to increase the duration of response. Ferrara et al.[80] demonstrated a significant reduction in relapse in patients given IFN-α after cytotoxic chemotherapy. In addition, two patients who received a partial remission with chemotherapy subsequently had a complete remission with IFN-α therapy. This experience is consistent with observations that IFN-α works best in patients with low tumor burden.

INTRAVENOUS IMMUNOGLOBULIN

Infection as a result of hypogammaglobulinemia is a major cause of morbidity and mortality in patients with CLL.[3] Low IgG levels have been reported in up to 70% of unselected patients with CLL. The decline in IgG concentrations correlate with the stage and duration of disease; patients with advanced disease or disease of long duration have the lowest IgG levels. The efficacy of administering intravenous IgG preparations to CLL patients with hypogammaglobulinemia was reported in a randomized, placebo-controlled, double-blind clinical trial of intravenous IgG dosed at 400 mg/kg every 3 weeks for 1 year.[81] There was a significant reduction in bacterial infections with the intravenous IgG group, with 14 bacterial infections versus 36 infections in the placebo arm. However, a cost-effectiveness study based on this experience demonstrated that its routine use is difficult to justify on a cost-utility basis.[82]

Infections cause morbidity and mortality in about 50% of CLL patients. Severe and persistent autoimmune-related decline in red blood cells and platelets is a significant source of morbidity and mortality in about 20% to 30% of CLL patients.[3] Although corticosteroids are considered the therapy of choice for autoimmune blood disorders associated with CLL, intravenous IgG may be helpful in patients who are not receiving benefit from prednisone or are unable to receive prednisone.[3]

Intravenous IgG has demonstrated the ability to improve disease parameters in CLL, leading to a reduction in lymphocyte numbers and lymphadenopathy and organomegaly. These are observations that will require further study to determine any potential role of intravenous IgG in the treatment of this malignancy.[83]

EVALUATION OF THERAPEUTIC OUTCOMES

For the past several decades, allogeneic BMT has been the only curative therapy for CML. Recently, cytogenetic responses have been obtained with IFN-α, leading to an improved duration of survival. However, there is no indication that IFN-α can permanently eliminate the malignant clone. Chemotherapy in chronic-phase CML is used to maintain a normal WBC count and consists of oral doses of hydroxyurea or busulfan with patients who are canditates for BMT receiving hydroxyurea. Although chemotherapy can produce hematologic remissions, it is unable to produce permanent cytogenetic responses. It is likely that improved cure rates in CML will come by increasing the number of patients who can receive BMT by using matched unrelated donors and by improving supportive care posttransplant so BMT can be offered to the older patient. Donor lymphocyte infusions may allow long-term survival in patients who have relapsed after BMT. Because CLL is often an indolent disease that occurs in older patients, an important goal should be to optimize quality of life rather than using aggressive relatively toxic therapy. Chemotherapy that initially involves the administration of chlorambucil and prednisone combinations may be used to reduce tumor bulk and relieve symptoms. Later, as the tumor becomes less responsive to initial chemotherapy, fludarabine is able to achieve subsequent responses. In younger patients with more aggressive CLL, dose intensification including BMT may offer long-term disease-free survival.

▶ PRINCIPLES OF PHARMACOTHERAPY

- Hydroxyurea has become the drug of choice to maintain white blood cell counts in CML patients in chronic phase.
- Busulfan should be avoided in patients who are being evaluated for transplantation.
- Allogeneic stem cell transplantation is the only method currently available to permanently cure patients with CML.
- In patients less than 50 years of age with a matched related or unrelated donor, transplantation should be considered within the first year of diagnosis.
- Interferon-α is the only nontransplant method of inducing patients into cytogenetic remission.
- Patients who achieve cytogenetic remission have improved survival.
- Chronic lymphocytic leukemia is managed by maintaining tumor load and preventing and treating infectious and hematologic complications.
- The combination of chlorambucil and prednisone remains adequate therapy for patients requiring tumor-load reduction.
- Fludarabine and 2-Cda are important new nucleoside drugs that can achieve responses in tumors resistant to chlorambucil.
- Allogeneic stem cell transplantation may have a role in younger patients, although no data exist on curative potential of transplant.

REFERENCES

1. Paker SL, Tong T, Bolden S, et al. Cancer statistics, 1997. CA Cancer J Clin 1997;47:5–27.
2. Cortes JE, Talpaz M, Kantarjian H. Chronic myelogenous leukemia: A review. Am J Med 1996;100:555–570.
3. Deisseroth AB, Kantarjian H, Andreeff M, et al. Chronic leukemias. In: Devita VT, Hellman S, Rosenberg SA, eds. Cancer: Principles and Practice of Oncology, 5th ed. Philadelphia, Lippincott, 1997:1965–1980.
4. Rowley JD. Molecular cytogenetics: Rosetta stone for understanding cancer—twenty-ninth G.H.A Clowes Memorial Award Lecture. Cancer Res 1990;50:3816–3825.
5. Butturini A, Gale RP. Age of onset and type of leukemia. Lancet 1989; 2:789–791.
6. Daley GQ, Van Etten RA, Baltimore D. Induction of chronic myelogenous leukemia in mice by the p210 *bcr-abl* gene of the Philadelphia chromosome. Science 1990;247:824–830.
7. Preisler H, Raza A. An overview of some studies of chronic myelogenous leukemia: Biological-clinical observations and viewing the disease as a chaotic system. Leuk Lymphoma 1993;11:145–150.
8. Canellos GP. Clinical characteristics of the blast phase of chronic granulocytic leukemia. Hematol Oncol Clin North Am 1990;4:359–367.
9. Preisler HD, Raza A, Baccarani M. Proliferative advantage rather than classical drug resistance as the cause of treatment failure in chronic myelogenous leukemia. Leuk Lymphoma 1993;11:303–306.
10. Estrov Z, Kurzrock R, Talpaz M. Role of interleukin-1 inhibitory molecules in therapy of acute and chronic myelogenous leukemia. Leuk Lymphoma 1993;10:407–411.

11. Cortes JE, Talpaz M, Beran M, et al. Philadelphia chromosome negative chronic myelogenous leukemia with rearrangement of BCR. Long term follow-up results. Cancer 1995;75:464–476.
12. Costello R, Sainty D, Lafage M, Gabert J. Clinical and biological aspects of Philadelphia negative and BCR negative chronic myelogenous leukemia. Leuk Lymphoma 1997;25:225–232.
13. Kantarjian HM, Keating MJ, Smith TL, et al. Proposal for a simple synthesis prognostic staging system in chronic myelogenous leukemia. Am J Med 1990;88:1–8.
14. Hehlmann R, Ansari H, Hasford J, et al. Chronic myelogenous leukemia: Progress in chemotherapy and evaluation of prognostic score. Semin Hematol 1993;30:44–48.
15. Sokal JE, Baccarani M, Russo D, et al. Staging and prognosis in chronic myelogenous leukemia. Semin Hematol 1988;25:49–61.
16. Ben-Yehuda D, Krichevsky S, Rachmilewitz EA, et al. Molecular follow-up of disease progression and interferon therapy in chronic myelogenous leukemia. Blood 1997;90:4918–4923.
17. Stock W, Westbrook CA, Peterson B, et al. Value of molecular monitoring during the treatment of chronic myelogenous leukemia: A Cancer and Leukemia Group B study. J Clin Oncol 1997;15:26–36.
18. Hehlmann R, Heimpel H, Kolb HJ, et al. The German CML study, comparison of busulfan versus hydroxyurea versus interferon-alpha and establishment of prognostic score 1. Leuk Lymphoma 1993;11: 159–168.
19. Kennedy BJ. The evolution of hydroxyurea therapy in chronic myelogenous leukemia. Semin Oncol 1992;19:21–26.
20. Clift RA, Appelbaum FR, Thomas ED. Treatment of chronic myeloid leukemia by marrow transplantation. Blood 1993;82:1954–1956.
21. Griesshammer M, Hehlmann R, Hochhaus A, et al. Interferon in chronic myeloid leukemia. Ann Hematol 1993;67:101–106.
22. Aulitzky WE, Despres D, Rudolf G, et al. Recombinant interferon beta in chronic myelogenous leukemia. Semin Hematol 1993; 30:14–16.
23. Kloke O, Wandl U, Opalka B, et al. A prospective randomized comparison of single-agent interferon-alpha with the combination of interferon-alpha and low-dose interferon-gamma in CML. Eur J Hematol 1992;48:93–98.
24. Freund M, Huber C. Interferon alpha has become a standard in the treatment of chronic myelogenous leukemia. Semin Hematol 1993; 30:1–5.
25. Dowding C, Gordon M, Guo A, et al. Potential mechanisms of action of interferon-alpha in CML. Leuk Lymphoma 1993;11:185–191.
26. Peschel C, Aman MJ, Rudolf G, et al. Regulation of the cytokine network by interferon: A potential mechanism of interferon in chronic myelogenous leukemia. Semin Hematol 1993;30:28–31.
27. Kantarjian HM, Smith TL, O'Brien S, et al. Prolonged survival in CML after cytogenetic response to interferon-alpha therapy. Ann Intern Med 1995;122:254–261.
28. Kantarjian HM, Talpaz M. Long-term follow-up results of alpha interferon therapy in chronic myelogenous leukemia at M.D. Anderson Cancer Center. Leuk Lymphoma 1993;11:169–174.
29. The Italian Cooperative Study Group on Chronic Myeloid Leukemia. Interferon-alpha-2a as compared with conventional chemotherapy for the treatment of CML. N Engl J Med 1994;330:820–825.
30. Morra E, Alimena G, Lazzarino M, et al. Evolving approaches with interferon alpha in chronic myelogenous leukemia. Semin Hematol 1993;30:26–27.
31. Schofield JR, Robinson WA, Murphy JR, et al. Low doses of interferon-alpha are as effective as higher doses in inducing remissions and prolonging survival in chronic myelogenous leukemia. Ann Intern Med 1994;121:736–744.
32. Alimena G, Morra E, Lazzarino, et al. Interferon-alpha 2a as therapy for Philadelphia chromosome positive chronic myelogenous leukemia: A study of 82 patients treated with intermittent or daily administration. Blood 1989;72:350.
33. Freund M, vonWussow P, Diedrich H, et al. Recombinant human interferon-alpha 2b in chronic myelogenous leukemia: Dose dependency of response and frequency of neutralizing interferon antibodies. Br J Haematol 1989;72:350.
34. Anger B, Porzolt F, Leichte R, et al. A phase I/II study of recombinant interferon-alpha 2a for chronic myelogenous leukemia. Blut 1989;58: 275.
35. Hehlmann R, Heimpel H, Hasford J, et al. Randomized comparison of interferon-alpha with busulfan and hydroxyurea in CML. Blood 1994;84:4064–4077.
36. Mahon FX, Montastruc M, Faberes C, Reiffers J. Predicting complete cytogenetic response in chronic myelogenous leukemia patients treated with recombinant interferon-alpha. Blood 1994;84:3592–3593.
37. Ohniski K, Ohno R, Tomonaga N, et al. A randomized trial comparing interferon-alpha with busulfan for newly diagnosed chronic myelogenous leukemia in chronic phase. Blood 1995;86:906–916.
38. Ozner H, George S, Schiffer C, et al. Prolonged subcutaneous injection of recombinant alpha-2b-interferon in patients with previously untreated Philadelphia chromosome positive chronic phase chronic myelogenous leukemia: Effect of remission duration and survival: Cancer Leukemia Group B Study 8583. Blood 1993;82:2975–2984.
39. Hehlmann R, Hasford AJ, Heimpel D, et al. Comparative analysis of the impact of risk profile and of drug therapy on survival in chronic myelogenous leukemia using Sokal's index and a new score. Br J Haematol 1997;97:76–85.
40. Kantarjian HM, O'Brien S, Anderlini P, Talpaz M. Treatment of chronic myelogenous leukemia: Current status and investigational options. Blood 1996;87:3069–3081.
41. Liberato NL, Quaglini S, Barosi J. Cost effectiveness of interferon-alpha in chronic myelogenous leukemia. 1997;15:2673–2682.
42. Kattan MW, Inoue Y, Giles FJ, et al. Cost effectiveness of interferon-alpha and conventional chemotherapy in chronic myelogenous leukemia. Ann Intern Med 1996;125:541–548.
43. Freund M, Hild F, Grote-Metke A, et al. Combination of chemotherapy and interferon alpha-2b in the treatment of chronic myelogenous leukemia. Semin Hematol 1993;30:11–13.
44. Guilhot F. Interferon alpha and low-dose cytosine arabinoside for the treatment of patients with chronic myelogenous leukemia in chronic phase. Semin Hematol 1993;30:24–25.
45. Guilhot F, Cahstang C, Michallet M, et al. Interferon-alpha 2a combined with cytosine arabinoside versus interferon alone in chronic myelogenous leukemia. N Engl J Med 1997;337:223–229.
46. The Italian Cooperative Study Group on Chronic Myeloid Leukemia. Results of a prospective randomized trial of early splenectomy in chronic myeloid leukemia. Cancer 1984;54:333–338.
47. Gratwohl A, Goldman J, Gluckman E, et al. Effect of splenectomy before bone marrow transplantation on survival in chronic granulocytic leukemia. Lancet 1985;2:1290–1291.
48. Bauder F, Delmer A, Blanc MC, et al. Treatment of chronic myelogenous leukemia in blast crisis and in accelerated phase with high or intermediate dose cytosine arabinoside and amsacrine. Leuk Lymphoma 1993;10:195–200.
49. Goldman JM, Szydlo R, Horowitz MM, et al. Choice of pre-transplant treatment and timing of transplants for chronic myelogenous leukemia in chronic phase. Blood 1993;82:223.
50. McGlave P, Bartsch G, Anasetti A, et al. Unrelated donor marrow transplantation therapy for chronic myelogenous leukemia: Initial experience of the National Marrow Donor Program. Blood 1993;81:543.
51. Lee SJ, Kuntz KM, Horowitz MM, et al. Unrelated donor bone marrow transplantation for chronic myelogenous leukemia: A decision analysis. Ann Intern Med 1997;127:1080–1088.
52. Beelen DW, Graeven U, Elmaagacli, et al. Prolonged administration of interferon-alpha in patients with chronic phase Philadelphia chromosome positive CML before allogeneic bone marrow transplantation may adversely affect transplant outcome. Blood 1995;85:2981–2990.
53. Soiffer R, Murray C, Fairclough D, et al. Low-dose IL-2 following T-cell depleted allogeneic bone marrow transplantation for chronic myelogenous leukemia. Blood 1994;84:213a.
54. Radich JP, Gehly G, Gooley T, et al. Polymerase chain reaction detection of the BCR-ABL fusion transcript after allogeneic bone marrow transplantation for chronic myelogenous leukemia: Results and implications in 346 patients. Blood 1995;85:2632–2638.

55. Collins RH, Shpilberg O, Drobyski WR, et al. Donor lymphocyte infusions in 140 patients with relapsed malignancy after allogeneic bone marrow transplantation. J Clin Oncol 1997;15:433–444.
56. Bhatia R, Verfaillie M, Miller JS, McGlave FB. Autologous transplantation therapy for chronic myelogenous leukemia. Blood 1997; 89:2623–2634.
57. DeFabritiis P, Amadori S, Calabretta B, Mandelli F. Elimination of clonogenic Philadelphia-positive cells using BCR-ABL antisense oligodeoxynucleotides. Bone Marrow Transplant 1993;12:261–265.
58. Dighiero G, Travade P, Chevret S, et al. B-cell chronic lymphocytic leukemia: Present status and future directions. Blood 1991;78:1901–1914.
59. Karmiris TD, Lister A, Rohatiner ZS. Chronic lymphocytic leukemia. Br J Hosp Med 1991;46:379–385.
60. O'Brien S, Giglio AD, Keating M. Advances in the biology and treatment of B-cell CLL. Blood 1995;85:307–318.
61. Rai KR, Han T. Pronostic factors and clinical staging in chronic lymphocytic leukemia. Hematol Oncol Clin North Am 1990;4:447–457.
62. Cheson BD, Bennett JM, Grever M, et al. National Cancer Institute sponsored working group guidelines for chronic lymphocytic leukemia: Revised guidelines for diagnosis and treatment. Blood 1996; 87:4990–4997.
63. Rozman C, Montserrat E. Chronic lymphocytic leukemia: When and how to treat. Blut 1989;59:467–474.
64. Han T, Rai KR. Management of chronic lymphocytic leukemia. Hematol Oncol Clin North Am 1990;4:431–445.
65. Han T, Ezdinli EZ, Shimaoka K, Desai DV. Chlorambucil versus combined chlorambucil-corticosteroid therapy in chronic lymphocytic leukemia. Cancer 1973;31:502.
66. Sawitsky A, Rai KR, Glidewell O, et al. Comparison of daily versus intermittent chlorambucil and prednisone therapy in the treatment of patients with chronic lymphocytic leukemia. Blood 1977;50:1049.
67. Keating MJ, O'Brien S, Kantarjian H, et al. Nucleoside analogs in treatment of chronic lymphocytic leukemia. Leuk Lymphoma 1993; 10:139–145.
68. Sorensen JM, Vena DA, Fallavollita, et al. Treatment of refractory chronic lymphocytic leukemia with fludarabine phosphate via the group C protocol mechanism of the National Cancer Institute: Five year follow-up report. J Clin Oncol 1997;15:458–465.
69. Keating MJ. Fludarabine phosphate in the treatment of chronic lymphocytic leukemia. Semin Oncol 1990;17:49–62.
70. Johnson S, Smith AG, Loffler H, et al. Multicenter prospective randomized trial of fludarabine versus CAP for advanced stage chronic lymphocytic leukemia. N Engl J Med 1996;347:1432–1438.
71. Tallman MS, Hakimian D. Purine nucleoside analogs: Emergency roles in indolent lymphoproliferative disorders. Blood 1995;86:2463–2474.
72. Pott-Hoeck, Hiddemann W. Purine analogs in the treatment of low grade lymphomas and chronic lymphocytic leukemia. Ann Oncol 1995;6:421–433.
73. Saven A, Carrera CJ, Carson DA, et al. 2-Chlorodeoxyadenosine treatment of refractory chronic lymphocytic leukemia. Leuk Lymphoma 1991;5:133–138.
74. Saven A, Lemon RH, Kosty M, et al. 2-Cda activity in patients with untreated chronic lymphocytic leukemia. J Clin Oncol 1995;13:570–574.
75. Juliusson G, Elmhorn-Rosenborg A, Liliemark J. Response to 2-chlorodeoxyadenosine in patients with B-cell chronic lymphocytic leukemia resistant to fludarabine. N Engl J Med 1992;327:1056–1061.
76. O'Brien S, Kantarjian H, Estey E, et al. Lack of effect of 2-chlorodeoxyadenosine therapy in patients with chronic lymphocytic leukemia refractory to fludarabine therapy. N Engl J Med 1994;330: 319–322.
77. Bandini G, Michallet M, Rosti G, Tura S. Bone marrow transplantation for chronic lymphocytic leukemia. Bone Marrow Transplant 1991; 7:251–253.
78. Heslop HE, Brenner MK, Ganeshagaru K, et al. Possible mechanism of action of interferon-alpha in chronic B-cell malignancies. Br J Haematol 1991;79:14–19.
79. Montserrat E, Villamor N, Urbano-Ispizua A, et al. Alpha interferon in chronic lymphocytic leukemia. Eur J Cancer 1991;27:S74–S77.
80. Ferrara F, Rametta V, Mele G, et al. Recombinant interferon-α2A as maintenance treatment for patients with advanced stage chronic lymphocytic leukemia responding to chemotherapy. Am J Hematol 1992; 41:45–49.
81. Cooperative Group for the Study of Immunoglobulin in Chronic Lymphocytic Leukemia. Intravenous immunoglobulin for the prevention of infection in chronic lymphocytic leukemia. A randomized, controlled clinical trial. N Engl J Med 1988;319:902–907.
82. Weeks JC, Tierney MR, Weinstein MC. Cost effectiveness of prophylactic intravenous immune globulin in chronic lymphocytic leukemia. N Engl J Med 1991;325:81–86.
83. Besa EC. Recent advances in the treatment of chronic lymphocytic leukemia: Defining the role of intravenous immunoglobulin. Semin Hematol 1992;29:14–23.
84. Fishleder AJ. Oncogenes and cancer: Clinical applications. Cleve Clin J Med 1990;57:723.

124

MELANOMA

Rowena N. Schwartz, PharmD

Cutaneous melanoma is increasingly becoming a more common disease. It is estimated that about 41,000 new cases of melanoma will be diagnosed in 1998. It is one of the few cancers in which both the incidence and the mortality are increasing every year. In the late 1970s, the incidence of cutaneous melanoma in the United States took a dramatic leap; the current lifetime risk of melanoma is approximately 1 in 100. Considering the rapid increase in incidence it is projected that 1 in 85 Americans will develop melanoma by the year 2000.[1,2] The incidence of melanoma increased by over 80% between 1973 and 1987, and the mortality increased by almost 30%.[3] The incidence of melanoma has increased during the past decade at a rate faster than that of any other malignancy except for lung cancer in women.

Worldwide, the incidence of cancer varies. The incidence is approximately 1 per 100,000 per year in the non-Caucasian population, but is as high as 30 per 100,000 per year for fair-skinned people living in the Queensland province of Australia.[4] The increase in incidence has most affected industrialized countries.

ETIOLOGY

The precise cause of melanoma is not fully understood. A number of host factors and environmental factors have been identified, and are likely to combine to increase the occurrence of cutaneous melanomas These factors are listed in Table 124–1.

Genetic factors have been strongly linked to the development of melanoma, but account for a small percentage of the overall incidence. Familial atypical multiple mole syndrome (FAMMS) or hereditary dysplastic nevus syndrome (HDNS) is a hereditary disease transmitted by an autosomal dominant gene, and is characterized by a predisposition to develop dysplastic nevi and cutaneous melanoma. In individuals with dysplastic nevus and a family history of cutaneous melanoma, the cumulative lifetime incidence approaches 100%.[5] Approximately 10% of cases of melanoma are associated with family history or HDNS. Dysplastic nevi are thought to be precursors of 20% to 40% of sporadic melanoma.

Sunlight is one of the most important environmental factors in the pathogenesis of melanoma, and radiation in the ultraviolet B (UVB) range (280 to 320 nm) is proposed to be a critical factor. There is increasing concern that prolonged exposure to ultraviolet A (UVA) is also a risk for the development of melanoma. A concern with use of UVB-blocking sunscreens is that these sunscreens allow individuals to sustain a more prolonged sun exposure without the ability to perceive erythema or pain, ultimately resulting in intense irradiation of the skin by UVA light.

The incidence of melanoma has been associated with latitude and the intensity of solar exposure among susceptible populations. Whites with fair hair (red and blond) and light-colored eyes (blue and green) who have a tendency to burn and rarely tan with exposure to sunlight are especially at risk. Nonmelanoma skin cancers, such as squamous cell and basal cell cancer, have long been shown to be directly related to the total sun exposure, and it was thought that melanoma was similarly related to lifetime exposure to the sun. Epidemiologic research has not been able to demonstrate such a relationship between cumulative exposure to sunlight and the occurrence of cutaneous melanoma. Studies have demonstrated a lower risk for the development of melanoma in outdoor workers when compared to indoor workers.[6] These findings suggests that the relationship of the sun to cutaneous melanoma is more complex than that of total exposure. Intermittent overexposure to sunlight, blistering sunburns, and the time of life of exposure to the sun are now believed to be the more critical factors for development of cutaneous melanoma.[4] Individuals who have a history of severe sunburns appear to have a higher risk of the development of melanoma than those individuals who have had chronic sun exposure without a history of burning. The risk with sunlight and ultraviolet radiation seems to be most active during childhood and adolescence. Intensive exposure to sunlight during infancy and early adolescence is more hazardous than exposure during adult life.

Immunocompromised patients are at increased risk for the development of cutaneous melanoma. Immunodeficiency includes those individuals with ataxia telangiectasia, chronic lymphocytic leukemia, Hodgkin's disease, and immunosuppression following organ transplant. Acquired immunodeficiency syndrome also has been shown to increase the risk of developing cutaneous melanoma.

PATHOGENESIS

The pathogenesis of melanoma has not been fully elucidated. Melanocytes are dendritic pigmented cells that arise from the neural-crest tissue during early fetal development and then migrate by 4 to 6 weeks to a variety of sites within the body. Melanocytes migrate to the skin, uveal tract, meninges, and ectodermal mucosa. In the adult, the majority of melanocytes are located at the epidermal–dermal junction of the skin and the choroid of the eye. Melanocytes are

TABLE 124–1. Risk Factors for Melanoma

Host Risk Factors
Adulthood (> 15 years)
History of cutaneous melanoma
Dysplastic nevi
Cutaneous melanomas in first-degree relative
Immunodeficiency/immunosuppression
High density of nevi
High degree of freckling
Sunburn easily/tan rarely
Blond or red hair
Blue or green or gray eyes
Socioeconomic status (higher > lower)
White (versus black) race
External Risk Factors
Intense intermittent sun exposures
History of sunburn
More than 4 painful sunburns before the age of 15
Outdoor leisure

From Refs. 1 and 4.

found in a variety of other tissues, such as the meninges and the alimentary and respiratory tract. Primary melanoma can, therefore, arise in any area of the body with melanocytes. The skin is the most frequent site of melanoma; cutaneous melanoma constitutes 90% of all melanoma. Primary melanoma can also arise in the eye, and less frequently in the meninges, respiratory tract, and gallbladder.

Melanocytes synthesize melanin to protect various tissues, such as the skin, from ultraviolet radiation-induced damage. Tyrosinase is the enzyme used in the melanosomes to synthesize melanin. Melanoma results from the malignant transformation of skin melanocytes or from the transformation of preexisting nevocellular nevi. Melanoma is a disorder of cell differentiation and proliferation.

Normal melanocytes arise from melanoblasts and undergo a series of differentiation events before reaching a final end-cell differentiation state. Normal melanocytes can be arrested in their differentiation process at any given state of maturation without loss of their proliferation capacity. The pathologic components of the progression in human melanoma appear to involve a series of morphologic stages: (1) an acquired or congenital melanocytic nevus, (2) melanocytic nevus with architectural atypia, (3) histologically dysplastic nevus with cytologic atypia and architectural atypia, (4) primary melanoma in radial growth phase, (5) primary melanoma in vertical growth phase with or without transit metastases, (6) regional lymph node metastatic melanoma (lymphatic), and (7) distant metastatic melanoma (hematogenous).[7] Primary melanoma is characterized by radial growth and limited vertical thickness (< 0.75 mm). Primary melanoma demonstrates little tendency to metastasize. Melanoma has a potential for metastasis formation with the onset of a vertical growth phase. Metastatic melanoma is seen with an increase in vertical thickness. Therefore the thickness of a primary melanoma is an important prognostic indicator, and is used in the staging classification of cutaneous melanoma.

Normal melanocytes require growth factors for proliferation, but melanoma cells are able to proliferate in the absence of growth factor supplementation. Melanoma cells secrete a variety of growth autocrine and paracrine factors that facilitate proliferation. The types of products that have been isolated from melanoma include various growth factors, proteases, protease inhibitors, cell adhesion proteins, and host response modifiers.[8] The identification of these biologically active substances has led to potential targets for cytotoxic therapy and immunotherapy of melanoma.

Immune factors appear to be involved in the progression of melanoma more than in most other solid tumors. Spontaneous cancer regressions are rare, but are a well-documented phenomenon seen in melanoma.[1] Focal regression in primary melanoma has also been reported. The regression of tumor appears to be associated with host immunity.

A number of different tumor antigens have been identified on melanoma cells by the use of monoclonal antibodies in both human and murine models. Melanoma-associated antigens (MAAs) have been identified in the cellular membrane and cytoplasm of melanoma cells. Ganglioside antigens have been of particular interest in the development of immunotherapy for melanoma. A large number of murine monoclonal antibodies to MAAs have been developed and are currently being used in clinical trials for the diagnosis and the therapy of melanoma.

The humoral and cellular responses of individuals with MAA have been described, and offer an insight into the potential of immunotherapy in the management of metastatic melanoma. Melanoma-directed antibodies have been isolated in the sera of patients with melanoma. The presence of antimelanoma antibodies in the sera of patients correlates with the clinical status of the patients, and the antibodies disappear from the serum as the disease progresses. This phenomenon may be explained by the possible formation of anti-idiotype antibody directed against the antimelanoma antibody, increase in the circulation of soluble tumor antigens that saturate all the antibody combining sites, increased levels of immunosuppression, or absorption of the antibodies on the tumor mass.

In recent years interest has focused on the role of cell-mediated immune response in melanoma. Specific cell-mediated responses may play a role in tumor regression, but the role of specific cells such as cytotoxic T lymphocytes (CTLs) is not fully understood. Tumor-infiltrating lymphocytes (TILs) have been shown *in vivo* and *in vitro* to possess antitumor reactivity. TILs contain a high frequency of mature tumor-specific lymphocytes and have been a target for manipulation in immunotherapeutic approaches for melanoma.

Specific genetic alterations have been demonstrated in the pathogenesis of melanoma. At least four genes have been identified on chromosome 1, 6, 7, and 9. Alterations in other genes located on other chromosomes may also contribute to the progression of melanoma. Alterations of chromosome 1 are seen in many forms of human cancer. The region of chromosome 1 that is involved in melanoma involves the tumor suppressor gene. The alterations seen in chromosome 6 potentially link melanoma and the major histocompatibility complex (MHC). A number of oncogenes have also been found to be activated in melanoma. The genetic influence to melanoma progression appears to involve a series of complex interactions. As these interactions are understood, the potential for gene therapy in melanoma expands.

HISTOLOGIC SUBTYPES OF MELANOMA

Cutaneous melanomas are categorized by growth patterns. The four histologic subtypes of cutaneous melanoma are distinctive in developmental phases and clinical features. The four major subtypes of cutaneous melanoma are superficial spreading melanoma, nodular melanoma, lentigo maligna melanoma, and acral lentiginous melanoma.[9] There is no difference in the clinical outcome of the four subtypes, if the comparison is controlled for depth of penetration. Uveal melanoma is considered a separate disease from cutaneous melanoma.

Superficial spreading melanoma is the most common morphologic type of cutaneous melanoma and accounts for about 70% of all melanoma. The lesions usually arise from a preexisting nevus, and evolve slowly over 1 to 5 years. At some point superficial spreading melanoma may progress to a more rapid growth phase. Early in the lesion development the superficial spreading melanoma is flat, but as the lesion develops the surface becomes irregular and asymmetrical. As the lesion develops a vertical growth phase it enlarges, and the edges appear notched or lacy. At times there are patches of regression within the lesion signified by amelanotic areas. This subtype of melanoma is more common in women. Superficial spreading melanoma usually occurs after puberty.

Nodular melanoma is the second most common growth pattern of melanoma and occurs in 15% to 30% of patients. Nodular melanoma is a "pure" vertical growth-phase disease. In nodular melanoma a small expansive nodule in the papillary dermis invades the reticular dermis and subcutis. Radial growth phase is absent at all times. Nodular melanomas are more aggressive, and develop more rapidly than superficial spreading melanoma. Nodular melanomas are dark blue-black and often uniform in color, although a small percentage of nodular melanomas are amelanotic and have a fleshy appearance. Nodular melanomas are raised and often symmetrical. They occur at any age, and are most common on the trunk, head, and neck. Nodular melanomas are more common in men.

Lentigo maligna melanoma represents a small percentage of melanomas and is unique from other histologic subtypes because it does not have the same propensity to metastasize. Lentigo maligna melanomas are generally large (> 3 cm), flat, and tan-colored lesions with shades of brown and black. This subtype of melanoma occurs in an older age group, and is typically located on the face of elderly Caucasians. Lentigo maligna melanoma is uncommon before the age of 50, and may have been present for over 5 years.

Acral lentiginous melanoma is characteristically seen on the palms of the hands, soles of the feet, and beneath the nailbeds. Most acral lentiginous melanomas are located on the sole of the foot and look like a large (> 3 cm) tan or brown stain. The lesions often have irregular, convoluted borders. Acral lentiginous melanoma includes subungual melanoma, and may present as a brown or black line in the great toe or the thumb nail. Acral lentiginous melanoma occurs in less than 10% of Caucasians with melanoma, but is the most common type of melanoma reported in blacks, Asians, and Hispanics.

Uveal melanoma is the most common primary intraocular malignancy seen in adults, but is an uncommon tumor. Unlike cutaneous melanoma, the frequency and mortality of uveal melanoma has remained steady. This melanoma arises from the pigmented epithelium of the choroid. Iris melanoma is a subset of uveal melanoma and tends to have a more benign course. The risk of metastasis varies with the histologic type and size of the tumor as well as the location in the eye. Metastases occur most frequently in the liver, but have been documented in a variety of tissues.

CLINICAL PRESENTATION

The initial clinical presentation of melanoma is often a melanoma lesion. The lesion can be located anywhere on the body, but is most common on the lower extremities in women, and the back and trunk of men. The clinical features used to describe or evaluate a questionable lesion are called the ABCDs of melanoma. Unlike benign pigmented lesions, the shape of a melanoma lesion is often (A) *asymmetric*. Benign lesions tend to have regular margins, whereas melanoma lesions often have irregular (B) *borders*. The (C) *color* of melanoma lesions are often variegated, ranging in color from tan to blue-black, and at times the lesion is intermingled with colors of red, purple, and white. The size or (D) *diameter* of a melanoma lesion is frequently 6 mm or greater when identified, whereas benign lesions are usually smaller. Early melanoma lesions may be diagnosed at a smaller size. Another warning sign of a potential melanoma is a change of a preexisting nevi. Some clinicians use the ABCDEs of melanoma, adding (E) for *evolution* of a mole. Changes such as a sudden or continuous enlargement of a lesion, an elevation of a lesion, or any change in the skin surrounding a nevi including redness or swelling are important clinical signs. Uncommonly, the sensation of the lesion may become itchy, or tender and painful. Friability of the lesion resulting in bleeding or oozing is also a danger sign.[10] Perhaps the most important warning sign of danger is the evolution in any characteristic of a lesion.

The clinical appearance of a melanoma depends on the histogenesis and the stage of development of the lesion. It is usually possible to distinguish three variants of cutaneous melanoma including flat melanoma, nodular melanoma, and a flat melanoma with a nodular area. Flat melanoma usually corresponds to the histologic classification of superficial spreading melanoma.

The diagnosis of melanoma is complicated by a number of pigmented moles (melanocytic nevi) and nonmelanocytic lesions that resemble melanoma. Ordinary nevi, found on the skin of white adults, average between 10 and 40 lesions. These lesions are usually absent at birth and increase in number through adult life, then gradually decline in number. They appear as tiny pinpoint macules and are usually uniform in color, but increase in size to a maximum of 4 to 6 mm. Nonmelanocytic pigmented lesions such as seborrheic keratoses, pigmented basal-cell carcinoma, and vascular lesions can also appear similar to a melanoma lesion.

SCREENING

Improved survival rates for melanoma have been the result of treatment of lesions at an earlier stage of development. Efforts to improve survival rates are concentrated on the diagnosis and treatment of the primary lesion. The cost-effectiveness of massive screening for all adults by a physician has never been demonstrated. A number of agencies, such as the American Academy of Dermatology and the American Cancer Society, have sponsored free annual screenings. Routine examination of the skin by physicians is recommended for individuals at high risk. The entire cutaneous surface should be examined including the scalp.

Self-examination of the skin places the responsibilities of identification on the individual. Identification of early melanoma allows the opportunity to treat the lesions when they are thin and curable. Educational pamphlets describing the method of self-examination (Table 124–2) for the public are available through the American Cancer Society, the American Academy of Dermatology, and the Skin Cancer Foundation. If a newly discovered pigmented lesion is identified or if a preexisting pigmented lesion changes, the individual should be evaluated by a physician immediately.

TABLE 124–2. Self-Examination of Suspicious Moles

1. Examine your body front and back in the mirror, and then right and left sides, arms raised.
2. Bend elbows and look carefully at forearms and upper arms and palms.
3. Look at the backs of the legs and feet. Look specifically in the spaces between toes and at the soles of the feet.
4. Examine back of neck and scalp with the help of a hand mirror; part hair (or use blow dryer) to lift and give you a closer look.
5. Check the back and buttocks with a hand-held mirror.

Derived from publications of the American Academy of Dermatology.

DIAGNOSIS

A biopsy is critical in establishing the diagnosis of melanoma. The subsequent histologic interpretation of the biopsy will determine the therapy and prognosis. An excisional biopsy with a margin of normal-appearing skin is recommended for a suspicious lesion, and should include a portion of underlying subcutaneous fat for microstaging.[11] Although a biopsy is recommended for large lesions where an excisional biopsy is impractical, an incisional biopsy can be performed but should include a core of full thickness of skin and subcutaneous tissue. When excisional biopsies may be inappropriate, as with the face or palmar surface of the hands, a full-thickness incisional or punch biopsy is preferred to a shave biopsy.

Evaluation of any individual with a suspected melanoma includes a complete history and total body skin examination. The focus of the patient history is to identify potential risk factors and must include a complete family history. Total dermatologic examination is necessary for staging. For patients with melanomas of 1.0 mm or more in thickness, a baseline chest x-ray and liver chemistries are generally recommended despite the fact that they are relatively insensitive at detecting clinically occult distant disease. Lactic dehydrogenase (LDH) should be evaluated, as it has been correlated with prognosis in some series. Any clinical indication of regional lymph node involvement should be confirmed with fine-needle aspiration or on biopsy of the enlarged lymph node. Additionally, any other signs or symptoms suggestive of metastatic disease should be completely evaluated.

STAGING

There is a definite association between the size of a primary melanoma lesion and the likelihood of metastases. The prognostic factor originally used to determining survival was based on the cross-sectional profile of the primary tumor; the cross-sectional profile could be evaluated if the deepest invasive tumor cells lay above or below the sweat glands.[12] This assessment was further clarified by Clark,[13] who described the relationship of depth of invasion of the cancer cells to the standard anatomic landmarks of the skin (Table 124–3). Clark's classification is a practical approach

TABLE 124–3. Clark Level

Clark Level	Anatomic Landmark
N	Epidermis
I	Dermo–epidermal junction
II	Papillary dermis
III	Interface between papillary dermis and reticular dermis
IV	Reticular dermis and subcutaneous fat

From Ref. 13.

for patients with more superficial tumors, because tumors classified as Clark's levels I through III seldom metastasize. Criticism of the Clark classification system is related to problems associated with practical measurements. Melanoma lesions that occur in the presence of lymphoid infiltration, fibrosis, or even the cells of preexisting nevi are difficult to assess with classical reference landmarks.

Breslow[14] replaced Clark's classification of reference landmarks with the use of thickness of the primary melanoma lesion. Tumor thickness is quantified to the nearest tenth of a millimeter with an ocular micrometer, measuring from the top of the granular layer of the overlying epidermis to the deepest contiguous invasive melanoma cell. The correlation between tumor thickness and probability of tumor metastases is strong, but does not include aspects such as tumor satellites and vascular invasion. There are a number of prognostic factors, in addition to tumor thickness and level of invasion that has been associated with a patient's probability of developing metastatic disease, although tumor thickness is often the only variable that is routinely used clinically to predict a patient's probability of survival.[15]

The American Joint Committee on Cancer (AJCC) has developed a staging system[16] for melanoma that divides patients with localized melanoma into four stages according to microstaging criteria of Breslow and Clark. In addition to consideration of the primary lesion, the AJCC staging system includes aspects of the tumor satellite, extent of lymph node involvement, and presence of metastatic disease. Patients with stages I and II include those patients with primary melanoma and/or satellite lesion(s); stage III includes patients with nodal and/or in-transit metastasis; and stage IV includes any patient with distant metastatic disease. Table 124–4 compares these three systems.

Recent analysis of several large databases worldwide has identified areas in which the current AJCC staging system may not reflect the natural history of melanoma. Issues such as the appropriate cutoff values for primary tumor thickness, ulceration of the melanoma, and the satellite lesions of the primary tumor may play a role in determining

TABLE 124–4. Staging of Cutaneous Melanoma

Stage	Description	TNM	Breslow	Clark
0	*In situ*	T_{is}	?	I
1A	Localized	T_1,N_0,M_0	≤ 0.75 mm	II
IB	Localized	T_2,N_0,M_0	0.76–1.5 mm	III
IIA	Localized	T_3,N_0,M_0	1.51–4.0 mm	IV
IIB	Localized	T_4,N_0,M_0	≥ 4.0 mm	V
III	Limited nodal or < 5 in-transit metastases but without nodal involvement	Any T,N_1,M_0		
IV	Advanced regional or distant metastases	Any T, any N, M_1		

Primary Tumor (T)

T_X	Primary tumor cannot be assessed
T_0	No evidence of primary tumor
T_{is}	Melanoma *in situ*
T_1	Tumor ≤ 0.75 mm thick, invading papillary dermis
T_2	Tumor > 0.75 mm and ≤ 1.5 mm thick, invading papillary reticular dermal interface
T_3	Tumor > 1.5 mm and ≤ 4.0 mm thick, invading reticular dermis
	T_{3a} Tumor > 1.5 mm and ≤ 3.0 mm thick
	T_{3b} Tumor > 3.0 mm and ≤ 4.0 mm thick
T_4	Tumor > 4.0 mm thick, invading subcutaneous tissue, or satellites within 2 cm of primary tumor
	T_{4a} Tumor > 4.0 mm thick
	T_{4b} Satellites within 2 cm of primary

Regional Lymph Nodes (N)

N_X	Regional lymph nodes cannot be assessed
N_0	No regional lymph-node metastasis
N_1	Metastasis ≤ 3 cm in greatest dimension in any regional lymph node
N_2	Metastasis > 3 cm in greatest dimension in any regional lymph node, and/or in-transit metastasis
	N_{2a} Metastases > 3cm in greatest dimension
	N_{2b} In-transit metastases
	N_{2c} Metastases > 3 cm in diameter AND in-transit metastases

Metastasis (M)

M_X	Distant metastasis cannot be assessed
M_0	No distant metastasis
M_1	Distant metastasis
	M_{1a} Skin, subcutaneous, or remote nodal metastases
	M_{1b} Visceral metastases

When the thickness and level of invasion criteria do not coincide within a T classification, thickness should take precedence.

From Ref. 16.

the natural history of the disease in an individual, and should be considered when making decisions about therapy. The cutoff values initially proposed by Breslow for primary tumor thickness are still used in the current AJCC staging system, but there is a suggestion that cutoffs of 1, 2, and 4 mm of thickness may better predict overall survival. The presence of ulceration of the primary lesion has been correlated with poorer survival in patients with very thin or thick lesions; but ulceration of the melanoma is not currently included in the AJCC staging system.

As with other solid tumors, the presence of regional lymph nodes is a powerful predictor of tumor burden and patient outcome. Until recently the primary method to determine nodal status was by surgical resection and analysis of the lymph nodes via a regional lymph node dissection (LND). In recent years, preoperative lymphoscintigraphy and intraoperative sentinel node mapping have become more prevalent methods to identify the first or sentinel lymph node in the direct pathway of lymph drainage from the primary cutaneous melanoma.[17,18] Lymphatic mapping and susequent sentinel node biopsy is based on the theory that regions of the skin have patterns of lymphatic drainage to specific lymph nodes in the regional lymphatic basin. The sentinel lymph node is believed to be the first node in the lymphatic basin into which the primary melanoma drains. Unlike other solid tumors, melanoma appears to progress in an orderly nodal distribution. The evaluation of sentinel nodes has been used for detection of micrometastases in breast cancer and is gaining popularity in melanoma. Sentinel lymph node biopsy provides an avenue to perform a more thorough examination of a single sentinel node than is possible when examining multiple lymph nodes with a lymph node dissection, and may be most useful in melanomas located in ambiguous drainage sites such as the head and neck areas. Additionally, the detection of clinically undetectable disease in a lymph node basin that is not directly adjacent to the primary lesion may allow for the upstaging of patients who are initially believed to have node-negative disease. Currently there is increasing interest in developing mechanisms to refine the detection of occult micrometastases in biopsied lymph nodes using more sensitive reverse transcriptase (RT)-PCR assays to detect the presence of tyrosinase messenger RNA, with the hope to eventually refine this technique for detection of occult melanoma cells in the blood of patients with small clinical lesions.[19]

TABLE 124–5. Prognostic Factors for Cutaneous Melanoma

Tumor Factors
Tumor thickness
Level of tumor invasion
Anatomic site of primary tumor (increased survival in tumors of extremities versus axial, neck, head, trunk)
Mitotic rate (correlated with decreased survival)
Angiogenesis
Occurrence of microsatellites
Area of tumor regression
Presence of tumor-infiltrating lymphocytes (correlated with increased survival)
Patient Factors
Age (decreased survival in patients > 60 yr)
Gender (survival: female > male)

From Ref. 15.

The stage of the melanoma at time of diagnosis is one of the primary indicators of natural history of the disease; other factors have been shown to influence survival of primary melanoma. Factors such as tumor growth phase, mitotic rate, density of TILs infiltrating the tumor tissue, anatomic site of the primary tumor, gender, and age have all been demonstrated to have an impact on survival (Table 124–5).[15]

▶ TREATMENT: Melanoma

The treatment and management of a patient with cutaneous melanoma is decided according to stage of the disease. Local disease is managed and cured with surgical ablation. Regional disease involves the surgical management of the lesion and possibly adjuvant therapy with interferon-α_{2b}. Treatment for disseminated melanoma is controversial and remains a challenge. Although the literature provides numerous clinical trials with single-agent and combination chemotherapy, endocrine manipulations, and immunotherapy, at this time there is no standard treatment regimen for metastatic melanoma.

SURGERY

Melanoma that is determined to be localized can be cured, in most cases, with surgical excision. The extent of margin to excise is important in the prevention of local recurrence and ultimate survival. Primary tumors less than 1 mm thick require a 1-cm margin.[20] This recommendation is a significant reduction from the 5-cm margin recommended in the past. Large primary tumors between 1 and 4 mm thick can also be surgically excised, but appear to require a more extensive margin of up to 2 cm.[21] Primary tumors more than 4 mm thick require at least a 2-cm margin, but it is not clear if a larger margin is beneficial.

When isolated regional lymph nodes are detected via physical exam in the absence of distant disease, therapeutic lymphadenectomy has been recommended. The extent of therapeutic lymph node dissection is often modified according to the anatomic area of the lymphadenopathy. The role of lymphadenectomy is not as established in situations in which the regional lymph nodes do not appear to be involved by clinical examination. Prophylactic regional lymph node dissection has not been shown to prolong survival or decrease time to relapse in large, randomized clinical trials, although a subgroup of patients with stage I melanoma will have microscopic metastatic disease in nonpalpable lymph nodes.[22,23] Selective regional lymphadenectomy performed after scintigraphic and dyelymphographic identification of the affected sentinel draining lymph node(s) is becoming increasingly common in major melanoma centers. If the sentinel node is found to have micrometastatic melanoma, regional dissection of the involved nodal basin is performed.

One of the most important aspects of the surgical management of cutaneous melanoma is the role of patient follow-up. Postsurgical follow-up of patients who have had a melanoma excised is essential. Even after excision there remains a risk of undetected metastatic disease, the risk of the development of a second primary cutaneous melanoma, and the risk of a second nonmelanoma primary malignancy. Scheduled screening in addition to routine surgical follow-up is required for any patient who has had a melanoma; the frequency and duration recommended is dependent on the stage of melanoma. The optimal duration of follow-up is controversial. Late recurrences seen in patients over 10 years following surgery have been documented, and the increased lifetime risk of developing a second primary melanoma supports lifetime dermatologic surveillance for all patients.

The role of surgery as curative is limited to that of early-stage disease in cutaneous melanoma. The role of surgery beyond that of cure is less defined, for surgery may offer a mechanism of palliation of isolated metastases. Resection of isolated lesions in the brain[24] and the lungs[25] may be appropriate in certain cases, and should be evaluated based on individual patient criteria. Surgery can be an option in situations when the lesion is accessible, and when the lesion may cause problems if not removed. Melanoma in the gastrointestinal tract can lead to obstruction, and appropriate resection or bypass may allow the patient significant relief of symptoms. Despite the lack of controlled clinical trials, the impact on palliative surgery should be evaluated in the context of a patient's comfort and quality of life. Surgery may be an appropriate option if the perceived outcome is to provide patient comfort. On the other hand, surgery may constitute a significant physical challenge or financial burden to a patient with a limited life expectancy. The clinical scenarios involving surgical resection should be fully evaluated in terms of overall quality of life.

PHARMACOLOGIC THERAPY

IMMUNOTHERAPY

Melanoma is considered one of the most immunogenic solid tumors; it appears to interact with and to respond to the immune system of the host in which it arises. The immune system can influence the pathogenesis of melanoma. Additionally, as melanoma is one of the tumors most resistant to standard modalities of radiation and chemotherapy, immunotherapy may offer an avenue of treatment if surgery fails or is not an option. The development of recombinant DNA technology combined with the growing understanding of the molecular basis of the immunologic defenses of melanoma give rise to new opportunities for the development of immune-based treatment for melanoma. Melanoma was an early target for immunotherapeutic trials, and has been a target for a variety of therapeutic management approaches. Although the complete response (CR) rate seen in patients treated with biotherapy is low, approximately half are durable. This has led to increasing research in the optimization of therapy for patients with metastatic melanoma, and for the role of biotherapy in the adjuvant setting.

The *interferons* consist of a group of antigenically and genetically distinct species and subspecies; the interferons have differing immunomodulatory activity and are directly cytostatic and cytotoxic. A number of studies have looked at various doses and schedules of recombinant interferon for the treatment of metastatic melanoma (Table 124–6). Response rates in metastatic melanoma range from 10% to 30%, but overall response rates are approximately 15% for interferon-α and interferon-β. Unfortunately the optimal dose, treatment schedule, and treatment combination have not been established for the management of metastatic melanoma.

TABLE 124–6. Interferon-α Therapy of Metastatic Melanoma

IFN	Dose (mU/m^2)	Route	Weekly Schedule	Response Rate (%)	Reference
α_{2a}	12	IM	3 × week	20	26
α_{2a}	50	IM	3 × week	23	27
α_{2a}	20	IV	Daily × 5	0	28
α_{2a}	50	IM	3 × week	11	29
α_{2a}	3–36	IM	Daily × 7	10	30
α_{2a}	18	IM	—	14	31
α_{2a}	18	IM	Daily × 7	8	32
α_{2b}	10–100	IM/IV	Daily × 7	22	33
α_{2b}	10	SC	3 × week	27	34
α_{2b}	30	SC/IV	3 × week	25	35
α_{2b}	10	IM	3 × week	14	36

Initial clinical trials with interferon in metastatic cutaneous melanoma demonstrate that the response rates are best in those patients with minimal disease. Additionally, responses are most frequent in subcutaneous, lymph node, and pulmonary metastases, but have been seen in all sites of disease. These facts led to the evaluation of interferon-α (IFN-α) in the adjuvant treatment of patients after surgical resection of the melanoma. Early trials of short-term use or low-dose regimens of IFN-α did not demonstrate survival benefit in the adjuvant setting.[37] In an attempt to deliver maximum tolerated doses of IFN-α in the adjuvant setting, a large, multicenter, cooperative group trial of IFN-α_{2b} versus observation was designed for patients with high-risk melanoma following surgical resection. IFN-α_{2b} was given intravenously as an induction therapy for 1 month at maximum-tolerated doses of 20 million IU/m^2/d 5 days per week for 4 weeks; treatment was continued for 48 weeks with subcutaneous IFN-α_{2b} 10 million IU/m^2/dose three times per week. Induction therapy was given in an outpatient setting, and maintenance therapy could be self-administered at home by patients. Analysis of the 280 patients demonstrated a disease-free survival and an overall survival advantage with IFN treatment for patients with stage IIb and III disease in the adjuvant setting.[38] The prolongation of overall survival was approximately 1 year, and the most significant reduction in melanoma recurrence was during the early treatment period. Subgroup analysis of this study indicated that patients with large primary tumors and node-negative disease ($T_4N_0M_0$) did not receive the same benefit from therapy, but the small number of patients in this group made it difficult to draw definite conclusions about treatment from adjuvant therapy. Whether the information from this trial should be extrapolated to patients with local recurrences, satellite lesions, or in-transit metastases is not known, and should be evaluated on a individual case basis.

Toxicities for the IFN-α therapy were common and severe in a majority of the patients at some point during therapy and necessitated dose reductions and/or delays during both the induction and maintenance phases of the study. Dose modifications were required for dose-limiting constitutional symptoms, hematologic toxicity, and hepatic toxicities, but 74% of the patients were able to complete the year of therapy in an outpatient setting. Guidelines for IFN dose modifications have been published based on the criteria used in the cooperative trial and the experience of investigators (Table 124–7).

The frequency and severity of toxicity seen with this therapy in an adjuvant setting has initiated interest in better understanding the mechanism(s) of IFN toxicity and to develop strategies for patient management. One of the categories of toxicities seen with IFN therapy is actually a diverse group of side effects referred to as constitutional symptoms; this can include acute symptoms

TABLE 124–7. Interferon-α Dose Modifications Guidelines

Symptom	Evaluation	Dose Modification
Anorexia	Calorie counts	33% to 50% with nutrition consultation
Weight loss	> 10% weight loss	33% to 50% with nutrition consultation
Fatigue	Thyroid function	33% to 50% after dose delay of 1 to 2 weeks
Depression	Beck's inventory	33% to 50% with psychiatric evaluation
AST	LFTs	33% to 50% when LFTs are < 3 × normal limits
WBC	ANC	33% to 50% when ANC < 250 /mm^3

From Ref. 39.

such as fever, chills, myalagia, and fatigue, and can encompass some of the more chronic toxicities such as fatigue, anorexia, and depression. Acetaminophen is used to prevent or minimize acute dose-related symptoms such as fever, myalgia, and chills. Opiates such as meperidine are required when patients experience severe chills or rigors, most commonly during the high-dose intravenous IFN induction phase. Nonsteroidal anti-inflammatory agents (NSAIDs) have been used to manage interferon-related myalgia, but may have overlapping side effects with interferon such as decrease in renal blood flow and nausea. NSAIDs, like acetaminophen, may mask a fever in patients who experience neutropenia while on therapy. Fatigue is one of the most frequently observed dose-limiting toxicities seen with IFN therapy. The mechanisms of interferon-induced fatigue are not fully understood at this time, and may be multifactorial in individual patients. It appears interferon-induced fatigue is dose related and may worsen with continued therapy. Pharmacologic (e.g., amantadine) and nonpharmacologic interventions (e.g., exercise, psychosocial techniques, distraction, energy management, dietary modifications) are currently being evaluated to treat cancer-related fatigue and now interferon-related fatigue.[40] Anorexia was reported in approximately 70% of patients receiving adjuvant interferon therapy for melanoma, and is thought to be mediated through direct effects on hypothalamic neurons, modification of normal hypothalamic neurotransmitter/neuropeptides, or effects from stimulation of other cytokines.[41] Taste alterations may contribute to anorexia. Investigational strategies for ameliorating interferon-induced anorexia include nutritional intervention, use of appetite stimulants such as megesterol acetate, and patient education. Glucocorticoids should not be used for an appetite stimulant or antiemetic effect as they may adversely effect the immunomodulatory effects of the IFN. Other toxicities such as hematologic or hepatic toxicities require monitoring and appropriate dose modification.

Because of the associated toxicity and adverse effects seen with IFN-α therapy, there has been concern about the usefulness of this intensive adjuvant therapy for melanoma despite the benefits in relapse-free and overall survivals. A subsequent report from the cooperative group study demonstrated a quality-of-life benefit with IFN therapy based on the quality-of-life-adjusted survival analysis (Q-TWIST).[42] This analysis calculates the quality of life adjusted years gained as a result of IFN-α treatment, or the clinical benefit of time without toxicities and without disease. The question remains if alternate dosing regimens may optimize benefit and/or minimize toxicities. Duration of therapy is also being evaluated in additional studies.

Interferon-α has been used as a single agent and in combination with other biotherapy with or without chemotherapy for metastatic melanoma. The role of IFN in advanced disease is not clear, especially for those patients who have recurred post-adjuvant IFN-α_{2b} therapy. Other toxicities that may be exacerbated by concomitant chemotherapy include renal insufficiency and neurologic toxicities. Hematologic toxicity is generally not dose limiting and correlates with dosage, schedule, and route of administration. In an attempt to limit systemic toxicity and to optimize local benefit, the regional administration of interferon has been evaluated in a variety of settings. Intralesional and perilesional application of interferon has been shown to have some efficacy in small lesions and appears to be well tolerated.[43]

Interleukin-2 (IL-2), a glycoprotein produced by activated lymphocytes, has been extensively studied in the management of metastatic melanoma. The precise mechanism of cytotoxicity of IL-2 is unknown; high concentrations of IL-2 have not been shown to have a direct antitumor effect on cancer cells *in vitro*. *In vitro* and *in vivo*, IL-2 stimulates the production and release of many secondary monocyte-derived and T-cell-derived cytokines—including IL-4, IL-5, IL-6, IL-8, tumor necrosis factor alpha (TNF-α), granulocyte macrophage colony-stimulating factor (GM-CSF), and interferon gamma (IFN-γ)—which may have direct or indirect antitumor activity. In addition, IL-2 appears to stimulate the cytotoxic activities of natural killer (NK) cells, monocytes, lymphokine-activated killer (LAK) cells, and cytotoxic T lymphocytes (CTLs). Although the clinical significance is not currently understood, preliminary studies have shown that several human melanoma cell lines express both α and β chains of the rIL-2 receptor that specifically bind to rIL-2.

Preclinical studies demonstrated a dose–response relationship between IL-2 and tumor response; therefore the initial clinical trials that evaluated the use of IL-2 in the treatment of patients with melanoma used relatively high doses of the drug as a single agent or in combination with LAK cells. The response rates seen in these trials ranged from 15% to 25%, and 2% to 5% of patients achieved complete responses, some of which were durable. Responses were seen at a number of metastatic sites such as lung, liver, bone, lymph node, and subcutaneous tissue. Based on the reevaluation of early clinical trials, rIL-2 (aldesleukin) was recently approved by the FDA for treatment of metastatic melanoma (Table 124–8). The doses used in the initial clinical trials and recommended in the labeling of the drug are associated with significant toxicities and may limit the practicality of therapy for individual patients. At the high doses (600,000 IU/kg/dose q8h × 14 doses) approved for treatment of metastatic melanoma,

TABLE 124–8. Aldesleukin ± LAK Cells in Patients with Malignant Melanoma

Reference	Route	N	CR	CR+PR (%)
44	Bolus	26	0	12
45	Bolus	46	2	22
46	Bolus	42	0	10
47	Bolus	27	0	26
48	Bolus	134	9	17
49	CI	10	0	50
50	CI	33	0	3
51	CI	33	0	12
52	CI	17	0	6
53	CI	15	0	0

LAK = lymphokine-activated killer; CR = complete response; PR = partial response; CI = continuous infusion.

cytokine-induced capillary leak syndrome is a common problem and may be accompanied by hypotension, visceral edema, dyspnea, tachycardia, and arrhythmias. Increased permeability of capillary walls allows for a fluid shift from the intravascular space into tissue. As the patient becomes intravascularly dehydrated, hypotension may occur, resulting in reflex tachycardia and arrhythmias. In addition, the decrease in blood volume may result in decreased renal blood flow and urine output, manifesting as an increase in blood urea nitrogen, serum creatinine, edema, weight, and a decrease in urine output (input > output). Visceral edema can result in pulmonary congestion, pleural effusions, and edema. The management of patients receiving high-dose rIL-2 requires careful monitoring and a staff trained in aspects of critical care such as hypotension management. Although some institutions manage patients receiving high-dose rIL-2 in an intensive care unit, these patients can be managed with intensive care on designated oncology units. Additional side effects seen with rIL-2 include constitutional symptoms, pruritis and eosinophilia, bone marrow suppression including thrombocytopenia, increase in liver function test, and nausea.

In an attempt to provide the benefit of interleukin-2 therapy without the limiting side effects, a number of studies have evaluated continuous-infusion IL-2 therapy, and lower-dose IL-2 alone[46] or with chemotherapy[54] and interferon therapy.[55–57] Response rates have been promising, but survival has not been significantly affected. At this time, direct head-to-head comparisons of various dosing schedules and regimens are needed to determine the optimum approach to rIL-2 therapy in metastatic melanoma. The coadministration of LAK cells with IL-2 does not appear to significantly improve clinical response. Although some studies have suggested improved response with coadministration of TILs with rIL-2, the therapy is technically difficult and costly, and overall clinical benefit has not been clearly demonstrated.

One of the greatest challenges in the management of patients with metastatic melanoma with immunotherapy is to determine on a patient-by-patient basis if the potential benefits of rIL-2 outweigh the substantial risk. It is obvious by the reports of long-term responses (> 10 years) in some patients that the risk is certainly worth the benefit for those individuals. A number of parameters such as human leukocyte antigen (HLA) expression and pretreatment immunologic status have been evaluated as potential predictors to therapy. Unfortunately, at this time it is difficult to determine which patients will respond to IL-2 therapy, as no biologic or immunologic parameters have been found that correlate with response.

Active immunization has become one of the most studied strategies for immunomodulation for melanoma. Current melanoma vaccines upregulate the antibody response of CTL to specific tumor antigens. Melanoma antigens are either tumor-associated antigens (TAAs) or melanoma-associated antigens (MAAs). TAAs are common to melanoma cells and other tumor cells, whereas MAAs are usually proteins or glycoproteins found predominately in melanomas and, at times, in normal melanocytes. The use of TAAs or MAAs for melanoma vaccines can be difficult, as the expression of antigens in melanoma cells is often heterogeneous and may change in response to the patient's immune response. Unfortunately, MAAs and TAAs also tend to be weakly immunogenics, although immunogenicity can be increased by physical alterations.

Melanoma vaccines range from complex antigen mixtures to purified antigens (Table 124–9). Complex vaccines are polyvalent and can stimulate an immune response to a number of tumor antigens, and are less susceptible to antigenic modulation by the cancer cells. Single-antigen vaccines can be problematic if a single-resistant-antigen-negative tumor cell develops.

Melanoma vaccines can be prepared from a patient's own tumor (autologous preparations) and will therefore target antigens from the patient's melanoma cell. Autologous vaccines may involve modification of the tumor cells with a hapten to increase immunogenicity of the preparation. Allogeneic preparations do not require patient tissue to prepare the vaccine. Allogeneic preparations often include a number of cell lines to increase the content of immunogenic TAA and MAA. Early results with one polyvalent whole-cell melanoma vaccine (PMCV) suggest a potential role in the adjuvant setting; currently a phase III clinical trial is underway comparing adjuvant PMCV versus IFN-α_{2b} for patients with surgically resected stage III melanoma.[58]

Melanoma vaccines may also be prepared with tumor cell lysate. Lysate vaccines can be prepared from the whole cells or from the cellular elements most likely to contain the antigens important for the induction of protective immune responses. Material shed from the melanoma cells is believed to be rich in cell-surface antigens and has been used for preparation of a melanoma vaccine. Melacine is a lysate vaccine prepared from two human melanoma cell lines administered with an adjuvant immunostimulant monophosphoryl lipid A (MPL) and purified mycobacterial cell-wall skeleton called DETOX. Initial reports from uncontrolled clinical trials with Melacine have suggested a role in treatment of metastatic melanoma.[59] The results of a large randomized controlled trial evaluating this vaccine are pending maturity and subsequent analysis.

An alternative approach to vaccine construction is to develop a vaccine from a single, highly specific antigen. Preparations currently in clinical trials include vaccines prepared from gangliosides, peptides such as MAGE or MART, and anti-idiotype monoclonal antibodies. Gangliosides GM_2, GD_2, GM_3, GD_3, and O-acetyl-GD_3 are present on the surface of many melanoma cells, but GM_2 is the most consistently expressed and immunogentic antigen. One vaccine composed of the ganglioside GM_2 coupled with KLH (keyhole limpet hemocyanine) is being evaluated in the adjuvant setting in a phase III intergroup study.[60] The vaccines from a single antigen have the advantage that they can be prepared in a reproducible manner on a large scale. The problem with this approach is that it is unclear if a single antigen or peptide will be sufficient to result in tumor cell kill.

Monoclonal antibodies have been used for the diagnosis and treatment of melanoma. Two strategies have been pursued: treatment with a monoclonal antibody to activate the host immune system[61,62] and treatment with a conjugated monoclonal antibody. Monoclonal antibodies have been conjugated to cytotoxic agents, radioisotopes, and toxins such as ricin A. Trials of monoclonal antibodies were initially limited secondary to the production of the monoclonal antibody. A problem seen in current studies is the induction of neutralizing antibodies to the murine monoclonal antibodies. Humanized murine or pure human monoclonal antibodies against melanoma-associated antigens could

TABLE 124–9. Melanoma Vaccines

Whole Melanoma Cells
Autologous cells
Allogeneic cells
Haptenized cells
Melanoma Cell Lysates
Viral oncolysates
Shed melanoma cell supernatant
Purified Antigens
Gangliosides (GM_2, GD_2)
Anti-idiotype Monoclonal Antibodies
Anti-GD_3 ganglioside

potentially avoid the problem with the human antimouse antibody (HAMA). Ferrone has developed a purified melanoma vaccine from an anti-idiotype mouse monclonal antibody.[63] This vaccine is composed of three monoclonal anti-idiotype antibodies that include the internal image of several determinants of the MAA. One of the problem with this antibody is the inability to directly induce a cell-mediated antitumor effect; therefore andjuvants are now being used to increase the ability of the anti-idiotype antibodies to induce a greater immune response.

Gene therapy of human melanoma is still in its infancy, but suggests several exciting approaches to the management of metastatic melanoma. Several strategies for gene therapy are currently under investigation for the treatment of melanoma.[64] One approach to gene therapy for melanoma is the modification of melanoma cells with the insertion of one or more cytokine genes, and then administering these altered allogeneic or autologous cells as a vaccine. Cytokine gene transduction has been accomplished with a number of cytokines including IL-2, TNF-α, IL-4, and IFN. The insertion of cytokine genes into melanoma cells is hoped to significantly increase the cells' immunogenicity.

Genes can also be transferred *in vitro* into TILs associated with melanoma in an attempt to potentiate the cytotoxicity of these cells. Rosenberg and colleagues were the first to attempt to transduce the gene coding for resistance to neomycin into human TILs.[65,66] This approach has since been used to transfer the tumor necrosis factor gene into TILs.

CHEMOTHERAPY

A number of cytotoxic agents have demonstrated *in vitro* activity to melanoma; only a few drugs have shown a response rate greater than 10% consistently in patients with melanoma. Chemotherapy has rarely cured a patient with melanoma; therefore the aim of chemotherapy is to palliate. The results of clinical trials are generally expressed in the term of response rates. The response rate often signifies the fraction of patients who experience a partial response plus those who experience a complete response. Partial response criteria vary, but may require a 50% reduction of the tumor for a minimum of 1 month. A complete response would require a total regression of all metastases for at least 1 month, and is uncommon (< 5%). It is essential to realize that these response rates do not reflect survival, and do not evaluate benefit to the patient. Response rates also do not represent the toxicities and the complications of therapy.

Dacarbazine (DTIC), a cytotoxic drug thought to exert its antitumor effect through alkylation, is currently the most effective single agent for the treatment of melanoma. DTIC is the only FDA-approved chemotherapeutic agent for the treatment of metastatic melanoma in the United States. In prospective controlled clinical trials, response rates of 20% to 25% have been seen,[67] with a average duration of response of 5 to 7 months. Early clinical trials demonstrate patients with skin, subcutaneous tissue, and lymph node involvement respond most frequently, whereas metastatic disease to the liver, bone, and central nervous system are often unresponsive.[9] Complete responses are uncommon, with a dismal 2% of patients treated with single-agent dacarbazine sustaining long-term complete responses.[68] The optimum dose schedule of dacarbazine has never been determined; therefore, single-dose regimens are often preferred for patient convenience. Common side effects of dacarbazine therapy include moderate myelosuppression, severe nausea and vomiting, and a flu-like syndrome after large doses. The nausea and vomiting can be prevented and managed with available antiemetics and is not a major complication. At this time there is no known role of DTIC in the adjuvant setting

Temozolomide is one of a series of imidazoletetrazine derivatives that was developed as a potential alternative to dacarbazine. Temozolomide is a prodrug of the active metabolite of dacarbazine. DTIC requires hepatic transformation to its active intermediate, whereas at physiologic pH, temozolomide chemically degrades to the cytotoxic triazene monomethyl 5-triazeno imidazole carboxamide (MTIC). Temozolomide is administered orally and appears to be less emetogenic than dacarbazine. Temozolomide appears to cross into the central nervous system and therefore may be beneficial for patients with CNS metastases.[69] Initial phase II trials in chemotherapy-naive metastatic melanoma suggest response rates similar to those seen with dacarbazine.[70]

The *nitrosoureas* have also been shown to be active against melanoma. Again, response rates for this group of alkylating agents tend to fall between 10% and 20%. Sites of responses are similar to those seen with dacarbazine.[71] It was initially thought that there may be an added benefit to the use of the lyophilic nitrosoureas in a malignancy that can metastasize to the brain. Unfortunately, despite the ability of these agents to cross the blood–brain barrier, the commercially available nitrosoureas have not been shown to produce an increased response in melanoma in the central nervous system. Fotemustine, an investigational nitrosourea, has shown preliminary responses in a limited number of patients with cerebral metastases.[72] The most common toxicity of the nitrosoureas is myelosuppression that can be delayed in occurrence and recovery. Leukopenia and thrombocytopenia may be seen as long as 3 to 5 weeks after drug administration, and may limit the application of these agents to multidrug regimens.

Cisplatin[73] and related compounds[74,75] have also been evaluated in the management of metastatic melanoma. The effectiveness of platinum compounds as single agents is limited, with response rates reported to be less than 10%.[76] The toxicities of cisplatin can be problematic, and include acute and delayed nausea and vomiting, renal toxicity, and neurotoxicity.

Taxanes[77] have demonstrated encouraging results in initial trials of metastatic melanoma, but require further evaluation to warrant the toxicities commonly seen.

COMBINATION CHEMOTHERAPY

In an attempt to extend the efficacy of dacarbazine, DTIC has been combined with other chemotherapeutic agents and, most recently, immunotherapy. The combination of dacarbazine with other chemotherapy, most commonly cisplatin, has been able to increase the response rates reported with dacarbazine alone, but the survival benefit has been minimal.[76,78,79] Again, responses were often limited to metastases in soft tissue, lymph nodes, and the lung—the sites most likely to respond to single-agent dacarbazine therapy. The concern with combination chemotherapy is increased toxicity, and any reports of an increase in response rates should be weighed with overall quality of life. The Dartmouth regimen is a combination chemotherapy regimen that includes carmustine, dacarbazine, cisplatin, and tamoxifen. Inital reports from uncontrolled phase II trials of this combination have demonstrated high response rates of 20% to 50%, but few patients achieve long-term survival. The benefit of tamoxifen to this regimen has been controversial, but a controlled clinical trial from the National Cancer Institute of Canada demonstrates no benefit from tamoxifen in this combination.[80] Careful analysis of the initial studies demonstrates that the criteria used to measure response were not consistent with standards used in large multicenter studies. Recently an intergroup study has been completed that compares the Dartmouth regimen without tamoxifen to single-agent dacarbazine therapy. The analysis of this study is anticipated in late 1998 and should help determine if there is a benefit with combination chemotherapy, and if the additional toxicities of the multidrug regimen are justified because of a response and/or survival benefit over chemotherapy with dacarbazine alone.

ENDOCRINE THERAPY

The role of endocrine therapy in the management of melanoma has been debated over the last decade. Initial reports that described high-affinity cytoplasmic estrogen receptors in patients with metastatic melanoma caused speculation about the possibility that anti-estrogens may be beneficial to modulate the biology of melanoma.[81] Additionally, estrogens have been shown to suppress T-lymphocyte activity and to suppress or stimulate the activities of B lymphocytes, macrophages, and natural killer cells, supporting a hypothesis that estrogens may influence the immunologic mechanisms that appear to be important in melanoma.

Tamoxifen was shown to have a response and survival benefit in one randomized trial[82] when combined with dacarbazine in 117 patients with metastatic melanoma; this benefit was most pronounced in women. As discussed previously, subsequent trials have not been able to confirm the initial reported benefit of the anti-estrogen when combined with chemotherapy, and tamoxifen is no longer routinely included in chemotherapy regimens.

Megestrol acetate, a synthetic progestin, has also been combined with chemotherapy in an attempt to influence patient responses and survival. In a small study of 19 patients with melanoma, the addition of megestrol 160 mg/d to dacarbazine, cisplatin, and carmustine suggested a response benefit.[83] Unfortunately the trial was small, and further investigation has not supported the routine use of progestins in the management of melanoma.

BIOCHEMOTHERAPY

The use of chemotherapy and immunotherapy alone has been limited by low overall response rates and toxicity. A new generation of multidrug combinations includes IFN-α and/or IL-2 with chemotherapy, and in initial trials has provided higher response rates. The phase I to III trials of biochemotherapy approaches include combinations of IFN and chemotherapy,[84,85] IL-2 and chemotherapy,[47,86–89] or the combination of IL-2, chemotherapy, and IFN.[90–94] Results to date suggest response rates similar to or slightly better than those seen with dacarbazine alone, with increased toxicity. Toxicities can be severe, and are consistent with the individual agents in the regimen.

LIMB PERFUSION

For recurrent melanoma of the limbs one approach to therapy is regional isolated perfusion with cytostatic drugs.[95–97] After regional perfusions, objective response rates have been reported to be as high as 80%. The role of hyperthermia (39°C to 40°C) with regional isolated perfusion is not clearly defined. Although most clinical trials have used melphalan, it is not known whether combination of melphalan with other agents may improve results. Recent work with the biologic response modifiers such as tumor necrosis factor have been encouraging.[98]

PREVENTION AND DETECTION

The results of early treatment emphasize the role for early detection and prevention.[99,100] The American Academy of Dermatology recommends monthly self-examination of skin to serve as a mechanism of recognizing moles or marks on the skin that may be melanoma. Patients with a strong family history should have a clinical examination, and in some cases screening photography to document size, shape, and location of moles.

Education and reeducation about the importance of sun protection has the potential to help decrease the rising incidence of this disease. Historically, patients have been counseled that the risk of skin cancer can be limited by the use of sunscreens with a sun-protection factor (SPF) of 15 or greater. It is important to include counseling about the appropriate use of sunscreens to optimize benefits from these products.[101] Additionally, sun protection beyond sunscreen may be beneficial for those individuals in the sun for prolonged periods of time or who are at high risk of burning.

▶ PRINCIPLES OF PHARMACOTHERAPY

- Cutaneous melanoma is becoming a common cancer, but it is a cancer that can be prevented and cured if detected early through surgical resection. Public education about screening and early detection provide one strategy for curbing the steady increase in this disease.
- Early-stage melanoma has excellent complete response rates with surgical resection.
- Patients with locally advanced disease now have the treatment option of adjuvant therapy with interferon-α_{2b}. The toxicities with this therapy are significant and require close patient monitoring and dose delay and/or reduction in a large percentage of the patients.
- Metastatic melanoma remains a clinical challenge. At this time there is not a standard therapy. Dacarbazine is considered one of the most active agents; the use of combination chemotherapy has not been shown in head-to-head comparative studies to be superior to single-agent therapy with dacarbazine.
- High-dose interleukin-2 has recently been FDA approved for the treatment of patients with metastatic melanoma. The toxicities with this regimen are high, but the potential benefit is that a small subset of patients may have a durable response.
- The results of chemoimmunotherapy look promising, but the definitive drug combination and/or schedules have not been defined. The role of biochemotherapy continues to be explored in the treatment of patients with metastatic melanoma.
- A number of melanoma tumor vaccines have been evaluated in clinical trials in metastatic melanoma and in the adjuvant setting. The role of specific melanoma vaccines has not been defined at this time.

REFERENCES

1. Koh HK. Cutaneous melanoma. N Engl J Med 1991;325:171–182.
2. Landis SH, Murray T, Bolden S, et al. Cancer statistics, 1998. CA Cancer J Clin 1998;48:6–29.
3. Rigel DS, Kopf AW, Friedman RJ. The rate of malignant melanoma in the United States: Are we making an impact? J Am Acad Dermatol 1987;17:1050–1053.
4. Autier P. Epidemiology of melanoma. In: Lejeune FJ, Chaudhuri PK, Das Gupta TK, eds. Malignant melanoma: Medical and surgical management. New York, McGraw-Hill, 1994:1–7.
5. Greene MH, Clark WH, Tucker M, et al. Acquired precursors of cutaneous malignant melanoma. N Engl J Med 1985;312:91–94.
6. Gallagher RP, Elwood JM, Yang P. Is chronic sunlight exposure important in accounting for increases in melanoma incidence? Int J Cancer 1989;44:813–815.
7. Kirkwood JM, Lotze MT. Melanoma. In: Kirkwood JM, Lotze MT, Yasko JM, eds. Current Cancer Therapeutics. Philadelphia, Current Medicine, 1994:131.
8. Dore JF, Carrel S. Biology of melanoma differentiation and progression. In: Lejeune FJ, Chaudhuri PK, Das Gupta K, eds. Malignant melanoma: Medical and surgical management. New York, McGraw-Hill, 1994:9–26.
9. Balch CM, Houghton AN, Peters LJ. Cutaneous melanoma. In: DeVita, Hellman S, Rosenberg SA, eds. Cancer: Principles and practice of oncology, 4th ed. Philadelphia, Lippincott, 1993:1613–1614.
10. Friedman RJ, Rigel DS, Silverman MK, et al. Malignant melanoma in the 1990's: The continued importance of early detection and the role of physician examination and self-examination of the skin. Ca Cancer J Clin 1991;41:201–227.
11. NIH Consensus Development Panel on Early Melanoma. Diagnosis and treatment of early melanoma. NIH Consensus Conference. JAMA 1992;268:1314–1319.
12. Cochran AJ. Histology and prognosis in malignant melanoma. J Pathol 1969;97:459–468.
13. Clark WH Jr. A classification of malignant melanoma in man correlated with histogenesis and biologic behavior. In: Montagna W, Hu F, eds. Advances in Biology of the Skin. The Pigmentary System. London, Pergammon, 1967:621–645.
14. Breslow A. Thickness, cross-sectional areas and depth of invasion in the prognosis of cutaneous melanoma. Ann Surg 1970;172:1902–1908.
15. Halpern AC, Schuchter LM. Prognostic models in melanoma. Semin Oncol 1997;24(suppl 4):2–7.
16. Flemming ID, Cooper JS, Henson DE, et al, eds. AJCC Cancer Staging Manual, 5th ed. Philadelphia, Lippincott-Raven, 1997:163–167.
17. Morton DL, Wen DR, Wong JH, et al. Technical details of intraoperative lymphatic mapping for early stage melanoma. Arch Surg 1992; 127:392–399.
18. Ross MI, Reintgen D, Balch CM. Selective lymphadenectomy: Emerging role of lymphatic mapping and sentinel node biopsy in the management of early stage melanoma. Semin Surg Oncol 1993:9: 219–223.
19. Hoon DS, Wang Y, Dale PS, et al. Detection of occult melanoma cells in blood with a multiple-marker polymerase chain reaction assay. J Clin Oncol 1995;13:2109–2116.
20. Veronesi U, Cascineli N. Narrow excision (1-cm margin): A safe procedure for thin cutaneous melanoma. Arch Surg 1991;126:438–441.
21. Balch CM, Urist MM, Karakousis CP, et al. Efficiency of 2-cm surgical margins for intermediate-thickness melanomas (1–4 mm): Results of a multi-institutional randomized surgical trial. Ann Surg 1993;218:262–269.
22. Balch CM, Soong SJ, Bartolucci AA, et al. Efficacy of elective regional lymph node dissection of 1 to 4 mm thick melanomas for patients 60 years of age and younger. Ann Surg 1996;224:255–266.
23. Cay CL, Sober AJ, Lew RA, et al. Malignant melanoma patients with positive nodes and relatively good prognosis: Microstaging retains prognostic significance in clinical stage I melanoma patients with metastases to regional nodes. Cancer 1981;47:955–962.
24. Somoza S, Kondziolka D, Lansford D, et al. Stereostatic radiosurgery for cerebral metastatic melanoma. J Neurosurg 1993;79:661–666.
25. Harpole DH, Johnson CM, Wolfe, et al. Analysis of 945 cases of pulmonary metastatic melanoma. J Thorac Cardiovasc Surg 1992; 103:743–750.
26. Creagan ET, Ahmann DL, Green SJ, et al. Phase II study of low dose recombinant leukocyte A interferon in disseminated malignant melanoma. J Clin Oncol 1984;2:1002–1005.
27. Creagan ET, Ahmann DL, Green SJ, et al. Phase II study of recombinant leukocyte A interferon (rIFN-alpha A) in disseminated malignant melanoma. Cancer 1984;54:2844–2849.
28. Coates A, Rallingsm, Hersey P, Swanson C. Phase II study of recombinant alpha 2-interferon in advanced malignant melanoma. J Interferon Res 1986;6:1–4.
29. Hersey P, Hasic E, MacDonald M, et al. Effects of recombinant leukocytes interferon (rIFN-alpha a) on tumor growth and immune responses in patient with metastatic melanoma. Br J Cancer 1985;51: 815–826.
30. Legha SS, Papadopoulos NE, Plager C, et al. Clinical evaluation of recombinant interferon alfa-2a (Roferon-a) in metastatic melanoma using two different schedules. J Clin Oncol 1987;5:1240–1246.
31. Elsasser-Beile U, Drews H. Interferon in the treatment of malignant melanoma. Results of clinical studies. Fortschr Med 1987;105:401.
32. Steiner A, Wolf C, Pehamberger H. Comparison of the effects of three different treatment regimens of recombinant interferons (r-IFN alpha, r-IFN gamma, and r-IFN-alpha + cimetidine) in disseminated malignant melanoma. J Cancer Res Clin Oncol 1987;113:459–465.
33. Kirkwood JM, Ernstoff MS, Davis CA, et al. Comparison of intramuscular and intravenous recombinant alpha-2 interferon in melanoma and other cancers. Ann Intern Med 1985;103;32–36.
34. Dorval T, Palangie T, Jouve M, et al. Clinical phase II trial of recombinant DNA interferon (interferon alfa 2b) in patients with metastatic malignant melanoma. Cancer 1986;58:215–218.
35. Robinson WA, Mughal TI, Thomas MR, et al. Treatment of metastatic malignant melanoma with recombinant interferon alpha-2. Immunobiology 1986;172:275–282.
36. Sertoli MR, Bernengo MG, Ardizzoni A, et al. Phase II trial of recombinant alfa-2b interferon in the treatment of metastatic skin melanoma. Oncology 1989;46:96–98.
37. Cascinelli N. Evaluation of efficacy of adjuvant rIFN alfa 2A in melanoma patients with regional node metastases. Proc Am Soc Clin Oncol 1995;14:1410.
38. Kirkwood JM, Straderman MH, Ernstoff MS, et al. Interferon alfa-2b adjuvant therapy of high-risk resected cutanteous melanoma: The Eastern cooperative oncology group trial EST 1684. J Clin Oncol 1996;14:7–17.
39. Borden EC, Parkinson D. A perspective on the clinical effectiveness and tolerance of interferon-alfa. Semin Oncol 1998;25(suppl 1):3–8.
40. Dalakas MC, Mock V, Hawkins MJ. Fatigue: Definitions, mechanisms, and paradigms for study. Semin Oncol 1998;25(suppl 1):48–53.
41. Plata-Salaman CR. Cytokines and anorexia: A brief overview. Semin Oncol 1998;25(suppl 1):64–72.
42. Cole BF, Gelber RD, Kirkwood JM, et al. A quality-of-life-adjusted survival analysis of interferon alfa-2b adjuvant treatment for high-risk resected cutaneous melanoma: An Eastern cooperative oncology group study (E1684). J Clin Oncol 1996;14:2666–2673.
43. Von Wussow P, Bock B, Hartmann F, Deicher H. Intralesional interferon-alpha therapy in advanced malignant melanoma. Cancer 1988; 61:1071–1074.
44. Hersh EM, Murray JL, Kong WK, et al. Phase I study of cancer therapy with recombinant interleukin-2 administered by intravenous bolus injection. Biotherapy 1989;1:215–216.
45. Parkinson DR, Abrams JS, Wiernik PH, et al. Interleukin-2 therapy in patients with metastatic malignant melanoma: A phase II study. J Clin Oncol 1990:8:1650–1656.

46. Whitehead RP, Kopecky KJ, Samson MK, et al. Phase II study of intravenous bolus recombinant interleulun-2 in advanced malignant melanoma: Southwest oncology group study. JNCI 1991;83:1250–1252.
47. Demchak PA, Mier JW, Robert NJ, et al. Interleukin-2 and high-dose cisplatin in patients with metastatic melanoma: A pilot study. J Clin Oncol 1991;9:1821–1830.
48. Rosenberg SA, Yang JC, Topalian SL, et al. Treatment of 283 consecutive patients with metastatic melanoma or renal cell cancer using high-dose bolus interleukin-2. JAMA 1994;271:907–913.
49. West WH, Tauer KW, Yannelli JR, et al. Constant-infusion recombinant interleukin-2 in adoptive immunotherapy of advanced cancer. N Engl J Med 1987;316:898–905.
50. Dutcher JP, Gaynor ER, Boldt DH, et al. A phase II study of high-dose continuous infusion interleukin-2 with lymphokine-activated killer cells in patients with metastatic melanoma. J Clin Oncol 1991; 9:641–648.
51. Dillman RO, Oldham RK, Tauer KW, et al. Continuous interleukin-2 and lymphokine-activated killer cells for advanced cancer: A national biotherapy study group trial. J Clin Oncol 1991;9: 1233–1240.
52. Perez EA, Scudder SA, Meyers FA, et al. Weekly 24-hour continuous infusion interleukin-2 for metastatic melanoma and renal cell carcinoma: A phase I study. J Immunother 1991;10:57–62.
53. Vlasveld LT, Horenblas S, Hekman A, et al. Phase II study of intermittent continuous infusion of low-dose recombinant interleukin-2 in advanced melanoma and renal cell carcinoma. Ann Oncol 1994;5: 179–181.
54. Flaherty LE, Redman BG, Chabot G, et al. A phase I-II study of dacarbazine in combination with outpatient interleukin-2 in metastatic malignant melanoma. Cancer 1990;65:2471–2477.
55. Richards JM, Mehta N, Schroeder. L, et al. Sequential chemotherapy in the treatment of metastatic melanoma. J Clin Oncol 1992;10: 1338–1343.
56. Keilholz U, Scheibenbogen C, Tilgen W, et al. Interferon-alpha and interleukin-2 in the treatment of metastatic melanoma. Cancer 1993; 72:607–614.
57. Atzpodien J, Korfer A, Fanks CR, et al. Home therapy with recombinant interleukin-2 and interferon-alpha 2b in advanced human malignancies. Lancet 1990;335:1509–1512.
58. Conforti AM, Ollila DW, Kelley MC, et al. Update on active specific immunotherapy with melanoma vaccines. J Surg Oncol 1997;66: 55–64.
59. Wallack MK, Sicanandham M, Balch CM, et al. A phase III randomized, double-blind, multi-institutional trial of vaccinia melanoma oncolysate-active specific immunotherapy for patients with stage II melanoma. Cancer 1995;75:34–42.
60. Livingston PO, Wong GYC, Adluris S, et al. Improved survival in stage III melanoma patients with GM2 antibodies: A randomized trial of adjuvant vaccination with GM2 ganglioside. J Clin Oncol 1994;12:1036–1044.
61. Carrasquillo JA, Abrams PG, Schroff RW, et al. Effect of antibody dose on the imaging and biodistribution of indium-111 9.2.27 antimelanoma monoclonal antibody. J Nucl Med 1988;29:39–47.
62. Murray JL, Rosenblum MG, Lamki L, et al. Clinical parameters related to optimal tumor localization of indium-111-labeled mouse antimelanoma monoclonal antibody ZME-018. J Nucl Med 1987;28: 25–33.
63. Ferrone S. Human tumor associated antigen mimicry by anti-idiotypic antibodies. Ann NY Acad Sci 1993;690:214–221.
64. Parmiani G, Colombo MP. Somatic gene therapy of human melanoma: Preclinical studies and early clinical trials. Melanoma Res 1995:5:295–301.
65. Rosenberg ST, Aebersold P, Cornetta K. Gene transfer into humans—immunotherapy of patients with advanced melanoma, using tumor-infiltrating lymphocytes modified by retroviral gene transduction. N Engl J Med 1990;323:570–578.
66. Rosenberg AS, Anderson F, Blaese, Hwu P. The development of gene therapy for the treatment of cancer. 1993;218:455–464.
67. Comis RL. DTIC in malignant melanoma. A perspective. Cancer Treat Rep 1976;64:1123.
68. Hill GJ, Krementz ET, Hill HZ. Dimethyl traiazenoimidazole carboxamide and combination therapy for melanoma. IV. Late results after complete responses to chemotherapy. Cancer 1984;53:1299–1305.
69. Newlands ES, Stevens MF, Wedge SR, et al. Temozolomide: A review of its discovery, chemical properties, pre-clinical development and clinical trials. Cancer Treat Rev 1997;23:35–61.
70. Bleehen NM, Newlands ES, Lee SM, et al. Cancer research campaign phase II trial of temozolomide in metastatic melanoma. J Clin Oncol 1995;13:910–913.
71. Ahmann DL. Nitrosoureas in the management of disseminated malignant melanoma. Cancer Treat Rep 1976;60:747.
72. Jacquillat C, Khayat D, Banzet P, et al. Final report of the french multicenter phase II study of the nitrosourea fotemustine in 153 evaluable patients with disseminated malignant melanoma including patients with cerebral metastases. Cancer 1990;66:1873–1878.
73. Mechl Z, Kreja P. Cis-diamminedichloroplatinum in the treatment of disseminated malignant melanoma. Neoplasia 1983;30:371–377.
74. Olver I, Green M, Peters W, et al. A phase II trial of zeniplatin in metastatic melanoma. Am J Clin Oncol 1995;18:56–58.
75. Evans L, Casper ES, Rosenbluth R. Phase II trial of carboplatin in advanced melanoma. Cancer Treat Rep 1987;71:171.
76. Steffens TA, Bajorin D, Chapman PB, et al. A phase II trial of high-dose cisplatin and dacarbazine: Lack of efficacy of high-dose, cisplatin-based therapy for metastatic melanoma. Cancer 1991;68:1230–1237.
77. Einzig AJ, Hochster H, Wiernik PH, et al. A phase II trial of taxol in patients with malignant melanoma. Invest New Drugs 1991;9:59–65.
78. Luger SM, Kirkwood JM, Ernstoff MS, Vlock DR. High-dose cisplatin and dacarbazine in the treatment of metastatic melanoma. J Natl Cancer Inst 1990;82:1934–1937.
79. Murren JR, DeRosa W, Durivage HJ, et al. High-dose cisplatin plus DTIC in the treatment of metastatic melanoma. Cancer 1991;67: 1514–1517.
80. Rusthoven JJ, Quirt IC, Iscoe NA, et al. Randomized, double-blind, placebo-controlled trial comparing the response rates of carmustine, dacarbazine, and cisplatin with and without tamoxifen in patients with metastatic melanoma. National Cancer Institute of Canada clinical trials group. J Clin Oncol 1996;14:2083–2090.
81. Adami HO, Bergstrom R, Holmberg L, et al. The effect of female sex hormones on cancer survival. JAMA 1990;263:2189–2193.
82. Cocconi G, Bella M, Calabresi F, et al. Treatment of metastatic malignant melanoma with dacarbazine plus tamoxifen. N Engl J Med 1992;327:516–523.
83. Nathanson L, Meelu MA, Losada R. Chemohormone therapy of metastatic melanoma with megestrol acetate plus dacarbazine, carmustine, and cisplatin. Cancer 1994;73:98–102.
84. Margolin KA, Doroshow JH, Akman ST. Phase II trial of cisplatin and alpha-interferon in advanced malignant melanoma. J Clin Oncol 1992;10:1574–1578.
85. Pyrhonen S, Hahka-Kemppinen M, Muhonen T. A promising interferon plus four-drug chemotherapy regimen for metastatic melanoma. J Clin Oncol 1992;10:1919–1926.
86. Mitchell MS, Kempf RA, Harel W, et al. Effectiveness and tolerability of low-dose cyclophosphamide and low-dose intravenous interleukin-2 disseminated melanoma. J Clin Oncol 1988;6:409–424.
87. Shiloni E, Pouillart P, Janssens J, et al. Sequential dacarbazine chemotherapy followed by recombinant interleukin-2 in metastatic melanoma. A pilot multicenter phase I-II study. Eur J Cancer Clin Oncol 1989:25(suppl 3):S45–S49.
88. Stoter G, Aamdal S, Rodenhuis S, et al. Sequential administration of recombinant human interleukin-2 and dacarbazine in metastatic melanoma: A multicenter phase II study. J Clin Oncol 1991;9:1687–1691.
89. Flaherty LE, Robinson W, Redman BG, et al. A phase II study of dacarbazine and cisplatin in combination with outpatient administered

interleukin-2 in metastatic malignant melanoma. Cancer 1993; 71:3520–3525.

90. Richards JM, Mehta N, Ramming K, Skosey P. Sequential chemoimmunotherapy in the treatment of metastatic melanoma. J Clin Oncol 1992;10:1338–1343.
91. Khayat D, Tourani JM, Benhammouda A, et al. Sequential chemoimmunotherapy with cisplatin, interleukin-2, and interferon alfa-2a for metastatic melanoma. J Clin Oncol 1993:11:2173–2180.
92. Bajetta E, Negretti E, Giannotti B, et al. Phase II study of interferon-2a and dacarbazine in advanced melanoma. Am J Clin Oncol 1990; 13:405–409.
93. Falkson CI, Falkson G, Falkson HC. Improved results with the addition of recumbent interferon alpha-2b to dacarbazine in treatment with patients with metastatic malignant melanoma. J Clin Oncol 1991;9:1403–1408.
94. Smith KA, Green JA, Eccles JM. Interferon alpha-2a and vindesine in the treatment of advanced malignant melanoma. Eur J Cancer 1992;28:438–441.
95. Kroon BBR. Regional isolation perfusion in melanoma of the limbs; accomplishments, unsolved problems, future. Eur J Surg Oncol 1998; 14:101–110.
96. Klaase JM, Kroon BBR, van Geel AN, et al. Prognostic factors for tumor response and limb recurrence-free interval in patients with advanced melanoma of the limbs treated with regional isolated perfusion with melphalan. Surgery 1994;115:39–45.
97. Klaase JM, Kroon BBR, van Geel AN, et al. A retrospective comparative study evaluating the results of a single perfusion versus double-perfusion schedule with melphalan in patients with recurrent melanoma of the lower limb. Cancer 1993;71:2990–2994.
98. Lejeuene FJ, Lienard D. Isolation perfusion of the limbs for in transit melanoma metastasized with cytokines and chemotherapy. In: Lejeune FJ, Chaudhuri PK, Das Gupta TK, eds. Malignant melanoma: Medical and surgical management. New York, McGraw-Hill, 1994:233–240.
99. Lober CW. Dysplastic (atypical) nevi: Significance and management. South Med J 1992;85:870–877.
100. Koh HK, Geller AC, Miller DR, Lew RA. Screening for melanoma and skin cancer in the United States. In: Miller AB, Chamberlain J, Day NE, et al, eds. Cancer Screening. New York, Cambridge University Press, 1990.
101. Westerdahl J, Olsson H, Masback A, et al. Is the use of sunscreens a risk factor for malignant melanoma? Melanoma Res 1995;5:59–65.

125
Bone Marrow Transplantation

Janelle B. Perkins, PharmD, BCPS, and Gary C. Yee, PharmD, FCCP

Bone marrow transplantation (BMT) is a process that involves intravenous infusion of hematopoietic stem cells from a compatible donor into a recipient with a life-threatening disease. Because of the widespread acceptance of peripheral blood rather than bone marrow as a source of hematopoietic stem cells for autologous transplants, BMT is sometimes referred to as hematopoietic stem cell transplantation (HSCT), and autologous BMT is sometimes referred to as autologous blood or marrow transplantation (ABMT) or blood cell transplantation (BCT). The rationale for BMT in the treatment of malignant disease is based on studies that show that most anticancer drugs have a steep dose–response relationship and that bone marrow suppression limits the chemotherapy dosage that can be safely administered. Although standard-dose chemotherapy can prolong survival in many cancer patients, most patients are not cured of their disease (Fig. 125–1). The infusion of hematopoietic stem cells allows oncologists to administer very high chemotherapy doses (as much as tenfold higher). Tumor cell kill will therefore be greatly increased, and the likelihood of cure higher, if we assume that most tumor cells that are resistant to standard doses would be sensitive to higher doses. The chemotherapy dose cannot be escalated indefinitely, however, because of the risk of death due to nonhematopoietic toxicity.

High-dose chemotherapy (HDC) with blood or marrow transplantation has become an important treatment modality for a variety of malignant and nonmalignant diseases. There are more than 100 active BMT programs in the United States. It is estimated that about 30,000 patients are currently transplanted worldwide (18,000 autologous, 12,000 allogeneic), and the number is expected to increase 15% to 20% each year. Historically the most common type of donor was a genetically nonidentical individual (referred to as allogeneic BMT) such as a histocompatible sibling. But the number of autologous transplants—in which the patient serves as his or her own donor—has increased dramatically, and the number of autologous transplants performed each year currently exceeds the number of allogeneic transplants. The rapid growth in the number of autologous transplants is related to the observation that this treatment modality results in long-term survival and probably cure in many patients with lymphoma and breast cancer. Although the use of HDC with autologous rescue in women with breast cancer remains controversial, this issue has greatly increased the awareness of the lay public and health care professionals to HDC as a treatment modality. Insurance coverage for HDC in women with breast cancer is now required in some states, and other states are considering similar mandates. Although this chapter focuses on the application of HDC with blood or marrow transplantation in the treatment of malignant disease, it is important to note that many nonmalignant diseases—including aplastic anemia, thalassemia, sickle cell anemia, immunodeficiency disorders, and other genetic disorders—are potentially curable with allogeneic BMT.

This chapter summarizes the current use of HDC with blood or marrow transplantation in the treatment of acute and chronic leukemia, lymphoma, multiple myeloma, breast cancer, and other solid tumors. More detailed information on HDC can be found in recently published reviews and books.[1–5]

DONORS AND HISTOCOMPATIBILITY TESTING

Three types of donors are used in HDC with blood or marrow transplantation. In autologous transplants, patients receive their own hematopoietic stem cells, which were collected and stored before intensive cytotoxic therapy. In syngeneic transplants, an identical twin serves as the donor. In allogeneic transplants, the donor is genetically not identical to the recipient but shares some common tissue antigens. Immunologic compatibility is evaluated with studies of cell surface antigens encoded by genes of the major histocompatibility complex (MHC), which in humans is located on the sixth chromosome and is referred to as the HLA (human leukocyte antigen) complex.[6,7] The genes of the HLA system are clustered in three distinct regions designated class I, class II, and class III. Class I and class II antigens function as major transplantation antigens, while products of class III genes play important roles in the immune system. The major class I loci in humans are referred to as HLA-A, HLA-B, and HLA-C. There is one major class II locus (HLA-D); this region is comprised of three sets of genes encoding HLA-DR, HLA-DQ, and HLA-DP molecules. HLA-D antigens are primarily DR specific, and the two are strongly correlated. Class I and class II antigens differ in their tissue distribution, structure, and function. Class I antigens are expressed on virtually all nucleated cells and serve as the primary targets for cytotoxic T lymphocytes. In contrast, class II antigens are expressed only on macrophages, B lymphocytes, and activated T lymphocytes, and serve as the primary targets for helper T lymphocytes. The relative importance of class I versus class II antigens as determinants of risk of acute graft-versus-host disease (GVHD) or graft failure is not clear.

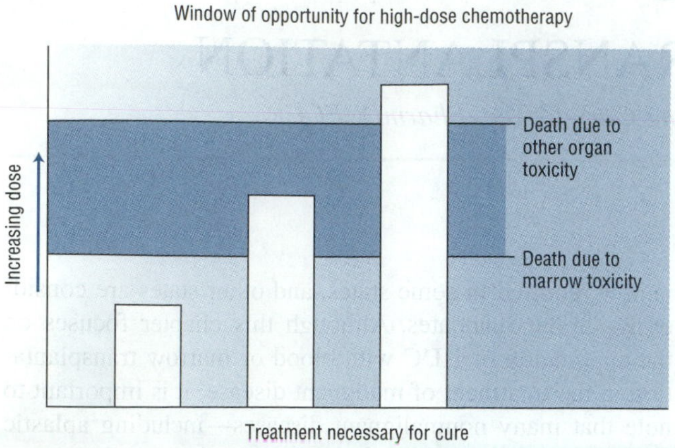

FIGURE 125–1. Patients represented by the middle column are the best candidates for bone marrow transplantation because this technique allows administration of chemotherapy or radiation in doses that would otherwise be intolerable due to severe myelosuppression. *(From Ref. 30. Reprinted by permission of Blackwell Science, Inc.)*

Historically, the most important HLA loci in allogeneic transplantation were HLA-A, HLA-B, and HLA-D (or HLA-DR). Typing for HLA-A, HLA-B, and HLA-DR is usually performed by serologic typing with standard microcytotoxicity assays. HLA types determined by this method are reported as the loci (A, B, or DR), followed by a number. A lowercase "w" is sometimes added before the number to indicate "workshop" or tentative designation based on American or international histocompatibility workshops. Typing for the HLA-D region also can be performed with cellular typing methods, such as the mixed lymphocyte reaction (MLR) or mixed lymphocyte culture (MLC). A "positive" MLR or MLC indicates incompatibility somewhere in the HLA-D region. Individuals who have a low degree of reactivity in the MLR or MLC (expressed as a low percent relative response) and who meet other selection criteria could serve as donors. However, recent studies indicate that MLR or MLC reactivity does not correlate significantly with the risk of acute GVHD, and some BMT centers no longer use this method to determine HLA compatibility.[8] In addition to serologic typing, some BMT centers use DNA-based techniques, such as polymerase chain reaction (PCR), for HLA-DR typing because of the extensive polymorphism in the HLA-DR subregion and the high error rate in serologic HLA-DR typing.[7] For example, although there are more than 100 DRB1 alleles, serologic reagents can distinguish no more than 15 different DR serotypes. Preliminary results indicate that the use of these DNA-based techniques to select unrelated donors may reduce the risk of severe acute GVHD in that setting.[9] Results of another study show that disparity at the HLA-C locus may be associated with graft failure in recipients of marrow from matched unrelated donors.[10]

The most common donor for allogeneic transplants is an HLA-identical sibling. However, only about 30% of Americans have an HLA-identical sibling. In an effort to offer allogeneic transplants to patients who lack an HLA-identical sibling donor, there is increasing interest in the use of alternative donors: a related donor who is partially HLA matched or a fully or closely HLA-matched unrelated donor. Rarely, a parent can be HLA identical with his or her child. A relative can be a zero- (rare), one-, two-, or three-loci mismatch (assuming testing for HLA-A, -B, and -DR antigens). It is estimated, however, that only an additional 10% of patients will have a closely HLA-matched related donor.

The most common type of alternative donor is an individual who is fully or closely HLA matched. To facilitate identification of these donors, the National Marrow Donor Program (NMDP) was started in 1986 with initial funding from a U.S. Navy contract.[11] Similar programs outside of the United States also have been started. To date, more than 3 million donors in the United States have been registered by the NMDP and more than 7000 matched unrelated donor (MUD) transplants have been facilitated by the NMDP. If we assume that testing is performed at three HLA loci (A, B, and DR) and that each patient has two phenotypes for each locus (one from each parent), matching is required for a total of six antigens. Therefore, a "completely" matched (i.e., 6/6 antigen match) unrelated donor is matched for HLA-A, -B, and -DR and is also MLC nonreactive. A "closely" matched unrelated donor is usually incompatible at one or two HLA antigens or is MLC reactive. The likelihood of any one unrelated individual being a match ranges from 1 in 100 to 1 in 1,000,000, depending on the prevalence of the patient's HLA type and ethnic background. With the current number of potential donors, the overall likelihood of finding a potential match on the NMDP registry is about 80%. This figure is lower than that predicted, probably because there appear to be more HLA types than previously recognized. Because most minorities are poorly represented in the program, the likelihood of finding a donor for patients from certain ethnic groups is lower. Another limitation is the time needed to search for a potential donor (average length of time from donor search to transplant is 135 days). Many patients with advanced leukemia will therefore relapse while waiting for completion of the search. Cost is also a concern, as the cost for donor search and marrow procurement ranges from $25,000 to $50,000.[12] About 75% of the matched unrelated transplants are performed in patients with some form of leukemia.

The clinical results of allogeneic BMT with alternative donors are encouraging. Although some patients who receive marrow from an alternative donor are probably cured of their disease, the risk of transplant-related mortality is high. In a study of 2055 patients with leukemia treated with allogeneic BMT, transplant-related mortality was significantly higher after alternative donor transplants than after HLA-identical sibling transplants.[13] The difference in mortality was primarily related to a higher risk of graft failure and acute GVHD.

With the increasing availability of donors other than HLA-identical siblings, patients with some types of leukemia who do not have an HLA-identical sibling donor may have to choose between allogeneic or autologous BMT. Each approach has advantages and disadvantages. Patients treated with allogeneic BMT have a lower risk of leukemic relapse because of the graft-versus-leukemia effect, but they are at higher risk for GVHD and its associated complications. Patients treated with autologous transplants have a lower risk of transplant-related complications, but may have a higher risk of leukemic relapse because of the lack of graft-versus-leukemia and the use of marrow that is potentially contaminated with residual leukemic cells.

COLLECTION OF HEMATOPOIETIC STEM CELLS

The most important transplanted cells in BMT are hematopoietic stem cells, which serve as "mother" cells for all blood cells including erythrocytes, leukocytes, and platelets (see Chap. 90.)[14] Stem cells have varying degrees of "stemness"; true totipotent stem cells are capable of replicating indefinitely and can differentiate into any of the different blood cells. Because of their capacity for self-renewal, these stem cells are capable of repopulating the marrow of the recipient. There is intense interest in stem cells because a single totipotent stem cell should be capable of permanently reconstituting the entire blood-producing and immune systems. Totipotent stem cells are rare cells, comprising less than 0.01% of all bone marrow cells. It has been extremely difficult to isolate stem cells because of their rarity, their similarity in appearance to other cells, and the lack of a rapid and direct method to quantitate the number of stem cells.

Figures 125–2 and 125–3 show the schemes for autologous and allogeneic BMT, respectively. Bone marrow from the donor is obtained by more than 100 separate aspirations from the anterior and posterior iliac crests.[15] The procedure takes about a hour and yields 200 to 1500 mL, depending on the size of the donor. The marrow is transferred into tissue culture medium containing preservative-free heparin. The pooled marrow is then passed through a series of stainless steel screens to break up aggregated particles, resulting essentially in a single-cell suspension. In allogeneic BMT, the marrow stem cells are given to the recipient within 12 to 24 hours after harvest. In autologous BMT, the marrow is frozen and stored until needed. After intravenous infusion over several hours, the marrow stem cells enter the systemic circulation and find their way to the bone marrow cavity, where they reseed and grow in the bone marrow microenvironment. Although the donor experiences local soreness for a few days, the procedure is usually well tolerated, with no delayed complications resulting from the marrow aspiration. The major risk of serving as a marrow donor is that of undergoing general anesthesia.

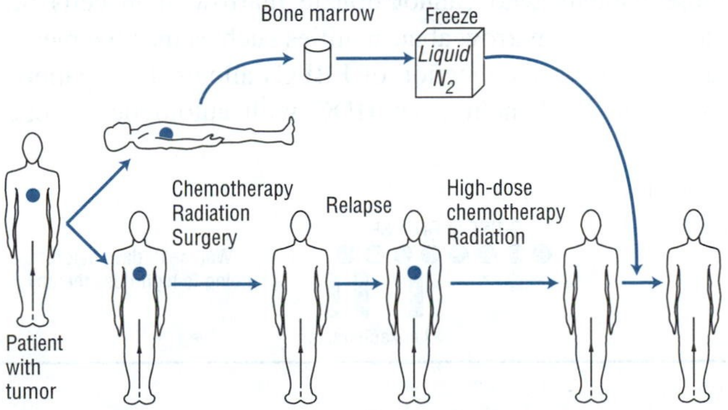

FIGURE 125–2. Scheme for autologous bone marrow transplantation. The patient with cancer typically undergoes marrow collection and cryopreservation early in the course of the disease. At a time when the disease is resistant to conventional treatment, intensive combined modality therapy is administered followed by reinfusion of the stored autologous bone marrow cells. *(From Champlin RE, Gale RP. Role of bone marrow transplantation in the treatment of hematologic malignancies and solid tumors: Critical review of syngeneic, autologous, and allogeneic transplants. Cancer Treat Rep 1984;68:146.)*

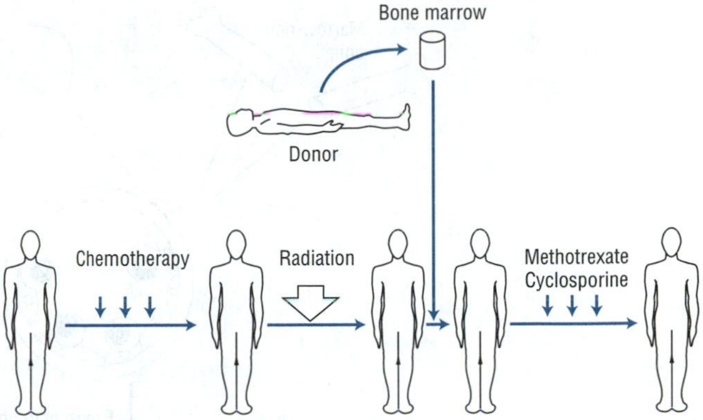

FIGURE 125–3. Scheme for allogeneic bone marrow transplantation in the treatment of cancer. The patient typically receives marrow ablative chemotherapy and/or total body irradiation to eradicate the malignancy and as immunosuppression to prevent transplant rejection. The bone marrow is administered as an intravenous infusion followed by posttransplant immunosuppression to prevent GVHD. *(From Champlin RE, Gale RP. Role of bone marrow transplantation in the treatment of hematologic malignancies and solid tumors: Critical review of syngeneic, autologous, and allogeneic transplants. Cancer Treat Rep 1984;68:146.)*

Hematopoietic stem cells also circulate in peripheral blood (peripheral blood progenitor cells [PBPCs] or stem cells [PBSCs]), where they can be harvested and used for transplantation.[16,17] PBPCs are found in the mononuclear (lymphocytes and monocytes) fraction of white blood cells and are collected by a procedure called *leukapheresis.* In this outpatient procedure, about 9 to 14 L of blood are processed over several hours during each leukapheresis. Most of the blood cells are returned to the donor, and each leukapheresis yields about 200 mL of cells.

The number of hematopoietic stem cells that circulate in peripheral blood is normally too low for this approach to be technically feasible.[16,17] Without mobilization techniques, at least six leukaphereses are usually required to collect a sufficient number of PBPCs. Two methods have been used clinically to "mobilize" hematopoietic stem cells

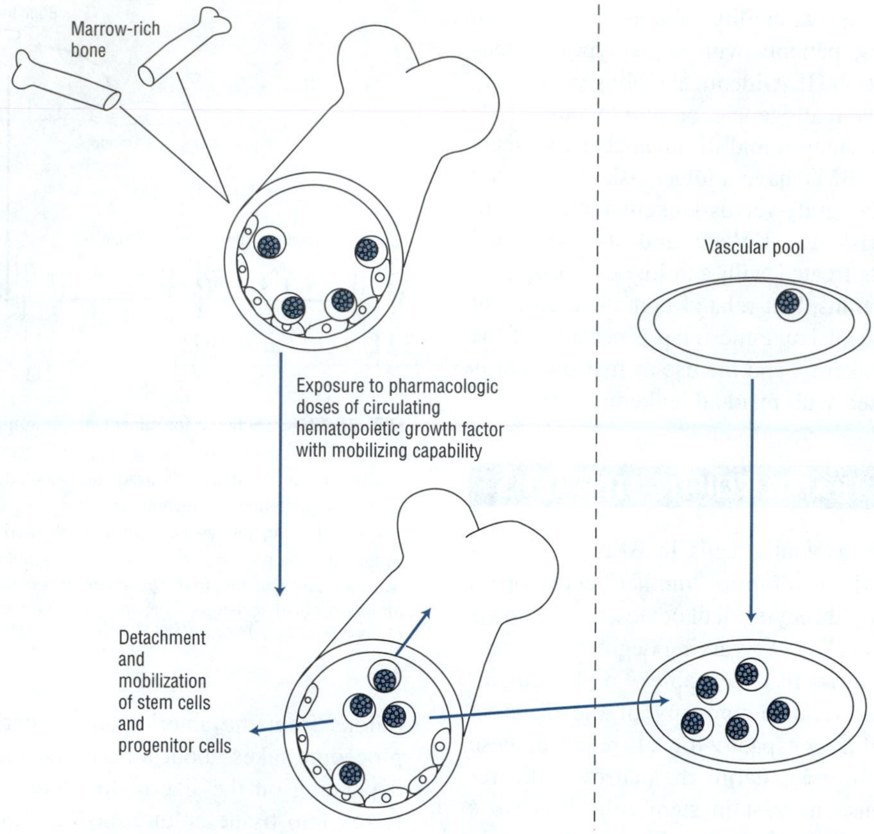

FIGURE 125–4. Hematopoietic growth factor-mediated mobilization of hematopoietic progenitor cells into the circulation. Many hematopoietic growth factors (G-CSF, GM-CSF, IL-1, IL-3, SCF, and likely others) have the ability to redistribute hematopoietic progenitor cells (and presumably true stem cells) from the bone marrow into the peripheral blood. *(Reprinted with permission from Demetri GD. Hematopoietic growth factors. Curr Probl Cancer 1992;16:238.)*

from the bone marrow into peripheral blood (Fig. 125–4). The first is to give chemotherapy, which can briefly increase the number of PBPCs as much as 100-fold. The second and most common method is to administer a recombinant hematopoietic growth factor such as granulocyte colony-stimulating factor (G-CSF) or granulocyte-macrophage colony-stimulating factor (GM-CSF) (both are FDA-approved for this indication). The combination of chemotherapy followed by administration of a growth factor appears to increase the number of PBPCs to a greater extent than either method alone. This approach is more expensive and is associated with more adverse effects than a growth factor alone, but the number of leukaphereses is reduced, and the additional chemotherapy may further reduce the tumor burden before transplant. With current mobilization techniques, many centers collect sufficient PBPCs with three or fewer leukaphereses. Figure 125–5 shows a representative protocol for mobilization and collection of PBPCs.

The use of peripheral blood instead of bone marrow as a source of hematopoietic stem cells for HDC with autologous rescue offers several advantages.[16,17] The most clinically important advantage is that patients who receive mobilized PBPCs experience more rapid hematopoietic engraftment. Although engraftment of all lineages is more rapid when PBPCs are used, the most significant effect is observed with platelet recovery. Patients who receive mobilized PBPCs experience platelet recovery as much as 2 to 3 weeks earlier than those who receive BMT. Another advantage is that the donor does not experience the discomfort associated with marrow aspirations and is not exposed to the risk associated with undergoing general anesthesia. For those patients who cannot donate marrow stem cells because of bone marrow abnormalities such as marrow metastases or fibrosis, collection of PBPCs allows these patients to potentially benefit from HDC with autologous rescue.

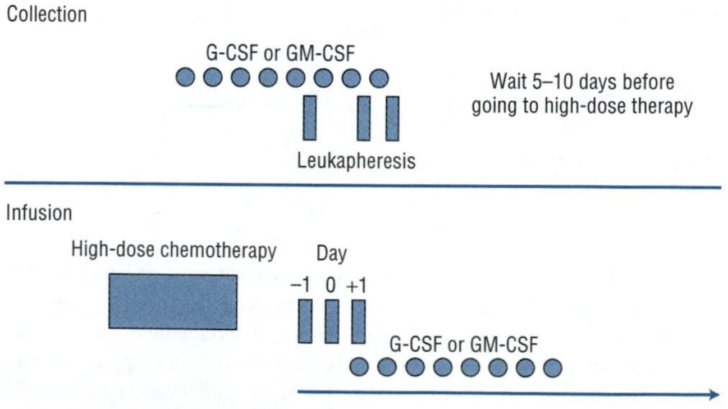

FIGURE 125–5. Schema for collection of PBPCs after full hematopoietic recovery from a previous course of chemotherapy.

Another theoretical advantage is that PBPCs may be less likely to be contaminated with malignant cells compared with marrow stem cells. Finally, because PBPCs are collected from the mononuclear cell fraction, a fraction that also contains immunocompetent cells, some investigators believe that infusion of PBPCs may represent a form of "adoptive immunotherapy." In this model, natural killer cells and lymphocytes targeted against tumor cells would help to kill residual tumor cells.[18]

Although studies have not reported a significant difference in disease-free survival between patients who receive mobilized PBPCs and those who receive BMT, the use of mobilized PBPCs is associated with other clinical and economic benefits. Patients who receive mobilized PBPCs have more rapid neutrophil and platelet recovery, require fewer platelet transfusions, and are usually discharged earlier from the hospital.[16,19,20] Many patients are discharged as early as 10 to 14 days posttransplant, and some BMT centers with intensive clinic support discharge patients even earlier posttransplant.[21,22] In an economic analysis of a randomized controlled trial, Smith and colleagues reported that the total average cost of a PBPC transplant was $13,521 lower than that of a BMT ($45,792 versus $59,314).[23] As a result of these clinical and economic advantages, PBPC transplants have replaced BMT in the autologous setting.

The quantity and type of cells collected during the leukapheresis procedure are important determinants in the rate of hematopoietic recovery early posttransplant. Because there is no currently available method to measure the number of hematopoietic stem cells, several different surrogate markers have been used to estimate the number of stem cells.[16,17] In the past, the number of mononuclear cells or colony-forming units granulocyte-macrophage (CFU-GM) was measured. However, these methods have been largely replaced by measurement of the number of cells expressing the CD34 antigen ($CD34^+$ cells), as determined by flow cytometry. CD34 is an antigen expressed on hematopoietic stem cells and other early progenitor cells. Several studies show that the number of $CD34^+$ cells correlates significantly with the rate of neutrophil and platelet recovery after HDC.[24,25] Prompt hematologic recovery is observed in most patients who receive at least 2×10^6 $CD34^+$ cells/kg. As a result, most transplant centers currently mobilize PBPCs to a target $CD34^+$ cell count of about 2×10^6 cells/kg body weight.[16,17]

There may be clinical and economic benefits associated with infusion of higher $CD34^+$ cell doses.[26,27] Although the difference in the median number of days to neutrophil or platelet recovery is usually no more than 1 to 2 days in patients who receive more than 5×10^6 $CD34^+$ cells/kg as compared to those who receive 2.5 to 5×10^6 $CD34^+$ cells/kg, fewer patients who receive more than 5×10^6 $CD34^+$ cells/kg have delayed engraftment. This small effect may be important, because patients with delayed engraftment can consume a disproportionate share of health care resources. These "outliers" tend to be overlooked, and changes in the values of these "outliers" would not change median values. Although changes in these "outliers" would change mean values, many studies report only median days to neutrophil or platelet recovery. Infusion of higher numbers of $CD34^+$ cells may reduce the percentage of the "outliers."[25] For example, Weaver et al. reported that the median day to neutrophil and platelet recovery was shortened by only 2 to 3 days as the number of $CD34^+$ cells increased from 2.5 to 5.0 to more than 12.5×10^6 $CD34^+$ cells/kg. However, the 95th percentile day to neutrophil and platelet recovery was shortened by 6 days and 15 days, respectively, as the number of $CD34^+$ cells increased from 2.5 to 5.0 to over 12.5×10^6 $CD34^+$ cells/kg. Not surprisingly, the range of days to neutrophil and platelet recovery was reduced with higher $CD34^+$ cell doses. The range of day to neutrophil and platelet recovery for patients who received 2.5 to 5.0×10^6 $CD34^+$ cells/kg was 5 to 26 and 0 to 53 (patient died on day 53 without platelet recovery), respectively. In contrast, none of the patients who received more than 10 $\times 10^6$ $CD34^+$ cells/kg had neutrophil and platelet recovery later than days 16 and 24, respectively.

Several methods can be used to mobilize higher $CD34^+$ cell doses: the use of G-CSF combined with chemotherapy, the administration of higher daily dosages of G-CSF (> 10 μg/kg), and the use of combinations of growth factors.[16,17] Preliminary results with the combination of G-CSF and recombinant stem cell factor show that the addition of stem cell factor increases the number of $CD34^+$ cells in the PBPC collection and leads to more rapid hematopoietic recovery after HDC in patients with breast cancer as compared with G-CSF alone.[28,29] Newer recombinant hematopoietic growth factors such as thrombopoietin (also referred to as megakaryocyte growth and development factor [MGDF]), flt-3 ligand, and danisplastim are also being investigated for potential use in mobilization regimens.[30,31] When given in combination with G-CSF, these agents may mobilize more PBPCs as compared with G-CSF alone. Each method has its advantages and disadvantages, but all have been shown to be effective in mobilizing higher $CD34^+$ cell doses. Although each of these methods increases the cost and sometimes the adverse effects of the mobilization procedure, they have the potential to reduce the overall cost of the HDC procedure.[26]

Although peripheral blood has replaced bone marrow as a source of hematopoietic stem cells for autologous rescue, bone marrow remains the major source of hematopoietic stem cells for allogeneic BMT, primarily because of concerns that the large number of T lymphocytes could increase the risk of GVHD. Recent studies suggest that patients who receive allogeneic PBPC transplants experience more rapid hematopoietic recovery and require fewer transfusions without any increase in their risk of acute GVHD, relapse, or transplant-related mortality when compared with those who receive allogeneic BMT.[32,33] Infusion of PBPCs may also be associated with more rapid immune reconstitution, which could translate into a lower incidence of infectious complications.[34] However, the Seattle BMT team has recently reported that the risk of chronic GVHD was significantly higher in patients who received allogeneic PBPC transplants as compared to recipients of allogeneic BMT.[35]

Another source of hematopoietic stem cells is umbilical cord blood.[14,17,36] Umbilical cord blood is an attractive source for several reasons. Because the stem cells are collected from placental blood, there is no risk to the mother or the baby. There is also very low risk of transmissible infectious diseases, such as cytomegalovirus and Epstein–Barr virus. Although the stem cells collected from umbilical cord blood could theoretically be used for either autologous or allogeneic transplants, they have been used primarily for allogeneic transplants. As of mid-1997, about two dozen blood banks worldwide have collected more than 14,000 umbilical cord blood units. The New York Blood Center has collected more than 7000 units.

Preliminary results with umbilical cord transplants have been encouraging.[36,37] In the 62 recipients of sibling umbilical cord blood transplantation reported to the International Cord Blood Transplant Registry, more than 90% of patients engrafted and only about 5% developed grades II to IV acute GVHD. The apparently lower risk of acute GVHD with umbilical cord blood suggests that cells from umbilical cord blood are less likely to mediate GVHD and that greater HLA disparities between donor and recipient may be tolerated. Most of the recipients of umbilical cord blood transplants in this series were children. Cord blood can also be used as a source of hematopoietic stem cells in patients who do not have a sibling donor. More than 450 unrelated donor umbilical cord blood transplants have been performed worldwide. The results of these transplants suggest that unrelated donor umbilical cord blood transplants are feasible in children and associated with a shorter search time. Patients have comparable myeloid engraftment but delayed platelet reconstitution when compared with unrelated donor BMT. About 20% to 25% of patients develop severe (grades III or IV) acute GVHD.

One of the major limitations to umbilical cord transplants is the limited volume of blood collected, usually 60 to 150 mL. Although the relatively low numbers of hematopoietic cells may be adequate for hematopoietic engraftment in children and small adults, it may not be adequate for larger recipients. The slow engraftment, particularly of platelets, is probably related to the low cell dose. Another limitation is that the effects of long-term cryopreservation are not known.

APPROACHES TO ERADICATE MALIGNANT CELLS

PRETRANSPLANT CHEMOTHERAPY

Nearly all patients who receive HDC must be prepared (or "conditioned") before infusion of hematopoietic stem cells.[38] In patients with malignant disease, the goal of the preparative regimen is to kill as many malignant cells as possible. Preparative regimens usually include commonly used anticancer drugs given at very high doses—doses that would be associated with severe and life-threatening bone marrow suppression if hematopoietic stem cells were not infused. In patients undergoing allogeneic transplantation, another purpose of the preparative regimen is to suppress the immune system of the recipient so that the graft is not rejected.

In some preparative regimens, the only drug given is cyclophosphamide, a drug with both immunosuppressive and cytotoxic effects. Because of the inadequate antitumor activity of cyclophosphamide in some types of cancers, other drugs are often added to the basic cyclophosphamide regimen. Examples of drugs that often are included in preparative regimens are cytarabine (ara-C), busulfan, thiotepa, etoposide (VP-16), carboplatin, cisplatin, and carmustine (BCNU).[39–42] Specific drug regimens are discussed in detail later.

Many patients also receive total body irradiation (TBI).[43] In patients with malignant disease, the rationale is to eradicate malignant cells located in areas inaccessible to the systemic circulation. TBI also has significant immunosuppressive activity. Historically, the standard total body irradiation regimen involves the administration of a midline tissue dose of about 1000 cGy (1 cGy = 1 rad), which is more than twice the lethal dose of radiation for a normal person. Many centers currently give fractionated rather than single-dose TBI to patients with malignant disease. The rationale for this approach is an improved therapeutic ratio—to destroy more leukemic cells and marrow stem cells while sparing other normal tissues. One randomized trial has demonstrated improved antileukemic activity with fractionated-dose TBI compared with single-dose TBI.[44] The nonmarrow acute toxicities of total body irradiation are generally mild, consisting of low-grade fever, nausea, vomiting, diarrhea, and tender swelling of the parotid gland.

The administration of HDC, either alone or combined with TBI, is associated with serious and sometimes life-threatening toxicities to organs other than the bone marrow (see "Regimen-related Toxicity" later in the chapter).

LEUKEMIA

In patients with leukemia undergoing allogeneic transplantation, the standard regimen is cyclophosphamide and TBI.[45] Cyclophosphamide is usually given first, as two 60 mg/kg doses, followed by TBI. TBI can be given as a single dose or fractionated over several days. Fractionated TBI appears to increase the therapeutic index compared with single-dose TBI.[44] The maximally tolerated dose of fractionated TBI is 1200 cGy, given as 200-cGy fractions daily for 6 days. Although higher TBI doses provide additional antileukemic activity, one randomized trial showed that survival is not improved because of increased mortality from causes other than relapse.[46] The cyclophosphamide–TBI regimen provides adequate antileukemic activity in patients with acute nonlymphocytic leukemia (ANLL) in first remission or chronic myelogenous leukemia (CML) in chronic phase, but it is associated with an unacceptably high relapse rate in patients with acute lymphocytic leukemia (ALL) or those with more advanced disease.

One variation of that regimen is to give hyperfractionated TBI first, followed by cyclophosphamide.[47] In that regimen, 11 TBI doses of 120 cGy are given; doses are given three times a day on days –7 to –5 (*note:* day 0 is designated as the day of transplant), and twice a day on the last day (day – 4). After TBI, two doses of cyclophosphamide are given intravenously once a day at a dosage of 60 mg/kg on days –3 and –2. This regimen appears to be more effective than the standard cyclophosphamide and TBI regimen in patients with ALL. It is not clear whether the increased effectiveness is related to the hyperfractionated TBI or the change in the sequence of TBI and cyclophosphamide administration.

Because many anticancer drugs do not have adequate immunosuppressive activity, most preparative regimens in allogeneic BMT include TBI or cyclophosphamide. Because of the many acute and chronic toxicities of TBI, it would be advantageous to omit it from the preparative regimen. One widely used preparative regimen that does not include TBI is busulfan and cyclophosphamide.[41] In that original regimen, busulfan was given orally at a dosage of 1 mg/kg every 6 hours (4 mg/kg/d) for 16 doses on days –9 to –6, followed by four doses of cyclophosphamide, given intravenously once daily at a dosage of 50 mg/kg on days –5 to –2. In one widely used modification of that regimen, the total cyclophosphamide dosage is reduced from 200 (50 × 4) to 120 (60 × 2) mg/kg. Some BMT centers monitor busulfan concentrations based on studies that suggest that busulfan systemic exposure may correlate with patient outcome.[48]

Several prospective randomized studies have compared cyclophosphamide (120 mg/kg) and either TBI or busulfan (16 mg/kg) in patients with leukemia. In patients with CML in first chronic phase, the busulfan–cyclophosphamide regimen had similar or greater antileukemic activity and was better tolerated than cyclophosphamide and TBI.[49,50] But in patients with ANLL in first remission or advanced leukemia (e.g., patients beyond first remission or first chronic phase), the cyclophosphamide–TBI regimen was associated with significantly better disease-free survival than busulfan and cyclophosphamide.[51,52] In contrast to the results of the study conducted by the Seattle BMT team,[49] one of those studies also reported that busulfan and cyclophosphamide was associated with more regimen-related toxicity than cyclophosphamide and TBI.[51]

Other allogeneic BMT groups have given other drugs in addition to or instead of cyclophosphamide in the preparative regimen, particularly in patients with ALL. Examples of other drugs that have been included in combination with TBI are cytarabine[53,54] or etoposide.[40,55] There are no convincing data to indicate that any of these regimens are superior to the standard regimen of cyclophosphamide combined with either TBI or busulfan. The same preparative regimens are usually given to patients undergoing autologous transplantation.[56]

LYMPHOMA

Based on experience in patients with leukemia, the initial regimen used in many patients with lymphoma was cyclophosphamide and TBI, particularly in allogeneic BMT. Most preparative regimens used in autologous transplantation for lymphoma include cyclophosphamide and at least one other drug.[57] TBI is usually not included in the conditioning regimen. One widely used regimen in autologous transplantation is the CBV regimen, which consists of cyclophosphamide, carmustine (BCNU), and etoposide (VP-16). In that original regimen, cyclophosphamide was given at a dosage of 1.5 g/m^2 on days –6 to –3, carmustine was given at a dosage of 300 mg/m^2 on day –6, and etoposide was given at a dosage of 100 mg/m^2 every 12 hours for six doses on days –6 to –4.[58] Various BMT groups have modified the original CBV regimen by changing the dosage of some of the drugs. Other BMT groups have added or substituted other drugs to the CBV regimen, including cytosine arabinoside, etoposide, melphalan, lomustine, and thioguanine. Other widely used regimens are BEAC (BCNU, etoposide, ara-C, and cyclophosphamide) and BEAM (BCNU, etoposide, ara-C, and melphalan).[57] No one preparative regimen has been shown to be clearly superior to other regimens in the treatment of lymphoma.

Although TBI is usually not included in the conditioning regimen, some form of radiation therapy is often given, depending on the type, location, and extent of disease. Instead of TBI, some patients receive localized radiation in high doses to areas of residual or bulky disease. Because many patients with Hodgkin's disease have received thoracic radiation as primary therapy for their disease, TBI is usually avoided in patients with Hodgkin's disease. Conversely, most patients with indolent non-Hodgkin's lymphoma receive TBI as part of their preparative regimen because of the known sensitivity of these tumors to low doses of radiation.

One novel approach is to substitute targeted radiotherapy for TBI. The goal of this approach is to deliver higher doses of radiotherapy to tumor sites, while exposing normal tissues to lower doses of irradiation. Monoclonal antibodies to antigens expressed on the malignant cells are used to deliver the irradiation (i.e., radioimmunotherapy). In studies conducted by the Seattle BMT team, ^{131}I-labeled anti-CD20 (B1) antibody was used to deliver maximally tolerated doses of radiotherapy (without chemotherapy) followed by autologous stem-cell rescue.[59] Results of phase I and II studies have been encouraging.

SOLID TUMORS

Initially, the conditioning regimens used in patients with solid tumors were similar to those used in patients with leukemia. Many patients with refractory disease also participated in phase I and II trials of single agents, in an attempt to determine the maximally tolerated dosage in the setting of BMT and the dose–response relationship in a selected solid tumor.[60,61]

Based on preclinical and clinical models, Frei[61] listed seven strategies for the development of an optimal conditioning regimen for solid tumors: (1) Three or more agents should be used; (2) agents should be individually effective in the treatment of metastatic disease; (3) agents should have a steep dose–response curve; (4) agents should have minimal or no cross-resistance; (5) agents should ideally exhibit synergism in preclinical or clinical models; (6) agents should have a tolerated dosage in the autologous transplant setting that is at least fivefold higher than the standard maximally tolerated dosage; and (7) agents should have sufficiently different nonhematologic dose-limiting toxicities to allow their use in combination in the autologous transplant setting without significant compromise in dose of individual agents. Several agents have been identified that satisfied these criteria, including cyclophosphamide, thiotepa, carmustine, melphalan, and carboplatin. Other anticancer drugs that modulated the activity of alkylating agents in a synergistic manner, such as etoposide, were also attractive drugs to include in high-dose preparative regimens. Most conditioning regimens in autologous transplantation include at least one alkylating agent because of their steep dose–response curve and other favorable characteristics. Many BMT groups include more than one alkylating agent, based on preclinical studies that show that resistance to a specific alkylating agent does not impart cross-resistance to other alkylating agents.

Breast cancer has served as a model for the development of intensive conditioning regimens in autologous transplantation. Table 125–1 shows the evolution of conditioning regimens at the Dana–Farber Cancer Institute.[42] STAMP I (solid tumor autologous marrow program) combined three alkylating agents at nearly full transplant dosages. Although that regimen continues to be used in some autologous BMT centers, the low activity of carmustine in breast cancer and its variable pharmacokinetics led investigators at the Dana–Farber Cancer Institute to develop a new conditioning regimen. Based on preclinical studies, STAMP III was developed, which combined cyclophosphamide, thiotepa, and melphalan. Because of severe mucositis, the dosage of melphalan could not be significantly escalated. This led to the development of STAMP V, where carboplatin is substituted for melphalan. In an effort to increase efficacy, decrease toxicity, and facilitate pharmacokinetic studies, these drugs are given as a continuous intravenous infusion. Based on phase I studies, the maximally tolerated dosages of these drugs in the autologous BMT setting are 6 g/m^2 of cyclophosphamide, 500 mg/m^2 of thiotepa, and 800 mg/m^2 of carboplatin.

The dose of nonalkylating agents with antitumor activity has also been escalated in patients with breast cancer. Mitoxantrone has been incorporated into high-dose regimens with intensification of three to four times the normal dose.[62,63] And paclitaxel doses up to seven times the standard dose have been given in combination with cyclophosphamide and cisplatin.[64] It is not clear whether these regimens offer any clinical advantages to those that include only alkylating agents.

MARROW PURGING

One disadvantage of the use of the patient as the donor (autologous transplantation) is that the marrow may be contaminated with residual malignant cells. Marrow harvest is usually performed when the patient has no evidence of tumor cells in the bone marrow by standard diagnostic techniques. However, because of our inability to detect small

TABLE 125–1. Schemata for STAMP[a] I, III, and V

	Day from Marrow Reinfusion								
Bone Marrow Reinfusion	−8	−7	−6	−5	−4	−3	−2	−1	0
STAMP I									
Cyclophosphamide		↑	↑	↑	↑				
Cisplatin	- - -	- - -	- - -	- - -	- - -				
BCNU					↑[b]				
Melphalan[c]				↑					
STAMP III									
Cyclophosphamide	- - -	- - -	- - -	- - -	- - -				
Thiotepa	- - -	- - -	- - -	- - -	- - -				
Melphalan		↑	↑	↑	↑				
STAMP V									
Cyclophosphamide	- - -	- - -	- - -	- - -	- - -				
Thiotepa	- - -	- - -	- - -	- - -	- - -				
Carboplatin	- - -	- - -	- - -	- - -	- - -				

[a]STAMP = Solid Tumor Autologous Marrow Program.
[b]The last 12 patients were given same total dose, divided over 4 days (administered twice a day).
[c]Dose levels 5 to 6 only.
Reproduced from Ref. 42.

numbers of malignant cells, residual malignant cells are probably present in most patients who serve as marrow donors. Several BMT teams are developing newer, more sensitive methods to detect "minimal residual disease."[65] Some of these methods can detect as few as one in a million cells.

Infusion of these malignant cells may theoretically result in tumor relapse. Many approaches are used by BMT teams to eliminate ("purge") the marrow of these tumor cells.[66] The most common approach is to add substances, such as chemicals or monoclonal antibodies, to the marrow while it is outside of the body (*ex vivo*) (Fig. 125–6). Because the substances are removed before marrow infusion, the advantage of this approach is that nonhematopoietic tissues are not exposed to the substances and therefore are not damaged. However, these substances can remove or damage pluripotent hematopoietic stem cells, which are essential for complete and rapid engraftment. *Ex vivo* marrow purging also is performed in allogeneic BMT in an attempt to eliminate T cells believed to be responsible for acute GVHD (Fig. 125–6). Results with this approach are discussed in the "Graft-Versus-Host Disease" section later in the chapter.

One approach is to add one or more monoclonal antibodies directed against specific antigens present on the tumor cells but absent on nearly all other cells.[67] Killing of tumor cells is usually achieved with the addition of complement. One novel approach is to add a monoclonal antibody against the cell surface product of the multidrug-resistant (MDR) gene, in an attempt to purge multidrug-resistant tumor cells. Another method to kill tumor cells is to use immunotoxins (monoclonal antibodies linked to a toxin). Although these approaches are theoretically attractive, they are limited by the observation that not all cells from patients with the same type of cancer will express a specific antigen. Furthermore, for some types of cancers, it has been difficult to identify antigens distinct from those present on normal hematopoietic progenitor cells. To date, this approach has been used most commonly in patients with lymphoid malignancies, either ALL or non-Hodgkin's lymphoma (NHL). Results are discussed in the "Clinical Results" section later in the chapter.

Another approach is to add chemicals or drugs to kill the tumor cells.[68] The advantage of this approach is that it can be used for a broader range of tumor types. However, this approach is not completely selective for tumor cells, and it is therefore important to add the precise amount of chemical or drug that kills sufficient numbers of tumor cells while sparing the largest number of hematopoietic stem cells. The chemical that is most commonly used for marrow purging is 4-hydroperoxycyclophosphamide (4-HC), a congener of cyclophosphamide. A stable compound, 4-HC enters cells and is rapidly reduced to 4-hydroxycyclophosphamide, which serves as the precursor to the reactive phosphoramide mustard. The level of aldehyde dehydrogenase, the enzyme that inactivates 4-hydroxycyclophosphamide, appears to be highest in early hematopoietic progenitors and decreases as these cells differentiate. This observation may explain why 4-HC appears to have an acceptable therapeutic index. Other analogs of cyclophosphamide and drugs also are being investigated as chemical purging agents.

A novel method to purge malignant cells is to identify, select, and concentrate hematopoietic stem cells, a process known as positive selection. Several different techniques are being commercially developed and one technique has recently received FDA approval for this indication. In this process, cells collected from marrow or peripheral blood

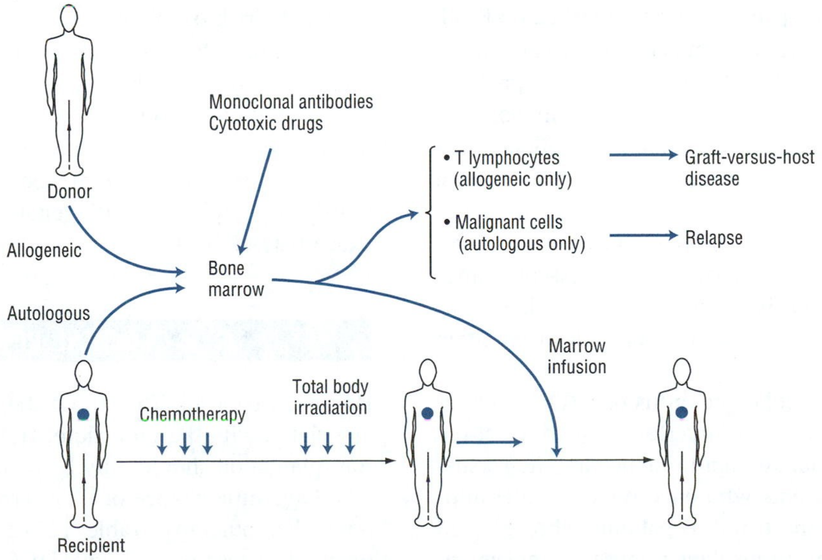

FIGURE 125–6. The use of *ex vivo* marrow purging to remove or destroy T lymphocytes (allogeneic only) or residual malignant cells (autologous only).

are treated *ex vivo* with monoclonal antibodies against CD34, an antigen expressed on hematopoietic stem cells and early progenitor cells. CD34 positive cells are therefore separated from those that are CD34 negative, including most malignant cells. The final volume of enriched cells that is infused back into the patient is remarkably small—only about 5 mL. Although preliminary results with one of these techniques show that a one- to four-log depletion of tumor cells can be achieved,[69] no significant difference in neutrophil recovery, immune reconstitution, or progression-free survival was observed.[70,71] In one study, patients who received the positively selected graft experienced significantly fewer dimethyl sulphoxide (DMSO) infusion-related reactions but also had delayed platelet recovery as compared to the unselected graft group.[71]

POSTTRANSPLANT IMMUNOTHERAPY

The rationale for posttransplant immunotherapy is based on observations that recovery of immune function can be impaired for months to years posttransplant and that the T lymphocytes that mediate GVHD can be directed toward leukemic cells.[45,72] This effect is referred to as the "graft-versus-leukemia" (GVL) effect. Evidence for a graft-versus-leukemia effect is based on retrospective studies that show that patients who developed acute or chronic GVHD had a lower risk of leukemic relapse than those who did not develop GVHD; overall survival, however, was not different because of the increased nonrelapse mortality associated with GVHD. Other anecdotal evidence supporting a GVL effect was the increased risk of relapse found with T-cell-depleted compared with unmodified marrow transplants and the difference in relapse rates between recipients of syngeneic and nontwin sibling transplants. However, because of the direct and indirect effects of GVHD, GVHD is usually associated with increased nonrelapse mortality during the early posttransplant period.

Based on these retrospective studies, the Seattle BMT team initiated a prospective randomized study to determine if a reduction in the intensity of acute GVHD prophylaxis or infusion of donor leukocytes (e.g., T lymphocytes) would reduce the risk of leukemic relapse in patients with advanced hematologic malignancies treated with allogeneic BMT.[73] Although the risk of acute GVHD was increased in patients randomized to receive short methotrexate or long methotrexate plus donor buffy coat cells, the risk of relapse was not decreased and survival was not improved. The incidence of chronic GVHD was similar in each of the three treatment groups.

Donor lymphocyte/leukocyte infusions (DLI), either alone or in combination with interferon-alpha (IFN-α), have also been given in an attempt to induce a graft-versus-leukemia reaction in patients who have relapsed after allogeneic BMT.[74,75] In a report of 140 patients who received DLI for treatment of posttransplant relapse, complete responses were observed in 60% of CML patients, with higher response rates in patients with cytogenetic and chronic phase relapse than in patients with more advanced disease.[76] Response rates in patients with acute leukemia were lower. The most serious complications of DLI are GVHD (60%) and pancytopenia (19%), and nonrelapse mortality at 1 year is about 14%. In an effort to reduce the morbidity and mortality associated with DLI, the BMT team at Dana–Farber Cancer Institute is investigating the administration of defined numbers of $CD4^+$ donor T cells after *ex vivo* depletion of $CD8^+$ cells to patients who had experienced posttransplant relapse.[77] They reported similar response rates in CML patients with a lower incidence of GVHD. Further studies will be necessary to determine the utility of DLI as well as the optimal method of delivery.

Based on reports that GVHD developed after cyclosporine was withdrawn in rats after syngeneic or autologous BMT, some BMT groups have induced autologous GVHD in an attempt to induce a graft-versus-leukemia effect.[78] The mechanism by which cyclosporine causes autologous GVHD is unknown, but the effector cells appear to be cytotoxic T cells aimed against MHC class II antigens. More recent studies show that the antitumor effect can be enhanced with IFN-α administration. In human studies, autologous GVHD is induced with administration of low doses of cyclosporine (1 mg/kg, given intravenously) for 28 days, beginning on the day of marrow infusion. With this regimen, about two-thirds of patients develop autologous GVHD of the skin while receiving the drug. Although generalized GVHD is observed in animals, autologous GVHD in humans does not appear to develop in extracutaneous organs. The skin rash either resolved spontaneously or with systemic corticosteroids. Preliminary results with this approach have been encouraging.[79,80]

Another approach is to administer a cytokine with immunomodulatory activity, such as interleukin-2 (IL-2) or interferons.[45,72,81,82] Early clinical experience indicates that IL-2 can be safely administered posttransplant and results in significant activation of immune effector cells and may reduce the risk of relapse.

Posttransplant immunotherapy would be particularly useful in patients undergoing autologous blood or marrow transplantation because these patients would not benefit from graft-versus-tumor reactions. Cytokines that directly or indirectly stimulate lymphocytes should be used cautiously in recipients of allogeneic BMT because they may exacerbate GVHD.

CLINICAL RESULTS

Because of the high cost and the morbidity and mortality associated with the procedure, HDC with blood or marrow transplantation should only be performed in cancer patients who have little chance of long-term survival with standard-dose chemotherapy. Table 125–2 lists the most common types of cancer treated with HDC. Many potential indications for HDC are controversial, and coverage for HDC is often denied if the payer believes that the likelihood for long-term survival and cure is low. High-dose chemother-

TABLE 125–2. Use of Bone Marrow Transplantation in Selected Malignant Diseases

Disease	Bone Marrow Transplantation		
	Preferred Type	*Potentially Curative in Advanced Disease*	*Standard Therapy*[a]
Acute leukemia	Allogeneic in most cases	Yes	Yes
Chronic myelogenous leukemia	Allogeneic	Yes	Yes
Chronic lymphocytic leukemia	Allogeneic in most cases	Uncertain	No
Multiple myeloma	Controversial	Uncertain	No
Non-Hodgkin's lymphoma			
Histologically aggressive	Autologous in most cases	Yes	Yes
Histologically indolent	Autologous in most cases	Uncertain	Yes
Hodgkin's disease	Autologous in most cases	Yes	Yes
Breast cancer	Autologous	Uncertain	No
Testicular cancer	Autologous	Yes	Yes
Neuroblastoma	Uncertain	Probably	Yes

[a]Standard therapy is defined as treatment that is widely accepted by physicians and routinely reimbursed by most third-party payers at some point in the course of the disease. As noted in the text, the designation of bone marrow transplantation as standard therapy is controversial. For example, although transplantation in patients with breast cancer is not routinely reimbursed by most third-party payers, the rate of reimbursement is approximately 75% at Duke University Hospital and 50% at the University of Nebraska Medical Center.
Reprinted from Ref. 2.

apy with autologous or allogeneic transplantation can be used at different times in the disease course (Table 125–3). Although HDC can cure a few patients with refractory disease, it is most effective when the tumor burden is low (i.e., when the patient is in remission). HDC is currently most often used as intensive consolidation therapy in patients who have responded to standard-dose chemotherapy but who have a low likelihood of long-term survival or cure. One example of this strategy is patients with ANLL who receive HDC during their first remission. High-dose chemotherapy is also commonly used in patients who experience relapse or recurrence of their cancer and respond to salvage chemotherapy (i.e., sensitive relapse). These patients undergo HDC with autologous or allogeneic transplantation during their remission. Examples of this strategy include patients with ALL or lymphoma who receive HDC during their second remission, or patients with metastatic breast cancer who receive HDC after responding to standard-dose chemotherapy. Finally, HDC with autologous or allogeneic transplantation is sometimes used as part of intensive adjuvant chemotherapy in high-risk patients, such as women with breast cancer with more than 10 positive lymph nodes.

TABLE 125–3. Possibilities for Timing of Bone Marrow Transplantation in the Treatment of Cancer

- Primary treatment
- Partial responders or slow responders (before progression)
- Initial complete remission (i.e., consolidation)
- Nonresponders (primary treatment failure)
- Relapse
  - Untested (i.e., no other salvage therapy)
  - Tested (i.e., after other salvage therapy)
    - Sensitive relapse (i.e., complete or partial remission)
    - Resistant relapse (i.e., no response or progression)
- End-stage patients

Modified from Armitage JO. Bone marrow transplantation in the treatment of patients with lymphoma. Blood 1989;73:1750.

ACUTE NONLYMPHOCYTIC LEUKEMIA

In ANLL, HDC with autologous or allogeneic transplantation is the only curative option for patients who fail initial induction therapy or those who have experienced leukemic relapse. The proportion of long-term survivors after autologous or allogeneic BMT when patients are transplanted while in untreated first relapse or in second remission is about 20% to 35% (Table 125–4).[45,83] Patients who are transplanted while in second complete remission have longer survival than those treated with standard chemotherapy, especially patients who are less than 30 years of age and those who had first complete remissions greater than 1 year in duration.[84] The proportion of long-term survivors

TABLE 125–4. Long-Term Results of High-Dose Chemotherapy with Allogeneic Bone Marrow Transplantation (BMT) Versus Intensive Chemotherapy in the Treatment of Leukemias

Disease[a]	Status	Long-Term Survival (%)	
		BMT	*Chemotherapy*
ANLL	1st remission	40–60	20–30
	2nd remission	20–30	0
	Multiple relapses	10–15	0
ALL	1st remission (high risk)	30–50	30–50
	2nd remission	25–40	<10
	Multiple relapses	10–15	0
CML	Chronic phase	50–60	0
	Accelerated/blast phase	15–30	0

[a]ANLL = acute nonlymphocytic leukemia; ALL = acute lymphoblastic leukemia; CML = chronic myelogenous leukemia.

decreases to about 20% when patients are transplanted while in chemotherapy-resistant first relapse, or to 10% to 15% when BMT is performed after patients have had multiple relapses.

For patients who achieve a complete remission with standard remission-induction therapy, however, the role of HDC with autologous or allogeneic transplantation is not clear. Response rates and median survival have steadily improved in patients with ANLL treated with intensive chemotherapy. About 20% to 40% of patients with ANLL survive for more than 5 years and are probably cured of their disease (see Chap. 122). In contrast, long-term survival is observed in 40% to 60% of patients with ANLL treated with allogeneic BMT from an HLA-identical sibling while in first remission (Table 125–4).[45,83] This difference in disease-free survival between patients treated with intensive chemotherapy versus autologous or allogeneic BMT has been confirmed in several prospective studies, but the difference is not statistically significant in all studies. In the largest series of more than 600 patients with ANLL, patients in the allogeneic BMT group had significantly better disease-free survival at 4 years than those in the intensive chemotherapy group (55% versus 30%).[85] Similar findings were reported in another study of 381 patients randomized to receive either autologous BMT or no further treatment.[86] Overall survival, however, was not significantly different between the two groups in either study. Some investigators argue that the better results reported with allogeneic BMT are related to patient selection. Patients undergoing allogeneic BMT are usually less than 50 years of age, while many patients who receive intensive chemotherapy are older than 50 years of age. Survival for patients treated with either intensive chemotherapy or allogeneic BMT is related to age, with better survival in younger patients.

Because patients treated with HDC as intensive postremission therapy have a longer disease-free survival than those treated with standard intensive chemotherapy, some investigators argue that all eligible patients should be offered HDC with autologous or allogeneic transplantation during first remission (Fig. 125–7). Other investigators argue that HDC should be delayed until the patient experiences a leukemic relapse, which would spare patients cured with standard chemotherapy from the risks of HDC. Because 20% to 35% of patients transplanted while in first relapse or second remission can be cured with HDC and BMT, the overall proportion of patients cured of their ANLL is similar regardless of whether BMT is offered to all patients as intensive postremission therapy or only after they have experienced leukemic relapse.[85]

The most commonly used conditioning regimens in ANLL are cyclophosphamide and TBI or busulfan and cyclophosphamide.[45,83] With either regimen, the leukemic relapse rate is about 20% in patients with ANLL who undergo allogeneic BMT while in first remission. Preparative regimens used in autologous transplants are similar to those used in allogeneic BMT. Patients with more advanced disease have higher relapse rates. Variations of that regimen or the addition of other drugs do not appear to provide superior antileukemic activity.[39] In an attempt to eliminate residual leukemic cells before infusion, marrow is sometimes "purged" in patients who receive autologous BMT. One common approach is to add a chemical such as 4-HC.[68] Although the value of marrow purging with 4-HC has not been proven in a controlled study, some investigators believe that this approach reduces the risk of leukemic relapse. This is supported by the observation that patients with adequate marrow purging, as measured by the number of hematopoietic progenitor cells, had significantly longer disease-free survival than those with inadequate marrow purging.[87]

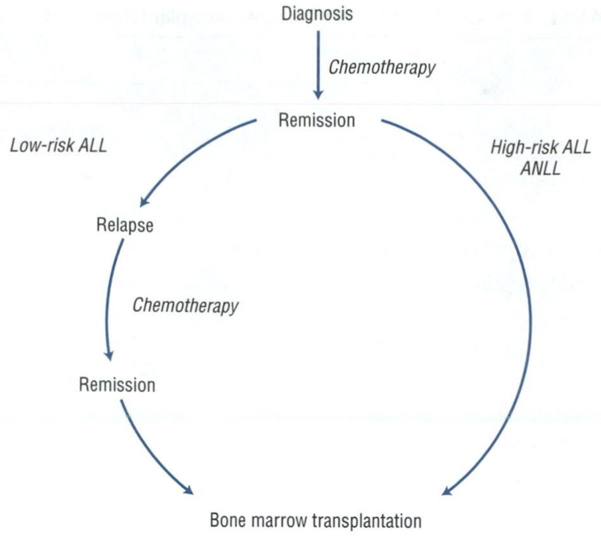

FIGURE 125–7. Current application of allogeneic bone marrow transplantation in the treatment of ANLL and ALL. *(Modified from Yee GC, McGuire TR. Allogeneic bone marrow transplantation in the treatment of hematologic diseases. Clin Pharm 1985;4:152. © 1985 American Society of Health-System Pharmacists, Inc. All rights reserved. Reprinted with permission.)*

Another controversy in the use of BMT as treatment for ANLL is whether patients should undergo allogeneic or autologous transplantation. As discussed earlier in the chapter, each approach has advantages and disadvantages. In one prospective study of more than 600 patients with ANLL transplanted while in first remission, disease-free survival at 4 years was similar in patients assigned to either autologous or allogeneic BMT.[85] The causes of death, however, differed depending on the type of transplant. The risk of leukemic relapse was higher in the autologous BMT group, while the risk of nonrelapse mortality—primarily related to GVHD—was higher in the allogeneic BMT group. Most of the patients in the autologous BMT group did not receive purged marrow. Ongoing trials for patients with ANLL compare allogeneic BMT from HLA-identical sibling donors with autologous BMT with 4-HC purged marrow.

Allogeneic BMT with closely or fully HLA-matched unrelated donors has been used to treat ANLL.[9,12,13] The major difficulty with this approach is that many patients will relapse during the time needed to find a donor.

MYELODYSPLASTIC SYNDROME

Myelodysplastic syndromes are a heterogeneous group of disorders associated with an increased risk of transformation to acute myeloid leukemia.[88] Hormones, chemotherapy, and differentiating agents (including recombinant hematopoietic growth factors) have been used as treatment for myelodysplastic syndromes.[88,89] None of these therapies has been shown to be curative or to increase survival. Allogeneic BMT is the only curative treatment for patients with this syndrome.[89] Long-term survival after allogeneic BMT is about 50%, but varies with the subtype of disease, presence of cytogenetic abnormalities, patient age, and percentage of blasts in the bone marrow.[88–90] Patients transplanted early in their disease course have a lower risk of disease recurrence.

ACUTE LYMPHOBLASTIC LEUKEMIA

With improvements in the therapy of ALL, most children and adolescents with ALL achieve long-term disease-free survival with chemotherapy. Although the cure rate in adults with ALL is lower than in children, many adults also can be cured of their disease with conventional chemotherapy (see Chap. 122). Therefore, HDC is usually reserved for patients with ALL who have experienced leukemic relapse, particularly if the duration of the first remission is short (less than 18 months) or in patients who do not respond to initial remission induction therapy (Fig. 125–7).[45,91] Although many studies show that chemotherapy can often induce a second or subsequent remission, the duration of remission is usually short and long-term survival is uncommon. In comparison, about 25% to 40% of patients with ALL transplanted while in second remission become long-term survivors (Table 125–4). In a large matched-pair analysis of children with ALL in second remission, children who received allogeneic BMT had significantly better disease-free survival at 5 years than those who received continued chemotherapy (40% versus 17%).[92] The difference in survival was related to a marked difference in the risk of relapse. Long-term survival after allogeneic BMT decreases to about 10% to 15% in patients who have had multiple relapses.

The application of allogeneic BMT as intensive consolidation during first remission in patients with ALL who are at high risk for leukemic relapse is controversial.[91] Examples of patients in this high-risk group are most adults and some children with high-risk features, such as those with high white blood cell counts or certain immunophenotypes or cytogenetic abnormalities, or those who require repeated courses to induce a complete remission. Long-term, disease-free survival is about 60% in children and 40% in adults transplanted while in first remission (Table 125–4).[45,91] Most of these patients were prepared with cyclophosphamide and TBI. In a prospective comparison of chemotherapy versus allogeneic BMT for adults with ALL in first remission, disease-free survival was higher in the BMT group (45% versus 31%), although the difference was of borderline statistical significance ($P = .1$).[93] In that study, significantly better survival was observed in those patients with high-risk ALL (39% versus 14%), which suggests that allogeneic BMT may be preferred over chemotherapy in certain patient groups. Although there is limited experience with closely or fully matched unrelated BMT in the treatment of ALL, clinical results have been similar to those reported with matched related siblings.[12,13,45] One of the difficulties with this approach in ALL is that many patients will relapse during the time needed to find a donor.

Most patients transplanted in these early studies were prepared with high-dose cyclophosphamide, followed by TBI. Because of the unacceptably high relapse rate with this regimen, some BMT groups are investigating new preparative regimens. As described earlier, preliminary results with the use of hyperfractionated TBI before cyclophosphamide in allogeneic BMT are encouraging.[47] With this regimen, estimated disease-free survival at 5 years is about 60% and 40% in children and adolescents with ALL transplanted while in second and third remission, respectively. Other BMT groups have reported promising results with preparative regimens that include high-dose cytarabine or etoposide, usually combined with TBI.[53–55]

Although there is less experience with autologous transplants, studies suggest that long-term survival with autologous transplants is slightly lower compared with allogeneic BMT.[94] Because of the widespread availability of monoclonal antibodies against antigens expressed on malignant lymphocytes, many patients have their marrow purged with monoclonal antibodies. Long-term survival is about 20% to 30% in children and adults with ALL treated with autologous BMT while in remission (primarily second or subsequent remission). High-dose chemotherapy with autologous transplantation has also been used as intensive postremission therapy in adults with ALL. Preliminary results of one study did not show a survival benefit of autologous BMT over maintenance chemotherapy.[95]

As with ANLL, there is controversy whether eligible patients with high-risk ALL should be treated with HDC as soon as possible after complete remission is achieved, or to delay HDC until leukemic relapse occurs. Because of the effectiveness of current chemotherapy protocols, many investigators recommend delaying HDC until leukemic relapse occurs.

CHRONIC MYELOGENOUS LEUKEMIA

With the possible exception of IFN-α, no currently available therapy is capable of eradicating the malignant clone associated with CML, measured clinically by the presence of cytogenetic markers (see Chap. 123). In contrast, many studies indicate that high-dose chemotherapy with allogeneic BMT from HLA-identical sibling donors can cure 60% to 70% of patients with chronic-phase CML (Table 125–4).[96,97] As a result, CML is currently the most common indication for allogeneic BMT in many BMT centers. In some series, the best results are achieved when BMT is performed early after diagnosis and in younger patients. For example, long-term survival in patients transplanted within 1 year of diagnosis is about 80%, compared with 40% to 50% when BMT is performed 1 to 3 years from diagnosis. Because busulfan may increase the risk of posttransplant interstitial pneumonitis and hepatic veno-occlusive disease, it has been recommended that pretransplant busulfan be avoided if patients are eligible for and considering BMT. Prolonged administration of IFN-α before BMT may adversely affect transplant outcome.[98] When allogeneic BMT is delayed until the patient is in accelerated or blast phase, survival is worse, but 15% to 30% of patients still can be cured (Table 125–4).[97]

The leukemic relapse rate is 10% to 30% in patients prepared with either cyclophosphamide and TBI or busulfan and cyclophosphamide and who are transplanted while in chronic phase.[97] Randomized studies show that busulfan and cyclophosphamide have similar or better antileukemic activity than cyclophosphamide and TBI.[49,50] When BMT is delayed until accelerated or blast phase, the relapse rate exceeds 50% in patients prepared with standard preparative regimens.[97]

Because of the relatively long duration of the chronic phase, there is usually adequate time to perform a search for a fully or closely matched unrelated donor for those patients with CML who lack an HLA-identical sibling donor. Therefore, CML has become the most common indication for allogeneic BMT from unrelated donors.[12,13,99] In a recent report from the Seattle BMT team of 196 patients with Philadelphia chromosome-positive CML treated with allogeneic BMT from unrelated donors, overall survival at 5 years was 57%.[100] In a multivariate analysis, survival was worse in patients who had an interval from diagnosis to transplantation of 1 year or more, an HLA-DRB1 mismatch, a high body-weight index, or were older than 50 years of age. Patients younger than 50 years old who received transplants from unrelated donors matched for HLA-A, B, and DRB1 within 1 year of diagnosis had a survival of 74% at 5 years, which compared favorably with patients transplanted at the same center with grafts from HLA-matched siblings. In the unrelated donor group, graft failure occurred in 5% of patients and grade III or IV acute GVHD was observed in 35% of patients receiving 6/6 HLA matched grafts. Nearly 40% of patients died without recurrent disease; the most common cause of death was GVHD.

Experience with autologous BMT is limited but it appears that autologous BMT is less effective in eradication of the malignant clone than allogeneic BMT.[101] Because the major cause of treatment failure is leukemic relapse, many BMT centers are investigating new preparative regimens and pharmacologic or immunologic approaches to purge marrow of malignant cells.

LYMPHOMA

Although most patients with Hodgkin's disease and some with aggressive non-Hodgkin's lymphoma (NHL) are cured with combination chemotherapy, the prognosis for those who relapse is poor. Similarly, most patients with indolent NHL are not cured of their disease with chemotherapy. In the United States alone, it is estimated that more than 10,000 patients with lymphoma are not cured with standard chemotherapy and are less than 60 years old. Although lymphoma is currently the second most common indication for HDC with autologous rescue, it is estimated that only a small proportion of the eligible patients are currently treated with this procedure.[102]

Based on the success of allogeneic BMT in leukemia, allogeneic or syngeneic BMT was used initially as salvage therapy in patients with relapsed or refractory Hodgkin's disease or aggressive NHL. Long-term results of these early studies show that some of these patients can be cured with HDC and BMT.[102] Although a graft-versus-lymphoma effect has been reported, there is no convincing evidence that survival is higher with allogeneic BMT compared with autologous BMT. Moreover, allogeneic BMT is not feasible in most patients and is associated with a higher risk of transplant-related complications due to GVHD. As a result, most eligible patients with lymphoma currently are treated with HDC and autologous rescue, usually with PBPCs.

High-dose chemotherapy with autologous rescue can be used at different times in the disease course (Table 125–3). It is most commonly used as initial salvage therapy in patients with Hodgkin's disease or aggressive NHL who experience their first relapse or as intensive consolidation therapy in relapsed patients who demonstrate a response to conventional-dose salvage chemotherapy. In that setting, HDC with autologous rescue produces a complete remission rate of 25% to 80%, with many patients in unmaintained, continuous complete remission for more than 5 years.[103,104] The best results have been observed in patients who had responded to conventional-dose salvage therapy and who received autologous rescue as intensive consolidation therapy. Results indicate that more than one-half of patients transplanted at a time when minimal disease was present are alive; many of these patients are likely to be cured of their disease. Although HDC has a high complete remission rate in newly diagnosed patients who never attained a complete remission or in those who had experienced multiple relapses, long-term survival in patients with refractory disease is poor.[103,104] Results from uncontrolled trials with the use of HDC as intensive consolidation therapy (i.e., during first complete remission) in high-risk patients are encouraging.[105] In a large prospective randomized trial of patients with aggressive non-Hodgkin s lymphoma in first complete remission, disease-free and overall survival did not differ significantly between patients who received high-dose CBV with autologous rescue as compared with those treated with standard-dose consolidation therapy.[106] But in high-risk patients, 5-year disease-free (59% versus 39%) and overall (65% versus 52%) survival was longer in patients treated with high-dose CBV as compared with those treated with standard therapy. Similar results have been reported in another study.[107]

Fewer patients with indolent NHL have been treated with HDC with autologous rescue and most of these have been patients who have relapsed following primary induction therapy. Early results are encouraging, and most patients have achieved a complete remission, although these remissions are generally not durable.[108] Several factors have been shown to be associated with prolonged survival after high-dose chemotherapy: transplant while in first remission, previous exposure to fewer courses of chemotherapy, and sensitive disease at the time of transplant.[109,110] Because of the indolent nature of the disease, longer follow-up is required before HDC with autologous rescue can be recommended for this group of patients.

One of the major problems in lymphoma patients is disease relapse. A variety of conditioning regimens have been used in these studies, and no one conditioning regimen has been shown to be clearly superior to other regimens.[57] One novel approach is targeted radiotherapy with a radiolabeled monoclonal antibody (radioimmunotherapy) in an attempt to deliver higher doses of irradiation to tumor sites.[59] Results of a phase II study in 25 patients given myeloablative doses of ^{131}I-labeled anti-CD20 (B1) antibody (without chemotherapy) show that targeted radiotherapy can produce complete responses of long duration in most patients with relapsed B-cell lymphomas.[59] Disease-free survival was significantly higher in patients who received more than 2000 cGy to the dose-limiting normal organ (with higher doses to tumor sites). Another approach is to eliminate residual malignant cells. Many patients treated with HDC and autologous BMT had their marrow purged with monoclonal antibodies, sometimes combined with 4-HC. The role of marrow purging is controversial. Although results of one study reported that *ex vivo* purging had no significant effect on disease-free survival,[111] another study reported that patients who had no detectable residual lymphoma cells after immunologic marrow-purging had increased disease-free survival compared with those who had residual lymphoma in their marrow.[112] In that study, a sensitive PCR method was used to detect the presence of residual lymphoma cells in the marrow. Other approaches that are being investigated include immunotherapy with IL-2 or interferon-α.[113] Preliminary results show that patients who receive cytokine therapy posttransplant have longer disease-free and overall survival as compared with historical controls.

MULTIPLE MYELOMA

Multiple myeloma is a relatively rare hematologic malignancy characterized by uncontrolled proliferation of plasma cells derived from a single malignant clone. Although combination chemotherapy induces a response in most patients, complete responses are uncommon and the disease is not curable with standard-dose chemotherapy. High-dose chemotherapy with autologous rescue induces a complete or partial response in 70% to 80% of newly diagnosed patients with multiple myeloma, and some of these patients may be cured of their disease.[114,115] In a randomized trial, patients randomized to high-dose melphalan and autologous BMT had signifcantly longer survival than those treated with standard-dose chemotherapy plus interferon-α.[116] However, patients in the autologous BMT group continued to relapse after 3 years of follow-up, which suggests that few, if any, patients will be cured. Several factors have been shown to be predictive of response to high-dose chemotherapy with autologous rescue: response to standard therapy, age less than 50 years old, β_2 microglobulin levels below 2.5 mg/L, and time from diagnosis less than 12 months. The most commonly used preparative regimen is high-dose melphalan, given either alone or combined with TBI. Some aggressive protocols include two transplants.

BREAST CANCER

Breast cancer has served as the model for the study of HDC with autologous rescue in the treatment of chemotherapy-responsive solid tumors.[61,117] Breast cancer was selected because of its high incidence and studies that demonstrated a correlation between dose intensity and objective response rate or median survival. Breast cancer is currently the most common indication for HDC with autologous rescue.

Table 125–3 shows the possibilities for timing of HDC with autologous rescue. Initially, HDC with autologous BMT was reserved for patients with metastatic disease who had failed prior chemotherapy. In that setting, the overall response rate was approximately 60%, which was about twofold higher than that achieved with conventional-dose salvage chemotherapy.[117,118] When HDC was used as initial treatment for metastatic disease following standard dose induction therapy, the objective response rate was 80% to 90%, of which 50% to 60% were complete responses. Some of the complete responders have remained in unmaintained remission for several years.

Based on the experience in leukemia and lymphoma, it was likely that HDC with autologous rescue would be most effective when used in patients with early or minimal disease (i.e., as consolidation therapy). This approach has been used in patients with metastatic disease or high-risk primary disease. In patients with metastatic disease, HDC is given after the patient has received induction with standard-dose chemotherapy. In that setting, the objective response rate is about 90% and the complete response rate is about 60%.[117,118] About one-half of the complete responders remain alive in unmaintained, continuous, complete remission with several years of follow-up.

The Autologous Blood and Marrow Transplant Registry (ABMTR) of North America recently reported results of more than 5800 consecutively treated women who received HDC with autologous rescue for breast cancer at over 130 centers between 1989 and 1995.[119] Various preparatory regimens were used; the combination of cyclophosphamide, thiotepa, and carboplatin (STAMP V) was used in more than 25% of all patients. Transplant-related mortality has gradually declined from 22% in 1989 to 5% in 1995. Median survival in the patients with metastatic breast cancer (n = 3450) was 19 months; overall and progression-free survival at 3 years were 30% and 18%, respectively. Most patients had chemotherapy-sensitive disease (complete or partial response before transplant), and women who achieved a complete response pretransplant had better survival (overall and progression free survival at 3 years of 46% and 32%, respectively) than those in partial remission or with resistant disease.

In an effort to determine the role of HDC, Bezwoda and colleagues randomized 90 patients with untreated metastatic breast cancer to either (1) high-dose cyclophosphamide, mitoxantrone, and etoposide with autologous stem cell support; or (2) conventional doses of cyclophosphamide, mitoxantrone, and vincristine.[62] The overall and complete response rates were significantly higher in the HDC group (overall 95% versus 53%; CR 51% versus 4%). In addition, patients who received high-dose chemotherapy had significantly longer median durations of response and survival. Although these results appear to support the use of HDC, the trial has been criticized and the results must be confirmed in larger trials. One large trial is ongoing as a joint effort by several cooperative oncology groups. In that trial, over 500 women with metastatic breast cancer are being treated with induction therapy and then randomized to either high-dose cyclophosphamide, thiotepa, and carboplatin or 2 years of maintenance therapy.[117,118]

Based on the initially encouraging results seen with metastatic disease, HDC with autologous stem cell rescue is also being used in patients with high-risk primary disease. In the ABMTR report discussed earlier, over 1700 women with high-risk primary disease (e.g., stage II or III, or inflammatory breast cancer) received HDC. Overall and progression-free survival at 3 years were 74% and 65% for stage II, 70% and 60% for stage III, and 52% and 42% for inflammatory disease, respectively.[119] The definition of "high-risk" varies in different BMT centers, but historically included women with stage II or III disease involving 10 or more axillary lymph nodes. Historical data indicate that 55% to 87% of patients with stage II or III disease involving 10 or more axillary lymph nodes will relapse within 5 years, despite standard-dose adjuvant chemotherapy.[117] Patients usually receive several courses of standard-dose adjuvant chemotherapy, followed by HDC with autologous rescue as intensive consolidation. Uncontrolled studies conducted at Duke University show that about 70% of women with high-risk primary disease treated with this approach are alive at 3 years.[120] High-dose chemotherapy is being investigated in patients with stage II/III disease with 4 to 9 lymph nodes positive for disease. In one uncontrolled report from the University of Colorado, 71% of women with 4 to 9 positive nodes were alive disease-free at 4 years, which compares favorably with historical controls treated with standard chemotherapy.[121] High-dose chemotherapy as intensive consolidation in women with high-risk primary disease is currently being evaluated by several cooperative oncology groups.[117,118]

Because of the large number of women with breast cancer, the use of HDC with autologous rescue has greatly increased the awareness of the lay public and health care professionals to BMT as a treatment modality. Although early results are encouraging, its use is controversial and there is variability in insurance coverage for the treatment.[118,122]

OTHER SOLID TUMORS

High-dose chemotherapy with autologous rescue has been used as salvage therapy for many adults with solid tumors, particularly chemotherapy-responsive tumors such as germ cell tumors, ovarian cancer, and small cell lung cancer.[60] Some patients with solid tumors not usually responsive to chemotherapy, such as colorectal cancer and malignant melanoma, also have been treated. Many children with neuroblastoma, Ewing's sarcoma, rhabdomyosarcoma, and brain tumors also have been treated, with varying success.[60]

TRANSPLANT-RELATED COMPLICATIONS

Although many patients with cancer treated with HDC and autologous or allogeneic transplantation experience long-term survival and cure of their disease, this modality is associated with many serious and potentially life-threatening complications. In the early 1970s, early posttransplant mortality was extremely high, and most BMT patients did not survive beyond 100 days. During those early years of allogeneic BMT, death was usually related to infection, GVHD, interstitial pneumonia, and leukemic relapse. The therapeutic armamentarium available at that time was limited. Today, largely because of the availability of new and potent drugs such as broad-spectrum antibiotics, immunosuppressive drugs, antiviral drugs, and hematopoietic growth factors and other biotechnology drugs, transplant-related mortality has been greatly reduced. Until recently, allogeneic BMT was usually restricted to patients less than 50 years old with an HLA-identical sibling donor. With advances in the prevention and treatment of transplant-related complications, allogeneic BMT is now being offered to more high-risk patients such as those who lack an HLA-identical sibling donor and those older than 50 years of age. Patients treated with HDC with autologous rescue have a very low risk for immune-mediated complications. The risk of transplant-related mortality after HDC with autologous rescue for lymphoma or breast cancer is less than 10% at most centers and less than 5% at many centers.

Unfortunately, similar progress has not been made in the eradication of malignant cells and tumor relapse remains the major cause of death posttransplant. The use of more sensitive methods to detect tumor cells, novel purging techniques, more effective conditioning regimens, and adoptive immunotherapy may lead to more effective tumor control.

REGIMEN-RELATED TOXICITY

Because myelosuppression is not a concern, dosages of anticancer drugs can be increased many times above those used in conventional chemotherapy. As a result, most patients treated with HDC experience regimen-related toxicity in nonhematopoietic tissues and some patients experience early death as a result of these toxicities. In this setting, these nonhematologic toxicities are dose limiting. Because of the severity of these regimen-related toxicities, toxicity grading scales used in cooperative oncology group trials are not appropriate. A toxicity grading system has recently been developed by the Seattle BMT team.[38] In that grading system, toxicities in eight different organs are graded on a scale of 0 (none) to 4 (fatal). If toxicity is related to another cause other than the preparative regimen, it is not considered regimen-related toxicity. After toxicity to individual organs is graded, the patient is assigned an overall grade of toxicity equivalent to the highest grade achieved in any organ.

In patients with leukemia, regimen-related toxicity is usually more severe in allogeneic BMT recipients compared with autologous BMT recipients, which suggests that GVHD or posttransplant immunosuppression contributes to regimen-related toxicity. Severe regimen-related toxicities are also more common in patients with advanced disease at the time of BMT. In the setting of autologous BMT, where graft rejection and GVHD do not occur, the mortality associated with severe regimen-related toxicity is about 10% to 20%. The dose-limiting nonhematologic toxicity varies according to the drugs included in the conditioning regimen. Table 125–5 lists the dose-limiting nonhematologic toxicity for several drugs commonly included in conditioning regimens. These toxicities may be uncommon or rare with the administration of conventional doses of a specific drug. Several unusual and severe manifestations of regimen-related toxicities are discussed in detail below.

The management of specific toxicities is supportive. The mechanism of toxicity probably varies according to the conditioning regimen and the organ involved. The clinical expression of regimen-related toxicity may be related to the release of tumor necrosis factor (TNF-α) and other inflammatory cytokines. Drugs that inhibit the release of inflammatory cytokines are being investigated to reduce regimen-related toxicity after BMT. Results of randomized controlled trials with pentoxifylline, an inhibitor of TNF-α production, have been disappointing.[123,124]

HEPATIC VENO-OCCLUSIVE DISEASE

Hepatic veno-occlusive disease (VOD), defined as an obliteration of the small intrahepatic central venules, is one of the most severe regimen-related toxicities.[125] Clinical signs of hepatic VOD include sudden weight gain, ascites, hepatomegaly, and increased serum bilirubin concentrations occurring within the first 3 weeks after transplant. The incidence of hepatic VOD ranges from 5% to 20% in most series. Factors reported to increase the risk of hepatic VOD include the use of TBI-containing conditioning regimens and the presence of elevated liver function tests or metastatic liver disease pretransplant. The use of some drugs, such as busulfan or carmustine, also may increase the risk of hepatic VOD. Busulfan concentrations have been correlated with the risk of hepatic VOD.[126,127] Patients with a high area-under-the-curve (AUC) for busulfan concentration had a greater risk of hepatic VOD than those with a low AUC. Based on these studies, some BMT centers adjust busulfan doses based on plasma concentrations. Hepatic VOD is frequently progressive, leading to death in 50% to 75% of patients. At many BMT centers, hepatic VOD is one of the leading causes of transplant-related mortality after high-dose chemotherapy with autologous rescue. Some studies suggest that prostaglandin E1, unfractionated and low-molecular-weight heparin, or ursodiol may be partially effective in the prevention of hepatic VOD.[125,128,129]

TABLE 125–5. Dose-limiting Nonhematologic Toxicities for Selected Chemotherapeutic Agents Included in Conditioning Regimens in Autologous Bone Marrow Transplantation

Drug	Conventional Dose[a] (mg/m^2)	ABMT[b] Dose (mg/m^2)	Dose-limiting Toxicity
Busulfan	2	450	Hepatic
Carboplatin	400	2000	Hepatic, renal
Carmustine	200	1200	Pulmonary, hepatic
Cisplatin	100	200	Renal, peripheral neuropathy
Cyclophosphamide	1000	7500	Cardiomyopathy
Etoposide	300–600	2400	Mucositis
Ifosfamide	5000	18000	Renal
Melphalan	40	225	Mucositis
Thiotepa	20–50	1125	Mucositis, CNS

[a]Doses are approximate and are for drugs as single agents. When combinations are used, doses may need to be decreased.
[b]ABMT = autologous bone marrow transplantation.
Modified from Eder JP, Elias A, Shea TC, et al. A phase I–II study of cyclophosphamide, thiotepa, and carboplatin with autologous bone marrow transplantation in solid tumor patients. J Clin Oncol 1990;8:1242.

Treatment is generally supportive. Recombinant tissue plasminogen activator is sometimes given to patients with severe VOD because of the possible role of the coagulation cascade in the pathogenesis of VOD.[130,131]

PULMONARY COMPLICATIONS

Pulmonary complications following HDC can be categorized as infectious and noninfectious; infections are discussed in Chapter 111; noninfectious complications are described as early (up to 3 months posttransplant) and late (after 3 months). Early complications include diffuse alveolar hemorrhage and idiopathic interstitial pneumonitis.[132] Diffuse alveolar hemorrhage is diagnosed by examination of bronchoalveolar lavage fluid.[132,133] Although it can be severe and life threatening, prompt treatment with high doses of corticosteroids has been reported to be beneficial. Idiopathic interstitial pneumonitis also is a severe form of regimen-related toxicity.[132,134] Patients with idiopathic interstitial pneumonitis are clinically indistinguishable from those with interstitial pneumonitis related to infection. The risk is similar in recipients of autologous or allogeneic marrow, but appears higher in patients who are conditioned with a TBI-containing regimen or who have acute GVHD. Mortality has been reported to be as high as 70% and treatment is supportive care only.

Late pulmonary complications cover a wide spectrum of disorders and include both obstructive and restrictive lung diseases. Included in these disorders are bronchiolitis obliterans with or without organizing pneumonia, diffuse alveolar damage, and lymphocytic interstitial pneumonia.[135] Therapy consists of steroids, which are about 50% effective; patients with mild to moderate airflow impairment appear to have the best response. Mortality from these disorders is approximately 40%.

GRAFT FAILURE

Initial engraftment usually occurs in the first 2 to 4 weeks posttransplant and is evidenced by rising peripheral blood counts and the presence of hematopoietic precursor cells in the marrow. In allogeneic BMT, the presence of donor cells is confirmed with cytogenetic markers. In most patients, engraftment is sustained with complete recovery of hematopoiesis.

Graft failure can occur after autologous, syngeneic, and allogeneic hematopoietic stem cell transplantation. Two syndromes have been observed.[136,137] Early graft failure is diagnosed clinically when the rate of neutrophil recovery is delayed (also referred to as primary graft failure or delayed engraftment), whereas late graft failure is characterized by a decline in the neutrophil count after temporary engraftment (also referred to as secondary graft failure). When graft failure occurs after allogeneic BMT and is characterized by the regrowth of immunocompetent host cells and a simultaneous loss of donor cells, it is referred to as graft rejection. Graft rejection occurs rarely in recipients of unmodified marrow from HLA-identical sibling donors who are conditioned with cyclophosphamide and TBI.[138] An increased risk of graft rejection has been observed in several groups of patients undergoing allogeneic BMT: recipients of marrow from partially HLA-mismatched donors, recipients of T-cell-depleted marrow (HLA-identical sibling donors), recipients of marrow from matched unrelated donors, and patients with severe aplastic anemia. With widespread use of PBPCs and posttransplant growth factors, graft failure is rare after autologous transplantation.

Graft failure not immunologically mediated also can occur in allogeneic BMT. It is usually difficult to determine the precise cause, although potential causes include infusion of low numbers of hematopoietic stem cells, viral infection (cytomegalovirus), or drug toxicity. Drug-induced graft failure can be caused not only by drugs that are known to be myelosuppressive (e.g., methotrexate, ganciclovir), but also by drugs that are not usually associated with neutropenia (e.g., ranitidine).[139] The use of chemicals or drugs, such as 4-HC, in *ex vivo* marrow purging in autologous BMT may damage hematopoietic stem cells and also increase the risk of graft failure.[68] Preliminary results of a randomized study suggest that amifostine may protect normal hematopoietic progenitors from 4-HC used in *ex vivo* marrow purging.[140]

Regardless of the cause, the long-term prognosis in patients with graft failure is poor.[141] Despite supportive care, death sometimes occurs from infection or bleeding. In some patients with an HLA-identical sibling donor, a second marrow transplant can be beneficial. The most effective therapy for graft failure is recombinant growth factors, such as G-CSF or GM-CSF. In one uncontrolled study, more than one-half of patients with marrow graft failure responded within 2 weeks to recombinant GM-CSF.[141] In many cases, responses were sustained without maintenance GM-CSF therapy. GM-CSF-treated patients had a better survival than historic controls.

The use of recombinant G-CSF or GM-CSF posttransplant dramatically reduces the incidence of early graft failure after autologous BMT.[142] Before the availability of recombinant growth factors, most patients required 3 to 4 weeks to engraft after autologous BMT. Recombinant G-CSF or GM-CSF given during the early posttransplant period significantly accelerates the rate of myeloid recovery in patients undergoing autologous BMT, defined as the number of days needed to reach a neutrophil count of 500 or 1000/mm^3.[142] The usual dosage of recombinant GM-CSF is 250 $mg/m^2/d$. Higher dosages (e.g., 10 μg/kg/d) of recombinant G-CSF can be given because of its more favorable adverse effect profile as compared with recombinant GM-CSF. Although recombinant growth factors were initially not given to patients undergoing allogeneic BMT because of concern that they may exacerbate GVHD, recent studies show that they accelerate the rate of hematopoietic recovery without increasing the risk of GVHD (both G-CSF and GM-CSF have received FDA approval for this indication).

Although recombinant G-CSF or GM-CSF clearly accelerates myeloid recovery after autologous BMT, its role is less clear in patients who receive mobilized PBPCs instead of bone marrow as a source of hematopoietic stem cells. Some investigators believe that PBPCs are primarily responsible for the rapid neutrophil and platelet recovery observed after HDC and that posttransplant administration of recombinant G-CSF or GM-CSF is less important and may not be necessary. However, in a prospective randomized trial, patients who received mobilized PBPCs and posttransplant recombinant G-CSF had significantly more rapid neutrophil recovery than those who received mobilized PBPCs alone.[143] Many different dosages of G-CSF have been used after PBPC transplantation. In one study of three different G-CSF dosages (5, 10, and 16 μg/kg/d), the rate of hematopoietic recovery was similar in each group.[144]

None of the commercially available recombinant growth factors has a significant effect on platelet recovery. Thrombopoietin (also called megakaryocyte growth and development factor) has recently been identified as the primary hematopoietic growth factor responsible for the growth and development of platelet precursors, megakaryocytes. Clinical studies are now ongoing to determine the role of thrombopoietin in the posttransplant setting.

GRAFT-VERSUS-HOST DISEASE

GVHD is caused by immunocompetent donor T lymphocytes reacting against antigens on host tissues.[136, 145–147] In that setting, donor T lymphocytes recognize histocompatibility antigens of the host as genetically foreign, become activated, proliferate, and attack recipient tissue, thereby producing the clinical syndrome of GVHD. Excessive or dysfunctional production of inflammatory cytokines such as IL-1 and TNF-α is probably responsible at least in part for the clinical syndrome of GVHD.[78,148] This hypothesis is supported by the observation that some patients with refractory acute GVHD respond to treatment with inhibitors of these cytokines (discussed later). Graft rejection can be viewed as a host-versus-graft reaction, an immune-mediated reaction in the opposite direction as GVHD. Two different clinical syndromes have been recognized, depending on the onset of GVHD. Acute GVHD occurs early while chronic GVHD occurs late in the posttransplant course.

ACUTE GRAFT-VERSUS-HOST DISEASE

Acute GVHD usually becomes clinically evident during the first 60 days posttransplant and is characterized by selective epithelial damage of target organs. The principal target organs for acute GVHD are the skin, liver, and gastrointestinal tract. Acute GVHD is classified into four grades, depending on the number of organs involved and the degree of involvement of each organ (Fig. 125–8).[145–147] Grade I disease involves only the skin while grades II through IV involve the skin and either the liver or gastrointestinal tract, or both. The initial sign of acute GVHD is usually a generalized maculopapular rash. Acute GVHD usually progresses, involving the liver, gastrointestinal tract, or both. Intestinal GVHD is manifested as diarrhea but may progress to abdominal pain and ileus. Hepatic GVHD is usually asymptomatic, consisting of hyperbilirubinemia and increases in serum aminotransferase and alkaline phosphatase levels.

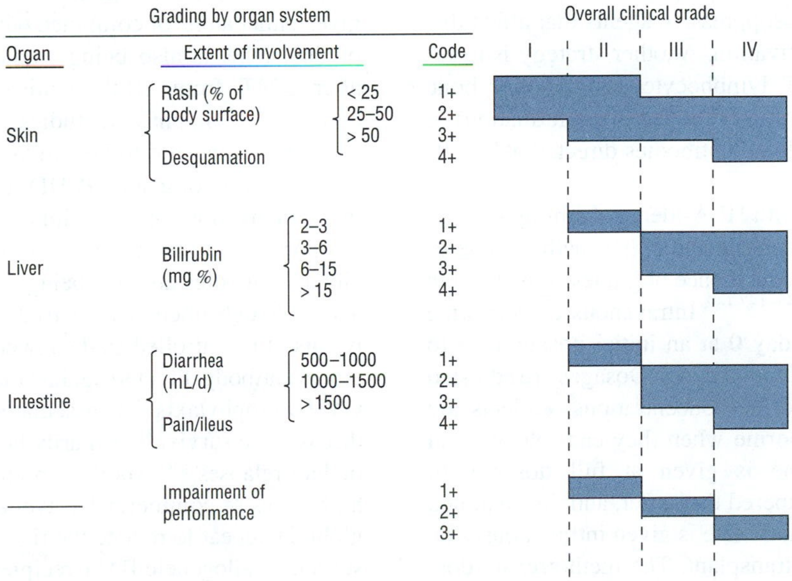

FIGURE 125–8. Clinical grading of acute GVHD. The left panel of the figure summarizes the grading by organ system; the right panel shows the overall clinical grade. With grade I, only the skin can be involved. With more extensive involvement of the skin or involvement of liver and intestinal tract and impairment of the clinical performance status, either alone or in any combination, the severity grade advances from II to IV. *(Reproduced, with permission, from the Annual Review of Medicine, Volume 35, © 1984, by Annual Reviews Inc.)*

The overall incidence of moderate to severe (grades II to IV) GVHD ranges from 10% to more than 80% after allogeneic BMT, depending on the degree of histocompatibility, number of T lymphocytes in the graft, patient age, and prophylactic regimen.[145–147] Other factors associated with an increased risk for acute GVHD in some studies are donor–recipient sex mismatch and the parity of female donors; the highest risk was observed in male recipients who received marrow from a previously pregnant female donor.[149] This observation suggests that alloimmunization against minor histocompatibility antigens may be important in the pathogenesis of acute GVHD. The reasons for the increased risk in older patients are not known, although many investigators believe that it is related to the gradual reduction in thymic function with increasing age. The most severe acute GVHD is observed in allogeneic BMT with non-HLA-identical related or HLA-identical unrelated donors. In that setting, the incidence of grades II to IV acute GVHD exceeds 50%, despite aggressive prophylactic immunosuppression with two or more drugs, sometimes combined with immunologic purging of T cells from donor marrow.[12,13]

Multiorgan acute GVHD and the drugs given to prevent or treat it are associated with delayed immunologic recovery and increased susceptibility to infections, particularly cytomegaloviral infection. Because treatment of established acute GVHD is unsatisfactory, aggressive preventive treatment is usually given. The most common strategy used to prevent acute GVHD is to block the activation of T lymphocytes by administration of immunosuppressive agents.[145–147] Several immunosuppressive agents have been used, including cyclophosphamide, methotrexate, cyclosporine, antithymocyte globulin, corticosteroids, and most recently tacrolimus or monoclonal antibodies directed at T lymphocytes. Most GVHD prophylaxis regimens combine two or more immunosuppressive agents that affect different stages of T-cell activation. Another strategy is to remove or deplete most T lymphocytes from donor bone marrow by physical separation (i.e., lectin agglutination) or by treatment with monoclonal antibodies directed at T cells (Fig. 125–6).[150]

In allogeneic BMT with HLA-identical sibling donors, the combination of cyclosporine and either methotrexate or corticosteroids reduces the incidence of grades II to IV acute GVHD to 25% to 40%.[145–147,149] Intravenous cyclosporine is usually started around day 0 at an initial dosage of 3 to 5 mg/kg/d, given in two divided doses. Dosages are adjusted based on trough cyclosporine concentrations. Patients are converted to oral cyclosporine when they can tolerate oral medications. Cyclosporine is given at full doses until about day 50, gradually tapered thereafter, and discontinued by day 180. "Short" methotrexate is given intravenously on days 1, 3, 6, and 11 posttransplant. The methotrexate dosage is 10 mg/m^2, except for the first dose given on day 1 (15 mg/m^2). Some protocols omit the day 11 dose because of adverse effects. When cyclosporine is given in combination with corticosteroids, methylprednisolone is usually started during the first 2 weeks posttransplant, given at full dosages for several weeks, and gradually tapered. Although the efficacy of cyclosporine–methotrexate and cyclosporine–corticosteroids appears to be similar, the use of methotrexate may increase the risk of early graft failure while corticosteroid administration has been associated with a higher incidence of infections.[147] It is not clear whether three-drug regimens are more effective than two-drug regimens. In one prospective randomized study conducted by the Seattle BMT team, the addition of methylprednisolone did not further increase the efficacy of the cyclosporine and methotrexate regimen.[151] Unexpectedly, patients who received cyclosporine, methotrexate, and methylprednisolone had a higher incidence of acute and chronic GVHD than those given cyclosporine and methotrexate. Subsequent analysis of that trial showed that patients who received three drugs as GVHD prophylaxis also had a significantly higher risk of infection early posttransplant compared with those who received cyclosporine and methotrexate.[152] But in another prospective randomized study, the three-drug combination of cyclosporine, methotrexate, and corticosteroids further reduced the incidence of grades II to IV acute GVHD to about 10%, compared with a 20% incidence in those randomized to receive cyclosporine and glucocorticoids.[153] It is not clear why the two trials reached different conclusions. In the trial conducted by the Seattle BMT team, methylprednisolone was given from days 0 to 35 posttransplant. In contrast, methylprednisolone was not started in the other trial until day 7 posttransplant. Some investigators speculate that early administration of methylprednisolone may have interfered with the antiproliferative effects of methotrexate on T lymphocytes.[151]

Newer approaches may increase the efficacy of GVHD prophylaxis after allogeneic BMT. Tacrolimus (FK506), given either alone or combined with methotrexate or methylprednisolone, is also being studied as GVHD prophylaxis after BMT from HLA-identical siblings and unrelated donors.[154–157] In phase II studies, the efficacy and toxicity of tacrolimus appeared to be similar to that of cyclosporine in the prevention of acute GVHD. Further studies to compare the combination of tacrolimus and methotrexate to cyclosporine and methotrexate are ongoing. Systemic monoclonal antibodies are also being studied in some clinical trials. Although uncontrolled trials suggest possible benefit, results of a controlled trial showed that addition of a monoclonal antibody directed against the IL-2 receptor to standard GVHD prophylaxis was associated with significantly lower disease-free survival, primarily because of an increased risk of late relapses.[158] Another interesting observation is that high doses of commercially available intravenous immunoglobulin appear to reduce the risk of acute GVHD in certain subsets of allogeneic BMT recipients.[159]

The role of *ex vivo* T-cell depletion from donor bone marrow is controversial (Fig. 125–6). Although the use of T-cell-depleted marrow can reduce the incidence and severity of acute GVHD, it is associated with an increased risk of graft failure, leukemic relapse, and Epstein–Barr virus (EBV)-related lymphoproliferative disorders post-BMT. This suggests that important cell populations (e.g., natural killer cells) are being eliminated in the depletion process.[136,150] As a result, survival in recipients of HLA-identical sibling donor marrow is not improved with this approach. Various approaches are being investigated to selectively remove the T cells responsible for GVHD while leaving those cells that mediate engraftment, antileukemic effect, and suppression of EBV-transformed lymphocytes. Another approach has been to add back the T cells originally depleted to prevent leukemic relapse.[160] Because of the higher risk of GVHD in allogeneic BMT with HLA-mismatched or matched unrelated donors, T-cell depletion is often included as part of the GVHD prophylaxis regimen in that setting (discussed later).

With allogeneic BMT with HLA-mismatched or HLA-identical unrelated donors, the risk of moderate to severe (grades II to IV) acute GVHD is 50% or higher with conventional prophylaxis with two immunosuppressive agents.[12,13] The combination of cyclosporine and corticosteroids is preferred by some investigators because of the bone marrow toxicity of methotrexate. Several approaches are generally used to reduce the risk of acute GVHD in this high-risk group of patients: three-drug GVHD prophylaxis (cyclosporine, methotrexate, and corticosteroids), *ex vivo* T-cell depletion of donor bone marrow (Fig. 125–6), or the addition of an intravenously administered monoclonal antibody directed at T cells to standard GVHD prophylaxis. In recipients of matched unrelated transplants, T-cell depletion has been associated with a significantly lower incidence of early graft failure and acute GVHD, with apparent preservation of the graft-versus-leukemia effect.[12,161]

Initial treatment of established acute GVHD usually consists of high-dose corticosteroids, given as intravenously administered methylprednisolone. The usual dosage is 2.0 mg/kg/d, given in two divided doses. The initial dosage is as high as 10 mg/kg/d in some protocols, although there is no convincing evidence that higher dosages are more effective. Results of one study suggest that a cumulative dose of 2000 mg/m^2 (about 50 mg/kg) of prednisone (or methylprednisolone) is needed for complete resolution of acute GVHD in most patients.[162] Antithymocyte globulin appears to be as effective as methylprednisolone, but difficulties in supply and toxicities have limited its usefulness. Overall complete or partial responses are observed in about 40% of patients.[145–147] Nonrelapse mortality is strongly correlated to response to initial treatment; mortality ranged from about 25% in patients who had a complete response to about 80% in those who had no response or progressive disease. A new immunosuppressive agent, mycophenolate mofetil, is also being evaluated for the treatment of acute GVHD.[163] In patients who fail initial treatment with corticosteroids, antithymocyte globulin or monoclonal antibodies directed at T lymphocytes can be given with some success.[164] In patients who experience a flare in their GVHD during the taper phase of corticosteroid therapy, therapy consists of increasing the steroid dose. A variety of biotechnology drugs have been shown to be effective in the treatment of refractory acute GVHD. Encouraging results have been reported with a humanized monoclonal antibody that binds to the IL-2 receptor, a monoclonal anti–TNF-α antibody, and recombinant IL-1 receptor antagonist.[147]

CHRONIC GRAFT-VERSUS-HOST DISEASE

Chronic GVHD usually occurs after day 100 and is the major determinant of late transplant-related morbidity and mortality.[145,165] Chronic GVHD is classified as limited or extensive, depending on pathologic findings and the extent of systemic involvement. Limited chronic GVHD indicates either localized skin involvement, mild hepatic dysfunction, or both. Most patients have extensive disease, with involvement of the skin, liver, eyes, mouth, esophagus, or other organs. The clinicopathologic findings of chronic GVHD are similar to those observed in various autoimmune diseases. Screening studies such as skin and lip biopsies and Schirmer's testing for lacrimal function done on day 100 have been shown to predict for the subsequent development of chronic GVHD.

The incidence of chronic GVHD in patients who survive more than 150 days ranges from 15% to 65%.[145,165] The risk of chronic GVHD increases with increasing patient age, and is higher in recipients of marrow from HLA-nonidentical related or unrelated donors, and in patients who had prior acute GVHD. In patients with aplastic anemia, the administration of donor buffy-coat transfusions also is associated with an increased risk of chronic GVHD. Most patients who develop chronic GVHD have a previous history of acute GVHD, although 20% to 30% develop the disease de novo.

If no functional impairment is present, patients with limited disease are not treated. Many patients with extensive chronic GVHD, if left untreated, will die of infections or become disabled. Long-term survival is worse in certain subgroups of patients, such as patients with thrombocytopenia or progressive onset of chronic GVHD, and those who fail to respond to immunosuppressive therapy.[166] Chronic GVHD is treated with immunosuppressive agents such as corticosteroids, cyclosporine, cyclophosphamide, or azathioprine. In patients without thrombocytopenia, treatment with prednisone alone (initial dosage: 1.0 mg/kg/d) is superior to prednisone and azathioprine.[166] Although control of chronic GVHD was similar in the two groups, patients treated with prednisone and azathioprine had more frequent bacterial and viral infections, which resulted in higher nonrelapse mortality (40% versus 21%). In patients with thrombocytopenia, an alternating-day cyclosporine and prednisone regimen appears superior to prednisone alone in the treatment of chronic GVHD.[167] In patients who fail initial treatment, azathioprine or alternating cyclosporine and prednisone have been used with some success. Thalidomide appears effective in some patients who fail initial treatment and is being investigated as primary treatment for high-risk chronic GVHD.[168] Oral trimethoprim–sulfamethoxazole is usually given as infection prophylaxis in all patients receiving treatment for chronic GVHD.

Treatment is continued until signs and symptoms of the disease have resolved, usually over a period of several months. As chronic GVHD improves, the immunosuppressive drug is discontinued, followed by gradual tapering of corticosteroid therapy. Because patients are usually leading fairly normal lives at this stage, it is important to minimize any unnecessary side effects of therapy.

INFECTION

Patients undergoing HDC with autologous or allogeneic transplantation are severely immunocompromised and therefore at high risk for bacterial, fungal, and viral infection. Management of these infections is discussed in detail in Chapter 111.

LATE COMPLICATIONS

With the success of HDC, the number of long-term survivors has grown. Many survivors experience delayed complications of transplantation. Major late complications include restrictive and obstructive pulmonary disease; cataract formation; endocrine dysfunction, including sterility; impaired growth; infections; and secondary malignancies.[169,170]

REFERENCES

1. Williams SF, ed. Autologous bone marrow transplantation. Hematol Oncol Clin North Am 1993;7:501–752.
2. Armitage JO. Bone marrow transplantation. N Engl J Med 1994;330: 827–838.
3. Forman SJ, Blume KG, Thomas ED, eds. Bone Marrow Transplantation. Boston, Blackwell, 1994.
4. Armitage JO, Antman KH, eds. High-dose Cancer Therapy: Pharmacology, Hematopoietins, Stem Cells, 2nd ed. Baltimore, Williams & Wilkins, 1995.
5. Appelbaum FR. The use of bone marrow and peripheral blood stem cell transplantation in the treatment of cancer. CA 1996;46: 142–164.
6. Dupont B, Yang SY. Histocompatibility. In: Forman SJ, Blume KG, Thomas ED, eds. Bone Marrow Transplantation. Boston, Blackwell, 1994:22–40.
7. Begovich AB, Erlich HA. HLA typing for bone marrow transplantation. JAMA 1995;273:586–591.
8. Mickelson EM, Bartsch GE, Hansen JA, Dupont B. The MLC assay as a test for HLA-D region compatibility between patients and unrelated donors: Results of a national marrow donor program involving multiple centers. Tissue Antigens 1993;42:465–472.
9. Petersdorf EW, Longton GM, Anasetti C, et al. The significance of HLA-DRB1 matching on clinical outcome after HLA-A, B, DR identical unrelated donor marrow transplantation. Blood 1995;89: 1606–1613.
10. Petersdorf EW, Longton GM, Anasetti C, et al. Association of HLA-C disparity with graft failure after marrow transplantation from unrelated donors. Blood 1997;89:1818–1823.
11. Stroncek D, Bartsch G, Perkins HA, et al. The National Marrow Donor Program. Transfusion 1993;33:567–577.
12. Kernan NA, Bartsch G, Ash RC, et al. Analysis of 462 transplantations from unrelated donors facilitated by the National Marrow Donor Program. N Engl J Med 1993;328:593–602.
13. Szydlo R, Goldman JM, Klein JP, et al. Results of allogeneic bone marrow transpants for leukemia using donors other than HLA-identical siblings. J Clin Oncol 1997;15:1767–1777.
14. Golde DW. The stem cell. Sci Am 1991;265:86–93.
15. Thomas ED, Storb R. Technique for human marrow grafting. Blood 1970;36:507–515.
16. Kessinger A. Reestablishing hematopoiesis after dose intensive therapy with peripheral stem cells. In Armitage JO, Antman KH, eds. High-dose Cancer Therapy: Pharmacology, Hematopoietins, Stem Cells, 2nd ed. Baltimore, Williams & Wilkins, 1995:196–210.
17. To LB, Haylock DN, Simmons PJ, and Juttner CA. The biology and clinical uses of blood stem cells. Blood 1997;89:2233.
18. Talmadge JE, Reed E, Ino K, et al. Rapid immunologic reconstitution following transplantation with mobilized peripheral blood stem cells as compared to bone marrow. Bone Marrow Transplant 1997; 19:161-172.
19. Beyer J, Schwella N, Zingsem J, et al. Hematopoietic rescue after high dose chemotherapy using autologous peripheral blood progenitor cells or bone marrow: A randomized comparison. J Clin Oncol 1995;13:1328–1335.
20. Schmitz N, Linch DC, Dreger P, et al. Filgrastim-mobilized peripheral blood progenitor cell translantation in comparison with autologous bone marrow transplantation: Results of a randomized phase III trial in lymphoma patients. Lancet 1996;347:353–357.
21. Peters WP, Ross M, Vredenburgh JJ, et al. The use of intensive clinic support to permit outpatient autologous bone marrow transplantation for breast cancer. Semin Oncol 1994;21(suppl 7):25–31.
22. Meisenberg BR, Miller WE, McMillan R, et al. Outpatient high-dose chemotherapy with autologous stem-cell rescue for hematologic and non-hematologic malignancies. J Clin Oncol 1997;15: 11–17.
23. Smith TJ, Hillner BE, Schmitz N, et al. Economic analysis of a randomized clinical trial to compare filgrastim-mobilized peripheral blood progenitor cell transplantation with autologous bone marrow transplantation in patients with Hodgkin's and non-Hodgkin's lymphoma. J Clin Oncol 1997; 15:5–10.
24. Bensinger W, Appelbaum F, Rowley, S, et al. Factors that influence collection and engraftment of autologous peripheral-blood stem cells. J Clin Oncol 1995;13:2547–2555.
25. Weaver CH, Hazelton B, Birch R, et al. An analysis of engraftment kinetics as a function of the CD34 content of peripheral blood progenitor cell collections in 692 patients after the administration of myeloablative chemotherapy. Blood 1995;86:3961–3969.
26. Yee GC. Peripheral blood progenitor cell transplantation: Economic issues. Pharmacotherapy 1998;18:9s–16s.
27. Ketterer N, Salles G, Raba M, et al. High $CD34^+$ cell counts decrease hematologic toxicity of autologous peripheral blood progenitor cell transplantation. Blood 1998;91:3148–3155.
28. Glaspy JA, Shpall EJ, LeMaistre CF, et al. Peripheral blood progenitor cell mobilization using stem cell factor in combination with filgrastim in breast cancer patients. Blood 1997;90:2939–2951.
29. Basser RL, To LB, Begley CG, et al. Rapid hematopoietic recovery after multicycle high dose chemotherapy: Enhancement of filgrastim-induced progenitor-cell mobilization by recombinant human stem cell factor. J Clin Oncol 1998;16:1899–1908.
30. Lyman SD and Jacobsen SEW. *c-kit* ligand and flt3 ligand: Stem/progenitor cell factors with overlapping yet distinct activities. Blood 1998;91:1101–1134.
31. Murray LJ, Luens KM, Estrada MF, et al. Thrombopoietin mobilizes $CD34^+$ cell subsets into peripheral blood and expands multilineage progenitors in bone marrow of cancer patients with normal hematopoiesis. Exp Hematol 1998;26:207–216.

32. Bensinger WI, Clift R, Martin P, et al. Allogeneic peripheral blood stem cell transplantation in patients with advanced malignancies: A retrospective comparison with marrow transplantation. Blood 1996; 88:2794–2800.
33. Przepiorka D, Anderlini P, Ippoliti C, et al. Allogeneic blood stem cell transplantation in advanced hematologic cancers. Bone Marrow Transplant 1997;19:455–460.
34. Ottinger HD, Beelen DW, Scheulen B, et al. Improved immune reconstitution after allotransplantation of peripheral blood stem cells instead of bone marrow. Blood 1996;88:2775–2779.
35. Storek J, Gooley T, Siadak M, et al. Allogeneic peripheral blood stem cell transplantation may be associated with a high risk of chronic graft-versus-host disease. Blood 1997;90:4705–4709.
36. Cairo MS, Wagner JE. Placental and/or umbilical cord blood: An alternative source of hematopoietic stem cells for transplantation. Blood 1997;90:4665-4678.
37. Gluckman E, Rocha V, Boyer-Chammard A, et al. Outcome of cord blood transplantation from related and unrelated donors. N Engl J Med 1997;337:373–381.
38. Petersen FB, Bearman SI. Preparative regimens and their toxicity. In: Forman SJ, Blume KG, Thomas ED, eds. Bone Marrow Transplantation. Boston, Blackwell, 1994:79–95.
39. Aurer I, Gale RP. Are new conditioning regimens for transplants in acute myelogenous leukemia better? Bone Marrow Transplant 1991; 7:255–261.
40. Blume KG, Forman SJ. High-dose etoposide (VP-16)-containing preparatory regimens in allogeneic and autologous bone marrow transplantation for hematologic malignancies. Semin Oncol 1992; 19(suppl 13):63–66.
41. Santos GW. The development of busulfan/cyclophosphamide preparative regimens. Semin Oncol 1993;20(suppl 4):12–16.
42. Antman K, Eder JP, Elias A, et al. High-dose thiotepa alone and in combination regimens with bone marrow support. Semin Oncol 1990;17(suppl 3):33–38.
43. Yahalom J, Fuks ZY. Strategies for the use of total body irradiation as systemic therapy in leukemia and lymphoma. In: Armitage JO, Antman KH, eds. High-dose Cancer Therapy: Pharmacology, Hematopoietins, Stem Cells. Baltimore, Williams & Wilkins, 1995; 69–98.
44. Thomas ED, Clift RA, Hersman J, et al. Marrow transplantation for acute nonlymphoblastic leukemia in first remission using fractionated or single-dose irradiation. Int J Radiat Oncol Biol Phys 1982; 8:817–821.
45. Appelbaum FR. Allogeneic hematopoietic stem cell transplantation for acute leukemia. Semin Oncol 1997;24:114–123.
46. Clift RA, Buckner CD, Appelbaum FR, et al. Allogeneic marrow transplantation in patients with chronic myelogenous leukemia in the chronic phase: A randomized trial of two irradiation regimens. Blood 1991;77:1660–1665.
47. Brochstein JA, Kernan NA, Groshen S, et al. Allogeneic bone marrow transplantation after hyperfractionated total-body irradiation and cyclophosphamide in children with acute leukemia. N Engl J Med 1987;317:1618–1624.
48. Slattery JT, Clift RA, Buckner CD, et al. Marrow transplantation for chronic myeloid leukemia: The influence of plasma busulfan levels on the outcome of transplantation. Blood 1997;89:3055–3060.
49. Clift RA, Buckner CD, Thomas ED, et al. Marrow transplantation for chronic myeloid leukemia: A randomized study comparing cyclophosphamide and total body irradiation with busulfan and cyclophosphamide. Blood 1994;84:2036–2043.
50. Devergie A, Blaise D, Attal M, et al. Allogeneic bone marrow transplantation for chronic myeloid leukemia in first chronic phase: A randomized trial of busulfan–cytoxan versus cytoxan–total body irradiation as preparative regimen: A report from the French society of bone marrow graft. Blood 1995;85:2263–2268.
51. Ringden O, Ruutu T, Remberger M, et al. A randomized trial comparing busulfan with total body irradiation as conditioning in allogeneic marrow transplant recipients with leukemia: A report from the Nordic bone marrow transplantation group. Blood 1994;83: 2723–2730.
52. Blaise D, Maraninchi D, Archimbaud E, et al. Allogeneic bone marrow transplantation for acute myeloid leukemia in first remission: A randomized trial of a busulfan–cytoxan versus cytoxan–total body irradiation as preparative regimen: A report from the group d'Etudes de la greffe de moelle osseuse. Blood 1992;79: 2578–2582.
53. Woods WG, Ramsay NKC, Weisdorf DJ, et al. Bone marrow transplantation for acute lymphocytic leukemia utilizing total body irradiation followed by high doses of cytosine arabinoside: Lack of superiority over cyclophosphamide-containing conditioning regimens. Bone Marrow Transplant 1990;6:9–16.
54. Coccia PF, Strandjord SE, Warkentin PI, et al. High-dose cytosine arabinoside and fractionated total-body irradiation: An improved preparative regimen for bone marrow transplantation of children with acute lymphoblastic leukemia in remission. Blood 1988;71: 888–893.
55. Snyder DS, Chao NJ, Amylon MD, et al. Fractionated total body irradiation and high-dose etoposide as a preparatory regimen for bone marrow transplantation in 99 patients with acute leukemia in first complete remission. Blood 1993;82:2920–2928.
56. Champlin R. Preparative regimens for autologous bone marrow transplantation. Blood 1993;81:277–280.
57. Mounier N, Gisselbrecht C. Conditioning regimens before transplantation in patients with aggressive non-Hodgkin's lymphoma. Ann Oncol 1998;9(suppl 1):s15–s21.
58. Jagannath S, Dicke K, Armitage JO, et al. High-dose cyclophosphamide, carmustine, and etoposide and autologous bone marrow transplantation for relapsed Hodgkin's disease. Ann Intern Med 1986;104:163–168.
59. Press OW, Eary JF, Appelbaum FR, et al. Phase II trial of 131I-B1 (anti-CD20) antibody therapy with autologous stem cell transplantation for relapsed B cell lymphomas. Lancet 1995;346:336–340.
60. Antman K, Elias A, Fine HA. Dose-intensive therapy with autologous bone marrow transplantation in solid tumors. In: Forman SJ, Blume KG, Thomas ED, eds. Bone Marrow Transplantation. Boston, Blackwell, 1994:767–788.
61. Frei E. Pharmacologic Strategies for High-dose Chemotherapy. In: Armitage JO, Antman KH, eds. High-dose Cancer Therapy: Pharmacology, Hematopoietins, Stem Cells, 2nd ed. Baltimore, Williams & Wilkins, 1995.
62. Bezwoda WR, Seymour L, Dansey RD. High-dose chemotherapy with hematopoietic rescue as primary treatment for metastatic breast cancer: A randomized trial. J Clin Oncol 1995;13:2483–2489.
63. Fields KK, Elfenbein GJ, Perkins JB, et al. Defining the role of high-dose chemotherapy regimens for the treatment of high risk breast cancer. Semin Oncol 1998;25(suppl 4): 1–6.
64. Stemmer SM, Cagnoni PJ, Shpall EJ, et al. High dose paclitaxel, cyclophosphamide and cisplatin with autologous hematopoietic progenitor cell support: A phase I trial. J Clin Oncol 1996;14: 1463–1472.
65. Negrin RS, Cleary ML. Laboratory evaluation of minimal residual disease. In: Forman SJ, Blume KG, Thomas ED, eds. Bone Marrow Transplantation. Boston, Blackwell, 1994;179–188.
66. Champlin R. Purging: Elimination of malignant cells from autologous blood or marrow transplants. Curr Opin Oncol 1996;8:79–83.
67. Gribben JG, Nadler LM. Antibody-mediated purging. In: Forman SJ, Blume KG, Thomas ED, eds. Bone Marrow Transplantation. Boston, Blackwell, 1994;149–163.
68. Rowley SD. Pharmacological purging of malignant cells. In: Forman SJ, Blume KG, Thomas ED, eds. Bone Marrow Transplantation. Boston, Blackwell, 1994;164–178.
69. Shpall EJ, Jones RB, Bearman SI, et al. Transplantation of enriched CD34-positive autologous marrow into breast cancer patients following high-dose chemotherapy: Influence of CD34-positive

peripheral-blood progenitors and growth factors on engraftment. J Clin Oncol 1994;12:28–36.
70. Schiller G, Vescio R, Freytes C, et al. Autologous CD-34-selected blood progenitor cell transplants for patients with advanced multiple myeloma. Bone Marrow Transplant 1998;21:141–145.
71. Shpall EJ, LeMaistre CF, Holland K, et al. A prospective randomized trial of buffy coat versus CD34-selected autologous bone marrow support in high-risk breast cancer patients receiving high-dose chemotherapy. Blood 1997;90:4313–4320.
72. Fefer A. Graft-versus-tumor responses: Adoptive cellular therapy in bone marrow transplantation. In: Forman SJ, Blume KG, Thomas ED, eds. Bone Marrow Transplantation. Boston, Blackwell, 1994; 231–241.
73. Sullivan KM, Storb R, Buckner CD, et al. Graft-versus-host disease as adoptive immunotherapy in patients with advanced hematologic malignancies. N Engl J Med 1989;320:828–834.
74. Giralt SA, Champlin RE. Leukemia relapse after allogeneic bone marrow transplantation: A review. Blood 1994;84:3603–3612.
75. Porter DL, Antin JH. Infusion of donor peripheral blood mononuclear cells to treat relapse after transplantation for chronic myelogenous leukemia. Hematol Oncol Clin North Am 1998;12:123–151.
76. Collins RH, Shpilberg O, Drobyski WR, et al. Donor leukocyte infusions in 140 patients with relapsed malignancy after allogeneic bone marrow transplantation. J Clin Oncol 1997;15:433–444.
77. Alyea EP, Soiffer RJ, Canning C, et al. Toxicity and efficacy of defined doses of $CD4^+$ donor lymphocytes for treatment of relapse after allogeneic bone marrow transplant. Blood 1998;91:3671–3680.
78. Vogelsang GB, Hess AD. Graft-versus-host disease: New directions for a persistent problem. Blood 1994;84:2061–2067.
79. Yeager AM, Vogelsang GB, Beveridge RA, et al. Induction of cutaneous graft-versus-host disease by administration of cyclosporine to patients undergoing autologous bone marrow transplantation for acute myeloid leukemia. Blood 1992;79:3031–3035.
80. Kennedy MJ, Vogelsang GB, Beveridge RA, et al. Phase I trial of cyclosporine to induce graft-versus-host disease in women undergoing autologous bone marrow transplantation for breast cancer. J Clin Oncol 1993;11:478–484.
81. Fefer A, Benyunes MC, Massumoto C, et al. Interleukin-2 therapy after autologous bone marrow transplantation for hematologic malignancies. Semin Oncol 1993;20(suppl 9):41–45.
82. Robinson N, Benyunes MC, Thompson JA, et al. Interleukin-2 after autologous stem cell transplantation for hematologic malignancy: A phase I/II study. Bone Marrow Transplant 1997;19:435–442.
83. Clift RA, Buckner CD. Marrow transplantation for acute myeloid leukemia. Cancer Invest 1998;16:53–61.
84. Gale RP, Horowitz MM, Rees JKH, et al. Chemotherapy versus transplants for acute myelogenous leukemia in second remission. Leukemia 1996;10:13-15.
85. Zittoun RA, Mandelli F, Willemze R, et al. Autologous or allogeneic bone marrow transplantation compared with intensive chemotherapy in acute myelogenous leukemia. N Engl J Med 1995;332:217–223.
86. Burnett AK, Goldstone AH, Stevens RMF, et al. Randomized comparison of addition of autologous bone marrow transplantation to intensive chemotherapy for acute myeloid leukemia in first remission: Results of MRC AML 10 trial. Lancet 1998;351:700–708.
87. Rowley SD, Jones RJ, Piantadosi S, et al. Efficacy of ex vivo purging for autologous bone marrow transplantation in the treatment of acute nonlymphoblastic leukemia. Blood 1989;74:501–506.
88. Appelbaum FR. Allogeneic bone marrow transplantation for myelodysplastic and myeloproliferative disorders. In: Forman SJ, Blume KG, Thomas ED, eds. Bone Marrow Transplantation. Boston, Blackwell, 1994;629–639.
89. Gassmann W, Schmitz N, Loffler H, de Witte I. Intensive chemotherapy and bone marrow transplantation for myelodysplastic syndromes. Semin Hematol 1996;33:196–205.
90. Runde V, de Witte T, Arnold R, et al. Bone marrow transplantation form HLA-identical siblings as first-line treatment in patients with myelodysplastic syndromes: Early transplantation is associated with improved outcomes. Chronic leukemia working party for the European group for blood and marrow transplantation. Bone Marrow Transplant 1998;21:255–261.
91. Chao NJ, Forman SJ. Allogeneic bone marrow transplantation for acute lymphoblastic leukemia. In: Forman SJ, Blume KG, Thomas ED, eds. Bone Marrow Transplantation. Boston, Blackwell, 1994.
92. Barrett AJ, Horowitz MM, Pollock BH, et al. Bone marrow transplants from HLA-identical siblings as compared with chemotherapy for children with acute lymphoblastic leukemia in a second remission. N Engl J Med 1994;331:1253–1258.
93. Sebban C, Lepage E, Vernant JP, et al. Allogeneic bone marrow transplantation in adult acute lymphoblastic leukemia in first complete remission: A comparative study. J Clin Oncol 1994;12: 2580–2587.
94. Kersey JH, Weisdorf D, Nesbit ME, et al. Comparison of autologous and allogeneic bone marrow transplantation for treatment of high-risk refractory acute lymphoblastic leukemia. N Engl J Med 1987;317:461–467.
95. Fiere D, Lepage E, Sebban C, et al. Adult acute lymphoblastic leukemia: A multicentric randomized trial testing bone marrow transplantation as postremission therapy. J Clin Oncol 1993;11: 1990–2001.
96. Gale RP, Hehlmann R, Zhang MJ, et al. Survival with bone marrow transplantation versus hydroxyurea or interferon for chronic myelogenous leukemia. Blood 1998;91:1810–1819.
97. Passweg JR, Rowlings PA, Horowitz MM. Related donor bone marrow transplantation for chronic myelogenous leukemia. Hematol Oncol Clin North Am 1998;12:81–93.
98. Beelen DW, Graeven U, Elmaagacli AH, et al. Prolonged administration of interferon-α in patients with chronic-phase Philadelphia chromosome-positive chronic myelogenous leukemia before allogeneic bone marrow transplantation may adversely affect transplant outcome. Blood 1994;85:2981–2990.
99. McGlave P. Unrelated donor transplant therapy for chronic myelogenous leukemia. Hematol Oncol Clin North Am 1998;12:93–105.
100. Hansen JA, Gooley TA, Martin PJ, et al. Bone marrow transplants from unrelated donors for patients with chronic myeloid leukemia. N Engl Med 1998;338:962–968.
101. Bhatia R, Forman SJ. Autologous transplantation for the treatment of chronic myelogenous leukemia. Hematol Oncol Clin North Am 1998;12:151–172.
102. Bishop MR, Kessinger A. Blood stem cell transplantation in non-Hodgkin's lymphoma. Cancer Invest 1997;15:138–142.
103. Stiff PJ, Dahlberg S, Forman SJ, et al. Autologous bone marrow transplantation for patients with relapsed or refractory diffuse aggressive non-Hodgkin's lymphoma: Value of augmented preparative regimens—A Southwest oncology group trial. J Clin Oncol 1998; 16:48–55.
104. Vose JM. High dose chemotherapy and hematopoietic stem cell transplantation for relapse or refractory diffuse large-cell non-Hodgkin's lymphoma. Ann Oncol 1998;9(suppl 1):s1–s3.
105. Nademanee A, Molina A, O Donnell MR, et al. Results of high dose therapy and autologous bone marrow/stem cell transplantation during remission in poor risk intermediate and high grade lymphoma: International index high and high intermediate risk group. Blood 1997;90:3844–3852.
106. Haioun C, Lepage E, Gisselbecht C, et al. Benefit of autologous bone marrow transplantation over sequential chemotherapy in poor-risk aggressive non-Hodgkin's lymphoma: Updated results of the prospective study LNH87-2. J Clin Oncol 1997;15:1131–1137.
107. Gianni AM, Bregni M, Siena S, et al. High dose chemotherapy and autologous bone marrow transplantation compared with MACOP-B in aggressive B-cell lymphoma. N Engl J Med 1997;336: 1290–1297.
108. Horning SJ. High dose therapy and transplantation for low grade lymphoma. Hematol Oncol Clin North Am 1997;11:919–935.

109. Freedman AS, Gribben JG, Neuberg D, et al. High dose therapy and autologous bone marrow transplantation in patients with follicular lymphoma during first remission. Blood 1996;88:2780–2786.
110. Bierman PJ, Vose JM, Anderson JR, et al. High-dose therapy with autologous hematopoietic rescue for follicular low-grade non-Hodgkin's lymphoma. J Clin Oncol 1997;15:445–450.
111. Weisdorf DJ, Haake R, Miller WJ, et al. Autologous bone marrow transplantation for progressive non-Hodgkin's lymphoma: Clinical impact of immunophenotype and *in vitro* purging. Bone Marrow Transplant 1991;8:135–142.
112. Gribben JG, Freedman AS, Neuberg D, et al. Immunologic purging of marrow assessed by PCR before autologous bone marrow transplantation for B cell lymphoma. N Engl J Med 1991;325:1525–1531.
113. Nagler A, Ackerstein A, Or R, et al. Immunotherapy with recombinant human interleukin-2 and recombinant interferon-alpha in lymphoma patients postautologous marrow or stem cell transplantation. Blood 1997;89:3951–3959.
114. Barlogie B, Jagannath S. Autologous bone marrow transplantation for multiple myeloma. In: Forman SJ, Blume KG, Thomas ED, eds. Bone Marrow Transplantation. Boston, Blackwell, 1994;754–766.
115. Attal M, Harousseau JL. Standard therapy vs autologous transplantation in multiple myeloma. Hematol Oncol Clin North Am 1997; 11:133–146.
116. Attal M, Harousseau JL, Stoppa AM, et al. A prospective, randomized trial of autologous bone marrow transplantation and chemotherapy in multiple myeloma. N Engl J Med 1996;335:91–97.
117. Peters WP. Autologous bone marrow transplantation for breast cancer. In: Forman SJ, Blume KG, Thomas ED, eds. Bone Marrow Transplantation. Boston, Blackwell, 1994;789–801.
118. Gradishar WJ, Tallman MS, Abrams JS. High dose chemotherapy for breast cancer. Ann Intern Med 1996;125:599–604.
119. Antman KH, Rowlings PA, Vaughan WP, et al. High-dose chemotherapy with autologous hematopoietic stem-cell support for breast cancer in North America. J Clin Oncol 1997;15:1870–1879.
120. Peters WP, Ross M, Vredenburgh JJ, et al. High-dose chemotherapy and autologous bone marrow support as consolidation after standard-dose adjuvant therapy for high-risk primary breast cancer. J Clin Oncol 1993;11:1132–1143.
121. Bearman SI, Overmoyer BA, Bolwell BJ, et al. High-dose chemotherapy with autologous peripheral blood progenitor cell support for primary breast cancer in patients with 4–9 involved axillary lymph nodes. Bone Marrow Transplant 1997;20:931–937.
122. Peters WP, Rogers MC. Variation in approval by insurance companies of coverage for autologous bone marrow transplantation for breast cancer. N Engl J Med 1994;330:473–477.
123. Clift RA, Bianco JA, Appelbaum FR, et al. A randomized controlled trial of pentoxifylline for the prevention of regimen-related toxicities in patients undergoing allogeneic bone marrow transplantation. Blood 1993;82:2025–2030.
124. Attal M, Huguet F, Rubie H, et al. Prevention of regimen-related toxicities after bone marrow transplantation by pentoxifylline: A prospective, randomized trial. Blood 1993;82:732–736.
125. Bearman SI. The syndrome of hepatic veno-occlusive disease after marrow transplantation. Blood 1995;85:3005–3020.
126. Grochow LB. Busulfan disposition: The role of therapeutic drug monitoring in bone marrow transplantation induction regimens. Semin Oncol 1993;20(suppl 4):18–25.
127. Dix SP, Wingard JR, Mullins RE, et al. Association of busulfan area under the curve with veno-occlusive disease following BMT. Bone Marrow Transplant 1996;17:225–230.
128. Reuven OR, Nahler A, Shpilberg O, et al. Low molecular weight heparin for the prevention of veno-occlusive disease of the liver in bone marrow transplant patients. Transplantation 1996;61: 1067–1071.
129. Essell JH, Schroeder MT, Harman GS, et al. Urosodiol prophylaxis against hepatic complications of allogeneic bone marrow transplantation. Ann Intern Med 1998;128:975–981.
130. Terra SG, Spitzer TR, Tsunoda SM. A review of tissue plasminogen activator in the treatment of veno-occlusive liver disease after bone marrow transplantation. Pharmacotherapy 1997;17:929–937.
131. Bearman SI, Lee JL, Baron AE, McDonald GB. Treatment of hepatic venoocclusive disease with recombinant human tissue plasminogen activator and heparin in 42 marrow transplant patients. Blood 1997;89:1501–1506.
132. Soubani AO, Miller KB, Hassoun PM. Pulmonary complications of bone marrow transplantation. Chest 1996;109:1066–1077.
133. Metcalf JP, Rennard SI, Reed EC, et al. Corticosteroids as adjunctive therapy for diffuse alveolar hemmorrhage associated with bone marrow transplantation. Am J Med 1994;96:327–334.
134. Clark JG, Hansen JA, Hertz MI, et al. NHLBI workshop summary. Idiopathic pneumonia syndrome after bone marrow transplantation. Am Rev Resp Dis 1993;147:1601–1606.
135. Palmas A, Tefferi A, Myers JL, et al. Late-onset noninfectious pulmonary complications after allogeneic bone marrow transplantation. Br J Haematol 1998;100:680–687.
136. Martin PJ, Hansen JA, Storb R, et al. Human marrow transplantation: An immunological perspective. Adv Immunol 1987;40: 379–438.
137. Quinones RR. Hematopoietic engraftment and graft failure after bone marrow transplantation. Am J Pediatr Hematol Oncol 1993; 15:3–17.
138. Anasetti C, Amos D, Beatty PG, et al. Effect of HLA compatibility on engraftment of bone marrow transplants in patients with leukemia or lymphoma. N Engl J Med 1989;320:197–204.
139. Agura ED, Vila E, Petersen FB, et al. The use of ranitidine in bone marrow transplantation. Transplantation 1988;46:53–56.
140. Cagnoni PJ, Jones RB, Bearman SI, et al. Use of amifostine in bone marrow purging. Semin Oncol 1996;23(suppl 8):44-48.
141. Nemunaitis J, Singer JW, Buckner CD, et al. Use of recombinant human granulocyte-macrophage colony-stimulating factor in graft failure after bone marrow transplantation. Blood 1990;76:245–253.
142. Dix SP, Gilmore SE. Cytokine therapy after bone marrow transplantation. Pharmacotherapy 1996;16:593–608.
143. Klumpp TR, Mangan KF, Goldberg SL, et al. Granulocyte colony-stimulating factor accelerates neutrophil engraftment following peripheral-blood stem-cell transplantation: A prospective, randomized trial. J Clin Oncol 1995;13:1323–1327.
144. Bolwell B, Goormastic M, Dannley R, et al. G-CSF post-autologous progenitor cell transplantation: a randomized study of 5, 10, and 16 μg/kg/day. Bone Marrow Transplant 1997;19:215–219.
145. Sullivan KM. Graft-versus-host disease. In: Forman SJ, Blume KG, Thomas ED, eds. Bone Marrow Transplantation. Boston, Blackwell, 1994;339–362.
146. Marcellus DC, Vogelsang GB. Graft-versus-host disease. Curr Opin Oncol 1997;9:131–138.
147. Lazarus HM, Vogelsang GB, Rowe JM. Prevention and treatment of acute graft versus host disease: The old and the new. A report from the Eastern cooperative oncology group (ECOG). Bone Marrow Transplant 1997;19:577–600.
148. Antin JH, Ferrara JLM. Cytokine dysregulation and acute graft-versus-host disease. Blood 1992;80:2964–2968.
149. Nash RA, Pepe MS, Storb R, et al. Acute graft-versus-host disease: Analysis of risk factors after allogeneic marrow transplantation and prophylaxis with cyclosporine and methotrexate. Blood 1992;80: 1838–1845.
150. Kernan NA. T-cell depletion for prevention of graft-versus-host disease. In Forman SJ, Blume KG, Thomas ED, eds. Bone Marrow Transplantation. Boston, Blackwell, 1994;124–135.
151. Storb R, Pepe M, Anasetti C, et al. What role for prednisone in prevention of acute graft-versus-host disease in patients undergoing marrow transplants? Blood 1990;76:1037–1345.
152. Sayer HG, Longton G, Bowden R, et al. Increased risk of infection in marrow transplant patients receiving methylprednisolone for graft-versus-host disease prevention. Blood 1994;84:1328–1332.

153. Chao NJ, Schmidt GM, Niland JC, et al. Cyclosporine, methotrexate, and prednisone compared with cyclosporine and prednisone alone for prophylaxis of acute graft-versus-host disease. N Engl J Med 1993;329:1225–1230.
154. Nash RA, Etzioni R, Storb R, et al. Tacrolimus (FK506) alone or in combination with methotrexate or methylprednisolone for the prevention of acute graft-versus-host disease after marrow transplantation from HLA-matched siblings: A single-center study. Blood 1995; 85:3746–3753.
155. Fay JW, Wingard JR, Antin JH, et al. FK506 (tacrolimus) monotherapy for prevention of graft versus host disease after histocompatible sibling allogeneic bone marrow transplantation. Blood 1996;87: 3514–3519.
156. Nash RA, Pineiro LA, Storb R, et al. FK506 in combination with methotrexate for the prevention of graft-versus-host disease after marrow transplantation from matched unrelated donors. Blood 1996;88:3634–3641.
157. Przepiorka D, Ippoliti C, Khouri I, et al. Tacrolimus and minidose methotrexate for prevention of acute graft versus host disease after matched unrelated donor marrow transplantation. Blood 1996;88: 4383–4389.
158. Blaise D, Olive D, Michallet M, et al. Impairment of leukaemia-free survival by addition of interleukin-2 antibody to standard graft-versus-host prophylaxis. Lancet 1995;345:1144–1146.
159. Sullivan KM, Kopecky KJ, Jocom J, et al. Immunomodulatory and antimicrobial efficacy of intravenous immunoglobulin in bone marrow transplantation. N Engl J Med 1990;323:705–712.
160. Barrett AJ, Mavroudis D, Tisdale J, et al. T cell-depleted bone marrow transplantation and delayed T cell add-back to control acute GVHD and conserve a graft-versus-leukemia effect. Bone Marrow Transplant 1998;21:543–551.
161. Drobyski WR, Ash RC, Casper JT, et al. Effect of T-cell depletion as graft-versus-host disease prophylaxis on engraftment, relapse, and disease-free survival in unrelated marrow transplantation for chronic myelogenous leukemia. Blood 1994;83:1980–1987.
162. Hings IM, Filipovich AH, Miller WJ, et al. Prednisone therapy for acute graft-versus-host disease: Short- versus long-term treatment. Transplantation 1993;56:577–580.
163. Basara N, Blau WI, Romer E, et al. Mycophenolate mofetil for the treatment of acute and chronic GVHD in bone marrow transplant patients. Bone Marrow Transplant 1998;22:61–65.
164. Martin PJ, Schoch G, Fisher L, et al. A retrospective analysis of therapy for acute graft-versus-host disease: Secondary treatment. Blood 1991;77:1821–1828.
165. Sullivan KM, Agura E, Anasetti C, et al. Chronic graft-versus-host disease and other late complications of bone marrow transplantation. Semin Hematol 1991;28:250–259.
166. Sullivan KM, Witherspoon RP, Storb R, et al. Prednisone and azathioprine compared with prednisone and placebo for treatment of chronic graft-versus-host disease: Prognostic influence of prolonged thrombocytopenia after allogeneic marrow transplantation. Blood 1988;72:546–554.
167. Sullivan KM, Witherspoon RP, Storb R, et al. Alternating-day cyclosporine and prednisone for treatment of high-risk chronic graft-versus-host disease. Blood 1988;72:555–561.
168. Vogelsang GB, Farmer ER, Hess AD, et al. Thalidomide for the treatment of chronic graft-versus-host disease. N Engl J Med 1992; 326:1055–1058.
169. Buchsel PC, Leum EW, Randolph SR. Delayed complications of bone marrow transplantation: An update. Oncol Nurs Forum 1996; 23:1267–1291.
170. Deeg HJ, Socie G. Malignancies after hematopoietic stem cell transplantation: Many questions, some answers. Blood 1998;91: 1833–1844.

126 ASSESSMENT OF NUTRITION STATUS AND NUTRITION REQUIREMENTS

Kathleen M. Teasley-Strausburg, MS, RPh, BCNSP, and Jan Dalke Anderson, PharmD, BCNSP

Nutrition assessment is performed to identify the patient who has or is at risk for developing malnutrition. Nutrition assessment may also quantify a patient's risk of malnutrition-associated complications (see Chap. 127). Nutrition assessment further establishes a baseline against which to measure the effect of nutrition therapy.[1]

The assessment of a patient's nutrition status initially involves the identification of the presence of risk factors for malnutrition. If the patient is at risk for malnutrition, a more comprehensive nutrition assessment is performed to identify the type and extent of malnutrition. This comprehensive evaluation includes a focused medical and dietary history, physical examination, anthropometric measurements, and laboratory data[2] and provides a basis for determining the patient's nutrition requirements, the optimal type of nutrition intervention, and when nutrition therapy should be initiated. Nutrition requirements will be dependent on the need for chronic maintenance versus acute repletion of nutrition status as well as the effect of organ function (e.g., renal function) on nutrient utilization. Nutrition assessment requires clinical skills, knowledge of objective measurements that reflect nutrition status, and the ability to apply general guidelines for nutrition requirements with a consideration for patient-specific factors.

This chapter is a critical review of the current markers used for nutrition screening and assessment. It also provides guidelines for developing a scheme for accurate, relevant, and cost-effective nutrition assessment including the determination of patient-specific nutrition requirements.

CLASSIFICATION OF NUTRITION DISEASE

Malnutrition, or more specifically undernutrition, is usually the result of starvation (inadequate nutrition intake) or altered metabolism (inappropriate utilization of ingested nutrients). In starvation states the problem is one of not getting adequate amounts of appropriate nutrients to the cells for tissue repair or new tissue synthesis. An alteration in nutrient metabolism exists when the cell has altered substrate demands or utilization characteristics. A clinically useful definition of malnutrition, therefore, is a state induced by alterations in dietary intake or nutrient utilization resulting in changes in subcellular, cellular, and/or organ function that expose the individual to increased risks of morbidity and mortality and that can be reversed by appropriate nutrition support.[3] In general, deficiency states can be categorized as those involving protein and calories [protein–energy malnutrition (PEM)] or those resulting from single nutrients such as individual vitamins or trace minerals. The three types of PEM are marasmus, kwashiorkor, and mixed marasmus–kwashiorkor:[4,5]

1. Marasmus is a chronic condition resulting from a deficiency in total intake and/or utilization of food. There is wasting of both somatic protein (skeletal muscle) and adipose stores (subcutaneous fat), but visceral protein production (e.g., serum albumin and transferrin concentration) is preserved. Weight loss usually exceeds 10% of well weight. When severe, cell-mediated immunity (measured by delayed cutaneous hypersensitivity) and muscle function are impaired. Patients with wasting diseases such as cancer commonly have marasmus and a starved, cachectic appearance.
2. Kwashiorkor is common in patients who have adequate calorie intake but a relative protein deficiency. These patients are often catabolic, usually secondary to trauma, infection, or burns. There is depletion of visceral (and to some degree somatic) protein pools with relative preservation of adipose tissue. Kwashiorkor is classically characterized by hypoalbuminemia and edema. This condition may develop rapidly in response to protein deprivation in the setting of metabolic stress and may be accompanied by impaired immune function.
3. Mixed marasmus–kwashiorkor is a form of severe PEM in chronically ill, starved patients who are undergoing hypermetabolic stress. It manifests as reduced visceral protein synthesis superimposed on wasting of somatic protein and energy (adipose tissue) stores.

Immunocompetence is lowered, the incidence of infection is increased, and there is poor wound healing.

These definitions of PEM are somewhat paralleled in the malnutrition codes used by the *International Classification of Diseases,* ninth edition, *Clinical Modification* (ICD-9-CM), which is a system for identification and coding of diseases and associated conditions.[6] These codes are used as part of the diagnosis-related group (DRG) payment system. Malnutrition is considered a comorbidity factor or complicating condition relative to a primary diagnosis. The use of the appropriate ICD-9-CM code for nutrition status based on the nutrition assessment can assure appropriate reimbursement for a given DRG. There is currently an effort underway to update the definitions for PEM used in these codes to make them more clinically useful.[7]

Coincident with PEM, single-nutrient deficiencies can and often do occur. Depletion of individual nutrients leads to symptoms related to that nutrient's function. Therefore, all potential nutritional deficiency states should be evaluated before an acute or chronic repletion plan is developed.

NUTRITION SCREENING

Nutrition screening provides a systematic way of identifying an individual at risk for PEM. Risk factors for malnutrition include any disease state, complicating condition, treatment, and socioeconomic condition that result in a decreased nutrient intake, altered metabolism, and/or malabsorption.[8,9] Nutrition screening can be done in the home by the patient or home health care professionals, in long-term care facilities, or in the hospital. Various rating and classification systems have been proposed to assess nutrition risk and guide subsequent interventions.[8–10] Checklists are often used to characterize a person's food and alcohol consumption habits, physical capability of buying and preparing food, and weight history. Depending on the specific criteria evaluated, three to four risk factors may put a person at "risk for malnutrition."

The Joint Commission on Accreditation of Healthcare Organizations (JCAHO) Standards call for developing, implementing, and monitoring a patient-specific nutrition care plan for all patients. For those patients "at risk for malnutrition" an interdisciplinary plan for nutrition therapy is required.[11] A nutrition screening process needs to take place within 24 hours of hospital admission to identify those patients "at risk for malnutrition." Nutrition screening in the hospital setting may use diagnosis and diet and weight histories.[10] Even in stable patients in the hospital setting, nutrition status should be reevaluated every 7 to 14 days to avoid deterioration secondary to changes in food intake during the course of hospitalization. By identifying individuals "at risk for malnutrition," nutrition screening can be a cost-effective way to help decrease complications and length of hospital stay.[12]

NUTRITION ASSESSMENT

Nutrition assessment is "a comprehensive evaluation to define nutrition status, including medical history, dietary history, physical examination, anthropometric measurements and laboratory data."[2]

CLINICAL EVALUATION

Clinical evaluation with a focused medical and dietary history and a physical examination remains the oldest, simplest, and probably most widely used method of evaluating nutrition status. Clinical evaluation of nutrition status has been well correlated with objective evaluations (e.g., laboratory parameters, anthropometric measurements).[13] When clinical evaluation is used as the sole method for identifying nutrition-related disease, it is referred to as subjective global assessment (SGA).[14] Laboratory parameters, however, provide additional objective data to confirm the diagnosis, quantify the degree of malnutrition, and identify the end-organ changes that occur with malnutrition. These objective parameters also provide a baseline from which to evaluate the response to nutrition therapy.

The medical and dietary history components of the clinical evaluation provide information about factors that predispose the patient to developing malnutrition (e.g., chronic diseases, gastrointestinal malfunction, alcohol abuse). The clinician should direct the interview to elicit any history of weight loss, anorexia, vomiting, diarrhea, and decreased or unusual food intake (Table 126–1). The physical examination focuses on an assessment of lean body mass and the

TABLE 126–1. Pertinent Data From Medical and Dietary History for Nutrition Assessment

Nutrition Intake and Dietary Habits
Anorexia; unusual or absent taste
Actual intake; special diets
Supplemental vitamin or mineral intake
Food allergies or intolerance
Underlying Pathology With Nutritional Effects
Chronic infections or inflammatory states
Neoplastic diseases
Endocrine disorders
Chronic illnesses including pulmonary disease, cirrhosis, renal failure
Hypermetabolic states: trauma, burns, sepsis
Digestive or absorptive diseases; nausea, vomiting, diarrhea
Hyperlipidemia
End-Organ Effects
Weight changes
Skin or hair changes
Activity and energy level, exercise tolerance, fatigue
Obesity
Gastrointestinal tract symptoms: diarrhea, vomiting, constipation
Miscellaneous
Catabolic medications or therapies: steroids, immunosuppressive agents, radiation, or chemotherapy
Other medications: diuretics, laxatives
Genetic background: body habitus of parents, siblings, and family
Alcohol or drug abuse

physical findings of vitamin, trace mineral, and essential fatty acid deficiency. The assessment should characterize the presence and degree of muscle wasting, edema, loss of subcutaneous fat, dermatitis, glossitis, cheilosis, and/or jaundice (Table 126–2).

ANTHROPOMETRIC MEASUREMENTS

Anthropometric measurements are gross measurements of body cell mass. The most common measurements are height, weight, and measurements of limb size, such as midarm muscle circumference, skinfold thickness, and wrist circumference. These parameters are used in two ways—to compare an individual with a population and as repeated measurements in an individual to indicate the response to dietary changes. Nutrition-related changes in anthropometric measurements occur slowly; several weeks are often required before detectable changes are noted. Acute changes in anthropometric measurements, specifically weight and skinfold thickness, usually reflect changes in fluid status, and fluid must be considered in the interpretation of these parameters.

BODY WEIGHT

Body weight is a nonspecific measure of body cell mass, representing skeletal mass, body fat, and the energy-utilizing component referred to as "lean body mass." Changes in weight over time, particularly in the absence of edema, ascites, and voluntary losses, are an important indicator of altered lean body mass. Interpretation of any actual body weight (ABW) measurement should take into consideration ideal weight for height, usual body weight, fluid status, and age. Dehydration from nausea, vomiting, or other fluid losses results in a decreased body weight but not a loss in body cell mass. The presence of edema or ascites indicates excess total body water, which will increase body weight. More subtle changes in fluid status may be detected by monitoring the patient's daily fluid intake and output and should be evaluated coincident with weight changes.

The ideal body weight for height (IBW) provides a population reference standard against which the ABW can be compared. The ideal weight for a given height is that weight correlating with maximum longevity. Numerous reference tables have been generated based on various population statistics.[15,16] In clinical practice mathematical equations are commonly used to determine IBW. A commonly used equation for adults (age 18 years and older) is based on gender and height:[17]

$$\text{Males: IBW (kg)} = 50 + (2.3 \times \text{height in inches over 5 feet})$$

$$\text{Females: IBW (kg)} = 45.5 + (2.3 \times \text{height in inches over 5 feet})$$

The change in weight over time can be calculated as the percentage of IBW or usual body weight (UBW) where % change = (ABW/IBW) × 100 or (ABW/UBW) × 100. Use of the patient's UBW as a reference point provides a more accurate reflection of clinically and nutritionally significant change in weight. Determining a patient's UBW, however, depends on patient recall, which may be inaccurate. The use of UBW avoids the problems of normative tables, and it documents comparative changes in body weight. The change in weight must be interpreted relative to time. An unintentional weight loss of more than 10% in less than 6 months has been correlated with a poor clinical outcome.[1]

TABLE 126–2. Physical Findings Suggestive of Malnutrition

General Appearance
Edema (especially ankle and sacral)
Cachexia or obesity
Ascites
Signs and symptoms of dehydration: skin turgor, sunken eyes, orthostasis, dry mucous membranes
Muscle-wasting; loss of subcutaneous tissue

Skin and Mucous Membranes
Thin, shiny, or scaling skin
Decubitus ulcers
Ecchymoses, perifollicular petechiae
Poorly healing surgical or traumatic wounds
Pallor or redness of gums, fissures at mouth edge
Glossitis; stomatitis; cheilosis

Musculoskeletal
Retarded growth
Bone pain or tenderness, epiphyseal swelling
Muscle mass less than expected for habitus, genetic history, and level of exercise

Neurologic
Ataxia, positive Romberg test, decreased vibratory or position sense
Nystagmus
Convulsions, paralysis
Encephalopathy

Hepatic
Jaundice
Hepatomegaly

BODY MASS INDEX

Body mass index (BMI), defined as body weight in kilograms/height in meters squared, is another way to compare weight to height. BMI has been used to categorize obesity and malnutrition. BMI values within a range of 18.5 to 25 have been associated with the least risk of early death; therefore, these values are generally considered to be a normal range for adults ages 18 to 65 years. Values greater than 25 are associated with obesity and values less than 18.5 are indicative of malnutrition.[18] It has been observed that BMI increases with age and that the ideal BMI for a 65-year-old is approximately 27.[19] This index is not a reflection of body composition, as demonstrated in the situation of a very muscular person who has a high BMI but a low percentage of total body fat. In this setting, the person may be falsely categorized as obese based solely on BMI.

SKINFOLD THICKNESS AND MIDARM-MUSCLE CIRCUMFERENCE

Skinfold thickness measurement provides an estimate of subcutaneous fat while midarm-muscle circumference estimates skeletal muscle mass. These anthropometric measurements are safe, simple, and easy tests for both population analysis and individual long-term monitoring. However, the results of individual anthropometric measurements should be cautiously interpreted because (1) standards do not account for individual variations in bone size, large muscle mass, hydrational status, or skin compressibility; (2) reference standards do not account for obesity, ethnicity, illness, and increased age; (3) technique is critical and interobserver error may be as high as 30%; and (4) these parameters are slow to change, often requiring weeks before significant alterations from baseline can be observed.

Triceps skinfold thickness (TSF) is the most common of the skinfold measurements, although reference standards also exist for subscapular and iliac sites. More than half of the total body fat is subcutaneous, and changes in subcutaneous fat have been assumed to reflect changes in total body fat. Careful technique in the use of pressure-regulated calipers is essential for reproducibility and reliability in measuring TSF. Midarm-muscle circumference is a calculated value based on the measurement of the circumference of the midarm and TSF.[18] These values, both measured and calculated, are then compared with population-based standards. Classification of the degree of malnutrition based solely on these values should be avoided since invalid categorization of malnutrition may occur.[20]

BIOCHEMICAL PARAMETERS OF LEAN BODY MASS

Lean body mass is representative of both structural proteins (skeletal muscle, somatic protein compartment) and functional proteins (circulating proteins, visceral protein compartment). It can be assessed by creatinine–height index and serum visceral protein concentrations in addition to body weight and midarm-muscle circumference measurements.

CREATININE–HEIGHT INDEX

Creatinine–height index (CHI) is based on creatinine, which is the metabolic end product of creatine, a complex molecule synthesized in the liver and concentrated mainly in body muscle. Creatinine is excreted unchanged in the urine; therefore, collection of a timed urine with measurement of total creatinine excreted indirectly reflects the total muscle mass. For clinical assessment, the creatinine production of an individual patient (obtained by the measurement of creatinine in 24-hour urine collection) is compared with the expected excretion by a healthy gender-matched individual of similar height and ideal weight. The CHI does not accurately reflect muscle mass in patients with impaired renal function or dehydration, and may be affected by a high dietary protein intake, steroids, age, or stress. Therefore, the clinical utility of CHI has been questioned[21] and variations of the index have been suggested.[22]

VISCERAL PROTEINS

The visceral protein compartment is assessed by measuring the concentration of serum transport proteins synthesized in the liver. It is assumed that a low serum protein concentration in states of malnutrition reflects the hepatic protein synthetic mass and, therefore, indirectly the functional protein mass of other organs such as heart, lung, kidney, and intestines. The visceral proteins currently thought to be of greatest relevance for nutrition assessment are serum albumin, transferrin, retinol-binding protein, and prealbumin (thyroxine-binding-prealbumin complex, transthyretin).[23,24] Many factors besides nutrition affect the serum concentration of these proteins, such as abnormal losses via the kidney (nephrotic syndrome) or gastrointestinal (GI) tract (protein-losing enteropathy), hydration status (dehydration may result in hemoconcentration, overhydration in hemodilution), and renal and hepatic function and metabolic stress (sepsis, trauma, surgery, and/or infection). Therefore, visceral protein data must be interpreted relative to the clinical status of the individual (Table 126–3).[25–27]

Albumin was one of the first biochemical markers of malnutrition and has long been used in population studies. Because of a large body pool size (4 to 5 g/kg body weight), a high extravascular distribution (60%), and a long biologic half-life (18 to 20 days), albumin is a relatively insensitive index of early protein malnutrition. However, chronic protein deficiency in the setting of adequate nonprotein calorie intake leads to marked hypoalbuminemia because of a net loss of albumin from the intravascular and extravascular pools (kwashiorkor malnutrition). Serum albumin concentrations also are affected by calorie deficiency, hepatic disease, renal disease, and infection. Although interpretation of serum albumin concentrations is difficult, data consistently indicate a positive correlation between depressed albumin levels and poor clinical outcome.[1,23]

Transferrin is the glycoprotein that binds and transports ferric iron to the liver and reticuloendothelial system for storage. As a surrogate marker of nutrition status it is more likely to respond to protein depletion before alterations in albumin are manifest because of its shorter biologic half-life (8 days) and smaller body pool (less than 100 mg/kg body weight).[28] Transferrin concentrations may be determined by direct measurement or can be estimated indirectly from measurement of total iron-binding capacity.[23] The serum transferrin concentration is affected by acute critical illness, hydration status, and iron stores. In iron deficiency, the hepatic synthesis of transferrin is increased, resulting in increased serum concentrations.[29]

Prealbumin is also referred to as thyroxine-binding prealbumin or transthyretin. It is the transport protein for thyroxine and a carrier protein for retinol-binding protein. It has a short biologic half-life (1 to 2 days) and a small body pool size (10 mg/kg body weight). Prealbumin may be reduced in as few as 3 days after calorie and protein intake is decreased.[28] Because of its short half-life, it is useful in monitoring the short-term effects of nutrition support.[30] However, prealbumin concentration also rapidly declines in acute stress, such as trauma or sepsis, in which there is increased protein catabolism. As with albumin and transferrin, prealbumin concentrations are depressed with

TABLE 126–3. Summary of Visceral Proteins Used for Assessment of Lean Body Mass

Serum Protein	Biosynthetic Site	Normal Value (range)[a]	Half-life (days)	Function	Factors Resulting in Increased Values[b]	Factors Resulting in Decreased Values[b]
Albumin	Hepatocyte	3.5–5.0 g/dL	18–20	Maintain plasma oncotic pressure; carrier for small molecules	Dehydration, anabolic steroids, insulin, infection	Overhydration, edema, renal insufficiency, nephrotic syndrome, poor intake, impaired digestion, burns, congestive heart failure, cirrhosis, thyroid/adrenal/pituitary hormones, trauma, sepsis
Fibronectin	Hepatocyte, fibroblasts, endothelial cells	210–300 μg/mL	0.5–1.0	A glycoprotein that in in blood has opsonic activity; may exert chemotactic activity & facilitate wound healing	None currently described	Trauma, shock, burns, sepsis, disseminated intravascular coagulation; inappropriate specimen handling
Prealbumin (transthyretin)	Hepatocyte	10–40 mg/dL	1–2	Binds T_3 and to a lesser extent T_4; carrier for RBP	Renal dysfunction	Cirrhosis, hepatitis, stress, inflammation, surgery, hyperthyroidism, cystic fibrosis, renal dysfunction
Retinol-binding protein (RBP)	Hepatocyte	2.0–6.0 mg/dL	0.5	Transports vitamin A in plasma; binds noncovalently to prealbumin	Renal dysfunction, vitamin A supplementation	Same as prealbumin; also vitamin A deficiency
Somatomedin C	Hepatocyte	0.4–2.0 IU/mL	0.1–0.3	An insulin-like peptide that has anabolic actions on fat, muscle, cartilage and cultured cells	None currently described	Growth hormone deficiency; psychosocial growth failure; hypothyroidism; renal failure; cirrhosis; drugs (estrogens, prednisolone)
Transferrin	Hepatocyte	200–400 mg/dL	8	Binds Fe in plasma and transports to bone	Iron deficiency, pregnancy, hypoxia, chronic blood loss, estrogens	Chronic infection, cirrhosis, enteropathies, nephrotic syndrome, burns, cortisone, testosterone

[a]Normal values represent pooled subjects; ranges vary between centers; check local values.
[b]All of the listed proteins are influenced by hydration and the presence of hepatocellular dysfunction.

liver disease because of decreased hepatic synthesis. Increased concentrations have been noted in patients with renal disease and are thought to result from impaired degradation of prealbumin by the kidney.[28]

Retinol-binding protein (RBP) is a specific protein for vitamin A alcohol (retinol) transport. It is filtered by the glomeruli and is metabolized by the kidney. RBP has a very short biologic half-life (12 hours) and a small body pool size (2 mg/kg body weight).[28] As a nutrition assessment parameter it has limitations. Its serum concentration will decrease with metabolic stress, liver disease, and vitamin A deficiency. However, its concentration will increase with chronic renal failure and vitamin A supplementation.[28]

These four serum proteins (albumin, transferrin, prealbumin, and RBP) are of greatest value in assessing uncomplicated semistarvation and recovery. In the setting of acute stress (trauma, burn injury, sepsis), these proteins become poor markers of nutrition status. Their synthesis is down-regulated as the liver reprioritizes hepatic protein synthesis in response to systemic injury. In this setting, the liver produces acute-phase reactants (APR), which are proteins such as C-reactive protein, α_1-acid glycoprotein, and α_1-antitrypsin.[31] Other serum proteins, such as fibronectin (an opsonic protein) and somatomedin-C (insulin-like growth factor-1, IGF-1), have been suggested as indicators of nutrition status.[27] However, the clinical availability of tests that measure these proteins is limited, and their relevance to nutrition status and the outcome of hospitalization has not been determined.

Plasma amino acid concentrations also have been used to assess lean body mass. Altered amino acid patterns have been identified in the setting of PEM and are characterized by a slight decrease in essential amino acid concentrations and an increase or no change in the nonessential amino acid concentrations. Consequently, the ratio of essential to nonessential amino acid concentrations decreases and has been used to characterize PEM. However, unless the nutrition depletion is severe, plasma amino acid concentrations are maintained fairly constant by the body's homeostatic mechanisms. The depletion state is clinically apparent before changes in amino acid concentrations become significant. Furthermore, plasma amino acid concentrations are altered in various disease states such as hepatic failure, renal failure, and sepsis. In addition to the lack of sensitivity and specificity, the measurement of plasma amino acid concentrations is not widely available and is expensive. Therefore, plasma amino acid concentrations are of limited usefulness in the assessment of lean body mass.

INDICES OF IMMUNE FUNCTION

The frequency with which immunocompetence is impaired and the high incidence of infection in malnutrition led to the suggestion that tests of immune function be used as markers of nutrition status[32] and as predictors of outcome.[33] The manner in which nutrition factors interact with immune status may be either direct, affecting primarily the lymphoid system; or indirect, affecting cellular metabolism or another organ system that is in turn involved with the regulation of immunocompetence.

The tests of immune function that have most frequently been used in nutrition assessment are total lymphocyte count (TLC) and delayed cutaneous hypersensitivity (DCH) reactions. Both are simple, readily available, and inexpensive tests. TLC reflects the number of circulating lymphocytes, most of which are T cells. Tissues generating T cells are very sensitive to malnutrition and undergo involution with a decrease in the production of T cells.[32] This eventually leads to lymphopenia.

DCH reactions represent an *in vivo* test of cell-mediated immunity. DCH may be assessed as a primary response to a mitogen such as phytohemagglutinin (PHA) or a chemical irritant such as dinitrochlorobenzene (DCNB). However, DCNB is no longer recommended because it leaves a scar in those with normal immunity. DCH is more commonly assessed as a secondary response using antigens to which the patient has been previously sensitized. The recall antigens that have been used in nutrition assessment are mumps, *Candida albicans,* streptokinase–streptodornase (SKSD), *Trichophyton,* coccidioidin, and purified protein derivative (PPD). Anergy is associated with malnutrition and may be restored with nutrition repletion. Other more sophisticated tests of immune function have also been used to evaluate nutrition status. These include lymphocyte surface antigens (CD4 and CD8 counts; CD4–CD8 ratio), T-lymphocyte responsiveness, and serum interleukin concentrations.[32] The impact of the timing of nutrition intervention has been evaluated using these tests.[34]

Tests of immune function may be affected by nonnutrition factors and, therefore, at best are nonspecific indicators of malnutrition.[1] For example, nonnutrition factors that affect TLC include infection, immunosuppressant drugs (corticosteroids, cyclosporine), and the presence of neoplasia. Factors that affect DCH include fever, critical illness, immunosuppressive drugs, and surgery. Though this lack of specificity currently limits the usefulness of these tests of immune function as markers of nutrition status and predictors of outcome, there may be a future role for these tests when a nutrition regimen includes nutritional immunotherapy.[35] Nutrients such as arginine, omega-3 fatty acids, and nucleic acids given in pharmacologic doses have been shown to improve immune function in a variety of settings.[36–38] Monitoring the efficacy of nutrition regimens that include these immunomodulating nutrients may need to include tests of immune function.

SPECIFIC NUTRIENT DEFICIENCIES

The assessment of nutrition status should include an evaluation of possible trace mineral, vitamin, and essential fatty acid deficiencies. Because of their key role in metabolic processes (as coenzymes and cofactors), the deficiency of any of these nutrients may result in altered metabolism and cell dysfunction and may interfere with processes necessary for repletion of PEM. The assessment of single-nutrient-deficiency states includes an accurate history to evaluate symptoms and the existence of factors predisposing the patient to developing a deficiency state, a physical examination for signs of deficiencies, and biochemical assessment to confirm the diagnosis. Ideally, biochemical assessment should be based on the function of the nutrient, for example, metalloenzyme activity, rather than simply measuring the concentration present in the assay sample. Unfortunately, few practical methods to assess micronutrient function are currently available, and most assays measure tissue or fluid concentration of a nutrient.

TRACE MINERALS

The trace minerals identified as essential to humans and for which deficiency states have been described are zinc, copper, manganese, selenium, chromium, iodine, molybdenum, and iron.[39] Each of these minerals participates in a variety of biologic functions and is necessary for normal metabolism.[40] Other trace minerals essential to humans but for which deficiency states have not been recognized include nickel, vanadium, cobalt, and silicon.

Zinc deficiency is clinically characterized by the development of a moist eczematous dermatitis most apparent in the nasolabial folds and around orifices.[41] Other presenting signs and symptoms may include hypogeusia (blunted sense of taste), alopecia, diarrhea, rash (which may vary from papular, scaly lesions to weeping, open erosions), apathy, and depression. Clinical zinc deficiency occurs most frequently in the setting of abnormal losses, such as in Crohn's disease, malabsorption states, and fistula losses, or from prolonged inadequate intake, such as with zinc-free parenteral nutrition. Zinc deficiency can be documented by the presence of low plasma zinc concentrations (Table 126–4).[26,39] However, plasma zinc concentration

TABLE 126–4. Assessment of Trace Mineral Status

Trace Mineral	Signs of Deficiency	Normal Plasma Concentration[a]	Factors Resulting in Altered Plasma Concentrations
Chromium	Glucose intolerance, peripheral neuropathy, increased free fatty acid levels, low respiratory quotient	0.12–2.1 μg/L	Not known
Copper	Neutropenia, hypochromic anemia, osteoporosis; decreased hair and skin pigmentation; dermatitis, anorexia, diarrhea	80–155 μg/L (female) 70–140 μg/L (male)	Decreased: serum ceruloplasmin concentrations, corticosteroid therapy, Wilson's disease Increased: infection, rheumatoid arthritis, pregnancy, oral contraceptive use
Iodine	Hypothyroid goiter, hypothyroidism	Assessed by T_4, TSH and free T_4 index	Assays are specific to hypo- and hyperthyroid states
Manganese	Nausea, vomiting, dermatitis, color changes in hair, hypocholesterolemia, growth retardation	0.6–2.0 ng/mL	Not known
Molybdenum	Tachycardia, tachypnea, altered mental status, visual changes, headache, nausea, vomiting	0.1–3.0 μg/L	Varies with assay method used
Selenium	Muscle weakness and pain, cardiomyopathy	46–143 μg/dL	Decreased: malignancy, liver failure, pregnancy Increased: reticuloendothelial neoplasia
Zinc	Dermatitis, hypogeusia, alopecia, diarrhea, apathy, depression	70–130 μg/dL	Decreased: infection, hypoalbuminemia, corticosteroid therapy, stress, inflammation, pregnancy Increased: tissue injury, hemolysis, contaminated collection tubes

[a]Normal values may vary between laboratories and will also depend on assay procedure.

decreases in acute stress states such as trauma, surgery, or sepsis. Also, since zinc is a normal contaminant of most blood collection tubes, special zinc-free collection tubes (e.g., Bio/Rad polypropylene micro test tube) must be used for plasma assays. Leukocyte zinc content is a better indicator of zinc status, but this assay is not widely available.[41]

Copper deficiency may present as hematologic changes (anemia, leukopenia, and neutropenia) and skeletal demineralization. In severe cases, such as in Menkes' syndrome, copper deficiency is further manifested as hypothermia, depigmentation of hair and skin, progressive mental deterioration, and growth retardation. Factors predisposing to copper deficiency include malabsorption states, protein-losing enteropathy, nephrotic syndrome, copper-free parenteral nutrition, and copper-deficient enteral nutrition.[42,43] Laboratory diagnosis of copper deficiency is made most frequently on the basis of plasma concentrations, although urinary concentrations also may be assessed. As with zinc, plasma copper concentrations may be altered by a variety of conditions and, therefore, may not accurately reflect copper nutrition (Table 126–4). Copper function may be assessed by measuring activity of cuproenzymes (erythrocyte superoxide dismutase or cytochrome-c oxidase in platelets or leukocytes). Enzyme activity is significantly decreased in copper deficiency. However, measurements of the activity of these enzymes are method and technique sensitive and not readily available.[44]

Chromium deficiency is characterized by glucose intolerance but also may include neuropathy, increased free fatty acid concentrations, and a low respiratory quotient (Table 126–4). Chromium deficiency has been identified in the setting of long-term parenteral nutrition where chromium intake was inadequate.[45] Plasma chromium concentrations do not accurately reflect chromium nutrition, presumably because the biologically active form of chromium is an organic chromium-containing substance known as glucose tolerance factor.

Manganese deficiency has been reported only in association with chemically defined manganese-deficient oral diets.[46] The symptoms include nausea, vomiting, dermatitis, color changes in hair, hypocholesterolemia, and growth retardation (Table 126–4). Manganese toxicity, however, has been described in several reports of patients receiving long-term parenteral nutrition.[47,48] Manganese appears to accumulate in brain tissue, especially in the setting of chronic cholestasis and short bowel syndrome. The clinical presentation of toxicity includes extrapyramidal symptoms mimicking Parkinson's disease. Serum concentrations of manganese do not correlate well with the clinical presentation, but magnetic resonance imaging (MRI) of the basal ganglia show hyperintensity areas, especially in the globus pallidus. In most cases, discontinuation of manganese added to the parenteral nutrition resulted in resolution of neurologic symptoms in 6 months with partial or total normalization of the MRIs after 1 to 2 years. Other methods of evaluating manganese status include measuring the manganese content of mononuclear blood cells[49] and the activity of manganese superoxide dismutase, a mitochondrial antioxidant enzyme.[50] These methods are good indicators of manganese status but are not widely available.

Selenium deficiency has been described in patients receiving long-term selenium-free total parenteral nutrition. Muscle pain and weakness are most frequently observed (Table 126–4),[41,51,52] but severe biochemical deficiency is not always accompanied by these symptoms.[53] A fatal cardiomyopathy has been reported in several cases. Selenium status may be assessed by plasma concentrations. Reduced concentrations may indicate selenium deficiency, but reductions have also been observed in patients with malignancies, liver failure, and pregnancy. Measurement of the activity of the selenium-containing enzyme glutathione peroxidase in erythrocytes or the plasma concentration of selenoprotein P may be more sensitive measurements of selenium status, although not widely available.[53]

Molybdenum deficiency in humans has rarely been observed.[54] There is one known case of molybdenum deficiency in a patient receiving long-term home parenteral nutrition who presented with symptoms that included tachycardia, tachypnea, headache, night blindness, nausea, vomiting, central scotomas, lethargy, disorientation, and ultimately coma.[55] Symptoms were reversed when molybdenum was added to the parenteral nutrition. Predisposing factors to molybdenum deficiency appear to be excessive loss via the gastrointestinal tract, as with short-bowel syndrome, and long-term inadequate intake, as with molybdenum-free parenteral nutrition. Assays of molybdenum concentration in tissues or fluids are not readily available.

Iodine deficiency may result in goiter formation (see Chap. 71). However, not everyone with an iodine-deficient diet will develop a goiter. Iodine is needed for synthesis of the thyroid hormones thyroxine (T_4) and triiodothyronine (T_3). Laboratory assessment of thyroid function is used to assess iodine status (Table 126–4). During parenteral nutrition iodine needs are generally adequately met by cutaneous absorption of iodine from germicides (e.g., povidone iodine) used in catheter care.[56,57] Therefore, intravenous supplements of iodine usually are not given during short-term courses of parenteral nutrition.

Patients with iron deficiency anemia present with fatigue, weakness, and pallor. The symptoms of iron deficiency may also include glossitis, headache, dysphagia, fingernail changes, gastric atrophy, and paresthesias. Inadequate intake of iron, malabsorption, and blood loss from any origin are the principal causes of iron deficiency anemia. Iron deficiency is confirmed on the basis of an assessment of body iron stores as reflected indirectly by measurement of hemoglobin, serum iron, iron-binding capacity, and serum ferritin, or directly by marrow staining and liver biopsy. The direct methods are the most accurate but are invasive. Therefore, the indirect measurements are more commonly used (see Chap. 91). Each indirect parameter may be altered by chronic illness independent of

TABLE 126–5. Indirect Assessment of Body Iron Stores

Parameter	Normal Values (Adult)[a]		Value in Iron Deficiency	Value in Specific Medical States
	Women	*Men*		
Hemoglobin (mg/dL)	11.7–15.5	13.2–17.3	Decreased	Decreased value in chronic illness
Serum iron (μg/dL)	50–170	65–170	Decreased	Decreased value in infection, nephrosis Increased value in hemolytic disorders, hemochromatosis, oral contraceptive use, acute liver disease
Total iron-binding capacity (μg/dL)	150–450	250–400	Increased	Decreased value in chronic disease, protein deficiency, liver disease Increased value in pregnancy
Serum ferritin (ng/mL)	10–120	20–250	<15	Decreased value in reticulo-endothelium cell damage Increased value in inflammation

[a]Normal values may vary between laboratories.

iron stores; thus, concomitant illness must be considered in their interpretation (Table 126–5).[26]

VITAMINS

A carefully performed history and physical examination may be the most valuable means of screening patients for risk factors as well as identifying symptoms that suggest physical findings of vitamin deficiency and toxicity (Table 126–6).[26,58] A thorough history focusing on dietary intake and enteral and parenteral nutrition is important in identifying people who are at risk for vitamin deficiencies and toxicities. It is uncommon to see a single vitamin deficiency; usually vitamin deficiencies occur with general malnutrition. However, single vitamin deficiencies do occur, as demonstrated by several cases of thiamin deficiency resulting in lactic acidosis and encephalopathy.[59]

Laboratory assessment is useful in confirming clinical suspicions. Laboratory assessment also identifies subclinical vitamin deficiencies; the first indication of a deficiency is usually a fall in circulating amounts of the vitamin or its coenzyme. Subsequently, there is a decrease in urinary excretion of the vitamin, which in turn is followed by diminished concentrations of the vitamin in tissue. The most common measurements of vitamin status are assays of circulating amounts in plasma or serum. Assays also may be performed to determine biochemical or metabolic function of the vitamin and are more likely to reflect body stores than are serum assays. Most of these functional assays use extracts of erythrocytes or leukocytes to determine activity of an apoenzyme, which is dependent on the vitamin coenzyme. Vitamin assays are summarized in Table 126–6.

ESSENTIAL FATTY ACIDS

In general, essential fatty acid (EFA) deficiency, or more specifically linoleic acid deficiency, is rare but can occur during prolonged use of continuously infused parenteral nutrition that does not include long-chain fatty acids. It also may occur with severe PEM. Symptoms of EFA deficiency include dermatitis (e.g., dry, cracked, scaly skin), alopecia, and impaired wound healing. In severe cases neurologic deficits, abnormal liver function, respiratory insufficiency, cardiac arrhythmias, and hemolysis may occur. A deficiency may appear as early as within 1 week of fat-free parenteral nutrition.[60]

Laboratory assessment of EFA deficiency is expensive and not readily available. Fatty acid composition of plasma may be measured: 5,8,11-eicosatrienoic acid and arachidonic acid are the primary fatty acids of interest. Eicosatrienoic acid is not normally present. With a deficiency of linoleic acid and, hence, decreased synthesis of arachidonic acid from linoleic acid, oleic acid metabolism to 5,8,11-eicosatrienoic acid becomes the primary metabolic pathway. The ratio of 5,8,11-eicosatrienoic (triene) acid to arachidonic acid (tetraene) reflects this derangement in metabolism. Normally, this ratio of triene to tetraene is less than 0.4. Values of 0.5 or greater define a deficiency state.

CARNITINE

Carnitine is a substance with vitamin-like properties; however, in states of normal nutriture there is no specific dietary requirement. Carnitine plays a role in lipid oxidation as the transport substance for the intramitochondrial transfer of long-chain fatty acids. Carnitine is available from dietary sources and can be endogenously synthesized from lysine and methionine. A deficiency of carnitine has been described in the setting of severe protein malnutrition, with inborn errors of metabolism, and in newborn infants with insufficient dietary carnitine intake.[61,62] Other predisposing factors to carnitine

TABLE 126–6. Assessment of Vitamin Status

Vitamin	Signs of Deficiency	Laboratory Assay	Normal Values	Comments
Niacin (B_5)	Pellagra: dermatitis, dementia, glossitis, diarrhea, loss of memory, headaches	Urinary niacin metabolites	2.4–6.4 mg/d	Varies with age, gender, pregnancy; blood levels not done
Folate (B_9)	Megaloblastic anemia, diarrhea, glossitis	Serum folate	3–16 ng/mL	Levels may be decreased in cases of increased cellular or tissue turnover (pregnancy, malignancy, hemolytic anemia)
Cyanocobalamin (B_{12})	Pernicious anemia, glossitis, spinal cord degeneration, peripheral neuropathy	Serum B_{12}	100–700 pg/mL	
Thiamine (B_1)	Paresthesias, nystagmus, impaired memory, congestive heart failure, lactic acidosis, Wernicke–Korsakoff syndrome	Red blood transketolase activity	850–1000 μg/mL/h	
Riboflavin (B_2)	Mucositis, dermatitis, cheilosis; vascularization of cornea, photophobia, lacrimation, and decreased vision, impaired wound healing, normocytic anemia	Urinary riboflavin	80–120 μg/g creatinine	Varies with age, pregnancy, exercise, nitrogen balance
Pyridoxine (B_6)	Dermatitis, neuritis, convulsions, microcytic anemia	Plasma B_6	5–30 μg/mL	Varies with age, gender
Pantothenic acid (B_3)	Fatigue, malaise, headache, insomnia, vomiting, abdominal cramps	Serum panthothenic acid	1.03–1.83 μg/mL	
Biotin	Dermatitis, depression, lassitude, somnolence	Urinary biotin	6–50 μg/d	
Ascorbic acid (C)	Enlargement and keratosis of hair follicles; impaired wound healing; anemia, lethargy, depression, bleeding, ecchymosis	Plasma ascorbic acid	0.5–1.5 mg/dL	
A	Dermatitis, night blindness, keratomalacia, xerophthalmia	Serum vitamin A	30–80 μg/dL	
D	Rickets and osteomalacia, muscle weakness	Plasma 25-hydroxy-vitamin D	13–50 ng/mL	Decreased in uremia, in cirrhosis, in individuals greater than 60 years old; may be decreased in winter
E	Hemolysis	Serum vitamin E concentrations	5.0–13 μg/mL	Decreased with low blood lipoprotein
K	Bleeding	Serum phyllo-quinone	0.13–1.19 ng/mL	Decreased with hepatic disease, anticoagulants

deficiency include chronic kidney disease, liver disease, and vitamin C deficiency.[62,63] The clinical presentation of carnitine deficiency includes generalized skeletal muscle weakness, fatty liver, and reactive hypoglycemia. Carnitine status may be assessed by measuring plasma, urine, or red blood cell concentrations using a radioisotope assay method.[63]

OTHER METHODS OF NUTRITION ASSESSMENT

Hand grip strength, or forearm muscle dynamometry, and stimulation of the ulnar nerve have been measured as indicators of muscle function and correlated with patient outcome.[1] Forearm muscle dynamometry is a relatively simple, noninvasive, and inexpensive procedure. Ulnar nerve stimulation causes measurable muscle contraction. In the setting of malnutrition, increased fatigability and a slowed muscle relaxation rate have been noted, with these indices returning to normal after refeeding.[64] Both of these parameters have the advantage of being an indicator of tissue function rather than composition. Their utility in clinical practice is currently hampered by a lack of appropriate reference standards and limited data confirming their sensitivity and specificity as nutrition assessment tools.

Bioelectric impedance analysis (BIA) is a simple, noninvasive technique used to measure lean body mass.[65] By placing electrodes on the wrist and ankle and applying an electrical current, impedance (resistance) to flow is measured. Lean tissue has a higher electrical conductivity (less resistance) because of its greater fluid and electrolyte content, whereas fat is a poor conductor of current. Assessment of body water and its distribution can also be determined with BIA.[66–68] Decreased impedance is seen with increased total body water. Therefore, it is important to evaluate fluid status along with BIA data. The potential limitations of the use of BIA include variability with electrolyte imbalance, interference by large fat masses, and the need for standards that reflect variations in individual body sizes.

Various methods to determine body composition have been used in the clinical research setting. These methods are generally complex, require expensive technology, and at present are limited mainly to experimental studies. Ultrasound and infrared interactance can be applied to measure subcutaneous fat. The latter uses an inexpensive and portable device, but the results of measurements have not been used extensively for nutrition assessment.[64] Dual-photon and dual-energy radiography, MRI, and computed tomography (CT) can measure subcutaneous, intra-abdominal and regional fat distribution.[69] Neutron activation is a means of measuring body nitrogen, calcium, sodium, chloride, and phosphorus. These measurements can then be used to calculate total body fat, bone, and protein.[66] Isotope dilutional methods determine total body water, and underwater weighing determines density. In addition, these methods can be used to estimate lean body mass and body fat. Furthermore, lean body mass can also be estimated via total body conductivity (TOBEC) and by measuring the naturally occurring isotope ^{40}K.[69]

ASSESSMENT OF NUTRIENT REQUIREMENTS

Nutrient requirements vary with age, gender, size, disease state, clinical condition, nutrition status, and level of physical activity. An assessment of nutrient requirements must, therefore, be made using guidelines interpreted in the context of these patient-specific factors. As a general reference point the U.S. recommended dietary allowances (RDAs) should be considered.[70] However, the RDAs are intended to represent the nutrition needs of healthy individuals and have been criticized as not accommodating the variability of health conditions in the American population. A new set of guidelines, the Dietary Reference Intakes, has been developed by the National Academy of Sciences and are scheduled for publication in early 1999.[71]

ENERGY

There are numerous methods for determining an individual's energy, or calorie (kcal), requirement.[72] The most commonly used methods to determine energy requirements are calories per body weight (kcal/kg), the Harris–Benedict equation,[73] or indirect calorimetry.

The simplest method to determine energy requirements is on the basis of population estimates of calories per body weight. This method requires that assumptions be made about the energy requirements associated with various disease states or clinical conditions as well as the additional requirements for repletion of a malnourished individual. It does not take into consideration age- or gender-related differences in energy metabolism in adults. In general, adult requirements determined by this method, using lean body weight, are as follows:

Healthy, normal nutrition status	~25 kcal/kg
Malnourished or mildly metabolically stressed	~30 kcal/kg
Critically ill, hypermetabolic	30–35 kcal/kg
Major burn injury	40+ kcal/kg

Clinical judgment as well as close monitoring is essential to ensure that the desired nutrition outcomes are attained.

The Harris–Benedict equation (HBE) has become a popular method during the last two decades to assess energy requirements. It has the advantage of taking into consideration the age, height, weight, gender, and clinical condition of the patient. The HBE was derived from oxygen consumption measurements made on normally nourished individuals who were in a fasting, resting state.[74] The HBE calculates basal energy expenditure (BEE), which is the amount of energy expended to perform only basal functions such as breathing, circulating blood, and fasting metabolic processes. The HBEs are:

$$\text{BEE (females)} = 655 + 9.6\,(\text{wt}) + 1.8\,(\text{ht}) - 4.7\,(\text{age})$$
$$\text{BEE (males)} = 66 + 13.7\,(\text{wt}) + 5\,(\text{ht}) - 6.8\,(\text{age})$$

where BEE is kcal/d, wt is weight in kilograms, ht is height in centimeters, and age is in years. Since this equation merely represents energy requirements to perform basal functions, it must be further modified by a factor that is most representative of the clinical situation. For example, an individual who is confined to bed may only require a 20% increase of the BEE whereas a person who is suffering from a severe burn injury may require up to a 130% increase of the BEE.[72] Controversy exists over the accuracy and reliability of predicting energy expenditure based on HBE[74,75] because clinical judgments will vary with each clinician.

The most accurate clinical tool for estimating energy requirements is indirect calorimetry.[76] Indirect calorimetry is based on the measurement of the oxygen and carbon dioxide content in expired air. In a noninvasive procedure, oxygen consumption (VO_2, mL/min) and carbon dioxide production (VCO_2, mL/min) are determined. Using the abbreviated Weir equation, resting energy expenditure (REE, kcal/d) can be calculated:

$$REE = [3.9(VO_2) + 1.1\ (VCO_2)] \times 1.44$$

This measured energy expenditure represents the actual energy expended by the patient for the point in time that the measurement was taken. It is extrapolated to a 24-hour period to represent approximate daily energy requirements. This measurement will reflect any alterations in energy requirements due to disease or clinical condition but does not include a requirement for repletion of nutrition status in a malnourished individual. Increasing energy intake by 20% to 25% may accommodate the need for additional calories for repletion.

The data obtained from indirect calorimetry can also be used to determine a respiratory quotient (RQ). The RQ reflects substrate oxidation and is calculated as follows:

$$RQ = VCO_2/VO_2$$

Each type of substrate produces a different RQ value. The following RQ values reflect the net substrate oxidation: fat, 0.7; carbohydrate, 1.0; mixed substrate (fat, carbohydrate, and protein), 0.85; and protein, 0.80. An RQ value of greater than 1.0 represents either lipogenesis or patient hyperventilation; an RQ value of less than 0.7 may indicate a ketogenic diet, fat gluconeogenesis, or ethanol oxidation. Values that fall outside of the 0.67 to 1.3 range raise serious doubts as to the validity of the test. Clinically, the RQ is used to determine if a patient is being overfed, which is indicated by an RQ value greater than 1.0.

PROTEIN

Adult protein requirements are based on nutrition status, disease state, and clinical condition.[72] The usual protein requirement for maintenance in a healthy individual is 0.8 g/kg/d. Protein metabolism is dependent on both kidney and liver function. Therefore, protein requirements will be altered with decreased kidney or liver function. In chronic renal failure, protein restriction may be necessary (see Chap. 42). If dialysis is part of the renal failure patient's care, protein requirements may be increased to 1.2 to 2.7 g/kg/d.[77] Critical illness (sepsis, burns, trauma) will result in a hypermetabolic state in which there is increased protein synthesis and degradation. Consequently, protein requirements will be increased to 1.5 to 2.0 g/kg/d. In burn patients, protein requirements may be as high as 3.0 g/kg/d. Liver failure typically results in the need for protein restriction (0.5 g/kg/d) except if a hypercatabolic state is also present in which case the requirement may be increased to 1.5 g/kg/d. The application of these guidelines requires both clinical judgment and frequent monitoring of renal and liver function, clinical condition, and nutrition outcomes (see Chap. 131).

An alternative method for determining protein requirements is to measure urinary nitrogen excretion. This method is occasionally used in clinical practice; however, it is more frequently used in nutrition research. This measurement indirectly reflects an individual's protein utilization or protein catabolic rate (PCR). An increase in PCR is one of the characteristics of hypermetabolism.[78] As the stress level increases, the concomitant increase in protein catabolism results in an increase in urinary nitrogen.[79] Usually in clinical practice the amount of urea nitrogen is measured in a 24-hour urine collection (UUN). The quantity of UUN accounts for 60% to 90% of the total urinary nitrogen (TUN) excreted.[24] Therefore, total nitrogen output is approximated by:

$$\text{Nitrogen output (g/d)} = (\text{UUN} \times 1.20) + 1$$

where 1 represents the estimated nitrogen losses from skin, fecal, and respiratory sources.[80] Alternatively, if it is available, TUN can be measured and may be more accurate.[81] In the setting of renal failure where measured urinary nitrogen does not represent nitrogen generation, protein turnover can be approximated by using equations based on the kinetics of urea to estimate the rate at which urea is being produced.[4]

FLUID

Daily adult fluid requirements are dependent on many factors but in general can be estimated as approximately 30 mL/kg or can be based on energy requirements and calculated as 1 mL/kcal. Increased fluid requirements are observed in individuals with increased insensible losses [e.g., fever, excessive sweating, increased metabolism (e.g., hyperthyroidism)] or with increased gastrointestinal losses (e.g., vomiting, diarrhea, high-output fistula). Decreased fluid requirements have been observed in patients with renal failure or with an expanded extracellular fluid volume (e.g., congestive heart failure) and in hypoproteinemia with starvation. When estimating fluid intake via a nutrition regimen, all nonnutrition sources of fluid intake must be taken into consideration (e.g., the fluid vehicle for intravenous medications).

MICRONUTRIENTS

Requirements for the micronutrients (electrolytes, trace minerals, and vitamins) vary with the route by which the nutrient is ingested (Table 126–7).[82,83] The variability is dependent on the extent to which the nutrient is absorbed via the GI tract versus intravenously. Nutrients administered intravenously bypass the GI tract, and their absorption is equivalent to 100%. Micronutrients poorly absorbed via the GI tract usually will be required in greater doses enterally than parenterally. However, many water-soluble micronutrients are more rapidly excreted via the kidneys when

TABLE 126–7. Recommended Adult Daily Maintenance Doses for Electrolytes, Trace Minerals, and Vitamins

Nutrient	Enteral	Parenteral
Electrolytes		
Calcium	800–1200 mg	10–15 mEq
Chloride	1700–5100 mg	—
Fluoride	1.5–4.0 mg	—
Magnesium	280–350 mg	10–20 mEq
Phosphorus	800–1200 mg	20–45 mmol
Potassium	1875–5625 mg	60–100 mEq
Sodium	1100–3300 mg	60–100 mEq
Trace Minerals		
Chromium	50–200 µg	10–15 µg[a]
Copper	1.5–3 mg	0.5–1.5 mg
Iodine	150 µg	70–140 µg
Iron	10–15 mg	(varies with age and gender)
Manganese	2–5 mg	0.15–0.8 mg
Molybdenum	75–250 µg	100–200 µg
Selenium	55–70 µg	40–80 µg
Zinc	12–15 mg	2.5–4.0 mg[b]
Vitamins		
Biotin	30–100 µg	60 µg
Cyanocobalamin (B_{12})	2.0 µg	5.0 µg
Folic acid	200 µg	400 µg
Niacin	13–19 mg NE	40 mg NE
Pantothenic acid (B_3)	4.7 mg	15 mg
Pyridoxine (B_6)	1.6–2.0 mg	4 mg
Riboflavin (B_2)	1.2–1.7 mg	3.6 mg
Thiamin (B_1)	1.0–1.5 mg	3 mg
Vitamin A	800–100 µg RE	600 µg RE (3300 IU)
Vitamin C	60 mg	100 mg
Vitamin D	5–10 µg	5 µg (200 IU)
Vitamin E	8–10 mg TE[c]	10 mg TE (10 IU)[c]
Vitamin K	60–80 µg	0.7–2.5 mg

NE = niacin equivalents; RE = retinol equivalents; TE = tocopherol equivalent.
[a]An additional 20 mg chromium/d is recommended in patients with intestinal losses.
[b]An additional 12.2 mg zinc/L of small-bowel fluid lost and 17.1 mg zinc/kg of stool or ileostomy output is recommended; an additional 2.0 mg zinc/d for acute catabolic stress.
[c]Recent data suggest that daily vitamin E requirements may be much greater, e.g., 135–150 IU.[83]
Adapted from Ref. 82, with permission.

administered IV versus being ingested enterally. In these situations the IV nutrient dose will be greater than the enteral dose. Other factors that affect micronutrient requirements include GI losses via diarrhea, vomiting, high-output fistula, and hypermetabolism. Cutaneous losses of micronutrients may also be significant in patients with major burn injury.[84,85] The electrolytes sodium, potassium, magnesium, and phosphorus are particularly dependent on renal function, and in the setting of renal failure intake may need to be restricted. Patients who are severely malnourished will have increased electrolyte requirements during early refeeding owing to preexisting deficiencies and/or rapid intracellular uptake with anabolism.[86] Failure to provide adequate electrolytes during refeeding has resulted in death.[87]

Several micronutrients—vitamins C and E—are also known to function as antioxidants.[88] These nutrients may have a beneficial role in the prevention or management of cancer (see Chap. 115), respiratory distress syndrome (see Chap. 26), acute head injury (see Chap. 54), and cardiovascular disease (see Chap. 12).

DRUG–NUTRIENT INTERACTIONS

The extent and clinical implications of drug–nutrient interactions will vary but may include drug-induced nutritient deficiencies, poor therapeutic response to a drug, enhanced drug toxicity, and interference with nutrition regimens if nutrition support is discontinued or withheld. With the potential for such problems to occur in the hospitalized patient the Joint Commission on Accreditation of Healthcare Organizations (JCAHO) has described a standard to ensure that patients are instructed and counseled on potential drug–food interactions. Therefore, to assure good patient outcomes and comply with JCAHO standards, it is important to establish a program for counseling and a method for screening medication profiles for potential drug-nutrient interactions.[89] As part of the screening process it is important to recognize the risk factors that influence drug–nutrient interactions. The potential for drug–nutrient interactions increases based on age (pediatric or elderly), poor nutrition status (obesity and marasmus), and chronic and/or multiple drug therapy.

Along with assessing the risk for interactions, an assessment of fluid and electrolyte status will prove beneficial in certain individuals. Mineral and electrolyte serum concentrations may change due to drug therapy.[90] For example, urine wasting of sodium, potassium, and magnesium may occur, causing the respective serum concentrations to decrease (see Table 126–8). Serum electrolyte concentrations may increase as a direct result of the mechanism of the drug (e.g., potassium-sparing diuretics) or due to the salt form of the drug (see Table 126–9). Medications may affect blood glucose concentrations. For example, steroids and cyclosporin are known to cause hyperglycemia as a side effect of drug therapy. Additionally, drugs are prescribed to pharmacologically lower blood glucose concentrations (e.g., insulin and oral hypoglycemics; see Table 126–10).

TABLE 126–8 Mineral and Electrolyte Depletion Caused by Drugs

Drug	Decreased Serum Concentration
Antacids	Phosphorus
Aminoglycosides	Magnesium
Amphotericin B	Potassium, magnesium, zinc
Cisplatinum	Magnesium, zinc, sodium
Cyclosporin	Magnesium
Diuretics (thiazide)	Potassium, magnesium, zinc
Diuretics (loop)	Potassium, calcium, magnesium, zinc
Glucocorticoids	Potassium, calcium
Laxatives	Potassium, calcium
Penicillamine	Zinc, copper
Sucralfate	Phosphorus

TABLE 126–9. Mineral and Electrolyte Increases Caused by Drugs

Drug	Increased Serum Concentration
Carbencillin (parenteral)	Sodium
Clindamycin (parenteral)	Phosphorus
Phosphate enemas	Phosphorus
Spironolactone	Potassium
Ticarcillin (parenteral)	Sodium

TABLE 126–11. Drug Effects on Vitamin Status

Drug	Possible Vitamin Effect
Antacids	Thiamin deficiency
Antibiotics	Vitamin K deficiency
Antineoplastics	Folic acid antagonism and malabsorption
Cathartics	Increased requirements for vitamins D, C, and B_6
Anticonvulsants	Vitamin D and folic acid impaired absorption
Isoniazid	Vitamin B_6 deficiency

From Ref. 40.

Vitamin status may be affected by drug therapies (see Table 126–11).[91] For example, sulfasalazine therapy has been noted to cause a decrease in folic acid, isoniazid therapy causes pyridoxine deficiency, and furosemide therapy may cause decreased concentrations of thiamin. Furthermore, drug therapies may be affected by vitamins. For example, large doses of folic acid will decrease the therapeutic effect of methotrexate, while increases in an individual's normal vitamin K intake have the potential to cause a reduction in the anticoagulation action of warfarin.

Furthermore, drug delivery systems may contain nutrients. Many intravenous therapies are delivered using dextrose in the admixture. For example, dextrose 5% in water (D_5W) is commonly used for hydration purposes as well as a means of administering medications and electrolytes (e.g., antibiotics and potassium). There are also drug delivery systems that use 10% lipid emulsion formulations (e.g., propofol), which may provide a large amount of calories to an individual. In these instances nutrition support regimens may be varied to accommodate the increase in calories from other sources.

PRACTICAL GUIDELINES FOR NUTRITION ASSESSMENT

The value of any given marker or group of markers used for nutrition assessment is only as great as its ability to accurately identify the patient with malnutrition and to correlate with malnutrition-associated complications. Most of the currently available markers of nutrition status were first used in epidemiologic studies to define large populations suffering from malnutrition caused by famine. The response of the various markers of nutrition status to nutrition therapy and the correlation between improvement in these markers and decreased morbidity and mortality further support their validity. However, when applied to an individual, most of these markers lack specificity and sensitivity, which makes the development of a clinically useful, cost-effective approach to individual patient nutrition assessment challenging.

The importance of the history and physical examination in both nutrition screening and nutrition assessment cannot be overemphasized. The least amount of objective data that can further substantiate the clinical impression and provide a baseline for subsequent monitoring are those markers that show the best correlation with outcome: *weight* and *serum albumin concentration.* The cost-effectiveness of the addition of further biochemical parameters is yet to be determined. The assessment of other anthropometric measures is probably most useful in the setting of anticipated long-term nutrition support in which these measurements will serve as a longitudinal marker of the individual response to therapy.

The assessment of nutrition requirements is best achieved with ongoing reassessment of nutrition goals and nutrition status. Initially, nutrition requirements are determined on the basis of assumptions made about clinical condition and the nutrition needs associated with repletion. Once nutrition intervention has been initiated, a periodic reassessment of nutrition status will determine the accuracy of the initial estimate of nutrition requirements. Also, nutrition requirements may be dynamic in the setting of acute or critical illness—as the patient's clinical status changes so may protein and energy requirements. This further emphasizes the need for periodic reassessment.

TABLE 126–10. Drugs That Alter Glucose Metabolism

Hyperglycemia	Hypoglycemia
Chlorpramazine	Anabolic steroids
Corticosteroids	Disopyramide
Dopamine	Clofibrate
Furosemide	Haloperidol
Phenytoin	Insulin
Theophylline	Oral hypoglycemics
Somatostatin	Propranolol
	Somatostatin

From Ref. 40.

TABLE 126–12. Principles of Nutrition Assessment

1. A focused physical assessment will help identify to the severity of PEM and the potential existence of micronutrient deficiencies.
2. A focused medical history will reveal the likelihood of PEM and micronutrient deficiencies.
3. Choose additional biochemical and anthropometric parameters based on their cost-effectiveness.
4. Laboratory tests used for nutrition assessment must be interpreted in the context of the physical findings and medical history as well as the limitations of each test.
5. When determining nutrition requirements, establish goals based on the need for maintenance versus repletion requirements.
6. When determining nutrition requirements, interpret the guidelines based on patient-specific, disease-specific considerations.

Better markers of nutrition status and methods for determining patient-specific nutrition requirements are definitely needed. Functional tests and simple, noninvasive tests for body composition analysis hold promise for the future. However, until better methods of assessment become clinically available and are demonstrated to be cost effective, the currently available battery of tests will continue to be the mainstay of nutrition assessment. The main principles of nutrition assessment are summarized in Table 126–12.

REFERENCES

1. Klein S, Kinney J, Jeejeebhoy K, et al. Nutrition support in clinical practice: Review of published data and recommendations for future research directions. JPEN J Parenter Enteral Nutr 1997;21:133–156.
2. ASPEN Board of Directors. Revised definition of terms used in ASPEN guidelines and standards. Nutr Clin Prac 1995;10:1–3.
3. Grant JP. Nutritional assessment in clinical practice. Nutr Clin Prac 1986;1:3–11.
4. Teasley-Strausburg KM. Nutritional/metabolic assessment. In: Teasley-Strausburg KM, ed. Nutrition Support Handbook: A Compendium of Products with Guidelines for Usage. Cincinnati, OH, Harvey Whitney Books Company, 1992:1–18.
5. Hill GL. The clinical assessment of adult patients with protein energy malnutrition. Nutr Clin Prac 1995;10:129–130.
6. International Classification of Diseases, 9th ed., Clinical Modification (ICD-9-CM). Ann Arbor, MI; National Center for Health Statistics, 1978:169–170.
7. Swails WS, Samour PQ, Babineau TJ, Bistrian BR. A proposed revision of current ICD-9-CM malnutrition code definitions. J Am Diet Assoc 1996;96:370–373.
8. White JV. The nutrition screening initiative: A 5-year perspective. Nutr Clin Prac 1996;11:89–93.
9. Council on Practice Quality Management Committee. Identifying patients at risk: ADA's definitions for nutrition screening and nutrition assessment. J Am Diet Assoc 1994;94:838–839.
10. Kovacevich DS, Boney AR, Braunschweig CL, et al. Nutrition risk classification: A reproducible and valid tool for nurses. Nutr Clin Prac 1997;12:20–25.
11. Dougherty D, Bankhead R, Kushner R, et al. Nutrition care given new importance in JCAHO standards. Nutr Clin Prac 1995;10:26–31.
12. McClave SA, Mitoraj TE, Thielmeier KA, Greenburg RA. Differentiating subtypes (hypoalbuminemic vs. marasmic) of protein-calorie malnutrition: Incidence and clinical significance in a university hospital setting. JPEN J Parenter Enteral Nutr 1992;16:337–342.
13. Elia M. Assessment of nutritional status and body composition. In: Rombeau JL, Rolandelli RH, eds. Clinical Nutrition: Enteral and Tube Feeding, 3rd ed. Philadelphia, W.B. Saunders, 1997:155–173.
14. Ottery FD. Instruments of proactive assessment and intervention in the context of outcomes-based research and clinical care. In: Improving Clinical Practice with Nutrition in a Managed Care Environment, Report of the Seventeenth Ross Roundtable on Medical Issues. Columbus, OH, Ross Products Division, Abbott Laboratories, 1997: 29–36.
15. Weight by height and age of adults 18–74 years: United States, 1971–74. Atlanta, GA, National Center for Health Statistics, 1979, series 11, no 9.
16. Metropolitan Life Insurance Company. Statistical bulletin, new weights and standards for men and women. Chicago, Metropolitan Life, 1983;64:2–9.
17. Anderson PO, Knoben JE, eds. Handbook of Clinical Drug Data, 8th ed. Stamford, CT, Appleton & Lange, 1997.
18. Heymsfield SB, Tighe A, Wang Z. Nutritional assessment by anthropometric and biochemical methods. In: Shils ME, Olson JA, Shike M, eds. Modern Nutrition in Health and Disease, 8th ed. Philadelphia, Lea & Febiger, 1994:827–828.
19. Mason JB, Russell RM. Parenteral nutrition in the elderly. In: Rombeau JL, Caldwell MD, eds. Clinical Nutrition: Parenteral Nutrition, 2nd ed. Philadelphia, W.B. Saunders, 1993:738–739.
20. Jeejeebhoy KN, Detsky AS, Baker JP. Assessment of nutritional status. JPEN J Parenter Enteral Nutr 1990;14:193S–196S.
21. Rosenfalck AM, Snorgaard O, Almdal T. Creatinine height index and lean body mass in adult patients with insulin-dependent diabetes mellitus followed for 7 years from onset. JPEN J Parenter Enteral Nutr 1994;18:50–54.
22. Van Hoeyweghen RJ, De Leeuw IH, Vandewoude FJ. Creatinine arm index as alternative for creatinine height index. Am J Clin Nutr 1992;56:611–615.
23. Charney P. Nutrition assessment in the 1990s: Where are we now? Nutr Clin Prac 1995;10:131–139.
24. Konstantinides FN, Kaproth PL, Cerra FB. Other aspects of metabolic monitoring in critically ill patients. Clin Chem 1990;36:1596–1603.
25. Veldee MS. Nutrition. In: Burtis CA, Ashwood ER, eds. Tietz Textbook of Clinical Chemistry, 2nd ed. Philadelphia, W.B. Saunders, 1994: 1236–1274.
26. Painter PC, Cope JY, Smith JL. Appendix: Table 41–20. Clinical chemistry and toxicology. In: Burtis CA, Ashwood ER, eds. Tietz Textbook of Clinical Chemistry, 2nd ed. Philadelphia, W.B. Saunders, 1994:2176–2211.
27. Mattox TW, Brown RO, Boucher BA, et al. Use of fibronectin and somatomedin-C as markers of enteral nutrition support in traumatized patients using a modified amino acid formula. JPEN J Parenter Enteral Nutr 1988;12:592–596.
28. Spiekerman AM: Proteins used in nutritional assessment. Clin Lab Med 1993;13:353–369.
29. Fairbanks VF. Iron in medicine and nutrition. In: Shils ME, Olson JA, Shike M, eds. Modern Nutrition in Health and Disease, 8th ed. Philadelphia, Lea & Febiger, 1994:190–191.
30. Erstad BL, Campbell DJ, Rollins CJ, Rappaport WD. Albumin and prealbumin concentrations in patients receiving postoperative parenteral nutrition. Pharmacotherapy 1994;14:458–462.
31. Peterson VM, Moore EE, Jones TN, et al. Total enteral nutrition versus total parenteral nutrition after major torso injury: Attenuation of hepatic protein reprioritization. Surgery 1988;104:199–207.
32. Chandra RK, Sarchielli P. Nutritional status and immune response. Clin Lab Med 1993;13:455–461.
33. Peck MD, Alexander JW. The use of immunologic tests to predict outcome in surgical patients. Nutrition 1990;6:16–19.
34. Sacks GS, Brown RO, Teague D, et al. Early nutrition support modifies immune function in patients sustaining severe head injury. JPEN J Parenter Enteral Nutr 1995;19:387–392.
35. Alexander JW, Peck MD. Future prospects for adjunctive therapy: Pharmacologic and nutritional approaches to immune system modulation. Crit Care Med 1990;18:S159–S164.
36. Moore FA, Moore EE, Kudsk KA, et al. Clinical benefits of an immune-enhancing diet for early postinjury enteral feeding. J Trauma 1994;37:607–615.
37. Kudsk KA, Minard G, Croce MA, et al. A randomized trial of isonitrogenous enteral diets after severe trauma: An immune-enhancing diet reduces septic complications. Ann Surg 1996;224:531–543.
38. Barton RG. Immune-enhancing enteral formulas: Are they beneficial in critically ill patients. Nutr Clin Prac 1997;12:51–62.
39. Baumgartner TG. Trace elements in clinical nutrition. Nutr Clin Prac 1993;8:251–263.
40. Mirtallo JM. Nutrient metabolism. In: Dipiro JT, Talbert FL, Yee GL, et al, eds. Pharmacotherapy: A Pathophysiologic Approach, 3rd ed. Stamford, CT; Appleton & Lange, 1997:2711–2734.
41. Shenkin A. Micronutrients. In: Rombeau JL, Rolandelli RH, eds. Clinical Nutrition: Enteral and Tube Feeding, 3rd ed. Philadelphia: W.B. Saunders, 1997:96–111.
42. Tamura H, Hirose S, Watanabe O, et al. Anemia and neutropenia due to copper deficiency in enteral nutrition. JPEN J Parenter Enteral Nutr 1994;18:185–189.

43. Wasa M, Satani M, Tanano H, et al. Copper deficiency with pancytopenia during parenteral nutrition. JPEN J Parenter Enteral Nutr 1994;18:190–192.
44. Milne DB. Trace elements. In: Burtis CA, Ashwood ER, eds. Tietz Textbook of Clinical Chemistry, 2nd ed. Philadelphia, W.B. Saunders, 1994:1317–1353.
45. Verhage AH, Cheong WK, Jeejeebhoy KN. Neurologic symptoms due to possible chromium deficiency in long-term parenteral nutrition that closely mimic metronidazole-induced syndromes. JPEN J Parenter Enteral Nutr 1996;20:123–127.
46. Jacob RA, Milne DB. Biochemical assessment of vitamins and minerals. Clin Lab Med 1993;18:371–386.
47. Alves G, Thiebot J, Tracqui A, et al. Neurologic disorders due to brain manganese deposition in a jaundiced patient receiving long-term parenteral nutrition. JPEN J Parenter Enteral Nutr 1997;21:41–45.
48. Fell JME, Reynolds AP, Meadows N, et al. Manganese toxicity in children receiving long term parenteral nutrition. Lancet 1996;347: 1218–1221.
49. Matasuda A, Kimura M, Takeda T, et al. Changes in manganese content of mononuclear blood cells in patients receiving total parenteral nutrition. Clin Chem 1994;40:829–832.
50. Malecki EA, Lo HC, Yang H, et al. Tissue manganese concentrations and antioxidant enzyme activities in rats given total parenteral nutrition with and without supplemental manganese. JPEN J Parenter Enteral Nutr 1995;19:222–226.
51. Abrams CK, Siram SM, Galsim C, et al. Selenium deficiency in long-term total parenteral nutrition. Nutr Clin Prac 1992;7:175–178.
52. Rannem T, Ladefoged K, Hylander E, et al. The effect of selenium supplementation on skeletal and cardiac muscle in selenium-depleted patients. JPEN J Parenter Enteral Nutr 1995;19:351–355.
53. Rannem T, Persson-Moschos M, Huang W, et al. Selenoprotien P in patients on home parenteral nutrition. JPEN J Parenter Enteral Nutr 1996;20:287–291.
54. Sardesi VM. Molybdenum: An essential trace element. Nutr Clin Prac 1993;8:277–281.
55. Abumrad NN, Schneider AJ, Steel D, Rogers LS. Amino acid intolerance during prolonged parenteral nutrition reversed by molybdate therapy. Am J Clin Nutr 1981;34:2551–2559.
56. Clugston GA, Hetzel. Iodine. In: Shils ME, Olson JA, Shike M, eds. Modern Nutrition in Health and Disease, 8th ed. Philadelphia, Lea & Febiger, 1994:252–263.
57. Nichoalds GE. Iodine. In: Baumgartner TG, ed. Clinical Guide to Parenteral Micronutrition, 3rd ed. Deerfield IL, Fujisawa USA, Inc, 1997: 361–374.
58. McCormick DB, Greene HL. Vitamins. In: Burtis CA, Ashwood ER, eds. Tietz Textbook of Clinical Chemistry, 2nd ed. Philadelphia, W.B. Saunders, 1994:1275–1316.
59. Silverman B, Franklin GM, Bolin R. Lactic acidosis traced to thiamin deficiency related to nationwide shortage of multivitamins for total parenteral nutrition—United States, 1997. JAMA 1997;278: 109–111.
60. Teasley-Strausburg KM. Lipid emulsions. In: Teasley-Strausburg KM, ed. Nutrition Support Handbook: A Compendium of Products with Guidelines for Usage. Cincinnati, OH, Harvey Whitney Books Company, 1992:81–89.
61. Borum PR. Carnitine in neonatal nutrition. J Child Neurol 1995; 10(suppl 2):S25–S31.
62. Broquist HP. Carnitine. In: Shils ME, Olson JA, Shike M, eds. Modern Nutrition in Health and Disease, 8th ed. Philadelphia, Lea & Febiger, 1994:459–465.
63. Borum PR. Carnitine. In: Baumgartner TG, ed. Clinical Guide to Parenteral Micronutrition, 3rd ed. Deerfield IL, Fujisawa USA, Inc, 1997: 629–641.
64. Lipkin EW, Bell S. Assessment of nutritional status. Clin Lab Med 1993;13:329–351.
65. Schroeder D, Christie PM, Hill GL. Bioelectrical impedance analysis for body composition: Clinical evaluation in general surgical patients. JPEN J Parenter Enteral Nutr 1990;14:129–133.
66. Jacobs DO, Scheltinga MRM. Metabolic assessment. In: Rombeau JL, Caldwell MD, eds. Clinical Nutrition: Parenteral Nutrition, 2nd ed. Philadelphia, W.B. Saunders, 1993:253–259.
67. Scheltinga MR, Jacob DO, Kimbrough TD. Alterations in body fluid content can be detected by bioelectrical impedance analysis. J Surg Res 1991;50:461–468.
68. Robert S, Zarowitz BJ, Hyzy R, et al. Bioelectrical impedance assessment of nutritional status in critically ill patients. Am J Clin Nutr 1993;57:840–844.
69. Forbes GB. Body composition: Influence of nutrition, disease, growth and aging. In: Shils ME, Olson JA, Shike M, eds. Modern Nutrition in Health and Disease, 8th ed. Philadelphia, Lea & Febiger, 1994:781–801.
70. Food and Nutrition Board, National Research Council. Recommended Dietary Allowances, 10th ed. Washington, DC, National Academy of Sciences, 1989.
71. Food and Nutrition Board, Institute of Medicine, National Academy of Sciences. Dietary Reference Intakes. Washington, DC, National Academy Press, 1999 (in press).
72. Mandt JM, Teasley-Strausburg KM, Shronts EP. Nutritional requirements. In: Teasley-Strausburg KM, ed. Nutrition Support Handbook: A Compendium of Products with Guidelines for Usage. Cincinnati, OH, Harvey Whitney Books Company, 1992:19–36.
73. Harris JA, Benedict FG. A Biometric Study of Basal Metabolism in Man, publication 279. Washington, DC, Carnegie Institute, 1919.
74. Garrel DR, Jobin N, DeJonge LHM. Should we still use the Harris and Benedict equations? Nutr Clin Prac 1996;11:99–103.
75. Osborne BJ, Saba AK, Wood SJ, et al. Clinical comparison of three methods to determine resting energy expenditure. Nutr Clin Prac 1994;9:241–246.
76. McClave SA, Snider HL. Use of indirect calorimetry in clinical nutrition. Nutr Clin Prac 1992;7:207–221.
77. Hynote ED, McCamish MA, Depner TA, Davis PA. Amino acid losses during hemodialysis: Effects of high-solute flux and parenteral nutrition in acute renal failure. JPEN J Parenter Enteral Nutr 1995;19:15–21.
78. Long CL, Lowry SR. Hormonal regulation of protein metabolism. JPEN J Parenter Enteral Nutr 1990;14:555–562.
79. Barton RG. Nutrition support in critical illness. Nutr Clin Prac 1994; 9:127–139.
80. Valesco N, Long CL, Otto DA, et al. Comparison of three methods for the estimation of total nitrogen losses in hospitalized patients. JPEN J Parenter Enteral Nutr 1990;14:517–522.
81. Konstantinides FN, Konstantinides NN, Li JC, et al. Urinary urea nitrogen: Too insensitive for calculating nitrogen balance studies in surgical clinical nutrition. JPEN J Parenter Enteral Nutr 1991;15:189–193.
82. Shronts EP, Lacey JA. Metabolic support. In: Gottschlich MM, Matarese LE, Shronts EP, eds. Nutrition Support Dietetics—Core Curriculum, 2nd ed. Silver Spring, MD, ASPEN, 1993:358.
83. Weber P, Bendich A, Machlin LJ. Vitamin E and human health: Rationale for determining recommended intake levels. Nutrition 1997; 13:450–460.
84. Berger MM, Cavadini C, Bart A, et al. Cutaneous copper and zinc losses in burns. Burns 1992;18:373–380.
85. Berger MM, Cavadini C, Bart A, et al. Selenium losses in 10 burned patients. Clin Nutr 1992;11:75–82.
86. Solomon SM, Kirby DF. The refeeding syndrome: A review. JPEN J Parenter Enteral Nutr 1990;14:90–97.
87. Weinsier R, Krumdieck C. Death resulting from overzealous total parenteral nutrition: The refeeding syndrome revisited. Am J Clin Nutr 1981;34:393–399.
88. Sardesai VM. Role of antioxidants in health maintenance. Nutr Clin Prac 1995;10:19–25.
89. Lasswell AB, Loreck ES. Development of a program in accord with JCAHO standards for counseling on potential drug–food interactions. J Am Diet Assoc 1992;92:1124–1125.
90. Townsend CE, ed. Nutrition and Diet Therapy, 6th ed. Albany, NY, Delmar, 1994:428.
91. Williams SR. Drug–nutrient interactions. In: Williams SR, ed. Nutrition and Diet Therapy, 7th ed. Chicago, Mosby, 1993:476–486.

127

PREVALENCE AND SIGNIFICANCE OF MALNUTRITION

Kathleen M. Teasley-Strausburg, MS, RPh, BCNSP, and Pamela D. Reiter, PharmD, BCPS

Malnutrition is a contributing factor in the poor outcome of many disease states. In this chapter the prevalence of malnutrition as defined by a variety of nutrition assessment parameters is documented, and the significant impact of abnormalities in these nutrition assessment parameters on the morbidity and mortality of selected disease states is presented. Interventional strategies for the prevention and management of malnutrition and the economic consequences of malnutrition are also presented.

PREVALENCE

Malnutrition occurs throughout the world. It is most prevalent in underdeveloped countries where food supply, ignorance, poverty, overcrowding, and poor sanitation are contributing factors. The most susceptible individuals are infants, especially premature infants, pregnant or lactating women, and the elderly. These individuals are also the most susceptible in developed countries. The factors that contribute to malnutrition in developed countries include a decline in breast-feeding, poor maternal nutrition before and during pregnancy, misconceptions about the use of certain foods, fad diets, and alcohol or drug abuse. In the United States poor nutrition in the community occurs mostly in lower socioeconomic groups but may be present throughout society when fad diets and alcohol or drug abuse are factors.

Malnutrition is most commonly associated with disease and illness and is prevalent in the hospital setting. The recognition of hospital malnutrition has occurred coincident with the systematic application of nutrition assessment techniques to hospitalized individuals in the last two decades. A review of adult patients from varying socioeconomic backgrounds hospitalized in a variety of institutions reported a high prevalence (40% to 55%) of previously unrecognized malnutrition.[1] There is evidence, however, that the prevalence of malnutrition has declined since the mid-1970s, and that there is a heightened awareness of nutritional disease and better in-hospital nutrition management.[2]

In children, malnutrition can have long-lasting effects, especially on cognitive development. Unfortunately, children have both limited body stores and high metabolic demands. These characteristics place them at particular risk for developing malnutrition, especially during illness. Recently, Hendricks et al. described the prevalence of protein–energy malnutrition in 224 hospitalized children.[3] A significant reduction from 33.6% to 24.5% was detected in the prevalence of acute malnutrition (weight-for-height < 90% of median) over the past 15 years. Likewise, the prevalence of chronic malnutrition (weight-for-height < 95% of median) also fell significantly from 46.8% in 1976 to 27.3% in the 1990s. Children with chronic disease and those younger than 2 years and older than 18 years had the highest prevalence of malnutrition.

In 1980, a publicly funded health and nutrition program known as the Pediatric Nutrition Surveillance System (PedNSS) was established.[4] This system generates data on the prevalence of malnutrition in children enrolled in a variety of federal and state programs. Children less than 5 years of age make up the majority of participants. The most recent published summary of PedNSS data includes surveillance from 1980 to 1991. The prevalence of shortness (height-for-age) in children less than 24 months old was 10%, which is more than twice the expected value. However, in older children aged 2 to 5 years, the prevalence was only slightly higher than expected. Thinness, or weight-for-height, has been stable at 2.5% to 5% since 1980 and indicates that prevalence of acute or severe malnutrition is low. Anemia, hematologic evidence of poor nutrition status and/or iron deficiency, was high between 1980 and 1985 (20% to 30%) but has rapidly declined and now approaches 5%.

EFFECT ON ORGAN AND CELLULAR FUNCTION

The outcome of malnutrition is an inappropriate reduction in lean body mass resulting in loss of structure and/or function (Table 127–1). Essentially every organ system is affected by malnutrition. The clinical significance of the effect will depend on the specific anatomic structure or system and on the degree of malnutrition. For example, with mild malnutrition, loss of skeletal muscle mass may be apparent as weakness or a decreased level of physical activity. However, alterations in cardiac function usually are not apparent until severe malnutrition is present.

Alterations in the immune system (Table 127–2) represent an end-organ or functional response to malnutrition and may reflect a decline in lean body mass as well as a deficiency in specific nutrients such as zinc.[5,6] Clinically, this is manifested as an increased incidence of infection.

Malnutrition also has an adverse effect on wound healing. Although wound healing occurs at the expense of other

TABLE 127–1. End-Organ Responses in Malnutrition

Organ	Anatomic Responses	Physiologic Response
Heart	Four-chamber dilation; atrophic degeneration with necrosis and fibrosis; myofibrillar disruption	QT prolongation, low voltage, bradycardia; decreased cardiac output, stroke volume, and contractility; preload intolerance; diminished responsiveness to drugs
Lung	Emphysematous changes; pulmonary infarcts; reduced bacterial clearance; muscle atrophy	Pneumonia; decreases in functional residual capacity, vital capacity, and maximum breathing capacity; depressed hypoxic/hypercarbic drives
Hematologic	Failure of stem-cell production; decreased PMN chemotaxis; decreased lymphocyte count with reduced helper T and increased suppressor T and killer cells; decreased blastogenesis to phytohemagglutinin	Anemia; anergy; decreased granuloma formation; impaired response to chemotherapy; increased infection rate
Renal system	Epithelial swelling; atrophy; mild cortical calcification; depressed erythropoietin synthesis	Reduced glomerular filtration rate and inability to handle sodium loads; polyuria; metabolic acidosis
Gastrointestinal system	Disproportionate mass loss; hypoplastic and atrophic changes; decrease in total mucosal height	Depressed enzymatic activity; shortened transit time; impaired motility; propensity for bacterial overgrowth; maldigestion and malabsorption
Liver	Mass loss; periportal fat accumulation	Decreased visceral protein synthesis; depressed microsomal activity; eventual hepatic insufficiency

From Cerra FB (ed.). Manual of Surgical Nutrition. St Louis, MO, CV Mosby, 1984, p 6, with permission.

tissues, in the setting of protein–energy malnutrition (PEM) the rate at which the wound heals and the tensile strength of the wound are decreased.[7] Wound healing may also be altered in the malnourished patient owing to the increased likelihood of wound infection from altered immunity. Deficiency of an individual nutrient may also affect wound healing. Those nutrients that are most critical to wound healing include arginine, copper, vitamin C, vitamin A, and zinc (Table 127–3). When given in pharmacologic doses, vitamin A and arginine have been shown to promote earlier wound healing.[7,8] Other nutrients, when ingested in excessive amounts, may impair wound healing. For example, excess vitamin E antagonizes the promotion of wound healing by vitamin A, and excess zinc will displace copper and interfere with lysyl oxidase (the enzyme necessary for collagen cross-link formation).[7]

TABLE 127– 2. Immune Response Mechanisms in Malnutrition

Parameter	Observation in Malnutrition
Cell-mediated immune response	
Delayed cutaneous hypersensitivity	Decreased
Lymphocyte transformation	Decreased
Polymorphonuclear leukocyte response	
Phagocytosis	Normal or decreased
Metabolism	Decreased
Bactericidal capacity	Decreased
Chemotaxis	Decreased
Total lymphocyte count	Decreased
T cells	
$CD4^+$	Decreased
$CD8^+$	Decreased
Helper:suppressor	Decreased
Humoral response	
Complement activity (CH50)	Decreased
Secretory IgA	Decreased
Serum complement	Decreased or normal
Serum immunoglobulins	Normal
Serum opsonization	Normal

DISEASE-SPECIFIC CONSEQUENCES

Malnutrition seldom exists as an isolated disease state but rather is usually found in patients with other preexisting illnesses. Often the primary disease or complications of the disease predispose an individual to the development of malnutrition. The primary factors that contribute to the likelihood of developing malnutrition include decreased dietary intake (e.g., due to nausea, vomiting, anorexia), malabsorption (e.g., due to short bowel syndrome, severe diarrhea, high-output fistula), and altered metabolism (hypermetabolic and catabolic states due to sepsis, trauma, cancer, AIDS). Those disease states or clinical conditions most commonly accompanied by malnutrition are discussed below. Malnutrition is also associated with major organ failure: renal, hepatic, cardiac, and pulmonary failure and multisystem organ failure (see Chap. 131).

CANCER

Patients with cancer have many factors that contribute to the likelihood of developing malnutrition (Table 127–4). The frequency is highest (> 80%) in patients with gastric and pancreatic tumors and lowest in patients with hematologic malignancies.[9] Weight loss, a sign of malnutrition, occurs in 30% to 80% of adult cancer patients. A significant relationship between weight loss and reduced survival has been demonstrated for some (lung, prostate, colon cancer) but not all tumor types.[9] The degree of reduction in median survival is statistically significant for some cancers and

TABLE 127–3. Nutritional Disorders and Wound Healing

Nutritional Disorder	Effect on Wound Healing
Arginine deficiency	Altered collagen formation
Copper deficiency	Impaired lysyl oxidase activity
Protein–energy malnutrition	Decreased wound strength because of reduced hydroxyproline content of wound; decreased rate of wound healing; increased incidence of wound infection
Vitamin C deficiency	Decreased fibroblast maturation with failure of collagen synthesis; decreased angiogenesis
Vitamin A deficiency	Decreased collagen accumulation; formation of abnormal collagen
Zinc deficiency	Impaired DNA and protein synthesis; impaired mitosis and cell proliferation

ranges from 49% to 79%. Malnutrition in children with cancer is common and is associated with tumor type,[10] disease progression and chemotherapy-related complications.[11] The prevalence of malnutrition is highest in Ewing's sarcoma (67%) and neuroblastoma (47%) and lowest in acute leukemias (6%) and non-Hodgkin's lymphomas (10% to 15%). Theoretically, early recognition and management of malnutrition in cancer patients may minimize the nutrition consequences, improve tumor response to therapy, reduce side effects of therapy, and improve survival. Cancer patients treated with bone marrow transplantation have shown improved tumor response and clinical outcome with parenteral nutrition (PN) compared to control groups not receiving PN.[12]

Improved nutrition status enhances survival and improves treatment tolerance in many but not all children.[13–15] Parenteral nutrition has been shown to be of benefit to malnourished children undergoing radiation therapy but failed to benefit well-nourished children.[16] Conversely, well-nourished children treated with PN at the initiation of therapy for metastatic neuroblastoma appeared to have longer remission and improved survival compared to their malnourished cohorts.[10] Malnutrition in cancer patients due to simple starvation, characterized by normal metabolism but inadequate nutrient intake or malabsorption, appears to be responsive to nutrition intervention.[17] However, malnutrition due to cancer cachexia, characterized by altered nutrient utilization in spite of adequate supply, does not.[18,19] Treatment of malnutrition due to cancer cachexia is controversial, especially in the absence of data showing an improved quality of life with nutrition therapy.

AIDS

One of the characteristics of AIDS is the generalized wasting and malnutrition.[20] In many patients weight loss and wasting may be one of the earliest symptoms along with opportunistic infection. The malnutrition is often progressive and may lead to death in some patients.[21,22] Poor nutrition status as indicated by weight loss and decreased serum albumin concentrations has been shown to be a predictor of survival in adult AIDS patients.[22–25] Growth and nutrition problems are also common in children with AIDS. Infants with perinatally acquired AIDS have normal birthweights but show signs of growth delay at as early as 4 months.[26] Impaired linear growth appears to correlate with periods of rapid viral replication during the first 18 months of life.[27] There is a direct

TABLE 127–4. Risk Factors for Malnutrition in Cancer Patients

Risk Factor	Nutrition Consequence
Primary disease	
Tumor type	Weight loss, anorexia, altered taste, altered metabolism
Complicating conditions	
Malabsorption	Impaired absorption of all or selected nutrients, diarrhea
Bowel obstruction	Nausea and vomiting, inability to ingest nutrients orally or by enteral nutrition
Infection	Increased energy expenditure and protein requirements, altered metabolism, anorexia, malabsorption
Psychological response	Anorexia, food aversion
Treatments	
Chemotherapy	Taste and appetite alterations, nausea and vomiting, mucositis, esophagitis, diarrhea, constipation
Surgery	
Radical resection of oropharyngeal region	Problems with chewing and swallowing
Esophageal reconstruction	Gastric stasis and hypochlorhydria secondary to vagotomy; diarrhea and steatorrhea
Gastrectomy	Dumping syndrome, malabsorption, lack of intrinsic factor, hypoglycemia
Intestinal resection	Malabsorption, renal oxalate stones, metabolic acidosis, diarrhea
Pancreatectomy	Malabsorption, diabetes mellitus
Radiation	
Head and neck	Stomatitis, dysgeusia, xerostomia
Abdomen and pelvis	Bowel obstruction, fistulae, radiation enteritis (diarrhea, protein-losing enteropathy, malabsorption)

relationship between these growth abnormalities and morbidity and mortality.[28] Up to 80% of older infants and children (4 months to 11 years) with AIDS or advanced HIV disease demonstrate evidence of retarded growth velocity with weight below the 25th percentile.[29] This growth velocity can be markedly improved with antiviral therapy.[29]

Many risk factors contribute to malnutrition in AIDS (Table 127–5). Poor oral intake frequently occurs and is often due to anorexia, depression, altered mental status, or oral and esophageal lesions. Hypermetabolism may be present if opportunistic infection and fever develop or if secondary malignancies such as Kaposi's sarcoma or lymphoma develop. Malaborption may occur if AIDS enteropathy develops.

The response to nutrition intervention has been variable. Kotler and associates[30] evaluated the effect of prolonged parenteral nutrition on body composition in 12 patients with AIDS. All patients gained body weight and increased body fat content. However, lean body mass improved only in the 5 patients with altered intake or absorption. The 7 patients with systemic disease, for example, systemic infection, did not have an improvement in lean body mass. Lean body mass repletion with enteral nutrition in AIDS patients with weight loss and inadequate food intake has also been reported.[31] In a retrospective review of home parenteral nutrition in 22 AIDS patients with weight loss greater than 10% of usual body weight, 15 patients gained weight, 6 stabilized, and 2 continued to lose weight.[32]

With earlier diagnosis and initiation of treatment for HIV-positive status prior to the onset of AIDS, the prevalence of malnutrition may decline. New treatment modalities for AIDS are also being developed that may affect the prevalence of malnutrition and the response to nutrition intervention in this patient population (see Chap. 114).

CRITICAL ILLNESS/TRAUMA/BURN INJURY

One of the characteristics of critical illness is hypermetabolism. Trauma, burn injury, and sepsis are all catalysts for the release of mediators that initiate and regulate the hypermetabolic response. The metabolic consequences of this response include altered carbohydrate metabolism, increased protein synthesis and degradation, and increased lipid oxidation, which ultimately result in loss of protein and lean body mass.[33,34] In a previously well-nourished individual, critical illness can result in the rapid onset of kwashiorkor-like malnutrition within 5 to 7 days. In a previously malnourished individual, critical illness can precipitate severe mixed marasmus–kwashiorkor in 3 to 5 days. In a recent prospective study of 129 patients admitted to the intensive care unit (ICU), 43% were malnourished.[35] The malnourished patients had an increased length of stay in the ICU (a mean of 27 vs 19 days) and a statistically significant increased incidence of complications (55% vs 40%) compared to well-nourished patients with a similar severity of illness.

The goal of nutrition support in critically ill patients is to prevent the development or worsening of malnutrition. Patient outcomes related to tissue repair and organ function may be improved through nutrition support in these patients.[34] Enteral nutrition initiated within 24 to 48 hours of injury may attenuate the hypermetabolic response.[36,37] Enteral nutrition has also been shown to result in fewer septic complications when compared to parenteral nutrition.[38–41] Critically ill patients appear to derive the greatest benefit when enterally fed an immune-enhanced formula that contains pharmacologic doses of immune-modulating nutrients such as arginine, glutamine, nucleic acids, and omega-3 fatty acids.[42,43]

INFLAMMATORY BOWEL DISEASE

Crohn's disease typically affects the terminal ileum but may occur anywhere in the gastrointestinal tract. Two-thirds to three-fourths of patients hospitalized with Crohn's disease are malnourished and exhibit weight loss, hypoalbuminemia, and vitamin deficiencies.[44] Growth failure occurs in 15% to 40% of prepubertal patients and is characterized by retarded skeletal maturation (which may be irreversible) and delayed development of secondary sex characteristics.[45] The nutrition consequences of ulcerative colitis tend to be less severe than those of Crohn's disease. Approximately 25% to 50% of patients with ulcerative colitis are hypoalbuminemic and 2% to 20% experience growth

TABLE 127–5. Risk Factors for Malnutrition in AIDS

Risk Factor	Nutrition Consequence
General factors: decreased oral intake, malabsorption	Anorexia, poor diet, esophageal/oral lesions, emotional stress, HIV wasting syndrome, diarrhea, enteropathy, medication side effects
Opportunistic infections: bacterial (MAI, TB); viral (CMV, herpes); fungal (*Candida albicans,* cryptococcus); protozoal (*Pneumocystis carinii,* microsporidia, isospora belli, cryptosporidia, *Giardia lamblia*)	Fever, hypermetabolism, anorexia, malabsorption
Malignancies: Kaposi's sarcoma, lymphoma	Anorexia, hypermetabolism, medication side effects
Medications: antibiotics, anticancer chemotherapy, antidepressants	Nausea, vomiting, diarrhea, anorexia, mucositis
Neuropsychiatric disorders: dementia, depression, anxiety, encephalopathy	Poor oral intake, anorexia, poor diet
Socioeconomic factors: IV drug abuse, low income	Poor oral intake, anorexia, poor diet

failure. The factors contributing to the risk of malnutrition in inflammatory bowel disease (IBD) include decreased food intake due to pain, anorexia, or altered taste; malabsorption due to mucosal abnormalities, bacterial overgrowth, and diminished absorptive surface after surgical resection of diseased bowel; and hypermetabolism from fever and infection.[44] Nutrition management of IBD may, therefore, require enteral and/or parenteral nutrition.[46] Enteral is the preferred route except in patients with a high-output fistula or obstruction or if enteral feeding exacerbates pain. Enteral or parenteral nutrition is likely to facilitate remission in 60% to 80% of patients with acute Crohn's disease. However, the course of ulcerative colitis is not influenced by the use of nutrition support, although nutrition status may be maintained in an acute exacerbation.

CHRONIC INTESTINAL PSEUDO-OBSTRUCTION

Pseudo-obstruction refers to a disorder of the gastrointestinal tract that presents with the symptoms of bowel obstruction, but no mechanical obstruction exists. The cause is thought to be a neuromuscular disorder of the smooth muscle and/or its innervation, which leads to hypomotility or dysmotility. Prolonged dysmotility can result in malnutrition and also in growth failure in children.[47] The primary factors contributing to a risk of malnutrition are anorexia, nausea, vomiting, and obstruction, which may recur over years. Approximately 15% to 30% of patients with pseudo-obstruction require nutrition support with either parenteral or enteral nutrition.[47]

SHORT BOWEL SYNDROME

Short bowel syndrome (SBS) is the result of the surgical resection of a large portion of the intestinal tract. The degree of nutrition impairment depends on the amount and location of excised bowel. Malabsorption is immediately present to some extent following surgery and may be temporary or permanent.[48] Bowel adaptation will occur over time (6 to 12 months) but may not result in restoration of the full absorptive capacity of the intestine. Intestinal adaptation occurs more frequently in children than adults.[49] In fact, the premature infant may have the best adaptive response to SBS owing to normal rapid intestinal growth during late gestation when the jejunum, ileum, and colon more than double in length.[50]

Adults who have 600 to 700 cm of ileum remaining after surgical resection (i.e., 100 to 200 cm of ileum resected) will require vitamin B_{12}, calcium, and magnesium supplementation. Massive resection of the small bowel leaving less than 60 cm in adults and 10 to 20 cm in children will result in severe malabsorption of all nutrients and will require total or supplemental PN for months or years postoperatively.[49,51,52] In the absence of nutrition support, malnutrition is inevitable and can be life threatening. For those children with extensive bowel loss or life-threatening complications from prolonged PN, innovative surgical procedures including bowel lengthening and transplantation can improve the gut's adaptive process and reduce the need for PN.[49,53–55]

SURGICAL PATIENTS

In general, malnourished patients have a greater risk of postoperative complications than well-nourished patients. Loss of weight was one of the earliest recognized nutrition factors associated with increased morbidity and mortality in surgical patients.[56] Several nutrition assessment parameters predict morbidity and mortality in surgical patients. Mullen et al.[57] examined the value of 16 nutritional and immunologic variables and found serum transferrin and albumin concentrations and delayed cutaneous hypersensitivity reaction to be the most reliable predictors of outcome. These factors have been shown by several authors to correlate with morbidity and mortality.[58–61] Other factors have been used to predict morbidity and mortality such as forearm muscle dynamometry,[62] total body potassium,[63] and total lymphocyte count.[64] A comprehensive study by Buzby et al.[63] confirmed the findings of Mullen et al.[57] and suggested that the measurement of triceps skinfold thickness was also a useful predictor. They developed a linear predictive outcome model, the prognostic nutritional index (PNI), which is a continuous quantitative nutritional index. Using this model, they accurately identified 87% of the patients who ultimately developed significant complications and 96% of the postoperative deaths. This predictive model has been validated in prospective studies of different patient groups by comparing the risk of morbidity and mortality predicted by the model with actual outcome.[65–67]

No studies have evaluated the effect of nutrition support on the PNI and the subsequent patient outcome. However, the use of preoperative parenteral nutrition in patients with malnutrition, particularly when associated with a low serum albumin concentration, has been demonstrated to reduce the incidence of major postoperative complications in several patient populations.[68] Furthermore, early postoperative parenteral nutrition has been shown to improve convalescence coincident with improvement in nutrition status after esophagogastrectomy[69] and radical bladder cystectomy.[70] Conflicting data were found in the multi-institutional VA Cooperative Study.[71] This prospective, randomized clinical trial in 395 malnourished patients evaluated the impact of perioperative parenteral nutrition on mortality and the rate of postoperative complications at 30 and 90 days. Differences in mortality at 30 and 90 days were not statistically significant, and there was no significant reduction in complication rate. The types of complications in the two groups were different. The parenteral nutrition group had a higher incidence of infectious complications and lower incidence of noninfectious complications. The incidence of noninfectious complications was higher in those with the greatest degree of malnutrition (determined by calculation of a Nutrition Risk Index using serum albumin concentration and weight). In the parenteral nutrition group, the highest incidence of infectious complications was in the borderline or mildly malnourished patients. The investigators concluded that preoperative parenteral nutrition did not result in an improved postoperative course except in patients who were severely malnourished preoperatively (i.e., a Nutrition Risk Index of < 83.5). In patients who were mildly to moderately malnourished, the incidence of infectious complications associated with the use of parenteral nutrition outweighed the benefits. As with critically ill patients, enteral feeding with immune-enhanced formulas appears to promote the best nutrition and clinical outcome with fewer metabolic and infectious complications.[72,73]

PEDIATRIC DISEASES

Regardless of the disease process, pediatric patients in general are at greater risk for nutrition disorders and more frequently develop the severe consequences associated with malnutrition. Nutrition deficiency in the young affects existing organs and cells, may impair normal development, and may result in permanent, irreversible damage. Pharmacologic and technologic advances in neonatal medicine have improved the survival of extremely premature infants (< 1000 g). However, with this survival rate has come morbidity owing to bronchopulmonary dysplasia and necrotizing enterocolitis, which may further complicate the infant's nutrition status.

BRONCHOPULMONARY DYSPLASIA

Bronchopulmonary dysplasia (BPD) or chronic lung disease (CLD) is a clinical, pathologic, and radiographic disease of the newborn resulting from prolonged exposure to positive pressure ventilation and elevated oxygen concentrations.[74] Risk factors for developing BPD include extent of prematurity, nutrition status, and immunologic status. Characteristics of BPD include pulmonary edema and tissue destruction with subsequent repair, fibrosis, and inflammation. These infants also have an elevated metabolic rate and growth failure.

Early evidence of growth failure and altered body composition is common in infants with BPD when compared to their peers without BPD.[75] The origin of this growth failure is multifactorial. An elevation in resting and total energy expenditure by as much as 25% has been reported.[76–78] Additionally, because pulmonary edema is common, fluid restriction is often necessary. This restriction further impedes provision of adequate calories and may contribute to poor growth.[79] Futhermore, there exists a direct relationship between growth retardation, severity of lung disease, and energy expenditure.[80] When infants with BPD receive appropriate oxygen therapy during the first year of life, growth patterns of matched infants without BPD can be attained.[81,82] Although early growth failure is a common finding in infants with BPD, the persistence of growth failure beyond the neonatal period is disputable and complex. Growth failure during the first 2 years of life, early childhood, and beyond has been reported,[74,83] but it appears that prematurity and sociodemographic factors rather than BPD are most predictive of future growth.[84,85]

NECROTIZING ENTEROCOLITIS

Necrotizing enterocolitis (NEC) is a complex disorder characterized by intestinal mucosal injury secondary to ischemia, bacterial overgrowth, and/or the presence of nutrients within the gut lumen. NEC typically occurs in premature infants (< 38 week gestational age), low-birth-weight infants (weighing < 2500 g), and in the first 1 to 10 days of life. The severe inflammation of the intestinal tract caused by the mucosal injury results in malabsorption of nutrients. Total bowel rest is the treatment of choice; hence, to prevent malnutrition, parenteral nutrition is indicated.[86] If NEC results in bowel perforation, necrosis, or stricture, surgery is required to resect the injured portion of the bowel. SBS may be a consequence if more than 70% of the bowel is resected, and long-term home parenteral nutrition will be required.[86] Additionally, those infants with advanced disease who require surgery are at increased risk of growth failure.[87] In the absence of significant intestinal resection, growth and nutrient absorption are normal.[88] Fortunately, the survival rate of NEC has increased over the past decade and now exceeds 70%.

CYSTIC FIBROSIS

The predominant clinical findings of cystic fibrosis (CF) are related to altered pulmonary function and pancreatic exocrine function. Growth retardation and failure to thrive are classic features of CF. According to the National Cystic Fibrosis Patient Registry data, malnutrition (height-for-age, or weight-for-age < 5th percentile) is very prevalent in infants (47%) and adolescents (34%) and in patients with newly diagnosed CF (44%).[89] The occurrence of malnutrition is closely related to the deterioration of lung function and contributes to the patient's poor clinical outcome.[90] Factors that contribute to the nutrition disorders associated with CF include an increased energy expenditure, malabsorption, anorexia, pharmacotherapy, and pulmonary toilet.[90,91] Increased energy requirements in CF patients are the result of the increased amount of work required to breath and an elevated resting energy expenditure (REE) during pulmonary exacerbation. Recent data suggest that children with only mild to moderate lung disease may be spared from this rise in REE during an acute exacerbation.[92] It is also theorized that the genetic defect that causes CF affects metabolism, causing an increase in energy requirements. Altered pancreatic function occurs in about 85% of patients with CF. Insufficiency of pancreatic enzymes secreted into the intestine reduces the absorption of fat and fat-soluble vitamins. Consequently, more than two thirds of the CF centers in North America use a hydrolyzed (semi-elemental) enteral formula for infants with CF. However, the nutrition benefits of this expensive hydrolyzed formula over a conventional cow's milk formula have recently been challenged. These data do not support the use of a hydrolyzed formula as part of routine nutrition care.[93,94] One of the treatments of CF patients is "pulmonary toilet." This treatment is the physical pounding on the back of the patient while in a partially inverted position in an attempt to loosen the thickened bronchial secretions that impair breathing. It may be performed numerous times throughout the day and may result in an increase in energy expenditure. It also interferes with the feeding schedule, which needs to be designed to ensure that the stomach is empty or nearly empty before the "pulmonary toilet" process begins to prevent pulmonary aspiration of stomach contents. Finally, the disease itself contributes to the development of anorexia in patients with CF. Nutritional management typically focuses on the use of oral pancreatic enzymes (e.g., Viokase, Pancrease), supplemental fat-soluble vitamins, and a high-protein, high-calorie diet.[89] If nutrition status cannot be maintained with these measures, supplemental enteral or parenteral nutrition may be indicated.

CHRONIC PROTRACTED DIARRHEA

Chronic protracted diarrhea is a major cause of fluid and electrolyte imbalance, as well as malnutrition, in infants and young children. This condition is defined as persistent diarrhea for more than 2 weeks with stool cultures negative for enteropathogens.[95] The etiology of chronic protracted diarrhea is diverse and includes microvillous atrophy, autoimmune enteropathy and small intestine enteropathy. Malnutrition is seen when food or a specific dietary product aggravates the intestinal malfunction, leading to malabsorption and worsening diarrhea. The extent of malabsorption will depend on the severity of the diarrhea and the underlying cause.

Failure to thrive, secondary to mucosal atrophy and malabsorption, will ensue unless prompt and effective nutrition intervention is initiated. Nutrition support, enterally or parenterally as tolerated, is indicated to prevent malnutrition and consequent growth failure.[96] Close attention to nutrition and use of refeeding protocols can reduce length of hospitalization and patient care costs in children with intractable diarrhea.[97]

MANAGEMENT

The increased awareness of the prevalence and significance of untreated protein–calorie malnutrition has provided a strong incentive for a more rigorous evaluation of abnormalities of nutrition status and prompt nutrition support of malnourished patients. If nutrition assessment (see Chap. 126) reveals no malnutrition, then the patient should be counseled on appropriate maintenance goals for nutrition intake. If mild to moderate malnutrition is present, an anabolic feeding regimen should be initiated using oral supplements. If anorexia is a major contributing factor, enteral tube feeding may be indicated. Intact nutrients can be administered enterally when normal bowel function is present, but a specially designed formula that has a modified fat content, is lactose-free, contains fiber, and/or is calorie or protein enriched may be indicated if intestinal function is compromised (see Chap. 129). If malabsorption is a major contributing factor, tube feeding using a disease-specific formula or, alternatively, supplemental or total parenteral nutrition may be indicated.

In the presence of severe malnutrition an anabolic feeding regimen should be initiated either enterally or parenterally depending on intestinal function and malabsorption (Fig. 127– 1).[94] When bowel obstruction, short bowel syndrome, or hypoperfusion of the gut is present, parenteral nutrition is indicated. The anticipated duration of the need for parenteral support will dictate the use of peripheral versus central vein administration of PN (see Chap. 128). Routine reevaluation of the response to nutrition therapy and attainment of nutrition goals should be incorporated into the overall patient care plan.

PHARMACOECONOMIC CONSIDERATIONS

Malnourished patients have increased complications during their hospital course, an increased length of stay (LOS), and thereby increased health care costs.[2,99–101] They are among the 10% of patients who disproportionately consume health care resources.[102] Robinson and associates[99] conducted a prospective study of 100 general medical patients with similar "diagnosis severity" to determine the relationship between nutrition status on admission to the hospital and length of stay and hospital costs. Nutrition status was defined using diet history, history of weight loss, anthropometrics, visceral protein measurements, and delayed cutaneous hypersensitivity. Of the 100 patients, 40 were identified as malnourished, 44 were well-nourished, and 16 were borderline. The diagnoses of malnutrition included kwashiorkor (12 patients), marasmus (1 patient), and mixed kwashiorkor–marasmus (27 patients). Malnourished patients had a significantly prolonged LOS compared to normal or borderline patients (15.6 ± 2.2, 8.2 ± 0.7, and 10.2 ± 1.7, mean ± SEM, respectively). Hospital charges were also significantly greater in the malnourished patients than the normal patients (\$16,691 ± \$4389 versus \$7692 ± \$687, mean ± SEM).

In a retrospective study, Reilly and associates[96] evaluated the effect of the likelihood of malnutrition (LOM) at admission on hospital length of stay, costs, and charges in medical and surgical patients. LOM was determined from diet history, physical examination, height-for-weight measurement, serum albumin concentration, and total lymphocyte count. LOM, defined as an abnormality in any one of the above criteria, was present in 59% of the medical patients and 48% of the surgical patients on admission. Across all major medical and surgical diagnosis related groups (DRG), patients with an LOM had a greater LOS. Consequently, hospital charges, which were also converted to direct variable costs, were greater for patients with LOM.

Although the evidence is strong that malnutrition is associated with increased health care costs, it has been more difficult to establish the cost–benefit or cost savings of nutrition intervention. Based on assumptions derived from the literature, Twomey and Patching[103] concluded that preoperative parenteral nutrition could be cost saving in patients undergoing surgery for gastrointestinal cancer. A similar conclusion applied to a broader patient population is supported by a model that examines the financial implications of malnutrition and nutrition therapy.[102] This model takes

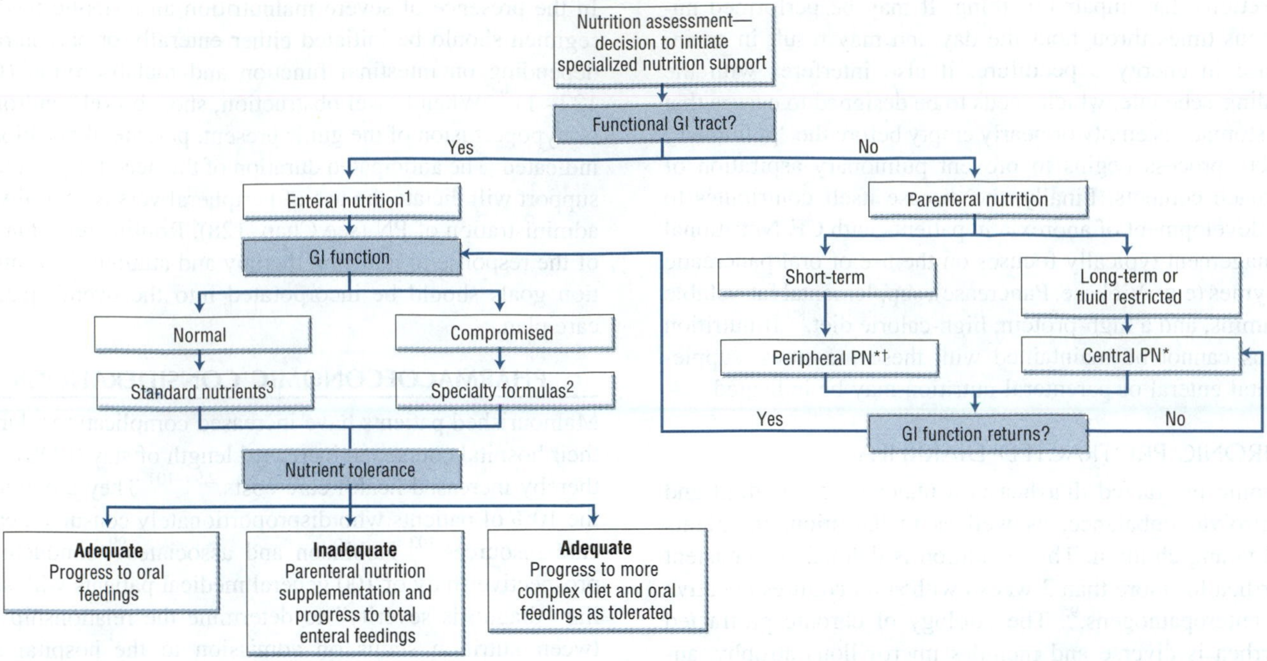

FIGURE 127–1. Routes to deliver nutrition support to adults: Clinical decision algorithm. *Formulation of enteral and parenteral solution should be made considering organ function (e.g., cardiac, renal, respiratory, hepatic). †In selected patients, peripheral parenteral nutrition may be considered to provide partial or total nutrition support for up to 2 weeks in patients who cannot ingest or absorb oral or enteral-tube delivered nutrients, or when central vein parenteral nutrition is not feasible. [1]Short-term: nasogastric, nasojejunal. Long-term: gastrostomy, jejunostomy. Feedings may be more appropriate distal to the pylorus if patient has increased risk of aspiration. [2]Formulas should be tailored to patient GI tolerance and includes elemental low/high fat content, lactose-free, fiber-rich, and modular formulas. [3]Polymeric, complete formulas are appropriate. *(From Ref. 98, with permission.)*

into consideration the increased costs associated with an increased LOS, morbidity and mortality caused by malnutrition as well as the costs of identifying patients at risk for malnutrition, providing nutrition support, and managing the complications associated with the nutrition support. Tucker and Miguel confirmed the association between poor nutritional status and prolonged length of hospital stay and also determined that when nutrition intervention occurred (oral, enteral, or parenteral nutrition), the average length of stay was decreased by 2.1 days.[97]

EVALUATION OF THERAPEUTIC OUTCOMES

Although the cost–benefit analysis of nutrition intervention is weak, the issue that seems clear is that malnutrition is associated with a significant morbidity and mortality in numerous disease states and clinical settings. Furthermore, it is likely that improved patient outcomes can be achieved by a systematic approach to identify the presence of risk factors for malnutrition, quantitate the degree of malnutrition, and initiate nutrition management.[104] The clinician's responsibilities in the management of nutrition disease include the following:

1. Assist in identifying patients at risk for malnutrition and/or candidates for nutrition intervention.
2. Assist in the design of patient-specific nutrition-support regimens.
3. Evaluate and manage all drug–nutrient interactions.
4. Evaluate laboratory data, especially parameters used to determine safety and efficacy of nutrition support.

REFERENCES

1. Gallagher-Allred DR, Coble Voss AC, Finn SC, et al. Malnutrition and clinical outcomes: The case for medical nutrition therapy. J Am Diet Assoc 1996;96:361–366.
2. Coats KG, Morgan SL, Bartolucci AA, Weinsier RL. Hospital-associated malnutrition: A re-evaluation 12 years later. J Am Diet Assoc 1993;93:27–33.
3. Hendricks KM, Duggan C, Gallagher L, et al.. Malnutrition in hospitalized pediatric patients. Arch Pediatr Adolesc Med 1995;149: 1118–1122.
4. CDC, Pediatric Nutrition Surveillance System—United States, 1980–1991. MMWR 1992;41(SS7):1–24.
5. Chandra RK. Nutrition and immunity: Lessons from the past and new insights into the future. Am J Clin Nutr 1991;53:1087–1101.
6. Bower RH. Nutrition and immune function. Nutr Clin Prac 1990;5: 189–195.
7. Albina JE. Nutrition and wound healing. JPEN J Parenter Enteral Nutr 1994;18:367–376.
8. Orgill D, Demling RH. Current concepts and approaches to wound healing. Crit Care Med 1988;16:8899–8908.
9. Dewys WD, Begg C, Lavin PT, et al. Prognostic effect of weight loss prior to chemotherapy in cancer patients. Am J Med 1980;69:491–497.

10. Rickard KA, Baehner RL, Coates TD, et al. Supportive nutritional intervention in pediatric cancer. Cancer Res 1982;42(suppl):766s–773s.
11. van Eys J. Malnutrition in children with cancer—incidence and consequence. Cancer 1979;43:2030–2035.
12. Weisdorf SA, Lysne J, Wind D, et al. Positive effect of prophylactic total parenteral nutrition on long-term outcome of bone marrow transplantation. Transplantation 1987;43:833–838.
13. Rickard KA, Detamore CM, Coates TD, et al. Effect of nutrition staging on treatment delays and outcome in stage IV neuroblastoma. Cancer 1983;52:587–598.
14. Mauer AM, Burgess JB, Donaldson SS, et al. Special nutritional needs of children with malignancies: A review. JPEN J Parenter Enteral Nutr 1990;14:315–324.
15. Holcomb GW, Ziegler MM. Nutrition and cancer in children. Surg Annu 1990:22:129–142.
16. Donaldson SS, Wesley MN, Ghavimi F, et al. A prospective randomized clinical trial of total parenteral nutrition in children with cancer. Med Pediatr Oncol 1982;10:129–139.
17. Klein S, Simes J, Blackburn G. TPN and cancer clinical trials. Cancer 1986;58:1378–1386.
18. Brennan MF. Uncomplicated starvation versus cancer cachexia. Cancer Res 1977;37:2359–2364.
19. Kern KA, Norton JA. Cancer cachexia. JPEN J Parenter Enteral Nutr 1988;12:286–298.
20. Raiten DJ. Nutrition and HIV. Nutr Clin Pract 1991;6(suppl):16S–52S.
21. ASPEN Board of Directors. Acquired immune deficiency syndrome. JPEN J Parenter Enteral Nutr 1993;17(suppl):13SA–14SA.
22. Kotler D, Tierney A, Wang J, et al. Magnitude of body-cell-mass depletion and the timing of death from wasting in AIDS. Am J Clin Nutr 1989;50:444–447.
23. Chlebowski RT, Grosvenor MB, Bernhard NH, et al. Nutritional status, gastrointestinal dysfunction, and survival in patients with AIDS. Am J Gastroenterol 1989;84:1288–1292.
24. Trujillo EB, Borlase BC, Bell SJ, et al. Assessment of nutritional status, nutrient intake, and nutrition support in AIDS patients. J Am Diet Assoc 1992;92:477–478.
25. Guenter P, Muurahainen N, Simons G, et al. Relationships among nutritional status, disease progression, and survival in HIV infection. J Acquir Immune Defic Syndr Hum Retrovirol 1993;6:1130–1138.
26. McKinney RE, Robertson JWR. Effect of human immunodeficiency virus infection on the growth of young children. J Pediatr 1993;123: 579–582.
27. Pollack H, Glasberg H, Lee E, et al. Impaired early growth of infants perinatally infected with human immunodeficiency virus: Correlation with viral load. J Pediatr 1997;130:915–922.
28. Brettler DB, Forsberg A, Bolivar E, et al. Growth failure as a prognostic indicator for progression to acquired immunodeficiency syndrome in children with hemophilia. J Pediatr 1990;117:584–588.
29. McKinney RE, Maha MA, Connor EM, et al. A multicenter trial of oral zidovudine in children with advanced human immunodeficiency virus disease. N Engl J Med 1991;324:1018–1025.
30. Kotler DP, Tierney AR, Culpepper-Morgan JA, et al. Effect of home total parenteral nutrition on body composition in patients with acquired immuno-deficiency syndrome. JPEN J Parenter Enteral Nutr 1990;14:454–458.
31. Kotler DP, Tierney AR, Ferraro R, et al. Enteral alimentation and repletion of body cell mass in malnourished patients with acquired immunodeficiency syndrome. Am J Clin Nutr 1991;53:149–154.
32. Singer P, Rothkopf MM, Kvetan V, et al. Risks and benefits of home parenteral nutrition in the acquired immunodeficiency syndrome. JPEN J Parenter Enteral Nutr 1991;15:75–79.
33. Barton RG. Nutrition support in critical illness. Nutr Clin Prac 1994; 9:127–139.
34. Cerra, FB, Benitez MR, Blackburn GL, et al. Applied nutrition in ICU patients: A consensus statement of the American College of Chest Physicians 1997:111:769–778.
35. Giner M, Laviano A, Meguid MM, Gleason JR. In 1995 a correlation between malnutrition and poor outcome in critically ill patients still exists. Nutrition 1996;12:23–29.
36. Peterson VM, Moore EE, Jones TN, et al. Total enteral nutrition versus total parenteral nutrition after major torso injury: Attenuation of hepatic protein reprioritization. Surgery 1988;104:199–207.
37. Chiarelli A, Enzi G, Casadei A, et al. Very early nutrition supplementation in burned patients. Am J Clin Nutr 1990;51:1035–1039.
38. Anderson JD, Moore FA, Moore EE. Enteral feeding in the critically injured patient. Nutr Clin Prac 1992;7:117–122.
39. Moore FA, Moore EE, Jones TN, et al. TEN versus TPN following major abdominal trauma—reduced septic morbidity. J Trauma 1989; 29:916–923.
40. Moore FA, Feliciano DV, Andrassy RJ, et al. Early enteral feeding, compared with parenteral, reduces postoperative septic complications. The results of a meta-analysis. Ann Surg 1992;216:172–183.
41. Kudsk KA, Croce MA, Fabian TC, et al. Enteral versus parenteral feeding. Effects on septic morbidity after blunt and penetrating abdominal trauma. Ann Surg 1992;215:503–513.
42. Kudsk KA, Minard G, Croce MA, et al. A randomized trial of isonitrogenous enteral diets after severe trauma. Ann Surg 1996;224: 531–543.
43. Jensen GL, Miller RH, Talabiska DG, et al. A double-blind, prospective, randomized study of glutamine-enriched compared with standard peptide-based feeding in critically ill patients. Am J Clin Nutr 1996;64:615–621.
44. Afonso JJ, Rombeau JL. Parenteral nutrition for patients with inflammatory bowel disease. In: Rombeau JL, Caldwell MD, eds. Clinical Nutrition: Parenteral Nutrition, 2nd ed. Philadelphia, W.B. Saunders, 1993:427–441.
45. Seidman EG, LeLeiko N, Ament M, et al. Nutritional issues in pediatric inflammatory bowel disease. Symposium report. J Pediatr Gastroenterol Nutr 1991;12:424–438.
46. ASPEN Board of Directors. Inflammatory bowel disease. JPEN J Parenter Enteral Nutr 1993;17(suppl):18SA–20SA, 45SA.
47. Vargas JH, Sachs P, Ament ME. Chronic intestinal pseudo-obstruction syndrome in pediatrics. Results of a national survey by members of the North American Society for Pediatric Gastroenterology and Nutrition. J Pediatr Gastroenterol Nutr 1988;7:323–332.
48. Thompson JS. Management of the short bowel syndrome. Gastroenterol Clin North Am 1994;23:403–419.
49. Thompson JS, Langnas AN, Pinch LW, et al. Surgical approach to short-bowel syndrome—experience in a population of 160 patients. Ann Surg 1995;222:600–607.
50. Touloukian RJ, Walker Smith GJ. Normal intestinal length in preterm infants. J Pediatr Surg 1983;18:720–723.
51. Bernard DKH, Shaw MJ. Principles of nutrition therapy for short-bowel syndrome. Nutr Clin Prac 1993;8:153–162.
52. ASPEN Board of Directors. Short bowel syndrome. J Parent Enteral Nutr 1993;17(suppl):19SA–20SA.
53. Figueroa-Colon R, Harris PR, Birdsong E, et al. Impact of intestinal lengthening on the nutritional outcome for children with short bowel syndrome. J Pediatr Surg 1996;31:912–916.
54. Thompson JS, Pinch LW, Vanderhoof JA, et al. Experience with intestinal lengthening for the short-bowel syndrome. J Pediatr Surg 1991;26:721–724.
55. Langnas AN, Shaw BW, Antonson DL, et al. Preliminary experience with intestinal transplantation in infants and children. Pediatrics 1996;97:443–448.
56. Studley HO. Percentage of weight loss: A basic indicator of surgical risk in patients with chronic septic ulcer. JAMA 1936;106: 458–460.
57. Mullen JL, Gertner MH, Buzby GP, et al. Implications of malnutrition in the surgical patient. Arch Surg 1979;114:121–125.
58. Rudman D, Feller AB, Nagraj HS, et al. Relation of serum albumin concentration to death rate in nursing home men. JPEN J Parenter Enteral Nutr 1987;11:360–363.

59. Meakins JL, Pietsch JB, Bubenick O, et al. Delayed hypersensitivity: An indicator of acquired failure of host defenses in sepsis and trauma. Ann Surg 1977;186:241–250.
60. Harvey KB, Ruggiero JA, Regan CS, et al. Hospital morbidity-mortality risk factors using nutritional assessment. J Clin Nutr 1978;26:251–257.
61. Kaminsky MV, Fitzgerald MJ, Murphy RJ, et al. Correlation of mortality with serum transferrin and anergy. JPEN J Parenter Enteral Nutr 1977;1:27A.
62. Kalfarentzos F, Spiliotis J, Velimezis G, et al. Comparison of forearm muscle dynamometry with nutritional prognostic index, as a preoperative indicator in cancer patients. JPEN J Parenter Enteral Nutr 1989;13:34–46.
63. Buzby GP, Mullen JL, Mathews DC, et al. Prognostic nutritional index in gastrointestinal surgery. Am J Surg 1980;139:160–166.
64. Halliday AW, Benjamin IS, Blumgart LH. Nutritional risk factors in major hepatobiliary surgery. JPEN J Parenter Enteral Nutr 1988;12:43–48.
65. Yamanaka H, Nishi M, Kanemaki T, et al. Preoperative nutritional assessment to predict postoperative complication in gastric cancer patients. JPEN J Parenter Enteral Nutr 1989;13:286–291.
66. Smale BF, Mullen JL, Buzby GP, Rosato EF. The efficacy of nutritional assessment and support in cancer surgery. Cancer 1981;47:2375–2381.
67. Dempsey DT, Buzby GP, Mullen JL. Nutritional assessment in the seriously ill patient. J Am Coll Nutr 1983;2:15–23.
68. Klein S, Kinney J, Jeejeebhoy K, et al. Nutrition support in clinical practice: Review of published data and recommendations for future research directions. JPEN J Parenter Enteral Nutr 1997;21:133–156.
69. Moghissi K, Hornshaw J, Teasdale PR, Dawes EA. Parenteral nutrition in carcinoma of the oesophagus treated by surgery: Nitrogen balance and clinical studies. Br J Surg 1977;64:125–128.
70. Askanazi J, Starker PM, Olsson C, et al. Effect of immediate postoperative nutritional support on length of hospitalization. Ann Surg 1986;203:236–239.
71. The Veterans Affairs Total Parenteral Nutrition Cooperative Study Group. Perioperative total parenteral nutrition. N Engl J Med 1991;325:525–532.
72. Daly JM, Lieberman MD, Goldfine J, et al. Enteral nutrition with supplemental arginine, RNA, and omega-3 fatty acids in patients after operation: Immunologic, metabolic, and clinical outcome. Surgery 1992;112:56–67.
73. Daly JM, Weintraub FN, Shou J, et al. Enteral nutrition during multimodality therapy in upper gastrointestinal cancer patients. Ann Surg 1995;221:327–338.
74. Northway WH. Bronchopulmonary dysplasia: Then and now. Arch Dis Child 1990;65:1076–1081.
75. deRegnier RA, Guilbert TW, Mills MM, Georgieff MK. Growth failure and altered body composition are established by one month of age in infants with bronchopulmonary dysplasia. J Nutr 1996;126:168–175.
76. Kurzner SI, Garg M, Bautusta DB, et al. Growth failure in infants with bronchopulmonary dysplasia: Nutrition and elevated resting metabolic expenditure. Pediatrics 1988;81:379–384.
77. de Gamarra E. Energy expenditure in premature newborns with bronchopulmonary dysplasia. Biol Neonate 1992;61:337–344.
78. Thureen PJ, Hay WW. Conditions requiring special nutritional management. In: Tsang RC, Lucas A, Uauy R, Zlotkin S, eds. Nutritional Needs of the Preterm Infant, Scientific Basis and Practical Guidelines. Pawling, NY: Williams & Wilkins, 1993:243–265.
79. Wilson DC, McClure G, Halliday HL, et al. Nutrition and bronchopulmonary dysplasia. Arch Dis Child 1991;66:37–38.
80. Kurzner SI, Garg M, Bautista DB, et al. Growth failure in bronchopulmonary dysplasia: Elevated metabolic rates and pulmonary mechanics. J Pediatr 1988;112:73–80.
81. Chye JK, Gray PH. Rehospitalization and growth of infants with bronchopulmonary dysplasia: A matched control study. J Paediatr Child Health 1995;31:105–111.
82. Tammela OKT, Koivisto ME. A 1-year follow-up of low birth weight infants with and without bronchopulmonary dysplasia: Health, growth, clinical lung disease, cardiovascular and neurological sequelae. Early Hum Dev 1992;30:109–120.
83. Yu VYH, Orgill AA, Lim SB, et al. Growth and development of very low birth weight infants recovering from bronchopulmonary dysplasia. Arch Dis Child 1983;58:791–794.
84. Robertson CMT, Etches PC, Goldson E, Kyle JM. Eight-year school performance, neurodevelopmental, and growth outcome of neonates with bronchopulmonary dysplasia: A comparative study. Pediatrics 1992;89:365–372.
85. Vrienich LA, Bozynski MEA, Shyr Y, et al. The effect of bronchopulmonary dysplasia on growth at school age. Pediatrics 1995:95:855–859.
86. ASPEN Board of Directors. Necrotizing enterocolitis. JPEN J Parenter Enteral Nutr 1993;17(suppl):SA37.
87. Walsh MC, Kliegman RM, Hack M. Severity of necrotizing enterocolitits: Influence on outcome at 2 years of age. Pediatrics 1989;84:808–814.
88. Abbasi S, Pereira GR, Johnson L, et al. Long-term assessment of growth, nutritional status, and gastrointestinal function in survivors of necrotizing entercolitis. J Pediatr 1984;104:550–554.
89. Lai H, Kosorok MR, Sondel SA, et al. Growth status in children with cystic fibrosis based on the national Cystic Fibrosis Patient Registry data: evaluation of various criteria used to identify malnutrition. J Pediatr 1998:132:478–485.
90. Roulet M. Protein-energy malnutrition in cystic fibrosis patients. Acta Paediatr 1994;395(suppl):43–48.
91. Ramsay BW, Farrell PM, Penchartz P, et al. Consensus report: Nutritional assessment and management of cystic fibrosis. Am J Clin Nutr 1992;55:108–116.
92. Stallings VA, Fung EB, Hofley PM, Scanlin TF. Acute pulmonary exacerbation is not associated with increased energy expenditure in children with cystic fibrosis. J Pediatr 1998;132:493–499.
93. Erskine JM, Lingard CD, Sontage MK, Accurso FJ. Enteral nutrition for patients with cystic fibrosis: Comparison of a semi-elemental and non-elemental formula. J Pediatr 1998;132:265–269.
94. Ellis L, Kalnins D, Corey M, et al. Do infants with cystic fibrosis need a protein hydrolystate formula? A prospective, randomized, comparative study. J Pediatr 1998;132:270–276.
95. Walker-Smith JA. Intractable diarrhoea in infancy: A continuing challenge for the paediatric gastroenterologist. Acta Paediatr 1994;395(suppl):6–9.
96. Kleinman RE, Galeano NF, Ghishan F, et al. Nutritional management of chronic diarrhea and/or malabsorption. J Pediatr Gastroenterol Nutr 1989;9:407–415.
97. Smith AE, Powers CA, Cooper-Meyer RA, Lloyd-Still JD. Improved nutritional management reduces length of hospitalization in intractable diarrhea. JPEN J Parenter Enteral Nutr 1986;10:479–481.
98. ASPEN Board of Directors. Routes to deliver nutrition support to adults: Clinical decision algorithm. In: Clinical Pathways and Algorithms for Delivery of Parenteral and Enteral Nutrition Support in Adults. Silver Spring, MD: ASPEN, 1998:5.
99. Robinson G, Goldstein M, Levine GM. Impact of nutritional status on DRG length of stay. JPEN J Parenter Enteral Nutr 1987;11:49–51.
100. Reilly JJ, Hull SF, Albert N, et al. Economic impact of malnutrition: A model system for hospitalized patients. JPEN J Parenter Enteral Nutr 1988;12:371–376.
101. Tucker HN, Miguel SG. Cost containment through nutrition intervention. Nutr Rev 1996;54:111–121.
102. Bernstein LH, Shaw-Stiffel TA, Schorow M, Brouillette R. Financial implications of malnutrition. Clin Lab Med 1993;13:491–507.
103. Twomey PL, Patching SC. Cost-effectiveness of nutritional support. JPEN J Parenter Enteral Nutr 1985;9:3–10.
104. ASPEN Board of Directors. Rationale for adult nutrition support guidelines. JPEN J Parenter Enteral Nutr 1993;17(suppl):5SA–6SA.

128

PARENTERAL NUTRITION

Todd W. Mattox, BCNSP

Maintenance of adequate nutrition status during illness has long been recognized as an integral part of the medical treatment plan for patients who are unable to use normal physiologic means of nourishment.[1,2] Successful techniques for providing intravenous nutrition support were introduced to clinical practice in the early 1960s.[3] Dilute nutrient solutions containing glucose with or without hydrolyzed protein were infused peripherally along with intravenous fat emulsion to provide adequate calories. However, early intravenous fat emulsions made of cottonseed oil were withdrawn from commercial availability in the United States in 1965 following several reports of serious adverse effects. Without lipid emulsions, larger volumes of nutrient solutions were required to provide the patient's energy requirements. Patients receiving intravenous nutrition solution volumes of up to 5 L/d were often given concomitant diuretic therapy to manage fluid status.[3] Metabolic complications associated with fluid overload and electrolyte imbalances stimulated the investigation of central venous access. These larger vessels permitted infusion of more concentrated formulas thus decreasing the fluid volume required and avoiding the phlebitis that commonly occurred when hypertonic infusions were given peripherally.

By the late 1960s, Rhoads and Dudrick[3] had documented continued growth and improvement in nutrition markers in humans with the use of central intravenous nutrition. As the use of intravenous nutrition became more widespread, reports of complications increased. During the subsequent 20 to 25 years, clinical experience and research resulted in the development of standard protocols, which promoted better patient care and a decline in complications associated with parenteral nutrition (PN) therapy.[4] The scope of practice for nutrition support clinicians has broadened as a result of increasing knowledge about the metabolic consequences associated with acute injury and chronic disease states and the increase in the number of products, techniques, and equipment designed for use in providing nutrition care. Depending on the level of nutrition intervention required, nutrition support clinicians may use specially formulated parenteral or enteral nutrients to maintain or restore optimal nutrition status.[5] The pharmacist's role in providing safe and effective nutrition support care requires a clear understanding of the principles of patient selection, initial therapy design, preparation and dispensing of the feeding formulation, and outcome monitoring[6–8] (Table 128–1). This chapter reviews indications for PN, components of PN formulations, routes of intravenous administration, practical aspects of regimen design, solution admixture, outcome monitoring, and management of complications.

The overall objective of nutrition support therapy is to promote positive clinical outcomes of an illness or improve a patient's quality of life. Four fundamental steps are key to providing optimal care for patients who require nutrition support: (1) definition of nutrition goals, (2) determination of nutrient requirements for achievement of the nutrition goals, (3) delivery of the required nutrients, and (4) subsequent assessment of the nutrition regimen.[9,10]

A patient's nutrition goals can be established after a thorough nutritional assessment (see Chap. 126). Nutrient requirements and an appropriate route for delivery of the required nutrients can then be determined (see Chaps. 126 and 127). Goals of nutrition support include correction of caloric and nitrogen imbalances, fluid or electrolyte abnormalities, and any known vitamin or trace element abnormalities without causing or worsening other metabolic complications. Specific caloric goals include energy equilibrium and preservation of fat calorie stores in well-nourished individuals and positive energy balance in malnourished patients with depleted endogenous fat stores. Obese patients with excess endogenous fat stores (> 120% ideal body weight) likely require less caloric support than nonobese patients within a range of negative energy balance to energy equilibrium depending on the clinical condition of the patient.[11] Specific nitrogen goals are positive nitrogen balance or nitrogen equilibrium and improvement in the serum concentration of a short half-life visceral protein marker such as transferrin or prealbumin.

The gastrointestinal (GI) tract is the optimal route for providing nutrients unless obstruction, pancreatitis, or other GI complications are present[12] (see Chap. 127, Fig. 127–1). Other considerations that may impact determination of an appropriate route for nutrition support include expected duration of nutrition therapy and risk of aspiration. Patients who have a nonfunctional GI tract or are otherwise not a candidate for enteral nutrition (EN) may benefit from PN. Use of the intravenous route for nutrition support is also commonly referred to as total parenteral nutrition (TPN) or hyperalimentation. Routine monitoring is necessary to ensure the nutrition regimen is suitable for a given patient as his or her clinical condition changes and to minimize or treat complications early.

INDICATIONS FOR NUTRITION SUPPORT

Although improvement in nutrition status as defined by various clinical nutrition markers has been reported in patients

TABLE 128–1. Scope of Practice for Nutrition Support Pharmacists

Assessment of the patient's nutrition care needs
- Determine nutrient requirements based on patient's data.
- Prevent and/or identify nutrient–nutrient, drug–nutrient, drug–drug, and drug–disease/condition interactions.
- Assess suitability for specialized nutrition support.

Development of a nutrition care plan
- Define goals and objectives of specialized nutrition support therapy.
- Select the preferred route for administration of nutrition support therapy.
- Design patient-specific feeding formulations.

Implementation of the nutrition care plan
- Obtain or write prescriptions for feeding formulations.
- Be proficient with techniques of compounding feeding formulations.
- Perform or supervise the compounding and dispensing of parenteral feeding formulations.

Monitoring the patient's response to the nutrition therapy
- Evaluate laboratory data to determine the patient's clinical, nutritional, and metabolic responses to specialized nutrition support.
- Prevent and/or identify nutrient–nutrient, drug–nutrient, drug–drug, and drug–disease/condition interactions.
- Evaluate continued need for specialized nutrition support.

Administrative management
- Participate in development of policy and procedures for patient care and operational aspects of specialized nutrition support.

Quality of care
- Develop and implement quality improvement activities directed at the process of nutritional and metabolic care.

Advancement of nutrition support pharmacy practice
- Contribute to the professional development of pharmacists and other health care professionals and to the education of patients through presentations, publications, and research.

Adapted from Ref. 6.

who received PN, the impact on clinical outcome has been difficult to demonstrate. Several investigations have reported a positive effect of PN on complications and mortality whereas others have failed to demonstrate any difference.[13] Early studies have been criticized for defects in study design such as small sample sizes, inappropriate randomization, and inconsistent baseline nutrition status among the study group, which hindered demonstration of the effectiveness of PN therapy. However, the association between malnutrition and development of complications and mortality has been well documented.[14,15] These conflicting data have complicated identification of the patient who is most likely to benefit from PN. Current guidelines are based on clinical experience and investigations of PN in specific patient populations where PN therapy is often prone to misuse, such as presurgical patients or patients receiving chemotherapy[10,16,17] (Table 128–2). The revised guidelines of the American Society for Parenteral and Enteral Nutrition (ASPEN) Board of Directors address the indications for PN.[17] This statement includes an evaluation of references reviewed in the report based on a strength-of-evidence grading system developed by the Agency for Health Care Policy and Research (AHCPR). Clinical guidelines are also graded based on an AHCPR code, which designates if the recommendation is based on good or fair research-based evidence, or if the recommendation is based on expert opinion. Although approximately 16% of the ASPEN guidelines were judged to be based on good research-based evidence, the majority are based on expert opinion rather than scientifically conducted studies.[18] However, these guidelines provide a degree of specificity, which should facilitate institutional development of appropriate PN usage guidelines. In a continued effort to define appropriate candidates for specialized nutrition intervention, representatives from the National Institutes of Health, ASPEN, and the American Society of Clinical Nutrition authored a critical review of the clinical use of nutrition support. The group focused on nutrition assessment; nutrition support in patients with gastrointestinal diseases, wasting diseases, and critical illness; and perioperative nutrition support.[19] The conclusions of the group were graded using a modified AHCPR format. Although the intent of the report is to identify future directions for research, this report may be useful in evaluating an institution's current practices based on the previous ASPEN guidelines.

PARENTERAL NUTRITION COMPONENTS

Parenteral nutrition solutions should provide the optimal combination of macronutrients and micronutrients to meet the specific nutritional requirements of the patient. Macronutrients include water, protein, dextrose, and intravenous lipid emulsion. Micronutrients include vitamins, trace elements, and electrolytes. Both macronutrients and micronutrients are necessary for maintenance of normal metabolism. In general, macronutrients are utilized for energy (dextrose, fat) and as structural substrates (protein, fats). Micronutrients are usually required in smaller amounts to support a variety of metabolic activities necessary for cellular homeostasis such as enzymatic reactions, fluid balance,

TABLE 128–2. Indications for TPN

1. Inability to absorb nutrients via the gastrointestinal tract because of one or more of the following:
   a. Massive small bowel resection.
      Usually patients with a jejunostomy and < 100 cm of jejunum or patients with an intact colon and < 50 cm of jejunum or ileum.
   b. Intractable vomiting when adequate enteral intake is not expected for 5–7 days.
   c. Severe diarrhea not expected to resolve in 5–7 days.
   d. Inflammatory bowel disease (Crohn's disease, ulcerative colitis)
      PN may benefit patients with acute exacerbations of ulcerative colitis when surgery is being considered and when preservation of lean body mass and functional capacity with enteral nutrition is impossible.
   e. Bowel obstruction
2. Cancer: antineoplastic therapy, radiation therapy, bone marrow transplantation
   Enteral tube feeding and parenteral nutrition support may benefit some severely malnourished cancer patients or those in whom gastrointestinal or other toxicities are anticipated to preclude adequate oral nutritional intake for more than 1 week. Patients who are candidates for nutrition intervention under these circumstances should receive nutrition support, if possible, in conjunction with the initiation of oncologic therapy. Specialized nutrition support is not routinely indicated for well-nourished or mildly malnourished patients undergoing surgery, chemotherapy, or radiation treatment and in whom adequate oral intake is anticipated.
   PN is unlikely to benefit patients with advanced cancer whose malignancy is documented as unresponsive to chemotherapy or radiation therapy.
3. Moderate to severe pancreatitis when adequate enteral intake is not expected for 5–7 days.
   PN should be used when enteral feeding exacerbates abdominal pain, ascites, or fistula output in patients with pancreatitis and limited oral intake.
4. Severe malnutrition[a] with a temporary (5–7 days) nonfunctional gastrointestinal tract.
5. Critical care
   Moderate to severe catabolism with or without malnutrition when the gastrointestinal tract is nonfunctional for 5–7 days. (e.g., major surgery, trauma, sepsis).
6. Organ failures (liver, renal, respiratory)
   Moderate to severe catabolism with or without malnutrition when enteral feeding is contraindicated.
7. Preoperative malnutrition[a] when the gastrointestinal tract is not functional and surgery is not expected for at least 7 days.
8. Hyperemesis gravidarum
9. Eating disorders
   PN should be considered for patients with anorexia nervosa who require nonvolitional feeding but who cannot tolerate enteral support for physical or emotional reasons.

[a]Malnutrition (upon initial assessment):
- 0–5% weight loss over past 6 months and serum albumin < 3.0 g/%.[61]
- 10–15% weight loss over past 6 months and serum albumin < 3.5 g/%.[61]
- Loss of 10% of pre-illness weight, decreased serum albumin concentration.[17]

and regulation of electrophysiologic processes. These components usually require individualized adjustments as the patient's clinical condition dictates because of changes in metabolic stress, organ function, fluid and electrolyte balance, and acid–base status.

AMINO ACIDS

Protein in PN solutions is provided in the form of crystalline amino acids (CAAs), which are utilized primarily for protein synthesis. Including the caloric contribution from protein when calculating calories provided by the PN regimen is controversial.[20] Although sufficient energy substrate should be provided to allow utilization of amino acids for protein synthesis rather than an energy source, oxidation of amino acids for energy has been demonstrated in critically ill patients and is thought to occur because of metabolic derangements seen during severe metabolic stress.[21] Hence, some practice settings may differ in expressing calories provided by a PN regimen as total calories (protein, carbohydrate, and fat calories) or nonprotein calories (carbohydrate and fat calories). When oxidized for energy, 1 g of protein yields 4 kilocalories (kcal).

Commercially available CAA solutions may be categorized as standard amino acid solutions or modified amino acid solutions. Standard CAA solutions are designed for use in patients with "normal" organ function and nutritional requirements (Table 128–3). Although commercially available CAA solutions differ in exact proportions of specific amino acids, they contain a balanced profile of essential, semiessential, and nonessential L-amino acids. Despite these differences, similar effects on markers of protein utilization have been reported.[22,23] These products also differ in total nitrogen content, electrolyte content, and commercially available concentrations. Differences in nitrogen content per gram of amino acids among CAA products may affect calculation of nitrogen amounts infused when determining nitrogen balance.[24] Because the nitrogen concentration of dietary protein is approximately 16%, 6.25 (100 g protein/16 g nitrogen) is commonly accepted as the conversion figure for calculating the amount of nitrogen provided by CAA protein when calculating nitrogen balance. However, the nitrogen

TABLE 128–3. Macronutrient Components of Parenteral Nutrition Solutions

Nutritional Substrate	Intravenous Source	Commercial Product (Manufacturer)		Comments
Fluid	Sterile water for injection USP	Various manufacturers		
Nitrogen	Crystalline amino acids			
	• Standard solutions	Aminosyn Aminosyn II FreAmine III Travasol Clinisol	(Abbott) (Abbott) (McGaw) (Travenol) (Clintec)	Contain a balanced profile of essential, semi-essential, and non-essential L-amino acids
	• Disease-specific solutions			
	Hepatic encephalopathy	Aminosyn HF Hepatasol Hepatamine	(Abbott) (Clintec) (McGaw)	Amino acid profile includes higher concentrations of BCAA and lower concentrations of AAA and methionine.
	Renal failure	Aminosyn RF RenAmine Aminess NephrAmine	(Abbott) (Clintec) (Clintec) (R & D Laboratories)	Amino acid profile includes higher concentrations of EAA and histidine.
	Metabolic stress/trauma	Aminosyn HBC BranchAmin[a] FreAmine HBC	(Abbott) (Clintec) (McGaw)	Amino acid profile provides standard essential, semi-essential, and non-essential amino acids with higher concentrations of BCAA
	Pediatrics	Aminosyn PF Trophamine	(Abbott) (McGaw)	Amino acid profile includes standard essential, semi-essential, and non-essential amino acids with lower concentrations of methionine, phenylalanine, and glycine. These solutions also contain taurine, glutamate, and aspartate.
	Intravenous dipeptides			
	• L-Alanyl-L-glutamine			Investigational
	• Glycyl-L-tyrosine			Investigational
	• L-Alanyl-L-tyrosine			Investigational
	• N-acetyl-L-tyrosine			Used in Trophamine (McGaw)
Energy				
Carbohydrate	Dextrose	Various manufacturers		
	Glycerol			Used in Procalamine (McGaw)
	Xylitol			Investigational
Fat	Intravenous fat emulsion			
	• LCT emulsions {oil source}	Liposyn II Liposyn III Intralipid Neutrilipid	(Abbott) (Abbott) (Clintec) (McGaw)	{soybean/safflower} {soybean} {soybean} {soybean}
	• LCT/MCT combination			Investigational
	• Short-chain fatty acids			Investigational
	• Omega-3 fatty acids			Investigational

BCAA = Branched-chain amino acids (leucine, isoleucine, valine); AAA = aromatic amino acids (includes phenylalanine and tyrosine).
EAA = essential amino acids (leucine, isoleucine, valine, phenylalanine, tryptophan, methionine, threonine, and lysine); LCT = long-chain triglycerides; MCT = medium-chain triglyceride.
[a]Used as a supplement to a standard amino acid solution to increase BCAA content.

content of commercially available CAA solutions varies from approximately 11% to 17% per gram of amino acid.[24] The clinical significance of these differences in calculations of nitrogen balance for routine clinical use is not known.[24,25]

Electrolyte composition of standard CAA solutions varies from small, obligatory amounts to the provision of maintenance requirement of most electrolytes for an adult. The contribution of electrolytes from CAA solutions must be considered when determining a patient's individual requirements. The availability of CAA in several different concentrations facilitates compounding of patient-specific PN regimens. Highly concentrated products (10% and 15%) are attractive for use in critically ill patients, who typically require fluid restriction but have large protein needs.[26] Modified amino acid solutions are designed for use in patients who have altered protein requirements such as those with hepatic encephalopathy, renal failure, metabolic stress/trauma, and neonates and pediatric patients (Table 128–3). These solutions tend to be more expensive than standard CAA solutions. The rationale for use and clinical efficacy of modified amino acids in disease-specific PN regimens is controversial (see Chap. 131). Commercially available CAA solutions have been altered by some to provide conditionally essential amino acids (CEAAs) in PN solutions. CEAAs are considered nonessential because they are produced from other amino acids during health. However, under certain physiologic conditions such as the perinatal period, or pathophysiologic conditions such as sepsis, these amino acids cannot be synthesized in sufficient quantities.[23] Because some amino acids are relatively unstable or poorly soluble, certain desirable alterations of the composition of CAA solutions may not be clinically feasible. Dipeptide amino acids have been investigated as a potential parenteral source for CEAAs that may provide a solution to overcoming these limitations. Dipeptides are synthesized by combining two amino acids with a peptide bond. The resulting protein is more soluble and stable than the individual amino acids.[27] Intravenous dipeptide formulations would be clinically advantageous since they incorporate higher concentrations of some specific amino acids, as well as some low-solubility, low-stability amino acids that are omitted or present in small quantities in current CAA solutions. In addition, use of dipeptides would allow formulation of CAA solutions with a higher nitrogen content. Further studies are needed to assess long-term safety and optimal combinations of amino acids in different disease states.[28] Examples of those amino acid combinations currently under investigation in humans or present in current CAA products are listed in Table 128–3.

DEXTROSE

The primary energy source in PN solutions is carbohydrate, usually in the form of dextrose monohydrate. This nutritional substrate is available in a variety of concentrations ranging from 5% to 70%. When oxidized, each gram of hydrated dextrose provides 3.4 kcal. Dextrose is oxidized at a maximum rate of 4 to 7 mg/kg/min in humans receiving TPN.[29] When the dextrose infusion rate exceeds 7 mg/kg/min, it is used by the liver for repletion of glycogen stores and lipid synthesis. Higher infusion rates may also contribute to development of metabolic complications such as hyperglycemia, excess carbon dioxide production, lipogenesis, and increased liver function tests secondary to fatty liver.[30] Recommended doses for routine clinical care rarely exceed 5 mg/kg/min.[10,31] Insulin is essential to transport dextrose into many cells such as skeletal muscle for oxidation to yield energy. Because critically ill patients tend to develop stress-related hyperglycemia, which may complicate the provision of PN, non-insulin-dependent sources of carbohydrate have been investigated[32] (Table 128–3). Those that have received the most attention are xylitol, sorbitol, fructose, and glycerol. Of these nutrients only glycerol is recommended for clinical use in humans as a carbohydrate source for PN. Glycerol is a sugar alcohol that provides 4.3 kcal/g and is commercially available as a 3% solution in combination with 3% amino acids and supplemental electrolytes (Procalamine, McGaw). This product is nearly isotonic so it may be infused peripherally. A major disadvantage with the use of this formula is the dilute concentrations of amino acids and carbohydrate. Most patients may require up to 3 to 4 L/d of Procalamine solution together with lipid emulsion as a caloric source to provide minimum energy requirements.[33]

LIPID EMULSION

Intravenous lipid emulsion (IVLE) may be used as a concentrated source of calories as well as a source of essential fatty acids. Current IVLE products differ in source of triglycerides (soybean oil or a combination of soybean oil and safflower oil), fatty acid content, and commercially available concentrations (10%, 20%, and 30%) (Table 128–3). These products also contain egg phospholipids as an emulsifying agent and glycerol to make the emulsion isotonic. Although the caloric contribution of fat is 9 kcal/g, the caloric content of IVLE is 1.1 kcal/mL for 10% emulsion, 2 kcal/mL for 20% emulsion, and 3 kcal/mL for 30% emulsion because of the caloric contribution of the egg phospholipid and glycerol.[34] The sources of triglyceride in IVLE differ in fatty acid composition. Soybean oil emulsions contain approximately 50% to 60% linoleic acid and 4% to 11% linolenic acid, whereas IVLEs that contain safflower oil consist of approximately 66% linoleic acid and 4% linolenic acid.[34] Linolenic acid, an omega-3 fatty acid, and linoleic acid, an omega-6 fatty acid, are both polyunsaturated long-chain triglycerides (LCTs).

Both types of IVLE are effective in the treatment or prevention of essential fatty acid deficiency (EFAD). EFAD is the result of a biochemical deficiency of linoleic acid and arachidonic acid, which are considered essential in humans. Although linolenic acid may not be essential, all commercially available IVLEs contain soybean oil as the predominant source of linolenic acid. These fatty acids are important for a variety of functions such as cellular integrity, platelet function, and wound healing.[35,36] Normally, linoleic acid is converted to the tetraene arachidonic acid. When linoleic acid is not present in sufficient amounts, oleic acid is converted to the triene 5,8,11-eicosatrienoic acid, a fatty acid of lesser physiologic integrity, and EFAD occurs. EFAD may be prevented by providing 2% to 5% of total calories as linoleic acid. This may be achieved in most patients by giving 500 mL of 10% fat emulsion two to three times weekly.[35]

As a caloric source, lipid emulsion is most useful in metabolically stressed patients, those with pancreatitis or diabetes, and carbon dioxide–retaining ventilator dependent patients.[37] The use of lipid emulsion may facilitate provision of adequate calories and minimize complications of nutrition therapy such as hyperglycemia, hepatotoxicity, or increased production of carbon dioxide (see Chap. 131). The dose of IVLE in adults should not exceed 2.5 g/kg/d or 60% of total daily calories. Lipid emulsion may be infused over a minimum of 4 to 8 hours. However, data in animals and humans suggest that rapid infusion of the current long-chain fatty acid formulations may negatively impact immunocompetence by saturating the reticuloendothelial system.[36,38] Provision of approximately 1 to 1.5 g/kg/d, not to exceed 30% to 40% of total calories infused over 24 hours, appears to be the best clinical strategy for providing IVLE because there is no clear consensus regarding the effect of IVLE on morbidity and mortality.[10,36,37]

The manufacturer's guidelines recommend initiating lipid emulsion infusions with a test dose of 0.5 mL/min for the first 15 to 30 minutes. In most patients, this is probably not necessary because of the relatively low incidence and benign nature of acute adverse reactions. In addition, infusions over 24 hours eliminate the need for a test dose because the infusion rate is less than the test dose rate recommended by the manufacturer. Commercially available 10% and 20%, IVLE products may be administered either by central or peripheral vein. They may be added directly to the parenteral nutrition solution as a total nutrient admixture (TNA) or 3-in-1 system (lipids, protein, glucose, and additives) or they may be piggybacked with the CAA/dextrose solution.[37] The more concentrated 30% IVLE is approved for use only in the preparation of TNA and is not intended for direct intravenous administration. In general, the use of IVLE is contraindicated in patients with an impaired ability to clear lipid emulsion such as patients with pathologic hyperlipidemia and hypertriglyceridemia associated with pancreatitis.[39]

Patients who are allergic to eggs should be carefully evaluated for the nature and severity of the reaction before deciding to initiate a lipid-based PN regimen. Most of the more toxic reactions such as impaired liver function, thrombocytopenia, prolonged clotting time, and spontaneous bleeding were reported in the early 1960s with the intravenous use of Lipomul, a cottonseed oil emulsion that was subsequently withdrawn from the market. Although the frequency of acute adverse effects is reported to be less than 1% with current formulations, patients receiving their first dose of lipid emulsion should be monitored for dyspnea, chest tightness, palpitations, and chills. Headache, nausea, and fever have also been reported and may be associated with a rapid infusion rate. Hepatic abnormalities such as elevated transaminases, hepatomegaly, and intrahepatic cholestasis have been reported with multiple infusions, although these alterations are transient and are usually associated with excessive doses.[37]

The negative effects of LCTs on immune function have stimulated a search for new sources of lipids.[36,37] Medium-chain triglycerides (MCTs) may offer several advantages, especially for critically ill patients. MCTs are more rapidly hydrolyzed and cleared than LCTs and do not accumulate in the liver. In addition, MCTs do not require carnitine for entrance into mitochondria for oxidation. However, MCTs are not a source of essential fatty acids. Furthermore, in early studies of pure MCTs in animals and humans, central nervous toxicities and other significant adverse effects such as dyspnea and vomiting, which appeared to be dose related, were reported.[36,40] Subsequent studies of intravenous MCT/LCT mixtures in a variety of patients have demonstrated safety and efficacy comparable to standard LCT emulsions.[36,38,40] Several MCT/LCT products are available in Europe, although no intravenous MCT formulations are currently commercially available in the United States. Other intravenous lipid formulations currently being investigated contain omega-3 polyunsaturated fatty acids (PUFAs).[41,42] Current IVLEs contains omega-6 PUFAs as linoleic acid and omega-3 PUFAs as linolenic acid. Omega-3 PUFAs are metabolized to cytokine mediators, which may be less inflammatory and immunosuppressive than those derived from omega-6 PUFAs.[36] Investigations of enteral solutions with a higher concentration of omega-3 PUFAs have reported decreased infections and improvement in *in vitro* immunologic indices in critically ill patients.[36,43] However, the optimal balance of omega-3 and omega-6 PUFAs required to achieve the greatest desired change in metabolism for different disease states is not known.[36,44]

Although IVLE products remain the most common source of parenteral lipids, a variety of drugs have been introduced that contain lipid as either a vehicle for delivery or a portion of the drug molecular formulation. Propofol, an intravenous anesthetic, is delivered in a soybean oil-in-water emulsion that is essentially the same as Intralipid 10%. This agent is commonly used for continuous sedation of ventilated patients and should be considered a potentially significant source of calories that may require adjustment of a patient's nutrition regimen.[45] The antifungal amphotericin B is available in several lipid-containing combinations such as liposomal and lipid complex formulations. The caloric contribution from these products when used in standard doses is generally small and is not clinically relevant.[46] Although use of amphotericin B with IVLE admixtures is controversial, the caloric contribution from these mixtures is significant and should be considered when determining a patient's nutrition regimen.[46]

VITAMINS

Vitamins are necessary for the maintenance of normal metabolism and cellular function. Fat-soluble vitamins (A, D, E, K) are extensively stored in the body's fat tissue, whereas water-soluble vitamins are stored in limited amounts by the body. Maintenance guidelines for daily parenteral vitamin supplements have been established by the Nutrition Advisory Group of the American Medical Association (NAG–AMA) for adults, children, and infants.[47] These guidelines are based on the recommended daily allowances (RDAs), which are designed to meet requirements of healthy people. Vitamin requirements during metabolic stress or specific organ failures have not been fully agreed upon.[10,48,49] Revised NAG–AMA recommendations for parenteral vitamin requirements in infants and children reflect data reported in pediatric patients who received currently available formulations.[50] The revised recommendations primarily focus on changes for preterm infants requiring PN.

Several commercially available adult and pediatric multiple vitamin products have been formulated to comply with the NAG–AMA guidelines. Parenteral multiple vitamin products for adults do not contain vitamin K to avoid a drug–nutrient interaction in patients receiving anticoagulants, which antagonize vitamin K. The NAG–AMA recommendation for vitamin K in adults is 2 to 4 mg weekly. However, others have recommended larger doses of 5 to 10 mg weekly.[49] Vitamin K may be given intramuscularly or subcutaneously or added to the PN solution.[51] Vitamin requirements may be altered in malnutrition and other specific disease states or with certain drug therapies. Individual and combination products are available to provide additional or tailored supplementation, which may be necessary to prevent development of vitamin toxicities or deficiencies caused by altered metabolism or drug therapy.

TRACE ELEMENTS

Trace elements are minerals that are required in very small amounts for a variety of biochemical and physiologic functions. Many trace elements are an important part of metalloenzymes and also function as cofactors in a variety of regulatory metabolic pathways.[52,53] Although 17 trace elements have demonstrated biologic importance, clear deficiency syndromes in humans have been described only for iron, iodine, cobalt (as vitamin B_{12}), zinc, and copper.[52–54] The NAG–AMA recognized zinc, copper, and chromium as being essential for intravenous supplementation in patients receiving PN.[55] Although a clear deficiency syndrome for manganese has not been reported in humans, the NAG–AMA considered manganese essential based on case reports of patients receiving PN with metabolic complications that corrected after manganese supplementation.[48,53,55] More recent reports of syndromes associated with selenium and molybdenum deficiency suggest that they may also be essential. However, recommendations for supplemental dosing of the two do not agree.[48,52,56] Recommendations for trace elements in pediatric patients receiving PN have been revised as well.[50]

Intravenous trace elements are available as single mineral solutions and as multiple mineral combinations with or without electrolytes. Most products were formulated to provide daily requirements for the trace minerals considered essential by the NAG–AMA (zinc, copper, chromium, and manganese), although some products may also include iodide, molybdenum, or selenium. Routine use of these trace elements during short-term PN is controversial. Currently, little evidence exists to support routine supplementation of the other trace elements in patients receiving PN. Requirements for trace elements are age specific and may change depending on the clinical condition of the patient. For example, higher doses of supplemental zinc are likely necessary in patients with high-output ostomies or diarrhea because the predominant route of excretion for zinc is via the GI tract. Manganese and copper are excreted through the biliary tract, whereas chromium, molybdenum, and selenium are excreted renally. Hence, these trace elements should be restricted or withheld from PN solutions in patients with cholestatic liver disease and renal failure, respectively. Although trace element requirements during organ failure are not clearly defined, a clinically practical method of empirically reducing trace element doses when using a multiple trace element solution is to give the recommended daily dose two to three times weekly instead of daily.[57]

ELECTROLYTES

Electrolytes such as sodium, potassium, calcium, magnesium, phosphorus, chloride, and acetate are necessary components of PN for the maintenance of numerous cellular functions, including acid–base balance and cellular growth. Electrolytes may be given to maintain normal serum concentrations or to correct deficits. Patients who have "normal" organ function and relatively normal serum concentrations of any electrolyte should receive normal maintenance doses of electrolytes on initiation of PN and daily thereafter. Requirements for specific electrolytes will vary according to the patient's disease state, organ function (see Chap. 131), previous and current drug therapy, nutrition status, and extrarenal losses such as nasogastric suction, vomiting, diarrhea, or fistulas (see Table 128–4). Electrolytes are commercially available as single-nutrient and multiple-nutrient solutions. Multiple-electrolyte solutions are useful in stable patients with normal organ function who are receiving PN. Concentrated multiple-electrolyte solutions designed for addition to PN solutions generally contain only sodium, potassium, calcium, and magnesium. Phosphorus must be added separately. Further information regarding metabolism and requirements of vitamins, trace elements, and electrolytes is given elsewhere.[48,49,58]

DESIGNING A PN REGIMEN

Several factors including available venous access, fluid status of the patient, and macronutrient and micronutrient requirements are important considerations when designing a patient-specific PN regimen. A patient's venous access and fluid status will determine how concentrated the PN solution may be compounded and, hence, will have impact on the amount of nutrient that may be provided. Parenteral nutrition solutions may be administered by central or peripheral venous access. The clinical condition of the patient will determine which route is most appropriate (Fig. 128–1).

ROUTES OF PN ADMISTRATION

PERIPHERAL ROUTE

Because of physical limitations of peripheral veins, peripheral parenteral nutrition (PPN) regimens are usually dilute solutions of amino acids, dextrose, and micronutrients. Although early PPN studies supported the use of amino acids alone as "protein-sparing" therapy, subsequent investigations have challenged this theory.[59,60] The rationale for

TABLE 128–4. Fluid, Electrolyte, and Acid–Base Abnormalities

Problem	Possible Causes	Intervention
Hypovolemia	Gastrointestinal fluid losses, osmotic diuresis	Increase fluid intake
Hypervolemia	Renal failure, excess fluid intake	Decrease fluid intake and diuretics
Hyponatremia	Gastrointestinal losses, fluid overload, diuretics	Varies with cause
Hypernatremia	Dehydration	Increase fluid intake
Hypokalemia	Gastrointestinal losses, diuretics, anabolism	Increase potassium intake
Hyperkalemia	Renal failure	Decrease potassium intake
Hypophosphatemia	Phosphate-binding antacids, anabolism, phosphate-free dialysate	Discontinue phosphate binders; increase phosphorus intake
Hyperphosphatemia	Renal failure	Decrease phosphorus intake
Hypomagnesemia	Diarrhea, malabsorption, anabolism	Increase magnesium intake
Hypermagnesemia	Renal failure	Decrease magnesium intake
Hypocalcemia	Hypoalbuminemia, chronic renal failure	Increase calcium intake (with chronic renal failure only)
Hypercalcemia	Rare	Decrease calcium intake
Metabolic acidosis	Diarrhea, high-output fistulae, renal failure, and excess amino acid intake	Treat underlying causes; increase acetate and decrease Cl in PN solution; decrease amino acid intake
Metabolic alkalosis	Gastric losses	Treat underlying cause; increase Cl and decrease acetate in PN solution

Adapted from Ref. 92, with permission.

protein-sparing PPN was based on the theory that the provision of dextrose in the setting of altered metabolism or stress would promote further increases in serum insulin concentrations and thereby hinder the utilization of endogenous fat stores and promote nitrogen catabolism.[59,60] Protein-sparing PPN is used for patients with marginal nutrition status and inadequate oral intake who are not candidates for central catheter placement and when the expected length of PN therapy is less than 1 week. However, two recent investigations of patients receiving postoperative PN suggest that some patients who meet criteria for protein-sparing PPN may not benefit from PN support.[17,19,61]

The addition of IVLE to PPN is referred to as "the lipid system." The lipid system is designed for use in mild to moderately stressed patients where central access is unavailable or undesirable and function of the GI tract is expected to return within 7 to 10 days. The addition of IVLE increases caloric support to levels more consistent with PN regimens administered centrally. Advantages of PPN include a lower risk of infectious, metabolic, and technical complications that may occur with central vein catheterization. However, several other factors may complicate use of PPN in many patient populations. Patients who have received multiple courses of chemotherapy, malnourished patients, elderly patients, and others with an illness of long duration who have already been subjected to multiple venous accesses for administration of fluids and medications are likely to have limited peripheral venous access. Use of PPN is also limited by relatively poor tolerance of peripheral veins to hypertonic solutions. Thrombophlebitis is a commonly reported complication in patients receiving PPN. Although the risk of developing phlebitis increases when solution osmolarities are greater than 600 to 900 mOsm/L,[59,60] peripherally administered total nutrient admixtures with much higher osmolarities have been associated with low infusion-site complications in some centers.[62] Efforts to minimize development of phlebitis in patients receiving PPN include addition of IVLE to the regimen as a possible venous lumen protectant, subtherapeutic doses of heparin (1000 U/L) to prevent thrombus formation, and/or small doses of hydrocortisone (5 mg/L) to minimize inflammation of the access site.[60] The osmolarity of a PN solution may be estimated by using the guidelines for osmolarities of selected PN components in Table 128–5. Because lower osmolarity solutions are relatively dilute, much larger volumes of solution are generally required to meet nutritional requirements. Finally, patients with large nutrition requirements who receive PPN will likely require the use of IVLE as a caloric source, so these patients should also be evaluated for lipid tolerance.

In summary, PPN is a relatively safe and simple method of nutritional support when patients are appropriately selected. Candidates for PPN include patients who do not have large nutritional requirements, are not fluid restricted, and are expected to regain function of the GI tract within 7 to 10 days.[59]

CENTRAL ROUTE

Central parenteral nutrition (CPN) solutions are highly concentrated, hypertonic solutions that must be administered through a large central vein. Unlike peripheral veins, central veins have a much more rapid rate of blood flow, which quickly dilutes hypertonic solutions. Central venous catheters are most commonly inserted percutaneously into

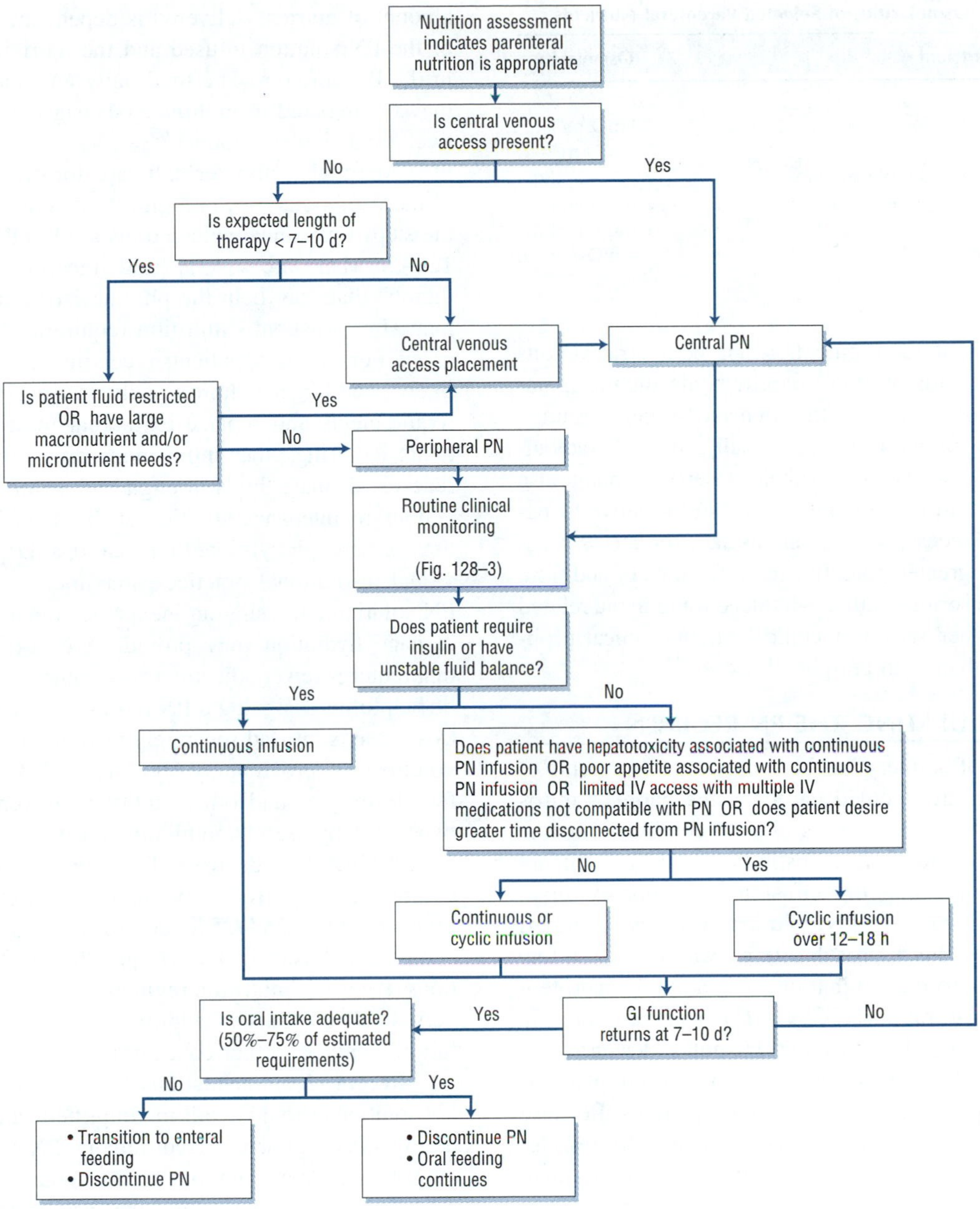

FIGURE 128–1. The route of parenteral nutrition and the infusion pattern (type) is dependent on the patient's clinical stature and the expected length of therapy.

the subclavian vein and advanced so that the tip is at the superior vena cava. If this approach is not possible, the internal jugular vein may be used. Radiographic verification of correct placement is necessary prior to infusion of the CPN solution. Catheterization may be performed either in the operating suite or in the patient's hospital room. Strict adherence to established protocols and catheter placement by an experienced clinician lessens the risk of complications (Table 128–6).[63]

Central venous catheters vary in composition, lumen size, number of injection ports, and other special features that affect ease or convenience of care and maintenance. Central venous catheters may be placed for short-term access or long-term access. Catheters are usually inserted by percutaneous venipuncture when therapy is expected to last less than 4 weeks. When therapy is expected to last longer than 4 weeks, the catheter is usually tunneled subcutaneously before entering the central vessel, secured initially with retaining sutures, and anchored in place with a felt cuff that promotes the growth of subcutaneous fibrotic tissue around the catheter.[64] The injection port may remain external or be entirely concealed beneath the skin. Implanted central venous catheters have a larger port or reservoir that is surgically placed beneath the skin surface and anchored in the muscle of the chest wall.

Central PN is predominantly used for patients who require PN for periods of greater than 7 to 10 days during hospitalization or indefinitely at home. These patients may

TABLE 128–5. Osmolarities of Selected Parenteral Nutrients

Nutrient	Osmolarity
Amino acid	100 mOsm/%
Dextrose	50 mOsm/%
Lipid emulsion	1.7 mOsm/%
Sodium (acetate, chloride, phosphate)	2 mOsm/mEq
Potassium (acetate, chloride, phosphate)	2 mOsm/mEq
Magnesium sulfate	1 mOsm/mEq
Calcium gluconate	1.4 mOsm/mEq

have large nutrient requirements, poor peripheral venous access, and/or fluctuating fluid requirements such as metabolically stressed patients with extensive surgery, trauma, sepsis, multiple organ failure, or malignancy. Disadvantages of CPN include risks of catheter insertion, routine use of the catheter, and care of the access site. Relative to peripheral venous access, central venous catheter access is associated with a greater potential for infection. In addition, the risk of more serious catheter-induced trauma and related sequelae and other serious technical or mechanical problems is greater than with peripheral access.

CALCULATING THE PN REGIMEN

Once the route of delivery has been chosen, components of the PN regimen are decided based on the patient's nutritional assessment. The patient's clinical condition and the compounding practices of an institution will have impact on decisions concerning PN infusion rates. For example, some institutions prepare PN solutions using a "standard formula" format. This approach offers a variety of base formulas (CAA/dextrose combination) with a fixed nonprotein calorie-to-nitrogen ratio (NPC:N). The standard formula format usually includes different formulas designed for mild to moderately stressed patients, renal failure patients, fluid-restricted patients, and liver failure patients. Because the NPC:N is fixed, the amount of nutrient delivered depends solely on the infusion rate. Other institutions may compound "individualized" formulas. This approach permits compounding of patient-specific solutions. Compounding of the PN solution is limited only by the concentrations of stock solutions and stability concerns. The amount of nutrient delivered is dependent on daily volume of the PN solution infused and the nutrient concentrations in the PN solution. The total daily amount of PN solution may be prepared in multiple, 1-L bags or more cost effectively in a single container.[65]

Although computer software for calculating volumes of base solutions for PN regimens is now widely available, the steps for manual calculations are briefly reviewed (Fig. 128–2). There are several guidelines or clinical "rules of thumb" that may help the pharmacist calculate a PN regimen after a patient's nutrition requirements have been decided. For example, patients receiving only PN therapy will likely need larger volumes of fluid to provide maintenance requirements and replace extrarenal losses. However, patients requiring other intravenous drug therapy will likely receive adequate fluids through the use of a standard intravenous maintenance solution such as 0.45% NaCl in 5% dextrose and piggybacked medications. Depending on individual institutional practices, maximally concentrating the PN solution and using an inexpensive maintenance fluid to manage hydration may provide a cost-effective regimen that requires fewer adjustments. Another guideline that may be helpful in designing a PN regimen where the CAA/ dextrose base is infused separately from the IVLE is to allow a volume of approximately 50 to 100 mL/L of base solution for electrolytes and other additives. Given this guideline, two clinically useful and highly concentrated base solutions are 7% CAA/15% dextrose (final concentration), which can be prepared from 10% CAA and 70% dextrose stock solutions, or 8% CAA/25% dextrose (final concentrations) compounded from 15% CAA and 70% dextrose stock solutions. Parenteral nutrition regimens for patients who require very small amounts of additives such as those with renal failure, may be further concentrated.

Recent recommendations for standardized labeling of PN solutions should result in simplified calculations for ordering a PN regimen.[66] Traditionally, PN solutions have required multiple calculations for compounding, since the orders were often based on the percentage of the final concentrations for base solution components, amount per liter concentrations for electrolytes and some medications, and amount per day for other micronutrients and medica-

TABLE 128–6. Complications of Central Venous Catheters

Complication	Description
Arterial injury	Puncture of subclavian or carotid artery during catheter insertion.
Pneumothorax	Perforation of the pleura or lung during insertion, which results in air collection in the pleural space.
Air embolism	Introduction of air into the catheter, which subsequently enters the venous circulation.
Catheter embolism	A portion of the catheter fragments and enters the venous circulation.
Venous thrombosis	Formation of thrombosis inside the lumen of the catheter and/or inside the vessel around the catheter, which may result in catheter or vessel occlusion.
Chylothorax	Injury to the thoracic duct during catheter insertion.
Brachial plexus injury	Injury to the nerve during catheter insertion, or injury secondary to catheter malposition or extravasation of a hypertonic solution.

Adapted from Ref. 63.

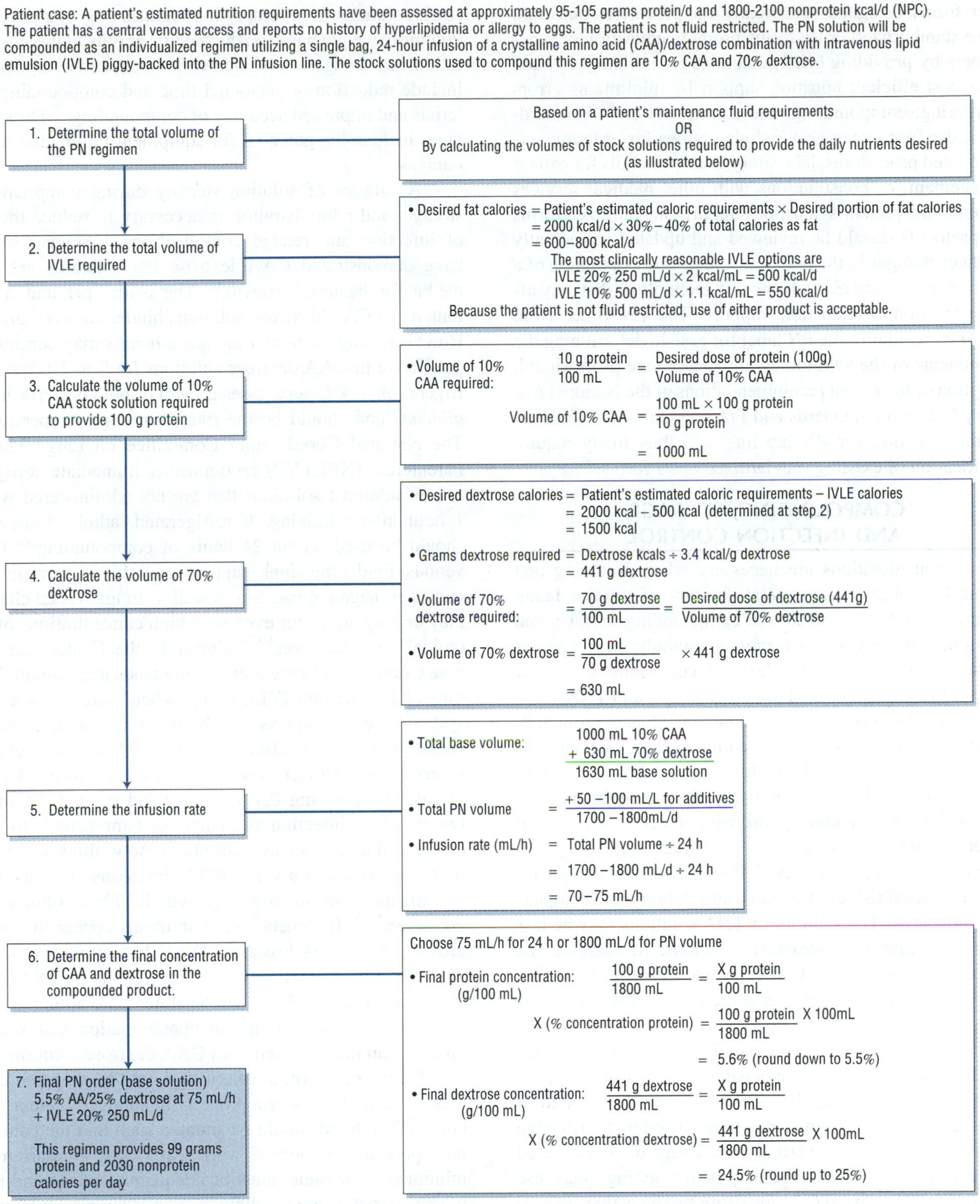

FIGURE 128–2. Calculation of a compounding plan for a parenteral nutrition regimen.

tions. To minimize the risk of compounding errors associated with misinterpretation of orders, the National Advisory Group on Standards and Practice Guidelines for Parenteral Nutrition (NAG SPGPN) recommends labeling the PN solution with amounts per day for the base solution, electrolytes, other micronutrients, and medications.[66]

ORDERING THE PN REGIMEN

Ordering PN solutions may be accomplished by several methods that are generally specific for each practice setting. Some health care systems may require the entire formula to be written in individual components and additives. More commonly, the ordering process has been simplified by the use of order forms designed specifically for parenteral nutrition. These standardized order forms promote education of practitioners by providing brief guidelines for initiating PN and foster cost-efficient nutrition support by minimizing errors in ordering, compounding, and administration.[67] Standardized order forms may also include options for ordering certain related procedures, laboratory tests, protocols for patient management, or consultations with other medical services related to the patient's nutrition support. Standardized forms and protocols should be reviewed and updated periodically to reflect changes in the practices and patient population of a practice setting and also advances in technology that may affect provision of nutrition support. The PN order form should be similar to the PN label for ease in determining the components of the solution by any health care professional. Adoption of the recent recommendations of the National Advisory Group on Standards and Practice Guidelines for Parenteral Nutrition for PN labeling will thus likely require modification of existing standardized order forms.[66]

COMPOUNDING, STORAGE, AND INFECTION CONTROL

Several considerations are necessary when preparing and storing PN solutions. In general, the type of solution being prepared will dictate methods of compounding, storage, and infusion. Currently, the two most commonly used types of PN solutions are the CAA/dextrose combination, with or without IVLE piggybacked into the PN line, and TNAs. Use of TNA solutions offers several potential advantages including reduced inventory (infusion pumps, tubing, and other related supplies), decreased time for compounding and administration, potential decrease in manipulations of the infusion line, which should correspond with a decreased risk of catheter contamination, and ease of delivery and storage for patients receiving home PN.[68] Potential disadvantages include increased risk of infections, and stability and compatibility concerns. The stability of TNA solutions may be less predictable than CAA/dextrose solutions. In addition, the opaque solution that results after the addition of IVLE makes detection of particulate matter difficult, and TNA solutions cannot be filtered with a bacterial-retentive 0.22-μm filter.[37,68,69] Methods for compounding PN solutions vary based on a health care system's patient population and medical practices and the number of PN solutions that need to be prepared. PN base solutions may be prepared by transferring CAA stock solutions to partially filled bags of concentrated dextrose stock solutions. Other practice settings may use commercially prepared CAA/dextrose products that are separated within a single bag and then mixed prior to use. Recent advances in compounding technology have facilitated use of automated compounders for preparing PN solutions. Automated compounders are computer-based systems that perform the calculations necessary to determine volumes of nutrient stock solutions for PN solutions. In addition, most automated compounder systems include software that directly communicates the determined calculations to a transfer pump device. The pump delivers appropriate volumes of stock solutions to an empty intravenous bag by converting volume to weight based on the specific gravity of the stock solution. Advantages associated with automated compounders include reduction in personnel time and compounding materials and improved accuracy of compounding.[70] Disadvantages include the potential for equipment failure and power outages.

Assurance of solution sterility during compounding, storage, and administration is necessary to reduce the risk of infection and related complications.[71] Several studies have demonstrated CAA/dextrose PN solutions are poor media for bacterial growth.[68] The acidic pH and hypertonicity of CAA/dextrose solutions hinder bacterial growth. However, fungi such as *Candida albicans* may continue to proliferate in CAA/dextrose solutions for 7 to 10 days. Refrigeration at 4°C suppresses growth of both bacteria and *C. albicans* and should be the routine storage temperature.[69] The National Coordinating Committee on Large Volume Parenterals (NCCLVP) recommends immediate refrigeration of admixed solutions that are not administered within 1 hour after admixing. If refrigerated, admixed solutions should be used within 24 hours of compounding.[72] Intravenous lipid emulsions support growth of gram-positive and gram-negative bacteria as well as fungi. Visual changes may or may not occur even with high concentrations of microbial contamination.[69,73] Currently the Centers for Disease Control and Prevention recommends a maximum hang time of 12 hours for IVLE except when used within a TNA system based on reports of substantial microbial growth in contaminated IVLE after 12 hours.[70] However, a clinical investigation of IVLE solutions infused for up to 24 hours in patients receiving PN, demonstrated no correlation between risk of infection and length of hang time.[74] In view of these findings, many institutions now allow expiration times up to 24 hours for IVLE infusions. Results from investigations of microbial growth in TNA solutions do not agree.[68,70] In general, TNA solutions appear to support growth of bacteria less than IVLE but more than CAA/dextrose solutions. However, investigations of TNAs used in a clinical setting have demonstrated safe administration over 24 hours with a risk of contamination that was no greater than that reported with CAA/dextrose solutions.[37,68]

Parenteral nutrition solutions should be prepared using aseptic technique under a properly maintained laminar flow hood.[75] The hood should be situated such that the contaminant potential of normal work traffic and air currents is minimized. Personnel must be adequately trained and must practice strict aseptic technique. Supervision by a pharmacist experienced in compounding intravenous solutions and knowledgeable about stability, compatibility, and storage of PN solutions is also necessary. Quality assurance procedures should be developed to maintain safe and accurate admixture preparation. The potential risk of sepsis associated with PN solution contamination can be greatly decreased when pharmacy-based admixture programs follow specific guidelines developed to ensure proper compounding of PN solutions.[71,75]

STABILITY AND COMPATIBILITY

Because of their complex compositions, PN solutions are prone to problems with stability and compatibility. Comprehensive sources of current information about compatibilities and stability of PN solutions are Trissel's *Handbook on Injectable Drugs,* which is published every 2 years with supplements during alternating years, and the *Guide to Parenteral Admixtures,* which is updated quarterly.[76,77] In many cases, the exact answer to a compatibility question may not be readily available and a review of the primary literature may be necessary. When information is not available, clinical judgment and experience must be used carefully to resolve the situation.

CAA/dextrose solutions are generally stable for 1 to 2 months if refrigerated at 4°C and protected from light.[78] Many studies have investigated stability of solutions containing various amounts of CAA, dextrose, and IVLE.[69] Several factors affect stability of TNA solutions including pH, electrolyte charges, temperature, and time after compounding. Because of differences in pH among various CAA products and differences in phospholipid content among IVLE products, specific manufacturers should be consulted for compatibility and stability information prior to routine mixing of components. In general, electrolytes (except phosphorus) and trace elements should be added to the dextrose solution, phosphate should be added to the CAA solution, and, finally, the amino acid solution should be added to the IVLE prior to or simultaneously with the dextrose solution. However, mixing components in a specific order and time sequence may not be possible with the use of automated compounders.[79] The compounder's manufacturer should be consulted for the optimal mixing sequence to ensure safe compounding of TNA solutions. Although TNA solutions should be infused within 24 to 48 hours after compounding, investigations of certain TNA solutions have reported acceptable stability for 10 to 28 days when refrigerated at 4 to 5°C.[69,71]

The precipitation of calcium and phosphorus is a common interaction that is potentially life threatening.[79] Factors that enhance the risk of precipitate formation include high concentrations of calcium and phosphorus salts, use of the chloride salt of calcium, decreased amino acid concentrations, increased solution temperature, increased solution pH, use of an improper sequence when mixing calcium and phosphorus salts, and the presence of other additives including IVLE.[76,79] Specific guidelines for avoiding a calcium–phosphorus interaction have been published elsewhere.[69,76,79] Electrolyte stability in TNA solutions is difficult to assess because of poor visualization of a precipitate should one occur. Alternative methods of delivering electrolytes or other medications should be pursued in clinical situations where compatibility information involving a TNA solution is lacking. Although some published compatibility data suggest otherwise, the addition of sodium bicarbonate to PN solutions is not recommended.[76,80] Addition of bicarbonate to acidic PN solutions may result in the formation of carbon dioxide gas and insoluble calcium and magnesium carbonates. Use of a bicarbonate precursor salt such as acetate is usually preferred.

Vitamins may be adversely affected by changes in solution pH, presence of other additives, storage time, solution temperature, and exposure to light.[58] Variable but significant losses of vitamin A have been reported secondary to adsorption to intravenous administration tubing and polyvinyl chloride intravenous bags.[69] Thiamine may be subject to degradation in solutions containing bisulfite. Because of variable stabilities of individual vitamins, intravenous vitamin solutions should be added to the PN solution as near to the time of administration as is clinically feasible and should not be in the PN solution longer than 24 hours.

Many patients receiving PN at home or in a hospital also receive other intravenous medications. The compatibility of these medications and other intravenous solutions is an important concern in delivering safe and effective drug and nutritional therapy. Intravenous medications are most often infused as a separate admixture piggybacked in the PN line. However, some medications may be added directly to the PN solution and administered at the same rate as the PN infusion. Because of the potential for ineffective drug therapy or other complications associated with physiochemical incompatibility and stability of the PN solution, specific criteria should be considered before one adds a medication directly to the PN solution.[81] The dosage regimen should be stable for each 24-hour period and should have pharmacokinetic properties appropriate for continuous infusion. There should be documented chemical and physical compatibility of the medication with PN mixture components and other medications that may be concomitantly piggybacked into the PN line. Finally, the PN regimen should be infused continuously over 24 hours. Advantages of using PN admixtures as drug vehicles include consolidation of dosage units, improved pharmacotherapy for certain drugs, conservation of fluid in volume-restricted patients, fewer venous catheter violations, and decreased compounding and administration time.[81] However, a major disadvantage to use of PN solutions as drug delivery vehicles is the lack of compatibility and stability data in the PN solutions that are commonly used in clinical practice. Original research reports should be carefully reviewed for experimental conditions and assay determination methods before extrapolating data into institution-specific guidelines.[69] Medications frequently added to PN solutions include albumin, aminophylline, hydrochloric acid, regular insulin, and histamine-2 antagonists such as cimetidine, ranitidine, and famotidine.[76,77,81]

SUMMARY

PN solutions should be administered with an infusion pump to ensure consistent and controlled delivery of the solution. The intravenous administration line may include an in-line filter at a point prior to connection to the catheter. A 0.22-μm filter is recommended for use with CAA/dextrose solutions to remove particulate matter, air, and any microorganism that may be present in the solution from prior manipulations of the admixture or the administration line. Because the average size of IVLE particles is approximately 0.5 μm, IVLE administered separately from the CAA/dextrose solution must be piggybacked into the PN line at a site beyond the in-line filter.[82] Routine use of in-line filters with TNA solutions is controversial.[83] However, the Food and Drug Administration recommends use of a 1.2-μm filter, which may be effective in preventing catheter occlusion due to precipitates or lipid aggregates.[81,84] This filter size is also reported to remove *C. albicans*.[78]

INITIATING THE PN INFUSION

The concentration of dextrose in the formula and the patient's history of glucose tolerance will dictate the infusion rate at which the PN solution should be initiated. Protocols for initiating PN differ widely depending on the practice setting. Many institutions begin infusions slowly and gradually increase the rate over 24 to 48 hours to the desired rate. The rate is also lowered in a stepwise fashion when PN therapy ends. This protocol is used to prevent development of hyperglycemia and rebound hypoglycemia, respectively. However, Krzyda et al.[85] investigated 18 patients who were initiated on PN solutions at the desired rate and discontinued without a taper schedule. Patients were monitored for clinical evidence of hyperglycemia or hypoglycemia at the initiation and discontinuation of a lipid-based PN regimen given over 24 hours of continuous infusion. The severity of illness of the patients ranged from stable condition postoperatively to multiple-system organ failure. Six patients had diabetes mellitus. None of the patients demonstrated clinical signs of hyperglycemia or hypoglycemia during the study period. The blood glucose concentrations of patients who received insulin from the PN infusion were less predictable when the PN infusion was stopped compared to those from patients who did not require insulin. While these investigators observed no adverse effects from abruptly initiating and discontinuing PN infusions, tapered scheduling has been recommended for patients receiving intermittent subcutaneous regular insulin, patients with severe renal or hepatic disease, patients with other disease states that may increase risk for development of hypoglycemia such as severe diabetes or pancreatic malignancy, and patients who are receiving concurrent drug therapy that may predispose development of hypoglycemia (oral hypoglycemics) or mask the cardiovascular symptoms of hypoglycemia (β blockers).[86]

CONTINUOUS VERSUS INTERMITTENT INFUSIONS

Parenteral nutrition solutions may be infused continuously or intermittently (Fig. 128–1). Continuous infusions are attractive for use in patients with unstable fluid balance or glucose control. Cyclic PN is the infusion of PN over a period of time less than 24 hours, usually for 12 to 18 hours each day.[87] Cyclic PN is useful in hospitalized patients with limited venous access where administration of multiple other medications requires interruption of the PN infusion. Cyclic PN may also prevent or treat hepatotoxicities associated with continuous PN therapy. In addition, cyclic PN allows patients receiving PN at home the ability to resume a relatively normal life-style.[87] Recommendations for administration of cyclic PN are similar to those for continuous PN. Various protocols have been reported that suggest incremental increases to the maximum infusion rate for a desired period of time followed by a gradual taper to discontinue the solution. However, metabolically stable patients receiving lipid-based PN regimens are likely candidates for abrupt initiation and discontinuation of the cyclic PN regimen.[85,86] Cyclic PN may not be well tolerated by patients with severe glucose intolerance or diabetes, or by those patients with unstable fluid balance.

EVALUATION OF THERAPEUTIC OUTCOMES

Thorough and consistent monitoring of patients receiving PN is necessary to ensure that the desired nutritional outcomes are achieved and to prevent the occurrence of adverse effects or complications. Routine evaluation should include the assessment of the patient's clinical condition with a focus on nutritional and metabolic effects of the PN regimen. Serial documentation of a patient's response to a particular regimen is a helpful guide for determining appropriate adjustments in fluid, electrolyte, and nutrient therapies.

A variety of biochemical and clinical measurements are necessary for effective monitoring of patients receiving PN. Important clinical laboratory measurements include serum concentrations of electrolytes, hematologic indices, and biochemical markers for renal function, liver function, and nutrition status. Other important clinical measurements include vital signs, weight, total fluid intake and losses, and nutritional intakes. The frequency of clinical laboratory measurements is usually dependent on the stability of a patient's clinical condition. Monitoring parameters considered important for patients receiving PN and the suggested frequency of measurement for each are outlined in Fig. 128–3. Appropriate assessment and evaluation of patient data can identify impending complications that may be avoided or treated early. Monitoring protocols should be developed and tailored for the patient population, medical practices, and resources of individual practice settings.

COMPLICATIONS OF PN

Parenteral nutrition can be a safe and effective therapy when appropriate patients have been selected and the course of therapy is correctly monitored and adjusted.

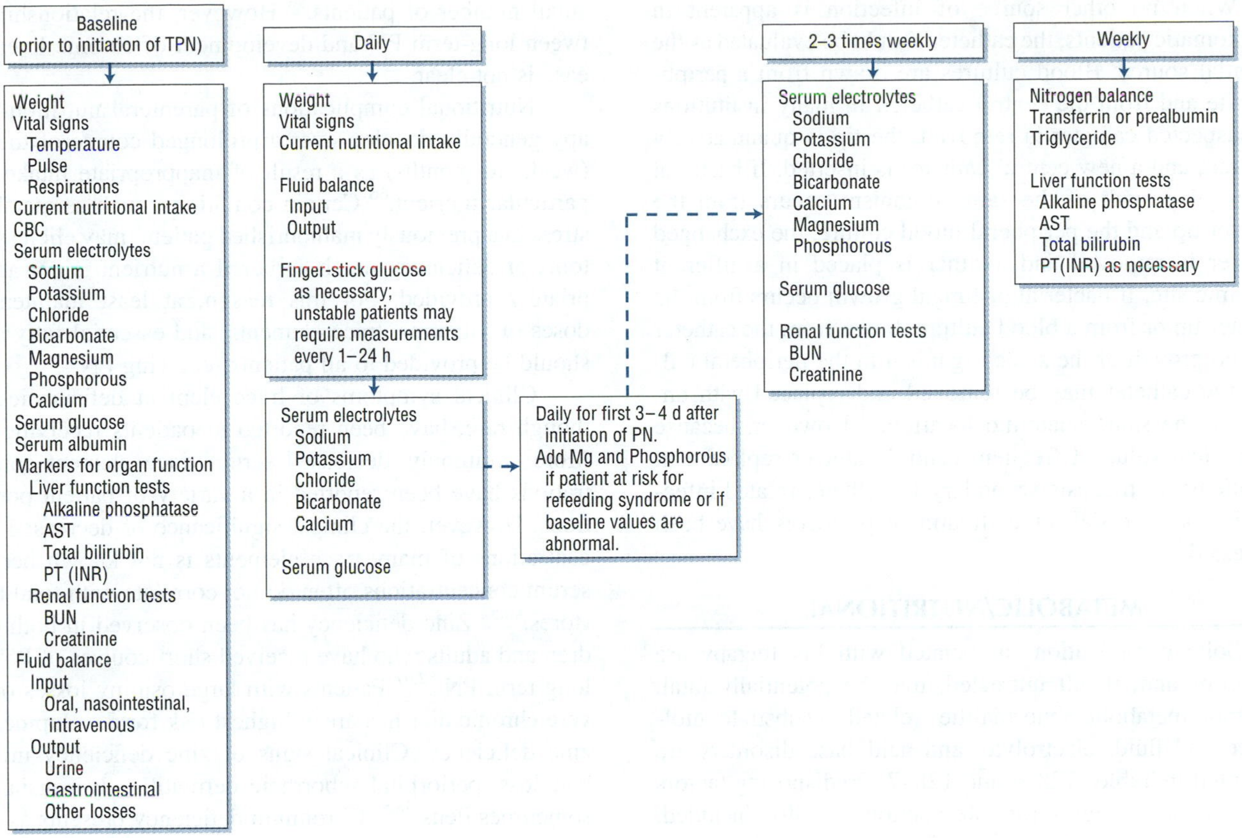

FIGURE 128–3. Monitoring strategy for patients receiving parenteral nutrition.

However, PN support is a complex therapy that is associated with numerous complications. These complications may be divided into four categories: mechanical or technical, infectious, metabolic, and nutritional.

MECHANICAL/TECHNICAL

Mechanical or technical complications include malfunctions in the system used for intravenous delivery of the solution. Examples of such malfunctions include infusion pump failure, problems with administration sets or tubing, and problems with the catheter. Catheter-related complications are potentially life threatening (Table 128–6). Pneumothorax, catheter misdirection into the wrong vein or ill-positioned within the cardiac chambers, arterial puncture, bleeding, and hematoma formation may occur during surgical placement of the catheter. Many of these complications in addition to venous thrombosis and air embolism may occur after insertion as well. Catheters occasionally occlude or break during use. If these problems cannot be easily rectified, the catheter may need to be surgically replaced.[63,88]

INFECTIONS

Infectious complications can be a major hazard in patients receiving central PN. Often these patients are predisposed to infection as a result of compromised immunity and/or concomitant infection already present in the urinary tract, wounds, or lungs. Frequent use of broad-spectrum antibiotic therapy and malnutrition are also predisposing factors for development of infection. Bacterial translocation across the wall of the GI tract has also been implicated as a source of sepsis in patients receiving PN for prolonged periods without enteral feeding.[89] Infection may develop secondary to solution contamination. However, strict adherence to specific protocols for preparation of PN solutions should minimize this occurrence.[71] A more common source of systemic infection is catheter-related infections. Catheter-related sepsis is defined as the presence of bacterial or fungal growth from the catheter tip and peripheral blood cultures. Catheter infection is defined as microbial growth from the catheter tip or from a blood culture drawn from the catheter with no growth of the same organism in the peripheral blood culture.[90] Patients with catheter-related infections may exhibit signs of sepsis syndrome such as fever, chills, mental status changes, hypotension, or glucose intolerance. These infections occur when the catheter becomes colonized by direct microbial invasion of the skin at the insertion site or at the infusion site of the catheter. For example, colonization may occur after multiple manipulations of the line used for PN administration, which can occur when the PN line is used to administer other medications. Other examples include failure of in-line bacterial filters, poor placement technique, and poor care of the insertion site.[88]

When no other source of infection is apparent in symptomatic patients, the catheter should be evaluated as the potential source. Blood cultures are drawn from a peripheral site and from the central catheter. In many institutions the suspected catheter is removed, the tip is quantitatively cultured, and a new central catheter is inserted. If bacterial or fungal growth of the same organism occurs from the catheter tip and the peripheral blood culture, the exchanged catheter is removed and another is placed in a different anatomic site. If bacterial or fungal growth occurs from the catheter tip or from a blood culture drawn from the catheter with no growth of the same organism in the peripheral culture, the catheter may be removed and replaced with another in the same anatomic location.[90] However, because the clinical value of frequent central catheter replacement in patients with sepsis secondary to catheter-related infection is controversial, other treatment protocols have been suggested.[91]

METABOLIC/NUTRITIONAL

Metabolic complications associated with PN therapy are numerous and, if left untreated, may be potentially fatal. Common metabolic abnormalities related to substrate intolerance and fluid, electrolyte, and acid–base disorders are presented in Tables 128–4 and 128–7. Predisposing factors and general strategies for intervention are also included. The etiology, mechanisms, and implications of individual metabolic abnormalities are multifactorial and have been summarized.[91–94]

Hepatic dysfunction, as evidenced by elevations in serum liver function measurements such as total bilirubin, AST, ALT, and alkaline phosphatase, is well documented in the literature. The most commonly reported abnormalities are fatty liver, cholelithiasis, and cholestasis.[95,96] In most patients, these complications are reversible by manipulations of substrate intake. Progressive liver injury in patients who have received long-term PN has been reported in a small number of patients.[96] However, the relationship between long-term PN and development of chronic liver disease is not clear.

Nutritional complications of parenteral nutrition therapy generally develop over a prolonged course of therapy (weeks to months) as a result of inappropriate intake of a particular nutrient.[66] Certain conditions, such as metabolic stress in a previously malnourished patient, may elicit symptoms of deficiency much earlier if a nutrient is not appropriately provided. For this reason, at least maintenance doses of vitamins, trace elements, and essential fatty acids should be provided to all patients receiving PN.

Clinical symptoms of trace element deficiencies, although rare, have been reported in patients receiving PN. More commonly, decreased serum trace element concentrations have been reported in a variety of patient populations. However, the clinical significance of decreased concentrations of many trace elements is not known because serum concentrations often do not correlate with total body stores.[48,52] Zinc deficiency has been observed in both children and adults who have received short courses of PN and long-term PN.[52,97] Patients with large ostomy losses or severe chronic diarrhea are at highest risk for development of zinc deficiency. Clinical signs of zinc deficiency include hair loss, periorbital seborrheic dermatitis, dysgeusia, and sometimes ileus.[48,52] Chromium deficiency presents as a diabetes-like syndrome, whereas copper deficiency may appear as a hypochromic, normocytic anemia with neutropenia. Selenium deficiency may develop during the course of PN therapy as cardiomyopathy and muscle pain.[48,52,56]

Patients receiving PN regimens without IVLE for extended periods of weeks to months are at risk for development of EFAD. Clinical signs of EFAD include hair loss, desquamative dermatitis, thrombocytopenia, and malabsorption and diarrhea resulting from changes in intestinal mucosa.[36,37] These manifestations may occur 1 to 3 weeks after initiation of fat-free TPN.[36] Biochemical evidence of

TABLE 128–7. Substrate Intolerance in Parenteral Nutrition

Complication	Possible Causes	Intervention
Hyperglycemia	Stress, infection, corticosteroids, pancreatitis, diabetes mellitus, peritoneal dialysis, excessive dextrose administration	Decrease dextrose load by decreasing infusion rate or dextrose concentration (may substitute fat calories); administer insulin
Hypoglycemia (rare)	Abrupt withdrawal of dextrose, insulin overdose	Increase dextrose intake; decrease exogenous insulin
Excess of carbon dioxide production	Excess dextrose intake	Decrease dextrose intake; balance calories from fat and dextrose
Hyperlipidemia (elevated cholesterol and triglyceride)	Stress, familial hyperlipidemia, pancreatitis	Decrease intake of fat or discontinue if indicated
Serum amino acid imbalance	Stress, hepatic failure	Modify amino acid intake if possible or decrease intake of amino acids
Abnormal liver function tests (elevated AST, alkaline phosphatase, and bilirubinw)	Stress, infection, cancer, excess carbohydrate intake, excess caloric intake, essential fatty acid deficiency	Decrease dextrose load (substitute fat); decrease total calories; provide essential fatty acids

AST = aspartate aminotransferase (SGOT).
Adapted from Ref. 92, with permission.

EFAD as demonstrated by a triene:tetraene ratio ≥ 0.4 may occur as early as 1 week after PN initiation in metabolically stressed patients.[36]

Occasionally patients may develop nutrient-induced toxicities, most commonly as a result of the accumulation of fat-soluble vitamins or trace elements. Toxic accumulation may be caused by either excessive intake or decreased excretion. Certain disease states (e.g., renal failure) may necessitate reduction in vitamin and trace element intake.[98] Patients receiving PN should be monitored closely by clinical observation and laboratory measurements, if indicated, to detect signs and symptoms of nutrient deficiency or excess. In either case, the PN regimen should be appropriately adjusted.

HOME PN

Advances in technology for the delivery of intravenous solutions have allowed medically stable patients who require extended PN therapy to be maintained indefinitely on intravenous nutrition. An increasing concern for cost containment of health care services has fostered use of sophisticated infusion devices to provide PN at home. Numerous programs are now available to support patients with various long-term or permanent medical conditions outside the traditional health care setting. Standards have been developed to promote safe and effective care.[99,100] Home PN services may be coordinated and administered through a hospital, by a commercially operated corporation, or through a joint venture between the two.[101]

Many factors are considered in selecting candidates for home PN therapy. Significant benefit must be expected from placing a patient into the program. Additionally, the patient and his or her caregiver must be willing to successfully complete training and assume numerous other responsibilities that are important for managing a new daily routine in the home. Other logistics such as funding, procurement of solutions and supplies, and clinical management and follow-up must be evaluated, resolved, and implemented for each patient to achieve the desired outcomes.[100,102]

Patients with Crohn's disease, ischemic bowel disease, severe GI motility disorders, extensive intestinal obstruction, radiation enteritis, and congenital bowel function have been successfully maintained with home PN.[103] Although patients with active cancer are the largest group of patients on home PN, the number of patients with AIDS on home PN is increasing rapidly.[103,104] In the past, patients or their caregivers may have been trained to mix PN solutions in the home. Today patients commonly receive premixed PN solutions from the hospital or a commercial vendor. Intravenous vitamins or other additives may be added daily by the patient or caregiver depending on the arrangement with the PN provider. The solution is generally administered through the night by infusion pump over 10 to 18 hours. A cycled regimen allows the patient time away from the pump during daylight hours and provides many patients with the freedom to have a reasonably normal daily routine. Clinical management and follow-up are performed periodically according to the needs of the patient and the protocol of the care provider. A coordinated effort among several health care professionals including physicians, pharmacists, nurses, social workers, and the patient and his or her caregiver, as well as the suppliers is paramount to providing safe and effective management. Home PN affords some patients the potential for an ambulatory life-style while maintaining an intravenous feeding regimen previously available only in the hospital setting. For others, home PN may contribute to a better quality of life in the comfort of their home.

PHARMACOECONOMIC CONSIDERATIONS

Methods of economic analysis such as cost–benefit analysis and cost-effectiveness analysis have been used to determine the financial and clinical utility of PN.[105] Because numerous variables have impact on the provision of PN support and the response to therapy, determining the true cost of PN is difficult. In general, PN is an expensive intervention according to a variety of published estimates.[105] Expenses associated with PN therapy may be categorized as direct and indirect costs[106] (Table 128–8.) Direct costs may be further categorized as fixed costs or variable costs. Fixed costs do not depend upon the volume of patients receiving therapy. For example, an automatic compounder and the tubing sets required to transfer volumes of stock solutions to the administration bag would be considered fixed costs in many practice settings. These costs tend to be relatively higher as the number of PN solutions declines. Variable costs such as PN administration bags are directly dependent upon the number of patients receiving PN.

Economic benefits and other clinical effects of PN (i.e., length of stay, frequency of complications) in some patient populations have been evaluated.[107,108] Few investigations have reported an economic assessment of the therapy. Attempting to measure the cost or cost savings associated with reported benefits of PN therapy and other clinical effects based on results of controlled clinical trials is difficult. Clinical outcomes measurements and, hence, economic outcomes are influenced by multiple factors including experimental design, sample size, and specific health-system practices. Several investigations used for determining costs and benefits of PN therapy have been criticized for such biases.[16,18,107]

Although the results of economic analyses of PN remain controversial, general similarities among several reports provide a basis for limiting the costs of PN therapy.[107] These include the following:

1. Use of PN in appropriate patients as described by institution-specific criteria based on current consensus statements. Determining appropriate candidates for PN therapy

TABLE 128–8. Costs Associated With PN Therapy

Type of Cost	Description
Direct	
• PN solution	
Components	Dextrose, AA, IVLE, other additives
Preparation	Dependent on system used for compounding: solution transfer sets, bags, syringes, technician time, pharmacist time
Administration	Administration sets, solution filter, pump, nursing time
• Catheter placement and site management	Venous access device *Central catheter:* site of procedure (bedside vs operating room), radiographic confirmation of placement, supplies used for site care *Peripheral line:* nursing time, supplies used for site care
• Monitoring	Routine laboratory and clinical measurements, changes in therapy to prevent complications or toxicities, nutrition support clinician time
• Complications	Mechanical: treatment of specific complication Infectious: cost of antibiotic therapy or venous access replacement Metabolic: increased clinical and laboratory measurements, possible waste of PN solution
Indirect	
• Morbidity	Quality-of-life expenses such as cost of patient discomfort, time lost from work or other activities as a result of PN therapy
• Mortality	Cost of premature death based, for example, on expected future wages

includes an initial evaluation of GI function and consideration of the patient as a successful enteral tube feeding candidate (see Chap. 129). The costs and complications associated with enteral nutrition have been repeatedly demonstrated to be less than those associated with PN.[105] If the patient is not considered a candidate for enteral feeding, PN therapy should be considered. In general, patients who are well nourished and not critically ill are at greater risk for potentially expensive complications that are not offset by potential clinical benefits of PN therapy.

2. Frequent evaluation of the necessity for standing laboratory measurements used for monitoring PN therapy. In general, the level of laboratory monitoring should decrease as a patient's clinical condition stabilizes (Fig. 129–3). Other practices should help minimize cost of PN to a lesser degree such as efficient purchasing practices for parenteral solutions and compounding supplies usually through contract purchasing, streamlining compounding procedures, minimizing PN waste by standardizing administration times and using 24-hour, single-bag PN solutions, and maximizing monitoring efficiency.

CONCLUSION

Parenteral nutrition is not a benign therapy. Appropriate patient selection, assessment, and monitoring are key to successful nutritional therapy and prevention of unnecessary complications or harm to the patient. Standardized order forms and monitoring protocols are useful tools to ensure appropriate administration and monitoring of PN therapy. Pharmacists have been involved in the provision of PN at many levels including direct patient care, education, and research. The field of pharmacy nutrition support has grown into a well-defined area of pharmacy practice with formally defined standards of practice.[7] These standards, although broad in scope, were considered to be focused and the demand for the services sufficient that specialty recognition by the Board of Pharmaceutical Specialties is now available for pharmacists.[109] The use of PN therapy and the role of the nutrition support pharmacist will be affected primarily by new insights from clinical research and economic challenges in the health care environment.

▶ PRINCIPLES OF PHARMACOTHERAPY

- Four steps to developing a successful nutrition plan include definition of nutrition goals, determination of nutrition requirements, determination of appropriate route of delivery of nutrients, and subsequent monitoring of the nutrition regimen to evaluate suitability of the regimen as a patient's clinical condition changes and to minimize or treat complications early.
- The appropriate route of nutrition support is dependent on the functional condition of the patient's GI tract, risk of aspiration, expected duration of nutrition therapy, and the clinical condition of the patient.
- Identifying the patient who is most likely to benefit from PN therapy is difficult. Indications for use of PN should be specific to a practice setting and based on current consensus statements.

- PN may be administered by peripheral or central venous access. Peripheral PN is useful in patients who do not have large nutrient requirements, are not fluid restricted, and are expected to regain function of the GI tract within 7 to 10 days. Peripheral PN is limited by the tolerance of peripheral veins to hypertonic solutions. Central PN is useful in patients who have large nutrient requirements and fluctuating fluid status and are likely to require parenteral support for > 7 to 10 days. Central PN is limited by the technical and infectious complications associated with establishing and maintaining central vascular access.
- PN solutions may be infused continuously or intermittently. Continuous infusions are useful in patients with unstable fluid balance or poor blood glucose control. Intermittent or cyclic PN is useful for patients with limited intravenous access who also require multiple intravenous medications not compatible with PN, those who developed hepatotoxicity while receiving continuous PN, or patients who desire more time disconnected from the PN infusion.
- Biochemical and clinical measurements considered necessary for effective monitoring of patients receiving PN include serum concentrations of electrolytes, hematologic indices, and biochemical markers for renal function, liver function, and nutrition status. Other important clinical measurements include vital signs, weight, total fluid intake and losses, and nutritional intake. The frequency of clinical laboratory measurements is usually dependent on the stability of a patient's clinical condition.
- Expenses associated with PN therapy may be minimized by using PN usage guidelines based on current consensus statements, frequent evaluation of the necessity for standing laboratory measurements used for monitoring PN therapy, maximizing efficient purchasing practices for parenteral solutions and compounding supplies usually through contract purchasing, streamlining compounding procedures, minimizing PN waste by standardizing administration times, and using 24-hour, single-bag PN solutions.

REFERENCES

1. Meguid MM, Campos AC, Hammond WG. Nutritional support in surgical practice: Part I. Am J Surg 1990;159:358.
2. Meguid MM, Campos AC, Hammond WG. Nutritional support in surgical practice: Part II. Am J Surg 1990;159:427–443.
3. Rhoads JE, Dudrick SJ. History of intravenous nutrition. In: Rombeau JL, Caldwell MD, eds Clinical Nutrition: Parenteral Nutrition, 2nd ed. Philadelphia, W.B. Saunders, 1993:1–10.
4. Wesley JR. Nutrition support teams: Past, present and future. Nutr Clin Pract 1995;10:219–228.
5. ASPEN Board of Directors. Definitions of terms used in ASPEN guidelines and standards. J Parenter Nutr 1995;19:1–2.
6. Holcombe BJ, Thorne DB, Strausburg KM, et al. Pharmacy practice insights. Analysis of the practice of nutrition support pharmacy specialists. Pharmacotherapy 1995;15:806–813.
7. American Society for Parenteral and Enteral Nutrition. Standards for nutrition support pharmacists. Nutr Clin Pract 1993;8:124–127.
8. American Society for Parenteral and Enteral Nutrition. Standards for nutrition support: Hospitalized patients. Nutr Clin Pract 1995;10: 208–218.
9. Foster GD, Knox LS, Dempsey DT, Mullen JL. Caloric requirements in total parenteral nutrition. J Am Coll Nutr 1987;6:231–253.
10. Cerra FB, Benitez MR, Blackburn GL, et al. Applied nutrition in ICU patients. A consensus statement of the American College of Chest Physicians. Chest 1997;111:769–778.
11. Amato P, Keating KP, Quercia RA, Karbonic J. Formulaic methods of estimating caloric requirements in mechanically ventilated obese patients: A reappraisal. Nutr Clin Pract 1995;10:229–232.
12. ASPEN Board of Directors. Routes to deliver nutrition support in adults. JPEN J Parenter Enteral Nutr 1993;17:7SA–8SA.
13. Buzby GP, Williford WO, Peterson OL, et al. A randomized clinical trial of total parenteral nutrition in malnourished surgical patients: The rationale and impact of previous clinical trials and pilot study on protocol design. Am J Clin Nutr 1988;47:357–365.
14. Giner M, Laviano A, Meguid MM, Gleason JR. In 1995, a correlation between malnutrition and poor outcome in critically ill patients still exists. Nutrition 1996;12:23–29.
15. Tucker HN, Miguel SG. Cost containment through nutrition intervention. Nutr Rev 1996;54:111–121.
16. Mattox TW. Drug use evaluation approach to monitoring use of total parenteral nutrition: A review of criteria for use in cancer patients. Nutr Clin Pract 1993;8:233–237.
17. ASPEN Board of Directors. Guidelines for the use of parenteral and enteral nutrition in adults and pediatric patients. JPEN J Parenter Enteral Nutr 1993;17:12SA–49SA.
18. Wolfe BM, Mathiesen KA. Clinical practice guidelines in nutrition support: Can they be based on randomized clinical trials? JPEN J Parenter Enteral Nutr 1997;21:1–6.
19. Klein S, Kinney J, Jeejeebhoy K, et al. Nutrition support in clinical practice: Review of published data and recommendations for future research directions. Summary of a conference sponsored by the National Institutes of Health, American Society for Parenteral and Enteral Nutrition, and American Society for Clinical Nutrition. JPEN J Parenter Enteral Nutr 1997;21:133–156.
20. Miles JM, Klein JA. Should protein be included in caloric calculations for a TPN prescription? Point-counterpoint. Nutr Clin Pract 1996;11:204–206.
21. Douglas RG, Shaw JHF. Metabolic response to sepsis and trauma. Br J Surg 1989;76:115–122.
22. Mirtallo JM, Schneider PJ, Mavco K, Ruberg RL. Clinical comparison of two 8.5% amino acid injection products. Am J Hosp Pharm 1981;38:83–89.
23. Furst P, Stehle P. Are intravenous amino acid solutions unbalanced? New Horizons 1994;2:215–223.
24. Miller SJ. The nitrogen balance revisited. Hosp Pharm 1990;25: 61–65, 70.
25. Grant JP. Administration of parenteral nutrition solutions. In: Handbook of Total Parenteral Nutrition, 2nd ed. Philadelphia, W.B. Saunders, 1992:171–202.
26. Broyles JE, Brown RO, Vehe KL, et al. Pharmacist interventions improve fluid balance in fluid restricted patients requiring parenteral nutrition. DICP Ann Pharmacother 1991;25:119–122.
27. Vasquez JA, Daniel H, Adibi SA. Dipeptides in parenteral nutrition: From basic science to clinical applications. Nutr Clin Prac 1993;8: 95–105.
28. Furst P, Stehle P. The potential use of parenteral dipeptides in clinical nutrition. Nutr Clin Prac 1993;8:106–114.

29. Wolfe RR. Carbohydrate metabolism and requirements. In: Rombeau JL, Caldwell MD, eds. Clinical Nutrition: Parenteral Nutrition, 2nd ed. Philadelphia, W.B. Saunders, 1993:113–131.
30. Freund HR. Abnormalities of liver function and hepatic damage associated with total parenteral nutrition. Nutrition 1991;7:1–5.
31. Goins WA, Wiles CE III, Cerra FB. Pharmacology, monitoring and nutritional support. Crit Care Clin 1993;9:689–713.
32. Dudrick PS, Souba WW. Special fuels in parenteral nutrition. In: Rombeau JL, Caldwell MD, eds. Clinical Nutrition: Parenteral Nutrition, 2nd ed. Philadelphia, W.B. Saunders, 1993:209–222.
33. Waxman K, Day AT, Stellin GP, et al. Safety and efficacy of glycerol and amino acids in combination with lipid emulsion for peripheral parenteral nutrition support. JPEN J Parenter Enteral Nutr 1993;16: 374–378.
34. Fat emulsions. In: McEvoy GK, ed. AHFS Drug Information 97. Bethesda, MD, American Society of Hospital Pharmacists, 1997: 2015–2016.
35. Sardesai VM. The essential fatty acids. Nutr Clin Pract 1992;7:179–186.
36. Gottschlich MM. Selection of optimal lipid sources in enteral and parenteral nutrition. Nutr Clin Pract 1992;7:152–165.
37. Warshawsky KY. Intravenous fat in clinical practice. Nutr Clin Prac 1992;7:187–196.
38. Ulrich H, Pastores SM, Katz DP, Kvetan V. Parenteral use of medium-chain triglycerides: A reappraisal. Nutrition 1996;12:231–238.
39. Sacks GS, Mouser JF. Is IV lipid emulsion safe in patients with hypertriglyceridemia? Nutr Clin Pract 1997;12:120–123.
40. Ball MJ. Hematological and biochemical effects of parenteral nutrition with medium-chain triglycerides: Comparison with long-chain triglycerides. Am J Clin Nutr 1991;53:916–922.
41. Manner T, Katz DP, Askanazi J, et al. Parenteral fish-oil administration in patients with cystic fibrosis. JPEN J Parenter Enteral Nutr 1993;17:24S.
42. Mashima Y, Tashiro T, Yamamori Y, et al. Effect of intravenous fish-soybean oil emulsion in serum fatty acid composition in total parenteral nutrition. JPEN J Parenter Enteral Nutr 1992;16:28S.
43. Bower RH, Cerra FB, Bershadsky B, et al. Early enteral administration of a formula (Impact) supplemented with arginine, nucleotides, and fish oil in intensive care unit patients: Results of a multicenter, prospective, randomized, clinical trial. Crit Care Med 1995;23:436–449.
44. Sanders TAB. Marine oils: Metabolic effects and role in human nutrition. Proc Nutr Soc 1993;52:457–472.
45. Roth MS, Martin AB, Katz JA. Nutritional implications of prolonged propofol use. Am J Health Syst Pharm 1997;54:694–695.
46. Sacks GS, Cleary JD. Nutritional impact of lipid-associated amphotericin B formulations. Ann Pharmacother 1997;31:121–122.
47. American Medical Association Department of Foods and Nutrition. Multivitamin preparations for parenteral use. A statement by the nutritional advisory group. JPEN J Parenter Enteral Nutr 1979;3: 258–262.
48. Demling RH, DeBiasse MA. Micronutrients in critical illness. Crit Care Clin 1995;11:651–673.
49. Demetriou AA, Keck-Jones L. Vitamins. In: Rombeau JL, Caldwell MD, eds. Clinical Nutrition: Parenteral Nutrition, 2nd ed. Philadelphia, W.B. Saunders, 1993:184–202.
50. Greene HL, Hambidge KM, Schanler R, Tsang RC. Guidelines for the use of vitamins, trace elements, calcium, magnesium, and phosphorus in infants and children receiving total parenteral nutrition: report of the Subcommittee on Pediatric Parenteral Nutrient Requirements from the Committee on Clinical Practice Issues of the American Society for Clinical Nutrition. Am J Clin Nutr 1988;48:1324–1342.
51. Schepers GP, Dimitry AR, Eckhauser FE, et al. Efficacy and safety of low-dose intravenous versus intramuscular vitamin K in parenteral nutrition patients. JPEN J Parenter Enteral Nutr 1988;12:174–177.
52. Solomons NW. Trace elements. In Rombeau JL, Caldwell MD, eds. Clinical Nutrition: Parenteral Nutrition, 2nd ed. Philadelphia, W.B. Saunders, 1993:150–183.
53. Leichtmann GA, Sitrin MD. Update on trace elements. Compr Ther 1991;17:42–48.
54. Mertz W. The essential trace elements. Science 1981;213:1332–1338.
55. American Medical Association. Guidelines for essential trace element preparations for parenteral use. A statement by the Nutrition Advisory Group. JPEN J Parenter Enteral Nutr 1979;3:263–267.
56. Levander OA, Burk RF. Report on the 1986 ASPEN Research Workshop on Selenium in Clinical Nutrition. JPEN J Parenter Enteral Nutr 1986;10:545–549.
57. Cerra FB. Parenteral nutrition. In: Pocket Manual of Surgical Nutrition. St Louis, Mosby, 1984:120–142.
58. Baumgartner TG, ed. Clinical Guide to Parenteral Micronutrition, 3rd ed. Deerfield, IL, Fujasawa USA, 1997.
59. Miller SJ. Peripheral parenteral nutrition: Theory and practice. Hosp Pharm 1991;26:796–801.
60. Payne-James JJ, Khawaja HT. First choice for total parenteral nutrition: The peripheral route. JPEN J Parenter Enteral Nutr 1993; 17:468–478.
61. Veterans Affairs Total Parenteral Nutrition Cooperative Study Group. Perioperative total parenteral nutrition in surgical patients. N Engl J Med 1991;6:336–337.
62. Kane KF, Cologiovanni L, McKiernan J, et al. High osmolality feedings do not increase the incidence of thrombophlebitis during peripheral IV nutrition. JPEN J Parenter Enteral Nutr 1996;20:194–197.
63. Grant JP. Vascular access for total parenteral nutrition: Techniques and complications. In: Handbook of Total Parenteral Nutrition, 2nd ed. Philadelphia, W.B. Saunders, 1992:107–138.
64. Lehmann S. Parenteral and enteral access devices. In: Teasley-Strausburg KM, ed. Nutrition Support Handbook: A Compendium of Products with Guidelines for Usage. Cincinnati, OH, Harvey Whitney Books Company, 1992:205–259.
65. Mirtallo JM, Jozefczyk KG, Hale KM, et al. Providing 24-hour nutrient infusions to critically ill patients. Am J Hosp Pharm 1986;43: 2205–2208.
66. National Advisory Group on Standards and Practice Guidelines for Parenteral Nutrition. Safe practices for parenteral nutrition formulations. JPEN J Parenter Enteral Nutr 1998;22:49–66.
67. Miller SJ, North GLT, Anderson WD. Parenteral nutrition order form to improve dextrose and lipid use. Am J Hosp Pharm 1990;47:2515–2518.
68. Campos ACL, Paluzzi M, Meguid MM. Clinical use of total nutritional admixtures. Nutrition 1990;6:347–356.
69. Dickerson RN, Brown RO, White KG. Parenteral nutrition solutions. In: Rombeau JL, Caldwell MD, eds. Clinical Nutrition: Parenteral Nutrition, 2nd ed. Philadelphia, W.B. Saunders, 1993:310–333.
70. Dickson LB, Somani SM, Hermann G, Abramowitz PW. Automated compounder for adding ingredients to parenteral nutrient base solutions. Am J Hosp Pharm 1993;50:678–682.
71. Thompson B, Robinson LA. Infection control of parenteral nutrition solutions. Nutr Clin Pract 1991;6:49–54.
72. National Coordinating Committee on Large Volume Parenterals. Recommendations to pharmacists for solving problems with large-volume parenterals. Am J Hosp Pharm 1976;33:231–236.
73. Keammerer D, Mayhall CG, Hall GO, et al. Microbial growth patterns in intravenous fat emulsions. Am J Hosp Pharm 1983;40:1650–1653.
74. Ebbert ML, Farraj M, Hwang LT. The incidence and clinical significance of intravenous fat emulsion contamination during infusion. JPEN J Parenter Enteral Nutr 1987;11:42–45.
75. AJHP Reports. ASHP technical assistance bulletin on quality assurance for pharmacy-prepared sterile products. Am J Hosp Pharm 1993;50:2386–2398.

76. Trissel LA. Handbook on Injectable Drugs, 9th ed. Bethesda, MD, American Society for Hospital Pharmacists, 1996.
77. King JC. Guide to Parenteral Admixtures. St. Louis, Pace Marq, 1997.
78. Parr MD, Bertch KE, Rapp RP. Amino acid stability and microbial growth in total parenteral nutrient solutions. Am J Hosp Pharm 1985;42:2688–2691.
79. McKinnen BT. FDA safety alert: Hazards of precipitation associated with parenteral nutrition. Nutr Clin Pract 1996;11:59–65.
80. Henann NE, Jacks TT. Compatibility and availability of sodium bicarbonate in total parenteral nutrient solutions. Am J Hosp Pharm 1985;42:2718–2720.
81. Driscoll DF, Baptista RJ, Mitrano FP, et al. Parenteral nutrient admixtures as drug vehicles: Theory and practice in the critical care setting. DICP Ann Pharmacother 1991;25:276–283.
82. Driscoll DF. Clinical issues regarding the use of total nutrient admixtures. DICP Ann Pharmacother 1990;24:296–303.
83. Mirtallo JM. The complexity of mixing calcium and phosphate. Am J Hosp Pharm 1994;51:1535–1536.
84. Driscoll DF, Bacon MN, Bistrian BR. Effects of in-line filtration on lipid particle size distribution in total nutrient admixtures. JPEN J Parenter Enteral Nutr 1996;20:296–301.
85. Krzyda EA, Andris DA, Whipple JK, et al. Glucose response to abrupt initiation and discontinuation of total parenteral nutrition. JPEN J Parenter Enteral Nutr 1993;17:64–67.
86. Dickerson RN. Question: How fast can I taper TPN in a hospitalized patient? Hosp Pharm 1985;20:620–621.
87. Bennett KM, Rosen GH. Cyclic total parenteral nutrition. Nutr Clin Prac 1990;5:163–165.
88. Evans NJ, Bamba M, Rombeau JL. Care of central venous catheters. In: Rombeau JL, Caldwell MD, eds. Clinical Nutrition: Parenteral Nutrition, 2nd ed. Philadelphia, W.B. Saunders, 1993:353–366.
89. Alexander JW. Nutrition and translocation. JPEN J Parenter Enteral Nutr 1990;14:170S–174S.
90. Cahill SL, Benotti PN. Catheter infection control in parenteral nutrition. Nutr Clin Prac 1991;6:65–76.
91. Grant JP. Septic and metabolic complications: Recognition and management. In: Grant JP, ed. Handbook of Total Parenteral Nutrition, 2nd ed. Philadelphia, W.B. Saunders, 1992:239–274.
92. Teasley-Strausburg KM, Shronts EP. Metabolic and gastrointestinal complications. In: Teasley-Strausburg KM, ed. Nutrition Support Handbook: A Compendium of Products with Guidelines for Usage. Cincinnati, OH, Harvey Whitney Books Company, 1992:295–303.
93. Apovian CM, McMahon MM, Bistrian BR. Guidelines for refeeding the marasmic patient. Crit Care Med 1990;18:1030–1033.
94. McMahon MM. Management of hyperglycemia in hospitalized patients receiving parenteral nutrition. Nutr Clin Pract 1997;12:35–38.
95. Freund HR. Abnormalities of liver function and hepatic damage associated with total parenteral nutrition. Nutrition 1991;7:1–5.
96. Briones ER, Iber FL. Liver and biliary tract changes and injury associated with total parenteral nutrition: Pathogenesis and prevention. J Am Coll Nutr 1995;14:219–228.
97. Wolman SL, Anderson H, Marliss EB, Jeejeebhoy KN. Zinc in total parenteral nutrition: Requirements and metabolic effects. Gastroenterology 1979;76:458–467.
98. Shuler CL, Wolfson M. Nutrition in acute renal failure. In: Rombeau JL, Caldwell MD, eds. Clinical Nutrition: Parenteral Nutrition, 2nd ed. Philadelphia, W.B. Saunders, 1993:667–675.
99. American Society for Parenteral and Enteral Nutrition. Standards for home nutrition support. Nutr Clin Prac 1992;7:65–69.
100. Joint Commission on Accreditation of Healthcare Organizations. 1995 Accreditation Manual for Home Care. Oakbrook Terrace, IL, Joint Commission on Accreditation of Healthcare Organizations, 1994.
101. Crocker KS. Current status of home infusion therapy. Nutr Clin Prac 1992;7:256–263.
102. Evans MA, Liffrig TK, Nelson JK, Compher C. Home nutrition support patient education materials. Nutr Clin Prac 1993;8:43–47.
103. Howard L, Heaphey L, Fleming CR, et al. Four years of North American registry home parenteral nutrition outcome data and their implications for patient management. JPEN J Parenter Enteral Nutr 1991;15:384–393.
104. Howard L, Blackburn G, Broviac J, et al. National trends in the use of home parenteral and enteral nutrition (HPEN) therapy. JPEN J Parenter Enteral Nutr 1994;18:22S. Abstract.
105. Eisenberg JM, Glick HA, Buzby GP, Kinosian B, Williford WO. Does perioperative total parenteral nutrition reduce medical care costs? JPEN J Parenter Enteral Nutr 1993;17:201–209.
106. Eisenberg JM, Glick H, Hillman AL, et al. Measuring the economic impact of perioperative total parenteral nutrition: Principles and design. Am J Clin Nutr 1988;47:382–391.
107. Twomey PL. Cost-effectiveness of parenteral nutrition. In: Rombeau JL, Caldwell MD, eds. Clinical Nutrition: Parenteral Nutrition, 2nd ed. Philadelphia, W.B. Saunders, 1993:401–408.
108. Trice S, Melnik G, Page C. Complications and costs of early postoperative parenteral versus enteral nutrition in trauma patients. Nutr Clin Pract 1997;12:114–119.
109. Task Force on Specialty Recognition and Certification of Nutritional Support Pharmacists. Executive summary of petition requesting recognition of nutritional support pharmacy as a specialty. Am J Hosp Pharm 1988;45:162–170.

129

ENTERAL NUTRITION

Douglas D. Janson, PharmD, BCNSP

Oral ingestion of food or the delivery of liquid formulas by a tube placed beyond the oral cavity are forms of enteral nutrition. "Enteral nutrition" and "tube feeding" are often used interchangeably to describe an artificial feeding method that includes the use of specialized feeding formulas, tubes, and pumps. Patients who are unable to chew or swallow because of a gastrointestinal (GI) obstruction, advanced neurologic or psychiatric diseases, or prolonged unconsciousness associated with critical illness benefit from nutrient delivery to the gut by tube feedings.

In this chapter the principles and practices related to the successful use of enteral nutrition support are described. Included herein is a review of digestive and absorptive physiology, the rationale for the use of the enteral feeding route whenever possible, indications for enteral nutrition, and a description of various enteral access and administration methods. Characteristics of commercially available formulas are presented, as well as initiation and monitoring guidelines to prevent complications. In addition, issues of drug compatibility, drug–nutrient interaction, and drug administration during enteral nutrition are discussed. Last, the effectiveness of enteral nutrition to enhance nutrition and disease outcome goals is reviewed.

GASTROINTESTINAL TRACT PHYSIOLOGY

Digestion and absorption are important and inseparably associated GI processes that generate the usable fuels for the body. Digestion consists of the stepwise conversion of a complex chemical and physical nutrient form into a molecular form acceptable to the intestinal mucosa. Absorption from the GI tract (GIT) consists of transfer of a nutrient across an intestinal cell membrane. The nutrient ultimately reaches the systemic circulation through the portal venous or splanchnic lymphatic systems provided that it is not excreted by the GI or biliary tract. Since the molecular forms of ingested nutrients are primarily large polymers that cannot be absorbed by the mucosal membrane unless they are broken down or transformed into an absorbable molecular form, digestion and absorption are inseparable. In addition, a coordinated interplay of gastrointestinal motility and neurohormonal secretion is required to facilitate adequate digestion and absorption.[1,2]

Nutrient digestion involves the complex coordination of multiple mechanical, enzymatic, and physicochemical processes. Mechanical dissolution of food occurs by chewing, mixing, and grinding of the stomach contents. Food stimulates the secretion of numerous neurohormones and enzymes from the salivary glands, stomach, liver and biliary system, pancreas, and intestines (Table 129–1). As food passes along the gut lumen, these neurohormones control GI motility and secretion among the organs of the digestive system. Nutrient digestion occurs within the gut lumen and also on the intestinal mucosa membrane. Absorption is a specific function of the intestinal mucosal membrane. The basic absorptive unit is a finger-like projection called the villus, which is made up of epithelial cells called enterocytes. The enterocyte surface contains special luminal projections called microvilli, which provide an increased surface area that is referred to as the brush border membrane.[1,2]

Digestible carbohydrates are presented to the small intestine as polysaccharides (starches) and oligosaccharides (sucrose and lactose). Enzymatic digestion within the gut lumen and at the surface of the brush border membrane produce simple sugars that are translocated across the membrane via active and passive transport mechanisms and are eventually released into the portal vein as shown in Fig. 129–1. Undigestible polysaccharides such as cellulose complexes and other fiber components are digested within the colon by bacterial hydrolases, disaccharidases, and enzymes to short-chain fatty acids (SCFAs). Subsequent to their rapid colonic absorption, SCFAs stimulate sodium and water reabsorption, serve as an energy source, and are trophic or nourishing to the cells of the intestinal mucosa.[3] Fat is primarily presented to the gut as long-chain triglycerides (LCTs) containing 14 to 24 carbons. LCT digestion includes lypolysis and the formation of mixed bile salt micelles to facilitate solubility and absorption across the mucosal membrane. Within the enterocyte cytosol, triglycerides are re-esterified and packaged into chylomicrons for release into the lymphatic system, as shown in Fig. 129–1. Chylomicrons eventually reach the venous system after transport through the thoracic duct. Medium-chain triglycerides (MCTs) containing 8 to 12 carbons do not require luminal lipolysis and can be absorbed intact by the mucosal membrane. Within the enterocyte, MCTs are acted on by intracellular lipase and the resultant free fatty acids pass directly into the portal vein.[4]

Protein is presented to the gut primarily as large polypeptides and to a small extent as amino acids owing to the denaturation of protein within the stomach. Subsequent to the luminal digestion of polypeptides to oligopeptides of two to eight amino acids, brush border membrane amino-oligopeptidases generate dipeptides and tripeptides. Membrane translocation of the resultant peptides occurs via a

TABLE 129–1. Gastrointestinal Enzymes and Hormones

Enzyme/Hormone	Site of Secretion	Main Actions
Amylase	Salivary glands	Converts carbohydrates, starch, and glycogen to simple disachharides
Cholecystokinin (CCK)	Duodenum, jejunum	Stimulates pancreatic enzyme secretion and gallbladder contraction
Chymotrypsinogen	Pancreas	Breaks down proteins into proteases and peptides
Enteroglucagon	Duodenum, small intestine	Inhibits pancreatic enzyme secretion and bowel motility
Gastric inhibitory peptide (GIP)	Small intestine	Decreases gastric motility and stimulates insulin secretion
Gastrin	Stomach, duodenum	Stimulates gastric acid secretion and mucosal growth
Glucagon	Pancreas	Stimulates hepatic glycogenolysis and inhibits motility
Lipase	Pancreas	Hydrolyzes short-chain and medium-chain triglycerides, involved in fat absorption
Pancreatic polypeptide	Pancreas	Inhibits gallbladder contraction and pancreatic and biliary secretion
Pepsinogen	Stomach	Converts large proteins into polypeptides
Secretin	Small intestine	Stimulates hepatic and pancreatic water and bicarbonate
Trypsinogen	Pancreas	Breaks down proteins into proteases and peptides
Vasoactive inhibitory peptide (VIP)	Small intestine, pancreas	Vasodilator; stimulates water and bicarbonate secretion, release of insulin and glucagon, and production of small intestinal juice

peptide transport system, and free amino acids are carried via specific amino acid transport systems. Amino acids and dipeptides are then passed into the portal vein as shown in Fig. 129–1. The digestive and absorptive physiology of these and other nutrients such as water, electrolytes, vitamins, and trace elements are discussed in detail elsewhere.[104] Under normal circumstances, almost 100% of carbohydrates and more than 80% of amino acids are absorbed within the proximal jejunum. The majority of fat absorption occurs within the jejunum and is completed in the ileum. The absorptive location of these and other nutrients within the GI tract is variable.[104]

Understanding the mechanisms of digestive and absorptive physiology can greatly enhance the rational use of enteral nutrition support during conditions of normal or altered GI function. Several circumstances may alter the efficacy of nutrient digestion and absorption (Table 129–2). These factors, as they relate to successful enteral nutrition practice, are discussed in detail throughout this chapter.

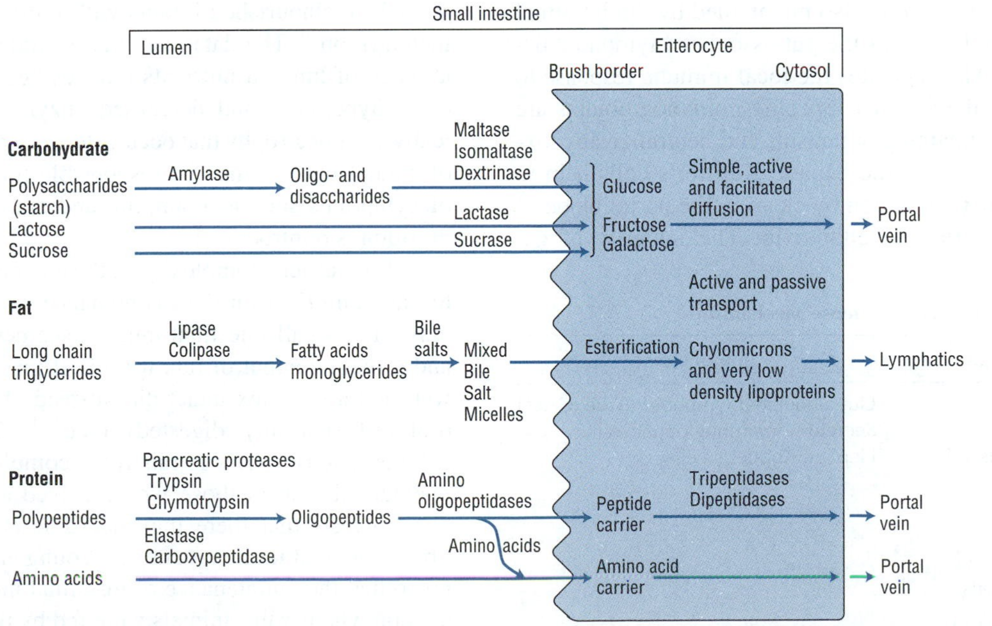

FIGURE 129–1. Schematic representation of carbohydrate, fat, and protein digestion and absorption within the small intestine. Subsequent to mechanical and enzymatic digestion of these substrates within the lumen and/or brush border of the enterocyte, smaller molecular forms are absorbed into the cytosol by numerous transport mechanisms. Then, nutrients are released from the enterocyte into the systemic circulation.

TABLE 129–2. Factors Affecting Intestinal Nutrient Absorption

Method of ingestion
Digestibility
Gastric emptying
Intraluminal digestive capacity of the pancreas and the bile
Transit time
Contact surface
Length
Surface of villi
Brush border enzyme content
Carrier function
Diffusion barrier thickness (unstirred layer)

GUT HOST DEFENSE MECHANISMS

Besides digesting and absorbing nutrients to maintain nutritional health, the GI tract is actively involved in defending the host from toxins and antigens by means of nonimmunologic and immunologic mechanisms (Table 129–3). These gut host defense mechanisms are also collectively referred to as the "gut barrier function."[5,6] The gut barrier acts to prevent the spread of intraluminal bacteria and endotoxin to systemic organs and tissues. Hydrochloric acid secreted by the stomach kills the majority of the bacteria ingested with food. Under normal circumstances a mucus gel layer coats the intestinal epithelium and thereby alters the adherence of bacteria to the cells of the GI tract and provides a favorable environment for anaerobic bacteria. Anaerobic bacteria, which normally colonize the mucus layer, aid in preventing tissue colonization by potential pathogens. Small bowel peristalsis further prevents bacterial stasis and overgrowth. The gut barrier function is also maintained by the intestinal immune system, known as the gut-associated lymphoid tissue (GALT). GALT regulates the local immune response to antigens within the GI tract. Specific immunoglobulins are secreted to kill remaining organisms and neutralize any toxins they produce. Last, the hepatic Kupffer's cells help to maintain gut barrier function by clearing the portal blood of gut-derived bacteria and endotoxin. The integrity of gut barrier function may be affected by numerous pathogenic insults such as physiologic stress, ischemia, and a variety of drugs including chemotherapeutic agents. The nutritional aspects that influence the maintenance of the gut barrier are discussed in the next section.

TABLE 129–3. Gut Host Defense Mechanisms

Nonimmunologic	Immunologic
Mechanical	Gut-associated lymphoid tissue (GALT)
Epithelial cell	Secretory immunoglobulin A
Epithelial mucus gel layer	Hepatic Kupffer's cells
Peristalsis	
Gastric acid	
Bile salts	
Salivary secretions	
Indigenous microflora	
Limits microbial proliferation	
Microbial antagonism	

RATIONALE FOR ENTERAL NUTRITION

Enteral nutrition is the preferred route of nourishment if the GI tract is functioning and accessible. A considerable body of laboratory and clinical evidence supports the importance and potential advantages of using enteral over parenteral nutrition. Advantages of enteral nutrition include maintaining the structure and function of the GI tract, fewer metabolic and infectious complications, and lower costs.

Experimental data derived predominantly from animal studies suggest that the maintenance of GI tract structure and function is dependent on the presence and composition of luminal nutrients as well as the presence of trophic hormones. A frequently cited benefit of enteral nutrition is that it preserves the process of intestinal crypt cell renewal necessary for the support of normal villi structure and associated enzymatic functions that are required for normal digestion and absorption. Rats who underwent an experimental small bowel bypass from the nutrient stream demonstrated a decrease in mucosal weight, protein, RNA, and enzyme activity.[7] Rats fed parenteral nutrition without enteral feeding for 7 or 12 days were also found to have a significant reduction in small bowel mucosal weight, height, protein, DNA content, and disaccharidase activity.[8,9] Mucosal atrophy and deficient disaccharidase and trypsin activities have also been documented in small bowel biopsies obtained from 16 malnourished infants with protracted diarrhea and malnutrition.[10] The data from these studies suggest that the absence of luminal nutrients induces "gut atrophy" or mucosal hypoplasia and decreased enzymatic activity. Clinically, the gut atrophy that occurs during a prolonged absence of enteral feeding may be responsible for the development of symptoms such as cramping and diarrhea when enteral nutrition is reintroduced.

The nutrient complexity of the enteral diet also appears to have an effect on the maintenance of intestinal mucosa mass. The small intestinal mucosa segment weights, DNA, and protein content of rats were best maintained when rats were fed a complex intact diet instead of an isocaloric hydrolyzed (partially digested) diet.[11,12] Furthermore, the colonic mucosal mass in rats fed a complex diet was better maintained than in those who received a hydrolyzed diet; this suggests that there may be some contribution of the fiber contained in the rat chow.[11] Young and coworkers also noted that the maintenance of intestinal mucosa was dependent on whether the animals were fed by the oral, gastric, or jejunal route.[12] The presence of luminal nutrients in animals also has been shown to stimulate the production of enteric hormones such as gastrin and enteroglucagon, which are trophic to the gut mucosa.[13–15] These hormones are found in humans, but have not been studied as intensively in humans as they have in animal models.

The intestine is an organ of protein synthesis as well as one of digestion and absorption. It therefore utilizes nutritional substrates directly. Glucose, glutamine, and L-leucine are examples of fuels used more efficiently when given via the enteral route as opposed to parenterally.[16,17] L-Leucine yields greater protein synthesis when given orally and is incorporated into the intestinal structure differently depending on the route of ingestion. Serum glutamine levels fall during stress, whereas intestinal uptake rises.[18] Glutamine and ketones are absent from parenteral solutions and may account for some of the intestinal structural deterioration seen during the administration of parenteral nutrition. The results from the aforementioned studies and others have stimulated several investigations into the effects of specific types of enteral diets, specific nutrients such as glutamine and fiber, and the interaction of trophic hormones on their ability to maintain the GI mucosa.

Maintenance of the functional integrity of the GI tract is intimately linked to proper gut barrier function. The immunologic and barrier functions listed in Table 129–3 prevent antigenic invasion of the gut mucosa, induction of local inflammation, and translocation of gut bacteria to the portal or lymphatic circulation. It has been suggested that bacterial translocation, the appearance of enteric organisms in the mesenteric lymph nodes, spleen, and liver, is promoted by parenteral nutrition and bowel rest. Since enteral nutrition better maintains the functional integrity of the gut, it may also prevent gut bacterial translocation. Animal studies comparing parenteral and enteral nutrient delivery supporting the theory of gut bacterial translocation include the following: enteral nutrition resulted in higher secretary IgA and biliary tract secretions,[19] less bacterial leak through intestinal mucosa,[20] greater maintenance of mucosal weight and thickness with lower secretion of catabolic hormones following a burn injury,[21] and reduced mortality following septic[22] or hypotensive insult.[23] The results of one human study among healthy volunteers also suggest the potential role of enteral nutrition in maintaining the gut mucosal barrier and preventing bacterial translocation. Subjects receiving total parenteral nutrition (TPN) and complete bowel rest for 7 days, compared to subjects receiving enteral feedings, had significantly higher levels of arterial epinephrine, glucagon, and hepatic venous tumor necrosis factor when given an equivalent dose of enteral endotoxin. Additionally, the parenterally fed subjects also had enhancement of acute-phase protein response, increased peripheral amino acid mobilization, and increased peripheral lactate production, a metabolic response expected to occur with systemic endotoxin effect.[24] The 1990 summary guidelines for the scientific review of enteral food products by the Life Sciences Research Office, Federation of American Societies for Experimental Biology, concluded that although available human data are insufficient to establish whether the atrophic changes in the gut that are associated with a lack of enteral nutrition lead to clinically significant translocation of gut bacteria, endotoxins, and antigenic macromolecules, these considerations seem to justify the use of at least partial enteral nutrition as one means of maintaining the gut mucosa or reducing such complications.[25] Prospective, randomized clinical trials among critically ill patients comparing enteral and parenteral delivery are unable to substantiate a direct cause and effect between the parenteral route and gut bacterial translocation. However, a recent critical review of several studies suggests that enteral nutrition may have a favorable impact on GI immunologic function and infectious morbidity.[26]

A metabolic advantage of enteral feeding compared to the parenteral route is improved glucose tolerance and markedly less hyperinsulinemia.[27,28] It has been proposed that better control of peripheral blood glucose levels occurs during enteral administration because the insulin released is absorbed with the glucose via the portal vein and is handled by the liver. The enteral feeding route is also as effective as the parenteral route in maintaining or promoting repletion of nutritional indices among several patient populations.[29] An additional physiologic benefit of enteral feeding is that it stimulates bile flow through the biliary tract and, hence, reduces the development of gallbladder sludge and stone formation, which has been associated with long-term parenteral nutrition and bowel rest.[30] Also, enteral nutrition removes the potential infectious or technical complications associated with the placement and use of a central venous access device required for parenteral nutrition. Finally, enteral nutrition is less costly than parenteral nutrition, as is discussed within the pharmacoeconomic considerations section of this chapter.

INDICATIONS FOR ENTERAL NUTRITION

Subsequent to assessing the patient's nutritional state and need for initiating specialized nutrition support, the clinician must assess the functional status of the GI tract and the optimal access site for tube placement. An algorithmic approach to nutritional management is shown in Fig. 127–1 of Chapter 127. Although enteral nutrition is indicated for many conditions or disease states (Table 129–4), its use is contraindicated for patients with a mechanical obstruction of the GI tract, diffuse peritonitis, severe diarrhea that makes metabolic management difficult, severe GI hemorrhage, intractable vomiting, chronic intestinal pseudo-obstruction, or severe malabsorption.

FUNCTIONAL STATUS OF THE GI TRACT

An assessment of the length, anatomy, and motility of the GI tract is required prior to the initiation of enteral therapy (see Table 129–2). The minimum length of functional small

TABLE 129–4. Potential Indications for Enteral Nutrition

Neoplastic disease	Gastrointestinal disease
Chemotherapy	Inflammatory bowel disease
Radiotherapy	Short bowel syndrome
Upper gastrointestinal tumors	Esophageal motility disorder
Cancer cachexia	Pancreatitis
	Fistulas
Organ failure	Neurologic impairment
Hepatic	Comatose state
Renal	Cerebrovascular accident
Cardiac cachexia	Demyelinating disease
Pulmonary	Severe depression
Multiple organ system failure	Failure to thrive
	Other indications
Hypermetabolic states	Acquired immune deficiency syndrome
Closed head injury	Anorexia nervosa
Burns	Complications during pregnancy
Trauma	Geriatric patients with multiple chronic disease
Postoperative major surgery	Organ transplantation
Sepsis	

bowel required for nutrient absorption is approximately 100 to 150 cm of jejunum and/or ileum. Enteral nutrient delivery may effectively nourish patients with less than 100 cm of small bowel, especially if the ileocecal valve and the colon are present and intact.[31] Increased small bowel motility, also referred to as an increase in transit time, occurs when the ileum and/or ileocecal valve are removed. The ileocecal valve acts as a brake and reduces the transit of the GI contents through the small bowel and into the colon. The colon maintains fluid and electrolyte balance in an enterally fed patient.

Hospitalized patients may have reduced gastric motility and emptying caused by sepsis, postoperative anesthetic agents, opioid analgesics, and underlying pathology such as diabetic gastroparesis. Reduced gastric emptying can place a gastrically fed patient at risk for nausea, vomiting, and subsequent pulmonary aspiration of gastric contents. Rather than resorting to parenteral nutrition, successful enteral nutrition can be initiated by placing the tip of the feeding tube beyond the pylorus into the duodenum or, preferably, more distal into the jejunum. Although there is some evidence that continuous feeding into the stomach or the duodenum increases the small bowel transit time, intestinal nutrient absorption is complete for either route.[32] Early enteral feedings started within 12 to 24 hours for the postoperative patient via the small bowel are frequently given, even in the absence of bowel sounds. However, during states of shock, borderline tissue oxygenation, and unstable cardiopulmonary hemodynamics, initiation of early GI feedings should be withheld since nutrient delivery and its associated oxygen requirement can further compromise oxygen tissue perfusion. Anecdotal reports and animal studies suggest that early enteral nutrition can be provided to the GI tract of a patient who has recently undergone a GI anastomosis without compromising the integrity of the anastomosis.[33]

Guidelines for the use of enteral nutrition have been established and published by the American Society of Parenteral and Enteral Nutrition.[34] Patients with neurologic impairment or psychological diseases who will not or cannot eat, but have functioning GI tracts, are candidates for enteral nutrition. Patients with organ failure, GI diseases, and patients in hypermetabolic states such as burns or trauma are frequently candidates for enteral nutrition. Enteral feeding is indicated during some clinical situations of GI fistulous disease such as colocutaneous or low-output ileal fistulas. Enteral nutrition is also favored for patients with an esophageal, gastric, duodenal, and proximal jejunal fistula when distal GI tract tube feeding access is possible. The use of enteral nutrition during severe pancreatitis or associated complications has increased over recent years. The precise effect of enteral nutrition on exocrine pancreatic secretion when infused into the jejunum is unclear because of conflicting data from human and animal studies. Nonetheless, clinicians have used the placement of a feeding tube into the jejunum for administering specialized enteral formulas to patients with severe and complicated pancreatitis. Based on case reports and uncontrolled retrospective series, jejunal tube feedings have been successfully used without aggravating the disease or associated complications. Prospective, randomized, and controlled trials are needed before concise recommendations for the use of enteral nutrition during severe pancreatitis can be proposed.[35] It has been recommended that TPN should be used when enteral feeding exacerbates abdominal pain, ascites, or fistulous output in patients with pancreatitis and limited oral intake.[34] Several clinical trials have shown that enteral nutrition is effective in supporting Crohn's patients with exacerbations of their disease. However, enteral nutrition is contraindicated in Crohn's disease with concomitant high-output fistula or high-grade obstruction, or when enteral feeding fails to normalize the nutritional status or results in unacceptable GI symptoms.[34] In patients with acquired immune deficiency syndrome (AIDS), enteral nutrition should be used unless situations of severe malabsorption develop because of GI infections such as cryptosporidium or cytomegalovirus or during complications of lymphoma involving the small bowel.[36]

ENTERAL ACCESS

Enteral nutrition support is distinguished in part from normal eating by the routes of nutrient intake and the equipment needed to administer it. Because the conditions necessitating specialized nutrition support are varied, multiple options are available to provide the therapy. All routes involve placement of a tube through which a liquid formula is infused. As the site of nutrient delivery moves further away from the mouth, the tube insertion becomes more difficult and invasive but, at the same time, more permanent. The technique and selection of enteral routes and access devices

TABLE 129–5. Options and Considerations in the Selection of Tube Feeding Access

Access	Indications	Tube Placement Options	Advantages	Disadvantages
Nasogastric or orogastric	Short-term Intact gag reflex Normal gastric emptying	Manually at bedside	Ease of placement Allows for intermittent bolus or continuous feeding Inexpensive Multiple commercially available tubes and sizes	Potential tube displacement Increased aspiration risk Small bore tube
Nasoduodenal or nasojejunal	Short-term Delayed gastric emptying (early postoperative period or diabetic neuropathy) High risk of gastroesophageal reflux or aspiration	Manually at bedside Fluoroscopic Endoscopic	Reduced aspiration risk Allows for early postoperative feeding Multiple commercially available tubes and sizes	Manual transpyloric passage requires greater skill Potential tube displacement Continuous (and cyclic) feeding only Attendant risks of complication for endoscopic placement Small bore tube
Esophagostomy or pharyngostomy	Long-term Nasopharyngeal access contraindicated Tumors of head or neck region	Bedside with local anesthesia or during surgery	Large-bore tube Easy tube placement	Dressing changes by patient more difficult owing to location Requires stoma site care
Gastrostomy	Long-term Normal gastric emptying Swallowing dysfunction owing to neuromuscular disease or central nervous system disorders Esophageal stricture or neoplasm	Surgically Endoscopically (percutaneous endoscopic gastrostomy [PEG]) Laparoscopically Fluoroscopically	Allows for intermittent, bolus, or continuous feeding Large-bore tube Multiple commercially available tubes and sizes Low-profile buttons available	Attendant risks for complication for each method of placement Higher cost, particularly with surgical placement Aspiration risk potential Requires stoma site care
Jejeunostomy	Long-term Impaired gastric emptying (diabetic neuropathy) Facilitate postoperative enteral feeding in trauma, malnourished or upper GIT surgery Inability to access upper GIT	Surgically Endoscopically (accessing jejunum via PEG) Laparoscopically Fluoroscopically	Allows for early postoperative feeding Reduced aspiration risk Multiple commercially available tubes and sizes	Attendant risks for complication for each method of placement Continuous (and cyclic) feeding only Requires stoma site care

have recently been extensively reviewed in the literature.[37,38] The indications, placement options, advantages, and disadvantages associated with the different tube feeding routes are summarized in Table 129–5.

The most frequently used short-term enteral feeding routes are those accessed by inserting a tube through the nose and threading it into the stomach or upper small bowel (Fig. 129–2). The names of these routes, nasogastric (NG), nasoduodenal (ND), and nasojejunal (NJ), indicate both the tube insertion point and the termination point. The oral gastric (OG) route is reserved for patients in whom the nasopharyngeal area is unaccessible or in infants unable to take food by mouth. These routes do not require surgical intervention and, therefore, are the least invasive. They are also temporary, because the tubes are frequently held in place by a piece of tape on the nose. One disadvantage is that they can easily be pulled out during routine patient care.

Dobbie and Hoffmeister[39] were the first to describe feeding through a flexible, weighted tube. Prior to their report, all enteral feedings were infused through heavy, large-bore, rigid rubber tubes. The use of the rigid tube was associated with loss of lower esophageal sphincter tone, otitis media, esophagitis, esophageal perforations, and mucosal injury.[40] Modern tubes patterned after Dr. Dobbie's prototype generally consist of small-bore pliable silicone rubber or polyurethane, which makes them lightweight and comfortable for the patient. The tube tip is either unweighted or weighted, frequently with inert tungsten. The weighted end is intended to help facilitate successful tube passage via peristalsis through the pylorus and into the small intestine after entering the stomach. Modern feeding tubes are available in varying lengths of 16 to 60 inches and small-bore sizes of 6 to 12 French, allowing for numerous options among pediatric and adult populations. A disadvantage of the small-bore tube is that it may become clogged, due to improper medication administration or tube-flushing techniques.

In general, the stomach is the least expensive and the least labor-intensive access site to use for enteral feeding; however, it is not necessarily the best. Patients who have delayed gastric emptying from complications of diabetes or

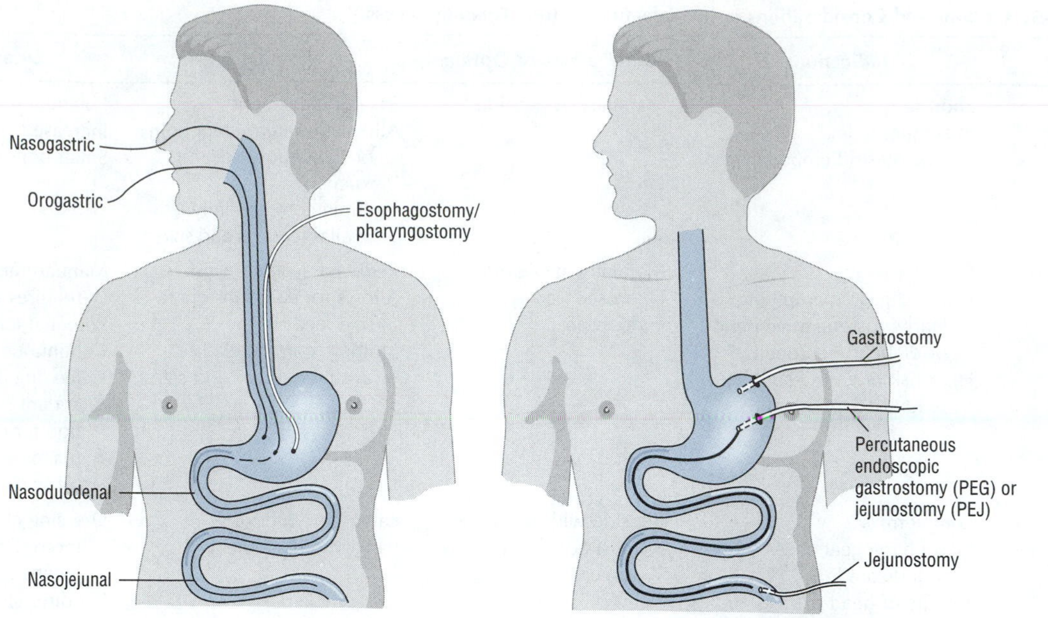

FIGURE 129–2. Access sites for tube feeding. Nasogastric, orogastric, nasoduodenal, and nasojejunal are generally short term (less than 6 weeks) enteral feeding routes. Esophagostomy/pharyngostomy, gastrostomy, PEG, percutaneous endoscopic jejunostomy (PEJ), and jejunostomy are longer term (months to years) enteral feeding routes. If the patient is at increased aspiration risk, the location of the enteral tube tip can be selected to deliver the feedings beyond the pylorus.

gastric atony during the postoperative period are at a higher risk for aspiration of gastric contents into the pulmonary system. Therefore, postpyloric tube placement may be required to enable successful enteral feeding. Studies have yet to prove definitively whether postpyloric tube feedings actually do decrease the risk of aspiration and pneumonia. The NG, OG, ND, and NJ tubes can all be placed manually at the patient's bedside. Greater skill is required to place the feeding tube beyond the pylorus at the bedside. Several techniques have been described in the literature to help facilitate manual placement at the bedside. These include the use of styletted tubes, that is, a wire in the tube to help guide its placement, weighted tubes, patient placement onto their right side, and/or use of metoclopramide. Even though success rates of 80% to 90% have been quoted in the literature using such techniques for postpyloric tube placement, this degree of success is not experienced by all clinicians.[37] Alternatively, it may be necessary to move the tube physically through the pylorus by using fluoroscopy or endoscopy, which also increases the cost of enteral therapy. X-ray verification of nasogastric or nasoenteric feeding tubes placed by manual techniques must be obtained routinely on all patients with altered consciousness or altered cough or gag reflex or those who are mechanically ventilated.[37]

More invasive, yet more permanent enteral feeding access includes esophagostomy or pharyngostomy, gastrostomy, and jejunostomy placement (see Fig. 129–2). Pharyngostomies and esophagostomies are indicated in patients with head and neck malignancies or maxillofacial anomalies that contraindicate nasopharyngeal access. Cervical pharyngostomy and esophagostomy are invasive as the tube is located in the neck and passes through the skin into the esophagus or the pharynx. Therefore, they are generally considered long-term enteral access devices. These routes use large-bore tubes, and tube replacement can be accomplished quite easily. As with any ostomy, site care is required. Dressing changes may be more difficult to perform by the patient owing to the location. Complications of these routes, though infrequent, include recurrent laryngeal nerve damage, aspiration, and infection.[38]

A feeding gastrostomy is another long-term enteral access device indicated for a patient with esophageal obstruction or impaired swallowing; however, the patient must have adequate gastric emptying. A gastrostomy can be placed surgically, under general anesthesia. The attendant risks of general anesthesia are hypotension and aspiration. However, if the patient requires surgery for another reason, a gastrostomy tube can also be placed at the time of surgery. The complication rates of surgical gastrostomy placement average less than 2% for such complications as wound infection or dehiscence, tube site problems including infection, continuous drainage or fistula formation, tube dislodgment or subsequent peritoneal contamination, and GI bleeding.[37]

The percutaneous endoscopic gastrostomy (PEG) is a popular nonoperative procedure that can be performed safely and cost effectively using local anesthesia. PEGs are generally placed in an endoscopy suite, eliminating costly operating room time. The results of a prospective randomized comparison between PEG and operative gastrostomy demonstrated similar complication rates, but the PEG had a higher benefit–cost ratio. More recently, two other techniques for gastrostomy placement have been described in the literature. They are laparoscopically and fluoroscopically placed gastrostomy tubes. Further investigation will be required to define the role of these two techniques. Gastrostomies use large-bore tubes, are associated with less tube clogging, and allow for all methods of tube feeding administration. Subsequent to the maturity of the surgical tract where the gastrostomy tube lies, a low-profile skin-level gastrostomy button may be placed for patient convenience and comfort. Gastrostomy sites require general stoma site care to prevent inflammation and infection.

Last, jejunostomies are long-term enteral access devices indicated during stomach or duodenal obstruction, impaired gastric emptying from diabetic neuropathy, or for the same situations as a gastrostomy tube. Frequently, jejunostomies are placed during a surgical procedure when the small bowel is readily accessible. This may allow for early postoperative enteral feeding since the small bowel is least affected by surgical manipulation, whereas gastric atony and colonic ileus may persist for a long time postoperatively. Delayed gastric emptying has been observed in 50% of patients undergoing pylorus-preserving pancreaticoduodenectomies.[41] Successful early enteral feeding of these patients requires gastric decompression while feeding into the small bowel through a jejunostomy tube. A jejunostomy tube may be placed surgically and has a complication rate of less than 1%, with intraperitoneal leakage of infusion as the major complication. Further, a jejunostomy tube may be created by conversion of a PEG to a jejunostomy (PEJ) by passing a feeding tube through the lumen of the PEG and then beyond the pylorus and into the jejunum. In addition, laparoscopically and fluoroscopically placed jejunostomies are also described in the literature.[37] Administration of enteral feeding into the jejunum should be done only by a continuous or a continuous-cyclic method of tube feeding. This is done to reduce the potential incidence of GI bloating, cramping, and diarrhea from tube feeding formula administered into the small capacity of the intestinal lumen.

ADMINISTRATION METHODS

The administration methods for tube feeding are continuous, continuous cyclic, intermittent, and intermittent bolus (Table 129–6). The choice of administration method is dependent on the anatomic location of the feeding tube, the clinical condition of the patient, the environment in which the patient resides, the intestinal function, and the patient's tolerance to the tube feeding.

CONTINUOUS FEEDING

Continuous tube feeding is characterized by the administration of enteral nutrition formula via a delivery system over 16 to 24 h/d. The delivery system includes a feeding reservoir or bag attached to an extension set that is connected to a pump. The delivery system is then attached to the patient's enteral access tube. Even though continuous infusion may increase nursing time to routinely check the enteral

TABLE 129–6. Administration Methods for Tube Feeding

Method	Equipment	Indication	Infusion Example
Continuous	Infusion pump generally recommended Enteral formula container Administration set	Gastric tube feeding Postpyloric tube feeding Critically ill patient Limited absorption capacity Limited feeding tolerance via intermittent and bolus methods	Full strength isotonic formula infused at 20 mL/h, advanced by 20 mL/h increments every 8 h to desired goal rate as tolerated
Continuous cyclic	Infusion pump generally recommended Enteral formula container Administration set	Gastric or postpyloric tube feeding Home tube feeding Rehabilitation patient Nocturnal tube feeding Potential transition to oral intake during daytime Limited feeding tolerance via bolus or intermittent method	Formula infused over 10–14 h daily at desired goal rate to achieve nutrient requirements
Intermittent	Infusion pump or gravity flow Enteral formula container Administration set	Gastric tube feeding Home tube feeding Rehabilitation patient Patient unlikely to make transition to oral intake Limited feeding tolerance via bolus method	240–480 mL formula infused over 20–40 min 4–6 times daily
Intermittent bolus	Large syringe (60 mL)	Gastric tube feeding Home tube feeding Rehabilitation patient Patient unlikely to make transition to oral intake	240–480 mL formula infused over <10 min 4–6 times daily

infusion, it does provide maximal tolerance by minimizing the side effects of abdominal distention or diarrhea. Infusion rates usually range from 50 to 125 mL/h, although rates of 150 mL/h have been reported without complications. Continuous delivery of nutrients is mandatory when the tube is placed in the duodenum or the jejunum. Continuous enteral feeding is widely practiced among critically ill patients.[41] A survey of nutritional support services compared the different techniques of administration of enteral feedings. The results indicated that 83% of enteral nutrition is given continuously whereas 17% is delivered by intermittent or bolus methods.[42] Continuous feeding is also beneficial for patients who have limited absorption capacity because of a rapid GI transit time or severely impaired digestion. Slow continuous administration in such patients allows greater time for digestion and absorption of nutrients as they pass through the intestine.

CONTINUOUS-CYCLIC FEEDING

Continuous-cyclic tube feeding uses the same delivery system as continuous feeding but the formula is administered over 10 to 14 h/d at the desired rate as specified by the tolerance of the patient and his or her nutrient requirements. Continuous-cyclic therapy is generally recommended for the noncritically ill patient, home tube feeding patient, or patients who are in rehabilitation settings. Cyclic enteral feedings allow a patient a physical and psychological break from being connected to the enteral infusion system and allow for greater rehabilitation and return to the activities of daily living. Frequently, continuous-cyclic enteral feeds are administered nocturnally, which may allow for transitioning a patient's diet to more oral intake during the daytime. Continuous-cyclic tube feedings may be administered into the stomach or small bowel. Cyclic feedings may require formulas of higher nutrient densities or higher infusion rates to compensate for the periods when the tube feedings are discontinued.[41] Therefore monitoring for GI tolerance is particularly important when patients are being initiated on a continuous-cyclic enteral feeding protocol.

INTERMITTENT FEEDING

Intermittent feeding consists of the administration of 240 to 480 mL of formula infused over 20 to 40 minutes four to six times daily. This method of delivery should be administered only to patients with feeding tube tips that lie within the stomach, because the stomach is capable of handling large and more rapid volumes of feeding formula. Since the stomach is the natural nutrient reservoir that controls the volume and osmolality reaching the small intestine, this prevents the dumping syndrome. The dumping syndrome occurs when a large quantity of a hyperosmolar solution is introduced too rapidly into the small bowel. Clinically this syndrome manifests as nausea, cramping, lightheadedness, and diarrhea. Intermittent enteral feeds may be administered by an infusion pump or via gravity flow with a roller clamp. Many authors advocate pump-assisted rate control, because roller clamps used to adjust the rate manually are known to be inaccurate and some patients may be acutely sensitive to even small variances.[43] However, gastric installation generally does not require such meticulous titration as long as gastric motility and the pyloric sphincter are intact. Intermittent enteral feeding is indicated for home tube feeding patients or patients in rehabilitation-type settings. Intermittent feeding is frequently selected for patients who are not able to eat normally on their own such as patients who have altered mental or cognitive function. Therefore, the tube feeding is given intermittently and is more physiologically consistent with normal eating patterns. Patients who receive intermittent feeding may be at higher risk for complications such as nausea, vomiting, and aspiration.

BOLUS FEEDING

Bolus feeding consists of the administration of 240 to 480 mL of formula infused over less than 10 minutes four to six times daily. It is used primarily for esophagostomy, pharyngostomy, or gastrostomy patients who have intact stomachs. The stomach then regulates the flow of formula into the intestine. Bolus feedings have the advantage of requiring little administration time and minimal equipment. Many times, only a large 60-mL syringe or bulb is needed to instill the feeding into the appropriate tube. Alternatively, bolus feedings can be infused via a complete infusion system consisting of an infusion reservoir, tubing, and possibly a feeding pump. Unfortunately, bolus feedings may not be well tolerated and can result in cramping, nausea, vomiting, aspiration, and diarrhea.

FEEDING EQUIPMENT

Feeding containers, administration tubing, and pumps should all be evaluated prior to their use. Feeding containers should be leak-proof, unbreakable, and easy to clean. They should be equipped with a reliable closure and have easy-to-read volume markings. The adaptability of the container to multiple infusion sets, its volume capacity, and ease of distinguishing it from an intravenous container should also be examined.[44] Administration sets consist of tubing that connects the feeding container to the feeding tube. These sets should be distinctly different from intravenous sets and adaptable to many feeding containers and feeding tubes. In addition, they should be long enough to connect the feeding container and patient easily. Last, the administration set should be equipped with an infusion control regulator that allows a reasonably accurate flow rate to within 20% of the expected rate. Pharmacists are sometimes asked to assist in evaluating enteral feeding pumps because of their familiarity with intravenous infusion pumps. Many considerations are the same for both types of pumps. They should be lightweight, easy to operate, have reasonably long battery life, and require little maintenance. The pump should have a useful alarm system that indicates low battery power, an empty container, or rising pressure in the set. Rising pressure indicates set occlusion. Last, the pump should be easy to operate by hospital or nursing home personnel and patients alike. Although delineation of the specific features of several manufacturers' enteral infusion pumps is beyond the scope of this chapter, they have been recently reviewed.[45]

CHARACTERISTICS OF ENTERAL FORMULAS

Since the introduction of enteral formulas in the 1940s, the composition and nutrient profile of enteral formulas have become highly sophisticated. Initially, enteral formulas were created to provide essential nutrients, and formula enhancements were made such as including fiber or modifying the specific amino acids to optimize the biologic value and utilization. Enteral formulas have also been modified in nutrient composition by changing the content of the amino acids, such as glutamine and arginine, changing the omega-3 polyunsaturated fatty acid content and adding ribonucleic acid, to promote a favorable physiologic effect that improves disease outcome. Modifying the enteral formula's nutrient content to improve disease outcome for a patient has been coined "nutritional pharmacology."[46] Currently, the U.S. Food and Drug Administration (FDA) describes enteral formulas as medical foods. The use of a medical food product is based on a need to provide energy and/or specific nutrients because of an underlying medical condition.[47] A lack of consensus exists as to whether medical foods should be components of supportive care and/or whether they ought to be categorized as pharmacologic treatment.[48] The Life Sciences Research Office has suggested that medical foods should "have documented evidence supporting claims of maintenance or improvement of nutritional status of patients . . . . and/or improvement of one or more specific nutrient-related disease manifestations significantly more than that observed from use of commercially available nutritionally complete formulas."[25] Currently the FDA has not developed any specific regulations for enteral formulas as to current food labeling requirements or to rules governing their health claims other than the regulatory statutes, which are designed to ensure good manufacturing practices for all processed foods.

The macronutrient content of enteral formulas (namely, protein, carbohydrate, and fat) varies in nutrient complexity (Table 129–7). Nutrient complexity refers to the amount of hydrolysis and digestion a substrate source requires prior to intestinal absorption. Polymeric or intact substrates are of similar molecular form as the food we eat. Those enteral formulas that contain partially hydrolyzed or elemental substrates are characterized as defined formula diets. The caloric contribution of each of the macronutrients is as follows: carbohydrates, 4 kcal/g; protein, 4 kcal/g; and fat, 9 kcal/g. The micronutrients, including electrolytes, vitamins, trace elements, and water, do not contribute to caloric content.

PROTEIN COMPOSITON

Important factors concerning the protein within enteral formulas are the quantity, quality, and the molecular form of protein. The essential amino acid content of the protein source determines the quality of the protein. The protein quality is frequently expressed in two standard ways, the biologic value and chemical score. It is desirable to have a protein source that is of high biologic value and chemical score because then less protein will be required to meet the patient's nitrogen requirements. Most of the readily available formulas contain proteins of high quality.[49] The molecular form of the protein source in enteral formulas will determine

TABLE 129–7. Enteral Formula Nutrient Complexity

Nutrient	Polymeric or Intact	Partially Hydrolyzed	Elemental

Carbohydrate	Starches
	  Fruit, vegetable, cereal solids
	Glucose polymers
	  Corn syrup solids
	  Polysaccharides
		Oligosaccharides
		Maltodextrins
		Disaccharides
		  Maltose, sucrose, lactose
			Monosaccharides
			  Glucose
			  Galactose

Fat	Long-chain triglycerides
	Polyunsaturated fatty acids
	  Corn oil
	  Safflower oil
	  Soybean oil
	  Butter fat
	  Menhaden
	  Fish oils
		Medium-chain triglycerides
		  Coconut oil
		  Palm kernel
		Free fatty acids
		  Linoleic	

Protein	Whole
	  Egg, milk, wheat, whey
	Isolates
	  Caseinate salts
	  Lactalbumin
		Oligopeptides
		Dipeptides
		Tripeptides
			L-Amino acids

the amount of digestion that is required for adequate absorption within the small bowel. Polymeric or intact protein sources require complete digestion to smaller peptides and free amino acids before they are absorbed from the GI tract. Therefore, enteral formula protein sources such as meat, milk, eggs, and caseinates require complete digestion by hydrochloric acid, specific protein enzymes, and pancreatic enzymes. Subsequent to these digestive processes, amino acids, oligopeptides, dipeptides, and tripeptides are presented to the enterocytes of the small bowel (see Fig. 129–1). The protein sources within enteral solutions have also been formulated with partially hydrolyzed proteins as peptides or elemental protein as L-amino acids (Table 129–7). The carriers for the peptides have proven to be very efficient in that they do not depend on sodium to function properly. Free amino acids, on the other hand, are absorbed via sodium-dependent mechanisms that appear to be slower and less efficient than peptide ones. Therefore, partially digested protein entities are the most readily absorbable form of nitrogen substrate.[2,32] As the molecular form of protein is reduced in size, the osmotic load within the enteral formula is increased. Also, as simplicity of the protein molecule increases, so does the prevalence of amino acids containing free sulfur; this in turn imparts a bitter flavor and foul odor to feeding solutions, making them less desirable for oral consumption.[50] Many commercially available enteral solutions contain combinations of intact and partially hydrolyzed protein sources.

CONDITIONALLY ESSENTIAL AMINO ACIDS

Glutamine and arginine have also been added to some enteral formulas. These amino acids are normally nonessential amino acids. However, during disease states of high physiologic stress, glutamine and arginine may become deficient and, therefore, have been characterized as conditionally essential. Glutamine is synthesized mostly in muscle and is used as the primary fuel for the enterocytes.[3] Therefore, during glutamine-deficient states, the utilization of glutamine increases beyond the synthesis or release of glutamine from the muscle tissue. Since glutamine is the primary fuel for the enterocyte, it has undergone investigation to determine its role in maintaining the integrity of the gut mucosa. Furthermore, it has been postulated that glutamine may play a role in preventing bacterial translocation. Free glutamine is not normally contained in TPN solutions. Two prospective, randomized clinical investigations of 0.57 g/kg of intravenous glutamine supplemented in TPN among bone marrow transplant patients have demonstrated conflicting results relative to the nutritional response and infectious complications. However, both demonstrated reduced length of hospital stay.[51,52] Glutamine-supplemented TPN in animals has been shown to increase the gut mass based on duodenal biopsies and reduced bowel permeability. Also in animal studies, glutamine-supplemented enteral amino acid diets have shown improved gut mass and function, whereas other investigators have found little benefit in supplementing glutamine to enteral diets.[3,53] The glutamine content of selected enteral formulas varies in the range of 1.8 to 14.2 g/L of formula. Enteral formulas containing glutamic acid also serve as an immediate precursor and eventually result in an increased production of glutamine. It has been questioned whether free glutamine is required to have a beneficial effect on the gut.[54] Some investigators have raised the concern whether glutamine may actually enhance some tumors in that it may act as a tumor stimulator. Obviously further research and investigation are required as to the potential benefits and harm associated with glutamine-enriched specialized nutrient formulas.[55]

Arginine is also a conditionally essential amino acid, in that it may not be synthesized in sufficient quantity during states of trauma or stress.[56] Data from animal investigations have demonstrated that arginine may have an antitumor effect, and among healthy subjects it has been shown to stimulate T-cell blastogenesis. In addition, supplemental arginine has been shown to decrease protein catabolism, enhance nitrogen retention following injury, and also accelerate wound healing. Arginine has been supplemented in selected enteral formulas in the range of 4.5 to 14 g/L of enteral formula. Diets enhanced with arginine have been studied in burn, cancer, and septic patients.

CARBOHYDRATE COMPOSITION

The carbohydrate content of enteral formulas is the major source of nonprotein calories. Polymeric or intact enteral formulas contain starches and numerous types of glucose polymers, which require complete digestion to the monosaccharide moieties prior to intestinal absorption (see Fig. 129–1). As the hydrolysis of carbohydrate increases within an enteral formula, the osmolality of the formula is also further increased. Elemental carbohydrates such as glucose and galactose contribute significantly to the osmolality of enteral formulas, which is directly correlated to enteral feeding intolerance. Therefore, partially digested entities, rather than elemental sugars, are the choice for inclusion in enteral formulas. Glucose polymers provide an especially useful carbohydrate source that is tolerated by most individuals (see Table 129–7). The polymers are large chains that provide a minimal osmotic load, yet are easily absorbed in the intestine. The one shortcoming of glucose polymers and oligosaccharides is that they are not as sweet as simple glucose and thus may decrease the palatability of orally consumed products. Finally, most commercially available enteral formulas are lactose free because some ethnic populations are lactase deficient and disaccharidase production within the gut lumen is reduced during illness or bowel rest.

FAT COMPOSITION

Fat is an important constituent in the diet because it provides a concentrated calorie source and serves as a carrier for fat-soluble vitamins. Sufficient linoleic acid is required to prevent essential fatty acid deficiency (EFAD), and should approximate 1% to 3% of total daily calories.[57] The most frequent sources of polymeric intact fat are vegetable oils (soy or corn) rich in polyunsaturated fatty acids. The digestion and absorption of LCTs are more complicated than those of either protein or carbohydrates. Fat digestion requires pancreatic enzyme release and formation of mixed bile salt micelles, which then facilitate absorption across the intestinal enterocyte as depicted in Fig. 129–1. The concentration of fat in enteral feeding formulas varies from less than 2 to 45% of total calories. The LCT fat sources have carbon chain lengths of 12 carbons. An alternative source of fat within enteral formulas is the MCTs, derived from palm kernel or coconut oils. MCTs are of 6 to 12 carbon lengths and have a caloric density between 8.2 and 8.4 kcal/g. MCTs do not contain the essential fats or linoleic acid. Therefore, most formulas contain some LCTs to provide essential fatty acids. Potential advantages of MCTs over LCTs are that they are more water soluble, they undergo rapid hydrolysis, and they require little to no pancreatic lipase or bile salt for absorption. They also do not require chylomicron formation for small bowel enterocyte absorption.

Also, some manufacturers have changed the source of long-chain fat (from omega-6 to -3 fatty acids) within enteral formulas to reduce the amount of the resultant physiologic products (i.e., prostaglandins, thromboxanes, and leukotrienes).[54,56] The omega-6 fatty acids are high in linoleic acid and are derived from vegetable oil, whereas the omega-3 fatty acids, derived from coldwater fish oils, are high in linolenic acid. The eicosanoid products of the omega-6 fatty acids have been shown to be potent inflammatory mediators and also decrease cell-mediated immunity. Therefore, if the fat content delivered from omega-3 is increased, the patient should experience less inflammation and immunosuppression.

NUTRITIONALLY COMPLETE FORMULAS

Most commercially prepared formulas contain micronutrients, including electrolytes, vitamins, trace elements, and water, to make them nutritionally complete. Nutritionally complete commercial formulas provide the recommended daily allowances (RDAs) of micronutrients for a patient receiving a sufficient volume of formula to meet their daily energy and macronutrient needs. A given predetermined nutrient complement, however, may not fit an individual's need because electrolyte, vitamin, and trace element requirements vary with disease state and organ function. One fairly common electrolyte abnormality occurring with enteral nutrition is hyponatremia.[58] Most formulas are made to mimic a low-salt diet, so hyponatremia could arise due to the limited sodium concentration. A low salt intake appears reasonable, because many patients who receive enteral nutrition are elderly and may have compromised cardiac function. However, patients who do not receive a sufficient volume of enteral formula to meet their RDA for micronutrients as the result of complications of fluid restriction or volume intolerance may require supplemental minerals and vitamins. Based on the adequate or high levels of vitamins in the blood of patients who have received long-term enteral therapy, the stability and absorption of vitamins that are contained in complete enteral formulas are felt to be adequate.[59] Patients who are fed enterally and have significant fat malabsorption may, over a long-term period, develop deficiencies of fat-soluble vitamins and therefore may need further supplementation of these vitamins. Most enteral feeding formulas contain the RDA of trace elements including iron, zinc, copper, and iodine, again based on receiving a sufficient volume of formula to meet the macronutrient needs of the patient. Selected enteral formulas also contain the RDA of selenium, molybdenum, and chromium. During deficiency states such as when diarrhea persists, supplementation of trace elements, namely, zinc, may be warranted.

FIBER CONTENT

Fiber, in the form of soy polysaccharide fiber, has been added to several enteral formulas in doses of 10 to 24 g of dietary fiber/L. Subsequent to bacterial degradation of fiber within the colon, the end products of fiber ingestion are SCFAs. Potential benefits of fiber are the trophic effects on the large bowel mucosa as well as promotion of sodium and water absorption within the colon. In addition, the resultant SCFAs are an excellent energy source. Fiber also has the ability to regulate bowel function by moderating intestinal transit time in individuals with altered motility conditions. The experimental evidence and clinical implications of fiber-enhanced enteral nutrition among healthy volunteers and several patient populations has been recently reviewed.[60] These authors concluded that even though there is good experimental evidence that fiber may play an integral role in normal human nutrition, the results of clinical studies have been disappointing. Fiber supplementation may be beneficial in long-term tube feeding of constipated patients. In intensive care units, however, drugs and stress seem to be more powerful determinates of bowel function than the addition of fiber to formulas.

OSMOLALITY AND RENAL SOLUTE LOAD

In addition to the macro- and micronutrient content within enteral formulas, the physical characteristics of formulas are important to the successful use of enteral nutrition. Patient tolerance and response to enteral formulas can be affected by the osmolality and the renal solute load. The osmolality of a given enteral formula is a function of the size and quantity of ionic and molecular particles, primarily related to the protein, carbohydrate, electrolyte, and mineral content within a given volume of formula. The unit of measure of osmolality is milliosmoles per kilogram (mOsm/kg). Enteral formulas with greater amounts of partially hydrolyzed or elemental substrates have a higher osmolality than formulas containing only polymeric or intact substrate forms. Therefore, formulas that contain sucrose or glucose, dipeptides and tripeptides, and amino acids are hyperosmolar. In general, enteral formulas range in osmolality from

300 to 900 mOsm/kg. Increased caloric density increases the hyperosmolar profile of an enteral formula. Symptoms of gastric retention, diarrhea, abdominal distention, nausea, and vomiting have been ascribed to the relative osmolality of the enteral feeding product. The results of clinical investigations to assess the relationship between osmolality and the incidence of GI side effects are conflicting.[61–63] Hospitalized patients administered hypotonic, isotonic, or hypertonic enteral formulas at a constant infusion rate demonstrated no significant differences in GI tolerance.[61] Other factors such as concurrent antibiotic therapy, which may alter the intestinal microflora; the method of delivery such as continuous versus bolus; and the appropriate selection of an enteral feeding formula for its composition play as much a role in the associated tolerance to the formula as the osmolality of the formula alone.[64]

The renal solute load is collectively made up of the protein, sodium, potassium, and chloride content of the enteral formula. Formulas that contain a greater solute load increase the obligatory water loss via the kidney. It is estimated that 40 to 60 mL of water is the minimal amount necessary to excrete 1 g of nitrogen.[49] Those receiving high-nitrogen enteral formulas, such as a geriatric patient or a patient with altered mental status unable to ingest more water, may be at risk for significant dehydration. Dehydration may be clinically detected as thirst, dry mucous membranes, depressed skin tugor, or an increased serum blood urea nitrogen or sodium level.

The rapid administration of hyperosmolar formulas reduces the gastric emptying rate.[49] Continuous administration into the stomach allows the pylorus to regulate the delivery of nutrient content into the duodenum and, hence, reduce gastric retention and associated symptoms of nausea and vomiting. When administering enteral formulas into the small bowel, products that are iso-osmolar can be initially administered at slow rates and advanced incrementally based on tolerance. Hyperosmolar formulas may require slower advancement to prevent the development of the dumping syndrome. As the lumen of the small bowel receives hypertonic enteral feedings, the small bowel secretes water to effectively dilute the formula and make it iso-osmotic, hence contributing to the diarrhea and further fluid and electrolyte depletion.

SELECTING AN ENTERAL FORMULA

The selection of an appropriate enteral feeding formula requires knowledge of several patient characteristics. First, the patient's medical history should be obtained. The length of small bowel, nutrient digestibility, and functional capacity help determine the appropriate formula complexity (see Table 129–7). In addition, the patient's underlying diseases, nutritional status, and fluid tolerance are required to determine nutritional goals. Knowledge of the feeding site will allow the selection of the appropriate delivery method of enteral feeding and reduce potential complications of therapy.

CLASSIFICATION OF ENTERAL NUTRITION FORMULAS

The proliferation of new enteral nutrition products continues, and it is easy to become overwhelmed with the variety of formulations available. Development of an enteral nutrition product formulary has been shown to be cost effective and to minimize confusion by identifying the rational use of prototype products.[65] Different criteria have been proposed to evaluate and categorize enteral nutrition products based on their unique characteristics.[25,54,55] The enteral formulas listed in Table 129–8 are categorized on the basis of the composition of the enteral formula with an emphasis on the general indication for product prototypes.

POLYMERIC FORMULAS

Polymeric solutions contain macronutrients in the form of intact protein, triglycerides, and carbohydrate polymers. They can be used orally or through a tube and provide complete nutrition.[55] An enteral formula is described as a "complete" product when it contains all of the micro- and macronutrients necessary to meet the RDAs for a patient. The majority of enteral products commercially available are lactose free, although there are enteral formulas available as oral supplements that do contain lactose. Frequently, the polymeric lactose-free tube feeding products are referred to as complete, "standard" enteral products. Describing enteral products as "standard" implies that these products require normal GI digestive and absorptive function for maintaining the nutritional status of a patient. Polymeric enteral feeding products are used in numerous settings including the critically ill, the noncritically ill, rehabilitation patients, and home enteral nutrition support patients. These polymeric enteral formulas or standard formulas are manufactured with variable caloric and protein densities ranging from 1 to 2 kcal/mL and 35 to 60 g/L protein, and have osmolalities ranging from 300 to 900 mOsm/kg. Products that are calorically concentrated generally have higher osmolalities. Fiber has also been supplemented in some of the standard formulas. The commercially available blenderized diets are made from natural whole foods. They are complete products with variable amounts of fiber and lactose. These products, owing to the nature of their composition, may have a higher viscosity and generally require an infusion pump and access through a large-bore feeding tube for successful administration

MONOMERIC FORMULAS

Monomeric enteral formulas have partially hydrolyzed and/or elemental components of protein, carbohydrate, and fat and, therefore, require less digestive and absorptive capacity. The major difference between polymeric and monomeric formulas is that monomeric formulas contain protein in small molecular forms. The chemically defined enteral

TABLE 129–8. Enteral Formula Classification System

Category	Subcategories	Indication	Features	Product Examples
Polymeric (normal GIT digestive and absorptive capacity required)	Lactose free	Standard oral supplement Complete tube feeding	Iso-osmolar, high nitrogen, fiber enhanced, and highly concentrated formulas available	Osmolite Resource IsoSource VHN Ultracal Deliver 2.0
	Lactose containing	Oral supplement Lactose intolerant	Palatable; hyperosmolar	Sustogen Meritene
	Blenderized	Complete tube feeding	May contain lactose; high viscosity and may require infusion pump	Complete modified
Monomeric (less digestion and absorption required)	Chemically defined	Complete tube feeding and some use as oral supplements Disease states that alter digestive or absorptive surface capacity	Nutrients hydrolyzed to varying degrees Osmolarity varies	Peptamen Reabilan HN
	Elemental	Complete tube feeding, rarely as an oral supplement Disease states that alter digestive or absorptive surface capacity Fat malabsorption	Free amino acids, >80% of kcal as oligosaccharides, <15% fat content as long-chain fat	Vivonex Plus Tolerex
Specialized (monomeric or polymeric)	Organ failure	Complete[a] tube feeding, rarely as an oral supplement Specific products for pulmonary, renal, hepatic, and endocrine failure	Composition varies; nutrient requirements modified to a specific disorder	Pulmocare Travasorb Renal Nutrihep DiabetiSource
	Immune support	Complete tube feeding, rarely as an oral supplement Enhance immune competency during critical illness or sepsis	Specific nutrients modified for immunopharmacologic function	Immun-Aid Impact
Modular (majority are polymeric)	Protein Carbohydrate Fat	Can be used to compound complete[a] formulas or to supplement enteral or oral feeding	May be labor intensive Micronutrients available to make complete formulas	ProMod Polycose MCT oil
Hydration	Glucose Electrolytes	Feeding tube or oral Dehydration, severe or chronic diarrhea		Equalyte

[a]May or may not be complete nutrient composition.

formulas are those in which the protein is in the form of oligopeptides, dipeptides, and tripeptides. The elemental products are those that can generally contain L-amino acids as the protein source (see Table 129–8). Carbohydrates are frequently in the form of oligosaccharides, sucrose, and glucose whereas fat sources are usually in the form of MCTs with small amounts of LCTs to provide essential fatty acid requirements. In general, the osmolality of monomeric products is higher, ranging from 500 to 700 mOsm/kg. The caloric density of monomeric formulas is generally 1.0 kcal/mL and they contain approximately 40 to 50 g protein/L. The intact protein of polymeric products must be digested to lower-molecular-weight peptides and/or free amino acids prior to absorption, whereas the monomeric enteral products, which already contain dipeptides and tripeptides, are more readily absorbed by the enterocyte.

The physiologic basis and clinical relevance for the use of monomeric enteral formulas in the clinical setting have been extensively reviewed.[32,55] The results from human and animal intestinal perfusion studies indicate that the partially hydrolyzed sources of protein have an absorptive advantage over those formulas that contain free amino acid. However, there are few controlled data on the nutritional efficacy of the protein hydrolysates or free amino acid formulations in humans. Even among pancreatectomized patients or those with severe short bowel, only slight differences in improved absorption have been shown to occur with the use of peptide-based diets. It has been hypothesized that the great reserve and adaptive capacity of the absorptive mucosa of the small bowel will still promote an adequate amount of nutrient absorption irrespective of the form of protein substrate delivered. Therefore, the relative indication for these products is currently controversial. Monomeric diets cannot be recommended for routine use in patients with normal GI function, those requiring early postoperative enteral feeding, or those with only mildly impaired pancreatic exocrine function, partial gastrectomy, and minor small intestinal resections. However, in pancreatectomized patients or those with markedly reduced GI surface area, the potential clinical benefit for the use of monomeric products warrants a therapeutic trial.[32,55] Monomeric products that have higher percentages of MCTs and small amounts of LCTs are generally recommended for patients with severe pancreatic insufficiency such as chronic pancreatitis and cystic fibrosis or severe abnormalities of the intestinal mucosa such as untreated celiac disease or extensive small bowel resection.[32]

DISEASE STATE–SPECIFIC FORMULAS

A third descriptive category of enteral feeding formulas is the specialized formulas based on specific metabolic needs such as organ failure and immune dysfunction. These specialized enteral formulas vary in their nutrient complexity composition (see Table 129–8). Specific nutrient concerns during organ failure are discussed in Chapter 131. The specialized enteral formulas that have been formulated to enhance immune competency during critical illness or sepsis provide substrates in pharmacologic doses that have experimentally been shown to enhance immune function.[56,66] These products contain more arginine and ribonucleic acids and an increased proportion of omega-3 polyunsaturated fatty acids. Glutamine has also been supplemented in some of these formulas to promote intestinal mucosal integrity and reduce infectious complications. A large prospective, randomized, double-blind multicenter clinical trial compared an immune-enhanced enteral product to a polymeric enteral product among patients in intensive care units after an event such as trauma, surgery, or sepsis.[67] Extensive statistical analysis of the aggregate data revealed that within a highly stratified subgroup of 37 septic patients, the intervention group had a decreased median length of hospital stay by 10 days (28 vs 18 days) and fewer infectious complications. Immune-enhanced products have also been studied among 85 patients who had major operations for cancer.[68] The length of hospital stay for the specialty formula group was reduced (15.8 ± 5.1 vs 20.2 ± 9.4 days), and favorable results from the *in vitro* tests of immune function were demonstrated. The nitrogen intake between the experimental and control populations in both of these studies was not controlled, and it is possible that the endpoints may have been affected by the nitrogen disparity between the groups.

Immune-enhanced enteral products have also been studied in small prospective, randomized, controlled trials among trauma patients. A comparison between an isonitrogenous, isocaloric standard diet and a modified diet containing glutamine, arginine, nucleic acids, and omega-3 fatty acids in 35 severely injured patients found that patients who received the immune-enhanced enteral product had significantly fewer major infectious complications (6% vs 41%, modified vs control).[69] Another trial with the same product in 98 patients with major torso trauma found significantly reduced intra-abdominal abscesses (modified, 0% vs control, 11%) and less multiple organ failure.[70] These data, however, provide no insight as to which nutrient(s) may have contributed to the improvement in clinical outcome.

MODULAR FORMULAS

A fourth category of enteral products is the modular nutrient components. Occasionally it is desirable or necessary to achieve a nutrient mix not supplied by a single commercially available product. Therefore, a single nutrient component such as carbohydrate, protein, and fat can be added to readily available solutions to enhance the specific substrate content. Protein modules may be singularly added to ready-made formulas when a higher nitrogen content is desired. These modules are marketed in powder form and may contain free amino acids, caseinates, or whole protein such as egg whites, solids, or whey. The module's nutrient complexity added to a commercial formula should be based on a patient's digestive capacity. Caloric enhancement of ready-made formulas may also be done by adding carbohydrate modules. Carbohydrate products such as glucose polymers are available in either solid or liquid forms and their caloric content varies.

HYDRATION FORMULAS

The last descriptive category of enteral products is hydration formulas. Oral rehydration formulas may be used in dehydrated patients to reduce diarrheal sequelae or replenish ostomy drainage fluid and electrolyte losses. Such formulas do not require intravenous access, are economical, and can be either purchased commercially or extemporaneously compounded. These formulas have been successfully used to manage mild to moderate dehydration in both children and adults. The oral rehydration solution is successful because of its glucose content. Glucose stimulates active transport systems, which in turn stimulate passive sodium and water uptake simultaneously with the glucose. Therefore, oral administration of several liters may actually decrease fecal water loss and generate a positive electrolyte balance.

FORMULARY AND DELIVERY SYSTEM CONSIDERATIONS

A practical issue that affects the enteral product selected for use in a patient is the product formulary of an institution. Obviously the selection of product should be based on patient characteristics and product features as previously discussed. However, such administrative concerns as cost, shelf life, ordering policies, product form, administration systems, and contract opportunities are frequently taken into account when an institution develops an enteral formulary. The majority of enteral products are available as ready-to-use, prepackaged liquids, whereas others are in a dehydrated, powdered state and require reconstitution prior to use. Advantages of ready-to-use liquid formulas are convenience and low susceptibility to microbiologic contamination. One of the disadvantages is that more storage space is required. The ease or convenience of packaging is especially important for patients involved in self-care, the disabled, and those who have difficulty receiving or following printed instructions.

Another practical issue that affects an institution's choice of an enteral delivery system is the potential complication of bacterial contamination. Both animal and human studies have demonstrated that contaminated enteral feeding formulas have been directly associated with infectious complications.[71–73] The GI tract may serve as a port of entry for bacteria into the systemic circulation, especially in patients who are receiving multiple antibiotics or who have undergone a surgical procedure. The contamination of enteral feeding formulas has been associated with the lack of attention to proper handling techniques, inability to disinfect preparation equipment, and nonsterile or contaminating tube feeding additives. Controversy exists as to how stringent handling procedures must be to ensure that the enteral feeding is safe for administration.[74] Nonetheless, controlling bacterial populations found in enteral feedings is warranted. Sterile enteral diets have been available in the form of the closed-administration systems, which are prefilled containers in volumes of 1 to 1.5 L of ready-to-feed enteral formula. This is in contrast to the more conventional open systems, which require cans or mixed powders to be decanted into larger volume delivery bags by institution personnel. The closed-administration system offers the advantage of requiring no mixing of formula and therefore lowers the risk of contamination and reduces time and labor required in preparing the formula.[75] Numerous types of enteral formulas are now available in the closed-administration system. The closed-administration system also offers the advantage of allowing hang times beyond 24 to 36 hours, whereas the conventional delivery system had hang times of generally 6 to 12 hours. A disadvantage of the closed-administration system is the inability to add minerals or color additives, for diagnostic or preventive purposes, without breaking the closed system.[54]

INITIATING AN ENTERAL NUTRITION REGIMEN

Subsequent to selecting the appropriate enteral access and feeding formula, the rate and strength of formula advancement must be determined. Schedules for progression of tube feeding delivery from initial to target rates are important and influence the maximum rate the patient can tolerate.[41] Frequently in the institutional setting, feeding into either the stomach or small bowel is begun with an infusion pump for slow continuous feeding. Although the advancement of enteral feeding should be individualized to specific patient issues, one may start half-strength dilution of the formula and administer it at a rate of 25 to 50 mL/h, regardless of the actual formula employed. This practice is used to prevent GI complications of enteral feeding such as diarrhea, abdominal cramping, bloating, and nausea. The rate is increased in 25 mL/h increments every 6 to 8 hours to a maximal rate with subsequent increase of the formula strength in the next day(s).[41] Such a progression should take no more than 3 days before the patient is at target feeding goals. However, many patients will tolerate more rapid advancement of a full-strength feeding formula from a rate of 20 to 25 mL/h with increments of 20 to 25 mL/h every 6 to 8 hours until the desired goal is achieved.

DRUG COMPATIBILITY WITH ENTERAL FORMULAS

Mixing of commercially available liquid medications with selected enteral nutrition products has been associated with several types of physical incompatibilities: granulation, gel formation, separation, and precipitation.[76,77] Not only can these physical incompatibilities inhibit the drug absorption within the small bowel of a patient, gel formation may potentially clog small-bore enteral feeding tubes. Physical incompatibility with medications is more common in formulas that contain intact protein than in those with hydrolyzed protein. Also medication and enteral formula incompatibilities are more common with the use of acidic pharmaceutical syrups. Liquid medications have osmolalities that range from 500 to 5000 mOsm/kg.[78] Subsequent admixture of liquid medications into enteral formulas can thus greatly enhance the final osmolality and result in the development of diarrhea. The most prudent recommendation for the mixing of commercial liquid medications and enteral nutrition formulas is to avoid the routine admixture whenever possible, especially the nonaqueous preparations and syrups. In the clinical setting, exceptions do exist, such as adding electrolyte injections of potassium or sodium to enteral formulas to assist in maintaining or repleting the electrolyte requirements for a patient.

COMPLICATIONS OF CONCOMITANT DRUG ADMINISTRATION

Enteral feeding tubes are frequently used as a route for the delivery of medications. However, the pharmacologic agent and its mode of delivery are modified when a feeding tube is placed. Concomitant administration of medications with enteral feedings delivered directly into the stomach through nasogastric or gastrostomy tubes allows the stomach to

TABLE 129–9. General Considerations for Medication Administration by Enteral Feeding Tubes

1. Administer medications by mouth when feasible; consider enteral feeding tube as an alternative route.
2. Determine location of the feeding tube tip, because pre- or post-pyloric drug instillation can alter effectiveness.
3. Liquid dosage forms should be used if available. Dosage and frequency adjustment are required if changing from a sustained-release drug to administer a non-sustained-release liquid form.
4. Hyperosmolar medications require dilution.
5. The contents of hard or soft gelatin capsules reconstituted with 10–15 mL of water and crushed compressed tablets reconstituted with 15–30 mL of water can be administered when a liquid form is unavailable.
6. Do not crush and administer sustained-release or enteric-coated medications.
7. Flush the feeding tube with water prior to administering a medication. Do not mix medications. Administer each medication separately, flushing with water between medications. Flush with water after medication administration completed.
8. In general, do not add medications to the enteral formula. Exceptions exist for the adding of hypertonic electrolyte injection to enteral formulas. Be aware of specific drug-enteral product incompatibilities.

function in its normal capacity for drug dissolution. However, placement of enteral tubes beyond the pylorus, such as with nasoduodenal, nasojejunal, and jejunostomy, alters drug dissolution because the stomach is bypassed. Therefore one must consider the anatomic location of the feeding tube tip when administering medications such as antacids or sucralfate, because their therapeutic effect is designed to occur within the stomach. Because many drugs are best absorbed in the fasted state, medications should be administered on an empty stomach as much as possible. Patients receiving bolus intragastric feedings may receive medications appropriately spaced between the feedings.[79,80] For those patients receiving continuous enteral feeding, the feedings may require interruption for drug administration, followed by prudent flushing of the tube with water. Pharmacists need to be aware of potential problems that may arise when medications are administered through enteral feeding tubes such as the degradation and/or inactivation of nutrient components or altered bioavailability of a drug that may compromise therapeutic efficacy[81–83] (Table 129–9).

Selecting the proper medication dosage form for administration by enteral feeding tubes is crucial to avoid drug inactivation and altered bioavailability (Table 129–10). Medications in sublingual form, sustained-released capsules or tablets, and enteric-coated tablets are designed not to be crushed and therefore should not be administered via enteral feeding tubes. An extensive list of oral dosage forms that should not be crushed is available in the literature.[84] For the most part, liquid drug preparations are the preferred dosage form when administering medications via enteral feeding tubes. In situations where a liquid medication is unavailable, compressed tablets or the contents of hard or soft gelatin capsules can be admixed with water and administered down enteral feeding tubes. Adherence to proper technique for administering the contents of tablets or capsules down feeding tubes such as flushing of the tube with water prior to and following the administration of medication is important to prevent clogging of the feeding tube.

DRUG–NUTRIENT INTERACTIONS

The most significant drug and nutrient interactions that can occur during continuous enteral nutrition are those in which the bioavailability of the drug is reduced and the desired pharmacologic effect is not achieved. Unfortunately, limited clinical studies are available to document the extent of

TABLE 129–10. Guidelines for Medication Administration by Enteral Feeding Tubes

Dosage Form	Administered by Enteral Feeding Tube	Comment
Sublingual or buccal tablets	No	Low dosage of drug not designed for gastric or intestinal administration Altered drug bioavailability and potency owing to first-pass effect
Sustained-release capsules or tablets	Not preferred Do not crush	Crushing a sustained-release dosage form destroys its time-release effect Altered therapeutic drug response and gastrointestinal irritation can occur
Enteric-coated tablets	Not preferred Do not crush	Crushing can result in gastrointestinal irritation and drug inactivation
Compressed tablets (sugar or film coated)	Yes	May be crushed and administered without altering therapeutic drug response May clog small-bore feeding tubes
Hard or soft gelatin capsules	Yes	Powders from hard capsules and oils from soft capsules may be administered without altering therapeutic drug response
Liquid preparations Solutions Suspensions Elixirs Emulsions	Yes Preferred	Frequently recommended; however, drug form can be hyperosmolar, requiring dilution Strong acid syrups may interact with enteral formulas and clog tubes

this problem with enteral feeding. Most of the observations are anecdotal case reports among few patients. A reduction in bioavailability of phenytoin has been demonstrated during continuous tube feeding, with subsequent subtherapeutic drug levels.[85] The exact cause for reduced phenytoin bioavailability during continuous enteral feeding is unclear; however, the results of *in vitro* studies suggest that protein and calcium chloride may bind the drug. A variety of methods to minimize this interaction for patients receiving continuous tube feedings have been suggested (Table 129–11). Little consensus exists as to the best method to prevent or reduce the impact of this interaction. Pharmacists must be aware that patients may require higher than normal doses of phenytoin while on enteral nutrition. The patient's clinical response and serum phenytoin levels should be closely monitored during continuous enteral feeding and after the discontinuation of enteral feeds.

Clinical studies documenting altered bioavailability with antibiotics during continuous enteral feeding are lacking. However, based on case reports and theoretical concerns, holding the tube feeding for 30 minutes before and 30 minutes after a selected antibiotic is administered is recommended (see Table 129–11). Warfarin resistance has also been documented during enteral feeding owing to the vitamin K content of the enteral feeding products. Prior to 1980, it was thought that the content of vitamin K in dosages of up to 1330 μg/1000 kcal of enteral feeding formula was contributing to the pharmacologic interaction with warfarin. Subsequently, the vitamin K content within formulas has been reformulated to less than 200 μg/1000 kcal. However, warfarin resistance has continued to be reported. Pharmacists should be observant of the vitamin K content within enteral formulas and adjust the warfarin dose based on monitoring the patient's coagulation parameters.

COMPLICATIONS AND MONITORING OF ENTERAL NUTRITION

A major advantage of enteral nutrition over parenteral nutrition is a reduced complication rate.[64] Major complications and potential causes for GI, technical, and infectious complications associated with enteral tube feeding are listed in Table 129–12. Several of the factors responsible for the metabolic complications seen among enteral nutrition patients are similar to those seen during parenteral nutrition and are presented in Tables 128–4 and 128–7 of Chapter 128. However, the GI, technical, and infectious complications seen during enteral nutrition are unique to this route of therapy.

METABOLIC COMPLICATIONS

The metabolic complications related to hydration and electrolyte and glucose control are more frequently observed in patients with underlying illnesses that cause organ dysfunction. The micronutrient and water content within enteral feeding formulas are in fixed amounts (RDAs) intended for the average patient. Therefore, the frequency of clinical and laboratory assessment to adequately monitor hydration, electrolyte, organ function, and glucose control for a patient

TABLE 129–11. Medications With Special Considerations for Enteral Feeding Tube Administration

Drug	Interaction	Comments
Phenytoin	Reduced bioavailability demonstrated when administered during continuous tube feeding. Results of in vitro studies suggest that protein (caseinate salts) and calcium chloride may reduce phenytoin bioavailability.[86]	Limited data from clinical studies and case reports provide basis for suggestions to overcome incompatibility. Suggestions include holding tube feeding 2 h before and after phenytoin;[85] administering phenytoin capsules rather than the suspension during continuous feeding;[87] and using a meat-based enteral formula rather than a protein hydrolysate-containing formula.[88] Monitor patient's clinical response and serum drug level closely.
Antibiotics (selected)	Reduced bioavailability demonstrated between food and penicillin, tetracycline, isoniazid, rifampin, enoxacin, norfloxacin, and ofloxacin.[89] Interaction also theoretically applied to continuous tube feeding.	Existence of clinical studies documenting enteral formula interaction with selected antibiotics is lacking. Holding tube feeding administration for specified time periods before and after drug administration has been recommended.[90] Monitor patient's clinical response closely.
Warfarin	Pharmacologic interaction demonstrated between warfarin and vitamin K contained in enteral feeding formulas, resulting in reduced anticoagulation effect.	Vitamin K is contained in most enteral products in doses less than 200 μg/1000 kcal. Adjust warfarin dose based on monitoring the INR and observing the vitamin K content of the enteral formula.
Antacids	Altered pharmacologic effect of antacid if administered into the small bowel. A physical incompatibility has been reported with aluminum-containing antacids causing an esophageal plug formation.	Administer antacids only into feeding tubes with the tip placed in the stomach. Administering aluminum-containing antacids after holding the tube feeding formula may prevent physical incompatibility formation.[91]

TABLE 129–12. Complications of Tube Feeding

Complication	Causes
Gastrointestinal	
Diarrhea	Drug related
	Antibiotic-induced bacterial overgrowth
	Hyperosmolar medications administered via feeding tubes
	Antacids containing magnesium
	Malabsorption
	Hypoalbuminemia/gut mucosal atrophy
	Pancreatic insufficiency
	Inadequate GIT surface area
	Rapid GIT transit
	Radiation enteritis
	Tube feeding related
	Rapid formula administration
	Formula hyperosmolality
	Low residue (fiber) content
	Lactose intolerance
Nausea and vomiting	Bacterial contamination
	Gastric dysmotility (surgery, anticholinergic drugs, diabetic gastroparesis)
	Rapid infusion of hyperosmolar formula
Constipation	Dehydration
	Drug induced (anticholinergics)
	Inactivity
	Low residue (fiber) content
	Obstruction/fecal impaction
Abdominal distention/cramping	Too rapid formula administration
Technical	
Occluded feeding tube lumen	Insoluble complexation of enteral formula and medication(s)
	Inadequate flushing of feeding tube
	Undissolved feeding formula
Tube displacement	Self-extubation
	Vomiting or coughing
	Inadequate fixation (jejunostomy)
Aspiration	Improper patient position
	Gastroparesis/atony causing regurgitation
	Feeding tube malpositioned
	Compromised lower esophageal sphincter
	Diminished gag reflex
Peristomal excoriation	Improper skin and tube care
	GIT secretions leaking peristomally
Infectious	
Aspiration pneumonia	Same as technical—aspiration comments
	Prolonged use of large-bore polyvinylchloride tube

who is critically ill is greater than for a stable patient residing in a rehabilitation unit or at home (Table 129–13). Patients receiving long-term home enteral nutrition should have clinical and laboratory monitoring done weekly to every 2 to 3 months, depending on the patient's clinical status. It is important to evaluate the actual content of water and micronutrients provided by the enteral formula for a patient at high risk for metabolic complications such as the critically ill. Additional hydration and electrolytes may need to be provided for patients being inadequately supported with an enteral formula. Conversely, for patients who have excessive fluid retention or increased serum electrolytes, the enteral formula may need to be changed to one that is more concentrated or provides less of a particular nutrient(s).

GI COMPLICATIONS

The GI complications associated with tube feeding include diarrhea, nausea and vomiting, constipation, abdominal distention, and cramping. In general, these GI side effects can be attributed to either drug-related, patient-related, or tube feeding–related factors. Diarrhea has been reported to occur in 2.3% to 30.6% of enterally fed patients.[64] It is speculated that the wide variability in incidence is caused, in part, by the multiplicity of clinical definitions for diarrhea. Monitoring of the patient for diarrhea includes evaluating stool frequency, consistency, and volume (see Table 129–13) and taking into consideration the patient's previous bowel habits and underlying disease state.[92] Drug-related causes of diarrhea include the administration of hyperosmolar medications or elixirs that contain high concentrations of sorbitol. Infec-

TABLE 129–13. Suggested Monitoring of Enteral Nutrition (EN) to Prevent Complications

Parameter	During Initiation of EN or for a Critically Ill Patient	During Stable EN Therapy or for a Rehabilitating Patient
Vital signs		
Temperature, respirations, pulse, blood pressure	Every 4–6 h	Every 12–24 h
Physical exam[a]		
Abdomen, lung fields, extremities, mucous membranes, skin turgor	Every 4–6 h	Every 12–24 h
Clinical assessment	Daily	Daily
Weight		
Total intake/output		
Urine, gastrointestinal and extraordinary fluid losses		
Stool frequency/consistency/volume		
Nausea or vomiting		
Concurrent medications and administration route	Daily	Daily
Verification of nasal or oral tube placement with x-ray	Done prior to initiating EN	N/A[b]
Ongoing assessment by tube placement	Every 6 h	Every 12 h
Gastric residual checks	Every 8–12 h	Every 8–12 h
Enterostomy tube site assessment for leakage and/or skin irritation/redness	Daily	Daily
Patient compliance with feeding procedures and feeding tube/ostomy care	N/A	Daily
Serum electrolytes, BUN/Cr, serum glucose[c]	Daily	2–3 times/wk
Serum calcium, magnesium, and phosphorous	4–5 times/wk	2–3 times/wk
Liver function tests	Weekly	Monthly
Urine glucose/acetone[c]	Every 6 h	Daily
Trace elements, vitamins	Frequently tailored to patient-specific situations	Frequently tailored to patient-specific situations

[a]Includes eyes, ear, nose, and throat exam for patients with nasoenteric feeding tubes.
[b]Not applicable.
[c]Frequency of glucose assessment for the nondiabetic patient.

tious causes, such as antibiotic-induced bacterial overgrowth by *Clostridium difficile* need to be considered when diarrhea develops. Diarrhea may also occur as a result of malabsorption, owing to such circumstances as severe malnutrition and related gut mucosal atrophy, exocrine failure such as chronic pancreatitis or cystic fibrosis, inadequate surface area or too rapid transit through the small bowel owing to radiation enteritis, short bowel syndrome, or celiac disease. During such clinical circumstances, a continuous infusion of chemically defined feeding formula may help improve the symptoms of malabsorption. Of the tube feeding–related factors that may contribute to diarrhea (see Table 129–12), the rate of infusion is a primary factor. Even hyperosmolar solutions can be infused without diarrhea or abdominal distention if the feeding is infused at a constant rate and incrementally titrated according to the tolerance of the patient.[64,92]

Occasionally pharmacologic intervention is indicated to control severe diarrhea. The primary agents employed are opiates, diphenoxylate, and loperamide.[93] Diphenoxylate acts by the same mechanism as the opioids, by decreasing GI motility and secretions. These actions decrease the amount of fluid to be reabsorbed in the small intestine and colon and increase the transit time to allow more absorption of exogenous fluids. Loperamide decreases GI motility and decreases small bowel output via the ileum. It is two to three times as potent as diphenoxylate and thus may be administered less frequently. Use of these agents should be limited, because overuse may produce constipation and paralytic ileus.

Nausea and vomiting in a patient receiving nasogastric tube feeding may be a result of gastric atony subsequent to recent surgery, anticholinergic side effect of drugs, and/or an underlying disease such as diabetic gastroparesis. Advancement of the feeding tube beyond the pylorus may reduce the associated symptoms of nausea and vomiting and enable successful enteral feeding. Constipation may also occur with tube feeding, particularly in the elderly and the long-term enteral nutrition patient. Multiple causes may contribute to the constipation (see Table 129–12). Using enteral formulas with enhanced fiber may improve the symptoms of constipation; however, the exact amount as well as the optional source of fiber is yet to be established.[60,94]

TECHNICAL COMPLICATIONS

The technical complications of enteral nutrition are frequently associated with the feeding tube. Occluded feeding tubes have been reported to occur in 10% of patients.[64] It is a common cause for feeding tube replacement and increases the cost of enteral feeding. Different techniques for clearing obstructed tubes have included instillation of water, meat tenderizer, pancreatic enzymes,[41] and passing of an endoscopic cytology brush.[64] Adherence to appropriate flushing protocols of the feeding tube during continuous tube feeding and medication administration is an extremely important variable in prevention of occluded feeding tubes (see Table 129–9). Inadvertent tube displacement has been reported to occur in > 50% of patients receiving enteral tube feeding.[64] Securing the tube and ongoing assessment of its appropriate placement may prevent tube displacement.

ASPIRATION OF GASTRIC CONTENTS

Bronchopulmonary aspiration of gastric contents is a potentially fatal complication of tube feeding. Patients who are mechanically ventilated or those with swallowing disorders are at higher risk for this complication. The incidence has been reported to be as high as 46%.[64] The use of small-bore feeding tubes preserves the lower esophogeal sphincter and, hence, patients are less prone to develop reflux in the esophagus with potential for aspiration. Aspiration can be further minimized by not allowing a large volume to accumulate in the stomach. The amount of liquid residing in the stomach is called the gastric residual. After holding the tube feeding for at least 30 minutes, gastric residuals can be checked by attaching a syringe to the open end of the tube and filling it with the liquid. In adults, the residuals should be less than 200 mL.[95] Small tubes often collapse easily when back-pressure is applied, making it difficult to measure residuals. Additionally, the risk of aspiration can be reduced by keeping the patient's head of the bed at a 30 to 45 degree angle during feeding and for 30 to 60 minutes after intermittent infusion. This makes it more difficult for fluid to migrate up the esophagus against gravity. Last, the aspiration risk may be decreased by infusing the feedings into the small intestine instead of the stomach. The passage of a small-bore feeding tube into the tracheobronchial passage with subsequent infusion of an enteral diet can also be fatal. Obviously patients with a diminished gag reflex are at risk for this complication. The small-bore tubes may not trigger the gag reflex, which indicates proper placement; therefore the tube position should always be verified with an x-ray to reduce the chance of infusion into the lung. Alleviation or prevention of bronchopulmonary aspiration involves meticulous tube insertion and tube maintenance. Other infectious complications besides bronchopulmonary aspiration, although less frequent, include acute otitis media or sinusitis. This complication has been associated with long-term use of polyvinylchloride tubes.[40]

THERAPEUTIC NUTRITION AND DISEASE OUTCOMES

Nutrition outcome goals of enteral tube feeding are to reverse protein–calorie malnutrition, promote growth and development of infants and children, or maintain an adequate nutritional state. Assessing the outcome of enteral nutrition includes monitoring objective measures of body composition, protein and energy balance as well as subjective outcome for physiologic muscle function and wound healing (Table 129–14). These nutritional outcome indices have improved with enteral feedings among critically ill,[29] rehabilitation,[96] and long-term home enteral patients.[97] Besides an improvement in nutrition outcome, another goal of enteral nutrition is to reduce disease-related morbidity and mortality. Measures of disease-related morbidity include the length of hospital stay, infectious complications, and the patient's sense of well-being. Such clinical outcome goals are extremely difficult to document with the use of enteral nutrition, in part because other factors such as age, underlying comorbidities, extent of injury, immunocompetence, and end-organ complications affect disease outcome.

Only a few prospective, randomized, controlled trials have demonstrated a change in disease outcome with the use of enteral nutrition. However, the results of clinical investigations of enteral nutrition in Crohn's disease suggest an improvement in some indices of clinical outcome. Historically, TPN and bowel rest were prescribed for patients with an active flare of their Crohn's disease. However, clinical investigation has established that for most patients with disease flare, bowel rest is not necessary to induce a clinical remission.[98] Short courses of nutrition support in hospitalized patients often demonstrate remission rates of 60% and 80% with either TPN or defined enteral diets, respectively. Polymeric and partially hydrolyzed formulas appear to be equivalent to the elemental formulas in clinical efficacy.[34,99] The contribution of enteral nutrition to the clinical outcome of patients with Crohn's disease will remain unanswered until prospective, randomized, controlled trials comparing enteral nutrition and placebo are performed.

The use of enteral nutrition over TPN has been evaluated for its effectiveness in reducing morbidity and mortality in critically ill patients. Heyland and colleagues[26] evaluated the role of enteral nutrition, particularly early enteral nutrition, on morbidity and mortality in critically ill patients. Of the eight randomized nonblinded clinical trials, three studies used objective criteria to define infectious outcomes. Although no differences were seen in the incidence of multiple-organ failure syndrome or mortality in the enteral versus the parenteral group,[100] patients who received enteral nutrition had a 17% sepsis rate, which included a 3% rate of major septic complications, compared to the parenteral group, which had a septic complication rate of 37% and a 20% rate of major septic complications.[29] In the third study, the septic complication rate was 15.7% in the enteral nutrition group compared to 40% in the parenteral group.[101] The enteral and parenteral study groups were comparable with respect to age, injury type, and their severity of illness scores.[29,101] Based on the results of the aforementioned studies and others reviewed, Heyland and colleagues conclude that sufficient data exist to suggest that critically ill patients benefit from early enteral nutrition and that enteral nutrition should be commenced as early as possible in the course of a patient's illness. Even if enteral nutrition may not meet all of the nutrient goals immediately, the role of

TABLE 129–14. Suggested Monitoring of Enteral Nutrition (EN) to Promote Nutritional Efficacy

Parameter	During Initiation of EN or for a Critically Ill Patient	During Stable EN Therapy or for a Rehabilitating Patient	During Long-Term Home EN Therapy
Anthropometrics			
Weight	Daily	Weekly	Weekly
Triceps skinfold	N/A[a]	N/A	Every 1–2 mo
Midarm muscle circumference	N/A	N/A	Every 1–2 mo
Muscle function			
Level of physical endurance	N/A	Weekly	Weekly to monthly, then frequency tailored to the patient situation
Metabolic			
Albumin	Monthly	Monthly	Monthly, then frequently tailored to the patient situation
Transferrin	Weekly	Weekly	Once to twice monthly, then frequency tailored to the patient response
24-h urine urea nitrogen	Weekly	Once or twice monthly	Frequently tailored to patient-specific situations
Indirect calorimetry	Frequently tailored to patient-specific situations	Frequently tailored to patient-specific situations	Frequently tailored to patient-specific situations
Nutritional intake			
Calories	Daily	2–3 times weekly	Weekly, then tailored to the patient situation
Protein, fluid, electrolytes, trace elements, vitamins	Daily	2–3 times weekly	Weekly, then tailored to the patient situation
Skin integrity	Daily	Daily	Weekly
Wound healing			
Pressure sore(s)			

[a]Not applicable.

tube feeding should be as a stimulant to the patient's GI immunologic function and mucosal integrity. Enteral nutrition may thus result in reduction of infectious complications in the critically ill patient. No prospective randomized controlled studies evaluating enteral nutrition in the critically ill have resulted in reduced mortality. Further clinical investigations are needed to establish the effect of specific nutrients on length of hospital stay and infectious complications. New enteral formulas with altered nutrient composition which include different enhancements of hydrolyzed protein sources (dipeptides, tripeptides), ribonucleic acid, increased omega-3 fatty acids, arginine, and glutamine may improve disease-related morbidity. Further prospective randomized clinical trials are warranted to assess the benefits and safety of these costly specialized formulas, to determine what components are most beneficial in reducing morbidity within specific disease states.

PHARMACOECONOMIC CONSIDERATIONS

Enteral nutrition has been shown to be consistently less expensive than TPN. A formal pharmacoeconomic analysis of nutrition support therapy should include an evaluation of therapeutic outcome relative to the cumulative cost associated with the nutrients, nonnutrient supplies, the time spent by professional staff in compounding, delivering and managing therapy, laboratory monitoring, and management of complications that results from therapy. Although none of the existing analyses has addressed all of these issues, selected comparisons of costs related to enteral and parenteral therapy derived from clinical research trials in institutional settings have been published. Nutritional support therapy costs can be divided into nutrient and nonnutrient supplies. Enteral nonnutrient supply costs include the specific enteral tube device, its related insertion technique, and infusion-related supplies as described in Tables 129–5 and 129–6. The distribution of nutrient and nonnutrient costs was found to be 87% and 13% for enteral nutrition and 57% and 43% for parenteral nutrition among VA Medical Center patients receiving nutrition support therapy.[102] The reported cost of enteral nutrition is thus 23% to 48% that of parenteral nutrition.[102,103] This broad range in reported cost is largely owing to the extent of data that were included in the analysis. Including the cost of managing complications related to each therapy greatly increases the overall cost of parenteral nutrition as compared to enteral nutrition.[103]

▶ PRINCIPLES OF PHARMACOTHERAPY

- The GI tract defends the host from toxins and antigens by both immunologic and nonimmunologic mechanisms, collectively referred to as the "gut barrier function." Thus when possible, enteral nutrition is preferred over TPN because it is as effective and may reduce infectious complications.

- Postpyloric placement of the feeding tube tip may prevent aspiration, and patients who are at high risk for aspiration (patients with gastric atony) should have the tube tip secured into the small bowel for successful feeding. Placement of a nasal feeding tube, at the beside, requires an x-ray to verify that the tube is not within the lung.
- Patients fed via a gastric (stomach) tube may be fed continuously via an infusion pump or by bolus feeding. Gastric residual volumes should be checked to reduce the risk of aspiration. Patients with small bowel feeding tubes should only be fed continuously via an infusion pump to avoid dumping syndrome. Infusion rates into the small bowel up to 150 mL/h can be successful in adults.
- Selection of the feeding formula depends on the nutritional goals, the patient's primary disease state and related complications, and nutrient digestibility and absorption. Polymeric or "standard" products containing 1 to 2 kcal/mL, and 35 to 60 g/L protein are commonly used for adult patients. Monomeric or partially hydrolyzed/elemental products that contain 1.0 kcal/mL and 40 to 50 g/L protein are indicated for patients who have severe pancreatic insufficiency or have undergone a total pancreatectomy or a major small bowel resection that markedly reduces GI surface area.
- Selection of a specialized product for patients with organ failure (pulmonary, renal, hepatic, endocrine) or immunologic impairment requires a knowledge of the achievable nutritional and disease-related outcomes and the circumstances of the particular patient.
- Liquid medications should not be added to an enteral product without prior review of the compatibility literature. Medications that are nonaqueous or are contained within syrups are often incompatible with enteral products.
- Prior to administering medications through a feeding tube, one must determine where the feeding tube tip is located (stomach vs small bowel) and whether the medication is in suitable dosage form. Suitable dosage forms include liquid preparations and gelatin capsules that may be opened and administered through the tube. Medications that should not be crushed and administered through a tube include enteric coated, sustained-release capsules or tablets, and sublingual or buccal tablets.
- Enteral feeding products can alter the bioavailability and/or change the desired pharmacologic effect of several medications including phenytoin, warfarin, and selected antibiotics and antacids.
- GI complications can be drug related (hyperosmolar medication–induced diarrhea), patient related (infection, malabsorption, dysmotility), or tube feeding–related (infusion rate and osmolality of the product). Bronchopulmonary aspiration may be prevented by checking gastric residuals, keeping the head of the bed at a 30 to 45 degree angle, or by placing the feeding tube tip postpylorically.

REFERENCES

1. Cashman MD. Principles of digestive physiology for clinical nutrition. Nutr Clin Prac 1986;1:241–249.
2. Caspary WF. Physiology and pathophysiology of intestinal absorption. Am J Clin Nutr 1992;55:299S–308S.
3. O'Dwyer ST, Smith RJ, Kripke SA, et al. New fuels for the gut. In: Rombeau JL, Caldwell MD, eds. Clinical Nutrition: Enteral and Tube Feeding, 2nd ed. Philadelphia, W.B. Saunders, 1990:548.
4. Record KE, Kolpek JH, Rapp RP. Long chain versus medium chain length triglycerides, a review of metabolism and clinical use. Nutr Clin Prac 1986;1:279–287.
5. Mainous MR, Block EFJ, Dietch EA. Nutritional support of the gut: How and why. New Horiz 1994;2:193–201.
6. Langkamp-Henken B, Glezer JA, Kudsk KA. Immunologic structure and function of the gastrointestinal tract. Nutr Clin Prac 1992;7:100–114.
7. Gleeson MH, Dowling RH, Peters TJ. Biochemical changes in intestinal mucosa after experimental small bowel by-pass in the rat. Clin Sci 1972;43:743–757.
8. Levine GM, Deren JJ, Steiger E, et al. Role of oral intake in maintenance of gut mass and disaccharide activity. Gastroenterology 1974; 67:975–982.
9. Thompson JS, Vaughan WP, Forst CF, et al. The effect of route on nutrient delivery on gut structure and diamine oxidase levels. JPEN J Parenter Enteral Nutr 1987;11:28–32.
10. Greene HL, McCabe DR, Merenstein GB. Protracted diarrhea and malnutrition in infancy: Changes in intestinal morphology and disaccharidase activities during treatment with total intravenous nutrition or oral elemental diets. J Pediatr 1975;87:695–704.
11. Morin CL, Ling V, Bourassa D. Small intestine and colonic changes induced by a chemically defined diet. Dig Dis Sci 1980;25:123–128.
12. Young EA, Cioletti LA, Winborn WB, et al. Comparative study of nutritional adaptation to defined formula diets in rats. Am J Clin Nutr 1980;33:2106–2118.
13. Johnson LR, Copeland EM, Dudrick SJ, et al. Structural and hormonal alterations in the gastrointestinal tract of parenterally fed rats. Gastroenterology 1975;68:1177–1183.
14. Sagor GR, Ghatei MA, Al-Mukhtar MYT, et al. Evidence for a humoral mechanism after small intestinal resection. Gastroenterology 1983;84:902–906.
15. Lickley HLA, Track NS, Vranic M, Bury KD. Metabolic responses to enteral and parenteral nutrition. Am J Surgery 1978;135:172–176.
16. Adibi SA. Leucine absorption rate and net movements of sodium and water in human jejunum. J Appl Phys 1970;28:753–757.
17. Souba WW, Scott TE, Wilmore DW. Intestinal consumption of intravenously administered fuels. JPEN J Parenter Enteral Nutr 1985;9: 18–22.
18. Souba WW, Wilmore DW. Postoperative alteration of arteriovenous exchange of amino acids across the gastro-intestinal tract. Surgery 1983;94:342–350.
19. Alverdy J, Chi HS, Sheldon G. The effect of parenteral nutrition on gastrointestinal immunity: The importance of enteral immunity. Ann Surg 1985;202:681–684.
20. Alverdy JC, Aoys E, Moss GS. TPN promotes bacterial translocation from the gut. Surgery 1988;104:185–190.

21. Saito H, Trocki O, Alexander JW, et al. Effect of route of administration on the nutritional state, catabolic hormone secretion and gut mucosal integrity after burn injury. JPEN J Parenter Enteral Nutr 1987;11:1–7.
22. Kudsk KA, Stone JM, Carpenter G, Sheldon GF. Enteral and parenteral feeding influences mortality after hemoglobin. *E. coli* peritonitis in normal rats. J Trauma 1983;23:605–609.
23. Zaloga GP, Knowles R, Black KW, Prielipp R. Total parenteral nutrition increases mortality after hemorrhage. Crit Care Med 1990;19: 54–59.
24. Fong Y, Marano MA, Barber A, et al. Total parenteral nutrition and bowel rest modify the metabolic response to endotoxin in humans. Ann Surg 1989;210:449–457.
25. Talbot JM. Guidelines for the scientific review of enteral food products for special medical purposes. JPEN J Parenter Enteral Nutr 1991; 15(suppl):99S–173S.
26. Heyland DK, Cook DJ, Guyatt GH. Enteral nutrition in the critically ill patient: A critical review of the evidence. Intensive Care Med 1993;19:435–442.
27. Vernet O, Christin L, Schultz Y, et al. Enteral versus parenteral nutrition: Comparison of energy metabolism in healthy subjects. Am J Physiol 1986;250:E47–E54.
28. McArdle AH, Palmason C, Morency I, Brown RA. A rationale for enteral feeding as the preferable route for hyperalimentation. Surgery 1981;100:616–621.
29. Kudsk KA, Groce MA, Fabian TC, et al. Enteral versus parenteral feeding—effects on septic morbidity after blunt and penetrating abdominal trauma. Ann Surgery 1992;215:503–513.
30. Messing B, Bories C, Kunstlinger F, Bernier JJ. Does total parenteral nutrition induce gall bladder sludge formation and lithiasis? Gastroenterology 1983;84:1012–1019.
31. Carbonnel F, Cosnes J, Chevret S, et al. The role of anatomic factors in nutritional autonomy after extensive small bowel resection. JPEN J Parenter Enteral Nutr 1996;20:275–280.
32. Silk DBA, Grimble GK. Relevance of physiology of nutrient absorption to formulation of enteral diets. Nutrition 1992;8:1–12.
33. McClave SA, Lowen CC, Snider HL. Immunonutrition and enteral hyperalimentation of critically ill patients. Dig Dis Sci 1992;37: 1153–1161.
34. American Society of Parenteral and Enteral Nutrition Board of Directors. Guidelines for the use of parenteral and enteral nutrition in adult and pediatric patients. JPEN J Parenter Enteral Nutr 1993; 17(suppl): 1SA–52SA.
35. Klein S, Kinney J, Jeejeebhoy K, et al. Nutrition support in clinical practice: Review of published data and recommendations for future research directions, summary of a conference sponsored by the National Institutes of Health, American Society for Parenteral and Enteral Nutrition, and American Society for Clinical Nutrition. JPEN J Parenter Enteral Nutr 1997;21:133–156.
36. Bell SJ, Mascioli EA, Forse RA, Bistrian BR. Nutrition support and the human immunodeficiency virus (HIV). Parasitology 1993;107 (suppl):63S–67S.
37. Minard G. Enteral access. Nutr Clin Prac 1994;9:172–182.
38. Lehman S. Parenteral and enteral access devices. In: Teasley-Strausburg KM, ed. Nutrition Support Handbook: A Compendium of Products with Guidelines for Usage. Cincinnati, OH, Harvey Whitney Books, 1992:205–257.
39. Dobbie RP, Hoffmeister JA. Continuous pump-tube enteric hyperalimentation. Surg Gynecol Obstet 1976;143:273–276.
40. Torosian MH, Rombeau JL. Feeding by tube enterostomy. Surg Gynecol Obstet 1980;150:918–927.
41. Clevenger FW, Rodriguez DJ. Decision-making for enteral feeding administration: The why behind where and how. Nutr Clin Prac 1995;10:104–113.
42. Martin D, Jastram CW. Enteral nutrition. Part II. Nutr Supp Serv 1987;7:8–10.
43. Leider Z, Sullivan L, Mullen MA, et al. Intermittent tube feedings: Pros and cons. Nutr Supp Serv 1984;4:59–62.
44. Orvieto A, Kirsch J, Goldberger J. Evaluation of enteral delivery systems. Nutr Supp Serv 1983;3:44–48.
45. Lehman S. Nutrient infusion devices. In: Teasley-Strausberg KM, ed. Nutrition Support Handbook: A Compendium of Products with Guidelines for Usage. Cincinnati, OH, Harvey Whitney Books, 1992:259–282.
46. Cerra FB, Holman RT, Bankey PE, et al. Omega-3 polyunsaturated fatty acids as modulators of cellular function in the critically ill. Pharmacotherapy 1991;11:71–76.
47. Mueller C, Nestle M. Regulation of medical foods: Toward a rational policy. Nutr Clin Prac 1995;10:8–15.
48. Heymsfield SB. Enteral solutions: Is there a solution? Nutr Clin Prac 1995;10:4–7.
49. MacBurney MM, Russell C, Young LS. Formulas. In: Rombeau JL, Caldwell MD, eds. Clinical Nutrition: Enteral and Tube Feeding, 2nd ed. Philadelphia, W.B. Saunders, 1990:149–173.
50. Smith JL, Heymsfield SB. Enteral nutrition support: Formula preparation from modular ingredients. JPEN J Parenter Enteral Nutr 1983;7: 280–288.
51. Schloerb PR, Almar M. Total parenteral nutrition with glutamine in bone marrow transplantation and other clinical applications (a randomized, double-blind study). JPEN J Parenter Enteral Nutr 1993;17:407–413.
52. Ziegler TR, Young LS, Benfell K, et al. Clinical and metabolic efficacy of glutamine-supplemented parenteral nutrition after bone marrow transplantation (a randomized, double-blind, controlled study). Ann Intern Med 1992;116:821–828.
53. Zaloga GP, MacGregor DA. What to consider when choosing enteral or parenteral nutrition. J Crit Illness 1990;5:1180–1200.
54. Shronts EP, Havala T. Formulas. In: Teasley-Strausberg KM, ed. Nutrition Support Handbook: A Compendium of Products with Guidelines for Usage. Cincinnati, OH, Harvey Whitney Books, 1992:147–186.
55. Shike M. Enteral feeding. In: Shils ME, Olson JA, Shike M, eds. Modern Nutrition in Health and Disease, 8th ed. Philadelphia, Lea & Febiger, 1994:1417–1429.
56. Kudsk KA. Clinical applications of enteral nutrition. Nutr Clin Prac 1994;9:165–171.
57. Mead J. Nutrients with special functions: Essential fatty acids. In: Alfin-Slater R, Kritchervsky D, eds. Human Nutrition, Vol 3A. New York, Plenum, 1980:213–238.
58. Vanlandingham S, Simpson S, Daniel P, et al. Metabolic abnormalities in patients supported with enteral tube feeding. JPEN J Parenter Enteral Nutr 1981;5:322–324.
59. Berner YN, Morse R, Frank D, et al. Vitamin plasma levels in long-term enteral feeding patients. JPEN J Parenter Enteral Nutr 1989;13: 525–528.
60. Scheppach WM, Bartram HP. Experimental evidence for and clinical implications of fiber and artificial enteral nutrition. Nutrition 1993;9: 399–405.
61. Keohane PP, Attrill H, Love M, et al. Relation between osmolality of diet and gastrointestinal side effects in enteral nutrition. Br Med J 1984;288:678–681.
62. Zimmaro DM, Rolandelli RH, Koruda MJ, et al. Isotonic tube feeding formula induces liquid stool in normal subjects: Reversed by pectin. JPEN J Parenter Enteral Nutr 1989;13:117–123.
63. Jones TN, Moore FA, Moore EE, McCroskey BL. Gastrointestinal symptoms attributed to jejunostomy feeding after major abdominal trauma—a critical analysis. Crit Care Med 1989;17:1146–1150.
64. Cabre E, Gassull MA. Complications of enteral feeding. Nutrition 1993;8:1–9.
65. Durfee DD, Skinner-Domet VM. Cost effectiveness of an enteral product's formulary. Am J Hosp Pharm 1984;41:2352–2354.
66. Gottschlick MM, Jenkins M, Warden GD, et al. Differential effects of three enteral dietary regimens on selected outcome variables in burn patients. JPEN J Parenter Enteral Nutr 1990;14: 225–235.

67. Bower RH, Cerra FB, Bershadsky B, et al. Early enteral administration of a formula (Impact) supplemented with arginine, nucleotides, and fish oil in intensive care unit patients: Results of a multicenter, prospective, randomized, clinical trial. Crit Care Med 1995;23:436–449.
68. Daly JM, Lieberman MD, Goldfine J, et al. Enteral nutrition with supplemental argenine, RNA, and omega-3 fatty acids in patients after operation: Immunologic metabolic, and clinical outcome. Surgery 1992;112:56–67.
69. Kudsk KA, Minard G, Croce MA, et al. A randomized trial of isonitrogenous enteral diets after severe trauma. An immune-enhancing diet reduces septic complications. Ann Surgery 1996;224:531–540.
70. Moore FA, Moore EE, Kudsk KA, et al. Clinical benefits of an immune-enhancing diet for early postinjury enteral feeding. J Trauma 1994;37:607–615.
71. Levy J, Laethen T, Verhaegen G, et al. Contaminated enteral nutrition solutions as a cause of nosocomial bloodstream infection: A study using plasmid fingerprinting. JPEN J Parenter Enteral Nutr 1989;13:228–234.
72. Thurn J, Crossley K, Gerdts A, et al. Enteral hyperalimentation as a source of nosocomial infection. J Hosp Infect 1990;15:203–217.
73. VanEnk R, Furtado D. Bacterial contamination of enteral nutrient solutions: Intestinal colonization and sepsis in mice after infection. JPEN J Parenter Enteral Nutr 1986;10:503–507.
74. Havala T, Shronts EP. Formula compounding. In: Teasley-Strausberg KM, ed. Nutrition Support Handbook: A Compendium of Products with Guidelines for Usage. Cincinnati, OH, Harvey Whitney Books, 1992:187–204.
75. Wagner DR, Emore MF, Knoll DM. Evaluation of "closed" vs "open" systems for the delivery of peptide-based enteral diets. JPEN J Parenter Enteral Nutr 1994;18:453–457.
76. Cutie AJ, Altman E, Lenkel L. Compatability of enteral products with commonly employed drug additives. JPEN J Parenter Enteral Nutr 1983;7:186–191.
77. Hardin TC, Reed M, eds. Nutrition and Drug Therapy: Clinical Pharmacology Drug Compatability and Stability—An Annotated Bibliography. Silver Spring, MD, ASPEN, 1992.
78. Dickerson RN, Melnik G. Osmolality of oral drug solutions and suspensions. Am J Hosp Pharm 1988;45:832–834.
79. Kumpf VJ, Barber JR. Enteral nutrition. US Pharm 1987;(June):H-1, 2, 5, 8–10, 15.
80. Bradley J. Principles of enteral nutrition. Hosp Pharm 1994;23:197–204.
81. Strom JG, Miller SW. Stability of drugs with enteral nutrient formulas. Drug Intell Clin Pharm 1990;24:130–134.
82. Gora ML, Tschampel MM, Visconti JA. Considerations of drug therapy in patients receiving enteral nutrition. Nutr Clin Prac 1989;4:105–110.
83. Thompson CA, Rollins CJ. Nutrient-drug interactions. In: Rombeau JL, Rolandelli RH, eds. Clinical Nutrition: Enteral and Tube Feeding, 3rd ed. Philadelphia, W.B. Saunders, 1997:523–529.
84. Mitchell JF. Oral dosage forms that should not be crushed: 1996 revision. Hosp Pharm 1996;31:27–37.
85. Bauer LA. Interference of oral phenytoin absorption by continuous nasogastric feedings. Neurology 1982;32:570–572.
86. Melnick G. Pharmacologic aspects of enteral nutrition. In: Rombeau JL, Caldwell MD, eds. Clinical Nutrition: Enteral and Tube Feeding, 2nd ed. Philadelphia, W.B. Saunders, 1990:472–509.
87. Nishimura LY, Armstrong RP, Plezia PM, Iacono RP. Influence of enteral feedings on phenytoin sodium absorption from capsules. Drug Intell Clin Pharm 1988;22:130–133.
88. Guidry JR, Eastwood TF, Curry SC. Phenytoin absorption in volunteers receiving selected enteral feeds. West J Med 1989;150:659–661.
89. Drug Facts and Comparisons. St. Louis, MO, Wolters Kluwer, 1995.
90. Gora ML, Tschampel MM, Visconti JA. Considerations of drug therapy in patients receiving enteral nutrition. Nutr Clin Prac 1989;4:105–110.
91. Valli C, Schulthess HK, Asper R, et al. Interaction of nutrients with antacids: A complication during enteral tube feeding. Lancet 1986;8483:747–748.
92. Eisenberg PG. Causes of diarrhea in tube-fed patients: A comprehensive approach to diagnosis and management. Nutr Clin Prac 1993;8:119–123.
93. Mirtallo JM, Fabri PJ. Concurrent therapy for complications of enteral nutrition support. Hosp Form 1982;17:945–953.
94. Shankardass K, Chuchmach S, Chelswick K, et al. Bowel function of long-term tube-fed patients consuming formulae with and without dietary fiber. JPEN J Parenter Enteral Nutr 1990;14:508–512.
95. McClave SA, Snider HL, Lowen CC, et al. Use of residual volume as a marker for enteral feeding intolerance: Prospective blinded comparison with physical examination and radiographic findings. JPEN J Parenter Enteral Nutr 1992;16:99–105.
96. Hebuterne X, Broussard JF, Rampal P. Acute renutrition by cyclic enteral nutrition in elderly and younger patients. JAMA 1995;273:638–643.
97. Newmark SR, Simpson MS, Beskitt MP, et al. Home tube feeding for long-term nutritional support. JPEN J Parenter Enteral Nutr 1981;5:76–79.
98. Greenberg GR, Fleming CR, Jeejeebhoy KN, et al. Controlled trial of bowel rest and nutritional support in the management of Crohn's disease. Gut 1988;29:1309–1315.
99. Fleming CR. Nutrition in patients with Crohn's disease: Another piece of the puzzle. JPEN J Parenter Enteral Nutr 1995;19:93–94.
100. Cerra FB, McPherson JP, Konstantinides FN, et al. Enteral nutrition does not prevent multiple organ failure syndrome (MOFS) after sepsis. Surgery 1988;104:727–733.
101. Moore FA, Moore EE, Jones TN, et al. TEN versus TPN following major abdominal trauma-reduced septic morbidity. J Trauma 1989;29:916–923.
102. Hamaoui E, Lefkowitz R, Olender L, et al. Enteral nutrition in the early postoperative period: A new semielemental formula versus total parenteral nutrition. JPEN J Parenter Enteral Nutr 1990;14:501–507.
103. McClave SA, Greene LM, Snider HL, et al. Comparison of the safety of early enteral vs parenteral nutrition in mild acute pancreatitis. JPEN J Parenter Enteral Nutr 1996;21:14–20.
104. Mirtallo JM. Nutrient metabolism. In: Dipiro JT, Talbert FL, Yee GL, et al, eds. Pharmacotherapy: A Pathophysiologic Approach, 3rd ed. Stamford, CT, Appleton & Lange, 1997:2711–2734.

130

PEDIATRIC AND GERIATRIC NUTRITION SUPPORT

Katherine Hammond Chessman, PharmD, BCNSP, BCPS, and Jan Dalke Anderson, PharmD, BCNSP

In the continuum from birth through old age, nutrition needs change. Although the principles of nutrition support may not be different based on age, the provision of nutrients to pediatric and geriatric patients must be based on the differences in metabolism, physiology, and organ function that are present at the ends of the age spectrum. In this chapter we will discuss the nutrition support needs of both children and older adults while differentiating them both from young to middle-age adults.

PEDIATRIC NUTRITION

Children have unique physiologic needs that make provision of nutrition support to them distinctly different from that for adults. The high incidence of protein–calorie malnutrition reported in hospitalized children[1] necessitates that all pediatric health care providers be familiar with pediatric nutrition support. Normally nourished children should in general be given appropriate specialized nutrition support after 5 to 7 days of suboptimal intake, term infants after 3 to 5 days, and preterm infants within 1 to 3 days.[2] Children with preexisting malnutrition may require earlier intervention.

PHYSIOLOGY

Body composition varies with age. A young child's body contains a higher percentage of water and lower calorie and protein reserves than does an adult's body. The percentage of body weight that is protein is approximately the same as in an adult; however, only about 50% of the protein is deposited in skeletal muscle compared to 90% in adults.

Caloric requirements per kilogram are higher because a child's basal metabolic rate (BMR), which is also termed basal energy expenditure (BEE) by some, is higher because the major metabolic organs, especially the brain, constitute a larger portion of the body. BMR is approximately 50 to 55 kcal/kg/d in infancy and declines to about 20 to 25 kcal/kg/d during adolescence. Equations used to estimate BMR in children are shown in Table 130–1.[3–6] When compared to measured resting energy expenditure (mREE) determined by indirect calorimetry in normal children, all these equations except the Harris–Benedict equations predict BMR within 10%.[7,8] Extrapolation of these values to sick children may not be appropriate. Chwals et al.[9] found that measured energy expenditure was only 52.6% of predicted energy requirements in 20 critically ill infants and children.

In children, normal growth and development depend on adequate nutrition. Thus growth is a primary screening and monitoring tool for nutrition adequacy. In healthy infants, 35% to 40% of energy is used for growth; by 2 years of age this drops to 25%. The second critical growth period that necessitates increased caloric intake is the adolescent years. Severe stress may impair growth even if adequate calories and protein are provided owing to increased production of catecholamines and counterregulatory hormones, which oppose insulin's anabolic effects, resulting in decreased endogenous tissue stores of protein, fat, and carbohydrate.[9–11]

Due to immature renal, hepatic, and gastrointestinal function, nutrients may be digested, absorbed, or metabolized differently, especially during the neonatal period. Neonates, especially premature ones, are more prone to hyperglycemia resulting from reduced insulin secretion, failure of glucose to suppress hepatic glucose output, and peripheral insulin resistance. Preterm infants also have a low renal threshold for glucose excretion; therefore, glycosuria may occur even at normal serum glucose concentrations.[12] Certain amino acids including cysteine, taurine, and tyrosine are considered essential in newborns because of their immature enzyme systems. Enzyme system immaturity allows accumulation of potentially toxic amino acids such as methionine and phenylalanine, if given in large concentrations. Plasma amino acid concentrations 2 hours postprandial in normally growing, 30-day-old breast-fed infants have been characterized and used for evaluating nutritional products.[13] Finally, gastrointestinal tract immaturity may result in decreased absorption of orally ingested nutrients.

NUTRITION ASSESSMENT

Nutrition assessment is a crucial aspect of pediatric patient care. Assessment goals are to quantify the degree of malnutrition if present, identify children at risk for developing malnutrition and its complications, and monitor nutrition support outcomes. Appropriate assessment includes a complete physical examination, medical and dietary history, anthropometric measurements, and appropriate laboratory studies. None of these tools is sensitive or specific enough for use alone. More sophisticated techniques, such as body composition and energy expenditure measurements, are used in some settings but are not routinely available.

Growth is evaluated by comparison of recumbent length (children less than 2 years of age), height (children older than 2 years of age), weight, head circumference (children less than 3 years of age), and growth rate to age- and

TABLE 130–1. Equations to Estimate Basal Energy Expenditure in Children

Harris–Benedict[3] (kcal/d):
Males: BEE = 66 + (13.7*W*) + [5*H* (cm)] − (6.8*A*)
Females: BEE = 655 + (9.6*W*) + [1.8*H* (cm)] − (4.7*A*)
Caldwell–Kennedy[6] (kcal/d):
Infants (< 3 years of age): BEE = 22 + (31*W*) + [1.2*H* (cm)]
Schofield[5] (MJ/d) (to convert to kcal/d multiply by 239.2):
3–10 years of age
Males: BMR = (0.08*W*) + [0.55*H* (m)] + 1.74
Females: BMR = (0.07*W*) + [0.68*H* (m)] + 1.55
10–18 years of age
Males: BMR = (0.07*W*) + [0.57*H* (m)] + 2.16
Females: BMR = (0.04*W*) + [1.95*H* (m)] + 0.84
FAO/WHO/UNU[4] (kcal/d):
3–10 years of age
Males: BMR = 22.7*W* + 495
Females: BMR = 22.5*W* + 499
10–18 years of age
Males: BMR = 17.5*W* + 651
Females: BMR = 12.2*W* + 746

Key: *W* = weight in kilograms; *H* = height in centimeters (cm) or meters (m), as indicated; *A* = age in years; BEE = basal energy expenditure; BMR = basal metabolic rate; FAO/WHO/UNU = Food and Agriculture Organization/World Health Organization/United Nations University.

gender-related standards as well as to previous measurements. Accurate and consistent measurements are important. Weight and height are evaluated by percentile according to age, by the weight-for-height percentile, and by growth velocity. These growth indices can be obtained by plotting the child's values on an appropriate National Center for Health Statistics (NCHS) growth curve, which was developed from a large population of normal children.[14] Special curves are available for assessment of short-term and long-term growth[15,16] of premature infants and children with Down syndrome.[17] For premature infants with corrected age of 40 weeks or more, the NCHS growth charts can be used; however, weight-for-age and height-for-age should be plotted according to corrected postnatal age until 2 years of age and 3.5 years of age, respectively.[18] Appropriate minimum time intervals between measurements for meaningful evaluation of growth are weight, 7 days; length, 4 weeks; height, 8 weeks; and head circumference, 7 days in infants and 4 weeks in children up to 3 years of age.[19] Adequate average weight gain is 10 to 12 g/kg/d in a term newborn and 20 to 36 g/kg/d in a premature infant. Weight gain per kilogram declines considerably after 2 to 3 months of age.

TABLE 130–2. Common Classifications of Undernutrition

	Degree of Undernutrition			
	Normal	*Mild*	*Moderate*	*Severe*
Weight-for-height	> 90	80–90	70–80	< 70
Weight-for-age	> 90	75–90	61–75	< 60

Growth failure or failure to thrive is defined as weight-for-age or weight-for-height below the 5th percentile or a fall-off of two or more major percentiles (major percentiles are defined as 95th, 90th, 75th, 50th, 25th, 10th, and 5th). Weight-for-height evaluation is age independent and helps differentiate the stunted child (chronic malnutrition) from the wasted child (acute malnutrition). Short stature, which is associated with many chronic diseases, is a manifestation of chronic undernutrition. Common classifications of undernutrition are shown in Table 130–2. These nutritional indices are primarily used to define risk of possible adverse effects of undernutrition rather than to quantify the degree of malnutrition.[20]

A medical and dietary history may identify variations from normal intake such as vegetarian diets, meal-skipping, sports fad diets, and anorexia/bulimia. In children, primary malnutrition or inadequate intake may be a result of an altered maternal–child relationship, lack of parental education, poverty, restricted allergy diets, and food fads. Secondary malnutrition is often caused by congenital malformation, infectious disease, trauma, malignancy, or chronic disease. The most accurate approach to obtain a diet history is to have the child or parent prospectively keep a 3- to 5-day diet diary. Parental 24-hour recall without warning is rarely accurate.

Laboratory studies used for nutrition assessment of children are similar to those used for adults; however, normal values may vary with age. Nitrogen balance studies are less reliable in infants and young children. Unless the child has an indwelling urinary catheter, it is difficult to get a complete 24-hour urine collection that is not contaminated with stool. Shorter collection times (6 hour), however, correlate with 24-hour collections.[21] Since urine urea nitrogen (UUN) represents an extremely variable proportion of total urine nitrogen (TUN), nitrogen balance studies in infants should measure TUN.

NUTRIENT REQUIREMENTS

Recommended dietary allowances (RDAs) for various nutrients have been established for healthy children.[22] RDAs for premature infants have not been established because desired intakes are less well defined for this population. Children should be encouraged to eat a variety of foods to ensure provision of RDAs and other nutrients for which no RDA has been established.

TABLE 130–3. Recommended Fluid Intakes for Newborns (mL/kg/d)

Birth Weight (g)	Days 1–2	Day 3	Days 4+
< 1000	105	140	150+
1001–1250	100	130	140+
1251–1500	90	120	130+
1501–1700	80	110	130+
1701–2000	80	110	130+
Term infant	70	80	100+

TABLE 130–4. Factors That Alter Fluid Requirements in Children

Increased Requirements	Decreased Requirements
Fever	Fluid overload
Radiant warmers	Cardiac failure
Diuretics	Decreased urinary output
Vomiting	Heat shields
Nasogastric suction	Relatively high humidity
Ostomy/fistula drainage	Humidified air via endotracheal tube
Diarrhea	
Glycosuria	
Phototherapy	
Increased ambient temperatures	
Hyperventilation	

FLUID INTAKE

Fluid requirements per kilogram are higher for newborns owing to their higher percentage of body water and higher BMR (Table 130–3). Premature neonates have increased fluid requirements due to greater insensible losses and the kidney's inefficiency in concentrating urine. The Holliday–Segar method as outlined below is a commonly employed, quick, and simple method for estimating minimum daily fluid needs. Infants or children who weigh less than 10 kg should receive at least 100 mL/kg/d. An additional 50 mL/kg/d should be provided for each kilogram between 11 and 20 kg and 20 mL/kg/d for each kilogram above 20 kg. Maintenance fluid needs for a child weighing 8 kg would be 800 mL/d, whereas 1350 mL/d would be the projected need for a 17-kg child. Alternatively, maintenance fluids may be estimated as 1500 mL/m^2/24 h in children weighing more than 10 kg. Factors that alter fluid needs are shown in Table 130–4.

Fluid status can be assessed by monitoring urine output and specific gravity, serum electrolytes, and weight changes. A urine output of 1.0 to 2.0 mL/kg/h or more is considered adequate. Urine output should be higher if large fluid volumes or high renal solute loads are being administered.

TABLE 130–5. Suggested Daily Caloric and Protein Intake for Normal Growth of Healthy Children—Recommended Dietary Allowances

Age(yr)	Total Calories (kg/day)	Protein (g/kg/d)
0–0.5	108	2.2
0.5–1.0	98	1.6
1–3	102	1.2
4–6	90	1.1
7–10	70	1.0
Boys		
11–14	55	0.9
15–18	45	0.8
Girls		
11–14	47	1.0
15–18	40	0.8

Source: Reproduced from Ref. 22.

TABLE 130–6. Stress Factors for Use in Children

Condition	Stress Factor[a]
Mild stress	
Postoperative recovery: uncomplicated surgery	1.0
Trauma: mild (e.g., long-bone fracture)	1.2
Moderate stress	
Sepsis (moderate)	1.3
Trauma: central nervous system (sedated)	1.3
Trauma: moderate to severe	1.5
Severe stress	
Sepsis (severe)	1.6
Trauma: central nervous system (severe)	up to 2.0
Burns (proportionate to burned area)	up to 2.0

[a]Multiply BMR by stress factor for approximate energy requirements.

Urine specific gravity depends on the kidney's concentrating and diluting capabilities. The neonatal kidney has limited ability to concentrate urine. A urine specific gravity of greater than 1.020 (1.015 in neonates) may indicate a need for more fluid whereas a urine specific gravity of 1.008 or less suggests fluid overload. Concomitant diuretic therapy owing to increased solute excretion will limit the usefulness of urine specific gravity as an index of fluid status.

CALORIC INTAKE

Suggested caloric intakes for maintenance and normal growth of healthy infants and children are shown in Table 130–5.[22] These maintenance energy requirements are approximately 150% of BMR. Caloric requirements increase with fever, sepsis, major surgery, trauma, burns, long-term growth failure, and in the presence of chronic conditions such as bronchopulmonary dysplasia (BPD) and congenital heart disease. Caloric needs may decrease with obesity and neurologic disability (e.g., cerebral palsy). The response to stress in children is similar to that seen in critically ill adults[23] and "stress factors" have been suggested for various conditions in children (Table 130–6).[11,24] Several formulas are available for determining caloric requirements of burned children. The revised Galveston formulas[25,26] correlated most closely with measured energy expenditure in children with greater than 30% BSA burns:

Children 0 to 12 years of age:

$$\text{kcal/day} = 1800\ \text{kcal/m}^2 + 1300\ \text{kcal/m}^2 \times \%\text{BSA burn}$$

Children older than 13 years of age:

$$\text{kcal/day} = 1500\ \text{kcal/m}^2 + 1500\ \text{kcal/m}^2 \times \%\text{BSA burn}$$

Energy needs of hospitalized children (stress factor times BMR) are slightly less than maintenance energy needs because of inactivity. Additionally, counterregulatory hormones present during acute stress may diminish and even stop growth, resulting in an overall decrease in energy needs.[9,11] Pharmacologic paralysis, sedation, and adequate analgesia may also decrease energy expenditure by decreasing activity, pain, and anxiety.

Premature infants with bronchopulmonary dysplasia often require more than the usual 120 to 150 kcal/kg/d. Their energy needs may decline as pulmonary function improves. Furthermore, children with BPD often have limited physical activity, and caloric needs after 6 months corrected age may be as low as 70 to 80 kcal/kg/d.[18] Energy needs in children with developmental disabilities (e.g., cerebral palsy) also vary from usual requirements. Several methods have been proposed for estimating the caloric requirements of these children. Caloric need may be estimated based on motor function: 14.7 kcal/cm of height or 77 kcal/kg for children without motor dysfunction, 13.9 kcal/cm or 75 kcal/kg for children with motor dysfunction but ambulatory; and 11.1 kcal/cm or 64 kcal/kg for nonambulatory children with motor dysfunction.[27] An alternative approach that adjusts for muscle tone has been suggested[28]:

$$\text{kcal/day} = [\text{BMR} \times \text{muscle tone factor (MT)} \times \text{activity factor (AF)}] + \text{normal growth factor (NGF)} + \text{catch-up growth factor (CGF)}$$

where BMR = basal metabolic rate; MT = 1.1 if hypertonic, 0.9 if hypotonic; AF = 1.15 if bedridden, 1.2 if wheel chair dependent, 1.25 if crawling, 1.3 if ambulatory; NGF = 5 kcal/g desired weight gain; and, CGF = 5 kcal/g desired catch-up weight gain.

Overfeeding may increase the risk of obesity, diabetes, cardiovascular disease, and respiratory compromise resulting from increased carbon dioxide production. Although measuring energy expenditure via indirect calorimetry is preferred, it is not widely available owing to technical problems in small children and cost. Furthermore, no studies to date have shown an improved patient outcome with the use of indirect calorimetry compared to traditional methods of estimating caloric need. A conservative approach to nutrition support of the critically ill child will help to avoid overfeeding complications.

To achieve catch-up growth after long-term growth failure, a child must receive and retain nutrients in excess of normal requirements. In general, children will require 1.5 to 2 times their age-appropriate intake to achieve optimal catch-up growth. Caloric needs for catch-up growth (CUG) may be estimated as:

$$\text{CUG caloric needs (kcal/kg/d)} = \frac{\text{kcal/kg for "wt age"} \times \text{"ideal wt (kg) for age"}}{\text{actual wt (kg)}}$$

where "wt age" is the age at which current weight is 50th percentile; and "ideal wt for age" is the 50th percentile weight for current age. Catch-up growth can be evident within 2 days to 2 weeks with appropriate refeeding.[29,30] Height usually lags behind weight but will recover if dietary treatment is not stopped prematurely because of an unwarranted fear of obesity. Energy must be provided as both glucose and fat. Glucose requirements per kilogram are higher in children due to the increased percentage of metabolic activity contributed by the brain, and lipid is essential for normal central nervous system (CNS) development. Dietary guidelines limiting fat intake should therefore not be imposed for children less than 2 years of age to avoid compromising CNS development. After that, fat should not exceed 30% of the total calories.[31] As in adults, children require approximately 1% to 2% of calories as linoleic acid to prevent essential fatty acid deficiency (EFAD). Newborns and small infants have limited fat stores; therefore, EFAD may develop more rapidly than in adults. Biochemical EFAD, evidenced by a rise in the triene:tetraene ratio, has been demonstrated within 72 hours after birth in preterm infants receiving fat-free intravenous solutions.[32]

PROTEIN INTAKE

Daily protein needs are based on the child's age and clinical condition. To maintain positive nitrogen balance, premature infants should receive at least 60 nonprotein kcal/kg/d with at least 2.5 g protein/kg/d; term infants at least 80 nonprotein kcal/kg/d with at least 2.5 g protein/kg/d. To attain postnatal growth rates approximately equal to in utero growth of 10 to 15 g/kg/d, premature infants must receive 120 to 150 kcal/kg/d. Protein requirements increase 25% to 50% with hypermetabolism and are altered by organ dysfunction (Table 130–7).[33,34] Protein must be increased in similar proportions to energy during CUG, and intake can be calculated as:

$$\text{CUG protein needs (g/kg/d)} = \frac{\text{g/kg for "wt age"} \times \text{"ideal wt (kg) for age"}}{\text{actual wt (kg)}}.$$

TABLE 130–7. Daily Protein Requirements of Children With Altered Organ Function

	Infants (0–1 yr)	Children (1–10 yr)	Children (>10 yr)
Renal failure			
Predialysis	0–0.5 yr: 2.2 g/kg 0.5–1 yr: 1.6 g/kg	1–6 yr: 1.2 g/kg 7–10 yr: 1 g/kg	11–14 yr: 1 g/kg 15–18 yr: 0.9 g/kg
Dialysis			
Hemodialysis	RDA[a]	RDA[a]	RDA[a]
Peritoneal dialysis[b]	2.5–4 g/kg	2–5 yr: 3 g/kg 5–10 yr: 2.5 g/kg	10–12 yr: 2 g/kg >12 yr: 1.5 g/kg
Transplant	3 g/kg	2–3 g/kg	2–3 g/kg
Severe hepatic failure	2–3 g/kg	0.5–1.5 g/kg	0.5–1 g/kg

[a]Based on height age—see Table 130–5.
[b]Varies with type of peritoneal dialysis.

RDAs for vitamins and trace elements are met with a well-balanced diet. Therapeutic supplementation may be needed in certain disease states and conditions including cystic fibrosis,[35] hepatic disease,[36] prematurity,[37] malabsorptive syndromes, and adolescent pregnancy.

ENTERAL NUTRITION

Most children have a sufficiently intact gastrointestinal tract to enable them to be fed enterally, and, whenever possible, oral intake is preferred. If oral intake is not possible or insufficient to meet nutrient needs, feeding tube placement should be considered. Gastric tubes (e.g., nasogastric, gastrostomy) are preferred if no contraindication exists to gastric feedings. Alternatively, transpyloric feeding tubes may be used. Table 130–8 lists common indications for tube feedings in children. Contraindications to enteral feedings include severe acute pancreatitis, bowel obstruction, and intestinal atresia. Enteral nutrition (EN) formulas are classified according to the age group for which they are indicated (premature infants, term infants to 1 year of age, children 1 to 10 years of age, children older than 10 years of age) and by their macronutrient composition. Formula selection depends on age, gastrointestinal tract function, metabolic needs, fluid requirements, and diagnosis.

FORMULAS FOR INFANTS

Human breast milk is the food of choice for newborns. Human milk contains unique biochemical, immunologic, and cellular components not duplicated in commercially prepared products. Contraindications to breast-feeding include galactosemia, phenylketonuria, urea cycle defects, and a few other rare inborn errors of metabolism. Maternal diseases, including tuberculosis, hepatitis, and AIDS, may also preclude breast-feeding. Additionally, some drug therapies may preclude a mother from nursing. Briggs et al.[38] have published an excellent reference guide for the use of drugs in pregnancy and lactation.

TABLE 130–8. Common Indications for Tube Feedings In Children

Oral Intake Contraindicated	Inadequate Oral Intake	Malabsorption/Altered Metabolism
Extreme prematurity	Anorexia nervosa	Intractable vomiting
Cerebral palsy	Cancer	Short bowel syndrome
Head injury	Cystic fibrosis	Chronic diarrhea
Coma	Chronic renal/hepatic disease	Pancreatitis
Facial trauma	Inflammatory bowel disease	Inflammatory bowel disease
Esophageal injury	Congenital heart disease	Inborn errors of metabolism
	Bronchopulmonary dysplasia	Pseudo-obstruction
	Gastroesophageal reflux	
	Burns/trauma	
	Sepsis	

The first modified cow's milk–based formula was marketed in 1919 as SMA (synthetic milk adapted). Today, many formulas are available in powder, concentrate, or ready-to-feed form for infants whose mothers do not want to or cannot breast-feed (Table 130–9). These formulas are all very similar, and the standard (20 kcal/oz) products provide approximately 67 kcal/dL with 1.5 g/dL of protein as either whey or casein, 3.5 g/dL fat (48% to 50% of total calories) as a mixture of vegetable oils, and carbohydrate as lactose. Vitamins and minerals are added to provide RDAs.

The daily protein intake provided by human milk is lower than formula; however, human milk contains a higher percentage (70%) of whey protein, a more easily digestible protein than casein, the predominant cow's milk protein (80%). Whey protein also supplies carriers for immunoglobulins, albumin, lysozyme, enzymes such as amylase, transaminases, proteases, lipases, vitamins, and minerals.

Iron absorption from human milk (20% to 50%) is significantly higher than from formula (4% to 7%), probably due to iron-binding proteins in human milk, lower protein and phosphorus content, and differences in lactose and ascorbate content. Historically, low-iron formulas were recommended until infants were approximately 4 to 6 months of age due to concerns that iron-fortified formulas contributed to colic, constipation, diarrhea, and regurgitation. Scientific investigations do not support these concerns. The American Academy of Pediatrics (AAP) recommends iron-fortified formulas starting from birth in all non-breast-fed infants, including preterm infants.[39] Whole cow's milk should not be introduced until 1 year of age to avoid milk protein sensitization, gastrointestinal blood loss, iron deficiency, dehydration caused by high renal solute load, and nutrient deficiencies.[40]

SPECIAL-NEEDS FORMULAS

A number of formulas are available for infants with special needs (see Table 130–9). Soy-based formulas are lactose free and indicated for the treatment of uncomplicated primary lactase deficiency, secondary lactose intolerance after gastroenteritis, protein–calorie malnutrition or other causes of mucosal injury, galactosemia, and cow's milk protein allergy. Soy formulas are considered nutritionally equivalent to cow's milk–based formulas.

Hydrolyzed or semi-elemental formulas (Table 130–10) are indicated for infants or children with altered digestion, absorption, or metabolism. Common indications include cow's milk and soy protein allergy, generalized malabsorption (e.g., short bowel syndrome), pancreatic insufficiency (e.g., cystic fibrosis), chylothorax, biliary atresia, chronic diarrhea, and acquired immunodeficiency syndrome (AIDS). Hydrolysate formulas cost three to four times or more than standard cow's milk– or soy-based formulas and

TABLE 130–9. Formulas for Infants and Children

Formula Type	Products (Mfr[a])	Indications
Cow's milk-based	Enfamil (MJ) 20, 22, 24 kcal/oz; Similac (R) 20, 24, 27 kcal/oz; Gerber Baby Formula (G); Carnation Good Start (C); Lacto*free* (MJ); Similac PM 60/40 (R)	Normal healthy infants Lactose intolerance (Lacto*free* only)
Soy-based	Isomil, Isomil DF,[b] Isomil SF[c] (R); Prosobee (MJ); Gerber Soy (G); Soyalac, I-Soyalac (LL); Alsoy (C)	Lactase deficiency or intolerance; galactosemia; cow's milk allergy
Premature	Similac Special Care (R) 20, 24 kcal/oz; Enfamil Premature (MJ) 20, 24 kcal/oz; Similac Neocare (R) 22 kcal/oz	Preterm infant less than 2–3 kg
Transition	Advance (R); Carnation Follow-Up, Carnation Follow-Up Soy (C); Next Step, Next Step Soy (MJ)	Transition from formula to cow's milk
Children 1–10 years of age	Pediasure, Pediasure with Fiber (R); Nutren Jr., Nutren Jr. with Fiber (N), Kindercal[d] (MJ)	Normal gastrointestinal tract function
Special diets	MSUD Diet Powder (MJ)	Maple syrup urine disease or branched-chain amino acid disorders
	Phenyl-Free (MJ)	Phenylketonuria
	Similac PM 60/40 (R)	Renal, cardiac, or endocrine disorders
	Protein Free Diet Powder (MJ) (Product 80056)	Altered amino acid metabolism
	RCF (R)	Intractable diarrhea; carbohydrate intolerance; ketogenic diet
	Product 3232-A (MJ)	Intractable diarrhea; carbohydrate intolerance

[a]Manufacturers: R = Ross Laboratories; N = Nestlé Clinical Nutrition; MJ = Mead Johnson Nutritionals; C = Nestlé Carnation Baby Formulas; G = Gerber; LL = Nutricia-Loma Linda.
[b]Diarrhea formula contains 0.77 g fiber/100 mL.
[c]Sucrose free.
[d]Contains soy fiber 5.9 g/1000 kcal.

thus should be used only when their benefit has been demonstrated.

Neither human milk nor standard cow's milk–based formulas are adequate to supply the premature infant's needs. Human milk fortifiers (see Table 130–9) are available to provide additional nutrients to human milk. Formulas designed for premature infants (see Table 130–10) are modified to compensate for alterations in absorption and digestion. Carbohydrate is provided as both lactose and glucose polymers; the protein quantities are increased, as well as the whey-to-casein ratio (60:40); and fat content is partially provided as medium-chain triglycerides (MCTs). Mineral and vitamin

TABLE 130–10. Semi-Elemental Formulas for Infants and Children

Product (Mfr[a])	Carbohydrate	Fat	Protein
Formulas for infants			
Nutramigen (MJ)	Sucrose, modified tapioca starch	Corn oil	Hydrolyzed casein
Pregestimil (MJ)	Corn syrup solids, modified tapioca starch	MCT 60%, sunflower oil	Hydrolyzed casein
Alimentum (R)	Sucrose, modified tapioca starch	MCT 50%; coconut, safflower, and soy oil	Hydrolyzed casein; free amino acids
Portagen (MJ)	Sucrose, corn syrup solids	MCT 86%; corn oil	Sodium caseinate
Neocate (SHS)	Corn syrup solids	Safflower, coconut, and soy oils	Free amino acids
Formulas for children 1–10 years of age			
Vivonex Pediatric (S)	Maltodextrin, modified starch	MCT 68%; soybean oil	Free amino acids
Peptamen Junior (N)	Maltodextrin, corn starch	MCT 60%; soybean oil; canola oil	Hydrolyzed whey
Neocate One+ (SHS)	Maltodextrin, sucrose	MCT 25%, coconut, canola, and high-oleic safflower oils	Free amino acids
Pro-Peptide for Kids (NM)	Maltodextrin, corn starch	MCT 40%; soybean oil; canola oil	Hydrolyzed whey

[a]Manufacturers: MJ = Mead Johnson Nutritionals; R = Ross Laboratories; S = Sandoz; N = Nestlé Clinical Nutrition; SHS = SHS International Ltd.; NM = Nutrition Medical, Inc.

content is also higher. These formulas are safe and produce improved growth rates, bone mineralization, and nitrogen retention compared to standard infant formulas. Healthy preterm infants may be weaned from premature formulas at approximately 2 kg. Preterm infants with BPD may benefit from preterm formulas until they reach 3 kg because of fluid restriction, increased energy needs, and diuretic therapy.[18]

FORMULAS FOR OLDER CHILDREN

Several products are available specifically to meet the mineral, vitamin, trace element, and protein needs of children 1 to 10 years of age. Standard products (see Table 130–9) are essentially lactose- and gluten-free but are not predigested and, therefore, are not suitable for children with malabsorption. Semi-elemental formulas (see Table 130–10) are used for children with malabsorption or intolerance to standard formulas. Formulas intended for adults (see Chap. 129) have also been used for older children (6 to 10 years of age) or children older than 1 year of age with nutrition needs not met by age-specific formulas.

Occasionally, commercial formulas fail to meet nutrient needs. The formula can be concentrated by adding less water to a powder or concentrate for children with increased caloric or protein needs who cannot tolerate the volume necessary to receive sufficient calories with standard products. A modular product (Table 130–11) may be added to the regimen for those children who have malabsorption of one or more nutrients.[41] Generally, infant formulas are first concentrated to 24 kcal/oz by adding less water or, if available, using pre-prepared 24 or 27 kcal/oz product. Modular components can be added to further increase the desired nutrient. Adding modules to 20 kcal/oz formula is usually avoided because this may dilute other nutrients to suboptimal levels. Mixing powdered or concentrated formulas with less water increases delivered quantities of all nutrients and may increase the renal solute load, predisposing the infant to dehydration.

TABLE 130–11. Modular Enteral Products

Primary Nutrient Supplied	Example Products (Mfr[a])
Carbohydrate	LC (C), PC (C), Moducal (MJ), Polycose (R), Sumacal (SM)
Protein	ProMod (R), Propac (SM), ProMix RDP (C), Casec (MJ), Gevral Protein (L), ProViMin (R)
Fat	High MCT Supplement (C), MCT Oil (MJ), Lipomul (RO), Microlipid (SM)
Human milk fortifier	Enfamil Human Milk Fortifier (MJ), Similac Natural Care (R)
Pectin/carbohydrate/potassium	Banana Flakes (K)

[a]Manufacturers: R = Ross Laboratories; MJ = Mead Johnson Nutritionals; SM = Sherwood Medical; L = Lederle; RO = Roberts Pharmaceutical Corporation; C = Corpak; K = Kanana.

FEEDING REGIMENS

Most approaches for initiating and advancing feedings are based on experience rather than controlled trials. In a stable, closely monitored child, it is reasonable to select an appropriate formula and to administer 100% of the therapeutic goal either by continuous or bolus feedings immediately.[42] This approach may be well tolerated and preferable to tapering either concentration or volume. Full feedings will be achieved more quickly, which may shorten hospital stay or time to recovery. Many, however, prefer gradual advancement of feedings, usually by increasing volume over hours to days depending on the child's condition and feeding tolerance. When intolerance is documented or expected (e.g., short bowel syndrome), gradual advancement often using a combination of parenteral and enteral nutrition is preferred. In premature infants, too rapid feeding advancement has been associated with the development of necrotizing enterocolitis. Intermittent bolus feedings are preferred because they more closely simulate normal feeding, are less expensive, and allow greater flexibility and mobility. However, children with severe intestinal disease may not tolerate this approach.[43]

Feeding intolerance is evidenced by the development of vomiting, abdominal distention, or diarrhea. Checking residuals, that is, the volume remaining in the stomach immediately prior to the next feeding, is not routinely recommended except in children at risk for aspiration.[44] If aspiration is a concern, residuals should be checked every 2 to 4 hours initially, then less often as tolerance is documented. Acceptable residual volume is variable. One rule of thumb is that the residual volume should be less than one-half of the previously administered volume. A single high residual should not result in feeding discontinuation. Holding a feeding or decreasing the rate for several hours may be adequate. Stool character is highly variable even in healthy children and is often related to formula type. Stool volume less than 15 to 20 mL/kg/d and absence of fecal reducing substances (unabsorbed sugars) or large amounts of fecal fat are indications of tolerance regardless of stool frequency, consistency, or color.

COMPLICATIONS

Complications of EN in children are similar to those seen in adults (see Chap. 129). Diarrhea is frequently associated with concomitant medications, carbohydrate malabsorption, or viral illness. Addition of large amounts of glucose to the diet in the form of modular additives or fruit juices may result in loose stools or diarrhea. Large quantities of added fat, especially MCTs, may result in diarrhea or delayed gastric emptying and gastroesophageal reflux. Constipation is frequently associated with long-term use of liquid formulas and may develop as a result of lack of sufficient fluid or bulk in the diet, medications, decreased muscle tone, or inactivity. Increased fluid intake, avoidance of constipating medications, and use of fiber-containing formulas or fiber supplements may be helpful in the management of constipation. Children fed exclusively via tube for extended periods, especially during the first year of life, may develop oral hypersensitivity, poor oral-motor skills, and food aversions. Making the transition from tube to oral nutrition often requires the involvement of an occupational or speech therapist, behavioral psychologist, or other trained individual. Avoidance of a strict nothing by mouth (NPO) status, if possible, is recommended to avoid this complication.

PARENTERAL NUTRITION

Central venous parenteral nutrition (PN) has been used for over 35 years to support normal growth and has resulted in decreased mortality for a number of patient populations, particularly those infants with surgical or other catastrophic gastrointestinal defects or diseases. PN is indicated only when a trial of EN has failed or when severely diminished intestinal function is anticipated due to underlying disease or treatment.[1] Common diagnoses necessitating the use of PN in children are similar to those of adults with the exception of extreme prematurity (see Chap. 128).

CENTRAL VERSUS PERIPHERAL ADMINISTRATION

Route selection, peripheral versus central, depends on expected length of therapy, caloric stores and needs, peripheral vein access, and inpatient or outpatient status. Peripheral administration is primarily limited by solution osmolality. In general, the osmolality of peripherally administered solutions should not exceed 900 mOsm/L to avoid complications. Central administration is limited primarily by catheter complications, including infection and thrombosis.

CALORIC NEEDS

Carbohydrate is generally administered as dextrose monohydrate. The maximum dextrose concentration recommended for peripheral PN ranges from 10% to 12.5% (osmolality 500 to 625 mOsm/L) depending on the solution's amino acid (AA) concentration (100 mOsm/L per %AA concentration). Phlebitis and other catheter complications may be increased when higher dextrose concentrations are utilized. Dextrose is usually advanced over several days to provide 40% to 60% of nonprotein calories. In neonates, dextrose is initiated at 5 to 8 mg/kg/min and advanced by 1 to 2 mg/kg/min daily to approximately 10 to 15 mg/kg/min. Older children usually tolerate larger daily increases in dextrose: increases of 2 to 4 mg/kg/min up to 6 to 9 mg/kg/min are generally well tolerated. Children older than 16 years of age should receive dextrose at 2 to 5 mg/kg/min as recommended in adults.[45] Dextrose tolerance is monitored by checking serum and urine glucose every 8 to 24 hours initially and less frequently once tolerance is documented.

Insulin must be used with caution because children, especially neonates, may have variable responses to insulin administration that can result in hypoglycemia.[46] If persistent hyperglycemia is present, it is prudent to administer insulin as a separate continuous infusion, 0.05–0.1 unit/kg/h initially, or as a sliding-scale subcutaneous injection, rather than adding insulin to the PN solution. This will allow titration of serum glucose concentrations until daily needs are established.

PROTEIN SOURCES

Amino acid solutions used in children are the same as those used in adults (see Chap. 128) with the exception of two products marketed specifically for neonates and infants: Aminosyn-PF (Abbott Laboratories) and TrophAmine (B Braun McGaw). Two studies compared outcomes in neonates who received these products versus standard AA solutions; improved weight gain and nitrogen balance and more "normal" AA patterns were observed in those who received the pediatric products.[47,48] Experience with the use of other specialty AA products in children is limited.

The optimal initiation and advancement of intravenous protein remains controversial. Starting at 0.5 to 1.0 g/kg/d and advancing by an equal amount daily has been recommended by some, but others initiate AA intake at full protein requirements. There is little evidence that gradual advancement is necessary; however, tapering may be appropriate for very-low-birth-weight neonates and in children with renal or hepatic dysfunction.

Carnitine, a quaternary amine required for transport of free fatty acids into the mitochondria for β-oxidation and energy production, can be synthesized from lysine and methionine. Synthesis is decreased in premature infants, and low plasma carnitine concentrations and/or overt carnitine deficiency have been documented in premature or surgical infants receiving PN or other carnitine-free diets.[49,50] Carnitine supplementation has not yet become standard therapy in all institutions, but intravenous doses of 8 to 16 mg/kg/d have been shown to improve intravenous fat emulsion utilization in premature infants.[51] Other studies, however, have produced conflicting results. Higher doses may be needed to reverse documented carnitine deficiency; doses of 50 to 100 mg/kg/d have been used for correction of carnitine deficiency.[52] Additionally, carnitine deficiency has been suggested as an etiologic factor in PN-induced hepatic disease.

FAT FORMULATIONS

Intravenous fat emulsions provide both essential fatty acids and a concentrated iso-osmolar calorie source and have been shown to prolong viability of peripheral intravenous lines when co-infused with dextrose and AA solutions.[53] Fat emulsions are usually started at 0.5 g/kg/d in neonates and 0.5 to 1 g/kg/d in older children and increased daily by an equal amount to a maximum of 3 to 4 g/kg/d[54] as long as triglycerides are not elevated. The reduced concentration of phospholipids in 20% emulsions enhances triglyceride clearance and lessens the accumulation of cholesterol and phospholipid in low-density lipoproteins.[37] Theroretically, gradual increases in the daily dose may improve tolerance by allowing time for increased lipoprotein lipase production. Many infants and children will, however, tolerate higher initial lipid doses. A test dose of 1 mL/kg given over 1 hour for children less than 5 kg and 0.1 mL/min for 10 to 15 minutes for children greater than 5 kg has been recommended owing to the potential for an immediate hypersensitivity reaction. Most institutions omit the test dose but monitor the patient carefully during the first hour of the initial lipid infusion. Fat emulsions generally supply 30% to 50% of calories but should not exceed 60% to prevent ketosis.

Adverse effects of intravenous fat emulsions administration in children are similar to those seen in adults (see Chap. 128). Hyperlipemia is uncommon and can be minimized by maintaining infusion rates less than 0.25 g/kg/h.[54] Brans et al.[55] demonstrated no adverse effects on pulmonary function when lipids were infused at 0.17 g/kg/d for 24 hours. Kernicterus remains a potential risk with the use of fat emulsions in hyperbilirubinemic neonates because free fatty acids (FFAs), the metabolic end product of lipid hydrolysis, compete with bilirubin for albumin binding sites. Bilirubin displacement depends on the relative concentrations of albumin, bilirubin, and unesterified fatty acids. Gutcher et al.[56] found that infants approximately 24 hours of age receiving 1 g/kg/d of intravenous lipid experienced a significant rise in free bilirubin concentration associated with increased FFAs. The measured FFA-to-albumin ratio, however, never exceeded 6, the level at which significant displacement is expected.[57] Caution is warranted, however, in infants whose bilirubin concentration exceeds 12 mg/dL. In these newborns, fat infusions should be limited to 0.5 to 1.0 g/kg/d, doses sufficient to prevent EFAD, and increased only when the bilirubin is consistently less than 12 mg/dL.

ELECTROLYTE, VITAMIN, AND TRACE ELEMENT REQUIREMENTS

Parenteral electrolyte requirements are shown in Table 130–12. Requirements may be altered with pathologic states such as necrotizing enterocolitis, peritonitis, prematurity, renal and hepatic dysfunction, and with drug therapy such as diuretics, amphotericin B, and corticosteroids. Of particular interest in pediatrics is the conditional solubility of calcium and phosphorus. Factors determining solubility include pH, time, temperature, order of mixing, and concentration of the two minerals. Pediatric-specific AA solutions have a lower pH and are particularly useful in neonates because they allow for improved calcium and phosphorus delivery.

Current recommendations for intravenous vitamin intake in children are based on revisions of the American Medical Association Nutritional Advisory Groups 1979 guidelines.[58] MVI-Pediatric (Lyphomed) is the only product marketed specifically to meet these needs. For children weighing more than 3 kg (up to 11 years of age), the recommended daily dose is 5 mL/d. Preterm infants should receive 2 mL/kg up to 5 mL/d. Children older than 11 years of age should receive an adult vitamin preparation. If MVI-Pediatric is unavailable, other multivitamin preparations may be used in children less than 11 years of age: Cernevit (Baxter) 0.8 mL/kg/d (maximum 2.5 mL/d) with vitamin K supplementation at a dose of 80 µg for infants weighing less than 2500 g and 200 µg for those weighing more than 2500 g; MVC (Fujisawa) 0.5 mL/kg/d (maximum 1 mL/d) plus vitamin K as above, folic acid 140 µg/d, and cyanocobalamin 100 µg/month; or MVI-12 (Astra or Multi-12

TABLE 130–12. Parenteral Electrolyte and Trace Element Requirements for Neonates, Infants, and Children

Recommended Intake	Preterm Neonates	Full-Term and Infants	Children
Sodium (mEq/kg/d)	3–6[a]	2–5	2–5
Potassium (mEq/kg/d)	2–3[a]	2–5	2–5
Chloride (mEq/kg/d)	3–6[a]	2–5	2–5
Phosphorus (mmol/kg/d)	1.5–2	1–2	1–1.5
Magnesium (mEq/kg/d)	0.5–1	0.5–1	0.25–0.5
Calcium (mEq/kg/d)	2–4	1–2	0.5–1
Acetate	—[b]	—[b]	—[b]
Zinc (µg/kg/d)	300–400	250 (< 3 months) 100 (> 3 months)	50 (max 5 mg)
Copper[c] (µg/kg/d)	20	20	20 (max 300 µg)
Chromium (µg/kg/d)	0.14–0.2	0.14–0.2	0.14–0.2 (5 µg)
Manganese[c] (µg/kg/d)	1	1	1 (50 µg)
Selenium (µg/kg/d)	1.5–2	2–3	2–3 (30 µg)
Molybdenum[d] (µg/kg/d)	0.25	0.25	0.25 (5 µg)
Iodide[d] (µg/kg/d)	1	1	1

[a]Newborns and low-birth-weight or very-low-birth-weight infants or with concomitant disease (e.g., necrotizing enterocolitis) may have higher requirements.
[b]As needed to maintain acid–base balance.
[c]May accumulate with cholestasis.
[d]Long-term PN only, if no topicals containing iodide or table salt are used.

(Sabex) 2 mL/kg/d (maximum 5 mL/d) plus vitamin K as above. Cernevit is the only product other than MVI-Pediatric that does not contain propylene glycol or polysorbate 80 and 20, and is therefore the only alternative product recommended for neonates less than 36 weeks' gestation or under 1500 g.[59]

Recommended parenteral intakes of essential trace elements are shown in Table 130–12.[58,60] Combination products are available specifically for children that provide manganese, copper, chromium, zinc, and selenium. Usual recommended intake is 0.3 mL/kg for children weighing less than 3 kg and 0.2 mL/kg (maximum 5 mL/d) for children weighing more than 3 kg. Children weighing more than 25 kg may receive the recommended adult product and dose. Owing to decreased elimination, trace elements may need to be decreased in children with renal disease (zinc, selenium, chromium) and/or cholestatic liver disease (copper, manganese). Children with high ostomy or stool output and burns will need extra zinc and possibly selenium.

Prematurity, acute illness, chronic gastrointestinal losses, and long-term, selenium-free total PN are associated with low selenium levels and decreased glutathione peroxidase activity.[61] The clinical significance of reduced selenium levels is unclear. Selenium supplementation is recommended for preterm and term infants after 2 weeks of PN[62] and for older children after 4 weeks[58] (see Table 130–12). Although iodine is not routinely added to PN solutions, many children have been maintained on iodine-free total PN without evidence of hypothyroidism.[63] Iodine absorption from topical povidone–iodine used during catheter dressing changes, the iodide contaminant in PN solutions, and the intake of iodized table salt provide apparently adequate intake.[63] Periodic assessment for signs of hypothyroidism is suggested but routine monitoring of thyroid hormone levels is not recommended. Aluminum contamination of PN solutions primarily through the calcium gluconate additive and other non-PN products (e.g., albumin, soy formulas) is a concern in premature infants, especially those with renal insufficiency. Aluminum toxicity may be associated with bone fractures, osteomalacia, encephalopathy, and microcytic hypochromic anemia.[64]

Oral iron supplementation is preferred to the use of parenteral iron–dextran since iron absorption from the proximal small intestine may occur even with bowel impairment. If oral therapy is not possible or ineffective, intravenous or intramuscular iron–dextran may be given. Hypersensitivity reactions, including anaphylaxis, can occur with parenteral iron–dextran administration. Local reactions, pain, and skin staining with intramuscular injection make the intravenous route preferred. Iron–dextran has been administered daily in PN solutions (10% of RDA/d) but monthly administration with the total monthly requirement given over one to several days is effective, less time consuming, less expensive, and, potentially safer.[65] Iron–dextran doses required for children with iron-deficiency anemia can be calculated as:

$$\text{Dose (mg Fe)} = [\text{wt (kg)}] \times (4.5) \times [(\text{Hgb}_d - \text{Hgb}_a)]$$

where hemogobin (g/dL) desired (Hgb_d) is 12 if < 15 kg or 14.8 if > 15 kg and Hgb_a is measured hemoglobin (g/dL).

The maximum recommended daily dose of iron–dextran is 25 mg for children weighing less than 5 kg, 50 mg for children weighing 5 to 10 kg, and 100 mg for children weighing more than 10 kg, infused no faster than 50 mg/min. Owing to the risk of anaphylaxis, a test dose of 0.5 mL (0.25 mL for infants) given over 1 hour has been recommended. When iron–dextran is added to PN solutions, many practitioners institute anaphylactic precautions for 1 hour after the infusion is started in lieu of a test dose. It is important to note that anaphylaxis can occur despite an uneventful test dose, and medications used for treatment of anaphylaxis (epinephrine, diphenhydramine, methylprednisolone) should be available whenever iron–dextran is administered.[65]

Metabolic and electrolyte abnormalities experienced in children receiving PN are similar to those seen in adults (see Chap. 128). Two complications with unique presentations in children are metabolic bone disease and cholestatic jaundice. The etiology of PN-associated cholestatic jaundice remains unclear. Toxic effects of AAs and lipids have been proposed but not substantiated. Excess energy intake probably contributes to cholestasis. Nutrient deficiencies (e.g., taurine, carnitine) have also been suggested as contributory factors in the etiology of cholestatic jaundice. Liver toxicity is usually not seen unless the child has received 6 to 8 weeks or more of total PN therapy. In the early stages, liver dysfunction is reversible but may be progressive, leading to fulminant hepatic failure. Premature infants, especially those experiencing necrotizing enterocolitis or sepsis, appear to develop liver dysfunction more commonly than others receiving long-term PN. Preventive strategies include early provision of enteral nutrients, cycling of PN solutions, avoidance of overfeeding, carnitine and L-glutamine supplementation, and ursodiol administration.

Due to the relative insolubility of calcium phosphate in PN solutions, the amount of calcium provided to premature infants may not be adequate for normal bone mineralization. However, serum calcium concentrations often remain normal despite inadequate intake as the result of calcium release from bone. Osteopenia, rickets, and collapsed vertebrae have been reported in both low-birth-weight and term infants requiring prolonged PN. Alkaline phosphatase activity is a good marker for metabolic bone disease. Quantification of alkaline phosphatase isoenzymes, however, may be necessary to distinquish bone disease from PN-induced liver disease.

Cyclic PN is used commonly in children, especially in the home, although there is little published information on the practice. The use of cyclic PN in infants less than 6 months of age (range 37 to 124 days) has been reported.[66] Cycling is usually begun with 1 to 2 hours off PN each day in infants and 2 to 4 hours off PN for older children. The time off PN is advanced to 4 to 6 hours for infants and 12 to 14 hours for older children, as tolerated. Tapering on and off PN in two or three steps by beginning at one-third to one-fourth the final rate for 30 minutes, increasing to two-thirds to one-half the final rate for 30 minutes, and then increasing to the final rate is generally well tolerated. Serum glucose should be checked 30 to 60 minutes after discontinuation or advancement to full rate until tolerance of the cyclic regimen is established. Hyperglycemia is uncommon; hypoglycemia, if it occurs, is usually transient and asymptomatic. Besides the increased mobility cycling offers, the incidence of cholestatic jaundice may be decreased with its use. If PN is expected to be used for longer than 1 month, early cycling should be attempted. Programmable infusion pumps are available to facilitate cycling in the home environment.

GERIATRIC NUTRITION

The elderly population in the United States is the fastest growing segment of the population. It is estimated that by the year 2000, 13% of the population will be older than 65 years old, with those older than 85 being in the highest proportion.[67] The elderly are the most heterogeneous group in our society in terms of socioeconomic, health, marital status, and educational background. Up to 85% of all older Americans are at risk of malnutrition[67] and its associated adverse effects such as increased rate of infection, poor wound healing, and increased morbidity and mortality (see Chap. 127). Nutrition is an integral component of the health maintenance needs of older adults. This portion of the chapter will present nutrition assessment issues, nutrition requirements, and nutritional regimen needs that have been specifically documented or proposed for the elderly.

PHYSIOLOGIC CHANGES

The human aging process is a continuum of biologic alterations. Changes in organ function, body composition, and physical performance are all part of this process and occur at varying rates in each individual. Factors that influence these changes include disease pathology, genetics, socioeconomic status, diet, and the environment. Nutrition plays a key role in maintaining biologic processes, preventing diseases, and aiding in the recovery from acute illness.

Body composition changes are the most obvious of the aging process. They include decreases in lean body mass (LBM), total body water (TBW), and bone density and an increase in total body fat. Unequivocally, the decrease in LBM or muscle tissue, which includes both skeletal muscle (somatic tissue) and smooth muscle (visceral/organ tissue), is the most outstanding. There is a progressive decline in LBM through the years. From the ages of 25 to 70 years, males will lose 16% to 19% of their LBM whereas females will lose 12%.[68] This decrease in muscle mass is secondary to decreases in protein synthesis and physical activity. Exercise can help minimize the amount of muscle lost as well as aid in rebuilding muscle mass in the elderly.

Corresponding with the decrease in LBM is an increase in adipose (fat) tissue. This occurs slowly from age 25 to age 70 years. During this time, body fat will increase by 18% in males and 12% in females.[68] Along with the increase in fat proportion there is also an alteration in fat distribution. As people age, fat tends to be located on the trunk of the body with internal fat deposited around the vital organs. This type of fat distribution has been associated with increased risk for cardiovascular disease, stroke, and cancer.[72] TBW decreases 10% to 20% by age 70 to 80 years.[68] Seventy-two percent of TBW is found in LBM as the intracellular compartment; hence, with a decrease in LBM there is a subsequent decrease in TBW. Decreases in TBW contribute to an increased likelihood of rapid dehydration under conditions of inadequate fluid intake. Bone mass peaks at 35 years of age and is determined by genetics, gender, exercise, and calcium intake. Bone loss occurs gradually over time, commencing between the ages of 40 and 50 years, with the degree of loss varying according to gender and anatomic site.[70]

Cardiovascular, pulmonary, hepatic, renal, and gastrointestinal function decline with age and ultimately affect nutrient and substrate requirements, tolerance, and utilization. Of these, gastrointestinal changes may be the most obvious to have an impact on nutrition status. A reduced rate of gastric emptying, with accompanying reductions in gastric acid, intrinsic factor, and pepsin secretion, all have a potential impact on nutrient utilization. Small intestinal changes include a diminished enzyme production and a decline in absorptive capacity. In addition, large intestine motility is frequently slowed, with constipation being a common complaint of the elderly. This constipative state is enhanced by a low-fiber diet, lack of exercise, and insufficient fluid intake. Finally, other age-related transformations of importance to nutrition include insulin resistance, depressed response to thirst, a decreased ability to sense odor, and an altered taste sensitivity.[71]

NUTRITION ASSESSMENT

Nutrition status plays an important role in the function of all muscle groups and organ systems and can be a factor in the length of hospital stay, wound healing, immune function, and mental status. However, accurately assessing the nutrition status of the elderly presents many challenges. Several factors, including those related to age, need to be evaluated and considered during the assessment process. Older adults tend to have chronic disease states, multiple drug regimens, and physiologic changes that have the potential to alter nutrition status. Body composition changes and lack of established anthropometric measurement standards all influence nutrition assessment parameters and their interpretation.

An accurate assessment combines data gathered from dietary, medical, drug, and social histories, physical exam, and appropriate anthropometric and laboratory measurements. During the process of evaluating nutrition status, risk factors associated with malnutrition can also be identified. Risk factors include inappropriate food intake, poverty, social isolation, dependency/disability, acute/ chronic diseases or conditions, chronic medication use, and advanced age.[72] Furthermore, a nutrition assessment has a predictive or prognostic value in certain settings. Elderly people with a subjective clinical diagnosis of malnutrition along with below-normal values in anthropometric measurements, visceral proteins (albumin, prealbumin, and transferrin), and vitamin A and C concentrations were shown to have increased mortality.[73] Nutrition assessments and screenings are of particular importance in the elderly because once malnutrition or the risk factors of malnutrition are identified, early intervention may preclude a poor response to injury or disease.

ANTHROPOMETRIC MEASUREMENTS

Anthropometric measurements are used to estimate body fat and LBM. Typically they include weight, height, limb circumference, and various skinfold thickness measurements. These parameters are used to compare an individual with a population standard, and repeated measurements in the same person can indicate response of an individual to changes in nutrition. Limitations of their utility in the elderly include lack of age-appropriate standards and reliability of the measurement process.[69] There are standards, based on frame size, for skinfold thickness (triceps and subscapular) and bone-free upper arm muscle area for people aged 55 to 74 years.[74] However, the current national standards for those older than 74 years of age are extrapolations of data from younger populations. With no national standards, researchers have focused on defining anthropometric values and reference ranges in the elderly population.

The reliability of triceps skinfold thickness measurements in the elderly is compromised because skin becomes less resilient and muscle becomes softer with advancing age. This makes it difficult to differentiate from the fat fold. Furthermore, triceps fat folds tend to decline in elderly women more than in men owing to redistribution of adipose tissue. Midarm muscle circumference is reflective of somatic protein stores. However, neuropathology and unilateral wasting secondary to stroke may compromise the accuracy of this measurement.

Weight history should include weight changes over time and as a percentage of ideal body weight (IBW). IBW is generally based on height, which may be difficult to determine in the elderly. Accurate height measurements depend on the person's ability to stand erect. Older people may be bedridden or have spinal curvature, which prevents this upright posture. In these situations, estimating height, or stature, is based on the measurement of long bones. By measuring from the knee to the heel, with the knee flexed at a 90 degree angle and beginning measurement 2 inches proximal to the patella, stature can then be approximated:[75]

Stature for men (cm) =

$$[2.02 \times \text{knee ht (cm)}] - [(0.04 \times \text{age (yr)}] + 64.19$$

Stature for women (cm) =

$$[1.83 \times \text{knee ht (cm)}] - [(0.24 \times \text{age (yr)}] + 84.88$$

CLINICAL ASSESSMENT

Physical exam and medical history should focus on the identification of major and minor indicators of poor nutritional status[76] (Tables 130–13 and 130–14, respectively). These indicators were developed to allow for prioritization and categorization of observations and are not absolute indicators of malnutrition. The physical exam should focus on assessing muscle wasting, edema, loss of subcutaneous fat, and physical findings of vitamin, trace element, and essential fatty acid deficiencies (see Chap. 126). Examining the mouth is a crucial part of the physical exam.[71] Poor dentition, mouth lesions, or infections have an impact on the type and quantity of food selected and consumed.

MEDICATION HISTORY

A complete medication history should include nonprescription medication (e.g., vitamin/mineral supplements and laxatives) as well as prescription drug regimens and compliance. Drug–nutrient interactions are a serious problem in this population because the use of multiple drugs increases the potential for such interactions. Drugs that are of importance include those agents that induce gastrointestinal changes (e.g., narcotics) and/or that alter electrolyte concentrations (e.g., diuretics) and nutrient absorption (e.g., cholestyramine, antacids).[77]

FUNCTIONAL STATUS

Activities of daily living (ADLs) and instrumental activities of daily living (IADLs) are a means of assessing functional status. ADLs include bathing, dressing, toileting, and feeding. IADLs are the skills needed to buy and prepare food. A change from independence to dependence in these activities is a potential indicator of poor nutrition status.[67] Chronic disease states such as arthritis, and Parkinson's and Alzheimer's diseases usually have detrimental effects on functional status, which may be progressive.

BIOCHEMICAL PARAMETERS

Visceral protein status indicators are albumin, transferrin, prealbumin (transthyretin), and retinol-binding protein. As

TABLE 130–13. Major Indicators of Poor Nutritional Status in Older Americans

Weight loss over time	5.0% in 1 month 7.5% in 3 months 10% or 10 lb in 6 months
Low or high weight for height	20% below or above desired body weight
Reduced serum albumin	Serum albumin concentration <3.5 g/L
Change in functional status	Change to dependent in 2 of the ADLs or 1 of the nutrition-related IADLs
Inappropriate food intake	Failure to eat minimum U.S. dietary guidelines from more than one basic food group Failure to observe moderation in salt and sugar intake Failure to observe saturated fat limitation Alcohol consumption above 1 oz/d (women) or 2 oz/d (men)
Reduction in midarm circumference	< 10th percentile of NHANES[a] standard
Increase or decrease in skinfold	< 10th percentile > 95th percentile
Obesity	> 120% of desirable weight
Nutrition-related disorders	Osteoporosis Osteomalacia Folate deficiency Vitamin B_{12} deficiency

[a]National Health and Nutrition Examination Surveys.

Reprinted with permission by the Nutrition Screening Initiative, a project of the American Academy of Family Physicians, the American Dietetic Association, and the National Council on the Aging, Inc., and funded in part by a grant from Ross Products Division, Abbott Laboratories. (Ref. 72.)

with the anthropometric standards, normal values for those older than 74 years of age are unknown with the exception of serum albumin, which decreases slightly with increasing age.[78] Hepatic function, stress metabolism, trauma, and hydration status need to be considered when interpreting serum albumin concentrations. Albumin concentrations appear to be a strong prognostic indicator in the elderly, and increased mortality has been associated with decreased albumin concentrations.[79] However, values appear to be maintained in the elderly who are well and are responsive to nutritional repletion over time. Transferrin values are not reliable nutrition markers in the elderly. They tend to have increased iron stores and therefore less circulating transferrin.[71] Prealbumin and retinol-binding protein concentrations are maintained in the elderly, with prealbumin being the more discriminant biochemical marker of nutrition status.[80]

OTHER MARKERS OF PROTEIN STATUS

Creatinine height index is a measure of somatic muscle mass. It is dependent on a 24-hour urine collection, which may be problematic in the elderly without bladder catheterization. It is not an accurate reflection of muscle mass in cachectic individuals, those with impaired renal function, or those in states of dehydration. It is also important to remember that creatinine excretion and LBM decreases in the elderly offset each other, and as a result serum creatinine values may appear to be normal even in individuals with moderate renal insufficiency (see Chap. 40).

Nitrogen balance studies rely on a 24-hour urine collection to determine urine urea nitrogen and total urine nitrogen excretion. Inactivity (immobility, bedridden) leads to an increase in nitrogen excretion secondary to muscle breakdown. Providing increased protein may not reverse this process, and thus a negative nitrogen balance results. To preserve muscle mass, or at least decrease the loss, exercise and adequate protein intake are required.

HEMATOLOGIC INDICATORS

Nutrition-related anemias secondary to deficiencies in iron, folate, and vitamin B_{12} are more prevalent in the elderly and appear to be related to dietary intake, pathology, and malabsorption. Chronic iron deficiency is often caused by gastrointestinal blood loss as the result of peptic ulcer disease or carcinoma of the colon or stomach. Medications such as aspirin, nonsteroidal anti-inflammatory drugs, or anticoagulants also increase the risk of bleeding and thus

TABLE 130–14. Minor Indicators of Poor Nutritional Status in Older Americans

Concurrent syndrome	Alcoholism Cognitive impairment Chronic renal insufficiency Multiple concurrent medications Malabsorption syndromes
Symptoms	Anorexia Nausea Early satiety Dysphagia Change in bowel habits Fatigue, apathy, memory loss, and new-onset falling
Physical signs	Cheilosis, angular stomatitis Glossitis Dehydration Poor dental status Poor wound healing, skin ulcerations Loss of subcutaneous fat Loss of muscular mass Fluid retention
Laboratory deficiencies and decreases	Serum albumin, transferrin, or prealbumin Folate Iron Ascorbic acid Zinc

Reprinted with permission by the Nutrition Screening Initiative, a project of the American Academy of Family Physicians, the American Dietetic Association, and the National Council on the Aging, Inc., and funded in part by a grant from Ross Products Division, Abbott Laboratories. (Ref. 72.)

iron loss. Folic acid deficiency may be due to low dietary intake, malabsorption, or altered folate metabolism as seen with alcoholism.[81] Common causes of vitamin B_{12} deficiency in the elderly are decreased absorption secondary to atrophic gastritis or ileal resection. Megaloblastic anemia is characteristic of vitamin B_{12} deficiency.

IMMUNOLOGIC MARKERS

Immune status indicators are affected similarly by age and malnutrition. It is thus difficult to separate the effects of nutrition on the immune system from the normal effects of aging. Quantitative assessments of cell-mediated immunity include skin testing or delayed cutaneous hypersensitivity (see Chap. 126). The incidence of anergy does increase with age, but anergy due to malnutrition can be reversed in the elderly with nutritional repletion. These markers are generally not used in routine monitoring but serve as additional indicators of nutrition status.

METABOLIC REQUIREMENTS

ENERGY

Age, gender, stature, physical activity, health status, and environment all influence individual nutrient and energy requirements. There is a decrease in basal metabolic rate with a decline in LBM and less physical activity. Therefore, total caloric requirements may be reduced in the elderly. Basal energy expenditure (BEE) can be estimated from the Harris–Benedict equations, which use weight, height, and age in gender-specific equations. These equations were developed over 75 years ago and their application in clinical settings has been questioned.[82] Therefore, other equations, have been developed for individuals over age 60:

$$\text{Men: BEE (kcal/d)} = 8.8W + 1128H - 1071$$
$$\text{Women: BEE (kcal/d)} = 9.2W + 637H - 302$$

where W is actual weight in kilograms and H is the height in meters.[82] Increases in energy requirements above the BEE are estimated to be 1.2 to 1.5 times the calculated BEE in active healthy elderly.[83]

The utility of the RDAs to accurately reflect the requirements of the elderly is controversial.[84] The controversy arises because the RDA categories are based on age and gender. The uppermost age category is "51 years and older," and thus there is no differentiation between a 51-year-old and a 90-year-old. The RDAs state that both males and females over 51 years of age require 30 kcal/kg body weight.[22] The RDAs should be viewed as a guideline with modifications employed based on disease state and activity level of the individual.[22]

PROTEIN

Unlike energy requirements, protein requirements do not decrease with age. The RDA for protein for individuals over 15 years of age is 0.8 g/kg/d.[22] However, there is some controversy as to whether this is an adequate estimation in the setting of normal renal function. Therefore, protein intake may need to be greater than the RDA to help decrease the LBM loss. It appears that 1 g protein/kg/d is appropriate in the elderly increasing up to 1.5 to 2.0 g/kg/d in states of metabolic stress such as infection, trauma, and surgery.[85] In general, protein intake should be 12% to 14% of total calories in the diet.

CARBOHYDRATE AND FAT

Carbohydrate is the major component of the American diet and should be 50% to 60% of total calories. Glucose tolerance decreases with age and simple sugars are not well tolerated; hence, complex carbohydrates (e.g., starch) should be used, whenever possible. Fiber is a form of carbohydrate that adds bulk, not calories, to the diet. With fluids and exercise, fiber aids in the normalization of bowel function. As with the younger population, dietary fat intake should be 30% of total calories to provide energy, essential fatty acids, and fat-soluble vitamins. Limiting the saturated fat to less than 10%, monounsaturated to 10% to 15%, and polyunsaturated fatty acids to 10% appears to be a prudent recommendation.[86]

FLUID

Dehydration is likely to occur with increased fluid loss secondary to a compromised urine concentrating ability, an increased insensible fluid loss via fragile skin, and a decreased thirst response. Hence, water is of importance in the elderly. Fluid requirements are estimated to be 30 mL/kg body weight/d or 1.5 to 2.0 L/d.[85]

MICRONUTRIENTS

Vitamin and mineral requirements change slightly with increasing age. Decreases in thiamine, riboflavin, and niacin needs in healthy adults correspond with the decrease in total kilocalories for both males and females 51 years and older.[22] Iron requirements for postmenopausal women also decrease. Vitamin A intake may need to be decreased to avoid toxicities in the setting of decreased renal and hepatic function, but specific requirements have not been determined. Vitamin A toxicity may present as dry skin, bone pain, cracking at the corners of the mouth, and anorexia. Vitamin D requirements increase if sunlight exposure is decreased because a large part of vitamin D is synthesized by the skin upon exposure to sunlight. Vitamin B_6 deficiency has been noted in several elderly populations, and hence intake may need to be higher than what is stated in the RDAs.[87] Finally, vitamin B_{12} requirements may need to be increased because absorption is decreased in the elderly who have atrophic gastritis, which leads to the inability to digest protein substances, which contain vitamin B_{12}.[87]

NUTRITION SUPPORT

The decision to initiate nutrition for the elderly person should be the same as for a younger individual in similar circumstances. Nutrition support in the setting of terminal disease states may require ethical decisions on whether to institute or withdraw nutrition care. In this situation, living wills and advance directives are of value in knowing the patient's attitude toward such endeavors. Once nutrition support is indicated, the route of administration (e.g., oral, enteral, or parenteral) is based on the same criteria as in the younger adult population (see Chaps. 128 and 129). However, the initiation of nutrition support in the setting of an acute illness should not be postponed. The reserve capacity of the elderly patient is less than that of a younger adult, and the older adult may not respond to the nutrition regimen as quickly. Furthermore, weight loss has been associated with increased morbidity and mortality in the elderly population.[1] In the setting of long-term care, it is essential that metabolic and nutrient requirements be met constantly and that chronic undernutrition be avoided.

ENTERAL NUTRITION AND ORAL NUTRITION SUPPLEMENTS

Enteral nutrition should be administered via the same techniques as with younger adults. Small bore nasoenteric feeding tubes should be placed for shorter lengths of therapy and gastrostomy or jejunostomy tubes may be placed when chronic therapy is indicated.[1] Complications associated with EN include agitation, extubation, and aspiration pneumonia. These do not differ significantly from the younger adult population.[88]

Selection of standard, specialty, or disease-specific products is also similar to that of the younger adult population (see Chap. 131). When choosing a standard enteral formula it is prudent to begin with a lactose-free product until lactose tolerance is determined owing to a higher incidence of lactose intolerance in the elderly. The majority of enteral products are lactose-free despite the milky appearance. Fiber is known to be physiologically helpful in maintaining stool regularity and formation. However, the optimal amount and type of daily fiber the elderly should receive remains controversial.[88] Whole protein and products containing oligopeptides have been shown to be efficacious as compared to free amino acid–based products.[88]

Often the elderly receive EN volumes that meet protein and calorie requirements but do not meet the RDAs for vitamins. In general, when micronutrient RDAs are not being met, supplemental multivitamins and minerals are recommended to avoid chronic decreased intake. Enteral feeding access also provides a means to deliver fluid to the elderly patient. Close monitoring of fluid status is important in the elderly patient because of the increased risk of dehydration.

Oral supplements when taken ad libitum have been shown to improve nutritional status in moderately malnourished nursing home residents and elderly who are dependent on home-delivered meals.[89] In general, these oral supplements are not needed in healthy individuals who are able to ingest and absorb nourishing meals.

PARENTERAL NUTRITION

The decision to implement a parenteral nutrition regimen either via peripheral or central venous access is the same as with younger adults (see Chap. 128). However, peripheral access may be less of an option in the elderly owing to the limited availability of accessible veins. PN formulations need to be designed to meet an individual's metabolic, nutrient, and fluid requirements.

Substrate tolerance (carbohydrate, fat/lipid, and protein) differs in the elderly patient as compared to younger adults. With dextrose infusion, hyperglycemia is more likely to occur, especially in patients with a prior diagnosis of diabetes. Therefore, it is prudent to closely monitor blood glucose concentrations and advance the dextrose concentration in the PN solution as tolerated.[1] The elderly are more susceptible to hypertriglyceridemia following lipid infusion. Hence, a serum triglyceride concentration should be obtained prior to the initiation of lipid therapy and rechecked as needed to verify lipid tolerance.[90] Protein tolerance is dependent on organ (hepatic and renal) function as in the younger adult population. In the setting of renal insufficiency, excessive protein intake accelerates azotemia, and hence, blood nitrogen concentration monitoring is required.[90]

▶ PRINCIPLES OF PHARMACOTHERAPY

- Adequate nutrition is essential for a child's normal growth and development and the maintenance of health in the elderly.
- Nutrition assessment should be incorporated into each pediatric and geriatric patient care encounter.
- Nutrition assessment should include determination of nutrition needs and adequacy of current nutrition regimen.
- Numerous enteral formulas are marketed for children, and selection should be based on age, clinical condition, gastrointestinal function, and cost.
- Parenteral nutrition should be reserved for those who do not tolerate enteral nutrition or in whom enteral nutrition is inadequate to meet nutrition needs.
- Established guidelines should be followed to ascertain when to initiate and advance enteral and parenteral nutrition solutions to avoid complications.
- Patients of all ages receiving either enteral or parenteral nutrition should be routinely monitored to ensure appropriate outcomes.

REFERENCES

1. American Society for Parenteral and Enteral Nutrition, Board of Directors. Guidelines for the use of parenteral and enteral nutrition in adult and pediatric patients. JPEN J Parenter Enteral Nutr 1993; 17(suppl):1SA–52SA.
2. American Society for Parenteral and Enteral Nutrition. Standards for nutrition support: Hospitalized pediatric patients. Nutr Clin Prac 1989;4:33–37.

3. Harris J, Benedict F. A biometric study of basal metabolism in man. Washington, DC, Carnegie Institute of Washington, publication no 279, 1919.
4. World Health Organization. Energy and protein requirements: Report of a joint FAO/WHO/UNU expert consultation. Geneva, World Health Organization, WHO technical report series, no 724, 1985.
5. Schofield C. Predicting basal metabolic rate, new standards and review of previous work. Hum Nutr Clin Nutr 1985;39c(suppl 1):5–42.
6. Caldwell MO, Kennedy CC. Normal nutritional requirements. Surg Clin North Am 1981;61:491–498.
7. Firouzbakhsh S, Mathis RK, Dorchester WL, et al. Measured resting energy expenditure in children. J Pediatr Gastroenterol Nutr 1993;16: 136–142.
8. Thomson MA, Bucolo S, Quirk P, Shepherd RW. Measured versus predicted resting expenditure in infants: A need for reappraisal. J Pediatr 1995;126:21–27.
9. Chwals WJ, Lally KP, Woolley MM, Mahour GH. Measured energy expenditure in critically ill infants and young children. J Surg Res 1988;44:467–472.
10. Marks KH, Maisels MJ, Moore E, et al. Head growth in sick premature infants: A longitudinal study. J Pediatr 1979;94:282–285.
11. Dimand RJ. Parenteral nutrition in the critically ill infant and child. In: Baker RD, Baker SS, Davis AM, eds. Pediatric Parenteral Nutrition. New York: Chapman & Hall, 1997:273–300.
12. Kien CL. Carbohydrates. In: Tsang RC, Lucas A, Uauy R, Zlotkin S, eds. Nutritional Needs of the Preterm Infant: Scientific Basis and Practical Guidelines. Baltimore, Williams & Wilkins, 1993: 47–64.
13. Wu PYK, Edwards NB, Storm MC. The plasma amino acid pattern of normal term breast-fed infants. J Pediatr 1986;109:347–349.
14. Hamil PVV, Drizd TA, Johnson CL, et al. Physical growth: National Center for Health Statistics percentages. Am J Clin Nutr 1979;32: 607–629.
15. Shaffer SG, Quimoro CL, Anderson JV, Hall RT. Postnatal weight changes in low birth weight infants. Pediatrics 1987;79:702–705.
16. Lair CS, Kennedy KA. Monitoring postnatal growth in the neonatal intensive care unit. Nutr Clin Prac 1997;12:124–129.
17. Cronk C, Crocker AC, Pueschel SM, et al. Growth charts for children with Down syndrome: 1 month to 18 years of age. Pediatrics 1988; 81:102–110.
18. Reimers KJ, Carlson SJ, Lombard KA. Nutritional management of infants with bronchopulmonary dysplasia. Nutr Clin Prac 1992;7: 127–132.
19. Klish WJ. Nutritional assessment. In: Wyllie R, Hyams JS, eds. Pediatric Gastrointestinal Disease: Pathophysiology, Diagnosis, Management. Philadelphia, W.B. Saunders, 1993:1090–1109.
20. Wright JA, Ashenburg CA, Whitaker RC. Comparison of methods to categorize undernutrition in children. J Pediatr 1994;124:944–946.
21. Lopez AM, Wolfsdorf J, Raszynski A, Contijoch-Serrano V. Estimation of nitrogen balance based on a six-hour urine collection in infants. JPEN J Parenter Enteral Nutr 1986;10:517–518.
22. Food and Nutrition Board. Recommended Dietary Allowances, 10th ed. Washington, DC; National Academy Press, 1989.
23. Weise K, Zaritsky A. Endocrine manifestations of critical illness in the child. Pediatr Clin North Am 1987;34:119–130.
24. Pollack MM. Nutritional support of children in the intensive care unit. In: Suskind RM, Lewinter-Suskind L, eds. Textbook of Pediatric Nutrition, 2nd ed. New York; Raven Press, 1993:207–216.
25. Hildreth MA, Herndon DN, Desai MH, Broemeling LD. Current treatment reduces calories required to maintain weight in pediatric patients with burns. J Burn Care Rehabil 1990;11:405–409.
26. Mayes T, Gottschlich MM, Khoury J, Warren GD. Evaluation of predicted and measured energy requirements in burn children. J Am Diet Assoc 1996;96:24–29.
27. Zemel BS, Stallings VA. Energy requirements and nutritional assessment in developmental disabilities. In: Walker WA, Watkins, JB, eds. Nutrition in Pediatrics: Basic Science and Clinical Applications. Hamilton, Ontario: B.C. Decker, 1997:169–177.
28. Krick J, Murphy PE, Markham JFB, Shapiro BK. A proposed formula for calculating energy needs of children with cerebral palsy. Dev Med Child Neurol 1992;34:481–497.
29. Udall JN. Malnutrition and re-feeding. In: Baker SB, Baker RD, Davis A, eds. Pediatric Enteral Nutrition. New York: Chapman & Hall, 1994:205–216.
30. Ellerstein NS, Ostrov BE. Growth patterns in children hospitalized because of caloric-deprivation failure to thrive. Am J Dis Child 1985;139:164–166.
31. American Academy of Pediatrics, Committee on Nutrition. Statement on cholesterol. Pediatrics 1992;90:469–473.
32. Foote KD, MacKinnon MJ, Innis SM. Effect of early introduction of formula versus fat free parenteral nutrition on essential fatty acid status of preterm infants. Am J Clin Nutr 1991;54:93–97.
33. Mandt JM, Teasley-Strausburg KM, Shronts EP. II. Nutritional requirements. In: Teasley-Strausburg KM, ed. Nutrition Support Handbook: A Compendium of Products with Guidelines for Usage. Cincinnati, OH; Harvey Whitney Books, 1992:19–36.
34. Swinford RD, Elenberg E, Ingelfinger JR. Persistent renal disease. In: Walker WA, Watkins JB, eds. Nutrition in Pediatrics: Basic Science and Clinical Applications. Hamilton, Ontario: B.C. Decker, 1997:493–515.
35. Ramsey BW, Farrell PM, Pencharz P, Consensus Committee. Nutritional assessment and management in cystic fibrosis: A consensus report. Am J Clin Nutr 1992;55:108–116.
36. Kaufman SS, Murray ND, Wood RP, et al. Nutritional support for the infant with extrahepatic biliary atresia. J Pediatr 1987;110:679–686.
37. Pereira GR. Nutritional care of the extremely premature infant. Clin Perinatol 1995;22:61–75.
38. Briggs GG, Freeman RK, Yaffe SJ. A Reference Guide to Fetal and Neonatal Risk: Drugs in Pregnancy and Lactation, 4th ed. Baltimore, Williams & Wilkins, 1994.
39. American Academy of Pediatrics, Committee on Nutrition. Iron-fortified infants formulas. Pediatrics 1989;84:1114–1115.
40. American Academy of Pediatrics, Committee on Nutrition. The use of whole cow's milk in infancy. Pediatrics 1992;89:1105–1109.
41. Davis A, Baker S. The use of modular nutrients in pediatrics. JPEN J Parenter Enteral Nutr 1996;20:228–236.
42. Fuchs GJ III. Enteral support of the hospitalized child. In: Suskind RM, Lewinter-Suskind L, eds. Textbook of Pediatric Nutrition, 2nd ed. New York: Raven Press, 1993:239–246.
43. Thureen PJ, Hay WW Jr. Conditions requiring special nutritional management. In: Tsang RC, Lucas A, Uauy R, Zlotkin S, eds. Nutritional Needs of the Preterm Infant: Scientific Basis and Practical Guidelines. Baltimore, Williams & Wilkins, 1993:243–265.
44. Davis A. Indications and techniques for enteral feeds. In: Baker SB, Baker RD, Davis A, eds. Pediatric Enteral Nutrition. New York, Chapman & Hall, 1994:67–94.
45. Teasley-Strausburg KM. Parenteral nutrition. II. Carbohydrate solutions. In: Teasley-Strausburg KM, ed. Nutrition Support Handbook: A Compendium of Products with Guidelines for Usage. Cincinnati, OH: Harvey Whitney Books, 1992:73–79.
46. American Academy of Pediatrics, Committee on Nutrition. Nutritional needs of preterm infants. In: Barness LA, ed. Pediatric Nutrition Handbook, 3rd ed. Elk Grove Village, IL, American Academy of Pediatrics, 1993.
47. Heird WC, Dell RB, Helms RA, et al. Amino acid mixture designed to maintain normal plasma amino acid patterns in infants and children requiring parenteral nutrition. Pediatrics 1987;80:401–408.
48. Helms RA, Christensen ML, Mauer EC, Storm MC. Comparison of a pediatric versus standard amino acid formulation in preterm neonates requiring parenteral nutrition. J Pediatr 1987;110:466–470.
49. Smith R, Sacha DS, Plattsmier J, et al. Plasma carnitine alterations in premature infants receiving various nutritional regimens. JPEN J Parenter Enteral Nutr 1988;12:37–42.
50. Greene HL, Tibboel D, Delemarre FMC, et al. Carnitine deficiency in surgical neonates receiving total parenteral nutrition. J Pediatr Surg 1990;25:418–421.

51. Helms RA, Mauer EC, Hay WW. Effect of intravenous L-carnitine on growth parameters and fat metabolism during parenteral nutrition in neonates. JPEN J Parenter Enteral Nutr 1990;14:448–453.
52. Breningstall GN. Carnitine deficiency syndromes. Pediatr Neurol 1990;6:75–81.
53. Phelps SJ, Cochran EB. Effect of the continuous administration of fat emulsion on the infiltration of intravenous lines in infants receiving peripheral parenteral nutrition solutions. JPEN J Parenter Enteral Nutr 1989;13:628–632.
54. Committee on Nutrition, American Academy of Pediatrics. Use of intravenous fat emulsions in pediatric patients. Pediatrics 1981;68: 738–743.
55. Brans YW, Dutton EB, Andrew DS, et al. Fat emulsion tolerance in very low birth weight neonates: Effect on diffusion of oxygen in the lungs and on blood pH. Pediatrics 1986;78:79–84.
56. Gutcher GR, Farrell PM. Intravenous infusion of lipid for the prevention of essential fatty acid deficiency in premature infants. Am J Clin Nutr 1991;54:1024–1028.
57. Innis SM. Fat. In: Tsang RC, Lucas A, Uauy R, Zlotkin S, eds. Nutritional Needs of the Preterm Infant: Scientific Basis and Practical Guidelines. Baltimore, Williams & Wilkins, 1993:65–86.
58. Greene HL, Hambidge KM, Schanler R, Tsang RC. Guidelines for the use of vitamins, trace elements, calcium, magnesium, and phosphorus in infants and children receiving total parenteral nutrition: report of the Subcommittee on Pediatric Parenteral Nutrient Requirements from the Committee on Clinical Practice Issues of the American Society for Clinical Nutrition. Am J Clin Nutr 1988;48: 1324–1342.
59. Center for Disease Control and Prevention. Lactic acidosis is traced in thiamine deficiency related to nationwide shortage of multivitamins for total parenteral nutrition—United States, 1997. MMWR 1997;46:523–528.
60. Zlotkin SH, Atkinson S, Lockitch G. Trace elements in nutrition for premature infants. Clin Perinatol 1995;22:223–240.
61. Lockitch G, Jacobson B, Quigley G, et al. Selenium deficiency in low birth weight neonates: An unrecognized problem. J Pediatr 1989;114:865–870.
62. Heird WC, Gomez MR. Parenteral nutrition. In: Tsang RC, Lucas A, Uauy R, Zlotkin S, eds. Nutritional Needs of the Preterm Infant: Scientific Basis and Practical Guidelines. Baltimore, Williams & Wilkins, 1993:225–242.
63. Moukarzel AA, Buchman AL, Salas JS, et al. Iodine supplementation in children receiving long-term parenteral nutrition. J Pediatr 1992; 121:252–254.
64. Solomons NW, Ruz M. Essential and beneficial trace elements in pediatric parenteral nutrition. In: Baker RD, Baker SS, Davis AM, eds. Pediatric Parenteral Nutrition. New York: Chapman & Hall, 1997: 175–196.
65. Kumpf VJ. Parenteral iron supplementation. Nutr Clin Prac 1996; 11:139–146.
66. Collier S, Crouch J, Hendricks K, Caballero B. Use of cyclic parenteral nutrition in infants less than 6 months of age. Nutr Clin Prac 1994;9:65–68.
67. Dwyer JT. Screening older Americans' nutritional health: Current practices and future possibilities. Washington, DC, Nutrition Screening Initiative, 1991.
68. Kuczmarski RJ. Need for body composition information in elderly subjects. Am J Clin Nutr 1989;50:1150–1157.
69. Forbes GB. Body composition: Influence of nutrition, disease, growth and aging. In: Shils ME, Olson JA, Shike M, eds. Modern Nutrition in Health and Disease, 8th ed. Philadelphia, Lea & Febiger, 1994:781–801.
70. Johnston CC, Slemenda CW. Changes in skeletal tissue during the aging process. Nutr Rev 1992;50:385–387.
71. Chernoff R. Physiologic aging and nutritional status. Nutr Clin Prac 1990;5:8–13.
72. Posner BM, Jette AM, Smith KW, Miller DR. Nutrition and health risks in the elderly: The Nutrition Screening Initiative. Am J Public Health 1993;83:972–978.
73. Volkert D, Kruse W, Oster P, Schlierf G. Malnutrition in geriatric patients: Diagnostic and prognostic significance of nutritional parameters. Ann Nutr Metab 1992;36:97–112.
74. Frisancho AR. New standards of weight and body composition by frame size and height for assessment of nutritional status of adults and the elderly. Am J Clin Nutr 1984;40:808–819.
75. Chumlea WC, Steinbaugh ML, Roche AF, et al. Nutritional anthropometric assessment in elderly persons 65 to 90 years of age. J Nutr Elderly 1985;4:39–51.
76. Chumlea WC, Roche AF, Mukherjee D. Nutritional assessment of the elderly through anthropometry. Columbus, OH, Ross Laboratories, 1987.
77. Roe DA. Drugs and nutrition in the elderly. In: Roe DA, ed. Geriatric Nutrition, 3rd ed. Englewood Cliffs, NJ, Prentice-Hall, 1992: 182–207.
78. Morrow FD. Assessment of nutritional status in the elderly: Application and interpretation of nutritional biochemistries. Clin Nutr 1986; 5:112–120.
79. Corti MC, Guralnik JM, Salive ME, Sorkin JD. Serum albumin level and physical disability as predictors of mortality in older persons. JAMA 1994;272:1036–1042.
80. Kergoat MJ, Leclerc BS, PetitClerc C, Imbach A. Discriminant biochemical markers for evaluating the nutritional status of elderly patients in long-term care. Am J Clin Nutr 1987;46:849–861.
81. Lipschitz DA. Impact of nutrition on the age-related declines in hematopoiesis. In: Chernoff R, ed. Geriatric Nutrition. Gaithersburg, MD, Aspen Publishers, 1991:271–287.
82. Makk LJK, McClave SA, Creech PW, et al. Clinical application of the metabolic cart to the delivery of total parenteral nutrition. Crit Care Med 1990;18:1320–1327.
83. Young VR. Macronutrient needs in the elderly. Nutr Rev 1992;50: 454–462.
84. Blumberg JB. Changing nutrient requirements in older adults. Nutrition Today 1992;Sept/Oct:15–20.
85. Carter WJ. Macronutrient requirements for elderly persons. In: Chernoff R, ed. Geriatric Nutrition. Gaithersburg, MD, Aspen Publishers, 1991:11–24.
86. Ausman LM, Russell RM. Nutrition in the elderly. In: Shils ME, Olson JA, Shike M, eds. Modern Nutrition in Health and Disease, 8th ed. Philadelphia, Lea & Febiger, 1994:770–780.
87. Russell RM. Micronutrient requirements of the elderly. Nutr Rev 1992;50:463–464.
88. Karkeck JM. Nutrition support for the elderly. Nutr Clin Prac 1993;8:211–219.
89. Gallagher-Allred CR, Voss AC, Finn SC, McCamish MA. Malnutrition and clinical outcomes: The case for medical nutrition therapy. J Am Diet Assoc 1996;96:361–367.
90. Mason JB, Russell RM. Parenteral nutrition in the elderly. In: Rombeau JL, Caldwell MD, eds. Clinical Nutrition: Parenteral Nutrition, 2nd ed. Philadelphia, W.B. Saunders, 1993:737–747.

131
Nutritional Considerations in Major Organ Failure

Renee M. DeHart, PharmD, and Rex O. Brown, PharmD

Because organ failure may alter absorption, use, and excretion of nutrients, administration of "standard" nutrients to patients with organ dysfunction may be inappropriate. Individualization of a nutritional regimen for these patients often requires a planned, disease-specific approach. Different laboratory tests or more frequent monitoring of traditional markers may be necessary to ensure that the desired therapeutic goals are achieved. For example, it is impossible to collect a 24-hour urine specimen to measure urea nitrogen and nitrogen balance in an anuric patient. In this situation, an alternative method of calculating urea nitrogen appearance is required.

Patients with acute organ failure requiring nutrition support are often hospitalized in intensive care units. With advances in treating chronic organ failure, increasing numbers of older, chronically ill patients will require nutrition support on a long-term basis. It will therefore become increasingly common for nutrition support to be provided in community and ambulatory settings. Regardless of the setting, the clinician needs a firm pathophysiologic foundation upon which to build a pharmaceutical care plan to assure appropriate outcomes for patients requiring nutrition support.

In this chapter, nutritional needs of patients with acute and chronic renal, hepatic, pulmonary, and gastrointestinal failure are presented. The predominant approaches to ensure delivery of safe and efficacious nutrients to patients with these disorders are critically reviewed.

RENAL FAILURE

Patients with end-stage renal disease (ESRD) and concurrent malnutrition have an increased risk of morbidity and mortality.[1,2] The adequacy of dialysis and the serum albumin concentration are strong predictors of mortality in hemodialysis and peritoneal dialysis (PD) patients.[1–6] Energy expenditure in these patients appears to be similar to normal subjects.[7] Unfortunately, intake of nutrients is often markedly decreased (66% and 50% of recommended protein and energy intake).[8] The provision of appropriate nutrition is especially challenging in patients with oliguric or anuric renal failure due to the fluid intake limitations. Major differences exist between the metabolic, fluid, and electrolyte management of patients with acute versus chronic renal failure. For example, positive nitrogen is more difficult to achieve in patients with acute renal failure due to the increased rate of protein catabolism. Additionally, patients with acute renal failure are more likely to develop hyperglycemia during nutritional support and are frequently dialyzed by modalities that are not commonly used in the ESRD patient. Because of these differences, the nutritional management of acute and chronic renal failure are discussed separately.[9,10]

ACUTE RENAL FAILURE

Epidemiology

Acute renal failure (ARF) occurs in approximately 5% of all hospitalized patients. The mortality rate of ARF patients who require renal replacement therapy ranges from 40% to as high as 80%.[11] Unfortunately, this rate has not significantly changed over the last 20 years.[12] This may be due in part to a reduction in the number of patients with uncomplicated ARF, as well as an increase in the incidence of multiple organ system failure (MOSF). The two main advances made in the treatment of ARF patients during the last 20 years are the introduction of continuous renal replacement therapies (CRRT) (see Chap. 41) and advances in the provision of nutritional support.[12]

Pathophysiology

ENERGY REQUIREMENTS

Patients with ARF typically require 30 to 35 kcal/kg/d.[12] Energy requirements in this patient population should ideally be measured by indirect calorimetry (see Chap. 126).[13] Energy expenditures of ARF patients are highly variable. In one study of mechanically ventilated acute renal failure patients, measured energy expenditure ranged from 70% to 170% of predicted resting energy expenditure.[14]

CARBOHYDRATE

Hyperglycemia and peripheral insulin resistance are common in ARF. These patients usually have a superimposed illness that may cause glucose intolerance. The etiology of glucose intolerance in ARF is thought to be due to increased levels of glucagon, growth hormone, and catecholamines, all known antagonists of insulin.[15] Other proposed mechanisms include an elevated glucagon-to-insulin ratio secondary to impaired degradation of these hormones and elevated secretion of inflammatory cytokines.

Intolerance to intravenous lipid emulsion (IVLE), evidenced by increased serum triglyceride concentration, is common in ARF. Hypertriglyceridemia is thought to be caused by decreased catabolism of triglycerides and increased synthesis from free fatty acids (FFAs).[16] Hepatic triglyceride lipase and peripheral lipoprotein lipase activity may be significantly reduced in ARF patients.[17] Insulin resistance and metabolic acidosis may contribute to this process by inhibiting lipoprotein lipase.[18] Triglyceride concentrations should therefore be measured before administering IVLE to patients with ARF. FFA concentrations are also elevated in ARF. This aberration, however, is not appreciated by measurement of the triglyceride concentration.

PROTEIN

Urea, the end product of nitrogen metabolism, accumulates rapidly in ARF. Most patients with ARF have a primary stressful illness that results in ureagenesis, and thus the protein catabolic rate (PCR) is markedly increased.[9,11] PCRs of 1.4 to 1.8 g/kg/day are frequently reported.[19–21] This increase in PCR may be the result of stimulation by interleukins, tumor necrosis factor, and circulating proteolytic enzymes.[22] This stimulation may affect protein metabolism both directly (via modulation of protein synthesis) and indirectly (by inhibiting the action of anabolic hormones).[23] In addition to this increased catabolism of proteins, significant amounts of protein and amino acids are removed by dialysis. Amino acid losses of 5.2 g per conventional hemodialysis (HD), 7.3 g per high-flux HD, and 13 to 16 g/d during continuous arteriovenous hemodialysis (CAVHD) or continuous venovenous hemodialysis (CVVHD) have been reported.[24,25] The clearance of some amino acids are enhanced (histidine and tryptophan), while the clearance of phenylalanine and valine were reduced in nondialyzed patients with ARF.[26]

FLUID, ELECTROLYTES, AND ACID–BASE DISORDERS

The volume status of patients with ARF is primarily dependent on residual urine output and the type of dialysis received, if any. The patient with oliguric ARF will have impaired excretion of sodium and water. In nonoliguric ARF, considerable sodium may be lost in the urine, necessitating replacement to maintain sodium balance. This also applies to the patient who is losing considerable gastric fluids. Patients on CRRT will lose sodium via hemofiltration or dialysis and should be given sodium as part of their CRRT replacement fluid regimen.

Hyperkalmeia is frequently observed in ARF secondary to protein catabolism and intracellular potassium release. Hyperkalemia also results from the impaired secretion and excretion of potassium by the kidney, and the endogenous release secondary to tissue breakdown. If this is severe, emergent dialysis may be indicated.

Because phosphorous is excreted renally, hyperphosphatemia is common in ARF. Like potassium, large amounts of phosphorous are released into the circulation secondary to tissue breakdown during ARF. Control of hyperphosphatemia is important because as the calcium–phosphorous product (serum calcium in mg/dL multiplied by serum phosphorous in mg/dL) exceeds 70, the risk of developing metastatic calcification increases.[27]

Hypermagnesemia is common in ARF secondary to impaired excretion and endogenous release from tissue breakdown. Serum magnesium concentrations do not decrease as quickly as potassium concentrations in patients receiving electrolyte-free nutrition regimens.

Patients with ARF usually have metabolic acidosis because of impaired excretion of organic acids. If potassium and sodium are needed in the parenteral nutrition (PN) regimen, they should be added as acetate salts, which will be converted to bicarbonate in the liver. This increase in bicarbonate will partially compensate their metabolic acidosis. Dialytic therapies may also help improve the metabolic acidosis accompanying ARF by increasing the removal of these endogenously generated acids.

TRACE ELEMENTS

The requirements for trace elements during nutrition support of ARF are not well established because trace element accumulation or losses during ARF have not been rigorously characterized. Zinc and chromium are excreted by the kidney and theoretically can accumulate due to reduced excretion and increased intake secondary to impurities in dialysate or intravenous fluids. This has been documented with chromium in patients on chronic dialysis.[28] Trace elements such as rubidium can be removed by dialysis if concentrations in the dialysate are adequately low; the clinical significance of this is unknown.[29] Some clinicians advocate elimination of trace elements from the PN formula of patients with ARF. However, because manganese and copper are excreted in bile, and zinc and copper are removed by PD and HD,[30] patients with ARF receiving PN should receive trace element supplementation.[31]

VITAMINS

Little information is available concerning vitamin requirements in ARF. Traditional HD clears several water-soluble vitamins such as folic acid, vitamin C, and pyridoxine, but not the highly protein-bound vitamins A, D, and B_{12}.[30,32] The clinical significance of these findings in ARF is unknown. Currently, it seems prudent to administer vitamins as recommended by the NAG-AMA for patients receiving PN (see Chap. 128). If the enteral route is used for nutritional support, vitamin adminstration to meet the recommended daily allowances (RDAs) is reasonable.

▶ TREATMENT: Acute Renal Failure

ADMINISTRATION ROUTES

Most patients with ARF have a superimposed illness that requires nutritional support by the parenteral route. Enteral nutrition (EN) should be considered when patients with ARF have functional gastrointestinal tracts. The products frequently used during EN in ARF are the calorically dense, electrolyte-free or electrolyte-reduced formulas (Table 131–1). These formulas are useful in patients with fluid overload, hyperkalemia, and hyperphosphatemia. Unfortunately, EN is impossible for many patients with ARF because they are critically ill and have an ileus.

SPECIALTY PRODUCTS

Improved survival and return of renal function were observed in the 1970s when essential amino acids (EAAs) plus glucose were compared with glucose alone in patients with ARF.[33] This lead to the marketing of parenteral amino acids containing predominantly or soley EAAs (NephrAmine, RenAmin, Aminosyn-RF, and Aminess). These products were formulated on the hypothesis that significant nitrogen reuse ("urea recycling") occurs during ARF to synthesize nonessential amino acids. Subsequently, several prospective, double-blinded studies indicate no significant reduction in mortality when the EAA formulations are used.[33] Thus urea recycling in the presence of uremia has been disproven. Based on the available data, it appears appropriate to use standard mixed amino acids rather than EAA solutions in ARF. An example of an initial PN solution to be used in ARF appears in Table 131–2.

DESIGN AND INITIATION OF NUTRITIONAL REGIMEN

Patients with ARF typically require 30 to 35 kcal/kg/d. In the absence of dialysis, the nutritional formula should be concentrated in a small volume and contain minimal sodium. In the oliguric patient receiving PD or HD, these restrictions may be lessened, but the formula will generally need to be concentrated (final dextrose concentration ≥ 30%). When using these high dextrose concentration formulas, careful monitoring of glucose homeostasis by glucose fingersticks every 6 hours is important because of the predisposition toward hyperglycemia in ARF. Additionally, CRRT, which is increasingly popular in the treatment of ARF (see Chap. 41), contributes significant calories to a nutritional regimen. This is a direct result of the absorption of glucose from the dextrose-containing fluids frequently used as the dialystate or ultrafiltrate replacement fluids during CRRT. During continuous arteriovenous hemofiltration (CAVH), a net uptake of up to 300 g/d was reported when a 1.5% peritoneal dialysis fluid or 5% dextrose in saline was used as the ultrafiltrate replacement fluid at a mean rate of 1.39 L/h.[34,35] Other studies of CAVHD with dextrose-containing dialysates and blood flow rates of 150 mL/min report glucose absorption of 35% to 45% (140 to 355 g/d).[36,37] Thus, these calories must be factored into the nutritional plan for the patient with ARF treated with these modalities.

Lipid administration during ARF is driven by serum triglyceride concentration monitoring. When the serum triglyceride level is less than 300 mg/dL, low doses of IVLE (3 to 7 kcal/kg/d over 24 hours) are recommended to prevent essential fatty acid deficiency and to provide a balanced caloric intake. IVLEs containing a combination of medium-chain triglycerides (MCTs) and long-chain triglycerides (LCTs) are available in Europe. MCTs are readily used for energy, not stored, and are carnitine independent, all attractive features for a fuel source. MCT and LCT clearance when given parenterally is reduced by more than 60% in ARF.[38] Therefore, both LCT- and MCT-containing IVLEs need to be used with caution in ARF.

An even or positive nitrogen balance is desired but is difficult to achieve in patients with ARF. In one study, the nitrogen balance deficit was reduced from 8 to about 3 g/d when patients were provided 1.5 to 1.74 g/kg/d of amino acids versus 0.7 g/kg/d.[39] In another study of critically ill patients with ARF on CAVHD or CVVHD, a negative mean nitrogen balance of 1.92 g/d was recorded, despite provision of 2.5 g/kg/d of protein.[40]

The question therefore arises of how much protein a patient with ARF requires. Although individual patient assessment of PCR and dialytic losses is necessary, it is not uncommon for patients to require 1.5 to 2.5 g/kg/d of protein or more to approach nitrogen balance. Patients not receiving dialysis who have a low urea nitrogen appearance (UNA) rate (less than 5 g/d) may be appropriately managed with a nutrition regimen low in protein (20 to 30 g/d or 0.6 g/kg/d) to minimize urea nitrogen appearnace from exogenous protein.[9] This plan should be used for short periods only, while the evaluation for dialysis is pursued. For patients with moderate UNA rates (5 to 10 g/d), more liberal amounts of protein should be provided (0.8 to 1.2 g/kg/d).[9] If dialysis therapy is instituted, protein intake should be liberalized: 1 to 1.2 g/kg/d for HD patients, and 1.2 to 1.5 g/kg/d for PD patients. CRRTs remove large quantities of extracellular fluid and thereby allow infusion of the required substrates in a normal volume. Patients with ARF treated with CRRT should be provided with up to 2.5

TABLE 131–1. Enteral Nutrition Products for Patients with Chronic Renal Failure or ESRD

Product	Form	Flavors[a]	Caloric Density (kcal/mL)	Protein (g/L)	Electrolytes
AminAid (R & D Laboratories)	Powder	O,S,B	2.0	19	None
Renalcal (Nestlé Clinical Nutrition)	Liquid	C,SB,A	2.0	34.5	Low
Suplena (Ross Laboratories)	Liquid	V	2.0	30	Low
Magnacal Renal (Mead Johnson Nutritional)	Liquid	V	2.0	70	Low
Nepro (Ross Laboratories)	Liquid	V,Ch,BP	2.0	70	Low
Deliver 2.0 (Mead Johnson Nutritional)	Liquid	V	2.0	75	Low
Nutren 2.0 (Nestlé Clinical Nutrition)	Liquid	V	2.0	80	Normal
NuBasics 2.0 (Nestlé Clinical Nutrition)	Liquid	V	2.0	80	Normal
TwoCal HN (Ross Laboratories)	Liquid	V,BP	2.0	84	Normal

[a]O = Orange; S = strawberry; B = berry; C = citrus; SB = strawberry–banana; A = apricot; V = vanilla; Ch = cherry; BP = butter pecan.

TABLE 131–2. Examples of Initial Parenteral Nutrition Formulas for Patients with Organ Failure

	Acute Renal Failure	Chronic Renal Failure	Hepatic Failure	Hepatic Transplant	Pulmonary Failure	Short Bowel
Dextrose (%)[a]	40	30	25	15	20	20
CAAs (%)	Variable	4	5[b]	5	5	5
Lipids (%)	1	2	2	2	3	2
0.45 NaCl (L/d)	—	—	—	—	—	0.5–2
NaCl (mEq/L)	0	0	0	0	0	80[c]
Na acetate (mEq/L)	0	30	0	0	0	0
Na phosphate (mEq/L)	0[d]	7.5	15	15	30	7.5
K acetate (mEq/L)	0[d]	0	50	0	20	60
K chloride (mEq/L)	0	10	0	40	20	0
Ca gluconate (mEq/L)	5	5	5	10	5	10
Magnesium sulfate (mEq/L)	0	6	16	20	5	10
Multivitamins (mL/d)	10	10	10	10	10	10
Zinc (mg/d)	3	3–6	8	3–6	3	10
Copper (mg/d)	1.2	1.2	<1.2	1.2	1.2	1.2
Manganese (µg/d)	300	300	<300	300	300	≤300
Chronium (µg/d)	12	12	<12	12	12	20
Selenium (µg/d)	—	40	40	40	40	60

[a]Final concentrations after admixture.
[b]Hepatamine 4% when criteria for use are met.
[c]Does not include 0.45% sodium chloride injection or lipid.
[d]The continuous renal replacement therapies frequently require variable additions of potassium and phosphate salts.

g/kg/d of protein (as indicated by UNA plus nonurinary urea losses) as their blood chemistries tolerate. Although this can be done safely while providing a greater percentage of patients with a positive nitrogen balance,[40] the clinical value of this practice has been questioned.[41]

Several electrolytes (phosphorous, magnesium, and potassium) warrant special attention when designing the initial nutritional regimen/formula for the ARF patient. During early ARF, PN solutions should not contain potassium unless the patient is hypokalemic. After several days, the serum potassium concentrations tend to decrease, often necessitating cautious addition of potassium to the PN solution. If the enteral route is used, formulas with minimal potassium may be needed. Serum potassium concentrations may decrease more rapidly in patients receiving the continuous dialysis therapies. Potassium losses in CVVHD and CAVHD are proportional to the potassium gradient between blood and dialysate. Potassium losses up to 129 mEq/d were noted when no potassium was added to the dialysate. However, when dialysate potassium concentrations were 3 to 5 mEq/L, the losses were only 57 mEq/day.[37] Therefore, cautious additions of potassium may be considered earlier in the course of ARF for those patients treated by CAVHD or CVVHD. Serum magnesium concentrations do not decrease as quickly as potassium concentrations in patients receiving electrolyte-free nutrition regimens. As serum concentrations decrease toward normal and/or renal function returns, magnesium should be added to the parenteral solution in small amounts (4 to 6 mEq/L). An empiric PN formula for the patient with ARF is highlighted in Table 131–2.

Phosphorous can be omitted from the nutritional formula of patients receiving PN until the phosphorous level approaches normal (less than 5.0 mg/dL). It is prudent to monitor phosphorous concentrations daily and to add phosphorous in small doses once the serum concentration is below 4.0 mg/dL. Failure to do so can lead to severe hypophosphatemia, despite continued renal failure. Patients with persistently high serum phosphorous levels who have a functional gastrointestinal tract can be prescribed phosphate-binding antacid therapy (see Chap. 42) and enteral feedings low in phosphorous to minimize the absorption of exogenous phosphorous.

EVALUATION OF THERAPEUTIC OUTCOMES

Acute renal failure, despite recent advances in treatment, is still associated with a 40% to 80% mortality rate.[11] The evaluation tools used in monitoring ARF patients are similar to other patients receiving PN and EN (see Chaps. 128 and 129). However, there is no clear consensus on the benefit of nutritional supplementation on the outcome parameters of renal recovery or mortality. Some advocate protein malnutrition as a predictor of outcome in patients with multiple organ dysfunction syndrome,[12] while others have not shown a survival benefit from aggressive nutritional support.[40] A recent preliminary report suggests that malnourished ARF patients experienced a statistically significant difference in mortality (48% versus 29%) compared to ARF patients without malnutrition.[42] While promising, these results need confirmation before it can be concluded that nutritional intervention significantly impacts patient survival in ARF.

CHRONIC RENAL FAILURE

Chronic renal failure (CRF), as evidenced by the inability of the kidneys to excrete nitrogenous and other waste products, usually develops over months to years (see Chap. 42). Malnutrition secondary to reduced oral nutrient intake is frequently evident when glomerular filtration rate (GFR) drops below 20 to 25 mL/min. Patients with CRF are considered to have end-stage renal disease when glomerular filtration rate falls below 10 mL/min, or 15 mL/min in the patient with diabetic nephropathy (see Chap. 44). Malnutrition is also a common occurrence in ESRD, not only because of decreased oral intake but also due to increased nutrient losses via the various renal replacement therapies. Because of its chronicity, malnutrition in these patients is most frequently treated in the ambulatory setting with EN.

EPIDEMIOLOGY

The prevalence rate of protein–energy malnutrition in the ESRD patient population is approximately 40%.[43] Approximately one-third of ESRD patients experience mild to moderate malnutrition, while 6% to 8% experienced severe malnutrition. More importantly, protein–energy malnutrition is a significant predictor of morbidity and mortality in these patients. In one study lasting 7 years, patients with a serum albumin less than 3.5 g/dL had a twofold increase in mortality risk relative to those patients whose serum albumin was greater than or equal to 4.0 g/dL.[44] In another study that compared long term (10 to 15 year) and very long term (15 to 30 year) to average (less than 5 year) ESRD survivors, expected survival was significantly greater in patients with baseline serum albumin concentrations greater than 3.5 g/dL. Serum albumin concentrations additionally increased in the long and very long term survivors during the study. Conversely, serum albumin concentrations decreased among those patients who survived less than 5 years.[45] Thus, nutrition support appears to be a critical intervention in the care of the ESRD patient.

PATHOPHYSIOLOGY

CARBOHYDRATE

In general, CRF and ESRD patients are not as stressed as patients with ARF; however, more than one-half of CRF patients have insulin resistance and hyperglycemia. This has been attributed to the increased glucagon-to-insulin ratio, resulting in protein breakdown and gluconeogenesis. Patients with ESRD who require PN and receive continuous ambulatory peritoneal dialysis (CAPD) absorb substantial amounts (approximately 500 kcal/d) of glucose.[33] This can worsen existing hyperglycemia and contribute significantly to the patient's energy intake. Therefore, kwashiorkor-type malnutrition is common. Insulin can be added to CAPD bags to control hyperglycemia;[46] however, glucose control is not problematic unless the patient is diabetic, infected, or subjected to operative stress.

FAT

Type IV hypertriglyceridemia is present in more than one-half of all CRF patients. This is mainly due to decreased catabolism of triglycerides secondary to decreased hepatic lipoprotein lipase activity.[16] Most ESRD patients receiving HD also receive heparin, which activates lipoprotein lipase and converts triglycerides to FFAs and glycerol. Carnitine, an amino acid necessary for the transport of long-chain fatty acids across mitochondria where oxidation results in energy production, is removed by HD and CAPD, and therefore serum carnitine concentrations are typically reduced in ESRD.[30] The effect of carnitine supplementation on plasma lipid profiles is controversial. Oral supplementation of 2.4 g of carnitine for 30 days significantly reduced serum triglyceride concentrations.[47] Intravenous supplementation of 0.5 to 1 g three times weekly also reduced serum triglyceride concentrations.[48] More recent trials of 20 mg/kg intravenous carnitine postdialysis for up to six months have failed to confirm these findings.[49] Additionally, if FFAs are not used by the body properly (as in carnitine deficiency), serum triglyceride measurements will not identify this defect. Patients receiving long-term dialysis treatment have also been shown to accumlate remnants of triglyceride-rich lipoproteins. This lipoprotein abnormality can result in type III hyperlipidemia with increased intermediate-density lipoprotein.

PROTEIN

For those CRF patients not yet receiving dialysis, early data suggested that protein restriction would slow the rate of decline in GFR and progression to ESRD.[50] Data from large-controlled trials have supported this intervention, particularly for those patients with a GFR less than 50 mL/min.[51–53] These studies are discussed in further detail in Chapter 42.

Because assessment of urinary nitrogen loss is impossible in anuric ESRD patients, nitrogen balance must be estimated on the basis of UNA. This method (Fig. 131–1) estimates protein catabolism as the sum of losses in the dialysate fluid and the change in the amount of urea nitrogen in the body.

When nitrogen intake in known, nitrogen balance can then be estimated, as previously discussed.[9] These calculations may be helpful in adjusting protein intake in ESRD patients.

UNA is calculated as follows:

$$\text{UNA (g/d)} = \text{urinary UN (g/d)} + \text{change in body UN (g/d)}$$

$$\text{Change in body UN (g/d)} = [\text{serum UN}_{t2} - \text{serum UN}_{t1}\text{ (in g/L)}] \times [\text{BW}_{t1}\text{ (kg/d)} \times 0.6\text{L/kg}] + [(\text{BW}_{t2} - \text{BW}_{t1}) \times \text{serum UN}_{t2}\text{ (g/L)} \times 1.0\text{ L/kg}]$$

where t1 and t2 are the starting and final values during the measurement period; BW is body weight in kg; 0.6 is percent body water; and 1.0 is the volume of distribution of urea associated with the change of body weight over the measurement period.

$$\text{Total nitrogen output (g/d)} = 0.97\text{ UNA (g/d)} + 1.93\text{ g/d (nonurinary losses)}$$

Nitrogen balance is then calculated as usual:

$$\text{Nitrogen balance} = \text{nitrogen intake (g/d)} - \text{nitrogen output (g/d)}$$

FIGURE 131–1. Calculating urea nitrogen appearance (UNA). *(From Ref. 9.)*

ESRD patients receiving continuous ambulatory peritoneal dialysis require special attention due to protein losses via the peritoneal dialysate. Recent investigations reveal that peritoneal protein losses average over 6 g/d in patients treated by CAPD.[54] PD protein losses, however, do not predict risk for malnutrition (as measured by serum albumin) in all patients.[55] Nonetheless, these losses should be taken into consideration when designing the PN or EN formula for the CAPD patient.

Dialysate protein losses must also be examined for the ESRD patient undergoing HD. The amount of protein lost via HD depends on the dialysis membrane used and whether the membrane is being reused. Low-flux polymethylmethacrylate membranes on first use are associated with a loss fo 6.1 g of amino acid per treatment. High-flux polysulfone membranes on first use are associated with an 8.0 g/dialysis amino acid loss. Amino acid losses also increased by 50% after reuse of the high-flux polysulfone membrane.[56] As in the case with CAPD, these losses should be considered when designing the protein regimen of the ESRD patient treated with HD.

FLUID AND ELECTROLYTES

Hyponatremia, often due to overhydration, is common in CRF but usually does not require additional administration of sodium. Regular dialysis is the principal means for control of body water and serum sodium concentration in the ESRD patient.

Patients with CRF or ESRD who develop hyperkalemia have generally ingested excessive potassium relative to the potassium-removing capacity of the failing kidney (and dialysis, in the case of ESRD). The undernourished CRF or ESRD patient receiving PN may, however, require considerable potassium as new body cell mass is synthesized. When inappropriately low amounts of potassium are given during refeeding, hypokalemia may develop.

Patients with CRF or ESRD are often treated for hyperphosphatemia with phosphorus-restricted diets and calcium-containing antacids as phosphate binders (see Chap. 42). When these patients receive aggressive nutrition support, the combination of refeeding (cellular uptake of phosphorus for synthesis of body cell mass) and vigorous phosphate binding therapy can result in hypophosphatemia.

Clinically significant hypermagnesemia is less common in patients with CRF and ESRD compared to ARF. It is usually added to the PN solution in reduced doses (4 mEq/L or less), and serum concentrations need to be monitored.

TRACE ELEMENTS

There is considerable data regarding trace element requirements in patients with ESRD.[30] Decreased zinc concentrations in dialysis patients have been linked to taste disturbances and sexual dysfunction.[28] Zinc supplementation, however, has not universally reversed these anomalies. Although serum concentrations of this trace element are decreased, total body stores of zinc in ESRD are often increased.[28] This suggests a redistribution of zinc or increased need to maintain normal enzymatic function in ESRD. It appears that HD and CAPD patients have depressed serum concentrations of zinc.[31] One study found that zinc supplementation for 6 months improved nerve conduction velocity in dialysis patients.[57] The clinical relevance of these finding are difficult to interpret because they have not been confirmed.

Chromium serum concentrations are elevated in chronic HD and CAPD patients.[28] Both the needles used during HD and the dialysate itself are sources of chromium.[58] The clinical significance of these findings is unknown. Manganese serum concentrations are normal in the HD patient and those patients undergoing PD.[59] Copper concentrations are also unchanged in HD patients.[59] There are conflicting data with regard to selenium in CRF patients.[28] Although deficiencies of selenium have been linked to cardiomyopathy,[60] the prevalence of selenium deficiency in CRF is unclear.

The trace element disorder with the most established significance in ESRD is aluminum toxicity. This toxicity is linked to aluminum in the dialysate or excessive use of aluminum-containing antacids. Consequently, significant quantities of aluminum have been removed from currently available dialysis solutions and calcium antacids have virtually replaced aluminum as phosphate binders. Aluminum toxicity can be treated with deferoxamine, as discussed in Chapter 42.

VITAMINS

CRF patients are prone to develop water-soluble vitamin deficiencies because of decreased dietary intake secondary to anorexia and restriction of certain foods because of their protein, potassium, or phosphorous content. Additionally, in the ESRD patient, HD losses of ascorbic acid, folic acid, and pyridoxine are common. The highly protein-bound vitamins (A, D, and B_{12}) are not significantly removed by HD.[30] Vitamin A concentrations are often elevated in CRF and ESRD and can lead to hypervitaminosis A and its cirrhotic-like syndrome.

▶ TREATMENT: Chronic Renal Failure

ADMINISTRATION ROUTES

CRF and ESRD patients who require nutrition support rarely need PN because their gastrointestinal tract is usually functional. The calorically dense low-electrolyte enteral formulas in Table 131–1 are particularly useful. Even though ESRD patients receive regular dialysis, many are anuric between dialysis sessions, so excess fluid intake is a potential problem. Nepro® is marketed specifically (due to its high caloric density and low electrolyte content) for the ESRD patient who receives regular dialysis. Suplena,

RenalCal, and AminAid, which are lower in protein and some electrolytes than Nepro, can be used in CRF patients not yet undergoing HD or CAPD. If there is superimposed illness that precludes EN, standard mixed amino acids should be used as the protein component of the PN solution.

The association of poor nutritional status and increased morbidity and mortality in ESRD has led to the development of alternative nutritional delivery systems for the ESRD patient. One such approach is intradialytic parenteral nutrition (IDPN), or the provision of glucose/amino acid/lipid admixture during HD. IDPN allows for the infusion of 600 to 700 kcal/session.[61] At least two studies have documented decreased mortality in malnourished chronic HD patients who were receiving IDPN.[61,62] Unfortunately, one of these studies was nonrandomized[61] and one was retrospective.[62] Other studies have failed to demonstrate a morbidity or mortality benefit of IDPN.[63] As a result of these conflicting data, the Health Care Financing Administration has made the qualification for reimbursement of this therapy quite stringent.[64] Until further data are available, IDPN should be reserved for those malnourished patients who have failed enteral feedings and other interventions. Recently, Charzot et al.[65] demonstrated that the addition of amino acid to the hemodialysate may prevent amino acid losses and, if provided in sufficient quantities, actually be a means for nutritional supplementation.

Amino acid dialysate (AAD) is the IDPN counterpart for the CAPD patient. This technique entails using a 1.1% amino acid solution in place of one or two of the dextrose-containing PD exchanges/day (see Chap. 44). Studies have demonstrated improvements in serum transferrin and total protein concentrations; however, no beneficial effect has been noted on patient morbidity or mortality.[66,67] Adverse effects of this therapy have included exacerbations of uremic symptoms (due to increases in blood urea nitrogen [BUN]) and metabolic acidosis.[66,67] Not all studies have demonstrated benefits from this intervention.[68] In summary, AAD may be useful in the treatment of malnourished CAPD patients, but better designed, longer studies are needed.

Recombinant human growth hormone (rhGH) has been used experimentally in adults with ESRD to enhance anabolism.[43] It may play a future role in the treatment of ESRD patients who still have inadequate oral intake despite appropriate dietary counseling and oral supplements. Additional study is needed before this can be advocated in general practice.

DESIGN AND INITIATION OF NUTRITIONAL REGIMEN

Current recommendations that factor in concurrent illnesses and the likelihood of preexisting malnutrition advocate 1.2 g/kg/d protein for chronic HD patients and 1.2 to 1.3 g/kg/d protein for CAPD patients.[43] This is higher that the spontaneous dietary protein intake in most dialysis patients.[8] Therefore, dietary counseling of the chronic dialysis patient is important in the ambulatory setting.

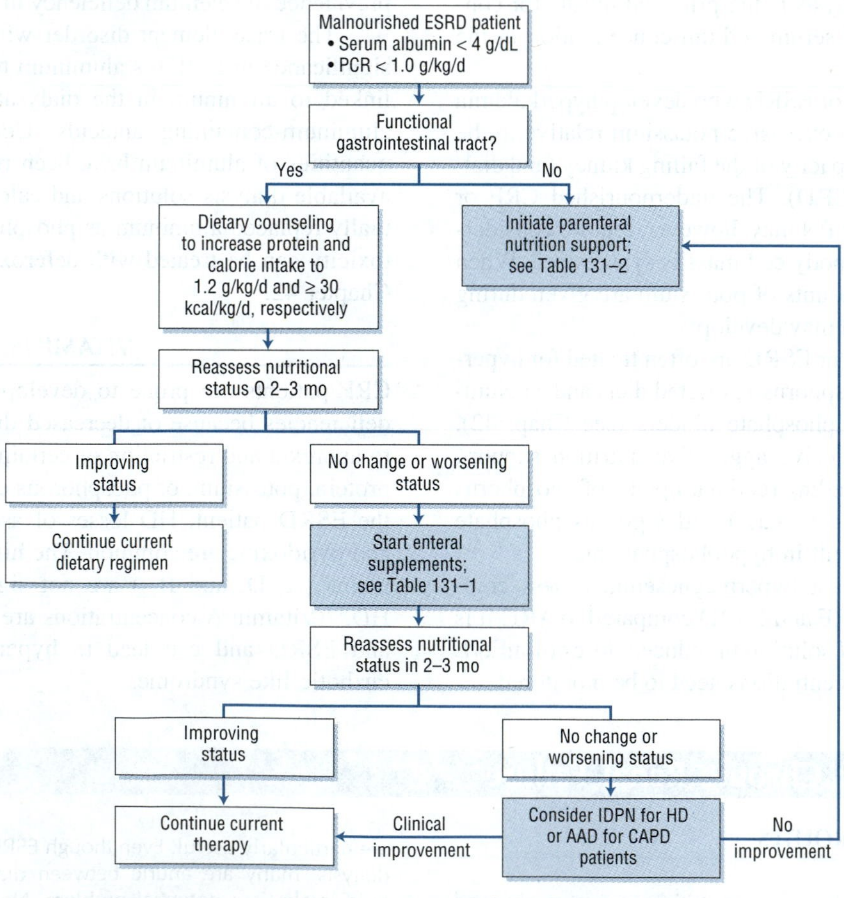

FIGURE 131–2. Algorithmic approach to nutrition support in the ESRD patient.

Several electrolytes warrant special attention when providing PN or EN to a patient with CRF or ESRD. Generally, sodium should be adminstered to CRF patients during nutrition support only to replace losses in order to avoid overhydration. Although these patients are also predisposed to hyperkalemia, once anabolism is attained in CRF patients, potassium requirements may be as high as 40 to 80 mEq/d. This dose needs to be given carefully and requires serum potassium concentration monitoring. Clinically significant hypermagnesemia is less common in patients with CRF compared to ARF. It is usually added to the PN solution in reduced doses (4 mEq/L).

Patients with CRF or ESRD are often treated for hyperphosphatemia. With agressive nutrition support, the combination of refeeding and phosphate-binding therapy can result in hypophosphatemia. Decreasing or temporarily discontinuing the phosphate-binding therapy is appropriate if this occurs. Thereafter, conservative amounts of phosphorus may need to be administered.

Some practitioners advocate withholding trace elements from CRF and ESRD patients receiving PN. The NAG-AMA guidelines do not offer specific guidelines for the use of trace elements in these patients.[31] Because serum concentrations of certain trace elements are normal in ESRD patients (copper and manganese), and others may actually be decreased (zinc and selenium), the standard dietary intake of these trace elements should be recommended and standard trace element supplements should be added to PN regimens.[30]

During PN in CRF or ESRD patients, elimination or reduction of the dose of vitamin A is recommended. Supplemental administration of the highly protein-bound vitamins is not warranted in the ESRD patient, as these vitamins are not significantly removed by dialysis. Dialytic losses of ascorbic acid, folic acid, and pyridoxine are common. Thus, ESRD patients should receive ascorbic acid 50 to 100 mg/d, pyridoxine 5 to 10 mg/d, and folic acid 1 mg/d in addition to the other essential vitamins.[30] An example of a PN solution for use in ESRD patients is presented in Table 131–2.

Successful enteral nutritional interventions are dependent on the patient's understanding of the need, and the sensitivity of the clinician regarding cultural variations in eating preferences and habits. Dietary counseling adaptations for African American and Mexican-American patients with ESRD have been proposed.[69,70] Other adaptations should be sought as patient situation dictates.

EVALUATION OF THERAPEUTIC OUTCOMES

The short- and long-term monitoring plan for the CRF or ESRD patient receiving PN or EN needs to be carefully tailored. Special attention should be paid to maintenance of fluid and electrolyte homeostasis. This can be achieved via frequent (daily) monitoring of serum electrolyte concentrations (sodium, potassium, phosphorous, magnesium, and calcium) and fluid balance. Serum glucose concentrations should be followed frequently (four times daily) in the CRF or ESRD patient who develops hyperglycemia. UNA can be monitored to estimate nitrogen balance, with which protein provision can be adjusted to maintain a positive nitrogen balance.

Because protein–energy malnutrition is a significant predictor of morbidity and mortality in ESRD patients, monitoring to assure the effectiveness of the long-term nutritional plan becomes critical. Albumin is perhaps the most studied marker of nutritional efficacy in this patient population. Increased serum albumin concentrations are correlated with increased survival. Thus, monitoring of serum albumin concentrations should be considered a critical component of the monitoring plan to assure patient longevity. An algorithmic approach to improve nutritional status and assure optimal outcomes is presented in Figure 131–2.[10]

HEPATIC FAILURE

The liver is the primary organ involved in the digestion, metabolism, and storage of nutrients. When functional capacity is depressed, profound nutrient intolerance (hyper- or hypoglycemia, hypertriglyceridemia, and hepatic encephalopathy) may result. Other sequelae that accompany the failing liver are fluid and electrolyte imbalances, vitamin deficiencies, and malnutrition. Nutritional supplementation provided to patients with alcoholic cirrhosis has reduced the frequency of hospitalizations.[71] Some information is also available now that suggests a survival benefit of nutritional supplementation in liver failure. In a study of oxandrolone and an enteral formula rich in branched-chain amino acids (BCAAs), severe protein–calorie malnutrition (PCM) was associated with a 6-month mortality rate of 45%, while moderate PCM was associated with a 6-month mortality rate of 29%.[72] Thus, nutrition support has become an important component of the overall care of the patient with liver disease.[73]

PATHOPHYSIOLOGY

ENERGY

Patients with alcoholic hepatitis or cirrhosis are hypermetabolic (up to 50% greater than expected) when their resting energy expenditure (REE) is normalized for lean body mass and compared with normal controls.[74,75] It must be emphasized, however, that providing excess calories should be avoided as this may promote liver dysfunction and increased production of carbon dioxide and an associated increased work of breathing.

CARBOHYDRATE

In healthy adults, approximately 60% of absorbed glucose is taken up by the liver and used for glycogen synthesis, triglyceride synthesis, and glycolysis. In general, glycogen synthesis and glycolysis are enhanced by insulin, while gluconeogenesis and glycogen breakdown are controlled by glucagon.

Hyperglycemia is common in cirrhosis as a result of peripheral insulin resistance, which is mediated by a decreased binding to insulin receptors and defective postreceptor signal handling in peripheral tissues.[76] Plasma concentrations of insulin are elevated with or without a glucose stimulus. This makes administration of large doses of glucose problematic, because of administration of insulin to control hyperglycemia may not improve use substantially.

Patients with fulminant hepatitis are prone to hypoglycemia,[77] because hepatic glucose production is depressed secondary to decreased glycogen stores and diminished gluconeogenesis. Also, impaired degradation of insulin by the damaged liver may contribute to this disorder. A continuous intravenous infusion of glucose usually prevents hypoglycemia in acute hepatitis, but concentrations greater than 10% glucose may be needed in the more severe cases.

FAT

The liver is responsible for synthesis of cholesterol, high-density lipoproteins, and very-low-density lipoproteins. The enzymes lipoprotein lipase and lecithin–cholesterol acyltransferase also are synthesized in this organ. Increased serum triglyceride and FFA concentrations are encountered in patients with hepatic failure. Chronic alcohol ingestion is linked to increased circulating triglycerides and fatty infiltration of the liver.[77] Ingestion of high-fat diets may exacerbate these alterations in metabolism.

Diarrhea and steatorrhea are common in patients with hepatic cholestasis because of intestinal malabsorption (due in part to mucosal edema from hypoalbuminemia), inadequate bile acid delivery to the duodenum, and pancreatic dysfunction with decreased secretion of lipase.[77] Micelle formation is impeded and thus the long-chain fatty acids pass through the colon, resulting in a foul-smelling, soapy diarrhea.

PROTEIN

Nitrogen requirements for the patient with liver failure are not unlike those of normal subjects, but intolerance to protein is well described in cirrhotic patients, and protein restriction has been used successfully as part of the therapy. A dilemma arises when the diet becomes so restrictive that malnutrition results and the patient becomes susceptible to infection and other complications. Overzealous use of protein to correct nutritional deficits invariably results in hepatic encephalopathy.

Because the liver metabolizes the aromatic amino acids (phenylalanine, tyrosine, tryptophan), methionine, and glutamine, the plasma concentrations of these amino acids are elevated in cirrhotic patients. Plasma concentrations of the branched-chain amino acids (valine, leucine, isoleucine) often are depressed because these amino acids are metabolized by skeletal muscle. This altered plasma aminogram is thought to be involved in the etiology of hepatic encephalopathy. In health, the ratio of branched-chain amino acids to aromatic amino acids is approximately 3.5 to 1, while ratios of 1 to 1 have been associated with hepatic encephalopathy in patients with cirrhosis.[78]

FLUID AND ELECTROLYTES

Patients with severe cirrhosis often have ascites and peripheral edema. The excess of total body sodium in the presence of an even greater excess of total body water results in hyponatremia. Salt and fluid restriction are required so as not to exacerbate this overhydrated state. Caution must be exercised, however, as severe sodium and fluid restriction during intravascular depletion may cause or exacerbate hepatic encephalopathy.

Hypokalemia is common in the patient with liver failure who has normal renal function. Poor nutritional intake and vomiting may initiate this disorder. Severe vomiting may lead to volume contraction metabolic alkalosis, with increased renal excretion of potassium. Secondary hyperaldosteronism, seen in the liver failure patient with intravascular depletion, also increases renal excretion of potassium. Loop diuretic therapy causes increased renal excretion of potassium, while diarrhea from lactulose therapy increases fecal excretion of potassium. All these conditions can lead to profound hypokalemia. Therefore, potassium requirements in the liver failure patient receiving specialized nutrition support are often substantially increased.

Poor nutritional intake secondary to alcohol abuse and increased excretion of magnesium secondary to diuretic therapy contribute to hypomagnesemia.[79] During nutrition support, requirements for phosphorus may also be supranormal as synthesis of body cell mass occurs. Therefore, this population is at risk for developing hypophosphatemia during refeeding.

TRACE ELEMENTS

Many patients with liver failure have a malabsorption syndrome and chronic diarrhea. Chronic diarrhea causes zinc deficiency because stool contains substantial quantities of zinc. Cytokines such as tumor necrosis factor (TNF)-α, interleukin (IL)-1, and IL-6 may stimulate metallothionein, an intestinal zinc-binding protein, thereby inhibiting zinc absorption.[80] Considering the importance of zinc in metalloenzyme reactions, wound healing, immunocompetence, and the senses of taste and smell, patients with chronic diarrhea or large ostomy losses should be suspected of having zinc deficiency; measurement of serum concentrations may be used to confirm such deficiencies. Patients receiving a protein-restricted diet may be at additional risk as substantial amounts of zinc are found in red meat.

Because copper and manganese are excreted in the bile, it has been recommended that these two trace elements not be administered or be administered in reduced doses to patients with serious cholestasis (see Table 131–2).[81] Increased manganese whole blood concentrations have been associated with the magnetic resonance imaging (MRI) findings in chronic hepatic encephalopathy.[81,82] It would be appropriate to provide reduced quantities of manganese in the nutritional formulation to avoid potentially exacerbating encephalopathy in the patient with chronic liver disease.

An association between alcoholism and low serum selenium concentrations have been reported.[83] Serum concentrations of selenium were lowest in patients who had decompensated alcoholic cirrhosis. Because selenium is important in maintaining the enzyme glutathione peroxidase, a deficiency of this trace element has been implicated as a cause of hepatic injury in the alcoholic patient. However, because human serum contains at least three fractions of selenium, the use of serum selenium concentrations as an accurate marker for selenium deficiency is controversial. Therefore, care must be used in the interpretation of serum selenium concentrations.[80]

VITAMINS

Poor intake and malabsorption are the principal causes of vitamin deficiencies in patients with chronic liver disease. Depletion of hepatic stores of vitamin A, pyridoxine, folic acid, riboflavin, pantothenic acid, vitamin B_{12}, and thiamine have been reported in patients with hepatic failure. Folic acid deficiency, the most common vitamin deficiency, may lead to megaloblastic anemia, while thiamine deficiency may result in Wernicke's encephalopathy after rehydration with intravenous glucose.

Hepatic stores of vitamin A have been reported to be depleted in the patient with alcoholic liver injury.[84] Because vitamin D is metabolized to one of the active forms, 25-hydroxyvitamin D, in the liver, low concentrations of this vitamin are seen in patients with biliary cirrhosis. Impaired absorption of dietary vitamin D also may contribute to these low serum concentrations. It is unclear whether vigorous supplementation of these fat-soluble vitamins should be given to these patients during nutrition support, but therapeutic doses are indicated when a deficiency is documented.

▶ TREATMENT: Hepatic Failure

ADMINISTRATION ROUTE

If the gastrointestinal (GI) tract is functional and accessible, EN should be attempted. The indications for PN in the patient with liver failure are similar to those for general hospitalized patients. In most cases, PN in the patient with liver failure can be accomplished via the administration of standard mixed amino acids (Fig. 131–3).

Currently, two enteral products are marketed as supplements for patients with hepatic encephalopathy (Hepatic-Aid II, and NutriHep). Both supplements have increased amounts of branched-chain amino acids (BCAAs) and reduced amounts of aromatic amino acids (AAAs) and methionine, but differ with regards to micronutrient composition. Hepatic-Aid II is virtually electrolyte and vitamin free, necessitating supplementation if tube feeding is used as the sole source of nutrient intake. Nutri-

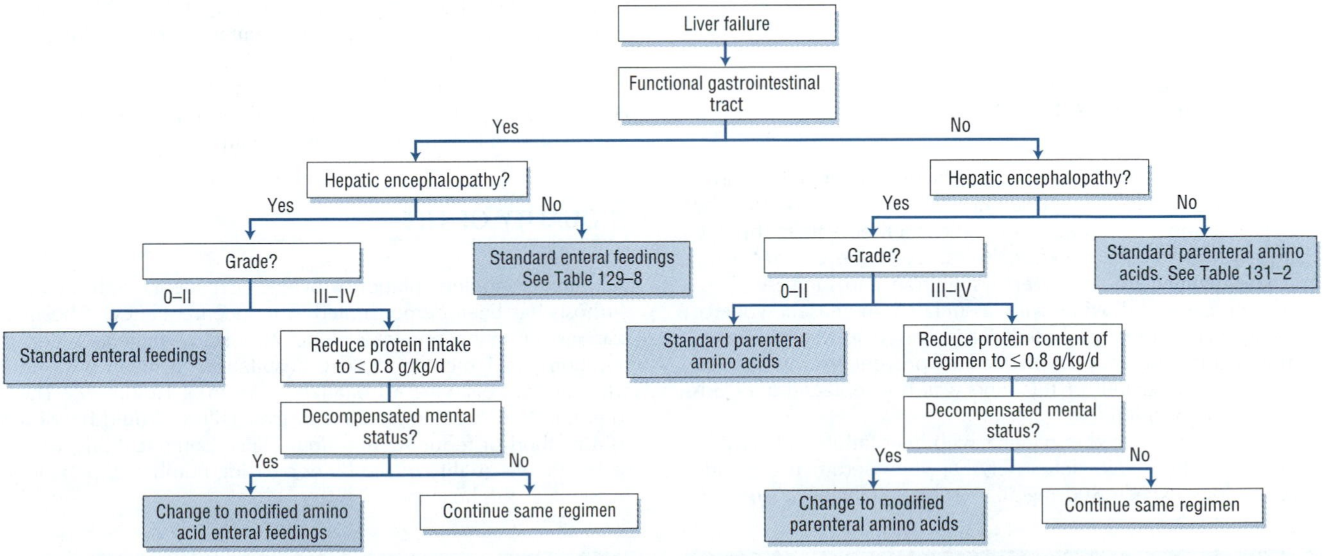

FIGURE 131–3. An algorithmic approach to nutrition support for the patient with hepatic failure.

Hep meets the U.S. RDA vitamin and mineral requirements, contains a high percentage of MCTs, and is supplemented with carnitine. The clinical trials using these products have yielded inconsistent outcomes.[73] At least two studies demonstrated improvements in hepatic encephalopathy with use of BCAA formulas. However, the remaining studies did not find improvement in hepatic encephalopathy.[78] Whether enteral feeding interventions improve mortality is perhaps even more controversial. At least three studies have demonstrated a significant improvement in early mortality, but one of these studies used a historical control,[85] and one used concurrent anabolic steroid therapy.[78]

There has been considerable interest in the use of vegetable-protein diets in the chronic management of patients with cirrhosis and hepatic encephalopathy. Enthusiasm for this therapy is based on the reduced amounts of AAAs and methionine in vegetable protein. The beneficial effects of vegetable protein may also result from decreased nitrogen absorption in response to decreased gastrointestinal transit time or an increased fecal nitrogen excretion by colonic bacterial flora.[86] Although these diets are somewhat more difficult to adhere to, preliminary results justify further study of this concept.

SPECIALTY PRODUCTS

The major controversy in nutrition support of the patient with liver failure has centered around the use of protein products. A modified amino acid solution for PN (HepatAmine) is marketed for patients with liver failure and hepatic encephalopathy. It is enriched with BCAAs and has reduced amounts of AAAs and methionine. The product was formulated on the basis of the false neurotransmitter hypothesis, which concludes that hepatic encephalopathy may be due to increased AAA concentrations in the central nervous system.

Branched-chain amino acid products have not universally improved nitrogen balance. Standard amino acid mixtures can be used successfully without worsening encephalopathy. Studies examining improvement in encephalopathy or mortality rates with use of these modified amino acids have yielded conflicting results. This, coupled with the increased cost of these products, has led most clinicians to reserve these products for patients with severe encephalopathy that decompensate on standard amino acids despite continued lactulose–neomycin therapy.

DESIGN AND INITIATION OF NUTRITIONAL REGIMEN

Patients with alcoholic hepatitis or cirrhosis are generally hypermetabolic. However, indirect calorimetry quantification may be preferred to empiric estimates of caloric requirements in this setting to avoid providing excess calories. Excessive calorie provision may actually promote liver dysfunction and increased production of carbon dioxide with associated increased work of breathing. When dextrose-based PN is started in these patients, additional thiamine may be needed to prevent Wernicke's encephalopathy, especially if thiamine was not replaced after admission to the hospital.[78]

IVLE should be used in patients with liver failure only to prevent essential fatty acid deficit (EFAD) when serum triglyceride concentrations exceed 300 mg/dL. If serum triglyceride concentrations are low or normal, IVLE also may be used as a calorie source. Monitoring serum triglyceride concentration and FFA oxidation (not available in all facilities) to ensure that lipid is both cleared and oxidized appropriately has been suggested. Triglyceride concentrations are the only available marker in most clinical practices at this time. Although not an indicator of use, this can help prevent marked hypertriglyceridemia and associated disorders (such as pancreatitis). Assessment of the GI tract is necessary before large amounts of lipid (beyond what is needed to prevent EFAD) are administered by the oral route. Oral MCTs have been used occasionally with success because they do not require pancreatic enzymes or micelle formation before absorption.[87] These products do not, however, provide essential fatty acids.

Most clinicians routinely use standard mixed amino acids and reserve branched-chain amino acid products for patients with severe encephalopathy who decompensate on standard amino acids despite continued lactulose–neomycin therapy. This is because modified amino acid products containing only branched-chain amino acids have been shown to not improve nitrogen balance. Second, standard amino acid mixtures can improve plasma aminograms without worsening encephalopathy as previously discussed. Careful monitoring and recognition that a therapeutic window for protein intake exists (40 to 80 g/d), however, are essential.

The electrolytes that warrant the most careful monitoring in liver disease include sodium, potassium, phosphorous, and magnesium. During fluid and salt restriction, patients (especially those receiving concurrent lactulose therapy) should be observed for symptoms of volume depletion (e.g., pulse rate, blood pressure, dry mucous membranes). The magnesium dose should be individualized to maintain concentrations in the normal range. This often requires magnesium concentrations as high as 24 mEq/L in the PN solution, which is two to three times the standard daily dose.

Trace elements that warrant individual attention include zinc and chromium. Oral supplementation of zinc sulfate capsules or intravenous zinc chloride can be used to prevent deficiency or correct deficits. Oral supplementation with zinc sulfate 600 mg/d in cirrhotic patients has been reported to improve serum zinc concentrations and psychometric tests.[88] For patients receiving PN, withholding copper from the solution until a copper serum concentration in the normal range is documented, or the cholestasis resolves, is appropriate. Patients who have chronic cholestasis may require copper in reduced doses (e.g., 0.6 mg/d); however, they should have serum copper concentrations checked regularly (once per month in the acute care setting and every 6 months in the ambulatory setting). For those patients with liver failure and a nonfunctioning GI tract, Table 131–2 gives and example of an empiric central PN formula for a patient with cirrhosis.

QUALITY OF LIFE

Nutritional supplementation provided to patients with alcoholic cirrhosis has been demonstrated to reduce frequency of hospitalizations. During a one-year ambulatory study, patients receiving nutrition supplementation were hospitalized a mean 0.85 times whereas controls were hospitalized a mean of 1.6 times.[71] Therefore, nutrition supplementation in liver failure should be viewed as a method of reducing nutrition-related complications, as well as improving quality of life by decreasing number of patient admissions to the hospital.

HEPATIC TRANSPLANTATION

Orthotopic liver transplantation (OLT) has become an important intervention for the patient with end-stage liver disease. Many patients receive PN support following this operation because of their poor preoperative nutritional status and the postoperative stress. Although hypermetabolism—36% to 38% above the basal energy expenditure (BEE) in the early postoperative period has been reported,[89]—a caloric intake of only 1.2 times BEE has met caloric needs immediately and for up to 28 days after transplantation.[90] Increased protein catabolism and urinary 3-methylhistidine levels have also been noted in response to the stress of liver transplantation and the administration of large doses of corticosteroids following surgical intervention.[90]

EPIDEMIOLOGY

The percentage of OLT patients requiring nutrition support has been well documented. In one report of 427 OLT patients, 32.7% received at least one form of nutrition support: 8.9% received tube feedings alone, 11.9% of patients received PN alone, and a combination of tube feedings and PN was provided to 11.9% of OLT patients. Thus, nutrition support is a frequently used therapy in the OLT patient population.

PATHOPHYSIOLOGY

CARBOHYDRATE AND PROTEIN

Postoperative hyperglycemia is common during the first day after OLT. Cyclosporine, which is often given to these patients to prevent organ rejection, has been reported to suppress insulin synthesis and secretion.[91] Administration of this drug may thus contribute to the hyperglycemia observed during the postoperative period.

Most patients will tolerate standard amino acids following OLT because the new liver is functioning properly and hepatic encephalopathy is not problematic. The excessive nitrogen losses associated with this procedure warrant the provision of at least 1.2 g/kg/d of protein.[90] One study demonstrated that at least 0.25 g/kg/d of nitrogen (1.38 g/kg/d of protein) is required to maintain a balanced plasma aminogram when OLT patients were fed 27 kcal/kg ideal body weight/d.[92] Modified amino acids should be reserved for those patients with marginal hepatic function associated with rejection or hepatic encephalopathy.

FLUID, ELECTROLYTES, AND ACID–BASE DISORDERS

Patients undergoing OLT receive a substantial amount of crystalloid and blood products during the operative procedure. This often results in an edematous state in the postoperative period, especially in patients who had ascites preoperatively. The large citrate load from administered blood products has been implicated in causing hypocalcemia (citrate binding of ionized calcium) and metabolic alkalosis (conversions of citrate to bicarbonate) in the postoperative period. Low serum concentrations of magnesium are common in the postoperative period. Reduced intake from restricted diets and increased urinary excretion secondary to cyclosporine therapy contribute to hypomagnesemia.

TRACE ELEMENTS AND VITAMINS

Low serum concentrations of zinc are common in the postoperative period. Restricted diets before surgery and hyperzincuria secondary to liver disease both contribute to hypozincemia in this population. These findings led investigators to recommend oral zinc supplementation pretransplant. Serum zinc concentrations have been found to rapidly recover posttransplant, obviating the need for further supplementation.[93] On the other hand, patients who have severe cholestasis before and after OLT should have copper and manganese restricted, as they are excreted in the bile and serum concentrations may thus be elevated.

Low serum vitamin A concentrations are present in many patients with chronic liver disease. Mean serum vitamin A concentrations measure less than one-half normal in pre-OLT patients.[84] These abnormally low serum concentrations, however, were found to increase one week posttransplant, and to normalize two weeks posttransplant.[84] Water-soluble vitamin E preparations have been used in an attempt to economically maintain therapeutic cyclosporine concentrations early in the posttransplant setting.[94]

▶ TREATMENT: Hepatic Transplantation

ADMINISTRATION ROUTES

Several studies have investigated the effect of route of feeding the OLT patient on patient outcome. Hasse and associates[95] compared nasointestinal feedings to maintenance IV fluids in the immediate postoperative period. Both groups were advanced to oral diets as tolerated posttransplant. Cumulative caloric and protein intakes were greater and nitrogen balance was better in the tube-fed patients. Additionally, 17.7% of patients given maintenance IV fluids developed viral infections compared to none in the tube-fed group.[95] Wicks and coworkers[96] demonstrated comparable efficacy between jejunal enteral feedings and PN in maintaining midarm muscle circumference and tricep skinfold thickness 10 days postoperatively. Another study demonstrated that patients fed via jejunostomy tube reached goal oral nutrition quicker and had less postoperative ileus than patients treated with PN post-OLT.[97] Based on the current literature, OLT patients can be successfully fed enterally; however, small bowel access is needed for this to occur. This would necessitate the placement of a nasoduodenal or nasojejunal tube during or immediately after surgery.

DESIGN AND INITIATION OF NUTRITIONAL REGIMEN

OLT patients should be given a nutritional formula that provides at least 1.2 times BEE/d. Because of the significant incidence of hyperglycemia immediately postoperatively, it is recommended to wait 24 hours before starting PN, or to begin very slowly with a relatively low concentration of dextrose (e.g., $D_{10}W$ or $D_{15}W$). These patients should also be provided with at least 1.2 g/kg/d of protein. Because OLT patients are frequently edematous postoperatively, this can be achieved with higher concentrations of amino acids (using a 10% or 15% stock solution). Also due to postoperative edema, sodium rarely needs to be added to the PN solution in these patients. Citrate-containing blood products bind ionized calcium, mandating supplemental doses of calcium. Additionally, OLT patients receiving cyclosporine therapy will often require magnesium in amounts that exceed standard doses during postoperative nutrition support. An example of a PN formula specific for OLT appears in Table 131–2.

EVALUATION OF THERAPEUTIC OUTCOMES

The monitoring plan of the OLT patient needs to be individualized. Those patients receiving cyclosporine should be monitored closely (at least every 6 hours) for hyperglycemia. Following successful OLT, hepatic encephalopathy is no longer problematic. Thus, nitrogen balance should be evaluated to determine the optimal amount of protein to be provided. Fluid balance (daily or more frequently) should be carefully followed to avoid volume overload, especially in those patients who received large volumes of fluids intraoperatively. Daily (or more frequent if deficiency documented) monitoring of magnesium is necessary, especially in those patients receiving cyclosporine therapy. Zinc and vitamin A serum concentrations should return to normal after successful OLT, requiring less aggressive monitoring than was needed preoperatively.

The prognostic importance of pretransplant nutrition status has perhaps been overlooked in the past. A strong correlation between pretransplant nutrition status and posttransplant survival exists. Perhaps the most striking results are reported in a 1997 study by Selberg and colleagues.[98] Better nutrition status in this study was associated with an 88% (versus 54%) survival rate. Optimum nutrition status should therefore be assured pretransplant as well as posttransplant. It appears this will assist OLT patients in achieving the best therapeutic outcome possible.

Advances in nutrition support for the post-OLT patient have additionally led to restoration of nitrogen balance, enhancement of host defense mechanisms, and decreased time on the ventilator and in the ICU.[99] Therefore, the clinician should throughly evaluate global outcome parameters (time on mechanical ventilation and in the ICU), as well as more traditional paramenters of nutrition efficacy (nitrogen balance and visceral protein markers). These global parameters should improve with the provision of more aggressive nutrition support in the post-OLT setting.

PULMONARY FAILURE

Substantial information documents the interaction between nutrition and respiratory function. Decreased body weight in the National Institute of Health sponsored intermittent positive-pressure breathing trial, involving 779 men with chronic obstructive pulmonary disease (COPD), was associated with decreased pulmonary function and increased mortality.[100] Impaired gas exchange has been associated with depressed visceral protein markers of nutritional status (e.g., albumin, prealbumin). Also, undernourished patients with chronic tracheostomy have demonstrated increased bacterial binding in the lower respiratory tract with enteric gram-negative bacilli.

Although patients with pulmonary failure do not have the severe metabolic alterations observed in patients with renal or hepatic failure, there is substantial information to aid the practitioner in providing safe and efficacious nutrition support.[101]

EPIDEMIOLOGY

Nutritional abnormalities were reported in 46.8% of COPD patients assessed for body mass index and pulmonary function.[102] A significant positive correlation was reported between the body mass index and both forced expiratory volume in one second and diffusing capacity for carbon monoxide.[102] In another report, a low body mass index and the use of home oxygen were both significantly correlated with reduced survival.[103] The major predictors of respiratory mortality in this cohort of patients were elevated $Paco_2$, decreased body mass index, decreased maximum inspiratory pressure, and decreased diffusing capacity.[103]

PATHOPHYSIOLOGY

ENERGY

In most disease states, undernutrition and weight loss results in hypometabolism. Hypermetabolism (increased REE), however, is a common finding in stable, undernourished patients with COPD.[104] This may account in part for the nearly universal weight loss seen in patients with these pulmonary disease states, even when nutritional intake appears adequate. Patients with clinically stable COPD who had a body mass index (expressed as weight in kg divided by height in m^2) of 21 or less demonstrated a depleted fat-free mass and an increased extracellular to intracellular water ratio.[105] These data strongly suggest that COPD patients who are losing weight have a primary deficit in their protein stores.

Nonsurgical patients who have acute respiratory failure requiring mechanical ventilation and sepsis have demonstrated a 20% increase in measured REE over the BEE predicted by the Harris–Benedict equation.[106] Other patients in this report who required mechanical ventilation and were not septic did not demonstrate hypermetabolism.[106] Thus, nonseptic patients with acute respiratory failure may require only 10% to 20% above calculated BEE to meet nutrition needs. Those patients with acute respiratory failure who are septic, however, may require energy at a level of 30% to 40% above BEE.

CARBOHYDRATE

Semistarvation in normal subjects (less than 500 kcal/d of carbohydrate) has been shown to blunt the normal response to hypoxia; however, refeeding can restore this response. This would suggest that early feeding of the mechanically ventilated patient improves the hypoxic response and is one reason why practitioners should institute nutrition support early in the course of respiratory failure. Stable patients with COPD in the ambulatory setting who have weight loss should be considered candidates for oral nutrition supplementation.

Oxidation of the major nutritional substrates can be represented by a respiratory quotient (RQ). The respiratory quotient is the ratio of the amount of CO_2 produced to the amount of O_2 consumed. Carbohydrate, protein, and fat oxidation have RQs of 1.0, 0.8, and 0.7, respectively.[101] Thus, oxidation of carbohydrate generates 1 mole of carbon dioxide for every mole of oxygen consumed. Fat synthesis (from carbohydrate) produces an RQ of 8.0. When a subject is overfed with glucose, net fat synthesis occurs and the amount of CO_2 produced markedly exceeds the amount of O_2 consumed.

The inability to wean mechanically ventilated patients because of overfeeding with glucose-based PN is a real problem. It is presumed that excessive infused carbohydrate is used for fat synthesis, resulting in substantial liberation of carbon dioxide.This would make weaning difficult secondary to respiratory acidosis. Significant increases in $V\text{CO}_2$ and RQ occur when glucose-based PN is administered to either depleted or severely stressed patients at approximately 50% above measured REE. Because of this potential problem, glucose-based PN should be administered in moderate doses (25 to 30 total kcal/kg/d) to patients with respiratory disease or mechanical ventilation unless they have sepsis.

FAT

Significant decreases in $V\text{CO}_2$ have been recorded when ventilated patients were switched from a high-carbohydrate to a high-fat formula.[107] A reduction in pulmonary membrane diffusion capacity, increased pulmonary artery pressure, and increased venous admixture, however, may occur when large doses of intravenous fat are given rapidly (e.g., 500 mL 10% intravenous lipid over 4 hours). Rapid infusion of IVLE is also associated with increased synthesis of prostaglandin $F_{2\alpha}$, a known pulmonary vasoconstrictor; whereas slow, continuous infusion results in synthesis of prostaglandin E_2 and prostaglandin I_2, known pulmonary vasodilators. The clearance of triglycerides from IVLE is actually increased in critically ill patients when compared with normal subjects. One report suggested that patients who have adult respiratory distress syndrome (ARDS) with a disrupted alveolar capillary membrane are more prone to develop ventilation–perfusion inequalities during IVLE than other patients receiving mechanical ventilation.[108] Studies of IVLE administration in septic patients with ARDS indicate significant decreases in $P\text{O}_2/F\text{IO}_2$ (an index of oxygenation) and increases in mean pulmonary arterial pressure and pulmonary vasculature resistance.[109]

PROTEIN

Undernourished patients have demonstrated a blunted response to hypercapnia that improves after one week of adequate nutrition support. This response is thought to result from protein administration as evidenced by decreased $P\text{CO}_2$, increased minute ventilation, and improved breathing patterns after the start of PN. An increase in neuromuscular ventilatory drive following protein administration has also been observed. Even though increased neuromuscular drive from protein administration can be beneficial, it can be detrimental in patients who are unable to increase their minute ventilation. In other words, excessive protein intake might increase pulmonary workload, resulting in muscle fatigue and respiratory failure.

FLUID AND ELECTROLYTES

It is desirable to keep these patients slightly "dry." Mortality has been reported to be significantly lower in those patients who have ARDS or pulmonary edema who have a negative fluid balance.[110] Therefore, excessive infusions of salt and water should be avoided, as they may exacerbate already compromised pulmonary function, and parenteral and enteral formulas should be relatively low in sodium. Losses of sodium from nasogastric suction or abdominal drains should be replaced.

The incidence of hypophosphatemia is higher in patients with pulmonary disease than in the general hospitalized population. It is well known that phosphorus is essential for adenosine triphosphate (ATP) and 2,3-diphosphoglycerate (2,3-DPG). Hypophosphatemia can cause reduced erythrocyte concentrations of these two compounds. Hemoglobin does not release oxygen during hypoxia appropriately without adequate 2,3-DPG, and respiratory muscles may be weakened without adequate stores of ATP. It has been shown that hypophosphatemia impairs diaphragmatic contractility in patients with acute respiratory failure.

Mechanical ventilation can actually cause hypophosphatemia, because the correction of the acidosis will cause potassium and phosphorus to move intracellularly. These data, combined with the problems of hypophosphatemia from refeeding,[111] emphasize the importance of phosphorus homeostasis in this patient population during nutrition support. Most patients with moderate to severe hypophosphatemia with respiratory failure are treated with intravenous sodium or potassium phosphate. Correction of hypophosphatemia using a graduated dosing scheme of phosphorus for intensive care unit patients receiving nutrition support has been reported (Table 131–3).[112]

ACID–BASE DISORDERS

Ventilator-dependent patients and those with stable COPD often have respiratory acidosis. A balanced mixture of chloride and acetate salts is often appropriate in these patients. The acid–base status of the patient with pulmonary compromise should be monitored daily for those in the intensive care unit (less often in the stable COPD patient).

TABLE 131–3. Acute Correction of Hypophosphatemia in the Critically Ill Patient

Serum Phosphorous Concentration (mg/dL)	Dose of Phosphorous (mmol/kg)
2.3–3.0	0.16
1.6–2.2	0.32
≤ 1.5	0.64

TRACE ELEMENTS AND VITAMINS

There are no significant alterations in trace element and vitamin metabolism in patients with pulmonary disease. Patients receiving PN should receive vitamins and trace elements as recommended by the NAG-AMA. Patients receiving EN should receive the RDA for vitamins, zinc, and selenium, and the recommended amounts for the other trace elements.

▶ TREATMENT: Pulmonary Failure

ADMINISTRATION ROUTE

Patients with pulmonary failure should receive nutrition support by the enteral route unless the GI tract is not functional or accessible. EN is more physiologic, and septic morbidity is decreased in trauma patients fed enterally when compared to those patients given PN. Data also suggest that PN decreases the immunity of the upper respiratory tract when compared to EN.[113] Most general EN formulas contain a balance of nonprotein energy between carbohydrate and fat. Elemental or chemically defined products are the exception as they are intended to be high-carbohydrate, low-fat formulas to enhance absorption and digestion. In general, administration of a high-carbohydrate formula will result in a significant increase in minute ventilation, heat production, and $\dot{V}CO_2$ when compared to a high-fat formula. Because most general formulas contain balanced nonprotein calories, moderate doses of these products are appropriate in most patients with pulmonary disease. An approach to the patient with respiratory failure who requires nutrition support appears in Figure 131–4.

Investigators have begun to measure changes in pulmonary function and respiratory muscle strength in patients with lung diseases receiving nutrition support. Undernourished patients with COPD who received supplemental tube feeding (1000 kcal/d) for a mean of 16 days demonstrated significant weight gain, increases in maximal expiratory pressure, and increases in mean sustained inspiratory pressure.[114] This short-term study showed overall improvement in respiratory muscle function with refeeding.

Several enteral products (Pulmocare, Ross Laboratories; Nutrivent, Nestlé Enteral Nutrition, Respilor, Bristol-Myers) are marketed for the patient with pulmonary failure. These products contain a substantial amount of fat and a lower amount of carbohydrate than standard enteral products. Several nutrition support studies have been conducted in patients with COPD or acute respiratory failure. Ten stable COPD patients received a 920 kcal meal as a high-fat formula, or a high-carbohydrate formula, or a calorie-free control liquid in a randomized, crossover design.[115] Administration of the high-fat formula to these patients resulted in a significant decrease in minute ventilation, VCO_2, VO_2, RQ, and $PaCO_2$. Also, the patients were able to walk farther in 6 minutes and have higher Borg scores (perception of effort to breathe by the patient) when they received the high-fat formula.[115] In a similar study, 12 COPD patients were given a meal (1.3 × BEE divided by 3) as a high-fat or high-carbohydrate diet.[116] Administration of the high-fat diet to the patients resulted in a significant increase in VCO_2, VO_2, minute ventilation, and RQ when compared to the high-carbohydrate diet.[116] Thirty-two patients with acute respiratory failure were randomized to either a high-fat or high-carbohydrate formula at 1.5 times the BEE.[107] The patients receiving the high-fat formula demonstrated a significant decrease in RQ during mechanical ventilation, and RQ and VCO_2 during weaning. The median time to receive mechanical ventilation was lower in the high-fat group (4 versus 6 days); however, this difference was not statistically significant.[107] Thirty-six patients with stable COPD were given 530 kcal as either a high-fat or moderate-fat diet in a randomized, double-blind, crossover study.[117] Gastric emptying time as well as pulmonary measurements were done in this protocol. Gastric emptying was significantly better with the moderate-fat diet, and VO_2 and VCO_2 were increased without demonstrating a difference in pulmonary function. These data suggest that the lower RQ in previous studies could be attributed to retardation of gastric emptying (and obviously delayed absorption of nutrients) instead of the change in dietary content of fat.[117] Taken together, there now appears to be some limited data supporting the use of high-fat or moderately high fat enteral formulas in pulmonary patients. We suggest using the algorithm in Figure 131–4 as a guideline for when to use these products. Concentrated enteral formulas (e.g., 2 kcal/mL) would be helpful in feeding patients with severe ARDS or pulmonary edema, and in others who may require fluid restriction.

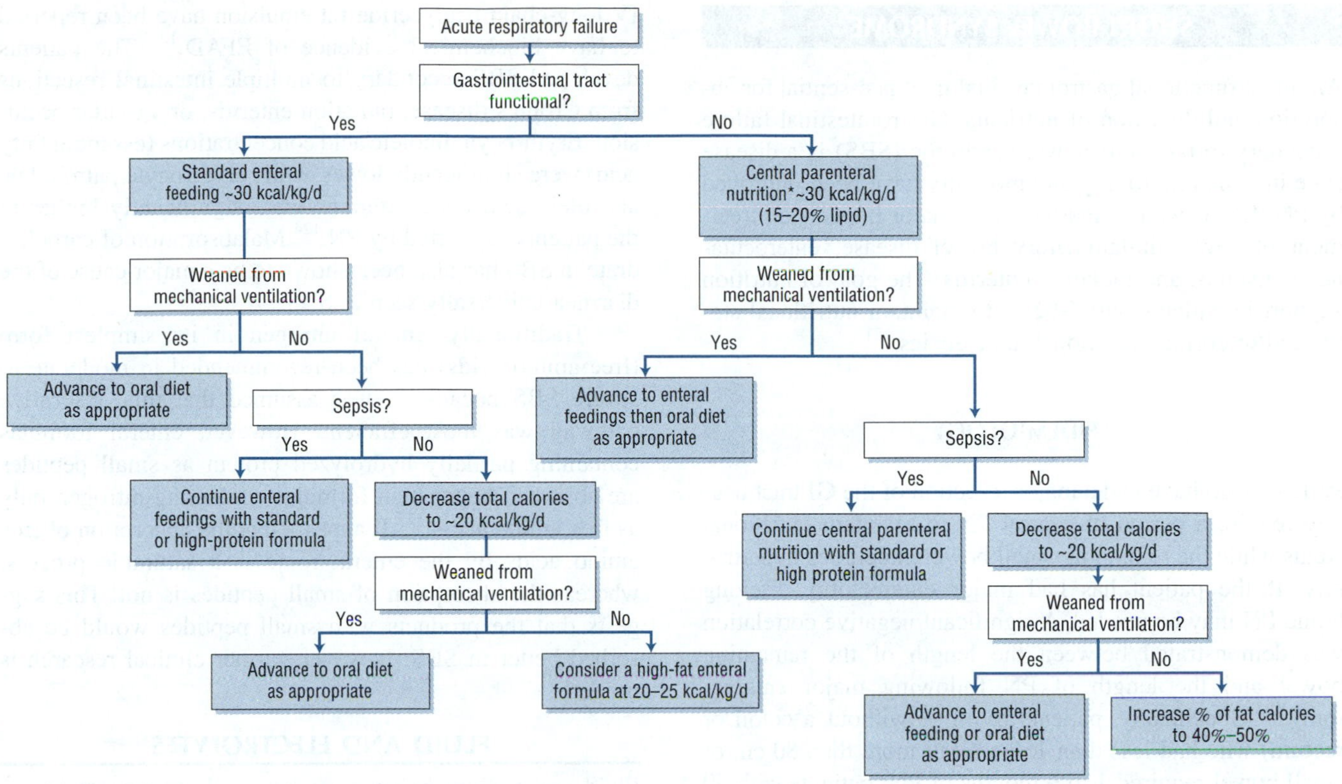

FIGURE 131–4. An algorithmic approach to nutrition support for the patient with acute respiratory failure. *(*Some centers would consider peripheral parenteral nutrition, especially if the patient would require nutrition support for ≤ 1 week.)*

There are some data addressing anabolic agents as adjunctive therapy to EN support in pulmonary patients. Improved lean body mass, maximal inspiratory pressure, and maximal exercise capacity have been reported in a small group of the COPD patients receiving growth hormone plus EN.[118] Studies focusing on improved clinical outcome will need to be conducted before expensive biotechnology products can be widely used as adjunctive therapy to nutrition support in undernourished patients with respiratory disease.

DESIGN AND INITIATION OF NUTRITIONAL REGIMEN

As there are no major alterations in substrate disposition among patients with pulmonary failure, moderate doses of intravenous carbohydrate, fat, and protein are appropriate in most conditions. Nonprotein calories should be administered as glucose and fat in a range from 55% to 80% carbohydrate and 20% to 45% lipid in ventilator-dependent patients because the oxidation of fat produces less CO_2 than glucose. Patients with sepsis and ARDS should be monitored closely during IVLE.[109] Moderate doses of lipid (e.g., 1 g/kg/d) should be infused over a 24-hour period each day in these patients.[119] A reasonable protein dose is 1.0 to 1.5 g/kg/d for the patient with stable COPD. Patients who are mechanically ventilated with superimposed illness may require higher doses of protein (1.5 to 2.5 g/kg/d). An approach to nutrition support in the patient with respiratory failure is shown in Figure 131–4.

Overfeeding with total calories is probably as important to avoid as overfeeding with carbohydrate. Talpers and colleagues[120] demonstrated a significant rise in V_{CO_2} in mechanically ventilated patients as total calories were increased from 1.0 to 1.5 and 2.0 times the BEE. When total calories were fixed at 1.3 times BEE, caloric composition (40% to 70% carbohydrate, 5% to 40% fat) had little effect on V_{CO_2}. In patients where fluid restriction is essential (e.g., severe ARDS) and PN is required, the use of the more concentrated amino acids and IVLE is indicated. The use of dextrose 70%, amino acids 15%, and lipid 20% or 30% can deliver substantial calories in 1.5 L/d. An empiric PN formula for the patient with respiratory failure is shown in Table 131–2.

EVALUATION OF THERAPEUTIC OUTCOMES

It is clear that undernutrition is highly correlated with both impaired pulmonary function and mortality. Clearly, interventional studies of sufficient magnitude and length are needed to measure the impact of improvement in nutrition status on major clinical outcome indicators. Measurements like the Borg score, where the patient's perception is assessed, will also be extremely important.

SHORT-BOWEL SYNDROME

An intact functional gastrointestinal tract is essential for absorption and digestion of nutrients. Gastrointestinal failure secondary to the short-bowel syndrome (SBS) is a disease state in which morbidity and mortality have been improved by PN. EN as well as PN have had major impacts on treatment of severe inflammatory bowel disease, enterocutaneous fistulas, and radiation enteritis. The goal of nutrition support in patients with SBS is to maintain nutritional status and/or correct nutritional deficiencies.[121]

EPIDEMIOLOGY

Patients who have had a major resection of the GI tract usually require a period of central PN to maintain nutritional status while the remaining small bowel undergoes hypertrophy. If the patient has had major enterectomy, lifelong home PN may be needed. A significant negative correlation was demonstrated between the length of the remaining bowel and the length of PN following major enterectomy.[122] Specifically, patients (with or without a colon or rectum) who had less than 150 cm but more than 80 cm of small bowel required 1 to 6 months of PN; patients with 50 to 70 cm of small bowel required 1 to 6 months of PN if they had an intact colon and rectum; patients with less than 70 cm and more than 40 cm of small bowel with a hemicolectomy required 6 to 12 months of PN; and patients with less than 60 cm of small bowel without a colon, or patients with less than 30 cm of small bowel with a colon, needed PN indefinitely.[122]

PATHOPHYSIOLOGY

CARBOHYDRATE, FAT, AND PROTEIN

Once absorbed, the macronutrients are processed normally in patients with gastrointestinal failure. If enteral nutrients cannot be absorbed appropriately, PN will be required temporarily or, in patients with extreme SBS, indefinitely. EN can often be used for provision of part of the required nutrients, with PN supplying the balance. In some patients with malabsorption managed solely on oral nutrition, doses of energy of 40 to 60 kcal/kg/d have been used to maintain nutrition status.[123]

Fat malabsorption has received the most attention in SBS because this process is complex. It involves pancreatic secretion of lipase, micelle formation with bile acids, absorption of micelles, and recycling of bile acids. Some patients with fat malabsorption have been treated with MCTs, which do not require pancreatic enzymes or bile acids for absorption. However, MCTs do not provide essential fatty acids, which could lead to EFAD. Long-chain fatty acids would need to be given orally or parenterally to prevent this disorder. Even patients with SBS receiving chronic PN with IV long-chain triglyceride fat emulsion have been reported to have biochemical evidence of EFAD.[124] The patients developed SBS secondary to multiple intestinal resections from Crohn's disease, radiation enteritis, or vascular occlusion. Erythrocyte linoleic acid concentrations (essential fatty acid) were significantly lower, while erythrocyte palmitoleic and oleic acid concentrations were significantly higher in the patients supported by PN.[124] Malabsorption of carbohydrate in SBS has also been shown to be a major cause of the diarrhea universally seen in SBS.

Traditionally, enteral nitrogen in its simplest form (free amino acids) has been recommended in moderate to severe SBS because it was assumed that this absorptive pathway was most efficient. However, enteral formulas containing partially hydrolyzed protein as small peptides are absorbed better than formulas containing nitrogen only as free amino acids.[125] It appears that the absorption of free amino acids by the enteral route is a saturable process, whereas the absorption of small peptides is not. This suggests that the products with small peptides would be absorbed better in SBS; however, further clinical research is needed.

FLUID AND ELECTROLYTES

Fluid and sodium balance are extremely important in patients with gastrointestinal failure because of significant extrarenal losses. Diarrhea is a hallmark disorder of SBS, and losses are difficult to measure. Stool frequency and consistency may aid in the calculation of the amount of replacement needed. Serum sodium concentration may not reflect sodium status, especially in dehydrated patients who may have elevated serum sodium values.

Losses of potassium from an ostomy in SBS can be as high as 200 mEq/d. Diarrheal fluid contains a high concentration of potassium, and patients may require fluid and potassium replacement if it cannot be controlled. Metabolic alkalosis, which may occur when a patient becomes dehydrated, accelerates the renal excretion of potassium, as all hydrogen ions are conserved in an attempt to correct the acid–base disorder. As bicarbonate ions are excreted renally, potassium is taken with them to maintain osmotic balance.

Patients with severe SBS invariably have fat malabsorption. Complexation of both dietary and secreted calcium in the remaining bowel by unabsorbed free fatty acids renders the ion unabsorbable, leading to negative calcium balance. Also, long-term PN has been associated with metabolic bone disease resulting in osteomalacia and osteoporosis. Excessive aluminum loading from protein hydrolysates (no longer used), parenteral vitamin D, and excessive infusion of protein all have been shown to cause hypercalciuria, a potential etiology of this disorder.

Considerable amounts of magnesium can be lost if diarrhea is severe and ostomy losses are large. Serum magnesium concentrations to assess magnesium status continue to be a problem, because only 1% to 2% of total body magnesium is found in the serum. Thus, patients with magnesium deficiency can maintain normal serum concentrations. The urinary excretion of magnesium over a 24-hour period has been suggested as a superior way to document magnesium deficiency in patients with gastrointestinal failure.[126] Sixteen outpatients with gastrointestinal failure (12 with SBS, 4 with diffuse small bowel disease) had a mean serum magnesium concentration of 1.7 mg/dL, with a mean urinary excretion of 19 mg/24 h. The sixteen age- and gender-matched controls had a mean serum magnesium concentration of 2 mg/dL, with a mean urinary excretion of 127 mg/24 h. These data suggest that urinary magnesium may be a superior way to assess magnesium status in outpatients who have gastrointestinal failure.[126]

ACID–BASE DISORDERS

Patients with severe SBS are at risk of developing dehydration and metabolic alkalosis. They can lose substantial amounts of chloride (60 to 140 mEq/L) and sodium (80 to 160 mEq/L) from ostomies and daily losses of fluid may vary from 0.5 to 10 L/d. Dehydration occurs when there are stable losses from an ostomy that are not replaced or when the patient is noncompliant with a restricted diet resulting in loss of more fluid than is taken in. Noncompliance with the infusion of appropriately prescribed fluids can also lead to dehydration. Patients who have SBS complicated by a pancreatic fistula lose considerable bicarbonate and may develop metabolic acidosis. Patients with severe diarrhea who have an intact colon will conserve sodium and chloride, resulting in considerable loss of potassium and bicarbonate and the development of metabolic acidosis. Quantifying fluid losses with particular attention to the sources of loss will aid in the acid–base management of these patients.

TRACE ELEMENTS

Much of the information that has been gained about trace element balance during specialized nutrition support has come from patients with gastrointestinal failure on long-term PN. This can, in part, be explained by the length of time required for a deficiency in a trace element to develop or be recognized (months to years). Also, signs or symptoms of deficiency may be underappreciated, and biochemical analysis is not available in all hospitals.

In patients receiving long-term PN, there are more data on zinc balance than for the other trace elements. Zinc replacement therapy for patients with extrarenal losses via the GI tract can be estimated as:

$$\text{ZN replacement (mg/d)} = 2 + 17.1a + 12.2b$$

where 2 represents normal urinary losses in mg, a is kilograms of stool or ileostomy output, and b is kilograms of small-bowel fluid from stoma/fistula or colostomy.

Because copper is excreted primarily in the bile, excessive losses of gastrointestinal fluid can have an impact on copper balance. Copper balance during PN also has been studied in patients with GI disease. Although requirements for patients with excessive GI losses were higher (0.4 to 0.5 mg/d) than those for patients with normal losses (0.3 mg/d), recommendations by the NAG-AMA exceed both of these doses. It is clear, however, that administration of PN without copper will result in depressed serum copper concentrations and eventually copper deficiency, which can lead to anemia.

A few patients with major enterectomy and gastrointestinal losses have developed chromium deficiency during long-term PN. It was suggested that these GI losses contributed to the chromium deficiency and glucose intolerance experienced by these patients.

Selenium should be administered to all patients receiving chronic PN, because an RDA has been established and there are several cases of cardiomyopathy reported in association with documented or presumed deficiency of this trace element during the administration of selenium-free PN. Decreased absorption of oral selenium has been reported in patients with SBS.[127]

VITAMINS

Most water-soluble vitamins (except vitamin B_{12}) are absorbed in the jejunum, so unless the patient has severe SBS, these can be maintained with an oral diet. Because patients with resection of the distal ileum cannot absorb vitamin B_{12}, the parenteral form of this vitamin needs to be administered. Patients with SBS who have fat malabsorption are prone to malabsorb the fat-soluble vitamins (A, D, E, and K). These vitamins can be supplemented orally if there is sufficient GI tract left. An aqueous form of vitamin E in a polyethylene glycol base was absorbed adequately after oral administration in a patient with SBS who had symptomatic vitamin E deficiency.[128] The patients with severe SBS who will be receiving PN should receive intravenous vitamins daily in virtually all cases.

▶ TREATMENT: Short-Bowel Syndrome

ADMINISTRATION ROUTES

After major gastrointestinal resection, EN should be introduced soon, as food is the stimulus for secretion of pancreatic enzymes and other trophic hormones thought essential for small-bowel hyperplasia. Historically, elemental diets or chemically defined formulas were initially used during EN in patients with SBS because the substrates are in the simplest, most easily digestible form. Currently, patients with SBS who are allowed to eat should receive standard diets with or without fat restriction.[129] These guidelines profoundly decrease the use of elemental or chemically defined formulas in the management of patients with SBS. As more patients with SBS are successfully transitioned to oral or enteral therapy, the need for long-term home PN would be reduced considerably. The degree of energy malabsorption is a measure of GI failure in patients with SBS and may be a useful guide for appropriate long-term therapy. For instance, a patient with SBS could have sequential measurements of total energy, carbohydrate, fat, and protein absorption to determine the dose of PN to meet nutritional needs. As small bowel adaption occurs, some patients could be weaned from PN. Weaning of chronic PN can be accomplished by gradually decreasing the volume of PN and IV solutions over several days to weeks. Once patients have been weaned to 1 liter, the frequency of administration can be decreased (e.g., every other day) until patients can support themselves entirely by the oral route. Another method of weaning would be to decrease the number of days of infusions per week.

Traditionally, patients with SBS who can maintain nutritional status by the oral route have been prescribed low-fat diets because fat malabsorption is a common disorder in these patients. More recent data have challenged this traditional approach and the patients have been given regular diets. Patients with SBS have demonstrated little change in ostomy output, monovalent cation loss, and in many cases, divalent cation loss when they were changed from a low-fat to a high-fat diet.

Some success has been reported in the treatment of severe SBS patients who were PN dependent using a combination of growth hormone, glutamine, and a high-carbohydrate diet.[130] Patients receiving this combination, in the initial 3- to 4-week study period, demonstrated a significant decrease in stool output and an increase in protein absorption. Forty-seven patients who had an average jejunal–ileal length of either 50 cm with all or part of a colon, or 102 cm with no colon, were further studied while receiving glutamine and the modified diet at home. After an average of 1 year of treatment, 40% of the patients were completely weaned from PN and 40% were receiving a reduced dose of PN.[130]

SURGICAL THERAPY

Currently, small bowel transplantation is in its infancy and many patients with SBS will become potential candidates for this procedure as more experience is gained.[131] As more patients with SBS survive with the administration of specialized nutrition support or are treated with small bowel transplantation, the management of these patients' pharmacotherapy will need to be addressed and studied. There will undoubtedly be a period in the immediate postoperative period where the patient will require PN. As oral nutrients are introduced and the gastrointestinal graft becomes "functional," medications will invariably be changed to oral dosage forms. Currently, only limited information on pharmacotherapy in patients with SBS is available.[132]

DESIGN AND INITIATION OF NUTRITIONAL REGIMEN

There are usually no substrate alterations in these patients, so standard crystalline amino acids, glucose, and intravenous lipids may be used either to maintain nutrition status or to correct nutritional deficits. An example of a PN formula for the patient with SBS is given in Table 131–2.

Often, the only modification to standard PN or EN regimen is an increase in fluids to replace losses and maintain a urine output above 1000 mL/d. Substantial losses of any fluids (e.g., from jejunostomy or colostomy) need consideration when preparing the nutritional formula.

Losses of potassium from an ostomy in SBS can be as high as 200 mEq/d. If these losses are stable, they can be replaced by adding supplemental potassium into the PN formula. Magnesium is also usually replaced in the PN formula in patients with severe SBS. Oral replacement of magnesium with gluconate or oxide salts may be used in less severe cases, but excessive use of oral magnesium results in diarrhea, which may exacerbate the deficit.

Patients on long-term PN will need additional calcium added to their formula to maintain calcium balance. It therefore appears reasonable to measure a 24-hour urine excretion of calcium before a patient is sent home with PN. This will help identify patients who may have trouble maintaining calcium balance. It appears that bone resorption during PN is greater during the first few months of therapy.[133] For patients with SBS who are able to maintain nutrition status on oral nutrition, calcium supplementation (1 to 4 g/d) often is required.

Excessive zinc losses via the GI tract can be well quantified. Therefore, patients with SBS who require PN should have zinc added to their formula in doses that are typically above the NAG-AMA recommendations. Patients with extensive GI losses should also be given chromium 20 μg/d during PN instead of the standard dose of 12 μg/d due to documented cases of chromium deficiency in this patient population.

QUALITY OF LIFE

Chronic use of PN or EN in patients with gastrointestinal failure results in both physical and life-style changes. First, patients who are to receive chronic intravenous therapy usually have a permanent access device placed into a large vein. Implanted ports (e.g., Portacath) or permanent central venous catheters (e.g., Hickman catheter) are most commonly used for long-term administration of PN. These are placed so that the tip of the catheter resides in the superior or inferior vena cava, and they exit at the midline of the chest. Patients receiving long-term EN usually have a permanent feeding enterostomy placed for ease of administration. The most commonly used enterostomies for enteral feeding are the gastrostomy and jejunostomy (see Chap. 129). All of these access devices are visible at the point that they exit through the skin, and have the potential of causing public embarrassment.

PN is very expensive (average of $100,000/y) and becomes a huge economic burden when needed for a prolonged period. Quality of life issues have been tabulated for patients receiving prolonged PN.[134] The patients' mean depression scores were higher (suggesting mild depression) than the caregivers' scores for those patients. The Quality of Life Index mean score was similar to those patients who were receiving chronic hemodialysis or peritoneal dialysis. Self-esteem was generally reported as normal by both patient and caregiver. Fatigue was a major problem in these patients, and it caused them to miss several important events. Two-thirds of the patients reported difficulties with the PN management, their physical condition, embarrassment, or emotional reactions.[134]

EVALUATION OF THERAPEUTIC OUTCOMES

The most comprehensive and thorough analysis of the clinical outcome of patients receiving home PN or EN comes from the Medicare and the North American Home Parenteral and Enteral Patient Registry.[135] It was estimated that 40,000 and 152,000 patients in the United States were receiving home PN and EN support, respectively. The number of patients receiving either PN or EN at home more than doubled between 1989 and 1992. Patients with GI failure—which included those with Crohn's disease, ischemic bowel disease, motility disorders, and congenital bowel defects—had relatively good outcomes, especially when compared to the groups with cancer or AIDS. The patients with GI failure had a 87% annual survival rate and a 50% to 75% likelihood of complete rehabilitation. Sepsis, metabolic disorders, and mechanical problems with catheters resulted in one to two hospitalizations per year for all patients.[140]

▶ PRINCIPLES OF PHARMACOTHERAPY

- Carbohydrate calories absorbed via continuous renal replacement therapy must be accounted for when designing the PN/EN regimen of the patient with acute renal failure.
- Lipid intolerance is common in ARF, requiring careful monitoring of serum triglyceride concentrations before and during IVLE administration.
- Protein requirements of the patient with ARF are highly variable and depend on PCR and dialytic losses of protein.
- Standard mixed amino acids should be used rather than essential amino acid preparations in ARF.
- The nondialyzed patient with oliguric ARF should receive a PN/EN formula concentrated in a small volume.
- Empiric PN formulations for patients with ARF will typically contain minimal potassium, phosphorous, and magnesium. With refeeding, additional amounts of these electrolytes may need to be added.
- Sodium and potassium salts, if added to the PN formula for the patient with ARF, should be added as acetate salts.
- More than one-half of chronic renal failure patients experience hyperglycemia. Patients with ESRD who receive CAPD absorb substantial amounts (approximately 500 kcal/d) of glucose from their peritoneal dialysate.
- Dialysate protein losses must be accounted for and added into the PN/EN nutritional plan for CRF patients. Peritoneal protein losses in patients treated by CAPD range from 6 to 7 g/d. The amount of protein lost via HD depends on membrane used and presence of reuse (typical range is from 6 to 12 g/dialysis).
- Although hyperkalemia and hyperphosphatemia are common early in the course of PN/EN with CRF patients, refeeding of these patients can result in hypokalemia and hypophosphatemia, warranting careful addition of these electrolytes to the PN/EN regimen.
- Calorically dense, low electrolyte enteral formulas may prove helpful in providing EN to the CRF or ESRD patient with preexisting electrolyte disturbances or volume overload. Likewise, the PN formula for these patients can be volume restricted by using higher concentrations of dextrose and amino acids ($D_{35}W$ and 7.5% amino acid final concentrations).
- Patients with alcoholic hepatitis or cirrhosis are hypermetabolic.
- Hyperglycemia is common in cirrhosis. Patients with fulminant hepatitis are prone instead to hypoglycemia.
- Increased serum triglyceride and FFA concentrations are encountered in patients with hepatic failure. IVLE should be used in patients with liver failure only to prevent EFAD when serum triglyceride concentrations exceed 300 mg/dL.
- Overzealous use of protein in patients with liver disease invariably results in hepatic encephalopathy. A therapeutic window (40 to 80 g/d) for protein intake exists.
- Patients with liver disease may require zinc supplementation, while receiving restricted amounts of copper and manganese.
- Folic acid and thiamine supplementation is important in patients with liver disease for the prevention of anemia and Wernicke's encephalopathy, respectively.
- For the OLT patient, energy provision of 1.2 times BEE with at least 1.2 g/kg/d of protein is appropriate.
- The high prevalence of postoperative hyperglycemia in the OLT patient mandates starting PN/EN slowly and with a low dextrose concentration formulation.
- Sodium rarely needs to be added to the PN solution of an OLT patient.
- Supplemental doses of calcium and magnesium are frequently required for the OLT patient.
- Pre-OLT patients frequently demonstrate depressed serum concentrations of zinc and vitamin A; these usually normalize post-OLT, obviating the need for further supplementation.
- Nonseptic patients with acute respiratory failure require only 10% to 20% above BEE to meet nutritional needs, whereas patients who are septic need to be given energy at 30% to 40% above BEE.
- High-fat or moderately high-fat enteral formulas should be considered in pulmonary patients.
- Undernourished pulmonary patients have a blunted response to hypercapnia that improves with nutritional support. However, excessive protein intake

should be avoided, as it may increase pulmonary workload.

- Excessive infusions of salt and water should be avoided in pulmonary patients, as they may exacerbate already compromised pulmonary function.
- The incidence of hypophosphatemia is higher in patients with pulmonary disease than in the general hospitalized population.
- Protein and energy requirements are relatively unchanged from normal in the short-bowel syndrome patient who requires PN.
- The nutritional regimen in SBS should include extra fluid to replace GI losses and maintain urine output.
- Complexation of calcium by unabsorbed FFAs renders the ion unabsorbable. Thus, SBS patients require increased amounts of calcium in their PN formula, or supplemental calcium orally.
- Considerable GI losses of potassium and magnesium also occur. Thus, SBS patients frequently require above-normal doses of these electrolytes.
- Above-normal doses of zinc and chromium should be given to SBS patients with extensive GI losses.
- SBS patients with resection of the distal ileum require parenteral vitamin B_{12} administration.
- As small bowel adaptation occurs, some SBS patients receiving PN can be successfully transitioned to EN.

REFERENCES

1. Kopple JD. Effect of nutrition of morbidity and mortality in maintenance dialysis patients. Am J Kidney Dis 1994;24:1002–1009.
2. Yang CS, Chen SW, Chiang CH, et al. Effect of increasing dialysis dose on serum albumin and mortality in hemodialysis patients. Am J Kidney Dis 1996;27:380–386.
3. Owen WF, Lew NL, Liu Y, et al. The urea reduction ratio and serum albumin concentration as predictors of mortality in patients undergoing hemodialysis. N Engl J Med 1993;329:1001–1006.
4. Lowrie EG, Lew NL. Death risk in hemodialysis patients: The urea reduction ratio and serum albumin concentrations as predictors of mortality in patients undergoing hemodialysis. Am J Kidney Dis 1990;15:458–482.
5. Spiegel DM, Breyer JA. Serum albumin: A predictor of long-term outcome in peritoneal dialysis patients. Am J Kid Dis 1994;23:283–285.
6. Struijk DG, Krediet RT, Koomen GC, et al. The effect of serum albumin at the start of CAPD treatment on patient survival. Perit Dial Int 1994;14:121–126.
7. Schneeweiss B, Graninger W, Stockenhuber F, et al. Energy metabolism in acute and chronic renal failure. Am J Clin Nutr 1990;52:596–601.
8. Ikizler TA, Greene JH, Yenicesu M, et al. Nitrogen balance in hospitalized chronic hemodialysis patients. Kidney Int 1996;50(suppl):S53–S56.
9. Molina MF, Riella MC. Nutritional support in the patient with renal failure. Crit Care Clin 1995;11:685–704.
10. Ikizler TA, Hakim RM. Nutrition in end-stage renal disease. Kidney Int 1996;50:343–357.
11. Ikizler TA, Himmelfarb J. Nutrition in acute renal failure. Adv Ren Replace Ther 1997;4:54–63.
12. Kierdorf HP. The nutritional management of acute renal failure in the intensive care unit. New Horiz 1995;3:699–707.
13. Alvestrand A. Nutritional aspects in patients with acute renal failure/multiorgan failure. Blood Purif 1996;14:109–114.
14. Bouffard Y, Viale JP, Annat G, et al. Energy expenditure in the acute renal failure patient mechanically ventilated. Intensive Care Med 1987;13:401–404.
15. Fougue D. Insulin-like growth factor 1 resistance in chronic renal failure. Miner Electrolyte Metab 1996;22:133–137.
16. Keane WF. Lipids and the kidney. Kidney Int 1994;46:910–920.
17. Gupta KL, Majumdar S, Sakhuja V. Postheparin lipolytic activity in acute and chronic renal failure. Ren Fail 1994;16:609–615.
18. Maheux P, Azhar S, Kern PA, et al. Relationship between insulin-mediated glucose disposal and regulation of plasma and adipose tissue lipoprotein lipase. Diabetologia 1997;40:850–858.
19. Chima SC, Meyer L, Hummel C, et al. Protein catabolic rate in patients with acute renal failure on continuous arteriovenous hemofiltration and total parenteral nutrition. J Am Soc Nephrol 1993;3:1516–1521.
20. Ikizler TA, Greene JH, Wingard RL, et al. Nitrogen balance in acute renal failure (ARF) patients. J Am Soc Nephrol 1995;6:466. Abstract.
21. Macias WL, Alaka KJ, Murphy MH, et al. Impact of the nutritional regimen on protein catabolism and nitrogen balance in patients with acute renal failure. JPEN J Parenter Enteral Nutr 1996;20:56–62.
22. Zamir O, Hasselgren PO, Kunkel SL, et al. Evidence that tumor necrosis factor participates in the regulation of muscle proteolysis during sepsis. Arch Surg 1992;127:170–174.
23. Cooney RN, Kimball SR, Vary TC. Regulation of skeletal muscle protein turnover during sepsis: Mechanisms and mediators. Shock 1997;7:1–16.
24. Hynote ED, McCamish MA, Depner TA, Davis PA. Amino acid losses during hemodialysis: Effects of high-solute flux and parenteral nutrition in acute renal failure. JPEN J Parenter Enteral Nutr 1995;19:15–21.
25. Frankenfield DC, Badellino MM, Reynolds HN, et al. Amino acid loss and plasma concentration during continuous hemodiafiltration. JPEN J Parenter Enteral Nutr 1993;17:551–561.
26. Druml W, Fischer M, Liebisch B, et al. Elimination of amino acids in renal failure. Am J Clin Nutr 1994;60:418–423.
27. Packman KS, Demeure MJ. Indications for parathyroidectomy and extent of treatment for patients with secondary hyperparathyroidism. Surg Clin North Am 1995;75:465–482.
28. Gallieni M, Brancaccio D, Cozzolino M, Sabbioni E. Trace elements in renal failure: Are they clinically important? Nephrol Dial Transplant 1996;11:1232–1235.
29. Gallieni M, Pietra R, Canavese C, et al. Trace elements in serum and tissues of dialysis patients. J Am Soc Nephrol 1995;6:530. Abstract.
30. Wolk R. Micronutrition in dialysis. Nutr Clin Prac 1993;8:267–276.
31. Guidelines for essential trace element preparations for parenteral use. A statement by an expert panel. AMA Department of Foods and Nutrition. JAMA 1979;241:2051–2054.
32. Frankenfield DC, Reynolds HN. Nutritional effect of continuous hemodiafiltration. Nutrition 1995;11:388–393.
33. Seidner DL, Matarese LE, Steiger E. Nutritional care of the critically ill patient with renal failure. Semin Nephrol 1994;14:53–63.
34. Monaghan R, Walters JM, Clancey SM, et al. Uptake of glucose during continuous arteriovenous hemofiltration. Crit Care Med 1993;21:1159–1163.
35. Frankenfield DC, Reynolds HN, Badellino MM, Wiles CE. Glucose dynamics during continuous hemodiafiltration and total parenteral nutrition. Intensive Care Med 1995;21:1016–1022.

36. Bellomo R, Martin H, Parkin G, et al. Continuous arteriovenous haemodiafiltration in the critically ill: influence on major nutrient balances. Intensive Care Med 1991;17:399–402.
37. Sigler MH, Teehan BP. Solute transport in continuous hemodialysis: A new treatment for acute renal failure. Kidney Int 1987;32:562–571.
38. Druml W, Fischer M, Sertl S, et al. Fat elimination in acute renal failure: Long chain versus medium chain triglycerides. Am J Clin Nutr 1992;55:468–472.
39. Kierdorf H. Continuous versus intermittent treatment: Clinical results in acute renal failure. Contrib Nephrol 1991;93:1–12.
40. Bellomo R, Seacombe J, Daskalakis M, et al. A prospective comparative study of moderate versus high protein intake for critically ill patients with acute renal failure. Ren Fail 1997;1:111–120.
41. Sponsel H, Conger JD. Is parenteral nutrition therapy of value in acute renal failure patients? Am J Kid Dis 1995;25:96–102.
42. Fiaccadori E, Lombardi M, Leonardi S, et al. Outcome of malnutrition in acute renal failure. J Am Soc Nephrol 1996;7:1372. Abstract.
43. Kopple JD. McCollum Award Lecture, 1996: Protein–energy malnutrition in maintenance dialysis patients. Am J Clin Nutr 1997;65: 1544–1557.
44. Avram MM, Mittman N, Bonomini L, et al. Markers for survival in dialysis: A seven-year prospective study. Am J Kid Dis 1995;26:209–219.
45. Avram MM, Bonomini LV, Sreedhara R, Mittman N. Predictive value of nutritional markers (albumin, creatinine, cholesterol, and hematocrit) for patients on dialysis for up to 30 years. Am J Kid Dis 1996;28:910–917.
46. Chan E, Montgomery PA. Administration of insulin by continuous ambulatory peritoneal dialysis. Pharmacotherapy 1993;13:455–460.
47. Lacour B, DiGiulio S, Chanard J, et al. Carnitine improves lipid anomalies in hemodialysis patients. Lancet 1980;2:763–764.
48. Guarnieri GF, Ranieri F, Toigo G, et al. Lipid-lowering effect of carnitine in chronically uremic patients treated with maintenance hemodialysis. Am J Clin Nutr 1980;33:1489–1492.
49. Golpher TA, Wolfson M, Ahmad S, et al. Multicenter trial of L-carnitine in maintenance hemodialysis patients. I. Carnitine concentrations and lipid effects. Kidney Int 1990;38:904–911.
50. Zeller KR, Whittaker E, Sullivan L, et al. Effect of restricting dietary protein on the progression of renal failure in patients with insulin-dependent diabetes mellitus. N Engl J Med 1991;324:78–83.
51. Teschan PE. Effects of dietary protein restriction on the progression of advanced renal disease in the modification of diet in renal disease study. Am J Kid Dis 1996;27:652–663.
52. Effects of dietary protein restriction on the progression of moderate renal disease in the modification of diet in renal disease study. J Am Soc Nephrol 1996;7:2616–2626.
53. Locatelli F, Buccianti G, Alberti D, et al. Prospective randomized multicenter trial of effect of protein restriction on progression of chronic renal insufficiency. Lancet 1991;337:1299–1304.
54. Kabanda A, Goffin E, Bernard A, et al. Factors influencing serum levels and peritoneal clearances of low molecular weight proteins in continuous ambulatory peritoneal dialysis. Kidney Int 1995;48: 1946–1952.
55. Harty JC, Boulton H, Venning MC, Gokal R. Is peritoneal permeability an adverse risk factor for malnutrition in CAPD patients? Miner Electrolyte Metab 1996;22:97–101.
56. Ikizler TA, Flakoll PJ, Parker RA, Hakim RM. Amino acid and albumin losses during hemodialysis. Kidney Int 1994;46:830–837.
57. Bonomini M, Di Paolo B, De Risio F, et al. Effects of zinc supplementation in chronic hemodialysis patients. Nephrol Dial Transplant 1993;8:1166–1168.
58. Gallieni M, Padovese P, Pietra R, et al. Chromium overload in dialysis patients. J Am Soc Nephrol 1994;5:447. Abstract.
59. Thomson NM, Stevens BJ, Humphrey TJ, et al. Comparison of trace elements in peritoneal dialysis, hemodialysis, and uremia. Kidney Int 1983;23:9–14.
60. Bonomini M, Albertazzi A. Selenium in uremia. Artif Organs 1995; 19:443–448.
61. Capelli JP, Kushner H, Camiscioli TC, et al. Effect of intradialytic parenteral nutrition on mortality rates in end-stage renal disease care. Am J Kid Dis 1994;23:808–816.
62. Chertow GM, Ling J, Lew NL, et al. The association of intradialytic parenteral nutrition administration with survival in hemodialysis patients. Am J Kid Dis 1994;24:912–920.
63. Siskind MS, Lien YH. Effect of intradialytic parenteral nutrition on quality of life in hemodialysis patients. Int J Artif Organs 1993;16: 599–603.
64. Kopple JD, Foulks CJ, Piraino B, et al. Proposed health care financing administration guidelines for reimbursement of enteral and parenteral nutrition. Am J Kidney Dis 1995;26:995–997.
65. Chazot C, Shahmir E, Matias B, Laidlaw S, Koppel JD. Dialytic nutrition: Provision of amino acids in dialysate during hemodialysis. Kidney Internat 1997;52:1663–1670.
66. Kopple JD, Bernard D, Messana J, et al. Treatment of malnourished CAPD patients with an amino acid based dialysate. Kidney Int 1995; 47:1148–1157.
67. Arfeen S, Goodship THJ, Kirkwood A, Ward MK. The nutritional/metabolic and hormonal effects of 8 weeks of continuous ambulatory peritoneal dialysis with a 1% amino acid solution. Clin Nephrol 1990; 33:192–199.
68. Dombron NV, Prutis K, Tong M, et al. Six month overnight intraperitoneal amino acid infusion in continuous ambulatory peritoneal dialysis (CAPD) patients—no effect on nutritional status. Peritoneal Dial Int 1990;10:79–84.
69. Patel C, Nicol A. Adaptation of African-American cultural and food preferences in end-stage renal disease diets. Adv Ren Replace Ther 1997;4:30–39.
70. Murrell KF. Nuances of the Mexican-American renal diet. Nephrol News Issues 1995;9:35–36.
71. Hirsch S, Bunout D, Maza P, et al. Controlled trial on nutrition supplementation in outpatients with symptomatic alcoholic cirrhosis. JPEN J Parenter Enteral Nutr 1993;17:119–124.
72. Mendenhall CL, Moritz TE, Roselle GA, et al. Protein energy malnutrition in severe alcoholic hepatitis: Diagnosis and response to treatment. JPEN J Parenter Enteral Nutr 1995;19:258–265.
73. Nompleggi DJ, Bonkovsky HL. Nutritional supplementation in chronic liver disease: An analytical review. Hepatology 1994;19: 518–533.
74. Muller MJ, Loyal S, Schwarze M, et al. Resting energy expenditure and nutritional state in patients with liver cirrhosis before and after liver transplant. Clin Nutr 1994;13:145–152.
75. Muller MJ, Boker KH, Selberg O. Are patients with liver cirrhosis hypermetabolic? Clin Nutr 1994;13:131–144.
76. Petrides AS, DeFrenzo RA. Glucose and insulin metabolism in cirrhosis. J Hepatol 1989;8:107–114.
77. Schenker S, Halff GA. Nutritional therapy in alcoholic liver disease. Semin Liver Dis 1993;13:196–209.
78. Marsano L, McClain CJ. Nutrition and alcoholic liver disease. JPEN J Parenter Enteral Nutr 1991;15:337–344.
79. Salem M, Muhoz R, Chernow B. Hypomagnesemia in critical illness: A common and clinically important problem. Crit Care Clin 1991;7:225–252.
80. McClain CJ, Marsano L, Burk RF, Bacon B. Trace metals in liver disease. Semin Liver Dis 1991;11:321–339.
81. Hauser RA, Zesiewicz TA, Rosemurgy AS, et al. Manganese intoxication and chronic liver failure. Ann Neurol 1994;36:871–875.
82. Krieger D, Krieger S, Jansen O, et al. Manganese and chronic hepatic encephalopathy. Lancet 1995;346:270–274.
83. Korpela H, Kumpulainen J, Luoma PV, et al. Decreased serum selenium in alcoholics as related to liver structure and function. Am J Clin Nutr 1985;42:147–151.

84. Janczewska I, Ericzon BG, Eriksson LS. Influence of orthotopic liver transplantation on serum vitamin A levels in patients with chronic liver disease. Scand J Gastroenterol 1995;30:68–71.
85. Ichida T, Shibasaki K, Muto Y, et al. Clinical study of an enteral branched-chain amino acid solution in decompensated liver cirrhosis with hepatic encephalopathy. Nutrition 1995;11(suppl 2):238–244.
86. Bianchi GP, Marchesini G, Fabbri A, et al. Vegetable versus animal protein diet in cirrhotic patients with chronic encephalopathy: A randomized cross-over comparison. J Intern Med 1993;233:385–392.
87. Record KE, Kolpek JH, Rapp RP. Long chain versus medium chain length triglycerides. Nutr Clin Prac 1986;1:129–136.
88. Marchesini G, Fabbri A, Bianchi G, et al. Zinc supplementation and amino acid-nitrogen metabolism in patients with advanced cirrhosis. Hepatology 1996;23:1084–1092.
89. Delafosse B, Faure JL, Bouffard Y, et al. Liver transplantation—Energy expenditure, nitrogen loss, and substrate oxidation rate in the first 2 postoperative days. Transplant Proc 1989;21:2453–2454.
90. Plevak DJ, DiCecco Sr, Wiesner RH, et al. Nutritional support for liver transplantation: Identifying caloric and protein requirements. Mayo Clin Proc 1994;69:225–230.
91. Dresner LS, Andersen DK, Kahng KU, et al. Effects of cyclosporine on glucose metabolism. Surgery 1989;106:163–170.
92. Iapichino G, Radrizzani D, Bonetti G, et al. Early metabolic treatment after liver transplant: Amino acid tolerance. Intensive Care Med 1995;21:802–807.
93. Pescovitz MD, Mehta PL, Jindal RM, et al. Zinc deficiency and its repletion following liver transplantation in humans. Clin Transplant 1996;10:256–260.
94. Pan SH, Lopez RR, Sher LS, et al. Enhanced oral cyclosporine absorption with water-soluble vitamin E early after liver transplantation. Pharmacotherapy 1996;16:59–65.
95. Hasse JM, Blue LS, Liepa GU, et al. Early enteral nutrition in patients undergoing liver transplantation. JPEN J Parenter Enteral Nutr 1995;19:437–443.
96. Wicks C, Somasundaram S, Bjarnason I, et al. Comparison of enteral feedings and total parenteral nutrition after liver transplantation. Lancet 1994;344:837–840.
97. Mehta PL, Alaka KJ, Filo RS, Leapman SB. Nutritional support following liver transplantation: Comparison of jejunal versus parenteral routes. Clin Transplant 1995;9:364–369.
98. Selberg O, Bottcher J, Tusch G, et al. Identification of high- and low-risk patients before liver transplantation: A prospective cohort study of nutritional and metabolic parameters in 150 patients. Hepatology 1997;25:652–657.
99. Reilly J, Mehta R, Teperman L, et al. Nutritional support after liver transplantation: A randomized prospective study. JPEN J Parenter Enteral Nutr 1990;14:386.
100. Wilson DO, Rogers RM, Wright EC, Anthonisen NR. Body weight in chronic obstructive pulmonary disease. Am Rev Resp Dis 1989; 139:1435–1438.
101. Mowatt-Larssen CA, Brown RO. Specialized nutrition support in respiratory disease. Clin Pharm 1993;12:276–292.
102. Sahebjami H, Doers JT, Render ML, Bond TL. Anthropometric and pulmonary function test profiles of outpatients with stable chronic obstructive pulmonary disease. Am J Med 1993;94:469–474.
103. Gray-Donald K, Gibbons L, Shapiro SH, et al. Nutritional status and mortality in chronic obstructive pulmonary disease. Am J Respir Crit Care Med 1996;153:961–966.
104. Schols AM, Fredrix EW, Soeters PB, et al. Resting energy expenditure in patients with chronic obstructive pulmonary disease. Am J Clin Nutr 1991;54:983–987.
105. Baarends EM, Schols AM, Lichtenbelt WD, Wouters EF. Analysis of body water compartments in relation to tissue depletion in clinically stable patients with chronic obstructive pulmonary disease. Am J Clin Nutr 1997;65:88–94.
106. Liggett SB, Renfro AD. Energy expenditure of mechanically ventilated nonsurgical patients. Chest 1990;98:682–686.
107. Van den Berg B, Bogaard JM, Hop WC. High fat, low carbohydrate, enteral feeding in patients weaning from the ventilator. Intensive Care Med 1994;20:470–475.
108. Hwang TL, Huang SL, Chen MF. Effects of intravenous fat emulsion on respiratory failure. Chest 1990;97:934–938.
109. Venus B, Smith RA, Patel C, Sandoval E. Hemodynamic and gas exchange alterations during Intralipid infusion in patients with adult respiratory distress snydrome. Chest 1989;95:1278–1281.
110. Simmons RS, Berdine GG, Seidenfeld JJ, et al. Fluid balance and the adult respiratory distress syndrome. Am Rev Resp Dis 1987;135: 924–929.
111. Marik PE, Bedigian MK. Refeeding hypophosphatemia in critically ill patients in an intensive care unit. Arch Surg 1996;131:1043–1047.
112. Clark CL, Sacks GS, Dickerson RN, et al. Treatment of hypophosphatemia in patients receiving specialized nutrition support using a graduated dosing scheme: Results from a prospective clinical trial. Crit Care Med 1995;23:1504–1511.
113. Kudsk KA, Li J, Renegar KB. Loss of upper respiratory tract immunity with parenteral feeding. Ann Surg 1996;223:629–638.
114. Whittaker JS, Ryan CF, Buckley PA, Road JD. The effects of refeeding on peripheral and respiratory muscle function in malnourished chronic obstructive pulmonary disease patients. Am Rev Resp Dis 1990;142:283–288.
115. Efthimiou J, Mounsey PJ, Benson DN, et al. Effect of carbohydrate rich versus fat rich loads on gas exchange and walking performance in patients with chronic obstructive lung disease. Thorax 1992;47: 451–456.
116. Kuo CD, Shiao GM, Lee JD. The effects of high-fat and high-carbohydrate diet loads on gas exchange and ventilation in COPD patients and normal subjects. Chest 1993;104:189–196.
117. Akrabawi SS, Mobarhan S, Stoltz RR, Ferguson PW. Gastric emptying, pulmonary function, gas exchange, and respiratory quotient after feeding a moderate versus high fat enteral formula meal in chronic obstructive disease patients. Nutrition 1996;12:260–265.
118. Burdet L, deMuralt B, Schutz Y, et al. Administration of growth hormone to underweight patients with chronic obstructive pulmonary disease. A prospective, randomized, controlled study. Am J Respir Crit Care Med 1997;156:1800–1806.
119. Skeie B, Askanazi J, Rothkopf MM, et al. Intravenous fat emulsion and lung function: A review. Crit Care Med 1988;16:183–194.
120. Talpers SS, Romberger DJ, Bunce SB, Pingleton SK. Nutritionally associated increased carbon dioxide production. Excess total calories vs. high proportion of carbohydrate calories. Chest 1992;102: 551–555.
121. Shanbhogue LK, Molenaar JC. Short bowel syndrome: Metabolic and surgical management. Br J Surg 1994;8:486–499.
122. Gouttebel MC, Saint-Aubert B, Astre C, Joyeux H. Total parenteral nutrition needs in different types of short bowel syndrome. Dig Dis Sci 1986;31:718–723.
123. Messing B, Pigot F, Morin MC, et al. Intestinal absorption of free oral hyperalimentation in the very short bowel syndrome. Gastroenterology 1991;100:1502–1508.
124. Abushufa R, Reed P, Weinkove C, et al. Essential fatty acid status in patients on long-term home parenteral nutrition. JPEN J Parenter Enteral Nutr 1995;19:286–290.
125. Brinson RR, Hanumanthu SK, Pitts WM. A reappraisal of the peptide-based enteral formulas: Clinical applications. Nutr Clin Pract 1989;4:211–217.
126. Fleming CR, George L, Stoner GL, et al. The importance of urinary magnesium values in patients with gut failure. Mayo Clin Proc 1996; 71:21–24.
127. Sandstrom B, Davidsson L, Bosaeus I, et al. Selenium status and absorption of zinc (^{65}Zn), selenium (^{75}Se), and manganese (^{54}Mn) in patients with short bowel syndrome. Eur J Clin Nutr 1990;44: 697–703.

128. Traber MG, Schiano TD, Steephen AC, et al. Efficacy of water-soluble vitamin E in the treatment of vitamin E malabsorption in short-bowel syndrome. Am J Clin Nutr 1994;59:1270–1274.
129. Lennard-Jones JE. Review article: Practical management of the short bowel. Aliment Pharmocol Ther 1994;8:563–577.
130. Byrne TA, Persinger RL, Young LS, et al. A new treatment for patients with short-bowel syndrome: Growth hormone, glutamine, and a modified diet. Ann Surg 1995;222:243–255.
131. Vanderhoof JA, Langnas AN. Short-bowel syndrome in children and adults. Gastroenterology 1997;113:1767–1778.
132. McFadden MA, DeLegge MH, Kirby DF. Medication delivery in the short-bowel syndrome. JPEN J Parenter Enteral Nutr 1993:17: 180–186.
133. Pironi L, Maghetti A, Zolezzi C, et al. Bone turnover in patients on home parenteral nutrition: A longitudinal observation by biochemical markers. Clin Nutr 1996;15:157–163.
134. Smith CE. Quality of life in long-term total parenteral nutrition patients and their family caregivers. JPEN J Parenter Enteral Nutr 1993;17: 501–506.
135. Howard L, Ament M, Fleming CR, et al. Current use and clinical outcome of home parenteral and enteral nutrition therapies in the United States. Gastroenterology 1995;109:355–365.

132

OBESITY

John V. St. Peter, PharmD, BCPS, and Mehmood A. Khan, MD, FACE

Obesity, a state of excess body fat stores, is considered a disease by some, and predominantly a social problem by others. Each year millions of Americans—an estimated 15% to 35% of the population—resolve to lose weight, especially at the start of the calendar year.[1–4] Within months, weeks, or even days, the vast majority give up on this resolve without any weight loss. Many others will ultimately regain the weight that they lost initially. An estimated $30 to $50 billion is spent each year by Americans with little or no documented improvement.[5,6] Prospective evidence to support weight loss programs is scanty, inconclusive, and often controversial. Observational epidemiologic studies show that overall mortality parallels body weight increases above an optimal level.[7] This evidence is strongest for adults between the ages of 30 and 44 years. In older age groups, excess body weight increases the risk of death, but the degree of impact diminishes with age.[8] In this chapter we review the epidemiology, pathophysiology and therapeutic approaches for obesity. Although nonpharmacologic treatment modalities are discussed, the pharmacotherapy of obesity is highlighted and the role of pharmacotherapy relative to therapeutic options is discussed.

DEFINITION OF CLINICAL OBESITY

Much of the confusion in interpreting studies by various investigators is due to their use of differing definitions and cutoff points to define obesity.[9] Furthermore, obesity can be defined epidemiologically based on health insurance data or physiologically based on body fat content. A clear distinction has been made between obesity and overweight by the National Center for Health Statistics (NCHS), yet researchers often use the two terms interchangeably.[10] "Overweight" refers to an excess body weight relative to a person's height. The body mass index (BMI) is a measure that attempts to correct weight changes for height. It is defined as weight in kilograms divided by height in meters squared (kg/m^2). In contrast, obesity refers to a state of excess body fat as determined by the various methods. These include measures of skinfold thickness, body density using underwater body weight, bioelectric impedance and conductivity, dual energy x-ray absorptiometry (DEXA), computed tomography (CT), and magnetic resonance imaging (MRI). Many of these measurement techniques that determine body fat directly are too expensive and time consuming to be used in population studies.

It is not clear what the criterion for "normal" weight should be. Should normal weight be associated with low mortality, low morbidity, or both? In the absence of better sources, life insurance data were used in the past to develop tables of normality. These tables provide weight ranges for height and frame size (small, medium, and large), and are associated with the greatest longevity in individuals who were healthy at the time of initial examination when their height and weight were measured. These data predominantly represent information compiled from the upper middle class white population. They are specific for height and weight but not age. Indeed, they essentially predict longevity in young persons weighed in their early 20s. The weight range provided by these tables is known as desirable or ideal body weight. Overweight is then defined as a weight greater than 10% above the ideal weight for a person's height, and obesity is defined as greater than 20% above this ideal body weight.

The NCHS has conducted large national surveys in the United States of health including body habitus and nutrition over the past three decades.[11] These surveys have been conducted in three samples, known as the National Health and Nutrition Examination Surveys (NHANES). The data have been used to establish norms for BMI, height, weight, and gender in Americans of all ages. The normal BMI for males and females is 20 to 24.9. Overweight was defined as a BMI of 27.8 or more in men and 27.3 or more in women. The overweight criteria correspond to approximately 124% and 120% of the midpoints of the ranges of weights recommended, respectively, for men and women of medium frame in the 1983 Metropolitan Life Height and Weight tables as adjusted for clothing weight and heel height.[12] Severe overweight corresponds to a BMI of over 31.1 in men and over 32.3 in women.[13] The relationship between BMI and mortality is shown in Figure 132–1. Excess weight relative to height (BMI) is an acceptable measure of obesity; however, it does not always correspond to excess fat.

Neither the BMI nor the ideal body weight reflects true body composition or distribution of body fat. Body composition is a more direct measure of degree of adiposity and therefore mass of fat stores. The gold standard to determine body composition historically has been underwater weighing (body density). The formulas used in this technique were developed using healthy young males and therefore may not be applicable for obese and older individuals. Newer techniques have improved our ability to measure body composition. Wang and colleagues[14] have proposed five levels of modeling for body composition: atomic, molecular, cellular, tissue system, and whole body. Techniques have been developed to estimate body composition at all these levels. Body weight, BMI, body volume, body surface area, height, skin

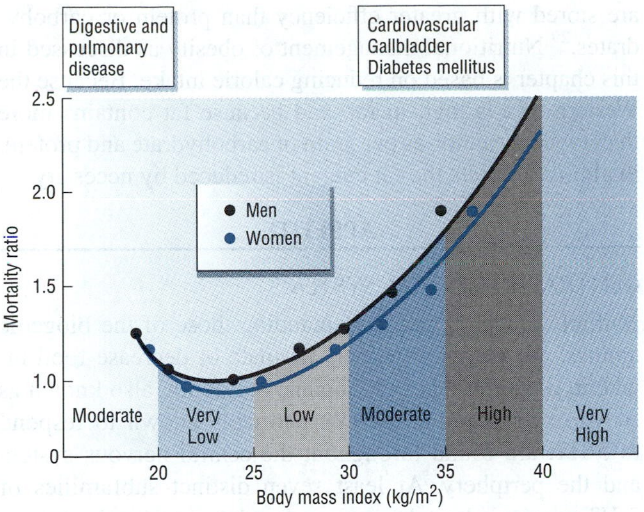

FIGURE 132–1. Mortality ratio and body mass index (BMI). This represents composite data for men and women demonstrating the relationship of body mass index to overall mortality. A J-shaped relationship exists wherein a BMI < 20 kg/m^2 and < 25 kg/m^2 correlates with an increase in relative mortality. The major causes of mortality are listed relative to BMI groupings. *(Adapted with permission from Bray GA. Obesity. In: Brown ML, et al, eds. Present Knowledge in Nutrition, 6th ed. Washington, DC, International Life Sciences Institute–Nutrition Foundation, 1990.)*

fold thickness, and body density are all measures of body composition at the whole-body level.[14,15] In addition to the absolute excess fat mass, the distribution of this fat regionally in the body has an important effect on the mortality of obese individuals. A number of studies have demonstrated excess mortality associated with a central or android distribution of body fat.[15,16] Generally, central obesity reflects high levels of intra-abdominal or visceral fat. Intra-abdominal fat is best estimated by imaging techniques such as CT or MRI. This pattern of obesity is associated with an increased prevalence of cardiovascular risk factors such as hyperlipidemia and glucose intolerance. These risk factors in part explain the high cardiovascular mortality rate of these individuals.[17] In contrast, a gynecoid (gluteofemoral) distribution of fat with low waist to hip ratios (WHR) or low waist circumference (WC) has a lower risk of mortality for the same degree of adiposity. Clinically, WC is the narrowest circumference measured in the area between the last rib and the top of the iliac crest.[18] The hip measurement is the maximal circumference around the buttocks.[18] Central obesity is associated with increased risks when WHR is 1.0 or more for men or 0.9 or more for females.[19] WC is an easier measurement to obtain in the clinical setting and is also independently associated with increased risks when 40 or more inches for males or 35 or more inches for females.[17]

EPIDEMIOLOGY

Obesity is increasing in prevalence in the United States. The NHANES II data (1976 to 1980) estimated a prevalence of overweight persons in the United States at 25.4% of adults, representing 34 million individuals. During NHANES III (1988 to 1991), the prevalence had increased to 33.3%, representing 55 million American adults.[20] The prevention of obesity is therefore a public health priority. This has been further emphasized by the current lack of any safe and effective long-term therapy for obesity. Individuals who were "fat" as children tend to remain overweight as adults.[21–23] Recent data from a large British study have provided further evidence for the relationship between an overweight childhood and subsequent excess weight as an adult.[24] In contrast to body weight, adult BMI was not well predicted from childhood weight. The fattest children had the highest risks of adult obesity. However, most obese adults had not been fat at earlier ages: only 17% and 18% of obese 33-year-old men and women, respectively, had been fat at age 7 years. Thus most obese adults were not fat children. In contrast, early adulthood may be an important time for intervention to prevent future obesity. Of 4519 men and 4806 women in the study by Power and associates, obesity increased in prevalence from 2% to 11% in men and from 3% to 12% in women during the 10-year period between ages 23 and 33 years.[24] This is consistent with historical data from the U.S. ten-state nutrition survey.[25]

The prevalence of overweight varies between races within the United States. Mexican-American women and black women had the highest prevalence, 48.1% and 49.1%, respectively. The prevalence of obesity also increases with age, reaching a maximum by the sixth decade in women and the seventh decade for men. Beyond this age, the prevalence progressively falls for both genders. Socioeconomic status also affects the prevalence of obesity in those between the ages of 25 and 54 years. The prevalence of overweight in nonpregnant women for each respective decade of life—25 to 34 years, 35 to 44 years, and 45 to 54 years—is 30.8%, 49.1%, and 54.1% of women with income below the poverty line, versus 18.4%, 23.7%, and 30.3% of those above the poverty line.[26] Educational achievement, which is linked to socioeconomic status, is also correlated with the fraction of people who are overweight; prevalence of overweight is greatest in those with less than a high school education versus those with some college education.

ETIOLOGY

The etiology of obesity in the vast majority of individuals is unknown. It is likely multi-factorial in origin, with environmental, genetic, and physiologic factors contributing to various degrees in different individuals. A definitive diagnosis of an underlying medical condition can be made in only a small minority of individuals. Even then, the diagnosed condition may or may not be treatable. One of the current controversies is the extent that genetic traits influence the risk of developing obesity as well as how these genetic traits interact with environmental factors to cause obesity.[27]

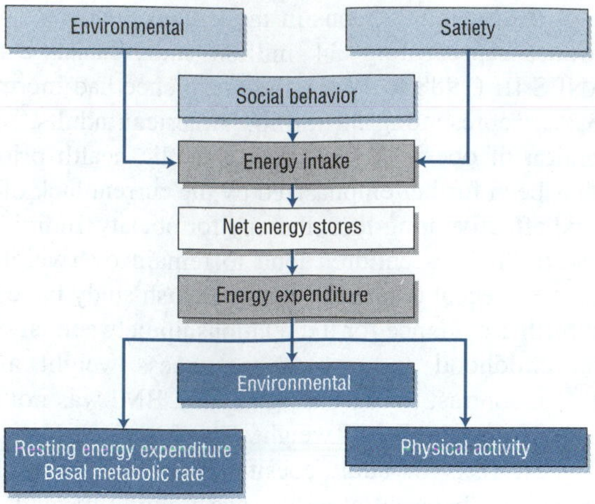

FIGURE 132–2. Net energy stores, determined by various inputs and outputs. Simply stated, obesity occurs when imbalance occurs between energy intake and expenditure. (REE = resting energy expenditure; BMR = basal metabolic rate).

ENVIRONMENTAL FACTORS

Economic development is associated with life-style changes that contribute to the observed rise in the prevalence of obesity throughout the world. These include reduced physical activity or work (sedentary life-style), abundant and readily available food supply, increased fat intake, increased consumption of refined simple sugars, and decreased ingestion of vegetables, fruits, and complex carbohydrates. These changes in our environment likely contribute to a state of positive energy balance in many individuals (Fig. 132–2).[28] Observations from public health studies support this concept. For example, the prevalence of obesity in Copenhagen remained stable during the period between 1925 and 1942 at approximately 0.1%. However, since the end of World War II, there has been a steady increase in the prevalence of obesity.[28] These observational data suggest an environmental role for the development of obesity.

NUTRITION

Decades of research have led to several thousand publications regarding nutrition therapy for obesity. Yet the appropriate diet that leads to long-term weight loss in ambulatory self-sufficient individuals is not known. The consensus is that weight regain is almost always inevitable. It is clear that excess caloric intake is a prerequisite to weight gain and obesity, but not all individuals with high caloric intake gain weight. There is an ongoing debate whether the primary consideration is total calorie intake or macronutrient composition of the diet (i.e., percent of calories as carbohydrates, protein, or fat). Of the three macronutrients, dietary fat has received the most attention. Both animals and humans prefer and often will seek out foods high in fat. High-fat foods have a desirable texture and sensory characteristic in the mouth. Though fat is itself tasteless, fats enhance the flavor of other foods. Clearly one way that fatty foods promote weight gain is by increased energy intake, because fat is more energy dense than other macronutrients. Furthermore, fats are stored with greater efficiency than protein or carbohydrates.[29] Nutritional management of obesity as discussed in this chapter is based on reducing calorie intake. Because the Western diet is high in fat, and because fat contains more than twice the calories per gram of carbohydrate and protein, in almost all diets the fat content is reduced by necessity.

APPETITE

CENTRAL RECEPTOR SYSTEMS

Multiple receptor systems, including those of the biogenic amines, are known to either stimulate or decrease food intake in both animals and humans. Serotonin, also known as 5-hydroxytryptamine (5-HT), and cells known to respond to 5-HT, are found throughout the central nervous system and the periphery. At least seven distinct subfamilies of 5-HT receptors have been cloned to date, with each of these seven exhibiting one or more subtypes.[30] Currently two major noradrenergic receptor subtypes are recognized (α and β) each with multiple subtypes.[31] Histamine and dopamine also demonstrate multiple receptor subtypes, but their role in regulation of human eating behaviors and food intake is less well documented. Direct stimulation of 5-HT_{1A} and noradrenergic α_2-receptors will increase food intake, while the opposite occurs with 5-HT_{2C} and noradrenergic α_1- or β_2-receptor activation. In animal models, stimulating histamine receptor subtypes 1 or 3, and dopamine receptor subtypes 1 or 2, results in lowering of food intake. Table 132–1 summarizes the major effects of direct receptor stimulation, inhibition, or changes in synaptic cleft amine concentrations on food intake.

PEPTIDES

Since the 1950s it has been conjectured that weight is controlled via a hormone interaction at the level of the hypothal-

TABLE 132–1. Effects of Various Neurotransmitters, Receptors, and Peptides on Food Intake

Neurotransmitter/ Receptor/Peptide	Action	Food Intake
Norepinephrine	Increase concentration	Decrease
α_1	Stimulate receptor	Decrease
α_2	Stimulate receptor	Increase
β_2	Stimulate receptor	Decrease
Serotonin	Increase concentration	Decrease
5-HT_{1A}	Stimulate receptor	Increase
5-HT_{1B}	Stimulate receptor	Decrease
5-HT_{2C}	Stimulate receptor	Decrease
Histamine		
H_1	Stimulate receptor	Decrease
H_3	Stimulate receptor	Decrease
Dopamine		
D_1	Stimulate receptor	Decrease
D_2	Stimulate receptor	Decrease
Leptin	Increase concentration	Decrease
Neuropeptide Y	Increase concentration	Increase
Galanin	Increase concentration	Increase

amus.[32] The protein product of the mouse obese gene (*ob*) described in 1994 appears to be the signaling mechanism between peripheral energy storage and hypothalamic feeding centers.[32,33] This protein was called leptin (after "leptos," the Greek term for thin). The *ob/ob* genetically obese mouse does not produce leptin, and this animal's marked hyperphagia subsides with leptin supplementation. The human leptin homologue has been cloned and various animal studies have demonstrated that leptin is produced in the periphery by white and possibly brown adipocytes.[34] Additionally, it appears that the sympathetic nervous system (SNS), via β_3-adrenoceptors, inhibits leptin expression. (Fig. 132–3).[34] Unlike the leptin deficient *ob/ob* mouse, obese human serum leptin levels increase as fat cell mass increases. There is a direct relationship between serum leptin concentrations and various markers of obesity such as percent body fat, BMI, and serum insulin concentrations.[35] Thus, humans appear to be resistant to the satiety effects of leptin and it is unknown whether leptin supplementation in humans will decrease obesity. Figure 132–3 shows the peripheral link that leptin appears to provide in signaling the central nervous system about the status of fat cell mass. A second peptide, neuropeptide Y (NPY), is being intensely studied for its effects on feeding. NPY elicits many effects both peripherally and centrally including appetite stimulation. Most recently, messenger RNA for two new appetite-stimulating proteins called "orexins" has been observed to be concentrated in the lateral hypothalamus.[36] An understanding of the relationships between the sympathetic nervous system, leptin, NPY, orexins, and other hormones such as insulin and glucocorticoids is still evolving.[37] Exogenous manipulation of these proteins may provide future pharmacotherapeutic approaches to obesity management.

ACTIVITY

It is generally accepted that increased physical activity is an important component in the management of obesity. Similarly, a sedentary life-style predisposes to weight gain and obesity. Yet, the question whether obese individuals are less physically active compared to age-matched lean individuals remains unanswered. Some studies show no difference in physical activity between lean and obese individuals while others suggest that obese persons are less active.[38] Even when studies suggest obese persons are less active, it cannot be determined whether less physical activity leads to obesity or physical inactivity is itself secondary to the physical effects of obesity. Physical activity includes voluntary work, recreational activity, and spontaneous physical activity including involuntary movements. Some authors have suggested that obese individuals have reduced levels of spontaneous physical activity leading to a lower daily energy expenditure.[39] However, results from studies designed to measure total daily energy expenditure remain controversial.[38]

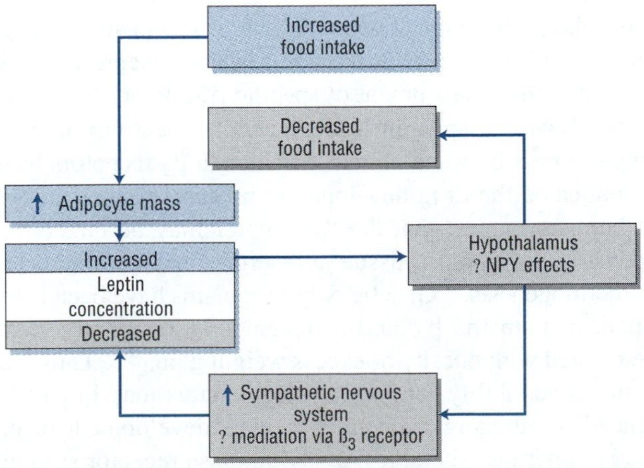

FIGURE 132–3. Effects of food intake on leptin concentrations and proposed feedback loops controlling intake and leptin concentration. (NPY = neuropeptide Y.)

WEIGHT GAIN SECONDARY TO MEDICAL CONDITIONS

Occasionally patients present with obesity secondary to an identifiable acquired medical condition. The commonest endocrine condition associated with weight gain is hypothyroidism[40] (Chap. 71). These patients lose significant weight within weeks of thyroxin replacement therapy. However, many patients will not achieve a normal or ideal body weight despite adequate thyroid hormone replacement. Indeed, it is not uncommon for patients to request higher than physiologic replacement doses of thyroxin to artificially suppress their weight. It is important to remember that excess thyroid therapy can be associated with complications including osteoporosis and cardiac disorders (see Chap. 71). Cushing's syndrome, another cause of obesity, is most commonly seen in patients receiving exogenous glucocorticoid therapy. These agents are often prescribed for a chronic condition such as chronic obstructive airway disease (COPD), postorgan transplantation, or arthritis. Idiopathic Cushing's disease due to excess endogenous steroid secretion is in contrast very rare. In both iatrogenic and idiopathic Cushing's disease the weight gain is in part due to fluid retention as well as increased adiposity. The adiposity associated with glucocorticoid excess has a particular body distribution in that it is central with relative loss of body muscle mass and thinning of the skin, leading to the characteristic purple skin striaie and a buffalo hump behind the neck.

Occasionally patients can present with lesions of the hypothalamus that lead to hyperphagia and obesity.[41] This disorder is rare and should not be confused with behavioral disorders of eating that are associated with psychopathology. These include binge eating disorders, which may respond to psychotherapy and in some cases pharmacotherapy (see Chap. 60). Obesity is itself associated with a higher prevalence of affective disorders, which if untreated may impair the success of any weight loss program. The clinician managing obesity must be aware of the presence of psychosocial disorders both as a cause and effect of obesity. Furthermore, medications used to manage affective disorders, such as the serotonin reuptake inhibitors, have not been extensively studied with regard to combination use with appetite suppressant agents.

GENETIC SYNDROMES

Syndromes in which obesity is a major component are extremely rare. Prader–Willi, Simpson–Goabi–Behmel, Cohen's, Bardet-Biedl, Carpenter's Börjeson's, and Wilson–Turner syndromes have all be associated with obesity.[18] Of these, Prader–Willi syndrome is the commonest and has a frequency of 1 in 20,000 live births. Other phenotypic features include changes in stature, mental retardation, and developmental abnormalities (e.g., hypogonadism). Because the incidence of these syndromes is rare, even collectively they contribute very little to the incidence of obesity. The clinician evaluating a patient for obesity needs to be aware of their existence, and the physical examination of obese patients should always include an assessment for secondary causes of obesity including genetic syndromes.

GENETIC PREDISPOSITION

Family studies show a clear correlation of body weight between parents and children. The correlation between siblings is even higher.[42,43] In monozygotic twins, BMI is almost always identical and there is a strong correlation in the accumulation of visceral fat. These twin studies demonstrate the strong role of genetics in determining both obesity and distribution of body fat.[43] The incidence of obesity in adopted individuals relative to their adopted parents provides insight into the role of genetics versus family environment. These studies show a clear correlation between the BMI of adult adoptees and their biologic parents. This relationship does not exist between an adoptee and his or her adoptive parent. These observations further support the notion that genes are primarily responsible for determining adult body weight. The relative impact of genetic versus environmental factors varies between persons. In some individuals, genetic factors are the primary determinants of obesity, while in others the obesity may be primarily caused by environmental factors. The actual variance in body fat between individuals determined by genes is not known. Estimates for this variance range from 20% to a high of almost 80%. Yet clearly without adequate caloric intake, obesity cannot occur. Thus the role of the environment is to facilitate expression of an underlying genetic trait for obesity. However, the specific gene or genes that code for obesity are unknown.[44] Most investigators would agree that more than one gene is involved in the development of human obesity.

PHYSIOLOGY

ENERGY BALANCE

The net balance of energy ingested relative to energy expended by an individual over time determines the degree of obesity. Figure 132–2 represents the interplay between energy intake and expenditure. Energy stores will increase if there is imbalance between intake and expenditure. An individual's metabolic rate is the single largest determinant of energy expenditure. It is important to determine metabolic rate under standardized conditions, giving rise to terms such as resting energy expenditure (REE) and basal metabolic rate (BMR). REE is defined as the energy expended by a person at rest under conditions of thermal neutrality. BMR is more precisely defined as the REE measured soon after awakening in the morning, at least 12 hours after the last meal. Metabolic rate increases after eating, based upon the size and composition of the meal. It reaches a maximum approximately 1 hour after the meal is consumed and is essentially back to basal levels 4 hours after the meal. This increase in metabolic rate is known as the thermogenic effect of food.[45] The REE may include the residual thermic effect of a previous meal and may be lower than BMR during quiet sleep. In practice, BMR and REE differ by less than 10%, and the terms are frequently used interchangeably.

PERIPHERAL STORAGE AND THERMOGENESIS

Adipose tissue is generally divided into two major types, white and brown.[46] The primary function of white adipose tissue is lipid manufacture, storage, and release. Lipid storage occurs in response to insulin and release during periods of calorie restriction, when insulin levels are suppressed. Brown type tissue is notable for its ability to dissipate energy via a process of uncoupled mitochondrial respiration.[46] Currently, the exact roles of each of these tissue subtypes are better defined in animal models than in humans. Adipose tissue is highly innervated by the sympathetic nervous system, and adrenergic stimulation is known to activate lipolysis in fat cells as well as increase energy expenditure in adipose tissue and skeletal muscle. These properties provide a potential pharmacologic avenue for altering energy balance and changing weight status. A major focus of research in obesity pharmacotherapy has centered on the activity of adrenergic receptors and their effect on adipose tissue with respect to energy storage and expenditure or thermogenesis.[46,47] All three subtypes of β-adrenergic receptors (β_1, β_2, and β_3) appear to be active in fat cell function. The β_3-receptor appears to be less responsive than β_1 and β_2 with respect to activation via norepinephrine. This has led to the development of specific β_3-adrenoceptor agonists. However, apparent differences in selectivity and responsiveness between animal and human β_3-receptors have complicated the drug development process. *In vivo* studies in humans suggest that the β_3-receptor may be largely responsible for adipose tissue adrenergic-mediated increases in thermogenesis.[48] Genetic polymorphisms have been identified, in both the β_2- and β_3-receptor systems, which are associated with obesity or excess weight gain.[49,50] Thus, genetic susceptibility for excess weight status may in part be related to adrenergic dysfunction. The development of effective pharmacotherapies involving these receptor systems may be delayed pending definitive identification of receptor subtype contributions.

COMORBIDITIES

Obesity is associated with serious health risks and increased mortality (see Fig. 132–1). Several disease states and/or conditions are more prevalent in obese patients (Table 132–2). Increased body fat, increased total body weight, and a central distribution of body fat are all associated with an increased incidence of mortality, primarily due to cardiovascular disease. Hypertension, hyperlipidemia, insulin resistance, and glucose intolerance are all known cardiac risk factors that tend to cluster in obese individuals. Therefore the obese individual is exposed to multiple risk factors. Epidemiologic studies have confirmed the relationship between obesity and increased risk of stroke and coronary heart disease in both men and women.[51,52] This increased mortality is seen even with modest excess body weight. The American Cancer Society study of 750,000 men and women found an increased cardiac mortality even at body weights only 10% above average.[53] Blood pressure is frequently elevated in obese individuals and may in part explain the increased incidence of stroke and cardiovascular disease observed with obesity. Hypertension in lean individuals is associated with concentric hypertrophy due to an increased afterload, which increases the risk of cardiac ischemia. In contrast, with obesity eccentric dilatation is observed, leading to an increased volume load. This dilated cardiomyopathy is associated with a reduction in ventricular ejection fraction and a high-output cardiac state. The combination of obesity and hypertension is associated with thickening of the ventricular wall, ischemia, and increased heart volume. This leads more rapidly to heart failure.[54] Alterations in pulmonary function are common in patients with obesity. Most significant and costly in terms of morbidity and mortality is sleep apnea.[18] This disorder is more common in men. The exact mechanism by which obesity leads to sleep apnea is unknown, but weight loss often results in significant and sometimes dramatic improvements in sleep apnea.

Diabetes mellitus and impaired glucose tolerance is associated with insulin resistance and obesity. The cellular mechanism by which obesity causes insulin resistance is unknown. Proposed mechanisms include down-regulation of insulin receptors, abnormal postreceptor signals, circulating antagonists to insulin such as fatty acids or cytokines, and impaired gene transcription in insulin-responsive cells. Regardless of the mechanism of the insulin resistance, as insulin response becomes impaired, the pancreatic β-cells respond by increasing insulin, resulting in a state of relative hyperinsulinemia. Though hyperinsulinemia is known to be associated with an increased risk of cardiovascular disease, it is not known whether the increased insulin levels directly contribute to cardiac disease or if they are just a marker for the underlying defect of insulin resistance and glucose intolerance. Insulin resistance in turn also frequently leads to impaired lipid metabolism (increased cholesterol, increased triglycerides, and a low HDL) and hypertension. As with cardiovascular disease, fat distribution is an important factor in determining the risk of developing type 2 diabetes. Central obesity has been shown to increase the risk of diabetes.

TABLE 132–2. Obesity and Comorbid Conditions

Cardiovascular	**Musculoskeletal**
Hypertension	Degenerative joint disease
Left ventricular hypertrophy	**Skin**
Congestive heart failure	Acanthosis nigricans
Coronary artery disease	Stretch marks
Pulmonary	Hirsutism
Obstructive airway disease	**Gastrointestinal**
Sleep apnea	Cholelithiasis
Pulmonary hypertension	Esophageal reflux
Metabolic	Hiatus hernia
Hypercholesterolemia	**Psychological**
Hypertriglyceridemia	Eating disorders
Low serum HDL	Depression
Diabetes mellitus and glucose intolerance	Affective disorders
	Social stigma
Hyperinsulinemia	**Neoplasm**
Polycystic ovary syndrome	Breast cancer
Increased serum urate	Colon cancer

Osteoarthritis in weight-bearing joints, such as the knees, may be directly related to the mechanical effects of excess body weight and the resultant forces exerted on these joint surfaces. The increase of osteoarthritis in non-weight-bearing joints, however, suggests that obesity may lead to altered cartilage, collagen, and even bone metabolism. Osteoarthritis and its symptoms, such as pain, are a significant barrier to physical activity, and a key impediment to sustained weight loss.

Obesity affects the human reproductive system in a number ways. Obesity is associated with earlier menarche in girls and hyperandrogenism, hirsutism, and anovulatory menstrual cycles in women. In some women this disorder manifests as overt polycystic ovary syndrome (PCOS).[18] Insulin resistance is common in these women. Weight loss, and more recently therapy with insulin-sensitizing drugs such as troglitazone, can restore normal ovulation in some women.[55] These observations suggest that insulin resistance plays a part in the causation of PCOS associated with obesity.

▶ TREATMENT: Obesity

GENERAL APPROACH TO TREATMENT

The success of obesity therapy has most often been measured as weight loss over study periods of up to 12 months. Successful obesity treatment plans have incorporated diet, exercise, behavior modification (with or without pharmacologic therapy), and/or surgical intervention. Figure 132–4 shows the sites of action of these therapies within the energy intake, storage, and expenditure cycle.

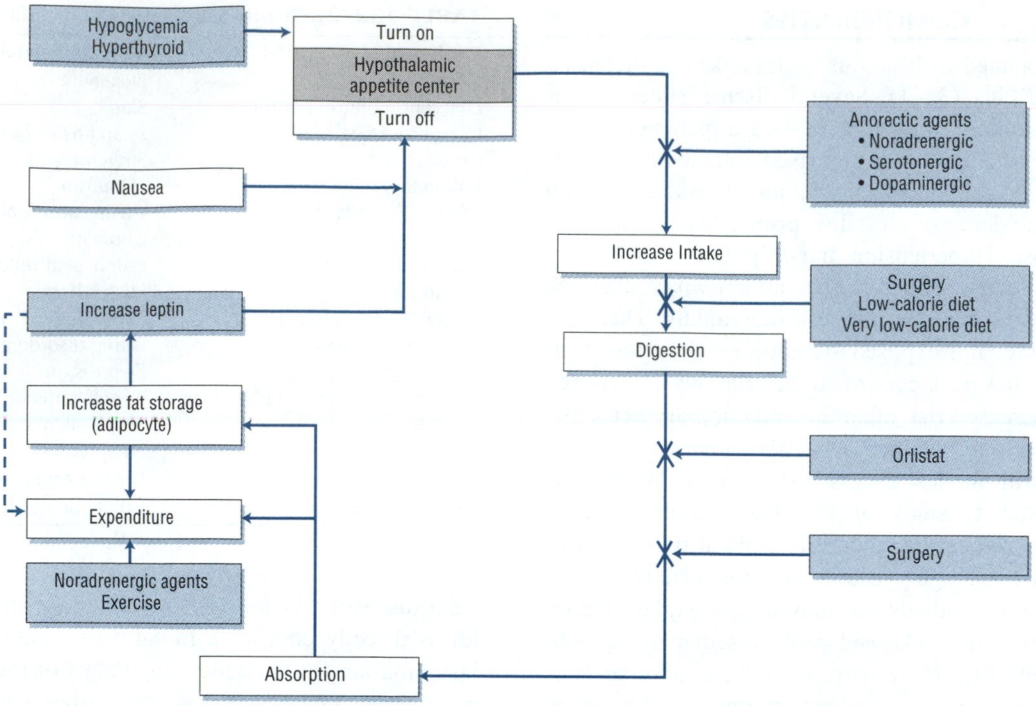

FIGURE 132–4. Hypothalamic appetite centers in the brain modulate both central and peripheral signals. This figure demonstrates the sites of action for various obesity treatment modalities within the cycle of energy intake and storage. Leptin, while signaling the central nervous system of the status of peripheral fat cell mass, may also have functions with regard to energy expenditure. Some appetite-suppressant agents, alone or in combination, also modulate energy expenditure.

Patients seeking help for obesity do so for many reasons, including improvement in their quality of life, a reduction in associated morbidity, and to prolong their life. Yet numerous individuals seek therapy for obesity primarily for cosmetic purposes and often have unreasonable goals and expectations. Aggressive marketing of weight loss programs, therapies, and diets—parallel to the fashion industry's standards of desirable body profiles—has led many individuals to set impossible goals and expectations. In some cases these persons will go to extreme measures to achieve weight loss, even at the risk of injury to themselves. Clinicians therefore must be careful not only to fully discuss risks of therapies but also clearly define achievable benefits and magnitude of weight loss. Criteria for weight loss vary from the most aggressive goal of trying to achieve an "ideal weight" to the more reasonable goals of modest (e.g., loss of 5% of body weight) but sustained weight loss. In practice the goal has to be set based on many factors including initial body weight, patient motivation and desire, presence of comorbid conditions, and age. For example, in patients with diabetes, even modest weight loss can significantly improve glucose control,[56] yet in individuals with osteoarthritis, significantly more weight reduction may be required to improve symptoms. Indeed, dietary modification and exercise have been shown to ameliorate hyperglycemia, hyperlipidemia, and hypertension with weight loss of less than 5% of initial body weight.[57] These data emphasize the importance of defining end points and measures of success in any weight loss plan.

Most weight loss interventions consist of a combination of life-style changes, diet, drug therapy if indicated, and in some cases surgery. Prior to recommending any therapy, the clinician must evaluate the patient for the presence of secondary causes of obesity. If a secondary cause is suspected, then a more complete diagnostic workup and appropriate therapy are paramount. The next step in the patient evaluation is to determine the presence and severity of other medical conditions either directly associated with obesity (e.g., diabetes) or those that impact therapeutic decision making (e.g., history of liver disease or cardiac arrhythmia). Appropriate laboratory tests to exclude and or quantify the degree of specific conditions such as diabetes, liver dysfunction, and nephropathy should be done as indicated by the history and physical examination. Based on the outcome of this medical evaluation, the patient should then be counseled on treatment options, benefits, and risks. The ultimate goals of treatment must be clearly defined. These goals may be absolute weight loss if obesity is present without other comorbid conditions. If improvement in blood glucose, blood cholesterol, and hypertension are primary goals, then these must be defined appropriately such as target levels for LDL cholesterol, glycosylated hemoglobin, or blood pressure. For these patients weight loss goals may be as little as 5% of starting weight.[56] In contrast, if obesity is causing physical problems such as impaired mobility, osteoarthritis, or sleep apnea, then 10% to 20% of starting weight may be more appropriate. All too often patients expect to lose weight "overnight," only to be disappointed. Thus it is important to set a time course for the plan. A reasonable rate of weight loss is typically about 0.5 kg/wk.

NONPHARMACOLOGIC THERAPY

BEHAVIORAL MODIFICATION

Behavior modification is common to almost all weight loss interventions. The primary aim is to help patients choose life-styles that are conducive to safe and sustained weight loss. Behavioral therapy is based on principles of human learning and therefore attempts to substitute learned undesirable habits with desirable behaviors using a combination of stimulus control and reinforcement. Most such programs use self-monitoring of diet and exercise both to increase patient awareness of behavior and as a tool for the clinician to determine patient compliance as well as patient motivation.[58] Behavior is reinforced by techniques including behavioral contracting, social support, relapse prevention, and in some cases booster treatments. Behavioral contracts are written agreements jointly developed by the patient and clinicians. Components of these agreements include goals of therapy, methods to achieve these goals, and rewards for successfully achieving these goals. Social support requires the active participation of a close friend or relative who is involved in monitoring compliance and reinforcing behavior. Relapse prevention is geared at identifying high-risk situations for relapse such as social events, and training the individual to avoid these circumstances. Eventually the patient is trained to actively deal with these situations such as refusing high-fat foods assertively rather than avoiding these social events.

DIET

Numerous diet or nutrition plans exist to aid in weight loss.[59,60] Whichever "diet" program is selected, it is clear that energy consumption must be less than energy expenditure to achieve weight loss (see Fig. 132–2). The challenge has been to develop a diet plan that leads to compliance by the patient and therefore sustained weight loss. Two broad categories of diet have been used in practice: low calorie and very low calorie. Low-calorie diets allow the consumption of less than 800 kcal/d. Very-low-calorie diets generally contain approximately 500 to 800 kcal/d. These highly restrictive diets often result in early weight loss but have been disappointing in the long term, in part because it is difficult for individuals to maintain compliance.[61] Other investigators have proposed total or modified fasts.[62] The obvious problem with total fasts is that both fat and lean body mass is lost. In addition, because of diuresis, significant mineral losses occur. Because of the problem with total fasting, alternate regimens called protein supplemented modified fasts (PSMFs) became popular. With a PSMF, the protein is given in the form of either formula or natural foods such as fish or lean meat. The consensus is that it is dangerous to allow these diets to be continued for longer than 16 weeks at a time.[61] Patients may lose 1.5 to 2.3 kg/wk on these diets. All these types of severe calorie-restricted diets need vitamin and mineral supplementation.[62]

A more reasonable goal for individuals is weight reduction of about 0.5 kg/wk achieved by a negative calorie balance of approximately 500 kcal/d. This translates into a diet of approximately 20 kcal/kg of desirable body weight for most adults. The dietary regime should be well balanced in fat, carbohydrates, and proteins as well as micronutrients. Generally 0.8 grams of protein per kg desirable body weight is recommended, with at most 30% of calories from fat.

SURGERY

Surgery remains the most effective intervention for moderate to severe obesity. Surgical procedures either reduce the absorptive surface of the alimentary tract resulting in some degree of malabsorption or reduce the stomach volume. In some cases a combination of these two approaches is used. The most common procedure performed in the past was some form of intestinal bypass.[63] This type of procedure reduces the surface area available for nutrients and in particular calories to be absorbed, resulting in malabsorption and subsequent weight loss. The early procedures of jejunocolic bypass (anastamosis of jejunum to colon) had serious side effects as well as an unacceptable mortality. Further developments in bypass procedures subsequently led to the use of a safer and more acceptable bypass procedure known as a jejunoileal bypass (jejunum to ileum anastamosis).

Jejunoileal bypass was the standard surgical procedure for obesity in the 1970s, until the advent of gastric restriction surgery. The operative risk of jejunoileal procedures was less than 1% and resulted in weight loss of approximately one-third of preoperative weight. Although these procedures did result in a state of malabsorption and loss of ingested calories in the stool, up to 75% of the weight loss observed in these patients could be accounted for by a reduction in caloric ingestion. In addition, animal studies suggest that bacterial overgrowth in the blind loop of the procedure may contribute to the weight loss observed. Unfortunately the complications of this procedure, which may in part be secondary to this bacterial colonization and overgrowth, resulted in hepatic steatosis, cirrhosis in up to 4% of patients, and in some cases liver failure.[61] Other long-term complications include arthritis, skin lesions, vasculitis, enteritis, electrolyte abnormalities, osteomalacia, renal stones and in some cases renal failure, an increased risk of tuberculosis, and systemic fungal infection.[63] These complications have led to this procedure becoming obsolete.

Gastric bypass is a procedure in which a loop of bowel is attached the stomach in a Roux-en-Y method. This procedure may ultimately result in the loss of approximately one third of body weight. Common complications include gallstone formation, prolonged nausea and vomiting, and ulceration and stenosis at the site of anastamosis.[63] Very rarely, hepatic failure has been reported. Many gastric reduction procedures have been described including numerous versions of gastroplasty and gastric balloon procedures. All are designed to reduce the volume of the stomach by either surgically reducing the volume of the stomach or the insertion of a silicone balloon into the stomach cavity so that it acts like a bezoar. The most successful of these procedures has been the vertically banded gastroplasty.[63] The complications of this procedure are similar to those seen with gastric bypass. Both gastric bypass and gastroplasty result in maximum weight loss around 18 months postsurgery. However, late weight gain and the need for surgical revision is greater in patients undergoing vertically banded gastroplasty.

It is clear that great attention needs to be paid to the selection of the appropriate patient for surgery and subsequently identification of the correct procedure. The input of an experienced surgeon working with a multidisciplinary team is invaluable (Table 132–3)

PHARMACOLOGIC THERAPY

Strategies for the pharmacologic management of obesity have revolved around impacting both central and/or peripheral sites that regulate human energy balance. Figure 132–4 shows sites of

TABLE 132–3. Surgical Procedures, Outcomes, and Complications

Procedure	Weight Loss (% of initial weight)	Operative Mortality (%)	Complications
Jejunoileal bypass	33	< 1	Hepatic steatosis, cirrhosis, bacterial overgrowth, nephrolithiasis, renal failure
Gastric bypass	30–35	< 1	Cholelithiasis, prolonged nausea, stomal ulceration and stenosis, anemia
Gastroplasty	20–25	< 1	Cholelithiasis, nausea, stomal ulceration and stenosis; weight regain is more common

TABLE 132–4. Obesity Pharmacotherapeutic Agents

Class	Availability	Daily Dosages (mg)
Noradrenergic Agents		
Methamphetamine HCl (desoxyephedrine HCl)	Rx[a]	5–15
Amphetamine sulfate	Rx[a]	5–30
Dextroamphetamine sulfate (Dexedrine)	Rx[a]	5–30
Amphetamine/dextroamphetamine mixtures (Adderall)	Rx[a]	5–30
Benzphetamine (Didrex)	Rx[a]	25–150
Phendimetrazine (Prelu-2, Bontril, Plegine, X-Trazine)	Rx	70–105
Phentermine (Fastin, Oby-trim, Adipex-P, Ionamin)	Rx	15–37.5
Diethylpropion (Tenuate, Tenuate Dospan)	Rx	75
Mazindol (Mazanor, Sanorex)	Rx	1–3
Phenylpropanolamine (Accutrim, Dexatrim, others)	OTC	75
Ephedrine (various)	OTC/unlabeled use	20–60
Serotonergic Agents		
Fenfluramine (Pondamin)	Removed from market	60–120
Dexfenfluramine (Redux)	Removed from market	15–30
Fluoxetine (Prozac)	Rx/unlabeled use	60
Sertraline (Zoloft)	Rx/unlabeled use	200
Noradrenergic/Serotonergic Agent		
Sibutramine (Meridia)	Rx	5–15
Gastrointestinal Lipase Inhibitor		
Orlistat (RO-18-0647)	Rx/pending release	150–360

[a]High abuse potential, not recommended for routine use.

action and Table 132–4 lists the most common classes of agents currently in use or of recent use. Since the 1970s numerous studies of the effects of central appetite suppressant agents on weight status have been completed.[64,65] The quality and interpretability of some of the data have been questioned.[66] The National Task Force on the Prevention and Treatment of Obesity concluded that short-term anorexic agent use was difficult to justify because of the predictable weight regain that occurs upon discontinuation of pharmacotherapy. However, long-term pharmacotherapy may have a place in the treatment of obesity for patients who have no obvious contraindications to available drug therapy.[67] Additionally, guidance for a multidisciplinary obesity team approach to therapy has been presented in a joint statement by the American Association of Clinical Endocrinologists (AACE) and the American College of Endocrinology (ACE).[68] Routine implementation awaits the development of medications that are effective and safe with long-term exposure. Recent discovery of cardiac valve disease in relation to serotonergic appetite suppressant use affirms the task force's warning for further study of available therapies prior to widespread implementation of routine obesity pharmacotherapy.[69–71] The next sections outline the current status of pharmacologic agents for obesity therapy, focusing on proposed mechanisms, dosing recommendations, potential side effects, and monitoring parameters.

NORADRENERGIC AGENTS

Amphetamines

Appetite suppressant effects of the amphetamines were well recognized in the 1930s. Amphetamines activate central noradrenergic receptor systems as well as dopaminergic pathways, at higher doses, by stimulating neurotransmitter release. Increases in blood pressure and mild broncodilation are attributed to peripheral α- and β-receptor activation. The central nervous system (CNS) stimulant and addiction potential of amphetamine relative to other compounds has been described as amphetamine > methamphetamine > phentermine > mazindol > diethylpropion.[72] The powerful stimulant and addictive potential of the amphetamines relative to other available agents has resulted in their general avoidance for the treatment of obesity.[68,73]

Phentermine

Phentermine is structurally similar to amphetamine but it has less severe central nervous system stimulation and a lower abuse potential. Its mechanism of action is related to enhanced norepinephrine and dopamine neurotransmission. Phentermine is available in both immediate-release and sustained-release formulations. However, the value of sustained-release formulations can be questioned based upon the reported phentermine plasma half-life of 12 to 24 hours.[64] A single dose of 30 mg once daily in the morning provides effective appetite suppression throughout the day. Divided doses of 8 mg immediately prior to meals, however, are common. Doses above 30 mg daily do not improve effectiveness.[74] Evening or nighttime dosing should be avoided because of insomnia. Significant increases in blood pressure, palpitations, and arrhythmias can occur with phentermine administration. Use is not advisable in hypertensive patients and those with unstable cardiovascular function. The potential for hypertensive crisis with coadministration of phentermine and monoamine oxidase (MAO) inhibitors is noted in product labeling because of the documented cases of this syndrome seen with coadministration of amphetamine or noradrenergic derivatives and MAO inhibitors.[75] Similar warnings have been noted regarding concomitant use of tricyclic antidepressants, but this is less well documented.[76] With MAO inhibitors, a minimum washout time of 14 days prior to use of any adrenergic agent is suggested to avoid excessive adrenergic stimulation syndromes. Phentermine use is contraindicated in patients who are abusers of substances such as cocaine, phencyclidine, and methamphetamine, again because of the potential for excessive adrenergic stimulation syndromes and abuse potential. Mydriasis from adrenergic stimulation can worsen glaucoma, and patients diagnosed with glaucoma should not receive phentermine. Diabetic patients may experience altered insulin or oral hypoglycemic dosage requirements soon after beginning therapy and prior to any substantial weight loss.

Phentermine is an effective adjunct to diet, exercise, and behavior modification for producing weight loss in excess of that seen with placebo.[64,77] Intermittent phentermine therapy appears to elicit comparable weight loss when compared to continuous use.[78] However, most individuals experience weight regains, during therapy and generally always after discontinuing use.[64] In spite of its recent extensive off-label use in combination with the fenfluramine derivatives and the occurrence of cardiac valvulopathy, phentermine currently remains on the market as a short-term pharmacotherapy for obesity.

Mazindol

Although chemically distinct from amphetamines and phentermine, mazindol's tricyclic structure results in amphetamine-like appetite suppression. Direct stimulation of hypothalamic activity and norepinephrine reuptake inhibition are potential mazindol mechanisms.[79] Mazindol undergoes extensive hepatic metabolism, and approximately 50% of an administered dose is recovered in urine, mostly as conjugated metabolites. The pharmacokinetics of mazindol have not been extensively described; however, dosing is based upon an elimination half-life of 10 hours.[64] Clinically, the drug is given once daily, 1 to 3 mg, prior to the morning or noon meal. However, some clinicians employ multiple small doses, 1 mg, given just prior to meals. Efficacy trials of single versus multiple daily doses are not available. Dry mouth commonly occurs with mazindol use and difficulty with urination is possible. Mazindol use results in fewer CNS stimulant complaints than either phentermine or the amphetamines. Additionally, fewer cardiovascular adverse effects have been reported, and thus obese patients with mild to moderate hypertension may be treated with mazindol. Contraindications for use are similar to phentermine and include concurrent MAO inhibitors, glaucoma, symptomatic cardiovascular disease, and stimulant substance abuse. Mazindol has been noted to cause lithium toxicity with concurrent use.[80] Early studies in type 2 diabetic patients treated with mazindol demonstrated no need for changes in oral hypoglycemic therapy.[81] More recently, improved insulin sensitivity with mazindol treatment was documented using euglycemic clamp studies.[82] Caution and close monitoring of insulin or oral hypoglycemic dosage needs are advisable when treating obese diabetic patients with this therapy. Several placebo-controlled trials have demonstrated the effectiveness of mazindol as a short-term therapy for weight reduction.[64]

Diethylpropion

Diethylpropion stimulates norepinephrine release from presynaptic storage granules. Increased adrenergic neurotransmitter concentrations activate hypothalamic centers, which results in decreased appetite and food intake. This drug undergoes extensive first-pass hepatic metabolism. Active metabolites are renally eliminated and account for approximately 70% of administered dose. The elimination half-life of these metabolites is approximately 8 hours.[74] Less than 10% of the parent compound is recovered in urine. No specific dosing recommendations exist for use in patients with renal or hepatic insufficiency. Diethylpropion can be taken in divided daily doses, generally 25 mg three times daily before meals. An extended-release formulation is also employed by some clinicians, usually as 75 mg taken once daily in the morning or midmorning. Both dosing regimens are effective in achieving short-term weight loss in excess of placebo.[64] Complaints of insomnia increase if late afternoon dosing is used. Diethylpropion causes less CNS stimulation than mazindol and generally causes less insomnia than phentermine. Patients with severe hypertension or significant cardiovascular disease should not receive diethylpropion. However, it is one of the safest noradrenergic appetite suppressants, and its use has been recommended in patients with mild to moderate hypertension or angina pectoris.[83] Diabetic patients may experience decreased insulin or oral hypoglycemic dosage requirements soon after beginning therapy and prior to any substantial weight loss. More frequent blood glucose self-monitoring and medical follow-up is warranted when treating diabetic patients with diethylpropion.

Phenylpropanolamine

Although commonly classified as a noradrenergic anorexic, phenylpropanolamine (PPA) is atypical with regard to its mechanism and site of action. PPA racemates, D- and L-norephedrine, have chemical structures quite similar to amphetamine.[84] The levo enantiomer has more potent anorexic effects. Centrally, PPA appears to stimulate α-adrenergic receptors without additionally activating the dopaminergic or β-adrenergic systems as seen with amphetamine.[84] PPA appears to preferentially activate medial as opposed to lateral hypothalamic regions.[84] Although PPA-induced increases in brown adipose tissue thermogenesis have been seen in animals, this is less evident in humans.[85] PPA exhibits an elimination half-life of 4 to 6 hours in humans with approximately 90% of an administered dose recovered unchanged in urine.[86] Both immediate-release and extended-release formulations are available in the United States over the counter. The extended-release formulations are generally used in weight management products and commonly employ a daily dose of 75 mg.

PPA use can result in nervousness, insomnia, headache, nausea, and dizziness. Most adverse effects are self-limited, but there are case reports of severe side effects such as hypertensive crisis, intracranial hemorrhage, and seizure.[87] A meta-analysis of PPA clinical trials has indicated that PPA use results in weight loss in excess of placebo and somewhat less than that seen with prescription anorectics.[88] Differences in weight loss versus prescription agents were most apparent in studies of greater than 4 weeks duration. The adrenergic action of PPA can elevate blood glucose in patients with impaired glucose tolerance, including overt diabetes, by increasing gluconeogenesis and glycogen breakdown. Patients with diabetes mellitus, hypertension, or heart disease should be intensely monitored when PPA therapy is started. Some products contain combinations of caffeine and PPA. Concurrent use of caffeine and PPA results in elevations of caffeine plasma levels and potentially excess adrenergic stimulation.[89] As with the other adrenergic agents, concurrent use of PPA and MAO inhibitors should be avoided because of accelerated hypertension.[75] A case-control study is underway to help determine whether PPA use is related to serious adverse events, specifically hemorrhagic stroke. The United States FDA intends to reclassified PPA from category I (safe and effective) to category III (needs more data to prove safety).[90] Currently, available information cannot implicate or refute PPA as a cause of hemorrhagic stroke, and further guidance regarding routine use is pending the cohort study results.[90]

Ephedrine

Chemically related to PPA (± norephedrine), ephedrine may be a viable obesity pharmacotherapy. It appears to suppress appetite and increase energy expenditure via release of presynaptic norepinephrine and direct stimulation of thermogenic β-adrenergic receptors.[91] The efficiency of ephedrine stimulation is somewhat blunted by physiologic feedback systems involving adenosine and various prostaglandins.[92] This notion has stimulated research to characterize the effect of ephedrine in the presence of adenosine and prostaglandin antagonists such as caffeine and aspirin.[93,94] Ephedrine in combination with caffeine has enhanced appetite suppression and thermogenesis as compared to placebo and other anorectics over time periods of up to 6 months.[65,91,95] Oral doses of 20 mg ephedrine and 200 mg caffeine up to three times daily have been studied.[96,97] The spectrum of side effects with ephedrine and ephedrine/caffeine combinations is similar to that seen with other noradrenergic agents. Side effects are more notable at higher doses and most commonly include tremor, agitation, nervousness, increased sweating, and insomnia; palpitations and tachycardia have also been reported. Patients with diabetes, hypertension, or cardiovascular disease (including arrhythmic conditions) should not self-medicate with ephedrine-containing products without evaluation by a qualified physician.

Ephedrine is available both with and without a prescription; neither form is labeled by the FDA for use as an obesity therapy.[98,99]

SEROTONERGIC AGENTS

Serotonin is an important neurotransmitter involved in many human physiologic systems. Sleep–wake cycles, sensitivity to pain, blood pressure, mood, and eating behaviors have links to serotonin activity. Increasing central serotonin levels decreases the amount of food consumed and prolongs the time between food intake.[73] Some serotonergic agents increase central serotonin concentrations via stimulating release of presynaptic stores and/or inhibition of reuptake into storage granules. Additionally, either the parent compound or metabolites of these agents may also directly stimulate postsynaptic 5-HT receptors.[100] Peripheral serotonin effects that impact appetite, such as slowing gastric motility, have also been described.[73] A major distinction between serotonergic and noradrenergic anorexiants is that serotonergic agents lack the central stimulant effects and abuse potential seen with the noradrenergic compounds.[64,101] Conversely, decreased wakefulness, altered sleep patterns, and changes in affect can be seen.

Fenfluramine

Fenfluramine is an orally active, racemic mixture (D,L-fenfluramine), was used extensively as monotherapy for appetite suppression for many years. Fenfluramine increases synaptic serotonin concentration via reuptake inhibition and possibly by increasing serotonin release. An early, double-blind, placebo-controlled trial in obese patients demonstrated that fenfluramine, 20 mg three times daily, had similar efficacy to daily phentermine, 30 mg.[102] Average weight loss after 20 weeks of therapy ranged from 7.5 to 10 kg. Both medications were more effective than placebo, which attained 4.4 kg average loss.[102] Additionally, this trial was one of the first to include a treatment arm employing the combination of fenfluramine (30 mg prior to the evening meal) and phentermine (15 mg in the morning). Combination dosages were half that used in the monotherapy arms and achieved average weight loss of 8.5 kg with fewer reported side effects. Subsequently, Weintraub and colleagues completed classic placebo-controlled studies in a small cohort of obese patients that stimulated widespread interest and use of the combination of fenfluramine and phentermine (fen/phen) for weight management.[103–111] The combination provided, in most cases, enhanced anorexia with weight loss in excess of placebo.[64,112] Additionally, it appears that phentermine coadministration decreased some of the anxiety and confusion sometimes associated with fenfluramine.[101] Weight loss with this combination was associated with improvements in blood pressure, lipid profile, and glucose tolerance.[109,110,113] The long-term effectiveness of this combination was never clearly documented and weight regain, while less than that lost, occurred during the second year of use in many patients.[113,114] Fenfluramine was withdrawn from worldwide markets in 1997 due to a relationship with cardiac valvular insufficiency and valvular structural abnormalities (see "Severe Adverse Effects" later in the chapter).[69–71,115]

Dexfenfluramine

The D-isomer of fenfluramine was used extensively in Europe prior to its release in the United States in 1996. Dexfenfluramine increased synaptic serotonin concentrations via reuptake inhibition. Additionally, *in vitro* observations demonstrated that its metabolite, dexnorfenfluramine directly stimulated 5-HT_{2C} receptors.[100] This compound was the first in the United States to receive labeling for chronic use. Dexfenfluramine was more effective than placebo in promoting weight loss as part of a program in conjunction with diet and exercise.[64,65] Additional effectiveness with the addition of phentermine was also noted with this agent.[116] As a derivative of fenfluramine, it was also removed from worldwide markets because of potential cardiac valve problems (see "Severe Adverse Effects" later in the chapter).[71,115]

Antidepressants: Selective Serotonin Reuptake Inhibitors (SSRI)

It is interesting to note that some of the serotonergic appetite-suppressing agents were first studied as antidepressants and then subsequently noted to have effects on weight. As a class, the serotonin reuptake inhibitors are generally weight-neutral as opposed to other commonly used compounds such as the tricyclic antidepressants.[31,117] The National Task Force on the Prevention and Treatment of Obesity has reviewed multiple randomized, double-blinded, placebo-controlled weight-loss clinical trials using fluoxetine and one with sertraline.[67,118] Patients receiving fluoxetine (60 mg/d) demonstrate initial weight loss of up to 2 to 4 kg on average, but weight regain occurs in spite of continued medication use such that no difference is noted between fluoxetine and placebo over periods of up to 1 year.[119] Similar findings are noted using sertraline (200 mg/d) as an adjunct to help maintain weight lost with VLCD.[118] A direct relationship exists between amount of weight lost and the sum of fluoxetine and norfluoxetine plasma concentrations. Higher plasma concentrations are associated with greater weight loss.[120] The antidepressant serotonin reuptake inhibitors are not approved by the FDA as weight management agents and are not currently recommended for routine treatment of obesity.[67,68] Some practitioners continue to prescribe these agents for the treatment of obesity, "off-label" either alone or in combination with phentermine.[121] The safety and efficacy of phentermine–SSRI combinations are currently unclear. A recent case report of adverse experiences (impaired mentation, tremor, hyperreflexia, and gastrointestinal symptoms) with unintentional concurrent use of phentermine and fluoxetine reinforces the need for caution by prescribers of unlabeled combination therapy.[122] Serious adverse effects such as primary pulmonary hypertension and cardiac valve abnormalities (see "Severe Adverse Effects" later in the chapter) in excess of background prevalence have not been reported in relation to SSRI use for obesity therapy.

NORADRENERGIC/SEROTONERGIC AGENT

Sibutramine

An orally active racemic mixture, sibutramine became available in the United States in early 1998. The parent compound and two active metabolites appear to increase synaptic concentrations of serotonin (5-HT), norepinephrine (NE), and dopamine via reuptake inhibition. The active metabolites (M_1 and M_2) are more potent than the parent sibutramine. Reuptake inhibition appears to be greatest for norepinephrine, followed by serotonin, with dopamine the least inhibited. Sibutramine, M_1, and M_2 do not directly stimulate serotonergic (5-HT_1 or 5-HT_2), noradrenergic (α_1, α_2, β_1, β_2, β_3), or dopamine receptors.[123] It is thought that sibutramine induces weight loss by both decreasing appetite and maintaining or increasing thermogenesis via the combined effects on 5-HT and NE reuptake inhibition.[123] In humans, the degree to which these effects can be attributed to central versus peripheral activity is currently unknown. Sibutramine is subject to hepatic first-pass metabolism via $CYP3A_4$.[124] Moderate changes in sibutramine and/or metabolite disposition have been seen with ketoconazole coadminstration.[124] M_1 and M_2 area-under-the-curve increased by 58% and 20%, respectively, with concurrent ketoconazole (200 mg twice daily for 7 days). Smaller changes have been noted with concurrent erythromycin and cimetidine. The active metabolites M_1 and M_2 exhibit elimination half-lives of 14 and 16 hours, respectively.[124,125] Further metabolism of the active metabolites results in conjugates that are renally eliminated. The pharmacokinetics of sibutramine allows for single daily oral dosing.

Sibutramine has been studied in clinical trials in doses from 1 to 30 mg daily and demonstrates a relatively clear dose–response relationship. Weight loss from daily doses of 1 mg is, on average, no different than placebo. The recommended starting dose is 10 mg daily, with a recommended dose range of 5 to 15 mg daily. Dry mouth, anorexia, insomnia, constipation, appetite increase, dizziness, and nausea were noted two- to threefold more frequently in sibutramine-treated subjects than in placebo-treated subjects.[124,125] Significant increases in both systolic and diastolic blood pressure and pulse rate have been noted with sibutramine use.[124] Baseline blood pressure should be established prior to beginning therapy and close monitoring is required when using this agent. Sibutramine product labeling indicates that it should not be used in patients with a history of coronary artery disease, stroke, congestive heart failure, or arrhythmias.[125] Like other centrally acting appetite suppressants, sibutramine should not be used in patients receiving MAO inhibitor therapies. Sibutramine is listed as a schedule IV prescription substance in spite of being noted as having no street value by recreational substance users.[125] Primary pulmonary hypertension has not been reported with sibutramine use. Echocardiographic assessments of a small cohort of patients from clinical trials, with approximately 6 months exposure, do not demonstrate the cardiac valve problems seen with the fenfluramine derivatives.[124] Based upon 12-month clinical trials, weight loss with sibutramine therapy appears to be most significant during the first 6 months of therapy. Twenty-nine percent of placebo-treated patients in these trials attained a 5% reduction in total body weight after 12 months.[125] Using sibutramine at 10 and 15 mg/d resulted in 56% and 65% of patients, respectively, achieving at least a 5% reduction in total body weight.[125] A 10% reduction in body weight was achieved by 8% of placebo-treated patients, while 30% and 39% of those taking sibutramine 10 and 15 mg/d, respectively, obtained this level of weight reduction. There is, on average, a tendency for weight regain after 6 months of treatment. As with other centrally active appetite suppressants, weight regain occurs with cessation of therapy.[126] Safety and efficacy beyond 1 year of exposure to sibutramine are currently uncertain.

LIPASE INHIBITORS

Orlistat

The percentage of dietary intake as fat has been implicated as a contributing factor in the development of obesity. Fat represents an extremely dense energy source, providing 9 kcal/g as compared to approximately 4 kcal/g from protein or carbohydrate. In humans, most of accumulated body fat excess is derived from dietary sources because of a limited capacity to synthesize fat from carbohydrate. Gastrointestinal (gastric, pancreatic, and carboxylester) lipases are essential in the absorption of the long-chain triglycerides commonly found in Western diets. Additionally, lipase is known to play a role in facilitating gastric emptying and secretion of other pancreaticobiliary substances.[127] Orlistat (Xenical, RO 18-0647) is a synthetic derivative of lipstatin, a natural lipase inhibitor produced by streptomyces toxyticini. Orlistat is minimally absorbed and selectively inhibits gastrointestinal lipases.[128] Lipase inhibition results in decreased formation of free fatty acids from dietary triglyceride. Additionally, lower luminal free fatty acid concentrations result in malabsorption of cholesterol.[66] Orlistat induces weight loss by a persistent lowering of dietary fat absorption. Clinical studies employing orlistat as an adjunct to diet therapy demonstrated dose-dependent reductions in fat absorption. Pharmacodymanic modeling using early clinical trial data demonstrated half-maximal inhibition of fat absorption from orlistat doses of 98 mg/d, with maximal effects at around 400 mg/d.[129] Clinically, as much as a 30% reduction in fat absorption occurs with daily doses of 360 mg.[129,130] No additional decreases in fat absorption occurs with doses above 400 mg/d.[129] The drug must be taken with foods that contain fat in order to exert its effect. However, varying either meal content with regard to fat/fiber ratio or timing of drug ingestion relative to meal demonstrated little effect on the inhibition of fat absorption.[131,132]

At least one gastrointestinal complaint (soft stools, abdominal pain/colic, flatulence, fecal urgency, or incontinence) is initially reported in up to 80% of individuals using orlistat.[133,134] These complaints are most common in the first 1 to 2 months of therapy, are mild to moderate in severity, and tend to improve with continued orlistat use. Orlistat in addition to a low-calorie diet over a 1-year time period resulted in a small cohort of obese subjects who maintained a 7% to 9% decrease in body weight as opposed to placebo-treated subjects who experienced weight regain at 6 to 7 months of therapy.[135] Orlistat-induced malabsorption of fat-soluble vitamins has been documented.[135,136] Therefore, vitamin supplementation should be considered during therapy with this agent. Despite its definite effects on fat absorption and gastrointestinal motility, orlistat does not appear to change the pharmacokinetic or dynamic profiles of numerous other agents. Controlled studies of concurrent administration documenting minimal effects include oral contraceptives, digoxin, glyburide, phenytoin, pravastatin, warfarin, extended-release nifedipine, captopril, atenolol, furosemide, and ethanol.[128] This agent may prove to be an acceptable long-term medication supplement in medically supervised weight loss programs. Most recently, a 1-year, randomized, double-blind, placebo-controlled trial of orlistat in obese type 2 diabetics was completed.[137] This trial demonstrated that prolonged use of orlistat results in significant sustainable weight loss with improvements in glycemic control and lipid profile. Additionally, a significant number of orlistat-treated diabetics either decreased or discontinued oral sulfonylurea therapy during and throughout the trial. Although unanimously recommended for approval by an FDA advisory committee in 1997, the FDA subsequently requested further information regarding the occurrence of breast cancer during clinical trials. An overall breast cancer incidence of 0.6% (9 cases, all female) was noted in the orlistat treatment versus 0.1% (1 case, female) with placebo. In retrospect, evidence of malignancy prior to study participation was apparent in 8 of the 9 orlistat-treated patients. Clarification of this issue resulted in orlistat approval by the FDA in 1998, and its arrival in U.S. markets is due sometime in 1999.

PEPTIDES

Multiple different endogenous peptides, which play a role in the regulation of food intake, have been identified in animals and humans. Leptin originates in the adipocyte and is proposed to function as a peripheral feedback messenger with respect to fat storage (discussed earlier in the chapter). Neuropeptide Y (NPY) and galanin are two central nervous system peptides that appear to similarly stimulate food consumption but have differing effects on preference to carbohydrate or fat as well as substrate metabolism.[138] Currently, NPY and galanin are thought to exert minimal effects on protein intake, but a third less well described central nervous system peptide, growth hormone-releasing factor, stimulates protein ingestion. Carbohydrate ingestion and use are related to NPY hypothalamic activity, specifically in the arcuate and medial paraventricular nucleus. Galanin activity, centering in the lateral paraventricular nucleus and medial preoptic areas, increases both carbohydrate and fat intake with preferential effects on fat consumption and utilization.[138] NPY enhances fat synthesis via increased respiratory quotient and use of carbohydrate. Galanin appears to slow energy expenditure.[138] NPY and galanin modulate the release of insulin, corticosterone, and vasopressin, further affecting nutrient intake behaviors and substrate metabolism. NPY is associated with increased levels of insulin, corticosterone, and vasopressin while decreases are seen with galanin.[138]

The macronutrient intake, energy use, and endocrine effects of NPY are most consistent with those seen in chronic obesity. Future pharmacotherapies may develop based upon knowledge of the effects of these endogenous peptides.

Currently, recombinant leptin has been administered subcutaneously to humans.[139] A phase I tolerability and dose ranging study demonstrated some initial prospects for exogenous leptin administration. Participants were randomly assigned to receive either leptin or placebo and were given exercise and nutrition counseling. The placebo-controlled study was not designed to demonstrate efficacy, but preliminary data analysis of 165 male and female participants showed that 19% of placebo-treated patients versus 30% to 45% of leptin-treated subjects lost at least 2 kg over 28 days of study. Thirty obese participants remained on the study through 90 days of therapy. Not all of the leptin doses studied elicited weight loss. Placebo-treated individuals lost an average of 1.5 kg and subjects exposed to some of the leptin doses lost 2 to 4 kg. These potentially effective doses are being used in phase II trials involving obese patients with and without type 2 diabetes. Some study participants suffered local injection site reactions, and systemic antibodies were detected at higher leptin doses in some patients. Second-generation leptin molecules are being developed to reduce injection site reactions, which will potentially improve tolerability for higher doses.

HERBAL, NATURAL, AND FOOD SUPPLEMENT WEIGHT LOSS THERAPIES

Many individuals, whether or not clinically overweight or obese, choose to undertake weight loss regimens without medical monitoring and incorporate the ingestion of herbal, natural, or food supplement products. It is important to remember that the FDA does not strictly regulate the manufacture and labeling of these products. Table 132–5 lists some of the common constituents found in many of these products.

CHROMIUM

The inclusion of chromium as an effective agent for weight loss is unclear. The hexavalent form of this trace element is thought to be carcinogenic, while the trivalent form found in human food sources is essentially nontoxic.[140] Chromium is considered an essential nutrient, and experimentally in animals is an insulin cofactor active in carbohydrate, protein, and lipid metabolism.[140] In humans, insulin resistance has been reported in a few cases of apparent severe chromium deficiency during long-term total parenteral nutrition (see Chap. 128). Currently, there is no reliable means of assessing total body chromium status, making diagnosis of deficiency difficult. The tryptophan metabolite, picolinic acid, forms a complex with trivalent chromium, which improves bioavailability. Food sources with highly available chromium include brewer's yeast, calf liver, American cheese, and wheat germ.[140] A recent double-blind, placebo-controlled study of chromium picolinate as a supplement to aerobic exercise in the treatment of obesity failed to demonstrate any effectiveness.[141]

TABLE 132–5. Weight Loss Agents in Herbal, Natural, and Food Supplements[a]

Herbal/Natural/ Food Supplements	Active Moiety	Proposed Effect
Chromium picolinate	Chromium	Mechanism unclear
Ma huang	Ephedrine derivatives	Noradrenergic
St. John's wort	Hypericin	Serotonergic/MAO inhibition
White willow bark	Salicylate	Inhibit norepinephrine breakdown
Calcium pyruvate	Pyruvate	Mechanism unclear
Guarana extract	Caffeine	Noradrenergic
Various tea extracts	Caffeine	Noradrenergic
Garcinia gambogia extract (citrin)	Hydroxycitric acid	Mechanism unclear

[a]Safety and efficacy not documented.

MA HUANG

Ma huang is a traditional Chinese medicine manufactured from various plant parts of the *Ephedraceae* species. This species is known to produce L-ephedrine, D-pseudoephedrine, L-norephedrine, D-norpseudoephedrine, L-*N*-methylephedrine, and D-*N*-methylpseudoephedrine.[142] The FDA Center for Food Safety and Applied Nutrition completed an analysis of several products labeled as containing ma huang; ephedrine-type alkaloids were detected in concentrations ranging from 0 to 56 mg/g.[142] Although it is quite difficult to determine actual exposure to active entities when using ma huang, side effects and cautions would be similar to those listed earlier for ephedrine. Recently, the FDA proposed constraints on allowable ephedrine alkaloid concentrations, and combinations with other stimulants such as caffeine in dietary supplements.[143] From 1994 through July 1997, the FDA received over 800 reports of serious adverse events, including seizures, stroke, and death coincident with ephedrine-containing dietary supplement use. These preparations are probably best avoided in patients with diabetes, hypertension, and other cardiovascular disease. The problem with many marketed products is the lack of consistency in labeling versus actual product content.

ST. JOHN'S WORT

A perennial flowering plant (*Hypericum perforatum*) St. John's wort has been employed as a medicinal herb for thousands of years. Its use in weight loss and herbal supplements is probably based upon the proposed effects of its constituent naphthodianthrones (hypericin and pseudohypericin). These are thought to be inhibitors of monoamine oxidase, and would be expected to increase synaptic concentrations of monoamines such as serotonin and norepinephrine. Consistent with these assumptions, hypericum extracts appear to be more effective than placebo in the treatment of depression.[144] However, *in vitro* studies have not been able to substantiate direct monoamine oxidase inhibition at physiologic hypericin concentrations and recognized antidepressant effects may be due to other constituents.[145,146] The risks of concurrent use of *Hypericum* derivatives and other adrenergic and serotonergic compounds have not been characterized. Currently, St. John's wort has not been studied with respect to its role in obesity management, and its safety and efficacy as a treatment modality in the self-management of obesity are unclear.

WHITE WILLOW BARK

White willow bark is a source of salicylate, a prostaglandin inhibitor. Prostaglandin inhibition may enhance adrenergic stimulation via inhibition of norepinephrine breakdown (see the eariler discussion of ephedrine).

GUARANA EXTRACT AND VARIOUS TEA EXTRACTS

Guarana and tea are sources of caffeine that have inherent adrenergic properties as well as increasing the effects of stimulant substances such as ephedrine or ephedra alkaloids (see the earlier discussion of ephedrine).

SEVERE ADVERSE EFFECTS

Severe adverse effects have been reported with almost all of the appetite-suppressant agents discussed in this chapter. Because of combination use or multiple use patterns by many patients, it is often difficult to identify direct causal relationships. Therefore, all practitioners dealing with patients who are current users of or have been exposed to anorectic agents should maintain a high index of suspicion for the occurrence of severe adverse effects. Primary pulmonary hypertension and cardiac valvulopathy, discussed next, appear to occur most frequently with the use of fenfluramine derivatives.

PRIMARY PULMONARY HYPERTENSION

Primary pulmonary hypertension (PPH) is a condition in which high pressures of unknown etiology in the pulmonary vasculature result in increased right ventricular afterload. Various causal relationships have been suggested including recent pregnancy, cocaine use, cirrhosis, genetic susceptibility, oral contraceptive use, and infection with the human immunodeficiency virus. Afflicted individuals have an impaired ability to increase cardiac output in response to exertion and can present with vague complaints of dyspnea, chest pains, and sometimes syncope. Progression of this disorder causes right-sided heart failure and death. About 50% of cases may spontaneously remit. In the unremitting cases, the condition responds poorly to medical management and patients have a median survival from diagnosis of about 2.5 to 3 years. The estimated annual incidence of this condition is 1 to 2 cases per million population. In Europe during the 1960s an increase in the incidence of PPH was noted during the same time period that an adrenergically active appetite suppressant, aminorex fumarate, was marketed. A return to the baseline incidence of PPH was observed after aminorex was removed from use. Overall, an increased risk of developing PPH appears possible with use of some of the noradrenergic and serotonergic appetite suppressants, either alone or in combination.[147–150] Specifically, the estimated odds ratio for occurrence of PPH with use of fenfluramine derivatives is stated as about 6 and possibly greater than 20 with use over 3 months duration.[149,150] The 20-fold increased PPH prevalence is similar to the rate of fatality from penicillin anaphylaxis (10 to 20/million exposures).[151] To date, PPH has not been identified as a problem with PPA, sibutramine, or the SSRI compounds.

CARDIAC VALVULOPATHY

Cardiac valve disease is known to occur coincident with serotonergic compounds (methysergide and ergotamine) and disease states (carcinoid disease) that result in systemic elevations of serotonin.[152,153] A form of cardiac valvular disease has been recognized coincident with the use of serotonergic appetite suppressants. Clinician investigators recently described 24 cases of symptomatic valvular heart disease in women, mean age 44 years, with no previous history of cardiac disease and a common association with exposure to the combination of fenfluramine-phentermine (fen/phen).[69] Cardiac ultrasonography demonstrated multivalvular regurgitation and abnormal valve morphology. Eight of the 24 cases demonstrated newly documented pulmonary hypertension with right ventricular systolic pressures ranging from 52 to 93 mm Hg. Mitral valve replacement was required in 5 of the 24 cases. Three of these five were concurrently exposed to SSRI or TCA compounds. Average exposure to fen/phen was 11 months (range, 1 to 28 months). Subsequently, a prevalence study using echocardiography was performed in 233 appetite suppressant exposed patients and 233 control subjects matched for age, gender, and BMI.[71] A significantly increased prevalence of mostly aortic insufficiency was observed in the exposed patients who had been treated with dexfenfluramine alone, dexfenfluramine/phentermine, or fen/phen for an average of 20.5 months. The investigators found that 1.3% of control subjects versus 22.7% of exposed patients demonstrated mild or greater aortic insufficiency. This study demonstrated a highly significant risk for cardiac valve insufficiency with appetite suppressant use (odds ratio, 22.6; $P < .001$; 95% confidence interval, 7.1 to 114.2). Fewer individuals demonstrated mitral or tricuspid insufficiency than the original case reports. Of note, this study demonstrates that the background prevalence of mild or greater aortic insufficiency in unexposed obese patients is similar to that of the general population under 50 years of age.

Three additional studies have reported risk estimates for this drug-related valvular insufficiency.[154–156] The differing study designs, populations, and duration of exposure can, in part, explain the variability of these risk estimates. Weissman and colleagues studied patients from a prematurely terminated, placebo-controlled, dexfenfluramine treatment trial.[155] The average exposure to dexfenfluramine at the time of study termination was 2.5 months. Using cardiac ultrasound, they demonstrated a significantly higher prevalence of aortic insufficiency in those exposed (17%) versus those in the placebo arm (11.8%), $P = 0.03$.[155] A population-based, follow-up study with nested case-control analysis by Jick and colleagues evaluated the prevalence of significant valve regurgitation in patients who used fenfluramine or dexfenfluramine for less than 3 months versus 4 or more months.[154] Those with 4 or more months of use demonstrated a significantly greater odds ratio (7.4; $P = 0.01$) for valve insufficiency. Two research groups have estimated the incidence of this drug-related disease by documenting valve disease prior to and after fenfluramine or dexfenfluramine exposure in small numbers of patients.[156,157] They reported a valve insufficiency incidence of 4% to 16.5% with periods of exposure less than 1 year. Although a relationship between fenfluramine-like drug use and valve insufficiency seems certain, the exact incidence and possible risk factors for developing the problem are not well-defined.[158,159] The long-term clinical significance of fen/phen or dexfenfluramine-related valve disease remains a topic of further research.

Valvular insufficiency is not readily appreciated on physical exam in many patients with appetite suppressant-related valvular disease, but is detectable via cardiac ultrasonography. An understanding of risk factors, etiology, progression, and natural history of this drug-related valve disease is evolving. The U.S. Department of Health and Human Services has issued interim recommendations for health care providers to deal with this valvulopathy. These include antibiotic prophylaxis for some dental and surgical procedures depending upon the degree of valve incompetence.[115] Most of the current research regarding this valvulopathy has centered around serotonergic pharmaceuticals. Interestingly, significant aortic insufficiency has been reported in women who have consumed "Chinese herbs" as part of a weight loss routine.[160] However, direct causal relationship with the herbal preparations is unclear, as these weight loss routines also included use of fenfluramine and diethylpropion.[160]

SEROTONIN SYNDROME

Concern regarding the potential occurrence of the serotonin syndrome has been heightened with the ever-increasing number of serotonergic agents being employed, in the treatment of obesity, depression, and migraine headache. The serotonin syndrome is defined by a spectrum of symptoms that develop coincident with the administration of multiple serotonergic agents.[161] Excess peripheral and central serotonergic stimulation may be involved, leading to a constellation of symptoms.[162] Specific diagnostic criteria include the presence of at least three of the following: fever, shivering, confusion, agitation, tremor, ataxia, hyperreflexia, sweating, or diarrhea. Although the syndrome is generally mild, severe episodes can include seizures, dyspnea, hypotension, hypertension, arrhythmias, renal failure, disseminated intravascular coagulation, and death. The syndrome occurs most commonly in patients consuming combinations of serotonergic agents. The largest number of reported cases center around MAO inhibitors taken concurrently with SSRIs, dextromethorphan, meperidine, and tricyclic antidepressants.[161] Case reports also include combinations of SSRIs with tryptophan, lithium, pentazocine, and dextromethorphan. Sumatriptan, a popular therapy for migraine headache, has been linked to syndrome development in a small number of patients who were also receiving an SSRI.[163] Interestingly, this review compiled a number of cases of SSRI–sumatriptan, and MAO inhibitor–sumatriptan, use without problems. No information regarding the safety of sumatriptan and noradrenergic or serotonergic obesity therapies was given. The apparent unpredictable nature of combination serotonergic therapy dictates extreme caution in these polypharmacy situations.

MONITORING THE PHARMACEUTICAL CARE PLAN

OUTCOME MEASURES

Specific weight goals should be established that are consistent with medical needs and patient personal desire. For most obese patients, a weight-loss goal of 5% to 10% to no more than 30% of initial weight is reasonable. An average rate of weight loss after the first month of therapy is around 1 pound per week. Patients should not be allowed to attain weight less than their estimated ideal weight. Assessment of patient progress should be documented in a health care setting once or twice monthly for 1 to 2 months, and then monthly thereafter.[68] Each encounter should document weight, WC, BMI, blood pressure, medical history, and patient assessment of obesity medication tolerability.[68] Chronic use of obesity medications should be consistent with the approved product labeling. Medication therapy should be discontinued after 3 to 4 months if the patient has failed to demonstrate weight loss or maintenance of prior weight. The recent AACE/ACE statement on obesity provides a patient evaluation checklist, a validated survey of general well-being, and sample informed consent that could be used in screening and follow-up of patients receiving obesity pharmacotherapy as part of a weight loss program.[68] The Short Form 36 (SF-36) has also been used as a quality of life evaluation tool for obese patients undergoing programmatic weight loss. Quarterly assessments of well-being and quality of life using validated assessment tools can be helpful in objectively quantifying the effectiveness of therapy as well as potential drug-induced side effects (e.g., depression).[68]

Diabetic patients receiving weight loss medication require more intense medical monitoring and self-monitoring of blood glucose. Some centrally acting weight loss agents, such as the serotonergic agents, have direct effects that immediately improve glucose tolerance, even prior to significant weight loss. Insulin therapy may therefore need to be adjusted with the start of obesity medication therapy. Peripherally active agents, such as orlistat, have also be shown to decrease oral hypoglycemic agent requirements in type 2 diabetic patients.[137] However, this effect was noted later in therapy and more directly correlated with weight loss. Some diabetic patients may require daily telephone contact with a health care provider to assist in adjusting their hypoglycemic therapy. Weekly patient visits to a health care setting may be necessary for 1 to 2 months until the effects of diet, exercise, and weight loss medication become more predictable. As frequent as quarterly assessment of hemoglobin A_{1c} may be appropriate in type 2 diabetics who lose weight, to aid in adjustment of hypoglycemic therapy. Lipid profiles can normalize or improve with weight loss. Lipid status should be assessed semiannually or annually in patients with hyperlipidemia to determine need for continued hyperlipidemia therapies. Weight loss can also result in normalization of blood pressure in hypertensive obese patients. Assessment of appropriateness of antihypertensive therapy should occur with each follow-up visit.

PHARMACOECONOMIC CONSIDERATIONS

There are few data regarding economic consequences of treating obesity. One study evaluated the savings in prescription costs following a 12-week weight reduction program in 40 type 2 diabetic patients.[165] Patients lost an average of 33.7 pounds over the study period. A cost analysis was completed on 32 of 40 patients who were taking antihypertensive and or antidiabetic medications using the out-of-pocket costs for these medications at the beginning of the study and after 1 year. The patients sustained a mean weight loss of 19.8 pounds over the next year. The average cost of these prescriptions at the beginning as compared to the 1-year follow-up was $63.30 versus $32.50 per month. The estimated annual average saving in prescription costs per patient was $443. *Money* magazine caught consumer eyes with a 1997 article entitled, "Shrink your weight while keeping your wallet plump."[166] This analysis evaluated out-of-pocket expenses per pound lost for several different diet options including Weight Watchers, Ultra Slim Fast, Redux (dexfenfluramine), Jenny Craig, and Optifast. Jenny Craig costs included purchase of food products, and Redux and Optifast costs included physician monitoring. Weight Watchers and Ultra Slim fast were lowest at $8 to $9 per pound lost, while Jenny Craig and Optifast came in high at $59 and $84, respectively, per pound lost. Redux fell in the middle at $28 per pound lost. Cost of side effects, quality of life parameters, and probability of long-term weight loss with the various products/services were not included in this analysis.

Finally, Martin and colleagues compared the costs associated with medical and surgical treatment of obesity.[167] Medical therapy groups received diet therapy only (no medications) and cost included weekly clinic visits for behavioral modification. A successful outcome was defined as loss of at least one-third of excess body weight above ideal body weight. They monitored all patients for 2 years and some for as long as 7 years so that long-term weight control could be addressed. As expected, the costs of surgery were much higher than medical therapy over the first 2 years ($24,000 versus $3000). However, when costs were extrapolated out to 6 years, the cost per pound lost for medical therapy exceeded surgical therapy (about $313 versus $261 per pound lost). It is clear from the data above that weight loss can be expensive for the consumer. Prospectively designed cost-benefit or cost-effectiveness analyses are needed to determine if costs of weight loss therapy or surgery are balanced by lower costs of hospitalizations for other medical problems associated with obesity or the additional life years gained. Quality of life measures also need to be taken into consideration when evaluating this type of data.

EVALUATION OF THERAPEUTIC OUTCOMES

An expert committee of the National Institutes of Health, Heart, Lung, and Blood Institute has completed and extensive summary of clinical guidelines for the assessment and treatment of obesity.[164] This report provides guidance with evidence-based, graded assessment and treatment recommendations from an extensive meta-analysis of the available obesity literature to date. The evaluation and management of a patient with obesity requires careful clinical, biochemical, and if necessary psychological evaluation. The evaluation must include an assessment of current medical conditions and medications the patient uses. Clearly, a multidisciplinary team including but not limited to a

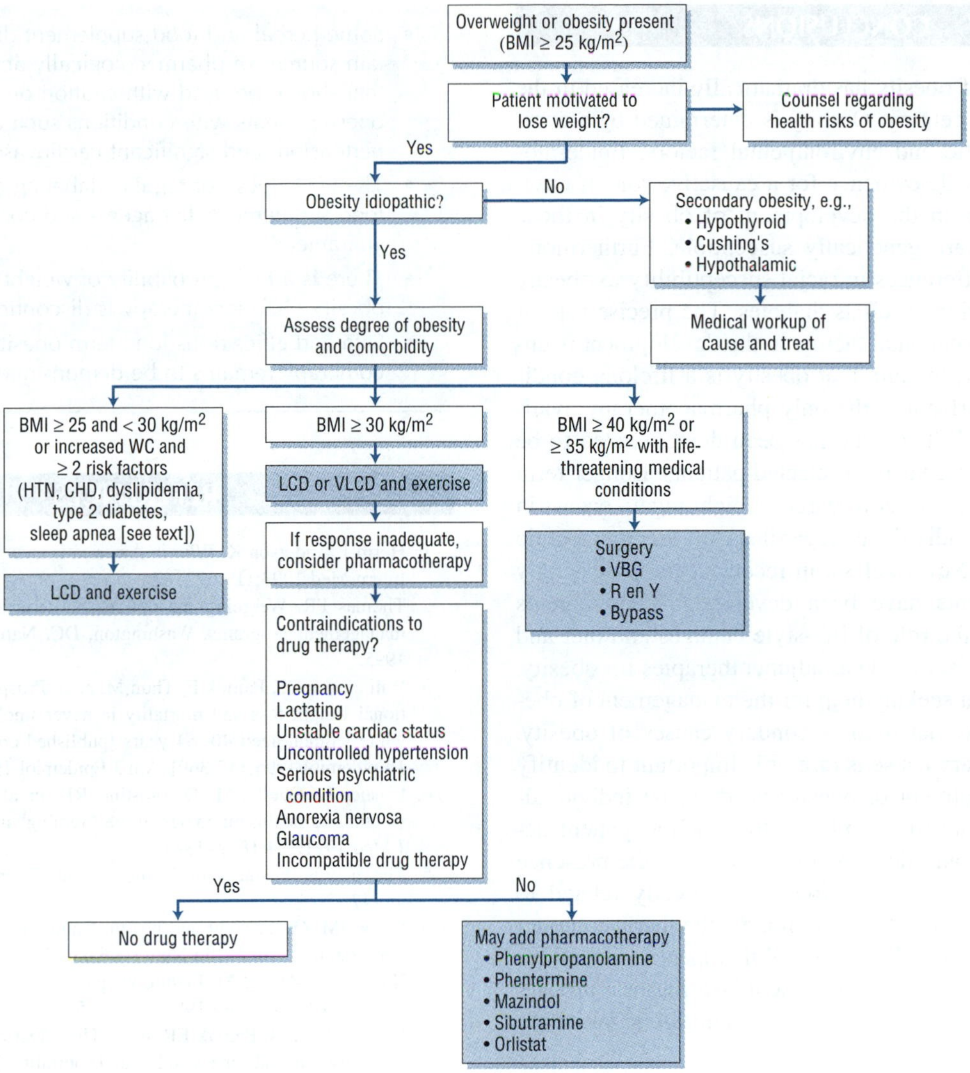

FIGURE 132–5. Pharmacotherapy treatment algorithm. A select population of individuals may benefit from medication therapy as an adjunct to a program of weight loss that includes diet, exercise, and behavioral modification. Increased WC > 40 inches for males and > 35 inches for females. (BMI = body mass index; CHD = coronary heart disease; LCD = low-calorie diet; VLCD = very-low-calorie diet; VBG = vertically banded gastroplasty; R on Y = Roux-en-y; WC = waist circumference.) [a]Pending approval.

physician, nutritionist, psychologist, and pharmacist best achieves this. The algorithm in Figure 132–5 shows an approach to determining appropriate types of treatment for the overweight individual. The decision to treat any overweight/obese patient is dependent upon the degree and distribution of obesity present, the motivation of the patient to lose weight, and the potential benefits and risks of weight loss. The initial step in this process should be to verify the presence of clinically significant excess body weight. In the clinical setting this is most often done by measuring height, weight, and WC of the individual and calculating BMI. If the BMI is greater than 25 kg/m^2 and/or waist circumference is greater than 40 inches for males or 35 inches for females, it is likely that the patient will benefit from weight loss. The next step is to assess whether the patient is actually motivated to lose weight. No matter what the treatment options are, they all require significant effort on the part of the patient to change life-style and comply with the management plan. If it is clear the patient is not yet ready to meet these expectations, then early counseling will reduce the chance of frustration for the patients, clinicians, and in some cases other family members. This does not exclude the possibility of educating the patient about potential risks of obesity and the benefits of weight loss. This type of basic information in certain cases can lead to a significant change in motivation and desire to lose weight and improved compliance.

Pharmacotherapy may be appropriate for some overweight individuals, those with a BMI of 30 kg/m^2 or more without weight-related, immediate life-threatening medical conditions. It should also be considered for those with BMI ≥ 27 or increased WC who have 2 or more risk factors. From the health care providers' perspective, drug therapy for obesity should always be considered as a supplement to an integrated program of diet, exercise, and behavior modification (including group support). A complete medical and medication history is essential in determining appropriate obesity drug therapy. Consideration must be given to alcohol, nicotine, caffeine, and herbal or food supplement use as well as prescription and nonprescription drugs.

CONCLUSIONS

The prevalence of obesity has dramatically increased in the latter part of this century. Obesity is determined by a combination of genetic and environmental factors. Epidemiologic studies provide evidence for a causative role of environmental factors in the development of obesity in those individuals who are genetically susceptible. Furthermore, there are clear differences in racial susceptibility to obesity and its complications such as diabetes. The precise role of genetic and environmental factors in the development is unknown. It is clear, though, that obesity is a lifelong condition. Currently, orlistat is the only pharmacotherapy available in the United States that has been demonstrated to be effective, for up to 2 years in selected patients. Longer-term results will require further research. Weight regain occurs in the majority of individuals regardless of the therapeutic modalities used. Nevertheless, in recent years increasingly effective treatments have been developed. These agents have augmented the role of life-style changes and diet and therefore serve a useful role as adjunct therapies for obesity.

Every patient seeking help for the management of obesity should be evaluated for secondary causes of obesity. Though a secondary cause is rare, it is important to identify and manage. Treatment of obesity needs to be individualized. It is important to consider factors such as patient desires, age, degree and duration of obesity, and the presence or absence of medical conditions both directly related to obesity as well as those that may impact the therapeutic decisions. Whatever combinations of therapeutic modalities are used, it is clear that management is a lifelong process requiring patient support and careful monitoring for safety and efficacy.

▶ PRINCIPLES OF PHARMACOTHERAPY

- A sufficient degree of obesity (BMI ≥ 30 kg/m^2 height or WC ≥ 40 inches for males or 35 inches for females or BMI ≥ 27 ≤ 30 with obesity risk factors) should be present before pharmacotherapy-facilitated weight loss is considered.
- Medication therapy for obesity is appropriate only as an adjunct to a regimen of diet, exercise, and behavioral modification.
- Concurrent use of noradrenergic and serotonergic obesity medications is contraindicated in the presence of monoamine oxidase inhibitors, and extreme caution is needed with other serotonergic combinations.
- Exposure to some appetite suppressants (fenfluramine derivatives) can result in cardiac valve disease.
- Obese individuals with concurrent diseases such as diabetes and hypertension require intensive monitoring when undertaking a weight loss program.
- Some herbal and food supplement diet agents contain sources of pharmacologically active substances that should be used with caution or avoided in obese patients with conditions such as diabetes, hypertension, and significant cardiovascular disease.
- The FDA does not regulate labeling of herbal and food supplement diet agents and content is not guaranteed.
- There is a high probability of weight regain when obesity pharmacotherapy is discontinued.
- Safe and efficacious long-term obesity pharmacotherapy remains to be demonstrated.

REFERENCES

1. Horm J, Anderson K. Who in America is trying to lose weight? Ann Intern Med 1993;119:672–676.
2. Thomas PR. Weighing the options: Criteria for evaluating weight management programs. Washington, DC, National Academy Press, 1995.
3. Williamson DF, Pamuk E, Thun M, et al. Prospective study of intentional weight loss and mortality in never-smoking overweight U.S. white women aged 40–64 years [published erratum appears in Am J Epidemiol 1995;142:369]. Am J Epidemiol 1995;141:1128–1141.
4. Lissner L, Odell PM, D'Agostino RB, et al. Variability of body weight and health outcomes in the Framingham population. N Engl J Med 1991;324:1839–1844.
5. The painful business of losing weight. Economist January:1997; 45–47.
6. Rippe JM. Overweight and health: Communications challenges and opportunities. Am J Clin Nutr 1996;63:470S–473S.
7. Kassirer JP, Angell M. Losing weight—an ill-fated New Year's resolution. N Engl J Med 1998;338:52–54.
8. Stevens J, Cai J, Pamuk ER, et al. The effect of age on the association between body-mass index and mortality. N Engl J Med 1998; 338:1–7.
9. Kuczmarski RJ. Prevalence of overweight and weight gain in the United States. Am J Clin Nutr 1992;55:495S–502S.
10. Abraham S, Carroll MD, Najjar MF, Fulwood R. Obese and overweight adults in the United States. Vital Health Stat 1983;11:1–93.
11. McDowell A, Engel A, Massey JT, Maurer K. Plan and operation of the second national health and nutrition examination survey, 1976–1980. Vital Health Stat 1981;1:1–144.
12. Metropolitan Life Insurance Company. Metropolitan Height and Weight Tables. Stat Bull Metrop Life Ins Co 1983;64, 2–9.
13. Williamson DF. Descriptive epidemiology of body weight and weight change in U.S. adults. Ann Intern Med 1993;119:646–649.
14. Wang ZM, Pierson RN Jr, Heymsfield SB. The five-level model: A new approach to organizing body-composition research. Am J Clin Nutr 1992;56:19–28.
15. Harsha DW, Bray GA. Body composition and childhood obesity. Endocrinol Metab Clin North Am 1996;25:871–885.
16. Bray GA. Topography of body fat. Adv Endocrinol Metab 1994;5: 297–322.
17. Pouliot MC, Despres JP, Lemieux S, et al. Waist circumference and abdominal sagittal diameter: Best simple anthropometric indexes of abdominal visceral adipose tissue accumulation and related cardiovascular risk in men and women. Am J Cardiol 1994;73:460–468.
18. Flier JS, Foster DW. Eating Disorders: Obesity, anorexia nervosa, bulimia nervosa. In: Wilson JD, Foster DW, Kronenberg HM, Larsen PR, eds. Williams Textbook of Endocrinology, 9th ed. Philadelphia, W.B. Saunders, 1998:1061–1097.

19. Bray GA. Overweight is risking fate. Definition, classification, prevalence, and risks. Ann NY Acad Sci 1987;499:14–28.
20. Kuczmarski RJ, Flegal KM, Campbell SM, Johnson CL. Increasing prevalence of overweight among US adults. The National Health and Nutrition Examination Surveys, 1960 to 1991. JAMA 1994;272: 205–211.
21. Abraham S, Collins G, Nordsieck M. Relationship of childhood weight status to morbidity in adults. HSMHA Health Rep 1971; 86:273–284.
22. Guo SS, Roche AF, Chumlea WC, et al. The predictive value of childhood body mass index values for overweight at age 35 y. Am J Clin Nutr 1994;59:810–819.
23. Sorensen TI, Sonne-Holm S. Risk in childhood of development of severe adult obesity: Retrospective, population-based case-cohort study. Am J Epidemiol 1988;127:104–113.
24. Power C, Lake JK, Cole TJ. Body mass index and height from childhood to adulthood in the 1958 British born cohort. Am J Clin Nutr 1997;66:1094–1101.
25. Garn SM, Clark DC. Trends in fatness and the origins of obesity ad hoc committee to review the ten-state nutrition survey. Pediatrics 1976;57:443–456.
26. Van Itallie TB. Health implications of overweight and obesity in the United States. Ann Intern Med 1985;103:983–988.
27. West DB. Genetics of obesity in humans and animal models. Endocrinol Metab Clin North Am 1996;25:801–813.
28. Hill JO, Peters JC. Environmental contributions to the obesity epidemic. Science 1998;280:1371–1374.
29. Lissner L, Levitsky DA, Strupp BJ, et al. Dietary fat and the regulation of energy intake in human subjects. Am J Clin Nutr 1987;46: 886–892.
30. Baez M, Kursar JD, Helton LA, et al. Molecular biology of serotonin receptors. Obes Res 1995;3(suppl 4):441S–447S.
31. Bloom FE. Neurotransmission and the central nervous system. In: Hardman JG, Gilman AG, Limbird LE, eds. Goodman and Gilman's The Pharmacologic Basis of Therapeutics, 9th ed. New York, McGraw-Hill, 1996:267–293.
32. Caro JF, Sinha MK, Kolaczynski JW, et al. Leptin: The tale of an obesity gene. Diabetes 1996;45:1455–1462.
33. Misra A, Garg A. Leptin, its receptor and obesity. J Investig Med 1996;44:540–548.
34. Giacobino JP. Role of the beta-3-adrenoceptor in the control of leptin expression. Horm Metab Res 1996;28:633–637.
35. Considine RV, Sinha MK, Heiman ML, et al. Serum immunoreactive-leptin concentrations in normal-weight and obese humans. N Engl J Med 1996;334:292–295.
36. Barinaga M. New appetite-boosting peptides found. Science 1998; 279:1134–1134.
37. Woods SC, Seeley RJ, Porte DJ, Schwartz MW. Signals that regulate food intake and energy homeostasis. Science 1998;280:1378–1383.
38. DeLany JP, Lovejoy JC. Energy expenditure. Endocrinol Metab Clin North Am 1996;25:831–846.
39. Roberts SB, Savage J, Coward WA, et al. Energy expenditure and intake in infants born to lean and overweight mothers. N Engl J Med 1988;318:461–466.
40. Larsen PR, Davies TF, Hay ID. The thyroid gland. In: Wilson JD, Foster DW, Kronenberg HM, Larsen PR, eds. Williams Textbook of Endocrinology, 9th ed. Philadelphia, W.B. Saunders, 1998:389–515.
41. Pi-Sunyer FX. Obesity. In: Bennett JC, Plum F, eds. Cecil Textbook of Medicine, 20th ed. Philadelphia, W.B. Saunders, 1998:1161–1168.
42. Bouchard C, ed. The genetics of obesity. In: Bouchard C, ed. Boca Raton, CRC Press, 1994.
43. Bouchard C, Perusse L, Leblanc C, et al. Inheritance of the amount and distribution of human body fat. Int J Obes 1988;12:205–215.
44. Comuzzie AG, Allison DB. The search for human obesity genes. Science 1998;280:1374–1377.
45. Garrow JS. Energy Balance and Obesity in Man, 2nd ed. New York, Elsevier/North Holland Biomedical Press, 1978.
46. Lowell BB, Flier JS. Brown adipose tissue, beta 3-adrenergic receptors, and obesity. Annu Rev Med 1997;48:307–316.
47. Vidal-Puig A, Solanes G, Grujic D, et al. UCP3: An uncoupling protein homologue expressed preferentially and abundantly in skeletal muscle and brown adipose tissue. Biochem Biophys Res Commun 1997;235:79–82.
48. Liu YL, Toubro S, Astrup A, Stock MJ. Contribution of beta 3-adrenoceptor activation to ephedrine-induced thermogenesis in humans. Int J Obes Relat Metab Disord 1995;19:678–685.
49. Large V, Hellstrom L, Reynisdottir S, et al. Human beta-2 adrenoceptor gene polymorphisms are highly frequent in obesity and associate with altered adipocyte beta-2 adrenoceptor function. J Clin Invest 1997;100:3005–3013.
50. Clement K, Vaisse C, Manning BS, et al. Genetic variation in the beta 3-adrenergic receptor and an increased capacity to gain weight in patients with morbid obesity. N Engl J Med 1995;333:352–354.
51. Hubert HB, Feinleib M, McNamara PM, Castelli WP. Obesity as an independent risk factor for cardiovascular disease: A 26-year follow-up of participants in the Framingham heart study. Circulation 1983; 67:968–977.
52. Manson JE, Colditz GA, Stampfer MJ, et al. A prospective study of obesity and risk of coronary heart disease in women. N Engl J Med 1990;322:882–889.
53. Garfinkel L. Overweight and cancer. Ann Intern Med 1985;103: 1034–1036.
54. Messerli FH. Cardiovascular effects of obesity and hypertension. Lancet 1982;1:1165–1168.
55. Ehrmann DA, Schneider DJ, Sobel BE et al. Troglitazone improves defects in insulin action, insulin secretion, ovarian steroidogenesis, and fibrinolysis in women with polycystic ovary syndrome. J Clin Endocrinol Metab 1997;82:2108–2116.
56. Barnard RJ, Ugianskis EJ, Martin DA, Inkeles SB. Role of diet and exercise in the management of hyperinsulinemia and associated atherosclerotic risk factors. Am J Cardiol 1992;69:440–444.
57. Appel LJ, Moore TJ, Obarzanek E, et al. A clinical trial of the effects of dietary patterns on blood pressure. DASH collaborative research group. N Engl J Med 1997;336:1117–1124.
58. Williamson DA, Perrin LA. Behavioral therapy for obesity. Endocrinol Metab Clin North Am 1996;25:943–954.
59. National Institute of Diabetes and Digestive and Kidney Diseases (NIDDK). Health information: Nutrition and obesity. Available at: http://www.niddk.nih.gov/health/nutrit/nutrit.htm. Accessed October 1998.
60. Weight-control information network. Available at: http://www.niddk.nih.gov/health/nutrit/win.htm. Accessed October 1998.
61 Wadden TA, Stunkard AJ, Brownell KD. Very low calorie diets: Their efficacy, safety, and future. Ann Intern Med 1983;99:675–684.
62. Pi-Sunyer FX. Obesity. In: Shils ME, Olson JA, Shike M, eds. Modern Nutrition in Health and Diesease, 8th ed. Philadelphia, Lea & Febiger, 1994:984–1006.
63. Greenway FL. Surgery for obesity. Endocrinol Metab Clin North Am 1996;25:1005–1027.
64. Bray GA. Use and abuse of appetite-suppressant drugs in the treatment of obesity. Ann Intern Med 1993;119:707–713.
65. Cerulli J, Lomaestro BM, Malone M. Update on the pharmacotherapy of obesity. Ann Pharmacother 1998;32:88–102.
66. Drent ML, van der Veen EA. Lipase inhibition: A novel concept in the treatment of obesity. Int J Obes Relat Metab Disord 1993;17: 241–244.
67. National task force on the prevention and treatment of obesity. Long-term pharmacotherapy in the management of obesity. JAMA 1996; 276:1907–1915.
68. Bray GA. AACE/ACE obesity statement. Endocr Pract 1997;3: 163–208.
69. Connolly HM, Crary JL, McGoon MD, et al. Valvular heart disease associated with fenfluramine–phentermine. N Engl J Med 1997;337: 581–588.

70. Graham DJ, Green L. Further cases of valvular heart disease associated with fenfluramine–phentermine. N Engl J Med 1997;337: 635.
71. Khan MA, Herzog CA, St. Peter JV, et al. The prevalence of cardiac valvular insufficiency assessed by transthoracic echocardiography in obese patients treated with appetite-suppressant drugs. N Engl J Med 1998;339:713–718.
72. Craddock D. Anorectic drugs: Use in general practice. Drugs 1976; 11:378–393.
73. Noach EL. Appetite regulation by serotoninergic mechanisms and effects of D-fenfluramine. Neth J Med 1994;45:123–133.
74. Silverstone T. Appetite suppressants. A review. Drugs 1992;43: 820–836.
75. Dawson JK, Earnshaw SM, Graham CS. Dangerous monoamine oxidase inhibitor interactions are still occurring in the 1990s. J Accid Emerg Med 1995;12:49–51.
76. Lasagna L. Safety. In: Lasagna L, ed. Phenylpropanolamine: A Review. New York, Wiley, 1988:191–300.
77. Valle-Jones JC, Brodie NH, O'Hara H, et al. A comparative study of phentermine and diethylpropion in the treatment of obese patients in general practice. Pharmatherapeutica 1983;3:300–304.
78. Truant AP, Olon LP, Cobb S. Phentermine resin as an adjunct in medical weight reduction: A controlled, randomized, double-blind prospective study. Curr Ther Res Clin Exp 1972;14:726–738.
79. Angel I. Central receptors and recognition sites mediating the effects of monoamines and anorectic drugs on feeding behavior. Clin Neuropharmacol 1990;13:361–391.
80. Amdisen A. Lithium and drug interactions. Drugs 1982;24:133–139.
81. Sanders M, Breidahl H. The effect of an anorectic agent (mazindol) on control of obese diabetics. Med J Aust 1976;2:576–577.
82. Nishikawa T, Iizuka T, Omura M, et al. Effect of mazindol on body weight and insulin sensitivity in severely obese patients after a very-low-calorie diet therapy. Endocr J 1996;43:671–677.
83. American Medical Association. Drugs Used in Obesity. Chicago, American Medical Association, 1995.
84. Wellman PJ. Overview of adrenergic anorectic agents. Am J Clin Nutr 1992;55:193S–198S.
85. Alger S, Larson K, Boyce VL, et al. Effect of phenylpropanolamine on energy expenditure and weight loss in overweight women. Am J Clin Nutr 1993;57:120–126.
86. Lasagna L. Basic Pharmacology. In: Lasagna L, ed. Phenylpropanolamine: A Review. New York, Wiley, 1988:84–190.
87. Lake CR, Gallant S, Masson E, Miller P. Adverse drug effects attributed to phenylpropanolamine: A review of 142 case reports. Am J Med 1990;89:195–208.
88. Greenway FL. Clinical studies with phenylpropanolamine: A metaanalysis. Am J Clin Nutr 1992;55:203S–205S.
89. Lake CR, Rosenberg DB, Gallant S, et al. Phenylpropanolamine increases plasma caffeine levels. Clin Pharmacol Ther 1990;47: 675–685.
90. United States Food and Drug Administration. OTC Weight Control Drug Products for Human Use. Comment #PR7, Docket #81N-0022, Division of OTC Products, Office of Drug Evaluation V, Rockville, MD, March, 1993.
91. Astrup A, Breum L, Toubro S. Pharmacological and clinical studies of ephedrine and other thermogenic agonists. Obes Res 1995;3 (suppl 4):537S–540S.
92. Dulloo AG. Ephedrine, xanthines and prostaglandin-inhibitors: Actions and interactions in the stimulation of thermogenesis. Int J Obes Relat Metab Disord 1993;17(suppl 1):S35–S40.
93. Dulloo AG, Seydoux J, Girardier L. Paraxanthine (metabolite of caffeine) mimics caffeine's interaction with sympathetic control of thermogenesis. Am J Physiol 1994;267:E801–E804.
94. Dulloo AG, Seydoux J, Girardier L. Potentiation of the thermogenic antiobesity effects of ephedrine by dietary methylxanthines: Adenosine antagonism or phosphodiesterase inhibition? Metabolism 1992; 41:1233–1241.
95. Breum L, Pedersen JK, Ahlstrom F, Frimodt-Moller J. Comparison of an ephedrine/caffeine combination and dexfenfluramine in the treatment of obesity. A double-blind multi-centre trial in general practice. Int J Obes Relat Metab Disord 1994;18:99–103.
96. Astrup A, Breum L, Toubro S, et al. The effect and safety of an ephedrine/caffeine compound compared to ephedrine, caffeine and placebo in obese subjects on an energy restricted diet. A double blind trial. Int J Obes Relat Metab Disord 1992;16:269–277.
97. Astrup A, Toubro S, Cannon S, et al. Thermogenic synergism between ephedrine and caffeine in healthy volunteers: A double-blind, placebo-controlled study. Metabolism 1991;40:323–329.
98. Williams DM, Self TH. Asthma Products. In: Covington TR, Berardi RR, Young LL, eds. Handbook of Nonprescription Drugs, 11th ed. Washington, DC: American Pharmaceutical Association, 1996: 157–177.
99. Tietze KJ. Cold, cough, and allergy products. In: Covington TR, Berardi RR, Young LL, eds. Handbook of Nonprescription Drugs, 11th ed. Washington, DC: American Pharmaceutical Association, 1996: 133–156.
100. Curzon G, Gibson EL, Oluyomi AO. Appetite suppression by commonly used drugs depends on 5-HT receptors but not on 5-HT availability. Trends Pharmacol Sci 1997;18:21–25.
101. Brauer LH, Johanson CE, Schuster CR, et al. Evaluation of phentermine and fenfluramine, alone and in combination, in normal, healthy volunteers. Neuropsychopharmacology 1996;14:233–241.
102. Weintraub M, Hasday JD, Mushlin AI, Lockwood DH. A double-blind clinical trial in weight control. Use of fenfluramine and phentermine alone and in combination. Arch Intern Med 1984;144: 1143–1148.
103. Weintraub M. Long-term weight control: The National Heart, Lung, and Blood Institute funded multimodal intervention study [published erratum appears in Clin Pharmacol Ther 1992;52:323]. Clin Pharmacol Ther 1992;51:581–585.
104. Weintraub M, Sundaresan PR, Madan M, et al. Long-term weight control study, I (weeks 0 to 34). The enhancement of behavior modification, caloric restriction, and exercise by fenfluramine plus phentermine versus placebo. Clin Pharmacol Ther 1992;51:586–594.
105. Weintraub M, Sundaresan PR, Schuster B, et al. Long-term weight control study, II (weeks 34 to 104). An open-label study of continuous fenfluramine plus phentermine versus targeted intermittent medication as adjuncts to behavior modification, caloric restriction, and exercise. Clin Pharmacol Ther 1992;51:595–601.
106. Weintraub M, Sundaresan PR, Schuster B, et al. Long-term weight control study, III (weeks 104 to 156). An open-label study of dose adjustment of fenfluramine and phentermine. Clin Pharmacol Ther 1992;51:602–607.
107. Weintraub M, Sundaresan PR, Schuster B, et al. Long-term weight control study, IV (weeks 156 to 190). The second double-blind phase. Clin Pharmacol Ther 1992;51:608–614.
108. Weintraub M, Sundaresan PR, Schuster B, et al. Long-term weight control study, V (weeks 190 to 210). Follow-up of participants after cessation of medication. Clin Pharmacol Ther 1992;51:615–618.
109. Weintraub M, Sundaresan PR, Cox C. Long-term weight control study, VI. Individual participant response patterns. Clin Pharmacol Ther 1992;51:619–633.
110. Weintraub M, Sundaresan PR, Schuster B. Long-term weight control study, VII (weeks 0 to 210). Serum lipid changes. Clin Pharmacol Ther 1992;51:634–641.
111. Weintraub M. Long-term weight control study: Conclusions. Clin Pharmacol Ther 1992;51:642–646.
112. Tuominen S, Hietola M, Kuusankoski M. Double-blind trial comparing fenfluramine, phentermine and dietary advice on treatment of obesity. Int J Obes 1980;14:138.
113. Hartley GG, Nicol S, Halstenson C, et al. Long-term results from phentermine, fenfluramine, diet, behavior modification, and exercise for treatment of obesity. Obes Res 1997;5:58S.

114. Spitz AF, Schumacher D, Blank RC, et al. Long-term pharmacologic treatment of morbid obesity in a community practice. Endocr Pract 1997;3:269–275.
115. Cardiac valvulopathy associated with exposure to fenfluramine or dexfenfluramine: U.S. Department of Health and Human Services interim public health recommendations, November 1997. MMWR 1997;46:1061–1066.
116. Khan MA, St. Peter JV, Hartley GG, et al. The effect of adding phentermine to weight management therapy in patients with declining response to dexfenfluramine alone. Obes Res 1997;5:22S.
117. Fluoxetine (Prozac) and other drugs for treatment of obesity. Medical Lett Drugs Ther 1994;36:107–108.
118. Wadden TA, Bartlett SJ, Foster GD, et al. Sertraline and relapse prevention training following treatment by very-low-calorie diet: A controlled clinical trial. Obes Res 1995;3:549–557.
119. Goldstein DJ, Rampey AHJ, Enas GG, et al. Fluoxetine: A randomized clinical trial in the treatment of obesity. Int J Obes Relat Metab Disord 1994;18:129–135.
120. Goldstein DJ, Rampey AHJ, Roback PJ, et al. Efficacy and safety of long-term fluoxetine treatment of obesity—maximizing success. Obes Res 1995;3(suppl 4):481S–490S.
121. Anchors M. Fluoxetine is a safer alternative to fenfluramine in the medical treatment of obesity. Arch Intern Med 1997;157:1270.
122. Bostwick JM, Brown TM. A toxic reaction from combining fluoxetine and phentermine. J Clin Psychopharmacol 1996;16:189–190.
123. Stock MJ. Sibutramine: A review of the pharmacology of a novel anti-obesity agent. Int J Obes Relat Metab Disord 1997;21(suppl 1):S25–S29.
124. Knoll Pharmaceutical Company. Sibutramine hydrochloride monohydrate (Meridia) product information. Mount Olive, New Jersey, Knoll Pharmaceutical Company, 1997.
125. Lean ME. Sibutramine—a review of clinical efficacy. Int J Obes Relat Metab Disord 1997;21(suppl 1):S30–S36
126. Bray GA, Ryan DH, Gordon D, et al. A double-blind randomized placebo-controlled trial of sibutramine. Obes Res 1996;4:263–270.
127. Schwizer W, Asal K, Kreiss C, et al. Role of lipase in the regulation of upper gastrointestinal function in humans. Am J Physiol 1997; 273:G612–G620.
128. Guerciolini R. Mode of action of orlistat. Int J Obes Relat Metab Disord 1997;21(suppl 3):S12–S23.
129. Zhi J, Melia AT, Guerciolini R, et al. Retrospective population-based analysis of the dose-response (fecal fat excretion) relationship of orlistat in normal and obese volunteers. Clin Pharmacol Ther 1994; 56:82–85.
130. Hauptman JB, Jeunet FS, Hartmann D. Initial studies in humans with the novel gastrointestinal lipase inhibitor Ro 18-0647 (tetrahydrolipstatin). Am J Clin Nutr 1992;55:309S–313S.
131. Guzelhan C, Odink J, Niestijl Jansen-Zuidema JJ, Hartmann D. Influence of dietary composition on the inhibition of fat absorption by orlistat. J Int Med Res 1994;22:255–265.
132. Hussain Y, Guzelhan C, Odink J, et al. Comparison of the inhibition of dietary fat absorption by full versus divided doses of orlistat. J Clin Pharmacol 1994;34:1121–1125.
133. Tonstad S, Pometta D, Erkelens DW, et al. The effect of the gastrointestinal lipase inhibitor, orlistat, on serum lipids and lipoproteins in patients with primary hyperlipidaemia. Eur J Clin Pharmacol 1994;46:405–410.
134. Drent ML, Larsson I, William-Olsson T, et al. Orlistat (Ro 18-0647), a lipase inhibitor, in the treatment of human obesity: A multiple dose study. Int J Obes Relat Metab Disord 1995;19:221–226.
135. James WP, Avenell A, Broom J, Whitehead J. A one-year trial to assess the value of orlistat in the management of obesity. Int J Obes Relat Metab Disord 1997;21(suppl 3):S24–S30.
136. Melia AT, Koss-Twardy SG, Zhi J. The effect of orlistat, an inhibitor of dietary fat absorption, on the absorption of vitamins A and E in healthy volunteers. J Clin Pharmacol 1996;36:647–653.
137. Hollander PA, Elbein SC, Hirsch IB, et al. Role of orlistat in the treatment of obese patients with type 2 diabetes. Diabetes Care 1998; 21:1288–1294.
138. Leibowitz SF. Brain peptides and obesity: Pharmacologic treatment. Obes Res 1995;3(suppl 4):573S–589S.
139. Amgen announces leptin causes weight loss in humans and plans for two phase 2 trials. Available at http://www.Amgen.com. Accessed June, 1997.
140. National Research Council. Trace elements. In: Recommended Dietary Allowances, 10th ed. Washington, DC, National Academy Press, 1998:195–246.
141. Trent LK, Thieding-Cancel D. Effects of chromium picolinate on body composition. J Sports Med Phys Fitness 1995;35:273–280.
142. Betz JM, Gay ML, Mossoba MM, et al. Chiral gas chromatographic determination of ephedrine-type alkaloids in dietary supplements containing ma huang. J AOAC Int 1997;80:303–315.
143. FDA proposes constraints on ephedrine dietary supplements. Am J Health Syst Pharm 1997;54:1578.
144. Linde K, Ramirez G, Mulrow CD, et al. St John's wort for depression—an overview and meta-analysis of randomised clinical trials. BMJ 1996;313:253–258.
145. Cott JM. *In vitro* receptor binding and enzyme inhibition by *Hypericum perforatum* extract. Pharmacopsychiatry 1997;30(suppl 2): 108–112.
146. Bladt S, Wagner H. Inhibition of MAO by fractions and constituents of hypericum extract. J Geriatr Psychiatry Neurol 1994;7(suppl 1): S57–S59.
147. Brenot F, Herve P, Petitpretz P, et al. Primary pulmonary hypertension and fenfluramine use. Br Heart J 1993;70:537–541.
148. Thomas SH, Butt AY, Corris PA, et al. Appetite suppressants and primary pulmonary hypertension in the United Kingdom. Br Heart J 1995;74:660–663.
149. Abenhaim L, Moride Y, Brenot F, et al. Appetite-suppressant drugs and the risk of primary pulmonary hypertension. International primary pulmonary hypertension study group. N Engl J Med 1996;335: 609–616.
150. McCann UD, Seiden LS, Rubin LJ, Ricaurte GA. Brain serotonin neurotoxicity and primary pulmonary hypertension from fenfluramine and dexfenfluramine. A systematic review of the evidence. JAMA 1997;278:666–672.
151. Chambers HF, Neu HC. Penicillins. In: Mandell GL, Bennett JE, Dolin R, eds. Principles and Practice of Infectious Diseases, 4th ed. New York, Churchill Livingstone, 1995:233–246.
152. Redfield MM, Nicholson WJ, Edwards WD, Tajik AJ. Valve disease associated with ergot alkaloid use: Echocardiographic and pathologic correlations. Ann Intern Med 1992;117:50–52.
153. Robiolio PA, Rigolin VH, Wilson JS, et al. Carcinoid heart disease. Correlation of high serotonin levels with valvular abnormalities detected by cardiac catheterization and echocardiography. Circulation 1995;92:790–795.
154. Jick H, Vasilakis C, Weinrauch LA, et al. A population-based study of appetite-suppressant drugs and the risk of cardiac-valve regurgitation. N Engl J Med 1998;339:719–724.
155. Weissman NJ, Tighe JFJ, Gottdiener JS, Gwynne JT. An assessment of heart-valve abnormalities in obese patients taking dexfenfluramine, sustained-release dexfenfluramine, or placebo. Sustained-Release Dexfenfluramine Study Group. N Engl J Med 1998;339: 725–732.
156. Wee CC, Phillips RS, Aurigemma G, et al. Risk for valvular heart disease among users of fenfluramine and dexfenfluramine who underwent echocardiography before use of medication. Ann Intern Med 1998;129:870–874.
157. Ryan DH, Bray GA, Helmcke F, et al. Echocardiographic abnormalities in patients treated with fenfluramine (F) or dexfenfluramine (D). Int J Obes 1998;22:S77. Abstract.
158. Devereux RB. Appetite suppressants and valvular heart disease. N Engl J Med 1998;339:765–766.

159. Parisi AF. Diet-drug debacle. Ann Intern Med 1998;129:903.
160. Reginster F, Jadoul M, van Ypersele de Strihou C. Chinese herbs nephropathy presentation, natural history and fate after transplantation. Nephrol Dial Transplant 1997;12:81–86.
161. Sporer KA. The serotonin syndrome. Implicated drugs, pathophysiology and management. Drug Saf 1995;13:94–104.
162. Brown TM, Skop BP, Mareth TR. Pathophysiology and management of the serotonin syndrome. Ann Pharmacother 1996;30:527–533.
163. Gardner DM, Lynd LD. Sumatriptan contraindications and the serotonin syndrome. Ann Pharmacother 1998;32:33–38.
164. Clinical guidelines on the identification, evaluation, and treatment of overweight and obesity in adults—the evidence report. National Institutes of Health. Obes Res 1998;6(suppl 2):51S–209S.
165. Collins RW, Anderson JW. Medication cost savings associated with weight loss for obese non-insulin-dependent diabetic men and women. Prev Med 1995;24:369–374.
166. Shrink your weight while keeping your wallet plump. Money 1997; February:162–167.
167 Martin LF, Tan TL, Horn JR, et al. Comparison of the costs associated with medical and surgical treatment of obesity. Surgery 1995; 118:599–606.

INDEX

Note: Page numbers followed by *f* refer to illustrations; page numbers followed by *t* refer to tables.

C

D

H

I

J

K

L

N

P

Q

R

S

V

U

V